Acknowledgments

In the four years of compiling, editing, sorting and updating th information contained in this book I have received inspiration and assis tance from many people and I would like to deeply thank everyone who ha participated in any way in the publication of this repertory. Special thank are due to the following individuals: Rochelle Domenick, Robert Macrorie Lawrence Galante, Henrietta Stern, David Little, Gerald Gewiss, Hakeem Lewis, Crystal Lewis, Cindy Lohan, Jim Klemmer, Jack Tips, Luc D Schepper, Louis Dion, Cindy Rounsaville, Mitzi Lebensorger, Colleen Nicholson, Wayne Nicholson, Chris Keser, Moshe Frenkel, Richard Fiske Steven Gorney and Neil Miller.

Also, I would like to thank all the students attending the HANA classe in 1991 and 1992 who helped with the repertory and joined with me t research Samuel Hahnemann's LM prescribing methods as outlined in hi masterpiece the sixth edition of " The Organon of the Healing Art ".

Homeopathic Medical Repertory - First Edition 1993

by Robin Murphy, ND

Published by :

Hahnemann Academy of North America (HANA)
60 Talisman Drive, Suite 4028
Pagosa Springs, Colorado, USA 81157

Printed in the United States by
R. R. Donnelley & Sons Company

ISBN 0-9635764-0-2

This book is dedicated to Kirpal Singh

Homeopathic Medical Repertory

by

Robin Murphy, ND

A Modern Alphabetical Repertory

First Edition

Hahnemann Academy of North America

Preface

The Homeopathic Medical Repertory was designed to be a modern, practical and easy to use reference guide to the vast homeopathic materia medica. To achieve these goals a completely new repertory had to be created. The alphabetical format was chosen as the most natural method to organize large amounts of information, thus bringing the repertory in line with all the large homeopathic materia medicas which are also alphabetically arranged.

T. F. Allen addressed this issue of whether our repertories should be organized in a hierarchical order (Kent's Repertory) or an alphabetical one in his introduction to the Index of the Encyclopedia of Pure Materia Medica. He states *"We venture to hope that future standard works will present a new scheme free from theoretical ideas concerning the physiological action of remedies, classifying our symptomatology in a form which will permit ready reference and enabling numerous provings to be condensed."*

All of Kent's Repertory and sections of Knerr's Repertory were used as the foundation for building the new repertory. Sixty seven different chapters were created and arranged in alphabetical order from the original thirty seven chapters. Next, all the rubrics (topics or entries) and sub-rubrics within each chapter were sorted into an alphabetical format. Thus simplifying Kent's complicated system for arranging rubrics and sub-rubrics, (sides, time, modalities, extensions, etc.).

Then the editing of the manuscript was done which involved adding modern terminology, cross references and correcting errors. The final step was to systematically survey the homeopathic literature for reliable additions to add to the alphabetical repertory. The highest priority was to find clinical information revelant to modern homeopathic practice and to fill in the areas where Kent's Repertory is weak in information (mental disorders, emergencies, infections, pathologies and major organs).

The result is the Homeopathic Medical Repertory which contains thirty new chapters, consistent formatting (alphabetical chapters, rubrics and sub-rubrics), modern terminology, modern disorders, with 39,000 new rubrics, 200,000 new additions and updates, in a small lightweight size for convenience.

The formatting for the Homeopathic Medical Repertory is similar to Kent's Repertory with the strongest remedies designated in bold-capitals, **ACON.,** (3 points), next, bold-italics, ***acon.,*** (2 points) and plain-type, acon., (1 point). Abbreviations used in this book are agg. = aggravates, worse from or symptoms increased by, and amel. = ameliorates, better from or symptoms decreased by.

The Word Index is used to find particular words and clinical references such as influenza or hepatitis. Common words found in most chapters such as burning, are not included in the Word Index because they are easily accessible alphabetically within each chapter (Abdomen, burning). The Table of Contents includes the major sections written after the chapter title for easy reference (Eyes, cornea or Fever, infections). At the end of the repertory is found the Homeopathic Remedies list which includes the abbreviations used in the Homeopathic Medical Repertory, plus the full Latin names and common names for many homeopathic remedies.

The modern practice of numbering all additions as to their author is a commendable one but was avoided in this work to keep the repertory as small as possible and in one volume. (check the Kunzli Repertory, Synthetic Repertory or the Complete Repertory, all excellent reference books).

Homeopathic References

Major Sources of Additions and New Rubrics

1. Allen, H. C., Keynotes and Characteristics with Comparisons, The Materia Medica of the Nosodes, Therapeutics of Fever.
2. Allen, J. H., Diseases and Therapeutics of the Skin.
3. Allen, T. F., The Encyclopedia of Pure Materia Medica, Handbook of Materia Medica and Homeopathic Therapeutics, Symptom-Register.
4. Anschutz E. P., New, Old and Forgotten Remedies.
5. Barthel H., and Klunker, W., The Synthetic Repertory.
6. Bell J. B., Therapeutics of Diarrea.
7. Boenninghausen, C.M. and Boger, C.M., Boenninghausens Characteristics and Repertory, Boenninghausen's Therapeutic Pocket Book.
8. Boericke, Wm. and O. E., Manual of Hom. Materia Medica and Repertory.
9. Boger, C. M., A Synoptic key of the Materia Medica, Additions to Kent's Repertory, Moon Phases, Times of Remedies.
10. Borland, D. M., Childrens Types, Homeopathic Practice.
11. Burnett, J. C., Fifty Reasons for being a Homeopath, Organ Diseases of Women, Diseases of the Liver and Spleen, Vaccinosis.
12. Clarke, J. H., Clinical Repertory, A Dictionary of Practical Materia Medica., The Prescriber.
13. Dewey, W. A., Essentials of Homeopathic Materia Medica, Practical Homeopathic Therapeutics, Twelve Tissue Remedies.
14. Eizayaga, F. X., El Moderno Repertorio de Kent.
15. Farrington, E. A., Clinical Materia Medica, Comparative Materia Medica.
16. Foubister, D., Carcinosin Research, Tutorials on Homeopathy.
17. Gallavardin, J., Repertory of Psychic Medicines & Materia Medica.
18. Gentry, W. D., The Concordance Repertory.
19. Gibson, D., Studies of Homeopathic Remedies.
20. Guernsey, H. N., Keynotes to the Materia Medica, Obstetrics.
21. Gupta, B. P., Encyclopedia of Homeopathy.
22. Hahnemann, S., Materia Medica Pura and Chronic Diseases.
23. Hale, E. M., Homeopathic Materia Medica of New Remedies, Diseases of the Heart.
24. Hansen, O., A Textbook of Materia Medica and Therapeutics of Rare Remedies.
25. Hering, C., Analytical Repertory of Symptoms of the Mind, The Guiding Symptoms of our Materia Medica.
26. Hughes, R. & Dake, J. P., A Cyclopaedia of Drug Pathogenesy.
27. Imhauser, H., Homeopathy in Pediatric Practice.

Homeopathic References

Major Sources of Additions and New Rubrics

28. Jahr, G. H. G., A New Manual of Homeopathic Practice.

29. Julian, O. A., Materia Medica of New Homeopathic Remedies, Dictionary of Materia Medica.

30. Kent, J. T., Repertory of the Materia Medica, (as well as his handwritten corrections of the last American edition of the Repertory), Lectures on Homeopathic Materia Medica, Lesser Writings, New Remedies.

31. Kichlu and Bose, A Textbook of Descriptive Medicine.

32. Knerr, C. A., Repertory of Herings Guiding Symptoms of our Materia Medica.

33. Kunzli, J., Kent's Repertorium Generale.

34. Lathoud, J. A., Homeopathic Materia Medica.

35. Lilienthal, S., Homeopathic Therapeutics.

36. Lippe, C., Repertory to the More Characteristic Symptoms of the Materia Medica.

37. Minton H., Uterine Therapeutics.

38. Murphy, R., Homeopathy and Cancer, Fundamentals of Materia Medica, (Transcribed Lectures and Notes) Fundamentals of Classical Homeopathy, (Home Study Course, Taped Lecture Series).

39. Nash, E. B., Leaders in Homeopathic Therapeutics.

40. Patel, R. P., Word Index with Rubrics of Kent's Repertory.

41. Phatak, S. R., Concise Repertory of Homeopathic Remedies, Materia Medica of Homeopathic Remedies.

42. Roberts, H. A., Sensations as if, Studies of Remedies by Comparison.

43. Royal, G., Textbook of Homeopathic Materia Medica.

44. Schussler, W., The Biochemic System, The Twelve Tissue Remedies.

45. Sirker, C., A Keynote Repertory of Materia Medica.

46. Sheppard, D., Homeopathy in Epidemic Diseases, Magic of the Minimum Dose., More Magic of the Minimum Dose.

47. Stephenson, J., A Materia Medica and Repertory, Hahnemannian Provings.

48. Tyler, M. L., Homeopathic Drug Pictures, Pointers to Common Remedies.

49. Underwood B. F., The Diseases of Childhood and Their Homeopathic Treatment, Headaches and Its Materia Medica.

50. Van Zandvoort., The Complete Repertory. (Computer Repertory)

51. Von Lippe, A., Keynotes and Redline Symptoms of the Materia Medica.

52. Vithoulkas, G., Additions to Kent's Repertory.

53. Ward, J. W., Unabridged Dictionary of the Sensations As If.

54. Warkentin, D. K., MacRepertory. (Computer Repertory)

55. Yingling, W. A., The Accoucheurs Emergency Manual.

Similia Similibus Curentur

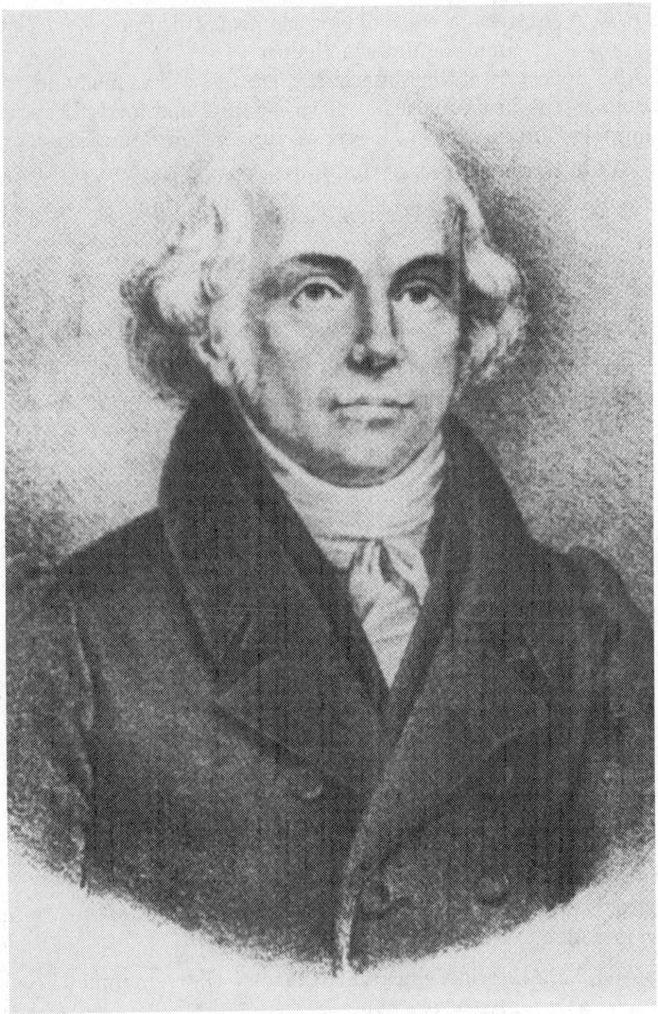

Samuel Hahnemann

April 10, 1755 - July 2, 1843

Founder

" The Healing Art of Homeopathy "

HOMEOPATHIC MEDICAL REPERTORY

by

Robin Murphy, ND

Abdomen to Wrists

First Edition

Hahnemann Academy of North America

Homeopathic Medical Repertory
Table of Contents

Chapters | Pages

Homeopathic Medical Repertory
Table of Contents

Chapters — Pages

Abdomen

ABSCESS, walls, in - crot-h., ***hep.,*** merc., rhus-t., ***sil.,*** sulph.
as if in and around anus - cycl.
abscess, inguinal - **HEP.,** ***merc.,*** sil., syph.

ACHING, pain (see Pain, Abdomen)

ADHESION, sensation - mez., ***sep.,*** verb.

ALIVE, sensation of something - arund., calc-p., cann-s., conv., **CROC.,** cur., ***cycl.,*** hyos., ign., kali-i., lac-d., lyc., merc., ***nat-c.,*** nux-v., op., phos., puls., sabad., sabin., sang., sep., spong., stram., stront-c., ***sulph.,*** ther., **THUJ.,** verat.
left side - croc.

ANXIETY, in - acon-f., agar., aloe, am-m., **ARS.,** aur., ***bar-c.,*** calc., carb-v., carl., cham., cupr., euph., gran., inul., ***kali-c.,*** merc., mez., mur-ac., nat-p., nit-ac., nux-v., olnd., phos., plat., sep., stram., ***sulph.,*** sul-ac., ***tarent.,*** verat., vesp.
adhere to chest, as if, would - mez.
burst, as if it would, better during sleep - am-m.
cramp, as from - lyc.
eating, after - bar-c.
evening - cham., tarent.
extending, head, into - laur.
stomach into, after midnight - phel.
flatus, amel. - mur-ac.
griping, as if intestines would be constricted - spig.
morning - sul-ac.
bed, in - sul-ac.
breakfast, after - ***ign.***
night - nit-ac.
puffed, in childbed - ***ambr.***
rigid, as if would become - ***mez.***
rising from - agar., stram.
breakfast, after - ign.
morning - bry.
spasmodic, contractive, cutting - plb.
stool, after - ***apoc.,*** **ARS.,** carb-v., dios., **HYDR.,** lept., mur-ac., ***nat-p., petr., ph-ac.,*** **PHOS.,** ***pic-ac.,*** plat., **PODO.,** rhod., ***sep., sul-ac., verat.***
amel. - mur-ac.
before - calc., merc.
diarrhea - merc.
during and before - calen.
involuntary, would pass, as if - sep.
supper, after - arg-n.
tearing - ***cham.***
anxiety, epigastrium - calc-ac., ***dig., kali-ar.,*** kali-c.
children, in - ***calc-p.***
gastralgia, with - ***lyc.***
oppression of breathing, with - sabad.
pressure, with, in hysteria - nux-v.
anxiety, hypochondria - acon., anac., ***arn.,*** cham., dig., dros., grat., ***nux-v.,*** ph-ac., staph.
left - phos.

APPREHENSION, sensation of - ***asaf.,*** merc-c., rhus-t.
lower, abdomen - merc-c.

ASCITES, dropsy - ***acet-ac.,*** acon., ***adon., agn.,*** alco., ant-c., **APIS, APOC.,** ***arg-n.,*** **ARS.,** asaf., ***aur., aur-m.,*** aur-m-n., bell., ***blatta-a., bry.,*** cahin., ***calc.,*** camph., cann-s., ***canth.,*** carb-s., ***card-m.,*** caust., ***chel., chim., chin., chin-a.,*** coca, ***colch.,*** coloc., cop., crot-h., cur., ***dig., digin., dulc.,*** ferr., ferr-ar., ***fl-ac., graph., hell.,*** helon., hep., iris, iod., kali-ar., kali-br., ***kali-c., kali-chl.,*** kali-p., kali-s., kalm., lact., ***led.,*** **LYC.,** mag-m., med., ***merc.,*** mill., mur-ac., nat-ch., nux-v., op., oxyd., ***phos.,*** plb., ***prun.,*** ptel., puls., rhus-t., sabin., sac-alb., samb., sars., ***senec.,*** sep., sil., sol-t-ae., spong., squil., ***sulph.,*** **TER.,** uran-n., urea
anxiety, with - ***fl-ac.***
diarrhea, chronic, with - ***apoc.,*** oena., sil.
edema - anan., ***apis, ars., graph.,*** tarent., thuj.
liver, induration, with - aur., lact.
menses, suppressed - senec.
quinine, after the abuse of - cann-s.
suffocation, lying on left side - ***apis.***
urination, with scanty - apis, squil.

ASLEEP, as if, about hypochondrium - dig.

BALL, as if, ascending to throat - ***arg-n.,*** raph.
rolling in - aur-s., lach., ***lyc.,*** sabad., sep.
ball, hypochondria, left - brom., cupr.

BAND, around - crot-c.

BAR in, as if - gins.

BEARING down, pain - apis, aq-pet., bell., elaps, nux-v., ox-ac., ***plat.,*** sabin., sars., **SEP.,** stry., sumb.
crampy, night, 2 a.m. - nux-v.
diarrhea, during - arund.
evening - ptel.
extending, anus, towards - ***sulph.***
colon, towards, dinner agg. - **SULPH.**
inguinal canal, into, and pelvic cavity - agar.
flatus, after collection of, amel. - plat.
laborlike - eug., sep.
menses, during - **SEP.**
after - kreos.
as before - phys.
as before, vaginal discharge, before - nat-m.
before - eupi.
night, 2 a.m. agg. - nux-v., sep.
waking, on - **SULPH.**
periodical, extending to small of back, movement of chest or lower limbs agg. - hedeo.
sleep, in - ptel.
stool, during - trif-p.
urging - corn.
warm drinks, especially coffee or tea agg. - elaps.
warmth, external amel. - nat-c.
bearing down, hypogastrium - bell., dict., lil-t., lyc., nux-v., plat., puls., ***sep.,*** sulph.

BLOOD, flowed back into, as if - elaps.

BOARD, across hypogastrium, sensation of - nux-m.

BODY, stiff, sides sensations - sep.

BOILS - am-m., phos., rhus-t., sec., zinc.
burning, smarting and throbbing - rhus-t.

boils, inguinal - ars., merc., ***nit-ac.,*** phos., rhus-t., stram.

BUBBLING, sensation - ant-c., cham., hell., **LYC.,** nat-m., ph-ac., ***puls.,*** stann., ***sul-ac.,*** tarax.
burst, as if would - phos.
bursting - nat-m.
lying on the back, while - ***sul-ac.***
night, 9.30 p.m. - com.
rhythmical with pulse, after eating - merc.
rising and bursting before emission of flatus - hell.
upwards - gent-l.
strings of air, running transversely over external abdomen - merc-i-f.

bubbling, inguinal - aeth., berb., kali-c., lyc.

bubbling, sides - arg-m., cham., cupr., nux-v., squil., sul-ac.
left - carb-v., cupr., lyc., sumb.

bubbling, umbilicus - aeth., berb., hyper., mez.

BUBO - alum., ant-t., anthr., ***ars.,*** ars-i., aur., aur-m., aur-m-n., bad., bapt., bar-m., bell., **BUFO,** ***carb-an.,*** carb-v., chel., chin., **CINNB.,** clem., ***crot-h.,*** **HEP.,** ign., iod., kali-chl., ***kali-i.,*** lac-c., ***lach.,*** lyc., ***merc.,*** merc-i-r., naja, ***nit-ac.,*** oper., ***phos.,*** phyt., ***pyrog.,*** rhus-t., ***sil.,*** sulph., ***tarent-c.,*** zinc.
burning, with - ars., ars-i., bell., ***carb-an., tarent-c.***
gonorrhea, after suppressed - ***aur.,*** aur-m., bar-m., bufo, hep., med., merc., zinc.
suppurating - ***aur.,*** bufo, ***carb-an.,*** chel., **HEP.,** ***iod.,*** kali-chl., ***kali-i.,*** **LACH.,** ***merc., merc-i-r.,*** nit-ac., ***sil., sulph.,*** tarent-c.
refuses to heal, old - ***carb-an., sulph.***

BURNING, pain - acet-ac., **ACON.,** agar., ail., aloe, alum., alumn., am-c., am-m., anac., anan., ant-t., ***apis,*** arn., **ARS.,** ***ars-i.,*** asaf., asc-t., bar-m., ***bell.,*** berb., ***bov.,*** bry., cact., calad., ***calc., calc-p.,*** calc-s., ***camph.,*** cann-s., ***canth.,*** **CAPS.,** carb-an., carb-s., **CARB-V.,** ***caust.,*** cham., chel., chin-a., cocc., colch., coloc., ***con.,*** cop., crot-h., crot-t., cub., cupr., ***cupr-ar.,*** cur., dios., dor., dulc., ***euph.,*** euphr., gamb., gels., glon., ***graph.,*** grat., hydr-ac., iod., ign., ***iris,*** jatr., jug-r., ***kali-ar.,*** kali-bi., kali-c., kali-i., kali-n., kali-p., kali-s., ***kreos., lac-c.,*** lach., ***laur., lil-t.,*** lyc., lyss., mag-s., ***manc.,*** merc., ***merc-c.,*** merc-sul., merl., ***mez., nat-a.,*** nat-c., ***nat-m.,*** nat-p., ***nat-s., nux-v.,*** ol-an., ***ox-ac.,*** phel., ph-ac., **PHOS.,** phyt., plat., plb., ***ran-b.,*** raph., rat., rhus-t., rumx., ruta, ***sabad., sars.,*** **SEC.,** sel., seneg., ***sep.,*** sil., spig., ***stann.,*** stront-c., stram., sulph., tab., tarent., **TER.,** thuj., **VERAT.,** vip.
afternoon - alum., ars.
blowing, nose - canth.

BURNING, pain
breakfast, after - agar.
chilliness, during - nat-c.
coughing - canth.
eating, after - ***hydr-ac.***
eating, while - phos.
evening - dirc., rhus-t.
down leg - **LIL-T.**
to lumbar region - kali-n.
ice cream, after - **ARS.**
lying, amel. - ***podo.***
abdomen on, amel. - ***acet-ac.***
menses, during - ***ars.,*** bry., canth., carb-v., caust., merc., nux-v., ph-ac., phos., rhus-t., sep., sulph., tarent.
morning - canth., rat.
motion, agg. - caps., kali-n.
noon - ars.
paroxysmal - plb.
radiating - ***graph.***
sitting, while - calc., sep.
bent - kali-n.
sneezing - canth., carb-v.
standing, while - ***sulph.***
stool, after - cupr-ar., jug-c., kali-bi., nat-a., sabad., sep.
amel. - ars.
before - aloe.
during - eug., sul-ac.
stooping - caps.
waking - caust.
walking, while - caps., carb-an., sulph.
air, in open - agar., sep.

burning, hypochondria - acon., aeth., ***apis,*** aur., aur-m., bell., bor., bov., ***bry.,*** bufo, cann-s., carb-s., caust., **CHEL.,** euphr., gamb., ***graph.,*** grat., ign., kali-c., kali-i., kali-n., ***lach.,*** laur., lept., merc., ***mur-ac.,*** nat-c., nat-m., ox-ac., plat., seneg., spig., stann., ***staph.,*** sul-ac., tab., ***ter.,*** thuj., zinc.
afternoon - alum., am-m., kali-c.
1 p.m. - sars.
eating, after - stann.
evening - mur-ac., nat-m.
extending to right, scapula - mag-m.
forenoon - tell.
left - am-c., bor., caust., chel., ***coc-c., graph.,*** grat., kali-i., lac-c., plat., ruta., sep., sulph., tab., verat.
deep breathing, on - bor.
lying on painful side, agg. - ***coc-c., graph.***
lying, amel. - ***lac-c.***
morning - dios., sang.
motion, amel. - ***graph.***
pressure, amel. - mur-ac.
right - am-m., ***ars.,*** aur., ***aur-m., bry.,*** chel., ***crot-c., gamb.,*** **KALI-C.,** ***lac-c., lach.,*** laur., mag-c., mag-m., ***med.,*** mur-ac., ***nit-ac.,*** ph-ac., phos., plb., sang., stann., sulph., ter., ***ther.,*** thuj., zinc.
rubbing, amel. - phos.
sitting, while - graph., sul-ac., tell.
standing, when - ***lac-c.***
touch - ther.

burning, hypochondria
walking, while - am-m.
amel. - grat.

burning, hypogastrium - agar., all-c., alumn., arund., bar-c., ***calad., camph.,*** card-m., crot-h., grat., helon., hep., kali-n., ***kreos.,*** lac-c., ***lach., lil-t.,*** ph-ac., stann., stram., sulph., tarent., tarax.
across - ***lil-t.***
cough, after - arund.
dinner, after - kali-n.
evening - kali-n.
left side - am-c., graph., lac-c., plat., ruta., sep.
menses, during - nat-m.
motion, amel. - bar-c., kali-n.
agg. - kali-n.
night - crot-h., phos.

burning, inguinal - alum., ***arn.,*** ars., aur., bar-c., ***berb.,*** bov., bry., canth., fl-ac., graph., grat., kali-c., kali-i., lil-t., lyc., mag-c., mang., mur-ac., phos., ruta., sep., stront-c., sulph.
extending, to testes - staph.
forenoon - alum.
left - mag-m., pall.
menses, during - kali-n., nat-m.
right - am-m., ***berb.,*** bry., fl-ac., kali-c., kali-n., mang., stront.
rising, from sitting - kali-c.
sitting, while - am-m., bar-c.
bent over - kali-n.
stooping, amel. - graph.
stretching, out agg. - graph.
urination, during - ***nat-m.,*** merc.

burning, sides - all-c., am-c., ars., carb-v., graph., grat., olnd., petr., plat., rat., ruta, sep.
afternoon - am-m.
cough, during - sul-ac.
dinner, after - bov.
flank, in - mag-c., plat., seneg., stann.
sneezing, on - carb-v.
left - hep., iod., ***lac-c., plat.***
right - caust., petr., plat., sep., stann.
sitting, on - am-m.
spots, in - graph., hyos., ox-ac., plat.
walking, while - sep.

burning, umbilical, region of - **ACON.,** ars., berb., bov., calc., calc-p., camph., canth., carb-v., cham., chel., clem., cocc., crot-h., cub., dios., dor., fl-ac., ***ham.,*** iod., kali-c., kali-i., lach., lyc., mag-s., merc., merc-i-f., nat-a., nat-c., nat-m., ox-ac., ph-ac., ***phyt.,*** plat., plb., raph., sabad., sang., sep., sul-ac., til.
afternoon - calc.
dinner, during - kali-c.
evening, dinner, after - lyc.
stool, before - ars.
urination, during - til.
walking, while - ph-ac.
sleep, amel. - nux-m.

burning, umbilicus - aesc., carb-v., kali-i., lach., nux-m.
above - kali-n.

BURROWING, pain - agar., dig., dulc., graph., hell., mag-m., spig., sulph.
bending, forward, amel. - coloc., grat.
rest, amel. - grat.

burrowing, hypogastrium - coc-c., nit-ac., sep., spig.

burrowing, inguinal - coc-c., spig., spong.

burrowing, sides, left - con., spong.
right - ars.

burrowing, umbilical, region - alum., coloc., grat.

BURSTING, pain - bar-c., calc., caust., coff., hyos., lac-c., lyc., phos., puls., sulph.
coughing, on - anac., caust.
drinking, after - carb-v.
eating, after - carb-v., dulc.
rigor, during - sulph.

BURSTING, pain
stool, before - spig.

CANCER, omentum, of - lob-e.

CLAWING, pain - alum., ars., ***bell.,*** carb-an., coloc., hep., ***ip.,*** lyc., mosch., sep., zinc.
menses, before - ***bell.***

clawing, hypochondria - **BELL.,** nat-m., rhod.
extending to back - nat-m.
right - **BELL.,** ***nat-s.***

clawing, hypogastrium - **BELL.,** lyc., puls.

clawing, inguinal - kali-i.

clawing, sides - hep., petr.

clawing, umbilical, region - acon., ***bell., hep.,*** kreos., petr., stann.
menses, before - kreos.
paroxysmal - petr.

CLOTHING, sensitive to - ***apis,*** **ARG-N.,** benz-ac., **BOV., CALC.,** caps., ***carb-v., caust., chin.,*** coff., **CROT-C.,** ***crot-h.,*** eup-per., ***graph., hep., kreos., lac-c.,*** **LACH., LYC.,** merc-c., ***nat-s.,*** **NUX-V.,** puls., raph., ***sars., sep., spong., stann.,*** sulph.
amel. - fl-ac., nat-m., nit-ac.
cannot bear - cupr-ac., phos.
eating, after - ***graph.***
groin, region - hydr.
pressing upon - cinnb., ***sulph.***
uncover, wants to - tab.

CLUCKING - bar-c., calc., chin., dig., graph., kali-c., mag-c., merc., plat., rheum., sars., stann., sulph., verb.

COBWEB, sensation - rhus-t.

COLD, sensitive to - caust.
easy taking - caust.
touch, on - kali-s., merc.

COLDNESS - acon., ***aeth.,*** agar., aloe, alum., **AMBR.,** amyg., arg-n., ***ars.,*** asaf., ***asar.,*** bell., berb., bov., calad., ***calc.,*** calc-s., ***camph.,*** caust., cham., chel., chin., chin-a., cic., ***cist.,*** colch., coloc., crot-h., ***crot-t.,*** cupr-s., dulc., eug., ***grat., hell.,*** hydr-ac., jatr., kali-ar., ***kali-bi., kali-br., kali-c.,*** kali-n., kali-p., ***kali-s., kreos., lach., laur.,*** mang., **MENY.,** meph., ***merc., merc-sul.,*** merl., mez., nat-m., nit-ac., olnd., op., ***par., petr.,*** phel.,

COLDNESS - ph-ac., ***phos.,*** plan., plb., podo., ***puls.,*** rat., ruta, sabad., ***sars., sec.,*** seneg., ***sep.,*** staph., ***sulph., tab., ter., tub.,*** **VERAT.,** zinc.
afternoon - alum., chel., lyc.
drinking water, on - chel.
air, as from a draft - sulph.
entrance of open, amel. - ph-ac.
alternating with, heat - cham.
heat, moving about - coff.
burning, with - phos.
chill, during - ***aeth.,*** apis, ars., **CALC.,** cham., chel., chin., chin-a., ***ign.,*** **MENY.,** ***mez., ph-ac.,*** puls., sec., sep., sulph., verat., zinc.
cold, drinks, after - ***ars., chel., rhus-t.***
wind, in - lyc.
colic, after - haem.
as if would become - hell.
with - calc., kali-s.
creeping - bov.
drinking, after - asaf., chel., ***chin.***
alcohol, spirituous, after - phel.
water, on - chel.
eating, after - ***chel., chin.,*** **PULS.,** sulph.
evening - ars., plect., zinc.
extending, across - eug., euphr., lil-t., sep.
back, to - puls.
back, to, lower, around to - **PULS.**
cheek, to - coloc.
chest, to - camph.
chest, to, afternoon - carl.
fauces, into - phos.
feet, to - calad.
intestines, around in, noon - gels.
loins, into - kali-i.
rising up into mouth - ***carb-an.***
stomach, to - phel.
upward - calc-p.
external - aeth., cupr-s., med., merc., merc-c., mez., op., sec., **VERAT.,** zinc.
heat of cheeks, during - chin.
night - cupr-s.
water, as if dashed with cold - mez.
fever, during - zinc.
flashes, like - coca.
heartburn, like, after breakfast - par.
extending to chest, in morning - arg-m.
hip-region - caust.
inside, of - anth.
inspiration, on every - ***chin.***
menses, during - kali-c.
morning - meny., plect.
rising from bed, on - meny.
warm room, in - plect.
nausea, like, extending to chest after breakfast - par.
night - cupr-s., sulph.
bed, in - sulph.
midnight - calad.
waking from anxious dreams, after colic - haem.
pains, during - phyt.
paroxysmal - plb.
pinching, 10 a.m. - nat-a.
pressure - meny.

COLDNESS,
rash, about - cham.
rising to cheeks during colic, amel. after more severe pain - coloc.
sitting quiet amel. - plect.
sparks, like electric 8 p.m. to 10 p.m. - phel.
stool, after - graph., phel., plect.
before - cop., graph.
uncovered, as if - ***lach.,*** ter.
dinner, after - ter.
uneasy - hydr.
upper part - ars., camph., kali-c., mang., olnd., ox-ac., sec., sulph.
uterus, as if in - sul-ac.
waist, around, as if wringing out cold water out of a cloth - lath.
walking in open air amel. - dulc., plect.
wandering, in evening - nat-s.
warmth of stove, agg. - plect.
amel. - meph.
water, as if cold, running through - cann-s., ***kali-c.***
dashed, with water, as if - mez.

coldness, hypochondria - cadm-s., nux-v.

coldness, hypogastrium - plb.

coldness, inguinal - plb.
burning, becoming - berb.

coldness, sides - all-c., ambr., merl., olnd., sulph.
left - ***ambr.***
one side, only - ***ambr.***

coldness, umbilical, region of - coloc., kreos., phos., rat., ruta., ter.
stool, after - coloc.

coldness, umbilicus - apis, coloc., ran-b., rat.
walking, while - coloc.

COLLAPSE, as if body would, from waist to lower pelvis - vib.

COMPRESSION, sensation, pressing tranversely across external abdomen - thuj.
iliac region, while walking - kali-n.

CONGENITAL growth, like a wart, scabby, sensitive and sore - nit-ac.

CONGESTION, feeling - aloe.
rise to head, seems to - crot-t.

CONSTRICTION - aesc., ***alum., alum-m.,*** alumn., ***arg-m., arn.,*** ars., aur-m., bell., berb., ***cact., calc.,*** camph., carb-an., carb-v., ***carl.,*** cench., ***chel.,*** chin., clem., cocc., coc-c., **COLOC.,** crot-c., cupr., dig., euph., ferr-ar., ferr-m., hydrc., kali-bi., kali-n., laur., ***lyc.,*** merl., mez., mosch., nat-m., nat-s., nit-ac., nux-m., ***nux-v.,*** petr., phos., ***plat., plb.,*** sars., ***sec., sep.,*** sil., sulph., sul-ac., thuj., zinc.
bandage, as from a - acon., dros., ign., nux-v.
bed, in, amel. - aur-m.
breathing - caust.
string, as by a, when - caust.
convulsive - chin., nit-ac.
convulsive, extending
to, chest - sulph.
to, genitals - sulph.
to, groin - sulph.

CONSTRICTION,
convulsive, extending
to, lower limbs, after stool - agar-ph.
cough, during - lach.
cramplike clawing - ***nux-v.***
eating, before - hep.
evening, towards - nat-m.
expectoration, from difficult - dros.
extending to, back, small of - calc.
bladder, to - **PULS.**
chest, to - ***calc.***, nat-s.
chest, to, before stool - nat-s.
chest, to, morning - calc.
side to side - elaps.
stomach, to - coc-c., ol-an.
uterus, towards - calc.
fasting - carb-an., hep.
flatus, passing, amel. - sars. sil.
forenoon - kali-n.
griping, extending to back - plat.
iron hoop, as from, preventing respiration - upa.
lying, while - zinc.
side, on, or back agg. - prun-p.
menses, as before, morning - nat-m.
menses, during - cact., cocc., croc., ***sulph.***
morning - ambr., calc.
night - phos., sulph.
4 a.m - nat-m.
pressive - carb-s.
pressure amel. - plb.
rhythmical - caust.
ring around, as if, deep respiration agg. - ***carl.***
rising agg. - zinc.
stool, desire for, during - ars., nat-m., nat-s.
diarrhea, before - laur.
during - sulph.
string, as by a - caust., **CHEL.**
as if, in intestines - elaps, verat.
tensive, as though she should vomit water, rising towards stomach, towards close of menses - cocc.
vomiting, before - colch.
walking, while - nat-m.
air, in open air, - nux-v.

constriction, hypochondria - ***acon.***, ***arg-n.***, **CACT.**, ***calc.***, ***chel.***, ***con.***, **CROT-C.**, dig., ***dros.***, kreos., **LYC.**, ***nux-v.***, puls., sep., staph., sulph., tarent.
bandage, as if - alum., ***cact.***, ***calc.***, chel., ***cocc.***, **CON.**, graph., ***lyc.***, ***sec.***
supper, after - ***sep.***
cough, during - ***dros.***
extending to umbilicus - mag-c.
laced, as if - ***calc.***
morning - ign.
right - ***lach.***
menses, during - bufo.

constriction, hypogastrium - bar-c., ***bell.***, carb-an., ***chel.***, clem., coloc., euon., ***hydr.***, sars., thuj., verb.
evening - sars.
forenoon - sars.

constriction, inguinal - bov., cact., gamb., kali-n., mag-c., rat.
extending around pelvis - ***cact.***
right - mag-c.
stretching out amel. - bov.

constriction, sides, below short ribs, extending to abdomen - camph.

constriction, umbilicus - bell., **COLOC.**, plb., plat., puls., sil., verb.
region of - coloc., mag-m., nat-m., nit-ac., petr., ***plat.***, plb., thuj., verb.

CONTRACTION - acon., am-c., ant-t., apis, arg-m., ars., aur., ***bell.***, carb-v., caust., ***cham.***, chel., colch., con., ***cupr.***, dig., dros., ferr., hep., hydrc., ign., kali-c., kali-i., lach., laur., ***lyc.***, ***mag-m.***, merc., merc-c., mur-ac., naja, nit-ac., ***nux-v.***, ***olnd.***, ph-ac., phos., ***plb.***, rhus-t., sabad., ***sars.***, sep., sil., sulph., sul-ac., tab., tarent.
bed, on going to - naja.
board, like a - plb.
breathing, expiration - dros.
colic, like in lead - sul-ac.
convulsive - act-sp., plb., sul-ac.
coughing, on - ***chel.***, dros., squil.
cramplike - aesc., lyc.
morning, towards - kali-bi.
diarrhea, before - mag-c.
evening in bed - dros.
extending to chest - con., mang.
chest - con., mang., nat-s.
stomach, region of, compression and by lying amel. - am-c.
throat - plb.
forenoon - am-c.
walking in open air - am-c.
hour glass - rhus-t.
lying, menses, after - con., nat-m.
menses, before - am-c., eupi., ***nat-m.***
lying, on abdomen, amel. - am-c.
morning - ph-ac.
bed, in - nat-m.
rising, after - mag-c.
waking, on - colch.
muscles - arg-m., ferr., nat-m., sabad., squil.
exertion, on - ferr.
stooping, on - ferr.
walking, while - arg-m.
night - sil.
pinching, only when sitting - dig.
pressure amel. - am-c.
rhythmic with palpitation - caust.
sitting, while - dig.
stool, after - arg-m., sulph.
during - ph-ac.
touch, on - colch.
twitching - nat-c., nat-m.
extending towards chest - con.
noon - caust.
walking, in open air must - con.
walking, while - apis, arg-m.

contraction, hypochondria - ip., mag-c., mang.
left - bar-c.
right - sulph.
menses, during - bufo.

contraction, inguinal - arg-n., carb-an., laur., rat., rhus-t.
dinner, after - laur.
evening - kali-n.
extending downward - laur.
menses, during - arg-n.
stool amel. - kali-n.
stretching out leg, on - carb-an.
urination, during - ars.
walking, while - kali-n.

contraction, sides, left - dulc., phos.
left, lying on right side - spong.
sitting - spong.
right - sep.

contraction, umbilicus - anac., ***bell.***, ***chel.***, cocc., **COLOC.**, gamb., graph., kreos., mag-m., ***mang.***, nat-c., ***ph-ac.***, phos., ***plat.***, plb., sulph., thuj.
as of a hard twisted ball - kreos.
below umbilicus - graph., phos.
inspiration, on - anac.
sleep, during - ***plat.***

CONVULSION, external abdomen - ran-s.

CONVULSIVE, pain - agar., ant-t., bov., cupr-am-s., dios., ferr., kali-c., lyc., ***nux-v.***, plb., ran-s., sars.
6 p.m., during urging for stool, while eating - tell.
abdomen, drawing in, and inspiration agg. - bov.
afternoon - stry.
dinner, after - bry.
flatus, as from incarcerated, afternoon amel. - tela
menses, during - ***am-c.***, carl.
periodic - ars.
pressure of clothes, from, and from touch, after a long walk - nux-v.
spot, in one - euph.
stool, during - crot-t.

CORD, as if, connecting, anus and navel, sensation of, with cutting on straightening up when bent forward - ***ferr-i.***, plb.

COVERING, agg. - camph., ***sec.***, ***tab.***

CRACKING, and crackling - caust. coloc.
evening - nat-m.

CRACKS, on surface of abdomen - ***sil.***

CRAMP, turning body - dros.

CRAMPING, pain - ***abrot.***, acet-ac., ***acon.***, aesc., aeth., **AGAR.**, ail., all-c., **ALOE**, ***alum.***, ***alumn.***, ambr., ***am-c.***, **AM-M.**, ***anac.***, anan., ang., ***ant-c.***, ***ant-t.***, ***apis***, aran., arg-m., ***arg-n.***, arn., ***ars.***, ars-i., ***asaf.***, ***asar.***, ***aur.***, aur-m., bar-c., bar-i., ***bar-m.***, **BELL.**, ***berb.***, ***bism.***, ***bor.***, ***bov.***, brom., ***bry.***, bufo, cact., calad., **CALC.**, ***calc-p.***, calc-s., camph., cann-s., canth., caps., ***carb-ac.***, ***carb-an.***, **CARB-S.**, **CARB-V.**, card-m., carl., caul., ***caust.***, cedr., **CHAM.**, **CHEL.**, ***chin.***, chin-a., ***cic.***, ***cina***, cinnb., clem., cob., coc-c., **COCC.**, ***coff.***, ***colch.***, **COLOC.**, ***con.***, ***cop.***, corn., croc., ***crot-t.***, cub., **CUPR.**, ***cupr-ar.***, ***cycl.***, ***dig.***, **DIOS.**, dros., **DULC.**, echi., elaps, ***elat.***, erig., ***eup-per.***, ***euph.***, ***euphr.***, eupi., ***ferr.***, ferr-ar., ferr-p., gamb., ***gels.***, gent-c., glon., gnaph., ***gran.***, **GRAPH.**, ***grat.***, guai., ***ham.***, ***hell.***, ***hep.***, ***hydr.***, hydrc., ***hyos.***, hyper., **IGN.**, iod., **IP.**, ***iris***, jab., jatr., jug-r., kali-ar., ***kali-bi.***, ***kali-br.***, ***kali-c.***, kali-i., kali-n., kali-p., ***kali-s.***, ***kreos.***, ***lac-c.***, ***lach.***, lact., ***laur.***, lec., ***led.***, ***lil-t.***, lob., **LYC.**, lycps., lyss., ***mag-c.***, **MAG-M.**, **MAG-P.**, mag-s., manc., mang., meny., ***merc.***, merc-c., merl., ***mez.***, ***mosch.***, ***mur-ac.***, naja, ***nat-a.***, ***nat-c.***, ***nat-m.***, nat-p., ***nat-s.***, ***nit-ac.***, ***nux-m.***, **NUX-V.**, olnd., ol-j., onos., **OP.**, ox-ac., paeon., pall., ***par.***, ***petr.***, phel., **PH-AC.**, phos., ***phyt.***, ***pic-ac.***, plan., ***plat.***, **PLB.**, **PODO.**, prun., psor., ptel., **PULS.**, ***ran-b.***, ran-s., ***raph.***, rat., ***rheum***, rhod., ***rhus-t.***, rhus-v., ***rumx.***, ruta, sabad., sabin., samb., sars., ***sec.***, senec., seneg., **SENN.**, ***sep.***, **SIL.**, ***spig.***, **SPONG.**, squil., **STANN.**, ***staph.***, ***stram.***, ***stront-c.***, **STRY.**, **SULPH.**, ***sul-ac.***, sumb., tab., tarax., ***tarent.***, tell., ***ter.***, teucr., ***thuj.***, trom., ***valer.***, **VERAT.**, verb., vib., viol-t., vip., ***zinc.***, **ZING.**

afternoon - agar., alum., bism., bry., carb-s., carb-v., coloc., corn., grat., kali-n., laur., lyc., mag-c., nat-c., nat-m., nat-s., nicc., op., par., phyt., sil., senec., sulph., ***verat.***
1 p.m. - mag-m.
3 to 10 pm - lyc.
4 p.m. - caust., coloc., hell., **LYC.**
4 to 9 p.m. - ***coloc.***
5 p.m. - aran., tell.

air, cold in - ***am-c.***, lyc.
open, in - ign.
amel. - nat-c.

alternating, pain in chest, with - ***ran-b.***
vertigo, with - verat.

ascending, steps - hell.

bed, in - alum., dig., dios., kali-c., lact., nat-m., nux-v., psor., rhus-t., sabin., valer.

belching, amel. - carb-v., kali-c., sep., ***sulph.***

bending, backward amel. - bell., ***dios.***, nux-v., onos.
forward amel. - ***acon.***, am-c., ***caust.***, ***chin.***, coff., ***colch.***, **COLOC.**, ***kali-c.***, ***lach.***, ***mag-p.***, phos., ***plb.***, prun., ***rhus-t.***, sars., senec., ***stann.***, stram., zinc.

breakfast, after - agar., eupi., grat., ham., kali-bi., lyc., nux-m., stront-c., **ZINC.**

breathing, on inspiration - aesc., am-m., brom., guai., ***sulph.***

chill, during - **COCC.**, led.
before - ars., ***spong.***

chilliness, during - rhus-t., sep.

coffee, from - ***cham.***, ign., nat-m., ***nux-v.***

cold, after taking - ***all-c.***, alum., alumn., ***dulc.***, nat-c., nit-ac.
as after taking cold - hep., petr., stann.

constipation, during - merc., ***op.***, ***plb.***, ***podo.***, sil.

convulsions, with - ***cic.***

coughing, when - chel., plb., tarent.

CRAMPING, pain

diarrhea, with - ars., petr., phos., sep., zinc.

before - ars., kali-n., mag-c., mag-m., phos., sulph.

dinner, during - am-c., kali-c., mag-s., zinc.

after - agar., alumn., caps., cocc., crot-t., gent-c., kali-c., **MAG-C.,** naja, phos., ***ran-b.,*** thuj., trom., valer., **ZING.**

drinking, water, after - cham., **COLOC.,** ***crot-c., manc.,*** nat-m., nit-ac., ***nux-v., puls.,*** raph., ***rhus-t.***

eating, while - carb-v., caust., dulc., kali-p., ***nux-v.***

2 hours, after - sil.

after - ***all-c., ant-t.,*** bell., carb-v., caps., caust., chin., cic., cocc., coc-c., ***colch., coloc.,*** con., cupr., gamb., ***graph.,*** grat., hell., kali-c., kali-p., lyc., ***nat-c.,*** nux-m., ***puls., rhus-t.,*** sars., ***sulph., verat.,*** zinc.

amel. - ***bov.,*** psor.

extending to,

chest, left side - kali-n.

lumbar region - alum., guai., kali-n., nat-m.

stomach - kali-n.

upward - mag-m.

evening - alum., am-c., bism., calad., **CALC.,** carb-v., cast., chin., cycl., grat., ***iris,*** kali-n., led., mag-c., mag-m., mag-s., merc., nat-m., petr., ph-ac., plan., plb., ***puls.,*** sars., senec., stann., sulph., sul-ac., tarent., thuj., ***valer.,*** zinc.

bed, in - alum., ars., hyos., ***valer.***

fever, during - caps., carb-v., elat., rhus-t., rob.

flatus, from - euph., graph., kali-c., mang., phos., sulph.

passing, while - aur., canth., ***chin.,*** mur-ac., nit-ac., spig., ***squil.,*** staph.

amel. - ***acon., am-c.,*** cimx., ***coloc., con., echi., graph., hydr.,*** lyc., mag-c., merc-c., nat-a., ***nat-m.,*** nux-m., ol-an., psor., rumx., sil., spong., squil., sulph.

before - ars., graph., guai., mez., mur-ac., rheum., sil., spig., tarax.

forenoon - agar., am-c., am-m., coloc., **DIOS.,** kali-bi., kali-n., lyc., mag-c., ***nat-c.,*** paeon., sars., sulph., tell., xan.

9 a.m. - mag-c.

10 a.m. - carb-s.

11 a.m. - corn.

fruit, after - calc-p., ***chin., coloc., puls.***

holding abdomen, amel. - mang.

humiliation, from - ***coloc., staph.***

hysterical - ars., bell., bry., ***cocc., ip., mag-m., mosch.,*** nux-v., ***stann., stram., valer.***

ice cream, after - **ARS.,** ***calc-p., ip., puls.***

indignation, after - **STAPH.**

jerking - graph., mur-ac., plat.

kneading, abdomen amel. - ***nat-s.***

leaning, on a sharp edge - ran-b., samb.

CRAMPING, pain

lying, while - ***phos., spig.***

abdomen on, amel. - am-c., chion., ***coloc.,*** der.

amel. - cupr., ferr.

back, on, from - phys.

with limbs drawn up amel. - ***rhus-t.***

right side, on, amel. - phys.

side, on - coloc., ign.

amel. - nat-s.

melons, from - **ZING.**

menses, during - acon., alum., ***am-c.,*** anac., ars., bar-c., ***bell., bor.,*** brom., calc., ***caul., caust., cham.,*** chel., ***chin., chin-s., cimic., cinnb.,*** clem., **COCC.,** ***coff., coloc., con., cupr.,*** form., gran., ***graph.,*** ign., ***kali-c.,*** kali-n., kali-s., mag-m., ***mag-p.,*** mosch., nat-c., ***nat-m.,*** nat-s., nicc., ***nit-ac., nux-v., plat., puls.,*** sabin., sars., ***sep.,*** stront-c., **SULPH.,** vib., zinc.

after - ***am-c.,*** cocc., kreos., merl., puls.

before - aloe, alum., ***am-c.,*** bar-c., ***bell.,*** brom., ***calc-p.,*** carb-v., ***caust., cham.,*** chin., ***cinnb., cocc., coloc., croc., cupr.,*** cycl., hyper., ***ign.,*** **KALI-C.,** ***lach.,*** mag-c., ***mag-p.,*** manc., nux-v., ph-ac., ***plat., puls., sep.,*** spong.

hip to hip, from - thuj.

midnight - alum., **COCC.,** coloc., lyc., **NIT-AC.,** petr., rhus-t., ***zinc.***

after - am-m., aur., sulph.

milk, after - bufo., cupr., ***lac-d.,*** mag-s., raph.

hot amel. - ***crot-t.***

warm, amel. - ***crot-t.,*** op.

morning - agar., am-c., calc., carb-s., **CAUST.,** coc-c., coloc., colch., con., cupr., **DIOS.,** dulc., euphr., graph., hep., kali-bi., kali-c., kali-n., lact., lob., ***lyc.,*** mag-m., mang., nat-c., nat-m., nit-ac., **NUX-V.,** phos., plan., psor., ***puls.,*** rat., ruta, sabin., sars., sep., staph., sulph., tarent., xan., zinc.

bed, in - agar., euph., kali-c., lact., mag-c., nat-m., **NUX-V.,** psor., ***puls.,*** sabin.

fasting, from - dulc.

uncovering, on - rheum.

morning, rising, on - nat-m., ruta

after - am-m., ars., mag-m., nit-ac.

amel. - nat-m.

morning, on waking - agar., cob., colch., lyc., mang., nat-m., rheum., xan.

5 a.m. - cob.

6 a.m. - ***coloc.***

motion, on - alum., brom., **COCC.,** corn-f., **IP.,** mag-p., ***mur-ac., nit-ac., nux-v.,*** phys., ran-b., raph., rhus-t., ***zinc.***

amel. - bov., ***gels.,*** rhus-t.

night - alum., arg-n., bry., **CALC.,** calc-s., carb-s., ***chin.,*** cupr., ***cycl.,*** dig., euphr., graph., ign., ***iris,*** kali-c., kali-s., mez., myric., nat-c., ***nat-s., nit-ac.,*** osm., ***podo., rhus-t.,*** senec., sep., stront-c., ***sulph.,*** sul-ac., ***valer.***

1 a.m. - ***mag-m.***

2 a.m. - nat-s., phos.

3 a.m. - carb-v.

CRAMPING, pain
night, at
bed, in - dig., rhus-t.
uncovering, on - bry.
noon - alumn., carb-v., kali-c., mag-c., sulph.
pressure, amel. - am-c., brom., bry., **COLOC.,** ***mag-p.,*** mang., ***podo., stann.***
riding, while - psor.
rising, from a seat - kali-c.
amel. - chin., spong.
rubbing, from - sulph.
sex, during - graph.
sitting, while - chin., dig., elaps, ferr., par., rhus-t., spong.
amel. - bell., mur-ac.
bent, while - carb-v., dulc.
head on knees, with amel. - euph.
sleep, during - kali-n.
amel. - alum., mag-m.
smoking, after - bufo., brom.
soup, after - zinc.
standing, while - bell., gent-c., mur-ac., zinc.
amel. - chin.
bent, amel. - spong.
stool, during - ***agar., aloe, am-c.,*** anac., ***apis,*** asc-c., aur., bapt., ***bor.,*** canth., caust., coc-c., colch., con., corn., crot-t., cupr-ar., cycl., dig., dulc., ferr., grat., hep., hydr., iris, kali-bi., kali-c., ***lil-t., mag-c.,*** mang., ***merc., nux-v.,*** op., phel., phos., plan., podo., puls., ***rheum,*** rhus-t., sec., senn., sep., **SULPH.,** sul-ac., zinc.
after - agar., ***aloe,*** **AM-C.,** ***ars.,*** carb-an., carb-s., ***carb-v., coloc.,*** con., cupr., eup-per., glon., graph., grat., kali-bi., kali-c., lil-t., lyc., mag-m., nat-c., ***nat-m.,*** nit-ac., ***op.,*** plb., rheum., rhod., **SULPH.,** sul-ac.
amel. - agar., aloe., carb-s., cinnb., coc-c., **COLOC.,** ferr., ***gamb., gels.,*** indg., ***mag-c.,*** naja, nat-a., **NAT-S., NUX-V.,** puls., seneg., sulph., ***verat.***
before - aesc., ***agar.,*** **ALOE,** alum., **AM-C.,** ***am-m.,*** ang., **ARG-N.,** ***ars.,*** arum-d., arum-i., arum-m., aur., bell., ***bry.,*** calc., ***calc-p.,*** camph., cann-s., canth., carb-an., carb-s., **CHIN.,** ***chin-s.,*** cina, coc-c., ***colch., coll.,*** **COLOC.,** ***crot-t.,*** cupr., cupr-s., cycl., dig., ferr., ferr-ar., ferr-i., ***gamb.,*** gels., glon., gran., grat., guai., hep., hyper., ign., ***jatr.,*** kali-ar., kali-bi., kali-c., kali-n., kali-s., lact., ***lil-t.,*** lycps., **MAG-C.,** mag-m., ***mag-p.,*** mang., meny., ***merc.,*** merc-i-r., ***mez.,*** mur-ac., nat-a., nat-c., nat-m., nat-p., nit-ac., ***nux-v.,*** **OP.,** petr., phel., ***phos.,*** phys., **PODO.,** puls., rat., rhod., rhus-t., rhus-v., sep., spig., stram., **SULPH.,** ***thuj., trom., verat.,*** zinc.
hard - meny., ***op.***
stooping, agg. - am-c., dulc., nux-v., ***sulph.***
supper, after - alum., calc., coff., gels., grat., ol-an., ***zinc.***

CRAMPING, pain
suppressed, hemorrhoidal flow - **NUX-V.**
tea, after - hyper.
turning, amel. - euph., mag-c.
urination, on - bar-c., ***cham., merc.,*** sul-ac.
amel. - tarent.
vaginal, discharge, before - con., mag-c., mag-m., sulph.
discharge, with - zinc.
vegetables, after - cupr.
vexation, after - cham., **COLOC.,** ***staph.***
waking, on - alum., coc-c., colch., euphr., ferr., lyc., mez., nat-m., stann., ***stront-c.,*** xan., ***zinc.***
walking, while - ang., bell., chin., ***coloc.,*** cupr., gent-c., graph., kali-bi., mur-ac., nat-p., phos., ph-ac., prun., ***ran-b.,*** stann., ***zinc.***
air, in open - agar., am-c., bry., ph-ac., rhus-t., sil., sulph.
amel. - chin., cycl., dig., elaps, ferr., par., puls., ***sulph.***
wandering - mur-ac., spig., staph.
warm room, amel. - am-c.
warmth, amel. - alum., am-c., cupr-s.
wet, getting feet - ***all-c.***
wine, after - lyc.
yawning - zinc.

CRAMPING, pain, hypochondria - aesc., aloe, am-m., arg-m., bar-c., bell., bry., bufo, calc., ***calc-s.,*** camph., caust., cupr., dios., ign., iod., ***ip.,*** kali-bi., ***kali-c.,*** kali-i., ***lact., lyc.,*** mag-c., ***mur-ac.,*** nat-m., nit-ac., ph-ac., phos., plat., sep., sil., stann., sulph., ***zinc.***
alternating, with oppression of chest - zinc.
belching, amel. - sep.
bending forward agg. - dig.
coughing, on - lyc.
evening - calc-s., dios.
extending, across back - **SIL.**
downward - hell.
hips, to - sil.
lumbar vertebrae, to - camph.
umbilicus, to - ph-ac.
upward - mag-c.
flatus amel. - mur-ac., sep.
intermittent - mag-c.
left - plat., zinc.
extending to stomach - phos.
menses, before - sulph.
morning - teucr.
motion agg. - zinc.
night - calc-s.
paroxysmal - nit-ac., sep., sil.
periodic - ph-ac.
respiration, deep - croc.
right - carb-an., iod., kali-c., mag-c., nat-m., ph-ac., phos., rhus-t., samb., staph., sulph., verb., zinc.
rubbing amel. - phos.
sitting - carb-an., rhus-t.
stepping - caust.
stool, during - sul-ac.
after - caust.

CRAMPING, pain, hypochondria
stooping, on - lyc.
turning the body - lyc.
walking, while - sulph.
after - ph-ac.

CRAMPING, pain, hypogastrium - ***acon., agar.,*** aloe, am-c., am-m., ***ars.,*** aur., ***bell.,*** bism., ***bry.,*** calc., carb-an., carb-s., ***carb-v., chel.,*** chin., cimic., ***cocc., coll.,*** coloc., ***con., cupr-ar.,*** cycl., dig., ***dios., gels.,*** guai., helon., kali-c., kreos., lil-t., lyc., mag-c., mez., meny., ***nat-c.,*** nit-ac., ***nux-v., prun.,*** psor., ran-b., rhus-t., ruta., sep., ***sil.,*** spig., spong., squil., stann., ***stry.,*** **SULPH.,** sul-ac., thuj., zinc.
bending double, compelling - ***prun.***
to left agg. - bell.
daytime - stram.
diarrhea, with - ars.
eating, after - con., ran-b.
evening - dulc., lyc.
flatus amel. - kali-c., mez., squil.
forenoon - agar.
left - lyc.
lying agg. - sulph.
on back - ambr.
menses, during - ***agar.,*** **AM-C.,** ***ars.,*** **COCC.,** ***con.,*** **GRAPH.,** ***mag-p.,*** nat-m., sulph.
after - kreos.
before - cimic., ***cocc.,*** **KALI-C.,** ***mag-p.,*** manc., ***nat-m., nit-ac.,*** sars., **SULPH.,** ***vib.,*** zinc.
metrorrhagia, with - mag-c.
morning - ambr., ars., dios., fago., hyos.
night - chel.
1 a.m.- mang.
menses, before - mang.
paroxysmal - chin., sep.
pressure amel. - fago.
retracting abdomen agg. - bell., kali-c.
right - ambr.
sit upright, must - sulph.
sitting - chin.
upright, amel. - sulph.
standing - chin.
stepping - calc.
stool, during - ***ars.***
after - agar., lyc.
before - agar., anac., ***ars., coll., gels.,*** meny., stram.
stooping, on - am-c.
supper, after - ran-b.
touch, on - cycl.
urination, during - bar-c., sul-ac.
after - sul-ac.
before - ***chel.,*** sul-ac.
vaginal, discharge, before - sulph.
walking - sulph., zinc.
in open air - agar., calc.
wandering - chin.
warmth, amel. - ***ars.***

CRAMPING, pain, inguinal - ***aloe,*** am-c., am-m., bov., ***bry.,*** calc., carb-v., ***chel.,*** cimic., ***gamb.,*** indg., kali-c., kali-i., ***kreos.,*** mag-c., nat-s., petr., phos., rat., stann., sulph., sul-ac., zinc.
afternoon, 3 p.m. - mag-c.
4 p.m. - nicc.
ascending stairs - alum.
dinner, after - nat-c.
extending to knee - aloe.
face, causing face to flush - cimic.
forenoon, 11 a.m. - mag-c.
inspiration, on - sulph.
intermittent - nat-c.
left - chel., kali-n., sars., stann.
menses, during - kali-c.
after - bor., kreos., plan.
morning - rat.
paroxysmal - nat-m.
right - aloe, bov., carb-v., dig., gamb., indg., mag-c., nat-c., sul-ac., zinc.
rising, from sitting - zinc.
rubbing, on - ***sulph.***
amel. - mag-c.
sitting, while - kali-c., petr., spong.
stool, during - nicc.
stooping - sulph.
stretching, on - am-c.
talking - calc.
walking, while - kali-n., mag-c., ***sulph.***

CRAMPING, pain, sides - acon., alum., ant-c., bell., bry., calc-p., canth., carb-v., caust., chin., coloc., cupr., ***ign.,*** kali-n., lach., laur., ***led., lyc.,*** mag-c., manc., mur-ac., naja, nat-c., nat-m., ***nat-s., nux-v.,*** petr., ***phos.,*** plat., puls., rat., rhod., ruta, sars., seneg., sulph., sul-ac., thuj., zinc.
afternoon - ant-c.
bind, must bind the abdomen - puls.
eating, after - mez.
evening - ant-c., nicc.
expiration, on - mur-ac.
flank - ambr., bell., carb-s., carb-v., cocc., coff., mag-c., mur-ac., ph-ac., sars., stann.
flatus, amel. - plat.
inspiration, agg. - mur-ac.
deep agg. - sars.
left - ang., ant-c., bry., calc-p., canth., chin., coloc., cupr., dulc., naja, nat-m., nux-v., puls., sars., seneg., staph., sulph., sul-ac., thuj.
to right - asar., carb-v.
lying - nat-m.
menses, during - ars.
motion, agg. - ant-c., zinc.
night - sulph.
pulse, synchronous, with - ant-c.
right - acon., ant-c., bell., carb-v., caust., hell., lach., **LYC.,** mag-c., manc., mez., nat-m., ***nat-s.,*** phos., rhus-t., sep., zinc.
extending to back - phos.
lying on left - nat-m.
sitting, while - carb-an.
bent, while - carb-v.
standing, agg. - kali-n.

CRAMPING, pain, sides
stool, during - mang., nicc.
before - mag-c., mang.
stooping - stram.
walking - bell., nat-m.

CRAMPING, pain, umbilical region - acon., agar., ***aloe,*** alum., am-m., anac., ant-c., ant-t., arn., aspar., bar-c., ***bell.,*** berb., ***bry.,*** calc., ***camph., carb-an.,*** carb-s., caul., caust., ***chel.,*** cham., ***chin.,*** cimic., ***cocc.,*** coc-c., **COLOC.,** ***crot-t.,*** cycl., **DIOS.,** dulc., euphr., fl-ac., ***gamb.,*** gent-c., gran., graph., grat., guai., ham., hyos., ign., ***iod.,*** **IP.,** jug-c., kali-bi., kali-i., kali-n., kreos., ***laur.,*** lec., led., lyc., mag-c., mag-m., mang., meny., merc-c., ***mez., mur-ac.,*** myric., naja, ***nat-c.,*** nat-m., nicc., nit-ac., nux-m., ***nux-v.,*** ox-ac., petr., ***ph-ac.,*** phos., ***phyt., plat., plb., podo., ptel., raph.,*** rheum, rhus-t., sabad., samb., sang., senec., sil., spig., squil., stann., staph., stront-c., ***sulph.,*** tab., tarent., thuj., ***verat.,*** verb., ***zinc.***
afternoon - euphr., nat-c., plb., **SULPH.**
4 p.m. - sulph.
5 p.m. - mag-c., sang.
below, umbilicus - kali-c., kali-n., mag-c., mag-m., nat-c., nat-m., phos., zinc.
supper, after - calc.
bend, body, must - lyc.
bending, body - nit-ac.
forward - con.
forward amel. - ***aloe,*** **COLOC.,** senec.
breakfast, during - alum.
after - agar., kali-bi.
cold, after taking - ***bry.***
as after taking - stann.
diarrhea, with - kali-n.
before - coloc., mag-c., plat.
dinner, during and after - ant-t., bry., calc., **COLOC.,** ham.
eating, after - bell., carb-v., graph., kali-n., mag-m., ***nux-v.,*** plat., sulph.
evening - alum., caust., phos., plat., **SULPH.**
bed, in - nux-m.
stool, during - inul.
extending, to
abdomen - calc.
anus - nat-m.
back - plat.
chest - kali-n.
downward - plat.
groin - thuj.
hip - mag-c.
sacrum - mag-c.
stomach - carb-v., mag-c., sulph.
throat - kreos.
flatus, amel. - bar-c., carb-v., mag-m., mez., sulph.
as from - plat., zinc.
forenoon - agar., lyc., nat-c.
fruit, after - **COLOC.**
inspiration, on - anac.
menses, before - ***kreos.***
morning - aeth., bor., bov., lyc., mag-c., nat-m.
bed, in - caust., lyc.
rising, after - aeth.
waking, on - bov.

CRAMPING, pain, umbilical region
motion - bar-c., nit-ac.
night - bry., cycl., lyc., nux-m., ***podo.***
bed, in - nux-m.
waking, on - cycl.
noon - mag-m., ***sulph.***
periodical - ph-ac.
rising, from stooping - chin.
sitting, while - ***all-c.,*** chin., ph-ac., sulph.
bent - ant-t.
soup, after - kali-n.
sour food, after - asaf.
standing - bry., gent-c.
stool, during - cocc., ***corn.,*** indg., iod., phos.
before - ***coloc.,*** graph., ***ham.,*** kali-n., lec., mag-m., mur-ac., phos., plb., psor.
amel. - meny.
stooping - am-m., phos.
supper, after - gels.
urination, after - mag-c.
vaginal, discharge, with - mag-c.
before - sil.
walking, while - ***all-c.,*** gent-c., zinc.
amel. - bar-c.

CREEPING, warm sensation, runs over - alumn.

CUTTING, pain - **ACON.,** aeth., ***agar.,*** agn., **ALOE,** ***alum., ambr.,*** am-c., am-m., anac., ***ant-c., ant-t., apis,*** arg-m., ***arg-n.,*** arn., **ARS.,** ***ars-i.,*** arum-t., asaf., asar., aur., bapt., ***bar-c.,*** bar-i., ***bar-m.,*** bell., berb., ***bol., bor., bov., bry.,*** bufo, cact., ***calc.,*** calc-p., calc-s., cahin., calad., camph., cann-s., **CANTH.,** ***caps., carb-an.,*** carb-s., carb-v., card-m., ***carl.,*** cast., caust., ***cham., chel.,*** **CHIN.,** chin-a., chin-s., chion., cic., cimic., ***cina,*** clem., ***cocc.,*** coc-c., ***colch.,*** **COLOC.,** ***con.,*** crot-t., cub., ***cupr.,*** cupr-ar., cycl., ***dig.,*** **DIOS.,** dros., ***dulc.,*** echi., elaps, ***elat.,*** euon., eupi., glon., graph., grat., hell., ***hep.,*** hydr., **HYOS.,** hyper., ***ign.,*** indg., ***iod.,*** **IP.,** ***iris,*** jatr., ***kali-ar., kali-bi.,*** **KALI-C.,** kali-i., ***kali-n.,*** kali-p., **KALI-S.,** kreos., ***lach.,*** lact., ***laur., led.,*** lept., lil-t., lob., ***lyc.,*** **MAG-C.,** ***mag-m., manc.,*** mang., ***merc., merc-c.,*** merc-i-f., merc-p-r., mez., ***mur-ac.,*** murx., naja, ***nat-a., nat-c., nat-m.,*** nat-p., **NAT-S.,** nicc., **NIT-AC.,** nux-m., **NUX-V.,** ***ol-an.,*** **OP.,** ***ox-ac.,*** paeon., par., ***petr.,*** phel., ph-ac., ***phos.,*** phyt., plat., plb., psor., ptel., **PULS.,** ran-s., ***rheum, rhus-t.,*** pob., rumx., ruta, ***sabad.,*** sabin., ***sars., sec., sel., seneg., sep., sil.,*** **SPIG.,** squil., stann., ***staph., stront-c.,*** **STRY.,** **SULPH.,** ***sul-ac.,*** sumb., ter., thuj., valer., **VERAT.,** verat-v., verb., ***viol-t.,*** vip., zinc.
afternoon - agar., berb., calc-s., chel., coloc., grat., kali-n., laur., mag-m., nat-c., nat-m., sars., sep., stront.
1 p.m. - grat.
2 to 4 p.m. - laur.
4 to 11 p.m. - alum.
5 p.m. - sars.
air, while, in - graph.
air, open, in - mang., merc-c.
air, open, in - ***aloe,*** kali-i.
ascending, on - merc.

CUTTING, pain
belching, amel. - rat.
bend, backward, must - kali-c.
bending, backward - sulph.
double amel. - **COLOC., KALI-C.,** petr., rheum., rhus-t., staph.
breakfast, after - bor., cahin., hydr., mag-m., spong., thuj., **ZINC.**
chill, during - ars.
after - ars., con.
before - ars.
cold, as from taking a - mur-ac., petr.
from a cold - camph.
cold, water, drinking, after - calc-p.
amel. - calc., cann-s.
coughing, on - ***arn.,*** cham., chin., valer., **VERAT.**
daytime - nat-m.
diarrhea, during - ars., kali-c., kali-n., mag-c., mag-m., petr., nit-ac., sep., sulph.
after - mag-c., mag-m.
before - ars., kali-n., petr., phos., sars., sulph.
dinner, during - lact., zinc.
after - cahin., cham., coloc., grat., hydr., lact., lyc., mag-m., nat-m., rheum, sil., sulph., **ZINC.**
before - hydr., lyc.
drawing, in abdomen, on - valer.
up feet amel. - ***coloc.***
drinking, after - ars., ***calc-p., nat-m.,*** staph.
eating, while - aloe, caust., grat., zinc.
after - ant-t., ars., cahin., calc-p., ***chel.,*** **COLOC.,** ign., ***kali-bi.,*** nat-m., olnd., ***petr.,*** spong., ***staph.,*** sul-ac., ***zinc.***
amel. - bov., calc.
electric shock darting through the anus, like - **COLOC.**
evening - agar., aloe, ambr., ant-t., bar-c., bell., calc., carb-v., dig., ***dios.,*** fago., hep., kali-n., led., mag-c., mang., merc., mez., nat-m., nicc., ox-ac., ***petr.,*** phos., ph-ac., puls., rat., rhus-t., sel., staph., stront-c., sulph., thuj.
5 p.m., lasting all night - canth.
7 p.m. - elaps, sulph.
in bed - ars.
sitting still agg. - ***puls.***
exercise, from - sep.
extending, anus, to - ***coloc.***
backwards and upwards during labor - ***gels.***
chest, to - phos.
groin, to - am-m.
left to right, from - ***ip.***
lumbar region, to - mag-m.
right to left from - **LYC.**
sacrum, to - am-m.
thigh, to - ***coloc.,*** ter.
fasting - dulc.
fever, during - rhus-t.
amel. - ***sulph.***
flatus, from - coloc., kali-c.
as from - sep.

CUTTING, pain
flatus, before - chin., con., lyc.
flatus, passing, with - iod., kali-c., petr., spig.
amel. - anac., ars-i., bapt., bov., bry., calc-p., **CON.,** eupi., gamb., ***hydr.,*** kali-n., laur., plb., psor., sel., sulph., viol-t.
forenoon - agar., carb-an., lyc., nat-c., nat-m., ***rhus-t.***
honey, after - calc-p.
humiliation, after - puls.
inspiration, on - cocc., guai., ***lyc.***
labor, during - phos., puls.
false labor, pains, like - kali-c.
lead, colic - **COLOC.**
lifting, after - sil.
lying - nat-m.
menses, during - alum., am-c., ars., bar-c., ***calc.,*** carb-v., ***caust.,*** **COCC.,** ***eupi.,*** ferr., graph., iod., ip., **KALI-C.,** ***kreos.,*** **LACH.,** ***lyc.,*** mag-c., nicc., ***ol-an., phos., senec., sulph.,*** zinc.
after - graph., kali-c.
appearance of, on - ***caust.,*** gels., graph., lyc., **PLAT.,** staph.
as if, would appear - laur.
before - alum., ***cham.,*** lach., ***lil-t.,*** mag-c., nat-c., nat-m., ol-an., staph.
from hip to hip - thuj., ust.
midnight - ambr., bar-c., lyc., nat-m., sep., sulph.
after - ambr., elaps., sars., sep., sulph.
milk, after - zinc.
warm, after - ***ang.***
morning - alum., ambr., bov., calc., caust., con., ***dios.,*** dulc., graph., kali-n., lyc., mag-m., nat-c., nat-m., nicc., **NIT-AC.,** nux-v., ox-ac., ***petr.,*** puls., sep., spong., stry., zinc.
bed, in - nat-m., **NIT-AC.,** spig., sulph.
rising, after - ars., nat-m.
stool, during - ambr.
waking, on - calc., petr.
motion, on - aloe, ***bry.,*** caps., ***cocc.,*** merc-c., puls., rhus-t., stann., staph.
amel. - nicc., ***puls.,*** sep.
night - ambr., bar-c., calc., camph., canth., fago., kali-c., kali-n., lyc., mag-c., mag-m., merc., nat-c., nat-m., nit-ac., ph-ac., ran-s., sars., sep., sil., sulph., sul-ac., zinc.
1 a.m. - phos.
2 a.m. - am-m., mag-m., sep.
3 a.m. - phos.
4 a.m. - **PETR.,** sulph., verat.
5 a.m. - nat-m., ox-ac.
bed, in - fago., zinc.
pressing to urinate, when - graph.
waking - coloc., sulph.
noon - mag-c., sang.
soup, after - ambr., mag-c.
paroxysmal - calc., coloc., grat., lyc., ph-ac., sep., sil., stann.
pressure, amel. - kali-c.
pork, after - acon.

CUTTING, pain
rising, after - dig., nit-ac.
sitting, while - alum., asaf., dros., mur-ac., nat-c., nicc., ***puls.,*** spig., staph.
amel. - mur-ac.
bent, while - alum.
standing, on - ***bry.,*** mur-ac.
step, on every - ***arn., sil.***
stool, during - acon., agar., **ALOE,** alum., ambr., am-c., ant-c., ***arn.,*** **ARS.,** ***ars-i., asar.,*** calc-s., ***canth.,*** caps., caust., cham., chel., cob., coloc., dig., dulc., ferr., iod., iris, kali-c., kali-n., kalm., laur., mag-m., merc., ***merc-c.,*** nit-ac., plb., rheum, rhus-t., sars., sec., **SULPH.,** verat.
after - ***am-c.,*** ars., ***canth.,*** carb-v., **COLOC.,** gels., kali-n., lept., ***merc., merc-c.,*** ox-ac., ***podo.,*** rheum, staph., ***sulph.***
amel. - am-m., bry., ***calc-p.,*** caust., dig., hell., mag-m., mur-ac., nat-c., nat-m., **NUX-V.,** plb., ***rhus-t.,*** sil., sulph.
before - acon., aesc., aeth., agar., **ALOE,** am-c., am-m., ant-c., **ANT-T.,** ***ars., asar.,*** bar-c., bor., brom., ***bry.,*** cahin., ***calc-p.,*** calc-s., caps., carb-s., carb-v., chel., cina, cob., **COLOC.,** con., crot-t., dig., **DULC.,** gamb., gels., graph., grat., hell., hep., hydr., ign., kali-n., kalm., lact., laur., lyc., ***mag-c.,*** manc., ***merc., merc-c.,*** merc-i-f., nat-a., nat-c., ***nat-m.,*** nicc., ***nit-ac.,*** nux-m., nux-v., petr., ***puls.,*** rheum, ***rhus-t.,*** rumx., sang., sec., sep., ***staph.,*** sulph., ***thuj.,*** valer., verat., viol-t., zinc.
causing urging to - ***calc-p.,*** dig., ***lept., nux-v.,*** staph., ***sulph.***
diarrhea, during - bov., ***crot-t.,*** ferr., gamb., kali-n., jug-c., mag-m., ***merc.,*** **SULPH.**
stooping, amel. - puls.
stretching, on - aloe.
supper, after - calc., coloc., ox-ac., ***puls.,*** sep.
urination, during - chin., eupi., lyc., mag-c., merc.
after - chin., stann., staph.
before - mag-c., sulph., sul-ac.
vaginal, discharge, before - nat-c., sulph., zinc.
vinegar, after - aloe
walking, while - asaf., coloc., ***dios.,*** kali-c., laur., lyc., naja, mur-ac., phos., ph-ac.
wandering - bell., card-m., dulc., led., stront.
warm, wraps amel. - sulph.
warmth, of bed amel. - ***ars.,*** coloc., staph., symph.

cutting, hypochondria - arg-m., arg-n., ars., ars-i., ***aur.,*** bar-c., ***bell.,*** bor., brom., ***bry.,*** calc-f., chel., coc-c., colch., coloc., crot-h., dios., ***dulc., graph.,*** hydr., iod., kali-ar., ***kali-bi., kali-c.,*** lyc., mag-c., meny., merc-i-r., nat-m., nat-p., nicc., phos., ptel., puls., ***ran-b.,*** stann., stry., sulph., trom.

cutting, hypochondria
afternoon - chin-s.
breakfast, after - bor.
coughing - bry.
extending, back, to - ran-b., sul-ac.
downward - bor.
upward - bar-c.
umbilicus, to - bor.
left - arg-m., ***arg-n.,*** bar-c., bor., dulc., kali-c., mag-m., sul-ac., sulph., ter.
walking rapidly - bor.
morning - cast., mag-m.
motion - ang., ter.
night - stry.
right - ang., ***aur.,*** bry., ***carb-ac.,*** crot-c., dulc., iod., kali-c., ptel., stann., stry.
sitting, while - ter., viol-t.
bent, while - stann.
stooping - arg-m.
stretching agg. - lyc.
touch agg. - ars.
walking - phos.
rapidly - bor.

cutting, hypogastrium - aeth., agar., ***all-c.,*** am-c., ang., ***ars.,*** asar., ***bar-c.,*** **BELL.,** bry., cact., calc., carb-an., carb-s., ***cimic.,*** coc-c., ***coll., coloc., croc.,*** cycl., elaps, euon., ***hydr.,*** **HYOS.,** iris, kali-c., ***kali-bi.,*** laur., ***lept., lil-t., mag-m.,*** mag-s., mang., med., ***merc.,*** mur-ac., nat-c., nicc., nux-v., ol-an., **PULS.,** sep., ***sil.,*** **SPIG., SQUIL., STANN., SULPH.,** ter., ***thuj., verat.,*** zinc.
afternoon - sep.
bending backward - sulph.
double amel. - coloc., puls.
coughing on - bry., chin., verat.
diarrhea, with - ars.
dinner, after - lyc., zinc.
eating, after - cic., spong., ***verat.***
evening - agar., spong.
extending, to back - ***croc.***
to left chest - spong.
to spermatic cord - med.
flatus, after - zinc.
amel. - kali-c., mag-m.
left - zinc.
lying amel. - nux-v.
menses, during - arg-n., calc., carb-v., ***caust.,*** **KALI-C.,** nat-m., ***senec.,*** sulph.
after - kali-c., plat., puls.
as though menses would reappear - ***kreos., lyc.,*** plat., ***puls.***
before - ***caust.,*** nat-c., senec., sulph.
milk, after - ang.
morning - sars.
bed, in - mag-m.
motion amel. - nicc.
night - lyc.
pressure agg. - sulph.
retraction of abdomen agg. - kali-c.
sit, has to sit bent - mag-m.
sitting - mur-ac., nicc., spig.
standing - mang., mur-ac.
step, at every - nux-v., ***sil.***

cutting, hypogastrium
stool, after, amel. - pall.
agg, pressing for - sulph.
transverse - stann.
urination, before - sulph.
vaginal, discharge, before - lyc.
walking, while - coloc., mang., mur-ac., ***sil.***

cutting, inguinal - aesc., all-c., alum., am-m., arg-m., ***arg-n.,*** aur., berb., ***bry.,*** calc., calc-p., ***canth.,*** carb-an., caust., ***coloc.,*** cycl., gamb., iod., kali-bi., lyc., mag-c., merc., nat-m., ph-ac., spig., tell., ter., thuj., valer.
breathing deep amel. - carb-an.
draws up leg must - aur.
evening - am-m., dios., lyc.
extending, to, through urethra extending, to glans penis - asar., lyc.
to back - am-m.
to testes - calc.
forenoon - alum.
inspiration, on - ***bry.***
left - aesc., tell.
menses, during - ***arg-n., nat-m., senec.***
motion, on - caust.
night - mag-c.
pregnancy, during - podo.
retract, must, abdomen - aur.
right - ***bry.,*** podo., ter.
extending to left - lyc.
sitting, agg. - carb-an.
urination, on - nat-m.
walking, while - canth., caust., par.
amel. - carb-an.

cutting, sides - arn., ars., calc., carb-an., caust., clem., con., crot-t., dulc., ign., kali-bi., ***lach.,*** laur., mag-c., mur-ac., par., ruta, sars., ***stront-c.,*** thuj., zinc.
dinner, after - phos.
evening - lyc., nicc.
flank, in - ang., sulph.
flatus, passing, amel. -laur.
inspiration, on - phos.
left - calc., **KALI-C.,** mag-c., phos., sars., thuj.
to right - ***ip.***
lying on the back, while - sulph.
menses, during - ars.
morning, in bed - bell.
night - sulph.
paroxysmal - kali-bi.
right - clem., con., ***lach.,*** nit-ac., stront.
side, lain on - bell.
sitting, while - carb-an.
stool amel. - calc.
touch agg. - ars.
walking - clem., phos.
amel. - carb-an.

cutting, umbilical, region of - aesc., agar., aloe, ammc., am-m., ant-t., arn., bell., bov., brom., cact., calad., calc-p., camph., canth., caps., cast., cham., chin., cocc., **COLOC.,** con., crot-t., ***cupr.,*** **DIOS.,** ***dulc.,*** graph., grat., hell., hyos., hyper., ign., iod., **IP.,** kali-bi., ***kali-c., kali-i., kali-n.,*** kreos., led., lyc., ***mag-c.,*** mag-m., ***mang., merc-c.,*** merl., mur-ac., naja, ***nat-m.,***

cutting, umbilical, region of - **NUX-V.,** ol-an., ***op.,*** paeon., petr., plan., plat., psor., ptel., puls., raph., ***rheum,*** rhus-v., ***sars.,*** senec., ***sil.,*** sol-n., spig., ***stann.,*** staph., sulph., ***sul-ac.,*** tab., ust., valer., verat., verat-v., verb., zinc., zing.
afternoon - lyc., naja, ptel., spig.
4 p.m. - lyc.
bed, when going to - nat-m.
below region of umbilicus - mez.
below region of umbilical, after stool - nat-c.
cold drinks, after - calc-p.
weather - ***dulc.***
daytime - stann.
diarrhea, after - cupr., nat-m.
dinner, after - cham.
dinner, before - mang.
eating, after - ***coloc.***
evening - bar-c., bry., nat-m., staph.
expiration, during - rhus-t.
extending to lumbar region - bell.
flatus, as from - coloc., plat.
flatus, passing, amel. - ***mag-c.,*** sars.
forenoon - sars.
10 a.m. - verat-v.
menses, during - mag-c.
ice cream, after - calc-p.
inspiration, during - arn., coloc., ***mang.***
labor, during - **IP., NUX-V.**
lying bent amel. - hell.
menses, during - mag-c.
as if, would appear - ip.
midnight - sulph.
morning - hell., mang., petr., sars., sulph.
motion, during - caps.
noon - mag-m.
night - sil.
paroxysmal - mag-m.
pressure, agg. - chel., ip.
amel. - nat-m., ***stann.***
rising, after - sulph.
sitting, while - rhus-t.
step, at every - arn.
stool, after - ***aloe,*** cact., **COLOC.**
before - ***gamb.,*** graph., grat., nat-c., **NUX-V.**
stooping agg. - caps., sulph.
touch, agg. - ip.
vaginal discharge, before - sil.
waking, on - sulph.
walking, while - arn., caps., dios., sul-ac.
yawning, on - sars.

cutting, umbilicus - ant-t., bol., bov., cact., calad., cast., ***chin-s.,*** cimic., coc-c., crot-t., dios., indg., ***ip.,*** laur., ***nux-m.,*** plb., puls-n, rhus-t., rhus-v., sil., ter.
afternoon - cimic.
bending forward amel. - bov., calad., ***rhus-t.***
evening - nux-m.
extending to, back - sil.
to, stomach - crot-t.
forenoon - ***rhus-t.,*** sil.
night - nux-m.

DEPRESSION, canal-like, from ensiform cartilage to pubes - plb.

DESQUAMATION - merc., vesp.

DIARRHEA, sensation as if, would come on - act-sp., aeth., agar., ail., ***aloe,*** am-c., am-m., ant-c., apis, apoc., ***asaf.,*** bar-c., ***bell.,*** bol., ***bor.,*** **BRY.,** calc., ***camph.,*** carb-an., carb-s., carb-v., caust., cham., cimic., cob., colch., coloc., ***con., crot-t.,*** dig., **DULC.,** eupi., ferr., form., graph., hell., helon., **HYDR.,** hyos., kali-bi., ***kali-c., lach.,*** laur., led., lil-t., lith., lob., mag-m., mag-s., meny., meph., merc-i-f., naja, ***nat-s.,*** nit-ac., **NUX-V.,** olnd., onos., ox-ac., petr., ***ph-ac., phos.,*** phys., phyt., plan., ***plat.,*** prun., ptel., ***puls.,*** **RAN-S.,** rhus-t., rumx., sabin., sars., ***seneg., sep., stry.,*** sulph., sumb., ter., verat., zinc.

alternating, with nausea - squill.
as after - ant-c.
belching, amel. - sep., ***sulph.***
flatus, passing, after - plat.
amel. - plat., sep., ***sulph.***
stool, after a normal - ***iod., kali-s.,*** ph-ac., ***sep., sulph.***
smoking tobacco, after - bor.

DISAGREEABLE, sensation, in - apoc., lach., nicot., tet.

DISCHARGE, umbilicus, from - ***abrot., calc., calc-p.,*** hydr., ***kali-c., lyc.,*** med., morg., ***nat-m.,*** nux-m., stann., tub.

bloody fluid - abrot., ***calc., calc-p., nux-m.***
yellow, from suppressed gonorrhea - nat-m.

DISCOLORATION, general

black-bluish - aeth.
blackness - vip.
spots, in - vip.
blotches - aloe, crot-t.
blue spots - ***ars.,*** mosch.
brown spots - ars., carb-v., ***cob.,*** hydr-ac., kali-c., ***lach.,*** **LYC.,** nit-ac., ***phos.,*** sabad., **SEP.,** ***thuj.***
greenish - rob.
inflamed spots - ars., bell., canth., ***kali-c., lach.,*** led., lyc., nat-m., **PHOS.,** sabad., ***sep.***
purple - vesp.
redness - anac., plb., plb-chr., ***rhus-t.,*** sang.
streak, curved above umbilicus - par.
redness, spots - bell., caps., crot-t., kali-bi., ***lach.,*** led., manc., ***merc.,*** rhus-t., sabad., sep.
air, open agg. - sabad.
coppery red - carb-o.
eruption, after - crot-t.
white spots - chlol.
yellow - cob., phos.
yellow, spots - ars., berb., canth., carb-v., ***kali-c., lach., phos.,*** sabad., sep., ***thuj.***
brown and yellow - ***cob.,*** **LYC.**
white patches between - chlol.

discoloration, epigastrium, redness - lyc., nat-m.
spots - lyc., nat-m.

discoloration, umbilical, region of, redness - phys.

DISTENSION, (see Intestines, Distension, flatus) - ***abrot.,*** acet-ac., **ACON.,** acon-c., aesc., ***aeth.,*** **AGAR.,** ***all-c.,*** **ALOE,** ***alum.,*** alumn., ambr., am-c., am-m., ***anac.,*** anan., ***ant-c., ant-t., apis, apoc., arg-m.,*** **ARG-N.,** ***arn.,*** **ARS.,** ars-i., ***asaf.,*** asar., aur., aur-m., ***bapt., bar-c., bar-i., bar-m.,*** bell., ***berb.,*** bism., bor., ***bov., brom., bry.,*** bufo, cact., cahin., calad., calc., calc-p., calc-s., ***canth., caps., carb-ac., carb-an.,*** **CARB-S., CARB-V.,** card-m., carl., cast., ***caust.,*** cedr., ***cham., chel.,*** **CHIN.,** ***chin-a., chin-s.,*** **CIC.,** cimic., ***cina,*** cinnb., ***cist.,*** clem., coc-c., **COCC.,** coff., **COLCH.,** coll., **COLOC.,** ***con.,*** cop., ***corn., croc., crot-h., crot-t., cupr., cycl., dig.,*** dulc., euph., ***eup-per.,*** fago., ferr., ferr-ar., ferr-i., ferr-p., ***gamb.,*** gins., gran., **GRAPH.,** grat., ***hell.,*** **HEP.,** ***hyos.,*** hyper., ictod., ign., ***iod.,*** ip., ***jatr.,*** jug-r., ***kali-ar., kali-bi.,*** **KALI-C.,** kali-chl., ***kali-i., kali-n., kali-p., kali-s., kreos., lac-c.,*** lac-d., **LACH.,** lact., laur., led., ***lil-t.,*** lob., **LYC.,** ***mag-c., mag-m.,*** mag-p., mag-s., manc., mang., ***meny.,*** **MERC.,** ***merc-c.,*** **MERC-D.,** ***mez.,*** mosch., ***mur-ac., murx.,*** nat-a., **NAT-C., NAT-M., NAT-P.,** ***nat-s.,*** nicc., ***nit-ac.,*** nux-m., ***nux-v.,*** ol-an., ***op.,*** ox-ac., pall., ***petr.,*** **PH-AC., PHOS.,** ***plat.,*** plb., podo., prun., ***psor.,*** ptel., ***puls.,*** pyrog., **RAPH.,** rheum, ***rhod., rhus-t.,*** rhus-v., rob., sabin., samb., sang., sars., ***sec., sep., sil.,*** spig., spong., squil., ***stann., staph., stram., stront-c.,*** **SULPH.,** sul-ac., sumb., tab., tarent., **TER.,** ***thuj., til.,*** uran., ***valer.,*** verb., ***verat.,*** vip., ***zinc.,*** zing.

afternoon - ***calc.,*** calc-s., ***carb-v., cast.,*** caust., cham., chin-s., con., fago., kali-n., mag-c., mag-m., nat-c., osm., petr., rat., sep., stann., stront-c., ***sulph.***
1 p.m. - grat.
4 p.m. - ***lyc.,*** sep.
4 p.m to 8 p.m. - **LYC.,** ***sulph.***
5 pm., emission of flatus, stool and sour urine, amel. - nat-a.
eating, after - bry., ***lyc.***
4 p.m - ***lyc.***
flatus, emission of, amel. - nat-c.
all day - plan.
alternating with, decrease of size - aesc.
sinking sensation - aster.
beer, after - ***nat-m.***
belching, amel. - ***carb-v.,*** sep., thuj.
before - sep.
do not amel. - phos.
bellows, like a pair of, set in motion - cahin.
breakfast, during - alum.
after - agar., chin-a., nat-m., sin-a.
hindering - con.
children, in - **BAR-C., CALC., CAUST.,** ***cina,*** cupr., **LYC.,** sil., staph., **SULPH.**
chill, during - ars., ars-h., cina, ***kali-c.,*** lach., lyc., mez., puls., rhus-t.
clothing, feels tight - mosch.
coffee, amel. - phos.
colic, during - colch., thuj.

DISTENSION,

constipation, during - alum., am-c., bry., ery-a., graph., hyos., iod., ***lach.,*** mag-m., nit-ac., phos., ph-ac., ter.

cramp-like, in several places, like blisters - plat.

diarrhea, before - chin-s., mag-s.

dinner, after - alum., anac., calc., carb-an., **CARB-V.,** euphr., grat., hep., iod., lyc., mag-c., mag-m., ***nat-m.,*** nicc., ***nux-m.,*** phos., ***sep.,*** sulph., ***thuj.,*** til.
before - all-c., euphr.

drinking, after - ambr., ars., calc., coloc., ***carb-v.,*** **CHIN.,** hep., petr., nat-m., ***nux-v.***

eating, while - dulc., graph., ign.
after - agar., aloe, alum., ambr., anac., ***ant-c.,*** ars., asaf., ***bor., bry.,*** calc., calc-s., caps., carb-ac., ***carb-an.,*** carb-s., **CARB-V.,** caust., ***cham.,*** **CHIN.,** chin-a., ***colch.,*** con., dulc., ***graph.,*** ign., jug-r., kali-ar., **KALI-C.,** kali-p., kali-s., ***kreos., lil-t.,*** **LYC.,** mag-c., mag-m., mag-s., mur-ac., nat-a., ***nat-c., nat-m.,*** nat-p., ***nux-m.,*** **NUX-V.,** petr., phos., plb., psor., ***puls.,*** raph., rheum, ***rhus-t., sep., sil.,*** **SULPH.,** tarent., ter., ***thuj., zinc.***
frozen things - psor.
herring, piece of - nat-m.
satiety, to - ***lyc.***
agg. - ***colch.,*** graph., ***nat-c.,*** petr., ***sil.,*** tarent.
flatus, with - ambr.

epileptic attack, before - cupr., ***lach.***

evening - acon., am-m., ***ant-c., bry.,*** calc., carb-v., caust., cedr., cham., con., crot-t., ***hell.,*** hyper., kali-n., lyc., lyss., mag-c., mag-m., mag-s., mur-ac., nat-c., nat-m., nux-m., osm., petr., plat., rhod., ruta, ***sep.,*** stram., ***sulph.,*** zinc.
6 p.m - sulph.
7 p.m. - caust., nicc.
agg. - caust., sep., ***sulph.***
dinner, after - yuc.
eating, while - ign.
after - con.
lying, while - hyos.
amel. - mur-ac.
pickled fish, after - calad.
sleep, before - meli., petr.
stool, before soft - ***sulph.***

fever, during the - ars., sil.

flatus, (see Intestines, Distention, flatus, from)

forenoon - croc., lil-t.

grief, after - calc., coloc.

hard - ***kali-c.***

here and there - carb-an., mag-m.

hot - merc-d.

humiliation, after - ***calc., coloc.,*** lyc.

hysterical - tarax.

irritability, with - aeth.

labor, during - kali-c.
after - ***lyc.,*** **SEP.**

DISTENSION,

large, pot-bellied, flabby - am-m., ***calc., calc-p.,*** mez., podo., sanic., sars., ***sep., sil.,*** sulph., thuj.
girls at puberty - calc., ***graph.,*** lach., sulph.
protrudes here and there - croc., nux-m., sulph., thuj.
women, pendulous in, who have many children - aur., aur-m., bell., frax., ***helon.,*** phos., ***sep.***

leaning against something amel. - ars.

loosening clothes, amel. - sep.

lying, agg. - carb-v.
lying down, amel. - mur-ac.

menses, during - aloe, alum., berb., brom., carb-an., ***chin.,*** **COCC.,** coff., croc., cycl., graph., ham., hep., ign., ***kali-c.,*** kali-p., kreos., lac-c., lachn., lyc., mag-c., ***nat-c., nicc.,*** nit-ac., nux-v., rat., **SULPH.,** zinc.
after - cham., kreos., lil-t., mag-c., rat.
before - am-m., apoc., aran., arn., berb., carb-an., carb-v., carl., cham., ***cocc.,*** cycl., hep., kali-c., kreos., ***lach., lyc.,*** mang., nux-v., ***puls., zinc.***
late menses, during - **SULPH.**
suppressed, from - cast., cham., rat.

mental exertion, from - hep., lyc., ***nux-m.***

midnight - bov., **COCC.**
after - ambr., phos.

milk, after - carb-v., **CON.**

morning - aloe, ars., asaf., ***cham.,*** chin., chin-a., grat., nat-s., nit-ac., ***nux-v.,*** ol-an., rhod., ***sulph.***
5 a.m. - bov.
6 am., on waking - corn.
11 am. loosening clothes amel. - fago.
fasting, while - dulc.
waking, on - mur-ac., nat-c., nit-ac., plan., raph., sulph.

mothers, in - iod., nat-c., ***sep.***

motion, confined, after a - bell.
constant amel. - rein.

night - alum., arg-m., haem., hyper., ***mag-c.,*** merc-c., nat-c., ptel., ***sulph.,*** valer.
10 p.m. - absin.
amel. - mag-s.
flatus, emission of, amel. - franz.
waking, on - gent-l.

noon - sulph.
sleep, after - con.
soup, after - mag-c.
walking, while - coloc.

operation, after - carb-an., carb-v., chin., hyper.

painful - **ACON.,** alum., ant-t., arg-m., **ARS.,** ***bar-c.,*** bell., **BRY.,** calad., canth., **CAUST.,** cham., chin., hell., ***hyos.,*** kali-i., **LACH.,** **MERC.,** merc-c., mez., nat-c., nat-m., nux-v., **RHUS-T.,** sep., stann., sulph., verat.
on touch - hyos., squil.

paroxysmal - plb.

perspiration, amel. - aesc.

puerperal - ter.

riding, on - sep.

DISTENSION,
sitting, while - nat-s.
soup, after - mag-c., sep.
spots, in - ***mag-m.,*** manc., plat.
stool, during - stram.
after - agar., ars., asaf., aur., ***carb-v., graph.,*** hep., **LYC.,** nat-m., petr., sulph.
amel. - alum., am-m., asaf., calc-p., caust., con., corn., hyper., nat-m., sulph.
before - ars., ***corn.,*** fl-ac., phyt., sulph.
sudden - kali-i., ***nat-m.***
supper, after - alum., ***arg-n.,*** arn., bor., calc., ***chin.,*** sep.
tympanitic - aeth., agar., ail., anan., ant-c., ***ant-t.,*** **ARG-N.,** ***arn.,*** **ARS.,** ars-i., bell., ***brom., bry., calc.,*** calc-ar., calc-p., ***canth.,*** carb-s., **CARB-V., CHAM., CHIN.,** ***chin-a.,*** **COCC., COLCH.,** ***coloc.,*** crot-h., crot-t., ***cupr.,*** euph., ***eup-per.,*** fago., ***graph.,*** **HYOS.,** iod., ***kali-bi., kali-p.,*** kali-s., kreos., laur., **LACH., LYC.,** mang., ***merc.,*** merc-c., mez., ***morph., mur-ac., nat-s., op., ph-ac.,*** **PHOS.,** ***podo.,*** rhus-t., ***sec.,*** sep., sil., ***stram.,*** sulph., ***sumb.,*** **TER.,** ***thuj.,*** til.
urination, before - chin-s.
vaginal discharge, during - graph.
walking in open air - calc., sep.

DIGGING, pain - alum., am-m., mag-c., mag-m., nat-c., sep., stann., sul-ac.

DRAGGING, pain, (see Bearing down) - aesc., agn., ***aloe,*** alet., ant-c., ***apis,*** arg-m., ***arg-n.,*** asaf., **BELL.,** ***bry.,*** calc., calc-s., carb-ac., carb-s., ***carb-v.,*** caul., caust., cham., chin., chin-a., coc-c., ***con.,*** corn., ***crot-t.,*** cycl., dig., ***ferr.,*** ferr-p., ***gels.,*** gran., ***graph., hedeo,*** hyos., iod., ip., ***kali-c.,*** kali-i., lac-ac., ***lac-c.,*** **LIL-T.,** lyc., lyss., mag-c., mag-m., mag-s., mang., ***merc.,*** merl., mur-ac., ***murx., nat-c.,*** **NAT-H.,** ***nat-m.,*** nat-s., ***nicc., nit-ac., nux-m.,*** **NUX-V.,** ***op.,*** ox-ac., ***pall.,*** phos., ***phyt., plat.,*** plb., psor., **PULS.,** rhus-t., sabin., sars., ***sec.,*** **SEP., STRY., SULPH.,** tarent., teucr., thuj., ***tril.,*** ust., vib., xan.,dragging, extending, anus, toward - crot-t., ***sulph.*** zinc.
afternoon - mag-m., **SEP.**
crossing limbs amel. - **LIL-T.,** ***murx.,*** **SEP.,** zinc.
dinner, after - sulph.
eating, after - carb-v., thuj.
amel. - sep.
extending to, anus, toward - con., crot-t., lyc., ***sulph.***
to, genitalia - graph.
to, lumbar region - mag-m.
to, sacrum - con.
to, testes - dig.
to, thighs - nit-ac., nux-v., vib.
fever, in low - ***cact.***
flatus, after, amel. - zinc.
forenoon - sep.
menses, during - am-c., **BELL.,** bor., ***calc-p., cham., chin., con., ferr.,*** graph., ***kali-c.,*** kali-i., **LIL-T.,** ***mag-c.,*** mag-m., med., ***murx., nat-c., nat-m., nit-ac.,*** nux-m.,

DRAGGING, pain
menses, during - ***nux-v.,*** **PLAT.,** ***podo.,*** **PULS., SEC., SEP.,** ***sulph., vib.,*** zinc.
after - kreos.
as if menses would come on - nat-c., plat.
before - alum., ***apis,*** **BELL.,** ***cina, chin., con.,*** eupi., ***gels.,*** iod., lac-c., mag-c., mosch., ***phos., plat.,*** sabad., sec., ***sep.,*** sulph., tarent., ust., ***vib.,*** zinc.
morning - ***bell.,*** hyos., mag-c.
9 a.m. to 6 p.m. - **SEP.**
motion agg. - ***kreos.,*** ph-ac.
night, 9 p.m. - ***sep.***
in bed - mag-c., **SULPH.**
riding in a carriage - asaf.
spermatic cords, through - **PULS.**
standing - con., graph., ***murx.,*** nat-m., pall., rheum, rhus-t., **SEP.**
stepping - calc.
stool, during - arg-n., ***bell.,*** iod., ***lil-t., podo., stann.***
after - ***carb-v., graph.***
before - mag-m., nat-c., nit-ac.
difficult, scanty, amel. after flatus - zinc.
urging to, with - ***con., corn.,*** **NUX-V.,** plat.
supper, after, amel. - ***sep.***
thighs, into - nit-ac., nux-v.
urinate, with urging to - nux-v., ***pall.***
walking, agg. - calc., ***chin., con.,*** kali-i., ***nux-v.,*** rhus-t., **SEP., TRIL.**
amel. - ***sep.***
warmth, amel. - nat-c.,

dragging, hypochondria, right - calc., cham., coc-c., podo., ptel.
right, when lying on left side - ***card-m., mag-m., nat-s., ptel.***
pressure amel. - plat.
sides - phos.

dragging, inguinal - am-m., ***apis,*** brom., bry., calc., canth., carb-an., ***cham., chel.,*** clem., coc-c., ***con.,*** ferr., gent-c., gran., ham., helon., kali-c., kali-i., kali-n., lac-d., ***lach., lil-t.,*** mag-c., mag-m., mag-s., med., murx., ***nat-c.,*** phos., ***plat.,*** rat., ***sep.,*** ter., teucr.
afternoon - mag-c., mag-m.
alternating sides - ter.
with pressing genitalia - plat.
colic, during - phos.
evening - teucr.
extending, forward - caust.
outward - con., kali-c.
to testicles - hydr., teucr.
lying amel. - gent-c.
menses, during - bor., mag-c., mag-m., plat.
before - phos., plat.
night - mag-c.
sitting, while - caust.
amel. - gent-c.
standing, while - **LIL-T.**
stool, during - kali-c., rat.
before - carb-an.

dragging, inguinal
urination, after - sul-ac.
walking, while - ***lil-t.,*** med.

DRAWING, pain - abrot., acet-ac., acon., agar., agn., ang., alum., alumn., am-c., am-m., ***anac.,*** ant-t., arg-n., ars., ars-i., asaf., aur., aur-m., bar-c., bar-i., ***bell.,*** berb., bor., ***calc.,*** calc-s., ***calad.,*** **CAPS.,** carb-s., ***carb-v., card-m.,*** caust., cham., chel., chin., clem., cocc., colch., ***coloc.,*** con., ***cupr.,*** cupr-ac., dig., dros., gels., ***gran.,*** hell., ***hep.,*** hyos., ***ign.,*** iod., jug-r., kali-ar., kali-c., kali-n., kreos., lach., ***laur.,*** led., ***lyc.,*** lyss., mag-c., ***mag-m.,*** mag-s., mang., merc., mez., mosch., murx., nat-a., ***nat-c.,*** nat-m., nat-s., ***nit-ac., nux-v.,*** op., par., petr., phos., ***plat., podo.,*** ptel., rhus-t., sabin., sars., sec., seneg., **SEP.,** spig., squil., stann. staph., stram., sulph., sumb., tarax., thuj., valer., verat., verat-v., zing.
afternoon - grat.
chill, during - bov.
cold, as from a - sars.
dinner, after - con.
drinking, after - caust., con.
amel. - aur-m.
eating - mang.
after - caust.
amel. - aur-m., mang.
evening - bor., bry., kali-n., mag-m.
walking - verat.
extending to,
arms - con.
calves - lyc.
hypogastrium - con.
inguinal - plat.
thighs - sul-ac.
upward - mag-m.
urethra - zinc.
flatus, as from - ars., staph.
flatus, before - nit-ac.
inspiration, during - rhus-t.
lying amel. - phos.
menses, during - calc., carb-v., croc., kreos., mosch., ***plat.,*** plb., sep., staph., ***stram., sulph.***
after - puls.
at beginning of - ***mag-c.***
before - carb-v., ***ign.***
morning - calc.
motion, on - bry., jug-r., mag-m.
amel. - aur-m.
night - graph., ***mag-m.,*** zing.
sitting, while - asaf., chin., con., phos.
sitting, after - con.
stool, during - ***arg-n.,*** chin.
amel. - aur-m.
before - cact., ***nit-ac.,*** zing.
supper, after - kali-n.
walking, while - con., squil.
amel. - phos.
warmth, amel. - **MAG-P.**

drawing, hypochondria - agar., all-c., aur., bapt., ***berb., calc., carb-v.,*** caul., cham., ***coc-c.,*** coloc., ***con.,*** gels., lact., mag-m., merc-i-r., nat-a., nat-m., petr., ***puls.,*** rhus-t., sil., squil., sulph., teucr., zinc.

drawing, hypochondria
bed, in - cham.
evening - ars., ***carb-v.***
extending,
downward - nat-m.
hip - **CUPR.,** sil.
leg - ***carb-v.***
small of back - carb-v., plb.
spine - sil.
symphysis- calc.
thighs - nux-v.
upward - ***rhus-t.***
forenoon - sulph.
left - ***ars.,*** coc-c., coloc., **CUPR.,** gels., plat.
extending to chest, when clearing the throat - ars.
extending to hip - **CUPR.**
morning - merc-i-r.
night - ***coc-c.***
right - agar., alum., aur., bry., calc., cham., con., mag-m., nat-m., sep., stann., sulph., zinc.
sitting - alum., ars.
walking - alum., bapt., phos.

drawing, hypogastrium - **AGAR.,** aur., bell., canth., carb-v., ***card-m.,*** chin., coc-c., coloc., con., lyc., meny., nit-ac., plb., sabad., spig., stann., thuj., valer.
extending to sacrum, before menses - carb-v.
to thighs - nat-m.
night - ph-ac.
vaginal discharge, after - sep.

drawing, inguinal - aeth., agar., aloe, alum., ammc., aspar., aur., bapt., bov., bry., cact., calc., calc-p., ***chel., clem.,*** coc-c., cocc., gamb., gran., kali-c., kali-i., lil-t., ***lyc., lyss., merc.,*** mez., nat-m., ***plat.,*** rat., ***rhod.,*** sil., stann., ter., thuj., valer., zinc.
alternating with prickling - zinc.
convulsive - chel.
dancing, while - alum.
evening - bor.
extending to,
pelvis, around - coloc., plat.
thighs - aur., rhod.
knee - thuj.
pubis - lil-t.
testicles - arg-m., ham., nat-m., plat., staph.
glands - mez., thuj.
inspiration agg. - plat.
left - aeth., alum., ammc., gamb., lyc., stann.
urination, during - ars.
menses would come on, as if - cocc., lyc., ***plat.***
night - zinc.
noon - thuj.
periodical - aloe
right - agar., aloe, bapt., bar-c., bov., card-m., gran., sil., thuj.
sitting, while - caust., chin., thuj., zinc.
spasmodic - agar., ***chel.***
standing - thuj.
stretching - coc-c., merc-c., nat-m.
amel. - bov.

drawing, inguinal
urination, during - agar., ars., card-m., caust.
walking - alum., chel., thuj.
drawing, sides - am-m., ant-t., camph., cupr., lyc., nat-c., phos., ran-b., sep., staph.
dinner, after - zinc.
flank, in - alum., ambr., ang., calc., carb-v., card-m., caust., chin., cocc., coff., colch., crot-t., kali-c., plat., puls., sabad., sabin., samb., sars., seneg., stann., staph., sulph.
left - zinc.
menses, as before - staph.
morning - phos.
night - lyc.
pressure agg. - zinc.
right - camph., cupr., med.,
sitting amel. - zinc.
standing - arg-n.
together - zinc.
walking - chin., zinc.
drawing, umbilicus - acon., aloe, anac., ars., bar-c., bell., calc-p., carb-s., ***chel.,*** clem., con., eupi., gamb., gent-c., grat., ign., kali-c., mang., mez., mosch., nat-c., nit-ac., nux-m., nux-v., phos., ***plb.,*** rat., rhus-t., ruta., sep., sulph., tab., zinc.
bending body - nit-ac.
eating, after - con.
extending to,
anus - nat-m.
pubis - rhus-t.
thighs - nat-m.
vagina - calc-p.
menses, during - nux-m.
morning - con., mang., nat-c.
motion, on - nit-ac.
paroxysmal - sep.
rising, after - con.
sitting - kali-c.
stool, before - nat-c.
walking - anac.
walking amel. - kali-c.

DRAWN in, upper - thuj.
involuntarily - valer.

DROPSY, (see Ascites)

DRYNESS - dig., plb.
evening, in bed - bov.

ECCHYMOSIS - phos.

ECZEMA - arn.
eczema, umbilical region - merc-p-r., sulph.

ELECTRIC shock passing through, like - coloc.

ELEVATIONS - bell.

EMACIATION, muscles of - fuc., plb.

EMPTINESS, sensation - ***agar.,*** ant-c., **ARG-N.,** arn., arum-m., ***calc-p., carb-v.,*** caust., ***cham., cina,*** cob., **COCC.,** ***coloc.,*** croc., ***crot-t., dig., dulc.,*** euph., euphr., fl-ac., ***gamb.,*** gels., guai., hep., jab., ***kali-c.,*** kali-p., ***lach.,*** lil-t., ***merc.,*** mez., ***mur-ac.,*** naja, ***nat-p.,*** nicc., **OLND.,** ***petr., ph-ac.,*** **PHOS.,** phys., plan., **PODO.,** ***psor.,*** ptel., **PULS.,** ruta, ***sars.,*** seneg., **SEP.,** squil., **STANN., SUL-AC., TAB.,** ***verat.,*** zinc.

EMPTINESS, sensation
belching amel. - ***carb-v., sep.***
breakfast, after - arum-m., phos., sars.
burning between shoulders - **PHOS.**
diarrhea, as after - myric.
dinner, after - nat-p., zinc.
amel. - dios.
before - nux-v.
eating, after - arum-m., nat-p., sars., ***stann.,*** zinc.
amel. - ant-c.
extending to,
esophagus, through, to throat - aq-pet.
stomach, at noon, after stool - gall-ac.
vagina, vulva - puls.
flatus, after - phos.
flatus, passing, amel. - ***kali-s.***
gnawing - ox-ac., wild.
lying on abdomen amel. - puls.
menses, during - ***phos.,*** sulph.
morning - euph., gall-ac., mez., sars.
5 a.m., agg. by rising and moving around - pic-ac.
eating, after - arum-m.
rising, after - mag-c.
stool, after - mur-ac.
night - puls.
noon - dios.
dinner, amel. - dios.
eating, after - nat-p., stann., zinc.
stool, after - paeon.
pressure amel. - caust., naja, **PULS.**
side - pall., sep.
smoking, as after excessive, amel. after sleep - phos.
stool, after - ***agar.,*** apoc., ***arg-n., carb-v.,*** caust., cob., coloc., jab., ***kali-c., kali-s., lach., mur-ac., nat-p., olnd.,*** **PETR.,** ***ph-ac.,*** **PHOS.,** ***pic-ac.,*** **PODO.,** ***psor., puls.,*** rhod., ***sep., stann.,*** sulph., **SUL-AC.,** verat.
after, diarrhea - coloc.
amel. - mur-ac.
before - verat.
tightening clothing amel. - ***fl-ac.***
walking agg. - carb-v., ***phos.***
wrapping up the abdomen amel. - puls.
emptiness, hypogastrium - kali-s., sec.
flatus passing amel. - kali-s.
emptiness, umbilical, region - fl-ac.

ENLARGED - alum., ***bar-c., bar-i.,*** **CALC.,** carb-v., caust., chel., colch., ***coloc., iod., iris, lyc.,*** ol-j., podo., ***psor.,*** **SANIC.,** sec., **SEP.,** sil., **SULPH.,** syph., ***thuj.,*** tub., vario.
children, in - alum., **BAR-C., CALC.,** calc-p., caust., cupr., mag-m., ***psor., sanic., sars.,*** **SIL.,** ***sulph.***
marasmus, with - **CALC.,** ***sanic., sars., sil.***
swelling, glands of, with - mez.
fat - ***am-m., calc.,*** **CHEL.**
girls, at puberty - calc., ***graph.,*** lach., lyc., sulph.
mothers, in - ***iod.,*** nat-c., **SEP.**

ERUPTIONS - agar., anac., ***apis,*** ars., bar-m., bry., calc., ***graph.,*** kali-ar., kali-bi., kali-c., ***merc.,*** merc-c., ***nat-c.,*** nat-m., phos., rhus-t., ***sulph.***
blotches - crot-t., merc., nat-c., ***sulph.***
hip region, red - hura.
burning - rhus-t.
crusts - anac., arn., kali-c.
desquamating - merc., vesp.
elevated - merc.
itch-like, scabies - merc., ***nat-c.***
itching - agar., calc., merc., rhus-t., ***sulph.***
miliary - manc.
moist - merc.
nodules - nat-c.
petechial - chol.
pimples - agar., aloe, arn., ars., ars-h., bar-m., bry., dulc., fl-ac., merc., nat-c., nat-m., petr., rhus-t., staph.
bleeding easily - agar.
burning - bry.
burning on touch - petr.
burning, scratched off, when - staph.
cold water agg. - tell.
flattened - rhus-t.
itching - aloe, bry., dulc., nat-c., ***staph.***
moist when scratched off - staph.
pimples, desquamating - chlol.
pointed - ars., pers.
raw - aloe
red - chlol., tell.
red, areola, with - aloe, lipp.
suppurating - chlol.
vesicating - chlol.
watery fluid, containing - ars.
whitish - ars.
pustular - crot-c., crot-t., kali-bi., merc., nat-m., puls., squil.
areola, with bright red - crot-t.
dark point in centre - kali-bi.
elevated - crot-t.
evening - bart.
itching - squil.
tips pale - crot-t.
scabs - arn.
scales - arn., kali-c.
yellow spots - kali-c.
scarlet - anac.
scurf-like - bar-m.
sore - merc.
sudamina - hydrc., merc.
rash, itching violently - ***calc.***
itching, red rash over the region of liver - sel.
menses, before - ***apis,*** ars.
red - merc.
red, fine - merc-i-f.
ringworm - nat-m., sep., tell.
roseola in patches - oena.
urticaria - merc., nat-c.
vesicles - arn., crot-t., kali-bi., caust., ***merc.,*** merc-c., rhus-t.

eruptions, inguinal - alum., cupr-ar., ***graph., merc.,*** sulph.
excoriations - ***ars.,*** arum-t., ***bov., graph.***
menses, during - bov.

eruptions, inguinal
pustular - puls., sep.
scales - merc.

ERYSIPELAS - graph.

EXCORIATION - arn.
as if, on strong pressure - coloc.
mons veneris - sil.

EXCRESCENCE, umbilicus, moist - ***calc.***

FALLING, down, sensation of - laur., ***nux-v.,*** plb.
extending into small of back - laur.
from side to side, as if intestines were falling, on turning in bed - ***bar-c., merc., merc-c.***

falling, out, sensation of - ***alum.,*** coloc., ferr., ***kali-br.,*** nat-m., ***nux-v.,*** ran-b., ***sep.***
cough, from - carb-an.
dinner, after - ran-b.
menses, before - alum.
standing, on - aur-s.
stool, during - kali-br.
walk carefully, obliging him to - ***nux-v.***
walking, while - ferr., nat-m.

falling, asleep, as if - calc-p.
sitting down, on - merc.

FAT - ***am-m.,*** calc., **CHEL.**

FEAR, (see Apprehension)

FORMICATION - aloe, ars., calad., calc., camph., carb-v., caust., colch., coloc., crot-t., cycl., ***dulc.,*** mag-m., nux-v., paeon., pall., petr., pic-ac., **PLAT.,** stann., zinc.
extending to urethra - zinc.
night - ars.
purgative, as after a - caust.
rumbling - ***puls.***
sitting, while - ant-t.
voluptuous - **PLAT.**
waist - aesc.

FULLNESS, sensation of - agar., all-c., **ALOE,** alum., alumn., ambr., am-c., am-m., ***anac.,*** ant-c., ant-t., ***apis,*** arn., ars., arum-t., asaf., asar., ***aur., bapt.,*** bar-c., bar-m., bell., cahin., calad., calc., calc-s., camph., cann-s., canth., caps., carb-ac., **CARB-S., CARB-V.,** carl., cast., caust., chel., **CHIN.,** chin-a., cimic., cinnb., clem., cocc., coc-c., coff., colch., coloc., com., con., corn., croc., ***crot-t., cycl.,*** **DIG.,** dor., dulc., echi., eup-per., fago., ferr., ferr-ar., ferr-i., ferr-p., ***gels.,*** glon., **GRAPH.,** grat., haem., hell., hep., hyos., hyper., indg., jug-r., kali-ar., **KALI-C.,** kali-i., kali-n., kali-s., ***lach.,*** lact., laur., lec., led., lil-t., **LYC.,** mag-c., mag-m., mag-s., ***meny.,*** merc-c., mez., ***mur-ac.,*** myric., naja, nat-a., nat-c., nat-m., nat-p., ***nat-s.,*** nux-m., **NUX-V.,** olnd., ol-an., onos., op., petr., **PH-AC., PHOS.,** phys., phyt., pic-ac., plan., plb., puls., raph., rhod., rhus-t., rumx., sarr., sars., ***sep.,*** sil., spig., stann., stram., stront-c., **SULPH.,** sumb., tab., ter., valer., verb., zinc.
afternoon - carl., clem., coca, con., mag-c., phyt., plb.
2 pm., when walking, amel. - mag-c.
5 p.m. and 11 pm., before eating - myric.
walking, while, in open air - plan.

FULLNESS, sensation of
bed, on going to - rumx.
belching amel. - rhod.
breakfast, during - alum.
after - carb-s., ***carb-v.,*** cic., sin-a., ***sulph.***
coffee, after - canth.
constipation, during - bry., dios., ery-a., graph., hyos., iod., lach., nit-ac., nux-v., phos., ter.
daytime - nux-m.
diarrhea, during - nat-s.
diarrhea, as if, were forming - rumx.
dinner, during - ant-c.
after - alum., cob., petr., thuj.
drinking, after - ***carb-v.,*** caust., nux-v., sars., sin-a.
eating, as after, too much - carb-v., coc-c., ***lyc., meny.,*** ter.
4 p.m. to 9 p.m. - clem., ***lyc.***
one hour after eating - graph.
eating, while - cham., ***chin.***
after - agar., arn., calc., calc-s., ***carb-v.,*** caust., chin., ***cob., cocc.,*** colch., hep., ign., kali-bi., **KALI-C.,** kali-p., kali-s., lach., **LYC.,** mag-m., mag-s., ***mur-ac.,*** myric., nat-a., nat-h., ***nit-ac.,*** **NUX-V.,** par., ph-ac., ***phos., puls.,*** rhod., sars., ***sep.,*** sil., spig., spong., stann., ***sulph., zinc.***
after, agg. - calc.
amel. - rhus-t.
evening - bry., calc., caust., dios., graph., hyper., **LYC.,**
after soup - cast.
belching amel. - fago.
eating, after - ign.
smoking agg. - **MENY.**
flatus, passing, amel. - alum., grat., hell., rhod., sulph.
flatulence, as from - **GRAPH.,** mez.
10 p.m. - cimic.
pressing forward towards stomach, agg. bending forward, amel. bending backward, and by walking - bry.
food, at sight of - **SULPH.**
forenoon - sulph.
11 a.m., after stool - gels.
stool, after - pip-m.
hunger, during - asar.
limpid secretion from cathartics, as of - tanac.
lying, while - rumx., spig.
bed, in - spig.
midnight, before stool - gent-l., grat.
morning - dios., phos., plat., sulph.
on waking - sulph.
night - graph., nat-m., phos.
noon, eating, after - sin-a.
pants or drawers, opening, amel. - nat-a.
puffy, to sternum - sumb.
respiration, compelling deep - cann-s.
sitting amel. - plan.
smoking, after - **MENY.**
stool amel. - colch., rein.

FULLNESS, sensation of
supper, after - agar., ***arg-n.,*** coff., colch., coloc., tell.
waking, on - ferr., myric., sulph.
walking amel. - mag-c.

fullness, hypochondria, sensation of - acon., aesc., ant-c., aran., arg-n., aur., bell., brom., ***carb-v.,*** card-m., ***cham.,*** chel., coc-c., colch., con., eup-per., ferr., glon., grat., ign., ***merc.,*** merc-i-f., phos., ***podo.,*** **SEP.,** sulph., tell.
eating, after - nat-m.
left - stict.
morning - con.
right - aesc., aloe, ***chel.,*** eup-per., kali-c., nat-m., ***podo.,*** sang., thuj.
stool amel. - ferr.

fullness, hypogastrium, sensation of - ***aesc.,*** bar-c., ***bell.,*** carb-v., sulph.
daytime, 10 a.m. until evening - sulph.
eating, after - hep.
evening - bell.

fullness, inguinal, sensation of - am-c., ***cocc.,*** nat-s., sep.

fullness, sides, sensation of - am-c.

fullness, umbilicus and ilium, between, while riding - rumx.

GALLBLADDER, general, (see Liver, chapter)

GANGRENE - **ARS.,** ***canth., phos., plb., sec.***

GAUCHER, morbus - med.

GLANDS, (see Inguinal, Mesenteric)

GNAWING, pain - am-c., ars., aur-m., calc., canth., colch., ***coloc.,*** cupr., cycl., dig., dulc., elat., ***gels.,*** olnd., plat., plb., ruta, seneg., sulph.
bend forward, obliging to - **COLOC.**
dinner, after, agg. - ***coloc.***

gnawing, hypochondria - bufo, ***ruta.***

gnawing, hypogastrium - gamb., kali-c., seneg., sumb.
right - ***sumb.***

gnawing, umbilical, region - nat-m., ruta.

GOOSEBUMPS - jab., sec.
stroked with something cold, at noon, motion agg. - sulph.

GOUT, metastasis, to abdomen - ant-c.

GURGLING, in - acon., ***agar.,*** **ALOE,** am-c., ang., ant-t., arg-n., ***ars.,*** bov., bry., canth., carb-an., carb-s., chel., ***cocc.,*** coc-c., coloc., con., **CROT-T.,** dig., dros., eupi., ferr., ferr-ar., ferr-p., ***gamb.,*** graph., ***hell.,*** hyos., ign., kali-bi., kali-i., lach., ***lyc.,*** mag-c., merc., mur-ac., nat-a., nat-c., ***nat-m.,*** nat-p., ***nux-v.,*** **OLND.,** op., par., ***ph-ac., phos.,*** phys., plat., **PODO.,** ***psor.,*** **PULS.,** ***raph.,*** rhod., rhus-t., ruta, ***sil.,*** spig., squil., staph., stront-c., **SULPH.,** sul-ac., tab., ter., thuj., valer., verb., zinc.
afternoon - lyc., ox-ac.
3 p.m - bry.
breakfast, after - agar.
coffee, and - ox-ac.
cramps, as in, on inspiration, morning and evening, eating amel. - mag-c.

GURGLING, in
deep - agar.
dinner, after - ***laur.,*** grat.
drinking, after - ***phos.***
eating, while - nit-ac.
amel. - sul-ac.
emptiness, as from - guai.
evening - lyc.
7 p.m. - nicc.
8 p.m. to 11 p.m. - phys.
extending towards sacral region - phos.
flatus, emission of, amel. - acon.
fluid, as from - ***carl., crot-t.,*** jatr., sin-a.
mixed with air - asim.
morning, fasting - plat.
moving body by breathing, on, while lying - sul-ac.
forenoon - ferr., mag-c.
waking, on - ferr.
hollow - ars.
inspiration, on - mag-m., sul-ac., tab.
lying, while - sul-ac.
morning - ***nux-v.,*** plb., ter.
7 a.m. - acon.
bed, in - ***nux-v.***
rising, after - plb.
stool, before - ferr-i.
motion, on - bar-c.
amel. - nat-m.
of breathing - sul-ac.
night - ***raph., sulph.***
1 a.m. - ferr.
noon - ox-ac.
pressure, on - plb.
purge, as after a - ***nat-m.***
respiration, on deep - tab.
rest agg., after breakfast or coffee - nat-m.
stool, during - calc-ac., rham-f.
after - bry.
before - acon., **ALOE,** coloc., merc., **OLND., PODO.,** rat.
swashing of water, as from, on touch, and on bending forward or backward - ph-ac.
walking, while - ***lyc.***
water, as from - sul-ac.
gurgling, hypochondria - kali-c., lyc., puls.
left - ***lyc.***
gurling, sides - calc., con., ***crot-t.,*** graph., kali-c., ***lyc.,*** meny., nat-m.
left - ***crot-t., lyc.***
pressure, on - kali-c.

HANDS, supports abdomen during urination - **LYC.**

HANGING, or falling down, as if - acet-ac., laur., nat-m., phos., podo., ***sep.***
walking, agg. - nat-m.
bent - carb-v.
walks carefully - nux-v.

HARD - alum., ***anac.,*** arn., ***ars.,*** ars-i., **BAR-C., BAR-M.,** bell., calad., **CALC.,** caps., ***carb-s.,*** caust., cham., ***chel.,*** chin., ***cina,*** clem., coff., colch., con., cupr., cupr-ar., dig., dirc., dulc., eup-pur., ***ferr.,*** ferr-ar., ferr-p., gels., ***graph.,*** grat., hep., hyper., ign., jug-r., kali-ar., ***kali-c.,***

HARD - kali-p., kali-s., lac-c., lach., laur., ***mag-m.,*** mag-s., **MERC.,** merc-c., merc-i-f., merc-i-r., ***mez.,*** nat-a., ***nat-c.,*** nat-m., nat-p., ***nit-ac.,*** nux-m., nux-v., ***op.,*** paeon., phos., plb., puls., ***raph.,*** sec., sars., ***sep.,*** **SIL.,** sol-t-ae., spig., spong., stram., sulph., sumb., tab., valer.
body, sensation of, moving in - bor., ***lyc.***
turning to right side, when - ***lyc.***
children - calc., sil.
diarrhea, amel. - cupr-ac.
dinner, after - calc.
eating, after - calc., con., phos.
evening - caust., cedr., cham., con., hyper., ***lac-c.,*** sep., sulph.
iliac region - phos.
menses, during - ign., nat-m., puls., ***sep.***
before - mang.
night - graph., mez.
paroxysms, between - plb.
rising, on - sep.
sensation - hyos.
touch agg. - cupr.
sides, right - mag-m.
stool, after - carb-v.
hard, hypochondria - bor., brom., bry., chin-s., **IOD.,** mag-c., phos.
intermittents, in - ***ars., iod.***
left - ***iod.***
right - ***calc-p.***
hard, hypogastrium - clem., graph., mang., sep.
hard, inguinal - ant-c., dulc., ***lith.***
hard, umbilicus - bry., plb., rhus-t.
above - sil.
region of - puls.
sensation - camph.

HEAT, in - abrot., ***acon.,*** agar., **ALOE,** all-c., ***am-c.,*** ant-t., ***ars.,*** ars-h., ars-i., **ASAF.,** aur., ***bell.,*** bov., brom., bry., cact., ***camph.,*** cann-i., ***canth.,*** caps., carb-an., caust., ***chin.,*** cic., cina, cocc., coc-c., coff., coloc., crot-h., crot-t., **CUPR.,** cycl., dig., dios., euph., ferr., ferr-ar., ferr-i., fl-ac., form., graph., gymn., hell., hep., hydr., hyos., iod., iris, jatr., kali-ar., kali-bi., **KALI-C.,** kali-i., kali-p., ***kali-s.,*** lac-c., lach., lachn., lact., ***laur.,*** lyc., mag-m., manc., mang., meny., ***mez.,*** nat-m., ox-ac., par., phos., phys., plb., ***podo.,*** ptel., puls., raph., rheum, ruta, sabad., sang., sars., ***sec.,*** **SIL.,** spig., spong., squil., stann., stram., stry., sumb., tarent., ***tab.,*** thuj., zinc.
abdominal paroxysms, during - plb.
afternoon - all-c.
4 p.m. - dios.
5 p.m. to 5 a.m. agg. - tarent.
coffee, after - all-c.
alternating with coldness - coff.
ascending to chest - bell.
bend up, obliging her to, and press with hands - coff.
burning - abies-c., ***acon.,*** aloe, alst., ant-c., ***apis,*** arg-n., ars., ***bell.,*** bry., ***camph.,*** cann-i., ***canth.,*** carb-v., colch., crot-h., ***iris,*** kali-bi., kali-s., ***lim.,*** lyc., manc., ***merc-c.,*** nat-s., nux-v., ***ox-ac.,*** ph-ac.,

HEAT, in
burning - ***phos.,*** podo., raph., rhus-t., sang., sec., sep., sulph., verat.
congestion of bowels, as from, afternoon - colocin.
forepart of abdomen - tarent.
spirituous drinks, as after - tell.
clothes, as if hot, on - nit-ac.
constipation, during - plb.
croup, in - cub.
dinner, during - hyper.
after - grat.
eating, after - **KALI-C.**
eruption, before - nat-m.
evening - ferr-i., laur.
8 p.m. to 11 p.m. - phys.
extending to
body, over - stry.
chest - alum., ***bry.,*** coloc., ip., lact., ***lyc.,*** stram.
chest, over to head - lyc.
head - alum., carb-o., indg., ***kali-c.,*** lyc., mag-m., nat-s., plb., sumb.
head, throat, and - sumb.
mouth - sabad.
shoulders - laur.
stomach - ill., mang.
stomach, forenoon - kali-c.
stomach, stool, after, noon - gall-ac.
upward - stram.
external - ang., cori-r., meny., ox-ac., plb., thuj., tong.
alternating with shivering creeping - cham.
creeping - chin.
dry - samb.
fever, during - apis, cact., calad., canth., chin., ***cic.,*** ferr., lach., sel., spig., stann.
flashes of - ***cact.,*** cinnb., ***kali-c.,*** ptel., sumb.
as if hot water pouring into abdomen from chest followed by diarrhea - sang.
as of hot water flowing in - ***sumb.***
coldness of limbs, during - ars-h.
forenoon - am-c., kali-c., phys.
internal, after walking in open air - stann.
iron, as from a hot - bell.
laughing, caused by - spira.
menses, during - ***graph.***
before - cycl., graph.
before and during - graph.
morning - nux-v., phos.
10 a.m. - phys.
night - ***bry.,*** fl-ac.
smoking while - spong.
soup, after - ol-an.
stool, during inclination for - ***podo.***
supper, after amel. - dios.
uncovering amel. - camph., ***sec., tab.***
walking, in open air - stann.
walking, amel. - ferr.
water flowing, as if - sang., sumb.

heat, hypochondria - aloe, aur., bapt., kali-c., plb., podo., sabad., thuj.
flushes rise from - glon.

heat, hypochondria
left - ***glon.***
right - aur., ***kali-c.***

heat, hypogastrium - aur-m., bry., camph., ferr., hydrc., kali-i., lil-t., mang.
menses, during, must have it uncovered - kali-i.

heat, inguinal - arund., aur., calc-p., sulph.

heat, umbilicus - aur-m., canth., chin., hyos., mang., plb., sul-ac.
extending to chest - mang.

HEAVINESS, as from a load, etc. - agar., ***agn.,*** **ALOE,** alum., ***ambr.,*** am-c., am-m., ars., ***asaf.,*** apis, aur., bell., bov., bry., ***calc.,*** calc-s., carb-an., ***carb-s., carb-v.,*** carl., chel., ***cham.,*** chin., chin-a., ***cimic.,*** cop., croc., crot-t., cupr-s., dor., dios., ferr., ferr-ar., ferr-p., gels., **GRAPH.,** ***hell.,*** ip., kali-ar., kali-bi., ***kali-c.,*** kali-p., kali-s., ***lac-d., lach.,*** lact., lil-t., **LYC.,** ***mag-c., mag-m.,*** mag-s., ***mez., murx.,*** nat-a., nat-c., ***nat-m.,*** nux-v., ***op.,*** phos., plb., ***podo.,*** ptel., ***rhod.,*** rhus-t., ruta, sabin., **SEP.,** sil., **STAPH.,** ***sulph.,*** sumb., tab., tep., ter., til., trom., zinc.
afternoon - alum., carl., dios.
breakfast, after - agar., kali-c.
dinner, after - agar., alum.
drinking, after - ***asaf.***
water - carl.
eating, after - kali-c., lyc.
evening - bry.
4 p.m. - dios.
flatus, amel. - carb-an.
forenoon - trom.
gas, as if full of - hydr.
inspiration, on - spig.
lump, like a - carb-an., ***rhus-t.***
lying on left side amel. - ***pall.***
menses, during - aloe apis, bell., glyc., graph., kali-s., nat-m., ***puls., sep.***
before - **PULS.**
first day of - graph.
impending, with - carl.
metrorrhagia, during - apis.
morning - ambr., dios., **SEP.**
motion, during - ***nat-m.,*** **SEP.**
night - mag-m., nat-m., zing.
noon, after nap - ter.
pressure and touch agg. - sin-a.
right, side - calc., camph., tab.
rising, on - **SEP.**
sitting, while, amel. - bell.
sitting, while - bry., rhus-t.
sleep amel. - am-m.
standing agg. - bell.
stone, as from a - lac-d., op., nux-v., ***puls.,*** sin-a.
afternoon, after eating - chin.
menses, before - **PULS.**
stool, after - agar., ***mur-ac., sep.***
before - yuc.
supper, after - ***arg-n.,*** coloc.
amel. - dios.
walk, bent must - carb-v.

HEAVINESS, as from a load
walking, while - ***alum.,*** bell., ery-a., ferr., kali-c., nat-m.
heaviness, hypochondria, as from a load, etc - acon., bell., ***coc-c.,*** kali-c., lact., merc-i-r., nux-m., ph-ac., podo., ptel., sulph., ***zinc.***
night - ***kali-c.***
walking, while - ptel.
heaviness, hypogastrium, as from a load, etc - agar., aloe, all-s., ***ammc.,*** am-m., aran., ars., bar-c., coloc., crot-c., crot-t., graph., kali-c., lil-t., ***pall., podo.,*** **SEC.,** sulph.
eating, after - all-s.
lying on left side amel. - pall.
menses, during - bar-c.
amel. - vib.
standing - pall.
tool, after - agar.
walking, agg. - kali-c.
heaviness, inguinal, as from a load, etc - bor., calc., carb-an., ***croc.,*** dios.
heaviness, sides, as from a load, etc - asaf., lil-t., **LYC.,** nat-s., rhus-t.
left - **LYC.**
right - calc., camph.
heaviness, umbilicus - camph.
sensation in - agar., camph., canth., carb-v., graph., nit-ac., op., ptel.

HEAVY, as if something lying on left side of - **LYC.**

HERNIA, inguinal - aesc., ***all-c., alum.,*** am-c., ***apis, asar., aur.,*** berb., ***calc.,*** calc-ar., caps., ***carb-an., carb-v., cocc., coff.,*** coloc., ***dig.,*** lach., **LYC.,** ***mag-c.,*** mill., ***mur-ac., nit-ac.,*** **NUX-V.,** ***op.,*** petr., phos., prun., psor., ***rhus-t.,*** sars., ***sil., spig.,*** staph., ***sulph., sul-ac.,*** ter., thuj., ***verat., zinc.***
children, in - **AUR.,** ***calc.,*** cina, lyc., ***nit-ac.,*** nux-v., sil., sulph.
left side - nux-v.
right side - aur., lyc.
incarcerated - lob., ***mill.,*** nux-v., ***op.,*** plb.
inflammation - acon., bar-c., iod., nux-v., op., sulph.
vomiting, with - acon., ars., bell., lach., ***tab.,*** verat.
left - nux-v.
painful - aesc., ***alum.,*** aur., cic., cocc., phos., ***sil.***
right - lyc.
sensitive - ***bell.,*** **LACH.,** ***nux-v., sil.***
stitching - sep.
strangulated - acon., ***all-c.,*** alum., ars., **BELL.,** ***carb-v., cocc., coff., dig.,*** lach., mill., **NUX-V., OP.,** ***plb.,*** rhus-t., ***sulph., sul-ac., tab.,*** verat.
hernia, sensation as if, would protrude - ***sul-ac.***
hernia, umbilicus - ***calc., lach., nux-m.,*** **NUX-V.,** ***op.,*** **PLB.**

HERPES, simplex - ***sep.***
herpes zoster, shingles - ars., graph., iris., merc., ***rhus-t.,*** sulph., thuj.
right, side - **IRIS.**
warmth of bed agg. - merc.
herpes zoster, inguinal - **GRAPH.**

HOLD, must - agn., lil-t., merc., rhus-t., sep., staph.
hypochondrium - dros.

HOLLOW, (see Emptiness)

HORRIPILATION, (see Goosebumps)

HYPEREMIA - arn.

ICTERUS, newborn - chel., chion., coll., merc., nux-v.

ILL, as if - asaf.

IMMOVABLE, almost, during respiration - op.
sensation as if, afternoon - tong.

INACTIVITY - cadm-s.
feeling of - sars.

INDURATION, (see Hardness)

INFLAMMATION, enteritis, (see Peritonitis)
inflammation, umbilicus - hydr., kali-n.
infants, of - calc.

INGUINAL, glands
aching - am-m., ***ars.,*** berb., bov., ***brom., calc.,*** **CLEM.,** cop., dig., dulc., graph., gymn., hell., kreos., lyss., mag-m., ***merc.,*** merc-c., mez., nit-ac., ran-b., rhus-t., ***sil.,*** stann., sumb., ter., thuj.
burning - ***ars.,*** ars-i., bell., ***carb-an.,*** tarent-c.
constriction - bov., cact., gamb., kali-n., mag-c., rat.
eruptions - alum., cupr-ar., ***graph., merc.,*** sulph.
excoriations - ***ars.,*** arum-t., ***bov., graph.***
fistulae - hep., ***lach., phos., sil.,*** sulph.
heaviness - bor., calc., carb-an., ***croc.,*** dios.
inflammation- apis, ars., aur., bac., ***bar-c.,*** bar-m., bell., bufo, ***calc.,*** carb-an., clem., dulc., graph., hep., kali-i., ***merc., merc-i-f., merc-i-r., nit-ac.,*** oci., pall., pin-s., ***puls., rhus-t., sil.,*** sulph., xero.
sore, bruised, tenderness - ***clem.,*** caps., gels., hep., merc., ***sil.,*** sumb., thuj.
suppuration - ars., aur., bar-m., bufo, ***carb-an.,*** chel., crot-h., **HEP., IOD.,** ***kali-i.,*** **LACH., MERC.,** ***nit-ac.,*** phos., ***sil.,*** sulph., thuj.
swelling - alum., am-c., anan., ant-c., ***apis,*** ars., ***aur.,*** **BAD.,** bapt., ***bar-c., bar-m., bell.,*** brom., ***bufo,*** **CALC.,** calc-ar., ***calc-p., carb-an.,*** carb-v., caust., ***chel.,*** **CLEM.,** cocc., cop., crot-h., ***cupr.,*** **DULC.,** elaps, eupi., ***ferr.,*** gels., ***graph.,*** **HEP.,** ***hippoz., iod., kali-c., kali-i.,*** lac-c., **LACH.,** lyc., ***lyss.,*** **MERC., MERC-C.,** ***merc-i-f., merc-i-r.,*** nat-a., ***nat-c.,*** nat-m., **NIT-AC.,** ph-ac., phos., ***phyt., puls., rhus-t.,*** sep., ***sil.,*** sin-n., spong., stann., ***staph.,*** stram., **SULPH.,** sumb., ***syph.,*** tarent., tep., ***thuj., tub.,*** zinc.
chancroidal - ars-i., ***merc.,*** merc-c., ***merc-i-r.,*** sil.
indurated - alum., bad., ***carb-an.,*** merc.

INGUINAL, glands
swelling, phagedenic - ***ars.,*** graph., hydr., ***kali-i.,*** lach., ***merc., merc-i-r., nit-ac.,*** sil., sulph.
tension, of - **AGAR.,** am-c., am-m., ***apis, arg-m.,*** benz-ac., berb., calc., canth., carb-an., ***clem.,*** coc-c., ***coloc.,*** crot-t., cycl., dig., ***dulc.,*** gamb., graph., jatr., kali-i., kreos., ***lac-c.,*** mag-s., merc., nat-m., nat-s., nit-ac., sars., spig., stront.

ITCHING - agar., ambr., anac., ***arn., ars.,*** aur., bell., ***bov.,*** carb-ac., carb-s., chel., cist., coc-c., com., con., ferr-ar., ferr-ma., form., ***graph.,*** jug-r., kali-ar., kali-bi., kali-c., kali-s., lac-ac., lach., ***merc.,*** merc-i-f., mez., nat-c., nat-m., nit-ac., ol-an., petr., phos., puls., rhus-t., rhus-v., ***sars., sep., sulph., thuj.,*** zinc.
biting - ***merc.***
burning - ***ars.,*** sars.
evening while undressing - nux-v.
morning while dressing - nux-v.
night - nux-v.
daytime - nat-c.
dinner, after - ***sulph.***
evening - cact., merc., stront-c., thuj.
and night agg. - ***thuj.***
undressing, while - cact., ***nux-v.***
fleabites, as from, at night - zinc.
internally - petr.
scratching amel. - cann-i.
morning - rat.
dressing, while - nux-v.
night - agar., crot-t., ***nux-v.,*** phos., **SULPH.,** ***thuj.,*** zinc.
on going to bed - thuj.
perspiration, as after, morning on waking and after rising - coloc.
rising and washing with cold water, after - carb-s.
scratching amel. - arn., ferr-ma., mez., sars.
sleep amel. - cact.
spots, in, on perspiration - wies.
steam, exposure to, agg. - kali-bi.
sticking in evening - merc.
tickled with a feather, as if - morph.

itching, hypochondria - agar., tab.
night - agar.

itching, hypogastrium - agar., anac., ***carb-ac.,*** elaps, indg., kali-c., merc., nat-c., nat-m., ph-ac., rhus-t., rhus-v., zinc.
afternoon - nat-c.
scratching amel. - ph-ac.
walking agg. - elaps.

itching, inguinal - agar., agn., ammc., bar-c., camph., cycl., form., laur., lyc., mag-c., mag-m., merc., rhus-t., rumx., spig., spong., ter.
bed, in - sep., verat-v.
evening - pall., sep.
extending to knee - ars-m.
left - cycl., pall., spig.
mons veneris - eup-per.
right - ammc., mag-c., mag-m., rhus-t., ter.
rubbing agg. - sep.

itching, inguinal
scratching, amel. - laur., mag-c., mag-s.
does not amel. - mag-m.
tickling amel. - sep.

itching, sides - alum., berb., coloc., hura, led., nat-c., phos., sars., tarax.
scratching, after - olnd.
amel. - phos., sars.

itching, umbilicus - aloe, aur-m., bell., carb-v., cist., ign., kali-c., phos., puls., ***sulph.***
evening - aloe
scratching, painful after - puls.

JERKING, pain - bell., carb-s., chin., ruta.
flank - chin.

KNOTTY, sensation - nux-m., ***plb.***

LABOR-like, pain - aur., coff., kali-c., merc-c., **PULS.,** sul-ac.
extending into hips - sul-ac.
menses, before - eupi.
morning - ferr.
riding in a wagon, while - ***nat-m.***

LANCINATING, pain - anan., ars., aur-s., bufo, cadm-s., ***carb-an., carb-v.,*** clem., con., cur., elaps, gels., kali-i., manc., murx., plat., plb., raph., ***zinc.***
respiration - clem.
right - ***gins.***
urination - clem.

lancinating, hypochondria - aeth., bad., bufo, ***cadm-s.,*** calc-f., coloc., lach., manc., phys., stann., sulph., tab., tarent.
doubling up amel. - calc-f.
extending to, ilium - lil-t.
to, right side - stann.
left - ***cadm.***
motion agg. - bufo
lying, on painful side agg. - calc-f.
amel. - calc-f.
right - aur-s., aeth., bufo, calc-f., caust.
sitting agg. - calc-f.
walking amel. - calc-f.

lancinating, hypogastruim - aur-s., elaps, plb.

lancinating, inguinal - ars., aur., elaps, ***mag-c.,*** manc., spong.
extending to perineum - ars.
to seminal cord - ars.
menses, after - ***bor.***
menses, during - ***bor.***

lancinating, sides - ign.
right - cahin.

lancinating, umbilicus - elaps, plb.
extending to uterus - elaps

LIFTING, agg. - cub.

lifting, sensation as after, lying on side, on - ***carb-v.***
raising arm and on touch, on - carb-v.

LIME boiling in, as if - caust.

LIVER, (see Liver)

LOATHING, rising into stomach, after midnight - phel.

LOOSE sensation - aran-s., nux-v.
walking, while - nat-m.

LUMP, sensation in - abrot., anac., ant-t., ars., bism., bor., bry., ign., kreos., nit-ac., nux-m., ***nux-v.,*** plb., ***rhus-t.,*** sabad., sec., sep., sulph., ***thuj.,*** ust., verb.
gathered into a, as if, before menses - inul.
globus hystericus, 1 a.m. - mag-m.
moving rapidly - sabad.
rising to throat - **ARG-N.,** raph.
on coughing - kali-c.
side, right - med.

lump, umbilicus, sensation in - acon., anac., bell., kali-bi., kreos., nat-c., nux-m., nux-v., ran-s., rhus-t., ***sep., spig.,*** zinc.
behind - ran-s.

MESENTERIC, glands
enlarged - ***ars., ars-i., aur., bar-c., bar-i.,*** bar-m., **CALC.,** ***carb-an., con., form., hep., iod.,*** nat-s., ***ol-j.,*** sulph.
hardness - ***ars.,*** aur., ***bar-c., bar-m.,*** **CALC.,** con., ***lyc., nat-s.***
inflammation - ***ars.,*** ars-i., bac., bar-c., bar-m., ***calc.,*** calc-f., ***calc-i.,*** con., graph., ***iod.,*** iodof., lap-a., ***merc.,*** mez., tub.
swelling - ***ars., aur.,*** bar-c., bar-m., ***calc.,*** cist., ***con.,*** dros., ***grat., hep., iod.,*** kreos., lyc., merc., nat-s., sul-i., sulph., tub.

MOVEMENTS, in abdomen - aesc., aloe, am-c., am-m., anac., arn., asaf., asar., berb., bov., ***bry.,*** calc., ***calc-p.,*** cann-s., canth., caps., ***carb-an., carb-v., card-m.,*** cast., caust., cham., chel., cina, coff., colch., ***coloc.,*** **CROC.,** crot-t., cur., ***cycl.,*** dig., dulc., euph., ***gran.,*** grat., hell., hyos., ign., iod., jatr., kali-bi., kali-c., kali-chl., kali-i., kali-n., lact., laur., led., lob., ***lyc.,*** lyss., ***mag-c.,*** mag-m., mag-s., mang., merc., ***nat-c.,*** nat-m., nat-s., nicc., nit-ac., ***nux-m.,*** ol-an., op., osm., par., phel., phos., plb., ***puls., ran-b.,*** rat., rhus-t., ***sabad.,*** sabin., sang., ***sars.,*** seneg., sep., sil., stann., stram., stront-c., sulph., tarax., ter., **THUJ.,** til., ***zinc.***
afternoon - camph., chel., coloc., grat., laur., mag-c.
1 p.m - grat., mag-c.
1:30 p.m. - chel
3:30 p.m. - laur.
3:30 p.m., flatus, emission of amel. - bov., grat., laur., mag-c.
diarrhea would follow, as if - chin-s.
audible - aloe.
breakfast, after - cycl., polyg.
bubbles, as from, breaking of - coloc.
child were bounding, as if - nat-c., tarent., ther.
colic, as if would have - ***nux-m.***
convulsive, menses, at beginning of - nux-v.
diarrhea, as if would ensue - caust., colch., gran., mez., phos., sars., tab., ter.
dinner, after - coloc., franz.
drawing - verat.
eating, while - ferr-ma.
after - nat-m., sil.
epileptic spasms, during - sulph.

MOVEMENTS, in abdomen
evening - plb., puls., ran-b., ***zinc.***
6 p.m. - sumb.
11 p.m. through night - merc-i-r.
lying, while - puls., ran-b.
stool, before - coloc., sin-a.
extending, bladder, into - iod.
breast, below left, after drinking - ol-an.
downward - mill.
pubis, into - iod.
sacral region, to - phos.
fasting, as from, afternoon - coloc.
fetus, like movement of - nat-c., tarent.
disturb sleep - con., thuj.
first movement - carl.
intolerable - sep.
lively - lyc., op.
nausea and vomiting, cause - arn.
painful - ***arn.,*** con., croc., op., puls., **SIL.**
rawness, from - sep.
somersault, like - lyc.
tympanitic abdomen, with - psor.
urinate, with desire to, pain, in bladder and cutting pain - thuj.
violent - croc., ***lyc.,*** op., psor., ***sil.,*** thuj.
violent, with vomiting - psor.
fist of a fetus, like - ***nat-c., sulph.,*** **THUJ.**
flatus, amel. - mag-m.
accumulation of, like - plat.
frees itself, as of - mez.
forenoon - cast-eq., cast., grat., mag-m., sars.
stool, before - mang.
griping - kali-n., stann.
herring, after - nat-m.
jumping - brach., ***croc.,*** cycl., nux-m., ***op.,*** sabad., sulph., ***thuj.***
living thing, as from - arum-t., calc-p.
menses, during - ***croc.,*** nicc.
before - calc-p., croc., cycl., ferr., sabin.
occur, as if would - inul.
morning - nat-c., nux-v., rat., rumx.
4.30 a.m., before stool - ant-t., mang.
bed, in - nat-c.
waking, on - rumx.
night - merc-i-r.
painful - iod., stann.
diarrhea, before - kali-n.
periodic, after eating agg. - aloe.
pressive - merl.
stool, after - chel., colch., ol-an.
as before - bry., nux-v., rumx.
before - aeth., colch., grat., kali-i., mag-c., nat-c., nat-s., ol-an., phos., plb., **PULS.,** sil., thuj.
before, diarrhea - kali-i., mag-c., plb., thuj.
soft amel. - caust.
up and down, of something - **LYC.**
convulsion after - bufo.
vermicular - crot-t.
waking, on - colocin.
walking, while - cast.
amel. - gent-c.
water, as from - hell., ph-ac.

MOVEMENTS, in abdomen
worm, as from - nat-c., zinc.
movements, hypochondria, in - bad.
left - nit-ac., phos.
menses, during - inul.
movements, hypogastrium, in - coloc., sabad., thuj.
after, dinner and after stool - coloc.
movements, inguinal, in - kali-i.
movements, sides, in - meny., rat.
left - kali-n., stann.
right - stann.
movements, umbilical, in, region - aloe, cham., coloc., crot-t., hyos., plb., sul-ac., zinc.
expiration, as of - card-m.

NEURALGIC pain - cupr., sul-ac.
paroxysms, in - cod.

NODES - nat-c., plb.

NOISES, in - dig.
creaking - cycl.
gurgling, hip-region - sep.
purring - merc-i-r.
quacking - sars.
raging - plb., vip.
purge, as from a, in evening after milk - mag-s.
screaming as of animals in - stram.
whistling - ferr-ma., mur-ac., sep.

NUMBNESS - acon., bry., ***calc-p.,*** dig., ferr-i., merc., petr., ***plat., podo., puls.,*** sars., tarent., tell.
left, side - sulph.
sacrum and lower limb - ***calc-p.***

OPPRESSION - am-m., arum-m., carl., con., corn., euphr., iber., ign.
clothing, from tight - eup-per.
coughing, when - aur.
eating, after - bell.
amel. - carl.
extending upward - rhus-t.
oppression, hypochondrium - ail., iber.

PAIN, abdomen - acet-ac., acon., ***aesc., aeth.,*** agar., agn., ail., ***all-c., aloe, alum.,*** alumn., ambr., ***am-c., am-m.,*** anac., anthr., ant-c., ant-t., ***apis,*** arg-n., arn., **ARS.,** ars-i., ***asaf., asar.,*** asc-t., aster., aur., aur-m., bapt., bar-c., bar-i., bar-m., ***bell.,*** berb., bism., ***bol.,*** bor., bov., ***brom.,*** **BRY.,** bufo, cact., calad., ***calc., calc-p., calc-s.,*** camph., cann-s., **CANTH.,** ***caps.,*** carb-ac., carb-an., ***carb-v.,*** caust., cedr., **CHAM.,** ***chel., chin.,*** chin-a., chin-s., chlor., cic., ***cina, cimic.,*** clem., coc-c., **COCC.,** ***coff.,*** **COLCH., COLOC.,** con., ***cop.,*** crot-t., cub., **CUPR., CUPR-AR.,** cycl., dig., ***dios.,*** dor., dros., **DULC.,** elaps, eug., euon., eup-pur., ***euph.,*** euphr., eupi., fago., ***ferr.,*** ferr-ar., ferr-i., ferr-m., ferr-p., gels., gins., ***gran.,*** **GRAPH.,** grat., gymn., hell., hep., ***hydrc.,*** hyos., ign., ind., indg., iod., **IP.,** ***iris,*** jac-c., jatr., jug-r., **KALI-AR.,** kali-bi., kali-br., **KALI-C.,** kali-chl., kali-i., ***kali-n.,*** kali-p., kali-s., kreos., ***lac-d.,*** lach., ***laur., led.,*** lept., lil-t., lith., lob., lyc., lycps., lyss., ***mag-m.,*** mag-s., manc., mang., ***meph.,*** merc., ***merc-c.,*** merc-i-f., merc-i-r., merl., ***mez.,*** morph., mosch., murx., mur-ac., myric., naja, nat-a., ***nat-c., nat-m.,*** nat-p., **NAT-S.,** nicc., nit-ac., ***nux-m., nux-v.,*** olnd., **OP.,** ***ox-ac.,*** paeon., pall., par., ***petr.,*** ph-ac., **PHOS.,** phyt., pic-ac., plan., plat., plb., **PODO.,** prun., ***psor.,*** ptel., **PULS.,** ***ran-b.,*** ran-s., ***raph.,*** rat., ***rheum, rhus-t.,*** rhus-v., rob., ***rumx.,*** ruta, sabad., ***sabin.,*** sang., sars., **SEC.,** senec., ***seneg., senn.,*** **SEP.,** ***sil.,*** spig., spong., squil., ***stann., staph.,*** stram., ***sry., sulph.,*** sul-ac., sumb., tab., tarax., ***tarent., ter., thuj.,*** til., urt-u., ust., valer., **VERAT.,** verat-v., zinc., zing.
acids, from - dros., ph-ac.
acute - ars., bell., bol., calc-p., cedr., ***cham.,*** chin., **COLOC.,** dig., dirc., ery-a., ferr., gels., iris, lept., merc-c., naja, ***nux-v.,*** phos., ***plb.,*** polyp-p, puls., rumx., squil., tarent., trio., zinc-s.
afternoon - dios.
evening - dios., ptel., rumx.
6 p.m. - iris, murx.
walking agg. - dios.
flatus, as from - acon.
inspiration, on - morph.
agg. - rumx.
night - cedr.
pressure, firm amel. - plb.
like a, of diaphragm towards thorax - euon.
slight, agg. - plb.
retiring, after - fago.
rising, on - calc-s.
sleep amel. - ptel.
stool, during - cimic.
before diarrhea - plb.
loose amel. - puls.
straining, pressure or walking, on - nat-a.
afternoon - agar., all-c., ***alum.,*** am-c., ammc., am-m., ***ars.,*** bism., bov., canth., carb-s., carb-v., cast., caust., cham., chel., chin-s., ***coloc.,*** dios., dirc., fago., gels., grat., hura, ***iris, kali-n.,*** laur., **LYC.,** mag-c., mag-m., myric., nat-c., nat-p., nat-s., nux-v., petr., phos., plb., rat., sang., sep., sil., sulph., tell., verat.
1 p.m. - dios., dirc., mag-m., nux-v.
bending forward amel. - dirc.
stool amel. - dirc.
1:30 p.m. - dirc.
2 p.m. - chin-s., dirc., verat-v.
3 p.m. - hura, tell.
before and during stool - phys.
4 p.m. - caust., coloc., hell., **LYC.,** mag-m., phys.
to 5 p.m. - coloc., kali-br., lyc.
5 p.m. - elaps, fago., hura, nat-m., spig., sulph.
after - sulph.
cold beer amel., after - coca
resting hands on hips amel. - elaps
sitting, while - elaps
stool, emission of gas and sour urine amel. - nat-a.
walking amel. - elaps.

PAIN, abdomen
afternoon
5 p.m. to 6 p.m., during diarrhea - spig.
air, in cool, amel. - lyc.
amel. - nat-s.
bed, warmth of, amel. - ***coloc.***
coffee, after - all-c.
diarrhea, during - carb-s.
and after - ars.
before - canth.
eating, after - puls-n
pear - puls-n
motion amel. - fago.
sleep, after short amel. - bor.
stool, amel. - nat-a., plect.
urging, during - bov.
walking, while - lyc.
air, cool, amel. - lyc.
every draft - ***sulph.***
fresh agg. - ***puls.***
open, agg. - ign., ***nux-v.,*** puls.
amel. - kali-i.
touches abdomen, if - caust., ***sulph.***
alternating with
chest problems - rad-br., ran-b.
coryza - calc.
delirium - plb.
ear problems - rad-br.
eyes, affections of - euphr.
headache - aloe, bry., calc., cina, plb., podo., thuj.
joints, in - plb.
limbs - vip.
other organs - bry., coloc., nux-v., rad-br., ran-b.
pain, back, in - cham., ***lyc.,*** morph., puls., samb.
chest, in - aesc., ***ran-b.***
teeth, in - agar.
vertigo - coloc., spig.
anger, after - ***cham.,*** cocc., **COLOC.,** ***nux-v.,*** **STAPH.,** ***sulph.***
agonizing - ***coloc.,*** merc-c., merc-p-r., naja, plb.
annual, at first hot weather - vip.
anxiety, causing - cupr.
aphthae in children, with - kali-br.
arm resting on abdomen, from - carb-s.
ascending, stairs - asc-t., hell.
bandaging, amel. - cupr., fl-ac., nat-m., nit-ac.
beer, after warm - sil.
bed, in - alum., cedr., dig., dios., kali-c., lact., mag-c., nat-m., **NUX-V.,** psor., rhus-t., valer.
on going to - dios., nat-m.
belching, amel. - ***bar-c.,*** carb-v., jug-r., kali-n., lach., sep., sil.
do not amel. - ***chin.,*** lyc.
bending, general
backward, on - anac., thuj.
amel. - ***bell., dios., lac-c.,*** nux-v., onos.
double - am-c., bell., cocc., dios., dulc., ***lac-c.,*** lyc., onos., sulph.

PAIN, abdomen
bending, general
double, amel. - aloe, ars-h., ars-i., ***bell., bov.,*** cast., ***caust., chin.,*** cimic., **COLOC.,** ***colch., cop.,*** cupr., euph., eupi., ***iris,*** **KALI-C.,** ***lach.,*** lyc., mag-c., ***mag-p.,*** mang., merc-c., nux-v., petr., phos., podo., prun., **PULS.,** ***rheum,*** senec., ***stann.,*** staph., stram., sulph., tarent., verb., zinc.
must - alum., aur-m., ars., bar-c., bell., bor., bov., ***bry.,*** calad., calc., ***caps., caust., cham.,*** chel., cimic., **COLOC.,** crot-t., eupi., grat., ***iris,*** kali-p., ***mag-p.,*** merc, nat-m., nit-ac., petr., **PULS.,** plb., ***rheum, rhus-t.,*** sabad., sep., spong., sulph., ter., thuj., zinc.
while lying on side amel. - podo.
forward, agg. - aran-s.
causing - bov., ***cham., coloc.,*** digin., plb., puls., ***rhus-t.,*** sep., sulph., ter., thuj.
paroxysmal, soft stool amel. - **COLOC.**
stool, amel. - cimic.
up amel. - cast., cupr., iris, **KALI-C.,** lyc., merc-c., phos., tarent.
lying on side, while - podo.
blowing, nose, on - canth., eupi., stront.
brandy, after - ign.
agg. - arum-i.
breakfast, during - alum., apoc.
after - am-c., calc-s., cycl., gels., kali-p., nux-v., phos., raph., thuj.
breathing, on - ***anac.,*** arg-m., ars., ***bell.,*** berb., ***bry., coloc.,*** dig., hyos., kreos., lyc., mag-c., mang., mosch., seneg., ***stann.,*** sulph., ***thuj.***
and on touch - sin-a.
deep, on - ferr-i.
agg. - calc., con.
amel. - card-m., fl-ac., thuj.
expiration, on - brom., dig.
inspiration, during - aesc., agar., am-m., ***anac.,*** brom., ***bry.,*** calc., carb-s., caust., ***nux-v.,*** rhus-t., rumx., ***sulph.,*** thuj.
deep amel. - ***card-m.***
long agg. - dor.
urging for deep, after - card-m.
cataplasm, amel. - anthr.
changing, about in - dios., mur-ac., nux-v.
cherries, after - mag-m., merc-c.
chill, during - aran., ars., ***bov.,*** bry., calad., calc., **CHIN.,** chin-a., ***cocc.,*** coff., **COLOC.,** eup-per., ign., ip., lach., led., meph., merc., merc-c., nit-ac., nux-v., phos., podo., puls., ***rhus-t.,*** rumx., ***sep.,*** sulph.
and with, suppressed menses - ***puls.***
before - ars., elat., eup-per., ***spong.***
clothing agg. - arg-n., ***bell.,*** bov., calc., **LACH.,** ***lac-c., lyc., nux-v.***
clutching, with nails, as if - bell., ip.
clyster of water, after - carl.

PAIN, abdomen
coffee, after - canth., ***cham.***, ign., nat-m., ***nux-v.***
agg. - canth., coca.
amel. - **COLOC.**
black - ***coloc.***
cold, general
air, in open - ***nux-v.***
as from taking - all-c., alum., bell., ***carb-v.***, **CHAM., CHIN.,** ***coloc.***, **DULC.,** graph., ***hep.***, lyc., ***merc.***, nat-c., nit-ac., ***nux-v.***, petr., ruta., samb., **VERAT.**
becoming, from - alum., **ARS.,** camph., hell., merc., **NUX-V.,** ***phos.***, ***plb.***
drinks after - calc., ***calc-p.***, calc-s., dulc., manc., ***nux-m.***, ***rhus-t.***, trom.
amel. - elaps.
water, amel. - gran.
evening - junc.
flatus passing, amel. - ***carb-v.***
food - mang., sep.
morning during perspiration - ***nux-v.***
stool, after - aloe.
taking hold of cold things - merc.
walking in open air, while - merc.
weather, morning, in bed, before stool - mez.
sitting, while - dig.
coldness of limbs, with - ars.
comes gradually and goes gradually - bell., plat., ***stann.***
quickly and goes quickly - **BELL.,** ***vib.***
concussion, agg. - bry.
constipation, from - all-s., ***aloe***, ***alum.***, ars., bell., carc., cocc., coll., con., cupr., grat., kali-c., lyc., merc., op., plb., podo., sil., sul-ac., thuj.
as from - cham.
constricting, pain below short ribs extending to abdomen - ***camph.***
constriction - cact., lyc.
coryza, after - calc.
cough, during - aloe, ambr., am-c., am-m., ***anac.***, apis, ***arn.***, ars., ***asc-t.***, aur., **BELL., BRY.,** calc., camph., canth., caps., ***carb-an.***, cench., cham., ***chel.***, cocc., ***colch.***, coloc., con., croc., crot-t., **DROS.,** eupi., ***ferr.***, ferr-ar., ferr-p., hell., hep., ***hyos.***, ip., kali-ar., kali-bi., kali-c., ***kali-n.***, kali-p., kreos., ***lach.***, lact., ***lyc.***, ***nat-m.***, nit-ac., **NUX-V.,** pall., ph-ac., ***phos.***, plb., psor., ***puls.***, ***ran-b.***, rhus-t., ***sep.***, sil., **SQUIL.,** ***sulph.***, tarent., verat.
covering, lifting up, amel. - bell., lac-c., ***lach.***, lil-t., phos., sec., staph., tab.
cracking, at night - hyper.
cucumbers, from - all-c.
cut away, as if abdomen from chest - ars.
damp weather, from - ars., ***dulc.***, **MANG.,** ***nat-s.***
daybreak - podo.
daytime - nuph., plan., sulph.
deep - stry.
extending into chest - aran.
despair, driving to - ***coff.***

PAIN, abdomen
diarrhea, amel. - apoc., bry., coloc., dirc., gels., grat., op., seneg., sulph., trom.
before - alum., ant-t., arg-n., astac., bond., ***bry.***, cact., canth., chim., colch., cycl., fl-ac., gran., jug-r., olnd., op., ***psor.***, rob., ***rumx.***, stram., stront-c., thuj.
causing - ***bry.***
rising, after - colch.
diarrhea, sensation as if, would come on - act-sp., aeth., agar., ail., **ALOE,** alum., am-c., am-m., ang., ant-c., apis, ***apoc.***, arg-m., ***asaf.***, ***bar-c.***, ***bell.***, bol., ***bor.***, **BRY.,** calc., ***camph.***, carb-an., carb-s., carb-v., caust., cham., chin., cimic., cob., colch., coloc., ***con.***, crot-t., cycl., dig., **DULC.,** eupi., ferr., form., graph., hell., helon., **HYDR.,** kali-bi., ***kali-c.***, kali-n., ***lach.***, laur., led., lil-t., lith., lob., mag-m., mag-s., meny., meph., merc-i-f., mez., naja, nat-c., ***nat-s.***, **NUX-V.,** olnd., onos., ox-ac., ***ph-ac.***, ***phos.***, ***phys.***, phyt., plan., ***plat.***, prun., ptel., ***puls.***, **RAN-S.,** rhus-t., rumx., sabin., ***seneg.***, squil., stann., staph., ***stry.***, sulph., sumb., ter., verat., zinc.
4 p.m. - vichy-g.
5 a.m. - nat-n.
9 p.m. - puls-n
10 p.m. - carb-s., ptel.
cold, from taking - nux-v.
colic, during - agar., **ALOE,** alum., am-c., am-m., ant-t., apoc., aran., ***arg-n.***, ***ars.***, asaf., bapt., ***bell.***, bov., ***bry.***, cact., calc., calc-p., canth., caps., carb-s., carb-v., cench., **CHAM.,** ***chin.***, chin-a., cob., ***colch.***, **COLOC.,** com., ***cop.***, crot-t., cupr., cycl., **DIOS.,** dulc., ferr-p., fl-ac., **GAMB.,** gels., ***gran.***, graph., hell., hep., iod., ***ip.***, kali-ar., ***kali-c.***, kali-i., kali-n., kali-p., kali-s., ***lyc.***, lycps., ***mag-c.***, med., merc., mez., mur-ac., ***nat-s.***, nit-ac., nux-v., ox-ac., petr., phos., plb., **PODO.,** puls., ***rheum***, rhus-t., rumx., sanic., sars., sec., sep., sil., stram., stront-c., ***sulph.***, tab., ter., thuj., ***trom.***, ***verat.***, zing.
after - mag-c., stann.
eating, after - bor.
evening - cund., digin., piloc., vichy-g.
flatus, emission of, amel. - cham., crot-t.
headache, during - seneg.
sitting, while - puls-n
stool, before hard - gymn.
supper, at - helon.
digestion, during - chin., cupr-ac., spira.
dinner, during - bry., cedr., mag-s., seneg., zinc.
after - agar., alum., asc-t., bov., bry., carb-s., cob., cocc., colch., ***coloc.***, con., crot-t., gent-c., grat., jug-c., kali-bi., kali-c., lyc., **MAG-C.,** ***naja***, nat-m., ***nux-v.***, ped., phos., ***ran-b.***, sed-ac., sulph., thuj., trom., valer., zinc.
walking, while - cocc.
drawing in abdomen - valer., zinc.

PAIN, abdomen

drinking, after - ars., ***bell.,*** caust., cham., chin., **COLOC.,** con., croc., dor., ferr., ***manc.,*** nat-m., nit-ac., ***nux-m.,*** nux-v., ***podo., puls.,*** rhus-t., **STAPH.,** sulph., teucr.

when overheated - ars., **COLOC.,** kali-c.

dysentery, like - ***arn.***

eating, while - ***calc-p.,*** carb-v., colch., dulc., mur-ac., nux-v., plan.

after - agar., ***all-c., alum.,*** am-m., ant-t., arn., ***ars.,*** ars-i., asc-t., aur., bar-c., bar-i., bar-m., bell., bor., bry., bufo, carb-s., ***carb-v.,*** caust., ***cham., chin.,*** chin-a., cic., cob., ***cocc.,*** coc-c., ***colch., coloc.,*** con., crot-t., cupr., dor., euon., ***ferr.,*** ferr-ar., ferr-i., ferr-p., ***gran.,*** **GRAPH.,** grat., ign., iod., kali-ar., kali-bi., ***kali-c., kali-p.,*** kali-s., lach., ***lyc., mag-c.,*** merc., mur-ac., nat-a., ***nat-c., nat-m.,*** nat-p., nit-ac., ***nux-m., nux-v.,*** par., petr., ***ph-ac., phos.,*** plb., podo., ***psor., puls.,*** raph., ***rhod., rhus-t., sars.,*** sec., sep., sil., spong., ***stann.,*** **STAPH.,** ***stront-c., sulph., sul-ac., thuj.,*** **VERAT.,** ***zinc.***

2 hours - ***nux-v.,*** ox-ac., sil.

agg. - all-c., com., cot., dor., ferr-i., hedeo, lob., lyc., plb.

amel. - anac., aur-m., ***bov., chel.,*** fago., ***graph.,*** hep., ign., iod., kali-p., lach., mag-m., mang., med., mez., ***nat-c.,*** petr., plan., ***psor., zinc.***

on every attempt to - ***calc-p.***

too much - ant-c., coff., ip., lyc., nux-v., ***puls.***

evening - acon., agar., aloe, alum., alumn., ambr., am-c., ant-c., aran., bar-c., ***bell.,*** bor., bry., ***calc.,*** calc-p., carb-s., carb-v., ***chin.,*** cob., coloc., com., con., cop., crot-t., dig., dios., dirc., ***dulc.,*** ferr., ferr-p., fl-ac., gels., ham., hep., hura, hyper., ign., ***iris,*** kalm., lach., led., ***lyc.,*** mag-c., ***mag-m.,*** mang., meph., merc., merc-i-r., ***mez.,*** murx., myric., naja, nat-s., nicc., nit-ac., nux-m., nux-v., ox-ac., par., ***petr.,*** ph-ac., ***phos.,*** phys., phyt., plan., plat., plb., psor., ptel., **PULS.,** ***rhus-t.,*** rumx., senec., ***seneg., sep.,*** stann., stram., ***stront-c.,*** stry., ***sulph.,*** sul-ac., tarent., ter., thuj., ***valer.,*** verat., ***zinc.***

6 p.m. - verat-v.

before and during stool - phys.

8 p.m. - hura.

9 p.m. - dirc., ped., phyt., sulph.

coffee with milk agg. - lyc.

walking, on - dirc.

7 p.m. - stry.

air, in - ***merc.***

bed, in - alum., ign., par., ***valer.,*** zinc.

coffee, after - hyper.

diarrhea, during - bor., rhus-t.

amel. - coloc.

before - meph., tab.

drinking, after - ***puls.***

eating, after - alum., ant-t., coloc., ***gran.,*** phos.

agg. - ferr-i.

amel. - psor.

PAIN, abdomen

evening, eating, before - puls.

ice-cream, after - calc-p.

lying, while - ***puls.,*** zinc.

amel. - kali-i.

menses, before - calc.

milk, after - mag-s.

sitting, while - chin.

standing - chin.

stool, during - bor., grat., rhus-t., zinc.

amel. - chel.

before - mag-c., stann., tab.

stooping, on - plan.

urination, after - fago.

walking, while - verat.

excitement, after - acon., ***cham.,*** **IGN.,** ***staph.***

exercise, from - aloe, arn., berb., cocc., cycl., dig., ip., kali-n., kreos., nat-m., nux-v., ol-an., plb., puls., sep., stram.

amel. - coloc.

exertion, after - ***calc.,*** pall.

extending legs, amel. - phys.

extending, across - ***aloe,*** alum., am-c., arg-m., ***arn.,*** canth., carb-v., caust., cham., **CHEL.,** chin., colch., cupr-ac., euphr., guai., ip., kalm., phos., phys., prun., sep., stann., staph., zinc.

ilium to ilium - asar., ***cimic.,*** lil-t.

all parts of body, to - **PLB.**

ankles, to - kali-n.

anus, to - aloe, ***coloc.,*** **CROT-T.,** hydr., ***ip.,*** led., mag-m., ***nat-m., nux-v.,*** ox-ac., rhus-t., sang., ***sulph.***

axilla, to - com., con.

back, to - calc., canth., caust., cocc., coc-c., kali-bi.

small of, to - ***aesc.,*** agar., carb-v., chel., ***coloc.,*** croc., fago., ***gels.,*** iod., laur., lyc., naja, plb., ptel., sil.

backwards - arn., **ARS., BELL.,** bor., carb-v., chel., con., cupr., ferr., kali-p., lyc., nux-v., **PHOS.,** plb., puls., sep., sulph., ***tab.***

towards umbilicus - verat.

behind, forward, to - verat.

bladder, to - brom., carb-v., cham., cic., plb.

breasts, to - ferr-m.

right, to - coloc.

chest, to - ***acon.,*** aeth., alum., caust., ***cham.,*** chel., coloc., con., cupr., dios., ign., kali-c., ***lach.,*** lat-m., mang., nat-p., nat-s., ***nux-v., plb.,*** sep., spig., spong., tarent.

menses, during - chin-s., cupr., mang.

stool, during - **ACON.**

clavicle, to - laur.

distant parts, to - ***dios.***

downward, to - aloe, alumn., bar-c., brom., chin., crot-h., **CROT-T.,** elaps, ferr-i., guai., **IP.,** kali-c., kali-i., nux-v., plat., plb., puls., ran-s., samb., sep., til., verb., zing.

left, and to - nux-m.

esophagus, to, as if belching and heartburn would occur - merc.

through - aq-pet.

feet, to - plb.

PAIN, abdomen
  extending, forward - thuj.
    genitals, to - alumn., calc., crot-t., dig., ***lyc.,*** plb., **PULS.,** rhus-t., ***sep.,*** tep., teucr., verat.
      menses, with impending - carl.
      sitting bent amel. - crot-t.
    groin, to - tarent.
    head, to - ars., mang.
    heart region, to, in forenoon, stooping amel., deep pain - fago.
    hips, to - kali-c., lyc., xan.
      thighs and legs - xan.
    hypochondria - stann.
    inguinal region, to - arg-n., bar-c., kali-i., puls., tarent., thuj.
    kidney, to - nux-m., ***plb.***
    leg, to - **CARB-V.,** ter., thuj.
    loins, to - kali-bi., kali-i.
    lower limbs, to - bar-c., **CARB-V.,** kali-i., ***plb.,*** sang., ***sep.***
      left, to - **CARB-V.**
    outward - itu
    pelvis, to - carb-v., coloc.
    penis, to - alumn., carb-v., coloc., lyc., puls.
    perineum, to - phos.
    pubic region, to - **COLOC.,** ***sep.***
      when coughing - ***sep.***
    rectum, to - ***aloe,*** ars., brom., cann-i., dios., eupi., guai., ign., lyc., mag-m., meny., nat-m., ***nux-v.,*** sang., spong., stront-c., tarax.
    scrotum, to - verat., verat-v.
    shoulder, to - lach.
    sides, to - ars., coca, ***ip., lach., lyc.,*** stann., tarent.
      left - ars., coca, ***lyc.***
      right - ***ip., lach.***
    spermatic cord, to - brom., verat.
      when coughing - verat.
    spine, to - iod., lyc., sil.
    stomach, to - both., ***carb-v.,*** crot-t., lyc., nat-p., nux-m., ol-an., stann., sulph.
      12 a.m. after stool - gall-ac.
      region of - gins.
      sides beneath ribs, and, on pressure on umbilical region - stann.
    testicles, to - dig., plb., **PULS.,** sec., sil., teucr.
      evening, while eating - sil.
      when coughing - sec.
    thigh, to - ***aloe,*** alum., apis, bar-c., bry., cact., calc., cham., cimic., cob., coloc., con., kali-i., lil-t., mag-p., nat-m., nux-m., nux-v., plb., podo., sabal., sabin., ***sep.,*** spig., ***staph.,*** stram., ter., thuj., thyr., ust., vib., xan.
    throat, to - caust., kali-bi., kreos., merc.
    transversely - arn., **CHEL.,** cina, ip.
    umbilicus, to - crot-c.
    upward - aloe, anac., ars., canth., chel., com., ferr-m., ***gels.,*** merc., naja, plb., ruta, sep., spong., sulph.
      diagonally - lach.

PAIN, abdomen
  extending, upward, left - alum., ign., ***naja,*** nat-s., spong., zinc.
      right - acon., kali-c., mag-m., ***murx.,*** seneg., sep.
    urethra, forward in - zinc.
    uterus - elaps, ***ip.***
    vagina - ***ars.,*** berb., calc-p., ***kreos.,*** nit-ac.
  exertion, after - alum., cadm-s., ***calc.,*** cupr., pall., petr.
  external - cann-i.
  eye symptoms, with - arg-n.
  farinacious food, after - coloc.
  fasting amel. - caust., sil.
  fat, agg. - carb-v., ***puls.***
  fever, during - **ANT-C., ARS.,** caps., **CARB-V.,** ***cham., cina,*** elat., ign., nux-v., **RHUS-T.,** sulph., valer.
    after - sil.
  fish and vinegar, after eating - fl-ac.
  flatulence, with - all-c., ***alum.,*** arn., arum-d., carb-v., cham., ***chin.,*** euph., gran., iber., ign., iod., kali-c., ***lyc.,*** mill., nat-c., ***nat-m., nat-s.,*** ox-ac., phos., puls-n, rhod., senec., **VERAT.**
    as from - zinc.
    beer, after brown - teucr.
    bladder, on, causing urination - nat-p.
    breakfast, after - asc-t.
    constipation, during - merc.
    daytime - stann.
    diarrhea, before and during - com.
    dinner, after, motion and walking amel. - zinc.
    disposition to - am-c.
    eating, after - aur., ***puls.***
    evening, in bed - ign.
    extending to chest, after drinking water, passing of flatus amel. - carl.
    fall out of bottom, as if everything would, when walking - asc-t.
    flatus passing amel. - ***nat-s.***
    hernia would occur, as if - phos.
    midnight - aur., **COCC.,** coloc.
      amel., lying on one side and on the other - **COCC.**
      diarrhea, during, after eating sugar - **ARG-N.**
    morning - cedr., hyos., stann.
      7 a.m. - crot-t., mim-h., murx., nuph., phys.
      agg., lying quiet - euph.
      bed, in - euph., mang.
      rising, after - nit-ac.
      waking, on - puls.
    motion agg. - ***nat-m.***
    night - bry., cist., ferr., ign., nat-m., sulph.
      bed, in, before going to sleep - naja
    pressing in evening - zinc.
    resting head on elbows and knees amel. - euph.
    sexual excitement, during, hindering sex - graph.
    stones, as by, after stool - ***nux-v.***
    supper, after - bry., ***puls.***

PAIN, abdomen
flatulence, with
walking, when - graph.
dinner, after - asaf.
wandering, evening, after lying down - **PULS.**
flatus, incarcerated, as from - arn., cast-v., colch., cupr-ar., dulc., lam., lyc., ***nux-v.,*** sarr., tell., til.
3 p.m. - trom.
eating, after - rhus-t.
evening - fl-ac., lyc.
eating, before - ***puls.***
morning, on waking - nat-m.
sleep amel. - nat-m.
stool, after - puls.
moving, as if, before stool - apoc.
passing, agg. - aur., canth., fl-ac., graph., nat-a., squil., zinc.
after - graph.
amel. - all-c., aloe, am-c., arn., ***calc-p., carb-v.,*** cham., ***cimx.,*** coloc., ***con.,*** com., crot-t., dulc., der., ***graph.,*** grat., ***guai.,*** iris, jatr., kali-n., ***lyc.,*** mag-c., merc-c., **NAT-A.,** nat-m., ***nat-s.,*** nux-m., phyt., plb., ***psor., rumx., sep.,*** sil., spong., sulph., ***tarent.***
as from - kali-n., mang., nit-ac.
before - calc-p., **CHIN.,** kali-n., ***nit-ac.,*** rheum., sil.,
on passing - ***chin.***
flexing, limbs amel. - ***bell., bry.,*** chel., **COLOC.,** grat., nit-ac., ph-ac., ***podo.,*** puls., rheum, ***sep.,*** sulph.
food, as from improper - coloc.
stale, agg. - ars.
stomach, in, during presence of, before diarrhea - arum-i.
forenoon - agar., am-c., am-m., asc-t., bapt., bry., coloc., dios., kali-bi., lach., lith., lyc., mag-c., mag-m., ***nat-c.,*** nat-m., nat-s., phos., pic-ac., ptel., sars., ***sep.,*** sulph., thuj.
9 a.m. - dios., pip-m., **SEP.**
breakfast, after - grat.
stool, before - phys.
10 a.m. - fago., pip-m., ptel.
stool, before - phys.
stool amel. - nat-a.
stool amel., and gas - nat-a.
10 a.m. to 11 a.m. - digin.
11 a.m. - mit., trom.
amel. - phyt.
soup, after, amel. - nat-c.
stool, after, amel. - phys.
chill, during - bov.
evening, till - kali-a.
menses, during - mag-c., nicc.
stool, after - pip-m.
walking in open air - am-c., sulph., thuj.
fright, from - plat.
as from - plat.
fruit, after - ars., ***calc-p., chin.,*** **COLOC.,** mag-m., ***merc-c., puls.,*** **VERAT.**
full - sep.

PAIN, abdomen
gouty - daph.
gruel, after, amel. - crot-t.
grumbling - lil-t.
all afternoon - myric.
hand on, agg. - psor., zinc-chr.
hard - iod.
headache, with - con., lept.
heart symptoms, with - merc-i-f.
heat, during, bed, of - elat.
after - hell., sil.
heavy - ***coc-c.,*** zinc.
hemorrhoids, from - ***aesc.,*** carb-v., coloc., lach., ***nux-v.,*** puls., ***sulph.,*** valer.
as from - acon-l.
hiccough, suffocative, with - verat.
hips, region of - arum-t., calc., chel., con., fl-ac., phos.
injured as if - phos.
extending from hip to hip before menses - thuj., ust.
walking, while - con.
holding, right hand on stomach, left on lumbar region, amel. - med.
holds - dros.
hot food and drinks amel. - lyc., mag-p., ***nux-v.,*** sul-ac.
humiliation, after - cham., ***coloc., staph.***
hunger, during - merc., stram.
yet refuses food - bar-c.
hysterical - stann.
ice cream, after - **ARS.,** calc-p., ***puls.,*** sep.
indescribable - phos.
lying amel. - merc.
indignation, after - **STAPH.**
inflammatory, coughing agg., sneezing and blowing nose amel. - eupi.
motion, during - eupi.
inflating abdomen amel. - plb.
inspiration, during, deep - ptel.
itching of nose, with - ***cina,*** fil.
jerking, causing - dulc.
kidney, as if from, compelling to stretch, after urinating amel. - tarent.
kneading, hand by, amel. - nat-s.
labor, during - ***sep.***
laughing, from - ars., con., nux-v.
lead, from - **ALUM., ALUMN.,** ***ars.,*** **COLOC.,** nat-s., **OP.,** ***plat., plb.,*** podo., ***sul-ac., zinc.***
leaning, on the side - raph.
left to right - ip., kali-p.
lifting, from - arn., bry., ***calc.,*** coloc., kali-n., sil.
lightning-like, afternoon - digin.
lying, while - apis, bar-c., ***bell.,*** coloc., dios., ***phos., puls.,*** spig.
amel. - am-c., bry., canth., cupr., dios., gran., merc., nux-v., phys.
abdomen, on - aloe, ambr., am-c., ars-h., **BELL.,** ***bry.,*** chin-a., chion., ***coloc.,*** ind., ***phos.,*** plb., rhus-t., ***stann.***

PAIN, abdomen
lying, while
back, on - ***ars.,*** mag-p., phys., podo., ptel., sulph.
amel. - coloc., ***kalm.,*** mez., onos.
with knees drawn up amel. - bry., coloc., lach., rhus-t.
knees drawn up, with, amel. - coloc., lach.
side, on - bry., ***carb-v.,*** cocc., coloc., ***kalm.,*** par., phos.
amel. - nat-s.
left, amel. - pall., sec.
right - acon., caust., ***merc.,*** stann.
right, amel. - nux-v., phos., phys.
making sick - nat-a.
meat, after - tub.
menopause, during, with sadness - ***psor.***
menses, during - acon., agar., alet., aloe, alum., ***am-c.,*** am-m., apis, arg-n., ars., ***ars-i.,*** aur., bapt., ***bar-c., bar-i., bell., bor., brom.,*** bry., bufo, cact., **CALC., CALC-P.,** ***canth.,*** **CARB-S.,** carb-v., cast., caul., ***caust., cham.,*** chel., ***chin.,*** **CIMIC.,** cina, cinnb., clem., ***cocc., coff., coloc., con.,*** croc., crot-h., ***cupr., cycl.,*** eupi., fago., ferr., ferr-ar., ferr-i., ferr-p., form., **GRAPH.,** hyos., ***ign.,*** inul., iod., ip., kali-ar., ***kali-c., kali-n.,*** kali-p., kali-s., kreos., ***lac-c., lach.,*** lyc., ***mag-c.,*** mag-m., mag-s., mang., merc., ***mill.,*** mosch., ***murx.,*** nat-c., ***nat-m., nat-s., nicc., nit-ac., nux-m.,*** **NUX-V.,** ol-an., petr., ***phos.,*** phyt., ***plat.,*** plb., **PULS., RAT., SABIN.,** ***sars., sec.,*** **SEP.,** ***sil.,*** stann., staph., ***stram.,*** **SULPH.,** sul-ac., thuj., ust., verat., **VIB.,** xan., zinc.
exercise amel. - ***sulph.***
flow becomes free, amel. ., when - bell., kali-c., kali-p., ***lap-a., lach.,*** mosch., sep., sulph.
hard, steady - ***ust.***
heat amel. - **ARS.,** coloc., ***nux-m., nux-v.,*** pall., puls., rhus-t., ***sil.***
rubbing back amel. - ***mag-m.***
after - ***am-c.,*** bor., cham., cocc., con., graph., iod., kali-c., ***kreos., lach.,*** lyc., mag-c., merl., ***nat-m., nit-ac.,*** plat., ***puls.,*** ust.
appear, as if, would - act-sp., ***aloe,*** ambr., am-m., ***apis, aur.,*** bry., cina, cocc., ***croc.,*** ferr., ferr-p., inul., kali-c., kreos., laur., ***lil-t.,*** lyc., ***mag-c., med.,*** mosch., ***murx.,*** mur-ac., ***nat-c.,*** nat-m., onos., phos., ***plat., puls.,*** sang., ***sep.,*** stann., sul-ac., til., vib.
evening in bed amel. - plat.
midnight - canth.
morning - ferr., plat.
morning, vaginal discharge, before - nat-m.
amel. - aster.
as during - act-sp., kali-fer.
as before - act-sp., ter.
at beginning of - ***calc., caust.,*** graph., ***kali-c.,*** lap-a., lyc., mag-c.

PAIN, abdomen
menses, before - aloe, ***alum., am-c.,*** bar-c., bar-i., ***bell.,*** brom., ***calc.,*** **CALC-P.,** carb-s., carb-v., ***caust., cham.,*** chin., cinnb., ***cocc., coloc., croc., cupr.,*** cycl., eupi., graph., hep., hyper., ***ign.,*** iod., **KALI-C.,** ***kali-p.,*** kali-s., ***lach., lyc., mag-c.,*** mag-m., ***mag-p.,*** manc., merc., mosch., nat-c., nat-m., nux-m., ***nux-v.,*** petr., ph-ac., ***phos., plat.,*** **PULS.,** sang., sars., ***sep., sil., spong.,*** sulph., sul-ac., ***tarent.,*** thuj., ust., zinc.
extending from hip to hip - thuj.
extending to chest - cupr., graph.
delay of, during - sul-ac.
suppression of, from - acon., agn., ***cham.,*** cocc., coloc., graph., ***puls., spong.***
midnight - **ARG-N.,** aur., ***chin.,*** **COCC.,** coloc., gels., lyc., ***nit-ac.,*** nux-v., phos., rhus-t., sulph.
after - gent-l., rhus-t.
amel. - fago.
sitting down after rising from bed - nux-v.
stool, before - ferr.
waking, on - gent-l.
milk, after - ang., bell., bry., bufo, carb-v., con., lac-d., mag-s., sul-ac.
amel. - graph., merc., mez., ***nux-v.,*** ruta, verat.
hot amel. - chel., crot-t.
warm, amel. - ***chel., crot-t.,*** op.
miscarriage, as before - tarent.
morning - agar., all-c., aloe, alum., ambr., apis, bar-c., bar-m., berb., bor., bov., ***calc.,*** calc-s., carb-s., ***caust.,*** cedr., cham., cob., coloc., con., crot-t., dor., ***dios.,*** ferr., ferr-p., gels., glon., graph., ham., hell., ***hep.,*** hyos., kali-i., kali-n., kreos., ***lyc.,*** mag-c., ***mag-m.,*** mur-ac., naja, nat-c., nat-m., ***nat-s.,*** nit-ac., nux-m., **NUX-V.,** op., ox-ac., petr., ***phos., plat.,*** plb., ***podo., ptel., puls.,*** ran-b., ran-s., ***sars.,*** **SEP.,** sil., spong., stann., ***sulph.,*** tab., tarent., ***verat.,*** zinc.
6 a.m. - ***coloc.,*** corn., dirc., fago., ox-ac., sapo.
moving, on - sep.
stool amel. - phys.
stool, before and after - petr.
waking, on - dirc.
7 a.m. - am-c., gnaph.
diarrhea, after - ox-ac.
diarrhea, before - ox-ac.
diarrhea, during - hura
waking, on - pic-ac.
8 a.m. - dirc., fago.
agg. - acon., aloe, bov., nat-a., phos., plb.
bath, after - calc-s.
bed, in - acon., agar., ambr., berb., cham., dios., lyc., mang., mez., mur-ac., nat-c., **NUX-V.,** pall., phos., plat., psor., ptel., sep.
uncovering, on - rheum
breakfast, before - ***nat-s.***
diarrhea, during - bov., hura, op.
before - ang., bar-c., nat-p., nux-v., ox-ac.
doubling up amel. - cham.

PAIN, abdomen
morning
eating, after - con., grat., nux-m.
fasting - dulc., gran., hell.
menses, during - sulph.
motion, on - gent-l.
rising, on - calc-s., caust., nat-m., ***nat-s.,*** phos., plat., ruta, ***sep.***
after - crot-t., ferr., lyc., mag-c., mag-m., mang., nat-m., nit-ac., ox-ac.
before - cham., ptel.
rubbing amel. - dios.
stool, during - dios.
after - agar.
amel. - ferr.
before - graph., verat.
urging, during - apis, mag-m.
sunrise - ***cham.***
turning on back amel. - morph.
waking, after - verat.
waking, on - agar., bry., ***calc.,*** cast-eq., colch., coloc., corn., dios., dirc., ery-a., hep., kali-i., ***lyc.,*** nat-a., nat-m., nux-m., pic-ac., ***puls.,*** xan.
stool, before - glon.
motion, on - alum., ant-t., bar-c., **BELL.,** brom., **BRY.,** carb-an., carb-s., caust., ***cocc.,*** colch., con., dig., eupi., ***gels.,*** graph., **IP.,** iris, jug-r., kali-c., kali-s., ***kalm.,*** kreos., mag-m., mag-p., mang., merc., nat-m., ***nit-ac.,*** **NUX-V.,** ox-ac., puls., ran-b., raph., ***rhus-t.,*** sep., stann., ***sulph.,*** thuj., zinc.
amel. - aur-m., bov., cycl., kali-n., ***petr.,*** phos., ptel., rhus-t., sulph.
continued amel. - gels.
sudden - ptel.
violent, and - bell., card-m., coloc.,
violent amel. - card-m., coloc.
nausea, during - ars., crot-t., ***gran., ip.,*** nux-v., sulph.
after - lat-m.
nervous colic, as in, affecting uterus - tarent.
neuralgic - cupr., sul-ac.
paroxysms, in - cod.
night - abrot., acon., ambr., am-c., am-m., ***arg-n.,*** ars., asc-t., ***aur.,*** bar-c., ***bell.,*** bor., bov., bry., **CALC.,** calc-s., carb-s., carb-v., cedr., cist., cob., cocc., ***coc-c.,*** colch., coloc., ***cycl.,*** dulc., ***ferr.,*** ferr-ar., ferr-p., gnaph., ***graph.,*** hell., ign., iris, kali-ar., kali-c., kali-p., kali-s., kreos., lach., lyc., mag-c., ***mag-m.,*** mag-s., **MERC.,** merc-i-r., mez., mur-ac., naja, nat-a., nat-c., nat-m., nat-p., ***nat-s.,*** **NIT-AC.,** ***nux-m.,*** ox-ac., ***petr.,*** phos., plan., ***plb.,*** prun., ptel., ***puls.,*** rhus-t., sang., sars., ***sep., sil.,*** sol-t-ae., ***sulph., sul-ac.,*** tab., tarent., thuj., valer., verat., zinc., zing.
10 p.m. - abrot., dirc., ferr-i.
eating, after - puls-n
stool, before - phys.
11 p., through night, during diarrhea - merc-i-r.

PAIN, abdomen
night
1 a.m. - asc-t.
had to lie crooked and uncovered - ***mag-m.***
2 a.m. - fl-ac., sep., rhus-v.
after - gent-l.
lying on side amel. - nat-s.
waking - nat-s.
2 to 3 a.m. - lyc.
3 a.m. - am-c., iris, ox-ac., podo., sapo.
menses, before - am-c.
pressure amel. - podo.
stool, before - petr.
waking, on - phys., podo.
waking, on, stool, before - cob.
4 a.m. - cob., phos., ***podo.***
watery stool amel. - cob.
5 a.m. - bov., cob.
waking, on - hell., nat-m., nat-s., ptel.
bed, in - bry., ***con.,*** kali-c., naja, ptel., rhus-t., sulph.
back, lying on - sulph.
movement, on - kali-c.
bending up amel. - iris
diarrhea, during - bov., carb-s.
before - **ARG-N.,** sol-t-ae.
menses, during, agg. - inul.
retiring, on - sapo.
stool, during - graph.
uncovering - bry.
vomiting, after - lach.
waking, on - mag-m., nat-c., zinc.
noon - calc-s., chin., coloc., kali-c., lyc., nat-s., ran-b., sulph., thuj.
amel. - chin-s.
eating, after - coloc., lyc.
before - chin.
standing, while - verat.
walking, while - ***coloc.,*** nat-s., ran-b., verat.
obscure, shooting through - cupr.
operation, from - arn., bism., ***calen.,*** hep., nux-v., op., raph., ***staph.***
pain in limbs, with - aeth.
paroxysm, during febrile - arund.
paroxysmal - ***alum.,*** ant-t., ars., asaf., ***bell.,*** berb., calad., carb-v., ***cham.,*** chel., ***cocc.,*** coff., colch., **COLOC., CUPR.,** ***cupr-ar., cycl.,*** dig., ***dios.,*** ferr., ferr-ar., ferr-p., ***gels.,*** gent-c., graph., ***ign.,*** ip., kali-ar., kali-c., kali-p., kalm., lac-c., lyc., mag-c., mag-m., ***mag-p.,*** merl., nat-c., nat-p., ***nux-v.,*** ol-an., olnd., ox-ac., ph-ac., plat., ***plb.,*** puls., ran-s., ***raph.,*** samb., sang., sars., sec., ***stann.,*** staph., teucr., thuj., verb., zinc.
11 a.m. - fago.
diarrhea, during - plb.
dinner, after - thuj.
menses, before - thuj.
night agg. - plb.
pressure, from - plb.
firm amel. - plb.
sitting, agg. - fago.
walking, amel. - fago.

PAIN, abdomen

paroxysmal, white discharge from vagina, with - eupi.

peaches, after - psor.

perforated, as if - kali-i.

periodical - ***ars.,*** cahin., ***calc.,*** **CHAM.,** ***chin., cimic., coloc.,*** **CUPR.,** ***cupr-ar., gels.,*** ign., ill., ***ip.,*** lac-c., **NUX-V.,** sulph.

every day - aran., arn., nat-m.

fever, during - hep.

heat, during, stool amel. - cimic.

plums, after - rheum

potatoes, after - alum., ***coloc.,*** mag-s., merc-c.

peritonitis, like - colch.

perspiration at night amel. - anthr.

pregnancy, during - arn., ***ars., bell., bry., cham., coloc., con.,*** hyos., ***ip., kali-c.,*** lach., **NUX-V.,** plb., puls., sep., ***verat.***

dragging, in, during - ***kali-c.***

lying on abdomen amel. - podo.

sore, bruised, in, during - arn., ***nux-m.,*** sep.

pressure, agg. - acon., agar-se., aloe, anac., ant-t., ars., **BELL.,** bry., calc., canth., ***carb-s.,*** carb-v., carl., chel., chin-s., cic., cina, cob., ***coff.,*** con., cupr., cupr-ac., cycl., cyt-l., dirc., eup-per., graph., jac-c., kali-bi., kali-chr., ***lac-c.,*** lac-d., ***lach.,*** led., merc-c., ***mez., nit-ac., nux-v.,*** plb., puls., ***ran-b.,*** ric., samb., sars., scroph-n., stann., ***sulph.,*** trom., yuc., ***zinc.***

amel. - agar., alumn., am-c., arg-n., asaf., ***bell.,*** bov., brom., cast., cina, **COLOC.,** dios., dulc., gamb., graph., grat., kali-c., kali-n., ***mag-p.,*** mag-m., mang., meny., nat-c., nat-m., ***nat-s., plb., podo.,*** ptel., ***stann.,*** sul-ac., tarent., thuj.

clothes, of - fl-ac., nat-m.

forcible - plb.

gentle - ant-t.

gradual - ***plb.***

pulse beat, with every - hep.

radiating - dios., ***ip.,*** **MAG-P.,** ***plb.***

to all parts of body - **PLB.**

umbilicus, from - benz-ac., senec.

raising, arm - carb-v.

reaching, high - alum., ***rhus-t.***

rest, agg. - bov.

retention of urine, on coughing, as in - ip.

retiring, after, amel. - sin-n.

retraction, agg. - ant-t., asar., nux-v., zinc.

amel. - ign.

umbilicus, of the, with - bar-c., plb.

rheumatic - caust., plb., polyp-p

riding, in a carriage - calc-f., ***carb-v., cocc.,*** nat-m., psor., ***sep.***

rising, on - bry., senec.

after - chin., coloc., ***lyc.***

amel. - dios.

before - pall.

from a seat amel. - chin., spong.

lying amel. - arg-m., bar-c.

rolling, on the floor amel. - coloc.

PAIN, abdomen

room, in, agg. - kali-i.

rubbing, amel. - ***aran.,*** lyc., mag-c., nat-s., pall., phos., plb., ***podo.***

gently with warm hand, amel. - lil-t.

rumbling - cast., phos., polyg., squil., ust.

7 a.m. on waking - pic-ac.

dull - aran-s.

scorbutic - chin.

sex, during - graph.

after - caust., ph-ac., ther.

sexual excitement, during - graph.

sharp, hips, region of - ***agar.,*** ambr., bry., calc., kali-c., ***lyc.,*** mag-c., ***mez.,*** nat-c., samb., sep., sulph.

shattered, sensation - carb-an., kreos., squil.

singing, agg. - puls.

amel. - calc-s.

sitting, while - all-c., asaf., bar-c., ***calc.,*** chin., ***con., dig.,*** dios., ferr., ***nat-m.,*** op., ***petr.,*** ph-ac., puls., rhus-t., ruta, ***sep.,*** spong., ***sulph.***

amel. - alum., apis, bar-c., bell., ferr., gent-l., ***kalm.,*** lepi.

bent - alum., ant-t., carb-v., dulc., ***lyc.,*** sulph.

amel. - ***bell., coloc.,*** merc., sars., sulph.

has to sit - kali-c.

erect amel. - ***gels.***

sleep, during - cina, kali-n.

amel. - alum., am-m., mag-m.

before going to - sulph.

interrupting sleep - mez., tab.

smoking, from - meny.

amel. - coloc.

sneezing, on - bell., canth., cham., eupi., ind., pall.

after - ind.

spots, in - jug-c., ran-s.

soup, after - acon., zinc.

speaking, after - brom.

standing, while - aloe, ***bell.,*** chin-s., ptel., sulph., zinc.

amel. - thuj.

still - coloc., tarent.

stomach becomes empty, as - fago.

step, at every - mur-ac.

hard, on - gent-l.

sticking - sil.

sticks, hard, like - bor.

stone, as from a - nux-v., sabad.

stones, like sharp, rubbing together - apis, ***cocc., coloc.,*** staph.

as if squeezed between two stones - ***coloc.***

stool, during - aeth., ***agar.,*** alum., ***aran.,*** arn., asc-t., bell., bor., **BRY.,** bufo, ***carb-an., carb-v.,*** cham., chin., cob., ***con.,*** crot-t., dios., ***dulc.,*** ferr., ***graph.,*** grat., guare., indg., iod., ip., jug-c., kali-ar., kali-bi., ***kali-c.,*** kalm., laur., ***lil-t., lyc., mag-c.,*** merc., ***mur-ac.,*** naja, nat-m., nux-v., osm., petr., phos., phys., plb., ***podo.,*** ptel., puls., ***rheum, rhus-t., rhus-v.,*** sec., senec., ***sep.,*** sil., stram., **SULPH.,** sul-ac., ***tab.,*** tarent., thuj., ***zinc.***

PAIN, abdomen
stool, after - agar., ***aloe,*** alum., ambr., am-c., am-m., arg-m., aur., bov., carb-an., ***carb-v., chin.,*** colch., ***coloc.,*** cop., crot-t., cupr., cupr-ar., dig., dios., dros., fago., graph., grat., ip., kali-bi., kali-c., lept., lyc., mag-m., ***merc.,*** merc-c., mez., nat-a., ***nat-m.,*** **NIT-AC.,** op., osm., pall., phos., ***pic-ac.,*** plb., ***podo., puls., rheum,*** rhod., sep., sil., staph., stront-c., **SULPH.,** ***sul-ac.,*** trom., ***zinc.***
as after, stool - alum.
amel. - agar., aloe, apoc., ars., bapt., bor., bov., bry., ***calc-p., carb-v.,*** chin-s., cimic., cinnb., coc-c., **COLCH., COLOC.,** dig., dios., ferr., **GAMB.,** gels., grat., helon., mag-c., nat-a., nat-c., ***nat-s.,*** **NUX-V.,** ***rheum, rhus-t.,*** senec., sil., sulph., thuj., trom., zinc.
before - aesc., agar., ail., **ALOE,** alum., **AM-C.,** ***am-m.,*** ant-t., apoc., **ARG-N.,** ars., ***bar-c., bar-m.,*** bell., ***bry.,*** cact., calc., ***calc-p.,*** camph., cann-s., canth., carb-an., carb-v., caust., cham., ***chin.,*** chin-a., chin-s., cimx., cina, coc-c., ***colch., coll., coloc.,*** cop., ***crot-t.,*** cupr., cycl., ***dig.,*** dulc., fago., ferr., ferr-i., ferr-p., fl-ac., form., gamb., gels., glon., graph., grat., guai., hell., hep., ign., ind., jug-r., kali-bi., ***kali-c.,*** kali-i., ***kali-n.,*** kali-p., ***lyc.,*** **MAG-C.,** mag-m., ***mang.,*** merc., merc-i-r., ***mez., mur-ac.,*** naja, nat-a., ***nat-c.,*** nat-m., nat-p., ***nat-s.,*** nicc., ***nit-ac., nuph., nux-v., olnd., op.,*** ox-ac., petr., ***phos.,*** plan., plb., **PODO.,** prun., ***psor.,*** **PULS.,** ran-b., raph., rat., ***rheum,*** rhod., ***rhus-t.,*** rhus-v., ***rumx.,*** sabad., ***sang., sep., stann.,*** stram., **SULPH.,** tax., ***thuj., trom.,*** verat., zinc., zing.
between - phos.
diarrheic, during - ***aeth., agar.,*** aloe, alum., ***anac.,*** ang., ***arg-n.,*** arn., ***ars.,*** ars-i., asaf., bapt., bov., canth., caps., carb-s., ***cham.,*** cimic., ***coc-c., colch., coloc.,*** cop., ***crot-t.,*** cupr., cupr-ar., euph., ***gamb., gran.,*** ham., hep., hura, iod., iris, jug-r., kali-bi., kali-c., kali-n., lact., ***med., merc., merc-c.,*** merc-i-r., ***nux-v.,*** op., plb., ***podo.,*** rhus-t., rhus-v., sars., senec., ***sulph.,*** tab., **THUJ.,** zinc-s.
straining while - acon., ***aloe,*** bell., bry., podo.
urging during - apis, bar-c., dulc., elaps, hydr., mag-m., ***nux-v., plb.***
after - nit-ac.,
before - brach., colch., crot-t.
stooping, agg. - am-c., sep., stann., stront-c., sulph., verb.
amel. - ant-t.
stretching, out - mag-s., rhus-t.
amel. - dios., mez., plb.
sudden - cyt-l.
sugar, after - ***arg-n.,*** ign., ox-ac., ***sulph.***
in tea or coffee, agg. - ox-ac.
summer - guai.

PAIN, abdomen
supper, after - alum., bry., calc., ***chin.,*** coff., ferr., gels., kali-n., ***puls.,*** zinc.
agg. - coloc.
walking, while - nat-p.
suppressed, hemorrhoidal flow - **NUX-V.**
swallowing liquids, after, agg. - plb.
sweets, from - arg-n., fil., sulph., zinc.
swollen, as if - stram.
talking unbearable - caust., helin., kali-c., laur.
tension - acon., lyc.
tobacco, after - bor., ign.
amel. - coloc.
touch, agg. - carb-an., cupr., kali-c., mag-m., nat-c., stann., sulph.
side agg., of - stram.
turning, the body - ambr.
violently - rhus-t.
uncovering, from - ***bry.,*** nux-v., rheum.
amel. - camph., med., sec., tab., vip.
limbs, from - rheum.
urethra, after smarting in, while urinating - plb.
urging, to urinate, with - lach., nit-ac., puls.
to stool, amel. - alum.
urination, during - bar-c., bry., ***cham.,*** chin., coloc., ip., ***merc.,*** nat-m., plb., til.
after - ars., chin., clem., mag-c., ph-ac.
amel. - carb-an., dios., merc., ***sep.,*** tarent.
before - ***puls.,*** sul-ac.
prevents - ***cham.***
vaginal discharge, with - bell., con., inul., merc-c.
after amel. - calc-p.
before - con., mag-c., nat-m., zinc.
vexation, after - **COLOC.,** *staph.*
violent - aloe, ant-t., ***apis, ars., bell.,*** cact., canth., cast., ***cham., colch.,*** **COLOC.,** ***cupr.,*** cycl., dig., euph., ***kali-ar.,*** kali-c., kali-n., ***mag-c.,*** mag-p., merc-c., ***nux-v., phos.,*** **PLB.,** sil., **SUL-AC.**
vomiting, with - agar., ***ars.,*** bism., cadm-s., hell., ***ip., nux-v.,*** sant.
after - ***ant-t.,*** ars., graph., lach., merc., staph., verat.
amel. - arg-n., ars., asar., dig., hyos., nat-c., plb., tab., tarent.
before - plb.
waking, on - aeth., alum., bar-c., coc-c., colch., ferr., lyc., merc-i-f., mez., morph., nat-a., nat-c., nat-m., pic-ac., ptel., sil., sol-t-ae., stann., stront-c., zinc.
walking, while - alum., alumn., asaf., bar-c., ***bell.,*** bry., carb-an., chin., ***coloc.,*** con., crot-t., ferr., ferr-p., gent-c., graph., grat., hep., hyos., lac-c., lach., lob., lyc., ***merc.,*** nat-c., ***nat-m., nux-v., ph-ac.,*** phos., phyt., prun., ptel., puls., ***ran-b., sil.,*** squil., stann., ***sulph.,*** tarent., ***thuj.,*** verat., zinc.
after - bar-c.
amel. - chin., coloc., ***con., cycl.,*** dios., fago., ferr., mag-c., ***puls.,*** sulph.

PAIN, abdomen
walking, bent, amel. - aloe, coloc., nux-v., rhus-t.
compels - calc., ***coloc., nit-ac., rhus-t.,*** sulph.
eating, after, in open air - mez.
rapidly - bor., ***chin.***
room, while in a - nat-p.
wandering - acon., ***aesc.,*** alum., am-m., arn., ars., arund., bar-c., cahin., calc-s., cimic., colch., cop., dulc., fl-ac., iris, ***manc.,*** mur-ac., nat-s., phyt., plb., podo., ***puls.,*** sang.
5 p.m. - podo.
diarrhea, during - ars.
forenoon - fl-ac.
morning on getting out of bed - nat-a.
pressure, on - plb.
shift suddenly to distant parts - **DIOS.**
stool, before - phyt.
stooping, on - dulc.
warm, drinks amel. - acon., ***chel., mag-p., spong.***
food, after - kali-c., ol-an.
amel. - mag-c., ***ph-ac.***
milk amel. - ***chel., crot-t.,*** op.
room amel. - am-c., sul-ac.
soup amel. - acon., ***ph-ac.***
warmth, amel. - ***aeth.,*** alum., am-c., **ARS.,** ars-i., ***bar-c., carb-v.,*** canth., cast., caust., **CHAM.,** ***coloc.,*** cupr., ferr-ar., kali-ar., **MAG-P.,** mang., meph., **NUX-M., NUX-V.,** pall., plb., ***podo., puls.,*** **RHUS-T.,** ***sabin., sep.,*** **SIL.,** stront.
moist, amel. - ***nux-m.***
watermelon, after - fl-ac.
wet feet, from - all-c., cham., dol., dulc.
wine, after - lyc.
agg. - arum-i.
amel. - chel.
yawning, amel. - ign., lyc., nat-m.

PAIN, hypochondria - abrot., acon., aesc., aeth., ***agar., aloe,*** ambr., am-c., am-m., arg-m., ***arg-n.,*** arn., ***ars.,*** ars-i., asaf., asc-t., aur., bapt., bar-c., bar-i., bar-m., ***bell.,*** berb., bov., brom., ***bry.,*** bufo, calc., ***calc-s.,*** camph., ***canth.,*** carb-ac., carb-an., carb-s., ***carb-v.,*** caul., ***chel., chin.,*** cimic., ***cinnb.,*** cist., clem., coc-c., coff., coloc., ***con.,*** cop., crot-t., cupr., ***dig., dios.,*** dros., elaps, ferr., ferr-ar., ferr-i., ferr-p., gels., glon., ***graph.,*** grat., ***hep., hyos.,*** ign., indg., ***iod., ip., iris,*** jatr., jug-c., ***kali-ar.,*** kali-bi., ***kali-c.,*** kali-i., kalm., kreos., lact., laur., lil-t., **LYC.,** lyss., mag-c., mag-m., manc., meph., **MERC.,** merc-i-f., merc-i-r., mur-ac., nat-a., ***nat-c., nat-m.,*** nat-p., **NAT-S.,** nit-ac., nux-v., op., ox-ac., petr., phos., phyt., plan., plb., prun., ***ptel., puls.,*** **RAN-B.,** rhod., ***rhus-t., rumx.,*** sang., seneg., sep., sil., ***stann.,*** stram., ***sulph.,*** tarent., thuj., trom., verat., ***zinc.***
afternoon - bov., calc-s., **LYC.**
2 p.m. - ptel.
3 p m - dios., tarent.
alternating with oppression of chest - zinc.
band around, as if - ***sep.***
bed, in - cedr., cham., chin-s., coc-c., dios., ox-ac.

PAIN, hypochondria
belching amel. - mez., sep.
bending body forward - cocc.
forward, amel. - ***aloe,*** chin.
forward, to that side amel. , left - agar.
forward, to that side amel. - nat-m.
blowing - sulph.
breakfast, after - graph.
breathing - asaf., ***bry.,*** ign., **LYC.,** kali-c., ran-s., staph.
coughing, from - ambr., ***bell.,*** bor., ***bry.,*** caps., chin-s., cimx., ***cocc., dros.,*** grat., kali-bi., lach., ***lyc.,*** nit-ac., psor., sang., spong., sulph., sul-ac., til., zinc.
dancing, after - anac., aur., cham., **LYC.,** ptel., sulph., zinc.
drinking, after - aur.
eating, after - agar., anac., aur., cham., ***nux-v.,*** rhod., trom., zinc.
amel. - ***chel.***
evening - calc-s., ***carb-v.,*** caust., ***chin-s.,*** coloc., dios., lact., mag-c., mang., phyt., plan., ptel., **RAN-B.,** sep.
exercising, on - sep., zinc.
expiration - tarax.
extending to,
abdomen - euphr., petr.
back, across the - sil.
backward - ***aesc.,*** agar., ***berb.,*** calc., camph., carb-v., **CHEL.,** dios., euphr., graph., kali-c., lact., laur., **LYC.,** naja, nat-m., plb., puls., ***ran-b.,*** sil.
chest - aloe, chin-s.
downward - ars., bapt., ***chel.,*** hell., lil-t., nat-m., nux-v.
forward - laur.
genitals - carl.
hips - alum., cupr.
ilium, to - alum., lil-t.
lumbar region - carb-v., plb.
outward - lyc., sulph.
sacrum - thuj.
scapula - ***aesc.,*** **CHEL.,** bov., hydr., ***mag-m.***
shoulder - cupr., laur., ***nux-v.***
spine - sil.
stomach - cupr., nat-c.
thighs - nux-v.
umbilicus - carl., kali-chl.
upward - agar., ***apis,*** mur-ac., ***rhus-t.***
forenoon - alum., fago., ptel., ***sulph.***
inspiration - ***aesc., agar., anac.,*** bar-c., cimic., con., kali-bi., **LYC.,** ***rumx.***
jarring agg. - **BELL.,** ***calc.,*** **LYC.,** ***nat-s.,*** sil.
left - agar., aur., brom., ***calc.,*** caust., cimic., ***coc-c.,*** gels., glon., iod., mag-c., meph., merc-i-f., nat-m., pall., phos., rhod., rhus-t., ruta, sang., syph., tarent.
blow, as from - kali-n.
chill, during - ***chin-s.***
coughing, on - ambr., ***caust.,*** chin-s., grat., sang., sulph., til.
eating, amel. - mag-c., rhod.

PAIN, hypochondria
left, extending, to back - coc-c., nat-m.
extending, to right - alum.
lying, amel. - sang., ***sulph., tarent.***
lying, on left side agg. - coc-c., mag-c., nat-m.
lying, on right side - phos.
motion agg. - sulph.
pressure from - nat-c.
pulsating - sul-ac.
stooping agg. - phos.
lying on back - caust.
on left side, agg. - arn., coc-c., colch., mag-c., **MAG-M.,** ***nat-s., ptel.***
on left side, amel. - sang.
on back, amel. - mag-m.
on painful side, agg. - coc-c., mag-c., phyt., sil.
on painful side, amel. - bry., sep., tarent.
on right side agg. - ***lyc., mag-m., merc.,*** nat-m., sil.
menses, during - nit-ac.
after - bor.
before - sulph., tarent.
morning - agar., asar., bov., dios., lact., sars., staph., tarent., teucr.
motion from - aur., bar-c., cimic., dios., ***iris,*** plan., ptel., ran-b., sil.
rapid - ptel.
night - aur., calc., calc-s., cedr., coc-c., fago., kali-c., ***mag-c.***
3 a.m. - sulph.
bed, in - calc-s., cedr., cham., ***coc-c.,*** mag-c.
midnight - phyt.
midnight, while lying on side - phyt.
waking, on - ***coc-c.,*** ruta.
noon - plan.
paralytic - mag-c.
paroxysmal - alum., am-m., chel., ***kali-bi., mur-ac., ph-ac.,*** rhod., ***stann.,*** zinc.
pressure, from - brom., clem., mez., phos., ruta., zinc.
amel. - dros., mag-m.
clothing agg. - am-c., ***bry.,*** calc., carb-v., caust., ***chin.,*** coff., hep., nat-s., nux-v., spong., sulph.
riding, from - bor., ***sep.***
right - ***aesc.,*** agar., ***aloe, alum.,*** ambr., am-c., arn., ***ars.,*** bapt., **BELL.,** bov., brom., ***bry., bufo,*** cahin., calc-f., ***calc-p., carb-ac.,*** carb-an., carb-v., ***card-m.,*** cedr., **CHEL.,** chen-a., chim., ***chin-s.,*** cinnb., clem., ***colch., con., crot-c.,*** crot-h., echi., fago., hydr., ***iod., iris, kali-bi.,*** kali-c., kalm., ***lept.,*** **LYC.,** lyss., ***mag-m., merc., nat-c., nat-m.,*** **NAT-S., NUX-V.,** ***ol-j., phos.,*** phyt., plan., **PODO.,** ptel., rhus-t., ***sang.,*** sep., sil., stram., stry., ***sulph.,*** tarent., thuj., trom.
bending to left agg. - agar.
coughing, on - bor., caps., chin-s., cimx., cocc., kali-bi., lach., psor., sulph.
eating, amel. - ***chel.***
eating, to satiety, after - **LYC.**

PAIN, hypochondria
right, extending, to back - ***aesc.,*** **CHEL.,** euphr., ***iod.,*** jug-c., ***kali-c.,*** **LYC., MAG-M.,** ***nat-m.,*** yuc.
extending, to back, sitting for long, while - calc-p.
extending, to inguinal region and testes - ars.
extending, to left - brom., ***nux-m.***
extending, to left scapula - ***lept.***
lying, amel. - ***ambr.,*** crot-h., ptel., sep.
lying, can lie only on abdomen - ***lept., phyt.***
lying, on painful side agg. - **BELL.,** ***lyc., mag-m., nat-m.,*** phyt., sil.
lying, on painless side amel. - calc-f., ***ptel.***
motion agg. - sep.
sitting for long - **CALC-P.**
rising, on - cedr., hydr., ptel.
rubbing amel. - phos.
running, after - tab.
sitting, while - brom., calc-f., mur-ac., ph-ac., rhus-t.
bent forward - agar.
standing, on - ***aloe,*** chin., ran-b.
standing, amel. - prun.
stool, after - zinc.
amel. - grat.
before - anac., ars.
stooping, on - alum., clem., cocc., fago., lyc., rhod.
touch, on - carb-an., carb-v., dros., iod.
turning the body - lyc.
waking, on - ***cist.,*** coc-c.
walking, while - ***aesc.,*** ars., ***aur.,*** bapt., ***calc.,*** iris, ***kali-bi.,*** lyss., manc., nat-m., phyt., ***rumx.,*** sars., sulph., ***zinc.***
amel. - brom., calc-f., sars.
writing, while - chim.

PAIN, hypogastrium - acon., aesc., ***agar.,*** ail., ***all-c.,*** aloe, alumn., am-c., ammc., apis, arg-m., ***arn.,*** **ARS.,** ars-i., arund., aur., bapt., ***bell., bry., cact.,*** calc., ***calc-p.,*** canth., carb-an., carb-s., ***carb-v., card-m.,*** caust., ***chel.,*** chin., chin-a., cimic., clem., ***cocc.,*** coc-c., coll., ***coloc., con.,*** cop., ***croc.,*** crot-t., cupr-ar., ***dios.,*** dor., ***euph.,*** ferr., ferr-ar., ferr-i., ***gels., gins.,*** graph., ham., hell., iod., kali-ar., ***kali-c.,*** kali-p., ***kreos.,*** lec., lept., ***lil-t.,*** lith., ***lyc.,*** mag-m., ***med., merc.,*** murx., nat-a., ***nat-c.,*** nat-m., ***nat-p., nux-v.,*** onos., ***phos.,*** **PLAT.,** plb., prun., ptel., **PULS.,** ran-b., rhus-t., rhus-v., ruta., sabad., ***sec.,*** **SEP.,** ***sil.,*** sol-t-ae., squil., stann., stry., **SULPH.,** sumb., tarent., tell., ter., thuj., valer., **VERAT.,** ***zinc.***
afternoon - dios., mag-m., rhus-t.
2 p.m. - rhus-t.
breathing, on - asaf., **BELL.,** spong.
deep - nat-c.
cold drinks, after - crot-c.
coryza, during - calc.
coughing, on - caps., carb-an., dros., ***ip.,*** lyc., nux-v., ph-ac., phos., sil., squil., verat.
dinner, after - cham.
doubling up - ***prun.***

PAIN, hypogastrium
eating, after, amel. - mag-c., ran-b., ter.
evening - pall., pic-ac., sec., sumb.
amel. - **SEP.**
exertion, on - ***calc.***
extending to,
back - carb-v., ***croc.,*** sabin., vip.
groin - ***gins.,*** nat-m.
loins - carb-v.
lower limbs with painful tingling - ***gins.***
right to left - gins.
sacrum - sep.
sides - carb-v.
spine - iod.
stomach - ars., elaps
symphysis - mang.
thighs - con., nux-v., sep.
umbilicus - lach., lyc., phos., sep.
vagina - ars.
flatus, as from - caps.
forenoon - agar., com., ***phos.,*** **SEP.**
inspiration, on - bry., graph.
jar, as from - calc.
jarring agg. - am-c., **BELL.**
lying, while - ***sep., sulph.***
abdomen amel., on - chel.
back agg., on - ambr., bar-c.
side with limbs drawn up amel. - ***sep.***
menses, during - ***agar., am-c., ars., bell., bov.,*** bry., **CALC.,** ***calc-p., carb-an., carb-v.,*** caust., ***cimic., con.,*** crot-h., graph., ***kali-c.,*** lac-ac., lac-d., ***lach.,*** lil-t., lyc., ***mag-c.,*** mag-m., manc., merc., mur-ac., ***murx.,*** nat-c., ***nat-m.,*** nit-ac., ***nux-m., phos., plat.,*** **PULS.,** ***sars.,*** **SEC.,** senec., **SEP.,** sil., ***stront-c.,*** **SULPH.,** sul-ac., verat., ***xan.***
after - cham., iod., kreos., mag-c., merc., nat-m., ***plat.,*** puls.
menses, before - aloe, carb-v., cimic., com., crot-h., **LACH., LYC.,** manc., mang., ***merc.,*** **NAT-M.,** ***nit-ac., phos.,*** plat., raph., sars., **SEP., SULPH.,** tep., ***vib.,*** zinc.
extending to back - carb-v., vib.
extending to umbilicus - lach., lyc., phos., sep.
metrorrhagia, with - mag-c.
morning - alumn., ambr., ***bell.,*** dios., fago., mag-c., sep., sol-t-ae.
motion - **BELL.,** bry., **FERR.,** lil-t.
night - ***aesc.,*** bell., caust., carb-an., chel., lyc., mang., prun., ***sep.,*** sil., ***sulph.***
overlifting, from - carb-v.
paroxysmal - am-c., bry., camph., carb-v., cham., cocc., con., dig., ferr., hyos., ign., iod., ip., mur-ac., nux-v., **PULS.,** stann.
riding in a carriage - agar.
right - ***carb-an., gins.,*** graph.
sex, after - ***all-c.***
sitting, while - all-c., card-m., valer.
erect - glon.
standing, while - chin., puls.
stepping - am-c.

PAIN, hypogastrium
stool, during - ptel., rhus-v.
after - agar., ambr., coloc., iod., ***pic-ac.***
before - ***coll.,*** gels., haem., mag-m., nat-m., stram., tarent.
stooping, on - am-c., kali-c.
supper, after, amel. - **SEP.**
touch, on - sulph.
touch of clothing - lil-t.
ulcerative - nit-ac.
urinate, desire to, if be delayed - lac-c., ***lac-ac.,*** prun., phos., puls., ruta., sep., sul-ac.
urination amel. - dios., ***sep.***
preventing - phos.
walking - acon., calc., graph., nat-m., ***puls.***
walking amel. - sep.
in open air - agar., calc.
wandering - dig.
warmth, amel. - ***ars.,*** nux-m., ***nux-v.***
weight, as from a - nat-m.
yawning - nat-c.

PAIN, ileo-cecal region - **BRY.,** ***carb-s., card-m.,*** chel., **CHIN.,** ***cocc.,*** colch., con., cop., ***crot-h.,*** dulc., ***echi.,*** gnaph., ***hydr.,*** iris-t., ***lach.,*** lyc., **MERC-C.,** morg-g., ***nit-ac.,*** **PHOS.,** ***plb., ter., thuj.,*** tub., verat.

PAIN, inguinal - aesc., aeth., **AGAR., ALL-C.,** aloe, alum., am-c., am-m., ant-c., ***apis,*** ars., ars-i., aur., bapt., bar-c., bar-i., **BERB.,** bor., ***bov.,*** brach., brom., **BRY.,** calc., calc-p., cann-s., canth., carb-s., carb-v., cast., caul., caust., ***chel.,*** cimic., ***clem.,*** cob., ***cocc.,*** coc-c., ***coloc., con.,*** croc., crot-t., dios., dulc., ferr-i., fl-ac., ***gamb.,*** gins., graph., ham., hura, hydr., indg., iod., jatr., kali-bi., kali-c., kali-i., kali-n., kali-s., kreos., ***lac-c., lach.,*** lept., ***lyc.,*** lyss., lycps., ***mag-c.,*** mag-m., mag-s., manc., ***med., merc.,*** mez., murx., naja, ***nat-m.,*** nat-s., nit-ac., ***nux-v.,*** petr., phos., phys., phyt., pic-ac., ***plat.,*** psor., raph., rat., sec., sil., spig., spong., stann., ***sulph.,*** sul-ac., ***tarent., thuj.,*** verat-v., zinc., zing.
after-pains - ***cimic.***
ascending, on - pic-ac.
childbirth, during - cimic.
coughing - alumn., bor., brom., ***calc., nat-m.,*** petr., tarent.
dancing - alum.
dislocated, as if - agar., am-m., euph., tarax.
drawing, up knee amel. - ***coloc.,*** mez., pall.
up the leg, when - ther.
up the leg, when, pain in abdomen - kali-c.
evening - alum., bor., sil.
walking - hydr.
extending to,
axilla, left - nat-s.
back - am-m., sep., ***sulph.***
calf - sec.
crest of ilium - lac-c.
down leg - aloe, caust., dios., sec.
genitals - ***alum., lach., plat.***
hip - am-m., murx.
hypogastrium, across - ***ferr-i.***

PAIN, inguinal
extending to,
knee - aloe, ***kali-c.***
nipple, right - crot-t.
pelvis - ***chel.***
pelvis, around - coloc.
pubes - lil-t.
inguinal ring, coughing, on - arn., ***bry., cocc., nat-m.,*** nux-v., ***sil.,*** sulph., verat.
inguinal ring, coughing, on, into testes - ***nat-m.***
shoulder blade, right - bor.
spermatic cord, along - all-c., ***nat-m.***
testicles - arg-m., ***dios.,*** ham., ***hydr.,*** lept., ***nat-m.,*** sep.
thigh - aloe, arg-m., ars., aur., berb., bry., coloc., laur., lil-t., plat., rhod., sec., sep., thuj.
flatus, from - graph.
hernia, as from a - all-c., guai., kali-c., lycps., nit-ac., spong., tarent.
walking, agg. - lycps.
walking, amel. - nit-ac.
hernia, as from a would appear - alum., arn., ars., aur., bar-c., berb., ***calc.,*** calc-ar., camph., cann-s., ***carb-an.,*** caust., cham., chin., ***clem.,*** **COCC.,** ***coloc., con.,*** cupr., dig., gent-c., ***gran.,*** hell., ***ign.,*** kali-bi., ***lyc.,*** nit-ac., **NUX-V.,** petr., ph-ac., phos., ***phyt.,*** prun., rhus-t., sil., spong., stann., ***sulph.,*** sul-ac., ter., verat., zinc.
coughing, on - carb-an., cocc., nat-m., nux-v., petr., sil., squil., sulph., tarent., ***verat.***
morning, on waking - sul-ac.
sitting, while - aur., ***cocc.***
stool, after - sul-ac.
stooping amel. - graph.
walking - ph-ac., rheum.
inspiration - plat.
left - alum., am-m., arg-m., ars., berb., brach., brom., ***bry.,*** calc., ***chel.,*** cob., crot-t., ***lac-c.,*** med., nit-ac., phos., ***pic-ac.,*** sars., sep., stann., sulph.
desire to urinate be postponed, if - ***lac-ac.***
extending, into testicles - sep.
extending, to axilla - nat-s., ***thuj.***
extending, to glans - asar.
morning - ***bry.***
then right - dios., lach.
urination, during - ars.
lying, while - **MERC.**
on back with legs extended - nat-m.
menses, during - am-m., ant-t., apis, ***arg-n.,*** arn., ***bor.,*** bov., carb-an., cast., iod., ***kali-c.,*** kali-i., kali-n., kreos., lyc., mag-s., nat-m., phos., ***plat.,*** senec., sep.
after - ***bor., plat.***
as if would come on - cocc., lyc., plat.
before - ***ant-t.,*** bor., ***carb-an.,*** chin., ***sars.,*** sul-ac., tab.
motion, on - berb., ther.
noon - thuj.

PAIN, inguinal
paroxysmal - aloe, ***bell.,*** caul., chel., dig., ign., nat-m.
pressure agg. - ant-c., caust., mag-m., ph-ac.
pulsating - alum.
right - aesc., aloe, am-m., ars., bar-c., bov., ***carb-an.,*** carb-v., cast., cop., gent-c., hell., helon., iod., kali-c., kali-bi., lyss., **MERC.,** mez., nat-s., psor., sil., sul-ac., zinc.
flexing the thigh - ***lyc.***
then left - calc-p., hydr., lyc., phys.
rising from a seat - ***cocc.,*** lyc., nat-m., stront.
sex, after - ther.
sitting, while - alum., am-m., calc-ar., caust., mag-s., petr., spong., sul-ac., thuj., zinc.
sprain, as from - calc., euph., hydr., nat-m.
standing - berb., camph., euph., mag-s., mez., nat-s., thuj.
stepping, on - pall.
stool, during - nicc.
after amel. - ***lac-c.***
before - nat-s., phos., ***trom.***
stooping, on - ars., kali-n.
stretching, on - am-c., cocc., merc-c., nat-m.
leg after sitting - euph.
swollen, as if - con., kali-c.
touch, on - mang.
ulcerous - am-m., cic., con.
urinate, urging to - ***bell.,*** carb-an., nat-s., rhod.
urinating, while - agar., ars., caust., mez.
after - lyc.
walk bent, must - am-m.
walking, while - agar., alum., am-m., berb., brom., calc-ac., caust., chel., ***clem.,*** ferr-i., helon., kali-n., ***lyc.,*** lycps., mag-c., ***merc.,*** nat-m., pic-ac., sulph., thuj., ust.
amel. - nit-ac., psor.
yawning, when - ***bor.***

PAIN, sides - acon., agar., all-c., ***aloe,*** alum., ant-t., ars., asar., bell., ***bor.,*** brom., bry., calc., carb-an., carb-v., cast., ***cham.,*** chin., coloc., com., con., cupr., elaps, eupi., eup-pur., ferr., ferr-ar., fl-ac., grat., haem., hep., ign., iris, kali-n., kalm., lach., laur., lith., lyc., mag-c., manc., med., mur-ac., murx., naja, nat-c., nat-m., ***nat-s., nux-v.,*** par., phos., plb., prun., rhus-t., rhus-v., sars., seneg., sep., sulph., sul-ac., tarent., thuj., valer., zinc.
afternoon - nit-ac., ox-ac.
breathing, on - calc., raph.
coffee, after - ***cham.***
coughing, on - ***bor.,*** caust., con., eupi., lyc., squil.
amel. - carb-an.
dinner, during - am-c.
eating, after - alum., kali-n.
evening - chin-s., fl-ac., nicc.
exertion - alum.
extending, bladder - plb.
downwards - med.
inspiration, on - con., mur-ac., sel., thuj.
lain on, side not - ***graph.***

PAIN, sides
left - ***berb.,*** brom., ***carb-v., card-m.,*** cast., ***caust., eupi.,*** eup-pur., ferr., grat., mag-c., ***meny.,*** naja.
above crest of ilium - ***eupi.***
coughing, on - ***caust.***
extending to vagina - bor.
menses, during - ***nux-v.***
morning - am-c., merc., merc-c., sulph.
waking, on - sulph.
motion, on - asar., eupi., stront.
night - nat-s., prun.
midnight - ***sulph.***
noon - ptel.
pressure amel. - bov., **NAT-S.**
protrude, as if something would - petr.
raising arms - eupi.
riding, while - card-m., hep., rumx.
right - ***card-m., bor.,*** kali-n., lec., lith., **LYC.,** ***merc.,*** nat-m., sel., sep., sil., sulph., tarent.
flatulence, from - ***colch.,*** **NAT-S.**
to left - med.
sitting, while - calc., carb-an., carb-v., sulph.
standing - arg-n.
stool, during - nicc.
after - rhus-t.
with urging to - bar-c.
stooping - sep.
supper, after - sulph.
touch, on - sil.
ulcerative, petr.
ulcer, as if an ulcer would form - alum.
walking, while - calc., con., eupi., mag-c., nat-c., squil., sulph.
yawning, when - spig.

PAIN, umbilical, region - ***aesc.,*** agar., ***all-c., aloe, am-m.,*** ant-c., ant-t., apis, arg-n., arn., ars., bapt., bar-c., ***bell.,*** berb., bov., ***bry.,*** calc., ***calc-p., carb-an.,*** carb-v., ***cham., chel., chin.,*** chin-a., cina, clem., coc-c., ***colch.,*** **COLOC.,** crot-h., ***crot-t.,*** cupr., dig., **DIOS.,** dulc., erig., fl-ac., ***gamb.,*** gels., graph., gymn., hell., hydr., indg., ***iod., ip., iris,*** jatr., jug-c., kali-bi., kali-i., kreos., lac-ac., ***laur., lept.,*** lyc., mag-c., mang., merc., merc-c., merc-i-f., mez., mur-ac., nat-a., ***nat-c., nat-m.,*** **NAT-S.,** nit-ac., nux-m., ***nux-v.,*** onos., op., ox-ac., petr., phel., ***ph-ac.,*** phos., phys., ***phyt., plat.,*** **PLB.,** ***ptel., raph.,*** rat., rhod., ***rhus-t.,*** rhus-v., sabin., sang., sarr., senec., seneg., spig., stann., stront-c., ***sulph.,*** sumb., tab., tarent., teucr., ***thuj., verat.,*** verat-v., ***zinc.***
afternoon, - alum., euphr., nat-c., ox-ac., seneg., **SULPH.**
2 p.m. - lyc., verat-v.
3 to 4 p.m. - chel.
4 p.m. - ***sulph.***
5 p.m. - mag-c., ptel., sang.
bending backward - lyc.
bending backward, amel. - onos.
cold, drinks, from - calc-p.
wet weather, in - ***dulc.***
coughing, on - ambr., ip., nit-ac., sep.
after - nit-ac.

PAIN, umbilical, region
diarrhea, during - fl-ac., iris, lach.
before - coloc., plat.
dinner, after - all-c., bry., carb-s., **COLOC.,** ham.
eating - bov., bry., carb-v., cob., ***coloc.,*** con., graph., nux-v., ox-ac., plat., ***sulph.***
evening - calc-p., coloc., con., ***ox-ac.,*** pic-ac., plat., spig., **SULPH.**
5 to 6 p.m. - spig.
extending to,
abdomen - coloc.
downward - nat-m., plat., thuj.
genitals - sep.
rectum - nat-m.
thighs, into - bar-c.
uterus - ***calc.,*** elaps, **IP.,** ind.
forenoon - agar., lyc., nat-c., verat-v.
10 a.m. - verat-v.
ice cream, after - calc-p.
inspiration, deep - bapt.
hernia, as if a, would protrude - dulc.
menses, as if, would appear - sang.
menses, before - ***ip.,*** kreos.
morning - aeth., aloe, ant-t., bar-m., bov., bry., dios., lach., lyc., mag-c., mang., ***nat-s.,*** nux-v.
6 a.m. - bry.
waking, on - bov.
motion agg. - phyt., ptel.
night - acon., ***aesc.,*** arn., bar-c., bry., ***calc., cham., chin.,*** coc-c., ***coloc.,*** cycl., graph., hep., mag-m., merc., nux-m., ***ox-ac.,*** podo., ***puls., rhus-t.,*** sep., sil., ***sulph.,*** zing.
midnight - ***chin.,*** fl-ac.
midnight, stool, after - **ARS.**
midnight, stool, during - fl-ac.
noon - colch., dios., sulph.
paroxysmal - nat-m., ***plb.***
pressure, agg. - mag-c., mang.
amel. - plb.
rising, after - plat.
sitting, while - nat-s., ph-ac., sulph.
sour food - asaf.
stool, during - cocc., fl-ac., gamb., iod., ***kali-bi.,*** nat-c., nat-m., phos.
after - aesc.
before - aloe, **AM-M.,** caps., crot-t., dulc., fl-ac., gamb., grat., kali-n., nux-v., ox-ac., psor.
touch, on - kali-c., lyc., sep., sil.
transversely across - **CHEL.,** ip., lach., paeon., ***prun.***
tumor, as from a - spig.
ulcerative - mag-c.
violent - aloe, ***bell.,*** crot-t., ***dios.,*** ip., jatr., ***plb.***
walking, while - all-c., bry., ***coloc.***
warm soup amel. - mag-c.

PAIN, umbilicus - ***aesc.,*** agar., ***all-c., aloe, apis, ars.,*** ars-i., arund., asaf., bapt., bar-c., bar-i., bol., bry., cahin., calc., ***calc-p.,*** carb-s., caul., **CHEL.,** ***chin.,*** cimic., ***cina,*** coc-c., ***coloc.,*** con., crot-t., ***dios.,*** dulc., echi., ferr-i., fl-ac., gels., ign.,

PAIN, umbilicus - indg., iod., ***ip.,*** kali-bi., kali-n., kalm., kreos., laur., lec., ***lept.,*** lyc., mag-c., mang., merc-c., merl., mur-ac., nat-m., nit-ac., nux-m., ***ox-ac.,*** ph-ac., phos., phyt., ***plat.,*** plb., ***ptel.,*** rhus-v., senec., sep., sil., squil., stann., stram., sul-ac., sumb., ter., ust., verb.
afternoon - chel., plb., sil.
bending, double amel. - aloe, **COLOC.,** echi.
breakfast, after - gels., raph.
cough, during - ip., ***lyc.,*** sep.
diarrhea, during - calc-p., rhus-v.
before - rhus-t.
dinner, during - calc.
eating, 2 hours after eating - ox-ac.
eating, after - calc-p., cina, cob.
evening - nux-m., ptel.
extending, across abdomen - **CHEL.**
anus, to - aloe, **CROT-T.,** ip., led., nat-m., nux-v.
bladder, to - cic.
breast region, to - kreos.
chest, to - ***ang.,*** chin-s.
downward - aloe, crot-h., **CROT-T.,** ferr-i., nux-v., plat., plb., sep.
ilium, to - coc-c.
inguinal region, to - thuj.
lumbar region, to - plb.
pudendum, to - ***sep.***
pudendum, to, coughing when - sep.
rectum, to - nat-m.
spine, to - lyc., sil.
sternum, to - ***ang.***
stomach, pit of - carb-v., crot-t., lyc., ol-an., sulph.
throat, to - kali-bi., kreos.
uterus - elaps, ***ip.***
vagina - calc-p.
fasting - indg.
flatus, passing, amel. - calc-p., caul., coloc.
forenoon - gymn.
inspiration, deep, on - bapt., indg., lyc.
lying on back - ***ars.***
menses, during - nux-m.
before - chin-s., ip., ruta.
morning - agar., aloe, ***apis, dios.,*** nat-c., nat-m., verat-v.
motion - phyt., ptel.
paroxysmal - bell., calad., ph-ac., verb., zinc.
pregnancy, aching, during - plb.
pressure amel. - cina, dios., ***ptel.***
radiating from - ***dios., plb.,*** senec.
rising, after - coloc.
sitting, while - ***all-c.,*** indg.
stool, during - kali-bi., ox-ac.
after - puls-n
before - aloe, bry., ***ham.,*** mag-m., nat-c., plb., ust.
stooping, on - sep., ***verb.***
supper, after - zinc.
walking, while - bry.
walking, amel. - ***all-c.***

PANCREAS, (see Glands)

PENDULOUS - bell., croc., plat., podo., ***sep.,*** zinc.
mothers, of - iod., nat-c., ***sep.***

PERFORATION, umbilicus, sensation of - aloe.

PERITONITIS, inflammation, enteritis - ***acet-ac.,*** **ACON.,** aloe, alumn., **ANT-T., APIS,** ***arn.,*** **ARS.,** ars-i., atro., ***bapt.,*** **BELL., BRY.,** bufo, ***cact., calc., canth., carb-v.,*** card-m., ***cham.,*** cocc., coff., **COLCH.,** ***coloc., crot-c., crot-h.,*** cupr., ***echi., ferr.,*** ferr-ar., ferr-p., gamb., ***gels.,*** **HYOS.,** iod., ***ip., kali-c., kali-chl.,*** kali-i., ***kali-n.,*** kali-p., **LACH., LAUR., LYC.,** ***merc., merc-c., mez., nux-v., op., ox-ac.,*** **PHOS.,** plb., ***puls.,*** **PYROG., RHUS-T.,** sabin., ***sec., sil.,*** spong., squil., ***sulph.,*** **TER.,** thuj., ***uran.,*** urt-u., ***verat., verat-v.***
chronic - apis, ***lyc.,*** merc-d., sulph.
puerperal - acon., ***bell.,*** bry., ***merc-c.,*** pyrog., sulph., ter.
pseudo-peritonitis, hysterical - bell., coloc., verat.
spots, in - rhus-t.
tubercular - ***abrot.,*** ars., ars-i., calc., carb-v., ***chin.,*** iod., psor., sulph., ***tub.***

PERSPIRATION - **AMBR., ANAC., ARG-M.,** ***arg-n., caust.,*** **CIC., COCC.,** ***dros.,*** merc., **PHOS.,** plb., rhus-t., **SEL.,** staph., thuj.
cold - ***dros.***
dinner, during, amel. - phos.
embrace, after - agar.
exercise, during - ***ambr.***
forenoon - arg-m.
griping, during - coloc.
night - anac., cic., dros., staph., sulph.
only abdomen and chest - **ARG-M., COCC., PHOS., SEL.**
sex, after - agar.
walking, after - caust.

perspiration, hypochondria - caust., conv., ign., iris, verat.

perspiration, hypogastrium, sitting, while - ***sel.***

perspiration, inguinal - ambr., canth., iris, sel., sep., thuj.

perspiration, umbilicus, spreading from - rhus-t.

PLUG, umbilicus, sensation of, behind navel - ran-s.
sides - sep.
press in, intestines - anac.

PRESS, desire to - cupr-ac., cycl.

PRESSING, pain - acon., aloe, alum., ***ambr.,*** am-m., ***anac.,*** ant-c., ***ant-t.,*** apis, arg-m., ***arg-n.,*** arn., ars., asar., ***aur.,*** bar-c., ***bell., bism.,*** bry., bufo, **CALC.,** calc-p., calc-s., camph., ***caps.,*** carb-an., carb-s., carb-v., ***carl.,*** cast., ***caust., chel.,*** chin., cimic., coff., colch., ***coloc., con.,*** croc., crot-t., ***cupr.,*** dig., elaps, ***euph.,*** euphr., ferr., ferr-p., ***grat.,*** hep., hyper., ign., iod., kali-c., kali-i., kali-n., ***kali-s.,*** lac-c., ***lach.,*** **LYC.,** lyss., ***mag-c.,*** mang., meny., meph., ***merc., mez.,*** mur-ac., ***nat-m., nat-n.,*** nit-ac., nux-m., **NUX-V.,** ***op.,*** paeon., ***par., petr.,*** phos., ***plat.,*** plb., prun., ***puls.,*** rhus-t., ruta, sabin., samb., sars., sec., **SEP.,** ***sil., spig.,*** stann., staph., stram., **SULPH.,** tab., tarax., tarent., ***ter.,*** thuj., verat., ***zinc.***

PRESSING, pain
afternoon - caust., chel., spig.
5 p.m. - sulph.
air, in open - mang.
belching amel. - mez.
bending forward - coloc., sep.
breakfast, after - calc-s., kali-c.
breathing - lyc.
deep - caust.
cold, as from, petrol., sars.
dinner, before - lyc.
dinner, after - cast-v., grat., iod., sulph.
drinking, after - ars., ferr.
eating - mang.
eating, after - agar., alum., ars., caps., caust., coloc., ***ferr.,*** kali-c., lyc., ***mag-c.,*** mez., ***nux-v.,*** phos., sep., sil., thuj., zinc.
amel. - mang.
anything cold - mang., sep.
erections, with - zinc.
evening - bar-c., bell., caust., chin., coloc., ferr., kali-c., mez., phos., zinc.
in bed - nat-m.
eating, after - chin., phos.
stool, during - ***zinc.***
walking - verat.
exertion, on - ***calc., pall.***
extending, to,
anus, towards - crot-t., ***sulph.***
chest - nat-m.
genitals - graph., tep.
pit of stomach, to - nux-m.
rectum - mag-m., nat-m.
sacrum - phos.
stomach - hep.
throat - caust. kali-c.
umbilicus - crot-c.
upward - ars., con.
forenoon - cupr., lyc., phos.
lying, while - bar-c., bell.
amel. - bar-c., petr., rhus-t.
on back amel. - mez.
on left side amel. - ***pall.***
menses, during - am-m., calc., graph., nit-ac., plat., **PULS., SEP.,** sulph.
after - nat-m.
before - graph., nux-m., sep.
morning - mag-c., nat-m., sil.
9 a.m. - **SEP.**
motion, on - bar-c., kali-c., zinc.
night - ign., mez., phos., sep., sulph.
outward - nit-ac., zinc.
peaches, after - psor.
protrude, as if something would - nit-ac.
retracting abdomen - lyc.
sitting, on - chin., coloc., hell., iod., op., rhus-t., stront.
amel. - bar-c.
standing - graph.
amel. - chin.
stone, as from - bell., ***cupr., merc.,*** op., thuj.
stool, during - arn., brom., hep., nat-m., ***zinc.***
after - dulc., grat., ***iod.,*** kali-c., ol-an., ***pic-ac.,*** zinc.

PRESSING, pain
after normal stool - ***iod.***
amel. - dig., meny., sep., ***spig.***
before - dig., dulc., grat., zinc.
touch agg., - cupr., lyc.
urination, during - chin., nat-m.
after - chin., ph-ac.
at the close of, pressing toward genitals - ph-ac.
walking, while - bar-c., chin., cupr., mez., ph-ac., zinc.
after - grat.
amel. - chin.
warm drinks agg. - elaps

pressing, hypochondria - ***acon.,*** aeth., ***agar., aloe,*** alum., ***ambr.,*** am-c., anac., ant-t., arg-n., arn., ars., aur., ***aur-m.,*** bar-c., ***berb., bor.,*** bov., brom., ***bry.,*** cahin., calc., calc-p., camph., caps., carb-v., carl., ***cham., chel., chin.,*** cocc., ***con., crot-t.,*** dig., dios., elaps, ferr., graph., hep., ign., iod., kali-chl., lil-t., ***lyc.,*** lyss., ***mang.,*** meny., merc., ***mur-ac.,*** nat-c., nat-m., nit-ac., petr., ph-ac., plb., ***podo.,*** rhod., rhus-t., ***sep., sil.,*** spong., staph., stann., sulph., verat., ***zinc.***
afternoon - bor.
bending body, forward, agg. - ***cocc.***
forward, amel. - ***chin.***
to left - agar.
to side - lyc.
breakfast, after - carb-v.
breathing, on - **LYC.,** ***lyss.***
coughing, on - ***cocc.***
dinner, after - sulph.
drinking, after - aur.
eating, after - anac., aur., cham., ***mag-m., nux-v.,*** **ZINC.**
amel. - nat-m.
evening - all-c., lact., mang., sep.
expiration, on - tarax.
extending, abdomen, to - graph., petr.
left side of abdomen, to - con.
lying, when, on right side - calc-f.
outward - cast., lyc.
scapula, to - bor., bov.
spleen, to - merl.
umbilicus - ph-ac.
upwards - agar.
exertion, amel. - nat-m.
flatus, as from - kali-c., zinc.
amel. - nat-m.
forenoon - alum.
inspiration, on - bar-c., cocc.
left - aeth., agar., arg-n., ***aur., berb.,*** bor., bov., carb-an., carb-v., con., crot-t., dig., iod., kali-c., nat-c., nat-m., nit-ac., phyt., ***plat.,*** sep., stann., sulph., tarax., thuj., ***zinc.***
left, breathing deeply - bor.
lying amel. - sep.
menses, during - graph., nit-ac.
after - bor.
morning - agar., sars.
motion, from - aur., bar-c., mang.

pressing, hypochondria
night - calc.
3 a.m. - sulph.
riding, while - bor.
right - acon., agar., all-c., aloe, anac., arn., bar-c., bell., brom., ***calc., calc-p.,*** carb-v., ***card-m., chel., chin., cocc., con.,*** elaps, ferr., hep., iod., ***laur.,*** lil-t., **LYC.,** ***lyss.,*** **MAG-M.,** merc., ***nat-m.,*** nit-ac., ph-ac., plb., rhus-t., sars., sep., ***sil.,*** staph., sul-ac., sulph., ***tarent.,*** thuj., zinc.
lying on painful side - ***mag-m.***
sitting, while - calc., ph-ac., phyt., rhus-t.
standing, on - ***chin.,*** ph-ac.
amel. - prun.
step, on every - ***calc.***
stool, after, amel. - zinc.
stooping - thuj.
talking, amel. - nat-m.
touch, agg. - bar-c., mang.
walking, while - ***aur., calc., mag-m.,*** nat-m., ***zinc.***
after - ph-ac.
amel. . - sars.
open air, in - ars.
open air, in, amel. . - ars.

pressing, hypogastrium - agar., agn., alum., ambr., am-c., am-m., ant-t., ***apis,*** aran., arg-m., ars-i., asaf., ***aur.,*** bar-c., bar-i., **BELL.,** bism., bry., ***calc.,*** calc-p., canth., carb-s., carb-v., caust., cham., chel., chin., cina, cocc., ***colch.,*** coloc., con., croc., cupr., dig., elaps, gins., ***helon.,*** ign., iod., kali-c., kali-i., kali-s., kreos., **LIL-T., LYC.,** ***mag-m.,*** med., merc., merc-i-f., ***mez., nat-c., nat-m.,*** nat-p., nit-ac., **NUX-V.,** pall., ***ph-ac., phos.,*** **PLAT., PULS.,** ruta., ***sec.,*** seneg., **SEP.,** spig., squil., ***stann., sulph., tab.,*** tarax., tarent., ***thuj.,*** til., valer., verb., ***zinc.***
asunder - spig.
chill, during - chin.
colic, during - ***thuj.***
crampy - sulph.
dinner, during - am-c.
downward - aloe., ***con.,*** cupr., lil-t., merc., ***pall., psor.,*** **PULS.,** ***sars.,*** **SEP.,** sulph.
eating - arg-m.
after - alum., arn., phos., sep., sulph.
amel. - mag-c.
evening - euphr., kali-c., phos., sec., spig.
exertion, on - ***calc.***
flatus amel. - kali-c.
forenoon - ***phos.***
genitals, toward - **BELL.,** caust., coloc., dig., **LIL-T.,** ***nat-c.,*** nit-ac., **NUX-V.,** ***plat.,*** **PULS., SEP.,** sulph.
groin, toward - ***plat., sars.,*** teucr.
hemorrhage, during - sec.
inward - cycl.
lie, must lie down - lyc.
left - lyc., nat-m., sulph.
lying, while - ***sulph.***
back, on the - bar-c.

pressing, hypogastrium
menses, during - calc., calc-p., carb-an., con., ***kali-c.,*** kali-i., ***mag-c.,*** mag-m., ***murx., nat-c., nat-m., plat.,*** **PULS., SEC., SEP.**
before - ***plat., sep.***
menses, would come on, as if - ambr., am-m., ***apis, aur.,*** bry., cina, cocc., ***croc.,*** kali-c., kreos., ***lil-t., lyc., nat-c.,*** nat-m., phos., **PLAT., PULS., SEP.,** stann., til.
morning - bar-c., ***bell.,*** **NAT-M.,** ***plat.,*** sep.
9 a.m. to 6 p.m. - **SEP.**
bed, in - mag-c., phos.
lying on the back - bar-c.
waking, on - phos.
motion agg. - sep.
amel. - am-c.
night - phos., ruta., sep., ***sulph.***
9 p.m. - **SEP.**
noon - merc-i-f.
outwards - ang., **BELL.,** ***carb-an., kali-c.,*** **LIL-T.,** lyc., ***nat-c., nat-m., plat.,*** **PULS., SEP.**
paroxysmal - iod., kali-c., ***tab.***
pressure agg. - stann.
rignt - lyc., sep., sulph., zinc.
sit bent, has to - kali-c.
sitting, while - am-c., ang., iod.
bent - ***bell.***
standing - arn., sulph.
stool, during - arg-m., calc., **LIL-T.,** ***nat-m.,*** nux-m., ***podo.***
after - arg-m., ambr., iod., zinc.
amel. - zinc.
before - nat-m., spig., thuj.
stooping - kali-c., lyc., sep.
stretching amel. - iod.
supper, after amel. - ***sep.***
touched, when - cycl., nat-c., nit-ac., thuj.
agg. - cupr.
turning to side in bed - sulph.
urination, during - ***lil-t., nux-v.***
after - ph-ac.
walking, while - kali-i., ***lil-t.,*** merc., nat-c.
against wind - sulph.
amel. - am-c.
bend, compelled to - ***lyc.,*** sulph.
open air, in - kali-c., meny., ***nux-v.***

pressing, inguinal - agar., ***alum.,*** am-c., arg-n., ars., ***aur.,*** bell., berb., bor., ***dulc.,*** cann-s., euph., graph., hell., iod., kali-c., kali-bi., ***kali-i.,*** lyc., merc., mez., nat-s., petr., ***plat.,*** ruta., sulph., sul-ac., ***thuj.,*** zinc.
afternoon - all-c.
coffee, after - all-c.
bending agg. - mez.
downward - ***plat.***
drawing - sulph.
up leg amel. - mez.
evening - alum.
expiration agg. - mez.
extending to genitals - ***alum., plat.***
to thighs - sep.
flatus amel. - kali-c.
glands - dulc., meny., stann.

pressing, inguinal
laughing - sep.
left - ***all-c.,*** berb., calc., sulph., zinc.
menses, during - ***bor., carb-an.,*** cast., kali-c., ***plat.,*** sep.
after - plat.
morning - sul-ac.
motion, on - bar-c., sep.
outward - ***alum.,*** anac., aur., bar-c., **BELL.,** camph., caust., ***cocc.,*** con., euph., gran., graph., ign., kali-c., lyc., nux-m., ph-ac., rhus-t., sep., sul-ac., ter., teucr., thuj.
pressure agg. - ph-ac.
right - aur., carb-v., clem., hell., iod., lyc., mez., nat-s., sep.
sitting, while - aur., caust., chin., petr., spong.
bent - ***bell.***
standing, while - camph., nat-s.
amel. - aur.
stool, during - bar-c.
before - ***trom.***
stooping - meny., sep.
amel. .- graph.
stretching out, on - am-c., aur., graph., mez.
touch agg. - arg-n.
urinating, when - mez.
after - euph., lyc.
walking - dig., ph-ac., sep.
wavelike - sep.

pressing, sides - alum., am-c., am-m., anac., ars., ***asaf.,*** asar., ***aur.,*** berb., carb-v., chin., dios., ign., kali-c., kalm., lyc., mag-m., merc., mur-ac., nat-c., ***nat-m.,*** **NAT-S.,** ***nit-ac., nux-v.,*** ph-ac., ***phos., sep.,*** staph., tarax., ***thuj.,*** zinc.
coughing, on - spong.
drawing - laur., nat-m., sulph.
drawing in the abdominal muscles, on - ***asaf.***
eating, after - sep.
evening - fl-ac.
extending to navel - aloe.
flank, in - ambr., coff., colch., sabad., sars.
inspiration, deep - thuj.
agg. - con., sars.
kneading amel. - **NAT-S.**
left - am-c., anac., berb., camph., carb-an., carb-v., kali-c., kali-n., led., lyc., mag-m., ***nat-c.,*** nat-m., ***nit-ac.,*** sars., sul-ac., sulph., tarax.
lying on right side - prun.
menses, during - ***nux-v.***
midnight, after - thuj.
morning - bar-c., merc.
bed, in - bell.
motion, on - asar.
outward - calc., coloc., lyc., ***nux-v.,*** sul-ac.
periodic - ph-ac.
pressing on stomach - bell.
riding, while - ***card-m.,*** hep.
right - ang., ars., bar-c., cahin., calc., ***card-m.,*** con., lyc., ***merc.,*** **NAT-S.,** prun., sep., stann., thuj., zinc.
side lain on - bell.

pressing, sides
sitting, while - am-c., calc.
stooping - kali-c.
touch, on - nat-c.
walking, while - cast., kali-n. led., nat-c., zinc.

pressing, umbilical, region - acon., alum., ambr., am-c., **ANAC.,** arn., bell., bry., camph., carb-v., chel., ***chin.,*** chin-s., cina, cocc., colch., ***coloc.,*** crot-h., crot-t., cupr., dig., ***dios.,*** dulc., grat., hell., hyos., ign., ***lach.,*** lact., lyc., mang., meny., ***nat-m.,*** nit-ac., olnd., petr., ***ph-ac., ran-s.,*** raph., rheum, samb., seneg., sep., ***spig.,*** stann., staph., sul-ac., ***sulph.,*** tab., teucr., ***verb.,*** zinc.
above umbilicus - kali-c.
afternoon - alum.
4 p.m. - ***sulph.***
standing, while - alum.
belching amel. - ambr.
below umbilical, morning - calc.
button, as from - am-c., ***anac.***
coughing, on - ambr.
eating, after - anac., chin., ***coloc.***
evening, bed, in - chin., valer.
extending to, anus - ox-ac.
chest, left - chel.
epigastrium - crot-t.
evening - nat-m.
bed, in - chin., valer.
flatus, as from - coloc., zinc.
hernia, as if, would form, here and there - carb-an., ign., nat-c., ***thuj.***
left side - dig.
protrude - dulc.
inspiration agg. - anac., coloc.
morning - mang.
night - carb-v., sep., sulph.
paroxysmal - nat-m., sep.
periodical - ***chel.,*** ph-ac.
pressure agg. - anac., zinc.
plug, like a - ***anac., verb.***
retraction of abdomen agg. - zinc.
standing - alum.
stool, during - anac.
after - anac.
stooping, on - ***verb.***
walking - anac., zinc.
fast - chin.
in open air, while - bry.

PRICKLING - verat., zinc.

PROTRUSION - plb.

protrusion, umbilicus - calc., con., dulc., lyc., nat-m., sulph., sul-ac.
hernia, as if, would form, here and there - carb-an., ign., nat-c., ***thuj.***
left side - dig.
protrude - dulc.

PROUD, umbilicus, flesh - **CALC.**

PULSATION - **ACON.,** aesc., aeth., aloe, ***alum.,*** **ANT-T.,** ars., ars-i., cact., cadm-s., cahin., calad., **CALC.,** calc-s., cann-s., caps., card-m., caust., colch., coloc., fl-ac., gels., ***ign., iod.,*** kali-ar., ***kali-c.,*** kali-s., kreos., ***lac-c.,*** lach., ***lyc.,*** med., merc., naja, nat-s., ***nux-v.,*** op., ***ph-ac.,*** plb., ptel., ***sang.,*** **SEL.,** sep., stront-c., sul-ac., sumb., tarent.
alternating with increased beating of heart - sabin.
aneurism, from - bar-m.
breakfast, after - manc.
deep - aesc., coloc.
extending to small of back - ars.
eating, after - cahin., **SEL.**
evening - ferr-i., ptel.
tea, after - brach.
extending to, back, to small of - fago.
to, head - rheum.
to, limbs - quas.
fever, during - **KALI-C.**
heat, after internal - calad.
heavy, seeming to lift abdomen upward while sitting still after dinner, in evening - naja
here and there - cann-i., cann-s.
lying, while - aloe, ***coloc.,*** plb.
agg. - carl.
menses, during - aesc., kreos.
morning, 5 a.m. - kreos.
menses, during - kreos.
night - aloe.
lying, while - aloe
palpitation, like, during rest, night agg. on lying down - aloe.
pregnancy, during - sel.
shattering, after yawning - calc.
sleep, amel. - ptel.
preventing - sel.
spots, in - bar-c., sep.
stool, after - agar., ***ph-ac.***
supper, after - cahin.
touch, on - fl-ac.

pulsation, epigastrium, in - ***asaf.,*** eucal., ***hydr.,*** nat-m., ***puls.,*** sel., ***sep.***

pulsation, hypochondria - acon., act-sp., anan., asc-t., bell., brach., brom., calc., calc-p., chel., cimic., cinnb., graph., kali-i., laur., lyss., nux-v., puls., ran-b., sars., sep., sil., sulph.
belching amel. - calc-p.
evening - apoc., brom.
left - agar., asc-t., calc., cann-s., cinnb., gels., ruta., sars.
morning - stry.
night - graph.
right - act-sp., bell., brach., brom., ***calc-p., chel.,*** kali-i., laur., med., nat-s., nux-v., ptel., sarr., sep., sil., sulph.
walking, while - nat-s.

pulsation, hypogastrium - ang., cina.
female, in - aesc., calc-p.

pulsation, inguinal - alum., brach., lyc., nat-c., stann., stront-c., sul-ac.
deep in - stann.
evening - lyc.
morning - brach.

pulsation, sides - chin., graph., hura, kali-c., nat-s.
flank, in the on inspiration - seneg.
night on waking - graph.
right - lyc.
walking, while - cinnb., nat-s.

pulsation, umbilicus - acon., aloe, ars., dulc., ptel., zinc.

PUSHING, in - thuj.

RASH, menses, before - ***apis,*** ars.
itching, red rash over the region of liver - ***sel.***
violently - ***calc.***

RELAXED, feeling - agar., ail., alum., ***am-m., carb-v., cast-v., ign.,*** lob., lyc., mag-m., mang., ***merc., op.,*** phos., ***psor.,*** ptel., rhus-t., rumx., ***sep., staph.,*** sumb.
internally, while walking - rhus-t.
loose, everything were, after eating and drinking - nat-m.
lying on back amel. - cast-v.
stool, after - mag-m., ***phos., sep.,*** sul-ac., sulph.
walking, while - alum., merc., ***nat-m.,*** rhus-t.

RESTLESSNESS - agar., alum., am-c., ***ant-t.,*** apis, apoc., ***arg-n.,*** **ARS.,** ***ars-i., asaf.,*** asc-t., aur., ***bell.,*** bry., **CALC.,** carb-an., cinnb., cist., colch., com., corn., crot-t., cycl., dirc., ***dulc.,*** euph., fago., ferr-ar., ferr-ma., gran., grat., gymn., hell., iod., **IP.,** jatr., kali-ar., ***kali-c.,*** merc-i-r., mez., ***mur-ac.,*** nat-a., nat-c., ***nat-m., nat-s., nit-ac.,*** par., **PHOS.,** plan., plat., ***podo., puls.,*** **SEP.,** vesp., ***zinc.***
afternoon - grat.
anxious - alum.
breakfast, during - plan.
after - grat., plan.
after, flatus passing amel. - sep.
cold, as from a - plat.
night, at - plat.
drinking, after - caust., sul-ac.
eating, after - aur., caust., kali-c., sul-ac.
agg. - grat.
evening - am-br., gnaph.
5 p.m. - phys.
6 p.m. before stool - euph-a.
extending to head - mang.
forenoon - cimic.
griping - plat.
morning - calc., nit-ac., sep.
rising, amel. - chr-ac.
rising, before - chr-ac.
waking, on - calc.
night - caust., kali-i., nit-ac., plat.
rest, during - ars.
retiring, after - bol.
sleep, after - sulph.
smoking, as after - mang.
stool, during - ind., kali-c.
after - ars., graph.
before - ind.
before, diarrhea - plan., plat.

RESTLESSNESS,
stool, as if before, 7 a.m., before eating - plan.
as before, diarrhea, 10 a.m. - plan.
as in diarrhea, all morning - phys.
waking, on - vichy-g.
restlessness, hypochondria - aloe, chin., equis., manc.
stool, before - aloe.

RETRACTION - agar., ***alum.,*** am-c., ***apis,*** ars., ***bar-c.,*** bell., bry., ***calc-p.,*** camph., canth., ***carb-ac., cocc.,*** colch., crot-t., ***cupr.,*** cupr-ac., cupr-s., dig., ***dros.,*** elat., euph., gamb., **HYDR.,** ***iod.,*** iodof., jatr., kali-bi., kali-br., laur., led., lob., lyc., merc., merc-c., mez., mur-ac., ***nat-m.,*** nat-n., op., paeon., phos., plat., **PLB.,** podo., ptel., puls., sil., staph., stram., sul-ac., ***tab.,*** thuj., ***verat., zinc.***
cholera, in - kali-br.
constipation, with - carb-ac.
evening - sulph.
6 p.m., supper amel. - dios.
faint, as if, before stool - graph.
forenoon, flatus passing amel. - sulph.
inclination to - valer.
lying on back - acet-ac.
motion, following loose, after breakfast - sulph.
spasmodically - kiss., plat., stram.
spots - plat.
at certain, distended at others - plb.
stool, during - agar.
string, as by a - chel., ***plb.,*** podo., tab.
vomiting - dros.
retraction, sensation of - abrot., carb-ac., phos., sabad., sulph.
retraction, umbilicus - acon., ***alum.,*** bar-c., calc-p., carb-s., ***chel.,*** grat., kali-c., mosch., nat-c., **PLB.,** podo., ran-b., tab., ter., zinc-s.
colic, with - nat-c.
lying, while - ter.
morning - acon.
sitting - kali-c.
stool, before - crot-t.
stooping, on - tab.

RHEUMATIC pain - caust., plb., polyp-p

RIGIDITY, side left - nat-m.

RINGWORM - nat-m., sep., tell., thuj.

RISING, sensation, in
eating, after - merc.
flatulence to throat, like, belching amel. - phos.
hot, air into chest - carb-o.
evening, towards, amel. - ol-an.
sensation of, of a substance rising to throat and pressing on it - bell.

ROLLING, something, in - lyc.

ROUGHNESS - dig.

RUMBLING, (see Intestines, Rumbling)

RUBS, abdomen - aran., cycl., kali-c., mag-c., nat-c., **PHOS.,** plb.

SENSITIVE, skin, of - bar-c., bell., bov., canth., coff., crot-c., **LYC.,** sars.

SHAKING, of - **CROT-T.,** mang., merc., sil., staph.
cough, from - ***carb-an.,*** kali-c., lact., ***sil.,*** squil.
morning - mez.
walking, while - mang., merc., mez., nux-v., rhus-t.

SHARP, pain - ***acon.,*** aeth., ***agar.,*** aloe, ***alum.,*** am-c., anac., ang., ant-t., apis, arg-m., ***arg-n., arn., ars.,*** asaf., bapt., ***bell.,*** berb., ***bov.,*** **BRY.,** ***calc., calc-s.,*** canth., caps., carb-an., ***carb-s.,*** carb-v., ***card-m., caust.,*** cedr., ***cham.,*** chel., chin., chin-a., cic., ***cimic.,*** cocc., ***colch., coloc.,*** con., ***croc.,*** cupr., ***cycl., dig.,*** ferr-i., fl-ac., graph., ***grat.,*** hell., hep., **IP.,** kali-ar., kali-bi., ***kali-c.,*** kali-n., ***kali-p., kali-s.,*** kreos., lach., lac-c., laur., led., lyc., lyss., mag-m., ***mag-s.,*** med., merc., mez., naja, nat-a., nat-c., nat-m., nat-n., nat-p., nit-ac., ***nux-v.,*** op., pall., ***ph-ac., phos.,*** phys., pic-ac., ***plb.,*** psor., ***puls.,*** rhod., ruta, samb., sel., sep., ***sil., spig.,*** stann., stram., **SULPH.,** sumb., ***tarax.,*** tarent., ***ter.,*** thuj., trom., ***verb.,*** verat., viol-t., zinc.
afternoon - sep.
bed, in - nat-m.
bending, forward - verb.
burning - lyc., spig., zinc.
coughing, on - acon., am-m., ars., ***bell.,*** bry., chin., lach., lyc., nit-ac., phos., sabad., samb., sep., staph., sulph., sul-ac.
dinner, after - sars.
eating, after - alum., thuj.
electric, shocks, like - arg-n.
evening - ***caust.,*** kali-n., ***plb.,*** tarent.
6 p.m.,. - mag-s.
expiration, on - coff.
extending, across - cupr.
body, into, on every step - mur-ac.
anus, to - rhus-t., sulph.
back, to - calc., canth., cocc., coc-c., kali-bi.
bladder, to - brom., cic.
chest, to - ***cham.,*** clem., ***con.,*** ign.
clavicle, to right - laur.
downward - alumn., brom., chen-a., chin., **IP.,** kali-c., puls., ran-s., samb., sil., verb.
hypochondria region, to - coc-c.
left to right - ***ip., ter.***
lower limbs, to - sang., ter.
lumbar region, to - kali-n.
pelvis, to - alumn., puls.
penis, into - alumn.
perineum, to - phos.
rectum, to - brom.
right to left - nux-m.
right to left, toward - fl-ac.
shoulders, to - lach.
spermatic cord, to when coughing - brom., verat.
testicle, to when coughing - sec.
vagina, to - ***ars., kreos.***

SHARP, pain
extending, to
transversely - ***arn.,*** calc., cham., colch., ip., phos., sep.
upwards - aloe, ***bry.,*** naja, ph-ac., ruta, spong.
flatus, from - coloc., nat-m.
amel. - zinc.
before - spig., sulph.
flexing thighs, amel. - podo.
forenoon - mag-s.
fright, at every - cham.
inspiration, on - agar., ***bry.,*** calc., chin., clem., tab.
inward - phos.
lying, while - caust.
crooked amel. - brom.
on abdomen amel. - phos.
menses, during - ars., bor., brom., calc., kali-c., mosch., **NUX-V.,** sul-ac.
before - brom., con., ***kali-c.,*** puls.
midnight - sulph.
before - cham.
waking, on - coloc., sulph.
milk, warm, after - ***ang.***
morning - agar., dig., kali-n., plat., ***ran-b.,*** sulph.
bed, in - chin.
walking, while - ran-b.
motion, on - caps., cycl., kali-c.
night - kali-c., ***sulph.***
on waking - coloc.
noon - lyc., phos., rhus-t.
paroxysmal - ***ip.***
periodic - caust.
potatoes, after - mag-s.
pressure, on - aur., nit-ac.
amel. - ***card-m.***
sitting while - bry., caust., chin., cina, nat-s., **NUX-V.,** phos., ruta, ***thuj.***
sneezing, while - carb-v.
step every - ***mur-ac.***
stinging - ***apis, ign., lach., sep., thuj.***
stool, after - zinc.
before - aloe, calc-s., kali-n., mang.
driving to - ***nux-v.***
urging to, with - spig.
stooping - am-c., bov., calc., caps., cocc.
straightening up while sitting - ph-ac.
touch, on - nit-ac.
urination, during - clem., nit-ac.
waking, on - agar., nat-m., podo.
walking, while - arg-n., caps., cham., mur-ac., olnd., ran-b., sel., thuj., zinc.
eating, after - zinc.
hindering walking - am-c.

sharp, hypochondria - ***acon., aeth.,*** aesc., ***agar.,*** aloe, ***alum.,*** ammc., am-c., am-m., anac., arg-m., arg-n., arn., ars., ars-i., asaf., aur., aur-m., bar-c., bar-i., bar-m., ***berb.,*** brom., ***bry.,*** calc., calc-p., cann-s., caps., ***carb-s., carb-v.,*** caust., cedr., cham., ***chel.,*** chin., ***chin-s.,*** cist., clem., colch., coloc., ***con.,*** cop., cupr., dig., dulc., euphr., fago., ferr., form., ***glon.,*** goss., ***graph.,*** guai., hep., hyper., hyos., iod., ip., kali-ar., ***kali-bi., kali-c.,*** kali-i., kali-n., kreos., ***lach.,*** lact., laur., lob-c., ***lyc.,*** mag-c., mag-m., mag-s., mang., merc., merc-c., mosch., mur-ac., naja, nat-a., ***nat-c., nat-m.,*** nat-s., nicc., ***nit-ac.,*** nux-v., ol-an., ox-ac., par., petr., ph-ac., phos., plan., plb., podo., psor., ptel., puls., ***ran-b., ran-s.,*** raph., rat., rhod., rhus-t., rumx., sabad., senec., ***sep.,*** **SIL.,** sulph., sul-ac., sumb., tab., tarent., tep., thuj., zinc.
afternoon - aeth., alum., am-m., aur., caust., laur., kali-c., mag-c., mag-m., nat-m., plb., sil., valer.
2 p.m. - mag-c., valer.
3 p.m. - lyc.
air, open - ol-an., staph., sulph.
alternating sides - thuj.
belching, during - caps., zinc.
amel. - sep.
bending, forward - agar., ***lyc.***
to left - agar.
to right - sars., sul-ac.
breathing deeply amel. - spig.
cold drink, after - ***nat-c.***
coughing, during - acon., am-m., ars., aur., ***bell., bry.,*** cann-s., caps., chin., nat-s., puls., rhus-t., rumx., sep.
dinner, after - coloc., grat., kali-bi., lact., kali-c., mag-c., nat-m., sars., thuj., zinc.
eating, while - ***podo.***
after - brom., lact.
evening - am-c., kali-bi., lyc., mag-m., mag-s., rat., rhod., sep., sumb., thuj., zinc.
exertion, on - petr.
expiration, on - chin., cic.
extending, to
abdomen - carb-v., euphr.
back - agar., ***berb.,*** calc., camph., euphr., graph., lact., laur., naja, plb., ran-b.
chest - aloe, carb-v., chin-s.
downward - ptel.
forward - laur.
front - fago.
hips - sil.
outward - calc., sulph.
sacrum, to - thuj.
shoulder, right - rhus-t.
stomach - cupr., nat-c.
flatus, as from incarcerated - iod.
flatus, from - sulph.
forenoon - calc., nat-s., sars., thuj.
inspiration, on - acon., agar., anac., ***bell.,*** calc., calc-p., cann-i., carb-v., cic., con., kali-c., lyc., mag-m., mang., ***merc.,*** mosch., ***nat-s.,*** ph-ac., **RAN-B.,** ran-s., sul-ac., tab., tarax., zinc.
deep - ***bell., calc-p.,*** form., nat-s., sil.
jumping, on - spig.
laughing, on - acon., aesc.
leaning to right - sul-ac.
left - aeth., alum., am-c., am-m., arg-m., arn., ars., ***asaf.,*** aur., bell., ***cann-s.,*** carb-an., carb-v., caust., chin., cic., chel., colch., con., dig., ferr., gran., ***guai.,*** hep., iod., ip., kali-c., kali-bi., kalm., lil-t.,

sharp, hypochondria
left - mag-c., ***mag-m.,*** mag-s., mang., mez., ***nat-c.,*** nat-m., nat-s., ph-ac., phos., puls., rat., ***sars.,*** sep., sil., spig., stann., sulph., ***sul-ac.,*** tarax., verb., zinc.
to chest when clearing throat - ars.
to epigastrium - nat-c.
to right - alum.
lying, down, after amel. - mag-s.
on back amel. - mag-s.
side, on - ars., ***bell.***
menses, during - mag-m., sul-ac.
before - puls.
morning - agar., ammc., am-m., con., graph., hep., kali-c., nat-m., nat-s., stry., tarent.
8 a.m. - kalm.
bed, in - carb-v., con.
motion, on - alum., graph., ***nit-ac., nux-v.,*** sep.
needles, like burning - anac.,
night - coloc., con., ***kali-c.,*** zing.
pressure, agg. - ***berb.,*** carb-v., ***crot-h., nux-v.***
amel. - mag-m., mag-s., meny., sul-ac.
pulsating - dulc., spig.
rhythmical - kali-n.,
riding in a carriage, while - caust.
right - acon., ***aesc., agar.,*** alum., am-m., anac., brom., ***bry.,*** **CALC.,** ***calc-p.,*** carb-an., carb-v., ***card-m.,*** **CAUST.,** cham., **CHEL.,** chin., ***cob., cocc., coloc.,*** **CON.,** ***crot-h.,*** euphr., fago., form., hyper., iod., ***kali-bi., kali-c., kreos.,*** lact., ***laur.,*** lyc., mag-c., mag-m., ***merc., merc-c.,*** mez., mur-ac., naja, ***nat-c.,*** nat-m., ***nat-s., nit-ac.,*** nux-v., ol-j., ph-ac., phos., podo., psor., ***ptel.,*** **RAN-B.,** ***ran-s.,*** rhus-t., sars., ***sep.,*** spig., spong., staph., sul-ac., ***sulph.,*** sumb., tab., tarent., tep., verb., ***zinc.***
bending to left - agar.
extending, to back - **CHEL.,** euphr.
extending, to chest - mag-c.
extending, to heart - zinc.
extending, to thigh - cob.
to left - brom.
rising from stooping - alum.
sitting, while - bry., carb-an., con., dulc., mag-s., meny., nat-c., phos., thuj.
amel. - alum., mag-m.
bent, while - agar., bov., ***sulph.***
sneezing, on - grat.
spinning, while - am-m.
standing, while - alum., arn., cham., glon., zinc.
stool, during - ***calc.***
stooping, on - arg-m., mag-c., mur-ac., sep.
after - **CALC.**
stretching, on - mang.
supper, after - zinc.
tearing - ars.
touch, on - nat-c.
transverse - sep.

sharp, hypochondria
walking, while - am-m., arg-n., cham., hep., mag-m., nat-c., nat-m., ***nat-s.,*** sep., spig., stann., staph., sulph., sumb., thuj., zinc.
amel. - carb-an., mag-c., plb.
yawning - aur.

sharp, hypogastrium - acon., all-c., aloe, ambr., am-c., ammc., ***anac.,*** ang., ant-t., arg-m., ***ars.,*** arund., aur., ***bell., bry.,*** calc., cann-i., carb-s., carb-v., ***caust.,*** cham., chel., chin.,

sharp, hypogastrium - cimic., coloc., elaps, graph., jug-r., ***kali-c.,*** kali-n., ***kali-p.,*** lyc., mang., mez., mur-ac., nat-m., nit-ac., ***nux-v., ph-ac.,*** phos., plb., podo., ptel., ran-b., sabad., samb., sep., spig., stann., sul-ac., sulph., tarax., tarent., thuj., verb., viol-t., zinc.
across - kali-p.
afternoon - lyc., plb.
changing position, on - ph-ac.
coughing, on - ars., sep., verat.
crampy - graph.
dinner, after - kali-n.
drawing in abdomen, when - ambr., kali-c.
eating, after - verat.
evening - lyc., sabad.
extending, to
epigastrium - elaps.
groin - nat-m.
hypochondrium - ran-b.
ilium - mez.
perineum - bell., phos.
spermatic cord - verat.
vagina - ***ars.***
flatus amel. - kali-c.
flatus after - zinc.
forenoon - thuj.
region of - bry., sulph.
left - zinc.
menses, during - bor.
after - ars.
morning - phos., sep.
motion, on - jug-r., kali-n., ph-ac., sul-ac.
pressure, on - ambr.
sitting - viol-t.
standing, while - am-c.
stool, after - carb-v.
before - mang.
touch, on - lyc., nit-ac.
transverse - am-c.
urination, during - nit-ac.
amel. - carb-an.

sharp, inguinal - agn., ***alum.,*** am-m., ammc., arg-m., ***ars.,*** arund., bar-c., bar-m., ***bell., berb., bor., bov., bry.,*** calc., calc-s., ***canth.,*** carb-ac., **CARB-AN.,** carb-s., cast-eq., caust., cham., chin-s., cocc., coc-c., con., ***cycl.,*** dros., euphr., gamb., graph., grat., hell., indg., kali-ar., ***kali-c.,*** kali-i., kali-n., kali-s., laur., lil-t., lyc., ***mag-m.,*** mang., ***merc.,*** merl., ***mez., mur-ac.,*** nat-a., ***nat-c.,*** nat-m., ***nat-s.,*** nicc., pall., prun., psor., rat., sabad., senec., sep., spig., ***stann.,*** staph., ***stront-c.,*** stry., ***sulph.,*** sul-ac., tarent., tell., ***thuj., vib.,*** viol-t., zinc.
afternoon - chin., laur., rat.
4 p.m. - sulph.

sharp, inguinal
afternoon,
walking in open air - nat-s.
ascending steps - alum.
bending toward painful side - ptel.
burning - sulph.
cough, during - lach., thuj.
dinner, during - mur-ac.
eating, after - kali-bi.
emission, after - petr.
evening - am-m., cast., kali-n.
expiration agg. - nat-c.
extending, to
abdomen - bar-c.
axilla, left - nat-s.
back, small of - am-m.
breast, left - **MURX.**
downward - berb., caust.
hip, behind - am-m.
outward through ilium - kali-n.
testicle - euphr., phys., staph.
thighs - ***ars.,*** laur., lyc., sep., thuj.
vagina - ars.
upward - sep.
forenoon - calc., thuj.
glands - bell., dulc., nit-ac., psor., rheum., ***thuj.***
hawking after rising from a seat - nat-c.
hernia, in - ***lyc.,*** nit-ac.
inspiration, on - **BRY.,** merc.
left - bell., calc-s., cast-eq., coc-c., ***cycl.,*** euphr., graph., kali-n., mag-m., merc., nat-s., nicc., plb., tarent., tell.
to axilla - nat-s.
menses, during - ***bor.,*** brom., goss.
after - ars., bor., brom.
morning - zinc.
moving, on - ***ars.,*** kali-c.
night - carb-an.
paroxysmal - berb., sabad.
pressing - nat-c.
amel. - caust., prun.
pulsating - berb., sabad.
right - ammc., am-m., ***ars.,*** bar-c., bov., **BRY.,** cham., cocc., dros., ferr-i., hell., kali-c., kali-i., kali-n., laur., lyc., mang., mez., **MURX.,** nat-c., nat-m., prun., sabad., sulph., thuj.
extending to left breast - **MURX.**
extending to thigh - podo.
rising, on - con., euphr.
amel. - stann.
sitting, while - am-m., chin-s., mag-s.
bent - ***ars.***
down - thuj.
standing amel. - thuj.
stool, during - calc-s., carb-an., kali-c., nicc., sep.
after - gamb.
before - kali-n.
stooping, on - am-m., laur., plb., stann.
stretching out, on - am-c., kali-c.
walking - chin., con., dig., kali-n., merl.
amel. - mag-s., thuj.

sharp, inguinal
walking open air, in - ***merc.,*** nat-s., thuj., sep., spig.

sharp, sides - abrot., acon., ***agar., all-c.,*** aloe, alum., am-c., am-m., arg-n., ***asaf.,*** asar., bar-c., bar-i., ***bell.,*** berb., bov., bry., calc., calc-p., carb-an., carb-s., carb-v., **CAUST.,** cham., cocc., coloc., con., crot-t., dig., dulc., ferr-i., graph., grat., hyos., ign., iod., ip., kali-c., kali-n., kali-s., laur., lyss., meny., mez., naja, nat-c., nux-m., nux-v., op., petr., ph-ac., phos., phys., plat., plb., psor., puls., ***ran-b.,*** rhus-t., sabad., sang., ***sars.,*** seneg., sep., sil., spig., spong., ***stann.,*** stram., stront-c., sul-ac., ***sulph.,*** tab., tarax., tarent., thuj., zinc.
bending, body to left - nat-c.
double amel. - coloc., kali-n.
blowing nose, on - stront.
boring - dros.
breathing - alum., caps., stann., zinc.
buring - sulph.
coughing, on - alum., arn., ars., bell., bor., carb-an., sep., stann., ***sulph.***
daytime - sulph.
eating, after - asaf.
evening - ***caust.,*** sil., ***sulph.***
expiration, on - dig.
extending, to
chest - alum.
downward - plat.
flank, in - acon., ambr., ***arg-m.,*** bar-c., caps., carb-s., carb-v., cham., chin., cocc., coc-c., **COLOC.,** croc., nat-c., ***nat-s.,*** sabad., squil., stann., stram., sulph.
flank, right - alum.
flank, left breast
groin - naja.
outward - asaf., cann-s., lach.
sacrum - caust.
small of back - calc.
spermatic cords - lac-ac.
umbilicus, lying on right side - plat.
upward - bell.
forenoon - nat-s., ***ran-b.***
hiccoughing, on - bar-c.
inspiration, on - carb-v., mez., ph-ac., **RAN-B.,** stann., stront-c., sulph., sul-ac.
laughing - kali-c.
left - aloe, alum., am-c., am-m., ang., ars., ***asaf.,*** bell., bry., calc., caust., chin., coloc., ***graph.,*** hep., hyos., lach., kali-n., laur., meny., mez., nicc., op., ph-ac., plb., ran-b., samb., ***sars., sep.,*** sil., staph., ***sulph.,*** sul-ac., ***tarax.,*** thuj., zinc.
to right - **IP.**
lying - caust.
left side, on, amel. - nicc.
left side, on, agg. - plat.
on sides - sul-ac.
right side - ***thuj.***
menses, during - ars.
morning - sars.

sharp, sides
motion, on - bry., ***kali-c.,*** nat-s., nux-v., sul-ac.
amel. - ars.
pressure amel. - ***asaf.,*** mag-c., thuj.
agg. - dulc., mez., zinc.
raising arms - ferr-i.
respiration - bar-c., caps., carb-v., nux-v., stann., ***sulph.,*** zinc.
right - agar., bar-c., bell., berb., bov., camph., ***caust.,*** cham., chel., cycl., dros., **KALI-C.,** lyss., mez., nat-c., nat-s., nux-m., petr., ph-ac., plat., rhus-t., spig., spong., stann., zinc.
sitting, while - am-m., asaf., carb-an., dros., grat., laur., meny., nat-c., nicc., phos., sabad., sars.
amel. - cinnb.
standing, while - alum., meny., nicc.
stool, during - nicc., ***zinc-s.***
on - alum., am-c., am-m., calc.
amel. -mag-c.
stretching out - kali-c.
supper, after - ***ran-b.***
tearing - ars.
touch, amel. - meny.
turning, body - bar-c., calc.
walking, while - ***asaf.,*** cham., cinnb., dros., ferr-i., meny., mez., ***nat-s.,*** ran-b., sil., spig., sulph.
amel. - sars.
open air, in - ***nat-s.,*** sulph., thuj.
wine, agg. - bor.
yawning - bar-c.

sharp, umbilical, region - aesc., ambr., am-m., anac., arn., asaf., bell., bov., bry., chin., ***coloc.,*** cycl., dig., dulc., eupi., gels., grat., lyc., merc-c., mur-ac., nat-m., ***nux-v.,*** olnd., ph-ac., plb., ruta., sep., spig., spong., staph., sulph., verb., zinc.
burning - sulph.
eating, after - bov.
eating, while - dig.
evening in bed - staph.
extending to uterus - **IP.**
upward - con.
inspiration, on - spig.
motion agg. - zinc.
pulsating - staph.
sides - crot-t., dulc., grat., kali-c., kali-i., lyc., psor., raph., spig.
left - anac., cina., con., crot-t., dulc., kali-i., sul-ac.
right - dulc., grat., kali-c., lyc., nat-m.
touch, agg. - zinc.
walking - spig.

sharp, umbilicus - acon., **AGAR.,** aloe, alum., ammc., ***anac.,*** ant-t., asaf., ***bell.,*** cic., cocc., colch., coloc., ***cycl., dig.,*** dulc., grat., gymn., hyos., **IP.,** kreos., laur., mag-s., merc-i-f., nux-v., pall., pic-ac., ***plat.,*** **PLB.,** raph., rhus-t., sep., sil., sulph., verb.
above - aur., bell., chel., dig., grat., kali-c.
afternoon - alum.

sharp, umbilicus
below - bar-c., chel., chin., coloc., kali-bi., olnd., plb.
extending, to
bladder - cic.
breast region - kreos.
breasts - ***pall.***
pelvis - pall.
pudendum when coughing - sep.
back - ptel.
uterus - **IP.**
inspiration, deep, on - ***hyos.,*** sil., verb.
left side of - jac-c.
morning - agar.
motion, on - cycl., mag-s.
pulse, synchronous with - rhus-t.
radiating from - ***plb.***
sneezing - aloe
standing, while - alum.
stooping - verb.
waking, on - agar.
walking - sulph.
fast - chin.

SHOCKS - arg-n., arn., bell., calc., camph., caust., clem., kali-c., nat-m., pip-n., plat., puls., squil., tab., thal.
cough, during - kali-c.
daytime - tab.
electric like, extending to fingers - caust.
to limb - camph.
extending to, whole body, when falling asleep - ant-t.
electricity, as of, when ascending and descending currents of cold met - sapo.
extending to chest - mag-arct.
fetus, as from - con.
inspiration, on - act-sp.
left, to right, from - stann.
lying, on side, while - camph.
motion, on - pip-n.
night, getting into a drowse - tab.
paralysis of lower limbs - thal.
pressing on right agg. - stann.
spasms, during - stry.
tingling - mag-m., petr.

shocks, hypogastrium - arn., cann-s.
coughing, when - nat-m., squil.

shocks, umbilicus at left from - anac.

SHORT, as if muscles to short - sulph.

SHRIVELED, or wilted appearance - ***bor.***

SHUDDERING, in - cann-s., ***coloc.***
extending over body - ***coloc.***

SICKENING, pain about the umbilicus after stool - ***ph-ac.***

SOFT - amyg., brom., piloc., kali-i., kreos., merc-cy., nat-m., phos., sec., stram.
sensation of - ptel.

SORE, pain - acet-ac., **ACON.,** ***aesc.,*** aeth., aloe, alum., ***alumn.,*** ambr., am-c., am-m., ant-t., **APIS,** ***arg-m., arg-n.,*** **ARN., ARS.,** arund., atro., asaf., aur., aur-m., ***aur-m-n.,*** **BAPT.,** bar-c., **BELL.,** bism., bol., bov., **BRY.,** bufo, cact., cadm-s., cahin.,

SORE, pain - calad., ***calc.***, calc-s., cann-s., ***canth.***, ***carb-ac.***, ***carb-an.***, carb-s., carb-v., caust., **CHAM.**, ***chel.***, chin., ***chin-a.***, cimic., ***cina***, cinnb., ***cocc.***, **COLCH.**, ***coloc.***, ***con.***, **CROT-C.**, ***crot-h.***, crot-t., **CUPR.**, cupr-ar., ***cycl.***, ***dios.***, euph., eup-pur., fago., ***ferr.***, ***ferr-ar.***, ferr-p., ***gels.***, gnaph., gran., ***graph.***, grat., gymn., ***ham.***, hell., ***hep.***, ***hydr.***, ***hyos.***, ign., ***ip.***, iris, jatr., ***kali-ar.***, kali-bi., kali-c., ***kali-chl.***, kali-i., kali-n., ***kali-p.***, kali-s., ***kreos.***, ***lac-d.***, **LACH.**, ***lec.***, led., ***lil-t.***, lob., **LYC.**, ***mag-m.***, ***manc.***, meny., **MERC.**, **MERC-C.**, merc-i-r., ***mez.***, murx., nat-a., nat-c., nat-m., nat-p., nat-s., **NIT-AC.**, ***nux-m.***, **NUX-V.**, onos., ***op.***, ox-ac., ***pall.***, paeon., petr., **PHOS.**, phys., phyt., plb., ***podo.***, ptel., ***puls.***, **PYROG.**, ***ran-b.***, ***raph.***, **RHUS-T.**, rhus-v., ruta, sabad., sabin., samb., ***sang.***, ***sars.***, sec., **SEP.**, sol-t-ae., squil., ***stann.***, staph., stram., stry., **SULPH.**, sul-ac., tab., tarent., **TER.**, til., ***ust.***, valer., ***verat.***, xan., zinc.
- afternoon - coloc., fago., osm., lyc.
  - 1 p.m.,. - nux-v.
- bending, double amel. - mag-c.
- clothing, agg. - apis, ***ars.***, benz-ac., **CALC.**, ***carb-v.***, coff., ***graph.***, ***kreos.***, ***lac-c.***, **LACH.**, ***lyc.***, merc-c., ***nux-v.***, puls., raph., ***spong.***, zinc.
- coughing, from - ars., ***bry.***, ***carb-an.***, ***caust.***, crot-t., ***ferr.***, hyos., ***nux-v.***, ***pic-ac.***, plb., ***puls.***, ***stann.***
- eating, after - ***sang.***
- evening - cast., fago., ferr., ham., sabin., sep.
  - menses, during - cast.
- forenoon - nat-m., sulph.
  - every step, on - ***sulph.***
- jarring, on - **BELL.**, **BRY.**, colch., ferr., kali-s., ***lach.***, ***lil-t.***, **NUX-V.**, **PHOS.**, phyt., prun., raph.
- lying, on abdomen amel. - phos.
  - on right side agg. - ***merc.***
- menses, during - ***bell.***, brom., bry., cast., ***cocc.***, ***ham.***, lac-d., nat-m., ***nux-v.***, pic-ac., ***puls.***, sulph.
  - after - cham., cycl., lil-t., pall.
  - as from - nat-c.
  - before - bell., bry., lac-c., lach., mang., sep.
  - pressing, amel. - cast.
- morning - apis, ***asaf.***, dios., ***hep.***, lil-t., lyc., **NUX-V.**, raph., **SEP.**, trom.
  - in bed - ign., nat-m., **NUX-V.**
- motion, on - **BELL.**, bov., **BRY.**, nux-v., **PHOS.**, podo., rob., stram.
- night - mang., ***nat-m.***, sep., tab.
- pregnancy, during - arn., ***nux-m.***, sep.
- riding, horseback - arn., nat-c.
  - in a carriage agg. - ***arg-m.***
- stool, during - ***arn.***, carl., ***sulph.***
  - after - am-m., crot-t., nat-m., puls., ***sulph.***, sul-ac., tab.
  - amel. - ***podo.***
  - before - nat-m., ***sulph.***, tab.
  - straining at, from - **SIL.**
- touch, on - phos., stann., sulph.

SORE, pain
- walking, while - ***bell.***, ***carb-ac.***, coloc., ***ferr.***, hep., kali-s., phos., phyt., puls., ran-b., sulph.
  - on stone pavement - con.
- warmth, amel. - nat-c.
- yawning - ruta.

sore, hypochondria - act-sp., aesc., ***agar.***, ail., alum., ***ambr.***, am-c., ant-t., **APIS**, ***arn.***, ***ars.***, ars-i., bapt., **BELL.**, brom., **BRY.**, bufo, **CALC.**, ***calc-p.***, cann-s., carb-ac., carb-an., carb-s., ***carb-v.***, ***chel.***, clem., ***cocc.***, ***corn.***, cupr., cupr-s., dros., ***eup-per.***, ferr-i., iod., kali-ar., kali-bi., ***kali-c.***, kali-n., kreos., ***lach.***, lact., **LYC.**, lycps., mag-c., mang., **MERC.**, mur-ac., nat-a., nat-m., ***nat-s.***, ol-j., ox-ac., ***phos.***, phyt., plb., ptel., **RAN-B.**, **RHUS-T.**, sec., stront-c., ***sulph.***, tab., tarent., vip., zinc.
- afternoon - phyt.
- chill, during - phos.
- coughing, on - ***bry.***, carb-v., cimx., lach., nux-v.
- diarrhea, during - **ARG-N.**
- eating, after - agar.
- evening - **RAN-B.**
- extending, into stomach - nat-c.
  - to shoulder - laur., ***nux-v.***
- jarring, on - **BELL.**, **BRY.**, colch., hep., ***lach.***, ***nat-s.***, **NUX-V.**, sil.
- left - ***apis***, ***brom.***, ***calc.***, cupr., ***iod.***, lycps., nat-c., nat-m., sars., stann., zinc.
  - humiliation, after - ign.
- lying on left side - ptel.
  - lying on painful side agg. - fago., phos.
- morning - cist., dios., lact., sulph.
  - 10 a.m. - fago.
- motion, agg. - ***bry.***, carb-ac., mang., ***ran-b.***, ***sil.***, sulph.
  - amel. - phys.
- night, mag-c.
  - lying on painful side - fago.
- pressure, amel. - bry.
- pulsating - zinc.
- right - act-sp., ***aesc.***, ***ambr.***, arn., ars., bapt., **BRY.**, ***calc-p.***, carb-ac., carb-v., ***card-m.***, ***chel.***, ***chin.***, chion., ***clem.***, ***con.***, **DIG.**, eup-per., fago., ***fl-ac.***, ***iod.***, ***kali-i.***, ***kreos.***, lact., **LYC.**, ***mag-m.***, ***mur-ac.***, **NAT-S.**, **NUX-V.**, ***ol-j.***, ***phos.***, ***phyt.***, **RAN-B.**, sec., ***sep.***, ***sil.***, sulph., tarent.
  - exertion, after - ***kali-i.***
  - lying on right side - ***sil.***, ***mag-m.***, ***merc.***
- side lain on agg. - **RHUS-T.**
- sitting - mur-ac.
- spots, in - kali-c.
- step, on every - ***bell.***, ***hep.***
- stooping, on - alum.
- touch, on - mag-c., mang.
- walking, while - **NAT-S.**, ***sil.***

sore, hypogastrium - ***acon.***, asc-t., ***arg-n.***, ***ars.***, aur., calad., **CALC.**, canth., carb-v., caust., cycl., euph., fago., ferr-ar., ferr-m., jac-c., ***hyos.***, kali-n., **LACH.**, ***lyss.***, mag-m., mang., merc., ***nat-m.***, nit-ac., onos., ***op.***, ***pall.***, ***phos.***, phys., pic-ac., prun., psor., puls., ***rhus-t.***,

sore, hypogastrium - sabin., ***sars.,*** sep., stann., ***sulph.,*** **TER.,** ***valer.,*** **VERAT.,** verb.
cough - carb-an.
drawing up leg amel. - aur.
flatus, before - nat-m.
night - sep.
rising from seat amel. - aur.
sitting bent agg. - coloc.
stool, before - nat-m.
touch, on - lyc.
walking while - ***prun.***

sore, inguinal - alum., am-c., ***apis, arg-m.,*** **ARN.,** bar-m., calc., calc-ar., calc-p., carl., caust., chin., ***clem.,*** cocc., coc-c., dig., dios., elaps, ferr-i., ***graph.,*** iod., kali-c., mag-m., mag-s., mez., mur-ac., nicc., nit-ac., ***pall.,*** ran-b., rhus-t., sars., spig., ther., ***valer.,*** zing.
afternoon - mag-s.
bed, in - dios.
bending agg. - mez.
evening - dios.
expiration agg. - mez.
glands - ***clem.,*** caps., gels., hep., lyc., merc., ***sil.,*** sumb., thuj.
hernia - sulph.
left - dios., elaps, ***lach.***
menses, during - kali-i., sars.
riding horseback, after - spig.
right - ***apis,*** calc-p., iod., sars., ***sulph.***
touch, on - am-m.
walk bent, must - **ARN.**
walking, while - arg-m., calc., caust., ferr-i.
amel. - nit-ac.

sore, sides - arg-m., arn., bad., camph., caust., chin., colch., eup-pur., ferr., lil-t., nux-v., ran-b., stront-c., zing.
below the floating ribs - ***sil.***
flank in - calc., caust., ***sil.,*** staph.
left - ***arg-m.,*** colch.
right - ang., camph., zing.

sore, umbilical, region - agar., ***carb-v.,*** caust., cina, cinnb., ***coloc.,*** con., gent-c., hep., ***hydr.,*** **IP.,** jatr., kali-bi., ***kali-c.,*** lyc., mag-c., ***merc., merc-i-f., nux-v.,*** ox-ac., plat., ***plb., puls.,*** stann.

sore, umbilicus - aesc., aeth., ***aloe,*** anac., calc., ***calc-p.,*** chin., cina, cinnb., con., crot-t., dulc., fago., form., kali-c., nat-m., phys., plan., ***rhus-t.,*** stront-c., thuj., verat.

SPASMS, muscles - ars., caust., ***cham.,*** **COLOC., CUPR.,** cupr-ac., guare., ***kali-br.,*** kali-i., ***kreos.,*** **MAG-P.,** mosch., ***plb.,*** sabad., ***tab.***
hysterical women, in - ***bry.,*** cocc., ***mosch.***
evening, after lying down, before stool and emission of flatus - ars.
night - sep.

SPLEEN, (see Glands, chapter)

SPONGE, in hypochondria, sensation of, alternating sides - lac-c.

SPRING, hypochondria, sensation as if a, were unrolled in left - sol-t-ae.

STABBING, knife, as with a - lach.
needle, as with a - lyc.
extending to mons veneris - rhus-t.

STIFFNESS - ars., lil-t., mag-s., rhus-t.

STIRRED up, sensation - dios.
afternoon, 4.20 p.m., after supper amel. - dios.
6 p.m., after supper amel. - dios.

STINGING, pain - **APIS,** asaf., bry., ***canth.,*** chel., chin., ign., kali-c., ***lyc., phos., puls.,*** sep., spig., verb.

STONE, in, sensation of - aloe, ant-t., ***calc., cocc.,*** coloc., hydr., nux-m., ***nux-v.,*** osm., **PULS.,** scop., sep.
long sitting, after - ant-t.
lying on abdomen - aloe
seems full of stones - ***ant-t.,*** **CALC.,** ***cocc., coloc.***
sharp - cocc., coloc.

stone, umbilicus, in, sensation of, about - ***cocc.***

STOPPED, sensation - bism., bry., cham., chel., ***chin.,*** guai., meny., nat-c., ***nux-m.,*** **OP.,** phos., puls., rhus-t., sep., spig., spong., verb.

STRING, about - chel.

STRUCK, sensation as if, pointed stick, as by a - manc.
pressure agg. - cupr.

STUFFED sensation, from food - laur., ***lyc.***

SUPPURATION, sensation of - cinnb., kreos.
last day of menses, on - bov.

suppuration, umbilicus - phos.

SWASHING - acon., ***aloe,*** bar-c., **CROT-T.,** kali-c., merc., mez., ***nat-m.,*** nux-v., **PH-AC.,** rhus-t.
bending forward and backward - ph-ac.
night, during diarrhea - crot-t.
walking - mang.

SWELLING, hypochondria, hard - bry.

swelling, inguinal - am-c., am-m., ant-c., ***apis,*** ars., ***clem.,*** con., gran., ***graph.,*** jac-c., kali-c., ***lyc., puls.,*** rhus-t., sil., ***ther.,*** thuj.
afternoon, 2 p.m. - lyss.
elastic - am-c.
evening, 8 p.m. - phys.
hard - clem., dulc., puls.
left - am-c., sil.
painful - clem., puls.
right - ***apis,*** ars., **CLEM.,** con., lyss.

swelling, umbilicus - bry., caust., plb., prun., ptel., puls., sep.
around, like ring - puls.
painful - caust.

TABES, mesenterica, tuberculosis - ***ars.,*** ars-i., ***aur.,*** aur-m., ***bar-c., bar-i., bar-m.,*** **CALC.,** ***calc-p., calc-s., carb-an., carb-s.,*** caust., ***con., hep., iod., kreos., lyc.,*** merc., merc-i-f., ***nat-s.,*** ol-j., sulph., ***tub.***

TEARING, pain - aloe, alum., ***am-c.,*** anan., ant-t., **ARS.,** bar-c., benz-ac., berb., ***bry.,*** bufo, ***cact.,*** calc., canth., carb-an., carb-s., **CHAM.,** chin., chin-s., cic., cocc., ***colch.,*** **COLOC.,** con., ***cop.,*** crot-t., cupr., cupr-ar., ***cycl., dig.,*** dulc., ***graph.,*** hell., ***kali-c.,*** kali-i., kali-n., ***lach., lyc.,*** lyss., ***mag-m.,*** med., ***merc., mez.,*** naja, nat-m., nux-m., ***nux-v.,*** op., ***phos.,*** plb., ***puls., rhus-t.,*** sec., sil., squil., stram., sulph., tab., tarent., verb., ***zinc.***
- afternoon - nux-v., sep.
- cramp-like - samb.
- eating, while - crot-t.
- evening - alum., bry., mag-m.
- extending, to,
  - downward - kali-i., verb.
  - genitals - calc.
  - left to right - lyss.
  - loins - kali-i.
  - right breast - coloc.
  - upward - ***chin-s.,*** mag-m.
- forenoon - mag-m.
- heat amel. - alum.
- hiccough, on - plb.
- hunger, during - stram.
- inspiration, on - ***calc.***
- left to right - lyss.
- menses, during - agar., am-c., bov., ***caust., chin-s.,*** cinnb., **GRAPH., LACH.,** ***merc.,*** sec., tep.
  - before - ***cinnb.,*** nat-m., tep.
- morning - alum., dig., naja
- motion, during - ***bry.,*** rhus-t.
- night - mag-m., merc., tab.
- outward - sep.
- pressure - cic.
  - amel. - plb.
- rising from a seat - dig.
- sleep amel. - mag-m.
- step, at every - all-s.
- stool, during - aloe, cop.
  - after - mag-m.
  - before - dig., hep., stram.
  - driving to - ***nux-v.***
- warmth amel. - alum.

tearing, hypochondria - alum., canth., carb-v., colch., ***con.,*** cupr-s., kali-bi., kali-c., lyss., nux-v., plb., teucr., thuj., ***zinc.***
- coughing on - ambr.
- evening - ars., caust.
- extending to hip - alum.
- forenoon - alum.
- inspiration, on - cupr., cupr-s.
- left - ars., canth., colch., kali-c., lyss., plb., sil.
- right - alum., ***con.,*** kali-c., mez., ***nux-m.,*** zinc.
- sitting - ars.

tearing, hypogastrium - anac., canth., carb-v., chin., ***colch.,*** con., iod., kali-n., lach., nat-c., spig., verb., zinc.
- extending to inguinal region - zinc.
  - to urethra - nat-c.
- menses, during - ***agar., am-c., lach., manc.***
- motion amel. - kali-n.

tearing, inguinal - am-m., ***ars., berb.,*** calc., chin., crot-t., cycl., euph., ***lach., lyc.,*** mez., ***plat.,*** sep., sil., stront-c., sul-ac., tarent., thuj.
- bending back amel. - chin.
- coughing agg. - tarent.
- evening - kali-c., sil.
- extending to, right nipple - crot-t.
  - to, thighs - ***ars.,*** lyc., plat., sep.
  - upward - thuj.
- glands - calc., sulph.
- inspiration agg. - plat.
- jerking - thuj.
- left - sul-ac.
- right - kali-c., mez., thuj.
- rising from a seat - stront.
- sitting, while - calc., spong., sul-ac.
- standing, while - euph.
- walking, while - am-m., calc., sep.

tearing, sides - alum., aur., bry., calc., crot-t., kali-c., ***lach.,*** lyc., mag-c., plb.
- bend, must bend double - aur.
- evening - kali-c.
- exertion, on - alum.
  - walking, while - mag-c.
- extending to bladder - plb.
- flank, in - crot-t., samb.
- left - bry., mag-c., samb., sulph.
- right - aur., ***lach.,*** mez.

tearing, umbilical, region - agar., arn., ***cham.,*** chin., coloc., con., crot-t., cupr., dig., grat., ip., jatr., mag-c., ***nat-s., plb.,*** psor., stram., tep., verb., zinc.
- breakfast, before - **NAT-S.**
- dinner, after - crot-t.
- expiration agg. - coloc.
- laughing aloud agg. - coloc.
- morning - dig.
- paroxysmal - ***plb.***
- pressure - plb.

tearing, umbilicus - chin., crot-t., cycl., laur., nux-v., plb., stram.
- afternoon, 2 p.m. - laur.

TENDERNESS, pressure, to - bry., ran-b.
- ensiform cartilage and umbilicus, between - sul-ac.

TENSION - acon., ***agar.,*** aloe, alum., ambr., am-c., ant-t., arg-m., ***arg-n., ars.,*** **BAR-C.,** ***bar-i.,*** bar-m., bell., ***bov.,*** bry., **CALC.,** calc-s., canth., caps., carb-ac., ***carb-s.,*** **CARB-V.,** caust., ***cham.,*** chel., chin., ***chin-a.,*** clem., ***cocc.,*** **COLCH.,** coloc., com., con., crot-h., crot-t., **CUPR.,** cycl., dig., ferr., ferr-ar., ferr-p., ***gamb.,*** gins., ***graph.,*** **HEP.,** hyos., hyper., iod., jatr., jug-r., ***kali-ar.,*** kali-bi., ***kali-c.,*** kali-n., kali-p., kreos., ***lac-c.,*** lach., lact., laur., **LYC.,** mag-c., mag-m., mag-s., manc., mang., meny., merc., merl., ***mez.,*** mosch., ***mur-ac.,*** naja, nat-a., nat-c., ***nat-m.,*** nat-p., nat-s., nit-ac., ***nux-v., op.,*** par., petr., ph-ac., ***phos., plat., plb.,*** ptel., puls., ***rheum,*** rhod., sabin., samb., sec., **SEP., SIL.,** spong., squil., stann., ***staph.,*** stram., stront-c., **SULPH.,** sul-ac., ***tab., ter., thuj.,*** verat., vip., zinc.

TENSION,

afternoon - bry., calc., carb-v., mag-c., petr., stront-c., sulph.
1 p.m. until evening - mag-c.
eating after - bry.
flatus passing amel. - nat-m.
siesta, after - cycl.
belching amel. - nat-m.
board, like a - cupr.
children - sil.
clothes were too tight, as if - op.
colic, during - onis.
contractive - caust.
convulsive - sec.
diarrhea, with - mag-c.
dinner, after - cycl., nit-ac., plat., sulph.
drawing - ant-t.
drinking, after - ambr., ***cocc.***
eating, on - phos.
after - ambr., asaf., bry., ***carb-v.,*** ign., lyc.
roast lamb., after - lyc.
emission, after - sep.
evening - arg-n., gent-l., hyos., lyc., mag-c.
exertion, during - calc.
extending to,
across - petr., tax.
chest - caps., con.
groins, down to - arg-n.
heart, toward - naja.
sacrum - stann.
fever, during - sil.
flatus, from - carb-v., nat-m., **SULPH.**
passing, amel. - ant-t., calc., mang., mez.
forenoon - nat-m.
menses, during - ***cocc., graph.,*** nicc., **NUX-M.**
morning - cinnb., sep., ***sulph.***
motion, on - clem., phos.
night - chin., nat-c.
noon until evening - sulph.
painful - acon., cadm-s., carb-an., carl., coloc., inul., ***op.,*** puls.
dinner, after, agg. - carl.
drawing - nux-v.
dull, pressure amel. - coloc.
extending, chest, to - caps.
extending, spermatic cords, through, into testicles - **PULS.**
menses, with impending - carl.
walking, when - inul.
pinching, spasmodic - hep.
pressive - ant-t., carb-s.
expiration amel. - merc.
motion agg. - caps.
pressure amel. - coloc.
reaching high, from - alum.
respiration, deep, on - ***cocc.,*** con.
sitting, while - calc., crot-t., kali-c., spong.
stool, during - apis, grat., plat.
amel. - gent-c., sulph.
amel., diarrhea - sulph.
stooping agg. - nat-c., spong., stann.
straightening up - dig.

TENSION,

waking, on - ferr.
walking, while - arg-m., nat-c., spong.
amel. - bry., ferr., ***kali-c., lyc.,*** nat-c.

tension, hypochondria - ***acon.,*** agar., ***aloe,*** ant-c., ant-t., ars., bell., bor., ***bry., calc., carb-v.,*** caust., cham., ***chin-s.,*** cimx., clem., coc-c., coff., colch., con., dig., eup-per., ***graph.,*** hyper., lact., ***lyc.,*** mang-m., mosch., murx., mur-ac., nat-a., nat-c., ***nat-m., nat-s.,*** nit-ac., ***nux-v.,*** puls., sep., staph., stry., ***sulph.,*** verat., vip.
afternoon - ars., nat-m.
2 p.m. - ars.
breathing, from - led.
emission, after - agar.
evening - murx.
extending, to
back - nat-m.
left side of abdomen - con.
upwards - mur-ac.
flatus amel. - mur-ac.
forenoon - nat-m.
fruit, after - nat-c.
fever, during - ***ars.***
left - ***ars.,*** con., eup-per., lyc., nat-m., nit-ac., plat., rhod.
lying on back, while - ***caust.***
lying on side, agg. - ars.
motion, on - sep.
right - aloe, ant-t., bry., calc., card-m., ***carb-v., ferr.,*** hyper., lact., ***lyc.,*** mag-m., mur-ac., nat-m., ***nat-s.,*** nit-ac., sulph.
lying on left side - ***card-m.,*** mag-m., nat-s., ptel.
sitting, while - mur-ac.
stool, after - plat.
before - ars.
stooping, on - nat-c., rhod., sep.
waking, on - ***carb-v.***
walking - sep.
in open air, while - nat-c., ***nat-s.***

tension, hypogastrium - agar., ars., ***aur., bell.,*** **CALC.,** chin., coc-c., gins., kali-c., merc., ***nat-m., op.,*** phos., ***SEP., stront-c.,*** sumb.
bending backward - calc.
eating, after - phel.
extending to rectum - spong.
to seminal cord - sep.
inspiration, deep, agg. - sumb., thuj.
morning - ***bell.***
rising, on - dulc.
sex, after - sep.
sitting - ruta.
standing erect - calc.
stool, before - haem.
vaginal discharge, with - am-m.

tension, iliac region, arg-m., chel., grat.
fossa - chel.
left - arg-m., grat.

tension, inguinal - **AGAR.,** am-c., am-m., ***apis, arg-m.,*** benz-ac., berb., calc., canth., carb-an., ***clem.,*** coc-c., ***coloc.,*** crot-t., cycl., dig., ***dulc.,*** gamb., graph., jatr., kali-i., kreos., ***lac-c.,*** mag-s., mang., merc., nat-m., nat-s., nit-ac.,

tension, inguinal - sars., spig., stront.
afternoon - cycl.
sleep, after - cycl.
ascending stairs - coloc.
bending over - coloc.
drawing up limb amel. - agar., ***lac-c.***
evening - nat-m.
glands - calc., nat-m.
left - arg-m., calc., lac-c., merc., merc-c., nat-m.
morning - coloc.
3 a.m. - merc-c.
motion, on - nat-m.
pressure - coloc.
raising arms - ***apis.***
right - am-m., sars., stront.
rising from a seat - dulc.
sitting, while - agar., calc.
stool amel. - nat-m.

tension, inguinal
stretching out limb - agar., carb-an.
standing, while - gamb., lac-c.
tendon, as from a swollen - mang.
touched, when - spig.
walking, while - am-m., ***clem.,*** graph., kreos., lac-c., nat-m.
amel. - agar.

tension, sides - agar., ***aur.,*** camph., caust., crot-t., cycl., ***lach.,*** merc., nat-m., rhus-t., zinc.
belching, amel. - zinc.
breathing deep - con.
left lower - phos., rheum.
night - kali-c., nit-ac.
right - con.

tension, umbilical, region - cham., crot-t., mang., nat-c., **SULPH.,** thuj., zinc.
lying, while - crot-t.
midnight - sulph.

tension, umbilicus - anac., crot-t., nat-m., verat.
below umbilicus - nat-c.

THREAD, sensation, moving rapidly - sabad.

TICKLING, sensation, shoots upward through - croc.

TINGLING, sensation - verat.

TREMBLING - ant-t., arg-n., bov., chel., colch., ***con., croc.,*** grat., ***hydr.,*** iod., kali-c., ***kali-s.,*** lil-t., mosch., **NUX-V.,** phos., raph., staph., **SUL-AC.**
eating, after - arg-n.
lying on the back, while - ***sul-ac.***
flatus passing amel., after, at 10 a.m. - bor.
menses, during - arg-n.
morning - colch.
waking, on - colch.
night - raph.
waking, on - hydr.
waking, on, anxious dreams, from - phos.
sensation of - lil-t., pip-m.
stool, after - carb-s.
before diarrhea-like - merc.

trembling, hypogastrium - calc-p., ***lil-t.***

trembling, inguinal region - agar., ***chel.,*** guai., merc., nat-c.
left - agar.

trembling, umbilicus - verb.

TUBERCLES, linear - bomb-pr.

TUMORS - ***con.***
sensation as if, right side - med.

TURNING, sensation - caps., ign., lact., mag-c., ***sabad.,*** sep.
around, as of a serpent - cact.
inside out, as if they would - sep.

TWINGING, pain - ***bov., carb-an.,*** cast., crot-t., grat., mag-c., ***mag-m.,*** merl., mur-ac., nat-c., nit-ac., sil., sul-ac., zinc.
eating, after - sil.
flatus, before - zinc.

twinging, hypochondria - laur., nux-v.
left - laur.
right - nux-v.

twinging, inguinal - cast., indg., lyc.
extending to chest - indg.

TWISTING, pain - ***agar.,*** alum., anac., anan., ant-t., ars., aur., bov., cact., calad., calc., ***caps.,*** caust., chin-s., dig., ***dios.,*** dros., elaps, eupi., eup-pur., grat., hura, lyc., mag-s., merc., ***mez.,*** pall., ***plat.,*** plb., prun., rhus-t., sep., sil., ***staph.,*** stram., sul-ac., sumb., **VERAT.**
evening - calad.
stool, before - ars., caust., mez.

twisting, hypochondria - dios., nat-m., podo.
evening - dios.
left - dios.
right - podo.
stool, during - nat-m.

twisting, umbilical, region - all-c., aloe, berb., bry., calc., caps., ***cina,*** coloc., crot-t., dulc., hell., mez., naja, nat-c., nux-m., ox-ac., plat., ***plb.,*** ran-b., ruta.
extending downward - nux-m.
flatus amel. - mez.
morning - hell.
night - ruta.
vaginal discharge, before - nat-c.

TWITCHING and jerking, of - **AGAR.,** alum., alumn., ambr., anac., ars., ***bry.,*** cann-s., caust., chel., con., cupr., dros., graph., guai., hyos., kali-ar., kali-c., lyc., manc., merc., murx., nat-m., ***nux-v.,*** op., phos., plat., ran-s., rhus-t., sul-ac., verat.
convulsive - ars.
eating, after - gaul.
evening, in bed - agar.
extending, across - rhus-t.
whole body, to, as soon as he fell asleep - ant-t.
external, like dull thrusts in a spot - plat.
flatus, from - rhus-t.
griping, after drinking water - croc.
midnight - manc.
night - caust.
pulsating - con.
spots, in - nux-m.

TWITCHING and jerking, of
stool, during - calc.
evening - nat-c.
left - thuj.
right - acon., mag-c., merc., nat-c., valer.
wandering - dulc.
twitching, hypochondria - acon., berb., carb-s., croc., lact., mag-c., merc., nat-c., nux-v., puls., stann., thuj., valer.
evening - nat-c.
left - thuj.
right - acon., mag-c., merc., nat-c., sep., valer.
coughing - lyc.
twitching, hypogastrium - arn., nat-c., phos., sul-ac.
twitching, inguinal - abrot., ammc., calc., cann-s., clem., cycl., ph-ac., psor., sulph., zinc.
extending, to
back - abrot.
penis - zinc.
pubis - rhus-t.
glands - clem.
twitching, sides - alum., chin., fl-ac., graph., meny., nat-c., nicc., sul-ac.
right - kali-c., sep.
left - aur., caust., stann.
walking, while - sul-ac.

TYPHUS abdominalis - plb.

ULCERS - ***arg-n.,*** **ARS.,** bar-m., ***calc.,*** **CARB-V.,** chin., ***coloc.,*** cupr., ***hep., kali-bi.,*** lach., ***lyc.,*** merc., **NIT-AC.,** ***phos.,*** plb., ***sil.,*** sulph., **TER.**
spreading - ***ars.***
ulcers, hypochondria - ars., nat-c., phos.
ulcers, inguinal region - anan., bad., bar-m., ***carb-an., chel., hep.,*** kali-c., ***kali-i., merc.,*** nat-m.
ulcers, umbilicus, spreading about - abrot., ***aesc.,*** apis, ***ars.,*** **CALC.,** calc-p., lach., lyc., ***nux-m.,*** petr., ***rhus-t.,*** sep., sil., sulph., thuj.
above - ars.
infants - petr.
newborn - apis

ULCERS, sensation of - carb-an., guare., kali-n., merc.
bending forward amel. - coloc.
morning after rising, when stretching - rhus-t.
moving, on - dig., eupi.
pressure, on - hell., ran-b.
respiration, on deep - kali-n.
upright position, agg. - coloc.

UMBILICUS, ailments in region of - bry., ***coloc.,*** dios., ***dulc.,*** ip., kreos., lept., nux-v., ***ph-ac., rhus-t.,*** spig., ***verat.,*** verb.
extending to,
navel - coloc., lach.
pelvis - pall., rumx., sep.
rectum - aloe, ars., crot-t., dios., ferr-i., lyc.
uterus - ip.
flatus amel. - mag-c.
sitting agg. - symph.

UMBILICUS, ailments in
stool, agg. - lept.
amel. - senec.
bleeding from, in newborn - abrot., ***calc-p.,*** phos.
proud flesh - ***calc.,*** kali-c., nat-m.
urine, oozing from - hyos.

UNCERTAINTY, feeling of - **ALOE.,** gast.

UNDULATING, sensation - lyss.
anxious, ascending and accelerating respiration - rhod.

UNEVEN - plb.

URGING - aloe., alum., caust.

URTICARIA - merc., nat-c.

VEINS, distended - adon., ***aesc., aloe,*** arn., ars., aur., bell-p., berb., calc., calc-hp., camph., ***carb-an., carb-v.,*** chin-s., ***coll.,*** conv., ***dig.,*** fl-ac., ***ham.,*** lept., lyc., ***nux-v.,*** op., plb., ***podo., puls., sep.,*** spong., stel., ***sulph.,*** verb.
portal system - aesc., ***aloe, coll.,*** lept., lyc., ***nux-v., sulph.***
varicose - ***ham., sulph.***
sore - ham.
veins, inguinal distended - ***berb.***

VESICLES - arn., crot-t., kali-bi., caust., ***merc.,*** merc-c., rhus-t.
vesicles, inguinal - nat-c.

WATER, cold, as if seated in, as far as abdomen - plb.
column of, were poured into, through tube, which closed suddenly as by a valve - elaps
full of, as if - casc., crot-t., hell., ***kali-c.,*** ol-an., ph-ac., sul-ac.
drank large quantities, as though he - apoc.
hot, were flowing through, as if - sumb.
sounds as if full of, on pressure, 10 a.m. - urt-u.

WEAKNESS, sense of - **ALOE,** alum., alumn., apoc., **ARG-N.,** bor., ***calc-p.,*** chin., colch., gels., **IGN.,** kali-c., led., lil-t., **LYC.,** mag-m., ***merc.,*** myric., ***nat-m.,*** olnd., ox-ac., ***petr.,*** **PHOS.,** phyt., ***podo., plat., psor.,*** ptel., rhod., sapo., ***sep.,*** spong., ***staph.,*** **SUL-AC.,** ***verat.,*** zinc.
belching, amel. - ***kali-m.***
breathing, on deep - carb-v.
diarrhea, as if, would come on - **ALOE,** ant-c., bor., crot-t., eucal., ferr-m., form., nux-v., opun-f., ran-s.
dragging into hips and small of back, with - sul-ac.
drop, as if it would - sep., **STAPH.**
evening - anac., carb-an.
extending, into throat - kalm.
faint, as if about to, evening, sitting down amel. - tarent.
menses, as if, would come on - **SUL-AC.**
menses, before - phos.
morning - chel., dios., hell.
6 a.m. to 3 p.m. - merc-i-r.
muscles - ars., cocc., con., sulph.

WEAKNESS, sense of
perspiration, after - ***ferr-ma.***
purgatives, as from abuse of - acon.
stool, during - form., ip.
after - ***arg-n.,*** carb-s., chin., dios., ***iod.,*** lept., mag-m., ***nat-p.,*** **PETR.,** ***phos., pic-ac.,*** plat., **PODO.,** ***sep.,*** stann., sulph., **SUL-AC., VERAT.**
before - verat-v.
diarrhea, as during - myric.
hard - ***plat., sep.***
upper abdomen after urination - ars.
walking, while - caust., hep.
after - ***phos.***

weakness, hypochondria - carb-an.

weakness, hypogastrium - am-c., apoc., calc., chion., phos., plb., sulph., verat.
stool, before - merc-i-f.

weakness, inguinal - aloe, aur., calc., nux-v., raph., tab.

WEIGHT, hypogastrium, falling, sensation of, on inspiration - spig.

WHIRLING, senation of - hep.

WHISTLING - mur-ac., sep.

WRENCHING - lyss.
sneezing, while - ind.

WRITHING, sense of - agar., aloe, alum., berb.
evacuation, before - stram.

Ankles

ABSCESS, ankle joint - ang., guai., ***ol-j.,*** sil.

ACHILLES tendons
aching, pain - ***cimic.***
boring, pain - aur-m-n.
contraction, of muscles and tendon - acon., ***calc., cann-s., carb-an.,*** cimic., ***colch.,*** euphr., ***graph., kali-c.,*** ruta, ***sep.,*** zinc.
cramps - ***calc., caust.***
night in bed - calc., ***caust.***
drawing, pain - aesc., alum., benz-ac., berb., ***calc., carb-an.,*** chel., graph., ***kali-bi.,*** lyc., mag-c., mur-ac., nat-m., nat-s., sulph., thuj., ***zinc.***
evening - carb-an.
motion, amel. - alum., **VALER.**
walking, fast - mag-c., thuj.
inflammation - ruta, ***sep., zinc.***
injuries to - ***calen.,*** ruta.
jerking, evening - rat.
pain - aesc., aur-m-n., benz-ac., berb., bry., calad., ***calc., cann-s.,*** carb-ac., ***carb-an.,*** cimic., ***cinnb.,*** coc-c., ***colch.,*** euphr., ign., ***kali-bi.,*** laur., ***led., merc.,*** merl., mill., mur-ac., nat-s., rat., rhod., rhus-t., ruta, thuj., ***zinc.***
exertion, on - ***ign.***
morning - sulph.
night - mur-ac.
rheumatic - bry., cimic.
stairs, when going up - rhus-t.
standing - benz-ac., berb.
walking, while - berb., bry., cimic., ***cinnb.,*** coc-c., ***ign.***
after - cinnb., coc-c., merc.
continued amel. - ***kali-bi., rhod., rhus-t.***
when stepping on the toes - kali-bi.
pulsation - prun., zinc.
sharp, pain - am-c., aur., berb., camph., cimic., hep., mur-ac., nat-m., rhus-t., sil., sul-ac., tarent., thuj.
limb hangs down, when - berb.
rest, during - aur.
sore, pain - ***aesc., bry.,*** carb-ac., ***cimic.,*** coc-c., mill.
sprained, as if - kreos.
stiffness - cimic.
swelling - berb., kali-bi., ***mur-ac., sep., zinc.***
tearing, pain - ***alum.,*** bell., berb., ***calc., caust.,*** cic., ***colch., ign., kali-c.,*** mez., nat-s., rat., thuj., ***zinc.***
evening - ***alum.***
exertion, on - ***ign.***
extending upwards - rat.
insertion, at the - colch.
standing, when - rat.
walking, while - ***ign.***
tension - berb., ***caust.,*** cimic., graph., mag-c., mur-ac., phos., ran-b., ***sep.,*** sulph., teucr., ***zinc.***

ACHILLES tendons
torn, tendons - ***calen.***
twitching - cedr., merc., tab.
visible - merc.
weakness - lyc., valer.
morning - lyc.
sitting, while - valer.

ACHING, pain - ***agar.,*** cann-i., carb-ac., cast-eq., coloc., con., dios., hell., jug-c., ***lac-d.,*** laur., ***led.,*** naja, nat-p., ox-ac., plan., ***podo.,*** ptel., puls-n, ***rhus-t.,*** rhus-v., sep., sin-n., stront-c., stry., sul-i., tab., zinc.
menses, after - nat-p.
morning - carb-ac.
motion amel. - plan., **RHUS-T.**
sitting, while - bry., chel., phys., **RHUS-T.**
amel. - cycl.
standing - cycl., stront.
walking, while - calc-p., cycl., stront.
after - ***rhus-t.***

BANDAGED, sensation, as if - acon., calc., helo., petr.

BOILS - merc.

BORING, pain - agar., am-c., ang., apis, aur., aur-m-n., bufo, chel., clem., coloc., graph., grat., hell., led., ***mez.,*** nat-s., plan.
anterior part - chel., merc-i-f.
bones - ***mez.***
evening, on lying down - plan.
inner sides - spig.
morning - mez.
waking, on - mez.
motion agg. - bufo, mez.
outer side - arg-n.
rheumatic - plan.
sitting - agar., coloc., grat., led.
standing - aur-m-n., ***mez.***
walking, while - coloc., ***mez.***

BROKEN, sensation as if - calc., carb-s., caust., graph., hep.
morning in bed - carb-s.
walking, while - calc., caust., hep.

BURNING, pain - agar., berb., euph., kreos., laur., manc., nat-c., nit-ac., plat., ***puls.,*** sulph., verat., ***zinc.***
bones - ruta.
evening - sulph.
extending over the soles to the toes - kreos.
malleolus, internal - berb., laur., spig., zinc.
behind - rheum.
outer - kali-n.
when standing - ruta.
side - all-c., ang.
over heel - agar.
rubbing agg. - sulph.
top of - ***puls.***
walking, while - agar.

COLDNESS - ***acon.,*** agar., berb., caust., chin., lach.
malleolus, inner, in spots - berb.
walking in open air - chin.

COMPRESSION, sensation - chlf., led., nat-m., nat-s., sep., thuj.
walking in open air, after - sep.

CONSTRICTION - acon., cham., graph., helo., petr., ***plat.***
as if tied with a string - acon., am-br.

CONTRACTION, tendons - sep., spig.

CRACKING, joints, in - am-c., ant-c., aster., ***camph.,*** **CANTH.,** carb-s., caust., hep., kali-bi., mag-s., ***nit-ac.,*** nux-v., petr., ph-ac., rhus-t., sars., ***sep.,*** sulph., thuj.
bending - ant-c.
side to side - caust.
evening - am-c.
false step - caust.
stepping - euphr.
stretching, on - ant-c., thuj.
walking, while - carb-s., ***nit-ac.,*** nux-v., sulph.

CRAMPS - agar., calc-p., carl., cupr., dulc., ***plat.,*** sel.
evening - sel.
evening, lying, while - sel.
extending, calf - cupr.
over heel - agar.
to toes - nat-c.
night - iod.
waking - dulc.
walking amel. - dulc.
sleep, with feeling as if limbs were going to - ***plat.***

CUTTING, pain - arg-m., benz-ac., ***coloc.,*** eup-per., hyos., iodof., lyss., merc-i-f., rhus-t., sang., stry., tell., tep.
outer - meny.
walking in open air - benz-ac., iodof.

DECAY, bones, of - asaf., ***calc., guai.,*** plat-m., ***puls., sil.***
internal malleolus - ***sil.***

DISCOLORATION
blue spots - ***sul-ac.,*** sulph.
dark, spreading up the limb - naja
purple - arn., ***lach.***
spots - **SUL-AC.**
redness - apis, ars-h., calc., ***cham.,*** lac-ac., ***lach.,*** lyc., rhus-t., sul-ac.
spots, in - calc., lyc., **SUL-AC.**
spots, in, in afternoon - lyc.
streaks - ferr-ma.
tetter - all-s.
white in spots - ***calc.***

DISLOCATION - arn., ***bry.,*** nat-c., nux-v., ruta, sulph.
left - kali-bi.
dislocation, as if, feeling - ***bry.,*** calc-p., kali-bi., verat-v.

DRAWING, pain - abrot., ***agar.,*** alum., ambr., anac., ang., arg-m., ***ars.,*** aster., aur-m-n., bapt., cact., camph., cann-s., ***caul.,*** caust., cham., chel., coloc., com., cupr., dig., dios., erig., fl-ac., indg., kali-bi., kali-c., kreos., ***led.,*** lyc., mang-m., med., mez., naja, nat-m., nat-s., nit-ac., ptel., puls-n, rhod., rhus-t., rhus-v., sil., spig., spong., staph., stram., stront-c., sulph., tarax., thuj., **VALER.,** zinc.
afternoon - indg., ptel.
cramp-like - arg-m., sulph.
daytime - mang-m.
evening - fl-ac., indg., kali-c., lyc., nat-s., ptel., stram., sulph.
walking, while - fl-ac.
extending upward - ars., fl-ac., guai., kreos., phos., rhus-v., spong.
forenoon - cham., kali-c.
lying, while - aur-m-n.
morning - lyc., sulph.
waking, on - sulph.
walking, while - ang.
motion - fl-ac., staph.
amel. - arg-m., bism., indg., ***valer.***
night - cham., nat-m.
waking, on - kali-c., nat-m.
outer malleous - am-c., kali-n.
paralytic - phos.
paroxysmal - coloc.
rheumatic - stram.
rising, after - coloc.
sitting, while - ang., caust., dig., indg., nat-s., **VALER.,** verat.
standing, while - anac., camph., kali-n., spig.
stepping, on - kali-c., nat-s.
tearing - clem., kali-bi., spong., tarax.
walking, while - ang., coloc., erig.
amel. - arg-m., **VALER.**

ECZEMA - ***chel.,*** nat-p., ***psor.***

ERUPTIONS - cact., ***calc.,*** calc-p., ***chel.,*** osm., ***psor.,*** puls., rhus-v., sel., sep., stront-c., tep.
dry - cact.
maleolus - ***cact.***
moist - chel.
patches - ***calc.***
pimples - calc-p., sep., stront-c., sulph.
pustules - cupr-ar., ***lach.***
red - calc., chel., sars.
spots - puls.

ERYSIPELAS - ***lach., rhus-t.,*** tep.

FISTULOUS, opening - ***calc-p.***
joints - ***calc.,*** hep., ol-j., **PHOS., SIL.,** ***sulph.***

FORMICATION - ars-i., meph., pall., rhus-v.
extending to os calcis - rhus-v.

GNAWING, pain - berb., graph., laur., sars., sulph.
anterior part - berb.
bones - graph.
morning, on waking - sulph.
outer behind - meny.

HEAT - ang., cycl., euph., hyos., ***kali-bi.,*** laur., lyc., osm., rat.

HEAVINESS - alum., caust., cupr., kali-c., nat-m., nit-ac., sil., sulph.

HERPES - cact., cycl., ***kreos.,*** nat-c., ***nat-m., petr.,*** sulph.

INFLAMMATION - arn., bry., kali-c., ***mang.,*** phyt., rhus-t.

INJURIES - **ARN.,** bell-p, **BRY.,** ***calc.,*** hyper., ***led.,*** nat-c., **RHUS-T., RUTA.,** ***stront-c., symph.***

ITCHING - agar., ambr., apis, aur., berb., bor., bov., cact., calc., carb-ac., ***chel.,*** cocc., com., cycl., dios., hep., jug-c., kali-c., ***lach.,*** **LED.,** lith., lyc., ***nat-p.,*** olnd., osm., pall., ph-ac., ran-b., rhus-t., rhus-v., ***sel.,*** sep., sulph., thea., vinc.
biting - berb.
below - ant-c.
burning - berb., calc., ***lith.,*** petr., staph.
on falling to sleep - mur-ac.
corrosive - dig.
evening - rhus-v., ***sel.,*** sep., sulph.
inner - tarax.
right - staph.
morning - sep.
bed, in - kali-c.
night - hep.
outer - petr.
red from scratching - ph-ac.
scratching, agg. - ***led.***
spots - vinc.
sticking - berb.
tingling - com.
walking, while - aur., cocc., dios.
warmth, agg. - **LED.,** rhus-v.
amel. - cocc.

JERKING - ***calc.,*** stann.

LAMENESS - abrot., aesc., ***arn.,*** bry., caps., cedr., com., dios., fl-ac., laur., lil-t., lyss., plb., **RUTA.**
evening, walking, while - fl-ac.
morning - dios., plb.
rising, after - caps.
sitting, while - ***nat-m.***
sprain after - ***rhus-t.,*** **RUTA.**
sudden - com.
walking, while - ***nat-m.***
in open air - com.

NUMBNESS - caust., cycl., glon., hep., ***lac-c.,*** nat-m., rhus-t., sulph.
night - ***sulph.***

PAIN, ankles - abrot., acon., agar., ***all-c.,*** alum., alumn., ant-c., ***ant-t., arn.,*** ars., asc-t., aster., bapt., bell., benz-ac., berb., ***bol.,*** bov., **BRY.,** cact., cann-i., ***carb-an., caul., caust., cham., chel.,*** colch., con., ***cop.,*** dios., dros., ferr., ferr-ar., ferr-p., form., gels., graph., ***guai.,*** jatr., kali-n., ***kalm., lac-ac.,*** lac-c., lach., **LED.,** lil-t., ***lith.,*** lyss., lob-s., ***lyc.,*** med., merc., ***mez.,*** nat-m., nat-p., nat-s., osm., ph-ac., ***phos., phyt.,*** plat., plb., podo., puls., ran-b., rhus-v., rumx., ***sal-ac.,*** seneg., sep., sin-n., spig., spong., stict., stry., sul-ac., thuj., valer., verat., xan., zinc.
afternoon - dios., rhus-v., verat.
3 p.m. - lyc., tab., tax.
anterior part - acon., berb., calc-p., chel., ruta.
burning - berb.
pulsating - ruta.
rheumatic - acon.
ascending, stairs - alumn., ***plb.***
dislocated, as if - arn., bry., ***calc-p., ruta.***
as if it would dislocate - calc., ruta.

PAIN, ankles
evening - dios., led., nat-c., nat-s., plan.
lying, while - nat-s., plan.
extending, outward - ***lith.***
soles - stann.
toes, to - lil-t.
upward - bell., ferr., nat-s., phos., plb., puls.
gonorrhea, suppressed, after - ***med.,*** thuj.
gouty - cimic., **LED.,** petr.
inner side - ang., com., dios., hyper., lob-s., merc., trom.
jarring - lil-t.
malleolus - bry., calc., coloc., plb., sulph., verat-v.
internal - berb., bov., chel., hura, kali-bi., mez., verat-v.
internal, as from a blow - hell.
internal, right - tarent.
outer - am-c., carb-ac., cic., lach., laur., thuj.
outer, walking - arg-m.
menses, after - nat-p.
morning - all-c., alumn., carb-ac., carb-s., dios., ***led.,*** mez., sep., sulph.
stepping - rheum.
walking - alumn., mez., plb., psor.
walking, amel. - sulph.
motion - ***arn.,*** bol., bry., bufo, ***cham., chel.,*** cocc., ***guai., kalm., led.,*** lil-t., sulph., zinc.
motion, amel. - aur-m-n., dios., nat-s., plan., valer.
night - lyc., petr., ***sulph.***
11 p.m. to 7 a.m. - sulph.
2 a.m. - agar.
outer, side - abrot., arg-n., fl-ac., rhus-t., verat.
evening - fl-ac.
paralytic - caust., nat-p., par., ph-ac., plb.
paroxysmal - coloc., hep., sil.
pulsating - lith-m., ***ruta.***
rheumatic - am-c., bapt., cact., ***chel.,*** chin-s., clem., colch., gnaph., ***guai., kalm., lac-c., lyc., ol-j.,*** plan., sang., stict., syph., urt-u., verat-v., viol-o., zinc.
running, while - mez.
sitting - arg-n., aur-m-n., bry., ***caust.,*** led., nat-s., **VALER.**
standing - cycl., led., rhus-v., stront-c., ***sulph.,*** **VALER.**
step, from a false - caust., chel., coloc., **LED.**
stepping, when - bor., bry., **LED.,** ***mez.,*** nat-m., rhus-t., sil.
stunning - thuj.
touch - ars., graph., kali-n., lyc., nat-m., sep.
ulcerative - am-m., kali-n., nat-m.
waking, on - ambr., mez.
walking, while - alumn., ambr., am-m., aster., bry., calc-p., caust., chel., cycl., ***dros.,*** fl-ac., kali-n., ***kalm., led.,*** lith., mez., nit-ac., ***phos.,*** puls., rhus-v., ruta., stront-c., stry., sulph.
amel. - ambr., caust., ph-ac., ***rhus-t.,*** sulph., **VALER.**

PAIN, ankles
warmth, agg. - ***guai.,*** lac-c., **LED., PULS.**
amel. - chel.

PARALYSIS - ***abrot.,*** ang., nat-m., ruta.
sitting, while - nat-m.
walking, while - nat-m.
paralysis, sensation of - ***dros.,*** nat-m.
walking - ***dros.***

PINCHING, pain - osm., sulph.
right - osm.

PRESSING, pain - ***agar.,*** all-c., ambr., arg-n., aur., aur-m-n., berb., brom., camph., ***chel.,*** clem., coloc., crot-t., dig., gins., graph., hell., ign., indg., lac-c., ***led.,*** mang-m., mez., nat-m., nat-s., nit-ac., seneg., sep., spig., sul-ac., verat., verb.
below - zinc.
bones - ***bism.,*** cupr., ***led.,*** sabin., staph.
cramp-like - verb.
daytime - mang-m.
dinner, after - indg.
evening - crot-t., nat-s.
after lying down - nat-s.
midnight, motion agg. - ***led.***
waking, on - ambr.
morning - ang., ***led.***
waking, on - mez.
motion, agg. - lac-c., ***led.,*** nat-s.
amel. - aur-m-n., indg., nat-s.
paroxysmal - coloc., indg.
sitting - agar., arg-n., aur-m-n., coloc., led., nat-s.
stepping - bor.
standing - spig.
waking, on - ambr., mez.
walking - ang., camph., coloc., gins., merc., nat-s.
after - sep.

PULSATION - am-m., arg-m., dros., kali-c., ruta.
lying - dros.
night - dros.

RASH - osm., tep.

SENSITIVE - ars-h., graph., sars.

SHARP, pain - abrot., ***acon.,*** agar., ***alum.,*** ambr., ang., ant-c., apis, apoc., arg-n., arn., ars-i., asar., aur., bapt., bar-c., berb., ***bov.,*** bufo, ***calc.,*** calc-p., cann-s., carb-s., carb-v., caust., cham., chel., chin-s., clem., coff., colch., coloc., con., crot-t., dios., dros., ferr-p., form., gins., gran., graph., guai., ham., ***hell.,*** hep., ign., indg., iod., kali-c., kreos., lach., led., ***lith.,*** lyc., mang., merc., mosch., naja, nat-c., nat-m., nit-ac., nux-v., ol-an., osm., petr., ph-ac., phos., psor., puls., rhod., ***rhus-t., ruta.,*** sang., sep., sil., spig., stann., staph., stront-c., sulph., thuj., trom., verat., verb., viol-t., xan., zinc.
above - meny.
anterior part - berb.
below, outer ankle, walking - nat-c.
bones - aur., puls.
cramp-like - rhus-t.
evening - kali-c., merc., stront.
bed, in - lyc., zinc.

SHARP, pain
extending to, calf - con.
to, foot - hell., kreos.
to, heel, over - agar.
to, knee - guai.
to, outward - lith., mosch.
to, tibia - ph-ac.
to, toes - graph., hell., kreos.
to, upwards - aur., caust., guai., mang., nux-v.
forenoon - chin-s., kali-c.
inner side - berb., ph-ac.
itching - stann.
malleolus - bapt., berb., iod., kali-c., lach., nit-ac., phos., valer.
internal - berb., chel., coc-c., coff., indg., nat-m., rhus-t., spig., tarax.
sitting, while - berb., par., tarax.
walking - puls.
morning, on every step - graph., psor.
motion, on - bar-c., bufo, kreos., sulph.
amel. - ***cham.***
night, lying, while - dros.
outer - agar., apis, arg-m., arg-n., ***bov.,*** bry., chin-s., clem., dios., mang., sars., sil., sulph., thuj.
burning - thuj.
sitting, when - agar., arg-m.
walking - mang., sulph.
running, on - berb.
sitting - ang., con., guai.
standing - berb.
stepping, on - alum., graph., kali-c., phos., psor., sil.
stretching foot - sulph.
sudden - indg.
tearing - caust., guai.
waking - con.
walking, while - agar., berb., kali-c., ***lach.,*** lyc., mang., sulph.
rapidly - con.
washing with cold water amel. - cann-s.

SHOOTING, pain- ***acon.,*** apis, aur., berb., bufo, ***calc-p., ferr-p.,*** naja, nux-v., osm., sep., trom., xan.
extending to knee - guai.
motion agg. - bufo.
over the heels - agar.
upwards - aur., guai., nux-v.

SHUDDERING- lyc.

SORE, pain - agar., agn., am-m., arg-m., ***arn.,*** ars., berb., cann-s., cham., chlf., cinnb., clem., con., dig., hep., hyos., mag-c., ***mez.,*** nat-m., plat., rhus-v., ruta., sel., sil., spig., valer.
afternoon - hyos., ***valer.***
below - mur-ac.
jarring agg. - ***valer.***
malleolus, inner - ***arg-m.***
morning - mag-c.
motion amel. - mez.
outer malleolus - valer.
sitting, while - arg-m., gins.
standing, while - mag-c., mez., valer.
stepping - mag-c., nat-m.

SORE, pain
sudden - valer.
touch - ars., mur-ac., nat-m., plat.
walking, while - am-m., mag-c., mez., nat-m.
long amel. - mag-c.

SPRAINED, as if - agar., all-s., aloe, **ANAC.,** ang., ant-c., **ARN.,** ars., asc-t., bar-c., **BRY.,** ***calc.,*** camph., carb-v., caust., chel., chin., chin-s., coca, cocc., cycl., dig., dros., eup-per., fl-ac., gran., graph., hell., hep., ign., laur., **LED.,** kali-bi., kali-n., lyc., ***merc.,*** mosch., nat-m., nat-s., nit-ac., nux-v., ph-ac., ***phos.,*** plat., plb., ***prun.,*** psor., puls., **RHUS-T., RUTA.** sep., ***sil., stront-c.,*** sulph., tep., thuj., ***valer.,*** verat., zinc.
bending from side to side - caust.
edema, with - ***stront.***
evening - gran.
evening, walking, while - verat.
false step - caust.
flexion - chin-s.
lying in bed - aloe.
morning - plb.
rising, on - dig., nat-s., nit-ac.
rising, on, after - rheum.
rising, on, after walking - camph.
standing - coca.
walking, preventing - dig., nat-s.
walking, while - ign., nux-v., plb., psor.
motion, on - ***bry.,*** cocc., sulph., zinc.
night, standing - coca.
outer - kali-n., mez.
paroxysmal - hep.
room, amel. - graph.
running, up stairs - **VALER.**
sitting, amel. - cycl.
standing, when - chin-s., cycl., sulph., **VALER.**
stepping - ars.
on left foot - **ANAC.**
stooping, on - cycl.
stretching, when - dig.
turning foot outward - ant-c.
walking, while - caust., cycl., ***dros.,*** fl-ac., hep., ***phos.,*** psor., puls., sep., sulph.
amel. - **VALER.**
in open air - graph.

STIFFNESS - ars., carb-an., **CAUST., CHEL.,** cocc., ***coloc.,*** con., dios., dros., graph., hep., ***hyper.,*** kali-c., lath., led., ***lyc.,*** med., nat-m., ***petr.,*** plb., **RHUS-T.,** ***ruta.,*** sep., **SIL., SULPH.,** sul-ac., ter., verb., ***zinc.***
evening - sep.
exercise amel. - dios., sulph.
morning, on rising - caps., carb-an.
sitting, after - zinc.
walking, while - led., sul-ac., sumb.

SUPPURATION - arn., hep.

SWELLING - ambr., ant-s., **APIS,** apoc., arn., ***ars., asaf.,*** aur-m., benz-ac., ***cact., calc., cench., chel., coloc., cop., dig., eup-per., ferr.,*** ferr-ar., ***graph., hep., hydr.,*** hyos., ***lac-c.,*** lac-d., ***lach., led.,*** lil-t., ***lyc.,*** manc., mang., **MED., MERC.,** merc-sul., ***ol-j.,*** onos., plb., ***phos., phyt.,*** podo., prun., ***psor., puls., rhus-t.,*** rhus-v., ***ruta.,*** sal-ac., samb., sep., sil., stann., stict., sulph., verat-v., xan., zinc., ziz.
bones - merc., staph.
cold - asaf.
dyspnea, with - hep.
evening - sep., stann.
walking, while - merc.
hot - kali-c.
menses, during - eup-per.
painful - ars., ***led.,*** plb.
rheumatic - cact., ***chel., kalm., lach.***
sharp - phos.
sudden - stann.
tendons, of - phos.
veins of - ***lac-c., lyc.,*** sars.
swelling, sensation of - laur., ox-ac., ***phos.,*** plat.

TEARING, pain - ***acon., agar.,*** alum., ambr., am-c., am-m., ammc., ***arg-m., arn., ars.,*** bar-ac., **BELL.,** berb., bism., calc., ***calc-p.,*** camph., carb-an., carb-s., cham., ***chin.,*** chin-a., cic., clem., ***colch.,*** coloc., con., ***dros.,*** euph., ***guai.,*** gins., hell., indg., kali-bi., **KALI-C.,** kali-n., lac-c., lact., led., ***lyc.,*** mang-m., mez., nat-a., nat-c., ***nat-s.,*** puls., rat., **RHUS-T.,** rumx., sabin., samb., sil., spong., stann., staph., stront-c., sulph., tarax., tep., ***teucr.,*** thuj., trom., ***zinc.***
afternoon - carb-s., con., trom.
5 p.m. - lyc.
anterior - agar., berb., rumx.
bed, before going to - ammc.
constrictive - stront.
cramp-like - kali-c.
drawing - dulc.
evening in bed - samb.
extending to, knee - ars., ***guai.,*** kreos., spong.
to, toes - am-c., hell., stann.
upwards - **BELL.,** caust., con., samb.
inner side - dulc., mez., thuj.
lying, while - ars., sep.
amel. - sil.
malleolus - alum., ambr., am-c., arn., berb., grat., mez., nat-m., par., phos., sil., spong.
inner - ***agar.,*** arg-m., berb., puls., zinc.
outer - arn., canth., con., kali-n., mag-m., par., rhod., samb., stront-c., zinc.
midnight - stront.
waking, on - coloc.
morning - puls.
motion of foot, on - puls.
waking, on - nat-s.
motion, agg. - ars., bry., kali-bi., puls.
amel. - arg-m., cham., dros., **RHUS-T.,** sulph.
night - phos.
waking, on - kali-c., ***lyc.,*** nat-m.
noon - con., kali-bi.
until evening - con.
outer side - berb., bism., caust., dulc., kali-n., merl., nat-c., rat., thuj.
paralytic - dros., til.
pulsative - ol-an.
right - agar., dros., kali-n., nat-m., rat.
rubbing - zinc.

TEARING, pain
sitting, while - agar., am-m., arg-m., coloc., con., kali-n., sep., stann., teucr.
standing, while - kali-n., rat.
walking - camph., ***dros.,*** plan., puls.
amel. - ***bell.,*** teucr.
wandering - lact.
warm feet amel. - kali-c.
warmth amel. - am-c., ars.

TENSION - aesc., aur., bell., bry., calc., carb-v., ***caust.,*** con., lyc., mang-m., med., ***merc.,*** nat-m., ***phos.,*** seneg., sep., sil., sulph., tep., thuj., vip., zinc.
drawing, pressive - calc.
inner - calc., ph-ac.
morning - con., lyc.
motion - **BRY.**
amel. - calc., zinc.
outer - euphr.
painful - seneg.
rheumatic - zinc.
sitting, while - nat-m., sil.
walking, while - phos., sep., sulph., thuj.
in open air - bell.

TINGLING, prickling, asleep, night, on waking - bar-c.

TUMORS- cupr-ar.

TWITCHING - agar., asaf., carb-s., iod., mag-m., mez.

ULCERS - ***calc-p.,*** carb-ac., cist., ***hydr.,*** merc-i-f., merc-sul., puls., rhus-t., sars., sep., sil., sulph., ***syph.***
chronic - ***carb-ac.***
fetid - ***carb-ac., calc-p., lyc.,*** sulph.
fistulous - ***calc-p.,*** sil.
malleolus - ***calc-p.***
painful - ***lach.,*** rhus-t.
painless - ***calc.***
spreading - ***merc.***

URTICARIA- ***nat-m.***

VESICLES - aster., rhus-v., sel.

WEAKNESS - abrot., agn., aloe, arg-n., arn., ars., ***calc.,*** calc-s., **CARB-AN.,** carb-s., ***caust.,*** chlf., cic., com., dios., ***ferr.,*** ferr-ar., glon., kali-c., ***lac-d.,*** med., merc., mez., **NAT-A., NAT-C.,** ***nat-m.,*** **NAT-P., NAT-S., NIT-AC.,** nux-v., phos., phys., plb., puls., **RHUS-T.,** ***rhus-v.,*** **RUTA,** ***sep.,*** **SIL., STRONT-C.,** ***sulph., sul-ac.,*** valer.
bath, warm, after - calc.
children learning to walk - **CARB-AN.,** nat-p.
morning - agn., coca.
walking, while - agn., valer.
motion on - laur., nux-v.
night - sulph.
outer - petr.
running, while - mez.
sitting, while - paeon.
walking, after - caust.
standing, while - calc.
stepping - phos.
sudden - com.

WEAKNESS, ankles
walking while - agn., aloe, carb-an., com., med., ***nat-c.,*** **NIT-AC.,** nux-v., plb., sulph.
air, in open - mez.
amel. - caust.
begining to walk - mez.

Arms

ABSCESS - anan., sil.
gangrenous - anan.
wounds, dissecting, after - ***ars., lach., sil.***
abscess, forearms - plb.
abscess, upper arms - agar.
deltoid - agar.

ACHING, pain - alum., arg-n., ***ars.,*** asaf., benz-ac., berb., ***bry., cact., calc.,*** calc-p., cann-i., ***carb-ac.,*** carb-s., caust., cham., chin-s., com., croc., dios., dirc., dol., ***dulc.,*** euphr., **EUP-PER.,** fl-ac., gamb., gels., glon., ham., ip., jug-c., kalm., lac-c., lach., lil-t., lob-s., lyss., lyc., merc., merc-i-f., mosch., myric., naja, nat-a., ***nit-ac.,*** ph-ac., phyt., pip-m., puls., raph., rhod., staph., ***sumb.,*** tarax., thuj., verat-v., zing.
afternoon - erig., verat-v.
bones - apis, calc-p., **EUP-PER.,** glon.
eating, after - cocc.
extending, down - sumb.
into forearm - dios.
to fingers - calc-p., euphr.
forenoon - jac-c., jug-c., verat-v.
left - sumb.
morning - fago.
motion agg. - nat-a.
singing, when - stann.
touch agg. - ip.
wandering - plan.
writing, while - merc-i-f.
aching, forearms - agar., aloe, bell., ***calc-p., carb-ac.,*** carb-an., carb-s., chlor., cic., cinnb., cocc., corn., dios., elat., **EUP-PER.,** fl-ac., hell., hyos., jatr., ***merc., merc-i-f.,*** merc-i-r., nux-m., phys., phyt., ***rhus-t.,*** sabad., ***sabin.,*** sep., sil., spig., sulph., tarent., trom., verat-v.
afternoon - lycps., nat-s.
4 p.m. - sulph.
bending the arm - sabad.
evening - com., dios.
bed, after going to - phyt.
extending, outward - nux-v.
to hand - elat., fl-ac., nit-ac., trom.
forenoon - trom.
intermittent - trom.
left - ***carb-ac.***
morning - nat-a.
motion, during - sabad., ***sabin.***
amel. - **RHUS-T.,** spig.
night - aloe.
11 p.m. - com.
posterior part - berb., chin-s.
forenoon - chin-s.
radius - ***sabin.***
sitting, while - led., **RHUS-T.**
touch agg. - ***sabin.***
ulna - verat-v.
waking, on - lycps.
writing, while - anac.
aching, upper arms - abrot., anac., arg-m., arg-n., calc., cinnb., com., cupr., **EUP-PER.,** gels., kali-n., kali-p., led., lob., merc-i-r., mez., paeon., **RHUS-T.,** rumx., sabad., sabin., stram., tep., vesp., zinc.
bone - hyos., iod., mag-s., ox-ac., phyt., rhod., sulph.
about the elbow - still., verat.
evening - ox-ac.
external condyle - asaf., sil., verat-v.
motion agg. - phyt.
evening - anac., ox-ac.
sitting - anac.
walking in open air - anac.
forenoon - com.
morning, in bed - euph.
motion, agg. - sabad., ***sabin.***
amel. - kali-p.
posterior part - jatr.
riding, while - abrot.
singing, when - stann.
touch, on - arg-m., sabin.

AIR, passing down from shoulder to finger, sensation as if - ***fl-ac.***

ALIVE, sensation of something, in arms - ***ign.***

ARTHRITIC, nodosites, forearm - am-c.

BEND, irresistible desire to - **FERR.**

BLOOD, rush of to, arms - calc., ***nux-v.,*** rhod., sil., **SULPH.**

BOILS - aloe, am-c., ars., bar-c., ***bell., brom., calc.,*** carb-an., carb-v., cob., coloc., elaps, graph., guare., iod., iris, ***kali-n., lyc.,*** mag-m., ***mez.,*** **PETR.,** ph-ac., **RHUS-T.,** ***sil.,*** sulph., syph., ***zinc.***
boils, forearms - ***calc.,*** carb-v., cob., ***iod., lach.,*** lyc., mag-m., ***nat-s.,*** petr., sil.
boils, upper arms - aloe, ***bar-c.,*** carb-v., coloc., ***crot-h.,*** iod., jug-r., mez., ***sil., zinc.***

BORING, pain - aran., aur., bar-c., bov., carb-v., carb-an., caust., coloc., gran., mang., mez., nat-c., ***nat-m.,*** phos., plb., ***rhod.,*** stann., ***thuj.***
afternoon - coloc.
bones - ars., kali-bi., sabad.
extending to fingers - gran.
morning - aran., plb.
lying on arm amel. - carb-an.
boring, forearms - am-c., arg-n., asaf., aur., aur-m-n., bov., calc., caust., coloc., dulc., hell., hep., led., mez., nat-c., ***ph-ac.,*** plan., plb., ran-s., spig., spong., thuj.
anterior part - asaf., plb., spong.
bones - nat-c., ***ph-ac.,*** rhus-t.
motion, on - rhus-t.
night - arg-n.
sitting, while - led.
ulna - arg-n.
boring, upper arms - aur., aur-m-n., canth., carb-an., ***cina, mang.,*** merc-i-f., mez.
bones - ***carb-v.,*** cocc., kali-bi., ***mang.,*** tep.
deltoid - stann.
lying on painful side - mang.

boring, upper arms
morning - mez.
waking, on - mez.
motion amel. - cina, mang.
night - mang.
right - merc-i-f.

BOUND, left arm feels as if bound to the side - cimic.

BROKEN, sensation as if - chel., nat-m., ***puls.,*** verat.
bones - nat-m.
left - cahin.
motion agg. - ***puls.***
pressure agg. - ***puls.***

broken, forearms, sensation as if - arn., calc-p., cupr.
radius - gymn.

broken, upper arm, sensation as if - bar-ac., cocc., cupr., puls., samb., sulph.
as if would break - bor., cinnb.
raising it, on - **COCC.**

BUBBLING, sensation, left - caust.

bubbling, forearms - spong., zinc.

bubbling, upper arms - berb., colch., cupr., nux-m., petros., squil., zinc.
left - zinc.
posterior part - colch.
right - berb.

BURNING, pain - agar., alum., ***ars.,*** ars-h., arum-t., arund., ***asaf., aur.,*** aur-m., aur-m-n., ***bell.,*** berb., bry., bufo, calc., ***carb-v.,*** chin., ***com., con.,*** corn., crot-t., ***cur.,*** dig., graph., hep., jug-c., jug-r., kali-bi., kali-c., lith-m., lyc., lyss., mag-m., med., merc., mez., mur-ac., nat-c., nat-m., petr., ***ph-ac.,*** phos., plat., plb., puls., ***rhus-t.,*** rhus-v., sil., spong., stann., stram., sulph., thuj., ***urt-u.,*** zinc.
covering agg. - rhus-v.
evening - ***puls.***
extending, over body - apis
to fingers - mag-m.
to hand - fl-ac.
forenoon - cast.
joints - ***carb-v.,*** graph., ***nat-c.,*** stront.
left - cocc.
morning - agar.
motion, on - crot-t.
night - chin., til.
bed, in - chin.
paralytic - calc.
paroxysmal - cocc., ***plb.***
right - plat., plb.
rubbing - crot-t.
scratching, after - kreos., led., merc., til.
amel. - jug-c.
sore - dig.
spots - am-c., bry., merc., ph-ac.
steam, exposure to, agg. - kali-bi.
touch agg. - crot-t.
uncovering agg. - crot-t.
vexation, after - nat-m.
washing, after - bov.

burning, forearms - ***agar.,*** alum., am-c., am-m., asaf., aur., aur-m., aur-m-n., bell., ***berb.,*** bor., bov., calad., carb-an., carb-s., carb-v., card-m., ***caust.,*** chel., con., ***graph., kali-bi.,*** laur., lyc., mag-m., mang., merc., mez., mosch., mur-ac., nat-m., nat-s., ol-an., osm., ph-ac., phos., plb., prun., ran-s., rat., rhus-t., rhus-v., ***spong.,*** staph., stram., ***sulph.,*** tarax., tarent., ***thuj., urt-u.,*** vip., zinc.
anterior part - agar., am-c., berb., calad., chel., ol-an., plb.
external - aur-m-n., con., mur-ac.
motion, during - thuj., zinc.
near the wrist - agar., bov., caust., kali-bi., rhus-v., zinc.
night - graph., ***zinc.***
lying on it - graph.
outside - osm.
right - osm.
posterior part - berb., euph., ol-an., osm., prun.
pressure agg. - bell.
rubbing amel. - ol-an.
scratching, after - am-c., caust., bor., clem., laur., sulph.
spots - am-c., graph., sulph.
stinging in spots - ran-s.

burning, upper arms - ***agar.,*** alum., am-c., arg-n., arn., berb., bor., carb-s., carb-v., caust., colch., coloc., dig., dulc., graph., hura, kali-bi., kali-c., mang., mur-ac., nat-c., nat-m., nat-s., ph-ac., rhus-t., sep., sulph., thuj., zinc.
anterior surface - zinc.
biceps, in bed - rhus-t.
deltoid - nux-v.
dinner, after - zinc.
extending downwards - all-c.
externally - fl-ac.
inner side - berb., tarent.
lower part - agar., kali-c., led., mez.
night, in bed - arg-n.
posterior part - mur-ac., zinc.
pricking on motion - coloc.
scratching, after - mosch.
skin - arg-n., aur., nat-c., phos., sep., sulph.
spots, in - am-c., berb., graph., sulph.

CARBUNCLES, forearm - hep.

CHILLINESS - astac., bar-c., ***bell.,*** berb., ***calc.,*** carb-ac., ***caust.,*** cham., cinnb., euphr., ign., mez., petr., ***plat., puls.,*** sars., sil., thuj., zinc.
afternoon - sil.
anterior surface - puls.
evening after lying down - ***nux-v.***
extending to back and legs - mez.
left - stann.
posterior surface - raph.
right - phys., plat.
in open air - lyss.
stool, after - plat.
walking in open air - chin.

chilliness, upper arms - chel., puls.

CHOREA, left arm - cimic.

CLAWING, pain - lach.

CLUCKING - ambr.

COLDNESS - acon., am-c., amyg., ant-t., ars., arund., asaf., aster., bar-ac., **BELL.**, berb., bry., ***calc.***, ***camph.***, carb-s., carb-v., ***caust.***, chel., chin., chin-a., cic., cimic., con., crot-h., euphr., dig., ***dulc.***, fl-ac., ***graph.***, hell., hep., hyper., ign., iod., ip., kali-bi., kali-c., kali-chl., kali-s., kreos., ***led.***, lyc., merc-c., merl., ***mez.***, mosch., naja, nat-c., nat-m., nux-v., ***op.***, ox-ac., pall., **PHOS.**, ***plb.***, **PULS.**, ***rhus-t.***, ruta., sars., sec., sep., ***sil.***, spig., staph., sulph., sumb., tep., thuj., verat., vip., zinc.

afternoon - euphr., nux-v., sil.
2 p.m. - euphr.
5 p.m. - chel.
air, cold - kali-c., lyss.
as if blew upon left arm - aster.
as if passing down to fingers - fl-ac.
chill, during - bell., dig., hell., mez.
cough, during - ars., calc., ferr., ***hep.***, kali-c., ***rhus-t.***, rumx., sil.
eating, after - ars., camph.
evening - nux-v.
lying down, after - nux-v.
fever, after - sil.
forenoon - berb.
internal - ruta.
left - ars., aster., ***carb-v.***, fl-ac., naja, nux-m., rhus-t., sumb.
lying on the back - ign.
menses, during - mang.
before - mang.
morning - aur., caust., chel., dulc., hep., staph.
night - am-c.
1 a.m. - mang.
1 a.m, before menses - mang.
pain, during - chel., fl-ac.
paralyzed arm - am-c., ***dulc.***, ***rhus-t.***
raising them - verat.
rest, during - ***dulc.***
rheumatism, in - ***sang.***
right - am-c., ant-t., berb., chel., dulc., hell., merl., pall.
sitting, while - chin.
stiffness, and numbness, with - aster., sulph.
thrill, a cold, down arm - ***lyss.***
walking in a warm room - squil.
in a open air - sil.
water, as if dashed with cold - mez.
wind, as from cold - aster.

coldness, forearms - ***arg-n.***, ars., bry., ***brom.***, ***calc.***, caust., ***cedr.***, con., ***crot-c.***, **GRAPH.**, hydrc., kali-chl., nux-v., **PHOS.**, plb., rhus-t., verat-v.
icy cold - **BROM.**, rhus-t., thuj.
menses, during - ***arg-n.***
morning - nux-v.
after rising - nux-v.
right - caust., med.

coldness, upper arms - coloc., graph., ***ign.***, mez., nat-m., ph-ac., puls., ran-b., rhus-t., sulph., sumb., tep.
burning, with - graph.

coldness, upper arms
dinner, after - ***puls.***
eating, after - coloc.
safter - ran-b.
wind, as if, blew on them - nat-m., tep.

COMPRESSION, forearms - led., nat-s.
left - led., nat-s.

compression, upper arms - am-m., brom., led., nat-s.

CONSTRICTION - alumn., brom., ***chin.***, coloc., nit-ac., ***nux-m.***, raph.
bones - con.
right - cupr.
spasmodic while writing - sul-ac.

constriction, forearms - cupr., gins.
right - cupr.
vise, as in - brom.
walking in open air - mez.

constriction, upper arms - alumn., bism., manc., mez., phys., plat.
above the elbow - phys.
near shoulder - alumn.
right - ***alumn.***

CONTRACTION, muscles and tendons - agar., all-s., ant-t., ***ars.***, atro., bell., ***calc.***, cann-i., carb-s., ferr., ***hydr-ac.***, ***ip.***, ***lyc.***, merc., merc-c., nux-v., olnd., op., ox-ac., phos., plb., ran-b., rhod., ***rhus-t.***, sec., tab.
drink, on attempting to - atro.
extensor muscles when writing - nat-p.
flexor tendons - crot-h., sil.
paralysis, during - carb-s.
spasmodic - ***ip.***, tab.
walking, while - viol-t.
writing - sul-ac.

contraction, forearms, muscles and tendons - calc., calc-ar., ***caust.***, cina, coloc., con., hydrc., ***meny.***, mez., nat-c., plb., rheum, rhod., sep., stann., verat.
near the wrist - ***caust.***, sil.

contraction, upper arms, muscles and tendons - calc., **CAUST.**, ***nat-m.***, rhod., stram., sulph.
tendons - **CAUST.**

CONVULSION - acon., agar., am-c., apis, ars., arum-t., **BELL.**, bry., camph., cann-i., caust., ***cham.***, chin-a., ***cic.***, ***cocc.***, ***crot-c.***, cupr., cupr-s., hydr-ac., hyos., ***ign.***, ***iod.***, ***ip.***, jatr., kali-i., lyc., lyss., meny., ***merc-c.***, nat-m., ***op.***, phos., ***plat.***, plb., ruta., sabad., ***sec.***, ***sil.***, squil., ***stram.***, **STRY.**, ***sulph.***, sul-ac., tab., verat., verat-v.
clonic - cupr-s., sec., stry., sul-ac., zinc.
on attempting to use them - plb.
drawing, limb backwards - ***am-c.***
here and there - nit-ac.
epileptic, starting from - ***sulph.***
extending to, finger - acon.
to, trunk - agar-ph.
to, up and down after exertion - caust.
left - caust.
miscarriage, after - ruta.
more than legs - camph., ***stram.***

CONVULSION
night - bell., nux-v., sulph.
1 to 4 a.m. - tab.
one-sided - sabad.
prosopalgia, in - plat.
right to left - visc.
rotation, convulsive - ***camph.***
tetanic - anthr., camph., cann-s.
working hard with hands amel. - agar.
convulsion, forearms - chen-a., sec., zinc.
tetanic - zinc.
flexor muscles of - carb-o., cham.
radial side - merc.

CRACKED, skin - ***graph.,*** kali-ar., sil.

CRACKING, joints of - anac., ant-t., benz-ac., brach., chin-s., ***croc.,*** kali-bi., merc., mur-ac., sep., thuj.
when leaning on arm - thuj.

CRAMPS - agar., alum., **AM-C.,** ars., ant-t., ***bell.,*** bufo, cact., **CALC.,** caps., carb-s., carb-v., caust., cimic., cit-v., **COLOC.,** crot-c., cupr., dios., eupi., fl-ac., graph., guare., hura, hyper., iod., ***jatr.,*** kali-i., kali-s., lach., lyss., lyc., **MAG-P.,** merc., ***nat-m.,*** nux-v., phos., plb., sec., sulph., ***tab.,*** tril., valer.
evening 9 p.m. - lyc.
left - cact., caps.
midnight, after - sulph.
on waking - caust.
morning - fl-ac.
right - bufo
cramps, forearms - am-c., anac., arn., berb., ***calc.,*** calc-p., cina, coloc., corn., ferr-ma., graph., kali-i., lyc., mur-ac., ph-ac., plat., plb., ruta., sep.
afternoon - lyc.
anterior part - berb., plat., plb.
extensor muscles - merc.
flexing - arn., mur-ac.
flexor muscles - chin-s.
morning - calc.
motion agg. - kali-i., plb.
night, in bed - anac.
outer side - nat-c.
resting elbow - plat.
walking, while - sep.
cramps, upper arms - agar., arg-m., bell., com., kali-bi., lil-t., lyc., mag-c., mur-ac., petr., ***ph-ac.,*** rhus-t., sulph., valer.
biceps - ruta., valer.
deltoid - petr.
exertion, on - mur-ac.
holding something in hand, on - petr., rhus-t., valer.
inner side - sulph.
motion agg. - petr.
raising arm., on - arg-m.

CUTTING, pain - am-c., ***anac.,*** apis, ars-h., arund., bell., caust., con., dig., kali-c., manc., mang., mur-ac., ***nat-c.,*** ox-ac., petr., ph-ac., sars., stann., stry., sul-ac.
cutting, forearms - ars-m., bism., ***bov.,*** mosch., mur-ac., ***teucr.***
cutting, forearms
extensor muscles - mur-ac.
elbow, near - bell., mur-ac.
wrist, near - bell., dros., ***teucr.***
cutting, upper arms - anac., bar-c., caust., ***chel.,*** lac-c., manc., ***plat.,*** spig.
bending arm - anac.
biceps - hydr., iris.
deltoid region - caust., spig.
extending the arm - anac.
writing, while - ars-i.

DECAY, bones, of - ***sil.***
decay, upper arms, humerus - ***sil.***

DISCOLORATION
black - vesp.
in spots - vip.
blotches - chlol., rhus-v.
blue - ***apis,*** arg-n., bism., elaps, morph., sulph.
hanging down, while - sep.
in spots, both - **SUL-AC.**
reddish - vip.
with asthma - ***kali-c.***
brown spots - guare., ***lyc., petr.,*** thuj.
copper colored spots - ***nit-ac.***
ecchymoses - vip.
liver spots - ant-c., guare., lyc., ***mez.***
becoming dark - ***mez.***
itching - lyc.
livid - agar-ph., amyg., ***ars.,*** crot-h., ***lyc.,*** naja, ox-ac., vip., zinc-m.
marbled spots - berb.
mottled - amyg., ***lach.,*** naja, nat-m.
orange colored - cinnb., kali-i., rhus-t., vip.
petechiae - berb., cop., cupr., phos., phys.
purple - naja, vesp.
in spots - ars.
purpura haemorrhagica - ***lach., phos., sec., sul-ac.,*** ter.
redness - acon., ant-c., apis, arn., ars., ***bell.,*** bry., chin-s., chlol., cit-v., cupr., hydr-ac., jac-c., jug-c., ***kali-bi.,*** merc., merc-c., rhus-v., **RUTA.**, stram., sulph., vesp., vip.
drinking warm drinks - phos.
evening - fago.
streaks - apis, euph.
redness, spots - apis, aster., berb., bry., cop., ***cupr.,*** dulc., elaps, ***graph.,*** kali-bi., kali-i., ***lach.,*** led., merc., oena., ***phos.,*** phyt., plat., ***rhus-t.,*** sabad., sep., ***sulph., thuj.***
burning - sulph.
washing, after with soap - sulph.
spots - am-c., ant-c., berb., bry., crot-h., led., oena., tep., vip.
spots, livid - ***hell.,*** lyc.
white - berb.
,in spots - apis
yellow, in spots - petr., vip.
rings - nat-c.
discoloration, forearms
blotches - cimx., hura.
blue - apis, arg-n., bism., plat., sep.

discoloration, forearms
bluish spots - **SUL-AC.**
dark - acon., ant-c., ***ars.,*** caust., com., sep.
lividity - ***ars.,*** vesp., vip.
mottled - ***crot-h.,*** **LACH.**
purple spots - ***kali-c.,*** kali-p.
red - hura, kreos.
redness - anac., ***apis,*** arn., bell., colch., kreos., mang., rhus-t.
in spots - ***ars.,*** berb., bor., chel., ***euph.,*** kali-n., mang., ***merc.,*** olnd., rhus-v., sulph., tarent., tax., thuj., vesp.
redness, streaks - anthr., euph.
itching on touch - euph., kali-n.
spots - carb-o., mang., mill., nat-m.
white - ***berb.***

discoloration, upper arms
blue spots - plat.
ecchymoses - vip.
red spots - rhus-t.
redness - anac.

DISLOCATION, as if, feeling - ***ant-t.,*** merc., rhus-t.
joints - caps., ign., puls.
left - cahin.

DRAWING, pain - acon., aesc., ***agar.,*** am-c., anac., ant-c., apis, ***arg-m., arg-n., ars.,*** ars-h., asaf., aster., bapt., ***bar-c.,*** bell., bry., calad., cact., ***calc.,*** calc-p., camph., caps., carb-ac., carb-an., carb-s., ***carb-v.,*** carb-h., cast-eq., **CAUST.,** ***chel.,*** chin., chin-a., cic., cimic., ***cina,*** cinnb., cist., cit-v., ***clem.,*** cocc., ***coloc.,*** con., crot-h., crot-t., ***cupr.,*** cycl., dig., dulc., elaps, euph., ferr., ferr-ar., form., gins., gran., graph., grat., ***guai.,*** ign., indg., kali-bi., kali-c., ***kali-n.,*** kali-p., kalm., kreos., lach., laur., led., ***lyc., mag-c.,*** mag-m., mang., meph., merc., merc-c., merl., mez., nat-m., nat-s., ***nit-ac.,*** nux-m., ***nux-v.,*** ol-an., pall., petr., ph-ac., phos., ***phyt., plat.,*** plb., ***puls., rhod.,*** **RHUS-T.,** ***rhus-v.,*** sang., sec., seneg., ***sep., sil.,*** sol-n., stann., staph., stry., sul-ac., ***sulph.,*** tab., ***teucr.,*** tell., ***thuj.,*** til., ***valer.,*** verat., zinc., zing.
afternoon - elaps, thuj., zinc., zing.
alternating sides - sulph.
bones - alum., bar-c., carb-an., caust., cham., cocc., coloc., lyc., mag-c., nat-m., nit-ac., ***rhod.,*** sep., ***thuj., valer.***
chill, during - ars-h.
cramp-like - anac., elaps, kali-n., nux-m.
downward - agar., apis, aur., con., cycl., form., kali-c., lyc., ***nux-v.,*** pall., ph-ac., puls., rhus-t., rhus-v., seneg., ***sep.,*** sil.
to fingers - agar., apis, cist., cycl., lyc., ol-an., puls., rhus-t., rhus-v., ***sep.,*** sil.
to hand - kali-c., rhus-v.
draft - chin., verat.
drawn forward, sensation of, when hanging down limbs - phos.
epilepsy before - cupr.
evening - crot-t., kali-n., phos., staph., thuj., zing.
extending, into chest - lach.

DRAWING, pain
extending to fingers - aesc., bry., chel., crot-h., cycl., ***lyc., rhus-t., sep.,*** thuj.
to fourth finger - sil.
to hand - kali-c.
to wrist - am-c., ***puls.***
fever, catarrhal, during - sep.
flexor muscles - asaf., bol., ham.
forenoon - sulph.
forward, on attempting to raise arm - plb.
hanging down - ***cina,*** kali-n.
internal - euph., sulph.
inward - laur.
jerk-like - nux-m.
joints of - caul., kali-bi., kreos., ***mang.,*** rhod.
lain on, the one - **CARB-V.,** cina.
left - **RHUS-T.**
lying, arm under head - staph.
on back - cham.
sore, side amel. - cham.
menses, during - spong., ***stram.***
morning - lyc.
motion, agg. - con., meph., sulph.
amel. - arg-m., aur., bell., camph., coloc., lyc., ***rhod.,*** **RHUS-T.,** ***valer.***
night - acon., ***ars., calc.,*** **CARB-V.,** caust., phos., puls., **RHUS-T.**
lying on it - acon., ***carb-v.***
paralytic - am-c., arg-n., chel., chin., cina, cist., mag-m., meph., ***nux-v.,*** **RHUS-T.,** ***rhus-v.,*** seneg., sep., staph., sul-ac.
part lain on - cina.
raising arm, when - cocc., sulph.
rheumatic - elaps, gran., ***phyt.,*** puls.
right - ***arg-n.,*** bar-c., caust.
sitting, while - **VALER.**
sprained - nit-ac.
sticking - am-c.
stormy weather - ***rhod.***
stretch, must - nat-m.
arm - sulph.
tearing - ***ars.,*** carb-v., ***caust.,*** cham., ***cina,*** colch., coloc., grat., hell., ol-an., puls.
tensive - arg-m.
thread, as by a - plat.
touch agg. - staph.
upward - ***ars.,*** con., mag-c., nux-v., plat., sep.
up and down on motion - con.
walking amel. - **VALER.**
wandering - rhus-v.
warm room - zing.
wet weather - ***rhod., rhus-t.***
writing, while - **MAG-P.,** sul-ac.
after - thuj.

drawing, forearms - acon., ***agar.,*** aloe, alum., ambr., am-c., am-m., anac., ang., ***ant-c.,*** arg-m., arg-n., ars., asaf., bar-c., bell., berb., brom., bry., bufo, **CALC.,** calc-p., canth., carb-s., ***carb-v.,*** **CARD-M., CAUST.,** cham., ***chel.,*** chin., cimic., cina, cist., ***clem.,*** coc-c., coloc., com., con., croc., crot-t., cupr., ***cycl.,*** dios., ***dulc.,*** euph., ferr-ma., fl-ac., gels., gins., gran., graph., hell., hep., ind., kali-bi., kali-c., kali-chl., kalm., kreos., laur., led., lyc., mag-c.,

drawing, forearms - ***mag-p.,*** mang., ***meny.,*** merc-i-f., ***mez.,*** mosch., mur-ac., nat-c., nat-m., nat-p., nat-s., nit-ac., ***nux-v.,*** op., osm., pall., petr., phos., ***phyt., plat., puls.,*** ran-s., ***rhod.,*** **RHUS-T.,** ***rhus-v.,*** ruta., seneg., ***sep.,*** sil., spong., stann., staph., ***sulph.,*** tarax., tell., ***thuj., valer., verat.,*** zinc., zing.
afternoon - ind., sulph., thuj.
air, open, amel. - pall.
alternating with pressure - gins.
anterior part - aloe, ant-c., arg-m., asaf., berb., carb-v., ***hep.,*** meny., nat-s., thuj., sars.
morning - thuj.
bones - acon., ***arg-n.,*** arn., bar-c., calad., canth., carb-v., chin., kali-bi., led., ***merc-i-f.,*** puls., sabin., zinc.
left - merc-i-f.
radius - carb-v., euph., indg., samb., sulph., thuj.
radius, below elbow - staph.
ulna - chin., ***cycl.,*** dulc., euph., lyc., kreos., nat-m., phyt.
cramp-like - anac., ang., arg-m., calc-p., cina, graph., kalm., laur., lyc., ***meny.,*** mur-ac., nat-c., plat., ***rhod.,*** zinc.
elbow, near - carb-v., eupi., hell., staph., sulph.
evening - alum., bufo, kali-c., op., sulph.
in bed - mosch.
exertion, on - berb.
after - berb.
extending to,
downward - am-m., ant-c., calc., cham., chel., clem., cocc., com., cupr., ind., kali-c., kreos., nat-m., phos., ***rhod.,*** sulph., thuj.
extensor muscles - hep., mur-ac.
fingers - agar., am-m., carb-v., clem., kreos., ind., mur-ac., phos., sars.
fingers, little finger - ***cist.***
flexor muscles - com., ***hep.***
hand - alum., carb-v., cocc., kali-c., lyc., mag-c.
palm - chel., ***meny.***
thumb - cupr.
upward - anac., ars., brom.
wrist - cham., carb-v.
flexing arm - dulc., mur-ac.
forenoon - sil.
headache, with - verat.
intermittent - croc., lyc., nat-c.
left - ***agar.,*** chel., kali-c.
lying - laur.
morning - bry., eupi., lyc., thuj.
on waking - alum.
motion, agg. - carb-v., staph.
amel. - alum., am-m., ***arg-m.,*** calc., cina, con., mag-c., mosch., **RHUS-T.,** thuj.
paralytic - ant-c., arg-n., ferr-ma., kali-c., mosch., nit-ac., petr., ran-s., ***rhus-v.***
periodic - cist., gran.
plaster, as from - nat-c.
posterior part - acon., mang., petr.

drawing, forearms
radial side - **CARD-M.,** ***thuj.***
rheumatic - chel., chin-s., lyc., ***phyt.,*** **RHUS-T.**
riding, while - bry.
right - ant-c., coloc., ferr-ma., mag-c.
tendons - hep., nat-c.
ulnar side - arn., aster., cham., chin-s.
ulnar side, afternoon, while writing - chin-s.
upper arms, side - nat-c.
warmth applied amel. - ***chel., chin., dulc.,*** ferr., gran., ***kali-c.,*** kalm., lyc., ***nit-ac.,*** **NUX-V., RHUS-T.,** sil., ***zinc.***
wrist, near - ant-c., indg., mez., olnd., zing.
writing, when - **MAG-P.**

drawing, upper arms - acon., ***agar.,*** aloe, alum., am-m., anac., ang., ant-c., ant-t., arg-m., arg-n., ***ars.,*** ars-h., asaf., aster., aur., aur-m., aur-m-n., ***bell., berb.,*** bry., bufo, ***calc.,*** camph., canth., carb-ac., carb-s., ***carb-v.,*** card-m., ***caust.,*** clem., cocc., coc-c., coloc., com., con., dig., ***dulc.,*** ferr-ma., ferr-p., gins., graph., grat., hep., indg., ip., kali-bi., kali-c., ***kali-n.,*** lach., lact., led., **LYC.,** mag-c., mag-m., mang., mez., mur-ac., nat-m., nat-s., nit-ac., ***nux-v.,*** ol-an., par., petr., ***ph-ac., phos.,*** phyt., ***plat.,*** plb., ***rhod., rhus-t.,*** sabin., sanic., ***sep., sil.,*** sin-n., spong., ***stann.,*** stram., ***sulph.,*** sul-ac., ***thuj., valer.,*** vinc., zinc.
air, draft agg. - ant-c.
biceps - mang., ruta., ***valer.***
bones - agar., alum., aur., bar-c., carb-v., caust., cocc., euph., ip., kali-bi., mez., nit-ac., plb., sabin., ***sulph.,*** ter., verat., zinc.
condyles - arg-m., coc-c.
condyles, night - coc-c.
forenoon - agar.
lying down, after - ip.
midnight, after - ***sulph.***
morning - ter.
motion amel. - aur.
cramp-like - grat., mag-c., nat-m., ruta., ***valer.***
daytime - coloc.
deltoid region - arg-m., asar., bell., card-m., caust., kali-n., sanic., spig., stann., staph.
dinner - canth.
epilepsy, before - cupr.
evening - com., kali-bi., sulph., zinc., zing.
in bed - led., lyc., staph.
extending to,
downward - ***agar.,*** anac., berb., carb-ac., carb-v., kali-bi., lach., ***lyc.,*** sulph.
upward - ph-ac.
wrist - lyc.
forenoon - agar., com.
inner side - bell., bry., carb-v., camph., con., led., ***lyc.,*** mang., nat-s., rhus-t.
left - ***agar.,*** alum., coloc.
lower portion - agar., caust., grat., sil., zinc.
lying down, after - ip.
midnight - sulph.
morning - lyc.

drawing, upper arms
motion amel. - ***arg-m.,*** aur., camph., cocc., coc-c., con., ***valer.***
night - ***ars.***
outer side - ***sanic.***
paralytic - aloe, arg-m., arg-n., **BELL.,** bry., ***caust.,*** cina, cocc., con., kali-c., ***phos.,*** rhus-v., sabin., sep.
paroxysmal - ant-t., mag-c.
posterior part - acon., con., lyc.
pressure, agg. - ***arg-m.,*** spig.
amel. - mag-c.
pulsating - ign.
raising arms, on - ***rhus-t.***
rheumatic - anac., card-m., chel., dulc., nat-m., sanic.
right - arg-m., arg-n., **BELL.,** ***caust.,*** coloc., ferr-p., staph.
rising, after - arg-n.
sitting, while - calc., dig.
sticking - spong.
waking, on - agar., kali-c.
walking, while - camph.
warmth amel. - ant-c.
wet weather agg. - rhod., sanic.
writing, while - anag., ***valer.***

DRAWN, inwards - nit-ac.

ECZEMA - ***canth.,*** graph., hell., ***merc.,*** mez., phos., ***psor., sil.***
eczema, forearms - ***graph., merc., mez., sil.,*** thuj.

ELECTRICAL, current, sensation of - bol., dor., gels.

EMACIATION - ars., carb-an., chin., cupr., graph., ***iod., lyc.,*** **PLB.,** sel., syph., thuj.
inner side - plb.
right - carb-an., cupr., ***plb.,*** thuj.
vaccination, after - maland., ***thuj.***
emaciation, forearms - ***phos.,*** **PLB.**
emaciation, upper arms - ***nit-ac.,*** plb.

ENLARGEMENT, sensation of - ***cupr.,*** hyos., ***lyc.,*** manc., ptel., sep., verat.

ERUPTIONS - agar., alum., alumn., ***ant-c.,*** ant-t., arn., **ARS.,** brom., bov., **CAUST.,** chel., cimic., cinnb., cob., com., con., cop., crot-h., cupr., elaps, euph., fl-ac., graph., guare., hep., jug-r., kali-ar., kali-br., lach., **LYC.,** mag-s., merc., mur-ac., **MEZ.,** nat-c., **NAT-M.,** nux-v., nit-ac., oena., petr., ph-ac., phos., ***psor.,*** **RHUS-T.,** ***rhus-v.,*** rumx., sars., **SEP., SIL., SULPH.,** tab., thuj., til., valer., vip., zinc.
black - sec.
bleeding, after scratching - cupr-ar.
blotches - cimx., hura, mur-ac., nat-m.
bran-like - ***bor.***
burning - con., merc., ***nat-c.,*** **RHUS-T.,** spig.
chicken-pox, like - led.
clusters - rhus-t.
confluent - cop., phos.
cracked - phos.
crawling - lach.

ERUPTIONS, general
desquamating - agar., ***am-c.,*** am-m., arn., bar-c., calc., chin-s., crot-t., ferr., hydr., led., ***merc.,*** **MEZ., RHUS-T.,** ***rhus-v.,*** sep., ***sulph.***
thick whitish scales - crot-t.
dry - dol., hyper., merc., **PSOR.**
elevations - alumn., anac., carb-v., cic., crot-h., crot-t., dros., graph., hep., kali-br., kreos., merc., nat-m., nit-ac., plb., sul-ac., urt-u.
bleeding after scratching - cupr-ar.
shiny - crot-t.
spots - syph.
tips become white and scaly - merc.
whitish - crot-t.
excoriation - arn., ruta., sul-ac.
excrescences - ***ars., lach., thuj.***
exuding, thin water - crot-h.
yellow water - cupr., hell., ***rhus-t.,*** sol-n.
hard - caust., mez., sep., sil.
itch-like - alum., berb., graph., ***lach.,*** merc., nit-ac., phos., rhus-t., sars., sel., ***sep., sulph.***
itching - agar., anag., ant-c., ant-t., berb., bov., calad., carb-an., carb-v., ***caust.,*** cupr., dulc., ***jug-c.,*** kali-c., kali-chl., kali-i., kreos., lach., ***laur., led.,*** lyc., mag-c., mag-s., mang., ***merc., mez.,*** nat-m., nat-s., nux-v., phos., psor., ***puls.,*** **RHUS-T., SEP.,** spig., ***sulph.,*** tab., til., urt-u., zinc.
leprous - ***meph., phos.***
lumps - phos.
hard bluish, oozing and scabbing - ***calc-p.***
measles, like - cop., rhus-v.
miliary - alum., ant-t., bry., cop., merc., nux-v., rhus-v., sel., sulph.
scratching, after - kali-c.
moist - alum., bov., con., kreos., rhus-t.
purulent discharge - lyc., rhus-t.
nodules - hippoz., petr., sep.
painful - ars., kali-c., lyc., merc., petr.
papules - ***crot-h., kali-bi.***
petechiae - berb.
pimples - acon., ***agar.,*** am-c., am-m., anac., ant-t., arg-n., arn., **ARS.,** arum-t., asc-t., bar-c., bell., berb., bry., bov., buf-s., ***calc-p.,*** calc-s., cann-s., canth., ***carb-an.,*** carb-s., ***carb-v.,*** **CAUST.,** chel., chin., chin-s., cob., com., crot-c., cupr-ar., dulc., elaps, ***fl-ac.,*** hura, jatr., ***iod.,*** kali-ar., kali-bi., kali-c., kali-chl., kali-n., kreos., lac-ac., lach., lyc., mag-c., mag-m., mang., merc., mez., mur-ac., nat-s., nit-ac., ol-an., op., osm., ph-ac., plat., psor., puls., rat., **RHUS-T.,** rhus-v., sabad., sars., sel., **SEP.,** spig., staph., ***sulph.,*** tab., tarax., thuj., til., valer., ***zinc.***
bleeding, when scratched - cob.
burning - agar., am-c., bov., mag-m., nat-s., ***rhus-t.***
disappear from scratching - mag-c.

ERUPTIONS, general
pimples, hard - arg-n., bov., calc-s., rhus-t., rhus-v., valer.
head, black, with depressed - calc-s.
indolent - chel.
inflamed - calc-s.
itching - acon., agar., am-c., am-m., asc-t., bar-c., cann-s., carb-an., carb-s., caust., hura, iod., kreos., lyc., mag-c., ***mag-m., merc.,*** sabad., sel., sulph., ziz.
menses, during - sulph.
painful - kali-chl., thea.
red - acon., anac., ars., bov., chel., com., elaps, hura, iod., kali-chl., mag-s., rhus-t., sulph., til.
scratching, after - canth., carb-an.
sensitive - ***calc-s.***
stinging - acon., arg-n.
white - til., valer.
white scratching, after - kali-c.
pustules - anac., ant-c., arg-n., ***ars.,*** asc-t., arund., bor., calc., chel., cocc., chlor., cop., crot-h., cupr., elaps, fl-ac., iris, jug-c., ***kali-bi., kali-br., merc., mez., nat-m.,*** phos., ***psor., rhod., rhus-t.,*** rhus-v., ruta., sars., sec., ***sep., sil.,*** spig., squil., ***staph.,*** still., **SULPH.,** tab., tarent.
black - anthr., ***ars.,*** lach., sec.
ecthyma, like - phos.
hair in centre, with a - kali-br.
heal very slowly - ***psor.***
inflamed halo, with - chlor., rhus-v., sep.
large - sep.
point dark in centre - kali-bi.
red - crot-t., mez.
red - am-c., ant-c., arg-m., cycl., dulc., gins., jug-r., mag-c., mag-s., ***merc., mez.,*** nat-m., phos., ***staph.,*** sep., ***sulph.,*** valer.
scarlet fever, like - cocc.
scabs - ***alum.,*** am-m., ***ars., calc.,*** cit-v., ***jug-c., jug-r., mez.,*** mur-ac., phos., plb., podo., ***rhus-t.,*** rhus-v., ***sep., staph., sulph.,*** sul-ac.
itching - sep.
moist - alum., staph.
serum, of - rhus-t., rhus-v.
white - mez.
yellowish brown - rhus-t.
scales - agar., anthr., arn., **ARS.,** berb., cupr., ***fl-ac., iris, kali-s., merc., phos.,*** pip-m., puls., ***rhus-t.,*** sec., ***sil., sulph.***
fall off on scratching - sulph.
spots, in - merc.
scratching, after - staph., til.
scurfs brownish - am-m., cinnb.
smarting - anag., hyper., urt-u.
stinging - mag-c., puls.

eruptions, forearms - ***alum.,*** ant-t., ars., bry., calad., ***carb-an., caust.,*** cinnb., con., cupr., ***graph.,*** mag-s., mang., ***merc., mez.,*** phos., rhus-t., sel., spong., ***tarax.,*** zinc.
crusts - ***mez.***
desquamation bran-like - agar.

eruptions, forearms
excoriated - rhus-t.
itching - carb-an., kali-n., mang., mez.
moist - ***alum., merc., mez.,*** rhus-t.
nodules on the flexors of - hippoz.
red itching - nat-m.
pimples - am-c., am-m., ant-t., ars., asc-t., bell., bor., bry., calad., calc-p., ***carb-s., caust.,*** cit-v., fago., gamb., iod., ***kali-bi.,*** kali-n., lach., laur., lyc., mag-c., ***mag-s.,*** mang., merc., nat-m., ***nat-s.,*** ol-an., osm., ph-ac., rat., rhod., sabad., sars., staph., ***sulph., tax.,*** thuj., valer., ***zinc.***
afternoon - mag-c.
alternating with asthma - calad.
burning - am-c., calad., mang., nat-s.
evening - am-c., fago.
itching - am-c., am-m., calad., carb-s., caust., gamb., lyc., mag-c., nat-s., sabad., staph., sulph., ***zinc.***
itching, daytime - zinc.
menses, during - sulph.
morning - mang.
scratching, after - am-m., kali-n., mag-c.
scratching, after, oozing - kali-n.
washing, from - mag-c.
purulent discharge - rhus-t.
pustules - anac., ant-t., ***calc.,*** cop., lyc., rhod., rhus-t., ***staph.,*** tarent.
painful - tarent.
rash - am-c., ant-t., bry., calad., merc., mez., rheum, sel.
rash, alternating with asthma - calad.
raw - petr., rhus-t.
red - petr., ph-ac.
rupia - kali-i.
scales - alum., merc., petr.
smelling like cheese - ***calc.***
whitish - ***merc.***
yellow - rhus-t.
scratching agg. - mang., ***mez.***
stitching, on touch - petr.
sun exposure - **SULPH.**
tubercle - ***agar.,*** am-c., jug-r., kali-n., lach., mur-ac., ph-ac.
after scratching - agar.

eruptions, upper arms - ant-t., cinnb., grat., led., merc., nux-v., sep.
blotches - sep.
blotches, scaling off - berb.
crawling - lach.
crusts - anac.
itching - mag-s., sep.
pimples - anac., ant-c., ant-t., arn., carb-v., dulc., iod., ***kali-c.,*** lach., ***laur.,*** mang., mosch., sep., sulph., tax., til., valer.
bleeding, after scratching - mosch.
itching - carb-v., kali-c.
pustules - anac., merc.
rash - ant-c., bry., mez., rheum
scaly, white - ars-i.
tubercles - ars., caust., cocc., dulc., mang.
vesicles - aran., sep.

ERYSIPELAS, forearms - anan., ant-c., apis, bufo, ***kali-c.,*** **LACH.,** merc., petr.

EXOSTOSES, forearms - ***dulc.***

EXTEND, the arms, desire to - am-c., bell., sabad., tab., verb.

EXTENDED, arms - benz-n., ***chin.,*** dig., nux-v., sep., ***stram.,*** stry.
alternately flexed and extended - carb-o., ***cic., cupr.,*** hyos., **LYC.,** nux-v., sec., ***tab.***
every seven days - lyc.
sitting, while - nit-ac.
as if he had intended to take hold of something - dulc., phos.
paroxysms, during - ***cic.,*** **CINA,** stry.
rigidly - merc.

FLEXED, arms - acon., ars., carb-o., hydr-ac., morph., plb., stry., tax.
alternately flexed and, extended, - carb-o., ***cic., cupr.,*** hyos., ***lyc.,*** nux-v., ***plb.,*** sec., ***tab.***
sitting, while - nit-ac.
backward - acon., lyc.
chest, over - olnd., morph., tab.
elbow, at - lyc.
left - caust.
sleep, in - ***ant-t.***
spasmodically - caust., hydr-ac., nux-m., nux-v., plb., stry.

FLUTTERING, upper arms in, while resting it on the table - phyt.

FORMICATION - **ACON.,** ***alum.,*** apis, arn., atro., arum-t., arund., ***bell.,*** cact., caps., carb-s., caust., chin., cic., ***cocc.,*** con., ***graph.,*** guare., ***hep.,*** kali-n., lach., nat-c., nat-m., nat-p., nux-m., pall., phos., plat., plb., ***rhod.,*** rhus-v., rumx., sarr., **SEC.,** stry., sulph., urt-u., vip.
daytime - ***arg-n.***
evening - nat-c.
in bed - ***sulph.***
walking, while - ***graph.***
heat of bed agg. - rhod.
left - nat-m.
lying down - rumx.
mercury, after abuse of - hep.
midnight before, on waking - caust.
right - nat-c.

formication, forearms - acon., alum., arn., carb-an., carb-s., ***caust.,*** chin., chlor., con., lach., merc., plb., ***sec.***

formication, upper arms - sep., thuj.

FULLNESS - alumn., verat.

GANGRENE - **ARS.,** ***crot-h., sec.***
cold - ***sec.***

GNAWING, pain - alum., ***ars.,*** bry., canth., dros., dulc., graph., kali-bi., laur., mag-c., mang., phos., ran-s., sars., stront-c., sulph.
daytime - sulph.

gnawing, forearms - bry., ***graph.***
bones of - ***graph.***
evening - stront.
ulna - stront.

gnawing, upper arms - canth., ferr., laur., mang., phos.
bone - canth., mang.

gnawing, upper arms
left - ***ferr.***
motion agg. - ***ferr.***
night - mang.
pressure amel. - laur.
right - canth.

GOOSEBUMPS - chin-s., merl., phel., phos., sanic., spig., stann.
forearms - ign., ran-b.
upper arms - ham., sulph.

HANG, down, letting, arms amel. - ***acon.,*** anac., ***bar-c.,*** bor., bry., caps., chin., **CON.,** cupr., ***ferr.,*** graph., lac-d., lach., ***led.,*** lyc., phos., plb., ran-b., ***rhus-t., sulph.,*** thuj.

HEAT - aesc., alum., alumn., arund., aur., cann-i., chin., cic., con., graph., guare., ***lach.,*** lil-t., lyc., mez., ***nat-m.,*** nux-v., ol-an., par., ***phos.,*** phys., rhus-t., ruta., spong., stram., tarent., verat., vip., zinc.
burning, heat - guare., urt-u.
external - mez., ***petr.,*** rhus-v., ruta., stram.
flashes - caps., nux-v., rhod., sil.
left - rhus-t.
morning - alumn.
night - ***lach.,*** phos.
prickly - apis
water, hot, as if were running through - ***rhus-t.***

heat, forearms - anac., apis, aur-m-n., bry., nit-ac., ***rhus-t.,*** tarent.
anterior part, sensation of - lyc.
posterior part - bell.

heat, upper arms - calc-p., cic., nat-m.

HEAVINESS, tired arms - acon., aesc., ***agar.,*** aloe, ***alum., am-c., am-m.,*** anac., ***ang.,*** ant-c., ***ant-t., apis,*** **ARG-N.,** arn., ars-h., ***ars-m.,*** arund., aster., aur., bar-c., ***bell.,*** benz-ac., berb., bism., brach., bry., bufo, cadm-s., cact., ***calc.,*** camph., cann-i., ***carb-ac.,*** carb-an., carb-s., carb-v., **CAUST.,** chel., cic., cinnb., cocc., colch., **CON.,** corn., cor-r., croc., crot-h., crot-t., ***cur.,*** cycl., dig., dulc., ***ferr.,*** ferr-p., fl-ac., **GELS.,** ***glon., ham.,*** hura, kali-i., **KALI-P.,** ***lach.,*** laur., ***lec.,*** led., ***lyc.,*** lyss., manc., ***merc., merc-c., mez.,*** mur-ac., ***nat-c.,*** **NAT-M.,** nat-p., nat-s., nit-ac., ***nux-m.,*** nux-v., ***onos.,*** op., par., petr., ***ph-ac., phos.,*** phys., ***pic-ac.,*** pip-m., plan., plat., **PLB., PULS.,** rhod., rhus-t., ***sabad.,*** sarr., sep., ***sil.,*** sol-n., spig., spong., ***stann., stram., sulph.,*** sul-ac., ***sumb., tarent.,*** tep., teucr., thuj., til., valer., verat., zinc., zing.
afternoon - nux-v.
3 p.m. - plan.
ascending steps - ***nux-v.***
bed, in - staph., til.
daytime - sulph.
dinner, after - plect.
emissions, after - staph.
evening - ***am-m.,*** mur-ac.
exertion, on - ***phos., pic-ac., stann.***
forenoon, 11 a.m. - zing.
hanging down, while - ang., valer.

HEAVINESS, tired arms
left - arg-n., arund., bar-c., ***calc.,*** camph., carb-v., ***dig.,*** merc-i-f., plat., spig.,thuj.
menses, suppressed, during - graph.
morning - ant-s., ***iod., sulph.***
waking, on - fl-ac., ***iod.***
washing, on - ***phos.***
writing - phos.
motion, on - carb-v., grat., nat-c., ***stann.***
amel. - ***apis,*** camph., led., ***rhod.***
night - ***merc.,*** stann.
noon - sulph.
numbness, with - ***ambr., apis, bufo,*** cham., croc., fl-ac., graph., kali-c., lyc., mag-m., ***nux-v.,*** puls., ***sep.,*** sil.
playing piano agg. - ***cur., gels.,*** merc-i-f.
raising them, on - cic., cocc., mag-c., merc., mur-ac., phos.
right - ***am-c.,*** **AM-M.,** anac., ***apis, caust., fl-ac.,*** mag-c., nat-c., rhod.
walking, while - anac., ang., spig.
washing, on - phos.
writing, while - caps., ***carb-v., caust.,*** ferr-i., fl-ac., kali-c., mez., phos., spig.

heaviness, forearms - acon., aeth., alum., am-m., anac., aran., **ARG-N.,** aur., berb., cann-i., ***croc.,*** laur., lyc., ***mur-ac.,*** nux-v., ph-ac., sabad., spig., spong., sulph., ***tell.,*** teucr., thuj.
forenoon - lyc.
night, 10 p.m. - tell.
rest, during - aur.
sex, after - sabin.
waking, on - aran.

HERPES - alum., bor., **BOV.,** calc., caust., ***con.,*** cupr., dol., ***dulc., graph.,*** kali-c., kreos., ***lyc.,*** mag-s., ***manc., mang.,*** **MERC.,** ***nat-c., nat-m.,*** nux-v., ***phos., psor.,*** sars., sec., ***sep., sil.***
crusty - con., thuj.
furfuraceous - merc., phos.
joints, on the - ***calc.,*** merc.

herpes, forearms - ***alum., con.,*** mang., mag-s., **MERC.,** nat-m., sulph.

herpes, upper arms - kali-c., mang., nat-m., sulph.

INCOORDINATION - bell., cupr., ***gels., merc., onos.,*** plb.
talking, while - hyos.

INDURATION, muscles - mag-c., petr., tab.
forearms sitting - ***sil.***

INFLAMMATION - arg-m., crot-h., cupr., kali-bi., kali-i., lach., merc., petr., ran-b., ***rhus-t.,*** rhus-v., sep.
erysipelatous - am-c., ***apis,*** arn., ***ars.,*** bell., ***carb-ac.,*** bufo, form., ***hippoz., kali-c.,*** kalm., **LACH.,** petr., ***ph-ac.,*** **RHUS-T.,** rhus-v.
burning - petr.
lymphatics of arms - **BUFO.**
phlegmonous - rhus-t., rhus-v.
spots, in - merc-c.

inflammation, forearms - ***ars.,*** lyc., ***rhus-t.***
erysipelatous - anan., ant-c., apis, bufo, ***kali-c.,*** **LACH.,** merc., petr.
periosteum of - ***aur.***

inflammation, upper arms erysipelatous - bell., petr.

INSENSIBILITY, forearms, heat of stove, to - ***plb.,*** thuj.
pain, to - kreos., ***plb.***

ITCHING - ***agar.,*** aloe, alum., alumn., ambr., am-c., am-m., anac., ang., anthr., ant-c., ant-t., apis, arg-m., arn., ars., ars-i., asc-t., aur., aur-m., bar-c., benz-ac., bor., **BOV.,** bry., calad., calc., calc-i., calc-p., camph., cann-s., canth., carb-ac., carb-an., carb-s., carb-v., **CAUST.,** chel., chin., chin-s., cimic., cina, cinnb., cit-v., cob., cocc., coc-c., coloc., colch., com., con., cop., corn., cycl., dig., dios., dulc., euph., eupi., fago., fl-ac., form., gels., glon., gran., graph., grat., ham., hep., hydr., hydr-ac., hura, ign., ind., iod., jatr., jug-c., jug-r., kali-bi., kali-br., kali-c., kali-i., kali-n., kali-p., lach., lachn., lact., laur., led., lyc., ***lyss.,*** mag-c., mag-m., mag-s., manc., mang., merc., merc-i-f., merc-i-r., mez., mill., morph., mur-ac., myric., nat-a., nat-c., nat-m., nat-p., nat-s., nicc., nit-ac., ***nux-v.,*** ol-an., olnd., osm., op., pall., per., petr., ph-ac., phos., phys., phyt., plan., plat., plb., podo., prun., psor., ptel., puls., ran-b., rat., rhod., ***rhus-t.,*** rhus-v., rumx., ruta., sabad., sars., sel., ***sep., sil.,*** sin-a., sol-n., spig., spong., staph., stront-c., stry., **SULPH.,** tarent., tax., **TELL.,** teucr., ***thuj.,*** til., ***urt-u.,*** verb., vesp., verat., zinc.
afternoon - aloe, cimic., coc-c., fl-ac., form., jug-r., mag-c., nat-m., sulph.
2 p.m. - ol-an.
menses, during - mag-c.
bed, in - ***alum.,*** cinnb., cupr-ar., kali-bi., kali-br., mag-c., mur-ac., nat-m., ph-ac., phos., rhus-v., sars., **SULPH., TELL.**
biting - ***berb.***
burning - ***agar.,*** berb., calc., cupr., dulc., mez., nux-v., ran-b., spig., stann.
cool, when - thuj.
corrosive - chel., hell., led., merc., ruta.
crawling - berb., thuj.
daytime - calc.
evening - am-m., bov., calc-p., chin., cimic., dios., fago., fl-ac., hura, mag-c., merl., ol-an., sin-a., ***sulph.,*** thuj.
in bed - hell.
flea bites, as from - ***led.,*** nat-c., tab.
forenoon - mag-c., sulph.
gnawing, erosive - hell.
here and there - plat.
hot water amel. - ***rhus-t.,*** rhus-v.
lying down, after, agg. - calad.
menses, during - mag-c.
mercury, after abuse of - ***hep.***
midnight - rhus-t.
morning - am-m., ham., hell., mag-c., ol-an., rhus-v., sulph., tax.
dressing, while - mag-m., nux-v., rhus-t., ***sulph.***
washing - bov.

ITCHING,
motion, agg. - crot-t.
amel. - com., sars.
nettles, as from - lach., nit-ac., **URT-U.**
night - agar., am-m., anac., ars., asc-t., canth., carb-v., chin., cupr., dig., hydr., kali-br., merc., phos., rhus-v., ruta., sabad., sulph., ***thuj.,*** til.
9 p.m. - asc-t., calc-p., hydr.
10 p.m. - mag-c.
rubbing, agg. - crot-t., ***nat-m.,*** rhus-v.
amel. - ang., berb., cupr-ar., ham., mag-s., ol-an.
scratching, agg. - ars., ham., ph-ac., rhus-v., stront-c., **SULPH.**
amel. - alum., ant-t., bov., camph., chel., coloc., graph., jug-c., led., mag-c., mang., merc., ol-an., olnd., ph-ac.
sitting in church - com.
spots - berb., cop., kali-bi., kali-n., merc., nat-m., psor., sulph.
sticking - berb., caust., lach., merc-i-f.
stinging - ars-i., phos., ran-b., ran-s.
sudden - phos.
suppressed eruptions, after - ***hep.***
tickling - kali-n., staph.
touch agg. - crot-t., psor.
undressing, while - crot-t., cupr-ar., kali-br., mur-ac., nux-v., ph-ac.
voluptuous - merc., ***sulph.***
warm room agg. - nux-v.
warmth agg. - chin., sulph.
water, immersing in - rhus-v.

itching, forearms - ***agar.,*** anac., am-c., am-m., berb., bol., bor., bov., ***carb-an.,*** carb-s., caust., chin-s., cit-v., clem., colch., cop., dulc., euph., gels., hura, kali-bi., kali-n., laur., mag-c., mag-m., mag-s., mang., merc-i-f., mez., mur-ac., myric., ol-an., psor., ***puls.,*** rat., ***rhus-t.,*** rhus-v., rumx., sars., spig., stront-c., sulph., tax., til., verb.
anterior part - am-c., am-m., berb., bor., carb-an., ol-an., mag-c., sars.
burning - agar., calad., ***kali-bi.***
evening - am-m.
bed, in, agg. - sars.
lying down, after - kali-bi.
morning - am-m., mag-c., tax.
night - am-m., anac., asc-t., ***mez.***
amel. - tax.
scratching amel. - mag-c., mill., ol-an.
spots, in - kali-n.
voluptuous - merc.

itching, upper arms - acon., anac., anag., arn., berb., bov., bry., canth., carb-s., chel., cocc., dulc., euph., kali-bi., kali-i., kali-n., lach., laur., led., lyc., mang., mez., ***nux-v.,*** olnd., pall., ph-ac., ***psor.,*** ruta., sep., spong., stront-c., thuj.
burning - berb., dulc., nux-v.
coldness, during - spong.
corrosive - led.
crawling - thuj.
evening, while undressing - nux-v.
inner side - acon., bov., carb-v., kali-i.

itching, upper arms
morning, dressing, while - nux-v.
motion, on - anac.
outer part - mang.
scratching amel. - chel., mang.
posterior part - tax.
scratching, agg. - stront.
amel. - chel., led., mang., pall.
spots - berb.
stinging - euph., led., ran-s.

JERKING - aesc., ***alum.,*** amyg., ***anac.,*** aran., ***arg-n.,*** ars., asaf., aur., aur-m., ***bar-m.,*** bell., berb., camph., cham., chel., **CIC., CINA,** cocc., coff., crot-h., ***cupr.,*** dulc., ***graph., hyos.,*** hyper., ***ign.,*** inul., ***ip.,*** kali-br., kali-c., ***lil-t., lyc.,*** meny., mez., mygal., nat-c., nit-ac., onos., plat., ***puls.,*** ran-b., sil., ***stann.,*** **STRAM.,** stront-c., ***stry.,*** **SULPH.,** sul-ac., ***tarent., thuj.,*** valer., verat., verat-v., ***zinc.***
air, in windy weather - sulph.
backwards - alum.
daytime - ***thuj.***
evening - graph., sil.
falling asleep, on - alum., graph., kali-c., hyper., sil., stront-c., ***stry.***
left - ***cic.,*** stann.
motion of arm on - dulc.
night - am-c., bar-m., graph., lyc.
paralyzed arm - arg-n., ***merc., nux-v.,*** phos., sec.
right - aesc., sep.
sleep, during - ip., ***lyc.,*** nat-c.
talking - cic.
warm room amel. - sulph.

jerking, forearms - caps., **CIC.,** ***cupr.,*** hyper., ***ign.,*** jal., staph.
evening - ***ign.***

jerking, upper arms - anac., ant-c., kali-bi., ***lyc.,*** meny., nat-m., nit-ac., ph-ac.
evening - kali-bi.
left - cupr.
right - am-c., kali-n., ran-b.

LAMENESS - abrot., ***agar.,*** alum., ars., **BELL.,** berb., bism., bov., ***brom.,*** **CALC.,** calc-p., carb-v., carl., ***caust., cinnb., cocc.,*** com., ***cycl.,*** dig., ***dulc., ferr., fl-ac.,*** glon., graph., hyper., kali-c., kreos., lyc., ***mag-c.,*** merc-i-f., mez., nat-s., ol-an., ***phyt.,*** plb., ***psor., rhus-t., sep.,*** **SIL.,** stann., sul-ac., thuj., verat.
afternoon - agar.
beaten, as if - plat., verat.
cold wet weather agg. - **RHUS-T.**
exercise, on moderate - sil.
forenoon - ***fl-ac.***
left - agar., brom., hyper., kali-c., lach., ***rhus-t.***
lying on it - fl-ac.
morning - fl-ac.
waking, on - abrot.
neuralgia, after - ars.
night, 10 p.m. - fl-ac.
raising the arm - syph.
rheumatic - ***calc-p.,*** carb-v., **RHUS-T.**

LAMENESS,
right - acet-ac., **FERR.**, fl-ac., kali-c., merc-i-f., nit-ac., **SANG.**
spot, in - plat.
waking, on - abrot.
walking, while - dig.
writing, after - ***agar.***, fl-ac., ***merc-i-f.***
lameness, forearms - agar., bell., berb., ***caust.***, colch., dulc., fl-ac., merc-i-f., myric., nat-m., ***sil.***, stront-c., sulph., thuj.
near the wrist - myric.
lameness, upper arms - abrot., act-sp., ***agar.***, bell., bry., colch., com., iris, plat., puls-n, thuj., zing.
extending to back of neck - iris.
left - agar.
raising it, on - bry.
riding, while - abrot.
writing, from - agar.

MOTION, general
agitated, lower limbs quiet - stram.
arm, difficult - coc-c.
automatic - ***cocc.***, ***hell.***, op.
of one - ***alum.***, apis, bell., ***hell.***
backward and forward - morph.
beating with one, groping with the other - ***stram.***
constant - ***bell.***
convulsive - apis, ***arg-n.***, aur-m., ***bell.***, caust., con., ***merc-c.***, mez., ***mygal.***, ***op.***, plb., ***stram.***, sul-ac., tab., zinc-s.
difficult - ars., aur., cinnb., clem., con., eupi., glon., merc., stann., ter., thuj.
walking in open air, while - anac.
dry, as if joints were - thuj.
face, toward - stry.
fiddling, as if - clem.
forward, over chest during clonic cramp - atro.
thrown violently - ip.
hurried - ***agar.***, ***bell.***
idiotic manner - merc.
involuntarily - ***cocc.***, hell., op.
irregular - ***agar.***, ***bell.***, merc., tab., tarent.
left arm - ***cimic.***
side to side, from - cupr-ar.
stretching, upward - alum.
turning - alum.
up and down - cupr-ar.
slowly - ars.
upward and outward - ***arg-n.***

MOUSE, sensation of, running up - **BELL.**, ***calc.***, ***sulph.***
before epilepsy - **BELL.**, calc., **SULPH.**
running down - lyss.

NODULES, forearms - calc., mur-ac.

NUMBNESS - abrot., ***acon.***, aesc., ***aeth.***, ail., ***alum.***, ***alumn.***, ***ambr.***, am-c., am-m., amyg., aran., **APIS,** arg-m., ars., ars-i., aur., bar-c., bell., berb., bor., both., ***bufo,*** calc-p., ***cact.***, cann-i., canth., caps., carb-o., **CARB-S.**, ***carb-v.***, cast-eq., caust., cedr., cham., chel., chin-a., chr-ac., cic., cimic., cinnb., **COCC.**, cod., colch., ***con.***, ***croc.***, ***crot-c.***, ***cupr.***, cupr-ar., ***cur.***, dios., ***dulc.***, euphr., fago., ***fl-ac.***, ***gels.***, glon., **GRAPH.**, helo., hell., ***hep.***, hura, iod., kali-ar., kali-bi., ***kali-c.***, **KALI-N.**, kali-p., ***kali-s.***, kreos., lac-c., ***lach.***, led., **LYC.**, lyss., ***mag-m.***, med., meph., merc., merc-c., merc-i-f., nat-m., nat-p., nat-s., nit-ac., ***nux-v.***, ***onos.***, ol-j., **OX-AC.**, ***pall.***, petr., ***phos.***, phys., **PLAT.**, ***plb.***, ***psor.***, ***puls.***, ***rhod.***, **RHUS-T.**, sarr., ***sec.***, ***sep.***, sil., **SPIG.**, stann., stront-c., ***sulph.***, sumb., tep., ***thuj.***, urt-u., verat., vip., xan., **ZINC.**
afternoon - calc-p., carl., nicc., teucr.
anterior part - plan.
bed, in - carb-an., ***ign.***, mag-m., phos.
on going to - psor.
carrying anything, when - ***ambr.***
cold, becoming - sumb.
cold, weather - ***kali-c.***, ***sumb.***
colic, with - aran.
covers, under - sep.
daytime - ambr., anac.
during rest - ambr.
eating, while - cocc.
after - cocc., ***kali-c.***
epilepsy, between attacks - cupr.
evening - bor., bry., lyss., merc-c., phos., plb.
7 p.m - phys.
8 p.m. - cinnb.
on lying down - mag-m.
exercise, after - sulph.
even after violent - ***kali-c.***
exertion, during cramp-like numbness - alum.
extending to thumb - sumb.
forenoon - fl-ac., mill., zing.
10 a.m. - zing.
grasping anything firmly - am-c., **CHAM.**, chin., cocc.
hanging down, when - berb.
holding anything in hands - ***apis,*** com., puls.
intermittent fever, in - agar., am-m., ars-s-r., cocc., merc-sul., zinc.
laying arm on table - bar-c.
leaning on it - hep., petr., sil., sumb.
left - ***acon.***, aesc., ail., ambr., anac., apis, ***bar-c.***, bufo, **CACT.**, cham., cinnb., cupr-ar., glon., ***graph.***, kali-c., kali-n., kalm., kreos., ***lach.***, lac-c., lat-m., ***med.***, mill., naja, nat-m., nux-v., petr., ***phos.***, rhod., sumb., tarax., tarent., xan.
arm and right leg - tarent.
from lying on it - cact., ***nat-m.***
in heart disease - **ACON.**, **CACT.**, cimic., dig., ***glon.***, kalm., ***lach.***, lat-m., ***naja,*** phos., **RHUS-T.**, ***spig.***, ***sumb.***
lying, while - aur., merc., rumx., sulph.
on back - kali-n.
on a table - bar-c.
on it - ***ambr.***, arg-m., ars., ***bar-c.***, bufo, ***calc.***, carb-an., ***carb-v.***, cop., ***graph.***, hep., ign., ***kali-c.***, ***lach.***, ***nat-m.***, pall., petr., ***phos.***, **PULS.**, **RHUS-T.**, sep., ***sil.***, ***spig.***, sumb.

NUMBNESS,
measles, in - zinc.
menses, during - graph., kali-n., sec.
morning - am-c., crot-h., fl-ac., mag-m., nux-v., phos., psor., puls., zinc.
bed, in - ***kali-c.***
lying on - arg-m.
lying on, arm under head - ph-ac.
pain in region of heart - pall.
waking, on - aur., calad., fl-ac., kali-c., ***mag-m.,*** mag-s., nit-ac., psor., teucr., zinc.
motion, agg. - plb., ruta.
amel. - ***ambr., aur., apis,*** dros., merc., phos., rumx., sep., sulph.
night - ***ambr.,*** am-c., carb-v., cop., ***croc.,*** hep., hyper., ***ign.,*** kali-c., kali-n., ***lyc.,*** mag-m., merc., nit-ac., ***nux-v., pall.,*** petr., ph-ac., phos., puls., sep., sil.
10 p.m. - fl-ac.
lying on it - cop., hep., petr.
sleep, in - croc.
pain in arm, with - kali-n., phos.
raising them - phos.
upright - ***puls.,*** sep.
upright, amel. - ars.
resting, head on it - ph-ac., ***phos., rhus-t.,*** sep.
on it - ambr., carb-an., fl-ac.
riding in a carriage - form.
right - am-c., am-m., ars., carb-an., cast-eq., chel., ***hep.,*** kali-bi., kali-n., lach., ***lil-t., lyc.,*** lyss., mag-m., merc-i-f., nat-p., nit-ac., phos., phys., ***sil.,*** thuj.
in heart disease - lil-t.
lying, on left side - ***mag-m.***
lying, on the right side - ***am-c., ars., carb-v.,*** fl-ac., petr., ***spig.***
scratching, after - sulph.
side not lain on - fl-ac., mag-m.
siesta, during - graph.
sitting, while - ***graph.,*** lyc., nicc., ***teucr.***
using it - ***puls., spig.***
writing, while - cer-b., ***merc-i-f.,*** spig.

numbness, forearms - **ACON.,** aesc., agar., ail., aloe, alum., am-m., ars-m., bapt., carb-an., ***carb-s.,*** carb-v., cedr., ***cham.,*** chin., chin-a., cinnb., ***cocc.,*** coloc., com., ***crot-c., cupr.,*** dios., euphr., ***fl-ac., gels., glon.,*** **GRAPH.,** helo., hydrc., ***kali-c.,*** kali-n., ***lyc.,*** lyss., mag-m., med., merc., merc-sul., ***nat-m., nit-ac.,*** nux-v., ***psor., op., pall., plb.,*** puls., rheum, rhus-t., sec., sep., stront-c., ***sulph.,*** tell., thuj., zinc.
afternoon, 5 p.m. - phys.
anterior part - aloe, cham., fl-ac.
bending, when - chin.
edematous - chel.
evening, 10 p.m. - tell.
extending to end of little finger - cinnb.
to finger - pall.
forenoon - fl-ac., zinc.
grasping anything - **CHAM.**
hangs down, when - berb.

numbness, forearms
left - **ACON.,** alum., cinnb., fl-ac., kali-c., med., onos.
lying, while - puls.
lying, while, on table when writing - lyc.
morning - mag-m., nux-v.
5 a.m. - fl-ac.
5 a.m., lying on right side - fl-ac.
after rising - mag-m., nux-v.
waking, on - kali-c.
motion amel. - ***cinnb.,*** puls.
night - rhus-t.
painful - com.
posterior part - berb., caj., plb.
radial side - fl-ac.
raising arm agg. - ***puls.,*** sep.
right - ***am-m., chin.,*** coloc., euphr., hep., ***nit-ac.,*** sulph.
sitting, while - fl-ac., merc.

numbness, upper arms - am-c., bry., carb-ac., carb-s., croc., fl-ac., hura, kali-c., merc., plat.
deltoid region - plb.
morning, bed in - merc.
sitting, on - merc.

PAIN, arms - abrot., acon., ***aesc.,*** agar., ***alum.,*** alumn., ammc., aml-n., apis, apoc., arg-n., arund., ***ars.,*** ars-h., ars-i., asaf., asc-t., aur., aur-m., bad., bapt., ***bar-c.,*** bar-m., bell., berb., ***bol.,*** bov., **BRY.,** bufo, ***cact.,*** caj., calc., ***calc-p.,*** calc-s., camph., carb-an., carb-s., carb-v., cast-eq., caul., ***caust., cham.,*** chel., chin-a., cina, cinnb., cimic., cit-v., cocc., ***coff.,*** **COLCH.,** coloc., com., crot-c., crot-h., cupr., cupr-ar., ***cycl.,*** dios., dirc., dros., dulc., elaps, **EUP-PER.,** ferr., ferr-ar., ferr-i., fl-ac., form., ***gels., glon.,*** gran., ***graph., guai.,*** gymn., ham., hell., ***hep.,*** hura, hydr., ign., iodof., ind., kali-bi., kali-n., kali-p., ***kalm.,*** lach., ***led.,*** lil-t., lyc., ***mag-p.,*** mag-s., mang., ***meph.,*** merc., merc-c., merc-i-f., mez., mill., morph., mosch., mur-ac., myric., naja, ***nat-a.,*** nat-m., ***nux-v.,*** ol-j., op., ox-ac., pall., par., petr., ph-ac., ***phos.,*** phys., ***phyt., pip-m.,*** plan., plat., ***plb.,*** ptel., **PULS.,** ***ran-s.,*** rhod., **RHUS-T.,** rumx., ***sang.,*** sarr., sil., ***spig.,*** staph., stram., stry., ***sulph.,*** tab., ***tarent.,*** tax., tep., thuj., trom., urt-u., ***verat.,*** vip., wye., xan., zinc.
afternoon - calc-p., chel., coloc., fago., naja, rumx., thuj., zinc.
air, cold - ***ars.,*** ign., nit-ac., ***ran-b., rhod.***
open amel. - cham.
alternating, sides - **LAC-C.,** sulph.
with lower, limbs - merc-i-r.
amputation, after - all-c., calen., ***hyper.***
annual - vip.
autumn, in - rhus-t.
bed, in - cycl., ***ferr.,*** ign., iodof., ***sulph.,*** verat.
weight of bedcovers - ferr.
bending arm, with - aeth.
bending, arm, amel. - ferr.
bones - apis, ars., calc-p., ***iod.,*** kali-bi., **LYC.,** mag-c., merc., plat., sabad., teucr.
hammering, in - nit-ac.

PAIN, arms
chill, during - bry., chin., lyc., nux-v., ph-ac., phos., puls., rhus-t.
before - ***eup-per., phel.***
cold, amel. - thuj.
weather agg. - agar., **CALC-P.,** kali-c., kalm.
cough, during - dig., ***puls.***
damp, weather - ***dulc., phyt., ran-b., rhod., rhus-t.,*** verat.
daytime - bor., plb., sulph.
dinner, during - kali-n.
eating, while - cocc.
eating, after - ars., ***indg.***
epileptic, before - ***calc-ar.***
evening - calc., cimic., fl-ac., hyos., kalm., led., merc-c., merc-i-f., nat-a., phos., psor., **PULS.,** rhus-t., stann., staph.
6 p.m. - arg-n., elaps
bed, in - carb-v., kreos., mag-m.
exertion, during - alum., cimic., iod., ***merc.,*** sulph.
after - gels., ruta., ***sep.,*** sil.
extending, arms - carb-s., hura, lyc., sulph.
arms, amel. - merc.
downward - aran., ***arn., aspar.,*** carb-an., ***guai.,*** kalm., nat-a., **RHOD.**
extending, to
back - ars., caust., dios.
chest - vip.
face to fingers - ***coff.***
fingers from heart - ***aur., cocc., cycl., guai.,*** lat-m.
little finger - hura, nat-a.
little finger from axilla - nat-a.
extensor muscles - bufo, ***iod.,*** plan., plb.
fatigue, as from - mez., nit-ac.
forenoon - bry., carb-s., cham., fago., kalm., sulph.
flexors, when grasping something - ***nat-s.***
hanging down, on - alum., am-m., ang., berb., ***bry.,*** canth., ***cina,*** ign., kali-n., nat-m., nux-v., ol-an., par., ph-ac., phos., plat., ruta., sabin., sep., stront-c., sulph., sul-ac., thuj., valer.
jerking - ***arn.,*** bell., ran-b., rhus-v., ***valer.***
joints - aur-m-n., **CALC.,** caust., cupr., led., mang., nat-m., plb., teucr.
bending - stann.
evening - ign.
left - nit-ac.
motion, on - nat-m.
motion, on, amel. - aur-m-n.
paroxysmal - mang.
rheumatic - anan., asaf., bry., hep., kali-bi., lach., ***led., lyc., merc., petr., phos.,*** rhod., ***rhus-t.,*** sabin., sars., spig., stann.
side lain on - ***ign.***
writing, while - cinnb.
leaning, when - ruta., sil., thuj.
left - ***aesc.,*** agar., asc-t., aster., arg-n., aur., cur., fl-ac., ***guai.,*** ind., iod., jac-c., ***kalm., lach., lat-m.,*** meny., merc-i-r., **RHUS-T.,** tab.

PAIN, arms
left, angina pectoris, in - cimic., dig., ***lat-m.***
epilepsy, before - calc-ar.
heart symptoms, with - acon., agar., aur., **CACT.,** calc-ar., chim., ***cimic., crot-h., dig.,*** iber., **KALM.,** ***lat-m.,*** lyc., med., **RHUS-T.,** spig., ***tab.***
left to right - ***calc-p.,*** form.
lifting, a load - ruta., sep.
lifting, a load amel. - spig.
lying, on it - acon., **ARS.,** ***calc., carb-v.,*** cocc., dros., ***graph., ign., iod.,*** **KALI-C.,** ***spig.,*** urt-u.
menses, during - agar., bry., ***calc.,*** elaps, eup-per., nux-v., spong., stram., verat.
morning - ars., ars-i., chel., crot-h., dios., dulc., fago., jac-c., merc-i-f., ptel., rhus-t., stict., staph.
motion, on - ars., crot-h.
rising - merc-i-f., phos., staph.
waking, on - ***aur.,*** chel.
motion - aml-n., ***ant-t.,*** berb., **BRY.,** bufo, cann-s., ***cham.,*** chel., chin., cimic., cinnb., **COLCH.,** ***coloc.,*** dros., ferr., ***guai.,*** hyos., iod., iris, kali-c., ***kalm.,*** led., mag-c., mag-m., meph., merc-i-r., mez., ***nux-v.,*** op., ***ox-ac.,*** ph-ac., phys., ***phyt., plb.,*** ran-b., sil., staph., sulph.
amel. - abrot., acon., agar., aur-m-n., camph., cina, cupr., cycl., ***dulc.,*** kali-p., ***lyc.,*** meph., phos., ***puls., rhod.,*** **RHUS-T.,** spig., stel., thuj.
impeding - nux-v.
slow amel. - ***ferr.***
neuralgic - ***acon.,*** aesc., arn., ars., crot-h., ***crot-t., ferr.,*** graph., ign., iod., lyc., phos., ran-b., ***rhus-t.,*** sep., ***staph.,*** sulph., ter., verat.
night - ambr., am-m., aran., ***ars.,*** asaf., bry., ***carc.,*** calc-s., carb-s., ***carb-v.,*** cast-eq., caust., cham., cit-v., coloc., croc., crot-t., dig., ***dulc.,*** gels., ign., ***iod.,*** kali-n., ***lyc.,*** mag-c., ***merc.,*** merc-i-f., mur-ac., nux-v., phos., phyt., puls., **RHUS-T., SANG.,** ***sil.,*** staph., sulph.
2 a.m. - ***ferr.***
3 a.m. - dios.
3 to 4 a.m. - gels.
3 to 6 a.m. - thuj.
4 a.m. - verat.
lying on it - acon., ***ars., carb-v., iod.***
midnight, after - nux-v.
noon, walking, after - pall.
palpitation, with - agar., ***cact., calc.,*** cimic.
paralytic - alum., arg-n., ***calc.,*** carb-s., ***chel.,*** cimic., cina, cocc., **COLCH.,** coloc., crot-h., cur., guai., kalm., mang., ***merc.,*** phos., ***rhus-t.,*** staph., sul-ac.
paralyzed, arm - agar., ***ars.,*** bell., calc., caust., ***cocc.,*** crot-t., ***kali-n.,*** lat-m., plb., sil., sulph.
paroxysmal - arg-m., ***caust., cina, kalm.,*** lach., lyc., ***mag-p.,*** meny., ***ran-b.,*** sul-ac.
perspiration, amel. - thuj.
piano, playing - ***gels.***

PAIN, arms
pressure, agg. - berb., merc-i-f., rhus-v., sil., ***spig.***
pronation, during - petr.
raising, arm - ***apis,*** caj., calc., cocc., eup-pur., **FERR.,** kali-p., lac-c., olnd., phos., phyt., ***sang.,*** sulph., syph., tab., zinc.
rest, during - cupr.
right - cast-eq., ***caust.,*** cimic., cina, ***cycl.,*** eupi., fl-ac., kalm., ***lyc., merc-i-f.,*** pall., phos., ***phyt.,*** pip-m., **SANG.,** ***spig.,*** xan.
heart symptoms, with - ***lil-t.***
left lower - asc-t.
then left - fl-ac.
rubbing, agg. - berb., kalm., merc-i-f.
leaves and goes to rubbing, lower limbs - ***kalm.***
scratching, when - berb., lach.
sewing, when - eupi.
siesta, during - lyc.
sleep, after - morph.
stormy, weather - **RHOD., RHUS-T.**
stretching out, when - alum., caust., sulph.
supinating, forearm - cinnb.
swollen, axillary glands, with - **BAR-C.**
taking, hold of anything - am-c., arn., calc., carb-v., caust., cham., dros., led., plat., puls., **RHUS-T.,** sil., verat.
amel. - lith.
taking, off coat - nat-c.
thinking, about it - ***ox-ac.***
tired, as if - ***lach., nux-v.,*** verat.
touched, when - agar., berb., **CHIN.,** carb-an., cocc., euph., lob., lyc.
turning, amel. - spig.
in bed - ***sang.***
ulcerative - berb., thuj.
uncovering, amel. - lac-c., **LED., PULS.,** sulph.
vibrating - berb.
waking, on - abrot., iod.
walking, after - pall.
amel. - daph., ***valer.,*** verat.
slow amel. - ***ferr.***
while - arg-n.
wandering - ars., asaf., cact., cast-eq., ***caul.,*** chel., ery-a., fl-ac., ***lac-c.,*** med., ***phyt., pip-m., puls.,*** sol-n., sulph.
warmth, agg. - ant-t., apis, bry., calc., caust., cham., dulc., ***guai., lac-ac.,*** **LED.,** nux-v., ***puls.,*** sabad., ***stel.,*** stront-c., ***sulph.,*** thuj., zinc.
amel. - **ARS.,** cinnb., ***graph., mag-p., sil.***
washing - am-c., ***sulph.***
cold water - am-c., ***ars.***
winter, in - petr.
writing, while - cer-b., cer-s., ***cycl.,*** **MAG-P.,** ***merc-i-f., pip-m.,*** sul-ac.
yawning, when - nux-v.

PAIN, forearms - acon., ***aesc.,*** agar., all-c., alum., am-c., am-m., anag., apis, apoc., ***arg-n.,*** ars., ars-i., arum-d., asaf., asc-t., aur., aur-m-n., bapt., bar-c., berb., bism., bor., bry., calad., calc., ***carb-v.,*** cast-eq., caul., cedr., ***cham.,*** chel., chin., cimic., coca, cocc., **COLCH.,** coloc., cor-r., croc., cupr., ***cycl.,*** dios., euph., fl-ac., gels., hell., hura, hyper., iod., kali-bi., kali-chl., lach., led., lil-t., ***mag-p.,*** mang., med., merc., merc-i-f., ***mez.,*** murx., nat-m., ***nit-ac.,*** ph-ac., phys., phyt., plat., plan., plb., ***podo.,*** prun., puls., **RHOD.,** ***rhus-t.,*** sabin., sars., sil., spig., spong., ***staph.,*** still., stront-c., sulph., tarent., tep., teucr., thuj., trom., upa., verat-v., verb.
afternoon - agar., nat-s., sulph., thuj.
anterior part - asaf., gels., plb., spong., tarent.
bed, in - aloe, am-c., am-m., ***mez.,*** sulph.
bending arm - chin., sabad.
between bones - calad.
daytime - plb., sulph.
evening - all-c., alum., am-c., calc-s., cast-eq., fl-ac., stront-c., sulph.
8 p.m. - phys.
extending to, elbow - spig.
to, finger - asc-t., cocc., con., ***cycl.,*** puls.
to, finger, little - agar., kreos.
to, thumb - agar., croc.
extensor muscles - coloc., hep., mur-ac., sil.
flexor muscles - arn., ***calc.,*** gels., nux-v.
radial side - chin-a., chin-s.
forenoon - sil., trom., verat-v.
grasping, on - chel., lach.
hanging down - berb., nat-m., zinc.
jerking - led., sil.
left - agar., ***med.***
lying, while - aur-m-n.
morning - ars., bar-c., bry., chin-s., coloc., dios., kali-bi., ***lyc.,*** nat-a., thuj.
waking, on - alum., kali-bi.
motion, on - anac., ***calc.,*** chel., croc., led., rhus-t., sabin., ***staph.***
amel. - alum., aur-m-n., bar-c., ***bism.,*** camph., cocc., **RHUS-T.,** spig., stront.
moving finger - asaf.
near the wrist - asc-t., ***calc.,*** cham., com., mez., olnd., zing.
neuralgic - chin-s., iod.
night - agar., aloe, ***arg-n., lyc., mez.,*** plan.
11 p.m. - trom.
noon - cedr., trom.
paralytic - aeth., bar-c., berb., caust., ***cham.,*** **COLCH.,** graph., ***med.,*** ph-ac., sil., ***staph.,*** sulph.
paroxysmal - ang., arg-m., berb., calc., ferr., kreos., mosch., mur-ac., ***ph-ac.,*** plat., plb., ruta., verb.
posterior part - berb.
pulsating - merc-i-f.
radial side - agar., fl-ac., merc., rhus-t.
morning - merc.
radius - all-c., fl-ac., gymn., ***lyc., mez.,*** nat-c., nat-m., osm., rhus-t., sabin., verat-v.
hang, letting arm - nat-m., osm.
head of - fl-ac.
periosteum - cycl., ***merc., mez.,*** phos.

PAIN, forearms
rheumatic - ***aesc.,*** agar., asc-t., bapt., chel., chin-s., ***colch.,*** form., ***hydr.,*** hyos., iris, lycps., merc., merc-i-f., ***nit-ac., phyt., podo., rhus-t.,*** stry.
right - ***cycl., merc-i-f.***
sitting, while - aur-m-n., led.
tendons - ***calc.,*** chel., chin., chin-s., sil.
touch, agg. - cupr., sabin., ***staph.***
amel. - bism., meny.
ulna - ***arg-n.,*** calc., ***caust.,*** calc-s., cham., chin., form., plat., ***podo.,*** verat-v.
lower part of, when writing - chin-s.
waking, on - agar., lycps.
wandering - nat-a.
warm applications amel. - ***chel., chin., dulc.,*** ferr., gran., ***kali-c.,*** kalm., lyc., ***nit-ac.,*** **NUX-V., RHUS-T.,** ***sil., zinc.***
writing, while - acon., anac., ***cycl.,*** fago., fl-ac., **MAG-P.,** ***merc-i-f.***

PAIN, upper arms - abrot., alumn., **ANAC.,** anag., ang., ant-c., apis, aran., arg-m., arg-n., ars-h., ars-i., ars-m., asaf., aspar., aur., ***bar-c.,*** **BELL.,** berb., bov., brach., bry., cact., calc., canth., card-m., cham., chel., chim., ***chin.,*** chin-s., cic., cinnb., clem., colch., crot-h., crot-t., ***cycl.,*** dulc., euon., euph., eupi., ***ferr.,*** ferr-i., fl-ac., form., gels., ham., ign., ***iod.,*** iris, Jal., kali-bi., ***kali-c.,*** kali-p., ***kalm.,*** lach., led., lil-t., lyc., mag-c., ***mag-p., mang.,*** merc-i-f., mez., mosch., mur-ac., murx., nat-a., nat-c., nat-m., nit-ac., nux-m., osm., paeon., phos., phyt., plb., plumbg., ***puls., rhod., rhus-t.,*** sabad., sabin., ***sang.,*** sarr., sil., ***staph.,*** stry., sulph., sumb., tarax., tarent., tep., thuj., urt-u., ***verat.,*** verat-v., xan.
afternoon - abrot., fl-ac., phos., stry.
1 p.m., while riding - hydr.
2 p.m. - **RHUS-T.**
3 p.m. - dios., phos., **RHUS-T.,** sarr.
bed, in - dulc., led., ***rhus-t.***
bending arms - ant-c.
bending arm backwards - **RHUS-T.**
biceps, after lifting - berb., chin-a., **RHUS-T.,** stict.
morning - agar.
blow, as from - ***anac.,*** bar-ac., hell., plat.
bone - alumn., anac., arum-d., ars-s-r., aur., bar-c., berb., bry., carb-v., euon., ferr., ***fl-ac.,*** ham., hyos., ign., iod., kali-bi., ***lyc.,*** mag-s., mang., merc., ***mez.,*** murx., nit-ac., osm., ox-ac., phos., phyt., rhod., rhus-t., sarr., staph., sulph.
afternoon - fl-ac.
afternoon, 3 p.m. - sarr.
lain on - ***iod.***
nightly - dros.
paralyzed, as if - nit-ac.
rheumatic - ***ars-i., ferr.,*** fl-ac.
touch agg. - staph.
ulcerative - bar-c.
chill, after - ars-h.
cold after taking - phos.
cold air - ***kalm.***
damp weather - ***phyt.,*** rhod., rhus-t., sanic.

PAIN, upper arms
deltoid region - ***asar.,*** aur., ***bar-c.,*** bufo, calc., caul., chel., coc-c., ***colch.,*** **FERR.,** kali-bi., ***kalm.,*** lac-c., merc-c., nat-m., nux-v., phos., phyt., rhod., ***rhus-t.,*** **SANG.,** stram., verat., viol-o., zinc.
hand lies on table, while - asar.
inner side - bov., chel., crot-t., led., sil., tarent.
left - nux-m.
left, to right - ox-ac.
lifting something - nat-m.
right - agar., card-m., ***cedr., kalm.,*** lob., ***urt-u.***
electric shocks, like - tarax.
evening - anac., chin., colch., kali-bi., ox-ac., stry., sulph., zinc.
bed, in - dulc., led.
excitement - coloc.
extending arm - phyt., plat.
downward - agar., berb., carb-v., chin., dros., kali-bi., lach., ***lyc.,*** sulph.
into hand and thumb - kali-bi., ***puls.***
to finger - chel.
to neck, during menses - berb.
forenoon - agar., bov., com.
heart affections - cact.
inner side, extending to fingers - chel.
intermittent - asaf., led., sars.
jerking - anac., chin., kali-bi., lact., puls., ***ran-b.,*** rhus-t., ruta., sil., tarax., valer.
left - **RHUS-T.**
lifting, after - berb.
lying, on painful side - ***mang.***
when lying on it - carb-an., ***nat-m.***
menses, during - berb.
morning - ars-i., chel., euph., lyc., mez., rhus-t.
rising, after - dulc.
waking, on - ars-s-r., mez.
motion, on - anag., berb., ***bry.,*** bufo, calc., ***cocc., colch.,*** crot-t., euph., ***ferr.,*** ferr-p., fl-ac., iris, kali-c., ***kalm.,*** lac-c., ***led.,*** mag-c., ***merc.,*** nat-m., nux-v., phyt., plat., sabad., sabin., sep., staph.
amel. - ***arg-m.,*** aur-m-n., cina, cocc., cupr., ***dulc.,*** kali-bi., meph., ox-ac., paeon., **RHUS-T.,** thuj.
slow, amel. - ***ferr.***
neuralgic - hyper.
night - ars., ***cact.,*** cham., crot-t., ***ferr.,*** mang., ***merc.,*** nat-m., nux-v., ***phyt.,*** puls., ***sang.,*** stry., sulph.
4 a.m. - verat.
lying on it - nat-m.
sleep, during - sep.
noon - sulph.
lying down, after - ***rhus-t.***
outer side - phyt.
paralytic - aloe, alum., ant-c., arg-m., arg-n., ***bell.,*** bry., cham., ***chel., chin.,*** cina, cocc., con., ferr., kali-bi., kali-c., mur-ac., nit-ac., ***phos.,*** sep., ***staph.,*** thuj.
paroxysmal - gels., mur-ac.
perspiration amel. - thuj.

PAIN, upper arms
posterior part - hyos., ***stict.,*** stry.
pressure, amel. - bov., indg., laur.
pressure, on - berb., calc., phyt., sil.
pulsating - ign., **KALI-C.,** mur-ac., nat-m.
putting it, across the back - calc.
on coat - bry., chel., rhus-t., sang.
raising arm - agar., ***bar-c., bry.,*** bufo, calc., ***calc-p.,*** cocc., colch., ***ferr.,*** nat-c., nat-m., olnd., phos., plb., ***rhus-t., sang.,*** syph., teucr., zinc.
rheumatic - alumn., ***ars.,*** aspar., bry., calc., calc-p., carb-s., chel., ***chim.,*** coff., ***colch.,*** crot-t., dulc., **FERR.,** ***ferr-i.,*** ferr-p., ***fl-ac.,*** hyos., iod., iris, ***kalm.,*** merc., nat-m., phos., ***phyt.,*** ptel., ***rhod.,*** **RHUS-T., SANG.,** stram., urt-u., verat., zinc.
right - canth., crot-h., ***cycl.,*** eupi., fl-ac., nat-c., zinc.
singing, when - stann.
sleep, worse on going to - ***kali-c., kalm.***
spasmodic - agar., lact., mosch., olnd., valer.
splinter, as of - agar., ***nit-ac.***
stooping - sep.
touch agg. - agar., agn., arg-m., ***chin.,*** puls., sabin., ***staph.***
triceps - ***stict.***
turning in bed agg. - ***sang.***
walking, while - arg-n., merc-c.
wandering - phyt.
warmth amel. - ferr.
writing, while - ars-i., ***cycl., fl-ac., valer.***

PARALYSIS - ***acon.,*** aesc., **AGAR.,** ant-t., ***apis,*** arg-m., arn., ***ars., bar-c.,*** bar-m., ***bell.,*** both., bry., ***calc.,*** calc-p., calc-s., **CANN-I.,** carb-o., **CAUST.,** chel., chin., ***cocc.,*** colch., ***con., crot-c.,*** cupr., ***dulc.,*** ferr., ferr-i., ***gels., hell.,*** hep., kali-ar., ***kali-c.,*** kali-n., kalm., led., ***lyc.,*** mag-c., ***merc., merc-c.,*** morph., ***nit-ac., nux-v., op.,*** phos., phyt., plat., **PLB., RHUS-T.,** sec., sep., sil., ***stann., sulph.,*** tep., verat., verat-v., vip.
coldness, with - caust., cocc., ***dulc.,*** nux-v., plb., ***rhus-t.,*** zinc.
icy, during rest - ***dulc.***
diphtheria, after - ***caust.***
fright, from - stann.
insensibility, with - plb., ***rhus-t.,*** zinc.
lead, from - alumn., plb.
left - brom., cact., ***calc.,*** **DIG.,** lac-c., lat-m., pall., par.
and numbness, of right - tarent.
hysteria, in - sep.
stroke, after - ars.
vertigo, during - arg-n.
meningitis, during - ***acon.***
mercury, after abuse of - ***hep., nit-ac.***
neuralgia of brachial plexus, after - crot-t.
night - ***nux-v.***
pain in heart, with - crot-h., ***lat-m.,*** pall.
partial - atro-s., cic., kali-a., lac-c., ***lat-m.,*** merc., ***nux-v.,*** phos., plb.

PARALYSIS, arms
right - ***aesc.,*** **AM-C.,** arn., ars-s-r., bell., bism., cann-i., ***caust.,*** colch., ferr-i., **LYC.,** nit-ac., nux-v., ***plb.,*** sang., sil., **SULPH.,** ter.
arm and left leg - ter.
paralysis, of tongue, with - ***caust.***
shaking, after - nit-ac.
shocks, with - **NUX-V.**
sleep, during - mill.
stroke, after - aesc., ars., bar-c., op., **PHOS.**
sudden - ***nux-v.***
suppressed eruptions, from - hep.
writing, from - cocc.

paralysis, forearms - bar-c., calc-p., caust., colch., phos., plat., ***plb.,*** **SIL.**
extensor muscles - colch., merc., **PLB.**
flexor muscles - ars., ***gels.***
flexor muscles, when supinated - plb.
left - bar-c., calc-p.
pressure, as from - cham.
right - ***plb., rhus-t.***

paralysis, upper arms - agar., arg-m., calc., calc-p., chel., nux-v.
biceps - plb.
deltoid muscle - ***caust., cur.***
evening - am-m.
morning - am-m.
partial - calc.

PARALYSIS, sensation of - ***abrot.,*** acon., **AESC.,** agar., ***alum.,*** am-c., **AM-M.,** ang., ***ars.,*** ars-i., bell., berb., brom., bufo, ***calc.,*** camph., ***caust.,*** cham., chel., ***chin.,*** cina, **COCC., COLCH.,** coloc., croc., ***crot-c.,*** crot-t., ***cycl.,*** dig., dros., dulc., eupi., ***ferr.,*** ferr-i., ***gran.,*** graph., grat., hyper., ***ign., iod.,*** kali-c., ***lach., lith.,*** lob., meny., mez., nat-m., nat-s., ***nux-v.,*** ol-an., par., ***phos., plat.,*** plb., psor., rhod., rhus-v., sars., sec., ***sep., sil.,*** stann., sulph., sul-ac., ***tab.,*** tep., thuj., ***verat., zinc.,*** zing.
afternoon, nap, after - phos.
walking, while - brom.
eating, after - cocc.
evening - ferr-i., grat.
leaning arm on chair agg. - plat.
left - ***calc.,*** nux-v., ***plat.,*** sep.
left, arm and right foot - hyper., stann.
morning - chel., ***nux-v.,*** sil.
bed, in - chel.
waking, on - sulph.
motion, during - arg-m.
amel. - dulc.
night - ***nux-v.,*** **RHUS-T.,** til.
10 p.m. - carb-s.
right - aesc., **AM-C., AM-M.,** ***caust.,*** cina, fl-ac., sil.
sleep, during - plat.
stretching arm - ang.
writing, while - cocc., sul-ac.
from much writing - agar., ***caust.***

paralysis, forearms, sensation of - acon., all-s., ambr., apis, bism., bov., chel., cocc., fl-ac., kreos., par., prun., **RHUS-T.,** seneg., staph., stront-c., sulph.

paralysis, forearms, sensation of
writing, while - cocc., ferr-i.
paralysis, upper arms, sensation of - **BELL.,** ***chin.,*** ferr-i., ***plat.,*** sulph., zinc.
alternating, with drawing, tearing - sulph.
evening - sulph.
on raising the arm in bed - mez.
morning, after rising - sulph.
motion amel. - dulc.
sitting, while - cycl.
writing, while - agar., ***caust.,*** dulc.

PEMPHIGUS - sep., ter.

PERSPIRATION - agar., asaf., asar., bry., caps., guare., hyos., ip., jab., merc., **PETR.,** stann., stront-c., zinc.
cold and clammy - ***zinc.***
inner side of - arn.
night - ol-j.
sex, after - agar.
perspiration, forearms - ***petr.***

PINCHING, pain, forearms - calad., dulc., fl-ac., mang., nat-m., osm., ph-ac., spig., sulph.
evening - fl-ac.
posterior part - berb., merc-i-f.
pressure amel. - mang.
rest, during - spig.
pinching, upper arms - arg-m., calc., cina, kali-n., nat-c., nux-m., olnd., osm., ph-ac.
bone - gamb.
motion amel. - cina.
rubbing amel. - nat-c.
walking in open air - calc.

PRESSING, pain - ***anac.,*** arg-m., asar., bell., berb., bism., calc., camph., carb-v., ***caust.,*** cham., clem., coloc., ***cycl.,*** dig., dros., ***dulc., fl-ac.,*** ind., iod., kali-c., ***kalm.,*** lach., led., lil-t., lyc., manc., mur-ac., nat-s., nit-ac., petr., phos., puls., sars., sil., stann., staph., ***sulph.,*** tarent., thuj.
afternoon - thuj.
bones - ***anac.,*** cham., ***coloc.,*** con., kali-c., ***mez.,*** phos., sil., thuj.
motion amel. - coloc.
cough, during - dig.
cramp-like - dros., petr.
drawing - thuj.
evening - fl-ac.
forenoon - tarent.
inward - lach.
joints - anac., calc., cham., kali-c., mez., nit-ac., sep., sulph., zinc.
left - **KALM.,** sil.
lying, while - iod.
motion, agg. - led., staph., sulph.
amel. - camph., dulc.
motion, of arm, on - dig.
night - ***dulc.,*** merc.
outward - lil-t., thuj.
paralytic - cham., coloc., staph.
raising arm - sulph.
rheumatic - dulc.
right - ***caust., cycl.,*** nit-ac.
spots - nux-v.
stretching arm - sulph.

PRESSING, pain
tearing - asar., led.
touch agg. - staph.
pressing, forearms - agar., am-m., ***anac.,*** ant-c., arg-m., asaf., **AUR.,** aur-m-n., ***bell.,*** berb., bism., brom., bry., calc., camph., cocc., coloc., con., clem., crot-t., ***cycl.,*** dig., ferr-ma., fl-ac., gins., graph., hell., hep., hyper., indg., jatr., ***led.,*** lil-t., lyc., **MANG.,** meny., ***merc.,*** mez., mosch., mur-ac., nat-s., ***olnd.,*** osm., ph-ac., ***plat.,*** prun., puls., rhod., ruta., sabin., ***sars.,*** sep., stann., ***staph.,*** stront-c., tarax., ***verat.,*** verb.
bed, in - am-m.
cramp-like - ***anac.***
evening - fl-ac.
extending to fingers - con., ***cycl.***
grasping agg. - prun.
lying, while - am-m., aur-m-n.
morning - bry.
motion, on - anac., led., ***staph.***
amel. - am-m., aur-m-n., ***bism.,*** camph., cocc.
paralytic - ***cycl.,*** graph., staph.
paroxysmal - arg-m.
right - ***cycl.***
sitting, while - aur-m-n.
touch, amel. - bism., meny., ***staph.***
writing, while - am-m., anac., ***cycl.***
pressing, upper arms - acon., ***agn.,*** **ANAC.,** asaf., **AUR.,** aur-m-n., **BELL.,** berb., bism., bry., ***calc.,*** camph., carb-s., ***caust.,*** chel., cic., clem., colch., coloc., con., crot-t., cupr., ***cycl.,*** euph., fl-ac., gins., hell., indg., jatr., kalm., ***led.,*** **MEZ.,** mosch., mur-ac., nat-s., nux-m., petr., ph-ac., ***sabin.,*** sars., **STANN.,** ***staph.,*** teucr., zinc.
anterior part - bell.
bone, in - ***anac.,*** ang., bry., con., mez., stann.
burrowing - clem.
constrictive - coloc.
cramp-like - anac., asaf.
deltoid - staph., sulph.
evening - anac.
evening, in bed - staph.
extending to elbow - fl-ac., mez.
to neck during menses - berb.
inner side - spig., stann.
intermittent - anac., asaf., led.
leaning on it - am-m., carb-s.
left - ***asaf.,*** carb-s., tarax.
menses, during - berb.
morning - con., fl-ac., mez.
in bed - euph.
morning, waking, on - euph., mez.
motion, agg. - ang., berb., ***colch.,*** fl-ac., led., ***sabin., staph.***
amel. - am-m., aur-m-n.
move, on beginning to - mez.
paralytic - **BELL.,** bism., chel., mez., ph-ac., staph.
periosteum - aur., phos., staph.
posterior part - acon., aur., camph., stann.
right - ***cycl.***

pressing, upper arms
sitting - anac.
amel. - cycl., jal.
tearing - arg-m., aur., bell., camph., led., stann., thuj.
touch - ***agn.,*** arg-m., ph-ac., sabin., spig., ***staph.***
as if - clem.
walking in open air - anac.
amel. - thuj.

PRONATED, arm - cupr., plb.

PSORIASIS - ***iris,*** kali-ar., ***kali-s.,*** rhus-t., sil.
psoriasis, forearms - ***rhus-t.***

PULLING - agar., hura, plb., raph.
pregnancy, during - plb.
pulling, forearms hairs of, as if, were pulled - thuj.

PULSATION - alum., anac., asc-t., aster., berb., carb-v., caust., coloc., con., dig., hura, iod., ***kali-c.,*** lach., lyss., mag-c., mag-m., manc., merc-i-f., merc-sul., mur-ac., nat-c., nat-m., nux-v., petr., phys., sep., sil., sulph., thuj., zinc.
burning - phys.
eating, after - sil.
heartbeat, with - graph.
left - nux-v., xan.
raising arm - sil.
right - sil.
pulsation, forearms - bell., bufo, hura, kali-bi., lyss., olnd., plat., sabad.
inner side, near wrist - olnd.
pulsation, upper arms - ars-h., dig., ***kali-c.,*** kali-n., rhod., sars., squil., tarax.
deltoid - nat-m.
intermittent - kali-c., tarax.
near shoulder - sars.
night - kali-c.

PURRING - sep.

RAISED, difficult to raise - dig., gran., mag-c., phys.
impossible to raise - alum., cann-i., ferr., glon., lyc., mag-m., merc., nat-c., nat-m., nux-v., plb., sol-t-ae., ***sulph.***
sleep, in - sep.
raised, upper arms - ferr., nit-ac., ***sang.***

RASH - alum., ant-t., bell., berb., bry., calad., chlol., cupr., daph., dig., elaps, form., kali-ar., led., mag-p., ***merc., mez.,*** nux-v., phyt., ***puls.,*** rheum, ***rhus-t.,*** sec., ***sep., sil.,*** stram., ***sulph., sul-i.,*** tep.
alternating with asthma - calad., mez.
brownish - mez.
itching - alum., caust., nux-v., rheum, sep., sul-i.
red - mez., stram.

RELAXATION - guai., hell., nux-m., plat.
laughing, when - carb-v.

RESTLESSNESS - acon., agar., ars., aster., atro., brom., bufo, canth., **CAUST.,** cham., cina, coloc., dig., dirc., ferr., ***glon.,*** lac-ac., lyc., ***meph.,*** merc., ***mur-ac.,*** naja, nat-a., nat-c., nux-v., op., phos.,

RESTLESSNESS - phys., psor., rumx., sep., sil., stram., ***tarent.,*** zinc.
evening - mur-ac., nux-v.
forenoon - cham.
motion amel. - cham.
open air amel. - cham.
joints - calc.
morning - alum., glon.
on waking - nit-ac.
night - caust., kali-bi., merc., nux-v.
sleep, during - abrot., **CAUST.,** merc.
right - sil.
restlessness, upper arms - agar.

RHEUMATIC, pain - abrot., ***aesc.,*** alumn., ammc., ***ant-c., ant-t.,*** arg-n., ars., ars-i., astac., bell., berb., **BRY.,** ***cact.,*** **CALC-P.,** ***chel.,*** chin., ***cimic.,*** **COLCH.,** ***coloc.,*** com., dros., ***dulc.,*** **FERR.,** ferr-ar., ***ferr-i.,*** fl-ac., grat., ***guai.,*** ham., iod., kali-bi., ***kalm.,*** lach., ***led., lyc.,*** med., meph., **MERC.,** ***merc-i-f.,*** mez., ***nat-a.,*** nat-c., nit-ac., ***nux-v.,*** phel., phos., ***phyt.,*** podo., ***puls., ran-b., rhod.,*** **RHUS-T.,** rhus-v., **SANG.,** squil., stel., stict., ***sulph.,*** teucr., thuj., ust., ***valer.,*** viol-o., verat.

ROLLING, arm, down the - rhus-t.

ROUGHNESS - crot-h.
roughness, forearms - rhus-t.
evening - peti.

SCRAPING, pain - sulph.
scraping, forearms - bry.
styloid process of ulna, on - asaf.

SENSITIVE, to cold - agar., calc-p.

SEPARATED, sensation - cinnb., daph., ***stram.***
driving a horse, while - daph.
writing, while - cinnb.

SHAKING - ***agar.,*** bell., bry., bufo, merc., op., **PLB.**

SHARP, pain - acon., aesc., all-c., alum., am-c., ang., ant-c., ant-t., ***apis,*** arg-m., arn., ars-h., asaf., asar., aur., aur-m., benz-ac., berb., bov., brach., bry., bufo, calc., calc-p., cann-s., canth., carb-o., ***carb-s.,*** carb-v., cast-eq., caust., cham., chel., chlor., **CIC.,** ***cina,*** cinnb., cist., clem., ***cocc.,*** coloc., ***con., crot-t., cupr.,*** cycl., dor., dros., ***dulc.,*** elaps, euphr., eupi., fago., ***ferr.,*** ferr-p., fl-ac., form., glon., graph., guai., hell., hyper., ind., iod., kali-bi., ***kali-c.,*** kali-i., lac-c., lach., led., lept., ***lith., lyc., mag-m.,*** manc., mez., nat-c., nat-m., nit-ac., nux-v., ol-an., ox-ac., pall., petr., phel., ph-ac., ***phos.,*** phys., ***phyt.,*** pic-ac., plat., plb., psor., puls., ***ran-b.,*** raph., rat., rheum, ***rhod.,*** **RHUS-T.,** rhus-v., ruta., sac-alb., sabad., sabin., ***sars.,*** senec., ***sep.,*** sil., sol-n., spong., stann., staph., ***stict., still.,*** stry., ***sulph., tarent., thuj.,*** urt-u., valer., viol-t., zinc.
asleep, as if - ***sil.***
bending arm - petr.
bones - bufo, calc., dros., merc., mez., petr., ***sars.***
chill, during - ars-h.
cold, catching, while sweating - ***dulc.***
coughing, on - ***puls.***

SHARP, pain
cramp-like - ***cina.***
drawing -rhus-t.
evening - ***ars.,*** fl-ac., gamb., lact., sep., sulph.
5 p.m. - phys.
7 p.m. - sulph.
exertion, on - sep.
extending, to chest - caust.
downward - aesc., cann-s., caust., cupr., daph., ***ferr.,*** fl-ac., ***manc.,*** petr., phos., pic-ac., puls., **RHUS-T.,** still.
to finger tips - cist., puls.
to wrist - asc-t.
upward - petr.
flexor muscles - asaf.
inner side - arn., benz-ac., carb-o., chel., lept.
joints - bry., ***calc.,*** dros., ferr., graph., kali-n., laur., led., lyc., phos., puls., sars., ***sep., stann.,*** staph., ***sulph., sul-ac.,*** tab., thuj., viol-t.
morning 7:30 a.m. - fago.
motion, on - phos., urt-u., zinc.
amel. - arg-m., ars., dros., dulc., sep.
night - alum., calc., cham., dulc., phos.
10 p.m. - fl-ac.
outer surface - benz-ac., tarax.
periodical - cist.
raising arm - cic.
right - ***caust.,*** phos.
walking, while - ant-c.
wandering - arg-m., ars-h., cast-eq., lac-c., ***puls.,*** sulph.

sharp, forearms - ***acon.,*** aesc., aeth., alum., anac., ant-c., apis, arg-m., asaf., asar., aur-m., bapt., bell., benz-ac., ***berb.,*** bor., ***bov.,*** bufo, calc., camph., ***carb-an.,*** carb-s., ***caust.,*** cham., chel., **CIC.,** clem., coloc., cupr., cycl., ***dig.,*** dios., ***eupi.,*** fl-ac., form., graph., ***guai.,*** ham., iris, kali-i., kalm., lyc., mag-c., mag-m., merc., mez., myric., nat-c., ox-ac., ***ph-ac.,*** plb., ***ran-b., ran-s.,*** raph., rhod., sabad., sabin., ***sars.,*** senec., ***sil.,*** spig., ***spong.,*** staph., still., stram., stront-c., sul-ac., tab., tarax., ***thuj.,*** trom., viol-t., ***zinc.***
acute - berb., cast., merc., ph-ac.
burning - ***berb.,*** spig.
drawing - clem.
evening - fl-ac., thuj.
exertion, on - tab.
extending, downward - chel., ***ran-s.,*** sars.
to fingers - eupi., plb., still., thuj.
upward - asaf., zinc.
extensor surface - agar.
fine - stram., tarax.
flexors - tarent.
forenoon - mag-c.
left - aesc.
morning - mez.
on waking - kali-bi.
motion, on - acon., spig.
near elbow - arn., eupi., ol-an., meny., thuj.
night - alum.
noon, before eating - senec.
radius - bapt.

sharp, forearms
right - mag-c.
sitting, while - sabin., thuj.
touch agg. - cupr.
ulnar side - berb., cham., chin-s., con., ox-ac., thuj.
writing, while - berb., lyc., ox-ac., thuj.

sharp, upper arms - abrot., agar., agn., all-c., ***alum.,*** anac., ant-c., arg-m., arn., ars-m., asaf., aur-m-n., bar-c., bell., berb., ***bry.,*** calc., calc-p., cann-s., canth., ***carb-s.,*** caust., chel., chin., chin-a., cina, ***cocc.,*** coc-c., coloc., con., dig., dulc., elaps, euphr., ***ferr.,*** form., graph., grat., ***guai.,*** hell., ind., indg., ***kali-c.,*** kali-n., lact., laur., ***led.,*** lyc., mag-c., mang., merc-i-f., mez., nat-s., nux-m., olnd., ph-ac., plb., ***plat.,*** puls., rhod., ***rhus-t.,*** rumx., sabad., sabin., ***sars.,*** sil., stann., staph., stry., sulph., tarax., tep., ther., ***thuj.,*** zinc.
afternoon - form.
bone - agar., bry., calc., canth., caust., coloc., mez., sars., sulph.
condyles - ant-t., brom., indg., mang., merc., ***sabin.***
condyles, evening - chin-s.
condyles, external - chin-s., stram.
boring - asaf., mang., rhus-t.
burning - arg-m., asaf., berb., calc-p., dig., rhus-t., zinc.
carrying something - caust.
cramp-like - cina.
deltoid - agar., caust., meny., ox-ac., puls., stann., thuj.
dinner, after - canth., zinc.
drawing - plb., thuj.
dressing - zinc.
evening - calc., elaps, sulph., stry.
amel. - nat-s.
extending arm agg. - ind.
to, elbow - lyc.
to, fingers - ***rhus-t.***
to, forearm - chel.
to, shoulder - mang., ther.
holding a book - coc-c.
inner side - asaf., berb., carb-v., chel., con., led., mang., nux-m., rhus-t., samb., rumx., tarax.
itching - ph-ac.
jerking - ***carb-s.***
morning - zinc.
motion - **BRY.,** caust.
amel. - chin., ***cocc., kali-c.,*** **RHUS-T.,** sabad., tarax.
night - caust.
outer side - caust., tarax.
paroxysmal - carb-s., tarax.
posterior part - acon., tarax.
raising arm - agar., bry., caust.
right - caust., ***cocc.,*** sulph.
rubbing amel. - caust., tarax.
sitting, while - calc.
tearing - calc-ac., dig.
touch, amel. - thuj.

sharp, upper arms
walking, while - dig., sulph.
amel. - cina
in open air - thuj.
wandering - lyc.

SHOCKS - ***agar.,*** aloe, apis, ***arg-m.,*** arn., aur-m., **CIC.,** fl-ac., lyss., manc., nat-m., ***nux-v.,*** op., phos., phyt., puls., tarax.
evening - manc.
extending to hands - fl-ac.
left - agar., arg-m., ***cic.,*** manc.
paralyzed part - ***nux-v.***
shocks, upper arms - ***agar.,*** arg-m., ruta., tarax., ***valer.***
writing, while - manc.

SHOOTING, pain - aesc., brach., calc-p., cann-s., cinnb., ***con., crot-t.,*** cupr., daph., ***ferr.,*** hyper., ***lith.,*** phos., pic-ac., ***rhus-t.,*** sep., sol-n., ***still.,*** sulph., valer.
coughing, while - puls.
evening - sep., sulph.
extending, down - aesc.
downward - aesc., cann-s., daph., ***ferr., manc.,*** phos., pic-ac., still.
to wrist - aesc.
periodical - cinnb.
rest, during - sep.
shooting, forearms - ***acon.,*** bell., form., ham., plb., still., thuj., trom.
extending to fingers - plb., still., thuj.
motion, on - acon.
shooting, upper arms - ***ferr.,*** sulph., tep.
bone, in - arum-d., sulph.
evening - sulph.
posterior part - acon.
walking, while - sulph.

SHORT, sensation as if - aeth., alum., bell., sep.
short, forearms, sensation as if - cham.

SINKING, down, arm - acon., ***nat-m.***

SORE, pain - acon., aesc., agar., all-c., alum., am-c., ammc., aml-n., anac., ang., apis, arg-m., ***arn.,*** ars., asaf., aster., berb., bor., ***bry., calc.,*** calc-p., calc-s., cann-s., ***carb-ac.,*** carb-s., carb-v., card-m., cast-eq., **CAUST.,** chlf., chin-s., cist., clem., cocc., coloc., com., ***con., croc.,*** crot-h., crot-t., ***cur., dulc.,*** **EUP-PER.,** ***ferr.,*** ferr-ar., graph., grat., hep., hyper., indg., kali-bi., kreos., ***lach.,*** laur., led., lyc., lyss., mag-c., meph., merc., merc-i-f., merc-i-r., mez., nat-m., nat-s., ***nit-ac.,*** nux-v., ol-an., ***ph-ac.,*** phos., pip-m., ***plat.,*** plb., plumbg., ***puls., rhus-t.,*** rhus-v., rob., ***ruta.,*** sang., sarr., ***sep.,*** sil., spong., stry., ***sulph.,*** sumb., tep., ***verat.,*** vip., zinc.
air, open amel. - caust.
daytime - sulph.
eating, after - clem.
evening - mag-m., zinc.
amel. - merc-i-r.
heat amel. - ***ferr.***
joints of - alum., alumn., aur-m-n., ph-ac.
joints of, when bending backwards - ign.
left - merc-i-f., sumb.

SORE, pain
lying, on affected side - merc-i-f.
on arms - anac., cocc.
morning - ign., nux-v., ***ph-ac.,*** tab., zinc.
motion, on - arg-m., ***calc.,*** croc., ferr., kali-bi., plb., sulph.
amel. - caust., ***dulc.***
motion, passive motion agg. - merc-i-f.
night - anac., merc-i-f., plb.
noon - merc-i-r.
paralytic - alum., coloc., dulc.
pressure, on - ***cina, merc-i-f.***
putting on coat - merc-i-r.
raising it agg. - ***nit-ac.,*** verat., zinc.
right - ***merc-i-f.,*** nit-ac.
rubbing - ***merc-i-f.***
sitting, while - berb., bry., caust., coloc.
taking hold of them - ***calc.***
waking, on - chel., mag-s., rumx., sulph.
walking, while - dios.
amel. - verat.
work amel. - caust.
writing, while - ***merc-i-f.***
sore, forearms - acon., ail., aloe, **ARN.,** ars-m., aur-m-n., bar-ac., ***calc.,*** calc-p., camph., canth., carb-an., **CAUST.,** cedr., chel., ***cic.,*** coca, com., con., croc., crot-t., cupr., ***cycl.,*** dig., **EUP-PER.,** ham., hep., hura, iod., kali-bi., led., lyc., merc., merc-i-f., merc-i-r., mur-ac., nit-ac., ol-an., ***ph-ac.,*** phos., plan., prun., ***rhus-t.,*** ruta., sabin., sal-ac., sil., sulph., sul-ac., thuj., ***zinc.***
extending to fingers - iod.
forenoon - led.
lying on table - ph-ac.
motion, on - nit-ac., zinc.
amel. - aur-m-n.
night - cycl.
posterior part - con.
radius - phos., ***rhus-t.,*** sil.
right - ***cycl.,*** merc-i-f.
sex, after, on flexing - sabin.
turning arm - zinc.
ulna - ars., ruta.
near elbow - mez.
near wrist - ***calc.***
sore, upper arms - aesc., agar., ***agn.,*** am-m., ammc., anac., arg-m., ars-h., arum-t., asaf., bar-c., bell., bov., ***calc.,*** canth., cedr., cina, cinnb., cocc., coff., crot-h., cupr., cycl., eupi., **EUP-PER.,** ferr-i., fl-ac., graph., grat., ham., hell., ***hep.,*** ign., indg., iod., iris, kali-c., kreos., laur., led., lyc., lyss., mag-m., mez., mur-ac., nat-c., ***nat-m.,*** nicc., ***nit-ac.,*** ox-ac., petr., ***ph-ac., phos.,*** phyt., plan., plat., sarr., ***sep., stann.,*** stry., ***sulph., sumb.,*** tep., thuj., verat., zinc.
ascending steps - ***calc.***
biceps - brach., ham.
bones, in - ang., bov., ***cocc.,*** croc., ham., **HEP.,** phos., sarr., ***sil.,*** thuj., zinc.
condyles - glon., graph., laur., phos., thuj.
cold hands, with - nit-ac.
deltoid - petr.

sore, upper arms
dinner, after - thuj.
evening - stry.
extending it, on - phyt.
to shoulder - laur.
to wrist - verat.
extensor muscles of - mur-ac.
left - sulph.
lifting - nat-m.
morning - bov., ham.
motion, on - cocc., cycl., grat., ham., nat-c., plan., plat., sep.
amel. - cupr., kali-c., ***lyc.,*** mur-ac.
motion, arm backward and forward - ***nat-m.***
night - sep.
pressure amel. - bov.
raising arms, on - grat., kali-c., nat-m., nit-ac., plan.
right - cinnb.
sitting, while - phos.
sleep, during - sep.
stretching limb agg. - plat., verat.
touched - cycl., kreos., mag-c., mez., nat-c.
waking - fl-ac.

SPRAINED, as if - ***ambr., arn.,*** aur-m., bell., bor., bov., ***ign.,*** jug-c., lach., lact., merc., mez., nit-ac., olnd., petr., ***phos.,*** prun., ter., thuj.
forenoon - petr.
joints - stann.
left - nit-ac.
motion agg. - mez.

sprained, forearms, as if - aur-m., nat-c., tab.
near wrist - ***calc.***

sprained, upper arms, as if - alum., caust., euph., ***rhus-t.,*** ter.
biceps - agar.
paralytic - acon.
rheumatic - anac.

STIFFNESS - agar., ***am-c.,*** am-m., anac., ars-h., aur-m., bell., calc., camph., canth., caps., ***caust., cham.,*** con., dulc., ***ferr.,*** ferr-ar., ***ham.,*** hyos., kali-bi., kali-c., kali-i., kali-n., lil-t., lyc., manc., meny., merc., merc-i-r., nat-c., nat-m., ***nux-v., op.,*** par., petr., ph-ac., phos., plat., puls-n, ***rhus-t.,*** sars., ***sep.,*** sil., stann., thuj., verat., zinc.
chill, during - eup-per.
cold, on becoming - am-c., kali-c., phos., ***tub.***
epilepsy, before - ***bufo.***
evening - am-m., petr.
extension impossible - caps.
grasping anything - am-c., cham.
hanging down - sep.
manual labor, after - **RHUS-T.**
morning - ***petr.***
motion, on - sars.
after - kali-c., ***rhus-t.***
amel. - kali-n.
night - am-c., bell., caust., kali-c., ***nux-v.***
paralytic - ***caust.,*** kali-i., nit-ac., plat.
raising arm impossible - nat-c.
over head - caust.
right - **AM-M.,** arn., bell., kali-bi., kali-c.
writing, while - ***caust.***

stiffness, forearms - aur-m., bry., calc-s., ***caust., cham.,*** coloc., hydr-ac., plat., prun., ***rhus-t.,*** stann., thuj.
cramp-like - plat., stann.
grasping anything - ***cham.***
painful - **RHUS-T.,** thuj.
writing, while - ***caust.,*** prun.

stiffness, upper arms, paralytic - acon.
rheumatic - anac.
biceps - agar.

SUPPURATION, forearms - lyc., plb.

SWELLING - acon., agar., alum., anac., ***anthr., apis, aran., ars.,*** bar-c., ***bell.,*** both., ***bry., bufo,*** cadm-s., ***chin.,*** chin-s., chlol., cinnb., colch., cop., ***crot-h.,*** crot-t., ***cur.,*** dig., dor., dulc., elaps, ferr., ferr-ar., ***ferr-p.,*** form., graph., ***hydr.,*** iod., kali-bi., kali-i., ***lach., lyc.,*** manc., merc., merc-c., ***mez.,*** naja, nat-s., ***phos.,*** **RHUS-T.,** rhus-v., sep., sil., sol-n., stry., ***sulph.,*** sul-ac., vario., verat., vesp., vip.
afternoon - nat-c.
black - ***carb-v., mur-ac.***
blisters, black, putrid - ***ars.***
bluish - ars., bufo, elaps, **LACH.,** samb.
bone - calc., dulc., lyc., mez., ***sil., sulph.***
burning - mur-ac., olnd., sulph.
cold - lach., ***puls.***
cramps, after - graph.
edematous - ***apis, aur.,*** aur-m., cact., calc-ar., crot-h., ***ferr., lach., lyc., merc-c., phos.,*** sil.
evening - ***cur.,*** rhus-t., stann.
hard - ars., carb-an., graph., lach., led., sulph.
heart affection - lycps.
hot - ant-c., ***apis,*** bry., bufo, ***cocc., hep., merc.,*** mez., rhus-t., sulph.
joints - calc.
lymphatic - berb.
night - ***aran.,*** dig., kali-n., phos.
nodular swellings - ***agar., ars.,*** carb-an., ***caust.,*** dulc., lyc., ***mag-c.,*** mag-m., mang., ***mez.,*** mur-ac., nat-m., nit-ac., sil., stann., zinc.
painful - ant-c., chin., hep., kali-c., ***lach., mosch.,*** nux-v., sep., ***sulph., thuj.***
painless - euphr., lyc.
pale - ***apis,*** bry., nux-v.
paralysis, after - sulph.
periosteum - ***aur., merc.,*** mez.
red - alum., ant-c., **BELL.,** ***bry., bufo,*** graph., ***hep.,*** lac-d., ***lyc.,*** mag-c., ***merc.,*** sep., spong., ***thuj.***
rigidity, with - sulph.
shining - bry., sulph.
stooping, on - sil.
uncovering amel. - chin.
white - ***apis.***

swelling, forearms - anac., ant-c., apis, aran., arn., ***ars.,*** aur., berb., bufo, calc., cadm-s., caust., crot-c., crot-t., dig., ***ferr-p., graph., lach.,*** lyc., ***merc.,*** nux-v., op., plb., ***rhus-t.,*** sep., sulph., vesp., vip.
dark blue - samb.
elbow, near - lyc.

swelling, forearms
gangrenous - **LACH.**
nodular - eupi., mez., mur-ac., nat-m., zinc.
posterior part - plb.
radius - ***calc.***
red - lac-d., sep., **SIL.**
line - ***lach.***

swelling, upper arms - acon., anac., ***apis,*** aran., arn., berb., ***bry.,*** calc-p., coloc., ***graph.,*** kali-c., puls., sang., sep., sulph., tep., vip.
bone of - guare., tep.
hard - ***sulph.***
hot - ***sulph.***
nodular swellings - ars., nat-m., zinc.
painful - ***puls.***
vaccination, after - ***apis,*** **SIL.,** ***sulph.,*** **THUJ.**

TEARING, pain - ***acon.,*** aesc., agar., ***alum., ambr.,*** am-c., ***am-m.,*** anac., ang., ant-t., ***arg-m., arg-n.,*** arn., ***ars.,*** ars-h., asaf., asar., aur., aur-m., ***bell.,*** benz-ac., berb., bism., bor., bov., brom., bry., bufo, ***cact., calc., calc-p.,*** camph., canth., ***caps.,*** carb-an., carb-s., carb-v., **CAUST.,** cham., chel., ***chin.,*** chin-a., cic., cinnb., ***cina,*** clem., ***cocc.,*** coff., ***colch., coloc., con.,*** crot-h., crot-t., ***cupr.,*** dig., dulc., ***ferr.,*** ferr-i., ferr-m., form., grat., ***guai.,*** hep., ***hyper.,*** ign., indg., iod., ***kali-ar., kali-bi., kali-c., kali-n., kali-p.,*** kali-s., kalm., kreos., lach., lachn., ***led., lyc.,*** lyss., ***mag-c.,*** **MAG-M.,** mag-s., mang., meny., ***merc.,*** mez., mur-ac., nat-a., **NAT-C.,** nat-m., ***nat-p.,*** **NAT-S.,** nicc., ***nit-ac.,*** nux-v., ol-an., par., phel., ***ph-ac., phos.,*** plat., **PLB.,** ***psor.,*** puls., ran-b., raph., ***rhod.,*** **RHUS-T.,** ruta., sabin., ***sars.,*** sep., **SIL.,** stann., staph., stront-c., stry., **SULPH.,** sul-ac., tep., ***teucr., thuj.,*** **VALER.,** verb., ***zinc.***
afternoon - kali-n., sars.
alternating sides - lac-c., sulph.
bones - ang., aur., benz-ac., cact., carb-v., caust., ***chin.,*** hell., iod., ***kali-bi., merc.,*** mez., phos., ***rhod.,*** ruta, stront-c., sulph., ***zinc.***
chill, during - ***ars.,*** ars-h., ***rhus-t.***
cold, air, from - ign.
food and drink - ***cocc.***
cramp-like - aur., nat-c., ruta.
daytime - ***sulph.***
evening - alum., hyper., kali-n.
by exposure to air - cham.
extending, downward - ***aesc.,*** calc., camph., caust., cham., ***chin.,*** crot-t., kali-c., kali-n., lach., lyc., nat-c., puls., sabin.
to all parts - chin.
to back - caust.
to fingers - alum., am-m., camph., caps., cham., ***chin., coloc.,*** crot-t., lyc., kali-n., mag-m., nat-c.
to fourth finger - aur-m.
to index finger - aesc.
to thumb - camph., cham., lyc., sil.
to wrist - kali-n., nat-c.
ulnar nerve, along - aesc., thuj.
upward - arn., ***ars.,*** sep.
forenoon, 11 a.m. - sars.

TEARING, pain
intermittent - kali-n.
jerking - **CHIN.,** puls., sil.
joints - alum., am-c., bov., cact., calc., carb-v., caust., cham., chin., coloc., con., dig., **GRAPH.,** grat., iod., kali-bi., **KALI-C.,** kali-n., lact., ***lyc.,*** nat-c., nit-ac., **PH-AC.,** phos., puls., sep., sil., stram., ***stront-c., sulph., teucr., zinc.***
morning - stront.
sitting - stront.
wandering - kali-bi.
left - asar., cic., kali-c., kali-n., phos., puls.
lying, while - sabin.
on left side - ***phos.***
painful side agg. - ***ars.***
side, on the - kali-n.
while still - ***rhus-t.***
manual labor, from - iod., ***rhus-t.***
menses, during - bell., kali-n.
morning - cham., hyper., thuj.
bed, in - carb-v., eupi., mag-m.
waking - cact.
motion, on - chel., dros., kali-n., nit-ac., sep., ***sil.,*** stann.
amel. - ***agar.,*** am-m., arg-m., ***ars.,*** cina, ***lyc.,*** **RHUS-T.,** thuj.
night - alum., am-c., ars., ***calc., ferr.,*** hyper., kali-n., merc., nat-c., plb., sep., stront.
10 p.m. - form.
3 a.m. - am-c.
bed, in - stront.
noon, during menses - nux-v.
numbness, with - sep.
outer side - mag-m.
paralytic - ***cham., chin., cina, ferr-m.,*** mag-m., stann.
paroxysmal - **CALC.,** kali-n., sep.
pressure, on - plb.
rest, during - ang., nat-c.
right - calc., chel., ***cina,*** nat-c., phos., **SULPH.**
while lying on left side - ***mag-m.***
rising amel. - nat-c.
sitting, while - nicc., **VALER.**
stretching them, on - hipp.
touch - ***chin.***
twitching - ph-ac., sul-ac.
walking amel. - arg-m., ***kali-s., rhod.,*** **RHUS-T., VALER.**
wandering - ***kali-bi.***
writing, while - cinnb.

tearing, forearms - ***acon., aesc.,*** aeth., ***agar., alum., ambr.,*** am-c., am-m., arg-m., ***ars.,*** asaf., aur., aur-m., bar-c., bell., ***berb., bism.,*** bor., bov., brom., ***bry.,*** cact., **CALC.,** calc-p., camph., canth., ***carb-s.,*** **CARB-V., CAUST.,** ***cham.,*** chel., ***chin.,*** cic., ***cina,*** cinnb., clem., cocc., ***colch., coloc.,*** crot-t., cupr., cycl., ***dig., graph., grat., guai.,*** hell., hyos., ***hyper.,*** indg., ***kali-bi.,*** **KALI-C.,** kali-chl., kali-n., kali-p., kalm., lach., lact., laur., led., lyc., mag-c., ***mag-m.,*** mag-s., mang., meny., ***merc., merl., mez., mur-ac.,*** myric., nat-c., nat-m., **NAT-S.,** ***nicc., nit-ac.,*** ol-an., op., par., phel.,

tearing, forearms - ph-ac., ***phos.,*** plb., ***puls.,*** ran-b., rat., rheum, ***rhod.,*** ***rhus-t.,*** ruta., sabin., ***sars.,*** sep., ***sil.,*** stann., staph., ***stront-c.,*** ***sulph.,*** tab., tarax., tep., teucr., ***thuj.,*** til., ***valer.,*** verb., ***zinc.***
afternoon - ***nat-s.,*** nicc., thuj.
while driving - thuj.
bending finger, on - asaf.
cold, when - phos.
cramp-like - cina, gran., ruta.
evening - alum., brom., nat-s., op., rhod.
extending to, finger, joints - ***coloc.***
to, finger, tips - alum., asaf., aur-m., sep.
to, hand - ***agar.,*** alum., am-m., ***berb.,*** ***carb-v.,*** caust., cham., coloc., grat., lyc., mag-m., mur-ac., rat., zinc.
to, ring finger - rat.
to, wrist - bar-c., ***calc.***
extensor muscles - mur-ac.
flexors - ***colch.***
forenoon - agar., ol-an.
11 a.m. - mag-s.
grasping anything - ***calc.***
hang down, letting arm - stront.
left - ***asaf.,*** camph., ***carb-v.,*** coloc., rat.
morning - alum., mez., phos.
waking, on - alum., cact.
motion, amel. - ***agar.,*** am-m., arg-m., bism., cina, cocc., ***lyc.,*** ***rhod.,*** ***rhus-t.,*** sars., ***valer.***
of fingers - asaf.
violent amel. - am-m.
night, in bed - ***ars.,*** ***merc.,*** ***rhod.***
paralytic - ***bism.,*** cocc., ***colch.,*** nat-m., phos., stann.
paroxysmal - arg-m., aur., ***calc.,*** cocc.
pressure amel. - sulph.
radius - agar., arg-m., berb., calc., camph., carb-v., caust., kali-bi., ***zinc.***
right - arg-m., aur., ***bism.,*** canth.
then left - arg-m.
sitting, while - cina, nat-s.
styloid process - kali-c., kali-n.
tendons of - ***calc.,*** caust., coc-c., kali-n., mag-s., tab.
touch agg. - nit-ac.
ulna - ***agar.,*** bry., caust., chin., cupr., kali-bi., kali-chl., lyc., mez., sars., verb., ***zinc.***
middle of, forenoon - thuj.
middle of, forenoon, while writing - thuj.
near the elbow - phel., sil.
posterior part of - dig., thuj.
warmth of stove amel. - cinnb.
wet weather - ***rhod.***
writing while - cic., cinnb., ***ran-b.***

tearing, upper arms - aesc., ***agar.,*** ***alum.,*** am-c., ***am-m.,*** arg-m., arn., **ARS.,** ars-h., aur., **BELL.,** ***berb.,*** bism., bov., ***bry.,*** calc., camph., canth., carb-an., carb-s., ***carb-v.,*** card-m., cast., caust., chel., ***chin.,*** cic., cimic., cina, clem., coc-c., colch., coloc., con., crot-t., dig., eupi., ferr., ferr-ar., ferr-p., ***grat.,*** guai., hyos., hyper., ign., ***indg.,*** ***kali-ar.,*** kali-bi., ***kali-c.,*** kali-n., kali-p., kalm., ***lach.,*** lachn., laur., ***led.,*** lil-t., ***lyc.,*** ***lyss.,*** mag-c., ***mag-m.,*** mag-s., mang., meny., ***merc.,*** merl., mez., ***mur-ac.,*** myric., ***nat-c.,*** nat-m., nat-p., **NAT-S.,** ol-an., olnd., petr., phel., ph-ac., phos., **PLB.,** psor., ***puls.,*** ***rat.,*** rheum, ***rhus-t.,*** rhus-v., ruta., sabin., sars., sec., sep., **SIL.,** ***stann.,*** ***staph.,*** ***sulph.,*** sul-ac., tep., ***thuj.,*** ***valer.,*** **ZINC.**
afternoon - bov., canth., nat-s., thuj.
alternating with tearing pain in hip - bry.
anterior part - sulph.
bed, in - caust., con., ***lyc.,*** mag-s., sulph., til.
bent, while, agg. - rat.
bone - acon., agar., alum., ***am-m.,*** ang., arn., bell., berb., bov., canth., carb-an., caust., ***chin.,*** cocc., eupi., kali-n., led., mag-m., merc., nat-c., ***nat-s.,*** phos., psor., rhus-t., ruta., ***valer.,*** zinc.
afternoon - nat-s.
evening - sulph.
extending to elbow - caust.
forenoon - agar., alum., nat-s.
morning - eupi.
motion amel. - cocc., psor.
night, 11 p.m. - am-m.
noon - nicc.
paralytic - phos.
pressure, amel. - canth.
sitting, while - ***am-m.,*** indg.
walking, while - psor., sulph.
chill, during - ***rhus-t.***
cold, on becoming - phos.
condyles, in - thuj.
constrictive - merl.
coughing, when - alum.
cramp-like - meny.
deltoid - kali-n., nat-c., staph., zinc.
drawing - bry., cina, coc-c., mur-ac., ***thuj.***
evening - agar., alum., clem., con., kali-c., lyc., sars., sulph.
amel. - nat-s.
lying down amel. - am-m.
exertion, from - **RHUS-T.**
extending, down arm - alum., am-m., canth., cast., caust., ferr., guai., ***lach.,*** mag-c., merc., merl., mur-ac., ol-an., ***rat.,*** til., ***zinc.***
to axilla - ars.
to elbows - rat.
to fingers - alum., am-m., aur-m.
to scapula - alum.
to shoulder - kali-c., lachn.
to wrist - am-m., mag-c., ol-an., sars.
upward - **ARS.,** kali-c., lach., led.
forenoon - agar., alum., chel.
hanging down amel. - rat., ***rhus-t.***
holding a book, while - coc-c.
increasing and decreasing rapidly - stann.
inner side - berb., camph., laur., lyc., mang., merl., nat-s., phel., spig., zinc.
intermittent - zinc.
jerking - ***chin.,*** mag-c., ph-ac., sulph.
left - agar., ***am-m.,*** aur., bov., caust., puls.
lying, on it - carb-an., cast.
lying, on well side, amel. - cast.

tearing, upper arms
morning - eupi., mag-s., sulph.
6 a.m. - bry.
11 a.m. - bry.
motion, agg. - carb-v., ferr., ferr-p., ***sil.,*** thuj.
amel. - am-m., ***arg-m.,*** coc-c., con., ***lyc.,*** psor., ***rhus-t.,*** sars., staph., thuj., valer.
preventing - tep.
moving arm amel. - mur-ac., sulph.
night - am-m., caust.
11 p.m. - am-m.
3 a.m. - nat-c.
in side not lain on - kali-bi., puls.
midnight, after - carb-an.
warm bed, in - caust.
noon - nicc.
outer side - mag-m., phos.
paralytic - **BELL.,** carb-v., ***chin.,*** phos.
paroxysmal - carb-v., led., ***zinc.***
periodic - grat.
posterior part - agar., alum., camph., hyos., nat-c., sil., sul-ac., zinc.
pressive - arg-m., aur., merl., stann.
pressure amel. - cina, indg.
raising when - ***agar.,*** carb-an., ***ferr.,*** mag-c.
rheumatic - ferr-p., nat-m.
right - canth., coc-c., eupi., ign., petr., ***ran-b.***
rising amel. - bry., nat-c., sulph.
rubbing amel. - nat-c.
side, lain on - cast.
not lain on - kali-bi.
sitting, while - ***am-m.,*** mur-ac., ***staph.***
sneezing, when - alum.
standing - nat-c.
stretching out amel. - mur-ac.
sudden - crot-t., kali-c., meny.
touch, on - thuj.
agg. - spig.
twisting - cham.
twitching - camph., mag-c., merc., merl., sulph.
uncovering it - aur.
walking, while - bry., dig., led., sulph.
amel. - mur-ac.
open air, in - calc.
open air, amel. - sulph.
wandering - merl.
warm bed - caust.
work agg. - ***rhus-t.***
writing, while - mur-ac., ***valer.***

TENSION - ***alum.,*** anac., arg-m., aur., bar-c., berb., carb-v., caust., chin., cic., coloc., **DIG.,** dulc., graph., hyper., kali-c., lach., mag-p., mang., meny., mez., mur-ac., nat-c., nat-p., nat-s., nit-ac., petr., phos., prun., puls., rhus-t., rhus-v., sep., sil., ***sulph.,*** tab., thuj., vip., zinc.
cold, as from - alum.
elevation agg. - kali-c.
extending to, finger tips - puls.
to, neck, during menses - berb.
joints - mang.
left - kali-c.
numbness, with - sep.
stretching, on - anac., cimx.

TENSION,
walking, on - cic.
writing, when - **MAG-P.**

tension, forearms - agar., ant-c., cadm-s., calc., camph., ***caust.,*** coloc., com., ***crot-h.,*** crot-t., kali-c., lach., mag-p., mang., nat-c., rat., stront-c., teucr., thuj., zinc.
evening - camph.
extensors, while writing - **MAG-P.,** thuj.
motion, on - calc.

tension, upper arms - agar., alum., berb., bry., bufo, carl., crot-t., prun., rhus-t., spig., sulph., zinc.
air, open, in - rhus-t.
biceps - agar.
extending to, fingers - crot-t.
to, forearm - phos.
lower part of - kali-c.
morning, in bed - crot-t.
motion, during - carl.
certain, during - agar.
walking, while - spig.

THRILLING, sensation - **CANN-I.**

TIED, sensation as if - abrot., alum., caj., nux-m.

TINGLING, prickling, asleep - ***acon.,*** acet-ac., ail., ***alum., ambr.,*** am-c., am-m., apis, arn., ars., ***aur.,*** bapt., bell., cann-i., cann-s., caps., ***carb-an., carb-s., carb-v.,*** caust., chel., ***cocc.,*** con., corn., ***dig.,*** fl-ac., **GRAPH.,** hyos., ign., kali-c., kali-n., ***mag-m.,*** merc., mez., mill., morph., nat-s., ol-an., paeon., ***ph-ac.,*** **PHOS.,** plat., puls., rhod., rhus-v., sabad., ***sec.,*** **SIL.,** stry., sulph., thuj., ust.
carrying anything, when - ***ambr.***
extending to fingers - carb-ac.
forenoon - mill.
left - elaps
lying on the back, while - kali-n.
midnight, before - caust.
morning - ail., ***mag-m.***
waking, on - ail., ***mag-m.***
right - am-c., am-m., carb-an., kali-bi., sil.
arm and left leg at night - kali-c.
when lying on the left side - mag-m.
side, lain on - ambr., arg-m., ars., ***bar-c.,*** bufo, ***calc.,*** carb-an., ***carb-v., chin.,*** cop., ***croc.,*** glon., ***graph.,*** hep., ***ign.,*** kali-c., ***lach., phos.,*** **PULS.,** ***rheum,*** **RHUS-T.,** samb., sep., sil.
not lain on - fl-ac., mag-m.
sitting, while - ***graph.,*** teucr.
writing, while - spig.

tingling, forearms, prickling, asleep - aesc., alum., am-m., ars., caps., ***cham., cocc.,*** coloc., con., croc., ***gels.,*** lac-c., ***lyc.,*** mag-m., merc., nat-m., ***nit-ac.,*** nux-v., ***ph-ac.,*** phys., pip-m., psor., puls., sec., sep., sulph.
extending to fingers - carb-ac., pip-m., phys.
left - alum.
right - am-m., coloc.

tingling, upper arms, prickling, asleep - sep.

TREMBLING - acon., ***agar.,*** alumn., ambr., anac., ***arg-n., ars.,*** bar-c., bell., bry., calc., ***calc-p.,*** caps., ***carb-s.,*** caust., chel., ***cic., cocc.,*** coff., colch., com., crot-h., ***cupr.,*** dor., eupi., ferr-m., graph., ***hyos.,*** hyper., ind., iod., kali-ar., kali-c., kali-s., lil-t., lyc., manc., med., meph., **MERC.,** murx., **NIT-AC.,** ol-an., onos., **OP.,** paeon., petr., ph-ac., ***phos.,*** phys., plan., **PLB.,** rhod., ***rhus-t.,*** sabad., sabin., seneg., ***sil., spig.,*** spong., ***stram.,*** sulph., tab., thuj., verat., viol-o., zinc.
convulsions, during - sulph.
eating, when - sec., stram.
after - bism.
epilepsy, before - ***sil.***
evening - ***hyos.,*** phys., plan.
7 p.m. - phys.
exertion of mind - vinc.
moderate, after - ***hyos.,*** **RHUS-T.,** sil.
fine work, with - sulph.
forenoon - paeon.
11 a.m. - phys., plb.
holding anything - coff., led., lyc., phos.
holding anything with abducted arm - caust.
internal - petr.
lain on - ***camph.***
leaning on it, when - astac., meph.
left - hyper., puls., sulph.
morning - ***sil.,*** sulph.
motion, on - bell., led., plb.
after - hyos.
amel. - com., **RHUS-T.**
on slight - bell., gels., iod., ***mag-p.***
night, on waking - verat.
brandy, night, amel. - plb.
paroxysms, in - ***op.***
right - eupi., sil., sulph.
rising, after - alumn.
sitting, while - merc.
sleep, during - merc.
standing, on - merc.
taking hold of anything - verat.
urinary difficulty - dulc.
work, fatigue - ***cupr., plb.***
writing, while - agar., ant-c., bar-c., caust., chin., cimic., colch., coff., hep., kali-c., **MERC.,** nat-m., nat-s., olnd., ph-ac., sabad., samb., sep., sulph., thuj., valer., zinc.
after - thuj.

trembling, forearms - agar., bar-c., ***calc-p.,*** carb-s., caust., cimic., colch., fl-ac., merc., nit-ac., onos., plb., spong., zing.
anything is grasped, when - verat.
extending to thumb - agar.
right - ***dulc., nit-ac.***
writing, while - ***caust.,*** com., **MERC.**

trembling, upper arms - agar., ant-c., aran., asaf., carb-s., fl-ac., nit-ac.
motion, amel. - asaf.

TUBERCLES - ars., crot-h., ***nat-c.,*** phyt., rhus-t.
painful - ars.
ulcerate - ***nat-c.***

tubercles, forearms - ***agar.,*** am-c., jug-r., kali-n., lach., mur-ac., ph-ac.

TWINGING, pain - pyrus, ***rhus-t.,*** teucr.

twinging, forearms - chin-s., mang.
extending to fingers - stram.
extensor muscles - stram.

twinging, upper arms - chin-s., hipp., sulph.
bone, condyles - merc.
evening - chin-s.
writing, while - chin-s.

TWISTING, sensation - **BELL.,** cit-v., graph., iod., stry.

TWITCHING - aesc., agar., aloe, alumn., ambr., am-c., ***ant-t.,*** ars., ars-i., ***asaf.,*** atro., bar-c., bar-m., bell., berb., brom., bry., calc., carb-ac., carb-v., cast., ***caust., chel.,*** chlf., **CIC.,** ***cina, coff.,*** con., ***cupr.,*** dulc., fl-ac., ***graph.,*** hell., hep., hyos., ign., iod., ***kali-c.,*** kali-n., lach., lact., ***lyc.,*** mag-c., mag-m., ***meny., merc., merc-c.,*** mez., morph., mosch., mygal., nat-a., nat-c., nat-m., nit-ac., ***nux-v.,*** olnd., ***op.,*** petr., phos., phyt., plan., plat., plb., ran-b., rheum, ***rhod.,*** rhus-t., rumx., sabad., sant., sep., sil., squil., ***stann.,*** stram., stry., sul-ac., tarax., tarent., teucr., **THUJ.,** ***valer.,*** verat., zinc., zing.
backward and inward - cupr.
bending, on - dulc.
daytime - nat-c.
evening, bed, in - carb-v., graph.
on falling asleep - cast., kali-c., sil.
forenoon - fl-ac.
grasping, on - nat-c.
left - zinc,
morning - caust., rheum.
in bed - zinc.
rising, after - alumn.
sleep, during - zinc.
moving the limb - chel.
night - aloe, bar-c., bar-m., calc., mag-c.
bed, in - hyos.
bed, in, on falling asleep - con., nat-c., stry.
outward - nat-m.
painful - meny.
sleep, during - con., cupr., graph., kali-c., lyc., nat-c., puls.
working hard with hands amel. - agar.

twitching, forearms - agar., aloe, alum., ars., asaf., atro., bar-c., calc., caps., cast., caust., fl-ac., graph., ***led.,*** merc., mez., nat-c., nat-m., nit-ac., nux-m., nux-v., olnd., plat., plb., puls., rhod., rhus-v., sabad., sars., sil., ***spig.,*** staph., stram., stry., ***tarax.,*** thuj., zing.
chill, during - nux-m.
cramp-like - asaf.
evening, 4 p.m. - zinc.
grasping anything - ***nat-c.***
morning, after walking - puls.
rest, during - asaf., ***spig.,*** staph.
sneezing, when - cast.
writing, while - caust., ox-ac.

twitching, upper arms - agar., am-c., arn., asaf., ***calc.,*** caust., ***cina,*** clem., cocc., crot-t., cupr., dig., dulc., hell., kali-bi., kali-c., kali-n., ***lyc.,*** mag-m., mang., meny., merc., mez., mur-ac., nat-m., nit-ac., olnd., ph-ac., phos., phyt., ***ran-b., sep.,*** sil., spig., squil., stann., tarax., teucr., thuj., zing.
bending - dulc.
biceps - mag-m., sep., teucr.
deltoid - ant-c., ign., nit-ac., ***sulph.***
drawing it backwards - dulc.
extensor, muscles of - tarax., zing.
inner side - caust., stann.
laying arm on something - stann.
left - kali-c., lyc.
motion amel. - ph-ac., stann.
outer side - mang., tarax.
right - am-c.
siesta, during - mez., seneg.
touch agg. - mez.
warmth amel. - ant-c.

ULCERS - ***anan.,*** kali-bi., kali-i., rhus-t., sil., stront.
malignant - lach.
painless - carb-v., plat., ***ran-b.,*** sep.
phagedenic - rhus-v.
syphilitic - phyt., rhus-v.
ulcers, forearms - kali-bi.

UNCOVER, inclination to, limbs - con., zinc.
sleep, during - con.

UNSTEADINESS - phos.

URTICARIA - acon., ant-c., ***apis,*** berb., calad., ***carb-v.,*** chin-s., ***chlol.,*** cop., hep., hydrc., hyper., indg., kali-i., lach., lyc., merc., ***nat-c., nat-m.,*** nat-s., ***phos.,*** rhus-v., **SULPH.,** thuj., ***urt-u.***
urticaria, forearms - am-c., calad., chin., clem., lyc., ***nat-m.,*** sil.
evening - lyc.
fever, during - calad.
morning - chin.
scratching, after - calad., calc., chin.

VARICOSE, upper arms - ***nux-v., plb.,*** **PULS.,** stront.

VESICLES - am-m., anac., anag., ***ant-c., ant-t.,*** arn., ***ars.,*** asc-t., bell., bov., brom., bruc., bufo, calad., calc., calc-p., canth., caust., chin., chlor., cinnb., cit-v., com., ***crot-h.,*** cupr-ar., cycl., daph., dulc., elaps, fl-ac., hipp., hura, indg., iod., iris, ***kali-ar.,*** kali-bi., ***kali-c.,*** kali-chl., ***kali-i., lach., mag-c.,*** mang., ***merc.,*** merc-c., mez., ***nat-c., nat-m.,*** phos., psor., ***puls., ran-b.,*** **RHUS-T.,** ***rhus-v.,*** ruta., sars., **SEP.,** ***sil.,*** sol-n., ***spong., staph., sulph.,*** ter., vip.
air, cold - dulc.
black - ***ars.***
discharging acrid serum - rhus-t.
itching - daph.
periodical every 4 to 6 weeks - ***sulph.***
putrid - ***ars.***
red, small - ***nat-m.***
scratching, after - ***calc.***
shooting, pain - mag-c.
ulcers, change into - calc.

VESICLES,
washing in cold water agg. - clem.
white - agar., kali-c., kali-chl., merc., nat-m.
vesicles, forearms - anac., ant-t., arn., ars., calad., carb-o., caust., chin., cit-v., hura, merc., petr., phos., rhus-r., rhus-t., rhus-v., sars., sil., spong., ***staph.,*** sulph.
burning - sil.
scratching, after - sars.
stinging - rhus-t.
transparent - rhus-t.
white - calad.
vesicles, upper arms - aran.

VIBRATION, sensation - am-c., dig., mosch., nit-ac., olnd., sep.

WARTS - ars., bov., **CALC.,** carb-an., ***caust.,*** dulc., kali-c., lyc., merc., **NAT-C.,** nat-m., ***nat-s., nit-ac.,*** petr., phos., rhus-t., **SEP.,** ***sil., sulph., thuj.***
warts, forearms - ***sil.***

WEAKNESS - abrot., ***acon.,*** **AESC.,** agar., ***all-c., alum.,*** alumn., ***am-c.,*** ammc., ***anac.,*** ant-c., ***apis,*** arg-m., arn., ***ars.,*** ars-i., asar., aur., arund., bapt., **BELL.,** berb., ***bism.,*** bor., bov., brach., brom., bry., bufo, cact., ***calc.,*** calc-p., ***calc-s.,*** camph., ***carb-s.,*** carb-v., ***caust.,*** cham., ***chel., chin.,*** chin-a., chin-s., **CIC.,** coloc., com., **CON.,** corn., ***crot-c., crot-t., cupr., cur.,*** **DIG.,** dios., dros., euph., eupi., ferr-m., ***gels.,*** gins., ***glon., gran.,*** graph., grat., ***guai.,*** ham., hep., hura, hyper., ign., ***iod.,*** kali-ar., kali-bi., **KALI-C.,** kali-i., kali-n., kali-s., ***kalm., lach.,*** lact., led., lil-t., ***lyc.,*** lyss., mang., merc-i-f., merc-sul., mez., nat-a., nat-c., ***nat-m.,*** nat-p., nat-s., nit-ac., ***nux-v.,*** par., ***petr., ph-ac., phos.,*** phyt., plat., plb., psor., ***rhod., rhus-t.,*** ruta., sabad., sars., sec., ***sep., sil.,*** spong., **STANN.,** ***staph.,*** stict., stram., stront-c., ***sulph.,*** sumb., tab., tarent., ter., til., ***thuj.,*** valer., verat., zinc.
afternoon - chin-s., nux-v.
2 p.m. - sarr.
anger, after a fit of - nat-m.
ascending steps, on - nux-v.
chilliness, during - gins., ***ph-ac.***
clenching hands, on - chin.
cold, from exposure to - ***rhod.***
dinner, after - grat.
eating, after - bar-c.
emissions, after - staph.
evening - brach., ferr-i., nat-m.
bed, in - phos.
vomiting, after - sulph.
exertion, after slight - ***cic., lach., stann.***
forenoon - indg., ph-ac.
hanging down amel. - asar.
laughing - carb-v.
left - agar., alumn., arn., brom., ***calc., dig.,*** nat-s., ***nux-v.,*** plat., sars., ***tab., sumb.***
morning - carb-s., dulc., ***kali-c.,*** lyc., ***nux-v.,*** sil., sulph., valer.
bed, in - kali-c., sil.
rising, on - caj., card-m.
waking, on - arg-m., nit-ac., sep.

WEAKNESS,

motion, on - carb-v., ***stann.***

amel. - acon., ***lyc.,*** plat., ***rhod.,*** stront.

night - ambr., lyc.

noon - colch., con.

paralytic - ph-ac., stann.

playing piano - gels.

right - am-c., ***bism.,*** carb-v., ***caust.,*** rhod.

spasms, after - **CIC.**

stormy weather - ***rhod.***

sudden - calc.

taking hold of something - arn., **ARS.,** bov., carb-v., cina, colch., nat-m., sil.

writing, while - acon., agar., brach., carb-v., ***caust.,*** cocc., kali-c., merc-i-f., mez., sabin.

weakness, forearms - aeth., agar., ang., arg-m., **ARS.,** aur., aur-m-n., **BELL.,** bufo, camph., cham., coloc., con., ***dig.,*** dulc., indg., kali-n., merc., mez., nat-m., nit-ac., nux-v., op., osm., phos., plb., rhod., **RHUS-T.,** sabin., stront-c., sumb., thuj., verat.

evening - dig.

knitting, while - aeth.

morning, on waking - arg-m.

night - kali-n.

right - arg-m., ***sil.***

writing, while - agar., arg-m., coloc.

weakness, upper arms - acon., ***arg-m.,*** arg-n., bell., brach., bry., carl., cic., clem., colch., crot-t., gins., guai., jatr., kali-n., lact., mang., nat-m., ***phos.,*** phyt., sep., sil., stann., ***sulph., thuj.***

exertion, after - ***arg-m.***

extending to the hand - crot-t.

flexion agg. - phyt.

morning, on waking - arg-m.

motion, on - grat., phyt.

amel. - arg-m.

night, during sleep - sep.

paralytic - ***arg-m.,*** bell., kali-n.

raised, when - grat.

rising, on - thuj.

sudden - mang.

waking, after - arg-m.

writing, while - carl., cic., con.

WIND, cold, blowing on it, as if - aster.

wind, upper arms, extensor muscles, coldness, as if - phos.

Back

ABSCESS - asaf., ***hep.,*** iod., lach., mez., ***ph-ac., sil.,*** staph., ***sulph., tarent-c.***
abscess, lumbar - ***calc-p.***

ACHING, pain - abies-n., abrot., ***aesc.,*** aeth., agar., ail., all-s., ***aloe,*** alum., am-c., am-m., ant-c., ***ant-t.,*** apis, apoc., arg-m., ***arg-n.,*** arn., ***ars., asaf.,*** asc-t., aur-m., ***bapt.,*** bar-c., bar-m., **BELL.,** bell-p., benz-ac., ***berb., bism.,*** bol., **BRY.,** but-ac., calad., ***calc., calc-f.,*** calc-p., calc-s., ***cann-i.,*** canth., cann-s., ***cann-i.,*** carb-ac., ***carb-an., carb-s., casc.,*** caul., caust., cham., ***chel.,*** chin-s., ***cimic.,*** cinnb., ***cob., cocc.,*** coc-c., colch., com., ***con.,*** conv., crot-t., ***cupr-ar.,*** dig., dios., ***dulc.,*** elaps, eug., euon., **EUP-PER., EUP-PUR.,** eupi., ferr., ferr-ar., ferr-i., ferr-p., ***gels.,*** glyc., **GRAPH., *ham.,*** hell., ***helon.,*** hyos., hyper., ind., inul., **IP.,** ipom., iris, kali-ar., ***kali-bi., kali-c.,*** kali-i., kali-n., ***kali-s., kalm.,*** kreos., lac-c., lach., lac-ac., laur., ***lil-t.,*** lob., ***lyc.,*** lycpr., lycps., ***lyss.,*** med., meph., merc-i-f., mez., ***morph.,*** **MUR-AC.,** nat-a., ***nat-c.,*** **NAT-M., *nat-p.,*** nit-ac., nux-m., **NUX-V.,** ol-an., ***ol-j.,*** olnd., op., osm., ***ox-ac.,*** pall., petr., ***ph-ac., phos.,*** phys., ***phyt., pic-ac.,*** plat., plb., ***psor.,*** ptel., **PULS., *pulx., rad.,*** **RAN-B.,** raph., rhod., ***rhus-t.,*** rhus-v., rumx., ***ruta,*** sabin., sang., sanic., ***sarcol-ac., sec.,*** senec., seneg., **SEP., *sil.,*** sin-n., solid., ***staph., still.,*** stront-c., stry., ***sulph.,*** sul-ac., ***symph.,*** syph., tarent., **TELL., *ter., tril.,*** upa., vario., ***vib.,*** visc., zinc., zinc-m.
afternoon - abrot., agar., cham., chel., equis., glon., hyos., pall., plb., ptel., rumx., sep., zing.
air, cool, amel. - kali-s.
open - ***nux-v.***
bar, as from a - ars., lach.
bed, confines him to - ars-s-f.
bending, backward amel. - aeth.
breathing, when - inul., raph.
arresting - asar., cann-s.
deep - nat-c.
carrying, a basket, when - phos.
chill, during - ***ant-t.,*** caps., ***eup-per., ip.***
before - carb-v., daph., ***dios.,*** **EUP-PER.,** ip., **PODO.,** rhus-t.
coffee, agg. - cham.
cold, after taking - nit-ac.
washing, amel. - vesp.
colic, in abdomen, with - sars.
confinement, after - ***hyper.***
coughing, on - am-c., kali-n., merc., puls., sep.
dinner, after - agar., cob.
eating, while - crot-c.
after - agar., ant-t.
emission, after - ant-c., cob., kali-br., ph-ac., sars., ***staph.***
evening - acon., agar., alumn., ***ars.,*** cham., cist., ferr-i., kali-s., led., lil-t., phys., sarr.
exertion, after, amel. - ruta.
extending to feet - cob.
fasting, while - kali-n.
fever, during - eug., ziz.

ACHING, pain
forenoon - equis., ptel.
10 a.m - am-m.
leaning, against something, amel. - eupi., zing.
left - bism., carb-an., cocc., mez., tarent.
lying - ***berb., cur.***
abdomen, on amel. - nit-ac.
back, on the - carb-an., nit-ac.
back, on the, amel. - equis., ***nat-m.***
menses, during - acon., agar., am-m., ***bell.,*** berb., bry., calc-p., caul., cimic., crot-h., eupi., ferr., graph., inul., ***kali-c.,*** mag-m., nat-c., nat-h., nat-p., ***phos.,*** phys., rhus-t.
after - berb., ***kali-c.,*** mag-c., ***verat.***
before - berb., brom., calc., ***caust.,*** eupi., ***gels.,*** hyos., hyper., nux-v., **PULS.,** spong.
beginning, at - piloc.
suppressed - **AESC., *kali-c., sep., sil.***
midnight, after, spasmodic, worse when inspiring - ***nit-ac.***
morning - berb., dios., equis., eug., euph., eupi., mag-s., phyt., rhod., thuj.
bed, in - ang., berb., euph., kali-n., mag-s., petr.
rising, on - caust., cedr., hep., graph., ran-b.
waking, on - berb., cham., ptel.
motion, on - ***aesc.,*** agar., am-c., equis., ferr., gent-l., ox-ac., ***petr.,*** sil., stry.
amel. - graph.
shoulders, of - cocc.
night - agar., aloe, ***am-m., arg-n.,*** berb., helon., lycps., mag-c., mag-m., nat-c., phys., senec., **SULPH.**
11 to 12 p.m - ***am-m.***
menses, during - am-m.
sleep, after - am-m.
noon - dios., eupi., rhus-t.
palpitation with - tub.
paroxysmal - asaf., phos.
pressure, amel. - **KALI-C., *nat-m., sep.***
prostration with - berb.
rheumatic - arn., ind., kali-c., plb., stram., stry.
evening - colch.
night - gels.
riding, in a carriage, after - **NUX-M.**
horseback, on - **ARN.,** ars.
right - asaf., bell., bar-c., benz-ac., blatta, dios., lyc., merc-i-f.
rising, from a seat - ***aesc.,*** ars., bell., calc.
sexual excess, from - symph.
sitting, while - berb., bism., bor., cann-i., cham., cob., cocc., equis., euphr., helon., nat-c., nux-v., ox-ac., pic-ac., plb., podo., puls., **SEP.,** thuj., **ZINC.**
bent over, while - sep.
down, when - cob.
long, after - lith-m., phos., **PULS.**
standing, on - lyc., tus-p.
step, false, on - ***sulph.***

ACHING, pain
stool, during - manc.
after - rheum
difficult - ***puls.***
stooping, on - ***agar.,*** bor., bov., caps., ***cham.,*** kali-n., ***sulph.***
after - **AESC.,** agar., chel.
supper, after - sulph.
swallowing, on - kali-c., raph.
turning, on, must sit up to turn over in bed - **NUX-V.**
urinating, amel. - **LYC.**
urination, painful, during - vesp.
vaginal discharge with - alet.
amel. - eupi.
waking, on - hep., myric., ptel.
walking, while - **AESC.,** bapt., bor., cham., euphr., iris, **KALI-C.,** lyc., **PSOR.,** sep.
after - ***nat-c.,*** phos., stry.
warm, room - kali-s.
working impossible - asaf.
writing, after continued - lyc., mur-ac., sep.

aching, lumbar - acon., **AESC.,** aeth., aloe, alum., am-c., am-m., aml-n., anth., ant-t., ***apis,*** apoc., arg-n., arn., ***ars., ars-h.,*** ars-m., arum-t., asaf., asar., asc-t., bad., bapt., ***bar-ac.,*** bar-c., bell., **BERB.,** bol., brach., ***brom.,*** **BRY.,** bufo, **CALC.,** ***calc-ar.,*** calc-f., calc-p., camph., cann-s., ***canth.,*** carb-an., ***carb-ac., carb-s., carb-v.,*** carl., casc., caul., ***caust.,*** cham., ***chel., chin.,*** chin-s., cic., cimx., ***cimic.,*** cinnb., ***clem.,*** cob., ***coc-c.,*** coff., colch., ***coloc.,*** com., con., crot-t., cupr., cupr-ar., cycl., dig., dios., ***dor.,*** **DULC.,** eup-per., equis., fl-ac., **GELS.,** glon., gnaph., ***graph.,*** gymn., ham., hell., ***helon.,*** hep., hipp., ***hura, hydr.,*** hyos., ***hyper.,*** ign., iodof., ***ind.,*** iris, jatr., jug-c., kali-bi., kali-br., ***kali-c.,*** kali-chl., ***kali-n., kali-p., kalm., kreos., lac-ac.,*** lach., lept., ***lil-t.,*** lob., lyc., lyss., mag-m., mag-s., merc., merc-i-f., mez., morph., ***mur-ac.,*** murx., myric., naja, nat-a., nat-c., nat-p., nat-s., nicc., nit-ac., nux-m., **NUX-V.,** ol-an., op., osm., ***ox-ac.,*** petros., ***phos.,*** phys., ***phyt., pic-ac.,*** plan., plb., ***podo.,*** prun., ***psor.,*** ptel., ***puls.,*** raph., rhod., rhus-t., rumx., sabin., samb., sang., sarr., ***sars., sec., senec.,*** **SEP.,** ***sil., staph.,*** stram., stront-c., ***stry., sul-ac.,*** **SULPH.,** sumb., tab., ***tarent.,*** thuj., trom., ust., verat., vip., ***zinc.,*** zing., ziz.
afternoon - calc-f., coc-c., dios., erig., fago., jug-c., kali-c., lycps., ptel., rhus-t., ***sep.,*** stry.
deep inspiration, on - sars.
fever, during - trom.
sitting, while, 2 p.m. - hura.
alternating with, headache - aloe, brom.
pain in thighs - am-c.
ascending, stairs - tus-p.
bending, amel. - caust., psor.
backward - asaf., con., kali-c., puls., sabin., sel.
backward, amel. - fl-ac., puls., sabad., sabin.
forward - asaf.

aching, lumbar
chill, during - gamb., myric.
constipated, when - kali-bi., tep.
cough, during - arund., kali-n., merc., tell.
daytime - ant-c., ox-ac.
rest, while at - am-c.
dinner, after - phos., sulph.
eating, while - coc-c.
elbows and knees, on, amel. - coloc.
emissions, after - ham.
erect, becoming - nat-m.
erections, violent, after - mag-m.
evening - alum., apoc., cob., coc-c., dios., dirc., erig., ferr., hura, kalm., lycps., murx., naja, nux-m., pic-ac., stry., sulph., sumb., tanac.
7:30 p.m., on waking - sep.
flatus, after, amel. - coc-c.
forenoon - jug-c., stront-c., sulph.
11 a.m. - lac-ac.
sitting - jug-c., sulph.
hip, above - bell., dulc., kali-bi.
jarring, on - carb-ac., podo.
kneeling - euphr.
labor-like - acon., ***kreos.,*** nux-v., **PULS.**
laughing, when - **CANN-I.,** tell.
leaning, against something amel. - zing.
side, on the, amel. - raph.
lumbo-sacral region - **AESC.,** asc-t., aspar., ***cimic.,*** colch., dios., gels., hura, lil-t., **ONOS.,** ***phos.,*** sil.
night - ***aesc.***
lying, while - agar., aml-n., mag-m., ***nux-v.,*** tab.
amel. - cob.
abdomen, on, can only - nit-ac.
back, on the - ign., lyc.
menses, during - aloe, ***am-m.,*** berb., cast., caust., ***coc-c.,*** cop., eupi., graph., iod., ***lach.,*** lyc., mag-c., mag-m., nit-ac., prun., rat., **SULPH.,** tarent., zing.
after - berb., calc-p., kali-n., puls.
before - am-c., arum-d., berb., caust., ***mag-c.,*** phos.
delayed - sul-ac.
on appearance of - acon., aloe, berb., nit-ac.
misstep - carb-ac., podo.
morning - aml-n., bufo, chel., cimic., cinnb., cop., croc., ***dios.,*** hura, ign., ***kali-bi.,*** lac-ac., lyc., mag-m., mur-ac., naja, nicc., **NUX-V.,** plan., ***puls.,*** ran-b., **RHUS-T.,** sang., sars., ***senec.,*** stann.
bed, in - chr-ox., ***nux-v.***
rising, on - aloe, calc., cedr., hipp., lyc., ox-ac.
rising, on, after, amel. - nat-s.
waking, on - carb-s., erig., op., plan.
motion, on - **AESC.,** alum., am-c., asar., canth., chel., colch., croc., hydr., ign., iris, kali-bi., kali-n., lyc., nit-ac., ***ox-ac., phyt., pic-ac.,*** plan., podo., ***psor.,*** **RHUS-T.,** sars., ***sep.,*** tep., ziz.
amel. - alum., calc-caust., calc-f., kali-n., kreos., nux-v., rhod., staph., stront.

aching, lumbar
motion, commencing, on - dig., ***led.,*** tab.
sudden - rumx.
night - ***aesc.,*** agar., arg-n., coc-c., fl-ac., lyc., mag-c., mag-m., nicc., nit-ac., ***nux-v.,*** podo., sang., senec., **SEP.,** sil., sulph.
bed, in - croc., lac-ac., naja
bed, on going to - bapt., sin-n.
bed, on turning in - zinc.
noon - lycps.
paralytic - carl., ***cocc.,*** kalm., nat-m., ran-s., ***sabin.,*** sel., zinc.
periodic - ars.
pressure, agg. - canth., ***graph.***
amel. - carb-ac., fl-ac.
riding, while - calc., carb-ac.
rising, up, on - aesc., agar., am-m., ant-c., ***ars., calc.,*** carb-an., led., nat-m., petr., phos., puls., ***sil.,*** sulph., tus-p., verat.
amel. - cob., ferr., ptel., ***ruta.,*** sulph.
walk, and beginning to - tab., zinc.
sewing - iris
sex, after - cann-i.
sitting, while - ***agar.,*** carb-an., caust., chin-s., ***cob.,*** equis., hura, lyc., mag-c., mag-m., mur-ac., nux-v., ol-an., pall., ***phos., prun.,*** puls., rhod., **RHUS-T.,** ***sulph.,*** tab.
amel. - mag-c., meny.
bent - chin-s., phos.
walk, after a - ruta.
sneezing - ***sulph.***
standing - kali-c., meny., mur-ac., phos., podo., stry., verat.
standing, amel. - ***arg-n.***
stepping agg. - acon., carb-ac., spong.
stool, during - nicc., squil., sulph., tab.
after - colch., dros.
amel. - coc-c.
before - kali-n., ox-ac.
hard, during - stront.
hard, amel. - ox-ac.
stooping, when - ***aesc.,*** alum., am-caust., cham., con., dig., dios., ***dulc.,*** hura, hyos., jug-c., kali-bi., lyc., mang., meny., nat-m., plb., puls., rhod., sabad., sars., ***sil.,*** **SULPH.,** ***thuj.,*** zinc.
after work in the garden - agar., ***arn., bell-p.***
amel. - chel., puls., sang.
straightening up, agg. - carb-ac., kali-bi.
amel. - nat-m.
touch, on - bry.
turning, must sit up to turn over in bed - **NUX-V.**
suddenly - mag-m.
urinate, during urging to - raph.
urinating, while - sulph.
after, amel. - **LYC.**
urine, after a large flow of - caust.
waist, line - calc., mur-ac., rumx., sars., sil., tarent.

aching, lumbar
walking - ***aesc.,*** agar., alum., am-c., am-m., apoc., bapt., brach., coff., colch., con., dios., grat., hyos., kali-bi., mez., nat-c., podo., rhus-v., sep., spong., stry., ***sulph.,*** tab., tus-p., ust., verat., zinc.
amel. - ant-c., ***arg-n.,*** cob., ***kali-p.,*** kreos., phos., ***ruta.,*** staph., tab.
bent, amel. - ***sulph.***
continued, amel. - zinc.
menses, during - mag-m.
wanting, as if third vertebra were - ***psor.***
warm applications, amel. - calc-f., caust., ***rhus-t.***
room, on entering - gels.
washing, after - aloe, aml-n., calc-caust., equis., gamb., myric., ***podo.,*** ptel., ***sulph.***

aching, scapula - aeth., asaf., calc-p., ***chin.,*** cor-r., hell., jug-c., lil-t., merc-i-f., mur-ac., phyt., petr., verat-v.
right - ol-an.
writing, while - mur-ac., petr.

aching, scapula, under - agar., arn., bell., calc., **CHEL.,** cupr., ind., kali-bi., kreos., laur., merc., myric., nat-m., phys., rumx., ***sulph.,*** tarent.
arm - led.
evening - seneg., ***sulph.,*** tarent.
7 p.m. - gels.
expiration, on - ***sep.***
left - aeth., ant-t., cench., crot-h., dios., equis., kali-bi., lach., lob., med., naja, nit-ac., ol-an., polyp-p, rumx., sabin., seneg., verat-v., xan.
motion, on - chel., tarent.
night - tarent.
riding - phyt.
right - ***chel.,*** ind.
sitting, while - seneg.
walking, while - led., med.

aching, spine - **AGAR.,** asaf., ***carb-v., chel.,*** chin-a., ***lac-c., lach.,*** lycps., lyss., ***nux-m.,*** ol-j., ***sil.,*** **TELL.,** ***zinc.***
base of brain to coccyx, from - lac-ac., ***lac-c.***
dull sensation as from fullness of blood - phos.
jar of bed, from - **BELL., GRAPH.**
sitting - helon.
waves, in, extending to occiput - crot-h.

aching, thoracic - **AESC.,** bol., calc., ***calc-ar., cann-s.,*** pic-ac., rhus-t., tep.
afternoon - calc-s., erig.
evening - calc-s., erig.
morning - calc-p.
night, latter part of - calc-p.
spine - ail., arund., calc., phos.
spine, respiration agg. - calc.

aching, thoracic, middle of - ***aesc.,*** ail., arn., arum-t., ***bell.,*** calad., calc-ar., calc-caust., carb-an., clem., dros., dulc., kali-p., lac-c., lob., merc., naja, ***nux-v.,*** ox-ac., phos., plb., ran-s., rhod., rhus-t., rhus-v., seneg., ***sep.,*** staph., tab.
coughing, on - calc., kali-bi., stram.

aching, thoracic, middle of
expiration agg. - sep.
leaning back amel. - lac-c.
morning - staph.
standing - rumx.
stepping hard - seneg.
walking - bell.
warm, becoming - lac-c.

ACNE - carb-v., nit-ac., rumx.

AIR, cannot bear a draft of, on nape - ***hep., merc., sil.***
cannot bear a draft of, spine - ***sumb.***
sensation of cold over spine and body before convulsions - agar.

ANKLOSING spondylitis - **AESC.,** agar., caust., cimic., ***con.,*** kali-c., **KALM.,** ***nat-m., rhus-t.***

ASLEEP, sensation, scapula - anac.

BAR, feeling as though a, in the back - ars., lach.

BIFIDA, spinal, (see Spinal Bifida)

BLOOD, lumbar, extravasation of, in - crot-h.

BLUISH, right side of back - vip.

BOILS - caust., coloc., ***crot-h.,*** graph., kali-bi., **KALI-I.,** ***lach.,*** mur-ac., ph-ac., ***phyt.,*** sanic., sulph., sul-ac., tarent-c., ***thuj.,*** zinc.
blood - ***carb-an., caust., graph.,*** hep., iris, kali-bi., murac., nat-m., sul-ac., thuj., zinc.
groups, in - berb.
shoulders, between - iod., tarent-c., zinc.
stinging, on touch - mur-ac.

boils, lumbar, region - ***hep.,*** psor., rhus-t., thuj.

boils, scapula, over - am-c., bell., led., lyc., ***nit-ac.,*** zinc.

BORING, pain - acon., agar., ang., asaf., bar-c., ***bism.,*** brom., carb-ac., cocc., ***ham.,*** laur., ***lyc.,*** mag-p., nat-c., psor., thuj.
as with a gimlet - ***lyc.***
spots, in - thuj.

boring, lumbar - agar., asaf., bor., canth., ***carb-ac.***
right - ***carb-ac.***

boring, scapula - acon., aur-m-n., corn., dig., mag-m., meny., paeon.
deep inspiration, on - acon.
left - aur., berb., dig., hyper., meny., mez., nat-c., par., ***ph-ac.,*** ruta, spig., spong.
tip of - nat-c.
motion, amel. - paeon.
right - acon.
to front of chest - acon.
to sternum - nat-c.

boring, thoracic - ***lil-t.***
thoracic, middle of - ***ph-ac.,*** psor., thuj.
shoulders, between - laur., mag-m., ph-ac.
rest, during - laur.
spine - ***lyc.,*** mez., naja, phos., psor.

BREAK, lumbar, as though the back will - aloe, arg-m., **BELL.,** chel., ***ham., kali-c., kreos.,*** **LYC.,** nat-m., nux-v., plat.
motion, amel. - kreos.
stooping, when - **CHEL.**

BROKEN, pain, as if - arn., agar., ***bell.,*** cina, cocc., conv., **EUP-PER.,** ham., ip., ***kali-c.,*** lyc., mag-arct., mag-aust., merc., ***nat-m., nux-v.,*** **PHOS.,** plat., ruta, senec., verat., vib.
hemorroids, with - bell.
lying on the back, while - cina.
on the side, while - cina.
stool before - ***nux-v.***
stooping and on rising up - verat.
walking, after - plat.

broken, lumbar, as if - aesc., arg-m., ***ars., bell.,*** bry., ***carb-an., cham.,*** chel., clem., con., cor-r., eup-per., ferr-i., ***graph., ham., kali-c.,*** kali-i., kreos., **LYC.,** mag-c., mag-m., meli., **NAT-M.,** ***nux-m.,*** ox-ac., **PHOS.,** plan., plat., psor., ***rhus-t.,*** ruta, senec., ***sep.,*** staph., sulph.
air, from a draft of - ***nux-v.***
bending back agg. - plat.
coughing - ***rhus-t.***
evening, during rest - nux-m.
exercising - con.
knocked away, sensation as if - arg-m.
lying, on - carb-an.
morning, in bed - ***staph.***
moving, on - chel., con., kali-c., ***rhus-t.***
amel. - ***kreos.,*** nux-m.
night - ferr-i., ***mag-c.***
sitting, while - meli.
standing - carb-an.
amel. - meli.
stool, during - **LYC.**
stooping - clem., mag-m.
stretching - mag-m.
touching, on - ***graph.***
vertebra - graph.
walking, after - carb-an., plat., sep.
amel. - meli.

broken, scapula, as if - crot-c., hell., kreos., lil-t., ***mag-c.,*** merc-i-f., nat-m., plat., ran-b., sil., verat.

BROWN, spots on shoulders - ant-c.
spots on - sep.

BUBBLING, sensation in - berb., lyc., petros., tarax.

bubbling, lumbar, sensation in, - ***berb.,*** lyc., sep.
agg., when lying and rising from a seat - berb.

bubbling, scapula, sensation in - berb., lyc., ***tarax.***
left scapula - spig.
right - ***tarax.***
under scapula - lyc., squil.

BURNING, pain - acon., ***alum.,*** alumn., ***agar.,*** am-c., ant-t., apis, arn., **ARS.,** asaf., asar., aur-m., aur-s., ***bar-c.,*** bell., berb., ***bism.,*** bor., bry., calc., calc-f., cann-i., ***carb-an.,*** carb-s., carb-v., carl., chel., clem., cocc., coloc., chr-ac., com., cupr., daph., dulc., ***glon.,*** helo., helon., hyper., kali-bi., ***kali-c.,*** kali-i., kali-n., ***kali-p.,*** kali-s., ***kalm., kreos., lach.,*** lachn., lil-t., lob., ***lyc.,*** lyss., mag-c., mag-m., ***med., merc.,*** mez., mur-ac., naja, nit-ac., nux-m., ***nux-v.,*** olnd., ***ph-ac.,*** **PHOS.,** phys.,

BURNING, pain - ***pic-ac.,*** rhus-t., rumx., sec., sel., seneg., ***sep., sil.,*** **SULPH.,** tab., ter., ***thuj.,*** ust., verat., xero, ***zinc.***
emissions, after - ***merc.,*** phos.
burning, forenoon - kali-bi.
grief, after - naja.
lying, while - kali-n., ***lyc.***
on the back - ars.
menses, before - kreos.
mental exertion - ***pic-ac.,*** sil.
morning - mag-m., zinc.
3 a.m., amel. by rising - nat-c.
after sex, agg. by rest, amel. by motion - mag-m.
on rising amel. on motion - rat.
motion amel. - mag-m., ***pic-ac.,*** rat.
night - helon., ***ph-ac.***
noon - rhus-t.
scratching, after - mag-c.
amel. - rhus-v.
sex, after - ***mag-m.***
sitting, while - apis, ars., asar., bor., cist., kali-n., **ZINC.**
sleep. during - zinc.
spots, in - agar., nit-ac., ***ph-ac.,*** **PHOS.,** ran-b., sulph., ***zinc.***
steam, exposed to agg. - kali-bi.
touched, when - carb-an., cist.
walking in open air - arn., kali-c., ***sil.***
amel. - kali-n.
warm in bed, when getting - sil.

burning, lumbar - acon., aesc., alumn., am-c., ant-s., arg-m., ars-i., arund., asar., aur., bar-c., bell., ***berb.,*** bor., carb-an., cedr., chel., cham., clem., ***coloc.,*** cupr., guare., ***helon., kali-c.,*** kali-p., ***kalm., kreos.,*** lac-d., ***lach.,*** lachn., mag-c., ***mag-m., med., merc-c.,*** mur-ac., murx., nat-c., nat-p., ***nit-ac., nux-v., ph-ac., phos.,*** pic-ac., ***ran-b., rhus-t., sep.,*** sil., spig., stann., sulph., sul-ac., **TER.,** thuj., verat., zinc., ziz.
afternoon - mag-m.
breathing deeply, when - sep.
deep-seated - clem.
evening - mag-m.
5 p.m. - dios.
after lying down - sulph.
extending, across abdomen - bar-c.
chest, to - berb., sulph.
right side and shoulder, to - clem.
up the spine to between scapula - ars., phos., sep., sil., thuj.
last lumbar vertebra - acon., aesc., cham., pic-ac.
lying - lac-d.
menses, during - med., phos.
before - kreos.
delayed - phos.
morning - zinc.
night - bar-c., mag-m., ***phos.***
3 a.m. - ***kali-c.***
pregnancy, during - rhus-t.
pressure or rising, on - arg-m.
rib, near last - kali-bi., lyss.
rising from sitting - arg-m., bar-c., berb.

burning, lumbar
sitting - asar., bor.
sleep, during - zinc.
spot - bar-c., mang., ***ph-ac.,*** rhus-t., zinc.
sudden, as from hot needle - aeth.
walking - nux-v., ***ran-b.***
amel. - bar-c.

burning, scapula - alum., ***ars.,*** **BAR-C.,** carb-s., ***carb-v.,*** caust., cund., echi., iod., kali-c., lachn., laur., lyc., ***lyc.,*** mang., med., **MERC.,** mez., mur-ac., nux-v., nat-c., nat-m., ***phos.,*** rob., seneg., ***sep., sil.,*** stann., sulph., sul-ac., verat., ***zinc.***
angle of, inferior - sulph.
upper - alum.
left - ambr., bar-c., card-m., com., euphr., fl-ac., nat-m., sil., teucr., zinc.
and itching on place below and to right of - pall.
and pricking - fl-ac.
levator anguli walking and writing - agar.
night - bar-c.
superior angle, amel. by friction - ***alum.***
under - bry., ***cund.,*** echi., mez., tab.
margin, lower - nat-c., ran-b.
motion, amel. - nat-c
sewing, from - ran-b.
right - bar-c., cann-s., ***carb-v.,*** caust., iod., lachn., laur., ***lyc.,*** plb., seneg., sulph., verat., zinc.
under - bry., cann-s., lob., pall., staph., tab.
sewing, while - ran-b.
tip of - plb.
upper part - bar-c., carb-v., chel., stann.
walking amel. - bar-c.
writing, while - ran-b.

burning, spine - acon., agar., **ARS.,** ***asaf., bell.,*** cham., ***gels.,*** glon., helon., ***kalm.,*** **LACH.,** lachn., ***lyc.,*** mag-m., ***med., nat-c., nat-p., ph-ac.,*** **PHOS.,** ***pic-ac.,*** plb., puls., **SEC.,** ***sep., thuj., verat., zinc.***
above, small of back - ***zinc.***
as if, a hot iron were thrust through lower vertebrae - ***alum.***
lying, while - ***lyc.***
mental, exertion - ***pic-ac., sil.***
night - ***ph-ac.***
rubbing amel. - phos.
sharp - mag-m., zinc.
motion amel. - mag-m.
shooting - acon.
spots, in - agar., ***phos.***
sitting, while - **ZINC.**
small place, in - agar.
walking, amel. - zinc.

burning, thoracic - caps., dios., lyc., mang., ***zinc.***
needle work or writing, from - ran-b., ***sep.***
spine - ars-m., lach., ***graph.,*** pic-ac., sep., ***sil.***

burning, thoracic, middle of - acon., alumn., ars-m., ***berb.,*** bry., calc., cur., glon., graph., helon., **KALI-BI.,** kali-c., **LYC.,** mag-m., ***med.,*** merc., ***nux-v.,*** ox-ac., ph-ac., **PHOS.,** sabad., senec., ***sil.,*** sul-ac., ***sulph., thuj., zinc.***
afternoon,1 p.m. - chel.
evening, lying down - sulph.
on bed - ferr.
extending, down the back - kali-c., merc.
to nape - ***nat-s.***
itching, and stinging - calc.
mental exertion - helon., ***pic-ac., sil.***
paroxysmal, agg. by motion - plb.
pulsating - ***phos.***
rubbing amel. - phos.
scratching, after - mag-c.
sitting, while - thuj., ***zinc.***
stinging, and - rumx., sabad.
summer, in - ***lyc.***

BURROWING, pain, lumbar - dulc., kreos.
walking, amel. - dulc.

BURSTING, pain, between shoulders - thyr.

CARBUNCLE - **ANTHR.,** ars., ***crot-h., lach., sil.***
carbuncle, thoracic - ***hep., lach.,*** tarent.

CLAWING, pain - arg-n.
clawing, lumbar - calc., ign., ***merc.***

COLDNESS - ***abies-c.,*** acon., aesc., agar., alum., am-br., am-c., ***am-m.,*** anac., anag., ant-c., aphis., apis, ***arg-m.,*** arn., ***ars., asaf.,*** asar., aur., aur-m-n., bapt., bar-c., ***bell.,*** benz-ac., berb., **BOL.,** bor., brom., ***bry.,*** **CACT.,** calad., ***calc.,*** calc-s., ***canth., camph.,*** **CAPS.,** carb-an., carb-s., carb-v., caust., cedr., ***cham.,*** chel., chin., chin-a., chlf., cic., cocc., coc-c., coff., colch., com., ***con.,*** croc., ***crot-t., dig.,*** dios., ***dulc.,*** elaps, euph., **EUP-PER., EUP-PUR.,** ferr., ferr-ar., ferr-p., ***gels.,*** gins., grat., ***ham.,*** hell., hep., hipp., hydr., ***hyos.,*** hyper., ign., ip., jatr., kali-ar., kali-bi., kali-c., kali-i., kali-n., kali-p., kali-s., kalm., ***lac-d.,*** **LACH.,** lachn., lact., laur., ***led., lil-t., lob.,*** lyc., mag-c., ***meny.,*** merc., merc-c., merc-i-r., ***mez.,*** mur-ac., nat-a., **NAT-M., NAT-S.,** ***nit-ac.,*** nit-s-d., ***nux-v.,*** op., ox-ac., ***phos.,*** phys., plat., **PULS.,** quas., ***raph., rhus-t.,*** rhus-v., ruta., sabad., sang., sanic., sarr., sars., ***sec.,*** seneg., sep., **SIL.,** spig., ***spong., stann.,*** staph., ***stram., stry.,*** **SULPH.,** sumb., tarent., thuj., valer., **VERAT.**
afternoon - alum., apis, asaf., carb-an., cast., cic., cimic., ***cocc.,*** fago., guai., hyos., ***kali-ar.,*** lyc., nat-a., rumx., stram., thuj.
2 p.m - cic., nat-s.
3 p.m - ***apis,*** lyc.
4 p.m - mag-c.
5 p.m - nat-m.
stool, after - fago.
air, open - acon., dulc.
as from cold air - benz-ac., camph., caust., coff.

COLDNESS,
air, as from cold, spreading from spine over body, like an aura epileptica - agar., nicc.
cold, when in - ***stront.***
cold, water spurted on, as if - caps., caust., croc., lyc., ***phos.,*** **PULS.,** vario.
coughing, agg. - carb-an.
dinner, after - cedr., cycl.
dressing, when - anth.
eating, during - raph.
after - crot-c., sil., staph.
evening - alum., ***ars.,*** bapt., berb., caps., cast., cimic., ***cocc.,*** coff., ***dulc.,*** graph., kali-c., kali-n., kreos., ***lyc., mur-ac.,*** nat-m., nux-v., ***rhus-t.,*** **PULS.,** sang., sep., ***stann.,*** **SULPH.,** tab., thuj.
6 p.m., in a warm room - lyc.
7 p.m - cast., lyc.
9 p.m - cast., kreos.
lying down, after - ***coff., lyc.,*** nat-c., ***nux-v.,*** sang.
extending, to, abdomen - cham., crot-t., ***phos., sec., spig.***
arms, into - gins., verat.
body, over whole - amyg., bell., ***lyc.***
body, over whole, 6:30 p.m - lyc.
extending, down back - abies-c., acon., **AGAR.,** ***all-c.,*** alum., arg-n., ars., asaf., bar-c., bell., bor., brom., bry., canth., carl., cedr., chel., **CINA,** ***cocc.,*** coff., ***colch.,*** crot-t., ***eup-per., eup-pur.,*** glon., hep., ***hyper.,*** iris, lac-c., lil-t., ***lob.,*** lyc., mag-c., ol-an., phos., pic-ac., **PULS.,** pyrus, ruta., sabad., ***samb.,*** sep., ***sil.,*** staph., **STRAM.,** stry., valer., ***zinc.***
as if cold water, poured down the - agar., alumn., anac., ars., ***gels.,*** lil-t., ***lyc.,*** **PULS.,** sabad., stram., vario., zinc.
as if cold water, trickling down - ars., caps., caust., ***gels.***
feet, to - croc.
limbs, to - gins.
lower limbs, to - acon., ferr., ham.
motion, on - rumx.
night, 9 p.m - all-c.
night, 10 p.m - sep.
extending, up the back - aesc., am-m., arg-n., ars., bar-c., bol., ***calc-p.,*** carb-an., ***cina, colch.,*** con., ***eup-per., gels.,*** hyos., ip., kali-bi., kali-i., kali-p., **LACH.,** lil-t., mag-c., merc-sul., ***nat-s.,*** ol-an., ol-j., ox-ac., phos., phys., ***puls.,*** ruta., rhus-v., **SULPH.,** thuj.
afternoon, 2 p.m - nat-s.
afternoon, 4 p.m - mag-c.
air, open, agg. on coming from - arg-n.
eating, after - arg-n.
evening - kali-p., sulph.
menses, during - kreos.
motion, from - sulph., thuj.
shivering, after urinating, with - ***sars.***

COLDNESS,
extending, up and down the back - abies-c., aesc., all-c., aphis., bapt., bell., caps., **EUP-PUR., GELS.,** hell., ***ip.,*** lach., med., puls., ruta, ***sulph.***
afternoon - rumx.
external - coc-c., lyc.
forenoon - ang., asaf., berb., cham., con., graph., hydr., lyc.
10 a.m - con.
11 a.m - cham.
walking in the room, while - ang.
walking in the room, while, in open air - hydr.
ice, as from - ***am-m.,*** cocc.
icy, coldness running down back before epilepsy - ***ars.***
itching, ending in - ***am-m.***
lying, down amel. - cast., kali-n., sil.
menses, during - bell., kreos.
after - kali-c.
motion - asaf., ***eup-pur.,*** phys., sulph., thuj.
morning - arn., bry., con., ferr., mez., nit-s-d., **NUX-V.,** sumb.
7 a.m - ferr.
8:30 to 9 a.m - asaf.
9 a.m - mag-c.
menses, after - kali-c.
rising, on - meny.
waking, on - con.
night - ***ars.,*** arum-t., chin., chin-a., chin-s., coc-c., lil-t., lyc., nat-a., nat-m., ***puls.,*** stront-c., thuj.
bed, on going to - coc-c., lil-t., phos.
noon - arg-n., rhus-t.
siesta, after - cycl.
sitting, while - brom.
stool, during - colch., ***trom.***
after - fago., ***puls.,*** sumb.
before - ars.
sudden - croc.
urinating, after - ***sars.***
waking, on - dig.
walking, while - asaf., hyos., nit-s-d.
air, in open - chin.
warm, stove, near - jug-c.
warmth, agg. - apis

coldness, lumbar - asaf., bapt., ***camph.,*** cann-i., canth., ***carb-an.,*** carb-s., carb-v., cham., chin., cupr., ***dulc.,*** **EUP-PUR.,** hell., **LACH.,** led., med., nat-m., nux-m., ox-ac., podo., psor., ***puls., sanic.,*** spong., ***sulph., sumb.,*** tarent.
air, as if cool, passed over it - stann., ***sulph., sumb.***
draft of cold, agg. - tarent.
cough, with - ***carb-an.***
evening, while sitting, agg. - canth.
extending to abdomen after urinating - sulph.
fanned, as if - ***puls.***
morning - cham., ***sumb.***
motion agg. - podo.
night - nat-m., podo.
dinner, during - hell.
right side - ***med.***
sitting, while - chin.

coldness, lumbar
starts, in - gels., hyos., lach., ***nat-m.,*** stroph., sulph.
stool, after - ***puls.***
before - nux-m.
walking agg. - ***camph.***
warmth of stove amel. - hell.

coldness, scapula - alum., ars., camph., ***caps.,*** caust., chin-s., croc., dios., nat-c., phos., pyrog., rhus-t., ***sep.***
under - agar., camph.

coldness, spine - acon., agar., ***aesc.,*** atro., bol., bry., canth., chlf., coc-c., ***crot-c., gels.,*** gins., ***hyos.,*** jug-c., kali-n., lept., meny., merc., ***mez.,*** mosch., op., ruta., ***sanic.,*** stry., ***sumb.,*** tab., trom., thuj.
extending down - canth., ***ruta.,*** stry.
stool, during - trom.
thoracic - am-m., cham., haem., ir-foe., ***meny.***
walking - gins.

coldness, thoracic - agar., croc., ***sil.,*** spong., thuj.

coldness, thoracic, middle of - abies-c., agar., ***am-c., am-m., arg-m.,*** arg-n., aur., **BOL., CAPS.,** carl., cann-i., caust., chel., ***eup-per.,*** helo., hyos., lac-d., ***lachn.,*** led., med., nat-c., nat-m., petr., ***puls., rhus-t.,*** sarr., sec., ***sep., sil.,*** sulph., tab., tub., viol-t.
cold water, as from - abies-c.
cough, with - ***am-m.***
extending upwards - ox-ac.
ice, like - agar., am-m., arg-m., ***lachn.***
an ice cold hand - sep.
wind, as from - caust., hep., sulph.

COMPRESSING, pain - con.
compressing, lumbar - bell., bov., ***caust.,*** stront-c., ***thuj.***

COMPRESSION, lumbar region - aeth., caust., thuj.

CONSTRINGING - canth., cocc., mag-m., ***nux-v.,*** sabad.

CONSTRICTING, lumbar - am-c., arund., hell., lach., lyc., meny., ***puls.,*** tanac.
evening - alum.
extending, into side - nux-v.
to rectum and vagina, amel. standing - kreos.
going to bed, on - naja.
stool, after - tab.
takes away the breath - **PULS.**
constricting, thoracic, sitting, when, amel. ., bending back, agg. bending forward - ***rhus-t.***

CONSTRICTION, or band - alum., anac., arg-n., aur., bor., ***cham.,*** clem., ***cocc., dulc.,*** graph., guai., guar., kali-c., mez., nit-ac., puls., rhus-t.
constriction, lumbar region - mag-c., puls.
as from a tight band - cina, **PULS.**
constriction, scapula - mag-m.

CONTRACTING, pain - ***bry.,*** cham., ***graph.,*** **GUAI.,** kali-c., mez., viol-t.
contracting, lumbar - mag-m.
menses, during - am-m.

contracting, thoracic - guai.
contracting, thoracic, middle of - chin., **GUAI.**, mag-m.

CONTRACTION - cimic., hydr-ac., kali-c., ***rhus-t.***

CRACKING, lumbar - calc., ***rhus-t.,*** ruta, sec., sulph.
extending to anus - sulph.
stooping, when - agar., rhus-t.
walking, while - **ZINC.**
cracking, scapula, lifting arm, on - anac.
cracking, spine, moving, on - ***agar.,*** cocc., kali-bi., sec.
cracking, thoracic vertebra, upper - kalm.
last - zinc.
cracking, vertebra - nat-c., ol-an., ***rhus-t.,*** sulph.

CRAMP - arg-n., bell., calc-p., caust., ***chin.,*** con., iod., kali-bi., led., lyc., mag-m., mag-p., naja, nux-v., petr., plb., verat.
rising, from sitting - led.
turning, body - dros.
walking - mag-m.
cramp, lumbar region - ant-c., ***caust., chin.***

CRAMP-like, pain - ***arg-n.,*** bell., bry., calad., chin., cimic., ***coloc.,*** con., euph., ***euphr.,*** graph., iris, lyc., ***mag-p.,*** mez., nit-ac., nux-v., sep., viol-t.
paroxsmal - lyc.
cramp-like, lumbar - am-c., ant-c., ***bell., calc.,*** **CAUST., CHIN.,** ***chin-s.,*** graph., ***iris,*** lyc., mag-m., merc., oci., ph-ac., sil.
buttocks, and - caust.
evening - dios., iris, led.
extending, to bladder and groins - bell.
to epigastric region at night - lyc.
menses, during - bell., calc., ***nux-v.***
motion, during - **CHIN.,** plb.
moving foot, on, after, standing - thuj.
nursing, while - arn., ***cham., puls.***
paroxysmal - plb.
pressure amel. - plb.
sitting, while - ***caust.***
standing - merc.
stooping amel. - am-c.
walk, when attempting to, after long standing - thuj.
walking, amel. - merc.
slow, amel. - bell.
cramp-like, scapula - grat., phos., verat.
angle, inner - ***chel.***
inner border - chel.
left - bar-c.
motion, during - ip.
night - nit-ac.
right - chel.
inner border of - chel.
cramp-like, thoracic, middle of - bell., ip., **PHOS.**
left - bar-c.
motion, during - ***ip.***

CRUSHED, as though, lumbar region - **BERB., CHIN.,** phos.
motion, on - **CHIN.**

CURVATURE of spine - **ASAF.,** aur., bar-c., ***bar-m.,*** **CALC., CALC-F.,** calc-i., **CALC-P., CALC-S.,** carb-s., ***carb-v., con.,*** dros., ferr-i., hecla, hep., ***lyc., merc.,*** **MERC-C.,** op., **PH-AC., PHOS.,** psor., ***puls.,*** sep., **SIL., SULPH.,** tarent., ther., thuj.
lies on back with knees drawn up - **MERC-C.**
pain in - ***aesc.,*** hecla, **LYC., SIL.**
curvature, neck - ***calc.,*** phos., ***syph.***
curvature, thoracic - bar-c., bufo, ***calc., calc-s., con., lyc.,*** plb., ***puls., rhus-t., sil., sulph., syph.,*** thuj.

CUTTING, pain - ail., ***alum., arg-n.,*** aur., aur-m., ***bell.,*** calc., ***calc-p.,*** canth., caust., ***coloc., con.,*** cupr., elaps, ***eup-pur., gels.,*** graph., guai., guare., helon., hyper., ign., iod., ***kali-bi., lith.,*** mag-p., **NAT-M.,** ***nat-s.,*** nux-v., petr., plat., sars., seneg., sep., sil., staph., stry.
evening - nat-m., nat-s.
extending, up - ***coloc.***
to uterus - helon.
left side - cupr., stry.
menses, during - ars., ***con.***
midnight - caust.
morning - all-s.
sitting - nat-s.
stool, during - ***coloc.***
cutting, lumbar - all-s., ***alum., arg-n., arn.,*** aur., ***bell.,*** calad., calc-p., cann-s., canth., ***chel.,*** dig., ***dulc., eup-per.,*** gels., hep., kali-bi., ***kali-c.,*** mag-m., mez., nat-c., ***nat-m.,*** petr., psor., rheum, senec., stry., ***sulph.,*** zinc.
afternoon - canth., naja, petr.
moving, on - petr.
stooping - petr.
extending to, back - ***chel.***
to, calves and feet on motion - zinc.
to, hips - gels.
to, outward - ang.
to, pubis - mag-c.
to, upward agg., on stooping - arn.
to, uterus - helon.
labor, during - kali-c.
lying, while - ***arn.***
menses, during - ***arg-n.,*** caust., helon., zinc.
before - ***ol-an.***
while sitting, amel. by walking - mag-c.
morning - petr.
moving, after - petr.
rising, after - petr.
stooping, on - petr.
motion, on - kali-bi., zinc.
night - sulph.
pressure amel. - dig., ***dulc.***
deep, amel. - ***dulc.***
rising, from sitting - bell.
sitting, while - aur., canth., mag-c.
standing erect amel. - petr.
stool, during - rheum
before - nat-c.
turning agg. - kali-bi.
urinating, before - graph.
walking, while - thuj.

cutting, scapula - alum., alumn., ang., canth., dios., lac-c., med., merc-i-f., nat-s., rhus-t., spig., thuj., zinc.
edge of - ran-b.
left - carb-s., daph., hyper., ***lac-c.,*** lyc., thuj.
extending into chest - ***lyc.***
inspiration, on - carb-s.

cutting, scapula, under - asaf., thuj.

cutting, spine, whole - ang., cina, ***elaps,*** mang., nat-s., polyg.
articulations of, motion agg. - cocc.
circle, in a, from spine to abdomen - acon.
extending to abdomen - meny.
to stomach - ***thuj.***
stabbing in vertebrae - bell.

cutting, thoracic - agar., asaf., asc-c., daph., hyper., ***kali-bi.,*** nat-s., staph., stry.
extending to sternum - kali-bi., lac-c.
spine - arg-m., euon., thuj.

cutting, thoracic, middle of - alum., arn., bov., ***calc., hyper.,*** kali-n., meny., **NAT-S.,** sul-ac.
afternoon - bov.
rest, during - ***calc.***
straightening up amel. - bov.

DECAY, of, spine - arg-m., aur., calc., calc-i., ***calc-p.,*** con., ***iod.,*** kali-i., merc-i-r., ***ph-ac., phos.,*** pyrog., ***sil.,*** still., sulph., ***syph.,*** tub., vitr.

decay, of, vertebrae - calc., dros., nat-m., ph-ac., sil., stict., syph.
inferior maxilla - phos.
lumbar spine, vertebrae - ***sil.***

DIGGING, pain - acon., ***dulc.,*** sep., ***thuj.***
splinter, as with a - agar.
raising right arm - thuj.
right side - stann., ***thuj.***

digging, lumbar - arg-n., berb., dulc.
on sitting and standing, amel. by walking - ***ruta.***
spine - kali-i.

DISKS, syndrome, slipped or ruptured - **AESC.,** arn., **AGAR.,** ***berb.,*** **BRY.,** ***coloc.,*** **HYPER.,** kali-c., mag-p., ruta.., tarent., ***tell.,*** zinc.

DISLOCATIONS, of vertebrae - **ARN., BRY., CALC.,** calc-f., caust., ***coloc.,*** hyper., lyc., nux-v., phos., **RHUS-T.,** ***ruta.,*** stront-c., sulph., zinc.

dislocations, lumbar, as if - bell., con., eup-per., lach.
night, 10 p.m. - carb-s.
exercising, on - con.
last lumbar vertebra, in - sanic.

dislocations, thoracic, as if - ***thuj.***

DRAGGING, pain - agar., calc., canth.
motion, during - agar.

dragging, lumbar - arn., bar-c., coc-c., colch., ***con.,*** ery-a., ***ferr., ham.,*** kali-chl., merl., myric., phos., ***pic-ac.,*** plb., **SABIN.,** ***sep.***
extending to buttocks - helon.
to groin during menses - ***sulph.***
to rectum - calc.
menses, during - ***kali-c.,*** sulph., zinc.
after - ust.
as if would come on - ***apis,*** sulph.

dragging, lumbar
menses, as if would come on, while sitting - mag-c.
before - canth.
morning, on exertion - ust.
on waking - myric.
pregnancy, during - aran., ***bell., kali-c.,*** nux-v., puls., rhus-t.
urinating, when - sulph.
before - graph.

dragging, thoracic, middle of - naja.

DRAWING, pain - ***agar., alum.,*** ambr., am-c., anac., ***ang.,*** ant-t., arg-n., ***ars.,*** asc-t., aster., aur., bad., bar-c., bell., ***berb.,*** bol., ***bry.,*** calc-p., calc-s., ***canth., caps., carb-an., carb-v.,*** **CARD-M.,** ***caust., cham., chel., chin.,*** **CIMIC.,** cina, cocc., coc-c., ***colch.,*** con., crot-c., crot-h., cupr., cycl., dig., dros., dulc., eupi., ***graph., guai., hep., hyper.,*** ign., kali-bi., ***kali-c.,*** kali-m., kali-p., kali-s., kalm., ***lach.,*** lact., ***lil-t., lyc., merc.,*** mez., mill., mosch., nat-a., nat-c., ***nat-m.,*** nat-p., **NUX-V.,** op., ***petr., phos.,*** pic-ac., psor., ***puls.,*** rat., rhod., rhus-r., rhus-t., ruta., sabad., sang., seneg., stann., stel., stram., ***stront-c., sulph.,*** sul-ac., ter., teucr., ***thuj.,*** valer., verat., viol-t., zinc., zing.
bending backward - calc-p., **CIMIC.**
amel. - petr.
chill, during - lyc., ***puls.***
dinner, after - rat.
draft, from every - verat.
evening - agar., ***calc-p.,*** carb-v., chel., ***lach.,*** lyc., nit-ac., rhus-t.
extending, to
anus - nat-c.
groin, agg. walking or rising from seat - ***sulph.***
arms - carb-v.
back, small of and abdomen - caust.
chest - merc.
downwards - ars., bry., con., merc.
esophagus - agar.
head, amel. after exertion - nat-m.
hips - ***lach.,*** mosch., ***nat-m.***
legs - ars., bell., lach., ***phos.***
neck - sang.
occiput and vertex, during chill - **PULS.**
sacrum - con., tep.
testes, agg. walking or rising from seat - ***sulph.***
upward - ars., lach., nat-m.
upward, on stooping - sulph.
forenoon - ars.
laughing, when - phos.
left - carb-v., cupr., rhod., til.
lying still, when - colch., nat-c.
menses, during - ***sil.,*** zinc.
before - hyos.
suppressed, from - con.
morning - calc-p., ***cimic.,*** hep., zinc.
4 a.m. on waking - calc-p., chel.
bed, in - hep., rhod.
rising, after - ***hep.***
motion, on - caps., carb-v., eupi., sul-ac.
amel. - alum., bry., colch., **RHUS-T.**

DRAWING, pain
night - ars., chel., hep., nat-m.
turning frequently amel. - nat-m.
paroxysmal - nat-c., nit-ac.
reading, while - nat-c.
right - bad., carb-v., cupr., sep.
sexual excess, after - ***ars.***
sitting, while - ***bry.,*** calc., ***carb-v.,*** lyc., nat-c., ph-ac., **RHUS-T.,** ter., ***thuj.***
sleep, during - zinc.
standing - caps., con., ign.
stepping - sul-ac.
stool, during - ***puls.***
after - caps.
urging to, with - zing.
stooping, on - ***carb-v.,*** sulph., sul-ac.
throwing shoulders backward amel. - cycl.
turning, agg. - ***bry.,*** hep.
amel. - nat-m.
urinate, urging to, with - ***lach.***
walking amel. - bry., **RHUS-T.,** ***sulph.***
in open air - ter.
yawning, when - calc-p.

drawing, lumbar - acon., agar., aloe, ambr., am-c., am-m., ***arg-m.,*** arg-n., arn., ***ars., aur., bar-c., berb., bell.,*** benz-ac., ***bry., calc.,*** calc-s., ***carb-an.,*** carb-s., carb-v., card-m., carl., ***caust., cham., chel., chin.,*** cinnb., clem., ***cocc.,*** coc-c., colch., ***coloc., con.,*** cycl., dig., ***dulc.,*** eupi., hep., hipp., hura, hyos., indg., ign., ***kali-bi., kali-c.,*** kali-n., kali-p., kreos., ***lach., led., lyc.,*** mag-m., ***mez., mur-ac., nat-m., nit-ac., nux-v.,*** **PH-AC.,** plb., psor., ***puls., rhod.,*** rhus-v., **SABIN.,** ***sep., sil., stram., stront-c., sulph.,*** sul-ac., ter., ***thuj.,*** verat., ***zinc.,*** zing.
afternoon - bry., carb-s.
ascending stairs - carb-s.
bending backward - bar-c., sabin.
amel. - acon., am-m., hura
breathing, when - coloc.
crampy - sil., sul-ac.
downward - bar-c., caps., staph.
eating, after - bry.
evening - ***bar-c.,*** meny., nit-ac., stront-c., sulph., zing.
extending, abdomen, walls of - cham.
arms, into - carb-v., kali-bi.
back, up - ***ars.,*** kali-c., ***lach.,*** led., nux-v.
buttocks, to, morning on rising - thuj.
calves, to - tep.
coccyx, to - carb-v.
groin, to, after urinating - sul-ac.
groin, to, in evening - lact.
hips, to - lach., rhus-v.
legs, to - am-c., cinnb., ***lach.,*** sep.
pelvis, to - tep.
penis, into - dros.
pubic bone, to - **SABIN.**
rectum, to - coc-c.
shoulders, to - ***ars.,*** indg.
stomach - nit-ac., puls.
testes - erig.

drawing, lumbar
extending, thighs - agar., berb., cinnb., ***dulc.,*** kali-bi., kreos.
thighs, during labor - bell.
thighs, during stool - stann.
flatulence, obstructed, as from - nat-c.
hip, above, on moving in bed - lil-t.
inward - am-m.
jerking - ph-ac.
leaning forward - hura
lie down, must - sil.
lying, while - carb-an., colch.
amel. - ***kali-c.***
on the back - **COLOC.,** sep.
quietly, amel. by motion - colch.
menses, during - am-m., calc., carl., cham., mag-c., sep.
before - ***hyos.***
morning - carb-s., dios., hipp., sulph., thuj., zinc.
in bed - hep., nux-v.
moving - acon., caps., colch., kali-n., sul-ac.
amel. - am-c., colch., ***dulc.,*** indg.
night - ars., bry., cinnb., eupi., colch., sulph.
noon - sulph., thuj.
paroxysmal - ph-ac.
pressure amel. - dig., led., ph-ac.
rising, on - bar-c., ***sulph.***
sex, after - nit-ac.
sitting, while - ang., calc., ***caust.,*** meny., stront-c., sulph., ***thuj.***
amel. - aeth., ph-ac., staph.
after long, could not stand erect - ***thuj.***
erect - zing.
sleep, during - zinc.
standing, while - caps., ***carb-an.,*** con., led., ph-ac.
stool, during - stann.
after - ***chin.,*** mag-m.
stooping, on - clem., meny., staph., zinc.
amel. - mag-c., ph-ac.
stretching, on - mag-c.
turning, in bed - bry., lil-t.
the trunk - thuj.
urinating, after - sul-ac.
waking, on - bry., colch.
walking, while - acon., aeth., arg-m., ***carb-an.,*** cocc., sulph., thuj.
amel. - am-c., ph-ac., thuj.

drawing, scapula - acon., ars., asaf., ***berb.,*** bor., ***calc.,*** camph., ***carl., caust.,*** cham., ***chel., chin.,*** cimic., ***coloc.,*** con., hep., ind., kali-c., kali-n., lyc., med., mez., mur-ac., ***nux-v.,*** rhod., ruta., sars., seneg., sep., sil., ***squil.,*** sulph., tell., thuj.
breath deep, must - nat-m.
evening - chel., lyc., sulph.
extending to neck - mang.
left - asaf., card-m., con., mez., ptel., sep., ***squil.***
motion, on - caps.
paroxysmal - sil.
right - **COLOC.,** con., lyc., nat-m., sulph., tell.

drawing, scapula
extending to right hand - plat.
inner margin of - ***card-m.***
sitting - ph-ac.
waking, on - rhod.
walking, while - asaf.

drawing, scapula, below - asaf., ***card-m.,*** cimx., cocc., con., mez., nat-s., ph-ac., rhus-t., ruta., stann., sulph., thuj.
extending to fingers - cimx.
raising arm - con.
right, scapula - calc., sep.
sitting - sep.
standing - cocc.
walking - cocc.

drawing, spine - ***bell.,*** berb., ***caps.,*** carb-v., chin., chin-a., **CIMIC.,** ***cina,*** colch., ***con.,*** cycl., daph., mosch., ***nat-m., ruta.,*** sulph., ***thuj.,*** verat., ***zinc.***
afternoon, while walking - stront.
evening in bed - kali-bi.
extending, downward, agg. throwing shoulders forward, amel. by throwing them backward - cycl.
upward on stooping - sulph.
joints of spine - staph.
midnight, after - ant-s.
sex, after - nit-ac.
sitting and stooping, like a painful weakness, while - zinc.

drawing, thoracic - alum., ***ars.,*** aur-m., bell., ***card-m.,*** **CIMIC.,** coloc., **GUAI.,** ind., med., mur-ac., nit-ac., ph-ac., stann., staph.
motion, amel. - alum.

drawing, thoracic, middle of - acon., ***alum.,*** am-c., ***ars.,*** bell., bor., bry., **CALC.,** carb-an., chel., **CIMIC.,** coloc., ***dros.,*** eupi., graph., grat., **GUAI.,** ***hep.,*** kali-bi., kali-n., lob., ***lyc.,*** mur-ac., nat-c., nat-m., ***nat-s.,*** nux-v., ***ph-ac., phos., puls., rhus-t.,*** sep., ***sil.,*** stann., stram., thuj., viol-t., ***zinc.***
afternoon - chel.
air, open - nat-c.
bending, backward amel. - sil.
forward - **CIMIC.**
evening - bell., kali-n., lyc., zing.
6 p.m. - kali-n., zing.
forenoon - alum.
lying amel. - ***ars.***
menses, during - ***am-c., sil.***
morning in bed - ang.
motion, on - bry., stann., sulph.
night - rhus-t., sil.
rubbing amel. - carb-an.
stooping, on - bor., nux-v.
straightening up agg. - coloc.
walking, while - coloc.

ECCHYMOSIS, lumbar - merc-c., vip.

ECZEMA - arn., merc., ***sil.***

EMACIATION - tab.
emaciation, lumbar - plb., sel.
emaciation, scapula, muscles - plb.

EMPROSTHOTONOS - ***canth., ip.,*** lach., nux-m.

ERUPTIONS - alum., am-m., ant-c., ant-t., arg-n., arn., ***ars.,*** bar-c., bell., berb., bry., calc., calc-s., cann-s., carb-s., ***carb-v., caust.,*** chin., chin-a., cina, cist., clem., cocc., con., dulc., euon., fago., hep., ***jug-r.,*** kali-p., lach., led., ***lyc., merc.,*** **MEZ.,** nat-m., ***nit-ac., petr.,*** ph-ac., phos., **PSOR.,** puls-n, rumx., ***rhus-t.,*** rhus-v., ***sep., sil.,*** squil., staph., stram., **SULPH.,** sumb., tab., til., zinc.
biting - bry.
blotches - lach., mez., phos., zinc.
burning - am-m., cist., lyc., rhus-t.
scratching, after - til.
crusts - arn., graph., nat-m.
fine - con., rhus-v.
fish scales, like - ars-i., ***mez.***
flea bites, like - phys.
itch-like, scabies - arg-n., bar-c., psor., sulph.
itching - bar-c., bar-m., ***bry.,*** calc., cann-s., ***caust.,*** carb-v., cham., con., lyc., ***mez.,*** puls., rat., rhus-t., sep., squil., staph., tab., til., thuj., zinc.
evening, in - fago.
evening, in, and night - ***sep.***
evening, in, on going to bed - rumx.
scratching, after - mez.
spots - zinc.
warm, when - cocc.
maculae - syph.
miliary - ant-c., ant-t., bry., caust., **CHEL.,** cocc., hydrc., nat-s., ph-ac., prun., psor., sec., sumb., valer.
moist - ***clem.,*** nat-m., psor.
painful - led., lyc., spig.
to touch - cist., hep., ph-ac., psor., spig., squil., verb.
patches - calc., kali-ar., mez.
menses, during - nux-m.
pimples - agar., alum., arg-n., arn., bell., berb., calc., cann-s., carb-v., cham., chel., chlor., cocc., con., crot-h., dig., fl-ac., hura, hyper., jug-r., iod., kali-bi., ***kali-c.,*** kali-p., lach., led., lyc., mag-m., mag-s., meph., ***nat-m.,*** nicc., petr., ph-ac., psor., ***puls.,*** rhus-v., rumx., sars., ***sel.,*** sil., ***squil.,*** staph., tab., tep., til., vesp., zinc.
evening - cocc., fl-ac., ph-ac., rumx.
itching - arg-n., asc-t., calc., cann-s., carb-an., carb-v., crot-t., fl-ac., iod., led., mag-m., mill., rat., rhus-t., sel.
itching, after scratching - psor.
itching, evening in bed - nat-m.
red - ph-ac.
sore, pressing pain when touched - zinc.
suppurating - chlor., kali-bi.
prickly heat - ***apis.***
pustules - agar., aur-m-n., bell., berb., calc., chin., chlor., clem., crot-t., dulc., kali-bi., kali-br., ***lach.,*** nat-c., nat-m., petr., rhod., ***sep., sil.,*** sulph.
black points, with - kali-bi.
painful - ant-t., **SIL.**
sensitive - nat-c.
small-pox, like - ant-t., sil.
red - bell., ***bry.,*** calc., **CHEL.,** cocc., rhus-t., spig., tab., verb.

ERUPTIONS, general
scabs, bloody - rhus-v.
scales - am-m., ars-i., ***mez.***
scapula, right - am-m.
smarting - bry., spig.
warm, when - cocc., stram.
eruptions, lumbar - arund., rhus-t.
itching - arund., lyc.
pimples - ars-h., calc., chel., chin., clem., kali-c., nat-c., nicc.
burning - lyc.
inflamed - sulph.
itching - lyc., tab.
oozing when scratched - sulph.
painful - lyc.
red at night on scratching, better morning - apoc.
scratching, after - chin., nicc.
pustules - calc., chlor., clem., nat-c.
eruptions, sacral region - jug-c.
eruptions, thoracic, pimples - am-m., berb., ***cic., cist.***
middle of - zinc.
shoulders, between - carc., gels., lyc., mag., ph-ac., rat., squil.
undressing, while - carc.

ERYSIPELAS - ***apis,*** graph., kali-i., ***merc.,*** ph-ac., ***rhus-t.***
shoulders, across the - ***apis.***
erysipelas, lumbar - ***merc.***

FISTULA - ***calc-p., hep., ph-ac.,*** **PHOS., SIL., SULPH.**

FALLING apart sensation, relieved by bandaging tightly - tril.

FLOWING sensation, scapula, right - hep.

FLUTTERING, lumbar - berb., chim.
fluttering, thoracic, shoulders, between - ***cupr.***

FORMICATION - **ACON.,** aesc., **AGAR.,** agn., ***all-c.,*** alum., anan., apoc., arg-m., ***arn., ars.,*** ars-m., arund., asaf., atro., bar-c., berb., bell., bov., carc., carl., caust., ***cham., cocc.,*** con., crot-h., euon., graph., hyper., lac-c., ***lach.,*** lact., mag-s., manc., merc-c., ***nat-a., nat-c., nux-v., osm.,*** ox-ac., pall., ***ph-ac.,*** **PHOS.,** ran-s., rat., rhod., sabad., sal-ac., sars., **SEC.,** sulph.
afternoon - asaf., mag-s.
cold - ars., lac-c.
down the back - carl.
evening - ***lyc.,*** mag-s., osm.
extending, to fingers and toes - sec.
to limbs - **PHOS.**
morning - ars-m.
night - bar-c., bov., zinc.
shoulders, between the - carl., laur., viol-t.
up and down - ***crot-h., lach.,*** manc.
formication, lumbar - acon., ars., arund., buf-s., canth., crot-t., meny., merc-c., ph-ac., stann., tarax., thuj.
extending to, face - arund.
shoulders - arund.
paroxysms - thuj.
sitting - canth.
formication, scapula - ***anac.,*** sil., zinc.
left - arg-m., med.
right during urination - hep.
formication, spine - **ACON., AGAR.,** arn., ***ars.,*** arund., con., kali-p., ***lach.,*** nat-c., rhus-t., ***sal-ac.***

GNAWING, pain - agar., ***alum.,*** hell., lil-t., stry.
dinner, after - sep.
extending to neck after lying down - mag-m.
spot , in small - sulph.
walking, while - ***canth.,*** stront.
gnawing, lumbar - alum., ***alumn.,*** am-c., ***berb.,*** canth., hura, lil-t., mag-m., nicc., ph-ac., ***psor.,*** plb., stront-c., ***sulph.***
evening after lying down - mag-m.
extending to cervical region - alum.
night - am-c.
in bed - lil-t.
rubbing amel. - ***phos.***
walking, while - stront.
amel. - am-c.
gnawing, scapula - alum., ph-ac.
below - agar.
gnawing, spine - **BELL.,** mag-m.
gnawing, thoracic, middle of - nat-c.

GRUMBLING, spine - sulph.

HAIR, on back - tub.

HEAT - aesc., ***agar.,*** alum., alumn., ***alum-m., apis, ars.,*** asaf., aur., bapt., bar-c., berb., calc., calc-s., camph., carb-an., carb-v., carl., caust., cham., chin., ***coff.,*** con., dig., ***dulc.,*** gels., ***glon.,*** hell., helon., hyos., laur., ***led.,*** lob-s., ***lyc.,*** mag-m., mang., ***med.,*** meny., ***merc.,*** nat-c., nat-m., ol-an., op., par., ph-ac., **PHOS.,** ***pic-ac.,*** plb., rhus-v., sars., sec., ***sil.,*** sol-n., spig., stann., staph., ***sulph., sumb.,*** verat., ***zinc.***
afternoon - phos.
alternating with, cold - carl., cham., verat.
shivering - cham.
boiling water, like - ust.
eating, after - staph.
evening - cham., ph-ac., phys., verat.
excitement - pic-ac.
extending, down back - calc-p., coff., con., laur., par., phys., sulph.
extending, up the back - ***ars.,*** bapt., cann-i., hyos., ***lyc.,*** **PHOS.,** ***podo.,*** sarr., verat.
menses, during - ***phos.***
stool, during - podo.
forenoon - hell.
menses, during - ***phos.***
mental exertion - ***pic-ac., sil.***
morning, on waking - con.
reading exciting news, while - ***gels.***
sitting, while - mang., meny., phos., ***zinc.***
streams up - ***ars., lyc., verat.***
walking, while - verat.
in open air - chin., merc., ph-ac., sil., sol-n.
warmth of bed - pic-ac.
wine, after - gins., ***zinc.***

heat, lumbar - ars-i., arund., aur., aur-s., bapt., ***berb.,*** colch., hura, hyos., kalm., lac-c., ***nat-m.,*** nit-ac., ***nux-v., phos., pic-ac.,*** plb., raph., sarr., sel., sep., sulph., thuj.
air, in open - hyos.
breath, deep, on - sep.
eating, after - sel.
extending to, face - arund.
rectum - colch.
externally - clem.
flushes, in spine - calc-p., sumb.
hot water flowing in - sumb.
riding in a carriage, after - hura
sitting, while - colch., hyos.
sleep, after mid-day nap - sel.
walking in a room - hyos.

heat, scapula - ***chel.,*** mur-ac.

heat, spine, in - ***alum., ars.,*** bry., cann-i., carb-v., coloc., hyos., ***lyc., med., nat-m.,*** op., ***phos., pic-ac.,*** plb., sarr., ***sil.,*** sin-n., spig., ***sumb.,*** verat-v., ***zinc.***
extending upward - ***ars., lyc., phos., podo.,*** sarr., sumb.
hot water flowing in - ***sumb.,*** ust.
spots - ***phos.***

heat, spine, in, flushes - ***acon.,*** bapt., **BOL.,** brom., clem., dig., ***mang.,*** merl., spig., **SUMB.,** yohim.
evening - ph-ac., sol-n.
stool, after - ***podo.***
supper, after - spig.
walking, on continued - glon.
extending to body - **SUMB.**
in waves, up - ***lyc.***
lower back - staph.
morning - lil-t.
stool, during - ***podo.***
after - ***podo.***
warm air streaming up spine into head - ***ars., sumb.***

heat, thoracic - merc., ***phos.,*** **PIC-AC.**
limbs, spreads to - ***camph.***
middle of - arg-n., kali-c., **LYC.,** ***naja, phos., pic-ac.,*** puls.

HEAVINESS, weight - aesc., ***aloe, am-m.,*** ambr., anac., ant-c., arg-m., arg-n., arn., **BAR-C.,** benz-ac., ***berb., bov.,*** carb-v., **CIMIC.,** colch., coloc., crot-c., equis., ***eup-pur.,*** euphr., ***helon., hydr.,*** kali-c., kali-chl., kali-p., ***kreos., lil-t.,*** mag-s., mang., nat-c., ***nat-m.,*** nat-p., nat-s., ***par.,*** petr., ph-ac., ***phos., pic-ac.,*** puls., rhod., ***rhus-t.,*** sapo., ***sep.,*** sulph.
forenoon - sulph.
sitting, while - nat-c.
lying - phos.
morning - petr.
bed, in - ant-t., euphr., pic-ac., ***sep.,*** sulph.
rising, on - ant-t., euphr., sulph.
waking - phos., pic-ac., ***sep.***
motion amel. - rhod.
night - carb-v.
rising agg. - ant-t.

heaviness, lumbar - ***arg-n.,*** arn., ***bar-c.,*** bov., carb-ac., **CIMIC.,** colch., coloc., ***con., hydr., kali-c.,*** kali-p., ***lil-t.,*** mag-s., ***merc.,*** nat-c., ***ph-ac., phos.,*** **PIC-AC.,** ***phyt.,*** **RHUS-T.,** syph.
hips, down thighs - cimic.
midnight - ***pic-ac.***
lying on left side amel. - ***coloc.***
menses, during - ***cimic., kali-c.***
before - bov.
motion, agg. - ***phos., pic-ac.***
amel. - nat-c.
sitting - nat-c.
turning, in bed agg. - ***corn.***
waking, on - ***pic-ac.***

heaviness, scapula - calc., chin., gran., lach., ***nux-v.,*** phyt., rhus-t., sil.
below - puls.
between, as from a load - ***carb-s.,*** meny.

heaviness, spine - ***arg-n.,*** arn., ***bar-c.,*** bov., carb-ac., **CIMIC.,** colch., coloc., ***con., hydr., kali-c.,*** kali-p., ***lil-t.,*** mag-s., ***merc.,*** nat-c., ***ph-ac., phos.,*** **PIC-AC.,** ***phyt.,*** **RHUS-T.,** syph.
lying on left side amel. - ***coloc.***
menses, during - ***cimic., kali-c.***
before - bov.
midnight - ***pic-ac.***
motion, agg. - ***phos., pic-ac.***
amel. - nat-c.
turning in bed agg. - ***corn.***
waking, on - ***pic-ac.***

heaviness, thoracic - carb-s., phyt., sil.

HERPES, simplex - all-s., ars., lach., lyc., nat-c., sep., zinc.
herpes zoster - ***cist., lach., merc.,*** rhus-t.

HYPERSENSITIVE, skin - merc., petr., plat., tarent.

IMPETIGO - ***petr., nat-m.***

INFLAMMATION, spinal cord - acon., ***alum-m.,*** agar., ***apis, ars.,*** bar-m., ***bell., benz-ac.,*** calc., camph., canth., caust., cedr., cic., cocc., colch., crot-h., ***dulc.,*** **GELS.,** hyos., kali-i., ***lach.,*** lath., lyc., merc., nat-m., ***nat-s., nux-v.,*** **OP.,** ox-ac., ***par.,*** **PHOS.,** phys., ***pic-ac.,*** plb., rhus-t., sec., sil., stry-p., sulph., tarent.
chronic - ***ars., crot-h.,*** lath., ***ox-ac., plb.,*** stry., thal.
abuse of mercury, after - ***kali-i.***
eruptions do not develop, when - bry., dulc.
membranes, spinal meningitis - ***acon.,*** **APIS, BELL.,** ***bry., calc., cic., cimic.,*** cocc., crot-h., cupr., dulc., **GELS.,** ***hyos.,*** hyper., kali-i., ***ip.,*** merc., ***nat-m., nat-s.,*** nux-v., ***op.,*** ox-ac., ***plb., rhus-t.,*** sec., verat-v., ***zinc.***
scarlet fever, or measles, during, eruptions do not develop - dulc.
suffocation, worse in warm room - **APIS,** op.

INJURIES, ailments, after - aesc., **ARN.,** ***bell-p.,*** **BRY.,** ***calc.,*** cic., **HYPER.,** ***kali-c., lyc.,*** mag-p., ***nat-s.,*** nit-ac., **RHUS-T., RUTA.,** ***thuj.***

INJURIES, ailments, after
dislocations - **ARN., BRY., CALC.,** calc-f., caust., ***coloc.,*** hyper., lyc., nux-v., phos., **RHUS-T.,** ***ruta.,*** stront-c., sulph., zinc.
lifting, from - **ARN., BRY., CALC., HYPER.,** ***lyc.,*** **RHUS-T.,** ruta.
aching after - anag., **ARN.,** bell-p., bor., bry., **CALC., GRAPH., LYC.,** ***nux-v.,*** ph-ac., **RHUS-T., RUTA.,** sang., ***sep.***
lumbar, remains sensitive to jar of walking - arn., **BRY.,** ***thuj.***
pain, after - **ARN., BRY.,** calc., ***con.,*** **HYPER.,** ***kali-c., nat-s.,*** **RHUS-T.,** ***ruta, thuj.***
straining, easy - bor., **CALC.,** calc-f., ***calc-p.,*** con., **GRAPH.,** ham., **LYC.,** mill., ***nux-v.,*** ph-ac., **RHUS-T., RUTA.,** sang., ***sep.,*** sil.
injuries, spine, to - aesc., ***apis,*** **ARN.,** bell-p., ***calc., con.,*** dam., **HYPER.,** kali-c., ***led.,*** **NAT-S.,** ***nit-ac., rhus-t., ruta., sil.,*** tell., ***thuj.,*** zinc.
bleeding in spinal cord - acon., ***arn., bell.,*** lach., nux-v., sec.
concussion, from - ***arn.,*** bell-p., cic., con., **HYPER., NAT-S.,** phys.
lies on back, jerking head backward after, injury - cic., ***hyper.***
lifting, from - ***arn.,*** bor., **CALC., GRAPH., LYC.,** ***nux-v.,*** ph-ac., **RHUS-T.,** ***ruta.,*** sang., ***sep.***
lumbar region remains sensitive to jar of walking - ***thuj.***
old injuries - ign.
shock, of - ***arn., hyper.,*** **NAT-S.,** ***nat-m., nit-ac.***
spasms, from - zinc.
wounds - calen., ruta, symph.

IRRITATION, of spine - aesc., **AGAR.,** ***ang.,*** ant-c., apis, ***arn.,*** ars., ***atro.,*** bapt., **BELL.,** ***benz-ac.,*** berb., ***calc., carb-ac.,*** caust., ***chel., chin.,*** chin-a., **CHIN-S.,** ***cimic., cocc., crot-c.,*** crot-h., ***cupr., dios.,*** eup-per., gels., ***glon.,*** **GRAPH.,** ***hep.,*** hyper., iod., iodof., ***kali-ar., kali-c.,*** kali-i., **KALI-P.,** ***lac-c.,*** **LACH.,** ***lec.,*** lil-t., **LYSS.,** mag-m., ***med.,*** merc-i-r., ***naja, nat-a., nat-c.,*** **NAT-M., NAT-P.,** ***nat-s.,*** nicc., **NUX-V.,** ***ol-j.,*** ox-ac., ***ph-ac.,*** **PHOS.,** phys., ***phyt.,*** plan., ***plat.,*** podo., ***puls., ran-b., rat., rhus-t.,*** **RUTA.,** sabad., ***sang., sars.,*** sec., ***sep.,*** **SIL.,** spig., squil., stram., sulph., ***tarent.,*** tanac., ***tell.,*** **THER.,** ***thuj.,*** verat., ***vib.,*** **ZINC.**
slight - stram.
fever, during - ***chin-s., cocc.***
footsteps - ***nux-v.,*** **THER.**
jar., of bed - **BELL.,** ***graph., lach.,*** **SIL., THER.,** ***thuj.***
leaning against a chair agg. - **AGAR.,** plb., **THER.**
lying, back, on - mag-m.
flat on the back with firm pressure, amel. - ***nat-m.***
on something hard, amel. - ***nat-m.***
menses, during - thuj.

IRRITATION, of spine
morning - agar., mag-m.
night - mag-m.
pressure, agg. - ther.
pressure, on - plat.
sewing, machine, from using - ***nux-v.***
sitting - ruta.
stretching - med.
thunderstorm, before - ***agar., phos.***
walking, while - ***ruta.,*** verat.

ITCHING - agar., all-s., aloe, ***alum.,*** am-m., **ANT-C.,** arn., arg-m., ars-i., asc-t., aur., ***bar-c.,*** calc., calc-s., carb-ac., carb-s., carb-v., **CAUST.,** chel., cist., clem., cocc., coc-c., corn., dios., daph., fago., fl-ac., glon., ***graph.,*** guai., hep., hura, kali-bi., ***kali-c.,*** kali-n., kali-p., lac-ac., ***lyc.,*** mag-c., mag-m., mag-s., med., ***merc.,*** merc-i-f., **MEZ.,** mill., mur-ac., ***nat-c.,*** nat-m., nat-p., ***nat-s.,*** nicc., **NIT-AC.,** ol-an., osm., pall., ph-ac., phos., ***puls.,*** raph., ***rhus-t., sars.,*** seneg., ***sep., sil.,*** spig., spong., **SULPH.,** tell., ther., ***thuj.,*** zinc.
afternoon - fago., sars.
burning - agar., alum., berb., ***calc.,*** daph., kali-c., mag-c., mez., ***nux-v.,*** raph.
evening while undressing - nux-v.
morning while dressing - nux-v.
night - nux-v., spong.
scratching, after - alum., squil.
walking in open air, while - merc.
cold, air, in - rhus-v.
when feeling - lyc., spong.
evening - con., fago., fl-ac., kali-c., lyc., rat., sulph., thuj.
bed, in - calc., lyc., merc., nat-m.
undressing, while - cocc., hyper., mag-m., nat-c., ***nat-s.,*** osm., puls.
forenoon - fl-ac.
morning - asc-t., kali-c., lyc.
6 to 10 a.m - kali-bi.
7 a.m - pall., rhus-t.
bed, in - rhus-t.
night - agar., ail., apoc., ars., asc-t., fl-ac., ***mez.,*** phos., rhus-v., zinc.
lying down - mag-c.
warmth of bed, in - nat-a., rhus-v., sulph.
scratching, amel. - mag-c., mag-m., mez., nat-c., pall., rat., rhus-v.
changes place, after - mez., pall.
pain, after - kali-c., nit-ac.
stinging - alum., anac., arn., caust., squil.
scratching amel. - anac.
scratching, unchanged by - nat-c.
sudden, amel. by scratching - ph-ac.
itching, lumbar - alum., ***bar-c., berb.,*** buf-s., carb-v., caust., chin., con., dig., fl-ac., hep., iod., kali-bi., kali-c., kali-n., lach., led., lyc., mag-c., ***mag-m., merc.,*** merc-c., mez., morph., ***nat-m.,*** nicc., ol-an., phyt., psor., ***puls.,*** sulph.
burning - alum., mag-c.
extending to abdomen and thighs - nat-m.
corrosive - ph-ac.
evening, bed, in - nat-m.
scratch it raw, must - ***bar-c.***

itching, scapula - alum., am-m., arn., asaf., bar-c., bell., calc., com., crot-h., cund., dios., form., laur., merc., merc-i-f., mez., olnd., petr., phel., rat., ruta., seneg., sil., spig., stront-c., ther., viol-t., zinc.
border, outer, right - dulc.
rubbing amel. - grat.
spots, in - fl-ac.

itching, thoracic, middle of - all-s., alum., am-m., arg-m., calc., calc-s., caust., chin-s., dios., ***hipp.,*** laur., mag-c., mag-m., mosch., rat., ruta., stront-c., ***zinc.***
evening - dios., mag-m., zinc.
night - am-m., cocc.
night, while undressing - sulph.
scratching, amel. - mag-c.
burning, after - rat.

JERKING - petr.
side, left - agar.

jerking, lumbar - sulph.

jerking, scapula - sep.

JERKING, pain - ang., calc., calc-p., chin., cinnb., euph., ***ferr.,*** laur., nat-m., petr., ran-s., sulph.
attempting to open mouth, on - stry.
extending toward heart - nat-m.
involuntary when pressing on dorsal vertebrae - arn.
motion amel. - petr.
night - staph.
sleeping, while - am-c.
sticking, when bending backward - chel.
swallowing, on - petr.

jerking, lumbar - alum., am-c., asar., euph.
lifting - nat-c.
raising thigh - agar.
sharp, stitching - rhus-t.

jerking, scapula - calc-p.

jerking, spine, middle of - cina.
lower spine - mag-c.

LABOR-like, pain - acon., ***aloe, carb-v., cocc., coff.,*** eup-pur., ferr., **KALI-C.,** ***kreos., lyc., nux-v.,*** **PULS., SABIN.,** sec., ***sep.***
extending to groin and thighs - ***sabin.***

labor-like, small of back - acon., ***kreos., nux-v., lil-t.,*** **PULS.,** sabin.
extending, to glutei muscles - **KALI-C.**
to loins and pubes - ***vib.***
to pubes - ***sabin.***
menses, during - agar., am-m., ***calc., cham., cimic., cycl.,*** graph., kreos., ***lyc., nit-ac.,*** **PULS.,** ***sulph.***
urging to stool, with - kreos., **NUX-V.**

LAMENESS, pain - acon., ***aesc.,*** abrot., agar., am-m., bell., **BERB.,** ***bry.,*** calc., camph-br., ***caust., cimic., cupr-ar., dios., dulc.,*** fl-ac., get., ***helon., hyper., kali-c.,*** kali-p., kalm., lachn., led., lyc., lyss., **NAT-M.,** ***nux-v.,*** phys., ***phyt.,*** plb., puls-n, ***rhus-t.,*** **RUTA.,** sabad., sarcol-ac., ***sep.,*** spong., staph., ***stry.,*** sul-ac., ***sulph.,*** zing.
cold from taking - **DULC.**
evening - cupr-ar.
morning - dios.
moving head, on - bapt., cupr-ar.

LAMENESS, pain
rising, on - nat-m.
rising up, on - ptel.
sitting, a while, after - cupr-ar.
long, or as from lifting - calc., ***lyc.,*** mur-ac., olnd., **RHUS-T.,** valer.
waking on - abrot., **AESC.,** ptel., puls-n
walking after - zing.

lameness, lumbar - agar., ***aesc.,*** ang., ***caust.,*** con., ***cupr-ar.,*** cur., dios., ***dulc., hyper.,*** iris, ***kali-c.,*** hep., **LACH.,** ***lept., nat-m., nux-v.,*** **PHOS.,** ptel., puls-n, **RHUS-T.,** ***ruta.,*** sel., sil.
childbirth, after difficult - ***nux-v.***
cold, from taking - **DULC.**
drawing - cham.
evening - alum., bart.
in bed - ***kalm.***
exertion, on - phys.
extending to thighs - cham.
morning - dios., sel.
on rising - nat-m., sil.
motion - cupr-ar.
amel. - dios.
pulling agg. - dios.
rising up, on - ptel.
standing - agar., coff., zing.
stooping - ang., cur., dios.
turning in bed almost impossible - dios.
waking, on - puls-n
walking, while - agar., zing.
wet, after getting - **DULC.**

LANCINATING, pain - alum., ant-ox., asc-t., ***berb.,*** colch., ***coloc.,*** elaps, kali-c., kali-i., kali-m., lyc., ***nat-s., nit-ac.,*** nux-v., sep., sil., stel., ***stry.***

lancinating, lumbar - anac., asaf., aur-s., **COLOC.,** cupr., ***elaps,*** ign., ***kali-c.,*** lac-c., plb., ***senec.,*** **VERAT-V.**
as from hot iron, morning - bufo
evening, 9 p.m. - hura.
extending, down thighs and legs - ***aesc.,*** aur-m., bapt., carb-ac., cocc., ***coloc.,*** cur., ham., ***helon.,*** kali-c., kali-m., lac-c., ***ox-ac.,*** phyt., ***stel.,*** tell.
downwards - ***elaps.***
legs, down - ***aesc.,*** aur-m., bapt., carb-ac., cocc., ***coloc.,*** cur., ham., ***helon.,*** kali-m., lac-c., ***ox-ac.,*** phyt., ***stel.,*** tell., xero
pubis, to - ***sabad.,*** vib., xan.
to coccyx - hura.
upwards - aspar., ***coloc., gels.***
injury, after - nat-s.
inspiration - aur., **COLOC.**
lying, while - berb.
on back - **COLOC.**
motion, on - plb.
amel. - ***nat-s.***
paroxysmal - plb.
pressure, amel. - plb.
raising arms - ***elaps***
rubbing amel. - nat-s.
standing amel. - berb.
thrusts, like - anan., **VERAT-V.**

lancinating, thoracic - bad., ***gins.,*** hura, rob.
lower vertebrae through chest - berb.
thoracic, middle of - ***gins.***
thrusts, like - euon., ran-b.

LUMP, sensation of, in - anac., ***arn.,*** berb., ***carb-v.,*** cinnb., phos., sars.
lump, scapula, on - am-m.
left - prun.

LUMPS, thoracic, middle of - calc., mag-s.

MOUSE, as if a, running up the back - ***sulph.***

MOVEMENTS, clucking, left side - ars.
up and down, shoulders, when speaking - ran-b.

NEEDLES, icy, sensation, in - agar., cocc.

NODULES, painless, red - petr.

NUMBNESS - ***acon., agar.,*** bell., ***berb.,*** bry., calc., ***calc-p., cocc.,*** cupr-ar., kali-bi., nux-v., ***ox-ac.,*** oxyt., phos., phys., ***plat.,*** pop-c., sec., sep., sil.
creeping down - phys.
nap, after - phos.
part lain on - calc.
numbness, lumbar region - **ACON.,** apis, ars., **BERB.,** carb-v., frax., graph., kali-bi., lappa-a., **PLAT.,** ***sil.,*** spong.
evening - alum., mag-m.
extending to lower limbs - ***acon.***
loss of sensation - ***ars.,*** bry., con., cupr-ac., kali-n., zinc.
morning, on rising - ***nat-m.***
numbness, scapula - anac., arg-m., bry.

OPISTHOTONOS - ***absin.,*** acon., agar., amyg., ang., apis, ***ars.,*** art-v., **BELL.,** berb., both., brach., bry., ***camph.,*** calc-p., ***canth.,*** carb-an., ***cham., chen-a.,*** **CIC.,** cina, cor-r., **CUPR.,** ***cupr-ar.,*** dig., **HYOS.,** hyper., ***ign., ip., lach.,*** led., med., merc., ***morph.,*** mosch., nat-s., **NUX-V., OP.,** oena., petr., phos., ***phyt., plat.,*** plb., ***rhus-t., sec., stann.,*** **STRAM., STRY.,** ***tab.,*** ter., verat., ***verat-v., zinc.***
epilepsy, in - ars., stann.
vertigo, with - cic.

OPPRESSION, between scapula - petr.

PAIN, back - abies-n., abrot., acon., **AESC.,** ***aeth., agar.,*** ail., aloe, **ALUM.,** ***alumn.,*** ambr., am-c., ***am-m.,*** anac., anan., ***ang.,*** ant-c., ant-t., ***apis,*** aran., ***arg-m., arg-n.,*** **ARN.,** ars., ars-i., asaf., asar., ***atro., aur.,*** aur-m., **BAR-C., BELL.,** ***berb., bism., bol.,*** bor., brach., brom., **BRY.,** cahin., **CALC., CALC-P.,** calc-s., ***camph., cann-i.,*** cann-s., canth., ***caps.,*** carb-ac., ***carb-an.,*** **CARB-S.,** ***carb-v.,*** card-m., ***caul., caust., cham., chel.,*** chen-a., chin., chin-a., ***chin-s.,*** chr-ac., cic., ***cimic.,*** cina, cinnb., clem., cob., coc-c., ***cocc., colch., coloc., con.,*** cor-r., ***crot-h., cub.,*** cupr., cycl., dios., ***dor.,*** dros., dulc., elaps, **EUP-PER., EUP-PUR.,** ***euph.,*** euphr., ***ferr.,*** ferr-ar., ferr-p., ***form.,*** gamb., ***gels.,*** **GRAPH.,** grat., ***gua.,*** **GUAI.,** gymn., ham., hell., ***helon., hep., hydr.,*** hyos., ***hyper., ign.,*** ind., iod., **IP.,** ***ipom.,*** kali-ar., ***kali-bi.,*** **KALI-C.,** ***kali-i.,***

PAIN, back - kali-m., ***kali-n.,*** kali-p., ***kali-s., kalm.,*** kreos., **LAC-C.,** ***lach.,*** lact., laur., ***led.,*** lil-t., lith., ***lob.,*** **LYC.,** lyss., mag-c., ***mag-m.,*** mag-p., mag-s., manc., ***med.,*** meph., ***merc., merc-c., mez.,*** **MUR-AC.,** ***murx., naja,*** nat-a., ***nat-c.,*** **NAT-M.,** nat-p., **NAT-S.,** ***nit-ac.,*** **NUX-M., NUX-V.,** ol-an., oena., ol-j., op., ox-ac., pall., **PAR.,** paraf., ***petr.,*** ph-ac., **PHOS.,** phys., phyt., ***pic-ac.,*** plat., ***plb.,*** podo., **PSOR., PULS.,** ***rad.,*** ran-a., rat., ***ran-b., rhod., rhus-r.,*** **RHUS-T.,** ***ruta.,*** sabad., sabin., ***samb.,*** sang., sarr., sars., ***sec.,*** sel., senec., seneg., **SEP., SIL.,** ***sol-n.,*** spig., spong., stann., ***staph., stel.,*** stram., ***stront-c.,*** stry., **SULPH.,** ***sul-ac.,*** tarax., tarent., ***tell.,*** tep., ther., thuj., torula., trio., ***upa.,*** valer., ***variol.,*** verat., viol-t., wye., xero, ***zinc.,*** zinc-m., zing.
acids, after - ***lach.***
afternoon - abrot., agar., bov., canth., caust., cham., chel., equis., glon., hyos., mag-c., mag-m., nicc., pall., plb., ptel., rumx., ruta., ***sep.,*** zing.
air, cold, in - acon., agar., bar-c., bry., ***dulc.,*** merc., nit-ac., ***nux-v.,*** rhod., ***rhus-t.,*** sabad., sep., sulph.
cold, in, amel. - **KALI-S.**
draft of, every - ***nux-v.,*** verat.
open, amel. - acon., nux-v., ***vib.***
alternating with, abdomen, pain in - vario.
headache - acon., aloe, alum., brom., ign., meli., sep.
alternating sides - agar., bell., ***berb.,*** calc., calc-p., kali-bi., kalm.
apyrexia, during - arn., ars., ***calc.,*** caps., cham., chin., ign., ***nat-m.,*** nit-ac., nux-v., petr., samb., sep., sil., spig., stram., thuj., verat.
ascends - agar., ***alum.,*** arn., ars., ***chin-s.,*** clem., ***cocc., coloc.,*** corn., cycl., dirc., eup-pur., **GELS.,** kalm., kreos., ***lach.,*** led., mag-m., meny., nat-m., **NIT-AC.,** nux-m., nux-v., ox-ac., ***petr.,*** phos., ***phyt.,*** plb., podo., sep., sil., stann., staph., sulph., ust.
constriction, of anus, with - ***coloc.***
descends, and ascends - kali-c.
labor, during - **GELS.,** ***petr.***
lying down, after - mag-m.
sitting, while - meny.
spreads upwards like a fan - ***lach.***
step, during every - sep.
stool, during - phos., podo.
stooping - arn., ***sil.***
twinges up the, better by drawing shoulders back - cycl.
belching, amel. - ***sep.,*** zinc.
bending, backwards, agg. - arg-m., bar-c., ***calc., calc-p., chel., cimic.,*** con., dios., kali-c., lam., mang., plat., puls., sel., stann.
amel. - aeth., acon., am-m., bell., cycl., eupi., fl-ac., hura, ign., lach., petr., puls., rhus-t., sil., sabad., sabin.
forward, agg. - ***pic-ac.***
amel. - chel., kali-c., meny., nat-a., ph-ac., puls., sang., sec., sep., thuj.

PAIN, back

breathing, when - acon., aesc., alum., alumn., ***am-m.,*** apis, arn., asar., ***aur.,*** berb., calc., cann-s., carb-an., carb-s., carb-v., cham., chel., cinnb., **COLOC.,** ***cop.,*** conv., cupr-ar., cupr., dig., dulc., inul., kali-bi., ***kali-c.,*** kali-n., kali-p., kali-s., kalm., led., lob., merc., mur-ac., nat-a., nat-c., nat-m., nux-v., par., petr., prun., ***psor.,*** ptel., puls., raph., ruta., sabin., sang., sars., seneg., ***sep.,*** spig., stann., ***sulph.,*** thuj.

deep - sars.

chill, during - ant-t., apis, ***arn., ars., bell.,*** **BOL.,** calc., ***caps.,*** carb-s., carb-v., caust., ***cham.,*** chin., chin-a., **CHIN-S.,** elat., ***eup-per.,*** gamb., hyos., ign., ***ip.,*** lach., lac-ac., lyc., mosch., myric., ***nat-m.,*** **NUX-V.,** phos., podo., ***puls.,*** sang., sep., sulph., verat., zinc.

extending to occiput and vertex - **PULS.**

before - **AESC.,** aran., ***ars.,*** bry., carb-v., daph., ***dios., eup-per.,*** eup-pur., ***ip.,*** **PODO.,** rhus-t.

coffee, agg. - ***cham.***

cold, exposure to, from - acon., ***bry., rhod.,*** sulph.

taking - ***dulc.,*** mag-p., nit-ac., sars.

weather, change to - **CALC-P., DULC.,** rhod., ***rhus-t.***

colic, with - sars.

convulsions, with - acon.

coughing, when - ***acon., am-c.,*** arn., arund., **BELL., BRY.,** ***calc.,*** calc-s., ***caps.,*** carb-an., chin., chin-s., cocc., cor-r., ***kali-bi.,*** kali-c., kali-n., kreos., ***merc.,*** nat-m., ***nit-ac.,*** ph-ac., phos., puls., rhus-t., rumx., seneg., ***sep.,*** stram., sulph., tell., tub.

damp, weather - **CALC., DULC.,** ***nux-m., phyt., rhod.,*** **RHUS-T.,** sep.

daytime - ***camph.***

descends - acon., ***aeth.,*** alum., am-c., chel., cimic., cina, cocc., con., cur., elaps, ferr-s., ***glon.,*** kali-bi., ***kali-c., kalm.,*** lil-t., mag-c., mang., merc., nat-m., nat-s., ***nux-m.,*** nux-v., ox-ac., ***phyt.,*** phys., ***pic-ac.,*** podo., psor., rat., sang., sep., thuj., ust., zing.

labor, during - ***nux-v.***

dinner, after - agar., cob., indg., phel., phos., sep., sulph.

drinking, while - chin.

eating, while - chin., coc-c.

after - agar., am-m., ant-t., bry., cham., cina, ***daph., kali-c.***

amel. - kali-n.

emissions, after - ant-c., cob., kali-br., ph-ac., sars., ***staph.***

amel. - zinc.

evening - acon., agar., alumn., ***ars., calc-p.,*** carb-v., cham., chel., cist., cocc., coloc., cupr-ar., ferr-i., gels., graph., kali-ar., kali-n., ***kali-s., kalm., lach.,*** led., lil-t., ***lyc.,*** mag-c., mag-m., ***naja,*** nat-a., nat-m., nat-s., nit-ac., nux-v., phys., psor., ***rhus-t.,*** ruta., sarr., sin-n., ***sep., sulph.,*** thuj., ter., zing.

lying down, after - thuj.

PAIN, back

evening, sunset to sunrise - **SYPH.**

everything agg. - bry., kali-c., lach., sep.

excessive, during labor - bell., cimic., coff., kali-c.

exertion, from - ***agar.,*** asaf., ***berb.,*** calc., calc-p., cann-i., caust., cocc., ferr., hyper., kali-c., kali-p., lyc., ox-ac., ph-ac., ruta, sec., sep., ***stry.,*** sulph., thymol., verat.

amel. - ruta., ***sep.***

mental - thymol.

extending, to

abdomen, to - cham.

anus - nat-c., phos.

arms - ars., berb., ***calc.,*** calc-ar., phos.

chest - arn., berb., camph., kali-n., laur., petr., samb., sars.

left - bar-c., ***bry.,*** mez., plat., zinc.

right - acon., calc-p., kali-c., lyc., merc., sep.

downward - agar., cocc., phos., pic-ac., puls., stram., tab., tell.

ears, to - gels.

feet - alum., berb., bor., cob., sep.

groin - ***sabin., sulph.,*** vib.

head, to - ***calc., chin-s.,*** hell., nat-m., sep., sil.

after exertion - nat-m.

on every step - sep.

heart, toward - nat-m.

heels, to - colch., ***sep.***

hips, to - ***bol.,*** cimic., ***lach., lyss.,*** mosch.

knees, to - arn., ***kali-c.***

lower limbs, to - agar., ars., bell., ***calc., calc-ar.,*** camph., ***kali-c.,*** lach., lob-c., ***phos.,*** **RHUS-T.**

lumbar region - ***berb.,*** cham., ***kali-c.,*** kreos., **SABIN.**

neck, to - sang.

to nape in evening after lying down - nat-c.

occiput, to - ***gels.,*** ol-j., ***puls.***

and vertex during chill - **PULS.**

pelvis, to - ***eupi.***

pubis - sabin., sep., vib.

sacrum, to - con., lyc., tep.

scapular region - bry.

left - phos., sulph., zinc.

shoulder, to - chel., chin., ***kalm.,*** lyc.

stomach, to - berb., **CUPR.,** lyc., nicc., nit-ac., puls., rhod., thuj.

on pressure - ***bell.***

while sitting - bry., nicc.

testes - kreos., sulph.

thighs - cimic., ***kali-c., lyc., nux-v.,*** ox-ac.

down - berb., caust., ***cimic.,*** hep., kali-c., ***nit-ac.,*** ox-ac., ***sep.,*** vib.

upward - ars., gels., lach., lil-t., nit-ac., phos., rad-br., sulph., zinc-valer.

uterus - sep., vib.

fasting, when - kali-n.

PAIN, back

fever, during - alst., ***arn.,*** ars., ***bell.,*** calc., ***caps.,*** carb-v., caust., chin., chin-s., cocc., eug., ***eup-per.,*** hyos., ign., kali-ar., kali-c., lach., laur., ***lyc., nat-m.,*** nat-s., **NUX-V.,** ***puls., rhus-t.,*** sulph., ziz.

flatus, amel. - berb., coc-c., ruta.

forenoon - ars., ***cham.,*** equis., ***nat-m.,*** nat-s., ptel.

10 a.m - am-m.

hard, bed, as from - bar-c.

injury, after - **ARN., BRY.,** calc., ***con.,*** **HYPER.,** ***kali-c., nat-s.,*** **RHUS-T.,** ***ruta, thuj.***

jarring, agg. - acon., **BELL.,** berb., ***bry., carb-ac., carb-an.,*** **GRAPH.,** kali-bi., ***lob.,*** mez., petr., podo., seneg., ***sep.,*** **SIL.,** sulph., tell., ***ther., thuj.***

kidneys, agg. - cadm-met., senec., solid.

kneeling, when - euphr., ***sep.***

laughing, agg. - ***camph.,*** **CANN-I.,** ***con.,*** phos., plb., tell.

labor, during - ***caust.,*** cimic., cocc., coff., **GELS., KALI-C.,** ***nux-v., petr.,*** **PULS.,** ***sep.***

downward - cimic., nux-v.

violent, want it pressed - caust., ***kali-c.***

laughing, agg. - **CANN-I.,** phos., plb., tell.

leaning, back against chair, agg. - ***agar., plb., ther.***

amel. - eupi., sarr., zing.

left - dros., glon., sil.

to right - bell., cund., dros., glon., nat-c., ox-ac., sil.

lifting, from - anag., ant-t., bor., **CALC., GRAPH., LYC.,** med., ***nux-v.,*** ph-ac., **RHUS-T.,** ***ruta,*** sang., ***sep.,*** sulph.

lying, while - agar., ***arn.,*** bar-c., bell., ***berb.,*** calc., carb-an., ***chin.,*** coloc., ***cur.,*** daph., dulc., euph., ***ferr.,*** hep., ***ign.,*** kali-c., kali-i., kali-n., ***kreos.,*** lyc., mag-m., mang., naja, nat-m., nicc., ***nux-v., puls., rhus-t.,*** samb., spig., staph., tab., tarax., vib.

abdomen, on, amel. - ***acet-ac.,*** chel., mag-c., ***nit-ac.,*** sel.

amel. - agar., ars., asar., bry., cob., kali-c., ***nat-m., nux-v., phos., ruta.,*** sars., sep., sil.

back, on - am-m., ap-g., apis, bell., berb., bry., carb-an., ***chin.,*** cina, **COLOC.,** cur., euph., euphr., hyos., ign., kali-n., lyc., mag-s., nat-m., ***nit-ac.,*** prun., psor., puls., sep., staph., tell., zinc.

amel. - aesc., ambr., bufo, casc., chin., ***cob.,*** colch., equis., gnaph., ign., ***kali-c.,*** lach., **NAT-M.,** nux-v., ***phos.,*** puls., ***rhus-t.,*** **RUTA.,** sanic., sep., abdomen, on - arg-n., ust.

hard, on something, amel. - am-m., bell., eupi., ***kali-c.,*** lyc., **NAT-M.,** puls., ***rhus-t.,*** sanic., ***sep.,*** stann.

pillow, amel. - ***carb-v.,*** sep.

side, on, agg. - cina, ign., ***nat-s.,*** puls., staph.

PAIN, back

lying, while, side on

amel. - kali-n., nat-c., nux-v., ***puls.,*** zinc.

left, agg. - ph-ac.

must lie on - nat-c.

right, amel. - kali-n., nat-s., ust.

manual, labor, from - arn., bry., calc., rhus-t., ruta, ***sulph.***

masturbation, after - nux-v., ph-ac., staph.

menses, during - acon., agar., aloe, ***am-c., am-m.,*** arg-n., arn., ars., ars-i., bar-c., ***bell., berb.,*** brom., **BRY.,** ***calc., calc-p.,*** calc-s., carb-s., carb-v., caul., **CAUST.,** cham., ***chel., cimic., coc-c.,*** croc., crot-h., eupi., ferr., ferr-ar., ferr-i., ferr-p., ***graph.,*** ham., ***hell., hydr., ign., iod.,*** kali-ar., ***kali-c.,*** kali-n., ***kali-p.,*** kali-s., ***kalm.,*** kreos., ***lac-c.,*** lac-d., ***lach.,*** lachn., ***lob., lyc.,*** mag-c., ***mag-m.,*** mag-s., nat-c., nat-p., nicc., ***nit-ac., nux-m.,*** nux-v., ol-an., ***phos.,*** plat., phys., prun., podo., ***puls.,*** rat., rhus-t., ***sabin.,*** sang., ***sars.,*** seneg., sec., sep., ***sil.,*** **SULPH.,** tarent., ***thuj.,*** vib., xan., zinc., zing.

after - berb., bor., calc-p., kali-c., mag-c., puls., verat.

amel. - senec.

as if, would come on - apis, calc., calc-p., cocc., mosch., ***vib.***

before - acon., am-c., asar., bar-c., ***berb.,*** bor., brom., ***calc.,*** carb-an., ***caust.,*** cinnb., cocc., dig., eupi., ***gels., hydr.,*** hyos., hyper., **KALI-C.,** ***kali-n., kreos., lach., lyc., mag-c.,*** mag-m., nit-ac., ***nux-m., nux-v.,*** ol-an., phos., plat., ***podo.,*** **PULS.,** ruta., sang., ***spong., ust., vib.,*** zinc.

on appearance of - acon., aloe, ***asar.,*** berb., caust., nit-ac.

suppressed - **AESC.,** am-c., apis, ***bell., cocc.,*** graph., ***kali-c., nux-m.,*** nux-v., podo., **PULS.,** sang., ***sep., sil.***

mental exertion - cham., con., nat-c.

midnight, after - mag-s.

before midnight - kalm.

waking him - ***chin-s.,*** nat-c.

morning - ***agar.,*** all-s., aur., berb., bor., bry., calc-p., canth., caust., cimic., cinnb., dios., dros., equis., eug., euph., eupi., hep., ign., kali-c., mag-s., naja, ***nux-v.,*** phyt., podo., puls., ***ran-b.,*** rhod., ruta., stront-c., sulph., thuj., zinc.

bed, in - ang., berb., carb-v., euph., hep., kali-n., mag-s., nat-m., nit-ac., ***petr.,*** puls., rat., rhod., ***ruta.,*** staph.

rising, on - am-m., calad., caust., cedr., graph., ***hep., lyc., nat-m.,*** nit-ac., ran-b., stann., sulph., thuj., verat.

amel. - ***lach.,*** nat-c., nat-m., nit-ac.

waking, on - aeth., ***agar.,*** arg-m., berb., calc-p., cham., chel., grat., kali-bi., lac-c., ***lach.,*** mag-m., mag-s., myric., nat-m., nit-ac., ptel., ran-b.

PAIN, back

motion, on - acon., **AESC.,** **AGAR.,** aloe, alum., am-c., ang., ***ant-t., arn.,*** asar., **BELL.,** brom., **BRY.,** bufo, calc., calc-p., calc-s., caps., carb-s., ***carb-v., caust.,*** cham., ***chel., chin.,*** cimic., cinnb., ***cocc.,*** **COLCH.,** ***coloc., croc.,*** cupr-s., ***dig.,*** dios., equis., eupi., ferr., ferr-p., ***guai., graph.,*** ign., iris, ***kali-bi., kali-c.,*** kali-i., ***kalm.,*** lach., **LED.,** lob., lyc., mang., meph., ***merc.,*** mez., mur-ac., naja, ***nat-c.,*** nat-p., nat-s., nit-ac., **NUX-V.,** ox-ac., paraf., ***petr.,*** phel., ***phos., phyt., pic-ac.,*** plan., podo., ***psor.,*** ptel., puls., ran-a., ***ran-b., rhus-t.,*** ruta., samb., ***sars.,*** sep., sil., stann., stram., **SULPH.,** sul-ac., ***tarent.,*** tell., ***zinc.***

amel. - aesc., aloe, alum., am-c., ***am-m.,*** arg-m., arg-n., bell., bry., calc-f., calc-p., caust., cina, ***cob.,*** coloc., cupr., dios., **DULC.,** ferr-m., fl-ac., graph., ***helon., kali-c.,*** kali-m., kali-n., kali-p., ***kali-s.,*** kreos., lach., laur., **LYC.,** mag-c., mag-m., mang., merc., nat-a., nat-c., ***nat-s.,*** nux-m., ox-ac., ***ph-ac.,*** phos., ***puls.,*** rad., rat., ***rhod.,*** **RHUS-T.,** samb., ***sep.,*** sin-n., ***spig.,*** staph., stront-c., sulph., tab., ust., vib., zinc-m.

beginning - lac-c., ***rhus-t.***

gentle by, amel. - bell., ***calc-f.,*** ferr., ***kali-p.,*** **PULS.**

move, beginning to - bry., **CAPS.,** ***carb-v.,*** caust., **CON., FERR.,** ***kali-p.,*** **LYC.,** ***phos.,*** **PULS., RHUS-T.,** sep., sil., tab., zinc.

compelled to, no relief - ***lach.,*** **PULS.**

constantly in bed - phos., ***puls.,*** **RHUS-T.**

music, from - ambr.

night - abrot., acon., agar., aloe, ***am-m.,*** ang., apis, arg-m., ***arg-n., ars., berb.,*** bry., calc., calc-s., carb-an., carb-s., carb-v., ***cham.,*** chel., cinnb., ***dulc., ferr-ar., ferr.,*** ferr-i., ferr-p., hell., ***helon.,*** hep., ign., kali-i., kali-n., ***kalm., kreos.,*** lil-t., lyc., ***mag-c.,*** mag-m., mag-s., mang., ***merc.,*** **MERC-C.,** mez., ***naja, nat-a., nat-c., nat-m.,*** nat-p., ***nat-s., nit-ac., nux-v.,*** ph-ac., phos., phys., plb., podo., rhod., sars., senec., ***sil.,*** staph., **SULPH., SYPH.,** tab., visc.

3 a.m - **KALI-C.,** kali-n., nat-c.

driving him out of bed - **KALI-C.**

4 a.m - ***nux-v.,*** ruta.

driving him out of bed - ***nux-v.***

between 11 and 12 p.m., violent headache - ***am-m.***

noise, agg. - ars., **THER.**

running water, of, agg. - ***lyss.***

noon - dios., eupi., rhus-t.

nursing, while - cham., crot-t., puls., **SIL.**

paralytic - ***cocc.,*** kalm., nat-m., ran-s., ***sabin.,*** zinc.

pregnancy, during - ***aesc.,*** kali-c.

paroxysmal - asaf., kalm., lyss., nat-c., pall., phos.

periodical - ***ars., chin-s.,*** kali-s., phos.

perspiration, during - carb-v., **MERC.**

PAIN, back

pressure - acon., aesc., agar., ang., arn., ars., bell., canth., chel., chin-s., cimic., cocc., coloc., ***colch.,*** crot-t., ***hep.,*** lac-c., lach., phos., plat., plb., ruta., sil., sulph., tarent., ther., thuj., verb.

amel. - aur., **BRY.,** camph., carb-ac., cimic., ***dulc.,*** fl-ac., **KALI-C.,** led., mag-m., ***nat-m.,*** ph-ac., plb., ***rhus-t.,*** ruta., **SEP.,** verat., vib.

by end of stick - sep.

pregnancy, during - caust., ***kali-c.***

pressure, pain in remote parts on - sil., tarent.

pulling, agg. - dios.

pulsating - am-c., ars., mez., sil.

puerperal, with debility and sweat - kali-c.

raising, arms, on - ***graph.,*** nat-m., rhus-t., sanic.

thigh, while sitting - agar.

reaching, up - **RHUS-T.**

reading, while - nat-c.

riding, in a carriage - calc., carb-ac., fl-ac., kali-c., lac-c., **NUX-M.,** ***petr.,*** sep., sulph., ust.

horseback, on - **ARN.,** ars.

right - calc., cic., fl-ac., ***sulph.,*** tell.

rising, from sitting (see straightening up) - aesc., **AGAR.,** alum., ant-c., apis, aran., arg-n., ***ars.,*** **BERB.,** bry., ***calc., calc-s.,*** cann-i., ***canth.,*** carb-an., **CAUST.,** con., ferr., ferr-p., iris, ***kali-bi.,*** kali-p., ***led.,*** lyc., **MERC.,** merl., petr., **PHOS.,** ptel., **PULS.,** rhod., **RHUS-T.,** ruta., sep., ***sil., staph.,*** **SULPH.,** tell., thuj., tus-p., tab., ***zinc.***

after amel. - kali-c., ruta, staph.

sitting, from, long, almost impossible - ***aesc., agar.,*** am-c., ***bell., berb., calc., phos.,*** **PULS., RHUS-T.**

stooping, from - ***aesc.,*** agar., am-m., ***berb.,*** bism., chel., ***eupi.,*** kali-bi., lach., ***lyc.,*** med., mur-ac., ***nat-m.,*** ph-ac., ***phos.,*** **PULS.,** ***rhus-t.,*** sars., ***sil., sulph.,*** verat., ***zinc.***

prolonged - ***nat-m.,*** **PULS.**

rubbing, amel. - aeth., kali-n., lach., lil-t., nat-m., nat-s., **PHOS.,** plb., puls., thuj.

sewing, while - iris, sec.

sex, after - cann-i., cob., ferr., kali-c., mag-m., nat-m., **NIT-AC.,** ***sabal.,*** staph.

amel. - zinc.

sexual excesses - ars., calc., carb-v., ***chin.,*** croc., ***nat-m., nat-p.,*** **NUX-V., PH-AC.,** ***phos., puls.,*** sel., ***sep.,*** **STAPH.,** ***sulph.,*** upa.

sitting, while - **AGAR.,** aloe, alum., ambr., am-m., ***ant-t.,*** apis, **ARG-M.,** arg-n., asaf., asar., aspar., bar-c., bell., ***berb.,*** bism., bor., ***bry., calc.,*** calc-f., ***cann-i.,*** carb-an., carb-s., ***carb-v., caust.,*** cham., chin., chin-s., cimx., cist., cob., cocc., coff., con., cycl., dros., dulc., equis., euphr., ferr., ferr-m., ferr-p., fl-ac., helon., hep., hura, hyos., kali-bi., ***kali-c.,*** kali-i., kali-n., kali-p., kali-s., kreos., ***lac-c.,***

PAIN, back

sitting, while - ***lach., led., lyc.,*** mag-c., mag-m., meny., merc., mur-ac., nat-a., nat-c., nat-m., nat-p., ***nat-s., nux-v.,*** ol-an., ox-ac., pall., ***par.,*** phel., ***ph-ac., phos.,*** pic-ac., podo., ***prun., puls., rhod.,*** **RHUS-T.,** ***ruta.,*** sabad., **SEP.,** sil., spong., stann., ***sulph.,*** tab., ter., ***thuj.,*** ust., **VALER., ZINC.**

amel. - ***aesc.,*** aeth., bell., bor., caust., ***colch.,*** mag-c., meny., mur-ac., nux-v., plb., sars., sep., sil., staph.

bent - chel., chin-s., kali-i., laur., nat-c., phos., ran-b., sec., sep., thuj.

has to sit - **KALI-C., SULPH.**

long, after - aloe, asaf., berb., ***calc., cupr-ar., led.,*** lith., ***ph-ac., phos.,*** **PULS.,** ***rhod., rhus-t.,*** thuj., valer.

dyspnea, with - lyc.

erect - **KALI-C.,** lyc., spong., **SULPH.**

sleep, during - ***am-m.,*** ars., kalm., lach., puls., zinc.

on going to - mag-m.

sound, after falling into - ***am-m.,*** kalm., ***lach.***

sneezing, when - arn., arund., ***sulph.***

before - anag.

speaking, when - cocc.

spot - agar., ***alum.,*** caust., chel., chin., kali-bi., ***lach.,*** nit-ac., ox-ac., ph-ac., ***phos.,*** plb., rhus-t., stram., thuj., zinc.

standing, while - ***aesc., agar.,*** agn., asar., bell., berb., ***bry.,*** cann-i., ***calc.,*** caps., cocc., coff., ***con.,*** dios., hep., ign., ind., kali-bi., kali-c., kali-m., kali-p., ***kali-s.,*** lil-t., lith., lyc., meny., merc., mur-ac., nat-m., nit-ac., nux-v., petr., ***ph-ac., phos.,*** phys., plan., plb., podo., puls., rumx., ***ruta.,*** sarcol-ac., ***sep.,*** spong., **SULPH.,** thuj., tus-p., **VALER.,** verat., zinc.

amel. - ***arg-n., bell.,*** calc., caust., mur-ac., sulph., thuj.

erect almost impossible after sitting - ***thuj.***

leaning sideways, while - thuj.

stepping, when (see jarring) - acon., carb-ac., carb-an., sep., spong., ***sulph., ther., thuj.***

false stepping, when - podo., ruta, ***sep., sulph., ther., thuj.***

stool, during - ***aesc.,*** apis, ***ars.,*** caps., carb-an., colch., coloc., cupr., cycl., ***dulc.,*** ferr., ferr-ar., kali-i., ***lyc.,*** manc., nicc., nux-v., phos., ***podo., puls.,*** rheum, squil., stront-c., sulph., tab., zing.

after - aesc., aloe, alum., asaf., berb., caps., colch., dig., dros., ***ferr.,*** mag-m., nat-m., podo., ***puls.,*** rheum, tab.

amel. - ox-ac., nux-v., puls.

before - bapt., cic., kali-n., ***nux-v.,*** petr., puls., verat.

urging to - zing.

stooping, when - ***aesc.,*** **AGAR.,** ***alum.,*** arn., berb., bor., bov., ***bry.,*** bufo, caps., ***carb-v., cham., chel.,*** clem., ***cocc.,*** con., corn., daph., dig., dios., ***dulc.,*** gua., hep., hura, hyos., kali-bi., ***kali-c.,*** kali-n., lyc., mang., meny., nat-m., nux-v., ol-an., par., plb., puls., ***rhus-t.,*** ruta., pic-ac., rhod., sabin., sars., **SEP.,** ***sil.,***

PAIN, back

stooping, when - stront-c., sul-ac., ***sulph.,*** tell., thuj., verat., ***zinc.***

impossible - bor.

prolonged, from - **NAT-M.**

as after - agar., bism., sulph., thuj.

straightening, up the back - aeth., agar., bufo, calc., ***cann-i.,*** carb-ac., chel., ***kali-bi.,*** kali-c., lach., nat-c., ***nat-m.,*** nux-v., ***psor., sep., sulph., thuj.***

amel. - bov., laur.

stretching - calc., mag-c.

struck with a hammer, as if - bell., cic., **SEP.,** stann.

stumbling - sep.

summer, in - lyc.

supper, after - sulph.

swallowing, on - ***caust., kali-c.,*** raph., ***rhus-t.***

talking, prevented - cann-i.

throwing, shoulders backward, amel. - cycl.

thunderstorm, during, agg. - agar., rhod.

turning, when - ***agar.,*** am-m., bov., ***bry.,*** dios., hep., kali-bi., merc., ***nux-v., sanic.,*** sars., sep., sil., thuj., verat.

bed, in, when - acon., am-c., ***bry.,*** calad., hep., ign., kali-bi., kali-n., mag-m., merc., nat-c., ***nux-v., staph.,*** sep., sulph., zinc.

amel. - nat-m.

compels - phos., **RHUS-T.**

must sit up to turn over - bry., kali-p., **NUX-V.**

head agg. - ***caust.,*** lachn., sanic.

suddenly - mag-m.

to left, pain in trapezius - bry.

ulcerative, pain in back - kreos., puls.

unbearable - phos.

urinate, with the desire to - clem., eupi., ***lach.,*** nat-s.

urinating, during - ***ant-c., ip., kali-bi.,*** phos., ***sulph.***

after - caust., ***syph.***

amel. - **LYC.,** med.

before - graph., ***lyc.***

urine, on retaining - arn., con., ***nat-s.,*** rhus-t.

uterine origin, of - cimic., kali-c., sep., visc.

vexation, after - nux-v.

waking, on - abrot., aesc., arg-m., berb., calc-p., chel., hep., ***lach.,*** mag-m., mag-s., myric., ptel., puls., rhod.

walking, while - **AESC.,** ***agar.,*** aloe, alum., am-c., am-m., ***ant-t.,*** arg-n., arn., ***asaf.,*** bapt., bell., bor., ***bry.,*** canth., carb-an., ***caust.,*** cham., ***chel.,*** chin., ***cocc.,*** coff., ***colch.,*** coloc., con., dios., euphr., ferr., ferr-p., grat., hep., hyos., hyper., iris, kali-bi., **KALI-C.,** kali-p., lyc., ***mag-m.,*** meny., mez., mur-ac., nat-a., nat-c., nux-v., ox-ac., paraf., petr., phos., phyt., plat., podo., ***psor.,*** ran-a., **RAN-B.,** rhus-t., ***ruta., sars.,*** sep., spig., spong., stront-c., ***sulph.,*** tab., ***thuj.,*** verat., zinc., zing.

after - alum., ***nat-c., phos.,*** stry.

air, in the open - nit-ac., ter., ***zinc.***

PAIN, back

walking, while, amel. - am-c., ant-c., ap-g., **ARG-M.,** ***arg-n.,*** arn., ars-m., asar., bar-c., ***bell.,*** bry., calc-f., cob., **DULC.,** ferr., gamb., kali-n., kali-s., kreos., mag-s., merc., nat-a., nat-m., ***nux-v., ph-ac.,*** phos., ***puls.,*** **RHUS-T.,** ***ruta., sep.,*** staph., stront-c., tell., thuj., vib., ***zinc.***

bent, compelled to - ***cann-i., kali-c.,*** psor., ***sep., sulph.***

preventing - phos.

slowly amel. - **FERR.,** ***puls.***

wandering - ang., ***berb.,*** chel., cimic., dros., kali-bi., ***kali-s., mag-p.,*** sang., sec., senec., tarent.

warm, bed agg. - lil-t., sulph.

room, agg. - gels., ***kali-s.***

warmth, external, agg. - guai., ***kali-s.,*** puls., sulph.

amel. - calc-f., caust., cinnb., ***nux-v.,*** **RHUS-T.**

weakness, with, before or during vaginal discharge - ***aesc., eupi.,*** graph., ***helon.,*** kali-bi., kreos., mag-s., ***murx.,*** nat-ch., ***nat-m.,*** ovi-g-p., psor., ***stann.***

wrestling - symph.

writing, while - laur., lyc., mur-ac., sep.

continuous, after - lyc., mur-ac., sep.

yawning - calc-p., plat.

PAIN, lumbar - acon., act-sp., **AESC.,** aeth., ***agar.,*** all-c., all-s., aloe, ***alum.,*** ambr., am-c., ***am-m.,*** anag., anan., ang., ant-c., ***apis,*** apoc., **ARG-M.,** ***arg-n., arn.,*** ars., ars-m., arund., asaf., asar., asc-t., aur., aur-m., aur-s., **BAR-C.,** ***bapt.,*** bell., **BERB.,** ***bol.,*** bor., bov., brom., **BRY.,** bufo, cahin., **CALC.,** ***calc-ar.,*** calc-f., ***calc-p.,*** calc-s., camph., cann-i., cann-s., **CANTH.,** caps., ***carb-ac., carb-an., carb-s., carb-v., card-m.,*** carl., ***caul., caust., cham.,*** chel., **CHIN.,** chin-a., chr-ac., ***cimic., cimx.,*** cina, cinnb., cinnam., clem., cob., ***cocc.,*** coc-c., coff., ***colch., coloc., con.,*** cop., cor-r., corn., croc., crot-h., crot-t., cund., cupr., cupr-ar., ***cur.,*** cycl., dig., dios., **DULC.,** ***echi.,*** elaps, **EUP-PER.,** eupi., ***ferr.,*** ferr-ar., ferr-i., ***ferr-p.,*** fl-ac., gamb., ***gels., gins., gnaph.,*** **GRAPH.,** grat., ***guai., ham.,*** hell., ***helon., hep.,*** hura, ***hydr.,*** hydrc., hyos., hyper., ign., ind., iod., ***ip.,*** ipom., iris, jug-c., kali-ar., ***kali-bi., kali-c., kali-i., kali-n., kali-p., kali-s., kalm.,*** kreos., ***lac-c., lac-d., lach.,*** lact., lath., lec., **LED.,** ***lil-t.,*** lob., lyc., lycps., ***lyss.,*** mag-c., ***mag-m., mag-p.,*** mag-s., mang., med., meli., ***meny.,*** merc., merl., ***mez.,*** murx., ***mur-ac.,*** naja, nat-a., ***nat-c., nat-m., nat-p., nat-s.,*** nicc., ***nit-ac.,*** **NUX-M., NUX-V.,** ol-an., ol-j., onos., ***op.,*** osm., ox-ac., petr., ***ph-ac.,*** **PHOS.,** ***phyt., pic-ac., plat.,*** plan., plb., ***podo., psor.,*** ptel., **PULS.,** rad., ran-b., ***ran-s.,*** rat., rham-cal., rheum, ***rhod.,*** **RHUS-T.,** rhus-v., rob., ***ruta., sabal.,*** sabin., samb., sang., sanic., ***sec.,*** sel., senec., **SEP.,** ***sil.,*** sin-n., solid., spira., stann., ***staph.,*** stram., ***stront-c., stry.,*** **SULPH.,** ***sul-ac.,*** sul-i., syph., tarax., tarent., ter., thuj., ***valer.,*** **VARIO.,** verat., vib., ***zinc.,*** zinc-ar.

PAIN, lumbar

affected by everything - kali-c., sep.

afternoon - bry., carb-s., coloc., hyos., kali-n., mag-c., mag-m., naja, nicc., petr., plb., **SEP.**

air, a draft of - nux-v.

cold, in - ***bar-c., nit-ac.,*** sep.

open, in - agar., lyc.

alternating with, headache - aloe, brom.

hemorrhoids - aloe.

pain in thighs - am-c.

pinching in abdomen - kali-n.

ascending, stairs - alum., carb-s.

bending, backward - bar-c., cina, con., kali-c., ***mang.,*** plat., puls., rhus-t., sabin., sel., thuj.

backward, amel. - acon., am-m., fl-ac., hura, puls., sabad., sabin.

forward while sitting - cocc., lac-c., pic-ac., puls.

amel. - caust., chel., psor., puls.

to left - plb.

blowing, nose - dig., calc-p.

breathing - alum., am-c., carb-an., carb-v., coloc., kali-bi., ***kali-c.,*** merc., prun., ***sulph.***

deeply - arn., asar., aur., conv., kali-n., nat-m., phel., sars.

sitting bent, while - dulc.

chill, during - ars., ***calc., nux-v.,*** ph-ac., phos., puls., rhus-t., sep., sil.

before - aesc., ***eup-pur.,*** podo.

chronic tendency - aesc., berb., ***calc-f., rhus-t.,*** sil.

cold, from taking - **DULC.,** ***nit-ac.,*** **RHUS-T.**

coughing, when - acon., ***am-c.,*** arn., bell., bor., bry., calc., ***calc-s.,*** caps., carb-an., ***kali-bi.,*** kali-n., merc., nit-ac., ph-ac., ***puls.,*** sep., sulph.

daytime - agar.

diarrhea, with - bar-c., kali-i.

dinner, after - phos., sulph.

drawing, up the limbs agg. - arg-m.

eating, after - am-m., bry., cina, kali-bi., kali-c., ran-b.

erection, after - mag-m.

evening - alum., ***bar-c.,*** bell., ***coloc.,*** dios., iris, kali-n., lach., mag-c., mag-m., meny., naja, nat-c., ***nat-s.,*** nit-ac., nux-m., pic-ac., ***sep.,*** sin-n., stront-c., **SULPH.,** zing.

7:30 p.m., on waking from a nap - sep.

lying down, after - alum., kalm., mag-m., naja

menstruation, during - kali-n.

exertion - ***agar., calc-p.,*** phys., zinc-ar.

amel. - rad.

extending

abdomen, to - ***berb.,*** bry., cham., kreos., lach., ruta, sulph.

around - **BERB.**

forward, or - coc-c., lil-t., lyc., nat-c., puls., sabin., sep., sulph., vib.

to, over ilium to ovaries and uterus - vib.

arms, to - rhod.

to right upper and left lower - alum.

back, up the - ars., dirc., nat-a., nux-v.

PAIN, lumbar
extending, bladder and groin, to - bell.
body, around the - acon., caust., cham., ***cimic.***
over the whole - mez.
buttocks, to - **KALI-C.,** thuj.
chest - berb., sulph.
left - kali-c.
coccyx, along - carb-v., equis., hura
downward, and upward - ***kali-c.***
worse walking - hep.
downward, worse stooping - staph.
epigastric region, to - sulph.
at night - lyc.
feet, to - ***bor.,*** lyc., lyss., sep., still.
forward, in - ***berb.,*** cham., ***kali-c.,*** kreos., **SABIN.**
genitals, to the - ***carl.,*** dros., erig., sars.
glutei muscles, to and thighs - **KALI-C.**
groins, to - ***bell.,*** phos., sabin., ***sulph.,*** vib.
and down legs - plat.
evening - lact.
menses, during - sulph.
hip, to - ***aesc.,*** am-c., ***am-m., bol.,*** carb-v., gels., kali-bi., ***lach.,*** mosch., ***nux-v.,*** pall., ***sep., sil.***
morning on rising - euphr., thuj.
over the, to umbilical region, better by rubbing - lil-t.
and legs, during menses - nit-ac.
and legs, to the, in afternoon - ars., dios.
hypochondrium, to the, morning on waking - kali-n.
knee, to - plb., psor., ruta., sulph.
legs, down the - agar., ***berb.,*** bor., carl., coloc., dios., ign., **KALI-C.,** lyc., lyss., nat-a., nit-ac., ox-ac., ph-ac., pic-ac., plat., sep., ***sil.,*** stann., stry., tarent.
during stool - agar., grat.
to calves - berb., ph-ac., tep.
worse from motion - pic-ac.
limbs, to, on bending backward and on raising the body - carl.
lung, left, to - sep.
patella, to, and back - tarent.
pectoral muscles and arms, to, after riding - brach.
pelvis, around - sabin., sep., vib.
pelvis, to - aloe, tep.
posterior portion and thighs - **BERB.**
perineum, to the - canth.
pubis, to - mag-c., **SABIN.**
rectum, to - aloe, calc., coc-c., lyc.
sacrum, to - cimic., ***nux-m.***
and thighs - kali-bi.
coccyx - sulph.
scapula, to - sulph.
shoulders, to - ars., indg.
side, toward the right, after rising from bending - ox-ac.
spermatic cords, down the, after emission - sars.
stomach, to - nicc., nit-ac., puls., thuj.
testes, to - abrot., sulph.
on coughing - osm.

PAIN, lumbar
extending,thighs, to - agar., am-m., **BERB.,** carb-ac., coloc., dulc., hep., ***kali-bi., kali-c.,*** kreos., ***lyc.,*** nat-m., nit-ac., nux-v., sep.
posterior portion of - **BERB.**
breath, with every - carb-an., nat-m.
stoolduring - stann.
umbilicus, to - prun., rhus-v.
upward - alum., ars., clem., dirc., kreos., lach., led., nux-v.
like a fan - ***lach.***
sitting, while - meny.
stooping, worse - arn., ***sil.***
uterus, to - elaps, helon., ***nat-m.***
vagina - kreos.
fatigue, as from - aur., hep., kali-c., sep.
flatus, passing amel. - am-m., bar-c., coc-c., kali-c., **LYC.,** ***pic-ac., ruta.***
with obstructed - calc.
flesh, were loose, as if - lyc.
forenoon - jug-c., kali-n., stront-c., sulph.
hemorrhoids, with - aesc., bell., ham., nux-v.
hot, cloth, as if, on fire - ars-i.
iron, as if - act-sp., alumn., cann-i., cann-s., graph.
humiliation, after - nux-v.
injury, after - ***arn., bry., hyper.,*** kali-c., rhus-t., ruta.
jarring - carb-ac., cocc., podo., ***thuj.,*** zinc-ar.
laughing - **CANN-I.,** ***con., phos.,*** plb., tell.
leaning, backward against the chair - hep.
forward - hura, lac-c.
kidney diseases, in - calc-ar., senec., solid., visc.
lifting - ant-t., ***calc., calc-p.,*** hura, med., nit-ac., ***nux-v.,*** ph-ac., rhus-t., sep., ***sang., staph.***
lumbo-sacral, region - **AESC.,** carb-ac., carb-an., carb-s., ***cimic.,*** coloc., helon., lil-t., **ONOS., PULS.,** sil.
coughing, on, agg. - phos.
extending, over ilium ending in cramp in uterus - sep., vib.
to uterus - helon.
lifting, too heavy a weight, as if from, when standing and when walking - phos.
lying, on back amel. - puls.
on side - puls.
morning - carb-s., ign.
night - carb-ac.
stooping - ***aesc.***
turning in bed - sulph.
lying, while - agar., ***arn.,*** **BERB.,** bry., ***calc., carb-an.,*** cham., ign., kali-i., kali-n., mag-m., nux-v., prun., ***puls.,*** **RHUS-T.,** tab., vib.
amel. - bry., ***cob.,*** cop., colch., euon., kali-c., ***nat-m.,*** nux-v., ruta., sars., sep.
abdomen, on amel. - chel., nit-ac., sel.
back, on - bry., carb-an., ***chin., coloc.,*** ign., kali-n., ***lyc.,*** mag-s., nit-ac., prun., **RHUS-T.,** sep., zinc.
amel. - ambr., cob., colch., ***kali-c., nat-m.***

PAIN, lumbar

lying, on something hard amel. - **NAT-M., RHUS-T.**
bent backward amel. - cahin.
down, on - bell., murx.
side, on the, amel. - zinc.
can only, on the right - nat-s.
left agg. - agar., **SULPH.**

masturbation, from - nux-v.

menses, during - acon., agar., aloe, **AM-C.,** ***am-m.,*** arg-m., ***arg-n.,*** ars-i., bar-c., ***bell., berb., brom., bry., calc.,*** calc-s., ***cann-i., carb-an.,*** carb-s., carb-v., carl., caul., ***caust., cham.,*** **CIMIC.,** ***cocc.,*** coc-c., cycl., eupi., ferr., ferr-i., ***ferr-p., graph.,*** ham., ***helon.,*** hyos., ign., iod., ***kali-c.,*** kali-i., kali-n., ***kali-p., kali-s., kalm.,*** kreos., **LACH.,** lachn., lac-ac., ***lyc., mag-c., mag-m.,*** mag-s., mang., nat-c., nat-p., ***nicc., nit-ac.,*** **NUX-M.,** ***nux-v., phos.,*** plat., plb., prun., **PULS.,** rat., sabin., senec., sep., **SULPH.,** sul-ac., ***tarent., thuj.,*** ust., ***xan.,*** zinc., zing.
after - berb., calc-p., kali-n., mag-c., puls., ***sep.,*** ust.
as if would come on - ***apis, calc-p.,*** carb-an.
before - acon., am-c., apis, ***asar.,*** bar-c., berb., brom., ***calc., calc-p.,*** canth., ***caul.,*** caust., cimic., ***ham.,*** hyos., iod., kali-n., ***mag-c.,*** nat-m., ***nit-ac.,*** nux-m., ol-an., phos., puls., sabin., **SEP.,** ***spong., sulph.,*** tril., ust., ***vib.***
beginning, at the - acon., aloe, ***asar.,*** berb., ***caust., kali-s.,*** **LACH.,** mag-c., ***nit-ac., vib.***
preceded by tickling - graph.
instead of - ***spong.***
suppressed - kali-c., ***nux-m.,*** **PULS.**

misstep - carb-ac., cocc., podo., thuj.

morning - alum., ang., arg-n., bor., bufo, ***carb-s.,*** carb-v., chel., ***cimic., colch.,*** dios., ***eup-pur., hep.,*** kali-c., ***kali-p.,*** naja, **NUX-V.,** onos., ***petr.,*** plan., ran-b., sang., senec., staph., stront-c., ***stry.***
bed in - carb-s., cocc., form., hep., ***nux-v.,*** petr., puls., ruta., staph.
bending forward, on - cocc., puls.
to left - mang.
rising from bed, on - arg-n., ***calc.,*** chel., graph., ***kali-c., lyc.,*** nat-m., petr., rat., ***sil.,*** thuj., valer.
after amel. - cocc., form., kali-p., staph.
waking - kali-n., mag-m.

motion, during - acon., **AESC.,** ***agar.,*** alum., ambr., am-c., arg-m., ***arn.,*** asar., **BRY.,** calc., calc-p., canth., caps., ***caust.,*** chel., **CHIN.,** cimic., colch., ***coloc.,*** conv., croc., dulc., ign., iris, kali-bi., kali-c., kali-i., kali-n., kalm., lach., ***lyc.,*** meph., mez., nat-c., ***nat-s.,*** nit-ac., **NUX-V.,** phos., phyt., pic-ac., plan., plb., podo., ***psor.,*** ptel., ***puls., ran-b.,*** **RHUS-T.,** ***sars., sep.,*** stann., **SULPH.,** tep., zinc., ziz.
after, agg. - ***rhus-t.***

PAIN, lumbar

motion, amel. - aesc., agar., alum., am-c., bry., calc., calc-f., cupr., dios., ferr., ***fl-ac.,*** graph., kali-c., kali-n., kali-p., ***kreos.,*** nat-a., nat-s., nux-m., nux-v., ox-ac., ph-ac., phos., podo., puls., rat., ***rhod.,*** **RHUS-T.,** ***ruta., staph.,*** stront-c., vib.
arms - ***kreos.***
beginning of, on, after lying down or sitting - anac., con., dig., glyc., ***rhus-t.***
beginning, on, after lying down - dig.
continued amel. - calc-f., ***rhus-t.***
gentle, amel. - prun.
least - bufo, lyc.
gives retching and cold sweat - lath.
sudden - rumx.

move, compelled to - mag-m.
but no relief - bry., ***puls.***

night - am-c., **AM-M.,** ***ars.,*** bry., ***cham., chin.,*** eupi., ***ferr.,*** ferr-i., fl-ac., kali-n., lac-ac., laur., ***lil-t., lyc.,*** mag-c., mag-m., mag-s., ***nat-s.,*** podo., rhus-t., sars., ***sep., sil.,*** staph., ***sulph.,*** zinc.
1 to 4 a.m. - am-m.
2 a.m. - kali-n.
3 a.m., driving him out - **KALI-C.,** kali-n.
bed, in - **AM-M.,** lil-t., kalm., ***naja,*** puls., zinc.
driving him out - mag-c.
midnight, before - laur., rhus-t.
sleep, during - **AM-M.**
wakes at 4 a.m. - staph.

noon - thuj.

numbness in lower part of with - gnaph.

operations, after - calen., berb.

paralytic - ***cocc.,*** kali-c., kalm., nat-m., ran-s., sabin., sel., sep., sil., verat., zinc.
labor, difficult, after - nux-v.

periodical - ars.

pregnancy, during - aran., ***bell., kali-c.,*** nux-v., puls., rhus-t.

pressure - acon., canth., colch., cycl., plat., plb.
amel. - aesc., arg-m., aur., carb-ac., dig., dulc., fl-ac., led., ***nat-m.,*** ph-ac., plb., ***rhus-t.,*** ruta., sabad., ***sep., vib.***

pulled, down, from, as if - visc.

pulling, agg. - dios.

pulsating - am-c., mez., nux-v.

raising, the thigh, when - aur.

radiating, from - bapt., berb., laur., sep.

raises, with the help of arms - bufo, hydr.

raising the thigh, when - aur.

raw, as if - nat-c.

rheumatic - acon., ***ant-c.,*** **BERB., BRY.,** cact., ***carb-an.,*** **CIMIC.,** ***colch., coloc., dulc., ferr.,*** iod., **NUX-V.,** ***phyt.,*** rhod., **RHUS-T.,** spong., stram., stry., ***sulph.,*** ter.

riding - calc., sep.

right - sil.

rising, amel. - ***cob.,*** ferr., ptel., ***ruta.,*** sulph.

PAIN, lumbar

rising, seat, from a - **AESC.,** agar., am-m., ant-c., ***arg-n.,*** ars., bar-c., **BERB., CALC.,** ***calc-s.,*** canth., carb-an., **CAUST.,** ***cham., cob.,*** cycl., hydr., iris, ***lach., led.,*** merl., nat-m., ***petr.,*** **PHOS.,** ptel., **PULS., RHUS-T.,** sep., ***sil., staph.,*** **SULPH.,** tab., tus-p., ***thuj.,*** verat., zinc.

sitting, after long - am-c., carb-an., thuj.

stooping, after - am-m., berb., chel., kali-bi., ***lyc.,*** mur-ac., nat-m., ph-ac., ***phos.,*** verat.

rubbing, amel. - kali-c., kali-n., nat-s., **PHOS.,** plb., lil-t.

sciatica, in - ***rhus-t.***

sewing - iris, ***lac-c.***

sex - cann-i., cob., nit-ac.

sick feeling, all over, with - solid.

sitting, while - **AGAR.,** ambr., ang., **ARG-M.,** ***arg-n.,*** asaf., asar., aur., bar-c., **BERB.,** bor., ***bry., calc.,*** calc-f., calc-s., canth., carb-an., carb-s., ***carb-v.,*** caust., chin-s., ***cimx., cob.,*** coff., coloc., dig., dulc., hep., hura, hyos., kali-c., kali-i., kali-n., kali-p., kali-s., led., ***lyc.,*** mag-c., mag-m., meli., meny., merc., mur-ac., nat-a., nat-c., ***nat-m.,*** nux-v., ol-an., pall., petr., phel., ph-ac., ***phos., prun., puls., rhod.,*** **RHUS-T.,** ***ruta.,*** sabad., stann., stront-c., ***sulph.,*** sul-ac., tab., ***thuj., zinc.,*** **VALER.**

amel. - aeth., bor., caust., mag-c., meny., ph-ac., plb., sars.

bent, agg. - chin-s., kali-i., ***lac-c.,*** phos.

amel. - chel., ***ran-b.***

down - zinc.

erect - conv., zing.

long, after - ***phos.***

raising thigh, while - agar.

sleep - am-m.

before - nat-m.

on going to - mag-m.

sneezing - arund., ***con., sulph.***

snowstorm, before a - ferr.

spine, lumbar - bell., cact., ***calc., calc-p., chel.,*** kali-i., ***kalm.,*** kreos., plb., psor., sarr., sabin., thuj.

forenoon - bry.

motion, on - lyc.

standing - agar., berb., ***bry.,*** caps., ***carb-an.,*** coff., ***con., kali-c.,*** led., ***lyc.,*** meny., mur-ac., ph-ac., phos., plan., plb., podo., puls., ***ruta.,*** sep., ***sulph.,*** sul-ac., tarax., thuj., tus-p., **VALER.,** verat., zing.

amel. - ***arg-n.,*** kreos., meli.

bent over - sulph.

erect, impossible - agar., ***bry.,*** cocc., ***petr.,*** phos., ***sulph.***

leaning sideways - thuj.

stepping, when - acon., carb-ac., ***carb-an.,*** spong., ***sulph.***

stool, during - agar., ***arg-n., carb-an.,*** coloc., grat., ox-ac., rheum, spong., squil., sulph., tab.

PAIN, lumbar

stool, after - aesc., ***carb-v.,*** colch., dig., dros., lyss., mag-m., nat-m., ***podo.,*** sil., tab.

amel. - ox-ac.

amel. - indg.

before - berb., carb-v., kali-n., nat-c., ***puls.,*** sulph.

hard, during - bry., stront.

soft, during - nicc., ***podo.,*** rheum, tab.

urging at, when - colch., sin-a.

with as if there would be - rat.

stooping - ***aesc., agar.,*** alum., am-c., ang., ars., bor., bry., ***cham., chel.,*** clem., colch., con., cur., cycl., dig., dios., ***dulc., echi.,*** graph., hyos., kali-bi., kali-n., kreos., lac-ac., lyc., mag-m., mang., meny., nat-a., nat-c., nat-m., nux-v., ol-an., petr., plb., puls., rhod., ruta., sabad., sars., ***sil.,*** **SULPH.,** ***thuj.,*** tus-p., verat., zinc.

amel. - chel., meny., ph-ac., puls., sang.

as after long - chin., **DULC.,** graph.

straightening, up - carb-ac., kali-bi., nat-c., nat-m., ***sulph.***

can not, straighten - cob.

stretching, when - ***calc.,*** mag-c.

tickling - kali-c.

touch, on - cimic., lil-t., sil.

turning - **BRY.,** bov., kali-bi., ***nux-v.,*** sars., sil., sulph., thuj., zinc.

bed, in - staph.

almost impossible - bor., **BRY.,** dios., kali-n., ***nux-v., zinc.***

body, when - alum., mag-m., ***nux-v.,*** sars., thuj.

while walking - hep.

ulcerative - cann-s., kreos., nat-s., prun.

upward, from - rad.

urinating, during - phos., sulph., syph.

after, agg. - syph.

amel. - **LYC.,** med., nat-s.

before - graph., ***nat-s.***

frequent, with - sep.

urging, during - nat-s., raph.

vaginal discharge, with - eupi., gels., kali-c., kali-n., syph.

vertebrae, of - kreos., stann., zinc.

dislocated, or, as if - sanic.

gliding over each other, as if - sanic.

vexation, after - nux-v.

waking, on - aesc., aeth., alum., anac., arg-m., arg-n., berb., bry., calc-f., calc-p., ***card-m.,*** chel., colch., equis., erig., ham., hyper., kali-bi., kali-m., kreos., lycps., mag-m., merc., merc-i-f., myric., naja, ox-ac., plan., psor., ptel., puls., ran-b., ***sep.,*** sil., spong., sulph., verat., zinc.

walking, while - **AESC.,** aeth., ***agar.,*** alum., am-c., am-m., arg-m., arn., bor., ***bry.,*** canth., ***carb-an.,*** caust., ***cham.,*** chel., ***cocc.,*** coff., coloc., con., ferr., hep., hyos., ***kali-c., kali-i., kali-s.,*** mag-m., meny., mez., nat-a., nat-c., nit-ac., onos., ol-j., plat., podo., puls., ***ran-b.,*** ran-s., sars., **SEP.,** stront-c., ***sulph., thuj.,***

PAIN, lumbar
walking, while - tus-p., verat., ***zinc.***
after - con., nat-c.
amel. - am-c., ant-c., apoc., **ARG-M.,** ***arg-n.,*** ars-m., asaf., cob., dulc., gamb., kali-n., mag-c., meli., nat-a., phel., ***ph-ac.,*** phos., puls., ***ruta.,*** sabad., **SEP.,** ***staph.,*** sulph., thuj., vib., ***zinc.***
bent compelled to - am-m., kali-c., murx., sep., ***sulph.***
cane, with, pressed across the back amel. - vib.
slowly, amel. - **FERR.,** ***puls.***
uneven ground, on - podo., ***thuj.***
warmth, amel. - ***calc-f.,*** caust., ***rhus-t.***
weight in pelvis, with - gnaph.
wet weather, in - ***calc.,*** **DULC.,** ***ran-b.,*** **RHOD.,** ***rhus-t.***
writing, while - laur.

PAIN, scapula - acon., aesc., aeth., alum., anac., apis, arn., ars., ***aspar.,*** bell., berb., bor., ***calc.,*** calc-p., camph., ***carb-v.,*** caust., cham., **CHEL.,** ***chin.,*** chin-a., ***cimic.,*** cic., cina, cocc., ***coloc.,*** con., cor-r., cund., ***dig.,*** elaps, graph., hell., hep., ***hydr.,*** kali-ar., ***kali-c.,*** ***kali-chl.,*** kali-p., kalm., ***kreos.,*** lach., laur., lil-t., led., lob., lyc., meny., merc., merc-i-f., ***mez.,*** naja, nat-a., nat-c., nat-m., nit-ac., ***nux-v.,*** ph-ac., ***phyt.,*** plb., sang., seneg., ***sep.,*** sil., spong., sulph., ***ran-b.,*** ran-s., rhod., rhus-t., rumx., ruta, ***tarent.,*** **TELL.,** tep., ***valer.,*** verat-v., vesp., zinc.
adherent - ran-b.
air, on blowing - caust., hep.
angle, of - iod.
inferior - alumn., apis, arn., calc., chel., kali-bi., led., rhus-t., sulph.
inferior, breathing, while - alumn., chel., clem.
inferior, motion amel. - alumn.
inferior, raising shoulders, when - rhus-t.
superior - kali-bi.
belching amel. - zinc.
bending arm - carb-v.
body backward- aur., sep.
breathing, when - ***aesc.,*** alumn., am-m., calc., sang.
hindering, breathing - calc., cann-s., kali-n., ***puls.,*** sulph.
chill, during - chin., rhus-t., **SEP.**
colic, with - am-c.
coughing, when - cor-r., sulph.
evening - chel., lyc., nat-p., ran-b.
extending, arm, to - aeth., coc-c.
back, whole - verat.
chest, to - bar-c., kali-c., sars., sep.
clavicle, to - mag-m.
epigastrium - bry.
forward, from - bar-c., phos., sulph.
forward, from, left - mez., phos., ran-b.
forward, from, right - merc.
heart - bry., sulph.
shoulders, to, and face - valer.
sternum, to - ***chel.***

PAIN, scapula
extending, stomach, to - bor.
gasping on - berb.
hang down, arm - ign.
inspiration, on - dulc., ferr-m., sep.
left - agar., aloe, ambr., anac., am-m., asaf., ***cact.,*** carb-v., card-m., cimic., colch., coloc., con., cund., dig., ***gels.,*** graph., hell., led., lil-t., mang., merc-c., nat-p., phos., phyt., ptel., sang., ***squil.,*** sulph., thuj., zinc-chr.
bending head back, on - sanic.
border of - brom.
edge of, worse on breathing - ***sang.***
inner angle of left - aphis., chel., chr-ac., ***ran-b.,*** sanic.
motion, on - hell.
riding - agar.
then right - cund.
left, under - ail., ***aphis.,*** arund., bry., ***cact.,*** ***cench.,*** chen-v., ***cimic.,*** corn., ***crot-h.,*** cund., cupr-ar., daph., dol., **GELS.,** hydr., ***ind.,*** ***kreos.,*** ***lac-c.,*** ***lach.,*** led., med., ***merc.,*** ***naja,*** ***ox-ac.,*** par., phyt., ***psor.,*** sabin., sang., seneg., ***sep.,*** sulph., tarent., thuj., xan., zinc.
cough, during - ***stict.***
expiration agg. - sep.
lying with the shoulder on something hard amel. - agar., kreos.
motion - kreos., ***psor.***
pressure amel. - kreos.
rheumatic - alumn.
riding in a carriage - kreos., phyt.
riding in a carriage, evening - phyt.
sitting, worse in evening - seneg., sulph.
margin, lower - seneg.
spinal - alumn.
morning - **CHEL.,** kali-p., ***mez.,*** nat-m., nat-s.
4 a.m. - ***chel.***
moving - calc., cina, hell., mez., naja, petr.
amel. - am-m., sabin.
arm - chel., ign.
head - cupr., merc., nat-s.
neck - ant-t.
nursing, when - crot-t.
pressure, agg. - ***chin.,*** sil.
amel. - ol-an.
raising, arm to head impossible - lyc.
rheumatic - aesc., alumn., ambr., asaf., ***bry.,*** calc., carb-v., chin-s., colch., ferr-m., graph., hyos., lyc., mag-s., ***mez.,*** ***ran-b.,*** rhod., ***rhus-t.,*** valer.
right - ***aesc.,*** ***ail.,*** ***all-c.,*** ambr., anac., arn., cahin., **CHEL.,** **COLOC.,** con., cund., Jug-c., ***kali-c.,*** lyc., lob., plb., ran-b., ***sep.,*** sulph., tell., zinc.
bending forward agg. - lob.
bending shoulders backward amel. - conv.
breathing, on - ***aesc.,*** ***chel.,*** kali-c.
edge of, near spine - alumn., ***card-m.,*** ***chel.,*** nat-c.
extending to shoulder - ***chel.***

PAIN, scapula
right, lying, while - ***all-c.***
motion of arm - ail., con., ruta
motion of arm, of right - ***chel.***
moving, when - calc., petr.
pulsating - merc-i-f.
sitting bent double, as if from - anac.
stooping - jug-c.
then left - kali-p., tell.
ulcer, like from an - cic.
waking, on, 4 a.m. - ***chel.***
right, under - ***abies-c.,*** aesc., ***all-c.,*** bad., bry., ***card-m.,*** **CHEL., CHEN-A.,** con., conv., cupr., ind., jug-c., kali-c., lac-c., ***lycps.,*** malar., med., nat-m., nux-v., phos., phys., ***podo., pic-ac.,*** rhod., ***ruta, senec.,*** vario.
bending, forward - ***lob.***
coughing, when - seneg.
sitting, after - ***all-c.***
throwing, shoulders back - bad.
sitting, while - ant-c., ind., mang.
stooping - cham., sulph.
swallowing - caust., kali-c., rhus-t.
turning, body to left - am-m.
walking, while - asaf., coloc., ***kali-p.,*** nat-s., nit-ac.
writing, when - carb-v.
continued, after - mur-ac.
pain, under, scapula - apis, asaf., brom., **CALC.,** ***calc-p.,*** card-m., cimic., con., ***elat.,*** fl-ac., hell., kali-bi., kali-n., lyc., mez., nat-s., nit-ac., ***puls., ran-b.,*** rhus-t., rumx., stann., ***sulph.,*** verat.
afternoon - cedr.
arms agg. - con.
chill, during - sang.
left - crat., gels.
morning - apis
moving, agg. - apis, hell., stann.
neuralgic - ter.
night, at - kali-bi.
rest, during - con., sabin.
right - chel., coloc., podo.
sewing - ran-b.
sitting, while - psor.
under, right, hot - lycpr.
writing - ran-b.

PAIN, spine - acon., aesc., ***aeth.,*** **AGAR.,** ***ang.,*** aran., ***arn.,*** ars., aur., aur-s., ***bell., berb.,*** benz-ac., brach., cact., camph., ***caps.,*** carb-v., ***caust.,*** **CHEL.,** chin., chin-a., **CIMIC.,** ***cina,*** cinnb., cob., ***cocc.,*** colch., coloc., ***con., crot-c.,*** cur., cycl., daph., dios., elaps, ***gels.,*** glon., hura, hyper., ign., iodof., jatr., kali-a., kali-bi., ***kali-p., kalm.,*** lac-ac., ***lach.,*** lact., led., lycps., mag-c., mag-m., mang., med., meph., ***merc.,*** morph., mosch., mur-ac., ***naja,*** **NAT-M.,** nit-ac., ***nux-m., nux-v.,*** oena., ol-j., olnd., par., ***petr., ph-ac.,*** **PHOS.,** plb., ran-b., **RUTA., SIL.,** spig., spong., staph., sulph., sul-ac., stry., tanac., tarent., ***tell.,*** ther., thuj., upa., valer., vario., verat., xan., **ZINC.**
afternoon - stront.
bending backward - ***calc., chel.,*** dios., mang., peti.

PAIN, spine
breathing deeply - ***chel.,*** led., ***ruta.***
convulsions, after - acon.
cough, during - **BELL.**
dinner, after - ***agar.,*** cob.
eating, after - ***agar., kali-c.***
evening in bed - kali-bi., mag-m.
extending, down - **BERB.,** cur., cycl., glon., mang., nat-m., phys., ust.
coccyx to occiput, from drawing head backward - ***phos.***
epigastrium, to - nicc., rat., thuj.
lower extremities, to - agar.
occiput, to - petr., ***phos.,*** plb.
on stooping - sulph.
up and down - gels., phyt.
up spine - agar., caust., mag-m., nux-v., petr., phos., sulph.
fall, as from - ruta.
jarring agg. - acon., **BELL., GRAPH.,** podo., ***sulph., ther., thuj.***
lying, down, on - ***nat-m.***
on back - ***nat-m.***
midnight, after - ant-s.
morning - aur., euphr.
rising, after - sulph.
waking, on - euphr.
motion on - ***agar.,*** meph., ***merc.***
amel. - euphr., ***ph-ac.***
night, with weakness of extremities - arg-n.
noise agg. - ars.
pressure, agg. - agar., arn., bell., ***chin.,*** kali-c., ***phys.,*** sep., **SIL.,** ther.
amel. - verat.
pulsating - ***lach.***
relieving the headache - kali-p.
sex, after - nit-ac.
shock, as from a, on riding in a carriage - petr., ***ther.***
sitting, while - helon., ***ph-ac., ruta.,*** spong., ***zinc.***
amel. - mur-ac.
spots - agar.
standing, while - nit-ac., ***ph-ac.,*** zinc.
amel. - mur-ac.
stimulants - ***zinc.***
stool, during - ***phos.***
stooping, while - ***agar.,*** zinc.
swallowing, while - caust., kali-c.
walking, on - ***mur-ac.,*** par., ***ruta.,*** sep., stront-c., verat.
amel. - gels., hydr., ***ph-ac.***

PAIN, thoracic - aesc., ***agar.,*** am-c., ***alumn.,*** apis, arg-m., asaf., aur., aur-m., ***bell.,*** berb., brom., ***bry.,*** calc., calc-ar., ***calc-p.,*** cann-i., ***cimic.,*** cocc., coloc., daph., dios., ferr-i., guai., hura, ***hyper.,*** ind., iodof., ***kali-c.,*** kali-p., ***kali-s., kalm.,*** lach., led., lil-t., lob., lyc., ***merc., naja,*** nat-c., ***nat-m.,*** nat-p., ***nat-s.,*** onos., petr., ***ph-ac., phos.,*** pic-ac., psor., ***ran-b.,*** rhus-t., ruta, sang., seneg., ***sep.,*** stann., staph., stram., **SULPH.,** verat., ***zinc.***
bending, backwards - aur.
forward - **CIMIC.**
breathing, hindering - apis, berb., ***bry.,*** phys., psor., sulph., thuj.

PAIN, thoracic
chill, during - ***chin-s.,*** sang.
clothing, tight - sep.
coughing - calc., caps., ***kali-bi.,*** merc., sil., stram.
extending to, arms and legs - ***calc.***
to, left nipple - ***asaf.***
to, occiput - ***cocc.,*** ind., ***kalm.,*** petr.
to, sternum - ***kali-bi.,*** laur.
to, stomach - bry., rhod.
to, stomach, on pressure - bell.
inspiration, on - bry., ***chel.,*** mur-ac.
labor, during - petr.
morning - sep.
motion, on - agar., bry., cupr-ar., psor., zinc.
of head - agar., sang.
night - zinc.
rheumatic - **CIMIC.,** ***dulc., rhus-t.,*** ruta
riding, while - fl-ac., ind.
sitting down, while - ***arg-m.,*** bry., fl-ac., kali-c., mang., ph-ac., ***phos.,*** tub.
sitting down, on - hura, lach.
stepping hard agg. - seneg.
turning head, on - ***bry.,*** ind.
walking, while - ***agar.,*** bell., coloc., nat-c., ***psor.,*** seneg., ***sulph.***

pain, thoracic, middle of - ***acon.,*** aesc., ***agar.,*** alum., ***am-c.,*** am-m., ambr., anac., ***ang.,*** apom., arg-n., arn., **ARS.,** arum-t., asc-t., bar-c., ***bell.,*** berb., bol., bov., ***bry.,*** calad., **CALC.,** calc-p., ***calc-s.,*** camph., cann-i., canth., caps., carb-an., carb-s., carb-v., caust., ***chel., chin.,*** chin-a., ***cimic.,*** cob., coc-c., colch., coloc., com., ***con.,*** crot-t., cupr., cur., ***dros.,*** echi., elaps, eupi., ***eup-per., ferr., ferr-ar.,*** ferr-p., glon., ***graph.,*** gua., ***guai.,*** hell., helon., ***hep.,*** hura, hyper., ind., ip., jug-c., ***kali-ar., kali-bi.,*** kali-br., kali-c., kali-n., ***kali-p.,*** kali-s., ***kalm., kreos.,*** lac-c., ***lach.,*** lap-a., laur., led., lil-t., lob., lyc., mag-m., mag-s., meny., med., merc., mur-ac., ***naja, nat-a.,*** nat-c., nat-m., nat-p., **NAT-S.,** nit-ac., ***nux-m., nux-v.,*** **NIT-AC.,** ox-ac., ***par.,*** petr., ***ph-ac., phos., plb., podo.,*** psor., ***puls.,*** rad., ran-b., rhod., ***rhus-t., rhus-v.,*** ruta, seneg., **SEP.,** ***sil.,*** sol-n., stann., stict., ***sulph.,*** syph., tab., tell., ter., ther., thlaspi, ***thuj., verat., zinc.,*** zinc-m.
afternoon - alum., canth., caust., chel., ruta.
air, open - nat-c.
beer, agg. - phos.
bending, backward - stann.
backward, amel. - sil.
forward - lac-c.
forward, amel. - nat-a.
breathing - berb., ***guai.,*** nit-ac., nux-v., prun., ***puls.,*** stann.
chill, during - sang.
cold air - rhus-t.
cold damp weather - ***nux-m.***
cough, during - calc., stram., sul-ac.
eating, after - ***arg-n.***
evening - bell., cocc., kali-n., lac-c., lyc., nat-a., sulph., thuj.
expiration, during - raph., sep.

pain, thoracic, middle of
extending to, back of neck - stict.
to, down arms - echi.
to, downward - ***verat.***
to, loins - ox-ac.
to, lumbar region - dros.
to, over head into temples - ***kalm.***
to, sacrum - ***zinc.***
to, shoulders - ***kalm.,*** valer.
to, shoulders, and face - valer.
to, sternum - ***kali-bi.,*** lac-c.
inspiration, during - nat-a., puls.
lifting - stann.
lying - nat-m.
amel. - ars.
back, on - kali-n.
left side agg. - ph-ac.
right side amel. - kali-n.
menses, during - ***am-c.,*** sil.
midnight, after - mag-s.
morning - nat-c., podo., **RAN-B.,** staph.
on waking - aeth., arg-n., kali-bi., ran-b.
moving, on - bry., ***calc.,*** colch., dros., ip., kali-bi., nux-v., ox-ac., petr., podo., puls., rhod., sil., stann., sulph.
amel. - kali-c., laur., ph-ac., sulph.
arms - colch., naja, sil.
head - nux-v.
night - podo., rhus-t., sil., tab.
paralytic - nat-c.
pulsating - merc-i-f., ***phos.***
rheumatic - aspar., calad., dros., lob., lycps., mag-s., ***rhus-t., rhus-v.,*** sil., staph., verat.
rising, after stooping - puls.
up, on - carb-v.
sitting, while - bell., bry., calc-caust., nat-m.
bent - bov.
standing, while - rumx.
stool, before - verat.
stooping, while - bor., cham., nux-v., prun.
as after prolonged - puls.
straightening up amel. - bov.
swallowing, on - ***rhus-t.***
turning, on - calad., merc., verat.
walking, while - bell., coloc., seneg.
amel. - bry., ferr., puls.
warmth, amel. - mag-p., ***rhus-t.***
wine agg. - ph-ac.

pain, spine, thoracic - ail., **ALUM.,** am-c., arn., asaf., ***calc., chel.,*** cina, cinnb., com., crot-t., gins., hell., ***kalm.,*** lob., mez., ***naja,*** nat-m., **NAT-S.,** ***nux-m., nux-v.,*** par., ***ph-ac., phos.,*** psor., ***ruta.,*** sabin., seneg., ***sep.,*** **SIL.,** stann., ***thuj., verat.,*** zinc.
between scapula and - ran-b.
deep inhalation - alum.
fall, as from a - ***ruta.***
motion - cocc.
sitting - ***ph-ac.***
stoop, compelling to - **CANN-I.**
touch, to - calc.

PARALYSIS, muscles of back, ***cupr., gels., led.***

paralysis, spine - **AESC.,** xan.
sensation of, muscles - **AESC.**

PARALYTIC, pain - cocc., kali-p., nat-m., sil., xan.

PERSPIRATION - acon., **ANAC.,** ars., ***calc.,*** calc-s., camph., casc., caust., **CHIN., CHIN-S.,** coff., dig., ***dulc.,*** guai., hep., hyos., ip., kali-bi., lac-c., lach., laur., ***led., lyc.,*** morph., ***mur-ac.,*** nat-c., nat-p., nit-ac., **NUX-V.,** par., ***petr., ph-ac., phos., puls., rhus-t.,*** sabin., **SEP.,** sil., stann., stram., ***sulph.***
chill, during - cann-s.
cold - acon., chin., colch., cub., ph-ac., ***sep.***
during and after coughing - cub.
daytime, while at rest - petr.
eating, after - card-m., par.
emissions, after - sil.
evening - mur-ac.
menses, during - ***kreos.***
before - ***nit-ac.***
morning - chim.
motion, on - **CHIN.**
night - anac., ars., calc., coc-c., coff., guai., lyc., ***sep.,*** sil.
3 a.m - **RHUS-T.**
after midnight - **HEP.**
woke him at 4 a.m - petr.
sleep, during - tab.
stool, during, effort at - ***kali-bi.***
waking, on - hep.
walking, on - ***caust.,*** lac-ac., lach., nat-c., petr., phos., ***rhus-t., sep.***
rapidly - nit-ac.

perspiration, lumbar - asaf., clem., hyos., naja, **SIL.**
cold - plan.
menses, before - ***nit-ac.***
night - sil.

POLYPS - calc., ***con.,*** thuj.

POTT'S disease, (see Tuberculosis)

PRESSING, pain - acon., ***aesc.,*** aeth., ***agar.,*** ambr., am-c., anac., ant-c., apis, arg-n., arn., aur., aur-m., **BELL.,** benz-ac., berb., bor., calc., calc-s., caps., carb-an., carb-s., carb-v., card-m., caust., ***chel.,*** cocc., colch., con., cycl., ***dulc.,*** elaps, euph., euphr., graph., hep., hyper., ***kali-c.,*** kali-n., kali-p., lach., led., lyc., mag-m., merc., ***mur-ac.,*** nat-m., nat-s., nit-ac., ***nux-m., nux-v.,*** ol-an., pall., petr., ***phos.,*** plat., ***psor.,*** puls., rhod., sabin., ***samb.,*** sars., seneg., ***sep.,*** sil., spong., ***stann.,*** staph., sulph., tarax., tell., ***thuj.,*** ust., verat., ***zinc.***
chill, with - sil.
extending, downwards - nit-ac.
to shoulders - chel.
forenoon, pressing - nat-m.
hemorrhoids, before protusion alum.
left - mur-ac., nat-m.
lying agg. - kali-n.
on a pillow amel. - ***carb-v.***
menses, during - agar., ***nux-m.,*** phys.
before - nux-m., podo.
morning - petr., verat.

PRESSING, pain
morning, in bed, amel. after rising - nat-m.
on waking - nit-ac.
motion, on - ***zinc.***
plug-like sensation - anac., ***carb-v.,*** lach., plat.
pulsating - sil.
right - lyc.
rising, from stooping - verat.
sitting, while - am-m., bor., cocc., kali-n., puls., thuj.
amel. - mur-ac.
bent, better erect - chel.
spots - thuj.
standing, while - nit-ac., puls.
amel. - mur-ac.
stool, during, difficult - ***puls.***
stooping - bor., sars., verat.
swallowing - nit-ac.
upwards - puls.
vise, as in a - aeth., am-m.
walking, while - bor., ***caust.,*** mur-ac., ***psor.***
air, in open - kali-c.
amel. - kali-n., puls.
weight, as from a - anac.

pressing, lumbar - acon., aeth., agar., all-c., ambr., anag., ang., arg-m., arn., ars., asaf., aur., ***bell.,*** berb., bor., bry., ***calc.,*** calc-p., calc-s., ***camph.,*** canth., ***carb-an.,*** carb-s., ***carb-v.,*** **CAUST.,** chel., clem., cocc., coc-c., coloc., con., cycl., elaps, euph., graph., ***kali-c., kali-i.,*** kali-n., lach., ***led., lyc.,*** mag-m., merl., mez., ***mur-ac.,*** nat-m., ***nit-ac., nux-v.,*** ol-an., osm., ph-ac., ***phos., plat., plb.,*** **PSOR., PULS.,** ran-s., rat., ***rhus-t.,*** ruta., **SABIN.,** samb., sep., sil., ***spong.,*** stann., ***stront-c.,*** **SULPH.,** tarax., thuj., ***zinc.***
air, open - lyc.
bending body backward - rhus-t.
coughing agg. - kali-n.
eating, while - bry.
evening - meny., puls., zinc.
extending to, below the short ribs - **LYC.**
bladder and groins - bell.
coccyx - carb-v.
feet - bor.
groin - **SULPH.**
hips - lyc.
lower limbs - berb.
testes on coughing - osm.
upward - clem.
flatus, obstructed from - coc-c., ***kali-c.,*** **LYC.**
inward - am-m.
menses, during - am-m., ***carb-an.,*** carb-v., ***ferr-p., kali-c., lach.,*** plat., plb., **PULS., SULPH.**
as if, would come on - ***apis, calc-p.***
morning - kali-c.
bed, in - cocc.
bending to left - mang.
rising, after, amel. - cocc., form., staph.
motion, during - mez., **PSOR.**
night, 4 a.m., wakens - staph.
outward - am-m.
paralytic - cocc., zinc.

pressing, lumbar
plug, like a, puts pillow under - ***carb-v.***
position, from lying in wrong - zinc.
pressure agg. - cycl.
rising, from sitting - zinc.
from stooping - chel.
sitting - ang., bor., carb-v., caust., coloc., meny., mur-ac., puls., **RHUS-T.,** sulph.
sleep, before - nat-m.
standing - mur-ac., ph-ac., puls., rhus-t., samb., tarax., verat.
bent over - sulph.
erect impossible - caust.
stepping - acon.
stool, during - spong.
after - dig.
before - berb., ***carb-v.***
hard, during - bry.
stooping - bor., chel., clem., cycl., meny., sabin., sulph., thuj.
thumb, as by a - meny.
turning body - bor.
urinating, before - graph.
vertebra, fourth lumbar - puls.
vise, as if in a - ***kali-i.,*** zinc.
walking - kali-n.
after - puls.
amel. - am-c., kali-n., puls., rhus-t., sulph.
weight, as from - chin.
yawning - am-m.

pressing, scapula - anac., arg-n., arn., aur-m-n., bell., bry., ***calc.,*** camph., caust., chel., chin., ***cocc.,*** cor-r., elaps, graph., ind., kali-c., kalm., lach., laur., led., lyc., mez., nat-m., nat-s., nit-ac., nux-v., phyt., ran-s., rhus-t., ruta., seneg., sep., sil., tell., zinc.
bending backward, upper arm and head - caust.
extending, to clavicle - mag-m.
to lumbar region - bor.
to sacrum - coc-c.
to small of back when riding - kali-c.
to sternum - ***chel.***
to stomach - bor.
inferior border - ant-c., mur-ac., plat.
inner edge - anac.
left, as from a plug - phos.
morning - sil.
in bed - nat-m., nat-s.
motion, agg. - caust., mag-m.
moving, arm agg. - camph., mag-m.
pressure, amel. - mag-m.
right - bism., bor., ***chel.,*** lyss., mag-m., ruta.
outer margin - plat.
sitting, while - ind.
turning head to left - caust.

pressing, scapula, under - anac., apis, brom., **CALC.,** card-m., chel., con., ind., lyc., lyss., nat-c., nat-s., phos., rhus-t., stann., sulph., zinc.
angle of - ruta.
and inner side - anac.
left - anac., bell., ind., nat-c., zinc.
moving arm - con.

pressing, scapula, under
right - con., cupr., nat-m., sep., staph., zinc.
sitting - sep.

pressing, spine - benz-ac., led., phos., samb., sep., spong.
fist, lower part of, as from a - lyc.
inspiring - led.
plug, as from a, middle of spine - plat.
pressure amel. - verat.
sitting amel. - mur-ac.
erect, while - spong.
standing, while, amel. - mur-ac.
thoracic - ail., asaf., **BELL.,** gins., mur-ac., sabin., sep., zinc.
on inspiration - mur-ac.
walking, while - mur-ac., verat.

pressing, thoracic - asar., con., kali-c., mur-ac., sep., zinc.
flatus, as from - zinc.
inspiration agg. - mur-ac.

pressing, thoracic, middle of - am-c., ant-s., ***arn.,*** **BELL.,** bry., **CALC.,** carb-an., carb-v., ***chin., cocc.,*** coc-c., crot-t., elaps, graph., hura, indg., kali-bi., kali-br., kali-c., lach., laur., led., lob., lyss., ***nux-v.,*** petr., psor., seneg., sep., sil., stann., ter., thuj.
menses, during - am-c.
morning, on waking - anac., arg-n.
motion, on - ***calc.,*** stann.
moving arm - carb-an., sil.
obstructing respiration - **CALC.**
rheumatic - sil.
rising, on - carb-v.
sitting - bell., bry.
stooping, as if plug were forced inward - prun.
waking - sil., thuj.
walking - coc-c.
amel. - bry.

PRICKLING - acon., aesc., apis, aur., aur-m., ox-ac., ran-s., sol-t-ae., verat.
in back - acon., aesc., lact., ox-ac., ran-s.
sleep, during - sol-t-ae.

prickling, scapula - ***mez.***

PSORIASIS, patches - calc., kali-ar., ***mez.***

PULSATING - agar., aloe, arg-n., ars., asc-t., **BAR-C.,** bell., berb., calc-ar., calc-p., cann-i., cann-s., carb-s., chin., cimic., cur., daph., ***eup-per.,*** ferr., ferr-ar., glon., iod., ***kali-c.,*** lac-c., ***lach.,*** lyc., **NAT-M.,** ***nit-ac., phos.,*** puls., sep., ***sil.,*** sumb., ***thuj.***
alternating with pains in back - ***kali-c.***
coughing, agg. - ***nit-ac.***
emotional, excitement, after - bar-c.
evening - tab.
express an idea, when wishing to - raph.
motion, during - phos.
amel. - bar-c.
sitting, while - calc-p., cur., thuj.
stool, after - alum., caps.

pulsating, lumbar - am-c., **BAR-C.**, ***bry.***, cann-s., ***caust.***, cimic., colch., ***coloc.***, graph., hura, kali-c., lach., **LAC-C.**, ***nat-m.***, ***nit-ac.***, ruta., **SEP.**, **SIL.**, sulph., sumb., thuj., vib.
alternating with pain - kali-c.
chill, during - nux-v.
evening, after lying down - nat-m.
fever - hura.
hips, above - ***coloc.***
inspiration, on deep - benz.
menses, before - ***nit-ac.***
motion, amel. - am-c., bar-c.
night - ars.
pressure amel. - ruta.
sitting - colch.
stool, after - alum.

pulsating, scapula - bar-c., calc-p., kali-c., merc., ph-ac., phos., zinc.
rising from stooping - kali-n.

pulsating, scapula, under left - zinc.
right - merc-i-f.

pulsating, spine - agar., bar-c., carb-s., cur., **LACH.**, thuj.

pulsating, thoracic - calc-p., carb-s., cur., phos.
thoracic, middle of - ***bar-c.***, hura, kali-i., merc-i-f., ***phos.***, plan., sumb., ter.
spine - dulc., ***lach.***, **PHOS.**

RASH - ***calc.***, con., merc., mez., psor., stram., tab.
rash, lumbar - cham.
rash, thoracic, middle of - caust.

RESTLESSNESS, lumbar - ***bar-c.***, ***calc-f.***, cedr., chin-s.
passing flatus. amel. - ***bar-c.***

RHEUMATIC, pain - acon., ambr., anac., ant-t., ***ars.***, asar., aspar., aur., bar-c., bapt., bell., **BRY.**, ***calc.***, ***calc-p.***, calen., ***carb-v.***, cham., ***chel.***, **CIMIC.**, ***colch.***, com., ***corn.***, cycl., dros., ***dulc.***, ***ferr.***, graph., ***guai.***, ***hep.***, iod., ***kali-bi.***, ***kali-i.***, lach., lyc., ***lycps.***, mez., ***med.***, **NUX-V.**, ol-an., petr., ***phyt.***, ***puls.***, ran-b., **RHOD.**, **RHUS-T.**, ***ruta.***, ***sang.***, squil., stram., ***sulph.***, teucr., ust., valer., verat., zinc.
pregnancy, during - acon., alet., ***cimic.***, op., rhus-t.

rheumatic, lumbar - acon., ***ant-c.***, **BERB.**, **BRY.**, cact., ***carb-an.***, **CIMIC.**, ***colch.***, ***coloc.***, ***dulc.***, ***ferr.***, iod., **NUX-V.**, ***phyt.***, rhod., **RHUS-T.**, spong., stram., stry., ***sulph.***, ter.

rheumatic, scapula - aesc., alumn., ambr., asaf., ***bry.***, calc., carb-v., chin-s., colch., ferr-m., graph., hyos., lyc., mag-s., ***mez.***, ***ran-b.***, rhod., ***rhus-t.***, valer.

SENSITIVE, between vertebra - agar., ther.
sensitive, lumbar, hot sponge, to - ***agar.***
skin, of - mag-m., squil.
left to touch - zinc.

SHARP, pain - acon., **AGAR.**, ail., all-c., all-s., aesc., aloe, ***alum.***, alumn., ambr., am-c., am-m., anac., apis, arg-m., arg-n., arn., arund., asaf., asar., asc-t., aur., aur-m., bar-c., ***bell.***, **BERB.**, bor., brom., ***bov.***, **BRY.**, ***calc.***, calc-ar., calc-s., calad., cann-s., carb-an., carb-s., carb-v., **CAUST.**

SHARP, pain - ***cham.***, chel., ***chin.***, ***cimic.***, cinnb., cocc., ***colch.***, coloc., com., ***con.***, corn., cycl., ***dulc.***, dig., dros., elat., eug., euon., ferr., ferr-i., ferr-p., form., gamb., graph., ***guai.***, hell., ***hep.***, hura, hyos., hyper., ***ign.***, iod., ***kali-bi.***, **KALI-C.**, kali-i., kali-n., ***kali-p.***, **KALI-S.**, kalm., ***kreos.***, ***lach.***, laur., **LYC.**, led., lob-s., lyss., mag-c., mag-m., ***mag-p.***, manc., mang., meph., ***merc.***, merc-i-f., ***mez.***, ***mur-ac.***, ***nat-c.***, nat-m., nat-p., nicc., **NIT-AC.**, ***nux-v.***, olnd., paeon., ***par.***, phos., ***phyt.***, ***plat.***, plb., psor., ***puls.***, rat., ***rhus-t.***, sabad., sabin., ***sanic.***, ***sars.***, sec., ***sep.***, ***sil.***, ***spig.***, spong., ***stann.***, staph., stram., stront-c., ***sulph.***, sul-ac., tarax., tell., **THUJ.**, verb., verat., ***zinc.***
afternoon - lyc., nicc., plb., stry.
ascending, stairs - alum.
bending, forward while sitting - pic-ac.
breathing - am-m., arn., berb., ***calc.***, lyc., ***merc.***, nat-m., nat-p., psor., ***sulph.***
burning - plat.
cold, exposure, to while sweating - ***dulc.***
coughing - ***acon.***, **BRY.**, ***caps.***, chin., kali-bi., kali-c., ***merc.***, nit-ac., puls., ***sep.***
cramp-like - cina, lyc., mag-c.
daytime - agar., nicc.
digging - stann.
downward - paeon.
drinking, when - chin.
eating, while - chin.
evening - bor., cham., lach., nat-c., rhus-t., stront.
extending, outward - stann.
to arms and legs - calc-ar.
to chest - bor., ***kali-c.***, mez., nat-c., sars.
to head - kalm., petr., sep.
to head, on every step - sep.
to head, stool, during - ***phos.***
to hypochondrium, on lying or coughing, amel. by standing or sitting - cinch.
to knees - arn.
to left side, while walking - spig.
to middle or left upper arm - nat-m.
to pit of stomach, while sitting - nicc.
to ribs - alum.
to sacrum - lyc.
to scapula - lyc., ***puls.***
to shoulder, right - alum.
to sternum, into - laur.
to vertex - rhus-t.
forenoon - cham.
herpes zoster, after - ***lach.***
inspiring, when - acon., alum., arn., calc., cham., mez., nat-c., sars., sulph.
itching - mang., spig., sulph.
leaning back - kali-p.
left - mur-ac., plat., stann.
lifting, on - ph-ac., rhus-t., ***sep.***
after - ***bor.***
lying, while - ***kali-c.***, tarax.
on abdomen - ***arg-n.***, tarax.
on back - kali-p., stann.
menses, during - ars.

SHARP, pain
morning - bor., bry., nat-p.
in bed on bending forward - puls.
rising amel. - nat-c.
motion - am-m., **BRY.,** colch., dig., lach., lyc., meph., nit-ac., phel., phos., ***rhus-t., sars.***
amel. - ***dulc.,*** kali-i., mur-ac., staph.
of head - acon.
night - apis, ars., bry., dulc., nat-c., nit-ac., phos., puls.
3 a.m., must get up and walk - **KALI-C.**
paroxysmal - lyc.
pulsating - chin., dulc., kali-c.
right - plat., stann.
rising from, a seat - canth., rhus-t.
stooping - mur-ac., ***rhus-t.***
rubbing - mang.
sitting, while - ambr., ang., asar., caust., ***chin.,*** dulc., kali-i., kali-n., lyc., mur-ac., nat-c., nicc., par., ph-ac., ruta., ***zinc.***
sneezing - arund.
standing - con., zinc.
amel. - calc.
stinging - ***apis,*** cham., chlor., rumx., sulph., ***zinc.***
stool, during - ***coloc.,*** nicc., ***phos.***
stooping, on - caj., ***rhus-t.,*** sabin., verat., zinc.
striking foot - ***sep.***
stubbing toe - ***sep.***
touch - calc., merc., mur-ac.
turning the body - bov., ***nux-v.,*** sars., sep.
upward - staph.
walking - arn., calc., canth., chel., kali-p., ran-b., rhus-t., sulph., thuj., zinc.
amel. - ***kali-c.***
warmth of bed amel. - rhus-v.

sharp, lumbar - **ACON.,** aeth., **AGAR.,** all-c., aloe, ***alum.,*** ambr., am-c., am-m., ***anac.,*** ant-s., ***arg-m.,*** arn., arund., ***asaf.,*** aspar., ***aur.,*** aur-m., ***bar-c., bell.,*** **BERB.,** bor., bov., **BRY.,** ***calc.,*** calc-ar., calc-caust., ***calc-p.,*** calc-s., cann-i., canth., caps., carb-an., carb-s., carb-v., ***caust.,*** cham., ***chel.,*** chin., cina, clem., ***cocc., coc-c., colch., coloc., con.,*** cupr., cycl., dios., dig., dulc., elat., euph., eupi., form., gamb., graph., hep., hyos., ***hyper.,*** ign., indg., iod., jatr., jug-c., ***kali-bi.,*** **KALI-C.,** ***kali-i.,*** kali-n., kali-p., kalm., kreos., lac-ac., ***lach.,*** laur., ***led., lil-t., lyc.,*** mag-c., ***mag-m., mag-p., merc.,*** mosch., ***nat-c., nat-m.,*** nat-p., ***nicc., nit-ac., nux-v.,*** ol-an., par., ***ph-ac., phos., plat., plb., prun., puls., ran-b.,*** rat., ruta., sars., ***sec., sep., sil.,*** spig., spong., staph., stram., ***stront-c., stry.,*** **SULPH.,** tarent., tarax., ***thuj.,*** til., verat., ***zinc.,*** zing.
afternoon - coloc., mag-c., nicc., plb.
ascending stairs - alum.
bending, forward while sitting - pic-ac.
to left - plb.
between ribs and ilium - caust.
breathing, on - ammc., arg-m., carb-an., dulc., ***merc.,*** prun.
deeply - arn., cycl., kali-n., nat-m., phel.

sharp, lumbar
breathing, expiration, on - spig., ***sulph.***
inspiration - alum., aur., ***coloc.,*** cycl., spig.
inspiration, while sitting bent - dulc.
burning - mag-c.
coughing - ***acon.,*** am-c., arn., bell., bor., ***bry.,*** caps., merc., ***nit-ac.,*** puls., pyrog., sep., sulph.
crawling - lyc.
dinner, after - zinc.
eating, after - kali-bi., ***ran-b.***
evening - kali-n., lach., nat-c., pic-ac., stront-c., zinc.
evening, in bed - alum.
extending to, abdomen - kali-c., puls., ***ran-b.***
to, along spine in zig-zags to scapular region - euon.
to, axilla - canth.
to, buttocks, 3 a.m. - **KALI-C.**
to, chest - kali-c., zinc.
to, downward - aloe, ***kali-c.***
to, extremities - ***ign., kali-c.***
to, gluteal regions and hips - **KALI-C.**
to, groin when walking - coloc.
to, groin when walking, right - ran-b.
to, knee - psor.
to, legs, down - eupi., ***kali-bi.,*** ox-ac., ***sil.,*** stry.
to, liver - ***lach.***
to, lung - sep.
to, outward around abdomen - **BERB.**
to, penis - dros.
to, pit of stomach - nicc., rat., thuj.
to, pubis and inguinal, region - carl., kreos.
to, rectum - lyc.
to, ribs - caust.
to, stomach - nicc.
to, thighs, into - ***kali-bi., kali-c.,*** nit-ac., ***nux-v.***
to, thighs, into, on every breath - carb-an., nat-m.
to, toes - eupi.
to, umbilicus - prun.
to, urethra - lach.
to, uterus - ***nat-m.***
to, vagina - kreos.
flatulence, from - sil.
hips, above - caust., thuj.
intermittent - zinc.
itching - mag-c.
jerking - ph-ac.
laughing, when - plb.
left - lyc.
lifting, on - nit-ac., ph-ac., sep.
lying - sil.
down amel. - ruta.
on back - ***coloc.,*** prun.
on face amel. - chel.
on right side agg. - sep.
menses, before - ***nat-m.***
morning - bor., kali-n.
3 a.m. - **KALI-C.**
in bed, on bending forward - puls.

sharp, lumbar
morning, rising - chel.
motion, on - ambr., arg-m., chel., **COLOC.,** dig., ***kali-bi.,*** kalm., lach., meph., mez., nat-c., ptel.
amel. - asaf., ***dulc.,*** ox-ac., ph-ac., ***staph.***
night - ars., bor., bry., laur., rhus-t.
before midnight - laur., rhus-t.
pressure amel. - arg-m., aur., dulc., ***kali-c.,*** mag-m., plb., ruta.
radiating - **BERB.**
raising thigh while sitting - agar.
rib, last - ***caust.,*** merc.
right - sep.
rising from, a seat - canth.
squatting - ph-ac.
stooping - ***lyc.,*** mur-ac.
rubbing, amel. - plb.
sitting - ambr., ang., arg-m., asar., bar-c., dig., dulc., euphr., kali-i., kali-n., lyc., ***nat-c.,*** ph-ac., ruta., sil., spig., stann., ***zinc.***
amel. - bor., plb.
sneezing - arund.
standing - ***con.,*** plb., zinc.
and leaning sideways - thuj.
stepping - sulph.
stinging - ***aur-m.***
stool, during - coloc., nicc.
amel. - indg.
stooping - bor., caj., lac-ac., puls., ruta., sabin., verat.
touch, on - calc.
amel. - cycl.
turning body - bov., nux-v., sars.
in bed - bor.
walking - arn., bor., canth., chel., coloc., ferr., ***merc., ran-b.,*** ran-s., ruta., sulph., thuj., ***zinc.***
amel. - asaf., ***dulc.,*** gamb., ***kali-c., staph.***
erect impossible - arg-m., ***kali-c.,*** sep.

sharp, scapula - agar., alum., alumn., ambr., am-c., am-m., **ANAC.,** ang., ***bar-c., bell.,*** berb., ***bov., bry., calc., camph.,*** cann-s., ***carb-an.,*** carb-s., ***caust.,*** cham., chin., ***cocc.,*** coc-c., colch., ***coloc.,*** cycl., ***dulc.,*** ferr., ferr-m., graph., ***guai.,*** hep., hyos., hyper., iod., ***kali-bi., kali-c.,*** kali-n., kalm., kreos., lach., lact., laur., lyc., manc., med., meny., merc., merc-i-f., ***mur-ac., nat-c.,*** nat-m., **NIT-AC.,** nux-v., op., ox-ac., paeon., ***par., phos., plb.,*** prun., puls., ***ran-b.,*** samb., ***sars.,*** seneg., ***sep.,*** sil., spig., spong., ***stann.,*** stram., ***sulph.,*** tab., tarax., tarent., ***thuj.,*** verb., ***zinc.***
afternoon - mez., sep., thuj.
air, open, agg. - seneg.
angle of - ruta.
inferior - apoc., chin-s., kali-bi., kali-n., lach., mur-ac., sulph.
bending backward amel. - lach.
breathing, deep - kali-n.
extending through chest - chel.
morning - sulph.
sitting long - lach.

sharp, scapula
belching agg. - zinc.
bending the arm - carb-v.
when leaning on it - sulph.
blowing nose, on - hep.
breathing, deep - hep., nat-m.
coughing, on - med.
cramp-like - ant-c.
evening - canth., kali-n., sep.
extending, to breast - grat.
to chest - bar-c., camph., kali-c., sars., sep.
to heart - thuj.
to occiput - ***grat., guai.,*** **PETR.**
to ribs - asaf.
hawking - caust., hep.
inspiration, on - dulc., ferr-ma., mill., sep.
left - ambr., am-m., **ANAC.,** bar-c., calc., graph., grat., kali-c., meny., mill., sep., spig., ***sulph.,*** zinc.
border of - dulc., zinc.
breathing or coughing - dulc., sep.
extending, to shoulder and breast - grat.
extending, to throat - zinc.
rest, during - am-m., ***kalm.,*** manc., ***sep.,*** verb.
resting, on left arm - sulph.
left, under - anac., carb-s., cupr., kali-bi., lac-ac., mez., nat-c., nat-m., ***sulph.,*** tarent.
brething deep - kali-n.
coughing, during - sulph.
drawing scapula toghter - nat-m.
through to heart - ***bry.,*** staph.
lifting - iod.
lowering the shoulder, on - am-m.
lying, on scapula impossible - nit-ac.
manual labour - ferr.
menses, during - phos.
morning - calc., hyper., ran-b.
9 a.m. - calc.
walking, while - ran-b.
motion, on - kali-c., mez., sulph., tarent.
amel. - am-m., samb.
arms, of - camph.
night - kali-bi., puls., ***sulph.***
in bed - nat-m., ***sulph.***
pressure amel. - sep.
respiration, on - acon., guai.
right - am-m., ***asaf.,*** bar-c., ***kali-c.,*** merc., nit-ac., phos., samb., ***sep., sil.,*** spig., spong., tarax.
coughing - sep.
dinner, after - nat-c.
extending, down back - sep.
extending, through chest - kali-c., ***merc.***
extending, to last false rib - sep.
extending, to left - cocc.
inner angle - samb.
inner margin - guai.
inspiring, when - am-m., **CHEL.,** kali-c., sars., sep.
walking in open air amel. - sep.

sharp, scapula
right, under - aur., ***bad.,*** **CHEL.,** coloc., ***guai.,*** kali-c., kali-bi., kali-n., samb., thuj., zinc.
agg. by throwing shoulders back - ***bad.***
breathing, deep agg. - ***guai.***
breathing, inspiring, on - coloc.
pulsating - samb.
sitting - samb.
sitting - ant-c., colch., sep.
speaking loud - caust.
stooping, on - sulph.
swallowing, when - caust.
turning body to left - am-m.
walking - coloc., nit-ac.
fast - sep.
slowly amel. - sep.

sharp, scapula, under - agar., all-s., aloe, arum-t., asar., aur., bad., bism., bry., calc., cann-s., canth., **CHEL.,** cimic., corn., cupr., guai., ***jug-c.,*** kali-bi., kali-c., kali-n., ***kreos.,*** lach., lyc., mez., nat-c., nat-m., olnd., par., ***phos.,*** pic-ac., plb., stann., **SULPH.,** tarent., thuj., zinc., zing.
afternoon, 3 p.m. - kreos.
breathing, deep - plb.
inspiration - cupr., guai.
left - anac., cupr.
motion, on - tarent.
amel. - olnd.
sitting, while - samb.
stooping, when - asaf.
agg. - sulph.
upper part - stann.

sharp, spine - **AGAR.,** ***bell.,*** **BERB.,** bor., caps., chin., ***cocc.,*** dulc., elaps, ***hyper.,*** ign., kali-bi., led., meph., mez., ***nit-ac.,*** olnd., ***petr., phos.,*** rat., sul-ac., tanac.
breathing - dulc.
inspiration - led.
evening - mag-c., mez.
extending, down small of back to region of bladder - **BERB.**
to anterior superior spinous process of left ilium - dros.
upwards - cocc., ***petr.***
jerking - ph-ac.
morning, on waking - euphr.
motion, on - meph.
moving about amel. - euphr.
pulsating - dulc.
sitting - ruta.
standing - nit-ac.
thoracic - **AGAR.,** ang., arg-m., crot-h., dig., euon., hura, merc., **PETR.,** raph., ruta., sabin., stann.
extending to sternum - kali-bi., **LAC-C.**

sharp, thoracic - ***agar.,*** arg-m., ***asaf.,*** bor., ***bry., cact.,*** calc., ***colch.,*** dros., fl-ac., kali-bi., kali-c., kali-p., ***lach.,*** nat-s., **PETR.,** rat., sabad., sabin., stann., ***zinc.***
breathing, arresting - berb., ***sulph.***
deeply, on - alum., aur., carb-an., kali-n., psor., sabin., spig., ***sulph.***
burning - stann.

sharp, thoracic
coughing - caps., **MERC.**
evening - mez.
extending to, arms - ***calc.***
to, occiput - ***cocc.,*** kali-c.
to, occiput, during labor - **PETR.**
to, pit of stomach - rhod.
to, ribs - ***asaf.***
inspiration, on - calc.
labour, during - petr.
lying amel. - ***psor.***
motion, amel. - mez.
stooping - arg-m., ***cocc.***
walking - ***asaf., cocc.,*** psor.

sharp, thoracic, middle of - acon., aeth., ***agar.,*** aloe, alum., alumn., ang., arg-m., asaf., asc-t., ***berb.,*** bov., ***bry., calc., camph.,*** cann-s., carb-an., carb-v., carl., cham., chel., chin., ***cocc., coc-c., colch.,*** coloc., con., cop., cupr., dig., dulc., ferr., guai., hep., hura, hyper., indg., kali-c., kali-n., kreos., **LAC-C.,** lach., laur., lyc., mag-m., mag-s., mang., mez., mill., nat-a., nat-c., **NIT-AC.,** nux-v., ol-an., ***par.,*** **PETR.,** plb., psor., prun., ***puls., ran-b.,*** ruta., sars., ***seneg.,*** sep., sil., stann., tab., thuj., verat.
afternoon - bov.
belching, during - sep.
before - nit-ac.
breathing, when - acon., berb., caps., carb-v., cop., ***guai.,*** kali-c., nit-ac., nux-v., prun., psor., puls., stann.
deep - acon., nat-a., prun.
dinner after - indg., phel.
evening - sulph.
in bed - thuj.
extending to stomach - bry.
inspiration - berb., nat-a., nat-c.
lacing corsets, on - laur.
lying, while - bry.
on back while - ***kali-n.***
morning - psor., ran-b.
motion, on - ang., arn., canth., ip., nux-v., ***puls.,*** stann., verat.
amel. - calc., mag-m., mez., nicc.
of trunk - bry.
night - carb-v.
in bed - ang.
outward - calc.
sitting, while - kali-c., thuj.
amel. - cann-s., chel.
sleep, waking from - kali-n.
standing, while - nicc.
stooping, while - nit-ac.
straightening up amel. - ***bov.***
turning around - verat.
walk, bent, must - coloc.
walking, agg. - coloc.

SHIVERING - acon., agar., all-c., anac., apis, ars., bell., bry., bar-ac., bor., calc., caps., carb-v., carl., cast., cham., clem., cocc., coff., ***colch.,*** crot-t., dig., eup-per., gamb., ***gels.,*** guai., ign., kali-bi., lach., lyc., mag-c., mang., meny., ***mez.,*** nat-m., nicc., osm., phos., puls., rumx., rhus-t., ruta., sabad., sang., sec., seneg., sep., spong., ***stann.,***

SHIVERING - staph., stram., stront-c., ***sulph.,*** verat.
afternoon - carb-an., guai., mag-c.
evening - apis, bry., canth., caps., cham., cocc., mag-m., mag-s., nat-m., verat.
bed, in - sang.
extending, down the back - agar., all-c., bry., calc-caust., chel., ***colch.,*** mag-c., rhus-v.
up the back - canth., carb-an., dig., puls., rhus-v.
forenoon - graph., mag-c.
lying down, on - nat-c.
morning - apis, cham., meny., staph.
bed, in - kali-c.
rising, after - staph.
night - carb-v.
bed, in - raph.
stool, during - coloc., trom.
warm, room - petr.
stove amel. - nicc.
shivering, lumbar - coff-t., jatr., lyc., petr.
stool, after - ***puls.***
warm room - petr.

SHOCKS, electric like, spine, along - agar., ang., cic., corn.
flank, left - stann.
shocks, left side of back - plat.
shocks, lumbar region - plat.
shocks, thoracic - bell., cic.
middle of - bell.
left - anac.

SOFTENING, spinal cord, of - alum., alum-sil., arg-n., ***aur-m.,*** bar-m., carb-s., crot-h., **KALI-P.,** merc., naja, ox-ac., ***phos.,*** phys., pic-ac., plb., ***sulph.,*** zinc.
amyotrophic lateral sclerosis, with - ***arg-n.,*** cupr., hyper., lath., plb.
multiple sclerosis, with (see Nerves) - ***arg-n., atro., aur.,*** bar-c., bell., calc., caust., chel., ***crot-h.,*** gels., ***lath.,*** lyc., nux-v., ox-ac., ***phos., phys., plb.,*** sil., ***stry.,*** sulph., tarent., thuj.

SOLID, as if, sacrum - sep.

SORE, pain - ***acon.,*** aesc., ***agar.,*** **ALUM.,** alumn., am-m., anac., ang., ant-t., ***apis,*** **ARN.,** ***ars.,*** ars-i., asar., bar-c., ***berb.,*** bry., ***calc.,*** calc-s., camph., carb-ac., carb-s., carb-v., caust., ***cham.,*** chin., cic., ***cina,*** cinnb., clem., coc-c., coloc., ***con.,*** conv., corn., cor-r., dig., ***dros.,*** dulc., **EUP-PER.,** gins., graph., grat., ***ham.,*** hep., hyos., kali-ar., **KALI-C.,** kali-n., kali-p., kali-s., lyss., mag-c., ***mag-m.,*** mag-s., ***merc.,*** myric., nat-a., ***nat-c.,*** **NAT-M.,** nat-p., ***nat-s., nux-m.,*** **NUX-V.,** ox-ac., ph-ac., **PHOS.,** ***phyt.,*** **PLAT.,** ***psor., puls.,*** rat., ***ran-b., rhod., rhus-t.,*** **RUTA.,** sabad., ***sang.,*** sil., sol-n., ***spig., stann.,*** stram., stront-c., **SULPH.,** sul-ac., tell., tep., ther., ***thuj.,*** verat., vib., ***zinc.***
air, in open - ***merc.***
chill, during - cham.
evening - psor.
evening after lying down - nat-c.
extending, to, abdomen - nat-c.

SORE, pain
extending, to, nape of neck extending to, sacrum - gins.
to, shoulders to loins on waking - ox-ac.
to, small of back and abdomen - caust.
left - petr., plat.
lying, while - hep., nat-m., ***puls.***
amel. - asar.
on side - ign.
on side, amel. - nat-s.
on the back, when - am-m., bry., hyos.
menses, during - ***mag-m.,*** phos., ***thuj.***
as if in the bones, during - carb-v.
before, worse at night - ***berb.***
midnight, waking from sleep - nat-c.
morning - ***dros.,*** ox-ac.
bed, in - nat-m.
motion amel. - am-m.
rising, on - am-m., calad., nat-m., stann., thuj.
rising, on, after amel. - nat-m., ***rat.***
waking, on - arg-m., grat., mag-m., mag-s.
motion, on - chel., chin., merc., ran-b., stram.
amel. - ***am-m.,*** **KALI-C.,** mag-c., rat.
night - ***am-m.,*** cham., mag-c., mag-m., ***nat-c.***
3 to 4 a.m., agg. - **NUX-V.**
in bed, amel. by motion - mag-c.
pregnancy, during - lyss.
pressure, on - sulph.
amel. - vib.
rising after sitting - apis, ***psor.,*** **SULPH.**
after long stooping - ***nat-m.***
shivering, during - **ARN.**
sitting, while - ***calc.,*** hep., hyos., nat-m., ph-ac., plat., ***ruta.,*** sabad.
standing, while - asar., ***calc.,*** hep., thuj.
stooping, while - cham., lec., stront.
turning the body - thuj.
waking, after - mag-s.
walking, while - hyos., ***ruta.***
amel. - ***puls.,*** thuj.
in open air - merc., ***zinc.***
sore, lumbar - acon., aesc., **AGAR.,** ***alum.,*** am-c., ***am-m.,*** ang., ant-ox., apoc., arg-m., ***arg-n.,*** **ARN.,** ***ars.,*** **AUR.,** aur-m., bar-c., bell., **BERB.,** brom., **BRY.,** calad., calc., ***calc-p., caps., carb-ac.,*** carb-s., ***caust., cham., chel.,*** **CHIN.,** ***cimic., cimx., cina,*** cinnb., clem., cocc., coc-c., ***colch., coloc.,*** conv., corn., cor-r., cupr-ar., cur., **DULC., EUP-PER.,** ***ferr.,*** ferr-ar., gamb., ***graph.,*** grat., hell., ***hep.,*** hura, hydrc., indg., jatr., kali-br., kali-i., ***kali-n.,*** lac-c., lact., lept., ***lil-t.,*** lob., lyc., ***mag-m.,*** mag-s., med., ***meny., merc., naja,*** nat-c., ***nat-m., nat-s., nux-m.,*** **NUX-V.,** ox-ac., phos., phys., pic-ac., ***plat.,*** plb., ptel., ***ran-s.,*** **RHOD., RHUS-T.,** ***ruta., sil.,*** stann., staph., stry., sul-i., **SULPH.,** ***sul-ac., tab., thuj.***
afternoon - cob., mag-c., plb., ***sulph.***
after pain - sang.
bending backward - nux-v., plat.
blowing nose - dig.
breathing deeply agg. - conv., sang.

sore, lumbar
chilbirth, during - ***caust.***
cold, from taking - **DULC.**
evening - caust., cob., ***coloc.,*** kali-n., mag-c., meny., sars., stront-c., ***sulph.***
extending, to abdomen - bar-c., nat-c.
to lower limbs - berb., hep.
to thighs - lyc.
forenoon - nat-c.
hips, above - ars., dulc., staph.
kidneys, over - apis, berb., helon., merc-c., phyt., solid.
leaning against chair - plb.
left - zinc.
lying, while - agar., berb., ***bry.,*** cham., puls., **RHUS-T.**
on back - am-m., ***ars., bry.,*** ign., ***rhus-t.***
on side, agg. - am-m.
on side, right amel. - nat-s.
menses, during - am-c., bar-c., carb-v., caust., ***cimic.,*** kali-i., mag-c., mag-m., mag-s., thuj.
after - mag-c.
before - mag-c., spong.
morning - alum., ***arg-m.,*** calc-p., colch., dios., sil.
3 a.m. - ***nux-v.***
bed, in - ***agar.,*** aur., ***nux-v., ruta.***
rising, on - ***calc-p.,*** kali-c., ***nat-m.,*** rat., ***stry.,*** thuj., valer.
rising, on, amel. - aur., nat-s., staph.
until 2 p.m, evening - nat-s.
until 2 p.m. - mag-c.
waking, on - kali-n.
motion, amel. - aur., bry., rat., **RHOD., RHUS-T.,** ***ruta.***
motion, on - arg-m., bufo, ***calc.,*** **CHIN.,** conv., dig., eup-per., nux-v., sul-ac., verat.
on beginning, after lying down - dig.
night - **AM-M.,** ***naja,*** **SIL.,** staph., **SULPH.**
2 a.m. - ***nat-s.***
3 a.m. - kali-n.
pressure, agg. - plat., sulph.
amel. - verat.
rib, last - **RAN-B.,** ph-ac.
rising agg. - ferr., sulph., thuj., verat.
from stooping - nat-m., ***sulph.,*** verat.
sitting, while - agar., berb., bry., kali-c., mag-c., mag-s., meny., merc., nat-m., phel., **RHUS-T.,** stront-c., sul-ac.
amel. - caust.
bent - ***kali-i.***
erect - conv.
sleep, on awaking from - berb.
spine - agar., ***arg-n.,*** bar-c., bell., ***chel.,*** colch., ***graph., lil-t.,*** lyc., mag-m., med., ***phos.,*** pic-ac., ***plat.,*** tab., **THUJ.**
leaning against chair, when - plb.
lumbo-sacral region - nat-p.
menses agg. - thuj.
stepping, when - berb., ***carb-an.,*** **THUJ.**
standing, while - agar., mag-s., ruta, sul-ac., thuj., zinc., zing.
stepping - berb., ***carb-an., thuj.***

sore, lumbar
stool, after - nat-m.
stooping, on - alum., aur-m., cham., graph., lec., ***meny.,*** nat-m., nux-v., ***sil., sulph., thuj., verat.***
touch agg. - graph., kali-c., phos., sep.
amel. - meny.
turning, when - alum., sil., ***thuj.***
vaginal discharge, with - caust., kali-n.
vertebra, last - acon., aesc., cham., ***nat-s., plat.***
walking, while - alum., caust., hep., hyos., kali-c., ***meny., thuj.,*** zinc., zing.
after short walk - grat.
amel. - apoc., aur., bry., mag-c, mag-s., phel., puls., ruta., thuj.
slowly amel. - ***puls.***
wet weather - **RHOD., RHUS-T.**

sore, scapula, in - anac., ant-t., ***arn.,*** ars., bar-c., berb., calc-p., chel., con., dios., graph., hell., kali-c., ***kreos.,*** lyc., merc., merc-i-f., nat-m., nux-v., phos., ran-b., sil., spong., thuj., verat., vesp., zinc.
extending down the back - chel.
lain, on - graph.
left - card-m., coloc., phyt.
edge, inner - ran-b.
morning in bed - con., nat-m.
motion, on - chin., cocc., kali-c.
amel. - coloc.
right arm, of - caust.
right - ars., caust., ***cic.,*** chel.
outer margin - plat.
spot, in - berb., chel.
tip, of - cimx.
turning body - con.
head - caust., merc.
head to right - caust.
yawning, when - nat-s.

sore, scapula, under - cist., cund., led., nat-a., nat-c., ol-j., sul-i., thuj.
burning, between paroxysms of - plb.
morning - ox-ac.
wheezing, with - ars.

sore, spine - aesc., **AGAR.,** ***ang.,*** ant-c., apis, ***arn.,*** ars., ***atro.,*** bapt., **BELL.,** ***benz-ac.,*** berb., ***calc., carb-ac.,*** caust., ***chel., chin.,*** chin-a., **CHIN-S.,** ***cimic., cocc., crot-c.,*** crot-h., ***cupr., dios.,*** eup-per., gels., ***glon.,*** **GRAPH.,** ***hep.,*** hyper., iod., iodof., ***kali-ar., kali-c.,*** kali-i., **KALI-P.,** ***lac-c.,*** **LACH.,** ***lec.,*** lil-t., **LYSS.,** mag-m., ***med.,*** merc-i-r., ***naja, nat-a., nat-c.,*** **NAT-M., NAT-P.,** ***nat-s.,*** nicc., **NUX-V.,** ***ol-j.,*** ox-ac., ***ph-ac.,*** **PHOS.,** phys., ***phyt.,*** plan., ***plat.,*** podo., ***puls., ran-b., rat., rhus-t.,*** **RUTA.,** sabad., ***sang., sars.,*** sec., ***sep.,*** **SIL.,** spig., squil., stram., sulph., ***tarent.,*** tanac., ***tell.,*** **THER.,** ***thuj.,*** verat., ***vib.,*** **ZINC.**
slight - stram.
fever, during - ***chin-s., cocc.***
footsteps - ***nux-v.,*** **THER.**
jar., of bed - **BELL.,** ***graph., lach.,*** **SIL., THER.,** ***thuj.***

sore, spine
leaning against a chair agg. - **AGAR.,** plb., **THER.**
lying, back, on - mag-m.
flat on the back with firm pressure, amel. - ***nat-m.***
on something hard, amel. - ***nat-m.***
menses, during - thuj.
morning - agar., mag-m.
night - mag-m.
pressure, agg. - ther.
pressure, on - plat.
sewing, machine, from using - ***nux-v.***
sitting - ruta.
stretching - med.
thunderstorm, before - ***agar., phos.***
walking, while - ***ruta.,*** verat.

sore, thoracic - ***apis,*** calc-p., nat-m., ***nat-s.,*** pall., ph-ac., plb., sep., stann.
morning on waking, amel. by exercise - calc-p.
spine - acon., aesc., ***agar.,*** ail., arn., ars-m., asaf., ***bell.,*** brach., cact., ***card-m., chel.,*** **CHIN-S.,** ***cimic., cocc.,*** colch., ***coloc., cupr.,*** gins., ***graph., hell.,*** hyper., merc., nux-v., ph-ac., **PHOS.,** plb., podo., ***ruta.,*** sec., ***sil.,*** **TELL., THER.,** ***zinc.***

sore, thoracic, middle of - ***acon.,*** am-m., ars., bar-c., chin., crot-c., dig., ***gran., hell.,*** kali-c., lach., mag-m., mag-s., ***meny.,*** merc-i-f., nat-m., nux-v., ***phos.,*** podo., rhus-t., ***sil.,*** sulph., ther.
coughing, when - sul-ac.
left and spine, amel. by pressure, rest and warmth, agg., by lifting, working during menses and vexation - ***phos.***
lying, while - nat-m.
motion amel. - kali-c.
sitting, while - nat-m.
stooping, when - cham., nux-v.
tip of - cimx.

SPASMODIC, drawing, sensation between shoulders, morning - apis, cham., meny., staph.
walking, while - calad.

SPASMS - acon., arn., ***ars.,*** bell., bry., calc., ***calc-p.,*** cham., cic., ***cimic., coloc., crot-c.,*** hyper., ***lach.,*** kali-c., **MAG-P.,** ***mygal., nat-m., nat-s., nux-v.,*** oena., ***phys.,*** rhus-t., ruta, sep., stram., syph., tab.
nursing, while - arn., ***cham., puls.***
spinal cord, from - pic-ac.
touch, on - acon.

SPOTS - calc., cist., lach., ***lyc.,*** sep., spong., sulph., sumb., zinc.
brown - thuj.
red - ant-c., bell., carb-v., cist., cocc., lach., sep., stann., vip.

SPINAL bifida - arn., ars., asaf., bar-c., bry., ***calc., calc-p., calc-s.,*** carb-v., dulc., graph., hep., lach., lyc., merc., mez., nit-ac., phos., ***psor.,*** ruta., **SIL.,** staph., sulph., syph., tub.

SPINAL, curvature, (see Curvature)

SPOTS, scapula, on - calc., cist., lach., sumb.

SPRAINED, as if - agar., am-m., arg-n., ***arn., bell.,*** **CALC.,** con., **GRAPH.,** kali-c., lyc., mur-ac., nux-v., olnd., petr., ***puls.,*** rhod., **RHUS-T.,** sep., sulph.
extending to left hypochondrium - lyc.
left - con., lyc.
nap, after - phos.
right - bell.
writing, after - mur-ac.

sprained, lumbar, as if - agar., arg-m., arg-n., **ARN., CALC.,** ***con.,*** gamb., ***lach.,*** mur-ac., ol-an., **PULS.,** ***rhod.,*** **RHUS-T.,** ***sep., staph.,*** sulph., **VALER.**
afternoon - sep.
evening, in bed - sep.
extending, above hip sitting and standing - **VALER.**
to abdomen - lach.
to gluteal muscles - ***aesc.***
to hips, afternoon and evening - sep.
morning - arg-n., petr.
bed, in - petr.
rising, on - arg-n.
motion, on - caust., kali-bi., **PULS.**
sitting, while - hep., petr., **VALER.**
sneezing - sulph.
standing, while - **VALER.**
stepping - ***sulph.***
stool, when urging - sin-a.
stooping, on - ars., ol-an.
stretching - calc.
turning body, while walking - hep.
walking amel. - staph.

sprained, scapula, , as if - bar-c., chel., chin., coloc., kali-c., mur-ac., nux-v., petr., sulph.
between scapula - am-m., bar-c., bell., chin., chel., coloc., kali-c., mur-ac., nux-v., petr., sulph.

sprained, thoracic, middle of, as if - am-m., bell., nux-v., petr., sep., stann.

STIFFNESS - abrot., acon., aesc., ***agar., alum., am-m., anac.,*** anan., ***ang., apis,*** arg-n., ***ars.,*** aur., aur-m., ***bar-c., bapt., bell., benz-ac.,*** **BERB.,** bol., ***bry., calc., calc-s.,*** caps., camph-br., ***carb-an.,*** carb-s., ***carb-v., carl.,*** **CAUST.,** cedr., ***chel., cic.,*** **CIMIC.,** cocc., con., cop., cupr., cupr-ar., dig., dios., dulc., get., gins., ***guai., helon.,*** hydr., hyper., ***ign.,*** ind., iris, Jac., ***kali-ar.,*** kali-bi., ***kali-c., kali-p., kali-s.,*** kalm., ***lach.,*** lachn., **LED.,** ***lyc., manc.,*** med., nat-a., nat-m., nat-s., ***nit-ac.,*** **NUX-V.,** ol-an., olnd., op., ***petr., phos.,*** phys., ***phyt., prun., puls.,*** rheum, **RHUS-T.,** rhus-v., ruta, sanic., sarcol-ac., **SEP., SIL.,** spong., ***staph., stram., stry.,*** **SULPH.,** sul-ac., tab., tub., ***thuj.,*** verat., zinc., zing.
ascending - ars.
bending backwards impossible - stram.
chill, during - ***lyc., nat-s., tub.***
cold, as from taking - sulph.
cramp-like - ***nit-ac.***
draft, from a - **RHUS-T.**
evening - dios., bar-c., lyc., petr.
exertion, after - lyc.
lying, while - puls.

STIFFNESS,
menses, before - mosch.
morning - ang., calc., carb-v., ox-ac., ***phyt.***, **RHUS-T.**, ***sep.***, sul-ac., stry., ***zinc.***
bed, in, amel. on rising - anac.
rising, on - bar-c., calc-s., ***carb-v.***, ferr-i., ign., mag-c., rhus-t., staph., sul-ac.
waking, on - calc., ***lach.***, ***led.***, ***sep.***
moving - acon., ***aesc.***, ***calc.***, ***cupr-ar.***, ***guai.***, led.
amel. - **RHUS-T.**, sul-ac.
on beginning - ***aesc.***, anac., con., cupr-s., ind., ***lyc.***, **RHUS-T.**
shoulders - cocc., guai.
night - ***lyc.***
noon - valer.
painful - ***am-m.***, ars., ***calc.***, **CAUST.**, ***helon.***, ***manc.***, ***nit-ac.***, ***puls.***, **RHUS-T.**, sanic., tub.
rising - ***agar.***, ***bry.***, cham.
from a seat - **AESC.**, ***agar.***, **AMBR.**, am-m., anac., ang., ***bar-c.***, **BELL.**, berb., bry., carl., **CAUST.**, ***hydr.***, ind., ***led.***, ***lyc.***, med., ***petr.***, ***puls.***, **RHUS-T.**, ***sil.***, ***sulph.***
sitting, after - **AMBR.**, am-m., ***bar-c.***, ***bell.***, caust., cham., con., cupr-ar., ind., led., ***phos.***, **RHUS-T.**, ***sil.***, ***sulph.***
bent amel. - anac.
side, onesided - guai.
standing - stry.
erect - bry.
erect impossible - sil.
stool, after - ferr., sep.
amel. - asaf.
stooping - ***berb.***, cic., caps., kali-c.
after - bov.
as after prolonged - thuj.
turning in bed - ***sulph.***
turns whole body to look around - sanic.
walk, must walk about some time before he can straighten up - hydr.
walking - aur., stry.
amel. - bry., calc-s., cop., **RHUS-T.**, sep., ***sulph.***
wet weather - ***phyt.***, **RHUS-T.**
writing - laur.

stiffness, lumbar region - bar-c., calc-f., carb-v., caust., lach., hyper., nat-m., ***rhus-t.***, ***ruta.***
thigh, cannot raise - aur.

stiffness, lumbo-sacral region - **AESC.**, ambr., anac., arg-n., ars., **BAR-C.**, bell., carb-an., carb-v., cham., dios., guai., ign., kali-c., nat-m., nit-ac., nux-v., petr., ***rhus-t.***, ruta, staph., valer.

STRAINING, easy - bor., **CALC.**, calc-f., ***calc-p.***, con., **GRAPH.**, ham., **LYC.**, mill., ***nux-v.***, ph-ac., **RHUS-T.**, **RUTA.**, sang., ***sep.***, sil.

STRUCK, with a hammer, as if, pressing against something hard amel. - **SEP.**

SWELLING, thoracic, of - am-m., **CALC.**, ***carb-an.***, ***kali-c.***, lyc., sil., spig., spong.

TEARING, pain - ***aesc.***, agar., alum., alumn., am-c., ant-c., ***arn.***, ***ars.***, asar., asc-t., aster., ***berb.***, calc., ***calc-p.***, ***canth.***, ***caps.***, carb-s., carb-v., caust., ***cham.***, ***chel.***, ***chin.***, ***cina***, cinnb., cocc., colch., coloc., cupr., dros., ferr., ferr-ar., ferr-p., gad., guai., kali-c., kali-m., kali-n., kali-p., led., ***lyc.***, ***mang.***, merc., mez., **NIT-AC.**, ***nux-v.***, op., petr., ***ph-ac.***, **PHOS.**, puls., sabin., sep., ***sil.***, ***stann.***, stel., ***stry.***, sulph., zinc.
bending, backwards - ***chel.***
forward - camph.
chill, with - sil.
cramp-like - bell.
drawing - cham., nux-v., op., stram.
eating, after - cham.
evening, in bed - sulph.
extending, down back - berb., ***cina***, mag-c., ***mang.***, nat-s.
to abdomen - cham.
to limbs - ***ars.***, ***chel.***, **PHOS.**
to nape, while walking - nat-s.
to thighs - chin.
upward - stann.
left - stann.
lying, while - ferr.
menses, during - agar., am-c., bell., ***caust.***, phos., **SEP.**
cramp-like - bell.
morning - ***canth.***, kali-c., mag-c., mez., puls., stry.
after rising - am-m.
motion, on - alum., am-m., ***caust.***, cinnb., dig., nit-ac.
amel. - alumn.
night - cinnb., nit-ac., ph-ac., rhod.
sharp, stitching - stann.
sitting - alumn., ***berb.***, ***ferr.***, ***lyc.***, spong.
standing, on - ***berb.***, bry., stann.
sticking, amel. pressing back against something hard - sep.
stooping, on - bry., ***chel.***
touch, on - chel.
walking - canth., ***chel.***
warmth of stove amel. - cinnb.

tearing, lumbar - acon., ***aesc.***, ***agar.***, **ALUM.**, ambr., ant-c., arn., ***ars.***, ***berb.***, brom., ***bry.***, calc., ***calc-p.***, canth., carb-s., ***carb-v.***, carl., ***caust.***, ***chel.***, chin., cina, cinnb., cocc., coc-c., ***colch.***, croc., cupr., dig., eupi., ***ham.***, hura, ign., ***kali-c.***, kali-p., lyc., mag-c., ***mag-m.***, mag-s., merl., ***mez.***, mur-ac., nat-c., ***nat-s.***, nux-v., ph-ac., ***phyt.***, ***rhod.***, rhus-t., sabin., sep., spig., ***stann.***, stront-c., thuj.
afternoon - mag-m.
standing - plb.
bending forward, when - chel.
breathing agg. - ***kali-c.***
evening in bed - alum.
extending, between ribs and ilium - ***teucr.***
in a circle to linea alba - caust.
occiput - led.
to hips - carb-v.
toes - eupi.
jerking - alum., chin.

tearing, lumbar
lying, while - berb.
amel. - ***bry.,*** nux-v.
on back - mag-s.
on back, amel. - ambr.
menses, during - guare., ***caust.,*** lachn.
before - eupi.
on appearance - ***caust.***
morning - stront.
4 a.m. - ruta.
9 a.m., amel. - ruta.
motion, on - alum., brom., ***bry.,*** calc-p., ***caust.,*** croc., dig., stann., sulph.
amel. - kali-c.
night - mag-m., mag-s.
pressure, amel. - aur., mag-m., ph-ac.
pressure, on - acon.
right - lyc.
rising, on - iris.
from a chair - merl.
from stooping - berb., chel., ph-ac.
sitting, while - asaf., berb., bry., kali-c., ***lyc.,*** nux-v.
amel. - ph-ac.
standing, while - berb., bry., ph-ac.
amel. - berb.
as from something alive - ph-ac.
stooping - ***bry.,*** chel., sabin.
amel. - ph-ac.
walking - agar., ***aesc.,*** asar., chel., nux-v.

tearing, scapula - ***acon., alum.,*** am-m., ***anac., aur.,*** berb., bov., camph., carb-v., ***caust.,*** chel., chin., cycl., dios., dulc., ***guai., kali-c.,*** kali-n., lach., led., ***mag-m.,*** manc., merc., mez., nat-c., nat-m., nat-s., nicc., nit-ac., ph-ac., phos., plb., psor., ptel., rhus-t., sars., ***sep.,*** stann., ***sulph.,*** thuj., zinc.
below - agar., alumn., dig., lyc., ***sil.***
on walking - ***sil.***
bending body backwards - aur., sep.
breathing deep, must - nat-m.
drawing - stann.
evening - alum., olnd.
extending, to arm - coc-c.
to sides - anac.
inner edge of - aur.
bending back or to left agg. - aur.
inspiration, on - chin.
left - alum., ambr., **ANAC.,** arg-m., carb-v., card-m., mang., sep., stann., thuj.
bending back the arm - carb-v.
cold, after taking - sep.
evening - alum.
sitting, while - arg-m., mang., sulph.
morning - ***kali-c.***
moving, arm agg. - camph.
head - nat-s.
right - anac., ***kali-c.,*** mag-m., nat-m., plb., sars., zinc.
on breathing - kali-c., sars.
on spine, between - zinc.
under - calc., dig.
rubbing amel. - phos.
sitting, while - mang.
bent - bov., ph-ac.

tearing, scapula
tip of - alumn., berb., mez.
motion amel. - alum.
waking, on - nicc.
walking, while - nat-s., nit-ac.

tearing, spine - aur-s., berb., camph., caps., chel., chin., chin-s., ***cina,*** cocc., **HYPER.,** mag-c., ***mang.,*** nat-m., ***nat-s.,*** nux-v.
anterior superior spinous process of left ilium - dros.
extending downward - ***cina, mang.,*** nat-m.
lower part - ars., chel., mag-c.
thoracic region - ***berb.,*** bor., mag-m., nat-c., ***nat-s.,*** psor., ***sil.,*** zinc.
upper part - cina.

tearing, thoracic - aur., berb., brom., ***calc.,*** guai., ***kali-c.***
bending body backward - aur.
burning - kali-c.
rubbing amel. - phos.
sitting down, on - arg-m., hura.

tearing, thoracic, middle of - agar., anac., bar-c., ***berb.,*** bor., ***calc.,*** calc-caust., canth., ***caust.,*** cocc., ferr., kali-c., kali-n., ***lach.,*** mag-m., meny., nat-c., ***nat-s.,*** petr., psor., puls., rhus-t., ***sil.,*** thuj., zinc.
afternoon - canth., caust.
breathing, deep - meny.
evening - cocc., sulph.
in bed - thuj.
midnight, after - mag-s.
morning, 4 p.m. - caust.
on waking - ***kali-bi.***
motion, on - petr.
stooping, agg. - bor.
turning, on - verat.
walking, on - ferr., meny.

TENSION - aeth., ***agar.,*** am-c., am-m., arg-n., ***ars.,*** aur., bar-c., berb., bry., coloc., con., hep., hyos., ign., ***lil-t., lyc.,*** med., mez., mosch., nat-c., nat-m., olnd., ol-an., ***puls.,*** rat., sars., sep., ***sulph.,*** tarax., teucr., thuj., tub., zinc.
breathing, inspiration agg. - lyc.
dinner, after - nat-c.
before - nicc.
extending, to anus while lying and sitting - nat-c.
to chest, agg. stooping - chel.
to neck - laur.
forenoon - bry.
left - nat-m., sulph.
lying on other side agg. - sep.
motion, during - colch.
amel. - am-m.
moving, arm - sulph.
trunk, amel. walking in evening - nat-c.
night - nat-c.
on turning the body - hep.
paroxysmal - nat-c.
right side - sep.
sitting, while - am-m., nat-c.
bent - nat-c., sulph.
standing, on - ign.

TENSION,
straighten up, on attempting to - bell.
amel. - nat-c.
tension, lumbar - acon., ***agar.,*** ambr., am-c., am-m., ars., aur-m., ***bar-c.,*** **BERB.,** bov., brom., bry., caps., ***carl.,*** carb-s., carb-v., caust., ***chin.,*** clem., coc-c., ***colch.,*** cycl., lyc., mag-c., merl., ***nat-m.,*** nit-ac., ***nux-v., phos., puls.,*** rheum, sep., sil., ***sulph.,*** thuj., verat., ***zinc.***
air, open - lyc.
ascending steps - carb-s.
bending backward - bar-c.
backward amel. - acon.
evening - ***bar-c.***
standing - agar.
stepping - acon.
extending to right hypochondrium - bar-c.,
to left hip - sars.
morning, in bed - sulph.
in bed, 4 a.m., on waking - sulph.
motion, on - brom., sars.
rising up - bar-c., sulph.
sitting - zinc.
standing - agar., lyc.
erect - ign.
stool, after - berb., plat.
stooping - bar-c., sabin., **SULPH.**
stretching agg. - agar.
touch agg. - agar.
walking - bry., lyc.
tension, scapula - alum., ***bar-c.,*** **CARB-AN.,** caust., cic., colch., ***coloc.,*** con., kali-c., lyc., mag-m., merc., merc-c., ***mez.,*** mur-ac., nat-c., ***nux-v.,*** op., ***rhus-t.,*** sep., sil., sulph., zinc.
below - con., kali-c., zinc.
raising arm - con.
evening - sep.
extending to neck - mang.
motion, on caust.
turning the head - caust., merc.
tension, thoracic - ang., aur-m., crot-c., lyc., mag-s., mur-ac., ***rhus-t., zinc.***
left - sep.
walking, amel. - mag-s.
tension, thoracic, middle of - alum., anac., ant-c., carb-an., ***colch.,*** ferr., ***hep., mag-m., mur-ac., nat-c., nux-v.,*** sep., zinc.
excitement, after - phos.
extending down back - mag-m.
to shoulder - sulph.
lying - sulph.
menses, during - am-c.
moving - sulph.
stooping - ant-c.
rubbing - carb-an.

TICKLING, pain - sumb.

THROBBING, pain, lumbar - bar-c., lac-c., sep., sil.
throbbing, scapula - plan., sulph.
scapula, left - mag-m.

THREADS, as if extending to limbs - lach.

THRUSTS, stinging - ther.

TREMBLING - apis, carb-v., cimic., ***cocc.,*** eup-per., lil-t.
fever, during - ***eup-per.***
morning - apis
paroxysmal - carb-v.
trembling, lumbar - benz-ac., berb., cimic., merc., oci., thuj.
trembling, scapula - sulph.
forenoon - sulph.
trembling, spine - lil-t.

TUBERCLES - am-c., am-m., caust., iod., lyc., nicc., squil.
tubercles, scapula, non-suppurative in the right - am-m.

TUBERCULOSIS, of vertebrae, or Pott's disease - aur., calc-p., iod., ph-ac., phos., stann., syph., tub.
lies on, with drawn up knees - merc-c.

TUMORS, cyst - phos.
pediculated bluish as large as a cherry - ***con.,*** thuj.
sarcoma - ***bar-c.***
spine, of - tarent.
vertebra - lach., tarent.

TWITCHING - ***agar.,*** alum., calc., carb-v., carc., chel., jatr., kali-bi., merc., mez., morph., mygal., nat-m., petr., phys., spig., stry., sulph., ***zinc.***
breathing - alum., calc.
like electric shocks - ***ang., nux-v.***
lying on back, while - agar.
opening the mouth, on - stry.
right - calc., meny.
twitching, lumbar - ***agar., alum.,*** calc., ***coloc.,*** con., crot-t., dulc., lach., mag-c., petr., rat., sumb.
afternoon, 1 p.m. - mag-c.
evening - agar.
in bed - sulph.
extending to rectum - calc.
lifting, after - nat-c.
lying, while - bry.
motion, on - petr.
pulsating - con.
sitting - bry., meny.
stooping - kali-c.
walking - rhus-t.
twitching, scapula - calc., calc-p., lyc., merc., mez., nat-c., phos., rhus-t., sep., squil., thuj.
twitching, thoracic - nat-ac., ***stry.***
lower thoracic - ruta.
manual labor - nit-ac.

ULCERS - ***cist., merc-c.***
ulcers, scapula - kali-bi., merc.

URTICARIA - apis, lach., lac-ac., sulph.
scratching, after - lyc.

VERTEBRAE, general
absent, as if - mag-p., psor.
cracking, in - ol-an.
heat, single sensitive to - agar.
loose, as if - calc.
rub against each other, as if - ant-t.
slipping, as if - sanic., sulph.

VESICLES - arn., bry., calc-caust., caust., cist., graph., hura, ***kali-c., lach.,*** nat-c., petr., rhus-t., ***sep.,*** wies.
evening, itching when undressing - nat-c., nat-s.
painful - caust.
red elevated base, on a - kali-bi.
shoulders, between the - sep.
surrounded by red areola - crot-h.
vesicles, scapula, on - am-c., am-m., ant-c., caust., cic., lach., vip.

WARM, sense of warm air steaming up spine into head - ***ars.,*** sars.

WARTS - nit-ac., sil., thuj.

WAVE, like sensation going up back - laur.

WEAKNESS - abrot., ***aesc., aesc-g.,*** aeth., ***agar.,*** alum., alum-sil., alumn., anan., ant-t., apis, arg-n., arn., **ARS.,** bar-c., berb., ***brach.,*** but-ac., **CALC.,** ***calc-p.,*** calc-s., carb-ac., carb-s., carb-v., ***casc.,*** cast., ***chin.,*** chin-a., ***cic.,*** cimic., ***cocc.,*** coloc., ***con.,*** cupr-ar., cur., ***eup-per., gels.,*** gins., glyc., **GRAPH.,** gua., guai., ***helon.,*** hep., hydr., ign., irid., iris, jac., ***kali-c.,*** kali-cy., kali-p., ***lach.,*** lob., ***lyss.,*** med., merc., ***murx.,*** nat-a., **NAT-M.,** nat-p., nit-ac., **NUX-V.,** ol-j., ox-ac., pall., petr., **PH-AC.,** ***phos.,*** phys., ***pic-ac.,*** plb., podo., psor., ***puls.,*** raph., **RHUS-T., RUTA,** sarr., **SEL., SEP.,** ***sil.,*** staph., ***stry.,*** **SULPH.,** sul-ac., tell., ther., verat-v., **ZINC.**
breathing, deep, on - carb-v.
cough, in whooping - verat.
eating agg. - ***nat-m.***
emissions, from - **SEL.**
evening - nat-p.
exertion, from - agar., kali-c., lach., nat-m., par., sil.
forenoon - calc-s.
left - sulph.
lying down - cic., phos.
amel. - ***casc., nat-m.***
manual labor - ***lach.,*** **NAT-M.,** ***sil.***
mental exertion, after - ***calc.***
morning - coloc., dios., ox-ac., pall., petr., ther.
on rising - nat-m.
motion of arms, on - clem., ***par., sil.,*** sulph.
night - petr.
riding - calc-s.
sex, after - nat-p.
sexual excesses - agar., ***calc., nat-m.,*** **NUX-V., PH-AC.,** ***phos.,*** **SEL.**
sitting, while - agar., bar-c., **CALC.,** cic., ***graph., lyss.,*** **SULPH., ZINC.**
after - ***sil.***
standing almost impossible - ox-ac., sul-ac., verat.
stool, after - sumb.
support body, can not - ox-ac.
typhoid fever, after - **SEL.**
vaginal discharge - graph.
walking, while - ***graph.,*** sabad., sep., **SULPH.**
after - bapt., petr.
amel. - ***hydr.***

WEAKNESS
writing - lyc.
weakness, lumbar - ***aesc., agar.,*** all-s., ***alum.,*** alumn., ambr., am-c., ***arg-n.,*** arn., **ARS.,** asar., aur., aur-m., bar-c., ***bell.,*** benz-ac., berb., **CALC., CALC-S.,** camph., carb-ac., carb-s., carl., chel., cimx., cimic., ***cina,*** clem., **COCC.,** ***coloc.,*** con., dios., ***eup-per.,*** gels., ***graph., helon., hep.,*** hura, hydr., ***kali-bi., kali-c.,*** kali-cy., kali-i., kali-s., ***lach.,*** laur., ***lec., led.,*** lil-t., ***lycps.,*** lyss., manc., ***merc.,*** merc-i-f., meph., morph., ***murx., mur-ac.,*** naja, nat-c., **NAT-M.,** nat-p., ***nux-m.,*** nux-v., ***nym., ox-ac., pall.,*** petr., ***phos.,*** phyt., **PIC-AC.,** plan., ***psor.,*** ptel., **PULS.,** raph., **RHUS-T.,** ***rhus-v.,*** rumx., **RUTA,** sabin., sanic., ***sec.,*** **SEL.,** senec., **SEP.,** ***sil.,*** **SULPH.,** sul-ac., sul-i., thuj., tub., ***zinc.***
eating agg. - nat-m.
emissions, after - ham., ***nat-p.,*** phos.
evening - alum., alumn., ***coloc.,*** hura, petr.
exertion, after - phys., plan.
fever, during - hura.
lying on back, while - calc-s., nat-p.
amel. - nat-m.
morning - hura.
rising, on- nat-m.
motion, on - pic-ac., ***sulph.***
reaching up agg. - zinc.
riding - berb., cer-b.
rising, from seat - phos.
sitting - alum., canth., ferr-p., graph., helon., hep., ir-foe., ***phos.,*** thuj., zinc.
standing - ***chel., cic.,*** **SULPH.**
stooping - am-c.
urinating, when - puls.
vaginal discharge, during - ***con.,*** **GRAPH.**
walking - brach., camph., **COCC.,** graph., petr., sep., ***zinc.***
child does not learn to walk - all-s.
on beginning to walk - ***zinc.***
weakness, scapula - agar., alum., ***apis, cocc.,*** kali-i., ***nat-m.,*** rad-br., raph., sars., sul-ac., thlaspi
leaning on something, amel. - sarr.
stooping, amel. - alumn.
weakness, thoracic, middle of - ***agar.,*** sarr.

WET, sensation as if clothes are - tub.

WIND, as if blowing, lumbar region - sulph., ***sumb.***

WOOD stretched across, as if - nux-m.

WOUNDS, spinal - ***calen.,*** **HYPER.,** ruta, symph.

Bladder

ABSENT, sensation, urethra, when urinating - ail., ***apis,*** apoc., **ARG-N., CAUST.,** cedr., chlol., ***cupr.,*** grat., hell., kali-br., **MAG-M.,** mag-s., merc., nux-v., ***sars.***

ACHING, pain - ***all-c.,*** arn., bell., ***berb.,*** calc-p., **CAPS.,** carb-v., ***carb-s.,*** chel., cop., crot-t., ***equis.,*** erig., ***eup-pur., fl-ac., hell.,*** lach., lyc., ***nux-v.,*** pall., phos., pop., ***puls.,*** sabin., ***sep.,*** sulph., ter.
heavy - sabal.
lying, while - ***nux-v.***
menses, during - sep.
sex, after - all-c.
urination, during - carb-v., fl-ac.
after - berb., calc-p., **CANTH.,** conv., ***fl-ac.,*** lith.
before - berb., ***fl-ac., nux-v.,*** pall.

aching, bladder, neck, of - acon., calc-p., con., cop., puls., sep., sulph.
afternoon, 3 p.m - sulph.
morning, 11 a.m - sulph.
urination, after - apoc., fl-ac., ***sep.,*** stann.

aching, urethra - bry., cahin., canth., eup-pur., lob., sulph.
meatus, urinating, when not - cocc., ***nux-v.***
urination, after - puls.
urination, during - canth.
nephritic colic, with - coc-c.
urination, after - apoc., lob., puls.

AGGLUTINATION, urethra, meatus, of - anag., bor., bov., calc-p., ***camph., cann-s.,*** canth., ***cupr.,*** cupr-ar., gamb., graph., ***med., nat-m., petros.,*** puls., tab., ***thuj.***
morning - canth., ***phos.,*** **SEP.,** ***thuj.***

AGONIZING, pain, with urination - acon., ***canth., sars.***

agonizing, urethra, clots of blood passing, from - canth.

AIR, passes from the female urethra during urination - sars.

APPREHENSION, in, region of - merc-c.

ATONY - ars., **CAUST.,** op., plb., ***sep.,*** stann., stram.
retention, from long - canth.

BALL, in, sensation of - anac., crot-h., kali-br., kreos., ***lach.,*** naja
forced from behind neck of, sensation of - kali-br.

ball, urethra, rolling through, sensation of - lach.

BEDWETTING, (see Urination, involuntary) - acon., ***aeth.,*** alum., ***am-c.,*** anac., anan., **APIS,** ***apoc., arg-m.,*** **ARG-N., ARN., ARS.,** ***aur.,*** aur-m., aur-s., bar-c., bar-m., **BELL., BENZ-AC.,** bry., cact., ***calc.,*** canth., ***carb-s., carb-v.,*** **CAUST.,** ***cham.,*** chin., ***chlol.,*** cimx., ***cina,*** coca, con., ***crot-c.,*** cub., cupr., dulc., **EQUIS.,** ***eup-pur.,*** **FERR.,** ***ferr-ac.,*** ferr-i., ferr-p., ***fl-ac.,*** **GRAPH.,** ***hep.,*** hyos., ign., kali-br., kali-c., ***kali-p.,*** **KREOS., LAC-C.,** lac-d., ***lyc.,*** mag-aust., mag-c., ***mag-m.,*** **MAG-P.,** mag-s., ***med., merc.,*** mur-ac., ***nat-a., nat-c.,*** **NAT-M.,** ***nat-p.,*** **NIT-AC.,** nux-v., ***op.,*** ox-ac., ***petr.,*** ph-ac., ***phos.,*** physal., ***plan., podo., psor.,*** **PULS.,** quas., rhus-a., **RHUS-T.,** ***ruta.,*** sabal., ***sanic.,*** sant., ***sars.,*** sec., sel., ***seneg.,*** **SEP., SIL.,** spig., squil., staph., ***stram.,*** **SULPH.,** ***syc-co.,*** tab., ter., ***thuj.,*** **THYR.,** ***tub., uran., urt-u.,*** uva., verat., ***verb., viol-t.,*** zinc.
adolescence - ***lac-c.***
children, in - aesc., ***bell.,*** benz-ac., ***caust.,*** chin., ***cina,*** **EQUIS.,** ***kreos., lyc.,*** med., nat-m., phos., puls., sep., sil., thuj.
difficult to waken the child - ***bell.,*** chlol., **KREOS.,** thuj.
dreaming of urinating, while - ***kreos.,*** lac-c., lyc., merc-i-f., ***seneg., sep.,*** sulph.
first sleep - benz-ac., **CAUST.,** cina, ***kreos., ph-ac.,*** **SEP.**
habit, when there is no tangible cause except - **EQUIS.**
midnight to morning - plan.
morning, toward - am-c., cact., chlol., zinc.
night, after 5 a.m. - cact.
spasmodic enuresis - **ARG-M.,** bell., canth., caps., cast., cina, coloc., ***gels.,*** hyos., ign., lach., lyc., ***nux-v.,*** op., puls., rhus-t., verat.
weakly children, in - ***chin.***

BITING, pain, urethra - alum., ars., berb., caps., ***clem., graph.,*** guai., ip., prun., rhus-t., teucr., thuj., zinc-ac.
anterior part - ***petros.,*** rhus-t., zinc.
rest agg., walking amel. - rhus-t.
evening, burning - chin.
extending backward - phos.
fossa navicularis - **PETROS.**
itching, and, before urination - cop., tab.
morning - rhus-t.
on waking - alum., sep.
posterior part - ***camph., petros.***
urinating, when not - cann-s., teucr., zinc.
urination, during - act-sp., ***canth.,*** carb-v., cham., chin., clem., ***equis., graph.,*** ign., kali-c., kali-n., lyc., mag-c., ***merc.,*** **MERC-C.,** nat-m., nit-ac., phos., rhus-t., sep., thuj.
after - bor., ***caps., chin-s., clem.,*** con., cop., ***equis.,*** kali-c., petros., rhus-t.
after, as if a drop were forcing its way out - sel.

biting, urethra, meatus - sep., staph.
evening - coc-c., kali-c., petros.
morning - kali-c., petros.
urination, during - bor., **CANN-S.,** echi., merc-c.
after - kali-c., zinc.
after, sticking - mur-ac.
waking, on - alum.

BLEEDING, from (see Urine chapter, bloody) cact., carb-v., crot-h., ***erig., ferr-p., ham.,*** lyc., mill., ***nit-ac.,*** **PHOS.,** rhus-a., ***sec.,*** ter., ***thlaspi.***

bleeding, urethra - aloe, ambr., am-c., ant-c., ant-t., ***arg-n.,*** arn., ***ars.,*** arum-m., bell., bry., ***cact., calc., camph., cann-s., canth., caps.,*** carb-s., ***caust., chel., chin., chin-s., con., crot-h.,*** cur., erig., ***euphr., ferr-m.,*** ferr-p., graph., ***ham.,*** hell., ***hep., ip.,*** kali-ar., kali-c., ***kali-i.,*** kali-s., ***lyc., merc.,*** **MERC-C.,** mez., ***mill.,*** mur-ac., murx., nat-m., ***nit-ac., nux-v., phos.,*** plb., ***puls.,*** sars., ***sec.,*** senec., seneg., sep., squil., ***sulph., ter.,*** thuj., zinc.
  burning, with - ambr., chin., coch., graph., kali-c., kali-i., merc., ***nux-v.,*** puls., seneg., ***sulph.,*** ter.
  constipation, with - lyc.
  cut, from a, hemorrhagic diathesis - ***phos.,*** ter.
  erection, during - ***canth.***
  first part of urine, with - ***con.***
  gonorrhea, after suppressed - **PULS**.
  menses suppressed - zinc.
  painful - canth., merc., zinc.
  painless - ars-h., lyc., merc., psor., sec.
  pains in, bladder, with - ant-t.
    kidneys and bladder, with - ip., puls.
    stomach, and vomiting - ip.
  paralysis of legs, with - lyc.
  pure blood - bry., ***canth.,*** caps., ham., hell., mez., **PHOS.**
    clotted - cact., ***caust., chin., coc-c., nux-v.***
    urinating, when not - bry.
  sex, during - ***caust.***
  stool, during - ***lyc.,*** puls.
  urination, after - dulc., **HEP**., merc-c., mez., puls., sars., sulph., ***thuj.,*** zinc.
    first part of - con.
  vicarious - ***phos.,*** zinc.

BORING, pain, region of - thuj.

bubbling, urethra, while sitting - berb.

BURNING, pain - ***acon., all-c., apis, ars.,*** bell., **BERB.,** camph., cann-i., **CANTH., CAPS.,** card-m., cham., chel., chin., clem., coff., colch., coloc., cop., erig., ***eup-pur.,*** fl-ac., hydrang., indg., lach., lyc., lyss., merc-c., nit-ac., nux-v., petr., phos., pip-n., ***prun., puls.,*** rheum, rhus-t., sabin., senec., ***sep.,*** sil., ***staph.,*** **TER.,** thuj., uva., zinc-ar.
  evening - lyss., nux-v., puls.
  lying, while - fl-ac.
  menses, during - sep.
  morning - berb., ***nux-v.***
    10 a.m - all-c.
  night - bell.
  standing, agg. - ***eup-pur.***
  urination, during - aloe, ***canth.,*** caps., cham., eup-pur., kali-bi., lyc., nux-v., phos., prun., rheum, ***ter.***
    after - alum., apis, ***berb.,*** calc-p., canth., ***fl-ac., lyc.,*** sep., sil., thuj.
    before - ***apis, berb.,*** bor., bry., calc., cann-i., ***canth., caps.,*** chel., clem., colch., ***fl-ac.,*** lach., nat-c., rheum, rhod., seneg., thuj., zinc.
  walking in open air amel - **TER.**

burning, bladder, neck, of - acon., ***berb.,*** **CANTH.,** ***cham.,*** con., ***cop., elat.,*** ign., mit., ***nux-v.,*** op., petr., ph-ac., plb., ***prun., puls., staph.,*** zinc-ar.
  extending through urethra - **CANTH.**
  lying bent up amel - staph.
  urinating, when not - acon., berb., canth., staph.
  urination, during - acon., ***aloe, apis,*** berb., **CANTH.,** ***cham., cop.,*** **NUX-V.,** petr., ph-ac., prun., puls., ***ran-b.,*** staph., sul-ac., thuj., trinit.
    after - ***apis,*** canth., merc., ***puls., sars.***

burning, urethra - acon., aesc., agar., agn., ***all-c.,*** all-s., aloe, alum., ambr., ammc., am-c., ***ant-c., ant-t., apis, arg-n.,*** **ARS.,** aspar., asar., aur., aur-m., bell., benz-ac., **BERB.,** bor., brom., bov., ***bry.,*** cact., calad., ***calc.,*** calc-f., calc-s., **CAMPH.,** cann-i., **CANN-S., CANTH.,** ***caps.,*** carb-an., carb-s., carb-v., ***card-m., carl., caust.,*** cedr., cham., chel., chim., ***chin.,*** chin-s., cinnb., clem., cimic., cob., coc-c., ***colch.,*** coloc., con., ***cop.,*** crot-t., cub., cupr., der., ***ery-a.,*** eup-pur., ferr-ar., ferr-i., ***fl-ac.,*** gins., graph., hep., hipp., ign., ip., piloc., kali-ar., kali-c., ***kali-i.,*** kali-n., kali-p., lac-c., laur., lil-t., ***lith., lyc.,*** lyss., mag-m., manc., **MERC., MERC-C.,** merl., mosch., ***nat-c.,*** nat-m., nat-p., ***nit-ac.,*** **NUX-V.,** ox-ac., op., par., ***petr., ph-ac., phos.,*** polyg., **PRUN.,** ptel., ***puls., rhod.,*** rhus-t., ***rhus-v.,*** sabin., ***sars.,*** senec., ***sep.,*** **SIL.,** stann., ***staph.,*** still., stry., **SULPH.,** ***tarent., ter.,*** teucr., **THUJ.,** thymol., thyr., uran-n., zinc.
  anterior part - canth., coff., ***nit-ac.,*** puls., ***sep.,*** stann., tep., thuj.
    emission, after an - carb-v., ***sep.***
    urinating, when not - asaf., bry., ***cann-s.,*** caps., kali-bi., nux-v., ***stann., sulph.,*** zinc.
    urination, during - ars., calc., caps., ***cann-s.,*** carb-v., coch., ery-a., ign., kali-bi., kali-n., ***merc.,*** nat-c., nux-v., ***phos.,*** raph., rhus-t., seneg., stann., ***sulph.,*** teucr., verat.
    urination, after - cann-s., kali-bi., lyc., mez., nit-ac., puls.
  at all times - calad., canth.
  discharge of thin liquid after urination, from - ***nat-m.***
  discharged, when semen is - ***agar., ant-c.,*** arg-n., ***berb.,*** bor., ***calc., canth.,*** clem., ***kreos.,*** merc., nat-m., ***nit-ac.,*** sars., sep., **SULPH.,** sul-ac., tarent., thuj.
    stricture in, during sex - ***clem.***
  drops of urine passing, as if - ambr., ox-ac.
  emission, during - ***ant-c.,*** bor., clem., sars., sep., **SULPH.,** thuj.
    after - carb-an., carb-v., caust., cob., dig., merc., sep., sulph., thuj.
  erections, during - anag., cahin., calc-p., ***canth.,*** carb-s., ferr-i., mag-m., mosch., nat-m., ***nit-ac.***
    ceases during sex - anag.

burning, urethra
evening - chin., lyc., nat-c., ox-ac., petr., phos., sulph.
as if a drop of acrid urine would pass - ox-ac.
exercise, during - alum.
extending to rectum - rhus-t.
flatus passing agg. - lyc., mang.
fossa navicularis - acon., cann-s., cub., ***petros.***
burning drops - thuj.
urination, before - senec.
urination, during - clem., ***kali-bi.,*** mez., nat-m., petros., thuj.
glandular portion, urination, during - apis, camph., dig., kali-bi., nux-v., rhus-t.
urination, during, and for long time after - apis, dig., ***kali-bi.***
menopause, during - ***berb.***
menses, before, (see Urine, burning)
menses, during - ***nat-m.***
morning, erections after - ***nat-m.***
urination, after - con.
urination, during - anag., con., ***fl-ac.,*** ign., seneg., teucr., thuj.
waking, on, after emission - carb-an.
motion agg. - alum.
night - berb., canth., caust., cinnb., ***merc.***
posterior part - cann-s., carb-an., kali-bi., staph.
emissions, after - carb-an.
urination, during - ***cann-s.***
rising, after - thuj.
root, at - camph.
sex, during - agar., ant-c., calc., ***canth.,*** kreos., merc., ***sulph.,*** thuj.
after sex - berb., ***canth.,*** nat-p., ***sep.,*** **SULPH.,** sul-ac.
after sex, urination, during - ***caust.***
shooting, and increased gonorrhea - arg-n., cann-s.
sitting, while - ***card-m.,*** par.
stool, after - ***nat-c.,*** nat-p.
stool, during - ***coloc.***
stream is interrupted, when - clem.
touching, on - berb., bor., merc.
effort is made to pass urine, when - calad., prun.
urging to urinate - ant-c., ant-t., **CANTH.,** con., ***nit-ac.,*** phos., ***prun.,*** sabad., ***sulph.***
urinating, when not - asaf., ***berb.,*** bov., ***bry.,*** calad., cedr., clem., ***graph.,*** **MERC.,** ***merc-c., nat-c.,*** nit-ac., sabad., ***staph., sulph.,*** teucr., thuj.
urination, during - ***acon., aesc., agar.,*** aloe, alum., ***ambr.,*** anag., anth., ***ant-c.,*** aphis., apis, apoc., **ARG-N.,** ars., asc-c., aur-m., ***bapt., bar-c.,*** **BELL.,** benz-ac., ***berb.,*** bov., ***bry.,*** cact., cahin., calad., **CALC.,** calc-f., ***calc-p.,*** calc-s., **CAMPH., CANN-I., CANN-S., CANTH.,** ***caps., carb-an.,*** carb-s., ***carb-v.,*** **CAUST.,** cedr., ***cham., chel., chim.,*** chin., chin-s., **CLEM.,** cob., coc-c., ***con., colch.,*** **COP.,** crot-t., **CUB.,** cupr., cupr-ar., cur., dig., dulc., ***echi., equis., ery-a.,*** eug., ***eup-pur., ferr.,*** ferr-ar., ferr-i., ferr-p., fl-ac., ***gels.,*** glon., graph., grat., hell., helon., ***hep.,*** hydr-ac., ***ign., ip.,*** kali-ar., kali-bi., ***kali-c., kali-n.,*** kali-p., kali-s., lach., laur., **LIL-T.,** lob., ***lyc., mag-c.,*** mag-m., ***mang.,*** med., ***merc.,*** **MERC-C.,** mez., mur-ac., ***nat-a.,*** **NAT-C.,** ***nat-m.,*** nat-p., ***nat-s.,*** **NIT-AC.,** ***nux-m.,*** **NUX-V.,** op., ox-ac., par., pareir., petr., ***petros.,*** ph-ac., ***phos.,*** pic-ac., plb., ***psor.,*** ptel., ***puls.,*** raph., rat., rheum, rhod., rhus-t., sabad., sabin., ***sars.,*** sec., ***sel., seneg., sep., sil., staph.,*** **SULPH.,** ***sul-ac.,*** tab., tarent., **TER., THUJ.,** ***uran-n.,*** **UVA.,** verat., viol-t., zinc.
after - alum., ang., ant-t., apis, apoc., arg-n., arund., aspar., benz-ac., ***berb., bor.,*** bov., brom., bufo, calc., calc-p., **CANN-I.,** ***cann-s.,*** **CANTH.,** ***caps., carb-an., card-m., caust., chel.,*** chin., ***clem.,*** cob., coc-c., colch., coloc., ***con.,*** cop., dig., ***fl-ac.,*** grat., iris, ***kali-bi., kali-c.,*** kali-p., led., ***lil-t., lyc.,*** lyss., mag-c., ***mag-m., merc., mez.,*** mur-ac., **NAT-C., NAT-M.,** nat-s., ***nit-ac.,*** nux-v., phel., ***phos.,*** pic-ac., plb., ptel., ***puls.,*** rhus-t., sars., seneg., sep., spig., ***staph.,*** tarent., tab., ***thuj.,*** zinc.
amel. - berb., bry., cocc., ***merc.,*** staph.
anterior part - ***mez.***
before - alum., ***apis,*** aspar., ***berb.,*** **BOR.,** ***bry., calc.,*** **CANN-I., CANTH.,** caps., chel., coc-c., colch., cop., dig., ery-a., fl-ac., ***merc., merc-c., nat-c., nit-ac., nux-v.,*** ph-ac., phos., ***prun., puls.,*** rhod., seneg., ***sulph.,*** zinc.
beginning to urinate, when - apis, ars., ***cann-s., clem.,*** **MERC.,** nat-a., ***prun.,*** teucr.
beginning to urinate, when, morning - ars.
close, at - ***cann-s.,*** clem., ***equis.,*** kali-n., ***mez.,*** **NAT-C.,** ph-ac., ***sars.***
constriction, and, extending to bladder - lyc.
last drops cause violent burning - arg-n., carb-v., ***clem.,*** colch., coloc., lyc., ***merc., mez.,*** nux-m., sel., tell.
menses, during, while urinating - zinc.
preventing urination - ph-ac.
walking, while - stry.

burning, urethra, meatus - ***acon.,*** agar., ambr., am-c., aphis., apis, ***berb.,*** bor., bry., ***calc.,*** calc-f., ***cann-s., canth., caps.,*** chel., ***chin.,*** clem., cic., cob., coch., coff., cupr., cupr-ar., ***dulc.,*** gamb., ***gels.,*** graph., iod., kali-c., ***kali-s.,*** lact., lyc., mag-s., med., menthol, ***merc-c., nat-m.,*** nicc., nit-ac., par., ***petros.,*** ph-ac., phos., puls., ran-s., sel., seneg., sep., ***spig.,*** staph., **SULPH.,** ***thuj.,*** verat., zinc., zing.

burning, urethra, meatus
evening - nat-m.
extending backward - cann-s.
morning - kali-c.
night - ***agar.,*** calc.
quiet, when - canth., par.
rubbing cloths agg. - chin.
sex, after - ***calc.,*** nat-p.
sitting, while - par.
urination, during - acon., ***agar.,*** aphis., ***calc.,*** cann-i., ***cann-s.,*** canth., caps., ***chin.,*** cupr., cupr-ar., ***dulc.,*** gamb., kali-n., merc., merl., nat-s., nicc., ***nux-v.,*** ph-ac., ***puls.,*** spig., ***sulph.,*** thuj.
after - ***cann-i.,*** caps., card-m., casc., chin., coloc., cupr-ar., graph., kali-c., lyss., nat-s., puls., tell.
before - ***caps.***
violent, very - ***berb.***
walking, while - nat-m.

BURSTING, pain - pareir., zinc.

CALCULI, (see Stones)

CANCER, of - con., crot-h.

CARTILAGINOUS, induration - pareir.

CARUNCLE, vascular bleeding from tumor of - arg-n., ars., ***cann-i., cann-s., eucal.,*** eup-pur., hep., nit-ac., sul-i., sulph., teucr., thuj.

CATARRH, muco-pus (see Urine chapter, Sediment, purulent) - alumn., ***apis, ant-c.,*** aspar., **BENZ-AC.,** ***calc.,*** calc-s., cann-s., ***canth.,*** carb-ac., ***carb-s., carb-v., caust., chim.,*** chin-s., coff., coll., **COLOC.,** ***con., cop.,*** cub., **DULC.,** ***equis.,*** erig., ***eup-pur.,*** eucal., ***ferr., gels.,*** ham., ***hydr.,*** indg., kali-c., ***kali-chl.,*** kali-p., kali-s., ***lach.,*** **LYC.,** med., mill., nat-m., **NUX-V.,** pareir., ***petr., ph-ac., phos.,*** plb., pop., **PULS.,** rhod., rhus-t., ***sars., senec., seneg., sil.,*** **SULPH.,** ***ter.,*** **UVA.**
elderly people, in - ***alumn., carb-v.,*** sulph., ***ter.***
gonorrhea, from suppressed - benz-ac., cub., ***med.,*** nat-s., ***puls.,*** sil., ***thuj.***
hemorrhoidal subjects, in - coll.

CHORDEE, urethra - **ARG-N.,** aur-m., bry., ***camph., cann-i.,*** **CANN-S., CANTH., CAPS.,** chlol., ***colch.,*** con., cop., ***cub.,*** cur., dig., ery-a., fl-ac., hep., kali-br., **KALI-CHL.,** kali-i., ***merc.,*** merc-c., ***mygal.,*** nat-c., ***nit-ac., nux-v., petros.,*** phos., pip-n., **PULS.,** sabad., sep., **TER.,** ***thuj.,*** zing.
burning, in with - calc-p.
extreme sensitiveness of urethra - ***caps.***

CHILLS, spread from the neck of the bladder after urinating - ***sars.***

CLAWING, pain - led., mez., valer.

CLOGGED, urethra, by pieces of coagulated mucus - cann-s., graph., ***merc., sep.,*** uva.

COLD, agg., complaints after - acon., all-c., alum., ant-t., apis, ***calc.,*** calc-p., canth., ***colch.,*** cop., **DULC.,** ***eup-pur., ip., kali-c., kreos.,*** lyc., merc-c., nux-v., **PULS.,** rhus-t., **SARS.,** sep., ***sulph.,*** ter.

COLD, sensation in - lach., lyss., sabal., syzyg.
alternating with heat - coc-c.
extending to genitals - sabal.

COLDNESS, urethra - clem.
painful shoots, during - ***sulph.***

CONGESTION - acon., ars., canth., kali-bi., scop., solid., ter.

CONSTRICTING, pain - ***berb.,*** calad., calc-p., coc-c., con., lach., ***led.,*** lyc., ***mez.,*** nit-ac., ph-ac., plb., prun., ***sars.,*** valer., zinc.
constricting, bladder, neck of - ant-c., carb-s., coc-c., ***lyc., mez.,*** op., petr.
beginning to urinate, on - kali-i.
urination, after - sulph.

CONSTRICTION - alum., ***berb., cact.,*** caps., caust., chel., cocc., cub., dig., hydrc., lyc., petr., ph-ac., ***puls., sars.,*** thuj., verat.
afternoon - ***chel.***
urination. during - berb., bry., dig., petr., thuj.
before - ***chel.***
after - cub., ***nat-m.***
constriction, bladder, neck, of - ant-c., ***cact.,*** canth., caps., colch., con., elaps, kali-i., mag-p., ***op.,*** paeon., petr., phos., plb., ***ruta.,*** sulph.
morning - caps.
urination, during - colch., kali-i., petr., polyg.
after - bry., ***cann-s.,*** cub., sulph.
constriction, urethra - cann-s., ***clem.,*** lyc.
convulsive - berb.
extending, backward, while reflecting - nux-v.
extending, bladder, to - lyc., op., phos.
sensation, as if - arg-n., dig.
sensation, of, behind the glans - verat.
smarting - berb.
urination, during - ***apis,*** arg-n., bry., ***clem.,*** cop., dig., graph., nit-ac., nux-v., op., puls., stram.
after - cub.

CONTRACTING, urethra - bry., ***canth., chin., clem.,*** dig., indg.
urination, after - camph.

CONTRACTION, sensation of - ant-c., ***berb.,*** carb-s., coc-c., hyos., kali-i., ***lyc., mez.,*** op., petr., ruta., verat.
contraction, urethra - asar., ***canth.,*** carb-an., carb-v., ***chin., clem., cop.,*** dig., indg., nux-v., petr., phos., **PULS.,** stram., verat., zinc.
extending backward after urination - camph.
gonorrhea, suppressed - **PULS.**
internally - **CANTH.**
meatus - coc-c., thuj.
morning - carb-v.
erection, during - ***canth.***
stool and urination, before - ***nat-m.***
urging to urinate, with - ***nat-m.***
urination, during - bry., ***clem.,*** dig., indg.
after - ***nux-v.***

CRACKS, urethra, in meatus - ***nat-c., nit-ac.,*** phos., ph-ac., thuj.

CRAMP, in - ***berb., caps.,*** carb-s., ***carb-v.,*** coc-c., mag-p., ***nux-v.,*** ph-ac., plb., prun., ruta., ***sars.,*** sep., zinc.
causing him to bend double - prun.
night - prun.
urination, during - carb-s.
after - caust., ***nat-m.***
cramp, urethra - canth., chel., chin., clem., nit-ac., phos.

CRAMPING, pain, bladder, morning - alum.

CRAWLING, in - sep.
urination, after - ***lyc.***
crawling, urethra - agar., ambr., berb., chin., ferr-i., ign., junc., ***lyc.,*** merl., mez., ***petros., ph-ac.,*** ran-s., tarent., thuj., tus-p.
fossa navicularis - **PETROS.**
meatus - agar., puls., ran-s., staph.
sticking - ***mez.***
urinating, during - ign., petros., ph-ac.
after - canth., ***lyc.***
when not - ph-ac.

CUTTING, pain - ***aeth.,*** am-c., ***berb., canth.,*** caps., coc-c., ***coloc.,*** dig., eup-pur., ***kali-c.,*** lach., ***lyc.,*** mang., nux-v., ***puls.,*** **TER.,** thuj.
extending to urethra - ***berb.***
sitting, while - mang.
standing - mang.
stool, amel. - pall.
urination, during - calc., canth., dig., eup-pur., kali-c., ***nat-c.,*** polyg., sec., ***ter.,*** thuj.
after - calc-p., ***canth.,*** cub., nat-c., petr., phos., polyg.
before - bry., calc-p., dig., mag-p., ***manc.,*** ph-ac., phyt., sulph., thuj.
close of, at the - nat-c., petr., sars., thuj.
walking, agg. - mang., thuj.
open air, in, amel., rest agg. - **TER.**
cutting, bladder, neck, of - berb., **CANTH.,** caps., ***con., kali-c.,*** lach., lyc., mez., nux-v., op., petr., polyg., puls., ter.
extending through urethra - **CANTH.**
morning in bed - caps.
urination, during - canth., kali-c., polyg.
before - ***canth.,*** ph-ac.
before, beginning to urinate, on - manc., petr.
close of, at the - petr., sars., sulph., thuj.
walking in open air, while - mez., thuj.
cutting, urethra - anac., ant-c., arg-n., asc-t., aspar., ***berb.,*** bry., bufo, ***calc.,*** **CALC-P., CANTH.,** ***caps.,*** caust., ***chel.,*** colch., **CON.,** ***dig., equis.,*** eup-pur., fago., guai., hura, ***ip., kali-c.,*** kali-s., ***lach., lyc.,*** mang., ***merc.,*** mur-ac., nat-m., ***nit-ac.,*** nux-m., nux-v., ***op.,*** ph-ac., psor., puls., sars., ***sep., sulph.,*** ter., thuj., zinc.
anterior part - alum., colch., lach., lyc., nux-v., thuj., zinc.
urination, after - alum., coc-c., mez.
urination, after, and lancinating - coc-c.
urination, during - alum., cann-s., colch., nat-s., rhus-t.

cutting, urethra
emission, during - bor., con., nat-m.
after - nat-m.
evening, lying down, after - fago., gran.
extending, backward - arg-n., caps.
from within outward - plan.
to anus when passing last drops - arg-n., thuj.
flatus, while passing - lyc., mang.
forenoon - caps.
fossa navicularis, urination, after - **PETROS.,** thuj.
ineffectual urging, with - puls.
meatus - arn., bad., chel., cupr., iod., mez., nit-ac., par., ***zinc.,*** zing.
sitting, while - zinc.
urination, after - arg-n., coc-c., mez., nat-s.
urination, at the close - arn., nat-s., zing.
urination, during - aur-m-n., con., cupr., nat-a.
menses, before, when urinating - canth.
midnight - equis.
morning - alum., graph., merc.
motion, on - chel.
paroxysmal - eup-pur., kali-c.
posterior part - mur-ac.
extending to abdomen - lyc.
stool, during - mur-ac., ***sulph.***
after - staph.
before - mur-ac., sulph.
urinating, when not - berb., calc-p., caps., kali-c., mag-s., mang., nux-v., staph., thuj.
urination, during - alum., ant-c., arg-n., bor., bry., calc., ***cann-s.,*** **CANTH.,** caps., carb-s., carb-v., caust., chel., colch., **CON.,** cub., cupr., graph., ***guai.,*** hell., hep., iris, led., ***merc.,*** mur-ac., ***nat-m.,*** nat-s., ***nux-m.,*** op., ph-ac., ***phos., psor., puls.,*** rhus-t., sars., sil., ***staph., sulph.,*** sul-ac., ***thuj.,*** tril.
and, growing worse towards end of, even to last drop - ***merc.***
pressure in rectum, with - ph-ac.
stool, and - mur-ac.
urination, after - alum., ***berb.,*** calc-p., **CANTH.,** chel., coc-c., con., cub., dig., ***lyc.,*** **NAT-M.,** ***petros.,*** rhus-t., staph., ***sulph.***
urination, amel., glans penis, - canth.
urination, before - bry., calc-p., **CANTH.,** dig., merc., ph-ac., sel.
urination, beginning to urinate, on - iris, merc., petr., sec.
urination, close of, at - arg-n., clem., med., merc-ac., ***nat-m.,*** nit-ac., petr., ***sulph.,*** sul-ac., thuj.
walking, while - thuj.

CYSTITIS, inflammation of bladder - **ACON.**, all-c., am-c., ***ant-t.,*** **APIS,** ***arg-n., arn., ars.,*** aspar., ***bar-m.,*** **BELL.,** benz-ac., ***berb.,*** cact., ***calad.,*** calen., ***calc.,*** camph., ***cann-i.,*** cann-s., **CANTH.,** ***caps.,*** carb-an., ***caust., chim., chin-s.,*** colch., coloc., ***con., cop., cub., dig., dulc.,*** elat., **EQUIS.,** ***ery-a.,*** eucal., ***eup-pur.,*** ferr-ac., ferr-p., ***gels., hep., hydr., hyos.,*** kali-ar., kali-bi., kali-c., kali-chl., **LACH.,** lil-t., lith., **LYC., MED.,** ***merc., merc-c., nit-ac., nux-v., ol-sant.,*** pareir., petr., petros., ph-ac., pip-m., polyg., pop., prun., **PULS.,** ***rhus-t.,*** sabal., **SARS.,** ***sabin.,*** senec., seneg., **SEP.,** solid., squil., **STAPH.,** ***stigm.,*** stram., ***sulph.,*** tarent., **TER., THLASPI,** thuj., tritic., tub., uva., verat-v.

burning, shooting pain and increased gonorrhea, with - ***arg-n.,*** cann-s.

cantharis, from abuse of - apis, camph., canth.

cold, from taking - acon., ant-t., ***apis,*** canth., **DULC.,** lyc., op., **PULS.,** rhus-t., ***sulph.,*** ter.

catherer, after - acon., ***calen.,*** camph., canth., ***staph.***

chronic - ***ars.,*** bals-p., ***benz-ac.,*** berb., ***cann-s., canth.,*** carb-v., ***chim.,*** cob., coloc., ***cop.,*** cub., ***dulc., epig.,*** ery-a., eucal., ***eup-pur., fab.,*** grin., ***hydr.,*** iod., juni., ***kali-m.,*** lith., lyc., ***med., merc-c.,*** nit-ac., ***pareir.,*** pip-m., ***pop.,*** prun., ***puls.,*** rhus-a., ***sabal.,*** sant., seneg., ***sep.,*** silphu., **STAPH.,** ***stigm., sulph., ter.,*** thlaspi, thuj., tritic., ***tub., uva.***

fever, with, in strangury - ***acon.,*** bell., ***canth.,*** gels., hydrang., stigm.

gonorrhea, from - bell., benz-ac., ***cann-s., canth., cop.,*** cub., merc-c., puls., sabal.

injuries, after - ***arn.,*** **CALEN.,** canth., ***staph.***

menses, before and during - senec.

miscarriage, from - rheum., staph.

neck, of bladder inflammed - ***apis,*** aspar., ***canth., caps., chim., clem., cop., dig.,*** elat., hyos., ***merc-c., merc-i-r., nux-v., petros., puls., sars., senec.***

pus-like discharge after lithotomy, with - mill.

recurrent - canth., lyc., puls., sep., staph.

scarlatina, after - ***canth.***

suppression of menses or hemorrhoidal flow, after - ***nux-v.***

surgery, from, and during pregnancy - pop.

throbbing all over, with - sabin.

violent pain and almost clear blood, with - canth., ***nit-ac.***

cystitis, bladder, neck, of - ***apis,*** aspar., ***canth., caps., chim., clem., cop., dig.,*** elat., hyos., ***merc-c., merc-i-r., nux-v., petros., puls., sars., senec.***

CYSTOCELE - calen., staph.

DISCHARGE, urethra

acrid - **ARG-N.,** aur-m., caps., cop., kreos., **MERC-C.,** ***nat-m., petros.,*** sars.

albuminous - canth., nit-ac., petros.

DISCHARGE, urethra

bloody - ***arg-n.,*** bell., **CALC.,** cann-s., **CANTH.,** ***caps.,*** cop., cub., cur., kali-i., lith., lyc., ***merc., merc-c.,*** mill., ***mur-ac., nit-ac., psor., puls.,*** thuj., zinc.

diarrhea, in chronic - euph.

urethra painful to touch - caps.

urination, after - zinc.

cheesy - hep.

clear - brom., cann-i., cann-s., canth., cub., elaps, lyc., mez., ***nat-m.,*** nit-ac., petros., ph-ac., phos.

colorless - canth., ***nat-m.,*** nit-ac., petros.

cream-like - **CAPS.,** nat-p.

fetid - bar-c., ***benz-ac., carb-v., hep.,*** psor., puls., ***sil.,*** sulph., thuj.

flocculent, urination, after - kali-bi.

gleety - ***agar.,*** **AGN., ALUM., ALUMN.,** aur-m., bar-c., ***bar-m.,*** **BENZ-AC.,** ***bov.,*** bry., ***calad., calc., calc-p.,*** calc-s., ***cann-i.,*** cann-s., canth., ***caps.,*** carb-s., ***carb-v.,*** cedr., chim., ***cinnb., clem., cob., cop., cub.,*** cupr., dulc., erig., ery-a., ***ferr.,*** ferr-p., fl-ac., gamb., ***graph., hep., hydr., iris, kali-bi., kali-c.,*** **KALI-CHL., KALI-I.,** ***kali-s., lyc.,*** **MED.,** ***merc.,*** merc-c., ***mez.,*** mill., mur-ac., **NAT-M.,** ***nat-s., nit-ac., petr.,*** **PETROS.,** ***ph-ac., phos., phyt., plb., psor.,*** sang., **SEL.,** senec., **SEP., SULPH.,** tell., ***ter.,*** **THUJ.,** zinc.

impotency, with - agn.

morning - aur-m., ph-ac., phos., **SEP.**

night - ***fl-ac., sep.***

painless - ***agar., alum., arg-m.,*** bar-c., ***cann-s., cop., ferr., hep., hydr.,*** **KALI-I.,** ***med., merc., mez.,*** **NAT-M., NAT-S.,** petr., ***psor., puls., sang.,*** **SEP.,** ***sulph.,*** **THUJ.**

protracted - caps.

gluey - ***graph., kali-bi.***

gonorrheal - acon., ***agn.,*** aloe, ***alum., alumn.,*** am-m., ***anag., ant-c.,*** apis, ***arg-n.,*** ars., ars-s-f., aur-m., ***bar-m., bism., bor., calad., calc.,*** **CALC-S.,** cann-i., **CANN-S., CANTH.,** caps., ***caul., cedr., cham., chel.,*** chim., ***cinnb., clem.,*** **COCH.,** ***cob., cub.,*** cupr-ar., **DIG.,** dor., erig., ery-a., eucal., ***ferr-i.,*** **FERR-P.,** fl-ac., gels., ***hydr.,*** **KALI-CHL.,** ***kali-i., kali-s.,*** lac-c., lachn., led., **MED., MERC.,** ***merc-c., mez.,*** mill., ***nat-m.,*** **NAT-S., NIT-AC.,** ***pareir., petr.,*** **PETROS.,** ph-ac., ***phos., phyt., plb., psor.,*** **PULS.,** rhod., sabad., sabin., sars., senec., **SEP.,** ***sil.,*** still., ***sulph., tarent.,*** **TER., THUJ.**

chronic - ***alum., alumn., arg-m.,*** brom., **CALC., CALC-P., CALC-S.,** chim., **CHLOR.,** ***cinnb.,*** **COCH.,** cub., ***cupr., ferr.,*** hydr., ***kali-s., med., mygal., myric.,*** **NAT-M., NAT-S.,** ***petr., petros., plb., psor., sep., sil., sulph.,*** **THUJ.**

increase after having decreased - bry., lil-t., ***sep., sulph., thuj.***

night - ***merc.,*** merc-c., sep.

only - sep.

DISCHARGE, urethra

gonorrheal, syphilitics, in - **AUR-M.**, cinnb., merc., ***merc-c.***

gray - ***arg-m.***, bufo

greenish - ***bry., cinnb., cob.***, cop., ***hydr., kali-i.***, kali-s., **MERC**., ***merc-c., nat-m.***, **NAT-S.**, ***nit-ac.***, ter., **THUJ.**

chronic - ***cinnb., cob.***, kali-i., **NAT-S.**

night - **MERC**., merc-c.

thick - kali-i., ***merc.***, **NAT-S.**

yellow - anan., ***arg-m., cinnb., cob., cub.***, cur., ***hydr.***, kali-i., kali-s., lith., lyc., **MERC., NAT-S.**, nux-v., phyt., **PULS**., ***sep.***, ter., ***thuj.***

thick, with priapism - ***anan., nat-s.***, **PULS**.

jelly-like - ***kali-bi.***

milky - ***cann-s., caps., cop., ferr., iod., kali-c., kali-chl., lach., merc.***, **NAT-M.**, ***nux-v., petros.***, **SEP**.

pasty - canth.

sticky - ***nat-m.***, thuj.

urination, before - mez.

stool, after - ***iod.***

urination, after - cop., kali-c., lach., nat-m., petros., sep.

mucous - agar., ***agn.***, ant-c., ant-s., ***arg-n.***, bell., ***benz-ac.***, brom., bry., ***calc., cann-s., canth., caps.***, cedr., ***chim., clem., cob.***, con., ***cop., cub.***, dulc., **ELAPS**, ***ferr.***, ferr-p., ***graph., hep.***, hydr., kali-i., kali-s., lyc., mag-p., ***merc.***, merc-i-f., ***mez.***, nat-c., ***nat-m., nit-ac., nux-v., pareir.***, petr., petros., phos., rhod., sabin., sars., **SEP**., ***sulph., thuj.***

bloody - canth., **NIT-AC**., puls.

evening, chill, after a - ferr.

urination, after - nat-m., nit-ac., nux-v., ***ph-ac.***

gelatinous, urination, after - nat-m.

glutinous - ***agar.***, kali-bi., thuj.

milky white - ***kali-chl.***

moving about, on - mez.

relaxation of genitals, during - ***phos.***

urinating - phos.

at close of, - carb-v., nat-c.

urination, after - nit-ac.

viscid, urination, after - nit-ac.

purulent, urination, after - nux-v.

night - sep.

painless - ferr., nat-s., thuj.

persistent - alum., arg-m., kali-bi., phos., sulph.

urination, after - sars.

profuse - apis, arg-m., arg-n., ars-s-f., bufo, ***cann-i.***, chim., ***cop., cub.***, cur., ***ferr., hydr., kali-bi.***, **MED.**, ***petros., sep.***, **THUJ**.

purulent - agn., arg-n., ***arn., bar-c.***, bov., ***calc.***, **CALC-S.**, ***cann-s., canth., caps., carb-v., chel.***, chim., ***clem., con., cop., cub.***, cupr-ar., ip., ***kali-i., kali-s., led., lyc., med., merc., merc-c.***, nat-m., nat-s., **NIT-AC.**, nux-v., phos., ***ph-ac.***, psor., ***puls.***, sabad., ***sabin.***, sars., ***sil.***, sulph., ***thuj.***

drop of pus before urination - tus-p.

semen, like - puls.

DISCHARGE, urethra

slimy - cann-s., caps., cub., dulc., ***ferr.***, fl-ac., hep., ***merc., nat-m., nit-ac.***, puls., sulph., ***thuj.***

spotting linen - ***nat-m.***

stringy - kali-bi.

thick - ***alum.***, anan., ***arg-m.***, arg-n., ***cann-s.***, caps., ***clem., cub.***, ferr., ***hep., hydr., kali-bi., kali-i.***, med., ***merc., merc-c., nat-s.***, nux-v., ***psor., puls.***, sil., ***sulph.***, thuj.

thin - apis, caps., ***kali-s.***, lyc., med., merc-c., ***nat-m.***, nit-ac., nux-v.

gleety, with formication over body - cedr.

transparent - cann-s., mez., petros., phos.

viscid - agar., agn., bov., dig., ham., nit-ac., ***nux-v.***, ph-ac., phos.

watery - apoc., cann-s., canth., ferr-p., ***fl-ac., hydr., kali-s.***, lyc., merc., merc-c., ***mez., mur-ac., nat-m.***, ph-ac., phos., sumb., **THUJ**.

meatus glued up in morning with a watery drop - ***phos.***

moving about, on - mez.

silver nitrate, after injections of - nat-m.

painless - cann-s.

white - ant-ox., arg-n., cann-i., ***cann-s.***, canth., ***caps.***, chim., cinnb., cob., ***cop.***, cupr-ar., ***ferr., gels., iod., kali-c., kali-chl.***, lach., med., merc., ***mez.***, **NAT-M**., nit-ac., petr., ***petros.***, ph-ac., sars., **SEP**., sulph., thuj., zinc.

morning, prostatic discharge evening - ***ph-ac.***

white, chronic - caps., chim., cinnb., ferr., merc., merc-c., ***mez.***, **NAT-M**., nit-ac., ***sel., sep.***, sulph., thuj., zinc.

anemic subject, in - **CALC-P.**

impotence, with - ***agn., calad.***, cob.

and fetid urine - calad.

silver nitrate, after injection of - ***nat-m.***

urination, after - cop., lach., petros., sep.

yellow - agar., ***agn.***, **ALUM**., anan., **ARG-M**., ars-s-f., ***bar-c.***, bell., ***calc., calc-s.***, cann-s., ***canth., caps.***, con., ***cop., cub.***, cur., ***fl-ac., hep., hydr.***, kali-bi., ***kali-s.***, lyc., ***med.***, **MERC**., ***nat-m.***, **NIT-AC**., petr., petros., ***psor.***, **PULS**., sars., **SEL., SEP.**, sil., sulph., **THUJ**., tus-p., zing.

chronic - **ALUM**., ***alumn.***, **ARG-M**., ***calc-s., fl-ac.***, hep., hydr., lyc., ***med.***, merc., ***nat-m., psor.***, **PULS**., ***sel., sil.***

evening - lyc.

morning, drop - fl-ac., ***med.***

night - ***merc.***, zinc.

spots on linen - ***alum., nat-m., psor.***

yellowish-white - cann-i., sulph.

painless - cann-i.

DISTENDED, feeling - stict.

DRAGGING, pain - ***canth., chel.***, cop., dig., fl-ac., lact., ***lyc.***, mosch., nat-c., psor., sep.

hold urine, on attempting to - calc-p., lac-c.

lying, horse-back riding amel - ***lyc.***

morning - sep., sulph.

night, lying down, while - ***lyc.***

siesta, after - cycl.

DRAGGING, pain
suppression of urine, with - hyos.
urination, during - arg-n., cycl., op., rheum, ruta.
after - arund., bry., ruta., sulph.
dragging, urethra - arg-n., eup-pur., ***lyc.,*** ph-ac., sabad., sel., ter., til.
extending as far as the tip, in evening, during urination - sabad.
into bladder after urination - lyc.

DRAWING, pain - apis, ***berb.,*** calad., card-m., coc-c., dig., rhod.
neck, of - alum., berb., cop., jatr., mez., rhod.
riding in a carriage, while - agar.
sitting, while - card-m.
upward - calc-p., ***phyt.***
urination, during - calc-p., dig., phyt., rhus-a.
drawing, urethra - alum., arg-n., asar., ***berb.,*** bry., cahin., ***cann-s.,*** caps., carb-v., cic., colch., con., cop., fl-ac., gran., hipp., iod., ***kali-bi.,*** kali-c., lyc., ***merc., mez., petros.,*** ph-ac., phos., pic-ac., puls., sabad., sep., ***thuj.,*** zinc.
anterior part - bry., ***kali-c., lyc.,*** par., zinc.
evening, urination, after - am-c.
urinating, when not - bry., puls., zinc.
evening, urination during - seneg.
urination, after - am-c.
extending, from anus through urethra - hipp.
perineum into urethra - kali-bi.
to anus - ph-ac.
fossa navicularis - cic., ***petros.***
meatus - arg-n., cop., phos.
morning, urinating, after - carb-v.
waking, on - alum., carb-v., sep.
posterior part - lyc.
urination, after - nat-m.
urination, during - con.
walking, while - thuj.
in open air, on - mez.

DRIPPING, from urethra, sensation of - ambr., cedr., lact., **sel**.
urination, after - ***thuj.***
urination, burning, drops run along, after - arg-n., ***thuj.***

DROPS, came out of, sensation as if, rest agg. - sep.
drops, urethra, sensation, passed, as if a few - ambr., aspar., cedr., lact., petros., sel., sep., vib.
flowing along - lact., sel., staph., thuj.

DRYNESS, urethra, sensation of - alum., cop.

EMPTINESS, sensation of - colch., dig., ***stram.,*** sumb.
distended, when - lycps.
pain, with - calc-p.

ERUPTION, urethra, meatus, about - caps.

EVERTED, urethra, meatus - caps.

EXCORIATION of meatus, urethra - stann.

EXCRESCENCES, urethra - teucr.

FALLS, to side lain on, sensation as if - puls., ***sep.***
sensation as if, forward - nux-m., sep.

FULLNESS, sensation of - abrot., all-c., ***apis, arg-n., arn., ars.,*** bell., ***calad., chim.,*** coc-c., conv., cub., **DIG.,** eup-pur., **EQUIS.,** gels., guai., ***hell.,*** hep., ***kali-i.,*** lac-ac., lyc., lycps., med., merc., merc-c., ***nux-v., op.,*** ox-ac., pall., petr., phys., plb., ***puls., ruta., sep., staph.,*** stann., ***stram., sulph.,*** thuj., ***zinc.***
motion, up and down, with - ruta.
sensation, without - lac-d.
urination, after - alumn., calc., con., conv., **DIG.,** ***eup-pur.,*** gnaph., lac-c., ***lycps.,*** merc., ***ruta.,*** sars., staph., sulph.
scanty - pall.
without desire to urinate - **ARS.,** calad., **CAUST.,** fl-ac., hell., ***op.,*** pall., ***phos.,*** stann., ***stram.,*** verat.

ENURESIS, (see Bedwetting)

FUNGUS-LIKE, growths - ***calc., thuj.***
fungus-like, growth, urethra - **CALC.,** con., graph., lyc., thuj.

GANGRENE - canth.

GAS, passes from - ***sars.***

GNAWING, urethra, when not urinating - bov.

GONORRHEA, infection - acon., ***agn.,*** aloe, ***alum., alumn.,*** am-m., ***anag., ant-c.,*** apis, ***arg-n.,*** ars., ars-s-f., aur-m., ***bar-m., bism., bor., calad., calc.,*** **CALC-S.,** cann-i., **CANN-S., CANTH.,** caps., ***caul., cedr., cham., chel.,*** chim., ***cinnb., clem.,*** **COCH.,** ***cob., cub.,*** cupr-ar., **DIG.,** dor., erig., ery-a., eucal., ***ferr-i.,*** **FERR-P.,** fl-ac., gels., ***hydr.,*** **KALI-CHL.,** ***kali-i., kali-s.,*** lac-c., lachn., led., **MED., MERC.,** ***merc-c., mez.,*** mill., ***nat-m.,*** **NAT-S., NIT-AC.,** ***pareir., petr.,*** **PETROS.,** ph-ac., ***phos., phyt., plb., psor.,*** **PULS.,** rhod., sabad., sabin., sars., senec., **SEP.,** ***sil.,*** still., ***sulph., tarent.,*** **TER., THUJ.**
acute, urethral discharge, with - ***agn.,*** aloe, ***alum., alumn.,*** am-m., ***anag., ant-c.,*** apis, ***arg-n.,*** ars., ars-s-f., aur-m., ***bar-m., bism., bor., calad., calc.,*** **CALC-S.,** cann-i., **CANN-S., CANTH.,** caps., ***caul., cedr., cham., chel.,*** chim., ***cinnb., clem.,*** **COCH.,** ***cob., cub.,*** cupr-ar., **DIG.,** dor., erig., ery-a., eucal., ***ferr-i.,*** **FERR-P.,** fl-ac., gels., ***hydr.,*** **KALI-CHL.,** ***kali-i., kali-s.,*** lac-c., lachn., led., **MED., MERC.,** ***merc-c., mez.,*** mill., ***nat-m.,*** **NAT-S., NIT-AC.,** ***pareir., petr.,*** **PETROS.,** ph-ac., ***phos., phyt., plb., psor.,*** **PULS.,** rhod., sabad., sabin., sars., senec., **SEP.,** ***sil.,*** still., ***sulph., tarent.,*** **TER., THUJ.**
burning, shooting pain and increased, with - ***arg-n.,*** cann-s.
chronic, urethral discharge, with - ***alum., alumn., arg-m.,*** brom., **CALC., CALC-P., CALC-S.,** chim., **CHLOR.,** ***cinnb.,*** **COCH.,** cub., ***cupr., ferr.,*** hydr., ***kali-s., med., mygal., myric.,*** **NAT-M., NAT-S.,** ***petr., petros., plb., psor., sep., sil., sulph.,*** **THUJ.**
increase discharge after having decreased - bry., lil-t., ***sep., sulph., thuj.***

GONORRHEA, infection
night - ***merc.,*** merc-c., sep.
only at - sep.
suppressed, gonorrhea - ***acon.,*** agn., ant-t., aur., benz-ac., brom., ***calc.,*** **CANTH.,** ***chel., clem., coca,*** crot-h., dam., daph., graph., kali-i., kalm., **MED.,** merc., mez., **NAT-S.,** ***nit-ac.,*** phyt., psor., ***puls., sars.,*** sel., sep., sil., ***staph.,*** **SULPH., THUJ.,** verat., viol-t., ***x-ray,*** zinc.
syphilitics, in - **AUR-M.,** cinnb., merc., ***merc-c., nit-ac.***

HARD, node, urethra - alum., bov.
sensation, as if - cann-i.

HARDNESS, urethra - ***arg-n., clem., hyper.***
meatus, of - cann-s.

HEAT, in - ***all-c.,*** canth., ***puls., senec.***
heat, urethra - all-c., alum., aur-m., cact., canth., kali-bi., merc., rhus-t., sulph.
emission of semen, during - tarent.
sensation - alum.
voluptuous - canth.

HEAVINESS - bell., cann-s., ***canth.,*** coc-c., dig., kali-i., ***lyc., nat-m.,*** puls., **SEP.**
menses, during - nat-m.
heaviness, urethra - eup-per., sabad., til.

HEMORRHOIDS, of - acon., ant-c., bor., ***canth.,*** carb-v., euph., ***ham., nux-v., puls.,*** sulph.
bleeding - ars., **CALC.,** carb-v., ferr., ***ham.,*** lyc., merc., ***nit-ac.,*** nux-v.

HOT wire, in urethra, sensation, of - nit-ac.

INACTIVITY, of - acon., ***ars.,*** **CAUST.,** ***op.,*** plb.

INDURATION, cartilaginous - pareir.
induration, urethra, chronic - ***arg-n.,*** bov., calc-p., clem., hyper., merc-i-r., nit-ac.
whip cord, like - clem.

INFLAMMATION, (see Cystitis)
inflammation, urethra, (see Urethritis)

INSENSIBILITY - caust., ham., op., stann.

IRRITATION, urethra - bell., cact., chim., cub., ***clem.,*** helon., hydrc., ***lil-t.,*** pop., pyrus, **STAPH.,** stram.
meatus - kali-bi., kali-s.

ITCHING, bladder, in region of, with urging to urinate, agg. night - ***sep.***
neck of, itching - ign.
morning, in bed - ***nux-v.***
itching, urethra - acon., agar., alum., ambr., anac., ang., ant-t., apis, arg-n., arn., aur-m., bell., ***berb.,*** bov., ***cann-s.,*** canth., carb-s., caust., ***chim.,*** chin., clem., cocc., coc-c., coloc., con., cop., cub., ***ferr.,*** ferr-i., gins., graph., hydr., ign., indg., kali-c., kali-chl., laur., ***led.,*** lith., ***lyc.,*** lyss., merc., ***merc-c., mez., nat-m., nit-ac., nux-v.,*** ol-an., pareir., ***petr., petros.,*** rhus-t., sel., sep., sil., staph., **SULPH.,** ***sul-i.,*** tab., ***thuj.,*** tus-p., vesp., zinc.
afternoon - ferr.

itching, urethra
anterior part - ***arn., cann-s.,*** cocc., ferr-i., ***ign., laur.,*** lob., merc-c., nux-v., ***thuj.***
urination, when not - arn., euph., ***sulph.***
desire to urinate, with - coloc.
erections, during - nux-v., ***sel.***
evening - hydr., mez., sulph.
extending to bladder - ferr.
female - petr., ***sep.,*** thuj.
fossa, navicularis - agar., cic., ***clem.,*** cocc., colch., cub., ferr., gins., **PETROS.,** ***thuj.***
shooting, and, evening - sulph.
urination, after - ***colch.***
voluptuous - ***petros., thuj.***
gleet, with - ***nat-m., nit-ac., nux-v.,*** **PETR.**
gonorrhea, with - ***agar.,*** **MERC-C.,** ***nat-m., petr.,*** **PETROS.**
following - ***nit-ac.***
morning - arg-n.
preceding discharge of pus - con.
urination, during - agar., ***ambr.,*** arg-n., cop., graph., ***lyc., mez.,*** nat-m., ***nux-v.,*** ol-an., pareir., petr., rheum, sars., tab., thuj.
after - arg-n., arund., carb-an., canth., clem., colch., cop., lyc., lyss., nux-v., petr., tab., ***thuj.***
before - cop., ferr., nux-v., tab.
voluptuous - alum., ***ambr.,*** arg-n., carb-an., colch., ***thuj.***
itching, urethra, meatus - agar., alumn., ambr., arum-t., brom., cann-i., canth., **CAUST.,** chel., cic., ***clem.,*** **COC-C.,** colch., coloc., cop., gins., hydr., iod., kali-c., kali-n., lach., led., merc-c., ***nat-m.,*** petr., petros., plan., ran-s., samb., ***sulph.,*** syph.
evening - alumn., hydr., nat-m.
sex, after - nat-p.
touched, when - jac.
urging, during - anthro., petr.
after - clem., ***merc.,*** plan., verat.
before - nat-m.
constant - brom.
urging to urinate, as if - chel.
voluptuous - chlol., gins., led.
walking - nat-n.**JAR,** sensitive to - ***bell.***

JERKING, urethra - ***alum.,*** ambr., cann-i., ***cann-s., lyc.,*** nat-c., nat-m., nux-v., ***petr., phos.,*** pic-ac., ***sars., thuj.***
standing, while - cann-s.
urination, after - ***lyc.***
voluptuous formication in fossa navicularis - ***thuj.***

KNOTTY, urethra, sensation - alumn., ***arg-n.,*** bov., cann-s.

MENSES, ailments before and during - calc-p., ***canth.,*** cocc., ***gels.,*** hyos., mag-p., med., nux-v., plat., puls., pulx., ***senec.,*** sep., verat-v., vib.

MOISTURE, urethra, meatus - nat-m., phos.
glutinous - dig.
yellow stain, causing a - phos.

MOTION, in - alum., bell., lach., ruta., sep.
up and down - ruta.

MUCUS, urethra, clogged up with coagulated - cann-s., graph., ***merc.,*** sep.

NARROW, urethra, as if, too - ***arg-n.,*** bry., dig., graph., stram.

NUMBNESS, urethra - apoc., **CAUST.,** ***cedr.,*** kali-br., **MAG-M.,** nux-v., sars.
uneasy feeling - ***cedr.***

OBSTRUCTION, sensation of, neck, urinating, while - sulph.

OPEN, urethra, as if - cop.

PAIN, bladder - acon., aeth., agn., all-c., alumn., ambr., ant-t., aphis., ***apis,*** arn., ars., **BELL.,** benz-ac., ***berb.,*** brach., brom., ***cact.,*** calad., calc., calc-f., ***calc-p.,*** cann-i., cann-s., **CANTH.,** ***caps.,*** carb-an., ***carb-s., carb-v.,*** caul., ***caust., chel., clem.,*** coc-c., coloc., ***con.,*** cop., der., dirc., ***dulc.,*** elat., **EQUIS.,** ***ery-a., eup-pur., ferr.,*** ferr-ar., ferr-p., ***fl-ac.,*** gall-ac., ***hyos.,*** indg., ip., kali-bi., kali-br., lach., lil-t., ***lith., lyc.,*** merc., ***merc-c.,*** morph., naphtin., nat-a., nux-m., nux-v., pall., pareir., ph-ac., phos., phyt., pic-ac., piloc., ***plb.,*** polyg., ***pop.,*** prun., ptel., ***puls.,*** pulx., rhod., rhus-a., rhus-t., ruta., ***sabal.,*** sabin., sang., ***sars.,*** sep., ***staph.,*** stict., stigm., stry., sulph., sul-ac., sul-i., tarent., ter., thuj., tritic., ***uva.,*** verat., ***zinc.***
alternating, with pain in umbilicus - ter.
cold, from taking - caust., ***dulc., eup-pur.,*** puls., sulph.
coughing, when - caps., ip.
desire be postponed, if - lac-c., ***lac-ac.,*** prun., phos., ***puls.,*** ruta., sep., ***sul-ac.,*** tub.
distension, as from - anth.
drinking agg - ***canth.***
evening - ip., morph., pall., pic-ac., uva.
urination, after - sep.
extending to
back - sars.
kidney - ***aesc.,*** apis, ***canth.***
pelvis and thighs, after urination - puls.
spermatic cords - anth., clem., lith., puls., spong.
thighs - fl-ac., ***puls.***
uterus - merl., tarent.
flatus, from - kali-c.
jarring - **BELL.**
lithotomy, after - arn., ***calen.,*** **STAPH.**
lying, on abdomen, amel. - chel.
menses, during - **SEP.**
morning - alumn., cop., morph., sin-n.
moving, on - **BERB.**
up and down at every step after urination - ruta.
night - bell., carb-an., lyc., prun.
paroxysmal - ***caul.,*** chel., ***cop.,*** **PULS.**
pulsating - ***dig.***
rectum, with pain in - ambr.
resting amel. - con.
retarding urination - phos.
riding in a carriage - agar.
sex, after - ***all-c.***

PAIN, bladder
sitting, while - card-m.
standing agg. - ferr-p., puls.
turning over in bed, as if bladder would fall to side lain on - puls.
urging to urinate, during - berb., calc-p., eup-pur., hell., ***nux-v., phyt.,*** puls., rhod., rhus-t., ruta., sul-ac., zinc.
urinating, during - ant-t., brach., calc., calc-p., carb-v., dig., fl-ac., indg., lil-t., ***manc., phyt., puls.,*** rhus-a.
after - ***brach., canth.,*** caust., epig., lith., sep., uva.
after a few drops pass - berb., calc-p., **CANTH.,** ***caust.,*** fl-ac., lith.
amel. - coc-c., hedeo.
before - berb., ***fl-ac., lith.,*** manc., ***nux-v.,*** pall., ***phyt.,*** prun.
beginning - acon., ***apis, ars.,*** cann-s., **CANTH.,** ***cast.,*** **CLEM.,** cop., manc., **MERC.**
beginning, when urine starts he is amel - prun.
walking, on - acon., con., prun., ***puls.***
air, open in, amel. - ***ter.***
amel. - ign., ter.

pain, bladder, neck - acon., alum., ant-ox., apis, arn., **BELL.,** ***berb.,*** brach., cact., ***calc-p., cann-s., canth.,*** cham., ***cop.,*** con., ***dig., ferr-p.,*** guai., hyos., lith., lyc., lyss., mez., ***nux-v.,*** op., pic-ac., puls., ruta., sars., sep., spong., sulph., ter., ***zinc.***
attempting to urinate, on - ***cop.***
beginning to urinate, on - ***clem.***
close of urination - ***cann-s.,*** caust., con., dig., equis., med., ***puls.,*** ruta., **SARS.**
evening - lyss.
urging to urinate, on - anth., bell., berb., ***calc-p.,*** canth., dig., ferr-p., sep., spong.
urination, after - ***apis,*** apoc., cann-s., con., fl-ac., nux-v., petr., ***puls.,*** ruta., sars., sep., stann.
urination, before - canth., ***lith., nux-v.***
urination, when last drops are voided - med., sars.
walking, while - ign.

pain, urethra - ***agar.,*** agn., ***arg-n.,*** asc-t., bry., cann-i., cann-s., ***canth.,*** caps., ***card-m.,*** chel., ***ferr-i.,*** lith., lyc., ***med.,*** phos., ***prun., puls.,*** sabin., seneg., still., ***sulph., thuj.***
acute, urination, during - hep.
anterior part, urination, after - ran-s., rhus-t.
urination, during - nux-v., phos., rhus-t.
when not urinating - berb., bry.
backward along - arg-n., ***berb.,*** cann-s., canth., caps., fl-ac., merc-c., nux-v., phos., plan., psor., squil., sumb., thuj., zinc.
daytime - still.
down along - lyc., merc., phos., sulph.
emissions, from - cob., pip-m., sars.
morning on waking - carb-an.
erections, during - nit-ac.
after - cann-s.
evening - caust., seneg.
extending to abdomen - sars.

pain, urethra
flatus passing agg. - mang.
fossa navicularis, urination, before - bar-c.
paroxysmal - eup-pur., kali-c., op., prun.
riding agg. - staph.
standing, while - cob.
stool, before - sulph.
touch, on - caps., clem., nit-ac.
urging, to urinate, on - ***agar.,*** cocc., con., hyper.
urinating, when not - **BENZ-AC.,** ***berb.,*** bry., cedr., cocc., nux-v.
urination, during - ***aesc.,*** aran., bar-m., ***berb.,*** bov., ***calad.,*** ***cann-i.,*** ***cann-s.,*** **CANTH., CAUST.,** chel., ***cinnb.,*** colch., ***con., dor.,*** elaps, ferr-i., hep., lyc., med., ***op.,*** phos., plat-m., prun., sabad., senec., seneg., still., til., zinc., zing.
after - agn., bor., bov., brach., caust., ***nux-m.,*** nux-v., **PULS.,** stann., sulph.
close of, at - apis, arg-n., arn., ***berb.,*** ***cann-s.,*** canth., carb-v., caust., clem., con., dig., echi., ***equis.,*** kali-n., ***lith.,*** lyc., med., ***merc., mez.,*** **NAT-C.,** ***nat-m.,*** nat-s., nit-ac., petr., petros., ph-ac., phys., pic-ac., ***puls.,*** ruta, **SARS.,** spig., staph., sul-ac., sulph., thuj., zing.
urging to stool, with - aloe, alum., aphis., canth., cycl., dig., **NUX-V.,** prun., staph., sumb.
waking, on - carb-an., ***card-m.,*** sars.
wet, after getting - calc.
walking agg. - staph.

pain, urethra, meatus - ***bor., cann-s.,*** **CANTH.,** chel., clem., cop., nux-v., puls-n, rhod., ***sars.,*** zing.
after urinating - ***bor., lac-c., sars.***
extending backward - **CANN-S.,**
woman, in a - ***lac-c., sars.***

PARALYSIS - acon., agar., ***alum.,*** apoc., arg-n., ***arn.,*** **ARS.,** aur., ***bell., cact., camph.,*** cann-i., ***cann-s., canth., carb-an.,*** carb-s., carb-v., **CAUST.,** ***cic.,*** con., ***cupr.,*** dig., **DULC.,** ***equis.,*** eucal., ***ferr-m.,*** ferr-p., form., **GELS.,** hell., helon., ***hyos.,*** kali-p., ***lach., laur.,*** mag-m., ***merc.,*** morph., mur-ac., nat-p., **NUX-V., OP.,** phos., ***plb.,*** psor., ***puls., rhus-t., sec., sil.,*** staph., ***stram., stry., sulph.,*** tab., thuj., **ZINC.**
anxiety, with - ***cic.***
childbirth, after, no desire - **ARS.,** canth., **CAUST.,** ferr., ***hyos.,*** kreos., nux-v., phos., zinc.
daytime - thuj.
elderly people, in - **ARS.,** ***cann-s., cic.,*** con., ***equis., gels.,*** kali-p., ***sec.,*** thuj.
forcible retention seems to paralyze the - ***ars., canth.,*** **CAUST.,** ***gels.,*** hell., hyos., ***rhus-t., ruta.***
hysterical subjects, in - **ZINC.**
over-distension, after - ars., ***canth.,*** **CAUST.,** hell., hyos., ***nux-v., rhus-t., ruta.,*** stry., ***sulph.***
surgery, after - calen., op.

PARALYTIC, weakness - **CAUST.,** cod., ***morph.,*** op., ***sep.,*** **SULPH.**
neck, of - agar., atro., bar-c., cadm-s., canth., ***caust.,*** cub., op., sep., stram.
sphincter, of - agar., apoc., ars., ***bell.,*** canth., **CAUST.,** chlf., cic., ***dulc., gels., hyos.,*** ign., jug-r., lach., laur., nat-m., op., ***phos.,*** plan., puls., sulph., ***tab.,*** thuj., ***zinc.***

paralytic, weakness, sensation of, evening, so that he fears he will wet the bed - alum.

PINCHING, pain - am-m., ***berb.,*** lyc., mez., sep.
lying, while, with stitching - am-m.

pinching, urethra - carb-v., cinnb., kali-c., lyc., thuj.
meatus - cinnb., thuj.
urinating, when not - verat.
urination, before - nat-m.

POLYPS - ant-c., **CALC.,** con., graph., lyc., merc., phos., puls., sil., **TEUCR.,** ***thuj.***

PRESSING, pain, pressure in - **ACON.,** all-c., alum., am-c., am-m., ant-t., aphis., **APIS,** arn., ***aur.,*** bell., berb., bor., brach., ***calc., calc-p., camph.,*** cann-s., ***canth.,*** caps., carb-an., carb-s., ***carb-v., card-m.,*** chel., ***chim.,*** chin-a., coc-c., coff., colch., ***coloc., con.,*** cop., cub., cycl., dig., ***dulc., equis., eup-pur.,*** fl-ac., graph., hep., hyos., ign., ***kali-c.,*** kali-p., kali-s., kreos., lach., lachn., lact., laur., **LIL-T., LYC.,** med., merc-i-r., mosch., nat-c., ***nat-m.,*** nat-p., **NUX-V.,** ol-an., pall., petr., ***ph-ac.,*** pop., ***puls.,*** raph., rhus-t., ***ruta., sars.,*** **SEP.,** sil., spig., squil., ***staph., sulph.,*** tarent., thuj., til., verat., zinc.
coughing, when - caps., colch., ***ip.,*** kreos.
cramp-like - con.
cystitis, in - **LYC.**
eating, after - arn.
evening - puls., ***sep.***
ineffectual desire for stool, with - aphis.
lying, while - ***lyc.***
morning - puls., ***sep.***
10 a.m - all-c.
motion, agg. - nux-v.
night - ***bell.,*** carb-an., fl-ac., kreos., ***lyc.,*** phos., sulph.
retention, with - aur., ***bor., hyos., sars.***
riding horseback amel - lyc.
sitting, amel - bry., con., ign.
sitting, cross-legged, compelled to, amel - sep., zinc.
standing - arn.
stool, after, urging to - chin.
stool, before - ***carb-v., nat-m.,*** sulph.
urination, during - asar., berb., calc-p., ***camph., chim.,*** dig., dulc., ***hep.,*** hyos., ***lach.,*** lachn., lact., nat-c., ***nat-m.,*** **NUX-V.,** op., ph-ac., ***sil.,*** verat.
after - asar., berb., brach., ***calc-p., camph.,*** canth., chin., ***dig.,*** dulc., **EQUIS.,** lac-c., lith., merc., nat-m., ruta, sep., sulph., ***uva.***
after, deep in left side - calc-p.
amel. - spig.

PRESSING, pain
urination, before - ang., arn., calc-p., chim., ***chin.,*** con., graph., ***kali-s.,*** nat-p., ***nux-v.,*** petr., phyt., ***puls.,*** ruta., ***sep.,*** spig.
desire resisted, if - sep.
walking, while - bry., con., ign., phos., puls.
pressing, bladder, neck of - alum., apis, brach., ***canth.,*** carl., coc-c., jatr., ***nux-v.,*** sul-ac., ter., thuj.
hold the urine, on attempting to - lac-ac.
sex amel. - sul-ac.
sitting, agg. - ter.
stitches, with, walking agg., sitting amel - con., ign.
thighs together, must press - sul-ac.
urination, during - ign., rhus-a., stann., thuj.
after - con., nat-m., ruta., uva., stann.
before - apis, arn., calc-p., chim., ***nux-v., phyt., puls.***
walking in open air, while - con., ign., nux-v., puls.
pressing, urethra - agn., aphis., bry., colch., cop., ***dulc.,*** graph., ***lach.,*** lyss., nux-v., petros., ***ph-ac.,*** puls., teucr., thuj., til.
evening, urination during - seneg.
meatus - chel., nux-v., puls.
when not urinating - nux-v.
urination, during - dig.
after - brach., ***puls.,*** stann.
between the acts of - nux-v.
voluptuous, extending to anus - sulph.

PRICKING, pain, urethra - cann-i., iris.
urination, before - ***nux-v.***
pricking, urethra, meatus - coloc., cycl., ***nit-ac.,*** rhod.

PROLAPSE - hyos., pyrus, ***sep.,*** staph.

PULSATING, urethra urinating, when not - cop.

PULSATION - berb., canth., ***dig.,*** epig.
neck, of - epig.
urination, before - ***dig.***
pulsation, urethra - benz., brom., canth., chin., cop., dulc., merc., **MERC-C.,** petr.
fossa navicularis, sharp, and beating - thuj.

RASPING, urethra, urination, during - carb-v., lyc., mag-c., nit-ac., phos., sep.

RAW, urethra, sensation - ph-ac.

REDNESS, urethra, meatus - cact., cann-s., cinnb., cub., cupr-ar., ***gels., hep., led.,*** nit-ac., petr., ***sulph.,*** thuj.
meatus, spots - bry.

RETENTION, of urine - **ACON.,** aesc., agar., all-c., alum., **AM-C.,** ant-t., **APIS,** ap-g., ***apoc.,*** arg-m., **ARN., ARS.,** ***ars-i.,*** aspar., atro., aur., ***bar-c.,*** bar-m., **BELL.,** bism., ***bor.,*** bufo, ***cact., calc.,*** calc-s., ***camph., cann-i., cann-s.,*** **CANTH.,** ***caps.,*** carb-s., card-m., **CAUST.,** chel., ***chim.,*** chin., chin-a., ***cic.,*** cimic., cinnb., ***clem.,*** coc-c., coch., ***colch., coloc.,*** **CON.,** cop., ***crot-h., cupr., dig.,*** dios., ***dulc.,*** elaps, erig., ***euph.,*** **GELS.,** graph., ***hell.,*** helon., ***hep., hyos.,*** hyper., ign., ***iod., ip.,*** iris, kali-ar., ***kali-chl.,*** kali-i., kreos., ***laur.,*** led., **LYC.,** ***mag-p.,*** mag-s., merc.,

RETENTION, of urine - merc-c., merc-cy., mez., morph., mur-ac., ***nit-ac.,*** nux-m., **NUX-V., OP.,** ox-ac., **PAREIR.,** petr., ph-ac., phos., ***phyt., plb., polyg., prun., puls.,*** ran-s., ***rhus-t.,*** ruta., ***sabin., sars., sec.,*** sep., sil., stann., ***staph., stigm., stram., sulph.,*** sul-ac., **TARENT., TER.,** ***thuj.,*** trinit., tub., urt-u., ***verat., zinc.***
air, from exposure to cold - ***caust.***
atony of fundus, from - ter.
beer, after - ***nux-v.***
birth, at - ***acon.,*** apis.
children, in - ***acon.,*** **APIS,** ***art-v.,*** bell., ***benz-ac., calc., caust., cop., dulc.,*** eup-pur., ferr-p., ***gels.,*** ip., ***op.***
every time child catches cold - **ACON.,** cop., ***dulc.,*** puls., sulph.
child, cries all night from retention - acon., apis.
chill, in - apis, arn., canth., hyos., lyc., op., puls., stram.
cholera, in - ***camph., canth.,*** carb-v., lach., op., **VERAT.**
chronic - ***calc., iod.***
clots, in the bladder, from - cact., caust.
in the vagina, from - coc-c.
cold, from catching - ***acon., caust., cop., dulc.,*** gels., ***puls.,*** rhus-t., sulph.
exposure to, and wet, from - ***acon., dulc.,*** gels., rhus-t.
standing on cold pavement - ***calc.,*** carb-v.
colic - arn., ***coloc.,*** **PLB.,** thuj.
confinement, during - plb.
after - ***arn.,*** **ARS.,** ***bell.,*** canth., **CAUST.,** ***equis., hyos.,*** ign., lyc., ***nux-v., op., puls.,*** rhus-t., sec., sep., stann., ***staph.,*** stram.
contraction of sphincter, sensation as if urine retained by - sulph.
coughing, on, sensation of retention with urging - ip.
dysentery - **ARN.,** merc.
elderly men - chim., dig., morph., ***solid.,*** zinc.
evening - bor.
exertion, after - **ARN., CAPS., RHUS-T.**
fever, from acute illness - acon., apis, ferr-p., op.
fright, after - acon., **OP.**
headache, in - con.
hysteria, in - ign., **ZINC.**
illness, in acute - ferr-p., lyc., op.
infants, in new born - **ACON.,** ***apis,*** arn., ***ars.,*** benz-ac., ***camph., canth., caust.,*** erig., hyos., ***lyc., op.,*** puls.
newborn, fails to urinate - acon., arn.
inflammation, from - ***acon.,*** apis, cann-i., ***canth.,*** nux-v., puls.
injuries, after - arn., calen.
locomotor ataxia - ***arg-n.***
menses, during - ham., kali-bi.
music amel. - tarent.
night, 3 to 6 a.m - pareir.
pain, in abdomen, when - cham.

RETENTION, of urine
painful - acon., ***arn.***, ars., ***aur.***, bell., bor., calc-p., **CANTH.**, caps., **CAUST.**, cop., crot-h., cupr., ***dulc.***, ***lyc.***, ***nit-ac.***, **NUX-V.**, ***op.***, ***pareir.***, ***puls.***, sabin., ***sars.***, sul-ac., ***ter.***
urging, with, while lying on the back - ***puls.***
painless - nit-ac.
paralysis, from - ***caust.***, dulc., hyos., nux-v., ***op.***, ***plb.***, stry.
paraplegia, with - apoc.
pregnancy, in - equis., hep.
presence of others, in - **NAT-M.**
prostate, from enlarged - ***apis***, bell., benz-ac., ***cact.***, canth., ***chim.***, con., **DIG.**, ferr., hyos., kali-i., merc-d., pareir., ***puls.***, sep., **STAPH.**, stram.
puerperal - acon., ***arn.***, ***bell.***, equis., ***hyos.***, ***op.***, staph., stram.
sitting bent backwards amel - ***zinc.***
sleepiness, with - ter.
suppressed eruptions or discharges, from - camph.
surgery, from - calen., caust.
unable to pass urine in presence of company - **NAT-M.**
urging, without - ***ars.***, ***caust.***, phos., plb.
water, noise of running, amel. - hyos., lyss., tarent., zinc.
wet after getting feet - ***all-c.***, ***rhus-t.***
whistling amel. - cycl., tarent.

retention, of urine, sensation of, urination, after - berb., hep.
retained by contraction of sphincter - bell., cact., camph., canth., ***hyos.***, lyc., ***nux-v.***, op., puls., rhus-t., stram., sulph., thlaspi

RHEUMATIC, affections, bladder - clem., dulc., merl.

SHARP, pain - acon., ant-t., aur., ***berb.***, calad., canth., carb-s., ***chel.***, ***clem.***, coc-c., coloc., ***con.***, ***kali-c.***, kali-p., kali-s., ***lith.***, ***lyc.***, ***nat-m.***, pall., rhus-t., sabad., ***sulph.***, thuj.
alternating between bladder and rectum - coloc.
cough, during - ***caps.***
dinner, after - nux-v.
extending, to kidneys - coc-c., oci.
to urethra - am-m., berb., carb-s., cycl., dig., phos., thuj.
lying, while - am-m.
respiration, during - aur.
sitting amel - con.
stool, during - gamb.
urging to urinate, when - canth., rhus-t.
ineffectual urging - ***guai.***
urination, during - carb-s., ***nat-m.***, sep.
after - bufo.
before - apis, ***lith.***, ***manc.***, puls., sep.
beginning to urinate, on - ***manc.***
walking, while - con., nat-m.

sharp, bladder, neck, of - acon., ant-t., ***bell.***, berb., ***calc-p.***, ***canth.***, caps., ***carb-s.***, ***cham.***, chel., con., dig., ***guai.***, jatr., ***lith.***, ***lyc.***, ***op.***, ***puls.***, ***stry.***, sulph., ***thuj.***
afternoon - sulph.
anus, and - lyc.
coughing, when - ***caps.***
desire be delayed, if - prun.
evening - phos.
extending to end of penis - dig., phos., stry.
ineffectual effort to urinate, after - ***guai.***
lying on face amel. - chel.
morning - sulph.
sitting, amel. - ***con.***
urinating, when not - ***cham.***
urination, during - carb-s., sulph.
after - con., dig., guai.
before - apis, ***canth.***, dig.
walking agg. - con.

sharp, urethra - acon., agar., alum., ant-t., ***apis***, arg-m., ***arg-n.***, arn., asaf., asar., asc-t., aspar., aur., ***bell.***, ***berb.***, bor., bov., brom., bry., ***calad.***, ***calc.***, ***cann-i.***, cann-s., ***canth.***, ***caps.***, chel., ***chin.***, chlf., cic., ***clem.***, cocc., coc-c., colch., coloc., con., crot-t., cupr., cycl., dulc., equis., ***hep.***, ign., indg., jatr., kali-p., ***lach.***, ***lyc.***, mang., ***merc.***, ***merc-c.***, mygal., nat-c., nat-m., nit-ac., nux-v., pall., par., petr., ***ph-ac.***, phos., plan., psor., ***sars.***, ***sep.***, sil., squil., stry., **SULPH.**, sumb., ***thuj.***, til., viol-t., zinc.
afternoon - thuj.
anterior, part - bell., bry., cann-s., ***caps.***, chel., cic., coc-c., cycl., euph., ign., ***lach.***, lyc., mag-c., ***merc.***, merc-c., nit-ac., pall., ***par.***, phos., sil., **SULPH.**, thuj.
urinating, when not - asaf., cann-s., ***caps.***, euph., ***merc.***, teucr.
urination, after - coc-c.
burning - agar., cann-s., merc., nit-ac., spig.
urination, during - cop.
cutting - ***calc.***, coc-c., ***lach.***, lyc., sars.
ineffectual desire to urinate, with - ***calc.***
drawing, when not urinating - merc.
dull - cic., merc.
shooting, on quiet emission of flatus - mang.
urinating, when not - viol-t.
erections - cann-s., clem., ***nit-ac.***, thuj.
evening - ***calad.***, canth., mez., nit-ac., sulph., thuj.
extending, abdomen, towards evening - merc.
anus, to - arg-n., canth., nux-v.
anus, to morning, urinating, after - thuj.
backward - berb., canth., con., **MERC-C.**, ***nux-v.***, plan., psor., squil., sulph., sumb., zinc.
bladder, to - berb.
forward, to - arg-m., arg-n., aspar., bell., berb., clem., dulc., jab., nat-c., nat-m., plan., sars., thuj., zinc.
forward, urinating, when not, urinating amel. - thuj.
forward, urination, after - sars.
glans, to - asar., equis., lyc., pall.

sharp, urethra
extending, hypogastrium, to - alum., sulph.
meatus, to - bell., brom., con.
meatus, to, from root of penis after urination - sars.
fine - agar., bry., nat-m., par.
fine, meatus - aspar.
flatus, after - lyc.
when passing - ***mang.***
forenoon - caps.
fossa navicularis - acon., ***caps.,*** chel., ***cic.,*** coc-c., gins., merc., nat-m., ***petros.,*** squil., sulph., thuj.
urination, on - acon.
itching, with, when not urinating - euph.
jerking - con.
morning - cimic., seneg., sumb.
motion, on - bell., chel.
night, erections, during - thuj.
rigors, with - sulph.
sex, after - calc., nat-m.
sitting - plan., thuj.
passing flatus, while - ***mang.***
splinter-like - ***arg-n.,*** coloc., ***nit-ac.***
standing, on - aur-m., cann-s.
stinging, gonorrhea, with - **MERC.,** ***mez.***
sex, during - calc.
stool, during - coloc., ol-j., ***nat-c.,*** squil.
sudden, sitting agg. - plan.
synchronous, with pulse - con., dulc.
tickling - calc.
twinging, like lightning, from before backward - ***berb.,*** zinc.
twitching, when not urinating - thuj.
urging, with - agar., cahin., cann-i., calc-p., ***canth., caps., phos.,*** spig., sulph.
urinating, when not - bell., bry., ***calc-p., cann-s., caps., cham.,*** coff., cop., euph., **MERC.,** ***nat-m., nux-v.,*** ph-ac., sep., ***sulph.,*** teucr., thuj., til.
urination, during - **CANN-I., CANN-S.,** caps., chel., chin., ***clem.,*** coc-c., cupr., cycl., equis., ***graph.,*** iris, mag-c., merc., merc-c., mygal., nat-c., nux-v., petr., ***puls.,*** seneg., ***sulph.,*** thuj.
after - apis, arn., ***berb.,*** **CANN-I.,** caps., con., kali-bi., led., merc., mur-ac., nat-c., nat-m., rhod., seneg.
after, and after sex - nat-m.
before - aspar., ***cann-i.,*** **CANN-S.,** coc-c., nat-c., nux-v., thuj.
before, urging, when - thuj.
close, of - ph-ac.
walking, while - acon., bell., chel., ign.
walking, open, air, in - alum., merc-c.

sharp, urethra, meatus - acon., aesc., agar., asc-t., **ASPAR.,** aur-m-n., bad., ***berb.,*** brom., cann-i., cann-s., caps., chel., cic., clem., coc-c., con., iod., kali-bi., led., mang., mez., nat-m., nat-s., **NIT-AC.,** pareir., ph-ac., psor., rhod., squil., sulph., thuj., zinc.
copious urine, with - agar.
evening - canth., rhod.
night - canth.

sharp, urethra, meatus
urinating, when not - cann-s., ***caps.,*** mang., thuj.
urination, during - cupr.
after - caps., mur-ac., pareir., verat.

SHOCKS, electric, extending to right thigh - fl-ac.

SMARTING, pain - apis, berb., ***canth.,*** eup-pur., phos.
extending to meatus - ***chim.***
standing agg - ***eup-pur.***
walking, while - phos.

SORE, pain - acon., ***all-c.,*** apis, arn., ***ars., bell., benz-ac.,*** berb., brach., ***calad., calc-p.,*** cann-s., **CANTH.,** ***carb-v., chim.,*** coff., dirc., **EQUIS.,** erig., eup-pur., lac-ac., lac-d., ***lith.,*** lycps., ***merc.,*** nat-a., ***puls., sars., sec., sep.,*** squil., sulph., **TER.,** thuj., uran-n.
motion agg - ***bell.,*** berb., ***canth.***
neck, of - ***atro.,*** brach., ***calc-p., carb-v., nux-v., puls.***
neck, urination, after - calc-p.
urination, during, agg - nat-a., puls.
after amel - nat-a.
profuse, with - stict.

sore, urethra - apis, ***arg-n., berb., cann-s., canth., caps., clem.,*** cop., cupr., ***ferr., hep., hyper.,*** ign., ***lach., med.,*** merc., mez., ***nat-m., nit-ac.,*** phys., ***prun.,*** ptel., sep., teucr., thuj., til., zinc.
erection, during - canth.
fossa navicularis - nux-v.
meatus - ***arg-n., bor.,*** bry., ***chin.,*** clem., cop., equis., nux-v., puls., stann.
sex, after - ***bor.,*** casc.
pressure agg. - mez., nat-m.
urinating, when not - teucr., zinc.
urination, during - ***apis,*** bov., brach., calc., canth., carb-an., cinnb., ***cinnam.,*** colch., daph., ***ferr.,*** ferr-i., hep., ign., ***lyc., mez.,*** nit-ac., nux-v., sil.
after - ***arg-n.,*** bor., lil-t., nux-v.

SPASM - ***ant-t.,*** asaf., ***bell.,*** berb., calad., ***calc., canth., caps.,*** caul., chim., chin., ***coc-c., cop.,*** dig., eup-pur., ***gels.,*** guar., hell., hydr., ***ip., nux-v.,*** op., ***ph-ac., prun., puls., sars., sep.,*** tarent., ter., uva., ***vib.,*** zinc.
surgery, following, on orifice - ***bell.,*** calen., coloc., ***hyper.***
urination, during - ***asaf.,*** cann-s., carb-s., colch., op.
after - asaf., ***prun.,*** puls.
before - manc., uva.

spasm, bladder, neck, of - arg-n., **ARN.,** cact., cann-s., ***colch.,*** cop., hyos., kali-br., mag-p., ***prun.,*** puls., ruta.
night - prun.
sexual excesses, after - ***nux-v.***
spasmodic stricture - mag-p., ruta.

spasm, urethra - nit-ac., prun.
spasm, without fissure of rectum - nit-ac.

SPASMODIC, pain - alum., ***berb., canth.,*** caps., ***caul., chel.,*** coc-c., cop., ph-ac., prun., ter.
action of - calc-p., tarent.

SPASMODIC, pain
extending to chest - alum.
morning - ***cop.***
night - prun.
spasmodic, bladder, neck, of - jatr., phos.
closure at - cann-s., caust., con., dig., med., ***puls.***, ruta., ***sars.***
extending to thighs, after urination - ***puls.***

STABBING, pain, region of - ***chel.***

STICKING, pain, urethra, urinating, when - camph., cann-s., caps., chel., clem., iris, nat-c., ***nux-v.***

STINGING, pain, urethra - ***apis,*** bov., cann-s., erig., sabal., sars., staph., thuj.

STONE, in, sensation - puls., **SEP.**
stone, in, sensation, urethra, as of a - coc-c.

STONES, bladder, calculi - ant-c., arg-n., **BENZ-AC., BERB.,** cact., **CALC.,** ***calc-renal.,*** **CANTH.,** card-m., ***chin., coc-c.,*** colch., ***eup-per., lach., lith.,*** **LYC.,** mez., ***mill.,*** naja, nat-m., nat-s., ***nit-ac., nux-m., nux-v., pareir., petr., phos., puls., raph., ruta.,*** **SARS., SEP.,** ***sil.,*** tarent., thuj., zinc.
calculi, deposits - vario.
surgery for, after - ***arn.,*** **CALEN.,** cham., chin., cupr., mill., nux-v., **STAPH.,** verat.

STRAW thrust, back and forth, urethra, sensation, as if - dig.

STRICTURE, urethra - acon., agar., ant-t., ***apis, arg-n.,*** arn., bell., ***berb., calc.,*** calc-i., ***cann-s.,*** **CANTH.,** ***chim.,*** chin., cic., cinnb., **CLEM.,** ***con., dig., dulc.,*** eucal., ***graph., indg., iod., kali-i.,*** lob., ***merc., nat-m.,*** nat-s., **NIT-AC.,** op., **PETR.,** ***petros.,*** phos., **PULS.,** sep., ***sil., sul-i., sulph.,*** tarent., thios., thuj.
alcoholics, in - op., sec.
dilatation, after - ***calen.,*** mag-m.
gonorrhea, after - sul-i.
sensation of - bry., coc-c., dig., graph., thuj.
spasmodic - ***acon.,*** apis, ***bell.,*** berb., camph., **CANTH.,** carb-v., ***cic., clem.,*** con., cop., ***dios.,*** ery-a., eucal., ***gels.,*** hydrang., indg., **NIT-AC.,** ***nux-v., op.,*** petros., ph-ac., ***plb., prun., sec.,*** stram.
morning - carb-v.

SUPPURATION - ***canth.,*** sars., ter.

SWELLING - apoc., atro., bell., chlor., dig., kali-bi., ***kali-i.,*** merc-c., op., ox-ac., petr., plb., tarent.
bladder, neck, of - **APIS,** ***puls.***
swelling, urethra - alum., ***arg-n., canth., cop.,*** gran., led., ***merc., merc-c.,*** **MIT.,** nit-ac., op., ph-ac., ***rhus-t., sulph.,*** **THUJ.**
anterior part - ***merc.***
meatus - acon., alum., arg-n., cann-i., **CANN-S.,** canth., ***cop.,*** gels., hep., jac., led., ***merc., nit-ac., ol-sant.,*** ph-ac., phos., **SULPH., THUJ.**
swelling, urethra, sensation of - ***arg-n.,*** cann-s., card-m., led., nit-ac., rhus-t., til.

TEARING, pain - ***kali-c.,*** berb., bry.
tearing, bladder, neck, of - canth., ***kali-c., nux-v.***
pressing during urination, when - ***kali-c.***
urination, during - kali-c., ***nux-v.***
tearing, urethra - alum., arg-n., ars., aur., ***bry.,*** calc., **CANN-S.,** clem., ***colch.,*** coloc., ign., ***kali-c.,*** kali-i., ***mez., nat-c.,*** **NUX-V.,** ***ruta., sars.,*** sep., ***sulph.,*** thuj., zinc.
afternoon, when seated - ign., thuj.
anterior part - ambr., ant-t., clem., coff., kali-c., sep., thuj., zinc.
urinating, when - aur.
urinating, when not - bry., zinc.
erection, during - agar., cann-s., canth., mur-ac.
extending forward - zinc.
goes through the body, when urinating, that - jac.
meatus - kali-c., lyc., pareir., zinc.
female - berb.
morning, after urination - carb-v.
shooting, and, ascending through hypogastrium, when walking in open air - alum.
urinating, when not - bry., ***clem., helon.,*** ign., kali-c., nux-v., zinc.
urination, during - aur., ***carb-v.,*** cur., nat-c., **NUX-V.,** ***ruta.,*** sulph.
after - ars., carb-v., tarent.
from root of penis to glans - sars.
walking in open air - alum.
zig-zags - ***cann-s., sars.***
toward hypogastrium, when walking in open air - alum.

TENEMUS, ineffectual straining to urinate - ***acon.,*** **AGAR.,** ***alum.,*** am-c., am-m., anac., ***ang., ant-c., apis, arn.,*** **ARS.,** aur-m., ***bell.,*** calc., ***camph.,*** cann-i., ***cann-s.,*** **CANTH.,** ***caps.,*** carb-s., caust., ***chim., clem., coc-c.,*** colch., ***coloc.,*** cop., crot-h., cub., ***cupr.,*** **DIG.,** dulc., elaps, epig., ery-a., ***equis.,*** eug., ***eup-pur.,*** ferr., ferr-ar., ferr-i., ferr-p., ***gels.,*** hydrang., hyos., ***ip., lach.,*** **LIL-T.,** ***lith., lyc., med., merc.,*** **MERC-C.,** ***mez.,*** morph., ***mur-ac.,*** nat-c., ***nit-ac., nux-m.,*** **NUX-V.,** ol-an., ***onis.,*** op., **PAREIR.,** phos., phys., plan., **PLB.,** ***podo.,*** polyg., pop., **PRUN.,** psor., **PULS.,** rheum, ***rhus-t.,*** sabad., ***sabal.,*** sabin., ***sars., senec.,*** sep., ***sil.,*** squil., staph., ***stigm.,*** sulph., tarent., **TER.,** tax., **THUJ.,** ust., uva., verat., viol-t.
after - canth.
evening, walking in open air - ***lith.***
forenoon - agar., phos.
icy, cold feet, with - ***elaps.***
lying, down agg - lyc.
menses, during - **TARENT.**
morning - par., ***senec.***
4 a.m - am-m.
night - ant-c., lith., ***merc.***
pregnancy, during - ***bell., canth., caust.,*** equis., ferr., nux-v., pop., ***puls.,*** staph.
rectum, with - canth., caps., erig., merc-c.
sitting, while - ter.
stool, during - ***alum.,*** canth., **CAPS.,** lil-t., ***merc-c.,*** **NUX-V.,** ***rhus-t., staph.***

TENEMUS,
urination, during - med.
after - ang., alum., ferr., squil.
vomiting, purging and urination - **CROT-H.**

TENSION - ACON., ant-t., coc-c., eup-pur., nux-v., phos.
tension, urethra - **bor.,** junc., lyc., phos.
erections, during - **CANN-S., CANTH.**

THICKENING, walls of - dulc., pareir.

TINGLING, urethra - apoc., ***clem.,*** cupr-ar., ***petros.,*** sep., staph.
fraenum, culmination at - ***clem.***
meatus - agar., anag., cann-i., clem., coc-c., ***petros.,*** plat., sep., staph.
sitting - staph.
urination, during - petros.

TRICKLING, urethra - arg-n., kali-bi., petros., staph., thuj.

TUMORS - ***calc.,*** thuj.
tumor, urethra, small - lach.
vascular - cann-s., ***eucal.***

TWINGING - ter.
twinging, urethra - arg-n., ***cann-s.,*** carb-v., clem., lyc., ***sel.,*** zinc.
extending from behind forward - sel.
meatus - berb., zinc.
during a bath - bart.
standing - clem.

TWISTING, neck - coc-c.
sensation - agar., bell.

TWITCHING, pain - agar., lith., op
neck, of, during urination - op.
twitching, urethra - alum., ambr., ant-s., ***cann-s., canth.,*** clem., coc-c., kali-chl., nat-c., nux-v., petr., ***phos.***
anterior part - coc-c.
seminal vesicles to glans penis - ***mang.***
ejaculation of semen, as if - petr.
urinating, when not - phos., thuj.

ULCERATION - all-s., canth., ***eup-pur., merc-c.,*** merc-i-r., petr., **PULS.,** ran-b., sep., ***sulph.***
stones, calculi, caused by - all-s.
symptoms of - ***hydr.***
ulceration, urethra - canth., **NIT-AC.**
chancres - ***arg-n.,*** **NIT-AC.**
meatus - abrot., eucal., lac-c., **MERC-C., NIT-AC.**
sticking, with - **NIT-AC.**
urine retained, with sensation as if - canth.
ulcerative, urethra, ulceration, as from sub-cutaneous - arg-n., lac-c., ***nit-ac., rhod.***
urination, during - arg-n.
between acts of - ***arg-n., prun.***

UNCONSCIOUS, urethra insensible - ail., ***apis,*** apoc., **ARG-N., CAUST.,** cedr., chlol., ***cupr.,*** grat., hell., kali-br., **MAG-M.,** mag-s., merc., nux-v., ***sars.***
mania, in - **CUPR.**
urine and stool - aloe, arn., bell., ***mur-ac.,*** psor., ***rhus-t.,*** sulph.

UNEASY feeling, urethra - cedr.

URETHRITIS, inflammation, urethra - ***acon.,*** apis, **ARG-N.,** ***ars., aur.,*** bov., ***cact.,*** camph., **CANN-S., CANTH.,** caps., caust., ***chim., cop., cub.,*** dor., ***gels.,*** gran., ***hep.,*** kali-bi., ***kali-i.,*** **MED.,** ***merc-c., nux-v.,*** pareir., ***petr., petros., sabin., sulph.,*** tab., **TER.,** teucr., **THUJ.** yohim.
burning, shooting, pain and increased gonorrhea, with - ***arg-n.,*** cann-s., canth., med.
meatus - alum., bov., ***calc.,*** calc-p., cann-i., **CANN-S.,** canth., ***cop.,*** erig., eup-pur., ***hep.,*** jac-c., kali-bi., led., ***med.,*** nat-m., ***nit-ac.,*** pareir., ph-ac., rhus-t., **SULPH.,** tab., ***thuj.***

URGING, to urinate, (see Tenesmus) - ***acon.,*** aesc., agar., alf., aloe, alum., ***alumn., am-c.,*** am-m., anac., ant-c., ***ant-t.,*** **APIS,** arg-m., **ARG-N.,** ***arn.,*** ars., ars-i., aspar., ***aur-m., bar-c.,*** bar-m., **BELL.,** ***benz-ac.,*** **BERB.,** bor., bov., **BRY.,** ***cact., calc.,*** **CAMPH., CANN-I., CANN-S., CANTH.,** ***caps.,*** carb-an., carb-s., carb-v., ***card-m.,*** cast., **CAUST.,** ***cham.,*** chel., **CHIM.,** ***chin.,*** chin-a., chin-s., cimic., cina, ***clem., coc-c.,*** coch., coff., ***colch., coloc., con., cop.,*** croc., crot-t., ***cub.,*** cupr., cycl., ***dig., dros., dulc.,*** equis., euph., ery-a., ***eup-pur., ferr.,*** ferr-ac., ferr-p., ***graph., guai.,*** ham., ***hell.,*** hep., hydr., ***hyos., ign.,*** iod., ***ip.,*** kali-ar., ***kali-bi.,*** **KALI-C.,** ***kali-chl.,*** kali-i., ***kali-n.,*** kali-p., kali-s., ***kreos.,*** lach., laur., led., **LIL-T.,** ***lyc., lyss.,*** mag-c., mag-m., mang., meny., meph., ***merc.,*** **MERC-C.,** mez., mit., morph., ***mur-ac.,*** nat-c., **NAT-M.,** nat-p., nat-s., ***nit-ac.,*** **NUX-V.,** olnd., oxyt., par., petr., **PH-AC.,** ***phos., plan.,*** plb., ***podo.,*** prun., **PULS.,** rhus-a., ***rhus-t.,*** ruta., sabad., ***sabal.,*** **SABIN.,** samb., sarr., **SARS.,** ***sec.,*** sel., ***senec., seneg.,*** **SEP.,** sil., ***spig.,*** spong., **SQUIL.,** stann., **STAPH.,** ***stigm.,*** stram., stront-c., **SULPH.,** tarax., **THUJ.,** ***tritic.,*** valer., verat., verb., ***vesp.,*** vib., ***viol-t., zinc.***
abdomen, on touching - acon.
absent, urging to - **ARS.,** bell., calad., **CAUST.,** ferr., hell., ***hyos., lac-c.,*** op., ***ox-ac.,*** pall., ***phos., plb.,*** stann., verat.
distended bladder, with - **ARS.,** ***calad.,*** **CAUST.,** fl-ac., hell., ***hyos.,*** op., pall., ***phos., plb.,*** stann., verat.
urine flows freely - phos.
after - am-m., anac., ang., apis, aur., bar-c., ***berb., bov.,*** bry., cact., ***calc., cann-i.,*** carb-an., caust., ***chim.,*** con., cop., crot-t., dig., ***equis.,*** graph., ***guai., hep.,*** iod., lac-c., lach., laur., merc., nat-c., pareir., phos., ***puls., ruta.,*** sabad., sabin., ***seneg., stann., staph.,*** sumb., thuj., verat., viol-t., zinc.
afternoon - bell., chin-s., cic., equis., ferr., hyper., indg., lil-t., merc., ***nux-v.,*** petr., sabad., ***sulph.***
agg., when not attended to - puls., sul-ac.
bus, train or car, in - dys-co.
children, in - ***bor.,*** sars.

URGING, to urinate

anxious - **ACON.**, ***ars.***, **CARB-V.**, ***cham.***, cur., **DIG.**, graph., ph-ac., phyt., sep., til.

urinate, on beginning to - **ACON.**, sars.

apples, after - mang.

apyrexia - ant-t., dros., hell., hyos., lyc., ph-ac., phos., thuj.

chill, during - ***ant-t.***, bry., chin., dulc., lyc., meph., nux-v., ph-ac., phos., puls., sulph.

coffee, after - cahin., cob., ign.

constant - absin., ***acon.***, agar., all-s., am-c., am-m., anac., anan., ant-c., **APIS**, apoc., aran., ***arn.***, ars., ars-i., asar., aur., ***aur-m.***, bar-c., bar-m., ***bell.***, ***berb.***, brach., brom., ***cact.***, cahin., calc., cann-i., ***cann-s.***, **CANTH.**, carb-s., carb-v., ***caust.***, cean., chel., ***chim.***, coc-c., ***colch.***, **CON.**, ***cop.***, crot-t., ***cycl.***, **DIG.**, ***dios.***, ***dulc.***, **EQUIS.**, **ERY-A.**, eup-pur., ***ferr.***, ferr-ar., ***ferr-m.***, ferr-p., gels., graph., ***guai.***, ham., ***hell.***, hep., ign., iod., kali-ar., ***kali-bi.***, ***kali-c.***, kali-p., kali-s., kreos., **LAC-C.**, **LIL-T.**, ***lyc.***, lyss., **MERC.**, **MERC-C.**, merc-i-r., mill., morph., mur-ac., ***murx.***, nat-a., nat-c., nat-m., nat-p., ***nux-m.***, ***nux-v.***, op., **PAREIR.**, petr., ph-ac., phos., ***prun.***, ***puls.***, rumx., ruta., sabad., ***sabal.***, sang., sec., ***senec.***, ***sep.***, ***sil.***, ***squil.***, ***staph.***, **STRY.**, **SULPH.**, sul-ac., sulfon., sumb., tab., tarent., ***thuj.***, ***tritic.***, urea, valer., verat., viol-t., zinc.

bladder, distended, with passing only a few drops - all-s.

cold, from becoming - ***dulc.***, lyc.

daytime - kali-bi.

evening, while lying - lyc.

night - ***apis***, **DIG.**, ***ery-a.***, ***lil-t.***, ***merc.***, ***sabal.***, thuj.

erections, with - mosch., ***rhus-t.***

every other - bar-c.

pain in liver, chest and kidneys, with - ***ferr.***

prolapsus of uterus, during - **LIL-T.**, **SEP.**, uva.

running water, at sight of - lyss.

sex, after - staph.

sitting, while - caps., chim.

coughing, while - ip.

daytime - ferr-p., kali-bi., led., mag-m., ***mang.***, phos.

dragging, down in pelvis, with - lac-c., ***lil-t.***, sep.

drinking, after - podo.

drops, only a few pass until the next stool, when it flows freely - all-s., am-m.

eating, during - mang.

after - bar-c., lyc.

elderly, women - cop.

erections, with - hep., kali-p., mosch., nat-c., ***rhus-t.***, sil.

evening - aloe, alum., am-c., ***bell.***, ***coloc.***, guar., kreos., ***lyc.***, nat-m., nux-m., ***puls.***, ***sabad.***, ***sep.***, ***sulph.***, thuj., ***zinc.***

lying, while - lyc., zinc.

waking, 9 p.m. - mag-c.

URGING, to urinate

fever, during - acon., ***ant-t.***, **APIS**, ***bell.***, bry., canth., caust., dulc., graph., hell., hyos., kali-c., lyc., nux-v., ph-ac., ***puls.***, rhus-t., sabin., sars., squil., staph., sulph.

forenoon - aloe, mez.

10 a.m. - am-m., ***equis.***

frequent - ***acon.***, act-sp., ***aesc.***, aeth., agar., ***aloe***, ***alum.***, alumn., am-c., am-m., anac., ang., ant-c., ***ant-t.***, **APIS**, aran., **ARG-M.**, ***arg-n.***, **ARN.**, ars., ***ars-i.***, ***aspar.***, ***aur-m.***, **BAR-C.**, **BAR-M.**, **BELL.**, ***benz-ac.***, ***berb.***, ***bor.***, ***bov.***, ***bry.***, ***cact.***, ***calc.***, ***calc-p.***, ***cann-s.***, **CANTH.**, ***caps.***, ***carb-an.***, carb-s., ***carb-v.***, **CAUST.**, cedr., ***cham.***, ***chel.***, **CHIM.**, ***chin.***, chin-a., chin-s., ***chlol.***, cic., ***cimic.***, ***cina***, ***clem.***, cob., ***cocc.***, **COC-C.**, coff., **COLOC.**, ***con.***, conv., ***cop.***, corn., ***cub.***, ***cupr.***, cur., ***cycl.***, daph., **DIG.**, ***dios.***, ***dros.***, dulc., echi., ***equis.***, erig., ***ery-a.***, euph., euphr., ***eup-pur.***, ferr-p., ***fl-ac.***, ***gels.***, ***guai.***, ***guare.***, ham., **HELL.**, ***hep.***, ***hyos.***, ***ign.***, ***indg.***, iod., kali-ar., kali-bi., ***kali-c.***, ***kali-i.***, **KALI-N.**, ***kali-p.***, kali-s., kalm., **KREOS.**, **LAC-AC.**, **LAC-C.**, lac-d., ***lach.***, ***led.***, **LIL-T.**, ***lith.***, **LYC.**, ***mag-m.***, ***mang.***, ***meny.***, meph., **MERC.**, **MERC-C.**, ***merc-i-r.***, mez., morph., ***mur-ac.***, murx., nat-a., ***nat-c.***, **NAT-M.**, nat-p., ***nit-ac.***, nux-m., **NUX-V.**, ***olnd.***, ol-an., ox-ac., pall., ***pareir.***, par., ***petr.***, ***petros.***, ***ph-ac.***, ***phos.***, plb., podo., prun., ***psor.***, **PULS.**, raph., rat., rhod., ***rhus-r.***, **RHUS-T.**, ***rumx.***, ruta., ***sabad.***, ***sabin.***, ***samb.***, ***sars.***, ***sel.***, ***sep.***, sil., ***spig.***, ***spong.***, **SQUIL.**, ***stann.***, **STAPH.**, stram., **SULPH.**, sul-ac., sumb., syph., tab., ***tarax.***, ***ter.***, **THUJ.**, ***tril.***, ***uva.***, verat., verb., ***vesp.***, viol-t., zinc., zing.

afternoon - aloe, equis.

cold, dry air, in - acon.

from taking - ***dulc.***, ***eup-pur.***, ***ip.***, ***lyc.***, puls.

cutting, pain from umbilical to ovarian region - coloc.

desire, increases as the quantity of urine diminishes - ***equis.***

evening - guare., kreos., ***lyc.***, sabad., sep., ***sulph.***, ***thuj.***, zinc.

flatus, when passing - ***puls.***

with, upward and downward - cycl.

horse riding, during - cahin.

infant screams before the urine passes - ***bor.***, lach., ***lyc.***, nux-v., ***sars.***

loss of tone of sphincter, from - apoc., jug-r.

menopause, at - sars.

menses, during - calc., nux-m.

after - cham., puls., sars.

before - ***alum.***, apis, asar., kali-c., **KALI-I.**, nux-v., phos., ***puls.***, ***sars.***, ***sulph.***

suppressed, with - ***canth.***, cham., ***dig.***, dros., ***gels.***, ign., nat-m., **PULS.**, sulph.

motion, the slightest, agg. - ***berb.***

URGING, to urinate

frequent,

night and day - aloe, apis, ***aur-m.,*** carb-v., chim., ***ery-a., lyc.,*** mag-m., nit-ac., ***rhus-t.,*** senec.

prolapsus, with - alum., aur., lac-c., **LIL-T., SEP.,** uva.

sitting amel. - phos.

standing - phos.

travelling - cahin.

urinate immediately, if he does not, a feeling as if urine passed involuntarily, which is not so - bry.

without passing any, then while sitting involuntary, flow - ***caust.***

heart affections, with - dig.

ineffectual - ***acon.,*** alum., am-m., ***apis,*** **APOC.,** aran., arg-n., **ARN., ARS.,** atro., aur., bar-m., ***bell., bor., cact., calc., camph., cann-i.,*** **CANTH.,** ***caps.,*** carb-ac., ***carb-an.,*** carb-s., **CAUST.,** cedr., ***cham.,*** chel., **CHIM.,** ***chin.,*** chin-a., ***cimx., clem.,*** coc-c., coff., colch., ***coloc., con., cop., cupr., cycl.,*** **DIG.,** dol., dulc., **EUP-PUR.,** ferr-i., gels., graph., ***guai.,*** **HELL.,** hep., **HYOS.,** ***ip., kali-ar., kali-c., kali-p.,*** kali-s., kreos., ***lach., laur., lyc.,*** merc., **MERC-C.,** morph., mur-ac., myric., nat-m., **NIT-AC., NUX-V., OP.,** ***pareir.,*** petr., ***petros.,*** phel., **PH-AC., PHOS.,** ***plb.,*** podo., prun., **PULS.,** rhus-t., ruta., sabin., ***samb.,*** **SARS.,** sec., senec., ***sep.,*** sil., squil., staph., **STRAM.,** sulph., sumb., tarent., thuj., verat., zinc.

but as soon as he ceases to strain stool and urine pass involuntarily - ***arg-n.***

children - **ACON.,** ***apis,*** camph., eup-pur., ***lyc.***

chill, during - arn., ars., canth., nux-v., phos., puls., sulph.

cramps in rectum with - ***caust.***

diarrhea, with - cupr.

fever, during - ars., canth., dig., hyos., nux-v., ***puls.,*** rat., sars., sulph.

headache, with - **CON.**

menses, during, agg. - ***aur.***

night - coc-c., nat-m., ***sep.***

perspiration, during - **ARS.,** camph., ***canth.,*** caust., dig., dulc., hyos., ***nux-v., puls.,*** sulph.

pregnancy, during - ***lyc.***

standing, while - phos.

then while sitting urine flows involuntarily - ***caust.***

stool, with urging to - alum., ***canth., dig.,*** nat-m., ***nux-v.,*** sumb.

labor, after - op., ***staph.***

lifting, after - ***bry.***

lying - ham., lyc., nux-v.

back, on - prun., ***puls.***

amel. - dig.

right side, on - phos., prun.

married women, newly - canth., **STAPH.**

URGING, to urinate

menses, during - alum., ant-t., apis, calc., cham., chin., kali-i., nux-m., nux-v., phos., puls., rat., ***sars.,*** sep.

after - cham., puls.

before - alum., apis, asar., aur., canth., kali-c., **KALI-I.,** lac-c., nux-v., phos., ***puls.,*** sabin., sars., ***sulph.***

mental exertion - calc., kali-c.

morning - ***alum.,*** ambr., am-m., berb., cocc., coff., graph., lil-t., ruta., senec., ***sep.,*** **SULPH.**

8 a.m. - puls.

8 to 9 a.m. - ferr.

early - carb-v.

rising, on - berb., mez., plan., **SULPH.**

waking, on - apoc., chin-s., hep., merc., mez., ***sars.***

motion, from - berb., bry.

night - agar., ***alum.,*** am-c., anac., ant-c., ant-t., apis, ***arn., ars., ars-i., aur-m., bell., bor.,*** bry., ***calc.,*** carb-ac., carb-s., carb-v., ***caust.,*** chim., cina, clem., coc-c., ***con.,*** croc., cupr., **DIG.,** equis., ***ery-a.,*** euphr., ferr., ***ferr-pic.,*** glyc., ***graph.,*** hep., hyper., iod., kali-ar., ***kali-bi., kali-c.,*** kali-p., kali-s., ***kreos., lach.,*** **LYC.,** lycps., mag-c., ***mag-m.,*** med., meph., ***merc.,*** mez., mur-ac., murx., nat-a., nat-c., ***nat-m.,*** nat-p., nicc., ***nit-ac.,*** nux-m., ***nux-v.,*** petr., ***ph-ac., phos.,*** phys., pic-ac., ***puls., rhus-t.,*** sabal., sabin., ***samb.,*** sang., sars., sec., sep., **SIL.,** spig., squil., stram., **SULPH.,** sul-ac., syph., tab., ter., ***thuj.,*** xero, zinc.

2 a.m. - anth., con., hyper., puls., uran.

3 a.m. - ***dig.,*** sarr.

3:30 a.m. - canth.

4 a.m. - mag-c., merc.

12 and 3 a.m., between - acon.

day, and - ***apis,*** arg-m., cact., ***carb-v.,*** cast., kali-c., kali-i., mag-c., mag-m., merc., nat-c., nat-m., ***rhus-t.,*** sars., sil., sulph., thuj.

midnight - ant-t., nat-c., sulph.

sex, after - ***nat-p., staph.***

waking, on - ant-c., ant-t., caust., dig., euph., hep., mag-m., murx., sil., staph.

painful - **ACON.,** ***agar.,*** alumn., anth., ant-t., ***apis,*** berb., bov., ***cann-s.,*** **CANTH.,** ***carb-an.,*** carb-s., ***chim.,*** con., ***dig., eup-pur.,*** graph., hell., ip., kali-i., ***lac-c.,*** laur., ***lil-t., lyc.,*** **NUX-V., PAREIR.,** ***phyt., prun., puls.,*** raph., ***rhus-a.,*** rhus-r., sec., ***sulph.,*** thuj., ***uva.,*** verat.

child cries - **CANTH., BOR.,** lach., **LYC.,** ***nux-v.,*** **SARS.**

jumps up and down with pain, if cannot be gratified - ***petros.***

children grasp the genitals and cry out - **ACON.,** merc.

disappears when menstrual flow starts - ***kali-i.***

pains in hypogastrium, during - spig.

URGING, to urinate

painful, stool, with urging to - aloe, ***alum., aphis.,*** canth., cic., cub., cupr-ar., cycl., ***dig.,*** kreos., nat-m., **NUX-V.,** ***prun., rhus-t., staph.,*** sumb.

pains, from - ter.

perspiration, during - ***ant-t.,*** apis, arn., **BRY.,** canth., ***caust.,*** dulc., graph., hell., hyos., lyc., **MERC.,** mur-ac., ***nux-v., ph-ac.,*** phos., puls., rhus-t., squil., staph., sulph., **THUJ.**

pregnancy, during - acon., lyc., ***puls.,*** sulph.

pressure, in rectum, with - nat-n.

prolapse of uterus, from - ***lil-t., sep.***

riding, horseback amel. - lyc.

seminal, emissions, after - bor., sulph.

sex, after - ***nat-p., staph.***

shuddering, with - hyper.

sitting, while - caps., caust., chim., clem., phos.

amel. - bar-c., canth.

standing - canth., cop., ferr-p., phos.

amel. - sep.

stool, with - ferr.

after - abrot., carb-an., ***cic.,*** phos.

amel. - alum., am-m.

sudden - agar., ***aloe,*** ambr., ***arg-n.,*** arn., ***bar-c., bor.,*** bov., ***bry., calc., cann-s.,*** **CANTH.,** carb-an., carb-s., caust., chel., clem., coc-c., ***ferr., ferr-p.,*** graph., ***ign.,*** kali-br., **KREOS.,** ***lith., merc.,*** nat-c., ***nat-m., nit-ac.,*** nux-v., ox-ac., petr., **PETROS., PH-AC.,** ***phos., prun., puls., rhus-t., rumx., ruta.,*** sanic., **SEP.,** spong., ***squil.,*** **SULPH.,** ***thuj.,*** trinit.

attended to, if the desire be not, feels as if urine had escaped, which is not so - ***bry.***

busily occupied, when, she has to run and pass a few drops of urine - ***calc., kali-c.***

hasten to urinate, must, or urine will escape - acon., ***agar.,*** aloe, ant-c., ***apis, arg-n.,*** **ARN.,** ars., bar-c., bell., bor., brom., ***bry., camph.,*** cann-s., **CANTH.,** cic., **CLEM.,** ***coc-c., colch.,*** dulc., equis., ***ferr-p.,*** hedeo, ***hyos.,*** ign., kali-br., kali-c., **KREOS.,** lath., ***merc., merc-c.,*** murx., naphtin., **NUX-V.,** ol-an., ***pareir., petros.,*** ph-ac., ***phos.,*** plan., plb., ***pop.,*** prun., **PULS.,** quas., rumx., ruta, sanic., sant., scut., **SEP.,** ***squil.,*** staph., ***stram.,*** **SULPH.,** ***thuj.,*** verat., zinc.

menses, during - bor., nat-m.

morning - phos.

waking, on - hep., sulph.

night - caust., ***sulph.***

child wakes but cannot get out of bed soon enough - kreos.

running water, on seeing or hearing, or putting hands in - ***canth.,*** kreos., **LYSS.,** ***sulph.***

sticking forward in urethra, with - nat-c.

urine seems to pass into glands, and then return and cause pain in urethra - ***prun.***

thinking of it, when - hell., ***ox-ac.,*** oxyt.

thirst, with - ant-t., cast., caust., ph-ac., verat.

URGING, to urinate

urination, after - am-m., anac., ang., apis, aur., bar-c., ***berb., bov.,*** bry., cact., ***calc., cann-i.,*** carb-an., caust., ***chim.,*** con., cop., crot-t., dig., ***equis.,*** graph., ***guai., hep.,*** iod., kali-c., lac-c., lach., laur., merc., mur-ac., nat-c., pareir., phos., ***puls., ruta,*** sabad., sabin., ***seneg., stann., staph.,*** sulph., sumb., thuj., verat., viol-t., zinc.

violent - ***acon.,*** ant-c., arg-n., ***arn.,*** bar-m., berb., bor., **CANTH., DIG.,** kreos., led., merc., ***nat-m., petros.,*** phos., phyt., ***sabin.,*** sep., ***squil.,*** sulph.

after urinating - berb.

menses, during - ant-t., chin., kali-i., nux-v., rat., sars., ***sep.***

night - bor., ***sulph.***

walking, while - ***alum.,*** bry., calc., ***canth.,*** caust., ferr., lith., nat-m., nat-s., ***phos.,*** puls., ruta., ***sep.,*** zinc.

water, hearing, running or putting hands in - asim., canth., kreos., **LYSS.,** sulph.

pouring out liquid - ham.

women, in - apis, berb., caps., cop., cub., dig., ***eup-pur.,*** gels., hedeo, kreos., lil-t., ***sabin.,*** senec., ***sep.,*** staph., verat-v., vib.

URINATION, general

amel., after - ***eug.,*** gels

dribbling, of urine, bladder - ***agar., all-c.,*** all-s., am-m., anan., ang., ant-c., ant-t., apis, ***arg-n., arn.,*** ars., ars-i., atro., aur., ***bell.,*** bor., brom., bry., ***cact.,*** calc., ***camph.,*** cann-i., ***cann-s.,*** **CANTH.,** caps., carb-s., ***caust.,*** chel., chin., cic., **CLEM.,** coff., colch., ***con., cop., dig., dros., dulc.,*** equis., erig., ***ery-a.,*** euph., gamb., ***gels.,*** graph., ham., hell., ***hyos.,*** iod., kali-ar., kali-c., ***kali-chl.,*** kali-m., kali-p., kali-s., ***lac-d.,*** lach., **LIL-T.,** ***lyc.,*** mag-aust., ***mag-m.,*** mag-s., **MERC., MERC-C.,** nat-m., ***nux-m.,*** **NUX-V.,** ox-ac., ***pareir.,*** petr., ph-ac., phos., pic-ac., **PLB.,** polyg., prun., **PULS.,** ***rhus-t., sabin., sars.,*** sec., sel., sil., spig., ***staph., stram.,*** **SULPH.,** tab., tarent., **TER., THUJ.,** thymol., ***verb.,*** vip., zinc.

afternoon, rising from seat, on - spig.

rising from seat, on, 4 p.m. - **LYC.**

beginning, to urinate, on - clem., euph., kali-n., sulph.

then free with stool - all-s., am-m.

enlarged, prostate, with - ***aloe,*** arn., bar-c., bell., cop., ***dig.,*** mur-ac., ***nux-v.,*** pareir., petr., ***puls.,*** sabal., sel., sep., ***staph.***

evening - lyc., zinc.

lying, while - lyc.

involuntary - ***agar., all-c., arg-n.,*** **ARN.,** ***ars.,*** ars-i., ***bell.,*** brom., bry., ***camph.,*** **CANTH., CAUST.,** chin-a., **CLEM.,** coc-c., ***dig., dulc., gels., hyos.,*** iod., jug-r., ***mur-ac., nux-v., petr.,*** plat., ***puls., rhus-t.,*** sant., ***sel., spig., staph., stram., sulph., tab.,*** thuj., ***verb.,*** zinc.

angry, when - puls.

boys, in - ***rhus-t.***

URINATION, general
dribbling, of urine, involuntary
day and night - ***arg-n.,*** ars., gels., iod., ***nux-v.,*** petr., ***verb.***
delayed, if - plan.
labor, after - ***arn.***
menses, during - cact., ***canth.***
not a drop flows on making the greatest effort, but, bladder distended, no pain - gels.
stool, after - chin-a.
labor, after - ***arn.,*** tril.
morning - coff.
night - caust., lyc., ox-ac.
drops flow from urethra, coloring shirt red - lachn.
perpendicularly, urine drops out - alumn., **HEP.**
retention, with - acon., alum., arg-n., arn., bell., canth., **CAUST.,** chim., ery-a., ***gels.,*** **NUX-V.,** op., ***pareir.,*** sabin., sep., staph., sulph.
rising from a seat, when - spig.
senile - all-c., bar-c., cic., con., equis., nux-v.
sharp, in glans penis, with - pareir., thuj.
sitting, while - merc-c., ***puls., sars.***
amel. - caust.
when standing urine passes freely - ***sars.***
spurts, in, then - caps., thlaspi.
stool, after - caust., kali-br., laur., nat-c., nat-m., petr., ***sel.,*** stram., sumb.
pressure in rectum, with - nat-m.
urination, after - agar., ant-c., apoc., arg-n., bar-c., brom., bry., calc., calc-p., **CANN-I.,** cann-s., ***caust., chin-s.,*** **CLEM.,** ***con.,*** dig., ***graph., helon.,*** **HEP.,** ***kali-c.,*** kali-p., ***lach.,*** lyc., nat-c., ***nat-m., petr., petros.,*** phos., pic-ac., psor., ran-s., rhod., ***sel., sep.,*** sil., ***staph.,*** stram., ***thuj.,*** verb., zing.
women, in, winter agg. - rhus-t.
feeble, stream, slow, urination - agar., **ALUM.,** alumn., am-m., ***apis,*** apoc., **ARG-N., ARN.,** atro., ***bell., berb., calc-p., camph.,*** cann-i., carb-s., carb-v., ***caust.,*** cham., chim., chin., chin-s., **CLEM.,** coc-c., cop., ***dig., gels.,*** graph., **HELL., HEP.,** hipp., hura, iris, ***kali-bi., kali-c.,*** kali-n., ***kali-p.,*** kreos., lath., ***laur., lyc.,*** mag-aust., ***med.,*** **MERC., MERC-C., MUR-AC.,** nat-m., ***nit-ac.,*** olnd., **OP.,** ***petr., ph-ac.,*** phos., plat., plb., ***prun.,*** psor., puls., raph., ***rhus-t.,*** **SARS.,** sec., sel., ***sep.,*** sil., spong., staph., ***stram.,*** **SULPH.,** syph., thuj., zinc.
copious, but - plb.
difficulty of breathing and heart symptoms, with - **LAUR.**
drops vertically - arg-n., caust., gels., ***hep.***
morning on waking - **ALUM.,** arn., hep., ***sep.***
night - kali-c., ***sulph.***
pain in the bladder, with violent - calc-p.
retention, from long - calc-p., ***caust.,*** rhus-t., **RUTA., SULPH.**

URINATION, general
feeble, stream, slow, urination
rising, after - merc-ac., mez., sal-ac., ***sulph.***
sleep, after - op.
slow after stool, only dribbling - sel.
forcible, stream, urination - agn., ant-c., carb-an., chel., ***cic.,*** coc-c., cycl., ***nux-v.,*** op., prun., spig., staph., sulph., verat-v.
forked, stream, urination - anac., anag., arg-n., ***cann-s., canth., caust.,*** chim., clem., ***merc.,*** **MERC-C.,** petr., prun., ***rhus-t.,*** **THUJ.**
frequent, urination - abies-n., acon., ***aesc.,*** aeth., agar., ***all-c., alum., alumn.,*** **AM-C.,** am-m., anac., ang., ***ant-c., ant-t.,*** **APIS, ARG-M., ARG-N.,** arn., ars., ars-i., arum-t., asc-t., aspar., aur., **BAR-C.,** ***bar-m., bell.,*** benz-ac., ***bism., bor.,*** bov., brom., ***bry.,*** bufo, ***cact.,*** **CALC., CALC-AR.,** ***camph., cann-i., cann-s.,*** **CANTH.,** ***caps., carb-ac.,*** carb-an., carb-s., ***carb-v.,*** casc., **CAST., CAUST.,** cedr., chel., ***chim.,*** chin., chlol., ***cic.,*** cimic., ***cina,*** cinnb., ***clem.,*** cob., cocc., coc-c., ***coff., colch., coloc.,*** con., cop., crot-c., crot-h., crot-t., ***cupr.,*** cur., ***cycl., daph., dig.,*** dros., dulc., equis., ***ery-a.,*** **EUPHR.,** ***eup-pur., ferr.,*** ferr-i., ***ferr-p., fl-ac.,*** **GELS.,** glon., **GRAPH.,** grat., guai., ham., hell., hydr., ***hyos.,*** **IGN.,** indg., ***iod., ip.,*** iris, jatr., ***kali-bi., kali-c.,*** kali-chl., kali-i., kali-p., kali-s., ***kalm.,*** kreos., **LAC-AC.,** lac-c., ***lac-d.,*** **LACH.,** lact., laur., ***led., lil-t., lith.,*** **LYC.,** lyss., ***mag-c.,*** mag-m., ***mag-p.,*** mang., med., meli., meph., **MERC., MERC-C.,** ***mez., murx., mur-ac.,*** nat-a., ***nat-c., nat-m.,*** nat-p., ***nat-s.,*** nicc., nit-ac., **NUX-V.,** ***olnd., op.,*** ox-ac., pall., pareir., par., ***petr., ph-ac.,*** **PHOS.,** ***plan.,*** plat., ***podo.,*** plb., ***psor.,*** **PULS.,** rheum, **RHUS-R.,** ***rhus-t.,*** ruta., ***sabin.,*** samb., ***sang., sars., sec., sel., seneg., sep.,*** sil., ***spig.,*** spong., **SQUIL.,** ***stann.,*** **STAPH., SULPH.,** sul-ac., sul-i., tab., ***ter., thuj., uva., valer.,*** verat., verb., vesp., vib., ***viol-t.,*** zinc.
acids agg. - sep.
afternoon - alum., alumn., bov., chlol., coc-c., petr., sars., sep., sulph.
busily occupied, when, must run and pass a little urine - calc., kali-c.
chill, during - **ARS.,** canth., hyper., lec., meph., **MERC.,** petros., ph-ac., phos., sulph.
coffee, after - cahin., cob., ign., olnd.
daytime - ham., ***mag-m.,*** nat-m., ***psor.,*** **RHUS-T.,** staph., uran.
daytime - ham., kreos., ***mag-m.,*** nat-m., ***psor.,*** **RHUS-T.,** staph., uran-n.
and night - ***alum.,*** apis, cahin., ***calc., canth., caust., colch.,*** hyos., jug-r., kali-c., lac-ac., mag-m., **MERC.,** nat-a., ***nat-m.,*** phos., ***plan., rhus-t.,*** sars.
dinner, after - cycl., nat-m.
drinking, after - podo.
elderly, people - ***bar-c.***
emission of water-colored urine in small quantity - ***dig.***

URINATION, general

frequent, urination

evening - alum., am-c., calc-p., cann-i., cic., euphr., ferr-i., grat., kreos., lyc., ox-ac., sabad., sep., sulph., zinc.

every, other day - bar-c.

10 to 18 minutes - bor.

hour - calc-ar.

exertion, after - aeth.

exposure to cold and wet - alum., ***calc.,*** calc-p., cop., **PULS., SARS.,** sulph.

fever, during - arg-m., bell., ***kreos.,*** lyc., merc., ph-ac., rhus-t., staph., stram.

drinking, after - cimx., eup-pur.

forenoon - ant-t., arg-n., ***kreos.,*** lyc., nat-m., sulph.

headache, with - ***bell.,*** **GELS.,** jug-r., ***lac-d.,*** scut., sel., ***verat.,*** vib.

hysterical - gels.

indigestion, with - nux-v.

labor, during - cham.

lying agg. - puls.

menses, during - alum., alumn., apis, aur., canth., caust., hyos., ***kali-i.,*** med., nux-v., plat., puls., ***sars.,*** sulph., vib.

before - ***alum., apis,*** asar., canth., dig., kali-c., kali-i., nux-v., phos., puls., ***sars., sulph.***

morning - ambr., am-m., anac., bar-ac., bell., calc-p., caust., coca, con., kreos., ***mez., phos.,*** pic-ac., sil., ***sul-i.***

morning, rising, after - ambr., phos.

nervous origin, of - cub.

night - agn., ail., aloe, ***alum., alumn.,*** ambr., ***am-c., am-m., anac.,*** ant-c., anth., ***apis, arg-m.,*** arg-n., arn., ars., ars-i., atro., **BAR-C.,** ***bar-m.,*** **BELL., BOR.,** bry., bufo, ***cact.,*** **CALC.,** ***calc-f.,*** cann-i., ***canth., carb-ac.,*** **CARB-AN.,** ***carb-s.,*** carb-v., ***caust.,*** chin., chlol., cinnb., clem., cob., coca, coff., coloc., ***con.,*** cop., ***cupr., cycl.,*** daph., dig., dros., ***equis., eug.,*** fl-ac., ***glon., graph.,*** hell., hep., ***hyos.,*** iod., kali-ar., ***kali-bi., kali-c.,*** kali-p., kali-s., **KREOS.,** ***lac-c., lach.,*** lil-t., ***lith.,*** **LYC.,** mag-c., mag-m., mag-p., **MED.,** ***meph.,*** **MERC.,** murx., mur-ac., nat-a., ***nat-c., nat-m., nat-p., nat-s.,*** nicc., ***nit-ac., nux-v.,*** op., petr., ***ph-ac.,*** **PHOS.,** plan., plb., ***podo.,*** prun., psor., ***puls.,*** ran-b., ***rhus-t., rumx.,*** ruta., ***sang., sars.,*** sel., ***senec.,*** **SEP.,** ***sil.,*** spig., ***squil.,*** stann., staph., ***stram.,*** **SULPH.,** tab., **TER.,** ther., ***thuj., uran.,*** zinc.

cries before urine passes - ***bor.***

midnight, after - zinc.

more than day - ther.

seldom during the day - ***bor., ther.***

pain, with - thuj.

in face, with - ***calc.,*** thuj.

perspiration, during - ant-c., bar-c., bar-m., **CALC.,** ***caust.,*** ign., kali-c., lach., **LYC.,** ***merc.,*** mur-ac., nat-c., nat-n., nat-p., ***ph-ac., phos.,*** **RHUS-T.,** ***sel.,*** squil., staph., **SULPH.,** thuj.

URINATION, general

frequent, urination

pregnancy, night, during - podo.

prostate affections, with - apis, ferr-pic., sabal., staph., thuj.

riding, in a carriage - phos.

amel. - lyc.

urine, with scanty - hell.

weather, change of - tub.

incomplete, urination - am-m., ***berb.,*** bry., ***calc.,*** cann-i., carl., ***caust.,*** **CLEM.,** cub., ***gels., helon.,*** **HEP.,** ***kali-c.,*** kali-chl., lac-c., **LACH.,** ***lyc.,*** **MAG-M.,** ***nat-c., nat-p.,*** nux-v., petr., phos., **SEL.,** sil., ***staph.,*** stram., ***thuj.***

bladder full, urging to urinate but scanty urine - abrot.

obliged to urinate five or six times before the bladder is empty - ***thuj.***

infrequent, urination - acon., agar., aloe, alum., alumn., ***arg-n., arn.,*** ars., ***aur.,*** bar-c., bell., bry., camph., **CANTH.,** carb-v., cast., chel., coc-c., cupr., ***cycl.,*** dig., grat., ***hep.,*** hyos., iris, kali-c., lac-c., ***laur.,*** led., ***lyc.,*** mag-m., merc-c., mez., nat-s., nicc., nit-ac., ***nux-v., op., plb.,*** prun., psor., ***puls., ruta.,*** sars., sec., stann., staph., ***stram.,*** sul-ac., stront-c., ***syph.,*** thuj., zinc.

daytime - ***lyc.***

interrupted, urination - ***agar.,*** aloe, ammc., ant-c., ant-t., apis, arg-n., bell., bov., cann-i., cann-s., caps., ***carb-an., caust.,*** chin-s., **CLEM., CON.,** ***dulc.,*** gamb., ***gels., graph.,*** hep., ***iod., kali-c.,*** kali-p., ***led., lyc.,*** mag-s., med., meph., ***op.,*** pareir., ***ph-ac.,*** phos., ***puls.,*** pulx., rhus-t., ***sabal.,*** sars., sed-ac., ***sulph., thuj.,*** vesp., zinc.

burning in urethra, by - ph-ac.

evening - ***caust.***

painful erections, with - ***ant-c.***

sex, after - ***ph-ac.***

spurts, in swelled prostate, with each spurt cutting, pain - **PULS.**

strains a few drops, then full flow follows - clem.

stream, after which the urine flows out drop by drop - mag-s., rheum

suddenly, then followed by pain - pulx.

urine flows better when standing - ***con., ph-ac.***

so thick, with cheesy masses like curdled milk - **PH-AC.**

violent contraction, in region of bladder, by - petr.

involuntary, urination - acet-ac., ***acon.,*** agar., **AIL.,** ***alet., alum.,*** alumn., am-c., anac., anan., ant-c., **APIS, ARG-N.,** ***arn.,*** **ARS., ARS-I.,** atro., aur-m., ***bar-ac., bar-c.,*** bar-m., **BELL.,** ***bry., bufo,*** cact., ***calc., calc-p., camph.,*** cann-i., ***canth.,*** carb-an., carb-s., ***carb-v.,*** **CAUST.,** ***cedr.,*** cham., chen-a.1, ***chin.,*** chin-a., chlol., ***cic., cimx., cina, colch., con.,*** crot-h., cupr., dam.1, ***dig.,*** dros., **DULC.,** ***echi., equis.,*** ery-a., eup-per., ***eup-pur., ferr.,*** ferr-ar., ferr-i., ***ferr-p., fl-ac., gels.,*** graph.,

URINATION, general

involuntary, urination - ***guare., hell., hep., hydr., hydr-ac.,*** hydrang., ***hyos., ign., iod.,*** kali-ar., ***kali-br., kali-p., kreos.,*** lac-c., lac-d., ***lach.,*** lath., ***laur.,*** led., ***lina.,*** lup., **LYC.,** mag-aust.1, mag-c., mag-m., mag-p., ***merc.,*** merc-c., mill., ***mosch., mur-ac., nat-a., nat-c.,*** **NAT-M.,** nat-p., ***nit-ac.,*** **NUX-M.,** ***nux-v., olnd.,*** ol-j., ***op.,*** ox-ac., ***petr., ph-ac.,*** **PHOS.,** phys., physal., pic-ac., ***plan.,*** plb., ***podo.,*** **PSOR., PULS.,** rat., ***rhus-a.,*** **RHUS-T.,** rumx., ***ruta, sabal.,*** sang., ***sanic.,*** sant., sapo., ***sec., sel.,*** seneg., **SEP.,** sil., ***spig., spong., squil.,*** **STAPH.,** ***stram.,*** **SULPH.,** tab., tarent., ***ter., thuj.,*** thyr., trinit., tritic., ust., ***uva., verat., verb.,*** vesp., vib., viol-o., zinc.

acute illness, after - psor.

adolescence - ***lac-c.***

blow, from, on the head - sil.

blowing, nose, when - **CAUST.,** nat-m., puls., zinc.

boys, in - ***rhus-t.***

catheterization, after - mag-p.

childbirth, after - arn., ***ars.***

children, in (see Bedwetting) - aesc.

nervous and irritable - thyr.

weakly - kali-p., thyr.

chill, during - caust., dulc., puls., rhus-t., sulph.

before - ***gels.***

cold, becoming - ***alet.,*** bell., **CAUST.,** ***dulc., rhus-t.***

constipation, with - tarent.

convulsions, during - art-v., **BUFO,** ***caust.,*** cocc., colch., cupr., **HYOS.,** nux-v., ***oena., plb.,*** stry., ***zinc.***

cough, during - ***alet., alum.,*** anan., ***ant-c.,*** **APIS,** ***bell., bry., calc.,*** canth., ***caps.,*** carb-an., **CAUST.,** ***cench., colch.,*** dulc., ferr., ***ferr-m., ferr-p.,*** hyos., ign., kali-c., ***kreos.,*** lach., laur., ***lyc.,*** mag-c., mur-ac., murx., **NAT-M.,** nit-ac., ***nux-v.,*** orig., ***ph-ac.,*** **PHOS.,** psor., **PULS.,** rhod., rhus-t., ***rumx.,*** sel., seneg., ***sep., spong.,*** **SQUIL.,** staph., sulph., tarent., ***thuj.,*** verb., ***verat.,*** vib., xero, ***zinc.***

pregnancy, during - cocc.

daytime - ***arg-n., bell.,*** caust., equis., ***ferr., ferr-p.,*** **FL-AC.,** sec., thuj.

and night - ***arg-n.,*** **ARS.,** bell., **CAUST.,** ***gels., hyos.,*** iod., ***nux-v.,*** petr., ***rhus-a.,*** ruta., ***verb.***

sleep, during - ***bell.***

walking, while - ferr., thuj.

delayed, if - ***lach.,*** phos., plan., ***sep.,*** squil., sulph., thuj.

desire is resisted, if - calc., dig., merc., nat-m., ***puls.,*** sep., squil., ***sulph., thuj.***

difficult to waken the child - ***bell.,*** chlol., **KREOS.,** thuj.

digestive disturbances, with - benz-ac., ***nux-v.,*** puls.

effort, during, no urine flows - ***gels.***

URINATION, general

involuntary, urination

elderly people, in - ***all-c.,*** aloe, ammc., apis, apoc., arg-n., ***ars., aur-m.,*** benz-ac., cann-s., canth., carb-ac., ***cic.,*** dam., equis., gels., ***iod.,*** kali-p., nit-ac., phos., rhus-a., ***sec.,*** seneg., ***thuj.***

men, with enlarged prostate - ***all-s., aloe,*** apoc., ***bar-c., cic.,*** dig., ***iod.,*** kali-p., nux-v., ***pareir., sec., thuj.***

empty, when bladder feels - helon.

excitement, from - ***gels.***

exertion, during - ***bry.,*** caust., ***nux-v.,*** ph-ac., rhus-t., tarent.

flatus, expelling when - mur-ac., ***puls.,*** sulph.

forenoon - phys.

fright, from - op., sep.

headache, with - gels.

hurry, when in - lac-d.

hysteria, in - ign.

inattention, from - sep.

jar, by - caust.

labor, after - ***arn.,*** **ARS.,** bell., caust., hyos., tril.

laughing - caps., **CAUST.,** ***nat-m., nux-v., puls.,*** **SEP.,** tarent.

lying, while - bell-p., ***kreos.,*** lach., lyc., pic-ac., ***puls.,*** uva.

mania, during - ***cupr.***

measles, after - puls.

menses, during - cact., calc., ***canth.,*** hell., ***hyos.***

moon, agg. - cina., sil.

at full, agg. - cina, ***psor.,*** sil.

morning - am-c., cina, phos., phys., til.

toward - am-c., cact., carb-v., chlol., cina, zinc.

motion, during - ***bell., bry.,*** calc., ***ph-ac., phos.,*** ruta., staph., tarent.

amel. - ***rhus-t.***

movement, sudden - ferr.

night - acon., ***aeth.,*** alum., ***am-c.,*** anac., anan., **APIS,** ***apoc., arg-m.,*** **ARG-N., ARN., ARS.,** ***aur.,*** aur-m., aur-s., bar-c., bar-m., **BELL., BENZ-AC.,** bry., cact., ***calc.,*** canth., ***carb-s., carb-v.,*** **CAUST.,** ***cham.,*** chin., ***chlol.,*** cimx., ***cina,*** coca, con., ***crot-c.,*** cub., cupr., dulc., **EQUIS.,** ***eup-pur.,*** **FERR.,** ***ferr-ac.,*** ferr-i., ferr-p., ***fl-ac.,*** **GRAPH.,** ***hep.,*** hyos., ign., kali-br., kali-c., ***kali-p.,*** **KREOS., LAC-C.,** lac-d., lyc., mag-aust., mag-c., ***mag-m.,*** **MAG-P.,** mag-s., ***med., merc.,*** mur-ac., ***nat-a., nat-c.,*** **NAT-M.,** ***nat-p.,*** **NIT-AC.,** nux-v., ***op.,*** ox-ac., ***petr.,*** ph-ac., ***phos.,*** physal., ***plan., podo., psor.,*** **PULS.,** quas., rhus-a., **RHUS-T.,** ***ruta.,*** sabal., ***sanic.,*** sant., ***sars.,*** sec., sel., ***seneg.,*** **SEP., SIL.,** spig., squil., staph., ***stram.,*** **SULPH.,** ***syc-co.,*** tab., ter., ***thuj.,*** **THYR.,** ***tub., uran., urt-u.,*** uva., verat., ***verb., viol-t.,*** zinc.

adolescence - ***lac-c.***

URINATION, general

involuntary, urination

night, children, in - aesc., ***bell.,*** benz-ac., ***caust.,*** chin., ***cina,*** **EQUIS.,** ***kreos., lyc.,*** med., nat-m., phos., puls., sep., sil., thuj.

difficult to waken the child - ***bell.,*** chlol., **KREOS.,** thuj.

dreaming of urinating, while - ***kreos.,*** lac-c., lyc., merc-i-f., ***seneg., sep.,*** sulph.

first sleep - benz-ac., **CAUST.,** cina, ***kreos., ph-ac.,*** **SEP.**

habit, when there is no tangible cause except - **EQUIS.**

midnight to morning - plan.

morning, toward - am-c., cact., chlol., zinc.

night, after 5 a.m. - cact.

spasmodic enuresis - **ARG-M.,** bell., canth., caps., cast., cina, coloc., ***gels.,*** hyos., ign., lach., lyc., ***nux-v.,*** op., puls., rhus-t., verat.

weakly children, in - ***chin.***

noise, sudden - caust., puls., sep.

onanists, in - sep.

pregnancy, during - **ARS.,** bell., canth., caust., clem., kreos., ***nat-m.,*** podo., **PULS.,** ***sep., syph.***

prolapse of uterus, from - ferr-i.

prostate enlargement, with - iod.

putting, hands in cold water - ***kreos.***

retain, great pain on attempting to - uran.

riding, while - lac-d., thuj.

amel. - lyc.

rising, from a seat, when - ***mag-c.,*** petr., spig.

running, while - ***arn., bry., lac-d.***

sex, after - cedr., staph.

fright for, with - lyc., staph.

sitting, while - ***caust., nat-m.,*** **PULS.,** ***rhus-t., sars.,*** sil., spig., stram.

amel. - zinc.

retention while standing - ***caust.***

she must swing her foot constantly or the urine will escape - zinc.

sleep, in first part of - benz-ac., **CAUST.,** cina, ***kreos., ph-ac.,*** puls., **SEP.,** tub.

sleepy, when - bell.

sneezing, when - alet., caps., **CAUST.,** colch., ***lac-c., nat-m., nux-v.,*** orig., petr., ***ph-ac.,*** phos., ***puls., sep.,*** zinc.

standing, while - bell., caust., ferr., lyc., ***nat-m., puls., rhus-t.,*** sep.

stool, after - acon., apis, ***arg-n., ars.,*** atro., aur., bar-c., bell., bry., calc., camph., carb-v., caust., chin., chin-a., cina, colch., con., dig., ***hyos.,*** kali-br., ***laur.,*** mosch., **MUR-AC.,** nat-m., petr., ***ph-ac., phos.,*** puls., rhus-t., sec., ***sel.,*** stram., sulph., verat., ***zinc.***

dysenteric, each - alum.

fully conscious, while supposing it to be flatus - ***ars.***

straining at, while - ***alum., lil-t.***

URINATION, general

involuntary, urination

stool, straining, when not, voluntary defection impossible - arg-n.

surprise, pleasurable, agg. - puls.

sycosis, history of - med., thuj.

thirst, and fear, with - **ACON.**

train catching, while - lac-d.

tumors, brain or spinal, with - calc-p.

typhoid, fever - ***arg-n.,*** arn., ***ars., colch., hell.,*** **HYOS.,** ***lach., lyc., mosch., mur-ac.,*** op., ***ph-ac., phos.,*** psor., ***rhus-t., stram.,*** sulph., ***verat., verat-v.***

urging, with - chin.

urination, after - agar., cann-i., **CLEM.,** helon., ***sel.,*** sil., ***staph.***

vomiting, while - ars., ***canth.,*** crot-h., merc., merc-sul., ***pareir.***

walking, while - alet., alum-sil., anan., ***arg-n.,*** arn., bell., ***bry., calc., caust.,*** **FERR.,** ferr-p., kali-s., ***lac-d., mag-c.,*** mag-m., **NAT-M.,** ***ph-ac.,*** phos., **PULS.,** ruta., ***sel.,*** sep., stram., tarent., thuj., vib., ***zinc.***

amel. - ***rhus-t.***

fast, while - alet.

yet on attempting to, when standing still, nothing passed - mag-m.

water running from a hydrant, on seeing - ***lyss.,*** sulph.

weakly children, in - ***chin.***

women, in - ***sil.***

worm affections, with - sil.

painful, urination - **ACON.,** aesc., aeth., ***agar., all-c.,*** all-s., aloe, ***alum.,*** ang., ant-c., ant-t., ***apis, apoc.,*** **ARG-N.,** ***arn.,*** **ARS.,** atro., aur., aur-m., bar-c., bar-m., **BELL.,** benz-ac., ***berb.,*** cact., calc., ***calc-p., camph., cann-i.,*** **CANN-S., CANTH.,** ***caps.,*** carb-s., caul., casc., ***caust., cham.,*** chel., ***chim.,*** cic., ***clem., coc-c.,*** coff., colch., ***coloc., con.,*** **COP.,** corn., cub., cuc-c., ***cupr.,*** **DIG.,** ***dor.,*** dros., ***dulc., epig., equis.,*** erig., euph., ***eup-pur., fab.,*** ferr-p., ***gels.,*** gum., ***hell., hep.,*** hydrang., ***hydr., hyos.,*** hyper., ind., jatr., ***kali-ar., kali-c.,*** kali-chl., kali-n., kali-p., kali-s., ***kreos., lac-c., laur.,*** **LIL-T.,** ***lith.,*** **LYC.,** mag-aust., mag-m., med., meph., ***merc.,*** **MERC-C.,** mit., morph., mur-ac., nat-a., nat-c., ***nat-m.,*** nat-p., ***nit-ac.,*** nux-m., **NUX-V.,** oci., **OP.,** ***ol-sant.,*** **PAREIR.,** petr., **PETROS.,** ph-ac., phos., plat., **PLB.,** podo., ***polyg.,*** pop., ***prun.,*** psor., **PULS.,** ran-b., ***rheum, rhus-a., rhus-t.,*** ruta, ***sabal., sabin.,*** sang., ***sant., sars.,*** sars., sec., sel., ***senec., sep.,*** spig., stann., ***staph.,*** stigm., stram., **SULPH.,** sumb., tab., ***tarent.,*** tax., **TER.,** thlaspi, ***thuj., tritic., uva.,*** verb., ***verat.,*** vib., zinc.

aching, in back, with - vesp.

after, agg. - **EQUIS.**

afternoon, walking amel. - lith.

alternating with bedwetting - ***gels.***

alcoholic drinks, from - nux-m.

apyrexia, during - caps., caust., dig., staph.

URINATION, general
painful, urination
attempting to urinate, on - plb.
children, in - apis.
child cries before urine starts - **BOR.,** lach., ***lyc., nux-v.,*** sanic., **SARS.**
childbirth, delivery, after - apis, equis.
chill, during - canth., ***cham.,*** lyc., merc., nux-v., ph-ac., puls., sulph., thuj.
close of urination - equis., sars.
coldness, numbness, and twitching, down left leg, with - agar.
dances around the room in agony, so that he - **APIS,** cann-i., ***cann-s.,*** **CANTH.,** ***petros.***
dentition, during - erig.
dinner and supper, after - nux-m.
dribbling, with - thlaspi.
dysentery, in - arn.
dysmenorrhea, during - nux-m., senec., verat-v.
erection, then - rad-br.
effort to urinate agg. - plb.
feet, from wet - all-c.
fever, during - ant-c., cann-s., canth., ***cham.,*** colch., dulc., nit-ac., nux-v., staph., sulph.
first portion - chim.
headache, with, children - con., senec.
hysterical - nux-m.
last portion - arg-n.
lying amel. - kreos.
married women, newly - cann-s., ***canth.,*** ery-a., **STAPH.**
menses, before - sars.
suppressed and drawing, pains in abdomen, with - ***puls.***
morning - corn., ***sep.***
elderly men, in - ***benz-ac., corn.***
neuralgic - prun.
night - ***cic., merc.,*** spig.
midnight, after, 3 to 5 a.m. - pareir.
pain in the sphincter of bladder, with hyperaesthesia of the skin down the course of the left sciatic nerve, pain in the left popliteus and heel, with coldness creeping over the whole course of the nerve, especially in the heel - ***agar.***
perspiration, during - **CANTH., CHAM.,** hep., lyc., ***merc.,*** nit-ac., puls., sulph., ***thuj.***
position, knee-elbow amel. - med., pareir.
must lie down - kreos.
must sit bend backward - zinc.
pregnancy, during - equis., eup-pur., ph-ac., plb., staph.
presence of others, in - ***ambr.,*** hep., mur-ac., nat-m., tarent.
prostate enlargement, with - apis, med., petros.
renal colic, with - coc-c.
riding on rough ground, from - eup-pur.
sleep, after - op.
spasm of the bladder, from - colch.
spasmodic closure of the sphincter while finishing - ***cann-s.***

URINATION, general
painful, urination
tenesmus of rectum, with, and spasm of urethra - ***prun.***
evening - ferr.
thinking of it agg. - ***hell.,*** nux-v.
urine, with profuse - equis.
uterine complaints, with, displacement - senec.
women, in plethoric - chim.
paroxysmal, urination - chel., cycl., merc-i-f., nux-v.
pressing, with urination - hyos., lyc.
retarded, urination - agar., ***alum.,*** alumn., am-m., ***apis,*** aran., arg-n., **ARN.,** bell., ***cact.,*** cadm-s., calc., ***cann-i.,*** canth., **CAUST.,** chel., ***clem.,*** coc-c., **COP.,** ***dig.,*** eucal., **HEP.,** hydr-ac., ip., kali-br., ***kali-c., kali-n.,*** lath., laur., **LYC.,** med., ***mur-ac.,*** nat-c., ***nat-m.,*** nat-p., ***nit-ac.,*** nux-v., ***op., pareir.,*** par., ***petr., prun.,*** puls., ***raph.,*** **RHUS-T.,** ***sars.,*** sec., ***sel.,*** **SEP.,** ***sil.,*** staph., ***stram.,*** sulph., tax., ter., ***thuj., zinc.***
alone, can only pass urine when - ***ambr.,*** hep., ***lyc.,*** mur-ac., ***nat-m.,*** tarent.
before, a cutting, with ineffectual straining, that stops the flow - ph-ac.
bending backward amel. - alum.
doubling up amel. - canth., prun.
great, straining, after a few drops of urine pass, which are followed by a full stream, with pain, after this sometimes dribbling urine - clem.
knees, on the, and pressing, head against floor, can pass urine only when - pareir.
lie down, must - kreos.
lying, can only pass urine while - kreos.
listening to, music, can pass urine only when - ***tarent.***
water running, can pass urine only when - lyss., tarent., zinc.
whistling, can pass urine only when - cycl., tarent.
last, few drops - caust.
long, while, and then only a little urine passes - caust.
and then only a little urine passes, especially if others are near him - ***nat-m.***
lying, can only pass urine while - kreos.
odd position amel. - zinc.
pain, by - con., phos.
in the fundus of bladder - phos.
pregnancy, in - equis.
presence of others agg. - ***ambr.,*** hep., mur-ac., **NAT-M.,** tarent.
press, must, a long time before he can begin - abies-n., ***acon.,*** agar., aloe, **ALUM.,** ***apis, arn., bell., cact.,*** cann-i., **CAUST.,** ***chim., coc-c.,*** equis., **HEP.,** ***hyos., kali-c., kreos., laur.,*** lil-t., lyc., **MAG-M., MUR-AC.,** nat-c., nat-p., ***nit-ac.,*** nux-v., **OP.,** ***pareir.,*** plb., ***prun.,*** raph., rheum, ***rhus-t., sabal.,*** sars., sec., stram., tax., thuj., tub., zinc.

URINATION, general
retarded, urination
a long time before he can begin, morning - **ALUM.,** ***arn.,*** **HEP., OP.,** ***sep.***
continue to, must, if he stops to breathe the urine ceases to flow until he strain again - nat-p., ***stram.***
continue to, must, to pass the last part - rheum
frequent pressing to urinate, with, with small discharges - stict., thuj.
long pressing, after, urine passes guttatim - bell., plb.
long time, must, which is painful - ***laur.***
painful and frequent with disposition to sit and strain a long time after which few drops pass - abies-n.
pressure, the more, the less it flows - ***kali-c.***
so hard, must, to start the urine that anus protrudes - **MUR-AC.**
stand and press a long time, must, before urine will start - nit-ac.
stand, must, with feet wide apart, body inclined forward - chim.
sitting, while agg. - puls., sars.
amel. - caust., zinc.
bent forward - pareir., sulph.
bent, backward - zinc.
can only pass urine, while - **ZINC.**
spasm, of sphincter, on account of - **OP.**
standing, amel. - alum., caust., con., hyper., ***sars.,*** syph.
can only pass urine, while - alum., hyper., **SARS.**
daytime agg. but at night flows freely - sars.
feet, wide apart, with, and body inclined forward, can only pass urine while - ***chim.***
flows, better, while - con.
flows, involuntarily while sitting - ***caust.***
pavements, on cold, agg. - carb-v.
urine will not flow, while, but passes involuntarily while walking - mag-m.
stool, while pressing, at, can pass urine only - aloe, ***alum.,*** am-m., apis, laur., mur-ac., nat-p., sel., stram., tub.
stooping amel. - canth., pareir., prun.
strangers, presence of - ambr., hep., mur-ac., ***nat-m.***
urging, to urinate, with, but can pass no urine until an enormous clot of black blood has passed from the vagina - ***coc-c.***
seldom - acon., agar., aloe, alum., alumn., apis, ***arg-n., arn.,*** ars., ***aur.,*** bar-c., bell., bry., camph., **CANTH.,** carb-v., cast., chel., coc-c., cupr., ***cycl.,*** dig., grat., ***hep.,*** hyos., iris, kali-c., lac-c., ***laur.,*** led., lob., ***lyc.,*** mag-m., merc-c., mez., nat-s., nicc., nit-ac., ***nux-v., op., plb.,*** prun., psor., ***puls., ruta,*** sars., sec., squil., stann., staph., ***stram.,*** sul-ac., stront-c., ***syph.,*** thuj., zinc.

URINATION, general
seldom, urination
daytime - bor., ***lyc.,*** ther.
twice - pyrog.
twice, scanty, but - pyrog.
once a day, but profuse - lac-c., syph.
difficulty, with - lac-c.
slender stream (see thin, stream) - ***clem., cop.,*** eup-pur., graph., nit-ac., ol-an., staph.
thread, like - prun.
spraying stream - kreos.
spurting stream - calc-p., cic., clem., con., helon., puls., spig., thlaspi, tub.
after - helon.
coughing, when - kreos., ***squil.,*** staph.
thin, stream, of urination - agar., apis, bell., ***camph., canth.,*** chim., chin., **CLEM., COP.,** eup-pur., gins., ***graph.,*** gymn., hell., ***merc., nit-ac., petr.,*** prun., ***puls.,*** samb., ***sars., spong., staph.,*** stram., ***sulph.,*** tax., ***thuj., zinc.***
twisted stream - sul-i.
unsatisfactory, urination - ***alum., arg-n.,*** arn., **ARS.,** aspar., aur., bell., ***berb.,*** brach., bry., cact., ***calc.,*** camph., canth., **CAUST.,** ***cic., clem.,*** cocc., colch., con., ***cub., gels.,*** gins., **HEP.,** ***hyos.,*** kali-ar., ***kali-c.,*** kali-p., lach., ***laur.,*** lyc., ***mag-m.,*** merc., nat-a., nat-c., nat-p., ***nux-v.,*** op., petr., ***ph-ac.,*** phos., plb., puls., rhod., rhus-t., ruta., ***sars.,*** sec., ***sel.,*** sil., stann., ***staph.,*** stram., ***sulph., thuj.,*** verat.
bladder were not emptied, as if, with dribbling - sep., ***staph.,*** thuj.
feeling as if urine remained in urethra - agar., all-c., alum., ambr., ***arg-n.,*** aspar., ***berb.,*** cedr., clem., dig., ery-a., eup-pur., gels., ***hep., kali-bi.,*** petr., rhus-t., ruta, sec., ***sel., sep.,*** sil., ***staph.,*** tell., ***thuj.***

URINE, sensation as if, in fossa navicularis, after urination (see Urine, chapter) - all-c., ferr-i., ***thuj.***
cold drop of urine passing, as if - agar.
cold, were, as if - nit-ac.
drops passed, as if a few - ambr., lact.
remained in, after urinating as if some - agar., all-c., alum., ambr., ***arg-n.,*** aspar., carb-s., cedr., clem., dig., ery-a., ***kali-bi.,*** lact., med., petr., rhus-t., ***sel., sep.,*** tell., ***thuj.***
still flowing, sensation of, urethra - aspar., vib.
stops at fossa navicularis - ferr-i., prun.
urine, feeling as if, remained in urethra - agar., all-c., alum., ambr., ***arg-n.,*** aspar., caust., cedr., clem., dig., ery-a., ***kali-bi.,*** petr., rhus-t., ***sel., sep.,*** tell., ***thuj.***
urine, still flowing, sensation of, urethra - aspar., vib.
stops at fossa navicularis - ferr-i., prun.

VESICLES, urethra, meatus - stann.
meatus, forming ulcers - ***nit-ac.***

VOLUPTUOUS, sensation
urination, during - ox-ac., thuj.
after - thuj.
voluptuous, sensation, urethra - anag., lith., nat-c., ox-ac., thuj.

WEAKNESS - ***all-c.,*** aloe, ***alum., alumn.,*** anan., ***apoc., ars.,*** aur., aur-m., ***bell., benz-ac.,*** brach., ***camph., cann-i., canth.,*** carl., **CAUST.,** ***cham.,*** clem., ***con.,*** dulc., ***equis.,*** erig., euphr., gels., hell., **HEP.,** ***hyos.,*** ipom., kali-c., laur., lycps., **MAG-M.,** mill., **MUR-AC.,** nat-p., ***nux-v.,*** **OP.,** pall., petr., ***ph-ac.,*** phyt., pic-ac., plb., puls., pulx., rheum, ***rhus-a., rhus-t.,*** sabal., sant., ***sars.,*** sel., **SEP.,** ***sil.,*** squil., ***stann., staph.,*** stram., ter., thuj., thymol., trib., uva., ***verb.,*** vib., xero, zinc.
childbirth, after - **ARS.,** caust., **SEP.**
elderly people - alum., ***ars., benz-ac.,*** carb-ac., clem., con., ***gels., pop.,*** sel., ***staph.***
evening - ***alum.***
press, must press to pass urine completely - caust., rheum.
sphincter - agar., alumn., apoc., bell., ***caust.,*** con., ***ferr-p.,*** gels., jug-r., nux-v., pall., rhus-a., sabal., sec., **SEP.,** sil., squil., stry., zinc.

WORM in, sensation of - bell., cina, ***sant.,*** sep., sulph.

Blood

ACETONEMIA, blood, in child - phenob.

ACIDOSIS - ***nat-p.***

AGRANULOCYTOSIS - lach.

ANEMIA - abel., ***acet-ac.,*** acon., agar., agn., ***alet.,*** aloe, alum., alum-p., alum-sil., am-c., ambr., anil., ant-c., ***ant-t., apis,*** apoc., aq-mar., ***arg-m., arg-n., arg-o., arn.,*** **ARS.,** ***ars-i.,*** **ARS-S-F.,** aur-a., ***bell.,*** benz-d-n., berb., beryl., bism., bol., **BOR.,** bov., ***bry.,*** cadm-m., **CALC.,** calc-ar., calc-i., calc-lac., **CALC-P.,** calen., calo., carb-an., ***carb-v., carb-s.,*** casc., ***caust.,*** cedr., cham., **CHIN.,** chin-a., ***chin-s.,*** chlol., chloram., chlorpr., cic., cina, cob-n., ***cocc.,*** coff., colch., coloc., ***con.,*** cortico., cortiso., crat., ***crot-h., cupr.,*** cupr-ar., cupr-s., ***cycl.,*** dig., eucal., **FERR.,** ferr-ac., **FERR-AR.,** ferr-c., ferr-cit., ***ferr-i., ferr-m.,*** ferr-o-r., ***ferr-p.,*** ferr-pic., ***ferr-r.,*** goss., **GRAPH.,** ***ham.,*** **HELL.,** ***helon.,*** hep., ***hydr., ign.,*** iod., ip., ***irid.,*** **KALI-AR.,** ***kali-bi., kali-br., kali-c.,*** kali-fer., kali-n., **KALI-P.,** kalm., kres., lac-ac., lac-d., ***lach.,*** led., lyc., mag-c., mag-m., **MANG., MED., MERC.,** ***merc-c.,*** mez., **MOSCH.,** nat-a., ***nat-c.,*** **NAT-M.,** nat-n., ***nat-p., nat-s.,*** **NIT-AC.,** nux-m., ***nux-v.,*** ol-j., ***olnd.,*** ozone, petr., ***ph-ac.,*** **PHOS.,** ***phyt., pic-ac.,*** **PLAT., PLB.,** ***plb-a.,*** psor., **PULS.,** rhod., ***rhus-t.,*** ric., rub-t., ruta, sabin., sac-alb., ***sec., senec., sep.,*** sil., spig., **SQUIL.,** ***stann.,*** **STAPH.,** stroph., **SUL-AC.,** sulfa., sulfonam., **SULPH.,** tab., ther., ***thyr.,*** trinit., tub., urt-u., valer., vanad., verat., ***x-ray, zinc.,*** zinc-ar., zinc-s.

- **bleeding,** after - ***arg-o., ars., calc., carb-v.,*** **CHIN.,** crot-h., **FERR.,** ***helon.,*** hydr., ign., ***lach.,*** nat-br., ***nat-m., nux-v., ph-ac., phos.,*** sabin., staph., ***sulph.***
- **brain,** of - alum., ambr., calc., calc-p., calc-s., chin., chin-s., con., dulc., **FERR.,** fl-ac., hell., kali-c., lyc., mag-c., mosch., mur-ac., nat-c., nat-m., nit-ac., nux-v., petr., **PH-AC., PHOS.,** sang., sel., sep., sil., stry., sulph., zinc.
- **face,** chlorotic - acet-ac., **ARS.,** bar-c., bell., **CALC., CALC-P.,** carb-an., **CARB-S.,** carb-v., caust., chin., chin-a., **COCC.,** con., crot-h., cycl., dig., **FERR.,** ferr-i., **FERR-M.,** ferr-p., **GRAPH.,** helon., hell., ign., kali-ar., **KALI-C.,** kali-p., kali-s., **LYC.,** mang., merc., **NAT-M., NIT-AC.,** nux-v., olnd., ph-ac., phos., **PLAT.,** plb., **PULS.,** sabin., **SENEC., SEP.,** spig., staph., **SULPH.,** sul-ac., valer., zinc.
- **exhausting** disease, from - acet-ac., alst., ***calc-p., chin.,*** chin-s., ***ferr.,*** helon., kali-c., ***nat-m., ph-ac., phos.,*** sec.
- **grief,** from - nat-m., ***ph-ac.***
- **heart** disease, from - ars., crat., stroph.
- **hemolytic,** chlorosis - ***abrot., absin., acet-ac., alet., alum.,*** alum-p., alumn., ***am-c., ambr., ant-c., ant-t.,*** aq-mar., ***arg-m.,*** arg-n., **ARS.,** ars-i., ars-s-f., aur-a., bar-c., **BELL.,** bry., cadm-m., **CALC.,** calc-ar., **CALC-P.,** carb-an., **CARB-S.,** ***carb-v.,*** caust., ***chin., chin-a.,*** chlor., cob-n., cina, **COCC.,** coch., ***con., cupr.,***

ANEMIA,

- **hemolytic,** chlorosis - ***cycl.,*** dig., **FERR., FERR-AR.,** ***ferr-i.,*** **FERR-M.,** ferr-p., ***ferr-s.,*** franz., **GRAPH.,** ***guare., hell., helon., hep.,*** ign., ***ip., kali-ar.,*** kali-bi., ***kali-c., kali-fer., kali-p.,*** kali-per., kali-s., lac-c., lach., **LYC.,** ***lyss.,*** **MANG., MED.,** merc., ***mill., nat-c.,*** nat-hchls., **NAT-M.,** nat-p., **NIT-AC.,** ***nux-v.,*** olnd., ***petr.,*** ph-ac., **PHOS.,** phyt., pic-ac., **PLAT.,** ***plb.,*** **PULS.,** sabin., sac-l., **SENEC., SEP.,** ***sin-n., spig.,*** staph., **SULPH.,** sul-ac., thuj., ust., valer., vanad., ***xan.,*** zinc., abies-c.
  - alternate days, symptoms agg. - alum.
  - winter, in - ***ferr.***
- **malaria,** from - alst., ***ars., nat-m.,*** ost., rob.
- **menorrhagia,** from - arg-o., ars., ***calc.,*** calc-p., ***cann-i.,*** chin., crat., ***cycl., ferr., graph., hydr., kali-c.,*** mang., ***nat-m., puls.,*** sep.
- **nutritional** imbalance, from - alet., alum., ***calc-p., ferr., ferr-p.,*** helon., nux-v.
- **pernicious** anemia - ***ars.,*** calc., ***carc., crot-h.,*** mang., nat-m., ***phos.,*** pic-ac., ***thyr.,*** trinit.
  - family, in - carc.

BLEEDING, general - abies-n., acet-ac., ***acon., adren., agar.,*** aloe, ***alum.,*** alumn., ambr., am-c., am-caust., am-m., ***ammc.,*** anac., ***ant-c.,*** ant-t., anthr., ***apis, aran.,*** arg-m., ***arg-n.,*** **ARN.,** ***ars.,*** ars-i., arum-t., asar., aur., aur-m., bapt., ***bar-c.,*** bar-m., **BELL.,** bell-p., bism., bor., ***bov.,*** **BOTH.,** brom., bufo, ***bry., cact.,*** **CALC.,** calc-f., **CALC-S.,** cann-s., **CANTH.,** ***caps.,*** carb-an., ***carb-s.,*** **CARB-V.,** casc., caust., cina, ***cham.,*** **CHIN.,** chin-a., clem., cinnb., ***cinnm.,*** cocc., coc-c., ***coff.,*** coff-t., colch., coll., ***coloc.,*** con., ***croc.,*** crot-c., **CROT-H.,** ***cupr.,*** dig., ***dros., dulc., elaps,*** equis., **ERIG.,** euphr., **FERR.,** ***ferr-ar., ferr-i., ferr-m., ferr-p., ger.,*** glon., ***graph.,*** **HAM., HELL.,** hep., hydr., ***hyos.,*** ign., ***iod.,*** **IP.,** kali-c., ***kali-chl.,*** kali-i., kali-n., ***kali-p.,*** kreos., **LACH.,** lat-m., ***led., lyc., lycps.,*** mag-arct., mag-aust., mag-m., **MELI., MERC., MERC-C.,** ***mez.,*** **MILL.,** mosch., mur-ac., **MURX.,** nat-c., **NAT-M.,** ***nat-s.,*** nux-m., **NUX-V.,** op., petr., ***ph-ac.,*** **PHOS.,** ***plat.,*** plb., ***psor.,*** **PULS.,** pyrog., rhod., ***rhus-t.,*** ruta, sabad., **SABIN.,** sal-ac., sang., sars., **SEC.,** ***senec.,*** **SEP.,** sel., ***sil.,*** squil., stann., staph., ***stram., stront-c.,*** sulfa., **SULPH., SUL-AC.,** syph., tarax., ***ter.,*** thlaspi, thuj., til., ***tril.,*** urt-u., ust., valer., verat., vib., vinc., vip., wies., x-ray, xan., zinc.

- **acrid,** blood - am-c., ars., bar-c., bov., canth., carb-v., graph., hep., ***kali-c., kali-n.,*** rhus-t., sars., ***sil.,*** sul-ac., sulph., zinc.
- **after,** agg. - **CHIN.,** ***ferr.,*** ip., ***nat-m., ph-ac.,*** sep., stict., sul-ac.
- **amel.** - ars., bov., brom., bufo, calad., card-m., coloc., ferr., ferr-p., ***ham.,*** kali-n., ***lach.,*** mag-c., meli., sars., sel., tarent., thiop.
- **anxiety,** with no mental - ham.
- **arterial** and venous, blood same color - aml-n.
- **black,** blood - am-c., anthr., arn., ars., asar., bapt., benz-n., both., canth., carb-v., ***chin., croc.,*** crot-h., elaps, ***ferr.,*** fl-ac., graph., ham., kali-n., kreos., lach., led., ***mag-c.,*** mag-m.,

BLEEDING, general

black, blood - mag-s., nat-c., ***nat-m.,*** nat-s., nit-ac., ol-an., op., ***puls.,*** sec., stram., sulph.
coagulated - ***camph.***
lumpy, fetid - ***graph.***
tar, like - anthr.

bright red, blood - abrot., **ACON.,** am-c., ant-t., ***arn., ars.,*** bar-c., ***bell.,*** bor., bov., bry., calc., canth., carb-an., carb-v., chin., cinnam., ***crot-h.,*** dig., dros., ***dulc.,*** erech., ***erig., ferr., ferr-p., graph., ham., hyos.,*** **IP.,** kali-n., ***kali-p.,*** kreos., laur., led., ***mag-aust.,*** mag-m., meli., **MILL.,** nat-c., ***nat-m.,*** nit-ac., nux-m., phos., plb., sabin., stront-c., ***tril.,*** ust.

brownish, blood - benz-n., bry., calc., ***carb-v., con.,*** ferr., puls., rhus-t., sul-h.

chronic, effects from - chin., ferr., stront-c.

clots, with - am-m., arn., ars., ***bell.,*** bry., calc., canth., carb-an., caust., **CHAM.,** ***chin.,*** con., ***croc.,*** erig., ***ferr.,*** ferr-p., ***hyos., ign., ip., kali-m.,*** kali-n., ***kali-p.,*** lach., mag-m., ***merc.,*** nat-s., nit-ac., nux-v., ph-ac., phos., **PLAT.,** ***puls.,*** rat., **RHUS-T.,** rhus-v., **SABIN.,** sec., sep., stront-c., sul-ac., sulph., ***thlaspi,*** ust.
fluid partly - erig., plat., puls., rat., ***sabin.,*** ust.
dark clots - alum., anthr., chin., **CROC.,** crot-h., ***elaps,*** ferr., ham., kali-m., lach., mangi., merc., merc-cy., mur-ac., plat., ***puls.,*** sabin., sang., ***sec., sul-ac.,*** ter., ***thlaspi,*** tril.
venous - sec., ham., mangi.

coagulate, blood does not - ***adren.,*** ail., alum., alumn., am-c., anthr., ***apis,*** aran., ***arn.,*** ars., ars-h., bell., **BOTH.,** ***bov., cact.,*** calc., calc-lac., calc-p., canth., carb-an., ***carb-v., chin.,*** chin-s., chlol., ***cinnam.,*** cortico., croc., **CROT-C.,** ***crot-h.,*** dig., dor., ***elaps,*** erech., ergot., ***erig.,*** **FERR.,** ferr-m., ***ferr-p.,*** fic., gall-ac., ***ger., ham., ip.,*** kali-c., ***kali-p.,*** kreos., **LACH., LAT-M.,** led., meli., merc., merc-cy., ***mill.,*** mur-ac., nat-m., nat-n., ***nat-s., nat-sil.,*** **NIT-AC.,** op., ph-ac., **PHOS.,** puls., rad-br., ***sabin., sec.,*** sil., ***sul-ac.,*** sulph., ***ter.,*** thlaspi, til., ***tril.,*** ust., verat., vip., visc., x-ray, xanth.
intermittent - phos.
thin, dark - ***crot-h.,*** elaps, ***lach., sec.,*** sul-ac.

coagulation, clots, formation of, causes plugs - ***kali-m.***
clots, loose - anthr.
clotted, partly, in hemorrhage - ***ferr.***
difficult - phos.
easy - ***merc.***
to a gelatinous mass - ferr-p.
slow, or not at all - dig.
sycotic pneumonia, in - ***nat-s.***

dark, blood - **CROC.,** ***cupr.,*** ham., kreos., lach., mag-c., ***merc.,*** naja, sec., ust., verat.
nosebleed, with - crot-h.
cherry red - anthr.
yellow fever, in - crot-h., **LACH.**

BLEEDING, general

decomposed, blood - cic., ***crot-h., lach., vip.***
rapidly - acet-ac., am-c., anthr., ***crot-h.,*** lach., ter.

exertion, after - bell-p., ***mill.,*** **NIT-AC.**

exudates, hemorrhagic - anthr.

fainting, tinnitus, with, loss of sight, general coldness, even convulsions - ***chin.,*** ferr., phos.

hot - acon., anac., ***bell.,*** dulc., sabin.

hysterical - bad., croc., hyos., ign., kali-i., merc., stict., sulph.

injury, after - ***mill.***

internally - abrot., acon., alumn., ***bell.,*** bry., cham., ***chin.,*** cic., con., dulc., euph., ferr., ferr-p., ham., hep., hyper., iod., ip., kali-c., lach., laur., mill., nux-v., par., petr., phos., plb., puls., rhus-t., ruta, sabin., sec., sul-i., sulph., thlaspi

light, blood in hemorrhage - ***merc.***

menopause period, in - ***phos.***

mucous membranes, from - calc-sil., ham.

offensive, blood - ars., bapt., ***bell., bry., carb-an.,*** carb-v., caust., ***cham.,*** chin., ***croc.,*** ign., kali-c., ***kali-p.,*** merc., mur-ac., phos., plat., rheum, sabin., sec., sil., sulph.

orifices of the body, from - anthr., aran., **BOTH.,** carc., ***chin.,*** **CROT-H.,** elaps, ***ip., lach.,*** **PHOS.,** ***sul-ac.***

painless, no fever - mill.

pale, blood - apis, carb-ac., carb-an., carb-v., ferr., graph., kreos., ***phos.,*** sabad., sulph., tarent.

passive, oozing - ars-h., bov., bufo, carb-v., ***chin.,*** crot-h., ferr-p., ham., ph-ac., sec., tarent., ter., ust.

plasma, coloring matter escapes into blood - arg-n.

prolonged, agg. - **CHIN.,** plat.

putrescence, with, tingling in limbs, debility - sec.

ropy, tenacious, blood - anthr., apis, **CORI-R.,** kali-chl., ***kali-m.***

sex, after - arg-n., kreos., nit-ac., sep.

slight, agg. - bufo, ***carb-an., chin.,*** ham., **HYDR.,** sec.

stringy, blood - croc.

suppression of - thlaspi

surgery, after, with coldness and prostration - ***calen., stront-c.***

thick, blood - agar., bov., carb-v., cham., chin., ***croc.,*** cupr., ***ferr-m.,*** kali-n., kreos., lach., laur., mag-c., mag-s., ***nux-m.,*** plat., ***puls.,*** rhus-t., sep., sulph.

thin, pale - ant-t., both., carb-v., crot-h., ***ferr.,*** ham., lach., laur., nit-ac., phos., ***sec.,*** sul-ac., til., ust.

traumatism, from - aran., ***arn.,*** bov., euph-pi., ham., ***mill.,*** tril.

vicarious - abrot., acet-ac., bry., ham., ip., kali-c., ***phos.***

BLEEDING, general

watery, blood - alum., am-c., ant-t., ***berb.,*** bor., bov., carb-v., crot-h., dulc., ***ferr., graph.,*** kali-c., kreos., lat-m., laur., mang., nat-m., nat-s., nit-ac., phos., prun., ***puls.,*** rhus-t., sabin., sec., stram., sulph.

mixed with clots - arn., bell., caust., puls., sabin.

BLOOD vessels, general, (see Blood, Veins) - acon., apis, ***arn., bell.,*** **CARB-V.,** chin., ferr., ***fl-ac.,*** gels., glon., graph., **HAM.,** ***hyos., lach.,*** lyc., nat-m., ***phos.,*** **PULS.,** sang., ***sec., sep.,*** sul-ac., sulph., ***thuj.,*** vip., zinc.

aneurism - ***aur., bar-c.,*** cact., calc-f., ***calen.,*** carb-v., kali-i., lach., ***lyc.,*** puls., sulph., thuj.

capillary - ***calc-f.,*** fl-ac., tub.

abdomen - ***bar-m., sec.***

anastomosis, by - cact., carb-v., caust., lyc., ***phos.,*** plat., plb., thuj., verat-v., zinc.

anastomosis, from - thuj.

aorta - ***calc.,*** calen., spong.

arch of - kali-i.

descending, of - **RAN-S.,** spong.

arteries, of the large - ***acon.,*** ambr., arn., ars., ars-i., aspar., aur., ***bar-c., bar-m., bell.,*** **CACT., CALC.,** calc-f., calc-p., ***calen.,*** cann-s., carb-an., ***carb-v.,*** caust., ***dig.,*** ferr., ***ferr-p.,*** glon., graph., guai., iod., kali-c., ***kali-i.,*** kalm., ***lach.,*** lith., ***lyc.,*** lycps., morph., nat-m., plb., puls., ran-s., **SPIG.,** ***spong., sulph.,*** thuj.***verat-v.***

bleeding violently from least wound - ***carb-v.***

flat - ***carb-v.***

heart, of - **CACT.,** ***carb-v.***

large vessels near - lycps.

left carotid and aorta, dilatation of - lach.

pains, of - cact., gall-ac., sec.

round - ***carb-v.***

small, all over body - plb.

syphilitic - iod., kali-i.

vagus and its branches, involving pressure on - eucal.

aorta, inflamed, acute - acon., apis, glon., tub.

chronic - adon., ***adren., ant-a., ars-i.,*** aur., aur-a., ***cact.,*** chin-s., crat., cupr., glon., kali-i., lyc., spig., stroph.

ulcerative - adon., ***adren., ant-a., ars-i.,*** aur., aur-a., ***cact.,*** chin-s., crat., cupr., glon., kali-i., lyc., spig., stroph.

arteriosclerosis - adren., am-i, am-van., aml-n., ant-a., arg-n., ***arn.,*** ars., ***ars-i., aur.,*** aur-br., ***aur-i.,*** aur-m-n., ***bar-c.,*** bar-i., bar-m., bell-p., benz-ac., cact., cal-ren., ***calc.,*** calc-ar., calc-f., card-m., chin-s., chlol., con., crat., ***cupr.,*** ergot., fl-ac., form., form-ac., fuc., ***glon.,*** hed., hyper., iod., ***kali-i.,*** kali-sal., kres., lach., lith., mag-f., man., naja, ***nat-i.,*** nit-ac., phos., ***plb., plb-i., polyg-a.,*** rad-br., rauw., ***sec.,*** sil., solid., ***stront-c., stront-i.,*** stroph., sumb., ***tab.,*** thlaspi, thyr., ***vanad., visc.,*** zinc-p.

BLOOD vessels, general

atheroma - aur-m., bell., brom., ***calc., calc-f.,*** caps., ***graph.,*** kali-i., ***lach., lac-ac.,*** lyc., phos., ***plb., sil.,*** sulph.

elderly people, in - ***lach.***

morbus brightii, in - ph-ac.

obese persons, in - caps.

pulmonary arteries, dilatation of right heart - phos.

burning, in - agar., ***ars.,*** aur., **BRY., CALC.,** ***hyos.,*** med., nat-m., nit-ac., ***op., rhus-t.,*** sulph., syph., verat.

calcareous deposits, in, (see arteriosclerosis) - vario.

capillaries, aneurism - ***fl-ac.***

contraction, causes - kali-br.

engorged with discharge of bloody serum - ***hyper.***

erethism, following wounds with or without hemorrhages and great nervous depression - hyper.

fill slowly after pressure on skin, in scarlatina - ***lach.***

hemorrhage, disposition to, oozing of dark, thin blood - ***sul-ac.***

injected - ***bell.***

net like appearance - ***caust.***

cold, sensation, in - abies-c., **ACON.,** ant-c., ant-t., **ARS.,** bell., led., lyc., op., plb., pyrog., **RHUS-T.,** sulph., sul-ac., ***verat.***

clucking, pulsation in some of larger arteries - caps.

distention, of - acon., aesc., agar., alum., alum-p., alum-sil., ***am-c.,*** ambr., ant-t., apoc., ***arn.,*** ars., aur., ***aur-m.,*** aur-s., ***bar-c., bar-m.,*** **BELL.,** bov., bry., calc., calc-f., calc-sil., ***camph., carb-s., carb-v.,*** caust., celt., ***chel.,*** **CHIN.,** chin-a., ***chin-s.,*** cic., clem., cocc., coloc., con., ***croc.,*** cycl., dig., **FERR.,** ferr-ar., ferr-i., ferr-p., fl-ac., ***graph., ham.,*** hep., **HYOS.,** ***lac-d.,*** lach., laur., ***led., lil-t.,*** lyc., mag-c., meny., merl., mosch., nat-c., nat-m., nit-ac.1, ***nux-v.,*** olnd., op., ph-ac., ***phos.,*** piloc., ***plb., podo.,*** **PULS.,** rheum, rhod., rhus-t., ruta, sars., sec., sel., sep., sil., spig., ***spong.,*** staph., stront-c., sul-ac., ***sulph.,*** **THUJ.,** vip., zinc.

arteries - aml-n., bell.

cerebral congestion - bell., glon., ***verat-v.***

and temporal - ***glon.***

carotids - ***bell., glon.,*** verat-v.

evening - **PULS.**

fever, during - ***agar.,*** **BELL.,** ***camph.,*** **CHIN.,** ***chin-s.,*** **HYOS., LED., PULS.**

head, especially those of, face and feet - bell., ***ferr.***

motion, on - spong.

nosebleed, with, relaxed, in old people - ***agar.***

superficial, of, extreme - ***bell.***

swollen, in stroke - ***hyos.***

tone, lack of, after congestion - lycps.

BLOOD vessels, general
heat, sensation, in - agar., **ARS.,** ***aur., bry., calc., hyos.,*** med., nat-m., nit-ac., op., **RHUS-T.,** ***sulph., verat.***
hot water, as if, were flowing through - ***ars.***
with sweat, disappearing when nausea comes on - sin-n.
inflammation, of - acon., ***ant-t.,*** apis, **ARN., ARS.,** ars-i., **BAR-C.,** calc., cham., chin., ***cupr., ham., kali-c.,*** kreos., ***lach.,*** lyc., **PULS.,** ***spig., puls.,*** sil., **SULPH.,** thuj., vip., zinc.
arteritis - ars., ***calc.,*** echi., hist., ***kali-i.,*** lach., ***nat-i.,*** sec., sulfa.
aorta, acute - acon., apis, glon., tub.
chronic - adon., ***adren., ant-a.,*** arn., ***ars-i.,*** aur., aur-a., ***cact.,*** chin-s., crat., cupr., glon., kali-i., lyc., merc., ***nat-i., puls.,*** ruta, spig., stroph.
ulcerative - acon., ars., chin-s.
injuries, to - arn., ham., hyper., led., mill., phos.
shot, rolling through the arteries, sensation - nat-p.
stenosis, of aorta, alleviates sufferings - hydrc.
swelled - apis, arn., ham., paeon., ***puls.***
tumors, of - calc-f.
veins, (see Blood, Veins)
vibrating, in - phel.

CIRCULATION, general - ***acon., adon.,*** am-c., am-m., ***aml-n.,*** apoc., arn., ***ars., ars-i.,*** aur., aur-m., bar-c., bell., benz-ac., ***bry., cact., calc-ar.,*** calc-f., carb-v., chin., cimic., coca, colch., ***coll., conv., crat., crot-h., dig., digin.,*** ferr-m., ferr-p., gels., ***glon.,*** grin., ***hydr-ac., iber.,*** ign., iod., kali-c., kali-chl., ***kalm.,*** **LACH.,** laur., lepi., ***lil-t.,*** lith., ***lycps.,*** merc-c., mosch., ***naja,*** nat-m., nux-v., ***ox-ac., phase.,*** **PHOS.,** piloc., ***saroth., sep., spig., spong.,*** squil., ***stroph., stry.,*** sumb., thyr., valer., verat-v.
agitated, easily - lach., sil.
blood to quick, sensation - ars.
coughing, symptoms worse sitting bent forward and - ***spong.***
diminished flow to parts remote from heart - calc., ***camph.,*** sep.
distribution, rapid deviations in - ***glon.***
disturbed, in intermittent fever - ***ferr.***
disturbance due to sudden and violent implication of solar plexus, with cyanosis and threatened suffocation - ***op.***
excited, easily - all-s., aml-n., ***bell.,*** berb., chin-s., ***corn.,*** ferr-i., **VERAT-V.,** zing.
acute enteritis, with - ***vera***t-v.
cholera infantum, in - ***kali-br.***
erysipelas traumatic, in - apis.
evening, with restlessness and trembling - ***lyc.***
hemorrhages, in - ***croc., ferr.***
hypochondriasis, in - valer.
menses, during - ***sulph.***
metrorrhagia, in - ***hyos.***
motion, by every - ***nat-m.***

CIRCULATION, general
excited, easily
pulse, with small, rapid - ***ran-b.***
sex, after - am-c.
walking in open air, when - ambr.
impaired, in renal congestion - crot-h.
impeded, gives rise to oedema - ***cocc.***
irregular - bor.
lying down, symptoms worse after, and lying on right side - ***spong.***
menses, symptoms worse before - ***spong.***
menopause, in, affected - **LACH.**
quickened, easily - ***glon.***
rheumatic, with - acon., aur., benz-ac., ***bry.,*** cact., caust., cimic., ***colch.,*** ign., ***kalm.,*** led., lith., lycps., naja, phyt., ***rhus-t., spig.,*** verat-v.
sluggish - aeth., ***calc., calc-p.,*** carb-an., ***carb-v.,*** cimic., cinnam., ferr-p., ***gels.,*** led., nat-m., ***rhus-t.,*** **SEP.,** ***sil.***
hemorrhoids, with - cact., ***coll.,*** dig., ham.
smoking, symptoms agg. from - ***spong.***
stagnation, threatened - ***carb-an.***
stoppage, sensation of, at night, with fright and then sweat - ***lyc.***
stopped, as if, eight a.m., tingling to tongue and finger-tips, with anxiety - ***bar-c.***
suspended, as if - ***gels., lyc.,*** sabad.
symptoms worse going upstairs - ***spong.***
weakness, of - acet-ac., ***adon.,*** adren., agar., ***am-c., am-m.,*** ant-a., ***ars., ars-i.,*** aur., ***cact., calc., calc-ar.,*** **CALC-P.,** camph., carb-ac., ***carb-v., chin.,*** chin-a., chlf., ***conv., crat., crot-h., dig.,*** dios., eucal., euph., ***ferr.,*** grin., helo., ***hydr-ac., iber.,*** kali-c., kalm., lach., lil-t., lycps., morph., mosch., nit-ac., nux-m., phase., plb., prun., psor., ***puls.,*** pyrog., sang., sarcol-ac., **SEP.,** spig., squil., ***stroph.,*** tab., thyr., ***verat.***
diminished, propelling power injures muscular fibres - chin-s.
edema, with - ***adon., apoc., ars.,*** ars-i., cact., coll., ***conv., dig.,*** iber., lach., lycps., olnd., squil., ***stroph.***
muscular debility, with - adon., adren., aether, ***alco.,*** amn-l., ant-t., atro., cocaine, conv., crat., ***dig., glon.,*** ser-ang., stroph., verat.
nervous debility, with - adren., cact., ***iber.,*** ign., ***lil-t.,*** lith., ***mosch., naja,*** piloc., ***spig.,*** tab., ***valer.***
dyspepsia, , with - ***hydr-ac.***
paleness and constant chilliness, with - ***puls.***
palpitations, with - olnd.
quickened, but - aml-n.
sensitive, nervous subjects, in - kali-p.
typhoid malarial fever - ***ham.***

COLD, sensation, as if - abies-c., **ACON.,** ant-c., ant-t., **ARS.,** bell., led., lyc., op., plb., pyrog., **RHUS-T.,** sulph., sul-ac., ***verat.***

CONGESTION, of blood - **ACON., AESC.,** act-sp., agar., agn., ***aloe, alum.,*** alum-p., ambr., aml-n., am-c., am-m., ang., anis., ant-c., ant-t., ***anthr., apis,*** aq-mar., arist-cl., ***arn.,*** ars., asaf., aster., ***aur.,*** aur-a., aur-i., aur-s., bar-c., **BELL.,** ***bor.,*** bov., brom., ***bry.,*** **CACT.,** ***calc.,*** calc-sil., camph., cann-s., canth., carb-an., ***carb-s., carb-v.,*** caust., cent., cham., chel., **CHIN.,** chin-s., cinnb., clem., cocc., ***coff.,*** colch., coloc., con., conv., croc., cupr., cycl., dig., dulc., erig., eucal., euphr., **FERR.,** ***ferr-i.,*** ferr-p., ***ferr-s.,*** fl-ac., gad., gels., **GLON.,** ***graph.,*** guai., ***ham., hell.,*** hep., hydr., hypoth., ***hyos.,*** ign., iod., kali-c., kali-i., kali-n., ***lach.,*** laur., led., lil-t., ***lyc.,*** mag-c., mag-m., mang., **MELI.,** merc., mez., mosch., nat-c., ***nat-m.,*** nat-s., ***nit-ac.,*** nux-m., **NUX-V.,** op., petr., ph-ac., **PHOS.,** piloc., plat., plb., podo., ***psor.,*** **PULS.,** ***ran-b.,*** rhod., ***rhus-t.,*** sabin., samb., ***sang.,*** sars., sec., sel., ***seneg., sep., sil.,*** spig., ***spong.,*** squil., staph., ***stram., stront-c., stront-i.,*** **SULPH.,** sul-ac., tarax., thuj., ust., valer., verat., verat-v., **VIOL-O.,** vip., zinc.
- bleeding, after - mill.
- coldness of legs, with - ***bell., nat-m., stram.***
- internally - ***aloe, apis,*** ars., **CACT.,** ***camph.,*** canth., ***colch.,*** conv., cupr., ***glon., hell.,*** **MELI.,** ***phos.,*** sars., sep., ***verat.,*** verat-v.
- menopause, during - acon., ***aml-n.,*** calc., ***glon.,*** lach., sang., sep., ***sulph., ust.***
- sudden - acon., bell., ***glon.,*** verat-v.

DISORGANIZATION, blood, of - ail., am-c., ***anthr.,*** arn., ***ars.,*** ars-h., ***bapt.,*** carb-ac., ***crot-h., echi.,*** kreos., ***lach., mur-ac.,*** phos., psor., ***pyrog., rhus-t.,*** tarent-c.

GUSHING, blood, as if - ox-ac.

HEAT, sensation, in - agar., **ARS.,** ***aur., bry., calc., hyos.,*** med., nat-m., nit-ac., op., **RHUS-T.,** ***sulph., verat.***

HOT, blood, as if - med., sec.
- hot water, as if, were flowing through - ***ars.***
  - with sweat, disappearing when nausea comes on - sin-n.

HYPERTENSION, high blood pressure - acon., adon., ***adren.,*** agar., aml-n., aran., arg-n., ars., asar., aster., ***aur.,*** aur-i., aur-m., aur-m-n., ***bar-c.,*** bar-m., cal-ren., ***calc.,*** calc-f., calc-p., caust., chin-s., coff., con., cortiso., **CRAT.,** cupr., cupr-ac., cupr-ar., dig., fl-ac., ***glon., grat.,*** ign., iod., iris, kali-ars., kali-c., kali-m., kali-p., **LACH.,** lat-m., lyc., lycps., mag-c., naja, **NAT-M.,** nit-ac., ***nux-v.,*** ph-ac., phos., pic-ac., pituit., ***plb.,*** psor., puls., rad-br., reser., ***rauw.,*** rhus-t., sang., scop., ***sec.,*** sep., sil., squil., ***stront-c.,*** stroph., ***sulph., sumb.,*** tab., thal., thlaspi, thuj., valer., vanad., **VERAT.,** verat-v., visc.
- sudden rise of - coff., ***glon.***

hypotension, low blood pressure - acon., agar., aran., cact., ***carb-v.,*** cur., gels., halo., hist., lach., lat-m., lyc., naja, ph-ac., ***phos.,*** rad-br., rauw., reser., ***sep.,*** staph., sulfa., ther., ***thyr.,*** verat., visc.
- diastolic - bar-m.

LEUKEMIA - acet-ac., acon., ***aran.,*** **ARS.,** ***ars-i.,*** bar-i., bar-m., bry., ***calc., calc-p., carb-s.,*** carb-v., ***cean., chin.,*** chin-s., con., cortiso., crot-h., ***ferr-pic.,*** ip., ***kali-p.,*** merc., **NAT-A.,** ***nat-m., nat-p.,*** **NAT-S.,** nux-v., op., phos., ***pic-ac.,*** sulfa., sulph., syph., thuj., tub., ***x-ray.***
- acute - ***ars.,*** lach., merc., merc-c., ***nat-m.,*** nit-ac., phos.
  - children, in - **ARS.**
- lymphoid - **ARS.,** ***ars-i.,*** carb-s., carb-v., **CEAN.,** kali-s., mur-ac., nat-a., nat-m., **PHYT.,** pic-ac., thuj.
- spleen, involvement - ***cean.,*** nat-m., nat-s., querc., succ.

ORGASM, of blood - **ACON.,** aloe, alum., alum-p., alum-sil., alumn., ***ambr., am-c., am-m., aml-n.,*** ant-c., ant-t., arg-m., **ARG-N.,** ***arn.,*** ars., ***ars-i., asar.,*** **AUR.,** aur-a., ***aur-i.,*** aur-s., bar-c., bar-s., **BELL.,** berb., bor., ***bov., bry.,*** **CALC.,** ***calc-ar.,*** calc-i., calc-s., cann-i., cann-s., carb-an., **CARB-S.,** ***carb-v., caust.,*** cench., ***cham.,*** chin., cina, cocc., coff., ***con.,*** corn., ***croc., cupr.,*** dig., dulc., erig., **FERR.,** ferr-ar., ***ferr-i.,*** ferr-p., ***gels.,*** **GLON.,** ***graph.,*** guai., ***hep.,*** hyos., ign., ***iod.,*** piloc., kali-bi., kali-br., ***kali-c.,*** kali-p., kali-s., kiss., **KREOS., LACH.,** ***lil-t.,*** **LYC.,** mag-c., mag-m., mang., ***meli., merc.,*** merl., ***mill.,*** mosch., nat-c., ***nat-m.,*** nat-p., nit-ac., ***nux-m., nux-v., op.,*** ox-ac., ***petr.,*** **PH-AC., PHOS.,** plb., rhod., ***puls., rhus-t.,*** sabad., sabin., ***samb.,*** sang., ***sars., sel., seneg., sep., sil.,*** **SPONG.,** ***stann.,*** staph., **STRAM.,** ***stront-c.,*** stroph., ***sul-ac.,*** sul-i., **SULPH.,** tab., ***thuj.,*** tell., ust., valer., ***verat.***
- anxiety, with - ***acon.,*** aloe, am-m., ***bar-c.,*** chel.
- ascending stairs, on - thuj.
- asleep, on falling - petr., sep.
- burning in hands, with - **SULPH.**
  - skin, of - ***sang.***
- eating, amel. - alum., chin.
  - warm food, while - mag-c.
- emotions, after - ***acon.,*** apis, ***aur., bell.,*** bry., calc., **CHAM.,** coff., colch., ***coloc., con.,*** cupr., **HYOS., IGN.,** kali-c., ***kali-p., lach.,*** lyc., mag-c., nat-m., ***nat-p., nit-ac., nux-v.,*** op., ***petr., ph-ac., phos.,*** plat., **PULS.,** ***sep., staph.,*** stram., teucr., thuj., verat.
- evening - arn., ***asar., caust.,*** dig., kali-c., lyc., ***merc.,*** petr., phos., rhus-t., sars., thuj.
  - lying down, after - ign., samb., sars., sil.
  - sexual excitement, during - clem.
  - sitting amel. - thuj.
- everything were moving in body, as if - croc.
- faintness, with - petr.
- lying, on left side - ***bar-c.***
- menses, during - ***calc., merl.***
  - before - ***alumn., cupr.,*** merc.
- morning, after restless sleep - calc.
  - rising, on, amel. - nux-v.
  - sleep, in - ang.
  - waking, on - calc., graph., kali-c., lyc., nux-v.

ORGASM, of blood
motion, on - nat-m.
motion or speaking agg. - iod., nat-c.
nervousness, from - ambr., ***bell.***, calc., ferr., kali-n., ***merc., nit-ac., phos., ph-ac.***, sep.
news, from bad - lach.
night - ***am-c.***, arg-n., ***calc., carb-an., carb-v.***, hep., ign., mag-c., ***merc.***, mur-ac., ***nat-c.***, nat-m., ***phos., puls.***, ran-b., raph., senn., ***sep., sil., sulph.***
bed, drives him out of - iod.
beer, after - sulph.
palpitation, with - kali-c., phos., sul-ac.
restlessness, with - aloe, ph-ac.
sensual impressions, from - ***phos.***
sex, after - am-c., ***sep.***
sitting, while - ***mag-m.***
sleep, on falling to - petr., sep.
tobacco, on smoking - phos.
vertigo, during - nat-c.
vexation, after - ***acon.***, **CHAM.**, coloc., ign., merc., ***petr.***, **SEP.**, staph.
vomiting, after - verat.
walking, after - arg-n., berb., ***petr.***, sul-i.
after a long - ***arg-n.***
amel. - mag-m.
wine, after - sil.

PHLEBITIS - **ACON.**, agar., ***all-c.***, ant-c., ***ant-t.***, apis, arist-cl., ***arn., ars., bell.***, both., **BRY.**, ***bufo***, **CALC.**, calc-ar., ***calc-f.***, carb-s., carb-v., ***cham., chin.***, chlorpr., **CLEM.**, crot-h., graph., ***ham.***, hecla., hep., hir., ***iod., kali-c.***, kali-m., kreos., **LACH.**, ***led., lyc., lycps.***, mag-c., mag-f., merc., merc-cy., merc-i-r., ***nat-s.***, nux-v., phos., ***puls.***, rhod., **RHUS-T.**, ruta, ***sep., sil.***, spig., stront-br., stront-c., sulfa., ***sulph.***, thiop., thuj., verat., **VIP.**, vip-a., zinc.
childbirth, after, forceps with - all-c.
contractions, with - ***sil.***
injuries, after - rhus-t.

PORTAL congestion, with hemorrhoids, and dysmenorrhea - **COLL.**

POLYCYTHEMIA, blood - phos.

PURPURA hemorrhagica - aln., ***arn.***, ars., ars-i., bell., berb., both., bov., bry., ***carb-v.***, chin-s., chlol., cor-r., ***crot-h., cupr.***, ferr-pic., ***ham.***, hyos., iod., ip., ***kali-i.***, **LACH.**, **LED.**, merc., merc-c., mill., naja, nat-n., nux-v., ***ph-ac.***, **PHOS.**, ***rhus-t.***, rhus-v., ruta, **SEC.**, sil., stram., sulph., **SUL-AC.**, **TER.**, thlaspi.
discoloration, legs - kali-i., ***lach.***, **PHOS.**, ***sec.***
limbs, upper and lower - ***lach., phos., sec., sul-ac.***, ter.
formication, with - phos.
idiopathica - acon., ***arn., ars.***, bapt., bell., bry., carb-v., chin-s., chlor., ***crot-h., ham.***, jug-r., kali-i., ***lach.***, merc., ph-ac., ***phos.***, rhus-t., sal-ac., sec., ***sul-ac.***, sulfon., ter., verat-v.
colic, with - bov., coloc., cupr., merc-c., thuj.

PURPURA hemorrhagica
idiopathica,
debility, with - arn., ***ars.***, carb-v., lach., merc., sul-ac.
itching, with - phos.
miliaris - acon., am-c., am-m., arn., bell., coff., dulc., sulph., sul-ac.
rheumatica - acon., ars., ***bry.***, merc., ***rhus-t.***, rhus-v.
senilis - ars., bar-c., bry., con., ***lach.***, op., rhus-t., **SEC.**, sul-ac.

RED blood cells, decay, rapid - ***kali-p.***
disorganize, as after snake bite - dor.
dissolution, of - sec.
irregular, smaller and - ***apis.***

RESTLESSNESS, blood, in - iod.

RUSHES, blood of - bell., ferr., glon., lach., sang., spong., sulph.,
downward - aur., meph., thyr.,
upward - acon., arn., bell., bry., ferr., glon., kali-i., meli., phos., sang., stront-c.,

SEPTICEMIA, blood poisoning - ***achy., acon.***, agar., ***ail.***, am-c., ***anthr.***, ap-v., ***apis***, arg-m., arg-n., ***arn.***, **ARS.**, ars-i., arum-t., atro., ***bapt., bell.***, bor-ac., both., ***bry.***, bufo, calc., calc-ar., calen., ***carb-ac.***, **CARB-V.**, ***cench., chin., chin-a., chin-s.***, chlorpr., colch., conch., crot-c., **CROT-H.**, dor., ***echi.***, elaps, ***ferr.***, ferr-p., gels., gunp., hell., ***hippoz.***, hydroph., hyos., ***ip.***, irid., kali-bi., kali-br., ***kali-c., kali-p.***, kreos., **LACH.**, lat-h., lob-p., ***lyc.***, mag-c., ***merc., merc-cy.***, methyl-b., ***mur-ac.***, naja, ***nat-m.***, nat-s-c., ***nit-ac.***, nux-v., op., paro-i., ph-ac., ***phos.***, phyt., ***puls.***, **PYROG.**, rad-br., raja-s., ***rhus-t., sal-ac., sec.***, sieg., sil., stram., strept., sul-ac., sulfonam., ***sulph.***, tarax., tarent., tarent-c., ***ter.***, trach., vario., ***verat., verat-v., vip.***, zinc.
absorption of deleterious substances, from - anthr.
ailments, from - **LACH.**, sal-ac., ***tarent.***
childbed, in - **ARS.**
diphtheria, in - ***crot-h.***
dissolution, general - ***phos.***
drowsiness, during, fever and great prostration - gels.
erysipelas - ***apis, crot-h.***
morbid ferments - ***nat-s.***
nosebleed, with - ***crot-h., lach.***
pyemia - **ANTHR.**, ***ars., crot-h., hipp***oz., **LACH.**, verat.
childbed fever, with - ***arn.***
gangrenous carbuncles - ***anthr.***
rapidly, decomposing - anthr.
scarlatina, in - ***apis***, carb-v.
scorbutus, in - ***nat-m.***
septic fever - acet-ac., **ANTHR.**, ***apis***, **ARN.**, **ARS.**, ***bell.***, berb., **BAPT.**, **BRY.**, ***cadm-s., carb-v.***, **CROT-C**, **CROT-H.**, ***cur.***, **ECHI.**, **KALI-P.**, **LACH.**, **LYC.**, ***merc.***, **MUR-AC.**, op., ***ph-ac.***, **PHOS.**, ***puls.***, **PYROG.**, ***rhus-t., rhus-v.***, **SULPH.**, **TARENT-C.**
tendency to typhoid - **ARN.**

SEPTICEMIA, blood poisoning
typhus, in - ***ars., cupr-m.***
vomiting, with - crot-h.
yawning, with - crot-h.

SERUM, increase of watery elements and decrease of solids - ***ferr.,*** **NAT-M.**
venous system, regulates water capacity of - nat-s.

STAGNATED, sensation as if - acon., bar-c., bell., bry., ***carb-v.,*** caust., croc., crot-t., dig., gels., hep., ign., ***lyc.,*** nit-ac., nux-v., olnd., ***pic-ac.,*** puls., rhod., ***sabad.,*** seneg., **SEP.,** sulph., zinc.

STASIS, of (see Weakness) - bell-p., calc., ***carb-v., ham.,*** puls., ***sep.,*** sulph.

STILL, stands, as if - acon., lyc., sabad., ***sep.,*** zinc.

STREAMING, sensation, of - ***ox-ac.***

SYSTOLE, extra - dys-co.

THIN, sensation as if - hell.

THROMBOSIS - acetan., ***apis, ars., both.,*** calc-ar., carb-v., cortico., ***kali-m.,*** kres., ***lach., nat-s.,*** sec., ***vip.***
albuminuria, in - ***calc-ar.***
collateral veins, circuit unusually developed - ***apis.***
great veins of region of groins, of - ***ars.***
hard thrombosis of veins - card-m., fl-ac.
heart clot, suspected, with pneumonia - am-c.
hydrogenoid constitutions, in, particularly with affections of glands - ***nat-s.***
middle of bend of thighs, a thick sensitive string all along inner side of thighs - ***apis***
pneumonia, in - am-c.
wet agg. - ***nat-s.***

TYPHOID, hemorrhagic - carb-v., **CROT-H.,** ***lach., mill.,*** **PHOS.,** ***sul-ac.***
oozing of dark thin blood from capillaries - crot-h., ***sul-ac.***

UREMIA - ***am-c., apis,*** apoc., ars., asc-c., bapt., ***bell., canth., carb-ac.,*** cic., ***cupr.,*** cupr-ac., dig., gels., ***glon., hell.,*** hydr-ac., ***hyos.,*** kali-br., ***kali-s., morph.,*** mosch., ***op.,*** phos., pic-ac., piloc., ***plb.,*** queb., ser-ang., ***stram., ter.,*** urea, **URT-U.,** verat-v.
convulsions, with - apoc., cic., crot-h., ***cupr.,*** cupr-ar., ***dig.,*** hydr-ac., ***kali-s.,*** merc-c., ***mosch., plb., ter.***
head, congestion, with - am-c., apis, ***bell.,*** con., ***cupr., gels., glon.,*** merc-c., ***stram.,*** tab., ter., verat-v.

VARICOSE, veins, general - acet-ac., aesc., alum., alum-sil., ***alumn., am-c., ambr.,*** ang., ***ant-t.,*** apis, arist-cl., **ARN.,** ***arg-n., ars.,*** ars-s-f., asaf., ***bar-c., bell.,*** bell-p., ***berb.,*** brom., ***bry.,*** **CALC.,** ***calc-f., calc-i.,*** calc-p., calc-s., calen., camph., ***carb-an.,*** **CARB-V.,** carb-s., carc., card-b., ***card-m., caust.,*** chel., ***chin.,*** chin-s., cic., clem., coll., coloc., con., ***croc., crot-h.,*** cycl., ***ferr.,*** ferr-ar., ferr-p., **FL-AC.,** form., form-ac., ***graph.,*** **HAM.,** hecla., ***hep.,*** hyos., kali-ar., kali-n., ***kreos.,*** lac-c., lach., ***lyc.,*** **LYCPS.,** mag-aust., mag-c., mag-f., man., mangi., meli., meny., merc-cy.,

VARICOSE, veins, general - mez., mill., morg., mosch., mur-ac., ***nat-m., nux-v.,*** olnd., op., ***paeon.,*** petr., ph-ac., ***phos., plb.,*** polyg., **PULS.,** pyrog., ***ran-s.,*** rhod., ***rhus-t.,*** ruta, sabin., sars., scirr., sec., **SEP.,** sil., sol-n., ***spig.,*** spong., ***staph.,*** stront-br., stront-c., sul-ac., ***sulph.,*** thuj., ***vip., zinc.***
alcohol, from - crot-h.
angina tonsillaris, with - ***bar-m.***
bleeding - ***ham., puls.***
blue - ***carb-v.,*** **HAM.,** ***lycps., mur-ac.,*** **SEP., PULS.**
bluish, affected parts, soreness and stinging - **PULS.**
burning - ***apis,*** **ARS.,** ***calc.***
like fire, particularly at night - **ARS.**
bursting, as if - vip.
constricting, sensation - ang.
distended, engorged, phletoric veins - adon., ***aesc.,*** aloe, arn., ars., aur., bell-p., calc., camph., ***carb-an., carb-v.,*** chin-s., ***coll.,*** conv., ***dig.,*** fl-ac., ***ham.,*** lept., lyc., ***nux-v.,*** op., plb., ***podo., puls., sep.,*** spong., stel., ***sulph.,*** verb.
extensive, painful, with numbness or sticking itching in skin - petr.
groin down thighs, from - berb.
highly inflamed - ***puls.***
inflamed - arn., ***ars., calc., ham.,*** kreos., lyc., ***lycps., puls.,*** sil., spig., sulph., zinc.
itching - ant-t., barb., brucin., ***caps.,*** carb-v., caust., ***graph.,*** lach., mag-aust., nux-v., plb., puls., ***sep.,*** sil., sul-ac., ***sulph.***
jar, agg. - ham.
large, from slight cause, in weakly individuals - ***sulph.***
network in skin - berb., ***calc., carb-v., caust.,*** clem., ***crot-h., lach.,*** lyc., nat-m., ox-ac., plat., sabad., thuj.
night - **ARS.**
painful - ***brom., caust., ham., lyc., mill.,*** petr., **PULS.,** sang., thuj., vip., zinc.
evening, towards, bluish - ***puls.***
warmth agg. by - **FL-AC., SULPH.**
painless - calc.
pimples, covered with - ***graph.***
pregnancy, during - acon., apis, ***arn., ars.,*** **CARB-V.,** ***caust.,*** **FERR., FL-AC.,** ***graph., ham., lyc., lycps., mill., nux-v., phos.,*** **PULS.,** ***sep., zinc.***
attributable to high living - **NUX-V.**
heartburn, with - ***zinc.***
pressure, agg. - ham.
prickling, with - **HAM.**
sensitive - ***fl-ac.,*** graph., ***ham.,*** lach., puls.
soreness - am-c., ang., bar-c., ***caust.,*** graph., grat., **HAM.,** hep., ign., ***kali-c.,*** kali-n., ***nux-v., phos.,*** puls., rhus-t., sil., sul-ac., ***sulph.,*** vip.
stinging - ***apis,*** graph., **HAM., PULS.**

VARICOSE, veins, general,
stitching - alum., ***ant-t., ars.,*** bar-c., ***caust.,*** grat., kali-c., ***kali-n.,*** lyc., merc., nat-m., nux-v., phos., ***sil.,*** sul-ac., sulph.
swollen - ***apis, berb.,*** **PULS.**
thighs, on - ***calc.***
tumid, bluish - ***ham.***
ulcers, ulcerated - ***aesc.,*** alumn., anac., ant-t., arist-cl., arn., ***ars., calc.,*** calc-f., ***carb-v.,*** **CARD-M., CAUST.,** cecr., ***cham.,*** cinnb., crot-h., crot-t., des-ac., ***fl-ac., graph.,*** grin., ***ham.,*** hydr., hydr-ac., kali-s., kreos., **LACH., LYC.,** merc., merc-c., mez., ***nat-m.,*** parat., **PULS.,** pyrog., raja-s., ***rhus-t.,*** rib-ac., sars., sec., ***sil.,*** sul-ac., ***sulph.,*** syph., thuj., ***zinc.***
bleed easily - ***sulph.***
burning - ***sulph.***
crusts, half transparent, like thick glue - ***arn.***
deep, flat, circular - ham.
dirty, bluish bottom - ***arn.***
elderly people, in - ***sec.***
fetid - ***sulph.***
hypertrophy, with granulating, with a syphilitic dyscrasia - cund.
itch - ***sulph.***
painful - ***arn.***
torpid - ***arn.***
watery, fetid secretion - ***arn.***
women, especially in, who have borne many children, obstinate - ***fl-ac., sep.***
young persons, in - ferr-p., phos.

VEINS, general
broken - card-m., ham., phos., sep.
burning, of, in metritis - ***ars.***
runs through - ***ars.***
distended - alum., **CHEL.,** ***chin.,*** chin-b., ***ham., hyos., phos.,*** ph-ac., ***puls.,*** sang., sars., ***spong., sulph.***
arms and legs, of - eucal.
burst, as if they would - am-c.
chill, with - ***chel.***
cutaneous - ***ferr.***
diarrhea, with - **SULPH.**
dry heat in evening, with - **PULS.**
dysentery, in - ***arn.***
elderly people - ***sec.***
engorged - ***hep.***
evening, during - **PULS.**
feet, of - ars., ***nat-m.***
fever, in prevailing - ***am-m.***
forehead and hands, of - ***abrot.***
hard, black cords in persons of robust health and accustomed to standing much on feet or sedentary habits - ***nux-v.***
hands, of - bar-c.
head and neck, about - ***chin-s.***
hyperemia of veins, chronic cases of choroiditis in persons subject to - puls.
venous, slightest irritation causes bleeding - ***carb-v.***
malaria, in - ***lycps.***
plethora, venous - ***carb-an.,*** sul-ac.

VEINS, general
distended,
superficial - ***bell.***
indicating impairment of innervation of sympathetic system of nerves - ***podo.***
swelling - agar., thuj.
cutaneous veins, of - ***ferr.***
heat, with - nit-s-d.
traced out by discolored lines over œdematous part - anthr.
typhoid pneumonia, in - ***phos.***
hard, knotty - ham., nux-v.
hot water, as if in - syph.
inflammation, of - ***ant-t., apis, arn.,*** cham., ***ferr-p.,*** **HAM.,** lach., lyc., nux-v., **PULS.,** spig., zinc.
contusion, from - ***arn., con.,*** hep., ***kali-c.***
cutaneous, hard, knotty and painful, swollen - ***ham.***
low, debilitated, erysipelatous state of system, in - crot-h.
metritis, with - ***phos.***
particularly when pus is formed - ***hipp***oz.
parts bluish, soreness and stinging - **PULS.**
prickling, pains - ***ham.***
typhoid symptoms, with - apis, ***ars., bapt.,*** lach., ***mur-ac.,*** phos., ***rhus-t.***
vena cava, superior - phos.
pulsations - ***asaf.***
sore - arn., ***ham.,*** puls.
swollen, in evening - carb-v.
undulatory motion, jugular veins, in - amyg.
pregnancy, during - ***phos.***
whipcord, like a - calc-hp.

VENESECTION, ailments from - chin., ***led.,*** hyper., senec., squil.

VENOSITY, general - carb-v., ***ham.,*** puls., ***sep.,*** sulph.

VIBRATE, blood vessels, as if - phel.

WEAKNESS, (see Circulatory)

WHITE blood cells,
disorganize, as after snake bite - dor.
dissolution, of - sec.
irregular and smaller - ***apis.***
prolification of, stimulate - calen.

WRITHING, in blood vessels- bell., hydr-ac.

Bones

ABSCESS - ang., arg-m., arg-n., asaf., ***aur.***, calc-f., ***calc-hp.***, calc-p., fl-ac., guai., mang., merc-aur., ***phos.***, puls., sec., ***sil.***, staph., sulph., symph.
accompanied by eczema on scalp, behind ears and in bends of elbows - **PSOR.**

ACHING, pain - ***arg-m.***, asc-t., ***aur.***, ***bell.***, ***crot-h.***, ***cupr-m.***, cycl., daph., **EUP-PER.**, form., guai., hep., ign., **IP.**, kalm., ***lyss.***, ***merc.***, ***mez.***, ***mur-ac.***, nit-ac., olnd., ***puls.***, ***rhus-t.***, ***sabin.***, ***staph.***, ***tub.***
catarrh, in nasal - eup-per.
chill, during - ***arn.***, ***ars.***, chin., **EUP-PER.**, ***ferr.***, **IP.**, mag-c., mur-ac., nat-m., ***puls.***, ***pyrog.***, ***rhus-t.***
9 a.m. to 3 p.m. - ***ip.***
chilliness, with - dios.
cold, as after taking - ***all-c.***
with sensation as if she had taken a severe - med.
diphtheria, in, and chronic otorrhea - ***lyc.***
fever and headache, followed by - verat-v.
influenza, in - **EUP-PER.**, ***merc.***, ***rhus-t.***
intermittent fever, in - podo.
measles, in - ***euph.***
nodes, with, in long bones - ***still.***
swelling, with - ***guai.***
aching, periosteum, - **ARN.**, ***ruta.***

BONE spurs (see Exostoses, Tumors) - ***arg-m.***, **AUR.**, **AUR-M.**, calc., **CALC-F.**, crot-c., ***dulc.***, ***fl-ac.***, **HECLA.**, ***kali-i.***, lap-a., maland., ***merc-c.***, ***mez.***, ***nit-ac.***, **PHOS.**, ***puls.***, rhus-t., ***ruta.***, **SIL.**, sulph.
face - ***aur-m.***, ***hecla.***, phyt.
head - **ARG-M.**, **AUR.**, ***calc.***, **CALC-F.**, ***fl-ac.***, ***kali-i.***, **MERC.**, ***mez.***, **PHOS.**, ***phyt.***
jaw, lower - **ANG.**, **CALC-F.**, ***hep.***
right cheek bones - ***aur-m.***

BORING, pain - agar., ***asaf.***, arn., **AUR.**, ***bar-c.***, ***bell.***, brom., ***calc.***, carb-an., clem., dulc., hell., hep., lach., ***lyc.***, mang., **MERC.**, ***mez.***, nat-c., nat-m., ph-ac., phos., ***puls.***, rhod., rhus-t., sabad., sabin., ***sep.***, ***sil.***, ***spig.***, staph., sulph., ***thuj.***
worse at night - **AUR.**

BRITTLE, bones - bufo, ***calc.***, calc-f., **CALC-P.**, carc., ***lac-ac.***, sil., symph.

BROKEN, bones (see Injuries)

BROKEN, sensation, as if - ***aur.***, ***bry.***, cupr., **EUP-PER.**, hep., ***nat-m.***, puls., ***pyrog.***, ***ruta.***, sep., ther., valer., ***verat.***, ***vip.***
as if about to fall asunder - ther.
long bones, in - ruta.
rheumatism, in - ***merc.***
supraorbital, feel shattered - lyss.

BRUISED, pain - arn., ***cocc.***, ***crot-h.***, **EUP-PER.**, **IP.**, kali-bi., lyss., ***ruta.***
awaking, worse on - crot-h.
beaten, as if - ***bry.***, dros., ***ign.***, kreos., ***lith.***, nit-ac., ***nux-v.***, ***rhus-t.***, sulph., thuj.
headache, with pressive, over left eye - ***nux-v.***

BRUISED, pain
morning, in, in bed, after awaking, disappears after rising - viol-o.
long, in - cann-s.

BURNING, pain - ars., ***asaf.***, ***aur.***, bry., ***carb-v.***, caust., con., ***euph.***, form., ***hep.***, ign., ***lach.***, lyc., mang., merc., **MEZ.**, nat-c., nit-ac., par., phos., ***ph-ac.***, puls., ***rhus-t.***, ***ruta.***, sabin., ***sep.***, sil., staph., ***sulph.***, thuj., **ZINC.**
menses, during - ***carb-v.***
night - ***mez.***, ph-ac.

CANCER, of - aur-i., aur-m., cadm-m., calc-f., con., hecla., ***phos.***, ***symph.***

COLD, sensation, in - ***aran.***, ***ars.***, ***berb.***, ***calc.***, calc-p., elaps, eup-per., kali-i., lyc., merc., per., pyrog., sep., sulph., ***verat.***, zinc.

CONSTRICTING, pain - alum.

CONSTRICTION - am-m., anac., aur., chin., cocc., ***coloc.***, ***con.***, ***graph.***, kreos., lyc., merc., nat-m., **NIT-AC.**, nux-v., petr., phos., **PULS.**, rhod., ***rhus-t.***, ***ruta.***, sabad., sep., sil., stront-c., **SULPH.**, zinc.

CREEPING, pain - cham., plb., rhus-t., sec.

CURVATURE, of - am-c., asaf., bell., **CALC.**, hep., lyc., ***merc.***, nit-ac., ***phos.***, puls., rhus-t., sep., ***sil.***, staph., **SULPH.**

CURVING, and bowing of - ***calc.***, ***calc-p.***, lyc., ***sil.***

CUTTING, pain - anac., dig., sabad.
long bones - calc., osm., sabad.

DECAY, of, (see Necrosis) - **ANG.**, ***anthro.***, ***arg-m.***, ***arn.***, ***ars.***, **ASAF.**, ***aur.***, aur-a., aur-i., ***aur-m.***, **AUR-M-N.**, bell., bry., ***calc.***, ***calc-f.***, calc-hp., ***calc-p.***, calc-s., caps., carb-ac., caust., chin., cinnam., ***cist.***, clem., con., ***cupr.***, dulc., euph., ferr., **FL-AC.**, graph., ***guai.***, ***guare.***, hecla., **HEP.**, ***iod.***, kali-bi., **KALI-I.**, kreos., lach., **LYC.**, mang., **MERC.**, ***mez.***, nat-m., ***nit-ac.***, ***ol-j.***, op., petr., ***ph-ac.***, ***phos.***, ***psor.***, ***puls.***, rad-br., rhod., rhus-t., ruta, sabin., sal-ac., sec., ***sep.***, **SIL.**, spong., ***staph.***, ***stront-c.***, ***sulph.***, symph., syph., tarent., tell., ter., **THER.**, thuj., tub., tub-k.
adhesion of skin in - asaf.
appetite, loss of - ***merc.***
broken down, easily, by probe - ***staph.***
crumble off, pieces of bone - ***ang.***
decomposition, putrid - ***nit-ac.***
marrow, penetrates to - **ANG.**
mercury, especially after abuse of - **AUR-M.**
pains worse and better periodically - ***aran.***
predisposing to, in children - coff-t.
psoric or syphilitic, especially if, or from abuse of mercury - **FL-AC.**
pus foul smelling - ***hep.***
watery - ***hep.***
scrofulous conditions after abuse of mercury or necrosis - asaf.
and after abuse of mercury - ***asaf.***
syphilitic - **AUR-M.**
after, and abuse of mercury - **KALI-I.**
nodes, following, in broken-down patients - ***staph.***

DECAY, of,
tetter, with, crusty, in rheumatic or gouty subjects - ***rhus-t.***
tubular bones, longing for coffee, touchy, sensitive mind - **ANG.**
decay, periosteum - ant-c., **ASAF.,** aur., bell., ***chin.,*** cycl., hell., ***merc.,*** mez., **PH-AC.,** puls., rhod., rhus-t., ruta., sabin., ***sil.,*** staph.

DIGGING, pain - aran., asaf., calc., ***carb-an., cocc.,*** dulc., ***mang.,*** rhod., ruta., sep., spig., thuj.
night - mang.

DISLOCATED, feel as if out of joint, in getting up shakes herself to get them in place - med.

DRAWING, pain - cham., ***chin., cocc.,*** gels., graph., kali-c., led., merc., ***mez.,*** petr., sulph., zinc.
as from a thread through shafts - bry.
awaking, worse on - crot-h.
long bones - ***led.***
long, in - arg-m., sabin.
lying, when, better for the moment, but soon returns - ***chin.***
painful in parts, when they lie near surface - cycl.
paralytic condition of limbs - ***cocc.***
drawing, periosteum - mur-ac.
chill, before - ***arn.***
heat in head, with - ***merc-c.***
pressing, where skin covers bones - cycl.
rheumatic, of long bones - cann-s.
tearing, worse at night, in wet stormy weather and rest, better in motion, worse in forearms and lower legs - ***rhod.***

EPIPHYSIS, acts on - ***calc.***

EXOSTOSES, (see Bone spurs, Tumors) - **AUR., AUR-M.,** ***calc., calc-f.,*** calc-p., ***dulc.,*** ferr-i., graph., ***hecla., kali-i.,*** **MERC.,** ***mez., sars.,*** **SIL.**
nightly pain - ***fl-ac.***
scrofulous - **RUTA.**
syphilis, in - ***phos.***
with feeling of soreness when touched, pain at night in bed - **MERC.**

FISTULA, of - ang., ***asaf.,*** aur., bufo, ***calc-f.,*** calc-hp., calc-p., calc-sil., fl-ac., ***hep.,*** lyc., merc., ***nat-s., ol-j.,*** phos., **SIL.**

FORMICATION - acon., arn., cham., colch., ign., kali-bi., merc., mez., nat-c., nat-m., nux-v., ph-ac., plat., ***plb.,*** puls., rhod., ***rhus-t.,*** sabad., sec., ***sep.,*** spig., sulph., zinc.

FULLNESS - cinnb., ham.

GNAWING, pain - am-m., arg-m., **BELL.,** brom., canth., ***con., dros.,*** graph., kali-i., lyc., ***mang.,*** phos., ***ph-ac.,*** puls., ***ruta.,*** samb., ***staph.,*** stront.

GROWING pains - acon., agar., bell., calc., **CALC-P.,** ***ferr-ac., guai.,*** mang., ol-an., **PH-AC.,** phos., sil.
legs, in - bell., **CALC-P.,** cimic., ***eup-per.,*** **GUAI.,** kali-p., mag-aust., mag-p., mang., nat-p., **PH-AC.**
night, at - calc-p.

GROWING, too fast - ***calc.,*** **CALC-P.,** ferr., ferr-ac., iod., irid., kreos., **PH-AC., PHOS.**

HEAVY, sensation, in - sarac.

INFLAMMATION, bones (see Osteomyelitis) - ***acon.,*** ars., ars-i., ***asaf., aur., aur-m., bell.,*** bry., **CALC.,** chin., clem., coloc., con., cupr., dig., euph., **FL-AC.,** guai., hecla., hep., iod., kreos., lach., ***lac-ac., lyc.,*** mag-m., ***mang.,*** **MERC., MEZ.,** nat-c., ***nit-ac.,*** **PH-AC.,** ***phos., phyt.,*** plb., ***psor.,*** **PULS.,** rhus-t., sep., **SIL.,** spig., **STAPH.,** ***sulph., symph.,*** thuj., verat.
inflammation, periosteum (see Periostitis)

INJURIES, bones, broken, fractured, bruised, blows etc. - acon., ang., **ARN.,** asaf., bell-p., **BRY.,** ***calc., calc-f.,*** **CALC-P.,** ***calen.,*** **CARB-AC.,** con., croc., crot-h., ***eup-per.,*** ferr., hecla., hep., ***hyper.,*** iod., kali-i., ***lach.,*** lyc., nit-ac., ***petr., ph-ac.,*** phos., ***puls.,*** rhus-t., **RUTA.,** ***sil.,*** staph., stront-c., ***sul-ac.,*** sulph., **SYMPH.,** ***thyr.,*** valer.
bare, or crushed and splintered - **CARB-AC.**
fractures, to promote union - arn., asaf., **CALC-P.,** calen., lyc., nit-ac., ruta, sil., sulph., **SYMPH.**
children, in - **ARN.,** bry., ***calc., calc-f.,*** **CALC-P.,** sil.
compound - ang., **ARN.,** ***calc., calen.,*** con., crot-h., hep., hyper., iod., ***lach., petr.,*** ph-ac., phos., puls., rhus-t., **RUTA,** sil., staph., symph.
often, in brittle bones - calc., **CALC-P.,** ***merc., sil., symph.***
slow healing of broken bones - asaf., **CALC.,** calc-f., **CALC-P.,** ***calen., ferr.,*** fl-ac., iod., lyc., mang., merc., ***mez.,*** nit-ac., ***ph-ac.,*** phos., puls., **RUTA.,** sep., ***sil.,*** staph., sulph., **SYMPH.,** ***thyr.***
sphacelus, after fracture of tibia - **ANTHR.**ailments from - calc-p., hecla., ruta, symph.
injuries, periosteum - arn., bell-p., kali-iod., **RUTA.,** ***symph.***

JERKING, pain - **ASAF.,** aur., bell., ***calc.,*** caust., ***chin.,*** clem., ***colch.,*** lyc., merc., ***nat-m.,*** nux-v., petr., phos., ***puls.,*** rhod., rhus-t., sep., sil., **SULPH.,** ***symph., valer.***
sudden cracking, at night, depriving one of sleep - plb.

NECROSIS, (see Decay) - **ARS.,** ***asaf., aur-m.,*** bell., ***calc., calc-f., carb-ac.,*** con., euph., **FL-AC., KALI-I.,** kreos., ***merc., merc-c., phos.,*** ph-ac., plb., ***sabin.,*** sal-ac., **SIL.,** ***sulph.,*** ther., thuj.
expulsion, promotes, of necrotic - fl-ac.
assisted, after fracture of head of femur - ***cocc.***
syphilis, after, and abuse of mercury - **KALI-I.**
threatened - asaf.
tibia, especially of - sal-ac.

OSGOOD-schlatter's disease - ***calc-p., sil.***

OSTEITIS, deformans, paget's disease - calc-p.

OSTEOGENSIS, imperfecta - calc-f., ***calc-p.,*** sil.

OSTEOMALACIA, softening of - am-c., **ASAF.,** ***bell.,*** **CALC.,** calc-f., ***calc-i., calc-p.,*** cic., con., ferr., ***ferr-i.,*** ferr-m., ***ferr-p.,*** fl-ac., guai., hecla., ***hep.,*** iod., ip., ***kali-i., lac-c., lyc.,*** **MERC.,** merc-c., mez., ***nit-ac.,*** nux-m., ***ol-j.,*** parathyr., petr., ph-ac., ***phos.,*** plb., ***psor., puls.,*** rhod., ruta., ***sep.,*** **SIL.,** staph., ***sulph., symph.,*** syph., ther., thuj.

OSTEOMYELITIS - **AUR.,** ***calc.,*** **CALC-P.,** ***fl-ac., mez., nit-ac., ph-ac., ruta., sil., staph., still.,*** symph.

OSTEOPORUS, brittle bones - bufo, ***calc.,*** calc-f., **CALC-P.,** carc., sil., symph.

PAIN, bones - abies-n., acon., ***agar.,*** agn., am-c., am-m., anac., ***arg-m.,*** arn., ars., ars-i., **ASAF.,** ***aur.,*** bar-c., bell., ***berb.,*** bism., bry., ***calc., calc-p.,*** calc-s., cann-s., canth., ***caps.,*** carb-an., carb-s., carb-v., caust., ***cham.,*** chel., ***chin.,*** chin-s., cic., ***cinnb.,*** clem., ***cocc.,*** colch., ***coloc., con., cupr.,*** cycl., dig., dios., dros., dulc., **EUP-PER.,** euph., ferr., ***fl-ac.,*** glon., graph., guai., hell., ***hep.,*** ign., iod., **IP.,** kali-bi., kali-c., kali-s., kreos., lach., led., ***lyc., lyss.,*** mag-c., mag-m., mang., **MERC.,** merc- i- f., ***mez.,*** nat-c., nat-m., **NIT-AC.,** olnd., op., petr., **PH-AC.,** ***phos.,*** plb., **PULS.,** ran-s., ***rhod., rhus-t.,*** **RUTA.,** sabad., ***sabin.,*** samb., ***sars.,*** sec., ***sep., sil.,*** spig., spong., ***staph.,*** still., stront-c., ***sulph.,*** teucr., ther., thuj., valer., verat., viol-t., zinc.

- air, worse in cold, especially in knees - sarac.
- awakened by, does not want to live - **AUR.**
- bed, in - calc-p.
- cold, as after taking, copious sweat, with pressing in forehead - ***nux-m.***
- condylomata, with - ***ph-ac.***
- deep, especially at night - ***merc***-i-f.
- despair, driving to, intolerable nocturnal - **KALI-I.**
- digging, dull, in all parts of body, more in humerus, forearm and fingers - aran.
- drinks, with longing for cold acid - eup-pur.
- excessive - puls.
- fever, in bilious - ***eup-per.***
- fever, intermittent - **EUP-PER.,** polyp-p
- hoarseness, with - uva.
- influenza, in - ***eup-per.***
- joints, with weak feeling in - ***staph.***
- mercurial, or after checked gonorrhoea, worse at night, in damp weather, or after taking cold in water - **SARS.**
- middle of long - bufo, ***phyt.***
- morning - sil.
  - early in - ***eup-per.***
- moving head and tongue, with difficulty on - **COLCH.**
- night - ***asaf.,*** **AUR.,** caust., ***cham.,*** cinnb., ***fl-ac., guare.,*** kalm., **KALI-I.,** ***mang.,*** **MERC.,** ***merc-i-f., mez.,*** **NIT-AC.,** ***ph-ac., phyt., sars.,*** thuj., verat.
  - downward, from above - ***mez.***
  - headache, with - mez.
  - keratitis, in, pustulosa - ***merc***-sol.
  - mercury, after abuse of - ***kali-i.***

PAIN, bones
- night, at
  - scraped, as if being, with a knife - ***ph-ac.***
  - sleep, preventing - ***merc.***
  - syphilis, in - asaf., iod.
- periodical - ***kali-bi.***
- syphilis, in - ***phos.***
  - in secondary - still.
  - mercurial - ***ph-ac.***
  - eruption, with, advanced stage - ***nit-ac.***
- touch, on - sulph.
- walking, in cold air - sep.
- wandering - ***kali-bi.***
- weather changes - am-c.

pain, periosteum - ant-c., **ASAF.,** aur., bell., bry., ***camph., cham., chin.,*** colch., coloc., ***cycl.,*** graph., hell., ign., ***kalm.,*** led., ***mang., merc., mez.,*** **PH-AC.,** ***phyt.,*** puls., ***rhod.,*** rhus-t., **RUTA.,** sabad., sabin., ***sil.,*** spig., staph.

PARALYTIC, pain - **AUR.,** bell., chin., ***cocc.,*** cycl., dig., led., mez., nat-m., nux-v., petr., puls., rhus-t., sabin., ***sil.,*** staph., verat., zinc.

PERIOSTITIS, inflammation of periosteum - ***acon.,*** agar., ant-c., ***apis, ars., asaf., aur., aur-m., bell.,*** chin., ***ferr-i., ferr-p.,*** **FL-AC.,** ***kali-i.,*** led., ***mang., merc., merc-c.,*** **MEZ.,** ***nit-ac.,*** **PH-AC.,** ***phos.,*** phyt., ***psor.,*** puls., rhus-t., **RUTA.,** ***sil., staph., symph.***

- articulating extremities, of, at night pains insupportable, worse on touching parts, better in open air - ***mang.***
- blow on shin, from a, leaving ulcer on spot size of a shilling, skin and cellular tissue inflamed - ***kali-bi.***
- burning at night - ph-ac.
- chronic - ***lac-ac.***
- erysipelatous inflammation of parts, with - ***ruta***
- long, bones of - ***rhus-t.***
- mercurial - ***staph.***
- night, at, pains are insupportable, worse on touching parts, better in open air - ***mang.***
- pains, tearing, burning, gnawing - ***ph-ac.***
- scrofulous - hecla., ***staph., still.***
- shafts, especially, after abuse of mercury and venereal disease - **MEZ.**
- spots, red, on skin, children are unable to walk - mang.
- strumous - ***ol-j.***
- synovitis, with - ***apis***
- syphilitic - hecla., ***kali-bi., kali-i.***
- throbbing and burning, with - con.

PINCHING, pain - bell., calc., cina, ign., mez., osm., petr., ***ph-ac.,*** plat., **VERB.**

PRESSING, pain - ***alum.,*** anac., ***arg-m.,*** ars., asaf., aur., ***bell., bism.,*** bry., cann-i., canth., carb-s., cham., cocc., colch., ***coloc.,*** con., ***cupr., cycl.,*** dros., graph., ***guai.,*** hell., hep., ign., ***kali-c.,*** kali-n., merc., mez., nux-m., ***olnd.,*** petr., phos., plat., puls., rhod., ***rhus-t., ruta., sabin.,*** sil., spong., stann., ***staph., thuj.,*** valer., verat., viol-t., zinc.

PRESSING, pain
asleep, on falling to - graph.
in parts where they lie near surface - cycl.
long bones, in - **ARG-M.**
painful, in ileum - ***guai.***
sticking - mez., staph.
tearing - arg-m., bell., cham., coloc., thuj.

PULSATION, internally - ***asaf., calc.,*** carb-v., lyc., ***merc.,*** nit-ac., phos., rhod., ruta., sabad., sep., sil., ***sulph.,*** thuj.

RHEUMATISM - abies-n., daph., ***merc.***
pains, after mercury, and checked gonorrheal discharge - sars.

RICKETS, rachitis - am-c., arg-m., ars., **ASAF.,** bar-c., ***bell.,*** bufo., **CALC., CALC-P.,** caust., cic., con., ***ferr., ferr-i.,*** ferr-m., ***ferr-p., guai.,*** hecla., hed., ***hep.,*** iod., ***ip.,*** iris., ***kali-i., lac-c., lyc.,*** **MERC.,** mez., ***nit-ac.,*** nux-m., ***ol-j.,*** op., petr., ***ph-ac.,*** **PHOS.,** plb., ***psor., puls.,*** rhod., ***rhus-t.,*** ruta.., sacch., sanic., ***sep.,*** **SIL.,** ***staph., sulph.,*** tarent., ther., thuj.
abdomen puffed, tense - **BELL.**
atrophy - ***kali-p.***
curvature - ***asaf., puls.***
curvature, especially spine and long bones - **CALC.**
curve, tendency to - ***calc-p.***
extremities deformed, crooked - **CALC.**
growing imperfectly - ***calc.***
head, abscess of - ***merc***-sol.
limbs crooked - graph.
pelvis, affecting female - ***ol-j.***
protracted, ill treated, hectic, profuse, fetid suppuration - petr.
scrofulous persons, in, malformation - ***calc.,*** iod.
soften or bend, disposed to - ***ferr.***
softening - ***calc., guai.,*** **LYC.,** ***sulph.***
vertigo, with - ***sil.***

SCRAPING, pain - asaf., berb., chin., ***ph-ac.,*** puls., **RHUS-T.,** sabad., spig.
as if, in long - bry., ***sabad.***
intense, especially in joints, as if interior were scraped and cut with a sharp knife - sabad.
evening, worse in - par.
motion, worse from, excitement, using eyes - ***par.***

scraping, periosteum - ***asaf.,*** **CHIN.,** coloc., **PH-AC.,** puls., **RHUS-T.,** ***sabad.,*** spig.

SENSITIVE - ***arg-n.,*** asaf., ***aur.,*** bell., bry., bufo, calc., carb-an., chel., chin., ***chin-s.,*** cupr., **EUP-PER.,** guai., hyper., lach., lyc., merc., ***merc-c.,*** mez., nat-c., **PHOS.,** ***puls.,*** rhus-t., ***sil., stram.,*** sulph., **TELL.,** zinc.
ankles particularly affected, children are unable to walk - mang.
tenderness - ***arg-n.***
touch, to, in typhus - ***mang.***
prominent projections sore to - ***rhus-t.***

sensitive, periosteum - ant-c., aur., bell., ***bry., chin.,*** ign., **LED.,** merc., ***mez., ph-ac., puls.,*** rhus-t., ***ruta.,*** sil., spig., staph.

SHARP, pain - acon., agar., agn., am-c., anac., ant-c., arg-m., ars., ***asaf.,*** aur., **BELL., BRY., CALC.,** canth., carb-v., **CAUST.,** cedr., chel., ***chin.,*** cocc., colch., **CON.,** ***dros.,*** dulc., euph., graph., **HELL.,** iod., kali-c., ***kalm., lach.,*** lyc., mag-c., mang., **MERC.,** mez., nit-ac., nux-v., par., petr., ph-ac., phos., **PULS.,** ***ran-s., ruta.,*** sabin., samb., **SARS., SEP.,** sil., spig., staph., stront-c., **SULPH.,** ***thuj.,*** valer., verb., viol-t., zinc.
flying along long bones, with nervous rheumatism or rheumatic neuralgia, worse at night - ***mez.***
needles, as from sharp - kali-bi.

SHOOTING, pain - lyss.

SMARTING, pain, at night - ph-ac.

SORE, pain - acon., ***agar.,*** am-m., anac., **ARG-M.,** ***asaf.,*** aur., bar-c., bov., ***calc.,*** cann-s., carb-v., chin., **COCC.,** ***con., cor-r., crot-h., cupr.,*** **EUP-PER., GELS.,** graph., **HEP.,** ***ign.,*** **IP.,** ***kali-bi., led., lith., lyss.,*** mag-c., ***mang., mez.,*** nat-m., ***nit-ac.,*** **NUX-V.,** ***par.,*** petr., ***ph-ac., phos., puls.,*** **RUTA.,** sabad., sep., ***sil., spig.,*** sulph., symph., valer., verat., zinc.
long bones - agar., ***calc., calc-p.***
menses, during scanty - carb-v.
morning in bed - **NUX-V.**
paralytic - ***calc.***
sitting - am-m.

sore, periosteum - bry., ***ruta.***
as of rheumatic origin - ***phyt.***

STINGING, pain - ***calc., sep.***
long, in - dros.

stinging, periosteum, boring, worse in cool air - ***hell.***

SUPPURATION - calc-p., ***hep., staph.***
chronic - **AUR-M-N.**
long bones suppurate and get better and worse periodically, pains worse at night, with great prostration - ***fl-ac.***
profuse sweat with - ***chin.***

SWELLING - am-c., **ASAF.,** ***aur.,*** bell., bry., **CALC.,** ***calc-p.,*** carb-an., clem., coloc., con., dig., dulc., euph., ferr., fl-ac., guai., hep., iod., ***kali-i.,*** kreos., lach., ***lac-ac., lyc.,*** mang., ***merc., mez.,*** nat-c., nat-m., ***nit-ac.,*** petr., **PH-AC., PHOS.,** plb., **PULS.,** rhod., rhus-t., ***ruta.,*** sabin., sep., **SIL.,** spig., **STAPH., SULPH.,** thuj., verat.
interstitial distension - **ASAF.,** aur., ***calc.,*** fl-ac., **LYC., MERC.,** ***mez., phos., ph-ac., sil.,*** sulph., **STAPH.**
mercurial, syphilitic or scrofulous - ***ph-ac.***
pains worse night - **KALI-I.**
long, of - ***rhus-t.***
mercurial - ***staph.***
night, worse at - ***mez.***
nodes - ***calc-f., caust., hep.***
painful, syphilitic - ***kali-i.***
nodosities, burning - ***hep.***
gouty - agn., dig.
hard and painful - ***phyt.***
osteophyte - calc-p.

SWELLING,
pains, nocturnal - **KALI-I.**
shafts, especially, after abuse of mercury and venereal disease - **MEZ.**
spongeous affection - ***guai.***
syphilis, mercurial - ***ph-ac.***
tophi - ***kali-i., lyc., mez.***
tumors, following mercury, or syphilis - ***nit-ac.***
ulcers, scrofulous - ***psor.***
swelling, periosteum, of - ant-c., **ASAF.,** ***aur.,*** bell., bry., chin., ***kali-i.,*** mang., ***merc.,*** mez., ***nit-ac.,*** **PH-AC.,** ***puls.,*** rhod., rhus-t., **RUTA.,** sabin., ***sil.,*** staph.

SUTURES, affected along - **CALC-P.**

SYPHILIS, ailments from - **AUR.,** fl-ac., **KALI-I., MERC.,** ***ph-ac., phyt.***
iritis - ***asaf.***
pains - ***nit-ac.***
secondary - ***still.***

SWOLLEN, sensation - ant-c., ars., bell., chel., guai., ***puls.,*** rhus-t., spig.

TEARING, pain - acon., ***agar.,*** alum., ***am-m.,*** anac., ***arg-m.,*** arn., ars., asaf., **AUR.,** ***aur-m., bar-c., bell., berb.,*** bism., bor., bov., bry., calc-p., cann-s., canth., ***caps., carb-v., caust.,*** cham., chel., **CHIN.,** ***cina, cocc.,*** coloc., con., crot-t., ***cupr., cycl.,*** dig., ***dros.,*** dulc., ***ferr.,*** graph., hell., hep., ign., iod., **KALI-C.,** ***kali-n.,*** **LACH.,** laur., ***lyc., mag-c.,*** mag-m., mang., **MERC.,** ***merc-c., mez.,*** nat-c., nat-m., ***nit-ac.,*** nux-v., ***ph-ac., phos.,*** plb., puls., **RHOD.,** rhus-t., ***ruta., sabin.,*** samb., sars., sep., **SPIG.,** spong., stann., ***staph., stront-c.,*** sulph., sul-ac., ***tab., thuj.,*** valer., verat., verb., ***zinc.***
arthritic - vinc.
burning - sabin.
cramp-like - aur., olnd., ***valer.***
dry, with, spasmodic cough, during chill - ***sabad.***
epiphysis, in arg-m.
feeling as if flesh were torn from - ***nit-ac.,*** **RHUS-T.**
jerking - ang., ***bry.,*** **CHIN.,** cupr., mang.
long, especially in - **ARG-M.,** bar-c., zinc.
middle of - ***zinc.***
paralytic - **BELL.,** ***bism.,*** chel., chin., ***cocc.,*** dig.
pieces, as if being torn to, with vomiting and pain in bowels - ***ip.***
pressive - **ARG-M.,** arn., asaf., bism., bry., coloc., **CYCL.,** staph., teucr.
skull, in exostosis of - **ARG-M.**
sticking - bell., cina, mur-ac., sabin.
sudden, at night, depriving one of sleep - plb.
surface, in parts near - cycl.
tearing, periosteum - bry., ***mez.,*** ph-ac., ***rhod.***

TENSION - agar., ***asaf.,*** **BELL.,** bry., cimic., cocc., ***con.,*** crot-h., dig., dulc., kali-bi., merc., nit-ac., rhod., ***ruta., sulph., valer.,*** zinc.
better for the moment when lying, soon returns - ***chin.***

TENSION,
long bones, in - bar-c.

THROBBING - ***calc.***

THICKENING, periosteum, with scrofulous ulcer on leg - ***mez.***

TINGLING, periosteum - ***puls.***

TUBERCULOSIS, of - ***dros.,*** phos., puls., stann.

TUMORS, bones - ***arg-m.,*** **AUR., AUR-M.,** calc., **CALC-F.,** crot-c., ***dulc., fl-ac.,*** **HECLA.,** ***kali-i.,*** lap-a., maland., ***merc-c., mez., nit-ac.,*** **PHOS.,** ***puls.,*** rhus-t., ***ruta.,*** **SIL.,** sulph.
cystic - mez.
face - ***aur-m., hecla.,*** phyt.
head - **ARG-M., AUR.,** ***calc.,*** **CALC-F.,** ***fl-ac., kali-i.,*** **MERC.,** ***mez.,*** **PHOS.,** ***phyt.***
jaw, lower - **ANG., CALC-F.,** ***hep.***
right cheek bones - ***aur-m.***

ULCERATIVE, pain - am-c., am-m., ***bry.,*** caust., cic., graph., ign., mang., nat-m., ***puls.,*** rhus-t.

ULCERATION, mercurio-syphilitic - ***sil.***

ULCERS, after abuse of mercury - ***aur.***
painful - **ANG.**
structure involved by - ***kali-i.***

WEAKNESS, of - **ASAF., CALC., CALC-F.,** ***calc-i.,*** **CALC-P.,** cic., con., ferr., ***ferr-i.,*** ferr-m., ***ferr-p.,*** fl-ac., guai., hecla., ***hep.,*** iod., ip., ***kali-i., lac-c., lyc.,*** **MERC.,** merc-c., mez., ***nit-ac.,*** nux-m., ***ol-j.,*** parathyr., petr., ph-ac., **PHOS.,** plb., ***psor., puls.,*** rhod., ruta., ***sep.,*** **SIL.,** staph., ***sulph.,*** **SYMPH.,** syph., ther., thuj.

Brain

BRAIN, general - acon., ***alum.,*** apis, arg-n., bar-c., ***bell.,*** bov., calc., **CON.,** dulc., ***gels.,*** **HELL.,** hyos., lach., ***nux-v.,*** **PHOS.,** pic-ac., stram., sulph., syph., tub., zinc.

ABSCESS - arn., bell., crot-h., iod., lach., op., vip.

ACHING, pain, deep in - ***acon.,*** aloe, alum., am-c., anac., arg-m., arg-n., ***ars.,*** asaf., asar., aur., bar-c., bell., bov., calc., camph., canth., carb-v., caust., cham., ***chin., chin-s.,*** cina, ***coloc.,*** coc-c., con., com., croc., daph., dros., ***dulc.,*** glon., graph., hyos., ign., kali-n., lach., laur., lyc., mag-c., mang., ***med.,*** merc., ***mosch.,*** mur-ac., nat-m., ***nit-ac.,*** nux-v., olnd., petr., ***ph-ac.,*** phos., phys., prun., ***psor.,*** ran-b., rhod., ruta., sabad., sars., sil., ***spig.,*** stann., ***staph.,*** sulph., sul-ac., ther., thuj., zinc.
afternoon - bar-c., hell., iris, lact., mag-s., merc-i-f., uran.
eating, after - canth., ign., ran-b.
evening - agn., all-c., nat-m., par., phos., ran-b., zinc.
exercise on - merc.
extending out through forehead - viol-t.
forenoon - fl-ac., indg., ran-b.
lying, while - ther.
morning - kali-bi., lach., ruta., spig.
rising, after - ruta., staph.
motion agg. - iod.
of upper lids - ***coloc.***
rising after stooping - laur.
shaking the head - ***caust., spig.***
thinking - daph.
touch, from - all-c., arg-m., bry., chin., cinnb., grat., kali-bi., lact., laur., mag-s., merc., merc-i-f., mez., mur-ac., nat-m., par., sabin., sars., staph., sulph., viol-t.
amel - sars.
waking, on - ***chin.,*** mang., phys.
walking, while - gran.
wandering - am-c., chin.

AIR, as if cold air passed over - anan., meny., ***petr., sanic.***
air or wind, cold, blowing on - cimic.

ALIVE, sensation as if something were in brain, as if an ant-hill - agar.

ANEMIA, of - alum., ambr., calc., calc-p., calc-s., chin., chin-s., con., dulc., **FERR.,** fl-ac., hell., kali-c., lyc., mag-c., mosch., mur-ac., nat-c., nat-m., nit-ac., nux-v., petr., **PH-AC., PHOS.,** sang., sel., sep., sil., stry., sulph., zinc.

ATROPHY, of - alum., ***aur., bar-c.,*** con., fl-ac., iod., ***phos., plb.,*** zinc.

BALL, sensation as of a, beating fast against skull - staph.
rolling in - anan., bufo, hura, lyss.

BANDAGED, as if - bry., lac-c., nat-m., nit-ac., sulph.

BURNING, pain - ***acon.,*** arn., bell., ***canth.,*** carb-ac., ***glon.,*** hydr-ac., ph-ac., **PHOS.,** ***verat.***
sitting upright, on - hell.
fire, were on, as if - ***canth.,*** hydr-ac., ***phos.***

BURSTING, pain, as if brain would burst out - alum., arg-n., cimic., con., ***glon.,*** sol-n., verat.

CEREBELLAR, disease - helo., sulfon

CEREBRAL hemorrhage, (see Stroke) - **ACON.,** ***arn., aur., bar-c.,*** **BELL., BOTH.,** ***camph.,*** carb-v., ***chin.,*** **COCC., COLCH.,** coff., con., ***cupr., crot-h., ferr.,*** ferr-p., **GELS.,** glon., helon., ***hyos.,*** **IP., LACH.,** laur., ***lyc.,*** merc., ***nat-m.,*** nit-ac., ***nux-m., nux-v.,*** **OP.,** ***phos.,*** plb., ***puls.,*** stram.
subarachnoid - gels.

CEREBRAL palsy - arn., hell., ign., op.

CEREBRO-spinal axis, ailments of - agar., arg-n., chin., cocc., ***gels.,*** ign., ***nux-v.,*** phos.

CHEWING, motion of jaw, in brain affections - bry.

CLOUD, going over - cimic., hydr-ac.

COLDNESS, in - mosch., phos.
cold cloth around the, as if - glon., ***sanic.***
frozen, as if - indg.

COMA, unconsciousness - absin., acet-ac., **ACON.,** act-sp., adel., aesc., aesc-g., aeth., agar., agar-cit., agar-pa., agar-ph., agar-pr., agar-se., agar-st., agar-t., agn., agro., ***ail.,*** alco., alet., ***alum.,*** am-caust., ambr., am-c., am-m., ***aml-n.,*** amyg., ***anac.,*** ang., anil., ant-m., anthr., ant-c., ant-t., ***apis,*** apoc., apom., aq-mar., arg-m., ***arg-n., arn., ars.,*** ars-h., art-v., ***arum-t.,*** asar., astac., ***aster.,*** atro., ***bapt.,*** **BAR-C.,** ***bar-m.,*** bar-s., **BELL.,** benz-n., benz-ac., bism., both., bov., brom., ***bry.,*** bufo, ***cact., calad.,*** cadm-s., calc., calc-mur., calc-s., calc-sil., ***camph.,*** **CANN-I.,** cann-s., ***canth.,*** caps., carb-ac., carb-an., ***carb-h., carb-o., carb-s., carb-v., caust., cedr.,*** cench., ***cham., chel.,*** chen-a., ***chin.,*** chin-s., chlf., ***chlol., chlor., cic.,*** cic-m., cimic., ***cina,*** cit-l., clem., **COCC.,** ***coff.,*** coff-t., ***colch.,*** coloc., ***con.,*** cor-r., cori-r., cortico., croc., ***crot-c., crot-h., cupr., cupr-ac.,*** cupr-s., ***cycl.,*** cyt-l., dat-m., dat-s., der., ***dig.,*** dirc., dor., dub., dulc., elaps, ether, euph., euphr., ferr., ferr-ar., ferr-m., ferr-p., fil., fl-ac., gaul., ***gels., glon.,*** graph., grat., guai., ham., **HELL.,** ***helon., hep.,*** home., **HYDR-AC., HYOS., IGN.,** iod., ip., jasm., jatr., jatr-u., juni., kali-bi., ***kali-br., kali-c.,*** kali-chl., kali-cy., kali-i., kali-m., kali-n., keroso., kreos., ***lac-d.,*** **LACH.,** lact., ***laur., led., lil-t., lyc.,*** lyss., mag-c., mag-m., manc., meli., merc., ***merc-c.,*** merc-n., merc-p-r., merl., meth-ae-ae., mez., **MOSCH.,** ***mur-ac.,*** naja, nat-c., nat-f., ***nat-m.,*** nat-p., nit-ac., ***nit-s-d.,*** **NUX-M.,** ***nux-v.,*** oena., oeno., ***ol-an., olnd.,*** **OP.,** ox-ac., ***par.,*** past., ***petr.,*** **PH-AC.,** ***phos.,*** phyt., piloc., ***plat., plb.,*** psor., **PULS.,** ran-b., rheum, rhod., ***rhus-t.,*** rumx-a., russ., ruta, sabad., sabin., sang., sapin., sars., ***sec.,*** sel., ***seneg.,*** sep., ***sil., sol-n.,*** sphing., spig., squil., stann., staph., ***stram.,*** sul-ac., sul-h., ***sulph.,*** tab., tanac., tarax., ***tarent.,*** tax., ***ter.,*** tere-ch., tub., uran-n., valer.,

COMA, unconsciousness - verb., ***verat.***, verat-v., verin., vesp., viol-o., vip., vip-a., visc., wies., xero, ***zinc.***, zinc-p.

afternoon, 1 p.m. - ol-an.
2 p.m. - nux-m.
air, in open - ferr., mosch., nux-v.
amel. - tarax.
alcoholic - gels., ***glon.***, hyos., ***kali-br.***, ***stram.***
delirium tremens, in (see Mind, Alcoholism) - **NUX-V.**
alone, when - ph-ac.
alternating with, convulsions - agar., aur.
dangerous violence - absin.
delirium - ***atro.***
escape, desire to - ***coloc.***
excitement - ***kali-br.***
rage - aloe
restless, melancholy - thyr.
restlessness - ***acon.***, **ars.**
fever, during - ***ars.***
answers correctly when spoken to, but delirium and unconsciousness return at once - ***ant-t.***, ***arn.***, ***bapt.***, diph., ***hell.***, ***hyos.***, ***nux-v.***, ***op.***, ***ph-ac.***, phos., sulph., ***ter.***
asphyxia, with (see Respiration) - **ANT-T.**, carb-v.
becoming, as if - cupr.
blood, sight of - nux-m.
burning, in - ***calen.***
candle-light, from - cann-i.
childbirth, during - ***chin-s.***, ***cimic.***, ***coff.***, ***gels.***, ***lach.***, **NUX-V.**, ***puls.***, **SEC.**
chill, during - ***ars.***, ***bell.***, camph., caps., cic., ***con.***, ***hep.***, kali-c., **NAT-M.**, nux-v., op., puls., ***spong.***, stram., valer.
before - ***ars.***, ***lach.***
cold, after taking - ***sil.***
surface, with - ***canth.***
water, dashed in face amel. - glon.
poured over head amel. - tab.
coma, vigil - acon., hydr-ac., ***hyos.***, laur., mur-ac., ***op.***, phos.
concussion, of brain, from - **ARN.**, nat-s., ***op.***
conduct, automatic - anac., anh., bufo, calc-sil., camph., cann-i., caust., cic., con., croc., cur., elaps, hell., hyos., lach., lyc., ***nat-m.***, ***nux-m.***, oena., ***phos.***, ***sil.***, ***vesp.***, ***visc.***
convulsions, after (see Nerves, convulsions) - ***art-v.***, atro., ***bell.***, **BUFO**, canth., carb-ac., ***cic.***, cori-r., ***glon.***, ***oena.***, plb., ***sec.***
prolonged - bell.
cough, from - cadm-s., kali-c.
attacks of, between - ***ant-t.***, cadm-s.
stiffness, and - cupr., ip.
cries, with howling - camph.
crowded room, in a - ambr., ars., bar-c., con., ign., ***lyc.***, nat-c., nat-m., ***nux-m.***, ***phos.***, **PULS.**, sulph.
daytime - euph., phos.
delirium, after - atro., bry., ***chel.***, phos.
delirium tremens, in (see Mind, Alcoholism) - **NUX-V.**

COMA, unconsciousness
diarrhea, after - ars.
dinner, after - cast., til.
diphteria, in - ail., ***nat-m.***, ***sul-ac.***
dream, as in a - ambr., anac., carb-an., cann-i., con., **NUX-M.**, phos., rheum, stram., valer., ***verat.***
does not know where he is - atro., cic., cortico., ***glon.***, merc., ***nux-m.***, op., ***petr.***, plat., ran-b.
night - bov.
from a dream - ***cann-s.***
waking, on - aesc., alum., puls.
eating, after - caust., ***mag-m.***, ***nux-v.***, ***ph-ac.***
emotion, after - ***acon.***, am-c., camph., ***caust.***, ***cham.***, **COFF.**, **IGN.**, **LACH.**, mosch., ***op.***, nux-m., ***ph-ac.***, phos., verat.
epilepsy, after (see Nerves, Convulsions) - ***ars.***, **BUFO**, ***kali-bi.***, **OP.**, plb.
erect, if he remained - chin.
eruptions, suppression of, after - ***zinc.***
evening - acon., ars., bry., calc., caust., coloc., lyc., merl., nux-m., oena., ol-an., puls., stry., thea., zinc.
8 p.m. - stry.
when lying down - mag-c., mag-m.
exanthema, is slow to appear, when - **ZINC.**
excitement, after - amyg., chlf., nux-m.
exertion, after - ***ars.***, calc., calc-ar., ***caust.***, cocc., hyper., ***senec.***, ***ther.***, ***verat.***
eyes, cannot open - gels.
closing, on - ant-t., cann-i., cann-s.
fixed, with - aeth., ars., bov., camph., canth., ***caust.***, cupr., op., stram.
open, with - ***cic.***
swallowing agg, during, sore throat - ter.
pressure in, and obstruction of sight, with - seneg.
face, with red - ***canth.***, ***glon.***, ***mur-ac.***
fever, during - ***acon.***, aeth., ***agar.***, ail., **APIS**, **ARN.**, ***bapt.***, ***bell.***, bor., bry., ***cact.***, ***calad.***, calc., ***camph.***, ***caps.***, ***chlor.***, cic., ***clem.***, ***colch.***, ***crot-h.***, dor., ***dulc.***, eup-per., ***gels.***, ***hyos.***, ***ip.***, ***iris***, kali-br., ***lach.***, ***laur.***, ***lyc.***, manc., meli., **MUR-AC.**, **NAT-M.**, ***nit-s-d.***, ***nux-m.***, nux-v., **OP.**, per., ***ph-ac.***, ***phos.***, ***puls.***, samb., sol-n., ***stram.***, sulph., ***ter.***, ***verat.***, zing.
frequent, spells - **ARS.**, ***bapt.***, ***hyos.***, ign., merc-cy., ***nat-m.***, op., ***phos.***
head, bending forward, on - cortico.
moving, on - calc., carb-an., nat-m., rhus-t.
turning, on - ***rhus-t.***
hydrocephalus, in - **APIS**, ***apoc.***, ***clem.***, ***hell.***, ***hyos.***, ***lyc.***, ***nat-m.***
incomplete - ars., chlor., crot-h., carb-ac., cupr., cupr-ar., glon., ign., morph., nat-c., nitro-o., op., sec., sol-t., stram., sul-ac.
interrupted, by screaming - bell.
jaundice, in - **CHEL.**
jaw, dropping - ***lyc.***, **OP.**, ***sulph.***

COMA, unconsciousness
kneeling, in church, while - **SEP.**
knows no one but answers correctly when touched or spoken to - cic.
lies, as if dead - arn., ***carb-v., op.***
looking, downward, on - salam.
upwards, on - lach.
lying, while - ***carb-v.,*** colch., mag-c., ***mag-m.***
stretched out - ***aeth.***
with outstretched arms, screaming and tossing - ***canth.***
meningitis, in - ***ant-t., apis,*** apoc., ***gels., hell., merc., rhus-t., sulph., verat.***
menses, during - apis, cocc., ***ign.,*** **LACH.,** ***nux-m.,*** nux-v., plb., puls., ***sars.,*** sep., sulph., verat., zinc-p.
after - chin., cupr., ***lach., lyc.***
before - ***nux-m., murx.***
suppression of - acon., cham., chin., con., lyc., **NUX-M.,** nux-v., verat.
from fright - ***op.***
mental, insensibility - bufo, con., cycl., ***hell., hyos.,*** laur., ***nux-m.,*** oena., op., phos., ph-ac., sabad., sec., stram.
morning - agar., anac., ang., ant-t., ars-m., ***bell.,*** **BRY.,** bov., ***calc.,*** carb-an., carb-v., caust., chel., ***chin-s.,*** clem., cocc., **CON.,** croc., dig., euphr., glon., **GRAPH.,** hep., hyos., ign., kali-c., kali-n., ***led.,*** lyc., ***mag-c.,*** merc., nat-c., nat-m., **NUX-V.,** ph-ac., phos., psor., puls., ran-b., spig., stram., stry., sulph., verat., zinc.
alone, when - ***ph-ac.***
rising, on - **BRY.**
waking, on - chel., nat-c.
motion, on least - **ARS.,** ***verat.***
head, of - calc., carb-an.
music, from - cann-i., sumb.
muttering - ***cocc.,*** dor., ***phos.,*** rhus-t.
night - arg-n., bell., cann-i., chel., nat-m.
1 a.m. - stry.
amel. - ferr.
waking, on - canth., con., cot., digin., hep., mag-c., phos.
noon - glon., zinc.
afternoon, and - euph.
odors, from - **NUX-V.,** ***phos.***
old age, in - ***bar-c.***
pain, from - agar., aloe, anac., ***hep., nux-m.,*** phyt., plat., stann., ***valer.,*** verat.
periodical - alum-p., bar-s., ***cic.,*** fl-ac., lyc.
perspiration, during - samb.
cold, with - sulph.
piano, listening to - cann-i.
pneumonia, in - carb-v., ***chel., phos.***
pregnancy, during - cann-i., ***nux-m., nux-v., sec.***
prolonged - ***cic., gels.,*** hydr-ac., laur.
raising, arms above head, on - ***lac-d.,*** lach.
reading, from - asaf., cycl., tarax.
remains, fixed in one spot - nux-m.
motionless like a statue - hyos., nux-m., stram.

COMA, unconsciousness
restlessness, with - ter.
riding, while - berb., grat., ***sep.,*** sil.
rising, up, on - ***arn.,*** **BRY.,** ***carb-v., croc., op., verat.***
rubbing, soles of feet amel. - chel.
sex, after - ***agar.,*** asaf., ***dig.***
scarlatina, in - ***ail., am-c., apis, cupr-ac., gels., lyc., mur-ac., sulph.***
screaming, with - ***tub.***
interrupted by - ***apis,*** bell., ***rheum.***
semi-consciousness - ***carb-v.,*** chin-s., coca, cocc., ign., kali-br., ***laur., stram.,*** tarax., ***verat.,*** verat-v., zinc.
sensation, of - mag-c.
sexual, excitement, with - ***orig., stram.***
shock, from injury, in - ***arn.,*** chlf., ***op.***
sighing, with - glon.
sinking, down - glon., hydr-ac.
sitting, while - aesc., asaf., bell., carb-an., ***caust.,*** mosch., nat-m., sil., tarax.
upright - ***colch.,*** stram.
snoring, involuntary urination and stool, with - amyg., ***op.***
somnolency, without snoring and eyes being closed - ph-ac.
standing, while - ant-t., aur., bov., chin., lyc., nux-m., rhus-r., sars.
having dress fitted - nux-m.
starts, up in a wild manner, but could not keep the eyes open - ***stram.***
stool, during - aloe, ox-ac., ***sulph.***
after - calc., cocc., ***phos., ter., verat.***
before - ***ars.,*** dig.
stooping, when - calc., hell.
stroke, in - ***acon.,*** **ARN.,** ***bar-c., crot-h.,*** cupr., cupr-ac., cupr-ar., ***hyos., lach., laur., oena.,*** **OP.,** ***phos., plb., puls.,*** sol-n., ***stram.***
sudden - absin., cann-i., ***canth.,*** carb-h., carb-o., ***cocc.,*** glon., ***hydr-ac.,*** kali-c., ***laur.,*** oena., op., plb.
sunstroke, in - ***bell.,*** cact., camph., **GLON.,** lach., **OP.**
swallow, inability to, with - aml-n.
talking, while - lyc.
trance, as in a - cann-i., **LACH.,** ***laur.,*** op., tab.
transient - asaf., bov., bufo, calad., calc., cann-i., canth., carb-an., chel., chim-m., hep., **IGN.,** kali-c., lyss., med., ***mosch., nat-m.,*** ol-an., **PULS.,** rhus-r., sec., sil., zinc.
afternoon, in warm room - **PULS.**
morning on rising, drowsiness in head - rhod.
trifles, at - ***sep.***
turning, in a circle, during - calc.
twitching, of limbs, with - ***bell., canth., cupr.,*** **HYOS., STRAM.**

COMA, unconsciousness

uremic, coma - ***am-c., apis,*** apoc., ars., asc-c., ***bell.,*** cann-i., ***canth., carb-ac.,*** cic., cupr., ***cupr-ar., glon.,*** hell., hydr-ac., hyos., kali-br., ***morph., op.,*** phos., ***pic-ac.,*** piloc., queb., ser-ang., stram., ***tab., ter.,*** urea, urt-u., ***verat-v.***

vertigo, during - acon., aeth., agar., arg-n., arn., ***ars.,*** bell., bor., bov., canth., carb-an., chel., chin-s., cocc., con., crot-h., ferr., grat., iod., jatr., ***kali-br., kali-c.,*** kreos., lach., laur., lyc., mag-c., manc., mez., mill., mosch., merc., nat-c., nat-m., nux-m., nux-v., op., ran-s., sars., sec., sep., sil., stann., stram., tab., zinc.

alcoholics, of - ***phos.***

vomiting, with - ail., ars-h., dor.

amel. - acon., tab., tanac.

wakes, often, but only for a short time - achy., ***ars.***

waking, on - aesc., aster., chel., chin., cod., mag-c., mez., nat-br., nat-c., phos.

after - con., kali-br., sel., stram.

walking, while - calc., carb-an., grat., vesp.

air, in open - canth., caust., hep., sulph.

warm, room - ***acon., lach., lyc.,*** paeon., **PULS.,** tab.

COMPRESSED, as if whole, was - ***asaf.***

CONCUSSION of, commotion, (see Emergency) - ***acon.,*** **ARN.,** bell., bry., **CIC.,** con., ham., ***hell.,*** hep., ***hyos.,*** **HYPER.,** kali-i., kali-p., led., merc., nat-s., op., ph-ac., ***rhus-t.,*** sep., sul-ac., sulph., zinc.

knocking foot against any, when - bar-c.

misstep, from - led.

CONGESTION - aur., spong.

CONTRACTED, hard, painful - laur.

CONVULSIONS, from

brain tumors, from - plb.

cerebral, softening - ***bufo, caust.***

commotion of the brain, from - **ARN., CIC.,** ***hyper., nat-s.***

numbness of brain - bufo, indg.

scleroses, brain tumor, from - plb.

waving sensation in brain, begins as - cimic.

CRACKING, in - calc., coff., puls.

CRAZY, feeling, in - med., vario.

CUTTING, pain, brain were cut to pieces, on stopping, as if - nicc.

DULL, sensation, base of - gels., hyos., staph.

EMPTY, as if between forehead and brain - caust.

ENCEPHALITIS, inflammation of brain (see Meningitis) - ***acon.,*** aeth., apis, apoc., arn., ars., bapt., **BELL.,** ***bry.,*** cadm-s., calc., calc-p., ***camph.,*** canth., carb-ac., cham., chin., chin-s., chr-ox., cic., cina, ***con.,*** crot-h., ***cupr., cupr-ar.,*** dig., gels., glon., ***hell.,*** hydr-ac., ***hyos.,*** hyper., iod., iodof., kali-i., kreos., lach., ***merc.,*** merc-c., merc-d., mosch., nux-v., ***op.,*** ox-ac., par., ***phos.,*** phys., plb., puls., rhus-t., ***sil.,*** sol-n., stram., sulph., ***tub.,*** verat-v., vip., zinc.

ENCEPHALITIS,

basilar - ***cupr-cy.,*** dig., hell., iod., tub., ***verat-v.***

cerebro-spinal - ***agar.,*** ail., ***apis,*** arg-n., atro., ***bell.,*** bry., ***cic., cimic., cocc., cupr-ac.,*** cyt-l., echi., ***gels.,*** glon., ***hell.,*** hyos., ip., kali-i., nat-s., op., oreo., phys., sil., stram., sulph., verat-v., zinc-cy., zinc-m.

sopor, with - bor.

traumatic - acon., ***arn.,*** bell., ***hyper.,*** nat-s., sil.

tubercular - ***apis, bac.,*** bell., bry., ***calc., calc-p.,*** cocc., dig., glon., ***hell.,*** hyos., ***iod., iodof.,*** kali-i., ***lyc., merc.,*** nat-m., op., ***sil.,*** stram., ***sulph., tub., verat-v., zinc.,*** zinc-oc.

ENLARGED sensation - cimic., form., glon.

ERUPTIONS, brain ailments after suppressed - cic.

EXPANDED, on stooping - spig.

FAINTING, concussion, from - ***hyos.,*** nat-s.

FALLING, forward, sensation, in - ***alum.,*** am-c., ant-t., bar-c., berb., bry., carb-an., cham., coff., ***dig.,*** grat., hipp., kali-c., kreos., laur., mag-s., nux-v., ***rhus-t.,*** sabad., sul-ac.

pain, as if fell forward and came up again - sul-ac.

raising head, amel. - alum.

stooping, on - alum., ant-t., bar-c., ***carb-an.,*** chel., coff., dig., kali-c., laur., mag-s., nat-m., ***nat-s., nux-v.,*** rhus-t.

falling, down - laur.

forehead, from - rat.

side, lain on - phys.

falling, side, to side, in - nicc., sul-ac.

FATIGUE, in, with mental torpidity, after male seminal emissions - ph-ac.

FOREIGN, body in, right side of, as if - con.

moving, sensation of - phos.

FORMICATION - hyper., puls.

FROZEN, as if brain were - indg.

head and brain, as if - ***indg.***

FULLNESS, fluid of - cur.

HEAT - bell., kali-c.

boiling, in - acon.

HOT vapor, as if, coming from below - ant-t., sars., sulph.

swallowing, when - form.

HEAVINESS - form., hyper., mag-c.

falls, down, as if would - alum., bell., berb., hipp.

forward, as if brain would - carb-an., laur., rhus-t., sul-ac.

pressed feels compressed - hyper.

forward, as if brain were - bry., canth., laur., thuj.

weight on brain, like a - chel., nux-v., sil.

HEMATOMA - ***arn.***, calc-f., merc., nat-s., sil.

HYDROCEPHALUS - ***apis,*** apoc., ***calc.,*** calc-p., hell., iodof., merc., ***sil.***, sulph., tub., ***zinc.***
diarrhea, after - zinc.
vision, loss of, with - apoc.

INFLAMMATION, of brain, (see Encephalitis)
inflammation, of meninges, (see Meningitis)

INJURIES, concussion, after - **ARN.,** bell., calen., chin., **CIC.,** ***cocc.,*** **HELL.,** hep., ***hyos., hell.,*** **HYPER.,** ***kali-p., led., lob.,*** mang., merc., **NAT-S.,** ***nat-m.,*** **OP.,** ph-ac., rhus-t., sep., stram., sul-ac., ***teucr.,*** zinc.

KNOCKING, against skull, as if brain were - ars., chin., daph., glon., hydr-ac., laur., mez., nat-m., nux-m., rheum, stann., sulph., sul-ac.
brain against skull, as of, motion, on - nux-m., ***rhus-t.***

LANCINATING, base of - aesc.

LACHRYMATION, of eye, in brain affections - dig., kali-i., zinc.

LARGE, feels - arg-n., berb., chin., cimic., clem., echi., form., ***glon.,*** hell.

LIGHTNESS, in - thyr.

LIQUID, as if - mag-p.

LOOSENESS, sensation of - acon., am-c., ***ars., bar-c.,*** bar-m., ***bell.,*** bry., ***carb-an.,*** caust., **CHIN.,** cic., cocc., con., croc., dig., elaps, genist., glon., graph., guai., ***hep., hyos., kali-c.,*** kali-m., kali-n., kali-s., kalm., lac-f., lach., lact., laur., ***lyc.,*** lyss., mag-s., mur-ac., ***nat-m.,*** nat-s., nicc., ***nux-m.,*** **NUX-V.,** phys., ***rhus-t.,*** rob., sep., sol-n., **SPIG.,** stann., staph., sul-ac., sulph., tell., tub., verat., xan.
ascending steps - lyc.
carrying a weight, while - mur-ac.
coughing, on - acon., bry., carb-an., sep., sul-ac.
diagonally across top, when turning - kalm.
falling laterally - bell., bry., rhus-t., sul-ac.
feels as if brain fell to side on which leans - am-c.
forehead in - chel., con., laur., nat-m., ***sul-ac.***
hot weather, during - ***nux-m.***
morning - cic., guai.
on waking - cic.
motion, on - am-c., ars., carb-an., ***caust.,*** croc., mag-s., tell.
occiput - staph.
rising from stooping - phos.
shaking the head - ars., bar-c., con., glon., nat-m., ***nux-m., rhus-t.,*** stann., sul-ac., Xan.
stepping, on - bar-c., guai., led., lyc., **RHUS-T.,** sep., **SPIG.,** stann., sul-ac.
stooping, on - bry., dig., kali-c., laur., nat-s.
straining at stool - spig.
temples - sul-ac.
when stooping feels as if brain fell toward left - nat-s.
turning the head - kali-c., kalm., **SPIG.**
waking, on - cic.

LOOSENESS, sensation of
walking, while - acon., bar-c., carb-an., cob., croc., guai., led., lyc., mag-s., nux-m., nux-v., ***rhus-t.,*** sep., **SPIG.,** staph., sul-ac., verat.
in open air - caust., sul-ac.

LUMP, right side, as if - con.

MADDENING, feeling in - plan.

MARBLE, feels as if, brain changed to - cann-i.

MEDULLA problems- acon., agar., cupr., naja, verat-v.

MENINGITIS - acon., aeth., ***agar.,*** ail., **APIS,** apoc., arg-n., ***arn.,*** ars., atro., bapt., **BELL.,** ***bry., calc.,*** calc-br., ***calc-p.,*** camph., canth., carb-ac., chin., chin-s., chr-ox., ***cic.,*** cimic., ***cina, cocc.,*** crot-c., crot-h., ***cupr., cupr-ac., cupr-m.,*** dig., echi., ***gels., glon.,*** **HELL.,** ***hippoz., hydr-ac., hyos.,*** hyper., iod., iodof., ip., ***kali-br.,*** kali-i., kreos., ***lach.,*** med., ***merc.,*** merc-c., merc-d., mosch., ***nat-m.,*** nat-s., ***op.,*** oreo., ox-ac., ***phos.,*** phys., ***plb., rhus-t., sil.,*** sol-n., **STRAM.,** ***sulph., tub.,*** verat-v., vip., **ZINC.,** ***zinc-c., zinc-m.***
cerbro-spinal - acon., aeth., agar., am-c., ant-t., **APIS,** ***arg-n.,*** arn., ars., bapt., **BELL.,** bry., cact., camph., canth., ***cic., cimic.,*** cocc., crot-h., cupr., dig., **GELS.,** glon., hell., hydr-ac., hyos., ***ign.,*** lyc., ***nat-m.,*** **NAT-S.,** ***nux-v.,*** **OP.,** ***phos.,*** plb., ***rhus-t.,*** sol-n., tarent., verat., **VERAT-V.,** ***zinc.***
suppressed ear discharge, from - stram.
urine, with pale, clear - bell., hyos., lach., phos.
meningitis, spinal - ***acon.,*** **APIS, BELL.,** ***bry., calc., cic., cimic.,*** cocc., crot-h., cupr., dulc., **GELS.,** ***hyos.,*** hyper., kali-i., ***ip.,*** merc., ***nat-m., nat-s.,*** nux-v., ***op.,*** ox-ac., ***plb., rhus-t.,*** sec., verat-v., ***zinc.***

NEEDLES, at - tarent.

NOISES, humming or roaring - kreos., lach., phos.

NUMBNESS, in - apis, bufo, calc., graph., hell., kali-br., nat-a., plat., staph.
affections, with brain - fl-ac.
convulsions, before - bufo.
morning - apis, bufo, ***con.,*** kali-br., mag-c., ***plat.***

PARALYSIS, of - alumn., con., cupr., gels., hell., lyc., op., ***plb., sec., zinc.***
incipient - am-c., ars., carb-v., hyos., **LYC.,** op., phos., plb., zinc.

PAROTID gland, inflammation, metastasis to brain - apis, bell., hyos.

PRESSING, pain, as if bound up - acon., aeth., am-br., ant-t., arg-m., asar., aur., **BRY.,** calc., camph., ***carb-v.,*** cham., chin., cimic., ***cocc.,*** colch., ***crot-c.,*** cupr., cycl., gels., graph., guai., hell., hyper., indg., **LAC-C.,** ***lach.,*** laur., mag-s., manc., meny., ***merc.,*** morph., ***mosch.,*** mur-ac., **NAT-M., NIT-AC.,** ***olnd.,*** op., par., petr., ***ph-ac.,*** plat., prun., ***psor.,*** puls., rhus-t., sars., sil., ***spig., staph.***

PRESSING, pain
cloth, by a - cycl.
forward - ***acon.,*** asar., bell., ***bry.,*** ip., kali-c.
forward, out of eyes - nat-m.
inward - asar., cupr., glon.
iron helmet, by an - ***crot-c.***
membranes were too tight - ***acon.,*** carb-v., op., par., psor.
outward - agar., bell., bry., glon., guai., hep., hydr., indg., laur., lil-t., ***nat-m.,*** phys., stann.
reading - arg-m.
middle of brain - phos., zinc.
on the brain - ars., ***cann-i.,*** glon., ign., manc., meny., ph-ac., phos., ruta., sep.
sharp corners, against, as if - sabad.
side lain on - ph-ac.
skull against the, as if - mez., rhod., rhus-v.
too small, as if - ***glon.,*** morph., scut.
spot - zinc.
standing - arg-m.

PRESSING, sides, as if something were lying on the brain - grat.
against the bone - mez.

PULSATING, brain seems to be - ***bell., chin.,*** cycl., dig., glon., hyos., kali-n., ***lyc.,*** nit-ac., op., rhus-t.
beating of, against skull - ars., ***bell.,*** **CHIN.,** daph., ***glon.,*** hydr-ac., laur., mez., nat-m., nux-m., psor., rheum, stann., ***sulph.,*** sul-ac.
deep-seated - cic.
hammers, like little - **NAT-M., PSOR.**
leaning back, on - **LYC.**
shooting, ending in - ***bell.***
throbbing pain in middle of every morning, lasts all day - calc.
transient, in one-half of - cham.
waves, as of - **CHIN.,** dig.

QUIVERING, sensation, as if brain were shaking while walking - rhod.

RISING, sensation, raised several times in succession, as if - thuj.
stooping, on - cob.

ROLLING, in, were rolled into small bulk, as if - ***arn., coc-c.***
rolling, over - plan.

SENSES, general
acute - ***acon.,*** alco., ambr., anac., ***arn.,*** **ARS.,** asaf., ***asar.,*** atro., ***aur.,*** bar-c., **BELL.,** bor., cann-i., caps., cast., caust., ***cham., chin.,*** cimic., cina, clem., **COFF.,** ***colch.,*** con., cupr., ferr., graph., hydr-ac., ***ign.,*** kali-p., lach., ***lyss.,*** morph., mur-ac., nit-ac., **NUX-V., OP., PHOS.,** plb., pyrog., sang., sil., ***stry.,*** sulph., tarent., thea., valer., verat., zinc.
confused - arg-n., bell., glon., lil-t., mang.
dullness of - acon., aeth., agar., agn., all-c., alum., alum-p., alum-sil., ambr., am-c., anac., ant-t., arg-n., ***arn.,*** ars., ars-i., asaf., asar., aur., ***bapt., bell.,*** bov., bry., calc., calc-i., calc-sil., ***camph.,*** canth., caps., carb-v., caust., cedr., ***cham.,*** chel., ***chin., chin-s., cic.,*** con.,

SENSES, general
dullness of - ***cycl.,*** dig., dros., dulc., gels., graph., **HELL.,** hep., ***hydr-ac., hyos.,*** ign., indg., iod., iris, ***kali-br.,*** kali-c., ***kali-p., lach.,*** lact., laur., led., ***lyc.,*** mag-arct., mag-aust., mag-c., mag-m., mang., meny., merc., mez., morph., mosch., nat-c., ***nat-m.,*** nit-ac., **NUX-M.,** ***nux-v.,*** ol-an., olnd., **OP.,** paeon., petr., ***ph-ac., phos., plb.,*** **PULS.,** ran-b., ran-s., rhod., rhus-t., sabad., ***sec.,*** sel., ***sil.,*** spong., stann., staph., stram., sul-i., ***sulph.,*** tab., ther., verat., vip., zinc., zinc-p.
perverted - arg-n., op.
vanishing, of - alum., anac., ant-t., asar., ars., bell., bor., bov., bry., bufo, calc., ***camph.,*** cann-i., cann-s., canth., carb-an., carb-o., cham., ***chel.,*** cic., coff., croc., crot-h., ***cupr.,*** glon., graph., hep., hyos., kali-c., kali-sil., kreos., ***lach.,*** laur., merc., mez., mosch., nit-ac., ***nux-m., nux-v.,*** ol-an., ph-ac., ***plat., plb., puls.,*** ran-b., rhod., rhus-t., sec., stann., staph., stram., verat.
pains, from - plb.

SENSITIVENESS, of - **BELL.,** ***bov.,*** brom., ***bry.,*** calc., ***carb-v.,*** **CHIN.,** ***con.,*** crot-t., dros., **GELS.,** gent-c., **GLON.,** hyos., iod., **IP.,** kali-c., kali-p., ***lach.,*** lact., led., lyc., ***mag-m.,*** **MEZ.,** ***nat-m.,*** **NIT-AC., PHOS.,** ***phyt.,*** raph., ***sil., spig., staph.,*** stram., zinc.
brushing hair, from - ***acon.,*** apis, **ARN.,** ars., aza., ***bell.,*** bov., ***bry.,*** carb-s., ***carb-v.,*** caust., ***chin.,*** **CINA,** coff., dys-co., euon., ***eup-per., gels., hep., ip.,*** kali-bi., ***kreos.,*** lachn., mang., meli., merc., nat-m., ***nit-ac.,*** nux-m., ***nux-v.,*** olnd., ***par., rhus-t.,*** sars., ***sep.,*** **SIL.,** stry., ***sulph.,*** vib.
external - ***agar.,*** am-c., bell., bor., bov., ***carb-an.,*** chin., chin-s., grat., lach., lyc., mag-c., merc., nat-m., nux-v., phos., sabin., tong.
hat, to - nit-ac., sil.
jar, to the least - **BELL.,** calc., cob., ferr-p., ***glon.,*** hep., ip., kali-p., lac-d., lyc., ***mag-m.,*** mang., nat-ac., **NIT-AC.,** ph-ac., phyt., raph., ***sil.,*** spig., stram., ***sulph., ther.,*** vib.
menses, during - **BELL.,** ***calc.,*** carb-v., con., gels., ***hyos.,*** ip., ***kali-c., mag-m., phos., sil., zinc.***
before - **CALC.,** ***carb-v., con., hyos., nat-m., phos.,*** sil., sulph., zinc.
stepping, to - **BELL.,** ***calc.,*** calc-p., ***carb-v.,*** chin., dros., gels., **GLON.,** ***ip., led.,*** lyc., ***nat-m., nit-ac.,*** raph., rhus-t., ***spig.,*** stann., ***sulph.***
when ascending - ***rhus-t.***
touch, to - iod., sep.
gentlest, after anger - mez.

SEPARATED, from skull, brain were - staph.

SHAKING sensation, as if, suddenly - upa.

SHARP, pain - ***agn.,*** **ALUM.,** am-c., bar-c., bell., ***bry.,*** calc., cham., cina, colch., cycl., dulc., euphr., gran., ***guai.,*** hyper., kali-c., laur., lyc., mag-c., mill., nat-m., petr., plb., ***puls.,*** sabin., sil., thuj.
  stooping - cycl.
  upward - sil.

SHOCKS, electric-like, in body, from concussion of brain - **CIC.**

SMALLER, brain feels smaller than skull - acon., glon.
  feels too far from skull - staph.

SOFTENING, of - agar., **ALUM.,** ambr., ***arg-n., aur., bar-c.,*** cann-i., ***caust., con.,*** fl-ac., kali-br., kali-i., kali-p., lach., lyc., nux-m., nux-v., **PHOS.,** pic-ac., ***plb.,*** salam., sil., stry., sulph., syph., vanad., ***zinc.,*** zinc-p.

SORE, pain, in - anac., ***arn.,*** aur., bar-c., **CHIN.,** coff., ***cupr.,*** **GELS.,** glon., hell., ***ign.,*** ind., iod., ***ip.,*** merc., mur-ac., ***nat-m., nux-v., ph-ac.,*** phos., phys., phyt., plan., rumx., stann., tell.
  afternoon - phos.
  paroxysmal - ***verat.***

STIFFNESS, sensation of, in open air - phos.

STIRRED, with a spoon, feels as if - arg-n., iod.

STRIKING, against the skull, sensation as though brain were - alum., ***ars.,*** **CHIN.,** ***nux-m.,*** plat., ***rhus-t.,*** rob., ***sep.,*** stann., ***sulph.,*** sul-ac.
  nodding the head, on - ***sulph.***

STROKE, apoplexy - **ACON.,** agar., ***alco.,*** **ANAC.,** ant-c., ant-t., apis, **ARN.,** ***ars.,*** ars-s-f., asar., ***aster., aur.,*** bapt., **BAR-C., BELL.,** brom., **BRY.,** bufo, cact., cadm-br., cadm-s., calc., ***camph.,*** carb-h., carb-s., carb-v., caust., chen-a., ***chin.,*** chin-a., chlol., **COCC.,** ***coff.,*** con., croc., ***crot-h., cupr.,*** cupr-ac., dig., erig., ***ferr.,*** fl-ac., ***form.,*** gast., **GELS.,** ***glon.,*** guare., hell., hep., **HYDR-AC.,** ***hyos.,*** ign., iod., **IP.,** juni., kali-br., kali-cy., kali-i., kali-m., kali-n., kreos., **LACH.,** ***laur.,*** lim., lith-br., lol., ***lyc.,*** merc., ***mill.,*** morph., nat-m., nat-n., nat-ns., nit-ac., ***nux-m.,*** **NUX-V.,** ***oena.,*** olnd., **OP.,** ox-ac., ph-ac., ***phos.,*** plb., ***puls.,*** ran-g., rhus-t., sabad., samb., sars., sec., sep., ***sil.,*** sin-n., sol-a., ***stram.,*** stront-c., sulph., tab., thuj., verat., ***verat-v.,*** viol-o., vip.
  mental, symptoms, from - **BAR-C., CROT-H.,** hell., ***ip.,*** **NUX-V.**
  paralysis, from - ***alum.,*** anac., apis, ***bar-c.,*** cadm-s., ***caust., cocc., crot-c., crot-h., cupr., gels.,*** **LACH.,** ***laur., nux-v.,*** **OP.,** ***phos., plb.,*** sec., stann., ***stront-c.,*** zinc.
    one-sided - anac., arn., ***bar-c.,*** bell., con., lach., laur., nux-v., **PHOS.,** stann., stram., zinc.
  post-hemiphlegia - ***arn.,*** ars., ***bar-c.,*** bell., both., ***caust., cocc.,*** cupr., cur., lach., nux-v., phos., ***plb.,*** rhus-t., vip., zinc-m.
  pulse irritable, with - acon.
    slow full, face red, pupils small - ***op.***
    small weak, face bluish pale - lach.
  speech, impairment, causes - ***bar-c.,*** caust., crot-c., ***crot-h., ip.,*** lach., ***laur.,*** **NUX-V.**
  subarachnoid - gels.

STROKE
  threatening, predisposition for - ***acon.,*** **ARN.,** ars., ***aster.,*** bar-c., ***bell.,*** calc-f., **COFF.,** ***fl-ac., gels., glon.,*** hyos., ign., kali-n., ***lach., laur., nux-v.,*** **OP.,** ***phos.,*** prim-v., stront-c., ***stront-c.***
  waves of congestion, holds head - glon.

SUNSTROKE - ***acon.,*** agar., **AML-N.,** ***ant-c.,*** apis, arg-m., ***arn., ars.,*** **BELL.,** bry., ***cact., cadm-met., camph., carb-v.,*** crot-h., cyt-l., euph-pi., ***gels.,*** **GLON.,** hydr-ac., hyos., kalm., **LACH.,** lyc., lyss., **NAT-C.,** nat-m., nux-v., ***op.,*** pop-c., rhus-t., **SOL.,** stram., syph., ***ther.,*** thuj., usn., valer., **VERAT.,** ***verat-v.***
  chronic effects - nat-c.
  sleeping in sun, from - acon., ***bell.***

SWASHING, to and fro - chin., hell.

TICKLING, in - laur., phos.
  night - hyper.

TONGUE, protruded, in brain affections - apis, hydr-ac.

TORN, pain, as if, torn to pieces, aches, morning on rising, agg. motion, amel. rest and warmth, passes off with much yawning - staph.

TUMOR, encephaloma - acet-ac., arn., ***ars., ars-i.,*** art-v., ***bar-c.,*** bell., bufo, ***calc.,*** carb-ac., ***carb-an.,*** caust., **CON.,** ***croc.,*** gels., glon., graph., hydr., hyper., ***kali-i., kreos., lach.,*** merc., nit-ac., nux-v., **PHOS.,** ***plb.,*** sep., ***sil.,*** stram., sulph., ***thuj., tub.***
  convulsions, in - plb.
  scleroses, from - plb.

TWITCHING, in, as if - aster., bar-c., bov., bry., calc., cann-s., nit-ac., rat.

UNCONSCIOUSNESS, (see Coma)

VERTIGO, (see Vertigo, chapter)

VOICE, male, affects - bar-c.

VOMITING, in brain affections - bell.,carc., glon., kali-i., plb.

WAVING, in as if - cimic., glon., phys.

WRAPPED, as if - cycl., op.

WRINKLED, forehead, with brain, symptoms - grat., ***hell.,*** **STRAM.**

Breasts

ABSCESS - apis, ***bell.***, ***bry.***, bufo, ***camph.***, ***cist.***, ***crot-h.***, crot-t., graph., **HEP.**, kreos., ***lach.***, **MERC.**, **PHOS.**, **PHYT.**, sars., **SIL.**, **SULPH.**, tarent-c.
fistula discharging serum or milk - ***sil.***
left, in - ***arn.***, ***cist.***
scars, hard, remaining with retarded flow of milk - **GRAPH.**
old scars, threatening in - calen., **GRAPH.**, **PHYT.**, ***sil.***
abscess, nipples - cast-eq., cham., ***merc.***, ***sil.***

ACHING, pain - apis, con., eupi., lil-t., mosch., stram., zinc.
empty, when - ***bor.***
left - lil-t., mosch.
nursing amel. - phel.
region of - berb., rhus-t.
sitting bent, while - rhus-t.
right - zinc.
under - carb-v., eup-per.
aching, nipples - ***calc-p.***

AIR, sensitive to cold - cact.
streaming from nipples, sensation of - cycl.

APHTHAE, nipples, bleeding - ***bor.***

ATROPHY, of - anac., anan., ars., bar-c., cham., ***chim.***, chin., **COFF.**, **CON.**, dulc., fago., ferr., **IOD.**, **KALI-I.**, ***kreos.***, lach., lac-d., **NAT-M.**, ***nit-ac.***, ***nux-m.***, onos., plb., ***sabal.***, sac-alb., sars., ***sec.***, sil.
and ovaries with infertility - iod.
decrease in size - lac-d.
dropsy, ovarian - ***iod.***
dwindling with small hard painful lumps in them - ***kreos.***
rapid - ***chim.***
skin, leaving a flaccid, bag-like - ***con.***
small hard painful lumps, with - ***kreos.***
atrophy, nipples - ***iod.***, sars.

BALL, sensation of, under left - hura.

BLEEDING, nipples, from - bufo, ***ham.***, ***lyc.***, med., ***merc.***, ***merc-c.***, ***sep.***, sil., ***sulph.***
child draws so much blood, when it vomits it seems to vomit blood - ***lyc.***
discharge of blood and water - ***lyc.***
easily - ***lyc.***
nursing, when - ***sulph.***
after - ***sulph.***
soreness, with great - ***ham.***
suppurate, seem about to - ***sep.***

BOILS - chin., mag-c., phos.

BORING, pain - bufo, ind., plb.
extending to back - plb.
pressure agg. - plb.

BREAST-feeding - acon., agn., ***ars.***, ***bell.***, **BOR.**, ***bry.***, **CALC.**, ***calc-p.***, carb-an., carb-v., ***cham.***, chel., ***chin.***, ***cina***, con., crot-t., ***dulc.***, ferr., graph., ***ign.***, iod., ***ip.***, kali-c., lach., lyc., ***mag-c.***, merc., nat-c., nat-m., **NAT-P.**, ***nux-v.***, phel., ***ph-ac.***, phos., phyt., **PULS.**, rheum, ***rhus-t.***, samb., sec., sel., **SEP.**, ***sil.***, spig., ***squil.***, stann., ***staph.***, stram., ***sulph.***, zinc.
aching, from cold, all over - **BRY.**
back, pain, during - **SIL.**
breast pain, nurses, while child - ***crot-t.***, ***puls.***, **SIL.**
ache, after nursing, being empty, is obliged to compress with hand - bor.
nurses, while child, wandering pains - ***puls.***
opposite breast, in, when child nurses - ***bor.***
sharp pain - **SIL.**
blood, pure, flows every time child nurses - **SIL.**
breathing, suffocative attacks - ***calc-p.***
cold, bad effects of taking - **BRY.**
distended breasts, milk scanty, feels cold air readily, is cold, want of vital activity to secrete milk - **CALC.**
eruptions - ***sep.***
fever - acon., arn., ***bell.***, **BRY.**, coff., rhus-t.
anger, after - ***cham.***
delirium, with - ***acon.***, ***bell.***
rheumatic pains in breast - **BRY.**
hair falls out - ***nat-m.***
headache after nursing infant - bell., bry., ***calc.***, cham., chin., dulc., phos., ***puls.***, ***sep.***, sil., staph.
as if head would burst, from cold - **BRY.**
neuralgic, during and after - ***chin.***
hemoptysis - **CHIN.**
induration of right, burning pain - ***con.***
lochia, increased - ***rhus-t.***, **SIL.**
mania - ***hyos.***
menses - ***chin.***, ***rhus-t.***, sil.
menorrhagia, blood pale or bright - ***phos.***
profuse - ***calc.***
sensation as if menses would appear, in afternoon - pall.
painful, nipples, sore and cracked, during - agar., arg-n., ***arn.***, calen., **CAST-EQ.**, ***cham.***, ***graph.***, ***ham.***, ***hydr.***, ***lyc.***, ***merc.***, ***mill.***, phos., ***phyt.***, ***puls.***, **RAT.**, ***sep.***, sulph.
aphthous - ***bor.***
bleeding - ***ham.***
complains every time she puts child to breast - **SIL.**
pain from nipple through to back - ***crot-t.***
sensitive, cannot bear clothing to touch - ***helon.***
crys every time child is put to breast - ***puls.***
weaning, after - dulc.
ulcerated - ***calc.***, **CAST-EQ.**
swollen heavy from a cold - **BRY.**
uterus, sharp pain in - **SIL.**
weakness, and deterioration of health in mother, after nursing - ***calc.***, ***calc-p.***, ***carb-an.***, **CARB-V.**, **CHIN.**, lyc., olnd., ***phos.***, **PH-AC.**, sep., ***sil.***, sulph.

BREAST-feeding
weaning - **BELL.**, carb-an., frag., lac-c., lac-d., puls., urt-u., vinc.
ailments, after in mother - con., bry., cycl., frag-v., ***lac-c.***, puls.
arrest, flow, to - **BELL.**, **LAC-C.**, urt-u.
breasts swell, feel stretched, tense, intensely sore - ***puls.***
left - ***bry.***
child, for the - **BELL.**, carb-an., ***cham.***, frag-v., lac-c., lac-d., **PULS.**, urt-u., vinc.
complaints after - ***cycl.***
diarrhea - arg-n.
eruptions - dulc.
secretion continues - carb-an., ***puls.***

BREAST-milk
absent - ***acon.***, ***agn.***, alf., apis, ***asaf.***, ***bell.***, bor., **BRY.**, **CALC.**, carb-an., card-m., ***caust.***, cham., ***chel.***, ***coff.***, **DULC.**, ***form.***, frag., ***ign.***, **LAC-C.**, ***lac-d.***, lach., **LACT.**, ***lec.***, merc., ***mill.***, nux-v., ***ph-ac.***, phos., phyt., piloc., **PULS.**, rheum, rhus-t., ***ric.***, samb., ***sec.***, ***sil.***, stict., sulph., ***thyr.***, **URT-U.**, ust., x-ray, **ZINC.**
suppressed, lochia and fever, with - ***mill.***
stinging in breast, with - ***sec.***
depression, with - agn.
nightwatching, from - caust.
altered - bell., merc.
bad milk - acet-ac., aeth., ***bor.***, bufo, **CALC.**, ***calc-p.***, carb-an., **CHAM.**, cina, crot-t., lach., lec., ***merc.***, nux-v., op., puls., sil., stann.
anger, from - calc-p., ***cham.***
bitter - rheum
bloody - bufo, ***cham.***, hep., ***lyc.***, ***merc.***, ***phyt.***, ***sep.***, ***sulph.***
blue - acet-ac., ***calc.***, ***lach.***, lyc., puls.
caking, of - nux-v.
ceased a few days after confinement - phyt.
cessation, sudden, in puerperal fever - ***verat-v.***
changeable, from alkaline to neutral or acid - ***calc-p.***
cheesy - ***bor.***, ***cham.***, ***phyt.***
child refuses mother's milk - ***acet-ac.***, ***bor.***, ***calc.***, **CALC-P.**, cina, lach., mag-c., ***merc.***, ***ph-ac.***, rheum, sabal., **SIL.**, stann., sulph.
vomits milk after nursing - acet-ac., aeth., ***ant-c.***, calc., calc-p., ***nat-c.***, ***ph-ac.***, ***sanic.***, **SIL.**, ***valer.***
copious, with depression - chin.
curdles, sour after being drawn - bor.
disappearing - agar., ***agn.***, ***arn.***, ***asaf.***, aur., bry., ***calc.***, ***camph.***, ***caust.***, cham., ***chel.***, chin., ***chion.***, coff., **DULC.**, hecla., ***ign.***, ***lac-c.***, ***lac-d.***, lyc., merc., mill., ***phel.***, ph-ac., phos., phyt., ***plan.***, ***plb.***, ***puls.***, ***rhus-t.***, ***sec.***, sep., sulph., ***tub.***, **URT-U.**, ***ust.***, ***verat-v.***, ***zinc.***
anger, after - cham.
brain troubles, with - ***agar.***
cold, after taking - dulc., ***puls.***
confinement, after - ***asaf.***
excitement, after - caust.

BREAST-milk
flow, milk, will not - ***sec.***
flowing - acon., ant-t., ***bell.***, ***bor.***, ***bry.***, **CALC.**, cham., chin., ***con.***, ***iod.***, ***kali-i.***, kreos., lac-c., ***lach.***, ***lyc.***, nux-v., ***phos.***, ***puls.***, ***rhus-t.***, ***sil.***, stann., staph., ust.
sensation of - dict., kreos., nux-v., puls.
increased, too profuse - ***acon.***, anan., arund., asaf., **BELL.**, ***bor.***, **BRY.**, **CALC.**, cham., chim., chin., ***con.***, erig., iod., lac-c., lact., ***medus.***, nux-v., parth., phos., phyt., pip-m., **PULS.**, rheum, ***rhus-t.***, ric., sabal., ***sabin.***, ***salv.***, ***sec.***, ***sol-o.***, spira., stram., ust., yohim.
insanity, during - bell., stram.
involuntary flow - **BELL.**, ***bry.***, **CALC.**, ***cham.***, chim., ***chin.***, ***con.***, ***iod.***, jab., ***kali-i.***, lac-c., ***lach.***, ***lyc.***, ***phos.***, ***rhus-t.***, ***sil.***, stram., ***uran-n.***, ust.
coagulates - ***bor.***
women who are not nursing, in - ***puls.***
menses, during - calc., calc-p., merc., pall., ***puls.***, ***tub.***
absent, with - bell., bry., calc., lyc., phos., puls., rhus-t., sabin., stram.
before - cycl., ***tub.***
instead of - merc.
suppressed - ***chin.***, cycl., lyc., ***merc.***, phos., puls., rhus-t., ***tub.***
metastasis - agar.
mother's milk agg. - acet-ac., ant-c., ***bor.***, calc., **CALC-P.**, ***cina***, lach., ***merc.***, ***nat-c.***, ***ph-ac.***, ***sanic.***, **SIL.**, stann., ***valer.***
non-nursing, women, in - ars., ***asaf.***, bell., bor., ***cycl.***, lyc., ***merc.***, phos., **PULS.**, rhus-t., stram., thlaspi., ***tub.***, ***urt-u.***
puberty, at - merc., ***puls.***
profuse, too, confinement, second day after - phyt.
hectic fever, with - **CALC.**
mania, in - ***hyos.***
several, for, days, causing prostration - ***phyt.***
thin, watery - ***iod.***
weakening - **CALC.**
watery, child refuses it - ***calc.***
salty - calc-p.
scanty - acon., apis, ***asaf.***, ***bell.***, ***bry.***, ***calc.***, carb-an., card-m., ***caust.***, **CHAM.**, ***chel.***, ***chin.***, ***coff.***, dulc., ***form.***, ***ign.***, jab., ***lac-d.***, lach., merc., ***mill.***, nux-v., puls., rheum, rhus-t., samb., sec., stict., sulph., **URT-U.**, ust., **ZINC.**
anxiety and night watching, from - ***caust.***
breasts small - **CALC.**
childbirth, after - ***asaf.***
debility, with, and great apathy - ph-ac.
emaciation, with - ***plb.***
fatigue, from - ***caust.***
mastitis, in - ***merc.***
metritis, in, from suppression of menses, or getting feet wet - **PULS.**
spoiled, child refused it - **MERC.**

BREAST-milk

stringy - bor., ***kali-bi.,*** kali-c., ***phyt.***

masses and water, has appearance of being composed of - ***kali-bi.***

suppression, of mother milk, ailments from - ***acon.,*** agar., ***agn.,*** aur., aur-i., aur-s., bell., **BRY.,** calc., calc-sil., camph-br., ***carb-v.,*** **CAUST.,** ***cham., chim.,*** cimic., cycl., dulc., frag., ***hyos.,*** ign., ***iod.,*** lac-d., ***lach., merc.,*** mill., phyt., **PULS.,** ***rhus-t., sec.,*** senec., ***sil.,*** sul-i., ***sulph., urt-u.,*** verat., zinc.

anger, after - ***cham.***

cold, from - **BRY.,** dulc.

comes back in twelve to twenty-four hours - lac-d.

fever, in puerperal - ***cham.***

heat, with general - ***rhus-t.***

mastitis, in - ***bry.***

suddenly - ***puls.***

tastes, bad - bor., ***calc-p.,*** cham., ***kali-bi.,*** lyc., ***phyt.***

bitter - cetr., ***rheum.***

disagreeable, nauseating, child will not nurse and cries much - ***calc.***

horseradish, like - coch.

salty - carb-an.

thick and tastes bad - ***bor., kali-bi.,*** lyc., ***phyt.***

stringy - phyt.

thin - ***calc-p.,*** carb-an., cham., ***con., lach.,*** lyc., merc., nux-v., ***sil., tub.***

and blue - acet-ac., ***calc., lach.,*** lyc., puls.

and salty - carb-an.

and watery - ***calc., con., iod., plb., puls., tub.***

long after weaning - ***con.***

yellow - phyt., ***rheum.***

BULLET, or rivet, feeling of, in region - lil-t.

BURNING, pain - aesc., ambr., anan., ***apis,*** **ARS.,** bell., bry., ***bufo,*** calc., ***calc-p.,*** carb-an., chin-a., ***cimic.,*** com., con., indg., iod., lach., laur., led., ***lyc., mez.,*** ol-an., ***phos., phyt.,*** sang., sel., tarent-c.

between, breasts - mez.

left - chin-a.

menses, during - indg.

pregnancy, during - ***calc-p.***

rubbing, from - con.

under, left - laur., mur-ac., rumx.

left, sitting, while - mag-c.

motion, amel. - ars.

right - aeth., phos.

burning, nipples - ***agar., ars.,*** arund., benz-ac., cast., cic., con., ***crot-t., graph., lyc.,*** onos., orig., petr., phos., psor., puls., sang., sep., ***sil.,*** **SULPH.**

around - psor.

fire, like - ***sulph.***

left, in - senec., ***sil.***

nursing, after - sang., ***sulph.***

rubbing, after - con.

sore, and - phos.

CANCER, of - alum., alumn., anag., ***apis, arg-n.,*** arn., ***ars., ars-i.,*** **ASTER.,** ***aur-a., aur-m-n., bad.,*** bapt., bar-i., ***bell., bell-p., brom.,*** bry., **BUFO,** calc., calc-i., ***calen., carb-ac., carb-an.,*** carb-s., carb-v., ***carc.,*** caust., cham., ***chim.,*** cic., cist., ***clem.,*** coloc., **CON.,** ***cund.,*** dulc., ferr-i., form-ac., ***gali.,*** **GRAPH.,** ***hep.,*** ho., ***hydr.,*** kali-c., ***kali-i.,*** kreos., ***lach.,*** lap-a., ***lyc.,*** **MERC.,** ***merc-i-f.,*** nat-cac., ***nit-ac.,*** ol-an., ***ox-ac., phos.,*** **PHYT.,** plb-i., ***psor.,*** puls., ***sang., scirr.,*** sem-t., ***sep.,*** **SIL.,** ***sulph.,*** tarent-c., ***thuj.,*** tub.

axilla - ***aster.,*** con., phyt.

axillary glands indurated - ***carb-an.***

bleeding - ho., kreos., lach., ***phos.,*** sang., thuj.

burning, of edges, smells like old cheese - ***hep.***

open tumor - **APIS.,** ***hydr.***

pains, better from external warmth - **ARS.**

towards axilla - ***carb-an.***

contusion, from - ***bell-p.,*** **CON.,** phyt.

discharge of blood and fetid ichor from livid red spot on tumor - ***aster.***

drawing pain toward axilla - ***carb-an.***

epithelioma - ***arg-n., ars., ars-i.,*** brom., **BUFO,** calc., calc-p., ***clem.,*** **CON.,** ***hydr., kreos., lach.,*** merc., ***merc-i-f., phos., phyt., sep., sil.,*** sulph., thuj.

epithelioma - ***hydr.***

face gray, earthy, oldish - **BROM.**

hen's egg in, size of - phyt.

hot, nipples in cancer - ***phos.***

indurations inflamed, very painful, worse by exposure to air - ***phos.***

itching, with - sil.

lancinating - **ASTER.,** ***lach.***

bleeding easily - ***phos.***

large as a small egg, as - ***hydr.***

left feels drawn in - aster.

open - ***hydr.***

nightly, pains - ***aster.***

occult - **BUFO**.

pains, with - ***hydr.***

red spots on skin - ***carb-an.***

right - ***apis.***

open, with burning pain - ***hydr.***

scars, in old - **GRAPH.,** sil.

which had remained, after repeated abscesses - **GRAPH.**

sharp pains, in shoulders and uterus, with - clem.

sleep from pain, cannot - ***aster.***

sore pain, a sort of raw feeling - **MERC.**

stinging of edges, smells like old cheese - ***hep.***

stony hard, large as tea cup - **CON.**

ulceration - ***calc., hep., phos.,*** **PHYT., SIL.,** sulph.

cancer, scirrhus - ***arg-n.,*** ars., ***aster., brom.,*** **BUFO,** ***carb-an.,*** **CON,** cund., hydr., kreos., lap-a., phyt., sars., ***scirr., sil.,*** sulph.

burning - ***sep.***

discharge, ulceration with fetid sanious, and sloughing - cund.

cancer, scirrhus
emaciated and cachectic - cund.
hard as cartilage and uneven, which has grown to size of a hen's egg, during menopause - ***con.***
heaviness - ***con.***
injury, caused by - ***con.***, hyper.
left, of - ***carb-ac.***
occasionally twitching in affected part, the mass is immovable - ***con.***
very painful, worse in cold weather and during night - ***clem.***
painful of right, about an inch in diameter, hard but movable, nipples drawn in - ***chim.***
purple, skin, in spots and wrinkled - cund.
right, in - cund.
adhering by entire base to thoracic walls - ***aster.***
with itching - sil.
sharp shooting pain - ***con.***
skin and axillary glands involved - cund.

CHILLINESS, in, shivering in - ***cocc., guai.,*** nux-v., petr.

CICATRICES, (see Scars)

COLDNESS - cimic., ***cocc.,*** dig., ***med.,*** rhus-t.
icy, before menses - med.
left feels cold - nat-c.
cough, during - nat-c.
region of - chin-s.
coldness, nipples - med.

CONGESTION - acon., apis, ***bell.,*** calc., ferr., ***kali-c.,*** lac-c., phos.
milk, with insanity, in - bell., stram.

CONSTRICTION, sensation of - lil-t., sang., stram., verat.
below right breast - alum., am-m.
deep inspiration - sang.
left, when child nurses from right - ***bor.***

CRACKS, nipples - aesc., anan., ***arn.,*** ars., ***aur-s.,*** calc-ox., ***calen.,*** carb-an., carb-v., ***cast.,*** **CAST-EQ., CAUST.,** cham., ***con., crot-t., cund.,*** cur., ***eup-a., fl-ac.,*** gali., ger., **GRAPH.,** ham., hep., hipp., ***hydr., lyc.,*** merc., ***merc-c., mill.,*** nit-ac., ***paeon.,*** **PETR.,** ***phel.,*** phos., **PHYT.,** **RAT., SARS.,** ***sep.,*** **SIL.,** ***sulph.***
across crown - ***sep.***
base, at, as if they would drop off - ***sulph.***
herpes around, with - caust.
pain, with intense, on putting child to breast - ***phyt.***
painful - ***graph.,*** phyt.
nursing, during - agar., arg-n., ***arn.,*** calen., **CAST-EQ.,** ***cham., graph., ham., hydr., lyc., merc., mill.,*** phos., ***phyt., puls.,*** **RAT.,** ***sep.,*** sulph.
aphthous - ***bor.***
bleeding - ***ham.***
complains every time she puts child to breast - **SIL.**
pain from nipple through to back - ***crot-t.***
sensitive, cannot bear clothing to touch - ***helon.***

CRACKS, nipples
nursing, during,
crys every time child is put to breast - ***puls.***
ulcerated - ***calc.,*** **CAST-EQ.**
weaning, after - dulc.

CRAMP, gradually increasing and decreasing in - plat.

CRAMPY, pain - ***lil-t.,*** plat.

CUTTING, pain - am-c., aster., bell., bufo, calc., calc-p., cham., chin-s., ***colch.,*** hura, ***iod.,*** lach., lil-t., olnd., phyt., sabin.
left - com., ***lach., lil-t.***
extending to scapula - lil-t.
lying on left side - lil-t.
nursing, while - **SIL.**
extending to back - colch.
under - rob.
left - bry.
right - ***chel.,*** kali-p.
cutting, nipples after menses - thuj.
extending to scapula, male - tell.
to left scapula, from left nipple - spig.
to left upper arm, from left nipple - spig.

DEFORMED, nipples - iod., merc., sars.

DISCHARGE, nipples, from - phyt., phel., phos.
bloody water, from - ***lyc., phyt.,*** sil.
milky, from right - thlaspi.
pure blood at every nursing - **SIL.**

DISCOLORATION, of
blueness of ulcerated - ***lach.,*** phos.
bluish red - kreos., ***lach.***
livid - plb.
redness - am-c., cocc., led., sabad.
streaks - bell., phos., rhus-t., sulph.
yellow - chel., thuj.
spots - ars., carb-v., chlor., kali-c., lyc., manc., ***phos., sep.,*** sulph., tab.
discoloration, nipples - agar., cast-eq., ***colch., fl-ac.,*** psor.
red - psor.
white spot in centre - nux-v.

DISTENSION, (see Congestion, Swelling) - apis, aster., calc., kali-c., zinc.

DRAWING, pain - carb-v., kreos., ***lil-t.,*** plb., stann., sumb.
inward - aster.
left, under - stann.
when child nurses right - ***bor.***
drawing, nipples - crot-t.
as with a string when child nurses - **CROT-T.**
extending to, back, to, during nursing - crot-t.
to, all over body during nursing - phyt., puls., sil.
to neck - mur-ac.
to scapula - rhus-t.
left - crot-t., euon., til., zinc.
morning - ***rhus-t.***
right - sumb.
below - mur-ac.

DRYNESS, nipples - cast-eq.

ECZEMA - anac., graph.
nipples - ***graph.***

EMACIATION - ars-i., cham., chim., **COFF., CON.,** ferr., **IOD.,** ***kali-i.,*** nat-m., nit-ac., ***nux-m., onos.,*** sabal., sec., sil.
lump, hard, small, painful, with - kreos.
one breast, smaller than the other - lach., **SABAL.**
ovary complaints, with - bar-c.

EMPTINESS, sensation of, after child nurses - ***bor.***

ENLARGED, as if - calc-p., cycl., sep.

ERUPTIONS - aster., ***caust.,*** graph., grat., hep., led., lyc., psor., staph., tab., valer.
burning - ars., grat., phos., rhus-t.
scratching, after - grat.
furfuraceous, between breast - aster.
itching - kali-c., staph., tab.
heat, from - staph.
mealy - petr.
miliary - ant-t., led., staph.
painful - lyc.
to touch - hep., ph-ac.
pimples, stinging - hep.
pustules - euon., hep.
red - staph.
rubbing, from - kali-c.
squamous - kali-c., ***kreos.,*** petr.
stinging - hep.
eruptions, nipples - caust., ***graph.,*** lach., psor., rhus-t., tell.
blisters, small bluish, with fluid discharge - ***graph.***
herpes, surrounded with - **CAUST.**
mealy - ***petr.***
moist, itching - ***sulph.***
pimples - agar.
pimples itching violently, oozing a fluid - psor.
scaly - ***lyc.***
scurf, covered with - ***lyc.***
scurfy - ***lyc., petr.***
vesicles - ***graph.***
yellow scaly spots, moist when scratched - ***kali-c.***

ERYSIPELAS, of - anan., **APIS,** arn., ***bell.,*** cadm-s., ***carb-an., carb-s., carb-v., cham.,*** coll., graph., ***phos.,*** plan., ***sulph.***

EVERYTHING, affects breasts - phyt.

EXCORIATION, nipples - alumn., anan., arg-n., ***arn.,*** calc., calc-p., cast-eq., **CAUST.,** ***cham.,*** crot-t., dulc., **FL-AC.,** ***graph., ham., hell.,*** hyper., ign., ***lyc., merc., nit-ac.,*** phos., **PHYT.,** puls., rhus-t., ***sang., sep., sil., sulph.,*** zinc.
rubbing, from - con.

FISTULOUS, openings, in - ***caust., hep., merc., phos.,*** **PHYT., SIL.**
callous edges and continuous suppuration, with - phos.
discharge thin and watery, or thick and offensive - **SIL.**

FISTULOUS, openings
large, gaping and angry, discharging a watery fetid pus - ***phyt.***
openings, downward and backward - phyt.

FLABBY - bell., **CALC.,** cham., **CON., IOD.,** onos.
except during menses - calc., con.

FORMICATION, in - calc., con., mang., ran-s.
cold - guai.
left - ant-t.
nipples, in - sabin.

FULLNESS, (see Congestion, Swelling) - bell., ***bry., calc., calc-p.,*** clem., ***con.,*** cycl., ***dulc.,*** **KALI-C.,** ***lac-c.,*** lact., merc., nux-v., ***phyt.,*** sabal., sec., ***sep.,*** zinc.
menses, during - ***con.***
sensation of - carb-an., ***sep.***

GURGLING, in - crot-t.

HEAT, right, in - bell., calc.
nipples - phos.

HEAVINESS - bry., chin., iod., lac-c., phyt.

HERPES - ars., ***caust.,*** dulc., graph., ***lach.,*** petr., psor., staph.
nursing women, in - dulc.
herpes, nipples - **CAUST.**
cracks of, with - caust.

HYPERTROPHY, of - ***calc.,*** chim., ***con., phyt.***
menopause, at - sil., sulph.

INDURATION - alumn., anan., apis, ***aster.,*** bar-i., ***bell.,*** bell-p., ***bry.,*** bufo, ***calc., calc-f.,*** calc-p., **CARB-AN.,** ***carb-s.,*** carb-v., **CHAM.,** ***cist., clem.,*** coloc., **CON.,** ***crot-h., crot-t., cupr.,*** dulc., ***graph., hydr., iod., kreos., lac-c., lap-a., lyc., merc.,*** nit-ac., ***phos., phyt., plb., plb-i.,*** puls., ruta., ***sep.,*** **SIL.,** ***sulph., thuj.,*** tub., ust., vip.
abscess, after - ***con., graph.***
scars, cicatrices, in - **GRAPH.**
contusion, after - ***bell-p., con.,*** phyt.
left - con., **SIL.**
mastitis, in - ***apis,*** bry., phos.
menses, during - carb-an., con.
absent, with - dulc.
before - ***con.,*** lac-c., sang.
miscarriage, after - lac-c.
painful to touch - con.
right - ***arn.,*** **CON.,** ***phyt.,*** vip.
breast-feeding, during, burning pain - ***con.***
painfulness to touch, and nightly stitches in it, with - **CON.**
stony hard, painful - con., ***phyt.***
sore pains, with - ***merc.***
stone, hard as a, after weaning - phyt.
stony hardness - ***bry., con., phyt.***
swelling, painful, about size of a walnut - ***con.***
tender to touch, very - ***cham.***
induration, nipples - ***bry., calc., carb-an., merc., sulph.***
harder than usual - ***merc.***
nodules, uneven, in left - ***carb-an.***
painful indurations below, size of hazelnut - ***carb-an.***

induration, nipples
stony, hardness, of left - ***carb-an.***

INFLAMMATION, breasts, (see Mastitis)
inflammation, nipples - arn., ***cadm-s.,*** calc., cann-s., ***cham.,*** helon., med., ***phos.,*** phyt., pic-ac., ***sil.,*** sulph.
erysipelatous - arn.
painful, and swelling followed by pus formation - phos.
tender to touch - ***cham.,*** helon., ***phyt.***

INJURIES - ***arn., bell-p.,*** **CON.,** phyt.
contusion, from - ***bell-p.,*** **CON.**

INSENSITIVITY, nipples - sars.

INVERTED, nipples - apis., graph., nat-s., phyt., ***sars.***

ITCHING - agar., alum., anac., ang., ant-c., arn., ars., bar-c., berb., bov., calc., canth., carb-s., carb-v., cast-eq., ***caust.,*** **CON.,** dulc., hipp., jug-r., ***kali-c.,*** led., lyc., mez., nat-m., nicc., phel., ***phos.,*** plb., rhus-t., sabad., sep., spong., squil., staph., sulph.
between - ph-ac., puls.
itching, nipples - ***agar.,*** anag., ***ars.,*** arund., cast., con., ***crot-t.,*** fl-ac., form., ***graph., hep.,*** lyc., onos., orig., ***petr.,*** puls., rhus-t., sars., ***sep.,*** sil., stann., ***sulph.,*** tarent., zinc.
menses, during - hep.
pimples around - psor.
right, of - ***fl-ac.***
skin, it red scaly, burning after rubbing - con.
voluptuous - sabin.

JERKS, in - croc.
left - croc.
as if drawn backward by a string - croc.

LACTATION, (see Breast-feeding)

LANCINATING, pain - ***aster.***

LUMPS, in (see Tumors)
lumps, sensation of - ambr., cic., sulph.
between - raph.

MASTITIS, infection - ***acon.,*** anan., ant-t., ***apis,*** arn., ars., **BELL., BRY.,** bufo, ***cact.,*** calc., ***carb-an., carb-s., carb-v., card-m., cham., cist.,*** clem., ***con., crot-t.,*** cur., ferr-p., galeg., graph., **HEP., LAC-C.,** ***lach., lyc., merc., phel., phos.,*** **PHYT.,** plan., plb., ***puls.,*** rhus-t., sabad., **SIL., SULPH.,** ust., verat-v.
bruises, from - ***arn., bell-p., con.***
chronic - carc., fl-ac.
cold air, with sensibility to - ***cist.***
confinement, a few days after - phyt.
dark color - phos.
erysipelatous - **APIS,** arn., cadm-s., ***carb-v., cham.,*** plan.
confinement, during - carb-an.
heat, swelling, pain - ***bell., plan.***
heaviness - ***bry.***
left, of - ***cist.***
childbirth, after, with fever and prostration - ***crot-h.***

MASTITIS, infection
pregnancy, during, and painful - ***bell., bry.***
pus, before formation of - ***kali-m.***
begins to form - calc-s.
brownish, dirty looking, with heavy odor - kali-p.
rose-colored, radiating, stinging, tearing - ***bell.***
stitches, with - ***con.***
streaks, in, or rays, diverging from center to circumference - ***bell.***
suppressed milk - ***bry.***
suppuration, to prevent - calc-s.

MEALY coating - ***petr.***

MENSES, before agg. - bry., ***calc., con., kali-c.,*** **KALI-M., LAC-C.,** lyc., ol-an., ***phyt.,*** puls.
after, with milky secretion - cycl.

MILK, (see Breast-milk)

NIPPLES, complaints of - ***arn.,*** calen., cham., ***graph.,*** lyc., puls., rat., ***sars.,*** sil., ***sulph.***
air, from - cycl.
areola, leaden cast - ***con.***
covered with yellowish scales, oozing acrid fluid, itching and burning in night - ***sulph.***
red, as in erysipelas - cast-eq.
backward, from - crot-t., phel.
left - sulph.
dark - ***colch.***
darting, in left - ***sil.***
discharge, purulent - ***phel.***
scant, watery - phos.
dry - cast-eq.
erect - lach.
gummy secretion, drying on orifice, when picked off, nipples bleed freely - med.
hanging - cast-eq.
left - nat-s., pyrog., rumx.
left, under - asc-t., rumx.
palpitation, with - asc-t.
nursing, when - calen., crot-t.
tender to touch - ***cham.,*** helon., ***phyt.***

NODULES - aster., ***bell-p., bry., bufo,*** calc-f., calc-p., calen., **CARB-AN.,** ***carb-v.,*** cham., ***chim.,*** chin., clem., ***coloc.,*** **CON.,** crot-t., cund., dulc., foll., ***graph., iod.,*** kali-m., kreos., ***lac-c., lyc.,*** mang., ***nit-ac., phos.,*** **PHYT.,** ***puls.,*** ruta., **SIL.,** ***sulph.,*** thuj., tub.
dry black points at tip - ***iod.***
girls, puberty, before - puls.
knots, in axilla, with - merc-i-f.
left - ***arum-t., calc-p., lyc.***
menses, during - ***lac-c.***
movable, tender, moving arms, agg. - calc-i.
neonatus in - cham.
old - chim.
painful, old fat men, in - bar-c.
pregnancy, during - ***fl-ac.***
purple - ***carb-an.***
right - ***sil.***
skin, on - iod.
soft, tender - kali-m., puls.
touch, agg. - ars-i.

NUMBNESS - graph.
  numbness, nipples - sars.
NURSING, (see Breast-feeding)
PAIN, breasts - acon., all-c., ambr., apis, arg-n., ***aster.,*** aur-s., **BELL.,** ***bor.,*** brom., ***bry.,*** ***bufo,*** cact., calad., ***calc.,*** calc-p., canth., ***carb-an.,*** carb-v., ***cham.,*** ***chim.,*** chin-a., ***cimic.,*** clem., ***coloc.,*** **CON.,** cot., croc., ***crot-t.,*** cycl., ***dulc.,*** eupi., grat., ***hep.,*** hydr., hyper., ind., iod., kali-bi., kali-m., kreos., ***lac-ac.,*** **LAC-C.,** ***lap-a.,*** lepi., lil-t., lyc., med., **MERC.,** merl., mosch., ***murx.,*** nat-m., nit-ac., oci., onos., orig., pall., ped., ***phel.,*** ***ph-ac.,*** ***phos.,*** ***phyt.,*** plb., ***plb-i.,*** polyg., prun., psor., puls., rheum, ***rhus-t.,*** sabal., ***sang.,*** **SIL.,** stann., stram., ***sulph.,*** sumb., urt-u., verat., zinc.
  afternoon - sang.
  alternating sides - **LAC-C.,** puls.
    with pain in teeth - kali-c.
  chill, after - ign.
  coldness agg. - sabal.
  cough, during - con.
  descending, on - bell., calc., carb-an., ***hep.,*** ***lac-c.,*** lyc., nit-ac., phos.
  empty, soon as - ***bor.***
  evening - ***con.,*** ***lac-c.***
  extending to,
    abdomen - phel., sang.
    arms - lith.
      inner side, to fingers - aster.
      left, to fingers - aster.
    axilla - aster., brom., lac-ac.
    back - **CROT-T.,** laur., lil-t., ***phel.,*** plb., tell., til.
      drawn - croc.
      left - form.
    fingers - aster., lith.
    hand - lac-ac.
    head - lac-ac.
    outward - arg-m., clem., ol-an.
      menses, during - grat.
    shoulder, between, left - sang.
  infra mammary - ***chin.,*** puls., ***ran-b.,*** raph., sumb., ust., zinc.
    menopause, during - cimic.
  lactiferous tubes, in, when child nurses - ***phel.***
  left - aster., bor., bov., chin-a., croc., lac-c., ***lach.,*** ***lil-t.,*** ***lyc.,*** mosch., ph-ac., ***phel.,*** sil.
    below - apis, bry., cimic., phos., sulph., thlaspi, ust.
    cough during - ***con.***
    dysmenorrhea, with - caust.
    extending to, scapula - com.
    head, to - glon.
    meals, after - rumx., stroph.
    menses, during - graph.
      during and between - graph., ust.
      between - ust.
    swollen, hard - cist.
    under left, waking her at night - graph.
    right side, while child nurses on - bor.
  lying, while - bell.

PAIN, breasts
  menses, during - calc., ***con.,*** dulc., helon., indg., kali-m., lac-c., ***merc.,*** murx., ***phel.,*** ***phos.,*** ***phyt.,*** sang., syph., thuj., tub., ***tub-k.,*** zinc.
    before - **CALC.,** **CON.,** ***kali-c.,*** kali-m., **LAC-C.,** nat-m., nux-v., sang., spong., **TUB.**
    suppressed, during - zinc.
  morning - ***lil-t.***
  motion of arm - hep.
  neuralgia in left - sumb.
  nurses, while child - ant-t., bor., bry., ***crot-t.,*** lac-c., lil-t., phel., phyt., ***puls.,*** **SIL.**
    amel. - phel.
    cramps - cham.
    opposite breast, in - bor.
  pregnancy, during - calc-p., cimic., ***sep.***
    burning, during - ***calc-p.***
    inflammatory pain - ***bell.,*** ***bry.***
    neuralgic pain - ***con.,*** puls.
    nipples, under, during - ***cimic.***
    sore, during - ***calc-p.***
  presses hard, with hand - cimic., con.
  pressure agg. - plb.
  radiating, from - phyt.
  raising, arms, when - bry.
  region of - berb., chel., lac-ac., nat-s., ran-s., rhus-t.
    evening - ran-s.
    hawking, when - nat-p.
    rivet or bullet feeling - lil-t.
    sitting bent, while - rhus-t.
  right - am-c., calc., colch., grat., ***ign.,*** kali-bi., **PHEL.,** phos., sang., **SIL.,** zinc.
    below - carb-an., caust., chel., **CIMIC.,** ***graph.,*** laur., lil-t., merc-i-r., ***phos.,*** ***sulph.,*** ust.
    extending to scapula - merc.
  step, every - ***con.***
  supporting amel. - ***bry.,*** ***lac-c.,*** phyt.
  touch, on - am-c., hep.
  under - carb-v., cean., cimic., eup-per., graph., lach., lil-t., ***puls.,*** ***ran-b.,*** sumb., zinc.
    extending to fingers - aster.
      left scapula - com.
    left - ***aster.,*** cimic., com., con., lil-t., puls., ran-b., sumb., ust.
    lying on left side - phos.
    menopause, during - ***cimic.***
    right - hura, merc., phos.
  urination, agg. - clem.
  uterus, with - sil.
  wandering - ***puls.***

PAIN, nipples - arund., ***calc-p.,*** calen., cast-eq., crot-t., cur., ferr-i., ***graph.,*** ***helon.,*** ***lac-c.,*** lach., ***merc-c.,*** nux-v., rheum, sang., sulph., thuj., zinc.
    back, through to - ***crot-t.***
    child, on each application of - ***phel.***
    constant - ***lac-c.***
    evening - con., ferr-i.

PAIN, nipples
extending, outward - berb., ***bry.,*** gels., kali-bi., lappa-a., lyc., mez., ***ol-an.,*** spig., stann.
flatuence, as from - rheum.
left, on - cast-eq.
menses, after - berb., thuj.
morning - ***rhus-t.***
neuralgic - plan.
nurse, when attempting to - ***merc-c.***
nursing, while - **CROT-T.,** ***merc-c., nux-v., phyt.***
pain, all over body - **PHYT.**
through to scapula of same side - **CROT-T.**
pregnancy, during, under nipples - ***cimic.***
pulsating - zinc.
radiating over whole body - ***phyt.***
respiration, during - sulph.
scapula, to - com., ***crot-t., rhus-t.,*** tell.

PERSPIRATION - arg-m., arn., bov., calc., hep., kali-n., lyc., plb., rhus-t., sel., sep.
between, fetid - ***nux-m.***
morning - bov., cocc., graph., kali-n.
night - agar., bar-c., calc., kali-c., lyc., sil., stann., sulph.

PRESSING, pain, in - ambr., ***bell.,*** carb-s., carb-v., euph., ph-ac., sulph., zinc.
left - ph-ac.
region of - chel., nat-s.
right - phos., zinc.
under - carb-v., lach., zinc.

pressing, nipples, in - mez.
behind left - berb.
left side of sternum - bism.
menses, after - berb.
under left - verb.
right - bell., calc., led., mur-ac., stann.

PULSATION - bor.

RED, nipples - agar., ***fl-ac.,*** psor.
as in erysipelas - cast-eq.
brownish - ***colch.***
right - ***fl-ac.***

RETRACTION, nipples, of - apis, ***ars-i.,*** carb-an., con., cund., graph., hydr., lach., lap-a., ***nat-s., nux-m.,*** phyt., **SARS.,** ***sil., thuj.,*** tub.
scirrhus - cund.
cancer of left breast - ***hydr.***
drawn in like a funnel - ***sil.***
from scirrhous tumor of right breast - ***chim.***
inverted - ***apis, con.***
skin smooth and adherent, around - ***aster.***

SCARS, old, in - calen., carb-an., **GRAPH.,** ***phyt., sil.***

scars, nipples, old - calen., carb-an., **GRAPH.,** ***phyt., sil.***
suppurating - **SIL.**

SENSITIVE - calc., ***kali-c.,*** **LAC-C.,** sep.
menses, before - kali-c., lac-c.

sensitive, nipples - calen., ***cham.,*** crot-t., ***helon.,*** **LAC-C., LACH.,** med., nux-v., ***phyt.,*** sil.
left - zinc.
nursing produces intense suffering, seeming to start from nipples and radiate over whole body, going to backbone and streaking up and down it - phyt.
painful, tender, cannot bear least pressure of dress - ***helon.***
tender - ***helon.,*** lac-c., ***sil.***
excessively, cannot bear touch of clothing - **CAST-EQ.,** lac-c.
particularly during menses - ***helon.***
touch, to - ***con.,*** **CROT-T.**
inflamed - med.
pain on slightest, by child - ***colch.***

SHAKING of, during cough - cocc., guai.

SHARP, pain - aeth., alum., ambr., am-c., anan., **APIS,** arg-m., arg-n., bar-c., bell., berb., ***bor.,*** bov., brom., ***bry., calc.,*** **CARB-AN.,** cimic., clem., **CON.,** cycl., graph., grat., indg., iod., kali-bi., ***kali-c.,*** kali-i., ***kali-p.,*** kreos., lap-a., ***lach.,*** laur., ***lyc.,*** mez., murx., ***nat-m., nit-ac.,*** ol-an., olnd., ***phel., phos., phyt.,*** plat., plb., polyg., psor., ***puls.,*** rheum, sabin., sang., ***sec., sep.,*** **SIL.,** spong., stry., zinc.
between - ph-ac.
cold, becoming - sep.
cough, during - bor., con.
dysmenorrhea, with - caust.
nursing, when - calc.
extending, from left nipple downward - ***asc-t.***
to back - **PHEL.,** stry.
flow of milk, on - ***kali-c.***
inspiration, during - con., pall.
left - bor., kali-n., ***lach.,*** lil-t.
while child nurses right - bor.
menses, during - berb., con., grat.
after - ***lach.***
morning - plb., sang., zinc.
night - ***con.,*** graph.
on waking - graph.
nursing, while - ***calc.,*** **SIL.**
outward - mez., ol-an.
pressure amel. - ***con.***
region of - grat., sil.
left - grat., sil.
right - grat., **PHEL.,** sang., sep., stry.
during menses - am-m.

sharp, breasts, under - am-m., brom., canth., hyper., kali-n., kalm., lach., mag-c., murx., nat-c., ol-an., phos., ***phel.,*** plb., zinc.
afternoon - kali-c.
1 p.m., when yawning - mag-c.
2 p.m., on expiring - sil.
lifting after - kali-c.
sitting, while - mag-c.
walking amel. - carb-an.
coughing - sulph.
inspiring - bry., mag-c.

sharp, breasts, under
left - am-c., arund., berb., bry., ***caust.,*** carb-v., ***kali-c.,*** kali-n., laur., mag-c., mez., mur-ac., nat-c., nicc., phel., zinc.
extending to sternum - mag-c.
extending upward - kali-c., stann.
menses, during - caust.
rubbing amel. - caust.
menses, during - am-m., caust.
morning - plb.
morning, after rising amel. - plb.
morning, in bed - plb.
night - nit-ac.
right - aloe, bruc., cast., carb-an., chel., gamb., ***kali-bi.,*** mag-m., nicc., ***phel.,*** plb., sulph.
coughing - sulph.
extending, downward - mag-c.
extending, to back - ***kali-bi.***
extending, to scapula - plb.
extending, to shoulder - mag-c.
menses, during - am-m.
rising from a seat - phos.
sitting - carb-an.
bent - am-m.
walking - kali-n.
yawning - mag-c.

sharp, nipples - agar., am-c., ***asaf.,*** bapt., ***berb.,*** bism., ***bor.,*** calc., ***camph.,*** cann-i., cast-eq., cham., chel., cocc., coc-c., ***con.,*** ign., ***kali-bi.,*** lach., ***lyc.,*** mag-m., mang., ***mur-ac.,*** ran-b., ***rheum,*** sabin., sang., ***sil., sulph.,*** ter., verb., zinc.
below - agar., mur-ac.
inspiration, on - con., ign., par., verb.
itching - mang.
left - ***asc-t.,*** bapt., berb., form., phyt., ran-b., rhus-t., sabin., ***sil.***
extending to scapula - rhus-t.
menses, after - thuj.
morning - ran-b., rhus-t.
outward - ***asaf.***
region of - bism., bor., caust., chin., spig., verat.
ending in itching - verat.
extending to back - ***kali-i.***
extending to umbilicus - caust.
sitting erect amel. - spig.
right - ***bor.,*** chel., con., grat., mag-m., sang., zinc.
to left - card-m.
sitting, while - nat-s.
walking, while - con.

SMALLER, one breast than the other (see Atrophy, Emaciation) - iod., lach., **SABAL.**

SORE, pain - ambr., ant-c., apis, arg-n., ***arn.,*** arum-t., ***aster., bell., bry.,*** calad., ***calc., calc-p.,*** carb-an., **CHAM.,** cic., clem., ***con.,*** dulc., graph., hell., ***helon., hep., iod.,*** kali-m., **LAC-C.,** lach., lyc., ***med., merc.,*** mosch., ***murx.,*** nat-m., nit-ac., onos., phos., ***phyt.,*** plb., rad., ***ran-s., puls.,*** rhod., sabal., sang., sep., **SIL.,** symph., syph., tab., ***zinc.***
axillary glands, enlargement, with - lac-ac.
bath, cold, agg. - sabal.

SORE, pain
dysmenorrhea, with - canth., sars.
infants - cham.
menopause, at - sang.
menses, during - arum-t., bry., calc., canth., ***con.,*** dulc., graph., ***helon.,*** kali-c., ***lac-c.,*** mag-c., med., merc., ***murx., phyt., puls.,*** sang., syph., thuj., ***zinc.***
absent, with - dulc., zinc.
before - **CALC., CON.,** kali-s., ***lac-c.,*** ol-an., ***puls.,*** sang., spong., ***tub.***
beginning, at the, of - tub.
nursing, amel. - phel.
pregnancy, during - ***calc-p.***
rubbing, hard, amel. - rad.
sneezing, agg. - hydr.
stairs, going up and down - **BELL.,** calc., carb-an., ***con.,*** **LAC-C.,** lyc., ***nit-ac.,*** phos.
under - am-c., am-m., caust.
urination, agg. - clem.
yawning, agg. - mag-c.

sore, nipples - ***alum.,*** ap-g., arg-n., **ARN., BAPT.,** bor., calc., ***calc-p.,*** calen., ***cast.,*** **CAUST.,** ***cham.,*** cist., colch., ***con.,*** **CROT-T.,** dulc., ***eup-a.,*** **FL-AC.,** ***graph., ham.,*** helon., ***hep.,*** hydr., lac-c., **LACH.,** ***lyc.,*** med., ***merc.,*** mill., ***nit-ac.,*** nux-v., oci., orig., paraf., ***phel.,*** phos., ***phyt.,*** pyrog., ***rat.,*** rhus-t., sang., seneg., ***sep., sil.,*** sulo-ac., ***sulph.,*** zinc.
abraded in nursing women - ***hydr.***
blisters, with small corrosive, or ulcers oozing limpid serum or a thick glutinous fluid, which forms crust that is removed by nursing, but forms again - ***graph.***
cancer, in - ***phos.***
confinement, after - rhus-t.
constantly - lac-c.
cracked, end, exuding limpid serum - ***graph.***
excoriation - ***anan., calen.,*** **PHYT.**
mastitis, in - ***merc.***
and raw - ***merc.***
menses, during - ***helon.***
particularly during - ***helon.***
morning - sulph.
nursing, during - crot-t.
pinching, after - arn., phos.
touch of clothing - calc., **CAST-EQ.,** ***con.,*** **CROT-T., LAC-C.,** zinc.
under - sang.
weaning, after - dulc.

STINGING, pain, nipples - bism., cast-eq., ***con.,*** ign., lyc., mang., mur-ac., sabin., ***sulph.***
fine - ***camph.***

SWELLING - aeth., all-s., anan., ***apis,*** arn., ars-i., ***asaf., aster.,*** asaf., aur-s., ***bell.,*** bell-p., brom., ***bry.,*** bufo, **CALC.,** ***carb-an.,*** cast., ***cham., crot-t., clem., con., cupr.,*** cur., cycl., ***dulc., graph., helon., hep.,*** **KALI-C., LAC-C.,** ***lach.,*** lyc., lyss., ***merc.,*** merc-c., merl., naja, nat-c., oci., onos., ped., ***phos.,*** **PHYT.,** psor., **PULS.,** ***rhus-t.,*** sabin., samb., **SIL.,** sol-o., ***sulph.,*** tarent., urt-u., vip., ***zinc.***
bath, cold, agg. - sabal.
glands - calc.

SWELLING,
hot - ***bell.***, bry., ***calc.***, ***merc.***, ***phos.***
inguinal glands, with - oci.
menopause, at - sang.
menses, during - bry., calc., canth., ***cham.***, ***con.***, dulc., graph., ***helon.***, kali-c., ***lac-c.***, mag-c., merc., ***murx.***, ***phyt.***, ***puls.***, sang., thuj., ***tub.***
after - cycl.
after, with secretion of milk - cycl.
before - **CALC.**, **CON.**, ***kali-c.***, kali-s., **LAC-C.**, murx., ***tub.***
instead of - dulc., rat.
milk, secretion of, from - ***asaf.***, ***cycl.***, ***tub.***
neuralgia of uterus, with each attack of - nux-v.
nursing, during - puls.
scars, of - calen., ***graph.***, phyt., **SIL.**
sensation, as if - calc-p.
vaginal discharge, with - dulc.
weaning, after - all-s., puls.
swelling, nipples - calc., ***cham.***, ***lach.***, lyc., ***merc.***, **MERC-C.**, orig., phos., sulph.
below, on right side, size of filbert, stabbing, darting pain - eucal.
glandular, about - merc-c.
morning - fl-ac., sulph.
right - ***fl-ac.***, sulph.

TEARING, pain - ***am-c.***, am-m., bar-c., ***bry.***, bufo, carb-v., chin-a., con., crot-t., kali-c.
extending to back - colch.
to ilium - camph.
left - chin-a., ***phel.***, stry.
menses, during - calc.
milk breasts, in - kali-c.
right - camph., colch.
tearing, nipples - bism.
around left - bism.

TINGLING, in - sabin.

TUMORS - ars-i., ***aster.***, ***bell.***, **BELL-P.**, berb-a., ***brom.***, bry., calc., ***calc-f.***, calen., ***carb-an.***, cham., ***chim.***, clem., **CON.**, ***cund.***, ferr-i., gnaph., ***graph.***, hecla., ***hydr.***, ***iod.***, kali-i., kali-m., ***lach.***, lap-a., lyc., ***merc-i-f.***, murx., nit-ac., ***phos.***, **PHYT.**, ***plb-i.***, psor., ***puls.***, sabin., sang., ***scirr.***, ***scroph-n.***, sec., **SIL.**, skook., **THUJ.**, ***thyr.***, tub.
burning - ***carb-an.***
fibroid - ***phos.***, **THYR.**
hard - ***carb-an.***, ***con.***, ***phyt.***
incompressible, knobby, immovable, lancinating pains - cund.
left, in, painful - ***cund.***
nodular - sil.
right, in, grew until milk was secreted - cact.
sensitive, painful - sec.
stony, nodulated, not attached to skin, movable and as large as a filbert, lancinating pains - ***hydr.***
indurated - ***carb-an.***, ***con.***
injury, after - bell-p., con.
lancinating, deprived her of rest, especially at night - aster.
left - skook., thuj.

TUMORS,
low-spirited, night sweat - ***carb-an.***
male, like a walnut in left - calc-p.
pain extending down arms - phyt.
painful to touch - ars-i.
painless, in right - ***carb-an.***
pains drawing towards axilla - ***carb-an.***
with piercing, worse at night - ***con.***
right - ***phyt.***
scirrhous - **CON.**
of right, size of hen's egg, hard, nodulated, tender to touch, stinging pain - sep.
sensitive to touch, and painful - ***ars-i.***
skin loose - ***carb-an.***
small, painless, near nipple - ***con.***
smarting, deprived her of rest, especially at night - aster.
tumors - ***ars-i.***, chim., **CON.**, ***kali-i.***, ***lach.***, phyt.
uneven - ***carb-an.***
young married woman, in a - ***chim.***
tumors, nipples - carb-an.
left, under, large as hen's egg, moving freely under superficial fascia, and hard and painful on pressure - ***con.***
right, in, hard, large as a hen's egg - ***carb-an.***

ULCERATION, of - aster., ***calc.***, calen., clem., ***hep.***, ***merc.***, paeon., ***phos.***, **PHYT.**, **SIL.**, sulph.
right - ***com.***
ulceration, nipples - abel., ***arn.***, ars., ***aur-s.***, ***calc.***, calc-ox., calen., carb-v., ***cast.***, **CAST-EQ.**, caust., cham., ***con.***, ***crot-t.***, ***cund.***, ***eup-a.***, gali., ger., ***graph.***, ham., hep., hipp., ***merc.***, ***paeon.***, ***phel.***, phos., ***phyt.***, ***rat.***, ***sep.***, ***sil.***, sulph.

ULCERATIVE, pain - **CALC.**

ULCERS - calen., hep., phyt., sil.
granulations, bottom covered with reddish, pale, edges hard, everted, sensitive - ***aster.***
unhealthy, with fetid discharge - ***phyt.***
indurated tumors - ***oena.***
inoculated by ichorous secretion producing similar sores around nipple - ***jug-c.***
itching, with - ***hep.***
left, in, sharp stitches through to back in left - ***aster.***
schirrous, stinging, burning, odor of old cheese - **HEP.**
serpiginous - bor.
sloughing, in right - ***com.***
ulcers, nipples - ***calc.***, cham., ***merc.***, ***sil.***, sulph.
nearly ulcerated off, hanging by strings - **CAST-EQ.**

UNDEVELOPED, small - iod., lyc., nux-m., onos., sabal., sil., syph.
one, smaller than the other - lach., **SABAL.**

VESICLES - aeth.

WARTS, nipple, on - morg-g., thuj.

Breathing

ABDOMINAL - **ANT-T.**, arg-n., am-m., ***aur-m.***, bry., ***ferr.***, ***mur-ac.***, ***phos.***, ***spong.***, ***stram.***, ter., thuj.

ACCLERATED - absin., acet-ac., **ACON.**, ***acon-f.***, aesc., ***agar.***, ***ail.***, alumn., am-c., aml-n., anthr., **ANT-T.**, apis, ***apoc.***, aral., ***arg-n.***, ***arn.***, **ARS.**, ars-i., ***asaf.***, ***aspar.***, ***aur.***, bar-c., bar-m., **BELL.**, bor., ***brom.***, **BRY.**, calc., ***calc-p.***, ***camph.***, cann-i., cann-s., ***canth.***, carb-ac., carb-s., **CARB-V.**, cast., ***cedr.***, ***cham.***, **CHEL.**, ***chin.***, chin-a., ***chin-s.***, chlor., cimic., ***cina***, clem., ***coca***, cocc., ***coc-c.***, coff., ***colch.***, coloc., con., ***cop.***, crot-h., cub., **CUPR.**, cupr-ac., cur., cycl., ***dig.***, dulc., ***ferr-p.***, **GELS.**, ***glon.***, hell., ***hep.***, hippoz., hydr., hydr-ac., ***hyos.***, ***ign.***, ***iod.***, **IP.**, kali-ar., ***kali-bi.***, kali-c., ***kali-i.***, kali-n., lach., ***lact.***, laur., led., lob-p., **LYC.**, lyss., mag-p., meny., ***merc.***, merc-c., merc-cy., ***merc-sul.***, mez., ***mur-ac.***, naja, nat-a., nat-c., ***nat-m.***, nat-s., ***nux-m.***, ***nux-v.***, ***op.***, ox-ac., petr., ph-ac., **PHOS.**, ***phyt.***, ***plan.***, plb., prun., ***puls.***, rhod., ***rhus-t.***, ***samb.***, ***sang.***, sel., seneg., **SEP.**, ***sil.***, spong., squil., stann., ***stram.***, **SULPH.**, sul-ac., tab., tub., ***verat.***, ***verat-v.***, ***vesp.***, vinc., ***zinc.***
- anxiety, during - acon., ars., kali-ar., nux-v., seneg.
- ascending - lycps.
- bed, first lying down - sulph.
- coma, during - stram.
- cough, during paroxysm of - **DROS.**
- drinking, while - nat-m.
- epigastrium, from pressing, stitching in - coloc.
- evening - merc-c., petr., stann.
- exercise, during - lycps.
- headache, during - **NUX-M.**
- lying down, while - ant-t., carb-v., tarent.
- mental exertion, by - ***plan.***
- morning - **ARS-M.**, asaf.
- night - apis, spong., thuj.
- rising from sitting - agar.
- sleep, during - chel., cocc., con., merc.
  - going to - ***hydr-ac.***
  - on awaking from - ***cimic.***
- standing - nat-m.
- waking, on- cimic.

ANXIOUS - abrot., **ACON.**, aeth., alumn., ***am-c.***, ***anac.***, ant-t., ***apis***, ***arn.***, **ARS.**, aur-m., bar-c., **BAR-M.**, ***bell.***, bov., bry., bufo, calc., calc-ar., ***camph.***, cann-s., ***carb-an.***, ***cham.***, **CHEL.**, ***chlor.***, chin-s., cina, ***cocc.***, ***coff.***, colch., ***coloc.***, ***crot-c.***, ***crot-h.***, crot-t., cupr., ***dig.***, ferr., gins., hell., ***hep.***, hydr-ac., ***hyos.***, ***ign.***, **IP.**, kali-ar., kali-bi., ***kali-c.***, kreos., ***lach.***, ***laur.***, lob., mang., mez., **NAT-M.**, nit-ac., nux-v., olnd., ***op.***, ph-ac., **PHOS.**, ***plat.***, plb., **PRUN.**, ***psor.***, **PULS.**, ran-b., ***rhus-t.***, sabad., ***samb.***, sars., **SEC.**, spig., **SPONG.**, **SQUIL.**, **STANN.**, staph., ***stram.***, tab., ter., thuj., valer., verat., viol-o., vip., zinc.
- afternoon - bell.
- evening - bar-c., mez., ***phos.***, stann.
  - after formication - cist.

ANXIOUS, breathing
- exertion, physical amel. - nat-m.
- headache, during - **NUX-M.**
- lying, while - apis, ***puls.***
  - on the back - aeth.
- mental exertion - phos.
- morning - ***phos.***
  - in bed - nat-c.
- oppression heart, with - bell.
- pulsating in epigastrium, from - chel.

ARRESTED, (see Breathing, Stopped)

ASPHYXIA, (see Emergency, Asphyxia)

ASTHMATIC, breathing (see Lungs, Asthma)

BREATH, cold - acon., ant-t., ars., **CAMPH.**, carb-o., **CARB-V.**, ***cedr.***, ***chin.***, chin-s., cist., colch., ***cop.***, cor-r., ***helo.***, jatr., merc., ***phos.***, rhus-t., ***tab.***, ter., **VERAT.**
- chill, during - **CARB-V.**, verat.

breath, hot - **ACON.**, aeth., agar., anac., ***ant-c.***, apis, ***ars.***, asaf., asar., ***bell.***, calc., calc-p., cann-s., **CARB-S.**, ***cham.***, chel., coc-c., coff., ***ferr.***, kali-br., mag-m., ***mang.***, med., merl., mez., naja, ***nat-m.***, ***phos.***, ptel., raph., ***rhus-t.***, ***rhus-v.***, ***sabad.***, squil., ***stront-c.***, ***sulph.***, sumb., trif-p., zinc.
- afternoon - ***bad.***, ***rhus-t.***
- as if - rad-br.
- chill, during - anac., camph., cham., **RHUS-T.**
- cold limbs, with - cham.
- coryza, during - mag-m.
- evening - mang., sumb.
- fever, during - zinc.
- morning, on waking - sulph.

CATCHING - ***arg-n.***, ***brom.***, calad., ***calc.***, carb-ac., ***caust.***, cina, gels., kreos., led., lil-t., merc-c., nit-ac., ***phos.***, sant., **SIL.**, stry., sulph.
- bending, on - ***calc.***
- cough - bry., ***cina.***
  - after - arn., ***ars.***, bry., hep., ***nat-m.***, ***puls.***
- dancing, after - ***spong.***
- fever, during - **SIL.**
- menses, before - bor.
- morning - sars.
- night - **SIL.**
- sharp, in abdomen to back - ***calc.***
  - in hemorrhoids - **SULPH.**
- sleep, during - lyc.
- working - sars.

CEASED, breathing (see Arrested)

CHEYNE strokes (see Irregular) - acon., ***acon-f.***, am-c., ang., antipyrin., atro., bell., ***camph.***, cann-i., ***carb-v.***, chlol., coca, cocaine, crot-h., ***cupr.***, cupr-ar., ***dig.***, ***grin.***, ***hydr-ac.***, ***ign.***, iod., ip., kali-cy., lach., ***laur.***, led., lob., nux-v., olnd., ***op.***, ***morph.***, parth., ***saroth.***, spong., sul-ac., sulph., vanad., verat.

CROAKING - cham., lach.

CYANOSIS - absin., acetan., acon., agar., alum., ***am-c.,*** amyg., ang., anil., ant-c., ***ant-a., ant-t., arg-n.,*** arn., ***ars.,*** asaf., asar., aur., bar-c., ***bell.,*** bism., both., benz-n., ***bor.,*** bry., calc., calc-p., **CAMPH.,** canth., carb-an., carb-o., **CARB-V.,** caust., cedr., cham., chel., chin., chin-a., cic., cina, cocc., cod., ***con., crot-h.,*** **CUPR.,** cupr-ar., **DIG.,** dros., ferr., glon., hep., ***hydr-ac.,*** hyos., ign., iod., ***ip., kali-chl.,*** kali-n., **LACH., LAUR.,** led., lyc., lycps., mang., merc., merc-c., merc-cy., meth-ae-ae., mez., mosch., mur-ac., ***naja,*** nat-m., nat-n., nit-ac., nux-m., nux-v., **OP.,** ox-ac., petr., ph-ac., phenac., phos., phyt., piloc., plb., puls., psor., ran-b., ***rhus-t.,*** ruta, sabad., ***samb.,*** sant., sars., ***sec.,*** seneg., sil., spong., staph., stram., stry., sulfon., sulph., sul-ac., tab., thuj., **VERAT., VERAT-V.,** vip., xan., zinc., zinc-m.
- fever, during - arund., crot-h.
- infants, in - arn., ars., ***bor., cact., camph., carb-v.,*** chin., **DIG., LACH., LAUR.,** ***naja,*** op., ***phos.,*** psor., rhus-t., sec., sulph.

DEEP, breathing - ***acon., agar., ail.,*** am-m., ant-c., ant-t., **ARG-N.,** arn., ars., **AUR.,** bar-c., bar-m., bell., bor., bov., ***brom.,*** **BRY.,** ***cact., calc.,*** calc-p., ***camph.,*** cann-s., **CAPS.,** carb-v., ***cast., caust.,*** cham., chel., chin., chin-a., chlor., cic., cimx., colch., croc., ***cupr., dig.,*** dros., euon., ***euph.,*** fl-ac., gamb., glon., hell., **HEP.,** ***hydr-ac.,*** hyos., ictod., **IGN.,** ***ind.,*** **IP.,** kali-ar., kali-c., kreos., **LACH.,** lachn., lact., laur., lob., ***lyc.,*** mag-c., merc., mez., ***mur-ac.,*** nat-a., nat-c., nat-m., **NAT-S.,** nicc., nux-v., olnd., **OP.,** ox-ac., par., **PHOS.,** ***plat.,*** podo., prun., ***ran-b.,*** ran-s., ***rhus-t.,*** sars., ***sec.,*** **SEL., SIL.,** spig., spong., squil., stann., ***stram.,*** stry., ***sulph.,*** sul-ac., tab., ther., thuj., ***zinc.***
- agg. - **ACON.,** ***agn.,*** am-m., arg-m., ***arn.,*** asaf., asc-t., ***bell., bor.,*** brom., **BRY.,** calad., calc., ***canth.,*** caps., carb-an., caust., cina, dros., dulc., fl-ac., ***graph., hell.,*** hep., hist., hyos., ign., ip., ***kali-c., kali-n.,*** kreos., lach., lyc., merc., ***phos.,*** ran-b., rhus-t., ***rumx.,*** sabad., sang., spig., squil., sulph.
- abdomen, from - alumn., cann-s.
- ameliorates - acon., asaf., bar-c., ***cann-i.,*** chin., ***colch., cupr.,*** dig., dros., ***ign.,*** iod., ***lach.,*** meny., olnd., osm., puls., rhus-t., ***seneg.,*** sep., ***spig.,*** **STANN.,** staph., viol-t., ter.
- chill, during - cimx.
- desire to breathe - acet-ac., acon., adon., agar., alum., alumn., am-br., arg-n., ***aur.,*** bapt., ***bor.,*** brom., **BRY., CACT., CALC.,** ***calc-p., caps., carb-ac., carb-v.,*** **CARC.,** ***card-m., caust.,*** cedr., ***chin.,*** cimx., coca, cocc., croc., ***crot-t., dig.,*** euon., eup-per., ***glon.,*** hep., hydr., ***hydr-ac.,*** ictod., **IGN.,** ***ind., kali-c., kreos.,*** **LACH.,** ***lact.,*** lil-t., ***lyc.,*** mag-aust., med., ***merc.,*** mez., mosch., **NAT-S.,** nux-m., op., ***par., phos.,*** plan., podo., prun., ran-b., samb., ***sang.,*** **SEL.,** ***seneg.,*** sep., squil., stann., stram., **SULPH.,** ther., tub., verb., xan.

DEEP, breathing
- desire to breathe
  - chill, during - cimx.
  - dinner, after - hep.
  - enough, cannot get - aur., ***carb-v.,*** crot-t., lach., prun., rad-br.
  - lying, while - ***ind.***
  - oppression in the stomach - nat-m.
- dinner, before - chin., rhus-t.
- eating, after - ant-c., rhus-t., sars.
- evening - eupi., ***ran-b.***
- heat, with - ph-ac.
- heart, from heaviness at - croc.
- impossible - alumn., ambr., ant-c., **ARS.,** ***aur.,*** bry., calc-p., ***cocc., crot-t.,*** dig., euph., euphr., ferr., kali-n., ***lob.,*** morph., plat., sep., sil., stann., sulph.
- lying down, while - ***ind.***
  - back, on, amel - ind.
  - left side agg - ind.
- menses, before - sulph.
- midnight, on waking - cann-i.
- oppression, in epigastrium, from - bell.
- running, after - ***hep.***
- sitting, while - cic., lach.
- sleep, during - ign.
- slow, wheezing - sep.
- walking, while - bell.
- writing, while - fl-ac.

DIFFICULT, breathing - abies-n., abrot., absin., acet-ac., ***acon., acon-f.,*** adren., ***aesc., aeth., agar., agn.,*** ail., ***all-c.,*** all-s., aloe, alum., alumn., ***ambr., am-c.,*** am-m., aml-n., **ANAC.,** ***ant-a., ant-c.,*** **ANT-T., APIS,** apoc., ***aral.,*** arg-m., ***arg-n., arn.,*** **ARS.,** ***ars-i.,*** arum-t., arund., ***asaf., asar., asc-t.,*** aspar., astac., ***aur.,*** aur-m., aur-m-n., aur-s., ***bac., bad.,*** bar-c., ***bar-m., bell., benz-ac.,*** bism., ***blatta,*** bor., ***bov., brom.,*** **BRY.,** bufo, **CACT.,** cahin., caj., calad., ***calc., calc-ar., calc-f., calc-p., calc-s., camph.,*** cann-i., cann-s., canth., ***caps.,*** carb-ac., carb-an., ***carb-o., carb-s.,*** **CARB-V.,** ***carl.,*** cast., **CAUST.,** ***cedr., cench., cham.,*** **CHEL.,** chen-a., **CHIN.,** ***chin-a., chin-s.,*** **CHLOR.,** chlol., ***cic.,*** cimic., ***cimx.,*** **CINA,** cist., ***cocc., coc-c., coca,*** coff., ***colch.,*** coll., ***coloc., con., conv.,*** cop., cor-r., crat., croc., ***crot-c., crot-h.,*** **CROT-T.,** ***cub.,*** **CUPR.,** ***cupr-ac.,*** **CUPR-AR.,** cupr-s., cur., ***cycl., dig.,*** dios., dirc., ***dros., dulc.,*** equis., ery-a., eup-per., euph., euphr., **FERR.,** ***ferr-ar., ferr-i., ferr-p., fl-ac., formal., gels.,*** gins., ***glon., graph., grin., guai.,*** ham., ***hell.,*** **HEP.,** hippoz., hura, hydr-ac., hydrc., hydr., hyos., hyper., ictod., ***ign.,*** indg., ***iod.,*** **IP.,** ***iris,*** jab., jatr., jug-c., ***just.,*** **KALI-AR.,** ***kali-bi.,*** **KALI-C.,** ***kali-chl.,*** **KALI-I.,** kali-m., kali-n., ***kali-p., kali-s., kalm.,*** kreos., lac-c., **LACH.,** ***lact., lat-m., laur.,*** led., ***lil-t., lith.,*** **LOB., LYC.,** ***lycps., lyss.,*** mag-c., mag-m., mag-s., manc., mang., ***med.,*** meli., meny., **MEPH.,** ***merc.,*** **MERC-C.,** merc-cy., merc-p-r., ***merc-sul.,*** merl., ***mez.,*** morph., ***mosch., mur-ac.,*** murx., mygal., **NAJA,** ***naphtin.,*** nat-a., ***nat-c., nat-m., nat-p.,*** **NAT-S.,** nicc., ***nit-ac.,*** **NUX-M.,** ***nux-v.,*** oena., ol-j., **OP.,** osm., ***ox-ac.,*** par., ped., petr., phel., ***ph-ac.,*** **PHOS.,** ***phys., phyt., plat., plb.,*** podo.,

DIFFICULT, breathing - ***prun., psor.,*** ptel., **PULS.,** queb., ***ran-b.,*** ran-s., raph., rat., rheum, rhod., ***rhus-t.,*** rumx., ruta., sabad., sabin., ***samb., sang.,*** sarr., sars., ***sec.,*** **SEL.,** senec., ***seneg., sep.,*** ser-ang., **SIL.,** ***spig.,*** **SPONG., SQUIL., STANN.,** staph., ***stram., stroph.,*** **STRY., SULPH.,** sul-ac., ***sumb., tab.,*** **TARENT.,** tax., ***ter.,*** thuj., tril., ***tub.,*** upa., valer., **VERAT.,** verat-v., viol-o., vesp., vib., ***visc.,*** xan., ***zinc.,*** zing.

abdomen, from distension and tension in - caps., caust., iod., mag-m., mez.

afternoon - act-sp., all-s., alumn., ***ars.,*** aur., bapt., bell., cahin., calc., carb-v., chel., dig., elaps, ***fl-ac., lach.,*** lyc., ***merc-sul.,*** nat-m., op., ped., phos., puls., sabad., ***samb., sang.,*** sep., ***sulph.,*** tril.

1 p.m - cact., squil.

2 p.m - chel.

3 p.m. when running - am-c., lyc.

3:30 p.m. while sitting - mag-c.

4 p.m - phos.

5 p.m., sudden - ign.

5 to 7 p.m - nat-m.

6 p.m - bapt.

6 to 9 p.m - cast.

6:30 p.m - chel.

air, amel - ***am-c., arg-n.,*** bell., ***bry., carb-s., carb-v.,*** cham., cist., lac-c., ***op., puls.,*** ust.

cold, in - apis, ***ars.,*** aur., graph., **LOB.,** ***lyc., merc.,*** nux-v., petr., puls., sel., seneg., ***spong.,*** sulph.

humid, agg. - aur., bar-c., ***nat-s.***

air, in open - ***bor.,*** caust., crot-c., phys., plat., **PSOR.,** rhus-t., sel., seneg., sulph.

amel - alum., ***am-c.,*** ant-t., **APIS,** arg-n., ars-i., bapt., bell., ***bry., cact.,*** calc., chel., ***chin-a.,*** cist., dig., fl-ac., ***gels., ip., kali-i., kali-s., lach.,*** lil-t., **NAT-M.,** nux-v., **PULS.,** stram., **SULPH.,** ***tub.***

alternating, with,

cough - ant-t.

pain in hypochondria - ***zinc.***

rattling - hyos..

sopor - plb.

urticaria - ***calad.***

uterine hemorrhage - fl-ac.

anger, after - arn., ars., **CHAM., IGN.,** ran-b., ***rhus-t., staph.***

children, in - arn., cham., ign.

anxiety, palpitation, with, waking after midnight - **SPONG.**

arms apart, amel. - lach., laur., nux-v., psor., spig., tarent.

ascending - acet-ac., agn., aloe, ***am-c.,*** ang., ***apis, arg-n.,*** **ARS.,** ***ars-i.,*** arund., aspar., aur., ***aur-m.,*** bar-c., berb., ***bor., brom.,*** bufo, ***cact.,*** **CALC., CALC-AR.,** calc-s., cann-i., canth., ***caps., carb-ac.,*** carb-s., carl., cast., cist., ***clem.,*** **COCA,** crot-t., cupr., dirc., ***elaps,*** graph., grat., hyos., ***iod.,*** **IP.,** kali-n., ***kali-p.,*** led., lil-t., ***lob., lyc., lycps.,*** **MERC.,** nat-a., **NAT-M.,** ***nat-s.,*** **NIT-AC.,** nux-v., ol-an., petr., ***pic-ac., plb.,*** puls., ran-b., rat., ***rhus-t.,*** ***ruta., sars., seneg.,*** sep., **SIL.,** spig., ***spong.,***

ascending - squil., ***stann.,*** sulph., tab., ther., thuj., til., zinc.

alcoholics - coca.

autumn - chin.

beer, after - cocc.

belching, amel. - am-m., ambr., ant-t., ***aur.,*** **CARB-V.,** cast., mosch., ***nux-v.***

bending, arm backwards, on - **SULPH.**

backward - apis, cupr., psor.

amel - cupr., fl-ac.

forward - apis, seneg., ***spig.***

amel - ars., cench., coc-c., colch., kali-bi., kali-c., lach., spong.

head backwards - bell., cham.

must rise up and bend head backwards - hep.

amel. - hep., lach., ***spong.,*** verat.

shoulders backwards, amel. - calc-ac.

breath, on taking a deep - phos.

as if the next would be the last - apis

breathing, deep amel. - sulph.

change, of weather - chel., ip.

children - ***ambr.,*** ars., calc., calc-p., lyc., **NAT-S.,** phos., ***puls.,*** samb., ***sil., tub.***

lifted, on being - bor., calc-p.

chill, during - **APIS,** ars., bry., cimx., gels., gins., guare., kali-c., mez., ***nat-m.,*** nux-m., nux-v., puls., sep., seneg., ***thuj.,*** zinc.

closing, eyes, on - carb-an., ***carb-v.***

clothing agg. - ars., chel., lach.

tight around waist agg. - nux-v.

coffee, from - ***bell., cham.,*** dig.

cold, after taking - dulc., ip., ***kali-i.,*** puls.

water, after drinking amel - cham.

ice water, agg. - meph.

when heated, after - ***kali-c.***

weather - apis, arg-n.

wet weather - ars., ***dulc., mang.,*** nat-s., ***sil.***

colic agg. - arg-n., berb.

constriction, of, larynx - **APIS,** bell., cocc., **CROT-H.,** hell., **LACH.,** sars., spong.

stomach, region of - guai.

trachea - petr.

convulsions, during - con., ***lyss., op.,*** stry., sulph., tanac.

after - sulph.

tetanic - mill.

coryza, with - ars., ars-i., calc., ip., mang., nat-m., nit-ac., phos., sulph.

cough, with - acon., all-s., **ALUM.,** am-c., am-m., anac., **ANT-T.,** aral., arn., **ARS.,** ***ars-i.,*** aspar., bar-c., bar-m., ***bell.,*** brom., bry., calad., calc., calc-p., calc-s., carb-an., ***carb-v., caust.,*** chin., chin-a., ***cina,*** coc-c., con., cor-r., **CUPR.,** dig., dol., **DROS.,** eup-per., euphr., ***ferr.,*** ferr-ar., ferr-p., guai., ***hep.,*** hydr-ac., ign., **IP.,** just., kali-ar., ***kali-bi.,*** kali-c., kali-n., ***kali-s., kreos.,*** lac-c., ***lach.,*** lachn., lact., laur., led., lob., ***lyc.,*** merc., merc-cy., mez., mur-ac., naja, nat-m., ***nat-s.,*** nicc., nit-ac., ***nux-m.,*** **NUX-V., OP.,** phel., **PHOS.,** rhus-t.,

DIFFICULT, breathing

cough, with - samb., ***sep., sil.,*** spig., spong., squil., **STANN.,** sulph., sul-ac., tarent., tub., viol-o., zinc., zing.
before - ant-t., caust., lyc.
drinking, or, with - anac.
covering, nose or mouth - ***arg-n.,*** cupr., ***lach.***
crowded, room - ***arg-m.***
dark, in the - aeth.
daytime - ***chel.***
deep breathing, agg. - thuj.
amel. - caps., sulph.
dinner, during - mag-m.
after - ***chel.,*** nat-m., ***nux-v., puls.,*** sars.
diseased, conditions of distant parts not involved in act of breathing - puls.
drawing shoulders back amel. - calc., calc-ac.
dreams, during - sang., zinc.
after frightful - ***chel.***
dressing, while - ***stann.***
drinking, when - anac., ***arg-n.,*** bell., ***cimx., kali-c.,*** kali-n., meph., nat-m., plb., thuj.
after - nux-v., thuj.
dropsy, in - eup-pur.
dust, as from - ars., ars-i., aur-m., bell., ***brom., calc.,*** cycl., dulc., ***hep., ictod.,*** ip., nat-a., nux-v., phos., **SIL.,** sulph.
eating, while - mag-m.
after - ***anac.,*** ant-a., ant-c., apoc., ars., ***asaf.,*** asc-t., ***aur.,*** calc., calad., carb-an., ***carb-v.,*** cham., chel., chin., dig., kali-p., **LACH.,** ***mag-m.,*** merc., nat-m., nat-s., ***nux-m., nux-v.,*** **PHOS., PULS.,** ran-b., rhus-t., sanic., sang., sars., ***sulph.,*** syph., viol-t., ***zinc.,*** zinc-valer.
amel - ambr., cedr., ***graph.,*** iod., med., ***spong.***
edema, pulmonary - **AM-C., ANT-T.,** ***carb-s., ferr-i.***
elderly, people - ant-t., ***bar-c., calc.,*** carb-v., ***chin.,*** seneg., ***sil., stann.***
emission, after - ***phos.,*** **STAPH.**
emphysema, in - am-c., ant-t., sars., sil.
epigastrium, from oppression in - ***ars.,*** chin., cocc., guai., lach., nat-m., ***phos.,*** rhus-t., sulph.
epilepsy, before - am-br.
eruptive, diseases, with - ***apis.***
evening - acon., aeth., agn., anac., ant-t., ***all-c., ars.,*** bell., ***calc-p.,*** calc-s., carb-an., ***carb-s., carb-v., chin.,*** chin-a., cist., clem., coloc., con., cycl., dig., elaps, ***ferr.,*** ferr-ar., ferr-p., ***fl-ac.,*** graph., ***hell.,*** hyper., ip., ***kali-ar., kali-c.,*** kali-s., ***lach., lob.,*** mag-c., merc., mez., nat-m., nux-m., ***nux-v.,*** ox-ac., petr., ***phos., psor., puls., ran-b.,*** raph., rhod., ***rhus-t.,*** sep., ***stann.,*** **SULPH.,** verb., ***zinc.***
6 p.m - mag-c., **RHUS-T.**
9 p.m - bry.
amel - lyc.

DIFFICULT, breathing

evening, bed, in - am-c., ant-t., ***ars.,*** bor., carb-an., ***carb-v.,*** chin., ***cist.,*** con., crot-h., ***ferr., graph.,*** merc., nat-m., ***nat-s.,*** par., ***phos.,*** podo., ***sep., sulph.,*** sul-ac., zinc.
amel - ***chel.***
excitement, agg. - ambr., ars., ***coc-c.,*** ferr., ***puls., sep.***
exertion, after - am-c., am-m., ***apis, arg-n.,*** arn., **ARS.,** ***ars-i.,*** asaf., ***aur-m.,*** benz-ac., bor., bov., brom., **CALC.,** ***camph.,*** carb-s., ***carb-v.,*** cimic., ***cench.,*** **COCA,** con., dirc., ***dig., ferr-m., iod.,*** **IP.,** ***kali-ar., kali-c., kali-i.,*** **LACH.,** ***laur., led.,*** **LOB., LYC., LYCPS.,** ***merc.,*** **NAT-M.,** ***nat-s., nit-ac., nux-m., nux-v.,*** ox-ac., ph-ac., ***phos., puls.,*** rat., sars., sep., **SIL.,** ***spig.,*** **SPONG.,** squil., ***stann., staph., sulph.,*** sumb., ter., tub., ***verat.***
athletics - arn., carb-v., coca.
hands and arms, with - am-m., berb., bov., **LACH.,** ***nat-m., nit-ac., sil.,*** spig., tarent.
least, after - calc., con., kali-c., nat-s., sil.
expectoration, amel. - ail., **ANT-T.,** aral., aur., ***grin.,*** guai., hyper., ip., lach., manc., nit-ac., ***sep., zinc.***
checked, after - ***sep.***
expiration - am-c., ***arg-m.,*** ars., ***caust.,*** chin., **CHLOR.,** dros., ***ip.,*** kali-i., ***med., meph.,*** puls., **SAMB.,** seneg., sep.
cough, during - meph.
falling down due to - petr.
fanned, wants to be - ant-t., apis, ars., bapt., cann-i., **CARB-V.,** chin., chlor., ***ferr.,*** kali-n., lach., ***med.,*** naja, ***puls.,*** sec., sulph., zinc.
wants to be, slowly and distant - lach.
flatulence, from - arg-n., **CARB-V.,** cast., cham., ***lyc., nat-s.,*** nux-v., ol-an., osm., puls., sang., ***zinc.***
forenoon - alum., bry., chin-a., hyper., ***ip.,*** nat-c., ***nat-s.,*** ox-ac., sulph.
8 a.m - dios.
9 a.m - chel., chin., nat-a., tarent., valer.
after breakfast - valer.
10 a.m - ***ferr.,*** iod.
11 a.m - agar., squil.
standing, while - kali-n.
walking - cocc.
in open air - ferr.
writing, while - mag-s.
foreign bodies, from - ant-t., sil.
fright, after - ***cupr., samb.***
formication, preceded by - cist.
gasping, with - acon., apis, ***carb-v.,*** cor-r., hydr-ac., ign., kali-n., lat-m., laur., lob., lyc., meph.
bleeding, with - ip.
chorea, with - laur.
spasms, before during or after - caust., laur.
gastric origin, from - ars., carb-v., ip., lob., nux-v., zing.

DIFFICULT, breathing

handkerchief, cannot bear to have, approach the mouth as it will cause dyspnea - am-c., ***arg-n.,*** cupr., ***lach.***

hands, on using - bov.

hang down, legs, amel. - ***sul-ac.***

headache, with - sep.

heart, pain, during - ***arg-n., aur., cact.,*** carb-v., cimic., cinnb., ***kalm., psor.,*** sep., ***spig., spong.,*** stroph., sumb., ***tarent.,*** vip.

heart, problems, with - acon., ***acon-f.,*** adon., ***adren.,*** am-c., apis, arn., ars., ars-i., aur., ***cact., calc-ar.,*** carb-v., ***chin-a.,*** cimic., coll., conv., crat., ***dig., glon., iber.,*** kali-n., kalm., lach., laur., lycps., magn-gr., naja, op., ox-ac., ***queb.,*** spig., spong., stroph., stry-ar., sumb., visc.

and ovarian troubles - **TARENT.**

and urinary troubles - **LAUR.,** ***lycps.***

hydropericardium - ant-a., apis, apoc., ars., iod., lach.

heartburn, from - carb-v., lyc.

heat, with - anac., **APIS,** arn., ars., ***cact.,*** carb-v., chel., cimx., cina, cinnb., con., **KALI-C.,** ***lach.,*** lyc., nat-m., phos., **PULS.,** ***sep., sil., tub.,*** zinc.

heated, when overheated - **APIS,** kali-c., ***puls.***

after - sil.

heavy - glon., verat-v.

hemoptysis, with - arn.

hiccough, with - aeth.

holding to something amel. - graph.

humiliation, after - puls.

hurried, if - caust.

hysterical - ***arg-n.,*** ars., asaf., ***ign.,*** gels., ***lob.,*** mosch., nux-m., valer.

injury, from - petr.

inspiration - ***acon., arg-n.,*** arn., ***ars., brom.,*** cact., calad., ***calc.,*** camph., **CAUST.,** chel., chin., chlor., con., euphr., ***ferr.,*** hep., ***ign., iod.,*** kali-c., meph., ***nux-m., ox-ac., phos.,*** **SAMB.,** staph., zinc.

agg. - crot-h., ip., kali-n., lob., mez., nux-m., spong., sumb.

amel. - ***colch.,*** cupr., ***ign.,*** lach., ***spig.,*** stann., verb.

cold air, amel. - sel.

expiration, hot - sulph.

did not reach the pit of stomach - prun.

double - led.

nose, through, expiration through mouth, while lying on back - chlol.

rapid expiration - chin., ign., ***kali-c.,*** meph., ***nux-m.,*** nux-v., ***sang.***

slow, expiration quick - stram.

itching, with - sabad.

knocked down, when - petr.

kyphosis, in - acon., ant-c., asaf., aur., bar-c., bell., bry., calc., camph., cic., clem., coloc., dulc., hep., ip., rhus-t., ruta, sabin., sep., sil., staph., sulph., thuj.

labor pain, with every - **LOB.**

DIFFICULT, breathing

laughing - ars., aur., ***bry.,*** cupr., lach., lyc., plb.

lips, with redness of - spig.

liver, from stitches in - acon., con.

lung, cannot expand the - ***crot-t.***

from heaviness in left - ferr.

lower, lung - lob-s., nux-v.

lying, while - abies-n., acon., acet-ac., act-sp., ***ant-a., ant-t.,*** **APIS,** apoc., aral., **ARS.,** ***ars-i.,*** asaf., ***aur., bapt.,*** bar-m., bor., brom., bufo, cact., cahin., calc., calc-s., ***cann-s.,*** carb-ac., ***carb-s.,*** **CARB-V.,** cast., caust., cedr., cench., cham., ***chin.,*** chin-a., cist., con., ***crot-t., dig.,*** euph., ***ferr., ferr-ar.,*** ferr-p., ***fl-ac.,*** **GRAPH.,** grin., ***ham.,*** hell., ***hep., kali-ar., kali-bi.,*** **KALI-C.,** ***kali-n.,*** kali-s., lac-c., lach., lact., ***lyc.,*** **LOB.,** ***meph., merc.,*** merc-sul., ***naja,*** nat-m., nux-v., olnd., phel., ***phos., plb.,*** podo., ***puls.,*** rumx., ***samb.,*** sang., sars., ***seneg.,*** sel., ***sep., sil., spig., spong., sulph.,*** syph., ***tarent.,*** tarax., ter., **TUB.,** zinc., zing.

amel - bry., ***calc-p., chel., dig.,*** euphr., ***hell.,*** kali-bi., kali-c., lach., ***laur.,*** nat-s., ***nux-v.,*** **PSOR.,** sabad., ter.

enlargement of the tonsils, from - bar-c.

back, on the - acet-ac., aeth., alum., ***ars., aur.,*** cast., ***hyper., iod.,*** **LYC.,** med., nat-m., ol-an., ***phos.,*** ptel., ***puls., sil., spig., sulph.***

amel - **CACT.,** dig., ind., kali-i., ***kalm.,*** nux-v.

arms outstretched amel - ***psor.***

with shoulders elevated amel - **CACT.**

down - nat-m.

face, on, amel., with protruding tongue - med.

head low, with the - **APIS, CACT.,** ***carb-v., chin.,*** colch., cop., eup-per., ***hep.,*** **KALI-C.,** kali-n., puls., rumx., ***spig., spong.***

impossible - acon., ***ant-t.,*** **APIS,** ***apoc.,*** **ARS.,** ***aur.,*** bar-m., bor., brom., bufo, ***cact.,*** cann-s., chin., ***crot-t., hep., kali-c., lac-c., lach., lyc., merc., nux-v., puls., seneg., sep.,*** stann., staph., ***sulph., tab., ter., tub.***

knees, on and elbows amel - med.

left side - absin., ***apis,*** cann-i., ***hydr.,*** ind., ***kali-c.,*** med., merc., naja, ***phos.,*** plb., ***puls., spig., tarent.,*** visc.

amel. - cast.

right side - cast., scroph-n., squil., visc.

amel. - ant-t., naja, ***spig.***

amel., head high, with - cact., spig., spong.

going to sleep - bad.

side, on - ars., carb-an., ***puls.***

amel. - alum., lyss., sang.

manual, labour - am-m., ***bov., lach., nat-m., nit-ac., sil.***

measles, from suppressed - **CHAM., PULS.,** ***zinc.***

menorrhagia, from being suppressed - fl-ac.

DIFFICULT, breathing
menses, during - cact., ***calc.,*** chin., cocc., ***coloc.,*** graph., ign., ***iod.,*** ip., kali-c., ***lach.,*** laur., lyc., plat., puls., sep., **SPONG.,** sulph., zinc.
after - am-c., ferr., ***nat-m., puls.***
before - brom., bor., ***cupr., nat-s., sulph.,*** **ZINC.**
suppressed with - **PULS.,** spong.
mental, exertion - ferr., phos., sep.
metrorrhagia, with - fl-ac.
midnight - ***acon.,*** **ARS.,** calc., ***chin.,*** ferr., puls., ***rhus-t.,*** samb.
morning - ambr., ant-t., aur., bell., ***brom.,*** carb-an., carb-v., ***caust.,*** chel., ***con., dig., kali-bi., kali-c.,*** kali-chl., kali-i., ***lach.,*** lyc., mang., merc., nit-ac., ***nux-v., phos.,*** puls., rhod., ***sang., sep., sil.,*** sulph.
bed, in - alum., ant-t., carb-an., com., con., led., mag-s., nux-v., puls., sulph.
breakfast, amel. - sulph.
chest, from anxiety in - puls.
exertion, from - lyc.
expectoration amel - ***sep.***
rising, on - calc-p., ***kali-bi.***
after - bell., carb-v., caust., dig., ran-b.
amel - con., led., puls., sulph.
standing, while - con.
waking, on - con., kali-i., nit-ac., seneg., ***sep.,*** sil.
motion - ***apis, arg-n.,*** arn., ***ars.,*** ars-i., aspar., bapt., **BRY.,** calc., cann-s., caps., ***carb-v., con.,*** ferr., ferr-i., graph., iod., ip., kali-ar., ***kali-c., kali-i., led., lob., lyc.,*** merc., ***nat-s.,*** nux-v., ox-ac., ***phos.,*** plb., puls., rhod., rhus-t., sabad., ***sep., spig.,*** **SPONG., STANN.,** sulph., ***tarent., verat.***
amel. - arg-n., ***aur.,*** bell., brom., calc., coff., **FERR.,** lob., nat-m., phos., puls., rhus-t., samb., seneg., sep., sil., sulph., vib.
arms, of - ***am-m.,*** **LACH.,** nat-m., ***nit-ac., sil.,*** spig., sulph.
quick agg. - merc.
slow motion agg - ***sep.***
mountains, in (see Emergency, Altitude sickness) - calc., carb-v., coca, mag-m., sil.
mucus, in the trachea, from - alum., ammc., **ANT-T., ARS.,** asar., aur., bov., ***cact.,*** camph., cina, **HIPPOZ.,** ***ip.,*** sel., thuj., verat.
bronchials, in - nat-m.
nausea, with - ip., kali-n., lob.
nervous causes, from - ambr., ***arg-n., ars., caj.,*** carb-an., **IGN.,** lob., ***mosch.,*** nux-m., puls., ***valer.,*** viol-o.
night, during - acon., alum., am-c., am-m., ***ant-t.,*** apis, arg-n., **ARS.,** ars-i., asar., aspar., ***aur.,*** aur-m., aur-s., bar-c., berb., bell., brom., bry., bufo, cact., ***calc.,*** calc-s., cann-i., carb-ac., carb-an., **CARB-S.,** ***carb-v.,*** cast., ***cench.,*** cham., chel., ***chin.,*** chin-a., ***coca, colch.,*** coloc., con., ***crot-t.,*** cupr., daph., ***dig.,*** elaps, ***ferr.,*** ferr-ar., ***ferr-i., ferr-p., graph., guai.,*** ign., ***iod., ip.,*** **KALI-AR.,** ***kali-bi., kali-c.,*** kali-i., kali-p., kali-s., **LACH.,** lact., ***lob., lyc.,*** mag-s., med., merc., **NAJA,** nat-c., nat-m.,

DIFFICULT, breathing
night, during - nit-ac., ***nux-v., op.,*** petr., ph-ac., **PHOS.,** plb., podo., ***psor., puls.,*** ran-b., ran-s., ***rhus-t.,*** **SAMB.,** sel., seneg., ***sep., spong., stann.,*** stict., **SULPH.,** ***sul-ac., ter., thuj., tub.,*** zinc., zing.
1 to 2 a.m - ***spong.***
1 to 4 a.m - ***syph.***
2 a.m - ars., ***kali-bi.,*** rumx.
2 to 3 a.m - **KALI-AR., KALI-C.**
3 a.m - am-c., **ANT-T.,** bufo, cupr., **KALI-C.,** nat-m., **SAMB.**
4 a.m - kali-bi., lil-t.
5 a.m - kali-i.
10 p.m - ip., ***phos.,*** phys., valer.
10 p.m, to 10 a.m - ip.
11 p.m - cact., nat-m., ***squil.***
11 p.m, to 3 a.m - colch.
bed, in - apis, **ARS.,** ***graph.,*** plb., spong.
amel - ***chel.***
midnight - ***acon.,*** **ARS.,** calc., ***chin.,*** puls., ***rhus-t.***
before - coloc., ***squil.***
frequent attacks until 4 a.m - **SAMB.**
midnight, after - ars., ***dros.,*** ferr., ***graph.,*** lyc., **SAMB.,** ***spong.***
on waking - arund., cann-i., sil., squil.
on waking, at 1 a.m - ptel., ***spong.,*** squil.
noon - gels., hura.
nose, felt in - ars., euphr., hell., kreos., lach., merc., phos., puls.
itching, after - sabad.
nosebleed, with - acon., bell., bry., carb-v., ip., phos., puls., spong., sulph.
odor, caused by - ars., ign., ph-ac., sang.
open, mouth with inspiration - acon., squil.
must sit by the window - ***chel., cann-s.***
wants doors and windows - **APIS,** ***arg-n.,*** aspar., bapt., ***cann-s., carb-v.,*** chin-a., ***chel.,*** cist., ***dig., ip.,*** **LACH.,** ***nat-s.,*** plb., **PULS., SULPH.**
pain, during - ***ars.,*** bry., carb-v., cocc., kalm., nat-m., prun., ***puls.,*** ran-s., sep., sil., sulph.
gastric, during - arg-m., arg-n., berb.
hypochondrium, in right, with - sep.
labor, with every - **LOB.**
night, from a blood boil - nat-m.
palpitation, during - ***acon.,*** am-c., ars-i., **AUR.,** bell., brom., ***cact.,*** cadm-s., ***calc.,*** calc-ar., carb-ac., ***carb-v.,*** caust., ***colch.,*** dig., ***glon.,*** glyc., grat., iod., ***kali-ar., kali-c.,*** kalm., lach., manc., merc-i-f., naja, olnd., ox-ac., ***phos.,*** plb., nit-ac., ***psor.,*** puls., sep., ***spig., spong.,*** tab., ***verat.,*** verat-v., viol-o., zinc-m.
11 to 3 a.m - colch.
periodic attacks - ars., **CACT.,** ***calc-p.,*** colch., plb., sulph.
seven days - chin., ign., sulph.
perspiration - ars., arund., lach., nux-v., samb., ***sep., sulph.***
anxious face and sleeplessness - eup-per.
pork, after - nat-c.

DIFFICULT, breathing
pregnancy, during - apoc., lyc., nux-v., puls., ***viol-o.***
pressing, on spine - ***chin-s.***
pressure, in stomach, with - kali-c.
pricking, with - lob.
raising, arms agg. - am-m., **BERB.,** cupr., lach., pop., **SPIG.,** tarent.
reading, while - hell., nit-ac.
amel - ferr.
rest, from - sil.
retraction of shoulders, amel - am-c., ars., ***calc.***
rheumatism of heart - ***abrot.,*** aur., ***cact.,*** cimic., ***kalm., psor.,*** sep., ***spong.***
riding, while - lyc.
amel - ***psor.***
horseback on, agg. - meph.
rising, after - ***coc-c.***
on, amel - olnd.
up in bed - laur., lyc., nat-c.
rocking amel. - kali-c., sec.
running, after - bor., hyos., ***sil.***
does not agg., slow motion agg - ***sep.***
sex, during - aeth., ***ambr.,*** arund., asaf., con., sep., ***staph.***
after - ***cedr., dig.***
desire for, with - nat-c.
toward end of - ***staph.***
singing, when - arg-m.
sinking sensation in abdomen, from - acet-ac.
sitting - alum., alumn., anac., calc., carb-v., caust., cedr., dig., dros., euphr., ***ferr.,*** gins., indg., ***lach., laur.,*** led., ***lyc.,*** mag-c., mez., nat-s., nicc., petr., ***phos., psor.,*** rhus-t., sep., sulph., verat.
amel. - acon-f., ***ant-t., apis,*** apoc., ***ars.,*** asaf., aspar., cann-s., ***crot-t.,*** dig., hep., ip., ***kali-c.,*** laur., merc-p-r., merc-sul., nat-s., nux-v., ***puls., samb.,*** sulph., ter., ***verat.,*** xan.
bent, backwards - psor.
bent, forward - dig., rhus-t., sep.
amel - ars., bufo, chin-a., **LACH.,** ***spong.***
half sitting amel - spig.
upright amel - acon., bar-m., caps., **KALI-C.,** nat-c., ***lach., laur., lyc., seneg.,*** sulph., ***ter.***
with head bent forward on knees amel. - coc-c., **KALI-C.**
sleep, during - acon., agar., bell., calc., ***carb-v., cench.,*** cham., con., dig., ***grin.,*** guai., hep., hyos., ign., ***kali-bi., kali-c.,*** **LACH.,** ***lact., lyc.,*** manc., meph., merc., nux-v., phos., ***op.,*** rhus-t., samb., sep., spong., stram., ***sulph.***
after - alum., apis, bell., cedr., lac-c., **LACH.,** nit-ac., ***phos., sep.,*** **SPONG.**
awakened to avoid suffocation, must be - **OP.,** sulph.
sleep, falling asleep, when - am-c., ars., ***arum-t.,*** bapt., bell., bry., cadm-s., carb-an., ***carb-s., carb-v., cench., crot-h., cur.,*** dig., gels., ***graph.,*** **GRIN.,** hep., kali-c., kali-i., ***lac-c.,***

DIFFICULT, breathing
sleep, falling asleep, when - **LACH.,** merc-i-r., ***merc-p-r.,*** morph., naja, nux-m., **OP.,** phos., ***samb., spong.,*** stront-c., sulph., tab., teucr., valer.
lying on right side - ***bad.***
smoke, as from - ars., bar-c., ***brom.,*** chin., cocc., ***ign.,*** lach., lyc., nat-a., puls.
sneezing, with - ambro., ars-i., phos.
agg. - naja, phos.
amel. - naja, sul-ac.
spasmodic - asaf., caust., ***chlor., cupr., laur.,*** plb., ***puls.,*** valer.
speaking, rapidly, when - caust.
stand, compelled to stand erect - cedr.
standing - aur-m., cina, kali-n., phel., ***sep.***
amel. - bapt., cann-i., cann-s., sil., spig.
can only breathe when - cann-s.
water, in - nux-m.
sternum, from pressure on - all-s., cann-s., ph-ac., phos., rhus-t., squil., thuj.
upper part of - bry.
stimulants, agg. - lach.
stomach, as from - caps.
stool, during - ***alumn., calc., rhus-t.***
after - caust., crot-t., rhus-t., sep.
bloody - kali-c.
amel. - ictod.
before - ictod.
stooping, on - ***am-m., calc.,*** caust., chin., dig., laur., mez., nit-ac., phos., seneg., sep., sil., sulph.
stormy weather - ars., ***nat-s., sep.***
stretching arms apart amel. - psor.
sudden - graph., ign., ***gels.,*** iod., ***sulph.***
5 p.m - ign.
sulphur, as if he inhaled, fumes of - brom., canth., camph., croc., kali-chl., **LYC.,** meph., ***mosch.,*** **PULS.,** sulph.
summer agg. - arg-n., syph.
supper, during - ant-c.
after - alumn., ant-c., mag-m., sanic.
suppressed, eruptions, from - **APIS.**
swallowing - atro., ***bell.,*** **BROM.,** ***calc.,*** chen-a., ***cupr.,*** thuj.
talking, after - apoc., ***ars.,*** bry., ***caust., dros.,*** laur., **LACH.,** meph., ***nat-ac.,*** ph-ac., ***sil., spig.,*** **SPONG., SULPH.,** thuj.
amel - ***ferr.***
fast, after - caust.
loud - petr.
tension, in epigastrium, with - phos.
throat-pit, constriction, at - cocc.
lump in - lob.
tickling in, from - sil.
thunderstorm, before - sep., ***sil.,*** syph.
tongue, with red - mosch.
touching, larynx - apis, bell., **LACH.**
tuberculosis, in - carb-v., ip., phos.
turning, in bed - ars., ***carb-v., sulph.***
to left side disappeared on sitting up - ***sulph.***
to right side - euph.

DIFFICULT, breathing

ulcer, with - kali-n.

uncovering, chest amel. - stann.

uremia, with - solid.

uterine displacements, from - nit-ac.

vertigo, with - kali-c.

vexation, after - ars., ***cupr.***

waking, with - alum., am-c., ***ant-t., apis, arg-n., arn., arum-t.,*** bad., bapt., bell., benz-ac., ***cadm-s.,*** calc., ***carb-v., cench., chel., chin.,*** crot-h., cur., ***dig.,*** euphr., ***graph.,*** **GRIN.,** guai., ***hep., kali-bi., kali-c., kali-i., lac-c.,*** **LACH.,** lact., med., ***naja,*** nit-ac., ***nux-m.,*** nux-v., **OP.,** ***phos.,*** ph-ac., puls., rhus-t., ***samb.,*** seneg., sep., sil., spong., sulph., tab., valer., vesp.

walking - ***acon.,*** agar., ***am-c.,*** am-m., ***apis,*** apoc., **ARS.,** arund., aur., bell., ***brom., cact.,*** **CALC.,** ***calc-s., caps., carb-v.,*** cast., ***caust.,*** chel., coca, coc-c., ***con., dig., ign.,*** ip., ***kali-ar., kali-c., kali-i.,*** kali-s., ***lach.,*** lact., ***laur.,*** led., lil-t., lyc., lycps., mag-c., ***merc.,*** nat-c., nat-m., ***nat-s., nit-ac.,*** nux-v., olnd., petr., phel., ***phos.,*** plat., ***prun., puls., psor.,*** ran-b., rhus-t., sel., seneg., ***sep.,*** sil., stront-c., **STANN., SULPH.,** thuj.

air, in the open - ***am-m., ars., aur., carb-v.,*** caust., graph., ***lyc.,*** nit-ac., zinc.

amel - brom., bry., ***dros., ferr.,*** indg., nicc., sep.

beginning to walk, on - petr., ph-ac., plat.

on level ground but not when ascending - ***ran-b.***

over uneven ground - clem.

rapidly - ang., ***aur., caust., cupr.,*** ign., ***kali-c., lob.,*** meli., merc., **NAT-M.,** ***nat-s.,*** **PHOS., PULS.,** seneg., ***sil., sulph.***

amel - ***sep.***

slowly, about, amel - **FERR.**

wind, against the - ***calc., cupr.,*** lyc., ***phos.,*** plat., psor., rhus-t., sel.

warm, bath - ***iod.,*** nit-ac.

clothing, from - ***ars.***

drinks, after - phos.

food - ***lob.***

room, in a - am-c., ant-t., ***arg-n.,*** ars., **APIS,** ***carb-s., carb-v.,*** chlor., fl-ac., ***iod.,*** ip., ***kali-i.,*** **KALI-S.,** kreos., ***lil-t., lyc.,*** **PULS.,** sep., **SULPH.,** thuj., tub.

becomes deathly pale and must remain quiet - ***am-c.***

entering warm room from open air - ***bry.***

water, when standing in - ***nux-m.***

weakness - ars., lach., sep.

respiratory organs, of - act-sp., ars., lach., plat., **STANN.**

wet weather - am-c., aran., bar-c., chin., cupr., ip., **NAT-S.**

windy, weather - ars., calc.

work, during - nit-ac.

DIFFICULT, breathing

writing, while - aspar., dig., kali-c.

amel - ***ferr.***

yawning, agg. - brom.

amel. - croc., prun.

EXPIRATION, during amel., general - **ACON.,** agar., am-m., anac., ang., arg-m., arn., asaf., asar., bar-c., ***bor.,*** **BRY.,** calc., cann-s., canth., caps., carb-an., caust., cham., chel., chin., cina, clem., croc., cycl., euphr., guai., hell., hep., ip., kali-c., kali-n., kreos.

FORCIBLE - brom., cann-s., hydr-ac.

expiration - bell., caps., cham., ***chin., gels.,*** ign., ***ox-ac.,*** stram.

GASPING - ***acon.,*** acet-ac., ***am-c., ant-t.,*** **APIS,** ***apoc., arg-n., ars.,*** ars-h., ***brom.,*** camph., canth., carb-an., **CARB-V.,** cast., ***chlor., cic., coff., colch., coloc.,*** cub., cupr., ***dig., dros.,*** gels., ***hell., hydr-ac.,*** hydrc., ***hyper., ip.,*** lat-m., ***laur.,*** **LYC.,** ***med.,*** merc., ***mosch., naja,*** op., ***phos.,*** phyt., puls., samb., ***spong., stram.,*** stry., ***tab.,*** thuj., tarent.

afternoon - nicc.

cough, during - ***ant-t., cor-r.,*** sul-ac.

before - ant-t., bry., ***brom.,*** coc-c.

dozing, when - naja

inspiration, expiration long and slow - ***ant-t., op.***

morning, 5 a.m - tarent.

night - lach.

2 a.m., with cough - chin-s.

HOARSE, hissing - acet-ac.

HOLDING, agg. - cact., ***kali-n.,*** led., merc., ***spig.***

amel. - ***bell.***

HOT air, ailments from inspiration of - carb-v.

HOT breath, as if - rad-br.

IMPEDED obstructed - ***abrot.,*** acon., anac., ant-t., arn., ***ars.,*** ars-h., aur-m., bar-c., bell., berb., bism., brom., ***bry., cact.,*** calc., calc-p., ***camph.,*** cann-s., canth., caps., carb-an., carb-v., caust., cham., chin., chlor., cimx., **CINA,** clem., ***cocc.,*** con., ***croc.,*** crot-c., cub., ***cupr.,*** dig., dol., euph., grat., ***hell.,*** hydr-ac., ***ign., iod.,*** kali-bi., ***lach.,*** laur., ***led.,*** lyc., ***merc., merc-c.,*** nat-m., nicc., **NIT-AC.,** ***nux-m.,*** nux-v., ***ol-an., op.,*** phos., plb., pic-ac., ***podo., psor.,*** puls., ran-s., rumx., ruta., sabad., samb., sant., sel., ***sil., spong.,*** squil., ***stann.,*** stram., ***sulph.,*** sul-ac., valer., ***verat.,*** verb., vesp.

abdomen, from disagreeable feeling in - ars.

afternoon - nux-v.

anxiety, with - acon., ars., verat.

chest in - phos.

coffee, after - ***cham.***

constriction, chest, of - bell., brom., **CACT.,** ***caps., chel.,*** cic., ***cupr-ac.***

stomach, in - anan., guai.

contraction, in stomach - sulph.

cough, during - ***cupr.,*** cupr-s., dig., ferr., ign., ***ip., nux-m.,*** sil., squil.

descending, on - **BOR.**

dreams, anxious from - graph.

IMPEDED obstructed
eating, while - mag-m.
after - cham.
evening - dig., sars.
bed, in - ***ant-t.***
eating, after - lach.
flatulency, from - caps., **CARB-V.,** ol-an., zinc.
forenoon - nat-m., phos.
fullness, in abdomen - phos.
gagging in oesophagus - ***cimx.***
lying, while - ***samb.***
on the back - ol-an., sil., ***sulph.***
on the back, amel - sumb.
side, left - ***puls.***
midnight - ign.
morning - bufo, sars.
in bed - ant-t.
night - ***kali-c.,*** sel., stann., ***sulph.***
sleep, during - ***guai.***
noon - hura.
oppression, from, epigastrium - chin., guai.
from heart - bell.
in occiput - kali-n.
pain, in abdomen - ars.
in back - sep.
in diaphragm - ip., spig.
in chest - brom., **BRY.,** caps., carb-v., colch., croc., merc., plb., ran-s., ruta., spong., sulph., valer., verb.
in epigastrium - ars.
in liver - con., sep.
pains, take away the breath - berb., **BRY.,** dios.
raising the arm - berb.
shooting in chest - canth., nux-m., ***ox-ac.***
spasms, of chest - hyos., petr., stram.
sharp pains
in abdomen - calc., mez.
in back - cann-s., mez.
in chest - aloe, arn., arg-m., asar., aur., berb., ***bry.,*** caps., carb-an., carb-v., chin., chin-s., dros., graph., kali-n., ***kreos.,*** lyc., mez., nat-m., nit-ac., ph-ac., rhod., squil., stann., sul-ac., thuj., verb.
in heart - ***cact., calc.,*** calc-p., mag-m., merc-i-f., ***naja,*** petr., ***staph.***
in hypochondria - arn.
in hypochondria and epigastrium - kali-c.
in liver - nat-m.
in neck - sep.
in occiput - nit-ac.
in scapula, between - nit-ac.
in scapula, under - sulph..
in sternum - nat-m., phos.
stooping, from - ***calc.,*** sil.
amel. - petr.
swallowing, on - **BROM.**
talking, while - ***caust.***
thinking, of past troubles - nat-m., sep.
thrust in left, toward heart - ***sulph.***

IMPERCEPTIBLE - acon., amyg., ***ars.,*** benz-ac., carb-ac., ***carb-v.,*** chlor., cic., ***cocc.,*** gels., hydr-ac., merc., morph., naja, nux-v., ***op.,*** petr., stram., verat.
sleep, during - caust.

INSPIRATION, during amel., general - - ant-t., asaf., bar-c., bry., cann-s., caust., ***chin.,*** cina, **COLCH.,** ***cupr., dig.,*** dros., dulc., **IGN.,** iod., ***lach.,*** mang., meny., nux-v., ***olnd.,*** ph-ac., ***puls.,*** ruta, sabad., sep., **SPIG.,** squil., ***stann.,*** staph., tarax.

INTERMITTENT, unequal - ang., **ANT-T.,** bell., calad., carb-ac., carb-an., carb-h., ***cham.,*** chlor., cina, coc-c., ***colch.,*** ign., **NIT-AC.,** ***op.,*** plb., stry., ter., ***verat.***
lying down agg - ant-t.
night - bell.
midnight on waking - cann-i.
sleep, during - ***ant-t.,*** bell., op.

INTERRUPTED, (see Arrested)
expiration - ars.
inspiration - **CINA,** ***led.***

IRREGULAR, (Cheyne strokes) - absin., acet-ac., **AIL.,** ambr., **ANG.,** ***ant-t., ars.,*** ars-i., aur., **BELL.,** calad., ***camph.,*** canth., ***cham.,*** chin-s., chlor., cic., ***cina,*** clem., coca, cocc., ***colch.,*** crat., ***crot-h.,*** **CUPR., DIG.,** dros., gels., hell., hippoz., hydr-ac., hyos., ***ign., iod.,*** laur., led., lyss., merc., **MORPH.,** mosch., nicc., ***nux-v.,*** olnd., **OP.,** plb., phos., ***puls.,*** sep., sol-t-ae., stram., ***stry.,*** sulph., sul-ac., tab., tax., ter., tril., valer., verat-v., zinc.
agg. - cact., rumx.
at one time slow, at another time hurried - acon., bell., grind., ***ign.,*** nux-v., op., spong.
cough, during - clem., cupr-s.
drinking, when - anac.
sleep, during - ant-t., cadm-s., ***ign.***
standing, while - arn.

JERKING - asar., bell., ***cact., calad.,*** crot-h., ***cupr.,*** gels., ***ign., iod.,*** laur., merc., nicc., op., ox-ac., tab.
expiration - ars.
inspiration - **OX-AC.**
by two distinct efforts - led.

LONG - ant-t., cham., ***chlor.,*** lob., ***op.***

LOUD, breathing - acon., agar., alum., am-c., ***ant-t., arn.,*** ars., bov., ***brom.,*** **CALC.,** carb-s., ***carb-v.,*** **CHAM., CHIN.,** chin-s., ***chlor., cina, colch.,*** con., ***cor-r.,*** cupr., ferr., ferr-m., gamb., guare., ***hep.,*** hydr-ac., ***hyos., ign.,*** **KALI-BI.,** ***kali-c., kalm.,*** **LACH.,** merc., morph., nat-m., ***nat-s.,*** nux-v., ***op.,*** **PHOS.,** ***puls., rhus-t.,*** **SAMB.,** ***seneg.,*** **SPONG.,** squil., ***stram.,*** **SULPH.,** sul-ac., **VERAT.**
expiration - ant-t., bell., mag-s., meph., ***nux-v.,*** op.
forenoon - hell.
inspiration - ***bell.,*** caps., cham., ***chin.,*** cina, coloc., hyos., ***ign.,*** mag-s., ***nux-v.,*** puls., rheum, sep.
lying on right side - sulph.
midnight, on waking - ant-s.
paroxysms, during - plb.

LOUD, breathing
sitting quiet, while - ***ferr.***
sleep, in - carb-v., cham., ign., rheum, **PULS.**
through nose - arn.
spasms, of glottis, as from - kalm.
walking - calc.
through nose - calc.

MOANING - acon., aeth., ***ant-t., ars.,*** bell., cina, coff., ***colch.,*** con., cupr., ***hydr-ac.,*** kali-c., ***lach.,*** laur., ***lyss., mur-ac., op.,*** phos., phyt., plb., ***puls.,*** rhus-t., sec., sel., spong., squil., tab.
expiration - bell.

PAINFUL - aeth., apis, ***ars.,*** asc-t., brom., ***bry.,*** chin., cimx., coff., crot-t., jug-c., led., nit-ac., ol-j., phos., plb., **RAN-B.,** sang., viol-o., zing.
inspiration, on - aesc.
morning - phos.
night - sang.

PANTING - **ACON.,** anac., ***ant-t., apoc.,*** arg-n., ***arn.,*** ars., bufo, calad., camph., ***carb-an.,*** **CARB-V.,** caul., cham., chin., chlor., ***cina, cocc.,*** con., cop., ferr., hyos., ***ip.,*** jatr., kali-bi., ***lyc.,*** laur., ***nit-ac., nux-m.,*** op., **PHOS.,** ***phyt.,*** plan., plb., prun., sec., ***sil., spong.,*** stram., ***tarent.,*** **VERAT-V.**
ascending stairs - arn., **CALC.,** ***carb-v.,*** plan., phos., sil.
motion, on - tarent.
reading, when - nit-ac.
running rapidly, as from - hyos.
stooping, on - nit-ac.
waking, on - kali-bi., rad-br.
walking, rapidly - sil.

PAROXYMAL - ars., arund., brom., ***cor-r., cupr., gels.,*** hydr-ac., ***ign., ip.,*** kali-c., kali-cy., led., ***mag-p.,*** mez., mill., mosch., mur-ac., nat-m., oena., op., ***ox-ac.,*** phos., plb., puls., pyrus, ***samb.,*** stann., sulph., tab., **VALER.,** ***verat.,*** verat-v.
evening - stann.
night - nat-m.

QUICK, expiration - cham., ***chin.,*** stram.
inspiration - cham.

RATTLING - acet-ac., ***acon.,*** agar., ***all-c.,*** all-s., alum., ***ammc.,*** am-caust., ***am-c., am-m.,*** anan., ang., ***ant-a.,*** ant-ox., **ANT-T.,** ***apis,*** **APOC.,** arg-n., **ARS.,** ***ars-i., art-v.,*** asaf., ***asc-t.,*** bals-p., ***bar-c., bar-m., bell., brom.,*** bry., bufo, **CACT.,** ***calc.,*** calc-ac., ***calc-p., calc-s.,*** camph., cann-i., ***cann-s., carb-an., carb-h.,*** carb-s., ***carb-v.,*** **CAUST.,** ***cham., chel.,*** chen-a., **CHIN.,** ***chin-a.,*** chin-s., chlor., cic., ***cina, coc-c.,*** cop., crot-t., cub., **CUPR.,** dig., **DULC.,** ***euphr., ferr.,*** ferr-ar., ferr-i., ferr-p., ***graph.,*** grin., **HEP., HIPPOZ.,** hydr-ac., ***hyos., iod.,*** **IP.,** kali-ar., ***kali-bi., kali-c., kali-chl.,*** kali-i., kali-p., kali-m., kali-n., **KALI-S.,** ***lach.,*** lact., laur., lob., **LYC.,** lyss., ***manc.,*** meph., merc., morph., mosch., ***mur-ac.,*** nat-c., ***nat-m., nat-s., nit-ac., nux-m., nux-v.,*** oena., ***op.,*** ox-ac., petr., ***ph-ac.,*** **PHOS.,** phyt., pix., plb., podo., **PULS.,** ***pyrog., ran-b.,*** rumx., sabin., ***sang.,*** sanic., sant., sars., sel., senec., **SENEG.,** ***sep., sil., spong.,*** squil., ***stann., stram.,*** stry., ***sulph.,*** sul-ac., syph., tab., thuj., ***tub., verat., zinc.,*** zing.
coarse - ant-t., cupr., kali-s.
cold drinks agg. - phos.
convulsion, during - tab.
cough, during (see Coughing, Rattling)
after - ant-t., carb-v.
amel. - squil.
before - dros., sep.
evening, in bed - carb-an., petr., sul-ac.
lying down - con.
expectoration, amel. - sulph.
before - sep.
without - am-c., ***ant-t.,*** carb-v., caust., hep., ip., lob., phos., sep., sulph., tub., verat.
expiring, when - calc., chin.
fine - ip.
loose - seneg.
lying, agg - **CACT.,** calc.
on back agg - agar., kali-c.
on side agg - anac.
midnight, before - ***stram.***
morning - agar.
night, and day - **CACT.**
elderly people - ***ammc.,*** **ANT-T.,** ***bar-c.,*** **HIPPOZ., KALI-BI., LYC.,** ***seneg.***
sitting upright amel - nat-c.
sleep, during - bell., con., ***hep.,*** stram., tab.
walking, while - cina.
in open air - ang., cina.

ROUGH - am-c., ***ant-t.,*** **BRY.,** ***hep., kali-bi.,*** nit-ac., plb.
crowing - **BRY.,** ***chlor., chin.,*** cor-r., ***cupr., gels.,*** **SAMB., SPONG.,** stann., verat.
sawing - ***ant-t.,*** **BROM.,** ***con.,*** **IOD.,** ***kaol.,*** lac-c., lac-ac., samb., ***sang.,*** **SPONG.**

SHORT, inspiration - bry., camph., ***op.***

SHRILL - bell., gels., ign., mosch.

SIGHING - ***acon.,*** agar., ail., am-c., ant-c., apis, apoc., ***arg-m., arg-n., ars., aspar.,*** bell., ***bor.,*** **BRY.,** cact., **CALAD.,** ***calc.,*** **CALC-P.,** ***camph.,*** carb-ac., carb-an., **CARB-V.,** ***caust.,*** cer-b., ***cham., chin-s., cimic.,*** cupr., **DIG.,** eup-pur., ***ferr-m., gels., glon.,*** gran., ***hell.,*** hura, **IGN., IP.,** jab., lach., lac-ac., lact., led., lil-t., ***lyc., lyss., merc-c.,*** morph., naphtin., nat-a., nat-p., nit-ac., nux-m., nux-v., **OP.,** phase., ***phos., phyt.,*** plb., phys., podo., prun., ***puls.,*** ran-s., sang., **SEC., SEL.,** sil., ***spong.,*** **STRAM.,** sulfon., sulph., tab., tarent., tax., ther., verat-v., vip.
afternoon - ant-c.
convulsions, after - ***cocc.***
cough, after - led.
dinner, after - arg-n.
eating, after - ***ant-c.***
evening - chin.
7 p.m - lycps.
forenoon, 9:30 a.m - hura.
menses, during - nat-p.
morning - sang.
night - bry.
2 a.m - ign.

SIGHING,
sleep, during - anac., ***aur.,*** calc., camph., puls., ***sulph.***
quickened on waking - cimic.
typhoid, in, jerks - calad.
unconsciousness, during - glon.
vaginal discharge, with - phys.

SLOW - ***acon.,*** am-c., ant-t., ***apis,*** arn., ars., ***asaf.,*** aur., **BELL.,** benz-d-n., ***brom.,*** bry., cact., ***camph.,*** cann-i., ***caps., cast.,*** chin., chin-s., chlol., cic., clem., ***cocc., colch., coloc.,*** con., cop., ***crot-c.,*** crot-h., crot-t., cub., cupr., ***dig., dios.,*** dros., ferr., gad., ***gels., glon., hell., hep., hydr-ac., hyos., hyper., ign., ip., lach., laur., lob-p.,*** lyc., ***merc-c.,*** mez., morph., nit-ac., nux-m., ***nux-v.,*** oena., ***olnd.,*** ox-ac., **OP.,** phase., piloc., plat., plb., phos., ***phyt.,*** sec., ***spong.,*** squil., stram., sul-ac., tab., verat-v.
alternating, with short, during sleep - ign.
with suffocation - cocc.
brain, from concussion of - arn., hell., nat-s., op.
convulsions, during - **OP.**
cough, during - clem.
evening, while lying quiet, agg - con., ferr.
expiration - ant-t., ***arn.,*** apis, bor., lob., ***op., sep.***
during sleep - chin., ign.
inspiration - cham., chin., ***ign.,*** stram.
morning - merc., ***lach.***
night - coloc., ***lach.***
palpitation, during - bell.
sleep, during - acon., chin., **OP.**
walking amel - ***ferr.***

SNORING - acon., aeth., amyg., ***ant-t.,*** arn., ars., bapt., benz-ac., bell., ***brom.,*** calc., ***camph., carl., cham., chin., cic.,*** con., cund., ***cupr.,*** cycl., dros., dulc., fl-ac., glon., ***hep.,*** hydr-ac., hyos., ***ign.,*** kali-bi., kali-chl., **LAC-C.,** ***lach., laur.,*** lyc., mag-m., mez., mur-ac., nat-m., nit-ac., nux-m., ***nux-v.,*** **OP.,** petr., rat., rheum, ***rhus-t.,*** sabad., samb., sep., sil., stann., ***stram.,*** stry., ***sulph.,*** teucr.
adenoids removal, after - carc., kali-s.
afternoon, nap, during - alum.
awake, while - chel., sumb.
children, in - chin., mez., op.
chill, during - ***chin.,*** laur., **OP.**
delirium, after - sec.
evening in bed - sil.
expiring, while - arn., camph., chin., ***nux-v., op.***
fever, during - apis, con., ign., laur., **OP.**
insensible, while - ***op.***
inspiration in sleep - bell., caps., cham., chin., hyos., ign., rheum.
lying on the back, while - dros., dulc., kali-c., mag-c., sulph.
midnight - mur-ac., nux-v.
morning, while sleeping - petr.
nose, through - puls.
sleep, in restless - chin., laur., ***op.,*** sil., stram., tub., ***zinc.***
swoon, during - stram.

SOBBING - acon., aeth., am-m., ang., ant-c., asaf., ***aur., bry., calc., cupr-ac.,*** gels., ***guare., ign.,*** laur., ***led., mag-p., merc.,*** nit-ac., ran-s., ***sec.,*** sil., stram., ther.
in sleep - **AUR.,** ***calc.***
paroxysmal - ***mag-p.***

SPONGE, dry, breathing as through - spong.

STERTOROUS - absin., acon., **AM-C.,** amyg., anac., **ANT-T.,** ***apis, arn., ars.,*** bell., bry., bufo, ***camph.,*** cann-i., ***carb-ac.,*** carb-an., cham., chen-a., ***chin.,*** chlol., cic., cocc., cupr., ferr-m., ***gels., glon.,*** hell., ***hippoz.,*** hydr-ac., hyos., jab., kali-bi., ***lach., laur.,*** lob-p., ***lyc.,*** merl., naja, nat-sal., ***nit-ac., nux-m., nux-v., oena.,*** olnd., **OP.,** petr., phase., phos., plb., ***puls.,*** sabad., sarr., sec., ***spong.,*** stann., ***stram.,*** sul-ac., ***sulfon.,*** tab., tanac., ter., trio., verat-v., visc.
brain, concussion of - arn., hell., hyos., nat-s., op.
convulsions, after - ***oena.,*** **OP.**
evening in bed - carb-an.
involuntary stools and urine - amyg.
lying on the affected side - anac.
puffing expiration, with - bufo, ***chin., lach., nux-v., op.,*** plb., tab.
sleep, during - ***brom.,*** chin., ign., nux-v., **OP.,** puls.
stupefaction and crying out as with a sharp pain - **APIS.**

STOPPED, (see Emergency, Asphyxia) - acet-ac., alum., anac., ang., apis, arn., ars., bar-c., bell., bor., bov., **BRY.,** ***cact., calc., camph.,*** cann-s., caps., carb-an., carb-s., **CARB-V.,** cast., ***caust.,*** chin., ***cic., cina,*** cocc., con., crot-c., **CUPR.,** ***cur.,*** euphr., guai., hydr-ac., ***ign.,*** iod., kalm., kali-c., kali-i., ***lach., lat-m., led., lyc.,*** lyss., merc., merc-c., ***mosch.,*** naja, nat-m., nat-s., nit-ac., ***nux-m.,*** nux-v., oena., **OP.,** ***phos.,*** plat., plb., ***puls., ruta.,*** **SAMB.,** sars., sep., ***sil.,*** stann., stram., ***sulph.,*** tab., tanac., ter., thea., ther., upa., ***verat.,*** verb.
afternoon - cham., dios., kreos., thuj.
3 p.m. stitches under right scapula - kreos.
4 p.m - dios.
air, in fresh - psor.
hot, as from - arg-n.
in open - caust.
anger from, children in - arn.
ascending steps - mag-c., nit-ac., thuj.
cannot breathe again - apis, bell., coca, dros., helon., lat-m., laur., rumx.
constriction, of, chest, during - carb-v., hell., sep., spig.
convulsions, during - ***cic., cina,*** coff., ***sant.,*** sars., ***stry.***
coughing - acet-ac., ***acon.,*** **ALUM.,** am-c., am-m., anac., **ANT-T.,** aral., arg-n., arn., **ARS.,** bar-c., bell., brom., bry., cahin., calad., calc., canth., carb-an., carb-v., caust., **CINA,** clem., cocc., coc-c., con., cop., ***cor-r.,*** **CUPR.,** dol., **DROS.,** euphr., ferr., ferr-ar., guai., hep., hyos., iod., **IP.,** kali-bi., kali-c., kali-chl., kali-n., ***kreos.,*** lach., lact., led., lob., ***lyc.,***

STOPPED, breathing
coughing - merc., mosch., mur-ac., nat-m., nat-s., nicc., nit-ac., ***nux-m.,*** **NUX-V.,** op., phel., phos., puls., rhus-t., ***samb.,*** sang., sarr., ***sep., sil.,*** spig., spong., squil., staph., sulph., sul-ac., verat., zinc., ziz.
before - led.
desire to stop breathing - calc.
drinking, from - am-m., anac., ***cimx.***
falling (child) - petr.
drinking, from - anac., ***cimx.***
evening, griping in inguinal region - nat-m., nicc., plan.
fever, during - ruta.
forenoon, stitches in side - stann.
knocking, against something - petr.
lying, while - apis, ***bor.,*** nat-m., ***puls.***
amel - ***psor.***
on the back - sil.
morning - lyc.
night - guai., ***kali-c.,*** **LYC.,** ruta., samb.
air, in fresh - **PSOR.**
cough, during - nat-m.
midnight - cinnb.
pain, during - ars., kalm., nat-m., nux-v., plb., prun., puls., ran-s., sep., sulph.
sleep, going to - ***am-c.,*** cadm-s., carb-v., cench., dig., **GRIN.,** lac-c., merc-p-r., ***op.,*** **LACH.,** samb.
swallowing, when - anac.
rubbing amel - mur-ac.
sitting, while - ***caust.,*** nat-s., psor.
sleep, during - am-c., cadm-s., ***carb-v.,*** **CENCH.,** dig., **GRIN.,** guai., ***kali-c., lac-c.,*** **LACH.,** lyc., **OP.,** samb., ***sulph.***
on going to - carb-v., cench., **GRIN.,** ***op.,*** **LACH.**
when going to sleep on the right side - bad.
smoking - tarax.
standing still, when - sep.
in water - nux-m.
stooping - psor., sil.
suddenly, in children - cham.
suppressed eruptions - ars., ***sulph.***
talking, when - ***caust.,*** mez., plan., ***sulph.***
turning in bed - carb-v.
walking, while - am-m., ***calc., caust.,*** cham., ***chin.,*** ign., nat-c., ***nit-ac.,*** sep., thuj.
against the wind - ***calc.,*** plat.

STRIDULUS - am-caust., **BELL.,** ***chlor.,*** **GELS., IGN.,** ***lach.,*** laur., ***meph.,*** **MOSCH.,** nit-ac., ***nux-v., op.,*** plb., ***samb., sang.,*** sarr., verat.
evening, on falling asleep - **PHOS.**

SUFFOCATION, (see Emergency, Asphyxia)

SUFFOCATIVE, (see Difficult, breathing)

SUPERFICIAL - ***bell., chin., laur., nux-m.,*** ph-ac., **PHOS.,** puls.

TREMULOUS - ***ant-t.,*** zinc.

TUBE, breathing as through a metal - merc-c.

VEHEMENT, expiration - bell., caps., chin., ign., stram.

WHEEZING, (see Lungs, Asthma) - ail., aloe, ***alum., ambr.,*** am-c., ***ant-t., apoc.,*** aral., arg-n., **ARS.,** ***ars-i., brom.,*** calad., calc., calc-s., ***cann-s., caps.,*** carb-s., **CARB-V.,** card-m., ***cham., chin., chin-a.,*** chlol., ***cina,*** crot-t., ***cupr.,*** dol., ***dros.,*** erio., ferr., ferr-i., ***fl-ac.,*** graph., ***grin.,*** hep., hydr-ac., ***iod.,*** iodof., **IP.,** just., ***kali-ar., kali-bi.,*** **KALI-C.,** ***kali-s., lach.,*** **LOB.,** ***lycps., lyc.,*** manc., merc., murx., naja, ***nat-m., nat-s., nux-m.,*** nux-v., ***nit-ac.,*** ox-ac., phos., prun., sabad., ***samb.,*** sang., sanic., seneg., sep., spong., squil., stann., sulph., ***syph.***
afternoon - fl-ac.
daytime - ***lyc.***
evening - lycps., murx.
bed, in - nat-m.
lying down, on - ***ars.***
expectoration amel. - ip.
expiring, when - ***lyc.,*** nat-m., ***sep.***
inspiring, while - ***alum., caps., chin., kali-c.,*** spong.
midnight, after - ***ars., samb.***
night - ***ars.,*** kali-bi.
sitting up, while - nat-c.
sleep, during - nux-v.
smoking, on - calad., kali-bi.
warm room - ***kali-s.***

WHISTLING - acet-ac., acon., aeth., aloe, alum., ***ambr., ant-t.,*** arg-n., ***ars.,*** arund., aur., bell., benz-ac., brom., bufo, calc., cann-s., carb-s., ***carb-v.,*** caust., ***cham.,*** **CHIN.,** chin-a., coloc., cupr., graph., ***hep., iod., ip.,*** kali-ar., ***kali-c.,*** kali-i., kali-s., kreos., laur., ***lyc.,*** mag-m., ***manc.,*** nat-m., nit-ac., nux-v., osm., ph-ac., phos., sabad., ***samb.,*** sang., seneg., sep., ***sil., spong.,*** stann., stram., ***sulph.,*** sul-ac., sul-i., thuj.
ascending, agg. - sulph.
cough, during - lyc.
at begining of - asar.
evening - ***calc.,*** carb-v., psor.
after lying down - ars., ***calc.***
expiration, on - nat-m.
inspiration, during - aral., cina, crot-t., graph., ***kali-c.,*** nit-ac., sulph.
lying, while - ***calc.***
on left side - arg-n.
on the back - aeth.
morning - ***lach.***
night, 3 a.m., in sleep - sulph.
sleep, in - chel., sulph.
waking, when - psor.
whooping cough, in - ***brom., carb-v., cupr., hep.,*** samb., ***spong.***

Chest

ACHING, pain - acon., agar., ***ail.,*** alum., ant-c., arg-n., ***arn., asaf.,*** bapt., ***bell.,*** bor., ***bry.,*** cact., ***calc-p.,*** cann-i., cann-s., carb-ac., ***carb-an.,*** carb-s., ***carb-v.,*** cham., chel., chin., ***clem., coc-c.,*** colch., crot-t., cupr-s., cycl., dig., hydr-ac., iod., kreos., lach., ***lact.,*** led., ***lyc.,*** mag-m., merc., merc-c., nat-m., nat-p., naja, ***phos., phyt.,*** psor., ***ran-b.,*** rhod., rhus-t., ***rumx.,*** sang., ***seneg.,*** sep., stict., stram., stront-c., sulph., tarent., zinc.

afternoon - kali-n.
ascending, agg. - cact.
breath, on holding - merc.
coughing, when - chin., kali-c., mag-m., mang., phyt., raph., samb., stront.
paroxysmal - mag-m.
dinner, after - sulph.
eating, after - alum., nux-v.
belching, amel. - lyc.
evening - coloc., nux-m., ran-b., sulph.
deep breathing agg. - ran-b.
expectoration - asaf.
forenoon - puls.
hawking, after - spig.
inspiration, agg. - bapt., calc., jatr.
amel. - merc.
lower, part - croc., ***chin.,*** fl-ac., kali-bi., seneg., sep., ***sulph.***
eating, after - arg-n.
inspiration - ***sulph.***
lying, while, amel. - ***chin.***
sitting, while - ***chin.,*** seneg.
walking amel. - chin.
middle, of - crot-h., lith., sars.
extending to back - ***crot-h.***
motion amel. - seneg.
pressure, on - am-c.
morning - sulph.
8 a.m. - naja.
8 a.m., anterior part - naja.
bed, in - lact.
eating, after - sulph.
waking, on - ***seneg.***
motion, agg. - bapt., bry., sep., stront.
agg. of arms, anterior part of chest - carb-an.
amel. - ***seneg.***
night - ran-b.
on waking - ***seneg.***
noon, on walking - bry.
reading, while - stann.
rising, on - agar., chin-s., ***lach.***
sitting - bell., con.
standing - nat-m.
straight, on becoming, agg. - acon.
talking, excited - ***nat-m.,*** stann., stram.
throat, clearing - spig.
touched - dros.
walking - bell., bufo, ***cact.,*** stront.

aching, clavicles - dros., jatr., mag-m., rhus-t.
below - ***ail.,*** carb-ac., coca, dros., naja, sulph.
extending to scapula, during inspiration - dros.
inspiring agg. - dros., mez.
breathing, during - ant-c.
inspiration, on - dros.
waking from a nightmare - rhus-t.

aching, costal cartilages of short - staph.

aching, ribs, along, backward - aml-n., arg-m.

aching, sides - am-c., ***arg-n.,*** bry., chin., cop., ferr., fl-ac., hydrc., kali-bi., lil-t., mur-ac., naja, nux-m., op., pall., phyt., rhus-t., seneg., sep., sulph.
ascending agg. - kali-bi.
deep inspiration - chin-a., mez., ***oena.,*** phyt.
evening - sulph.
extending from left to right - carb-v., graph.
left - ***apis,*** berb., carb-an., clem., eup-per., ham., iod., kali-p., mez., oena., rhus-t., ***rumx., seneg.,*** sep., sumb., tarent., zinc.
extending to scapula - kali-p.
lying, while - caps.
left side, on - eup-per.
right side, on - phyt.
morning - fago., nit-ac.
night - iod.
bed, in - merc-i-f.
right - bism., caust., chin-a., dig., fago., merc-i-f.
turning chest - brom.
using arms - ham.
waking, on - ***arg-n.***
walking - brom.

aching, sternum - **BRY.**

ADHESION, sensation of - arn., aur., aur-m., bry., cadm-s., coloc., dig., euph., hep., kali-c., kali-n., ***merc., mez.,*** nux-v., par., petr., phos., ***plb.,*** puls., ***ran-b.,*** **RHUS-T.,** seneg., ***sep., sulph., thuj.,*** verb.

AIR, entering too much, or forced in - chlor., sabin., ther.

air, chest, sensitive to - ***ph-ac.***

ALIVE, sensation of something moving - ***croc.,*** led.
evening - colch.
eating, after - colch.
heart - cycl.

ALTERNATING, with
diarrhea and bronchitis - ***seneg.***
eye, symptoms - ars.
rectal, symptoms - calc-p., **SIL.,** verat.
skin symptoms - crot-h.

ANGINA, pectoris - acet-ac., ***acon.,*** adren., agar., **AM-C.,** ***aml-n.,*** anac., ang., **APIS,** arg-c., **ARG-N., ARN., ARS.,** ars-i., **AUR., AUR-M.,** bism., **CACT.,** camph., caust., cer-b., ***chel.,*** **CHIN-A.,** ***chin-s.,*** chlol., chr-ac., ***cimic.,*** coca, ***cocaine,*** conv., ***crat.,*** crot-h., ***cupr., cupr-ac., cupr-ar., dig., dios., glon., haem., hep., hydr-ac.,*** ip., ***jug-c., kali-c.,*** kali-i., kali-p., ***kalm.,*** **LACH.,** lact., **LAT-M.,** ***laur.,*** lil-t., lith., lob., ***lyc., mag-p.,*** magn-gr., morph., ***mosch.,*** **NAJA,** ***nat-i.,*** nat-n., ***nux-v.,*** olnd., **OX-AC.,** petr., **PHOS.,** phyt., pip-n., prun., **RHUS-T.,** ***samb.,*** saroth., sep., **SPIG., SPONG.,** staph., stict., ***stram.,*** stront-c., stront-i., stry., ***tab., tarent., ther.,*** thyr., ***verat.,*** verat-v., zinc-valer.
- abuse of, coffee, from - coff.
  - stimulants, from - nux-v., spig.
- drinking, water agg. - ars.
- heart disease, from organic - ***ars-i., cact.,*** calc-f., crat., kalm., nat-i., tab.
- hot drinks, amel. - spig.
- lies, on knees, body bent backwards - nux-v.
- muscular origin - cupr., hydr-ac.
- pain, excessive - agar.
- pseudo angina pectoris - aconin., cact., ***lil-t., mosch.,*** nux-v., tarent.
- rheumatism, from - cimic., lith.
- standing, amel. - ars.
- straining, overlifting, from - ***arn.,*** carb-an., caust.
- tobacco, from - calad., kalm., lil-t., nux-v., spig., staph., tab.

ANXIETY, in - **ACON.,** acon-f., aeth., agar., am-c., anac., ***ant-c.,*** arg-n., arn., **ARS.,** ***ars-i.,*** asaf., astac., aster., **AUR.,** ***aur-m.,*** bell., bor., brom., ***bry., cact.,*** **CALC.,** cann-i., cann-s., canth., caps., carb-an., carb-s., ***carb-v.,*** caust., ***cench., chel.,*** chin., chin-a., cinnam., cocc., ***colch.,*** con., cop., crot-t., ***cupr-ac.,*** cupr-s., ***dig.,*** ferr., ferr-ar., ferr-i., ferr-p., ***graph.,*** guai., ***guare.,*** hyos., hyper., ign., iod., ***ip.,*** jab., ***kali-ar.,*** kali-bi., kali-c., kali-cy., kali-n., kali-p., ***kali-s., kreos.,*** lach., laur., ***lob., lyc.,*** **MERC.,** merc-c., mez., mosch., ***nat-a., nat-c.,*** nat-m., nat-p., ***nit-ac., nux-v.,*** olnd., ol-an., op., petr., ph-ac., **PHOS.,** plat., ***plb.,*** prun., ***psor., puls., ran-b.,*** rhus-t., samb., sec., seneg., sep., ***spig.,*** spong., stann., staph., ***sulph.,*** tab., teucr., ***ther.,*** thyr., valer., vanad., verat., viol-o., ***zinc.***
- air, open, driving him into - anac.
- ascending steps - hyos.
- bending forward amel. - ***colch.***
- breakfast, after - valer.
- coughing, on - arund.
- eating, after - caps., carb-an.
- evening - anag., bor., chel., kali-c., kali-p., ***phos.,*** **PULS.,** seneg., stann.
  - amel. - ***zinc.***
  - bed, in - anag., bor.
  - undressing - chel.
- excitement agg. - **PHOS.**
- exertion, from - ferr.
- forenoon - ol-an.
- inspiration deep, after - chel., nat-m.

ANXIETY, in
- lying, while - ***cench., graph., tarent.***
  - on back, while - ***sulph.***
  - on left side, while - **PULS.**
- morning - bry., carb-an., hyper., puls.
  - 4 or 5 a.m. - alum.
- motion amel. - seneg.
- night - ***ars.,*** aster., ign., lyc., **PULS.,** ***ran-b.,*** sulph.
  - 2 a.m. - kali-c.
- playing piano, while - ***nat-c.***
- pressing, on left side agg. - plb.
- sitting, while - cupr., kali-c.
  - bent, while - chin.
- standing, while - meny.
- stool, after - calc., ***caust.,*** cund.
- straightening up amel. - chin.
- walking, while - meny.

APPREHENSION - carl., nat-m., ph-ac.

BALL, ribs, along, round, as if rolling to and fro - cupr.
- below ribs - cupr.

BAR, of iron, across the centre of chest - haem., vich-g.
- sensation of, around chest - arg-n.

BLEEDING, from lungs and chest - ***acal., acet-ac.,*** **ACON.,** ***all-s.,*** aloe, ***alum.,*** am-c., ***anan., ant-t., apoc., aran.,*** arg-n., **ARN., ARS.,** aur-m-n., aspar., ***bell.,*** brom., ***bry.,*** bufo, **CACT.,** ***calc., calc-p.,*** calc-s., canth., carb-an., carb-s., carb-v., ***card-m.,*** casc., caust., cham., **CHEL., CHIN.,** chin-a., chin-s., chlor., cinnam., ***coc-c., colch., coll.,*** con., ***cop., croc.,*** crot-h., cupr., cupr-s., ***dig.,*** dros., dulc., elaps, erech., ***erig.,*** **FERR.,** ***ferr-ac.,*** **FERR-AR.,** ***ferr-i.,*** ferr-m., ferr-p., ***gall-ac., ger.,*** **HAM.,** hyos., **IP.,** kali-ar., kali-bi., ***kali-c., kali-chl., kali-i.,*** kali-n., kali-p., kali-s., ***kreos., lach., lam., led.,*** lyc., ***lycps.,*** mag-c., mag-m., mang., meli., merc., ***merc-c.,*** **MILL.,** ***nat-a.,*** nat-n., **NIT-AC.,** ***nux-m., nux-v.,*** ol-j., op., ***ph-ac.,*** **PHOS.,** ***plb., puls., rhus-t., sabin., sang.,*** sarr., **SEC.,** ***senec.,*** sep., sil., **STANN.,** staph., ***stram.,*** stront-c., stroph., sulph., ***sul-ac.,*** tab., ***ter.,*** tril., tub., ***urt-u.,*** vanad., verat., verat., ***verat-v.***
- alcoholics, in - ars., hyos., led., **NUX-V.,** op.
- alternating with rheumatism - led.
- anger, from - ***nux-v.***
- coagulated - acal., acon., ***arn., bell.,*** brom., bry., canth., carb-an., caust., **CHAM.,** ***chin.,*** coc-c., coll., con., ***croc.,*** crot-h., dros., ***elaps,*** erig., ***ferr.,*** ferr-m., ham., ***hyos., ip.,*** kali-n., kreos., mag-m., ***merc., nit-ac.,*** nux-v., ph-ac., ***puls.,*** **RHUS-T.,** ***sabin.,*** sec., sep., stram., stront-c., sul-ac.
  - black - kreos.
  - brown - bry., rhus-t.
  - dark - arn., coll., ham., mag-c., puls.
- exertion, after - acon., ***arn.,*** ferr., ip., ***mill.,*** puls., ***rhus-t., urt-u.***
- frothy, foaming - acon., ***arn.,*** dros., ferr., ip., ***led.,*** mill., op., ph-ac., ***phos.,*** sec., ***sil.***
- full moon, during - kali-n.

BLEEDING, from lungs and chest
hemorrhoidal flow, after suppression of - acon., ***carb-v., led., lyc.,*** **NUX-V.,** phos., ***sulph.***
hot blood - acon., ***bell.,*** mill., psor.
lying-in women, in - ***acon., arn., chin.,*** hyos., ip., lach., ***puls.,*** sulph., tril.
menses, after suppression of - ***acon.,*** ars., ***bell., bry.,*** con., ***dig.,*** ferr., graph., ham., mill., ***phos.,*** **PULS.,** ***sang., senec.,*** sep., sulph., ust.
before - ***dig.***
nursing mothers - ***chin.***
pneumonia, results of - calc-s., ***sul-ac.***
puerperal fever - ham.
walking slowly amel. - ***ferr.***
whiskey, after - merc., puls.
whooping cough, in - con., ip.
wine, after - acon.

BOILS, on - am-c., chin., ***hep.,*** **KALI-I.,** lach., mag-c., mag-m., phos., **PSOR., SULPH.**

BORING, pain - alum., ***bism., brom.,*** cina, cupr., ***ferr.,*** indg., kali-c., lob., mag-m., med., ***mur-ac.,*** ph-ac., psor., rhus-t., ***seneg.,*** sil., tarax., thuj.
chill, during - med.
drawing - colch.
evening - alum.
inspiration, during - alum.
night agg. - sil.
paroxysmal, in - plb.
tension, during respiration - mur-ac.
walking, amel. - alum.

boring, sides - colch., kali-c., merc-i-f., mur-ac., plan., seneg., staph.
breathing deep, amel. - colch.
evening, 10 p.m. agg. - colch.
in bed - rhus-t.
left - merc-i-f., ph-ac., seneg., spig.
right - ***bism.,*** colch.

BROKEN, pain, as if ribs were - agar., ***bry.,*** caps., kali-bi., naja, petr., psor., sep., stram.

BURNING, pain - acet-ac., ***acon.,*** aesc., ail., agar., alum., am-c., am-m., ambr., anan., ant-c., ***ant-t.,*** **APIS,** arg-n., ***arn.,*** **ARS.,** ars-i., arum-t., ***asaf.,*** aur., bar-c., ***bell.,*** bell-p., berb., ***bism.,*** brom., bry., bufo, ***calc., calc-ar.,*** calc-p., calc-s., cann-i., **CANTH.,** caps., ***carb-an., carb-s.,*** **CARB-V.,** cast-eq., ***caust., cham.,*** chel., ***cic.,*** cina, clem., cocc., coc-c., colch., ***cop.,*** croc., ***crot-h.,*** crot-t., cub., cupr., ***dros.,*** euph., gels., ***graph.,*** ham., hep., ***hydr.,*** hyper., ign., iod., kali-ar., ***kali-bi.,*** kali-br., kali-c., kali-p., kali-s., ***kreos., lach.,*** lact., laur., ***led.,*** lob., ***lyc.,*** mag-m., mag-s., manc., ***mang., med., merc., merc-sul.,*** mez., mosch., ***mur-ac.,*** murx., ***nat-a.,*** nat-c., nat-p., nat-s., nit-ac., ***nux-m., nux-v.,*** op., ***ph-ac., phos., plat.,*** polyg., psor., puls., ran-b., raph., rat., rhus-t., ***sabad., sang., seneg.,*** sep., ***sil.,*** spig., ***spong.,*** stann., stry., ***sulph.,*** tab., ***ter.,*** thuj., vip., zinc-m., ***zinc.***
anterior part - **APIS,** kali-n., sulph.
scratching, agg. - cinnb.

BURNING, pain
coughing, during - agar., ail., ambr., am-c., ***ant-c.,*** ars., arum-t., bry., ***bufo,*** cann-s., carb-v., ***caust.,*** cina, dig., ferr., gels., hep., **IOD.,** kali-c., ***lach.,*** led., lyc., ***mag-m., mag-s.,*** ph-ac., phos., phyt., pyrog., rumx., ***seneg.,*** sep., **SPONG.,** syph., sulph., zinc., zing.
after - ***carb-v.,*** mag-s., ***seneg.***
dinner, after - agar.
dry cough - bry., ***caust.,*** **IOD.,** ***kali-c., mag-m.,*** **SPONG.**
evening - kali-n., kreos., murx., verat., zinc.
5 p.m. - hyper.
6 p.m. - puls.
evening, bed, in - bell., nat-p.
expectoration amel. - kali-n.
extending, to face - **SULPH.**
to mouth - ph-ac.
to throat - ***ant-t.,*** calc-p., kali-n., ***merc.,*** sabad.
upward - lob., **SULPH.**
external - agar., ambr., ars., bar-c., ***bell.,*** bov., dig., ***euph.,*** kali-n., ***mez., mur-ac.,*** nat-m., ph-ac., ***plat., seneg.,*** stront-c., ***sulph.,*** sul-ac., zinc.
fixed spot, in - ***led.***
forenoon - mag-s.
inspiration, during - ***laur.,*** sep.
lower, part - chel., phos.
lying down, on - puls.
menses, before - ***zinc.***
middle, of - agar., ***ars.,*** carb-s., cast-eq., ***dros.,*** graph., iod., kali-n., laur., mag-s., mez., ol-an., ph-ac., sul-ac., verat.
afternoon - mag-s.
breakfast, after - verat.
extending to throat - mez.
inspiration, during - graph.
vexation, after - ph-ac.
morning - caust., kali-n., zinc.
motion, agg. - crot-h.
amel. - euph.
mouth, extending into, during coryza - ph-ac.
night - ***lach.***
midnight till morning - ***ars.***
respiration, on - kali-c.
sitting agg. - phos.
salt, food - nit-ac.
sleep, after - nux-m.
spots, in - ***am-m., led.,*** mang., seneg., zinc.
walking, while - mag-s.
air, in the open - am-m.
air, in the open, after - sulph.

burning, clavicles - aur-m., berb., grat., sulph.
below - sang.

burning, ribs, between the - coc-c., plat.
costal cartilages during expiration - bell.

burning, sides - ***agar.,*** ail., all-c., iod., kali-bi., prun., rumx., sabin., seneg.
afternoon - alum., bar-c., seneg.
dinner, after - agar.
expiration, agg. - mang.
evening - bar-c., ***seneg.***
bed, in - nat-p., ***rumx.***

burning, sides
extending, to back - zinc.
upward - stront.
external - nat-c., sul-ac., thuj.
spots, in - am-m.
inspiration, during - lyss., ***rumx.***
left - all-c., ***ars.,*** bar-c., ***carb-s., carb-v.,*** cycl., ***euph.,*** graph., grat., ind., laur., mang., myrt-c., nat-c., ol-j., ph-ac., **PHOS., RAN-B., RUMX.,** sabad., ***seneg.,*** stront-c., sul-ac., zinc.
extending down to groin - fl-ac.
lying, while - ***rumx.***
back, on - ***rumx.***
left side, agg. - ***phos.,*** seneg.
left side, amel. - ***rumx.***
on right side agg. - ***rumx.,*** seneg.
morning - nat-c.
motion, agg. - mang.
amel. - ***euph., seneg.***
moving, arm agg. - ***bry.***
pressure, agg. - mang.
right - abrot., alum., ars., asar., ***bell.,*** **BRY.,** carb-an., coloc., mur-ac., nat-c., nat-p., raph., rumx., ruta., ***sang.,*** sulph., zinc.
rising in bed, on - nicc.
from stooping - kali-c.
rubbing, agg. - mang.
short ribs - sulph., thuj.
sitting, while - ph-ac., ***seneg.***
touch, agg. - ph-ac.

burning, sternum - agar., ars., bov., canth., cham., chel., clem., con., hura, ind., ***kali-bi.,*** laur., mag-s., ***merc.,*** mez., mur-ac., puls., sang., sep., sulph., tarax., ter., zinc.
coughing, after - ***ferr.***
dinner, after - phos.
drinking beer - sep.
expiration, on - tarax.
extending into shoulder during cough - ***kali-bi.***
left, side - rheum.
under - ***acon., asaf., ars., carb-v., cham.,*** clem., coc-c., cund., echi., ***lach.,*** mag-s., mang., mez., ***phos., sang.,*** seneg.
extending to left clavicle - phos.
extending to mouth - cham.
lower part - gels.
motion - seneg.
warm drinks, from - ter.

BURSTING, pain - ***aur-m.,*** bry., carb-an., cham., cina, coff., lach., lyc., merc., mur-ac., rhus-t., tarent., seneg., sulph., zinc.
ascending, when - arg-n.
coughing, on - ars., ***bry.,*** caps., cham., **LACT.,** ***merc.,*** mur-ac., ***sulph.,*** zinc.
expectoration - puls.
night - asaf., ***merc.***
sneezing - ol-an., sil.

CANCER, clavicles, fungus haematodes - sep.
cancer, sternum - sulph.

CAPILLARY, network, chest - carb-v.

CARTILAGES, affections, of the - ***arg-m.***

CHILLINESS, in - alum., ***ars.,*** bry., mez., nat-c., par., ***ran-b.,*** ruta.
eruption, with - staph.
evening - ***ars.***
left side - nat-c., nat-m.
stool, after - plat.
walking in open air - chin., ***ran-b.***

CICATRICES, (see Scars)

CLAWING, pain, chest - **SENEG.**
sensation, in chest - samb., stront.

CLOSE to back - cina.

CLOTHING, agg. - ail., aur-m., benz-ac., bov., calc., **CAUST.,** ***chel., con.,*** graph., ***kali-bi.,*** **LACH.,** lact., ***lycps., merc., tarent.,*** zinc.
wet, as if - ran-b.

CLUCKING, sound - cina, kali-c., nat-m., ruta.

COATED, sensation, as if - ant-t., bar-c., caust., ***nat-m.***

COLD, pain in, on coughing - ***med.***

COLDNESS - abies-c., aesc., ***am-m.,*** ambr., am-c., ***apis,*** arn., **ARS.,** berb., ***brom.,*** bry., bufo, ***camph., carb-an.,*** carb-s., cic., cist., cor-r., culx., dig., ***elaps,*** graph., helo., hydr., ign., ***kali-c.,*** lact., lil-t., lith., lyc., med., merl., nat-c., nat-m., nat-p., olnd., ***par.,*** petr., ***ph-ac., ran-b.,*** rhus-t., ruta., sabad., sep., spong., **SULPH.,** sul-ac., tep., ***zinc.***
air, cold, breathing - ***cor-r.,*** lith., **RAN-B.**
anterior part, below the clavicle, sensation of, cold water running to the toes - ***caust.***
cold water, sensation of running down the chest when drinking - verat.
chill during - ***caps.***
coughing, chest cold, on - med.
drinking, after - ***elaps.***
expectoration, after - ***zinc.***
external - **RAN-B.**
internal - **ARS.,** am-br., ***sulph.***
as if ice water were rising and descending through a cylindrical tube - elaps.
middle of - raph.
pain, at seat of - ***cact.***
respiration, on - arn., ***brom.,*** camph., chin., ***cist., rhus-t.,*** sulph.
right - med., ***sulph.***
walking in open air - **RAN-B.**
warmth of bed amel. - nat-c.
wind, from wind on the chest - chin-s., phos., ***ph-ac.***
wrap up the chest, must - bor., nux-v., ***ph-ac.***

coldness, sides - olnd.
left - ferr-ma., nat-c., nat-m.
as if a lump of ice, in - sulph.
right - berb., merc., sulph.

coldness, sternum - apis, ***camph.,*** cupr-ac., **RAN-B.**

CONGESTION, hyperemia of, lungs - **ACON.,** adren., ***aesc.,*** aloe, alum., ambr., ***aml-n.,*** ammc., ***am-c., apis, arn.,*** ars-i., ***aur.,*** **BELL.,** both., brom., **BRY., CACT.,** ***calc.,*** **CAMPH.,** carb-s., ***carb-v.,*** cent., ***chin.,*** chlor., cimic., ***coc-c.,*** cocc., conv., ***cupr.,*** cycl., **DIG.,** ***ferr.,*** ferr-i., ferr-m.,

CONGESTION, hyperemia of, lungs - ***ferr-p.,*** gad., ***gels., glon., graph., iod.,*** **IP.,** ***kali-c.,*** kali-chl., kali-i., kali-n., **LACH.,** lact., lil-t., ***lyc.,*** mag-m., ***meli., merc.,*** merl., ***mill.,*** nat-m., ***nit-ac.,*** **NUX-V.,** ol-an., ***op.,*** **PHOS.,** ***puls.,*** rat., rhod., **RHUS-T.,** ***sang.,*** sarr., sec., ***seneg.,*** **SEP.,** ***sil.,*** **SPONG.,** squil., stel., stroph., sulfon., **SULPH., TER.,** ***thuj., verat-v.***
- afternoon - seneg.
- alternating with congestion of head - ***glon.***
- coldness of body, with - carb-v.
- desire to urinate, if not obeyed - **LIL-T.**
- excitement - ***phos.***
- exertion, after - ***spong.***
- exposure to cold air - cimic., ***phos.***
- lying down impossible - **CACT.**
- menopause, at - arg-n., **LACH.**
- menses, during - glon.
  - before - kali-c.
  - delayed - graph., nux-m., ***puls.***
  - suppressed, with - acon., calc., sep.
- morning - elaps, pall.
  - on waking - carb-v., phos., sulph.
- motion, after - ***spong.***
- night - ***ferr.,*** nit-ac., ***puls.***
- pregnancy, during - ***glon., nat-m., sep.***
- sea, bathing - ***mag-m.***
- sensation as of blood stopping - sabad., ***seneg.***
- sleep, during - mill., puls.
- urination, desire, if not attended to - lil-t.
- uterine hemorrhage, after - **AUR-M.,** ***chin., phos.***
- waking, on - **LACH.**
- walking in open air - mag-m., ***phos.***
- weakness and nausea - ***spong.***
- writing, after - am-c.

CONSTRICTION - **ACON.,** ***aesc.,*** aeth., ***agar.,*** ail., ***all-c., alum.,*** alumn., ambr., am-c., am-m., anac., ***ang., ant-t.,*** apis, aral., ***arg-n., arn.,*** **ARS.,** ***ars-h., ars-i., asaf.,*** asar., asc-t., aspar., **AUR.,** ***aur-m., bapt., bar-c.,*** **BELL.,** bism., ***bor.,*** bov., **BROM., BRY.,** bufo, **CACT.,** ***cadm-s.,*** cahin., **CALC.,** ***calc-p.,*** calc-s., ***camph.,*** cann-i., cann-s., canth., ***caps., carb-ac., carb-an., carb-o.,*** **CARB-S., CARB-V.,** carl., **CAUST.,** ***cham.,*** **CHEL.,** chin., chin-a., ***chlor.,*** chlol., ***cic., cimx.,*** cina, cinnb., clem., ***cocc., coc-c.,*** coff., ***colch., coloc.,*** **CON.,** cop., ***crot-c.,*** crot-h., ***crot-t., cupr.,*** cupr-s., cycl., ***dig.,*** dios., ***dros., dulc.,*** elaps, ***euph., ferr.,*** ferr-ar., ferr-i., ferr-p., gamb., ***gels.,*** gins., ***glon.,*** **GRAPH.,** ***hell., hep.,*** hydr-ac., ***hyos., hyper.,*** ictod., **IGN.,** ***iod., ip.,*** iris, jatr., ***kali-ar., kali-bi., kali-c., kali-chl.,*** kali-i., ***kali-n.,*** kali-p., kali-s., kreos., **LACH.,** ***lact.,*** lappa-a., lat-m., ***laur.,*** lec., ***led.,*** lith., **LOB., LYC.,** ***lycps., mag-c., mag-m., mag-p., manc.,*** mang., ***merc., merc-c.,*** merc-i-r., ***mez.,*** morph., mosch., mur-ac., ***naja, nat-a., nat-c.,*** **NAT-m.,** nat-p., ***nit-ac., nux-m., nux-v.,*** olnd., ***op.,*** osm., ox-ac., petr., ph-ac., **PHOS.,** phys., pic-ac., ***plat.,*** plb., podo., psor., ***puls.,*** ran-b., rat., ***rhod., rhus-t.,*** ruta., sabin., samb., ***sars.,*** **SENEG.,** ***sep.,*** **SIL.,** ***spig., spong.,*** squil., **STANN.,** ***staph., stram.,*** stront-c., stry., sulo-ac., **SULPH.,** sul-ac., sul-i., sumb., ***tab.,*** tarent., ter., thea., thuj., ***thyr.,*** tub., upa., verb., **VERAT.,** xan., zinc.
- afternoon - bapt., eupi., kali-n., lac-c., mag-c., nat-m., petr., ph-ac., sulph.
- alternating with
  - distension of abdomen - lyc.
  - drawing in occiput and nape of neck - kali-n.
  - pain in abdomen - ***calc.***
  - sudden expansion - sars.
- anger, from - ***cupr.***
- armor, as if from an - **CACT.,** ***crot-c.***
- arms, from bringing, together in front - ***sulph.***
- ascending - **ARS.,** ang., **CALC.,** led., ***mag-c.,*** nux-v.
- asthmatic - ang., ars., coff., ***led.,*** mez., naja, nux-v., sulph.
- band, as from - **ACON.,** aeth., ***aml-n.,*** anag., arag., ***arg-n., ars.,*** bry., **CACT.,** chlor., helon., ign., led., ***lob., lyc.,*** op., **PHOS.,** pic-ac., sil., stann., sulph., zinc.
  - walking, on - cocc.
  - yawning, with - stann.
- belching, amel. - lyc., mag-c.
- bending, backwards - nit-ac.
  - backwards, amel. - caust.
  - forward - dig.
- breakfast, after - agar., sulph.
- breathing, agg. - bor.
- breathing deep, during - agar., aspar., ***caust.,*** cham., ***cic., coc-c.,*** dulc., euon., ***ferr.,*** ham., kali-bi., kali-n., lact., lyc., mag-m., mosch., nat-c., nat-m., nux-v., ***puls.,*** sang., seneg., stry., ***sulph.,*** tab., tarax., thuj.
  - amel. - sulph.
  - must, to expand lungs - xan.
- burning - bism., mag-m.
- chill, during - ***ars., cimx., kali-c.,*** mez., **NUX-V.,** ***phos.***
- coat of mail, as from - chel.
- cold, from, air - bry., ***phos.,*** sabad.
  - bathing - nux-m.
  - becoming - mosch., ***phos.***
- convulsive - **ASAF., BELL., CUPR.**
- cough, during - am-c., calc., ***cham.,*** cimx., ***con., cupr., form., hell.,*** lyc., ***mag-p.,*** merc., ***myrt-c.,*** **PHOS.,** ***puls.,*** stram., ***sulph.***
  - amel. - con.
  - inclination to, from - ***sep.***
  - spasmodic, during - ***mosch.***
  - whooping, during - ***caust.,*** mur-ac., spong.
- covering of bed agg. - ***ferr.***
- crying, amel. - anac.
- daytime - mez., phos.
- dinner, after - am-m., carb-s., hep., phel.
- drawing, shoulders back amel. - **CALC.**
- drinking, after - ***cupr.***
- eating, after - arn., carb-an., cupr., hep., phel., ***puls.,*** sil.
  - amel. - sulph.

CONSTRICTION,

evening - ***ars., bry.,*** calc-p., carb-s., carb-v., hyper., kali-n., lyc., mag-c., phos., ***puls.,*** raph., rhus-t., sep., ***stann.,*** sulph., verb., ***zinc.***
bed, in - ***ars.,*** bell., verb.
exertion, from - ***ars., calc.,*** ferr., ***nat-m.,*** nux-v., ***spong., verat.***
expectoration amel. - ***calc., manc.***
expiring, during - bor., ***caust.,*** chel., ***kali-c.***
falling asleep, when - bry., ***graph., lach.***
fever, during - sep.
flatulence, from - lyc., **NUX-V.,** ***rheum,*** sil.
forenoon - kali-n.
heart disease, acute rheumatic - asaf.
hot - bism.
hydrothorax, in - ***apis,*** apoc., asaf., colch., lact., merc., psor., ***spig.,*** stann.
inspiration, during - agar., asaf., aspar., cham., chel., con., dros., mez., raph., sabad., seneg., ***sulph.***
lumbar, pain, from - lyc.
lungs, as with a wire - asar.
lying, while - aral., lach., nat-m., nux-v.
amel. - ***calc-p.***
head high amel. - ***ferr.***
on left - myric.
on right, agg. - ***lycps.***
quiet agg. - caps.
manual labor, from - ***calc.***
menses, during - sep.
before - phos.
morning - ***arg-n.,*** calc., carb-v., cycl., lyc., nat-m., phos., ***puls.,*** sars., sep.
fasting - sulph.
lying - kali-n.
waking, on - dig., sep.
motion, agg. - agar., ang., ***ars.,*** caps., ***ferr., led.,*** lyc., nux-v., ***spong., verat.***
motion, amel. - ***seneg.***
night - alum., aral., ***bry.,*** coloc., ***ferr.,*** kali-n., ***lach., mez.,*** myric., ***puls.,*** seneg., sep., sil., stram., ***tab.***
bed, in - ***ferr., nux-v.***
noon - agar.
painful - dig., cupr., sars., ***sulph., verat.***
paroxysmal - sep.
perspiration, amel. - sulph.
sex, after - staph.
sit up, must - dig.
sitting, while - agar., ars., mag-c., mez., nit-ac.
amel. - nux-v.
bent - alum.
bent, amel. - lach.
sneezing - phos.
spasmodic - am-c., **ASAF.,** ***aur.,*** calc., carb-s., carb-v., ***caust., cupr.,*** glon., ***hep.,*** **IGN.,** ip., ***kali-c.,*** kali-p., lact., led., nat-m., ***op., phos.,*** sars., sec., ***sep., spong., sulph.,*** verat.
standing, while - am-m., kali-n., spig., verat.
amel. - mez.
stitching - spig.
stool, during - coloc.

CONSTRICTION,

stooping - alum., laur., merc., mez., seneg.
straightening up - sars.
amel. - mez.
stretching - nat-m.
sulphur, as from - kali-chl.
supper, after, agg. - mag-m., mez.
suppressed, foot-sweat, after - **SIL.**
swallowing - ***kali-c.***
talking, after - ***hep.***
preventing - ars., ***cact.***
touch agg. - arn., cupr.
upper part - ang., carb-an., cham., nit-ac., phos., rhus-t., spig., stann., tab.
vomiting, after - verat-v.
before - ***cupr.***
waking, on - alum., carb-v., cocc., dig., ***graph.,*** **LACH.,** ***lact.,*** seneg., sep.
after - dig., psor.
walking, while - am-c., ***anac.,*** **ARS.,** ang., ***dig.,*** ferr., ***jug-c., kali-c.,*** led., ***lyc.,*** mag-c., nit-ac., nux-v., puls., sil., sulph., ***verat.***
air, in open - am-c., ***calc.,*** lith., lyc., zinc.
air, in open, amel. - alum., chel., dros., ***puls.***
amel. - ferr.
rapid - ***puls.***
warmth, of bed amel. - phos.

constriction, lower part - aesc., agar., am-m., bry., **CACT.,** chlor., ***dros., gels., ham.,*** lact., lil-t., lycps., ***nux-v., puls., ran-b., spig., sulph.,*** thuj.
band, as from - agar., chlor., cocc., cupr., ***plat.,*** thuj.
lying on the right side agg. - lycps.

constriction, middle - cact., lob., ol-an.
evening, 6 p.m. - mag-c.
string, as from a - led.

constriction, sides - ***acon.,*** aeth., aloe, alum., asar., bell., carb-v., colch., kali-n., lil-t., lyc., meny., mez., myric., nat-m., nit-ac., plat., puls., sil., spig., thuj.
forenoon - nat-m.
inspiration, on - lyc.
left - graph., lyc., nat-m., plat., sep., sil., sul-ac., sumb., zinc.
straightening up - dig.
lying, down agg. - lil-t., plat.
one-sided - cocc., zinc.
right, side - am-m., cina, cocc., lyc., mag-m., nat-m., puls., sulph., zinc.
sitting, while - nit-ac.
turning, body - nat-m.
right to - euph.

constriction, sternum - acon., cann-s., lob., mur-ac., nux-m., ***phos.,*** puls., rhus-t., sabin., staph., sulph., zinc.
breathing, hindered - mur-ac.
coughing, on - **PHOS.**
eating, while - led.
motion, on - **CACT.,** op.

CONVULSIONS - acon., ang., **ARS.,** bell., ***calc.,*** cic., **CUPR.,** ***hydr-ac.,*** hyos., ip., merc-n., ***nat-s.,*** op., phos., sep., stram., stry., sul-ac., verat.
night - phos., sep.
waking, on - ***ars.***

CRACKING, sternum, in, on bending chest backwards - am-c.
motion, on - nat-m., sulph.

CRAMP - alumn., arg-n., ars., asaf., bell., bov., cact., calc., ***cocc.,*** coff., con., cupr., dig., ***ferr.,*** graph., ham., ign., iod., ***kali-c.,*** kali-i., lact., ***lyc., mez.,*** mosch., nit-ac., nux-m., nux-v., ***petr., plat.,*** plb., puls., rad-br., sang., ***sars.,*** sec., sep., ***sulph.,*** tab., tarent., vip., ***zinc.***
air, open - iod.
belching - dig.
coughing, on - ***kali-c.,*** laur.
eating, after - nat-m.
pork, after - ham.
evening - phos.
riding, while - phos.
warm room, in a - sulph.
exertion, after - plb.
lying, down amel. - sulph.
menses, during - ***cocc.***
motion, agg. - ferr., sulph.
night - alum., lyc., phos., sep.
1:30 a.m. - nat-a., sep.
walking - ***ferr.***
warm, room, in - ***sulph.***

CRAMPY, pain - aesc., ***cact., cocc.,*** lact., mez., petr., ***puls., sang., spong.***
belching, amel. - kali-c.
blowing, nose, on - sumb.
cough, with - bell., kali-c., laur.
eating, after - petr.
forenoon, 10 to 11 a.m. - aesc.
menses, during - ***cocc.***
morning, 5 a.m., with cough - kali-c.
night - kali-c., nit-ac.
sleep, during - bell.
waking, from - nit-ac.
sitting - mez.
stooping, amel. - petr.
walking, air, in open, while - mez.
amel. - mez.
crampy, sternum - dig.
belching amel. - phos.
bending, forward agg. - dig.

CRUSHING, sternum, behind on ascending - **AUR., AUR-M.**

CUTTING, pain - ***acon.,*** aloe, ang., ***ant-t., apis,*** arg-m., ***ars.,*** ars-i., ***asc-t., aur., bad.,*** bapt., ***bell.,*** benz-ac., bov., ***bry., cact.,*** cahin., ***calc., calc-p.,*** calc-s., cann-s., carb-s., carb-v., cedr., chel., chin-s., cimic., ***colch.,*** con., crot-c., dig., ***dios.,*** dros., dulc., glon., hell., hyos., ***iod.,*** kali-ar., **KALI-C.,** ***kali-i., kali-n.,*** kali-s., lac-ac., laur., led., ***lyc., mag-c.,*** manc., mang., ***merc.,*** merc-i-r., ***mur-ac.,*** nat-a., nat-c., **NAT-M.,** nat-p., ol-an., petr., phos., plb., ***psor., puls., ran-b.,*** rat., rhus-v., ***rumx.,*** ruta., sabin., seneg., sep., spig., spong., ***stann.,*** stry., ***sulph.,*** sumb., tab., tarax., thuj., verat., xan., zinc.
afternoon - bad.
anterior part - colch., coloc., dulc.
below clavicle - dulc.
bending forward - arg-m.
amel. - chin-s.
chill, after - **ACON.**
before - ars.
coughing - ***bry.,*** calc., colch., kali-n., lachn., mag-c., mag-s., mang., ***nat-m.,*** nat-n., ox-ac., raph., ***sulph.***
eating, after - ***nux-v.,*** sumb.
erect, on becoming, from stooping - aloe
evening - bad., cahin., **KALI-C.,** kali-i., kali-n., ***mag-c.,*** nicc., ol-an.
evening, after lying down - **KALI-C.**
extending to, abdomen - berb.
liver - ran-b., upa.
pit of throat - thuj.
scapula - **NAT-M.**
shoulders - ox-ac., ***verat.***
upward - stann.
flatus, as from - dulc., kali-c.
inspiration - ***asc-t.,*** aur., **BRY.,** ***calc.,*** con., ***guar.,*** hell., naja, phos., stann.
deep - bapt., com., kali-n., naja, spong.
lower, part - ***kali-c., ox-ac.,*** stry.
dragging feeling - phos.
extending to abdomen - kali-c.
lying on, left side agg. - ***phos.***
right side agg. - ***kali-c.***
with arms close to side amel. - lac-ac.
middle, of chest, amel. in p.m. - mag-c.
extending to abdomen - berb., sulph.
morning - caust., **KALI-C.**
moving, on - kali-c.
motion, agg. - bad., **BRY.,** chin-s., lac-ac., ox-ac.
amel. - phos.
arms, of - ***asc-t.,*** sumb.
night - ***syph.***
when bending to the right - rhod.
respiration, during - arg-m., bapt., ***colch.,*** raph.
short ribs - sulph.
sitting, amel. - alum.
bent - chin.
smoking, while - merc.
stooping, on - ***asc-t.***
upper part through apex of both lungs - elaps, ind.
walking amel. - elaps.
walking fast - alum.
air, in open, after - sulph.
cutting, clavicles - calc-p., ruta.
above - bad.
below - dulc., kali-c.
pressure amel. - dulc.
cutting, costal cartilages of short ribs - arg-m.
inspiration, on - cimic.
intercostal muscles - bor., kreos., ***mez.***
cutting, ribs - stann.

cutting, sides - all-s., ang., arg-m., aur., cedr., ***con.,*** dulc., hura, kali-c., kali-n., laur., nat-a., ph-ac., plb., sumb.
bending backward - rhod.
coughing - nat-m.
evening - mang.
inspiration - ***asc-t.,*** aur., con., thuj.
deep - arg-m., ph-ac., spong., sumb., tab.
left - ***agar.,*** arg-m., ars-h., ***asc-t.,*** aur., ***brom., calc.,*** colch., dulc., kali-c., lac-c., ***lil-t.,*** lyc., manc., **NAT-M.,** ***ox-ac.,*** ph-ac., polyg., rhod., rumx., spig., spong., stann., sumb., tarent., verat.
coughing, when - ox-ac.
extending to scapula - **NAT-M.**
noon - rumx.
right - agar., aur., bell., cahin., chin-s., colch., con., guar., iod., lyc., sang., sep., stann., thuj., trom.
coughing when - colch., lachn.
bending to left - petr.
right, to left - petr.
side to side - ***cimic.***
sitting - ph-ac.
standing - stann.
still amel. - thuj.
walking - stann., thuj.
cutting, sternum - ***calc-p.,*** manc., nat-c., petr., phos., rhus-v., stram., verb.
behind, cough, during - kali-n.
swallowing - cann-i.
emission, of flatus amel. - stram.
extending, to right scapula - phos.
to spine - dulc.
inspiration, amel. - nat-c.
motion, amel. - nat-c.
night, on lying down - stram.

CYANOSIS, (see Lungs) - ***ant-t., bor.,*** carb-an., ***dig., ip.,*** **LACH., LAUR.**
region of clavicle - thuj.

DECAY, clavicles - sil.
decay, sternum - con.

DIGGING, pain - acon., cann-s., carb-an., carb-s., cina, **DULC.,** lach., mang., meny., olnd., petr., seneg., stann., stram., tarax.
extending to abdomen - stann.
motion, amel. - ***seneg.***
night - graph.
digging, clavicles - mang.
digging, sternum - led.

DIAPHRAGM, general
cramping, pain - lyc., nat-m., nux-v., stann., verat., verat-v., zinc.,
drawing, pain, region of - agar.
inflammation, of - acon., atro., bell., bism., ***bry., cact., cupr.,*** dulc., ham., ***hep.,*** hyos., ign., mosch., ***nux-m., nux-v., ran-b., stram., verat.,*** verat-v.
rheumatism, in - ***bry.,*** cact., ***cimic.,*** spig., stict.

DIAPHRAGM, general
neuralgic, pain - bell., stann.
oppression, in region of - ***agar.***
pain, region of - echi., nux-m.
forenoon - nux-m.
inspiration - nux-m.
painful and inflammed - asaf., bism., ***bry.,*** cact., ***cimic.,*** nat-m., nux-v., sec., spig., ***stann.,*** stict., ***stry.,*** verat., zinc-oc.
paralysis - bell., cact., cimic., cupr., mosch., rhus-t., mez., sil.
pressing, pain - **IP.**
sharp, pain, on speaking - ptel.
spasms, of - ***bell., chel.,*** cic., cupr., gels., ***lob., mosch.,*** oena., ph-ac., staph., stram.

DISCOLORATION, of
blueness clavicle, near - ***ars., cupr.,*** lach., thuj.
copper, colored - stram.
livid - ars.
redness - am-c., aster., aur., bar-c., bell., chin-s., ***graph.,*** iod., kali-ar., ***lac-c.,*** rhus-t., rhus-v., sulph., tarax., vesp.
blotches - apis, chlol., cinnb.
burning - am-m., mez.
coppery - stram.
erythematous - ***apis.***
itching - am-m.
redness, spots - am-m., ant-c., arn., ***bell.,*** cinnb., cocc., led., mag-c., manc., ***merc.,*** mez., puls., raph., sil., sabad., tab.
spots - am-c., am-m., ars., ***bell.,*** carb-v., cinnb., cocc., crot-c., ***crot-h.,*** ery-a., ip., ***lach.,*** **LED.,** lyc., ***mag-c.,*** mez., ***nit-ac.,*** **PHOS.,** phyt., sabad., ***sep.,*** squil., sulph., vip.
black, mottled - vip.
brown - cadm-s., ***carb-v., lyc., mez., petr., phos.,*** **SEP.,** thuj.
brown, breasts, on - cadm-s., carb-v., lyc., phos., ***sep.***
brown, itching - hydr., lyc., sulph.
dark - phos.
ecchymoses - ***lach.,*** phos., ***sul-ac.***
freckles - nit-ac.
itching - nit-ac.
liver - **LYC.**
mottled - **CROT-H., LACH.,** naja, vip.
yellow - ars., ***phos.***
yellow, become dark - mez.
yellow, itching in the evening - sulph.

DISTENSION - ars., bell., benz-ac., cadm-s., carb-v., **LACH.,** lil-t., petr., rhus-t., thuj., vip.
convulsions, during - ars.
distension, sensation, of - alum., ***ars.,*** brom., cadm-s., caps., chin., coca, olnd., sil., stann., ter., thuj., zinc.
breathing, on - bry.
cough, from - tarent.

DRAWING, pain - abrot., acon., agar., ***anac.,*** arn., asaf., aster., aur-m., ***bor., cadm-s.,*** camph., ***caps.,*** carb-v., ***cham.,*** chel., ***chin.,*** com., con., crot-t., dig., dulc., euon., ***ferr.,*** iod., ***kali-c.,*** lact., lyc., ***mur-ac.,*** nit-ac., **NUX-V.,** olnd., petr., plat.,

DRAWING, pain - ***seneg.,*** sep., squil., ***stann.,*** stront-c., zinc., zing.
afternoon - chel.
anterior part - berb., card-m., carl., com., dulc.
midnight - chel.
pectoral muscles - berb., card-m.
chilliness, during - sep.
coughing - caps., crot-t., dig., merc.
crampy - nit-ac.
downward, on expiration - am-c.
downward, standing - am-c.
evening - nat-c.
evening, in bed - cahin., con.
7 p.m. agg. - zing.
when lying on the left side - cahin.
extending, across - kali-c.
back and forth - apis.
before backwards, from - ***aster.***
to groins - plat.
to lower jaw - apis
to arms - ***aster.,*** com.
to axilla - aur., seneg.
umbilicus - chel.
upward - lach., mang.
external - bry., cadm.
inspiration, on - calad., ***camph.,*** lact., led., raph., stann.
deep - zing.
inward - cham.
lower, chest - arg-m., chel., mang., verat.
lying, on side, while - con.
menses, during - ***sep.***
morning - nat-c.
bed, in - lact.
bed in, after rising agg. - lact.
motion, from - abrot., seneg.
paroxysmal - nit-ac., stront.
pulse, synchronous, with - iod.
sitting, while - ***chin.***
standing, while - calc., spig.
amel. - ***chin.***
walking - lact., led.
amel. - ***chin.***
fast - seneg.

drawing, clavicles - caps., coc-c., led., sars., stann., tarax., zinc.
below - brom., chel., zinc.
left - coc-c.
right - com.
extending to tips of fingers - caps.

drawing, costal cartilages - stann.
ribs - cupr., stann.
false right - sep.

drawing, sides - agar., aur-m., berb., bor., bry., cadm-s., ***caps.,*** chel., cocc., kali-bi., led., petr., rhus-t., sil., spong., thuj.
afternoon - alum.
bending to right - cocc.
breathing, on - puls.
coughing - caps.
evening - seneg.
extending to, abdomen - chel.
axilla - card-m., meny., sil.
back - chel., zinc.

drawing, sides
extending, fingers - com.
hypogastrium - stann.
neck - caps., mur-ac.
scapula - brom.
shoulder joint - cact.
submaxillary gland - ***calc.***
left - anac., brom., cact., calad., ***calc.,*** card-m., cic., clem., dulc., mang., med., petr., phos., ruta, stann., sul-ac., zinc.
morning - lil-t., nux-v., sang.
motion, amel. - sep.
right - asar., ***bell.,*** bor., cham., cocc., com., dig., meny., mur-ac., ruta., sang., ***stront-c.,*** sul-ac., thuj.
rubbing, amel. - sep.
sitting - china., nit-ac.
walking - cocc.

drawing, sternum - dig., dulc., nit-ac. puls.
behind - chin.

DRAWN, toward back, chest feels - ind., syph.
heart, downwards - thuj.
lungs, downwards - am-c.

DROPSY - acet-ac., ***adon., am-c., ant-t.,*** **APIS, APOC., ARS.,** ***ars-i., asaf., aspar., aur-m.,*** **BRY.,** calc., ***canth., carb-s., carb-v.,*** chin., chin-a., **COLCH.,** ***crot-h., dig., dulc.,*** ferr-m., ***fl-ac.,*** **HELL.,** ***iod., kali-ar.,*** **KALI-C.,** ***kali-i., lach., lact.,*** **LYC.,** ***merc.,*** **MERC-SUL.,** mez., mur-ac., ***nat-m.,*** op., phase., phos., piloc., ***psor., ran-b.,*** rat., ***sang., seneg., sil., spig., squil.,*** stann., ***sulph., ter.,*** tub., uran-n., visc., ***zinc.***
asthma, with - psor.
disease, with organic - ***apoc.,*** spig.
side, can lie only on, affected side - ***ars.***
left side - visc.
right side with head low - ***spig.***

DRYNESS - alum., con., ***ferr.,*** kali-chl., ***lach., merc.,*** osm., phos., ***puls.,*** stram., zinc.

DULL, pain in sternum - mang.

ECZEMA - anac., ***calc.,*** calc-s., ***carb-v.,*** cycl., **GRAPH.,** hep., kali-s., ***petr.,*** **PSOR., SULPH.**

EMACIATION - kali-i., petr., senec.
emaciation, clavicles, under - tub.

EMPTINESS, sensation of - all-s., aspar., bov., ***calad.,*** carb-an., chin., chr-ac., ***cocc.,*** crot-t., ferr-ma., graph., ***guare., ign., kali-c.,*** med., nat-p., nat-s., olnd., ph-ac., phos., phyt., plat., rhus-t., sars., ***sep.,*** **STANN.,** sulph., vinc., zinc.
cough, during - ***sep., stann.,*** sulph.
after - ill., kali-c., nat-s., sep., stann., zinc.
eating, after - nat-p., olnd.
expectoration, after - calad., ruta, ***stann., zinc.***
faint, feeling - sulph.
left - naja.
night - ***sep.***
palpitations, with - olnd.
sing, on beginning to - ***stann.***

emptiness, sensation of, sternum, behind - zinc.

ERUPTIONS - agar., ***alumn.,*** am-c., am-m., anac., ant-c., **ARS.,** arund., asar., ***bar-c.,*** berb., bov., cadm-s., ***calc.,*** calc-s., camph., cann-s., **CARB-AN.,** ***carb-s., carb-v., caust.,*** chel., chin., cic., ***cinnb.,*** cist., cocc., con., cycl., dulc., fl-ac., **GRAPH.,** ***hep.,*** hippoz., hydr., hydr-ac., hydrc., hyper., iod., jug-c., kali-ar., kali-bi., kali-br., ***kali-c., kali-i.,*** kali-s., lach., ***led., lyc.,*** mag-c., ***mag-m., merc-c.,*** mez., nat-a., nat-c., nat-p., ***nat-s.,*** **PETR.,** ph-ac., ***phos.,*** plb., **PSOR.,** puls., rhus-t., ***sep.,*** sil., staph., stram., **SULPH.,** ***syph.,*** tab., thuj., urt-u., valer., zinc.

- blisters, blood - ***ars.***
- blotches - nat-c., sars.
- burning - alum., bov., ***cic.,*** mez., ***rhus-t.***
- crusts - anac., ars., ***fl-ac., hep., mez., nat-s.***
- desquamating - ***led.,*** mag-c., mez., sulph.
- dry - ***carb-v., petr.,*** **PSOR.,** ***sep., sulph.***
- hay, causes - ***graph.***
- itching - cann-s., ***graph.,*** led., ***rhus-t.,*** stram., urt-u.
- miliary - hydrc., mez.
- painful - lyc.
- pimples - am-m., ***ant-c.,*** arg-n., ***ars.,*** berb., bor., bov., calc., cann-s., canth., chin., cinnb., ***cist.,*** cocc., con., dulc., fl-ac., ***graph., hep.,*** hura, hyper., iod., kali-ar., ***kali-c., lach.,*** led., mag-m., mez., nat-a., nat-c., nat-p., ph-ac., plb., puls., ***rhus-t.,*** squil., staph., stront-c., tab., valer., verat., zinc.
  - acne - bar-c.
  - angry - sep.
  - bleed easily - ***cist.***
  - burning - agar., bov., staph.
  - elevated - valer.
  - flattening - rhus-t.
  - hard - bov., valer.
  - hard, under the skin - alum.
  - indolent - cund.
  - itching - ant-c., cann-s., dulc., gins., iod., mag-m., nat-c., tab.
  - painful - cist.
  - painful, on touch - con.
  - pointed with whitish semi-transparent vesicles, on - bry.
  - red - am-c., apis, arund., bov., cocc., iod., ***mez.,*** ph-ac., plb., stram., zinc.
  - red, evening - ph-ac.
  - red, like lichen simplex - ant-t.
  - white - valer.
  - white, red areola, with - bor.
- pustules - agar., ***ant-t., ars.,*** arund., asar., aur., bar-c., ***calc.,*** chel., chlor., cocc., euon., fl-ac., graph., ***hep.,*** hydr., ***hydrc.,*** kali-bi., kali-s., mag-m., merc-c., petr., ***psor., rhus-t., sil.,*** stront.
- red - mag-c., ***merc.,*** merc-i-f., ust., valer., vip.
  - red, coppery - merc., stram.
- roseola after abuse of mercury - ***kali-i.***
- spring, every - ***nat-s.***
- yellow, scaly, itching spots - kali-c.

EXOSTOSES, on - merc-c.

EXPANSION, of vessels, sensation - asaf.

FALLING, sensation of something, forward in chest when turning in bed - bar-c., sulph.

- drops were, in the chest - thuj.

FLUCTUATION, feeling of - plb.

FLUTTERING, in (see Heart, chapter) - naja, nat-m.

FOREIGN body, sensation, ascending - zinc.

FORMICATION - acon., alum., am-m., ars., arund., cadm-s., cahin., ***carl.,*** chin., coloc., cycl., guai., mag-m., ***ran-s., seneg., sep.,*** thuj., urt-u.

- house, on entering - phos.
- warm, food - ***mez.***
  - room - ***mez.***

formication, clavicles, region of - alum., arund., mez.

formication, sternum - ***ran-s.***

FULLNESS - **ACON.,** aesc., agar., ***ail.,*** aml-n., **APIS,** arg-n., ***ars.,*** arum-t., ***asaf.,*** aster., ***aspar., bar-c.,*** benz-ac., brom., bry., ***cact.,*** cadm-s., calc., calc-ar., ***canth., caps., carb-s., carb-v.,*** carl., caust., chin., ***cist., coff.,*** colch., con., cop., croc., ery-a., ***ferr.,*** ferr-ar., ***ferr-p., gels.,*** gent-l., ***glon., hydr.,*** ign., ***kali-bi.,*** **LACH.,** lact., lil-t., lyc., ***lob.,*** med., merc., mosch., ***nat-a.,*** nat-m., nat-p., ***nit-ac., nux-m.,*** nux-v., ***phos., puls., rhus-t.,*** rumx., ruta., sabin., sang., sac-alb., sel., sep., spong., ***sulph.,*** sul-ac., sumb., tax., ter., verat.

- afternoon - alumn., coca
- air, open - lyc.
- ascending - bar-c.
- belching, incomplete from - ang.
- coffee, after - ***canth.***
- eating, after - ant-c., caps., ***lyc.***
- evening - ***carb-v.,*** eupi., lact., **PULS.,** ***sulph.***
  - 5 p.m. - phos.
  - eating, after - alumn.
  - in bed - ***nat-s.,*** sulph.
- exertion, during - nat-a.
- expectoration amel. - ***ail.,*** calc.
- forenoon, walking, while - acon.
  - writing, while - fl-ac.
- inspiration, deep - kali-n., nat-a., sulph.
- menses, before - brom., **SULPH.**
- morning - calc., con., lyc., ***sulph.***
  - smoking, after - cycl.
  - waking - ph-ac.
- noon - lyc.
- sitting - anac., ***caps.***
- urinate, desire to, if delayed - **LIL-T.**
- waking - con., ph-ac.
- walking - ferr., verat.

GNAWING, pain - calc., calc-p., ***colch.,*** mang., mosch., nat-m., ran-s., ruta.

gnawing, clavicles - acon., mang.

gnawing, costal cartilages of short ribs - bell.

gnawing, sides, in - lil-t., olnd.

- left - arg-m., calc., ruta., stann.
- right - ruta.

gnawing, sternum - par.

GRIPING, pain - aesc., ***cact.***, ***caul.***, cast., cocc., ***dig.***, ***graph.***, ***nit-ac.***, pall., plat., spig., sulph., zinc.
- afternoon - sulph.
  - walking, while - sulph.
- coughing, when - ***sulph.***
- inspiration agg. - cina, mur-ac.
- left - cina, graph., upa.
- lying amel. - graph.
- menses, during - ***cocc.***
- right - acon., bov., coloc., mur-ac., sulph., verat.
- sitting, while - graph.
- standing amel. - graph.
- warm food, amel. - sulph.

griping, sternum - puls.
- behind, sternum - ***cact.***, led.

GURGLING, breathing, when - cina, ind., mur-ac.

gurgling, side, right - nat-m.

HEAT - acet-ac., **ACON.**, aesc., all-c., alum., am-c., am-m., anac., ***ant-t.***, ***apis***, aral., arg-n., ***arn.***, **ARS.**, ars-h., arund., asaf., aster., aur., aur-m-n., bar-m., **BELL.**, bism., bov., ***brom.***, ***bry.***, ***calc.***, ***calc-p.***, canth., carb-s., **CARB-V.**, cast., caust., cham., chin., chlol., ***cic.***, cist., clem., cocc., cop., crot-t., dig., dros., ***elaps***, eup-per., euph., ***ferr.***, ferr-ar., ferr-i., ferr-p., glon., grat., helo., ***hep.***, hyos., hyper., iod., ***kali-c.***, kali-m., kreos., ***lach.***, lachn., lact., ***lil-t.***, lith., ***lyc.***, mag-m., manc., mang., ***med.***, meny., merc., merc-sul., mez., myris., naja, nat-m., nit-ac., ***nux-v.***, ol-an., ol-j., ***op.***, osm., paeon., petr., **PHOS.**, plb., prim-v., ***psor.***, puls., ran-s., rat., rhus-t., rumx., ruta, samb., ***sang.***, ***sars.***, sel., ***seneg.***, ***sep.***, sil., spig., ***spong.***, ***stann.***, **SULPH.**, tax., tep., thuj., ***tub.***, ust., verat., verat-v., wye., zinc.
- afternoon, 1 p.m., on ascending a hill - clem.
  - 1 to 3 p.m. - plan.
  - 2 p.m. - hura.
  - 2:30 p.m. - laur.
  - walking, while - thuj.
- alternating with pain on internal surface of thigh - coc-c.
- bed, in - sars.
- burning - apis, paeon., puls., raph., ***sulph.***
- chill, during - sars., sil.
- cold, hands icy - thuj.
  - stomach, sensation - polyg.
- coughing, agg. - iod., phos., seneg., spong., thuj.
- desire to urinate be delayed, if - lil-t.
- eating, after - clem., sel.
- evening - mang., puls.
- excited talking, on - phos.
- expectoration, amel. - cham.
  - bloody, with - psor.
- external - dig., phos., thuj.
- flushes - alum., arg-n., bism., clem., ***coc-c.***, ***cupr.***, ***ferr.***, ***glon.***, kali-n., lact., ***lil-t.***, merc., nit-ac., nux-v., ol-an., ***phos.***, plb., rhod., **SENEG.**, ***sep.***, ***spong.***, **SULPH.**, ***thuj.***, yohim.
  - rising, to face - **SULPH.**
  - rising, to head - glon.

HEAT,
- glowing - bell., lach., ***spong.***
- hot stream, as of - kreos., merc., sang.
- inspiration, on - laur.
- left, on walking in sun, right cold - ***med.***
- morning, waking, on - apis, nat-m., sulph.
- motion, on - ***spong.***
- night - ant-c., arg-n., carb-an., sars.
- nosebleed, with - thuj.
- rising from stooping, on - rhus-t.
  - rising up - caust., ***sulph.***, thuj.
- siesta, after - clem.
- sleep, during - arg-n.
- smoking, agg. - cic.
- smoking, on - spong.
- speaking - phos.
- walking - naja.
  - air, in open - rhus-t.
  - air, in open, after - stann.
  - sun, in the - med.
- water, as if hot, poured into, abdomen from chest before stool - sang.
  - as if hot, poured into, lungs - acon., ***hep.***

heat, sternum - bell.

HERPES - ***ars.***, ***graph.***, ***hep.***, lyc., mag-c., ***petr.***, ***staph.***, ***syph.***
- herpes zoster - ars., dol., graph., lach., mez., nat-m., ran-b., ***rhus-t.***

IMMOVABLE - **PHOS.**

ITCHING - agar., ***alum.***, alumn., ***ambr.***, am-m., anac., ang., **ANT-C.**, arg-n., arn., ars., ars-i., arund., aster., bar-c., berb., bor., ***bov.***, bufo, cact., ***calc.***, calc-s., caps., carb-s., carb-v., caust., chel., chin., cic., clem., cocc., con., corn., dios., fl-ac., iod., jug-r., kali-ar., kali-bi., kali-br., kali-c., kali-n., kali-p., kali-s., ***lyc.***, mag-m., manc., merc-i-f., ***mez.***, nat-c., nat-m., nat-n., nit-ac., op., phos., phyt., puls., rhus-t., sep., sil., spong., stront-c., **SULPH.**, ***til.***, thuj., ***urt-u.***
- afternoon - nicc.
- air, in open - nat-m.
- biting - ***laur.***, spong.
  - cold agg. - nicc.
- burning, after - agar.
- evening - am-m., cact., chin., mez., stront-c., ***sulph.***
  - walking, while - fl-ac.
  - warm in bed, on becoming - puls., rhus-v.
- extending to nose - con., ***ip.***
- fleas as from - alum., cact., nat-c., led.
- morning - brom.
  - bed, in - rhus-t.
- night - ant-c., lith.
- scratching, agg. - con.
  - amel. - alum., nicc., phos.
  - returns after - berb., bov., chin., grat., mez., squil.
- spots, in - aster., nit-ac.
- sticking - caps., con., staph.
- tingling and - con.
- warm, when - bov., cocc.

itching, clavicles, region of - nicc.
- scratching, amel. - grat.

JERKING, pain - calc-p., con., lac-c., spig.

JERKS - ***agar.,*** anac., arg-m., calc-p., cina, ***con.,*** lyc., spong., squil., valer.

breathing, when - lyc.

moving the arm - anac.

night - am-c.

LOOSE, sensation - bry., rhus-t.

coughing on - kali-n.

flesh, as if, were loose - squil.

LUMPS, sensation of - ambr., am-m., ambr., ***anac.,*** cast., cic., cupr., ***kali-m.,*** lil-t., nat-c., nux-m., **PHOS.,** ***ran-s.,*** stict., sulph., tarax., thlaspi, zinc.

moving, up and down, swallowing empty, on - lil-t.

lumps, sternum, middle of - ***chin., puls.***

under - aur., bell., chin., echi., gels., lec., ***phos.,*** puls., ran-s., sil., thlaspi.

food, had lodged, as if - led., lyc.

MUCUS, in right - caust.

NAIL, deep in right - chel.

NARROW, as if too - agar., mez., seneg.

NAUSEA, felt in - rhus-t.

NECROSIS, sternum - con.

NODULES - ***bar-c., carb-an.,*** hippoz., hydr., ***merc-c.,*** nat-c., ***nat-s.***

sensitive - **CARB-AN.,** caust., mang.

NUMBNESS - bufo, carbn., chel., cupr-ar., ***glon.,*** graph., lat-m., merc., nux-m., physal., rhus-t., stict., urt-u.

and arm, down left - glon.

left - cupr-ar., ***cur.,*** plb.

right - chel.

numbness, clavicles - ferr.

OPEN, sensation as if - paull.

OPPRESSION - ***absin.,*** **ACON.,** ***aesc.,*** aeth., ***agar., ail., all-c., alum., alumn., ambr.,*** **AM-C.,** ***am-m., anac., ang., ant-c., ant-t.,*** **APIS, APOC.,** arag., ***arg-n., arn.,*** **ARS., ARS-I.,** ***asaf.,*** asar., asc-t., aspar., **AUR.,** aur-m., ***bapt.,*** bar-c., bar-m., **BELL.,** benz-ac., berb., bism., bor., ***bov.,*** brach., brom., **BRY.,** bufo, **CACT.,** cadm-s., cahin., ***calad.,*** **CALC.,** ***calc-ar., calc-s., camph., cann-s.,*** cann-i., canth., carb-ac., carb-an., **CARB-S., CARB-V.,** ***carl.,*** caul., ***caust., cedr., cham.,*** **CHEL.,** ***chin., chin-a.,*** **CHIN-S.,** chlol., chlor., chlf., ***cic., cimx., cina,*** cinnb., ***clem., cocc.,*** coc-c., ***coff.,*** **COLCH.,** ***coloc., con.,*** cop., cor-r., croc., **CROT-C.,** ***crot-h., crot-t.,*** **CUPR.,** ***cupr-ar., cupr-s., cycl., dig.,*** dor., ***dros., dulc., elaps,*** euon., ***eup-per.,*** **FERR., FERR-AR.,** ferr-i., ferr-p., ***fl-ac.,*** gamb., ***gels., glon., graph.,*** gran., grat., ***ham., hep.,*** hydr-ac., hydrc., hyos., hura, **IGN.,** ***iod.,*** **IP.,** jab., jug-c., jug-r., **KALI-AR., KALI-BI.,** kali-br., **KALI-C.,** kali-chl., ***kali-i.,*** kali-m., ***kali-n.,*** kali-p., ***kali-s., kalm., kreos., lach.,*** lachn., ***lact.,*** laur., led., lil-t., ***lob., lyc.,*** lyss., ***mag-c., mag-m.,*** mag-s., med., ***manc.,*** meli., meny., ***merc.,*** merc-c., merc-i-f., ***mez.,*** mill., mosch., mur-ac., ***mygal., naja,*** nat-a., nat-c., ***nat-m.,*** nat-p., **NAT-S.,**

OPPRESSION - ***nicc., nit-ac.,*** **NUX-M., NUX-V.,** ol-j., olnd., onos., ***op.,*** ox-ac., par., ***petr.,*** ph-ac., **PHOS.,** ***phyt., plat.,*** plb., podo., ***prun., psor.,*** **PULS.,** ***ran-b.,*** raph., rheum, rhod., ***rhus-t.,*** ruta., sabad., sabin., ***samb., sang.,*** sanic., sars., sec., **SEL., SENEG., SEP.,** ***sil., spig., spong.,*** squil., ***stann.,*** staph., stict., ***stram.,*** stront-c., stry., **SULPH.,** sul-ac., sumb., syph., ***tab., tarent.,*** teucr., ***thuj.,*** til., trinit., **TUB.,** valer., **VERAT.,** verat-v., verb., vesp., viol-o., viol-t., vip., xan., ***zinc.***

afternoon - agar., alum., bufo, caust., coloc., gels., lyc., nat-m., nicc., petr., ph-ac., seneg., staph., sulph., thuj.

2 p.m. - chin., sulph.

3 p.m. - am-c., arn.

4 p.m. - plan.

5 p.m. - med.

6 p.m. - chel.

sleep, after - calad.

air, cold, after sitting in - ***petr.***

in open - carb-s., ***lyc.,*** nux-v., ***psor.,*** seneg.

amel. - anac., chel., ***nat-m.,*** **PULS.,** sep.

alternating, with

back pain - sil.

headaches - glon.

palpitation after eating - alum.

urticaria - ***calad.***

anger, after - ***staph.***

anxiety, with - ***acon., dig.,*** ph-ac., phos., ***psor.***

ascending - **ACON.,** agn., apis, **ARS.,** bar-c., bufo, cact., **CALC.,** cann-i., ***elaps,*** gran., grat., lyc., ol-an., ran-b., ***seneg.,*** sulph., til.

bed, in - ***alum.,*** am-c., ***phos.***

belching, amel. - ***am-m.,*** **CARB-V.,** grat., ***lach.,*** **LYC.,** ***phos.***

bending, backward amel. - fl-ac.

backward amel., arm backward - **SULPH.**

forward amel. - ***colch.***

head forward agg. - **ALUM.**

breathing, on - chel., dulc., ferr., kali-c., kali-n., ***lyc., sil.,*** squil.

amel. - op., tab.

deep - agn., plb., ***lyc.***

changes, to cold, when weather changes - **ARS.**

chill, during - **APIS,** ars., ***bry.,*** cimx., daph., ***eup-per.,*** gels., ***ip., kali-c.,*** lach., merl., ***mez.,*** nat-m., ***puls.,*** sep.

clothing, agg. - **ARS.,** aur-m., bov., **CHEL., LACH.,** meli., ***merc-c.,*** mez., phos., ***sep.,*** tarent.

conversation, from - ***ambr.***

coryza, with - berb., ***calc., carb-v.,*** graph., lyc.

coughing, when - am-c., ***ars.,*** aur., bapt., **DROS.,** cocc., ***kali-bi., nit-ac.,*** **PHOS.,** ***psor., seneg., sil., stann.,*** **SULPH.,** tarent., ***verat.***

after - ars., cocc.

desires - am-c.

damp, weather - ***dulc., kali-c.,*** nat-s.

dancing, amel. - caust.

dinner, during - mag-m.

after - ***phos.,*** stram.

OPPRESSION,
drawing, shoulders back amel. - **CALC.**
drinking - cimx., ***verat.***
eating, after - alum., aran., ars., asaf., calad., ***caust.,*** chin., chin-s., chlol., cinnb., coloc., con., elaps, ip., lyc., ***mag-m.,*** nat-c., nat-s., ***nux-v.,*** ran-b., ***rhus-t.,*** ruta., sars., sil., stry., ***sulph.,*** thuj., ***verat.,*** viol-t., ***zinc.***
amel. - ambr.
erect, after rising, on sitting bent - nat-m.
evening - ***all-c.,*** am-m., ars., ***bry.,*** chin., clem., ***coloc.,*** crot-t., ***elaps,*** ferr., ferr-ar., hyper., lact., lyc., ***mag-c.,*** mur-ac., nat-c., nat-m., nux-m., nux-v., ***phos.,*** **PULS.,** ran-b., rhod., sars., seneg., **SEP.,** ***stann.,*** stront-c., sulph., ***zinc.***
9 p.m. - hura
bed, in - ***apis,*** bor., chel., ***chin., sep.,*** zinc.
sunset, after - nat-s.
expectoration, amel. - ***asaf.,*** calc., ***manc.***
expiration, during - am-c., anac., cina, chel.
amel. - staph.
fever, during - ***apis,*** ars., **BOV.,** cact., carb-v., cimic., elaps, ***ip.,*** **KALI-C.,** lach., ***nat-m.,*** plan., puls., sep.
flatus, as from - con., nat-c.
flatus, from - phos.
passing amel. - bry., ol-an.
upper abdomen, in - cham.
hang, down, unless his legs - ***sul-ac.***
headache, with - sep.
inspiration, on - asc-t., carc., cina, crot-t., ferr., ferr-m., graph., grat., ign., nat-a., ***phos.,*** **SPIG.,** zinc.
after - zinc.
amel. - acon., ***chel.,*** chin.
jerking - mez.
labor, during - ***chin-s.***
laughing - plb.
lying, while - alum., ambr., am-c., asaf., bar-c., cact., ***chin., colch.,*** fl-ac., ***graph., olnd., phos.,*** sabad., ***sep., spong., stann.,*** thuj.
affected side, on - phel.
amel. - alum., ***nat-s.,*** zinc.
back, on - alum., am-c., chin.
down - nat-m.
head low, with - ***chin.,*** **SPONG.**
left side, on - ***cact.,*** corn., magn-gr., naja, ***phos., puls.***
right side - kali-c.
menses, appearance of, on - phos.
menses, before - **BOR.,** ***lach.***
morning - ***alum.,*** am-m., ant-c., ***ars.,*** asaf., bapt., bry., calc-s., carb-v., chel., chin., ***ip.,*** lyc., mang., nat-c., ***nat-s.,*** nit-ac., ***nux-v., phos.,*** plb., ***psor., puls.,*** rhod., sars., **SEP.,** ***sulph.,*** sul-ac., zinc.
9 a.m. until 3 p.m. - sulph.
10 or 11 a.m. - cham.
forenoon - bry., calc., ***ip.,*** sulph., thuj.
rising, on - calc., clem., graph., verat., puls.
talking - bry., coc-c.

OPPRESSION,
motion, on - bapt., carl., led., nat-m., plb., ***stann.,*** sulph., tarent.
amel. - ***seneg.***
arm, of - am-m.
fast - **ACON., ARS.,** ***puls.***
night - ***alum.,*** ambr., ***apis,*** ars-m., ***aur.,*** aur-m., berb., ***bry., calc.,*** chin., ***coca, coloc.,*** gamb., ***lact.,*** lyc., nat-c., nat-s., nit-ac., ***nux-v., op.,*** petr., ph-ac., ***phos., rhus-t.,*** ruta., sars., sin-n., sulph.
2 a.m. - am-c., ***kali-bi.,*** lach.
3 a.m. - am-c., am-m., ant-t.
4 a.m. - chel., lil-t.
bed, in - am-m., ***nux-v.***
chill, during - ol-j.
dreaming - mag-m.
falling asleep - ***nux-m.***
midnight - ign., ***lach.***
before - ***coloc.,*** grat.
waking, on - cinnb., op.
painful - nat-m.
palpitation, with - ambr., glon., coca, grat., hyos., kali-n., ***phos.,*** sep., spig.
paroxysmal - mur-ac., sep.
perspiration, during - psor., sep.
pressure, of hand amel. - sep.
raising, arms agg. - tarent.
reclining, when - fl-ac.
rising, after - am-m.
amel. - olnd., nux-v.
as if something is, in the throat - stann.
from bed and walking about amel. - kali-bi.
sides - asaf., caust., mag-s., ***ox-ac.***
evening, while lying - calc.
left - arg-m., am-m., calc., crot-t., graph., samb., seneg., thuj.
right - acon., ***bry.,*** euph., mur-ac., staph.
upper - con.
sit up, must - sulph.
sitting - agar., anac., calad., carb-an., cham., cic., crot-t., kali-c., kali-n., mang., mez., ***nat-s.,*** phos., psor., sabad., staph.
amel. - alum.
erect, after sitting bent - nat-m.
motion, after - acon.
stooped - alum., coloc., dig.
sleep, during - all-s., **LACH.,** lact., nux-m.
before - berb.
falling asleep, on - ***nux-m.***
smoking - asc-t.
sneezing - sil., sulph.
standing - mang., olnd., phel., sep.
lower part of chest - am-m.
sternum, of - arg-n., ars., bry., calc., ***phos.,*** ran-s., rhus-t.
behind - ph-ac., samb., zinc.
eating, after - con., lac-ac.
night - am-c.
under, ascending agg. - aur.
stool, after - calc., **CAUST.,** sil.
stooping, when - alum., am-m., cop., mez., ***samb.***

OPPRESSION,
stormy, weather - **ARS.**
talking, while - ambr., **DROS.,** lach., nat-m., stram.
continued, from - ***chin.***
thinking, of it agg. - gels.
turning, in bed agg. - ***calc.***
vomiting, green amel. - ***cocc.***
waking, on - ***alum.,*** ant-c., ***ars., carb-v.,*** chin., ***cinnb., con.,*** kali-bi., **KALI-I.,** ***lach., lact., nat-s., nux-m.,*** op., phos., sep., tarent.
walking, while - agar., alum., aml-n., **ARS.,** bry., bufo, cact., calc., carb-an., chel., clem., colch., dig., ***kali-c.,*** led., lach., lyc., mag-s., mang., naja, olnd., paeon., ph-ac., phos., puls., ran-b., seneg., ***sep.,*** sil., staph., sulph., thuj., verat.
after - ***calc.,*** nux-m., **PHOS.**
air, in cool - ***lyc.,*** nux-m.
air, in open - am-c., am-m., ***aur.,*** calc., lact., lyc., ***phos.,*** spig., zinc.
amel. - ***alum.,*** anac., ***lyc.***
amel. by walking - gins., staph.
begining - ph-ac.
quickly - ang., **ARS.,** ***puls.,*** nat-m., nit-ac., ruta., ***spig.***
warm, room - alum., anac., **APIS,** ars-i., nat-m.
weather, changes to cold - **ARS.**
wine, amel. - acon.
writing, while - alum.
yawning, agg. - sulph.
amel. - croc.

ORGASM, of blood - acon., anac., alum., **AML-N.,** aur., bov., ***carb-v.,*** chel., chlor., colch., elaps, ***ferr.,*** **GLON.,** indg., iod., **LACH.,** lachn., ***lil-t.,*** mag-m., ***merc.,*** merl., ***mill.,*** nat-m., ***nit-ac.,*** ol-an., ph-ac., **PHOS.,** phyt., rhod., ***seneg.,*** **SEP.,** sil., **SULPH.,** ***thuj.***
evening - carb-v., kali-c.
exertion, least - **SPONG.**
flatus, from obstructed - carb-v.
left - sep.
menses, during - ***merl.***
morning - nux-v., sep.
motion, on - ***spong.***

PAIN, chest - abies-n., abrot., acal., ***acet-ac., acon., aesc., agar.,*** ail., all-c., alum., alumn., ambr., **AM-C.,** am-m., **AML-N., ANT-C.,** ***ant-t.,*** **APIS,** ***arg-m., arg-n.,*** **ARN., ARS.,** ars-i., arum-t., asc-t., **AUR., AUR-M.,** bapt., bar-c., ***bar-m.,*** **BELL.,** ***bism., bor.,*** brom., **BRY., CACT.,** ***cadm-s.,*** cahin., **CALC., CALC-P., CALC-S.,** camph., cann-i., cann-s., ***canth., caps., carb-an.,*** carb-s., ***carb-v., card-m.,*** cast., caul., **CAUST.,** ***cham., chel.,*** chin., chin-a., chin-s., chlor., ***cimic.,*** cina, ***cist.,*** colch., coll., coloc., com., con., corn., ***crot-c.,*** crot-h., crot-t., ***cupr.,*** cupr-ar., ***dig., dulc.,*** echi., elaps, erio., euon., ***eup-per.,*** euph., ***ferr., ferr-ar.,*** ferr-p., fl-ac., gels., gran., ***graph.,*** guai., ***hecla., hep.,*** hura, ***hydr.,*** hydr-ac., ictod., ign., ***iod.,*** ip., jab., jac., jug-c., just., kali-ar., kali-bi., ***kali-c.,*** kali-chl., ***kali-i.,*** kali-n., kali-p., kali-s., ***kalm.,*** kreos., ***lach.,*** lachn., ***lact., laur.,*** ***lob., lyc., mag-p.,*** mag-s., med., meli., meph., ***merc.,*** merc-i-f., merc-i-r., ***mez., mur-ac.,*** myris., ***myrt-c., naja,*** nat-a., nat-m., nat-p., nicc., nit-ac., ***nux-m., nux-v.,*** ol-an., ol-j., op., **OX-AC.,** paeon., ***ph-ac.,*** phel., **PHOS.,** ***phyt.,*** plan., plb., podo., ***psor., puls.,*** **RAN-B.,** ***ran-s.,*** raph., rhod., rhus-t., ***rumx.,*** sabad., ***sang., sars.,*** sec., senec., **SENEG.,** ***sep., sil.,*** sin-n., **SPIG., SPONG.,** ***squil.,*** **STANN.,** stict., ***stram.,*** stry-p., succ., ***sulph.,*** sul-ac., sumb., ***tab., tarent.,*** tep., ***ther.,*** tub., ***verat., verat-v.,*** verb., vinc., vip., visc., ***zinc.,*** zinc-s., ziz.
afternoon - am-m., bad., bar-c., canth., chel., coloc., eupi., fago., gamb., iod., kali-bi., kali-n., led., lyc., nicc., op., sang., sulph., tarent.
1 p.m. - sars.
2 p.m. - alum., chel., elaps, rhus-t.
3 p.m. - hura, nat-m., ol-an.
4 p.m. - asc-t.
4 to 5 p.m. right side - merc-sul.
6 p.m. lasting all evening - phos.
air, open amel. - nat-m.
alternating, with pain in
abdomen - aesc., ran-b.
stomach - ***caust.***
arms, near agg. - psor.
amel. - lac-ac.
ascending - acon., ars., bor., cact., crot-h., graph., kali-bi., ran-b., rat., sep., staph., stram.
bed, as from hard - bor.
belching, from - cocc., phos., staph.
amel. - ambr., ang., bar-c., canth., kali-c., lach., lyc., phos., sang., sep.
bending, backward - ars., bry., ***calc.,*** caps., carb-v., ***chel.,*** con., cupr., kali-bi., kali-i., lil-t., ***merc.,*** mez., nat-m., phos., rhod., sep., spig., ***sulph.,*** ther.
amel. - fl-ac.
forward - aloe, alum., alumn., arg-m., bor., brom., lact., nat-m., stann., sulph.
amel. - ***asc-t.,*** chel., chin-s., hyos., mag-c., **PULS.**
sideways agg. - acon., bor.
right - acon., ars., ***carb-v., chel.,*** dulc., guai., kali-bi., nit-ac., phel., phyt., rhod., sep., ***sulph.***
left - bry., kali-n., lil-t., ***lyc.,*** mur-ac., nat-m., phys., rhus-t., spig., sul-ac., ther.
blow, as from a - bor.
blowing nose - chel., sumb.
boots, putting on, agg. - arg-n.
breath, at every - am-m., arn., ***bry.,*** colch., menthol, nat-m., phos., ***ran-b.,*** seneg., sep., sil., sulph.
deep, agg. - nat-p.
amel. - chel.
breathing - acon., aesc., am-c., ***anac.,*** ant-t., arg-m., aur., bapt., **BOR.,** bov., **BRY.,** ***calc.,*** calc-p., cann-s., caps., card-m., ***cham.,*** chin., colch., crot-t., ***dig.,*** dros., elaps, **KALI-C.,** ***kali-p., kalm., kreos.,*** lob., ***lyc., manc.,*** meny., merc-sul., mez., mur-ac., nat-m., nicc., ph-ac., ***phyt.,*** **PSOR.,** raph., sabad., ***sep.,***

PAIN, chest

breathing - ***spig.,*** spong., squil., ***stann.,*** sulph., tab., verat.

deep - acon., aesc., aloe, arg-m., arn., bapt., bar-c., benz-ac., ***berb., bor.,*** **BRY.,** ***calc., calc-p.,*** carb-an., carb-v., ***caust.,*** chel., cob., crot-t., cycl., fl-ac., form., graph., ***guai.,*** hell., iod., ***kali-bi.,*** **KALI-C.,** ***kali-n.,*** lyc., merc-c., mez., mur-ac., naja, **NAT-M.,** nat-p., nit-ac., olnd., pall., ***phos.,*** ph-ac., phyt., plat., puls., **RAN-B.,** ran-s., raph., rhus-t., rumx., ***sang.,*** seneg., sil., ***spong., stann.,*** sumb., thuj., valer., zinc., zing.

amel. - ign., seneg., verb.

inspiration, during - **ACON.,** aesc., agar., alum., alumn., arg-m., arn., ***ars.,*** asaf., asar., aspar., aster., aur., aur-m., bapt., bar-c., **BOR., BRY.,** calad., **CALC.,** camph., canth., carb-an., carb-v., card-m., caust., ***cham., chel.,*** cina, clem., cocc., colch., coloc., com., con., cupr-ar., euon., ferr., ferr-p., grat., hyos., inul., iris, jatr., ***kali-ar.,*** kali-c., kali-n., kali-p., ***kreos.,*** lact., led., ***lyc., merc.,*** merc-sul., mez., mur-ac., ***naja,*** nat-m., nat-s., nicc., ***nux-m.,*** op., ***phos.,*** plat., plb., podo., ***psor., ran-b.,*** raph., rumx., sabad., samb., sang., ***seneg.,*** sep., ***sil., spig.,*** **SQUIL.,** stann., stront-c., sulph., sul-ac., tarax., tarent., thuj., valer., viol-t., zinc.

amel. - merc.

menses, before - puls.

sitting, while - chin.

carrying, a load, from - alum.

chill, during - ars., bell., **BRY.,** ***chin-s.,*** **KALI-C.,** lach., puls., ***rhus-t., sabad.,*** seneg.

chill, before - ars., plan.

chilliness, during - eupi., sep.

clothing, agg. - ars., ***caust.,*** chel., ***lach.***

cold, air - act-sp., ***calc-p.,*** petr., ***ph-ac.,*** ran-b.

air, amel. - ferr.

weather - petr., phos.

cough, during - ***acon.,*** aeth., ail., alum., ***ambr.,*** am-c., am-m., ***anac.,*** ant-c., ant-t., apis, arn., ars., aur., **BELL., BOR.,** brom., **BRY.,** ***calc., camph.,*** canth., caps., carb-an., **CARB-V., CAUST.,** ***cham.,*** chel., ***chin.,*** chin-a., cina, coff., ***con.,*** crot-t., cupr., ***dig.,*** **DROS.,** elaps, eupi., eup-per., ferr., ferr-ar., ferr-i., ferr-m., ferr-p., gels., iod., kali-ar., kali-bi., kali-c., kali-i., **KALI-N.,** kali-p., kreos., lach., led., **LYC.,** ***mag-m.,*** mang., meph., ***merc.,*** mez., mosch., mur-ac., naja, nat-a., nat-c., ***nat-m.,*** nat-n., nat-p., ***nat-s.,*** nit-ac., nux-m., nux-v., ol-j., ox-ac., petr., ph-ac., **PHOS.,** ***phyt.,*** psor., **PULS.,** ran-b., raph., ***rhus-t.,*** rumx., sabad., samb., ***sang.,*** sec., **SENEG.,** ***sep., sil.,*** spig., **SPONG., SQUIL., STANN.,** staph., stram., stront-c., **SULPH.,** tarent., upa., ***verat., zinc.,*** zing.

damp weather - ***cupr., kali-c.,*** **NAT-S.,** ***ran-b.,*** rhus-t., ***sil.,*** spig.

dancing, amel. - caust.

PAIN, chest

deep, in - all-c., arn., bry., dros., eup-per., kali-c., kreos.

desire to urinate be delayed, if - **LIL-T.**

dinner, after - bry., canth., cimic., carb-s., lob., mez., nat-p., rat., sulph., zinc.

drawing, on boots - arg-n.

shoulders back amel. - aster., calc., caust., mez.

drinking cold water, after - ***carb-v.,*** nit-ac., ***psor.,*** staph., thuj.

cold water, amel. - caust., cupr., phos., tab.

warm amel. - spong.

eating, while - kali-bi., led., ol-an.

after - alum., anag., arg-n., aspar., caust., chin., cimic., ***kali-c.,*** laur., mez., nat-c., nux-v., phos., sumb., sulph., thuj., verat., zinc.

amel. - anac., bism., chel., ferr., rhod., spong.

evening - acon., alum., ambr., ant-t., bad., bar-c., cahin., calad., calc., chel., coloc., dig., dios., euphr., gamb., hyper., kali-bi., **KALI-C.,** kali-i., kali-n., lyc., mez., mur-ac., nicc., nux-m., olnd., ***phos., ran-b.,*** ran-s., rumx., seneg., sulph., tab., thuj., verb., zinc.

6 p.m. - bry.

lasting until retiring - phos.

7 p.m. - ol-j., zing.

8 p.m. - canth., kali-n.

9 p.m. - lyss.

bed, in - benz-ac., cahin., ***kali-c.,*** nat-c., nit-ac., ran-b., sep.

excitement agg. - stann., stram.

exertion - alum., ang., caust., ferr., laur., plb., ran-b.

arms, with - ang., ant-c., led.

mental - cham., sep.

expanding, chest - carb-v.

expectoration, amel. - chel., euon., mag-s.

before - lyc.

expiration, on - chin., crot-t., spig., staph., tarax., ***viol-o.,*** zinc.

extending to

arms - ***alum.,*** bry., dig., dios., lat-m.

arms, right - phos.

downward - agn., kali-bi.

left - ***kali-c.,*** laur., phos., puls., squil., zinc.

right - dulc., nit-ac., sang., sep.

epigastrium - ox-ac.

forward - berb., bor., **BRY.,** cast., ***kali-c.,*** kali-n., psor., rat., ***sep.,*** sulph.

left - agar., bar-c., ***bry.,*** lac-c., naja, phos., ***sulph.,*** thuj., zinc.

right - acon., coloc., merc.

throat - apis, bell., calc., laur., phos., sulph., thuj., zinc.

transversely - caust., thuj.

upward - ars., calc., caust., lach., mang., mur-ac., thuj.

left - am-m., bov., ***coc-c.,*** kali-c., laur., med., spig., ***squil.,*** stann., zinc.

right - arn., plat., thuj.

PAIN, chest
extending,upward, right, to - calc., carb-v., graph., ign., lil-t.
right, to left - petr.
various directions - thuj.
fasting, from - ***iod.***
fever, during - **ANT-C.,** ars., canth., caps., carb-v., cina, ***guare.,*** kali-c., ***kalm.,*** nux-v.
fistula, operation for, after - abrot., berb., calc-p., sil.
flatuence, from obstructed - carb-v., verat.
flatus amel. - stram.
forenoon - agar., am-m., caust., cham., coloc., puls., ***ran-b.***
9 a.m. agg. - chel.
10 a.m. - cham., kali-cy.
11 a.m. - cham.
hands on chest amel., placing - ***bry.,*** caps., , dros., eup-per., lact., nat-s.
hanging legs, amel. - sul-ac.
hawking, during - calc., camph., kali-n., plb., rumx., spig.
after - asaf.
herpes zoster, after - ***mez.,*** morg., morph., ***ran-b.,*** vario., zinc.
hiccoughing - am-m., stront.
hot application, amel. - phos.
injuries, after - ruta.
laughing - acon., bry., laur., mez., nicc., psor.
lifting - alum., bar-c., phos., ***psor., sulph.,*** zinc.
as from - plat.
lower - arn., bism., chel., ***chin.,*** croc., kali-c., kali-p., lach., lyc., mang., nat-s., ol-j., **PULS.,** rhus-t., seneg., stann., tarent., teucr., valer., verat.
inspiration, deep - carb-s., chel., naja
left - ***cact.,*** carb-s., carb-v., colch., ***kali-p.,*** lith., **OX-AC., PHOS.,** rhod., tarent.
eating amel. - rhod.
lying, amel. - ***chel.***
on back amel. - ambr.
on left side - **PHOS.**
right - ***ambr., chel., kali-c., merc-c.,*** naja
sitting, while - ***chin.,*** seneg.
walking - bism., sep.
amel. - chin.
extending transversely - bism.
lying, while - alumn., asaf., bry., calc., caps., caust., con., kali-n., psor., puls., seneg.
abdomen on, agg. - asc-t.
abdomen on, amel., - ***bry.***
amel. - alum., bry., calc-p., ferr., gall-ac., mang., ox-ac., psor.
arms near, amel. - lac-ac.
back, on - alum., sulph.
amel. - ambr., bor., ***cact.,*** phos., sulph.
can lie only - ***acon.,*** bry., phos.
down, at night - calc., sep.
lying, side, on - ***canth., hydr.,*** ran-b.
affected side - ***ant-t., bell., calc.,*** nux-v., phos., sabad., stann.
amel. - alum.

PAIN, chest
lying, side, on, left - ***agar.,*** am-c., asc-t., cahin., calc., kalm., lyc., ***naja,*** **PHOS., SPIG.**
painful - **BELL.,** bry., ***nux-v., ran-b.,*** rumx.
amel. - ***ambr.,*** **BRY.,** calad., ***nux-v.,*** puls., stann.
right - ***bor., kali-c.,*** lyc., **MERC.,** phyt., ***seneg.***
right, can lie only on - ***kali-c., naja,*** **SPIG.**
sound - ambr., **PULS.,** stann.
menses, during - cocc., ***graph.,*** phos.
before - puls.
middle - acon., ***alum.,*** bell., ***bry.,*** calc., crot-h., dulc., ***gamb., graph.,*** jug-c., kali-bi., lith., ox-ac., phel., ***phos.,*** sars., sep., ***spig., sulph.,*** tell.
afternoon - ***am-m.***
cough, after - cina.
eating - alum.
evening - ran-b.
extending to shoulder - crot-h.
inspiration - sulph.
deep - thuj.
motion - equis., seneg., sulph.
pressure of hand amel. - **BRY.,** kreos.
raising the arms - sep.
sitting - ***seneg.***
walking in open air - lyc.
writing - ran-b.
morning - acon., am-m., bov., ***bry.,*** carb-v., caust., chel., chin., con., ferr-p., hep., kali-c., lyc., mang., merc., merc-c., nat-s., nit-ac., ox-ac., phos., puls., ***ran-b.,*** rhus-t., sang., sep., ***squil.,*** sulph., thuj.
bed, in - colch., lact., mag-s., phel., ***rumx.,*** seneg., sil.
motion, agg. - abrot., alum., ***arn.,*** bad., bapt., **BELL., BRY., CALC.,** caps., carb-s., card-m., ***chel.,*** chin., ***cimic.,*** equis., gamb., ***graph., hep.,*** hyos., kali-c., kali-p., ***kalm.,*** lac-ac., ***laur.,*** lyc., manc., meny., ***merc., naja,*** nat-m., nit-ac., ***nux-v., phos.,*** psor., ***ran-b.,*** sabad., sars., sec., sep., sil., **SPIG.,** ***squil.,*** stront-c., sulph., viol-t., zinc.
amel. - ign., lob., phos., puls., rhus-t., ***seneg.***
arms, of the - carb-an., card-m., caust., ***nux-m., seneg.,*** sulph.
head, of the - ***guai.***
muscles of chest - ant-c., bor., ***bry.,*** echi., merc., phos., rhus-t.
nausea, with - croc.
night - **ALUM.,** am-c., ant-t., apis, arg-n., **ARS.,** bor., ***caust.,*** chel., con., graph., ***lyc.,*** mag-s., merc-c., nit-ac., ***nux-v.,*** ran-b., ran-s., rhus-t., sabad., seneg., sil., sin-n.
4 a.m. - asc-t.
falling asleep, on - ***nux-m.***
going into open air - am-m.
midnight, after - rhus-t.
noon - dig., naja.
nosebleed, after - calc.
palpitation, during - sep., ***spig., spong.***
paroxysmal - caul., nit-ac., ***ox-ac.,*** plb., sep., stront-c., stry.

PAIN, chest

pleurisy, after - am-c., ***ars.,*** **BRY.,** kali-c., ***lach.,*** lyc., ***phos.,*** **RAN-B.,** ***sulph.***

pneumonia, after - am-c., ***ars.,*** **BRY.,** ***lach.,*** **LYC., PHOS., SULPH.**

pressure, agg. - am-c., ant-c., arn., ars., ***bry.,*** coch., meny., merc-i-f., nat-p., nux-v., ***phos.,*** ran-b., seneg., stann., sul-ac., tarax.

amel. - **ARN.,** ***bor.,*** **BRY.,** cimic., **DROS.,** dulc., ***eup-per.,*** kreos., merc., nat-m., ***nat-s., phos.,*** ran-b., ***sep.***

clothing, of, agg. - benz-ac., ran-b.

spine, on, agg. - sec., tarent.

pulsating - ***caps.,*** com., ***kali-c.,*** zinc.

raising of arm - ang., ant-c., berb., ***ran-b.,*** sel., sep., spig., ***sulph.,*** tarent., tell., thuj.

reading, while - stann.

rest, from - bry.

rheumatic - ***abrot.,*** ambr., ant-t., ***arg-n.,*** arn., berb., **BRY.,** ***cact.,*** cadm-s., carb-v., caust., ***chin., cimic., colch.,*** con., ***corn.,*** guai., hydr., iod., ***kali-i.,*** **KALM., LAC-AC.,** lach., lyc., ***nux-v., phos.,*** plb., **RAN-B.,** ***rhod.,*** **RHUS-T.,** ***rumx.,*** **SPIG.,** ***tarent.***

subcutaneous ulceration, as from - ran-b.

riding, in a carriage - alum., dig.

on horseback - nat-c., ol-j.

rising, on - agar., chin-s., lach., ran-b.

after - agar., lact.

sitting - kali-c., nat-c., sil.

stooping - aloe, nicc.

stooping, amel. - kali-c.

up in bed, on - am-c., ph-ac., **PHOS.**

rubbing, amel. - calc., ***phos.***

shoulders, throwing them back, amel. - calc.

singing, agg. - am-c.

sitting - agar., alum., alumn., bell., ***bry.,*** cact., ***caps.,*** chin., ***con.,*** dig., dros., graph., kali-i., mag-c., mez., nat-s., paeon., ph-ac., ***phos.,*** **SENEG.,** spong., staph.

amel. - alum., am-m., asaf., bry., crot-t., dros., hep., hyos., nat-s., phel., puls., sang.

bent - am-m., dig., meny.

long, as after - ph-ac.

sleep, during - cupr.

before going to sleep - carb-v., sulph.

smoking - ***seneg.***

sneezing - acon., ***bor.,*** **BRY.,** ***caust., chel.,*** coc-c., crot-h., ***dros.,*** hydr., lact., ***merc.,*** mez., rhus-t., seneg., sil., thuj.

spinal irritation, from - agar., ran-b.

splinter, as if - **ARG-N.**

spots - agar., anac., bufo, nat-m., ol-j., seneg., thuj., tub.

squatting, agg. - cadm-s.

standing - aur-m., bov., calc., nat-m., ***nat-s.,*** ran-b., spig., stann., zinc.

amel. - ***chin.,*** graph.

stool, after - agar.

stooping - am-c., ars., card-m., chel., fago., lyc., merc., merl., mez., nat-s., nit-ac., ran-b., rhod., ***seneg.***

PAIN, chest

straightening, up - acon., aloe, nicc.

stretching, the arm - ***ran-b.***

amel. - berb., puls.

swallowing - all-c., alum., ***calc-p.***

talking, while - am-c., **BOR.,** cann-s., **KALI-C.,** kali-n., ***nat-m.,*** prun., rhus-t., tab.

excitement of - stann., stram.

throat, clearing - spig.

touched, when - bor., calc., dros., ***phos., ran-b.,*** staph., sulph.

tuberculosis, in - acon., bry., calc., guai., kali-c., myrt-c., phos., pix.

turning - alum., plb., **RAN-B.**

in bed - caust., thuj.

uncovering, amel. - ferr., sars.

undulating - anac., dig., ***dulc.,*** spig.

ribs, along floating - zinc-i.

upper - anis., calc., iod., mang., myrt-c., pix., puls., stann., ther.

left - spig.

urination, delayed, when - lil-t.

vexation, from - phos.

vomiting, green, amel. - cocc.

waking, on - graph., kali-bi., merc-i-r., ***phos.,*** seneg., thuj.

walking, while - agar., am-c., bell., brom., ***bry.,*** bufo, cact., calc., camph., card-m., cham., chel., cimic., cinnb., cocc., colch., coloc., dig., hep., kali-i., lact., merc., merl., nat-m., olnd., ox-ac., **RAN-B.,** rhus-t., sars., spig., stann., stront-c., sulph., sul-ac., tarax., tarent., ***viol-t.,*** zinc.

air, in open - caust., lyc., ran-b., sulph., zinc.

amel. - ***chin.,*** dros., mez., nat-m., ph-ac., ***seneg.***

dressing and - alum.

rapid - alum., brom., chin., rhod., sulph.

slowly amel. - bor.

wandering - acon., ***all-c.,*** alum., arg-n., ars-h., bell., ***cact.,*** caust., colch., ***ferr., lyc.,*** lyss., mag-m., merc., nat-c., ***ol-j.,*** phos., ***puls., seneg.,*** sin-n., ***tarent.***

pressure, amel. - caust.

room agg. - mag-s., sil.

warm in bed, on getting - rhus-v.

warmth, amel. - ***ars.,*** bar-c., caust., **PHOS.**

covering head with bedclothes - hep., rhus-t., rumx.

washing, cold water, with, amel. - bor.

weather, changing - **RAN-B.**

wine, after - bor.

winter, returning every - ***arg-m., kalm.***

writing, while - mag-s., ran-b.

yawning - bell., ***bor.,*** gall-ac., graph., hep., nat-s., phel., sang., sulph.

PAIN, clavicles - acon., alumn., am-m., apis, brom., calc-p., caps., cham., chin-s., cinnb., crot-c., dros., gamb., hydr., jatr., kali-n., lac-c., led., lyc., mag-m., mang., nat-m., pic-ac., ***puls.,*** rhus-t., rumx., tell., zinc.

PAIN, clavicles
below - ail., arund., ***aspar.,*** berb., brom., ***calc., calc-p.,*** carb-ac., chel., crat., dros., naja, ptel., rumx., spig., sulph., tarent., zinc.
extending to scapula, during inspiration - dros.
inspiration, agg. - mez.
left - coc-c., ***con.,*** mez.
morning - ***sang.***
morning, on waking - ***sang.***
right - com.
coughing, on - apis.
extending to wrist - ***calc-p.***
inhalation - alumn., ant-c., dros., mez.
region of - apis, ***chel.,*** coc-c., kali-bi., led., plat., stann., tell., zinc.
region of, on coughing - apis
rheumatic - ***calc-p., colch.***
sitting - cham.
waking, on - rhus-t., sang.

PAIN, intercostal - ***acon.,*** aesc., ***am-c.,*** aml-n., arist-m., ***arn.,*** ars., ***asc-t.,*** aza., bor., ***bry.,*** caust., chel., ***cimic., colch.,*** echi., gaul., guai., ***kali-c.,*** mez., ***nux-v.,*** ox-ac., ***phos., puls., ran-b.,*** rham-cal., rhod., rhus-r., rhus-t., rumx., seneg., sil., sin-n., sul-ac., verb.
plug sensation - caust., cocc., lyc., ran-s., verat.
pain, cartilages, costal, perichondritis - arg-m., bell., cham., ***cimic.,*** guai., olnd., plb., ***ruta.***

PAIN, ribs
fifth and sternum, between, left - ox-ac.
right - mag-c., thuj.
floating - benz-ac.
left - ther.
right - berb.
last, left - arg-n.
boil, near - arg-m.
lower left, touch, on - sil.
stepping agg. - rat.
upwards, from - apis.

PAIN, sides - ***acon.,*** agar., all-s., alum., alumn., ***ambr.,*** am-c., anac., ang., arg-m., ***arg-n.,*** arn., ars., ars-i., asc-t., aur., aur-m., bad., bell., berb., bov., brom., ***bry.,*** cadm-s., ***calc.,*** calc-p., calc-s., cann-s., caps., carb-s., ***carb-v.,*** caust., cedr., ***chel.,*** chin., chin-a., ***cocc.,*** colch., ***con.,*** cop., ***cupr.,*** dig., dulc., euphr., ferr., ferr-ar., ferr-i., ferr-p., fl-ac., graph., hura, hyos., hydrc., iod., jug-c., kali-ar., kali-bi., ***kali-c.,*** kali-n., kali-p., kalm., lact., laur., led., lil-t., lob., **LYC.,** lycps., med., ***meny.,*** merc-i-f., mez., mur-ac., naja, ***nat-m.,*** nit-ac., nux-m., ***nux-v.,*** op., par., petr., phos., phys., phyt., plan., plb., ***puls.,*** **RAN-B.,** raph., rhus-t., ***rumx.,*** samb., seneg., sep., sil., ***spong.,*** stann., stram., **SULPH.,** sul-ac., sumb., thuj., til., verat., zinc.
afternoon - alum., bar-c., canth., chel., coloc., form., kali-bi., led., lyc., nicc.
1 p.m. - nicc., sars.
2 p.m. - elaps
3 p.m. - ol-an., nat-m.
4 p.m. - **LYC.**

PAIN, sides
air, open air - am-m.
amel. - nat-m.
alternating sides - ***agar.,*** apis, arn., ***calc., cimic.,*** dulc., graph., hyper., lac-c., lyc., mang., mosch., **PHOS.,** plb., ran-b., rumx., thuj.
ascending, steps - kali-bi., staph.
bending, backward - rhod.
forward - aloe, alum., alumn.
to right - cocc.
blood, entered forcibly, as if - zinc.
blowing, nose - sumb.
breathing - aesc., **BRY.,** ***chel.,*** nat-m., puls.
breathing, deep - ***acon., ant-c.,*** arg-m., ***arn.,*** aur., bar-c., bor., bufo, **BRY.,** calc., calc-p., canth., caps., carb-an., carb-v., cham., chel., chin., chin-s., cycl., ferr., ferr-p., form., fl-ac., graph., grat., **KALI-C.,** ***kali-n.,*** lyc., ***meny., mez.,*** nit-ac., oena., ph-ac., phos., phyt., plat., rhus-t., rumx., seneg., ***sil.,*** spong., sumb., stann., sulph., thuj., verat.
cough, during - apis, ***arn.,*** ars., ***bell.,*** **BRY.,** calc-caust., calc-s., caps., caust., ***chel.,*** coff., con., kali-c., kali-n., lact., lyc., **MERC.,** nat-s., psor., ***puls.,*** rhus-t., sabad., seneg., ***sep.,*** **SQUIL.,** stram., **SULPH.,** tarent., verat., zinc.
dinner after - bry., canth., nat-p., rat., zinc.
eating, after - arg-n., brom., caust.
erect, on becoming - dig.
evening - bar-c., calc., dig., dios., euph., hyper., lyc., mag-s., mez., mur-ac., nat-m., ran-b., ***seneg.,*** sulph., thuj., zinc.
8 p.m. - kali-n.
bed, in - nat-c., nit-ac., rhus-t.
excitement, agg. - phos.
exertion - alum., ferr.
of mind - cham.
expiration, during - ambr., carb-v., cina, raph., spig., staph., zinc.
forenoon - am-m., cham., coloc., ran-b.
11 a.m. - hydr.
heat, amel. - phos.
inspiration - acon., aesc., arn., ars., aspar., aur., benz-ac., bor., bov., brom., **BRY.,** calc-s., canth., caps., carb-s., caust., cham., **CHEL.,** cimic., cocc., colch., con., grat., ***kali-c.,*** kali-n., led., lyc., mez., nat-a., nat-s., nicc., oena., op., phyt., plat., plb., ***ran-b.,*** **RUMX.,** sang., sep., sil., spig., **SQUIL.,** sumb., tarax., viol-t.
jar, on - plat.
laughing - acon., **BRY.,** laur., nicc., plat., psor.
leaning, over - hell.
left - am-m., anac., ***apis,*** arg-m., ***arg-n.,*** arum-t., arund., aster., aur., benz-ac., berb., brom., cact., calc., carb-an., carb-s., card-m., cic., ***cimic.,*** clem., colch., con., ***cur.,*** dulc., euph., fago., ferr., fl-ac., graph., hep., ign., iris, kali-bi., kali-c., kali-n., ***lach.,*** laur., lyc., manc., mang., merc., mez., mur-ac., myric., **NAT-M.,**

PAIN, sides
left - ***nat-s.,*** nit-ac., ***nux-v., ox-ac.,*** pall., **PHOS.,** polyg., **RAN-B.,** rhod., rhus-t., ***rumx.,*** seneg., sil., ***spig.,*** stann., staph., ***sulph.,*** sumb., tarent., tub., ust., verat., vip., xan., zinc.
extending to, epigastrium, lower - ox-ac.
extending to, groin - fl-ac.
extending to, scapula - gels., ill., kali-c., lil-t., lyc., mag-c., pix., rhod., rhus-t., sil., spig., sul-ac., sulph., ther.
extending to, shoulder - ***verat.***
extending to, shoulder, right - carb-v., graph.
extending to, throat - sulph.
right, to - apis, calc., graph., ign., kali-bi., kreos., lil-t., ***lyc.,*** phos., plb., zinc.
lifting - alum., arn., bar-c., brom., phos.
lying, while - caps., ***puls.,*** ran-b., ***rumx.,*** seneg.
bed, in - calc., con.
back, on, amel. - ***phos.***
side, on, amel. - ***ambr., bry., kali-c.***
side, on, left side - am-c., eup-per., **PHOS.**
side, on, painful side agg. - ***bell., nux-v., ran-b., rumx.***
side, on, right side - lyc., lycps., phyt.
menses, before - puls.
menses, during - phos., puls.
morning - bov., bry., chin-s., con., elaps, fago., fl-ac., lil-t., lyc., merc-c., nat-s., nit-ac., nux-v., puls., ***ran-b.,*** sang., sep., sulph., sumb., thuj.
bed, in - colch., phel., rumx., sil.
motion, on - aster., bad., brom., **BRY.,** calc., **CHEL.,** gamb., graph., hell., hyper., lyc., phos., psor., ***ran-b.,*** sabad., sars., sulph., viol-t., zinc.
arm - nat-m.
arm, pain in opp. side of chest - dig.
amel. - aur-m-n.
night - am-c., ***chel.,*** con., graph., iod., myris., rumx.
10 p.m. - colch.
noon - rumx., naja
palpitation, during - sep.
paroxysmal - ***ox-ac., phos.***
pressure - brom., merc-i-f., meny., plat., sul-ac., tarax.
amel. - bor., ***bry.,*** cimic., ***phos.***
riding, on horseback - nat-c.
wagon, in a - dig.
right - abrot., ***aesc.,*** arn., ars., ***asaf.,*** asar., bar-c., **BELL.,** bism., blatta, bor., brom., ***bry.,*** cact., carb-an., ***caust.,*** cham., **CHEL.,** chim., chin., ***chin-a.,*** cimic., cocc., colch., coloc., crot-h., dig., elaps, ferr., ferr-i., form., gymn., hydr., ***iod.,*** ill., ***kali-c.,*** lach., ***lyc.,*** mur-ac., nat-a., psor., ptel., puls., ruta., ***sang.,*** sel., sep., squil., ***stront-c.,*** sulph., sul-ac., tarent., teucr., thuj., trom., verat., verat-v., xan., zinc.
apex of right lung - **ARS.,** cimic.

PAIN, sides
right, chest to right arm - hydr., kreos., lob., phos., phyt., plb., sang.
to left side - acon., lach., lachn., petr.
to scapula, worse 4-5 p.m. - merc-sul.
to shoulder - ***sang.***
rising, on - puls.
amel. ., after - kali-c.
seat, from, a - kali-c., nat-c.
stooping, from - nicc.
bed, in - am-c.
sitting, while - am-m., bry., chin., dig., graph., nat-s., nit-ac., paeon., ph-ac., plan., seneg., spig., staph.
bent, while - am-c., anac.
bent, while, amel. - ***chel., ran-b.***
sleep, before going to - sulph.
sleep, during - cupr.
sneezing, after - bor., cina, crot-h., merc., thuj.
standing - calc., ***nat-s.,*** stann., zinc.
stepping - plat.
stool, before - calc-s.
stooping, after - nat-s.
stooping, when - am-c., lyc., nit-ac., sep.
talking, while - **BOR.,** ***kali-n.,*** rhus-t., tab.
touch, on - sulph.
turning, to the right - rumx.
vexation - phos.
waking, on - ***arg-n.,*** graph.
walking - agar., am-c., brom., cact., camph., cham., cocc., colch., dig., merl., nat-m., olnd., ox-ac., **RAN-B.,** rhus-t., sars., seneg., spig., stann., sulph., sul-ac., tarent., tarax., viol-t., zinc.
amel. - nat-m.
amel. air, in open - kali-n.
warm, room agg. - mag-s., nat-m.
wine - ***bor.***
writing - fago.
yawning - nat-s.

PAIN, sternum - agar., apis, asaf., ***bell.,*** bor., ***bry.,*** calc-p., calc-s., caps., carb-an., cocc., con., dulc., ***ferr-ar.,*** fl-ac., hura, ***jug-c.,*** kali-i., kalm., lach., led., ***kreos., manc.,*** morph., mur-ac., nat-m., nit-ac., ox-ac., ***puls.,*** rhus-t., ***sulph.,*** tarax., ***ter.,*** zing.
afternoon - bor., fl-ac., kali-i.
ascending - ***jug-c.***
behind - ***agar.,*** am-c., ap-g., ***arg-n.,*** ars., ***asc-t.,*** aster., aur., aza., ***bry., cact.,*** calc., card-m., ***caust.,*** cham., ***chel., cimx.,*** con., ***dios., eup-per.,*** gels., ind., iod., jug-r., kali-bi., kali-n., ***kreos.,*** lact., lat-m., lob., morph., nit-ac., nit-s-d., osm., ph-ac., phel., ***phos.,*** psor., puls., ***ran-b.,*** ran-s., rhus-t., ***rumx.,*** ruta, samb., **SANG.,** sang-n., ***seneg.,*** sep., ***sil.,*** spig., sulph., ***syph.,*** ter., tril.
coughing, when - **BRY.,** carc., **CAUST.,** ***chel.,*** chin., cina, daph., ***euphr., kali-n.,*** hep., osm., ***phos.,*** rumx., ***sang.,*** staph.
drinking - kali-c.
extending to, axilla - kali-n.

PAIN, sternum
behind, extending to back - ***con.,*** **KALI-BI.,** stict.
food had lodged, as if - all-c., ***led.***
inspiration, on - ***chel., kali-c., manc.,*** sil.
sitting erect amel. - kalm.
swallowing, when - all-c., phos.
walking fast - **SENEG.**
breathing - caps., hep., manc.
deep - ***caust.,*** lyc., nat-m., psor.
convulsive - dig.
coughing, when - bell., **BRY.,** chel., ***chin.,*** cor-r., **KALI-BI.,** ***kali-i.,*** kali-n., ***kreos.,*** osm., ox-ac., ph-ac., ***phos., phyt.,*** psor., rumx., ***sang.,*** staph., ***sulph.,*** thuj.
drinking, when - sep.
eating, after - chin., con., ***jug-c.***
extending to, abdomen - stict.
to, back - ***kali-bi.,*** kali-i., merc-sul., ox-ac., phyt.
to, spine - con., stict.
to, throat - zinc.
to. back - ***kali-bi.,*** ox-ac., phyt.
inhalation, during - bry., caps., chel., laur.
lower, sternum, with cough - am-c.
motion, jaw, of - tarax.
neck, of - tarax.
motion, on - ***bry.,*** led., ph-ac.
night - chin.
paroxysmal - nat-m.
pressure, agg. - manc., ph-ac.
raising, arm - chin.
rubbing, after - led.
sitting, bent - chin., kalm., rhus-t.
smoking, after - thuj.
spots, in - carb-v., puls., ruta.
sprain, as from, in - rumx.
stooping, on - carb-v., dig., ***kalm.,*** ph-ac., ran-b.
stretching, agg. - staph.
talking, while - stram.
touch, on agg. - carb-v., mur-ac., ph-ac., staph., sulph.
upper, sternum - ars., sulph.
coughing - sep., sil.
walking, on - coc-c., ***jug-c.***

PERSPIRATION - agar., ambr., anac., ant-t., **ARG-M.,** arn., asar., bell., benz., **BOV., CALC.,** canth., ***cedr., chel.,*** chin., cimx., cina, **COCC.,** ***crot-c.,*** dros., **EUPHR.,** glon., graph., hep., ip., **KALI-N.,** laur., ***lyc.,*** merc., merc-c., nat-m., nit-ac., op., ***petr., ph-ac.,*** **PHOS.,** plb., rhus-a., rhus-t., ruta, sabad., sec., **SEL.,** ***sep.,*** sil., spig., stann., staph., ***stry.,*** tab., thuj., verat.
abdomen and chest, only - arg-m., cocc., phos., sel.
chilliness, during - sep.
cold - agar., ***camph.,*** canth., cocc., hep., lyc., merc., petr., ***sep.,*** stann.
daytime - petr.
evening, while walking - chin., sabad.
5 to 9 p.m. - chel.
forenoon - arg-n.
menses, during - ***bell.,*** kreos.

PERSPIRATION,
midnight - nat-m., ph-ac.
after - lyc.
morning - bov., ***cocc.,*** graph., kali-n.
4 a.m. - sep.
5 to 6 a.m. - bov.
night - agar., anac., arg-m., bar-c., bell., ***calc.,*** nit-ac., ***sep.,*** sil., stann.
sleep - euphr.
waking, on - canth.
offensive - ***arn.,*** graph., hep., **LYC.,** phos., **SEL.,** ***sep.***
oily - ***arg-m.***
red - arn.
sex, after - agar.
walking, rapidly - nit-ac.
perspiration, sternum - **GRAPH.**
morning - **GRAPH.**

PETECHIAE - ars., cop., stram.
purple - ars.
stellated - stram.

PINCHING, pain - agar., alum., ang., ant-c., bor., bell., carb-an., carb-v., cina, cupr., ***dulc.,*** graph., ip., ***kali-c.,*** lact., lyss., mag-c., mur-ac., par., ph-ac., ***phos.,*** ran-s., rhod., ***seneg.,*** sil., spong., stann., thuj., tub., zinc.
pectoral muscle, left, in - ther.

PLUG, sensation of - anac., aur., caust., coc-c., cocc., ***lyc., ran-s., verat.***

PRESSING, pain - ***abies-n.,*** abrot., acon., agar., ***ail., alum., ambr.,*** am-c., ***anac.,*** anag., ant-c., apis, arg-m., arg-n., arn., ars., ars-i., ***asaf.,*** asar., ***aur.,*** bar-c., ***bell.,*** berb., bism., ***bor., bov.,*** brom., ***bry., cact.,*** cahin., ***calc.,*** calc-p., caps., carb-ac., carb-an., ***carb-s., carb-v., caust.,*** cham., ***chel., chin.,*** chlor., cic., ***cimx., cist.,*** clem., cocc., coc-c., colch., ***coloc.,*** con., com., cor-r., crot-t., cupr., ***cur.,*** cycl., ***dig., dulc.,*** ferr-ac., fl-ac., graph., grat., gymn., ***hell., hydr-ac.,*** hyos., hyper., ign., ***iod.,*** ip., kali-bi., **KALI-C.,** ***kali-n., kreos., lac-d., lach., lact.,*** laur., ***lil-t.,*** lith., ***lob.,*** lyc., lyss., ***mag-m., mag-s.,*** mang., merl., ***merc.,*** merc-sul., ***mez., mill., mur-ac.,*** nat-a., ***nat-c., nat-m., nat-p., nat-s., nicc., nux-m., nux-v.,*** olnd., op., petr., ***ph-ac., phos., plat.,*** plb., prun., psor., ptel., puls., ***ran-b.,*** ran-s., ***rhod., ruta.,*** sabad., sabin., sang., sang-n., samb., ***sars.,*** **SENEG.,** ***sep., sil.,*** spig., spong., **STANN.,** staph., stram., ***stront-c.,*** **SULPH.,** ***sul-ac.,*** tab., tarax., ***thuj.,*** tub., **VALER.,** vanad., verat., verat-v., verb., viol-o., ***zinc.***
anterior, part, morning - nit-ac.
belching amel. - ambr., kali-c., lyc., sep., zinc.
bending head forward agg. - alum.
breathing, deep - caps., sep.
burning - chin.
chill, after - ***iod.***
constant - ***lyc.***
cough, during - alum., am-c., ***anac.,*** ars-i., bism., bor., **BRY.,** ***calc.,*** canth., chin., ***con.,*** cupr., dig., iod., ***kali-n.,*** mag-m., nicc., ph-ac., sil., squil., stront-c., ***sulph.***

PRESSING, pain
cough, after - mag-m.
when desiring to cough - sil.
damp, weather agg. - ***cupr., kali-c., nat-s., sil.***
dinner, after - caust., meny.
drawing, downwards - phos.
eating, while - alum., ars.
after - agar., con., nat-c., phos.
evening - ***ran-b.***
bed, in - sep.
expectoration, amel. - mag-s.
expiration, on - coloc., ruta.
flatus, amel. - ph-ac.
as from - zinc.
forenoon - alum.
hawking, after - spig.
inspiration - asaf., aur-m., ***bor., calc.,*** con., kalic., ran-b., stann.
deep, on - arg-m., **KALI-C.,** mez., ran-s., ***spong.***
deep, on, amel. - ***ign.***
inward - bell., chin.
lower, part - ***agar.,*** alum., arn., asar., bism., chin., dig., lact., phos., ***seneg.,*** teucr., valer., zinc.
night, waking - ruta.
asunder - euph.
lying - am-c.
amel. - alum.
on side, amel. - alum.
menses, during - cocc.
middle - agar., ***alum.,*** am-c., camph., carb-an., crot-t., ***gamb.,*** gymn., hyper., iod., ***kali-c.,*** lact., laur., lith., ph-ac., ***phos.,*** puls., ran-b., raph., sabad., sep., ***spig.,*** tell., thuj.
afternoon - ***am-m.***
as from a load - asaf., samb.
coughing, agg. - ph-ac.
evening - ran-b.
expiration, agg. - ph-ac.
pressure, agg. - ph-ac.
sitting - seneg.
walking in open air - lyc.
morning - ***ran-b.,*** sars., sulph.
bed, in - mag-s., phel., rhus-t., seneg., sil., sulph.
waking - ant-c., cupr.
motion, agg., at certain - sep.
amel. - dros., ***seneg.***
night - **ALUM.,** chel., mag-s., seneg.
asleep, on falling - ***nux-m.***
lying on back - alum.
paroxysmal - nat-m.
plug, as from a - anac.
outward - bell., dulc., seneg., **VALER.,** zinc.
scraping, after - spig.
sitting - anac., cact., ***chin.,*** mez., ***seneg.,*** stann.
amel. - alum.
stooped - bor., chin., ***dig.***
sneezing, while - sil.
standing - aur-m., ***ran-b.,*** spig.

PRESSING, pain
standing, after - nat-m.
amel. - ***chin.***
stone, like a - cor-r.
stooping, on - caust., ***ran-b.,*** sep.
talking - stram.
after - nat-m.
touch, agg. - mang.
touch, on - ruta.
turning - caps.
vise, as if in - am-m.
walking - caust.
air, in open - graph.
amel. - ***chin.,*** mez., ***seneg.***
writing, while - mag-s., ran-b.

pressing, clavicles - bism., led., puls., sars., zinc.
below - ant-c., plat., ***spig.,*** zinc.
extending to teeth - mag-m.

pressing, sides - alum., ***ambr.,*** ang., arn., aur., benz-ac., calc-p., carb-v., ***caust.,*** chin., con., ***cor-r.,*** hyos., iod., ***kali-c.,*** lact., ***lyc., meny.,*** mez., mur-ac., nat-m., par., ph-ac., phos., sars., sep., sil., sul-ac., verb.
belching, after - nit-ac.
amel. - kali-c., nux-v., sep.
breathing deep - arg-m., **KALI-C.,** ph-ac., spong., thuj.
breathing, on - ars.
dinner, after - iod.
evening - caust., dig., euph., mang., ran-b., zinc.
8 p.m. - kali-n.
lying - ant-c.
sitting - seneg.
expectoration, during - ***ang.***
expiration, during - ambr., aur., tarax., zinc.
finger, as from - phos.
flatus, as from - meny.
forenoon - ran-b.
inspiration, during - arn., con., grat., iod., kali-c., meny., mur-ac., squil.
intermittent - zinc.
lain on, side - caps.
leaning on table - con.
left - acon., ambr., am-m., anac., ang., arg-m., aur., calad., carb-s., carb-v., chel., crot-t., cycl., dig., dulc., ferr., graph., hep., ign., kali-c., lyc., mag-m., merc., nat-c., nat-m., ***nat-s.,*** nit-ac., nux-v., pall., petr., ph-ac., plat., ran-b., sil., spong., staph., sulph., sul-ac., tarent., verat., zinc.
lying in bed - calad., calc., con.
morning - thuj.
bed, in - phel., sil.
rising, after - ran-b.
motion, after - calc., viol-t.
arm, of - dig.
violent, on - alum.
night air, on going into open - am-m.
outward - ***asaf.,*** dulc., ***valer.,*** zinc.
plug, as from - ***anac.***
pulsating - asar., verat.

pressing, sides
right - ***anac.,*** ang., ant-c., arg-m., ars., ***asaf., bell.,*** bism., cact., calc., ***carb-v.,*** caust., com., con., cupr., kali-c., nit-ac., ph-ac., sep., squil., tarax., tarent., teucr., thuj., viol-t., zinc.
as from a plug - ***anac.***
extending to liver - kali-c.
lower - hyos.
morning - nit-ac.
sitting - chin., graph., paeon.
amel. - calad.
bent - anac., dulc., rhus-t.
standing, while - calc., ***valer.***
stool, after, amel. - thuj.
touch, on - carb-v.
walking - cact.
amel. - nat-m.
quickly - ang.

pressing, sternum - agar., agn., alum., anac., ***ant-t.,*** arg-m., arn., **ARS.,** asaf., astac., **AUR., AUR-M.,** bell., bor., bov., brom., ***bry.,*** calc., ***calc-p.,*** camph., canth., chel., cocc., coloc., con., cop., crot-t., ***cycl., euphr.,*** eupi., ***ferr.,*** gamb., gymn., ictod., ***kali-m., kreos.,*** lact., laur., led., lyss., mag-m., meny., mur-ac., nat-m., petr., **PHOS.,** ran-b., rheum., rhus-t., ***ruta.,*** sars., ***seneg.,*** sep., sil., staph., sulph., tab., thuj., verat., zinc.
afternoon - fl-ac., kali-i.
behind - acon., alum., **AUR., AUR-M.,** camph., caust., cham., ***chel.,*** dulc., ***euphr., phos.,*** mez., nat-c., ph-ac., rumx., samb., ***syph.,*** ter.
ascending, when - **AUR., AUR-M.**
belching, on - kali-c.
breathing - kali-c.
breathing deep - nat-c.
coughing, after - ***euphr.,*** hep.
intermittent - dulc.
morning - nat-c.
motion - bry.
sitting - con.
sitting, erect amel. - ***kalm.***
belching, amel. - petr.
breathing, deep -arg-m., bor.
dinner, after - verat.
eating, while - anac.
after - con., hyos., chin., verat., zinc.
evening - alum., mur-ac.
expiration, on - anac., tarax.
inspiration, agg. - agar., bor.
morning - petr.
motion agg. - arg-m., led., nat-m.
night - am-c., petr.
pressure, amel. - chin.
raising, arm - chin.
regular, intermittent - verat.
right, border, morning - kali-c.
sitting, while - euph., seneg.
bent - chin.
standing - camph., con., euph.
stooping, agg. - arg-m., ***kalm.***
talking - stram.

pressing, sternum
upper - plat., stann.
left - phos., ssep.
walk, begining to - sulph.
walking, while - alum., arn., cic., coc-c., sulph.
writing, while - asaf.
xiphoid process, coughing - kali-c.
inspiration, on - kali-c.
standing - spig.
stooping, on - carb-v.
swallowing - kali-c.

PULSATION - agar., alum., am-m., ars-h., asaf., ***aster., bar-c.,*** **BELL.,** ***cact.,*** calad., calc., ***calc-p., caps.,*** carb-v., caust., chel., cinnb., colch., crot-t., ***dig.,*** graph., hura, ***hydr.,*** ign., iod., ***kali-c.,*** kali-n., kali-p., lach., lact., lyc., mag-m., manc., mang., merc., nat-c., nux-m., nux-v., paeon., ***phos., puls.,*** rumx., **SENEG.,** ***sep., sil., spig.,*** sulph., thuj., trom., ***zinc.***
aorta - plb., sulph., tarent.
costal cartilages - plat.
coughing, when - manc.
eating, after - am-m., asaf.
evening, after lying - lyc.
in bed - mang.
left - am-m., cann-i., cann-s., gels., graph., ***meny.,*** nat-c., sep., thuj., zinc.
lying, while - meny.
down after, eating, when - asaf.
morning - am-m., ***cact.***
motion agg. - ***glon.,*** phos.
night - ***aster.,*** **PULS.**
interrupting sleep - **PULS.**
waking, on - **SULPH.**
right - asar., crot-t., ***dig.,*** ign., indg., paeon., phos.
short ribs - puls.
standing, while - am-m.
talking, while - manc.
trembling - ars., calc., kreos., ***nat-s., rhus-t.,*** sabin., ***spig.,*** staph.
walking, rapidly - nit-ac.
wine, amel. - nit-ac.
writing, while - mag-s.

pulsation, clavicles, region of - berb., bry., ***kali-c., myrt-c.,*** rhod.
night - nit-ac.

pulsation, sternum - ang., ars-m., chin., ***lach.,*** nat-c., ***sil.,*** sulph.
extending to abdomen - stict.

PURPURA - kali-i., phos.

RASH - ***am-c.,*** ant-t., ***bry.,*** calad., ***calc.,*** calc-s., **CHEL.,** cupr., ferr., ***ip.,*** lach., **LED.,** merc., mez., plb., ***sil., staph., sulph.,*** syph., ter.
alternating with asthma - ***calad.***
itching - calad., caust., sil., staph.
red - am-c., calc., ***camph.,*** **CHEL.,** corn., staph., stram., sulph.
itching rash over region of liver - ***sel.***
warmth, agg. - stram.
whitish, in typhus - ***apis,*** valer.

RASPING - carb-v.

RAWNESS, pain - abrot., acon., ***aesc.***, ***agar.***, alum., alumn., ***ambr.***, am-c., am-m., ***anac.***, anan., ant-t., apis, aral., **ARG-M.**, ***arn.***, ***ars.***, arum-t., ***asc-t.***, berb., ***bry.***, ***calc.***, calc-p., calc-s., calc-sil., cann-s., carb-s., ***carb-v.***, **CAUST.**, cham., chin., ***chin-a.***, cimic., ***cist.***, clem., ***coc-c.***, ***cop.***, cur., dig., ***eup-per.***, ferr-p., gamb., ***gels.***, ***graph.***, ham., ***hydr.***, iod., ***ip.***, kali-c., kali-i., kali-n., ***kaol.***, led., **LYC.**, meph., merc., ***mez.***, naja, naphtin., nat-a., nat-c., ***nat-m.***, nat-p., ***nat-s.***, ***nit-ac.***, **NUX-V.**, ol-j., ***petr.***, **PHOS.**, ***phyt.***, pop-c., psor., ***puls.***, ***ran-b.***, ***ran-s.***, ***rumx.***, ***sang.***, ***seneg.***, sep., sil., ***spong.***, **STANN.**, ***staph.***, ***sulph.***, thuj., zinc.

afternoon, speaking, after - lyc.
bifurcation of trachea, at, when speaking and singing - ***arg-m.***
cold air - apis, **PHOS.**
coryza, during - kreos., meph., sep., sulph.
coughing, when - alum., alumn., ambr., anac., ant-c., ***arg-m.***, arn., ***ars.***, ***calc.***, ***carb-v.***, **CAUST.**, chin-s., ***coc-c.***, ***graph.***, grat., ip., kali-c., kreos., lach., laur., mag-c., mag-m., mag-s., meph., merc., mez., nat-c., ***nat-m.***, nat-p., nat-s., nit-ac., nux-m., nux-v., petr., ***phos.***, ***rumx.***, ruta., sanic., ***sep.***, sil., spig., ***spong.***, ***stann.***, ***staph.***, sulph., thuj., zinc.
after - ***arn.***, ***carb-v.***, caust., lach., lyc., ***nat-m.***, ***phos.***, sep., spong., ***stann.***, staph., zinc.
dinner, after - nat-c.
eating amel. - nat-c.
evening - ***ars.***, calc., murx., nat-c.
8 p.m. - am-m.
hawking, while - rumx.
inspiration, on - ***acon.***, anac., ***calc.***
lying, while - coc-c.
amel. - nat-c.
morning - bor., caust., nat-c.
waking, on - sulph.
night - zinc.
cough, during - alum., ***calc.***, carb-v., nit-ac., nux-v.
singing, when - ***arg-m.***
speaking, after - ***arg-m.***, ***calc.***
temperature, after change of - ***acon.***
walking, after - calc.

rawness, sternum, behind - iod., kali-bi., kali-n.

RESTLESSNESS, in - bell., petr., seneg., thuj.

RHEUMATIC pain - ***abrot.***, ambr., ant-t., ***arg-n.***, arn., berb., **BRY.**, ***cact.***, cadm-s., carb-v., caust., ***chin.***, ***cimic.***, ***colch.***, con., ***corn.***, guai., hydr., iod., ***kali-i.***, **KALM.**, **LAC-AC.**, lach., lyc., ***nux-v.***, ***phos.***, plb., **RAN-B.**, ***rhod.***, **RHUS-T.**, ***rumx.***, **SPIG.**, ***tarent.***

subcutaneous ulceration, as from - ran-b.

RUMBLING, audible, left - cocc.

SCRAPING, pain - seneg.
talking, agg. - seneg.

SCARS, suppurating - **SIL.**

SCRATCHING, pain - arg-m., caust., kali-c., sil.

SENSITIVE - ang., helon., nat-c., nux-v., ph-ac., phos., seneg., stront-c., sulph., tub., zinc.
cold air, to - ***ph-ac.***

SHAKING, of, during cough - calc-ar., cench., hyos., ***lact.***, mag-s., rhus-t.
shuddering, with - mez.

SHARP, pain - **ACON.**, aesc., aeth., ***agar.***, ***ail.***, all-s., ***alum.***, alumn., aloe, ***am-c.***, am-m., ***anac.***, anan., ***ant-c.***, ***ant-t.***, ***apis***, ***arg-n.***, ***arn.***, ***ars.***, ***asaf.***, asar., ***asc-t.***, aspar., aster., ***aur.***, ***aur-m.***, bad., bar-c., ***bell.***, berb., **BOR.**, bov., brom., **BRY.**, bufo, ***cact.***, cahin., calad., **CALC.**, ***calc-p.***, calc-s., camph., cann-i., **CANTH.**, ***caps.***, ***carb-an.***, carb-s., ***carb-v.***, ***card-m.***, ***caust.***, **CHAM.**, ***chel.***, ***chin.***, chin-a., chin-s., cimic., cina, cinnb., ***clem.***, cocc., coc-c., **COLCH.**, ***coloc.***, ***con.***, corn., croc., crot-h., crot-t., cycl., dig., ***dros.***, ***dulc.***, elaps, elat., euon., eupi., ***ferr.***, ferr-ar., ferr-i., ferr-p., form., gamb., gels., gnaph., ***gran.***, ***graph.***, grat., ***guai.***, ham., hep., hydr-ac., ***hyos.***, ***ign.***, inul., ***iod.***, ***ip.***, jab., jug-r., kali-ar., ***kali-bi.***, **KALI-C.**, ***kali-i.***, kali-n., **KALI-P.**, ***kali-s.***, kalm., ***kreos.***, ***lach.***, ***lact.***, laur., led., ***lob.***, ***lyc.***, ***mag-c.***, mag-m., mag-s., manc., mang., med., meny., ***merc.***, **MERC-C.**, merc-i-f., ***mez.***, mill., mosch., ***mur-ac.***, myrt-c., ***nat-a.***, ***nat-c.***, **NAT-M.**, ***nat-n.***, nat-p., nat-s., ***nicc.***, ***nit-ac.***, **NUX-M.**, nux-v., ol-an., ol-j., olnd., ox-ac., ***paeon.***, par., ***petr.***, ***ph-ac.***, phel., **PHOS.**, phyt., plan., ***plat.***, plb., polyg., psor., ***puls.***, **RAN-B.**, ***ran-s.***, raph., rat., rheum, rhod., rhus-r., ***rhus-t.***, ***rhus-v.***, **RUMX.**, ruta., sabad., samb., ***sang.***, ***sars.***, **SENEG.**, ***sep.***, ***sil.***, sin-n., **SPIG.**, spong., **SQUIL.**, ***stann.***, ***staph.***, ***stict.***, still., ***stront-c.***, stry., **SULPH.**, ***sul-ac.***, sumb., ***tab.***, tarax., ther., ***thuj.***, tril., tub., ***valer.***, verat., ***verb.***, viol-t., vinc., ***zinc.***, zing.

afternoon - alum., coloc., iod., sulph.
2 p.m. - chel.

air, open amel. - sul-ac.

anger, after - arg-n., caust.

anterior part - ***canth.***, cann-s., card-m., kali-n., lyc., **MERC.**, nit-ac., ter., ther.
afternoon - am-m., gamb.
coughing, on - lyc., **MERC.**
deep breathing - gamb.
evening - gamb., nicc., zinc.
inspiration, during - kali-c.
forenoon - ***ran-b.***
sweat, during - ran-b.
inspiration - canth., ***card-m.***, ***lyc.***
morning - am-m.
night - caust.
sitting, amel. - am-m.
sneezing, on - ***merc.***
standing - bov.
stooping, agg. - nit-ac., card-m.
walking - card-m.

arm, below - canth., ***caust.***, laur.
evening - bell.
left - euon., petr.
right - plb.
standing - plb.

ascending, steps - bor., rat., ruta., stram.

SHARP, pain
autumn - ***kali-c.***
bending, backwards or forwards - agar.
compelling - sars.
forward, amel. - ***chel.,*** chin.
sideways, agg. - acon.
boring - meny., spong.
breathing, agg. - acon., aloe, am-c., ***anac.,*** ant-c., arg-m., arn., ***aur.,*** **BOR., BRY.,** bov., ***calc.,*** cann-s., caps., card-m., cham., ***chel.,*** chin., colch., ***coloc., dros.,*** elaps, euph., ***hep.,*** **KALI-C.,** ***kali-n.,*** kali-p., ***kreos., lyc.,*** mag-c., meny., mez., mur-ac., nat-c., nat-s., nicc., ***nux-m.,*** ox-ac., ph-ac., ***psor.,*** sabad., seneg., ***sep., spig., spong., squil., stann.,*** tab., verat., verb.
deep - ***acon.,*** aesc., aeth., arg-m., ***all-c.,*** ant-c., arn., asar., aur., bapt., benz-ac., ***berb.,*** **BOR.,** bov., brom., **BRY.,** ***calc., calc-p.,*** carb-s., card-m., ***caust., cham.,*** chel., ***cupr.,*** dros., ferr-p., ***guai.,*** hell., **KALI-C.,** ***kali-n.,*** mang., merc-c., mez., ***mur-ac.,*** **NAT-M.,** nit-ac., nux-v., olnd., pall., ***phos., puls., ran-b.,*** raph., ***rhus-t., rumx.,*** sep., sil., ***spong., sulph.,*** valer., zinc.
impeded - arg-m., ***bry.***
burning - ***all-c.,*** alum., ***ars.,*** bar-c., ***carb-an., carb-s., cina, crot-t.,*** mur-ac., sang.
change, of weather - **RAN-B.**
chill, during - **BRY.,** eup-per., kali-c., lach., phos., ***rhus-t., rumx.,*** sabad.
chilliness, during - eupi.
cold, air - ***kali-c.***
cold, drinks - staph., thuj.
coughing - ***acon.,*** am-c., am-m., ant-c., arg-m., ***arn., ars., asaf.,*** asc-t., aur., **BELL.,** berb., **BOR., BRY.,** cact., calc., ***calc-p.,*** cann-s., caps., carb-an., carb-v., card-m., caust., ***chel., chin.,*** chin-a., clem., ***coff.,*** con., ***corn.,*** crot-h., cupr., cur., **DROS.,** dulc., ***ferr.,*** ferr-ar., ferr-i., ***ferr-m.,*** guai., **IOD.,** kali-ar., ***kali-bi., kali-c.,*** kali-n., kali-p., ***kreos., lach., lyc.,*** **MERC.,** mez., myric., nat-m., nat-s., nit-ac., nux-m., nux-v., petr., ***phos., psor., puls.,*** ran-b., rhus-t., rumx., ruta., sabad., sel., seneg., ***sep.,*** sil., **SQUIL.,** ***stann.,*** stront-c., ***sulph.,*** verat., zinc.
descending, steps - alum.
dinner, after - carb-s.
eating, after - ***asaf.,*** bov., nat-c., sulph.
eating, while - bov.
erect, becoming, agg. - nicc.
evening - calad., kali-bi., ***kali-i.,*** kali-n., ***mag-c.,*** ran-s., rumx., verb.
6 p.m. - bry.
8 p.m. - canth.
bed, in - benz-ac., nat-c.
exertion - alum., bor., caust., ferr., led.
mental - sep.
expiring - ***ant-c.,*** calc., clem., ***colch.,*** crot-t., mang., spong.
compelling - chin.

SHARP, pain
extending, to back - agar., ambr., ***anac., apis, asaf., bry.,*** bov., calc., ***canth.,*** carb-v., ***card-m.,*** caust., ***chel., chen-a.,*** colch., ***con., crot-c.,*** crot-t., ferr., gamb., glon., hep., ***kali-bi., kali-c.,*** kali-n., lact., lyc., ***merc.,*** mez., nat-m., pall., ***phyt.,*** rhod., rhus-t., ***sep., sil.,*** **SULPH.,** sul-ac., tab.
back, 6 p.m. - laur.
downward - alumn., berb., com.
forward - agar.
inward - berb.
inspiration, during - tarax.
left arm - tarent.
liver - ***calc-p.***
lower part of abdomen - ***corn.***
neck, left - zinc.
outward - ***asaf.,*** bell., spig., thuj.
between scapula - calc.
scapula - acon., ***bry., ferr., hep.,*** ox-ac., seneg., ***sulph.***
shoulder - alum., bar-c., ***card-m., sang.,*** ther.
side to side - gnaph.
stomach - caust., ox-ac.
throat - anac., calc., ther.
transverse - nat-m., nit-ac.
upwards - gamb., mang., mur-ac., nat-c., stann., stront.
face, compelling to lie on - bry.
fever, during - acon., **BRY.,** ***kali-c.,*** nux-v.
forenoon - caust., mang., nit-ac., stann.
hawking, after - asaf.
heartbeat, every - calc-ac.
hiccoughs, with - am-m.
inspiring - **ACON.,** alum., am-m., ***arg-m., ars.,*** asaf., ***asar., aur.,*** aur-m., bar-c., **BOR., BRY.,** ***calc.,*** calc-p., canth., carb-an., card-m., ***chel.,*** clem., cob., coloc., ***con., dros.,*** grat., guai., ***hyos.,*** **KALI-C.,** ***kreos., lyc.,*** lyss., ***mag-c., merc., merc-c.,*** mez., **NAT-M.,** nat-s., op., ***phos.,*** plat., ***ran-b.,*** rhus-t., seneg., sep., ***sil.,*** spong., **SQUIL.,** stront-c., sulph., tarax., valer.
itching - calc.
laughing, while - acon., mez., nicc.
left, on the side - aeth., am-c., calad., **PHOS., SPIG.,** ***stann.***
apex - ther.
lower, part - agar., aloe, bry., ***chel.,*** coc-c., hep., **KALM.,** lach., ***naja,*** sang., seneg., sulph., valer.
extending to,
abdomen - ***chel.***
back - ***carb-s.***
shoulders - sang.
forenoon - agar.
inspiration, deep - cob., crot-t.
left - carb-s., cob., **OX-AC.**
respiration - kali-bi., lyc.
right - ***chel., chen-a.,*** crot-t., med.

SHARP, pain
lying, while - asaf., bry., chel., kali-n., psor.
back, on, agg. - kali-c., rumx., sulph.
can lie only on the - ***acon., bry., phos., plat.***
face, on the, amel. - bry.
side, on - acon.
menses, during - bor., ***croc.,*** kali-n., ***puls.***
before - ***kali-c.***
middle - agar., alum., ***am-m.,*** ant-c., benz-ac., bor., grat., hyper., indg., iod., ***kali-i.,*** kali-n., ***kreos., lyc.,*** mag-c., nat-m., nux-v., olnd., ox-ac., pall., phos., rumx., sars., seneg., zinc.
afternoon - crot-t., mag-c.
ascending - graph.
bending body forward - pall.
dinner, after - kali-n.
expiration, during - cham.
extending to back - ox-ac.
extending to right side - cham.
inspiration, during - ***alum., kreos.,*** zinc.
after - zinc.
amel. - seneg.
menses, during - kali-n.
moving, agg. - nux-v.
sitting, while - indg., pall.
stooping, on - zinc.
stretching the body - eupi.
walking - kali-i., kali-n.
amel. - kali-i.
morning - chin., hep., ***kali-bi.,*** mang., merc., rhus-t., ***squil.***
rising, on - ran-b.
motion, during - alum., aur-m., bad., **BRY.,** ***calc., chel.,*** chin., hyos., kali-n., meny., merc., mur-ac., nit-ac., ox-ac., phos., puls., ***ran-b.,*** **SPIG.,** ***sulph.***
amel. - con., ***dros., euph.,*** indg., ***kali-c.,*** phos., **RHUS-T.,** ***seneg.***
arms - ***camph., sulph.,*** sumb.
night - alum., am-c., ***apis, ip., lyc.,*** merc-c., nit-ac., phos., ran-s., ***rhus-t.,*** sabad., seneg.
bed, in - phos.
waking, on - seneg.
noon - agar.
outward - chin.
paroxysmal - nat-m.
periodical - acon., aloe.
pleurisy, after - bry., carb-an.
posterior part - arg-m., asaf., bor., bov., bry., canth., cast., chin., fl-ac., kali-n., mang., nicc., rhus-t., sabin., stront-c., tarax., verat.
deep inspiration, on - sabin.
pressure, from - ran-b.
amel. - asaf., ***bor.,*** **BRY., DROS.**
raising the arms - berb., bor., ol-j., puls., rhus-t., ***sulph.,*** thuj.
reading, while - euph.
rhythmical - am-m., ***calc.,*** chin., cocc.
right - act-sp., ***bor.,*** rumx., seneg., xan.
extending to scapula - xan.
only amel. - **SPIG.**

SHARP, pain
rising, from stooping - nat-c.
rubbing, amel. - calc., ***phos.***
running, agg. - bor., lyc.
side, affected, on the - ***calc., kali-c.,*** sabad.
painful, on the - am-c., stann.
amel. - calad., **BRY.**
sound, on the - stann.
singing, agg. - am-c.
sitting, agg. - agar., chin., ***con.,*** indg., phos.
amel. - asaf., chel.
crooked - am-m., bor., chel., ***rhus-t.***
sleep, on going to - carb-v.
sneezing agg. - acon., ***bor., bry.,*** chel., **DROS., MERC.,** rhus-t.
stooping - alum., am-c., ars., card-m., mang., merc., merl., nit-ac., ***ran-b.,*** zinc.
supper, after - am-c., lyc.
talking - bor., cann-s., carb-an., rhus-t.
touched, when - phos., **RAN-B.**
turning, by - caust., phos., **RAN-B.,** staph.
twitching - calc.
walking, while - am-c., ***asaf.,*** cinnb., coloc., cocc., ***con.,*** hep., ***kali-i.,*** kali-n., merc-i-r., olnd., rhus-t., spong.
air, in open - caust., ***merc., ran-b.,*** zinc.
amel. - pall., ***seneg.***
rapidly - brom., chin., sulph.
wandering - acon., carb-s., ***ferr.,*** **PULS.,** ***sulph.***
warm, on getting warm in bed - rhus-v.
writing, while - carb-an., rumx., spig.
yawning - aur., bell., ***bor.,*** mag-c., nat-s., phel.

SHARP, pain, clavicles - alumn., am-m., berb., bry., chel., guai., kali-n., lachn., lyc., mez., nat-m., ol-an., paeon., pall., phos., tarax., sabin., stann., zinc.
breathing, on - squil.
inhaling, when - alumn.
intermittent - sabin.
moving, head - am-m.
pulsating - berb.
region, of - berb., mang.
left - mang., meny., spig.
downward toward sternum - con.
right - berb., caust.
tearing - am-m.
twitching - chel.
under - ***ail.,*** ant-t., arund., aur-s., chel., cina, ***dulc.,*** sang., spig.
coughing, on - kali-c.
evening - lyc.
extending, to
deeply - mez.
elbow - kali-n.
scapula - **SULPH.,** ther.
sternum - ***ail.***
upward - nat-m.
inspiration - lyc.
itching - spig.

SHARP, pain, clavicles
under,
left - chel., colch., kali-c., mez., ***myrt-c., sulph., ther.***
morning - nat-m.
4 a.m. - nat-m.
motion - lyc.
noon - coca.
pressure agg. - cina.
pulsation - lyc.
right - alumn., **ARS.,** bell., ***dulc.,*** kali-c., ***lyc.,*** nat-m.
walking - bell.
walking, while - paeon.

SHARP, pain, costal cartilages - bell., staph.
between - staph.
of lower ribs, stooping - staph.
of short ribs near sternum - cina, plat., sul-ac.

SHARP, pain, ribs, between the - coc-c., kreos., mag-m., ***mez., ran-b.***
between the, right then left - coc-c.
lower - anac., bism., chin., hep., kali-i., mag-m., nat-c., rhus-t., squil., sulph.
afternoon - canth., stram.
coughing, on - bry., kali-n.
evening - mag-m., zinc.
inspiration, on - chin.
laughing - kali-n.
left - ***agar.,*** anac., canth., ***ran-b.,*** mur-ac., sang., sil., tarax., zinc.
morning - bov.
night, during inspiration - sil.
right - aesc., agar., calc., kali-c., kali-n., mang., merl., verat., zinc.
sitting, while - agar., mag-c.
sneezing - cast.
turning, on - plb.
walking, while - merc.

SHARP, pain, sides - ***acon.,*** aesc., agar., ***alum., am-c., am-m.,*** ang., ***apis, arg-m.,*** arg-n., ***arn., ars.,*** asaf., aur., ***bad., bar-c.,*** bell., ***bor.,*** **BRY.,** calad., ***calc., canth.,*** **CARD-M., CAUST.,** cedr., ***cham., chel., chin.,*** clem., cocc., ***coloc., con.,*** croc., ***cupr.,*** dig., ***dulc.,*** elaps, ferr-p., fl-ac., gamb., gran., graph., ***guai., hyos.,*** ign., indg., ***kali-bi.,*** **KALI-C.,** ***kali-i.,*** kali-n., ***kali-p., kalm., lach.,*** lachn., laur., lil-t., lyc., mang., med., ***meny., mosch.,*** nat-c., **NAT-M.,** nat-p., ***nat-s.,*** nicc., nit-ac., nux-v., ol-an., op., par., petr., ph-ac., ***phos.,*** pic-ac., plat., ***plb., puls.,*** **RAN-B.,** rhus-t., rumx., samb., sars., ***sel., sep.,*** sil., spig., ***spong.,*** **SQUIL.,** stann., staph., ***sulph.,*** sul-ac., sumb., ***tab., tarax.,*** thuj., verb., verat., ***zinc.***
afternoon - bar-c., canth., chel., coloc., kali-bi., led., lyc., nicc., sars.
1 p.m. - sars.
2 p.m. - elaps.
3 p.m. - ol-an., nat-m., rumx.
rising from stooping, agg. - nicc.
ascending steps - bor., ***staph., sulph.***

SHARP, pain, sides
bending, forward, agg. - aloe.
backward - staph.
breathing, agg. - calc., caps., cic., graph., lyc., meny., nat-c., phos., zinc.
deep - ***acon.,*** all-c., aloe, ant-c., arg-m., ***arn.,*** ars., aur., ***bad.,*** bar-c., bor., ***bry.,*** bufo, ***calc.,*** calc-p., canth., caps., carb-an., carb-v., cham., ***chel., chin.,*** chin-s., clem., ***colch., crot-c.,*** cycl., ***elaps,*** fl-ac., form., graph., grat., ***guai., kali-c., kali-n.,*** lyc., ***meny., mez., nicc.,*** nit-ac., olnd., ***ph-ac.,*** plat., ***ran-b.,*** rhus-t., **RUMX.,** seneg., ***sil.,*** stann., ***sulph.,*** thuj., verat.
inspiration - ***acon.,*** agar., alum., ***ars.,*** aspar., aur., ***bad., bar-c., bor.,*** bov., **BRY.,** ***calc.,*** canth., carb-v., caust., cham., ***chel.,*** cocc., colch., con., graph., iod., **KALI-C.,** kali-n., led., ***lyc.,*** lyss., meny., ***merc-c.,*** merl., **NAT-M.,** nat-s., nicc., op., plb., ***ran-b.,*** **RUMX.,** ruta., sabad., sep., sil., ***spig.,*** spong., **SQUIL., SULPH.,** sul-ac., tarax., viol-t.
cold, air - ***kali-c.***
coughing - acon., ant-t., ***arn., ars.,*** aur., ***bor.,*** **BRY.,** cann-s., ***caps.,*** **CARD-M.,** caust., ***chel.,*** chin., clem., coff., ***con.,*** crot-h., cur., dulc., ferr-p., ***kali-c.,*** kali-n., ***lyc.,*** **MERC.,** nat-s., phos., ***puls.,*** rhus-t., rumx., sabad., seneg., ***sep.,*** squil., ***stann., sulph.,*** zinc.
dinner, during - sil.
after - bry., canth., rat., zinc.
drawing - mang., spong.
eating, after - caust., rat.
evening - bar-c., calc., cocc., graph., hyper., kali-n., lyc., mur-ac., nat-m., ran-b., sars., ***sel.,*** seneg., sulph., thuj., zinc.
bed, in - calad., nat-c., nit-ac.
entering house from open air, on - mag-s.
excitement, agg. - phos.
exertion - alum., ***bor.,*** ferr.
of mind - cham.
expiration - ant-c., ars., chin., cina, iod., mang., mur-ac., sep., sil., spig., staph., stann., zinc.
extending, to
abdomen, lower - nit-ac.
arms, toward - brom., nat-m.
back - alumn., arum-t., bov., chel., ***chen-a.,*** guai., hep., ***kali-c.,*** kali-n., lyc., mez., nit-ac., ox-ac., par., sil.
lying, on left side agg. - ***kali-c.***
lying, on right side amel. - ***kali-c.***
elbow - sil.
hypochondrium - berb.
outward - ***arg-n.,*** asaf., spong.
precordial region - chin.
sacral region - thuj.
scapula - arum-t., ***chel., chen-a.,*** lact., ***nat-m.,*** seneg., **SULPH.**
shoulders - indg., ***kali-c.,*** nat-m., ***sang.***
sternum - laur.
submaxillary gland - calc.
upwards - gamb., mur-ac., nat-c., stann.
flatus, as from - nit-ac.

SHARP, pain, sides
forenoon - am-m., bov., cham., coloc., ***ran-b.***
11 a.m. - cham.
heat, amel. - ***phos.***
itching - chin., dig., spig.
laughing - acon., laur., nicc.
leaning on table - con.
left - aesc., aeth., agar., all-c., aloe, ***alum.,*** alumn., ***am-c.,*** am-m., anac., ant-c., ant-t., ***apis, arn., ars.,*** bad., bar-c., berb., bor., bov., calad., ***calc., calc-p.,*** camph., caps., ***carl., caust.,*** chel., ***chin., chin-s.,*** cic., ***cina,*** clem., ***coloc., croc., crot-c.,*** crot-h., ***crot-t.,*** cupr., cycl., dig., ***dulc.,*** echi., elaps, eupi., ***euph.,*** fl-ac., graph., guai., hell., ***hep.,*** hipp., hyper., hura, ***ign.,*** kali-a., ***kali-c., kali-n., lach.,*** lachn., lact., ***lyc.,*** lyss., ***mag-c.,*** mag-m., ***mang., merc., mez.,*** mur-ac., ***naja, nat-m.,*** nat-p., ***nat-s., nicc.,*** nit-ac., olnd., ***ox-ac.,*** plb., ph-ac., **PHOS.,** plan., ***plat.,*** psor., ***ran-b., ran-s.,*** rat., **RUMX.,** ruta., sabin., sabad., sang., sars., **SENEG.,** ***sep.,*** sil., ***spig.,*** spong., **STANN.,** staph., **SULPH.,** ***sul-ac.,*** tarax., tarent., ***ther., thuj.,*** trom., ***ust.,*** valer., ***zinc.,*** zing.
cough, during - agar., crot-h., iod., kali-c.
evening - kali-n., mur-ac., nat-m., nit-ac., sul-ac., zinc.
bending to left - calc.
carrying a weight - kali-n.
chill, during - sil.
cough, during - agar., bell., caust., crot-h., iod., kali-c., nit-ac., sep., sul-ac.
extending, to,
back - am-c., lyc., sul-ac., **SULPH.,** ***ther.***
groin - fl-ac.
hip - cupr.
right - aesc., calc., ***caust., kreos.,*** nat-c., ***rumx.***
right on inspiration - ***bry.***
scapula - caust., ***lact.,*** mag-c., ***nat-m.,*** **SULPH.**
shoulder - asc-t., calc-p., mag-c., nat-m., sang.
throat - calc.
upward - bar-c.
inspiration - calc., calc-p., lyc., kali-n., mag-c., nit-ac., ph-ac., **SULPH.,** sul-ac.
lying, in bed - nit-ac.
back, on - ***sulph.***
left side agg., on - am-c., camph., kali-c., ***lyc., phos., rumx.,*** sil., ***stann.***
right side amel., on - **PHOS.**
motion - calc., ***sulph.***
arm of - zinc.
pulsating - anac., verat.
sitting, bent - arg-m.
upper - sul-ac.
sitting bent, when - kali-i.
lifting - bar-c., phos.
lower, part of - am-c., carb-v., kali-n., led., ph-ac.
afternoon - gels.
evening - coc-c., dig.

SHARP, pain, sides
lower, part of
left - aesc., arg-m., berb., bov., ***calc-p.,*** canth., cham., ***colch.,*** eupi., gels., ***lact., nat-s.,*** ox-ac., sabad., squil., stry., tarax.
urination amel. - aesc.
menses, on beginning - kali-n.
morning - carb-an.
motion, agg. - **BRY.,** ***chel.***
right - aloe, bad., bry., ***cann-s., canth.,*** carb-v., ***card-m.,*** **CHEL.,** ***chen-a.,*** dig., ferr-p., **KALI-C.,** ***lach.,*** lyc., mag-m., ***merc., phos.,*** rumx., sep., sul-ac., ***thuj.,*** verat.
walking, amel. - ph-ac.
lying, while - ***puls., rumx., seneg.***
back, on - ***sulph.***
left side, on, agg. - am-c., camph., ***stann.***
amel. - ***rumx.***
painful side agg. - nat-c.
amel. - **BRY.,** calad.
right side, on, agg. - lyc., ***rumx.***
menses, during - bor., ***croc.,*** phos., sul-ac.
before - puls.
morning - bov., brom., ***bry.,*** colch., con., ferr., lyc., mang., merc-c., nat-s., nit-ac., puls., ***rumx.,*** sang., sars., sel., sep., sulph.
motion, during - alum., ***bad.,*** **BRY.,** calc., caust., ***chel.,*** chin., gamb., graph., hyper., lyc., mang., meny., ox-ac., phos., ***ran-b.,*** **RUMX.,** sabad., sars., ***sulph.***
amel. - euph., indg., ***kali-c., seneg.***
arm, of - led.
night - am-c., ***caust.,*** chin., **CON.,** graph., kali-c., **LYC.,** ***puls., rumx.,*** sil., ***sulph.***
4 a.m. - chel.
waking, on - graph.
noon - naja.
pressure - meny., merc-i-f., sul-ac., tarax.
amel. - chin., graph., mag-c., verb.
pulsating - con., lyc.
pulse, synchronous, with - dig.
raising arm - bor., nicc., ran-b.
reading - euph.
riding, in a wagon - dig., ***rumx.***
horseback, on - nat-c.
right - abrot., ***agar.,*** ambr., **AM-C.,** am-m., apis, apoc., ***arg-m.,*** **ARS.,** arum-t., ***asar.,*** aspar., ***bell.,*** benz-ac., **BOR.,** ***brom.,*** **BRY.,** bufo, cahin., calad., calc., ***canth., carb-v.,*** card-m., cham., **CHEL.,** ***chen-a., chin.,*** chin-s., cimic., coc-c., ***colch.,*** cop., croc., dig., equis., euon., euph., ferr., ferr-p., form., kali-bi., **KALI-C.,** ***kali-i.,*** kali-n., ***lyc.,*** mag-m., manc., mang., meny., merc., ***merc-c.,*** merc-i-f., ***mez.,*** mur-ac., murx., naja, nat-c., ***nat-m.,*** nat-s., ***nit-ac.,*** pall., ph-ac., phyt., plat., ***ran-b.,*** ran-s., sang., ***sars., sep., sil.,*** spong., ***staph., sulph.,*** sul-ac., tab., tep., verat., verat-v., ***zinc.,*** zing.
alternating, with stitching in the right abdomen - zinc.

SHARP, pain, sides
right,
apex - **ARS.**
to base - ***cimic.***
bending, body to the right - staph.
to left - petr.
breathing, during - aesc., ambr., ars., **BOR., BRY.,** calc., chin-s., ***cimic., mez.,*** psor.
deeper, amel. - tarax.
coughing, on - **BOR.,** cann-s., chel., sep., ziz.
dinner, after - zinc.
extending, to
back - ambr., calc., colch., merc., nit-ac., sil.
left - agar., alum., calc., petr.
left abdomen - rhus-t.
right groin - bor.
scapula - ***nit-ac.,*** phyt., **SULPH.**
stomach - sulph.
inspiration, on - arg-m., carb-v., graph., nit-ac., plat., sep., sil.
lower part - aesc., alumn., ***chel., chen-a., kali-c.***
lying, on back - ***sulph.***
left side - calad.
right side, when - ***acon., bor.,*** graph., ***kali-c.,*** kali-n.
lying, with head low - kali-n.
pressure, agg. - sul-ac.
amel. - ***bor.,*** graph., nat-m.
night - nit-ac.
raising, arms - bor.
sitting, while - bry., mur-ac.
sneezing or yawning - bor.
stooping, on - **AM-C.**
turning, body to right - zinc.
walking - am-c., nat-m., sep.
rising, after, amel. - kali-c.
bed, in - am-c.
seat, from a - kali-c., nat-c., phos.
stooping, from - kali-c.
scratching, amel. - plat.
screaming, from - cupr.
sitting, while - am-m., bry., chin., dig., euph., indg., kali-c., led., mur-ac., nat-s., ***seneg.,*** spong., staph.
bent - agar., spong.
sleep, during - cupr.
before - sulph.
sneezing, after - bor., crot-h., ***merc.,*** thuj.
standing, while - euph., ***nat-s.,*** sars., zinc.
stooping, on - ***am-c.,*** lyc., mang., nit-ac.
after - nat-s.
amel. - chin., mag-c.
stretching, on - nit-ac.
amel. - zinc.
talking, while - **BOR.,** rhus-t., ***kali-n.,*** tab.
tearing - led., nat-m.
touch, agg. - chin., crot-h., phos.
vexation, agg. - nat-m., ***phos.***

SHARP, pain, sides
walking, while - agar., am-c., ***brom., camph.,*** caps., cham., cocc., colch., dig., merl., nat-m., olnd., ox-ac., **RAN-B.,** rhus-t., sars., seneg., spig., spong., stann., ***sulph.,*** sul-ac., tarax., tarent., ***viol-t.,*** zinc.
air, in open - con., euph., sars., stann.
amel. - kali-n.
amel. - euph.
washing, with cold water amel. - bor.
wine, after - bor.
writing, while - ***rumx.***
yawning - nat-s.

SHARP, pain, sternum - acon., aesc., aeth., agar., alum., am-c., ang., arg-m., ***arn.,*** **ARS.,** aur., bism., bov., ***bry.,*** cact., ***calc., calc-p., canth.,*** carb-an., carb-s., **CAUST.,** cham., chel., ***con., crot-c.,*** crot-h., cycl., ***dulc.,*** ferr., gamb., graph., hep., hydr-ac., indg., ***kali-bi., kali-i.,*** kali-n., laur., lact., ***lyc.,*** mag-c., mag-m., ***manc.,*** mang., meny., mur-ac., nat-c., ***nat-m.,*** nit-ac., ***olnd.,*** ph-ac., ***phos.,*** plb., puls., rheum, ***rhus-t.,*** ruta., sars., ***seneg.,*** sil., spig., squil., stann., staph., stront-c., sul-ac., ***sulph.,*** tab., tarax., ***thuj.,*** viol-t., vinc., zinc.
afternoon - lyc., nux-v., plb.
4 p.m. - lyc.
ascending a hill - ran-b., rat.
breath, at every - ***manc., nat-m.***
coughing, on - am-c., ***ars.,*** bell., **BRY.,** con., petr., ***psor.,*** sil., sulph.
daytime - ***calc-p.,*** nux-v.
behind - alum., euphr., mur-ac., zinc.
belching, from - kali-c.
breathing, deep - arg-m., arn., bapt., bor., ***bry.,*** caps., carb-v., **CAUST.,** chin., cina, hep., lyc., ***manc., nat-m.,*** psor., rumx., sil.
expiration - caust.
inspiration - euphr., phos., sil.
dinner, after - bor., sil.
drinking, after - chin.
eating, while - zinc.
evening - acon., bov., lyc., mag-c., sul-ac.
bed, in - nat-c., sul-ac., thuj.
inspiration, on - kali-c.
sitting, while - mag-c.
exertion - ***caust.***
extending to,
axilla - kali-n.
back - chin., ***con.,*** dulc., **KALI-BI., *kali-i.,*** laur.
downwards - chel., squil.
elbow - thuj.
lumbar region - zinc.
scapula, right - phos.
shoulders - ***kali-i.***
upward - ***ars.,*** carb-s.
itching - staph.
lifting, from - **CAUST.**
morning - led., lyc., nat-m., sars., sulph.
motion - carb-an., ruta.
amel. - lyc., phos.
night in bed - ferr.

SHARP, pain, sternum
room, entering a, from open air - sul-ac.
sitting, while - ***con.,*** dulc., euph., ***indg.,*** kali-i.
bent, while - ***rhus-t.***
sneezing, agg. - bry.
standing - euph., plb.
sterno-costal, joints - chin.
stooping - zinc.
swallowing, liquids - kali-c.
talking - alum.
touch, agg. - sulph.
walking - arn., cinnb., hep., mag-c., psor.
xiphoid - stann., sulph.
yawning - bell.

SHOCKS, in - agar., alum., ang., ant-t., arn., calc., cann-s., clem., **CON.,** croc., dulc., ***graph.,*** hep., ind., **LYC.,** mang., meny., mur-ac., myrt-c., nux-v., ol-an., ***plat.,*** rhus-t., ruta., sec., sep., ***sulph.,*** zinc.
cough, with - con., **LYC.,** ***seneg.***
sleep, during - ***lach.,*** spong.

SHUDDERING - agar., aur.
right - aur.
yawning - aur.

SMALL, feels too - ign.

SMOKE, as if - ars., ***bar-c.,*** brom., bry., ***nat-a.***

SORE, pain - acon., aesc., agar., alum., ambr., ***am-m.,*** anac., ant-t., **APIS, ARN.,** ***ars.,*** arum-t., asc-t., ***bad.,*** bapt., bar-c., berb., brom., **BRY., CALC.,** calc-p., calc-s., canth., carb-an., ***carb-s., carb-v.,*** **CAUST.,** cham., **CHEL., CHIN.,** chlor., ***cic.,*** cimic., ***cina,*** cocc., ***coc-c.,*** colch., ***cop.,*** corn., crot-t., ***cur.,*** dig., ***dor.,*** echi., ***euon., eup-per., ferr.,*** ferr-ar., ferr-m., ferr-p., fl-ac., gamb., ***gels.,*** graph., ***guai., ham.,*** **HEP.,** ***hydr., hyos.,*** ign., iris, ip., kali-ar., **KALI-BI.,** ***kali-c.,*** kali-n., kali-p., kali-s., ***kreos., lac-d., lach.,*** lact., laur., ***led.,*** lob., ***lyc.,*** lyss., ***mag-c., mag-m.,*** manc., mang., med., meph., ***merc., mez., mur-ac.,*** nat-a., ***nat-c., nat-m.,*** nat-p., nat-s., nicc., ***nit-ac., nux-m.,*** nux-v., olnd., ol-j., ox-ac., ***petr.,*** **PHOS.,** ***phyt.,*** psor., **PULS., RAN-B.,** ran-s., rat., rhod., ***rhus-t.,*** rumx., samb., sang., sanic., **SENEG.,** ***sep., sil., spong.,*** **STANN.,** ***staph.,*** stront-c., ***sulph.,*** sul-ac., syph., tarent., thuj., tab., ***zinc.***
afternoon - alum., nicc.
air, open - spig.
anterior - con., merc., nux-m., sarr.
bed, in - iod.
belching, on - phos.
amel. - ambr.
bending, forward - mang., seneg.
breathing, agg. - **ARN.,** ***calc.,*** eup-per., ***kali-c.,*** lob., nit-ac.
deep - aesc., aloe, eup-per., ferr., ferr-i., hydr., iod., kali-c., nat-a., ***ran-b.,*** sang., ***stann.***
inspiring - anac., **BRY., CALC.,** ***camph.,*** cinnb., ***eup-per.,*** kali-c., nat-a., nat-m., nit-ac., nux-m., sang., seneg., sil.
chill, during - lach.

SORE, pain
coughing, from - acon., alum., ambr., am-c., **APIS,** arg-m., **ARN.,** ars., bar-c., ***bell.,*** berb., bor., brom., **BRY.,** ***calc.,*** calc-s., ***carb-s.,*** **CARB-V.,** ***caust.,*** chlor., chin., cina, cocc., colch., ***cop., cur.,*** dig., **DROS.,** eug., ***eup-per., ferr.,*** ferr-ar., ***ferr-m.,*** ferr-p., gamb., ***gels.,*** graph., guare., hep., hydr., ip., ***kali-bi.,*** kali-n., ***kreos.,*** lach., lact., lec., lyc., mag-c., ***mag-m.,*** meph., merc., mez., mur-ac., nat-a., ***nat-c., nat-m., nat-s., nit-ac.,*** nux-m., ***nux-v.,*** ol-j., **PHOS.,** psor., **RAN-B.,** rat., rumx., sanic., **SENEG.,** sep., ***sil.,*** **SPONG., STANN.,** ***staph.,*** stram., stront-c., ***sulph.,*** syph., thuj., verat., zinc.
crossing, arms - ang.
damp, weather - cur.
drinking, after - nit-ac.
eating - nit-ac.
evening - coc-c., dig., ***kali-i.,*** lyss., mur-ac., murx., nat-m., ran-b.
exercising - colch., lob.
expectoration, during - lyc., zinc.
forenoon - alum., ***bry.***
hawking - ***calc.***
holds chest with hands, during cough - **ARN.,** bor., **BRY.,** cimic., **DROS.,** ***eup-per.,*** kreos., merc., nat-m., ***nat-s., phos., sep.***
lifting - alum., kali-c.
lower, part - am-m., meph.
lying, agg. - **CHIN.**
amel. - alum.
menses, before and during - **ZINC.**
middle - ***sep.***
morning - alum., am-c., ang., calad., corn., crot-h., mur-ac., nat-a., seneg., staph., thuj.
eating, after - sulph.
motion, on - alum., ang., ***arn.,*** mag-c., ol-j., ***phos., ran-b., seneg.,*** staph., thuj.
amel. - tab.
arms - nat-c., ***seneg.***
percussion, agg. - **CHIN.,** seneg.
pressing, on - ang., **ARN.,** ***bar-c., crot-t.,*** dros., nat-m., phos.
amel. - bry., dros., eup-per., nat-m., nat-s.
riding in a carriage - zinc.
rubbing, after - ant-c.
sitting, bent - meny.
upright, amel. - **BRY.,** nat-c., ***nat-s.***
sneezing, on - carb-s., lact., mez., ***seneg.***
straining, lifting causes soreness - alum.
stooping, on - phos., seneg.
supper, after, amel. - phos.
talking - alum., ***kali-c.,*** lyc., puls.
throbbing - agar.
touch - am-c., arg-m., arg-n., **ARN.,** bry., **CALC.,** calc-p., canth., **CHIN.,** cist., colch., con., crot-t., ***kali-c., led.,*** lyc., med., nat-m., nux-v., psor., **RAN-B.,** ***seneg.,*** zinc.
turning in bed, on - alum., **RAN-B.**

SORE, pain
waking, on - merc-i-r.
walking, in open air amel. - nat-m.
sore, clavicles - alumn., am-m., ***calc-p.,*** coc-c., lyc., manc., nat-m., phos., phys., still., sumb.
above - **APIS,** ***con.***
below - coc-c., ***ferr.,*** **PULS.,** phos.
left, motion, agg. - coc-c.
sore, costal cartilages - ***arn.,*** calc-p., plb., **RAN-B.,** staph.
cartilages of short ribs - arg-m., ***arn.,*** calc-p., ***lyc.,*** **RAN-B.,** staph., sulph.
last true rib - ph-ac., sulph.
right - ph-ac.
morning, in bed - arg-m.
sore, ribs - ph-ac.
anterior part - nit-ac.
fourth left, before and during stool - spig.
joints - chin.
sore, ribs, short - calc., caust., ***chel.,*** hep., ***lyc.,*** med., meph., nat-a., nat-m., ***ph-ac.,*** **RAN-B.,** ***sulph., tarent.***
inspiration, on - ***arn.,*** sulph.
left - med.
motion, on - ***arn.,*** meph.
right - ***chel.,*** lyc.
sore, sides - agar., alum., am-c., am-m., arg-n., ***arn.,*** calc., ***carb-v., chin.,*** **CON.,** iod., kali-i., lac-ac., nit-ac., ph-ac., phos., ***puls., ran-b.,*** rhus-t., rumx., seneg., stram., zinc.
bending, when - alum., nat-m.
breathing - iod., nat-m.
inspiration, on - nat-a.
chill, during - tarent.
evening - ***ran-b.,*** seneg.
chill, during - tarent.
extending to shoulder - laur.
left - ***am-m., arg-n.,*** arund., bar-c., calc., calc-p., chel., ***eup-per.,*** lac-c., laur., merc., mur-ac., nat-m., phos., ran-b., ***rumx.,*** stram., zinc.
lying on painful side - ***rumx.***
then right - agar.
lying on left side - ***puls., rumx.***
morning - ran-b.
pressure, on - mag-m.
right - ***aesc.,*** am-m., ***caust.,*** **CHEL.,** con., cupr-ac., elaps, nat-a., ph-ac., rhus-t., sulph., thuj., urt-u., zinc.
breathing, when - ***aesc.***
last rib - ***ph-ac.***
stooping - nit-ac.
stretching - nit-ac.
touch - am-c., calc., carb-v., **CON.,** iod., kali-i., lac-ac., ***ph-ac.,*** **RAN-B.,** ***rhus-t.,*** sulph., tarent., verat.
turning to left - ***rumx.***
sore, sternum - acon., benz-ac., bry., ***calc-p.,*** dros., ***kreos.,*** led., mez., mur-ac., naja, nat-c., nat-m., ***osm.,*** rumx., ph-ac., ***ran-b.,*** sabin., sars., stront-c., sul-ac., zinc.
ascending - ran-b.
cough, during - ***mur-ac.***
inspiration amel. - nat-c.

sore, sternum
laughing agg. - mur-ac.
motion amel. - nat-c.
lower part of - ***cic., nit-ac.***
talking agg. - mur-ac.
touch, on - cann-s., cimx., cop., mur-ac., ph-ac., psor., ***ran-b.,*** stront-c., sul-ac.
under - con., ***eup-per.,*** **RUMX.**
coughing, on - am-c., **BRY.,** chel., cina, iod., osm., psor., ***rumx.,*** staph.
inspiration, on - ***eup-per.***
spot - anac.
turning body - ***eup-per.***
walking, while - ***cic.***
yawning agg. - mur-ac.

SPASMODIC, motion in - arn.

SPASMS, of - acon., ang., ***arg-n., ars.,*** **ASAF.,** ***bell., calc.,*** camph., ***cann-s., cham.,*** chin., ***cic.,*** cina, ***cocc., colch.,*** **CUPR.,** ***elat., ferr.,*** ferr-ar., ferr-p., ***gels., graph., hyos., ip., kali-c.,*** kali-p., ***lach.,*** lact., ***laur.,*** led., ***lyc., merc., mez., mosch.,*** nat-s., nit-ac., ***nux-v., op., ph-ac., phos.,*** plb., ***puls., samb., sang.,*** sars., sec., sep., spig., spong., staph., ***stram., sulph.,*** tarent., ***verat., zinc.***
breathing, stopped, from - ***cupr.,*** stram.
colic, with - ***cupr., sep.,*** verat.
compelling him to bend forward - hyos., ph-ac.
coughing, when - agar., am-c., ars., chlor., cina, cupr., kali-c., lach., merc., mosch., sep., ***sulph.***
exercise, agg. - ferr.
heat and congestion, with - puls.
hysterical - ars., **ASAF.,** bell., cic., ***cocc., mosch., stram.,*** zinc.
menses, during - ***chin., cocc.***
before - bov., ***lach.***
walking, agg. - ferr.

SPLINTER, pain, in right lower ribs - ***agar.***

SPOTS, itching - hydr-ac., lyc., sulph.

SPRAIN, as from - agar., ***arn.,*** aur-m., dulc., ***kalm.,*** lyc., petr., rhod., sulph., tell.
breathing, deep agg. - agar., ***arn.***
standing - aur-m.

SQUEEZING, sensation - brom., cina, dros., graph., lact., merc., ***ph-ac., plat.,*** seneg., teucr., thuj., verat.

STABBING, pain - kali-c., nat-m., spig.

STAGNATION, of blood - ***lob.***

STICKING, pain, lung, as if ribs into - kali-c.
sticking, in short ribs - **SEP.**
right - agar.

STIFFNESS - ox-ac., ***phos.,*** stry.
chest muscles - lyc., puls.

STINGING - laur., nat-m., ***phos.,*** plb.

STUFFED up, as if - ambr., lach., med.
lungs with cotton, as if - kali-bi., med.

SUPPURATION, deep in - ***phos.***

SWELLING - ars., calc., ***dulc.,*** iod., kali-m., merc., nat-c., rhus-t., sep., ***sil., sulph.***

swelling, clavicles - phos.

swelling, sternum, lower part of - sac-alb.

TEARING, pain - aesc., aloe, anac., ant-t., aur., aur-m., bar-c., bell., berb., bry., canth., carb-h., ***carb-s., carb-v.,*** caust., ***clem.,*** **COLCH.,** con., cub., cycl., ***dulc.,*** elaps, graph., hura, hyos., kali-bi., ***kali-c.,*** kali-i., kali-p., merc., nat-m., **NUX-V.,** petr., ***phos.,*** psor., ***puls., ran-b.,*** rumx., sang., sil., ***spig.,*** thuj., valer., ***zinc.***

afternoon, deep inspiration, during - sang.
yawning - sang.
air, open - caust.
anterior part - clem., kali-bi., mez.
pectoral muscles - berb.
arm, on moving the - carb-an.
raising, arm toward head - spig.
stretching, the - berb.
belching - sep.
breathing, agg. - bry., puls.
inspiration, on - aur-m., ***psor.***
inspiration, deep agg. - kali-n.
cough, during - ***ambr.,*** aeth., bufo, ***calc.,*** elaps, eupi., kali-c., ***nat-m.,*** nit-ac., nux-v., psor., ***rhus-t.***
drinking, after - nit-ac.
evening - ambr., kali-n.
bed, in - con.
externally - bar-c.
lifting, on - ***psor.***
lying on side - con.
motion - aur-m., bry., nit-ac.
night - am-c., nit-ac., sil.
standing - spig.

tearing, clavicles, of - am-m., brom., caps., cham., ***lyc.,*** stann.
fine - agar.
paralytic - ferr-m.

tearing, ribs, between the - ***sul-ac.***
costal cartilages of short - grat., merc-c.
lower ribs - bism., plb., sep.

tearing, sides - ***acon.,*** aur-m., berb., bry., cann-s., ***carb-v.,*** caust., chel., ***cocc.,*** euph., graph., grat., hydr-ac., kali-bi., kali-c., lact., laur., ***lyc.,*** plb., puls., ***sel.,*** sep., sil., sumb., zinc.
afternoon - nicc.
ascending stairs agg. - kali-bi.
blowing nose, on - sumb.
breathing, deep - spig.
cramp-like - con.
erect, on becoming - dig.
evening - kali-c.
extending to
left, upper arm - spig.
scapula - spig.
inspiration - ferr-ma., lyc., sang., spig.
left - ***ambr.,*** am-c., anac., berb., cann-s., ***carb-v.,*** chel., ***dig.,*** dulc., ferr-ma., graph., grat., kali-c., sil., spig., zinc.
upper - sep.
morning - sumb.
inspiration agg. - sumb.

tearing, sides
motion - ***bry.***
right - arg-m., ars., aur-m., ***bry.,*** caust., ***cocc.,*** con., elaps, iod., kali-c., lyc., plb., sang., sep., zinc.
apex of lung - elaps.
right, then left - aur-m.
sitting bent - anac.

tearing, sternum - aesc., aur., ***calc-p., dig.,*** dulc., ***lyc.,*** osm., phos., psor.
cough, with - chin., ***kali-i.,*** osm., ox-ac., ***phos.,*** psor.
midnight, after - merc-c.

TENSION, clavicles - ***lyc.,*** nat-m., ***zinc.***
left - zinc.
under - ***lyc.***

tension, lower, ribs - sulph.

THREAD, swaying by the - tub.

TICKLING, in - ***calc.,*** cham., coc-c., con., graph., ign., ***iod.,*** kali-c., ***lach.,*** merc., mur-ac., ***ph-ac., phos.,*** puls., ***rhus-t.,*** **RUMX.,** sep., sul-ac., verat., verb., visc., zinc.

ticking, in short ribs, right - agar.

TINGLING - acon., ars., cadm-s., colch., plb., puls., ran-b., ***rhus-t.,*** seneg., spong., stann.

TREMBLING - ambr., apis, ***arg-m., arg-n., ars.,*** benz-ac., bov., ***calc.,*** calc-p., ***camph.,*** carb-an., ***carb-v.,*** **CIC.,** ***cocc.,*** dig., kali-c., kali-n., ***kalm.,*** lac-c., lachn., lact., manc., nat-p., nicc., phos., ruta., sabin., seneg., **SPIG.,** ***staph.,*** ther., zinc.
chilliness, with - phos.
coughing, on - rhus-t.
crying, as from - stront.
dinner, after - zinc.
inspiration, on - ang.
moving the arms, on - ***spig.***
noon, toward - sulph.
painful - benz-ac.

TUBERCLES - am-c., caust., mang., nicc.

TURNING, over, chest, as if something were - apis, arn., cact., ***camph.,*** caust., crot-h., ***lach.,*** rhus-t., ***sep.,*** stram., tab., tarent.

TWISTING - ph-ac.

TWITCHING, muscles, in - agar., anac., asar., calc., chin., cic., cina, coloc., dros., dulc., kali-c., lyc., mez., nat-c., nat-m., plat., seneg., sep., spig., stann., tarax.
burning - nat-c.

ULCERATIVE, pain - bry., carb-an., kreos., ***lach.,*** mag-m., merc., psor., ***puls., ran-b.,*** spig., staph., sulph.
coughing, on - mag-m., psor.

ulcerative, sternum, under, as if - psor.

ULCERS - ***ars.,*** hep., ***sulph.***

ulcers, clavicle and over sternum - ***calc-p.***

URTICARIA - ***calad.,*** hydrc., sars., sulph., urt-u.

VAPOUR, in, as if - merc.

VELVETY, sensation, in chest - ant-t.

VESICLES - alum., arund., calc., calc-s., camph., carb-s., caust., ***graph.***, kali-i., led., ***merc.***, rhus-t., sep., stram., sulph.
burning - alum.

WARMTH, sensation of - alum., euph., hell., lact., ***mang.***, nat-m., ol-an., rhod., rhus-t., **SULPH.**, verat.

WARTS, sternum - nit-ac.

WATER, sensation of, in - bov., bufo, crot-c., hep., samb.
boiling, was poured into - **ACON.**
cold, running from clavicle in narrow line to toes - caust.
hot, in - **ACON.**, cic., ***hep.***

WEAKNESS - acon., ail., aloe, alum., alumn., ammc., am-c., am-m., **ANT-T.**, **ARG-M.**, ***arg-n.***, ***ars.***, ***ars-i.***, arum-t., asc-t., bapt., ***benz-ac.***, bor., brom., cadm-s., ***calc.***, calc-s., canth., ***carb-s.***, **CARB-V.**, carl., chin-a., coc-c., cocc., con., cycl., ***dig.***, ***hep.***, ***ign.***, iod., kali-ar., ***kali-c.***, kali-i., kali-p., kali-s., lact., **LAUR.**, lob., manc., mang., nat-m., nat-s., nit-ac., ol-j., olnd., ***ph-ac.***, **PHOS.**, ***plat.***, ***psor.***, **RAN-S.**, raph., rhus-t., ruta., **SENEG.**, sep., ***sil.***, ***spong.***, **STANN.**, ***staph.***, ***sulph.***, ***sul-ac.***, thuj., til., ***tub.***
bending forward amel. - nux-v.
breathing, deep - carb-v., ***plat.***
cough, from - graph., ***nit-ac.***, ***ph-ac.***, ***psor.***, ruta., sep., **STANN.**
impeding - ***stann.***
menses, before - graph.
eating, while - carb-an.
evening - ran-s.
lying, while - ***sulph.***
exertion, after - aloe, **SPONG.**
expectoration after - **STANN.**
lying amel. - alum.
amel., on side - ***sulph.***
morning on waking - **CARB-V.**, dig.
lasting until 3 p.m. - merc-i-r.
palpitations, with - olnd.
reading agg. - sulph.
aloud - cocc., ***sulph.***
singing, when - carb-v., stann., sulph.
on beginning to - **STANN.**
sitting long agg. - dig., ***ph-ac.***
speech, impeding - ***calc.***, dig., ***hep.***, ph-ac., rhus-t., ***stann.***, ***sulph.***, sul-ac.
talking, when - calc., ***ph-ac.***, rhus-t., sil., **STANN.**, ***sulph.***, sul-ac.
loud, when - calc., gels., kali-c., ***laur.***, **SULPH.**
waking, on - **CARB-V.**
walking - ***lyss.***, ***rhus-t.***
air, in open - nat-m., ***rhus-t.***
amel. - ***ph-ac.***
rapid - ***kali-c.***
rapid, in open air - nat-m.
sun, in - nat-m.

WEIGHT, weight seems to fall from pit of chest to abdomen - nat-h.

WINE, agg. - bor.

XYPHOID bone, absent - syph.

Children

CHILDREN, general - abrot., **ACON.,** ***aeth.,*** agar., alum., ***ant-c.,*** **ANT-T.,** arg-n., ***ars.,*** asaf., ***aur.,*** **BAR-C., BELL., BOR.,** ***bry.,*** **CALC.,** calc-f., **CALC-P.,** calc-s., **CAPS., CARC.,** caust., **CHAM.,** chel., chin., ***cic.,*** **CINA,** clem., ***cocc.,*** coff., dros., ferr., ***ferr-p.,*** hep., ip., ***kali-p.,*** **LYC.,** mag-p., **MED., MERC.,** mur-ac., nat-c., **NAT-M.,** ***nux-m., nux-v.,*** **OP., PHOS.,** ph-ac., phyt., ***podo.,*** psor., **PULS.,** ***rheum,*** rhus-t., ruta, sabad., ***samb.,*** sanic., senn., sep., **SIL.,** ***spong.,*** staph., stram., sul-ac., **SULPH., THUJ.,** thyr., **TUB.,** verat., zinc.
  constitutional, remedies - bar-c., **CALC.,** ***calc-p.,*** calc-s., ***lyc.,*** **PHOS., SIL.,** ***sulph.***

ABDOMEN, enlarged, in - alum., **BAR-C., CALC.,** calc-p., caust., cupr., mag-m., ***psor., sanic., sars.,*** **SIL.,** ***staph., sulph.***
    emaciation, with - **CALC.,** ***sanic., sars., sil.***
    girls, at puberty - calc., ***graph.,*** lach., lyc., sulph.
    swelling, glands of, with - mez.
  distension, in - **BAR-C., CALC., CAUST.,** ***cina,*** cupr., **LYC.,** sil., staph., **SULPH.**
  hard - calc., sil.
    hot, distended - ***sil.***
  tension, of - sil.

ABUSED, ailments from being - ***acon.,*** alum., am-m., **ANAC.,** ***arg-n.,*** ars., ***aur., aur-m.,*** bell., ***bry.,*** calc., calc-s., **CARC.,** caust., ***cham.,*** **COLOC.,** con., form., gels., grat., **IGN.,** ***lach.,*** **LYC.,** ***lyss.,*** med., merc., **NAT-M.,** ***nux-v., op.,*** **PALL.,** petr., **PH-AC.,** plat., ***puls.,*** rhus-t., ***seneg.,*** sep., sil., **STAPH.,** stram., ***sulph.,*** thuj., verat., zinc.
  anger, with - anac., carc., **COLOC.,** ***staph.***
  indignation, with - anac., **IGN., STAPH.**
  punishment, from - ***anac.,*** **CARC.,** cham., ign., lyc., nat-m., **STAPH.,** tarent.
  sexual abuse, from - **ACON.,** anac., **ARN., CARC., IGN.,** lyc., ***med.,*** **NAT-M.,** nux-v., **OP.,** ***plat.,*** **SEP., STAPH.,** thuj.
    shame, from - ign., ***nat-m.,*** **STAPH.,** thuj.
  violence, from - acon., ***anac.,*** **ARN.,** ***aur., bry.,*** **CARC.,** coff., lyc., nat-m., **OP., STAPH.**

ABUSIVE, children, who insult parents - am-m., calc-p., ***cham.,*** **CINA,** hyos., **LYC.,** nat-m., **PLAT., TUB.**

ACETONEMIA, in child - phenob.

ACROMEGALY - ***bar-c.,*** carc., pituit., thyr.

ADENOIDS, problems with - agra., ***bar-c., bar-m., calc.,*** calc-f., calc-i., calc-p., **CARC.,** chr-ac., iod., kali-s., lob-s., merc., mez., phyt., psor., sang-n., sulph., ***thuj.,*** **TUB.**
  post nasal - mez.
  removal, after - ***carc.,*** kali-s.

ANGRY, children - anac., ***calc-p.,*** **CHAM., CINA,** hep., nux-v., ***phos., sanic., tub.***

ANOREXIA nervosa - **ARS.,** calc., ***carc.,*** **CHIN.,** ***ign.,*** lach., levo., merc., ***nat-m.,*** perh., puls., rhus-t., staph., **SULPH.,** tarent., verat.

ANXIOUS, children - acon., ***ars., bor.,*** calc., calc-p., carc., ***cina, gels., kali-c., phos.***
  chest complaints, with - ***calc-p., phos.***
  infants, in - ***acon.,*** ars., ***cham.,*** phos.
  lifted from the cradle, when - calc., ***calc-p.,*** bor.
  rocking, during - **BOR.**
  waking, evening, in - **CINA**
    morning, in - ***chin.***
    night, at - ***dros.***
  watchful, who are on the look out for every gesture - phos.

ASTHMA - ***acon.,*** ambr., **ANT-T., ARS.,** ***carc.,*** **CHAM., IP.,** kali-br., kali-c., kali-i., **KALI-N., KALI-S.,** lob., **MED.,** ***mosch.,*** **NAT-S.,** nux-v., psor., **PHOS., PULS., SAMB.,** sanic., ***sil.,*** stram., sulph., ***thuj.,*** **TUB.,** vib.
  vaccination, after - **ANT-T.,** ***sil.,*** **THUJ.**

AUTISTIC, children - ***carc.,*** cann-i., ***nat-m.,*** op., thuj.
  vaccinations, after - carc., thuj.

BASHFUL, disposition - aloe, ***ambr.,*** anac., arg-n., ars-s-f., aur., ***bar-c.,*** bar-s., bell., **calc.,** calc-s., calc-sil., ***carb-an.,*** carb-v., caust., ***chin.,*** **COCA,** con., coff., ***cupr.,*** graph., hyos., ***ign.,*** iod., kali-bi., ***kali-p.,*** lil-t., manc., mang., meli., merc., mez., ***nat-c.,*** nat-p., nit-ac., nux-v., ***petr.,*** phos., **PULS.,** sil., ***staph., stram., sulph.,*** tab., tarent., ***zinc.***
  covering their face with their hands, but look through their fingers - bar-c.
  hiding - **ARS.,** ***bar-c.,*** **CUPR.,** ***hyos.,*** puls.

BATHING, dislike of - am-c., **SULPH.**

BEDWETTING - acon., ***aeth.,*** alum., ***am-c.,*** anac., anan., **APIS,** ***apoc., arg-m.,*** **ARG-N., ARN., ARS.,** ***aur.,*** aur-m., aur-s., bar-c., bar-m., **BELL., BENZ-AC.,** bry., cact., ***calc.,*** canth., ***carb-s., carb-v.,*** carc., **CAUST.,** ***cham.,*** chin., ***chlol.,*** cimx., ***cina,*** coca, con., ***crot-c.,*** cub., cupr., dulc., **EQUIS.,** ***eup-pur.,*** **FERR.,** ***ferr-ac.,*** ferr-i., ferr-p., ***fl-ac.,*** **GRAPH.,** ***hep.,*** hyos., ign., kali-br., kali-c., ***kali-p.,*** **KREOS., LAC-C.,** lac-d., ***lyc.,*** mag-aust., mag-c., ***mag-m.,*** **MAG-P.,** mag-s., ***med., merc.,*** mur-ac., ***nat-a., nat-c.,*** **NAT-M.,** ***nat-p.,*** **NIT-AC.,** nux-v., ***op.,*** ox-ac., ***petr.,*** ph-ac., ***phos.,*** physal., ***plan., podo., psor.,*** **PULS.,** quas., rhus-a., **RHUS-T.,** ***ruta.,*** sabal., ***sanic.,*** sant., ***sars.,*** sec., sel., ***seneg.,*** **SEP., SIL.,** spig., squil., staph., ***stram.,*** **SULPH.,** ***syc-co.,*** tab., ter., ***thuj.,*** **THYR.,** ***tub., uran., urt-u.,*** uva., verat., ***verb., viol-t.,*** zinc.
  adolescence - ***lac-c.***
  children, in - aesc., ***bell.,*** benz-ac., carc., ***caust.,*** chin., ***cina,*** **EQUIS.,** ***kreos., lyc.,*** med., nat-m., phos., puls., sep., sil., thuj.
  difficult to waken the child - ***bell.,*** chlol., **KREOS.,** thuj.
  dreaming of urinating, while - ***kreos.,*** lac-c., lyc., merc-i-f., ***seneg., sep.,*** sulph.
  first sleep - benz-ac., **CAUST.,** cina, ***kreos., ph-ac.,*** **SEP.**

BEDWETTING,
habit, when there is no tangible cause except - **EQUIS.**
midnight to morning - plan.
morning, toward - am-c., cact., chlol., zinc.
night, after 5 a.m. - cact.
spasmodic enuresis - **ARG-M.,** bell., canth., caps., cast., cina, coloc., ***gels.,*** hyos., ign., lach., lyc., ***nux-v.,*** op., puls., rhus-t., verat.
weakly children, in - ***chin.***

BIRTHMARKS, nevi - **ACET-AC.,** arn., ars., ***calc.,*** calc-f., carb-an., ***carb-v.,*** **CARC.,** cund., **FL-AC.,** lach., ***lyc.,*** med., nux-v., **PHOS.,** plat., rad., ***sep.,*** sol, ***sulph.,*** **THUJ.,** ust., vac.
smooth - con., phos., sep., sulph.
spidery - carb-v., lach., ***plat.,*** sep., thuj.
red - med.

BITING, of fingernails, habit - ***acon., am-br.,*** arn., ars., **ARUM-T.,** ***bar-c.,*** calc., ***carc.,*** **CINA,** hura, ***hyos., lyc.,*** lyss., med., ***nat-m.,*** nit-ac., phos., plb., sanic., senec., ***sil.,*** stram., ***sulph.***

BOTTLE-fed, marasmus, abdomen swollen, liver large, colic after eating, stomach containing undigested food - nat-p.

BREAST-feeding, ailments during - acon., agn., ***ars., bell.,*** **BOR.,** ***bry.,*** **CALC., CALC-P.,** carb-an., carb-v., **CHAM.,** chel., ***chin., cina,*** con., crot-t., ***dulc.,*** ferr., graph., ***ign.,*** iod., ***ip.,*** kali-c., lach., lyc., ***mag-c.,*** merc., nat-c., nat-m., **NAT-P.,** ***nux-v.,*** phel., ***ph-ac.,*** phos., phyt., **PULS.,** rheum, ***rhus-t.,*** samb., sec., sel., **SEP.,** sil., spig., ***squil.,*** stann., ***staph.,*** stram., ***sulph.,*** zinc.
mother's milk agg. - acet-ac., ant-c., ***bor.,*** calc., **CALC-P.,** ***cina,*** lach., ***merc., nat-c., ph-ac., sanic.,*** **SIL.,** stann., ***valer.***
refuses mother's milk - ***acet-ac., bor., calc.,*** **CALC-P.,** cina, lach., mag-c., ***merc., ph-ac.,*** rheum, sabal., **SIL.,** stann., sulph.
vomits milk after nursing - acet-ac., aeth., ***ant-c.,*** calc., calc-p., ***nat-c., ph-ac., sanic.,*** **SIL.,** ***valer.***
weaning, child - **BELL.,** carb-an., ***cham.,*** frag-v., lac-c., lac-d., **PULS.,** urt-u., vinc.

BULIMIA - ***carc.,*** ign., iod., nat-m., puls., staph.

CAPRICIOUS, children - calc-p., carc., ***cham., cina,*** ign., puls., sac-alb.

CARRIED, desires to be - acon., acet-ac., ant-c., ant-t., ***ars.,*** aspar., bell., benz-ac., bor., brom., **BRY.,** calc., carb-v., **CHAM.,** ***chel., cina,*** coff., coloc., ign., ip., kali-c., ***kreos., lyc., kali-c.,*** merc., podo., phos., **PULS.,** ***rhus-t.,*** sanic., stann., staph., sulph., vac., ***verat.***
aversion to be - ***bry., coff.***
wants to lie quiet - ***bry.***
caressed and carried, desires to be - acon., kreos., puls.
croup, in - brom.
fast - acon., **ARS.,** bell., brom., **CHAM.,** ***cina.,*** rhus-t., verat.
fondled, and - kreos., phos., ***puls.***
rocked, and - ***cina.***

CARRIED, desires to be
shoulder, over - ***cina,*** podo., stann.
sitting up - ant-t., ***puls.***
slowly - ferr., **PULS.**
will not be laid down - benz-ac.

CEPHALAHEMATOMA - ***calc-f., merc.,*** **SIL.**

CHOREA, in children who have grown too fast - calc-p., phos.

CLINGING, child awakens terrified, knows no one, screams, clings to those near - ***acon., ars.,*** **BOR.,** cham., cina, stram.
convulsions, before - **CIC.**
grasps at others - ***ant-t.,*** ars., ***camph.,*** op., phos.
bystanders - **ANT-T.**
the nurse when carried - ***ars.,*** bor., ***gels.,*** puls.
held, wants to be - acon., ***ars., cham.,*** gels., kali-p., lach., nux-m., nux-v., **PULS.,** sang., sep., stram.
amel. being - diph., **PULS.**
restlessness, with - ***ars., carb-v.***
take the hand of mother, will always - ars., bar-c., ***bism., phos.,*** puls.
to persons or furnitiure - ***bar-c.,*** bism., bor., coff., gels., phos., stram.

COMPLAINING, children - anac., ***ant-c.,*** **ARS.,** bell., ***bism.,*** bor., ***bry., bufo,*** **CALC-P.,** caps., caust., **CHAM., CINA,** ***coloc.,*** hep., hyos., ***ign., lach., lyc.,*** mag-p., ***merc.,*** **NIT-AC.,** ***nux-v.,*** psor., puls., rheum, rhus-t., sil., staph., ***sulph.,*** tab., tarent., **TUB.,** ***verat.,*** zinc.

CONCENTRATION, difficult - ***aeth.,*** am-c., **BAR-C.,** ***carc.,*** graph., lach., **MED.,** ph-ac., ***phos.,*** sil., zinc.
can't fix attention - ***aesc.,*** bov., hipp., hyos., ign., **MED.,** ***phos.,*** **SIL., SIN-N.,** verat.
studying, reading, while - acon., **AETH.,** agar., ***agn.,*** alum., ambr., ang., asar., ***bar-c.,*** bar-m., bell., calc-f., calc-sil., carb-ac., carb-s., caust., cham., coff., corn., ***dros.,*** fago., ferr-i., **HELL.,** iod., kali-bi., kali-c., ***kali-p.,*** kali-sil., lach., lyc., merc., mur-ac., nat-a., ***nat-c.,*** nat-p., **NUX-V.,** olnd., ox-ac., ***phos.,*** pic-ac., scut., **SIL.,** sin-a., spig., ***staph.,*** sul-i., sulph., ***syph.,*** tab., zinc-p.

CONFIDENCE, lacking of self esteem - ***anac.,*** arg-n., ars., aur., **BAR-C.,** ***calc.,*** **CALC-F.,** calc-p., calc-sil., carb-v., **CARC.,** caust., gels., hyos., ign., ***kali-p.,*** kali-s., ***lac-c.,*** lach., **LYC.,** ***med.,*** merc., nat-c., **NAT-M.,** nat-s., nit-ac., phos., ***psor., puls.,*** sant., **SIL., STAPH.,** stram., syph., ***thuj.,*** verat.

CONSCIENTIOUS, about trifles - **ARS.,** ***bar-c.,*** calc., ***calc-p.,*** calc-s., ***carc.,*** cham., hyos., **IGN.,** ***lyc.,*** nat-c., ***nux-v.,*** puls., **SIL.,** ***staph.,*** sul-i., ***sulph., thuj.,*** verat.

CONSTIPATION - acon., ***aesc.,*** **ALUM.,** ***ant-c.,*** apis, bell., **BRY., CALC.,** caust., ***cham., coll.,*** croc., ***graph., hep., hydr.,*** hydr-ac., kreos., **LYC.,** ***mag-m.,*** meph., ***nat-m., nit-ac.,*** **NUX-V.,** nyct.,

CONSTIPATION - **OP.**, ***paraf.***, ***plat.***, ***plb.***, ***podo.***, ***psor.***, sanic., ***sep.***, ***sil.***, sulph., verat.
infants, in - aesc., ***alum.***, bry., ***calc.***, caust., coll., lyc., mag-m., ***nux-v.***, ***op.***, plb., psor., sel., sep., verat.
bottle fed, from artificial food - alum., calc., nux-v., op.
newborn, in - alum., ***calc.***, caust., med., **NUX-V.**, **OP.**, ***sulph.***, verat., ***zinc.***

CONVULSIONS - absin., acon., ***aeth.***, agar., ***ambr.***, ***aml-n.***, ant-t., ***apis***, arn., ars., **ART-V.**, asaf., **BELL.**, bry., bufo, **CALC.**, ***calc-p.***, ***camph.***, canth., caust., ***cham.***, ***chlol.***, ***cic.***, cimic., **CINA**, cocc., ***coff.***, colch., ***crot-c.***, ***cupr.***, ***cupr-ac.***, ***cypr.***, dol., ***gels.***, glon., ***guare.***, **HELL.**, ***hep.***, ***hydr-ac.***, ***hyos.***, ***ign.***, ***ip.***, ***kali-br.***, kali-c., kali-p., kreos., ***lach.***, laur., ***lyc.***, ***mag-p.***, meli., merc., mosch., nux-m., ***nux-v.***, oena., **OP.**, passi., ph-ac., phos., plat., scut., sec., ***sil.***, ***stann.***, **STRAM.**, ***sulph.***, ter., upa., **VERAT.**, ***verat-v.***, **ZINC.**, ***zinc-cy.***, zinc-s., ***zinc-valer.***
approach of strangers, from - lyss., op., tarent.
dentition, during - ***acon.***, ***aeth.***, art-v., arum-t., ***bell.***, **CALC.**, ***calc-p.***, ***caust.***, **CHAM.**, ***cic.***, ***cina***, coff., ***colch.***, ***cupr.***, ***cupr-ac.***, ***cypr.***, gels., hyos., ***ign.***, ***ip.***, **KALI-BR.**, ***kreos.***, ***lach.***, mag-p., ***meli.***, merc., mill., nux-m., passi., ***podo.***, rheum, sin-n., ***stann.***, ***stram.***, sulph., thyr., ***verat-v.***, ***zinc.***
diarrhea, with - nux-m.
holding, when, amel. - nicc.
infants, in - ***art-v.***, **BELL.**, bufo, ***cham.***, ***cupr.***, **HELL.**, ***hydr-ac.***, ***mag-p.***, ***meli.***
newborns, in - ***art-v.***, ***bell.***, ***cupr.***, nux-v.
nursing, angry or frightened mother - bufo.
playing or laughing excessively from - coff.
strangers, approach of - op.

COWARDICE, (see Confidence) - ***acon.***, agar., anac., arg-n., ars., **BAR-C.**, bar-i., bar-m., calc., calc-s., ***calc-sil.***, carb-v., caust., cham., **GELS.**, graph., ign., iod., kali-p., **LYC.**, merc., nat-m., **OP.**, ph-ac., ***phos.***, ***puls.***, ***sil.***, staph., ***stram.***, thuj., ***verat.***

CRAWLS, child crawls into corners, howls, cries - camph.

CRETINISM - absin., ***aeth.***, ***anac.***, arn., bac., ***bar-c.***, bar-m., ***bufo,*** calc-p., hell., ign., iod., ***lap-a.***, lol., nat-c., oxyt., ph-ac., plb., sep., sulph., ***thyr.***

CROSS, disposition - cham., ***cina,*** lyc., ***nux-v.***, upa., tub.
waking, on - **LYC.**, **NUX-V.**

CRUELTY, children cannot bear to see cruelty at the movies - ***calc.***, ***carc.***, caust., cic., phos.

CRUSTA lactea - **STAPH.**

CRYING, children - ars., ***bell.***, ***bor.***, bry., camph., caste., caust., **CHAM.**, chin., cina, ***coff.***, ***graph.***, ***hyos.***, ***ign.***, ***jal.***, ***kali-c.***, ***lyc.***, nit-ac., **PULS.**, **RHEUM**, ***seneg.***, sil.
birth, since - acon., carc., cham., syph.

CRYING, children
cries piteously if taken hold of or carried - ***cina,*** sil.
difficult dentition, from - cham., ***phyt.***
his will is not done, when - calc-p., cham., **CINA.**, tub.
infants - ***acon.***, ars., bell., bor., calc., ***cham.***, coff., ign., ip., jal., ***puls.***, ***rhod.***, senn., syph., thuj.
night - arund., ***bor.***, ***lac-c.***, ***psor.***, ***rheum***
quiet only when carried - **CHAM.**, cina.
toss all night - ars., ***psor.***, ***rheum.***

CURSING, swearing - **ANAC.**, ***bell.***, hyos., ***lyc.***, lyss., nit-ac., nux-v., plat., ***stram.***, tarent., ***tub.***, ***verat.***

CURVATURE of spine - **ASAF.**, aur., bar-c., ***bar-m.***, **CALC.**, **CALC-F.**, calc-i., **CALC-P.**, **CALC-S.**, carb-s., ***carb-v.***, ***con.***, dros., ferr-i., hecla, hep., ***lyc.***, ***merc.***, **MERC-C.**, op., **PH-AC.**, **PHOS.**, psor., ***puls.***, sep., **SIL.**, **SULPH.**, tarent., ther., thuj.
lies on back with knees drawn up - **MERC-C.**
pain in - ***aesc.***, hecla, **LYC.**, **SIL.**
curvature, neck - ***calc.***, phos., ***syph.***
curvature, thoracic - bar-c., bufo, ***calc.***, ***calc-s.***, ***con.***, ***lyc.***, plb., ***puls.***, ***rhus-t.***, ***sil.***, ***sulph.***, ***syph.***, thuj.

CURVING and bowing of limbs - ***calc.***, ***calc-p.***, lyc., ***sil.***, ***syph.***
of leg bones - am-c., hep.

CYANOSIS, infants, in - arn., ars., ***bor.***, ***cact.***, ***camph.***, ***carb-v.***, chin., **DIG.**, **LACH.**, **LAUR.**, ***naja,*** op., ***phos.***, psor., rhus-t., sec., sulph.

DELICATE, puny, sickly - brom., ***calc-p.***, ***caust.***, irid., ***lyc.***, mag-c., phos., psor., **SIL.**

DENTITION, difficult teething - **ACON.**, ***aeth.***, am-c., ***ant-c.***, ***ant-t.***, ***apis***, ***arn.***, **ARS.**, arund., **BELL.**, ***bism.***, **BOR.**, ***bry.***, **CALC.**, calc-f., **CALC-P.**, ***canth.***, ***caust.***, **CHAM.**, cheir., chlor., cic., cimic., ***cina***, ***coff.***, ***colch.***, ***coloc.***, cupr., cypr., ***dol.***, ***dulc.***, ***ferr.***, ***ferr-p.***, ***gels.***, ***graph.***, ***hecla.***, ***hell.***, hep., hyos., ***ign.***, ***ip.***, ***kali-br.***, ***kreos.***, ***lyc.***, ***mag-c.***, **MERC.**, ***merc-c.***, mill., nat-m., nit-ac., op., passi., ***phyt.***, plat., ***podo.***, puls., ***rheum,*** scut., sec., sep., **SIL.**, sol-n., stann., **STAPH.**, **SULPH.**, syph., ***ter.***, tub., tub-k., zinc., zinc-br.
ailments from - ***acon.***, ***cham.***, ***coff.***, mag-c., mag-p., ***nux-v.***, rheum, ***rhus-t.***, stann., staph.
brain and nervous symptoms, with - acon., agar., ***bell.***, ***cham.***, cimic., cypr., dol., ***hell.***, kali-br., ***podo.***, sol-n., ter., ***zinc.***
compression of gums, with - cic., phyt., podo.
constipation, general irritation and cachexia, with - ***kreos.***, nux-v., op.
convulsions, with - ***bell.***, calc., ***cham.***, ***cic.***, cupr., glon., kali-br., ***mag-p.***, sol-n., stann.
cough, with - acon., bell., ferr-p., kreos.
deafness, otorrhea and stuffiness of nose, with - cheir.

DENTITION, difficult

diarrhea, with - acet-ac., aeth., apoc., arund., ***calc.,*** calc-ac., ***calc-p., cham.,*** ferr-p., ip., jal., kreos., mag-c., ***mag-p.,*** merc., olnd., phos., ***phyt.,*** podo., puls., rheum, ***sil.***

effusion of brain, with threatening - ***apis,*** hell., tub., ***zinc-m.***

eye symptoms, with - bell., calc., puls.

insomnia, with - bell., cham., ***coff., cypr.,*** kreos., passi., scut.

intertrigo, with - caust., lyc.

milk indigestion, with - aeth., calc., ***mag-m.***

salivation, with - bor.

slow - aster., **CALC.,** calc-f., **CALC-P.,** ***fl-ac.,*** mag-c., mag-m., mag-p., merc., nep., phos., **SIL.,** sulfa., ***sulph.,*** thuj., **TUB.,** zinc.

sour smell of body, pale face and irritability, with - kreos.

weakness, palor, fretfulness and must be carried rapidly, with - ars.

worms, with - ***cina,*** merc., stann.

DEPRESSED, children - abrot., ***ars.,*** aur., ***calc.,*** carc., caust., ***lach.,*** lyc., **NAT-M.,** rhus-t., sulph.

DESTRUCTIVE, behaviour - anac., ***bell.,*** cham., ***cina,*** hep., ***hyos.,*** lach., med., ***nux-v., staph.,*** **STRAM.,** tarent., **TUB.,** ***verat.***

DEVELOPMENT, arrested - aeth., ***agar.,*** bac., **BAR-C.,** bor., ***calc.,*** **CALC-P., CARC.,** caust., chin., cupr., des-ac., iod., kali-c., kreos., lac-d., med., ***nat-m.,*** nep., ph-ac., ***phos.,*** pin-s., ***sil.,*** sulfa., sulph., thyr., vip.

bones, of - ***calc.,*** calc-f., ***calc-p.,*** sil.

glands - bar-c., iod.

muscles, of - nat-m.

nutritional disturbances, due to - bac., ***bar-c., calc., calc-p.,*** caust., kreos., lac-d., med., nat-m., pin-s., ***sil.,*** thyr.

DIAPER, rash, buttocks - ***bapt., bor.,*** bry., ***kali-chl., merc., merc-c., mur-ac., nit-ac., sulph.,*** **SUL-AC.**

aphthous, anus, condition of - ***bapt., bor.,*** bry., ***kali-chl., merc., merc-c., mur-ac., nit-ac., sulph.,*** **SUL-AC.**

excoriation, between buttocks - arg-m., arum-t., ***berb.,*** bufo, calc., calen., ***carb-s.,*** carb-v., **GRAPH.,** ***kreos.,*** nat-m., ***nit-ac.,*** puls., ***sep., sulph.***

DIARRHEA - ***acon.,*** **AETH.,** ***agar.,*** agn., apis, ***arg-n.,*** **ARS.,** arund., bapt., bar-c., bell., ***benz-ac.,*** bism., ***bor.,*** **CALC.,** calc-ac., ***calc-p.,*** **CALC-S.,** camph., **CHAM.,** ***cina,*** chin., ***coloc.,*** colos., ***crot-t., dulc.,*** elat., ***ferr., form.,*** gamb., grat., hell., hep., **IP.,** ***iris,*** jal., kali-br., kreos., laur., lyc., lyss., ***mag-c.,*** **MAG-M.,** med., **MERC.,** ***merc-c., merc-d., mez., nat-m.,*** nit-ac., nux-m., ***nux-v.,*** olnd., paull., ***ph-ac.,*** **PHOS., PODO., PSOR.,** ***puls.,*** **RHEUM,** sabad., samb., senn., sep., **SIL.,** stann., ***staph.,*** **STRAM., SULPH.,** sul-ac., **TUB.,** ***valer.,*** verat., zinc.

nursing - arund., calc-p., cham.

DIRTINESS - **AM-C.,** bor., calc-s., ***caps., crot-h.,*** med., merc., ***nux-v.,*** petr., ***plat., psor.,*** sil., **STAPH., SULPH.,** verat.

dirting everything - am-c., bry., ***nat-m.***

dirty skin, with - am-c., ars., lyc., nux-v., ***psor., sulph.***

urinating and defecating everywhere - ***sep.,*** sil., sulph.

DISCONTENTED, children - calc-p., carc., ***cham., cina, tub.***

DISCOURAGED, feelings - calc-p., lyc., sil.

DISOBEDIENT, children - cham., ***chin., cina,*** med., thuj., ***tub.,*** verat.

DOMINATION, by others, ailments from (see Abused, Humiliation) - ***anac.,*** **CARC., LYC.,** med., nat-m., sil., **STAPH.,** thuj.

DOWN'S, syndrome (see Idiocy) - **BAR-C.,** ***bar-m.,*** calc., ***carc.,*** pituit., thyr.

DULLNESS, of mind - aeth., abrot., ***agar.,*** **ARG-N., BAR-C.,** ***bar-m.,*** bufo, ***calc.,*** **CALC-P.,** ***carb-s., carc.,*** iod., lach., ***lyc., med., merc., sil.,*** **SULPH.,** ***syph., tub., zinc.***

DYSLEXIA, (see Learning disabilities)

DWARFISHNESS - ambr., aster., bac., **BAR-C.,** ***bar-m.,*** bor., ***calc.,*** **CALC-P.,** ***carb-s., carc., con.,*** iod., lyc., mag-m., ***med.,*** merc., merc-pr-a., nat-m., nep., ***ol-j.,*** op., ph-ac., sec., ***sil.,*** sulfa., **SULPH.,** syph., ***thyr., tub.,*** zinc.

do not grow - **BAR-C.**

EARS, red - ***sulph.***

ECZEMA - carc., graph., nat-m., sulph.

EDEMA, newborn, in - ***apis,*** carb-v., coffin., dig., lach., sec.

EFFEMINATE, boys - ***calc.,*** **LYC.,** med., ***plat.,*** **PULS.,** ***sil.,*** staph., **THUJ.**

EMACIATION, (see Marasmus) - ***abrot.,*** **ACET-AC., AETH.,** alum., ant-c., ***apis, arg-n.,*** arn., **ARS., ARS-I.,** ars-s-f., **ARUM-T.,** aur., bac., bar-c., ***bar-i.,*** bell., bor., **CALC., CALC-P.,** ***calc-sil., carb-v.,*** caust., cham., chin., cina, coca, con., ***ferr.,*** hecla., hep., ***hydr.,*** **IOD.,** kali-c., kali-i., ***kreos., lyc., mag-c.,*** med., morg., **NAT-M.,** ***nux-m., nux-v., ol-j., op.,*** petr., ***phos., plb., podo., psor., puls.,*** sanic., sars., ***sel., sep.,*** **SIL.,** ***staph.,*** sul-i., ***sulph.,*** syph., ther., thyr., ***tub.***

emaciation - ***coff.***

appetite, ravenous, with - ***abrot.,*** ars-i., ***bar-c., bar-i.,*** **CALC.,** ***calc-p., caust., chin.,*** **CINA, IOD.,** ***lyc., mag-c.,*** **NAT-M.,** ***nux-v.,*** petr., ***sil.,*** sul-i., ***sulph.***

cholera infantum - ***ars-i.,*** coff-t., ***crot-t., manc., tab.***

especially about face and neck - **VERAT.**

dentition - **ARS.**

diarrhea during dentition - ***ars.***

diarrhea, with - teucr.

flesh soft, with debility - ***podo.***

glands, enlarged, with - iod., ther.

infants, bottle fed - nat-p.

legs, of - abrot.

EMACIATION,
nutritional problems, from - bac., ***bar-c., calc., calc-p.,*** caust., ***cina,*** kreos., lac-d., med., nat-m., ***ol-j.,*** pin-s., ***sil.,*** thyr.
old man, looks like an - ***nux-v.,*** stram.
rapid - ***kreos.***
rickets, with - **BELL.,** ***kali-p.***
summer complaint, in - coff.
after - med.
worms, from - ***cina, ol-j.***

EMBARASSMENT, ailments, after - anac., arg-n., coloc., gels., **IGN.,** kali-br., **LYC., NAT-M.,** ***op.,*** ph-ac., plat., sep., ***staph.,*** **SULPH.**

EXCITABLE, children - aloe, ambr., ***carc.,*** hyosin., lyc., ***med., phos.***

EYELASHES, delicate - ***phos.***

FAILURE, to thrive (see Marasmus)

FALLING, fear of - **BOR.,** cupr.

FAIR and plump - ***calc.***

FEARFUL, children - **ACON., ARS., BAR-C.,** ***calc.,*** **CARC.,** ***caust.,*** **LYC., PHOS.**
night, at - **ACON.,** arg-m., **ARS.,** ***aur-br.,*** **BOR., CALC.,** cham., ***chlol.,*** cic., ***cina,*** cypr., ***kali-br.,*** kali-p., **PHOS.,** scut., sol-n., ***stram.,*** tub., zinc.
dentition, during - kali-br.
worry, from - ars., calc., kali-br.

FEVER, blisters, lips (see Herpes) - **APIS.,** ars., brom., ***calc-f.,*** canth., ***crot-t.,*** graph., hyos., ***lac-c.,*** med., **NAT-M.,** phos., **RHUS-T.,** sep., urt-u.

FINGERS, in the mouth, children put - ***calc.,*** calc-ox., calc-p., ***cham.,*** **IP.,** lyc., med., nat-m., ***sil.,*** tarent., verat.
boring fingers in ears - arund., **CINA,** ***psor., sil.***

FLABBY - **CALC.**
thin - **CALC-P.**

FLESH, loose, will not stand, do not learn to walk - ***calc-p.***
softness of, with debility - ***podo.***

FONTANELLES, open - ***apis,*** apoc., **CALC., CALC-P.,** ***ip., merc., puls., sep.,*** **SIL.,** ***syph., sulph.,*** tub., zinc.
close and reopen - calc-p.
posterior - calc-p., sil.
sinking - mag-c.
reopening - calc-p.
sunken - ***apis,*** calc.

FRIGHT, ailments from, in highly exitable children, nervous - acon., ***arg-n.,*** carc., coff., gels., hyosin., ***ign.,*** op., phos.

GLOOMY, disposition - ***ant-c., ant-t.,*** ars., bor., calc., **CHAM.,** ***cina,*** graph., hep., psor., ***puls.,*** rheum, sac-alb., sil.
carried, desire to be - benz-ac., cham.
cry, when touched - **ANT-C.**
daytime - ***cina***
morning early - **STAPH.**
spoken to, when - ***nat-m.***

GROWING pains - acon., agar., bell., calc., **CALC-P.,** ***ferr-ac., guai.,*** mang., ol-an., **PH-AC.,** phos., sil.
legs, in - bell., **CALC-P.,** cimic., ***eup-per.,*** **GUAI.,** kali-p., mag-aust., mag-p., mang., nat-p., **PH-AC.**
night, at - calc-p.

GROWTH too fast - ***calc.,*** **CALC-P.,** ferr., ferr-ac., iod., irid., kreos., **PH-AC., PHOS.**
growth, in length to fast - ***calc., calc-p.,*** ferr., ferr-ac., iod., irid., kreos., ***ph-ac., phos.***
young people, in - ***calc-p.,*** hippoz., kreos., ***ph-ac.,*** **PHOS.**

HAIR, cutting, ailments after - ***bell.,*** glon., kali-i., phos.
child, refused - ***cina.***
hair, growth of on child's face - calc., morg., nat-m., ol-j., psor., sulph., tarent., thuj., thyr., tub.

HEAD, cannot hold up - abrot., ***cupr-m.***
large - **CALC.,** sil.
open sutures - **CALC-P.,** ***sil.***
much sweat about head, large bellies - **SIL.**

HELD on to, desires to be - **ARS.,** ***gels.,*** kali-p., lach., ***nux-m., nux-v., phos.,*** **PULS.,** ***sang., sep., stram.***

HERNIA, inguinal - **AUR.,** ***calc.,*** cina, lyc., ***nit-ac.,*** nux-v., sil., sulph.
left side - nux-v.
right side - aur., lyc.

HERPES, anus, about - ***berb., graph.,*** lyc., med., ***nat-m.,*** **PETR.,** ***thuj.***
herpes, mouth, around - am-c., anac., ars., ***bor.,*** cic., con., ***hep.,*** kreos., mag-c., med., nat-c., **NAT-M.,** ***par.,*** phos., **RHUS-T.,** ***sep.,*** sulph.
cutting - phos.
sharp, stitching - phos.
corners of - carb-v., ***lyc.,*** med., phos., ph-ac., sep., ***sulph.***
corners, below - ***calc-f., nat-m.***

HICCOUGH - bor., ign., ip.

HIDE, desire to - ars., ***bar-c.,*** **BELL.,** camph., chlol., ***chlor.,*** cupr., eug., ***hell.,*** hyos., ***ign.,*** lach., ***puls.,*** **STAPH.,** ***stram.,*** tarent.
child thinks all visitors laugh at it and hides behind furniture - ***bar-c.***
children, desire to - aur.
run away, and - meli.
strangers, from - bar-c.
fear, on account of - ***ars., bell.,*** cupr.
fear, on account of, assaulted, of being - tarent.
things - bell.

HIGH-spirited - ***carc.,*** hydr., hyos., ***med.,*** op., spig., spong., ***tub.,*** verat., verb.

HOMESICKNESS, ailments, from - ***caps., clem.,*** eup-pur., hell., ***ign.,*** mag-m., **PH-AC.,** senec.

HYDROCELE, boys, of (see Male) - ***abrot., ars., aur., calc., calc-s., graph., kali-chl.,*** **PULS., RHOD., SIL.,** sul-i., ***sulph.***
congenital - rhod.

HYDROCEPHALUS - acon., am-c., **APIS,** apoc., ***arg-n.,*** arn., ***ars., aur., bac.,*** bar-c., bell., ***bry.,*** **CALC.,** ***calc-p.,*** canth., carb-ac., chin., chin-s., ***con.,*** cupr-ac., cypr., ***dig., ferr.,*** ferr-i., gels., ***hell., hyos.,*** indg., ***iod., iodof.,*** ip., kali-br., ***kali-i.,*** kali-p., lach., ***lyc.,*** mag-m., ***merc., nat-m., op.,*** ph-ac., ***phos.,*** plat., podo., ***puls.,*** samb., **SIL.,** sol-n., ***stram., sulph.,*** **TUB.,** verat., zinc., zinc-m.
coldness, with, of face - agar., arg-n., **CAMPH.,** hell., ***verat.***
diarrhea, after - zinc.
headache, with - petr.
lies, with head low - apis, merc., sulph., zinc.
sweat, with - merc.
vision, with loss of - apoc.

HYPERACTIVE, children (see Restlessness) - anac., ***ars.,*** ars-i., calc-p., ***cina,*** coff., **HYOS.,** ***iod.,*** med., nux-v., **STRAM.,** ***tarent.,*** thuj., ***tub., verat.***

ICTERUS, newborn - chel., chion., coll., merc., nux-v.

IDIOCY, (See Mind) - absin., ***aeth.,*** agar., alum., anac., anan., ant-c., apis, ars., bac., **BAR-C.,** ***bar-m.,*** bell., bell-p., ***bufo,*** calc., ***calc-p.,*** caps., carb-o., ***carb-s.,*** carc., cent., cham., chlol., cic., ***hell.,*** **HYOS.,** lach., lyc., med., merc., morg., mosch., nat-m., nux-m., olnd., op., ph-ac., ***phos.,*** plb., sarr., sec., stram., sulph., tab., thuj., thyr., ***tub.,*** verat.
alternating with furor - aeth.
bite, desire to - **BELL., STRAM.**
cretinous - bac.
giggling - stry.
masturbation, with - bufo, med., orig.
pulling feathers out of bed - ant-c.
shrill shrieking, with - ***bor., lac-c.,*** **TUB.**

IMPRESSIONABLE, (See Sensitive) - ant-c., ***arg-n., carc.,*** con., croc., med., **PHOS.,** tarent., viol-o.

INCOORDINATION - ***agar.,*** **ALUM.,** arag., arg-n., bell., ***calc.,*** carb-s., caust., chlol., coca, cocc., **CON.,** ***cupr., gels.,*** merc., ***onos., ph-ac., phos., plb.,*** sec., ***stram., sulph.,*** tab., ***zinc.***

INDEPENDENT - ***calc.,*** calc-p., ***bell.,*** kali-c., nat-m., ***nux-v., sulph.***

INSOLENT, children - sac-alb.

INSOMNIA - ***absin., acon., ars.,*** arund., ***bell.,*** calc., **CARC., CHAM.,** ***cina,*** **COFF.,** ***cypr.,*** hyos., ***kali-br., mag-m.,*** passi., phos., ***puls., stict.,*** sulph., tub.
caressed, child must be caressed - ***kreos.***
carried, child must be - cham., puls.
evening - lyc.
fretful from bedtime to morning, next day lively - ***psor.***
laughing, with - cypr.
nervous children, during cough - stict.

INSOMNIA,
rocked, child must be - ***carc.,*** cham., cina, ***stict.***
wants to play and laughs, child - cypr.

INTELLECTUAL - **ACON.,** anac., aur., bapt., **BAR-C., BELL.,** cann-i., cann-s., **CARC.,** cocc., **HELL., HYOS.,** ign., **LACH.,** laur., **LYC.,** merc., nat-c., nat-m., nux-v., **OP., PH-AC., PHOS.,** ***plat., puls., rhus-t.,*** **SEP.,** sil., **STRAM., SULPH., VERAT.**

INTUSSUSCEPTION, intestines - ***acon., arn.,*** **ARS.,** ***bell., bry., colch., coloc., cupr.,*** kali-bi., kreos., ***lach., lob., lyc., merc., nux-v.,*** **OP.,** ***phos.,*** **PLB.,** ***rhus-t., samb.,*** sulph., tab., tarent., thuj., **VERAT.**

IRRITABLE, children - abrot., ant-c., ant-t., ars., benz-ac., bor., bry., ***calc-p., carc.,*** caust., **CHAM.,** ***chin.,*** **CINA,** cupr., dulc., gels., graph., ***iod.,*** ip., kali-br., kali-p., kreos., lac-c., lyc., **MAG-C.,** phos., puls., rheum, rumx., sanic., sep., ***sil., staph., tub.,*** zinc.
day and night, sleepless - ***psor.***
cross, good all night - **LYC.**
good, cross at night - ***jal.***
pushes nurse away - lyc.
scream by touch - **ANT-T.**
sick, when - ***cham., lyc.***
sleepless day and night - psor.

JAUNDICE, in newborn children - ***acon., bov.,*** cham., ***chel., chin.,*** chion., coll., elat., merc., merc-d., myric., ***nat-s.,*** nux-v., podo., sep.
stool, with bilious - elat.

JEALOUSY, ailments from - ***apis,*** **HYOS.,** ***ign., lach.,*** **NUX-V.,** ***phos.,*** **PULS.,** staph.
animals and objects, of - **CAUST.,** hyos., lach., nux-v.
between children - ars., lyc., ***nat-m., nux-v., puls.,*** sep.

JUMPING, chairs, on, tables and stove - ***bell.***
evening - **CINA.**
start, scream fearfully - nat-c., sulph.

KICKING, child - ***bell.,*** carb-v., ***cham.,*** cina, ***lyc.,*** nux-v., prot., ***stram.,*** stry., tarent., verat-v.
child is cross, kicks and scolds on waking - lyc.
legs, with - ign.
sleep, in - **BELL.,** cina, nat-c., phos., ***sulph.***
stiff and kicks when carried, becomes - ***cham.,*** cina,
worm affections, in - ***carb-v.,*** cina.

KNEES, knocked, together - agar., arg-m., ***arg-n.,*** bry., ***caust.,*** chel., clem., coff., ***colch., con., glon.,*** nux-v.

LEARNING, disabilities (see Mind, Mistakes) - **AGAR.,** agn., ***anac., ars.,*** **BAR-C., CALC.,** ***calc-p.,*** **CARC.,** caste., caust., cham., con., kali-sil., **LYC.,** mag-p., med., nat-m., olnd., okou., ph-ac., ***phos.,*** rib-ac., ***sil.***
understanding, difficult - agn., ***ail.,*** alum., ***anac.,*** **BAR-C.,** ***bapt.,*** **CARC.,** cocc., ***gels., hell.,*** kali-p., lyc., nat-c., ***nux-m.,*** olnd., ***op., ph-ac.,*** phos., plb., xero, ***zinc.***

LICE - am-c., ars., lach., ***lyc., merc.,*** nit-ac., olnd., ***psor., sabad.,*** staph., ***sulph.,*** vinc.
head, of - am-c., apis, ars., bell-p., ***carb-ac.,*** lach., led., lyc., ***merc.,*** nit-ac., olnd., ***psor.,*** **STAPH.,** sulph., tub., vinc.

LIPS, picking, of - apis, ***arn.,*** ars., **ARUM-T., BRY., CINA,** cob., con., hell., kali-br., ***lach.,*** **NAT-M.,** ***nit-ac., nux-v.,*** ph-ac., rheum, sanic., ***stram.,*** tarent., zinc., zinc-m.
upper - acon., kali-bi.

LIVER, enlarged, in - calc-ar., ***nux-m.***

LIVELY - ***arg-n.,*** bell., **CARC.,** cimic., coff., ***lach.,*** med., ***phos., rhus-t., sulph., verat.***

MALNUTRITION, (see Marasmus)

MARASMUS, (see Emaciation) - ***abrot., acet-ac.,*** **AETH.,** alf., ***ant-c., apis,*** arg-n., ***ars.,*** bac., ***bar-c., bell.,*** **CALC.,** ***calc-p.,*** caps., ***cham.,*** coca, ***con.,*** ferr-m., ***hydr., iod.,*** kreos., lac-d., ***lyc., mag-c.,*** med., **NAT-M.,** ***nux-m., nux-v., ol-j., op.,*** petr., pin-s., ***podo., sars.,*** **SIL.,** ***sulph.,*** thyr., tub.
abdomen, large - ***calc.***
angina pectoris, with - chin-s.
belching, with sour, worse during night - con.
bottle fed, children who are - nat-p.
buttocks emaciated - ***nat-m.***
exercise, averse to, hollow, wrinkled face, hair dry - ***calc.***
incipient - ***cham.***
irritability, child will be approached by no one - ***iod.***
jerking hiccough after nursing, and belching without bringing up food - ***teucr.***
incipient - ***cham.***
last stage, in - ***nuph.***
nervous, restless, weakly children - sul-ac.
nourishment, from defective - ***nat-m.***
nutritional disturbances, from - bac., ***bar-c., calc., calc-p.,*** caust., kreos., lac-d., med., nat-m., pin-s., ***sil.,*** thyr.
old man, like an, had not grown, limbs lax, skin wrinkled, bones of skull had lapped over during birth - op.
reduced weight - ***hydr.***
skin dry and wrinkled - ***calc.***
tendency to - ***iod.***

MASTURBATION, children, in - bell-p., ***carc.,*** dys-co., hyos., ***med.,*** orig., plat., ***scirr.,*** stann., staph., thuj.
girls, in - ***med.,*** orig., plat.
due to itching of vulva - ***calad., orig.,*** plat., zinc.

MASCULINE, habits of girls - carb-v., ***nat-m., sep.,*** petr., plat.

MOANING, children - bor., ***cham., cina,*** lach., mill., phyt., ***podo.,*** sac-alb.
carried, if desires to be - puls.
piteous, of child, because he cannot have what he wanted - **CHAM.**

MUSCULAR, weakness - ***calc.***

MUTINISM, childhood, of - agra., lyc.

NIGHTMARES, in - achy., ***acon.,*** bell., **CALC., CARC.,** ***phos., puls.,*** ter., tub.
monsters, of - aloe, bell., **CALC.,** ***carc.,*** hydr., phos., ped.
fear, followed by - ***acon.,*** alum., ***am-m., carc., chin., cocc., con.,*** hep., lyc., mag-s., mur-ac., nat-c., ph-ac., sil., sulph., zinc.

NOSEBLEEDS, in - bell., calc., chin-s., ***croc.,*** **FERR., FERR-P.,** ***ham.,*** merc., nat-n., **PHOS.,** ***sil., ter.***

NURSING, (see Breast-feeding)

OBESITY, in - ***ant-c., bad.,*** bar-c., bell., **CALC.,** ***caps., ferr., kali-bi.,*** sac-l., seneg.
young people, in - ***ant-c.,*** calc., calc-ac., lach.

OBSTINATE, children - abrot., am-c., ***ant-c.,*** arg-n., ars., arum-t., aur., bell., **CALC.,** ***calc-p., caps.,*** carc., ***cham., chin., cina,*** hyos., kreos., lyc., nux-v., psor., sec., ***sil.,*** syph., tarent., thuj., **TUB.**
annoy those around them - ***psor.***
chilly, refractory and clumsy - ***caps.***
inclined to grow fat - **CALC.**
masturbation, boys after - aur.
yet cry when kindly spoken to - sil.

OLD looking, hard to awaken - kreos.
like an old man, had not grown, limbs lax, skin wrinkled, bones of skull had lapped over during birth - op.
look, withered, dried up - ***arg-n.***

OSTEOGENSIS, imperfecta, bones - calc-f., ***calc-p.,*** sil.

PARALYSIS, infants, of - ***acon., aeth.,*** bung., ***caust.,*** chr-s., ***gels.,*** kali-p., lath., nux-v., phos., ***plb.,*** rhus-t., sec., sulph., vip.
dentition, during - kali-p.
paresis, after - olnd.

PEEVISH - ***calc-p.,*** **CHAM., CINA,** puls., psor., tub.
changeable, pale and chilly - ***puls.***
unhealthy looking, with a disagreeable odor - ***psor.***

PLAY, alternating with, sadness - psor.
aversion to - ***bar-c.,*** bar-m., carc., ***cina, hep., lyc.,*** nat-m., **RHEUM,** ***sulph.***
desire to play - ***con.,*** tarent.
dirty trick on others or their teachers, schoolboys p. a - lach., zinc.
grass, in the - elaps.
hide and seek, at - bell.
night - cypr., ***med.***
inability to - merc., nat-m., sulph.
sit in corner and play - bar-c., bar-m., calc.

PLAYFUL - aloe, bufo, cimic., cocc., croc., elaps, ign., lach., meny., naja, ox-ac., seneg., tarent.

PNEUMONIA, infants (see Lungs, chapter) - ***acon.,*** **ANT-T.,** ***bry., ferr-p.,*** **IP.,** ***kali-c., lob., lyc., merc., nux-v.,*** op., **PHOS.,** ***sulph.***
ailments after - ***carc., phos, tub.***

PRECOCITY, mental - **ASAR.,** calc., **CARC.,** lyc., merc., phos., **SULPH.,** tub., verat.

PROCRASTINATES - ***lyc.,*** med., sulph.

PUBERTY, ailments in - ***acon.,*** agar., ***ant-c.,*** apoc., aur., bell., ***calc., calc-p.,*** caust., cimic., croc., cupr., ferr., ***ferr-p.,*** **GELS.,** ***graph.,*** guai., hell., helon., ign., iod., ***jug-r.,*** kali-br., ***kali-c.,*** kali-p., ***lach.,*** mag-p., mill., ***nat-m., ph-ac.,*** **PHOS.,** plat., **PULS.,** ***senec.,*** sep., sil., stram., ther., verat., viol-o.

chlorosis, with longing for indigestible substances - alum.

retarded - ***ferr.***

girls, in - ***aur., bar-c., bell., calc-p., ferr.,*** fil., ign., **LACH.,** nat-m., ***phos., puls.,*** **SEP.**

melancholia - ***hell.,*** nat-m.

nervous palpitation - ***puls.***

school - ***calc-p.***

tall slim, epistaxis - ***phos.***

unduly delayed in, of mild disposition - ***puls.***

mental affections during - ant-c., hell., ***ign.,*** manc., ***nat-m., puls., sep.***

precocious, chlorosis, anemia, with excessive muscular debility - **PHOS.**

PUNISHMENT, ailments after - agar., ***anac., carc.,*** cham., ign., lyc., nat-m., ***staph.***

QUIETED, child cannot be - ars., calc-p., **CHAM., CINA.**

carried, only when - **CHAM.**

rapidly - ars., ***cham.***

REJECTED, feelings - ign., **NAT-M.,** puls., staph., thuj.

RELIGIOUS, affections in children - ***ars., calc.,*** carc., ***lach., stram., sulph.***

RESPONSIBILITY, aversion to - **LYC.,** ***med.,*** phos.

inability to realize - fl-ac., lyc.

over responsible - aur., ***calc.,*** calc-p., ***carc.,*** ign., nat-m., nat-s.

unusual agg. - aur., ***calc.,*** **CARC.,** lyc.

RESTLESSNESS, in children, (see Hyperactive) - absin., ambr., ***anac.,*** ant-t., ***arg-n.,*** **ARS.,** bor., bufo, calc-br., ***carc., cham.,*** cina, cypr., hyos., ign., ip., ***jal.,*** kali-c., mag-c., **MED., MERC.,** rheum, **RHUS-T.,** sulph., ***tarent., tub.,*** verat., zinc.

babies, in - ars., kali-p., sil.

dentition, during - **RHEUM.**

eruption, with skin - ***psor.***

night - acon., ars., kali-c.

but morning fresh and lively - ***psor.***

relieved by being carried about - ant-t., ars., ***cham.,*** cina, kali-c.

roving, wandering - bell., bry., nux-v.

RETARDED, mentally - absin., ***aeth.,*** agar., anac., anan., ant-c., **BAR-C.,** ***bar-m.,*** bell., ***bufo, calc-p.,*** caps., ***carb-s.,*** **CARC.,** cent., cham., chlol., ***hell.,*** hyos., ***med.,*** merc., nat-m., nux-m., ***phos.,*** plb., sars., tab., ***tub.***

RHEUMATIC, fever - acon., bell., kalm., rhus-t.

RICKETS, bones - am-c., arg-m., ars., **ASAF.,** bar-c., ***bell.,*** bufo., **CALC., CALC-P.,** caust., cic., con., ***ferr., ferr-i.,*** ferr-m., ferr-p., ***guai.,*** hecla., hed., ***hep.,*** iod., ***ip.,*** iris., ***kali-i.,*** lac-c., ***lyc., mag-m.,*** **MERC.,** mez., ***nit-ac.,*** nux-m., ***ol-j.,*** op., petr., ***ph-ac.,*** **PHOS.,** plb., ***psor., puls.,*** rhod., ***rhus-t.,*** ruta.., sacch., sanic., ***sep.,*** **SIL.,** ***staph., sulph.,*** tarent., ther., thuj., tub.

appetite, voracious - ***ol-j.***

bronchial affections - ***sil.***

crooked legs - **CALC., CALC-P.**

otitis with tenderness of head - ***kali-i.***

RUDE, children - ***ant-c.,*** cham., ***chin.,*** cina, dulc., ***merc.,*** nat-m., rheum, staph., sulph.

SEBACEOUS cysts, head - agar., ***bar-c., calc.,*** **GRAPH.,** ***hep., kali-c., lob.,*** lyc., nat-c., nit-ac., **SIL.,** sulph.

scalp, of - agar., ***bar-c., calc.,*** **GRAPH.,** ***hep., kali-c., lob.,*** lyc., nat-c., **SIL.**

SEBORRHEA, head - ***am-m., ars.,*** bry., bufo, calc., chin., graph., ***iod.,*** kali-br., kali-c., kali-s., lyc., merc., mez., nat-m., phos., ***plb.,*** psor., raph., rhus-t., sars., sel., sep., staph., sulph., thuj., ***vinc.***

SEXUAL, abuse, (see Abused)

SCREAMING, children - aeth., ail., anac., ***apis,*** bell., benz-ac., **BOR.,** calc., ***calc-p.,*** camph., ***carc.,*** caste., **CHAM.,** ***cina,*** coff., cupr., dor., dulc., ***glon., hell., ign.,*** ip., ***jal.,*** kali-br., ***kali-p., kreos.,*** **LAC-C.,** lyc., mag-c., ***nux-v.,*** puls., ***rheum, senn.,*** sil., stram., syph., **TUB.**

colic with - **CHAM.,** mag-p., ***nux-v.***

consolation, agg. - bell., cham., ign.

crying and - ***cham.,*** ign., nux-v.

day and night - calc., rheum

evening - ***cham.,*** **CINA,** cinnam., zinc.

night - ***cham., chlol.,*** jal., ***kali-p., lac-c.,*** nux-v., psor., rheum.

nursed, when being - bor.

playing at daytime, but - psor.

sleep, during - **APIS,** ***arn.,*** bell., bor., ***calc-p.,*** caste., ***ign.,*** inul., ***lyc., psor.,*** **PULS., SULPH.,** ***tub.***

dreams, from - acon., tub.

spoken to, when - sil.

stool, during - ***kreos.,*** **RHEUM**

urging for, on - **RHEUM.**

touched, when - ant-t.

urination, before - sars.

waking, on - bor.

SCROFULOUS - ***am-c., ant-c.,*** **BAR-C.,** ***bell.,*** **CALC.,** ***calc-p.,*** camph., cina, cur., dig., viol-t., ***ph-ac., sil., sulph.***

ascarides and lumbrici - spig.

caries of femur - ***stro***nt.

catarrhal ophthalmia - ***merc-d.***

cervical glands indurated and swollen - **CON.**

diarrhea - ***sec.***

hydrocele - **RHOD.**

indurations - ***carb-an.***

large bellies, sweat about head, worm fever slow and chronic - ***sil.***

SCROFULOUS,
mesenteric disease, teeth ill and irregular formation in lower jaw - ***phos.***
outrageously cross - ***hep.***
pale, inflamed, swollen tonsils - chen-a.
scrofulous and syphilitic, enuresis - ***kali-i.***
spasms - ***sulph.***
subacute and chronic hydrocephalus where effusion has not progressed too far - ***sulph.***

SENSITIVE, children - ***acon.,*** agar., ***ant-c.,*** ant-s., ant-t., ***bell.,*** bor., calc., ***calc-p.,*** calc-sil., **CARC.,** caust., **CHAM.,** chin., ***cina,*** coloc., croc., gels., **IGN.,** kali-c., ***kali-p.,*** lyc., med., **NAT-M.,** ***nux-v.,*** op., ph-ac., **PHOS.,** plat., ***puls.,*** stann., ***staph.,*** stram., tarent., ***teucr., tub.***

SEXUAL abuse, (see Abused)

SHAMELESS, behaviour, in children - hyos., med., plat., ***tub.***

SLEEP, will not, in the dark but soon fall asleep in lighted room - phos., **STRAM.**

SLEEPLESS, (see Insomnia)

SLOWNESS, of mind - alum., ***anac.,*** **BAR-C., CALC.,** carc., caust., con., cortiso., gels., ***graph.,*** **HELL.,** hyos., kali-bi., kali-br., lyc., merc., nat-m., ***op.,*** **PH-AC., PHOS.,** puls., ***sil.,*** thuj., ***verat.,*** zinc.

SNAPPISH - ***calc-p.,*** **CHAM., CINA,** lil-t., ***nux-v., sep.***

SNORING, children, in - chin., mez., op.

SOUR, smelling - ***calc.,*** **RHEUM,** sul-ac.
cry a great deal - ***rheum***
despite careful washing - sul-ac.

SPINAL bifida - arn., ars., asaf., bar-c., bry., ***calc., calc-p., calc-s.,*** carb-v., dulc., graph., hep., lach., lyc., merc., mez., nit-ac., phos., ***psor.,*** ruta., **SIL.,** staph., sulph., syph., tub.

STRANGERS, presence of, agg. - ***ambr.,*** ant-t., **BAR-C.,** ***bry.,*** bufo, carb-v., caust., cina, con., lyc., nat-m., petr., phos., ***sep., stram.,*** tarent., ***thuj.***
child coughs at sight of - ambr., ***ars.,*** bar-c., phos.

STRIKING, hitting, behaviour - **CHAM.,** chel., **CINA,** cur., lyc., ***tub.***

SWALLOWS, everything - ***sulph.***

THRUSH - arum-t., **BOR.,** iod., lac-c., ***kali-chl.,*** **MERC.,** merc-cy., mur-ac., **NAT-M.,** nit-ac., sang., sulph., **SUL-AC.,** syph., thuj.

THIN, sickly - brom., ***calc-p.,*** carc., ***caust.,*** irid., ***lyc.,*** mag-c., ***phos.,*** psor., **SIL.**

TIMID, school children, in - carc., lyc., puls., sil.

TOUCH, agg. - ant-t., apis, ***cina.***
touch things, impelled to - carc., ***cina.***

URINATION, painful, child cries - **CANTH., BOR.,** lach., **LYC.,** ***nux-v.,*** **SARS.,** staph.
jumps up and down with pain, if cannot be gratified - ***petros.***

URINATION, painful
children grasp the genitals and cry out - **ACON.,** merc.
urination, sudden, at night, child wakes but cannot get out of bed soon enough - kreos.
urination, urging to, in - ***bor.,*** sars.
ineffectual - **ACON.,** ***apis,*** camph., eup-pur., ***lyc.***

URINE, retention, in - ***acon.,*** **APIS,** ***art-v.,*** bell., ***benz-ac., calc., caust., cop., dulc.,*** eup-pur., ferr-p., ***gels.,*** ip., ***op.***
child, cries all night from retention - acon., apis.
every time child catches cold - **ACON.,** cop., ***dulc.,*** puls., sulph.
infants, in new born - **ACON.,** ***apis,*** arn., ***ars.,*** benz-ac., ***camph., canth., caust.,*** erig., hyos., ***lyc., op.,*** puls.
newborn, fails to urinate - acon., arn.

VACCINATIONS, ailments, from (see Toxicity, chapter)

WALK, slow learning to walk - ***agar., bar-c.,*** bell., **CALC., CALC-P., CAUST., NAT-M.,** nux-v., ***sanic., sil.,*** sulph.
child late learning to walk, weak legs - **CALC.**
child does not learn to walk, weak back - all-s.
unable to walk - mang.

WASHING, dislike of - am-c., **SULPH.**

WEAK, children - ars., bar-c., bell., calc., carb-v., ***carc.,*** cham., ***cina,*** ferr-p., kali-c., lach., ***lyc.,*** med., nux-v., **SIL.,** ***sulph.,*** thuj., tub.
delicate - calc-p., ***caust., phos., sil.***
excitable - **COFF.,** phos.
growing fast, after - calc-p., hipp., ph-ac.
sickly - cina, sil., ***staph., thuj.***
with well developed heads but puny, sickly bodies - ***lyc.***
without cause - sul-ac.

WORMS, in (see Intestines, chapter) - **CALC.,** ***carc.,*** cic., **CINA,** ***gaertner., ign., lyc.,*** **NAT-P.,** ***nux-m., ruta,*** **SPIG.**
behaviour problems, from - **CINA,**
dentition, with constipation - ***dol.***
difficult - **SIL.**
headaches, from - ***calc.,*** chin., **CINA,** graph., nux-v., plat., sabad., ***sil.,*** spig., ***sulph.***
masturbation, with - calad.

Chills

AFFECTED, parts, of - ars., bry., caust., cocc., colch., dulc., graph., lach., ***led.,*** merc., mez., nux-v., petr., plat., plb., rhod., ***rhus-t.,*** sec., ***sil.,*** thuj.

AFTERNOON, (see Time) - acon., alum., am-c., anac., ***ang.,*** ant-c., ant-t., **APIS,** ***arg-m.,*** arg-n., ***arn.,*** **ARS.,** arum-t., ***asaf.,*** bapt., bar-c., berb., ***bor., bry.,*** canth., caps., **CARB-AN.,** carb-s., ***caust.,*** cast., cedr., cham., ***chel.,*** **CHIN., CHIN-A., CHIN-S.,** cic., cimic., ***cina, cocc.,*** colch., ***con.,*** cop., croc., cur., dig., ***dros.,*** elaps, euphr., eup-per., **FERR.,** ferr-p., **GELS.,** ***graph.,*** ip., ***kali-ar.,*** kali-bi., kali-c., kali-i., kali-n., kali-p., kreos., ***lach.,*** laur., **LYC.,** mag-m., merl., nat-m., ***nit-ac.,*** **NUX-V.,** op., ox-ac., petr., ***ph-ac.,*** phos., plan., plb., podo., ***psor.,*** **PULS.,** ***ran-b., rhus-t., sabad.,*** sarr., ***sil., spig., staph., stram., sulph., thuj.,*** verat., zinc.
- 3 p.m. - kali-s., staph.
  - 3 p.m., lasting until bed time - puls.
- 4 p.m. - caust.
  - 4 to 5 p.m. - mag-m.
  - 4 to 6 p.m. - sulph.
  - 4 to 8 p.m., with icy coldness and goose flesh - nat-s.
  - 4 to 8 p.m., with numb hands and feet icy cold at 7 p.m. - ***lyc.***
- air, in open - caust.
- constantly increasing chilliness without subsequent heat or perspiration - lyc.
- diarrhea, after - ox-ac.
- dinner, after - **ANAC.,** bor., colch., ***carb-an.,*** caust., coc-c., cycl., mag-m., merc., nit-ac., nux-v., puls., spig., ***sulph.,*** thuj.
- heat, following - nux-v., **PULS.,** stram.
  - heat, following, and sweat, with, at 5 p.m. - nux-v.
- lasting, 4 hours - nux-v.
  - until falling asleep in the evening - graph.
  - until morning - canth., kali-i., sars.
- menses, during - nat-c., nat-m., ***nat-s.,*** phos.
  - first day of - nat-m.
- perspiration, with - dig., nat-m.
  - cold - gels., sarr.
- sleep, after - acon., anac., ***bry.,*** con., cycl., merc., sabad.
- violent chill with thirst and red face - **FERR.**
- walking, after - graph.
- warm room, even in a - mag-m., rhus-t.

AIR, open, in the - **AGAR.,** ***alum., am-c.,*** **ANAC.,** ***ant-t.,*** **ARS., ASAR., BAPT.,** ***bar-c.,*** bell., bol., bor., bov., brom., ***bry.,*** bufo, calad., **CALC.,** calc-p., calen., ***camph.,*** canth., cann-s., ***caps.,*** carb-ac., carb-an., carb-v., caust., ***cham., chel.,*** **CHIN.,** ***chin-a.,*** cocc., **COFF.,** colch., **CYCL.,** ***con.,*** dulc., ***euph.,*** guai., **HEP., IGN.,** ***kali-ar.,*** kali-c., ***kali-chl.,*** kali-n., kali-p., kreos., ***laur.,*** mag-m., mag-s., mang., **MERC.,** ***merc-c., mosch.,*** nat-m., ***nit-ac.,*** **NUX-M., NUX-V., PETR.,** ph-ac., phos., **PLAT., PLB.,** ***puls., ran-b.,*** rhod., ***rhus-t.,*** sars., ***seneg.,*** **SEP.,** ***sil.,*** spig., stram., stront-c., sulph., sul-ac., tab., ***tarax.,*** thuj., viol-t., ***zinc.,*** zing.
- amel. - acon., alum., ***ang.,*** ant-c., **APIS,** arg-m., **ASAR., BRY.,** cocc., **CAPS.,** ***graph.,*** **IP.,** ***mag-c., mag-m., mez.,*** nat-m., phos., **PULS.,** ***sabin., staph.,*** **SUL-AC.**
- cold, on going into the air - aesc., **AGAR.,** ***ars.,*** bry., ***calc., camph.,*** **CAPS.,** caust., **COFF.,** cham., **CYCL.,** dig., hell., hep., kali-ar., kali-c., **MEZ.,** mosch., nat-a., nat-c., nat-p., nux-m., **NUX-V.,** petr., phos., ***rhod., rhus-t.,*** sabad., sep., sil., spig., verat., ***zinc.***
- cold on going into the, from a warm room - ***puls.***
- draught, the least of air - ***bar-c.,*** bell., bry., **CALC.,** canth., **CAPS.,** carb-an., ***cham.,*** **CHIN.,** dulc., hep., kali-c., mag-c., ***merc.,*** **NUX-V.,** pyrus, rhod., sel., sil., sulph., ***zinc.***
- exercise in, amel. - alum., **CAPS.,** mag-c., mag-m., **PULS.,** spong., staph., sul-ac.
- walking in the - acon., anac., ***ant-t.,*** **ARS.,** bell., bor., bry., carb-an., carb-v., cham., **CHEL., CHIN.,** chin-a., cocc., colch., con., dig., **EUPH.,** hep., mag-m., mang., ***merc., merc-c.,*** nux-m., **NUX-V.,** ph-ac., sel., ***sil., spig., sulph.,*** sul-ac., tarax.
  - walking in the, after - am-c., anac., ***ars., bry.,*** cann-s., carb-v., kali-c., laur., nit-ac., nux-v., ***puls., rhus-t., sep.,*** spong., staph., zinc.
- warm feels cold - thuj.

ALCOHOL, abuse of - led., ***nux-v.***

ALTERNATING, sweat, with - ant-c., ars., calc., chin., euph., led., lyc., mez., nux-v., ***phos.,*** sabad., spig., sulph., thuj., verat.

ANGER, after - acon., ars., **BRY.,** ***cham.,*** **NUX-V.,** teucr.

ANNUAL, chill - ***ars.,*** **CARB-V., LACH.,** ***nat-m., psor., rhus-r.,*** **RHUS-V.,** ***sulph., thuj.,*** tub., ***urt-u.***
- semi-annual - lach., ***sep.***

ANTERIOR, part of body - stram.

ANTICIPATING - ant-t., ***arg-n.,*** **ARS.,** bell., **BRY.,** cham., chin., chin-a., **CHIN-S.,** eup-per., gamb., ***gels.,*** ign., **NAT-M., NUX-V.,** sep.
- about 2 hours each attack - ***chin-s.***
- every, day, 2 hours - cham.
  - one hour - ars., chin., ign., nat-m., nux-v.
  - other day - nat-m., nux-v.
  - tertian, several hours - ant-t.
  - two hours - nux-m.
- or postponing - ***bry.,*** chin., gamb., ***ign.***

ANXIETY, caused by - acon., ars., gels., ***tub.***

ARSENIC, abuse of - ip.

ASCENDING - ***acon.,*** am-m., ammc., ang., ars., bar-c., benz-n., calc., ***calc-p.,*** carb-an., canth., caust., cimx., ***cina,*** coff., croc., ***dig.,*** dulc., eup-per., ***gels., hyos.,*** kali-bi., kali-i., ***lach.,*** mag-c., mag-s., merl., nat-s., ox-ac., ***phos., puls.,***

ASCENDING - **SABAD.,** ***sars., sep.,*** spig., staph., **SULPH.,** verat.

AUTUMN - **AESC.,** ars., bapt., **BRY.,** chin., **COLCH., NAT-M.,** ***nux-v.,*** rhus-t., **SEP.,** verat.
and spring - ars., apis, **LACH.,** ***psor.,*** sep.

BACK, part of body - cham., ***cocc., gels.,*** **IGN.,** ***rhus-t.,*** stront.

BATHING - bell., calc., calc-s., eupi., sulph., ***tub.***
cold water, in - aran., cedr.

BED, in - acon., **ALUM.,** ambr., am-c., am-m., ***ang.,*** ant-t., arg-m., arn., ***ars.,*** ars-i., **AUR.,** bar-c., bar-m., ***bell.,*** bor., bov., ***bry.,*** calad., calc., canth., caps., **CARB-AN.,** carb-v., caust., **CHEL., CHIN.,** chin-a., clem., colch., coloc., dios., **DROS., FERR.,** ferr-ar., graph., guai., hell., **HEP., HYOS.,** iod., ip., ***kali-c.,*** kali-n., ***kali-p.,*** kreos., laur., ***lec., led.,*** **LYC.,** mag-c., mag-m., mang., meny., **MERC.,** ***merc-c., mur-ac.,*** nat-a., nat-c., nat-m., ***nat-s.,*** **NIT-AC.,** ***nux-v., par.,*** petr., ***ph-ac., phos.,*** plat., **PULS.,** ***rhod.,*** rhus-t., sabad., sabin., samb., sang., sars., sel., sep., **SIL.,** spig., spong., squil., stann., staph., stront-c., **SULPH.,** thuj., verat., ***zinc.***
amel., in - am-c., bry., canth., **CAUST.,** cimx., cocc., con., hell., **KALI-C.,** ***kali-i.,*** kali-n., ***lachn.,*** mag-c., **MAG-M.,** mag-s., mez., mosch., nat-c., nit-ac., ***nux-v., podo.,*** puls., **PYROG.,** ***rhus-t.,*** sars., ***squil.,*** stram., sulph.
coldness out of, heat in bed - mez.
putting hand out of bed - **BAR-C.,** ***canth.,*** **HEP.,** phos., **RHUS-T.,** ***sil.***
rising from, agg. - bar-c., bism., bor., **CALC.,** ***canth.,*** cham., ferr-i., mag-c., **MERC.,** mez., **NUX-V.,** ***phos., rhus-t., sil.***
amel. - ambr., am-c., ant-t., arg-m., ars., aur., bell., dros., euph., ferr., ign., **IOD.,** led., ***lyc.,*** mag-c., merc., merc-c., ***nat-c.,*** plat., ***puls.,*** rhod., rhus-t., sel., ***sep.,*** stront-c., sulph., ***verat.***
turning over in - acon., agar., ***bry.,*** caps., hep., lyc., nat-m., **NUX-V., PULS.,** sil., staph., ***stram.,*** sulph.

BEGINNING, in
abdomen to fingers and toes - calad.
and extending from - **APIS,** ***bell.,*** calad., calc., ***camph.,*** cann-s., coloc., cur., **IGN.,** merc., par., teucr., verat.
ankles - chin., lach., puls.
arms - **BELL.,** dig., **HELL.,** ***ign.,*** mez., plat., sulph.
and thighs - psor.
both at once - ***bell.,*** hell., mez.
left, and hand - ***carb-v.***
left, and lower limbs - ***nux-m.***
right, and right side - ***merl.***
back - ant-t., ***arg-m.,*** bapt., bell., ***bol.,*** bov., cact., canth., **CAPS.,** cedr., croc., **DULC.,** ***eup-per., eup-pur., gamb.,*** gels., ***hyos.,*** kali-i., **LACH.,** led., lept., ***lyc.,*** nat-m., ***nux-v.,*** puls., ***pyrog., rhus-t.,*** sarr., sep., spig., spong., staph., sulph., verat.

BEGINNING, in
back, between the scapula - bol., **CAPS.,** led., ***pyrog.,*** rhus-t., sarr., ***sep.***
lumbar region - ***eup-per.,*** hydrc., lach., **NAT-M.,** stront-c., tarent.
thoracic region - ***eup-per.,*** gels., **LACH.,** nat-m.
bladder, neck of, after urinating - sars.
body, left side of - ***carb-v.,*** caust.
body, right side of - bry., nat-m., rhus-t.
buttocks - puls.
calves - ***lach.,*** lyc., ox-ac.
chest - **APIS,** ars., ***carb-an., cic.,*** cina, kreos., lith., merl., nux-v., rhus-t., ***sep.,*** spig., sulph.
chest, right side of - ***merl.***
face - acon., arn., bar-c., berb., bor., calc., carb-ac., ***caust., cham.,*** ign., kreos., laur., merc., petr., phos., puls., ***rhod.,*** ruta., staph., stram.
feet - alum., apis, arn., bar-c., bor., calc., calc-s., ***chel.,*** cimx., dig., **GELS.,** ***hyos.,*** kali-bi., lyc., mag-c., **NAT-M.,** nux-m., ***nux-v.,*** puls., ***rhus-t.,*** sabad., sarr., ***sep.,*** spig., ***sulph.***
right foot - chel., lyc., sabin.
soles - dig.
toes - ***bry.,*** coff., **NAT-M.,** ***sep.,*** sulph.
fingers - ***bry.,*** coff., dig., **NAT-M.,** nux-v., ***sep., sulph.***
tips of - **BRY.,** nat-m., puls.
tips of and toes - **BRY.,** cycl., dig., meny., nat-m., **SEP.,** stann., ***sulph.***
hands - bry., ***chel.,*** dig., eup-per., **GELS.,** ip., puls., ***nux-v.,*** rhus-t., sabad., ***sep., sulph.***
and feet - apis, bry., carb-v., chel., dig., ***ferr., gels.,*** **NAT-M.,** nux-m., op., sabin., samb., sulph.
left hand - ***carb-v.,*** nux-m.
palms and soles - dig.
right hand - merl.
head - bar-c., mosch., nat-m., stann., valer.
vertex - arum-t.
knees - apis, benz-ac., puls., thuj.
legs - cedr., ***chin.,*** kali-bi., ox-ac., ***nux-m.,*** puls., rhus-t., sep., thuj.
lips - **BRY.**
neck - puls., staph., valer.
nose - nat-c., sabad., sulph., tarax., tub., zinc.
palms and soles - dig.
sacrum - bell., puls.
scalp - mosch.
scrobiculus cordis - ***arn.,*** bar-c., ***bell.,*** **CALC.,** cadm-s., caust., cur., ***helon.,*** merl., mez., spig.
thighs - cedr., ***cham., rhus-t.,*** ther., **THUJ.**
throat - sep.
toes - ***bry.,*** coff., **NAT-M.,** ***sep.,*** sulph.
umbilicus - puls.
wrist, left - ***nux-m.***

CHANGING, type - ***elat., eup-per.,*** **IGN.,** meny., **PULS.,** sep.

CHILLINESS, of body - abrot., acon., ***aesc.,*** aeth., ***agar., alum.,*** am-c., am-m., **ANAC.,** ang., ant-c., ant-t., ***apis, aran., arg-n.,*** **ARN.,** ***ars., asaf.,*** asar., asc-t., aur., aur-m., ***bapt.,*** **BAR-C.,** ***bar-m.,*** **BELL.,** bism., bol., bov., brom., **BRY.,** ***cact.,*** calad., **CALC., CAMPH.,** caps., ***carb-an.,*** **CARB-S., CARB-V., CAUST.,** cedr., ***cham.,*** **CHEL.,** ***chin., chin-s., cic.,*** cimx., cist., ***clem.,*** cocc., coff., **COLCH.,** con., corn., croc., crot-t., cupr., dig., ***dros.,*** dulc., euph., **EUPHR., FERR.,** ferr-p., gamb., ***gels.,*** **GRAPH., HEP.,** hydr., ***ign., ip.,*** kali-bi., kali-c., kali-p., ***kali-s.,*** kreos., lac-ac., lach., lachn., lact., ***laur., led.,*** lept., **LYC.,** meny., ***merc., merc-c.,*** **MEZ.,** mill., mosch., mur-ac., nat-a., nat-c., ***nat-m.,*** nat-p., ***nat-s.,*** **NIT-AC., NUX-M., NUX-V.,** ***olnd.,*** op., ox-ac., par., ***petr.,*** ph-ac., ***phos., plat.,*** **PLB.,** podo., **PULS.,** ran-b., ***rhus-t., sabad.,*** **SABIN., SEP.,** ***sil.,*** spig., squil., stram., stront-c., **SULPH., SUL-AC.,** sumb., **TARAX.,** ***tarent.,*** ter., **TEUCR.,** valer., viol-t., zinc.

afternoon - ***acon.,*** am-c., arg-m., ***bar-c.,*** carb-an., caust., chin-s., cina, con., ***croc.,*** cycl., dulc., graph., kali-chl., kali-n., ***lyc.,*** mag-m., meny., nat-c., nit-ac., petr., phos., ran-b., sil., stram., sulph.
- 4 p.m. - mag-c., sep.
- dinner, after - anac., ars., bell., carb-an.
- menses, during - nat-m.
- not relieved by heat of stove, but relieved by covering up warmly in bed - ***podo.***
- siesta, after - anac., ***bry.,*** merc.
- subsequent heat, without - nit-ac., ph-ac.

air, as if cold air were blowing on uncovered parts - mosch.
- chest, the well-covered is chilly in the - ran-b.
- draft, after air-draft - caust.
- open in the, and heat in the room - ***chin.***
  - while walking in the - acon., cham., chin., dig., euph., led., merc-c., plb.
- over the whole body, but not in cold air - caust.

apyrexia, during the - anac., ***ars.,*** bry., caps., cocc., daph., dig., ***hep.,*** led., nat-m., puls., ran-s., sabad., sil., verat.

attacks of, frequent, with intermediate sleep - **NUX-M.**
- attacks of, short - ferr.

bed, out of, heat in bed - mez.

coffee, abuse of - ***cham., nux-v.***

drinking, after - tarax.
- when - ars.

eating, after - ***ars.,*** asar., calc., carb-an., caust., kali-c., nux-v., rhus-t., sil., sulph., tarax., teucr., zinc.
- eating, while - carb-an., euph., ran-s.

evening - ***acon.,*** agar., all-c., alum., ambr., am-c., ***am-m.,*** apis, arg-m., arn., asar., aur., bell., bov., brom., bry., calad., ***calc.,*** canth., caps., carb-an., carb-s., carb-v., cham., cimx., cocc., colch., dulc., ***ferr.,*** graph., guai., hep., ign., kali-c., kali-i., kali-n., kali-s., kreos., lyc., mag-m., mag-s., mang., meny., merc.,

CHILLINESS, of body

evening - ***merc-c., mur-ac.,*** nat-c., nat-m., **NAT-P.,** ***nat-s.,*** nit-ac., petr., phos., podo., ***psor.,*** **PULS.,** ran-b., ***rhus-t.,*** sep., squil., sulph., ***tarent.,*** thuj., zinc.
- eating, after - croc., ***kali-c.***
- falling asleep, on - lyc., phos.
- flushes of heat in the face, with - nit-ac., petr.
- hair standing on end, sensation of - am-c., ***bar-c.,*** calc., ***dulc.,*** nit-ac.
- headache, with - ***acon.,*** bry.
- lasting all night, with cold legs - aur.
- lying in bed, on - am-m., aur., bov., bry., colch., lyc., ***merc.,*** merc-c., ***mur-ac.,*** podo., ***zinc.***
  - amel. - kali-i., kali-n., mag-m., mag-s.
- nausea and cold limbs, with - apis
- sleepiness, with - lycps., nat-m., op.
- wakes, as often as she - **AM-M.**
- walking, while - puls.
- warm stove agg. - merc.

forenoon - aeth., agar., ambr., arg-n., asar., bar-c., chin-s., gamb., guai., kali-c., laur., led., mag-c., mag-m., mur-ac., **NAT-M.,** plat.
- before dinner, amel. by eating - ambr.
- hair standing on end - mag-m.

frequent attacks of, short attacks of - ferr.
- intermediate sleep, with - **NUX-M.**

hair standing on end, sensation of - am-c., bar-c., calc., caust., dulc., grat., mag-m., mur-ac., nit-ac.

headache, during - agar., am-c., **CALC., CAUST.,** cist., coca., **COFF., COLOC.,** con., **CUPR.,** elat., ***ferr.,*** **KALI-C., LAC-D., MERC.,** mez., **MOSCH.,** nit-ac., ***nux-v.,*** **PULS., SANG., SIL., SULPH.,** ***thuj.,*** zing.
- after - alum., rhus-t.
- menorrhagia, during - chin-s.
- temple, right - ziz.

heat, before, flushes of - sang.
- without, subsequent - agn., lyc.

itching, with - petr., puls.
- abdomen - mag-c.

labor pain, after - ***kali-c., kali-i.***

lifting the bed clothes - agar.

menses, before - aloe, am-c., ***calc.,*** cimic., ***caul., kali-c., kreos.,*** **LYC.,** ***mag-c.,*** nat-m., nux-v., **PULS.,** ***sep.,*** **SIL.,** verat.
- menses, during - am-c., bell., berb., ***bry.,*** bufo, calc., ***carb-an.,*** carb-s., cast., ***caul.,*** cimic., ***cocc.,*** cycl., eupi., ***graph.,*** ip., kali-i., kreos., mag-c., nat-m., nat-p., ***nux-v., phos.,*** **PULS.,** ***sec.,*** **SEP., SIL., SULPH.,** ***tab.,*** zinc., zing.

morning - am-c., anac., ang., arg-m., ***arn.,*** asaf., bov., carb-an., chin., chin-a., con., euph., eup-per., ferr., hep., mag-s., mang., mur-ac., nat-m., nit-ac., rhod.
- lasting all day - ferr., mag-c., mang., mez., nat-m., sabin., **SIL.**
  - all forenoon - ***arn.***
- rising, on and after - acon., arg-n., mag-m., mang., mur-ac., nat-c., nux-v., sep.

CHILLINESS, of body
morning, waking, on - ang., ***arn.,*** chel., mag-s., rhod., zinc.
movement, slightest, of the bed-clothes - acon., **ARN.,** ***calc.,*** **NUX-V.,** rhus-t., stram., sulph.
news, bad, from - ***gels.,*** sulph.
exciting, from - gels., sulph.
night - acon., agar., aloe, am-c., bov., caps., carb-v., ***card-m.,*** caust., croc., kali-i., staph.
9:30 p.m. has to go to bed, followed by shaking chill - ***sabad.***
lasting all night - graph.
lying down, after, and as often as she wakes, without thirst - **AM-M.**
menses, during - ***lach.***
before - aloe.
sleep, during - am-c., grat., nat-c., sil.
undressing - acon., ***merc-c.,*** op.
noon - apis, lac-ac., lob.
sleep, after - bry.
pain, with - ***ars.,*** bar-c., bry., calc., caps., ***caust.,*** dulc., euphr., graph., kali-c., kali-n., led., lyc., mez., nat-m., ***puls.,*** rhus-t., sep., squil.
abdomen, in - merc.
burning - caps., mag-c.
burning, pains with - caps.
throbbing pains, with - hep.
part, touched - spig.
perspiration, with - acon., ail., am-c., aml-n., ant-c., arg-n., ars., bry., ***calc.,*** chin., ***caps.,*** dig., euph., **EUP-PER.,** eup-pur., led., **MERC.,** ***nat-m.,*** **NUX-V.,** petr., phos., psor., puls., ***pyrog.,*** sabad., sang., sulph., thuj., **TUB.**
as soon as he gets warm in bed - arg-n.
sex, after - nat-m.
stool, after - bufo, grat., mag-m., ***plat.***
stool, before - ***ars.,*** bapt., bar-c., benz-ac., calad., dig., ip., mang., ***merc., mez.,*** nat-c., phos., puls., verat.
stool, during - aesc., ***ars.,*** bell., calc-s., mag-m., mez., rheum, ***sil.,*** stann., **VERAT.**
urging, during - mag-m.
urination, during - ***lyc., nit-ac.,*** **PLAT.,** sep., ***stram.,*** thuj.
after - arn., **PLAT.,** puls., sep., sulph., thuj.
amel. - med.
before - ***med.,*** nit-ac.
urging to, on - hyper., ***med.***
after - caust.
followed by - senec.
vomiting, during - dulc.
waking, on - card-m., staph.
walking, after - gins.
warm room, going from the open air into, when - am-c., ars., bar-c., bry.
more in a warm room than in the open air - bry., grat., ***puls.***
when in a - carb-ac., cinnb., grat., iod., lact., ***puls.***
washing - bry., zinc.

COLD, damp weather - am-c., ***aran., calc., dulc.,*** lyc., mang., merc., **NUX-M.,** ***rhus-t.,*** sulph., verat.

COUGHING, from - ars., bry., calc., carb-v., con., cupr., hyos., mez., nat-c., nux-v., phos., **PULS.,** rhus-t., sabad., sep., sulph., verat.

CREEPING - acon., all-c., aloe, am-m., aml-n., anac., ***ang.,*** ant-t., apis, ars., ars-h., asaf., berb., bol., ***bry.,*** calad., calc., calc-p., camph., cham., chlor., cimx., clem., crot-h., crot-t., dig., dros., gels., grat., kali-i., lyc., meny., **MERC.,** merc-sul., mez., ***nat-m.,*** ph-ac., ***psor.,*** rhus-t., ruta., samb., sec., ***spig.,*** stram., ***sulph.,*** sul-ac., ***thuj.,*** til., ***tub.,*** valer., verat., zing.
afternoon - alum., arg-n., calc., calen., caust., carb-an., psor.
4 to 6 p.m. - alum., arg-n.
dinner, after - thuj.
siesta, after - bry.
alternating with heat - anthr.
cold air, in - anac., bufo
evening - am-m., ***ars.,*** ars-h., arg-n., bell., calc., chlor., gins., kali-i., lyc., nat-m., psor., ***puls.,*** rhus-t., sul-ac., thuj., ***tub.,*** zing.
forenoon - chlor.
on going in a warm room - aloe
morning - cina, lyc., spig., viol-t.
on rising from bed, creeping coldness of abdomen - meny.
motion, on - acon., sin-a.
night - hep., merc-c., puls., tub.
rising from sitting, when - coff.
standing, while - coloc., ham.
stool, during - nat-m.
after - ambr., grat.
before - ***mez.***
urinating, after - eug., plat., sars., sep.
warm room, in a - aloe, ran-b., ***puls.***

DAY, a cold, in summer - acon., aran., cham., dulc., rhus-t.
seventh - am-m., canth., ***chin.,*** lyc., plan.
fourteenth - am-m., **ARS.,** ***calc., chin., chin-s.,*** **LACH.,** plan., psor., ***puls.***
twenty-first - chin-s., mag-c., psor., sulph., ***tub.***
twenty-eighth - nux-m., **NUX-V.,** puls., **SEP.,** tub.

DAYTIME, (see Time) - alum., ant-c., ars., asar., arund., bapt., camph., carb-an., **CHIN.,** dros., gels., graph., kali-ar., kali-c., kali-p., lyc., mag-s., merc., mosch., nat-c., ***nat-m.,*** nat-s., nit-ac., plan., sabin., sars., ***sil.,*** tarent.
fever, with at night - alum.
sweat, with at night - ars.

DESCENDING - acon., **AGAR.,** am-m., aml-n., apis, ars., ars-h., arum-t., bar-c., ***bell.,*** bor., brom., calad., canth., carb-ac., caust., cedr., chel., ***cic.,*** cocc., ***coff.,*** colch., croc., ***eup-per.,*** eup-pur., kreos., lach., lil-t., lob., mag-c., ***mez.,*** **MOSCH.,** ***phos.,*** plat., ***psor., sabad., staph.,*** **STRAM.,** sulph., ***sul-ac.,*** thuj., ***valer.,*** **VERAT.,** zinc.
head to toes - verat.

DIARRHEA, during - aloe, ambr., apis, kali-n., sulph.

DIET, indiscretions, in - ant-c., cycl., **IP.,** ***nux-m.,*** **PULS.**

DISORDERED, stomach - ***ant-c.,*** **IP.,** ***puls.***

DRINKING, agg. - alum., ant-t., arn., **ARS., ASAR.,** bell-p., bry., cadm-s., **CALC.,** cann-s., **CAPS.,** ***chel.,*** **CHIN.,** ***chin-a.,*** cimx., cocc., ***con.,*** croc., ***elaps,*** **EUP-PER.,** hep., kali-ar., ***lob.,*** lyc., mez., nat-m., nit-ac., **NUX-V.,** phos., puls., ***rhus-t.,*** sep., sil., sulph., tarent., ***tarax.,*** tarent., thuj., **VERAT.**

amel. - bry., carb-an., **CAUST., CUPR.,** ***graph., ip.,*** mosch., nux-v., olnd., ***phos.,*** rhus-t., sil., spig., tarax.

as if ice-water were rising and falling through a cylindrical opening in left lung - elaps

cold water, agg. - bell-p.

is felt as if pouring over outside of thorax - ***verat.***

cough, causes - cimx., ***psor.***

hastens and increases the chill, and causes nausea - ***eup-per.***

increases the chill and causes vomiting - **ARS.,** cadm-s., nux-v.

makes headache, and all the other symptoms unbearable - **CIMX.**

warm drinks, agg. - ***alum.,*** cham.

amel. - bry., eupi.

are tolerated - ***ars.,*** casc., ***cedr., eup-per., lyc., nux-v., rhus-t.,*** sulph.

EATING, while - apis, bov., carb-an., carb-v., cocc., con., ***euph.,*** kali-c., lyc., nit-ac., ***ran-s.,*** raph., ***rhus-t.,*** sep., sil., staph.

after - agar., alum., am-c., am-m., anac., ***arg-n.,*** **ARS., ASAR., BELL.,** bor., ***bry., calc.,*** camph., **CARB-AN.,** carb-s., ***carb-v., caust.,*** cham., chin., coc-c., coloc., con., croc., cycl., dig., ***graph.,*** ign., ***ip.,*** kali-ar., **KALI-C.,** kali-p., lach., ***lyc.,*** nat-c., nat-m., nat-p., nit-ac., ***nux-v., petr.,*** ph-ac., phos., puls., **RAN-B.,** ***rhus-t.,*** sel., sep., sil., staph., ***sulph.,*** **TARAX.,** teucr., ther., verat., zinc.

amel. - acon., **AMBR.,** ***ars.,*** bov., cann-s., chel., cop., ***cur.,*** ferr., ign., **IOD.,** kali-c., laur., mez., ***nat-c.,*** petr., ***phos.,*** rhus-t., sabad., squil., stront.

before - graph.

warm things agg. - ***alum., bell.,*** bry., **PULS.**

EPILEPSY, after - calc., **CUPR.,** sulph.

EVENING, (see Time) - acon., agar., aesc., **ALUM., AM-C.,** ***am-m.,*** ant-t., **APIS,** aran., **ARN.,** arg-m., arg-n., ars., aur., bapt., bar-c., bar-m., **BELL.,** berb., ***bor., bov.,*** **BRY.,** ***calad., calc.,*** calc-s., ***canth., caps., carb-an., carb-s., carb-v.,*** cast., caust., ***cedr.,*** cham., ***chel.,*** **CHIN.,** chin-a., ***chin-s.,*** cimx., **CINA,** ***cocc.,*** colch., croc., **CYCL.,** dios., dulc., elaps, ***ferr.,*** ferr-ar., ***gamb., gels., graph.,*** grat., **HEP.,** hyos., hydr., ***ign.,*** kali-ar., kali-bi., ***kali-c.,*** kali-n., ***kali-p.,*** **KALI-S.,** ***lach.,*** lachn., laur., led., **LYC.,** mag-c., ***mag-m.,*** mag-s., mang., merl., **MERC.,** mez., ***mur-ac.,*** naja, nat-a., nat-c., nat-m., nat-p., nat-s., nicc., ***nit-ac.,*** nux-m., nux-v., ox-ac., ***petr., ph-ac.,*** **PHOS.,** phel., plat., plb., podo., psor., **PULS., PYROG.,** rat., **RHUS-T.,** sabad., samb., sarr., sel., **SEP.,** sil., spig., stann., ***staph.,*** **SULPH.,** ***tarent.,*** thuj., ***zinc.***

abdomen with burning, in the - nat-c., ***phos.***

asleep, before falling - carb-v., lyc., nux-v., ***phos.***

on falling - calc., graph., sil.

bed, in - **ALUM.,** am-c., agar., ars., aur., bry., ***calc.,*** calc-ar., carb-an., cast., ***chel., chin.,*** chin-s., coc-c., colch., ***dros.,*** ferr., guare., kali-n., lyc., mag-c., mag-s., ***merc.,*** mur-ac., nat-a., nat-c., nat-m., nat-p., ***nit-ac.,*** nux-v., op., petr., ***phos.,*** raph., rhus-t., sang., ***sil., sulph.,*** tarent., thuj., ***tub.***

amel. - chin-s., mag-c., mag-m., ***nat-s., rat.***

cold, from external - nux-m.

colic, with - led.

continuing, all night - bov., cina, gamb., hyos., ip., lyc., nux-v., puls., rhus-t., sarr.

until midnight - calad., ***merc.,*** phos., ***tub.***

drinking, after - nat-m.

eating, while - bov., con.

after - ***calc., kali-c.,*** nux-v.

evening, 7 p.m., as though dashed with ice-cold water, or as if the blood water running cold through the blood vessels, cold when he moves, increased by eating and drinking - ***rhus-t.***

followed, by convulsions and heat lasting all night - cina

followed, by sweat - carb-an., cedr., sabad.

heat, with flushes of - petr., thuj.

heat, without subsequent - calc., lyc., sabad., sulph.

lying down, after - acon., am-m., ***aur.,*** bov., bry., camph., caps., ***cham.,*** grat., hell., lac-c., lyc., merc., nat-c., nat-m., nit-ac., nicc., ***nux-v.,*** par., ph-ac., phos., ***podo.,*** **PULS.,** sabad., sars.

mingled with heat, then heat no sweat - ***kali-s.***

motion, during - apis, brom., bry., calad., colch., nux-v.

pains with the - cycl., ign., **PULS.**

rising, on - bor., canth.

sleep, with stupefying - lyc.

stool, during - alum., sulph.

sunset - ***ars., ign.,*** carb-ac., ***puls.,*** thuj.

tea, after drinking - ox-ac.

undressing - acon., calc., cocc., fago., mag-c., ***merc.,*** nat-a., nit-ac., op., plat., ***rhus-t.,*** spig., tarent., ***tub.***

waking, on - nat-c., nux-m.

walking, while - petr.

warm room, in a - arg-n., chlor., laur., nat-m., puls.

EVENING,
warmth, during external - ***mur-ac.***
external, not relieved by - calc., canth., chin., cina, laur., **NUX-V.,** rhus-t.
writing. while - sulph.

EXCITEMENT, after - calc., cic., **GELS.,** ign., teucr.

EXERTION, after - arn., ***ars.,*** bar-c., eup-per., kali-s., merc., nux-v., rhus-t., sil., sulph.

EXPOSURE, after - ***acon.,*** ang., ant-c., ***aran.,*** arn., ***ars.,*** bar-c., bol., ***bry.,*** cact., **CALC.,** canth., carb-v., **CEDR.,** ***chin., chin-s.,*** dros., ***dulc.,*** eucal., eup-per., ***hep.,*** kali-c., led., lach., nat-m., ***nat-s.,*** **RHUS-T.,** sep., spig., ***tarent.,*** zinc.
cold bathing too frequent - ant-c., ***calc., rhus-t., tarent.***
draught, to a, after - ***acon.,*** bar-c., ***calc.,*** canth., ***ferr., hep., merc., tarent.***
to a, when heated - acon., carb-v., sil.
living on water courses, from - ***calc., nat-m., nat-s., nux-v.***
malarial influences - **ARN.,** carb-ac., **CEDR.,** ***chin.,*** chin-a., ***chin-s., eucal.,*** **EUP-PER.,** ***ferr.,*** ip., ***nat-m., nat-s., nux-v.,*** **PSOR.,** ***sulph.***
rains, during - ***aran.,*** bell., ***calc.,*** cedr., cur., ***dulc., ferr.,*** **NAT-S., RHUS-T.,** zinc.
seashore, residing at - ***nat-m., nat-s.***
sleeping in damp rooms - aran., ***ars., calc.,*** carb-v., chin-a., lach., ***nat-s., rhus-t.***
soil freshly turned up - ***nat-m.***
standing in water - arn., ***calc.,*** led., ***rhus-t.***
sun, to the heat of - ***cact.,*** bell., glon., lach., nat-c.
swamps - ***ang., cedr.,*** chin., ***chin-s.,*** eucal., ***nat-m.,*** **NAT-S.,** nux-v.
tropical countries - ***ang., bry.,*** **CEDR.,** chin., ***nat-m.,*** **NAT-S.,** podo., ter.
wet, from becoming - acon., ***aran.,*** bar-c., bell., ***bry., calc., cedr., dulc., nat-s.,*** **RHUS-T.,** sep., ***tarent.***
from becoming, when overheated - acon., ***calc., clem.,*** colch., **RHUS-T.,** sep., sil.
wind, to violent - nit-ac.
working in clay - **CALC.**
in water - **CALC.,** ***rhus-t.***

EXTERNAL - **ACON.,** ***aeth.,*** agar., ***alum.,*** am-c., **AM-M.,** ***ant-t., apis,*** aran., arn., **ARS.,** ***ars-i.,*** bar-c., ***bar-m.,*** bell., bry., calc., **CAMPH.,** canth., caps., ***caust.,*** cham., chel., chin., cimx., cimic., cina, colch., con., cupr-ar., ***dig.,*** dulc., ***euphr.,*** ferr-m., gamb., gels., hyos., iod., ***ip.,*** **IGN.,** kali-ar., kali-bi., kali-c., kali-chl., kali-p., lach., laur., mag-c., meny., ***merc., merc-c., mez.,*** mosch., mur-ac., naja, nat-m., nat-s., **NIT-AC.,** nux-v., **OLND.,** petr., ***phos.,*** plb., rhus-t., ***sabad., sec.,*** sil., ***sulph.,*** sul-ac., til., **VERAT.,** ***verat-v., verb.,*** **ZINC.**
afternoon - chel., puls.
sweat, during - gels.
cholera, as in - **CAMPH.,** colch., ***sec.,*** **VERAT.**

EXTERNAL,
evening - am-c., calc., dulc., ***gamb.,*** ran-b., nux-m., rhus-t.
bed, in - nat-m.
lasting until 4 a.m. - gamb.
lasting 36 hours, with thirst, without desire for warmth or dread of open air, without subsequent heat - ***mez.***
morning - acon., aeth.
night - nit-ac., phos.
sleep, during - crot-h.
waking, after - bov., bry.
sensation as if the hair were standing on end, with - am-c., ***bar-c.,*** calc., cina, dulc., meny., nit-ac., puls., ***sil.***
spots, in - ***ambr.,*** ars., bell., bry., **CAUST.,** ***cham.,*** hep., **IGN.,** ***led.,*** lyc., merc., **MEZ.,** mosch., nux-v., ***par.,*** petr., **PULS.,** rhus-t., **SEP.,** ***sil., spig.,*** thuj.
stool, during desire for - ant-c.
stupor, during - hep.
uncovering, on - arg-m.

FORENOON - aeth., agar., alst., alum., ***ambr.,*** am-c., **ANG.,** ***ant-c.,*** ant-t., ***arn.,*** arg-n., **ARS.,** ***asar.,*** asc-t., bapt., bar-c., berb., bov., **CACT., CALC.,** calen., ***chin., chin-a.,*** chin-s., cimic., cocc., con., cop., **CYCL., DROS.,** ***eup-per.,*** eup-pur., euphr., gamb., graph., grat., guai., kali-ar., kali-c., kali-p., laur., ***led.,*** lyc., mag-m., merc-i-r., merl., mez., ***nat-a., nat-c.,*** **NAT-M., NUX-V.,** petr., ***ph-ac.,*** phos., podo., sars., senec., sil., stann., staph., ***stront-c.,*** **SULPH.,** thuj., ***viol-t.,*** zinc.
5 p.m., continuing until - sulph.
10 a.m., lasting until 5 p.m. - sulph.
11 a.m., with, disgust at even the smell of food - ***cocc.***
hot room, in a - sil.
sleep, during - phos.
stool, after - dios.
sudden chill, with goose skin and hair standing on end - bar-c.
waking, on - canth.
warm stove, by a - bapt., ferr-i., lyc.

FREQUENT, several times a day - bell.

FRIGHT, from - acon., ars., **GELS.,** ign., lyc., ***merc.,*** nux-v., ***op.,*** plat., ***puls.,*** sil., ***verat.***

GRIEF, from - ***gels., ign., ph-ac.***

HEADACHE in the forehead, with - mang.

HEAT, with (see Fevers, Chills, with)
external ars., mur-ac.
without subsequent - acon., agar., ***aran.,*** bov., calc., camph., chin., ***hep.,*** led., lyc., mez., ***mur-ac.,*** nit-ac., ph-ac., ran-b., sabad., sep., staph., sulph.

HEATED, overheated - acon., ***ant-c.,*** ant-t., bell., ***bry.,*** camph., **CARB-V.,** dig., ***kali-c.,*** nat-m., ***nat-s., nux-v.,*** op., phos., **PULS.,** rhus-t., sep., **SIL.,** ***thuj.,*** zinc.

HELD down, desire to be - ***gels., lach.***

ICY, coldness, of the body - acon-f., ant-t., **ARS.**, bism., ***bry.***, cadm-s., ***calc.***, **CAMPH.**, carb-s., **CARB-V.**, cic., **CUPR.**, con., hell., lachn., ***merc-c.***, nat-m., nat-s., nux-v., **SEC.**, ***sep.***, **SIL.**, stram., ***tarent.***, verat., zinc.
- clammy sweat and blueness, cannot bear to be covered, with - **SEC.**
- coldness, as if lying on ice - lyc.
- menses, during - ***sil.***
- single places, in - ars., calad., camph., ***meny.***
- skin, of and covered with a cold sweat, hands and feet livid - ***stram.***, verat.
  - dry and blue, yet wants to be uncovered - camph.
- spots, in - arg-m., par., petr., verat.
- uncover, with desire to - ***camph.***, **SEC.**
- whole body, with cold breath - **CARB-V.**, verat.

INTERNAL - ***acon.***, aeth., agar., ***agn.***, all-c., ***alum.***, **ANAC.**, ang., ant-c., **APIS**, ***arn.***, **ARS.**, ars-i., bar-c., ***bell.***, ***berb.***, bov., ***bry.***, **CALC.**, ***canth.***, ***caps.***, carb-an., carb-v., **CAUST.**, ***cham.***, ***chel.***, **CHIN.**, ***chin-s.***, cimic., ***coff.***, **COCC.**, colch., coloc., ***con.***, cor-r., croc., **DIG.**, ***dros.***, elaps, eupi., ***euphr.***, hell., **HEP.**, guai., ign., iod., ***ip.***, kali-ar., kali-c., kali-p., lac-c., lach., laur., lyc., mang., **MERC.**, merc-c., mez., nat-a., nat-c., ***nat-m.***, nat-p., ***nat-s.***, **NUX-V.**, paeon., par., petr., ph-ac., **PHOS.**, plat., plb., ***psor.***, **PULS.**, ran-b., ***rhus-t.***, ruta., sars., ***sep.***, ***sil.***, spig., squil., **SULPH.**, sul-ac., ***tarent.***, ther., thuj., verat.
- afternoon - ***ars.***, cocc., guai., phos., psor.
  - 3 p.m. - staph.
  - following heat - guai.
  - without subsequent heat - ang.
- coldness, as if, in blood vessels - **ACON.**, ant-c., ant-t., **ARS.**, **RHUS-T.**, lyc., **VERAT.**
- coldness, as if, in the bones - berb., elaps, merc., verat.
- evening - atro., caust., cocc., eupi., ***gamb.***, guai., lyc., mang., nit-ac., par., petr., phos., plb., psor.
  - on falling asleep - phos.
  - worse lying down - **HELL.**
- external heat agg. - ***ip.***
- forenoon - euphr., lyc., ***merc.***, sulph.
- lying down - **HELL.**, squil.
- morning - arg-n., ***con.***, ***lyc.***, merc., sulph.
  - bed, in - lyc., merc.
  - breakfast, during - ther.
- night - ambr., ***dros.***, nux-v., petr., ***sil.***, squil.
  - as if cold air were streaming through the bones - verat.
  - midnight - caust.
  - open air, in - anac.
  - sleep, first, during - dig.
  - waking, on - arn.
  - warm room, in a - ***anac.***, cist., kreos., puls.
- noon - kali-c., psor.

IRREGULAR, (see Periodicity)

LONG lasting, (see Shaking)

LYING, while - am-m., cham., ***cimx.***, nux-v., phel., podo.
- amel. - arn., asar., ***bry.***, canth., colch., kali-n., nat-m., ***nux-v.***, phos., sil., zinc.
  - after - kali-i., merl., nit-ac., rhus-t., sulph.
- down for sleep - graph.

MALARIA, chill, after exposure to malarial influences - **ARN.**, carb-ac., **CEDR.**, **CHIN.**, chin-a., ***chin-s.***, ***eucal.***, **EUP-PER.**, ***ferr.***, ip., ***nat-m.***, ***nat-s.***, ***nux-v.***, **PSOR.**, ***sulph.***

MENSES, during - aloe, ***am-c.***, ***bell.***, berb., bry., bufo, ***calc.***, carb-an., cast., caust., ***cham.***, coff., ***cycl.***, eupi., ***graph.***, ip., kali-i., kali-n., ***kreos.***, lach., ***led.***, lyc., mag-c., nat-c., nat-m., nat-p., ***nat-s.***, ***nux-v.***, ***phos.***, **PULS.**, ***sec.***, **SEP.**, **SIL.**, **SULPH.**, thuj., verat., ***vib.***, zinc.
  - constant - cast., cycl., ***kreos.***, rhus-t.
  - intermission, of - eupi.
  - uncovered, when - mag-c.
  - walking, while - mag-c.
- after - graph., jug-r., kali-c., ***nux-v.***, nat-m., phos., ***puls.***
- before - am-c., berb., ***calc.***, ***kali-c.***, ***kreos.***, **LYC.**, nux-v., **PULS.**, sep., **SIL.**, sulph., thuj., verat.

MENTAL, exertion, after - aur., colch., ***nux-v.***

MIDNIGHT, (see Time) - ars., cact., canth., **CAUST.**, ***chin.***, chin-a., grat., mez., mur-ac., nat-m., raph., sep., ***sulph.***
- after - **ARS.**, **CALAD.**, coff., dros., ***hep.***, merc., mag-s., ***op.***, petr., ***thuj.***, sil.
- before - alum., am-c., ***arg-m.***, arund., cact., carb-an., caust., ***mur-ac.***, nit-ac., ***phos.***, **PULS.**, sabad., sulph., verat.

MONTHLY, (see Day)

MORNING, (see Time) - acon., agar., am-c., am-m., **ANG.**, ***apis***, ***arn.***, ***ars.***, bar-c., bar-m., bell., berb., **BOV.**, **BRY.**, ***calc.***, calen., canth., carb-v., caust., cedr., chin., chin-a., cimx., cocc., **CON.**, ***cycl.***, dios., dros., **EUP-PER.**, ***ferr.***, ***ferr-ar.***, ***gels.***, ***graph.***, ***hell.***, ***hep.***, kali-ar., kali-c., kali-n., kali-p., ***led.***, ***lyc.***, mag-c., mag-m., mag-s., meny., ***merc.***, mez., ***mur-ac.***, nat-a., nat-c., **NAT-M.**, nat-s., **NIT-AC.**, nux-m., **NUX-V.**, petr., ***phos.***, phyt., **PODO.**, ***rhus-v.***, ruta., **SEP.**, sil., ***spig.***, ***staph.***, ***sulph.***, ***sumb.***, ther., thuj., **VERAT.**
- 3 a.m., on waking - cimic., **FERR.**
- 4 a.m., followed by sweat - **CEDR.**
- 5 a.m., after 36 hours, fever - apis.
- bed in - ***ang.***, apis, ***arn.***, ***bov.***, carb-s., caust., chin., chin-a., ***chin-s.***, con., ***graph.***, kali-c., kali-n., ***led.***, lyc., mag-s., **MERC.**, ***mur-ac.***, **NAT-M.**, ***nit-ac.***, **NUX-V.**, rhod., sars., staph., sulph., **VERAT.**
- breakfast, during - carb-an., eupi., gels., graph., verat.
  - after - calc-s., carb-an., eupi., gels., verat.
- continuing, through the forenoon - ***arn.***, ars., eup-per., ***nat-m.***, petr., plb.
  - until evening - bapt., hell., mag-c., nat-c., plb.

MORNING,
heavy chill morning of one day, light in afternoon of next - ***eup-per.***
menses, during, after faintness - **NUX-V.**
nightly emissions, after - merc.
perspiration, after - mag-s., op.
rising, after - acon., aloe, bor., **CALC.,** calc-p., canth., hep., mag-m., mang., meny., merc., nat-c., nat-s., nux-v., ***spig.,*** **VERAT.**
sleep, during - caust., nat-m.
uncovered, if - clem., **NUX-V.**
waking, on - ant-t., arn., ars., bry., canth., ***chel.,*** cimic., con., ***lyc.,*** mag-s., ***merc.,*** nat-c., nat-s., nit-ac., rhus-t., sep., sulph., tarent., trom., thuj., zinc.
warm stove, by a - ***ferr-i.,*** lyc., mag-c.

MOTION, during - ***acon., agar.,*** aloe, alum., ant-c., ***ant-t.,*** **APIS,** arn., ars., ars-i., asaf., asar., ***bell.,*** brom., **BRY.,** ***camph.,*** **CAPS.,** cann-s., casc., ***canth.,*** caust., cedr., cham., chin., **COFF.,** colch., con., crot-t., ***cur.,*** cycl., eup-per., gels., hell., ***hep.,*** iod., kali-ar., ***kali-c.,*** kali-n., merc., **MERC-C.,** mez., ***nat-m., nit-ac.,*** **NUX-V.,** petr., plan., ***plb.,*** podo., psor., **RHUS-T.,** rumx., sang., **SEP., SIL.,** ***spig.,*** **SQUIL.,** staph., sulph., sul-ac., ***thuj.***
after - agar., **ARS.,** cadm-s., kali-c., nux-v., phos., **PULS.,** rat., **RHUS-T.,** sep., stann., valer., zinc.
motion of hand - caust.
amel. - ***acon.,*** apis, arn., asar., bell., ***caps.,*** cycl., ***dros., kreos.,*** mag-m., merc., mez., nit-ac., nux-v., podo., **PULS.,** rhus-t., sep., sil., spig., staph., sul-ac., ***tarent.***

NEWS, sad, from - calc., cic., ***gels.,*** ign., teucr.

NIGHT, (see Time) - acon., ***alum.,*** ambr., ***am-m.,*** apis, ***ars., ars-i.,*** arum-t., bar-c., ***bell.,*** berb., bor., bov., bry., cact., calad., canth., caps., **CARB-AN.,** carb-s., carb-v., ***caust.,*** cham., chel., chin., chin-a., con., dros., **EUP-PER., FERR., FERR-AR., FERR-I.,** ferr-p., gamb., **HEP., HYOS.,** iod., ip., kali-ar., kali-c., kali-i., kali-s., ***lach.,*** lyc., mag-c., mag-s., meny., **MERC.,** merl., mur-ac., ***nit-ac.,*** **NUX-V.,** op., **PAR., PHOS.,** puls., rhus-t., sabad., sarr., sep., sil., stram., **SULPH.,** thuj., ***tub.,*** verat.
bed, in - canch., canth., **CARB-AN.,** dros., euphr., ***ferr-i.,*** ferr-p., mag-c., mag-s., meny., sars., ***sulph.***
hot head, with - colch.
nausea, after - phyt.
never at night - chin.
putting hand out of bed, on - ***canth., hep., sil.***
rising, on - ant-t.
room, warm, in a - rat.
sweat, during - eup-per.
waking, on - aloe, carb-an., chel., graph., sars., sil.

NOON, (see Time) - agar., alum., anac., ant-c., arg-m., ***arg-n.,*** apis, ***arn., ars.,*** bapt., bar-c., ***bor.,*** bry., chin-a., chin-s., chel., cic., cina, cocc., croc., colch., dig., ***elat., elaps, eup-per.,*** ferr., ferr-ar., ferr-i., gels., graph., kali-bi., kali-c., kali-p., lac-ac., lach., **LOB., LYC.,** merc., merl., **NAT-M.,** nit-ac., op., petr., ph-ac., phos., **PULS.,** ran-b., rob., sabad., samb., sarr., senec., sil., spira., staph., ***sulph.,*** thuj., tub., zinc.
bathing, after - sulph.
dinner, after - grat., mag-s.
heat, followed by - colch.
sleep, after - bry.

PAIN, with chills - ang., ***aran., ars.,*** asaf., aur., bar-c., **BOV.,** bry., caps., cocc., **COLOC.,** cycl., **DULC.,** ***euph., graph.,*** hep., ***ign., kali-bi.,*** kali-c., **KALI-N.,** lach., ***led.,*** lyc., **MEZ.,** nat-c., nat-m., petr., plb., **PULS.,** ran-b., ***rhus-t.,*** **SEP.,** sil., ***squil.,*** sulph.
after - kali-c.

PARTIAL, (see Sides)

PERIODICITY, regular and distinct - aesc., ang., apis, **ARAN.,** ***bov.,*** **CACT.,** ***caps.,*** **CEDR., CHIN-S.,** cina, ***ferr., gels., hell.,*** lyc., ***nat-s.,*** podo., ***pyrog., sabad., spig.,*** stann., staph., ***tarent.,*** thuj.
clock-like - ***aran.,*** cact., ***cedr.***
irregular - **ARS.,** ***eup-per.,*** ign., ***ip.,*** kali-ar., ***meny.,*** mill., **NUX-V., PSOR., PULS.,** samb., **SEP.**
not marked - acon., ambr., am-m., bell., camph., canth., carb-an., carb-v., caust., chel., cic., coloc., mag-c., **PSOR., SEP.**

PERNICIOUS - apis, **ARN.,** ***ars., bell., cact., camph., caps.,*** chin-s., cur., elat., **GELS.,** ***hyos., lyc., nat-s.,*** **NUX-V.,** ***op.,*** **PSOR.,** ***puls., stram.,*** sulph., sul-ac., tarent., **VERAT.,** verat-v.
red face, with delirium and bursting headache, pale face when lying down, red when sitting up - ***bell.***
violent congestion of head, cold body, with thirst, chill felt most severely in pit of stomach, body feels bruised - **ARN.**
suffocation in warm room, chill beginning in chest - ***apis.***

PERSPIRATION, chill, after - ant-c., ars., bry., calad., **CAPS.,** ***carb-v.,*** **CAUST.,** cham., dig., eup-per., kali-c., lach., **LYC.,** mag-s., mez., nat-m., op., petr., phos., ph-ac., puls., rhus-t., sabad., sarr., ***sep.,*** sulph., ***thuj.,*** verat.
after - bell.
colder he becomes, the more he sweats the - ***cinnb.***
with chill - alum., am-c., ***ars.,*** calc., cedr., **CHAM.,** cinnb., cupr., dig., ***eup-per.,*** euph., ferr., gels., kali-ar., led., lyc., nat-m., nux-v., **PULS.,** pyrog., ***rhus-t.,*** sabad., sang., sars., sulph., thuj., verat.

POSTPONING - alst., bry., chin., cina, **GAMB.,** ign., ***ip.***

PREDOMINATING - alum., am-m., **ANT-C.**, ***ant-t.***, ***apis***, **ARAN.**, **ARN.**, ars., aur., bor., bol., ***bov.***, **BRY.**, **CAMPH.**, **CANTH.**, **CAPS.**, carb-v., ***caust.***, **CEDR.**, **CHIN.**, **CHIN-S.**, cimic., cina, cycl., ***cocc.***, dros., elat., eup-per., ***gamb.***, graph., hep., kali-c., kali-n., laur., led., ***lyc.***, **MENY.**, meph., merl., merc., **MEZ.**, mur-ac., nat-c., **NAT-M.**, nicc., **NUX-V.**, ***petr.***, ph-ac., phos., plat., plb., podo., ***puls.***, ***rob.***, rhus-t., **SABAD.**, sarr., **SEC.**, sep., **STAPH.**, sulph., thuj., **VERAT.**

afternoon - apis, arn., **ARS.**, **LYC.**, plb., **PULS.**, ***rhus-t.***, thuj.

evening - alum., arn., ***cina***, cycl., ***hep.***, ***kali-s.***, mur-ac., ph-ac., ***phos.***, **PULS.**, **RHUS-T.**, ***sulph.***

long lasting chill, with little heat, no thirst - ***lyc.***, puls.

without heat, sweat or thirst - **ARAN.**, bov.

morning - bry., **EUP-PER.**, hep., **NAT-M.**, **NUX-V.**, ***podo.***, sep., **VERAT.**

night - apis, gamb., ***merc.***, phos.

noon - ***ant-c.***, elat., **SULPH.**

paroxysm consists only of chill - aran., bov., camph., canth., hep., led., ***lyc.***, mez., mur-ac., ran-b., sabad.

without heat or thirst - mur-ac., sep., staph., sulph.

QUARTAN - acon., anac., ant-c., apis, ***arn.***, **ARS.**, **ARS-I.**, bapt., bell., brom., bry., bufo, carb-v., chin., chin-a., chin-s., cina, **CIMX.**, clem., coff., cor-r., ***elat.***, **HYOS.**, ***ign.***, **IOD.**, ip., kali-ar., lach., **LYC.**, ***meny.***, mill., ***nat-m.***, nux-m., ***nux-v.***, plan., podo., **PULS.**, rhus-t., **SABAD.**, sep., sulph., thuj., **VERAT.**

double - ***ars.***, chin., **DULC.**, eup-per., ***eup-pur.***, gamb., lyc., nux-m., puls., rhus-t.

with constant diarrhea, on the days free from fever - **IOD.**

QUOTIDIAN - acon., aesc., agar., alum., anac., ***ang.***, ant-c., ant-t., apis, **ARAN.**, ***arn.***, **ARS.**, arund., asaf., bapt., bar-c., bell., bol., bry., **CACT.**, ***calc.***, camph., ***caps.***, carb-v., ***cedr.***, cham., chel., chin., chin-a., ***chin-s.***, cic., ***cina***, con., ***cur.***, cycl., ***dros.***, elaps, elat., ***eup-per.***, eup-pur., ***ferr.***, ferr-ar., gamb., ***gels.***, graph., hep., ign., **IP.**, ***kali-ar.***, kali-bi., kali-c., kali-s., lach., led., lob., ***lyc.***, mag-c., meny., **NAT-M.**, ***nat-s.***, nit-ac., **NUX-V.**, op., petr., ***phos.***, plan., ***podo.***, **PULS.**, ***pyrog.***, ***rhus-t.***, sabad., ***samb.***, sarr., sep., ***spig.***, stann., staph., stram., sulph., ***tarent.***, thuj., verat.

double - ant-c., apis, ars., bapt., ***bell.***, ***chin.***, dulc., **ELAT.**, **GRAPH.**, led., nux-m., ***puls.***, rhus-t., ***stram.***, ***sulph.***

heavy chill, morning of one day, light chill afternoon of next - eup-per.

RIDING, on horseback - kali-c.

RISING, rising, up, on - acon., arn., ars., ***bell.***, ***bry.***, cham., merc., **MERC-C.**, mur-ac., nux-v., phos., puls., ***rhus-t.***, squil., sulph., verat.

amel., on - ***rhus-t.***

bed, from, after rising - euphr.

SEWER, gas, from - ***pyrog.***

SHAKING, with chills - acon., ***aesc.***, agar., aloe, alum., ***am-c.***, anac., ang., ant-c., ***ant-t.***, ***apis***, arn., ***aran.***, arg-m., arg-n., **ARS.**, ***ars-i.***, asaf., asar., aster., aur., bapt., bar-c., bar-m., ***bell.***, berb., bol., bor., ***brom.***, ***bry.***, ***cact.***, calad., ***calc.***, calc-p., calc-s., **CAMPH.**, ***cann-s.***, ***canth.***, ***caps.***, ***carb-an.***, ***carb-v.***, **CAUST.**, cedr., cham., **CHEL.**, **CHIN.**, ***chin-a.***, **CHIN-S.**, ***cina***, ***clem.***, ***cocc.***, ***coff.***, **COLCH.**, ***coloc.***, con., croc., cupr., cycl., dig., ***dros.***, dulc., ***elaps***, ***euph.***, ***eup-per.***, ***eup-pur.***, eupi., **FERR.**, ferr-p., **FERR-I.**, ***gamb.***, guai., ***gels.***, graph., hell., **HEP.**, hyos., **IGN.**, ***iod.***, ***ip.***, kali-ar., ***kali-c.***, kali-chl., ***kali-i.***, kali-n., kali-p., kali-s., kalm., kreos., ***lach.***, ***laur.***, **LED.**, ***lob.***, **LYC.**, lyss., ***mag-c.***, mag-m., mag-s., mang., ***meny.***, **MERC.**, merc-c., ***mez.***, ***mosch.***, ***mur-ac.***, ***nat-a.***, ***nat-c.***, **NAT-M.**, nat-p., ***nat-s.***, nit-ac., nux-m., **NUX-V.**, olnd., ***op.***, par., ***petr.***, ***ph-ac.***, **PHOS.**, ***plat.***, plan., plb., ***podo.***, **PSOR.**, **PULS.**, **PYROG.**, **RHUS-T.**, **RUTA.**, ***sabad.***, sabin., ***samb.***, sang., sarr., **SEP.**, ***sec.***, ***sil.***, spig., spong., stram., ***staph.***, stann., **SULPH.**, sul-ac., ***tab.***, ***tarent.***, ***tarax.***, ter., **THUJ.**, verat., ***verb.***, zinc.

afternoon - ***ang.***, ARS., ***canth.***, cast., cham., chel., ***chin.***, chin-s., cocc., coff., con., croc., dig., **FERR.**, ip., kali-n., petr., ph-ac., **PHOS.**, psor., ***rhus-t.***, sabad., ***staph.***, sulph.

4 to 8 p.m. - zinc.

air, open, slightest contact with - nux-v.

as if dashed with cold water - sabad.

coldness and blue nails, with for 4 hours, followed by heat without subsequent sweat - ***nux-v.***

lasting until next morning - kali-i.

air, from a draft of - acon., bry., bar-c., ***caps.***, **CHIN.**, mosch., phys., verat.

open, in the, not ameliorated by covering - rhus-t.

bed, on putting hand out of - **HEP.**, phos., **RHUS-T.**

chill, before - ip.

cold, taking hold of anything - ***zinc.***

convulsions, during, rigors - ***hell.***

drinking, on - alum., arn., ars., calc., calc-s., **CAPS.**, cann-s., chel., ***chin.***, elaps, lyc., **NUX-V.**

eating, while - caps., graph., lyc., mag-m.

evening - acon., agar., **AM-C.**, **ARS.**, asar., bell., ***caps.***, ***carb-v.***, cham., **CHEL.**, ***chin.***, ***cocc.***, croc., cycl., ***elaps***, ***ferr.***, gamb., graph., grat., ***hep.***, hyos., **IGN.**, kali-i., kali-n., **KALI-S.**, ***lach.***, **LYC.**, mag-c., mag-m., mag-s., mang., ***merc.***, nat-m., nat-s., nit-ac., nux-m., ox-ac., ***petr.***, ph-ac., ***phos.***, puls-n, **PYROG.**, rat., sars., ***sep.***, ***sil.***, staph., stront-c., sulph., tab., ***tarent.***, thuj., ***zinc.***

7 p.m., lasting until 4 a.m. - gamb.

8 p.m., commencing in the feet with hair standing on end - bar-c.

9 p.m., lasting until 10 a.m. - mag-s.

air, in the open - mang.

SHAKING, with chills
bed, in - agar., am-c., ***chel.,*** chin., mag-c., ***merc., mez.,*** nat-m., rhus-t., sabad., ***sil.,*** sulph., tab., thuj.
bed, amel. - mag-m., mag-s., sars.
heat, without subsequent - ***led.***
house in the - mang.
sleep, on going to - am-c., phos., staph.
undressing, while - agar., mag-c.
undressing, after - spong.
walking in open air, while - **ARS.,** ***chin.***
face, livid - ***rhus-t.***
forenoon - ang., arg-n., carb-an., chin-s., kali-n., **NAT-M.**, nit-ac., ***nux-v.,*** op., ph-ac., **PHOS**., podo., puls., sars., staph.
11 a.m., lasting until 4 p.m. - sep.
flying heat, with - bov.
heat, without subsequent - kali-n., nat-c.
fright, from - gels., merc.
hair standing on end, with - ***am-c.,*** bar-c., calc., caust., cina, dulc., meny., nit-ac., puls., sil.
heat, with - **ARN**., ***ars., bell.,*** bry., cham., cann-i., ***chel., chin.,*** cocc., ***hell.,*** hep., hyos., ign., ***lach.,*** merc., mosch., puls., ***rhus-t.,*** sep., tab.
of face - staph., ***thuj.***
of head - **ARN., BELL.,** bry., ***cact.,*** mang.
of forehead - ant-c.
heat, without subsequent - **ARAN.,** bov., camph., canth., cocc., graph., hep., kali-c., kali-n., led., lyc., mez., mur-ac., **STAPH**., sulph., verat.
or sweat - **ARAN.,** bov., canth., cast.
or thirst - **SEP.,** ***staph., sulph.***
held, wants to be, so he would not shake so hard - ***gels., lach.***
house, on entering the, from open air - aeth., arg-n., caust., chin.
inspiring, on - **BROM.**
long-lasting - ant-t., **ARAN.,** ***ars.,*** bapt., bov., calad., camph., canth., caps., cina, ***gamb.,*** hell., hyos., kali-i., kalm., kreos., ***led., lyc., mez.,*** nat-c., ***nux-v.,*** podo., puls., ***rhus-t.,*** sec., ***sep., verat.***
12 hours - canth.
24 hours, without heat, sweat or thirst - ***aran.***
36 hours, with subsequent heat - mez.
little heat, no thirst - puls.
not relieved by anything - **ARAN.,** merc., ***nux-v.***
the whole day, with drawing, pains in throat and back - verat.
without heat or sweat - **ARAN.,** bov., canth., lyc.
without subsequent heat - **ARAN.,** bov., camph., hep., led., lyc., mez., verat.
maniacal delirium, with - cimx., tarent.
morning - ant-c., ars., carb-v., chin., cocc., coff., cor-r., caps., ***hell.,*** kali-n., ***mang., merc.,*** nat-a., nat-c., ***nat-m.,*** nux-m., ***podo.,*** rat., sarr., sep., spong., ***verat.***
bed, in - chin., coff., mag-s., nat-s.

SHAKING, with chills
morning, heat, without subsequent - cocc.
morning, 8 a.m. - sulph.
rising - acon., kreos., mag-s., nux-v.
waking, after - sep.
walking, while - sep.
motion, during - alum., ant-t., ***caps.,*** cedr., eup-per., sang., sil., sulph., thuj.
night - acon., ***calc.,*** dros., gamb., kali-c., kali-i., merc., nat-m., nat-s., petr., ***phos.,*** rhus-t., sars., sulph.
air, in the open - **ARS.,** calc., calc-p., caust., ***cham.,*** chel., chin., coff., lach., mag-m., nux-v., plat., rhus-t., tab.
bed, before going to - cocc., laur., nat-m., ***samb.***
lying down, on - ***acon.***
on waking - caust., phos., sulph.
noon - ant-c., ***sep.***
dinner after - mag-m.
dinner during - grat.
pain, during - ***ars.,*** sulph.
partial - ***ars., bry.,*** caps., caust., ***chin.,*** cocc., graph., hell., hep., ign., ***puls.,*** rhus-t., sabin., samb., spig., spong., staph., thuj., ***verat.***
perspiration, with - alum., cedr., cupr., ***eup-per.,*** **NUX-V**., ***rhus-r., rhus-t.,*** verat.
pulsating pain in occiput, with - bor.
siesta, during - sep.
skin cold and blue, with - ***camph.,*** carb-v., chin., nux-m., nux-v., ***rhus-t., sec.***
sleep, with deep, and snoring - ***op.***
stool, during - ***bell.,*** mag-m., nit-ac., stann.
after - carb-an., ***plat.***
before - carb-an., caust., chin-s., mag-m., merc., mez.
swallowing, during and after - merc-c.
vomiting, after - thuj., zinc.
walking in open air - chel., mang., tarax.
warm room, on going into - colch., plat., rhus-t.
yawning, on - arn., cina., plat.

SIDES, one-sided - alum., ambr., anac., ant-t., ***arn., bar-c.,*** bell., **BRY., CARB-V., CAUST.,** ***cham., chel.,*** chin., cocc., croc., dig., dros., elat., ferr., ign., kali-c., kali-p., ***lach.,*** **LYC.,** nat-c., nat-m., nat-p., **NUX-V.,** ***par.,*** ph-ac., ***phos.,*** plat., **PULS.,** ran-b., **RHUS-T.,** ruta., sabad., sabin., sars., ***sep.,*** **SIL.,** spig., stann., stram., ***sulph.,*** sul-ac., ***thuj., verb.,*** verat.
coldness of right side and heat of left - ***rhus-t.***
left - ant-c., ***bar-c.,*** **CARB-V., CAUST.,** elaps, ferr., **DROS.,** ***lach.,*** **LYC.,** nat-c., ***rhus-t.,*** ruta., spig., ***stann.,*** sulph., **THUJ.**
before epilepsy - ***sil.***
numbness - ***puls.***
right - arn., **BRY.,** caust., **CHEL.,** eupi., ***lyc., nat-m.,*** nux-v., ***par., phos.,*** puls., ran-b., **RHUS-T.,** sabin.
side not lain on - ant-c., ferr-ma.
on which he lies - arn., mur-ac.

SINGLE, parts - **AMBR.,** ars., asar., bar-c., bell., bry., calad., ***calc.,*** carb-v., ***caust.,*** cham., chel., chin., hep., **IGN.,** kali-c., ***led.,*** lyc., **MEZ.,** meny., ***mosch.,*** nux-v., **PULS.,** rhus-t., sec., **SEP.,** sil., spig., sulph., thuj., verat.

SITTING, amel. - ign., nux-v.
up in bed amel. - nit-ac.

SLEEP, during - ***am-c.,*** aeth., ***ars.,*** bell., **BOR.,** bov., bry., calc., cadm-s., carb-an., carb-s., carb-v., caust., cham., chin., grat., hep., hyos., ***ign.,*** indg., lyc., mur-ac., ***nat-m., op., ph-ac.,*** phos., ***puls.,*** sabad., samb., sep., sulph., zinc.
after - acon., ***agar.,*** **ALUM., AM-M.,** ***ambr.,*** arn., ars., bry., cadm-s., calc., caust., con., crot-t., cycl., ***lyc.,*** merc., nit-ac., nux-v., phos., puls., rhus-t., sabad., samb., sars., sep., sil., staph., sulph., thuj., tarent., verat., zinc.
amel - arn., ars., bry., calad., calc., caps., chin., colch., cupr., ferr., kreos., ***nux-v.,*** **PHOS.,** rhus-t., samb., sep.
alternating with attacks of coldness - ***nux-m.***
starting, from - ang.

SPRING, in - ***ant-t., ars.,*** canth., ***carb-v.,*** cham., ***gels.,*** **LACH.,** nux-m., **PSOR.,** sep., sulph.

STOOL, during - aloe, alum., ars., bell., bry., calc., cact., calad., caps., cast., coloc., con., ***ferr-m.,*** grat., ind., ip., jatr., lyc., mag-m., mang., ***merc.,*** nat-c., phos., plat., ***podo., puls.,*** rheum, ***rhus-t.,*** sec., sil., spig., stann., ***sulph.,*** trom., ***verat.,*** vib.
after - ambr., bufo, ***canth.,*** dios., grat., lyc., mag-p., merc-c., mez., ox-ac., paeon., petr., ***plat.,*** stront-c., sulph.
before - aloe, ant-c., ***ars.,*** bapt., ***bar-c.,*** benz-ac., calad., chin-s., dig., ip., mag-m., ***merc., mez.,*** nat-c., ***phos.,*** puls., ***verat.***

STORMY, weather - ***bry.,*** cham., **CHIN.,** nux-m., nux-v., phos., puls., rhod., ***rhus-t.,*** **ZINC.**

SUDDEN - graph.

SUMMER, in - caps., casc., cedr., lach., nat-m., **PSOR.**
hot weather of - ang., bapt., bell., bry., chin.

SUNSHINE, amel. - anac., con.

SUPPRESSED, swallowing agg. - ***merc-c.***

SWALLOWING, agg. - merc-c.

TALKING - ars.

TERTIAN - aesc., alum., anac., ant-c., ant-t., ***apis,*** **ARAN.,** arn., **ARS.,** ars-i., bar-c., ***bar-m.,*** bell., bol., bor., ***brom.,*** **BRY.,** ***calc., canth.,*** **CAPS.,** carb-an., carb-v., ***cedr., cham., chin., chin-a., chin-s.,*** cic., ***cimx.,*** cina, cor-r., dros., dulc., elat., **EUP-PER., EUP-PUR.,** ***ferr.,*** ferr-ar., gamb., gels., hyos., ign., iod., **IP.,** kali-ar., ***lach., lyc., mez.,*** mill., ***nat-m.,*** nux-m., **NUX-V.,** plan., petr., ***podo.,*** **PULS.,** ***rhus-t.,*** sabad., sarr., sep., staph., sulph., ***thuj.,*** verat.
double - aesc., apis, **ARS.,** chin., dulc., elat., eup-pur., gamb., lyc., nux-m., puls., **RHUS-T.,** thuj., verat.

THINKING, of the chill, agg. - chin-a.

TIME of, chills (see Afternoon, Forenoon, Morning, Night etc.)
1 a.m. - **ARS.,** canth., kali-ar., nat-m., puls., sil.
1 a.m. to 2 a.m. - aloe, dios.
2 a.m. - **ARS.,** canth., caust., hep., lach., nat-a., puls., rhus-t., sarr., sil., tax.
2 to 4 a.m. - bor.
3 a.m. - aloe, am-m., canth., ***cedr.,*** cimic., cina, eup-per., **FERR.,** led., lyss., nat-m., rhus-t., sil., ***thuj.***
4 a.m. - ***alum.,*** am-m., **ARN., CEDR.,** con., ferr., nat-m., ph-ac., sil.
4 a.m. and 4 p.m. - cedr.
4 a.m.to 5 a.m. - bry., ***nux-v., sulph.***
5 a.m. - ant-t., ***apis,*** bol., ***bov., chin.,*** coff., con., dios., dros., nat-m., sep., sil.
5 a.m. after fever lasting 36 hours - apis.
6 a.m. - ***arn., bov.,*** dros., eup-per., ***ferr.,*** graph., hura, ***hep., lyc.,*** nat-m., ***nux-v.,*** ph-ac., sil., stram., **VERAT.**
6 a.m. to 9 a.m. - bov., chin-s., eup-per., nux-v.
6:30 a.m. - hura.
7 a.m. - am-m., bov., dios., dros., **EUP-PER.,** ferr., graph., ***hep.,*** hura, nat-m., nux-v., **PODO.,** sil., stram.
7 a.m. to 9 a.m. - dros., **EUP-PER.,** nat-m., ***podo.***
7 a.m. to 9 a.m., one day hard chill 12 a.m., next, light one - **EUP-PER.**
7:30 a.m. - ferr.
8 a.m. - bov., chin-s., cocc., dios., dros., **EUP-PER.,** lyc., mez., nat-m., phos., podo., puls., sil., sulph.
8 a.m. to 9 a.m. - ars., asaf., dros., eup-per., hura
8:30 a.m. - chin-a.
9 a.m. - alst., ang., ant-t., asaf., carb-ac., dros., **EUP-PER.,** hydr., ip., kali-c., ***lyc.,*** mag-c., merc-sul., mez., ***nat-m.,*** ph-ac., rhus-t., sep., staph., sulph.
9 a.m. to 10 a.m. - bov., eup-per., ferr-i., rhus-t.
9 a.m. to 11 a.m. - ***alst.,*** bol., **NAT-M.,** ***stann.***
10 a.m. - alst., ***ars.,*** bapt., berb., bol., cact., carb-v., chin., chin-s., cimic., colch., eup-per., fago., ferr-i., gels., led., mag-s., merc., **NAT-M.,** petr., ph-ac., phos., puls., rhus-t., sep., sil., **STANN.,** sulph., thuj.
10 a.m. to 2 p.m. - merc-sul.
10 a.m. to 3 p.m. - sil., sulph.
10 a.m. to 5 p.m. - ***sulph.***
10 a.m. to 11 a.m. - agar., ***ars.,*** carb-v., lob., **NAT-M.,** ***nux-v.,*** sulph.
10:30 a.m. - cact., ***caps.,*** hura, lob., nat-m.
11 a.m. - ***bapt.,*** berb., bol., **CACT.,** calc., canth., cast., carb-v., cham., ***chin-s., cocc.,*** hyos., ***ip.,*** lob., nat-c., **NAT-M., NUX-V.,** op., podo., puls., ***sep.,*** sil., sulph.
11 a.m. and 11 p.m. - **CACT.**
11 a.m. one day, 4 p.m. next - ***calc.***
11 a.m. to 4 p.m. - ***cact.,*** gels.

TIME of, chills
11 a.m. to 12 a.m. - cob., ip., kali-c., sulph.
12 a.m. - agar., ***ant-c.***, apis, ***chin.***, colch., elat., ***elaps***, eup-per., ferr., ferr-i., gels., graph., ***kali-c.***, ***lach.***, lob., merc., nat-m., nux-v., petr., phos., senec., ***sil.***, ***sulph.***, thuj., zing.
12 a.m. to 2 p.m. - **ARS.**, bol., ***lach.***, sulph.
1 p.m. - **ARS.**, ***cact.***, canth., cina, chel., coff., colch., elat., eup-per., ferr-p., gels., ***lach.***, merc., nat-a., nux-m., phos., **PULS.**, sabad., sars., sil., sulph.
1 p.m. to 2 p.m. - **ARS.**, arg-m., eup-per., ferr., merc., nat-m., ***puls.***
2 p.m. - **ARS.**, ***calc.***, canth., caust., chel., cic., cur., ***eup-per.***, ***ferr.***, gels., hell., ***lach.***, laur., lob., nat-a., ***nit-ac.***, plan., ***puls.***, sang., sarr., sil., sulph.
2 p.m. to 3 p.m. - cur., ***lach.***
2 p.m. to 4 p.m. - gels.
2 p.m. to 6 p.m. - bor.
2:30 p.m. - led.
3 p.m. - **ANG.**, **ANT-T.**, **APIS**, **ARS.**, ars-h., asaf., ***bell.***, bol., calc., canth., **CEDR.**, ***chel.***, **CHIN-S.**, cic., coff., con., cur., ferr., kali-ar., kali-c., lyc., nux-v., petr., puls., sabad., ***samb.***, sil., **STAPH.**, **THUJ.**
3 to 4 p.m. - ***apis***, asaf., canth., ***lach.***, med., puls.
3 to 5 p.m. - **APIS**, ***con.***, ferr.
3 p.m. to 6 p.m. - ***ars.***, eup-per., ferr.
3 p.m. to 9 p.m. - cedr.
3 p.m. lasting 12 hours - **CANTH.**
4 p.m. - aesc., anac., **APIS**, ars., asaf., bol., bov., canth., caust., **CEDR.**, cham., chel., chin-s., con., eupi., gamb., gels., graph., ***hep.***, hell., ip., kali-ar., kali-c., kali-i., lec., **LYC.**, mag-m., nat-m., ***nat-s.***, ***nux-v.***, petr., phel., ph-ac., **PULS.**, samb., sep., sil., sulph.
4 p.m. to 5 p.m. - **APIS**, cob., graph.
4 p.m. to 6 p.m. - nat-m., sulph.
4 p.m. to 7 p.m. - kali-c., kali-i., nat-m.
4 p.m. to 8 p.m. - ***bov.***, graph., hell., hep., kali-i., **LYC.**, mag-m., ***nat-s.***, sabad., zinc.
4 p.m. to 10 p.m. - phel.
5 p.m. - alum., am-m., apis, ars., bov., canth., caps., carb-an., cast., ***cedr.***, chel., chin., cimic., coloc., con., dig., eup-per., ferr., gamb., gels., graph., hell., ***hep.***, hura, ip., **KALI-C.**, kali-i., kali-s., **LYC.**, mag-c., ***nat-m.***, nux-m., nux-v., phos., ***rhus-t.***, sabad., samb., sarr., sep., sil., sulph., ***tarent.***, **THUJ.**, ***tub.***
5 p.m. to 6 p.m. - am-m., caps., ***cedr.***, chel., hell., ***kali-c.***, phos., puls., sulph., ***thuj.***
5 p.m. to 7 p.m. - canth., ***hep.***
5 p.m. to 8 p m. - alum., ***carb-an.***, gamb., ***hep.***, ***nat-m.***, nat-s., sulph.
5:30 p.m. - ***nat-m.***

TIME of, chills
6 p.m. - am-m., ant-t., arg-n., ars., bell., bov., canth., caps., carb-an., ***cedr.***, cham., chel., gamb., graph., hell., **HEP.**, **KALI-C.**, kali-i., kali-n., kali-p., kali-s., lyc., mag-m., ***nat-m.***, nat-s., nux-m., ***nux-v.***, ***petr.***, phel., ph-ac., phos., puls., rhus-t., samb., sep., ***sil.***, sulph., tarent., thuj.
6 p.m. lasting until 4 a.m. - gamb.
6 p.m. lasting until 5 a.m. - gamb., **HEP.**, nicc.
6 p.m. lasting until 10 p.m. - kali-i., phel.
6 p.m. lasting until midnight - lachn.
6 p.m. to 7 p.m. - hep., mur-ac., nicc., stram., ***tub.***
6 p.m. to 8 p.m. - ars., ***hep.***, kali-i., mag-m., naja, sulph.
7 p.m. - alum., am-m., ars., ***bov.***, calc., canth., caust., carb-an., carb-s., cast., ***cedr.***, ***chin-s.***, chel., colch., elaps, ***ferr.***, ***gamb.***, graph., hell., **HEP.**, kali-i., kali-n., ***lyc.***, mag-c., mag-m., mang., nat-m., **NAT-S.**, nux-v., petr., phel., ph-ac., phos., ***puls.***, **PYROG.**, **RHUS-T.**, sil., ***sulph.***, ***tarent.***, thuj., ***tub.***
7 p.m. to 9 p.m. - chel., mag-c.
7 p.m. to 10 p.m. - bov., phos.
7:30 p.m. - calc., cast., caust., ***ferr.***, mag-s., thuj.
8 p.m. - alum., ars., bar-c., ***bov.***, canth., cast., carb-an., carb-s., chel., ***coff.***, ***elaps***, form., gamb., graph., hell., ***hep.***, kali-i., lyc., mag-c., mag-m., mag-s., naja, nux-v., phel., ph-ac., phys., pip-m., rat., ***rhus-t.***, sil., sulph., tarax.
9 p.m. - ***ars.***, bol., ***bov.***, ***bry.***, canth., carb-an., cedr., croc., cycl., gamb., gels., hydr., kali-n., laur., mag-c., mag-m., mag-s., merc., merl., nux-m., nux-v., phel., ph-ac., rat., sabad., sulph.
9 p.m. to 10 a.m. - ***mag-s.***
9 p.m. to 10 p.m. - elaps, mag-c., mag-m., sarr.
9 p.m. to 12 p.m. - am-c.
10 p.m. - ***ars.***, ars-h., ***bov.***, canth., carb-an., cact., ***chin-s.***, elaps, euph., hydr., ***kali-i.***, lach., mag-c., ***petr.***, phel., ph-ac., sabad.
10:30 p.m. - chel.
11 p.m. - ***ars.***, **CACT.**, canth., ***carb-an.***, euph., lec., naja, sulph.
12 p.m. - ***ars.***, cact., canth., **CAUST.**, ***chin.***, chin-a., grat., mez., mur-ac., nat-m., nit-ac., raph., sep., ***sulph.***

TOUCH, agg. - **ACON.**, ang., apis, bell., cham., **CHIN.**, colch., hep., hyos., ***lyc.***, **NUX-V.**, phos., puls., sep., spig., staph., sulph.

TREMBLING - acon., ***agar.***, ***agn.***, **ANAC.**, **ANT-T.**, apis, arn., ars., asaf., bell., berb., bor., bov., brom., bry., calc., cann-s., canth., caps., carb-an., cham., chin., chin-s., cic., cimic., cina, cocc., con., ***croc.***, ***eup-per.***, ferr., ferr-ar., **GELS.**, kali-n., ***led.***, **MERC.**, merc-i-f., mygal., nat-c., nat-m., nux-v., olnd., op., par., petr., ph-ac., phos.,

TREMBLING - **PLAT.,** psor., ***puls.,*** rhus-t., sabad., **SIL.,** stram., sulph., ***tarent.,*** teucr., ther., ***valer.,*** zinc.
afternoon - asaf., carb-an.
evening - nat-m., par., ph-ac., plat., teucr.
forenoon - lyc., par.
internal - par.
morning - anac.
night - bor.
noon - gels.

UNCOVERED, wants to be, with cold, dry skin, but desire to be covered with heat and sweat - ***camph.***

UNCOVERING - ***acon.,*** **AGAR.,** am-c., ***am-m., arg-m., arg-n.,*** **ARN.,** ***ars.,*** ars-h., asar., aur., ***bell., bor., calc.,*** canth., ***caps.,*** carb-an., card-m., **CHAM., CHIN.,** chin-a., ***clem.,*** cocc., colch., con., **CYCL.,** dig., dros., ***eup-per., ferr.,*** **HEP.,** kali-n., lach., ***mag-c.,*** merl., ***merc.,*** mez., ***mosch.,*** nat-m., nit-ac., ***nux-m.,*** **NUX-V.,** ***phos.,*** plat., ***puls.,*** rhod., **RHUS-T.,** samb., ***sep.,*** **SIL.,** spong., ***squil.,*** **STRAM.,** stront-c., ***tarent., thuj.***
amel. - ***apis,*** **CAMPH.,** ***ip.,*** med., puls., **SEC.,** ***sep.***

UPPER, part of body - arg-m., euph., ***ip.,*** mag-m., meny., plat.

URINATION, during - bell., eug., ***gels.,*** kali-ar., ***lyc.,*** merc., ***nit-ac.,*** nux-v., phos., **PLAT.,** puls., senec., sep., ***stram.,*** sulph., ***thuj.,*** verat.
after - ***arn.,*** calc., eug., hep., ***med.,*** nat-m., **PLAT.,** puls., rhod., sars., sep., sulph., thuj.
begins in neck or bladder and spreads upwards - sars.
before - arn., bor., bry., coloc., hyper., med., **NIT-AC.,** nux-v., puls., rhus-t., sulph., thuj.

VEXATION, after - acon., ars., bry., gels., merc., ***nux-v., rhus-t., tarent.***

VIOLENT, chill, with bluish, cold face and hands, mottled skin - **NUX-V.,** ***rhus-t.***
delirium, with - ***arn., ars., bell.,*** bry., cham., **CHIN., NAT-M.,** nux-v., puls., ***sep.,*** stram., sulph., ***verat.***
heat without subsequent - **ARAN.,** bov., camph., hep., ***led., mez.***
red face and thirst, with - **FERR.,** ***ign.***
unconsciousness, with - ***ars., bell.,*** camph., ***hep.,*** lach., **NAT-M.,** nux-v., op., puls., stram., valer.

VOMITING, before - kali-c.

WAKING, and on - **ALUM.,** ***ambr.,*** **ARN.,** ars., ***bry.,*** calc., card-m., caust., hep., ***lyc.,*** mag-c., merc., nit-ac., ***nux-v.,*** phos., puls., rhus-t., sabad., samb., sars., ***sep.,*** sil., staph., sulph., tarent., thuj., verat., zinc.
as often as he awakes - **AM-M.,** arn.

WALKING, after - calc., mag-c.
while - arn., asaf., cham., ***chin.,*** meny.

WARM, room, agg. - ***acon.,*** **APIS,** ***arg-n.,*** bry., cinnb., **IP.,** merc., nat-m., puls., **SEC.,** ***sep.,*** staph.

WARM, room, agg.
air, open, on coming in from - am-c., ***arg-n.,*** ars., bar-c., chin., plat., rhus-t.
room, amel. - ***aesc.,*** agar., am-c., **ARS.,** ***bar-c.,*** bell., brom., camph., canth., carb-an., carb-v., ***caust.,*** **CHEL.,** ***cic., chin.,*** chin-a., con., gels., hell., ***hep.,*** **IGN., KALI-AR.,** ***kali-bi.,*** **KALI-C.,** kreos., ***lach.,*** laur., mag-c., mang., **MENY.,** merc., merc-c., mez., nat-a., **NUX-M.,** ***nux-v.,*** petr., ***plat.,*** ran-b., rat., rhod., ***rhus-t.,*** **SABAD.,** sel., ***sep.,*** sil., spig., sulph., ***sul-ac., tarent., ther.,*** valer., zinc.
not amel. in, nor by a warm stove - ***acon., alum.,*** **ANAC.,** ***ant-c.,*** **APIS,** aran., arg-n., ars., ars-i., asar., ***bapt.,*** bell., **BOV., BRY.,** cact., calc., canth., carb-ac., ***chin., cina,*** cic., cinnb., clem., **COCC.,** colch., dios., dros., ***dulc.,*** euphr., ***ferr-i.,*** graph., guai., hell., hep., iod., **IP.,** kali-i., ***kreos.,*** lach., ***laur.,*** lyc., ***mag-m.,*** meny., ***merc.,*** **MEZ.,** ***nat-m.,*** nit-ac., nux-m., **NUX-V.,** ph-ac., ***phos., podo.,*** **PULS.,** ***ruta.,*** sabin., sars., ***sep., sil., spong., staph.,*** stry., sulph., ***sul-ac.,*** teucr., thuj., til., **VERAT.**
on coming in from open air - ***arg-n.***
smothering in - **APIS.**
stove, desire to be near - ***gels.,*** mosch., ***rhus-t.***
but it increases the chill - chin.
cold, and gets sick near - ***laur.***
weather, in - ant-c., ***ars.,*** bapt., ***bell., bry.,*** calc., **CAPS.,** carb-v., ***cedr.,*** chin., cina, ***ip.,*** **LACH.,** nat-m., puls., **SULPH.,** ***thuj.***

WARMTH, desire for, which does not relieve - acon., alum., **ARAN.,** bell., bov., calc., camph., ***chin.,*** cic., ***cina,*** cocc., colch., con., dros., ferr., ***hep.,*** kali-i., **LACH.,** lyc., meny., ***merc., nat-m.,*** **NUX-V.,** ***phos.,*** podo., ***pyrog.,*** sil., ***tarent.,*** verat.
bed, amel., but not by heat of stove - kali-i., kreos., podo., tarent.
external, amel. - ***aesc.,*** arg-m., **ARS.,** arn., ***bar-c.,*** **BELL.,** canth., ***caust.,*** **CAPS.,** carb-an., chel., ***chin., chin-a.,*** cic., cimx., cocc., colch., con., cor-r., ***eup-per.,*** ferr., ***gels., hell., hep.,*** hyos., **IGN., KALI-C.,** kali-i., ***lach., lachn.,*** laur., **MENY.,** ***mez.,*** merl., mosch., nat-c., **NUX-M., NUX-V.,** ***plat., podo.,*** **RHUS-T., SABAD.,** samb., sep., sil., ***squil.,*** stront-c., ***stram.,*** sulph., ***tarent., ther.***
hot irons amel. - ***caps.,*** **LACHN.**
but not by external covering - lachn.
sun, desire for - anac., con.
unbearable - **APIS,** ***camph.,*** **IP., PULS., SEC., SEP.,** staph.
wrapping up, amel., followed by severe fever and sweat - sil.

WATER, as if cold water were dashed over him - ***agar.,*** ail., ant-t., apis, **ARN.,** ars., ***bar-c.,*** bry., ***chel., chin., gels.,*** lyc., lil-t., merc., mez., nat-m., nux-v., phel., ***phos., puls.,*** **RHUS-T.,** ***sabad.,*** spig., thuj., ***verat.,*** verb.
getting wet, from - acon., ***aran.,*** bar-c., bell., ***bry., calc.,*** cedr., ***dulc., nat-s.,*** **RHUS-T.,** ***sep.,*** sil.
when overheated - acon., ***calc., clem.,*** colch., ***rhus-t.,*** sep., sil.
from the clavicles across the chest down to the toes, along the narrow space - caust.
poured over him - ***ant-t., anac.,*** ars., ***bar-c., chin.,*** cimx., ***led., mag-c.,*** **MERC.,** mez., ***rhus-t.,*** stram.
running down the back - agar., alumn., ars.
spurted upon the back - caust., lyc.
trickled down the back - ars., caps., caust., **GELS.**
working in, from - **CALC.,** ***rhus-t.***

WIND, as if it were blowing cold upon the body - asar., camph., ***chin.,*** caust., cimx., croc., cupr., hep., ***laur.,*** mosch., ph-ac., rhus-t., samb.
as if wind blowing upon soles while body sweating - acon.
between the shoulder blades - ***caust.***
sensation as if cold air were spreading from the spine over the body like an aura epileptica - agar.
when walking - chin.

WRITING, while - agar., zinc.

Coughing

ABDOMEN, seems to come from - ant-c., sep., verat.

ACIDS, agg. - ***ant-c.,*** brom., ***con.,*** lach., mez., nat-m., ***nat-p.,*** nux-v., sep., sil., sulph.

ACRID, fluid through post nasal, sensation of, from - kali-bi.

AFTERNOON - agar., all-c., alum., am-c., am-m., anac., ant-t., anth., arn., ars., asaf., astac., bad., bapt., ***bell.,*** bov., bry., calc., calc-p., caps., ***chel.,*** chin., chin-a., coca, coc-c., cupr., fago., ferr-i., gamb., kali-ar., kali-bi., kali-c., laur., lyc., mag-c., mez., mosch., mur-ac., nat-a., nat-c., nat-m., nat-p., nux-v., ol-an., phel., phos., ***sang.,*** stann., staph., sulph., thuj., zinc.

1 p.m. - nat-s.

1 p.m. to 1 a.m. - hep.

1 to 2 p.m. - ars.

1:30 p.m. - phel.

2 p.m. - coca, dios., laur., ol-an.

3 p.m - ang., calc-f., cench., hep., phel.

3 to 4 p.m. - calc-f., lyc.

3 to 5 p.m. - sal-ac.

3 to 10 p.m. - bell.

4 p.m. - calc-f., cench., ***chel.,*** coca, kali-bi.

4 p.m. until bedtime - ***mang.***

4 p.m. until morning - dol.

4 to 6 p.m. - lyc.

4 to 8 p.m. - ***lyc.,*** phel.

5 p.m. - cupr., mang., nat-m., sol-t-ae.

5 to 9 p.m. - caps.

bath, after - calc-s.

evening, until - nux-m.

midnight until - bell., sulph.

AGG. in general from coughing - ***bell.,*** cist., cocc., ***hep.,*** **IGN.,** raph., squil., stict., teucr., thyr., zinc-i.

AGITATION, from - ***cist.***

AIR, effects of

close, agg. - brom., nat-a.

cold - acon., agn., **ALL-C.,** all-s., alum., am-m., aphis., **ARS.,** aur., ***bad., bar-c.,*** bov., ***brom.,*** bry., ***calc., carb-an.,*** carb-s., ***carb-v.,*** **CAUST.,** cham., cimic., cina, cist., ***coca,*** cocc., coff., ***con.,*** cub., ***cupr.,*** cur., cycl., dulc., ***ferr., ferr-ar.,*** ferr-p., **HEP., HYOS.,** hyper., ip., ***kali-ar., kali-bi., kali-c.,*** kali-i., **KALI-N.,** kali-p., ***lach.,*** lac-ac., lyc., mez., mosch., naja, nat-s., nit-ac., nux-m., **NUX-V.,** osm., ph-ac., **PHOS.,** ***phyt.,*** plan., ***rhus-t.,*** **RUMX.,** sabad., samb., sang., ***seneg., sep., sil.,*** sin-n., spig., spong., squil., staph., stram., sulph., ***sul-ac.,*** verat., verat-v.

amel. - calc-s., ***coc-c.,*** kali-s.

walking in - ***ars.,*** cist., ip., ***kali-n.,*** **PHOS., RUMX.,** ***seneg.,*** spig., ***sul-ac.,*** verat.

AIR, effects of

damp, cold - ant-t., bar-c., ***calc.,*** carb-an., carb-v., ***chin.,*** cur., **DULC.,** ***iod., lach.,*** mag-c., merc., mosch., mur-ac., ***nat-s., nit-ac.,*** nux-m., phyt., rhus-t., sep., sil., ***sulph.,*** sul-ac., verat., zinc.

draft of - ***acon., calc.,*** caps., ***caust., chin., ph-ac.,*** sep.

dry - caust., sep.

cold - **ACON.,** brom., caps., cham., crot-h., **HEP.,** nux-m., ***phos.,*** rumx., samb., ***spong.***

night - calc-p., ***hep., merc.,*** phos., spig., sulph., sul-ac., trif-p.

open - ***acon.,*** all-s., alum., ang., aphis., **ARS.,** bar-c., bry., calc., carb-v., cham., cina, cocc., ***coff.,*** con., cycl., euphr., ferr., ferr-ar., ferr-p., ***hep.,*** ip., kali-bi., **KALI-N.,** ***lach.,*** lyc., mag-arct., mosch., ***naja,*** nit-ac., nux-v., osm., ph-ac., **PHOS.,** phyt., ***rhus-t.,*** **RUMX.,** sang., seneg., sil., spig., squil., staph., stram., ***sulph., sul-ac.***

amel. - ***all-c.,*** ambr., ant-c., anth., apis, ***arg-m., arg-n.,*** bov., ***brom.,*** **BRY.,** calc., cench., chel., **COC-C.,** cycl., dros., dulc., **IOD.,** ***kali-s., lil-t.,*** **MAG-P.,** ***nat-s.,*** nux-v., **PULS.,** pyrog., sanic., sulph.

walking in - acon., alum., ang., **ARS.,** carb-v., cina, dig., ferr., ferr-ar., ip., kali-n., lyc., mag-m., nux-v., osm., ox-ac., ph-ac., **PHOS.,** ***rhus-t., seneg.,*** sep., spig., staph., stram., ***sulph.,*** sul-ac.

ALTERNATING, (see Sciatica and eruptions)

ALCOHOL, from drinking - arn., ferr., ign., lach., led., ***spong.,*** stann., stram., zinc.

ALCOHOLICS, coughs of - ***ars., coc-c.,*** lach., nux-v., ***stram.***

ANGER, from - acon., ***ant-t., arg-m.,*** arg-n., ***arn.,*** ars., bry., caps., ***cham.,*** chin., ***coloc., ign.,*** nux-v., sep., ***staph.,*** verat.

ASCENDING, stairs - am-c., arg-m., arg-n., ***ars.,*** bar-c., ***bry.,*** calc., carb-v., cench., iod., kali-n., lyc., mag-c., mag-m., merc., nux-v., seneg., sep., sil., spong., squil., stann., staph., zinc.

ASTHMATIC, coughing - ***acon., alum.,*** ambr., ***am-c.,*** am-m., anac., **ANT-T.,** aral., arg-n., arn., **ARS.,** ***ars-i.,*** asaf., aspar., bar-c., bar-m., ***bell., brom.,*** bry., calad., calc., calc-s., carb-an., carb-s., ***carb-v.,*** caust., cham., ***chin.,*** chin-a., chlor., cic., **CINA,** coc-c., cocc., con., cor-r., croc., ***crot-t.,*** **CUPR.,** dig., dol., **DROS.,** dulc., ***euph.,*** euphr., ferr., ferr-ar., ferr-i., ferr-p., guai., ***hep.,*** hyos., ign., iod., **IP.,** ***kali-ar., kali-bi., kali-c.,*** kali-chl., kali-n., kali-p., ***kreos., lach.,*** lact., laur., ***led.,*** lob., lyc., merc., mez., mosch., mur-ac., nat-m., nat-s., nicc., nit-ac., ***nux-m.,*** **NUX-V.,** op., petr., phel., ***phos.,*** prun., psor., ***puls.,*** rhus-t., sabad., ***samb., sang., sep., sil.,*** spig., ***spong.,*** squil., stann., ***stram.,*** sulph., sul-ac., verat., viol-o., zinc., zing.

AUTUMN, agg. - caps., ***cina, iod.,*** kreos., lac-ac., verat.
and spring - cina, kreos., lac-ac.

BARKING - **ACON.,** all-c., ant-t., aur-m., **BELL.,** brom., caps., cimx., clem., ***coc-c.,*** cor-r., cub., **DROS.,** ***dulc.,*** **HEP.,** hipp., ***kali-bi.,*** lac-c., lact., lyc., lyss., merc., mur-ac., ***nit-ac.,*** nux-m., phos., phyt., ***rumx.,*** **SPONG.,** stann., stict., **STRAM.,** sulph., verat.
day and night - ***spong.***
deep breath, after - dulc.
dog, like a - bell., lyss.
drinking cold water, amel. - ***coc-c.***
barking, evening - ***nit-ac.***
loud - **ACON.,** aur-m., kali-bi., lyc., stann., verat.
morning - kali-bi., thuj.
night - bell., nit-ac.
11 p.m., wakens suddenly, face fiery red, crying - bell.
sleep, during - hipp., lyc., nit-ac.

BATHING, agg. - ant-c., ars., ***calc.,*** calc-f., ***calc-s., caust.,*** dulc., lach., ***nit-ac.,*** nux-m., ***psor.,*** **RHUS-T.,** sep., stram., sulph., sul-ac., verat., zinc.
chest, in cold water amel. - bor.
cold - bor., psor.

BED, in, changing position - ars., con., **KREOS.**
changing position, in amel. - bor., ign.
warm, on becoming, in, agg. or excites - ant-t., brom., **CAUST.,** ***cham.,*** dros., led., merc., naja, nat-m., ***nux-m.,*** nux-v., **PULS.,** ***verat.***
amel. - cham., ***kali-bi.***
evening - nux-m.

BEER, agg. - mez., nux-v., rhus-t., spong.

BELCHING, amel. - **SANG.**
excite - ***ambr.,*** bar-c., lac-ac., sol-t-ae., staph.

BENDING, forced to bend double - agar., ther.
head, backward agg. - ***bry.,*** cupr., hep., kali-bi., lyc., psor., ***rumx., sil.,*** spong.
head, forward, agg. - **CAUST.,** dig.
amel. - eup-per., ***spong.***

BLOOD, determination of, to chest, from - aloe
rush of, to chest, 11 a.m. - raph.

BRANDY - ferr.

BREAD - kali-c.
black - ph-ac.

BREAKFAST, during - alum., alumn., seneg.
after, amel. - alumn., aspar., bar-c., coc-c., kali-c., lach., murx.
before - alumn., kali-c., murx., seneg., sulph.

BREAST-feeding, during - ferr.

BREATH, holding - kali-n., prun.

BREATHING, agg. - am-c., asar., bell., coloc., dulc., graph., hep., ip., kali-n., mag-m., nat-m., sulph.

BREATHING, deep, agg. - ***acon., aesc.,*** am-c., am-m., apis, arn., ars., asar., **BELL.,** bism., ***brom.,*** **BRY.,** carb-an., chin., chin-a., cina, coc-c., **CON.,** ***cor-r.,*** crot-h., cupr., dig., dros., ***dulc.,*** euphr., ***ferr.,*** ferr-ar., ferr-p., graph., ***hep., iod.,*** ip., kali-ar., ***kali-bi.,*** **KALI-C.,** kali-n., kali-p., ***lac-c.,*** lach., lec., ***lyc.,*** mag-m., mang., meny., ***merc.,*** mez., mur-ac., naja, nat-a., nat-m., nit-ac., ph-ac., phos., plb., ***puls., rhus-t., rumx.,*** sabad., samb., seneg., sep., serp., sil., ***squil.,*** stann., stram., ***sulph.,*** zinc., ziz.
amel. - lach., ***puls., verb.***
morning, after lying down - **IP.**
deficient, being - am-c., ***ars., aur.,*** aur-m., carb-v., cina, cocc., coloc., con., ***cur., dros.,*** euphr., ferr., guai., hep., ign., ***ip.,*** lyc., nux-v., op., spig.
night, at - aur., coloc.
irregular, from - **RUMX.**

BRIGHT, objects - stram.

BRUSHING, teeth - carb-v., coc-c., dig., euphr., sep., staph.

BURNING, chest, in - am-c., caust., coc-c., euph., euphr., led., mag-m., ph-ac.
burning, larynx - acon., aphis., arg-n., ars., bell., bov., brom., bufo, caust., mag-s., ph-ac., phos., phyt., seneg., ***spong.,*** stict., tarent., urt-u., zing.
burning, throat-pit, from - ars.
burning, trachea, from - acon., ars., euphr.

CARBON, as from vapor of - arn., ***puls.***

CELLARS, air, of - ant-t., nat-s., nux-m., ***sep.,*** stram.

CHAGRIN and trouble - ign., ph-ac.

CHICKEN-pox, after - ant-c.

CHILDBIRTH, after - apis, cimx., nux-m., ph-ac., phos., ***samb.,*** rhus-t.

CHILL, during - acon., apis, ***ars.,*** bell., bor., ***bry.,*** calc., calc-p., carb-v., cham., ***chin., chin-a.,*** cimx., con., ***ferr.,*** hep., hyos., ip., kali-ar., kali-c., kali-p., kreos., lach., lyc., nat-c., nat-p., nux-m., nux-v., ph-ac., **PHOS.,** ***psor., puls.,*** **RHUS-T.,** ***rumx.,*** **SABAD.,** ***sep.,*** sil., spong., sulph., thuj., ***tub.***
before - apis, eup-per., **RHUS-T.,** rumx., ***samb., tub.***

CHOKING, (see Suffocative) - ***agar.,*** **ALUM.,** ars., carb-v., cina, **COC-C.,** crot-h., dros., ***hep.,*** iod., **IP.,** kali-ar., ***kali-bi., kali-c., lach.,*** lyc., mag-p., merc., nat-m., ***ruta., sep.,*** spong., ***sulph.***
evening - cina.
inspiration, from - cina.
lying on side, when - kali-c.
morning, rising, after - **CINA.**
night - carb-v., hep., ip., ruta.
midnight, about - dros., ***ruta.***
sensation, fauces from, to bifurcation of bronchia - syph.
sleep, as soon as one falls into a sound - **LACH.,** ***sulph.***

CHURCH, air of agg. (see Cellars)

CLEANING, the teeth (see Brushing)

CLOCK, like tick of, in its regularity - nicc.

CLOSING, eyes at night excites cough - **HEP.**

CLOTHING, tight, agg. - lach., stann.

COFFEE, agg. - caps., caust., cham., cocc., ign., nux-v., sul-ac.
odor of - sul-ac.

COLD, temperature
becoming, on - arn., **ARS.,** ***bad., bry., calc., calc-p.,*** carb-s., ***carb-v., caust., con., dulc.,*** **HEP.,** kali-ar., ***kali-bi.,*** **KALI-C.,** ***lach., mosch.,*** mur-ac., **NUX-V., PHOS., PSOR., RHUS-T., RUMX.,** ***sabad., sang.,*** **SIL.,** spong., ***squil., staph., sulph.,*** sul-ac., thuj., **TUB.**
arm or hand - ars., bar-c., calc., ***con.,*** ferr., **HEP.,** kali-c., **RHUS-T.,** ***sil.,*** sulph.
feet - ***bar-c., bufo, sil.,*** sulph.
single part - bar-c., **HEP., RHUS-T.,** sil.
drinks - am-m., ant-c., **ARS.,** ***bar-c.,*** calc., ***carb-v.,*** dig., hep., kali-ar., kali-c., lyc., ***merc., phos., ph-ac.,*** **PSOR.,** rhus-t., rumx., ***sil., spong., squil.,*** staph., stram., sul-ac., ***thuj., tub.,*** verat.
amel. - am-caust., bor., brom., caps., **CAUST.,** ***coc-c.,*** **CUPR.,** euphr., glon., iod., ip., kali-c., kali-s., onos., ***op.,*** sulph., verat.
dry air, (see air)
milk - ant-t.
food - am-m., ***carb-v.,*** dros., ***hep.,*** lyc., mag-c., ***ph-ac.,*** rhus-t., ***sil.,*** thuj., verat.
going from warm, to - ***acon., carb-v.,*** nat-c., ***nux-v., phos.,*** **RUMX.,** ***sang.,*** sep.
standing, cold water, in - nux-m.
wind on chest - ***phos., rumx.***

COLD, sensation in trachea - camph.

COMPANY, agg. - ***ambr.,*** bar-c.

CONSCIOUSNESS, loss of, with - cadm-s., carb-v., cina, ***cupr.***

CONSOLATION, agg. - ars.

CONSTANT - acon., ***agar.,*** ail., **ALUM.,** am-br., am-c., ant-t., apoc., arg-c., ***arn., ars.,*** bell., benz-ac., bry., calad., calc., cann-s., carb-ac., ***carb-v.,*** **CAUST., CHIN.,** chlor., cimic., cimx., cina, ***coff., con.,*** cor-r., cub., ***cupr.,*** cupr-s., dol., dros., elaps, euph., ***ferr.,*** ferr-p., guare., ***hep., hyos.,*** hyper., ***ign., ip.,*** kali-bi., kali-chl., kali-i., kali-ma., kali-n., kalm., kreos., ***lac-c., lach.,*** lac-ac., lact., laur., lob-s., **LYC.,** mag-arct., mang., med., merc., ***mez.,*** nat-m., nat-p., ***ph-ac.,*** phos., phel., phyt., plan., podo., ***puls., rhus-t.,*** **RUMX.,** sang., ***seneg.,*** sep., **SPONG.,** ***squil.,*** stict., tab., thuj., zinc.
day, and night - ign., lyc., nat-m., phos., spong., squil.
day, or night - ***squil.***
evening - acon., ***caust.,*** cub., **PULS.**

CONSTANT, coughing
lying, agg., sitting up amel. - **HYOS.,** ***laur.,*** **PULS.,** rhus-t., sang., **SEP.**
amel. - mang.
morning - cupr-s., phel.
night - anac., calc., ***con.,*** laur., lyc., med., **SEP.,** stict., stront-c., zinc.
lying down - **SEP.,** zinc.
sleep, on falling to - med.
waking - **SEP.**
vomiting, amel. - ***mez.***

CONSTIPATION, during - sep.

CONSTRICTION, chest, from - cact., carb-v., clem., dros., ip., mosch., samb., stram., sulph.

constriction, larynx, from - **AGAR.,** ant-t., arg-n., ars., asc-t., bell., brom., calc., carb-an., carb-s., cham., chlor., coc-c., coff., cor-r., **CUPR.,** dros., euphr., gels., hep., hyos., ign., iod., ip., kali-c., ***lach.,*** laur., lob., mang., meny., naja, nit-ac., **PHOS.,** puls., sil., spong., stram., sulph., verat.
eating - puls.
night, during sleep - agar., lach., nit-ac., phos., sulph.
sleep, in first, while lying on the side - kali-c., phos., spong.
sleep, on going to - agar., arg-n., **LACH.,** phos., spong., sulph.

constriction, trachea, from - cocc., mosch., stann., staph.

CONVULSIONS, with - ars., ***bell.,*** brom., calc., ***cham., cina,*** croc., **CUPR.,** ***dros., hyos.,*** led., ***meph., stram.,*** sulph., verat.

CRAMPS, in chest, from - bell.

CRAWLING, sensation of - aeth., apis, chin., caust., con., kreos., nux-m., ***psor.,*** rhus-t., squil.
air passages, in - aeth.
bronchials, in - eupi., kreos.
evening, bed, in - kreos.
night - aeth.
midnight, before - apis

crawling, chest - cahin., caust., con., kreos., nux-m., rhus-t., sep., squil.

crawling, larynx - am-m., ant-t., bry., calc-p., carb-v., ***caust.,*** colch., **CON.,** ***dros.,*** euph., iod., **KALI-C.,** kreos., lach., lact., led., mag-m., nux-m., prun., ***psor.,*** rhus-t., ***sabin.,*** sang., stann., stict., sulph.

crawling, throat, in - carb-v., euph.
throat-pit - apis, kreos., mag-m., **SANG.**

crawling, trachea, in - anac., arn., carb-v., caust., kreos., mag-m., prun., rhus-t.

CROAKING - acon., ant-t., lach., nit-ac., ruta., ***spong.***
daytime - nit-ac.

CROUPY, cough (see Larynx, Croup) - ***acet-ac.,*** **ACON.,** anac., ant-t., apis, ***ars., ars-i.,*** arum-d., ***bell., brom., calc-s., carb-ac.,*** cham., ***chin., chlor., cina,*** cinnb., cor-r., cub., cupr-s., dros., ***gels.,*** **HEP., IOD.,** ***ip.,*** **KALI-BI.,** ***kali-m.,*** kali-s., ***lac-c.,*** **LACH., PHOS.,** ***phyt., rumx., ruta.,*** **SAMB.,** ***sang.,*** **SPONG.,** staph., stict., **STRAM.**
eating, after - anac.
evening - cinnb.
expiration, on - acon.
midnight, after, agg. - ***ars.***
morning - ***calc-s.***
night - ars., carb-ac., ***hep., ip.,*** phyt., ***spong.***
sopor, stertorous breathing and wheezing, the child starts up, kicks about, suffocating turning black and blue in face, after which cough with rattling breathing sets in again, suffocation and paralysis of lungs appear unavoidable - ***samb.***
waking, only after - **CALC-S.**
winter, alternating with sciatica in summer - staph.

CROWING, (see Croupy)

CRUMB, feeling as of a, in larynx, from - ***bry.,*** coc-c., **LACH.,** pall., plb.

CRYING, agg. - ant-t., **ARN.,** ars., ***bell.,*** cham., cina, dros., ferr., guare., ***hep.,*** lyc., phos., samb., sil., sulph., ***verat.***

CUTTING, larynx in, stinging from coughing - ang., ***arg-m.***
thyroid gland in, from coughing - arg-n.

DAMP, room agg. (see Cellars) - bry., ***dulc., nat-s.***

DANCING, after - puls.

DAYTIME - ***agar.,*** ail., alum., **AM-C.,** am-m., anac., ang., ant-t., ***arg-m., arn.,*** arum-d., bar-c., bar-m., ***bell.,*** bism., bov., brom., ***bry.,*** bufo, calc., calc-p., cham., chin., cic., coc-c., coloc., com., con., cot., cupr., **EUPHR.,** ferr., ferr-p., gamb., graph., guai., hep., kali-bi., kali-br., ***kali-c.,*** kali-n., kali-p., **LACH.,** laur., lyc., manc., mez., mur-ac., nat-a., nat-c., nat-m., **NAT-S.,** nicc., nit-ac., nux-v., **PHOS.,** rhus-t., sars., sep., sil., sol-t-ae., spong., stann., ***staph.,*** sulph., sumb., thuj., viol-o., zinc.
amel. - bell., ***caust.,*** con., dulc., euphr., ign., lach., lyc., merc., nit-ac., sep., spong.
day, 6 a.m. to 6 p.m. - calc-p.
day, every other, violent coughs - ***anac.,*** lyc., ***nux-v.***
day, every third - anac., lyc.
expectoration copious, greenish, salty agg, morning - ***stann.***
hour, at the same - lyc., sabad.
menses, before - graph.
night, and - ars-i., ***bell.,*** bism., calc., calc-p., carb-an., cham., chin., cupr., dulc., euph., hep., ***ign.,*** indg., kali-bi., kali-n., ***lyc.,*** mez., mur-ac., nat-c., ***nat-m.,*** nit-ac., ***phos.,*** rhus-t., ***sep.,*** sil., **SPONG.,** ***squil.,*** stann., sulph., zinc.
night, and, expectoration, with - dulc., sil.

DAYTIME,
night, and, which makes boy quite breathless - nat-m.
only, during daytime - ***am-c., arg-m.,*** brom., bry., ***calc.,*** chin., cic., dulc., **EUPHR.,** ***ferr.,*** graph., hep., kali-n., ***lach.,*** laur., lyc., ***mang.,*** merc., nit-ac., nux-m., ***phos., rumx.,*** sep., sin-n., stann., ***staph.,*** thuj., viol-o.
long, lasting spells, dry, short, violent, with much dyspnea - viol-o.
morning on rising, continuing until lying down again - euphr.
or cough which wakens at night - sep.
or cough which wakens at night, morning after rising, and evening after lying down - thuj.
or cough which wakens at night, only at night - merc.

DEBAUCH, after - ***nux-v.,*** stram.

DEEP - ail., all-s., ***ambr.,*** am-br., am-m., ammc., anac., ang., ant-c., ***ars.,*** ars-i., bufo, ***carb-v.,*** chr-ac., ***dig.,*** dios., **DROS.,** eug., guare., ***hep.,*** iod., kali-bi., ***kali-c., lach.,*** lob., lycps., mag-m., ***mang.,*** med., meph., nat-a., ***nux-v.,*** petr., phos., ***sabad., samb.,*** sanic., sel., sep., sil., **SPONG.,** squil., **STANN.,** ***still.,*** **VERAT.,** ***verb.***
afternoon and evening - am-br.
evening - eug., **VERAT.**
inspiration, on - hep., ip.
deep amel. - ***verb.***
lying amel. - **MANG.,** sep., squil.
midnight, after - ars.
morning - ang., dios.
deep, enough, sensation as though he could not to start mucus - ars., bell., **CAUST.,** dros., lach., med., ***mez.,*** rumx.
deep-sounding - aloe, ***kali-bi.,*** mang., **SPONG., STRAM.,** ***verb.***
night - verb.

DENTITION, during - calc., calc-p., ***cham.,*** cina, cupr., hyos., ip., kreos., podo., rhus-t.

DESCENDING, on - lyc.

DIARRHEA, amel - bufo.

DIFFICULT - ant-t., ars., brom., cocc., chin., chlor., dig., kali-br.

DINNER, after - aeth., agar., anac., arg-n., bar-c., bry., calc-f., carb-v., coc-c., ferr., hep., kali-bi., lach., mur-ac., nux-v., phos., sil., sulph., syph., tab., tax., thuj., zinc.
before - arg-n.
sleeping, when - puls., staph.

DISTRACTING - ant-t., rumx.
day and night - ant-t.

DISTRESSING - agn., aspar., ***arum-t., brom.,*** **CAUST.,** iris, ***lach.,*** lyc., meli., ***nit-ac.,*** **NUX-V.,** ***sang., seneg., sep., squil., stann.***
daytime - lyc.
morning and evening, on going to sleep - agn., ***brom., lach.,*** lyc., nit-ac.

DOWN, sensation of, in throat-pit, from - calc., cina, ***ph-ac., sulph.***

DRAFT, (see air)

DRINKING, after - acon., am-caust., am-m., ant-t., arn., **ARS.,** ***bry.,*** calc., carb-v., ***chin., cimx.,*** cina, cocc., con., dig., **DROS.,** ferr., ferr-ar., ***hep.,*** hyos., kali-ar., kali-bi., kali-c., lac-c., ***lach.,*** laur., lyc., ***manc.,*** meph., nat-m., nat-p., nux-m., nux-v., op., ***phos.,*** **PSOR.,** rhus-t., sil., squil., staph., stram., sul-ac., tell., verat.
after, amel. - brom., bry., ***caust., coc-c., cupr.,*** euphr., iod., kali-c., ***op.,*** **SPONG.**

DRY, cough - acal., acet-ac., **ACON.,** aesc., ***agar.,*** ail., aloe, all-s., **ALUM.,** ***alumn., ambr.,*** am-br., ***am-c., am-m.,*** anac., anag., anan., ang., ant-c., ant-t., anth., apis, aphis., apoc., arg-c., arg-m., arg-n., ***arn.,*** **ARS., ARS-I.,** arum-t., asaf., asar., ***asc-t.,*** asim., atro., aur., aur-m., aur-m-n., aur-s., ***bar-c., bar-m.,*** **BELL.,** benz., benz-ac., berb., bor., bov., **BROM., BRY.,** ***bufo,*** cact., calad., **CALC.,** calc-p., **CALC-S.,** camph., cann-i., cann-s., ***canth., caps., carb-ac.,*** **CARB-AN.,** ***carb-s., carb-v.,*** card-m., casc., cast., ***caust.,*** cench., ***cham., chel.,*** **CHIN.,** chin-a., chlor., chr-ac., cimic., cimx., ***cina,*** cinnb., clem., cocc., ***coc-c.,*** cod., ***coff.,*** colch., coloc., ***con.,*** cop., corn., ***croc., crot-c.,*** crot-h., ***cupr.,*** cur., cycl., der., dig., dios., dros., ***dulc.,*** elaps, euph., euphr., eupi., eup-per., ***ferr., ferr-ar., ferr-i., ferr-p.,*** fl-ac., ***form.,*** gamb., gels., graph., grat., guare., ***guai.,*** gymn., ham., ***hell., hep.,*** hura, hydr., hydr-ac., **HYOS.,** ***hyper.,*** **IGN.,** ***indg.,*** inul., **IOD.,** ***ip.,*** iris, ir-foe., ***kali-ar., kali-bi., kali-br.,*** **KALI-C.,** ***kali-i., kali-p.,*** kali-s., kreos., lac-ac., lac-c., lac-d., **LACH.,** ***lachn.,*** lact., laur., lec., led., lil-t., lob., ***lyc.,*** mag-c., mag-m., ***mag-p.,*** mag-s., **MANG.,** med., meli., ***merc.,*** merc-c., ***mez.,*** mosch., mur-ac., murx., ***myrt-c.,*** naja, **NAT-A.,** ***nat-c.,*** **NAT-M.,** nat-p., nat-s., nicc., ***nit-ac., nux-m.,*** **NUX-V.,** olnd., ***op.,*** osm., ***ox-ac., par.,*** paull., **PETR.,** phel., **PH-AC., PHOS.,** ***phyt.,*** pic-ac., plan., ***plat., plb.,*** podo., polyg., ***psor.,*** ptel., **PULS.,** pyrus, ran-s., rat., rheum, ***rhod.,*** rhus-r., ***rhus-t.,*** **RUMX.,** ruta., sabad., sabin., sal-ac., ***samb., sang.,*** sarr., sars., sel., ***seneg., sep., sil.,*** sol-t-ae., spig., **SPONG.,** squil., ***stann., staph.,*** stict., still., stram., stront-c., stry., **SULPH.,** sul-ac., sumb., syph., tab., tarax., ***tarent.,*** tep., ter., teucr., thea., ***thuj.,*** til., tril., **TUB.,** valer., verat., verat-v., verb., viol-o., wye., ***zinc.,*** zing.
afternoon - am-m., anth., calc-p., cench., ***chel.,*** kali-bi., mez., nat-c., nat-m., ***nux-m.,*** phel., ***sang.,*** sulph., thuj.
1 p.m. - aesc.
3 p.m. - calc-p.
4 p.m. - cench., ***chel.***
5 p.m. - bov., nat-m.
entering warm room - anth., nat-c.
walking, while - ***thuj.***
air, dry cold air - crot-h.
cold, from - kali-c., phos., sang., ***seneg.***
open air - ***coff.,*** kali-c., mag-arct., ***seneg.,*** spig.

DRY, cough
air, amel. - iod., lil-t.
going from warm room to - ***acon., con.***
blood, ends in raising black blood - elaps
with discharge of - zinc.
breath, sudden loss of, with - ***nux-m.***
chill, during - ***ferr., rhus-t.***
after - nux-m., samb.
before - mag-c., **RHUS-T.,** ***samb., tub.***
chronic in pining boys - **LYC.**
scrofulous children, in - **BAR-M.**
constant, almost - **ALUM.,** ***arn.,*** euph., ***ign.***
constriction, throat from - aesc.
coryza, during - bell., graph., merc., nat-c., nat-m., nit-ac., sel., sep.
evening - ***dig.***
damp weather - cur.
daytime - ***alum.,*** bar-c., bell., calc., chel., coloc., con., euph., gamb., ign., ***kali-bi.,*** lyc., op., phos., puls., ***sep.,*** sol-t-ae., **SPONG.,** sulph.
loose at night - caust., sep., staph.
lying down amel. - sep.
menses, before - graph.
night, and - acon., bell., brom., carb-an., cimic., ***euph.,*** ign., ***kali-c.,*** kreos., laur., ***lyc.,*** mez., mosch., ***nat-m.,*** mur-ac., ***spong.,*** stram., verb.
dinner, after - aeth., agar., ***kali-bi.,*** lach., nux-v.
amel. - bar-c.
drinking, after - ars., hyos., kali-c., ***nux-m.,*** phos., staph.
amel. - brom., bry., ***caust., coc-c.,*** iod., kali-c., ***op.,*** **SPONG.**
cold drinks, from - ***sil.***
loose after eating - nux-m., staph.
dyspnea as from, day and night - euph.
eating, from - aeth., agar., all-s., ferr-ma., ***hyos., kali-c.,*** nux-v., ***sep.,*** sulph., ter.
amel. - **SPONG.**
night - ter.
emaciated boys, in - **LYC.**
evening - agn., aloe, alum., ***alumn.,*** am-br., am-m., ***arg-n., ars.,*** arund., bar-c., ***bell.,*** bor., bov., **BROM.,** bry., ***calc., caps.,*** carb-an., carb-v., chin., cimic., coca, com., ***con.,*** cop., dig., ***ferr.,*** ferr-ar., ***grat.,*** gymn., **HEP., IGN.,** indg., kali-ar., kali-bi., ***kali-c.,*** kreos., lach., lec., lith., **LYC.,** mag-c., ***mag-m.,*** mag-s., merc., merc-i-r., mez., nat-a., nat-c., nat-m., nat-p., nicc., nit-ac., ***nux-m., nux-v.,*** petr., phel., ***ph-ac., phos.,*** phyt., psor., **PULS.,** rheum, ***rhus-t., sang., seneg., sep.,*** sol-t-ae., ***spong.,*** **SQUIL.,** stann., ***stict.,*** still., stront-c., **SULPH.,** tab., teucr., thuj., verat., zinc., zing.
6 p.m. - am-m., ***con., nat-m.***
7 p.m. - grat., spira.
bed, in - petr., phos., sep., sulph.
entering warm room - nat-c., ***puls.***
inspiration agg. - dig.

DRY, cough
evening,
loose in morning - acon., alum., ***ambr.***, ant-c., ant-t., bar-c., ***bry.***, **CALC.**, ***carb-v.***, cupr., dros., euph., ***ferr.***, **HEP.**, ***hyos.***, ip., kali-c., lach., led., lyc., mag-c., mag-m., mez., mur-ac., nat-m., nit-ac., nux-v., ***phos.***, ***ph-ac.***, ***puls.***, rhus-t., seneg., ***sep.***, ***sil.***, spong., **SQUIL.**, stann., stram., sulph., ***sul-ac.***, zinc.
lying down - ***alumn.***, ***bell.***, bor., ***caps.***, carb-v., ferr., indg., **KALI-C.**, nat-m., nicc., ***nux-v.***, **PH-AC.**, **PULS.**, **SANG.**, **SEP.**, ***stict.***, **SULPH.**, teucr.
lying down, amel. - am-m., zinc.
midnight, until - ***hep.***, ***phos.***, ***rhus-t.***, sep., stann.
night, and, can neither sleep nor lie down - stict.
sleep, on going to - ***hep.***, ***sulph.***
smoking, from - thuj.
exertion, violent, from - ***ox-ac.***
expectoration, hawking, later copious green sputum - kali-i.
morning, only in - ***alum.***, ***am-c.***, bell., ***bry.***, ***calc.***, ***carb-v.***, coc-c., euph., ***ferr.***, ***hep.***, **KALI-BI.**, kali-c., led., lyc., ***mag-c.***, ***mang.***, mur-ac., nat-c., ***nat-m.***, nit-ac., nux-v., ph-ac., ***phos.***, **PULS.**, ***sep.***, ***sil.***, **SQUIL.**, stann., ***sul-ac.***
expiration, after every, with flush of heat and sweat - carb-v.
fever, during - **ACON.**, ang., ant-c., ***apis***, ***arn.***, ***ars.***, bell., brom., **BRY.**, calc., carb-v., caust., cham., chin., chin-a., cina, coff., **CON.**, cupr., dros., hep., ***hyos.***, ign., **IP.**, **KALI-C.**, kali-p., lach., lyc., **NAT-M.**, nit-ac., nux-m., **NUX-V.**, op., petr., **PHOS.**, plat., puls., rhus-t., **SABAD.**, samb., sep., spig., spong., squil., staph., sulph., sul-ac., tarent., verat., verb.
intermittent, before - eup-per., ***rhus-t.***, ***tub.***
flatus, discharge up and down, amel. must sit up also - **SANG.**
forenoon - agar., alum., ***am-m.***, ***camph.***, coc-c., sars., zing.
11 a.m. - ***rhus-t.***
gonorrhea, suppressed, after - benz-ac., sel.
inspiration, on - bell., brom., dig., ***hep.***, lach., nat-a., plb., rumx.
deep - aesc., ***brom.***, dig., ***ferr-p.***, ***hep.***, nat-a., plb., squil.
sleep, in - sep.
irritation in larynx - aphis., bell., carb-ac., cimic., kali-i., lach., lith., lyc., ***rumx.***, ***seneg.***, sulph., tab., thuj., ***zinc.***
lying, while - alum., cinnb., ***con.***, **HYOS.**, ip., ***kali-br.***, lyc., nit-ac., ***ph-ac.***, phos., **PULS.**, rhus-t., sabad., ***sang.***, sep., sil., sulph., ter.
amel. - am-c., **MANG.**, sep., zinc.
back, on - am-m., iod., nux-v., ***phos.***, rhus-t., sil.
amel. - ***mang.***
midnight - ***nux-v.***
side, on, amel. - ***nux-v.***

DRY, cough
lying, while
side, on, left, agg. - acon., bry., eup-per., kali-bi., par., **PHOS.**, puls., rumx.
right, agg. - acon., carb-an., ip., merc., phos.
measles, after - cham., ***dros.***, hyos., ign.
menses, during - ***bry.***, cast., cop., cur., ***graph.***, lac-c., phos., **ZINC.**
profuse sweat, during - graph.
before - graph., hyos., lac-c., plat., ***sulph.***, **ZINC.**
morning - **ZINC.**
suppressed, from - ***cop.***
midnight - ***am-c.***, grat., nicc., ***nux-v.***, phos.
after - ***ars.***, ***calc.***, bell., hyos., lec., nicc., **NUX-V.**
1 to 2 a.m. - zing.
2 a.m. - ***kali-c.***, ***op.***, ***rumx.***
3 a.m. - **AM-C.**, ***kali-c.***, op.
4 a.m., until - nicc.
loose - ***calc.***
before - arg-n., **CALC.**, ***lyc.***, ***nit-ac.***, phos., rhus-t., ***stann.***
10:30 p.m. - sol-t-ae.
sleep, during - ***nit-ac.***, ***rhus-t.***
daybreak, until - **NUX-V.**
lying, back, on - ***nux-v.***
on side amel. - ***nux-v.***
morning - agar., ***alumn.***, am-m., ant-c., ant-t., arg-m., ***arn.***, bar-c., bor., bov., brom., bry., carb-an., carb-s., ***carb-v.***, caust., chin., ***coc-c.***, con., cop., cur., dios., grat., gymn., hep., hyper., ign., **IOD.**, ***kali-c.***, kreos., lec., lyc., mag-s., ***mosch.***, **NAT-A.**, nat-c., nat-s., nux-v., ol-an., ***op.***, rhod., ***rhus-t.***, sang., sep., sil., stann., sulph., sul-ac., tab., tarent., thuj., verat.
early - alum., am-m., ant-c., chin., graph., grat., lyc., nux-v., ol-an., op., rhod., stann., sul-ac., verat.
loose, afternoon, in - am-m.
evening - arn., bov., chin., cina, crot-t., dig., ign., iod., nux-v.
menses, before - graph., **ZINC.**
suppressed - ***cop.***
rising, after - alum., ang., arg-m., arn., bar-c., bor., bov., ***carb-an.***, ***chin.***, dig., grat., nat-s., plb., sul-ac.
waking, on - caust., ign., mag-s., sil.
motion, on - bell., iod., seneg.
amel. - kali-c., phos.
night - acon., agar., aloe, ***alum.***, **AM-C.**, ***am-m.***, ***arg-n.***, **ARS.**, ***asaf.***, aur-m., **BELL.**, bry., calad., **CALC.**, calc-s., ***caps.***, **CARB-AN.**, ***carb-s.***, ***carb-v.***, card-m., caust., ***cham.***, ***chel.***, chin., chin-a., ***cimic.***, coc-c., coloc., ***con.***, ***crot-c.***, ***cupr.***, **DROS.**, euph., ***euphr.***, form., gamb., graph., grat., ***hell.***, **HEP.**, **HYOS.**, ***ign.***, ***ip.***, ***kali-ar.***, kali-br., ***kali-c.***, kali-p., **LACH.**, laur., lec., ***lyc.***, ***mag-c.***, ***mag-m.***, mag-s., mang., ***med.***, ***merc.***, ***mez.***, nat-a., nat-m., nat-s., ***nit-ac.***, ***nux-m.***, ***nux-v.***, ol-an., ol-j., op., petr., **PHOS.**, ***phyt.***, **PULS.**, rhod., ***rhus-t.***, ***rumx.***, ***sabad.***, samb., ***sang.***,

DRY, cough

night - sep., ***sil.***, sol-t-ae., **SPONG.**, squil., ***stict.***, stront-c., **SULPH.**, syph., tab., tarent., ***verat.***, verb., zinc., ***zing.***

falling asleep, on - med.

first, followed by profuse salty expectoration with pain as if something were torn loose from larynx - calc.

inspiration agg. - nat-a.

loose by day - acon., anac., ars., bry., ***calc.***, carb-an., caust., cham., chin., con., euphr., ***hep.***, hyos., kali-c., lach., ***lyc.***, mag-c., mag-m., merc., nit-ac., nux-v., phos., ***puls.***, sabad., samb., sil., **SULPH.**, verat., zinc.

lying, agg. - ***con., hyos.***, kali-br., laur., ol-j., ***phyt., puls.***, **SULPH.**, zinc.

agg., on right side only, while - carb-an.

amel. - ***mang.***

midnight, after (see midnight)

motion agg. - bell., ***seneg.***

sitting up amel. - **HYOS., PULS.**, sang.

smoking amel. - tarent.

sunset to sunrise - aur.

waking from sleep - graph., ***puls., sil.***, **SULPH.**, zinc.

noon - arg-n., naja, sulph.

reading, aloud - ***mang.***, meph., **PHOS.**

rising, on - grat.

room, heat of, agg. - coc-c., nat-a.

room, in - alum.

scraping, in larynx, from - alum., aur-m-n., ***bell.***, bor., bov., **BROM.**, bry., chel., ***coc-c.***, ***con.***, dig., gamb., hep., hydr-ac., laur., led., mang., naja, nit-ac., nux-v., op., osm., **PULS.**, ***sabad.***, seneg., til.

throat, in - graph.

sitting, while - agar., lach., phos., rhus-t.

amel. - arg-n., cinnb., ***sang.***

sleep, during - **CHAM.**, coff., mag-s., ***nit-ac.***, ***rhus-t.***, sep.

after every - puls.

disturbing, from - alum., calad., caust., ***kali-c.***, nux-v., ol-j., phos., rhod., rhus-t., ***sang.***, spong., squil., stict., sulph., syph., zinc.

smoke, from - acon., all-s., atro., coca, coc-c., hell., petr., thuj.

inhaling, from - kali-bi.

sneezing, and - ***cina.***

spasmodic, exhausting, especially in children, agg. night lying down and going to cold room to sleep - sang.

stomach, as if from - **BRY., SEP.**

stopped, up feeling in stomach, from - guai.

talking, on - atro., bell., cimic., crot-h., dig., ***hep., hyos.***, lach., ***mang., rumx.***, stann.

temperature, from change of - ***acon.***

DRY, cough

tickling, in larynx, from - ***agar., am-m., arg-n.***, asaf., aur-m., aur-m-n., bar-c., ***bell.***, bor., bov., ***brom.***, cact., calc-f., carb-ac., carb-an., ***caust.***, cimic., coca, colch., coloc., **CON.**, ***crot-c.***, cycl., hydr., hydr-ac., iod., ip., ir-foe., iris, kali-bi., ***kali-c., lach., lachn.***, led., **LYC.**, mang., mez., mur-ac., ***nat-m.***, nat-s., nit-ac., nux-v., ***op., ox-ac.***, phos., ***phyt., psor.***, **PULS.**, rat., rumx., ***sang., seneg., sep., zinc.***, zing.

waking, on - ***agar.***, bry., calc., caust., coc-c., dig., ign., mag-s., ***puls., sang.***, sil., sol-t-ae., **SULPH.**, ***thuj.***

walking - phel., ***seneg.***, thuj., verat.

air, in open, from - alum., sulph.

sharp, cold air, from - verat.

warm, room, on entering a - anth., com., ***nat-c.***

DRYNESS, of air passages, from - carb-an., lach., merc., petr., ***puls.***

dryness, chest - bell., benz-ac., kali-chl., lach., laur., merc., ***puls.***

dryness, fauces - **DROS.**, ***mez., phyt.***

dryness, larynx - ant-t., atro., bell., bry., ***calc.***, carb-an., carb-o., caust., colch., ***con.***, cop., ***crot-h., dros.***, eug., ip., ***kali-c.***, kali-chl., kalm., lach., lachn., laur., ***mang.***, mez., ***nux-v.***, petr., phyt., plan., ***puls.***, raph., rhus-t., **SANG.**, seneg., spong., stann., stram., ***sulph.***, verat., verat-v.

dry spot - cimic., **CON.**, crot-h., nat-m.

morning - phyt.

dryness, throat, in - mang.

spot, in - cimic.

dryness, trachea in, from - carb-an., cycl., laur., ***puls.***, stann.

DUST, as from - agar., ***alumn., am-c.***, **ARS.**, aur-m., ***bell., brom., calc.***, calc-s., chel., ***chin.***, cina, ***coc-c.***, crot-c., cycl., **DROS.**, ferr-ma., glon., ***hep.***, ictod., ***ign.***, iod., ***ip.***, **LYC.**, meph., nat-a., ph-ac., pic-ac., **PULS.**, teucr., **SULPH.**

throat-pit, in - ***ign.***

trachea, in - ferr-ma.

EATING, from - acon., aeth., agar., all-s., ambr., am-m., ***anac., ant-t.***, arn., ***ars.***, bar-c., bell., brom., ***bry.***, bufo, ***calc.***, calc-f., caps., carb-s., ***carb-v.***, caust., cham., ***chin., coc-c.***, cor-r., ***cupr.***, ***cur.***, dig., dros., euphr., ***ferr.***, ferr-ar., ferr-ma., ferr-p., ***hep.***, hyos., ***ip.***, **KALI-BI.**, kali-c., kali-p., kali-s., lac-c., lach., laur., lyc., mag-c., mag-m., med., ***mez.***, mosch., myos., nat-m., nit-ac., nux-m., **NUX-V.**, op., ph-ac., phos., puls., rhus-t., ***rumx.***, ruta., sang., ***sep.***, sil., squil., staph., sulph., tarax., ter., ***thuj.***, verat., zinc.

amel. - all-s., am-c., ammc., anac., carb-an., ***euphr.***, ferr., ferr-m., kali-c., sin-n., **SPONG.**, tab.

hastily agg. - sil.

satiety, from eating to - carb-v.

spicy, highly-seasoned food agg. - sulph.

vomits, until he - ***mez.***

ELDERLY people - alum., alumn., ***ambr., ammc., am-c.,*** ant-c., **ANT-T.,** ***bar-c.,*** camph., con., hydr., hyos., ip., kreos., **PHOS.,** ***psor., seneg., sil.***
morning, chronic - alumn.
night - hyos.
winter - kreos., psor.

ELONGATED, uvula, as from - alum., bapt., brom., hyos., merc-i-r., nat-m.
morning - brom.

ERUPTIONS, alternating with - ***ars., crot-t.,*** mez., ***psor., sulph.***
suppressed, from - dulc.

EVENING - acet-ac., acon., agar., agn., ail., ***all-c.,*** alum., alumn., ***ambr.,*** am-br., am-c., am-m., anac., anan., ant-c., ant-t., apis, apoc., arg-n., arn., **ARS.,** ars-i., arum-d., arund., aspar., bad., bar-c., bar-m., ***bell.,*** bism., bor., bov., ***brom.,*** bry., **CALC.,** calc-s., **CAPS.,** carb-an., carb-s., **CARB-V.,** ***caust.,*** cham., chel., chin., ***chin-a.,*** chin-s., chlor., cimic., cina, cinnb., coca, cocc., coc-c., coff., coloc., con., cop., crot-t., cub., dios., dol., ***dros.,*** eug., ***eup-per.,*** eup-pur., euphr., ***ferr.,*** ferr-ar., ferr-i., ferr-p., ***fl-ac.,*** graph., gymn., **HEP.,** hydr-ac., **IGN.,** indg., iod., ip., ir-foe., kali-bi., ***kali-c.,*** kali-i., ***kali-s.,*** kalm., kreos., lach., lact., laur., led., lith., **LYC.,** lycps., mag-c., ***mag-m.,*** mag-s., **MERC.,** merc-c., merc-i-r., mez., mosch., mur-ac., naja, nat-a., nat-c., ***nat-m.,*** nicc., **NIT-AC.,** nux-m., nux-v., ol-an., olnd., ox-ac., par., ***petr.,*** phel., ph-ac., ***phos.,*** prun., ***psor.,*** **PULS.,** ran-b., rheum, rhod., rhus-t., rumx., ruta., ***sang., seneg., sep.,*** sil., ***sin-n.,*** sol-t-ae., spong., squil., **STANN.,** staph., stict., still., stront-c., sulph., sul-ac., sumb., tab., tarent., teucr., thuj., upa., verat., verat-v., ***verb.,*** zinc., zing.
6 p.m. - am-m., chel., con., nat-m., phys., ***rhus-t.,*** sulph., sumb.
6:15 p.m. - ol-an.
6 to 7 p.m. - ip.
6 to 10 p.m. - hyper.
6:30 p.m. - dios.
7 p.m. - bry., cimic., com., grat., ***ip.,*** ir-foe., spira.
7 p.m. to 1 a.m. - ***cahin.***
7 p.m., after - ip., rumx.
7 to 8 p.m. - sin-n.
7:30 p.m. - cimic., raph.
8 p.m. - dios., nat-m., sep.
8 to 9 p.m. - ***sep.***
8 to 11 p.m. - nat-m.
8:20 p.m. - coca.
9 p.m. - apis, dios., lyc., ***sil.***
9 p.m., about, with fever, followed by burning, heat of head cramps in legs and feet, hands and arms and rapid pulse - lyc.
9 p.m., till morning - ***kali-c.***
9 p.m., to 4 a.m. - ***apis.***

EVENING,
bed in - acon., agn., **ALUMN.,** ***am-c.,*** am-m., anac., ant-t., **ARS.,** bell., bor., ***calc., caps.,*** carb-an., ***carb-v., caust.,*** coca, cocc., coff., **CON.,** dol., ***dros.,*** ferr., ferr-ar., graph., **HEP.,** hyos., **IGN.,** indg., ip., kali-ar., ***kali-c.,*** kali-p., ***kali-s., kreos., lach.,*** lact., **LYC.,** mag-c., mag-s., **MERC.,** naja, nat-c., **NAT-M.,** nat-p., nicc., ***nit-ac., nux-m., nux-v.,*** par., petr., ph-ac., ***phos.,*** phyt., ***puls.,*** rhus-t., ruta., **SEP.,** ***sil., stann.,*** staph., still., **SULPH.,** teucr., thuj., verat., verb.
menses, before - sulph.
going out, on - naja
midnight, until - arn., ***bar-c.,*** bell., carb-v., ***caust.,*** ferr., **HEP.,** led., mag-m., merc., mez., nit-ac., nux-v., **PHOS.,** ***puls., rhus-t., sep.,*** spong., stann., sulph., sul-ac., verat., zinc.
after - mag-m.
sleep, after going to - carb-an., ***caust., lach.,*** petr.
on going to - ***con., hep.,*** ign., **LYC.**
sunset to sunrise - aur.

EXCITEMENT - acon., ant-t., ars., asar., bry., bufo, ***cham., cist.,*** con., dig., dros., hyos., lach., lob., mag-c., nux-v., op., ph-ac., rhus-t., **SPONG.**

EXERTION, agg. - ail., arn., ars-i., ***bar-c., brom.,*** bry., camph., coc-c., dulc., ***ferr.,*** iod., ip., ***kali-c.,*** led., ***lyc., manc.,*** merc., mur-ac., naja, nat-a., ***nat-m., nux-v., ox-ac.,*** phos., **PULS.,** sil., spong., squil., sulph., verat.
mental - arn., ***ars.,*** asar., cina, cist., cocc., colch., ign., ***nux-v.***
violent - ***brom.,*** carb-v., ***ferr.,*** ox-ac., **PULS.,** verat.

EXHAUSTING - ail., alum., anan., ant-t., arg-m., arg-n., **ARS.,** ars-i., **BELL.,** benz-ac., ***brom., camph., carb-v.,*** **CAUST.,** cham., chel., chin., chin-a., chlor., ***cocc., coc-c.,*** coff., colch., cor-r., ***croc., cupr.,*** daph., dig., ***dros.,*** eup-per., ferr., ferr-ar., ferr-p., graph., ***hyos.,*** iod., ***ip., kali-ar.,*** kali-bi., ***kali-c.,*** kali-s., ***kreos., lach.,*** lyc., mag-s., ***merc.,*** merc-c., nat-a., nat-c., ***nux-v., phos.,*** plb., ***puls.,*** rhod., ***rhus-t., rumx.,*** sang., sarr., seneg., **SEP.,** ***sil.,*** spong., squil., **STANN.,** stict., ***still.,*** stram., sulph., sul-ac., tarent., tax., thuj., verat., zinc.
daytime - lyc.
evening - arg-n., ip., ***kali-c.,*** lyc., rhod., ***sil., still.***
going to sleep, on - lyc.
morning - rhod., squil., sulph., thuj.
going to sleep, on - lyc.
waking, after - mag-s., thuj.
night - ***caust.,*** nat-c., **PULS.,** rhod., tarent.
bed, in - ***caust.,*** tarent.
sitting up amel. - nat-c.
sleep, disturbing - **PULS.**
noon - arg-n.

EXPECTORATION, amel. - ail., alum., alumn., bell., calc., carb-an., caust., ***guai., hep., iod., ip.,*** kali-n., kreos., ***lach.,*** lob., meli., mez., ***phos.,*** phyt., plan., ***sang., sep.,*** sulph., zinc.

EXPIRATION - acon., cann-i., cann-s., ***carb-v., caust.,*** dros., iod., kreos., lach., merc., nux-v., ph-ac., staph.

EXPLOSIVE - ***caps.,*** rumx., sil., stry.
escape of fetid, pungent air, with - caps.
evening - sil.

FASTING - kali-c., mag-m.

FAT, food - mag-m.

FEARS, to cough and seems to avoid it as long as possible, in children with bronchial catarrh - bry., phos.

FEATHER, as from, sensation of, or awn of barley in trachea - rumx.

FEVER, during - **ACON.,** alum., anac., ang., ant-c., ant-t., ***apis,*** arg-m., ***arn.,*** **ARS.,** ars-i., bapt., ***bell.,*** bism., brom., ***bry.,*** **CALC.,** carb-v., caust., cham., ***chin., chin-a.,*** cic., cimx., cina, coff., **CON.,** cub., cupr., dig., ***dros.,*** dulc., eup-per., ***ferr.,*** ferr-ar., ferr-i., ***ferr-p.,*** hep., ***hyos.,*** ign., iod., **IP.,** ***kali-ar.,*** **KALI-C.,** kali-p., ***kali-s.,*** kreos., lach., lyc., **NAT-M.,** nit-ac., nux-m., **NUX-V.,** op., petr., ph-ac., **PHOS.,** plat., podo., puls., rhus-t., ruta., **SABAD.,** samb., sang., seneg., sep., sil., spig., spong., squil., staph., sulph., sul-ac., tarent., thuj., ***tub.,*** verat., verb.
intermittent, before, in spells - eup-per., ***rhus-t.,*** samb.
after - nat-m.
suppressed, from - eup-per.
remittent, during - podo.
scarlet, after - ant-c., con., hyos.

FILLING, up, sensation as of, in throat, from - apis, ars., sil.

FIRE, look into - ***ant-c., stram.***

FISH, from eating - lach.

FLATUS, passing, amel. - **SANG.**

FLUIDS, loss of animal, from - ***chin.,*** cina, ferr., ph-ac., staph.

FOG, agg. - sep.

FORCIBLE - acon., alum., bry., con., hep., lyc., ***phos.,*** ruta.
evening and night - ruta.

FOREIGN, body, sensation as of, in larynx - am-caust., ***arg-m.,*** **BELL.,** brom., ***dros., hep., lach.,*** lob., ***phos.,*** ptel., ***rumx., sil.***
larynx, in, awn of barley swaying in larynx - rumx.
trachea, in, from - hyos., ***kali-c.,*** **SANG.,** sin-n., staph.

FORENOON - agar., alum., am-c., ***am-m., bell.,*** bry., camph., chin-s., coc-c., dios., dros., glon., grat., hell., kali-c., lact., mag-c., nat-a., nat-c., nat-m., rhus-t., sabad., sars., seneg., sep., sil., stann., staph., sulph., sul-ac., zing.
9 a.m. to 5 or 6 p.m. - merc.

FORENOON,
9 to 10 a.m. - ars-h.
9 to 12 a.m. - staph.
10 a.m. from rawness, in air passages while lying - coc-c.
10 to 12 a.m. - coc-c., nat-m.
11 a.m. - lach., nat-m.
dry cough from tickling behind upper half of sternum, while sitting bent forward - ***rhus-t.***
rush of blood to chest, from - raph.
waking - dios., nat-m.
after - rhus-t.

FRETTING - ***cina.***

FRIGHT, from - acon., bell., ign., op., rhus-t., samb., stram.

FRIGHTENS, them, weak, nervous children arouse with a dry, spasmodic which causes them to cry out in terror - kali-br.

FROSTY, weather amel. - spong.

FRUIT, agg. - arg-m., mag-m.

FULLNESS, of chest - chin-a., ph-ac., sulph.
morning - chin-a., sulph.

GASTRIC - ant-c., bor., card-m., ferr., ***ip.,*** kali-ar., ***lob.,*** nux-v.

GONORRHEA, suppressed, after - benz-ac., ***med.,*** sel., ***thuj.***

GOUT, before an attack of - led.

GRASPING, larynx involuntarily at every feels as though larynx would be torn - all-c.
genitalia - zinc.
throat, during coughs - ***acon.,*** all-c., ant-t., arum-t., bell., dros., hep., iod., lach., ***samb.***

GREASE, sensation as if throat irritated by smoke of rancid - hep.

GRIEF, from - arn., asar., ***cham., ign.,*** ph-ac., phos.

HACKING, cough - acon., aesc., aeth., agar., ail., ***all-c., aloe,*** **ALUM.,** am-c., am-m., anac., ang., ***ant-c.,*** ant-t., apoc., arg-m., arn., **ARS.,** ***ars-i.,*** arum-t., asaf., ***asar.,*** asc-t., benz-ac., ***bor.,*** bov., brom., **BRY.,** bufo, ***calc., calc-f.,*** calc-p., calc-s., camph., cann-i., cann-s., ***canth., caps., carb-ac.,*** carb-an., carb-s., carb-v., caust., cham., ***chin.,*** chin-a., cimic., ***cina,*** clem., cocc., cob., coc-c., coff., colch., coloc., ***con., cupr-s.,*** cycl., dig., dios., ***dros.,*** dulc., eup-per., euph., eupi., ferr-i., ferr-p., gels., grat., guare., hell., hep., hydr-ac., ***hyos., hyper., ign.,*** ip., iris, jatr., ***kali-ar.,*** kali-bi., kali-br., kali-c., ***kali-i.,*** kali-ma., kali-n., kali-p., kali-s., **LACH.,** lact., laur., lil-t., lob-s., lyc., mag-s., mang., merc., merc-i-f., mur-ac., **NAT-A.,** nat-c., **NAT-M.,** nat-p., nicc., nit-ac., ol-j., onos., op., osm., ***par.,*** **PHOS.,** phyt., plan., plb., podo., prun., ***psor.,*** ptel., ran-s., ***rhus-t., rumx.,*** ruta., sabin., sal-ac., **SANG.,** ***seneg.,*** **SEP.,** ***sil.,*** sin-n., squil., ***stann.,*** staph., stict., ***still.,*** stront-c., ***sulph.,*** sul-ac., ***sumb.,*** tarax., ter., ***thuj.,*** til., trom., **TUB.,** ust., valer., verat-v., xan., zinc.

HACKING, cough
afternoon - calc-f., calc-p., cench., kali-c., laur., **SANG.**
2 p.m. - laur.
3 p.m. - calc-p.
3-4 p.m. - calc-f., calc-p., cench.
air, chill, during - calc-p.
cold agg. - **ALL-C.,** hyper.
open - osm., ***seneg.***
open, amel. - lil-t.
crawling in the larynx, from - carb-v., caust., colch., euph., lach., prun.
daytime - ***calc.,*** com., gamb., nat-m., ***sumb.***
deep inspiration - nat-a.
dinner, after - agar., calc-f., **HEP.**
dryness in larynx, from - carb-an., **CON.,** ***dros.,*** kali-c., laur., mang., plan., ***puls.,*** **SANG.,** ***seneg.,*** spong.
eating, while - nit-ac., sang.
after - anac., ***hep.***
evening - alum., am-br., am-m., ***bor.,*** bry., caps., carb-an., coloc., com., eup-per., eup-pur., **IGN.,** kali-bi., lach., lil-t., nit-ac., ol-an., phos., phyt., ***rhus-t.,*** rumx., **SANG., SEP.,** sil., sin-n., stront-c., ***sulph.,*** sumb., zinc.
6 p.m. - sumb.
7 p.m. - com.
bed, in - bry., carb-an., **IGN.,** lact., nit-ac., ***rhus-t.,*** **SEP.,** ***sulph.***
lying down, after - caps., **IGN.,** kali-bi., phyt., ***rhus-t.,*** rumx., **SANG., SEP.,** sil.
lying down, after, amel. - am-m.
smoking, from - coloc.
warm room - com.
forenoon - am-m.
irritation in larynx, from - hep., hyper., ***seneg., sumb.,*** thuj., trom.
lying down while - ***ars., bry., con.,*** **HYOS.,** ***ign., lach.,*** nat-m., par., phos., rhus-t., ***rumx.,*** **SANG.,** sep., sil., stann., sulph., vesp.
menses at beginning of - phos.
midnight, wakening - ruta.
morning - all-c., ant-t., arg-m., arn., ***ars.,*** calc., cina, con., iris, kali-c., kali-i., laur., mang., nit-ac., ol-an., par., phos., sil., sumb., thuj.
mucus from - laur.
rising, after - arg-m., ***arn., chin.,*** euph., ***ferr.,*** lach., nit-ac., ox-ac., par., staph., thuj.
talking, from - sumb.
waking, on - phos., sil.
motion - osm., ***seneg.***
night - aeth., calc., ***cina, con.,*** graph., kali-bi., ***kali-c.,*** mag-s., nat-m., phyt., senec., ***sil.***
and day - euph.
smothered feeling - asaf.
noon - arg-n., naja
rawness in larynx, from - alum., bry., ***caust., coc-c., dulc.,*** kali-bi., kali-i., laur., ***phos.,*** rumx., sil., stront-c., sulph.

HACKING, cough
rising, on - benz-ac.
amel. - rhus-t.
short, minute, guns, like - ***cor-r.***
sleep, when going to - agar., arn., brom., hep., lach., lyc., nit-ac., sep., sulph.
smoking, from - clem., coc-c., coloc., hell., ign., lach., nux-v., petr.
tickling in larynx, from - acon., **ALL-C.,** ***alum.,*** ang., **ARS.,** bor., ***bry., calc., carb-an.,*** carb-v., caust., **COC-C.,** colch., ***con.,*** dig., **DROS.,** hyos., ip., kali-bi., kali-c., kali-n., lac-c., **LACH.,** laur., lob-s., lyc., nat-s., **NAT-M.,** nit-ac., **PHOS.,** phyt., psor., rhus-t., ***rumx.,*** sabin., ***sang., seneg.,*** sep., sil., spira., spong., sumb.
waking, on - arum-t., phos., sil.
walking, fast - seneg.
open air, in - ang.

HAIR, sensation of, in trachea - sil.

HANDS, holding, abdomen amel. - carb-an., con., phos.
holds chest with both, must while coughing - **ARN.,** ***bor.,*** **BRY.,** cimic., **DROS.,** ***eup-per.,*** kreos., merc., nat-m., ***nat-s., phos., sep.***
holding head while coughing - **BRY.,** nicc., nux-v., sulph.
hypochondria - dros.
larynx - **ALL-C.**
pit of stomach - phos.
pit of stomach, amel. - ***croc., dros.***

HARD - alumn., apoc., ars., asc-t., aur-m., aur-s., **BELL.,** ***bor.,*** calc., cann-i., caps., ***carb-v., caust.,*** cench., chlor., chr-ac., cina, ***coc-c.,*** coll., ***cupr.,*** eup-per., eupi., gymn., ***kali-bi.,*** **KALI-C.,** ***lac-c., lach.,*** laur., ***lyc.,*** naja, ***nux-v.,*** osm., ***phos., phyt., puls.,*** rhus-t., sarr., sec., seneg., ***sep.,*** spong., **STANN.,** stict., syph., ziz.
evening - apoc., caps., ***puls.***
night - apoc., ars., syph.
night, 1 a.m., after - ars.
smoking, while - all-s., nux-v.
spells of, not ceasing until masses of offensive sputa are raised - ***carb-v.***

HAWKING - eug.
agg. - am-m.
choking and vomiting, when hawking up phelgm in morning - ambr.

HEART, affections, with - ado., cact., **LACH.,** ***laur.,*** lycps., **NAJA,** nux-v., ox-ac., spong., ***tab.***

HEARTBURN, from - carb-s., carb-v., staph.

HEAT, after - bell.
sensation of, bronchials - aeth., eup-per.
chest - carb-v.

HEATED, on becoming - acon., ant-c., ***brom., bry.,*** carb-v., caust., ***coc-c., dig.,*** iod., kali-c., mag-c., nux-m., nux-v., **PULS.,** rhus-t., sil., thuj., zinc.

HECTIC - bov., nux-v., ***phos.,*** puls., sil., ***stann.***
suppressed, intermittent, after - eup-per.

HEMORRHOIDS, after the appearance of - berb., euphr., sulph.

HISSING - ***ant-t., caust.***
hoarseness, with, raises hand to larynx, which is sensitive to touch - ***ant-t.***

HOARSE - **ACON.,** agar., agn., **ALL-C.,** aloe, ambr., anan., ant-t., apis, apoc., asaf., asc-t., **BELL.,** bov., **BROM.,** bufo, calad., ***calc.,*** calc-s., camph., cann-i., carb-an., carb-s., **CARB-V., CAUST.,** cench., chin., cina, cop., **DROS.,** ***dulc., eup-per.,*** gels., graph., **HEP.,** hydr., ign., **KALI-BI.,** ***kali-i.,*** kali-s., kreos., lac-ac., ***lac-c., lach.,*** laur., ***lyc.,*** merc., naja, nat-c., nat-m., nux-v., phyt., ***rhus-t., rumx.,*** sabad., samb., sec., ***sil.,*** **SPONG., STANN.,** sul-ac., verat., ***verb.***
evening - ***caust.,*** cina.
evening, until midnight - **HEP.**
midnight - dros.
after - **DROS.,** rumx.
barking, 2 to 5 a.m. - rumx.
before, barking, 11 p.m. - rumx.
morning - carb-an., ***caust.,*** hep.
night - dros., rumx., verb.

HOLD, cough obliges him to, himself inwardly - coff.

HOLDS, chest with hands etc., (see Hands)

HOLLOW - ***acon.,*** all-s., ***ambr.,*** anac., ant-t., apis, **BELL.,** brom., bry., bufo, carb-v., **CAUST.,** chel., cina, ***dig.,*** dros., euph., euphr., hep., ***ign., ip.,*** jatr., ***kali-i.,*** kreos., lach., lact., led., ***mag-c.,*** med., meph., merc., merc-c., myrt-c., nat-c., nat-p., nit-ac., nux-v., op., osm., ***phos.,*** samb., sanic., sil., spig., **SPONG.,** staph., ***stram.,*** **VERAT.,** ***verb.***
breathing deep amel. - ***verb.***
daytime - spong.
evening - ***caust.,*** **IGN.,** lact., verat.
lying down, after - lact.
midnight, until - bry., caust.
morning - ***caust.,*** cina, ***ign., phos.***
bed, in - ***phos.***
rising, after - cina
waking, on - **IGN.**
night - acon., anac., ant-t., ***caust.,*** nat-c., ***phos.,*** samb., spong., verb.
noon, toward - sil.
sitting up, amel. - med., nat-c., nit-ac., phos., sil.
stooping, agg. - spig.

HUNGER, from - kali-c., mag-c.
violent, with - nux-v., sul-ac.

HYSTERICAL, attack of, followed by crying, night - form.
women - cocc., der., ***gels., ign.,*** nux-m., plat., verat.

ICE cream, at first amel, then agg. - ars-h.

ICY, cold air, in air passages, sensation of, from - ***cor-r.***

INABILITY, to - ***ant-t.,*** bry., ***dros.,*** nat-s., ox-ac., sulph.
pain from - **BRY.,** dros., nat-s.
amel. by pressure of hand on pit of stomach - ***dros.***
side in, from - ox-ac.

INSPIRATION, agg. - acon., apis, asaf., asar., benz-ac., bell., ***brom., calc., camph.,*** chlor., cina, cist., coff., con., cor-r., croc., dig., dulc., graph., ***hep.,*** ip., lach., ***kali-bi.,*** mag-m., ment., meny., meph., merc-i-f., nat-s., olnd., op., plb., ***puls.,*** prun., **RUMX.,** squil., stict., ter., verb.
crowing, violent, spasmodic commencing with gasping for breath, and continuing with repeated crowing inspirations till face becomes black or purple and patient exhausted, agg. night and after a meal - ***cor-r.***

INTERMITTING, 6 a.m., drinking cold water amel. - ***coc-c.***

INTERRUPTED - agar., coff., kreos., sul-ac., thuj.
dinner, after - agar.
evening, smoking, from - thuj.
infiltration of lower chest, from - kreos.

IRRESISTIBLE, short, hawking - osm.
sudden, violent, in evening, while sitting - alum.

IRRITABLE - arg-m., ***bry.,*** chlor., clem., cocc., cod., coff., ign., hippoz., kali-c., lach., laur., ol-j., ozone, ph-ac., phos., phyt., plan., ***rumx,*** teucr.
morning, rising, after - arg-m.
night - ***cod.,*** phos.

IRRITATING, things, such as salt, wine, pepper, vinegar, immediately start cough - alum., sulph.

IRRITATION, air passages, coughing from - **ACON.,** ***agar.,*** agn., all-s., aloe, alum., am-br., am-c., am-m., aml-n., ***anac.,*** ant-t., aspar., bar-c., cahin., ***calc.,*** carb-ac., carb-s., ***carb-v., caust.,*** **CHAM.,** chin-s., chlor., clem., coc-c., coff., colch., coll., con., crot-t., dios., ferr-ar., ferr-p., ***gels.,*** hyos., **IOD.,** kali-bi., kali-c., kali-i., lob., lyc., mag-s., merc-i-r., mez., mosch., mur-ac., nat-a., nat-s., **NUX-V.,** osm., ox-ac., ph-ac., phos., plan., psor., ***puls-n,*** raph., **SEP.,** ***sulph.,*** sul-ac.
afternoon - bapt.
cardiac region - bar-c.
evening - chel., cimic., dios., petr., sulph.
7:30 p.m. - cimic.
bed in - agn., am-c., coff., kali-c.
extending to palate - dig.
forenoon - mag-c.
increases the more one coughs - ***bell.,*** cist., cocc., hep., **IGN.,** raph., squil., teucr.
morning, rising after - alumn.
night, on waking - thuj.

irritation, bronchials - aesc-g., ***anac.,*** arg-m., carb-s., chlor., cocc., con., cub., ***dros.,*** ind., ip., ***kali-bi.,*** kali-n., ***lach., lyc.,*** phyt., ***sang.,*** squil., trif-p., verat.
bifurcation of - bry., carb-s., dub., ***kali-bi., spong.***
right - kali-n.

irritation, chest, in - ***anac.,*** ant-ox., arn., ars., ars-h., ***bell.,*** bov., ***calc.,*** carb-s., ***carb-v., cham.,*** colch., dros., euph., ***ferr-p.,*** graph., grat., guai., guare., kali-n., kreos., mag-arct., mag-c., merc., mez., mur-ac., nat-c., nat-p., nux-m., ol-j., osm., petr., ***ph-ac.,*** **PHOS.,** puls., rhus-t., ***sang.,*** sanic., **SEP.,** spong.,

irritation, chest, in - **STANN.,** sul-ac., thuj., verat., zinc.
lower, in - kreos.
upper, in - ars-h., carb-v., myrt-c., nux-m., ol-j.

irritation, epigastrium, in, from - bar-c., bell., ***bor.,*** **BRY.,** cann-s., cench., cham., guai., ***hep.,*** ign., ***lach.,*** merc., nat-m., nit-ac., nux-v., ph-ac., **PULS.,** raph., **SEP.**

irritation, fauces - dios., lycpr., mag-s., ***mez.,*** sul-ac.

irritation, larynx, in, coughing from - ***acon.,*** **AGAR., ALL-C.,** ***alum.,*** alumn., ambr., am-c., am-m., anac., ang., ant-c., ant-t., aphis., ***arg-m., arg-n.,*** ars., ars-i., asaf., asar., bar-c., bar-m., **BELL.,** bov., ***brom., bry., calad., calc.,*** calc-f., camph., canth., caps., carb-ac., ***carb-an.,*** carb-s., ***carb-v.,*** card-m., ***caust.,*** **CHAM.,** chel., chin., chin-a., cimic., cina, coca, **COC-C.,** ***cocc.,*** coff., colch., ***coloc.,*** **CON.,** crot-h., ***cupr.,*** dig., dios., **DROS.,** euph., ***euphr.,*** ferr., ferr-i., form., ***gels.,*** graph., guare., **HEP.,** hyos., hydr-ac., hyper., **IGN.,** ***iod.,*** **IP.,** ***kali-ar., kali-bi.,*** **KALI-C.,** kali-chl., kali-i., kali-p., lac-ac., lac-c., **LACH.,** lachn., laur., lith., ***lyc.,*** mag-c., manc., mang., meny., ***merc.,*** merc-c., mez., mur-ac., myric., ***naja,*** nat-a., nat-c., **NAT-M.,** nat-p., nicc., nit-ac., **NUX-V.,** olnd., osm., ***petr., ph-ac.,*** **PHOS.,** ***phyt.,*** plan., ***psor.,*** **PULS.,** ***rhus-t., rumx.,*** sabad., sabin., sang., ***seneg., sep., sil.,*** **SPONG.,** ***squil.,*** stann., ***staph.,*** stront-c., sul-i., **SULPH.,** sumb., tab., tarax., teucr., thuj., trom., verat., verb., zinc., manc., mang., meny., ***merc.,*** merc-c., mez., mur-ac., myric., ***naja,*** nat-a., nat-c., **NAT-M.,** nat-p., nicc., nit-ac., **NUX-V.,** olnd., osm., ***petr., ph-ac.,*** **PHOS.,** ***phyt.,*** plan., ***psor.,*** **PULS.,** ***rhus-t., rumx.,*** sabad., sabin., sang., ***seneg., sep., sil.,*** **SPONG.,** ***squil.,*** stann., ***staph.,*** stront-c., **SULPH.,** sul-i., sumb., tab., tarax., teucr., thuj., trom., verat., verb., zinc.
afternoon - coca, ferr-i., phos.
2 p.m. - coca.
as if some fluid had gone the wrong way - **LACH.**
eating, while - ***rumx.***
evening, bed, in - cocc., coc-c.
lying, while - ***ign.***
midnight, before - ***spong.***
morning - ***sil.***
sleep, in first, when lying on side - ***kali-c., spong.***

irritation, lungs, in, from - dios., lach., lycps.
evening, 8 p.m. - dios.
right - carb-an., nux-m.

irritation, throat-pit, in, from - ***apis,*** bell., ***cann-s.,*** card-m., ***cham.,*** croc., **IGN.,** iod., kreos., lac-c., mag-c., nat-m., ph-ac., rhus-r., **RUMX., SANG.,** ***sil.,*** squil.

irritation, thyroid gland, in region of - mag-c.

irritation, trachea, in, from - acon., agar., alum., ang., ant-t., ***arg-m.,*** arg-n., ***arn.,*** ars., ars-i., asaf., bar-c., bar-m., ***bell., bov., bry., calc., cann-s.,*** carb-an., carb-s., ***carb-v., caust., cham.,*** chin., chin-a., cina, ***coc-c.,*** cocc., colch., coloc., ***con.,*** croc., dig., **DROS.,** euph., ***ferr., ferr-ar.,*** ferr-i., ferr-ma., ***ferr-p.,*** graph., grat., hep., hydr-ac., hyos., ign., ***iod.,*** ip., ***kali-ar.,*** kali-bi., **KALI-C.,** ***kali-i.,*** kali-n., kali-p., laur., led., **LYC.,** mag-c., ***mang., merc.,*** mez., mur-ac., nat-a., ***nat-m.,*** nicc., ***nit-ac.,*** nux-m., nux-v., ***petr.,*** **PHOS.,** plan., prun., psor., ***puls.,*** rhod., **RHUS-T.,** ***rumx.,*** sabin., seneg., **SEP., SIL.,** spig., ***spong.,*** squil., **STANN.,** staph., ***stict.,*** stront-c., **SULPH.,** teucr., ***thuj.,*** trif-p., verat., zinc.

ITCH, suppressed, after - psor.

ITCHING, in chest - agar., ambr., ars., carb-v., coc-c., con., iod., kali-bi., kali-c., mag-m., mez., ***nux-v.,*** ph-ac., phos., polyg., puls., sep., spig., stann.
chest, extending through trachea to tip of nose - iod.
larynx - ambr., ant-t., bell., cact., ***calc.,*** calc-f., carb-v., ***con.,*** dig., lach., laur., mang., ***nux-v.,*** puls., sil.
trachea, from - cham., con., kali-bi., laur., ***nux-v.,*** puls.

KNEELING, with face, toward pillow amel. - eup-per.

LABOR, following difficult, or abortion, with backache and sweat - kali-c.

LACTATION, (see Breast-feeding).

LAUGHING - ***arg-m., arg-n.,*** ars., ***bry.,*** **CHIN.,** con., cupr., cur., dros., dulc., hyos., kali-c., lach., mang., merc-i-f., mur-ac., nit-ac., ol-j., ***petr., phos.,*** rhus-t., ***sanic.,*** sil., sin-n., ***stann.,*** staph., zinc.

LIE, down, could not, sat bent forward - iod.

LIFTING, heavy weight - ambr.

LIQUIDS, swallowing, night - sul-ac.
touching back part of mouth, from - am-c.

LOOSE - acet-ac., agar., alum., ammc., am-m., anac., ant-t., apis, apoc., ***arg-m.,*** **ARS.,** ***ars-i.,*** arum-d., arum-t., asaf., aur-m., bell., bism., brom., bry., ***calc.,*** calc-s., carb-an., carb-s., ***carb-v.,*** carl., cench., cham., ***chel.,*** chin., chin-a., chin-s., cic., cina, cocc., ***coc-c.,*** coloc., ***con.,*** cub., cupr-n., dig., dros., ***dulc.,*** elaps, eup-per., euph., eupi., ferr., ferr-ar., ferr-i., ferr-p., graph., hep., hydr., ign., iod., jab., kali-ar., kali-c., kali-p., kali-s., kreos., lappa-a., lyc., mag-s., merc., merc-c., merc-i-f., mur-ac., nat-a., nat-c., nat-s., nit-ac., nux-m., ol-j., ph-ac., ***phos.,*** podo., **PULS.,** ruta., sabad., sac-alb., sec., ***senec.,*** seneg., ***sep., sil.,*** spong., squil., ***stann.,*** staph., stict., still., sulph., sul-ac., tarent., tell., thuj., verat-v.
afternoon - am-m.
dry in morning - am-m.
apyrexia, during - eup-per.
breakfast, after - coc-c.

LOOSE, cough
daytime, dry at night - ***calc.,*** euphr., lyc., puls.
night, and daytime - dulc., sil.
drinking cold water amel. - ***coc-c.***
eating, while - phos.
after - bell., nux-m., ***phos.,*** sanic., sil., staph., thuj.
after, dry after drinking - nux-m., staph.
evening - bov., eug., mur-ac.
7 p.m. - spira.
dry in morning - bov.
exercise and warm room agg. - brom.
expectoration, without - ammc., arn., arum-t., brom., ***caust., con.,*** crot-t., dros., ***kali-s.,*** lach., ***phos., sep.,*** stann., sulph.
fever, during - alum., anac., apis, ars-m., **ARS.,** bell., bism., brom., bry., **CALC.,** carb-v., ***chin.,*** cic., cub., dig., dros., dulc., ferr., iod., **KALI-C.,** kreos., lyc., ph-ac., phos., puls., ruta., seneg., sep., ***sil.,*** spong., squil., stann., staph., ***sulph.,*** thuj.
forenoon - **STANN.**
morning - ***agar., alum.,*** ars., bad., **BRY.,** ***calc., carb-s.,*** **CARB-V.,** cench., cham., ***chel.,*** coc-c., **HEP.,** meph., mur-ac., nat-m., nat-p., nat-s., nit-ac., nux-v., ***ph-ac., phos., psor.,*** **PULS., SEP.,** ***sil.,*** **SQUIL., STANN.,** stict., stram., **SULPH., SUL-AC.**
tight, afternoon - bad.
night - am-m., calc., eug., eup-per., puls., ***sep.,*** sil., stict.
less free during day - stict.
lying - arum-d.
midnight - phos., sep.
midnight, after - ***calc.,*** hep.
midnight, sitting up, amel. - phos.
skin hanging in throat, sensation of, from - alum.
tickling deep in chest from - graph.

LUMP, in throat, from - ***bell.,*** calc., coc-c., lach.

LYING, general
agg. - acon., aeth., agar., all-c., ***ambr.,*** am-br., am-m., ant-t., **APIS,** aral., arg-n., ***arn., ars.,*** bar-c., bell., bor., ***bry.,*** calc., calc-s., caps., carb-an., carb-s., ***carb-v.,*** **CAUST.,** cham., cinnb., cocc., ***coc-c.,*** colch., **CON.,** corn., ***crot-t.,*** dol., ***dros., dulc.,*** eupi., ferr-ar., ferr-p., hep., **HYOS.,** ign., ***iod.,*** ip., kali-br., ***kali-c.,*** kali-p., ***kali-s.,*** **KREOS.,** lac-c., ***lach.,*** lact., ***laur.,*** lith., ***lyc.,*** mag-c., mag-m., mag-p., mag-s., med., ***meph.,*** merc., ***mez.,*** nat-c., nat-m., nat-s., nicc., nit-ac., nux-v., ol-j., par., petr., ph-ac., ***phos.,*** phyt., plan., psor., **PULS.,** pyrog., ***rhus-t.,*** **RUMX.,** ruta., ***sabad.,*** **SANG.,** sanic., ***seneg., sep., sil., spong.,*** stann., staph., stict., ***sulph.,*** tarent., ter., teucr., thuj., verb., vesp., vip., zinc.
afternoon - calc-p., laur.
2 p.m. - laur.
3 p.m. - calc-p.

LYING, general
amel. - acon., am-c., am-m., arg-m., bry., coca, **EUPHR.,** ***ferr., hydr.,*** indg., kali-bi., **MANG.,** nit-ac., sep., sin-n., squil., sulph., ***thuj.,*** verat., zinc.
abdomen, on - aloe, alum., am-c., bar-c., calc., caust., eup-per., ***med.,*** phos., podo., rhus-t., syph.
back, on - agar., ***am-m., ars.,*** crot-t., eup-per., iod., kali-bi., ***nat-m.,*** nat-s., ***nux-v., phos.,*** plb., rhod., rhus-t., ***sep.,*** sil., spong.
amel. - ***acon.,*** bry., ***lyc., mang.***
better than either side, though worse lying on left side - ***phos.***
bed agg. - agn., ***alumn.,*** am-c., am-m., anac., ant-t., aral., arg-n., ***ars.,*** bry., cact., calc., ***caps.,*** cham., coca, coc-c., coff., **CON.,** ***crot-t.,*** dol., ***dros.,*** euphr., ferr-ar., ferr-p., hep., ***hyos.,*** ign., indg., iod., ip., ***kali-c.,*** kali-n., kali-s., kreos., lach., lachn., lact., lyc., mag-c., mag-m., mag-s., meph., mez., nat-c., nat-m., nit-ac., nux-v., **PHOS.,** psor., ***puls., rhus-t.,*** sabad., samb., sang., ***sep., sil.,*** squil., ***still.,*** **SULPH.,** verb.
must sit up, or sleep in chair from sense of suffocation - crot-t.
daytime amel. - ***dros.,*** nit-ac., sep.
evening - alum., **ARS.,** ***bell.,*** bor., bry., carb-an., carb-s., **CON., DROS.,** graph., ign., kali-ar., **KALI-C.,** kali-c., lach., lact., mez., nat-m., nicc., nux-v., petr., ***ph-ac., psor.,*** **PULS.,** rumx., **SANG.,** ***seneg.,*** **SEP.,** ***sil.,*** staph., stict., ***sulph.,*** teucr., thuj.
amel. - am-m.
must sit up - **ARS., CON., PULS., SANG., SEP.**
face, great rattling of mucus, while cough only reaches to throatpit, consequently hard cough does not reach phlegm unless he lie on his face when he brings up a greenish-yellow gelatinous mucus without taste - ***med.***
first lying down, on - arg-n., ***ars.,*** caps., con., ***dros.,*** hyos., laur., phyt., puls., sabad., sang.
hands and knees, on, amel. - eup-per.
head, with, low - am-m., ***bry.,*** carb-v., **CHIN.,** hyos., puls., rumx., samb., sang., spong.
head, with, raised, amel. - ***carb-v.,*** **CHIN.,** rumx., sep.
long in one position (or sitting) agg. - con., ph-ac.
night - am-m., ***ars.,*** arum-d., ***bell.,*** bor., ***carb-an.,*** carb-s., ***con.,*** dol., **DROS.,** ***dulc.,*** gamb., kali-bi., kali-br., **KALI-C.,** ***laur.,*** lyc., ***meph.,*** nat-s., nit-ac., ol-j., ***ph-ac., phyt.,*** **PULS.,** rhus-t., **RUMX., SANG.,** sanic., **SEP.,** sil., sulph., ***thuj.,*** zinc.
as soon as head touches pillow - caps., ***con.,*** **DROS.**
midnight, wakens him - **APIS.**
midnight, wakens him, after - nux-v.

LYING, general
night, before midnight, wakens him - ***aral., spong.***
sleep amel. - dulc., kali-bi.
waking, on - sanic.
noon, amel. - **MANG.**
only on lying - ***caust.***
when first lying down, was obliged to sit up and cough it out, then had rest - **CON.**
side on - ***acon.,*** am-m., bar-c., bry., carb-an., erig., kali-c., kreos., lyc., merc., phos., puls., seneg., sep., ***spong., stann.,*** sulph.
left - am-c., apis, arg-n., ars., ***bar-c.,*** bry., chin., eup-per., ip., kali-bi., lyc., merc., par., ***phos.,*** puls., rhus-t., ***rumx., seneg., sep., sulph., thuj.***
left, turning to right side amel. - ars., kali-c., ***phos., rumx., sep., sulph., thuj.***
painful, agg. - acon.
right - alum., am-m., ***carb-an., cina,*** ip., kali-c., lyc., **MERC.,** phos., plb., ***puls.,*** sil., ***spong.,*** **STANN.,** syph., tub.
right, night - ***carb-an.***

MANUAL, labor, from (see exertion) - led., nat-m.

MEASLES, during - coff., ***cop.,*** eup-per., spong., squil.
daytime - cupr.
daytime, eruption develops, which amel. - cupr.
after - ant-c., ***arn.,*** bry., ***calc.,*** camph., ***carb-v.,*** cham., chel., chin., coff., con., cop., cupr., **DROS.,** dulc., euphr., ***eup-per.,*** gels., hep., ***hyos.,*** ign., ***kali-c.,*** murx., ***nat-c.,*** nux-v., **PULS.,** stict., squil., ***sulph.***

MEAT, after - ***staph.***

MENSES, during - am-m., atro-s., bry., cact., ***calc-p.,*** cast., cham., coff., cop., cub., cur., ***graph.,*** iod., kali-n., lac-c., lachn., nat-m., phos., rhod., senec., ***sep.,*** sulph., thuj., ***zinc.***
coryza, with - cub., ***graph.***
evening, every - ***sulph.***
hysterical - hyos., plat.
morning - cop.
roughness in throat, from - cast.
menses, before - ***arg-n., graph.,*** hyos., lac-c., plat., ***sulph.,*** zinc.
beginning of, at - ***phos.***
daytime - graph., sulph., zinc.
evening - ***sulph.,*** zinc.
bed, in, sitting up amel. - ***sulph.***
hysterical - plat.
morning - graph., **ZINC.**
early - graph.
suppressed, from - mill., puls.

METALLIC - eupi., iod., ***kali-bi.,*** lac-c., rumx., sang., ***spong.***

METASTATIC, with the sound of croup - cupr.

MILK, agg. - ambr., ant-c., ant-t., brom., kali-c., spong., sul-ac., zinc.

MINUTE, guns, short, hacking cough, like - coc-c., cor-r.

MOIST, (see Loose)

MORNING - acon., ***agar.,*** agn., ail., all-c., all-s., **ALUM.,** alumn., ambr., am-c., am-m., anac., ang., ant-c., ant-t., apoc., arg-m., arn., **ARS.,** ***ars-i.,*** arum-d., aur., bad., bar-c., bar-m., bell., bor., bov., brom., bry., calad., **CALC.,** ***calc-p., calc-s.,*** canth., ***carb-an.,*** carb-s., carb-v., ***caust.,*** cham., ***chel.,*** **CHIN.,** ***chin-a.,*** chin-s., cina, coca, ***coc-c.,*** cod., colch., con., cop., cor-r., crot-t., cupr., cur., dig., dios., dirc., dros., dulc., erig., **EUPHR.,** ferr., ferr-ar., ferr-i., ferr-m., ferr-p., graph., grat., gymn., hep., hyper., ign., indg., ***iod.,*** ip., iris, **KALI-AR., KALI-BI., KALI-C.,** kali-i., kali-n., kali-p., ***kali-s.,*** kreos., lach., lachn., laur., ***led., lyc.,*** mag-c., ***mag-s.,*** mang., meny., ***meph.,*** merc., mill., **MOSCH.,** mur-ac., naja, nat-a., nat-c., ***nat-m.,*** nat-p., nat-s., nit-ac., nux-m., **NUX-V.,** ol-an., ol-j., op., osm., ox-ac., par., phel., ***ph-ac.,*** **PHOS.,** phyt., plb., ***psor.,*** **PULS.,** pyrus, rhod., rhus-t., **RUMX.,** sang., sars., sel., seneg., ***sep., sil.,*** spig., **SQUIL.,** stann., staph., stram., **SULPH.,** sul-ac., sumb., tab., tarent., tell., thuj., verat., vib., zinc., zing.
6 a.m. - ***alum., cedr., coc-c.,*** petr.
6 a.m. to 6 p.m. - calc-p.
6 to 7 a.m. - arum-t., calc-p., ***coc-c.,*** mez.
6 to 8 or 9 a.m. - ***cedr.***
7 a.m. - coc-c., dig.
7 to 10 a.m. - sil.
8 a.m. - dios., ham., ol-an.
8 to 9 a.m. - sil.
9 a.m. - sep., tarent.
until - sep.
amel. - agar., coc-c., grat.
bath, after - calc-s.
bed, in - am-c., aster., bry., ***caust.,*** coc-c., ferr., kali-n., **NUX-V.,** ***phos.,*** rhus-t.
daybreak amel. - syph.
dressing, while - seneg.
and - ***caust.***
rising, after - ail., all-s., alum., alumn., am-br., ang., ant-c., arg-m., arn., ***ars.,*** bar-c., bor., bov., bry., calc., canth., carb-an., carb-v., ***chel.,*** chin., chin-s., **CINA,** coc-c., dig., ***euphr.,*** **FERR.,** ferr-ar., ferr-p., grat., indg., lach., ***nat-m.,*** nat-s., nit-ac., nux-v., osm., par., **PHOS.,** plb., sep., ***sil., spong.,*** staph., sulph., thuj.
sleep, on going to - lyc.
waking, on - agar., ail., am-br., arn., aur., carb-v., ***caust., chel., coc-c.,*** cod., ferr., ***ign.,*** **KALI-BI.,** mag-s., **NUX-V.,** phos., plb., ***psor.,*** rhus-t., **RUMX., SIL.,** sulph., tarent., thuj.

MOTION, agg. - arn., ***ars.,*** ars-i., bar-c., bell., brom., **BRY.,** bufo, ***calc.,*** carb-o., ***carb-v., chin.,*** chin-a., cina, coc-c., cur., dros., eup-per., **FERR.,** ferr-ar., form., iod., ip., kali-ar., kali-bi., ***kali-c.,*** kali-n., kreos., lach., laur., led., lob., lyc., merc., mez., mosch., mur-ac., nat-m., nat-s., nit-ac., ***nux-v.,*** osm., ***phos.,*** plan., psor., pyrog., ***seneg.,*** sep., ***sil.,*** spong., ***stann.,*** squil., staph., sul-ac.,zinc.

1 p.m. - nat-s.
4 p.m. - calc-f., kali-bi.
arms, of - ars., calc., ***ferr.,*** kali-c., led., lyc., **NAT-M.,** nux-v.
chest, of - anac., bar-c., cocc., **CHIN.,** dros., ***lach.,*** mang., merc., mur-ac., nat-m., **NUX-V.,** ***phos.,*** sil., **STANN.**
rapid - ***nat-m.,*** puls.

motion, amel. - ambr., arg-n., ars., caps., coc-c., dros., dulc., euph., euphr., grat., hyos., ***kali-i.,*** mag-c., mag-m., nux-v., ph-ac., phos., psor., puls., rhus-r., ***rhus-t.,*** sabad., samb., sep., sil., stann., sulph., verb., zinc.

MOVE, on beginning to - nit-ac., plan., sil.

MUCUS, general, (see Lungs, Expectoration)

mucus, chest, in - **ANT-T.,** arg-m., ars., arum-t., asar., bar-c., ***calc.,*** caust., cham., cina, euphr., graph., guare., hydr., iod., ***ip.,*** **KALI-BI.,** kali-n., kreos., med., nat-m., plb., **PULS.,** sep., ***spong.,*** **STANN.,** sulph.
upper, in, agg. - plb.

mucus, larynx - aesc., am-br., am-c., am-caust., arg-m., arg-n., ***arum-t.,*** asaf., asar., atro., brom., caust., cham., chin-s., cina, cocc., coc-c., crot-t., ***cupr.,*** dig., dulc., euphr., grat., hyos., **KALI-BI.,** kreos., **LACH.,** laur., mang., ***nux-v.,*** osm., par., phel., plan., raph., seneg., ***stann.,*** stram., zinc.

mucus, trachea - arg-m., ***arum-t.,*** caust., cham., cina, crot-t., cupr., dulc., euphr., gels., hyos., ***nux-v.,*** rumx., seneg., ***spong.,*** squil., **STANN.**
ascending or descending, as from - coc-c.
sensation of, in, from - kali-c., **STANN.**

MUSIC, agg. - **AMBR.,** ***calc.,*** cham., kali-c., kreos., ph-ac.

NERVOUS - aur., **CAPS.,** cina, cocc., cor-r., crot-h., cupr., ***hep.,*** hydr-ac., ***hyos., ign.,*** kali-br., lach., nux-m., nux-v., phel., phos.
all night - ***hep.***
anyone enters the room, when - phos.
evening, sunset to sunrise, peculiar to women - aur.
lying, while - **HYOS.**

NIGHT - **ACON.,** aeth., ***agar.,*** alum., ***ambr.,*** **AM-BR., AM-C.,** ***am-m.,*** **ANAC.,** anan., ant-t., apis, apoc., aral., ***arg-n.,*** arn., **ARS.,** ***arum-d., asaf.,*** asar., ***aur.,*** aur-m., aur-s., bad., **BAR-C.,** bar-m., **BELL.,** bism., bor., bry., cact., calad., **CALC.,** calc-f., calc-s., ***caps., carb-an.,*** **CARB-S.,** carb-v., card-m., cast., ***caust.,*** cench., **CHAM.,** ***chel., chin., chin-a.,*** chin-s., cimic., cina, cocc., ***coc-c.,*** cod., coff., ***colch.,*** coloc., com., ***con.,*** cor-r., crot-t., ***cupr.,*** cur., ***cycl.,*** dig., ***dros.,*** dulc., erig., eug., eup-per., ferr., ferr-ar., ***ferr-p.,***

NIGHT - gamb., gels., **GRAPH.,** ***grat.,*** guai., ***hep.,*** **HYOS.,** ***ign.,*** indg., ***ip.,*** ir-foe., **KALI-AR.,** kali-bi., kali-br., **KALI-C.,** kali-n., kali-p., **KALI-S.,** kalm., ***kreos.,*** lac-ac., **LACH.,** lachn., led., lepi., **LYC.,** ***mag-arct.,*** mag-aust., ***mag-c., mag-m.,*** mag-p., mag-s., ***manc.,*** meph., **MERC.,** merc-c., ***mez.,*** mur-ac., naja, ***nat-a.,*** nat-c., ***nat-m.,*** nat-p., nat-s., ***nit-ac.,*** nux-v., oena., ol-an., ol-j., op., par., ***petr.,*** phel., phos., ***phyt.,*** psor., **PULS.,** rhod., ***rhus-t., rumx.,*** ruta., ***sabad.,*** samb., ***sang.,*** senec., seneg., **SEP., SIL.,** sol-t-ae., spig., spong., squil., stann., staph., stict., stront-c., **SULPH.,** sul-ac., ***syph.,*** tab., tarent., ther., thuj., ***verat., verb.,*** vib., vinc., ***zinc.,*** zing., ziz.

4 a.m., until - ***apis,*** nicc., sil.
only - ***ambr., caust.***
perspiration, with - chin., dig., eug., kali-bi., lyc., ***merc.,*** nat-c., nit-ac., psor., sulph.
rising, after - sulph.
two hours after sleep - ***aral.***
waking from the cough - am-m., ***bell., calc., caust.,*** cocc., coc-c., coff., hep., **HYOS., KALI-C.,** kali-n., lach., mag-m., nit-ac., phos., ***puls.,*** ruta., sang., **SEP.,** sil., squil., stront-c., **SULPH.,** zing.
1 a.m. - coc-c.
2 a.m. - cocc., ***dros., kali-s.,*** kali-n.
3 a.m. - ***kali-c.,*** kali-n.
4 a.m. - nit-ac.

midnight - am-c., ant-t., apis, arg-n., ars., bar-c., bell., bry., calc., caust., ***cham.,*** chin., cocc., coff., dig., dros., grat., hep., kali-c., kali-n., lyc., mag-m., manc., mez., mosch., naja, nit-ac., nux-v., phos., puls., rhus-t., ruta., samb., sep., ***sulph.,*** zing.

midnight, after - ***acon.,*** am-c., am-m., ant-t., ***ars.,*** ars-i., arum-d., bar-c., ***bell.,*** bry., calc., caust., cham., chin., chin-a., cocc., coc-c., coff., dig., **DROS.,** grat., hep., ***hyos.,*** iod., ***kali-ar.,*** kali-c., lyc., mag-c., mag-m., mang., merc., mez., nit-ac., ***nux-v.,*** phos., ph-ac., ***rhus-t.,*** rumx., samb., sep., spong., squil.

1 a.m. - coc-c., sulph.
1 to 2 a.m. - rumx., zing.
1 to 4 a.m. - bufo.
2 a.m. - am-c., am-m., ***ars.,*** caust., chin., chin-s., cocc., ***dros.,*** glon., **KALI-AR.,** ***kali-c.,*** kali-n., nat-m., op., petr., phos., rumx., sulph.
2 a.m., until - sulph.
2 and 2:30 a.m. - kali-p.
2 or 3 a.m - ant-t., ars., ***kali-c.,*** merc.
2 to 3 a.m. - am-c., ***kali-bi.***
2 to 3:30 a.m. - coc-c.
2 to 4 a.m. - eup-per.
2 to 5 a.m. - rumx.
3 a.m. - ***am-c., ars.,*** bapt., bufo, cahin., chin., cupr., **KALI-AR., KALI-C.,** kali-n., mag-c., mur-ac., nux-v., op., rhus-t., sulph., thuj.
3 a.m. - ant-t.
3 a.m., until - acon.
3 to 4 a.m. - ***am-c., bufo,*** cahin., ***kali-c.,*** lyc., op., rhus-t.

NIGHT,
midnight, after
4 a.m. - ***anac.,*** ant-t., asc-t., chin., kali-c., lyc., nat-s., nit-ac., nux-v., petr., phos.
4 a.m., until - nicc.
5 a.m. - ant-c., arum-t., ***kali-c.,*** rumx.
5 to 6 a.m. - kali-i.
5 to 12 a.m. - kali-c.
5:30 a.m. - ars.
amel. - brom., rhus-t.
daybreak, until - **NUX-V.**
morning, until - nux-v., sep., stict.
midnight, before - alum., ant-t., apis, aral., ***arg-n.,*** arn., ars., bar-c., bar-m., bell., brom., calc., carb-s., **CARB-V.,** caust., ferr., ferr-ar., graph., hep., kali-c., lach., led., ***lyc.,*** mag-c., mag-m., mez., mosch., mur-ac., nat-m., ***nit-ac.,*** nux-v., osm., ***phos.,*** puls., rhus-t., rumx., sabad., sep., spong., squil., **STANN.,** staph., sulph., sul-ac., verat., zinc.
10 p.m. - ***bell.,*** dios., nat-m.
10 p.m., to 1 p.m. - ***ant-t.,*** calad., cupr., hep., lach.
10:30 p.m. - carb-s., sol-t-ae.
11 p.m. - ***ant-t.,*** aral., ***bell.,*** hep., lach., rhus-t., ***rumx.,*** verat.
11 p.m., to 1 a.m. - cupr.
11 p.m., to 3 a.m. - squil.
11 p.m., to 12 p.m. - hep.
11:30 p.m. - **COC-C.**

NOISE, agg. - arn., ph-ac.

NOON - agar., arg-n., arund., bell., euphr., naja, sil., staph., sulph.
lying down, amel. - **MANG.**
sleep, in - euphr.

ODORS, strong - ***phos.,*** sul-ac.

OPPRESSION, epigastrium - kali-bi.
chest - lyc., ***phos.***
left, chest and hypochondrium - thuj.

OPPRESSIVE - ail., phel.

OVERPOWERING, as if larynx were tickled by a feather in evening before sleep - **LYC.**

PAIN, larynx, in, from - acon., ang., arg-m., bry., calad., caust., chin-s., euphr., ferr., grat., hep., iod., kali-c., sars., ***spong., stann.***
pain, trachea, in, from - acon., ang., arg-m., bry., calad., euph., grat., hep., indg., ip., sars., ***spong.,*** stann.

PAINFUL - acon., ***agar., ail.,*** **ALL-C.,** ant-ox., ant-t., apis, arn., brom., **BRY.,** calad., ***caps.,*** caust., chin., coc-c., cop., cor-r., ferr-p., ill., kreos., lact., ***merc.,*** merc-c., nat-c., nat-s., rhus-t., tarent., ust.
evening, in bed - bry.
midnight, waking before - ***rhus-t.***
night - caust., ***rhus-t.***

PANTING - calad., ***carb-v., dulc.,*** mur-ac., phos., rhus-t., sul-ac.
audible rumbling in chest from above downward - mur-ac.
preventing sleep - calad.

PAROXYSMAL - acon., aeth., ***agar.,*** alum., ***ambr., anan.,*** ang., ***ant-c.,*** anth., ***arg-n., arn., ars.,*** arum-t., ***bad.,*** **BELL.,** brom., bry., calad., ***calc.,*** calc-f., cann-s., ***caps., carb-h., carb-s.,*** **CARB-V.,** ***caust., cham., chel., chin.,*** cimx., **CINA,** coca, cocc., **COC-C.,** coff., ***con., cor-r.,*** croc., ***crot-c.,*** **CUPR.,** cycl., dig., **DROS.,** elaps, ***euphr.,*** ferr., ferr-m., ferr-p., gins., **HEP.,** hydr-ac., **HYOS.,** ign., indg., iod., **IP.,** jatr., kali-bi., ***kali-br., kali-c., kali-chl.,*** kali-n., ***kali-p.,*** kali-s., ***kreos., lach.,*** lact., laur., lob., lyc., ***mag-c., mag-m.,*** mag-p., mang., **MEPH.,** merc., merc-c., merc-i-r., morph., naja, nat-m., nicc., nit-ac., **NUX-V.,** op., ph-ac., phos., phyt., plb., ***psor.,*** **PULS., RUMX.,** sabad., sang., sarr., ***seneg.,*** **SEP.,** sil., ***spong.,*** squil., **STANN.,** staph., ***sulph., sul-ac.,*** **TARENT.,** thuj., **VERAT.,** zinc.
afternoon - agar., all-c., bad., ***bell.,*** bry., caps., ***chel.,*** coca, cupr., mosch., mur-ac., ol-an., phel.
1:30 p.m. - phel.
2 p.m. - ol-an.
4 p.m. - ***chel.,*** coca
5 p.m. - cupr.
5-9 p.m. - caps.
attacks, first the strongest, following ones weaker and weaker - ***ant-c.***
follow one another quickly - ***agar.,*** ant-t., cina, coff., ***cor-r.,*** **DROS.,** hep., ***ip.,*** merc., sep., sulph.
bread, or cake, from eating - kali-n.
breath, gasping for, commences with - ant-t., cor-r.
chill, after - phos.
consisting of, few coughs - bell., calc., laur.
long coughs - ambr., carb-v., **CUPR.,** ip., lob.
short coughs - alum., ant-t., asaf., bell., calc., carb-v., cocc., ***coc-c., cor-r., dros.,*** kali-bi., ***kali-c.,*** lact., squil.
three coughs - ***carb-v., cupr.,*** phos., stann.
two coughs - agar., cocc., grat., laur., merc., phos., plb., puls., sulph., sul-ac., thuj.
two in quick succession - merc-sul.
convulses, whole body in sudden paroxysms - caps.
crawling, in larynx, from - ***psor.***
daytime - ***agar., euphr., hep.,*** nit-ac., staph.
amel. - bell., ign., lyc., spong.
dinner, after - aeth., calc-f., phos.
evening - all-c., anan., bad., bar-c., ***bell.,*** bry., calc., ***carb-v.,*** chel., chlor., coca, ***coc-c.,*** grat., ***hep.,*** ign., indg., ip., lach., laur., led., mag-c., merc., mez., nat-a., nat-m., nit-ac., ***nux-v.,*** ol-an., ***phos.,*** ph-ac., puls., rhus-t., ***sep.,*** sil., stann., still., stram., tarent., verat-v.
6 :15 p.m. - ol-an.
7 p.m. - grat.
bed, in - cocc., nat-m.
cool wind, in - coca
lying down, after - ***nux-v.***

PAROXYSMAL,
evening, till midnight - bar-c., carb-v., ferr., ***hep.,*** led., mag-c., mez., nit-ac., ***puls.,*** rhus-t., sep., stann., zinc.
forenoon - ***agar.,*** cact., coc-c., grat., sabad., ***sep.***
lachrymation, is profuse with every attack - arn.
midnight - ***cham.,*** dig., mosch., naja, phos., ***sulph.***
after - bell., ***cocc.,*** dig., **DROS.,** hyos., kali-c., squil.
after, 2 a.m. - **DROS.**
after, 2 and 3:30 a.m. - coc-c.
before - ant-t., apis, aral., bell., ***hep.,*** lach., mosch., mur-ac., rhus-t., **RUMX.,** ***spong.,*** squil., sulph.
before, 11 p.m. - ant-t., bell., lach., **RUMX.,** spong., squil.
before, 11:30 p.m. - **COC-C.**
before, lying down, after - **RUMX.**
before, on falling asleep on either side - ***spong.***
before, sleep, after - aral., ***lach.***
before, swallowing mucus, amel. - apis
morning - ***agar., ant-c.,*** carb-v., coc-c., dig., ferr., ferr-m., ferr-p., ign., iod., ip., kali-c., kreos., nat-a., nat-m., nat-p., ***nux-v.,*** ol-j., ph-ac., puls., sang., squil., stram., sulph., sul-ac., thuj.
bed, in - coc-c., ferr., **NUX-V.**
eating amel. - ferr.
rising, after - ***ant-c.,*** ferr-p.
waking, after - ***agar., ambr.,*** **RUMX.,** thuj.
mucus, followed by copious - ***agar.,*** alumn., ***anan., arg-n.,*** **COC-C.,** kali-bi., seneg., stann., sulph.
night - ***agar.,*** anac., anan., ant-t., apis, aral., arg-n., aur., aur-m., aur-s., **BELL.,** bry., calc., calc-f., **CARB-V.,** ***chel.,*** chin., ***coc-c., con.,*** cor-r., ***dros.,*** ferr., ***hep.,*** **HYOS.,** ign., ***ip.,*** kali-br., kali-c., ***lach.,*** lyc., ***mag-c.,*** mag-m., ***meph., merc.,*** merc-c., naja, ***op., phos., puls.,*** **RUMX.,** sang., sil., ***spong.,*** squil., sulph., tarent., thuj., vinc.
bed, becoming warm, in - ***coc-c.,*** naja
bed, before going to - ***coc-c.***
every other, on falling asleep - merc.
noon, until midnight - mosch.
rinsing, mouth with cold water, amel. - coc-c.
sitting, up amel. - cinnb., phos.
smoking, while - all-s.
sneezing, with - **AGAR.,** carb-v., lyc.
spells, of hard coughing, not ceasing until masses of offensive sputa are raised - carb-v.
stomach, laying hand on pit of, amel. - ***croc.***
suffocation, suddenly on swallowing - **BROM.**
sun, walking in hot - coca.
temperature, change of - ***spong.***
uninterrupted, paroxysms - **CUPR.**
walking, in cool wind - coca.

PEPPER, from - alum., cina.

PERIODIC - anac., ars., aur., cocc., coc-c., colch., lach., lact., lyc., merc., ***nux-v.,*** sep., stram.
day, every other - anac., lyc., nux-v., sep.
daytime - anac.
evening sunset to sunrise - aur.
hour, every three hours - anac., dros.
same, every day - lyc., sabad.

PERIODIC,
morning - stram.
night - acon., cocc., merc.
every fourth - cocc.
every other - merc.
midnight - cocc.
midnight, after - acon., cocc.
midnight, after, 2 a.m. - cocc.
midnight, after, every half hour - acon.
speaking or smoking, from - atro.

PERSISTENT - acon., am-caust., **BELL.,** cact., crot-t., cub., **CUPR.,** dios., ***hyos.,*** ip., jatr., kali-n., lyc., mag-p., merc., mez., ***nux-v.,*** rumx., sang., squil.
midnight, lying on back agg., lying on side, amel. - ***nux-v.***

PERSONS, approaching or passing, agg. (see strangers) - carb-v.
many are present, where, agg. - ***ambr.***
other, coming into room, agg. - phos.

PIANO, when playing - ambr., **CALC.,** cham., kali-c., kreos., ph-ac.
when playing, every note she struck seemed to vibrate in her larynx - ***calc.***

PLEURISY, in - acon., ***ars.,*** **BRY.,** ip., ***lyc., sulph.***

PLUG, sensation of a, moving up and down in trachea, from - ***calc.***

POTATOES, agg. - alum.

PREGNANCY, during - calc., ***caust., con.,*** ip., kali-br., nat-m., ***nux-m.,*** phos., puls., sabin., sep., vib.
night, during - ***con.***

PRESSING, pain in larynx, from - agar.
pressing and straining, in child - agar.

PRESSURE, chest, in - iod., op., phos.
goitre, on the, from - psor.
larynx on, from - apis, ***bell., chin.,*** cina, crot-h., ferr., **LACH.,** rumx., tarax.
sensation between pressure and roughness, which gradually becomes a tickling, from - tell.
stomach, in - calad.
throat-pit, on - rumx.
trachea, from - bell., hydr., ***lach.,*** rumx.

PRICKLING, in trachea, from - hydr-ac.

PURRING - nat-c.

PUTTING, out the tongue, from - lyc.

RACKING - **AGAR.,** alumn., am-m., anac., anan., ang., ant-c., ***arn.,*** arg-n., ars., arum-t., aur., **BELL.,** brom., **BRY.,** calc., calc-ar., calc-s., cann-i., ***caps., carb-an.,*** **CARB-V., CAUST.,** cench., ***chel.,*** chin., chin-s., cocc., **COC-C.,** coll.,

RACKING - ***con.,*** cop., croc., cupr., cur., daph., ***dulc.,*** graph., gymn., ***hyos.,*** **IGN.,** ***ip.,*** ir-foe., kali-bi., **KALI-C.,** ***kali-p.,*** kali-s., kreos., lac-c., ***lach., lact.,*** led., ***lyc.,*** mag-m., mag-s., **MERC.,** merc-c., ***mez.,*** mur-ac., nat-a., nat-c., nat-m., nat-p., nicc., nit-ac., **NUX-V.,** olnd., op., osm., **PHOS., PULS.,** rhod., ***rhus-t.,*** rob., sarr., ***sec.,*** sel., ***seneg., sep., sil.,*** spig., ***spong.,*** squil., **STANN.,** staph., stict., **SULPH.,** sul-ac., sumb., syph., ***verat.,*** zinc.
afternoon, 3 p.m. - cench.
deep inspiration, on - con.
drinking water amel. - ***op.***
evening - anan., cench., ***ip.,*** ir-foe., led., lyc., nat-m., nit-ac., petr., ***puls.,*** rhus-t., stict.
10 p.m. - nat-m.
till midnight - led., nit-ac., ***puls.,*** rhus-t.
morning - caust., ***chel.***
waking, on - caust.
night - agar., anan., aur., **BELL.,** chin-s., ***hyos.,*** ir-foe., merc., nat-c., nit-ac., stict.
midnight, after - hyos.
sitting up amel. - arg-n., **HYOS., PULS.**

RAISED, child must be, gets blue in face, cannot exhale - meph., samb.
arms, agg. - ***bry., ferr.,*** lyc., ol-j.

RAPID, until patient falls back as limber as a rag - ***cor-r.***

RASPING - calc., **SPONG.,** stram.

RATTLING - alum., ***ammc.,*** ang., **ANT-T.,** aral., ***arg-m., arg-n.,*** arum-d., arund., ***bar-c.,*** bar-m., ***bell.,*** brom., ***bry., cact.,*** cahin., ***calc., calc-s., carb-an., carb-v.,*** **CAUST.,** ***cham., chel.,*** chen-a., ***cina, coc-c.,*** con., cupr., eug., ferr., ferr-p., gamb., ***hep., hippoz., hydr.,*** hydr-ac., ***iod.,*** **IP.,** ***kali-bi., kali-chl.,*** kali-p., **KALI-S.,** ***lach., lyc.,*** med., meph., merc., merc-c., merc-i-f., merc-i-r., mur-ac., nat-c., ***nat-m., nat-s., nux-v.,*** oena., ***op.,*** phos., podo., ***puls.,*** rumx., samb., ***sang., sanic.,*** sars., **SEP.,** ***sil., squil., stann., sulph.,*** sul-ac., verat., verat-v.
daytime - ***arg-m.,*** ferr.
eating, while - ***phos.***
after - hep.
elderly, people - ***ammc.,*** **ANT-T.,** ***hippoz., kali-bi., seneg.***
evening - caust., sil.
hoarseness, with - ***kali-chl.***
without - **KALI-S.**
morning - aral., hep., meph., stram.
night - anac., gamb.
open air amel. - arg-m., ***kali-s.***
spells in - cina.
wheezing or whistling with while lying on back, or on either side - med.

RAWNESS, in larynx excites - acon., ***alum.,*** ambr., bar-c., brom., ***bry.,*** cast., ***coc-c.,*** dulc., ***hep.,*** kali-i., laur., **NUX-V.,** ol-an., **PHOS., RUMX.,** sang., ***sil.,*** **SULPH.**
sternum, behind, excites - kali-n.

RE-echo, seems to, in stomach - cupr., ***spong.***

READING, aloud agg. - ***ambr.,*** cina, ***dros., mang.,*** meph., nit-ac., ***nux-v.,*** par., **PHOS.,** ***stann., tub.,*** verb.
aloud agg., evening - ***phos.***

REMITTENT, fever, during - podo.

RESONANT - kali-bi., ***spong.***

RIDING - staph., sulph., sul-ac.

RINGING, clear - acon., all-c., apis, ***ars.,*** asaf., dol., **DROS.,** ***kali-bi.,*** lac-c., spong., stram.

RINSING, mouth agg. - ***coc-c.***

RISING, on - acon., alum., alumn., ang., arg-n., arn., ars., bar-c., benz-ac., bov., bry., calc-s., canth., carb-an., carb-v., chel., chin-s., cina, cocc., con., dig., euph., euphr., ***ferr.,*** ferr-ar., ferr-p., grat., ign., indg., ***lach.,*** mag-c., nat-s., nit-ac., osm., ox-ac., par., phos., plb., sep., staph., stram., sulph., sul-ac., tarent., thuj., verat.
amel. - mag-c., mag-s., rhus-t.
bed, from - acon., ars., bar-c., bry., calc-s., canth., carb-an., carb-v., chel., cocc., con., ***euphr.,*** ferr-p., ign., **LACH.,** mag-s., nat-s., phos., plb., sep., sul-ac., tarent., thuj., verat.
before - ail., **NUX-V.**
stooping, from - phos.

ROOM, in - arg-m., brom., bry., croc., kali-n., laur., mag-c., mag-m., nat-c., nat-m., puls., spig., spong.

ROUGH - acon., bell., brom., cann-i., carb-an., carb-v., card-b., cop., dulc., ***eup-per.,*** eupi., ***hep.,*** iod., ip., mag-m., meli., ***merc.,*** mur-ac., nat-c., nat-m., ***rhus-v.,*** sep., sil., tarent., ust.
midnight - ***nit-ac.***
night - ***cham.,*** lyc., nat-c., ***nit-ac.***

ROUGHNESS, causes in larynx - ***alum.,*** ang., aur-m., bar-c., ***bry.,*** carb-an., carb-s., ***carb-v.,*** cast., ***caust.,*** coloc., con., dig., graph., ***kali-c.,*** kali-i., kalm., kreos., ***lach.,*** laur., mang., nat-s., **NUX-V.,** ol-an., plb., ***puls.,*** rhod., ***rhus-t.,*** sabad., sars., ***seneg., spong., sulph.,*** stront-c., verat-v.
palate, in, from - calc.
throat, in - phos.
trachea, causes in, from - bar-c., carb-an., dig., kreos., laur., sabad.

RUNNING, agg. - cina, iod., merc., seneg., sil., stann., sul-ac.

SALIVA, running in larynx - agar., spig.

SALT, and pepper in larynx, as if from - crot-h.
salt, food - alum., con., lach.

SCARLATINA, following - ant-c., con., hyos.

SCIATICA, alternating with, in summer - staph.

SCRAPING, from - ***alumn.,*** bell., calc., ***caust.,*** cham., cimx., coff., dros., eup-per., ***euphr.,*** eupi., grat., ***hep.,*** kali-c., kreos., lyc., merc., nat-c., nicc., nit-ac., ***nux-v.,*** plan., puls., rhod., sabad., samb., ***sel.,*** sep., sil., spong., **STANN.,** zing.
evening - bry., rhod., stann.
lying down, after - bry.
night - calc., cham., nat-m., rhod.
waking, on - calc.

scraping, chest, in - arg-m., bry., con., kali-bi., kreos., ***puls.***, ruta., staph., ***thuj.***
upper, in - ruta.
scraping, fauces - **DROS.**
scraping, larynx, from - aesc., ang., aloe, alum., ***alumn.***, ambr., ***am-c.***, arg-n., aur-m-n., bar-c., ***bell.***, bor., bov., **BROM.,** ***bry.***, cahin., camph., ***carb-s.***, **CARB-V.,** card-m., ***caust.***, chel., chin-s., ***coc-c.***, colch., ***con.***, croc., cycl.,
scraping, larynx, from - dig., **DROS.,** graph., **HEP.,** hydr-ac., kali-bi., kalm., kreos., laur., led., mag-c., mag-m., mang., naja, nit-ac., **NUX-V.,** ol-an., op., osm., paeon., petr., ph-ac., phyt., plat., prun., **PULS.,** ***sabad.***, **SEL.,** ***seneg.***, sil., sin-n., syph., ter., thuj., til., upa.
scraping, pharynx, in - arg-n., cycl., graph., hep., kali-bi.
scraping, trachea, in, from - bry., cycl., ***puls.***, sabad., thuj.

SCRATCHING - kali-c., rumx., zing.
larynx, in - ***acon.***, alum., alumn., ***am-c.***, ang., arg-n., arn., bart., dig., kreos., mag-m., nux-m., petr., ***phos.***, psor., puls., sabad., sul-ac., sil., staph., zing.
throat, in - ambr., carb-v., mag-m., phos., rumx.
trachea, in, from - acon., agar., cimx., dig., kreos., puls.

SCREECHING, shrill, in painless paroxysmal - stram.

SEA, wind, from - cupr., mag-m.

SERIES, in - ***coc-c.***, phos., sumb.
morning,10 to 11 a.m. - sumb.

SHARP - arn., calc-s., staph.
eating, after - staph.

SHOCKS, at heart, from - phos.

SHORT, coughs - **ACON.,** ***aesc.***, aeth., agar., ***alum.***, am-c., anac., ang., ant-c., ant-t., ***apoc.***, arg-m., arg-n., arn., ***ars.***, asar., aur., aur-m., ***bell.***, berb., brom., ***bry.***, cadm-s., ***calc.***, calc-s., camph., canth., carb-ac., carb-o., carb-s., carb-v., card-m., casc., ***caust.***, ***chel.***, ***chin.***, chin-a., chin-s., cimic., cina, cinnb., cob., cocc., **COC-C.,** ***cod.***, **COFF.,** colch., coloc., con., cop., croc., cupr., cur., dig., dros., dulc., eup-per., euph., eupi., ***ferr-i.***, ferr-p., fl-ac., ***graph.***, hep., hydr-ac., hyos., hyper., **IGN.,** iod., ip., iris, jatr., kali-ar., kali-bi., kali-c., kali-chl., kali-i., kali-ma., kali-n., ***kali-p.***, kreos., lac-d., ***lach.***, lachn., lact., laur., led., lob., ***lyc.***, mag-c., ***merc.***, ***mez.***, mur-ac., naja, nat-a., nat-c., ***nat-m.***, nat-p., ***nit-ac.***, ***nux-v.***, oena., olnd., osm., paull., ***petr.***, ***phos.***, pin-s., ***plat.***, ***plb.***, podo., puls., **RHUS-T., RUMX.,** sabad., seneg., **SEP.,** sin-n., spig., ***spong.***, ***squil.***, **STANN.,** stict., ***still.***, stront-c., sulph., ***sul-ac.***, tab., ***tell.***, tep., teucr., ***thuj.***, verat-v., viol-o., zinc., zing., ziz.
afternoon - anac., chin-s., laur., nat-m.
2 p.m. - laur.
5 p.m. - nat-m.
air, open, agg. - ang., seneg., spig.
breathing, deep - ***aesc.***

SHORT, coughs
daytime - arg-m., kali-bi., nat-c., phos.
daytime, and night - mez.
deep alternating with - apoc.
dinner, after - agar.
eating, after - anac., caust., ter.
evening - alum., bar-c., ***bell.***, carb-v., chel., cimic., **IGN.,** kali-bi., lyc., phos., ***sep.***, sulph., thuj.
bed, in - lyc., ***sep.***
sleeping sitting, while - sulph.
smoking agg. - thuj.
undressing, on - chel.
forenoon - agar., alum., coc-c., rhus-t.
forenoon, 11 a.m. - rhus-t.
frequent - fl-ac.
inspiration agg. - nat-a.
irritation, in larynx, from - am-c., seneg., spong.
lying, after eating - caust., ter.
morning - agar., am-br., arn., ars., croc., kali-bi., lyc., nit-ac., thuj.
rising, after - am-br., arn.
tea drinking, after - ars.
waking, on - dig.
moving when - carb-o.
night - arg-n., bell., ***calc.***, mez., rhus-t.
bed, in - arg-n., ***calc.***
midnight, before - ***rhus-t.***
wakens - ***rhus-t.***
wakens, 11 p.m. - rhus-t.
wakens, after - acon., ***ars.***
siesta, after - rhus-t.
sitting up amel. - ***arg-n.***, cinnb., nat-c.
smoking, when - coca, thuj.
swallowing, from - ***aesc.***
talking, while - ant-t.
tickling in larynx, from - ***acon.***, agar., ***ang.***, carb-an., croc., cimic., graph., iris, kali-bi., laur., led., mez., ***spong.***
walking fast - seneg.
open air, in - ang., sulph.

SHRILL - ant-t., sol-t-ae., stram.
waking, on - sol-t-ae.

SIBILANT - kreos., prun., ***spong.***
dry, like a saw driven through a pineboard - ***spong.***

SINGING, agg. - alum., ***arg-m.***, ***arg-n.***, ***dros.***, hyos., kali-bi., mang., meph., ***phos.***, rhus-t., rumx., sil., spong., ***stann.***, stram.
raising the voice, from - ***arg-n.***

SIT up, must - ***agar.***, ***ant-t.***, aral., ***ars.***, ***bry.***, caust., chin-s., ***coc-c.***, colch., **CON.,** crot-t., eupi., ***ferr.***, ferr-ar., gamb., hep., ***iod.***, ***kali-bi.***, kali-c., kreos., lach., mag-m., mag-s., nat-s., nicc., **PHOS., PULS.,** plan., ***sang.***, ***seneg.***, ***sep.***, staph.
as soon as cough commences - ars., ***bry.***, caust., ***coc-c.***, colch., **CON.,** hep., lach., plan.
cough it out, when had rest - **CON.**

SITTING, while - agar., aloe, alum., astac., euphr., ferr., guai., hell., kali-c., mag-c., mag-m., mur-ac., nat-c., nat-p., phos., ph-ac., puls., ***rhus-t.,*** sabad., ***seneg.,*** sep., spig., stann., zinc.
bent, agg. - rhus-t., spig., stann.
amel. - iod.
erect - kali-c., nat-m., spong.
amel. - ant-t.
long agg. - coc-c., ph-ac.
still, while - coca, rhus-t.
afternoon - coca

SITTING, while
amel. - verat.
up, when agg. - con.

SLEEP, during - ***acon., agar.,*** alum., ***apis, arn.,*** ars., arum-t., ***bell.,*** calc., carb-an., **CHAM.,** coff., ***cycl.,*** hipp., hyos., ip., kreos., **LACH.,** lyc., lycps., mag-s., merc., murx., nit-ac., ***petr.,*** phos., rhod., ***rhus-t.,*** samb., sang., sep., sil., stram., ***sulph.,*** tub., verb.
after - ***apis, aral., caust., kali-bi.,*** **LACH.,** lachn., nit-ac., puls., ***sep.,*** sulph.
before - ***coc-c.,*** lyc., merc., **SULPH.**
disturbing - ***agar.,*** alum., bism., calad., mez., nux-v., ol-j., phos., rhod., rhus-t., sang., sep., spong., squil., stict., **SULPH.,** syph., zinc.
falls asleep during dry cough - mag-s.
going to, on - ***agar.,*** agn., arn., brom., ***carb-v., con.,*** guare., ***hep.,*** ign., ***kali-c.,*** **LACH., LYC.,** med., merc., nit-ac., ***phos.,*** sep., **SULPH.**
lying on side, when - ***arg-n.,*** kali-c., ***lyc., psor., spong.***
one hour after - aral., arn., calc.
preventing - am-m., anac., apis, calad., carb-v., caust., daph., kali-bi., ***kali-c.,*** kali-cy., laur., **LYC.,** phos., **PULS.,** ***rhus-t.,*** sang., **SEP.,** stict., sulph., zinc.
starting in, on - apis, cina, hep.
wakens from - acon., ***agar.,*** alum., ***apis, aral.,*** arn., ***ars.,*** bell., calc., carb-s., **CAUST.,** cham., cocc., ***coc-c.,*** coff., con., daph., dros., graph., hep., hipp., ***hyos., kali-c.,*** kali-n., ***lach.,*** mag-m., med., merc., nit-ac., op., ***petr.,*** **PHOS.,** rhod., ***rhus-t., sang., sep., sil.,*** sol-t-ae., squil., **SULPH.,** stront-c., verb., zinc., zing.

SMARTING, (see burning)

SMOKE, of all kinds agg. - euphr., ment.
sensation of, in trachea, from - ***ars.,*** bry., nat-a.

SMOKING, agg. - ***acon.,*** agar., all-s., arg-n., atro., brom., bry., ***calad.,*** carb-an., cham., clem., coca, cocc., coc-c., ***coloc., dros., euphr.,*** ferr., hell., hep., **IGN.,** iod., lac-ac., mag-c., ment., nux-v., osm., petr., puls., spig., spong., staph., sul-ac., tarent., thuj.
dinner, after, on - acon., bry., coc-c., dros., ***lact.,*** petr.
evening - arg-n., coloc., thuj.
night amel. - tarent.

SMOTHERED - meli.

SMOTHERING, in throat, from - lach.

SNEEZING, with - all-c., alum., anac., ant-t., aspar., bad., ***bell., bry.,*** carb-an., carb-v., chin., ***cina, con.,*** eup-per., hep., iod., just., kali-c., kreos., lob., merc., ***nat-m.,*** nit-ac., nux-v., osm., sal-ac., sep., sil., squil., staph., ***sulph.***
amel. - osm.
ends in - **AGAR.,** ***arg-n.,*** bad., ***bell.,*** bry., caps., ***carb-v.,*** hep., lyc., psor., seneg., ***squil., sulph.***
from - seneg.

SNORING, with - ant-t., arg-m., bell., caust., ip., nat-c., nat-m., nux-v., puls., sep.

SNOWFALL, exposure to, in children, from - sep.

SOLID, food, from - cupr.

SOMETHING, sitting fast in trachea, from - staph.

SONOROUS - ***spong.,*** **STRAM.**

SOUR, food - ant-c., brom., con., lach., nat-m., nux-v., ***sep.,*** sulph.

SPASMODIC (see Paroxysmal) - acon., **AGAR.,** ***all-c.,*** **AMBR.,** am-br., am-caust., anac., ***anan.,*** apis, ***arg-n., ars.,*** ars-i., arum-t., asc-t., aur., ***bad.,*** bar-c., **BELL.,** brom., bov., **BRY.,** ***cact., calc.,*** calc-f., calc-s., ***caps., carb-an.,*** carb-s., **CARB-V.,** cast., ***caust., chel.,*** **CHIN.,** chin-a., ***chlol., chlor.,*** chlf., cimic., **CINA,** ***coc-c.,*** **COCC.,** coff., coll., coloc., ***con.,*** com., **COR-R.,** ***crot-c.,*** **CUPR.,** cur., ***dig.,*** **DROS.,** ***dulc.,*** euph., ***ferr.,*** ferr-ar., ferr-i., ferr-m., ferr-p., ***gels., hep.,*** hydr-ac., **HYOS.,** ***ign.,*** indg., ***iod.,*** **IP.,** kali-ar., kali-bi., **KALI-BR.,** ***kali-c., kali-chl.,*** kali-p., ***kreos.,*** **LAC-AC.,** lach., ***lact.,*** laur., ***led., lob.,*** lyc., ***mag-c., mag-m.,*** **MAG-P.,** meli., ***meph., merc.,*** merc-c., mez., mosch., nat-a., ***nat-m.,*** nit-ac., **NUX-V.,** oena., op., osm., petr., ph-ac., ***phos., plb., psor.,*** **PULS.,** ***rhus-t.,*** **RUMX.,** sal-ac., ***samb., sang.,*** **SEP.,** sil., **SPONG.,** ***squil.,*** staph., still., stram., stry., ***sulph.,*** sul-ac., tab., ***tarent., thuj., verat.,*** verat-v., verb., vinc., ***zinc.***
afternoon - agar., all-c., bad., **BELL.,** bry., mur-ac., zinc.
autumn - caps.
change of temperature - ***spong.***
cold drink amel. - ***ip.***
daytime only - ***agar.,*** staph.
amel - bell., euph., ign., lyc., spong.
deep inspiration amel. - verb.
drinking, after - ***bry., ferr.***
eating, after - carb-v., cocc., **FERR.,** hyos.
amel. - ***ferr-m.***
elderly, people - ***ambr., ip.***
evening - all-c., bad., bar-c., bell., bry., calc., carb-o., ***carb-v., coc-c., ferr.,*** ign., ***ip.,*** lach., laur., led., mag-c., merc., mez., nat-a., nat-m., nit-ac., ***phos.,*** ph-ac., ***puls.,*** rhus-t., **SEP.,** sil., stann., **STILL.,** stram., tarent., verat-v.
evening, after - mag-c., mag-m.

SPASMODIC, cough
evening, midnight, until - bar-c., carb-v., ferr., led., mag-c., mez., nit-ac., ***puls.,*** rhus-t., ***sep.,*** stann., zinc.
forenoon - ***agar.,*** lact., sabad., sep.
lying agg. - **COC-C.,** ***con., hyos.,*** meph., puls., ***sang.***
midnight - dig., mosch., ***sulph.***
after - bell., dig., ***hyos., kali-c.,*** squil.
afternoon, until - mosch., ***sulph.***
before - mur-ac., rhus-t., sabad., ***spong.***
before, 10:30 p.m. - carb-s., **COC-C.**
sunset to sunrise - aur.
morning - ***agar.,*** carb-v., dig., ferr., ferr-m., ferr-p., ign., iod., ip., kali-c., kreos., nat-a., nat-m., ph-ac., puls., squil., stram., sulph., thuj.
bed - ferr.
eating amel. - ferr., ferr-m.
rising, after - ferr-p.
waking - ***agar.,*** thuj.
night - ***agar.,*** anac., apis, arg-n., aur., bad., **BELL.,** ***bry.,*** calc., calc-f., cina, ***coc-c.,*** coll., con., cor-r., **DROS.,** euph., ***ferr., hep.,*** hyos., ***ip.,*** ign., kali-c., lyc., ***mag-c., mag-m.,*** meph., merc., ***op.,*** petr., ***phos., puls., sang.,*** sil., spong., sulph., tarent., thuj., vinc.
waking, on - thuj.
noon, until midnight - mosch.
smoking, agg. - lac-c.
amel. - tarent.
summer heat amel. - ars.
swallowing liquids agg. - sul-ac.
talking, after - dig.
vomiting, with - bry., carb-v., ferr., ip., puls.
waking, on - ***thuj.***
whooping cough, after - **SANG.**
winter - ars., psor.
women, peculiar to - aur., ***cocc., hyos., ign.***

SPICEY, food from, highly, seasoned - nux-v., sulph.

SPIRITS, (see Alcohol)

SPLENIC, troubles, from - card-m.

SPLITTING - aur.
night - aur.

SPOKEN, to, on being - ars.

SPOT, in larynx, as if from dry - cimic., **CON.,** crot-h.
chest, in, right, as if from - carb-an.

SPRING, in the - ambr., ***cina, gels.,*** kreos., lac-ac., verat.
autumn, and - cina, kreos., lac-ac.

SPRINGS, up, child, and clings to those around, calls for help in a hoarse voice, or bends backward and grasps at larynx - ***ant-t.***

STANDING, agg. - acon., aloe, euphr., ign., mag-s., nat-m., nat-s., sep., stann., sulph., zinc.
amel. - mag-s.
erect, while - acon., nat-m., stann.
sitting, after, and vice versa - aloe.
stopping still, during a walk - ign.

STERTOROUS - cact.
night - cact.

STICKING, in chest - iod.
in larynx, from - bufo, lyc., mur-ac., ***phos., sil.***
1 to 4 a.m. - bufo.

STINGING, in larynx, or burning, tickling, from - ***agar.,*** aphis., bufo.

SHARP, pain, with
sharp, chest in, from - acon., ars., bry., kali-c., nit-ac., nux-v.
epigastric region - rhus-t.
epiglottis - caps.
pharynx - caps.
throat - lyc., phos.
sharp, larynx in, from - acon., ***agar.,*** aphis., bufo, cham., ***cist.,*** hydr-ac., indg., kali-c., naja, ox-ac., sol-t-ae., stann.
evening - bufo.
sharp, trachea in, from - ***arg-m.,*** lach., stann.

STOMACH, seems to come from the - all-s., ant-t., bell., **BRY.,** cann-s., ery-a., lach., merc., ***nux-v.,*** puls., **SEP.**
turned inside out, feeling as if - ***puls.,*** ruta., tab.

STOOLS, frequent, amel. - bufo

STOOPING - all-s., arg-m., arg-n., arn., bar-c., **CAUST.,** chel., dig., ***hep.,*** kali-c., laur., lyc., phos., seneg., sil., ***spig.,*** spong., staph., verat.

STORM, before - phos.
thunder, before - phos., sil.

STRAINING - aspar., caust., ***chel.,*** cocc., croc., ***cupr.,*** ip., lach., led., nux-v., par., phos., rhod., rhus-t., sel., thuj.

STRANGERS, child coughs at sight of - ambr., ***ars.,*** bar-c., phos.

STRETCHING, followed by - merc.
out the arms - lyc.
the throat - lyc.

STUDENTS, of - nux-v., phos., sil.

SUDDEN - ***agar.,*** alum., am-br., apoc., bell., calad., coloc., ***cupr., ip.,*** kali-bi., kali-c., kali-p., naja, ***sep.,*** **SQUIL.**
daytime - agar., coloc.
evening - alum., ***am-br.,*** apoc.
sitting, while - alum.
forenoon - agar.
morning - am-br., **SQUIL.**
rising, on - am-br.
night - apoc.

SUFFOCATIVE - acon., ***agar.,*** **ALUM.,** ambr., am-m., anac., anan., **ANT-T.,** ***apis,*** apoc., ***arg-n., ars.,*** ars-i., bar-c., bell., ***brom., bry., carb-an.,*** carb-s., **CARB-V.,** ***caust., cham.,*** chel., **CHIN.,** ***chin-a.,*** **CINA,** cocc., coc-c., ***con.,*** crot-h., **CUPR.,** ***cycl.,*** der., **DROS.,** euphr., eupi., guare., **HEP.,** hydr-ac., **HYOS.,** ign., indg., ***iod.,*** **IP.,** kali-ar., kali-bi., ***kali-c.,*** kali-i., kali-s., kaol., kreos., ***lach.,*** lact., ***led.,*** lyc., mag-p., mang., meph., ***merc.,*** nat-m., ***nux-m.,*** **NUX-V.,** ***op.,*** petr., phel., ***puls.,***

SUFFOCATIVE - ruta., **SAMB.**, ***sep.***, sil., spig., ***spong.***, squil., stram., **SULPH.**, ***tab.***, tep., thuj., ***tub.***, verat., zinc.
child becomes stiff and blue in face - ***cupr.***, **IP.**, ***samb.***
daytime - anac.
eating and drinking, after - bry.
evening - ***carb-an.***, cina, indg., ***ip.***, ***lach.***, nat-m.
6 p.m. - am-m.
7 p.m. - **IP.**
bed, in - indg.
inspiration, from - cina.
lying, while - spong.
midnight - cham., ***dros.***, ***ruta.***, **SAMB.**
2 and 4 a.m. - chin.
5 a.m. - ***kali-c.***
after - ars., chin., ***kali-c.***, ***samb.***
morning - coc-c.
5 a.m. - ***kali-c.***
lying down, while - coc-c.
rising, after - **CINA.**
night - ars., bell., bry., carb-an., ***carb-v.***, cham., ***chin.***, coc-c., ***cupr.***, **HEP.**, indg., ip., lyc., ruta., sil., thuj.
noon - ***arg-n.***
sleep, during - aral., carb-an., **LACH.**
swallowing, on - **BROM.**
walking - ars.

SUGAR, agg. - arg-n., zinc.
amel. - sulph.
dissolving in larynx, as if was - bad.

SULPHUR, fumes or vapor, sensation of agg. - am-c., aml-n., **ARS.**, asaf., ***brom.***, bry., calc., ***carb-v.***, ***chin.***, cina, **IGN.**, ip., kali-chl., ***lach.***, **LYC.**, mosch., ***par.***, **PULS.**
evening, before sleep - ars.

SUN, agg. - ***ant-t.***, coca.

SUPPER, during - carb-v.
after - nat-a.

SUPRISES, happy, agg. - acon., merc.

SWALLOWING, agg. - ***aesc.***, **BROM.**, ***cupr.***, eug., kali-ma., lyc., lyss., ***nat-m.***, op., phos., puls., sul-ac.
amel. - apis, eug., spong.
empty - caust., lyc., ***nat-m.***, op.
amel. - bell.

SWEETMEATS, agg. - bad., med., spong., sulph., zinc.

SWOLLEN, feeling in larynx, from - ars., ox-ac.,
larynx, from - ***kali-i.***

SYMPATHETIC - ***carc.***, card-m., caust., dros., **LACH.**, **NAJA.**, **PHOS.**
night - card-m.

TALKING, agg. - acon., alum., ***alumn.***, ***ambr.***, anac., ant-t., arg-m., ***arg-n.***, arn., ars., atro., bar-c., ***bell.***, brom., bry., calad., calc., ***calc-s.***, carb-s., ***carb-v.***, ***caust.***, cham., ***chin.***, chin-a., ***cimic.***, cina, coc-c., ***cocc.***, con., crot-h., ***cupr.***, dig., **DROS.**, dulc., erig., ***euphr.***, ferr., ferr-ar., ferr-i., ferr-p., ***hep.***, hyos., ign., iod., ip., kali-bi., lac-c., ***lach.***, mag-c., mag-m., mag-p., mang.,

TALKING, agg. - ment., meph., ***merc.***, mez., mur-ac., myric., nat-m., nit-ac., par., ph-ac., ***phos.***, ***phyt.***, ***psor.***, rhus-t., **RUMX.**, **SANIC.**, ***sil.***, ***spong.***, squil., ***stann.***, stram., sulph., sul-ac., sumb., ***tub.***, verb.
evening - psor.
inability to speak with - ***am-m.***, brom., calad., ***cimic.***, ***cupr.***, ***lach.***, mag-p., ***merc.***, ***rumx.***
loud - ***ambr.***, ***arg-n.***, ***coc-c.***, mang., ***phos.***, ***tub.***
night - puls.

TALL, slender tuberculous subjects, in - ***phos.***

TEA, agg. - ferr., spong.
hot, agg. - spong.

TEARING - all-c., ***bell.***, bor., calc., med., phos., senec.
during - senec.
night - ***bell.***, senec.
sensation, cardiac region - elaps

TEDIOUS - form., tub.

TENSION, chest, in - ars., thuj.

THINKING, of it agg. - bar-c., ***ox-ac.***, nux-v.

THREE, coughs in succession - ***carb-v.***, coc-c., ***cupr.***, phos., stann.

TICKLING - acet-ac., **ACON.**, alum., alumn., ***ambr.***, am-c., am-m., anac., ang., ant-t., ***arg-m.***, arg-n., ***arn.***, ars., arum-t., ***asaf.***, atro., bar-c., ***bell.***, bov., ***brom.***, ***bry.***, cahin., ***calc.***, calc-p., canth., ***carb-an.***, ***carb-v.***, ***caust.***, **CHAM.**, chin., chin-a., cimic., cina, ***coca***, cocc., ***coc-c.***, colch., coloc., **CON.**, **CROT-C.**, cupr., dig., ***dros.***, ***euphr.***, ferr., ferr-ar., ***ferr-p.***, graph., ham., hep., **HYOS.**, ***ign.***, inul., ***iod.***, **IP.**, ***iris***, ***kali-bi.***, **KALI-C.**, kali-ma., kali-n., kali-p., kali-s., **LACH.**, lact., laur., led., **LYC.**, mag-c., mag-m., merc., mur-ac., naja, nat-c., **NAT-M.**, nat-p., nit-ac., **NUX-V.**, olnd., ol-an., ol-j., op., petr., ***ph-ac.***, ***phos.***, prun., ***puls.***, ***rhus-t.***, **RUMX.**, sabad., ***sabin.***, **SANG.**, sars., ***seneg.***, **SEP.**, sil., ***spong.***, ***squil.***, ***stann.***, **STAPH.**, sulph., ***tab.***, teucr., ***thuj.***, verat., zinc.
afternoon, 3 p.m. - hep.
air, in open - ***lach.***, ox-ac., **PHOS.**
breathing, deep, on - nat-m.
daytime - coloc., lyc., nat-m., staph.
daytime, and night - nat-m.
eating, after - kali-c.
evening - alumn., calc-p., carb-v., chin., cimic., coloc., lyc., merc., nat-m., ***ph-ac.***, rhus-t., sulph.
6 p.m., expectoration of mucus, amel. - sulph.
bed, in - calc-p.
falling asleep, before - merc.
going to sleep, on - lyc.
midnight until - rhus-t.
morning - alumn., cahin., carb-v., coloc., lyc., nat-m., sumb., thuj.
rising, after - alumn., ***arn.***
walking, after - carb-v.

TICKLING, cough
night - arg-n., ***asaf., calc.,*** coc-c., ***coloc., dros.,*** kali-bi., kali-c., lyc., myric., nat-m., rhus-t., rumx., sanic., sep., zinc.
3 a.m. - cahin.
precordial region - bar-c., verat.
smoking, from - atro., coloc.
talking, on - alumn., atro., **PH-AC.,** phos.
tonsils, below - ***am-br.***
waking, on - carb-v., ham.
walking - nat-m.
tickling, bronchials - ***ant-t.,*** arg-m., bar-c., cop., dios., ip., kali-bi., kali-n., merc., ph-ac., phos., rhus-t., sep., stict., tarent., ***verat.,*** verat-v.
bifurcation - kali-bi., **PH-AC.**
tickling, chest - arn., bar-c., bor., bov., bry., ***carb-an., cham.,*** chin., coc-c., ***con.,*** eup-per., euph., graph., ign., iod., ***kali-bi.,*** kali-n., kali-s., kreos., lach., ***merc.,*** mur-ac., myrt-c., nat-c., nat-m., nat-p., ***nux-v.,*** **PH-AC., PHOS.,** polyg., rhus-t., sars., sep., **STANN.,** squil., sulph., sul-ac., tell., ***verat.,*** verat-v., verb., zinc.
upper, in - merc., polyg., zinc.
tickling, epigastrium, from - bar-c., bell., bry., guai., hep., ***lach., nat-m., nit-ac., ph-ac., phos.,*** sang., tarax., thuj.
tickling, fauces - aloe, carb-ac., ***gels.,*** lact., til.
tickling, larynx, in, from - ***acon., aesc., agar.,*** **ALL-C.,** alum., ***alumn., ambr.,*** am-br., ***am-c., am-m.,*** anac., ***anan.,*** ang., ant-t., anth., apis, ***arg-m., arg-n., arn.,*** **ARS.,** ***asaf.,*** aspar., astac., aur-m., ***bad.,*** bar-c., **BELL.,** bor., bov., ***brom., bry.,*** bufo, cact., cadm-s., cahin., calad., ***calc.,*** **CALC-F.,** ***caps., carb-ac., carb-an., carb-s., carb-v.,*** carl., ***caust., cham., chel.,*** chlor., cimx., cimic., cinnb., ***cist.,*** **COC-C.,** cocc., colch., coloc., **CON.,** cop., **CROT-C.,** crot-h., crot-t., ***cupr., cycl.,*** dig., dios., **DROS.,** ***dulc.,*** euph., ***euphr.,*** eupi., ferr-ar., glon., graph., ***hep.,*** hydr., hydr-ac., ***hyos., ign.,*** **IOD., IP.,** ***iris, ir-foe., kali-bi., kali-c.,*** kali-n., kali-p., kali-s., kreos., ***lac-c.,*** **LACH.,** lact., laur., led., lob., lob-s., **LYC.,** mag-c., mag-m., mang., merc., merc-c., mez., mur-ac., naja, nat-a., nat-c., **NAT-M.,** nat-p., nat-s., nicc., ***nit-ac.,*** **NUX-V.,** olnd., onos., op., osm., ox-ac., par., ***ph-ac.,*** **PHOS.,** ***phyt.,*** plan., ***prun., psor.,*** **PULS.,** rat., rhus-t., ***rumx., sabin., sang.,*** sars., ***seneg., sep., sil.,*** sol-n., spira., **SPONG.,** ***squil.,*** stann., **STAPH.,** ***stict.,*** sulph., sumb., tab., tarent., tep., thuj., til., verb., ***vinc.,*** zinc., zing.
afternoon - anth., mag-c., naja
2 p.m. - arg-n., **COC-C.**
down, as from - calc., ***ph-ac.,*** sulph.
evening - ambr., carb-an., ***carb-v.,*** cimic., graph., lyc., nat-m.
extending, to chest - sil.
to midsternum - rumx.
lying, while - **DROS.**
tickling, larynx,
morning - iod.
rising, after - alumn., arn., ***op.***
night - agar., ***dros.***
3 to 4 a.m. - ***bufo.***
11:30 p.m. - **COC-C.**
12 p.m. - hep., phos.
small spot in, agg. - apis, cimic., con.
tickling, palate, in - cham., dig., nux-v., phos.
tickling, pharynx, in - anac., arg-n., ars., carb-s., cham., coca, coc-c., hydr-ac., lact., mag-s., olnd., sil.
night - anac., mag-s., ***sil.***
tickling, sternum, behind - zinc.
tickling, throat-pit, in, from - ***apis,*** aspar., bell., cann-s., ***caust.,*** **CHAM.,** cinnb., cocc., coloc., ***con.,*** crot-h., ***ign., inul., iod.,*** lac-c., lach., lith., nat-c., nat-m., ph-ac., puls., rhus-r., **RUMX., SANG.,** ***sil.,*** squil., tarax.
tickling, trachea, in, from - ***acon.,*** agar., ail., ambr., am-m., anac., ang., ***ant-t., arn.,*** ars., arum-t., asaf., aur-m., bar-c., bell., bov., ***brom.,*** bry., ***calc., caps.,*** carb-ac., ***carb-s.,*** casc., caust., cham., chin., chin-s., cina, coc-c., coloc., com., con., cop., dig., dulc., euph., ***euphr., ferr.,*** ferr-ar., ferr-i., gymn., hyos., indg., **IOD.,** ir-foe., iris, ***kali-bi.,*** **KALI-C.,** kali-n., kali-p., kali-s., kreos., lac-c., lach., lact., laur., mag-c., mag-m., med., ***merc.,*** mez., nat-a., nat-m., nicc., nit-ac., **NUX-V.,** ol-an., ox-ac., petr., **PH-AC.,** ***phos.,*** plat., prun., ***psor., puls.,*** rhod., **RHUS-T.,** rhus-r., rumx., sabin., **SANG.,** sanic., ***seneg., sep.,*** **SIL.,** spig., squil., ***stann.,*** staph., stict., ***still.,*** sulph., tarent., teucr., thuj., verat., zinc.

TIGHT - calc-s., ***caust.,*** cimx., ***con., cupr., form.,*** guai., ***hell., mag-p.,*** merc., ***mosch., myrt-c.,*** nat-a., **PHOS.,** ***puls.,*** stram., ***sulph.,*** ziz.
daytime - nat-a.
evening - calc-s.

TINGLING, chest - sep., squil.
larynx, from - ***agar.,*** caps., ***iod.,*** mag-m., sep.
trachea, from - stann.

TITILLATING - acet-ac., asaf., coloc., dros.

TONELESS - calad., cina, card-b., dros.

TORMENTING - alum., am-c., anac., ang., arg-n., **ARS.,** arum-t., asaf., bar-c., **BELL.,** benz-ac., berb., bor., brom., ***calc.,*** cann-s., carb-an., carb-v., **CAUST.,** chel., chin., cina, ***cocc., con.,*** cor-r., ***croc., cupr.,*** daph., **DROS.,** dulc., ferr-p., hep., hydr-ac., **IP.,** ***kali-c.,*** kali-n., kreos., ***lach.,*** lact., led., lob., merc., merc-c., ***mez.,*** mur-ac., ***nat-a.,*** nat-c., ***nat-m.,*** nit-ac., ***nux-v.,*** op., ***petr., phos.,*** phyt., rhod., rhus-t., rumx., ***sang.,*** sel., sep., spig., ***squil., stann., sulph.,*** verat.

TOUCHING, general
canal of ear, on - ***agar., arg-n., carb-s.,*** kali-c., ***lach.,*** mang., ***psor.,*** sil., ***sulph.,*** tarent.
larynx lightly agg. - ***bell.,*** chin., ferr-p., **LACH.,** ***rumx.,*** staph., stram.

TOUCHING, general
tonsils - phos.

TRUMPET-toned - verb.

TUBE, sounds as if he coughed in a - osm.

TURNING, from left to right side amel. - ars., kali-c., ***phos., rumx., sep., thuj.***
bed agg., in - kreos.
head agg. - spong.
side on, agg. - am-m.

TWITCHING, in hips - ars.

ULCERATION, deep in trachea, as if from an - stann.

UNCOVERING, agg. - ars., chel., **HEP.,** ***kali-bi.,*** nux-v., **RHUS-T., RUMX.,** sil.
feet or head - **SIL.**
hands - bar-c., **HEP., RHUS-T.,** sil.

VACCINATION, after - ant-t., carc., sil., ***thuj.***

VARIOLA, after - calc.
during - plat.

VEXATION, after - acon., ant-t., ars., bry., **CHAM.,** chin., ***cina,*** **IGN.,** iod., ***nat-m.,*** nux-v., ph-ac., sep., **STAPH.,** verat.

VINEGAR, after - alum., ant-c., ***sep.,*** sulph.

VIOLENT - **AGAR.,** alum., ambr., am-m., am-m., anac., anan., ang., ant-t., apis, arg-n., ars., **BELL.,** ***bor.,*** brom., bry., bufo, ***calc.,*** camph., carb-an., **CARB-V., CAUST.,** ***cham., chel.,*** chin., ***cimx., cina,*** clem., **COC-C., CON.,** cop., cor-r., croc., **CUPR.,** ***cycl.,*** **DROS.,** elaps, ***eup-per., euphr., form.,*** gamb., gels., guare., **HEP.,** hydr-ac., **HYOS., IGN.,** indg., **IP.,** kali-bi., **KALI-C.,** kali-chl., ***kreos.,*** **LACH.,** lact., led., lith., ***lob.,*** lycps., mag-p., manc., ***mag-c., meph., merc.,*** **MEZ.,** mur-ac., ***nat-a., nat-c.,*** nat-p., nicc., nit-ac., ***nux-v.,*** ol-j., olnd., ***op.,*** par., petr., **PH-AC., PHOS.,** plat., **PULS.,** ***rhus-t.,*** rumx., ruta., sabad., sang., seneg., **SEP.,** ***sil.,*** spig., ***spong.,*** **SQUIL., STANN.,** staph., stict., stront-c., sulph., ther., verat., viol-o., ***zinc.***
afternoon - ***nat-c.***
daytime - ***agar.,*** alum., ***euphr.***
dinner, after - anac., mur-ac.
evening - alum., anac., bor., ***calc.,*** con., indg., ***kali-c., mez., nat-c.,*** verat.
lying, after - am-m., ***kali-c., mez.,*** **SEP.**
laughing - mur-ac.
morning - ars., bry., cina, nux-v., ***puls.,*** **SQUIL.,** verat.
early, in bed - bry., ***mez.,*** **NUX-V.**
rising, before - **NUX-V.**
waking, on - ***agar.,*** **LACH.**
night - am-c., arg-n., bell., calc., **CON.,** cupr., ***cycl., hep., merc.,*** nicc., petr., verat.
night, 3 a.m. - **KALI-C.,** mur-ac.
noon - bell.
sitting or lying, while, not during motion - phos.
sleep, in - apis, cham., ***cycl., sulph.***
spasmodic jerking of head forward and knees upward - ther.
talking, from - mur-ac.

VIOLENT, cough
uninterrupted until relieved by vomiting - ***mez.***
waking, on - ***agar.,*** calc., carb-v., rhus-t.
yawning, on - mur-ac.
violin, playing on - kali-c.

WAKING, on - acon., ail., ambr., apis, ***aral.,*** arg-n., arum-t., bell., calc., carb-v., caust., ***chel., chin.,*** cina, **COC-C.,** cod., coff., crot-h., dig., euphr., ferr., ferr-p., ign., ***kali-bi.,*** kali-n., kreos., lac-c., **LACH.,** lachn., mag-s., nat-a., nit-ac., nux-v., ph-ac., phos., psor., puls., ***rhus-t.,*** rumx., ***sang.,*** sanic., sep., sil., sol-t-ae., spong., squil., stram., sulph., sul-ac., tarent., thuj.

WALKING - alum., ars., ***calc.,*** carb-v., cina, dig., **FERR.,** hep., iod., ip., lach., mag-m., mang., mez., nat-a., nat-m., rumx., ***seneg.,*** stram., stront-c., sul-ac., ***thuj.***
air, in open - ars., sulph., sul-ac.
amel. - astac., dros., grat., ign., phos.
fast - cench., coca, merc., nat-m., ***puls., seneg.,*** sep., sil., squil., stann.

WARM, becoming, on - caust., laur., nit-ac., nux-m., ***puls.***
fluids - ambr., ant-t., caps., ***coc-c.,*** ign., laur., mez., phos., ***stann.***
amel. - alum., **ARS.,** ***bry.,*** eupi., **LYC., NUX-V., RHUS-T., SIL.,** ***spong.,*** verat.
food - ***bar-c., coc-c., kali-c.,*** laur., ***mez., puls.***
amel. - ***spong.***
room - acon., ***all-c.,*** ambr., anan., ant-c., ***apis,*** arn., ars., brom., ***bry.,*** **COC-C.,** com., cub., dig., ***dros., dulc., iod., ip., kali-s.,*** laur., ***lyc.,*** mag-p., med., mez., nat-a., ***nat-c.,*** nit-ac., phos., **PULS.,** pyrog., sanic., ***seneg., spong.,*** sulph., ***tub.,*** verat.
entering, from open air - ***acon., all-c.,*** anth., **ANT-C.,** bov., ***brom., bry.,*** carb-v., ***coc-c., com.,*** con., cupr., dig., med., ***nat-c., nat-m., nux-v., puls.,*** sep., squil., ***sulph.,*** verat., verb.
going from, to cold air, or vice versa, agg. - acon., all-c., carb-v., lach., nat-c., nux-v., **PHOS.,** ***rumx.,*** sep., verat-v.
stove - coc-c.
warming abdomen amel. - sil.

WATER, (see Drinking)

WEATHER, change of - ***dulc.,*** erig., lach., nit-ac., phos., rumx., sil., spong., verat., verb.
damp - bar-c., calc., carb-v., cur., ***dulc.,*** iod., lach., ***mang.,*** nat-s., phyt., rhus-t., spong., sil., sulph.
hot - lach.
stormy - mag-m., phos., ***rhod., sep., sil.,*** sulph.
warm, wet - iod.

WEEPING, with (see Crying)

WET, getting - ant-c., calc., ***calc-s.,*** dulc., lach., nit-ac., psor., rhus-t., sep., sulph.

WHEEZING, (see Asthmatic)

WHINING, during - acon., ars., cina

WHISPERING, sound, has a - card-b.

WHISTLING - acon., ars., brom., carb-v., chlor., ***hep.,*** kali-bi., kali-i., kali-p., kreos., ***laur.,*** lyc., prun., samb., ***sang.,*** seneg., ***spong.***

WHOOPING, cough - acon., all-c., ***ambr.,*** am-c., ***anac., anan.,*** ant-c., **ANT-T.,** ***arg-n., arn., ars.,*** arum-t., asaf., asar., asc-c., bad., ***bar-c.,*** bar-m., ***bell., brom., bry., calc., calc-p.,*** caps., ***carb-ac., carb-an., carb-s.,*** **CARB-V.,** ***cast-v., caust., cham., chin.,*** chlol., ***chlor., cina, coc-c.,*** con., ***cor-r., crot-h.,*** **CUPR.,** cupr-ar., dig., **DIRC., DROS.,** ***dulc., euphr., ferr.,*** ferr-ar., ***ferr-p., graph.,*** guare., ***hep., hippoz.,*** hydr-ac., ***hyos.,*** hyper., ign., indg., ***ip., kali-bi.,*** kali-br., ***kali-c.,*** kali-chl., kali-i., ***kali-p.,*** **KALI-S.,** ***kreos., lact.,*** laur., ***led., lob., lyc., mag-m.,*** mag-p., ***meph.,*** merc., ***mez.,*** mosch., mur-ac., ***nat-m.,*** nicc., ***nit-ac., nux-v.,*** op., par., phel., **PHOS.,** podo., ***puls.,*** rhus-t., ***rumx.,*** ruta., ***samb.,*** **SANG.,** sec., ***seneg., sep., sil.,*** spig., ***spong., squil.,*** stann., stict., stram., ***sulph.,*** sul-ac., syph., ***tab., verat.,*** viol-o., ***visc.,*** zinc.
- afternoon - lyc., mur-ac., sulph.
  - midnight, until - sulph.
- ailments after - carc., per., sang.
- daytime - brom., cupr., ***euphr.***
- evening - ambr., arn., ars., bar-c., bell., bry., carb-v., chin., cina, coc-c., dros., hep., ign., ***laur.,*** lyc., mez., nat-m., puls., seneg., sep., spong., sul-ac., verat.
  - 6 to 10 p.m. - hyper.
  - midnight, until - arn., bar-c., carb-v., hep., mez., puls., sep., spong., sul-ac., verat.
  - night, and - ars., bry.
- face bluish during - ars., ***coc-c., cor-r.,*** crot-h., **CUPR.,** ***dros., ip., nux-v.***
- forenoon - sep.
- heart, as if would break after paroxysm - arn.
- midnight, after - acon., am-m., bell., chin., dros., ***hyos., kali-c.,*** samb.
  - after, 2 a.m. - dros.
  - after, 3 a.m. - ***kali-c.***
  - before - lyc., mur-ac., ***spong.***
- morning - ant-c., ***calc.,*** cina, verat.
- night - ambr., anac., ant-t., arn., ars., bar-c., bell., bry., carb-v., ***cham.,*** chin., coc-c., cor-r., cupr., dros., dulc., ***hep.,*** hyos., meph., ***merc.,*** mez., mur-ac., nat-m., nit-ac., puls., samb., seneg., sep., sil., spong., stann., sulph., sul-ac., verat.
- nosebleeds, with - **ARN.,** ***bry., cina, cor-r., crot-h.,*** **DROS., IP.,** ***led., merc., mur-ac., nux-v.,*** **PHOS.,** spong., stram.
- sequelae - ***sang.***

WIND, in the - ***acon.,*** caps., cham., coca, cupr., euphr., **HEP.,** lyc., lycps., samb., sep., spong., stram.
- cold, in - coca, **HEP.,** lyc., lycps.
- dry, in - **ACON.,** cham., **HEP.,** spong.
- east, in - **ACON.,** cham., cupr., **HEP.,** samb., sep., spong.
- north, in - **ACON.,** caps., cham., cupr., **HEP.,** sep., spong.
- sea, in - ***cupr.***
- sharp, in - caps.
- south, in - euphr.
- west, in - **HEP.**

WINE - acon., ant-c., arn., bor., ferr., ign., lach., led., ***stann.,*** stram., **ZINC.**
- amel. - sulph.

WINTER - acon., ars., cham., ***coc-c.,*** dulc., eupi., ***kreos., nit-ac.,*** plan., ***psor., rumx.,*** sep., ***stann.,*** staph.
- alternating with sciatica in summer - staph.
- elderly people - am-c., ***kreos.***

WORM, sensation as if a, crawled up from pit of stomach in throat, from - zinc.

WRITING - cina.

YAWNING - arn., asaf., cina, mur-ac., nux-v., puls., staph.
- yawning and coughing consecutively - ant-t., ***nat-m.***

Delusions

DELUSIONS, general - abel., ***absin.,*** acet-ac., ***acon., aeth., agar.,*** alco., alum., ***ambr.,*** **ANAC.,** anan., anh., ant-c., ant-t., ***antipyrin.,*** apis, aran., aran-ix., arg-m., **ARG-N.,** arn., ***ars.,*** ars-i., ars-m., ars-s-f., art-v., asaf., asar., atro., ***aur.,*** aur-a., ***aur-m., bapt., bar-c.,*** bar-i., **BELL.,** berb., bism., bry., ***calc.,*** calc-ar., calc-i., calc-s., ***camph.,*** **CANN-I.,** ***cann-s.,*** canth., carb-an., carb-v., carl., caust., cench., cham., chel., chin., chin-a., chlol., chlor., chloram., chlorpr., cic., cimic., cina, coc-c., coca, cocaine, **COCC.,** ***coff.,*** colch., coloc., con., convo-s., cortico., croc., ***crot-c.,*** crot-h., ***cupr.,*** cupr-ac., cyt-l., dat-a., dig., digin., dub., dulc., elaps, eup-pur., euph-a., eupi., fl-ac., form., ***glon.,*** gran., graph., ***hell., hep.,*** hoit., hura, hydr-ac., **HYOS., IGN.,** iod., kali-bi., ***kali-br.,*** kali-c., kali-p., kali-sil., lac-c., **LACH.,** lachn., led., levo., ***lol., lyc., lyss.,*** mag-m., ***mag-p., med.,*** meli., meny., meph., ***merc.,*** merl., mez., morph., mosch., mur-ac., murx., nat-c., nat-m., nat-p., nat-sal., ***nit-ac.,*** nux-m., ***nux-v., oena.,*** **OP.,** orig-v., ox-ac., oxyt., par., passi., past., **PETR., PH-AC.,** ***phos.,*** **PLAT.,** plb., psil., ***psor., puls., pyrog.,*** ran-b., rheum, rhod., rhus-g., ***rhus-t.,*** russ., ruta, **SABAD.,** sac-l., sal-ac., samb., sant., ***sec.,*** sel., sep., ***sil.,*** spong., stann., ***staph.,*** **STRAM.,** sulfonam., **SULPH.,** syph., tarent., ter., tere-ch., thea., ther., thuj., thyr., trio., tub., ***valer.,*** verat., verat-v., verb., verin., viol-o., visc., xan., ***zinc.,*** zinc-m.

ABDOMEN, is fallen in, his stomach devoured, his scrotum swollen - **SABAD.**

ABROAD, thinks he is - verat.

ABSURD, ludicrous - cann-i.
figures are present - ambr., arg-m., camph., cann-i., caust., cic., op., tarent.

ABUSED, being - ***bar-c.,*** cocaine, hyos., ign., lyss., pall., ***staph.***

ABYSS, behind him an - ***kali-c.***
fear of falling down an - alco.

ACCIDENT, sees - anac., ars.
relatives, of - phos.

ACCUSED, thinks she is - laur., zinc.

ACTIVE - ***bell., hyos., stram.***

AFFECTION, of friends, has lost - ***aur.,*** hura

AFTERNOON, that it is always - lach., stann.

AIR, that he is hovering in, like a spirit - ***asar.,*** calc., cann-i., ***dat-a.,*** hyper., ***lac-c.,*** lach., lact., lat-h., nat-a., op., pen., phys., rhus-g., ***stict.,*** tell., ***valer.,*** xan.

ALONE, that she is always - ***puls.,*** stram.
castaway, being a - ***phys.***
graveyard, in a - lepi., sep.
wilderness, in a - stram.
world, that she is alone in the - camph., cycl., hura, ***plat., puls.***

ANGELS, seeing - ether, cann-i., stram.

ANIMALS, of - absin., aeth., alum., am-c., am-m., arn., ***ars.,*** aur., aur-a., aur-s., **BELL.,** ***calc.,*** cham., cina, ***cimic.,*** colch., con., ***crot-h., hyos.,*** lac-c., lyc., lyss., mag-m., med., merc., mosch., nux-v., **OP.,** phos., puls., sant., sec., sil., **STRAM.,** sul-ac., sulph., tarent., thuj., valer., verat., zinc.
abdomen, are in - ***thuj.***
bed, on - ars., colch., ***plb.,*** stram., valer.
dancing on the - con.
under the - cham.
beetles, worms, etc. - ars., bell., cimic., hyos., nep., ***stram.***
black, on walls and furniture, sees - bell.
creeping of - lac-c.
in her - cycl., stram., thuj.
cup, moving in a - hyos.
dark colored - bell.
fire, in the - bell.
frightful - ***bell.,*** cham., ***crot-h., op., stram.,*** tarent.
grotesque - absin.
jump out of the ground - stram.
jumping at her - ***merc.***
passing before her - thuj.
persons are - hyos., stram.
rats, mice, insects, etc - ***aeth.,*** bell., ***cimic., med.,*** stram.
unclean - bell.
starting up - stram.

ANNIHILATION, about to sink into - calc., cann-i., carb-h.

ANSWERS to any delusion - anh., aster.

ANTS, bed seems full of - plb.
ants, letters seem - hyos.

ANXIOUS - ***acon., anac.,*** calc., carb-v., ign., mag-c., ***phos., puls.,*** sep., verat.

APPRECIATED, that she is not - ***pall.,*** plat., sulph.

ARGUMENT, making an eloquent - cann-i.

ARMS, bound to her body, are - caj., cimic.
cut off, are - bac.
do not belong to her - agar., bapt.
four, that she has - ***sulfon.***
many, has, as if - pyrog.
reach the clouds when going to sleep - pic-ac.
separated, from body - bapt., daph., psor.
three, that she has - petr.

ARMY passed him in the street, a silent - cann-i.

ARRESTED, is about to be - arn., ars., ***bell., cupr.,*** kali-br., meli., plb., ***zinc.***

ASSAULTED, is going to be - abel., tarent.

ASSEMBLED things, swarms, crowds etc. - acon., ambr., anac., ars., bell., cann-s., con., graph., hell., lyc., merc., nat-c., op., phos., plb., **STRAM.,** sulph., tab.

ASYLUM, that she will be sent to - cench., lach.

ATTACKS and insults, defend themselves against imaginary - lyss.

BABIES, are two in bed - petr.

BABY looks odious - ***puls.***

BALL, that he is sitting on a - cann-i., chim.

BATS, of - bell.

BEATEN, that he is being - bry., elaps.

BEAUTIFUL - anh., **BELL., CANN-I.,** coca, ***lach., op., sulph.***
atmosphere, in - dat-a.
landscape - ***coff., lach.***
rags seem, even - ***sulph.***
she is beautiful and wants to be - stram.
things look - bell., olnd., ***sulph.,*** tab.
urination, after, all things seem - eug.

BED, general
as if someone was in, with him - anac., apis, ***bapt.,*** carb-v., graph., nux-v., op., petr., ***puls.,*** rhus-t., sec., stram., valer.
some one was in, with him, bouncing her up and down - bell., canth.
two persons in bed with her - cycl.
bouncing her up and down, someone - bell., canth.
creases, is full of - ***stram.***
drawn from under her - stram.
evening, as if some one would get into and no room in it, or as if some one had sold it - nux-v.
feels as if not lying on, on waking 4 a.m. - hyper.
hard, too - **ARN.,** ***bapt.,*** bry., con., dros., gels., kali-c., ***morph.,*** nux-v., phos., plat., ***pyrog., rhus-t.,*** ruta, ***sil.,*** til.
hot, as if - op.
lumps, in - arn., mag-c.
motion, in - lac-c.
waking on - lac-c.
naked man is wrapped in the bedclothes with her - ***puls.***
occupied by another person - petr.
whole body, as if - pyrog.
raised, were - canth.
sinking, were - bapt., ***bell., benz.,*** bry., calc-p., chin-s., dulc., kali-c., ***lach.,*** lyc., rhus-t., sac-alb.
small, too, to hold him - sulph.
someone, drives him out - rhus-t.
over it - calc.
stands at the foot menacing - chlol.
tries to take away the bed clothes - bell.
someone, under it - am-m., ars., ***bell.,*** calc., canth., colch.
knocking - **BELL.,** calc., canth., colch.
strange objects, rats, sheep in - cimic.
swimming - bell.

BEES, sees - puls.

BEETLES, worms, etc. - ars., bell., ***stram.***

BEHIND, him, abyss, there is an - ***kali-c.***
walking, behind him, somebody - calc.

BELLS, hears, ringing of - ars., cann-i., ether., kres., ph-ac., thea.
door bell - thea.
his funeral - ether
numberless sweet toned - cann-i.

BELONG, to her own family, does not - ***plat.***

BETROTHAL, must be broken - fl-ac.

BETTER, than others, that he is - myric., plat.

BEWITCHED, thinks he is - cann-i.

BIER, is lying on a - anac., cann-i.

BIRD, he is a, runs about, chirping and twittering, until he faints - lyss.

BIRDS, sees - bell., kali-c., lac-c.
that he is picking feathers from - hyos.

BITTEN, will be - ***hyos.,*** stram.

BLACK objects and people - **BELL.,** ***plat., puls.,*** **STRAM.**
she is black - sulph.

BLIND, that he is - bell., mosch., verat.

BLOOD, does not circulate well - ***atro.***
rushed through like roar of many waters - alumn., cann-i.

BODY, general
adherent to woollen sack, night, while half awake - ***coc-c.***
able to go out of body and walk around, looking down upon - pyrus.
alive, on one side, buried on the other - stram.
only half alive - crot-h.
black, as if it were - sulph.
brittle, is - sars., ***thuj.***
covered the whole bed - pyrog.
the whole earth - cann-i.
dashed to pieces, being - calc.
deformed, some parts are - ***acon.,*** **SABAD.**
delicate - ***thuj.***
disintegrating - ars., ***lach.***
divided - cann-i., lil-t., ***petr.,*** sil., ***stram.***
erroneous ideas as to the state of his - **SABAD.**
expanded, is - xan.
feels every fiber in the right side - sep.
greatness of, as to - ***cann-i., plat.,*** staph.
headless, is - nux-v.
heavy and thick, has become - nat-c.
immaterial, is - anh.
lighter than air - asar., lach., ***op.,*** thuj., visc.
parts, absent - cocaine.
taken away - ***bapt., daph.***
pieces, in danger of coming in - thuj.
putrify, will - ***ars.,*** bell.
scattered about bed, tossed about to get the pieces together - ***bapt.,*** daph., petr., ***phos.,*** pyrog., stram.
limbs conversing with each other - bapt.
shrunken, like the dead - ***sabad.***
sink down between the thights, body will - bell.
spotted brown, as if - bell.
state of his, as to the - **SABAD.**
sweets, is made of - merc.
thick - nat-c.
thin, is - thuj.
threads, inside is made of - nux-v.
threefold, has a - ars., petr.
whithering, is - sabad.
would sink down between the thighs - bell.

BONES in fragments and cannot fit pieces together - phos.

BORN, feels as if newly, into the world and was overwhelmed with wonder at the novelty of his surroundings - cori-r.

BRAIN, cracking, is - nux-m.
hard, seems - mez.
possesses stomach - acon.
softening, has - abrot., ***arg-n.,*** cann-i.

BREASTS are too big or too small - bar-c.

BROTHER, fell overboard in her sight - kali-br.

BUGS and cockroaches, of - stram.

BUILDING, stones, appearance of - thuj.

BULLS, of - bell.

BUSINESS, fancies is doing - bell., ***bry.,*** canth., cupr., op., ***phos., rhus-t.***
occupied about - ***bry.,*** op.
thought they were pursuing ordinary - ars., atro., bell., plb., stram.
unfit for, that he is - ***croc.***

BUTTERFLIES, of - bell., cann-i.

CALLS, him, someone - ***cann-i.,*** rhod., ***sep.,*** sulph.
with name, the absent mother or sister - anac.

CALLS, to someone - anac., ant-c., bell., cann-i., dros., kali-c., ***plb.,*** ruta, thuj.
absent persons, for - hyos.
sleep, during - sep.
waking, on - ant-c., ars., bell., dulc., rhod., rhus-t., sep.

CANCER, has a - ars., carc., nit-ac., verat.

CARESSED, on head by someone - ***med.***

CASTLES, and palaces, sees - plb.

CATCHES at, imaginary appearance - ***hyos.,*** **STRAM.**
people - stram.

CATS, see - absin., ***aeth.,*** arn., ***bell., calc.,*** daph., hyos., op., puls., ***stram.***
black - bell., puls.

CAUGHT, as if he would be - bell.

CHAIR, is rising up - phos.
thinks he is repairing old - cupr., cupr-ac.

CHANGEABLE - hyos.

CHANGED, thinks everything - arg-n., bar-m., carb-an., ***nux-m., plat.,*** stram.

CHANGING, suddenly - cann-i.

CHARMED and cannot break the spell - ***lach.***

CHERRIES, sees - sant.

CHILD, childish fantasies, has - lyc.
companions of his youth, is with - ether.
not hers - anac.
thinks he is again a - bar-c., ***cic.***

CHILDBIRTH, of - verat.

CHILDREN, thinks he must drive, out of the house - fl-ac.

CHIN, too long, is - glon.

CHOIR, on hearing music thinks he is in a cathedral - cann-i.

CHOKED, by icy-cold hands - canth.
thinks he is about to be, night, on waking - cann-i., phos., ***plat.***

CHRIST, thinks himself to be - cann-i., verat.

CHURCHYARD, visits a - anac., arn., ***bell.,*** stram.
that he is dancing in - stram.

CIPHERS, sees - ***ph-ac.,*** phos., sulph.

CLEAR, everything is too - ambr.

CLIMBING, up - hyos.

CLOCK, hears strike - ph-ac.

CLOTHES, thinks beautiful - aeth., ***sulph.***
is clad in rags - ***cann-i.***
would fly away and become wandering stars, on undressing - cann-i.

CLOUDS, before the fancy - hep., mag-m., rhus-t.
clouds, and rocks as if looking over - mag-m.
heavy black enveloped her - arg-n., ***cimic., lac-c.,*** puls.
strange, settled upon patients, or danced about the sun - cann-i.

COCKROACHES, swarmed about the room - bell.

COMMANDER, being a - cann-i., cupr.

COMPANIONS, of his youth, with - ether
seemed half men, half plants - cann-i.

CONFIDENCE, in him, his friends have lost all - aur., hura

CONFUSION, imagines others will observe her - ***calc.***

CONSCIOUSNESS, belongs to another - alum.

CONSPIRACIES, against her father, thought the landlord's bills were - kali-br.
against him, there were - anac., ***ars., lach.,*** plb., puls.

CONTAMINATES, everything she touches - ars.

CONVENT, thinks she will have to go to a - lac-d.

CONVERSING, with - **BELL.,** nat-m., ***stram.***

CORNER, animals and figures coming out of, sees - stram.
people coming out of, sees - ***stram.***
something coming out of, sees - ***phos.***
and toward him - stram.

CORNERS of houses seem to project so that he fears he will run against them while walking in the street - ***arg-n.***

COUNCIL, holding a - arn., cham.

COWARDS, thinks persons leaving him to be - cann-i.

CRABS, of - hyos.

CREATIVE, power, has - cann-i.

CREEPING things, full of - stram.

CRIME, about to commit a - ***kali-bi.,*** kali-br.
as if he had committed - alum., ***anac.,*** ars., carb-v., chel., cina, ***ign., kali-bi.,*** kali-br., lach., med., merc., nux-v., ruta, sabad., staph., ***verat-v.,*** zinc.
5 p.m. to 6 p.m. - am-c.

CRIMINAL, about, there is a - alum., am-c., ***ars.,*** bell., carb-v., caust., ***chel.,*** cina, ***cocc.,*** coff., dig., ***ferr.,*** graph., ***hyos.,*** merc., nat-c., nit-ac., nux-v., puls., ruta., sil., stront-c., sulph., verat.
that he is a - cob., cycl., dig., hyos., ***ign., merc.,*** op., phos., sarr., thuj.
executed, to be - **OP.**
others know it, and - cob.

CRITICIZED, that she is - ***bar-c.,*** cocaine, hyos., ign., laur., lyss., pall., plb., rhus-r., staph.

CROWDED, with arms and legs, as if - ***pyrog.,*** pyrus.

CRYING, with - acon., dulc., lyc., merc., stram.

CUCUMBERS, sees on the bed - ***bell.***

CURSING, with - ***anac.,*** verat.

CUT, through, as if he were - ***stram.***
cut, in two - ***bell.,*** plat., ***stram.***

CYLINDER, seemed to be a - cann-i.

DANCING, satyres and nodding mandarins - cann-i.

DANGER, impression of - fl-ac., kali-br., ***stram.,*** valer.
life, to his - plb.
family, from his - kali-br.

DARK, objects and figures, sees - cimic.
dark, in the - carb-v.

DAY and night - aeth., ars., kali-c.

DEAD, corpse of
acquaintance of absent, on sofa and has dread - ars.
bier, on a - anac., cann-i.
dead brother and child - con., plb.
husband - plb.
mutilated - ant-c., arn., con., mag-m., merc., nux-v., sep.
sister - agar.
tall yellow, trying to share bed with him and promptly ejected - bell.

DEAD, everything is - mez.
all her friends are and she must go to a convent - ***lac-d.***
her child was - ***kali-bi.,*** kali-br.
mother is - lach., nat-m.
he himself was - anac., anh., apis, camph., cann-i., ***lach.,*** mosch., ***op.,*** phos., stram.

DEAD, persons, sees - agar., alum., am-c., ***anac.,*** arg-n., arn., ***ars.,*** ars-i., bar-c., bar-i., ***bell.,*** brom., bry., calc., calc-ar., calc-i., ***calc-sil.,*** canth., caust., cocc., con., fl-ac., graph., ***hep.,*** hura, ***hyos.,*** iod., kali-ar., ***kali-br., kali-c.,*** kali-p., kali-sil., ***lach.,*** laur., ***mag-c.,*** mag-m., nat-c., nat-m., nat-p., nit-ac., nux-v., op., paull., ***ph-ac., phos., plat.,*** plb., ran-s., sars., sil., stram., stry., sulph., sul-ac., sul-i., thuj., verb., zinc., zinc-p.

DEAD, persons, sees
midnight, on waking - cann-i.
morning on waking, frightened by images of - hep.

DEAF, and dumb - verat.

DEATH, approaching - agn.

DEBATE, of being in - hyos.

DECEIVED, being - dros., ruta.

DELIRIOUS, at night, expected to become - bry.
imagines he was - cann-i.

DEMONIACAL, thinks he is - **ANAC., HYOS.**

DESERTED, forsaken, being - **ARG-N.,** ***aur.,*** bar-c., camph., cann-i., carb-an., carb-v., chin., ***cycl.,*** hura, hyos., ***kali-br.,*** lil-t., lyss., nat-c., pall., ***plat., puls., stram.***

DESPISED, that is - **ARG-N.,** hura, lac-c., ***orig-v.***

DESTRUCTION of all near her, impending - ***kali-br.***

DEVIL, possessed of a, is - **ANAC.,** ***hyos., plat.,*** **STRAM.**
that everyone is - meli.

DEVILS, sees - ambr., **ANAC.,** ars., ***bell.,*** cann-i., cupr., dulc., ***hell.,*** hyos., kali-c., lach., nat-c., op., ***plat., puls.,*** stram., sulph., ***zinc.***
coming after her - ***zinc.***
blasphemous words, whisper - ***anac.***
present, are - anac., cann-i., op., phos., **PLAT.**
sit in his neck - ***anac.***
speaking in one ear, angel in the other, prompting to murder, or acts of benevolence - ***anac.***
that all persons are - meli., **PLAT.,** ***plb.***
he is a devil - anac., camph., cann-i., kali-br., stram.
he will be taken by - bell., manc., ***puls.***

DEVOURED, had been by animals - ***hyos.,*** stram.
of being - ***stram.***

DIE, thought he was about to - **ACON.,** agn., ***arg-n.,*** arn., bar-c., bell., cact., calc., cann-i., ***chel., croc.,*** cupr., hell., iris-t., kali-c., ***lach.,*** lac-d., lyc., mag-p., med., merc., ***nit-ac.,*** nux-v., petr., ***plat.,*** podo., rhus-t., stram., ***thuj., xan.***
heart trouble with rheumatism, in - ***cact.***
time has come to - ars., bell., lach., med., sabad., thuj.
walking while, thinks he will have a fit or die, which makes him walk faster - ***arg-n.***
would, and soon be dissected - cann-i.

DIMENSIONS of things, disturbed - agar., calc., ***cann-i.,*** cann-s., onos., plat., stram.
enlarged - agar., ***arg-n.,*** atro., bov., ***cann-i., gels.,*** glon., ***hyos.,*** op., par.
reversed - camph-br.
smaller - cann-i., cinnam., grat., lac-c., plat., sabad., sulph.

DIMINISHED - cann-i., cinnam., grat., lac-c., plat., sabad., sulph.
abdomen has fallen in - sabad.
body, whole, is - agar.
everything in room is, while she is tall and elevated - plat.
left side of body is smaller - cinnam.
short - lac-c.
shrunken, parts are - ***sabad.***
small - grat.
thin, is too - thuj.

DIRT, eating - verat.

DIRTY, that he is - ***lac-c.,*** lycps., rhus-t., ***thuj.,*** syph.
everything is, that - cur.

DISABLED, that she is - cit-v.

DISEASE, incurable, has - acon., alum., ***arg-n.,*** arn., ***ars.,*** cact., chel., ***ign.,*** lac-c., ***lach., lil-t.,*** mag-c., nit-ac., plb., ***sabad.,*** stann.
deaf, dumb and has cancer - verat.
every disease, that he has - ***aur-m.,*** stram.
heart disease - calc., ***kali-ar.***
unrecognized, has an - ars., nit-ac., raph.

DISGRACED, that she is - plat., sarr., staph., sulph.
he has disgraced the family of his absent friends - sarr.

DISORDER, objects appear in - glon., op.

DISSECTED, that he will be - cann-i.

DISTANCES - cann-i., cann-s., nux-m.

DISTINGUISHED - phos., stram., verat.

DIVIDED, or cut in two - bell., plat., stram.
and could not tell of which part he had possession on waking - thuj.
into two parts - ***bapt.,*** bell., cann-i., lil-t., petr., puls., sil., stram., thuj.

DIVINE, thinks he is - cann-i., glon., stram., ***verat.***

DIVISION between himself and others - nat-c., plat.

DOCTORS, thought three were coming - sep.

DOGS, sees - ***aeth.,*** arn., aur., **BELL.,** ***calc.,*** calc-ar., calc-sil., lyc., merc., puls., sil., ***stram.,*** sulph., verat., zinc.
attack him - **STRAM.**
biting his chest - stram.
black - ***bell.,*** puls.
he is a dog, growls and barks - bell., lyss.
others are dogs, barks at them to be understood - ***stram.***
swarm about him - bell., ***calc.,*** stram.

DOLLS, people appeared like - plb.

DOOMED, being - acon., ars., **AUR.,** bell., cycl., hell., hyos., ***ign., kali-br., kali-p., lach., lil-t.,*** lyc., med., meli., nat-m., op., ***plat.,*** psor., puls., stram., sulph., ***verat.***
alcoholics, in - aur., ***lach.***
expiate her sins and those of her family, to - ***lil-t.***

DOOMED, being
soul cannot be saved, cries and rages - aur., ***ign.***

DOOR, that some one was coming in at the, at night - con.

DOUBLE, of being - alum., arg-n., **ANAC.,** anh., arg-n., ***bapt.,*** cann-i., ***cann-i.,*** cann-s., cycl., ***gels.,*** glon., lach., lil-t., lyc., mosch., nat-m., ***nux-m.,*** op., ***petr.,*** phos., **PLAT.,** plb., psor., puls., pyrog., sec., sil., ***stram.,*** ther., thuj., ***trill.,*** valer., xan.
head and pairs of limbs are - sulfon.
nose, has a double - merl.
objects are - ***anh.,*** zinc.
one limb is - petr.
sensations present themselves in a double form - cann-i.

DRAGGED, from the lowest abyss of darkness, at night, on waking - thea.

DRAGONS, of - op.

DREAM, as if in a - ***anac.,*** **CANN-I.,** med., ***nux-m.***

DREAMING, when awake, imagines himself - bell.

DRINKING - bell.

DRIVING, sheep - acon.
peacocks - hyos.

DUMB, thinks he is - verat.

DYING, that he is - apis, cann-i., nux-v., rhus-t., stram.

EAT, she must not - kali-m.
cannot - myric.

ELDERLY, men, in, rags are as fine as silk - **SULPH.**
sees elderly men - laur.

ELEVATED, bed were raised - canth., lac-c.
air, in - asar., nit-ac.
carried to an elevation - oena.

EMACIATION - ***anh.,*** nat-m., sabad., sulph., ***thuj.***

EMPEROR, thought himself an - cann-i.
talked of - carb-s.

ENCAGED, in wires - cact., ***cimic.***

ENCHANTMENT, of - coff-t.

ENEMY, everyone is an, (see Schizophrenia) - lach., meli., ***merc.,*** plat.
surrounded by - ***anac.,*** carb-s., ***crot-h.,*** lach., ***merc.***
under the bed, is - am-m.
wait for an, lying in - alco.

ENGAGED, in some occupation, is - acon., ars., atro., bell., cann-i., cupr., hyos., lyss., plb., rhus-t., stram., verat.
ordinary occupation, in - ars., atro., bell., plb., stram.

ENLARGED - acon., alum., aran., arg-n., asaf., bapt., bell., berb., bov., caj., **CANN-I.,** coc-c., euph., glon., hyos., laur., nat-c., nux-v., ***op.,*** pic-ac., ***plat.,*** sabad., stram., zinc.
body is - mim-p.

ENLARGED,
body, parts of - alum., hyos., op., pic-ac., stram.
chin is - glon., sabad.
distances are - acon., agar., ***arg-n.,*** atro., bov., camph., **CANN-I.,** cann-s., ***gels.,*** glon., ***hyos.,*** nux-m., op., par., stann.
eye-lashes are - cann-i.
eyes are - bell., op.
forearm is - aran.
head is - acon., ***bapt.,*** berb., ***bov.,*** cann-i., ***gels.,*** glon., kali-ar., mang., nux-m., ***par.,*** pip-m., ***plat.,*** zinc.
objects are - acon., agar., ***anh., arg-n.,*** atro., bov., **CANN-I.,** ***gels.,*** glon., ***hyos.,*** op., par.
diminished, and, letters are - ***anh.***
one leg is longer - cann-i.
persons are - cann-i., caust.
scrotum is swollen - sabad.
tall, very, is - op., pall., plat., staph., stram.

ENTERING, someone is - con.

EPILEPSY, fancies he has - atro.

ETERNITY, lived an, he has - ether.
that he was in eternity - cann-i.

EVENING - bry., lach., lyc., sulph.
bed, in - alum., ambr., ***calc.,*** camph., carb-an., ***carb-v.,*** chin., graph., ign., merc., nat-c., nit-ac., nux-v., ph-ac., rhus-t., sulph.
falling asleep, on - bell., calc., guai., phos.

EXCITED - coff.

EXECUTE him, people want to - ***op.***

EXECUTIONER, visions of an - stram.

EXISTENCE, doubt if anything had - agn.
doubted his own - cann-i.
without form in vast space - cann-i.

EXISTENCES, to have two - cann-i.

EXPANDING, thought passers-by were - cann-i.

EXPERIENCED, before, thought everything had been - kali-br.

EYELASHES, prolonged - cann-i.

EYES, falling out - crot-c.
big eyes, of - ***lac-c.,*** op., ***puls.***

FACES, sees - ***ambr.,*** apis, arg-n., ars., aur., **BELL.,** ***calc.,*** calc-sil., cann-i., carb-an., carb-v., caust., cham., ***cupr.,*** kali-c., ***lac-c.,*** laur., med., merc., ***nux-v.,*** **OP.,** phos., samb., stry., ***sulph., tarent.***
closing eyes, on - aeth., anh., ***arg-n.,*** ars., **BELL.,** ***bry.,*** **CALC.,** carb-v., caust., chin., euphr., ***op.,*** samb., sulph., ***tarent.***
dark, in the - chin., **LAC-C.**
dark, in the - chin., **LAC-C.**
diabolical, can't get rid of them - ambr.
crowd upon him - ***ambr.,*** carb-an., caust., ***tarent.***
cannot get rid of them - ambr.
distinguished people, of - cann-i.

FACES, sees
distorted - lac-c.
daytime, on lying down - ambr., arg-n., cupr., laur.
elongated, it - stram.
everybodies face in a glass except his own - anac.
grows larger - acon., aur.
hideous - ***ambr., bell.,*** **CALC.,** calc-sil., cann-i., carb-an., caust., ***kali-c.,*** lac-c., lyc., merc., nux-v., **OP.,** phos., stry., sulph., ***tarent.***
mask-like - anh., op.
mirror, in except his own - anac.
reaching the clouds - pic-ac.
ridiculous - cann-i.
scheming - anh.
stooping, when - ***nat-m.***
ugly faces seem pleasing - cann-i.
wherever he turns his eyes, or looking out from corners - aur., med., ***phos.***

FAIL, everything will - act-sp., ***arg-n., aur.,*** carc., merc., nux-v., sil.
as if things would - hyos., stram.

FAILURE, he is a - aur., carc., naja, staph., sulph.

FAINTNESS, of - mosch.

FALL, as if things would - hyos., stram.

FALLING, asleep - bell., bry., ***calc.,*** camph., chin., guai., ign., merc-ac., ph-ac., phos., spong., sulph.
bed, out of - ***arg-n., ars.,*** ars-s-f., ***crot-h.***
bed, falling through bed and through floor - benz.
forward, that she is - alum-sil., elaps, mosch., stram.
he is - stram.
height, from a - mosch.
hole, in a - carb-s.
pieces, to, she is - ***lac-c.***
walls are - arg-n., cann-i.
of room seem to fall inward, before epileptic fit - carb-v., lyss.

FAMILY, does not belong to her own - plat.

FANCY, illusions of (see Fancies) - ***acon., aeth.,*** agar., alum., ***ambr.,*** anac., ang., anh., ant-c., ant-t., apis, arn., ***ars.,*** ars-i., ***aur.,*** bar-c., bar-i., ***bell.,*** berb., bism., bry., bufo, calc., calc-ar., calc-p., calc-sil., camph., **CANN-I.,** cann-s., canth., carb-an., carb-s., carb-v., caust., cham., chin., chin-a., chin-s., cic., ***cina, cocc.,*** coff., colch., coloc., con., croc., ***crot-c.,*** cupr., dig., dros., dulc., euphr., ***fl-ac.,*** graph., hell., hep., **HYOS., IGN.,** indg., iod., kali-ar., ***kali-br.,*** kali-c., ***kali-p.,*** kali-sil., lac-c., **LACH.,** led., lyc., ***lyss., mag-m.,*** mag-s., ***merc.,*** nat-c., ***nit-ac., nux-m.,*** nux-v., ***op.,*** par., ph-ac., phos., ***plat.,*** plb., puls., rheum, rhod., ***rhus-t., sabad.,*** samb., sec., sep., sil., spong., stann., ***staph.,*** **STRAM.,** sul-i., **SULPH.,** ***tarent.,*** thuj., valer., verat., verb., viol-o., visc., zinc., zinc-p.
air, amel. in open - ***plat.***
chill, during - kali-c., nit-ac., phos., sulph.
evening, in bed - calc., hell.
eyes, on closing - calc., led., sep.

FANCY, illusions of
heat, during - carb-v., hyos., mag-m., merc., phos., samb., stram.
sleep, on going to - puls.

FASTING - brom., euphr., iod.
afternoon - iod.

FEET, touching scarcely the ground - dat-a.
separated from body, are - stram.
walking, when - peti.

FEVER, during - bell., calc.

FIERY - bell.

FIGHTING, that people are - op., stram.

FIGURES, sees - acon., agar., anac., anh., ***bell.,*** bry., ***calc.,*** carb-v., chin., cic., cimic., cina, coca, cocc., cupr., hell., ***hyos.,*** kali-p., nat-c., nit-ac., nux-m., ***op.,*** ph-ac., plb., rhus-t., sant., sec., spong., ***stram.,*** sulph., tarent., valer.
closing eyes for sleep, as soon as - chin.
gigantic - atro.
hurled bottle, at - chlol., chlor.
large black, about to jump on him - mosch.
marching in the air, evening while half asleep - nat-c.
sleep, during - kali-c.
strange figures accompany him, one on his right, the other on his left - ***anac.***

FINGERS, cut off - mosch.

FINGER-nails, seem as large plates during drowsiness - cann-i.

FIRE, visions of - alum., am-m., anac., ant-t., ars., ***bell., calc.,*** calc-ar., calc-p., clem., croc., daph., ***hep.,*** kali-n., kreos., laur., lyss., mag-m., mez., nat-m., phos., plat., ***puls.,*** rhod., rhus-t., spig., spong., stann., stram., sulph., zinc., zinc-p.
distant home, on - bell.
every noise is a cry of fire, she thinks, and she trembles - bar-c.
flash, passing through him - **PHOS.**
head is surrounded by - am-m.
home, on distant - bell.
house, on - bell., hep., stram.
neighbor's house on, morning, waking in a fright - hep.
room is on - stram.
world is on - ***hep.,*** puls., verat.

FISHES, flies, etc. - bell., ***stram.***

FIT, thinks she will have a fit and walks faster - ***arg-n.***

FLASH, passing through him - **PHOS.**

FLATUS, everyone notices his - zinc-p.

FLIES, sees - lyc.

FLOATING, in air - ***acon.,*** agar., ***ambr.,*** anh., ***arg-m.,*** arn., ***asar.,*** bell., calc-ar., camph., cann-i., canth., chlf., ***euon.,*** hura, hyos., kali-br., **LAC-C.,** ***lach.,*** nat-m., ***nux-m., op.,*** phos., **SPIG.,** ***stach.,*** stict., ter., thuj., valer., visc.
bed - bell., stram.
is not resting in - ***lach.,*** stict.
suspended in - bell., stram.

FLOATING, in the air
evening - bell.
eyes, on closing - pen.
maze, in a wavy - keroso.
walking, while - asar.

FLOWERS, of gigantic - cann-i.

FLUID, etheral, surrounded by, resisting passage - cann-i.

FLYING, away, what he holds in his hands - coloc., dulc., **STAPH.**
sensation of - asar., bell., camph., ***cann-i.,*** euon., lach., oena., op.
from a rock into dark abyss, on going to bed - cann-i.
skin, out of his - thuj.

FOOLISH - ***bell.,*** cann-i., hyos., merc-ac., nux-v.

FOOTSTEPS, hears - canth., carb-v., crot-c., nat-p.
behind him - crot-c.
room, in next - nat-p.

FOREHEAD, she must look out under - ph-ac.

FORTUNE, that he was going to lose his - psor., staph.

FOUL, everything appears - cur.

FOWLS, sees - stram.

FRAGMENTS, being broken in, scattered about - ***bapt.,*** daph., ***petr.,*** phos., stram.

FRIEND, thinks she is about to lose a - hura.
affection of, has lost the - ***aur.,*** hura, hyos.
he had never seen them - stram.
met with an accident - ars.
offended - ars.
surrounded by, shaking hands and calling them by name - ***hydr-ac.***

FRIENDLESS, that he is - mag-m., sars.

FRIGHT, after - bell., ***op.,*** plat.

FRIGHTENED, being, by a mouse running from under a chair - ***aeth., cimic.,*** lac-c.

FURNITURE, imagines it to be persons, night on waking - nat-p.

GALLOWS, vision of, with fear of - ***bell.***

GATHERING objects from pictures and walls, making efforts at - bell.

GEESE, sees - hyos.
threw themselves into water, thinking themselves to be geese - con.

GENERAL, that he is a - cupr.

GHOSTS, spectres, spirits, sees - acon., agar., alum., ambr., am-c., ant-t., ***ars.,*** ars-m., atro., aur., **BELL.,** bov., brom., ***camph.,*** carb-v., cocc., ***cupr., cupr-ac.,*** dulc., hell., hep., hura, ***hyos.,*** hyper., ign., ***kali-br.,*** kali-c., kali-sil., lach., lepi., lyc., merc., ***nat-c., nat-m.,*** nit-ac., ***op.,*** phos., phys., plat., puls., sars., sep., sil., spig., ***stram., sulph.,*** tarent., thuj., verb., visc., zinc.
bed, in - atro.
behind him - lach.
black forms when dreaming - arn., ars., puls.

GHOSTS, spectres, spirits, sees
chill during - nit-ac.
closing eyes, on - apis, arg-n., bell., ***bry., calc.,*** chin., ign., ***lach.,*** led., nat-m., samb., sep., spong., stram., ***sulph., thuj.***
clutches at - hyos.
conversing with, he is - nat-m., plat.
day and night - ***ars.***
death, of, as a gigantic black skeleton - crot-c.
evening, feels as if spectre would appear - brom.
fire, in - bell.
hovering in the air - aur., lach.
morning on waking, continues to enlarge until it disappears - dulc.
night, sees at - atro., merc.
pursued by, is - lepi., plat., stram.
sleep, in - camph.
throng upon him - ***psor.,*** verb.
twilight, in - berb.
waking, on - dulc., zinc.

GIANTS, sees - bell.

GIRAFFE, imagines himself to be a - cann-i.

GLASS, that she is made of - thuj.
wood, glass, etc. being made of - eupi., rhus-t., ***thuj.***

GLOW-worms, of - cann-i.

GNOME, being a - cann-i.

GOD, sees - ether.
is the object of god's vengeance - anac., kali-br.
that he is in communication with - anac., stram., verat.
he is, then he is devil - ***anac.,*** **STRAM.**

GOITRE, imagines he has a - indg.
has one which he cannot see over when sitting down - zinc.

GOOSE, that he is a - con.

GRAVE, that he is in his - anac., ***gels.,*** lepi., stram.

GREAT, person, is - ***agar.,*** aeth., alum., bell., ***cann-i.,*** cupr., glon., ***hyos., lach.,*** lyc., lyss., phos., ***plat.,*** stram., ***sulph., verat.***

GRIEF and anger, from - bell.

GRIMACES, sees - ambr., caust., cocc., ***op.,*** stram., sulph.
falling asleep, on - sulph.

GROANS, fancies he hears - ***crot-c.***
groans, with delusions - bell., ***cham.***

GROTESQUE - cann-i., plb., sulph.
people appear - hyos.

GROWING longer and longer - plat.

GROWLING, as of a bear - mag-m.

GUN, uses a stick for a - bell.

HALL, illusions of a gigantic hall - cann-i.

HALVES, left half does not belong to her - sil.

HAND, midnight vision of something taking her - canth.
felt a delicate, smoothing her head - med.
passes over body - carb-v.
separated from body - stram.
visions, of white, outspread, coming toward face in the darkness - benz.

HANDS, bound with chains - hyos.

HANGING, sees persons - ars.
wants to hang himself - ***ars.***
hanging, or standing high, seems as if - phos.
three feet from the ground, on falling asleep - hura

HAPPEN, that something terrible is going to - ***lyss.,*** pall.
happened anything, of having - calc., nux-v., ***staph.,*** sulph.

HAPPY, that he will never be, in his own house - ars.

HARLEQUIN, as if he were a - hyos.

HAPPY, that he will never be, in his own house - ars.

HAT, is a pair of trousers which he tries to put on - stram.

HEAD, belongs to another - alum., cann-i., cann-s., nat-m., ther., thuj.
can lift it off - ther.
caressed on, by someone - med.
cold breeze blows on - petr.
deceased acquaintances of, without bodies at night - nux-v.
disease will break out of head - stram.
fall off - nux-m.
friend's head stick out of a bottle, sees - bell.
heavy, his own seemed too - bry.
large, head seems too - acon., sil.
lift it off, can - ther.
monstrous, on distant wall of room - aur., cann-i.
pendulum, seems an inverted, oscillating - cann-i.
shaking the - bell., cham.
transparent and speckled brown - bell.

HEADS, large, make grimaces evening on closing eyes - euphr.
two, thinks she has - nux-m.

HEALTH, he has ruined his - ars., chel., thuj.

HEAR, he thinks he cannot - mosch., verat.

HEARING, of - absin., acon., agar., am-c., ***anac.,*** anh., ***antipyrin.,*** ars., atro., bell., calc., **CANN-I.,** cann-s., canth., carb-o., carb-s., carb-v., ***cham.,*** cocaine, coff., colch., con., coni., crot-c., dros., elaps, eup-pur., hyos., kali-ar., kali-br., mag-m., manc., med., merc., naja, nat-p., ph-ac., phos., puls., stram., thea.
objects moving - ph-ac.
talk seems distant - aran.

HEAR, he cannot - hyos., mosch., verat.

HEART, diseases, is going to have, and die - arn., ***kali-ar.,*** lac-c., lach., podo.
disease, has a heart - calc., graph., ***kali-ar., nat-c.,*** podo.
fluttering, like a bird's wings - nat-m.
stops beating when sitting - ***arg-n.***
too large - bov., lach.
turning around, is - aur.

HEAT, has a furious, radiating from epigastrium - cann-i.

HEAVEN, is in - cann-i., op., ***verat.***
talking with god - ***verat.***

HEAVY, is - nat-c., thuj.

HELL, is in - camph., cann-i., lyss., merc., ***orig.***
at gate of, and obliged to confess his sins - agar.
going to, because he has committed a unpardonable crime - med.
in shadows of, midnight, on waking - cann-i.
suffers the torments of, without being able to explain - lyss., merc.

HELP, calling for - plat.

HEMORRHAGE, after - chin-a.

HERBS, gathering - bell., cupr.

HIPOPOTAMUS, being oneself a - cann-i.

HOLE, small, appears like a frightful chasm - agar.

HOLLOW, being, organs, in - ***cocc.,*** oxyt.
whole body - aur., ***kali-c.,*** pall.

HOME, thinks is at, when not - cann-i., hyos.
everything at, has changed - arg-n.
thinks is away from - acon., ***aster.,*** bell., **BRY.,** calc., calc-p., cic., cimic., ***coff., hyos.,*** lach., meli., ***nux-v., op.,*** par., plb., **RHUS-T.,** valer., verat., vip.
must get there - ***bry.,*** calc-p., cimic., hyos., ***op.***

HONEST, he is not - ***stram.***

HORRIBLE, everything seems - ***plat.***

HORRID - lac-c.

HORSES, sees - bell., mag-m., zinc.
horseback, is on - cann-i.

HOUSE, is full of people - ars., cann-i., con., lach., lyc., merc., nat-m., nux-v., sil., stram.
movable, seems - cann-i.
place, is not in right, while walking in the street after headache - glon.
surrounded, is - stram.

HOUSES, on each side would approach and crush him - arg-n.

HUMILIATION, after - ***aur.,*** bell., nux-v., ***puls.,*** staph.

HUMILITY, and lowness of others, while he is great - plat., staph.

HUNTER, thinks he is a - cann-i., verat.

HUSBAND, neglecting her - stram.
thinks he is not her - ***anac.***

HYDROTHORAX, that he has - alco., ***phos.***

ICHTHYOSAURUS, seeing an - cann-i.

IDEAS, floating outside of brain - dat-a.

IDENTITY, errors of personal - ***alum.,*** anac., ant-c., bapt., cann-i., cann-s., cic., hyos., lac-c., lach., mosch., nat-m., petr., phos., plat., plb., pyrog., pyrus, stram., thuj., valer., ***verat.***
thinks she is someone else - anac., ***cann-i.,*** cann-s., gels., ***lach.,*** mosch., phos., plat., plb., pyrog., stram., ***valer., verat.***

IMAGES, sees, of phantoms - acon., alum., ***ambr., apis, arg-n., ars.,*** bar-c., **BELL.,** berb., brom., calc., calc-ar., calc-s., camph., ***cann-s.,*** canth., carb-an., ***carb-v.,*** caust., cham., chin., chin-a., cic., cimic., coca, ***crot-h.,*** cupr., dros., dulc., graph., hell., ***hep., hyos.,*** ign., kali-ar., kali-c., kali-br., kali-p., lac-c., **LACH.,** lachn., led., ***lyc.,*** mag-m., med., ***merc.,*** nat-c., ***nat-m.,*** nat-p., nit-ac., nux-m., nux-v., ***op.,*** ph-ac., ***phos.,*** plat., puls., rhod., rhus-t., ruta, ***samb.,*** sep., sil., spong., ***stram.,*** sulph., tab., ***tarent., thuj.,*** valer., verat., ***zinc.***
afternoon - lyc.
all over - merc., ***sil.***
alone, when - fl-ac., lach.
black - arn., ars., ***bell.,*** caust., op., plat., puls., **STRAM.**
closing the eyes, on - anh., ***arg-n.,*** bell., **CALC.,** ***caust.,*** graph., nat-m., puls., samb., sep., ***sil.,*** sulph., ***tarent., thuj.***
in bed - cupr., samb., sulph.
dark, in the - ***bell., carb-v.,*** hell., petr., puls., stram.
disappearing and reappearing - nit-ac.
dozing during day, sees images, while - lachn.
dwells upon - arn., nux-m., sil.
evening - calc., carb-an., lyc., nit-ac.
in bed - nit-ac.
ever changing - carb-o.
past to present - mur-ac.
frightful - ***ambr.,*** anac., arg-n., arn., ars., atro., bar-c., ***bell.,*** **CALC.,** calc-s., camph., ***carb-an., carb-v., caust.,*** chin., chin-a., cina1, coca, con., croc., graph., gels., ***hep.,*** hyos., ign., kali-ar., ***kali-br.,*** kali-c., ***kali-p.,*** kali-sil., ***lac-c., lach.,*** laur., lyc., mang., ***merc.,*** mur-ac., nat-c., nat-p., nit-ac., nux-v., **OP.,** petr., ph-ac., ***phos.,*** puls., rhod., rhus-t., samb., sars., sec., sil., spong., ***stram.,*** sulph., tab., tarent.
night, while trying to sleep - calc-s., sil.
increasing and decreasing, sees - nit-ac.
moving up and down - zinc.
night - acon., ambr., arg-n., arn., bell., berb., calc., calc-sil., ***camph.,*** canth., carb-an., carb-v., cham., chin., crot-h., cupr., cur., graph., ign., ***kali-br.,*** kali-c., kali-sil., led., lyc., ***merc.,*** nat-m., nit-ac., nux-v., op., phos., puls., ***sep.,*** sil., spong., tab., ***thuj.,*** valer., zinc., zinc-p.
pleasant - bell., cann-i., cycl., ***lach.***
rising out of the earth - stram.
running, sees - nit-ac.

IMAGES, sees, of phantoms
sees, all over - merc., ***sil.***
side, at his - stram.
sleep, during - lyc.
before - carb-an., merc., nit-ac., sep.
hateful, during - lyc.
on going to - carb-an., chin., nat-m.
preventing - alum., arg-n., lyc., op., tab.
twilight, in - berb.
wall, on the - lyc., samb.

IMMORTALITY, of - anh.

INANIMATE, objects are persons - bell., calc., nat-p., stram.

INCUBUS, being weighed down by - cer-b.

INFERIOR, on entering house after a walk, people seem mentally and physically - ***plat.***

INFLUENCE, is under a powerful ***anac.,*** cer-b., ***lach., stram.***

INJURED, being - bry., cact., canth., elaps, kali-br., lach., lyss., phos., rhus-t., stram., sulph.
head, to the - naja.
surroundings, by his - ***hyos., lach.,*** naja.

INJURY, receive, is about to - arn., ars., bell., cann-i., carb-s., con., hyos., lach., lyc., merc., nux-v., ***op.,*** sil., stram., sulph.
his fingers and toes are being cut off - mosch.

INKSTAND, fancied he saw one on bed - lact.
he was one - cann-i.

INSANE, that she will become - ***acon.,*** alum., ambr., ars., **CALC., CANN-I.,** cann-s., ***chel.,*** chlor., **CIMIC.,** colch., ham., kali-br., lac-c., lam., lil-t., ***manc.,*** **MED.,** merc., nat-m., nux-v., pall., phys., plat., psor., ***syph.,*** tanac., tarent.
that people think her - **CALC.**

INSECTS, sees - **ARS., BELL.,** caust., dig., hyos., ***lac-c.,*** merc., phos., plb., puls., ***stram.,*** tarent.
shining - bell.

INSULTED, thinks he is - alco., bell., cham., ign., kali-br., lac-c., lyss., nux-v., ***pall.,*** puls., staph., tarent.
boarders in hotel, by - kali-br.

INSULTING, with - lyc.

IODINE, illusions of fumes of - iod.

ISLAND, is on a distant - phos.

JEALOUSY, with - ***hyos., lach.,*** stram.
lovers concealed behind stove, wife has - lach., ***stram.***

JELLY, as made of - ***eupi.***

JOURNEY, that he is on a - bell., brom., cann-i., cann-s., crot-h., hyos., lach., mag-m., nat-c., op., sang., sil.

JUGGLER, thinks himself a - bell.

JUMPED, up on the ground before her, all sorts of things - brom., ther.

KNEES, that he walks on - ***bar-c.,*** bar-m.

KNOWLEDGE, thought he possessed infinite - cann-i.

LABOR, pretends to be in, or thinks she has pains - verat.

LARGE, people seemed too during vertigo - caust., ***cham., trom., tub.***
parts of body seem too - acon., alum., aran., bov., ***hyos.,*** nux-m., op., pic-ac., stram.
grow too large - kali-br.
self seemed too - op., pyrog., staph., stram.
on entering the house after walking - plat.
surroundings seemed - ferr.

LASCIVIOUS - ambr., bell., calc., sil., ***stram.,*** verb.

LAUGHED, at, imagines she is - ***bar-c., ign.,*** nux-v., ***ph-ac., sep.***

LAUGHTER, with - op., sep., ***stram., verat.***

LAWSUIT, being engaged in a - ***nit-ac.***

LEG, tin case filled with stair rods, is - cann-i.

LEGS, conversing, are - bapt.
conversing, are, toe is conversing with thumb - ***bapt.***
cut off, are - bapt, bar-c., stram., tarent.
don't belong to her - ***agar., bapt.,*** op., sumb.
four, has - ***sulfon.***
three, has - petr., stram.
too long - cann-i.

LIE, thinks all she said is a - lac-c.

LIFE, careering from life to life - cann-i.
is threatened - kali-br.
symbols of, all past events revolve rapidly on wheels - cann-i.

LIFTED up, sensation as if - hyper., phos., stront.
sleep, during - stroph.

LIGHT, on falling to sleep, thinks there is too much in room - ambr.
incorporal, he is - agar., ***asar., cann-i., coff., croc.,*** dig., lac-c., lact., mez., op., phos., ***stict.,*** stram., thuj., valer., zinc.

LIMBS, separated from body, are - bapt., stram.
crooked - sabad.
four or eight, has - ***sulfon.***
many - pyrog.
not his own - agar., bapt., coll., ign., op.
talking together - bapt.

LIP, lower is swollen - glon.

LIVING, under ordinary relations, thinks is not - cic.

LOCOMOTIVE, imagines himself to be - cann-i.

LONGER, things seem - berb., camph., dros., kreos., nit-ac., sulph., zinc.
chin seems too long - glon.
one leg is long - cann-i.

LOOKED, down upon, that she is - ***lac-c.***

LOOKING, at her, that everyone is - aq-mar., **ARS.,** ***bar-c., calc., hyos.,*** meli., rhus-t.

LOST, fancies herself - ars., ***aur.,*** hell., hura, plb.
waking, on - aesc.
predestination, from - ***lach.***

LOW down, things beneath him seem - staph.

LUDICROUS - calc., cann-i., hyos., ***nux-m.,*** sulph.
antics - ***bell.,*** cic.

LYING, near him, fancies some one is - petr.
crosswise - stram.

MACHINE, thinks he is working a - plb.

MAELSTROM, seemed carried down a psychical - cann-i.

MAGICIAN, is a - bell.

MAN, in the room intending to perforate his throat with a gimlet - merc-i-f.
does all the things he does - ars.
elderly men with long beards and distorted faces, sees - laur.
naked man in bed - ***puls.***
same man walking after him that he sees walking before him - euph.
thinks men are on the bed at night - merc.
who hung himself, saw - ars.

MANDARIN, mistook friend for a - cann-i.

MARBLE, statue, felt as if he were - cann-i.

MARRIAGE, must dissolve - fl-ac.

MARRIED, that he is - ign.
is going to be - hyos.

MASKS, sees - bell., kali-c., ***op.***
laughing - ***bell.***

MELANCHOLY - alum., ***aur.,*** **KALI-BR.,** murx., nux-v., plat.
night, while half awake at - nux-v.

MELTING, away, sensation of, worse from change, better in recumbent position - sumb.

MESMERIZED, that she is, by her absent pastor - meli.

MICE, sees - ***aeth.,*** bell., ***calc., cimic.,*** colch., hyos., lac-c., lach., mag-s., med., op., stram.
running from under a chair - ***aeth., cimic.,*** lac-c.

MIND, and body separated - anac., sabad., thuj.
as if they would lose their - kali-br.

MISFORTUNE, inconsolable over fancied - calc-s., lil-t., ***verat.***

MONEY, as if counting - alum., bell., cycl., mag-c., zinc.
money, sewed up in clothing, is - kali-br.
talks of - calc., carb-s.

MORNING - bry., con.
bed, in - ambr., dulc., hell., hep., nat-c.

MOTION, all parts being in - anac., canth., kreos., ***op.,*** stram.
bed and ground, of - clem.
chair and table in different directions, of - chlf.
up and down, of - lach, plb., ***spong.***

MOUNTAIN, thought himself to be on the ridge of a - cann-i.

MOUTH, fancied living things were creeping into, at night - merc.
cannot open, lower jaw stiff and painful - lyss.
puts stones into - merc.

MOVE, hears things that are high up near him out of sight - canth., carb-v., ph-ac., phos.

MURDER, thinks she is about to, her husband and child - jab., kali-br.
family with a hatchet, that she will - jab., piloc.
someone, that he has to - anac., ars., hyos., lach.

MURDERED, that he would be - absin., am-m., ***bell., carc., hep., hyos.,*** ign., kali-br., kali-c., lact., lyc., mag-c., merc., ***op.,*** phos., plb., ***rhus-t.,*** staph., ***stram.,*** verat., zinc.
conspiring to murder him, are - ars., plb.
sees some one - calc.
someone, had - ars., phos.
that every one around him is a murderer - ***plb.***
he was killed, roasted and eaten - stram.
thinks persons were bribed to murder him - cann-i.
thought her mother had been - nux-v.

MUSHROOM, fancies he is commanded to fall on his knees and confess his sins and rip up his bowels by a - agar.

MUSIC, fancies he hears - anh., **CANN-I.,** croc., ether, ***lach.,*** lyc., merc., nat-c., plb., puls., sal-ac., ***stram.,*** thuj.
delightful - lach., plb., puls.
evening, hears the music heard in the day - lyc.
sweetest and sublimest melody - ***cann-i., lach.***
unearthly - cann-s., ether.

MUTILATED, bodies, sees - ant-c., arn., con., mag-m., merc., ***nux-v.,*** sep.

MYSTERY, everything around seemed a terrifying - cann-i.

MYSTIC, hallucinations - cann-i., ether., op.

NAKED, thinks is - stram.

NARROW, everything seems too - guai., plat.

NECK, is too large - kali-c.

NEEDLES, sees - merc., ***sil.***

NEGLECTED, his duty, that he has - ars., **AUR.,** cycl., hell., hyos., ign., ***lyc.,*** naja, nat-a., ptel., puls.
that he is - ***arg-n.,*** aur., naja, **PALL.,** puls.

NEW, everything is - stram.

NEWSPAPERS, thinks he sees - atro.

NIGHT - ***acon.,*** aeth., arn., ars., aur., ***bell., bry.,*** camph., cann-i., canth., carb-v., carl., cham., chin-a., coloc., con., dig., ***dulc.,*** kali-c., lyc., meny., ***merc.,*** nit-ac., nux-v., op., ***plb., puls., rheum,*** sec., sep., sol-n., sulph., tub., vip.

NOBLE, thinks he is a - phos., plat.

NOISE, hears - anh., bell., calc., ***cann-i.,*** carb-v., cham., coff., colch., con., hyos., mag-m., ph-ac., sulph., verat.
bed, under - bell.
clattering above the bed when falling asleep - calc.
knocking at door - ant-c.
under bed - calc., canth.
making a, delusions with - verat.
of shout, vehicles - ***cann-i.***

NOSE, has a transparent - bell.
has some one else's - lac-c.
takes people by - merc.
two noses, has - merl.

NUMB, being - alum.

NUMERAL, appeared nine inches long, night, on waking, better lying on other side - sulph.

NURSING, her child, that she was - atro.

NUTS, cracking - hyos.

OBJECTS, brilliantly colored - anh., bell., camph.
air, in open - atro.
animals, are - hyos.
appear different - nat-m.
on closing eyes - scroph-n.
blood covered - stront-c.
bright, from - anh., **STRAM.**
bright, of - canth.
crooked - glon.
different - nat-m.
flight from - **STRAM.**
glittering - bell.
immaterial, in room - ***cupr-ac.,*** lyss.
large - nux-m.
motion, in - ***anh.,*** phos.
new, all seem - hell., stram.
numerous in room, too - phys.
open air, in - atro.
seize, tries to - ars., atro., bell, hyos., oena.
sometimes thick, sometimes thin, on closing eye in slumber - camph.

OBSCENE - stram.
actions of which she had not been guilty, accuses herself - ***phos.***

OBSTRUCTED, being - ***chin.***

OFFENDED people, that he has - **ARS., HYOS.,** nit-ac.

OFFICER, that he is an - agar., bell., cann-i., ***cupr.,*** cupr-ac.

OLD men, sees - laur.
rags are as fine as silk - **SULPH.**

OPPOSED by everyone - mosch.

OUTSIDE his body, someone else saw or spoke - alum.

PARADISE, thought he saw - cann-i., coff.

PAINS, during sleep, he has - alum.

PARALYZED, being - syph.

PASS, cannot, a certain point - kali-br.

PAST, of events long - atro., hyos., op.
anxious thoughts and things past seem present - staph.

PEACOCKS, as if chasing - hyos.
frightening away - hyos.

PEOPLE, behind him, someone is - anac., bell., brom., calc., casc., cench., crot-c., crot-h., lach., led., mag-m., ***med.,*** ruta, sac-alb., sac-l., sanic., staph., sil., tub.
walking - calc.
fast, when - staph.
dark, in the - ferr., sanic., ***staph.***

PEOPLE, beside him, are - anac., apis, ***ars.,*** atro., bell., calc., camph., carb-v., cench., nux-v., petr., thuj., valer.
doing as he does - ***ars.***

PEOPLE, sees - anac., ***ars.,*** atro., ***bell.,*** brom., ***bry.,*** chin., con., ***hyos.,*** kali-c., lyc., lyss., mag-c., mag-s., med., merc., nat-m., op., petr., plb., ***puls.,*** rheum, sep., ***stram.,*** sulph., thuj., valer., verat.
closing eyes, on - ars., ***bell.,*** bry., **CHIN.,** nat-m.
converses, with absent - agar., aur., bell., calc., crot-c., dig., hyos., lach., op., ***stram.,*** thuj., ***verat.***
day and evening - lyc.
disagreeable, sees - calc-ar., calc-sil.
elderly, men, sees - laur.
entering the house at night - con.
front of him, in - con.
looking at him - bar-c., med., rhus-t.
night, at - med.
morning on waking - sulph.
noise, making - puls.
persons are looking at him - rhus-t.
prank with him, carry on all sorts of - **NUX-V.**
questions and he must answer, ply him with - **NUX-V.**
say "come" - med.
seize them, sees a number of strangers and tries to - stram.
threatening her, screams horrible - ars-m.

PERSECUTED, that he is, (see Schizophrenia) - abrot., absin., ***anac.,*** ars., aur., ***bell.,*** calc., **CHIN.,** cic., ***cocaine,*** con., crot-h., cupr., cycl., **DROS.,** hell., ***hyos.,*** **IGN.,** kali-br., **LACH.,** lyc., med., meli., merc., nat-c., nat-m., ***nux-v.,*** op., plb., puls., ***rhus-t.,*** sil., spong., staph., stram., stry., ***sulph.*** syph., thyr., verat., ***zinc.***

PERSON, that something hanging over chair is a, sitting there - calc.
another person in the room - anac., brom., cann-i., con., lyc.
waking, on - mag-p.
same person in front and behind - euph.
thinks she is some other - alum., cann-s., gels., ***lach.,*** mosch., phos., plb., syph., valer., verat.
three persons, that he is - ***nux-m.***

PIGEONS, flying in room which he tries to catch - ***kali-c.***

PINS, about - **NUX-M., SIL.,** spig.

PITIED, on account of his misfortune and he wept, he is - ***nat-m.***

PLACE, that he cannot pass a certain - ***arg-n.,*** kali-br.

PLACES, of being in different - cann-i., ***lyc.,*** plb., raph.
at night, on waking thought to find himself in strange and solitary - par.
two places, of being in, at the same time - ***cench., lyc., sil.***
wrong, in - hyos.

PLEASING - atro., cann-i., op., stram.
morning, after sleep - bell.

POISON, of - cocc.

POISONED, thought he had been - ars., caj., cimic., culx., ***hyos., lach.,*** plat-m., rhus-t., verat-v.
medicine or remedies are being - lach.
that he was about to be - ***hyos.,*** kali-br., lach., plb., **RHUS-T.,** verat-v.

POLICEMAN, called on him, officers - ***cupr.***
come into house, thought he saw - hyos., kali-br.
that physician is a - bell.

POOR, thinks he is - bell., calc-f., hep., mez., nux-v., ***sep.,*** stram., valer.

POSITION, she is not fitted for her - stram.

POSSESSED, as if - **ANAC.,** bell., canth., ***hyos.,*** man., op., ***plat.,*** sil., **STRAM.,** ***sulph.,*** verat.
as if, devil, by a - **ANAC.,** ***hyos.,*** ***plat.,*** **STRAM.**

POWER, over all disease, has - ***stram.***

PREGNANT, thought herself - apis, caul., ***croc.,*** cycl., ign., nux-v., ***op.,*** puls., ***sabad.,*** sulph., thuj., ***verat.***
thought herself, if there is distention of flatus - ign.

PRESENT, some one is - hyos., lyc., thuj.

PRESUMPTUOUS - lyc.

PRINCE, is a - verat.

PROSTRATION, cannot endure such utter - ***chin-a.***

PROUD - lach., plat., stram., verat.

PUMP-log, he was a - cann-i.

PURE, that she is - ***stram.***

PURSUED, thought he was - absin., ***anac.,*** ars., aur., bell., bry., con., cycl., dros., ***hyos., kali-br.,*** lach., med., plb., rhus-t., sil., ***staph.,*** stram., thuj., verat-v.
animals, by - nux-v.
enemies, by - absin., ***anac.,*** ars., aur., ***bell., chin.,*** cic., ***cocaine,*** con., crot-h., cupr., cycl., dros., hell., ***hyos.,*** kali-br., ***lach.,*** lepi., lyc., med., meli., merc., nat-c., nux-v., plb., ***puls.,*** rhus-t., sil., stram., stry., zinc.
fiends, by - plb.
ghosts, by - lepi., plat., stram.
murderers, robbers, by - alco.

PURSUED, thought he was
police, by - alco., ars., bell., ***cupr., hyos.,*** lach., ***kali-br.,*** meli., phos., plb., zinc.
robbing a friend, for - kali-br.
soldiers, by - absin., bell., bry., nat-c., plb.
some horrid thing - anac.
tormented by a frightful scene of some mournful event of the past, and - spong.

QUEEN, thinks she is - cann-i., plat.

RABBITS, sees - stram.

RAGS, as fine as silk - **SULPH.**
body torn into - phyt.

RAILWAY, train, thought he was obliged to go off by - atro.

RAIN, from having wet cloth on head, thought he had been out in - atro.

RANK, thinks himself a person of - cupr., phos., verat.

RATS, feels, running up legs - ail., ***calc.***

RATS, sees - ***aeth., ars.,*** bell., calc., ***cimic.,*** colch., hyos., med., op., stram.
all colors - absin.
running across the room - ***aeth.,*** ail., ars., cimic., med.
large, at night - med.

READING, after her, some one is, which makes her read the faster - mag-m.

REASON and sense, must lose - alum., ambr., ***calc.,*** cann-s., chel., chlor., ***cimic.,*** kali-br., ***lil-t.,*** manc., med., merc., nat-m., nux-v., plat.

RELIGIOUS - ***anac., ars.,*** aur., bell., croc., ***hyos., kali-br.,*** lach., lyc., med., merc., nux-v., plat., ***puls., stram., sulph., verat.***

REPROACH, has neglected duty and deserves - ***aur.***

REPUDIATED, by relatives, thinks is - arg-n., hura.

REPULSIVE, fantastic imaginations - ***fl-ac.***

RESIN, exuding from every pore - cann-s.

RIDING, an ox - bell.
a horse - cann-i.

RIGHT, does nothing - anac., arg-n., ***aur.,*** nat-c.

RISING, then falling, of - bar-c., lach.

ROAMING, in the fields - rhus-t.

ROBBED, is going to be - bar-c., bor., caust., nat-m., sep.

ROBBERY, had committed a - carb-s.

ROCKS in air - mag-m.

ROOM, garden, is a - calc.
foam, is like the, of a troubled sea, is - sec.
people in, sees at bedside - atro., con.
sees on entering - lyc.
walls, of, seem gliding together - cann-i.
sees horrible things on the - bell., cann-i., hyos., samb.
that the, will crush him - ***arg-n.***

RUINED, thinks that he is - calc., **IGN.,** verat.

SATYRS, vision of dancing - cann-i.

SAW, thought he was a huge, darting up and down - cann-i.

SAYS, something, it seems as if someone else has said it - alum.

SCALP, too small - stict.

SCORPIONS, sees - **OP.**

SCRATCHING, on linen or similar substance, thought some one was - asar.

SCREAM, with - canth., hyos., ***stram.,*** verat.
obliging to - ars., kali-c., plat., puls., stram.

SCROTUM, thinks his, is swollen - sabad.

SEASICK, that he is - der.

SEE, cannot - hyos., stram., verat.

SEES, thinks some one else sees for him - alum.

SEIZED, as if - canth., ***hyos.,*** phos.
thoughts are - sabad.

SENSATIONS, misrepresents his - bell.

SEPARATED, from the world, that he is - ***anac., anh., plat.,*** thuj.

SERPENT, a crimson, fastening on his neck - bell.

SERVANTS, thinks he must get rid of - fl-ac.

SEWING, imagines herself to be - atro.

SHEEP, sees - ***cimic.***
is driving - acon.

SHINING objects, of - canth.

SHIP, thinks they are on board of, in a storm - alco.

SHOOT, tries to, with a cane - bell., merc.

SHOPPING, with her sister - atro.

SHOULDER, thinks people are looking over his - brom.

SHOUTING, fancies himself to be - cann-i.

SICK, imagines himself - arg-n., **ARS.,** bar-c., bell., **CALC.,** caust., graph., ***iod., kali-c.,*** lac-c., ***lyc.,*** mosch., murx., nat-c., nat-m., nit-ac., petr., phos., podo., psor., ***sabad., sep.,*** stram., syph., ***tarent., thuj.***
friend, a beloved, is sick and dying - bar-c.
members of the family are - hep.
someone else is - gels.
that he was going to be - nat-p., podo.
and for that reason he will not work - ***calc., caust.,*** **NUX-V.,** sep.
two sick people were in bed, one of whom got well and the other did not - sec.

SIDE, imagined himself alive on one side and buried on the other - stram.
right, she can feel every muscle and fibre of her - sep.
that she did not own her left - sil.

SIGHT, and hearing, of - ***cham.,*** stram., eup-pur.

SIGHT and hearing, of - anac., bell., **CANN-I.,** ***cham.,*** phos., stram., eup-pur.

SIN, unpardonable has been committed - stram.

SINGING, fancied himself to be - cann-i.

SINKING, to be - bapt., benz., kali-c., lyc.
through the floor - benz., hyos., phos.

SKELETONS, sees - crot-c., op.

SKULL being raised and lowered - stict.

SLEEPING, while awake, insists that he was - acon., alco.

SMALL, body, limbs - agar., cact., calc., carb-v., croc., glon., kreos., tab., tarent.
objects appear in motion, small - anh.
sensation of being smaller - acon., agar., alum-sil., calc., carb-v., sabad., tarent.
before epileptic fit - carb-v.
things appear - aur., hyos., nat-c., **PLAT.,** puls., ***staph.,*** stram., thuj.
grow smaller - agar., cact., camph., carb-v., nit-ac., plat., stram., tab.

SMELL, of - ***agn., anac.,*** ars., cic., cina, euph-a., ***lach., op.,*** par., **PULS.,** ***sep.,*** sulph., zinc-m.

SMOOTH, being - alum.

SNAKES, in and around her - ail., anh., arg-n., bell., calc., cench., cund., gels., ***hyos.,*** ign., **LAC-C.,** lach., lachn., op., phys., phyt., stram., tub., viol-o.
black - arg-n., cund.
crawling up her leg, feels a - ail.
white - gels., ign.

SODA, water, thinks he is a bottle of - ***arg-n.***

SOLD, as if would be - hyos.
his bed, some one has - nux-v.

SOLDIER, being a - chel.

SOLDIERS, sees - bar-c., ***bell.,*** bry., nat-c., op.
bed, on his - lact.
cutting him down, better on getting cool - bry.
half asleep, in - nat-c.
march silently past - cann-i.
air, in the - nat-c.
surrounded by - ***nat-c.***

SOMETHING, else, appeared as if, objects - staph.
comes from above and oppresses his chest - sep.

SOOT, shower of, fell on him - cann-i.

SORROW, thinks everyone he meets has a secret - cann-i.

SOUL, fancied body was too small for, or that it was separated from - ***anac.,*** cann-i., nit-ac., sabad., ***thuj.***

SOUNDS, listens to imaginary - cann-i., hyos.

SPACE, fancied he was carried into, while lying - cann-i., coca, ***lach.***
expansion of - cann-i., nux-m.
that there is empty, between brain and skull - caust.

SPECTRES, (see ghosts)

SPHERE, thought himself a - cann-i.

SPIDERS - ***lac-c.***

SPIED, being - lach.

SPINAL, column a barometer - cann-i.

SPINNING, is - hyos., stram.

SPIRIT, that he is a - cann-i.

SPOTTED, brown, his body is - bell.

SQUANDERS money - ***verat.***

SQUARE, fancies of a colossal, surrounded by houses a hundred stories high - cann-i.

STABBED, that he had, a person who passed him on the street - ***bell.***

STANDING, by oneself - anh.
on head, with bed tilted - ***ph-ac.***

STARS, saw in his plate - cann-i.

STARVE, family will - ars., calc-sil., ***sep.,*** staph.
he must - kali-chl., kali-m.

STARVED, being - naja.

STEPPING, as if persons are - aloe.

STATUE, poses as, to be admired - ***stram.***

STOLEN, something, she has - lach.
somebody thinks it - lach.

STOMACH, thinks has corrosion of - acet-ac., ign., sabad.

STOVE, for a tree, mistakes - hyos.
heats in heat of summer the - merc.
climb it, wants to - hyos.

STRANGE, everything is - anac., ***bar-m.,*** cann-s., carb-an., cic., ***graph.,*** kali-p., ***med., nux-m.,*** petr., ***plat.,*** plb., staph., stram., tub., valer.
everything is, disagreeable, and - valer.
terrible, and - cic., plat.
familiar things, seem - arg-n., atro., bar-m., bell., bov., calc., ***cann-i., cann-s.,*** carb-an., ***carc.,*** cic., ***cocc.,*** croc., glon., ***graph.,*** hyos., kali-p., kali-per., lyss., mag-m., med., merc., mosch., ***nat-m., nux-m.,*** op., petr., phos., ***plat.,*** puls., ran-b., rhus-a., rhus-t., staph., stram., ***sulph., thuj., tub.,*** valer., verat.
horrible, are - plat.
ludicrous, are - cann-i., hyos., nux-m.
familiar places seemed - cic., hyos., plat., rhus-r., tub.
headache after - glon.
land, as if in a - bry., par., plat., verat.
notions - ***lyss.***
pregnancy, during - lyss.
objects seem - carb-s.
streets, loses his way in, the houses seem strange - ***glon.***
surroundings - cic., hyos., plat., tub.
voice, her own seemed - alum., ***cann-i.***

STRANGERS, seemed to be in the room - ***tarent., thuj.***

STRANGERS, about her, while knitting - mag-s.
control of, under - aster., bry.
friends appear as - bry., stram.
full of strange men, who snatch at her - ***bell.***
looking over shoulder - brom.
seemed to be in the room - bry., ***tarent., thuj.***

STRANGERS, about,
surrounded by - nit-ac., **PULS.**
thinks he sees - anac., cann-i., mag-s., nit-ac., nux-v., ***puls.,*** stram., ***thuj.***

STROKE, thought he would have - arg-m.

STUDY, after - hyos., nux-v.

SUCCEED, that he cannot, does everything wrong - anac., ***arg-n.,*** nat-c.

SUFFERED, fancies he has - **HYOS.,** lach., ***lyss.,*** naja.

SUICIDE, driving to - ars., hyos., verat.

SUN, is reeling - cann-i.

SUPERHUMAN, is - cann-i.
control, under, is - agar., ***anac., lach., naja,*** op., plat., ***thuj.***

SUPERIORITY, is - ***plat.***

SUSPENDED in air, he is - sep.

SURROUNDED, by friends, is - bell., cann-i.

SURROUNDINGS, capacious, are - ferr.

SWALLOW, cannot - lyss.

SWIMMING, is - cann-i., rhus-t.
air, in the - **LAC-C.**

SWINE, thinks men are - hyos.

SWOLLEN, is - acon., ***aran., arg-n.,*** asaf., bapt., ***bov., cann-i.,*** carb-s., glon., op., plat.
swollen, is, convulsion, before - kali-br.

SWORD, hanging over head - am-m.

TACTILE hallucinations - anac., canth., ***op.,*** stram.

TALKATIVE, loquacity, with - ***bell.,*** hyos., lach., op., rhus-t., ***stram., verat.***

TALKING, fancies herself - raph.
body, one part is talking to another part of - bapt.
dead, people, as with - bell., **CALC-SIL.,** canth., hell., ***hyos.,*** nat-m., stram.
in churchyard - bell.
sister, with his dead - bell., ***hyos.***
hears, he - elaps.
imaginary persons, loudly and incoherently to - atro., bell.
inanimate objects with names, talking to, but observes no one standing by him - stram.
insane - nit-ac.
irrationally - nit-ac.
persons, of, as though near, about midnight - sep.
rapidly, all around her are - ***sang.***
someone behind him, with - ***med.***
else is, when he speaks - alum., cann-s.
spirits, with the - bell., **NAT-M., PLAT.,** stram.

TALL, as if he were - cop., op., plat., stram.
fancies herself very - eos., op., plat., stram.
had grown while walking - pall.
things grow taller - berb., camph., dros., kreos., nit-ac., sulph.
pulse is throbbing, as the - camph.

TANKARD and chases with figures of dragons, looked an huge - cann-i.

TARTARS, of a band - cann-i.

TASTE, of - cina, ***staph.***

TETANUS, must die of, with pain in right leg - ***mag-p.***

THIEVES, sees - alum., arn., ars., aur., bell., cupr., cupr-ac., kali-c., kali-sil., lach., mag-c., mag-m., merc., nat-c., ***nat-m.,*** petr., phos., sil., sol-t-ae., verat., zinc.
dream, after a, and will not believe the contrary until search is made - nat-m.
of robbers, is frightened on waking, and thinks dream is true - verat.
house, in - ars., cann-i., con., ***cupr-ac., lach.,*** merc., ***nat-m.,*** sil., sol-t-ae.
and space under bed are full of - ***ars.***
jump out of window, therefore wants to - ***lach.***
night - ***ars.***
robbing, that he has been accused of - kali-br.
that he has been accused of robbing - kali-br.

THIN, is getting - sulph.
body is - thuj.

THINK, she cannot - ***chel.***

THINKING, coming from the stomach - acon.
someone else is, on her side - thuj.

THOUGHTS, were separated - sabad.
being outside of body - sabad.

THREE, persons, that he is - anac., bapt., cann-i., nux-m., ***petr.***

THROAT, some one with ice cold hands took her by the - canth.

THUMBS, fingers are - **PHOS.**

TIME, passes too slowly - ***alum.,*** ambr., anh., ***arg-n.,*** **CANN-I.,** cann-s., con., med., nux-m., nux-v., onos.
passes too quickly - ***cocc.,*** sulph., ther.
seems earlier - sulph.
space, and, lost or confused - anh., bor., ***cann-i.,*** caust., cic., ***glon.,*** lach., nux-m.

TOES, cut off - mosch.

TONGUE, made of wood - apis.
pulling out - bell.
seems to reach the clouds when going to sleep - pic-ac.
too long - aeth.

TORMENTED, thinks is - ***chin.,*** lyss.

TOUCH, everything - bell.
everything, could not, as if she - pall.
sensory - anac., canth., op., ***rhus-t.,*** stram., ***thuj.***

TOUCHED, her head, someone - **MED.**

TOUCHING, everything - bell.

TOWN, he is in a deserted - carb-an.

TOYS, fancies himself playing with - atro.
object seemed as attractive as - cic.

TRANSFERRED, to another room - coloc.
to another world - cann-i.

TRANSPARENT, seemed to be - anh., cann-i.
everything is - anh.
head and nose are - bell.

TRAVELLING, of - **BELL.,** cann-i.
through inner worlds - canni-i., ether, bell.

TREES, seem to be people in fantastic costume, afternoon, while riding - bell.

TREMBLING, of everything on him, at night, when only half awake - sulph.

TROUBLES, broods over imaginary - ***ign., naja.***

TURTLES, sees large, in room - bell.

TYPHOID fever, thought he would have - nat-p.

UNEARTHLY, of something - cann-i.

UNFIT for, the world, he is - ***aur.***
work, for - meph.

UNFORTUNATE, that he is - bry., caust., ***chin.,*** cub., graph., hura, ip., lyc., sep., staph., verat.

UNPLEASANT - alum., bell., carb-s., hep.
distinct from surrounding objects - bell., op.

UNREAL, everything seems - ail., ***alum.,*** aml-n., ***anac.,*** anh., aran., **CANN-I.,** cann-s., cic., ***cocc.,*** lac-c., lil-t., ***med.,*** staph.

UNSEEN, thing - tarent.

VAGINA, living things creep into at night - merc.

VANISH, seems as if everything would - lyc.
senses, will - plat.

VEGETABLE, existence, thinks he is leading a - cann-i.
thinks he is selling green - cupr.

VENGEANCE, thinks he is singled out for divine - **KALI-BR.**

VERMIN, sees crawl about - alum., am-c., ***ars.,*** bov., calc., kali-c., lac-c., mur-ac., ***nux-v.,*** phos., ran-s., sil., ***sulph.***
his bed is covered with - ars.

VEXATIONS, after - bell., ***plat.***
and offences, of - cham., chin., dros.

VIOLENCE, about - kali-br.

VIOLENT - ***bell.,*** hyos., sec., ***stram.***

VIRGIN, mary, thinks she is - cann-i., verat.

VISIONS, has - absin., alum., alum-sil., ambr., anac., anh., antipyrin., arg-n., arn., ***ars.,*** **BELL.,** calc., ***calc-s.,*** camph., **CANN-I.,** ***cann-s.,*** canth., carb-an., ***carb-s.,*** carb-v., caust., cench., cham., chlol., chlorpr., cic., cimic., ***cina,*** coff., con., convo-s., cortico., ***crot-c.,*** dros., graph., hell., ***hep., hyos.,*** kali-c., ***lach.,*** lyc., mag-s., merc., methys., naja, ***nat-m.,*** nit-ac., nux-m., ***nux-v., op., ph-ac.,*** phos., plat., ***puls.,*** rhod., rhus-t., sec., sep., ***sil.,*** spong., **STRAM.,** ***sulph.,*** tarent., ther., valer.
arches - chlol.
beautiful - bell., ***cann-i.,*** coca, lac-c., lach., olnd., **OP.**

VISIONS, has
closing the eyes, on - anh., apis, ***arg-n.,*** ars., ***bell., bry.,*** **CALC.,** camph., caust., ***chin.,*** cocc., cupr., graph., hell., ***ign., lach.,*** led., lyc., nat-m., plb., ***puls.,*** samb., sec., sep., spong., stram., ***sulph.,*** tarent., thuj.
clouds of colors - lach.
colorful - anh.
daytime - bell., lac-c., lyc., nat-m., stram.
evening - brom., carb-an., carb-v., chin., ***cina,*** cupr., ign., phos., puls.
fantastic - arn., ars., ***chlol.,*** hyos., lach., nit-ac., op.
grandeur, of magnificent - cann-i., carb-s., coff.
horrible - absin., atro., **BELL., CALC.,** calc-sil., camph., carb-an., carb-v., ***caust.,*** hep., ign., ***kali-br.,*** lac-c., lyc., merc., ***nux-v.,*** op., phos., ***puls.,*** rhod., samb., sil., ***stram.,*** sulph., tarent.
behind him - ***lach.,*** med.
beside him - ***stram.***
evening - calc., carb-v.
events, of past - spong.
in the dark - ***bell., carb-v.,*** hell., petr., puls., stram.
night - camph., nit-ac., phos., tab.
waking, on - zinc.
imaginary power of - cann-i.
monsters - ***bell.,*** camph., **CALC.,** cann-i., cic., lac-c., op., samb., ***stram.,*** tarent.
on falling asleep and on waking - ign.
morning, in bed - hep.
night - camph., canth., cham., spong., ***stram.,*** thuj.
power, of imaginary - cann-i.
rats and strange objects - cimic.
strikes at them and holds up the cross - ***puls.***
wonderful - calc., camph., cann-i., lach.

VIVID - ***absin.,*** acon., ether, agar., ambr., ***bell., calc., cann-i.,*** cham., dub., ***hyos.,*** kali-c., ***lach.,*** lyc., ***op.,*** phos., plb., puls., rhus-t., scop., spong., ***stram.,*** sulph., ***verat.***

VINDICTIVE - agar.

VITALITY, vivid consciousness of usually unnoticed operations of - cann-i.

VOICES, hears - abrot., acon., agar., **ANAC.,** anh., aster., bell., benz-ac., calc-sil., cann-i., ***cann-s.,*** carb-s., cench., **CHAM.,** chlol., coca, ***coff., crot-c.,*** crot-h., ***cupr-ac., elaps,*** hyos., ign., ***kali-br.,*** lac-c., lach., lyc., manc., med., nat-m., nit-ac., petr., ***phos.,*** plb., sol-n., stram., verat.
abdomen, are in his - thuj.
abusive and filthy language, voices from within him speaking in - anac., ***zinc.***
answers, and - calc-sil.
bed, in, ceases when listening intently - abrot.
calling him - ***sulph.***
him at night - ***sulph.***
his name - anac.
confess things she never did - lach.

VOICES, hears,
confused, swallowing or walking in open air agg. - benz-ac., petr., phos.
dead people - anac., ***bell.,*** calc-sil., ***hyper.,*** nat-m., stram.
distant - bell., cann-i., cham., nat-m., sabal., stram.
hears, that he must follow - anac., crot-c.
his own, sounds strange and seems to reverberate like thunder - cann-i.
night - ***cham., sulph.***
steal and kill, that she must - **ANAC.,** lach.
strangers, of - bell., ***cham.***
unpleasant, about, himself - coca.

VOW, that she is breaking her - ign., verat.
keep it, must - verat.

WAKING, on - aur., carb-v., colch., dulc., merc., nat-c., par., ph-ac.

WALK, cannot walk, must run or hop - apis, hell.
fancies he cannot - ign., stram.
he sees the same one walking after him that he sees walking before him - euph.
knees, that he walks on his - bar-c., bar-m.
some one walks behind him - crot-c., ***med., staph.***
beside him - calc., petr., sil., thuj.

WALLS, falling - arg-n., cann-i., lyss.
is surrounded by high - cann-i.

WANT, fancied that he would come to - calc-f., sulph.
that they had come to - cann-i.

WAR, being at - bell., ***ferr.,*** hyos., plat., ran-b., thuj., verb.

WARTS, thinks he has - mez.

WASHING, of - bell., syph.

WATCHED, that she is being - anac., aq-mar., **ARS.,** ***bar-c., calc., hyos.,*** lach., meli., rhus-t.

WATER - alum., am-m., ***ant-t.,*** ars., bov., dig., ferr., graph., ign., iod., kali-c., kali-n., mag-c., mag-m., meph., ***merc.,*** nat-c., ran-b., sep., sil.
disasters by, floods - cann-i.
drinking, thought it delicious nectar, when - cann-i.
illusion of blue - cann-i.
nectar, water is delicious - cann-i.
sees flowing - ***merc.***
spoonful, a, seems like a lake - agar.
talking of, with - sep.
wades in the - ant-t.

WEALTH, imaginations of - agn., alco., bell., calc., cann-i., kali-br., nit-ac., ***phos., plat., pyrog., sulph.,*** verat.

WEDDING, of a - alum., hyos., mag-m., nat-c.

WEIGHT, has no - cann-i., hyos., op.

WELL, thinks he is - ***apis,*** **ARN.,** ars., bell., cinnb., hyos., **IOD.,** kreos., merc., **OP.,** puls.

WHIMSICAL - cann-i.

WHISPERS, hears blasphemic - anac.

WHISPERING, - rhodi.
someone to him - anac., med.

WHISTLING, with - bell., stram.

WIFE, is faithless - hyos., ***lach.,*** stram.
will run away from him - staph.

WILL power, loss of - ***anac.,*** chin-s.
possessed of two wills - **ANAC.,** lach.

WIND, sighing in chimney sounded like the hum of a vast wheel, and reverberated like a peal of thunder on a grand organ - cann-i.

WIRES, is caught in - cact., cimic.

WITHERING, body is - sabad.

WOLVES, of - bell., stram.

WOMEN, fancies his mother's house is invaded by lewd - kali-br.
evil, are, and will injure his soul - puls., thuj.
illusions of old and wrinkled - calc-sil., cann-i.

WOOD, is made of - kali-n., petr., rhus-t., thuj.

WORLD, he is lost to the, beyond hope - ***arg-n.***

WORK, cannot accomplish the - bry.
hard at, is - bell., ***bry.,*** canth., phos., **RHUS-T.,** verat.
hindered at, is - ***chin.***
will do him harm - ***arg-n.***

WORMS, bed, are in - ars.
creeping of - alum., am-c., ars., bov., kali-c., mur-ac., ***nux-v.,*** phos., ran-s., sil.
imagined vomit to be a bunch of - cann-i.
imagines he is covered with - ***coca.***

WRETCHED, thinks she looks, when looking in a mirror - nat-m., tub.

WRONG, fancies he has done - ***ars., aur.,*** aur-a., chin., cina, cocc., cycl., dig., digin., ***hell.,*** hyos., ***ign.,*** lyc., merc., nat-a., puls., sarr., sil., sulph., thuj.
has suffered - chin., **HYOS.,** lach., ***lyss.,*** naja, sarr.

Dreams

DREAMING, general

asleep, on falling - ambr., ant-c., aur., bell., calc., chin., cocc., cor-r., ferr-ma., hep., hyos., ***kali-c.,*** kreos., laur., mag-arct., mag-m., mang., mur-ac., ***nat-m.,*** phos., rhus-t., ***sil., spong., staph.,*** tarax., ***thuj.,*** verat., zinc.

awake, while - ***acon.,*** all-s., am-c., anac., ang., ant-t., arn., ars., ***bell.,*** berb., bry., calc., camph., cedr., cham., chin., cinnb., graph., ham., hell., hep., hyos., ***ign.,*** lach., led., lil-t., mag-arct., merc., narcot., nux-m., ***nux-v.,*** olnd., ***op.,*** petr., ***ph-ac., phos.,*** puls., ran-s., rheum, samb., sel., sep., ***sil.,*** spig., spong., stram., ***sulph.,*** thuj., ust., verat.

bed, driving out of - sep.

beginning, of sleep - ambr., aur., bell., cycl., mang., puls., thuj.

chill, with - sil., spong., sulph.

closing eyes, on - graph., led., lyc., plat., ***sep., spong.,*** stann.

cold sweat, with - nat-m., nicc.

continued, waking, after - acon., all-s., anac., ant-c., arg-m., arn., bry., calc., carl., caust., ***chin.,*** euph., graph., ign., lach., led., ***lyc.,*** merc., nat-c., ***nat-m.,*** nit-ac., phos., ***psor.,*** puls., sep., sil., sulph., zinc.

going to sleep the former dream is - ars., calad., carl., lam., nat-c., nat-m., nit-ac., petr.

continuous - anac., bar-c., mosch., nat-s., ***phos.,*** plat., sabin.

daytime, periodically, during - cann-i.

sleep, during - aur., bism., carb-v., eug., ign., lach., lyc., nux-m., ***nux-v.,*** par., petr., plat., sel., stann., tarax., ther.

dreamless, sleep - sabad.

emotional causes, from - absin., ***acon., alf.,*** am-val., ***ambr.,*** aur., bry., ***cann-i.,*** cham., chin-a., chlol., ***cimic.,*** coca, ***coff.,*** coloc., ***gels., hyos.,*** hyosin., ***ign., kali-br.,*** mosch., nat-m., ***nux-v., op.,*** passi., ph-ac., plat., senec., ***sep., stram.,*** sulph., thea., valer., zinc-valer.

evening, bed, in - arn., aur., calc., chin., ferr-ma., hell., kali-i., merc., nat-c., nux-v., puls., ***sep.***

going to bed, before - ign., nat-m., nux-v., plat., sulph.

fever, during - ***acon.,*** bry., chin., ferr-ma., ign., lact., ***nat-m.,*** **NUX-V.,** ***ph-ac.,*** phos., **PULS.,** ***rhus-t.,*** sabad., sep., sil., **SPIG.,** staph., sulph.

forenoon - bism., lact.

falling asleep - nat-m.

lucid - fl-ac., nictot.

revealing a perplexed situation when waking - acon.

lying on back, on - ***arn.,*** kali-chl., mag-arct., mag-c.

side, on - ign., mag-c., thuj.

left - lyc., phos., puls., sep., thuj.

DREAMING, general

menses, during - agar., alet., alum., am-c., bell., cact., calc., cann-s., carb-an., cast., caust., con., ham., helon., ign., kali-c., laur., lyc., mag-c., mag-m., merc., nat-c., ***nat-m.,*** **NUX-M.,** ***phos.,*** plat., puls., rhus-t., senec., sep., spong., sulph., thuj.

before - alum., calc., canth., caust., con., kali-c., merc., spong., sul-ac.

falling asleep, after - ferr-ma., glon.

midnight - mag-arct., sep.

before - ambr., ant-c., arn., aur., bell., calc., ***chel.,*** chin., ferr-ma., hell., hep., hyos., ign., kali-c., kali-i., kreos., mag-arct., mag-m., merc., nat-c., nux-v., puls., sep., ***sil.,*** spong., staph., ***sulph.,*** tarax., teucr., thuj.

morning - ambr., ang., atro., aur., calc., chel., chr-ac., con., ***cycl., fl-ac.,*** glon., goss., hell., ***kali-m.,*** lact., led., lyc., mag-arct., mag-aust., mez., nat-m., nit-ac., ***nux-v.,*** ph-ac., phos., puls., ran-b., rhod., rhus-t., sabin., spig., zinc.

5 a.m. - ham., lycps.

nausea, followed by - sulph.

noon - ther.

afternoon, and - nux-v., sel., ther.

siesta, during - aur., eug., ign., lach., lyc., **NAT-M.,** ***nux-v.,*** par., petr., pip-m., plat., sel., ***ther.***

5 p.m., while sitting - nat-m.

palpitation, with - ign., merc., phos., rhus-t., ***sil.,*** zinc.

perspiration, with - acon., **ARS.,** bar-c., bry., chin., dulc., ferr-ma., ign., kali-n., kreos., ***led.,*** mag-s., mur-ac., ***nat-m.,*** nat-s., nicc., nit-ac., ***nux-v.,*** petr., ph-ac., **PHOS.,** ***puls.,*** rat., rhus-t., sabad., **SEP.,** ***sil.,*** spig., staph., ***sulph.,*** thuj., zinc-oc.

cold, when taking - sabad., sil.

sex, after - rhod.

thirst, followed by - mag-c., rat., sulph.

vomiting, followed by - verat.

ABDOMEN, as if were constricted - **NAT-M.**

covered with warts and ulcers - junc.

painful - apis.

ABSURD - apis, chin., cina, colch., coloc., ferr-m., ***glon.,*** mag-m., mygal., pip-m., plan., rumx., ***sulph.,*** thuj.

midnight, after - ***chin.***

ABUSED, being too weak to defend himself - ambr.

ACCIDENTS, of - allox., am-m., ant-c., arn., **ARS.,** bell., ***calc.,*** cham., chin., cinnb., con., ***dig.,*** **GRAPH.,** ind., iod., iodof., piloc., kali-c., kali-s., kreos., lyc., mag-m., man., nat-s., nit-ac., ***nux-v.,*** puls., rumx., sars., sil., sul-ac., sulph., thuj., verat.

boat, foundering - alum., lyc., sil.

drowning, of (see Drowing)

falling, (see Falling)

injuries, (see Injuries)

explosion - stann.

ACCIDENTS, of
struck by lightning, being - ***arn.***

ACCUSATIONS - clem., lach., nat-m., thuj.
crime, wrongful of - clem.

ACQUAINTANCES, distant - fl-ac., plat., plb., sel.
walking on water - ped.

ADVENTUROUS - bar-c., senec., sulph.

AFFECTIONATE - coc-c.

AIR, attacks, battles - visc.

ALTERNATING, with pain in head - ars.

ALARMS - hipp.

AMOROUS, sexual - acon., aesc., ether, agn., ***alum.,*** alum-sil., am-c., **AM-M.,** ambr., anag., ang., ***ant-c.,*** aphis., ***arg-n.,*** arn., ars., ars-i., astac., ***aur.,*** aur-a., bar-c., bar-i., ***bar-m.,*** bell., bism., bor., bov., cact., cahin., caj., ***calc.,*** calc-ar., calc-i., calc-p., calc-sil., ***camph., cann-i.,*** cann-s., ***canth., carb-ac.,*** carb-an., carb-s., carb-v., carl., cast., caust., ***cench.,*** cent., chel., chin., ***cic.,*** cinnb., clem., ***cob.,*** coc-c., coca, cocc., coloc., ***con.,*** cop., cycl., ***dig., dios.,*** dros., ery-a., euph., form., gall-ac., ***gels.,*** gins., goss., ***graph.,*** ham., hipp., hura, hydr., hyos., hyper., ***ign.,*** ind., inul., iod., ***iris,*** kali-ar., ***kali-br., kali-c.,*** kali-chl., kali-cy., kali-m., kali-n., kali-p., ***kalm.,*** kreos., lac-ac., **LACH.,** lact., led., ***lil-t.,*** linu-c., lith., ***lyc.,*** lyss., mag-arct., mag-c., mag-m., mag-s., meny., merc., merc-c., merc-i-f., merc-i-r., merc-sul., mez., mur-ac., myric., nat-a., **NAT-C.,** ***nat-m., nat-p.,*** nicc., nit-ac., nux-m., **NUX-V.,** olnd., **OP.,** orig., ox-ac., paeon., par., ped., pen., ***petr.,*** **PH-AC.,** ***phos.,*** phys., pic-ac., pip-m., plan., ***plat.,*** plb., ***psor., puls.,*** ran-b., raph., rhod., rhus-v., ***sabad.,*** samb., sanic., ***sars.,*** sel., senec., ***sep.,*** serp., ***sil.,*** sin-n., sol-t-ae., spig., spira., spirae., squil., stann., **STAPH.,** stram., sul-ac., sul-i., sulph., sumb., ***tarax., thuj.,*** thymol., trom., tub., ust., valer., verat., verat-v., vinc., viol-o., **VIOL-T.,** x-ray, yuc., zinc.
afternoon - par.
erections, with - aur., cact., camph., ***cann-i.,*** clem., coloc., kreos., lac-ac., led., merc., mur-ac., ***nat-c.,*** par., ***ph-ac.,*** pic-ac., plat., plb., ran-b., rhod., ***sars.,*** sep., sil., sin-n., ***spig.,*** stann., thuj.
priapism, with - ***camph., pic-ac.***
evening - coloc., puls., sil.
lying, back, on - coloc.
right side, on - sars.
menses, during - calc., goss.
before - ***calc., kali-c.***
midnight, after - cann-s., des-ac., paeon.
after, 3 a.m. - pip-m.
before - coloc.
morning - aloe, colch., grat., lil-t., plb., sabad., sil., sumb.
5 a.m. - merc-i-r.
night, 3 a.m. - pip-m.

AMOROUS, sexual
pollutions, with - ***alum.,*** ambr., ang., ***ant-c.,*** aphis., arist-m., arn., ars., ars-s-f., aur., bar-c., bell., bism., bor., bov., ***calad., calc.,*** calc-p., ***camph.,*** cann-i., cann-s., canth., carb-ac., carb-an., caust., chin., ***cic., cob.,*** coloc., con., cycl., dig., dios., euph., ferr., form., ***gels., graph.,*** grat., ham., hura, hydr., indg., iod., ***iris, kali-br., kali-c.,*** kali-chl., ***kali-m.,*** kali-s., lach., lact., led., ***lil-t.,*** lyc., lyss., merc-i-f., merc-sul., myric., ***nat-c.,*** nat-m., nat-p., **NUX-V.,** ***olnd.,*** op., paeon., par., ***ph-ac., phos., pic-ac.,*** plb., ***puls.,*** ran-b., rhod., sabad., samb., ***sars.,*** sel., senec., ***sep., sil.,*** sin-n., ***spig.,*** spira., stann., staph., stram., sulph., thuj., thymol., ust., ***viol-t.***
sex, after - kali-c.
vaginal discharge, with - ***petr.***

AMPUTATION of, arm - lob.
leg, of - atro.

ANGER - all-c., alum., am-c., ambr., ant-c., apis, ***arn.,*** asar., aster., aur., bell-p., brom., ***bry.,*** calc., calc-sil., canth., cast., carl., caust., cham., crot-c., crot-h., dros., kali-n., lach., ***mag-c.,*** mag-m., mag-s., mang., merc-i-r., mosch., myric., nat-a., nat-m., nicc., **NUX-V.,** paeon., peti., ph-ac., ***phos.,*** puls., rat., rheum, rumx., sabin., sars., sel., sep., sil., spong., stann., **STAPH.,** sul-ac., tarax., verat., zinc.

ANIMALS - aloe, am-c., ***am-m.,*** arg-n., **ARN.,** bell., bov., cham., cench., chlorpr., daph., gran., hura, hydr., hyos., lac-c., lyc., ***merc., nux-v., phos.,*** op., ***phos.,*** phys., ***puls.,*** ran-s., sil., staph., sul-ac., sulph., tarent.
bite, which - bov., calc., cench., daph., mag-aust., merc., ***phos.,*** puls., sulph., verat., zinc.
black - arn., ***puls.***
copulating - cench.
dead - ptel.
fights, with - staph.
wild animals - hyos., lyc., nux-v., sil., stram., sulph., tarent.
pursuing him - allox., alum., bell., cench., eupi., hipp., ind., led., nux-v., sil., stram., ***sulph.,*** tarent., tet., verat.

ANXIOUS - abies-n., abrot., **ACON.,** aesc., aeth., agar., agn., all-c., all-s., **ALUM.,** alum-p., alum-sil., ***ambr.,*** ammc., **AM-C., AM-M.,** aml-n., ***anac.,*** anag., anan., ang., ant-c., ant-ox., ant-t., apis, ***arg-m., arg-n.,*** **ARN., ARS.,** ***ars-i.,*** ars-s-f., asar., asc-t., astac., ***aur.,*** aur-a., aur-m., ***bapt.,*** **BAR-C.,** bar-i., ***bar-m.,*** bart., ***bell.,*** berb., bism., ***bor.,*** bov., brucin., ***bry.,*** bufo, calad., **CALC.,** calc-caust., calc-i., calc-p., calc-s., ***calc-sil., camph.,*** cann-i., cann-s., ***canth.,*** caps., carb-ac., carb-an., **CARB-S.,** ***carb-v.,*** carl., ***caust., cham.,*** chel., ***chin.,*** chin-a., chr-ac., cic., ***cimic.,*** cina, cinnb., ***cist.,*** clem., coc-c., **COCC.,** coca, coff., colch., coloc., com., ***con.,*** cor-r., cortico., ***croc.,*** crot-h., crot-t., cupr., cupr-ar., cycl., cyt-l., dig., digox., dios., ***dros.,*** elaps, euph., euph-l., euphr.,

ANXIOUS, - eupi., ery-a., ***ferr., ferr-ar.,*** ferr-i., ***ferr-p., gamb.,*** glon., guare., **GRAPH.,** guai., ***hell., hep.,*** hipp., hydr., hydr-ac., ***hyos., hyper., ign.,*** indg., ***iod.,*** ip., iris, jal., jug-c., ***kali-ar.,*** **KALI-C.,** kali-chl., kali-i., kali-m., kali-n., kali-p., kali-s., ***kali-sil., kreos., lach.,*** lachn., lact., lam., ***laur., led.,*** levo., lil-t., lob., **LYC.,** lycps., **MAG-C.,** ***mag-m., mag-s., mang., merc.,*** merc-c., merc-i-r., mez., ***mur-ac.,*** murx., ***nat-a.,*** **NAT-C., NAT-M.,** nat-p., ***nat-s.,*** nicc., **NIT-AC., NUX-V.,** ***ol-an., op.,*** orig., oxyt., paeon., palo., par., ***petr.,*** petros., ***ph-ac.,*** **PHOS.,** plan., ***plat.,*** plb., ***psor.,*** **PULS.,** ***pyrog., ran-b., ran-s.,*** raph., rat., ***rheum,*** rhod., **RHUS-T.,** rumx., sabad., sabin., sang., ***sars.,*** sec., sel., ***sep.,*** **SIL.,** sin-a., spig., **SPONG.,** squil., stann., staph., ***stram.,*** stront-c., ***sul-ac.,*** sul-i., **SULPH.,** tab., tarax., ter., teucr., **THUJ.,** til., ust., valer., ***verat.,*** verat-v., verb., ***zinc.,*** zinc-p., zing.
- afternoon - adlu.
- anxiety, amel. on waking - am-c., arg-m., bov., calc., cann-s., caust., ***chin., graph.,*** lach., led., nat-m., nit-ac., ***phos., sil., sulph.***
  - continued after waking - acon., zinc.
- armies, rising from their graves - ptel.
- children, in - ***ambr.***
- crying during sleep, with - ***nat-m.***
- falling asleep - ars., cori-r., dig., fl-ac., mez., ***nat-c.,*** nat-m., nit-ac., phos., puls., staph., thuj., zinc.
- lying on left side - lyc., phos., ***puls.,*** sep., ***thuj.***
- midnight - all-s.
- midnight, after - merc., ***sulph.***
  - 3.30 a.m. - nat-m.
  - toward morning - ***kali-m.,*** zinc.
- midnight, before - mez., sulph.
- morning - alum., calc., lyc., nit-ac., phos., puls., zinc.
- siesta, during - nat-m.

ARMS, amputated - lob.
- bitten, into - am-m., mag-aust., nicc.
- covered with blisters - cast.
- hurt, mother's arm - chin.
- painful - nicc.
- paralysed - nicc.

ARRESTED, of being - bov., clem., mag-c.
- imprisonment - bov.

ASTRAY, going - mag-c., mag-m., nat-c., sep.

ASPIRING - zing.

ASYLUM, of insane - lyss.

AUTOPSIES, seeing - rumx.
- dissecting dead bodies - cench., chel., iris, ped., sang.

BACK, burnt - mag-c.
- covered with warts - mez.
- pinched, back and breast are - phos.

BAFFLED, being - verat-v.

BALLS - mag-c., mag-s.

BANQUET, of being at a - mag-s., nit-ac., ph-ac.

BASEBALL, playing - atro.

BATHING in boiling water, child is - mag-c.
- boiling water, people are in - chin-b.

BAT, flying in room - ham.

BATTLES - ***all-c.,*** bell., bry., ferr., guai., hyos., ***meny.,*** nat-m., plat., ran-s., sil., stann., thuj., verb.

BEATEN, being - kali-c., kali-n., nat-m.

BED, too small - ferr-i.

BEES - puls.

BEETLES - coca, kres.

BEGGARS - mag-c.

BETRAYED, having been - sil.

BICYCLING, difficult - visc.

BIRDS - com.

BITTEN, by animals, being - bov., calc., daph., mag-aust., merc., ***phos.,*** puls., sulph., verat., zinc.
- arms, into - am-m., mag-aust., nicc.
- dogs, being bitten by - calc., lyss., merc., ***sulph.,*** verat.
- snakes, being bitten by - bov., cench.

BLACK, forms - arn., ars., puls.
- beasts - ***puls.***

BLEEDING - phos., sol-t-ae.

BLIND, that he was - phys.

BLISTERS, on arms - cast.

BLOOD - ***phos.,*** rhus-t., sol-t-ae.
- pools of - ***phos.,*** rhus-t., sol-t-ae.

BLOODSHED - plat.

BOARS, wild - merc.

BOASTING - asc-t.

BOAT, foundering - alum., lyc., sil.

BODY, disfigured - sep.
- emaciated, becoming - kali-n., kreos.
- embalmed - carb-ac.
- knees, swollen - cocc.
- limbs, broken - cimic.
- parts of - mag-c.
- pieces, in - dict.
- rash, covered - am-m.
- swollen - squil.

BOOSTING - mag-s.

BOUND, with chain across mouth, being - bapt.

BRUISING, himself - nicc.

BUGS, (see Insects)

BUILDINGS - hura, myris., pall.
- admirable - graph.

BULLS, chased by - ind., tarent.

BULLYING - peti.

BURIALS - alum., hura.

BURIED, alive, being - ***arn.,*** chel., ign.

BURNING, blisters - cast.
- hands, by washing - mag-m.

BUSINESS, of - ether, anac., apis, arist-m., asaf., bell., ***bry.,*** bufo, **CALC.,** calc-ac., calc-sil., camph., canth., carb-v., carc., carl., ***chel.,*** cic., croc., ***cur.,*** elaps, gels., hep., hura, hyper., kali-c., ***lach., lyc.,*** merc., **NUX-V.,** phos., psor., ***puls.,*** pyrog., **RHUS-T.,** sang., sars., sel., ***sil.,*** staph., tarent.
cannot accomplish - mag-m., ***phos.,*** sabad.
day, of the - acon., alum., anac., apis, arg-m., asaf., asc-t., bapt., bell., ***bry.,*** calc., calc-f., canth., carb-v., cham., chel., cic., cina, cur., euph., fl-ac., gels., graph., hep., kali-c., kali-chl., lach., lyc., mag-c., mag-m., merc., nit-ac., nux-v., ph-ac., phos., plat., ***puls.,*** rhus-t., sabin., sars., sel., sep., sil., stann., staph., sulph.
of the, morning - nit-ac., sul-ac.
falling asleep - rhus-t., staph.
forgot during day, he - sel.
neglected, of - hyper., myris., sil., stann.
succeed, don't - mag-m., ***phos.,*** sabad.

BUSY, being - ambr., anac., apis, bapt., bell., **BRY.,** ***calc.,*** camph., canth., carb-ac., ***carl.,*** coca, hydr., hyos., hyper., ign., kalm., lach., led., lil-t., lyc., mosch., osm., phos., pip-m., polyg., sabad., sabin., sang., sep., spig.

CANCER - halo.

CARES, full of - alum., am-m., ***ars.,*** caps., carl., cast., caust., crot-t., ign., laur., lyc., mur-ac., nat-c., nat-m., nux-v., op., phos., rheum, rhus-t., spong., stront.

CALCULATING - sel.

CALLED, that some one - ant-c., merc., sep.

CALLING out - kali-c., thuj.
help, for - kali-c., lil-s., plat.
someone is calling - ant-c., merc., sep.

CANNONADING - menis.

CAUTERIZING of arm - bomb-pr.

CAROUSING - graph., kali-c., lyc., nat-c., nat-m., nit-ac., nux-v., petr., sil., sulph., zinc.

CATS - arn., ars., calc-p., ***daph.,*** graph., hyos., lac-c., mez., nux-v., op., puls., thuj.
black - arn., daph.
pursuing him - ***nux-v.,*** sil., verat.

CELLAR, of being in, and walls falling in - bov.

CHANGING, places often - led., lyc.
objects - mang.

CHASED and had to run backwards - sep.

CHEEK, is swollen - kali-n.
burnt - mag-c.
swollen - kali-n.

CHEST, being pressed - am-m.
wished to open the chest and look in - paull.

CHILD, had been beaten - kali-c., kali-n., nat-m.

CHILDREN, about - ***absin., acon.,*** am-m., ars., ***bell.,*** calad., cas-s., ***cham., cina, cypr.,*** hura, hyos., kali-br., kali-n., lipp., mag-c., merc., oci., ***passi.,*** phos., puls., sulph.
murdered, being - thea.

CHILL, with - sil., spong., sulph.

CHOLERA - linu-c.

CHURCHES - asc-t., coc-c., lyss., zing.

CHURCHYARD - crot-h., hura.

CITIES - nat-m.
destroyed by fire - sol-t-ae.

CIVIL, war - op.

CLAIRVOYANT - **ACON.,** asaf., bov., ***cann-i.,*** cortico., mag-arct., mang., ph-ac., phos., rad., ***sulph.,*** ther.
drunkenness, during - lach.

CLIMBING, a step - brom., hyper., mur-ac., rhus-t.

CLOSET, being on - psor.

CLOSING eyes, on - graph., led., lyc., plat., ***sep., spong.,*** stann.

CLOTHES, did not wish to make up - mag-c.

COFFINS - brom., form., lipp., merc-i-f.

COLORED - nat-m., psil., saroth., sulph.

COMICAL - ***glon.,*** lach., mez., phos., ***sulph.***

COMPANIES - canth., phel.

COMPLICATED, and containing its explanation, dream - asc-t.

CONFUSED - ***acon.,*** agar., agar-ph., aloe, ***alum.,*** alum-sil., am-c., ammc., anag., ang., ant-t., apis, arg-n., asc-t., bar-c., bart., bism., brach., brucin., ***bry.,*** calad., ***calc.,*** calc-ac., calc-f., calc-sil., camph., ***cann-s.,*** canth., carb-an., carl., caust., cedr., cench., ***chel., chin.,*** chin-s., ***cic.,*** cina, clem., ***coff.,*** coff-t., con., coloc., ***croc.,*** cycl., cyt-l., dig., digin., digox., ***dulc.,*** erig., ery-a., equis., eug., euph., euphr., eupi., ***ferr.,*** ferr-i., ferr-ma., ferr-p., gast., ***glon.,*** grat., ***hell.,*** hydr., hydr-ac., hyper., ***ign.,*** iod., iodof., ***kali-br.,*** kali-cy., kiss., laur., led., lina., ***lyc., lyss.,*** mag-aust., mag-c., mag-s., mang., ***menis.,*** mez., nat-a., ***nat-c., nat-m.,*** nat-p., nicc., nit-ac., ***nux-v.,*** ped., petr., phos., plat., plb., podo., **PULS.,** rumx., ruta, ***sabad.,*** sabin., sel., senec., ***sep.,*** sil., sin-a., sol-t-ae., spig., spirae., ***stann.,*** stram., sul-i., ***sulph.,*** thuj., til., valer., verat., wild.
afternoon, 2 p.m. - sulph.
falling asleep, on - nat-c.
midnight, after - chin.
morning - chin-s., mag-c.
siesta, during - plat.

CONNECTED, dreams - acon., am-c., ammc., ars., calc., carl., coloc., ***ign.,*** lyc., nat-m., petr., plan., staph.

CONSPIRACIES - mosch., ped.

CONTEMPT - tarent.

CONTINUATION, of former ideas - ant-t., asaf., ign., puls., rhus-t.

CONTRABAND - mag-c.

CONVERSATIONS, previous day, of - nat-c.
women, with - cedr.

CONVULSIONS - calc-s.

COOKING - canth.

CORONATION - upa.

CORPSES, coming alive after funeral - allox.

COUGH - eupi.

COUNTRY - asc-t.
beautiful - ol-an.
foreign - ind., plat., sil.

CRAZY - aloe, apis.
man, a - apis.
man, for which he has held to answer - nat-m.

CRIMES - cocc., hura, nat-m., nat-s., nit-ac., petr., rumx.
accused wrongfully, that he was - clem., sil.
committed, that he had - cocc., nat-s., nit-ac., petr.
conscience acquits him of a - thuj.

CROCODILES - led.
pursuing him, by - led.

CRUELTY - ***ign.,*** lil-t., nat-m., nux-v., sel., sil., stann.

CRUSHED, that he would be - ***sulph.***

CRYING - ang., calc-f., elaps, fl-ac., ***glon.,*** kali-c., ***kreos.,*** mag-c., nux-v., plan., ***sil.,*** sol-m., spong., stram., tarent.

CUT, being - frax., guai., nat-s.
pieces, to - lil-s.

CUTTING - calc-f., chin., hura, mag-m., nat-c., nicc., op.
being cut with a knife - guai.
cutting a woman up for salting - calc-f.
ears cut off, having - nat-c.
face cut away, having one side of - mag-m.
hands being cut to pieces - sol-t-ae.
seeing a person cut up - merc.

DANCING - gamb., mag-c., mag-m., mag-s., zing.

DANGER - aloe, am-c., anac., ***ars.,*** ars-m., bell., calc-f., calc-p., ***cann-i.,*** carb-s., chin., con., graph., ***hep.,*** indg., iod., kali-bi., kali-c., kali-i., kali-n., ***lach.,*** linu-c., lyc., macro., mag-c., mag-m., mag-s., mang., nat-c., nat-s., nux-v., phos., psor., puls., ran-b., rumx., sin-a., sul-ac., sulph., tarent., thuj.
death, of - bell., mag-m., mang., ran-b., sul-ac., sulph., thuj.
drowning, of - bov.
escaping from a - hep.
fruitless efforts of - ind.
falling, of - alum., am-m., macro.
flood, into - am-m.
height, from a - alum.
fire, from - ant-t., bell., clem., merc-ac.
water, from - ars., ars-m., ***graph., kali-n., mag-c.,*** mag-m., merc., merc-ac., nat-c., nat-s., sulph.

DARKNESS - ars., aur.

DEAD, bodies - alumn., am-c., **ANAC.,** aur., bar-ac., bar-c., bry., ***calc., calc-sil.,*** cann-i., cann-s., carb-ac., ***chel., crot-c.,*** crot-h., dirc., elaps, grat., hura, hydr-ac., iod., iris, jac-c., kali-c., laur., mag-m., mag-s., merc., nat-c., nat-p., nit-ac., peti., ph-ac., phos., ran-s., rumx., sol-t-ae., sulph., tarent., ***thuj.,*** verb., zinc.

DEAD, bodies
dissecting - chel., iris, ped., sang.
returning to life - rumx.
smell of - calc., crot-h.

DEAD, people, of - alum., am-c., ***anac.,*** ange-s., ant-c., ***arg-n., arn.,*** **ARS.,** ars-i., ars-s-f., aur., aur-a., bar-ac., bar-c., bry., calad., calc-ar., ***calc.,*** calc-f., calc-i., ***calc-sil.,*** cann-i., carb-s., caust., cench., ***chel.,*** chin-a., chin-b., coca, cocc., cod., con., convo-d., ***crot-h.,*** culx., elaps, ferr., ferr-i., goss., ***graph.,*** iod., iris, kali-ar., ***kali-c.,*** kali-n., kali-sil., laur., lepi., lipp., lyc., **MAG-C.,** mag-m., mag-s., ***med.,*** mur-ac., nat-c., nat-p., nat-s., nicc., nit-ac., nux-v., ol-an., paull., ph-ac., ***phos.,*** plat., plumbg., ran-b., ran-s., rat., rauw., rheum, saroth., sars., sil., sin-n., spong., sul-i., ***sulph.,*** sul-ac., syc-co., **THUJ.,** verb., vip-a., zinc.
friends long deceased - arg-n., cedr., con., ferr., nat-c.
talking with deceased friends - lepi.
menses, during - goss.
relatives - caust., ferr., fl-ac., kali-c., mag-c., mag-s., rheum, sars.
wife - aran-ix.

DEATH, of - allox., alum., alum-p., alum-sil., alumn., am-c., anac., arn., ars., ars-s-f., aur., aur-a., brom., ***calc.,*** calc-f., calc-sil., camph., cast., chel., chin., chin-a., chin-b., cocc., coff., con., cortico., crot-c., crot-h., culx., ferr-i., fl-ac., grat., hura, kali-ar., kali-c., kali-chl., kali-m., kali-n., kali-s., kali-sil., **LACH.,** lyc., mag-m., mag-s., merc-c., nat-m., nat-s., nicc., nit-ac., paeon., plan., plat., raph., rat., rauw., rheum, rhus-v., saroth., sil., spong., ***sulph.,*** tarent., thuj., ven-m.
approaching - kali-c., kali-chl., sil., ***sulph.,*** tab.
dying, of - am-c., arn., bov., brom., camph., chel., cocc., cortico., dulc., fl-ac., kali-chl., rauw., sulph., ***thuj.***
lying on the left side, while - ***thuj.***
friend, of a - allox., coff., coff-t., con., cortico., fl-ac., kali-n., lach., nicc.
lying on the left side, while - ***thuj.***
morning - calc.
peril, of - bell., sul-ac., sulph., thuj.
relatives - alumn., aran-ix., ***calc-f.,*** cast., caust., chin., fl-ac., grat., levo., kali-c., mag-s., mur-ac., nicc., paeon., plan., plat.

DECLIVITIES - anac.

DEFAMATORY - mosch.

DELIBERATIONS - ***ign.***

DESERT - sil.

DEVILS - apis, arg-m., kali-c., lac-c., nat-c., nicc., op., sin-n.

DIARRHEA - allox., apis.

DIFFICULTIES - alum., **AM-M.,** anac., ant-t., **ARS.,** bell., cann-s., caps., croc., ***graph., mag-c.,*** mag-m., mur-ac., ***phos.,*** plat., rhus-t., sep.
bicycling, while - visc.
journeys, on - am-m., calc-p., mag-s., merc., mez., nat-c.

DIRT - kreos., prun.
linen - kali-n., ***kreos.***
roads - apis.
table - prun.

DISAPPOINTMENTS - cann-s., ign., rumx., ust.

DISASTER - sars.

DISCHARGE, watery, nose - ped.

DISCONNECTED - agar., ***apis, arn.,*** cadm-s., chel., chin., cina, cinnb., coca, crot-t., equis., grat., guare., hir., lyc., ***lyss.,*** myris., plan., plat., phos., ***puls.,*** sil., sol-t-ae., sulph.

DISEASE - am-c., am-m., anac., anan., apis, asar., bar-c., bor., ***calc.,*** calc-ac., calc-sil., caust., cocc., con., dros., eupi., fago., graph., hep., kali-c., kali-n., kali-s., ***kreos.,*** lac-c., ***lyc.,*** mag-c., meph., nat-m., nat-s., **NUX-V.,** peti., phos., prun., rat., sil., squil., sulph., sumb., syph., upa., ven-m., zinc.

DISGUSTING - alet., aloe, alumn., am-c., anac., arist-m., bor., cast-v., chel., ***chin.,*** chin-b., chr-ac., con., eupi., inul., kali-n., ***kreos.,*** lach., mag-m., mag-s., merc., mur-ac., nat-m., ***nux-v.,*** phos., plan., ***puls.,*** rheum, sil., sulph., zinc.
dirt - kreos., prun.
linen, about dirty - kali-n., ***kreos.***
morning - inul.
wading in excrements - iod.

DISSECTING, dead bodies - cench., chel., iris, ped., sang.

DISTANT, acquaintances - fl-ac., plb., sel.
strange things - plat.

DOGS - abrot., am-c., ***arn.,*** calc., cer-b., graph., hyos., lyc., lyss., merc., nux-v., op., paull., puls., rumx., ***sil.,*** stram., ***sulph.,*** verat., zinc.
bitten, by, of being - calc., lyss., merc., ***sulph.,*** verat.
black - ***arn.,*** puls., tub.
frightened by a black dog - puls.
killing a mad dog - abrot., rumx.
large dog following him - sil.
mad dog - abrot., rumx.

DRAGONS - op.

DRINKING - ars., dros., med., nat-m., phos.
impossible - arist-m.

DRIVING, out of bed - sep.

DROWNED, being - ign.

DROWNING - alum., bov., ether, ign., kali-c., lyc., mag-s., merc., merc-ac., merc-i-f., nicc., ran-b., rauw., rumx., samb., sil., verat., verat-v., zinc.
danger of - bov.
foundering boat, on a - alum., lyc.
man, of a - sol-t-ae.
mother had been drowned, that her - nicc., rauw.
people are drowning - mag-s., verat.

DRUNKEN, people - cench.

DUELS - asc-t.

DYING, of - am-c., arn., bov., brom., camph., chel., cocc., cortico., dulc., fl-ac., kali-chl., rauw., sulph., ***thuj.***
lying on the left side, while - ***thuj.***

EARS, cut off, of having - nat-c.

EARTHQUAKE - calc., rat., sil.

EATING - ***iod.***
dog flesh - alum.
human flesh - sol-t-ae.

EMACIATED, becoming - kali-n., kreos.
body in pieces - dict.

EMBARRASSMENT - allox., alum., ***am-m., ars.,*** graph., lyc., mag-c., phos.

ENTERTAINMENT - nat-c.

ENCIRCLED, tightly, being - ruta.

ENEMIES - arg-m., con., ptel.

ERRORS - am-m.

ERUPTION - am-c., am-m., anac., cast.

EVENTS, important - osm.
future, of - **ACON.,** asaf., bov., ***cann-i.,*** cortico., mag-arct., mang., ph-ac., phos., rad., ***sulph.***
unfortunate - cocc., sulph.

EVENTS, previous - ***acon.,*** aeth., am-c., anac., ***ant-t.,*** arg-m., asaf., aster., bov., ***bry.,*** calad., calc., ***calc-p.,*** **CAPS.,** carb-s., chel., chin., ***cic.,*** coca, cocc., ***croc.,*** crot-t., elaps, euph., ferr-i., fl-ac., graph., ind., jatr., kali-c., kali-chl., kali-m., kali-sil., ***lach.,*** nat-c., nat-p., nat-sil., nit-ac., nux-v., osm., ph-ac., phos., plan., ***rhus-t.,*** sang., sars., sel., senec., sep., **SIL.,** spig., sol-t-ae., sulph., sumb., thuj.
contorted - graph.
day, of - ***acon.,*** aeth., agav-t., arg-m., arg-n., bals-p., **BRY.,** calc-f., calc-p., chel., ***cic., croc.,*** cur., euph., ferr., fl-ac., graph., hep., ind., kali-c., kali-chl., lach., lyc., mag-c., merc., methys., nat-c., nit-ac., ***nux-v.,*** ph-ac., phos., ***puls.,*** rhus-t., sars., sel., senec., sep., sil., sol-t-ae., stann.
evening, of - ph-ac., thuj.
long past, forgotten - acon., am-c., anac., bov., calad., calc., cer-b., chin., ferr., ferr-i., nat-c., senec., **SIL.,** spig., sulph., sumb.
morning, of - ***camph.***
painful - osm.
previously read, talked or thought about - ***ant-t.,*** asaf., bov., bry., calc-p., carb-s., coca, fl-ac., jatr., nat-c., nux-v., ***rhus-t.,*** sars., thuj.
read - ***bry.,*** calc-f., ***calc-p.***

EXASPERATION - staph.

EXCELLING, in mental work - acon., anac., arn., ***bry.,*** camph., carb-an., graph., ***ign.,*** lach., ***nux-v.,*** puls., rhus-t., sabad., ***sabin., thuj.***

EXCITING - bell-p., carc., cob-n., cod., coloc., dicha., kali-cy., lyss., mag-s., nat-m., nux-v., orig., ***phos.,*** pip-m., saroth.

EXCREMENTS - aloe, cast-v., iod., psor., sars., zinc.
closets - psor.
smeared with being - zinc.
soiling himself with - aloe, cast-v., iod., sars., zinc.
wading in - iod.

EXCRESCENCES - mez.

EXERTION, mental - ***acon.,*** alum., ambr., ***anac., arn.,*** ars., aur., bell., berb., ***bry.,*** calc-p., camph., carb-an., cham., ***chin.,*** cic., clem., coff., coloc., dulc., ***graph.,*** **IGN.,** iod., kali-n., ***lach.,*** laur., led., mag-aust., mosch., ***nat-m.,*** **NUX-V.,** ***olnd.,*** op., par., ***ph-ac., phos.,*** plb., ***puls.,*** **RHUS-T.,** ***sabad.,*** sabin., sars., sec., spong., staph., ***sulph.,*** teucr., ***thuj., viol-t.,*** zinc., zinc-p.
exertion, physical - apis, arn., **ARS.,** atro., bapt., brom., ***bry.,*** dicha., echi., lil-t., med., nat-m., nux-v., phos., puls., **RHUS-T.,** sabin., sel., spong., staph.
making great, of - ***ars., rhus-t.***

EXHAUSTING - aeth., alum., ant-c., ant-ox., ant-t., arn., ars., asc-t., atro., aur., bell., bov., bry., carb-s., cina, croc., equis., ferr., graph., hyper., iod., lach., lyc., lyss., mag-c., mang., med., op., petr., phos., ph-ac., polyg., ***puls.,*** rhod., ***rhus-t.,*** ruta, sabin., sep., spig., spong., valer., verat., vichy-g., ***zinc.***

EXPECTORATION, purulent - hep.

EXPLOSION - stann.

EYELIDS, itching - upa.

EYES, stitches in - calc.

FACE, covered with pustules - anac.
cut away, having one side of face - mag-m.
disfigured - sep.
swollen - kali-n.

FAILURES - fago., ign., mosch., op.

FALLING, of - acon., allox., alum., alum-p., ***am-m.,*** ange-s., aur., **BELL.,** bism., ***cact.,*** cahin., calc., canth., caps., chel., chin., cimic., cob-n., ***dig.,*** dulc., elaps, eupi., ferr., ferr-p., ***guai.,*** hell., ***hep.,*** ign., kali-c., kali-i., kali-n., kali-p., ***kreos.,*** lyc., mag-arct., mag-m., ***merc.,*** mez., nat-s., nicc., nit-ac., nux-m., nux-v., op., ph-ac., phos., plb., ***puls.,*** rumx., sabad., sabin., sang., ***sars.,*** sep., sil., sol-t-ae., ***sulph.,*** sumb., tab., **THUJ.,** verat., zinc., zinc-oc., zinc-p.
danger of - alum., am-m.
hammac, from a - phos.
high places, from - acon., alum., am-m., anan., arn., aur., bell., calc., chin., cimic., ***dig.,*** guai., hep., kali-c., kali-n., ***kreos.,*** lyc., merc., merc-c., ***mez.,*** nat-s., nicc., nit-ac., nux-m., op., ph-ac., phos., sep., sil., sin-n., sol-t-ae., ***sulph.,*** sumb., **THUJ.,** verat., zinc.
men are killed by falling from a height - sabin.
horse, from - tarent.
loft, from - nicc.
pit, into a - elaps.

FALLING, of
water, into - ***am-m., dig.,*** eupi., ***ferr.,*** ign., iod., mag-m., mag-s., merc., nicc., ph-ac.
child is falling - eupi.
mother is falling - nicc.

FAMINE, being left in a dungeon to die of, escaping by crawling out - ped.

FAMILY, own - ant-c.

FANTASTIC - acon., ambr., am-c., ant-t., arg-n., ars., ars-h., bar-c., bufo, **CALC.,** calc-sil., **CARB-AN.,** ***carb-s., carb-v.,*** cench., ***cham., chin.,*** coff., ***con.,*** ferr-i., ***graph.,*** hell., ***ign.,*** kali-ar., ***kali-c.,*** kali-n., kali-sil., kalm., **LACH.,** lact., led., lyc., merc., morph., mur-ac., ***nat-c.,*** **NAT-M.,** ***nat-s.,*** nicc., nit-ac., nux-v., **OP.,** pen., petr., plan., prun., ptel., puls., ***sep.,*** sil., spong., ***sulph.,*** thymol., zinc., zinc-oc.

FARMING - mag-s., merc-i-r.

FEASTING - anan., ant-c., asaf., hura, mag-s., nit-ac., ph-ac., tril., zinc.

FEVER - kali-chl., sulph.

FEVERISH - euphr., lachn.

FIELDS, roaming over - **RHUS-T.**

FIGHTS - ***all-c.,*** aesc., allox., aza., bapt., bell., brom., bry., calad., coca, con., crot-c., ***culx.,*** elaps, ***ferr.,*** ferr-i., guai., guare., hyper., indg., iris, piloc., jac-c., kali-bi., kali-c., kali-n., lyc., lyss., mag-aust., mag-c., mag-s., mosch., nat-a., nat-c., ***nat-m.,*** nat-s., nicc., phel., phos., pip-m., plat., ptel., puls., ***ran-s.,*** rat., sars., senec., sil., sol-t-ae., stann., ***staph., stram.,*** verb.
conquers, and - bapt.
ghosts, with - sars., sep., sil.
robbers, with - ferr-i., jac-c., mag-c., nat-c., sil.
suggested by reading - coca.

FINGER, of being seized by a - sil.

FINGERS, stiff - calc-s.

FIRE - alum., am-c., **ANAC.,** ant-t., ***ars.,*** bar-c., ***bell.,*** calc., ***calc-p.,*** calc-sil., cann-i., cann-s., ***carb-ac.,*** carb-v., cas-s., cench., chin., clem., ***croc., cur.,*** daph., euphr., fl-ac., graph., **HEP.,** iris, kali-ar., kali-c., kali-n., kali-sil., kiss., ***kreos.,*** lach., **LAUR.,** ***mag-aust.,*** **MAG-C., MAG-M.,** ***mag-s., meph.,*** merc., merc-c., naja, nat-c., ***nat-m.,*** nat-p., nat-s., nit-s-d., osm., ***phos.,*** pip-m., plat., rhod., ***rhus-t.,*** sel., sil., sol-t-ae., spig., spong., stann., stront-c., ***sulph.,*** sul-ac., zinc., zinc-oc., zing.
come down from heaven - ***sulph.***
danger of - ant-t., bell., clem., merc-ac.
destroying a city - sol-t-ae.
lightning, from - euphr.
world on fire - ***rhus-t.***

FISHES - arg-n., chin., chin-b., kali-c., mag-c.

FISHING - arg-m., cinch., mag-c., verat-v.

FIT, that he had a - iris, mag-c., sil.

FIXED, upon one subject - acon., ign., puls., stann.

FLAYED, being - arn.

FLEEING, of - asc-t., zinc.

FLOATING - hell.

FLOOD - mag-c., merc., nat-c., ***sil.***

FLOWERS - mag-c., nat-s.

FLYING - ***apis,*** asc-t., atro., bell., convo-d., indg., ***lat-m.,*** lyc., nat-s., ***rhus-g.,*** stict., xan.
airplane - allox.
tops of houses, over - xan.

FOOD - ptel.

FOOT, stitching in the - asar.

FOREIGN, country - ind., plat., sil.

FOREST, of a, going astray in a forest - mag-m., sep.

FORMS - bry., calc., cina.
black - arn., ars., puls.
form, darkening the sun - ped.
horrid, presenting a bottle - merc-c.
grotesque, dancing before her - narcot.
sitting on chest - paeon.

FRACTURE of, jaw - rauw.
limbs - cimic.

FREEZING - grat.

FRIENDLY, being - ped.

FRIENDS - ferr., oci., rumx.
death of - allox., coff., coff-t., con., cortico., fl-ac., kali-n., lach., nicc.
dead friends - arg-n., cedr., coca, ferr., nat-c.
meeting friends - calc-p.
old - ant-c., ferr., rumx.
seeing friends - rumx.

FRIGHTFUL, (see Nightmares) - abrot., ***acon.,*** adon., aeth., ether, agar., agn., alco., alet., all-c., all-s., alum., alumn., am-c., **AM-M.,** ambr., ***ammc.,*** anac., ang., ***ant-c.,*** ant-t., apis, ***aran.,*** aran-ix., ***arg-m., arg-n., arn.,*** **ARS.,** ars-i., ars-s-f., asar., asc-t., atro., **AUR.,** aur-a., aur-m., aur-s., bad., ***bapt.,*** bar-c., bar-m., ***bell., bism.,*** bol., **BOR.,** bov., brucin., ***bry.,*** bufo, **CALC.,** calc-ac., ***calc-f., calc-p., calc-s., calc-sil., camph.,*** cann-i., ***cann-s.,*** canth., caps., carb-an., carb-s., **CARB-V., CARC.,** ***carl.,*** casc., cast., caust., ***cench., cham., chel., chin.,*** chin-a., chin-s., ***chol.,*** cimic., **CINA,** clem., **COCC.,** cod., coff., coloc., ***colch.,*** **CON.,** cop., corn., ***croc.,*** **CROT-C.,** crot-h., ***cycl.,*** dig., digin., digox., dios., dor., dros., dulc., elaps, ***erig., eup-pur.,*** euph., euphr., eupi., ferr., fl-ac., **GRAPH.,** grat., guai., ham., hell., hep., hipp., hydr., ***hyos.,*** hyper., iber., ign., indg., ip., iris, jac-c., jug-c., jug-r., **KALI-AR.,** kali-bi., **KALI-BR., KALI-C.,** kali-cy., ***kali-i.,*** kali-m., kali-n., kali-p., ***kali-s.,*** kali-sil., kalm., kiss., kreos., lach., ***laur.,*** led., lil-t., **LYC.,** lyss., ***mag-c., mag-m.,*** mag-s., man., manc., mang., ***med., merc.,*** merc-c., merc-i-f., merc-i-r., merc-sul., mez., mit., morph., mosch., mur-ac., myric., naja, ***nat-a., nat-c.,*** **NAT-M.,** ***nat-p., nat-s.,*** **NICC.,** ***nit-ac.,*** nux-m., ***nux-v.,*** op., ox-ac., paeon., ***par.,*** ped., petr., phel., ph-ac., **PHOS.,** plan., plat., plb., ***psor.,*** ptel., phys., **PULS.,** ***pyrog., ran-b., ran-s.,*** rat., rheum, rhod., rhus-t., sabad., sabin., sang., sarr., sars., scroph-n., scut., sec., sel., sep., serp., **SIL.,** sin-n., sol-n., spig., ***spong.,*** squil., stann., staph., stram., stront-c., ***sul-ac., sulph.,*** tab., ***tarax.,*** teucr., til., thea., thuj., ust., valer., verb., verat., verat-v., ***zinc.,*** zinc-p., zing.
afternoon - ign.
alternating with headache - chin.
closing eyes - chin.
dysmenorrhea, in - ***cycl.***
falling downstairs, after - ***rhus-t.***
fear, followed by - ***acon.,*** alum., ***am-m., chin., cocc., con.,*** hep., lyc., mag-s., mur-ac., nat-c., ph-ac., sil., sulph., zinc.
midnight - all-s.
after - dor., ph-ac., plan., stront.
monsters - aloe, **CALC.,** hydr., phos., ped.
morning - ***con.,*** ign.
sleep, on going to - chin.
true after waking, seeming - nat-m.
waking him - acon., bell., casc., corn., ***erig.,*** **LYC.,** ***meph., sulph.***

FRUIT - cast-eq., jac-c., mag-c.

FROG, in bed - allox.

FUNERALS - allox., alum., ange-s., bart., brom., ***chel.,*** form., mag-c., nat-c., nicc., rat.
corps coming alive after a funeral - allox.
funeral-knell, his own - ether.

GARDENS - com., nat-s., phel.

GARMENT, made the previous day - aeth.

GEESE, of being bitten by - zinc.

GHOSTS, spectres - aesc., alum., am-c., ***arg-n.,*** asc-t., atro., bell., bov., ***camph.,*** carb-s., ***carb-v.,*** cham., chlol., convo-d., ***crot-c.,*** eupi., ***graph.,*** ign., ***kali-c.,*** kali-s., kali-sil., lach., mag-s., manc., ***med.,*** nat-c., nat-m., ***ol-j.,*** op., paeon., puls., sars., sep., ***sil.,*** spig., ***sulph.***
black - ars., cerv.
fighting with - sars., sep.
pursued, by - sil.
white - sars.

GIANTS - bell., lyc.
pursued by - bell.

GIRL, that he is a - apis.

GRAVES - anac., ***arn.,*** hura, iris, mag-c., ptel.
armies rising from their graves - ptel.
thrown into a grave, being - mag-c.

GREATNESS - bufo.

GRIEF - alum., am-c., arn., ***asar.,*** calc-p., con., ***ign.,*** led., mag-m., mosch., mur-ac., **NAT-M.,** rheum, ***sil., staph.***

GRIMACES, horrible - op.

GROTESQUE - lil-t.

GROWING things - kreos.

GUILT - asar.

GUNS - hep.

GYMNASTICS - bell.

HAIR, of being obliged to dress hair in company - mag-c.
falling out - mag-c.

HANDS, burning by washing - mag-m.
cut to pieces, being - sol-t-ae.

HEADACHE - pip-m.

HEADS - glon., jac-c.
cut off - hura, nicc.

HEARING, talking - stram.

HELD, by finger, being - sil.
tightly by hand - am-m.

HEMOPTYSIS - hep., meph., phos.

HEMORRHAGE - phos., sol-t-ae.

HIDING, from danger, of - lyc.

HIGH, places - all-c., anac., brom., chin., cortico., laur., lyss., macro.
falling from high places - acon., alum., am-m., anan., aur., cimic., chin., ***dig.,*** guai., hep., kali-c., kali-n., ***kreos.,*** merc., merc-c., ***mez.,*** nat-s., nicc., nux-m., op., ph-ac., phos., sep., sin-a., sol-t-ae., ***sulph.,*** sumb., **THUJ.,** zinc.
men are killed by falling from a height - sabin.

HISTORIC - acon., am-c., ant-t., brom., caust., ***cham.,*** cic., croc., graph., hell., hyos., mag-arct., ***mag-c.,*** merc., ***phos.,*** sel., ***sil.,*** stram.

HOME - lach., mur-ac.

HOMELAND - ant-c., lach., mur-ac.

HOMESICKNESS - ***glon.***

HORSES - alum., am-c., am-m., asc-t., atro., crot-c., hyper., indg., mag-aust., mag-m., mag-s., merc., phos., senec., sul-ac., tarent., ther., zinc.
arm bitten by a - am-m.
changing into dogs - zinc.
falling from horse - tarent.
kicking - ***mag-s.***
pursuing him - allox., alum.
riding - nat-c., ther.
running - atro., indg., lipp.
stealing a horse - ether, rumx.
ugly - merc., phos.

HOUSE, loses his way in his - mag-c.

HOUSEHOLD, affairs - calc., bell., ***bry.***

HOUSES - pall.
looses his way in - mag-c.

HUMILIATION - alum., am-c., arn., ***asar.,*** con., ***ign.,*** led., mag-m., mosch., mur-ac., **NAT-M.,** rheum, ***sil., staph.***

HUNG, of being - am-m., ars.
persons, seeing them - merc-sul.

HUNGER - ***arg-n.,*** bry., calc., ign., iod.

HUNTING - hura, hyper., merc-i-r., verat.

HURRIED - coca, merc-c., zinc.

ILL-treatment - ambr., dros.

ILLUMINATIONS - crot-c.

IMPRESSIVE - acon., arn., camph., carb-an., graph., ign., lach., nux-v., puls., sabin., thuj.

IMPRISONMENT - bov., cerv.

INDIANS, that he is among - jug-c.

INJURIES - allox., am-m., ant-c., chel., chin., cortico., lob., ***mag-s.,*** nat-s., nicc., phos., sumb.
machinery, by - cortico.
self-inflicted - nicc.

INSANE, becoming - aloe, ferr-p.
man becomes insane - apis.

INSECTS - arg-n., hist., kreos., myric., spig.
stung by an insect - phos.
stinging insects - phos.

INSULTS - asar., ant-s., tarent.

INSURRECTIONS - ped.

INTELLECTUAL - all-s., anac., ars., buf-s., carb-ac., carb-an., cham., cinnb., coloc., ferr., fl-ac., guai., ign., ind., kali-n., lyc., nat-p., phos., sabin., ***senec.,*** sil., thuj., ust.
midnight, after - mag-c.
morning - ign.

INVENTION, full of - apis, kali-n., lach., sabin.

INTRIGUE, that his character is one of - lach.

ITCHING, eyelids - upa.

JEALOUSY - lyc.

JOKE, relating a - coca.

JOURNEY - all-s., am-c., am-m., anan., ***apis,*** bart., brom., bufo, calc-f., ***calc-p., carb-ac.,*** carc., chel., chin., chin-b., ***cortico.,*** crot-h., elaps, hyper., hura, hydr., ind., indg., **KALI-N.,** lac-c., lac-d., ***lach.,*** linu-c., ***mag-c.,*** mag-m., mag-s., merc., merc-c., merc-i-r., mez., ***nat-c.,*** nat-m., ***op.,*** pip-m., psor., rauw., ***rhus-t.,*** sang., sel., ***sil.,*** sin-a., ther., ***tub.***
difficulties, with - am-m., calc-p., mag-s., merc., mez., nat-c.
horseback, on - nat-c., ther.
long - nat-m.
railroad, by - apis, cortico.
water, by - alum., chin-b., nat-s., sang., valer.
anxious - op.

JOYOUS - ant-t., ars., asaf., caust., coff., ***croc.,*** dig., dros., grat., ***lach.,*** laur., mag-c., mag-m., mag-s., mez., **OP.,** palo., ph-ac., phos., squil., sulph.

JUMPING - calc-f., verat.
great leaps - apis.
water, men jumping into - mag-s.

KILLING, mad dog, a - rumx.

KNEE, painful - zinc.
swollen - cocc.

KNIVES - guai., lach., nat-c.
stabbed his antagonist with a knife - nat-c.

LATIN, speaking - lyss.

LAUGHING - alum., caust., coca, croc., hyos., kreos., lyc.

LEG, amputated - atro.

LEPER - paull.

LETHARGY - graph., op.

LEWD fancies even dreaming - ambr.

LICE - am-c., chel., gamb., mur-ac., ***nux-v.,*** ped., phos.

LIGHT - coff.

LIGHTNING - ***arn.,*** euphr., phel., phos., spig.
struck by lightning, being - ***arn.***

LION, that he was a - phys.

LITERATURE - ign.

LOATHSOME - anac., arg-m., nux-v., puls., zinc.

LONG - ***acon.,*** bry., calc., chin., ***coff.,*** euph., ***ign.,*** naja, nat-c., puls., spig., tarent., thuj.
object, of same - **PETR., SPIG.**

LOOKING, for someone and failing to find him - carc.

LOSS, disheartening - ***meph.***

LOST, as in a forest - am-m., ind., mag-c., mag-m., mag-s., sep.
mountains, in the - ind.

LOTTERY - mag-c., nat-s.

LUCID - fl-ac.
revealing a perplexed situation when waking - acon.

LUDICROUS - bell., cod., glon., grat., iber., jug-c., lach., merc-c., merc-i-r., mez., mygal., phos., sol-t-ae., ***sulph.***
lying left side, on - sep.
midnight, after - mez.

LUMP, in throat and ear - cinnb.

LYING, someone, under him - nit-ac.
in bed with another person - petr.

MAGIC - sol-t-ae.

MANY, dreams - abrot., acon., aconin., agar., agn., alco., all-c., **ALUM.,** ***am-c., am-m.,*** ambr., aml-n., ammc., anac., ang., ant-c., ant-s., ant-t., ***apis,*** arg-m., arg-n., arist-m., ***arn., ars.,*** asaf., asar., asc-t., astac., atro., aur., bals-p., bapt., bar-c., bart., **BELL.,** benz-ac., berb., bism., bol., bond., bor., bov., brach., brom., **BRY.,** buf-s., cact., caj., calad., **CALC.,** calc-caust., calc-f., calc-p., camph., cann-i., canth., caps., carb-ac., carb-an., carb-s., ***carb-v.,*** card-m., carl., casc., cast-eq., ***caust., cham.,*** chel., **CHIN.,** chin-s., chr-ac., cic., cimic., cina, cinnb., clem., cob., coc-c., coca, cocc., cod., coff., coff-t., colch., coloc., com., **CON.,** cor-r., cori-r., cortico., cortiso., croc., crot-t., cund., cupr., cupr-ac., ***cycl.,*** dig., digin., digox., ***ferr.,*** ferr-p., fl-ac., form., franz., gall-ac., gamb., gast., gels., gins., glon., ***gran., graph.,*** guai., hall, ham., ***hell., hep.,*** hipp., hydr., hyos., hyosin., hypo., ***ign.,*** ind., iod., ip., piloc., jal., jug-r., kali-bi., kali-br., **KALI-C.,** kali-cy., kali-n., kali-s., kiss., **KREOS.,** lac-ac., ***lach.,*** lact., laur., led., lil-t., lob., lob-c., **LYC.,** lycps., ***mag-arct., mag-c.,*** mag-m., mag-s., ***mang.,*** menis., meny., ***merc.,*** merc-i-r., merc-sul., merl., ***mez.,*** mosch., mur-ac., myric., naja, nat-a., nat-c., ***nat-m.,*** nat-p., ***nat-s.,*** nicc., **NIT-AC.,** nux-m., **NUX-V.,** olnd., op., ox-ac., paeon., ***par.,*** peti., petr., **PH-AC., PHOS.,** phys., pic-ac., pimp., pip-m., plan., plat., plb., prun., psor., ***puls., rhus-t.,*** rhus-v., ruta, sabad., sabin., samb., sars., sec., sel., senec., ***sep.,*** **SIL.,** sin-n., sol-n., spig., ***spong.,*** squil., ***stann., staph.,*** stram., stront-c., sul-ac., **SULPH.,** tab., tarax., tarent., ***ter.,*** teucr., ther., thuj., tril., **TUB.,** tus-p., valer., verat., verat-v., verb., viol-t., zinc.
children, in - valer.
crowding one upon another - kali-c., sep., ***sil.,*** thuj.
menses, before - alum.
nap, during - nat-m.

MARRIAGE, of - alum., mag-c., mag-m.

MASKS - kali-c., mag-c.

MEAT, thrust into mouth - alum.

MEDITATION, with - acon., anac., arn., bry., camph., carb-an., graph., ***ign.,*** lach., ***nux-v.,*** puls., rhus-t., sabad., sabin., thuj.

MEN - frax., nicc., ***puls.***
following to violate her - ***cench.,*** kali-n., kreos., sep.
green - sol-t-ae.
naked - eupi., ***puls.***

MERRY - ph-ac., squil.

MENTAL, exertion (see Exertion)

MERRY - ph-ac., squil.

MICE - colch., mag-s., sep.
yellow - mag-s.

MIND, affecting the - bry., chin., ***ign., lach.,*** nat-m., ***nux-v.,*** olnd., ph-ac., phos., sabad., sabin., sulph., thuj., viol-t.

MISCARRIAGE - mag-arct.

MISFORTUNE, of - alum., ***am-m.,*** anac., ant-c., ***arn., ars.,*** ars-s-f., aur-m., bar-c., bar-m., bar-s., ***bell.,*** cann-s., carb-an., ***cham., chin.,*** chin-a., clem., cocc., croc., **GRAPH.,** guai., ign., iod., ***kali-ar., kali-c.,*** kali-m., kali-n., kali-p., kali-s., kreos., laur., led., **LYC.,** ***mag-c.,*** mag-m., mang., ***merc.,*** mur-ac., nat-s., nicc., **NUX-V.,** op., petr., ph-ac., ***phos.,*** **PULS.,** ran-b., rhus-t., rhus-v., sars., sel., spong., stann., staph., ***sul-ac., sulph.,*** tarent., **THUJ.,** verat., verb., zinc., zinc-p.

MONEY - alum., ***cycl.,*** mag-c., mag-m., phos., puls., zinc., zinc-oc.
counterfeit - zinc-oc.
disputes about - chin.
gold, of - ***cycl.,*** puls.

MONSTERS - aloe, **CALC.,** hydr., phos., ped.

MONSTROUS - arg-n.

MOUTH, opening impossible - agar.

MOWING, people - glon.

MUD, walking in - iod.

MULE, driving a - cinch.
driving out of bed - sep.

MURDER - am-m., ***arn.,*** bell., calad., calc., calc-sil., carb-an., carc., cast., chel., crot-h., guai., hura, ign., kali-i., kali-s., kalm., kiss., ***kreos.,*** lach., lact., led., lyc., mag-arct., mag-m., man., merc., merc-c., naja, nat-a., nat-c., ***nat-m.,*** nicc., ol-an., ***petr.,*** puls., rhus-v., rhus-t., rumx., sanic., saroth., sedi., sel., ***sil.,*** sol-a., spong., ***staph.,*** sulph., thea., thuj., ven-m., zinc.
of seeing murdered men - rumx.

MURDERED, of being - am-m., chel., chr-ac., guai., ign., kali-i., ***kreos., lach.,*** lact., lyc., mag-m., merc., merc-ac., merc-c., phos., sil., zinc.

MURDERING, boys and girls - thea.
father, her - cast.

MUSIC - mag-s., sarr.

MUTILATION - ant-c., arn., con., hura, mag-arct., mag-c., mag-m., merc., ***nux-v.***

NAKEDNESS - erech., kali-p., rumx.

NAKED, people - cench.
men - eupi., ***puls.***

NATIVE country - ant-c., lach., mur-ac.

NEW, scenes, places - calc-f.

NIGHTMARE, (see Frightful) - achy., ***acon.,*** ether, aloe, ***alum., alum-sil.,*** alumn., ambr., ***am-c.,*** am-m., ammc., ange-s., ant-t., arg-n., arn., ars-s-f., arum-t., ars., ars-i., asar., ***aur-br.,*** aur-m., aur-s., ***bapt.,*** bell., berb., ***bor., bry.,*** bufo, cadm-s., **CALC.,** calc-i., calc-sil., ***camph., cann-i.,*** canth., **CARC.,** card-m., ***carl.,*** cast., cench., ***cham.,*** chel., ***chin.,*** chin-s., chlol., ***cinnb.,*** cina, clem., colch., ***con.,*** cot., ***crot-t., cycl.,*** cypr., daph., dig., dulc., elaps, ***ferr.,*** ferr-i., ferr-p., gels., gink-b., ***guai.,*** hep., hydr-ac., hyos., ign., ind., ***iod.,*** iris, kali-ar., kali-bi., ***kali-br.,*** kali-c., ***kali-i.,*** kali-n., kali-p., kali-s., kali-sil., kres., lach., lact., laur., ***led.,*** lob., lyc., lyss., mag-c., mag-m., mag-s., mang., med., meph., merc., ***merc-c.,*** merc-i-f., mez., murx., naja, nat-a., ***nat-c.,*** nat-m., nat-p., nat-s., nat-sil., ***nit-ac.,*** nitro-o., ***nux-v.,*** op., osm., **PAEON.,** pariet., **PHOS.,** pic-ac., plb., polyg., ptel., ***puls.,*** rhod., rhus-t., ruta, ***sars.,*** scut., sec., sil., sol-n., staph., stram., sul-ac., sul-i., **SULPH.,** tab., tell., ter., thea., thiop., thuj., valer., ***zinc.***
afternoon - mez.
amorous dreams, during - nit-ac.
children, in - achy., ***acon.,*** bell., **CALC.,** ***carc., phos., puls.,*** ter., tub.
falling asleep, on - am-c., ***cann-i.,*** canth., cycl., digin., gels., nit-ac., ter.
every night - cann-i.
fear, followed by - ***acon.,*** alum., ***am-m., chin., cocc., con.,*** hep., lyc., mag-s., mur-ac., nat-c., ph-ac., sil., sulph., zinc.
full moon, at - nat-c.
lying on the back - card-m., guai., ind., **SULPH.**
menses, after - thuj.
before - sul-ac.
midnight - merc-ac., mez.
after - cinnb., ***mez.***
before - cycl., kali-c.

NIGHTMARES,
monsters, of - aloe, bell., **CALC., CARC.,** hydr., phos., ped., stram.
morning - phos.
night, 4 a.m. - alum., kali-bi.
room must be searched before appeased - ***cham.***
tea, after - thea.
waking, on - ptel.

NOISE - atro., cer-b., lyc., stann.

NOSE, being pulled by the - nat-c.
own his - ***syph.?***

OBJECTS, desired - sil.

OCCURRENCES, in the next room - sumb.

OXEN, are pursuing him - eupi., hipp., tet.
pursuing him, putrid - hura.

PAIN, during dreams - ars., cann-i., ***cham.,*** coloc., mag-m., merc., passi., puls., sin-n.
pain, dreams of - asar., bry., cahin., carb-h., cocc., ***med.***
abdomen, in - apis.
arm, in - nicc.
knee, in - zinc.
maxillary joint, in - agar.
temples, in - lyc.

PARTIES - crot-c., ***hura, nat-c.,*** phel., pip-m.

PASSION, outburst of - mag-c.

PEACEFUL - nux-m., spig.

PENIS, breaking off - kali-n.
breaking off, glans penis - kreos.
prepuce sloughed off - linu-c.

PEOPLE, of - apis, ars-h., art-v., aster., bell., calc-ar., coc-c., dig., **EQUIS.,** gels., lyss., mang., merc., nat-m., ***puls.***
assembled - apis, cer-b.
companies - canth., phel.
crowd - ars-h., **EQUIS.**
elderly - ***acon.,*** ars., op., passi., ***phos.***
influential persons - lyss.
near to him - nat-m.
parties - crot-c., hura, nat-c., phel., pip-m.
picnics - nat-s.
seen for years, people not - calad., calc-ar.

PERIODICAL, every second night - chin., lach.

PERSISTENT - ***acon.,*** agav-t., anac., ant-t., ***arn.,*** asaf., bar-c., ***bry., calc., chin.,*** coff., euph., graph., **IGN.,** lach., merc., mosch., ***nat-c.,*** nat-m., nat-s., ***phos.,*** plat., ***puls.,*** sabin., sep., sil., staph., zinc.

PERSON, another lying in bed with him - petr.

PHYSICIAN - canna, mang.

PICNICS - nat-s.

PINCHED, of being - phos.
at back and at breast, being - phos.

PINS, of - merc.

PLACES - equis., lyc., merc-i-r.
changing often - all-s., led., lyc.

PLACES,
high, places - all-c., anac., brom., chin., cortico., laur., lyss., macro.
falling from high places - acon., alum., am-m., anan., aur., cimic., chin., ***dig.,*** guai., hep., kali-c., kali-n., ***kreos.,*** merc., merc-c., ***mez.,*** nat-s., nicc., nux-m., op., ph-ac., phos., sep., sin-a., sol-t-ae., ***sulph.,*** sumb., **THUJ.,** zinc.
men are killed by falling from a height - sabin.
new - calc-f.

PLAYING, baseball - atro.

PLEASANT - acon., ether, agar., agn., all-c., alum., alum-sil., ambr., am-c., am-m., ***ant-c.,*** ant-t., ***arn.,*** ars., ars-h., asaf., atro., ***aur.,*** bar-c., bar-m., bell., bism., bor., bov., bry., **CALC.,** cann-s., canth., ***carb-an.,*** carb-v., caust., cench., cham., chel., chin., cic., clem., cocc., cod., ***coff.,*** coloc., com., ***con., croc.,*** cycl., dig., dros., erig., eug., euph., fago., gins., ***graph.,*** grat., hell., hura, hyos., ign., ***kali-c.,*** kali-cy., kali-i., kali-m., kali-n., kali-p., kreos., ***lach.,*** laur., led., lyc., ***mag-c.,*** mag-m., mag-s., manc., mang., menis., meny., merc., mez., morph., mur-ac., nat-a., **NAT-C.,** ***nat-m., nat-p.,*** nat-s., nicc., nit-ac., nitro-o., nux-m., ***nux-v.,*** ol-an., olnd., **OP.,** ox-ac., par., ped., petr., ***ph-ac.,*** phel., ***phos.,*** phys., ***plat.,*** plb., **PULS.,** ran-b., rhod., ***sabad.,*** samb., saroth., sars., senec., **SEP.,** ***serp.,*** spig., spong., squil., stann., **STAPH.,** stram., stront-c., ***sulph.,*** sumb., tarax., tarent., tep., ***teucr.,*** thuj., valer., verat., **VIOL-T.,** zinc., zing.
afternoon - mez.
evening - zing.
midnight, before, pleasant, after frightful - ph-ac.
night, after 2 a.m. - tarent.

POETIC - ars-h., buf-s., lach., nat-m., til.

POISONED, of being - chr-ac., kali-n., ***kreos.,*** nat-m., oci.
by herself - kali-n.

POLICE - frax.

POLITICAL - asc-t.

POLLUTION which didn't take place - thuj.

PRAYING - ars-h., pip-m.

PREACHING - allox., anac., ant-t.
has to preach - anac.

PRECIPICES - ***all-c., lac-ac.***

PREGNANT - pic-ac.

PRISONER, being taken a - allox., nat-m.
release of prisoners - hura.

PROFOUND - saroth.

PROJECTS - anac., bufo, camph., rhus-t.
coming true - rhus-t.

PROPHETIC - arg-n., asaf., bor., ***cann-i.,*** cortico., mag-arct., mang., ph-ac., phos., rad., sulph.
prophesying death - kali-c., kali-chl.

PROVING, remedy - merc., pip-m.

PROVOKED, being - verat-v.

PRUDE, being - **TUB.**

PURCHASE, making - hura.

PURSUED by, of being - allox., arg-m., atro., bell., hir., hydr., kreos., mag-s., nux-m., nux-v., ped., ph-ac., sep., ***sil., sulph.,*** verat., ***zinc.***
animals, by - allox., alum., cench., eupi., hipp., ind., led., nux-v., sil., ***sulph.,*** tarent., tet., verat.
bulls, by - ind., tarent.
mad - ind.
cats and dogs, of being - ***nux-v.,*** sil., verat.
crocodiles, by - led.
enemies - con.
ghosts - sil.
giants - bell.
horses, by - allox., alum.
man - eupi., hipp., tet.
who will rape her (see Rape) - ***cench.,*** kali-n., kreos., sep.,
robbers - mag-m.
run backwards, must - sep.
soldiers - mag-s.
wild beasts - sil., ***sulph.***

PUS - hep.

QUARRELS - alum., alum-sil., am-c., am-m., anan., ant-c., apis, aran-ix., ***arn.,*** ars., aur., aza., ***bapt.,*** bar-c., ***bell.,*** brom., ***bry.,*** calc., calc-ac., canth., carl., cast., ***caust.,*** cham., chin., con., ***crot-h.,*** culx., ferr-p., guai., guare., hep., hydr., indg., kali-c., ***kali-n.,*** lyc., mag-aust., ***mag-c.,*** mag-s., ***merc.,*** mosch., nat-c., nat-m., nat-s., nicc., nit-ac., **NUX-V.,** op., paeon., ph-ac., ***phos.,*** plat., ***puls.,*** raph., rat., rheum, sabin., ***sel.,*** sep., sil., spig., ***stann., staph., stram.,*** tarax., verat., zinc.
dead relatives, with - kali-c., staph.
money, about - chin.

QUIET - atro.

RAIN, of being soaked in - mag-c.

RAINBOWS - coff-t.

RAPE - ***cench.,*** kreos., op., petr., sep., staph.
pursued by man for the purpose of - ***cench.,*** kali-n., kreos., sep.
seeing, of - ***cench.***
that he has committed - ***cench.,*** kreos., petr., sep.
threats of - sep.

RAPID, transit from place to place - all-s.

RASH, covered with - am-m.

RATS - allox., sep.
creeping under the clothes - menis.

RECALLING, things long forgotten - acon., am-c., anac., bov., calad., cer-b., chin., ferr-i., nat-c., sel., senec., **SIL.,** spig., sulph., sumb.

RECONCILIATION - mang.

REGIONS, beautiful - ol-an., rumx.
regions, of far off - sil.

RELATIVES - merc-i-r., oci.
dead - ferr., caust., fl-ac., kali-c., mag-c., mag-s., rheum, sars.
death, of the - alumn., aran-ix., ***calc-f.,*** cast., chin., fl-ac., grat., levo., mag-s., mur-ac., nicc., paeon., plan., plat.

RELIGIOUS - sol-t-ae.

REMEMBERED - ammc., bell., brom., bry., cann-s., carb-v., carl., casc., caust., cham., clem., cob., con., fl-ac., franz., gins., glon., graph., indg., lyc., mag-c., mag-s., mang., mez., ***nat-m., nuph.,*** nux-v., pall., phos., plat., sin-a., ***sulph.,*** tarent.

REMORSE, of - arn., ars., ether, elaps, fl-ac., hyper., lach., led., nat-c., nat-m., sanic.

REPEATING - ***arn.,*** cer-b., eupi., ign., nat-m., petr.

REPENTANCE - ars.

REPROACHING, himself - nat-m.

RESTLESS - ambr., anac., ange-s., arg-n., ***ars.,*** brom., bry., calad., calc., calc-caust., carb-s., carb-v., carl., caste., cham., cic., ***clem.,*** colch., esp-g., euph., graph., indg., ***iod.,*** jug-r., ***kali-c.,*** kali-n., ***led.,*** lith., lyc., mez., mosch., mur-ac., nat-c., nat-m., nux-v., ***olnd.,*** op., par., ph-ac., phos., psor., ptel., sabad., ***sil.,*** stann., staph., ***sulph., viol-t.,*** visc.

RESURRECTION - allox.

REVELLING, a perplexed situation when waking - ***acon.***

REVOLUTION - hura, merc.

RIDICULOUS - mez.

RIDING - chr-ac., nat-c., ther.
carriage, in - bell., indg., nat-s.

RIOTS - bry., con., guai., indg., kali-c., lyc., nat-c., nat-m., phos., puls., stann.

RISEN and dressed, having - sumb.

ROAMING, over fields - **RHUS-T.**

ROBBERS - allox., **ALUM.,** alum-p., ***arn., aur.,*** bell., calc-p., carb-v., cast., cench., ferr-i., jac-c., ***kali-c.,*** kali-s., lil-s., **MAG-C.,** mag-m., mag-s., ***merc.,*** merc-ac., nat-c., **NAT-M.,** petr., phel., phos., plb., psor., ptel., rumx., ***sanic.,*** sel., ***sil.,*** sin-n., tub., verat., ***zinc.***
cannot sleep until the house is searched - **NAT-M.,** sanic.
dissecting robbers - merc-i-r.
fighting with - jac-c., mag-c., ferr-i., nat-c., sil.
menses, during - ***nat-m.***
pursued by - mag-m.

ROMANTIC - am-c.

ROWDY, feeling disposed to act like a - caj.

ROWING - rhus-t.

RUBBISH is falling on her - mag-m.

RUNNING - bell.
after someone - cadm-met.
up and down - ambr.
vainly - croc., ind.

SAD - alum., ant-c., ***ars.,*** asar., asc-t., aur., aur-m., cann-i., caps., carb-an., carb-s., cast., caust., chin., crot-t., graph., guare., ign., junc., laur., lepi., lyc., mag-c., manc., mosch., mur-ac., nat-c., ***nat-m.,*** nit-ac., ***nux-v.,*** op., paeon., paull., peti., phos., plan., ***puls.,*** rat., ***rheum,*** rhus-t., ruta, spong., stront-c., tarent., ust., zinc.

SAILING - alum., chin., hura, nat-s., sang., senec., valer., verat-v.
dangerous sail in a small boat - nat-m.

SCENES, new - calc-f.
vulgar - chin-b.

SCHOOLMATE, seeing again an old - ant-c., ferr.

SCIENTIFIC - carb-an., carb-v., guai., ***ign.,*** mag-arct., spong.

SCREAM, unable to - ars., cast., mag-m., sil., tab.

SEA - all-c., chin., chin-b., murx.

SENSIBLE - aur.

SEX, of (see Amorous) - am-m., bor., ind., iod., lac-ac., lyc., sil., thuj., ***zinc-pic.***
unsuccessful - ind., iod.

SHAMEFUL - acon., alum., am-c., arn., ***asar.,*** con., erech., led., mag-m., ***mosch.,*** mur-ac., staph., tub.

SHED, being under a - merc-i-r.

SHOCKING - bell., hyos., ph-ac.

SHOOTING - ***am-m.,*** hep., mag-s., ***merc.,*** merc-i-r., spong.
being shot, of - bell., lact., lob., mag-s., mang.
hearing, of - hep.
soldier is shot, a - am-m.

SHOTS - cerv., hura.

SHUDDERING - calc-ac.

SICK, people - calc., calc-sil., cast-eq., ign., mosch., nat-s., peti., rat., rheum, staph.

SINGING, political songs - asc-t.

SKATING, in the water - ped.

SKELETONS - op.

SLEEP, comatose, of - graph.

SLEEPING, in air - acon.

SLEIGH-rides - sars., tril.

SMEARED with excrements, being - zinc.

SLEEP, comatose of - graph.
on begining to sleep - ambr., aur., bell., cycl., mang., puls., thuj.,

SMELLING, sulphur, tinder - anac.

SMOKING - tell.

SNAKES - alum., ***arg-n.,*** bov., carc., cench., daph., grat., iris, kali-c., kalm., **LAC-C.,** ***lach.,*** merl., op., ptel., ran-a., ***ran-b., ran-s.,*** rat., sep., sil., sol-n., spig., tab., teucr-s., tub.
bitten by, of being - bov., cench.

SNOW - art-v., bapt., kali-n., ***kreos.***
working in - bapt.

SOAKED, with rain, being - mag-c.

SOILING, himself - aloe, cast-v., iod., zinc.

SOLDIER - bry., chel., mang., nat-c.
being a - chel.
pursued by a - mag-s.
seeing a soldier shot - am-m.

SOLEMNITIES - ant-c.

SOLES, tickled on - phos.

SOMERSAULTS - zing.

SOMNAMBULISTIC - sil.

SOMNOLENCE - graph., op.

SORE, throat - bar-c., bor., pip-m.

SPEECH, giving - cham.
making a long - arn., cham.

SPIDERS - cinnb., crot-c., sars., ven-m.
as large as an ox - cinnb.

SPINNING - lachn., sars.

SPITTING, of blood - hep., meph., phos.
pus - hep.

SPLENDOR - stann.

SPOKEN to, of being - aur.

STAB others, will, his antagonist - nat-c.
friend, his - allox.

STABBED - chin., guai., lil-s., nat-c., op.
dread of being - lach.

STAGS - canth.

STARS, falling - alum.

STEALING, fruit - rumx.
horse, someone is stealing his - ether.

STIFFNESS, fingers - calc-s.

STITCHES, in eyes - ***calc.***
foot - asar.

STONE, lying on him - kali-c.

STOOL - aloe, cast-v., psor., sars., zinc.

STOPPAGE, throat - kreos.

STORMS - all-s., ***ars.,*** jac-c., mag-c., ***sil.***
at sea - all-c., sil.
snow storm - ***kreos.***
thunder - ***arn., ars.,*** euphr., nat-c., phel., spig.

STOVE, hot - apis.

STRANGE - acon., ant-t., bar-ac., chin-s., ***lach.,*** lact., nit-ac., ph-ac., sarr., stram.

STRANGLED, of being - ars., phos., sil., zinc.

STRANGURY - chr-ac.

STREAM - com.
crossing a stream on horseback - chr-ac.

STRIVING - cina, croc., graph., nux-v., rhus-t., sabin.

STRUCK, by lightning, that he was - ***arn.***

STUNG, by an insect - phos.

SUBJECT, of one and the same - ***ign.,*** puls.

SUBORDINATION, like a servant - lyss.

SUFFERING - cimic.

SUFFOCATION - arn., chel., ign., iris, kali-bi., kali-c., sang., xan.

SUICIDE - naja.

SUPERNATURAL, things - asc-t.

SWALLOWING, pins - merc.

SWEAR, disposed to - caj.

SWELLING of body - squil.
cheek - kali-n.
face - kali-n.

SWINGING - sang.

TALKING with someone - plb.

TALL, of being very - ferr-i.

TEETH, breaking off - kali-n., rauw., sul-ac., ther., thuj.
falling out - coca, cocc., convo-d., nicc., nux-v., tab.
filling is falling out - nux-v.
pulled out, being - cench., nat-m.

TEMPLES, painful - lyc.

THEATER, but could not get dressed, going to - mag-s.

THEFT, of being accused of - lach.
of having committed - alum., plb.

THINGS, black - nat-a.
fixed upon the same dreams - acon., ign., puls., spig., stann.
growing - kali-n., kreos.
small, seem - ferr-i.
strange - plat.
varied - am-c., cann-i., carl., coloc., equis., ***gran.,*** iber., ir-foe., lachn., mang., mez., ***nat-c., nat-m.,*** op., pip-m., plan., stram., zing.

THIRSTY - dros., mag-c., **NAT-M.**

THREATS - anac., ars., sep.

THROAT, having a lump in the - cinnb.
grows up - xan.
sore throat - bar-c., bor., pip-m.
stoppage of the throat - kreos.

THROW away, being to - rhus-t.?

THROWN from carriage, being - nat-s.
grave, into a - mag-c.

THUNDER, storms - ***arn., ars.,*** euphr., nat-c., phel., spig.

TICKLED, on the soles, being - phos.

TOAD, in bed - allox.

TOE, cut off - nat-s.

TONGUE, too large - tab.

TOSSING, someone out of the window - bry.

TREATMENT, medical - canna.

TREES - lyc.

TRIUMPH - bapt.

TOMBS - anac.
living in - nicc.
putting tapers on tombs - hura.

TREASON - sil.

TRUE, coming (see Prophetic) - ***mag-arct.,*** mang., rad., sulph.
dreams seem, on waking - am-m., anac., ***arg-m.,*** arn., caps., hyos., merc., nat-c., nat-m., verat.

TURNING, around - lact.

ULCERS, abdomen - junc.

UNCONSCIOUSNESS - graph.

UNIMPORTANT - alum., anac., arg-m., ars., bell., ***bry.,*** canth., cham., chel., ***chin.,*** cic., cina, clem., cocc., coff., con., euph., ferr-i., hep., ign., kali-c., kali-n., lach., lyc., lycps., ***mag-c.,*** merc., nat-m., ***nux-v.,*** peti., ***ph-ac.,*** phos., plat., ***puls.,*** rhod.

UNPLEASANT - abies-n., agar., alum., ang., ant-t., apis, arg-m., ars., asar., ***bell.,*** bry., calc., calc-caust., calc-f., cann-i., ***cann-s.,*** carb-s., cham., chin., chr-ac., cic., ***cimic.,*** cina, cit-v., cob., coca, coff., coff-t., con., ***corn.,*** fago., dig., ferr., ferr-i., fl-ac., ***gels.,*** glon., ham., iber., ign., iod., iris, kalm., kali-bi., ***lac-c.,*** lach., laur., levo., lil-t., lyc., lyss., merc., merc-c., merc-d., myric., nat-m., ***nat-s.,*** nux-m., nux-v., op., ox-ac., peti., ***petr.,*** plan., polyg., psil., ptel., rhus-t., rumx., sang., senec., sep., sil., staph., stry., **SULPH.,** tarent., tell., tep., til., ust., wild., ziz.
falling asleep, on - lyss.

UNREMEMBERED - agar., agn., aloe, arg-m., ***arn.,*** ars., ***aur.,*** bapt., ***bell.,*** bov., ***bry.,*** buf-s., cact., calc., calc-ar., calc-caust., canth., ***carb-ac.,*** carb-an., carb-v., ***carl., chel.,*** chr-ac., ***cic.,*** cinnb., cob., coca, cocc., con., croc., eupi., fl-ac., franz., goss., gran., ***hell.,*** hipp., hydr., hyper., ign., iod., ip., kali-i., lach., lact., laur., lipp., ***lyc., mag-arct.,*** mag-c., mag-m., mang., meny., merc., mez., mur-ac., myric., naja, nat-c., ***nat-m.,*** nat-s., nicc., nux-m., ol-an., ox-ac., paeon., peti., petr., phel., ph-ac., phos., pip-m., plan., plat., plect., rhus-t., ***sabad.,*** samb., sars., ***sel.,*** seneg., sin-a., ***spig.,*** spirae., stann., staph., stram., ***sulph.,*** sul-ac., ***tarax.,*** tarent., til., ***verat.***
morning sleep, in - nat-m.

UNSUCCESSFUL efforts to, do various things - am-m., cadm-m., calc., calc-f., cann-s., carl., cham., croc., dig., ign., mag-c., mag-s., mosch., mur-ac., nat-c., op., ph-ac., plat., stann., tab.
business, in - mag-m., ***phos.,*** sabin.
dress for a ball - mag-c., mag-s.
for theater, for going to - mag-s.
find way in his own house - mag-c.
open the mouth, to - agar.
reach a distant place - croc., plat.
running, of - croc., ind.
screaming, of - am-m., ars., cast., mag-m., sil., tab.
sex, in - ind., iod.
talk - mag-c.

URINATING, of, desire for - kali-n., kreos., merc-i-f.

VARIOLA - anac.

VERTIGO - ***sil.***

VENGEANCE - lach.

VERMIN, (see Insects) - alum., am-c., bell., chel., colch., gamb., lac-c., mag-s., mur-ac., ***nux-v.,*** ped., phos., sep., sil.
lice - am-c., chel., gamb., mur-ac., ***nux-v.,*** phos.
spiders - cinnb., crot-c.

VERTIGO - sil.

VEXATIOUS - acon., ***aeth.,*** agar., ***alum.,*** alum-p., alum-sil., ***ambr.,*** am-c., am-m., anac., ang., ant-c., ant-t., apis, arn., ars-s-f., **ASAR.,** ***ars.,*** asc-t., aur., aur-m., aur-s., bapt., bell-p., bor., bov., ***bry.,*** calc., calc-sil., ***cann-i.,*** cann-s., **CARB-S.,** ***caust.,*** cham., chel., chin., chin-a., ***cimic.,*** cina, cinnb., coca, cocc., coloc., ***con.,*** dig., dros., elaps, erig., ***gamb., gels.,*** **GRAPH.,** grat., hep., hydr., ***ign.,*** iris, jug-c., junc., kali-chl., kali-m., kali-n., kiss., kreos., lach., led., lil-t., linu-c., lyc., lycps., ***mag-arct.,*** mag-aust., mag-c., mag-m., mag-s., mang., merc-i-r., mit., ***mosch.,*** mur-ac., murx., nat-a., nat-c., ***nat-m.,*** nat-p., nat-s., ***nit-ac.,*** ***nux-v.,*** op., petr., ph-ac., phel., phos., plan., plat., plb., ptel., puls., rat., rheum, rhus-g., ***rhus-t.,*** rumx., ruta, sabad., sabin., sang., sars., scut., sep., sil., sol-t-ae., spong., ***staph.,*** stront-c., sul-ac., **SULPH.,** tarent., thuj., ust., zinc.
children, in - ambr.

VIOLENCE - apoc-a., aran-ix., arg-n., aur., led., ven-m.

VISIONARY - aloe, am-c., ambr., ***anh.,*** ant-t., arn., ars., bar-c., bell., bufo, ***calc.,*** calc-sil., camph., carb-an., ***carb-v.,*** cham., chin., coloc., ***con.,*** graph., hell., ***kali-c., kali-n., lach.,*** lachn., led., ***lyc.,*** merc., mur-ac., nat-c., ***nat-m.,*** nicc., nit-ac., ***nux-v., op., petr.,*** plan., prun., sep., ***sil.,*** ***spong.,*** sulph., zinc., zinc-oc.
frightful - bell.

VISITS, brother, from - nicc.
making - mag-s.

VIVID - ***acon.,*** agar., alco., all-s., ambr., am-c., **ANAC.,** ang., ***ant-t.,*** aran-ix., arg-m., ***arg-n.,*** ***arn.,*** ars., ars-i., ars-s-f., ars-s-r., asaf., aster., **AUR.,** aur-a., bapt., bar-ac., bar-c., bar-i., bar-m., bar-s., ***bell.,*** bism., brom., brucin., ***bry.,*** calad., ***calc.,*** calc-ac., calc-f., calc-i., ***calc-p.,*** calc-sil., cann-i., cann-s., canth., caps., ***carb-an., carb-s.,*** **CARB-V.,** carl., ***cench., cham., chel.,*** chin., chin-a., chr-ac., chr-ox., ***cic.,*** cinnb., clem., cob., coca, ***cocc.,*** coc-c., ***coff.,*** colch., coloc., ***con.,*** croc., ***cycl.,*** daph., dig., dios., dros., euph., ***ferr., ferr-i.,*** ferr-p., fl-ac., form., franz., gast., gins., **GRAPH.,** guai., ham., hydr-ac., ***hyos.,*** hyper., ign., ind., indol., ***iod.,*** ip., jug-c., kali-ar., kali-bi., kali-c., kali-cy., kali-m., kali-n., kali-p., kali-s., kali-sil., lach., lact., ***lam.,*** laur., led., lipp., lob., **LYC.,** ***mag-arct.,*** mag-aust., ***mag-c.,*** mag-m., mag-s., ***mang.,*** meny., meph., ***merc.,*** merc-c., merc-sul., mez., mosch., mur-ac., naja, nat-a., ***nat-c.,*** **NAT-M.,** ***nat-p.,*** **NAT-SIL.,** nit-ac., nux-m., ***nux-v.,*** ol-j., op., orig., ox-ac., paeon., ***petr.,*** ***ph-ac.,*** **PHOS.,** phys., pin-s., plan., plat., psor., ptel., ***puls.,*** pyrog., rad., ran-b., ran-s., raph., ***rheum,*** rhod., **RHUS-T.,** rhus-v., rumx., ***ruta,*** ***sabad.,*** samb., senec., ***sep.,*** **SIL.,** sin-n., spig.,

VIVID - spirae., squil., ***stann., staph.,*** stram., ***stront-c.,*** sul-i., sumb., **SULPH.,** tab., tarax., ***teucr.,*** til., thuj., tub., valer., verat., verat-v., viol-o., viol-t., visc., zinc., zinc-p., zing.
afternoon - ang., sin-a.
erections, with - sulph.
lying with head down - plat.
midnight - zinc.
after - coloc., mez., nat-m., ***puls.,*** zinc.
before - mez.
morning - chin-s., kali-bi., mag-c., mez., staph., sulph., sumb.
towards - mez., staph.

VOICE - rhus-t.

VULGAR scenes - chin-b.

WADING in excrements, water, in - ant-t., merc-i-r.

WAGONS - nux-v., senec.

WAKING, the patient - ***acon.,*** agar., am-c., ***am-m.,*** ang., ***ant-t.,*** arg-m., arg-n., ***arn., ars.,*** asc-t., atro., aur., bad., bar-c., ***bell., bov.,*** bry., cahin., calc., calc-f., ***camph.,*** cann-s., carb-v., carc., casc., cham., chel., ***chin.,*** chr-ac., ***cic., cina,*** cinnb., coca, coff., colch., coloc., cupr., cycl., dicha., ***dig.,*** dros., dulc., euph., ***ferr-ma.,*** gran., graph., grat., ***hep.,*** hyper., ***ign.,*** indg., ip., kali-bi., ***kali-c., kali-chl., kali-i.,*** kali-n., kreos., lob., lyc., lycpr., lyss., ***mag-arct.,*** mag-aust., mag-c., ***mag-s., mang., meph., merc., mez.,*** mur-ac., murx., ***nat-c.,*** nat-m., ***nat-s., nicc.,*** nit-ac., ***nux-v.,*** olnd., ***op.,*** par., ***petr.,*** ph-ac., phos., plan., plat., puls., rat., rheum, rhus-t., ruta, sabad., ***sabin.,*** sars., ***sep.,*** sil., ***spig.,*** spong., stann., staph., ***stront-c.,*** **SULPH.,** tab., ***teucr., thuj.,*** verat., verb., ***zinc.***
daytime, while sitting - acon.
evening - sulph.
forenoon, while sitting - ant-t.
frequently - alum., cina, euphr., lyc., stront-c., tab.
midnight - fl-ac., zinc.
after - mez.
morning - lyc.
6 a.m. - rhus-t.
night, after lying down - acon.
sensation of waking from a dream - glon.

WALKING, of - agar., bell., canth., elaps, med., nat-c., nat-s., pall., rhus-t.
apartments, through - pall.
dreamy state, in a - rheum.
floor, on hot - apis.
roads, over dirty - apis.
ruins, among - hura, iod.
staircases, in - pall.
water, acquaintances walking on - ped.

WANDERING - cench., stram., zing.

WANT - am-c.

WAR - ferr., ***meny.,*** plat., thuj., verb., visc.
civil war - op.

WARTS - junc., mez.
abdomen, on - junc.
back, on - mez.

WATER - ***all-c., all-s.,*** alum., **AM-M.,** arg-n., arn., ***ars., bell.,*** bol., bov., carb-v., chin., chr-ac., com., ***dig.,*** eupi., ***ferr., graph.,*** hura, ign., iod., ***kali-c.,*** kali-n., kali-sil., kalm., ***lyc.,*** mag-c., mag-m., mag-s., ***meph., merc.,*** merc-i-r., murx., nat-c., nat-m., nat-s., nicc., ox-ac., ran-b., rhus-t., sang., ***sil.,*** sol-t-ae., sulph., tarent., valer., verat., ***verat-v.,*** zinc.
black - ***ars.,*** lac-c.
boat foundering - alum., lyc., sil.
child bathing in boiling - mag-c.
danger from - ars., ***graph.,*** kali-n., ***mag-c.,*** mag-m., merc., nat-c., nat-s., sulph.
daughter is in, and crying for help - nat-s.
falling into - ***am-m., dig.,*** eupi., ***ferr.,*** ign., iod., mag-m., mag-s., merc., nicc.
her child - eupi., iod.
her daughter - iod.
her mother - nicc.
fishes swimming in - chin.
flood - mag-c., merc., nat-c., rumx., ***sil.***
men, jumping into - mag-s.
noon - nat-m.
people bathing - chin-b.
poured upon him - ox-ac.
putrid - arg-n.
rowing on - rhus-t.
sailing - chin., hura, nat-s., sang., senec., verat-v.
sea, of - all-c., chin.
stream, of - com.
swimming in - ***bell.,*** hura, iod., lyc., merc-i-r., ran-b., rhus-t., sol-t-ae.
wading in - ant-t., merc-i-r.
in which are serpents - alum.
yellow - hura.

WAY, loosing - nat-c.

WEAKNESS - ambr.

WEDDING - alum., chel., mag-c., mag-m., mag-s., nat-c., nat-s.
with two women - nat-c.

WEEPING, (see Crying)

WELLS, of being let down into - ***all-c.,*** merc-c.

WHIPPED, getting - ptel.

WILD - aloe, apis, cann-i., dor., glon., kalm., op., pip-m., tab.

WINDOW, broken - hep.
trying to get out of - calc-f.
jumping from - mag-m.

WIND-colic - fago.

WOMEN - ***dios.***
changed into animals - sol-t-ae.

WONDERFUL - chin-s., op., paeon., ph-ac.

WORK - ambr., ***calc.,*** carc., ***nux-v.,*** rhus-t., sel.

WORKING, in snow - bapt.

WORLD, on fire - ***rhus-t.***

WORMS, creeping - am-c., esp-g., mur-ac., nux-v., phos.
vomiting of - ***chin.,*** chin-b.

WOUNDED, of being - ant-c., chel., lob., ***mag-s.***
shot, by a - lob.

WITCHES - sol-t-ae., stram.

WRITING - senec.
table, on dirty and paper becoming smeared - prun.

WRONG, doing - cocc.

YOUTH, time of - sil.

VOMITING, worms, of - chin., chin-b.

Ears

ABSCESS, behind - anan., **AUR.,** ***bar-m., caps.,*** carb-an., hep., kali-c., ***nit-ac.,*** phyt., **SIL.**
below - nat-h.
every two weeks, ear forms a, and discharges - iris.
meatus, in, - **CALC-S., CALC-SIL.,** crot-h., **HEP.,** ***mag-c., puls.,*** **SIL.**
menses, during - puls.

ACHING, pain - all-c., aloe, asaf., bell., brom., cann-i., ***caps.,*** caust., **CHAM.,** chlf., ***cimic.,*** clem., colch., coloc., ***con.,*** cur., **DULC.,** ery-a., euphr., form., guai., ham., hyos., iod., ip., jatr., jug-r., kali-c., ***kali-s.,*** lach., lact., laur., lyc., mang., meny., merc-i-r., meph., mez., mosch., nat-m., nat-p., nit-ac., nux-m., nux-v., olnd., osm., ***phos.,*** psor., **PULS.,** ran-b., rhus-t., seneg., sep., sil., spong., **SULPH.,** tab., tarent., **TELL.,** thuj., ust.
above ear - dulc., mez., tell.
afternoon - euphr.
air, in open - euph., ***lyc.***
behind ear - arum-d., caust., cedr., con., glon., lyc., mang., mosch., nat-m., stry., viol-o.
extending to temples - cedr.
open air - mang.
shaking head - glon.
touch agg. - mang.
blowing nose - sil.
evening - berb., brom., kali-bi., lyc., nat-m., sep.
5 p.m. - dios., ham., sep.
evening, in open air - sep.
front of, in - anac., cupr., dios., merc-i-f.
afternoon, 3 p.m. - dios.
left - bell., ery-a., guai., mez., nat-m., sil., sulph.
then right - brom.
lying down, after - sang.
menses, during - aloe
midnight, after - sep.
morning, in bed - merc-i-r.
rising, on - ferr.
night - ***dulc., lach.***
wind, after walking in the - sep.
pressure amel. - ham.
right - asaf., berb., brom., ham., nat-p., psor.
swallowing, on - con., fago.
thunderstorm, before a - rhod.
warm room, on entering, amel. - sep.

ADHESIONS, in middle ear - iod., iris, thiosin.

AGGLUTINATION, of auricle to head - olnd.

AIR, sensitive to open, about ears - ***acon.,*** ars., bell., ***bor.,*** caps., caust., **CHAM., CAUST.,** ferr-p., ***hep.,*** **LACH.,** merc., ***mez.,*** nux-v., petr., tell.
cold - ***acon., caust.,*** dulc., ***mez.,*** plat., staph., vinc.
cold, about ear, to - **ACON., CAUST., CHAM.,** cinnb., clem., ***hep., lac-c.,*** **LACH.,** ***lyc.,*** merc., ***mez., sil., thuj.***
air, sensation of, in - graph., ***mez.***
bubble of air - ***nat-m.***
air, sensation of,
distension, meatus in evening - mez.
fanning before, sensation of - calc., mang., nit-ac.
forced into, belching, during - caust., graph.
blowing nose, when - puls., sulph.
rushing, in - lachn., mang., mez., staph.
belching, during - caust.
rushing, out, as if - ***chel.***
as of cold air - mill.
streaming into, on drawing jaw to other side - sarr.

ALIVE, sensation in ear - sil.

BALD, spot above - phos.

BITING, pain - caust., lyc., phel., psor.
behind the ear - lyc., ol-an.
boring into ear with finger agg. - phel.
8 to 10 p.m. - phel.
evening, electric sparks, like - phel.
itching - caust., phel.
left - psor.

BLOW, pain, as from - am-c., anac., arn., bell., cina, con., nat-m., nux-v., paeon., plat., spig.

BLOWING, sensation in - ail., rhus-t., ***sel.***
headache, during - ***sel.***
pulsative, at night - sep.
right - ail., rhus-t.

BOARD, before, sensation of - arg-m.
left - arg-m.

BODY, hard, behind the ear, sensation - graph.

BOILS - kali-c., sil., spong., ***sulph.,*** syph.
behind - ***ang.,*** bry., ***calc., con.,*** nat-c., ***phyt., sulph., thuj.***
below - ***calc.***
front of, in - bry., carb-v., laur., sulph.
inside, alternately one ear, then the other - carc., lac-c.
lobes, on - nat-m.
meatus, in - bell., bov., crot-h., hep., **MERC.,** ***merc-sul.,*** **PIC-AC.,** puls., rhus-t., ***sil.,*** **SULPH.**

BORING, fingers in - agar., arund., chel., ***cina,*** lach., mez., mill., phys., psor., rheum, ruta., sal-ac., ***sil.,*** spig., thuj.
amel. - chel., lach., ***mez.,*** par., rheum, spig.
children - arund., **CINA,** ***psor., sil.***
sleep, during - ***sil.***

BORING, pain, in - alum., am-c., am-m., ant-c., ***arund.,*** aur., aur-m-n., ***bar-c., bell.,*** cann-i., canth., carb-an., carb-s., caust., chel., ***cina,*** coc-c., colch., coloc., ***cupr.,*** cupr-ar., euph., euphr., gels., hell., hydr-ac., indg., kali-c., ***kali-i.,*** kali-s., lact., laur., mag-c., mag-m., mag-s., mang., **MERC.,** merc-c., ***merc-i-f.,*** mill., nat-m., ***ol-an.,*** phel., ***phos.,*** plat., plb., ran-s., rhod., ***ruta.,*** sil., ***spig.,*** stann., stront-c., stry., sulph., thuj.
about the ear - am-m., bell., rhod.
above the ear - arg-n., cann-i., rhod.
acute - merc-i-f.
afternoon - alum., gels., indg., merc-c.

BORING, pain
behind the ear - am-m., ***aur.,*** aur-m-n., cann-i., caust., coloc., ***cupr.,*** mez., mosch., nat-s., ran-s., rumx., sabad., ***sep.,*** spig.
evening - ran-s.
left - **AUR.,** caust., ***lach.***
reading - spig.
right - cann-i., coloc., ran-s.
writing - spig.
below the ear - caust.
bores into ear with finger - agar., mez., phys.
dinner, after - plb.
evening - phys., ran-s.
extending to left nostril - lac-c.
feet become cold, when - stann.
forenoon - mag-c.
front of ear - arg-n., aur-m-n., ***bar-c.,*** laur.
bending body, to right, on - mag-m.
lain on, one - am-m.
left - agar., canth., mag-s., med., merc-i-f., merc-c., stry.
morning - alum.
night - am-m., mang.
pressure on - alum.
right - am-m., bar-c., cann-i., carb-an., carb-s., caust., chel., colch., coloc., cupr-ar., gels., hell., mag-m., mez., nicc., plb., stann., stront.
sticking - mag-m.
tickling - nicc.
walking in open air, while - am-m.
warmth of bed, from - **MERC.**

BREATH, sensation as if it came from ear - psor.

BURNING, pain - acon., aesc., all-c., alum., alumn., am-c., am-m., aml-n., ang., ant-c., ant-t., ***apis,*** arg-m., arn., ***ars.,*** arum-t., arund., asaf., **AUR.,** bell., berb., brom., bry., camph., cann-i., ***caps.,*** carb-an., carb-v., **CAUST.,** chel., chin., chin-a., cic., con., cop., cycl., daph., dig., ***dros.,*** fago., ***ign.,*** jac-c., jatr., kali-ar., kali-bi., kali-n., kreos., laur., lob-s., lyc., lycps., lyss., mag-c., mag-m., ***mang.,*** **MERC.,** merc-sul., merl., mur-ac., naja, **NAT-M.,** nat-p., ol-an., op., phel., ph-ac., phos., pic-ac., plat., sabad., **SANG.,** spig., spong., staph., sulph., tab., **TELL.,** til., upa., zinc.
about the ear - ***calc.***
afternoon - stry.
open, agg. - acon.
behind the ear - aur., aur-m., calc-p., grat., nat-m., rhus-v., sabad., spong., thuj.
night - aur-m.
right - calc-p., grat., nat-m., thuj.
below, menses, during - mag-c.
concha - caust., kali-bi., merc., mur-ac., nat-m., op., phos., spig., staph.
dry warmth, from - bry.
eating, after, amel. - acon.
evening - ars., brom., ham., ol-an., zinc.
8 to 10 p.m., like electric sparks - phel.
bed, in - caust.
open air agg. - acon.
pressure amel. - ham.
rubbing, after - grat.

BURNING, pain
external ear - **AGAR.,** ***ars., clem.,*** dros., kreos., pic-ac., ***rhus-t.,*** sulph., **TELL.**
fever, during - ran-b.
left - acon., am-c., ant-c., arum-t., bry., cop., fago., **TELL.,** stry.
lobe - carb-an., carb-v., chel., kali-n., sabad., **TELL.**
meatus, in - anan., arund., aur-s., bor., brom., canth., caust., crot-t., jatr., mag-c., ***merc.,*** olnd., sep., spong., stry.
right - brom.
menses, during - agar.
night - stry.
sleep, before - still.
noon - stry.
perspiring, when - acon.
right - am-c., arum-t., bov., calc-p., carb-an., carb-v., chel., cycl., dros., ham., lycps., lyss., mag-c., nat-m., nat-p., sabad.
scratching, after - ol-an.
spots, in - calc-p.
touched, when - cop.
tragus - ***mur-ac.***
tympanum - ang.
walking in open air - am-m.
warm room, coming from cold air - kali-n.
yawning, when - acon.

BURROWING, pain - am-c., am-m., ant-c., coc-c., hell.
ear lain on - am-m.
right - am-m., hell.

BURSTING, sensation - calc-caust., ***caust., clem., dulc., guai.,*** hell., lyc., ***merc., mur-ac.,*** nit-ac., ***phos.,*** **PLAT.,** psor., ***stann.***
coughing, on - caps.
heart beat, with each - aml-n.
in front of - dros.
sneezing, on - ***puls.***

CALCAREOUS, deposit on tympanum - ***calc-f.,*** syph.

CARIES, (see Decay)

CATARRH, eustachian tube - alf., alum., ars-i., **ASAR.,** bar-m., **CALC.,** calc-i., calc-s., caps., ***caust.,*** cench., con., ferr-i., ferr-p., gels., graph., hep., ***hydr., iod., kali-bi., kali-chl., kali-i.,*** **KALI-M., KALI-S.,** kali-sil., lach., lob., ***mang.,*** menthol, ***merc.,*** **MERC-D.,** merc-sul., ***nat-m., nit-ac.,*** pen., **PETR.,** ***phos.,*** phyt., **PULS.,** ros-d., ***sang.,*** sang-n., sep., **SIL.,** thiosin., visc.

CHILDREN, chronic complaints of - bell., calc., calc-p., caust., ***cham., hep.,*** kali-m., lyc., ***merc.,*** phos., ***puls.,*** sil., thuj., ***zinc.***

CHILLINESS - calc.

COLDNESS, of - aeth., amyg., ars., bapt., berb., ***calc., calc-p.,*** carb-v., ***chel.,*** cic., ip., kali-ar., ***kali-c., lach.,*** lyc., ***mang.,*** meny., merc., ***nit-ac.,*** paeon., ***petr., plat.,*** psor., ran-s., seneg., stram., ter., thea., ***verat.,*** verat-v.
about the ear - aeth., bry.
above the ear - indg., lac-ac.
alternating with heat - verat.

COLDNESS, of
behind right ear - ***form.***
below the ear - aeth.
burning hot yet cold to touch - bapt., nat-n.
draft, as from a - mang., stann.
evening - mez., paeon.
5 p.m - paeon.
in warm bed - merc.
extending through - seneg.
fever, during - ***ip., lach.***
meatus, in - caust., ***merc., mez., plat.,*** staph.
wind, as from - caust., mang., ***mez.,*** sanic., staph.
one cold the other hot - chel., nit-ac.
right - ***kali-c.,*** lyc.
and burning of left - nat-n.
sensation of, in external ear - lachn., nat-n.
warmth of bed agg. - merc.
water, as if cold, had got in - meny.
cold, running out of ear - merc.

CONSTRICTION, of - thuj.

CONTRACTION - anac., asar., caust., dig., lach., sars.
below - aeth., dulc., zinc.
front, of, in - zinc.
meatus, in - anac., arg-n., bry.
sensation of - graph.
evening, after lying down, agg., sleeping on that side - caust.
spasmodic, afternoon on sitting - aeth.

CORROSIVE, pain in lobule - plat.

CRAMP, in - agar., aloe, ***anac.,*** anan., ang., ars., bry., calc., carb-an., ***cina,*** colch., croc., crot-t., dig., ***glon.,*** graph., kali-c., kali-n., kali-p., kreos., mang., ***merc.,*** mur-ac., nat-m., nit-ac., nux-v., olnd., petr., **PH-AC.,** ***plat.,*** ran-b., samb., ***sars., sil.,*** spig., spong., stann., staph., thuj., valer., zinc.
behind - calc-ac., mang., murx.
concha - staph.
evening - ran-b., thuj.
left - agar., mur-ac., nat-m., spong., zinc.
walking - mez.
lobule - zinc.
right - petr., samb., stann., thuj.
walking in open air - mang., spong.

CRAWLING - bar-c.

CUTTING, pain, in - anac., arg-m., cadm-s., canth., caust., cham., ***coloc.,*** cur., dros., ***ferr-i., form., hydr., hyos.,*** kali-i., kali-s., lach., mang., mur-ac., ***nit-ac.,*** nux-m., petr., ***puls., syph., zinc.***
above the ear - carb-v.
behind ear - sil.
extending to neck - mur-ac., sil.
boring with finger amel. - ***coloc.***
eustachian tubes when chewing - arg-m.
evening - lach.
in front - arg-m.
left - arg-m., petr.
mastoid process - bell., caust., con., mur-ac.
motion of jaw agg. - nux-m.
open air, on going into - mang.

DECAY, of mastoid process, threatened - **AUR.,** calc-f., **CAPS.,** carb-an., ***fl-ac., hep., lach., nit-ac.,*** **SIL.,** syph.
temporal - calc-f., caps.

DIGGING, pain - am-m., anan., colch., gels., kali-i., mang., merc-c., nat-m., plat., ***ruta.,*** stry.
afternoon - gels., merc-c.
as if an insect had got into them - kali-i.
extending to left nostril - lac-c.
left - merc-c., stry.
night - am-m., mang.
lying on it - am-m.
right - am-m., colch., ***gels.***

DILATATION, of meatus, sensation of - mez.
evening - mez.

DISCHARGES, from - absin., aeth., ***all-c., alum., alumn.,*** am-c., am-m., anac., anan., ***ant-c., apis,*** arund., ***ars., ars-i., asaf., aur.,*** bar-c., **BAR-M.,** ***bell., bor.,*** bov., brom., ***bry.,*** bufo, **CALC.,** ***calc-f.,*** **CALC-P., CALC-S.,** caps., ***carb-an.,*** **CARB-S., CARB-V.,** cast., **CAUST.,** ***cham.,*** chin., cic., **CIST.,** coc-c., colch., **CON.,** cop., ***crot-c., crot-h.,*** crot-t., cur., ***elaps,*** ery-a., ferr., ferr-ar., ferr-p., ***fl-ac.,*** **GRAPH., HEP.,** hipp., ***hydr.,*** iod., jug-r., ***kali-ar.,*** **KALI-BI., KALI-C.,** kali-p., **KALI-S.,** kreos., ***lach.,*** lachn., **LYC.,** meny., meph., **MERC.,** ***merc-c., nat-m., nat-s., nit-ac.,*** **PETR.,** phos., **PSOR., PULS.,** rhus-t., sal-ac., ***sang., sel., sep.,*** **SIL.,** spig., **SULPH.,** syph., tarent., **TELL.,** tep., thuj., vesp., zinc.
blood - am-c., ***arn.,*** arund., asaf., ***bell.,*** **BOTH.,** bry., bufo, ***chin., cic.,*** colch., con., **CROT-H.,** ***elaps,*** ery-a., ***ham.,*** merc., mosch., ***op., petr.,*** **PHOS.,** puls., ***rhus-t.,*** tell.
cough, during - bell.
menses, instead of - ***bry., phos.***
morning - merc.
prolonged suppuration, after - ***chin.***
bloody - am-c., ars., arund., bar-c., bell., bry., ***calc.,*** **CALC-S.,** cann-s., ***carb-s., carb-v.,*** caust., ***chin.,*** cic., con., **CROT-H.,** elaps, ery-a., ***graph.,*** ham., ***hep.,*** kali-ar., kali-c., kali-p., kali-s., ***lach.,*** lyc., **MERC.,** merc-i-r., mosch., ***nit-ac., petr.,*** phos., **PSOR.,** ***puls.,*** rhus-t., sep., **SIL.,** ***sulph., tell.,*** zinc.
brownish - ***anac.,*** carb-v., ***kali-s., psor.,*** tarent.
cheesy - ***hep.,*** **SIL.**
chronic - caust., sil., tub.
clear - bry.
cold, exposure to, agg. - graph.
copious - ***bar-m.,*** skook., tell.
decay, threatening - ***asaf.,*** **AUR.,** ***calc., calc-f., calc-s.,*** caps., nat-m., **SIL.,** sulph.
earwax - am-m., anac., hep., kali-c., lyc., merc., mosch., nat-m., nit-ac., phos., puls., ***thuj.***
eruption, suppressed, after - cist., ***sulph.***
every, seven days - ***sulph.***
excoriating - ars-i., calc-p., carb-v., fl-ac., hep., lyc., merc., nat-m., puls., rhus-t., **SULPH.,** syph., **TELL.**

DISCHARGES, from
fetid - ***ars., ars-i.,*** **AUR.,** ***bov., calc., carb-ac.,*** carb-s., ***carb-v.,*** **CIST.,** cub., ***elaps, hep., kali-ar., kali-bi.,*** kali-c., meph., **MERC.,** ***merc-c., nit-ac.,*** **PSOR.,** sal-ac., sep., **SULPH., TELL.,** thuj., zinc.
flesh colored - carb-v., kali-c., zinc.
gluey, sticky - **GRAPH.,** hydr., kali-bi., nat-m.
green - elaps, hep., kali-i., **LAC-C.,** lyc., merc.
morning - elaps
odorless - lac-c.
hot, as if - aeth.
ichorous - am-c., **ARS.,** calc-p., ***carb-an., carb-v.,*** **LYC.,** ***nit-ac.,*** **PSOR.,** sep., ***sil., tell.***
left - ferr., graph., psor., zinc.
measles, after - ***bov.,*** cact., ***carb-v.,*** colch., ***crot-h., lyc.,*** merc., ***nit-ac.,*** **PULS.,** ***sulph.***
mucous - bov., tarent.
night - sep.
in warm bed - merc.
offensive - ***ars.,*** asaf., **AUR.,** ***bar-m., bov., calc.,*** calc-s., ***carb-s., carb-v., caust., chin.,*** **CIST.,** crot-h., elaps, ery-a., ferr-ar., ***fl-ac., graph., hep., hydr., kali-ar., kali-bi.,*** kali-c., ***kali-p., kali-s.,*** kreos., lyc., mang., meph., merc., ***merc-c., nit-ac.,*** ol-j., psor., puls., sep., **SIL.,** ***sulph.,*** sul-ac., ***tell., thuj., tub.,*** zinc.
cadaverous, smelling - ***ars.***
fish-brine, like - ***graph.,*** sanic., **TELL.**
horse-urine, like - nit-ac.
persistent - tub.
putrid, purulent - aur., carb-an., psor.
putrid meat like - **KALI-P., PSOR.,** ***thuj.***
rotten cheese, like - ***bar-m., hep.***
sour - sulph.
painful - ***calc-s.,*** ferr-p., **MERC.**
periodic every seventh day - ***sulph.***
purulent - aeth., ***all-c., alum., alumn., am-c.,*** am-m., anan., arn., ***asaf., arund., aur., bar-m.,*** bell., ***bor., bov.,*** bufo, **CALC., CALC-S.,** ***caps.,*** carb-an., ***carb-s., carb-v., caust.,*** cham., ***chin., cist., con.,*** cop., cur., ferr-p., gels., ***graph.,*** **HEP.,** ***hydrc.,*** **KALI-BI., KALI-C.,** ***kali-p.,*** **KALI-S.,** kino, ***lach.,*** **LYC., MERC.,** ***merc-c., nat-m., nit-ac., petr.,*** phos., **PSOR., PULS.,** rhus-t., sac-alb., sal-ac., ***sep.,*** **SIL.,** sulph., syph., tell., tep., thuj., ***tub., zinc.***
eczema, with - ***calc., hep., lyc., merc., sulph.***
mercury, after abuse of - ***asaf., aur.,*** **HEP., NIT-AC.,** ***sil., sulph.***
offensive, and putrid - aur., carb-an., psor.
sulphur, after abuse of - ***calc.,*** merc., ***puls.***
right - aeth., elaps, ***lyc., nit-ac., sil., thuj.***

DISCHARGES, from
scarlet fever, after - apis, asar., aur., bar-m., bov., brom., calc-s., **CARB-V.,** crot-h., graph., hep., kali-bi., **LYC.,** merc., nit-ac., **PSOR.,** puls., sulph., tell., verb.
sensation of - acon., agar., calc., chr-ac., cinnb., dirc., graph., merc., sil., tell.
sequelae - **AUR.,** bar-m., ***cact., calc.,*** **CARB-V.,** ***colch.,*** crot-h., ***hep.,*** lach., ***lyc.,*** merc., ***nit-ac.,*** **PULS., PSOR.,** ***sulph.***
serous - elaps, tarent., ***tell.***
suppressed - alum., asaf., **AUR.,** ***calc.,*** **CARB-V.,** ***cast., graph., hep.,*** **MERC.,** petr., ***puls.,*** sil., sulph., zinc.
thick - **CALC., CALC-S.,** ***carb-v.,*** ery-a., **HYDR., KALI-BI.,** ***kali-chl., lyc.,*** nat-m., **PULS.,** sep., **SIL.,** tarent.
thin - ars., cham., elaps, ***graph.,*** **KALI-S.,** merc., petr., ***psor., sep., sil., sulph.***
watery - calc., ***carb-v., cist., elaps, graph.,*** **KALI-S.,** ***merc.,*** **SIL.,** ***syph.,*** **TELL.,** thuj.
white - ery-a., ***hep., kali-chl.,*** **NAT-M.**
white, milky - **KALI-CHL.**
yellow - aeth., ars., calc., calc-s., crot-h., hydr., kali-ar., **KALI-BI.,** kali-c., **KALI-S.,** lyc., merc., nat-s., petr., phos., **PULS.,** sil.
yellowish-green - ***cinnb., elaps, kali-chl., kali-s., merc.,*** **PULS.**

DISCOLORATION, ears
blue - sant., **TELL.**
brown, spots - cop.
livid - carb-o., op.
redness - acon., **AGAR.,** ail., ***alum., ant-c.,*** **APIS,** arn., asaf., astac., ***aur., aur-m., bell.,*** bry., calc-p., ***camph., caps., carb-s., carb-v., caust., cham.,*** **CHIN.,** cit-v., ***elaps, glon.,*** graph., hep., ***hydr., ign.,*** ind., jab., jug-r., ***kali-bi., kali-c.,*** kali-n., ***kreos.,*** lyc., ***mag-c.,*** manc., meph., ***merc., nat-m.,*** nat-p., ***nit-ac.,*** op., ***phos.,*** plat., plan., ***psor.,*** **PULS.,** ***rhus-t.,*** samb., ***sang., sulph.,*** tab., ***tell.,*** trom.
about the ear - arn.
afternoon - nat-m.
behind ears - acon-l., ant-s., ***hydr., nit-ac., petr.,*** ptel., rhus-v., tab.
chilblains - **AGAR.**
concha - arn., nat-m.
evening - ***alum., carb-v.,*** elaps, oena., raph., rhus-t., sep., tab., tarent., trom., vesp.
left - sep.
lobes - camph., ***cham.,*** chin., kali-n.
meatus - ***acon., cham., mag-c., pic-ac.,*** **PULS.**
menses, during - agar.
one-sided - alum., ant-c., carb-v., chin., ***ign.,*** ind., ***kali-c.,*** kreos., meph., nat-m., nat-p., sep., tab., tell.
right - calc.
touched or scratched, when - ail.

DISTENSION, sensation of, in - bell., kali-i., laur., ***mez.,*** nit-ac., ***puls.***
nose, on blowing - ***puls.***

DRAWING, pain, in - acon., aloe, anac., ang., ant-c., arg-m., arn., ars., asaf., asar., aur-m., ***bar-c.,*** bar-m., ***bell.,*** berb., bism., bov., bry., calc., carb-an., ***cham.,*** chel., coc-c., colch., ***con.,*** crot-h., ***cycl.,*** dros., dulc., ferr-ma., ferr-p., hell., kali-ar., kali-bi., ***kali-c.,*** kali-n., kali-p., kalm., kreos., lact., lyc., mag-m., mag-s., merc., mez., mill., mosch., mur-ac., ***nat-m.,*** nicc., ***nit-ac.,*** olnd., ol-an., op., petr., **PH-AC.,** ***phos., plat.,*** puls., ran-s., rhod., sars., ***sep., sil., spig.,*** spong., ***stann.,*** staph., sulph., sul-ac., ***tarax.,*** til., valer., ***verb.,*** zinc.
about the ear - asaf., grat., nit-ac.
afternoon - clem.
pressure, amel. - grat.
above the ear - asaf., chel., coloc., lach., mez., verat.
bed, in - chel.
scar, in an old - lach.
behind the ear - aloe, anac., arg-m., ars., asaf., bar-c., canth., chel., chin., coloc., crot-h., dig., kali-bi., kali-c., kali-n., laur., mang., merc., mur-ac., petr., ***prun.,*** sil., sulph., thuj., zinc.
daytime - kali-n.
extending, to
downward - arg-m.
front, in - ***bar-c.,*** sulph.
lobule - ***cham.,*** dros., phos.
lobule, under - arg-m.
jaw - ***zinc.***
mastoid process - chin.
nape of ear - mur-ac.
shoulder - ars.
motion, on - ***prun.***
rest, during - arg-m.
touch agg. - sil.
belching, during - sulph.
below the ear - arg-m., dig., sulph.
concha - sars., stann.
dinner, after - ant-c.
downwards - berb.
evening - coc-c., ran-s.
extending to
crown - lach.
eustachian tube, into - ant-c.
neck, to - bell.
neck, to, and shoulders - ***nat-m.***
teeth, to the - bell.
front of, in - ***bar-c.,*** dig., sulph.
left - arn., chel., con., dig., hyper., mez., mill., plat., spig., til., valer., ***verb.***
lobule - ars., cham., dros., phos., sars.
under - arg-m.
lying down, after - sulph.
mastoid to forehead - sars.
teeth, to - mez.
motion of lower jaw - stann., verb.
night - alum., bar-c., ***sil.***
cold, from taking - glon.
outwards - caust., ***con., euphr.,*** sul-ac.

DRAWING, pain,
paroxysmal - alum., ***ph-ac.***
pressing on ear - raph.
right - ant-c., aur-m., bry., ***caust.,*** coc-c., ***cycl.,*** dros., gamb., glon., mosch., nat-m., nit-ac., petr., sep., sil., spong.
rising from a seat, on - ***sil.***
sneezing, after, amel. - mag-m.
swallowing - alum., ferr-ma.
thread drawn through the ear, as if a - rhus-t.
tragus - mur-ac., ph-ac.

DRYNESS - aeth., arn., aur., berb., ***calc.,*** carb-s., ***carb-v.,*** cast-eq., colch., **GRAPH.,** ***lach.,*** nit-ac., ***nux-v., onos., petr.,*** phos., ***puls., sulph.***
meatus - sil.
sensation of - petr., phos.

EARDRUM, ruptured - ***calen.***

EARWAX - am-m., anac., con., hep., kali-c., lyc., merc., mosch., nat-m., nit-ac., phos., puls., ***thuj.***
black - elaps, **PULS.**
brown - calc-s., thuj.
red or dark - ***mur-ac.***
dry - ***elaps,*** lac-c., ***lach.,*** mur-ac., petr.
peeling off in scales - ***mur-ac.***
foul - caust.
red - con.
hardened - all-s., ***con.,*** elaps, lach., **PULS.,** sel.
increased - agar., am-m., anan., bell., ***calc.,*** **CAUST.,** ***con.,*** cycl., dios., ***elaps,*** helo., ***hep.,*** kali-c., ***lyc.,*** merc-i-r., merl., mosch., mur-ac., petr., sel., sep., sil., sulph., syc-co., tarent., **THUJ.,** zinc.
pale - **LACH.**
purulent - con., sep.
red - **CON.,** mur-ac., ***psor.***
reddish - ***psor.***
rotten paper, like - con.
soft - sil.
thick - chel., ***petr.***
thin - am-m., ***con., hep.,*** iod., ***kali-c.,*** lach., ***merc.,*** mosch., ***petr.,*** sel., ***sil.,*** sulph., ***tell.***
wanting - aeth., anac., ***calc., carb-v., cham., lach.,*** mur-ac., ***petr.***
whitish - chel., con., **LACH.,** sep.
mush, like - chel.
yellow - ***carb-v., kali-c.,*** lach.

ECZEMA - calc., graph., ***kali-bi.,*** lyc., ***kali-s., psor.,*** sulph.
about the ears - ***ars.,*** arund., bov., chrysar., clem., crot-t., ***graph.,*** hep., kali-n., ***mez.,*** olnd., petr., psor., ***rhus-t.,*** sanic., tell.
behind ears - ars., arund., bov., **CALC.,** ***chrysar.,*** **GRAPH.,** ***hep.,*** jug-r., kali-m., **LYC.,** ***mez., olnd., petr.,*** **PSOR.,** rhus-t., sanic., ***scroph-n.,*** sep., staph., sulph., tell., tub.
meatus, in - nit-ac., ***psor.***

ERUPTIONS - agar., alum., am-m., ant-c., apis, ars., **BAR-C.**, ***bar-m.***, bov., bry., calad., ***calc.***, calc-p., cann-s., carb-v., caust., chin., ***cic.***, ***cist.***, com., cop., elaps, ***fl-ac.***, **GRAPH.**, hep., kali-ar., ***kali-bi.***, kali-c., kali-p., kali-s., kreos., ***lyc.***, mez., mosch., mur-ac., nat-m., nat-p., ***olnd.***, ***petr.***, ***phos.***, **PSOR.**, ptel., puls., rhus-t., rhus-v., ***sep.***, spong., staph., ***sulph.***, tell., teucr., thuj., verb.
about the - ***cic.***, ***cist.***, hep., ***hyper.***, lach., ***mez.***, nat-p., olnd., ***sulph.***
moist - kreos.
rash - ***ars.***
spread to scalp - hep.
above the, pimples - cop., mur-ac.
antetragus - am-m., spong.
behind - ant-c., ars., arund., **BAR-C.**, bufo, **CALC.**, calc-s., ***carb-s.***, carb-v., **CAUST.**, chin., **CIC.**, cocc., **GRAPH.**, guare., ***hep.***, jug-r., kali-c., kali-i., ***kali-s.***, lach., **LYC.**, mag-m., mag-p., mag-s., ***merc.***, ***mez.***, mur-ac., nat-m., nit-ac., ***olnd.***, **PETR.**, **PSOR.**, ***puls.***, sanic., sel., ***sep.***, **SIL.**, **STAPH.**, **SULPH.**, teucr., tell., tub., ***viol-t.***, vinc.
excoriating - **GRAPH.**, kali-c., nit-ac., **PETR.**, **PSOR.**, sanic., sulph.
left then right - ***graph.***
moist, sticky - **GRAPH.**, sanic.
scratching, after - mag-m.
blisters - camph., ***kreos.***, meph.
blotches - berb., bry., calc., ***carb-an.***, caust., dros., lach., merc., nicc., phos., spong., staph.
behind ears - anac., ***bry.***, ***calc.***, carb-an., caust., chin., ***mur-ac.***, ***nit-ac.***, ***sabad.***, staph.
boils, (see Boils)
burning - anan., ***cic.***, mosch., puls., sars.
burning, behind - viol-t.
concha - am-m., ars., chin., phos.
crusts - mur-ac., nat-p.
pimples - mur-ac.
scurfy - iod.
confluent - cop., ***psor.***
cracked and desquamating a substance like powdered starch - ***com.***
cracks - calc., ***graph.***
behind the ears - chel., **GRAPH.**, ***hep.***, ***hydr.***, ***lyc.***, ***petr.***, ***sep.***, ***sulph.***
below ears, cracks - syc-co.
meatus, in - ***graph.***, petr.
desquamating - ***anac.***, bry., ***com.***, cop., ***graph.***, merc., phos., ***psor.***
excoriating - **KALI-BI.**, kali-c., kali-s., ***merc.***, ***petr.***, ***sulph.***
extending, to face - ***graph.***, ***sep.***
extending, to scalp - hep.
front of, in - berb., cic., olnd., ter., sep.
pimples - ant-c., nat-c., verb.
pustules - mag-c.
vesicles - cic.
herpes, (see Herpes)
itching - am-m., ***kali-bi.***, ***mez.***, mosch., pall., ***psor.***, puls., sars., ***staph.***

ERUPTIONS,
itching, behind - bufo, ***graph.***, mag-m., mag-s., mez., nat-m., ***petr.***, staph., viol-t.
lobes, on - bar-c., caust., puls., sars., tell., teucr.
lupus - nit-ac.
menses, during - mag-c.
pimples - lach., merc.
scabs - sars.
scurfs - sars.
scurfs, burning and itching - sars.
ulceration of earring hole - stann.
vesicles caused by discharge - **TELL.**
margins, moist - sil.
meatus, in - calc-sil., kreos., morg., ***nit-ac.***, ***psor.***
pimples - jug-r., kali-p.
pustules - cast-eq.
scurfy - all-s., **LYC.**, ***psor.***
moist - ant-c., bov., ***calc.***, **GRAPH.**, hep., ***kali-bi.***, kreos., ***lyc.***, ***merc.***, mez., morg., petr., ***psor.***, ptel., sanic., staph., tub.
behind - am-m., ant-c., aur., ***calc.***, carb-v., caust., **GRAPH.**, kali-c., ***lyc.***, ***mez.***, nit-ac., ***olnd.***, **PETR.**, phos., **PSOR.**, ptel., ***rhus-t.***, rhus-v., sanic., ***sep.***, sil., ***staph.***
behind, scratching, after - ***graph.***
pimples - agar., am-c., am-m., berb., ***calc-p.***, calad., cann-s., cic., coff., kali-c., ***kali-s.***, ***kreos.***, merc., merc-c., ***mur-ac.***, nat-m., petr., phos., ***psor.***, sabad., sel., spong., staph., ***sulph.***
behind - alum., calad., calc., cann-s., canth., caust., dros., graph., ham., mez., nat-m., nicc., ***pall.***, puls., rhus-t., sabad., sel., sulph.
behind, burning on touch - canth.
behind, itching - rhus-t.
itching - mur-ac.
stitching - phos.
purulent - cic., cycl., ***kreos.***, **PSOR.**, sep., ***sulph.***
pustules, behind - berb., cann-s., carb-v., cast-eq., crot-h., phyt., ***psor.***, ptel., **PULS.**, spong., sumb.
scabby - anan., bry., elaps, graph., ***hydr.***, iod., lach., lyc., mur-ac., nat-p., ***psor.***, ***puls.***, sanic., sars., sil., spong.
behind - aur-m., ***bar-c.***, **GRAPH.**, kali-c., lach., **LYC.**, **SIL.**, tell., thuj.
behind, exuding a glutinous moisture, sore on touch - thuj.
scaly - cop., ***petr.***, psor., teucr.
scurfy - aur-m., bov., calc., com., graph., hep., ***iod.***, ***lach.***, **LYC.**, mur-ac., **PSOR.**, puls., sars., sil.
behind - hep., **PSOR.**, puls., ***sil.***, staph.
right ear - cinnb.
sore, behind - ***graph.***, kali-c., nit-ac., **PETR.**, **PSOR.**
tragus - mur-ac., ***puls.***, sulph.
tympanum, scurfy - graph.

ERYSIPELAS - ***apis,*** ars., bell., calc-p., ***carb-v., crot-h., kali-bi., lach.,*** meph., ***merc., petr.,*** **PULS.,** ***rhus-t., rhus-v.,*** samb., ***sep., sulph.,*** tell., tep.

EXCORIATION, behind - ***graph.,*** kali-c., nit-ac., petr.

EXOSTOSIS - calc-f., hecla., puls.
meatus, in - calc-f., ***hecla.,*** kali-i.

FOREIGN body, in, as if - ang., phos., sil.
eustachian tube - ***nux-m.***

FORMICATION - ambr., am-c., ant-c., ***arg-m.,*** ars., arund., bar-c., calc., caust., chin., coloc., colch., cop., dros., grat., kali-c., lachn., laur., merc., mill., nat-m., nux-v., osm., phys., plat., rat., samb., sep., spig., stry., sulph., sul-ac., zinc.
about the ear - calad.
behind the ear - bry.
eating, while - lachn.
extending to lower jaw - am-c.
meatus, in - ambr., am-c., ant-c., calc., caust., kali-n., laur., med., plat., puls., samb., sulph.
morning - zinc.

FREEZING, easily - agar., zinc.

FROZEN, as if - **AGAR.,** caust., colch., crot-h., **PETR., PULS.,** sang.

FULLNESS, sensation of - aesc., ***arg-n.,*** arum-d., bell., berb., **CANN-I.,** carb-v., cham., chel., cinnb., com., ***crot-h.,*** cur., eup-per., ferr., ***glon.,*** hep., iod., jug-r., kali-i., kali-p., lac-c., laur., lyc., mang., ***merc.,*** **MEZ.,** nat-c., nat-p., nat-s., nit-ac., ***op.,*** pen., phos., ***puls.,*** phys., stry., sulph., ***thuj.,*** verat-v.
afternoon - stry.
1 p.m - com.
behind - glon., ther.
blowing nose, when - mang., ***puls.***
boring in, amel - mez.
eating, while - ***nat-c.***
evening - mez., nat-p.
excitement, from - dig.
morning - ham., thuj.
sharp, pains, after - iod.
swallowing, from - arum-d., ***mang.***

FUNGUS, excrescences - ***merc.***

GLUE-ear - hydr., kali-bi., kali-m., merc.

GNAWING, pain - dros., kali-c., kali-i., led., mang., mur-ac., sulph., tab.
afternoon - indg.
behind the ear - kali-i.
evening - mur-ac.
in front of - sulph.
left then right - indg.
night - mang.
right - mur-ac., tab.
rubbing, amel. - indg.

GRIPING, pain - carb-s.
left - carb-s.
right - carb-s.
waking, on - carb-s.

HAMMERING - kali-c., thuj.

HEARING, (see Hearing, Chapter)

HEAT - **ACON.,** aeth., agn., aloe, ***alum.,*** alumn., aml-n., anan., ang., ant-c., ***arg-m.,*** arn., ***ars.,*** ars-i., arund., asaf., asar., aur-m-n., ***bell.,*** berb., bor., bov., brom., ***bry.,*** **CALC.,** ***calc-p., camph.,*** cann-s., canth., ***caps.,*** carb-s., ***carb-v., carl.,*** casc., ***cham.,*** chel., chin., ***cic.,*** clem., coc-c., coloc., com., crot-h., ***elaps,*** fago., gran., ***graph.,*** hep., hyos., ***hyper., ign.,*** iod., jac., jatr., kali-ar., ***kali-bi., kali-c.,*** kali-n., kali-p., kreos., lach., ***lyc.,*** lyss., mag-m., manc., mang., meny., meph., ***merc.,*** mur-ac., nat-a., ***nat-m.,*** nat-n., nat-p., nat-s., ***nit-ac.,*** nux-m., oena., ol-an., op., paeon., par., petr., ph-ac., ***phos.,*** phys., pip-m., plat., psor., ***puls.,*** raph., ruta, sabin., sang., seneg., sep., sil., ***spong.,*** stry., sul-ac., ***sulph.,*** tab., tarent., ter., thuj., til., verat., zing.
afternoon - cann-s.
1 p.m - com.
after coffee - nat-m.
chill, during - acon., alum., ars., bell., merc., puls., rhus-t.
back, in - asaf.
cold alternating with - berb., ***cic.,*** verat.
coldness of body, during - acon.
lying, while - ars.
to touch - bapt.
eating, after - ***asaf.***
escaping, sensation of - aeth., calc., ***canth.,*** clem., ***kali-c.,*** mur-ac., ol-an., par.
as if hot water were running out of right - cham.
evening - ***alum.,*** bry., ***caps., carb-v.,*** cycl., nat-m., nat-n., ***nat-s.,*** sabin., sanic., sil.
10 p.m - stry.
lying - ars.
on going to bed - hyper.
sleep, before - ph-ac.
extending, occiput to nape of neck - spong.
over half of head - chel.
to pharynx, evening, while riding - nux-m.
flushes - arg-m., **LYC.**
inside - acon., asar., bell., ***calc.,*** calc-p., canth., casc., chel., euphr., ***lyc.,*** puls.
water, boiling, as if - mag-arct.
left - arn., ***asaf., carb-v., cycl., graph.,*** jac-c., nat-m., sep.
then right - mur-ac.
lobes - alum., ang., camph., hyos., kali-c., kali-n., nat-m., sil.
morning, in bed - cocc.
night - alumn., sulph.
midnight - alumn.
one-sided - alum., asar., carb-v., chin., ign., nat-m., nat-p., puls.
sensation of - arn., mang.
pressure in occiput, during - gran.
redness of one ear, with - alum., tab.
right - asar., com., ***kali-c.,*** lyss., ***nat-s.,*** samb., sep., ter.
red and hot, left pale and cold - ***kali-c.***
swallowing, from - arum-d.
water boiling, as if, inside - mag-arct.

HERPES - am-m., caust., cist., graph., kreos., mag-m., ***olnd.,*** phos., psor., rhus-t., sep., tell., teucr.
about the - olnd.
behind - am-m., bufo, ***caust.,*** cist., con., ***graph., mag-m.,*** mez., ***olnd., sep.,*** teucr.
front of, in - olnd.
lobes, on - caust., cist., ***sep.,*** teucr.
meatus, in - merc.
scabby, behind - kali-i.

HOLLOWNESS, sensation of - aur-m., ***nux-v.***
morning, in, amel., after dinner - nux-v.

INFLAMMATION, of - ***apis, bell.,*** bor., bov., ***bry., cact.,*** cadm-s., ***calc.,*** canth., ***fl-ac.,*** kali-bi., kali-c., kali-i., ***kreos.,*** mag-c., **MERC., MERC-C.,** ***pic-ac.,*** **PULS.,** ***rhus-t.,*** ter., verat.
concha - nat-m., sil.
lobe - kali-n.
margin - sil.
petrous portion temporal bone - caps.
right lobe - carc.
suppurative - arn., caps., sil.
inflammation, eustachian tube - am-m., **CALC.,** ery-a., ***gels., iod.,*** kali-chl., **KALI-M., KALI-S.,** ***mang., merc., merc-d., nat-m.,*** nit-ac., petr., ***phyt.,*** **PULS.,** ***sang.,*** **SIL.,** ***sulph.,*** teucr.
inflammation, inner ear infection, (see Otitis interna)
inflammation, mastoid (see Mastoiditis)
inflammation, middle ear, (see Otitis media)

ITCHING - acon., aeth., ***agar.,*** all-c., alum., ambr., ***am-c.,*** am-m., ***anac.,*** anag., ant-c., ***ars.,*** **AUR., BAR-C.,** bar-m., benz-ac., bor., ***bov., calad., calc., calc-s., caps., carb-s., carb-v., caust.,*** chel., cinnb., ***cist.,*** coc-c., ***colch., coloc.,*** crot-h., crot-t., cupr., ***cycl., elaps,*** ferr-ar., ***fl-ac.,*** form., ***graph.,*** ham., **HEP.,** hyper., ***ign., kali-ar., kali-bi.,*** **KALI-C.,** kali-n., ***kali-p., kali-s.,*** lach., lachn., ***laur., lyc.,*** mag-c., mag-m., manc., **MANG.,** med., meny., ***merc.,*** merc-i-f., merc-i-r., ***mez.,*** mill., mur-ac., nat-a., nat-c., nat-m., nat-p., nat-s., nit-ac., **NUX-V., PETR.,** ph-ac., ***phos., psor.,*** rat., rhod., rumx., ruta., sabad., samb., ***sars.,*** **SEP., SIL.,** ***spig.,*** stann., **SULPH.,** sul-ac., sul-i., tab., tarax., tarent., ***tell.,*** zinc.
about the ear, evening - phel.
afternoon - agar., laur., ol-an., puls.
alternating ear to ear - chel.
anus, with - sabad.
antitragus - coc-c.
behind ear - ***agar.,*** alum., aur., aur-m., brom., calc., carb-v., fago., **GRAPH.,** hura, lyc., mag-c., mag-m., merc-i-f., ***mez., mosch.,*** **NAT-M.,** ***nit-ac., petr.,*** rhus-v., ***ruta,*** sulph., ther., til., verat., verat-v.
burning, followed by - nat-m.
evening, in bed - merc-i-f., sulph.
night - ***aur-m.,*** mag-c., mag-m., merc-i-f., ruta.
noon - fago.
scratching amel. - brom., mag-c., mag-m., ruta.

INFLAMMATION, of
below ear - ars., caust., mag-c., ol-an., verat.
scratching amel. - mag-c.
boring with finger, amel. - aeth., agar., ***bov.,*** coc-c., ***coloc.,*** fl-ac., lachn., laur., mag-m., mill., ol-an., zinc.
does not amel. - agar., ***carb-v.,*** laur., mang.
burning - **AGAR.,** alum., ***arn.,*** **ARS.,** arund., bad., **BRY.,** calc., calc-p., carb-an., carb-v., ***caust.,*** corn., lach., ***lyc., mur-ac.,*** nat-p., ***nit-ac., nux-v.,*** **PETR.,** ***phos.,*** puls., stry., ***sulph.,*** thuj., zinc.
scratching, after - ***fl-ac.***
burning, warm room - calc-p.
concha - agar., ant-c., arg-m., calc., chel., paeon., raph., spig., sulph.
corrosive - ***arg-m.***
cough, from - lach.
deaf - sep.
eating, while - lachn.
eustachian tube - agar., arg-m., ***calc.,*** caust., coc-c., coloc., ign., ***kali-m.,*** **NUX-V.,** ***petr.,*** **SIL.**
compels swallowing - gels., **NUX-V.,** sil.
evening - acon., bor., calad., calc-p., elaps, graph., grat., mag-c., nat-m., psor., puls.
9 p.m - phel.
walking, while - bor.
extending into mouth - coc-c.
over whole body - am-c.
external ear - **AGAR.,** ***alum.,*** am-m., ant-c., apis, ***arg-m.,*** berb., calc-p., ***calc-s., carb-v., coloc., con.,*** fago., ***graph., kali-c.,*** mag-m., manc., nat-c., nat-m., ***petr.,*** ph-ac., pic-ac., plat., **PULS.,** rhod., **RHUS-T.,** sil., stry., **SULPH., TELL.,** trom., verat., zinc.
front of, in - alum., ol-an.
frozen, as if - **AGAR.,** colch., crot-h., hipp., **PETR.**
left - **ANAG.,** benz-ac., calc., caust., cist., coc-c., form., ham., mang., mur-ac., nat-s., phel., rhus-t., sars., stann., sulph., ***tell.,*** verat-v., zinc.
lobes - agar., alum., ***arg-m.,*** caust., graph., kali-bi., kali-c., laur., nat-c., nat-m., nux-v., ph-ac., sabad., sulph.
night, at - nux-v.
right - nat-p.
lying - kali-p.
meatus, external - tell.
meatus, in - arund.
menses, during - agar.
morning - am-c., arg-m., kali-n., nat-c., sars.
moving jaws, when - ph-ac.
night - ***merc-i-r.,*** sep., stry.
riding, after - calc-p.
right - carb-ac., chel., cinnb., meny., merc-i-r., mez., nat-m., nat-p., psor., rat., rumx., tarent.
lobe - nat-p.
rising, soon after - arg-m., trom.

INFLAMMATION, of
rubbing, agg. - alum.
amel - mez., ol-an., phel.
does not amel. - zinc.
scratching, amel. - caust., mag-c., nat-c.
does not amel. - am-m., ***arg-m.,*** fl-ac., ***sars.***
must scratch until it bleeds - alum., ***arg-m.,*** nat-p.
sharp - lach.
sleep, during - ***lyc.***
stooping, on - lepi.
swallowing - mang., ***sil.***
compelling - carb-v., **NUX-V.**
touch amel. - hyper., mur-ac., nat-m.
tragus - mur-ac.
walking, while - bor.
warm room - calc-p., coc-c.
entering from cold air - ***coc-c.***
yawning, while - acon.

JERKING, pain - all-c., anac., ang., ***calc.,*** calc-p., cann-s., carb-v., caust., ***cina,*** clem., dig., fl-ac., ***hep.,*** mag-aust., mag-m., mang., mur-ac., nux-v., paeon., petr., ph-ac., **PLAT.,** ***puls.,*** rhod., sabad., sil., spig., valer., zinc.
jerking, behind - kali-c., mang., merc., mez., sil.
evening - mang.
on lying down - mang.
on lying down, after lying in bed amel. - mang.
in front - dros.
morning - mang.

LACERATING, pain - calen., bell., cadm-s., **SULPH.,** tarent.
right - tarent.

LABYRINTHITIS, (see Otitis interna)

LANCINATING, pain - acon., aeth., all-c., alum., am-m., anac., arg-m., ***asaf.,*** aster., aur-s., ***bell.,*** berb., cadm-s., caps., caust., ***cham.,*** chin., cit-v., cur., der., ferr-i., ferr-p., gamb., hura, kali-c., kali-i., ***mag-p.,*** meny., nit-ac., nux-v., plb., ***puls.,*** raph., sil., ***spig.,*** tarent., teucr., viol-o., zinc.
behind ear - kali-c.
below ear - tarent.
evening - nux-v.
intermittent - ***asaf.***
morning - tarent.
outward - ***asaf.***

LUMPS, hard, behind ear - cinnb.

LUPUS, on the lobe - nit-ac.

MASTOIDITIS, infection - aur., calc-p., canth., **CAPS.,** ferr-p., hep., lach., ***phos.,*** sil.
decay, threatened of mastoid process - **AUR., CAPS.,** carb-an., ***fl-ac., hep., lach., nit-ac.,*** **SIL.**

MENIERE'S disease - alum., arg-m., ***arg-n.,*** arn., ars., asar., bar-m., bell., benz-ac., bry., calc., ***camph.,*** carb-v., carb-s., ***caust.,*** chen-a., chin., **CHIN-S.,** ***chin-sal., cic., cocc.,*** colch., com., con., crot-h., crot-t., ***dig.,*** eucal., ferr-p., gels., ***glon.,*** gran., hell., hydrobr-ac., jab., kali-c., kali-i., kali-m., kali-p., kalm., laur., mag-c., morg., myric., nat-a., nat-c., nat-m., nat-p., nat-s., ***nat-sal.,*** nux-v., onos., op., petr., ph-ac., **PHOS.,** pic-ac., psor., puls., rad-br., ***sal-ac., sang.,*** seneg., sep., ***sil.,*** stann., tab., ***ther.,*** thyr., zinc.
noises, before vertigo - lachn., sep.
seasick, as if - tab.

MOISTURE, behind the ears - calc., carb-v., caust., **GRAPH.,** hep., kali-c., lyc., nit-ac., ***olnd., petr.,*** phos., sil.
concha - sil., sulph.
margin - sil.

NARROW, sensation - lyc.

NAUSEA, in - dios.

NODES, on, copper-colored - arg-m., dros., graph., merc., staph.
copper-colored, behind - bar-c., ph-ac.

NOISES, in ears, (see Hearing chapter)

NUMBNESS - calc-i., irid., gels., fl-ac., lach., manc., nux-m., ***plat.,*** sulph., thuj., ***verb.***
about ear - ***fl-ac.,*** lach.
behind - ox-ac.
concha - lach.
front of, in - sulph.
left - tarax., thuj., ***verb.***
mastoid, in - **PLAT.**
meatus, in - lach., mur-ac.

ODOR, bad - graph.

OPEN, meatus seems open - aur-m., mez.
morning - mez.

OPENING, and closing, sensation like a valve - ***bar-c.,*** bor., graph., ***iod., nat-s., psor.***
step, at every - graph.

OPENING, sensation of, through which the air penetrates on opening and closing the mouth - thuj.

OTITIS interna, inflammation of inner ear - ***acon.,*** arund., ***bar-c., bar-m.,*** **BELL.,** bor., bov., bry., ***cact.,*** **CALC., CALC-S.,** canth., ***caps.,*** carb-s., carb-v., ***caust.,*** **CHAM.,** cur., ***con.,*** ferr-p., **GRAPH., HEP.,** ***kali-bi., kali-c., kali-chl., kali-i.,*** kino, ***lach.,*** led., **LYC.,** ***mag-c.,*** mag-m., **MERC.,** ***merc-c.,*** mez., ***nat-s., nit-ac., petr.,*** phos., ***pic-ac., psor., puls., rhus-t., sang.,*** sep., ***sil.,*** spig., **SULPH.,** ter., ther., ***thuj.,*** verb., verat-v., zinc.
otitis media, inflammation of middle ear - ***apis, arn., bar-c.,*** **BELL.,** ***bor.,*** **CALC., CALC-S.,** ***caps., carb-v., caust.,*** **CHAM.,** cur., ***dulc., ferr-p.,*** gels., **HEP.,** hydr., **KALI-BI.,** ***kali-c., kali-chl., kali-i.,*** **LYC., MERC., MERC-D.,** ***nat-c., nat-m., psor.,*** **PULS.,** rhus-t., **SIL., SULPH.,** ***tell., thuj.,*** tub., zinc.
chronic - calc., calc-f., ***carc.,*** caust., cham., hep., **MERC.,** ***merc-d., psor., puls., sil.,*** thuj.
with discharge - caust., ***sil.,*** tub.

PAIN, ears - ***acon.,*** act-sp., aesc., aeth., agar., ail., ***all-c.,*** aloe, alum., ambr., am-c., am-m., ***anac., ang., ant-c.,*** ant-t., ***apis,*** aran., arg-m., ***arg-n., arn., ars.,*** ars-i., arum-t., arund., asaf., ***asar., aur.,*** aur-m., aur-m-n., ***bar-c., bar-m.,*** **BELL.,** berb., bism., ***bor.,*** bov., brach., brom., bry., cact., calad., ***calc.,*** calc-f., ***calc-p., calc-s.,*** cadm-s., camph., ***cann-i.,*** cann-s., canth., ***caps.,*** carb-an., ***carb-s., carb-v.,*** carl., cast., ***caust.,*** **CHAM.,** ***chel.,*** chin., chin-a., chin-s., chlf., cic., ***cimic.,*** cinnb., clem., cob., coc-c., colch., coloc., com., con., croc., crot-h., crot-t., ***cupr.,*** cupr-ar., ***cur.,*** cycl., der., dig., dios., ***dros., dulc.,*** elaps, ery-a., euph., euphr., eupi., fago., ferr., ferr-ar., ferr-i., ferr-m., ferr-p., ***fl-ac., form.,*** gamb., ***gels.,*** glon., ***graph., guai.,*** ham., hell., **HEP.,** hura, hydr., hyos., hyper., ign., indg., iod., ip., jatr., kali-ar., ***kali-bi., kali-c.,*** kali-chl., kali-i., kali-n., ***kali-p., kali-s., kalm.,*** kreos., lac-ac., **LACH.,** lac-c., lact., laur., lil-t., lith., lob., lob-s., **LYC.,** lyss., mag-c., mag-m., ***mag-p.,*** mag-s., ***mang.,*** med., meph., **MERC.,** merc-c., ***merc-i-f., merc-i-r.,*** merl., ***mez., mill.,*** morph., mosch., ***mur-ac.,*** nat-a., nat-c., ***nat-m., nat-p., nat-s.,*** nicc., ***nit-ac.,*** nux-m., ***nux-v.,*** olnd., ol-j., op., osm., ox-ac., par., ***petr., phel.,*** **PH-AC., PHOS.,** phys., phyt., ***plan., plat., plb.,*** prun., ***psor.,*** ptel., **PULS.,** ran-s., raph., ***rhod., rhus-t.,*** rumx., ruta., sabad., sabin., samb., ***sang.,*** sarr., **SARS.,** seneg., ***sep., sil., spig., spong.,*** squil., ***stann.,*** staph., stram., stront-c., **SULPH.,** sul-ac., syph., tab., tarax., tarent., tell., teucr., til., ***thuj.,*** trom., ***tub.,*** ust., valer., verat., **VERB.,** xan., ***zinc.,*** zing.

- **about** the ear - am-m., arg-n., asar., bell., bry., coc-c., dulc., glon., grat., kali-c., merc-i-f., mez., nit-ac., ox-ac., ***petr., puls.,*** rhod., sabin., tell.
  - morning after rising - arg-n., brom.
  - morning after rising, walk, after a - pall.
- **above** the ear - ***arg-m.,*** arg-n., asaf., aur-m., aur-m-n., brom., camph., cedr., chel., cann-i., carb-v., chin-s., coloc., dios., dulc., hura, lach., merc., mez., nat-s., nux-m., ox-ac., ***puls.,*** rhod., sabin., sil., tell., verat.
  - evening - chin-s., dios.
  - extending to upper back teeth - chel.
  - morning - brom.
  - stool, during - ox-ac.
- **afternoon** - aeth., alum., aran., bov., brom., bry., carb-s., ***chel.,*** chin-s., dios., form., euphr., gels., lyss., ***merc-c.,*** nat-a., rumx., stry., sulph., tarent., trom.
  - 1 p.m. - graph.
  - 2 p.m. - chin-s.
  - 3 p.m. - phys.
  - 4 p.m. - kalm., nat-c.
  - 5 p.m. - berb.
- **air,** cold, in - agar., ***ars.,*** bry., calc-p., caps., ***cham.,*** colch., ***dulc., hep.,*** kali-m., lach., ***lyc.,*** mag-p., merc., ***mez.,*** nat-c., par., sang., ***sep.***
  - amel. - ***phos.***
  - draft - camph., ***dulc., hep., lyc., mez.***

PAIN, ears

- **air,** open, in - acon., bry., con., euph., ***hep., lyc., mang.,*** mez., ***sep.,*** sulph., tab.
  - amel. - acon., aur., cic., ferr-p., ***puls.***
- **alternating,** with eyes - bell.
- **antitragus** - mur-ac.
- **behind** ear - acon., aesc., agar., alet., all-c., aloe, alum., ***ambr.,*** am-c., anac., arg-m., arg-n., ars., arum-d., asar., asaf., ***aur., aur-m-n.,*** bar-c., ***bell.,*** bor., bry., cadm-s., ***calc-p., calc-s.,*** cann-s., canth., ***caps.,*** carb-ac., carb-v., cast., ***caust.,*** cedr., ***chel.,*** chin., cic., coc-c., colch., ***coloc.,*** con., croc., ***crot-h., cupr.,*** dig., dios., fl-ac., ***glon.,*** ham., ***hep.,*** hura, ign., indg., kali-ar., kali-bi., ***kali-c.,*** kali-i., kali-n., ***kali-p.,*** kalm., ***lach.,*** laur., led., lith., lyc., manc., mang., merc., merc-i-f., merl., mez., mosch., mur-ac., myric., nat-a., nat-c., nat-m., nat-s., ***nit-ac.,*** nux-v., paeon., par., phel., phos., phys., phyt., pic-ac., ptel., ran-s., rhus-t., rumx., sabin., sars., sep., **SIL.,** spig., stann., stry., ***sulph.,*** tab., thea., ther., ***thuj.,*** verb., verat-v., viol-o., xan., zinc.
  - afternoon - ham., iris, ptel.
    - 1 p.m. - nat-c., sil.
    - 3 p.m. - phel.
    - 4 p.m. - caust., grat.
    - on waking - ptel.
  - air, open - ***kali-p.,*** mang.
  - evening - ham., nat-m., ran-s.
  - extending, down neck - lith.
    - to eye - **PRUN.**
    - to left arm - staph.
    - to temple - cedr.
  - left - **AUR.,** kali-p., ***lach.***
  - lying on it - coc-c.
  - morning - dios., ptel., sulph.
    - 11 a.m. - ham.
  - moving head - am-c., ***kali-p.***
  - paroxysmal - aesc.
  - pressure, on - mur-ac..
  - pulsating - hura.
  - reading, while - aesc., spig.
  - rest, during - arg-m.
  - right - aesc.
  - shaking the head - glon.
  - sitting amel. - asar.
    - up in bed amel. - alum.
  - touch agg. - bar-c., mang., sil.
  - turning head - bar-c.
  - walk bent, must - lyc.
  - walking, on, agg. - asar.
    - in open air - mang.
  - warm bed - coc-c.
  - writing, while - spig.
- **belching,** during - sulph., tarent.
- **bell**-stroke, during - mag-m., ph-ac.
- **below,** the ear - acon., aloe, alum., am-c., asar., ***bar-c.,*** caps., chel., caust., ***merc.,*** nat-p., olnd., ol-an., phos., sep., sil., zinc.
  - extending to lower jaw - ***merc.***
  - moving head agg. - am-c.
  - rubbing amel. - phos.
  - sitting, while - phos.

PAIN, ears
below, the ear
swallowing, when - nat-h.
biting, teeth together - anac.
blowing, nose, on - act-sp., alum., bar-c., ***calc.,*** caust., con., dios., hep., lyc., ph-ac., puls., sil., spig., stann., teucr., trom.
boring, with finger, agg. - anac., mur-ac., ruta., ***tarent.,*** zinc.
amel. - agar., ***coloc.,*** fl-ac., lach., mez., mur-ac., ph-ac., phys., psor.
breathing, when - mang.
centering, at the ear, hard pains - mang.
changing, weather - ***mang.,*** rhod., ***rhus-t., sil.***
chewing, when - aloe, ***anac., apis,*** arg-m., bell., cann-s., hep., lach., nux-m., nux-v., seneg., verb.
chill, during - acon., apis, calc., gamb., graph., ***nux-v.,*** puls., sulph.
cleaning - sulph.
cold, applications, agg. - bor., bufo, calc., dulc., **HEP.,** sep., ***sil.***
applications, amel. - ***ferr-p.,*** merc., puls.
drinks amel. - bar-m.
weather in - asar.
cold, from taking - ***dulc., gels., kalm., merc., puls.,*** sep.
from taking, in head - ***bell.,*** gels., led., puls.
when feet become - stann.
concha - lyc., phos., spig.
cough, during - ***calc., caps.,*** dios., kali-bi., nux-v., sep., thuj.
damp, weather - ***calc., calc-p., dulc., nat-s., nux-m., petr., sil.***
day, and night - hell.
daytime - nat-m., rhod.
descending, steps - bad., chin-s.
dinner, after - agar., ant-c., bov., carb-an., plb.
drinking, while - con.
ear-wax, from - spig.
eating, while - apis, carb-an., carb-s., cinnb., phel., verb.
after - graph., mang.
amel. - mag-c.
eustachian tube - ant-c.
evening - acon., aloe, alum., ***ars.,*** berb., bor., brom., carb-s., carb-v., caust., chin-s., cob., dios., graph., ham., hyos., hyper., indg., kali-ar., ***kali-bi.,*** kali-c., kali-i., kali-s., lach., lyc., mang., merc., nat-c., nat-m., nux-v., ox-ac., par., psor., ran-b., rhus-r., sep., staph., sulph., tarent., thuj., verb., zinc.
7 p.m. - phys., zing.
7:30 p.m. - fago.
8 p.m. - nat-s.
8 to 10 p.m. - phel.
9 p.m. - carb-s., dios.
exertion, of vision, after - sil.
extending, to
chest, to - stram.
chin, to - bell.

PAIN, ears
extending, to
downward - **BELL.,** cur., verb.
eustachian tube, to - ant-c., carb-an.
eye, to - glon., hura, ***puls.,*** spig.
to left - hura.
face, to - anac., ***bell.,*** cann-s., ***merc.,*** nux-v., stram., thea.
finger ends, to - ham.
forehead, to - bell., dig., nux-v., ptel., spig.
from left to right - calc-p.
head, to - ***sulph.***
inward - arn., arg-m., bry., ***calc.,*** carb-an., carb-v., dros., hyos., kali-bi., kali-i., lob., lyss., med., nat-s., nux-v., rhus-t., thuj., verb.
jaw, to - bov., lyc., merl., phel., spig.
jaw, to lower - am-c., asar., com., kali-bi.
jaw, to upper - agar.
left arm - staph.
legs, to - cur.
lobule, to - phos.
malar bone, to - spig.
mouth, roof of, to - kali-bi.
neck, to - ars., **BELL.,** coc-c., ***crot-h., haem., kreos.,*** lith., lyc., mur-ac., ***nat-m.,*** sil., tarax., ***ther., zinc.***
to side of - ***carb-v.,*** coc-c., kali-bi., ***mag-p.,*** meph., ***nat-m.***
nose, to - sil.
occiput, to - ambr., ***bell.,*** fago., ***mur-ac.***
to side of - coc-c.
other ear, to - chel., ***hep.,*** laur., thuj.
outward - aeth., am-c., ***am-m., ars.,*** bar-c., berb., calc-p., cann-s., carb-v., con., dulc., glon., gran., ***kali-c.,*** kali-i., lyc., merc-i-f., nat-m., ***nat-s.,*** nicc., ***puls., sep., sil.,*** thuj., til.
palate, to - ***kali-bi.***
parietal bone, to - indg., ran-b.
parotid gland and mastoid process, to - ***kali-bi.,*** sep.
right to left - ***arn.***
shoulder, to - ***ars.,*** cann-s., ***kreos., nat-m.,*** rumx.
to left - nat-m.
side of neck and clavicular region and to last back teeth and side of occiput - coc-c.
spine, to - ptel.
teeth, to - chel., bell., lyss., mang., mosch., ol-an., ***spig.,*** xan.
temples, to - eupi., form., indg., lach., lac-c., ***nux-v.,*** puls., sars., tarent.
throat, to - carb-an., chel., fago., kali-bi., ***merc-i-f., spig.***
vertex, to - arn., chel., ol-an., psor., sars.
zygoma - hyper., spig.
faceache, with - **BELL.,** merc., ph-ac.
fainting with pain in ear - cur., ***hep., merc.***
forenoon - chin-s., hydr., ***mag-c.,*** nat-m., nux-m., plb., sars.
9 a.m. - elaps, nat-s.
9 a.m., after going out - tell.
10 a.m. - mag-s.
10:30 a.m. - hydr.

PAIN, ears
forenoon,
11 a.m. - dios., hydr.
sitting, while - phos.
standing, while - plb.
hammer, from sound of - sang.
headache, during - ham., lach., merc., phos., psor., puls., ran-s., sang.
fever, during - calad., calc., chin-s., graph.
front of ear, in - ang., anac., arg-n., aur-m-n., ***bar-c.,*** bov., ***calc-p.,*** colch., ***cupr.,*** dios., indg., kali-i., mag-c., mag-m., merc-i-f., nat-p., ol-an., ***phos.,*** rat., sep., stront-c., sul-ac., tab., zinc.
hiccough, from - bell.
inside - absin., agar., aloe, alum., ***anac.,*** ang., ant-c., apis, apoc., arg-m., arn., arund., ***asaf., asar., aur.,*** aur-m-n., bar-c., ***bar-m.,*** **BELL.,** berb., bism., bor., bov., brom., bry., ***calc., calc-p., canth.,*** caps., carb-an., carb-v., ***caust.,*** **CHAM.,** chel., chin., cic., coc-c., colch., croc., dig., dros., ***dulc.,*** ferr., ferr-p., ***fl-ac.,*** gamb., ***graph.,*** ham., hell., **HEP.,** ign., indg., ***kali-c.,*** kali-n., kreos., **LACH.,** ***lyc.,*** mang., meph., ***merc., merc-i-f., mez., mur-ac., nat-m.,*** nat-p., nat-s., ***nit-ac., nux-v.,*** olnd., op., ox-ac., par., petr., phel., **PH-AC.,** ***phos.,*** phys., ***plat.,*** plb., psor., **PULS.,** ran-b., ran-s., rheum, rhod., rumx., samb., sars., sep., ***sil., spig., spong.,*** stann., stry., ***sulph.,*** sul-ac., sumb., tab., tarax., tarent., ***tell., thuj.,*** upa., valer., verat., viol-t., ***zinc.***
intermittent - arn., nat-c., nat-m.
laughing, when - mang.
leaning on hand - arn., kali-n., lac-c., lach.
left - acon., asaf., calen., camph., coch., erig., ery-a., ***dulc.,*** form., ***graph.,*** guai., ***lac-c.,*** lach., mag-s., mang., mez., mur-ac., nat-m., petr., sep., spig., stram., tarax., ***verb.,*** zinc.
then right - aesc., arn., brom., merc.
lie, down, compelled to - cur.
lobule - cham., dros., mur-ac., nat-m., phos., ph-ac., plb., sabad., tab., zinc.
lying, in bed, while - ***caust.,*** kali-i., ***kali-p.,*** nux-v., sang., ***sulph.,*** thuj.
on ear - agar., am-c., am-m., ***bar-c.,*** bar-m., chin., hep., kali-n., lac-c., med.
on ear, amel. - lach.
on right side - ptel.
mastoid, extending to neck - lith., mur-ac.
operations, after - caps.
menopause, during - gels., sang.
menses, during - agar., aloe, ***kali-c.,*** kreos., mag-c., merc., petr.
suppressed - am-c., puls., sulph.
mercury, abuse of - asaf., nit-ac., staph.
midnight - kali-c.
after - sep.
driving her out of bed - ***mygal.***
walking in wind - sep.
moon, full, during - sil.

PAIN, ears
morning - all-c., alum., ars., bor., carb-v., ferr., form., lyss., ***mang.,*** merc., merc-i-f., ***nat-a.,*** nat-c., nat-s., nux-m., nux-v., rumx., sars., sep., tarent., trom., verat.
8 a.m. - dios., nat-c.
waking, on - sep., ***verb.***
motion, on - ***sil.,*** stann.
amel. - ***cham., psor.***
lower jaw - nux-m., ph-ac., stann., verb.
head, of - am-c.
music, from - ambr., cham., kreos., ***ph-ac.,*** tab.
nausea, with - ***dulc.***
night - ***acon.,*** alum., am-m., ars., bar-c., bell., ***bry.,*** calc-p., caps., ***cham.,*** cycl., **DULC.,** ferr-p., hell., ***hep.,*** kali-ar., ***kali-bi.,*** kali-c., kali-i., kali-n., lac-c., ***lach.,*** mang., **MERC.,** merc-i-f., nux-v., **PULS.,** ***rhus-t.,*** sep., ***sil.,*** stry., tell., ***tub.,*** vib.
10 p.m. - form.
noises, from - am-c., arn., ***bell.,*** carb-v., cham., **CON.,** gad., mur-ac., ***op., phos., sang., sil.,*** **SULPH.**
deaf ear, from, in the - am-c.
loud - spig.
noon - aloe, chin-s., gels., psor., sulph.
opening the mouth amel. - nat-c.
paroxysmal - alum., anac., crot-t., ***cham.,*** ferr-p., ***ph-ac.,*** stront-c., tarent.
periodical - arn., ***gels.,*** nat-c., ***nat-m.***
perspiration, during - ign.
pressing, forehead, on - nit-ac.
teeth together - anac.
pressure, on - cina, lac-c., raph., spong.
amel. - alum., bism., carb-an., caust., ham.
pulsating - bufo, kali-bi., rhus-t., ***tell.***
reason, pain which almost deprived him of - merc., ***puls.***
rhythmical - mur-ac.
right - aeth., ambr., ***am-m.,*** arg-n., asaf., aur-m., ***bar-c., bar-m.,*** **BELL.,** berb., brom., bry., ***caust.,*** chel., chin., colch., ***coloc.,*** cupr., ***cycl.,*** dros., ***elaps,*** eupi., **FL-AC.,** gels., hura, hyper., ***kali-c., kalm., lac-c.,*** lach., ***lyc.,*** mag-c., mag-m., ***merc.,*** merc-i-f., mur-ac., ***nat-s.,*** **NIT-AC.,** ***nux-v.,*** petr., prun., ***puls.,*** psor., seneg., sep., stront-c., sulph., tab., tarent., ***tell.,*** thuj., verb.
lying on it amel. - ***lach.***
then left - bar-c., ***lyc.***
then left, extending around back of head - helo.
room, on entering - nux-v.
rubbing amel. - aeth., mang., ol-an., phos.
singing, while - ph-ac.
sitting, while - berb., gels., indg., lach., nat-c., phos.
after long - ***sil.***
sleep amel. - sep.
sneezing, on - act-sp., calc., ph-ac., phos., ***sulph.***
amel. - mag-m.

PAIN, ears
sore throat, with - **APIS,** ***bar-m., cham.,*** **LACH.,** ***merc.,*** **NIT-AC.,** ***par.***
sounds, sharp - **CON.,** ***cop., sil.***
standing, while - mag-s., nat-c., plb.
stool, during - sep.
stooping, while - bry., ***cham.,*** graph., kreos., mag-arct., mang., merc., phos., rheum.
amel. - carb-v.
suppression of ague, after - ***puls.***
swallowing, on - ail., alum., anac., **APIS,** benz-ac., bov., ***calc.,*** carb-an., ***carb-s.,*** coc-c., ***con.,*** dros., ***elaps,*** fago., ferr-m., ferr-ma., jug-c., **LACH.,** lyc., mang., ***merc.,*** merc-i-f., mur-ac., nat-m., **NIT-AC., NUX-V.,** ***par., petr.,*** phos., ***phyt.,*** plb., sars., ***sulph.,*** thuj., trom.
left ear - carb-s., kali-bi., mang.
amel. - rhus-t.
right ear - brom.
talking, while - mang., nux-v., spig., teucr.
thunderstorm, before - rhod.
tobacco, from - raph.
toothache, with - clem., ***glon.,*** meph., merl., mur-ac., ph-ac., sep., ***plan.,*** **RHOD.**
after - mang.
touch, on - caust., chin., cop., ***lach.,*** mag-c., mang., ***mur-ac.***
tragus - fago.
traumatic, causes - arn.
turning, eyes outward, on - raph.
head, on - ***carb-v.,*** coc-c., chin-s., **MAG-P.,** meph.
urine, profuse - **THUJ.**
vexation, after - sulph.
waking, on - sep., tarent., ***tub.***
walking, while - am-c., bor., bry., con., kali-bi., ***lach.,*** mang., rumx.
air, in open - am-m., benz-ac., bry., ***chin.,*** con., ***mang.,*** nat-c., par., ***sep.,*** spong.
amel. - am-m.
warm room, in - ***nat-s., nux-v.,*** phos., ***puls.***
amel. - sep.
entering from cold air, agg. - ***nat-s.***
warmth, agg. - acon., anac., bor., calc-p., ***cham.,*** dulc., ***ign., merc.,*** nux-v., ***puls.,*** verat.
bed, of, agg. - **MERC.,** merc-i-f., ***nux-v.,*** phos., puls.
dry - bry.
wrapping up amel., and - ***bell.,*** caps., ***cham., dulc.,*** **HEP.,** kali-ar., lach., ***mag-p.,*** mur-ac., rhus-t., ***sep.,*** stram.
wind, in cold - ars-i., ***lac-c.,*** sep., spong.
cold wind, and rain, in - nux-v.
writing, while - phys.
yawning, on - acon., cocc., hep., rhus-r., verat.

PECKING - dros.

PERFORATION of eardrum, tympanum - aur., calc., **CALEN.,** caps., kali-bi., merc., ***sil.,*** tell., ***tub.***

PERSPIRATION - act-sp., puls., zinc.
behind ears - cimic.

PIERCING, pain - berb., calc., cench., con., glon., kali-i., ***nat-c., nat-s.***
inward - ***nat-s.***
outward - berb., glon.
right - glon., ***nat-s.***

PINCHING, pain in - am-c., ang., aran., asar., ***bell.,*** bry., carb-an., carb-v., caust., colch., ***con.,*** crot-t., der., dulc., ferr-ma., kali-c., kreos., laur., mang., meny., ***merc., mur-ac.,*** nat-c., nit-ac., nux-v., sabin., ***spig.,*** stann., staph., teucr., thuj.
about the ear - glon.
above the ear - carb-v.
afternoon - aran.
behind the ear - lyc., merc., paeon., sabin.
drinking, while - con.
evening - am-c.
hiccoughing, when - bell.
left - carb-an., carb-v., dulc., staph.
morning - nat-c.
night - bry.
right - nat-c., thuj.
then left - bell.
rubbing, amel. - mang.

POLYPS - anac., **CALC.,** calc-i., caust., kali-bi., kali-chl., ***kali-s., lach., lyc., merc.,*** petr., ***phos.,*** sang., staph., sulph., ***teucr., thuj.***
bleeding - calc., merc., thuj.
soft, easily bleeding - ***calc., merc.,*** **THUJ.**

PRESSING, pain - acon., aesc., **ANAC.,** aran., arn., asaf., ***asar.,*** aur., ***bell.,*** berb., bism., bry., calc., calc-p., camph., cann-s., ***caps.,*** carb-s., carb-v., carl., ***caust.,*** **CHAM.,** ***chel.,*** chin., ***clem.,*** coc-c., con., crot-t., ***cupr.,*** dig., ***dros., dulc.,*** eupi., fl-ac., form., glon., ***graph., guai.,*** hell., hydr-ac., hyper., indg., iod., ip., kali-c., kali-n., kali-p., kali-s., kreos., lach., laur., lyc., lyss., mang., **MERC.,** merc-i-r., merl., mosch., ***mur-ac.,*** nat-c., ***nat-m., nat-s.,*** nit-ac., nux-m., ***nux-v.,*** olnd., ***par.,*** petr., ***ph-ac., phos., plat.,*** prun., **PULS.,** rheum, rhod., ruta., sabad., **SARS.,** seneg., sep., ***sil., spig.,*** spong., ***stann.,*** sulph., tarax., ***thuj.,*** verat.
above the ear - arg-m., aur-m-n., brom., camph., cedr., dulc., hura, mez., nux-m., ox-ac., ***puls.,*** sabin.
morning - brom.
stool, during - ox-ac.
air, cold, amel. - phos.
asunder - spig.
behind - asar., ***bell.,*** bor., cadm-s., cann-s., canth., ***caust.,*** coc-c., coloc., ***crot-h.,*** hell., ip., kali-bi., led., manc., mang., merl., mez., mur-ac., nat-m., nat-s., ox-ac., ***plat.,*** stann., ther., ***thuj.,*** verb., viol-o.
drinking rapidly - nat-m.
evening - nat-m.
left - anag., bell., coloc., graph., ph-ac.
lying on it - coc-c.
sitting, amel. - asar.
touch, amel. - mang.
walking, agg. - asar.
walking, in open air, while - mang.

PRESSING, pain
below - asar., iod., sep., zinc.
blowing, nose - sil.
boring, with finger, agg. - anac., ruta.
boring, with finger, amel. - fl-ac.
chewing - seneg.
cold weather - asar.
concha - bell., bism., cupr., lyc., sars., staph.
coughing, when - ***caps.***
evening - berb., hyper., kali-bi., mang., sep., ***verb.***
extending to malar bone and teeth - spig.
temple - sars.
finger, like a - rheum.
forward in ear - ***cann-s.,*** caust., nat-s., nux-v., par., ***puls.,*** spong.
front of the ear, in - aur-m-n., caust., ***cur.,*** dios., ***phos.,*** sep., verb., zinc.
warm room, in - ***phos.***
hot - ruta.
intermittent - arn.
inward - nit-ac.
left - asaf., dig., sep., spig., tarax.
left, then right - arn.
lobule - phos.
lying on ear - bar-c., coc-c.
mastoid - mur-ac., plat.
menses, during - kreos.
morning - nat-s., nux-m., verat.
9 a.m. - nat-s.
10:30 a.m. - hydr.
waking, on - sep., ***verb.***
motion of jaw - nux-m.
out, as if something must be torn from within - ***con.,*** lil-t., nat-s.
outward - astac., calc-caust., ***caust.,*** chel., ***con.,*** graph., guare., hydr., iris, kali-n., kreos., lyc., ***merc.,*** mur-ac., nat-m., ***nat-s.,*** nit-ac., ***nux-v.,*** prun., **PULS.,** sep.
plug, like a - ***anac., spig.***
pressure amel. - bism.
rhythmical - mur-ac.
right - berb., chel., eupi., hyper., mur-ac., nat-s., prun., rhod., seneg., verat.
then left - bar-c.
sneezing, on - phos., ***sulph.***
stool, during - sep.
stooping, when - cham., kreos.
swallowing - nux-v., phos., ***sulph.***
tickling - ruta.
tragus - mur-ac., ph-ac.
walking in open air - mang.
warm room - phos., ***puls.***

PRICKING - **AUR.,** brach., dulc., merc., sil.
itching - spig.

PRICKLING - dulc.

PUFFING, in ears from pulsation of temporal arteries - benz-ac.

PULSATION - aloe, alum., alumn., am-c., am-m., aml-n., anac., anan., ars-s-r., bar-c., bar-m., **BELL.,** benz-ac., berb., brom., ***cact.,*** calad., **CALC.,** calc-p., ***calc-s.,*** **CANN-I.,** cann-s., carb-ac., carb-an., ***carb-o.,*** carb-s., ***carb-v., caust.,*** chel., chin., coca, cob., coc-c., ***coloc.,*** ***con.,*** crot-h., dig., ferr-m., gamb., ***glon.,*** graph., ***hep.,*** hydrc., ign., indg., kali-bi., kali-c., kali-n., kali-p., kali-s., ***lach.,*** lyc., ***mag-m., med., merc., merc-c.,*** merc-i-f., mez., ***mur-ac.,*** nat-c., ***nat-m.,*** nat-p., **NIT-AC.,** ol-an., op., **PHOS.,** phys., plan., ptel., ***puls.,*** rheum, rhod., ***rhus-t.,*** rumx., sang., sel., sep., ***sil.,*** spig., spong., sulph., ***tell.,*** thuj., zinc.
air, exposure to, agg. - ptel.
behind ear - ***aml-n.,*** anan., ang., calc-p., caust., glon., kali-c., lach., mez., phos., pic-ac., rhus-t.
cold air amel. - rhus-t.
lying on affected side - rhus-t.
moving head - kali-c.
walking amel. - rhus-t.
warmth agg. - rhus-t.
below ear - sang.
dinner, after - carb-an., indg.
eating agg. - graph.
evening - cob., indg., phys., zinc.
evening, in bed - hep., thuj.
evening, on falling asleep - sil.
forenoon - coca.
in front of ear - bar-c., calad., hep., lyc.
evening - lyc.
lying down, after - hep.
lying down, after, on ear - bar-c.
morning - lyc.
left - am-c., ***bar-c.,*** berb., carb-o., cob., gamb., ***merc-c.,*** nat-c., plan., rhod., spig.
lobes - ferr-m., phos.
lying, on the ear - am-c., bar-c., kali-c., nat-h., sil., ***spong.***
side - bar-c., nat-h.
morning - graph.
morning, after breakfast - zinc.
night - am-m., dig., ***kali-bi.,*** **PULS.,** ***rhus-t.,*** sep.
lying on the ear, when - am-c., ***bar-c.,*** kali-c., lec., sil.
warm in bed, when becoming - ***merc.***
pressure amel. - carb-an.
right - am-m., cact., calad., glon., hydrc., lec., mag-m., ol-an., phos., ptel., sel., sil.
sitting, while - am-m., indg.
standing, while - cann-s.
stooping, on - graph., rheum, zinc.
amel. - cann-s.
walking, after - phos.
wavelike - spig.
writing, while - rheum, zinc.

QUIVERING - bov., kali-c.

RASH, behind - ant-c., nat-m.

RELAXATION, eardrum, sensation - rheum.

RETRACTION, sense of - verb.

ROLLING, as of something, to and fro in ear on shaking head - ruta.

ROUGH, epidermis in ears - olnd.

RUSH, of blood to right ear - lyss.

SCRAPING - ruta.

SCRATCHING, sensation - mang., ruta.

SCREWING - bell., daph.
morning on waking - daph.
twisting, evening - nux-v.

SEBACEOUS cyst, behind ear - merc-i-r., verb.
on lobe - nit-ac.

SENSIBILITY, diminished - mur-ac.
increased - kali-i., ***lach., merc.,*** mur-ac., valer., zinc.
in deaf ear - ***am-c.***

SENITIVE, lobule - phos.

SHARP, pain, in - ***acon.,*** aesc., ***aeth.,*** agar., all-c., aloe, ***alum.,*** am-c., ***am-m.,*** anac., anan., ang., ant-c., apis, apoc., arg-m., ***arg-n., arn., ars.,*** ars-i., arum-d., ***asaf.,*** aur., aur-m., aur-m-n., ***bar-c.,*** bar-m., **BELL.,** benz-ac., ***berb., bor., bov.,*** brom., ***bry.,*** bufo, calad., ***calc., calc-p.,*** calc-s., ***camph.,*** canth., cann-s., ***caps., carb-an.,*** **CARB-S.,** carb-v., **CAUST., CHAM.,** chel., **CHIN.,** ***chin-a., chin-s.,*** cimic., ***cinnb.,*** coc-c., ***colch., coloc.,*** com., **CON.,** crot-c., cupr., cycl., dol., ***dros.,*** **DULC.,** echi., euph., eupi., ***ferr.,*** ferr-ar., ferr-p., fl-ac., form., gamb., ***gels.,*** glon., gran., **GRAPH.,** hell., ***hep.,*** hura, hyos., hyper., ign., indg., ir-foe., jatr., ***kali-ar., kali-bi.,*** **KALI-C., KALI-I.,** ***kali-n.,*** kali-p., ***kali-s., kalm., kreos., lach.,*** lact., laur., lob., lyc., lyss., mag-c., ***mag-m.,*** mag-s., ***mang.,*** meny., ***merc., merc-c.,*** merc-i-f., mez., mill., mur-ac., ***nat-a., nat-c., nat-m., nat-p., nat-s.,*** nicc., ***nit-ac., nux-m., nux-v.,*** olnd., ol-an., paeon., ***petr., ph-ac., phos., phyt.,*** pic-ac., plan., ***plat., plb.,*** psor., ptel., **PULS.,** ran-b., ran-s., raph., rat., rhod., ***rhus-t.,*** rhus-v., ruta., sabad., samb., sang., sarr., ***sars.,*** sep., ***sil.,*** spig., spong., stann., ***staph.,*** stry., stront-c., **SULPH.,** sul-ac., tab., tarax., tarent., tep., teucr., ***thuj.,*** til., valer., verb., vesp., viol-o., ***zinc.***
about the ear - asaf., clem., con., fago., nat-m., phos., viol-o.
above the ear - ars., asaf., coc-c., indg., kali-c., mag-c., merc., mur-ac., plan., sep.
afternoon, 4 p.m. - merc.
walking, while - ars.
afternoon - aeth., bry., carb-s., chin-s., clem., form., merc-c., nat-s., trom.
1 p.m. - graph.
3 p.m. - phys., trom.
4 p.m. - kalm., nat-c.
5 p.m. - berb.
air, cold - kali-ar.
draft, from - ***camph.***
open, agg. - acon., sulph., tab.
going into - am-m., bry., con.
antitragus, on touch - coc-c., kreos.
behind the ear - aeth., agar., ***arn.,*** aur., bar-c., bell., berb., brom., calc., calc-p., canth., cann-s., carb-an., ***caust.,*** cina, con., cop., dig., dios., euphr., gels., hep., ***kali-c., kali-n.,*** kali-p., ***kalm.,*** lyc., mag-c., meny., mur-ac., nat-c., nat-m., nat-p., nit-ac., ph-ac., phos., ptel., sabad., sabin., sars., stry., sulph., tab., tarax., thuj., verat., verb., viol-o., xan.
afternoon - calc.

SHARP, pain
behind the ear
1 p.m. - nat-c.
3 p.m. - mag-c.
evening - bell., berb., carb-an., nit-ac., sulph.
extending, to eye - **PRUN.**
to jaws - kali-n., lyc.
to neck - nat-m.
left - am-m.
morning - calc.
motion - nat-m.
pressure amel. - mag-c., nat-c.
rest, during - sabin.
right - berb., canth., euphr., thuj.
belches, with - bell.
bell-stroke, from - mag-m., ph-ac.
below the ear - apis, bar-c., bry., coc-c., crot-t., hell., mag-s., nit-ac., sars., viol-o., xan.
bending, body to right - mag-m.
blowing nose, when - ***calc.,*** con., hep., lyc., trom.
boring into ear with finger amel. - aeth., ***coloc.,*** mur-ac., ph-ac., psor.
chewing, while - cann-s., nux-v.
chill, during - gamb., graph., psor., puls.
chilliness, on beginning of - gamb.
closing, eyes amel. - calc.
mouth, on - nat-c.
cold, amel. - merc.
ice-cold needle - agar.
stitches - ferr-ma.
concha - ant-c., nat-c., rhus-t., stann., sulph., thuj.
margin of - caust.
cough, with - nux-v.
damp weather - ***nat-s.***
deaf ear, in the - ***mang.,*** sep.
descending stairs - chin-s.
drinking, while - con.
eating, while - verb.
eustachian tube - agar., coloc.
evening - ***alum., ars.,*** berb., bor., chin-s., clem., daph., graph., hyper., kali-c., kali-i., kali-n., merc., nat-m., ox-ac., phos., psor., ran-b., staph., sulph., tarent., thuj.
6 p.m. - phys.
8 p.m. - nat-s.
8 to 10 p.m. - phel.
9 p.m. - carb-s.
bed, in - caust., kali-c., kali-i., ***nux-v.,*** spong., thuj.
on going to - ferr-p.
eating, after - graph.
lying on it agg. - kali-n.
extending, to
backwards - mur-ac.
inwards - arg-m., carb-v., kali-bi., meny.
outward - ***ars.,*** calc-caust., canth., ***con.,*** kali-c., ***sil.***
brain - arg-m., chin.
chin - bell.
ear - ***hep.***

SHARP, pain
extending, to
eye - puls.
lobule - phos.
neck - nat-m.
roof of mouth - kali-bi.
shoulder - nat-m.
temples - ***nux-m.***
throat - sulph.
forenoon - chin-s., kali-bi., kali-i., mag-c., mag-s., nat-a., nat-m., nux-m., paeon., sars.
10 a.m. - mag-s.
headache, with - ***kali-bi.,*** kali-n.
fever, during - calc.
front of ear, in - arg-m., aur-m-n., caust., ***cham.,*** laur., mag-c., mag-m., plan., ran-s., sars., stront-c., ***thuj.,*** verb., zinc.
evening - con., mag-c., ran-s.
intermittent - plat.
inward - alum., arg-n., carb-v., dros., hyos., kali-bi., mag-c.
itching - mez., mur-ac., ph-ac.
laughing, when - ***mang.***
left - aesc., arg-m., bar-c., bor., bry., calad., carb-an., coc-c., colch., cop., dros., eupi., form., graph., **KALI-BI.,** kali-p., kali-n., mag-c., mag-m., mag-s., merc-c., merc-i-f., mill., nicc., psor., ptel., ***puls.,*** rhod., sabad., samb., sang., sep., sil., ***staph.,*** **SULPH.,** verat., verb.
left, then right - aloe, bor., staph.
lobes - nat-c., nat-m., ph-ac., phos., plb., sabad., tab., zinc.
pressure amel. - nat-c.
rubbing amel. - nat-c.
lying - kali-p.
on it - kali-n.
on left side - merc.
on right side - ptel.
mastoid - sars.
extending to forehead - sars.
menses, during - kali-c.
morning - all-c., ars., bor., ***ferr.,*** form., kali-c., ***nux-v.,*** sars.
bed, in - ***nux-v.***
waking, on - bor.
washing in cold water, when - bor.
moving jaw - ***nux-m.,*** ph-ac.
music, from - ***ph-ac.,*** tab.
night - ***alum., ars.,*** cop., cycl., hell., ***kali-bi.,*** kalm., ***phos.,*** thuj.
10 p.m. - form.
toothache, with - hell.
waking, on - carb-s.
noon - chin-s., gels., psor.
opening mouth - ***petr.***
amel. - nat-c.
outward - ***alum., ars., asaf.,*** berb., calc., ***con.,*** dulc., kali-c., mang., ***nat-c.,*** sep., ***sil.,*** stront-c., tarax.
paroxysmal - caust.
picking - clem.

SHARP, pain
pressing forehead - nit-ac.
pressure amel. - alum.
rest, during - phos., psor.
right - acon., ***aeth.,*** agar., all-c., brom., **CARB-S.,** ***caust.,*** clem., dros., ***echi.,*** ferr., ferr-p., glon., hell., hyper., kali-n., kalm., kreos., ***lyc.,*** lyss., med., nat-c., nat-m., ***nat-s.,*** nit-ac., phys., raph., rat., rhus-t., sars., sep., staph., tarent., thuj., trom., vesp., zinc.
right then left - ***arg-n.,*** laur., sulph.
rising from bed, amel. - coc-c.
rubbing amel. - mang.
scratching - mang.
shaking head amel. - kali-c.
singing, while - ph-ac.
sitting, while - gels., nat-m., phos.
sneezing, on - calc.
standing, while - mag-s.
stool, after - carb-s.
stooping, when - **CHAM.,** ***merc.,*** merc-c.
styloid process - agar., con.
swallowing, when - anac., con., ***gels.,*** lach., lyc., ***mang.,*** nat-m., **NUX-V.,** ***petr.,*** **PHYT.,** thuj., trom.
talking, while - ***mang.***
tickling - dros.
touch, amel. - mur-ac., sars.
tragus - cham.
turning head, when - chin-s.
waking, on - ***form.,*** spong.
walking, while - arg-n., bor., kali-bi., mang., merl.
warm room, on entering - ***nat-s., nux-v.***
warmth of bed agg. - **MERC.**
yawning, when - acon.

SHOCKS, on swallowing - con.

SORE, pain - ***arn.,*** bor., bry., ***calc-p., caust., chin.,*** cic., cupr-ar., ery-a., fago., jug-r., kali-bi., ***lac-c.,*** mag-c., mag-s., ***mang., merc.,*** merc-i-f., ***mur-ac.,*** phos., ptel., ***ruta.,*** sel., sep., spong., stry., ***sulph.,*** zinc.
about the ear - calc-p., coc-c.
behind - anac., bor., bry., calc-p., **CAPS.,** chel., cic., cupr-ar., **GRAPH.,** kali-c., lachn., lyc., merc., mur-ac., nit-ac., ***petr., psor.,*** ruta., ***sil.,*** verat.
both the ears - murx.
cough, with - phos.
below ear - **BAR-C.,** sars., ptel., zinc.
below ear, mastoid - **RUTA.**
boring with finger - bor.
concha - ruta, spong., zinc.
evening - bor.
external ear - ***acon.,*** bry., ***calc-p.,*** form., ***mang.,*** mur-ac., vib., ***zinc.***
in front - ***calc.,*** ptel., senec., zinc.
inside ear - anac., ***ang., caust.,*** croc., ferr., kreos., merc., mur-ac., petr., ***ph-ac., plat.,*** puls., ran-b., samb., thuj., valer.

SORE, pain
lobule - chel., crot-h., mur-ac.
behind - mag-c.
meatus, on touch - sep.

SPASMODIC, pain - chin., merc., murx., ol-an., ran-b., spig., ***thuj.***
behind the ear - murx.
inside ear - anac., ***ang., caust.,*** croc., ferr., kreos., merc., mur-ac., petr., ***ph-ac., plat.,*** puls., ran-b., samb., thuj., valer.

STEATOMA, behind ears - olnd.

STOPPED, up, sensation - acon., aeth., agar., alet., alum., ***anac.,*** anag., ant-c., arg-m., ***arg-n.,*** ars., ars-i., **ASAR.,** aur-m., ***bar-c.,*** berb., bism., bor., brom., bry., bufo, calad., calc., calc-s., cann-i., ***carb-s.,*** **CARB-V.,** ***caust.,*** cham., ***chel., chin.,*** chin-s., chlf., cinnb., coc-c., cocc., ***colch.,*** coloc., **CON.,** crot-h., cycl., dig., dios., ***glon., graph., guai.,*** guare., hura, hydr., hydrc., indg., ***iod.,*** jac., kali-bi., kali-c., kali-p., kali-s., ***lach.,*** lachn., ***led.,*** lob., **LYC.,** lyss., mag-m., manc., ***mang., meny.,*** **MERC.,** merc-c., merc-i-f., merl., ***mez., mill.,*** nat-a., ***nat-c.,*** nat-m., nat-p., ***nat-s., nit-ac., nux-m.,*** ol-an., op., petr., ***phos.,*** phys., phyt., plat., psor., **PULS.,** raph., rhus-t., rumx., sabad., sanic., ***sang.,*** sec., ***sel.,*** seneg., sep., **SIL.,** ***spig.,*** spong., stann., ***sulph., sul-ac.,*** symph., tab., tell., tep., teucr., thuj., til., tub., upa., ***verat., verb.***
afternoon - mill., nat-m.
3 p.m. - jac.
amel. - nat-m.
air open - spig.
alternating sides - cocc.
blowing nose - alum., calc., ***con., mang.,*** spig., ***sulph.***
amel. - ***merc.,*** stann.
boring with finger amel. - lob., mag-m., sel., spig.
cough, after - chel.
dinner, after - mill.
eating, while - ***sulph.***
eustachian tube, sensation - ***phyt.***
evening - ant-c., ham., kali-c., spig., thuj.
8 p.m. - dios.
bed, in - sel.
sitting, while - kali-c.
excitement agg. - dig.
forenoon - nat-m., psor., tell.
hawking, when - hyos.
left - acon., agar., aur-m., berb., coc-c., hydr., hydrc., jac., kali-bi., rumx., sel., spig., stann.
then right - ***verb.***
loud report, ears open, with - ***sil.***
lying, while, agg. - coc-c.
on it, after - sel.
menses, during - mag-m.
morning - ant-c., brom., caust., sil., teucr., thuj., ***tub.***
breakfast, after amel. - ant-c.
reading aloud - verb.
rhythmically - coloc.

STOPPED, up
right - aeth., ant-c., arg-m., cann-i., caust., colch., crot-h., cycl., nat-c., ***nat-s.,*** rhus-t., tell., til., thuj., ***tub.***
rising, on, amel. - stann.
swallowing, during - ars.
amel. - alum., calc., merc., ***sil.***
talking, while - meny.
valve, by a, as if - ***bar-c.,*** bor., graph., ***iod., nat-s.***
walking, while - colch.
writing, while - raph.
yawning amel. - nat-m., ***sil.***

STROKES, blows in ears - arn., nat-m., nux-v., paeon., plat.

SUPPURATION, behind ear (see Mastoid) - kali-c., ***nit-ac.,*** phyt.
front of ear, in - ***merc.***
middle ear - am-c., bar-c., ***calc.,*** **CALC-S.,** ***caps.,*** carb-an., ***carb-v., caust.,*** **HEP.,** hydr., **KALI-BI.,** ***kali-p.,*** lyc., **MERC.,** nat-m., olnd., ***puls.,*** sil., ***spong.,*** stann., sulph.

SURGING - kali-p.

SWELLING - ***acon.,*** alum., anac., ant-c., ars., ***apis,*** arn., bor., ***bell.,*** bry., **CALC.,** calc-p., ***carb-v.,*** caust., chlol., cist., ery-a., glon., **GRAPH.,** jug-r., kali-ar., ***kali-bi., kali-c.,*** kali-p., kreos., lyc., ***merc., nat-m.,*** nit-ac., ***petr.,*** ph-ac., phos., pic-ac., psor., ptel., **PULS.,** ***rhus-t.,*** rhus-v., samb., ***sep., sil.,*** spong., ***tell.,*** tep., urt-u., zinc.
about the ear - arn., form., ***phyt.***
glands, of - ***bar-c.,*** bar-m., bell., ***calc.,*** caps., carb-an., dig., graph., iod., ***merc., nit-ac.,*** tub.
sudden - dys-co.
antitragus - kreos., spong.
behind - ant-s., ***aur., bar-c.,*** bar-m., benz-ac., berb., bry., calc., ***calc-s.,*** **CAPS.,** ***carb-an.,*** caust., cist., colch., dig., ***graph., hep.,*** kali-c., ***lach.,*** lyc., ***nit-ac.,*** ph-ac., puls., rhus-t., rhus-v., ***sil.,*** tab.
hard and red - tab.
knotty - ***bar-c., graph.***
lymphatic glands - apis, ***bar-c.,*** dig., ***nit-ac.***
periosteum - caps., ***carb-an.***
shiny - con., lyc., rhus-v.
warmth of bed amel. - nit-ac.
below - all-c., **BAR-C.,** berb., ***caps.,*** cist., hura, nat-h., ptel., samb., sars.
concha - ant-c., arn., nat-m., phos., sil., tep.
in front of ear - anthr., bry., ***calc.,*** cist., iod., ***merc.***
glands - puls.
glands, of, about the - ***bar-c.,*** bar-m., bell., ***calc.,*** caps., carb-an., dig., graph., iod., ***merc., nit-ac.,*** tub.
behind ear, lymphatic glands - apis, ***bar-c.,*** dig., ***nit-ac.***
below ear - am-c., **BAR-C.,** ***cist.,*** dig., ***graph., nit-ac.,*** ptel., sars.

SWELLING,
inside - acon., bry., **CALC.**, calc-p., cann-s., ***caust., cist., cupr.***, graph., kali-c., lach., mag-c., mez., nat-m., ***nit-ac., petr.***, ph-ac., **PULS.**, ***sep., sil., tell.***, thuj., zinc.
evening - mez.
left - ant-c., ery-a., graph., nit-ac., rhus-t., ***tell.***
lobes - kali-n., puls., ***rhus-t.***
right - bell., calc., crot-c., glon., jug-r., ptel.

TEARING, pain, in - ***acon.***, aeth., ***agar., alum., ambr.***, am-c., am-m., ***anac.***, ang., ***arg-n.***, arn., ***ars.***, ars-i., arum-t., aur., ***bar-c.***, bar-m., **BELL.**, berb., bism., bor., bov., brom., calc., calc-p., camph., cann-i., ***canth., caps.***, carb-an., carb-s., ***carb-v.***, **CAUST.**, **CHAM.**, ***chel.***, **CHIN.**, ***chin-a.***, coc-c., colch., ***con.***, cupr., cycl., ***dulc.***, elaps, ery-a., eupi., gamb., gran., ***graph.***, grat., ***guai.***, hyos., indg., iod., kali-ar., kali-bi., **KALI-C.**, kali-i., kali-n., kali-p., kali-s., kalm., ***lach.***, lachn., laur., **LYC.**, ***lyss., mag-c., mag-m., mang.***, meph., **MERC.**, merl., ***mez.***, mur-ac., nat-a., nat-c., ***nat-p.***, nicc., ***nit-ac., nux-m.***, nux-v., par., petr., phel., ***ph-ac., phos., plat., plb.***, psor., **PULS.**, raph., rat., ***rhod.***, sabin., ***sars., sep.***, sil., spig., ***squil., stann.***, stram., stront-c., **SULPH.**, ***sul-ac.***, tab., tarax., tarent., teucr., ***thuj.***, til., ***verb., zinc.***, zing.
about the ear - aeth., am-c., canth., ***con.***, ery-a., grat., kali-c., mur-ac., nat-s., phos., plb., rhod.
above the ear - ***arg-m.***, camph., chel., nat-s., sil.
evening - chel.
left - arg-m.
right - chel.
afternoon - aeth., bov., ***chel.***, cast., indg., sars.
alternating with pressing - bell.
antitragus - anac., berb.
behind the ear - agar., alum., ***ambr.***, am-c., anan., ang., arg-m., arg-n., ars., ***bar-c.***, bar-m., bell., berb., brom., calc., canth., caul., ***caps.***, carb-v., ***caust.***, chel., coc-c., colch., dig., indg., kali-c., kali-n., laur., lyc., mang., meny., mez., mur-ac., nat-c., nit-ac., nux-v., petr., phel., rhus-t., rhus-v., sars., ***sep.***, **SIL.**, squil., tab., tarax., thuj., zinc.
afternoon - caust., nat-c., phel., sars., sil.
1 p.m. - nat-c., sil.
3 p.m. - phel.
4 p.m. - caust.
evening - canth., nit-ac., thuj.
9 p.m. - alum.
sitting up in bed amel. - alum.
extending to,
clavicle - petr.
nape of neck - mur-ac.
neck - chel., tarax.
shoulder - ars.
upward in afternoon - rat., sars.
vertex, occiput, nape and shoulder agg. moving head - am-c.
intermittent - petr.
left - ***ambr.***, caps.
moving, head - am-c.

TEARING, pain
behind the ear,
reading, while - aesc.
right - agar., bar-c., calc-caust.
touch, agg. - bar-ac.
below the ear - acon., alum., am-c., caust., iod., nit-ac., ol-an., phos., sil., tab., zinc.
moving, head agg. - am-c.
rubbing, amel. - ***phos.***
sitting, while - ***phos.***
bending, body to the right - mag-m.
boring with finger, agg. - anac.
cold air, agg. - agar.
concha - bell., bism., bov., ***caps.***, chin., cupr., guai., hyos., kali-c., lyc., mag-c., mang., ph-ac., sars., thuj.
dinner, after - bov., carb-an., phel.
eating, while - verb.
evening - alum., ***ars.***, indg., kali-i., mag-c., nat-s., thuj., zinc., zing.
7 p.m. - mag-c., zing.
bed, in - thuj.
lying down - mang.
in bed, after amel. - mang.
extending, to
downwards - **BELL.**, verb.
cheek - sul-ac.
head - sulph.
occiput - ambr.
teeth - chel.
temples - lach., ***nux-v.***, sul-ac.
upper jaw - agar., anac., mag-c.
vertex - phos.
forenoon - elaps, kali-i., mag-c., phos., plb.
9 a.m. - elaps.
front of ear, in - ang., ***bar-c.***, bov., ***carb-v.***, colch., dros., grat., indg., kali-i., kali-c., mag-c., mag-m., nat-p., ol-an., rat., stront-c., sul-ac., tab., verb., zinc.
evening - con.
extending to, cheek - sul-ac.
temples - kali-i., sul-ac.
intermitting - nat-c., psor.
left - ***acon.***, anac., apis, ***ars.***, bar-c., calc., camph., carb-an., caust., coc-c., elaps, ***graph.***, grat., mag-c., merl., mez., puls., sabin., ***sulph.***, sul-ac., teucr., ***verb.***
left, to right - aloe.
lobes - ambr., ars., carb-an., ***carb-v.***, cham., chin., mur-ac., zinc.
lobes, left - ars., mur-ac., stann., verat.
lying, on ear agg. - agar., am-m.
mastoid - mang.
menses, during - ***merc.***
morning - mang., sars., zinc.
8 a.m. - nat-c.
bed, in - carb-v.
moving, lower jaw agg. - ***nux-m.***, stann.
night - am-m.
noises, agg. - **SULPH.**
noon - sulph.
outward - ars.

TEARING, pain
paroxysmal - stront.
pressure of the hand amel. - alum., bism., carb-an., hyos.
right - aeth., agar., ambr., am-m., arg-n., cann-i., ***canth.,*** carb-v., con., cupr., eupi., iod., ***kali-c.,*** kali-i., ***lyc.,*** lyss., mang., plb., rat., rhod., sars., spig., stram., stront-c., tab., ***tarent.,*** til., zing.
to left - laur., sulph.
to right teeth - chel.
rising, from stooping - mang.
rubbing, amel. - aeth., phos.
sitting, while - indg., nat-c., phos.
standing, while - nat-c., plb.
swallowing, agg. - anac.
tragus, in the - anac., nit-ac.
warm, room agg. - ***nux-v.***

TENSION - alum., ambr., apis, dros., graph., kreos., lach., lyc., nux-v., thuj.
behind - am-c., caust., ***con., kali-n.,*** lyc., mag-c., mez., nit-ac.
below - thuj.
concha - bov.
inside - ***asar.,*** aur., cham., dig., euphr., kali-n., lact., ***merc.***

TINGLING - agar., ambr., am-c., am-m., anac., ant-c., arn., ars., asaf., aur-m-n., bar-c., bar-m., ***bell.,*** brach., ***calc.,*** camph., cann-s., carb-an., ***carb-v.,*** caust., cham., chel., ***chin-s.,*** cic., ***colch.,*** con., dig., dulc., ferr-ma., ***graph.,*** ign., kali-ar., kali-c., kali-n., kalm., lachn., ***laur.,*** lyc., mill., mag-c., ***mur-ac.,*** nat-m., nux-v., plat., puls., rhus-t., sars., ***sep.,*** stann., stry., ***sulph.,*** sul-ac., sul-i., thuj., verat.
boring with finger, amel. - lachn.
meatus - alum.
menses, before - ferr.
morning in bed - sulph.
night - carb-an.
noon - stry.
right - anac.
sitting, while - sulph.
sneezing, when - euph.
turning head - nat-c.
walking, while - rhus-t.
air, in open - carb-an.

TINNITUS, (see Hearing, chapter, Noises)

TREMBLING, in, after sad news - kali-c., sabin.

TUBERCLE, hard, behind left ear - nicc.
behind right ear - graph., ph-ac.
lobe, on the - merc.
posteriorly - nit-ac.

TUMORS, cystic - ***nit-ac.***
behind, small - berb., bry., caust., ***con.***
front of, in - bry., ***calc.***
lobe, on - merc., ***nit-ac.***
lobe, under - ***calc.***
steatoma - calc., nit-ac.
wen, behind ears - merc-i-r., verb.

TWINGING - aloe, anac., anag., aran., arg-n., asar., ***bar-c.,*** carb-v., caust., coc-c., coloc., ***crot-t.,*** dulc., ferr., graph., kali-n., kreos., merc., mez., par., plan., prun., staph.
afternoon - aran.
evening - aloe, carb-v., mez.
left - coc-c., crot-t., prun., staph.
morning in bed - ferr.
right - anag., arg-n., coloc., dulc., kreos.
spasmodic - crot-t.

TWITCHING - act-sp., aeth., ***agar.,*** am-c., am-m., anac., ang., ant-t., bar-c., bar-m., bor., bov., ***calc.,*** calc-ac., calc-p., cann-i., caust., chin., clem., dig., fl-ac., hep., kali-c., kali-p., mag-m., manc., mang., merc., mez., ***mur-ac.,*** nat-m., nicc., nit-ac., nux-v., petr., ph-ac., phos., plat., ***puls.,*** rhod., sars., sil., spig., sul-ac., thuj., zinc.
behind ear - bar-c., kali-c.
concha - agar., calc-ac., ph-ac., spig., upa.
evening - nux-v., mez.
blowing nose - act-sp.
rising, on - kali-c.
extending, below ear - elaps
outward - caust.
to eye and lower jaw - spig.
to lobe - phos.
to lower jaw - nit-ac.
to mouth - thuj.
to throat - spig.
front, in - ang., dros., mag-m.
left - am-c., bar-c., bov., sil.
lobe, in - kali-c., ph-ac., sars.
meatus - am-m., anac., carb-v., lyc., nit-ac., valer.
visible - sars.
morning - ant-t., mang., nux-v.
6 a.m. - nat-m.
waking, on - nux-v.
right - ant-t., calc., mag-m., ***mang.,*** nat-m., nit-ac., sul-ac., thuj.
sneezing, when - act-sp.

ULCERATION - ***anac.,*** bov., bry., bufo, ***calc., camph.,*** graph., hep., kali-bi., merc., mur-ac., ***olnd., petr.,*** sars., sep., sulph.
about the ear - calc-p.
eardrum, tympanum - ***calc., iod., kali-bi., kali-p.,*** **MERC.,** ***psor., sil., tub.***
ragged edges, with - tub.
front of ear, in - carb-v., merc.
fistulous opening - ***calc.***
inside - bov., ***calc., camph., carb-v., hep.,*** kali-bi., kali-c., ***lyc., merc., puls.,*** sep., ***sil.,*** sulph., tell.
left - camph., graph., mur-ac., sars.
lobe, in hole for earrings - ***lach.,*** med., stann.
right - bov.
swallowing, painful - anac.
tragus - graph.

ULCERATIVE, pain - anac., calc., ferr., kali-c., mag-c., mang., mur-ac., sars., sep.

VESICLES - alum., ars., meph., ***olnd.,*** phos., ptel., rhus-v., sep., ***tell.***
behind - am-m., calc., caust., chin., nat-m., phos., ***psor., rhus-t., rhus-v.,*** tell.
extends to face - ***graph.,*** sep.
below - ptel.
coalescing - ars.
concha - ars., phos.
discharging water - ptel.
below - ptel.
gangrenous - ars.
lobes, on, caused by the discharge - **TELL.**
meatus, in - nicc.
purulent - ptel.
serum, filled with - rhus-v.
surrounded by inflamed base - ars.
transparent - alum.
white - ptel.
on red base - ptel.

WARMTH, sensation - sul-ac.

WART-like, growth, behind ear, inflamed and ulcerated - calc.
ears, on the - bufo.

WATER, sensation of, in ear - ant-c., graph., meny., spig., ***sulph.***
cold, running out of ears - merc.
hot, in left ear - acon.
hot, running out of right ear - cham.
left ear - graph.
passing out of - calc., spig., sulph.
rushing into ears - rhod.
warm, in - calad.

WAX, (see Earwax)

WIND, sensation of, in - ail., ***bell.,*** carb-s., ***caust., chel.,*** eupi., led., mag-c., mang., ***merc., mez.,*** mosch., ***plat.,*** puls., rhus-t., sanic., ***sel.,*** stann., staph., stram., vinc.
cold, as if blowing against meatus of right ear - ***caust.,*** mang., sanic., staph.
passing into or blowing upon - ***caust.,*** mang., meny., mosch., plat., stann., staph., tell.
passing out of ears - abrot., ***aeth., bell., calc.,*** canth., ***chel.,*** meli., ***mill.,*** psor., stram.
putting finger in, amel. - chel.
puffing out of ears - meli., sil.

WIND, sensitive to - **ACON.,** ail., ***bell.,*** carb-s., **CAUST., CHAM.,** ***chel.,*** eupi., **LACH.,** led., ***lyc.,*** mag-c., mang., ***merc., mez.,*** mosch., ***plat.,*** puls., rhus-t., sanic., ***sel.,*** stann., staph., stram., vinc.
cold, about ear, to - **ACON., CAUST., CHAM.,** cinnb., clem., ***hep., lac-c.,*** **LACH.,** ***lyc.,*** merc., ***mez., sil., thuj.***

WORMS, sensation of - acon., calc., coloc., guare., med., pic-ac., puls., rhod., ruta.

Elbows

ABSCESS - crot-h.

ACHING, pain - aesc., ang., asaf., caul., coc-c., dios., fl-ac., gels., glon., gymn., ham., hydr., led., merc-i-f., ol-j., phos., ***podo.,*** rumx., ruta., sep., thuj., ust., xan.
about the elbows - gels.
alternating with pain in knees - dios.
bend of - arg-m., clem.
pressure amel. - arg-m.
stretching arm - clem.
evening - fl-ac., ***still.***
extending to forearm - dios., xan.
morning - sumb.
bed, in - sumb.
motion, during - hydr., prun.
amel. - ol-an., ust.
olecranon - spong.
motion, on - hep.
wet weather - erig.

ANCHYLOSIS - calc-f., sil.

ARTHRITIC, nosodities, above elbows - mag-c.
olecranon, on - still.
stiffness of - lyc.

BANDAGED, sensation as if - ***caust.***

BORING, pain - alum., am-c., aur., bufo, clem., crot-t., dulc., mez., nat-s., nux-m., nux-v., spong., thuj.
bend of - am-c., led.
extending to shoulder - phos.
to wrist - dulc.
lying on the opposite side, when - nux-v.
motion amel. - dulc.
noon - crot-t.
olecranon - alum., am-c., caust.

BROKEN, sensation as if - ***bry.,*** coc-c., phos.

BUBBLING, sensation - kreos., mang., rheum, spong.
bend of - bell.

BURNING, pain - agar., alum., ***arg-m.,*** arund., asaf., bell., berb., calc-p., carb-an., carb-v., coc-c., colch., coloc., kali-n., merc., mur-ac., ph-ac., phos., ***plat.,*** sep., sulph., ter.
bend of - kali-n., laur., led., rat., rhus-v., sulph., tep., teucr.
evening - arg-m., carb-an.
forenoon, 9 a.m. - sulph.
night - sep.
olecranon - arg-m., chel., ph-ac.

COLDNESS - ***agar.,*** cedr., gins., graph., ir-foe.
extending to hands toward noon - cedr.
olecranon - ***agar.***

COMPRESSION - chlor., nat-s.
evening - nat-s.

CONSTRICTION - agar., caust., lach., mang., petr., rat., sep.
as with a cord - rat.
bend of - elaps, rat.
bending, on - rat.
left - agar.

CONSTRICTION,
morning - petr.

CONTRACTION, of muscles and tendons - ars., glon., lyc., nux-v., tep.
bend of - ***caust.,*** elaps, graph., ***puls.,*** sars., sulph.
flexed, tendons, contracted as if - ***apis, caust.***

CRACKED, skin - graph.

CRACKING, in joints - am-c., ant-c., brom., cinnb., con., dios., ***kalm.,*** merc., mur-ac., nat-m., sulph., tep., thuj., zinc., zing.
afternoon - kalm.
stretching - thuj.

CUTTING, pain - caust., cedr., graph., hep., hydr., manc., med., ph-ac., tell.
bend of - con., mur-ac.
flexion, on - mur-ac.
moving, when - med.
paralysing - graph.
walking, while - bell.

DECAY, of bone - ***sil.***

DISCOLORATION, of
brown spots - cadm-s., ***lach.,*** sep.
red spots - ***phos.***
spots - calc., ***sep.,*** vip.

DRAWING, pain - acon., agar., aloe, ***arg-m.,*** **ARS.,** aur-m., aur-m-n., ***bell.,*** berb., ***bry.,*** canth., carb-s., carb-v., caul., caust., cham., chel., coc-c., coloc., com., con., dig., dios., dulc., elaps, euphr., graph., grat., hell., kali-bi., ***kali-c.,*** kali-n., lach., lact., led., lyc., ***mang.,*** mez., ***mur-ac., nat-c.,*** nat-s., petr., ph-ac., phos., rhod., ***rhus-t.,*** rhus-v., ruta., sabad., sec., seneg., sil., stann., staph., stront-c., ***sulph.,*** tab., thuj., viol-o., zinc.
afternoon - sulph.
3 p.m. - gels.
bend of - arg-m., ***caust.,*** chin., hell., kali-n., ***puls., rat.,*** thuj., valer., verat.
extending arm amel. - rat.
while writing - valer.
bending, on - chel., dulc.
bone, in - sil.
condyles - arg-m., coc-c.
cramp-like - ***rhus-t.***
evening, bed, in - mag-c., ***nat-c.***
lying, while - ***nat-c.***
extending arm - ruta.
downward - kali-bi., lach., mez., sec., seneg., thuj.
to axilla - **ARS.**
to wrist - dulc., guai., rhus-t., sulph.
upward - kali-n., stann.
left - agar.
morning - carb-v., lyc., thuj.
motion, during - **BRY.,** ***coloc.,*** rhus-t., sil., staph.
amel. - carb-v., dulc., graph., mez., ***rhus-t.***
night - ***ars., phos.***
olecranon - carb-an., lact.
paralytic - bell., cham.
paralyzing - graph.

DRAWING, pain
rheumatic - caust., euphr., mez., ***rhus-t.,*** zinc.
right - canth., phos., sulph.
sitting, while - ***rhus-t.,*** sulph.
touch agg. - sil.
turning, when - tab.
wind in - carb-v.

ECZEMA - brom.
bend of - ***cupr.,*** **GRAPH.,** ***mez.,*** **PSOR.**

ERUPTIONS - aster., berb., ***brom.,*** cact., cupr., hep., iris, ***kali-s.,*** kreos., lach., merc., ***phos., psor.,*** sabin., ***sep., staph.,*** sulph., tep., thuj., zinc.
blister - crot-h.
black - ars.
desquamation - sulph.
elevations - merc.
itchy and scaly - merc.
itching - merc., ***sep.,*** staph.
nodules - eupi., mur-ac.
olecranon - berb.
dry, furfuraceous - aster., sep.
pimples - berb.
painful - merc.
pimples - ant-c., asc-t., berb., bry., ***dulc., hyos.,*** kali-n., lach., merc., nat-c., ol-an., sabin., sep., ***staph.,*** sulph., tarax., thuj.
biting - kali-n.
burning - kali-n.
inflamed base, on - tarax.
pustules - eup-per., hep., jug-c., lach.
itching - hep.
yellow - jug-c.
red - cinnb., rhus-t.
scales - calc., jug-r., ***kali-s.,*** merc., ***sep., staph.,*** sulph.
suppurating - sulph.

eruptions, bend of - am-m., bry., calad., calc., ***cupr., graph., hep.,*** merc., ***mez.,*** nat-c., ***nat-m., psor., sep.,*** staph., sulph.
crusts - ***cupr., mez.,*** **PSOR.**
dry - ***mez.***
exudation - sulph.
fissures - ***kali-ar.***
itching - sulph., zinc.
corrosive - ant-c.
evening - cupr.
painful - am-m., ant-c., dros., dulc., hura, lachn., nat-c., ol-an., phos., rhus-t., sep.
pimples - am-m., ant-c., dulc., hyos., hura, ol-an., nat-c., phos., ***sep.,*** thuj.
evening, in warmth - dulc.
morning - dulc.
pustules - sulph.
red - ***cor-r.,*** rhus-t.
scabies - bry., merc.
scratching, after - nat-c.

GNAWING, pain - dulc., indg., mag-c., phos., ran-s., stront.
extending to shoulder - phos.
sitting, while - phos.

HEAT - alum., arg-m., arund., berb., kali-c., sep.

HEAVINESS, sensation - am-c., chin-a., con., phos., samb., sars.

HERPES - bor., cact., **CUPR.,** hep., ***kreos., phos.,*** psor., ***sep., staph., thuj.***
bend of - cupr., graph., kreos., **NAT-M.,** sep., thuj.

INFLAMMATION, of - ant-c., lac-ac., lach., sil.
erysipelatous - ars., lach., sulph.

INJURIES, to elbows - ***arn.,*** aur., bell-p., **BRY.,** ***hyper., rhus-t.,*** **RUTA.**

ITCHING - agar., alum., arg-m., berb., calc-i., caust., crot-h., cycl., fago., ign., indg., kali-n., lachn., laur., mang., med., ***merc.,*** merc-i-f., mur-ac., **NAT-C.,** nat-p., ol-an., pall., petr., phos., psor., rhus-v., ***sep., sulph.***
bend of - canth., carb-s., cupr., ***hep.,*** laur., nat-c., nit-ac., ol-an., petr., phos., psor., rumx., **SEP.,** spig., sulph., ter.
afternoon - sulph.
evening - cupr., sulph.
evening agg. - ***sulph.***
olecranon - agar., ars-m., mag-m., nit-ac., olnd., puls., sep.
rubbing, amel. - ol-an.
scratching, amel. - ol-an.

JERKING - nat-m., stram., zinc.

LAMENESS - ***all-c.,*** dios., dulc., hydr., iris, merc-i-f., mez., petr., sars.
morning - dios.

NUMBNESS - all-c., cinnb., dig., dios., jatr., kali-n., nat-s., phos., pip-m., puls.
bend of - hura, plb., sulph.
evening, lying down, when - phos.
extending to tips of fingers - jatr.
lain, on - graph.
motion agg. - all-c.

PAIN, elbows - abrot., acon., agar., agn., all-s., aloe, ***alum., alumn.,*** am-c., ant-c., ant-t., arg-m., ars-h., ars-i., aster., aur., bapt., ***bry.,*** calc., calc-p., calc-s., cann-i., carb-s., cast-eq., ***caust.,*** cedr., cham., chel., chin., cic., cimic., clem., ***coloc., corn.,*** crot-c., crot-h., cupr., cycl., dig., dios., dulc., elaps, fago., ferr., ferr-ar., ferr-i., fl-ac., form., gels., glon., grat., ***guai.,*** hep., hyos., hyper., ***iod.,*** iris, jac-c., jug-c., kali-ar., ***kali-bi.,*** kali-c., kali-n., kalm., ***lac-ac.,*** lach., lachn., laur., lept., lob., ***lyc.,*** lyss., mag-c., mag-s., manc., mang., merc., merc-i-f., mez., nat-a., nat-c., nat-s., nux-m., nux-v., osm., petr., ph-ac., phos., phys., phyt., pip-m., plan., plat., plb., prun., puls., ran-b., ***rhus-t.,*** rhus-v., rumx., ruta., seneg., sep., ***sil.,*** spong., stry., sulph., sul-ac., tarent., tell., tep., ter., thuj., valer., verat., xan., zinc.
afternoon - sulph.
4 p.m. - dios.
alternates, with pain in knees - dios.
in shoulder - kalm.
asleep, as if - caust.
bed, after going to - dios.
bending arm, when - all-s., chel., dulc., mag-c., mur-ac., puls., stann.
bones - graph., lyc.

PAIN, elbows
carrying a weight, after - ***cham.***
chill, during - ang., **PODO.**
cramp-like - bell., chel., verb.
evening - cast-eq., cop., dios., dulc., fl-ac., jac-c.
5 p.m. - stry.
7 p.m. - chin-s., dios.
9 p.m. - calc-p., lyc.
lying, while - nat-c., phos.
pulling the door bell - chin-s.
extending to, finger, the little - aesc., arund., jatr., lyc., phyt., puls., seneg.
to, fingers, joints - kali-n.
to, fingers, under nail - kali-n.
to, hand - kali-bi., lach., nicc., tarent.
to, shoulder - cycl., phos., still.
to, wrist - ars., guai., kali-n., phyt., prun., rhus-t.
forenoon - abrot., dios., plan.
gout - ars-h., caust., kali-i.
jerking - rhus-t.
leaning on it - camph.
lying, when - carb-an., kreos., nat-c., phos.
on opposite side, when - nux-v.
morning - brach., caust., dios., lyc., ran-b., sep., sumb., thuj.
6 a.m. - dios.
motion, agg. - agn., bell., **BRY.,** ***carb-s., guai.,*** kali-bi., led., plb., sil., sulph., ust.
amel. - ***arg-m., aur-m., aur-m-n.,*** bism., dulc., hyos., ***lyc.,*** mez., **RHUS-T.**
night - dig., gels., kali-n., lyc., merc-i-f., ***phos.,*** ter.
11 p.m. until morning - ***sulph.***
from putting arm out of bed - am-c.
waking - caust.
noon - arg-m., cedr.
olecranon - alum., am-c., carb-an., caust., chin-a., hep., kali-n., rhod., spong., verat.
motion, on - hep.
outer side - sil.
pain in side, with - fl-ac.
paralytic - ***bry.,*** cham., graph., lyss., prun., sil.
paroxysmal - kreos., rat.
periosteum - plat.
pronation - sars.
rash, after disappearance of - ***lept.***
rheumatic - acon., ammc., ars., ant-t., bapt., ***bry.,*** calc., ***carb-s., colch.,*** coloc., cupr., ***ferr.,*** form., grat., guai., hydr., hyper., iris, ***kali-bi.,*** kalm., lach., lob., mag-s., mez., nat-a., ***nat-c.,*** nicc., prun., ran-b., rhus-v., sal-ac., sep., ust., zinc.
riding, after - verat.
sitting, while - phos.
straightening the arm in front of him - am-c.
stretching arm - hep., kali-c., nit-ac., puls., ruta.
tendon, snapped from place, as if - sars.
touched, when - ambr., bell., calc-p., carb-v., dulc., hyos., mang., ph-ac.
walking, after - valer.

PAIN, elbows
wandering - cact.
warmth, agg. - ***guai.***
amel. - ***caust.,*** **RHUS-T.**
pain, bend of - alumn., anac., arg-m., aur-m-n., carb-an., caust., chel., cina, clem., cocc., gels., glon., graph., hep., hura, hyos., iod., lyc., merc-i-f., nat-c., plb., ***puls.,*** spig., still., thuj., valer., verat.
extending to, fingers - hura
to, palm - carb-an.
to, shoulder - plb.
hanging down - still.
morning - alum., lyc., merc-i-f.
motion, on - hura, plb., ***puls.***
amel. - coc-c.
paralytic - cina, cocc.
paroxysmal - plb.
pressure, amel. - arg-m.
stretching arm, on - alumn., **CAUST.,** clem., graph., ***hep., puls.,*** thuj.
touched, when - nat-c.
walking, while - gels.
writing, after - gels.

PARALYSIS - fago., petr., sabin.
paralysis, sensation of - ambr., arg-m., mez., samb., stront-c., sulph., valer.
afternoon - ***sulph.***
motion, during - arg-m.
night - stront.
raising the arm - mez.

PINCHING, pain - buf-s., merc-i-f., prun.

PRESSING, pain - acon., agar., agn., ang., aur-m-n., camph., ***caust.,*** clem., coc-c., coloc., cop., dig., gins., graph., hell., hep., indg., iod., ***led.,*** lyc., mang., mez., nat-s., rat., ruta., ***sars.,*** spong., ter., verb., verat., zinc.
bend of - anac., arg-m., aur-m-n., carb-an., clem., hyos., iod., rat., sep.
stretching out arm amel. - rat.
stretching out upper arm - clem.
walking, while - aur-m-n.
evening - cop.
extending to forearm - aur-m-n., verb.
to hand - camph.
hanging arm down - ang.
leaning upon - camph.
motion - agn., led., sulph.
motion, amel. - aur-m-n., bism., mez.
olecranon - hep.
paralytic - graph.
prickling - verat.
rheumatic - zinc.
siesta, after - graph.
sitting - gins.
stretching arm - ruta.
walking, while - ang.
after - acon.
air, in open - anac.
amel. - gins.
warmth amel. - ***caust.***

PSORIASIS, in patches - graph., ***iris,*** kali-ar., ***kali-s., phos.***
bends of - ***graph.***

PULSATION - agar., grat., hura, indg., rhus-t., ***still.,*** ter., thuj.
evening - still.
olecranon - agar.

RASH - calad., ***mez.,*** sulph.
bend of - calad., ***hep.,*** sep., zinc.

RESTLESSNESS, bend of, when covered - aster.

RHEUMATIC, pain - acon., ammc., ars., ant-t., bapt., ***bry.,*** calc., ***carb-s., colch.,*** coloc., cupr., ***ferr.,*** form., grat., guai., hydr., hyper., iris, ***kali-bi.,*** kalm., lach., lob., mag-s., mez., nat-a., ***nat-c.,*** nicc., prun., ran-b., rhus-v., sal-ac., sep., ust., zinc.

RINGWORM - cupr.

SCABIES, bend of - bry., merc., sulph.

SCRAPING, pain - coc-c.

SHARP, pain - acon., agar., alum., aloe, ammc., am-c., apis, ***arg-m., asaf.,*** aster., bell., berb., bov., brom., ***bry.,*** calc., ***calc-p.,*** calc-s., caps., caust., cedr., cham., chel., chin., cocc., coc-c., colch., com., con., cupr., eupi., graph., grat., guare., hell., hep., hura, hydr., indg., iris, kali-bi., kali-c., kali-n., kalm., laur., lyc., mag-c., mag-m., mang., ***merc.,*** mez., mur-ac., naja, phos., phys., plb., raph., rhod., sars., ***sep.,*** sil., ***spig.,*** spong., stry., tab., tarax., tep., ter., ther., ***thuj.,*** trom., viol-t., zinc.
afternoon - com., kali-n., naja
bend of - asaf., coc-c., coloc., grat., kali-c., led., merc-i-f., nat-c., rat., ***spig.,*** tarent.
chill, before - rat.
extending to tip of elbow - grat.
morning - kali-c.
itching - coloc.
rest, during - coc-c., coloc.
right - merc-i-f., rat.
burning - ***arg-m.***
chill, during - hell.
evening - bov., eupi., lyc., mag-m., thuj., zinc.
5 to 10 p.m. - chel.
extending, downward - acon., bov., caps., cupr., ***guai.,*** thuj.
fingers - bov., cupr., thuj.
shoulder - colch., indg.
wrist - acon., ***guai.***
forenoon - cham.
fright, after - phos.
left - kali-bi.
left, then right - ***calc-p.***
morning, 8 a.m. - mag-c., trom.
motion, during - mag-c., spong.
amel. - arg-m., cocc.
night - graph.
noon - cham., lyc., tarent.

SHARP, pain
olecranon - agar., arg-m., arg-n., bry., calc., carb-an., coc-c., mur-ac., nat-m., sep., spig., spong.
bending arm - bry.
itching - spig.
night - sep.
rest, during - arg-n.
outer side - thuj.
posterior surface - laur., sabad., thuj.
motion, amel. - sabad.
stinging - arg-m., berb., sil.
stretching arm - mez.
touch, amel. - thuj.
yawning - zinc.

SHOCKS - agar., nat-m., phos., verat.
to head - agar.

SHOOTING, pain - acon., bell., ***calc-p.,*** naja, plb., tep., tarent., trom.
afternoon - naja
alternating with shoulder - tep.
extending to, fingers - plb., thuj.
wrist - acon., ***guai.***
left then right - ***calc-p.***
morning - trom.
noon - tarent.

SORE, pain - all-c., agar., alum., am-c., ang., ***arn.,*** asaf., aur-m-n., bar-c., bov., brom., calc-p., camph., ***carb-v.,*** caust., cedr., cinnb., clem., colch., con., cycl., dros., dulc., hep., ind., iod., lach., led., mag-s., merc-i-f., nat-s., ***ol-j.,*** phos., plat., puls., ***ruta., sulph.,*** sul-ac., tell., ter., thuj., verat., zinc.
bend of - caust., valer., zinc.
extending arm, on - hep.
writing, when - valer.
bending it - dulc.
evening - am-c., still.
extending to forearm - led.
fist, making - sulph.
forenoon - thuj.
left - agar., phos.
lifting, on - sulph.
morning - carb-v., puls.
bed, in - ***carb-v.***
motion - puls.
motion - clem., cycl.
amel. - aur-m-n.
arm, of - ang.
night - merc-i-f.
olecranon - carb-an., hep., stann.
on bending arm - stann.
resting, on arm - ang.
touch, agg. - cycl., dros., dulc.
walking, after - tell.

SPRAINED, sensation, as if - ***ambr.,*** cur., ferr-m., gels., lach., mang., nicc., puls., tab., tell.

STIFFNESS - acon., aeth., alum., am-c., anac., ang., asaf., bell., **BRY.,** ***calc., chel.,*** ham., ***kali-c.,*** lach., lac-ac., ***led., lyc.,*** phos., pip-m., puls., ***sep.,*** spig., stann., sulph., thuj., zinc.
evening - com., sep., valer.
extending arm - kali-c.

STIFFNESS,
morning - dios.

SUPPURATION - dros., tep.

SWELLING - acon., agar., benz-ac., ***bry.,*** calc-f., chel., cic., colch., ***coloc.,*** con., dios., hydr., ***lac-ac.,*** lac-c., **MERC.,** petr., puls., sil., spig., tep., ter.
condyles - **CALC-P.,** ***mez.***
hot and red - **MERC.**
rheumatic - agar., **BRY.,** chel., coloc., com., lyc.
sensation of, in bend - verat.

TEARING, pain - acon., agar., ***alum.,*** ambr., am-c., am-m., arg-m., arg-n., **ARS.,** ars-h., ***ars-i.,*** **AUR.,** aur-m-n., bar-c., ***berb.,*** **BOV.,** bry., cact., ***calc., carb-s., caust.,*** chin., ***chin-a.,*** cina, clem., cocc., coc-c., colch., coloc., con., croc., cycl., euphr., graph., ***grat.,*** hyper., indg., **IOD., KALI-AR.,** kali-bi., **KALI-C.,** kali-i., ***kali-n.,*** kali-p., kalm., ***lachn.,*** lact., led., **LYC.,** mag-c., mag-m., mag-s., ***merc., mez.,*** mur-ac., nat-c., nat-p., ***nat-s.,*** nicc., nit-ac., par., phel., ph-ac., ***phos.,*** psor., puls., rat., **RHUS-T.,** rhus-v., ruta., sars., sep., sil., spong., ***stront-c.,*** **SULPH.,** tab., tell., tep., til., thuj., verb., ***zinc.***
afternoon, 1 p.m. - grat.
air, open - lact.
alternating with tearing, in shoulder - tep.
bend of - bar-c., canth., **KALI-C.,** laur., nat-s., olnd., rat., sep., zinc.
right - canth.
stretching out arm - hep.
bending arm - mez., puls., rat., spong., stront.
cramp-like - aur.
evening - alum., lyc., merc., mez., psor., rat., stront.
extending the arm - lyc.
extending, downward - am-c., berb., colch., kali-bi., kalm., lyc., merc., nat-c., nicc., nit-ac., rhus-t., rhus-v., ruta., sulph., thuj., til., zinc.
to axilla - ***ars.***
to fingers - am-c., am-m., kalm., nat-c., puls., thuj.
to forearm, middle of - mag-c.
to hand - am-c., berb., kali-bi., merc., phos.
to shoulder - lachn., phos., rhus-v.
upward - sulph., zinc.
to wrist - **CALC.,** colch., guai., lyc., nicc., nit-ac., **RHUS-T.**
forenoon - alum.
10 a.m., while knitting - mag-c.
while sitting amel. - indg.
hang down, letting arm, amel. - rat.
knitting, while - mag-c.
left - agar., ***iod.***
lying on left side - ***phos.***
morning - bov., lyc., ***zinc.***
motion, during - chin., graph., lyc., sil., thuj.
amel. - am-m., aur-m-n., cast., ***lyc.,*** **RHUS-T., SULPH.**
night - am-c., **ARS.,** ***phos.***
night, bed, in - ars.

TEARING, pain
olecranon - bov., lyc., mur-ac., nat-c., valer.
extending to bend - nat-c.
rest, during - agar.
posterior surface - mag-c.
raising arm - graph., rat.
rheumatic - ***ars., calc., lyc.,*** **RHUS-T.**
right - arg-n., coloc., phos., ***zinc.***
rubbing amel. - phos., ***zinc.***
taking hold of something - **CALC.**
twitching - rhus-t.
walking in open air, while - con.
warmth amel. - caust., **RHUS-T.**

TENNIS, elbow - arn., aur., bell-p., ***bry.,*** calc-f., hyper., ***rhus-t., ruta.***

TENSION - acon., all-s., alum., berb., dros., kali-c., kali-n., kreos., lach., laur., manc., mang., ***mez., mur-ac.,*** puls., rhus-t., ***sep.,*** stann., sulph., sul-ac., tab., ter., zinc.
bend of - arg-m., kali-n., nat-m., ***puls.,*** rhus-t., sep., sulph., thuj.
extending arm - **CAUST.,** ***rhus-t.***
morning - sulph.
writing, while - thuj.
bending agg. and on - berb., dros., ***merc.***
evening, on yawning - zinc.
olecranon - arg-m., stann.
bending arm - arg-m., stann.
raising arm - mez.
stretching arm - mang.

TINGLING, prickling, asleep - meny., verat.

TUBERCLE - am-c., caust., mag-c., mur-ac.

TUMORS, point of, steatoma - hep.
painful - puls.

TWINGING - carb-an.
evening - carb-an.

TWITCHING - agn., aloe, am-c., arg-m., bell., carb-s., caust., graph., lact., ***nat-m.,*** phos., rheum, ruta., sabad., sulph., zinc.
afternoon - nat-m.
3 p.m. - arg-m.
bend of - arg-m., bar-c.
extending to wrist - nit-ac.
morning - nat-m.
motion amel. - agn., arg-m.
noon, while lying - zinc.
resting on it - caust.
stretching arm amel. - nat-m.

ULCERS - ***calc.,*** hydr., lach., nat-s.
blisters change into - ***calc.***

URTICARIA - aran.

VESICLES - ***ars.,*** calad., nat-p., sulph.
bend of - ***calc., nat-c.,*** rhus-v., sulph.
red - ***nat-c.***
black - ***ars.***
suppurating - sulph.
white - sulph.
yellow - sulph.

WARTS, bend of - calc-f.

WATER, sensation of cold water dripping from - stry.

water running through - graph.

WEAKNESS, of - adeps., ang., chin-s., coloc., dios., fago., glon., hyper., led., nat-s., op., phos., plb., raph., ***ruta,*** sarr., staph., ***sulph.,*** thuj., valer.

afternoon, 5 p.m. - valer.

bend, of - cann-i.

dinner, after - nit-ac.

Emergency

ABSCESS, acute (see Generals) - acon., ***anan.,*** anthr., apis, ***arn., ars., bell.,*** calc-hp., ***calc-s.,*** calen., canth., ***carb-ac.,*** chin., chin-s., crot-h., fl-ac., **HEP.,** hippoz., ***kreos., lach.,*** lap-a., lyc., **MERC.,** ***merc-sul., myris., nit-ac.,*** ph-ac., phos., ***pyrog., rhus-t.,*** **SIL.,** sil-mar., ***sulph., sul-ac.*** syph., ***tarent-c.,*** vesp.
burning - **ANTHR., ARS.,** merc., ***pyrog.,*** **TARENT-C.**
foreign bodies, promotes elimination of - arn., ***hep., myris., lob.,*** **SIL.**
gangrenous - ***ars., asaf., carb-v., chin.,*** chin-s., ***hep., kreos.,*** **LACH.,** ***merc., nit-ac.,*** phos., ***sil., sul-ac.***
organs, of internal - calc-s., ***canth.,*** **LACH., PYROG.,** sil.

AIRPLANES, flying in, agg. - ***acon., arg-n.,*** arn., ars., bell., bor., cham., coca, cocc., gels., kali-m., petr., phos.
ear pain, from - cham., kali-m.
fear of flying - ***acon.,*** **ARG-N.,** ars., **CALC.,** ***gels.,*** nat-m., phos.
jet-lag - arn., cocc., gels.

ALLERGIC, reactions
anaphylaxis, allergic attack - acon., **APIS.,** ***ars.,*** ars-i., ***carb-ac.,*** caust., ***hist.,*** led., ***nat-m.,*** psor., ***rhus-t.,*** sulph., **URT-U.**
allergy injections, ailments from - carc., ***thuj.***
asthma - ambro., **ALL-C., ARS.,** ***ars-i., bad., carb-v.,*** chin-a., ***dulc., euphr.,*** **IOD.,** kali-i., lach., linu-u, ***naja,*** nat-c., ***nat-s., nux-v.,*** op., ***sabad.,*** sang., ***sin-n.,*** sil., stict., sulph., **THUJ.**
sneezing, with - ***ars., carb-v., dulc., euphr.,*** lach., ***naja, nat-s., nux-v.,*** sin-n., stict.
hives and swelling, with - ***acon.,*** agar., all-c., ***ant-c.,*** **APIS,** arn., **ARS., ASTAC.,** bell., ***bov., calad.,*** **CARB-AC.,** chlor., ***graph.,*** **HIST., LED.,** ***lyc., mez.,*** **NAT-M.,** ***nat-p.,*** nit-ac., ***psor., puls.,*** **RHUS-T.,** ***sal-ac.,*** **SULPH.,** ***sul-ac.,*** **URT-U.,** vesp.
rhinitis - **ALL-C., ARS.,** ars-i., carb-v., **EUPHR.,** iod., kali-i., ***nat-m.,*** **NUX-V.,** puls., ***sabad.,*** sang., sil., wye.

ALTITUDE, sickness - ***acon., arn., ars.,*** aur., bell., **CALC., CARB-V.,** caust., **COCA.,** con., conv., cupr., gels., kola., ***lach.,*** lyc., nat-m., olnd., ***op.,*** puls., **SIL.,** spig., verat.
ascending high, agg. - acon., bry., ***calc.,*** carb-v., **COCA,** ***conv., olnd., sil., spig.,*** sulph.

AMPUTATION, pain, after - ***acon., all-c.,*** am-m., ***arn., asaf.,*** bell., **CALEN., COFF.,** cupr., hell., **HYPER.,** ign., kalm., ***ph-ac.,*** **PHOS.,** rauw., spig., ***staph.,*** symph., verat.
compound fracture of left upper arm, after - ***calen.***
fingers, stump painful - ***calen.,*** **HYPER.,** phos., ***staph.***

AMPUTATION, pain
neuralgia of stump - ***all-c.,*** am-m., arn., **CALEN.,** ***coff., hyper.,*** kalm., ph-ac., symph.
burning, stinging - ***all-c.***
scars ulcerating, after - ***calc-p.***
thigh, after, neuralgia of stump - asaf.

ANESTHESIA, problems from - ***acet-ac.,*** am-c., am-caust., aml-n., ***carb-v., chlf.,*** hep., **PHOS.**

ANKLES, injury, sprain - **ARN.,** bell-p, **BRY.,** ***calc.,*** hyper., ***led.,*** nat-c., **RHUS-T., RUTA.,** sil., ***stront-c., symph.***

ANXIETY, panic attacks - **ACON.,** aloe, alum., **ARG-N.,** ***ars.,*** ars-i., bar-c., bell., calc., ***cann-i.,*** carb-v., caust., cham., cupr., ***gels.,*** **KALI-AR.,** kali-br., kali-c., lyc., ***med.,*** merc., nat-c., nit-ac., op., **PHOS.,** sep., sulph.
engagement, from upcoming - **ACON., ARG-N.,** ***ars., carb-v.,*** **GELS., LYC.,** med., **NAT-M.,** ph-ac., ***sil., thuj.***
fright, after - **ACON.,** ***ars., gels.,*** lyc., merc., nat-m., **OP.,** rob., ***sil.***
on going to, doctor or dentist, with fear - **ACON.,** ***arg-n., arn.,*** **GELS.,** ***ign.,*** nat-m., ***phos.***

ASPHYXIA, (see Death apparent) - ***acet-ac.,*** acon., **ANT-T.,** arn., ars., bell., ***camph., carb-s.,*** **CARB-V.,** chin., ***chlor., coch., coff.,*** coloc., crot-h., hydr-ac., laur., merc., nit-ac., **OP.,** ph-ac., phos., ***rhus-t., sin-n.,*** stram., sul-ac., tab.
carbon monoxide, from - acon., bell., ***carb-v.,*** op.
cholera - ***hydra-ac., laur.***
coal gas - ***carb-s.,*** carb-v.
drowned, persons, of - ant-t., lach.
hanged, strangled persons, of - ars., op.
new-born infant - acon., **ANT-T.,** ***arn.,*** bell., **CAMPH.,** carb-v., chin., **CUPR., LAUR.,** ***op.,*** upa.

AVIATOR'S, disease - ars., bell., bor., ***coca, cocc.,*** psor.

BACK, injuries, after - aesc., **ARN.,** ***bell-p.,*** **BRY.,** ***calc.,*** cic., **HYPER.,** ***kali-c., lyc.,*** mag-p., ***nat-s.,*** nit-ac., **RHUS-T., RUTA.,** ***thuj.***
lumbar, remains sensitive to jar of walking - arn., **BRY.,** ***thuj.***
dislocations - **ARN., BRY., CALC.,** calc-f., caust., ***coloc.,*** hyper., lyc., nux-v., phos., **RHUS-T.,** ***ruta.,*** stront-c., sulph., zinc.
disks, slipped, herniated, syndrome, or ruptured - **AESC.,** arn., **AGAR.,** ***berb.,*** **BRY.,** ***coloc.,*** **HYPER.,** kali-c., mag-p., ruta.., tarent., ***tell.,*** zinc.
lifting, ailments, from - **ARN., BRY., CALC., HYPER.,** ***lyc.,*** **RHUS-T.,** ruta..
aching after - anag., **ARN.,** bell-p., bor., bry., **CALC., GRAPH., LYC.,** ***nux-v.,*** ph-ac., **RHUS-T., RUTA.,** sang., ***sep.***
pain, after - **ARN., BRY.,** calc., ***con.,*** **HYPER.,** ***kali-c., nat-s.,*** **RHUS-T.,** ***ruta, thuj.***

BACK, injuries,
spasms - acon., arn., ***ars.,*** bell., bry., calc., ***calc-p.,*** cham., cic., ***cimic., coloc., crot-c.,*** hyper., ***lach.,*** kali-c., **MAG-P.,** ***mygal., nat-m., nat-s., nux-v.,*** oena., ***phys.,*** rhus-t., ruta, sep., stram., syph., tab.
spinal, injuries - aesc., ***apis,*** **ARN.,** ***calc., con.,*** **HYPER.,** ***led.,*** **NAT-S.,** ***nit-ac., rhus-t., ruta.,*** ***sil.,*** tell., ***thuj.***
concussion, from - ***arn.,*** cic., **HYPER., NAT-S.**
lies on back, jerking head backward after, injury - cic., ***hyper.***
lifting, from - ***arn.,*** **CALC., RHUS-T.,** ***ruta..***
lumbar region remains sensitive to jar of walking - ***thuj.***
shock, from - ***arn.,*** **HYPER., NAT-S.,** ***nat-m., nit-ac.***
wounds, spinal - ***calen.,*** **HYPER.,** ruta, symph.
straining, easy - bor., **CALC.,** calc-f., ***calc-p.,*** con., **GRAPH.,** ham., **LYC.,** mill., ***nux-v.,*** ph-ac., **RHUS-T., RUTA.,** sang., ***sep.,*** sil.
wounds, spinal - ***calen.,*** **HYPER.,** ruta, symph.

BITES, animals and insects, from - acet-ac., all-s., ***apis, arn., ars.,*** aur., ***bell.,*** calad., calen., ***cedr., echi.,*** grin., **HYPER.,** ***lach.,*** **LED.,** lyss., ***plan.,*** pyrog., seneg., stram., ***sul-ac.,*** tarent., ***thuj.***
animals, of poisonous or enraged - ***am-c.,*** anthr., ***apis,*** arn., ***ars.,*** aur., bell., calad., ***caust., cedr.,*** cist., ***echi.,*** hyper., ***lach.,*** **LED.,** ***lob-p., lyss.,*** mosch., nat-m., ***plan.,*** puls., pyrog., ***seneg.,*** stram., sul-ac., vip.
cats, of - acet-ac., **HYPER.,** ***lach.,*** **LED.**
cat scratch fever - hyper., led.
mad cat, lacerated wound, swollen leg - ***acet-ac.***
dogs, of (see Rabies) - acet-ac., am-c., am-caust., anthr., ***apis,*** arn., ***ars.,*** **BELL.,** calad., camph., ***cedr.,*** crot-h., ***echi., grin.,*** gua., gymne., hydr-ac., ***hyper.,*** kali-per., ***lach., led.,*** **LYSS.,** ***nat-m.,*** mosch., pyrog., sisy., spirae., ***ter.***
burning better by hot steam - ***lyss.***
headache, after - ***lyss.***
fleas - bapt., calad., calc., grin., hyper., ***led.,*** pulx., staph.
fever, with - ***pyrog.***
flies, itch and burn - calad.
insects - led., hyper.
leeches - alumn., sec.
application, of, agg. - sec.
gangrenous - ***lach.***
mosquitoes - calad., led., staph.
burn, itch intensely - ***calad.***
rats - hyper., led.
scorpions - hyper., led.
septic - hyper., lach., led., pyrog.
snakes, venomous - acet-ac., am-c., am-caust., anag., anthr., ***apis,*** arist-cl., arn., ***ars.,*** aur., **BELL.,** calad., ***camph., cedr., crot-h., echi., grin.,*** gymne., hydr-ac., ***hyper.,*** kali-per., **LACH., LED.,** lob-p., lycps., mosch., ***plan.,***

BITES, animals and insects, from
snakes, venomous - pyrog., seneg., sisy., spirae., stram., sul-ac., ***thuj., vip.***
chronic affects - lach., led., merc., ph-ac.
rattlesnake - ***crot-h.,*** hyper., led., ***plan.***
viper - ***camph.***
spiders, bites - apis., ***hyper.,*** lat-m., ***led.,*** lycps., tarent.
tarentula, of - hyper., led., lycps., tarent.
swelling, with - both., led.

BLADDER, burning, after catherer - acon., ***calen.,*** camph., ***canth., staph.***
injuries, after - ***arn.,*** bell-p., ***calen.,*** canth., ***staph.***
bladder, retention, of urine, painful - acon., ***arn.,*** ars., ***aur.,*** bell., bor., calc-p., **CANTH.,** caps., **CAUST.,** cop., crot-h., cupr., ***dulc., lyc., nit-ac.,*** **NUX-V.,** ***op., pareir., puls.,*** sabin., ***sars.,*** sul-ac., ***ter.***
children, in - ***acon.,*** **APIS,** ***art-v.,*** bell., ***benz-ac., calc., caust., cop., dulc.,*** eup-pur., ferr-p., ***gels.,*** ip., ***op.***
inactivity, of - acon., ***ars.,*** **CAUST.,** ***op.,*** plb.
new born infants, in - **ACON.,** ***apis,*** arn., ***ars.,*** benz-ac., ***camph., canth., caust.,*** erig., hyos., ***lyc., op.,*** puls.
bladder, stones, calculi - ant-c., arg-n., **BENZ-AC., BERB.,** cact., **CALC.,** ***calc-renal.,*** **CANTH.,** card-m., ***chin., coc-c.,*** colch., ***eup-per., lach., lith.,*** **LYC.,** mez., ***mill.,*** naja, nat-m., nat-s., ***nit-ac., nux-m., nux-v., pareir., petr., phos., puls., raph., ruta.,*** **SARS., SEP.,** ***sil.,*** tarent., thuj., zinc.
surgery for, after - ***arn.,*** **CALEN.,** cham., chin., cupr., nux-v., **STAPH.,** verat.

BLEEDING, blood does not coagulate, (see Wounds or Blood, chapter) - am-c., anthr., ***apis,*** ars., ***both., carb-v.,*** chin., chlol., **CROT-C.,** ***crot-h.,*** dig., dor., ***elaps,*** **FERR-P.,** ham., **IP.,** ***kali-p.,*** **LACH.,** lat-m., ***mill.,*** nat-m., **NIT-AC., PHOS.,** ***sec., sul-ac.***
passive, oozing - ars-h., bov., bufo, carb-v., ***chin.,*** crot-h., ferr-p., ham., ph-ac., sec., tarent., ter., ust.
surgery, after, with coldness and prostration - ***calen., stront-c.***
trauma, from - aran., ***arn.,*** bov., euph-pi., ham., ***mill.,*** tril.

BLISTERS - alum., am-c., ***anac.,*** **ANT-C.,** ***ars.,*** aur., bor., bry., ***bufo,*** canth., carb-an., carb-s., **CAUST.,** ***cham., clem.,*** crot-h., ***dulc., graph.,*** hep., ***kali-ar., kali-c.,*** kali-s., lach., ***mag-c., merc.,*** nat-a., ***nat-c.,*** nat-m., nat-p., nit-ac., ***petr.,*** phos., ***ran-b., ran-s.,*** **RHUS-T.,** rhus-v., ***sep., sil., sulph.,*** thuj., verat., vip., zinc.
burn, as from a - ambr., aur., bell., **CANTH.,** carb-an., clem., lyc., nat-c., phos., sep., sulph.

BLOOD, poisoning, septicemia - anthr., ***apis,*** arg-n., ***arn.,*** **ARS.,** ***bapt., bry.,*** **CARB-V.,** ***cench.,*** con., **CROT-H.,** echi., ***ferr., hippoz., kali-p.,*** **LACH.,** ***lyc., phos., puls.,*** **PYROG.,** ***rhus-t., sulph.,*** tarent.

BLOOD, vessels, injury to - arn., ham., hyper., ***mill.,*** phos.
rupture of - mill.

BLOWS, (see Injuries) - ***acon.,*** **ARN.,** ***aur-m., bad., bell-p., bry.,*** **CALEN.,** ***cic., con.,*** glon., ***ham., hep.,*** **HYPER.,** ***lach., led.,*** **NAT-S.,** puls., pyrog., ***rhus-t.,*** **RUTA,** ***sil., staph.,*** stront-c., sul-ac., ***symph.***
ecchymosis from slight - agar.
nosebleeds, profuse, sudden - arn., elaps., mill.
swelling - arn., kali-m., led.

BONES, broken or fractured, bruised, blows - acon., ang., **ARN.,** asaf., bell-p., **BRY.,** ***calc., calc-f.,*** **CALC-P.,** ***calen.,*** **CARB-AC.,** con., croc., crot-h., ***eup-per.,*** ferr., hecla., hep., ***hyper.,*** iod., kali-i., ***lach.,*** lyc., nit-ac., ***petr., ph-ac.,*** phos., ***puls.,*** rhus-t., **RUTA.,** ***sil.,*** staph., stront-c., ***sul-ac.,*** sulph., **SYMPH.,** ***thyr.,*** valer.
ailments from - calc-p., hecla., ruta, symph.
children, in - **ARN.,** bry., ***calc., calc-f.,*** **CALC-P.,** sil.
compound fracture - ang., **ARN.,** bry., ***calc.,*** calc-p., ***calen.,*** con., crot-h., hep., hyper., iod., ***lach., petr.,*** ph-ac., phos., puls., rhus-t., **RUTA,** sil., staph., symph.
fractured often, brittle bones - calc., **CALC-P.,** ***merc., sil.***
periosteum, injuries - arn., bell-p., calc., kali-iod., **RUTA.,** ***symph.***
slow healing of broken bones - asaf., **CALC.,** calc-f., **CALC-P.,** ***calen., ferr.,*** fl-ac., iod., lyc., mang., merc., ***mez.,*** nit-ac., ***ph-ac.,*** phos., puls., **RUTA.,** sep., ***sil.,*** staph., sulph., **SYMPH.,** ***thyr.***

BREASTS, injuries - ***arn.,*** **BELL-P., CON.,** phyt.
contusion, from - ***bell-p.,*** **CON.**
mastectomy, after - bell-p., ***calen.,*** x-ray.

BREATHING, imperceptible - acon., amyg., ***ars.,*** benz-ac., carb-ac., ***carb-v.,*** chlor., cic., ***cocc.,*** gels., hydr-ac., merc., morph., naja, nux-v., ***op.,*** petr., stram.
painful - apis, asc-t., ***ars.,*** brom., **BRY.,** chin., cimx., coff., crot-t., jug-c., led., nit-ac., ol-j., phos., plb., **RAN-B.,** sang., viol-o., zing.
panting - **ACON.,** anac., ***ant-t., apoc.,*** arg-n., ***arn.,*** ars., bufo, calad., camph., ***carb-an.,*** **CARB-V.,** caul., cham., chin., chlor., ***cina, cocc.,*** con., cop., ferr., hyos., ***ip.,*** jatr., kali-bi., ***lyc.,*** laur., ***nit-ac., nux-m.,*** op., **PHOS.,** ***phyt.,*** plan., plb., prun., sec., ***sil., spong.,*** stram., ***tarent.,*** **VERAT-V.**
ascending stairs - arn., **CALC.,** ***carb-v., sil.,*** plan.

BRUISES - absin., acon., agn., ant-c., ***arg-m.,*** **ARN.,** ***bad.,*** caust., ***cic., con.,*** croc., ***dros.,*** euph., ***form., glon.,*** **HAM.,** ***hep., hyper., iod.,*** kali-c., lach., **LED.,** ***lith.,*** teucr., mez., mosch., mill., ***olnd.,*** pareir., petr., **PHOS.,** plan., plat., polyg., ***puls.,*** rhod., rhus-t., **RUTA,** sep., sulph., **SUL-AC.,** ***symph.,*** verat., verb.

BRUISES,
blunt instruments, with - **ARN.**
contused - **ARN.,** ham., **LED.,** sul-ac., symph.
crushing, as mashed fingers, especially tips - ***hyper.***
discoloration remaining after pain and inflammation subsides - ***led.***
ecchymosed, when - ***sul-ac.***
laceration, without - **ARN.**
nervous tissues are mainly concerned - ***hyper.***
orchitis - zinc.
persistence of ecchymosis, with - arn., ham., led., ***sul-ac.***
riding on horseback, while - ***bar-m.***
spine, ill effects - ***con.***
suppuration, painful - ***croc.***
swelling remains - arn., ***kali-m., led.***
tension, in skin - samb.
tumors, after - ***con.***
ulcers, after - ***con.***

BURNS, general - acet-ac., ***acon.,*** agar., aloe, alum., alumn., ant-c., ***apis.,*** arist-cl., arn., **ARS.,** ***bar-c., bell., bry.,*** calc., calc-p., calc-s., ***calen.,*** **CANTH.,** carb-ac., ***carb-s., carb-v., caust.,*** chin., cic., crot-h., cycl., echi., euph., ferr., gaul., graph., grin., ***ham., hep.,*** hyos., ***hyper., ign.,*** piloc., ***kali-bi.,*** kali-c., ***kali-m., kreos.,*** lach., mag-c., ***mag-m., merc., nat-c., nux-v.,*** op., par., passi., petr., phos., pic-ac., ***plan.,*** plat., plb., ***puls.,*** rad-br., ran-b., ***rhus-t.,*** ruta, sabad., ***sec.,*** sep., ***sil.,*** **SOL,** spira., ***stram., sul-ac., ter.,*** thuj., **URT-U.,** verat.
ailments, from - carb-ac., caust., pic-ac.
blisters to prevent from arising - **CANTH.,** ***kali-m.***
chemicals, from - canth., carb-ac., caust., pic-ac.
cornea - ***canth.,*** ham.
delirium - calen.
diarrhea, chronic - ***calc.***
erysipelas or gangrene, threatening - ***crot-h.***
extensive - carb-ac.
fail to heal - carb-ac., caust.
gangrene, threatening - ***ars.,*** plb.
mustard poultice causes ulceration - ***calc-p.***
nettles, from - caust.
esophagus, of, with loss of substances - calen.
ophthalmia, from unslaked lime - ***apis***
painful - **CANTH.,** carb-ac.
pyaemia, hectic fever - ***crot-h.***
radiation, from - calc-f., fl-ac., phos., rad-br., ***sol,*** x-ray
scalds - **CANTH.,** ***carb-ac., carb-s.,*** **CAUST.,** ***crot-h.,*** petr., ***stram.***
laryngitis - ***crot-h.***
scars, from - ars., ***carb-an., graph.,*** lach.
shock, from - canth.
sunburn - acon., ***agar., ant-c., apis.,*** **BELL.,** bry., bufo, ***calen., camph.,*** **CANTH.,** clem., cortiso., euphr., ***hyos.,*** lach., lyc., ***mur-ac., nat-c.,*** op., **PULS.,** rob., sel., **SOL,** sulph., **URT-U.,** ***valer.,*** verat.

BURNS, general
suppuration, with - calc-s.
tongue, of - ***ars.,*** calen., ***caust.***
and lips, of - **CANTH.,** ham.
ulcerate, discharge offensive - ***carb-ac.***
ulcers, from burns - kali-bi.
unconsciousness, after - calen.
vapors, from hot - canth., kali-bi.

CARBON, gas poisoning - acet-ac., acon., am-c., bell., bry., **CARB-V.,** lach., op., phos.,
carbon monoxide, from - acon., bell., bry., ***carb-v.,*** op.

CARBUNCLES - agar., ***apis, anthr.,*** ant-t., ***arn.,*** **ARS., BELL.,** ***bufo,*** caps., carb-an., coloc., ***crot-c., crot-h., echi., hep., hyos.,*** jug-r., ***lach.,*** mur-ac., nit-ac., phyt., pic-ac., ***rhus-t., sec.,*** **SIL.,** ***sulph., tarent-c.***
burning - ***anthr., apis, ars., crot-c.,*** crot-h., coloc., hep., **TARENT-C.**
purple, with small vesicles around - ***crot-c.,*** **LACH.**
stinging - **APIS,** carb-an., ***nit-ac.***

CATHETER, bladder, ailments from - ***acon.,*** arn., **CALEN.,** ***camph., canth.,*** mag-p., nux-v., petr., **STAPH.**
burning, after - acon., ***calen.,*** camph., ***canth., staph.***
fever, from - ***acon.***
infection, from - ***camph.,*** canth., staph.
injury, from - ***calen.***

CAUTERY, antidote to - arg-n., ***nat-m.***

CHEST, pain, angina, pectoris - acet-ac., ***acon.,*** **AM-C.,** ***aml-n.,*** anac., ang., **APIS, ARG-N., ARN., ARS., AUR., AUR-M., CACT.,** caust., ***chel.,*** **CHIN-A.,** ***chin-s.,*** chr-ac., ***cimic.,*** coca, ***cupr., cupr-ar., dig., dios., hep.,*** ip., ***jug-c., kali-c.,*** kali-p., ***kalm., lach.,*** lact., **LAT-M.,** ***laur., lyc., mag-p., mosch.,*** **NAJA,** ***nux-v.,*** **OX-AC.,** petr., **PHOS.,** phyt., **RHUS-T.,** ***samb.,*** sep., **SPIG., SPONG.,** ***stram., tab., tarent., ther., verat.***
drinking, water agg. - ars.
standing, amel. - ars.

CHILL, violent, with bluish, cold face and hands, mottled skin - **NUX-V.,** ***rhus-t.***
delirium, with - ***arn., ars., bell.,*** bry., cham., **CHIN., NAT-M.,** nux-v., puls., ***sep.,*** stram., sulph., ***verat.***
heat without subsequent - **ARAN.,** bov., camph., hep., ***led., mez.***
red face and thirst, with - **FERR.,** ***ign.***
unconsciousness, with - ***ars., bell.,*** camph., ***hep.,*** lach., **NAT-M.,** nux-v., op., puls., stram., valer.

CHOKING, on swallowing - acon., ars., ***bar-c.,*** bell., bry., ***cic., cupr.,*** gent-c., ***graph., hyos.,*** kali-c., ***laur.,*** **LYC.,** mag-p., manc., meph., ***merc.,*** mur-ac., ***nat-m.,*** onos., par., ***plb.,*** **PULS.,** rhus-t., stry., tarent., verat., zinc.
convulsive - acon., ars., ***bell., calc., caps., carb-v., cic., con.,*** **HYOS.,** ***mag-p.,*** nat-s., puls., sars.

CHOKING, on swallowing
liquids - **HYOS.,** lyss., ***mag-p.,*** nat-s., rhus-t.
solids - ***carb-v.,*** **PULS.,** lach.

CHLOROFORM, agg. - ***chlf.,*** phos.

COAL gas, from - acet-ac., am-c., arn., bell., bor., bov., ***carb-s.,*** carb-v., coff., ip., lach., ***op.,*** phos., sec.

COCCYX, tailbone injuries - aesc., arn., bellis-p., ***carb-an.,*** **HYPER.,** led., ***mez.,*** **SIL.,** tell.
fall, after a - **HYPER.,** ***mez.,*** **SIL.**

COLD, body, severe from chills - acon-f., ant-t., **ARS.,** bism., ***bry.,*** cadm-s., ***calc.,*** **CAMPH.,** carb-s., **CARB-V.,** cic., **CUPR.,** con., hell., lachn., ***merc-c.,*** nat-m., nat-s., nux-v., **SEC.,** ***sep.,*** **SIL.,** stram., ***tarent.,*** verat., zinc.
clammy sweat and blueness, cannot bear to be covered, with - **SEC.**
coldness, as if lying on ice - lyc.
skin, dry and blue, yet wants to be uncovered - camph.
covered with a cold sweat, hands and feet livid - ***stram.,*** **VERAT.**
uncover, with desire to - ***camph.,*** **SEC.**
whole body, with cold breath - **CARB-V.,** verat.

COLLAPSE - acet-ac., acetan., ***acon.,*** aconin., adren., aeth., **AM-C.,** amyg., ***ant-t.,*** apis, arn., **ARS.,** ***ars-h.,*** bar-c., **CAMPH.,** cann-i., canth., ***carb-ac.,*** carb-an., **CARB-S., CARB-V.,** cench., **CHIN.,** cina, cit-l., colch., con., crat., croc., ***crot-h.,*** crot-t., ***cupr., cupr-ac.,*** cupr-s., ***dig.,*** diph., dor., euon., hell., ***hydr-ac., hyos.,*** iod., ip., piloc., kali-br., kali-chl., kali-chr., kali-cy., kali-n., ***lach.,*** lat-m., ***laur.,*** lob., lob-p., lol., lyc., ***med.,*** merc., merc-c., merc-cy., merc-n., merc-pr-a., morph., ***mosch.,*** mur-ac., naja, nicot., olnd., op., ox-ac., ***phos.,*** phys., plb., sabad., sant., scam., ***sec., seneg.,*** sep., stram., sul-ac., ***sulph.,*** tab., tarent., tarent-c., tax., ***verat.,*** verat-v., vip., ***zinc.***
diarrhea, after - ant-c., **ARS., CAMPH., CARB-V.,** ric., sec., **VERAT.**
flashes of light, photopsies, after - sep.
injury, from - acet-ac., arn., nat-s., op., sul-ac.
menses, at - ip., lach., merc., nux-v., sep.
moist - colch.
needle, prick of a - calc.
nervous - am-c., laur.
paralysis, at beginning of - con.
before - con.
sudden - **ARS.,** ***colch.,*** crot-h., graph., hydr-ac., phos., sep.
vomiting, during - ***ars., verat.***
after - **ARS.,** lob., phys., ***verat.***

COMA, unconsciousness, (see Brain, Coma)
alcoholic - gels., ***glon.,*** hyos., ***kali-br., stram.***
delirium tremens, in - **NUX-V.**
asphyxia, with - **ANT-T.,** carb-v.
blood, sight of - nux-m.
childbirth, during - ***chin-s., cimic., coff., gels., lach.,*** **NUX-V.,** ***puls.,*** **SEC.**

COMA, unconsciousness

chill, during - ***ars., bell.,*** camph., caps., cic., ***con., hep.,*** kali-c., **NAT-M.,** nux-v., op., puls., ***spong.,*** stram., valer.

before - ***ars., lach.***

coma, vigil - acon., hydr-ac., ***hyos.,*** laur., mur-ac., ***op.,*** phos.

concussion, of brain, from - **ARN.,** nat-s., ***op.***

convulsions, after (see Nerves, convulsions) - ***art-v.,*** atro., ***bell.,*** **BUFO,** canth., carb-ac., ***cic.,*** cori-r., ***glon., oena.,*** plb., ***sec.***

prolonged - bell.

diphtheria, in - ail., ***nat-m., sul-ac.***

emotion, after - ***acon.,*** am-c., camph., ***caust., cham.,*** **COFF., IGN., LACH.,** mosch., ***op.,*** nux-m., ***ph-ac.,*** phos., verat.

epilepsy, after (see Nerves, Convulsions) - ***ars.,*** **BUFO,** ***kali-bi.,*** **OP.,** plb.

excitement, after - amyg., chlf., nux-m.

exertion, after - arn., ***ars.,*** calc., calc-ar., ***caust.,*** cocc., hyper., ***senec., ther., verat.***

fever, during - ***acon.,*** aeth., ***agar.,*** ail., **APIS, ARN.,** ***bapt., bell.,*** bor., bry., ***cact., calad.,*** calc., ***camph., caps., chlor.,*** cic., ***clem., colch., crot-h.,*** dor., ***dulc.,*** eup-per., ***gels., hyos., ip., iris,*** kali-br., ***lach., laur., lyc.,*** manc., meli., **MUR-AC., NAT-M.,** ***nit-s-d., nux-m.,*** nux-v., **OP.,** per., ***ph-ac., phos., puls.,*** samb., sol-n., ***stram.,*** sulph., ***ter., verat.,*** zing.

hydrocephalus, in - **APIS,** ***apoc., clem., hell., hyos., lyc., nat-m.***

jaundice, in - **CHEL.**

meningitis, in - ***ant-t., apis,*** apoc., ***gels., hell., merc., rhus-t., sulph., verat.***

mental, insensibility - bufo, con., cycl., ***hell., hyos.,*** laur., ***nux-m.,*** oena., op., phos., ph-ac., sabad., sec., stram.

odors, from - **NUX-V.,** ***phos.***

old age, in - ***bar-c.***

pain, from - agar., aloe, anac., ***hep., nux-m.,*** phyt., plat., stann., ***valer.,*** verat.

pneumonia, in - carb-v., ***chel., phos.***

pregnancy, during - cann-i., ***nux-m., nux-v., sec.***

rubbing, soles of feet amel. - chel.

scarlatina, in - ***ail., am-c., apis, cupr-ac., gels., lyc., mur-ac., sulph.***

semi-consciousness - ***carb-v.,*** chin-s., coca, cocc., ign., kali-br., ***laur., stram.,*** tarax., ***verat.,*** verat-v., zinc.

stroke, in - ***acon.,*** **ARN.,** ***bar-c., crot-h.,*** cupr., cupr-ac., cupr-ar., ***hyos., lach., laur., oena.,*** **OP.,** ***phos., plb., puls.,*** sol-n., ***stram.***

sudden - absin., cann-i., ***canth.,*** carb-h., carb-o., ***cocc.,*** glon., ***hydr-ac.,*** kali-c., ***laur.,*** oena., op., plb.

sunstroke, in - ***bell.,*** cact., camph., **GLON.,** lach., **OP.**

COMA, unconsciousness

uremic, coma - ***am-c., apis,*** apoc., ars., asc-c., ***bell.,*** cann-i., ***canth., carb-ac.,*** cic., cupr., ***cupr-ar., glon.,*** hell., hydr-ac., hyos., kali-br., ***morph., op.,*** phos., ***pic-ac.,*** piloc., queb., ser-ang., stram., ***tab., ter.,*** urea, urt-u., ***verat-v.***

CONTUSIONS, (see Bruises) - **ARN.,** bell-p., con., ***ham.,*** hyper., led., rhus-t., ruta, sul-ac., symph., ter.

CONVULSIONS, from injuries - **ARN.,** art-v., **CIC.,** cupr., **HYPER., NAT-S.,** ***op.,*** oena., ***rhus-t.,*** sulph., ***valer., zinc.***

bone, in the throat, from - ***cic.***

fever, during - **BELL.,** ***cic., cina,*** cur., ***hyos.,*** **NUX-V.,** op., **STRAM.**

vaccination, after - apis., ant-t., bell., ***carc., cic.,*** **SIL.,** ***thuj.***

CUTS, (see Punctures, Stabs, Wounds) - anthr., apis., ***arn.,*** ars., **CALEN.,** ***carb-v., cic.,*** con., dig., ***ham.,*** hep., ***hyper.,*** kali-m., ***lach., led.,*** merc., nat-c., ***nit-ac.,*** ph-ac., ***phos.,*** plan., plb., puls., pyrog., ***sil.,*** **STAPH.,** sulph., ***sul-ac.***

dissecting - ***anthr., apis,*** **ARS., CALEN.,** crot-h., ***echi.,*** ham., hyper., kreos., **LACH.,** led., **PYROG.,** ***ter.***

gangrenous, become - anthr., **ARS., LACH.**

pyaemia, hectic fever - ***crot-h.***

gangrenous - plan.

incised - arn., **CALEN.,** ham., hyper., lach., led., ***phos.,*** puls., ***staph.,*** sul-ac.

inflammation - ***calen., plan.***

sharp instruments, from, glass, etc. - **CALEN.,** hyper., ***staph.***

suppuration, with thick yellow matter - calc-s.

swelling - ***kali-m.***

CYANOSIS - acon., agar., alum., ***am-c.,*** ant-c., ***ant-t., arg-n.,*** arn., ***ars.,*** asaf., asar., aur., bar-c., ***bell.,*** bism., ***bor.,*** bry., calc., **CAMPH.,** carb-an., **CARB-V.,** caust., cedr., cham., chel., chin., chin-a., cic., cina, cocc., ***con.,*** **CUPR., DIG.,** dros., ferr., hep., hyos., ign., ***ip., kali-chl.,*** **LACH., LAUR.,** led., lyc., mang., merc., mosch., mur-ac., ***naja,*** nat-m., nit-ac., nux-m., nux-v., **OP.,** ph-ac., phos., plb., puls., ran-b., ***rhus-t.,*** ruta., sabad., ***samb.,*** sars., ***sec.,*** seneg., sil., spong., staph., stram., sulph., sul-ac., thuj., **VERAT.,** xan.

fever, during - arund., crot-h.

infants, in - arn., ars., ***bor., cact., camph., carb-v.,*** chin., **DIG., LACH., LAUR.,** ***naja,*** op., ***phos.,*** psor., rhus-t., sec., sulph.

DEATH, apparent, (see Asphyxia, Dying) - ***acet-ac.,*** acon., **ANT-T.,** arn., ars., bell., ***camph., carb-s.,*** **CARB-V.,** chin., ***chlor., coch., coff.,*** coloc., crot-h., hydr-ac., laur., merc., nit-ac., **OP.,** ph-ac., phos., ***rhus-t., sin-n.,*** stram., sul-ac., tab.

carbon monoxide, from - acon., bell., ***carb-v.,*** op.

cholera - ***hydra-ac., laur.***

coal gas - ***carb-s.,*** carb-v.

DEATH, apparent
drowned, persons, of - ant-t., lach.
frozen persons, of - acon., ars., bry., carb-v.
hanged, strangled persons, of - ars., op.
hemorrhages, after - carb-v., chin.
injuries, after - arn., op.
lightning stroke, after - lach., nux-v.
new-born infant - acon., **ANT-T.,** ***arn.,*** bell., **CAMPH., CARB-V.,** chin., **CUPR., LAUR.,** ***op.,*** upa.

DEHYDRATION, loss of fluids - ***ars.,*** ars-i., ***calad.,*** **CALC., CALC-P.,** ***carb-an.,*** **CARB-V.,** caust., **CHIN.,** ***chin-a.,*** **CHIN-S.,** ***con., crot-h.,*** dig., ***ferr.,*** **GRAPH.,** ***iod.,*** ip., ***kali-c., kali-p.,*** led., lyc., mag-m., ***merc.,*** mez., nat-c., nat-m., ***nat-p.,*** nit-ac., ***nux-m., nux-v.,*** **PH-AC., PHOS.,** plb., **PULS.,** sec., **SEL., SEP.,** ***sil.,*** stann., **STAPH.,** ***sulph.,*** thuj., valer., **VERAT.,** zinc.
ailments from loss of fluids - ***calad.,*** **CALC.,** ***carb-an., carb-v.,*** caust., **CHIN.,** ***ph-ac.***
amblyopia - ***chin.***
dyspepsia - ***ph-ac.***
fainting - chin., ***ph-ac.***
hysterical attacks - cinnam.
locomotor ataxia - ***phos.***
vertigo - ***chin.***
weakness - ***ph-ac., sec.***

DISLOCATIONS, of joints - ***agn.,*** ambr., ***am-c.,*** ang., ***arn.,*** bar-c., ***bell.,*** bov., ***bry.,*** **CALC.,** cann-i., ***carb-an.,*** carb-v., caust., con., ***form.,*** graph., hep., ***ign.,*** kreos., **LYC.,** ***merc.,*** mez., mosch., **NAT-C., NAT-M.,** ***kali-n., nit-ac., nux-v.,*** **PETR., PHOS.,** ***puls.,*** rhod., **RHUS-T.,** ***ruta,*** sabin., sep., spig., stann., staph., ***stront-c., sulph.,*** zinc.
easy dislocation - am-c., ***bry., calc.,*** cann-i., ***carb-an.,*** carb-v., con., hep., ***lyc.,*** merc., **NAT-C.,** ***nat-m., nit-ac.,*** kali-n., ***nux-v., petr., phos.,*** **RHUS-T., RUTA,** ***stront-c., sulph.***
lameness of wrists and knees - rheum, ***ruta.***
parts, with injuries to soft - ***calen.***

DROWNED, persons, asphyxia, of - ant-t., carb-v., lach.

DRUG, overdose - ars., ***gels.,*** ip., ***nux-v., op.***

DYING, agony, while - ***acon.,*** alum., ***ant-t.,*** **ARS.,** cocc., cupr., **LAT-M.,** puls., ***rhus-t., op.,*** **TARENT.,** ***verat.***

ELBOW, injury - ***arn.,*** aur., bell-p., ***hyper., rhus-t.,*** **RUTA.**
tennis elbow - arn., aur., bell-p., ***rhus-t., ruta.***

ELECTROSHOCK, electricity, agg. - arn., hell., morph., nux-v., op., ***phos.***
ailments from - hell., morph., phos.
lightning strike, after - arn., crot-h., hell., lach., morph., nux-v., op., phos.

EXTRAVASATIONS, from injuries - **ARN.,** ***bad.,*** bry., cham., chin., cic., ***con.,*** dulc., euphr., ferr., ***hep.,*** iod., ***lach.,*** laur., led., nux-v., par., plb., ***puls.,*** rhus-t., ***ruta.,*** sec., ***sulph.,*** **SUL-AC.**

EYES, injuries - **ACON., ARN.,** calc., calc-s., **CALEN.,** ***euphr.,*** ham., hep., **HYPER.,** ***led.,*** sil., ***staph.,*** sulph., sul-ac., **SYMPH.**
black eye, ecchymosis - ***acon.,*** aeth., am-c., arg-n., **ARN.,** ***bell.,*** **CACT.,** cham., ***chlol., con., crot-h., cupr-ac.,*** erig., ***glon., ham.,*** kali-bi., ***kali-chl.,*** kreos., ***lach.,*** **LED.,** ***lyc.,*** lyss., ***nux-v., phos.,*** plb., ruta., ***sul-ac.,*** **SYMPH.,** ter.
blow, to - arn., led., ***symph.***
glaucoma, caused - phys.
foreign, objects, in - **ACON., ARN.,** ***calc.,*** calen., ***puls.,*** **SIL.,** sulph.
inflammation, after injuries - **ACON., ARN.,** calc., calc-s., **CALEN.,** ***euphr., ham., hep.,*** **HYPER., LED.,** ***puls.,*** sil., ***staph., sulph.*** sul-ac., **SYMPH.**
scratched, cornea - acon., ***calen., hyper.***
splinters, in - **ACON.,** ***calc.,*** **CALEN., HYPER.,** ***sil., sulph.***
wounds, from cuts, surgery, etc. - acon., arn., **CALEN.,** euphr., hyper., **STAPH.**

FAINTING, (see Nerves, chapter)
anger, after - ***cham., gels., nux-v.,*** phos., staph., vesp.
angina pectoris, in - ***arn., hep., spong.***
precordial, anguish with - ***aml-n., merc-i-f.,*** plb., tab.
bleeding, from - ***acon.,*** cann-s., crot-h., ***ip., lach.,*** verat.
childbirth, after - calc.
rectum - ***ign., nux-v.***
uterine - ***apis,*** **CHIN.,** ***coc-c., kreos.,*** merc., ***phys.,*** tril.
blood, at sight of - **ALUM.,** nux-m., nux-v., ***verat.***
childbirth, with - cimic., ***coloc.***
loss of fluids, from - **CHIN.,** ***ph-ac., tril.***
crowded, in a, room - ambr., ***am-c.,*** ars., bar-c., con., ***ign., lyc.,*** nat-c., ***nat-m., nux-m., nux-v., phos., plb.,*** **PULS.,** sulph.
street, in a crowded - asaf.
dehydration, loss of fluids, from - ars., bar-c., ***carb-v.,*** **CHIN., IP.,** kreos., merc., nux-m., nux-v., **PH-AC., TRIL.,** ***verat.***
blood loss - **CHIN.,** ***ferr.,*** ferr-p., ***ip.,*** op., tril.
fright, after - **ACON.,** ***gels., ign., lach., nux-v.,*** **OP.,** ***phos., staph., verat.***
grief, from - ***ign., staph.***
heated, when - ip., ***puls.,*** tab.
summer, from - ***ant-c., ip.***
hunger, from - cocc., croc., crot-c., **CULX.,** ***phos., sulph.,*** tub.
injury, from shock in - ***arn.,*** atro., ***camph., cham.,*** dig., ***hyper., nat-s.***
concussion of brain, from - ***hyos.,*** **NAT-S.**
injuries, from slight - verat.
pain, from - ***acon.,*** apis, ars., asaf., bism., bol., ***cham., cocc.,*** coff., coloc., ***gels.,*** **HEP.,** ign., iod., morph., mosch., ***nux-m., nux-v.,*** phos., phyt., ran-s., sil., ***stront-c.,*** stroph., ***valer., verat.,*** vib., vip.

FAINTING,
pulse, with imperceptible - ***chin., crot-h.,*** morph.
irregular - **DIG.,** morph.
slow - **DIG.**
shock, from - ***atro.***
wounds, from slight - ign., ***verat.***

FALLS, (see Injuries, general) - ***acon.,*** **ARN.,** ***aur-m., bad., bell-p., bry.,*** **CALEN.,** ***cic., con.,*** euph., glon., ***ham., hep.,*** **HYPER.,** ***lach., led.,*** lith., **NAT-S.,** puls., pyrog., ***rhus-t.,*** **RUTA,** ***sil., staph.,*** stront-c., ***sul-ac., symph.***
asphyxia, with shootings and jerkings - ***hyper.***
back painful after falling from a height - ***con.***
pain in small of - ***kali-c.***
bloodspitting - ***mill.***
deep hole in forehead - ***calen.***
glaucoma - phys.
groin, swelling in - ***aur.***
headache, with sore eyes - ***hyper.***
hernia, inguinal - eug.
internal injuries - arn., ***bell-p., mill.***
bleeding, from - arn., ***mill.***
nosebleed - acet-ac.
ovarian irritation - ham.
swelling - kali-m.
vertigo - acon., ***glon.***

FEVER, traumatic - ***acon., apis,*** **ARN.,** ***ars.,*** bry., cact., carb-v., ***chin., coff.,*** croc., euphr., hep., ***iod., lach., lyss.,*** merc., nat-c., nit-ac., ph-ac., phos., ***puls.,*** pyrog., ***rhus-t., staph.,*** sul-ac., ***sulph.***

FINGERS, amputated, stump painful - ***calen.,*** **HYPER.,** phos., ***staph.***
abscess, under nails from splinter - ***myris.,*** sil.
crushed, and lacerated finger ends - arist-cl., ***carb-ac.,*** coff., **HYPER.,** ***led.,*** phos., ***ruta.***
contusion - ***arn., ruta.***
dissecting, wounds - ***apis,*** **ARS., CALEN., LACH.,** ***pyrog.,***
fracture with laceration - ***hyper.***
lacerations - **CALEN.,** ***hyper.***
sprain - **ARN.,** ***calc., rhus-t., ruta.***

FINANCIAL, shock, loss of wealth, property - arn., **ARS., AUR.,** calc., ***calc-p.,*** caust., ***con., ign.,*** kali-br., lyc., ***psor.***

FRIGHT, acute - **ACON.,** ***arg-n., arn.,*** ars., ***bell.,*** calc., ***caust.,*** cham., ***coff.,*** **GELS.,** ***hyos.,*** **IGN.,** lyc., **OP.,** ***ph-ac., phos.,*** puls., sil.

FOOD, poisoning - ant-c., **ARS.,** bapt., bry., ***carb-v.,*** chin., ***coloc.,*** crot-h., ***ip.,*** lach., lyc., nat-p., ***nux-v.,*** ph-ac., ***podo.,*** psor., ***puls.,*** pyrog., sul-ac., ***urt-u.,*** zing.
bad, water - ***ars.,*** bapt., zing.
fish, spoiled - ars., ***carb-v.,*** chin., ***puls.***
fruit, acid, sour - ***ant-c., ip.,*** ox-ac., **NAT-P.,** ***ph-ac., psor.***
shellfish, agg. - ***aloe,*** ars., ***brom.,*** bry., fl-ac., **LYC.,** ***podo., sul-ac., urt-u.***

FOOD, poisoning
spoiled, fatty, rich - ars., ***carb-v.,*** chin., nux-v., **PULS.**
meat, agg. - **ARS.,** ***carb-v.,*** chin., ***crot-h., lach., puls., pyrog.***

FOREIGN, objects, from (see Punctures, Stabs) - acon., anag., calc-f., cic., ***hep., lob., myris.,*** **SIL.**
enteritis, cause - ***calen.***
expulsion of fishbones, needles, splinters, to promote - anag., ***cic.,*** hep., lob., ***myris., sil.***
glass, needles, etc. - **SIL.**
irritation and inflammation of eyes - **ACON.,** ***sil.***
lacerate esophagus - calen., cic.

FROSTBITE - **AGAR.,** alum., nat-c., nux-v., paeon., ***petr., puls., sil.,*** staph., sulph., ***zinc.***
ailments, from - agar., zinc.
nose - ***agar.***
frost-bitten easily - ***zinc.***

GALLSTONES, gallbladder pain, colic, from - ars., ***bapt.,*** **BELL., BERB.,** ***bry., calc.,*** **CARD-M.,** ***cham., chel.,*** **CHIN.,** ***chion., chlf., chlol.,*** **COLOC.,** cupr., dig., ***dios., ip., iris,*** kali-ar., ***kali-bi., kali-c., lach.,*** laur., ***lept., lith.,*** **LYC.,** mag-p., mang., merc., **NAT-S.,** ***nux-v.,*** podo., puls., rhus-t., ***sep.,*** tab., **VERAT.**

GASPING, for air - ***acon.,*** acet-ac., ***am-c., ant-t.,*** **APIS,** ***apoc., arg-n., ars.,*** ars-h., ***brom.,*** camph., canth., carb-an., **CARB-V.,** cast., ***chlor., cic., coff., colch., coloc.,*** cub., cupr., ***dig., dros.,*** gels., ***hell., hydr-ac.,*** hydrc., ***hyper., ip.,*** lat-m., ***laur.,*** **LYC.,** ***med.,*** merc., ***mosch., naja,*** op., ***phos.,*** phyt., puls., samb., ***spong., stram.,*** stry., ***tab.,*** thuj., tarent.
afternoon - nicc.
cough, during - ***ant-t., cor-r.,*** sul-ac.
before - ant-t., bry., ***brom.,*** coc-c.
dozing, when - naja
inspiration, expiration long and slow - ***ant-t., op.***
morning, 5 a.m - tarent.
night - lach.
2 a.m., with cough - chin-s.

GENITALIA, injuries to - **ARN., BELL-P.,** ***calen.,*** con., ***hyper.,*** mill., ***rhus-t., staph.***

GLANDS, injuries - ***arn.,*** aster., cann-s., ***bell-p.,*** cann-s., cic., ***cist.,*** **CON.,** ***dulc.,*** glon., ***hep., iod.,*** kali-c., kalm., merc., ***petr., phos., phyt.,*** puls., rhus-t., ***sil., sul-ac., sulph.***
bruised, induration of accompanied by a sensation of numbness - con.

GRIEF, acute - am-m., ***ambr., arn., ars.,*** **AUR.,** calc., ***calc-p., caust., cocc.,*** coloc., ***gels.,*** hyos., **IGN.,** kali-br., kali-p., ***lach.,*** lyc., **NAT-M.,** ***op.,*** **PHOS., PH-AC.,** ***plat., puls.,*** **STAPH.**

GUNSHOT, wounds - apis, **ARN., CALEN.,** chin., ***euph., gunp.,*** **HYPER.,** lach., **LED.,** ***nit-ac., plb.,*** puls., ruta.., ***staph., sul-ac.,*** sulph., symph.
abdomen - hyper.
hand, in - ***lach.***

GUNSHOT, wounds
lung, shot through, with collapse and hemoptysis - ***chin.***
perineum, to - symph.
soles and palms - ***hyper., led.***

HANDS, contusion - ***arn., ruta.***
dissecting wounds - ***apis,*** **ARS., CALEN., LACH.,** ***pyrog.,***
fracture with laceration - ***hyper.***
lacerations - **CALEN.**, hyper.
sprain - **ARN.,** ***calc., rhus-t., ruta.***

HANGED, strangled persons, asphyxia, of - arn., ars., op.

HANGOVER, reveling, from a night of - agar., ambr., ant-c., ***ars.,*** bry., ***carb-v.,*** coff., colch., ip., lac-d., ***laur.,*** led., nat-c., **NUX-V.,** ***puls.,*** ran-b., rhus-t., sabin., staph., sulph.

HEAD, injuries, blows, concussions etc. - acet-ac., acon., am-c., ***anac.,*** **ARN.,** aur., **BAD.,** ***bell.,*** bell-p., both., bry., ***calc., calc-p.,*** calc-s., calen., camph., cann-s., ***carc.,*** caust., chin., ***cic.,*** cina, ***cocc., con.,*** cupr., echi., euphr., ***glon., ham.,*** **HELL.,** ***hyos.,*** **HYPER.,** ***iod., kali-p.,*** kreos., lac-c., ***lach.,*** laur., ***led.,*** lyc., mag-arct., mag-m., ***mang.,*** merc., mez., nat-m., **NAT-S.,** nux-m., ***nux-v.,*** op., ph-ac., ***puls., rhus-t., ruta,*** seneg., ***sep., sil., spig.,*** staph., stram., stry., sul-ac., sulph., ***symph., teucr.,*** valer., ***verat.,*** verb., viol-t., zinc.
epilepsy, after - ***arn., cic.,*** hell., hyper., ***nat-s.,*** zinc.
mental, functionings altered - ***hell.,*** kali-p., ***nat-s.,*** op., stram.
scalp, of - ***calen.***
vertigo, after injuries - cic., **NAT-S.**

HEADACHES, severe, migraine - acon., **AGAR.,** ***anac.,*** **ANT-C.,** apis, ***arg-m.,*** arn., ***ars.,*** **ASAF.,** ***asar.,*** aur., bell., **BRY.,** ***cact.,*** calad., ***calc., calc-p.,*** caust., cedr., ***cham.,*** chel., **CHIN.,** cic., cimic., cina, cocc., **COFF.,** coloc., ***eup-per.,*** **GELS.,** glon., graph., **IGN., IP., IRIS,** kali-bi., ***kali-p.,*** lac-c., lach., lyc., **NAT-M.,** ***nat-s.,*** **NUX-V.,** op., **PHOS., PULS., SANG.,** scut., ***sep.,*** **SIL.,** spig., ***stram., sulph., tab.,*** tarent., ***ther.,*** **THUJ.,** ***valer.,*** **ZINC.**
blinding - asar., aster., ***bell., caust.,*** **CYCL.,** ferr-p., ***gels.,*** **IRIS, KALI-BI.,** lac-d., ***lil-t., nat-m., petr., phos., psor., sil., stram., sulph.***
head, injuries, after - **ARN.,** ***bell.,*** calc., calc-s., ***cic.,*** cocc., con., dulc., ferr-p., ***glon., hep., hell., hyper.,*** lac-c., lach., merc., ***nat-m.,*** **NAT-S.,** nit-ac., petr., ***phos.,*** puls., ***rhus-t., staph.,*** sulph., sul-ac.
sinus, headache - acon., ***all-c., alum., ars., aur.,*** bell., ***bry., calc.,*** **CALC-S.,** ***carb-v.,*** cham., chin., cina, **DULC., EUPHR.,** ***ferr.,*** ferr-p., ***gels.,*** **GRAPH., HEP., HYDR.,** ***iod.,*** **KALI-BI.,** ***kali-c.,*** **KALI-I.,** kali-m., ***kali-s., lach., lyc.,*** **MERC.,** mez., ***nat-m.,*** **NUX-V.,** ***phos.,*** **PULS.,** rumx., sabad., sang., sil., ***stict., sulph.,*** **THUJ.**

HEADACHES, severe
vascular, headaches - ***bell.,*** meli., ***glon.,*** lach., sec.

HEMATOMA, brain - ***arn.,*** calc-f., merc., nat-s., sil.

HIPS, injuries - **AESC., ARN.,** calc-p., con., ***rhus-t.,*** sil., tarent.

HIVES, urticaria (see Allergic)

INJECTION, painful, wound, from (see Puncture) - ***crot-h.,*** **HYPER.,** ***led.***

INJURIES, general (see Blows, Falls and Bruises) - ***acon.,*** **ARN.,** ***aur-m., bad., bell-p., bry.,*** **CALEN.,** ***cic., con.,*** glon., ***ham., hep.,*** **HYPER.,** ***lach., led.,*** **NAT-S.,** puls., pyrog., ***rhus-t.,*** **RUTA,** ***sil., staph.,*** stront-c., sul-ac., ***symph.***
blood vessel, rupture of - mill.
chest, to - ***ruta***
chronic effects of - ***arn.,*** carb-v., cic., ***con.,*** glon., ham., hyper., led., ***nat-s., stront-c.***
esophagus, to - ***cic.***
exudation of blood, fibrin or pus - **ARN.**
lungs, of - mill.
bleeding from - ***arn.,*** ip., ***mill.***
hyperaemia - ***ferr-p.***
internal, bleeding - mill.
meningitis, spinal, after - ***acon.***
mental symptoms, from - acon., bell., cic., ***glon., hell.,*** hyos., hyper., mag-c., **NAT-S.,** op., stram., verat.
neuralgia - ***chel., hyper.***
osseous growth - calc-f.
paralysis - cur.
periostitis of foot - ***aur-m.***
proud flesh - kali-m.
sore spot from - lith.
suppuration - asaf., calc-s., ***cham., hep., sil.***
suppurate, slight, skin unhealthy - ***bor.***
swelling of parts, with, proud flesh - kali-m.
tight boots, from - paeon.
ulceration, every hurt festers - sil.
ulcers, malignant, with blue border - mang.

INTESTINES, impaction - ***caust.,*** coloc., gels., lac-d., ***lach.,*** **OP.,** ***plb.***
intussusception - ***acon., arn.,*** **ARS.,** ***bell., bry., colch., coloc., cupr.,*** kali-bi., kreos., ***lach., lob., lyc., merc., nux-v.,*** **OP.,** ***phos.,*** **PLB.,** ***rhus-t., samb.,*** sulph., tab., tarent., thuj., **VERAT.**
paralysis - **OP.,** ***phos.,*** **PLB.,** ***sec.***

JET lag - alum., arg-n., ***arn., cocc.,*** con., ***gels.***

JOINTS, injuries, to - arn., bell-p., ***bry., rhus-t., ruta.***

KIDNEY, stones - ant-c., bell., **BENZ-AC., BERB., CALC.,** ***calc-renal., canth.,*** coc-c., coloc., equis., hydrang., lach., **LITH., LYC.,** mill., nat-m., ***nit-ac., nux-v.,*** oci., **PAREIR.,** ***petr., phos.,*** **SARS., SEP.,** ***sil.***
operation, after - ***arn.,*** **CALEN.,** cham., chin., cupr., nux-v., **STAPH.,** verat.

KNEE, injuries - apis., ***arn.,*** bell-p., ***bry.,*** calc., ***rhus-t., ruta.,*** thuj.

LACERATIONS, (see Wounds) - arist-cl., arn., **CALEN., CARB-AC.,** ***ham.,*** **HYPER.,** led., staph., sul-ac., symph.

LIFTING, straining of muscles and tendons, from - ***agn.,*** alum., ambr., **ARN.,** bar-c., ***bell-p., bov.,*** **BRY., CALC.,** calc-f., calc-p., ***calc-s.,*** calc-sil., **CARB-AN.,** calen., ***carb-v., caust.,*** chin., ***cocc.,*** coloc., ***con.,*** croc., dulc., ***ferr.,*** ferr-p., ***form.,*** **GRAPH.,** ***hyper.,*** iod., ***kali-c., kalm.,*** lach., ***lyc.,*** merc., ***mill.,*** mur-ac., ***nat-c.,*** nat-m., nit-ac., ***nux-v.,*** olnd., phos., ***ph-ac.,*** plat., podo., rhod., **RHUS-T., RUTA,** sep., **SIL.,** spig., stann., staph., stront-c., sulph., sul-ac., thuj., valer.
- arms, of - rhus-t., sul-ac.
- children - bor., calc-p.
- debility, causes great - **CARB-AN.**
- easily - **GRAPH.**
- headache, from - ambr., ***arn.,*** bar-c., ***bry., calc.,*** cocc., ***graph., lyc., nat-c.,*** nux-v., ***ph-ac.,*** **RHUS-T.,** ***sil.,*** sulph., valer.
- hernia, in general - cocc., ***nux-v.,*** sulph.
- overlifting, agg. - agn., ambr., carb-v., graph., sep.
- prolapsus uteri - aur., bell., **NUX-V.,** sep.
- reaching high - sulph.
- tendency to strain in lifting - arn., bry., ***calc.,*** carb-v., con., graph., lyc., ***nat-c.,*** nat-m., psor., ***rhus-t.,*** **SIL.,** ***symph.***

LIGHTNING strike, after - arn., crot-h., hell., lach., morph., nux-v., op., ***phos.***

LOCKJAW, (see Tetanus)

LUNGS, collapsed, atelectasis - **ANT-T.,** ***hyos.***

MENTAL, symptoms from injuries - acon., arn., calc-p., cic., ***glon.,*** hell., ***hyper.,*** mag-c., **NAT-S.,** ***stram.***

MOTION, sickness, riding in a car, bus or train, while - bor., ***calc., calc-p.,*** **COCC.,** ***cycl., hep., iris, lyc., mag-c.,*** naja, ***nux-m., nux-v.,*** **PETR.,** sel., **SEP.,** sulph., ***tab., ther.,*** zinc.
- nausea, with - ***carb-ac.,*** **COCC.,** colch., **CON., EUPH-C.,** ***glon.,*** hyos., ***kali-bi., kreos.,*** lac-ac., nat-m., **NUX-V., PETR.,** sanic., ***sep., staph.,*** **TAB.,** ther.
- vomiting while riding in carriage, car etc. - ars., bell., **CARB-AC., COCC.,** ***colch., ferr.,*** ferr-p., glon., ***hyos.,*** nux-m., **PETR.,** phos., sec., ***sil.,*** staph., sulph., **TAB.**

MOUNTAIN, sickness (see Altitude, sickness)

MUSHROOM, poisoning - ***absin.,*** agar., ***ars.,*** atro., ***bell.,*** camph., pyrog.

MUSCLES, cramps - ***ars.,*** **BELL., CALC.,** calc-s., camph., ***caust., cocc.,*** **COLOC., CUPR.,** ***dios., dulc., hyos., ign., kali-c.,*** kali-p., ***lyc.,*** **MAG-P.,** nat-m., nux-v., ***rhus-t., sep., sil.,*** staph., ***sulph.,*** tarent., ***verat., zinc.***
- injuries, soft parts - **ARN.,** bell-p., calc., ***calen.,*** cham., **CON.,** dulc., euphr., ham., hyper., lach., ***nat-c.,*** nat-m., phos., ***puls.,*** **RHUS-T.,** samb., sulph., ***sul-ac., symph.***
- tears or rupture of - ***calen.***

NAILS, injuries, fingernails - all-c., **ARN.,** calen., **HYPER.,** ***led.,*** rhus-t., sep.
- crushed, and lacerated fingernails - arist-cl., ***carb-ac.,*** **HYPER.,** ***led., ruta.***
- hangnail - ***calc.,*** lyc., ***merc.,*** **NAT-M.,** ***rhus-t.,*** sabad., sep., ***sil., stann.,*** **SULPH.,** ***thuj.***
  - inflamed - kali-chl.
  - painful - sel., stann.
- splinter of glass, from - calen., hyper., ***sil.***

NAUSEA, severe - all-c., ant-c., arg-n., ***ars., cadm-s., camph.,*** cocc., **CROT-H.,** ***dig.,*** ferr-p., hell., **IP., LOB.,** ***med., nux-v.,*** puls., **TAB.**
- vomiting, does not amel. - ***dig.,*** **IP.,** sang.
  - inability to - **NUX-V.**

NECK, injuries - ***arn.,*** bell-p., **BRY.,** ***calc.,*** calc-f., caust., cic., **HYPER.,** mez., ***nat-s.,*** **RHUS-T.,** ***ruta, symph.***
- brachial, neuralgia - acon., all-c., bell-p., **BRY.,** calc-f., cham., **HYPER.,** ***kalm.,*** merc., nux-v., ***rhus-t.,*** ruta., sulph., verat.
- spine, concussion, of - arn., mez., nat-s.
- whiplash - arn., **BRY.,** bell-p., ***calc.,*** caust., cic., **HYPER., RHUS-T.,** ***ruta.***

NERVES, injuries - all-c., bell-p., bry., **CALEN.,** ***coff., cur.,*** glon., **HYPER.,** led., ***mag-p.,*** meny., nit-ac., ***phos.,*** tarent., ter., ther., xan.
- ailments from - ***calen., hyper.,*** meny., xan.
- great pain, with - ***all-c.,*** arn., bell-p., bry., ***calen.,*** ceph., ***coff., cur.,*** glon., **HYPER.,** led., ***mag-p.,*** meny., ph-ac., ***phos.,*** tarent., ther., xan.
- jerking in muscles, with - ***hyper.***
- lacerated, with pains excruciating - ***hyper.***
- neuritis - calen., hyper., ***stram.***
- soreness, with - ***hyper.***

NEWS, shock from bad - ***apis,*** **CALC.,** calc-p., chin., cinnb., cupr., dros., form., **GELS., IGN.,** kali-c., kali-p., lach., lyss., ***med., nat-m.,*** nat-p., paeon., ***pall.,*** phos., puls., stram., ***sulph.***

NIGHTMARE, frightening dreams - **ACON.,** arn., ars., ***bapt.,*** bell., ***bor., bry.,*** bufo, **CALC.,** ***cann-i., carc., cham.,*** chel., cina, ***con.,*** dig., elaps, ***ferr.,*** ferr-p., gels., hep., ign., kali-ar., kali-c., lyc., mag-m., ***nat-c.,*** nat-m., ***nit-ac., nux-v.,*** **OP., PHOS.,** puls., rhus-t., ruta., ***sil.,*** **SULPH.,** tell., ter., thuj., ***tub.,*** valer.

NOSE, injuries - arn., bell-p., ham., led., mill., phos.

NOSEBLEED, blow, from a - acet-ac., **ARN.,** ***elaps,*** ferr-p., ***ham.,*** **MILL.,** phos., ***sep.***
- children, in - bell., calc., chin-s., ***croc.,*** **FERR., FERR-P.,** ***ham.,*** merc., nat-n., **PHOS.,** ***sil., ter.***
- fever, during - bry., carb-v., ***ferr-p.,*** ham., meli., phos.

ORGANS, injury, to internal - arn., ***bell-p., mill.***

OVEREXERTION - **ARN.,** ***ars., ham., mill., rhus-t.***

PAIN, (see Generals, Pain)

anxiety, from the - **ACON., ARS.,** carb-v., caust., kali-ar., ***nat-c.,*** **PHOS.**

despair, with the - acon., **ARS., AUR.,** aur-ar., calc., carb-v., ***cham., chin.,*** chin-ar., ***coff.,*** colch., hyper., lach., lil-t., mag-c., nux-v., stram., ***verat.,*** vip.

faintness, from - apis, asaf., **CHAM.,** ***cocc.,*** coloc., ***hep.,*** **IGN.,** ***nux-m., nux-v.,*** phyt., ***valer.,*** verat.

screaming, with the - **ACON.,** ***ars.,*** **BELL., CACT., CHAM., COFF.,** ***coloc.,*** kali-n., mag-c., mag-m., mag-p., op., **PLAT.,** puls.

unbearable - **ACON.,** ***ars.,*** **CHAM., COFF., HEP.,** ign., ***hyper., phyt., pip-m.***

violent behaviour, from pain - **AUR., CHAM., HEP.**

weakness, from - ***arg-m.,*** **ARS.,** carb-v., hura, kali-p., ***ph-ac.,*** plb., ***rhus-t., sil.***

PAINLESSNESS, of complaints, usually painful - **ARN.,** ***hell.,*** **OP., STRAM.**

PANTING, breathing - **ACON.,** anac., ***ant-t., apoc.,*** arg-n., ***arn.,*** ars., bufo, calad., camph., ***carb-an.,*** **CARB-V.,** caul., cham., chin., chlor., ***cina, cocc.,*** con., cop., ferr., hyos., ***ip.,*** jatr., kali-bi., ***lyc.,*** laur., ***nit-ac., nux-m.,*** op., **PHOS.,** ***phyt.,*** plan., plb., prun., sec., ***sil., spong.,*** stram., ***tarent.,*** **VERAT-V.**

ascending stairs - arn., **CALC.,** ***carb-v.,*** plan., phos., sil.

motion, on - tarent.

reading, when - nit-ac.

running rapidly, as from - hyos.

stooping, on - nit-ac.

waking, on - kali-bi., rad-br.

walking, rapidly - sil.

POISON, oak or ivy - agar., am-c., **ANAC.,** arn., ***bry.,*** **CLEM., CROT-T.,** cupr., ***graph., grin.,*** kali-s., led., lob., ***nuph.,*** plan., **RHUS-T.,** ***sang., sep.,*** sulph.

POISONING, general (see Toxicity, chapter)

PTOMAINE poisoning, ailments from - absin., acet-ac., all-c., ***ars.,*** camph., carb-an., carb-v., crot-h., ***cupr-ar.,*** gunp., kreos., lach., puls., ***pyrog.,*** urt-u., ***verat.***

PUNCTURE, wounds (see Splinters, Stab) - **APIS,** aran., arn., **CALEN.,** ***carb-v.,*** cic., hep., **HYPER.,** lach., **LED., NIT-AC.,** phase., ***plan.,*** plb., sil., sul-ac., sulph.

awls, rat bites, nails, etc., particularly if wounded parts feel cold to touch and to patient - **LED.**

brain, of - calen., ***hyper.***

injection, from painful - ***crot-h.,*** **HYPER.,** ***led.***

lumbar puncture, after - **HYPER.**

nails or splinters in feet - ***hyper.***

needles, from - ***hyper., led.,*** sil.

nervous tissues, of - ***hyper.***

pain, severe - **HYPER.**

palms and soles, of - **HYPER., LED.**

PUNCTURE, wounds

sore, feel very, from nails, needles, pins, splinters, rat bites, etc., to prevent lockjaw - **HYPER.**

RABIES, hydrophobia - acet-ac., aconin., agar., agav-a., anag., anan., ant-c., arg-n., ars., ***aspar.,*** **BELL.,** calc., cann-i., ***canth.,*** cedr., chlol., chlor., cocc-s., crot-h., cupr., ***cur.,*** fagu., gua., ho., ***hydr-ac.,*** **HYOS.,** iod., jatr., ***lach.,*** laur., **LYSS.,** merc., nux-v., perh., ***phel., phos.,*** plb., ran-s., ruta, sabad., sant., scut., spirae., **STRAM.,** sulph., tanac., tarent., ter., trach., verat., xan.

cannot hear the word "water" without shudder of fear - ***lyss.***

delirium, wth - ***bell., lyss., stram.***

idea of water causes paroxysm - lyss.

moaning and violent cries alternating with barking - canth.

pregnancy, during - phos.

prophylactic - ***bell.,*** canth., hyos., ***lyss.,*** stram.

screams or howls in a high voice - ***stram.***

RADIATION, sickness, for side effects, of - ars., **CADM-S.,** calc-f., chin., fl-ac., ***ip.,*** nux-v., phos., rad-br., **SOL.,** x-ray.

burns, from - calc-f., fl-ac., phos., rad-br., ***sol.,*** x-ray.

RAPE, victims, of - **ACON.,** anac., **ARN., CARC., IGN.,** lyc., ***med.,*** **NAT-M.,** nux-v., **OP.,** ***plat., sep.,*** **STAPH.,** thuj.

ailments, from - ***carc.,*** ign., nat-m., ***staph.***

image of rapist keeps returning - carc. ***op.,*** staph.

RIDING, horseback, agg. - **ARN.,** ars., ***bell.,*** bell-p., bry., ***graph., lil-t.,*** mag-m., meph., ***nat-c.,*** nat-m., **SEP.,** sil., spig., ***sul-ac.,*** valer.

SACRO-iliac, pain - **AESC.,** ant-t., apis, arg-n., ***arn.,*** bell-p., bry., ***calc-p., cimic.,*** coloc., dios., ferr., gels., hep., hyper., jug-c., nat-p., ol-j., plb., rhus-t., rumx., sabad., spong., sulph., symph., thuj.

SEASICKNESS, with nausea, (see Motion Sickness) - ***carb-ac.,*** **COCC.,** colch., **CON., EUPH-C.,** ***glon.,*** hyos., ***kali-bi., kreos.,*** lac-ac., nat-m., **NUX-V., PETR.,** sanic., ***sep., staph.,*** **TAB.,** ther.

closing eyes, agg. - ther.

amel. - cocc.

nausea, without - kali-p.

sensation as if - tab.

SHOCK, traumatic - ***acet-ac.,*** **ACON.,** ***am-c.,*** **ARN.,** ***ars.,*** bell., ***calc., calen.,*** **CAMPH.,** ***caps.,*** **CARB-V.,** ***cham., chin., chlf., cic.,*** cocc., ***coff., cupr.,*** cupr-ar., **DIG.,** ***gels.,*** hell., hep., ***hydr-ac.,*** hyos., **HYPER.,** ***ip.,*** **LACH.,** ***laur.,*** lyc., merc., ***nat-m.,*** nit-ac., ***nux-m.,*** nux-v., **OP.,** ***phos.,*** psor., ***ran-b.,*** sec., sep., ***staph.,*** stront-c., stry-p., sulph., ***tab.,*** **VERAT.**

mental - ***acon.,*** apis, ***arn.,*** carc., ***gels., ign.,*** mag-c., nit-ac., nux-m., **OP.,** ph-ac., pic-ac.

blood or fluid loss, from - ***carb-v., chin.,*** stront-c.

SHOCK, traumatic
fractures, from - acon., ***arn.,*** bry., stront-c.
surgical - acon., arn., **CALEN.,** camph., carb-v., **OP.,** pyrog., ***staph.,*** **STRONT-C.,** verat.

SHOULDERS, injuries - ***arn.,*** calc., bry., ***ferr-m.,*** **RHUS-T., RUTA,** sang., zinc.
straining, after - ***rhus-t.,*** ruta..
rheumatic, lameness, with - ***ferr-m.,*** rhus-t., ruta., sang.

SLOW, breathing - ***acon.,*** am-c., ant-t., ***apis,*** arn., ars., ***asaf.,*** aur., **BELL.,** benz-d-n., ***brom.,*** bry., cact., ***camph.,*** cann-i., ***caps., cast.,*** chin., chin-s., chlol., cic., clem., ***cocc., colch., coloc.,*** con., cop., ***crot-c.,*** crot-h., crot-t., cub., cupr., ***dig., dios.,*** dros., ferr., gad., ***gels., glon., hell., hep., hydr-ac., hyos., hyper., ign., ip., lach., laur., lob-p.,*** lyc., ***merc-c.,*** mez., morph., nit-ac., nux-m., ***nux-v.,*** oena., ***olnd.,*** ox-ac., **OP.,** phase., piloc., plat., plb., phos., ***phyt.,*** sec., ***spong.,*** squil., stram., sul-ac., tab., verat-v.
alternating, with short, during sleep - ign.
with suffocation - cocc.
brain, from concussion of - arn., hell., nat-s., op.
convulsions, during - **OP.**
cough, during - clem.
evening, while lying quiet, agg - con., ferr.
expiration - ant-t., ***arn.,*** apis, bor., lob., ***op., sep.***
during sleep - chin., ign.
inspiration - cham., chin., ***ign.,*** stram.
morning - merc., ***lach.***
night - coloc., ***lach.***
palpitation, during - bell.
sleep, during - acon., chin., **OP.**
walking amel - ***ferr.***
slow, pulse (see Pulse, chapter)

SPINAL, tap, pain after - arn., led., **HYPER.**

SPLEEN, injuries - arn., ***bell-p., cean., mill.***

SPLINTERS, wounds, from (see Punctures) - acon., ***anag., apis,*** **ARN.,** ***bar-c.,*** calen., ***carb-v.,*** **CIC.,** colch., ***hep.,*** **HYPER.,** iod., lach., **LED.,** lob., **MYRIS.,** ***nit-ac.,*** petr., plat., ran-b., **SIL.,** ***staph.,*** sulph.
abscess, under nails from splinter - ***myris.,*** sil.
expulsion of, to promote - anag., **SIL.**
eye, in - **ACON.,** ***calc.,*** **CALEN., HYPER.,** ***sil., sulph.***
panaritium, causes - ***led.***
throbs, ulcerates - bar-c.

SPRAINS, distorsions - ***agn., am-c.,*** **ARN.,** ***asaf.,*** bell., ***bell-p.,*** **BRY., CALC.,** calen., carb-an., carb-v., ***hyper.,*** ign., ***led.,*** lyc., ***mag-aust.,*** **MILL., NAT-C.,** nat-m., nit-ac., nux-v., petr., phos., polyg., puls., **RHUS-T.,** rhus-v., **RUTA,** sep., stront-c., sulph., ***symph.***
ankles and knees, of - arn., bry., **LED., RHUS-T., RUTA.**
lameness of ankles, wrists and knees - rheum, **RHUS-T., RUTA.**

SPRAINS, distorsions
lifting, from - agn.
lifting or stretching - **RHUS-T., RUTA.**
small weight, sprain easily from - ***carb-an.***
muscles, rupture of - ***calen.***
redness, bluish, intense soreness, swelling - **ARN.**
tendency to - nat-c., nat-m., psor., ***sil.,*** **RUTA.**

STAB, wounds (see Punctures) - acet-ac., ***all-c.,*** **APIS,** arn., **CALEN.,** ***carb-v.,*** cic., con., eug., hep., **HYPER.,** lach., **LED.,** nat-m., nit-ac., phase., ***phos.,*** plan., plb., puls., ***rhus-t.,*** sep., sil., ***staph.,*** sul-ac., sulph.
palms and soles, of - **HYPER., LED.**

STINGS, insects, of - acet-ac., acon., am-c., am-caust., ***anthr.,*** ant-c., **APIS,** ***arn.,*** ars., ***bell.,*** bry., bufo, ***calad.,*** camph., ***carb-ac.,*** caust., ***cedr.,*** coloc., ***crot-h., echi., grin.,*** gua., gymne., hydr-ac., **HYPER.,** ip., kali-per., kreos., ***lach.,*** lat-m., **LED.,** merc., mosch., ***nat-m.,*** pulx., pyrog., seneg., sep., sil., sisy., spirae., sulph., sul-ac., tab., tarent., **URT-U.**
bee stings to face, with swelling - **APIS.,** arn., ***carb-ac.,*** **HYPER.,** ***lach.,*** **LED.,** ***nat-m.,*** **URT-U.**
face, with swelling - **APIS.,** ***carb-ac., hyper., lach., led.,*** nat-m., urt-u.
eye - acon., **APIS.,** arn., ***cann-s.***
opacity of cornea - ***cann-s.***
tongue - acon., **APIS.,** arn., bell., merc.
jelly-fish - ***apis,*** hyper., urt-u.
scorpions - led., hyper.
swelling changes color - anthr., led.
wasps - ***acet-ac.,*** apis, carb-ac., hyper., ***led.,*** vesp.
burning - vesp.
yellow jacket, of - apis, hyper., ***led.***

STRAIN, from overexertion (see Lifting) - **arn.,** ***ars.,*** **CALC.,** calc-f., carb-an., carb-v., cocc., ***con., ham.,*** lyc., ***mill.,*** nat-c., ovi-g-p., **RHUS-T., RUTA,** sanic., sil., ter.
easily strained - **CALC.,** ***con., rhus-t., ruta.***
producing great debility - **CARB-AN.**

STRANGLED, victims of being - arn., ars., op.

STROKE, recent, or begining of - ***acon.,*** **ARN.,** ars., ***aster.,*** bar-c., ***bell.,*** calc-f., **COFF.,** ***fl-ac., gels., glon.,*** hyos., ign., kali-n., ***lach., laur., nux-v.,*** **OP.,** ***phos.,*** prim-v., stront-c., ***stront-c.***

SUFFOCATION, (see Asphyxia or Death apparent)

SUICIDAL, acute, depression - ***anac.,*** arg-n., ***ars.,*** **AUR., AUR-M.,** ***calc.,*** carc., caust., cic., crot-h., hell., ***hep., hyos.,*** kali-ar., ***kali-br., lac-d., lach.,*** lil-t., med., meli., ***merc.,*** morph., naja, **NAT-M., NAT-S.,** ***nux-m.,*** phos., plat., ***plb., psor., puls., sep., stram.,*** tarent., thea., thuj., verat., ***zinc.***
pains, from - **AUR.,** bell., lach., ***nux-v.,*** sep.

SUN, exposure, worse from - acon., ***agar.,*** **ANT-C.,** ***arg-m., bar-c., bell.,*** brom., ***bry.,*** cact., calc., cadm-s., ***camph., carb-v.,*** clem., cocc., crot-h., ***euphr.,*** gels., **GLON.,** graph., ign., iod., ip., ***kalm., lach., lyss.,*** mag-m., med., mur-ac., **NAT-C., NAT-M.,** ***nux-v., op.,*** prun., ***psor.,*** **PULS.,** ***sel.,*** **SOL.,** stann., stram., sulph., symph., syph., ***uva., valer.,*** **VERAT.,** verat-v., zinc.
ailments, chronic - nat-c., nat-m., ***sol.***
exertion, from, in - **ANT-C.**
head, congestion from exposure - ***acon., bell., cact., gels., glon.,*** verat-v.
headache, from - ***acon.,*** act-sp., ***agar.,*** aloe, **ANT-C.,** ***arum-t., bar-c.,*** **BELL.,** brom., bruc., **BRY.,** cadm-s., ***calc.,*** calc-s., ***camph.,*** cann-i., ***carb-v.,*** cast-v., ***chim.,*** chin-s., ***cocc.,*** euphr., ***gels.,*** genist., **GLON.,** hipp., hyos., ign., **LACH.,** manc., nat-a., **NAT-C.,** ***nat-m., nux-v.,*** **PULS.,** ***sel.,*** sol., ***stram.,*** syph., ***sulph., ther.,*** valer., zinc.
rashes, dermititis from sun - nat-m., ***sol.***

SUNBURN - acon., ***agar., ant-c., apis.,*** **BELL.,** bry., bufo, calen., ***camph.,*** **CANTH.,** clem., cortiso., euphr., ***hyos.,*** lach., lyc., ***mur-ac., nat-c.,*** op., **PULS.,** rob., sel., **SOL,** sulph., **URT-U.,** ***valer.,*** verat.
face, on - canth., sol., ***thuj.,*** urt-u.
sunburns, easily - nat-m., ***sol.***

SUNSTROKE, (see Sun) - ***acon.,*** agar., **AML-N.,** ***ant-c.,*** apis, arg-m., ***arn., ars.,*** **BELL.,** bry., ***cact., cadm-met., camph., carb-v.,*** crot-h., cyt-l., euph-pi., ***gels.,*** **GLON.,** hydr-ac., hyos., kalm., **LACH.,** lyc., lyss., **NAT-C.,** nat-m., nux-v., ***op.,*** pop-c., rhus-t., **SOL.,** stram., syph., ***ther.,*** thuj., usn., valer., **VERAT.,** ***verat-v.***
chronic effects - nat-c.
sleeping in sun, from - acon., ***bell.***

SURGERY, complications, from - acet-ac., ***acon.,*** all-c., apis., **ARN., BELL-P.,** berb., calc-f., calc-p., **CALEN.,** camph., ***carb-v., chin., chlf.,*** croc., echi., ferr-p., ham., hyper., kali-s., led., merc., mill., naja., nit-ac., nux-v., ***op.,*** ph-ac., ***phos., piloc.,*** pop., raph., rhus-t., ruta., **STAPH.,** ***stront-c.,*** sul-ac., verat., zinc.
adhesions, after - calc-f., calen., carc., sil., thiosin.
anesthesia, problems from - ***acet-ac.,*** am-c., am-caust., aml-n., ***carb-v., chlf.,*** hep., **PHOS.**
bleeding, after - calen., ***phos.***
cancer, for - ***coca***
colic, in lithotomy or ovariotomy - ***staph.***
fistula, operation of, after - berb., calc., calc-p., calen., caust., graph., sil., sulph., thuj.
gallbladder surgery, after removed, agg. - **CHIN.,** lyc.
healthy granulations, to promote, and to prevent or arrest gangrene - **CALEN.**
hernia, for pain in abdomen, after - ***hyper.***

SURGERY, complications, from
inflammation, from - acon., ***anthr.,*** arn., ars., ars-i., ***bell.,*** bell-p., calc-s., **CALEN.,** echi., gunp., ***hep.,*** hyper., iod., merc-c., merc-i-r., myrt-c., ***pyrog.,*** rhus-t., ***sil., staph.***
intestines, paralysis after laparotomy - ***op.***
joints, to - bry., calen., hyper.
mastectomy, after - calen., bell-p., x-ray.
orifices, on - calen., coloc., ***staph.***
sensitive, wounds painfully, fever - ***acon.***
skin is drawn tight over the wound, when - kali-p.
stretching of tissues, with - staph.
wounds, of - **CALEN.,** ***staph.***

SWELLING, from injuries - acon., ***apis., arn.,*** bell., bry., ***led.,*** nux-v., puls., rhus-t., sulph., sul-ac.

SYNOVITIS, joints - ***apis,*** bell., ***bry.,*** calc., caust., ferr-p., iod., kali-c., kali-i., led., lyc., merc., phyt., puls., rhus-t., sep., sil., sulph., verat-v.

TEETH, general
abscess, of roots - am-c., arn., ***bar-c.,*** bell-p., calc., calc-f., canth., caust., euph., ***hecla.,*** **HEP.,** lach., ***lyc.,*** **MERC.,** merc-i-f., petr., phos., plb., **PYROG., SIL.,** sulph., zinc.
dry, socket - plan., ruta.
extraction, bleeding, after - arn., calen., ferr-p., ***phos.***
pain, after - arn., ***hyper.,*** staph.
filling, pain, after - **ARN.,** hyper., merc., ***merc-i-f.,*** **NUX-V.,** sep.
nerve, exposed, as if - ***cham.,*** coff., ***hyper., kalm.***
injuries to from dental work - **HYPER.**
toothache, neuralgic, pain - **BELL.,** bor., ***carb-s.,*** **CHAM.,** ***chel.,*** chlol., cimic., **COFF.,** ***coloc.,*** gels., hyper., ***iris, kali-p.,*** **MAG-P.,** ***nux-m., plan., phyt.,*** rhod., ***sil.***

TENDONS, injuries - arn., ***anac., arg-m.,*** calen., **RHUS-T., RUTA.**
lumps and nodes after - ruta.
rupture of - rhus-t.
tendonitis - anac., ant-c., ***rhod., rhus-t.***

TETANUS, lockjaw - absin., acet-ac., ***acon.,*** act-sp., aeth., agar., alum., alumn., ambro., aml-n., amyg., anan., ***ang.,*** anthr., ant-t., ***arg-n.,*** arn., ars., art-v., aster., aur., aur-m-n., bapt., **BELL.,** bry., bufo, calc., ***calen., camph.,*** cann-i., ***canth.,*** carb-s., cast-eq., ***caust., cedr.,*** cham., chin-s., chlf., **CIC.,** cina, cob., ***cocc.,*** colch., con., ***crot-c.,*** crot-h., ***cupr., cupr-ac.,*** cur., dig., dios., dulc., ***gels., glon., hep.,*** hydr-ac., ***hyos.,*** **HYPER.,** ign., iod., ***ip.,*** kali-br., lach., ***laur.,*** **LED.,** ***lyc.,*** lyss., mag-p., mang., ***merc.,*** merc-c., merc-i-f., morph., ***mosch.,*** naja, ***nux-m.,*** **NUX-V.,** ***oena.,*** **OP.,** ox-ac., ***passi.,*** ph-ac., phos., phys., ***plan.,*** phyt., ***plat., plb.,*** podo., puls., rhus-t., ***sec.,*** sil., sol-n., spong., staph., ***stram.,*** **STRY.,** sulph., tab., tarent., ter., ther., ***upa., verat.,*** verat-v., vip., zinc-m.
injuries, after - all-c., ***hyper., led.,*** plan.

TETANUS, lockjaw
preventive, for - **ARN., HYPER., LED.,** phys., tetox., thuj.

TRAVELING, ailments from (see Jet lag) - alum., arn., ***cocc.,*** con., gels.

ULCERS, inflamed - **ACON.,** agn., ant-c., arn., **ARS.,** asaf., bar-c., ***bell.,*** bor., bov., ***bry., calc.,*** caust., ***cham.,*** cina, cinnb., cocc., colch., con., croc., cupr., dig., **HEP.,** hyos., ign., kreos., ***lac-c., lach.,*** led., ***lyc.,*** mang., **MERC.,** mez., nat-c., ***nat-m.,*** nat-p., ***nit-ac.,*** nux-v., petr., **PHOS.,** plb., ***puls.,*** ran-b., ***rhus-t.,*** ruta., sars., sep., **SIL.,** ***staph., sulph.,*** thuj., verat., zinc.
gangrenous - am-c., ***anthr.,*** **ARS.,** ***asaf., bapt.,*** bism., ***carb-v., chin., cinnb., con., crot-c., crot-h.,*** euph., ***kali-bi.,*** kali-p., ***kreos.,*** **LACH., LYC.,** mill., ***mur-ac.,*** rhus-t., sabin., ***sars.,*** **SEP.,** ***sil.,*** squil., sul-ac.
varicose, veins - ant-t., anac., ***ars., calc.,*** calen., ***carb-v., card-m.,*** **CAUST.,** cinnb., crot-h., ***fl-ac.,*** graph., grin., ham., hydr., kreos., ***lach.,*** **LYC.,** merc., mez., **PULS.,** pyrog., ***rhus-t.,*** sars., sec., ***sil., sulph.,*** sul-ac., thuj., ***zinc.***

UNCONSCIOUSNESS, (see Coma)

UTERUS, injuries, bleeding, from - ***arn., bell-p.,*** cinnam., ***mill.,*** phos., puls., ***rhus-t.,*** ruta., ***sec.,*** sulph.

VACCINATIONS, acute reactions (see Generals, chapter) - acon., apis., arn., bell., calen., cic., echni., hep., **HYPER., LED.,** plan., pyrog., thuj.,
preventive, for side effects - **HYPER., LED.,** sil., sulph., ***thuj.,*** vario.

VIOLENT, rage - agar., ***anac.,*** **BELL., HYOS., LACH.,** nux-v., **STRAM.**

VOMITING, violent - aeth., ant-t., apoc., **ARS.,** ars-i., bell., bism., **CARC.,** ***cic., cina,*** **COLCH.,** con., **CROT-T.,** ***cupr.,*** dig., ***ferr.,*** ferr-p., ***iod.,*** **IP.,** ***jatr.,*** kali-n., lach., lob., merc., mez., mosch., **NUX-V., PHOS.,** ***plb.,*** raph., **TAB., VERAT.**
nausea, without - ant-c., chel., lyc.
relief, without - ant-c., ip.

WOUNDS, general (see Cuts, Punctures, Stab) - anag., ***apis,*** arist-cl., ***arn., ars.,*** bell-p., bor., bor-ac., bov., bry., bufo, calc-p., **CALEN.,** carb-ac., carb-v., cham., cic., cist., con., croc., ***echi.,*** erig., ery-a., eup-per., ferr-p., ham., helia., hell., hep., **HYPER.,** iod., kali-p., kreos., ***lach., lappa-a.,*** **LED.,** merc., mez., mill., nat-c., nat-m., nit-ac., ph-ac., ***phos.,*** phys., plan., plb., ***puls.,*** **PYROG.,** rhus-t., ruta, sec., senec., seneg., sil., ***staph.,*** stront-c., sulph., ***sul-ac.,*** symph., zinc.
atrophy, of - ***form.***
black - ***chin., lach.,*** led., trach., vip.
bleeding, freely - ***acon.,*** am-c., ant-t., aran., ***arn.,*** ars., asaf., bell-p., bor., both., ***calen., carb-v.,*** caust., cench., ***chin.,*** clem., con., ***cop.,*** croc., ***crot-h., dor.,*** eug., ***euphr.,*** ferr., ***ferr-p.,*** ham., ***hydr., kreos.,*** **LACH., LAT-M.,** led., merc., mez., **MILL.,** ***nat-c.,*** nat-m., **NIT-AC.,** ***nux-m., nux-v., ph-ac.,*** **PHOS.,**

WOUNDS, general
bleeding, freely - plb., puls., rhus-t., ruta, sec., sep., sil., ***staph.,*** sul-ac., ***sulph.,*** vip., ***zinc.***
edges, from closed - ***mill.***
suppurate, and - phos.
bleed much, slight wounds - ***hydr., kreos., lach.,*** **PHOS.,** sec.
black blood - vip.
fall, after - ***arn.,*** ham., ***mill.***
small wounds - am-c., carb-v., hydr., kreos., lach., ph-ac., phos., sul-ac., ***zinc.***
bloody, open, and serous infiltrations of cellular tissues - calen.
bluish - ***apis, lach., led.,*** lyss., ***vip.***
boots, from tight - paeon.
break, and heal again - ***calen.,*** carb-v., phos.
burning - ***acon.,*** arn., ***ars.,*** bry., ***carb-v.,*** caust., hyper., merc., mez., nat-c., nat-m., rhus-t., ***sul-ac., sulph.,*** urt-u., zinc.
chronic, effects - ***arn.,*** carb-v., **CALEN.,** con., glon., hep., ***hyper., iod., lach.,*** **LED.,** nat-m., ***nat-s., nit-ac., phos.,*** puls., rhus-t., ***staph., stroph., sul-ac.,*** zinc.
cold, part becomes - ***led.***
cold to touch, parts feel, and to patient - **LED.**
corrosive, gnawing - mez.
crushed - arn., con., hyper., ruta, staph.
and lacerated finger ends - arist-cl., ***carb-ac.,*** **HYPER.,** ***led., ruta.***
crusts, hard yellow, healing - hyper.
cutting, burning, stinging pain - ***calen.,*** nat-c.
deep - bell-p., calen., hyper., led., staph.
depression, mental after - ***hyper.***
dissecting - ***anthr., apis,*** **ARS., CALEN.,** crot-h., ***echi.,*** ham., hyper., kreos., **LACH.,** led., **PYROG.,** ***ter.***
gangrenous, become - anthr., **ARS., LACH.**
pyaemia, hectic fever - ***crot-h.***
easily, wounded - phos., ***syph.***
fainting, cause - chin., ign., verat.
falling, height, from - ***arn., mill.***
fester - ***anthr., apis, ars.,*** calen., echi., led., pyrog.
fever, with - calen., ***pyrog.***
gangrenous - acon., am-c., ***anthr.,*** **ARS.,** ***bell., brom.,*** calen., ***carb-v., chin., eucal.,*** euph., **LACH.,** sal-ac., ***sec., sil.,*** sul-ac., trach., vip., vip-a.
gaping - calen., hyper.
granulations, proud flesh - alum., ***alumn., anac., ant-t.,*** **ARS.,** bell-p., ***calc.,*** **CALEN.,** carb-v., caust., crot-h., cund., **FL-AC., GRAPH.,** hep., hydr., hyper., iod., ***kali-m.,*** kreos., ***lach., merc.,*** nit-ac., nux-v., phos., phyt., psor., rhus-t., ***sabin.,*** **SIL.,** sul-ac., sulph., thiosin., thuj., tub., vip.
green, skin around - ***lach.***
greenish - senec.
heal, do not - all-c., calen., carc., sil.
with difficulty and easily suppurate - sil.

WOUNDS, general
inflammation, of - ***acon.***, arn., calc-f., ***calen.***, ***cham.***, ***con.***, hyper., kali-bi., lach., led., nat-m., plb., ***puls.***, ***rhus-t.***, ***sul-ac.***, ***sulph.***, vip.
lead, colored skin around the - ***lach.***, vip.
leeches - alum.
little, pains terribly - colch.
lymphatics, redness and swelling along course of - ***bufo.***
maggoty - ***calen.***
mental, effects - cic., ***glon.***, hyper., mag-c., ***nat-s.***
offensive - ***calen.***, ***pyrog.***
old, wounds - ***calen.***, ceph., symph.
neglected - ***calen.***
suppuration threatens - calen., ***sil.***
pains, in - ***calen.***, ceph., kali-i., sil., symph.
painful again, become - eug.
reopen and bleed - ***phos.***
painful - ***all-c.***, am-c., ***anthr.***, ***apis***, arist-cl., ***arn.***, bell., calc., calc-f., **CALEN.**, cham., con., croc., crot-h., eug., ***hep.***, **HYPER.**, led., nat-c., ***nat-m.***, ***nit-ac.***, nux-v., ***ph-ac.***, **STAPH.**, sulph.
as if bruised, in morning - calen.
open - ***hyper.***
picking at it - calen.
proud flesh, stinging, purplish - ***lach.***
suppuration, before - ***hyper.***
pains, returning - glon., kali-i., nat-m., ***nat-s.***, ***nit-ac.***, nux-v.
pelvic, organs, of - bell-p.
poisoned - ars., cist.
poisonous plants, from - echi.
pulsating - ***bell.***, ***cham.***, clem., ***hep.***, ***merc.***, mez., ***puls.***, ***sulph.***
raw - calc., calen.
painful, as if beaten - calc.
red, surroundings look - calen.
and bluish, around - ***lach.***
reactionless - ars., camph., carb-v., con., laur., op., ph-ac., sulph.
reopening, of old - asaf., **CALEN.**, ***carb-v.***, ***caust.***, ***croc.***, crot-h., fl-ac., ***glon.***, ***graph.***, kreos., ***lach.***, nat-c., ***nat-m.***, ***nit-ac.***, ***nux-v.***, ***op.***, **PHOS.**, ***sil.***, ***sulph.***, ***vip.***
scars, old, - asaf., ***bor.***, calc-p., calen., ***carb-an.***, carb-v., ***caust.***, con., croc., ***crot-h.***, fl-ac., glon., ***iod.***, ***lach.***, nat-c., ***nat-m.***, **PHOS.**, **SIL.**, sulph., ***vip.***
salt, sprinkled on, as if - sars.
scurfiness, with - ***calen.***, ***carb-ac.***, ***hyper.***
septic - ***anthr.***, ***apis***, **ars.**, **CALEN.**, ***crot-h.***, ***echi.***, ham., ***hyper.***, kreos., ***lach.***, led., **PYROG.**, ***ter.***
slight, wounds, agg. - valer., verat.
slow, to heal - ***all-c.***, alum., alum-p., alum-sil., am-c., ars., ***bar-c.***, ***bor.***, both., ***calc.***, calc-s., **CALEN.**, ***carb-v.***, **CARC.**, caust., ***cham.***, chel., clem., con., cortiso., croc., crot-h., echi., ***graph.***, ***gunp.***, hell., **HEP.**, hyper., kali-c.,

WOUNDS, general
slow, to heal - kreos., **LACH.**, lyc., lyss., mag-c., mang., ***merc.***, ***merc-c.***, mur-ac., nat-c., **NIT-AC.**, nux-v., **PETR.**, ph-ac., phos., plb., puls., psor., ***rhus-t.***, sars., sep., **SIL.**, squil., ***staph.***, **SULPH.**, ***tub.***, x-ray.
small, wounds bleed much - am-c., phos.
smarting - calen.
spasms begin in wound - ***led.***
stinging, in - acon., **APIS**, arn., bar-c., bell., bry., ***calen.***, caust., chin., clem., ***led.***, merc., mez., nat-c., ***nit-ac.***, sep., sil., ***staph.***, sulph.
fever, during - calen.
suppurating - arn., asaf., ***bell.***, bor., ***bufo***, ***calc.***, calc-f., **CALC-S.**, ***calen.***, caust., ***cham.***, ***chin.***, ***croc.***, echi., **HEP.**, ign., lach., led., ***merc.***, ***nat-m.***, plb., ***puls.***, **SIL.**, ***sulph.***, syph., vip-a.
excessive - bufo, calc-s., ***sil.***
suppurate, do not heal - calc., ***sil.***
throbbing, lancinating - bufo.
swelling, of - acon., ***arn.***, ***bell.***, ***bry.***, kali-m., nux-v., ***puls.***, ***rhus-t.***, sul-ac., ***sulph.***, vip.
twitching - led.
ulcerate and spread, small wounds - petr.
become very sore - bar-c.
yellow, skin around - ***lach.***

WRIST, injuries - ***arn.***, ***bry.***, ***calc.***, **HYPER.**, ***rhus-t.***, **RUTA.**, sil., ***stront.***

WRITER'S, cramp - brach., cupr., cycl., **MAG-P.**, **STANN.**, ruta, tril.

Environment

AIR, general

cold, agg. - ***abrot.,*** **ACON.,** ***aesc.,*** **AGAR., ALL-C.,** ***alum.,*** alum-p., alum-sil., ***alumn.,*** am-br., ammc., ***am-c.,*** anac., ant-c., apis, apoc., ***aran.,*** arn., **ARS.,** ars-i., ars-s-f., ***asar.,*** astac., **AUR.,** aur-a., aur-s., bac., **BAD.,** ***bapt.,*** **BAR-C.,** ***bar-m.,*** bar-s., ***bell.,*** bor., bov., brom., ***bry.,*** bufo, cadm-s., **CALC., CALC-P.,** calc-sil., calen., **CAMPH.,** canth., caps., ***carb-ac., carb-an., carb-s., carb-v., carl.,*** **CAUST.,** cham., chin., chin-a., cic., **CIMIC.,** cina, **CIST.,** clem., ***coc-c., coca, cocc.,*** coff., ***colch., coloc., con.,*** cupr., cur., ***cycl., dig.,*** **DULC.,** ***elaps, ferr.,*** ferr-ar., ferr-p., fl-ac., ***graph.,*** ham., **HELL., HEP.,** ***hyos.,*** **HYPER.,** ***ign.,*** ind., ***ip.,*** **KALI-AR.,** ***kali-bi.,*** **KALI-C.,** kali-m., kali-p., ***kreos., lac-d.,*** lach., lappa-a., lat-m., laur., **LYC.,** lycps., lyss., ***mag-c.,*** mag-m., **MAG-P.,** ***mang.,*** med., meny., ***merc., merc-i-r.,*** mez., **MOSCH.,** mur-ac., ***nat-a.,*** nat-c., nat-m., ***nat-p.,*** nat-sil., nit-ac., nit-s-d., **NUX-M., NUX-V.,** ***osm.,*** par., ***petr., ph-ac., phos.,*** phys., physal., ***plan.,*** plat., plb., psil., **PSOR.,** ptel., ***puls.,*** **RAN-B., RHOD., RHUS-T., RUMX.,** ruta, **SABAD.,** samb., sars., sel., senec., seneg., **SEP., SIL.,** sol-n., spig., spong., squil., staph., stram., **STRONT-C.,** ***sulph., sul-ac., sumb., tarent., thuj.,*** tub., urt-u., ***verat., verat-v.,*** verb., viol-o., viol-t., visc., ***zinc.,*** zinc-p., ***zing.***

amel. - ***acon.,*** aesc., aeth., ***all-c.,*** aloe, ***alum.,*** am-m., ambr., ***aml-n.,*** anac., anan., ang., ***ant-c.,*** ant-t., ***apis,*** aran., ***arg-n.,*** asaf., ***asar.,*** bar-c., bell-p., beryl., ***bry., bufo,*** cact., calad., calc., cann-i., ***carb-v.,*** cham., ***chin.,*** cina, cit-v., clem., ***coc-c.,*** coca, ***colch.,*** com., conv., crat., croc., dig., dios., ***dros.,*** dulc., euon-a., euph., euphr., foll., gels., ***glon.,*** iber., ign., ip., kali-bi., ***led.,*** luf-op., meph., merc., nep., ***nit-ac.,*** nux-v., ***op.,*** pituin., psil., rad-br., rauw., ***sel.,*** seneg., stront-c., tere-ch., teucr., thuj., tub., tub-r., visc.

aversion to cold air - am-c., ***aran., ars.,*** bart., bell., bry., ***calc.,*** caps., caust., ***cham.,*** chin., graph., grat., ***hep., kali-c.,*** nat-c., nat-m., nux-m., ***nux-v., petr.,*** sel., ***sil.,*** sulph., tub.

desire for cold air - achy., aloe, ***apis,*** arg-n., asaf., asar., ***aur.,*** camph., carb-v., cic., ***croc.,*** gran., ***iod.,*** kali-s., lil-t., ***puls., sec.,*** sul-i., sulph.

inspiring of agg. - aesc., alum., ***am-c.,*** ant-c., ***ars., aur., bell., bry., calc.,*** camph., **CAUST.,** cham., ***cimic.,*** cina, cist., dulc., ***hep.,*** hydr., **HYOS.,** ***ign.,*** kali-bi., ***kali-c.,*** **MERC.,** mosch., nat-m., ***nux-m.,*** **NUX-V.,** par., petr., phos., psor., ***rumx.,*** ruta, sel., seneg., sep., ***stront-c.,*** syph.

draft, of, agg. - acon., alum., anac., ***ars.,*** ars-s-f., **BELL.,** benz-ac., bov., brom., ***bry.,*** cadm-s., **CALC.,** calc-f., **CALC-P.,** ***calc-s.,*** calc-sil.,

AIR, general

draft, of, agg. - camph., ***canth., caps.,*** carb-an., ***carb-s., caust.,*** cench., ***cham., chin., cist.,*** cocc., colch., coloc., crot-h., dulc., ***ferr.,*** gels., ***graph., hep., ign.,*** kali-ar., ***kali-bi.,*** **KALI-C.,** kali-m., kali-n., kali-p., kali-s., kali-sil., lac-c., ***lac-d., lath.,*** led., **LYC.,** ***lyss., mag-c., mag-p., med., merc.,*** mim-p., mur-ac., ***nat-c., nat-m.,*** nat-p., nat-sil., ***nit-ac., nux-m.,*** **NUX-V.,** ***ol-j., petr., ph-ac., phos., psor.,*** **PULS.,** ***ran-b.,*** **RHUS-T.,** ***rumx., sanic.,*** sars., **SEL.,** senec., ***sep.,*** **SIL.,** ***spig., stann., stram.,*** stront-c., **SULPH.,** ***sumb.,*** tep., tub., valer., verb., x-ray, ***zinc.,*** zinc-p.

cold agg., when perspiring - dulc., merc-i-f.

ailments, from - cadm-s., lach.

amel. - ***ars.,*** bry., ***carb-v.,*** lycps., ***rhus-t., sil.***

frosty, agg. - ***agar., calc.,*** caust., ***con.,*** lyc., mag-m., merc., nat-c., nux-v., ph-ac., phos., ***puls.,*** rhus-t., ***sep.,*** sil., sulph., syph.

indoor, agg. - ***acon.,*** **ALUMN.,** am-c., am-m., ***ambr., anac., ang., ant-c., arg-m., arn.,*** ars., ***asaf., asar., aur., bar-c.,*** bell., ***bor., bov.,*** bry., calc., camph., cann-s., canth., caps., carb-an., ***meny.,*** merc., ***mez.,*** mosch., mur-ac., nat-c., ***nat-m.,*** nit-ac., nux-v., ***op., ph-ac., phos., plat., plb.,*** **PULS.,** ***ran-b., ran-s., rhod.,*** rhus-t., ruta, **SABIN.,** ***sars.,*** sel., ***seneg.,*** sep., spig., ***spong., stann.,*** staph., ***stront-c.,*** sul-ac., ***sulph., tarax.,*** thuj., ***verat., verb.,*** viol-t., ***zinc.***

amel. - ***agar.,*** alumn., ***am-c., am-m.,*** ambr., anac., ang., ***ant-c.,*** arn., ars., bar-c., ***bell.,*** bor., bov., bry., ***calad., calc., camph., cann-s., canth., caps.,*** dulc., ***euph., ferr.,*** graph., **GUAI.,** hell., hep., hyos., ***ign.,*** iod., ***ip.,*** kali-c., ***kali-n., kreos.,*** lach., laur., ***led.,*** lyc., mag-c., mag-m., mang., meny., ***merc.,*** mez., ***mosch., mur-ac., nat-c.,*** nat-m., ***nit-ac.,*** **NUX-M., NUX-V.,** oci-s., ***olnd.,*** op., ***petr.,*** ph-ac., phos., plat., plb., puls., ran-b., ***rheum,*** rhod., ***rhus-t., ruta, sabad.,*** sabin., sars., ***sel.,*** seneg., sep., **SIL.,** ***spig.,*** stann., ***staph., stram.,*** stront-c., ***sul-ac.,*** sulph., tarent., ***teucr., thuj., valer.,*** verat., verb., ***viol-t.,*** zinc.

night, agg. - acon., am-c., ***carb-v.,*** **MERC.,** nat-s., nit-ac., ***sulph.***

open, agg. - ***acon., agar.,*** agn., agre., alco., all-c., alum., alumn., ambr., ***am-c.,*** am-m., anac., ang., ant-c., ***ant-t.,*** aran., arg-m., arn., ***ars., ars-s-f.,*** asar., aur., aur-a., aur-s., aza., ***bar-c.,*** bar-m., ***bell.,*** benz-ac., berb., bor., bov., brucin., ***bry.,*** bufo, cact., cadm-s., calad., ***calc.,*** calc-i., ***calc-p., camph.,*** cann-s., canth., ***caps., carb-an.,*** carb-o., carb-s., ***carb-v., caust.,*** cedr., ***cham., chel.,*** **CHIN.,** chin-a., cic., cimic., cina, cist., ***clem.,*** **COCC.,** ***coff.,*** coff-t., colch., ***coloc., con.,*** cor-r., crot-h., crot-t., ***cycl.,*** dig., dros., ***dulc.,*** epip., euph., euphr., ***ferr.,*** ferr-ar., ferr-p., fl-ac., form.,

AIR, general

open, agg. - ***graph.,*** **GUAI.,** ***ham.,*** hell., ***helon.,*** **HEP.,** hyos., ign., iod., ip., ***kali-ar., kali-bi.,*** **KALI-C.,** kali-m., ***kali-n., kali-p.,*** kali-sil., kalm., ***kreos., lach.,*** laur., led., lina., ***lyc.,*** lycpr., ***lyss.,*** mag-arct., mag-c., mag-m., mag-p., ***mang.,*** meny., **MERC.,** ***merc-c.,*** mez., mosch., ***mur-ac.,*** nat-a., ***nat-c.,*** nat-m., nat-p., nat-sil., **NIT-AC., NUX-M., NUX-V.,** olnd., op., par., ***petr., ph-ac., phos.,*** phyt., plat., plb., ***psor.,*** puls., ran-b., rheum, rhod., ***rhus-t.,*** **RUMX.,** ruta, sabad., sabin., sang., sars., ***sel.,*** senec., ***seneg., sep.,*** **SIL.,** ***spig.,*** spong., ***stann.,*** staph., ***stram., stront-c.,*** **SULPH.,** ***sul-ac.,*** tarax., ***teucr.,*** thea., thuj., urt-u., ***valer.,*** verat., verb., viol-o., viol-t., x-ray, ***zinc.***

agg., and house air agg. - ars., aur., iod., mez.

open, amel. - abrot., ***acon.,*** aesc., aeth., agar., ***agn., all-c., aloe,*** **ALUM.,** alum-p., alum-sil., **ALUMN.,** am-c., ambr., ***am-m., aml-n., anac.,*** ang., ange-s., ***ant-c., apis,*** aran., aran-ix., ***arg-m.,*** **ARG-N.,** arist-cl., arn., **ARS.,** ars-i., ars-s-f., ***asaf., asar., atro., aur., aur-i.,*** aur-m., bapt., bar-c., bar-i., bar-s., bell., bor., ***bov., bry.,*** buni-o., ***cact.,*** caj., ***calad.,*** calc., calc-i., ***calc-s., camph.,*** **CANN-I.,** cann-s., canth., ***caps.,*** carb-ac., carb-an., ***carb-s., carb-v.,*** carc., caust., ***chel., chlor.,*** cic., ***cimic.,*** cina, ***cinnb.,*** coca, coc-c., ***coff.,*** colch., coloc., com., ***con.,*** **CROC.,** ***crot-c.,*** culx., dicha., dig., ***dios., dulc.,*** erig., euphr., ferr-i., ***fl-ac.,*** flor-p., ***gamb.,*** gels., glon., ***graph.,*** grat., hed., ***hell.,*** hep., hip-ac., ***hydr-ac., hyos., iber.,*** ign., ind., **IOD.,** ***ip., kali-bi.,*** kali-c., **KALI-I.,** ***kali-n., kali-s., lac-c., lach.,*** lact., laur., ***lil-t., lyc.,*** **MAG-C., MAG-M.,** mag-p., mag-s., mang., **MED.,** ***meli.,*** meny., merc., merc-i-f., merc-i-r., ***mez., mosch.,*** mur-ac., myrt-c., naphtin., nat-c., ***nat-m.,*** **NAT-S.,** nep., nicc., nit-ac., nux-v., op., ***osm.,*** ph-ac., ***phos., phyt.,*** pic-ac., pip-n., pituin., ***plat.,*** plb., pneu., **PSOR.,** ***ptel.,*** **PULS.,** rad-br., ran-b., ***ran-s.,*** rat., rauw., ***rhod.,*** **RHUS-T.,** ruta, **SABAD., SABIN.,** sal-ac., sang., ***sanic.,*** saroth., sars., ***sec.,*** sel., ***seneg., sep.,*** spig., ***spong.,*** stront-c., sul-ac., ***sulph., tab.,*** tarax., ***tarent., tell.,*** thiop., ***thlaspi,*** thuj., tril., **TUB.,** upa., valer., verat., verb., ***vib.,*** viol-t., visc., ***zinc.,*** zinc-p.

mental symptoms, amel. - agar., am-m., bar-c., bar-s., bell., ***bry.,*** calc., ***cann-i.,*** croc., dulc., ***laur.,*** mag-c., mag-m., meny., merc., nat-c., nit-ac., par., ***plat.,*** **PULS.,** ***rhus-t.***

riding in carriage, amel. - arg-n., naja

open, aversion to - agar., alum., **AM-C.,** ***am-m.,*** ambr., anac., ang., aran., arn., ***ars.,*** ars-s-f., aur., **BAPT.,** ***bell., bry.,*** **CALC.,** calc-ar., **CALC-P.,** calc-sil., camph., cann-s., canth., ***caps.,*** carb-an., carb-v., ***caust.,*** **CHAM.,** chel., ***chin.,*** cic., cina, ***cist.,*** **COCC., COFF.,** coloc., ***con., cycl.,*** dig., dros., ***ferr., ferr-ar., graph., guai., helon., hep.,*** **IGN.,** ip., kali-ar.,

AIR, general

open, aversion to - **KALI-C.,** kali-m., kali-n., kali-p., kali-sil., kreos., ***lach.,*** laur., led., ***lyc., lyss.,*** mag-m., mang., meny., ***merc.,*** merc-c., ***mosch.,*** mur-ac., **NAT-C.,** ***nat-m., nat-p.,*** **NAT-SIL.,** nit-ac., ***nux-m.,*** **NUX-V.,** op., **PETR.,** ph-ac., phos., plat., ***plb., psor.,*** puls., rhod., ***rhus-t.,*** **RUMX.,** ruta, sabin., sars., sel., seneg., ***sep.,*** **SIL.,** ***spig.,*** staph., stram., stront-c., ***sul-ac.,*** **SULPH.,** teucr., thuj., tub., valer., verb., ***viol-t.,*** zinc.

alternating with desire for - ars-s-f.

open, desire for - acon., ***agn.,*** all-c., aloe, ***alum.,*** alum-p., alum-sil., am-c., ambr., am-m., aml-n., anac., ang., ange-s., ***ant-c.,*** ant-t., ***apis,*** aran-ix., arg-m., **ARG-N.,** ***arn., ars., ars-i., asaf., asar.,*** aster., **AUR.,** aur-a., ***aur-i.,*** **AUR-M., AUR-S.,** ***bapt., bar-c.,*** bar-i., bar-m., bar-s., bell., ***bor.,*** bov., ***brom., bry.,*** bufo, calc., **CALC-I.,** ***calc-s.,*** cann-s., caps., carb-an., carb-h., ***carb-s.,*** **CARB-V.,** caust., chel., cic., cimic., cina, cit-v., clem., coca, **CROC.,** dig., ***elaps,*** ferr., ***fl-ac.,*** gels., glon., ***graph., hell.,*** hep., hyos., **IOD.,** ***ip.,*** kali-bi., kali-c., **KALI-I.,** kali-n., **KALI-S., LACH.,** lact., laur., ***lil-t.,*** **LYC.,** ***mag-c., mag-m.,*** mang., med., meny., ***mez.,*** mosch., mur-ac., nat-c., ***nat-m., nat-s.,*** op., ph-ac., phos., ***plat.,*** plb., prun., ***ptel.,*** **PULS.,** rad-br., rhod., rhus-t., ruta, ***sabad., sabin., sanic.,*** sars., ***sec.,*** sel., seneg., sep., ***spig.,*** spong., stann., staph., ***stram.,*** sul-ac., sul-i., **SULPH.,** ***tab., tarax., tarent., tell., teucr.,*** thuj., ***tub.,*** tub-r., verat., viol-t., zinc., zinc-p.

but draft agg. - acon., anac., ***ars.,*** bor., ***bry., calc-s.,*** carb-an., ***carb-s., caust., graph.,*** **KALI-C., KALI-S.,** ***lach.,*** **LYC.,** ***mag-c.,*** med., mur-ac., ***nat-c.,*** nat-m., ph-ac., phos., puls., rhus-t., sanic., sars., sep., spig., stram., sulph., zinc.

flatulency, with - kali-i., zinc.

pollution, ailments, from - am-c., ars., carb-v., sil., ***sul-ac.***

seashore, agg. - ***aq-mar., ars.,*** brom., ***carc.,*** iod., kali-i., ***mag-m.,*** mag-s., med., morbill., ***nat-m.,*** nat-s., rhus-t., **SEP.,** syph., ***tub.***

amel. - ***acon., agar.,*** ant-c., ant-t., ***bor.,*** brom., camph., ***carc.,*** eucal., ***hyos., iris,*** lyc., lyss., **MED.,** ***nat-m., op., ox-ac.,*** plat., ***stram., sul-ac., tub.,*** verat.

warm, agg. - agn., ***aloe,*** ambr., anac., ***ant-c., ant-t., arg-n.,*** ars-i., ***asar.,*** aur., aur-i., ***aur-m., bry.,*** calad., calc., calc-i., ***calc-s.,*** cann-s., ***carb-v.,*** cham., cina, ***coc-c.,*** cocc., colch., croc., dros., ***euph., fl-ac.,*** **GLON.,** ign., ***indg.,*** **IOD.,** ***ip.,*** kali-bi., **KALI-S., LACH.,** led., ***lyc.,*** **MERC.,** ***mez., nat-m., nat-s., nit-ac.,*** nux-m., nux-v., ***op., ph-ac.,*** phenob., ***phos., pic-ac.,*** plat., podo., **PULS.,** rhus-t., sabin., sars., ***sec.,*** sel., ***seneg., sep., sul-i., sulph.,*** teucr., thuj., xan.

AIR, general

warm, amel. - ***acon.,*** ***agar.,*** alumn., ***am-c.,*** anac., ant-c., arn., **ARS.,** asar., **AUR.,** ***bar-c.,*** ***bell.,*** bor., ***bov.,*** ***bry.,*** ***calc.,*** **CAMPH.,** canth., ***caps.,*** ***carb-an.,*** ***carb-v.,*** **CAUST.,** ***cham.,*** chin., ***cic.,*** ***cina,*** ***coc-c.,*** coff., ***colch.,*** ***coloc.,*** ***con.,*** dig., **DULC.,** ***ferr.,*** graph., **HELL., HEP.,** ***hyos.,*** ***ign.,*** ip., **KALI-C.,** kreos., lach., laur., led., ***lyc.,*** mag-c., mag-m., mag-p., ***mang.,*** meny., ***merc.,*** ***mez.,*** **MOSCH.,** mur-ac., nat-a., ***nat-c.,*** ***nat-m.,*** nat-s., ***nit-ac.,*** **NUX-M., NUX-V.,** par., ***petr.,*** ***ph-ac.,*** ***phos.,*** psor., ran-b., ***rhod.,*** **RHUS-T.,** ***ruta,*** **SABAD.,** samb., ***sars.,*** ***sel.,*** seneg., ***sep.,*** ***sil.,*** ***spig.,*** ***spong.,*** squil., staph., stram., **STRONT-C.,** sul-ac., ***sulph.,*** thuj., ***verat.,*** verb., viol-t., zinc.

becoming, in open air amel. - ***acon.,*** ***agar.,*** am-c., ant-c., ***arn.,*** **ARS.,** asar., ***aur.,*** ***bar-c.,*** ***bell.,*** ***bor.,*** bov., ***bry.,*** ***calc.,*** ***camph.,*** canth., ***caps.,*** carb-an., carb-v., ***caust.,*** ***cham.,*** ***chin.,*** ***cic.,*** clem., ***coc-c.,*** colch., ***con.,*** dig., ***dulc.,*** ferr., **GRAPH.,** ***hell.,*** ***hep.,*** ***hyos.,*** ***ign.,*** **KALI-C.,** ***kreos.,*** lach., ***lyc.,*** ***mag-c.,*** mag-m., ***mang.,*** meny., ***merc.,*** mez., **MOSCH.,** mur-ac., ***nat-c.,*** nat-m., ***nit-ac.,*** ***nux-m.,*** **NUX-V.,** ***petr.,*** ***ph-ac.,*** ***phos.,*** ran-b., rhod., **RHUS-T.,** ruta, **SABAD.,** samb., ***sars.,*** sel., ***sep.,*** ***sil.,*** spig., ***spong.,*** staph., thuj., ***verat.,*** ***verb.,*** viol-t., zinc.

AUTUMN, agg. in - all-c., ***ant-t.,*** aur., bapt., bar-m., bry., ***calc.,*** calc-p., ***chin.,*** cic., **COLCH.,** ***coloc.,*** **DULC.,** ***graph.,*** hed., hep., ign., iris, **KALI-BI., LACH.,** ***merc.,*** merc-c., nat-m., ***nat-s.,*** nux-v., rhod., **RHUS-T.,** ***stram.,*** ***verat.***

ailments since - kali-bi.

amel. - flav.

BAROMETER, sensitive to changes of - ***dulc.,*** merc., nat-c., ***phos.,*** ***rhod.***

CHANGE of weather

agg. - abrot., achy., acon., alum., alumn., ***am-c.,*** anh., ant-c., ***ant-t.,*** apis, aran., ars., asar., bar-c., ***bell.,*** benz-ac., bor., brom., **BRY.,** ***calc.,*** calc-f., ***calc-p.,*** carb-v., carb-s., ***caust.,*** ***cham.,*** ***chel.,*** chin., cinnb., colch., crot-c., crot-h., cupr., cur., ***dig.,*** **DULC.,** euph., galph., ***gels.,*** ***graph.,*** harp., ***hep.,*** hyper., ***ip.,*** kali-bi., ***kali-c.,*** kali-i., ***kalm.,*** lach., lept., mag-c., man., ***mang.,*** meli., ***merc.,*** merc-i-r., ***mez.,*** mosch., ***nat-c.,*** nat-m., nat-p., nat-sil., nit-ac., **NUX-M.,** nux-v., ***petr.,*** ***ph-ac.,*** **PHOS.,** phys., phyt., **PSOR.,** ***puls.,*** **RAN-B.,** ***rheum,*** **RHOD., RHUS-T.,** ***rumx.,*** ruta, sang., sep., **SIL.,** spig., stann., stict., stront-c., ***sulph.,*** tarent., ***teucr.,*** thuj., **TUB.,** ***verat.,*** ***vip.***

amel. - onop.

spring, in - all-c., ant-t., gels., kali-s., nat-s.

ailments from - carb-v., ***dulc.,*** merc-i-f., nat-s., ran-b., ***rhod.***

CHANGE of weather,

cold to warm, agg. - ant-c., brom., **BRY.,** carb-v., ***chel.,*** crot-h., ***ferr.,*** gels., **KALI-S.,** ***lach.,*** ***lyc.,*** nat-c., ***nat-m.,*** ***nat-s.,*** nux-v., **PSOR.,** ***puls.,*** sep., **SULPH., TUB.**

amel. - mang.

rapid, agg. - acon., sep.

warm to cold, agg. - acon., ***ars.,*** calc., calc-p., **DULC.,** hep., **MERC.,** nat-sil., nit-ac., ***nux-v.,*** puls., ***ran-b.,*** ***rhus-t.,*** sabad., ***sil.,*** stront-c., tub., **VERAT.**

CLEAR, weather, agg. - acon., asar., ***bry.,*** **CAUST.,** ***hep.,*** ***nux-v.,*** plb., sabad., spong.

CLOUDY, weather, agg. - aloe, am-c., ammc., aran., arn., ars., ars-i., ***aur.,*** bar-c., benz-n., bry., calc., calen., ***cham.,*** ***chin.,*** dulc., hyper., gels., lach., ***mang.,*** merc., naja, ***nat-c.,*** nat-m., ***nat-s.,*** ***nitro-benz.,*** ***nux-m.,*** phys., plb., ***puls.,*** rhod., **RHUS-T.,** sabin., sang., ***sep.,*** stram., sulph., verat., viol-o.

agg., mental symptoms - aloe, alum., am-c., **AUR.,** nat-c., ***phos.,*** sang.

amel. - caust., bry., kalm., lappa-a.

COLD, temperature, agg. - abrot., acet-ac., ***acon.,*** achy., ***act-sp.,*** adon., aesc., ***agar.,*** ***agn.,*** ***alum.,*** alum-p., ***alum-sil.,*** alumn., ***am-c.,*** am-m., ambr., anac., ***ant-c.,*** ant-t., ***apoc.,*** ***aran.,*** ***arg-m.,*** arg-n., arist-cl., arn., **ARS.,** ars-i., asar., ***aur.,*** aur-a., aur-s., ***bad.,*** **BAR-C.,** ***bar-m.,*** bar-s., ***bell.,*** bell-p., benz-ac., ***bor.,*** ***bov.,*** ***brom.,*** ***bry.,*** cadm-s., **CALC-AR., CALC., CALC-F., CALC-P.,** calc-s., **CALC-SIL., CAMPH.,** ***canth.,*** **CAPS.,** ***carb-an.,*** ***carb-s.,*** ***carb-v.,*** card-m., ***carl.,*** cast., ***caul.,*** **CAUST.,** ***cham.,*** chel., **CHIN.,** ***chin-a.,*** chin-s., ***cic.,*** ***cimic.,*** cinnb., ***cist.,*** clem., coc-c., ***cocc.,*** coch., ***coff.,*** ***colch.,*** coll., ***coloc.,*** ***con.,*** crot-c., ***cycl.,*** cyt-l., ***dig.,*** **DULC.,** elaps, ***eup-per.,*** ***euphr.,*** **FERR.,** ***ferr-ar.,*** ferr-p., ***form.,*** franz., gins., **GRAPH.,** ***guai.,*** gymn., ham., hed., ***hell.,*** ***helon.,*** **HEP.,** hydr., ***hyos.,*** **HYPER.,** hypoth., ***ign.,*** iod., ***ip.,*** ***iris,*** **KALI-AR.,** ***kali-bi.,*** **KALI-C.,** kali-i., kali-m., **KALI-P.,** ***kali-sil.,*** ***kalm.,*** ***kreos.,*** lac-ac., ***lac-d.,*** lach., lat-m., laur., ***led.,*** lob., **LYC.,** lycps., **MAG-C.,** ***mag-m.,*** **MAG-P.,** man., ***mang.,*** med., meny., ***merc.,*** ***mez.,*** mit., moly-met., **MOSCH.,** mur-ac., **NAT-A.,** ***nat-c.,*** ***nat-m.,*** ***nat-p.,*** nat-s., nat-sil., **NIT-AC.,** ***nux-m.,*** **NUX-V.,** oci-s., onop., ***ox-ac.,*** ***petr.,*** ***ph-ac.,*** **PHOS.,** phys., ***phyt.,*** pimp., ***plb.,*** ***podo.,*** polyg., polyg-p., **PSOR.,** ptel., ***puls.,*** **PYROG.,** raja-s., **RAN-B.,** rheum, ***rhod.,*** **RHUS-T., RUMX.,** ***ruta,*** **SABAD.,** samb., saroth., ***sars.,*** sec., sel., ***senec.,*** seneg., **SEP.,** sieg., **SIL.,** sol-n., sol-t-ae., **SPIG.,** spong., squil., ***stann.,*** staph., stram., **STRONT-C.,** stry., ***sulph.,*** ***sul-ac.,*** ***sumb.,*** syph., tab., ***tarent.,*** teucr., thala., ***ther.,*** ***thuj.,*** ***thyr.,*** ***tub.,*** upa., valer., verat., verb., vichy-g., ***viol-t.,*** visc., x-ray, xero, ***zinc.***

cold, ailments from - coloc., kali-c., rhod.

damp places - ant-t., ***aran.,*** ars., ars-i., calc., calc-sil., ***dulc.,*** ***nat-s.,*** nux-m., ***rhus-t.,*** ter.

COLD, temperature

cold, ailments fromdrinks, when overheated - bell-p., bry., rhus-t.
feet, from cold - con., ***sil.***
menses, during - bar-c., graph., mag-c., senec., sep.
spring, in - all-c.
wind, dry - ***acon.***, bry., caust., hep., ***rhod.***

cold, amel. - ***acon.***, aesc., all-c., aloe, alumn., am-m., ***ambr.***, ***anac.***, ***ant-c.***, ***ant-t.***, ***apis***, ***arg-n.***, arn., ***asar.***, ***aur.***, aur-i., bar-c., bell., bell-p., beryl., bor., ***bry.***, ***calad.***, calc., camph., ***cann-i.***, carb-v., caust., ***cham.***, chin., ***cina***, coc-c., cocc., ***colch.***, coloc., ***croc.***, cycl., ***dros.***, dulc., ***euph.***, fago., ferr., fl-ac., ***glon.***, guai., hist., **IOD.**, kali-i., kali-m., kali-s., ***lac-c.***, ***led.***, lil-t., ***lyc.***, mag-m., mag-s., med., merc., moly-met., mur-ac., ***nat-s.***, onos., ***op.***, psor., **PULS.**, rhus-t., sabin., ***sang.***, ***sec.***, spig., **SULPH.**, syph., tab., thuj., trio.
heat agg. - syph.
place, entering a - til.
rheumatic pains - fl-ac., guai., iod., kalm., led.
windows open, must have - ***aml-n.***, apis, ***arg-n.***, bapt., bry., calc., camph., ***carb-s.***, carb-v., glon., graph., iod., ***ip.***, ***lach.***, lyc., med., ***puls.***, sabin., sec., ***sulph.***, tub.

cold, becoming, agg. - acon., aesc., ***agar.***, ***alumn.***, ***am-c.***, ant-c., arg-n., ***arn.***, **ARS.**, ars-i., asar., **AUR.**, aur-s., ***bad.***, **BAR-C.**, bar-m., bar-s., bell., bor., bov., ***bry.***, ***calc.***, ***calc-p.***, calc-sil., ***camph.***, canth., ***caps.***, ***carb-an.***, ***carb-s.***, ***carb-v.***, ***caust.***, ***cham.***, chin., chin-a., cic., ***cimic.***, clem., ***cocc.***, ***con.***, ***dig.***, ***dulc.***, elaps, ***ferr.***, ferr-ar., ferr-p., ***graph.***, hell., **HEP.**, ***hyos.***, ***hyper.***, ign., ip., **KALI-AR.**, **KALI-BI.**, **KALI-C.**, kali-p., kali-s., ***kreos.***, lach., **LYC.**, ***mag-c.***, mag-m., ***mag-p.***, mang., ***med.***, meny., merc., merc-i-r., mez., **MOSCH.**, mur-ac., ***nat-a.***, nat-c., nat-m., ***nat-p.***, nicc., nit-ac., nux-m., **NUX-V.**, ***petr.***, **PH-AC.**, ***phos.***, ***psor.***, puls., **PYROG.**, **RAN-B.**, rhod., **RHUS-T.**, ***rumx.***, ruta, **SABAD.**, samb., sars., **SEP.**, **SIL.**, spig., spong., squil., staph., stram., ***stront-c.***, sulph., **SUL-AC.**, ***sumb.***, ***tarent.***, ***thuj.***, ***verat.***, verb., viol-t., ***zinc.***
after, agg. - ***acon.***, agar., ***alum.***, alum-p., alum-sil., ***alumn.***, ***am-c.***, anac., ***ant-c.***, ***ant-t.***, ***arg-n.***, arn., **ARS.**, ars-s-f., aur., aur-s., **BAR-C.**, bar-s., **BELL.**, bor., **BRY.**, **CALC.**, **CALC-P.**, calc-s., calc-sil., camph., ***carb-s.***, ***carb-v.***, ***caust.***, **CHAM.**, **CHIN.**, cimic., ***coc-c.***, cocc., ***coff.***, colch., ***coloc.***, ***con.***, croc., cupr., cupr-s., ***cycl.***, dig., dros., **DULC.**, ferr., ferr-ar., **FL-AC.**, **GRAPH.**, guai., **HEP.**, hydr., **HYOS.**, hyper., ign., ***ip.***, kali-ar., ***kali-bi.***, ***kali-c.***, kali-m., kali-p., ***kali-sil.***, kalm., led., ***lyc.***, mag-c., ***mang.***, ***med.***, **MERC.**, nat-c., ***nat-m.***, nat-p., ***nit-ac.***, ***nux-m.***, **NUX-V.**, op., ***petr.***, ***ph-ac.***, **PHOS.**, phyt., plat., polyg., ***psor.***, **PULS.**, **PYROG.**, **RAN-B.**, **RHUS-T.**,

COLD, temperature

cold, becoming,
after becoming, agg. - ruta, sabin., ***samb.***, sang., sars., sel., **SEP.**, **SIL.**, **SPIG.**, ***stann.***, staph., stront-c., sul-i., ***sulph.***, **SUL-AC.**, ***tarent.***, ***thuj.***, tub., valer., ***verat.***, ***xan.***, zinc-p.
ailments from - kalm., phyt.
heated, when - acon., bry., kali-s.
amel. - acon., aesc., agn., all-c., aloe, alum., alumn., am-c., am-m., ambr., anac., ang., ant-c., ant-t., ***apis***, ***arg-n.***, arn., asaf., asar., aur., bapt., bar-c., bell., bov., brom., ***bry.***, cadm-met., calad., calc., calc-i., cann-s., carb-v., ***cham.***, clem., coc-c., cocc., coff., colch., coloc., croc., ***dros.***, dulc., euph., fl-ac., ***glon.***, ***graph.***, guai., hell., ign., **IOD.**, ip., kali-c., kali-i., kali-s., kalm., ***lac-c.***, ***lach.***, ***led.***, lil-t., **LYC.**, mang., ***merc.***, mez., mur-ac., nat-c., ***nat-m.***, nit-ac., ***nux-m.***, nux-v., olnd., op., ***petr.***, ph-ac., phos., plat., **PULS.**, rhus-t., sabad., ***sabin.***, sars., ***sec.***, sel., seneg., sep., sil., spig., spong., staph., ***sulph.***, teucr., thuj., verat.
body, a part of agg. - agar., am-c., ***bar-c.***, ***bell.***, ***calc.***, cham., ***hell.***, **HEP.**, ip., ***led.***, ***nux-v.***, ph-ac., ***phos.***, psor., puls., **RHUS-T.**, ***sep.***, **SIL.**, tarent., thuj., zinc.
back - piloc.
feet - alum., am-c., ars., ***bar-c.***, bufo, cham., clem., ***con.***, ***cupr.***, kali-ar., kali-c., ***lach.***, lyc., mag-p., nit-ac., nux-m., ***nux-v.***, phos., phys., ***puls.***, sep., **SIL.**, stann., zinc.
hand, out of bed - acon., **BAR-C.**, canth., ***con.***, **HEP.**, merc., phos., **RHUS-T.**, ***sil.***
head - am-c., ant-c., arg-n., bar-c., ***bell.***, ***hep.***, hyos., led., nux-v., puls., rhus-t., ***sep.***, **SIL.**
limbs - aur., ***bry.***, con., **HEP.**, ***nat-m.***, **RHUS-T.**, **SIL.**, squil., stront-c., **THUJ.**
heated, when - ***acon.***, ars., bell., ***bell-p.***, brom., bry., dulc., ferr-p., ***hep.***, kali-ar., kali-c., merc-i-f., ***nux-v.***, phos., psor., puls., ran-b., rhod., **RHUS-T.**, sep., **SIL.**, zinc.
ailments from - acon., bry., kali-s.
part of body becoming cold, agg. - agar., am-c., ***bar-c.***, ***bell.***, ***calc.***, cham., ***hell.***, **HEP.**, ip., ***led.***, ***nux-v.***, ph-ac., ***phos.***, psor., puls., **RHUS-T.**, ***sep.***, **SIL.**, tarent., thuj., zinc.
back - piloc.
feet - alum., am-c., ars., ***bar-c.***, bufo, cham., clem., ***con.***, ***cupr.***, kali-ar., kali-c., ***lach.***, lyc., mag-p., nit-ac., nux-m., ***nux-v.***, phos., phys., ***puls.***, sep., **SIL.**, stann., zinc.
hand, out of bed - acon., **BAR-C.**, canth., ***con.***, **HEP.**, merc., phos., **RHUS-T.**, ***sil.***

COLD, temperature

cold, becoming,

part of body becoming cold, agg.

head - am-c., ant-c., arg-n., bar-c., ***bell.,*** ***hep.,*** hyos., led., nux-v., puls., rhus-t., ***sep.,*** **SIL.**

limbs - aur., ***bry.,*** con., **HEP.,** ***nat-m.,*** **RHUS-T., SIL.,** squil., stront-c., **THUJ.**

perspiration, during - **ACON.,** ***ars-s-f.,*** calc-sil., dulc., sul-i.

sitting on cold steps - chim., ***nux-v.,*** rhod.

cold, dry, weather - **ACON.,** ***ars.,*** **ASAR.,** bell., bor., ***bry.,*** carb-an., carb-v., **CAUST.,** cham., ***crot-h.,*** **HEP.,** ***ip.,*** **KALI-C.,** laur., mag-c., mez., mur-ac., **NUX-V.,** rhod., ***sabad.,*** sep., ***sil.,*** spig., ***spong.,*** staph., sulph., zinc.

cold, heat, and cold agg. - ***alum.,*** alum-p., ang., ***ant-c.,*** ant-t., arn., ***ars-i.,*** asar., aur-s., bar-s., calc., calc-s., caps., ***carb-s., caust.,*** cimic., cina, cinnb., ***cocc., cor-r.,*** ferr., **FL-AC.,** flav., ***glon., graph.,*** hell., ***ip.,*** kali-c., ***lach., lyc.,*** mag-c., mag-m., **MERC.,** nat-c., ***nat-m.,*** nux-v., ***ph-ac., phys., psor.,*** puls., ***ran-b.,*** rob., sanic., ***sep., sil.,*** sul-ac., ***sulph.,*** syph., tab., thala., thuj., **TUB.**

cold, hot days with cold nights - acon., dulc., merc-c., rumx.

cold, lying in bed - ***ign.***

cold, one part cold, with heat of another - apis, bry., cham.

cold, place, entering a, agg., - **ARS.,** bell., calc-p., ***camph.,*** carb-v., caust., con., ***dulc.,*** ***ferr., ferr-ar., graph., hep.,*** ip., **KALI-AR.,** kali-c., kali-p., kali-sil., mosch., nux-m., ***nux-v., petr.,*** phos., ***psor., puls.,*** **RAN-B.,** ***rhus-t., sabad.,*** **SEP.,** ***sil.,*** spong., stront-c., ***tub., verb.***

cold, taking cold, agg. - acon., ***bac.,*** bell., bry., calc., ***camph.,*** carb-an., cham., cist., coloc., dulc., kali-n., merc., phos., sil., ***tub.***

DARKNESS, agg. - acon., ***am-m.,*** anac., ang., arg-n., ***ars.,*** bar-c., **CALC.,** camph., ***cann-s.,*** ***carb-an., carb-v.,*** caust., con., ***gels., lyc.,*** nat-m., phos., ***plat.,*** **PLB.,** puls., ***rhus-t.,*** staph., **STRAM.,** ***stront-c.,*** sul-ac., valer., zinc.

aversion to - phos., sanic., stram.

desire for - achy.

to lie down in the dark and not be talked to - tarent.

DRY, general

dry, cold, agg. - abrot., **ACON.,** aesc., agar., alum., alumn., am-c., apoc., ***ars.,*** ars-i., **ASAR.,** aur., bac., ***bar-c.,*** bell., bor., ***bry.,*** calc., calc-i., calc-p., ***camph.,*** caps., ***carb-an.,*** carb-v., **CAUST.,** cham., ***chin., cist.,*** coc-c., cocc., coff., ***crot-h.,*** cupr., cur., daph., dulc., euph., ferr-ar., fl-ac., **HEP.,** ign., ***ip.,*** **KALI-C.,** kali-sil., kreos., lach., lappa-a., laur., lyc., mag-c., mag-p., med., mez., mur-ac., nat-c., nat-s., nit-ac., nit-s-d., nux-m., **NUX-V.,** ***petr.,*** ph-ac., phos., phys., physal., phyt., plat., plb., ***psor., puls.,*** rhod., rhus-t., ***rumx., sabad.,*** sel., sep., ***sil.,*** spig., ***spong.,*** staph., sulph., tub., urt-u., ***verat.,*** viol-o., visc., zinc.

cold, amel. - led., sil.

dry, weather, agg. - ***acon.,*** alum., alumn., ars., **ASAR.,** aur-m., ***bell.,*** bor., ***bry., carb-an.,*** carb-v., **CAUST.,** ***cham., fl-ac.,*** hep., ***hyper.,*** ***ip., kali-c., laur.,*** mag-c., med., ***merc.,*** mez., ***mur-ac., nit-ac.,*** **NUX-V.,** phos., ***plat.,*** ***rhod.,*** sabad., ***sep.,*** sil., spig., spong., staph., sulph., zinc.

dry, weather, amel. - agar., ***am-c., ant-c.,*** ***aur.,*** bar-c., bell., ***bor.,*** bov., bry., **CALC.,** canth., ***carb-an., carb-v.,*** cham., ***chin.,*** ***clem.,*** con., ***cupr.,*** **DULC.,** ***ferr.,*** hep., ip., kali-c., ***kali-n., lach., laur., lyc., mag-c.,*** magn-gr., ***mang., merc.,*** merc-c., mez., moly-met., ***mur-ac., nat-c., nit-ac.,*** **NUX-M.,** nux-v., petr., phos., ***puls., rhod.,*** **RHUS-T.,** ***ruta, sars., seneg.,*** sep., sil., ***spig.,*** stann., ***staph.,*** still., ***stront-c., sul-ac., sulph.,*** ***verat., zinc.***

dry, warm, agg. - ant-c., carb-v., cocc., kali-bi., lach.

amel. - alum., ***calc-p.,*** nat-s., nux-m., penic., rhus-t., ***sulph.***

FOGGY, weather agg. - abrot., aloe, ***aran.,*** ars., bapt., bar-c., bry., calc., calen., cham., chin., dulc., ***gels.,*** **HYPER.,** mang., merc., mosch., nat-m., ***nat-s.,*** nux-m., plb., ***rhod.,*** **RHUS-T.,** sep., ***sil., staph.,*** sulph., ***thuj.,*** verat.

FROSTY, weather agg. - ***agar., calc.,*** carb-v., caust., **CON.,** lyc., mag-m., merc., nat-c., nux-v., ***ph-ac.,*** phos., ***puls.,*** rhus-t., **SEP.,** ***sil., sulph.,*** syph.

HEATED, becoming agg. - acon., am-c., **ANT-C.,** ***arg-n., arn., bell.,*** bor., ***brom.,*** **BRY.,** calc., calc-s., calc-sil., caps., ***camph., carb-v.,*** coff., ***cycl., dig.,*** dros., dulc., ***ferr.,*** fl-ac., gels., ***glon.,*** ***graph.,*** hep., ign., **IOD.,** ip., kali-ar., **KALI-C.,** **KALI-S.,** lach., lyc., merc., mez., ***nat-m.,*** nux-m., nux-v., olnd., ***op., phos.,*** **PULS.,** ***ran-b.,*** rhus-t., ***sep.,*** **SIL.,** staph., sul-ac., sulph., ***thuj., zinc.***

alcoholics, old - ***bar- c.***

easily - brom., kali-n., nit-ac.

headache, from - ***acon., aloe,*** am-c., ***arum-t.,*** **ANT-C.,** ***apis,*** arg-n., arn., bar-c., **BELL.,** ***bry.,*** calc., calc-s., camph., caps., ***carb-s.,*** **CARB-V.,** con., dig., dros., form., **GLON.,** grat., ign., ***ip., kali-c.,*** kali-p., ***kali-s., kalm.,*** **LYC.,** nat-a., ***nat-m.,*** nux-m., op., phos., ptel., ***sep.,*** ***sil.,*** staph., ***stram., sulph., thuj.,*** zinc.

by a fire or stove - **ANT-C.,** ***apis, arn.,*** ***arum-t., bar-c.,*** bry., cimic., com., euph., **GLON.,** lac-d., ***manc.,*** merc., nux-v., ***phos., puls.,*** rhus-t., ***sanic.,*** ***zinc.***

sun, or fire, by, agg. - ***acon., ant-c.,*** **BELL.,** bor., ***bry.,*** carb-v., ***gels.,*** **GLON.,** iod., ip., kali-c., lach., lyss., merc., ***nat-c.,*** nat-m., op., puls., samb., sel., sil., ther., verat-v., zinc.

amel. - **ARS., IGN.**

HEATED, becoming agg.
weakness, causes - aster., ***carb-s.,*** coc-c., ***lach., nat-c.,*** nat-p., ***puls.,*** rhod., **SEL.,** ***sulph.,*** tab., vesp.
summer, in - alum., ***corn.,*** **IOD.,** ***lach.,*** **NAT-C.,** nat-m., **SEL.**

HOT, weather, agg. - ***acon.,*** aeth., aloe, ***ant-c.,*** ant-t., **APIS,** bapt., ***bell.,*** bor., brom., ***bry.,*** carb-v., cocc., croc., ***crot-h.,*** crot-t., ***cupr., gels., glon.,*** hep., ***iod.,*** kali-bi., **LACH.,** ***nat-c., nat-m., nat-s.,*** nit-ac., ***op.,*** phos., pic-ac., ***podo.,*** **PULS.,** sabin., sel., **SULPH.,** syph.
ailments from - ant-c., kali-bi., lach.

MOON, general
agg. - **ALUM., ARG-N.,** bry., **CALC.,** ***cina,*** cupr., ***lyc.,*** nux-v., ***phos.,*** sabad., **SIL.,** sulph.
agg. and amel. - clem., phel., tarent.
decreasing. agg. - alum., ***apis, ars.,*** bry., ***calc.,*** clem., ***daph., dulc.,*** gels., kali-bi., kali-c., ***lach., lyc., merc.,*** merc-i-r., ***nat-m., nux-v.,*** ph-ac., phel., **PHOS.,** phyt., plat., **PULS., RHUS-T., SEP.,** sil., sul-i., **SULPH.,** tab., thuj., tub., verat.
first quarter agg., increasing - ars., bry., nat-m.
full, agg., when - ***alum., anac., apis.,*** **ARG-N., ARS.,** bar-c., bell., bov., brom., bry., **CALC.,** calc-p., ***caust., cina., croc.,*** cupr., cycl., fl-ac., gels., ***graph., hep.,*** ign., kali-bi., kali-n., ***lach.,*** led., **LYC.,** ***merc.,*** nat-c., nat-m., nit-ac., nux-v., ph-ac., **PHOS.,** psor., **PULS.,** ***rhus-t.,*** sabad., sang., ***sep.,*** **SIL.,** sol-m., sol-t-ae., spong., sul-i., ***sulph.,*** teucr., thuj., verat-v.
every other - syph.
waxing - ***clem.***
increasing, agg. - ***alum.,*** apis, arn., **ARS.,** arum-t., bell., ***bry.,*** **CALC.,** calc-p., caust., chin., cimic., ***clem.,*** cupr., graph., ign., kali-bi., kali-c., ***lach., lyc., med.,*** merc-i-f., ***nat-m.,*** nit-ac., ***nux-v.,*** phel., **PHOS., PULS.,** ***rhus-t.,*** sang., **SEP.,** ***sil.,*** staph., sul-i., **SULPH.,** ***thuj.***
last quarter, decreasing, agg., - lyc., sep.
moonlight, mental symptoms from - ***ant-c., arg-n.,*** bell., calc., luna, meph., sil., thuj.
agg. - ***ant-c.,*** arg-n., bell., calc., luna, sep., ***sulph.,*** thuj.
amel. - aur.
new moon, when, agg. - ***agar.,*** alum., am-c., ***apis., arg-n.,*** arn., **ARS.,** ars-i., bell., ***bry.,*** bufo., ***calc.,*** calc-p., canth., ***caust.,*** chin., ***cina.,*** clem., croc., ***cupr.,*** daph., graph., hep., kali-bi., kali-br., ***lach.,*** lyc., merc., merc-c., merc-i-f., nat-m., **NUX-V., PHOS.,** phyt., **PULS., RHUS-T.,** sabad., ***sep., sil.,*** **SULPH.,** thuj.

MOUNTAINS, amel. in - prot., ***syph., tub.***

RAIN, agg. during - aran., elaps, erig., ***dulc.,*** glon., ham., lac-c., lach., mag-c., mang., merc., ***nat-s.,*** oci-s., phyt., plat., ran-b., ***rhus-t.,*** sabin., senn., ***sulph., thuj.,*** tub.

SEASHORE, general, air, agg. - ***aq-mar., ars.,*** brom., ***carc.,*** iod., kali-i., ***mag-m.,*** mag-s., med., morbill., ***nat-m.,*** nat-s., rhus-t., **SEP.,** syph., ***tub.***
amel. - ***acon., agar.,*** ant-c., ant-t., ***bor.,*** brom., camph., ***carc.,*** eucal., ***hyos., iris,*** lyc., lyss., **MED.,** ***nat-m., op., ox-ac.,*** plat., **PULS.,** ***stram., sul-ac., tub.,*** verat.

SNOW-air, agg. - agar., asar., ***calc., calc-p.,*** caust., cic., **CON.,** fl-ac., ***form.,*** lach., ***lyc.,*** mag-m., merc., nat-c., ***nux-v., ph-ac., phos., puls.,*** rhod., ***rhus-t.,*** **SEP.,** ***sil., sulph.,*** urt-u., vib.
ailments, from - con., sep.
brightness of - glon.
snowglare - acon., cic., glon.

SPRING, agg. - acon., all-c., **AMBR.,** ***ant-t., apis, ars-br., aur.,*** bar-m., **BELL.,** brom., ***bry.,*** **CALC.,** calc-p., ***carb-v., cench.,*** ceph., ***chel.,*** cina, ***colch.,*** con., ***crot-h.,*** dulc., **GELS.,** ham., hed., hep., ***iris, kali-bi.,*** **LACH., LYC.,** merc-i-f., nat-c., ***nat-m., nat-s.,*** nit-s-d., nux-v., ***puls.,*** rhod., ***rhus-t., sars.,*** sec., sel., ***sep., sil., sulph.,*** tarent., urt-u., ***verat.***
ailments since - con., kali-bi., merc-i-f.
amel. - flav.

STORMS, during, agg. - agar., aran., arg-m., aur., ***bry.,*** calc., carb-v., caust., cedr., conv., elaps, erig., ***gels.,*** glon., ham., hydr-ac., ***lach.,*** mag-c., man., mang., ***med.,*** morph., **NAT-C.,** nat-m., nat-p., nit-ac., nit-s-d., petr., **PHOS.,** phyt., prot., psor., puls., ran-b., ***rhod.,*** sabin., ***sep., sil.,*** syph., thuj., tub., visc.
after agg. - asar., calc-p., carc., rhus-r., rhus-t., sep., tub.
amel. - carc., psor., sep.
approach of a, agg. - ***agar.,*** arg-m., aur., ***bell-p.,*** caust., ***cedr.,*** dulc., ***gels.,*** harp., hyper., ***kali-bi., lach., lyc.,*** mag-p., man., mang., med., meli., ***nat-c.,*** nat-m., nat-p., ***nat-s.,*** nit-ac., petr., ***phos.,*** phyt., **PSOR.,** puls., ***ran-b.,*** **RHOD.,** ***rhus-t., sep.,*** sil., sul-ac., sulph., syph., thuj., ***tub.,*** zinc.
ailments from - crot-h., gels., morph., nat-c., nat-p., nit-s-d., phos., psor., puls., ***rhod.,*** syph.
amel. - carc., ***sep.***
enjoys, storms - ***carc., sep.***
storms, thunderstorm, during agg. - bor., bry., caust., lach., nat-c., nat-m., nit-ac., petr., ***phos., rhod.,*** sep., ***sil.***
amel. - carc., psor., rhus-r., sep.
before, agg. - bry., hyper., ***nat-c.,*** nat-m., petr., **RHOD.,** zinc.
loves to watch - bell-p., ***carc.,*** lyc., ***sep.***

STORMY, and windy weather agg. - ***acon., all-c., am-c.,*** arg-m., ars., asar., aur., aur-a., **BAD.,** bell., bry., carb-v., caust., ***cham.,*** chel., ***chin.,*** chin-a., con., erig., euphr., gels., graph., ***hep.,*** hydr-ac., hyper., ip., **KALM.,** ***lach.,*** lyc., mag-c., ***mag-p.,*** mez., ***mur-ac.,*** nat-c., nat-m., nit-s-d., **NUX-M.,** ***nux-v.,*** petr., ***phos.,*** plat., ***psor., puls.,*** ran-b., **RHOD.,** rhus-t., ruta, ***sep.,*** spig., sul-ac., sulph., tab., thuj.

SUMMER, agg. - ***acon., aeth.,*** aloe, ***alum.,*** alum-sil., **ANT-C.,** apis, arg-n., ars-i., bapt., bar-c., **BELL.,** bor., bov., brom., **BRY.,** calc., **CAMPH., CARB-V.,** ***carb-s.,*** cham., ***chion.,*** cina, cinnb., coff., croc., crot-h., crot-t., cupr., dulc., **FL-AC.,** ***gamb.,*** **GELS., GLON.,** graph., ***guai., iod.,*** iris, kali-bi., kali-br., kali-c., kali-i., **LACH.,** ***lyc.,*** mur-ac., **NAT-C.,** ***nat-m.,*** nit-ac., nux-m., ***nux-v., ph-ac., phos.,*** pic-ac., **PODO.,** ***psor.,*** **PULS.,** rheum, rhod., sabin., ***sel.,*** sep., sin-n., sul-i., syph., thuj., ***verat.,*** verat-v.

ailments since - podo., sin-n.

amel. - aesc., alum., ars-i., aur., aur-m., calc-p., calc-sil., caust., ferr., kali-sil., ***petr.,*** psor., sil., stront-c.

children, in - acon., ***ip.***

cool days in summer, after - **BRY.**

overcoat, wearing in - hep., psor.

solstice agg. - apis, **BELL.,** brom., ***bry., carb-v., gels.,*** iris, ***kali-bi.,*** **LACH.,** ***lyc.,*** nat-c., ***nat-m.,*** nux-v., ***puls.,*** rhod., sep., ***verat.***

SUN, exposure, worse from - acon., ***agar.,*** **ANT-C.,** ***arg-m., bar-c., bell.,*** brom., ***bry.,*** cact., calc., cadm-s., ***camph., carb-v.,*** clem., cocc., crot-h., ***euphr.,*** gels., **GLON.,** graph., ign., iod., ip., ***kalm., lach., lyss.,*** mag-m., med., mur-ac., **NAT-C., NAT-M.,** ***nux-v., op.,*** prun., ***psor.,*** **PULS.,** ***sel.,*** sol., stann., stram., sulph., symph., syph., ***uva., valer.,*** **VERAT.,** verat-v., zinc.

ailments, chronic - nat-c.

amel. - anac., con., crot-h., iod., kali-c., kali-m., pic-ac., ***plat.,*** rhod., rhus-t., ***stram.,*** **STRONT-C.,** tarent., ***thuj.***

exertion, from, in - **ANT-C.**

eyes sensitive to sunlight - **ACON.,** ***ars., asar.,*** berb., ***bry.,*** calc., camph., cast., **CHIN.,** ***cic., clem., euphr.,*** **GRAPH.,** ***hep., ign., kali-ar., lac-c., lith., merc.,*** merc-c., ***merc-sul.,*** **NAT-M.,** petr., ph-ac., ***phos.,*** **SULPH.,** zinc.

head, congestion from exposure - ***acon., bell., cact., gels., glon.,*** verat-v.

headache, from exposure - ***acon.,*** act-sp., ***agar.,*** aloe, **ANT-C.,** ***arum-t., bar-c.,*** **BELL.,** brom., bruc., **BRY.,** cadm-s., ***calc.,*** calc-s., ***camph.,*** cann-i., ***carb-v.,*** cast-v., ***chim.,*** chin-s., ***cocc.,*** euphr., ***gels.,*** genist., **GLON.,** hipp., hyos., ign., **LACH.,** manc., nat-a., **NAT-C.,** ***nat-m., nux-v.,*** **PULS.,** ***sel., stram.,*** syph., ***sulph., ther.,*** valer., zinc.

SUNBURN - acon., ***agar., ant-c., apis.,*** **BELL.,** bry., bufo, calen., ***camph.,*** **CANTH.,** clem., cortiso., euphr., ***hyos.,*** lach., lyc., ***mur-ac., nat-c.,*** op., **PULS.,** rob., sel., sulph., **URT-U.,** ***valer.,*** verat.

SUNSTROKE - ***acon.,*** agar., **AML-N.,** ***ant-c.,*** apis, arg-m., ***arn., ars.,*** **BELL.,** bry., ***cact., camph., carb-v.,*** cit-l., crot-h., cyt-l., euph-pi., ***gels.,*** **GLON.,** hydr-ac., hyos., kalm., **LACH.,** lyc., lyss., **NAT-C.,** nat-m., nux-v., ***op.,*** pop-c., rhus-t., stram., syph., ***ther.,*** thuj., usn., valer., **VERAT.,** ***verat-v.***

SUNSTROKE,

slept, from having, in sun - acon., ***bell., stram.***

TEMPERATURE, change, of agg. - acon., act-sp., aesc., alum., alumn., ant-c., ***ant-t.,*** **ARS.,** bar-c., bufo, calc., ***calc-p., carb-v.,*** caust., ***dulc.,*** **FL-AC.,** graph., ip., kali-i., ***lach.,*** lyc., ***mag-c.,*** meli., **MERC.,** merc-c., **NAT-C.,** nit-ac., ***nux-v., phos.,*** phys., ***puls.,*** **RAN-B.,** ran-s., rhod., rhus-t., rumx., sabad., ***sabin.,*** sang., sep., sil., ***spong.,*** stict., sul-i., sulph., thuj., verat., **VERB.**

THUNDERSTORM, general, (see Storms)

TIME, (see Generals, Time)

VAULTS, cellars, agg. - aran., **ARS.,** ***bry.,*** calc., ***carb-an.,*** carc., caust., dulc., ***kali-c.,*** lyc., merc-i-f., **NAT-S., PULS.,** ***sep., stram.***

WARM, temperature

warm, agg. - acon., adlu., ***aesc.,*** aeth., ***agar.,*** agn., ***all-c., aloe,*** **ALUM.,** alumn., ambr., ***anac., ant-c., ant-t.,*** **APIS,** aq-mar., **ARG-N.,** ***arn.,*** **ARS-I.,** ***asaf., asar.,*** aster., aur., ***aur-i., aur-m.,*** bar-c., bar-i., ***bell.,*** beryl., ***bism., bor.,*** brom., ***bry., calad., calc., calc-i., calc-s., camph.,*** cann-s., canth., carb-v., ***carb-s.,*** caust., cench., cham., chin., cimic., cina, clem., ***coc-c.,*** cocc., coff., colch., coloc., ***com.,*** conv., cortico., cortiso., ***croc., crot-h.,*** cycl., dig., ***dros., dulc.,*** euph., euphr., ferr., ferr-i., **FL-AC.,** flav., foll., **GELS.,** ***glon., graph., grat., guai., ham.,*** hed., helio., hell., hep., hip-ac., hist., hydroph., ***hyos.,*** iber., ign., ***ind.,*** **IOD.,** ***ip.,*** jug-c., just., kali-br., kali-c., **KALI-I.,** ***kali-m.,*** **KALI-S.,** ***lac-c.,*** **LACH.,** laur., **LED.,** ***lil-t., lyc.,*** mag-aust., mag-c., ***merc., mez.,*** mur-ac., nat-c., **NAT-M., NAT-S.,** nit-ac., nux-m., nux-v., ***op.,*** ph-ac., phenob., ***phos.,*** phyt., pic-ac., pituin., **PLAT.,** prot., **PULS.,** rat., rauw., rhus-t., sabad., ***sabin., sang.,*** **SEC.,** sel., ***seneg.,*** sep., sil., spig., ***spong.,*** staph., stel., sul-ac., ***sul-i.,*** **SULPH.,** tab., teucr., ***thuj.,*** trio., ***tub., verat., vesp.,*** visc., ***zinc.***

radiated - ant-c.

sun - cact., cadm-br., cob., cocc., murx.

water - stront-c.

warm, air, amel. - ***acon., agar.,*** alumn., ***am-c.,*** anac., ant-c., arn., **ARS.,** asar., **AUR.,** ***bar-c., bell.,*** bor., ***bov., bry., calc.,*** **CAMPH.,** canth., ***caps., carb-an., carb-v.,*** **CAUST.,** ***cham.,*** chin., ***cic., cina, coc-c.,*** coff., ***colch., coloc., con.,*** dig., **DULC.,** ***ferr.,*** graph., **HELL., HEP.,** ***hyos., ign.,*** ip., **KALI-C.,** kreos., lach., laur., led., ***lyc.,*** mag-c., mag-m., mag-p., ***mang.,*** meny., ***merc., mez.,*** **MOSCH.,** mur-ac., nat-a., ***nat-c., nat-m.,*** nat-s., ***nit-ac.,*** **NUX-M., NUX-V.,** par., ***petr., ph-ac., phos.,*** psor., ran-b., ***rhod.,*** **RHUS-T.,** ***ruta,*** **SABAD.,** samb., ***sars., sel.,*** seneg., ***sep., sil., spig., spong.,*** squil., staph., stram., **STRONT-C.,** sul-ac., ***sulph.,*** thuj., ***verat.,*** verb., viol-t., zinc.

WARM, temperature

warm, amel. - ***acon., agar.,*** alum-sil., alumn., ***am-c.,*** anac., ant-c., ***arg-m.,*** arist-cl., ***arn.,*** **ARS.,** asar., ***aur.,*** bad., ***bar-c., bell.,*** bell-p., ***bor., bov., bry.,*** calc., calc-f., calc-p., calc-s., **CAMPH.,** ***canth., caps., carb-an., carb-v.,*** cast., **CAUST.,** cench., cham., chel., ***chin., cic.,*** cimic., ***clem., cocc., coff., colch., coll., coloc., con.,*** cor-r., cupr-ac., cycl., cyn-d., ***dig.,*** dros., **DULC.,** ***ferr.,*** flor-p., form., gink-b., ***graph.,*** gymn., ***hell.,*** **HEP.,** ***hyos., ign.,*** ip., kali-ar., kali-bi., **KALI-C.,** kali-p., ***kreos.,*** lac-d., ***lach.,*** laur., led., levo., lob., lyc., lycpr., ***mag-c., mag-m., mag-p.,*** man., ***mang.,*** med., ***meny.,*** **MERC.,** ***mez.,*** moly-met., **MOSCH.,** ***mur-ac., nat-c.,*** nat-m., nid., nit-ac., ***nux-m.,*** **NUX-V.,** onop., ph-ac., ***petr., phos.,*** phyt., psor., puls., pyrog., ***ran-b., rheum,*** **RHUS-T.,** rumx., ***ruta,*** **SABAD.,** ***samb., sars.,*** seneg., ***sep., sil., spig., spong., squil., staph., stram.,*** **STRONT-C.,** ***sul-ac.,*** **SULPH.,** syph., thea., ther., thuj., tub., verat., verb., viol-t., xero, zinc.

radiated - mez.

sun - anac., cinnb., con., crot-h., iod., kali-m., phos., pic-ac., plat., rhod., ***stront-c.,*** tarent.

water, feet in, amel. - bufo.

warm, becoming, agg. - ***acon.,*** am-c., **ANT-C.,** bar-i., ***bell.,*** bor., brom., **BRY.,** calc., ***caps., carb-v.,*** coff., ***dig., gels., glon., hep., ign., ip.,*** **KALI-C.,** lach., lyc., mez., ***nat-m., nux-m., nux-v.,*** olnd., ***op., sep., sil.,*** staph., ***thuj., zinc.***

air, in open, agg. - acon., agn., alum., alumn., ambr., anac., ***ant-c.,*** asar., aur., aur-i., ***aur-m.,*** bar-c., ***bell.,*** bor., bov., **BRY.,** calad., calc., cann-s., ***carb-v.,*** caust., cham., chin., cina, cocc., coff., colch., coloc., croc., dros., ***dulc.,*** euph., **GELS.,** ***glon.,*** graph., ign., **IOD.,** ip., kali-c., lach., led., **LYC.,** mang., ***merc.,*** mez., nat-c., nat-m., ***nat-s.,*** nit-ac., nux-m., nux-v., olnd., ***op.,*** petr., ph-ac., ***phos.,*** plat., **PULS.,** rhus-t., ***sabad.,*** sabin., ***sec.,*** sel., ***seneg.,*** sep., ***sil., spig.,*** spong., staph., ***sulph.,*** teucr., thuj., ***verat.***

air, in open, amel. - ***acon., agar.,*** am-c., ant-c., ***arn.,*** **ARS.,** asar., ***aur., bar-c., bell., bor.,*** bov., ***bry., calc., camph.,*** canth., ***caps.,*** carb-an., carb-v., ***caust., cham., chin., cic.,*** clem., ***coc-c.,*** colch., ***con.,*** dig., ***dulc.,*** ferr., **GRAPH.,** ***hell., hep., hyos., ign.,*** **KALI-C.,** ***kreos.,*** lach., ***lyc., mag-c.,*** mag-m., ***mang.,*** meny., ***merc.,*** mez., **MOSCH.,** mur-ac., ***nat-c.,*** nat-m., ***nit-ac., nux-m.,*** **NUX-V.,** ***petr., ph-ac., phos.,*** ran-b., rhod., **RHUS-T.,** ruta, **SABAD.,** samb., ***sars.,*** sel., ***sep., sil.,*** spig., ***spong.,*** staph., thuj., ***verat., verb.,*** viol-t., zinc.

WARM, temperature

warm, bed, agg. - aeth., agn., ***alum.,*** alumn., ambr., anac., ***ant-c., ant-t.,*** **APIS,** arg-n., arn., ars-i., ***asaf.,*** asar., aur., aur-i., ***aur-m.,*** aur-s., bar-c., bell-p., bov., ***bry.,*** calad., calc., calc-f., calc-i., ***calc-s., camph.,*** cann-s., ***carb-v.,*** carb-s., ***caust.,*** cedr., **CHAM.,** chin., cina, cinnb., ***clem., coc-c., cocc.,*** colch., coloc., croc., daph., **DROS.,** dulc., ***euph., fl-ac., glon.,*** goss., ***graph.,*** hell., hyos., ign., ***iod., ip., kali-c., kali-chl.,*** kali-m., ***kali-s., lac-c., lach.,*** **LED.,** ***lyc., mag-c.,*** med., **MERC.,** ***mez.,*** mur-ac., nat-c., ***nat-m.,*** nit-ac., ***nux-m., nux-v.,*** **OP.,** ***ph-ac.,*** phenob., phos., phyt., ***plat.,*** psor., **PULS.,** ***rhod., rhus-t.,*** sabad., **SABIN.,** sars., **SEC.,** sel., ***seneg.,*** sep., ***sil.,*** spig., ***spong.,*** staph., stram., stront-c., ***sul-i.,*** **SULPH.,** teucr., ***thuj.,*** til., ***verat.,*** visc., x-ray.

amel. - agar., ***am-c.,*** arn., **ARS.,** ars-s-f., ***aur.,*** bapt., bar-c., bell., **BRY.,** ***calc-p.,*** camph., canth., ***caust.,*** cic., cocc., ***coloc.,*** con., ***dulc., graph.,*** **HEP.,** hyos., ***kali-bi.,*** **KALI-C.,** ***kali-i.,*** kali-p., lach., **LYC.,** ***mag-p.,*** mosch., nit-ac., **NUX-M., NUX-V.,** petr., ph-ac., ***phos.,*** **RHUS-T.,** ***rumx., sabad., sep.,*** **SIL.,** spong., squil., ***stann.,*** staph., stram., stront-c., sul-ac., sulph., ***tarent.,*** thuj., **TUB.,** verat.

cold limbs, with - **CAMPH., LED.,** ***mag-c., med.,*** **SEC.**

desire for warm bed - spig.

warm, clothing, agg., wraps - ***acon.,*** ant-c., ant-t., **APIS,** ***arg-m., arg-n.,*** arn., ***ars-i., asar.,*** aur., aur-i., ***aur-m.,*** aur-s., **BELL.,** ***bor.,*** brom., ***bry., calc.,*** calc-i., calc-s., ***camph.,*** carb-v., carb-s., ***cham.,*** chin., ***coc-c.,*** coff., ***crot-h.,*** cupr., ***ferr.,*** ferr-i., ***fl-ac.,*** glon., ign., **IOD.,** ***ip.,*** kali-bi., kali-i., **KALI-S.,** ***lac-c.,*** **LACH., LED.,** lil-t., **LYC., MAG-P.,** ***merc.,*** mosch., mur-ac., ***nat-m., nit-ac.,*** nux-v., op., phos., plat., **PULS.,** rhus-t., sabin., sanic., **SEC.,** ***seneg.,*** sep., ***spig.,*** staph., ***sul-i.,*** **SULPH.,** tab., thuj., ***verat.***

amel. - ars., colch., **HEP.,** ign., ***mag-c.,*** **NUX-V.,** psor., puls., rhod., rhus-t., sabad., ***samb.,*** **SIL.,** squil., ***stront-c.***

desire for warm, clothing - alum., ars., ***bar-c.,*** bell., calc., caul., graph., hep., kali-c., nat-c., nat-s., plb., psor., ***sabad.,*** sil.

afternoon - nux-v.

heat sensation of, in spite of - achy.

warm, desire for, warmth - alum., am-br., arg-m., ***ars.,*** bar-c., calc., caps., ***caust., colch.,*** con., ***hep., kali-c.,*** moly-met., ph-ac., psor., ***sabad., sil.,*** thuj., tub.

warm bed - ars., spig.

warm stove - bar-c., cic., ptel., ***sil.,*** tub.

warm, radiated warm, agg., - ant-c.

warm, room, agg. - acon., aeth., ***agn., all-c., alum.,*** alum-sil., ***alumn.,*** am-c., ambr., ***anac., ant-c.,*** ant-t., **APIS,** aran-s., ***arg-n.,*** ars-i., arn., ***asaf., asar.,*** aur., aur-i., ***aur-m.,*** aur-s., bapt., bar-c., bar-i., bell., bor., ***brom., bry.,*** bufo, calad., calc., calc-i., calc-p.,

WARM, temperature

warm, room, agg. - **CALC-S.,** cann-s., ***carb-ac., carb-v.,*** **CARB-S.,** caust., cina, ***coc-c.,*** cocc., colch., crat., **CROC.,** culx., ***dros.,*** dulc., euphr., ***fl-ac., glon.,*** **GRAPH.,** hell., hep., hip-ac., hyos., hyper., ign., ***ind.,*** **IOD.,** ***ip.,*** kali-c., **KALI-I., KALI-S.,** lach., laur., ***led., lil-t.,*** luf-op., **LYC.,** ***mag-m.,*** med., ***merc., merc-i-f.,*** mez., mosch., mur-ac., nat-a., ***nat-c.,*** nat-m., ***nat-s.,*** nit-ac., nux-v., ***op.,*** ozone, ph-ac., phos., ***pic-ac.,*** plat., pneu., ***ptel.,*** **PULS.,** ran-b., rhus-t., **SABIN.,** ***sanic.,*** **SEC.,** sel., **SENEG.,** sep., spig., ***spong.,*** staph., ***sul-i.,*** **SULPH.,** ***tab., thuj., til., tub., verat.,*** vib.

amel. - aur-a., carb-v., ***caust.,*** cham., chel., chin., chin-a., cocc., cycl., guai., ***hep.,*** mag-p., mang., merc., nux-m., nux-v., plat., rhus-t., ***rumx., sil.***

warm, stove, agg. - ***ant-c., apis, arg-n.,*** ars., ***bry.,*** bufo, ***cimic., cocc., con.,*** cupr., ***euph., iod.,*** **GLON.,** ***kali-i., laur.,*** mag-aust., mag-m., ***merc.,*** nat-m., nux-v., op., psor., ***puls.,*** **SEC.,** thiop., ***zinc.***

ailments from - glon.

amel. - acon., agar., am-c., **ARS.,** aur., bar-c., bell., bor., bov., camph., canth., caps., caust., cic., cocc., con., conv., ***dulc.,*** graph., hell., **HEP.,** hyos., **IGN.,** kali-c., lach., mag-c., **MAG-P.,** mang., meny., mosch., ***nux-m.,*** **NUX-V.,** petr., ran-b., rhod., **RHUS-T.,** rumx., sabad., **SIL.,** ***stront-c.,*** sulph., tub.

he is cold and stiff on approaching stove - ***laur.***

warm, sun, agg. - cact., cadm-br., cob., cocc., murx.

amel. - anac., cinnb., con., crot-h., iod., kali-m., ***phos.,*** pic-ac., plat., rhod., ***stront-c.,*** tarent.

warm, wet, weather, agg. - ***aloe,*** ars., bapt., bell., ***brom.,*** bry., calc-f., **CARB-V.,** ***carb-s.,*** caust., erig., ***gels.,*** ham., ***iod., ip., kali-bi.,*** **LACH.,** lath., lyc., lyss., man., mang., merc-i-f., ***nat-m.,*** **NAT-S.,** phos., puls., rhus-t., sabad., **SEP.,** ***sil.,*** **SYPH.,** tub., ***verat.,*** vip-a.

ailments from - carb-v., gels.

amel. - ***aloe,*** bell., brom., ***carb-v.,*** cham., ***gels.,*** ham., hep., ***ip.,*** kali-c., nat-m., sep., sil.

WATER, affects of, (see Generals, Water)

agg. - calc., cupr., stront-c.

cold agg. - aeth.

pouring out of, agg. - lyss.

seeing or hearing of running water agg. - ang., apis, arg-m., bell., brom., canth., **LYSS.,** nit-ac., ***stram.,*** sulph., ter.

thinking of it agg. - ham.

wading in, ailments from - ars., dulc., mag-p.

working in, agg. - ***calc.,*** calc-p., cupr., mag-c.

working, in water

ailments from - calc.

cold - bell-p., calc., cupr., mag-p., rhus-t.

hands in cold, agg. - calc., lac-d., mag-p.,

amel. - jatr.

WEATHER, change of, (see Change)

WET, general

wet, agg. - agar., **AM-C.,** ant-c., ***ant-t., aran.,*** arg-m., ***arg-n.,*** **ARS.,** ***ars-i.,*** aur., **BAD.,** bar-c., bar-m., bell., bor., bov., brom., bry., **CALC.,** ***calc-p., calc-s.,*** canth., ***carb-an., carb-v.,*** cham., chin., ***cist.,*** clem., ***colch.,*** con., cupr., **DULC.,** elaps, ***ferr., ham., hep.,*** hyper., ***iod.,*** ip., kali-c., ***kali-i.,*** kali-n., ***lach.,*** laur., ***lem-m., lyc.,*** mag-c., ***mag-p., mang.,*** meli., ***merc.,*** mez., mur-ac., ***naja, nat-a., nat-c.,*** **NAT-H., NAT-S.,** ***nit-ac.,*** **NUX-M.,** nux-v., paeon., petr., phos., ***phyt.,*** **PULS.,** ***ran-b.,*** **RHOD., RHUS-T.,** ***ruta.,*** sang., sars., seneg., ***sep., sil.,*** spig., stann., staph., ***stront-c., sulph.,*** sul-ac., sumb., teucr., ***thuj., tub., verat., zinc.***

wet, applications, agg. - **AM-C.,** am-m., **ANT-C.,** bar-c., ***bell.,*** bor., bov., bry., **CALC.,** cann-s., ***canth.,*** carb-v., **CHAM., CLEM.,** con., crot-h., dulc., ***kali-c., kali-n., lach.,*** laur., ***lyc.,*** mag-c., ***merc.,*** mez., mur-ac., nat-c., nit-ac., nux-m., nux-v., phos., puls., **RHUS-T.,** sars., ***sep.,*** sil., ***spig.,*** stann., staph., ***stront-c.,*** sul-ac., **SULPH.,** zinc.

ailments from - **AM-C.,** am-m., **ANT-C.,** bar-c., ***bell.,*** bor., bov., bry., **CALC.,** ***canth.,*** carb-v., **CHAM., CLEM.,** con., dulc., ***kali-c., kali-n.,*** laur., ***lyc.,*** mag-c., ***merc.,*** mez., mur-ac., nat-c., nit-ac., nux-m., nux-v., phos., puls., **RHUS-T.,** sars., ***sep.,*** sil., ***spig.,*** stann., staph., ***stront-c.,*** **SULPH.,** sul-ac., zinc.

amel. - ***alumn., am-m.,*** ant-t., ***ars.,*** **ASAR.,** bor., bry., caust., cham., ***chel., euphr.,*** laur., ***mag-c.,*** mez., mur-ac., ***nux-v.,*** **PULS.,** ***rhod., sabad.,*** sep., ***spig.,*** staph., zinc.

cold, agg. - **AM-C.,** am-m., **ANT-C.,** apoc., ***ars.,*** bar-c., ***bell., bor.,*** bov., ***bry.,*** cadm-met., **CALC.,** ***canth., carb-v., cham.,*** **CLEM.,** ***con.,*** dulc., graph., ***hep., kali-c., kali-n.,*** lach., ***laur., lyc.,*** mag-c., ***merc., mez.,*** mur-ac., nat-c., ***nit-ac., nux-m.,*** nux-v., ***petr.,*** ph-ac., ***phos.,*** puls., **RHUS-T.,** ruta, ***sars., sep., sil., spig.,*** stann., ***staph., stront-c., sul-ac.,*** **SULPH.,** syph., ***zinc.***

amel. - aloe, alum., aml-n., anac., ***apis,*** arg-n., arn., aur., asar., bell., bry., ferr-p., ***fl-ac.,*** glon., iod., kali-m., kali-p., ***led.,*** lyc., merc., nat-hchls., phos., pic-ac., ***puls.,*** sabin., sec., spig.

warm, agg. - ***apis,*** bry., ***fl-ac.,*** lach., ***led.,*** phyt., ***puls., sec.***

warm, amel. - alum-sil., anac., ant-c., ***ars.,*** ars-i., bry., calc-f., coloc., fl-ac., ***hep.,*** kali-bi., kali-c., ***lach., mag-p.,*** nux-m., paraph., ph-ac., phos., pyrog., rad-br.,

wet, applications
warm, amel. - ***rhus-t.,*** ruta, sep., ***sil.,*** sulfa., thiop., thuj., x-ray.

wet, getting, agg. - ***acon.,*** **ALUM.,** am-c., ant-c., ant-t., ***apis, arn.,*** ars., ***bell.,*** bor., ***bry.,*** **CALC.,** calc-p., ***calc-s.,*** camph., carb-v., **CAUST.,** cham., ***chin., colch., dulc.,*** euph., fl-ac., ***hep., hyos., ip.,*** kali-bi., ***kali-c.,*** lach., ***lyc.,*** malar., merc-i-r., nat-m., **NAT-S.,** nit-ac., ***nux-m.,*** nux-v., phos., phyt., **PULS.,** ran-b., rhod., **RHUS-T.,** ***sars.,*** sec., **SEP.,** ***sil.,*** sulph., thuj., tub., urt-u., verat., visc., xan., zinc.
feet - agn., ***all-c., bar-c.,*** bry., ***calc., camph.,*** caps., cham., ***colch.,*** cupr., ***dulc.,*** fl-ac., graph., guai., ***dulc.,*** fl-ac., graph., guai., ***lach.,*** lob., lem-m., ***lyc.,*** merc., nat-c., nat-m., nit-ac., ***nux-m.,*** **NUX-V.,** ***phos.,*** **PULS.,** ***rhus-t., sep.,*** **SIL.,** stram., ***sulph.,*** tub., xan.
amel. - calad., led., puls.
head - bar-c., **BELL.,** hep., hyos., led., phos., ***puls.,*** rhus-t., ***sep.***
heated, when - bell-p., rhus-t.
perspiration, during - ***acon.,*** ant-c., ars., ***bell-p., bry.,*** calc., ***clem., colch.,*** con., ***dulc.,*** nat-c., ***nux-m.,*** **RHUS-T.,** ***sep., verat-v.***
rooms, in wet - ***aloe,*** ant-t., ***aran.,*** **ARS.,** ars-i., atro., ***bry., calc.,*** calc-p., calc-sil., ***carb-an., carb-v.,*** caust., **DULC.,** form., lyc., nat-n., **NAT-S.,** nit-ac., nux-m., **PULS.,** rhod., ***rhus-t., sel., sep.,*** sil., ***stram.,*** ter., ***thuj.,*** verat.
sheets, ailments from wet - rhus-t.
sitting on the ground, ailments from - ***ars.,*** caust., ***dulc.,*** nux-v., ***rhus-t.***

wet, weather, agg. - achy., acon-c., agar., alum-sil., **AM-C.,** amph., anac., ant-c., ***ant-t.,*** **ARAN.,** arg-m., ***arg-n.,*** **ARS.,** ***ars-i.,*** ars-s-f., aster., aur., **BAD.,** bar-c., bar-m., bell., blatta, bor., bov., brom., bry., **CALC.,** calc-f., calen., canth., caps., carb-an., ***carb-s., carb-v.,*** caust., cham., chim., chin., chin-s., ***cist.,*** clem., ***colch.,*** con., crot-h., cupr., cur., **DULC.,** elaps, elat., erig., euphr., ***ferr.,*** form., ***gels., glon., graph., ham., hep.,*** hyper., ***iod.,*** ip., kali-c., ***kali-i.,*** kali-m., kali-n., ***lac-ac.,*** lac-c., lac-d., ***lach.,*** lath., laur., ***lem-m., lyc.,*** lyss., mag-arct., mag-c., ***mag-p.,*** magn-gr., ***mang.,*** meli., ***merc.,*** mez., mur-ac., ***naja, nat-a., nat-c.,*** nat-m., **NAT-S.,** ***nit-ac.,*** **NUX-M.,** nux-v., oci-s., onop., paeon., petr., phos., ***phyt.,*** **PULS.,** rad-br., ***ran-b.,*** rauw., **RHOD., RHUS-T.,** ***ruta,*** sabin., sang., sars., seneg., senn., ***sep., sil.,*** sin-n., spig., stann., staph., stict., still., sumb., **SYPH.,** teucr., ***thuj., tub., verat., zinc.,*** zinc-p., zing.
amel. - ***acon.,*** alum., alumn., ***ars.,*** **ASAR.,** aur-m., ***bell.,*** bor., bov., **BRY.,** ***carb-an., carb-v.,*** **CAUST.,** ***cham., fl-ac.,*** **HEP.,** ***ip.,*** laur., mang., **MED.,** mez., mur-ac., ***nit-ac.,*** **NUX-V.,** oci-s., ***plat.,*** rhod., ***sabad., sep., sil.,*** spig., ***spong.,*** staph., sulph., zinc.

wet, weather, cold, agg. - abrot., aesc., ***agar.,*** all-c., all-s., **AM-C.,** ***ant-c., ant-t., apis, aran., arg-m., arg-n.,*** arn., **ARS.,** ars-i., ars-s-f., asc-t., ***aster.,*** aur., aur-a., ***aur-m-n.,*** **BAD.,** ***bar-c.,*** bar-i., bar-s., bell., bell-p., bor., bov., bry., **CALC., CALC-P.,** calc-s., calc-sil., calen., canth., ***caps.,*** carb-an., ***carb-v., carb-s.,*** cham., chin., ***cimic.,*** clem., **COLCH.,** coloc., con., cupr., **DULC.,** elaps, erig., eucal., ***ferr., fl-ac., form., gels.,*** glon., ***graph., guai.,*** hep., ***hyper., iod.,*** ip., ***kali-bi.,*** kali-c., kali-i., kali-m., kali-n., kali-p., kali-sil., ***lach., lath.,*** laur., lept., ***lyc.,*** mag-c., mag-p., ***mang.,*** **MED.,** ***merc.,*** merc-c., merc-i-f., ***mez.,*** mur-ac., naja, ***nat-a., nat-c.,*** nat-m., **NAT-S.,** ***nit-ac.,*** **NUX-M.,** nux-v., onop., paeon., penic., ***petr.,*** phos., physal., ***phyt.,*** polyg., psor., ***puls.,*** **PYROG.,** ***ran-b.,*** **RHOD., RHUS-T.,** rumx., ***ruta,*** sars., seneg., sep., **SIL.,** ***spig.,*** stann., staph., ***still., stront-c., sul-ac., sulph., tarent.,*** teucr., ***thuj.,*** **TUB.,** urt-u., ***verat.,*** zinc., zinc-p., ***zing.***
elderly people, in - ammc.
night and warm days in autumn - dulc., merc., rhus-t.
ailments from - ant-t., ***aran.,*** ars., ars-i., calc., calc-sil., ***dulc., nat-s.,*** nux-m., phyt., ***rhus-t.,*** ter.
amel. - aur-m.

wet, weather, warm and wet, agg. - ***aloe,*** ars., bapt., bell., ***brom.,*** bry., calc-f., **CARB-V.,** ***carb-s.,*** caust., erig., ***gels.,*** ham., ***iod., ip., kali-bi.,*** **LACH.,** lath., lyc., lyss., man., mang., merc-i-f., ***nat-m.,*** **NAT-S.,** phos., puls., rhus-t., sabad., **SEP.,** ***sil.,*** **SYPH.,** tub., ***verat.,*** vip-a.
ailments from - carb-v., gels.
amel. - ***aloe,*** bell., brom., ***carb-v.,*** cham., ***gels.,*** ham., hep., ***ip.,*** kali-c., nat-m., sep., sil.

WIND, general, agg., from - ***acon.,*** anac., ***ars.,*** ars-i., arum-t., asar., **AUR.,** aur-a., ***bell.,*** bry., bufo, calc., ***calc-p.,*** canth., caps., carb-an., carb-v., caust., **CHAM.,** ***chin.,*** coff., colch., coloc., con., cupr., elaps, ***euphr.,*** graph., **HEP.,** hyos., ip., kali-c., kalm., ***lach.,*** **LYC.,** mag-c., mag-p., med., mur-ac., nat-c., nit-ac., ***nux-m.,*** **NUX-V.,** ph-ac., **PHOS.,** plat., ***psor.,*** **PULS.,** rheum, **RHOD.,** ***rhus-t.,*** sabad., samb., sel., sep., ***sil.,*** spig., **SPONG.,** squil., stram., stront-c., sul-ac., sulph., tab., thuj., tub., verb., zinc.
east, agg. - acon., ars., ***asar.,*** bell., bry., carb-an., ***carb-v., caust., all-c.,*** cham., **HEP.,** ip., ***nux-v.,*** **RHUS-T.,** sabad., sep., sil., **SPONG.,** verat.
amel. - arg-n., ferr., iod., nux-m., ***puls.,*** sec., tub.
cold, agg., from - ***acon., all-c.,*** apis, arn., ***ars.,*** ars-i., ***asar.,*** **BELL.,** bell-p., ***bry.,*** cadm-s., calc-p., carb-an., carb-v., **CAUST., CHAM.,** cupr., ferr-ar., **HEP.,** ip., ***kali-bi.,*** kalm., lach., ***mag-p.,*** nit-ac., **NUX-V.,** psor., ***rhod.,*** **RHUS-T.,** rumx., sabad., ***sep., sil.,*** **SPONG.,** thlaspi, tub., verat., zinc.

WIND, general
cold wet, agg., from - all-c., calc.
desire to be in - puls., ***tub.***
north, agg., - acon., ars., ***asar.***, bell., bry., carb-an., carb-v., ***caust.***, cham., ***hep.***, ip., ***nux-v.***, sabad., ***sep.***, sil., **SPONG.**, zinc.
riding, in, agg. - sang-n.
cold amel. - ***arg-n., tub.***
slight, agg., from - caps.
south, agg. - ***gels., ip.***
warm, agg., from - sel.
amel. - thuj.
south, agg. - ***ars-i.***, asar., bry., carb-v., euphr., ***gels., ip.***, lach., nat-c., rhod., sil.
warm, wet, agg., from - ***acon.***, **HEP.**
west, agg. - ***acon.***, **HEP.**
windy, and stormy weather, agg. - ***acon., all-c., am-c.***, arg-m., ars., asar., aur., aur-a., **BAD.**, bell., bry., carb-v., caust., ***cham.***, chel., ***chin.***, chin-a., con., erig., euphr., gels., graph., ***hep.***, hydr-ac., hyper., ip., **KALM.**, ***lach.***, lyc., mag-c., ***mag-p.***, mez., ***mur-ac.***, nat-c., nat-m., nit-s-d., **NUX-M.**, ***nux-v.***, petr., ***phos.***, plat., ***psor., puls.***, ran-b., **RHOD.**, rhus-t., ruta, ***sep.***, spig., sul-ac., sulph., tab., thuj.

WINTER, agg. - **ACON.**, ***aesc., agar., alum.***, **AM-C.**, ammc., ***arg-m.***, **ARS.**, **AUR.**, aur-a., aur-s., ***bar-c., bell.***, bor., bov., **BRY.**, ***calc., calc-p.***, calc-sil., **CAMPH.**, ***caps.***, carb-an., ***carb-v.***, carb-s., ***caust., cham.***, cic., cina, cist., ***coc-c., cocc.***, colch., ***con.***, **DULC.**, ***ferr.***, ferr-ar., **FL-AC.**, graph., **HELL.**, **HEP.**, ***hyos., ign., ip., kali-bi.***, **KALI-C.**, ***kali-p.***, kali-sil., ***kalm.***, **LYC.**, mag-c., **MANG.**, ***merc., mez.***, **MOSCH.**, nat-a., nat-c., nat-m., **NUX-M.**, **NUX-V.**, **PETR.**, ph-ac., ***phos.***, prot., **PSOR.**, **PULS.**, ***rhod.***, **RHUS-T.**, ruta, ***sabad.***, sang-n., sars., sec., ***sep., sil.***, spig., spong., stann., **STRONT-C.**, ***sulph.***, syph., **VERAT.**, viol-t., visc.
ailments since - sang-n.
amel. - glon., ilx-a., ilx-c., sul-i.
solstice agg. - ***aur.***, bry., ***calc.***, calc-p., cic., colch., ***dulc.***, graph., hep., ign., ***kali-bi.***, merc., nat-m., nux-v., ***rhod.***, **RHUS-T.**, ***verat.***

Eyes

ABSCESS, cornea, of - calc-hypo., calc-mur., hep., merc-c., sil., sulph.

ABRASION, cornea - ***acon.,*** arn., **CALEN.,** ham., hyper.

ACHING, pain - **ACON.,** aesc., ***agar.,*** ail., ant-t., apis, ***arg-m.,*** arn., ***ars.,*** aur., ***bad.,*** bapt., bar-c., ***bell.,*** bov., brom., ***bry., calc-p., calc-s., carb-s.,*** carb-v., ***carl.,*** caul., ***cer-b.,*** cham., chel., chin., chin-s., **CIMIC.,** ***cina,*** cob., coca, coc-c., colch., coloc., cop., cupr., dig., dios., ery-a., **EUP-PER.,** ferr., ferr-ar., ferr-p., form., gels., ***glon., graph.,*** grat., hell., ***hep.,*** hydrc., hydr-ac., iod., ip., kali-bi., kali-n., ***kali-p.,*** lach., laur., led., lept., lob., lyc., lyss., mag-m., mang., ***med.,*** merc., merc-i-r., ***mez.,*** myric., naja, nat-a., ***nat-m.,*** nat-p., ***nit-ac., nux-v.,*** onos., par., paeon., petr., phel., ph-ac., ***phos., phyt.,*** pic-ac., ***plan., podo.,*** psor., **PULS.,** ***rhus-t.,*** rhus-v., rumx., ***ruta.,*** sang., sep., sil., **SPIG.,** staph., stront-c., stry., ***sulph.,*** sumb., syph., tep., thuj., til., ust., valer., verat., verat-v., xan., zinc.

afternoon - staph.
air, open amel. - ***seneg.***
evening - dios., ferr., merc., myric., paeon., petr., **PULS.,** rhus-t., ruta., **SULPH.,** verat-v.
amel. - chel.
light, from - carb-an., petr., ***ruta.***
lying down, after - ***carb-v.***
extending to upper jaw - ***fl-ac.***
forenoon - cimic., sulph.
left - ***agar.***
light, bright, agg. - ***hep.,*** petr., phyt., ruta., thuj.
looking sharply, when - ***carb-v., chel.,*** nat-a., **NAT-M.,** ***psor., rhus-t.***
near objects, at - ***mang.***
straining sight - ***carb-v.,*** coloc., merc., ***nat-m.,*** **RUTA.**
up, when looking - ***chel.***
morning - ***form., graph.,*** podo., spig., stry., sulph.
breakfast, after amel. - naja.
waking, on - nat-a., sumb.
moving eyes agg. - ***bad.,*** **BRY.,** chel., ***gels., hep.,*** nat-a., phyt., pic-ac.
nausea, with - thuj.
night - ***bry.,*** cob., coloc., merc., merc-i-f.
closing lids - bell.
closing lids, amel. - nit-ac., pic-ac.
onanism, after - ***cina.***
pressure, after - ***bar-ac.***
amel. - pic-ac.
reading, while - cann-i., **DULC.,** ***jab.,*** nat-a., ol-j., olnd., ***puls.,*** **RUTA.,** staph.
riding, while - verat.
sleep, before - ***con.***
stooping - coloc.
sunlight agg. - ***nat-a.***
touching, when - dig.
walking in open air, while - pall., zinc.
warmth, amel. - ery-a., ***hep.***

ACHING, pain
writing, while - ***calc-f.***

aching, above the eyes - acon., aesc., aeth., agar., ail., all-c., aloe, alum., ambr., am-c., ang., ant-c., ***apis,*** arg-m., ***arg-n., arn., ars.,*** ars-i., asaf., aspar., aur-m., bapt., bar-c., ***bell.,*** berb., bor., bov., brom., ***bry.,*** cadm-s., ***calc., calc-p.,*** calc-s., cann-i., canth., caps., carb-ac., carb-an., carb-v., caust., **CEDR.,** chim-m., ***chel., chin., chin-s.,*** chlol., cimic., cina, cinnb., cist., coca, colch., con., cop., ***croc.,*** crot-h., cupr., dig., dios., dros., echi., elaps, ferr., ferr-ar., ferr-i., ferr-p., fl-ac., ***gels., glon.,*** gymn., ham., hell., ***hep.,*** hipp., hura, hydr., hydrc., hyos., hyper., ign., ind., iod., ip., ***iris,*** jug-r., kali-ar., ***kali-bi.,*** **KALI-C.,** kali-n., kali-p., ***kali-s.,*** kalm., **LAC-C.,** ***lac-d.,*** **LACH.,** lac-ac., lact., laur., lil-t., lith., lob., ***lyc.,*** lyss., mag-c., mag-p., mang., med., ***meph.,*** merc., merc-i-r., merl., mez., mosch., naja, nat-a., nat-c., ***nat-m., nat-p.,*** nit-ac., nux-m., **NUX-V.,** ol-an., onos., op., osm., ox-ac., ***petr.,*** ph-ac., ***phos., phys., phyt.,*** pic-ac., plan., plat., plb., ***psor.,*** ptel., **PULS.,** ran-b., raph., rheum, rhus-r., rhus-t., sabad., ***sang., sanic., sel., seneg., sep.,*** **SIL.,** ***sol-n.,*** **SPIG.,** spong., ***stann.,*** staph., sulph., sul-i., tab., tarent., tax., tell., ter., teucr., ther., thuj., urt-u., ***valer.,*** verat., viol-t., ***zinc.,*** zing.
afternoon - carb-v., cinnb., com., kali-bi., ***lac-c.,*** lyss., puls., sang., sulph.
1 p.m. - chin-s., dios., phys.
3 p.m. - hura, pip-m.
4 p.m. - com.
motion - cinnb.
air, cold, in - kali-bi.
open, in - calc., chel., colch., ham.
open, in, amel. - echi., kali-bi., pip-m., phos., ***sep.***
alternating sides - ***iris,*** **LAC-C.,** ***lil-t.***
bed, on going to - ferr.
breakfast, after - hyper., ***lyc.***
close the eyes, compels him to - ***bell.***
cold applications amel. - agn., cedr., chel., kali-bi., lac-d., ***lach., spig.***
damp weather - ***sil., spig.***
dry wind - **ACON.**
contraction, of brow - ***arn.***
coryza, as from - sulph.
coughing, after - ***ol-j., spig.***
dark, in the - onos.
daytime - phos., pic-ac., sulph.
eating, after - bry., colch., nit-ac., sulph.
amel. - chin.
evening - ars., chel., ferr., iod., kalm., lyss., nat-m., plan., ***puls.,*** ran-b., ***sep.,*** stry.
6 p.m. - colch., dios., lil-t.
8 p.m. - chin-s.
9 p.m. - lyss.
reading, while - ***chel.,*** lyss.
extending, outward - nat-c., sec.
temples - ***arn.,*** bor., dios., hell., nat-a., phys.
to ear - aur-m., glon., lac-c., osm.
to eyes - con., lil-t.

aching, above the eyes
extending to face - ***mag-p.***
to head - gymn.
to nose - all-c., bov., ***calc.,*** **LACH.,** phys., ran-b.
to occiput - bism., chel., cimic., dios., kali-p., kalm., kreos., ***lach.,*** lyc., naja, sep., zing.
to root of nose - **LACH.**
vertex - arg-n., gymn., phos., phys.
forenoon - cinnb., glon., ***mez.,*** rhus-t., sulph., thuj.
8 a.m. - hydr.
9 a.m. - lyss., petr., pip-m.
9 a.m. until 3 p.m. - ***caust.***
10 a.m. - crot-c., petr., stram., tell.
10 a.m. to 4 p.m. - ***stann.***
11 a.m. - mag-p., merc-i-r., myric., verat.
walking, while - thuj.
glasses, from wearing - sil.
heat of stove agg. - ***arn.***
left - acon., ***aesc.,*** aeth., ambr., ant-t., arn., ***ars.,*** arum-t., asaf., bar-c., berb., brom., **BRY.,** caj., calc-p., camph., cann-i., cedr., ***chel., colch.,*** cupr., echi., euph., ferr., glon., ham., hell., helo., hydr., ign., ***ip.,*** iris, ***kali-bi., kali-c.,*** kalm., lac-c., ***lach.,*** lil-t., lob., lyss., mag-c., mag-s., meny., merc-c., merc-i-r., mosch., mur-ac., naja, nat-p., nit-ac., ***nux-v.,*** onos., ox-ac., ***ph-ac., phos.,*** pip-m., psor., puls., ptel., rhus-r., ***sep.,*** **SPIG.,** stann., stram., sul-ac., tell., ter., uran., verat., verat-v., verb.
extending, over whole increasing and decreasing gradually - ***stann.***
extending, to occiput and finally over whole body - ***bry.***
extending, vertex, to - ferr-i.
lying on left side amel. - ***bry.***
periodical - sep.
sex, after - cast., cedr.
then right - kali-bi., ***lac-c., lach.,*** nit-m-ac., ***psor.,*** zing.
light, from - chel., chin-s., mez., nat-m., nux-v., pic-ac., spig.
looking, at bright objects - sol-n.
down - ***nat-m.***
intently at anything - puls.
lying down, after - chim-m., ***ran-b., sang.,*** tell.
amel. - cupr., kali-bi.
menses, during - cimic., graph., ***lach., lyc.,*** nat-p., sang.
after - mag-m.
amel., during - kali-bi.
before - bell., graph., hyper., nat-p., sil., xan.
mental exertion, during - ph-ac., **PIC-AC.,** ***puls.,*** sep., ***spig.***
morning - agar., alum., alumn., ***arg-n., chin.,*** chin-s., coc-c., dios., dros., ***kali-bi., lac-c., lach., mez.,*** nat-a., nux-m., **NUX-V.,** petr., phys., sol-n., ***stann.,*** sulph.

aching, above the eyes
morning, 4 a.m. - spig.
6 to 12 a.m. - ***glon.***
in bed - coc-c., ***nux-v.,*** sol-n., spig.
until 4 p.m. - ***mez.***
waking - bell., phos.
motion, during - ***bry.,*** cinnb., cupr., mag-m., onos., ***nux-v.,*** plb., ***sang.,*** sol-n., ***spig.,*** ther.
amel. - dios., ***puls.***
narrow line, in a - bry.
night - ars., ***chel., glon.,*** hyper., ***kali-bi.,*** lyss., ***mez.***
midnight after - ambr.
noise - chin-s.
noon - form., ham.
numbness, followed by - ***mez.***
periodical - ***chin-s., tub.***
pressure amel. - chin-s.
pulsating - ***bry.,*** caust., chel., dig., ***glon.,*** ham., ***kali-bi., lach., lyss.,*** mag-m., nat-m., ***pic-ac.,*** plat., ptel., **PULS.,** sep., ***spig.,*** ther.
reading - calc., chel., ph-ac.
right - acon., aesc., agar., am-m., anac., aran., arg-n., ars., aur-m., bapt., ***bar-ac., bell.,*** bism., bry., **CARB-AC.,** carb-an., **CHEL.,** ***chin.,*** cinnb., cist., coca, cocc., coc-c., com., cycl., daph., dig., dros., dulc., euon., ferr., fl-ac., ***gels.,*** gins., glon., graph., ham., hyos., ***ign.,*** iris, kali-n., lac-c., lach., ***lyc., mag-p.,*** mang., merc-i-f., mez., mur-ac., ***nat-m., nux-m., ol-an.,*** op., phys., phyt., **RAN-B.,** rhus-t., rumx., **SANG.,** ***spig.,*** staph., stront-c., tab., tarent., viol-t., xan., ziz.
then left - calc., ***lac-c., nat-m.,*** ptel., sep., sin-n.
sewing, while - **LAC-C.**
sex, after - cast., cedr.
sitting, while - ter.
sleep amel. - kali-bi.
sneezing, when - echi.
standing amel. - ***ran-b.***
stooping, when - dros., kali-bi., ***ign.,*** lyss., nat-m., petr., ***puls.,*** sin-n., sol-n., ***spig.***
sudden - ***mez.***
supper, during - chlor.
waking, on - bry., ***lac-c.,*** nat-a., sol-n., ***spig.***
walking, while - agar., chin., puls., thuj.
amel. - dros., ***ran-b.***
in open air, amel., while - bor., chel., hydr., nux-v., ***sep.***
warm applications amel. - ***arg-m.,*** **ARS.,** ***aur-m., mag-p.,*** sang., ***thuj.***
room agg. - mez., ***puls.***
warmth - chel., mez.

aching, behind - acon., asc-t., bad., ***bell.,*** berb., bism., cann-s., chel., cimic., cob., cop., daph., dig., fago., ***fl-ac.,*** gels., glon., kali-n., ictod., lach., led., merc-c., pall., phos., ***podo.,*** rhus-t., ***sel.,*** seneg., sep., ***ther.,*** ziz.

aching, between - **CUPR.,** ***hep.,*** ictod., lach., lyc., phos.

aching, canthi - mag-m.
inner - acon., mosch., ***puls.,*** rhus-t., stann.
outer - chin., dios., lyc.

aching, eyelids, on closing lids at night - bell.
closing lids at night, amel. - nit-ac., pic-ac.

AGGLUTINATED - ***aeth., agar., all-s., alum.,*** apis, ***arg-m.,*** **ARG-N.,** ***bar-c.,*** bar-m., bell., ***bry.,*** **CALC.,** calc-s., carb-an., ***carb-s.,*** carb-v., **CAUST., CHAM.,** chel., ***clem.,*** coc-c., colch., cycl., ***dig.,*** dros., euph., ***euphr.,*** **GRAPH.,** hydr., ***ign.,*** kali-ar., ***kali-c.,*** kali-n., kali-p., kali-s., **KREOS.,** lac-c., laur., led., lept., lil-t., **LYC.,** ***mag-c.,*** nat-a., ***nat-s.,*** nicc., ***nux-m., nux-v.,*** op., ph-ac., **PHOS.,** plb., ***phyt.,*** plat., **PULS.,** rhod., rhus-t., **SEP.,** ***sil.,*** spig., spong., ***stann., staph., sulph., thuj.,*** uran., valer., verat.
afternoon - nat-c.
air, in open - thuj.
evening - plat., plb., sep.
menses, during - ***calc.***
morning - aeth., ail., ***alum.,*** ambr., am-c., am-m., ang., ***arg-m.,*** **ARG-N.,** ***ars.,*** aur., aur-m., aur-s., bar-c., ***bell.,*** berb., bor., bov., bry., **CALC.,** calc-s., ***carb-v.,*** carl., **CARB-S.,** ***caust., cham., chel.,*** **CLEM.,** con., cop., ***dig., dios.,*** euph., ***euphr.,*** **GRAPH.,** ***hep.,*** hydr., kali-ar., ***kali-bi., kali-c.,*** kali-n., kali-p., led., lyc., mag-arct., ***mag-c.,*** mag-m., ***mang.,*** **MED.,** ***merc.,*** mill., mur-ac., naja, ***nat-a., nat-c., nat-m., nat-s.,*** nicc., nit-ac., nux-v., petr., phos., plb., ***psor., puls.,*** rheum, **RHUS-T.,** sanic., sars., ***seneg., sep.,*** sil., stann., **SULPH.,** sul-ac., tarax., ***tarent.,*** thuj., vip., ***zinc.***
menses, during - calc., mag-c.
night - **ALUM.,** am-c., ang., ***ant-c., apis,*** ars., ***arg-n.,*** bar-c., bell., ***bor., bov.,*** bry., calc., **CARB-S.,** ***carb-v.,*** cham., chel., cic., ***croc.,*** dig., ***euph., euphr.,*** ferr., ferr-ar., ***gamb.,*** **GRAPH.,** ***hep., ign.,*** kali-c., led., **LYC.,** mag-c., mag-m., merc-n., nat-m., nit-ac., nux-v., ol-an., phos., plb., puls., rat., rhod., ***rhus-t.,*** sars., **SEP.,** ***sil., spong., stann.,*** staph., stram., sulph., ***syph.,*** tarax., ***thuj.,*** verat.
sensation - carb-v., caust., plat.
sleep, after - rheum.

agglutinated, morning, inner canthi - mag-c., phos., staph., zinc.
morning, outer canthi - ars., sep.

AMAUROSIS, (see Vision, chapter, Blindness), optic nerve paralysis - acon., anac., anan., ***arg-m.,*** arg-n., ***ars.,*** aur., ***aur-m., aur-m-n.,*** bar-c., **BELL.,** ***bov.,*** both., bry., bufo, ***calc.,*** caps., ***caust., chel., chin.,*** chin-s., cic., cocc., **CON.,** croc., dig., dros., dulc., ***elaps,*** euphr., ***ferr.,*** ferr-ar., fl-ac., **GELS.,** guai., ***hyos.,*** kali-ar., kali-c., **KALI-I.,** kali-p., ***kali-s.,*** laur., ***lyc., meny., merc.,*** nat-a., nat-c., **NAT-M.,** nat-p., nit-ac., ***nux-v.,*** olnd., ***op.,*** petr., ***ph-ac.,*** **PHOS.,** ***plb., psor.,*** **PULS.,** ***rhus-t., ruta.,*** **SEC.,** ***sep.,*** **SIL.,** spig., staph., **STRAM., SULPH.,** syph., ***thuj.,*** verat., verat-v., vib., ***zinc.***

AMAUROSIS, optic nerve paralysis
left - phos., thuj.
right - ***bov.***
then left - ***chin.***

ANEMIA, conjunctiva, of - dig., plb.
anemia, retina, of - agar., chin., dig., lith.

ANESTHESIA of retina from looking at eclipse - hep., sol.

ARCUS senilis, (see Opacity, cornea)

ASTIGMATISM - gels., lil-t., phys., pic-ac., ***tub.***

ATROPHY, optic nerve - agar., arg-n., carb-s., iodof., kali-i., ***nux-v.,*** **PHOS.,** sant., syph., ***tab.***
tobacco, from - ars., con. phos.
atrophy, retina, of - nux-v.

AVERSION, to bringing objects near the eyes - fl-ac., mang.

BAND, around the eyeballs, sensation of - ***lac-d.,*** laur.

BLEEDING, from - acon., aloe, am-c., am-caust., calen., caust., ***arn.,*** bell., **BOTH.,** ***calc., calen.,*** camph., ***carb-v., cham.,*** cor-r., **CROT-H.,** dig., elaps, euphr., ***kali-chl.,*** **LACH.,** nit-ac., **NUX-V., PHOS.,** plb., raph., ruta., ***sulph.***
blowing nose, on - nit-ac.
burning, with - carb-v.
coughing, from - arn., carb-v., cham., nux-v.
inside, after injury - arn., sul-ac.
whooping cough, in - arn., nux-v.

bleeding, choroid - arn., bell., chin., crot-h., ham., lach., merc-c., phos.

bleeding, conjunctiva - sang.

bleeding, eyelids - arn., bell., ***hep., nat-m., nux-v.,*** **SULPH.**

bleeding, iris, iridectomy after - calen., led., phos.

bleeding, retina - acon., ***apis.,*** arn., ***bell.,*** both., croc., ***crot-h.,*** dub., ***gels.,*** glon., ham., **LACH.,** led., ***merc-c.,*** **PHOS.,** ***prun., sul-ac., sulph.,*** symph.

BLEPHARITIS, inflammation, eyelids - ***acon.,*** act-sp., anac., **ANT-C., ARG-M., ARG-N., APIS,** ***ars.,*** arund., bar-c., bell., berb., **CALC-S.,** ***carb-an.,*** **CARB-S.,** caust., ***cinnb., cocc.,*** com., con., crot-t., ***dig.,*** euph., euphr., **GRAPH.,** ***hep., hydr.,*** hyos., ***iris,*** kali-ar., kali-bi., ***kali-c.,*** kali-s., kreos., lach., lil-t., **LYC., MED.,** meph., **MERC.,** ***mez.,*** nat-a., ***nat-c., nat-m., nit-ac.,*** **PETR.,** phos., ***psor.,*** puls., **RHUS-T.,** ***sang., sanic.,*** sarr., sars., ***seneg., sep., sil., spig.,*** stann., **STAPH.,** stram., **SULPH., TELL.,** ***ter., thuj., uran.,*** verat., zinc.
lower - mag-c., sulph.
margins - ***aeth., arg-m., arg-n.,*** ars., ***aur-m.,*** bell., ***bor., bov., cham.,*** **CLEM.,** ***dig.,*** euphr., **GRAPH.,** ***hep., hydr.,*** lach., merc., ***merc-c.,*** nat-a., ***nat-m.,*** nat-s., nux-v., ***puls.,*** **SANIC.,** ***seneg., staph.,*** stram.

BLINDNESS, (see Vision)

BLINKING, (see Winking) - bell., ***carc.,*** chel., euphr., kali-bi., kalm., lyc., mez., nux-v., petr.
epilepsy, during - agar., anac., bell., cham., hyos., kali-bi., lyss., mag-m., stram.
reading, during and after - calc., croc.

BLOATED, eyelids, (see Swelling)

BLOODSHOT, (see Ecchymosis)

BLUENESS, canthi - aur., ham., sars
blueness, conjunctiva - bell., carb-o., plb., stram.
blueness, of eyelids - ***dig.***, dros., ***kali-c.,*** naja, zinc.
margins - ***bad., bov., phyt.,*** verat.
blueness, sclera - ars., calc., ***carc.,*** puls., tub.

BOILS, (see Pulstules) - phos., ***sil.***
orbital arch, on - phos.

BORING, pain - apis, arg-n., asaf., ***aur.,*** aur-m., bism., chin-s., ***crot-h.,*** coff., elaps, form., hell., kali-c., ***merc.,*** merc-i-f., nat-m., ***nux-m.,*** puls., spig., stry., thuj.
boring, canthi, inner, above - thuj.
boring, eyes, over - agar., arg-n., ***ars.,*** asaf., aster., aur-m-n., **BELL.,** calc-caust., cimic., colch., cupr-ar., dulc., ip., laur., led., lyc., mag-s., ol-an., sep., spig., sulph.
afternoon - sang.
closing eyes amel. - ip.
cold air, in - sep.
evening in bed - mag-s.
forenoon, 10 a.m. - cimic.
11 a.m. - ***spig.***
left - ***arg-n.,*** cimic., cupr-ar., kali-c., lyc., nux-m., spig.
morning - sulph.
pressure, amel. - ip.
right - ***aur.,*** colch., sulph.
thunderstorm, in - sep.
walking, while - aur-m-n.
amel. - ars.

BREAKING glass, sensation of, on opening eyes - meph.

BRILLANT, (see Glassy) - absin., acon., ***aeth.,*** ail., ***ars.,*** atro., bapt., **BELL.,** benz., **CAMPH.,** cann-i., cann-s., cedr., coca, ***coff., coloc.,*** cupr., ***eup-per.,*** euph., ***gels., hyos., lachn., lyc., lyss.,*** mill., ***op.,*** plb., puls., sant., ***stram.,*** tanac., ***zinc.***
sweat, during - op.

BURNING, pain - **ACON.,** aesc., ***aeth., agar.,*** agn., ail., **ALL-C.,** aloe, **ALUM.,** alumn., ambr., am-c., ***am-m.,*** anan., ang., aphis., **APIS,** ***arg-n.,*** aran., arn., arum-t., arund., **ARS.,** ***asaf.,*** asar., aur., aur-m., bapt., bar-c., bar-m., **BELL.,** berb., bism., bor., brom., ***bry.,*** bufo, buf-s., cahin., calad., **CALC.,** calc-s., camph., ***canth., caps.,*** carb-ac., carb-an., **CARB-S., CARB-V.,** card-m., ***carl., caust., cedr.,*** cham., ***chel.,*** **CHIN.,** ***chin-a., chlol., clem.,*** cob., coc-c., coff., ***colch., coloc.,*** **CON.,** cop., croc., ***crot-h., crot-t.,*** cupr., ***cycl., dig.,*** dios., dros., elaps, eug., ***euph.,*** **EUPHR.,** eupi., fago., ferr., ferr-ar., ferr-i., ferr-p., fl-ac., form., ***gamb.,*** gels., glon., gran., ***graph.,*** gymn., hell., ***hep., hydr.,*** hyos., hyper., ***ign., iod.,*** ip., jug-r., ***kali-ar., kali-bi.,*** **KALI-C.,** ***kali-i.,*** kali-n., kali-p., ***kali-s.,*** kalm., kreos., ***lach.,*** lachn., ***lac-c.,*** lact., laur., led., lil-t., ***lyc.,*** lyss., ***mag-c., mag-m.,*** mang., meph., ***merc., merc-c.,*** merc-i-f., ***merc-i-r., mez.,*** mosch., ***mur-ac.,*** nat-a., ***nat-c.,*** **NAT-M.,** nat-p., ***nat-s., nicc., nit-ac.,*** nux-m., ***nux-v.,*** ol-an., olnd., ***op.,*** osm., paeon., par., ***petr.,*** **PH-AC.,** ***phos.,*** phel., phys., ***phyt.,*** pic-ac., plb., plat., podo., psor., **PULS., RAN-B.,** ***ran-s.,*** raph., ***rhod., rhus-t.,*** rhus-v., **RUTA.,** sabad., sabin., ***sang.,*** sars., ***seneg., sep.,*** sil., ***sin-n.,*** sol-n., ***spig.,*** spong., ***stann.,*** staph., stram., stict., ***stront-c., stry., sul-ac.,*** **SULPH.,** syph., tab., tarax., ***tarent.,*** tep., ***teucr., thuj.,*** til., vesp., valer., verat., vib., viol-o., viol-t., **ZINC.,** zing.
afternoon - bor., caust., com., gamb., jug-c., kalm., merc-i-f., ***nat-c., nat-s.,*** nicc., ph-ac., rhod., stry., ***sulph., thuj.,*** **ZINC.**
menses, during - nicc.
air, in open - graph., kali-bi., ***merc.,*** merc-c., nat-a., ol-an., sul-ac., verat.
amel. - ***gamb., phyt.,*** **PULS.**
alternately - ***chin.***
around the eye - canth., chlor., cic., manc., nat-c., phos., spong., staph.
back of the eyes - form.
bathing, agg. - ***mur-ac.,*** sulph.
amel. - am-m, nicc.
amel., the eye - mur-ac.
candlelight - ***calc.,*** cor-r., graph., mag-s., ol-an., ph-ac., pic-ac., sulph.
amel. - am-m.
caruncle - bell.
chill, before - rhus-t.
cleaning eyes, when - phos.
closing lids - agar., am-m., calc., carb-v., ***clem.,*** ham., lyc., ***manc.,*** sars., sil.
must - spig.
cold, bathing amel. - ***apis, aur.,*** nicc., ***puls., sep.,*** thuj.
wind - **SEP.**
cough, with - agar., chin., bol.
daylight - mag-c.
daytime only - am-c., hep., ***mang.,*** nat-c., phos., sulph.
reading, while - sul-ac.
dim light agg. - am-m., stram.
dinner, after - carb-v., kali-bi., mag-m., nat-c., thuj., zinc.
evening - acon., agar., ang., ***alum.,*** am-br., am-c., am-m., ant-t., ars., bapt., cann-s., carb-s., ***caust.,*** con., dios., erig., eug., fago., gamb., graph., hura, kali-ar., kali-bi., laur., led., lyc., mag-c., mag-s., mur-ac., nat-a., nat-c., **NAT-M.,** ***nat-s.,*** nicc., ph-ac., phos., pic-ac., psor., **PULS.,** rat., **RUTA.,** seneg., **SEP.,** sil., ***sulph.,*** thuj., viol-o., **ZINC.**
6 to 8 p.m. - caust.
air, in open - kali-bi.
bed, after going to - op.
candlelight, by - calc., graph., ol-an., ph-ac., **RUTA.**
fire, on looking at - mag-m., ***nat-s.,*** phyt.

BURNING, pain
evening, gaslight - phyt.
lying down amel. - nat-c.
reading, while - agn., ***graph., nat-m.,*** **RUTA.,** sul-ac.
twilight - am-m., stram., sul-ac.
writing, while - ***nat-m.***
exertion of vision - bar-c., dros., **NAT-M.,** ***petr.,*** **RUTA.,** staph.
eyebrows - dros., sulph.
fever, during - cedr., chin., lyc., ***petr.,*** rhod., sul-ac.
fire, looking at the - ***apis,*** mag-m., ***merc., nat-s.,*** phyt.
forenoon - dios., gels., kali-bi., nat-c., phys., ***sulph.,*** ust., valer.
headache, during - ail., aran., carb-s., ***coff., eug.,*** hep.
itching - calc., ***kali-bi., lyc.,*** **PULS.**
lachrymation, with - chin., sulph.
left to right - mur-ac.
light, agg. - calc., cob., ery-a., iod.
light, bright - ery-a., ***kreos., mag-m., rhod.***
amel. - am-m.
looking sharply, when - bar-c., cast., mag-m., ***nat-m.,*** psor., rhod., sul-ac.
at the light - mag-m., nux-v.
upward - alum.
lying down agg. - ***nux-v.***
menses, during - cast., mag-c., nicc., ***nit-ac.***
moistening, eye amel. - nat-c.
morning - ***alum.,*** am-c., am-m., calc., calc-s., caps., carb-an., carb-s., ***chel.,*** dios., elaps, fago., ***ferr.,*** graph., hep., ***kali-bi.,*** kali-n., ***lyc.,*** mag-m., meph., ***mur-ac.,*** nat-a., **NAT-M.,** ***nat-s.,*** nicc., ***nit-ac.,*** **NUX-V.,** phel., phys., rat., rhod., ruta., sars., ***seneg., sep.,*** sil., stront-c., **SULPH.,** thuj., **ZINC.**
breakfast, after - ***sulph.***
rising, on - ars-m., fago., nat-c., nat-m., ***sulph.,*** thuj.
waking, on - alum., am-c., chel., elaps, iod., nicc., ol-an., rat., sars., sep., ***sulph.***
washing - kali-n., ***mur-ac., sulph.***
washing, amel. - alum., am-m., nicc.
motion agg. - berb., caust,
night - alum., am-m., **ARS.,** asaf., ***con., crot-t.,*** eug., fago., kali-ar., kali-c., merc., **RUTA.,** sanic., stry., sulph., ***tarent.***
like balls of fire - **RUTA.**
midnight, after - **SULPH.**
reading in bed, while - cycl.
noon - gymn., ***sulph.***
12:30 p.m. - nat-m.
one then the other - **CHIN.,** nat-c.
opening, the eyes, on - **ARS.,** ***kali-bi.,*** mag-m.
operations, after - asar., **CALEN.,** hyper., ***staph., zinc.***
periodic - asaf.
pressure, amel. - pic-ac.
upward amel. - bell.

BURNING, pain
reading, while - agn., ***ars.,*** asar., bar-c., ***calc., carb-v.,*** cob., ***con., croc.,*** cycl., ***graph.,*** kali-ar., ***kali-c.,*** lil-t., myric., ***nat-a., nat-c.,*** **NAT-M.,** ***olnd.,*** petr., phos., pic-ac., ***puls.,*** psor., rhod., ***ruta., seneg.,*** sep., ***staph.,*** sul-ac., ***sulph.,*** thuj., zinc.
fine print - ind., mur-ac., nat-m., psor., ***ruta.***
right - ambr.
rub, must - **ALL-C.,** chin., **PULS.**
rubbing, on - carb-an., carb-v., ***con.,*** kalm., ***puls.,*** sep.
amel. - am-m., mag-c., zinc.
sand in, as if - agar., ambr., **CAUST.,** con., ***euphr.,*** ign., iod., mag-m., merc., ***nat-m.,*** zing.
sleep, after - alum., canth.
amel. - chel.
smoke as from - aeth., ***all-c., croc.,*** lyc., mosch., nat-a., petr.
spots - nat-m., ***phos.***
stool, after - ***nat-c.***
stooping, on - bov.
surgery, after - **CALEN.,** hyper., ***staph., zinc.***
touch agg. - agar., ***caust.,*** thuj.
warm, bed agg. - ***merc.***
warm, room, in a - aeth., **APIS,** ***con.,*** **PULS.**
walking, in a, amel. - ***coloc.***
washing, amel. - kali-n.
work, during - graph., nat-c.
writing, while - cob., lact., ***lil-t.,*** nat-a., nat-c., ***nat-m.,*** rhod., ***seneg.,*** staph., zinc.
yawning - agar.

burning, canthi - aesc., ***agar.,*** alum., ***am-m.,*** ant-t., ***apis, asaf., aur.,*** bar-c., bell., berb., **BRY.,** cact., ***calc.,*** carb-an., ***carb-s., carb-v., caust.,*** cinnb., ***clem.,*** con., coloc., euphr., fl-ac., gels., gran., ***graph.,*** hell., hyper., iris, kali-bi., ***kali-c.,*** kali-n., lact., mag-c., mez., ***mur-ac.,*** nat-c., nat-m., nux-v., par., petr., ph-ac., phos., ran-b., ***ran-s.,*** rhod., ***rhus-t.,*** ruta., sanic., ***sep.,*** sil., spig., ***staph.,*** stront-c., ***sulph.,*** tab., teucr., ther., thuj., tril., zinc.
evening - ang., sulph., thuj.
inner - agar., alum., alum-sil., ant-t., asar., aur., bry., calc., calc-s., carb-an., carb-v., ***caust.,*** coloc., ***con.,*** dios., graph., mag-c., mez., mur-ac., nat-m., nicc., nux-v., ox-ac., ***petr.,*** ph-ac., ***phos.,*** phyt., ***puls.,*** sep., sil., stann., ***staph., sulph.,*** teucr., ***zinc.***
evening - mag-c.
morning - calc-s., **NUX-V.**
itching - alum., euphr.
morning - am-m., carb-an., rhod., sil., stront-c., sulph.
morning, waking, on - sep.
night - **BRY.**

burning, canthi
outer - **ANT-C.,** arg-n., aur-m., bry., camph., carb-an., carb-v., colch., dig., ***hep.,*** ign., kali-bi., kali-c., kali-n., lyc., mang., mur-ac., nux-v., phos., ***ran-b.,*** ran-s., ruta., sep., spig., squil., staph., sulph., thuj., zinc.
washing, after - am-m.
amel. - am-m.
writing - kali-bi.

burning, eyelids - alum., ambr., aur., calc., dros., kali-c., kali-n., lyc., phos., ph-ac., sars., sep., sil., spong., stann., sulph., tarax., zinc.

burning, eyes, over - acon., agar., **ARS.,** chel., coloc., dig., dros., meny., merc., nux-m., rhus-t., sil., sulph.
afternoon - sulph.
evening - chel.
night - **ARS.**

burning, margins of eyelids - alum., ***apis,*** arum-d., **ARS.,** asaf., asar., aur., aur-m-n., brom., bry., bufo, calc., camph., cann-i., carb-s., card-m., caust., clem., coc-c., ***colch.,*** crot-h., ***dig.,*** **EUPHR.,** fago., ferr-p., gins., hell., hura, jatr., kali-bi., kali-p., kreos., ***lach., led.,*** manc., med., meph., ***merc-c.,*** mez., ***nat-s.,*** nux-v., ***olnd.,*** ran-s., sanic., sep., sol-n., spig., ***sulph.***
afternoon - kali-bi., ***sang., sulph.***
daytime only - nat-m., ***sulph.***
evening - **ARS.,** ***thuj., zinc.***
forenoon - sulph.
gland - rheum.
morning - ***gamb., nat-s., nit-ac., nux-v.,*** seneg., **SULPH.,** ***zinc.***
reading, while - ign.
waking, on - agar., euphr., kali-bi., sulph.

BURNS, cornea - ***canth.,*** ham.

BURROWING, pain, eyes, over - dulc., kali-c., plat.
while walking - plat.

BURSTING, pain - asar., daph., ***gels., glon.,*** juni., lac-ac., mag-c., **PRUN.,** puls., ***seneg.,*** spig., ***staph.,*** stram.
bubble, like a - puls.
light - staph.
lying - ***gels.***
night - staph.
over, eyes - crot-c., kali-bi., mag-m., nit-ac.
reading, while - asar., staph.
stooping, agg. - lac-ac.
turning, head, agg. - lac-ac.
using, eyes - staph.

CANCER, eyes - aur-m-n., **CALC.,** con., ***lyc.,*** **PHOS.,** ***sep., sil.,*** thuj.

cancer, epithelioma - cund., ***lach.***
cornea - hep.
eyelids - hydr., lach., phyt., ran-b., thuj.
lower - apis, cund., thuj.

cancer, fungus - bell., **CALC.,** ***lyc.,*** **PHOS.,** ***sep., sil.,*** thuj.
medullaris - bell., **CALC.,** ***lyc., sil.***

cancer, lachrymal glands - ***carb-an.***

CATARACT - ***am-c., am-m.,*** ant-t., ***apis,*** arn., ***bar-c.,*** bell., **CALC., CALC-F.,** ***calc-p.,*** calc-s., ***cann-s., carb-an.,*** **CAUST.,** ***chel.,*** chim., chin., ***cine.,*** coch., ***colch., con.,*** dig., ***euph.,*** euphr., hep., hyos., iod., ***jab., kali-c.,*** kali-m., kali-sil., kreos., kali-s., lac-c., led., ***lyc.,*** **MAG-C.,** merc., naph., nat-m., ***nit-ac.,*** op., **PHOS.,** plb., psor., ***puls.,*** rhus-t., ruta., ***sant., sec.,*** seneg., ***sep.,*** **SIL.,** spig., **SULPH.,** tell., ***thiosin., zinc.***
capsular - ***am-m.,*** colch.
contusion, from - arn., ***con.***
cortical - **SULPH.**
footsweat, suppressed, after - **SIL.**
incipient - caust., ***puls.,*** sec., sep.
injury, after - con., tell.
lachrymation, with - euphr.
left - phos., ***sulph.***
menses, absent, with - lyc.
ocular lesions, from - tell.
perpendicular half-sight, with - caust.
reticularis - caust., plb.
right, eye - ***am-c., kali-c., nit-ac., sil.***
senile - ***carb-an., sec.***
soft - ***colch.,*** sec., merc.
surgery, after - arn., **CALEN.,** ***seneg.***
prolapse - alumn., staph.
viridis - colch., con., ***phos.,*** puls.
vision, better on a dark day - euph.
women, in - sep.

CHEMOSIS, edema of conjunctiva - am-caust., ***acon.,*** **APIS, ARG-N.,** ars., bell., bry., cadm-s., cham., ***con.,*** crot-h., dulc., ***euphr., guare., hep., ip., kali-bi.,*** **KALI-I.,** ***lach.,*** merc., merc-i-r., mez., ***nat-m.,*** nit-ac., phyt., **RHUS-T.,** sil., syph., ter., thuj., ***vesp.***
chill, during - bry.
evening, while at work - mez.
left - bell.
right - syph., vesp.
surgery, after, for cataract - ***calen.,*** guare., phyt.
yellow - am-caust., ***merc-i-r.***

chemosis, cornea - ***hep.***

CLAWING, pain, in - am-m.

CLOSE, eyes,general
desire to - agar., ant-t., bell., ***calc., caust., chel.,*** con., dios., elaps, gels., lac-ac., ***med.,*** ox-ac., ***sil.***
desire to, chill, during - bry.
evening while at work - mez.
difficult - aur-m., cadm-s., carb-s., carb-v., euph., **NUX-V., PAR.,** ***phos., sil.***
evening - bor.
headache, during - hep., lach., sulph.
involuntary - acon., alum., bov., carc., **CAUST.,** chin., **CHIN-S.,** chlor., cic., **CON.,** euph., eupi., ***gels.,*** graph., ***grat.,*** hura, mag-s., ***merc.,*** mez., ***nat-c.,*** phos., ***rhus-t., sep.,*** spong., **SULPH.,** viol-t.
afternoon - alum.
menses, during - phos.
morning - upa.

CLOSE, eyes,general
must - agar., arn., calc., ***canth.,*** carb-v., ***chel.,*** euph., ***kali-c., lyc.,*** petr., ph-ac., mez., sil., spig.
bathing, while - phos.
headache, during - carb-v., plat.
pain in eyes, with - hep., ph-ac., plat., spig.
close, eyes, spasmodic - acon., agar., ***alum.,*** apis, **ARS., *bell.,*** brom., ***calc.,*** cham., **COLOC., *con.,*** hep., ***hyos.,*** **MERC., *merc-c.,*** **NAT-M.,** nux-v., osm., ***psor., rhus-t.,*** sep., sil., spong., staph., stram.
abdomen, from pain in - coloc.
evening - con., ***hep.,*** nat-m., sep.
headache, with - calc-ac., ***nat-m.,*** sep.
looking, on - ***merc.***
morning - hep., nat-m., sep., spong.
night - alum., hep., nat-m.
walking in open air, while - calad.
weak feeling - cupr.

CLOSED, eyes (see Open unable to) - ***calc., cocc., grat.,*** hyos., ***lachn.,*** **RHUS-T.,** sep., stram., stry., sulph., urt-u.
evening - nat-m.
melancholia, in - **ARG-N.,** sep.

COLD, agg. - cob., ***clem.,*** hep., **MERC.,** sanic., ***thuj.***
amel. - acon., agar., ***apis, asar.,*** bry., led., ***nux-v., puls., sep.***

COLDNESS, in - aesc., alum., ambr., am-c., amyg., ***arg-n.,*** asaf., asar., berb., bufo, ***calc., calc-p.,*** chlor., ***con.,*** croc., ***euphr.,*** eupi., form., ***fl-ac.,*** graph., ***kali-c.,*** lachn., lith., ***lyc.,*** med., par., ***phyt., plat.,*** plb., raph., sep., seneg., sil., spig., spong., squil., stram., sulph., syph., ***thuj.***
above eyes - graph.
back of eyes - calc-p.
cold air blew in, as if - asaf., asar., berb., cinnb., ***croc., fl-ac.,*** med., mez., sep., sulph., syph., ***thuj.***
evening - lyc.
ice, as if lump of - lyc., mag-arct., mag-aust.
left - tarent.
painful eye, in the - ***thuj.***
right - plat.
swimming, in cold water, sensation as if - squil.
walking in cold wind - ***squil.***
in open air - alum., con., sil., squil.
coldness, canthi - asaf., euphr., lith.
coldness, eyelids - brom., hura, ***kali-c.,*** ph-ac.
edges of - kali-c.
closing on - ph-ac.

COLOR, blindness, vision - bell., carb-s., chlol., cina, sant.

CONDYLOMATA, growths - arund., ***calc.,*** cinnb., ***merc., nit-ac.,*** phos., staph., **THUJ.**
canthi - calc., nit-ac. psor.
cornea - ars.
eyebrows - anan., ***caust., thuj.***

CONDYLOMATA, growths
eyelids - ***caust.,*** cinnb., ***nit-ac.,*** sulph., **THUJ.**
bleeding when touched - nit-ac.
right, lower - ***nit-ac.***
irises - ***cinnb.,*** **MERC.,** staph., thuj.
sclerotics - arund.

CONGESTION, (see Redness)

CONICAL, cornea - ***euphr.,*** puls.

CONJUNCTIVITIS, infection - **ACON.,** act-sp., ail., ***all-c.,*** **ALUM.,** ant-c., ant-t., **APIS, ARG-N.,** arn., **ARS.,** ars-i., asc-t., **BELL.,** brom., bry., **CALC., *calc-f., calc-p.,*** **CALC-S.,** cann-i., ***canth.,*** **CARB-S.,** cedr., ***cham.,*** chin., ***chlol.,*** chlor., ***cinnb., clem.,*** coc-c., crot-h., ***crot-t., dig.,*** dub., dulc., **EUPHR.,** ferr-i., ***ferr-p.,*** guare., ***ham., hep., hydr., iod., ip., kali-bi.,*** kali-chl., kali-m., kali-p., led., ***lyc.,*** med., ***merc.,*** merc-c., ***nat-a.,*** nat-p., ***nat-s.,*** nit-ac., ***nux-v.,*** op., ***petr.,*** pic-ac., ***puls.,*** **RHUS-T.,** sep., ***staph.,*** stict., **SULPH.,** sumb., tell., tep., ***thuj.,*** tub., upa., ***zinc.***
croupous - acet-ac., apis, guare., iod., kali-bi., merc., ***merc-cy.***
gonorrheal - ***acon.,*** ant-t., apis, ***arg-n.,*** euphr., ***hep.,*** kali-bi., merc., merc-c., nit-ac., ***puls.,*** rhus-t., verat-v.
granular - ***alum., apis,*** **ARG-N.,** ars., aur-m., ***calc.,*** cinnb., dulc., ***ery-a., euphr.,*** graph., ***ham.,*** hep., ***kali-bi.,*** kali-m., ***merc.,*** nat-a., nat-s., ***petr., phyt.,*** psor., puls., rhus-t., sep., ***sil., sulph., thuj.,*** zinc.
cold applications amel. - ***apis,*** asar., ***puls.***
injuries, from - ***acon., arn.,*** bell., **CALEN.,** canth., euphr., ***ham.,*** led., symph.
menses, with absent - euph.
phlyctenular - ant-t., ars., ***calc.,*** con., euphr., graph., ign., merc-c., puls., ***rhus-t.,*** sil., sulph.
pouting - nit-ac.
purulent - ***arg-n.,*** hep., merc., ***merc-c.,*** puls., ***rhus-t.,*** sil.
pustular, (see Pustules)

CONSTRICTING - acon., amph., cham., chlor., elaps, lyc., naja, nit-ac.
evening - rat.

CONTORTED, (see Distorted)

CONTRACTIVE, pain - agar., bism., bor., crot-c., euphr., ***kali-n.,*** nat-c., plb., spig., ***verat.***
evening - agar., euphr., glon., rhus-t.
forehead and face concentrate in tip of nose - ***kali-n.***
morning - stry.

CONTRACTED, eyes, with headache - sulph.

CONTRACTION, eyelids - acon., agar., ***ant-t.,*** ars., ***bell.,*** bov., bry., carb-an., carc., **CHIN.,** cocc., cic., con., ***croc.,*** cupr., cycl., ferr., ign., kali-c., kali-n., lyc., merc., **NAT-M., *nux-m.,*** olnd., ph-ac., plat., sep., sil., spong., squil., stann., staph., **SULPH.,** tab., viol-o., viol-t.

CONTRACTION, eyelids
morning - sulph.
headache, with - kali-n., nit-ac., sep., sulph.

CONTRACTIVE, sensation - agar., alum., bell., bor., bov., kali-n., nat-c., ***nat-m.,*** nit-ac., phys., sep., squil., stann.
eyebrow, muscle - hell.
headache, during - ***carb-v.,*** kali-n., mag-c.
reading and writing by candlelight, while - sep.
right - hyper.
contractive, canthi, outer - graph.
contractive, eyelids - agar., bor., nux-v., rhus-t., staph., staph.

CORNEA, affections in general - **CALC.,** calc-f., ***cann-i.,*** con., ***euph.,*** hep., merc., merc-i-f., phos., ***puls.,*** sulph.

CRACKS, canthi, in - alum., ant-c., bor., **GRAPH.,** iod., **LYC.,** merc., ***nat-m.,*** nit-ac., petr., phos., plat., sep., sil., staph., ***sulph.,*** zinc.
outer - ***nat-m.,*** sulph., zinc.

CRAMPS, eyes - sil.
eyelids - meny., ruta.
lower - ruta.

CRAWLING - agar., asar., bell., chin., cina, colch., nat-c., ***nat-s.,*** seneg., sep., spig., sulph., verat.
canthi - plat.

CROOKED, objects seem - bufo.

CRUSHING, pain - acon., **BRY., PRUN.**

CUTTING, pain - act-sp., am-c., ***apis, asaf.,*** asar., atro., aur., ***bell.,*** bor., bufo, bry., cadm-s., ***calc., calen.,*** carb-s., caust., ***chel., chin.,*** cic., ***cimic., colch., coloc.,*** con., crot-c., ***cund.,*** dros., echi., ***euphr., ferr-i.,*** graph., ind., iod., ***lach.,*** lac-f., ***merc.,*** mur-ac., nat-p., ***nux-v.,*** ol-an., petr., phyt., puls., rhus-t., sang., sil., ***sulph.,*** tarent., verat., viol-t., zinc.
candlelight - ***calc.***
evening - calc., chr-ac.
exerting them - merc., petr.
inward - acon., act-sp., ***asaf.,*** bry., ***coloc.***
outward - cadm-s., ***lach.,*** sulph.
to head - coloc.
left - ***asar.,*** bor., caust., lac-f.
lying on left side - lac-f.
morning - hura.
moving, on - bry., ind.
night agg. - ***merc.***
opening eyes - ***bry.***
pressure, amel. - ***bry.,*** coloc.
reading, while - ***calc., merc.,*** petr., phyt.
rest, during - mur-ac.
right - ***coloc., sulph.***
stooping, on, agg. - coloc.
sunlight - ***graph.***
touching, from - ***asaf.***
walking in a warm room amel. - ***coloc.***
writing, from - cann-s., canth., phyt.
cutting, canthi - bell., brom.
outer - brom., hep., kali-i.
cutting, eyelids - calc., coloc., staph., spig.
margin, of - spig.

DEEP, as if too - ambr.

DEGENERATION, cornea - ***ars.,*** phos.
retina - ham., phos.
sclerotica - aur., bar-m., plb.

DERMOID, swelling, conjunctiva - nat-m.

DETACHMENT, choroid, of - acon., arn., nux-v.
retina, of - ***apis,*** aur., ***aur-m.,*** dig., ***gels.,*** naphtin., ***phos.,*** piloc., ruta.

DIGGING, pain - bell., bism., colch., phos., sep., spig.
canthi - anan.

DILATATION, (see Pupils)

DISCHARGES, mucus, pus - ***agar.,*** alum., am-c., ant-c., ***apis, arg-n.,*** ars., ***aur.,*** bar-m., bism., ***bry., cadm-s.,*** **CALC., CALC-S.,** ***carb-s.,*** carb-v., **CAUST.,** ***cham., chel., chin., chlor.,*** clem., ***con.,*** dig., dulc., ery-a., euph., **EUPHR.,** ***ferr.,*** ferr-ar., ferr-p., ***graph., hep., hydr., ip.,*** kali-ar., kali-bi., ***kali-c., kali-i.,*** kali-p., kali-s., ***kreos.,*** lach., lachn., lact., led., ***lith., lyc.,*** mag-c., mag-m., merc-n., **MERC.,** mez., mill., ***nat-a.,*** nit-ac., ***nat-m.,*** nat-s., ***nux-v.,*** petr., ph-ac., phos., phys., pic-ac., plb., **PULS.,** rhus-t., ***sanic.,*** seneg., sep., ***sil.,*** spig., staph., stict., stram., ***sulph.,*** **TELL.,** ***thuj.***
acrid - am-c., ars., ars-i., calc., ***carb-s., cham.,*** coloc., ***euphr.,*** fl-ac., ***graph., hep.,*** kali-ar., merc., merc-c., nit-ac., psor., rhus-t., ***sulph.***
bloody - ars., asaf., ***carb-s.,*** carb-v., ***caust.,*** cham., ***hep., kali-c.,*** kreos., lach., lyc., ***merc.,*** mez., nat-m., petr., ph-ac., phos., ***puls.,*** rhus-t., sep., ***sil.,*** sulph., thuj.
clear mucus - ip., kali-m.
evening - kali-p., phos.
green - merc.
lachrymal sac, from - arum-t., ars., ***con.,*** iod., ***hep., merc., nat-m.,*** **PETR.,** ***puls., sil.,*** stann., ***sulph.***
water - **CLEM.**
morning - arg-n., ars., cinnb., kali-bi., mag-c., plb., sep., staph., sil., ***sulph.,*** tarax.
night - alum.
offensive moisture - led.
purulent - ail., alumn., ***arg-m.,*** **ARG-N.,** bar-c., bell., **CALC.,** ***carb-s., carb-v., caust., cham., chlor.,*** euph., ery-a., ferr-i., ***graph., grin.,*** **HEP.,** ***kali-i., lach., led.,*** **LYC.,** ***lyss.,*** mag-c., mag-m., **MERC.,** nat-c., nit-ac., petr., ph-ac., phos., **PULS.,** rhus-t., ***sep.,*** spong., ***sulph.,*** tarax., tell., zinc.
daytime - phos.
morning - ars., bapt., bar-c., cham.
sensation of a, hanging over eyes which must be wiped away - croc., ***puls.***
thick - alum., arg-n., calc-s., ***chel., euphr., hep., hydr., kali-bi., lyc., nat-m., puls.,*** sep., ***sil.,*** sulph., thuj.
thin - ***graph.***
white - alum., hydr., lachn., ***petr.,*** plb.
milk-white - kali-chl.

DISCHARGES, mucus, pus
yellow - ***agar.,*** alum., ***arg-n.,*** ars., aur., ***calc., calc-s.,*** carb-s., carb-v., caust., chel., ***euphr., kali-bi.,*** kali-c., kali-chl., kali-s., kreos., ***lyc., merc.,*** nat-p., **PULS.,** ***sep.,*** **SIL.,** ***sulph., thuj.***
discharges, canthi - ***agar.,*** ant-c., bell., berb., bism., calc., dig., euph., euphr., graph., guai., kali-bi., lyc., nat-c., nat-m., ***nux-v.,*** pic-ac., psor., staph.
dry, in - calc., caust., cham., euphr., grat., ***hell.,*** nit-ac., viol-t.
morning - lyc.
forenoon - coff.
hard, in - dig., ***hep.,*** guai., ***ip.,*** nux-v., ***petr.,*** sabad.
morning - ant-c., calc-p., ***cham.,*** ruta.
night - seneg.
pus - cham., ***graph., kali-bi.,*** kali-c., kali-i., led., **NUX-V.,** ***ph-ac.,*** ran-b., ***zinc.***
sticky - euphr., kali-bi.
discharges, canthi, inner - agar., ant-c., euphr., mag-s., nicc., phos., **PULS.,** staph., ***stram.,*** thuj., ***verat-v., zinc.***
dry - hell., staph.
menses, during - mag-c.
morning - nicc., phos., **PULS.,** staph., zinc.
discharges, canthi, outer - ant-c., bar-c., bry., chin., ip., lyc., mez., nux-v., rhus-t., sep.
hard, in - euph., ***hep., ip.,*** nux-v., sabad.
morning - nux-v., rhus-t., sep.
night - bar-c., ***lyc.***
purulent - nux-v.

DISCOLORATION, around eyes
bluish, circles, around - abrot., ***acet-ac.,*** acon., agar., ail., ***anac.,*** ant-t., ***aran.,*** **ARS.,** ars-i., bad., ***bell.,*** **BERB.,** ***bism.,*** cadm-s., ***calc., calc-ar.,*** calc-p., ***camph., canth.,*** carb-an., cham., chel., **CHIN.,** ***cic.,*** cimic., cinnb., **CINA,** ***cocc.,*** corn., ***crot-h., cupr.,*** cycl., fago., ***ferr.,*** ferr-ar., ferr-p., ***graph.,*** ham., hell., ***hep.,*** hura, ***indg., iod.,*** **IP.,** ***iris,*** jatr., kali-ar., kali-bi., kali-c., ***kali-i.,*** kali-p., kreos., lach., **LYC.,** mag-c., merc., mez., ***naja,*** **NAT-A., NAT-C.,** ***nat-m., nat-p.,*** **NUX-M., NUX-V., OLND.,** op., pall., petr., **PH-AC., PHOS.,** ***phyt.,*** plat., plb., psor., ***puls.,*** raph., **RHUS-T.,** rhus-v., ***sabad.,*** sabin., **SEC.,** ***sep., stann., staph.,*** stram., sulph., tab., tarent., ter., upa., ***verat.,*** zinc.
brown, around - ***lach.***
greenish, about the eyes - ***verat.***
red, around, on crying - bor.
yellow, around eyes (see Yellow) - coll., mag-c., ***nit-ac.,*** nux-v., spig.
discoloration, conjunctiva, yellow, in spots - ph-ac.
discoloration, iris, of - ***aur.,*** coloc., ***euphr.,*** kali-i., merc-i-f., ***nat-m.,*** spig., syph.
discoloration, sclera, blue - ars., calc., ***carc.,*** puls., tub.
yellow - chin.

DISTENDED, feeling - acon., ant-t., ***asar.,*** **BELL.,** bism., ***bov.,*** **BRY.,** calc-p., cann-s., ***caust.,*** gels., ***guai.,*** hep., hyos., merc., nat-c., ***nat-m.,*** **NUX-V.,** op., ***par.,*** ph-ac., phyt., plb., prun., rhus-t., ***seneg.,*** **SPIG.,** staph., tarax., thuj., zinc.

DISTORTED - ***acon., agar., ars.,*** **BELL.,** cadm-s., calc-p., ***camph.,*** canth., carb-ac., carb-v., ***cham., chel., chin., cic.,*** cocc., colch., con., crot-h., ***cupr.,*** dig., ***hydr-ac., hyos.,*** kali-s., ***lach., laur., merc., mosch.,*** olnd., op., petr., ph-ac., ***plat.,*** plb., puls., ran-s., sant., sec., ***sil., stram., sulph.,*** sul-ac., tarent., verat., verat-v.
evening - bry., caust.
pneumonia, in - chel.
sleep, during - aeth., chin., cocc., cupr., hyper., ph-ac.
distorted, iris - apis, ***merc.,*** rhus-t.

DRAGGING, pain - apis, ***caust.,*** sep.

DRAWING, pain - ***agar.,*** apis, arn., ***ars.,*** asar., bell., bov., calc-p., ***camph.,*** cann-s., canth., carb-s., carb-v., ***caust.,*** cham., ***chel.,*** cic., ***colch.,*** con., cop., crot-c., ***cur., glon., graph.,*** hell., ***hep.,*** hyos., jug-c., kali-ar., kali-bi., kali-c., kali-p., **KALM.,** kreos., lac-d., lach., lil-t., lith., lyc., lyss., med., ***naja,*** **NAT-M.,** nit-ac., oena., petr., ***phys.,*** plat., podo., ran-s., **RUTA.,** ***seneg.,*** sep., sil., ***spig.,*** stront-c., sulph., tab., til., thuj., ***zinc.,*** zing.
afternoon - phys.
around eye - plat.
backward, the eyeball - agar., aster., aur-m., bov., bry., carb-s., cham., ***crot-t.,*** cupr., ***graph., hep., lach., mez.,*** nicc., olnd., **PAR.,** petr., phos., plb., ***puls.,*** rhod., sep., sil., stry., sulph., zinc.
below left eye - bell.
between eyes - caust.
bones - sulph.
closing eyes agg. - carb-v.
daytime only - ***kalm.***
dinner, after - agar.
downward - aeth.
evening - bov., phys.
extending to, ear - petr.
head - ***graph.,*** lach.
forehead - agar.
occiput - ***lach., naja.***
vertex - ***lach.***
forenoon - podo.
lamplight agg. - syph.
morning - grat., sep.
motion, on - **KALM.,** ***nat-m., puls.***
night - lyc.
open air amel. - sep.
outward - cop., crot-c., med.
pain in occiput, during - ***carb-v.***
sitting, while - merc.
standing, while - merc-sul.
sticking - ***lach.***
stiff sensation, in muscles - **NAT-M.**
string, as with a, to back of head or into the brain - ***crot-t.,*** hep., ***lach.,*** **PAR.,** sil.
together - lyc., **NAT-M.,** op., sep., ***sulph., zinc.***

DRAWING, pain
toward the temple - crot-c.
turning sideways - **KALM.**
walking, while - merc-sul.

drawing, above eyes - ***agar.,*** asaf., bry., calc., ***cann-i.,*** carb-an., ***chel.,*** colch., con., ***ign.,*** lyss., nat-m., nit-ac., ***puls.,*** seneg., sil., spig., stann., sulph., thuj., zinc.
blowing, nose agg. - mag-c.
extending, upwards - staph.
feel as if projecting, with sensation as if a thread were tightly drawn through eyeball and backward into middle of brain, sight weak - **PAR.**
left - chel., mag-c., nat-m., thuj., spig.
mental exertion - calc.
right - aur., carb-v., dulc., ign., lyss.

drawing, canthi in - ***aur.,*** sep.
outer - spong.

drawing, eyebrow - cic., caust., dros.

drawing, eyelids - graph., ph-ac.

DRAWN, backward - aster.
together, sensation of - lyc., **NAT-M.,** sep., ***sulph.,*** zinc.
upward, eyebrows and lids - lachn.

DRYNESS - **ACON.,** agar., **ALUM.,** arg-m., ***arg-n., arn.,*** **ARS.,** aur-m., ***asaf., asar.,*** bar-c., **BELL.,** berb., bry., carb-v., ***caust.,*** cedr., ***cham.,*** chin., cina, ***clem.,*** cocc., cop., ***croc.,*** crot-h., ***cycl.,*** dros., ***elaps, euphr.,*** fago., gamb., ***graph.,*** grat., hep., kali-ar., kali-bi., kali-c., kali-n., kali-p., kali-s., lach., lachn., laur., lec., lith., **LYC.,** ***mag-c.,*** mag-m., manc., ***mang., med., meny.,*** merc., merc-c., ***merl.,*** **MEZ.,** nat-a., nat-c., **NAT-M.,** nat-p., ***nat-s.,*** nicc., **NUX-M.,** ***nux-v.,*** **OP.,** paeon., pall., ***petr.,*** phel., phos., pic-ac., plb., **PULS.,** ***rhod., rhus-t.,*** rumx., ***sang.,*** sanic., sars., ***seneg., sep.,*** sil., spig., ***staph.,*** **SULPH.,** thuj., **VERAT., ZINC.**
afternoon - caust., ***nat-s.***
sleep, after - mag-m.
artificial light, in - ars., pic-ac.
evening - ***alum., caust.,*** cina, coloc., graph., ***lyc.,*** mang., nat-s., nicc., pall., ***puls.,*** sang., sep., sil., ***staph.,*** **ZINC.**
on going to bed - op.
on looking at fire - op.
looking at bright light - **MANG.**
menses, during - mag-c.
morning - acon., berb., ***caust.,*** graph., lachn., lyc., mag-c., mag-m., ***nux-v., puls., sil.,*** **ZINC.**
evening, and - mag-aust.
lachrymation, after - **SULPH.**
waking, on - arg-m., elaps, lyc., mag-arct., phos., sanic., ***staph.***
night - lyc., sanic., spig., sulph.
reading - aur., cina, graph., hyos., nat-m., phos.
waking, on - arg-m., elaps, phos., puls., sanic., staph., ***verat.***
warm room - **PULS.,** ***sulph.***

dryness, canthi - ***alum.,*** arg-m., asar., berb., ***nat-m.,*** **NUX-V.,** ***thuj.***
evening - nat-m.
outer - thuj.

dryness, eyelids - alum., ang., asar., cham., carb-v., cycl., euph., graph., ip., mag-m., nat-m., petr., sars., verat., zinc.
edges of - ars., cham., nat-m., sulph.

DULLNESS - abrot., acon., aesc., aeth., **ALL-C.,** ang., **ANT-T.,** arn., ars., asar., atro., bapt., bell., berb., bov., bry., bufo, calc., ***calc-ar.,*** camph., carb-s., ***carb-v., cedr., chel.,*** chin., ***chin-s., chlor.,*** cimic., coloc., com., con., cupr., cycl., daph., ferr., gels., ***glon.,*** graph., grat., hyos., iod., kali-bi., kali-br., kali-c., kali-p., ***kalm.,*** kreos., lach., ***lyc., merc.,*** merc-c., mez., mosch., ***nit-ac.,*** **NUX-V.,** op., ph-ac., phos., plb., podo., rheum, rhus-t., rumx., sabin., sang., spig., spong., squil., stann., ***staph.,*** stram., ***sulph.,*** sul-ac., valer., verat., zinc., zinc-s.
exertion, after - ferr.
menses during - mag-c.
morning - sep.
sexual excesses - **STAPH.**

dullness, iris - kali-bi., kali-i., sulph., syph.

ECCHYMOSIS - ***acon.,*** aeth., am-c., arg-n., **ARN.,** ***bell.,*** **CACT.,** cham., ***chlol., con., crot-h., cupr-ac.,*** erig., ***glon., ham.,*** kali-bi., ***kali-chl.,*** kreos., ***lach.,*** **LED.,** ***lyc.,*** lyss., ***nux-v., phos.,*** plb., ruta., ***sul-ac.,*** ter.
coughing, from - ***arn.,*** bell.
right - ***con.***

ecchymosis, conjunctiva - acon., ***arn.,*** calen., canth., ham., led., sang.

ecchymosis, eyelids - ***arn.,*** led.

ECZEMA, eyelids - bac., chrysar., clem., **GRAPH.,** ***hep.,*** kali-m., med., ***mez., petr.,*** staph., sulph., tell., **THUJ.,** tub.

EMBOLISM - croc.

ENLARGED, lens - colch.

ENLARGEMENT, sensation - **ACON.,** ant-c., ***ars.,*** benz-n., bufo-s., calad., calc-p., caps., caust., chel., chlol., chlor., cimic., colch., ***com.,*** con., ***daph.,*** hyos., kali-ar., lach., ***lyc., mez.,*** nat-a., **NAT-M.,** onos., ***op.,*** **PAR.,** ph-ac., ***phos., plb.,*** rhus-t., seneg., **SPIG.,** stram., tril.
evening - am-br.
headache, during - arg-n.
morning - nat-a.
night - chr-ac.
gaslight agg. - sulph.
right feels larger than left - **COM.,** ***phos.***

ERUPTIONS, about the eyes - agn., arn., ***ars.,*** calc., carb-s., ***caust.,*** con., crot-h., euphr., ***graph., hep.,*** ign., kali-c., ***kali-s.,*** **MERC.,** merc-c., olnd., petr., ***rhus-t., sel.,*** sil., spong., **STAPH., SULPH.,** ***syph.,*** thuj.
boils - sil.
fine - euphr.
inflamed - spig.
pimples - **HEP.,** merc., petr.
rash - sulph.

ERUPTIONS, about the eyes
above the eyes - ran-b.
bluish, black vesicles - ran-b.
below eyes - dulc., guai., sel., thuj.
eruptions, canthi - lact., syph.
external - ant-c., tax.
inner crusts - clem.
pustules - bell, bry., calc., kali-c., ***lach.,*** lyc., nat-c., petr., puls., sil.
left, inner - stann.
eruptions, cornea, pustules - aeth., ant-c., kali-m.
vesicles - ran-b.
eruptions, eyebrows, about the - bar-c., ***caust.,*** clem., ferr-ma., ***kali-c.,*** **NAT-M.,** par., ***phos.,*** ***sel.,*** sep., sil., stann., staph., sulph., thuj.
crusty - anan., fl-ac., nat-m., sep., spong.
dandruff - sanic.
itching - **NAT-M.**
pimples - fl-ac., guai., kali-c., sil., tarax., stann., thuj.
burning - stann.
pustules, between eyebrows - thuj.
spongy - fl-ac., nat-m.
yellow, about - fl-ac., nat-m., rhus-t., spong.
eruptions, eyelids - ant-t., ***bry.,*** carb-s., crot-t., dys-co., **GRAPH.,** guai., **HEP.,** kali-s., kreos., ***mag-m.,*** med., ***mez.,*** morg., ***nat-m.,*** petr., ***psor.,*** puls., ***sars.,*** sil., **THUJ.,** rhus-t., sulph., tub., upa.
blotches - aur., bry., calc., ran-s., staph., thuj.
crusts - ant-c., ***arg-n., ars., aur.,*** berb., bor., bufo, calc., dig., ***graph.,*** hep., kali-m., lyc., ***psor., sanic.,*** seneg., sep., ***sulph.,*** tub.
dry, burning, itching tetters - ***bry.***
itching - nit-ac., ***sars.***
pimples - alum., chel., guai., **HEP.,** ***lyc.,*** merc-c., nat-m., nit-ac., petr., rhus-t., sel., ***seneg.***
pustules - ***ant-c.,*** arg-m., carb-s., lyc., ***merc.,*** ran-b., sep., ***sil., sulph.,*** **TELL.,** upa.
left, inner - stann.
margins - ***arg-m.,*** puls., sep.
rash - sulph.
scales - ars., ***psor.,*** **SEP.**
scurfy - lyc., ***mez.,*** **PETR., SEP.,** tub.
spots, red - camph., sil.

ERYSIPELAS, (see Face) - ***acon., anac.,*** **APIS,** ***bell.,*** com., ***graph., hep., led., merc., merc-c.,*** **RHUS-T.,** vesp.
around eyes - acon., anac., **APIS,** ars., bell., com., ***graph., hep., led., merc., merc-c.,*** **RHUS-T.,** vesp.
insects bites, from - apis, led.

ESOPHORIA, (see Paralysis) - rhod., ***ruta.***

EVERSION, eyelids - alum., ***apis,*** **ARG-M., ARG-N.,** bell., ***calc., ham.,*** hep., graph., ***lyc., merc-c., merc.,*** mez., ***nat-m., nit-ac., staph., sulph.,*** psor., zinc.
lower, lid - ***apis.***
silver nitrate, after - ***nat-m.***

EXCORIATION, canthi - alum., apis, **ARS.,** bor., euph., hell., kali-c., nat-m.
outer - ant-c., bor., zinc.

EXERTION, (see Eyestrain) muscular, amel. - ***aur.***

EXCORIATION, eyelids - apis, **ARG-N., ARS.,** ***calc.,*** graph., ***hep., med., merc-c.,*** **MERC.,** ***nat-m., sulph.***

EXOPHORIA, (see Paralysis)

EXOPHTHALMUS, (see Protrusion) - aml-n., ars., ***aur.,*** bad., ***bar-c.,*** bell., cact., ***calc.,*** con., crot-h., dig., **FERR., FERR-I.,** ***ign.,*** **IOD.,** ***lycps., nat-m., phos.,*** **SEC.,** ***spong.***

EXPRESSIONLESS, (see Dullness)

EXUDATION of retina - kali-m.

EYE, gum - alum., am-c., ant-c., ***arg-n.,*** bism., ***calc.,*** caust., con., graph., hep., ip., nit-ac., nux-v., ***psor., seneg.,*** staph., thuj.
dry - bor.
eye, gum, canthi, on - aeth., ***agar., ant-c.,*** bism., ***calc.,*** caust., dig., ***euph.,*** guai., nat-a., nat-c., ***nat-m.,*** nit-ac., nux-v., sil., staph., ***sulph.***
outer - ars., chin., euph., kali-c., nat-a.
eye, gum, eyelids, on, morning - alum., berb., con., ***phos.,*** seneg.

EYEBROWS, hair, falling from - agar., ail., alum., ***anan.,*** aur-m., bor., hell., **KALI-C.,** med., merc., mill., ***nit-ac.,*** plb., sanic., sel., sil., sulph.
hair knits, in - viol-o.
white eyebrows - ars-h.

EYELASHES, hair, falling from - alum., ***apis, ars.,*** aur., bufo, ***calc-s., chel.,*** chlol., ***euphr.,*** med., ***merc.,*** ph-ac., psor., **RHUS-T.,** ***sel.,*** sep., sil., ***staph., sulph.***
ingrown - bor.
long and silken - phos., tub.

EYESTRAIN, exertion, of vision, agg. - agar., alum., ***am-c.,*** am-m., anac., ***apis,*** arg-m., **ARG-N.,** ***asaf.,*** asar., ***aur.,*** bar-c., bar-m., bell., bor., bry., **CALC.,** cann-i., canth., ***carb-v., caust.,*** chlol., ***cic.,*** **CINA,** cocc., coff., con., **CROC.,** cupr., dros., dulc., ferr., ***graph.,*** hep., ign., ***jab.,*** **KALI-C.,** kali-p., kali-s., kreos., led., **LYC.,** mag-c., mag-m., mang., merc., mez., mur-ac., ***naja,*** nat-a., ***nat-c.,*** **NAT-M.,** ***nat-p.,*** nicc., nit-ac., nux-m., ***nux-v.,*** olnd., **ONOS.,** par., petr., ***ph-ac., phos.,*** phys., ***phyt.,*** puls., ran-b., **RHOD.,** ***rhus-t.,*** **RUTA.,** sabad., ***sars.,*** sel., **SENEG.,** ***sep.,*** **SIL.,** ***spig., spong.,*** staph., stram., stront-c., sulph., sul-ac., ther., thuj., valer., verb., viol-o., zinc.
headaches, from - ***agar.,*** arg-n., ***aur.,*** bell., ***bor., cact., calc., carb-v., caust., cimic., cina,*** gels., ***ham.,*** jab., **KALI-C.,** kali-p., kali-s., **LYC.,** mag-p., mur-ac., ***nat-c.,*** **NAT-M.,** ***nat-p., onos.,*** par., **PH-AC.,** ***phos.,*** phys., **RHOD.,** ***rhus-t.,*** **RUTA.,** sep., **SIL.,** ***spong.,*** staph., sulph., ***tub.,*** valer., zinc.

FALLING of eyelids - acon., ***alum.,*** ant-t., apis, apoc., arn., ***bell.,*** cann-i., carb-s., caul., ***caust.,*** cham., chel., con., croc., crot-h., dulc., **GELS.,** graph., haem., helo., kali-br., kali-p., kalm., lach., ***lyc.,*** merc., ***morph.,*** naja, nat-a., nat-c., nit-ac., nux-m., nux-v., ***op.,*** phel., phos., plb., rhus-t., ***sep.,*** sil., spig., spong., stram., sul-ac., sulfon., sulph., syph., upa., verat., viol-o., ***viol-t.,*** tax., vip., zinc.

evening, in - am-br., am-m., bar-c.
falling out, sensation as if - lyc.
headache, during - ***sep.***
morning, after waking - bell.
reading - mez.
sleepiness, with - plat.
walking, in open air - graph.

FAT, sensation of, in eye - calc.

FILMY - lyc., nat-c.

FIRE, looking into, agg. - ***merc.,*** nat-s.

FISSURE, canthi, (see Cracks)

FISTULA, cornea, of the - ***sil.***

fistula, lachrymalis - agar., ***apis, arg-n., aur-m., brom.,*** **CALC.,** caust., chel., **FL-AC.,** graph., ***hep.,*** kreos., ***lach., lyc.,*** merc-c., mill., nat-c., ***nat-m., nit-ac.,*** **PETR.,** phos., phyt., **PULS., SIL.,** ***stann., sulph.***

discharging pus on pressure - nat-m., **PULS.,** ***sil., stann.***
eruptions on face, with - lach.
suppurating - ***calc.,*** **PULS.**

FIXED, look, (see Staring)

FRIGHTFUL, look, (see Face, Expression)

FOREIGN body, pain, as from - ***acon.,*** alum., am-m., ***anac.,*** **APIS,** arn., ***aur., bell.,*** bor., ***bov., calc.,*** **CALC-P.,** calc-s., ***caps.,*** carb-an., caul., ***caust., chel.,*** cinnb., ***cist.,*** coc-c., ***euphr., fl-ac., gels., hep.,*** hyos., ***ign.,*** kali-bi., ***lyc.,*** med., meph., ***merc., nat-m.,*** phos., plb., ***psor.,*** puls., rhus-t., ruta., sang., sars., sep., ***sil.,*** stann., staph., stram., ***sulph., thuj.,*** upa.

back behind lids - ***merc.,*** stann., ***staph.***
conjunctiva, under - tab.
evening - ***sulph.***
forenoon - am-m., dios., sulph.
hairs - ***coc-c.,*** sang.
little grains - ***euphr.,*** lith., sars., sep.
morning - ***sulph.***
right - sulph.

foreign body, canthi, in - alum.

inner - agar., berb.
outer - apis, bar-c., con., ***euphr.,*** ign., phos., ***sul-ac.***

foreign body, eyelids, behind - ***merc.,*** stann., ***staph.***

FRINGE, sensation as of a, were falling over the eyes - ***con.***

FULLNESS, sensation of - apis, ***arg-n.,*** bell., caust., cub., dulc., euph., gels., ger., ***guai.,*** gymn., hep., lac-ac., lyc., morph., nat-m., ***nux-m.,*** olnd., phys., plb., ***seneg.,*** sep., sulph., thuj., verat.

FUNGUS, oculi, (see Cancer)

GERONTOXON, (see Opacity)

GLASSY, appearance - acon., am-m., arn., ars., ***bell.,*** benz-n., bry., camph., cedr., ***cic.,*** chlor., cocc., coc-c., corn., croc., cupr., daph., elaps, eup-per., fago., ***glon., hell.,*** hydr-ac., hyos., iod., ***kali-ar., lach., lyc.,*** lyss., merc., mosch., **OP.,** ox-ac., petr., **PH-AC.,** ***plat.,*** psor., puls., sang., sec., sep., spig., ***stram.,*** sulph., tab.

chill, during - bell., cocc.
fever, during - bell., bry., glon., iod., op.
morning - sep.
perspiration - bell., cocc., puls.

GLAUCOMA - ***acon.,*** atro., arn., ars., asaf., aur., ***bell., bry.,*** camph., caust., cedr., cham., cinnb., coca, colch., coloc., com., con., croc., crot-h., crot-t., **GELS.,** ham., ictod., ***jab.,*** kali-i., lac-c., lach., lyc., mag-c., merc., mez., nux-v., op., ***osm., phos., phys.,*** plb., poth., prun., rhod., ***rhus-t.,*** sil., ***spig.,*** sulph.

afternoon and evening agg. - bell.
morning, agg. - nux-v.
pain, with - acon., ***phos.,*** mez.
motion agg. - bry., spig.
pressure amel. - coloc.
storm, before agg. - rhod.

GLAZED - apis, bell., cupr., hyos., op., ph-ac., podo., zinc.

GLIOMA, retina - cean.

GLISTENING, (see Brillant, Glassy)

GNAWING, pain - agn., ars., berb., kali-c., ox-ac., ***plat.***

eye, above right, morning - dros.

GRANULAR, eyelids - ***alum.,*** ant-t., ***apis, arg-n.,*** **ARS.,** ***aur.,*** bar-c., bell., ***bor., carb-s., caust., euphr.,*** fago., **GRAPH.,** ***kali-bi.,*** **LYC.,** ***merc-c., merc-i-f., merc-i-r.,*** mez., ***nat-a., nat-m., nat-s., nux-v.,*** ol-j., petr., phyt., ***puls.,*** rheum, rhus-t., ***sang., sep., sil., sulph., thuj., zinc.***

cold applications amel. - ***apis, puls.***
evening - ***nux-v.***
outer canthi - ant-t.
summer - nux-v.
water agg. - ***sulph.***

GREEN, color - canth., cupr-ac.

HAIR, (see Eyebrows, Eyelashes)

HAIR, sensation of, in eye - calc-f., ***coc-c.,*** euphr., kali-n., mag-p., nat-c., plan., **PULS.,** ***ran-b.,*** sang., sil., tab.

afternoon - sang.
lashes, on - spig.
ran inward, as if a hair - bor., tell.

HARDNESS - cann-i., coloc., con., ***phos.***

marble, sense of - cann-i.
meibomian glands, of - ***bad., lith.,*** staph.

hardness, eyelids - ***acon.,*** arg-m., ***calc., con.,*** med., ***merc-c., nit-ac., phyt.,*** psor., ran-s., sep., ***sil., spig., thuj.***

HEAT, agg. - ***apis, arg-n.,*** caust., clem., ***coff.,*** **MERC.,** ***puls.,*** til., ***zinc.***

HEAT, sensation in eyes - ***acon.,*** aesc., agar., anan., ang., aran., ***arg-n., ars.,*** aster., aur., bar-c., **BELL.,** benz-ac., berb., ***bov.,*** calc., ***canth., carb-s.,*** carb-v., **CHAM.,** ***chel.,*** caust., **CHIN.,** chlol., ***clem.,*** con., cor-r., ***cycl.,*** dig., ***glon., graph., ign., jab.,*** kali-ar., ***kali-bi.,*** **KALI-C.,** ***kreos.,*** lach., ***lil-t.,*** **LYC.,** mang., med., meph., ***merc., mez.,*** nat-a., nat-c., nat-m., ***nat-s.,*** nicc., ***nit-ac.,*** onos., ***op.,*** petr., ph-ac., ***phos.,*** plat., ***psor.,*** ran-b., rhus-t., **RUTA.,** sabin., ***sep.,*** sil., ***spig.,*** staph., **SULPH.,** ***tab.,*** tarent., tell., thuj., ***verat.,*** verb., viol-o., zinc.

afternoon - petr.
air, cold. agg. - zinc.
around eye - cic.
chill, after - petr.
closing eyes on - ***cor-r.,*** ust.
cold, after taking - kali-c.
daytime - ***ars.,*** phos.
eating after - caust.
evening - con., dios., kali-bi., nat-m., nicc., psor., ***puls.***
as if hot air streamed out - dios.
candlelight, with - graph.
exertion, during - aur., jab., **RUTA.**
fever, during - ***sep.***
flushes - ***gels.,*** phos., sep.
forenoon - con.
morning - apoc., ***hep., mez.,*** sep., sulph.
night - ***crot-t.,*** nat-c., zinc.
steaming out, sensation of - ***clem.,*** **CHAM.,** dios., nat-s.
using eyes - aur., jab., **RUTA.**
walking in open air, after - lyc.

heat, canthi - carb-v., phos., psor., thuj.
outer - cann-s., glon., thuj.

heat, choroiditis, in - ***coloc.***

heat, eyelids - acon., benz-ac., ***calc.,*** calc-p., chel., cimic., ***gels., glon., graph.,*** lil-t., ***med.,*** sep., syph., upa.
margins - par., phyt., ***sep., sulph.***

heat, iritis, in - ***arn.,*** puls.

HEAVINESS - ***aesc.,*** **ALOE,** all-s., anan., apis, ***arn.,*** ars-n., arum-t., bell., carb-s., ***carb-v.,*** caust., ***com.,*** gels., hep., hipp., lach., lyc., manc., plb., podo., rumx., stram., ***sulph.,*** vib.
menses, during - carb-an., lac-d., nat-m.
before - lac-d., ***nat-m.***

heaviness, eyelids - absin., acon., agar., anan., apis, arum-t., arund., asaf., bell., berb., brom., bufo, caj., ***calc.,*** cann-i., carb-s., ***caul.,*** **CAUST.,** cham., chel., chlol., cimic., cina, cinnb., ***cocc.,*** **CON.,** corn., crot-c., cupr., euph., ***ferr., form.,*** **GELS.,** ***graph., hell., hydr., kali-bi.,*** kali-p., ***lac-c., lac-d.,*** lachn., ***lyc.,*** mag-m., ***merl.,*** naja, nat-a., ***nat-c., nat-m.,*** nat-p., ***nat-s.,*** nit-ac., ***nux-m., nux-v.,*** onos., op., phel., ph-ac., ***phos.,*** phyt., pic-ac., **RHUS-T.,** ***sep.,*** sil., ***spong., sulph.,*** tarent., thuj., viol-o., ***verat-v., zinc.***
evening - bufo, cinnb., dig., pic-ac., sulph.
reading by lamplight, while - ***nat-c.***
frontal headache - sep.
headache, during - bell., gels.

heaviness, eyelids
morning - daph., ferr., myric., phos., ***sep.,*** ***upa.***
as if could not be held open - lach
nit-ac., ***sep.***
waking, on - ***kali-bi., sep.***
using the eyes - nat-c., ***nat-m.***
vaginal discharge, with - caul.

HEMORRHAGE, (see Bleeding)

HERPES - alum., ***apis,*** bry., calc-p., ***caust., co***
euphr., ***graph.,*** hep., kreos., lach., ***nat-m.,*** oln
ran-b., rhus-t., sep., spong., sulph., tell.
vesicular - ***apis, ars.,*** calc-p., euphr., nat-m.
ran-b., rhus-t., sep., tell.

herpes, cornea - apis, ***graph., hep.,*** ign., nat-m., ran-b., rhus-t.

herpes, eyelids - bry., com., ***graph.,*** kreos., ***psor., rhus-t., sep.,*** sulph., tarent., tub.
scaly - ***chel.,*** kreos., ***nat-m.,*** **PSOR.,** sep.
margins - ***apis,*** arg-n., ***aur.,*** aur-m., ***dulc.,*** **GRAPH.,** ***kali-chl., kali-s., merc., tub.***

HORDEOLEUM, (see Styes)

HYPERSENSITIVE, retina - ***bell.,*** cimic., ***con.,*** crot-h., ***ign.,*** lac-ac., lil-t., **NAT-M.,** ***nux-v., ox-ac.,*** phos., stry.

HYPERPHORIA, (see Paralysis)

HYPERTROPHY, conjunctiva, of - apis.

HYPOPION, (see Iritis)

IMMOBILITY, (see Fixed look, Staring, etc.)

INDURATION, (see Hardness)

INFANTS, eye complaints of (see Inflammation)

INFILTRATION, (see Hardness, Thickening)

INFLAMMATION, eyes - **ACON.,** ***act-sp., agar.,*** **ALL-C.,** ***alum., ambr.,*** am-c., ***ant-c., ant-t.,*** **APIS,** arg-m., ***arg-n.,*** **ARN., ARS.,** ars-i., ***asaf.,*** asar., ***aur.,*** aur-m., ***bad., bar-c., bar-m.,*** **BELL.,** benz-ac., ***bor.,*** brom., ***bry.,*** cadm-s., ***cahin.,*** calad., **CALC.,** ***calc-p.,*** **CALC-S.,** camph., cann-s., ***canth.,*** caps., carb-s., carb-v., ***caust., cham., chin.,*** chin-a., cimic., ***cinnb., clem.,*** coff., ***colch., coloc., con.,*** cop., croc., crot-t., cupr., daph., dig., dulc., elaps, ery-a., eug., ***eup-per., euph.,*** **EUPHR.,** ferr., ferr-ar., ferr-p., ***form., gels., glon., graph., grin., ham., hep., hydr.,*** hyos., ***ign., iod., ip., iris,*** kali-ar., ***kali-bi., kali-c., kali-chl., kali-i.,*** kali-p., kali-s., ***kalm.,*** kreos., ***lach., led., lith.,*** **LYC.,** ***lyss., mag-c.,*** mag-m., meph., ***merl.,*** **MERC.,** ***merc-c., merc-i-r., mez.,*** morph., mur-ac., nat-c., **NAT-M.,** nat-p., ***nat-s., nit-ac., nux-v.,*** op., ***petr.,*** ph-ac., ***phos., phyt.,*** plb., **PSOR., PULS.,** ran-b., rat., **RHUS-T.,** sang., **SEP., SIL.,** ***spig.,*** staph., ***stram.,*** **SULPH.,** ***sul-ac.,*** syph., tarax., tarent., ***ter.,*** teucr., ***thuj.,*** verat., ***zinc.***
acute - **ACON., APIS,** ***ars.,*** aur-m., ***bell., bry.,*** **CALC.,** calen., ***cham.,*** **EUPHR.,** ***ferr-p., hydr., merc., nux-v.,*** **PULS.,** ***sep.,*** **SULPH.**
afternoon, 4 p.m. - ***ars.***
air, open, amel. - asaf., ***asar.,*** **PULS.**

INFLAMMATION, eyes
alternating, with, a sore throat - par.
with swelling of feet - apis., ***ars.***
arthritic, (gouty and rheumatic) - ***ant-c.,*** **ANT-T.,** ***apis, ars.,*** arum-m., bell., ***bor., bry.,*** **CALC.,** cact., ***cham., chin., cocc., colch., coloc.,*** dig., ***euphr.,*** **FORM.,** ***graph., hep., kalm., led.,*** **LYC.,** ***merc., mez., nux-v.,*** **PHYT.,** ***psor., puls.,*** **RHUS-T., SEP.,** spig., ***staph., sulph.***
bee sting, acute, after - ***apis,*** sep.
burns, from - **CANTH.,** ham., kali-bi.
caruncles - bell., berb., cann-i.
catarrhal, from cold - **ACON.,** act-sp., **ALL-C.,** alum., alumn., ant-c., ant-t., ***apis, arg-m., ars.,*** ars-i., ***arund., aur.,*** bapt., **BELL.,** ***bry.,*** **CALC.,** ***calc-p., carb-s., cham.,*** chel., ***chlol.,*** com., con., ***dig.,*** **DULC., EUPHR.,** gamb., ***graph., hep., hydr.,*** iod., ip., ***iris,*** kali-ar., ***kali-bi.,*** kali-c., ***lyc.,*** **MERC.,** ***merc-c., mez., nux-v., petr., phyt.,*** **PSOR., PULS.,** ***sang., sep., staph., sulph., thuj.***
morning - hep., kali-bi., ***mez.***
night - all-s., ***cinnb., dulc.,*** **MERC.,** ***rhus-t.***
night, after 1 a.m. - chin-a.
night, when trying to read - all-s.
cold, agg. - ***ars.,*** sil.
amel. - apis, **ARG-N.,** asaf., ***asar., bry.,*** caust., **PULS.,** ***sep.***
water, agg. - sep.
wet, weather - **DULC., RHUS-T.,** ***sil.***
croupous - kali-bi.
dentition agg. - ferr-p.
dust, from - acon., calen., euphr.
fire, agg. - **ANT-C.,** ***arg-n.,*** **MERC.,** phos.
being over, cold air and cold applications amel. - **ARG-N.**
foreign, objects - **ACON., ARN.,** ***calc., calen.,*** hyper., ***puls.,*** **SIL.,** sulph.
gaslight, from - ***merc.***
gonorrheal - ant-c., ***ant-t.,*** arg-n., chin., clem., cor-r., cub., kali-br., ***med., merc.,*** **NIT-AC., PULS.,** ***spig., sulph., thuj.***
headache, with - apis, led., verat.
three days, during - med.
heat, agg. - **APIS, BAD., BELL.,** ***bry.,*** **GLON.,** ***kali-i.,*** med., ***merc.,*** still.
of fire, agg. - phos.
infants - **ACON.,** alumn., **APIS,** ***arg-m.,*** **ARG-N.,** arn., **ARS.,** arund., ***bell.,*** bor., ***bry.,*** **CALC.,** ***cham., dulc.,*** **EUPHR.,** ***hep., ign., lyc., merc., merc-c.,*** **NIT-AC.,** ***nux-v.,*** **PULS.,** ***rhus-t., sulph.,*** **THUJ.,** zinc.
injuries, after - **ACON., ARN.,** calc., calc-s., **CALEN.,** ***euphr., ham., hep.,*** **HYPER., LED.,** ***puls.,*** sil., ***staph., sulph.*** sul-ac., **SYMPH.**
light, reflected, from - acon.
measles, during - ***euphr., puls.***
after - arg-m., ***carb-v.,*** crot-h., ***euphr., puls.***

INFLAMMATION, eyes
menses, during - ***ars.,*** puls., **ZINC.**
absent, with - euph.
suppressed - ***puls.***
mercurial - ***asaf., hep., mez.***
pneumonia, in - ant-t.
recurrent - ars., bry., **CALC.,** med., ***sulph.***
sand, and dust, from - acon., calen., euphr, sil., sulph.
scrofulous - acon., alumn., ***ant-c., apis,*** **ARS.,** ars-i., ***arg-m.,*** arund., **AUR., AUR-M-N.,** ***bad., bar-c.,*** **BAR-M.,** ***bell., cadm-s.,*** **CALC.,** ***calc-p.,*** **CALC-S.,** cann-s., **CARB-S., CAUST.,** ***cham.,*** chin., chin-a., ***cinnb., cist., con.,*** dig., ***dulc., euphr.,*** ferr., ferr-ar., ***fl-ac.,*** **GRAPH., HEP.,** ***hyos., iod.,*** ip., ***kali-bi., kali-i., lith., lyc., mag-c.,*** **MERC.,** ***merc-c., nat-m., nat-p., nat-s.,*** **NIT-AC.,** ***nux-v.,*** ol-j., **PETR., PHYT., PSOR., PULS.,** ***rhus-t., sars.,*** **SEP., SIL.,** ***spig.,*** **SULPH.,** ***sul-ac., tell., viol-t., zinc.***
children, in, disposed to scaled head and inflammation of external ear - ars.
snow, sun, from - acon., calc-p., cic., kali-n., sol.
summer - ***sep.***
syphilitic - arg-m., arg-n., ***ars.,*** **ASAF.,** ***aur.,*** aur-m., aur-m-n., ***cinnb., clem., graph., hep.,*** **KALI-I., MERC., MERC-C.,** ***merc-cy., merc-i-f.,*** **NIT-AC., PHYT.,** ***staph., syph.,*** thuj.
vaccination, after - thuj.
warm, covering amel. - ***hep.***
warmth, of bed agg. - **MERC.**
washing, agg. - **SULPH.**
cold amel. - asaf.
wet, becoming, agg. - ***calc.,*** dulc., ***rhus-t.***
getting feet - ***chel.***
wind, dry cold - **ACON.**
wounds, from cuts etc. - ***acon.,*** arn., calad., **CALEN.,** hyper., **STAPH.**

inflammation, canthi - am-c., ant-c., apis, **ARG-N.,** ***bor.,*** bufo, ***calc.,*** calc-s., clem., euphr., ***graph.,*** kali-c., mag-c., merc., nat-c., sulph., zinc.
inner - ***agar., bor., clem.,*** mag-c., nat-c., ***nux-v.,*** petr.
morning, agg. - ***nux-v.***
outer - ***bor.,*** **GRAPH.,** ***kali-c.***
with ulceration - ***calc-ac.,*** upa.
ulceration, with - ***apis,*** bufo, ***kali-c.,*** zinc.

inflammation, choroid - agar., ***ars., aur., bell.,*** **BRY.,** ***cedr., coloc., gels., ip.,*** piloc., ***kali-chl., kali-i., merc., merc-c., merc-d.,*** merc-i-r., naphtin., ***nux-v.,*** phos., ***phyt., prun.,*** psor., puls., rhod., ruta, ***sil., spig., sulph.,*** tab., tell., ***thuj.,*** viol-o.

inflammation, conjunctiva, (see Conjunctivitis)

inflammation, cornea - acon., ***apis, ars.,*** ars-i., ***aur-m., bell.,*** **CALC.,** ***calc-p.,*** cann-s., ***cinnb., con., crot-h.,*** crot-t., ***euphr., graph., hep., kali-bi., kali-chl.,*** kali-m., ***kalm., lyc.,*** **MERC.,** ***merc-c., merc-i-f.,*** nux-v., phos., plat., plb., ***psor., puls., rhus-t.,*** sang., ***sep.,*** spig., **SULPH.,** syph., **THUJ.,** vac., vario.
bathing, cold amel. - syph.

inflammation, eyelids, (see Blepharitis)

inflammation, iris, (see Iritis)

inflammation, lachrymal glands - ***ant-c.,*** apis, brom., ***cupr.,*** fl-ac., hep., **PULS.,** sabad., **SIL.**
lachrymal, canal - acon., apis, ***calc., fl-ac.,*** hep., iod., kali-bi., ***nat-m.,*** nit-ac., **PETR., PULS.,** ***sil., stann.***
lachrymal, sac - apis, arum-t., fl-ac., ***graph.,*** hep., ***merc.,*** nat-c., **PETR., PULS., SIL.**

inflammation, meibomian glands - cham., ***colch., dig., euphr., hep.,*** indg., ***iod.,*** kreos., phos., puls., ***staph.,*** stram., sulph.
suppurative - ***con., phos.***

inflammation, optic nerve - ***apis,*** ars., ***bell.,*** carb-s., kali-i., merc., ***merc-c.,*** nux-v., ***phos.,*** pic-ac., plb., ***puls.,*** rhus-t., sant., tab., thyr.

inflammation, retina, (see Retinitis)

inflammation, retrobulbair - chin-s., iodof.

inflammation, sclera - acon., ars., aur-m., bell., bry., ***cocc.,*** hep., hura, kali-i., ***kalm., merc.,*** merc-c., ***psor.,*** rhus-t., sep., spig., ter., ***thuj.***
with stitches and aversion to sunlight - nux-v.

INJECTED - all-c., ant-t., astac., ***bell.,*** bufo, camph., cedr., ***clem.,*** con., ferr., ferr-ar., ferr-m., ferr-p., **GLON.,** ***hep., kali-bi.,*** merc.
headache, during - ***bell.,*** meli., nux-v.

injected, conjunctiva, full of dark vessels - ***apis,*** arg-n., ars-h., ars., bar-m., ***bell., calc., calc-p., camph.,*** cann-i., ***carb-s., chin-s., chlol.,*** clem., ***con., cop., crot-c., crot-t., euphr., ferr., graph., ham., hep., ip.,*** kali-ar., ***kali-bi.,*** kali-c., ***kali-i.,*** kali-p., kali-s., ***lach.,*** lyss., merc., ***merc-c., mez.,*** morph., ***nat-a.,*** **NAT-M.,** ***nux-v., op.,*** phos., podo., sang., sec., sep., ***sil.,*** spig., stram., stry., ***sulph.,*** tarent., thuj.
menses, before - puls.
morning - ***mez.***

injected, canthi, inner - laur., nat-p.
outer - sars.

injected, cornea - **AUR.,** ***graph.,*** hep., ***ign.,*** ip., ***merc.,*** plb.

INJURIES - **ACON., ARN.,** asar., calad., ***calc.,*** calc-s., **CALEN.,** canth., coch., ***euphr.,*** ham., hep., **HYPER.,** lach., ***led.,*** nux-v., phys., ***puls., rhus-t.,*** ruta, seneg., **SIL.,** ***staph.,*** sulph., sul-ac., **SYMPH.,** ***zinc.***
black eye, ecchymosis - ***acon.,*** aeth., am-c., arg-n., **ARN.,** ***bell.,*** **CACT.,** cham., ***chlol., con., crot-h., cupr-ac.,*** erig., ***glon., ham.,*** kali-bi., ***kali-chl.,*** kreos., ***lach.,*** **LED.,** ***lyc.,*** lyss., ***nux-v., phos.,*** plb., ruta.,

INJURIES, eyes
black eye - ***sul-ac.,*** **SYMPH.,** ter.
bloodshot - nux-v.
bone - ruta, symph.
cornea, scratched, (see Abrasions) - acon., **CALEN.,** ***hyper.***
foreign, objects, in - **ACON., ARN.,** ***calc.,*** calen., ***puls.,*** **SIL.,** sulph.
inflammation, after - **ACON., ARN.,** calc., calc-s., **CALEN.,** ***euphr., ham., hep.,*** **HYPER., LED.,** ***puls.,*** sil., ***staph., sulph.*** sul-ac., **SYMPH.**
retina, of - acon., ***arn.,*** bell., ***ham.,*** lach., led., phos.
surgery, complications of eyes after - arn., asar., bry., **CALEN.,** croc., ***hyper.,*** ign., led., rhus-t., senn., **STAPH.**
wounds, from cuts, surgery, etc. - acon., arn., **CALEN.,** euphr., hyper., **STAPH.**

INSENSIBILITY - carb-o., carb-s., crot-h., hyos., kali-br., op., ***stram.***

INVERSION of eyelids - anan., ***bor., calc., graph., merc., nat-m., nit-ac.,*** puls., sil., ***sulph.,*** tell., zinc.

IRITIS, inflammation, iris - ***acon., apis, arg-n.,*** **ARN.,** ***ars.,*** ars-i., ***asaf., aur., bell.,*** calc., ***cedr., chin., cinnb., clem., colch., coloc., com.,*** crot-h., ***crot-t.,*** dub., ***dulc., euphr.,*** ferr-p., gels., grin., ***hep.,*** iod., ***kali-bi., kali-i., merc.,*** **MERC-C.,** merc-i-f., merc-sul., mez., ***nat-m., nit-ac.,*** petr., plb., ***puls.,*** **RHUS-T.,** ***seneg., sil.,*** spig., ***staph., sulph., syph.,*** tell., ***ter.,*** thuj., zinc.
adhesions, with - ***calc.,*** calen., ***clem., merc-c., nit-ac.,*** sil., spig., staph., ***sulph., ter.***
hypopion, with - crot-t., **HEP.,** ***merc., merc-c.,*** plb., rhus-t., **SIL.,** sulph., ***thuj.***
night, agg. - ***ars., dulc.,*** **KALI-I., MERC., MERC-C.,** ***nit-ac., rhus-t., staph., sulph.,*** zinc.
prostate gland inflammation, with - sabal.
rheumatic - arn., ***ars., bry.,*** clem., ***colch.,*** coloc., ***dulc., euphr.,*** form., ***kali-bi.,*** kali-i., ***kalm.,*** led., merc-c., **RHUS-T.,** ***spig.,*** syph., ***ter.***
sharp pain, iritis, in - ***asaf.,*** **MERC., RHUS-T.,** ***thuj.***
syphilitic - ***ars., arg-n., aur., aur-m., asaf., cinnb.,*** clem., ***hep.,*** iod., kali-bi., **KALI-I.,** ***merc.,*** **MERC-C.,** merc-cy., ***merc-i-f.,*** **NIT-AC.,** petr., ***staph.,*** sulph., syph., ***thuj.,*** zinc.
bursting pain in eyeball, temple and side of face - **STAPH.**
tubercular - ***ars.,*** bar-i., kali-bi., sulph., syph., tub.

IRRITATION, to - apis, ***ars., caust.,*** con., fago., ign., iod., lyc., merc-i-f., nat-a., puls., ran-s., rhus-t., ruta., sang.
afternoon - bad.
candlelight, from - lyc.
daytime only - iod.
evening - iod., lyc., ***ruta.***

IRRITATION, to
looking through too sharp spectacles, as after - croc.
morning - apoc.
reading by lamp-light - ***apis.***
smoke in eyes, as if - croc., valer.
violent, as after crying - croc.
irritation, eyelids, amel. in cold air - coff.
irritation, optic nerve - phos.

ITCHING - absin., acon., ***agar., all-c., alum.,*** am-m., anan., ***ant-c., apis, arg-m., arg-n.,*** ars., arund., asc-t., aspar., aur., aur-m., ***bar-c., bar-m.,*** bell., berb., bor., bry., bufo, ***calc.,*** calc-p., calc-s., cann-s., canth., carb-an., ***carb-v.,*** casc., ***caust.,*** chel., chim., chin., clem., coloc., cop., cupr., cycl., elaps, eug., ***euphr.,*** fago., ferr., ferr-i., gels., hep., hura, ign., iod., ***kali-bi.,*** kali-c., kali-n., kali-s., ***kalm.,*** kreos., lach., lachn., lob., ***lyc.,*** lyss., mag-c., ***mag-m.,*** mang., meph., ***merc.,*** merc-c., ***mez.,*** mosch., ***mur-ac., nat-c., nat-m.,*** nat-p., nat-s., nicc., nit-ac., ***nux-v.,*** ol-an., osm., paeon., pall., ***petr., phel.,*** ph-ac., ***phos.,*** phyt., plat., **PULS.,** ran-b., rhod., rhus-t., ruta, sars., sep., sil., spig., squil., stann., stram., stront-c., **SULPH.,** tarent., verat., vesp., viol-t., ***zinc.***
about the eyes - agn., apis, ars., berb., ***carb-v.,*** con., lach., lyc., pall., sars., til.
air, open, agg. - staph.
amel. - **PULS.**
below the eyes - nat-m., spong.
biting, from rubbing - ruta.
cold, application amel. - ***puls.***
corrosive - ars.
coryza, during - caps., euphr.
dinner, after - mag-c.
evening - ***acon.,*** calc., calc-p., ***cupr.,*** dios., erig., eug., euph., ferr., ***gamb.,*** mag-c., meph., ***merc-c.,*** pall., phos., plat., **PULS.,** sil., **SULPH.,** vesp.
exertion, of vision - ***rhus-t., ruta.***
forenoon - ***sulph.***
11 a.m. - nat-c.
gaslight agg. - ***phyt.***
house, in - ran-b.
lachrymation from rubbing - nat-c., ruta.
light produces - anan.
moistening eye amel. - nat-c.
morning - agar., am-c., caust., dios., fago., meph., nat-c., ***nat-m., nat-s., sulph.***
rising, after - nat-m.
night - ars., sulph.
pressure upward amel. - bell.
rubbing, agg. - ***kalm.,*** kreos., sulph.
amel. - agar., am-c., ***caust.,*** euph., ***euphr.,*** mag-c., mag-m., nat-c., ***nux-v.,*** ol-an., phos., spig., spong., stann., stram., sulph., zinc.
warm, bathing - ***mez.***
room - ***puls., sulph.***

itching, canthi - agar., **ALUM.,** ***ant-c.,*** **ARG-M.,** ***arg-n.,*** arn., asc-t., ***aur.,*** bell., benz-ac., berb., bor., **CALC.,** carb-v., ***caust.,*** cina, cinnb., clem., ***con.,*** crot-c., ***euph., euphr.,*** ferr-m., ***fl-ac., gamb.,*** hell., hyos., iod., led., ***lyc., mosch., mur-ac., nat-m.,*** nux-v., petr., ph-ac., prun., ***puls.,*** ruta., sep., staph., ***stront-c., sulph.,*** trom., zinc.
air, open, agg. - staph.
amel. - gamb.
evening - mag-c., ph-ac., puls.
inner - **ALUM.,** ***apis, aur.,*** bell., bor., calc., carb-v., ***caust.,*** chel., cina, ***cinnb.,*** clem., ***con.,*** cycl., fl-ac., ***gamb., graph.,*** grat., hyos., lach., laur., led., ***lyc.,*** mag-c., **MAG-M.,** mez., mur-ac., ***nat-m.,*** nit-ac., osm., phos., ph-ac., ***psor., puls., ruta.,*** sep., stann., staph., ***stront-c., sulph.,*** syph., tab., ***zinc.***
evening - dios., fl-ac., ***puls.***
morning - sep.
outer - ant-c., aur-m., benz-ac., bry., carb-v., cinnb., com., euph., euphr., fago., form., mez., ***nat-m.,*** prun., rhus-t., sep., squil., ***sulph.,*** tax., tarent., upa.

itching, eyebrows - agar., agn., all-c., alum., ars., arund., berb., bry., caust., com., con., ferr., fl-ac., laur., manc., mez., nat-m., pall., par., rhod., sel., sil., spig., **SULPH.,** verat., viol-t.
evening - all-c.
morning - nat-m.

itching, eyelids - agar., alum., ambr., anag., ang., apis, **ARG-M.,** asaf., asc-t., aur., aur-m., bell., berb., bry., bufo, ***calc.,*** camph., carb-an., carb-s., ***caust.,*** chin., con., croc., ***crot-t.,*** cycl., dros., euph., ***euphr., graph., hep.,*** iod., kali-ar., ***kali-bi.,*** lob., lyc., mag-m., ***mez.,*** nat-c., nat-p., nux-v., paeon., pall., ***petr., ph-ac., phos.,*** **PULS., RHUS-T.,** ruta, ***sep.,*** sil., sin-n., spong., **SULPH.,** tarent., **TELL.,** vesp., vinc., zinc.
daytime only - ***phos.,*** **SULPH.**
evening - ***mez.,*** phos., **PULS.**
lower lids - sul-ac.
margin - am-c., asaf., bar-c., bry., ***calc., carb-v.,*** chin., con., euphr., fago., grat., jatr., kali-bi., kali-c., kreos., mez., nat-a., nat-p., ***nat-s.,*** nux-v., phos., **PULS.,** prun., sel., ***sep.,*** **STAPH.,** ***sulph.,*** zinc.
morning - carb-v., nat-c., nux-v.
orbital arch - kali-n.
rubbing amel. - staph.

JAGGED, iris - sil., staph., thuj.

JERK, eyelid, burning, right - sulph.

JERKING, pain - agar., ***asar.,*** lac-f., staph.
left - agar., lac-f.

LACHRYMAL duct, ailments of - apis, fago., hep., merc-d., ***nat-m., petr.,*** plb., sil., staph.
glands - brom., sabal.
obstructed - merc-d., ***nat-m.***
stricture, of - ***arg-m.,*** calc., euphr., ***fl-ac.,*** graph., hep., ***nat-m., puls., rhus-t.,*** **SIL.**

LACHRYMATION, general, (see Tears) - absin., acet-ac., ***acon.,*** act-sp., aesc., ***agar., ail.,*** **ALL-C.,** all-s., aloe, ***alum.,*** ambr., am-c., am-m., anac., ***apis, arg-n.,*** arn., ***ars.,*** ars-i., art-v., arum-t., arund., ***asar., aur.,*** bar-c., **BELL.,** berb., bor., ***brom.,*** bry., cadm-s., **CALC.,** calc-p., ***caps.,*** carb-an., ***carb-ac., carb-s., carb-v.,*** caul., ***caust., cham., chel.,*** chin., chin-a., chlol., chlor., cimic., cinnb., cina, clem., coc-c., ***colch.,*** coloc., ***com., con., croc., crot-c., crot-h., crot-t.,*** cupr-ar., daph., dig., dios., ***elaps,*** eug., ***eup-per., euph.,*** **EUPHR.,** ***ferr.,*** ferr-ar., ***ferr-i., ferr-p.,*** **FL-AC.,** gamb., gels., glon., ***graph.,*** grat., ***ham., hep.,*** hydr., ***ign., iod.,*** ip., kali-ar., ***kali-bi., kali-c., kali-i.,*** kali-n., kali-p., kali-s., kreos., ***lach.,*** lachn., ***led.,*** **LYC.,** ***mag-c.,*** mag-s., meny., **MERC.,** ***merl., mez.,*** mill., mosch., mur-ac., naja, nat-a., ***nat-c.,*** **NAT-M.,** nat-p., ***nat-s.,*** nicc., **NIT-AC.,** nux-m., ***nux-v.,*** olnd., ol-an., **OP.,** osm., ***par.,*** petr., ph-ac., **PHOS.,** phyt., ***psor.,*** **PULS.,** ran-b., ran-s., rheum, ***rhod.,*** **RHUS-T.,** ***ruta., sabad.,*** sabin., ***sang.,*** sars., sel., ***seneg., sep., sil.,*** sin-n., ***sol-n., spig., spong.,*** squil., stann., staph., ***stram.,*** stry., **SULPH.,** ***sul-ac.,*** sumb., ***tarax.,*** tell., teucr., ***thuj.,*** ust., ***verat., zinc.***

- afternoon - lyc.
- air, open, in - ail., alum., arn., bar-c., bell., bry., **CALC.,** camph., ***canth.,*** carb-s., ***caust.,*** chel., chlor., ***clem.,*** cob., coc-c., ***colch.,*** dios., dulc., euph., ***graph.,*** hyos., merc., nat-a., ***nat-m.,*** nit-ac., petr., phel., **PHOS.,** ***puls.,*** phyt., rheum, ***rhus-t., ruta., sabad.,*** senec., seneg., ***sep.,*** **SIL.,** staph., **SULPH., THUJ.,** ust., verat., zinc.
  - amel. - chin-s., ***croc.,*** phyt., plat., prun.
- bending head backwards, amel. - seneg.
- brain, affections in - dig., kali-i., zinc.
- breathing deep, on - graph.
- chill, during - elat., sabad.
- closed eyes, with - spong.
- closing, on - berb.
- cold air, in - cob., dig., echi., euphr., kreos., lyc., phos., **PULS.,** ***sep., sil.,*** sulph., thuj.
  - application, from - sanic.
- colds, during - all-c., carb-v., euphr., sang., tell., verb.
- contraction of upper eyelid, from - spig.
- coryza, during - acon., agar., **ALL-C.,** alum., ***anac.,*** anan., ***arg-n.,*** ars., ars-i., carb-ac., **CARB-V.,** ***chin.,*** dulc., **EUPHR.,** iod., jab., ***kali-c.,*** lach., lyc., **NUX-V.,** ***phos., phyt., puls.,*** ran-s., ***sabad., sang.,*** sin-n., ***spig.,*** squil., staph., **TELL.,** ***verb.***
- cough, with - acon., aloe, ***agar.,*** arn., brom., bry., calc., carb-ac., carb-v., cench., chel., cina, cycl., ***eup-per.,*** euph., **EUPHR.,** ***graph.,*** hep., ip., kali-c., kali-ma., kreos., merc., **NAT-M.,** op., ***phyt.,*** **PULS.,** rhus-t., ***sabad.,*** sil., **SQUIL.,** staph., sulph.
  - profuse lachrymation with every attack of cough - arn.
  - whooping cough, with - all-c., ***caps., graph., nat-m.***

LACHRYMATION, general

- damp weather - crot-t., graph.
- daytime only - **ALUM.,** lyc., sars., zinc.
- dreams, during - plan.
- eating - ol-an., zinc.
- evening - acon., all-c., asar., calc., eug., mag-m., merc., nicc., phos., rhus-t., ***ruta., sep.,*** ter., **ZINC.**
- fever, during - acon., apis, bell., calc., cham., eup-per., ign., lyc., petr., ***puls.,*** spig., spong., sulph.
- fire, looking at the - ant-c., chel., ***mag-m., merc.,*** sabad.
- forenoon - nat-c., squil.
- gushes, in - am-c., aur., chin-a., eug., ip., rhus-t.
- headache, during - agar., arg-n., asar., bell., bov., carb-an., carb-v., chel., com., con., eug., hep., ***ign.,*** ind., kali-c., kali-i., lac-c., lil-t., merc., osm., ***plat., puls.,*** rhus-r., spong., stram., tax.
- heart symptoms, with - am-c., spong.
- larynx, tickling, from - chel., cocc.
- laughing, when - carb-v., nat-m.
- left - carb-ac., carb-v., clem., ***coloc.,*** dios., ***ign.,*** mag-c., sin-n., thuj., uran.
- light, from - dig., kreos., puls., spong.
  - bright, from - ail., chel., ***chin-s., kreos., mag-m.,*** sabad., spong.
  - sun, from, of - bry., ign., graph., staph.
- looking steadily - ***apis,*** chel., cinnb., echi., euphr., ign., ip., kali-c., kreos., nat-a., osm., plat., ***seneg.,*** spong., tab.
  - broad day light, when - mag-m.
  - intently, agg. - chel.
- lying, agg. - euphr.
- menses, during - calc., phyt., zinc.
- morning - alum., am-m., bell., bor., ***calc.,*** carb-an., kali-n., kreos., lachn., mag-c., merc., nat-c., nat-m., nicc., phel., phos., **PULS.,** rat., rhus-t., ***sep.,*** staph., **SULPH.,** zinc.
  - waking, after - alum.
  - waking, on - nat-a., sep., zinc.
- music, hearing - graph.
- night - acon., all-s., am-c., am-m., ***apis,*** arn., ars., bar-c., chin., gels., hep., nit-ac., phos., ran-s., **ZINC.**
- nose, from biting pain in - aur.
  - itching, from - mag-m., plat.
- opening eyes, on - ***kali-bi.***
  - forcibly, on - ***apis, con., ip., merc-c., rhus-t.***
- pain, after - hep.
- pain, with, in the eye - calc., chel., cimic., ***coloc.,*** ferr., ip., mag-c., mag-m., meny., nat-c., rheum, sulph., thuj.
  - body, in other parts of - acon., chel., cinnb., ferr., lach., mez., nat-m., plan., ***puls.,*** ran-b., rhus-t., ***sabad.***
  - eyelid, in right - xan.
  - nose, in the - anac., aur., mag-m.
  - throat, in the - sep.

LACHRYMATION, general
reading, while - ***am-c., carb-s., croc.,*** grat., ign., nat-a., nit-ac., olnd., phos., ***ruta., seneg.,*** sep., still., sul-ac.
right - brom., calc., chin., ***hyos.,*** kali-n., lyc., mag-c., nit-ac., sang., verb., vesp.
room, in a - asar., caust., ***croc.,*** dig., phos.
rubbing, after - nat-c., ph-ac., ruta, sep.
side affected - lach., nat-m., nux-v., puls., spig.
sneezing, with - just., nat-m., sabad.
spasms, alternating with - alumn.
eyelids, lower, after - ruta.
stool, during - **PHOS.**
sun, looking at - staph.
from the light of - bry., ign., graph., staph.
swallowing, on - arg-n.
urination, during - **PHOS.**
vomiting, by - cupr.
warm room - ***all-c., phos.***
wind, in - calc., **EUPHR.,** lyc., ***nat-m.,*** phos., **PULS.,** rhus-t., sanic., ***sil.,*** sulph., ***thuj.***
writing, while - ***calc.,*** ol-an., staph.
after - ferr.
yawning, when - ant-t., bar-ac., bell., calc-p., ign., kali-c., kreos., meph., ***nux-v.,*** ph-ac., plat., rhus-t., ***sabad.,*** sars., staph., viol-o.

LENS, ailments of - ***calc-f.,*** euphr., phos., ***puls., sil., sulph.***

LIGHT, sensitivity to (See Photophobia)

LINE, in young, girls, hysterical children - asaf., lil-t., mosch., nat-m.

LIVID - lyss.

LOOKING, steadily (see Eyestrain) - agar., apis, cadm-s., caust., cina, croc., ***merc., ruta,*** spong., thuj.
all sides, agg. - kali-br.
around, agg. - calc., ***cic.,*** **CON.,** ip.
constantly in one direction - brom., hyos.
down, agg. - arg-n., bor., calc., kali-c., kalm., olnd., ***phos., spig., sulph.***
amel. - sabad.
eclipse, at, agg. - hep., sol.
either way, right or left, agg. - ***con.,*** spig.
intently agg. - cina, mur-ac., olnd., ruta.
amel. - agn., petr.
into distance agg. - dig., euphr., ruta.
amel. - bell.
long, anything, at agg. - acon., aur., nat-m., ruta, sep., spig.
amel. - dig., ***nat-c.,*** sabad.
mirror, in agg. - kali-c.
moving things, flowing water, at, agg. - agar., **BELL.,** brom., canth., ***con., ferr.,*** hyos., piloc., lyss., stram., sulph.
one eye only, with - phos.
point, at one, amel. - agn.
red objects, at agg. - lyc.
revolving objects, at agg. - lyc.
sideways agg. - ***bell.,*** merc-c., olnd.
amel. - chin-s., olnd., sulph.
snow, at, agg. - apis

LOOKING, steadily
straight forward, agg. - olnd.
amel. - ***bell.,*** olnd.
through sharp spectacles, as if - croc.
upward agg. - ***ars.,*** bell., carb-v., ***chel.,*** colch., sulph.
white objects, at, agg. - apis, ars., cham., lyc., nat-m., tab.
agg., yellow spots - am-c.
window, out of, agg. - camph., carb-v., **NAT-M.,** ox-ac.

LOOSE, sensation as if - ***carb-an.***

LUPUS, eyebrows - alumn., anan.
lupus, eyelids - alumn., kali-chl., phyt.
lower - ***apis.***

LUSTRELESS, (see Dullness)

MELANOSIS - ***aur.***

MELT, away, feel as would - ham.

MEMBRANE, sensation as if, drawn over eyes - apis, caust., daph., puls., rat.

MOONLIGHT, amel. eye symptoms - ***aur.***

MOVEMENT, of eyeballs
closed lids, under - benz-n., cupr., zinc.
constant - agar., ***bell.,*** benz-n., ***iod.,*** raph., sil., ***stram.***
convulsive - acon., ***agar.,*** **BELL.,** bufo, canth., chin-s., coff., hyos., ign., kali-cy., ***mag-p.,*** sulph., verat., zinc.
labor, during - chin-s.
light agg. - bell.
sleep, during - hell., op., ph-ac.
waking, when - coff.
involuntary - ***agar., calc.,*** canth., cupr., ***mag-p., nux-v.,*** spig., sulph.
staring, ahead, when - ph-ac.
pendulum like, from side to side - **AGAR.,** amyg., ***ars.,*** benz-n., ***carb-h.,*** cic., cocc., con., ***cupr., gels.,*** kali-c., puls., sabad., sulph., zinc.
rolling - aeth., ***agar.,*** amyg., arg-n., ***bell.,*** benz-n., ***bufo,*** camph., ***caust.,*** cham., ***cic., cocc.,*** colch., ***cupr., euphr., gels.,*** hell., ***hyos.,*** kali-br., kali-i., lyss., merc., merc-c., nat-a., op., petr., sant., sec., ***stram.,*** stry., tarent., ter., tub., ust., ***verat., zinc.***
downwards - ***aeth.,*** hyos.
drink, at sight of - bell.
sleep, during - ***apis,*** ol-an., puls.
up and down - benz-ac., sulph.
upward - ***acon.,*** anan., amyg., ***apis,*** bell., ***bufo,*** camph., ***cic.,*** cina, cub., ***cupr.,*** hell., ***laur., lact.,*** mur-ac., oena., plat., ter., ***verat.***
sideways - spig.

NAIL, in, as if - hell.

NARROWING, of intervals between eyelids - ***agar.,*** arg-n., dig., euphr., nat-m., nux-v., rhus-t.

NODULES, eyelids - ***con., sil.,*** **STAPH.,** sulph., ***thuj.,*** tub.

NODULES, eyelids
margins - aur., ***calc., con., sep.,*** sil., **STAPH.,** thuj.

NYSTAGMUS, (see Movement)

NUMBNESS, around eyes - **ASAF.**

ONYX, inflammation, iris - ***hep., merc.,*** rhus-t.

OPACITY, cornea, of (see Spots) - agn., ***apis,*** **ARG-N.,** ***aur., aur-m.,*** bar-c., ***bar-i.,*** **CADM-S., CALC.,** calc-f., calc-p., ***cann-s., caust., chel., chin., cine., cinnb., cocc., colch.,*** **CON.,** ***crot-t.,*** euph., ***euphr., hep., hydr., kali-bi.,*** kali-m., ***kali-s., lach., lyc., mag-c.,*** merc-c., ***merc-i-f., merc.,*** nat-s., ***nit-ac.,*** op., phos., puls., rhus-t., ***seneg., sil.,*** **SULPH.,** ***tarent.,*** thiosin., tub., ***zinc.***
arcus senilis - acon., ars., calc., ***cocc., coloc.,*** kali-c., ***kali-bi.,*** lyc., ***merc.,*** merc-c., mosch., phos., **PULS., SULPH.,** vario., zinc.
dense - kali-bi.
left - ***hep., sulph.***
punctuated - kali-bi., kali-chl., kali-i.
right - ***lyc., sil.***
smallpox, after - ***sil.***
spots - calc-f.
wounds, from - ***euphr.***

opacity, vitreous - colch., ***gels.,*** ham., hep., kali-i., merc-c., ***merc-i-f.,*** morg-g., ***phos.,*** prun., psor., seneg., ***sulph.,*** syc-co., thuj.
turbid - chol., ***kali-i.,*** phos., prun., ***seneg.,*** sulph.

OPEN, eyelids - ant-t., apis, ***caust., cocc.,*** crot-h., ***cupr., dol.,*** **GUAI.,** hydr-ac., ***hyos.,*** **IOD.,** ***laur.,*** **LYC.,** naja, nux-v., olnd., ***onos., op.,*** sol-n., squil., ***stram.***
and close in quick succession - agar., chlf., mygal.
attack, before an - ***laur.***
delirium, with - ***crot-h.,*** **STRAM.**
desire to keep eyes wide open - onos.
dislikes to open, them, fears it will agg. headache - phys.
half open - ***agar.,*** amyg., ***ant-t., apis, ars., art-v.,*** bapt., **BELL.,** ***bry.,*** cadm-s., cann-i., ***canth.,*** caps., ***carb-h., cham., coff., colch., coloc., crot-c., crot-h.,*** **CUPR.,** ***dig.,*** ferr., ferr-m., ferr-p., **GELS.,** ***hell., hydr-ac., ip., kreos., lach.,*** laur., ***lyc.,*** mag-m., ***merc., morph., nat-m., oena.,*** **OP.,** phel., ph-ac., ***phos.,*** plb., podo., ***rhus-t.,*** samb., ***stram., sulph.,*** ter., verat., ***zinc.***
dreams, during - bell., ***cham.,*** hyos., ip., ***op.,*** podo., ***zinc.***
hard to keep open - ars., bapt., ***bor.,*** bufo, caust., **GELS.,** hyos., naja, nat-a., ph-ac., pic-ac.
morning - hep.
must keep them open, and look into the light - puls.
one, only - ant-t.
right, more than the left - staph.

OPEN, eyelids
sensation as if wide - carb-v., onos., pip-m.
closed are wide open - phos., sep.
sleep, during - ant-t., apis, ars., ***bell.,*** bry., cadm-s., calc., chin., ***cocc.,*** con., cupr., ferr., ip., ***lach., lyc.,*** op., ph-ac., puls., samb., stram., sulph.
unable to - abrot., ***alum.,*** am-c., anan., ars., ***arg-m., aur.,*** bufo, cadm-s., carb-v., ***cham., chel., con.,*** gels., hell., hyos., kali-n., lach., lyc., mag-c., merl., nat-a., **NUX-M.,** ***nux-v.,*** oena., op., petr., ph-ac., sil., staph., sul-ac., ***tarent.,*** thuj.
headache, during - euph., nux-v., petr., ph-ac., ***tarent.***
menses, during - ***cimic.***
morning - ***lyc.,*** mag-m., petr., ph-ac., staph., thuj.
morning, from pressure in forehead - ph-ac.
night - ars., carb-v., cinnb., ***cocc.***
night, waking on - ***merl.***
sleeplessness, with - nat-c.
waking on - am-c., ***merl.***
unconsciousness, during - ***op.***

OPENING, eyelids difficult - ***agar.,*** alum., ambr., anan., ***arg-m.,*** arg-n., **ARS.,** ***bor.,*** caps., **CAUST.,** ***chel.,*** cina, ***con.,*** cupr., elaps, ***ferr.,*** ferr-ar., ***fl-ac.,*** **GELS.,** hell., hydr-ac., hyos., kali-ar., kali-c., ***lyc., mag-m., merc.,*** merl., ***nat-c.,*** nat-m., ***nit-ac., nux-v., phos.,*** sep., spig., samb., sul-ac.
morning - ambr., bar-c., bor., bov., ***caust.,*** con., ***lyc.,*** mag-c., mag-m., nicc., ***nit-ac., petr., ph-ac.,*** psor., rhus-t., ***sep.,*** sul-ac.
waking, on - ***cocc.,*** kali-c.
night - carb-v., chel., ***cocc.,*** mag-m., nat-m., rhus-t., ***sep.***

opening, eyelids, causes sneezing - **GRAPH.**

OPENNESS, spasmodic - aeth., ang., apis, arn., **BELL.,** camph., ***caust., cocc.,*** dol., ***guai.,*** hyos., **IOD.,** ***ip.,*** laur., lyc., lyss., naja, nat-m., **NUX-V.,** op., **STRAM.,** ***stry.***
delirium, during - ***op., stram.***

OPHTHALMIA, (see Inflammation, eyes) - xan.

PAIN, eyes - absin., ***acon.,*** aeth., agar., ***all-c., aloe, alum., ambr., am-c.,*** am-m., ***anac.,*** anan., ant-t., ***apis, arg-n., arn., ars.,*** ars-i., ***asaf.,*** asar., asc-t., **ASPAR.,** ***atro.,*** **AUR.,** aur-m., bad., bapt., ***bar-c.,*** bar-m., **BELL.,** ***berb., bor.,*** bov., brom., bufo, **BRY.,** calad., ***calc., calc-p., calc-s., carb-ac.,*** carb-an., ***carb-s.,*** carb-v., card-m., ***carl., caust., cedr.,*** **CHAM.,** ***chel., chen-a.,*** **CHIN.,** chin-a., chlor., cic., ***cimic.,*** cina, ***cinnb., clem., cocc., colch., coloc., com., con.,*** cop., cor-r., ***croc.,*** crot-c., ***crot-h., crot-t., cupr.,*** daph., ***dig.,*** echi., ***elaps,*** eup-per., ***euphr.,*** ferr., ***ferr-ar.,*** ferr-i., ***ferr-p.,*** fl-ac., gamb., ***gels., glon., graph., guar.,*** gymn., ***ham.,*** hell., ***hep., hydr.,*** hydrc., hyos., hyper., ***ign.,*** iod., ip., jab., ***kali-ar.,*** kali-bi., ***kali-c.,*** kali-i., ***kali-p.,*** kali-s., **KALM.,** kreos., ***lac-c., lach., lac-ac.,*** led., lil-t., lith., lob., **LYC.,** ***lyss.,*** mag-c., mag-m., ***mag-p.,*** manc., mang., ***med.,*** meph., **MERC.,** ***merc-c.,*** merc-i-f., merc-i-r., ***merl., mez.,*** naja, nat-a., **NAT-M.,**

PAIN, eyes - nat-p., **NIT-AC.,** ***nux-v.,*** osm., ox-ac., par., pall., ***petr.,*** phel., ***ph-ac., phos., phys., phyt.,*** pic-ac., ***plan., plat., plb.,*** podo., ***prun., psor., ptel., puls.,*** **RAN-B.,** ***rhod., rhus-t.,*** rhus-v., rumx., **RUTA.,** sabad., **SANG.,** sant., ***sars.,*** sec., ***sel.,*** **SENEG.,** ***sep., sil.,*** **SPIG.,** ***spong., stann., staph.,*** stram., stry., ***sulph.,*** tab., tarax., ***tarent., ter., ther., thuj.,*** tub., urt-u., ust., valer., verat., vesp., ***zinc.,*** zing.

afternoon - ars-m., ***cham.,*** chin., ***cimic.,*** grat., lachn., petr., phys., phyt., rhus-t., sang., seneg., sep., sil., staph.
1 p.m. - ars.
2 p.m. - dios., phys., sep.
2 p.m, after siesta - euphr.
3 p.m. - mag-c.
3 or 4 p.m. - ***com.***
4 p.m. - caust., gent-l., hura, **LYC.,** sil.
4 p.m., after beer - sulph.
4 to 8 p.m. - **LYC.**
5 p.m. - mag-c., nat-a., thuj.
6 p.m. - euph., phys.
closing eyelids, on - cimic.
rolling upward or outward agg. - sang.

air, agg. - ***acon.,*** chel., cinnb., ***clem.,*** cob., **HEP., SIL.,** ***spig.***

air, cold, agg. - ***acon.,*** asar., chel., cinnb., ***clem.,*** cob., **HEP.,** mag-p., **SIL.,** ***spig.***
amel. - ***arg-n.,*** asar., bism.

air, open, agg. - aur-m., benz-ac., berb., clem., glon., ***kalm.,*** kali-bi., merc-c., seneg., ***spig.***
amel. - **ARG-N.,** ars., **ASAF.,** ***lil-t.,*** nat-m., ***phos., puls.,*** sep.

alternates, with pain in, abdomen - ***euphr.***
left arm - plb.
ovary - sulph.

around, the eyes - ***cinnb., gels., ign.,*** **MAG-M.,** merc., merc-c., nit-ac., pall., phyt., puls., **SPIG.,** sulph., ter.

bathing, eye, agg. - ***sulph.***
amel. - aur., mur-ac., nicc., thuj.
cold water, in, amel. - ***apis, asar., phos., puls.***

bending, forward agg. - ***coloc.***

between, eyes - asc-c., carb-h., caust., dios., gymn.
eye and nose - mang.

blinking, amel. - bar-c.

blow, from a - **ARN., SYMPH.**

blowing, nose agg. - nit-ac..
amel. - aur.

center, of eyeballs - cimic.

change of weather - cadm-s.

changing, from dark to light, and light to dark - ***stram.***

chill, during - seneg.

ciliary - croc.

close, must - ***aur.,*** bar-c., ***calc.***

closing, agg. - ***bell.,*** canth., ***carb-v.,*** cimic., clem., con., fago., lac-ac., sil., staph., sumb.
closing, amel. - ***chel., lac-d.,*** nit-ac., ph-ac., pic-ac., plat., sin-n.

PAIN, eyes

cold, water amel. - acon., ***apis, asar., aur., form.,*** lac-d., nat-a., nit-ac., ***phos.,*** pic-ac., ***puls.***
wind agg. - acon., caust., **SEP.**

combing hair agg. - nux-v.

congestion, as from - nit-ac..

coughing, on - seneg., sul-ac., viol-o.

covering eyes with hand amel. - ***aur-m., thuj.***

crying, after - berb., tab.
as after, crying - stann.

dark amel. - bell., ***chin.,*** con., ***euphr.,*** lil-t., ***nux-m.,*** staph.

daytime, only - ammc., caust., cob., ***hep.,*** **KALM.,** lyc., mang., phos., **SANG.,** sep.

dinner, after - agar., mez., phos., seneg.

dryness, of eyeballs, with - nat-m., **SULPH.**

ear affection, in - viol-o.

eating, after - dig., lyc., sulph.

evening - aloe, alum., apis, ars-m., bov., ***calc., calc-s.,*** camph., carb-an., ***carb-s., carb-v.,*** cedr., coloc., con., croc., daph., dig., dios., euphr., ferr., graph., hep., ind., kali-chl., ***kalm.,*** lyc., mag-m., merc., mur-ac., nat-c., nat-m., nit-ac., op., ***petr.,*** phys., plat., **PULS.,** rhus-t., **RUTA.,** sars., seneg., ***staph.,*** stry., **SULPH.,** tarent., verat., **ZINC.**
7 p.m. - ***cedr.,*** glon.
8 p.m. - ham., lac-ac., stry.
air in open - glon., kali-bi.
amel. - chel.
gaslight, by - ***calc.,*** carb-an., petr., ***ruta.,*** seneg.
looking at light - amph., plat.
lying down - ***carb-v.,*** fl-ac., zinc.
reading, while - ***calc.,*** mill., phys., ***nat-s.,*** **RUTA.**
by light - mez., sars.
and writing, on - nat-a.
sewing, while - apis, mez., **RUTA.**
sitting, while - chin-s.
twilight - nat-m.
walking and driving - plan.
writing, while - sel., wild.

exertion of vision, from - bar-c., **BRY.,** calc., canth., carb-v., ***chel.,*** ign., ***mang.,*** mur-ac., naja, **NAT-M.,** ***nux-m., phyt.,*** plat., ***psor., puls., rhus-t.,*** **RUTA.,** sil., ***spig., staph.***
as from exertion of vision - graph.
fine work, from - ***carb-v.,*** coloc., ***con., jab.,*** merc., mur-ac., ***nat-m.,*** **RUTA.,** seneg., sulph.

extending, to
arm, to - rumx.
backward - ***aur.,*** cimic., colch., coloc., ***com.,*** crot-h., hep., lach., lil-t., mez., nat-m., ***par.,*** phos., phys., ***rhus-t., spig.,*** tarent., ***thuj.***
downward - ***aur.,*** bry., cahin., carb-v., coloc., ***gels.***
ear, to - bar-c., fago., petr., tub.
face, over side of - lyc., op.

PAIN, eyes
extending, to
forehead, to - agar., croc., hura, kalm., ran-b.
across - cedr., lac-ac.
frontal, sinus - **SPIG.**
occiput, to - ***bry.,*** coc-c., colch., com., crot-t., dios., kali-p., lach., ***nat-a.,*** pic-ac., sil., syph., tub.
outward - ***asaf.,*** aster., hydr-ac.
temples, to - anac., bad., bar-c., chel., coc-c., ip., phys.
vertex, to - cimic., ***croc.,*** kreos., lach., phyt., viol-o.
eye, and nose, between, in the afternoon - kalm.
eyeballs - thuj.
centre of - cimic., vib.
fever, during - ***guar.,*** hep., kali-c., ***led.,*** **LYC.,** ***nat-m., nux-v.,*** ph-ac., puls., rhod., rhus-t., ***sep., stram.,*** thuj., **VALER.**
fire, glare of - **MERC.**
forenoon - kali-bi., lach., lyc., nat-c., phyt., plat., podo., rumx., sulph., zinc.
8 to 9 - ***chin.***
10 a.m. till noon - ***chin.,*** stann.
11 a.m. - jac., phys.
glaucoma, in - acon., ***phos.,*** mez.
headache, during - ***agar.,*** ail., ***apis,*** aran., **BELL.,** carb-s., cimic., ***coff.,*** con., eug., hep., hipp., nit-ac., ***sel.,*** sep., seneg., stict., thuj., zinc.
after, stitching pain in eyes - gels.
occiput headache, in - carb-v., gels., **NUX-V.**
heart, at each beat of - atro.
increasing until noon - **KALM.,** ***nat-m., puls., stann.***
left - agar., ***anac., ars., asar.,*** asc-t., ***aur.,*** aur-m., ***caust., elaps, hep.,*** lac-f., ***lach.,*** lyc., mag-m., naja, onos., pic-ac., ***sulph.,*** zinc.
extending to vertex - viol-o.
headache, with left sided - apis.
light - ***apis, ars.,*** asc-t., atro., ***aur-m.,*** **BAR-C.,** ***bell., calc., chel.,*** **CHIN.,** cob., **CON.,** ***cupr.,*** euphr., ferr-i., ***hep.,*** iod., ***lac-d.,*** mang., ***merc.,*** nat-a., **NAT-M.,** ***nux-m., nux-v.,*** petr., ***phos., phyt.,*** sep., ***sil., staph.,*** sulph., syph., thuj.
artificial - ***calc., calc-p.,*** carb-an., ***chel.,*** cina, croc., ip., ***lith.,*** lyc., mang., nat-a., ***nat-m.,*** nux-v., petr., pic-ac., plat., sars., ***seneg.,*** sep., staph.
daylight, from - am-c., hell., hep., lac-ac., ***merc.,*** sars., ***sil.***
dim light agg. - am-m., ***apis,*** sars., ***stram.***
strong - ***asar.,*** com., ***hep., mang.,*** nat-a., petr., phos., pic-ac., ruta., ***sil., sulph.,*** thuj.
looking when - acon., anac., ***apis,*** caust., **NAT-M.,** ph-ac., ***phos.,*** rheum, ***ruta.,*** sars., sulph., tab.
candlelight, at - euphr., staph.
downward, agg. - nat-m.
amel. - bar-c.
sharply - sul-ac.
sideways - bar-c.

PAIN, eyes
looking, when
steadily - ***ars., apis, arund., carb-v., caust., chel., cina,*** nat-a., nat-c., **NAT-M.,** plat., ***psor.,*** rheum., ***rhus-t., ruta., seneg.***
at near objects - echi., ***mang.***
upward - ars., bar-c., ***carb-v., chel.,*** con., kali-c., mang., plb., sabad., sulph.
lying, while - ***carb-v.,*** cedr., ***gels.,*** nux-v., ***phos.***
back, on, amel. - puls.
amel. - chel., ***cimic.***
left side amel., on - nat-a.
painful side, on, agg. - syph.
amel. - lach., zinc.
masturbation, after - ***cina.***
menses, during - carb-an., croc., ***coloc.,*** nicc.
morning - ***ambr.,*** arg-n., ars-m., asar., ***aur.,*** bor., chel., cimic., elaps, euphr., form., graph., kali-c., meph., naja, ***nat-a.,*** nat-c., nat-m., nicc., ***nux-v.,*** paeon., phos., podo., ***puls.,*** rhus-t., seneg., ***sep.,*** **SPIG.,** stann., stry., sulph., tarent., thuj., valer., zinc.
4 a.m., on waking - ***nux-v.***
5 a.m. - stann.
7 a.m. - ***puls.***
begins in and increases till noon and ceases in evening - **KALM.,** ***nat-m.***
breakfast, after, amel. - naja
on opening - form., ph-ac.
rising, after - sep., sulph., thuj.
twilight - am-m.
waking - bry., ferr., ***form.,*** kali-p., ***lach.,*** nat-m., **NUX-V.,** ***sep.,*** sulph., upa.
walking, while - puls.
working amel. - ***form.***
motion of, on - agar., apis, arg-n., arn., ***ars.,*** astac., bad., ***berb.,*** brom., **BRY.,** camph., ***carb-s., carb-v.,*** caust., chel., ***chin.,*** cimic., clem., com., cor-r., crot-h., ***cupr., gels.,*** glon., grin., ***hep.,*** kali-ar., kali-c., kali-p., ***kalm., lac-d.,*** lach., lyc., ***mang.,*** med., meph., merc., nat-a., ***nat-m.,*** par., phos., phys., phyt., pic-ac., **PRUN.,** ***puls., ran-s.,*** **RHUS-T.,** sep., sil., ***spig.,*** stann., ***sulph.,*** sumb.
amel. - dulc., op.
quick - ran-s., stram.
night - acon., am-m., ars., ***asaf., aur., bry.,*** canth., chel., ***chin.,*** chin-a., cimic., cob., cocc., coloc., ***con., crot-t.,*** cycl., ***hep.,*** kali-ar., ***kali-i., led.,*** lyc., **MERC., MERC-C.,** merc-i-f., ***nux-v., plb.,*** **PRUN.,** ***sep., spig., staph., syph.,*** thuj., vesp., **ZINC.,** ziz.
11 p.m. - euphr., nat-m.
bed, in - arn., cimic., sil.
midnight - merc.
3 a.m. - spig.
after - ars., sulph.
throbbing - ***asaf.***
waking, on - chel., cycl.
noon, daily - cham., ***chin-s.,*** ign., sulph., valer., verat.
opening, lids, on - ars., croc., ***graph., hydr.,*** kali-bi., ***led.,*** ph-ac., upa.

PAIN, eyes

paroxysmal - ars., **BAD.,** ***chin., chin-s.,*** hep., nicc., plat., puls., sil.

periodic - aur-m., ***cedr., chin., chin-s., coloc., euphr., gels., nat-m.,*** **PRUN.**

every other day - ars.

press, should them - calc.

pressure, after - bar-ac.

agg. - brom., dros., ham., plan., sars.

amel. - ***asaf.,*** bapt., bry., ***calc., caust.,*** chel., chin-s., cimic., coloc., con., ham., mag-m., ***mag-p.,*** mur-ac., pic-ac.

pulsating - ***ars., asaf., chel.,*** petr., rheum., rhus-t.

raising, eyelids - ***nat-m.***

reading - ***agar.,*** alum., ammc., ***apis, arg-n., arn.,*** ars-i., ***ars.,*** ars-m., asar., aur., bapt., ***bry., calc.,*** calc-p., cann-i., caust., cic., **CON., DULC.,** ***echi.,*** ign., ***jab.,*** kali-ar., ***kali-c., kali-p., lac-c., lac-d., lach.,*** lac-ac., ***lith.,*** lyc., ***mang.,*** merc., ***merl.,*** mur-ac., ***nat-a.,*** nat-c., **NAT-M.,** nat-p., nat-s., nit-ac., ***nux-v.,*** ol-j., olnd., ***onos.,*** petr., phel., ***phos.,*** phys., phyt., pic-ac., ***puls., rhod.,*** **RUTA.,** sars., ***seneg.,*** **SEP.,** ***staph.,*** sulph., thuj.

candlelight, by - benz-ac., ***cina,*** lach., mang., nat-m., nux-v., staph.

light, by - kali-c.

other eye, with - kalm.

rest, agg. - ***coloc.,*** dros., dulc., merc-i-f., mur-ac., thuj.

amel. - asaf., berb., bry., cimic., pic-ac.

rheumatic - anac., ***apis,*** clem., ***dulc.,*** kali-c., ***led., mez., phyt.***

right - anan., ***apis,*** **BELL.,** calc-ar., **CARB-AC.,** card-m., coc-c., **COM.,** crot-h., dol., erig., ***kali-c., kalm.,*** med., ***nat-m.,*** pall., ***prun., ran-b.,*** **SANG.,** ***sil.,*** tarent.

extending, to forehead - kalm.

extending, to left - bad.

lying on left side - lac-f.

ring, as from a - sep.

rising, when - ars., cer-b., fago.

rubbing, agg. - carb-v., caust., euphr., kali-c., sep.

amel. - ***caust., ran-b.,*** zinc.

sand, as from - euphr., zing.

sewing, while - apis, ars-m., ***cina,*** dig., lyc., mez.

fine work, on - carb-v., coloc., ***con.,*** merc., ***nat-m.,*** **RUTA.**

sex, after - bart.

sitting, while - chin-s., merc., phos.

sleep, after - alum., canth., euphr., gels.

amel. - am-c., chel., **PHOS.**

before - ***con.,*** **PHOS.**

smoking, from - calad.

spark, as from - tarent.

step, at each - hep.

stool, during - ***crot-t.***

after - nat-c.

PAIN, eyes

stooping, when - berb., bov., ***coloc.,*** fl-ac., merc., seneg., spig.

storm, before - ***cedr.,*** **RHOD.,** ***sil.***

during - **RHOD.,** sep., ***sil.***

strained, as if - ***mez.,*** **RUTA.**

sunlight, agg. - aml-n., calc., ***clem., hep., kali-p., mang., nat-a., nat-m.,*** sulph.

sunrise, until sunset - ***kalm.***

swallowing, when - tarent.

thinking, of the pain agg. - ***lach., spig.***

thunderstorm, during - dig., sep.

touch agg. - ***agar.,*** arg-n., asaf., aur., ***bell., bry., caust.,*** chin., clem., cupr., dig., dirc., **HEP.,** mag-p., ***merc.,*** nat-c., phos., plan., psor., sil., sulph., thuj., tub.

turning, right, to - sep.

sideways - bad., bar-c., ***bry., crot-t., cupr.,*** **KALM.,** lyc., ***med.,*** phys., ***rhus-t., sil.,*** **SPIG.,** ***stict.,*** tarent., **TUB.,** ust.

upwards - ars., bar-c., ***carb-v., chel.,*** con., mang., plb., sabad., ***sulph.***

unbearable - zinc.

urination, profuse amel. - acon., ferr-p., ***gels., ign., kalm.,*** sang., sil., ter., verat.

using, eyes, when (see reading) - ***arg-n., arn., bry., calc.,*** carb-v., cimic., con., euphr., kalm., ***lach., merl.,*** **NAT-M.,** ***nux-v.,*** onos., phos., phys., puls., rhus-t., **RUTA,** ***spig.,*** staph., stront-c.

walking, while - anac., puls.

after - anac., bell., con., euphr., pall., puls., sep.

air, in open air - benz-ac., plan., sulph., zinc.

amel. - arn., carb-v., nat-m.

warm, room agg. - aeth., ***apis,*** **ARG-N.,** ***con., puls.***

room in, amel. - ***coloc.***

stove agg. - ***apis, com.***

weather agg. - sulph.

warmth, agg. - arg-n., arn., ***chel., com.,*** merc., nat-m., mez., ***puls.,*** sulph., thuj.

amel. - **ARS.,** ***aur-m., dulc.,*** ery-a., **HEP.,** kali-ar., ***lac-d., mag-p., nat-a.,*** nat-c., seneg., sil., spig., ***thuj.***

wet, weather agg. - ***calc., dulc., merc., rhus-t., spig.***

wind, agg. - ars-m., asar.

wine, after a glass - zinc.

writing, while - ***calc-f.,*** coff., con., euphr., ***merl., nat-a.,*** nat-c., **NAT-M.,** phyt., sep.

yawning - agar.

PAIN, canthi - ***agar.,*** calc., carb-v., chin., euphr., kali-n., lach., nat-m., nux-v., plb., ***puls., sil.,*** **SULPH.**

closing the eyes, on - ign.

inner - ***alum.,*** asc-t., bell., ***fl-ac., graph., lach.,*** sol-n., staph., syph.

extending around eyebrows - cinnb.

PAIN, canthi
inner, left - agar., alum., arg-n., ***aur.,*** aur-m-n., calc., cann-i., carb-an., clem., elat., nat-c., nat-m., nat-s., nit-ac., rhus-r., spong., stann.
right - arg-n., brom., coloc., eug., fl-ac., grat., ind., led., mag-s., sol-n., spig.
outer - calc., chin., ign., ran-b., sulph.

PAIN, conjunctiva - ***acon., all-c.,*** apis, **ARG-N.,** ars., ***bell.,*** **EUPHR.,** merc., **PULS.,** rhus-t., ***sulph.***
granular - apis, arg-n., ars., kali-bi.
pouting - nit-ac.
raw - kali-i., lyc.
saccular - apis, ars.
spring - cob., nux-v.

PAIN, eyebrows - acon., aeth., bell., caust., ***chel.,*** con., cupr., dros., elaps, ferr., fl-ac., hell., hyper., kali-c., lith., lyss., naja, nat-m., par., rhus-t., sel., thuj.
night agg. - hyper., lyss.
outward, along - cinnb., echi., kali-bi., mez., viol-o.
reading, while - ferr-p.
right - ***chel.,*** hyper., lyss.
touch, on - nux-v.
walking, after - lyss.

PAIN, eyelids - ***caust.,*** chel., chin., ign., ***lyc.,*** mez., sep., ***sulph.,*** vesp., xan.
afternoon - cimic.
1 p.m. - ars.
on closing lids - cimic.
closing, on - cimic., phyt., rhus-t.
evening - thuj., zinc.
margin of - phos., thuj., zinc.
morning - calc., lyc., nux-v., sep., sulph.
moving, eyelids - mang.
opening, lids, on - ars., croc., ***graph., hydr.,*** kali-bi., ***led.,*** ph-ac., upa.
paralytic - graph.
raising, eyelids - ***nat-m.***
touch, on - lyc.
using, when - cob.

PAIN, lachrymal, duct - all-c.

PALPEBRAL, fissure (see Narrowing)

PANNUS, cornea - alum., ***apis,*** **ARG-N.,** ***aur., bar-c., calc.,*** cann-s., ***caust., euphr., graph., hep.,*** kali-bi., kali-c., merc., ***merc-i-f., merc-i-r.,*** merl., ***nit-ac.,*** petr., rhus-t., ***sep.,*** sil., syph., ***sulph.***

PARALYSIS, of eyelids, esophoria - ***alum., ars.,*** bapt., bar-m., bell., ***cadm-s., cocc., con., graph., guare.,*** hydr-ac., ***merc-i-f.,*** nat-a., nit-ac., op., ***plb.,*** puls., **SEP., SPIG.,** stram., ***verat.,*** vip., zinc.
upper - ***alum.,*** apis, arn., ***ars.,*** bufo, ***cadm-s.,*** **CAUST.,** chlol., cina, ***cocc., con.,*** crot-c., crot-h., cur., ***dulc.,*** euph., **GELS.,** ***graph., led.,*** lyss., ***mag-p., med., merl., morph.,*** naja, nat-a., nat-c., **NIT-AC.,** ***nux-m.,*** op., ***phos., plb.,*** **RHUS-T.,** ***sec.,*** **SEP., SPIG.,** stann., ***syph., verat., zinc.***

PARALYSIS, of eyelids
upper, cold, from - **CAUST.,** ***rhus-t.***
injury, after - calen., hyper., ***led.***
left - ars., bar-c., caust., coloc., ***kali-p.,*** nux-v., plb., thuj.
morning - ***nit-ac.***
right - alum., ***apis, cur.,*** gins., mag-p., med., nat-m., phys., rad., rhus-t., sulph.

paralysis, iris - **ARS.,** kali-bi., ***par.***

paralysis, muscles of eyeball - arg-n., bell., **CAUST.,** ***con., euphr.,*** **GELS.,** gua., hyos., kali-i., lach., mang-o., merc-i-f., ***nat-m.,*** **NUX-V.,** oxyt., phos., phys., plb., ***rhus-t., ruta,*** sant., ***seneg.,*** syph., til.
ciliary - ***acon., arg-n., con., dub.,*** gels., graph., kali-br., nat-m., nux-v., par., phys., **RUTA.,** seneg.
external recti - ***caust.,*** chel., gels., ***kali-i.,*** sulph.
internal recti - ***agar.,*** alum., ***con.,*** graph., ***jab.,*** lil-t., merc-i-f., **MORPH., NAT-M.,** phos., rhod., ***ruta., seneg.***
superior oblique - ***arn.,*** cupr., ***seneg., syph.***

paralysis, optic nerve, (see Amaurosis)

PERSPIRATION, on brows and eyelids - calc-p.

PHOTOMANIA - ***acon.,*** am-m., **BELL.,** calc., **GELS.,** ***lac-c.,*** ruta., **STRAM.,** valer.
delirium, with - calc., stram.

PHOTOPHOBIA, light sensitivity - **ACON.,** aeth., agar., ***agn., ail., all-c., alum.,*** am-c., am-m., anac., ***anan.,*** ant-c., ***ant-t., apis,*** **ARG-N.,** ***arn.,*** **ARS.,** ***arum-t.,*** arund., ***asar.,*** aster., ***aur., aur-m.,*** aur-s., bapt., **BAR-C.,** ***bar-m.,*** **BELL.,** berb., bor., brom., ***bry.,*** bufo, cact., **CALC.,** ***calc-p.,*** calc-s., camph., cann-i., carb-ac., **CARB-S.,** cast., ***caust.,*** cedr., cer-b., ***cham., chel.,*** **CHIN.,** ***chin-a., chin-s., cic.,*** cimic., cina, cinnb., ***clem., coff.,*** coloc., **CON.,** ***croc., crot-h., crot-t., dig.,*** dros., elaps, ***eup-per.,*** **EUPHR.,** ferr-i., gamb., ***gels., glon.,*** **GRAPH.,** ***hell., hep., hyos., ign.,*** ip., ***kali-ar., kali-bi., kali-c.,*** kali-i., ***kali-n., kali-p.,*** **LAC-C.,** ***lac-d., lach., lac-ac., led., lil-t., lith.,*** **LYC.,** lyss., mag-c., ***mag-p.,*** mag-s., **MERC.,** ***merc-c., merc-i-f., merl.,*** mosch., mur-ac., ***nat-a., nat-c.,*** **NAT-M.,** nat-p., **NAT-S.,** nicc., nit-ac., nux-m., **NUX-V., OP.,** petr., ph-ac., ***phos., phyt., psor., puls.,*** **RHUS-T.,** ***sanic.,*** sec., seneg., ***sep., sil.,*** **SOL.,** sol-n., ***spig.,*** staph., ***stram.,*** **SULPH.,** sul-ac., ***sumb., tab., tarent.,*** tarax., ther., ***tub., verat., zinc.,*** ziz.
afternoon - zing.
artificial light - agar., ***arg-n.,*** aster., bor., ***calc.,*** calc-p., cast., chel., coff., ***con., crot-h.,*** cupr., dros., ***euphr.,*** gels., ***ip., lac-d.,*** lith., ***merc., nat-m.,*** phos., ***puls.,*** stram., ***sulph.***
blue light - tab.
candle light - hep.
chill, during - acon., apis, ars., **BELL.,** bor., cham., hep., lyc., nux-v., rhus-t., sep.
chronic - aeth., ***nat-s., sil.***
crusts are torn from nose, if - ***kali-bi.***

PHOTOPHOBIA, light sensitivity
daylight - ***acon.***, ant-c., **ARS.**, bell., berb., ***bry.***, camph., cast., ***caust.***, ***cic.***, **CHIN.**, ***clem.***, ***con.***, ***euphr.***, **GRAPH.**, hell., ***hep.***, ***ign.***, kali-ar., ***kali-bi.***, ***kali-c.***, kali-s., lac-c., ***lith.***, ***lyc.***, ***merc.***, merc-c., merc-sul., ***nat-a.***, nat-c., **NAT-M.**, nit-ac., nux-v., petr., ph-ac., ***phos.***, psor., ***sars.***, sep., sil., stram., ***sulph.***, ***zinc.***
lamplight, desires - stram.
more than gaslight - ***graph.***, kali-bi.
only - ***kali-bi.***, nit-ac.
dinner, after - ***calc.***
eating, after - sil.
evening - arund., bor., **CALC.**, carb-an., ***caust.***, eug., ***euphr.***, ***lyc.***, ***merc.***, ph-ac., sil., stram., sumb., ***zinc.***, zing.
6 to 8 - **CAUST.**
fire, light of - **MERC.**
foggy weather, in - cic.
gaslight - asc-t., ***calc-p.***, ***graph.***, ***med.***, **MERC.**, ***sulph.***
grief, after - ***nat-m.***
headache, during - ***ferr-p.***, kali-p., **NAT-S.**, tarent.
inflammation, without - **CON.**, hell.
menses, during - ferr-p., ign.
morning - am-c., am-m., ***ant-c.***, ***calc.***, kali-n., ***nat-s.***, **NUX-V.**, phyt., sil., verat.
rising, on - ant-c., calc.
waking, on - ***lach.***, rhus-v.
night - con., gels.
midnight, to 3 a.m. - chin-a.
onanism, after - cina.
rage, during - ***acon.***, ars., **BELL.**, hyos., merc., nux-v., phos., puls., **STRAM.**
sex, after - apis, calc., ***chin.***, ***graph.***, **KALI-C.**, kali-p., phos., sep., sil.
snow, from - ant-c., **ARS.**
straining the after - **ARG-N.**
sunlight - **ACON.**, ***ars.***, ***asar.***, berb., ***bry.***, calc., calc-f, camph., cast., **CHIN.**, ***cic.***, ***clem.***, ***euphr.***, **GRAPH.**, ***hep.***, ***ign.***, ***kali-ar.***, ***lac-c.***, ***lith.***, ***merc.***, merc-c., ***merc-sul.***, **NAT-M.**, petr., ph-ac., ***phos.***, **SOL.**, **SULPH.**, zinc.
sweat, during, shuns light - sulph.
vernal - cob.
walking, in open air - ***clem.***, ***psor.***
air, in open, amel. - ***gamb.***
warm, room agg. - **ARG-N.**
weather - sulph.

PINCHING, pain - arn., kali-c., nit-ac.

POLYPS, conjunctiva, of - ***kali-bi.***, ***staph.***, thuj.
polyps, canthus, outer - ***lyc.***
polyps, under surface of upper eyelid - ***kali-bi.***

PRESSING, pain, pressure in - acon., aeth., ***agar.***, aloe, ***alum.***, ***ambr.***, ***am-c.***, ***anac.***, ang., ant-t., ***apis***, arg-n., arn., ars., ***asaf.***, asar., ***aur.***, bapt., bar-c., bar-m., ***bell.***, berb., benz-ac., bism., bor., bov., **BRY.**, bufo, cahin., calad., **CALC.**, calc-s., camph., cann-i., cann-s., canth., caps., carb-an., ***carb-s.***, ***carb-v.***, card-m., ***carl.***, ***caul.***, ***caust.***, cer-b., **CHAM.**, ***chel.***, **CHIN.**, chin-a.,

PRESSING, pain, pressure in - cic., cimic., cina, cinnb., ***clem.***, coca, coc-c., ***cocc.***, colch., ***coloc.***, ***com.***, ***con.***, croc., crot-c., ***crot-t.***, ***cupr.***, ***cycl.***, daph., ***dig.***, dulc., ***euphr.***, fago., ferr-m., fl-ac., gels., ***glon.***, ***graph.***, grat., gymn., ham., hell., ***hep.***, hydr., ***ign.***, ind., indg., iod., kali-ar., ***kali-bi.***, ***kali-c.***, kali-chl., kali-i., kali-n., kali-p., kali-s., kalm., kreos., ***lac-c.***, ***lach.***, lachn., lac-ac., laur., ***led.***, lil-t., **LYC.**, lyss., ***mag-c.***, mag-m., manc., mang., med., meny., meph., **MERC.**, ***merc-c.***, merc-i-f., merc-i-r., ***mez.***, mosch., mur-ac., naja, nat-a., nat-c., **NAT-M.**, nat-p., ***nat-s.***, nicc., **NIT-AC.**, ***nux-v.***, olnd., ol-an., op., paeon., ***petr.***, ***ph-ac.***, ***phos.***, phys., ***phyt.***, ***plat.***, ***plb.***, ***prun.***, ***psor.***, ***puls.***, **RAN-B.**, ran-s., raph., ***rhod.***, ***rhus-t.***, ***ruta.***, sang., sant., ***sars.***, sec., sel., **SENEG.**, ***sep.***, ***sil.***, **SPIG.**, ***spong.***, ***stann.***, ***staph.***, ***stram.***, stry., stront-c., sul-ac., ***sulph.***, tab., ther., ***thuj.***, tub., valer., verat., viol-o., vip., ***zinc.***, zing.
afternoon - bor., ***cham.***, chin., coloc., grat., lachn., phyt., sil.
2 p.m., after a nap - euphr.
4 p.m., daily - sil.
air, in open - aur-m., ***clem.***, glon., kali-bi., seneg., sul-ac.
amel. - asaf., phos., puls.
around, eyes - bor., kali-n., mag-c., mez., phyt., staph.
backward - bism.
behind, eyes - caust.
below, right eye at night - ars.
between, eyes - caust.
burning, alternating with - sars.
candlelight - carb-an., croc., mang., petr., ***seneg.***, staph.
caruncle - bell.
closing, when - ***bell.***, con., sep., staph.
contractive - euphr.
coryza, with - lyc.
dark, agg. - ph-ac.
amel. - ***bell.***, euphr., staph.
daytime, only - caust., lyc., sep.
dinner, after - agar., mez., phos., seneg.
downward - anac., aur., carb-an., sulph.
eating, while - meny.
after - sulph.
evening - aloe, alum., ang., ant-t., ***calc.***, ***calc-s.***, camph., carb-an., carb-s., coloc., con., croc., euphr., graph., hep., ***kalm.***, led., lycps., mag-m., mur-ac., nat-c., ***nat-m.***, nit-ac., ***petr.***, rhus-t., sars., ***seneg.***, spong., ***staph.***, **SULPH.**, ***zinc.***
air, in open - glon., kali-bi.
bed, after going to - upa.
candlelight, in - carb-an., ***petr.***, seneg.
reading, by light - sars.
reading, while - alum., mill., ***nat-s.***
twilight, in - ***nat-m.***
extending, downward - ***aur.***, bry., cahin., carb-v., coloc.
into head - hep., nat-m.
to forehead - agar., croc., ran-b.
fever, during - kali-c., nat-c., sep., thuj.
fine, work, during - ***con.***, ***ruta.***

PRESSING, pain, pressure in
finger, as from a - nit-ac.
forenoon - kali-n., lach., lyc., plat.
hair, as if from - kali-n.
hard, substance in, as from a - olnd.
headache, during - carb-v., ***sel.,*** seneg., sulph.
inward - agar., anac., ***aur.,*** aur-m., bapt., bell., bor., **CALC.,** caust., ***crot-t.,*** hep., kali-c., olnd., par., ph-ac., spig., zinc.
left - agar., calc-s., ***coloc.,*** indg., ***puls.,*** sulph., zinc., zing.
light, agg. - aur-m., ***bell., con.,*** euphr., mag-m., ***phos.,*** sep., ***staph.,*** sulph.
light, change of - stram.
looking, when - acon., anac., caust., **NAT-M.,** ph-ac., ***phos.,*** rheum
as from looking at sun - nit-ac.
at candlelight - ***euphr.,*** staph.
at near objects - ph-ac.
at one point agg. - bar-c., ***nat-m.***
downwards amel. - bar-c.
inwards - mang.
sharply - sul-ac.
sideways - bar-c.
steadily - anac., caust., ***nat-m.,*** rheum., rhus-t.
up - ars., bar-c., mang., sabad.
menses, during - carb-an., ***croc.,*** nat-p.
morning - agar., bell., bor., calc., caust., con., euphr., graph., meph., ***nux-v.,*** phos., rhus-t., seneg., ***sep.,*** thuj., ***valer.,*** **ZINC.**
waking, on - agar., bry., nat-m., ***sep.,*** staph., thuj., upa.
waking, on, 5 a.m. - stann.
moving, eyes, when - agar., brom., **BRY.,** camph., ***carb-v.,*** chel., clem., crot-h., glon., ***hep., lach., mang.,*** merc., ***spig.,*** stann.
moving, amel. - op.
night - alum., chel., ***cocc.,*** croc., cycl., ***sep., staph.***
11 p.m. - euphr., nat-m.
open air, in - aur-m.
waking. on - chel., cycl.
noon - cham., ign., kali-c., valer., verat.
opening, eyes - alum., caust., croc., upa.
impossible - alum.
orbits of eyes - bell., caust., con., kali-c., phos., ph-ac., sep.
outward - agar., ***asaf.,*** asar., aur., bell., berb., ***bry.,*** camph., ***cann-s.,*** caul., caust., cham., cimic., crot-c., daph., eupi., fago., ***fl-ac., glon.,*** guai., guare., ***ham.,*** ign., ip., ***lac-c.,*** lach., **LED.,** lycps., mag-c., ***merc.,*** merc-c., merl., nat-m., ***nat-s.,*** **NUX-V.,** op., par., ph-ac., ***phos., phyt., psor.,*** puls., ***sang., seneg., sil.,*** **SPIG.,** staph., sulph., thuj.
headache, with - phos.
pressing throat, when - **LACH.**
periodical - aur-m., ran-s.
plug, like a - ***anac., ran-b.***
pressing, amel. - ***asaf., caust., ham.,*** mur-ac.

PRESSING, pain, pressure in
reading, while - ***agar.,*** alum., asar., cic., ***con.,*** dulc., ign., ***kali-c.,*** mang., merc., mur-ac., ***nat-m., nat-s., nux-v.,*** pic-ac., ***ruta.,*** sars., staph.
by light - mang.
rest, amel. - berb., pic-ac.
right - apoc., ***coloc.,*** crot-c., ***ferr., fl-ac.,*** kalm., nat-m., ***spig.***
rub, them must - chin.
rubbing, agg. - sep.
amel. - bor., ***caust., ran-b.***
sleep, after - kali-c.
as from loss of - chin.
smoke, as from - ran-b.
smoking, from - calad.
stooping, agg. - ***coloc.,*** fl-ac., merc., seneg.
straining, eyes - mur-ac., nat-m., ***ruta.***
stye, on lid, as from - stann.
sun, working in the - sulph.
throbbing, in temples, after - glon.
touching, agg. - ***aur., caust.,*** cupr., psor.
turning, eyes agg. - **SPIG.,** tub.
to right - sep.
upward - bism.
walking, while, in open air - carb-v., euphr., sep., sulph., zinc.
amel. - arn., nat-m.
walking, after - con., euphr.
warm, bed amel. - nat-c.
room agg. - ***apis.***
warmth, amel. - nat-c., seneg.
washing, in cold water amel. - ***apis, asar., phos., puls.***
weakness, causing - glon., staph.
writing, while - alum., con.

pressing, canthi, in - agar., alum., calc., ***carb-v., colch.,*** cycl., grat., lach., sil.
inner - anac., carb-an., ***caust.,*** cic., cycl., **EUPHR.,** gamb., hell., hydr-ac., iod., lach., laur., lyc., mag-m., nat-m., petr., ph-ac., puls., rhod., ***stann.,*** staph., tarax., zinc.
looking steadily - phos.
outer - anac., carb-v., chin., con., lach., ***mez.,*** op., staph., sul-ac., thuj.

pressing, eyebrow - camph., sul-ac.
above - sulph.
left - ambr.

pressing, eyelids - alum., am-c., bor., cupr., graph., hep., kali-c., lyc., nat-m., nit-ac., ph-ac., sars., sep., sil., sulph., zinc.
downward - zinc.
evening - sulph.
margin, of lids, glands - rheum.
lower - zinc.
reading - zinc.
stye, on lid, as from - stann.
under - kali-n., ph-ac., spong.
upper - graph., lyc., nat-c., ph-ac., phos., stann., staph., sulph.

pressing, eyes, over - ***acon.,*** aeth., agar., **ALOE,** alum., alumn., am-c., ***anac.,*** ang., ant-c., apis, arg-m., arg-n., arn., ars., ars-i., asaf., aster., bar-c., ***bell., bism.,*** bor., bov., brom., **BRY.,** calc., ***calc-p.,*** cann-i., carb-an., carb-s., ***carb-v., card-m.,*** caust., ***chel.,*** chin., chin-a., cist., con., ***crot-h.,*** dig., dros., dulc., euph., eupi., euon., fl-ac., ***glon.,*** grat., gymn., haem., hep., ***ign.,*** indg., iod., ***kali-ar., kali-c.,*** kali-n., kali-p., kalm., kreos., lach., lil-t., lith., lyc., lyss., mag-c., merc., merc-c., merc-i-r., merl., mez., morph., **NAT-M.,** ***nat-p.,*** nat-s., nit-ac., ***nux-m., nux-v.,*** op., paeon., petr., ph-ac., ***phos.,*** phyt., pic-ac., plan., plect., **PULS.,** rheum, ***rhus-t.,*** ruta., sabad., sant., seneg., sep., ***sil.,*** sol-t-ae., spig., spong., stann., staph., stront-c., ***sulph.,*** tab., teucr., ther., thuj., urt-u., ***valer.,*** zinc., zing.
- afternoon - ***acon.,*** cann-i., carb-v., ph-ac., sulph.
- air, in open - staph.
- close the eyes, compelled to - nux-v.
- closing the eyes, amel. - ip.
- daytime - sep.
- dinner, after - phos.
- evening - camph., iod.
- extending, eyes, into - con.
  - nose, to - bov.
  - outward - sec.
- eyes would be forced out, as if - cocc., gymn., ign., lachn., nat-m., phos., sabin., seneg., sep., sil., tarent.
- left - ***acon.,*** arg-m., bry., camph., cupr., mur-ac., ***nux-v.,*** phos., ***sep.,*** sulph., ***ther., thuj.,*** verb.
  - extending to right - thuj.
- light by - sep.
- margin of orbits to temples, from - cann-s.
- menses, during - lac-c.
  - before - sep.
- morning - alumn., kali-n., lach., mag-c., petr., sulph.
  - waking, on - alumn.
- motion agg. - **BRY.,** ***sep.***
- opening eyes agg. - sil.
- outward - ang., bell., ip., kali-c., lyc., phos.
- pressing down upon the eyes - arg-m., bell., hell., ***hep., phos.,*** plat., sabin., spig., zinc.
- pressive pain above left eye, followed by a dull, pressive pain in occipital protuberances, thence spreading over whole body, on quick motion and after eating, pain so severe that it seemed a distinct pulsation in head - ***bry.***
  - pressure amel. - apis., ip.
  - pressure so severe, when rising, could only half open eyes, could not look up - stram.
- raising, eyebrow agg. - nat-m.
- right - am-m., ant-c., caust., ***chel.,*** con., dulc., ***ign.,*** nat-m., plat., rhus-t., ***sang.,*** sil., spig., spong., staph., thuj., urt-u., zinc.
  - right, upward and inward - bism.
- stooping agg. - merc-c., spong., teucr.

pressing, eyes, over
- stunning - plat.
- walking after - con.
  - walking in open air - ***sep.***
- wavelike - plat.

pressing, lachrymal gland - staph.

PRICKLING - lyc., sep., zinc.

PROLAPSE of iris after cataract operation - alum., calen., staph.

PROTRUSION, (see Exophthalmus) - acet-ac., ***acon., aeth.,*** aloe, arn., ***ars., ars-i., aur., bar-c.,*** **BELL.,** brom., ***cact.,*** calc., calc-p., ***camph., canth.,*** caps., cedr., ***cham.,*** chin., chlor., ***cic., clem., cocc.,*** colch., **COM.,** con., ***coloc.,*** crot-h., cupr., dig., dor., ***dros.,*** dulc., ***ferr., ferr-ar.,*** **FERR-I.,** ***ferr-p.,*** fl-ac., ***glon.,*** **GUAI.,** gymn., ***hep.,*** hydr-ac., ***hyos., ign., iod.,*** kali-ar., kali-i., ***kreos.,*** lac-ac., lac-c., ***lach., laur.,*** morph., mosch., **NAT-M.,** ***nux-v.,*** oena., ***op., phos., plat., puls.,*** rhus-t., sang., sant., spig., ***spong., stann.,*** **STRAM.,** stry., sulph., sul-ac., tab., thuj., ***verat.,*** vip.
- coryza, during - spig.
- right - arn.
  - eye more than left - **COM.**

protrusion, sensation of - bell., bry., daph., guai., ham., ***med.,*** **PAR.**
- canthi, in - euphr.

PSORIASIS, eyebrows, about - ***phos.***

PTERYGIUM - ***am-br.,*** apis, ***arg-n., ars., ars-m.,*** bell., ***calc., cann-s.,*** chim., ***euphr., form.,*** guare., ***lach.,*** lyc., merc., ***nux-m., psor., rat.,*** spig., ***sulph.,*** tell., ***zinc.,*** zinc-s.
- pink color, of a - ***arg-n.***

PUCKERED, conjunctiva, (see Wrinkled)

PULLED out, pain, as if being - bell., ***glon.,*** med.
- headache, with - carb-v., cocc.
- shut, when - med.

PULLING, sensation, (see Drawing, pain) - crot-t., mur-ac., raph., sep.

PULSATION, in eyes - ammc., apis, ***ars.,*** asaf., asar., aur-s., **BELL.,** benz-ac., brom., bry., bufo, cact., ***calc., chel.,*** clem., ***coloc., gels.,*** glon., ***hep., hyos.,*** lil-t., lith., lyss., mang., ***merc., merc-i-f., nux-v.,*** petr., phys., pic-ac., rheum, seneg., ***sil.,*** stram., tarent., ter., ther.
- alternating with sharp pain - calc.
- around the eyes - ***ars.***
- evening - cycl., kreos.
- midnight, after - ***ars.***
- morning - ***nux-v.***
  - lying down - nux-v.
- night - ars., **ASAF., MERC.,** ***merc-i-f.***
- paroxysmal - calc., ***sil.***
- reading, while - ammc.

pulsation, eyebrows - petr.

pulsation, eyelids, upper - mang., stry.

PUPILS, general

alternately contracted and dilated in the same light - acet-ac., ***acon.,*** am-c., anac., ars., ***bar-c.,*** cann-s., ***carb-ac.,*** cham., cic., cycl., dig., dros., dulc., ***hell., lach.,*** oena., ***phys.,*** sol-n., zinc.

angular - acon., bar-c., ***cocc.,*** hyos., merc-c.

contract, difficult to - nit-ac.

contracted - ***acon.,*** aesc., agar., ***anac.,*** ang., ant-t., ***apis,*** arg-m., ***arn., ars., aur., bell., calc., camph.,*** canth., caps., carb-ac., carb-s., cham., ***chel.,*** chin., ***chin-s.,*** cic., cocc., con., crot-t., ***daph., dig.,*** dros., ***euphr.,*** fl-ac., gamb., gels., ***gins.,*** haem., ***hell., hyos.,*** ign., jab., kali-bi., kali-i., led., mang., ***merc., merc-c.,*** meny., ***mez., mur-ac.,*** nat-c., ***nat-m., nux-m.,*** nux-v., ol-an., **OP.,** ph-ac., phos., ***phys.,*** phyt., ***plb.,*** podo., ***puls.,*** rheum, ***rhus-t.,*** ruta, sabad., samb., sec., seneg., ***sep.,*** sil., sol-n., squil., ***stann.,*** staph., stram., sulph., sul-ac., tab., tarax., **THUJ.,** tub., ***verat., zinc.***

chill, during - bell., caps., nux-v., sep., sil., sulph.

convulsions, during - cic., ***op.,*** phyt.

dilated, then - arn., stann., staph.

fever, during - acon., arn., ars., bell., cham., cocc., ***gels.,*** hyos., mur-ac., nux-v., phos., sec., stram., verat.

headache, with - bell.

left - ***arg-m., tarent.***

right dilated - colch., lyss., rhod., ***tarent.***

one, the other dilated - cadm-s., rhod., tarent.

perspiration - bell., cham., cocc., mez., mur-ac., phos., puls., sep., sil., sulph., thuj., verat.

pinpoint, to a - cub., ***op.,*** phys.

right - anac., ***arg-n.,*** onos., verat-v.

dilated - acet-ac., ***acon.,*** aesc., ***aeth., agar., agn., ail.,*** alumn., ***anac., apis,*** **ARG-N.,** ***arn.,*** ars., ars-i., arund., astac., aur., bar-c., ***bar-m.,*** **BELL.,** brom., bufo, cadm-s., cahin., **CALC.,** ***camph.,*** caps., ***carb-an.,*** carb-s., caust., ***cedr., chel.,*** **CHIN.,** ***chin-s., cic.,*** cimic., ***cina,*** coca, ***cocc., coff., colch., coloc., con., cor-r., croc.,*** crot-c., crot-h., crot-t., cupr., ***cycl., dig.,*** dros., dulc., euph., **GELS.,** ***glon., guai., hell.,*** hep., hydr-ac., **HYOS.,** ***hyper.,*** ign., ***iod.,*** ip., ***kali-br., kali-i.,*** kali-n., lach., lachn., lac-ac., lact., ***laur., led.,*** lyc., lyss., **MANG.,** meny., ***merc., merl.,*** mez., ***mosch.,*** mur-ac., nat-a., ***nat-c., nat-p., nit-ac.,*** nux-m., ***nux-v., op.,*** petr., ***ph-ac., phos.,*** phys., phyt., pic-ac., ***puls.,*** ran-b., raph., rhod., samb., ***sang.,*** sars., **sec.,** sol-n., ***spig.,*** squil., staph., **STRAM.,** ***stry.,*** sulph., tarax., thuj., valer., ***verat.,*** verb., vib., zinc.

chill, during - aeth., apis, calc., carb-an., cham., cic., hyos., ip., lach., mez., nux-m., op., stram.

convulsions, before - arg-n., bufo.

PUPILS, general

dilated, epilepsy, during - aeth., ***bell.,*** calc., carb-an., cic., ***cina,*** cocc., cycl., hyos., ign., lac-ac., laur., led., oena., op., plb., stram., verat., verat-v.

before - **ARG-N.,** ***bufo.***

fever, during - ail., apis, ars., **BELL.,** bufo, chin., cic., cina, cocc., colch., hell., hyos., lyc., merc., nux-v.

left more than right - nat-a., urt-u.

menses, during - glon.

before - lyc.

one-sided - cadm-s., nat-p.

perspiration, during - acon., bell., bufo, calc., cina, cocc., hell., hep., hyos., op., stram.

reading agg. - ***ph-ac.***

reproaches, at - stram.

right more than left - cycl., mang., ***ph-ac.,*** plb., sil., ***tarent.***

stupor, during - sec.

toothache, during - mang.

vertigo, with - ***bell.,*** hell., teucr.

insensible to light - aeth., agar., arg-n., **ARN.,** ars., aur-m., ***bar-c., bar-m.,*** **BELL.,** bufo, cahin., ***camph.,*** carb-ac., carb-an., carb-v., cedr., ***chel.,*** chin., ***cic., colch.,*** **CUPR.,** ***dig.,*** dub., euph., gels., ***hell.,*** hep., hydr., hydr-ac., **HYOS.,** kali-bi., ***kali-br., kali-i.,*** laur., ***merc., merc-c.,*** naja, nit-ac., nux-m., **OP.,** ox-ac., par., phos., ***plat.,*** ran-b., rhus-t., sol-n., ***stram.,*** sulph., sul-ac., tab., ter., ***tub.***

irregular - acon., bar-c., chlor., cinnb., dub., hyos., nit-ac., **OP.,** plb., sil., sulph., tab.

sluggish - bell., carb-s., cham., cupr., dig., ***hell.,*** ip., jatr., merc., naja, nit-ac., phos., rumx., sec., seneg., sul-ac., tab., tax.

unequal - bell., cadm-s., cann-i., chlor., colch., dig., hyos., lyss., mang., merc-c., morph., nat-p., **OP.,** plb., rhod., sulph., tarent., zinc.

weak - spig.

PUSTULES, inflammation of conjunctiva (including cornea) - ***aeth.,*** agar., ant-c., **APIS,** ars., aur., bar-c., **CALC.,** calc-i., ***cham., chlol.,*** **CLEM.,** ***con., crot-t., euphr.,*** **GRAPH.,** hep., ***ip., kali-bi.,*** **KALI-CHL.,** ***kali-i., lach., merc., merc-c., merc-d., merc-i-f., nat-c., nat-m., nat-s., nit-ac.,*** **PETR., PSOR., PULS.,** rhus-t., **SEC., SEP.,** ***sil.,*** **SULPH.,** ***syph.,*** tell., ***thuj.,*** zinc.

pustules, cornea, on the - ***ant-c.,*** calc., con., crot-t., euphr., ***hep.,*** kali-bi., kali-i., merc-n., nit-ac.

QUIVERING - alum., ***am-m., apis,*** aran., carb-v., con., fl-ac., ***glon., hyos.,*** petr., ***phos., rat.,*** rhus-t., sars., ***seneg.,*** stann., sulph., zinc.

evening - alum.

left - alum.

looking, down, when - alum.

steady - ***seneg.***

night - ***apis,*** berb.

right - sars.

rubbing amel. - am-m.

quivering, canthi - phos., stann.

quivering, eyebrows - alum., caust., kali-c., ol-an., ruta., stront.

between, while reading - ang.

quivering, eyelids - aesc., **AGAR.,** alum., am-m., asaf., ars., **BELL.,** berb., **CALC.,** carb-an., ***carb-s., carl., caust.,*** **CIC.,** ***cocc.,*** con., croc., ***crot-c.,*** crot-h., cupr., ***cur.,*** grat., ***iod.,*** lyc., merc., mez., ***nat-m.,*** nat-p., ***ol-an.,*** par., petr., phel., ***phos., plat., rat.,*** rhod., rhus-t., sabin., sars., sep., sil., stront-c., ***sulph., verat.,*** zinc.

left - lyc.

upper - **ARUM-T.,** berb., ***croc.,*** mez., mur-ac.

painful - bell.

right - bell., nat-p., nit-ac., petr., sars.

upper - alum., bell., calc., nat-m., sars.

reading, while, by candlelight - berb.

RASH - sulph.

REDNESS - absin., abrot., acet-ac., **ACON.,** aeth., **AGAR.,** ail., **ALL-C.,** aloe, alum., ambr., am-c., am-m., aml-n., anac., ***ant-c.,*** **APIS,** apoc., **ARG-N.,** ***arn.,*** **ARS.,** ars-i., ars-h., ***asaf.,*** asar., aster., ***aur.,*** aur-m., bad., ***bar-c.,*** **BAR-M., BELL.,** ***berb.,*** bism., bov., bry., bufo, calad., ***calc., calc-p., calc-s.,*** camph., **CANN-I.,** ***caps., carb-an.,*** carb-h., ***carb-s.,*** card-m., ***caust.,*** cham., ***chel., chin.,*** chin-s., ***chlol., cimic., clem.,*** cob., coff., ***colch.,*** coloc., con., cop., ***crot-h., crot-t., cupr.,*** cycl., der., ***dig.,*** dor., dros., elaps, **EUPHR.,** fago., ***ferr., ferr-ar.,*** ferr-i., ***ferr-p.,*** **GLON.,** gran., ***graph., ham., hell., hep.,*** hura, ***hyos.,*** iod., ***ign., ip., iris,*** jab., jug-c., ***kali-ar., kali-bi., kali-br., kali-c.,*** kali-chl., ***kali-i., kali-p.,*** **KALI-S.,** kreos., ***lach.,*** lact., led., ***lith., lyc.,*** lyss., manc., ***mag-c., mag-m., meph.,*** merc., ***merc-c., merl., mez., mur-ac., nat-a.,*** **NAT-M.,** nat-p., ***nat-s.,*** nicc., ***nit-ac.,*** **NUX-V.,** oena., olnd., ***op.,*** osm., paeon., ph-ac., phos., phyt., pic-ac., ***plb.,*** podo., ***psor.,*** puls., ***rhus-t.,*** rhus-v., ***ruta.,*** sant., sec., ***seneg., sep., sil.,*** sol-n., ***spig., spong.,*** stann., ***staph.,*** **STRAM.,** stry., **SULPH.,** sul-ac., syph., tab., tarent., ter., ***teucr., thuj., verat.,*** vesp., vip., xan., zinc., ziz.

air, open, amel. - **ARG-N.**

carunculae - kali-c.

daytime - ***sulph.***

evening - apoc., dig., ***hyos.,*** kali-chl., lyc.

headache, during - arg-m., bell., carb-an., ***cimic.,*** glon., lach., mez., sang., spig., sulph.

before - phos., sulph.

injuries, after - **ACON.,** ***arn.,*** calen., ***euphr., hep., sil.***

megrim, during - ***kali-br., spig.***

menses, during - acon., bell., cham., euphr., glon., hep., ign., merc., nux-v., puls., zinc.

before - glon.

morning - ambr., apoc., bry., caps., dios., fago., ***mez.,*** nat-a., raph., ***rhus-t.,*** sang., sep., spig., **SULPH.,** valer.

4 a.m. - hyper.

9 a.m. to 3 p.m. - meny.

REDNESS, eyes

neuralgia, with - aml-n., chel., mag-p., nat-m.

reading, while - ammc., **ARG-N.,** lact., ***merl., nat-m.***

sewing, while - **ARG-N., NAT-M.,** ***ruta.***

sexual excesses, after - **STAPH.**

redness, canthi - agar., **ARG-N.,** ***aur.,*** bell., brach., ***bor.,*** bov., bry., ***calc-s.,*** crot-h., gran., iris, kali-bi., kali-n., ***mag-c., nat-m.,*** nux-v., sil., **SULPH.,** tab., teucr., upa., zinc.

dark - rhus-t.

inner - arg-n., aur., calc-p., chel., ***graph.,*** mag-c., nat-a., podo., rhus-t.

outer - **ANT-C.,** carb-s., nux-v., ran-b., ***sulph.***

pale - apis.

redness, eyelids - ***acon.,*** **ANT-C., APIS,** ***arg-m.,*** **ARG-N.,** ***ars.,*** ars-i., ***aur., aur-m.,*** bar-c., bar-m., ***bell.,*** berb., ***bry., calc.,*** cann-s., ***carb-s., caust.,*** cham., chel., ***chin-s.,*** cinnb., ***cocc.,*** colch., com., ***crot-t.,*** cupr., elaps, **EUPHR.,** ***ferr., ferr-ar.,*** ferr-i., ferr-p., **GELS.,** ***graph., hep.,*** iod., ***kali-ar.,*** kali-bi., ***kali-c.,*** **KALI-I.,** ***lac-d.,*** **LYC., MERC.,** ***merc-i-f., mur-ac., nat-m.,*** nicc., nux-v., **PETR.,** plb., podo., psor., ***puls.,*** rhod., ***rhus-t.,*** rhus-v., sanic., ***sep.,*** sil., ***sulph.,*** **TELL.,** teucr., upa., vinc., zinc.

edges of - ***arg-m., arg-n.,*** **ARS.,** aster., ***bor.,*** calc., **CARB-S.,** carb-v., ***chel.,*** coff., ***colch., coloc., con.,*** **EUP-PER., EUPHR.,** ***ferr-m., gels.,*** **GRAPH.,** hura, ***ip., kali-bi., kali-s.,*** kreos., ***lil-t., med., merc-c., nat-m.,*** nux-m., nux-v., par., ***ph-ac., puls., rhus-t.,*** sabad., sanic., stram., **SULPH.,** syph., upa., zinc.

lower lids - ph-ac.

menses, before - aur.

morning - bry., **SULPH.**

night - **MERC.**

spots - berb.

veins - ***acon.,*** aeth., ***alumn.,*** all-c., ***ambr., ant-t., apis, arg-n., ars.,*** bar-m., ***bell., calc-p., camph., carb-s., caust., clem.,*** con., ***crot-t.,*** elaps, ***euphr., graph., hep.,*** ign., kali-ar., ***kali-bi.,*** kali-c., ***kali-i., kali-s., lach., lyc.,*** mag-c., mag-m., meph., ***merc., merc-c.,*** **NAT-A., NAT-M.,** nat-p., onos., ph-ac., phos., ***sang.,*** sil., spig., ***stram., sulph.,*** ter.

RESTLESS, eyes - bell., ***chin-s.,*** kali-p., ***lach.,*** lyss., ***stram.,*** stry., valer., ***verat.***

RETINITIS, inflammation, retina - apis, ***ars.,*** asaf., aur., ***calc.,*** crot-h., ***gels., kalm., lach., merc., merc-c., phos., plb., prun.,*** puls., sal-ac., sec., ***sulph.***

albuminuric - gels., merc-c.

pregnancy, during - gels.

diabetic - sec.

hemorrhagic - merc-c.

overuse of eyes, from - sulph.

pigmentary - nux-v., phos.

ROLLING, (see Movement)

ROUGH, cornea - sil.
sensation on winking - ail., bell.

RUB, desire to - agar., all-c., apis, bor., carb-ac., ***caust., con., croc.,*** fl-ac., gymn., kali-bi., ***mez.,*** morph., nat-c., ***op.,*** phos., plb., ***puls.,*** rat., ***squil., sulph.***

SAND, pain, as from - agar., alum., ambr., am-br., ***apis,*** arg-n., **ARS.,** asaf., asc-t., ***aur.,*** bar-c., bell., berb., bry., **CALC.,** cann-s., caps., carb-s., ***carb-v.,*** **CAUST.,** ***chel.,*** **CHIN.,** cina, cob., cocc., con., ***cor-r., dig.,*** elaps, euph., **EUPHR.,** ***ferr.,*** ferr-ar., ferr-i., ferr-p., **FL-AC.,** form., graph., grat., ***hep., ign., iod.,*** kali-ar., kali-bi., kali-chl., kali-p., kreos., lac-d., lach., lachn., ***led.,*** lith., ***lyc.,*** mag-m., ***med.,*** merc., myric., **NAT-M.,** nat-p., nit-ac., ol-an., ***op.,*** ox-ac., paeon., petr., ph-ac., phos., ***phyt.,*** pic-ac., plat., ***psor., puls.,*** rhus-t., sars., ***sep., sil., spig.,*** sol-n., stram., stront-c., **SULPH.,** sumb., syph., tarent., ***thuj.,*** upa., urt-u., viol-t., ***zinc.***
afternoon - bry.
evening - ***ars., calc.,*** ferr., kali-bi., ox-ac., petr., ***puls.,*** **ZINC.**
forenoon - chel., con.
morning - apoc., lyc., **NAT-M.,** ***sil.,*** sol-n., ***sulph.,*** thuj.
night - calc., kali-bi., **ZINC.**
open air amel. - sars.
right - **SEP.**
sand, canthi, in - acon., dig., sumb., thuj.
outer - bar-c., con., crot-c., ***nit-ac.,*** staph., sulph.

SARCOMA - iod., phos.
conjunctiva, of - iod.

SCROFULOUS, affections - aeth., ***am-br., apis,*** ars., ***aur.,*** bell., **CALC.,** ***cann-s.,*** **CAUST.,** ***cham., chin-a.,*** cist., ***con., dulc.,*** **EUPHR.,** ferr., **GRAPH.,** ***hep.,*** mag-c., merc., nat-m., ***nux-v.,*** **PULS.,** rhus-t., **SULPH.,** zinc.

SENSITIVE, bathing, to - clem., ***sulph.***
brilliant objects, to - **BELL.,** bufo, ***canth.,*** **LYSS.,** ***stram.***
cold air, to - **ACON.,** cinnb., clem., ***hep., lac-c.,*** merc., ***sil., thuj.***
cold water, to - elaps, ***hep., sulph.***
heat, to - ***apis, arg-n.,*** caust., clem., con., ***merc.,*** puls.
light, (see Photophobia)
touch, to - ***acon.,*** arn., ars., aur., ***bell., bry.,*** cimic., clem., eup-per., ***ham., hep.,*** lept., rhus-t., sil., ***spig.,*** thuj.
sensitive, eyelids, to, cold air - **ACON.**
right upper lid - zinc.

SHARP, pain - ***acon.,*** aesc., agar., all-c., alum., am-c., anac., anan., ang., ant-c., **APIS,** aran., ***arg-m., arg-n.,*** arn., ars., ars-i., ***asaf.,*** aspar., aur., aur-m., aur-m-n., bapt., bell., ***berb.,*** bor., ***brom., bry.,*** calad., ***calc.,*** canth., caps., carb-an., carb-s., carb-v., ***caust., cham., chel.,*** chin., ***cimic.,*** cinnb., cist., cob., cocc., coloc., con., crot-h., crot-t., cycl., ***dig.,*** dios., dros., ***dulc., euphr.,*** eup-per., eupi., fago., ferr., ferr-i., ferr-p., form., ***gels., glon., graph., hell., hep., hyos.,*** hyper., ign., iod., ***ip., kali-bi.,*** **KALI-C.,** kali-chl., kali-i., kali-n., ***kali-p., kalm., lach.,*** lac-f., laur., led., ***lith., lyc.,*** lyss., mag-c., ***mag-m.,*** manc., mang., meny., ***meph., merc.,*** merc-i-r., merl., ***mur-ac.,*** naja, nat-a., ***nat-c., nat-m.,*** nat-p., nat-s., ***nit-ac., nux-m., nux-v.,*** ol-an., ***par., petr.,*** ph-ac., ***phos.,*** phys., phyt., pic-ac., plan., psor., **PRUN.,** ***puls.,*** **RHUS-T.,** rhus-v., sang., sars., sec., sel., ***senec.,*** seneg., ***sep., sil.,*** sin-a., **SPIG.,** spong., stann., staph., stram., stront-c., stry., **SULPH.,** tab., tarax., ***tarent.,*** ter., til., ***thuj.,*** verat., ***zinc.***
about the eyes - acon., aeth., ant-c., cinnb., coloc., hura.
encircles - cinnb.
afternoon - caust., dig., sin-n.
sitting, while - phos.
walking, while - bell.
air, cold - thuj.
open - ***hep.,*** kalm., phel., ***sil.,*** spig.
open, amel. - **ASAF.,** ***puls.,*** sars.
alternating with pulsation - calc.
bed, in - arn.
below the eyes - nat-m., rhus-t., spong.
burning - ***euphr.,*** stann., tarax.
candlelight, by - ***colch., sep.***
closing eyes - ***cimic.,*** clem., hell., sars.
coughing, when - ***seneg.***
daytime - cimic.
dinner, after - nat-c., ol-an.
downward - carb-an., hell.
eating, after - ambr., dig.
evening - bor., ***caust., crot-h.,*** hep., ***kalm.,*** **LYC.,** ***merc.,*** pic-ac., spong., ***stann.,*** tarent., thuj.
bed, in - hipp.
coryza, during - sep.
light, when looking at - **LYC.**
reading, while - caust., mill., pic-ac.
exerting them, after - staph.
extending, backward - bell., berb., cinnb., graph., hyper., lac-f., rhus-t., sep., **SPIG.**
forward - spig.
head, to top of - cimic., ***lach.,*** phyt.
inward - ***asaf., caust., cimic.,*** cinnb., ***coloc.,*** graph., lac-f., phos., phyt., **PRUN., RHUS-T., SPIG.,** stram., syph.
jaw, upper - agar.
nose, root, of - coloc.
occiput - ***bell.,*** cic., dios., ***ign., lach.,*** lac-f., ***prun.,*** rhus-t., uran.
outward - **ASAF.,** ***bell.,*** cadm-s., ***camph.,*** cocc., dros., ***kali-bi., mur-ac., nat-c.,*** rhod., senec., sil., ***spig.,*** sulph., ***thuj.***
side of head - tarent.
temples - kali-p., ***lach.***
fever, during - ***kali-c.,*** lyc.
forenoon - apis, ery-a.
headache, during - hipp., thuj.
after a - gels.
house, in - phel.
itching - cycl.
jerking - staph.

SHARP, pain
left - chim., chin., cimic., cist., ***croc.,*** lac-f., ***mur-ac.,*** sep., ***spig., thuj.,*** zinc.
lying on left side - lac-f.
to right - croc., mur-ac.
to vertex - phos., phyt.
light, bright, in - amph., ***calc.,*** cob., euphr., graph., iod., ***kali-c.,*** lyc., ***merc., puls.,*** thuj.
looking at anything, white or red, or at the sun - **LYC.**
fixedly - arund., lac-f.
lying down - dig.
amel. - cimic.
menses, during - calc.
midnight - ars.
morning - arg-n., croc., ***crot-h.,*** fago., ign., lyc., nit-ac., ***nux-v., sil.,*** tarent., thuj.
6 a.m. - arg-m.
waking, after - hell.
motion - **ACON.,** ***asaf.,*** brom., ***bry.,*** gels., ***prun.,*** rhus-t., ***spig.,*** sulph., viol-t.
amel. - ***coloc.,*** dros., **DULC.,** phys., thuj.
of eyes - stann.
night - acon., ***apis, caust., coloc., con., euphr.,*** hep., **MERC.,** prun., rhus-t., ***spig.,*** tarent., thuj., til.
10 p.m. - arg-m.
opening the on - **ARS.**
pannus, in - ***apis.***
presses eyelid down - spig.
pressure, agg. - brom., petr.
amel. - ***bry., coloc.,*** kali-p., phys., tarent.
pulsating - ***ars.,*** calc., rhus-t.
radiating from the eyes - **SPIG.**
reading, while - ***apis,*** carb-s., caust., ***kali-c.,*** lac-f., nat-c., ph-ac., pic-ac., phyt., rhod., sel., ***sulph.***
rheumatic - bry., ***merc., rhus-t.***
right - cic., dios., nat-m., phys., rhus-t.
shaking the head, on - puls.
sleep, on going to - **PHOS.**
stool, after - carb-s.
stooping agg. - brom., coloc., dros.
storm, before - ***cedr., rhod., sil.***
sudden - sil.
sunlight - ***calc.,*** graph., ***puls.***
swallowing - tarent.
talking, while - bry.
turning eye, on - ars.
walking in a warm room amel. - ***coloc.***
warm weather agg. - ***sulph.***
warmth - ***arn.***
amel. - ***hep., ign., sil.,*** thuj.
washing, while - ***mur-ac.***
wet weather - rhus-t.
writing, while - cob., lyc., ***phyt.***

sharp, canthi - agar., alum., ant-t., arg-m., bar-c., berb., brom., calc., chel., con., laur., nat-m., ph-ac., ***puls.,*** ruta., sulph., verat.

sharp, canthi
inner - agar., alum., ant-t., arg-m., arg-n., arn., ***aur.,*** aur-m-n., bar-c., ***bell.,*** brom., ***calc.,*** cann-i., carb-an., chel., ***cinnb.,*** clem., ***con.,*** elaps, elat., eug., fl-ac., grat., ***graph.,*** indg., led., mag-m., mag-s., meny., nat-c., nat-m., nat-p., nat-s., ***petr.,*** phos., plan., ***puls.,*** sang., sol-n., spig., stann., staph., sulph., ***thuj.,*** **ZINC.**
evening - ***puls.,*** sulph.
morning - carb-an., con., eug., phos.
open air, morning - phos.
outer - aur-m-n., cinnb., bar-c., euphr., kali-c., laur., mur-ac., nat-c., nat-m., nicc., ol-an., op., petr., spong., staph., ***sulph., thuj.***
extending to inner canthi - petr.

sharp, eyebrows - bov., cic., hell., mang., petr., thuj., zinc.

sharp, eyelids - alum., ang., aur., bar-c., camph., cycl., mang., mez., ph-ac., sil., spig., stann., sul-ac., zinc.
presses eyelid down - spig.

sharp, eyes, over - agar., aloe, alum., am-c., anac., ang., arum-t., bell., berb., bor., ***bov.,*** bry., calc., caps., ***cedr.,*** **CHEL.,** coc-c., colch., ***ferr.,*** ferr-p., kali-c., **KALI-I.,** kali-p., lach., ***lyc.,*** mag-p., mag-s., manc., mang., mez., nat-m., ol-an., paeon., petr., ph-ac., ***phos.,*** pip-m., rhus-t., sel., ***sep.,*** sil., ***spig.,*** sulph., tarent., valer.
blowing nose - mag-c.
coughing - hyos.
dinner - arn., am-c., bor.
eating, after - am-c.
evening - hep., inul., kali-bi., pip-m.
left - caust., ***lac-f.,*** **KALI-I.,** mag-c., ph-ac., ptel., **SEL.,** ***sep.,*** thuj., zinc.
extending to right - thuj.
morning - alum., nit-ac., sep.
night - lyc.
3 a.m. - pip-m.
right - anac., ***bov.,*** carb-v., ***cur., lyc., mag-p.,*** mang., tarent.
stooping - ip.
walking in open air amel. - ***phos.,*** sep.

sharp, lachrymal, duct - all-c.

SHORT, as if muscles are - sabin.

SHOOTING, over eyes - ***acon.,*** agar., am-c., ant-c., berb., bov., bry., caust., **CEDR.,** ***kali-bi.,*** kali-p., lyss., nat-a., nat-m., nit-ac., ph-ac., ***prun., sep.,*** sulph., zinc.
4 p.m, extending occiput, to - **PRUN.,** sol-n.
4 p.m. - sol-n.
afternoon - sulph.
left - ***acon.,*** agar., **CEDR.,** nat-a., pip-m., ***sep.,*** sulph.
3 p.m. - pip-m.
extending, occiput, to - **SEP.**
extending, vertex, to - phyt.
morning on waking - agar.
outward - bar-ac., bell., con., ferr., glon., gran., lyc., ph-ac., puls., senec., sep., sulph., verb.
pressure amel. - kali-p.

SHOOTING, over eyes
right - bry., nat-a., **PRUN.**
rubbing amel. - kali-p.
upward - ph-ac., scut.
violent shooting pains from root of nose along left orbital arch to external angle of eye, with dim sight, begins in morning, increases till noon, and ceases toward evening - kali-bi.

SICKLY, look around the eyes - **CINA,** guare.

SLEEPY, feeling in the eyes - ***gels.,*** phos., staph., thuj.

SMALLER, sensation of eyes - alum., bell., bry., croc., merl., mer-c., nat-m.

SORE, pain - ***acon.,*** aesc., ***agar.,*** alum., am-br., ant-c., ant-t., ***apis,*** arg-m., arg-n., ***arn., ars.,*** ars-i., ***aur.,*** bad., ***bapt.,*** bar-c., ***bell.,*** **BRY.,** cahin., calad., calc., ***calc-p., calc-s.,*** camph., canth., ***carb-s., carb-v.,*** caust., cedr., cham., ***chel., cimic.,*** clem., cocc., ***colch., com.,*** cor-r., ***corn., croc., cupr.,*** dios., dirc., dor., **EUP-PER.,** fago., ***gels., glon., gymn.,*** **HAM., HEP.,** hura, hyos., ***hyper.,*** iod., kali-bi., kali-p., ***lach.,*** lec., lil-t., lith., ***lyc.,*** lyss., manc., ***merc.,*** nat-a., nat-c., nat-m., nat-p., naph., ***nit-ac., nux-v.,*** onos., ox-ac., phos., ***phys.,*** phyt., pic-ac., plan., podo., **PRUN.,** psor., ***puls., ran-b.,*** **RHUS-T.,** rob., rumx., ***ruta.,*** sang., sars., ***sep., sil.,*** sin-n., ***spig.,*** stann., stry., sulph., sul-ac., ***symph.,*** ter., ***tub.,*** urt-u., ust., verat., vib., **ZINC.**
afternoon - dios., fago., nat-m.
4 p.m. - lyc.
air agg. - ***chel.***
cold - chel., ***sil.,*** zinc.
bending head down - chel.
blow, from - **SYMPH.**
chill, during - ***tub.***
closing eyes forcibly - sulph.
cold applications amel. - chel., ***puls.,*** sulph.
daytime only - sulph.
evening - am-br., calc-s., cinnb., com., dios., ***gels.,*** lyc., nat-p., stry., zinc.
walk, after a - **SEP.**
extending into the head - ***hep.***
eyebrows - ***kali-c.***
foreign body, as from - gels., hura.
headache, during - aloe, cedr., ***cimic., eup-per., gels.,*** hom., menthol, myric., nat-m., phel., ***scut.,*** sil., ***spig.***
infuenza, during - bry., gels., ***eup-per.***
light agg. - ***chel.***
menses, during - ***zinc.***
after, with throbbing headache - nat-m.
morning - dios., fago., myric., nat-a., sars.
motion, during - carb-s., ***cupr.***
moving, eyes - agar., ***bapt.,*** **BRY.,** ***carb-s., carb-v., com., crot-t., cupr.,*** gels., nat-a., ***nat-m.,*** phos., ***phys.,*** pic-ac., **RHUS-T.,** ***stict.,*** **TUB.**
eyelids - **BRY.,** glon., nat-a.
night - ***bry., cocc.,*** dios., gels.
opening, on - sil.
pressing, amel. - ***chel.,*** hyos., verat.
reading, while - ***croc., kali-bi.,*** nat-a., nat-p.

SORE, pain
right - ***chel., com.***
touch - bor., hep., sulph.
sore, canthi - ***apis,*** arg-n., ***carb-v., cham.,*** **GRAPH.,** ***nat-m., nux-v.,*** phos.
inner - bry., ***nux-v.,*** podo., ***puls.,*** sep., **ZINC.**
outer - **ANT-C.,** bor., calc-ac., cham., fago., form., ***kali-c., ran-b.,*** rhus-t., sep., ***zinc.***
with denuded lids - cham.
sore, eyebrows - dros., guai., ***kali-c.,*** stront-c.
sore, eyelids - ang., bell., cham., chim., cob., coloc., dios., ***euphr.,*** form., kali-a., kali-bi., kalm., lith., lyc., merc., myric., nat-p., ***phys.,*** phyt., pic-ac., plb., psor., sil., verat., zinc.
closing, on - dig., phyt., rhus-t.
cold air, in - rhus-t.
denuded, as if - cham., ***psor.***
margins of - ***acon., apis, bor.,*** dig., kalm., ***nux-v.,*** spig.
morning - nux-v., ***sulph.,*** valer.
moving, the lids - **BRY.,** glon., nat-a.
night - kali-c.
orbit, lower - sars.
orbital arch - nat-m.
rubbed, as if - verat.
sore, eyes, above - cann-i., gels., ***kali-c.,*** plan., plat., ***sil.***
opening eyes agg. - ***sil.***

SPARKS, burning on eyelids - sulph.

SPASMS, ciliary muscle - agar., ***arg-n.,*** aur., aur-m., caust., gels., ***jab., morph.,*** nat-m., nit-ac., ***nux-v.,*** phys., puls., ***ruta.,*** spig., sulph., tab.
orbicularis palpebrarum - chin-a., ***mez.***
spasms, of eyelids - agar., alum., ***bell., calc.,*** calc-p., camph., chin-a., croc., ***cupr., euphr., mag-p.,*** meny., ***merc-c., nat-m., nux-v.,*** plat., ***plb., puls.,*** ruta., sep., sil.
night - alum., croc., ***merc-c.***
right - hyper.

SPLINTER, as from a - apis, aur., ***hep.,*** merc., sulph., thuj.
left - elat.

SPOTS, cornea, on the (see Opacities) - agar., alumn., **APIS,** ***ars., aur.,*** bar-c., bell., ***cadm-s.,*** **CALC.,** ***calc-f., calc-p.,*** cann-s., ***caust., chel.,*** cina, ***colch.,*** **CON.,** cupr., ***euphr., form., hep.,*** kali-ar., ***kali-c.,*** kali-s., lyc., ***merc., nat-m., nit-ac.,*** nux-v., phos., psor., ***puls.,*** rhus-t., ***ruta., seneg.,*** sep., ***sil.,*** spong., ***sulph., syph.,*** thuj.
bluish - ***colch.***
brown - agar.
scars - ***apis, ars.,*** cadm-s., ***con.,*** euphr., kali-chl., ***merc., sil.***
spots, canthi, outer, humid spots, painful if sweat touches them - ***ant-c.***
white spots in - colch.
spots, sclera, yellow, in - agar., aur., ph-ac.
marked by a network of blood vessels of cornea - **AUR.**

STAPHYLOMA - ***alumn., apis, aur-m.,*** bar-m., ***caust., chel., euph., euphr., hep.,*** ilx-a., ***lyc., nit-ac.,*** puls., sil., ***thuj.***

STARING - ***acon., aeth., agar.,*** am-c., ***anac., ant-t., arn., ars., ars-i., art-v.,*** asar., atro., aur., **BELL.,** benz-n., bor., ***bov.,*** brom., bry., ***calc., camph.,*** cann-i., ***canth.,*** carb-ac., ***carb-s.,*** carb-v., caust., ***cham.,*** chin., ***chin-s., chlor., cic.,*** cina, clem., coca, ***cocc., colch., croc.,*** crot-c., ***cupr.,*** dor., eup-per., gels., ***glon.,*** grat., guai., ***hell., hep.,*** hydr-ac., **HYOS.,** ***hyper., ign.,*** **IOD.,** ip., kali-ar., kali-br., kali-c., ***kali-cy., kali-i.,*** kali-n., kali-p., kalm., ***kreos.,*** lach., lachn., ***laur.,*** **LYC.,** lyss., manc., med., **MERC.,** merc-c., ***mez.,*** morph., mosch., mur-ac., ***naja,*** nat-a., nat-c., nat-p., ***nux-m., nux-v.,*** oena., olnd., **OP.,** paeon., petr., ***ph-ac.,*** phos., ***phyt.,*** plat., plb., puls., ran-b., rhus-t., ruta., sang., sant., **SEC.,** seneg., sil., sol-n., ***spong., squil.,*** **STRAM.,** ***stry.,*** sulph., sul-ac., tab., tarent., ter., ***verat.,*** vip., ***zinc.***

chill, during - ***calc.***
cold, after being - cic.
convulsions, during - aeth., ars., bell., canth., cham., cupr., hydr-ac.
evening - chin.
  bed, in - sil.
  convulsions, during - ars.
  waking, on - ***ip.***
headache, during - **BELL., GLON., STRAM.**
menses, before - puls.
morning, in open air - nux-v.
music, on listening to - tarent.
night - corn., eup-pur.
  sleep, during - ant-t., corn., op.
pain in, with, forehead - spig.
  occiput - ***carb-v.***
sensation as though - med.
sleeplessness, with - eup-pur.
stupor, during - ars., ***hell.***
sunstroke - ***glon.***
unconsciousness - caust., hyos.
vertigo, during - hep.
waking, on - ***arn.,*** bell., ip., stram., ***zinc.***
  suddenly - sec., ***zinc.***
walking, in open air, after - alum.

STICKY, eyelids - acon., calc-ac., euph., ***puls.***

STIFFNESS of - agar., ars., asar., aur., bar-m., calc., calc-p., camph., caust., crot-c., cupr-s., gels., hep., **KALM.,** med., ***nat-a.,*** **NAT-M.,** onos., phos., rhus-t., seneg., spig., stry.

eyeballs - sil.
muscles about the eyes - agar., **KALM.,** ***nat-m.***
eyelids - **APIS,** arum-d., camph., gels., **KALM.,** nat-a., ***nux-m., rhus-t., sep., spig., verat.***

STINGING, pain - **APIS,** ***calc., caust., crot-t.,*** euphr., mag-s., meph., nat-c., nit-ac., ***puls.,*** spong., tarent., thuj.

about the eyes - aesc., spong.

stinging, canthi - ***apis,*** asar., carb-an., ran-s., spong., squil.

stinging, eyelids - ***apis, aur.,*** tarax.

STONES, little, around, as if - kali-n.

as if full of little - kali-n., lac-d.

STRABISMUS - agar., ***alum.,*** alumn., ant-t., **APIS,** apoc., ***arg-n.,*** ars., **BELL.,** benz-n., bufo, ***calc.,*** calc-p., cann-i., ***canth., chel., chin-s.,*** **CIC.,** ***cina,*** coloc., ***con.,*** cupr-ac., **CYCL.,** ***gels.,*** graph., ***hell., hyos.,*** jab., ***kali-br., kali-i.,*** kali-p., lil-t., ***lyc.,*** lyss., ***mag-p.,*** meny., ***merc., merc-c.,*** merc-i-f., morph., nat-a., ***nat-m.,*** nat-p., ***nux-v.,*** op., phos., plb., psor., puls., rhus-t., ruta, sec., ***spig., stram.,*** sulph., syph., ***tab.,*** thuj., tub., verat., ***zinc.***

alternate, days - ***chin-s.***
chorea, with - ***stram.***
convergent - alum., art-v., calc., **CIC.,** cina, **CYCL.,** piloc., mag-p., nux-v., spig., syph.
dentition, during - alum.
divergent - ***agar.,*** alum., ***coloc., con.,*** graph., ***jab.,*** lil-t., merc-i-f., **NAT-M.,** phos., rhod., ruta., seneg.
epilepsy, during attacks - tarent.
fever, with - bell., cycl.
left turned in - ***calc., cycl.***
mental emotions or fear agg. - ***cic., nux-m.,*** stram.
night - spig-m.
periodic - chin., ***chin-s., cic.,*** jab., ***nux-v.,*** piloc.
reading, while - tab.
right turned in - alumn.
sensation, of - meny., puls.
warmth, from - spig.

STRICTURE, lachrymal duct, (see Lachrymal duct)

STYES, eyelids - agar., alum., am-c., ant-t., ***apis,*** ars., ***aur.,*** bry., cahin., calc-f., **CARB-S.,** carc., caust., ***chel.,*** colch., **CON.,** cupr., dys-co., elaps, ferr., ferr-p., **GRAPH.,** hep., ***jug-c.,*** kali-p., lappa-a., **LYC.,** mag-aust., meny., ***merc.,*** morg., morg-g., nat-m., ***ph-ac.,*** phos., ***psor.,*** **PULS.,** pyrog., ***rhus-t.,*** seneg., **SEP.,** ***sil.,*** skook., stann., **STAPH., SULPH.,** ***thuj.,*** tub., upa., uran-n., valer.

induration from - ***calc., con.,*** **SEP.,** ***sil.,*** **STAPH.,** ***thuj.***
left - ***bar-c.,*** colch., elaps, hydr., ***hyper.,*** staph., sulph.
recurrent - alum., calc-f., carb-s., ***con., graph., psor., sil.,*** skook., **STAPH., SULPH.,** thuj., tub.
rheumatism, following attack of - skook.
right - am-c., cupr., cypr., ferr-p., ***nat-m.***

styes, canthi, inner - bar-c., ***nat-m.,*** stann., sulph.

  toward - kali-c., ***lach., lyc., nat-m.,*** petr., puls., sil.

outer - aur-s.

styes, lower lids - ***colch.,*** cupr., elaps, ferr-p., ***graph., hyper.,*** kali-p., ***phos.,*** puls., ***rhus-t.,*** seneg., thuj.

styes, upper lid - alum., am-c., bell., ferr., merc., ***ph-ac.,*** **PULS.,** staph., sulph., thuj., tub.

left, and edema of lower lids - uran-n.

SUNKEN - acet-ac., ***aeth.,*** agar., am-c., ***anac.,*** ant-c., **ANT-T.,** arg-n., ***arn., ars.,*** ars-i., aster., bar-m., bell., ***berb., bufo,*** cadm-s., calc., ***camph., canth., carb-s., carb-v., cedr.,*** chel., **CHIN.,** chin-a., chin-s., chlor., cic., cimic., **CINA,** coca, coc-c., ***colch., coloc.,*** crot-h., ***cupr., cur., cycl., dros.,*** ferr., ferr-ar., ferr-p., ***glon., graph.,*** haem., hell., iod., ***iris,*** kali-ar., ***kali-br., kali-c., kali-i.,*** kali-p., ***kreos.,*** lach., lith., ***lyc., merc.,*** merc-c., morph., naja, nit-ac., nux-v., oena., olnd., ***op.,*** ox-ac., petr., ***ph-ac., phos.,*** phyt., ***plat.,*** plb., podo., **PULS.,** raph., rob., sang., **SEC.,** sep., ***spong., stann., staph.,*** stram., stry., ***sulph.,*** tab., ter., teucr., thuj., til., upa., ***verat.,*** vip., zinc.
- afternoon agg. - iod.
- air, in open - kali-c.
- convulsions, before - ars., bufo, staph., stram.
- forenoon - lyc., ox-ac.
- menses during - ***cedr.***
  - pale face, with - cycl., ip., verat.
- morning - elaps, zinc.
- sensation of - ambr., ap-g., aur., chin., cinnb., iod., lac-f., lyc., teucr., zinc.

sunken, cornea - aeth.

SWELLING, sensation of - acon., arg-n., bapt., calc., calc-p., cann-i., caust., chel., **GUAI.,** ham., ip., mag-c., nat-a., phys., rhus-t., sarr., thuj.

SWOLLEN - ***acon.,*** **ANAC., APIS,** ***ars.,*** atro., bapt., bar-c., ***bry.,*** bufo, cann-i., carb-v., card-m., ***cedr., cham.,*** **CHLOL.,** coloc., croc., dulc., ery-a., fago., ferr., ferr-ac., gels., **GUAI.,** ***hep.,*** hura, ***ign., ip.,*** jug-c., ***kali-c.,*** kali-i., kali-p., lach., lyc., ***mag-c.,*** mang., merc., ***nat-a., nit-ac., nux-v.,*** oena., ol-j., par., phos., phys., plb., psor., puls., pyrog., raph., **RHUS-T.,** sars., **SEP.,** spig., ***stram.,*** stry., til., vesp.
- caruncles - agar., **ARG-N.,** bell., cann-i., ***kali-c.,*** zinc.
- evening - ***hep.,*** sep.
- forenoon - bry., ***euphr.,*** myric.
- headache, with - sep.
- left - carb-v., ***coloc.***
- meibomian glands - ***aeth.,*** bad., bor., ***clem., colch., con.,*** dig., graph., hep., merc., nicc., ***phyt.,*** puls., rhus-t., sil., ***staph., sulph.,*** thuj.
- morning - bar-c., bry., **CHAM.,** cocc., ***crot-h.,*** cupr., myric., naja, sarr., **SEP.,** sil., **SULPH.,** uran.
  - headache, after - ***cocc.***
  - waking, on - chel., kali-bi., mag-c., nat-a., nicc.
- night - ***hep.***
- orbital arch, temporal - spig.
- right - ***lyc.***

swollen, canthi - agar., ***arg-n.,*** aur., bell., bry., **CALC.,** cinnb., graph., merc., petr., sars., sil., stann., zinc.
- inner - calc-p., petr., sars., sep.

swollen, conjunctiva - ***apis, arg-n., ars.,*** bell., bry., cadm-s., cedr., cham., ***chel.,*** chlol., euph., ***graph., ip.,*** led., nat-a., ***nat-c.,*** nat-m., nux-v., sep.
- dermoid - ***calc., nat-c., nat-m.,*** thuj.

swollen, eyebrows, hard, over - sang.

swollen, eyelids - absin., ***acon.,*** agar., ***all-c.,*** alum., anac., **APIS,** ***arg-m.,*** **ARG-N.,** arn., **ARS.,** ars-i., aur., bar-c., ***bar-m., bell.,*** berb., bry., ***calc., carb-s.,*** card-m., ***carl., caust.,*** cham., ***chin-s.,*** cinnb., ***colch.,*** com., ***con., crot-t.,*** cupr., ***cycl., dig.,*** euph., **EUPHR.,** ***ferr., ferr-ar., ferr-i., ferr-p.,*** gels., ***graph.,*** ham., ***hep.,*** hyos., ign., iod., ***ip., kali-ar., kali-bi., kali-c.,*** **KALI-I.,** kali-p., kali-s., **KREOS.,** lach., ***lyc.,*** mag-m., manc., mang., **MERC.,** merc-c., merc-i-f., mez., ***mur-ac.,*** **NAT-A., NAT-C.,** ***nat-m.,*** nat-p., nat-s., **NIT-AC.,** nux-m., ***nux-v.,*** op., petr., ***phos., phyt.,*** plb., ***psor., puls.,*** **RHUS-T., RHUS-V.,** ruta., ***sanic.,*** sec., ***seneg., sep.,*** sil., spong., squil., stram., ***sulph.,*** sul-ac., syph., ***tell.,*** ter., ***thuj.,*** urt-u., valer., verat., vesp., vip.
- dogs, after bites of - lyss.
- edematous - anac., **APIS,** ***arg-n., arn.,*** **ARS.,** ars-i., colch., ***crot-t., cycl., graph., iod., kali-ar., kali-bi.,*** **KALI-C.,** ***kali-i.,*** kali-p., ***merc-c., nat-a., phos., phyt., psor.,*** puls., raph., **RHUS-T., TELL.,** urt-u., vesp., zinc.
- hard and red - acon., thuj.
- lower lids - aur., cahin., calc., crot-c., ***dig.,*** glon., mag-c., **KALI-AR.,** op., ph-ac., ***phos.,*** raph., rhus-t., sep.
  - left - calc., merc.
  - morning - calc.
- margins - arum-t., ***chel.,*** coc-c., ***con.,*** **EUPHR.,** ***graph., hep., kali-c., kreos., merc-c.,*** nux-m., ph-ac., ***phos.,*** psor., puls., sulph., syph., valer.
- menses, during - apis, cycl., kali-c.
  - suppressed - acon., arg-n., ***ars., calc.,*** cycl., ***kali-c.,*** merc., nux-v., rhus-t., sulph.
- morning - bar-c., cham., crot-h., sep.
  - headache, with - tub.
- orbital arch, temporal - spig.
- purple color - phyt.
- sensation of swelling - ***caust.,*** chel., cimic., coc-c., ***croc., cycl.,*** guai., mag-m., meny., psor., tarax., ***thuj.***
- under the lids - **APIS, ARS.,** ***hep.,*** **KALI-C.,** med., ph-ac., **PHOS.**
- upper lids - **APIS,** bry., ***con., cycl., ign.,*** **KALI-C.,** kali-i., ***med., nat-c.,*** nux-m., ***petr.,*** puls., ***squil.,*** sulph., syc-co., ***syph.,*** teucr., thuj., zinc.
  - headache, during - stront-nit.
  - left - asar., cahin., tell.
  - right - ***caust.,*** nat-c., phos., sep.
- watery, white - ***iod.***

swollen, lachrymal gland - ***agar.,*** anan., ***graph.,*** kali-i., **SIL.**
- lachrymal, canal - apis, bell., brom., ***calc., nat-m.,*** **PETR.,** ***sil.***
- lachrymal, sac - nat-c., nat-m., **PULS., SIL.**

swollen, retina - apis, kali-i.

TEARING, pain - acon., aeth., agar., all-c., alum., ambr., am-m., ***anac.,*** ant-t., apis, ***arn., ars.,*** asar., aur., aur-m., bar-c., ***bell.,*** berb., bor., bov., bry., cadm-s., ***calc.,*** canth., carb-s., carb-v., caust., ***cham., chel., chin-s.,*** cic., cob., ***cocc., colch., coloc.,*** con., croc., ***crot-h.,*** dros., gran., graph., grat., ***hyos.,*** hyper., ***ip.,*** kali-ar., ***kali-c.,*** kali-n., kali-p., kali-s., kreos., led., ***lyc.,*** mag-c., med., **MERC.,** merc-c., ***mez.,*** nat-s., nicc., ***nux-v.,*** paeon., par., ***phos.,*** plb., ***prun.,*** **PULS.,** rhus-t., ruta., sep., ***sil.,*** spong., squil., sulph., tax., thuj., valer., ***verat.,*** zinc.
afternoon - bor., calc., lyc., phos., sep.
2 p.m. - lyc., sep.
sitting - phos.
around eyes - iod., lyc.
bed, in, agg. - arn., mag-c., mag-s., **MERC.**
closing eyes - sil.
covering, with hand amel. - aur-m.
damp, weather - ***merc.***
evening - calc., ***chel.,*** coloc., crot-h., hyper., kali-c., nat-c., nat-m., thuj.
evening, after lying down - cocc., chel.
extending to, brain - ***thuj.***
forehead and cheeks - lyc.
occiput - colch.
teeth - ***chel.***
temples - anac., chel., ip.
zygoma - ***chel.***
forenoon - kreos.
left - agar., caust., ***chel.,*** coloc., nicc., sulph., thuj.
light, on looking at the - ***ars., aur-m.***
menses, during - ***coloc.***
morning - ***crot-h.,*** mag-c., mag-s.
walking, while - anac.
night - coloc., ***kali-c.,*** **MERC.,** nux-v., ***plb.,*** rhus-t.
around eyes agg. - ***acon.,*** coloc.
bed, in - **MERC.**
waking him - ***nux-v.***
noon - chin-s.
orbita - sep.
orbital arch - alum.
outward - sil.
paroxysmal - chin-s., nicc., ***sil.***
periodic - aur-m., chin-s.
right - ambr., bov., colch., croc., gran., mag-c., ***prun.***
in short jerks in and around right eye - ambr.
warmth, while - anac.
agg. - arn.

tearing, canthi, in - chin., hyos., nat-m.
inner - bell., calc-caust., kali-n., meny., nat-c., nicc., rat.
outer - am-m., aur

tearing, eyebrows - bell., ***cocc.,*** euph., kali-c., rhus-t., ***thuj.,*** zinc.

tearing, eyelids - alum., bar-c., kali-c., mag-c., nat-c.

tearing, eyes, behind - bism., squil.

tearing, eyes, over - agar., agn., ***ars.,*** aur., aur-m., calc., chel., ***chin.,*** ferr-i., iod., kali-ar., kali-c., kali-i., lach., laur., lyc., mag-p., mang., merc., mez., phos., sang., sep., sil.
afternoon - sang., sep.
air, open, amel. - aur-m., merc.
evening - agn.
intermitting - ***ars.***
left - aeth., arg-m., ***iod.,*** laur., merc., ***merc-c.,*** stann., verb., zinc.
morning - ***chin.,*** lyc.
motion agg. - agn.
night - ***lyc.***
opening eyes on - euph.
pressing the eye, when - arg-m., lyc.
pressure amel. - ***anac.***
right - agn., anac., bism., **CARB-AC.,** mag-p., mang.
walking about amel. - ***ars.***

tearing, lachrymal gland - staph.

TEARS, (see Lachrymation)
acrid - all-s., **ARS.,** bell., bry., ***calc., caust.,*** cedr., clem., ***colch., coloc.,*** dig., eug., ***euph.,*** **EUPHR.,** fl-ac., gamb., graph., ***ham., ign.,*** iod., kali-ar., kali-n., ***kreos., led., lyc., merc.,*** **MERC-C.,** ***nat-m., nit-ac.,*** ph-ac., pic-ac., plb., puls., rhus-t., sabin., spig., staph., **SULPH.,** syph., teucr.
night - ***merc.***
biting - com., con.
bland - **ALL-C.,** ***puls.***
bloody, newborn in - cham.
burning - **APIS,** ***arn., ars., ars-i., aur.,*** bell., cadm-s., ***calc.,*** canth., **CHIN.,** chin-a., eug., dios., **EUPHR.,** kreos., ***lyc., merc., nat-s., nit-ac.,*** nux-v., ph-ac., phos., ***phyt.,*** plb., psor., **RHUS-T.,** ***sang., sil.,*** spig., staph., stict., stront-c., **SULPH.,** ***verb.,*** zinc.
sun, looking, at - sang., staph.
cold - lach.
itching - ars., senec.
oily - sulph.
salty - bell., ***kreos., nat-m.,*** nux-v.
sensation as from - eupi., hyos., ign., lil-t., merc., nit-ac., pyrog., sep., sil., spig., staph., sulph.
sticky - plat.
suppressed - ***nat-m.,*** sec.
thick - tarent.
varnish mark, leave - euphr., graph., nat-m., petr., ***rhus-t.,*** thuj.

TENSION - apis, agar., asaf., ***aur.,*** bar-c., berb., ***calc.,*** camph., carb-v., carl., caust., chin., colch., ***coloc.,*** cop., croc., dros., dulc., euphr., ***gels.,*** glon., hyper., ***ip.,*** kreos., lach., led., ***lith.,*** merc., mez., ***nat-m., nux-m., nux-v.,*** onos., ***par., phos.,*** phys., plat., **RUTA.,** sabad., seneg., sep., ***sil.,*** sol-n., spig., stann., stram., tab., til.
around the eyes - alum., ***nux-m., nux-v.,*** par., spong.
closing eyes amel. - aur.
fixing eyes agg. - aur.

TENSION,
left - lyc.
looking upward - sulph.
morning - ang., merc., thuj.
waking, on - sulph.
motion, of eyes agg. - nit-ac.
pain in occiput, with - carb-v.
reading, while - calc., caust.
right - zinc.
sex, after - agar., ***calc.,*** phos., sep., ***sil.***
turning eyes - ***calc.***

tension, canthi, internal - bar-c., kali-cy.

tension, eyebrows - bov., hell.

tension, eyelids - acon., dros., hyper., merl., nit-ac., ***nux-m.,*** olnd., ph-ac., plat., sul-ac.
closing, on - phys.
lower - arum-t.
morning - sulph.
reading, while - calc., caust.
right - carb-v.

THICKENING, of conjunctiva - apis.

thickening, cornea - ***apis, arg-n.,*** asar., bell., ***nit-ac.,*** sil.

thickening, eyelids - **ALUM.,** apis, **ARG-M., ARG-N.,** calc., ***carb-s.,*** coloc., ***euphr., graph.,*** hep., **MERC.,** ***nat-m., phyt., psor., puls., sulph.,*** **TELL.,** thiosin.

TICKLING, periosteum of orbit - phos.

TINGLING - clem., phos., ***phyt.,*** pic-ac., spig.
bones, in - phos.

TIRED, expression - clem., cupr., ***gels.,*** kali-c., ***ph-ac.***
reading, from - ruta, sulph.
sensation - am-m., ars., bar-c., ***gels., graph.,*** iod., jab., lyc., nat-a., nat-m., petr., ***phos.,*** psor., ***ruta.,*** ***sep.,*** stann., stram., sulph., ***zinc.***

TUBERCLES - aur., bry., calc., ran-s., ***staph., thuj.***

TUMORS, on eyelids (see Polyps, Styes) - aur., ***calc.,*** caust., ***con.,*** graph., ***hep.,*** hydrc., kali-bi., lyc., ***nat-m., nit-ac., phos., puls., sil., staph.,*** sulph., teucr., ***thuj.***
cystic - ***benz-ac., calc., calc-f., graph.,*** iod., kali-i., ***merc.,*** morg., nit-ac., platan., ***sil.,*** staph., thuj.
sebaceous cyst, on - ***graph.***
meibomian glands - bad., prot., **STAPH.,** ***thuj.***
nodules in the lids - ***con., sil.,*** **STAPH.,** ***thuj.***
right, lower - zinc.
upper - zinc.
sarcoma - iod., ***phos.***
conjunctiva, of - iod.
tarsal tumors - ant-t., bar-c., calc., caust., con., ***kali-i.,*** platan., ***puls., sep., sil., staph., thuj.,*** **ZINC.**
recurrent - **CALC-F.,** ***puls., staph.***
repeated styes, after - **SEP.**

TURN, sensation, as if they would - petr., phos.

TURNED, (see Movement) - bell., caust., con., hipp., meph., nicc., **SPIG.**
downward - ***aeth.,*** canth., cham.
convulsion, during - aeth.
inwards - arg-n., bell., benz-n., ***calc.,*** plb., rhod., ruta.
left - amyg., bufo, dig., hydr-ac.
outward - bell., camph., ***crot-h.,*** dig., glon., morph., op., phos., stry., sul-ac., verat., zinc.
right - camph., ***ip.***
upward - acet-ac., ***acon.,*** agar., am-c., amyg., anan., ant-t., ***apis,*** arn., ars., art-v., bell., ***bufo, camph.,*** carb-ac., carb-an., chin., cic., cina, chlol., cocc., cub., ***cupr.,*** euph., ***glon., hell.,*** hyos., jatr., kali-cy., kalm., lach., ***lact., laur.,*** morph., mosch., nux-v., olnd., ***op.,*** plat., stry., tab., ter., verat.
convulsions, during - acon., cupr., glon., lach., oena., plat.
falling asleep, when - mez.
fever, during - hell.
left, to - amyg., bufo, dig., hydr-ac.
right, to - camph., stry.

TWISTED, sensation - chin., petr., phos., phys., pop-c., spong.

TWITCHING - acon., aesc., **AGAR.,** alum., am-m., apis, ***ars.,*** atro., bar-c., ***bell.,*** calc., carb-ac., carb-an., carb-s., cedr., cham., chin., cic., cod., croc., ***crot-t.,*** gels., ***glon.,*** guai., ***hyos.,*** ign., iod., kali-n., kali-p., kalm., ***lachn.,*** lith., lob-p., mag-p., mez., nat-m., nicc., ***nux-v.,*** petr., phys., phyt., ***puls.,*** rat., rhus-t., ruta, sel., ***stann.,*** stry., sul-ac., ther., upa., ust., vesp., xan.
cold, water amel. - agar.
daytime - aloe, nat-m.
left - apis, mez., sel.
looking fixed agg. - lach.
orbits - upa.
painful - agar.
paroxysms - ars., calc.
reading, while - agar.
right - rat., ther.
rubbing amel. - am-m.

twitching, canthi - agar., kali-chl., lachn., rhus-t.
inner - ***carl.,*** chel., kali-chl., rat., stann., sul-ac.
outer - am-c., bar-c., camph., ***cann-i.,*** mez., nat-m., nicc., ***phos.,*** seneg.
chewing, while - kali-n.
right - lachn.

twitching, eyebrows - carc., caust., cic., cina, echi., grat., hell., kali-c., ol-an., puls., ruta, sin-n., stront-c., zinc.

twitching, eyelids - aesc., **AGAR.,** alum., anac., ant-c., ***apis, ars.,*** ars-i., arund., asar., aster., bad., bar-c., bell., berb., calc., calc-s., camph., canth., carb-s., carb-v., ***caust.,*** cedr., ***cham.,*** chel., chin., **CIC.,** ***cocc.,*** croc., ***crot-t., cupr.,*** dulc., euphr., grat., hell., hydr-ac., ***ign.,*** indg., ind., ***iod., ip.,*** jatr., kali-bi., kreos., ***lach.,*** lachn., lyc., mag-c., ***mag-p.,*** meny., merc., merl., ***mez.,*** nat-c., ***nat-m.,*** nit-ac., ***nux-v.,***

twitching, eyelids - ol-an., par., petr., ***phos.***, **PHYS.**, ***plat.***, ***puls.***, ***rat.***, **RHEUM**, rhod., rhus-t., sabin., sel., seneg., sep., ***sil.***, spig., stront-c., **SULPH.**, verat-v.
closed, when - cupr-s., lachn., merc.
cold air - dulc.
eating, while - meny.
epileptic convulsions, before - agar.
left - aloe, bad., carc., ***caust.***, croc., merl., ***mez.***, puls., stront-c.
lower - am-c., coc-c., graph., ***iod.***, kali-i., lyc., nat-m., ph-ac., seneg., sulph., zinc.
left - am-m., lyc.
menses, before - ***nat-m.***
opening, on - kali-bi.
reading, while - agar., kali-bi., puls.
by lamplight - berb.
right - alum., chin., coloc., form., ***lach.***, nat-m., par., syph.
sleep, during - rheum
thunderstorm, before - ***agar.***
upper - alum., ars., ***aur.***, ***calc.***, cedr., lachn., lac-ac., ***merl.***, ***mez.***, mur-ac., nat-m., rat., stram., stront.
vertigo, during - chin-s.

ULCERATION, canthi - calc., phos.
external - bor., ***kali-c.***

ulceration, conjunctiva - **ALUM.**, **CAUST.**, coloc., ***crot-t.***, ***hydr.***, ***lyss.***, nit-ac.

ulceration, cornea - ***agar.***, **APIS**, ***arg-n.***, ***ars.***, ***asaf.***, ***aur.***, ***bar-c.***, bar-m., bufo, **CALC.**, calc-f., ***calc-p.***, ***calc-s.***, ***cann-s.***, cedr., ***chin.***, chin-a., chlol., cimic., ***clem.***, ***con.***, crot-c., ***crot-t.***, ***cund.***, **EUPHR.**, ***form.***, ***graph.***, ***hep.***, hippoz., ***ip.***, kali-ar., ***kali-bi.***, ***kali-c.***, kali-chl., kali-s., kreos., ***lach.***, ***lyss.***, ***merc.***, ***merc-c.***, merc-d., ***merc-i-f.***, nat-a., ***nat-c.***, ***nat-m.***, ***nit-ac.***, podo., ***psor.***, ***puls.***, ***rhus-t.***, ruta., ***sang.***, ***sanic.***, ***sil.***, ***sulph.***, ***thuj.***
one, then the other - ***ars.***
painful - ***merc-c.***
and without photophobia - kali-bi.
midnight to 3 a.m. - chin-a.
perforating - apis.
right to left - **CON.**
scars, from - cadm-s., calen., ***euphr.***, sil.
vascular - aur., calc., cann-s., hep., merc-c., merc-i-f., ***sil.***

ulceration, eyelids - anan., ***apis***, ***ars.***, ***bar-m.***, ***clem.***, ***graph.***, ***hep.***, kali-bi., kali-i., led., **LYC.**, ***merc.***, ***merc-c.***, nat-m., nat-p., phos., psor., rhus-t., sep., ***spig.***, ***stram.***, ***sulph.***, ***zinc.***

ulceration, eyelids
malignant - phyt.
margins - bufo, calc., **CLEM.**, crot-t., ***euphr.***, ***graph.***, ***merc.***, ***nat-m.***, psor., puls., **SANIC.**, spig., staph.
under surfaces - **ARS.**, bell., merc., nux-v., phos., puls., rhus-t., sil., sulph.

ulceration, lachrymal, canal - anan.

ulceration, meibomian gland - ***colch.***

UNSTEADY, look - aloe, anan., ***bell.***, camph., cedr., cupr., ***lach.***, **MORPH.**, par., ***stram.***

VESICLES, (see Herpes) above the eyes, bluish black - ran-b.

vesicles, cornea - ***agar.***, ars., ***aur.***, bar-c., bell., ***calc.***, cann-s., ***euphr.***, ***hep.***, ip., ***kali-bi.***, ***kali-chl.***, ***merc.***, ***merc-c.***, ***nat-c.***, ***nat-m.***, ***nit-ac.***, psor., ***puls.***, sulph.

vesicles, eyelids - berb., ***cimic.***, ***crot-t.***, mez., pall., ***psor.***, rhus-t., rhus-v., ***sars.***, sel.
margins, on - aur., pall., ***sel.***, urt-u.
yellow - dulc., ***psor.***, rhus-t.

vesicles, sclera - am-m.

VISION, general (see Vision, chapter)

WARMTH, sensation of - asar.

WEAK, eyes (see Vision, weak) - ***agar.***, alum., am-c., ***anac.***, ant-t., ***apis***, ars., asc-t., ***aur.***, bapt., bar-c., bov., calc., cann-i., ***cann-s.***, caps., ***carb-an.***, ***carb-s.***, ***carb-v.***, carb-o., caust., cham., chel., chin., chlor., cic., cina, cinnb., cob., **CON.**, croc., crot-t., cupr., cycl., daph., dig., dios., dor., dros., ***euphr.***, eupi., ***ferr.***, ferr-i., gels., ***graph.***, ham., hep., hura, hyos., hyper., iod., kali-bi., ***kali-c.***, kali-n., kali-p., kalm., kreos., lach., lact., ***lil-t.***, lyc., lycps., lyss., mang., meph., merc., merc-i-r., morph., naja, nat-a., ***nat-m.***, nat-s., nicc., nit-ac., nux-m., ***op.***, osm., ox-ac., par., petr., ***phos.***, ***phys.***, plat., plb., raph., rhod., rhus-t., **RUTA.**, sabad., sec., **SENEG.**, sep., ***sil.***, sin-n., spig., staph., stram., stront-c., stry., sulph., tab., tarent., ***thuj.***, urt-u., ust., verat., zinc.
afternoon - sin-n.
crying, as after - cycl.
daytime - stann.
dinner, after - valer.
emissions, after - jab., kali-c., lil-t., nat-m., puls., sep.
evening - alum., carb-an., nicc., psor.
after going to bed - op.
by the light - lyc., sep.
forenoon - ph-ac., squil., sulph., valer.
light - aster., gins., merc., nat-p.
candlelight - bell.
looking, intently, while - ***lyc.***
long - alum.
measles, after - euphr., ***kali-c.***, ***puls.***
menses, during - ***cinnb.***
morning - ars., bry., cina, dig., dios., phos., sang., upa.
noon - cinnb.
reading, while - agar., ***ammc.***, bell., kali-i., lyc., myric., ***nat-m.***, phys., **RUTA**, **SENEG.**, ***sep.***
after - am-c.
sex, after - **KALI-C.**, kali-p.

WEAK, eyes,
sexual excesses, after - ***calc.***, ***chin.***, gels., upa.
writing, while - bell., carl., ***nat-m.***, ***sep.***

WILD, look - acet-ac., ail., ***alumn., anac.,*** anan., arg-m., ***ars.,*** ars-i., **BELL.,** ***camph.,*** cann-i., ***carb-v., cimic.,*** con., ***cupr., glon.,*** hydr-ac., ***hyos.,*** iod., kali-i., ***lach.,*** **LYSS.,** ***nit-ac.,*** **NUX-V.,** op., plb., sec., **STRAM.,** stry., tab., valer., vip.

WIND, sensation of cool, blowing on it - med.

WINE, agg. - ***gels.,*** **ZINC.**

WINKING - agar., am-c., ***agar.,*** anan., ***apis,*** arg-n., astac., **BELL.,** ***caust.,*** chel., chin., con., ***croc.,*** cycl., **EUPHR.,** ***fl-ac.,*** glon., ***ign., mez.,*** nit-ac., ***nux-v.,*** op., petr., ph-ac., plat., ***spig.,*** sulph., sumb.

- air, open, in - merl.
- ameliorates - asaf., ***euphr.,*** croc., olnd., stann.
- epilepsy, during - kali-bi.
- looking at bright objects - acon., apis
- reading, while - ***calc., croc.,*** merl.
- sunlight - ***merl.***
- writing, after - hep.

WIPE, inclination to - agar., alum., arg-n., ***calc.,*** carb-an., ***croc.,*** kreos., lac-c., lyc., ***nat-c.,*** plb., ***puls.,*** rat., sep.

WRINKLED, conjunctiva - brom., nat-a.

YELLOWNESS, of - acon., agar., anan., ***ars.,*** ars-h., bell., ***canth.,*** carb-an., ***card-m.,*** caust., ***cham.,*** chel., **CHIN.,** ***chion.,*** clem., cocc., con., corn., **CROT-H.,** cupr-ac., cur., ***dig., dios., eup-per., ferr.,*** ferr-ar., ferr-i., ferr-p., ***gels.,*** graph., ***hep., hydr., iod., ip.,*** kali-ar., ***kali-bi.,*** **LACH.,** lyc., ***mag-m.,*** myric., nat-c., nat-p., ***nat-s.,*** nit-ac., **NUX-V.,** op., phel., ph-ac., ***phos.,*** pic-ac., ***plb., podo., sang.,*** sec., **SEP.,** sulph., ***verat.,*** vip.

- lower part - nux-v.
- spot on eye - agar., ph-ac.
- white of eyes is dirty yellow - nat-p.
- yellow, brown rings around - nit-ac.

Face

ABSCESS, (see Decay) - anan., ***bell.,*** **HEP.,** ***kali-i.,*** **MERC.,** ***phos., sil.***
antrum - kali-i., lyc., ***merc.,*** mez., **SIL.**
submental - staph.
vesicles, on - rhus-t.

ACHING, pain, (see, Pain, face)

ACNE, eruptions - agar., ambr., ***ant-c.,*** ant-s., ant-t., anthr., ***ars.,*** ars-br., ***ars-i.,*** ars-s-f., ars-s-r., asim., aster., **AUR.,** aur-a., aur-m., aur-s., bar-c., bar-s., ***bell.,*** bell-p., berb-a., bov., ***calc.,*** calc-p., **CALC-S., CALC-SIL.,** carb-ac., **CARB-AN., CARB-S., CARB-V.,** carc., **CAUST.,** chel., cic., cimic., clem., cob., ***con., cop., crot-h.,*** crot-t., **DULC.,** echi., ***eug.,*** **FL-AC.,** glon., gran., graph., **HEP.,** hydrc., ind., iod., jug-c., jug-r., kali-a., **KALI-AR.,** kali-bi., **KALI-BR.,** kali-c., kali-i., kali-m., ***kreos., lach.,*** lappa-m., led., lyc., mag-c., mag-m., med., merc., morg., mur-ac., nat-c., ***nat-m.,*** nat-p., ***nit-ac.,*** **NUX-V.,** olnd., ***ph-ac.,*** **PHOS.,** prot., ***psor., puls.,*** rad., **RHOD.,** rhus-t., rob., sabin., sang., sanic., **SARS.,** sel., **SEP., SIL.,** staph., ***sulph.,*** sul-i., sumb., **SYPH., TEUCR.,** ***thuj., tub.,*** uran-n., **ZINC.**
alcoholics, in - ant-c., bar-c., ***led., nux-v.,*** rhus-r., ***sulph.***
anemic girls, in, at puberty, with vertex headache, flatulent dyspepsia, amel. by eating - calc-p.
cheese, from - nux-v.
chocolate, from - arg-n., phos., sep.
cosmetics, from - bov.
emaciation, cachexia, with - ars., carb-v., nat-m., sil.
fire, near - ***ant-c.***
fleshy young people, in, with coarse habits, bluish red pustules on face, chest and shoulders - kali-br.
glandular swellings, with - brom., calc-s., merc-sul.
heated, becoming agg. - ***caust.***
indurated papules, with - agar., arn., ars-i., berb., bov., brom., carb-an., cob., con., ***eug.,*** iod., ***kali-br.,*** kali-i., ***nit-ac.,*** rob., ***sulph.,*** thuj.
menses, during - med.
menstrual irregularities, with - aur-m-n., bell., bell-p., berb., ***berb-a.,*** calc., ***cimic.,*** con., eug., ***graph., kali-br.,*** kali-c., kreos., nat-m., psor., **PULS.,** ***sang.,*** sars., **SEP.,** thuj., verat.
mercury, abuse of, from - kali-i., ***mez.,*** nit-ac.
potassium iodine, abuse of, from - aur.
pregnancy, during - bell., sabin., sars., sep.
rheumatism, with - led., rhus-t.
scrofulous people, in - bar-c., brom., ***calc.,*** calc-p., con., ***iod.,*** merc-sul., mez., sil., ***sulph.***
sexual excesses, with - ***aur.,*** calc., kali-br., ***ph-ac.,*** rhus-t., sep., thuj.
stomach, derangements, with - ***ant-c., carb-v.,*** cimic., lyc., ***nux-v.,*** puls., rob.
sweets, from - arg-n., lyc., phos., sep.

ACNE, eruptions
symmetric distribution, with - arn.
syphilis, from - aur., ***kali-i., merc-sul.,*** nit-ac.
tubercular children, in - tub.
chin - ***hydr.,*** prot., verat., ***viol-t.***
pregnancy, after - sep.
forehead - ant-c., ***ars.,*** aur., bar-c., bell., ***calc.,*** calc-pic., ***caps.,*** **CARB-AN., CARB-S., CARB-V., CAUST.,** ***cic.,*** clem., **HEP.,** ***kreos.,*** led., ***nat-m., nit-ac.,*** **NUX-V.,** ***ph-ac.,*** **PSOR., RHUS-T., SEP., SIL., SULPH.,** viol-t.
lips - bor., psor., sars., ***sul-i.***
nose - am-c., ars., ***ars-br.,*** aster., bor., calc-p., caps., cann-s., **CAUST.,** clem., elaps, graph., kali-br., nat-c., sel., ***sep.,*** sil., ***sulph., thuj.,*** zing.

ADHESION, of skin to forehead - sabin.

AIR, cool, seems blowing upon - coloc., mez., olnd., thuj.

ANGIOMA - abrot.

BARBER'S itch, ringworm of beard - ant-t., anthr., ars., aur-m., ***bac., calc.,*** calc-s., chrysar., ***cic.,*** cinnb., cocc., cypr., ***graph., kali-bi.,*** kali-m., lith., ***lyc.,*** mag-p., med., merc-p-r., nat-s., ***nit-ac.,*** petr., phyt., plan., ***plat.,*** rhus-t., sabad., sep., sil., ***staph.,*** stront-c., sul-i., ***sulph.,*** tell., **THUJ.**

BELL'S palsy, (see Paralysis)

BLACKHEADS, (see Comedones)

BLOATED (see Swelling) - **ACON.,** agar., ***ant-t., apis, apoc.,*** arn., **ARS.,** ***aur.,*** bar-c., ***bell., bry., bufo, cact.,*** calc., ***camph.,*** carb-s., ***cedr.,*** cham., ***chim.,*** chlor., ***cina, cocc., colch.,*** con., cop., ***crot-c., crot-h.,*** dig., dirc., dor., dros., ***dulc.,*** elaps, ferr., glon., graph., guare., hell., ***hippoz.,*** hura, hydr-ac., hyos., hyper., ip., kali-bi., ***kali-c., lach.,*** laur., led., manc., merc., ***nat-c., nat-m.,*** nux-v., oena., ***op., phos.,*** plb., puls., ***samb.,*** sang., senec., sep., sol-n., ***spig.,*** spong., stram., sulph., thuj., vesp., vinc.
eyebrows, between lids and - cench., **KALI-C.**
eyelids, upper, about - kali-c.
lower, about - ***apis,*** xero.
eyes, about the - ***am-be., apis, ars.,*** bor-ac., colch., elaps, ***ferr.,*** merc., ***merc-c.,*** nat-c., ***phos.,*** rhus-t., thlaspi, xero.
between the - lyc.
morning - nit-ac.
over the - ruta., sep.
under the - apis, ***ars., aur.,*** bry., kali-c., merc., nux-v., olnd., phos., puls.
fever, during - sil.
glossy, and - aur.
lying, while - apoc.
menses, before - bar-c., ***graph., kali-c., merc., puls.***
morning - crot-h., dirc., nat-c.
waking, on - agar., hura, ***spig.***
side lain on - phos.
speaking in company - carb-v.

BOILS - alum., am-c., anan., ant-c., arn., bar-c., ***bell.***, bry., ***calc.***, calc-s., carb-v., chin., cina, coloc., ***hep.***, hyos., iod., iris, kali-ar., kali-br., **KALI-I.**, ***lappa-a.***, led., ***mez.***, mur-ac., nat-c., nat-m., nit-ac., rhus-v., sars., ***sil.***, ***sulph.***
blood, small - alum., iris, ***sil.***
menses, during - med.
painful - hep.
repeating - alum.
boils, chin - am-c., cob., hep., lyc., nat-c., nit-ac., sil.
right side of - cob.
under - carb-v.

BORING, pain - arg-n., **AUR.**, bar-c., bell., bov., ***calc.***, camph., carb-v., ***cocc.***, dulc., euph., ***ign.***, indg., ***mag-c.***, ***mez.***, **PLAT.**, sil., ***thuj.***
left - aur., ***thuj.***
night, agg. - ***mag-c.***, ***mez.***, ***plat.***, ***sil.***
pressure, amel. - ***merc.***
rest agg. - ***mag-c.***
right - ***camph.***, ***plat.***, stront.
touch, amel. - ***thuj.***
boring, cheek bones - aur-m-n., bov., indg., ***mag-c.***, ***mez.***, nat-m., ***stront-c.***, ***thuj.***
night, agg. - nat-m.
boring, zygoma - ***aur.***, ***psor.***, thuj.
walking, agg. - ***aur.***

BURNING, pain - acon., aeth., ***agar.***, all-c., alum., anac., anac-oc., ***apis***, aran., ***arg-m.***, arg-n., ***arn.***, **ARS.**, asar., aspar., astac., bapt., ***bell.***, berb., brom., ***bry.***, calc., camph., cann-s., ***caps.***, carb-s., carb-v., ***caust.***, cedr., ***cham.***, chel., ***chin.***, chin-a., cimic., cist., clem., cocc., coloc., com., cop., corn., ***crot-t.***, cycl., dig., dros., dulc., elaps, ***euph.***, euphr., graph., guar., hyper., jac., jug-c., ***kali-ar.***, kali-bi., ***kali-i.***, ***kali-n.***, ***kreos.***, lach., laur., **LYC.**, mag-c., manc., merc., merc-c., merc-sul., ***mez.***, mur-ac., myric., mosch., nat-p., olnd., pall., phos., ***ph-ac.***, ***plat.***, psor., puls., raph., **RHUS-T.**, rhus-v., ruta, sil., ***spig.***, ***stann.***, staph., ***stront-c.***, **SULPH.**, ***thuj.***, til., ust., verat., vesp., zinc.
afternoon - fago., ***phos.***
air, open, amel. - kali-i.
burrowing - coloc.
chilliness, during - ***caust.***, mur-ac.
after - merc-sul.
cold, burning - sul-ac.
water amel. - ***ars-m.***
coldness, during - grat., nat-m.
cutting - chin.
daytime - manc., sulph.
decay, in - **AUR.**
dinner, after - grat.
eating, after - spig.
amel. - chin.
evening - bor., cham., com., mag-c.
exertion agg. - kreos.
frostbitten, as if - agar.
headache, during - stront.
left - arg-n., asar., bapt., **COLOC.**, ***hydr.***, murx., ***rhus-t.***, ***spig.***, thuj.
lying, when - chin., plb.
on painful side amel. - kreos.

BURNING, pain
malar bone - caust., cist., grat., nat-m., ol-an., par., spig., staph., sulph., thuj.
mental exertion - spig.
morning - corn., lyc.
9 to 4 p.m. - lyc.
to 3 p.m. - stront.
motion agg. - spig.
mouth, around - sulph.
corner of - ambr., bor., carb-an., cob., coloc., **DROS.**, ip., kali-chl., mez., nat-c., nat-s., ph-ac., zinc.
needles, like - **ARS.**, ***caps.***, spig.
night - chin., ***lach.***, ***mez.***
right - arund., chin., ham., ***merc.***, nux-v., pall., psor., puls.
rising from bed, after - nat-m.
rubbing, after - kali-c., sep.
shaving, after - aur-m.
spot - ph-ac.
standing - chin.
talking agg. - kreos.
toothache, with - sil.
touch agg. - ***chin.***
washing, with cold water after - sil.
burning, chin - anac., apis, berb., bov., canth., caust., mang., merc., mez., nat-c., ol-an., rhus-t., spong.
as from hot sparks - ant-c.
scratching, after - sulph.

BURSTING, pain - bov., ***thuj.***

CANCER - **ARS.**, ***aur.***, ***carb-an.***, ***con.***, ***kali-ar.***, kali-c., kali-i., lach., nit-ac., ***phos.***, sil., sulph., zinc.
antrum - aur., symph.
epithelioma - **ARS.**, cic., con., hydr., kali-ar., **KALI-S.**, ***lach.***, lap-a., ***phos.***, ***sep.***, sil.
lower - ***dulc.***
lupoid - ***hep.***, syph.
lupus - alumn., ***arg-n.***, **ARS.**, aur-m., carb-ac., ***carb-v.***, cist., **HYDRC.**, kali-ar., ***kali-bi.***, kali-chl., kreos., lach., psor., ***sep.***, ***sil.***
near wing of nose - ***aur.***
noli me tangere, on nose - cist., jug-c., phyt., thuj.
open, bleeding - cist.
scirrhus - ***carb-an.***, sil.
submaxillary glands - ***anthr.***, calc-s., carb-an., ferr-i.

CARIES, (see Decay)

CHAPPED - ***arum-t.***, ***graph.***, ***lach.***, kali-c., ***petr.***, ***sil.***

CHILBLAINS - agar.

CHILLINESS - ang., ars., brach., berb., camph., **CAUST.**, coloc., rhod.

CHLOASMA - cadm-s., card-m., caul., ***lyc.***, nux-v., rob., ***sep.***, ***sol.***
sun, agg. - cadm-s., sep., sol.

CHLOROTIC, greenish - ***acet-ac.,*** **ARS.,** bar-c., ***bell.,*** **CALC., CALC-P.,** carb-an., **CARB-S.,** ***carb-v.,*** caust., ***chin.,*** chin-a., **COCC.,** ***con., crot-h., cycl.,*** dig., **FERR.,** ***ferr-i.,*** **FERR-M.,** ferr-p., **GRAPH.,** ***helon., hell.,*** ign., kali-ar., **KALI-C.,** kali-p., ***kali-s.,*** **LYC.,** ***mang.,*** merc., **NAT-M., NIT-AC.,** ***nux-v.,*** olnd., ph-ac., ***phos.,*** **PLAT.,** plb., **PULS.,** sabin., **SENEC., SEP.,** spig., staph., **SULPH.,** sul-ac., valer., zinc.

CHOREA, (see Twitching and Distortion)

COBWEBS, sensation of - ***alum., bar-c.,*** bor., ***brom.,*** bry., calad., calc., carb-s., carl., con., **GRAPH.,** laur., ***mag-c.,*** mez., morph., ph-ac., plb., ***ran-s., sang-n.,*** sulph., ***sul-ac.,*** sumb.
- evening - ran-s.
  - 10 a.m. in bed - sumb.
- mouth, about - rat.
- tension, as from - ***bar-c.***

COLDNESS - abrot., acon., agar., ***ant-t.,*** aml-n., ***apis,*** **ARS.,** ***ars-i., bar-c.,*** bell., berb., bism., bry., ***cact., calc.,*** cann-i., ***camph.,*** canth., carb-s., **CARB-V.,** cedr., ***cham.,*** chel., ***cic.,*** **CINA,** cimic., ***cocc., coloc.,*** colch., crot-t., ***cupr.,*** dig., dros., ***graph., ham., hell., hep.,*** hydr-ac., ***hyos.,*** ign., ***iod.,*** ip., iris, kali-bi., ***kreos.,*** lil-t., lyc., merc., mez., morph., naja, ***nux-v.,*** oena., op., ox-ac., petr., ph-ac., **PLAT.,** plb., ***puls.,*** ran-s., rhus-t., ***ruta.,*** sabin., ***sec.,*** sep., ***stram.,*** stry., sulph., sul-ac., ter., upa., **VERAT.,** verat-v., zinc.
- afternoon - ars.
  - 2 p.m. - grat.
  - 5 p.m. - ars.
- alternating with heat - ***calc.,*** chel., lyc., merc.
- burning, with sensation of - bar-c., grat., nat-m.
- chill, with - asar., chel., **CINA,** ***dros., lyc.,*** nat-c., ***petr., plat.,*** puls., ***rhus-t.,*** sec., ***stram.,*** **VERAT.**
- cholera, with - ant-t., **CAMPH.,** ***carb-v., cupr.,*** iris, **VERAT.**
- cold wind, as from - coloc., mez., ph-ac.
- dinner, after - cann-i.
- drops, sensation as if, were spurting in face when going into open air - berb.
- dry, and - ***camph., carb-v.***
- extending to back - berb.
- forehead - anac., bar-c., ***calc., cimic.,*** cinnb., merc.
- forenoon - phos.
  - 10 a.m. - petr.
- headache, during - ars., ***carb-v.,*** ip.
- heat, of body, with - spong.
  - forehead, with - thuj.
  - internal, with - nat-m.
- hydrocephalus, in - agar., arg-n., **CAMPH.,** hell., ***verat.***
- icy, coldness - ***agar.,*** lyc.
- left - ars., dros., **GRAPH.,** lob., ruta
- menses, during - nat-m.
- morning - cedr., petr.
- mouth, corners of - aeth.
- night - ***lyc.***

COLDNESS,
- one side cold and red, the other hot and pale - ip., ***mosch.***
- one-sided - ph-ac., puls.
- pain, followed by - ***dulc.***
  - in occiput, with - ***carb-v.***
- painful - lyc., plat.
- palpitation, with - ***camph.***
- paroxysmal - sulph.
- right - gels., ph-ac., **PLAT.,** polyg.
  - when pain is most severe in left - polyg.
- sense of - acon., bar-c., ***merc., plat.,*** ran-s.
  - on one side - ph-ac., ***plat.***
- sleep, during - ign.
- spots, in - ***agar.***
- water, as from - sulph.

coldness, cheeks - coloc.

coldness, chin cold - aeth., chin., chin-s., kali-n., stram., verat.
- sense of - **PLAT.**

COMEDONES, blackheads - ***abrot., ars.,*** aur., ***bar-c., bell., bry., calc.,*** calc-sil., **CARB-S.,** ***carb-v.,*** chel., cic., dig., dros., ***eug.,*** **GRAPH.,** ***hep.,*** hydr., jug-r., mez., ***nat-a., nat-c., nat-m., nit-ac., sabad.,*** sabin., **SEL.,** ***sep., sil.,*** **SULPH.,** sumb., thuj., ***tub.***
- chin - dros., ***tub.***
  - and upper lip - sulph.
- forehead - ***sulph.***
- ulcerating - dig., ***sel., tub.***

CONGESTION, (see Heat) - acon., agar., **AML-N.,** ant-t., ***apis,*** arg-n., **AUR.,** bar-c., **BELL.,** ***bry., cact., calc.,*** cann-s., caust., chin., coc-c., coloc., cop., equis., eup-per., ***gels.,*** **GLON.,** hydr-ac., hyos., ign., ind., ***iod.,*** lac-ac., ***lach.,*** lil-t., meli., merc-c., mit., morph., oena., op., paeon., ***phos.,*** **PULS.,** sabin., **STRAM.,** ***stry.,*** tanac., thuj., ust., ziz.
- afternoon, 3 p.m. - sulph.
- air, open - phos.
- eating, during - ***cop.***
  - after - alum.
- hurrying, during - ign.
- rubbing, after - aesc.
- stool, during - aloe.
- walking, after - caust.

CONTRACTION - acon., ars., asar., ***bell.,*** cann-s., ***cham.,*** con., gels., kali-i., laur., lyc., ***merc.,*** morph., nit-ac., phos., phys., phyt., plb., rhus-t., sars., sec., tab., zinc., zinc-s.
- cheeks, sudden - eup-per.
- malar, bone - nit-ac.
- parotids - mang.
- right - eup-per., sars., stann.
- salivary glands - ambr., chin.
- skin of - cann-i.
- submaxillary gland - sil.

CONVULSIONS, of - acon., agar., ambr., amyg., anan., ant-t., arg-n., ***ars.,*** atro., bar-c., **BELL.,** bism., ***bov.,*** brom., ***bufo,*** calc., camph., canth., carb-s., ***caust., cham.,*** **CIC.,** ***cocc.,*** con., crot-c., **CUPR.,** dig., ***glon., hep.,*** hydr-ac., ***hyos., ign., ip.,*** kali-n., ***laur., lyc., lyss.,*** merc-c., morph., nat-c., nit-ac., nux-v., ***oena.,*** ol-an., ***op.,*** phos., ***phys.,*** plb., ***ran-b.,*** ran-s., rhus-t., sec., **STRAM.,** stry., sulph., sul-ac., tab., verat., vip., ***zinc.,*** ziz.

beginning in face - absin., ***bufo,*** cina, dulc., hyos., ign., sant., ***sec.***

beginning in left side - ***lach.***

chill, during - ars., bell., cham., cic., ign., op., stram.

extending to limbs - sant., sec.

masseters - ambr., ang., cocc., cupr., mang., nux-v.

menses, before - puls.

mouth - bell., cham., dulc., ign., ***ip., lyc.,*** merc., nit-ac., olnd., op., stram.

one-sided - dig., plb.

right - agar.

speaking, while - plb.

CRACKED, corners of mouth - ambr., am-c., ***ant-c.,*** apis, **ARUM-T.,** calc., caust., cinnb., **CUND.,** eup-per., **GRAPH.,** ***hell., hydr.,*** ind., ***iod.,*** lac-c., lyc., mag-p., ***merc.,*** merc-c., ***mez.,*** morg., ***nat-a., nat-m.,*** **NIT-AC.,** prot., psor., ***sep.,*** **SIL.,** ***thlaspi, zinc.***

right - ***lyc.,*** merc.

CRAMP-like, pain - calc., ***cocc.,*** hyos., ***mag-m., mag-p.,*** mang., mur-ac., plat.

burning - stann.

eating, after - mang.

opening, mouth - cham.

opening, and shutting mouth amel. - ang.

cramp-like, cheek, left - stann.

right - thuj.

cramp-like, malar bone - ***ang.,*** cina, cocc., ***coloc.,*** dig., hyos., ***mag-m.,*** mez., nit-ac., ruta., sep., valer.

extending to left eye - ***coloc.***

left - ol-an., ***plat.***

CUTTING, pain - arg-n., ars., ***bell.,*** calc-s., chin., clem., rhus-t., staph., til.

left - bell., senec.

maxillary, articulation - asar.

motion, of face, on - stann.

right - **BELL.**

standing - chin.

submaxillary gland - arg-m.

cutting, chin, in - caust., stann.

DECAY of bone (see Abscess) - **AUR.,** aur-m., caps., cist., fl-ac., hecla., hep., kali-s., mez., ***nit-ac., phos.,*** sil.

DIGGING, pain - aur-m., bov., cupr., euph., ***kali-bi., mag-c., plat.,*** sep., ***thuj.***

digging, cheek bones - ***mag-c.,*** mang., ***psor., thuj.***

DISCOLORATION, face

ashy - ***ars., bad., chlor., cic., ferr.,*** kali-bi., morph., ***phos., plb.,*** sec., sulph., verat.

black - camph., **CHIN.,** ***cor-r.,*** crot-h., hydr-ac., ***lach., oena.,*** op., stry., ***tarent.***

black, and blue spots - arn., crot-h., ***lach.,*** phos., rhus-t., **SUL-AC.,** ***tarent.***

mouth, around - ars.

bluish - absin., acetan., acon., ***agar., ail.,*** am-c., aml-n., ***ant-a.,*** ant-t., ***apis, arg-n.,*** **ARS.,** ***ars-i.,*** **ASAF.,** asim., ***aur.,*** bad., **BAPT., BELL.,** benz-n., bor., both., brom., **BRY.,** bufo, ***cact.,*** calc., calc-p., **CAMPH., CANN-I.,** ***canth., carb-an., carb-s.,*** **CARB-V.,** carl., ***caust., cedr., cench., cham.,*** chin-a., ***chol., chlor., cic.,*** cimic., ***cina,*** cinnb., ***cocc.,*** colch., **CON.,** cor-r., croc., crot-h., crot-t., **CUPR.,** cupr-ac., **DIG.,** ***dros., dulc.,*** ferr., ***glon., hep.,*** hydr-ac., **HYOS.,** ign., iod., **IP.,** ***kali-c.,*** kali-cy., ***kali-i.,*** kali-p., ***kreos.,*** **LACH.,** lachn., ***laur., lyc.,*** lycps., mag-p., meph., merc., merc-c., merc-cy., **MORPH.,** mosch., nat-a., ***nat-m.,*** nat-n., nat-p., ***nux-v.,*** oena., **OP.,** ox-ac., petr., phenac., phos., ***phyt.,*** piloc., plb., psor., prun., ***puls.,*** rhus-t., ***samb.,*** sang., sars., sec., sil., spig., ***spong., staph., stram., stry., sulph.,*** sul-ac., ***tab., tarent.,*** **VERAT., VERAT-V.,** vesp., ***vip.,*** zinc.

angry, when - ***staph.***

asthma, in - cupr., ***stram.,*** tab.

cheeks - cham.

chill, during - asar., bry., ***cact.,*** lach., nat-m., **NUX-V.,** petr., **STRAM.,** sulph., ***tub.***

chin - plat.

chloera, in - ***camph.,*** **CUPR., VERAT.**

convulsions, with - ***cic.,*** **CUPR.,** ***hyos., ip., oena.,*** phys., stry.

cough, during - ***apis,*** bell., caust., ***coc-c., cor-r.,*** cupr., **DROS., IP.,** ***mag-p., verat.***

whooping cough, during - ars., ***coc-c., cor-r.,*** crot-h., cupr., ***dros., ip., nux-v.***

dyspnea, with - bry., ***op., stram.***

eyes, circles around - abrot., ***acet-ac.,*** acon., agar., ail., ***anac.,*** ant-t., ***aran.,*** **ARS.,** ars-i., bad., ***bell.,*** **BERB.,** ***bism.,*** cadm-s., ***calc., calc-ar.,*** calc-p., ***camph., canth.,*** carb-an., cham., chel., **CHIN.,** ***cic.,*** cimic., cinnb., ***cina, cocc.,*** corn., ***crot-h., cupr.,*** cycl., fago., ***ferr.,*** ferr-ar., ferr-p., ***graph.,*** ham., hell., ***hep.,*** hura, ***indg., iod.,*** **IP.,** ***iris,*** jatr., kali-ar., kali-bi., kali-c., ***kali-i.,*** kali-p., kreos., lach., **LYC.,** mag-c., merc., mez., ***naja,*** **NAT-A., NAT-C.,** ***nat-m., nat-p.,*** **NUX-M., NUX-V., OLND.,** op., pall., petr., ***ph-ac., phos., phyt.,*** plat., plb., psor., ***puls.,*** raph., **RHUS-T.,** rhus-v., ***sabad.,*** sabin., **SEC.,** ***sep., stann., staph.,*** stram., sulph., tab., tarent., ter., upa., ***verat.,*** zinc.

menses, after - phos.

menses, before - tub.

eyes, under - lachn.

cholera, in - ***camph.,*** **CUPR., VERAT.**

DISCOLORATION, face

bluish, forehead - apis.

headache, during - cact., ***op.***

heart trouble - ***apis, cact.***

heat, during - lach.

laughing, when - **CANN-I.**

maniacal rage - acon., ars., bell., con., hyos., lach., merc., ***op.,*** puls., verat.

menses, at close of - verat.

before - ***puls.,*** tub.

morning - phos.

mouth, about the - ars., **CINA,** ***cupr.,*** kreos., ph-ac., sabad., stram., sulph., verat.

pain in abdomen, with - chin., fil.

pregnancy, during - ***phos.***

reddish - carb-v.

retching, from - bell.

spasm of glottis - ***bell., coff.,*** **LACH.,** ***mosch.***

speaking, in company - carb-v.

spots - ail., apis, ars., aur., ***bapt.,*** crot-h., ferr., hura, kali-br., kali-p., lach., led., mur-ac.

spots, following eruptions - ant-t., ferr., **LACH.,** thuj.

stool, during - rhus-t.

stool, after - rhus-t.

urinating, when - aspar.

vexation after - verat.

bluish, red - ***acon.,*** agar., ***ant-t., apis, ars.,*** asar., aur., **BELL., BRY.,** camph., **CANN-I.,** carb-ac., cham., cic., cina, ***con.,*** cor-r., ***crot-c., cupr.,*** dig., dros., grin., ***hep.,*** hydr-ac., hyos., ign., ip., kali-chl., ***lach.,*** lyc., meli., merc., morph., ***op., ox-ac.,*** petr., phel., phos., puls., sang., ***samb.,*** spong., staph., stram., verat., verat-v.

blushing - ambr., carb-an., carl., ***coca,*** ferr., sulph.

bronzed - ant-c., ars-h., nit-ac., sec., spig.

brown - ***arg-n.,*** ars., ars-i., ***bapt.,*** bry., carb-ac., caust., con., crot-h., gels., hyos., ***iod.,*** lyss., mag-m., ***nit-ac.,*** op., puls., rhus-t., samb., sars., ***sep.,*** staph., stram., ***sulph.***

angry, when - ***staph.***

eyes, around - ***lach.***

forehead - kali-p., phos.

spots - ***caul., nat-c., sep.***

spots, vaginal discharge, with - caul.

reddish - bry., hyos., nit-ac., ***op.,*** puls., samb., ***sep.,*** stram., sulph.

sleep, during - ***stram.***

spots - ambr., anan., ant-c., ars., ars-i., benz-ac., cadm-s., ***calc., carb-an., carb-s.,*** caust., ***colch.,*** con., ferr., hyos., iod., ***kali-c.,*** kali-i., kali-p., ***laur., lyc.,*** nat-a., ***nat-c.,*** nat-p., ***nit-ac.,*** petr., phos., ***sep., sulph.,*** sumb., thuj.

childbirth, after - crot-h., sep.

sun and wind agg. - cadm-s.

yellowish - phos., vac.

brownish-yellow, forehead, at hairline - caul., kali-p., med., nat-m.

DISCOLORATION, face

changing, color - ***acon., alum.,*** ars., bell., bor., bov., camph., ***caps., cham.,*** chin., ***cina,*** croc., ***ferr.,*** hyos., **IGN.,** iod., kali-c., laur., led., ***mag-c.,*** mag-s., nux-v., olnd., ***op.,*** ph-ac., **PHOS., PLAT.,** puls., ***sec.,*** spig., squil., ***sul-ac.,*** verat., zinc.

copper colored - alum., ***ars.,*** ars-h., calc., ***calc-p., carb-an.,*** cupr., ***kreos.,*** led., nit-ac., ***rhus-t., ruta,*** stram., verat.

spots - ***benz-ac.,*** carb-an., ***graph.,*** lyc., nit-ac.

cyanotic - anan., **ARS.,** ***aur., cact., cupr.,*** hydr-ac., lyss., merc-cy., **NAT-M.,** vesp.

dark - ***ail.,*** alum., ant-t., ***apis,*** ars., **BAPT.,** both., ***carb-s., carb-v.,*** colch., crot-h., cub., cupr., dub., elaps, ***gels.,*** hell., hura, hydr-ac., iod., kali-i., lach., morph., mur-ac., **NIT-AC.,** ***op.,*** ox-ac., ***phos.,*** plb., psor., stram., ***sulph.,*** thuj., trinit., tub., verat.

eyes, around - cimic.

dirty, looking - ***apis,*** **ARG-N.,** ***caps.,*** card-m., ***chel., cupr.,*** iod., kali-p., **LYC.,** ***mag-c., merc.,*** phos., **PSOR.,** ***sanic.,*** sec., **SULPH.,** thuj.

dusky, (see dark)

earthy - ***ant-t., arn., ars.,*** ars-h., ***ars-i.,*** ars-m., ***aster.,*** aur., bell., ***berb.,*** bism., ***bor., brom., bry., calc., calc-p., carb-an., carb-v.,*** **CHIN.,** chin-a., ***cic.,*** cimic., ***cina,*** cocc., con., ***croc.,*** der., **FERR.,** ***ferr-ar.,*** **FERR-I., FERR-P.,** gran., **GRAPH.,** hyos., hydr-ac., ***ign.,*** iod., ip., kali-ar., kali-bi., kali-chl., kali-p., kreos., ***lach., laur., lyc., mag-c., mag-m.,*** mag-s., ***med.,*** **MERC.,** ***mez.,*** mosch., nat-a., nat-c., ***nat-m.,*** nat-p., ***nit-ac., nux-v.,*** ol-an., **OP.,** pall., ***ph-ac., phos.,*** plb., psor., ***puls.,*** samb., sec., **SEP.,** ***sil.,*** sulph., tarent., ter., thuj., vip., zinc.

eyes, about - elaps, lappa-a., maland., ***puls.,*** sil.

fever, during - lach.

grayish - ***ars., berb., brom., bufo, cadm-s., carb-v., chel.,*** **CHIN.,** ***chlor., colch., cupr.,*** gels., ***hydr-ac.,*** kali-c., kreos., ***lach.,*** laur., **LYC.,** ***mez.,*** oena., phos., tarent., tab.

grayish, yellow - ***carb-v.,*** chel., ***kali-c.,*** kreos., **LYC.**

greenish, (see Chlorotic) - ***ars.,*** berb., **CARB-V., CHEL.,** crot-h., cupr., dig., ***ferr.,*** ferr-ar., ***iod.,*** kreos., ***med.,*** merc., merc-c., nux-v., ***puls.,*** verat.

about the eyes - ***verat.***

spots - ars.

hectic spots - acon., ***ars.,*** calc., ***chin.,*** ferr., iod., kali-c., kreos., lyc., ph-ac., ***phos.,*** puls., ***sang.,*** sil., stann., ***sulph.,*** tub.

lead-colored - **ARG-N.,** ars., benz-n., carb-an., carb-o., coca, cocc., crot-h., ***kali-i.,*** lach., merc., ***nat-m.,*** nit-ac., ***oena.,*** op., ***plb.,*** thuj., verat.

marbled - phos., sabad.

menopause, during - ***phys., sang.***

DISCOLORATION, face

mottled - ***ail., bapt., bell., cench., crot-h., dor., lach.,*** lachn., ***rhus-t.***

nosebleed, amel. - bapt., bell., erig., ferr., meli., nux-m.

one-sided - acet-ac., ***acon.,*** ant-t., ***arn.,*** ars., bar-c., bell., calc., cann-s., caps., **CHAM.,** ***chel., cina,*** coloc., ***ign.,*** **IP.,** ***lach., lyc., mosch., nat-m., nux-v., phos., plb., puls.,*** rheum, ***rhus-t.,*** sang., sulph., tab., tub., verat.

pain, when in - cimic., ter.

pale, (see Pale)

parchment, like - ars.

pink, spots - carb-an.

purple, (see bluish)

red, (see Red)

rising, on - verat.

ruddy, florid - arn., ferr.

sallow - ail., alum., alumn., ***apis, arg-m.,*** **ARG-N.,** ***arn., ars.,*** ars-h., ars-i., ***bapt.,*** berb., ***calc., calc-p., carb-ac.,*** **CARB-V.,** carl., **CHEL.,** ***coc-c.,*** cocc., ***coloc.,*** con., ***corn., croc., crot-c., crot-h., eup-per., ferr.,*** ferr-ar., ***ferr-i.,*** ferr-p., ***helon.,*** hydr., hydr-ac., ind., ***iod.,*** kali-c., kalm., ***lac-d., lach.,*** lept., **MED.,** ***merc.,*** myric., naph., **NAT-M.,** ***nat-s., nux-v.,*** op., ***pall.,*** plan., **PLB.,** podo., puls., ***sep.,*** **SULPH.**

sickly, color - acet-ac., aesc., aloe, alum., alumn., am-c., apis, ***arg-m., arg-n.,*** **ARS.,** ars-h., ***ars-i., bapt.,*** bism., bor., brach., **CALC.,** calc-s., carb-s., ***carb-v., caust., chel., chin.,*** chin-a., ***cina, clem.,*** con., ***crot-c., crot-h.,*** dig., eup-per., **FERR.,** ***ferr-ar., ferr-i., iod., kali-c.,*** kali-chl., kali-n., kali-p., kali-s., ***kreos.,*** lachn., **LYC.,** mag-c., ***mag-m., mang.,*** **MED.,** ***merc.,*** nat-s., ***nit-ac., nux-v., ph-ac., phos.,*** podo., psor., rhus-t., sil., ***spig., staph., sulph.,*** tab., teucr., thuj., til., **TUB.,** zinc.

sudden - calc., ferr., phos.

white, (see Pale) spots - ars., merc., nat-c.

nostrils - stram.

yellow, (see Yellow)

DISTORTION, of - absin., acon., am-m., ant-t., apis, ***ars.,*** bar-m., ***bell.,*** bism., ***bufo, camph.,*** cann-i., caust., ***cham., cic.,*** cina, cocc., ***coloc.,*** crot-c., ***crot-h.,*** cupr., dulc., ***graph., hell., hydr-ac.,*** **HYOS., IGN.,** ip., kali-i., kali-s., ***lach.,*** lact., ***laur.,*** lyc., lyss., ***merc-c.,*** mill., ***nux-m.,*** **NUX-V., OP.,** petr., phos., phyt., plat., plb., rhus-t., ***sec.,*** sep., ***sil.,*** sol-n., squil., **STRAM., STRY.,** sul-ac., tab., tarent., verat., vip.

abdomen, from pain in - ***coloc.***

chill, during - cann-s.

maniacal rage, with - ars., ***bell.,*** lach., nux-v., sec., **STRAM.,** ***verat.***

morning - olnd., ***mygal., spig.***

mouth, talking, when - caust., tell.

pain, with - coloc., phos.

side, on one - tell.

sleep, during - til.

after - cic.

speaking, on - ***ign.***

DISTORTION, of

supper, after - lyc.

swallowing, when - **NIT-AC.**

toothache - staph., tarent.

vomiting, while - ***verat.***

waking, on - crot-h.

distortion, mouth - agar., ***bell.,*** bry., camph., ***cocc., con., cupr.,*** cur., ***dulc., graph.,*** ign., kali-n., lach., ***laur., lyc.,*** merc., **NUX-V.,** op., ph-ac., plat., **PLB.,** puls., sec., stram., stry., sulph., tarent.

one-sided - dulc., graph.

one-sided, alternating sides - cham., lyc., nit-ac.

right corner outward - bell.

sleep, during - bry., cupr.

talking, when - caust.

DRAWING, pain - abrot., acon., acon-c., ***agar.,*** aloe, ***alum.,*** am-c., anac., ant-t., arg-m., **ARS.,** asaf., ***aur.,*** aur-m-n., bar-c., bar-m., bell., ***bry.,*** cadm-s., ***calc.,*** carb-s., ***carb-v., caust.,*** cham., ***chel.,*** cit-v., cocc., ***colch., coloc., con.,*** **DIG.,** dros., dulc., euon., euphr., graph., guai., hep., hyper., ***ign.,*** kali-ar., kali-bi., ***kali-c.,*** kali-chl., ***kali-n.,*** kali-p., kali-s., kreos., ***lach.,*** led., lob-c., lyc., mag-m., mang., **MERC.,** ***mez.,*** nat-h., nat-m., ***nux-v., ol-an.,*** ph-ac., ***phos., plat.,*** puls., ran-s., rhod., ***rhus-t.,*** rhus-v., ***sars., sep., sil., spig., stann., staph.,*** sulph., tep., ter., thuj., valer., ***verat., verb.,*** zing.

afternoon - alum., euphr., lyc., sulph.

masseter - ***sars.,*** verb.

cold air amel. - all-c., nat-h.

coughing - carb-v.

draft of air - ***verb.***

evening - anac., cist., thuj.

9 p.m. - zinc.

extending, into ear - ***acon., caust.,*** con., ph-ac.

to chin - phos.

left - arg-n., ***aur.,*** chel., nat-h., ph-ac., ***sulph., verb.,*** zing.

lying, while - chel.

morning - kali-bi., sulph.

rising, on - guai.

mouth to nose - thuj.

music, from - ph-ac.

paroxysmal - ***caust.,*** cocc., nat-h., sep.

rheumatic - caust., sul-ac.

right - agar., am-c., anac., arg-m., ***caust.,*** kali-chl., lyc., lyss., nit-ac., sars., ter., thuj., verat.

stooping, on - nux-v.

tighter and tighter and then suddenly let loose - ***puls.***

upward - ***ol-an.***

warmth amel. - **ARS.,** ***caust., coloc.***

drawing, cheek bones - am-c., anac., arg-m., carb-an., ***caust., chel., colch.,*** kali-chl., nat-c., nat-m., ***plat.,*** sil., stann., staph., ***verb.***

drawing, chin - agar., aur-m-n., caust., chin-s., cupr., hyper., olnd., stront-c., ***verb.***

drawing, zygoma - calc., chel., dig.

lying, while - chel.

DRAWN - ***acon.***, **AETH.**, ambr., am-c., **ANT-C.**, ***arg-n.***, **ARS.**, ***ars-h.***, ars-i., bar-c., **BELL.**, bism., ***bry.***, calc., ***camph.***, cann-s., ***canth.***, carb-h., carb-s., ***carb-v.***, **CAUST.**, ***cham.***, chel., ***cic.***, cocc., colch., crot-h., ***cupr.***, dig., dulc., gels., ***gran.***, ***graph.***, guai., hell., hep., hydr-ac., ***hyos.***, ***ign.***, iod., ***ip.***, kali-bi., kali-c., kali-s., lach., laur., **LYC.**, ***merc.***, ***merc-c.***, ***mez.***, mosch., nat-c., nit-ac., nux-m., nux-v., olnd., **OP.**, ph-ac., ***phos.***, ***plat.***, plb., puls., ran-b., ran-s., rheum, ***rhus-t.***, samb., **SEC.**, sep., sil., spig., spong., ***stann.***, staph., ***squil.***, **STRAM.**, ***sulph.***, **TAB.**, **VERAT.**, vip.
- lines, in - ars., lyc.
- lower jaw drawn backwards - bell.
- sleep, during - tab.
- to a point - brom.

DROPPING, corners of mouth - agar.
- jerks, pain, with - tell.

DRYNESS - **ARS.**, cimic., eup-per., hydr-ac., ***iod.***, jug-c., kali-c., merc-c., sulph.
- cheeks - euph.
- nose - carb-an., ***caust.***
- nose, wings - chlor., hell., ***sang-n.***

ECZEMA - alum., ***anac.***, ***ant-c.***, **ARS.**, bac., bar-c., ***bor.***, **CALC.**, ***calc-s.***, ***carb-ac.***, carb-v., ***caust.***, **CIC.**, clem., coll., corn., **CROT-T.**, cur., cycl., **DULC.**, ferr-i., ***fl-ac.***, **GRAPH.**, **HEP.**, hyper., ***iris***, ***kali-ar.***, kreos., lac-d., led., ***lyc.***, ***merc.***, merc-i-r., merc-p-r., ***mez.***, mur-ac., nat-m., ***petr.***, phos., **PSOR.**, ran-b., **RHUS-T.**, **SARS.**, ***sep.***, sil., staph., ***sul-i.***, **SULPH.**, sul-ac., ***syph.***, vinc., ***viol-t.***
- bleeding - alum., ***ars.***, dulc., ***hep.***, ***lyc.***, ***merc.***, ***petr.***, psor., sep., ***sulph.***
- burning - ***cic.***, ***viol-t.***
- ear, spreading from - ars.
- fetid - lyc.
- heat of stove - **ANT-C.**
- honey, like dried - ***ant-c.***, **CIC.**, mez.
- margins of hair - graph., mez., **SULPH.**
- moist - ***cic.***, **GRAPH.**, **LYC.**, ***petr.***, ***psor.***, ***rhus-t.***
- mouth, around - ant-c., ***mez.***, mur-ac., ***nat-m.***
- nursing mothers, in - sep.
- occiput, spreading from - ***lyc.***, sil.

eczema, chin - bor., ***cic.***, graph., ***merc-i-r.***, phos., rhus-t., sep.

EMACIATION - acet-ac., agar., alum., anac., ars., ars-i., bar-c., ***calc.***, carb-v., chin-s., cupr., ferr., ***guai.***, hura, iod., kali-bi., kali-i., ***lac-d.***, merc-c., mez., naja, nat-c., nat-m., nat-p., nux-m., plb., ***psor.***, ***sel.***, ***sep.***, sil., staph., sulph., sumb., tab., ***tarent.***, ***verat.***
- face and hands, of - grat., sel.
- neuralgia, after - plb.

EPULIS - thuj.

ERUPTIONS - agar., ail., ***alum.***, ambr., ***am-c.***, ***am-m.***, **ANT-C.**, ***ant-s.***, ***ant-t.***, apis, arg-m., arg-n., arn., ***ars.***, ars-i., asc-t., ***aur.***, aur-m., ***bar-c.***, ***bar-m.***, ***bell.***, berb., bor., ***bov.***, brom., ***bry.***, cadm-s., **CALC.**, ***calc-f.***, ***calc-p.***, ***calc-s.***, canth., caps., carb-an., ***carb-s.***, ***carb-v.***, **CAUST.**,

ERUPTIONS - cham., chel., chin-s., ***cic.***, cinnb., ***cist.***, clem., coloc., com., ***con.***, crot-h., ***crot-t.***, **DULC.**, elaps, eug., euph., ***fago.***, ferr-ma., ***fl-ac.***, gels., ***graph.***, guai., hell., ***hep.***, hydr., ign., iod., ip., kali-ar., ***kali-bi.***, **KALI-BR.**, **KALI-C.**, kali-chl., ***kali-i.***, kali-p., ***kali-s.***, **KREOS.**, lac-c., ***lach.***, lac-ac., **LED.**, ***lyc.***, mag-c., ***mag-m.***, mang., med., **MERC.**, merc-c., **MEZ.**, morph., ***mur-ac.***, ***nat-a.***, ***nat-c.***, **NAT-M.**, nat-p., nat-s., nicc., ***nit-ac.***, nux-v., pall., par., **PETR.**, ***ph-ac.***, ***phos.***, phyt., pic-ac., plan., **PSOR.**, **PULS.**, **RHUS-T.**, ***rhus-v.***, ruta., sang., sars., seneg., **SEP.**, sel., ***sil.***, spong., ***staph.***, **SULPH.**, sul-ac., tarent., ter., thuj., urt-u., valer., ***verat.***, ***viol-o.***, zinc.
- biting - bry., merc., nat-m., plat., sil.
- blackish - ars., spig.
- bleeding when scratched - ***merc.***, ***mez.***, par., ***petr.***, ***rhus-t.***, ***sulph.***
  - bleeding when touched, on nose - ***brom.***, ***merc.***
- blotches - alumn., apis, arg-n., ars., bar-c., calc., canth., ***carb-an.***, carb-v., chel., con., cop., dig., dulc., elaps, ***fl-ac.***, ***graph.***, ***guai.***, hell., ***hep.***, iod., ***kali-bi.***, kali-c., ***kali-i.***, lach., ***led.***, ***lyc.***, mag-c., mag-m., merc., nat-c., nux-v., op., ***phos.***, phyt., puls., rhus-r., ***rhus-t.***, sabin., sep., sulph., sumb., viol-t.
  - chin - bry., carb-an., euph., hep., mag-m., olnd.
  - forehead - nat-c.
  - itching - graph., sep.
  - menses, before, agg. - mag-m.
  - night agg. - ***mag-m.***
  - warmth of bed agg. - mag-m.
  - washing, after - am-c., phyt.
- brownish - dulc.
- burning - alum., am-m., ***anac.***, ant-c., apis, ***ars.***, bar-c., calc., ***caust.***, chin-s., ***cic.***, euphr., graph., kali-c., led., mag-m., merc., nat-m., phos., rat., ***rhus-t.***, samb., ***sars.***, seneg., ***sep.***, staph., sulph.
  - cannot sleep without cold applications - am-m.
  - open air, when in - ***led.***
  - scratched, when - nat-s., sars.
  - wet, when - euphr.
- carbuncles on chin - ***lyc.***
- cold, air agg. - ***ars.***, dulc.
- confluent - carb-v., cic.
- coppery - ***ars.***, **ARS-I.**, ***aur.***, benz-ac., calc., **CARB-AN.**, ***graph.***, ***hydrc.***, ***kali-i.***, ***lyc.***, merc., ***psor.***, rhus-t., ruta., verat.
  - chin, about - verat.
  - forehead - ***carb-an.***, ***lyc.***
- corrosive - dig.
- coryza, with - mez.
- crusty - ***anan.***, ***ant-c.***, **ARS.**, bar-c., bar-m., **CALC.**, ***carb-s.***, ***caust.***, ***chel.***, ***cic.***, ***cist.***, ***clem.***, ***con.***, **DULC.**, elaps, fl-ac., ***graph.***, ***hep.***, hyper., jug-c., ***kali-bi.***, lappa-a., ***led.***, ***lith.***, ***lyc.***, ***merc.***, merc-i-r., **MEZ.**, ***mur-ac.***, **PETR.**, ph-ac., ***psor.***, **RHUS-T.**, sars., ***sulph.***, sul-ac., syph., thuj., vac., ***viol-t.***, zinc.

ERUPTIONS, general
crusty, black - ***ars.***
cheek - ***ant-c., lyc.***
chin - ***cic.,*** **DULC.,** ***graph., mez., sep., sil., sulph.,*** syph.
chin, elevated white scabs - ***mez.***
forehead - ***ars., calc., dulc., mur-ac.***
greenish yellow - calc., ***merc., petr.***
offensive - ***psor.***
serpiginous - sulph.
white - ***mez.***
yellow - ***ant-c., calc., cic.,*** **DULC.,** ***hyper., merc., mez.,*** ph-ac., sulph., ***viol-t.***
zygoma - ars., ***cist.,*** mag-m.
desquamating - apis, ***ars., bell.,*** canth., chin-s., hydr., ***kali-ar.,*** lach., ***merc.,*** ol-an., phos., ***psor.,*** puls., ***rhus-t.,*** rhus-v., ***sulph.,*** thuj.
yellow, spot - kali-c.
dry - **ARS.,** kali-i., led., ***lyc.,*** psor., ***sep.***
elevations - bell., cic., cop., nat-a., pic-ac.
indurated - rhus-v.
reddish - phos., pic-ac., rhus-v.
excoriating - ***graph.,*** hell., **MERC.,** ***mez.,*** **PETR.,** ***phos., psor., sulph.,*** viol-t.
chin - ant-c., hep., mang., verat.
fissures - calc., **GRAPH.,** ***merc.,*** nicc., nit-ac., ***petr., psor.,*** sil., sulph.
bleeding - petr.
furuncles - alum., ***ant-c.,*** calc-p., ***hep., led.,*** med.
furfuraceous, in whiskers - kali-ar.
granular, honey colored, chin - ant-c.
hard - anac., crot-h., mag-c., puls., verat.
itching - agar., am-c., ***anac., ant-c., ars.,*** bufo, ***calc., calc-s.,*** caps., ***carb-s., caust.,*** chel., chin-s., ***cic.,*** con., dig., euphr., ***graph., jug-c., kali-bi., kali-c., kali-i.,*** led., ***lyc., mag-m., merc.,*** **MEZ.,** nat-c., ***nat-m.,*** nicc., ***nit-ac., olnd., petr., phos.,*** psor., **RHUS-T.,** sanic., ***sars.,*** **SEP.,** squil., stann., staph., stram., **SULPH.,** teucr., thuj., ***viol-t.,*** zinc.
chin - dulc., lyc., mag-m., nat-c., nat-m., nux-v., par., sars., sep., thuj., zinc.
forehead - caps., ***sars.***
night agg. - ***mez., sulph., viol-t.***
scratching unchanged by - am-c.
warmth agg. - ***ant-c.,*** euphr., ***mez., psor., sulph.,*** teucr.
leprous, spots - ***ant-t., graph.,*** phos., **SEC.**
leprous spots, chin, on - calc.
menses, during - am-c., calc., dulc., eug., graph., kali-c., nux-m., psor., sang., sars.
before - dulc., ***mag-m.,*** nat-m., nux-m., sars., sep.
menstrual troubles, with - sang.
miliary - ail., anan., ars., bell., cham., euphr., hep., hura, ip., manc., par., phos., sarr., tab., tarent., verat.

ERUPTIONS, general
moist - ant-c., ***ars., ars-i., calc., carb-s., carb-v.,*** caust., cham., cic., ***clem.,*** con., **DULC., GRAPH.,** ***hep.,*** kreos., **LYC.,** ***merc.,*** **MEZ.,** nat-a., nat-c., nit-ac., olnd., ***petr.,*** ph-ac., ***psor.,*** **RHUS-T.,** sars., ***sep., sil.,*** squil., ***sulph., thuj.,*** vinc., ***viol-t.***
fetid - cic., merc.
scratching, after - ***kali-c., sars.,*** sulph.
yellow - lyc., rhus-t., ***viol-t.***
mouth, around, (see Mouth)
night, agg. - ***ars., mag-m.***
warm room agg. - ***mag-m.***
nodular - bry., ***chel.,*** cic., kali-ar., rhus-t.
forehead - ars.
painful - alum., apis, ***bell., berb.,*** calc., cic., clem., eug., led., phos., plat., sep., staph., **SULPH.**
chin - **SULPH.**
night - viol-t.
touched, when - ant-c., bell., ***hep.,*** lach., led., nit-ac., par., sabad., sep., stann., sulph., valer.
papular - aur., bor., ***calc.,*** carb-v., ***crot-h.,*** dig., dulc., ***gels., hydrc., kali-c., kali-i., lyc.,*** ol-an., ***petr., pic-ac.,*** sep., sil., syph., zinc.
chin, on - calc., caust., ***crot-h., lyc.,*** merc., nit-ac., ***sars.***
painful - ***calc.***
patches - calc., ***graph.,*** lac-c., ***kali-bi., merc., nux-m.,*** phos., puls., sec., sep., stram., sumb.
menses, during - nux-m.
pimples - agar., alum., am-m., ambr., anan., ***ant-c.,*** apis, ***ars., ars-i.,*** arum-t., aster., ***aur.,*** bar-c., bar-m., ***bell.,*** berb., bor., ***bov.,*** **CALC.,** calc-p., ***calc-s.,*** **CARB-AN.,** ***carb-s., carb-v.,*** **CAUST.,** ***chel., cic.,*** clem., coloc., ***con.,*** crot-h., dros., **EUG.,** gels., ***glon.,*** **GRAPH.,** ***hep.,*** hura, hydr., ***hydrc.,*** indg., iod., jug-r., ***kali-ar.,*** **KALI-C.,** kali-chl., kali-n., kali-s., **KREOS.,** lach., ***led.,*** **LYC.,** lyss., ***mag-m.,*** meny., meph., **MERC.,** mosch., ***mur-ac.,*** nat-a., ***nat-c.,*** **NAT-M.,** ***nat-p., nat-s.,*** **NIT-AC., NUX-V.,** ol-an., pall., par., petr., ***ph-ac., phos., psor.,*** puls., ***rhus-t.,*** sabin., sanic., ***sars., sep., sil.,*** sol-t-ae., ***staph.,*** **SULPH.,** syph., tarax., tarent., thuj., til., vinc., zinc.
bluish - lyss.
burning - aphis., ***cic.,*** graph., kali-c., nat-c., sars.
burning, when touched - coloc., nat-s.
chin - alum., ambr., ant-c., aster., bor., calc., ***chel., clem.,*** crot-h., con., dulc., ferr-m., ***hep.,*** kali-chl., ***lyc.,*** mag-c., merc., nat-c., nat-s., nit-ac., par., ph-ac., ***psor., rhus-t.,*** sars., ***sep.,*** sil., thuj., zinc.
cold air agg. - ***ars.***
confluent - ***cic., psor.,*** tarent.
copper colored - kali-i.
elevated margins - verat.

ERUPTIONS, general
pimples, greenish - cupr.
inflamed - bry., ***chel.,*** sars., stann., sulph.
insects, as from - ant-c.
itching - agar., ***ant-c.,*** asc-t., calc., ***caust., con.,*** **GRAPH.,** ***hep., mur-ac.,*** ol-an., pall., ***psor.,*** sars., ***sep.,*** stann., staph., ***til.,*** zinc.
itching, moist after scratching - **GRAPH.**
itching, when warm - ***ant-c.,*** cocc., ***til.***
liver spot, on - con.
lower jaw - par., ***sil.***
menses, before, agg. - dulc., ***mag-m.***
menses, during - dulc., eug., graph., kali-c.
night agg. - ***mag-m.***
purplish halo with - **MERC.**
red - ph-ac., phos., zinc.
scratching, after - alum.
stitching - staph.
warm room agg. - ***mag-m.***
washing agg. - nux-v., ***sulph.***
whiskers - ***agar.,*** ambr., calc., calc-s., graph., lach., nit-ac., pall., sulph.
white - coloc., graph., mag-m., zinc.
pustules - am-c., ***anac.,*** **ANT-C.,** ant-t., arn., ***ars.,*** **AUR., BELL.,** bov., ***calc.,*** calc-p., calc-s., carb-s., ***carb-v., caust.,*** chel., chin., **CIC.,** cimic., clem., ***con., crot-t.,*** cund., dros., dulc., eug., eup-per., graph., grat., ***hep., hydr.,*** hyos., ind., ***iris,*** jug-c., ***kali-bi.,*** kali-c., ***kali-br., kali-i.,*** kali-n., kreos., lach., lyc., mag-c., mag-m., mag-s., ***merc., mez., nat-p., nit-ac.,*** nux-m., pall., ph-ac., phos., psor., puls., rhus-t., sars., sulph., tarax., thuj., **TUB.,** verat., ***viol-t.,*** zinc.
cheeks - am-c., calc., carb-an., iris, ***kali-bi.,*** lyc., pall.
cheeks, menses, during - am-c.
chin - am-c., camph., caust., ***clem., graph.,*** hyos., ***kali-bi.,*** kali-i., mang., merc., ***mez.,*** nit-ac., nux-m., olnd., petr., ***psor.,*** rhus-t., sars., ***tub., viol-t., zinc.***
confluent - ***cic.***
corners, of the mouth - bar-c.
forehead - am-c., anac., ars., carb-an., chel., chin., clem., cycl., eup-per., ***kali-bi.,*** kali-c., kali-p., ***merc.,*** mur-ac., ***nat-m.,*** rhod., sars.
itching - euph., ph-ac., sars.
menses, during - am-c.
sanious - iris.
ulcers, terminating in - crot-t.
red - alum., ant-c., aur., calc., calc-p., carb-an., carb-s., caust., cham., cic., euphr., fago., hyper., ***lac-c., led.,*** nit-ac., par., ***petr.,*** phos., psor., sep., sulph.
chin - mag-m., verat.
mouth, around - verat.

ERUPTIONS, general
rough - alum., anac., bar-c., ***berb-a.,*** kali-c., kalm., led., nat-m., ***petr.,*** puls., rhus-t., rhus-v., sep., stram., sulph., teucr.
forehead, on - pall., rhus-t., sars., sep., sulph., teucr.
forehead, on, spots - sars.
lips - merc., sulph., tab.
morning - nat-m.
mouth, around - anac., ars.
red - phos., sep., sulph.
summer - kalm.
scabby, (see crusty)
scurfy, scaly - alum., anac., **ANT-C.,** ant-t., **ARS.,** ***ars-i.,*** aur., **BAR-C.,** bell., ***bufo, calc.,*** calc-s., carb-an., carb-s., **CAUST.,** chin-s., ***cic.,*** coloc., crot-t., dulc., ***graph., hep., kali-ar.,*** kreos., **LACH.,** led., ***lyc.,*** mag-m., ***merc.,*** merc-i-f., ***mez.,*** mur-ac., nit-ac., ***nux-v., petr., ph-ac., phos., phyt.,*** plat., **PSOR.,** rhus-t., rhus-v., sars., **SEP.,** ***sil.,*** sulph., thuj., verat., ***viol-t.,*** zinc.
cheek - anac., bell., calc., ***cic.,*** kreos., lach., ***lyc.***
chin - am-c., ***cic.,*** dulc., ***graph.,*** kreos., merc., sep.
whiskers - calc., lach.
white - anac., ***ars.***
yellow - ***merc.***
smarting, (see Burning) - cic., ip., rhod., verat.
spots - acon., alum., ambr., am-c., ars., bar-c., bell., berb., bry., ***calc.,*** carb-an., carb-v., colch., croc., ferr., ferr-m., hyos., lyc., ***merc., nat-c.,*** nit-ac., par., phos., samb., sars., **SEP.,** sulph., tub., vip., zinc.
copper-colored - benz-ac., ***carb-an.,*** lyc., nit-ac.
red - ***berb-a.,*** euph., kali-bi., ***kali-c.,*** oena., petr.
yellow - nat-c., ***sep.***
stinging, painful - clem., dulc., led., plat., squil., staph.
suppurating - **ANT-C., CALC-S.,** ***cic.,*** lyc., ***psor., rhus-t.***
syphilitic - ***ars-i., aur., cinnb., fl-ac., hep., kali-bi.,*** **KALI-I.,** kreos., ***lach., lyc.,*** **MERC., MERC-C.,** ***nit-ac., phyt.,*** sep., ***sil., sulph.,*** **SYPH.**
warmth, agg. - euphr., mez., psor., sulph., teucr.
amel. - ***ars.***
washing, agg. - nux-v., sulph.
eruptions, cheeks - agar., alum., am-c., anac., **ANT-C.,** ***bell., bov.,*** bry., ***calc.,*** carb-an., ***caust.,*** cham., cic., con., dig., ***dulc.,*** **EUPH.,** ferr-ma., ***kali-chl.,*** kali-i., **KREOS.,** ***lach.,*** laur., ***lyc.,*** mag-m., merc., merc-i-r., mez., nat-c., ***nat-m.,*** nit-ac., phos., **RHUS-T.,** ***sep., sil.,*** spong., **STAPH.,** stront-c., ***verat.,*** verb., viol-t.
tubercles, cheeks, small - asaf.

eruptions, chin - alum., ambr., am-c., anac., ***ant-c.,*** arg-n., bor., ***bov., calc., carb-s.,*** carb-v., caust., ***chel., cic.,*** clem., cob., con., crot-h., crot-t., dig., ***dulc.,*** ferr-ma., ***graph., hep.,*** hydr., kali-bi., kali-c., kali-i., ***kreos., lach., lyc.,*** mag-c., manc., ***merc.,*** merc-i-r., ***mez.,*** nat-c., **NAT-M.,** nat-p., nat-s., nit-ac., nux-m., ***nux-v.,*** olnd., ***par.,*** ph-ac., phos., ***psor.,*** puls., **RHUS-T.,** sars., **SEP.,** ***sil.,*** spig., **SULPH.,** ***syph.,*** thuj., verat., viol-t., zinc.
painful - merc., rhus-t., sars., **SULPH.**
whiskers - ambr., ***calc.,*** graph., lach., nit-ac., thuj.

ERYSIPELAS - ail., anac-oc., anan., ***anthr.,*** **APIS,** arn., ars., ***astac., aur.,*** aur-m., **BELL.,** ***bor.,*** bufo, calc., ***camph., canth., carb-an.,*** carb-s., ***carb-v., caust., cham., chel., chin.,*** cinnb., cist., com., crot-h., crot-t., ***cupr.,*** dor., ***echi., euph.,*** gels., **GRAPH.,** gymn., ***hep.,*** hippoz., ***jug-c.,*** kali-ar., kali-c., kali-i., **LACH.,** ***led.,*** meph., ***mez.,*** naja, nat-s., ***nit-ac.,*** phos., plb., ***puls.,*** **RHUS-T.,** ***rhus-v.,*** sarr., sep., sol-t-ae., stram., ***sulph., sul-ac.,*** tep., ter., thuj.
bites of insects, from - ***led.***
ear, right, beginning in - sulph.
edematous - ars., **APIS,** chin., crot-t., hell., lyc., merc., ***rhus-t.,*** sulph., thuj.
erratic - arn., bell., mang., **PULS.,** rhus-t., sabin., sulph.
extending, to body - ***graph.***
to ear - ***jug-c.***
to head - ***chel.,*** op.
eye, around - acon., anac., **APIS,** ars., bell., com., ***graph., hep., led., merc., merc-c.,*** **RHUS-T.,** vesp.
gangrenous - **ARS.,** camph., **CARB-V.,** chin., ***hippoz.,*** **LACH.,** mur-ac., ***rhus-t.,*** **SEC.,** sil.
left - agn., ***bor., cham.,*** lach.
left, to right - lach., **RHUS-T.**
nursing, while - bor.
one side - apis, bor., nux-v., sep., ***stram.***
periodic - **APIS**
phlegmonous - ***acon., apis, arn., bell.,*** bry., bufo, carb-an., carb-s., cham., ***crot-h., hep., hippoz., graph.,*** **LACH.,** merc., phos., puls., **RHUS-T.,** sep., ***sil., sulph.***
pregnancy, during - ***bor.***
rays, spreading like - graph.
recurrent - **APIS,** ***crot-h.***
right - arund., ***bell.,*** stram.
right, to left - apis, arund., **GRAPH.,** lyc., sulph.
scalp, and face - ***lach.***
spots - ***apis.***
vesicular - ***ars.,*** bell., camph., canth., chin., cist., com., **EUPH.,** ***graph.,*** hep., lach., puls., ran-b., **RHUS-T.,** ***rhus-v.,*** sep., sulph., tep.

ERYTHEMA - ars-i., ***bell.,*** con., echi., ***graph.,*** nux-v.

EXCORIATED, menses, agg. - ***kreos.***
excoriated, corners of mouth - ant-c., ***ars.,*** **ARUM-T.,** bell., bov., brach., ***caust., cocc., cund., dios.,*** eup-per., form., ***hell.,*** ind., ip., ***lyc.,*** **MERC.,** mez., nat-c., nat-m., pall., phos., ***psor., sulph.,*** zinc.

EXOSTOSIS - ***aur-m.,*** calc-f., fl-ac., ***hecla.,*** phyt.
right, cheek bone - ***aur-m.***
lower, jaw - **CALC-F.**

EXPRESSION, facial
absent - camph., graph., mang.
anxious - **ACON., AETH.,** agar., **AIL.,** all-c., aloe, am-c., am-m., ***ant-t., apis,*** **ARS.,** ars-h., ***bapt.,*** bar-m., ***bell.,*** **BOR.,** ***cact., calc.,*** **CAMPH.,** cann-i., canth., carb-o., carb-s., ***carb-v., chel.,*** chin-a., **CHIN-S.,** chlol., cic., coff., colch., ***coloc., crot-h., cupr.,*** cupr-ar., ***cur., dig.,*** dulc., eup-per., ferr-m., iris, kali-ar., kali-bi., ***kalm.,*** **LAC-C.,** ***lat-m., lyc.,*** lyss., merc., merc-c., morph., mygal., naja, nit-ac., ***nux-v., plb.,*** sol-n., ***spig., spong., stram., stry., sulph.,*** sul-ac., **VERAT.,** vesp., vip., zinc.
cradle, when child is lifted from - calc.
croup, in - **SPONG.**
downward motion, during - **BOR.,** gels.
astonished - acon., bell., cann-s., carb-s., plb., stram.
besotted - ail., **BAPT.,** bell., ***bry., bufo,*** cench., ***cocc., crot-c., crot-h., gels., lach.,*** led., mur-ac., ***nux-m.,*** op., sol-n., ***stram.***
bewildered - ***aesc., bry.,*** carb-s., glon., ***lyc.,*** nux-m., ***ph-ac.,*** plb., ***stram.,*** zinc.
changed - acon., aeth., apis, arg-n., ***ars.,*** bell., bufo, ***camph.,*** caust., ***cham.,*** colch., ***cupr., gels., hell.,*** hyos., ign., lyc., mang., ***op.,*** ph-ac., phos., sec., squil., **STRAM.,** verat.
changing - squil.
childish - ***anac.,*** nux-m.
cold, distant - puls.
confused - ***aesc., ars., bufo,*** cupr-ac., hyos., **LYC.,** nat-m., phos., plb.
distressed - ***ail.,*** am-c., **ARS.,** ***aspar.,*** **CACT.,** ***crot-t.,*** cupr., ***iod., nux-m.,*** nux-v., phos., stry., ***stram.***
fierce - **BELL.,** hydr-ac., merc-i-r., op.
foolish - absin., acon., arg-n., ***bar-c.,*** **BUFO,** kali-br., ***lyc., phos., nux-m., stram.***
frightened - **ACON.,** apis, **ARS.,** atro., ***bapt., canth.,*** cimic., cocc., cupr., kali-ar., lyss., **PHOS.,** sol-n., **STRAM.,** stry., tab., tarent., vip., zinc.
aroused, when - ***ail.***
fuzzy - caust., psor.
haggard - am-c., **ARS.,** bell., ***camph.,*** canth., ***caps., carb-v.,*** colch., cupr., ***hydr., hyos.,*** kali-ar., **KALI-C.,** kali-p., ***lach.,*** merc., morph., naja, ***nat-m.,*** nit-ac., op., ox-ac., ***phos.,*** plb., sang., sec., ***sil.,*** staph., stram., tab., ***verat-v.***
happy - ***apis, op.***

EXPRESSION, facial

idiotic - **AGAR.**, ***calc.***, kali-br., ***lach.***, ***laur.***, ***lyc.***, plb., sec., stram., tarent., thuj.

incoherent - cub.

intoxicated - ***bufo***, cann-i., chlf., ***cocc.***, dor., eug., ***gels.***, hydr., hyos., kali-i., ***lach.***, ***led.***, merl., merc., mur-ac., ***nux-v.***, ***op.***, ruta., ***stram.***

less - kali-br., lycps.

looks, in a mirror, to see - nat-m.

mask-like - lycps., mang.

morose, and coughing - spong.

old looking - ***abrot.***, ***alum.***, ***ambr.***, **ARG-N.**, ***ars.***, ***ars-h.***, ***ars-i.***, ***aur-m.***, ***bar-c.***, **CALC.**, chlor., **CON.**, ***fl-ac.***, **GUAI.**, hydr-ac., ***iod.***, kali-fer., ***kreos.***, lyc., merc-c., **NAT-M.**, ol-j., **OP.**, plb., sanic., ***sars.***, ***sep.***, staph., ***sulph.***, syph., ter., tub.

few weeks old infant - op.

newborns, in - op.

sallow, and wrinkled - ***sep.***

pinched - ***acon.***, ***aeth.***, carb-an., ***carb-v.***, ***cina***, cocc., ***cupr.***, ferr., ***iod.***, kali-n., merc., phos., ***sec.***, staph., ***tab.***, ***verat.***, verat-v., zinc.

ridiculous, during sleep - hyos.

sickly - acon., aesc., aloe, alumn., ***anac.***, ***apis***, ***arg-n.***, **ARS.**, **ARS-H.**, ***ars-i.***, ***berb.***, bism., ***bor.***, ***calc.***, ***calc-p.***, cann-i., carb-ac., carb-an., carb-s., ***carb-v.***, carl., ***caust.***, ***chel.***, ***chin.***, chin-s., **CINA**, ***clem.***, colch., con., cop., corn., crot-h., cund., cupr., ***dig.***, ***eup-per.***, ***ferr.***, ferr-i., glon., ***gran.***, hura, ***iod.***, **IP.**, ***kali-ar.***, kali-bi., ***kali-c.***, kali-chl., kali-n., kali-p., kali-s., kreos., **LACH.**, lact., **LYC.**, ***mag-m.***, ***mang.***, ***merc.***, naja, ***nat-m.***, nat-s., nit-ac., nux-m., nux-v., op., ***ph-ac.***, ***phos.***, ***plb.***, phyt., psor., ptel., ***rhus-t.***, sep., ***sil.***, ***spig.***, ***stann.***, ***staph.***, ***sulph.***, tab., ***tub.***, thuj., til., zinc.

cough, during - cina.

evening - phos.

morning - sep.

sleepy - **CANN-I.**, laur., ***nux-m.***, **OP.**, phos., phys.

solemn, on waking - stram.

stupid - ***arg-n.***, ***arn.***, ***ars.***, ars-h., aster., bell., camph., **CANN-I.**, cann-s., chin-s., ***crot-c.***, cupr., ***ferr.***, ***gels.***, ***hell.***, hura, ***hydr.***, ***hyos.***, kali-br., lil-t., merc., ***nux-m.***, op., ox-ac., phos., phyt., plb., rhus-v., sec., ***stram.***, sulph., tab.

suffering - ***acon.***, aeth., ***am-c.***, ***anac.***, ***ant-t.***, arg-n., **ARS.**, ***bor.***, **CACT.**, ***calc-ar.***, ***canth.***, carb-s., ***carb-v.***, caust., ***chel.***, ***chin-s.***, ***cocc.***, coloc., ***colch.***, cupr., helon., hyper., kali-ar., kali-br., **KALI-C.**, kali-p., kali-s., ***kreos.***, ***lach.***, **LYSS.**, mag-c., ***mag-m.***, **MANG.**, ***mez.***, nat-m., nit-ac., ***nux-m.***, ph-ac., ***phos.***, ***phyt.***, plat., plb., ***puls.***, raph., sec., **SIL.**, stry., stram., **SULPH.**, sul-ac.

sullen - alum., mag-c., nux-v.

tired - acon., ***ars.***, cimic., hell., stram.

EXPRESSION, facial

vacant - ***anac.***, anan., arn., ***bell.***, ***camph.***, carb-s., cic., ***cocc.***, ***ferr.***, ***hell.***, hyos., ***kali-br.***, ***lach.***, ***mez.***, op., **PH-AC.**, ***phos.***, ***stram.***, sul-ac., zinc.

wild, (see Eyes)

withered - acon., cupr., kali-c., sep.

wretched - ars., nat-m.

young looking - puls., tub.

FEELING, face before attack - bufo.

FORMICATION - ***acon.***, acon-f., alum., agn., apis, arund., aster., bar-c., berb., brom., cadm-s., calad., calc., camph., coc-c., con., crot-c., ***crot-t.***, grat., gymn., lact., lachn., ***laur.***, lyss., mag-m., myric., nux-v., ol-an., ph-ac., **PLAT.**, **SEC.**, sul-ac., sulph., tab., thuj., til., urt-u.

following, pain - euph.

left - arg-n.

right side - alum., ***plat.***

formication, chin, on - stram.

formication, zygoma, towards - thuj.

FRECKLES - ***am-c.***, ***ant-c.***, ***calc.***, carc., ***dulc.***, ***graph.***, ***kali-c.***, **LYC.**, mur-ac., ***nat-c.***, ***nit-ac.***, ***nux-m.***, **PHOS.**, ***puls.***, ***sep.***, sil., sol., **SULPH.**, thuj.

FROWNING, (see Wrinkled)

FULLNESS - aeth., apis, cub., ferr., glon., kreos., lac-c., merc-c., nat-m., ox-ac., phos., plan., sang.

mental exertion, after - phos.

FUR, like, in hemiplegia - caust.

GANGRENE - merc., sul-ac.

erysipelas, gangrenous - **ARS.**, camph., **CARB-V.**, chin., ***hippoz.***, **LACH.**, mur-ac., ***rhus-t.***, **SEC.**, sil.

GLANDS, (see Swelling)

GLOWING, (see Discoloration)

GNAWING, pain - arg-m., bar-c., berb., eug., euph., ***glon.***, indg., lyc., lyss., ph-ac., stann., sulph.

mouth, around - puls.

right - ***lyc.***

right zygoma - ***lyss.***

GREASY - ***acet-ac.***, agar., apis, arg-n., ars., aspar., aur., ***bar-c.***, ***bry.***, bufo, calc., caust., ***chin.***, con., ferr-ar., hydr., iod., lyc., ***mag-c.***, med., ***merc.***, ***nat-m.***, phos., ***plb.***, ***psor.***, raph., ***rhus-t.***, sanic., ***sel.***, sep., sil., stram., sulph., thuj., ***tub.***

forehead - ***hydr.***, ***psor.***

HAIR, (see Generals, Hair)

chin, women in, on - ol-j.

growth of, child's face - calc., morg., nat-m., ol-j., psor., sulph., tarent., thuj., thyr., tub.

mustache, falling out, of - bar-c., kali-c., plb., sel.

women, in - cortico., nat-m., sep., thuj., thyr.

upper lip - ol-j.

HAIR, facial
whiskers, falling out, of - agar., ambr., anan., aur-m., ***calc.***, carb-an., ***graph.***, ***kali-c.***, ***nat-c.***, ***nat-m.***, nit-ac., ***ph-ac.***, plb., sanic., sil.
grief, after - ***ph-ac.***

HAIRS, sensation of - carl., chlol., ***graph.***, laur., sulph., sumb.

HARDNESS, (see Indurations)

HEAT - acet-ac., ***acon.***, ***aesc.***, ***aeth.***, ***agar.***, agn., ***ail.***, ***all-c.***, aloe, ***alum.***, ***am-c.***, ***am-m.***, ***aml-n.***, ***anac.***, ***ant-c.***, ***ant-t.***, ***apis***, aran., ***arg-m.***, arg-n., ***arn.***, ars., asaf., asar., atro., aur., ***bapt.***, bar-c., bar-m., **BELL.**, benz-ac., berb., ***bov.***, **BROM.**, **BRY.**, ***calc.***, calc-ar., ***calc-p.***, calc-s., calad., camph., cann-s., ***canth.***, ***caps.***, ***carb-an.***, carb-s., carb-v., card-m., cedr., **CHAM.**, ***chel.***, ***chin.***, ***chin-s.***, chlol., cimic., **CINA**, ***cinnb.***, cist., ***clem.***, coc-c., ***cocc.***, ***coff.***, colch., coloc., ***con.***, ***cor-r.***, corn., ***croc.***, crot-t., cupr., cycl., dig., ***dros.***, dulc., ***elaps***, equis., euph., euphr., eup-per., fago., ***ferr.***, ferr-ar., ferr-ma., ***ferr-p.***, ***fl-ac.***, form., ***gels.***, ***glon.***, gran., **GRAPH.**, ***grat.***, ***guai.***, ***gymn.***, hell., **HEP.**, hipp., hydr., hyos., hyper., hura, ***ign.***, ind., indg., inul., ***ip.***, jab., jatr., ***kali-ar.***, ***kali-bi.***, kali-c., kali-i., kali-n., kali-p., ***kreos.***, ***lach.***, lact., laur., ***led.***, lil-t., ***lyc.***, lyss., mag-c., manc., ***mang.***, meny., ***merc.***, merc-c., ***mez.***, morph., mosch., mur-ac., myric., narcot., naja, nat-a., ***nat-c.***, ***nat-m.***, nat-p., ***nit-ac.***, ***nux-m.***, **NUX-V.**, olnd., **OP.**, ***ox-ac.***, paeon., par., ***petr.***, phel., ***ph-ac.***, ***phos.***, ***phyt.***, pin-s., plan., ***plat.***, plb., psor., ptel., **PULS.**, ran-b., rat., ***rhod.***, ***rhus-t.***, ***rhus-v.***, rumx., ruta., sabad., samb., ***sang.***, sars., seneg., sep., ***sil.***, spig., spong., squil., ***stann.***, staph., ***stront-c.***, **STRAM.**, stry., ***sulph.***, ***sul-ac.***, ***tab.***, tarent., ***tarax.***, ***thuj.***, til., **TUB.**, ***urt-u.***, ***verat.***, ***xan.***, zinc.
afternoon - agar., alum., anac., **ARUM-T.**, bar-c., berb., cann-s., ***carb-an.***, carb-s., chel., chin-s., com., dig., gels., graph., grat., hyper., ip., kali-bi., lyc., mag-c., mag-m., mag-s., nat-m., nit-ac., petr., phos., ph-ac., phys., phyt., ***rhus-t.***, ruta, stront-c., zing.
1 p.m. - equis.
2 p.m. - ***chel.***, grat., lyc., phys.
2:30 p.m. - gels.
2 to 3 p.m. - phos.
3 p.m. - chin., sol-n.
4 p.m. - agar., anac., sol-t-ae.
5 p.m. - kali-bi., ***rhus-t.***, zing.
6 p.m. - cann-i., cedr., ferr-p.
air, in open - dig., hep., mur-ac., sulph., valer.
amel., in open - am-m., phos., stann.
side, exposed to, in open - ph-ac., viol-t.
alternating, with
chilliness - caust.
cold body - stram.
headache - coc-c.
anxiety, during - **CARB-V.**, graph.
bed, in - nux-v., sep., verat.
amel. - alum.

HEAT,
burning - acon., am-m., ant-t., apis, aran., ***bapt.***, **BELL.**, bor., ***bry.***, camph., caps., ***cham.***, chel., **CINA**, cist., ***clem.***, cocc., croc., grat., hyos., ign., iod., mag-c., mang., ***nat-c.***, nat-p., nux-v., paeon., petr., phos., plat., ***puls.***, rhus-t., ptel., sabad., samb., ***sang.***, sep., stront-c., sulph., tab., thuj., verat.
left side, burning, and redness of - alum., asaf., lac-c., murx., nat-m., ol-an., ph-ac., spig.
cheeks - ang., hell., hep., mang., rheum, sil., staph.
chill, during - acon., agar., ambr., alum., anac., ***apis***, **ARN.**, ars., aur., bell., ***bry.***, ***calc.***, ***calc-p.***, carb-s., cedr., **CHAM.**, chin., cina, **COFF.**, coloc., con., dig., ***dros.***, **FERR.**, gels., graph., hell., ***hyos.***, jatr., kreos., lach., led., lyc., ***merc.***, mez., ***mur-ac.***, nat-c., nat-m., nat-p., **NUX-V.**, **OLND.**, ph-ac., ***phos.***, plat., ***puls.***, ran-b., ruta., ***rhus-t.***, sabad., samb., sars., seneg., spong., staph., ***stram.***, sulph., tub.
after - ars., petr., sep., staph., sulph.
before - calc., chin., lyc., meny., staph., sulph.
chilliness, during - alum., asar., bor., dig., ferr., gels., ***hell.***, kali-c., **MERC.**, ***nux-v.***, ol-an., ran-b., samb., squil.
after - kali-c.
chin - canth., euphr., nat-m.
coffee, after - lyss.
cold, body, with heat in face - ***arn.***, ***calc-p.***, cann-s., ***cham.***, ***chin.***, dig., ***led.***, nit-ac., ***stram.***, tab., trom.
feet, with - acon., ars., aur., bell., caps., gels., graph., ign., kali-c., mag-c., petr., phos., samb., sep., sil., **STRAM.**, verat.
fingertips, with - thuj.
hands - **ARN.**, ars., asaf., aur., camph., caps., chin., con., cycl., ***dros.***, euph., euphr., graph., hyos., ign., kali-n., nat-c., nit-ac., phos., plat., ruta., sabin., sil., **STRAM.**, sumb., thuj.
limbs - ***arn.***, bell., ***calc-p.***, cham., chin., hell., ***stram.***
nose, with - arn.
one cheek cold and red, the other hot and pale - ***mosch.***
one side, the other hot - ***acet-ac.***, ***acon.***, **CHAM.**, **IP.**, ***kali-c.***, ***lach.***, ***mosch.***, ***nux-v.***
room, in - ***cocc.***, nat-c.
to touch - spig.
coryza, during - ars-m., **ARUM-T.**, croc., graph., **NUX-V.**
coughing, on - sulph.
daytime - petr., sulph.
dinner after and during - am-c., ***am-m.***, caps., carb-an., ***cor-r.***, grat., hell., hura, mag-m., phyt., ran-b., tell.
dinner during - am-c., am-m., mag-m.
drinking, after - **CHAM.**, cocc.
warm drinks, after - sabad.

HEAT,

eating, after - am-c., am-m., anac., ***asaf., calc.,*** carl., caust., **CHAM.,** ***coff.,*** cor-r., ***lyc.,*** merc., nat-m., nit-ac., nux-v., ***petr.,*** phos., phyt., sil., sep., sulph., viol-t.
eating, while - am-c., nat-c.
eruption, before - nat-m.
evening - ***acon.,*** agar., alum., anac., ***ang.,*** ant-t., apis, ***arn.,*** ars., aur., bry., ***calc-p.,*** carb-an., carb-s., ***cham.,*** chin-s., con., croc., dig., euphr., fago., fl-ac., graph., gran., ***guai.,*** **HEP.,** hura, ip., lob., lyc., mag-c., mez., naja, nat-c., nat-m., nat-p., nit-ac., nux-v., oena., ph-ac., phos., plat., puls., ran-s., rhus-t., rumx., sabad., sep., sil., ***sulph.,*** thuj., verat., zinc., zinc-s.
6 p.m. - cann-i., cedr., chin-s., ferr-p.
6 to 7 p.m. - phos.
7 p.m. - ***hep.***
7 to 8 p.m. - ars.
9 p.m. - ars., hura
10 p.m. - ***chr-ac.***
bed, in - sep.
chilliness, during - apis, graph.
lying, after - am-m., asar., nux-v.
sleep, before - ph-ac.
exertion, during - am-c., spig., spong., squil.
faintness, with - petr.
flashes - ***acon., aesc.,*** agar., alum., ***ambr., arg-m.,*** ars., asaf., bufo, ***cact.,*** calc., calc-s., camph., carb-ac., carb-an., **CARB-S.,** carl., cedr., cham., ***chel.,*** cic., cimic., ***cist.,*** clem., coc-c., ***cocc.,*** coff., colch., crot-c., crot-h., cub., dig., dros., ferr., ferr-ar., ferr-p., ***glon.,*** **GRAPH.,** hep., hydrc., inul., ***kali-bi.,*** kali-c., kali-chl., kali-p., kali-s., ***kreos.,*** **LACH.,** lob., **LYC.,** mang., med., meny., nit-ac., nux-v., ***petr.,*** ph-ac., ***phos.,*** plb., podo., ***psor.,*** ran-s., rhus-t., sabad., sabin., seneg., **SEP.,** ***sil.,*** spig., spong., ***stann.,*** stront-c., **SULPH.,** ***sul-ac.,*** tarent., tell., ***ter.,*** teucr., ***thuj.,*** til., valer.
afternoon - cedr., seneg.
alternating with chills - cedr., petr.
chilliness, with - nit-ac., petr., puls., sulph.
coughing - petr.
evening - alum., arn., cedr., nit-ac., nux-v., petr.
6 p.m. - cedr.
left - ***lac-d.,*** sulph.
menopause, during - aml-n., ***graph., kali-bi.,*** **LACH.,** ***lyc., psor.,*** **SUL-AC.,** ***ter.***
morning - lyc.
motion, on - ***stann.***
shivering, with - **SULPH.**
sudden - mang.
headache, with - agar., aloe, ang., aran., bell., calc., **CHIN-S.,** cop., ***glon.,*** grat., lac-ac., lith., nat-m., puls., rumx., ruta, sang., ***spong.,*** viol-t., xan., zing.
heart, constriction of - hydrc.
internal - chin., con., squil.
labor, during - ***arn., bell., coff., gels., op.***

HEAT,

left - alum., alumn., arg-n., arn., bor., euphr., inul., ***lac-d., olnd.,*** ph-ac., raph., verat.
lying, while - mang., phos., petr., plb.
after lying down - am-m., asar., ***cham.,*** nux-v.
maniacal rage, with - ***acon.,*** **BELL.,** kali-c., lach., lyc., merc., op., puls., ***verat.***
menopause, during - bell., carc., glon., kali-br.
menses, during - nat-m.
before - alum., lyc.
mental exertion - agar., ***am-c.,*** berb., lyc., lyss., tub.
midnight - alum., nat-m., sulph.
after - sulph.
morning - ail., bar-c., chel., croc., cycl., ferr., hep., kali-c., kali-n., nit-ac., nux-v., phos., ph-ac., ***sep.,*** sulph., til., verat.
8 a.m. - asaf., myric.
9 a.m. - asaf., lyc.
9 a.m. to 4 p.m. - lyc.
11 a.m. - equis., sol-n.
forenoon - lact., lyc., nux-m., ox-ac., zinc.
rising, on - coloc., lyc., nux-v., rhod.
until 3 p.m. - stront.
motion, during - chin., spig.
after - **SPONG.**
agg. - nux-v., spig.
movements, of first of child - sulph.
night - aloe, **HEP.,** ***mez.,*** ph-ac., rhus-v., sars.
waking, on - am-c., tarax.
noon - lyc., mag-c., sep., ***spig.***
nose, around - rheum.
blowing, amel. - acon.
one-sided - arn., asar., bar-c., benz-ac., cimic., chin., coff., ign., kali-c., lac-c., lac-d., mag-arct., murx., phos., spong., stann., sulph., upa., viol-t.
other side cold - cham., dros., ip.
pains, with - ars.
painful, part - spig.
palpitation during - ***arg-n., calc-ar., glon.,*** kali-n., mag-m.
parotid, gland - brom.
periodic - aloe, phos.
prickly - bell.
reading, while - arg-m.
right - alum., cham., lyss., nat-m., nicc., puls.
right, then left - brom.
rising, from a seat - nat-c.
room, entering, from open air, on - **CHIN.**
room, in - am-m., kali-n.,
sensation of - ang., bar-ac., ***bell.,*** euphr., hyper., mag-m., mang., ***merc.,*** nit-ac., petr., plat., rhus-t., stront-c., tarax., thuj.
when cold to touch - chin., grat.
shuddering, with - ars., thuj.
side, affected - tub.
not lain on - ph-ac., viol-t.
sitting, while - calc., carb-v., con., ferr-p., phos., viol-t., **VALER.**
sleep, during - meny.

HEAT,
smoking - ***calad.***
sneezing, when - nux-v., rhod.
standing, while - mang.
stool, during - gran., hep., merc.
after - caust.
stooping, after - rhus-t.
sudden - alum., euphr.
supper, after - alum., anac., ang., carb-v., chin-s.
symptoms, before other - bell., graph.
talking, after - fl-ac., sep., squil.
toothache, with - ferr-p., graph., nat-m., phos., sil., stann., staph.
vexation, after - ***cham., phos.***
waking, on - alum., bry., cham., nit-ac., sulph.
walking, while - mang., nux-v., stront-c., ***sulph.,*** tarax.
after - sep.
air, in open - ph-ac., tarax.
amel. - sabad.
warm, room - hyos., ***puls.***
wash, in cold water, desire to - ***fl-ac.***
washing, with cold water, after - camph., phos., sil.
wine, after - fl-ac.
writing, while - chin-s.
yawning, after - calc.

HEAVINESS, feeling - alum., cham., iod., kali-i., nicc.

HERPES - agar., alum., ***am-c.,*** am-m., anac., ***anan., ars., bar-c.,*** bell., ***bov.,*** bry., bufo, ***calc.,*** calc-f., ***calc-s.,*** caps., ***carb-an., carb-s., carb-v.,*** caust., chel., ***cic.,*** coloc., ***con.,*** crot-t., ***dulc.,*** elaps, ***graph., hep.,*** kali-ar., ***kali-bi., kali-c., kali-i.,*** kali-s., kreos., **LACH., LED.,** ***lyc., merc., nat-a., nat-c.,*** **NAT-M.,** ***nat-s.,*** nicc., ***nit-ac.,*** petr., ph-ac., phos., ***psor.,*** **RHUS-T.,** sabad., sarr., **SEP.,** ***sil.,*** spong., ***sulph.,*** tarent., thuj.
above, lips - phos.
mealy - **ARS.,** bry., cic., kreos., ***lyc.,*** merc., nit-ac., sulph., thuj.
mouth, around - am-c., anac., ars., ***bor.,*** cic., con., ***hep.,*** kreos., mag-c., med., nat-c., **NAT-M.,** ***par.,*** phos., ***rhus-t., sep.,*** sulph.
cutting - phos.
sharp, stitching - phos.
mouth, corners - carb-v., ***lyc.,*** med., phos., ph-ac., sep., ***sulph.***
corners, below - ***calc-f., nat-m.***
nose - **AETH.,** aloe, aur., ***calc.,*** chel., graph., gins., iod., lyc., ***nat-c., nat-m., nit-ac.,*** ph-ac., ***rhus-t., sep.,*** sil., spig., sulph.
nose, across the - sep., ***sulph.***
scurfy - anac., anan., calc., ***graph.,*** kreos., led., lyc., phos., ***rhus-t.,*** sep., ***sulph.***
whiskers - agar., calc., lach., ***nat-m., nit-ac.,*** sil.
whiskers, wing of nose - ***nit-ac.***

herpes, cheeks - ambr., alum., am-c., anac., ant-t., bov., caust., chel., **CON.,** dulc., graph., hep., kali-i., kreos., lach., merc., nat-m., nicc., ph-ac., sars., sil., ***spong.,*** staph., stront-c., thuj.
herpes, chin - am-c., ***bov.,*** carb-v., chel., dulc., ***nat-m.,*** nux-v., ph-ac., sars., ***sil.***
herpes, zoster, burning and itching, with - ***mez., rhus-t.***
facial neuralgia, with - mez., ***kalm., rhus-t.***

HIPPOCRATIC, (see Sunken) - acon., **AETH.,** agar., ***am-c., ant-c.,*** **ANT-T., ARS.,** asc-t., ***camph.,*** canth., carb-h., **CARB-V., CHIN.,** chlor., cic., ***colch., cupr.,*** dig., ferr., ferr-ar., ferr-i., ferr-p., iod., kali-bi., kali-n., ***lach.,*** lyc., merc., merc-c., mez., nux-m., op., ox-ac., ***ph-ac., phos.,*** phyt., ***plb.,*** rhus-v., **SEC.,** stann., staph., stry., sul-ac., **TAB., VERAT.,** vip., zinc.

IMPETIGO - **ANT-C.,** ars., calc., ***cic., con., crot-t., dulc., graph., hep., kali-bi.,*** kreos., ***lyc., merc., mez., nit-ac., rhus-t.,*** sep., ***viol-t.***
forehead - ant-c., kreos., led., ***merc., rhus-t.,*** sep., sulph., ***viol-t.***
lips, around - tarent.

INDURATIONS - ars., bry., clem., cob., ***graph.,*** led., mag-c., olnd., puls., rhus-t., sep., **SIL.,** sulph.
forehead - cic., con., led., olnd.
mouth, corners - aur-m., nat-a., sil.
nose, below - thuj.
red, hard lumps - cob.
submental gland - ***staph.***
temples - thuj.
indurations, cheeks - ***cham.,*** merc.

INFLAMMATION, bone, of - **AUR.,** aur-m., ***calc., fl-ac., mez., nit-ac., ph-ac., ruta, sil., staph., still.,*** symph.
periosteum - **AUR.,** ***calc., fl-ac., merc.,*** merc-c., ***mez.,*** **NIT-AC., PH-AC., PHOS.,** phyt., ***ruta.,*** sil., ***staph.,*** still., symph.

INVOLUNTARILY, mouth opens - ***ther.***

ITCHING, (see Skin) - acon., ***agar., agn., alum.,*** ambr., am-c., ***anac.,*** anac-oc., anan., ant-c., ***apis, apoc-a., arg-m.,*** arn., ***ars.,*** bell., berb., brach., ***brom.,*** buf-s., **CALC.,** ***calc-s.,*** cann-s., caps., carb-ac., carb-s., **CAUST.,** chel., chin-s., cod., colch., com., con., cycl., dol., euph., ferr-ma., ***fl-ac.,*** gels., glon., gran., ***graph.,*** grat., hydr., indg., kali-ar., kali-bi., kali-br., ***kali-c.,*** kali-i., kali-n., kali-p., kali-s., lach., lachn., ***laur.,*** lyc., meph., merc., morph., nat-a., ***nat-c.,*** nat-m., nat-p., ***nat-s.,*** nicc., nux-v., op., pall., par., petr., ph-ac., ***phos.,*** plan., ***rhus-t.,*** **RHUS-V.,** ruta., ***sars., sep., sil.,*** stram., stront-c., ***sulph.,*** sul-ac., tarent., til., ***urt-u.,*** verat., zinc.
afternoon - ***chel.,*** fago.
biting - ***agar.,*** agn., alum., calc., ***caust., euph.,*** hell., ***lach., lyc., merc., nat-c.,*** nat-m., nat-p., petr., ph-ac., phos., sep., sil., ***sulph.,*** urt-u., zinc.
burning - kali-c., sil.
after rubbing - con.
changes place on scratching - sars.

ITCHING,
evening - ph-ac., rhus-v., sabad., ***sulph.,*** zinc.
7 p.m. - fago.
eyes, under - apis, ***con.***
frostbitten, as if - ***agar., arg-m.***
morning, 10 a.m. - mag-c.
morning, 10 a.m, 11 a.m. - iod.
mouth, around - anac., calc., caust., ***hep.,*** rhus-t., sil., zinc.
mouth, below - mang.
mouth, corners, of - alum., hell.
night - dig., kalm., ***lach., mez.,*** rhus-v., stry.
pain, following - euph.
right - kali-p.
rubbing, amel. - rhus-v.
scratching, amel. - ***apis,*** caust., con., grat., mag-c., nat-c., rhus-t., squil.
spot - sulph.
stinging - agn., **APIS,** arn., ars., ***calc., calc-s., caust.,*** con., ***graph., kali-c.,*** kali-s., merc., nat-c., ***nat-m.,*** nat-p., ***rhus-t.,*** sars., ***sep., sil., sulph.***
touched, when - psor.
warm, on becoming - ***mez.,*** puls.
whiskers - agar., ambr., arg-m., ***calc.,*** cob., kali-bi., kali-p., mez., **NAT-C.,** nat-m., sil.
writing, when - chin-s.
zygoma - alum., hep., thuj.

itching, cheeks - agar., agn., alum., anan., ang., ant-c., asaf., bell., berb., dig., dulc., graph., hyper., kali-p., mag-m., nat-m., puls., rhus-t., ruta., spong., staph., sulph., ***stront-c.,*** thuj., viol-t.
cheeks, dinner, during - hep.

itching, chin - alum., am-c., berb., benz-ac., calc., carb-an., ***chlor.,*** con., dig., gamb., ***kali-c., lyc.,*** nat-c., nat-m., phos., puls., squil., ***stront-c.,*** **SULPH.,** ther., trom., zinc.
chin, under - alum., tarax.

JERKING, (see Twitching)

JERKING, pain - am-m., **BELL.,** bry., **CARB-V.,** ***cham.,*** cina, ***cocc.,*** colch., gels., indg., ***glon.,*** mang., puls., rhod., ***sep.,*** spig., stront-c., sul-ac., thuj., valer., ***zinc.***
cheek, bones - **CARB-V.,** cina, colch., mang., spig., stront.
laughing, on - mang.
pressure, amel. - am-c.
right - am-m., carb-v.
walking in open air - thuj.

jerking, zygoma - am-m., **CARB-V.,** chel.
evening - am-m., ***carb-v.***
left, in front of ear - carb-v.
right - chel.

LANCINATING, pain - ***agar.,*** acet-ac., alum., ***asaf.,*** aur., bufo, ***chin.,*** cocc., ***guai., kalm.,*** **MAG-P.,** ***plan.,*** senec., sil., sulph., verb.
below eye up through to vertex - tarent.
left - chin-s., sulph.
malar bone - alum., cimic., ***guai.***
morning - verb.
right - ***agar.,*** brach., ***guai., mag-p.,*** verb.

LARGE, sensation of being - **ACON.,** alum., arg-m., glon.
after dinner - alum.

LINEA, nasalis - aeth.

LOCKJAW, (see Emergency, Tetanus)

LONG, sensation as if elongated - stram.
chin - glon.

LUPUS - alumn., ***arg-n.,*** **ARS.,** aur-m., carb-ac., ***carb-v.,*** cist., **HYDRC.,** kali-ar., ***kali-bi.,*** kali-chl., kreos., lach., psor., ***sep., sil.***

MEMBRANE, on, corners of mouth - arum-t., ars-i., bry., iod., kali-bi.

MUSTACHE, in women - cortico., nat-m., ***sep.,*** thuj., thyr.

NEURALGIA, facial, (see Pain, face)

NODOSITIES - ***ars.,*** bry., cic., cund., ***hep., mag-c.,*** merc., ***merc-i-r.,*** still.
mouth, corners of - ***mag-c.,*** sil.
nodosities, chin, on - euph.

NUMBNESS - acon., ***asaf.,*** asar., bapt., bell., benz-ac., ***caust.,*** cham., cocc., gels., kalm., ***mez., nux-v.,*** **PLAT.,** rumx., ***ruta,*** samb., sep., tab., thuj., ***verb.***
affected side - bell., ***caust., nux-v., plat.,*** puls.
bones - ruta.
forehead - mur-ac., ***plat.***
left - graph.
morning, upper - phos.
zygoma - fl-ac.
mouth, about - plat.
right - ***chel., gels.,*** **PLAT.**
chill, during - **PLAT.**

numbness, cheek - asaf., ***caps., mez., nux-v., olnd.,*** plb., ***plat.***
following pain - ***caust., mez.***

numbness, chin - ***asaf., plat., spong.***

numbness, zygoma - fl-ac., **PLAT.**

PAIN, face - abrot., **ACON.,** ***agar.,*** all-c., alum., ambr., am-c., am-m., ***anac.,*** anan., apis, arg-m., ***arg-n., arn.,*** **ARS.,** ***ars-i., ars-m.,*** arund., asaf., asar., **AUR.,** aur-m., bar-c., **BELL.,** benz-ac., ***berb.,*** bism., bor., bov., brach., ***bry.,*** cact., ***cadm-s.,*** **CALC.,** ***calc-p.,*** calc-s., camph., ***caps., carb-an.,*** carb-s., ***carb-v.,*** casc., **CAUST., CEDR.,** ***cham., chel., chin.,*** chin-a., ***chin-s., chlol., cimic., cina,*** cist., clem., ***cocc.,*** coc-c., ***coff., colch.,*** **COLOC.,** ***con.,*** cor-r., crot-h., ***cupr., cupr-ar.,*** dig., dros., ***dulc.,*** echi., euon., ***euph.,*** euphr., ferr-ar., ferr-m., ferr-p., **GELS.,** ***glon.,*** graph., grat., ***guai., hep.,*** hura, ***hyos.,*** hydrc., ***hyper., ign.,*** iod., ***iris, kali-ar., kali-bi., kali-c., kali-i., kali-p., kali-s.,*** kalm., kreos., ***lach.,***

PAIN, face - lac-c., led., lepi., ***lith.***, lob., ***lyc.***, ***mag-c.***, ***mag-m.***, **MAG-P.,** mang., ***merc.***, ***merc-c.***, merc-i-f., ***mez.***, morph., naja, nat-a., ***nat-c.***, nat-h., **NAT-M.,** nat-p., nat-s., nicc., nit-ac., **NUX-V.,** ol-an., onos., ***paeon.***, ph-ac., **PHOS.,** ***phyt.***, **PLAT.,** ***plan.***, plb., psor., ***puls.***, ran-b., ran-s., ***rhod.***, ***rhus-t.***, rhus-v., ruta., sabad., sabin., sanic., sang., sars., sec., ***sep.***, ***sil.***, sol-t-ae., **SPIG.,** spong., **STANN., STAPH., STRAM.,** stront-c., ***sulph.***, sul-ac., tarax., ter., ***thuj.***, valer., ***verat.***, **VERB.,** viol-o., zinc.

afternoon - calc., cimic., ***cocc.***, hyper., kalm., lac-c., nux-v., sulph., ter., verb.
1 p.m. - ars., coff.
2 p.m. - mag-p.
3 p.m. - calc., ***chin-s.***, pip-m.
4 p.m. - chin-s., coloc., verb.
4 p.m. lasting all night - merc-c.
4 to 8 p.m. - **LYC.**

air open, agg. - alum., ***ars.***, ***bell.***, calc., carb-an., chin., chin-a., cocc., guai., ***hep.***, kali-ar., ***kali-c.***, ***kali-p.***, kreos., laur., mag-c., mag-p., ***merc.***, merc-c., ***phos.***, plat., puls., ***rhus-t.***, sars., sep., sil., spig., spong., **SULPH.,** thuj., valer.
amel. - all-c., am-m., hep., kali-bi., ***kali-i.***, ***kali-s.***, lac-c., nat-m., nat-s., ***puls.***, ***sulph.***

alone, when - pip-m.

alternating, with pain in
celiac region - coloc.
limbs - ***kali-bi.***
shoulder - mag-p.
stomach - bism.

bathing, agg. - am-c., coff., con.

bed, in, agg. - **CARB-V.,** ***mag-c.***, ***mag-p.***, puls., ***sil.***, spong., verb., viol-t.

bending, forward, agg. - lac-c.

binding, tightly, amel. - kali-c., sep.

blowing, nose agg. - **MERC.**

bones - aeth., alum., anan., arg-n., aur., ***caps.***, carb-an., caust., ***chin-s.***, ***cimic.***, colch., dulc., graph., guai., hell., ***hep.***, kali-c., kali-n., ***merc.***, merc-i-r., nat-c., nat-m., nit-ac., nit-s-d., nux-v., onos., ***phos.***, ***phyt.***, ruta, ***sil.***, sulph., zinc.
chewing, on - nat-m.
malar bones - tub.

change, of air - staph.
temperature - mag-c., ***verb.***
weather - ***rhod.***

chewing, when (see Motion) - acon., alum., am-m., anac., arg-n., ***bell.***, ***bism.***, ***bry.***, calc., ***cham.***, coca, coff., coloc., cur., euphr., graph., lach., ***nat-m.***, nit-ac., osm., phos., plat., puls., sep., sil., spig., ***staph.***, verat., verb.
amel. - cupr.

chill, during - acon., ***caust.***, chin., lach., mez., nux-v., rhus-t., spig.

chilliness with the pain - ***caust.***, coloc., rhus-t.

chin - mang., nux-m.

closing, eyes - cimic., med.

coffee, agg. - spig.
after abuse of - **NUX-V.**

PAIN, face

cold, air, agg. - ***acon.***, ***agar.***, **ARS.,** ***bell.***, ***carb-s.***, ***colch.***, ***dulc.***, kali-ar., kali-c., kali-p., ***mag-c.***, **MAG-P.,** ***merc.***, phos., ***rhod.***, **RHUS-T.,** ruta., sulph., verb.
amel. - ***all-c.***, **KALI-S.,** nicc., ***puls.***

cold, applications, agg. - aesc., ***bell.***, con., ***ferr.***, ***hep.***, ***mag-c.***, **MAG-P.,** ***phos.***, ***rhod.***, **RHUS-T.,** sanic., **SIL.,** stann.
amel. - apis, arg-m., ars-m., asar., ***bism.***, ***bry.***, ***caust.***, chin., **COFF.,** ***ferr-p.***, fl-ac., ***kali-p.***, ***lac-c.***, nicc., ***puls.***, sabad., sep.

cold, from exposure to, (see Wind) - acon., ***agar.***, arn., ***bell.***, ***calc.***, ***calc-p.***, ***caust.***, ***dulc.***, ***gels.***, ***graph.***, ***hep.***, ***kalm.***, ***mag-c.***, ***mag-p.***, ***merc.***, ***phos.***, ***rhod.***, ***rhus-t.***, ruta., ***sep.***, **SIL.,** ***sulph.***, verb.
from, or heat - merc., plan., sul-ac.
from becoming, cold - calc-s.
from becoming, body, agg. - mag-p.

cold, water holding in mouth amel. - clem.

contradiction, from - ***bell.***

cough, during - ***kali-bi.***

damp, weather, agg. - ***calc.***, ***calc-p.***, chin-s., dulc., ***merc.***, ***nat-s.***, ***sep.***, ***sil.***, spig., verat.

daytime - calc., ***cimic.***, kalm., mag-p., puls., **SPIG.,** ***stann.***, thuj.

diversion, of the mind amel. - pip-m.

draft, agg. - bell., calc-p., caps., chin., coff., hep., kali-p., ***mag-c.***, ***mag-p.***, ***merc.***, ***nux-v.***, ***sil.***, ***stram.***, sulph., ***verb.***

eating, while - bry., gels., mag-p., ***mez.***, phos., plan., spig., spong., syph.
after - agar., chin., iris, mang., nux-v., ***phos.***, zinc.
amel. - chin., kali-p., ***kalm.***, spig.
amel. - caj., rhod.

eruptions, after suppressed - ***dulc.***, ***kalm.***, ***mez.***, thuj.

evening - am-m., caps., ***chin-s.***, cist., cocc., guai., hyper., ign., kali-s., mag-s., ***mez.***, nit-ac., ***phos.***, pip-m., ***plat.***, ***puls.***, rhus-t., sep., spong., stram., ***sulph.***, ***thuj.***, ***verb.***, ***zinc.***
6 p.m. till morning - ***guai.***
7 to 8 p.m. - **CEDR.**
amel. - kali-bi., spig., stann., sulph., verat.
lying down after - stram.

excitement - cact., ***coff.***, cupr., lyc., sep., ***staph.***
amel. - kali-p., pip-m.

exertion, agg. - **BRY.,** ***cact.***, calc-p., lac-c., merc.
amel. - iris, sep.

extending to, arms - kalm.
to, bones - sulph.
to, chest - sil.
to, ears - **BELL.,** ***calc.***, carb-an., ***caust.***, ***coloc.***, ***hep.***, **LACH.,** lyc., ***mez.***, plan., **PULS.,** sang., ***sep.***, spig., thuj.
to, fingers - ***coff.***
to, neck - ***bell.***, ***coloc.***, ***guai.***, ***puls.***, sang., ***spig.***
to, nose - ***spig.***
to, other parts - calc-p., ***cocc.***

PAIN, face
extending, to, root of nose - phos.
to, teeth - merc.
to, temples - berb., hep., ***mez.,*** phos., spig.
eye, below - ***acon., arg-n., ars.,*** aur-m-n., ***bell.,*** chin., cina, coloc., ***gels.,*** hydrc., iris, mag-p., mang., mez., ***nux-v.,*** phos., plat., ***sil.,*** spig., sulph., verb., zinc.
left - arg-n.
eye symptoms, with - coloc.
open cannot - chel.
falling, asleep, on - ***caps.,*** lach.
fasting, from - ***cact.***
forenoon - ***chin-s.,*** lach., nat-m., plat.
7 a.m. to 12 - ***chin-s.***
9 a.m. - ***caust.,*** kali-bi., lac-c., nux-v., sul-ac., ***verb.***
9 a.m. to 4 p.m. - ***verb.***
9:30 - verb.
10 a.m. - ***chin-s.,*** gels., nat-m.
11 a.m. - mag-p., nux-v., puls.
11 a.m. to 2 p.m. - mag-p.
gradually increasing and ceases suddenly - arg-m., ***bell.,*** puls., sul-ac.
and, gradually decreasing - ***plat.,*** **STANN.**
heat, after over-heating - ***ferr.***
agg. - cedr., chin., glon., ***phos.,*** rhod.
amel., of stove - ***mez.,*** **SIL.**
hot needles penetrating, as if - ars., spig.
icy needles penetrating, as if - agar., spig.
inflammatory - ***acon.,*** arn., ***bar-c.,*** **BELL.,** ***bry.,*** cact., caust., ***ferr-p.,*** glon., ***lach.,*** **MERC.,** phos., plat., spig., thuj., verat.
intermittent - ***cedr.***
jar agg. - ***arn.,*** **BELL.,** chin., ***cocc., mag-c., spig.***
lachrymation and coryza, with - verb.
laughing, when - bor., mang., tab.
left - ***acon., ars.,*** arund., asar., ***cedr., chel., chin., chin-s., coloc.,*** cor-r., ***dulc.,*** echi., glon., ***guai.,*** hell., ***kali-bi.,*** **LOB.,** lyc., ***mag-c.,*** merc-c., nat-h., osm., ***phos.,*** plan., polyg., puls., sabad., sep., **SPIG.,** staph., stann., ***thuj.,*** **VERB.,** vesp.
left, to right - ***chin.***
light, agg. - ***ars., bell., cact., chel., con.,*** mag-p., spig.
lying, while - ail., ambr., arn., bell., carb-s., cham., chel., ***chin., coloc., ferr.,*** gels., graph., hep., ign., kalm., lac-c., ***mag-c.,*** phos., pip-m., plat., plb., ***puls.,*** ruta., sil., spig., sulph., syph., ***verb.***
amel. - ***cact.,*** calc-p., chin-s., coff., ***nux-v.,*** sep., spig.
affected side, on, agg. - acon., arn., chin., ***clem.,*** puls., spig., syph.
amel. - bry., cupr., ign., sul-ac.
face, on the, amel. - spig.
quiet, amel. - bry., sep.
head low agg., with - ***puls.***

PAIN, face
menses, during - am-c., caust., graph., lyc., mag-c., mag-m., ***nat-m.,*** sep., sil., stann., zinc.
after - spig.
before - am-c., mang., ***stann.,*** zinc.
suppressed - stann.
mental, exertion agg. - am-c., bry., calc-p., ***coff.,*** ign., kalm., lac-c., ***nux-v.,*** staph.
mental, foramen - ***mez.***
extending to ear - calc.
mercury, after - aur-m., carb-v., chin., **HEP., KALI-I.,** ***nit-ac., sulph.***
morning - agar., ***chin., chin-s., cupr.,*** mez., nat-h., ***nux-v.,*** rumx., sars., thuj., verat., verb.
5 a.m. - caj.
7 to 8 a.m. - rhus-t.
breakfast, after - ***iris.***
amel. - caj.
increases, till noon, then subsides - mag-c.
waking, on - agar., ***iris,*** sars., sep., sulph.
motion, agg. - ***acon.,*** **BELL., BRY.,** ***cact.,*** calc., calc-p., ***chin.,*** chin-a., ***colch., coloc., ferr-p., gels.,*** lac-c., mez., **NUX-V.,** phos., rhod., sep., **SPIG.,** squil., staph., ***verb.***
amel. - agar., ***bism.,*** ferr., iris, kali-p., lyc., ***mag-c.,*** mag-p., meny., ***plat., puls., rhod.,*** **RHUS-T.,** ruta., ***valer.***
eyes, of - bry., kali-c.
jaw, of lower, amel. - ***rhod.***
muscles, of face agg. - stann.
music, from - ***cact.,*** nux-v., ph-ac.
nerves - caps.
night - ***acon.,*** agar., aran., ***calc-p., caust.,*** chel., ***cocc., con., glon., guai., lach.,*** led., ***mag-c., mag-p.,*** **MERC.,** merc-c., ***mez.,*** nicc., phos., ***phyt.,*** plan., plat., puls., ***sep., sil.,*** spong., staph., ***sulph.***
2 a.m. - spig.
3 a.m. - ***sulph.,*** **THUJ.**
9 p.m. - sul-ac., urt-u.
9 p.m. to 3 a.m. - sulph.
10 p.m. - chin-s., coloc., ign.
amel. - cupr., ***staph.***
bed, driving him out of - ***mag-c., mag-p., rhus-t.***
rest, during - ***mag-c.,*** mag-p.
noise, agg. - acon., arn., calc-p., ***chin., cocc., coff., nux-v.,*** sep., **SPIG.**
noon - nat-m., spig., stram., sulph., verb.
numbness, with - acon., **CHAM.,** ***kalm., mez., plat.***
odors, agg. - sep.
one-sided - acon., am-c., caps., ***caust.,*** cham., colch., euon., grat., ***kali-bi.,*** kalm., kreos., led., mez., nux-v., ol-j., phos., puls., verat., verb.
opening, the eyes - bry.
the mouth (see motion) - alum., ang., cham., **COCC.,** dros., mag-p., merc., phos., sabad., spong., thuj., verat.
paralysis, with - acon., ***caust., cur., gels.,*** kali-chl., **NAT-M.**

PAIN, face

paroxysmal - acon., ***bell., caust., cedr., cham., chin.,*** chin-s., ***coloc.,*** cocc., dulc., plat., sabad., sep., stann., thuj., ***verb.***

periodical - ***ars., cact., cedr., chin.,*** chin-a., ***chin-s.,*** coll., glon., graph., ***guai.,*** kali-ar., ***mag-p.,*** **NAT-M.,** plan., **SPIG.,** thuj., verat., verb.

same hour morning and afternoon - verb.

pregnancy, during - ***ign.,*** mag-c., ***sep.,*** stram.

pressure, agg. - ***bell., caps., cina, coloc.,*** cupr., dros., gels., ***mag-c.,*** merc-i-f., nux-v., petr., ***verb.***

amel. - ail., aur., ***bry.,*** coloc., ***dig.,*** cupr., guai., lepi., ***mag-c.,*** **MAG-P.,** ***mez.,*** sang., sep., spig., stann., staph., syph.

hard, amel. - bell., ***bry.,*** chin., ***chin-s., rhus-t.,*** spig.

pulsating - **ACON.,** arg-m., ***arn., cact.,*** cupr-ar., ***ferr-p., glon., mag-c.,*** merc-i-f., nit-ac., ***plat.,*** puls., sabad., sep., spig., staph.

quiet, in a dark room amel. - ***mez.***

quinine, after - ***hep.,*** **NAT-M.,** ***nux-v., puls., stann.***

radiating - sang., spig.

fingers, to - cocc.

rheumatic - **ACON.,** act-sp., **ARS., BRY.,** ***calc-p.,*** **CAUST.,** ***chin., cimic., colch., coloc.,*** gels., ***hell., kali-ar.,*** kali-bi., ***kalm.,*** lach., ***lith.,*** mag-c., ***merc.,*** merc-i-f., mez., nux-v., phos., ***phyt., puls.,*** rhod., ***rhus-t., sil., spig.,*** verat.

right - agar., am-c., ***am-m.,*** anac., arn., ***aur.,*** **BELL.,** bry., ***cact., calc-p.,*** camph., ***carb-v., caust.,*** cedr., **CHEL.,** ***chin-s., cist., clem.,*** coff., ***cur.,*** dor., ***ferr.,*** ho., indg., ***iris, kali-i., kali-p., kalm.,*** lil-t., ***lyc.,*** lyss., ***mag-p., merc.,*** nux-v., ***plat.,*** psor., **PULS.,** rhod., ***rhus-t.,*** sanic., ***sep., spig.,*** spong., stront-c., ***sulph.,*** sul-ac., syph., ter., urt-u., ***verb.,*** zinc.

right, to left - calc-p., lyc., nat-m.

rising, from bed, agg. - chin., olnd., rhus-t., spig.

amel. - hep.

up again - chin.

room, in - am-m., chin., hell., mag-aust., ***puls.,*** ran-s.

rubbing, amel. - ant-c., ***caust.,*** **PHOS.,** plat., plb., ***rhus-t.,*** valer.

shaving, after - aur-m., carb-an., ox-ac.

shocks, in rapid succession - coff.

sitting, agg. - am-m., canth., graph., guai., ***mag-c., phos.,*** rhus-t., thuj.

up in bed amel. - bell., ***ferr.,*** hep., mag-c., ***puls.,*** sulph.

sleep, from - mez., verb.

amel. - mag-p., **PHOS.,** sep.

smoking, amel. - clem.

sneezing - chin., mag-c., ***verb.***

spring - ***lach., nux-v.***

standing, agg. - chin., guai., nux-v., spig.

stool, during agg. - spig.

PAIN, face

stooping, agg. - bry., canth., coloc., ferr-p., gels., kali-c., nux-v., petr., puls., ***spig.***

storm, before a - ***rhod.,*** sep., ***sil.***

stormy weather - ***caust.,*** phos., **RHOD., SIL.,** spig., verb.

stunning - ***mez., plat.,*** verb.

sudden - ***ign.,*** kalm., valer.

suddenly, coming and going - **BELL.,** ***spig., sulph.***

sun, come and go with - kali-bi., ***kalm., nat-m., spig., stann., verb.***

suppressed, ague, after - **NAT-M.,** sep., ***stann.***

swallowing, agg. - bell., kali-n., phos., staph.

talking, agg. - ***bry.,*** chel., coca, coloc., euphr., kali-chl., mag-c., ***mez.,*** phos., puls., rhod., spig., squil., tell., verb.

amel. - kali-p.

tea, agg. - ***spig.***

teeth, chattering, with - sul-ac.

thinking of it aggr - aur.

tobacco, from - ign., sep.

touch, agg. - arn., aur., **BELL.,** ***bry., caps., chel., chin.,*** chin-s., cina, cocc., **COFF.,** ***coloc.,*** cor-r., cupr., dig., dros., **HEP.,** kali-c., **LACH.,** lyc., mag-c., mag-p., nat-m., ***nux-v.,*** par., ph-ac., ***phos.,*** puls., ***sep.,*** spig., spong., staph., sulph., verb., zinc.

amel. - am-c., am-m., asaf., chin., euphr., kali-p., olnd., thuj.

urination, frequent, with - calc.

profuse, amel. - acon., ferr-p., **GELS.,** ign., kalm., sang., sil., ter., verat.

vexation - ***coloc.,*** kalm., staph.

waking, on - croc., hell., hep., ***lach.,*** nux-v., puls., sabad., sep., spig., verb.

walking, after - ran-s.

after, slowly amel. - chin., ***ferr., puls.***

after, warm, becoming - plan., **PULS.**

agg. - coca, coloc., guai., laur., mang., merc., mur-ac., petr., thuj.

air, in open - nat-c., nux-v.

air, in open, amel. - asar., ***coloc., mag-c.***

amel. - agar., ***mag-c.,*** rhus-t., sil., sulph.

wandering - acon., ***colch.,*** **GELS.,** graph., ***mag-p.,*** **PULS.**

warm, applications, agg. - cedr.

bed agg. - clem., glon., ***merc., mez.,*** plat., ***puls.,*** verat.

drinks, agg. - cham.

food agg. - mez., ***puls.,*** sep.

warm, room, agg. - am-c., **KALI-S.,** ***mez.,*** **PULS.**

amel. - ***calc., hep.,*** lac-c., laur., ***sep.,*** staph.

warmth, amel. - **ARS.,** ***calc., calc-p.,*** caust., ***cham.,*** chin-s., coloc., cupr., **HEP.,** kali-p., lach., **MAG-P.,** ***mez.,*** phos., rhod., ***rhus-t.,*** sanic., **SIL.,** spig., sulph., sul-ac.

washing, in cold agg. (see cold applications)

PAIN, face
wind, agg. - ***caust., dulc.,*** lac-c., mag-p., phos., ***rhod., sep.***
dry cold, agg. - **ACON.,** ***caust.,*** **HEP.,** lac-c., **MAG-P.,** rhod.
south, warm, moist agg. - ip., ***kali-s., puls.***
wine, agg. - bell., ***cact.***
writing, while - chin-s.
yawning - arn., ign., op., mag-c., rhus-t., sabad., staph.

PAIN, cheeks - acon., ***ang., bell., bism.,*** bry., ***caps., caust., chel., chin-s.,*** cimic., ***cina,*** cocc., ***coloc.,*** dig., dulc., ***hep.,*** hyos., ***kali-bi., kali-i., mag-c., mag-m., merc.,*** merc-i-f., mez., nat-m., onos., ***plat.,*** psor., rhus-t., ruta., sep., ***stann.,*** valer., **VERB.**
bones, with toothache - mur-ac.
coughing, when - ***kali-bi.***
coughing, when, extending to head - thuj.
daytime - cimic.
right - ***chel.***

PAIN, malar bones - ars-i., ***aur., calc-p.,*** caps., caust., chel., cinnb., coloc., glon., ***kali-bi.,*** kali-i., mag-c., mang., mez., ol-an., olnd., psor., sep., stann., stroph., thuj., tub., verb.
evening - lyc.
menses, before and during - stann.
neuralgic - stann.
night - kali-c.
amel. - cimic.
running, about, amel. - bism.

PAIN, zygoma - ***aur., calc-p.,*** caps., caust., chel., cinnb., ***kali-bi.,*** psor., verb.

PALE, face - absin., ***acet-ac., acon.,*** agar., ***aesc., aeth.,*** ail., aloe, all-s., alum., alumn., ambr., ammc., ***am-c., am-m.,*** amyg., aml-n., **ANAC.,** anan., ant-c., **ANT-T.,** ***apis,*** apoc., **ARG-M.,** ***arg-n., arn.,*** **ARS.,** ars-h., ***ars-i., aspar., aster., aur.,*** aur-m-n., aur-s., ***bad., bar-c.,*** bar-m., ***bell.,*** benz., benz-n., **BERB.,** bism., ***bor.,*** bov., brom., ***bry., bufo, cact.,*** cadm-s., **CALC.,** ***calc-ar.,*** **CALC-P.,** ***calc-s.,*** **CAMPH.,** cann-i., cann-s., ***canth.,*** caps., ***carb-ac., carb-an.,*** carb-h., carb-o., **CARB-S., CARB-V.,** ***caust.,*** cedr., ***cham., chel.,*** **CHIN.,** chin-a., **CHIN-S.,** chlol., chlf., ***chlor., cic.,*** cimic., **CINA, CLEM.,** ***cocc.,*** cod., coff., ***colch., coloc., con.,*** cop., ***croc.,*** crot-h., crot-t., **CUPR.,** cupr-ar., ***cycl.,*** der., **DIG.,** dirc., dor., ***dros., dulc., eup-per.,*** euph., euphr., fago., **FERR.,** ferr-ar., **FERR-I.,** ferr-m., **FERR-P.,** fl-ac., ***gels., glon.,*** gran., **GRAPH.,** grat., ham., ***hell., hydr-ac., hydr., hyos.,*** hura, ***ign., iod., ip.,*** jab., jatr., ***kali-ar., kali-bi.,*** kali-br., ***kali-c., kali-chl., kali-i., kali-p.,*** kali-n., kali-s., ***kalm., kreos., lac-d., lach.,*** lachn., lact., ***laur.,*** lec., ***led.,*** lept., **LOB., LYC.,** lyss., ***mag-c., mag-m., mag-p.,*** mag-s., manc., **MANG., MED.,** meli., ***merc., merc-c., merc-cy., merc-d., merc-sul., mez.,*** morph., mosch., ***mur-ac.,*** naja, **NAT-A., NAT-C., NAT-M.,** nat-n., **NAT-P.,** nat-s., nicc., ***nit-ac.,*** nuph., ***nux-m., nux-v.,*** oena., ol-an., olnd., **OP.,** ***ox-ac., par., petr.,*** **PH-AC.,** ***phos.,*** phys., ***phyt., plat.,*** **PLB.,** podo., ***psor.,*** ptel., ***puls., pyrog.,*** raph., ***rheum, rhus-t.,*** rhus-v., sabad., sabin., ***samb., sang.,*** sant., **SEC.,** sel., senec., **SEP.,** ***sil., spig., spong., stann., stram.,*** stry., **SULPH.,** ***sul-ac.,*** sumb., **TAB.,** tarent., tax., tep., ***ter., teucr.,*** thea., ther., thuj., til., **TUB.,** valer., **VERAT.,** verat-v., verb., vesp., vinc., vip., **ZINC.**
abdomen, with pain in - phos.
afternoon - hura, mag-c., nat-m.
2 p.m. - verat-v.
waking, on - spig.
air, damp agg. - ***nux-m.***
air, fresh amel. - cann-i., caust., ***gels.***
air, on going into cold - nux-m.
air, open, in - kali-c.
alternating with redness - **ACON.,** alum., am-c., aml-n., ars., aur., bell., ***bor.,*** bov., brom., ***camph.,*** caps., cham., ***chin.,*** cimic., cina, ***croc.,*** cub., **FERR.,** ferr-p., gins., ***glon., hell.,*** hyos., ***ign.,*** kali-c., **LAC-C.,** ***led.,*** lyc., mag-c., merc., mur-ac., nat-c., nat-p., nit-ac., nux-v., olnd., ph-ac., phos., plat., puls., rhus-t., sep., squil., sul-ac., tab., verat., zinc.
alternating with redness, menses, during - zinc.
anger, after - ***con.***
ascending, on - dirc.
chill, during - arg-m., bell., **BRY., CAMPH.,** canth., ***chin.,*** chin-s., **CINA,** coff., croc., ***dros., hep.,*** ign., ip., ***lyc., nux-v.,*** ph-ac., phos., ***puls., rhus-t., sec.,*** sep., ***sulph.,*** **VERAT.,** zinc.
chill, before - ars., cina, ferr.
damp weather - aloe, nux-m.
deathly, during vertigo - ***dub.,*** puls., tab.
dinner during - mag-m., nat-m., nit-ac., phel.
after - nit-ac.
eating after - ***kali-c.,*** mag-c., thuj.
evening - caust., kali-c., lyc., merc., olnd., ***phos.,*** sep.
7 p.m. - phos.
walking - phos.
exertion, from - spong.
eyes, about - ptel.
fever, during - ***ars.,*** **CINA,** cocc., **CROC.,** ***hep., ip., lyc.,*** nat-m., puls., rhus-t., sep., spong., thuj., tub., verat.
flushes easily - **FERR.**
headache, with - acon., aeth., ***alum.,*** ambr., am-c., anac., ***ars.,*** canth., ***carb-v., chin-s., echi., hell.,*** hydr., ign., ip., ***lach.,*** mag-c., ***phos., sep.,*** spig., ***stram.,*** valer., ***verat., zinc.***
heat, of head, during - hell.
heated, when - hep.
hot, and - cimic., cina, croc., hyos., op.
linea nasalis - ***aeth.,*** ant-t., carb-ac., ***cina,*** ip., merc-cy., ***phos., stram.,*** tarent.
lying, while - ***bell.,*** thea.
amel. - petr.
maniacal rage, with - anac., ars., croc., merc., phos., puls., ***verat.***

PALE, face
menses, during - am-c., apis, ***ars.***, cast., ***cedr.***, ***ferr.***, graph., **IGN.**, ***ip.***, lyc., ***mag-c.***, ***mag-m.***, puls., stann., verat.
absent, with - lob.
after - ***nat-m.***, puls., verat.
before - am-c., cycl., ip., mang., verat.
morning - aloe, ***bov.***, cod., con., lyc., mag-c., nat-m., olnd., op., **SEC.**, sep.
rising, after - ***bov.***, graph., ph-ac.
waking, on - nat-s.
mouth, around - aeth., arum-t., bell., ***carb-ac.***, cic., **CINA,** ferr-p., merc-c., sant., **STRAM.**
rest of face dusky red - carb-ac.
night - carb-v., mang., merc.
noon - kali-c., ox-ac., phos., sulph., ***verat.***
nosebleeds, with - carb-v., chin., ferr., ***ip.***, puls., verat.
one-sided - acon., arn., bell., ***cham.***, coloc., ign., ip., ***mosch.***, nux-v., tab., verat.
left red and hot, right pale and cold - upa.
one pale, and hot, the other red and cold - ***mosch.***
pain, abdomen, in, with - cina, fil.
after - ***ferr.***
heart, in, with - xan.
palpitation, with - ambr.
perspiration, during - mosch., sep.
reading, from - graph., sil.
red in spots - ***aur-m.***, ***ferr.***, ***sulph.***
rising up, on - ***acon.***, ***puls.***, ***verat.***, ***verat-v.***
sitting up, in bed - acon.
sleep, during - rheum
after - spig., tub.
spots, in - bell., calc., sil.
standing, when - chin., petr., rumx.
stool, during - ***calc.***, crot-t., ip., ***kali-c.***, ***rheum,*** verat.
stool, after - coloc., ***crot-t.***, ferr-m.
sudden - ***cimic.***, graph., phos.
vexation, after - ***ars.***
warm room - am-c., apis
amel. - nux-m.

PARALYSIS, facial - ***acon.***, ***agar.***, all-c., alum., ***am-p.***, anac., ***bar-c.***, ***bell.***, ***cadm-s.***, carc., **CAUST.,** ***cocc.***, crot-h., ***cupr.***, ***cur.***, ***dulc.***, form., ***gels.***, ***graph.***, hyper., ***ign.***, iod., ***kali-chl.***, ***kali-i.***, kali-p., merc., nat-m., ***nux-v.***, op., petr., phys., plat., plb., puls., ***rhus-t.***, ruta, seneg., solid., stry., syph., zinc., zinc-pic.
bathing, from - graph.
chewing difficult, with - syph.
cold, from - acon., ***cadm-s.***, **CAUST.,** ***dulc.***, ruta.
corners of mouth, drop and saliva runs out - agar., op., zinc.
distortion of muscles, with - graph.
eyes, close, cannot - cadm-s.
closed, with - apis.
goitre, suppression, from - iod.
left - ***all-c.***, cadm-s., ***cur.***, form., graph., ***nux-v.***, seneg., spig., sulph.
mouth opening aggr - caust.

PARALYSIS, facial
one-sided - ***bar-c.***, cadm-s., **CAUST.,** ***cocc.***, ***graph.***, ***kali-chl.***, kali-p., puls., sil., syph.
pain, after - kali-chl., kali-m.
riding in the wind, from - acon., bell., ***cadm-s.***, **CAUST.,** ign.
right - apis, ***arn.***, bell., ***caust.***, hep., kali-chl., kali-p., ***phos.***, plb., sil.
swallowing difficult - cadm-s.
talking difficult - cadm-s., syph.
twitching of muscles, with - kali-m.
eyelids, of, with - syph.
urine, profuse, with - all-c.
wet, after getting - **CAUST.**

PAROTID, gland, (see Glands, chapter)

PERSPIRATION - acon., aesc., aeth., ***agar.***, ***alum.***, ambr., ***am-m.***, amyg., ant-t., arg-m., ***arg-n.***, ***arn.***, ***ars.***, ars-h., aur., ***bapt.***, **BELL.,** benz-ac., bor., ***bry.***, ***bufo,*** **CALC.,** ***calc-p.***, calc-s., **CAMPH.,** ***caps.***, ***carb-ac.***, carb-an., ***carb-s.***, **CARB-V.,** cham., ***chin.***, chin-a., cic., **CINA,** ***cocc.***, ***coff.***, colch., coloc., con., crot-h., ***cupr.***, cupr-s., ***dig.***, ***dros.***, dulc., elaps, ferr., ferr-ar., ferr-p., fl-ac., ***glon.***, guai., ***hell.***, hep., hydr-ac., ***hyos.***, **IGN.,** ***ip.***, jab., ***kali-ar.***, ***kali-bi.***, kali-c., kali-i., kali-p., kali-s., kreos., ***lach.***, lachn., laur., **LYC.,** mag-c., med., **MERC.,** mez., morph., mosch., mur-ac., ***nat-m.***, ***nat-s.***, **NUX-V.,** ol-an., **OP.,** ox-ac., par., ***petr.***, ***phos.***, ***psor.***, **PULS.,** rheum, rhus-t., sabad., ***samb.***, ***sars.***, ***sec.***, ***sep.***, **SIL.,** spig., **SPONG.,** ***stann.***, staph., ***stram.***, stry., ***sulph.***, sul-ac., ***tab.***, tarent., tell., ***thuj.***, til., **VALER.,** **VERAT.,** verat-v., vip.
afternoon - com., ign., samb.
anxiety, with - nat-c.
bee sting, from - sep.
belching, during - cadm-s.
cold - acon., aeth., ant-c., ***ant-t.***, arn., **ARS.,** ***aur.***, bell., benz-ac., ***bry.***, **CACT.,** cadm-s., ***calc.***, ***calc-p.***, calc-s., **CAMPH.,** caps., carb-ac., carb-an., ***carb-s.***, **CARB-V.,** ***chin.***, chin-a., **CINA,** ***cocc.***, coc-c., crot-h., ***cupr.***, ***dig.***, ***dros.***, elaps, ferr., ***glon.***, hell., hep., hura, ***ip.***, ***kali-bi.***, ***lach.***, lachn., ***lob.***, ***lyc.***, ***merc.***, **MERC-C.,** morph., mur-ac., nat-m., ***nux-v.***, ***op.***, ox-ac., plat., ***puls.***, pyrog., ***rheum,*** rhus-t., ruta., sabad., ***samb.***, ***sec.***, sep., spig., **SPONG.,** staph., ***stram.***, ***sulph.***, sul-ac., ***tab.***, **VERAT.,** verat-v.
diarrhea, in - apoc.
mouth, around - **CHIN.,** rheum
convulsions, during - ***bufo,*** ***cocc.***
coughing, when - tarent.
dinner, during - carb-an.
after - sulph.
drinking, after - ***cham.***
eating, while - ***ign.***, ***nat-m.***, ***sulph.***
eating, after - alum., **CHAM.,** nat-s., psor., viol-t.
eating, warm food - sep.
evening - hura, psor., puls., sars., spong.
house, in - mez.
exertion, from slightest - sulph.

PERSPIRATION
except the face - ***rhus-t., sec.***
eyes, under - con.
face only - con., ign., phos.
except the - ***rhus-t.,*** sec.
fever, during - alum., ars., bell., ***cham., chel., dros.,*** dulc., ***lach., psor.,*** **PULS.,** sep., spong., valer.
flatus, when passing - kali-bi.
forenoon - phos.
morning - ars., chin., nit-ac., puls., ruta, sulph., verat.
motion, during - valer.
night - dros., hep., puls.
2 a.m. - ars.
midnight - plat., rhus-t.
noon - cic.
offensive - ***puls.***
palpitation - ars.
right - alum., puls.
scalp, and - puls., valer., verat.
side, lain on - ***acon.,*** act-sp., chin.
not lain on - thuj., sil.
one side - alum., ***ambr., bar-c.,*** **NUX-V., PULS.,** sulph.
sitting, while - calc.
sleep, during - med., prun., sep., tab.
before - calc.
asleep, on falling - sil.
small spots while eating - ign.
standing - eupi.
stool, during - alum., chin., nat-m., nux-m., nux-v., sil.
after - com.
supper, during - calc.
vomiting, during - cadm-s.
waking, on - puls.
walking, while - bor., valer., verat.
warm, food and drink - sep., sul-ac.

PICKING - lach.
chin, point of - arund.

POINTED, peaked - **ARS., CHIN.,** ***nux-v., ph-ac., rhus-t.,*** **STAPH., VERAT.**

PRESSING, pain - acon., ***anac.,*** arg-m., arg-n., asaf., bry., chin., ***cina, coca,*** cocc., ***dig.,*** dros., ferr-p., kali-c., merc., nat-c., nat-m., phos., rhus-t., ***sep., stann.,*** staph., sul-ac., tarax., verat., **VERB.,** zinc.
evening - ***verb.***
finger, as with a - sul-ac.
left - **VERB.**
motion, of face - stann.
opening, jaw agg. - ***cocc.,*** dros.
pressing, out - kali-i., merc.
pressure, agg. - ***cina,*** verb.
amel. - aur.
right - chel., iris, kalm., psor., spong., verb.
rubbing, amel. - phos.
walking, in open air - nat-c.
warm, room amel. - sep.

pressing, cheek bones - agar., am-c., anac., ant-t., arg-m., ***bell.,*** berb., ***bism., caps.,*** chel., ***cina,*** cocc., colch., ***coloc.,*** dros., hyos., kali-chl., ***kali-i.,*** mang., ***merc., mez.,*** nat-c., nat-m., ***olnd.,*** phos., ***plat.,*** sabin., samb., sep., spig., ***stann.,*** staph., sulph., teucr., **VERB.,** viol-o.
blowing, nose, on - ***merc.***
chewing, warm food - phos.
crampy - stann.
entering, warm room - phos.
extending, to teeth - nat-m.
intermittent - ***verb.***
night - mang.

pressing, chin - agar., anac., asaf., bov., fl-ac., plat.
between chin and lower lip - mag-c.
under - bar-c.

pressing, zygoma - caps., ***cinnb.,*** dulc., euph., lec., ***plat., verb.***
evening - caps., con.
outward - dros.
touch, agg. - caps.

PRICKLING, pain - lyc.

PRICKLING, sensation, (see Tingling)

PSORIASIS, of eyebrows - ***phos.***

PULSATION - acon., ***agar., arg-m.,*** arn., ars., bell., bry., bufo, ***calc.,*** cann-s., carb-an., caust., cham., clem., croc., ***ferr-p.,*** hura, kreos., mag-c., ***mur-ac.,*** myric., nit-ac., rumx., sabad., spong., staph., sulph.

pulsation, cheek bones - calc., carb-an., mag-c., merc-i-f., sulph.

pulsation, chin - stry.

QUIVERING - agar., chin., coloc., ***gels., kali-c.,*** lyss., mag-m., phel., plb., stront-c., thuj.

quivering, chin - coloc.

RASH - ***acon., ail.,*** anan., ***ant-c.,*** ant-t., ***ars.,*** **BELL.,** ***bry.,*** carb-s., caust., ***cham.,*** coff., con., ***euphr., graph., hep.,*** hydr., ***ip.,*** jab., kali-br., lach., ***merc., mez., nat-m.,*** nit-ac., phos., **PULS., RHUS-T.,** ***stram.,*** **SULPH.,** tab., tarent., teucr., verat.
bluish - ***lach., phos.,*** sulph.
burning - teucr.
chin - am-c.
itching - caust., teucr.
purple - hyos., sep.
scratching, after - alum.
syphilitic - syph.
warmth agg. - ***euphr., kali-i.,*** teucr.
washing, after - glon.

RED, face - acet-ac., **ACON.,** aeth., ***agar., ail.,*** aloe, alum., am-c., ***aml-n., anac., ant-c., ant-t.,*** **APIS,** arg-m., ***arg-n., arn., ars.,*** ars-h., ars-i., arum-t., ***asaf., astac., aster.,*** atro., aur., ***aur-m., bad.,*** **BAPT.,** ***bar-c.,*** bar-m., **BELL.,** berb., bor., ***bov.,*** brach., brom., **BRY.,** cact., calad., calc., ***camph.,*** cann-i., cann-s., ***canth.,*** **CAPS.,** carb-ac., carb-h., carb-o., carb-s., carb-v., ***carl.,*** cast., ***caust., cedr.,*** **CHAM., CHEL., CHIN.,**

RED, face - ***chin-s.,*** chlor., **CIC.,** cimic., **CINA,** clem., ***cocc., coc-c.,*** cod., ***coff., coloc.,*** com., con., cop., ***croc.,*** crot-c., ***crot-h., crot-t.,*** cub., ***cupr.,*** cur., ***dig.,*** dor., ***dros.,*** dub., ***dulc.,*** echi., ***elaps, eup-per.,*** eup-pur., euphr., fago., **FERR., *ferr-ar.,*** **FERR-I.,** ferr-m., ***ferr-ma.,*** ferr-p., gels., ***glon.,*** graph., ***grat., guai., hell., hep.,*** hippoz., ***hura,*** **HYOS.,** ***hyper., ign.,*** ind., indg., iod., ip., iris, ***jab.,*** jug-c., jug-r., kali-a., kali-bi., kali-br., kali-c., kali-chl., ***kali-i.,*** kali-n., kali-p., kali-s., kalm., kreos., **LACH.,** laur., led., lil-t., lob., ***lyc.,*** lyss., mag-c., mag-m., mag-s., mang., **MELI.,** meny., ***merc., merc-c.,*** merc-i-r., merl., **MEZ.,** mill., morph., mygal., ***mur-ac., naja,*** nat-a., ***nat-c., nat-m.,*** nat-p., nat-s., nicc., nit-ac., nux-m., **NUX-V.,** oena., olnd., **OP.,** ox-ac., paeon., ***petr.,*** phel., ph-ac., **PHOS.,** phys., phyt., ***plan., plat., plb.,*** podo., psor., ptel., ***puls., pyrog., ran-b.,*** raph., **RHUS-T.,** rhus-v., rumx., ruta., ***sabad.,*** sabin., ***samb.,*** **SANG.,** sant., sarr., sec., ***senec., sep., sil.,*** sol-n., sol-t-ae., ***spig., spong.,*** squil., ***stann.,*** staph., **STRAM.,** ***stront-c.,*** stry., ***sulph., sul-ac., tab., tarax.,*** tep., ***ter.,*** ther., ***thuj.,*** til., uva., valer., ***verat.,*** **VERAT-V.,** vesp., vib., zinc., zing.

afternoon - calc., meli., nat-c., phos., phys., sang., senec., **TUB.**

2 p.m. - nat-m.

3 p.m. - coff., meli.

4 p.m. - agar., sil., puls-n

5 p.m. - chel., mag-c.

5 to 7 p.m. - mag-c.

5 to 9 p.m. - plat.

6 p.m. - cann-s., sarr.

alternating with paleness - **ACON.,** alum., am-c., aml-n., ars., aur., bell., ***bor.,*** bov., brom., ***camph.,*** caps., cham., ***chin.,*** cimic., cina, ***croc.,*** cub., **FERR.,** ferr-p., gins., ***glon., hell.,*** hyos., ***ign.,*** kali-c., **LAC-C.,** ***led.,*** lyc., mag-c., merc., mur-ac., nat-c., nat-p., nit-ac., nux-v., olnd., ph-ac., phos., plat., puls., rhus-t., sep., squil., sul-ac., tab., verat., zinc.

menses, during - zinc.

anger, after - ***bry.,*** staph.

bleeding, preceding - meli.

chill, during - acon., aeth., all-s., alum., ***am-m.,*** apis, ***arn., ars., bell., bry., calc.,*** **CHAM.,** ***chin.,*** coc-c., dig., **FERR., *ferr-ar.,*** glon., hyos., ***ign., ip.,*** kali-n., kreos., ***led.,*** lyc., merc., merl., mur-ac., ***nux-v.,*** ox-ac., plb., puls., ***rhus-t., sep.,*** **STRAM.,** ***sulph.,*** thuj., ***tub.,*** zinc.

chill, before - cedr., chin.

circumscribed - acon., ***ant-t.,*** arg-n., ***ars.,*** ars-i., bar-c., benz-ac., bry., calc., carb-v., chel., **CHIN.,** chin-a., ***cina, colch.,*** con., croc., dol., dros., ***dulc.,*** **FERR.,** ***ferr-i.,*** ferr-p., hep., iod., ***kali-c.,*** kali-n., kali-p., kali-s., ***kreos., lach.,*** lachn., laur., led., **LYC.,** merc., nat-m., nit-ac., nux-v., op., ph-ac., **PHOS.,** ***puls.,*** pyrog., sabad., samb., ***sang.,*** seneg., sep., sil., spong., ***stann.,*** **SULPH.,** thuj., **TUB.**

red cheeks, with heart disease - aur-m.

RED, face

cold and - asaf., caps., chin., ***ferr.,*** mosch., ol-an., phos., psor.

colic, during - cham.

coma, with - chin., ***mur-ac.***

contradiction, from - ign.

convulsion, during - bufo, caust., **GLON., *oena.,*** **OP.**

cough, during - acon., am-c., **BELL.,** bry., cadm-s., caps., ***carb-v.,*** chr-ac., ***coc-c.,*** con., cor-r., ***cupr., dros.,*** eup-per., ferr., ***graph.,*** hep., hyos., ***ip.,*** kali-bi., ***kali-c.,*** lach., lyc., mag-p., mur-ac., nit-ac., sabad., samb., **SANG.,** sil., squil., staph., stram., sulph.

dark red - bar-c., cor-r., kali-c., squil., stram.

dark red, otherwise pale - kali-c.

deathly pale when not coughing - ***nit-ac.***

dark red - alum., ant-t., **BAPT.,** ***bar-c.,*** **BELL., BRY.,** ***camph., chel., coloc., gels., hyos.,*** kreos., **OP.,** ph-ac., ***sang., sec.,*** sil., stann., ***sulph., tarent., verat.***

dinner, after - cedr., grat., hell., nat-c., par.

dysmenorrhea, during - ferr-p., **XAN.**

eating, while - sep.

after - arum-t., caps., carl., caust., coff., cycl., ***lyc.,*** merc., nit-ac., nux-v., petr., puls., sil., sulph., vesp.

erysipelatous - **ACON.,** am-c., ***apis,*** ars., bar-c., **BELL.,** bor., bry., calc., camph., canth., carb-an., ***cham.,*** clem., **EUPH., GRAPH., HEP.,** ***lach.,*** lyc., merc., nat-c., ph-ac., phos., **RHUS-T.,** ruta., samb., sep., sil., stram., sulph., thuj.

extending to neck, back and perineum - med.

evening - bar-c., bell., calc., carb-an., ***croc.,*** elaps, **IGN.,** iod., kali-c., lyc., mag-c., mag-m., naja, nat-m., nux-v., oena., ox-ac., plan., plat., puls., rumx., scut., sep., sulph., thuj., trom., verat., zinc.

9 p.m. - phos.

excitement - ***coff.,*** **FERR.,** phos., sep., sulph.

exertion, after - **FERR.,** nux-v., squil.

eyes, about - elaps, lappa-a., maland., puls., sil.

around, on crying - bor.

fever, during - am-m., **BELL.,** brom., calc., carb-an., ***cedr.,*** chel., **CHIN.,** cina, ***cocc.,*** coff., dig., **EUP-PER.,** ferr., ferr-p., hell., hura, ip., lyc., merc., nat-m., ***nux-v.,*** phos., ***psor.,*** rhus-t., sang., **SEP.,** sil., sulph., ***tub., verat.,*** zinc.

fever, without - **CAPS., FERR.,** ol-an., phos., psor.

fiery - aml-n., coca, ***meli.,*** tarent.

flushes - aml-n., coca, ferr., stroph., tell.

anxiety, after - cupr.

menses, before - ***bell.,*** calc-p., ferr., ***ferr-p.,*** gels., ***sang.***

forenoon - lyc.

8 a.m. - myric.

9 a.m. - lyc.

11 a.m. - nat-c., sol-n., zing.

RED, face
glowing red - ***acon., apis,*** **ASTAC.,** aur., **BELL.,** ***calc., camph., carb-v.,*** **CINA,** cocc., croc., euph., ***ferr., glon., hep.,*** kali-c., ***lyc.,*** mur-ac., nat-c., ***plat., sabad.,*** sil., ***stram.,*** tab., ***thuj.***
headache, during - acon., agar., ail., alum., aur., **BELL.,** ***bufo,*** bov., bry., ***cact., calc.,*** camph., cann-s., canth., ***cic., coff., croc.,*** cycl., ferr., ***ferr-p.,*** **GLON.,** ign., ind., indg., ip., kali-i., ***kalm.,*** kreos., ***lach.,*** led., lyc., lyss., mag-c., mag-m., mag-p., **MELI.,** mur-ac., nat-c., ***nat-m., nux-m., op.,*** phos., plat., plb., ***psor.,*** ptel., puls., rhus-t., sil., spong., stront-c., sulph., tarax., thuj., zinc.
heart, with shocks at - phos.
heat of fire, during - **ANT-C.,** nat-m.
hot, and red - ***bell.,*** chin., hell.
hot, air, open, in - valer.
hypertension, with - ***stront-c.***
left - ***acet-ac.,*** aesc., agar., alumn., am-c., apis, asaf., bor., cham., chel., lac-c., ***lyc.,*** merc., murx., ***nat-m.,*** ol-an., ph-ac., **PHOS.,** ***rhus-t.,*** spig., stram., ***sulph.,*** thuj., verat.
left red, right pale - cann-s.
loss of vital fluids, from - chin.
lying, while - acon., lob-c., verat.
becomes pale on rising - ***acon., puls., verat., verat-v.***
on back - chlol.
on left side - ***calc.***
mahogany red - ***ail., arn.,*** eup-per., ***gels.***
maniacal rage, during - acon., ars., **BELL.,** cic., ***cupr., hyos.,*** lyc., merc., nux-v., ***op.,*** plat., puls., ***stram., verat.***
menopause, during - ***graph., kali-bi.,*** **LACH.,** lyc., phys., sang., **SUL-AC.,** ter.
menses, during - ind., ***puls.,*** xan.
morning - ail., dirc., kali-c., lyc., phos., ***podo.,*** rhus-t.
until 3 p.m. - stront.
waking, on - nat-m.
motion, at least - nux-v., squil.
mottled - ferr., ***lach.***
mouth, around - ip.
mouth, corners of - ars.
music agg. - ambr.
night - aloe, cedr., cic.
1 a.m. to 8 a.m. - lachn.
noon - apis, bell., lyc., mag-c., nat-m., phos., sep., sil., spig.
nosebleeds, amel. - bapt., bell., erig., ferr., meli., nux-v.
one-sided - ***acon.,*** ant-t., ***arn.,*** ars., bar-c., bell., calc., cann-s., ***cham., chel.,*** chin., cina, coloc., dros., ***ign.,*** ip., lac-c., lyc., mag-arct., merc., ***mosch.,*** nat-m., nux-v., ***phos.,*** plb., ***puls.,*** ran-b., rheum, rhus-t., sang., sep., spig., sulph., tab., tub., verat.
alternating sides - chel., lach., nat-p., ***phos.***
lung affection, same side as - tub.

RED, face
one-sided, one pale, the other red - acet-ac., ***acon.,*** caps., **CHAM.,** ***cina,*** **IP.,** ***lach., mosch., nux-v., puls.,*** rheum, sulph.
pain, when in - acon., ***bell.,*** caps., cham., cimic., **FERR.,** ferr-p., ign., meli., ter., verb.
before - graph.
palpitations, with - agar., aur., bell., glon.
purple - syph., tub.
riding, while - ferr.
right - ***ars., calc.,*** cham., elaps, lachn., mag-c., merc., mosch., nat-c., puls., sang., sul-ac., tab.
left waxy-yellow - canth.
without heat, paleness of the left with heat - mosch.
rising, on - naja, phys., verat.
up in bed - mag-s.
scratching, after - sulph.
shivering, while - **ARN.**
sitting, while - **BELL.,** phos.
sleep, during - ***arum-m.,*** bell., chlol., meny., viol-t.
spots - aeth., ail., alum., ambr., **AM-C.,** ***anan.,*** ars., aur., **BELL.,** berb., berb-a., ***bry.,*** canth., ***caps.,*** carb-an., ***carb-s.,*** croc., cycl., elaps, euphr., ***ferr.,*** hura, ictod., kali-bi., kali-c., lach., ***lac-c., lyc.,*** mag-arct., merc., nat-m., ***oena.,*** op., ox-ac., petr., **PHOS.,** rhus-t., rhus-v., **SABAD.,** samb., ***sil.,*** stroph., **SULPH.,** sumb., tab., tarax., tub.
burning - ***chel., croc.,*** tab.
eating, after - lyc., sil.
eruptions, after - dig.
fright after - am-c.
hot - bry.
painful - alum.
vexation, after - am-c.
washing, after - ***aesc., am-c., kali-c.,*** phos.
stool, during - caust.
before - manc.
stooping, on - ***bell., canth.***
sudden - alum., ***bell.,*** clem., euphr., ***mur-ac.,*** puls., thuj.
supper, after - carb-v.
talking - squil.
tea, drinking after - plan.
toothache, with - ***acon.,*** **BELL., CHAM.,** ***coff., ferr-p.,*** merc., nux-m., phos., puls., rhus-t., sulph.
unconsciousness, during - glon., ***mur-ac.***
vertigo, during - anan., ***bell., cact., cocc.,*** kalm., ***stram.***
waking, on - cimic., **CINA,** hura
walking, on - stront.
air, in open - mur-ac., sulph.
warm room - grat., ***sulph.***
washing, after - ***aesc., am-c., kali-c.,*** phos.
wine, the pale face becomes red, after - ***carb-v., ferr.***

red, cheek, bones - phos.
red, chin - ail., canth., colch., merc., nat-m., zinc.
spots - anac., ***caust.,*** crot-t., dig., sulph., sumb., zinc.
red, forehead - calc., hura, laur., lil-t., merc-i-r., mez., rhus-v., stram., vac., verat.
spots, in - aesc., berb., caps., cycl., mosch., sars., sulph., ***tell.***
reddish-yellow - ***chel.,*** gels., lach., **NUX-V.**
spots - kreos.

RHEUMATIC, pain - **ACON.,** act-sp., **ARS., BRY.,** ***calc-p.,*** **CAUST.,** ***chin., cimic., colch., coloc.,*** gels., ***hell., kali-ar.,*** kali-bi., ***kalm.,*** lach., ***lith.,*** mag-c., ***merc.,*** merc-i-f., mez., nux-v., phos., ***phyt., puls.,*** rhod., ***rhus-t., sil., spig.,*** verat.

RHUS poisoning - **ANAC.,** ***bry., crot-t., graph.,*** **RHUS-T.,** ***rhus-v.,*** sep., sulph.

RINGWORM, (see Barber's itch) - anag., ***bac.,*** bar-c., calc., cinnb., clem., dulc., ***graph.,*** hell., kali-chl., lith., lyc., ***nat-c., nat-m.,*** phos., **SEP.,** sulph., tarent., ***tell., thuj.,*** **TUB.**

RISUS sardonicus - **BELL.,** ***caust., cic., colch.,*** con., cupr-ac., hydr-ac., ***hyos.,*** ign., med., nux-m., ***oena.,*** op., plb., ran-s., ***sec.,*** sol-n., ***stram.,*** stry., tell., verat., zinc.

ROUGH, skin - alum., ***berb-a.,*** kali-c., ***petr.,*** sulph.
forehead - sep.
mouth, around - phos.
temples - nat-m.

ROUND - op.

RUBS, fist with, coughing while - caust., puls., ***squil.***
hand with - nux-v.

SADDLE across the nose - ***carb-an.,*** sanic., **SEP.,** syph., tril.

SCABBY - nit-ac.

SENSITIVE - acon., carb-an., ***carb-s.,*** chin-s., cod., kali-chl., ***lach.,*** nux-v., ***puls., zinc.***
air, to - colch., kali-i.
bones - aur., ***carb-v., hep., kali-bi., merc., merc-i-f.,*** mez., sulph.
shaving, when - carb-an., ox-ac.

SHARP, pain - ***acon.,*** aesc., aeth., agar., alum., am-c., am-m., ang., ant-c., apis, ars., arund., ***asaf.,*** asar., **AUR.,** aur-m., bar-c., **BELL.,** berb., calad., calc., camph., caps., ***carb-an.,*** carb-s., carb-v., cast-eq., ***caust.,*** cedr., ***cham.,*** chin., chin-s., ***cist.,*** clem., ***cocc., coloc.,*** con., cupr-ar., cycl., ***dig.,*** euphr., ferr-ma., ferr-p., fl-ac., ***gels., graph., guai., ham., ign.,*** indg., kali-ar., ***kali-bi., kali-c.,*** kali-chl., ***kali-i., kali-n.,*** kali-p., kali-s., ***kalm.,*** lach., lyc., lyss., ***mag-c.,*** mag-m., ***mag-p.,*** manc., ***mang.,*** meny., ***merc.,*** merc-c., merc-i-f., mez., naja, nat-c., nat-h., nat-m., nat-p., nit-ac., par., ***phos.,*** plan., ***plat.,*** psor., **PULS.,** ***rhod., rhus-t.,*** sabin., ***sang.,*** senec., **SEP.,** ***sil., spig.,*** spong., ***stann.,*** stict., still., stront-c., ***staph., stry., sulph.,*** sul-ac., tarax., tarent., thuj., valer., verb., vesp., ***zinc.***

SHARP, pain
bending forward with head to floor amel. - ***sang.***
burning - stann.
needles - **ARS.,** agar., ***aur.,*** caps., ***spig.***
change in temperature - mag-c.
chill, during - **CAUST.,** dros.
draft of air agg. - mag-c.
eating, while - ***mez.,*** phos.
evening - guai., lach., zinc.
extending to, ear - ***acon., bell., carb-an., coloc.,*** kali-bi., mur-ac.
to, eyes - chin., clem., naja
to, eyes, chewing, when - bell.
to, forehead - nat-c.
to, to neck - bell., nat-h.
to, to temple - alum., chin., mez., nat-h., naja
to, upwards - clem., sul-ac.
intermittent - ***asaf.***
itching - aur., cycl., plat., stann., staph.
jarring - chin.
jerking - zinc.
left - aesc., all-c., apis, asar., camph., chel., **COLOC.,** ***con.,*** dros., ***guai.,*** indg., ***kali-bi.,*** kali-i., ***mag-c., mang.,*** merc-i-f., ***nat-m.,*** par., ***plan.,*** puls., ***sang.,*** senec., sep., stict., ***sulph.,*** valer.
extending to left ear - ***coloc.***
light - chin.
mercury, after abuse of - kali-i.
motion - chin.
night - clem., ***guai., mag-c.***
noise - chin.
outward - **ASAF.**
right - am-m., ***bell.,*** cist., ***clem.,*** cupr., ***guai.,*** ham., ***kali-i.,*** lyss., ***mag-p.,*** nat-p., onos., ***phos.,*** sars., ***sep., spig.,*** spong., verb., verat., zinc.
extending to left ear - ***coloc.***
rubbing amel. - nat-c.
speaking - mez., ***phos.,*** verb.
touch - ***chin.,*** chin-s., cupr., mag-m., ***phos.,*** sep., staph., ***verb.***
vexation - nat-h.
walking, amel. - ***mag-c.***
walking, in open air - thuj.
warm, room agg. - ***mez.,*** nat-h.
warmth of bed - clem.
sharp, cheek bones - aesc., aeth., agar., alum., arg-m., ars., berb., ***carb-an.,*** con., euon., guai., ***kali-bi., kali-i.,*** merc., mez., par., phos., psor., sabin., sil., stann., staph., verb.
sharp, chin - agar., am-m., ant-c., bell., con., euphr., lact., stann., zinc.
sharp, zygoma - aur., rhus-t., verb., ***zinc.***

SHAVING, after agg. - calad., ***carb-an.,*** ox-ac., phos., ph-ac., **PULS.,** rad-br., stroph-s., thuj.

SHINY - acon., **APIS,** arg-n., ***aur.,*** caust., coff., cupr., der., eup-pur., hyos., ***lyc.,*** med., ***nat-m.,*** op., ***plb.,*** psor., rheum, rhus-t., sel., thuj.
as if oily - ***nat-m., plb.,*** thuj.
spots after eruptions - nat-m.

SHIVERING, in and spreading from - caust., mag-m.
chin - stram.

SHOCKS, followed by burning - ***thuj.***

SHRIVELLED, (see Wrinkled) - apis, ant-t., crot-t., kali-fer., merc., op., plb., rob., sin-n., ter., zinc-s.

SICKLY, (see Expression, and Discoloration)

SMUTTY, (see Skin, Filthy) - ***ant-t.***

SORE, pain - alum., anac., ant-t., ***arn.,*** **AUR.,** ***bry.,*** carb-s., caust., con., cor-r., cupr., graph., ham., ***ign.,*** kali-bi., ***kali-c.,*** **LACH.,** ***manc., merc-i-f.,*** mez., ***nat-m., phos.,*** plan., ***plat.,*** puls., ***ruta.,*** sars., stann., sulph., thuj., til., ***verat.,*** zinc.
bathing, after - con.
bones of face - bufo, ***carb-v.,*** cupr-ar., ***merc-i-f., kali-bi.,*** nat-m., tarent.
chewing, when - caust., ***nat-m.***
maxillary articulation, on chewing - sil.
on motion - rhus-t.
menses, during - stann.
morning - sars.
waking, on - sars.
mouth, around - plat.
opening - nat-m.,
corners, of - bell., graph., sul-ac.
pressure, on - caust., euph.

sore, malar-bones - cor-r., mang., merc-i-f., nat-m., nit-ac., ***rhus-t.,*** stann., sulph., sul-ac., zinc.
chewing - nat-m.
extending to forehead and side of head - merc-i-f.
left - cor-r., sul-ac.
right - ***merc-i-f.,*** sulph., zinc.

sore, zygoma - cor-r., sul-ac., zinc.

SPASMS, of - acon., agar., ambr., amyg., anan., ant-t., arg-n., ***ars.,*** atro., bar-c., **BELL.,** bism., ***bov.,*** brom., ***bufo,*** calc., camph., canth., carb-s., ***caust., cham.,*** **CIC.,** ***cocc.,*** con., crot-c., **CUPR.,** dig., ***glon., hep.,*** hydr-ac., ***hyos., ign., ip.,*** kali-n., ***laur., lyc., lyss.,*** merc-c., morph., nat-c., nit-ac., nux-v., ***oena.,*** ol-an., ***op.,*** phos., ***phys.,*** plb., ***ran-b.,*** ran-s., rhus-t., sec., **STRAM.,** stry., sulph., sul-ac., tab., verat., vip., ***zinc.,*** ziz.
beginning in face - absin., ***bufo,*** cina, dulc., hyos., ign., sant., ***sec.***
beginning in left side - ***lach.***
chill, during - ars., bell., cham., cic., ign., op., stram.
extending to limbs - sant., sec.
masseters - ambr., ang., cocc., cupr., mang., nux-v.
menses, before - puls.
mouth - bell., cham., dulc., ign., ***ip., lyc.,*** merc., nit-ac., olnd., op., stram.
one-sided - dig., plb.
right - agar.
speaking, while - plb.

SPLINTER, as from a - agar.

SPOTS, (see Discoloration) - ***all-s.,*** benz-ac., ***calc.,*** **CARB-AN.,** dor., ***guai.,*** kali-chl., ***lyc., nat-c.,*** nux-m., **RHUS-T.,** sabad., **SIL.,** sul-ac., syph., verb.
painful sensation - verb.
ulcerating - nat-c., staph.

STIFFNESS, muscles - absin., acon., agar., anac., arn., bapt., bry., ***caust.,*** gels., ham., helo., ip., ***nux-v.,*** plan., rhus-t., sang., staph., stry., ***verat.***
cough, during - **IP.**
pain, during - nit-ac.
in occiput, with - staph.

STINGING, pain - all-s., **APIS,** arn., **ARS.,** asar., berb., caust., ***chin., cinnb., clem.,*** **COLOC.,** con., dros., ***euph., ferr-p., graph., ind., kali-c.,*** kalm., merc-i-f., sars., spong., vesp., zing.
heat, during - olnd.
right - sars.

SUNBURN - canth., sol., ***thuj.,*** urt-u.

SUNKEN - acon., ***aeth.,*** aloe, ***ant-c.,*** **ANT-T.,** apis, ***arg-n., arn.,*** **ARS.,** ars-h., bell., **BERB.,** ***calc.,*** **CAMPH.,** canth., ***carb-s.,*** **CARB-V.,** ***cham., chel.,*** **CHIN.,** chlor., cina, ***colch.,*** con., ***cub.,*** cupr., **DIG.,** dirc., dros., eup-per., ***ferr.,***

SUNKEN - ***ferr-ma.,*** ferr-p., gels., gran., hell., hydr-ac., hyos., **IGN.,** iod., ***ip., kali-ar., kali-c.,*** kali-n., kali-p., kali-s., ***lach.,*** laur., ***lyc.,*** **MANG.,** ***merc.,*** merc-c., mez., morph., ***mur-ac., nat-s., nit-ac.,*** nux-v., olnd., ol-an., **OP.,** ox-ac., petr., ***ph-ac., phos.,*** phyt., ***plat., plb., rhus-t.,*** sabad., ***samb.,*** **SEC.,** sep., sin-n., squil., ***stann., staph., sulph.,*** sul-ac., ***tab.,*** ter., **VERAT.,** ***zinc.***
dinner, after - nat-m.
morning - lyc., nat-m., ol-an.
rage, during - ***ars.,*** canth., cupr., lach., nux-v., phos., sec., verat.
stool, after - ferr-m.

SWELLING - **ACON.,** aesc., aeth., agar., ail., aloe, alum., am-c., am-m., amyg., anac-oc., anac., anan., ***ant-t.,*** **APIS,** apoc., ***arn.,*** **ARS.,** ***arum-t., aur., aur-m., bar-c.,*** **BELL.,** bor., **BOV., BRY.,** ***bufo, cact.,*** **CALC.,** ***calc-ar., camph., canth.,*** caps., carb-h., ***carb-s., carb-v.,*** **CHAM.,** chel., ***chin.,*** chin-a., chlor., cic., ***cina, cocc., colch., coloc., com., con.,*** cop., ***crot-h.,*** crot-t., cub., cupr., dig., dol., dor., dros., ***elaps, euph.,*** fago., **FERR.,** ***ferr-ar.,*** ferr-i., ferr-m., ***ferr-p.,*** gels., glon., ***graph., guai.,*** guare., gymn., hell., helon., **HEP.,** hura, hydr-ac., hydrc., hyos., hyper., ip., kali-ar., kali-bi., ***kali-c.,*** kali-chl., ***kali-i.,*** kali-p., ***lach.,*** lachn., lac-c., laur., led., **LYC.,** mag-c., manc., **MERC.,** ***merc-c., mez., nat-a., nat-c., nat-h.,*** **NAT-M.,** nicc., ***nit-ac., nux-m., nux-v., oena.,*** **OP.,** ox-ac., ***phos.,*** plan., ***plat.,*** plb., psor., puls., **RHUS-T.,** ***rhus-v.,*** sabin., ***samb.,*** sang., sec., sel., senec., seneg., ***sep.,*** sil., sol-n., ***spig.,*** spong., ***stram., stann.,*** stry., sulph., tab., tarax., tax., ter., thuj., vac., ***verat.,*** vesp., vinc., vip., zinc-s.
afternoon - ***ars.,*** bell., phos.
bee stings, from - **APIS,** ***carb-ac., lach., led.***
bones - nat-a.
eating, after - merc.

SWELLING,
eating, while - sep.
edematous - aeth., ant-a., ***ant-t.,*** **APIS,** ***apoc.,*** **ARS.,** ars-h., ***ars-m., cact.,*** **CALC.,** carb-s., ***chel., chin., colch., crot-h.,*** cupr-ar., ***dig., dulc.,*** euph., ***ferr., ferr-p.,*** **GRAPH.,** ham., ***hell.,*** kali-ar., **LYC.,** ***merc., merc-c., nat-a., nat-c., nat-m., phos., plb., rhus-t.,*** thuj., ***vesp., xan.***
amenorrhea, in - xan.
evening - ars., lyc., rhus-t., sulph.
hard - am-c., ***arn.,*** ars., bell., bor., **HEP.,** ***merc., sil.***
hot - bor., rhus-t.
intermittents, in - ars., chin., lyc., nat-m.
itching - rhus-t.
left - anac., arg-m., arg-n., ***com., kali-c.,*** **LACH.,** lyss., nat-m., ***phyt.,*** zinc.
heat and burning, with - arg-m.
lying, while - apoc.
menses, during - aeth., ***sulph.***
menses, before - bar-c., ***graph., kali-c., merc., puls.***
menses, instead of - ***kali-c.***
mercury, after - ***kali-i.***
morning - **ARS.,** aur., calc., crot-h., dirc., graph., ***hep.,*** kali-c., ***kali-chl., kalm., lyc.,*** manc., merc., ***nit-ac., phos., sep., spig.,*** sulph.
waking, on - agar., hura, nat-a., rhus-t., spig.
mouth, around - carb-an., olnd., nux-v.
mouth, corner of - clem., vinc.
night - ***lach.***
nodular - alum.
one-sided - arn., ***ars., aur.,*** bar-c., ***bell.,*** bor., ***bry.,*** canth., ***cham.,*** graph., mag-arct., ***merc., merc-c.,*** nux-v., ***phos.,*** plb., puls., sep., spig., staph.
pale - ***apis, ars., calc.,*** graph., hell., lyc.
coughing, when - samb.
pregnancy, during - ***merc-c., phos.***
red - ***acon., arn.,*** ars., bell., bor., chin., cic., coloc., euph., ferr., guai., ***kali-c.,*** lach., merc., nat-c., nux-v., olnd., op., rhus-t., stram., sulph., verat.
right - act-sp., arn., ***ars., bor., calc.,*** elaps, merc., merc-i-f., nicc., ***plb.,*** polyg., rumx., sang.
scarlet fever - **APIS, ARUM-T.,** ***calc., lyc., hell., kali-s.,*** zinc.
shining - apis, arn., aur., spig.
stiff - rhus-t.
submental gland - am-c., graph., led., staph.
submental gland, painful - am-c.
toothache - all-c., am-c., ***ant-c.,*** aur., bor., ***calc., calc-s.,*** **CHAM.,** colch., ***euph.,*** graph., ***hep.,*** iod., ***kali-c.,*** **LACH.,** lyc., ***mag-c.,*** **MERC.,** nat-m., nit-ac., nux-v., phos., samb., **SEP., SIL.,** ***spig.,*** staph., stront-c., ***thuj., verat.***
washing, after - ***aesc.***
zygoma - con.

swelling, cheeks - am-c., am-m., apis, ***arn.,*** ars., ***aur.,*** bell., bor., bov., bry., ***calc.,*** caps., carb-an., carb-v., caust., ***cham.,*** dig., euphr., hep., kali-ar., ***kali-c., kali-i.,*** lyc., ***mag-c.,*** mag-m., **MERC.,** merc-c., nat-c., nat-m., nit-ac., nux-v., puls., sep., ***sil., spong., stann.,*** staph., sulph.
hard - am-c., calc-f.
left - sul-ac.
menses, during - graph., sep.
after - phos.
before - phos.
morning - nat-c.
red - sulph.
sense of swelling - acon., calc., ***chel.,*** samb.

swelling, chin - carb-v., caust.
left - chin-a.

swelling, eyes, above - chin., **KALI-C.,** ***lyc.,*** nat-a., puls., ruta., sep.
around - all-c., **APIS,** ***ars.,*** chin., colch., cupr., elaps, ***ferr.,*** **KALI-C.,** merc., nit-ac., ***phos.,*** **RHUS-T.,** sang., spig., stram., urt-u.
morning - ars., nit-ac.
right - ail., ***rhus-v.***
between - lyc.
under - **APIS,** apoc., **ARS.,** ***aur.,*** bry., calc., ***calc-ar., carb-ac.,*** cinnb., colch., ***fl-ac.,*** hep., **KALI-C.,** ***kali-i.,*** med., merc., nat-c., nit-ac., nux-v., olnd., phos., puls., ***raph., sulph.,*** syc-co., ***thlaspi.***
left - colch., ***sulph.***
morning - sep.
right - ***carb-ac.***

swelling, forehead - apis, ars., hell., lyc., ***nux-v., phos., rhus-t., ruta, sep.***
glabella - fl-ac., kali-c., sel., sil.

swelling, glands - am-c., am-m., arn., ***ars., ars-i.,*** **ARUM-T.,** asaf., aur., aur-m., bad., ***bar-c., bar-m.,*** **BELL.,** bov., brom., bry., calad., **CALC.,** camph., ***carb-an., carb-s.,*** cham., chin., cic., clem., cocc., con., cor-r., crot-t., dulc., graph., **HEP., IOD.,** jab., ***kali-c.,*** kali-i., ***lach.,*** led., ***lith., lyc.,*** **MERC.,** ***mur-ac., nat-c., nat-m.,*** nat-p., ***nit-ac.,*** nux-v., petr., ***phos.,*** plb., puls., **RHUS-T.,** ***sep.,*** **SIL.,** spig., spong., **STANN.,** ***staph.,*** **SULPH.,** ***sul-ac.,*** thuj., verat.
hard, painful - bar-c., ***bell.,*** calc., hell., iod., mur-ac., nat-m., petr., ***rhus-t.,*** **SIL.,** staph., ***sulph.***

swelling, sensation of - ***aesc.,*** aeth., alum., ***aran.,*** ars-m., bar-c., ***bell.,*** calc., ***chel., ferr., grat., gymn., lil-t., mez., nat-m.,*** nicc., ***nux-m.,*** phos., pip-m., puls., ***staph.,*** stram., ***sul-ac.***
air, in open - phos.
cheeks - acon., samb.
house, on entering - aeth.
malar bone - spig.

SYPHILITIC, eruptions - ***ars-i., aur., cinnb., fl-ac., hep., kali-bi.,*** **KALI-I.,** kreos., ***lach., lyc.,*** **MERC., MERC-C.,** ***nit-ac., phyt.,*** sep., ***sil., sulph.,*** **SYPH.**

TEARING, pain - act-sp., aeth., ***agar., alum.,*** ambr., am-c., am-m., ***anac., ant-t., arg-m., ars.,*** **AUR., BELL.,** berb., bor., bry., ***calc.,*** calc-ar., caps., carb-an., carb-s., **CARB-V., CAUST.,** ***chel., chin.,*** chin-a., cist., ***cocc., colch.,*** **COLOC.,** ***con.,*** dulc., euon., gels., ***graph.,*** grat., hep., indg., kali-ar., kali-bi., ***kali-c.,*** kali-chl., ***kali-n.,*** kali-p., kali-s., ***kalm.,*** **LACH.,** lachn., led., **LYC.,** ***lyss.,*** **MAG-C., MAG-P.,** mag-s., **MERC.,** ***mez.,*** mur-ac., ***nat-s., nit-ac.,*** **NUX-V.,** ***phos., plat.,*** plb., **PULS.,** ***rhod., rhus-t.,*** ruta., sars., ***sep., sil., spig.,*** spong., staph., stram., ***stront-c., sulph.,*** sul-ac., tab., teucr., thuj., ***verat.,*** vinc., viol-o., zinc.
afternoon - alum., calc.
change of weather - ***rhod.***
coffee, after abuse of - ***nux-v.***
cold, air - aeth., ***rhus-t.***
cold, applications amel. - **PULS.**
damp weather agg. - ***merc., rhod., rhus-t.,*** verat.
dinner, after - carb-an.
eating, agg. - phos.
amel. - chin., phos., rhod.
evening - am-m., carb-an., carb-v., cist., mag-s., phos., **PULS.,** rhus-t., zinc.
8 p.m. - ***guai., puls.***
in bed - kali-n.
extending to,
arms - ***kalm.,*** lyc.
ear - **COLOC., LACH.,** ***lyss.,*** plan., **PULS.,** ***sep.***
fingers - lyc.
forehead - zinc.
head - ***coloc.***
neck - ***puls.***
occiput - sep.
parietal bone - chin.
temples - zinc.
increases gradually and ceases suddenly - ***arg-m.***
jerking - agar., am-m., ***carb-v.,*** euph., ***puls.,*** rhod.
left - am-c., ars., ***aur., carb-v., caust.,*** **COLOC.,** gran., graph., ***guai., lach.,*** mag-s., ***mez.,*** plan., sars., ***spig.,*** spong., staph., ***thuj.,*** zinc.
lying, agg. - ail., ***chin.,*** **MAG-C.,** phos., ***puls.***
amel. - nux-v.
lying, on affected side amel. - kali-n..
back, agg. - ***arg-m.***
face, amel. - spig.
menses, after - spig.
morning - ***mez., nux-v.,*** thuj.
until sunset - ***spig.***
motion, agg. - **BELL.,** ***colch.,*** coloc., ***nux-v., spig.***
amel. - **MAG-C., RHUS-T.**
motion, of lower jaw amel. - phos.
mouth, corners of - bell., carb-v.
night - chin., ***cocc., con., mag-c., lach.,*** led., rhus-t.
nose and eyes, between - mang.
paroxysmal - **CAUST.,** ***coloc.,*** nux-v., puls.

TEARING, pain
periodic - guai., ***spig.***
pressure, amel. - aur., ***bry.,*** carb-an., kali-c., kali-n., **MAG-C., MAG-P.,** ***rhus-t.***
rheumatic - sul-ac.
right - agar., am-c., am-m., anac., anag., arg-m., ***bell., carb-v.,*** **CHEL.,** ***chin., con., kalm.,*** led., ***lyc., lyss., mag-c., mag-p.,*** phos., ***plat.,*** psor., sars., spig., spong., stram., ***sulph.,*** thuj.
rubbing, amel. - alum., nat-c., ***phos., rhus-t.***
spring - ***lach., nux-v.***
storm, before - ***rhod.***
swallowing, agg. - phos.
talking - phos.
touch, agg. - ***chin.,*** **COLOC.,** ***mag-p.,*** staph.
vexation, after - ***coloc.***
walking, amel. - ail., **MAG-C.**
wandering - colch., puls.
warmth, agg. - ***puls.***
amel. - ***coloc.,*** **MAG-P.,** ***rhod.,*** **RHUS-T.**
wind agg. - ***rhod.***

tearing, cheek bones - aeth., agar., alum., am-c., ***am-m.,*** ant-t., ***arg-m.,*** aur., berb., bor., bry., ***calc., carb-v., chel.,*** cina, ***colch., coloc.,*** graph., indg., kali-c., kali-n., **LYC.,** ***mag-c.,*** mag-s., **MERC.,** mez., mur-ac., ***nat-s.,*** nit-ac., nux-v., ***phos., rhus-t.,*** ruta., sep., sil., ***spig.,*** staph., stann., stront-c., sulph., sul-ac., tab., teucr., ***zinc.***
left - caust., kali-n., lyc., sul-ac.
left, extending to lower jaw - stann.
right - agn., calc-caust., ***chel.***

tearing, chin - agar., am-m., aur., ***caust.,*** plat., zinc.
chin, right - kali-n.

tearing, zygoma - alum., ***arg-m.,*** arg-n., **AUR.,** am-m., berb., bor., carb-an., **CARB-V.,** chel., con., ***graph.,*** mag-m., merl., mur-ac., nat-c., nit-ac., phos., spig., spong.
extending to head - mag-m.
left then right - arg-n.
right - arg-m., ***chel.,*** spong.

TENSION, of skin - acon., ***alum.,*** ambr., am-c., ant-t., ***asaf., bar-c.,*** bar-m., benz-ac., berb., bov., cann-i., canth., colch., ***euph., gels.,*** graph., ***grat.,*** hep., hyper., kali-c., kali-chl., kali-n., kali-p., ***lach.,*** laur., lyc., ***mag-c.,*** mag-m., ***merc.,*** merl., ***mez.,*** mosch., ***nat-m.,*** nit-ac., phel., ***ph-ac., phos., puls.,*** rheum, ***rhus-t.,*** sabad., samb., sep., squil., stann., staph., verat., viol-o., viol-t.
evening - alum.
eyes, below - nux-v., viol-o.
malar bone - aur., bar-ac., lec., lyc., mag-m., ***phos.,*** plat., verb.
across - verat-v.
masseter muscles - ***nux-v.,*** sars., verb.
morning - nit-ac.
on waking - am-c.
night - apis.
1 to 4 p.m. - apis

TENSION, of skin
one-sided - benz-ac., coloc., mag-c., phos.
as if muscles were drawn to one side - cist.
pain, before - ign.
prosopalgia, before - ign.
right - am-c., verat.
varnished, as if - ***lec.***
white of egg were dried on the as if (see Cobwebs) - ***alum., bar-c.,*** calad., graph., ***lec., mag-c.,*** nat-m., ol-an., petr., ph-ac., sulph., sul-ac.
tension, cheek, as from swelling - ambr.
tension, chin, below - staph.
chin, on - ***alum.,*** plat., ***verb.***
tension, forehead - am-c., cann-i., com., ***nit-ac.***
contracted, feels - bapt., bell-p., grat., hell., lyc., phos., prim-v.
tension, mouth, eyes and nose, around - nux-v.

TETANUS, lockjaw, (see Emergency)

THICK, skin - bell., viol-t.
spots - carb-an.

TICS, facial (see Twitching)

TINGLING - ***acon.,*** alum., ambr., apis, arund., aur., bar-c., bell., calc., cann-i., caust., ***colch.,*** crot-h., cycl., ***ferr-ma.,*** grat., hep., hyper., lach., lachn., lact., laur., lyc., nux-m., nux-v., ol-an., olnd., paeon., plat., ran-b., rhus-t., sabad., ***sec.,*** stront-c., sul-ac., thuj.
eyes, around - ambr.
forehead - ambr., stram.
left - euon., zinc.
right - aur., elaps, gymn.
whiskers - ambr.
tingling, cheeks and lips - agn., ***arn.,*** ars., berb., dros.
tingling, chin and nose - ran-b., verat.

TREMBLING - ***ambr.,*** merc., ***op.,*** plb., sabad., sec.
lower - ant-c., ***gels., ran-s.***
right, then left - ***plb.***
spasmodic - ambr., sec.
talking, when - merc.

TUBERCLES - ***alum.,*** ant-c., ***ars.,*** asaf., bar-c., calc., ***carb-v.,*** cic., con., dulc., ***fl-ac., graph.,*** hep., ***kali-bi.,*** kali-c., ***kali-i.,*** lach., ***led.,*** lyc., mag-c., mag-m., merc., ***nat-c.,*** nit-ac., olnd., phyt., puls., sil., sumb., thuj., zinc.
forehead - ***fl-ac., led.,*** olnd.
itching - kali-n.
mouth, about - ars., bar-c., bry., caust., con., mag-m., sep., sil., sulph.
painful - sep.
pregnancy, during - ***hyos.***
suppurating - ***fl-ac., nat-c., sil.***
wings of nose - hippoz.
tubercles, chin - carb-an., euph., hep., mag-m., olnd.

TUMOR, cystic
cheek, on - graph., thuj.
sebaceous - kali-br.
malar bone - mag-c.

TWITCHING, facial - acon., **AGAR.,** ***ambr.,*** am-m., ant-c., ***ant-t.,*** arn., ***ars., ars-i.,*** atro., aur-m., bar-c., bell., brom., bufo, calc., camph., cann-s., carb-ac., carb-v., ***caust., cham.,*** chel., chlol., cic., ***cina,*** cocc., colch., ***con.,*** crot-c., cupr-ar., dros., glon., graph., ***hell., hyos., ign., iod., ip.,*** kali-ar., kali-c., ***kali-chl.,*** kali-i., kali-n., kali-s., ***laur.,*** **LYC.,** lyss., mag-c., meny., ***mez., mygal.,*** nat-a., nat-c., ***nat-m.,*** nit-ac., nux-v., ***oena.,*** olnd., **OP.,** ox-ac., ***phos.,*** plb., puls., ran-s., sang., sant., sec., **SEL.,** sep., spig., stram., ***stront-c.,*** stry., sulph., ***sul-ac.,*** syph., thuj., valer., verat., verat-v., ***zinc.***
asthma, before - bov.
coughing, when - **ANT-T.,** kali-m.
eating, when - kali-m.
evening after lying down - ambr., ***nux-v.***
eyes, below - nit-ac.
right - bell.
eyes, left - ant-c., arg-n., bar-c., bell., brach., carb-v., chin., con., euph., ***glon.,*** kali-c., ***phel.,*** phos., sulph., ***tell., thuj.,*** valer.
eyes, right - am-m., bor., bry., calc., chel., kali-n., ***mag-c.,*** meny., mez., nux-v., phos., ***plb., thuj.***
flatulence, from - nat-c.
from obstructed - nat-c.
left - agar., ***calc.,*** tell.
mercury, after abuse of - ***kali-chl., nit-ac.***
morning - ***nux-v.,*** sulph.
motion, of head, on - sul-ac.
mouth, around - bry., ***chel.,*** guare., ***ign.,*** mag-p., mosch., **OP.,** phys., plat., ***rheum.***
sleep, in - anac.
corners of - anac., ant-c., bor., ***bry., chel., ign.,*** mag-p., olnd., ***op.,*** rheum, zinc.
upper molars - am-m., ***glon.,*** phos.
night, during sleep - nat-c.
painful - acon., aconin., anan., arg-n., ars., ***bell.,*** caps., ***colch., gels.,*** glon., graph., kali-c., kali-chl., ***kali-i., mag-p., mez.,*** nat-s., ***phos.,*** rhus-t., sep., stann., staph., ***stry.,*** sulph., ***thuj., verb.,*** zinc-m.
pressure, amel. - am-c., nux-m.
protruding tongue, on - hyos.
rest, during - meny.
right - ***caust.,*** puls.
rubbing, amel. - phos.
sleep, during - bry., nat-c., rheum.
spasmodic - agar., arg-n., ***bell.,*** caust., cham., ***cic., cina, gels., hyos., ign.,*** laur., meny., ***mygal.,*** nux-v., ***oena.,*** op., sec., stram., tell., visc.
talking, when - kali-m., plb., sep., sil.
vision, misty, with - mill.
twitching, chin - plat., sulph.
twitching, eyes, left - ant-c., arg-n., bar-c., bell., brach., carb-v., chin., con., euph., ***glon.,*** kali-c., phel., phos., sulph., ***tell., thuj.,*** valer.
below, left - thuj.
right - bell.
right - am-m., bor., bry., calc., chel., kali-n., mag-c., meny., mez., nux-v., phos., ***plb., thuj.***

twitching, mouth, one-sided, when speaking or smiling - cub.
upper molars - am-m., ***glon.,*** phos.
twitching, zygoma - kali-n., phos., spig., sulph.
zygoma, towards - thuj.

ULCERS - anan., ant-t., **ARS.,** aur-m-n., ***con.,*** cund., ***hep.,*** iod., ***kali-ar.,*** kali-bi., ***kali-chl., kali-i., lach.,*** merc., nat-m., ***nit-ac., phos., phyt., psor.,*** thuj., vesp.
burning - hep., nux-v.
eating - ***ars., con.,*** nux-v., ***phos.***
hard edges - ***kali-bi.***
mouth, around - nat-c., ***nit-ac.***
mouth, corners of - ail., ***am-m.,*** anan., ant-c., arn., aur-m-n., ***bell., bov.,*** **CALC.,** carb-an., carb-v., ***cocc.,*** **GRAPH.,** ***hep.,*** ign., ip., ***mang.,*** **MERC.,** mez., ***nat-m.,*** **NIT-AC.,** nux-v., ***phos., psor.,*** **RHUS-T.,** ***sil.,*** staph., ***sulph.,*** thuj., zinc.
itching - sil.
painful, on motion - ars., caps.
putrid - merc.
sensitive to air - **HEP.**
serpiginous - caust., ***staph.***
touch agg. - ars.
wart-like - **ARS.**
ulcers, cheek - ant-t., calc., iod., nat-m., phos.
ulcers, chin - **CUND.,** hep., merc., ***nat-m., nit-ac.,*** sep.
ulcers, zygoma - phos.

URTICARIA - anan., ***am-c.,*** **APIS, ARS.,** ***bell., calc., chel., chin-s.,*** **CHLOL., COP.,** crot-t., dulc., ***gels., hep.,*** hydr., ***kali-i.,*** lach., ***led.,*** mez., ***nat-m.,*** nit-ac., ***rhus-t., sep.,*** sil., **SULPH.,** ***urt-u.***
disappearing in open air - calc.
morning - chin.
winter, in - ***kali-i.***

VEINS, distended - bapt., **CHIN.,** ***ferr., glon.,*** **LACH.,** ***op.,*** sang., sars., thuj.
chin - ***plat.***
forehead - abrot., calad., camph., chin., cub., ***piloc., sulph.***
nets as if marbled - ***calc., carb-v., crot-h.,*** **LACH.,** lyc., thuj.
temples - ars., glon., sang.

VESICLES - aeth., ***agar.,*** alum., am-c., am-m., anac., ***ant-c.,*** ant-t., ***ars.,*** benz-ac., bor., calc-s., canth., carb-an., ***carb-s.,*** caust., cic., cist., ***clem.,*** **CROT-T.,** ***dulc., euph.,*** ferr-i., ***graph.,*** hep., indg., kali-ar., kali-bi., ***kali-i.,*** kali-n., lach., ***mag-c.,*** **MANC.,** mang., ***merc.,*** mez., nat-a., ***nat-c.,*** **NAT-M.,** ***nat-s., nit-ac.,*** ol-an., ***petr.,*** ph-ac., phos., plb., **PSOR.,** ran-b., **RHUS-T.,** rhus-v., samb., **SEP.,** ***sil.,*** stront-c., ***sulph.,*** stram., syph., valer., zinc.
acrid - caust., rhus-t.
burning - agar., ***anac.,*** aur., caust., cic., hep., nat-c., ***nat-m., ran-b.***
cold air - ***dulc.***
confluent - crot-t., ran-b., rhus-t., ***sulph.***
forehead - am-c., arn., bor., canth., kali-i., mez., nat-m., plb., ***psor.,*** rhus-v., stront.

VESICLES,
itching - ***anac.,*** ant-c., ***ars.,*** cic., mang., ***mez.,*** sars., sep.
mouth, around - ***bor., hell.,*** **NAT-M.,** ***nat-s.***
mouth, corners - agar., caust., ***cic.,*** mez., seneg., senn.
varioloid - ant-c.
white - clem., hell., mez., nat-c., sulph., valer.
yellow - ***agar.,*** ant-c., ars., cic., com., crot-t., ***dulc., euph.,*** kreos., ***manc., merc.,*** mur-ac., nat-c., ph-ac., **RHUS-T.,** ***rhus-v.,*** sep.
vesicles, chin, on - agar., anac., canth., ***cic.,*** crot-t., hep., ***manc., nat-c.,*** **NAT-M.,** ***nat-s., nit-ac., sanic., sars.***

WARTS - ***calc.,*** calc-s., cast., **CAUST., DULC.,** ***kali-c.,*** lyc., ***nit-ac., sep.,*** sulph., ***thuj.***
cheek - ars.
chin - ***lyc.,*** **THUJ.**
forehead - cast.
mouth, around - cund., ***psor.***

WASH, in cold water, desire to - ***apis, asar.,*** cann-i., ***fl-ac.,*** mez., sabad.

WAXY - ***acet-ac.,*** **APIS, ARS.,** ***aspar., calc.,*** calc-p., carb-v., con., ***ferr-ar.,*** ferr-m., lach., **MED.,** merc-c., nat-c., nat-m., nit-ac., ph-ac., ***phos.,*** sel., senec., ***sep., sil.,*** thuj., zinc.

WEAKNESS - cham.

WRINKLED - ***abrot.,*** aeth., alum., apis, ant-t., ***arg-n., ars.,*** bar-c., bell., bor., **CALC.,** calc-p., carb-h., con., crot-t., culx., ***fl-ac., hell.,*** iod., kreos., ***lyc.,*** merc., nat-c., nat-m., nit-ac., op., plb., ***psor.,*** rob., ***sanic., sars.,*** sec., sil., sin-n., stram., sulph., syph., ter., zinc., zinc-s.
deep - lyc., phos.
eyebrows - ox-ac., ***rheum,*** stram., ther., viol-o.
fine - calc.
wrinkled, forehead - acet-ac., alum., brom., ***caust., cham., cycl., graph.,*** grat., ***hell.,*** lachn., **LYC.,** mang., merc., nat-m., ox-ac., phos., plb., rheum, rhus-t., ***sep., stram., syph.,*** verat., zinc.
brain symptoms, in - grat., ***hell.,*** **STRAM.**

YELLOW - acon., aesc., agar., ail., alumn., ***ambr.,*** anan., ant-a., apis, **ARG-M., ARG-N.,** arn., **ARS.,** ***ars-h., ars-i.,*** asc-t., ***bapt., bell.,*** blatta, ***bry.,*** caj., **CALC., CALC-P.,** ***canth.,*** carb-an., ***carb-s., carb-v.,*** **CADM-S., CAUST.,** cedr., ***cham.,*** **CHEL.,** ***chin.,*** chin-a., ***chin-s., chion.,*** chlor., cimic., cina, coc-c., **CON.,** ***corn., croc., crot-c., crot-h.,*** cupr., ***dig.,*** dol., ***elaps,*** **FERR.,** ***ferr-ar.,*** **FERR-I.,** ***ferr-p., gels.,*** gran., ***graph., hell., hep.,*** hura, hydrc., ***iod., ip.,*** kali-bi., kali-br., ***kali-c.,*** kali-p., kali-s., **LACH.,** lachn., laur., ***lept.,*** **LYC.,** lyss., ***mag-c., mag-m.,*** manc., mang., ***med.,*** **MERC.,** merc-c., mez., ***myric.,*** naja, nat-a., nat-c., ***nat-m.,*** nat-p., **NAT-S., NIT-AC., NUX-V.,** ***op.,*** ox-ac., ***petr., phos., phyt.,*** **PLB.,** ***podo.,*** psor., ptel., ***puls.,*** raph., rhus-t., samb., ***sars., sec.,*** **SEP.,** ***sil.,*** spig., stram., **SULPH.,** sul-ac., upa., verat.

YELLOW, face
afternoon - gels.
anger, after - nat-s.
chloasma gravidarum - lyc., nux-v., sep.
eyes, around - coll., mag-c., med., ***nit-ac.,*** nux-v., spig.
fever, during - ***ferr.,*** lach., nux-v.
forehead - chel., phos.
hair, at the edge of - caul., kali-p., med.
intermittent, in - am-c., ***chin-s., con.,*** ferr., nat-c., nat-m., ***nux-v.,*** **SEP.,** ***tub.***
menses, during - ***caust.***
suppressed - chion.
morning - raph.
mouth, around - act-sp., hydrc., nux-v., ***sep.***
night - plb.
nose, around the - nux-v., sep.
rage, during - ***acon.,*** canth., lach., lyc., merc., ***nux-v.,*** phos., puls., verat.
saddle across cheeks - ***carb-an.,*** ictod., sanic., **SEP.**
uterine disease, in - sep.
spots - kreos., nat-c., ***sep.***
cheeks, on - cadm-s.
streaks, on upper lip - stram.
syphilis - **LACH.,** merc-c., nit-ac.
temples - ***caust.***
vexation, after - ***kali-c.***

Feet

ABDUCTED, toes, in spasms - camph., ***glon.***

ABSCESS, feet - ***merc.,*** sil., tarent.
abscess, heels - am-c., ars., lach.
abscess, toes - cocc.

ACHING, pain, feet - ang., bov., bry., calc., caust., clem., ***coloc., cur.,*** dios., fago., gymn., ham., ***kali-c.,*** kalm., lac-ac., mez., nit-ac., olnd., petr., phos., phyt., ptel., still., ***sulph.,*** verat., vip.
afternoon - ptel.
exercise amel. - dios.
extending to hips - nit-ac.
to thigh - ferr.
joints - clem., ***kali-c.,*** phos.
lying in bed - ***cur.***
night, sitting, while - olnd.
waking, on - bar-c.
periosteum, in - ***coloc.***
walking, while - phyt., stry.
aching, back of feet - asaf., chel., ***coloc.,*** jatr., lil-t., merc-i-f., mez., xan.
sitting, while - asaf.
aching, heels - agar., carl., calc-p., carb-s., ferr., kali-c., phyt., puls., spong., zinc.
elevating feet amel. - phyt.
previously frozen - carl.
standing long, after - zing.
walking, while - spong.
aching, soles - asaf., caust., croc., dios., hydr., kali-c., ***rhus-t.,*** stry., sul-i., sumb., viol-t.
hollow - rhus-t.
morning - dios., hydr.
sitting, on - asaf.
standing - croc., sul-i.
walking, while - kali-c., ***rhus-t.,*** viol-t.
aching, toes - arn., carl., coc-c., cupr., dios., euon., ham., hell., led., mez., mosch., puls-n, phos., pyrus, sulph.
ball of - sulph.
fifth - dios.
joints - coloc.
first - calc., carb-ac., coc-c., graph., ***kali-c.,*** mag-c., phys.
joints - ***cann-i.,*** cimic., nat-s.
joints, extending up limbs - cimic.
root of nail - calc-p.
previously frozen - agar., carl.
pulsating - arn.
walking, while - mez., phos.

ATHLETE'S foot, fungus - **BAR-C.,** carb-v., **GRAPH.,** ***nit-ac., sanic.,*** sep., **THUJ., SIL.,** zinc.

ARTHRITIC, nodosities, feet - bufo, ***kali-i.,*** **LED.,** ***nat-s.***
arthritic, toes - asaf., caust., ***graph.,*** ran-s., sabin., sulph., thuj.
fibrous, of first toe - ***rhod.***

BALLS, sensation of, heels, in, morning - kreos.

BANDAGED, sensation as if - mur-ac.
as with iron - ferr.
bandaged, toes, first - ***plat.***
ball, of first - petr.

BENDING, feet, soles - anac., ***nux-v., plb.***
bending, toes - ant-t., carb-v., chel., euph., ferr., ***graph., hyos.,*** kali-c., lyc., mag-m., merc., kali-n., ***nux-v., paeon.,*** sec., sulph.

BLISTERS, heels - calc., ***caust.,*** graph., ***lach.,*** led., ***nat-c.,*** nat-m., ***petr., phos.,*** sep., ***sil.***
blisters, soles - ars., calc.
blisters, toes - ars., nit-ac., ph-ac.

BLOOD, rush of to, while standing - graph.
first toe - led.

BLOWING, as of, toes wind issuing from toes - cupr.

BOILS - anan., calc., led., lyc., sars., sil., **STRAM.**
boils, heels - calc., lach.
boils, soles, of - rat.

BORING, pain - aesc., ang., ***bell.,*** bufo, ***caust.,*** cocc., merc., mur-ac., ***ran-s.,*** sulph., ***zinc.***
ball of - mur-ac., ran-s.
bones of - ***bism.,*** led., mez.
morning - led.
walking, while - mez.
joints of - coloc., ***hell.***
walking, while - mez.
motion, agg. - bufo.
os calcis, continued motion, amel. - aran.
sides, of - arg-m.
boring, back of feet - aesc., aur., aur-m-n., coloc., lil-t., mez., nat-s., spig.
walking, while - coloc.
boring, heels - agar., anac., aran., aur., aur-m-n., led., **PULS.,** ***zinc.***
evening - **PULS.**
wine, after - **ZINC.**
boring, soles - bell., mez., nux-m., ran-s., tarax.
morning - nux-m.
night - merc-i-f.
boring, toes - aesc., agar., coloc., merc., mez., ***ran-s.***
fifth - dios., ph-ac.
first - agar., aur-m-n., ind., **LED.,** ***nux-m., ran-s., sil.***
evening - ind.
joints - ind., nat-s.
lying down, after - ***nux-m.***
morning - **LED.**
rest, during - ind.
right - ***ran-s.***

BROKEN, sensation as if - kali-bi., kali-c., lac-d., psor.
broken, toes, sensation as if - cocc.

BUBBLING, sensation - bell., berb., chel., lach.
bubbling, first toe, left - rheum.

BUNIONS - am-c., **ANT-C.,** hyper., ***kali-chl.,*** ph-ac., ***phos.,*** plb., **SIL.,** zinc.
frost bite, after - ***calc.***
bunions, soles - calc.
ulcerated - ***calc.***

BURNING, pain - agar., ***am-c.,*** anac., ant-c., apis, ***arn., ars.,*** aster., aur-m., ***berb.,*** bor., bry., ***calc., calc-s.,*** cann-s., caps., ***carb-s., caust.,*** cham., chel., chin., chin-a., coloc., ***cocc.,*** con., corn., croc., eup-per., dulc., fago., ***graph., hep.,*** hyos., kali-ar., ***kali-c.,*** kali-i., kali-p., ***kali-s.,*** kreos., ***lach.,*** lachn., led., lil-t., ***lyc.,*** **MED.,** ***merc.,*** merl., ***mez.,*** nat-a., ***nat-c., nat-m., nat-s., nit-ac.,*** ox-ac., petr., ***ph-ac., phos.,*** phyt., plan., ***puls.,*** rat., rhus-t., rhus-v., sang., ***sec., sep., sil., spig.,*** squil., ***stann., staph., stram.,*** stront-c., **SULPH.,** tarax., thuj., vesp., ***zinc.,*** zing.

ball, of - mez., squil.

bones - ***ruta.***

evening - calc., ***nat-s.,*** sang., ***sulph.***

evening, in bed - calc., hep., merc., stront-c., **SULPH.**

menopause - sang.

morning, in bed - hep., ***nat-s.***

night - ars-m., coloc., lac-c., ***nat-c., sep.,*** sil., **SULPH.**

bed, in - nat-p., **SULPH.**

bed, in, during menses - nat-p.

sleep, during - ars-m.

noon - am-c., hura.

left one burning while the other is cold - hura.

perspiration, with - ***sil.***

touch agg. - bor.

uncovers - sulph.

walking, while - carb-an., ***nat-c.,*** nat-m., phyt.

after - kali-c., puls.

warmth of bed, from - agar., calc., merc., stront-c., **SULPH.**

burning, back of feet - agar., alum., bapt., berb., calc., canth., chin., hep., ign., lyc., mag-m., manc., **PULS.,** rhus-t., sil., spig., stram., ***sulph.,*** tarax., thuj.

evening - agar.

morning in bed - hep.

burning, heels - arg-m., arund., carl., ***cycl.,*** eupi., fago., ***graph., ign., kali-n.,*** puls., raph., rhus-t., sep., sul-ac., tep., verat., vip., zinc.

extending to tongue - vip.

morning - eupi.

bed, in - fago., ***graph.***

night in bed - kali-n.

stepping - con., zinc.

walking - cycl., zinc.

burning, soles - aesc., ail., all-s., aloe, alum., ***ambr.,*** am-c., ***anac.,*** ars., ars-s-f., ars-s-r., arum-d., aur-m., bar-c., bell., berb., bov., **CALC.,** ***calc-s., canth., carb-s., carb-v., caust., cham.,*** chel., clem., ***cocc.,*** coc-c., ***coloc.,*** con., cop., croc., crot-h., crot-t., ***cupr.,*** dulc., eup-per., fl-ac., ***graph.,*** guare., jal., hep., kali-ar., kali-bi., kali-c., kali-n., kali-p., ***kali-s.,*** kreos., lac-c., ***lach., lachn., lil-t.,*** **LYC.,** mag-c., ***mag-m., manc., mang.,*** med., merc., merl., mur-ac., myric., nat-a., ***nat-c.,*** nat-m., nat-p., ***nat-s.,*** nux-v., ox-ac., petr., ***ph-ac., phos.,*** phyt., ***plb., puls., sang.,*** sanic., sec., sep., ***sil.,*** squil., stann., **SULPH.,** ***sul-i.,*** tab., tarax., tep., ***zinc.***

burning, soles

afternoon - gels., ol-an.

bed, in - canth., **CHAM.,** hep., ***ph-ac., plb., sang.,*** **SULPH.**

amel. - nat-c.

cold to touch - ***sulph.***

eating, after - sil.

evening - berb., **LACH.,** lyc., mag-m., merc., nat-c., ph-ac., ***phos.,*** sulph., zinc.

scratching, after - am-c.

menses, during - carb-v., petr.

morning - ph-ac., phyt., zinc.

bed, in - hep.

night - aloe, bar-c., ***calc.,*** **CHAM.,** fl-ac., **LACH.,** lyc., mag-m., nat-s., petr., ***ph-ac., sang.,*** sil., **SULPH.**

palms and - ***lach.***

putting them to the ground - mur-ac.

putting, foot to ground agg. - mur-ac.

rubbing amel. - kali-n.

sick headache, with - ***sang.***

sitting, while - anac., carb-v., lyc., mur-ac., tarax.

standing, after - carb-v., merc., sul-i.

summer, in - vesp.

walking, while - carb-v., coc-c., graph., kali-c., lyc., ***nat-c.,*** **SULPH.**

after long sitting - **SULPH.**

air, in open - hep.

amel. - ol-an.

burning, toes - aesc., ***agar.,*** alum., ant-c., **APIS,** arn., ars., arund., ***asaf.,*** aur., ***aur-m., berb., bor.,*** calad., calc., carb-an., caust., ***con.,*** dulc., ***ferr-p.,*** fl-ac., ***hep.,*** ind., ***kali-c.,*** kali-p., lith., ***lyc.,*** merc., mez., mosch., mur-ac., nat-c., nit-ac., nux-v., paeon., ph-ac., phos., plat., ***puls.,*** sabin., sec., ***staph., tarax.,*** thuj.

ball, of - puls.

between the toes - ***nat-c.***

cold feet, with - apis

daytime - ind.

fifth - ars., carb-an., meph., staph., til.

walking, while - nat-c.

first - aesc., am-c., ant-c., ars., benz-ac., bor., ***cimic., colch.,*** con., form., lachn., ph-ac., plat., ***ran-s.,*** ruta, verat., vio-t.

ball, of - ant-c., ***caust., kali-c.,*** zinc.

freezing, as after - zinc.

joints, of - ***cimic.,*** ph-ac.

left - aesc., lachn.

morning in bed - ars.

nail, under - calc., ***nit-ac.***

night - form.

pressing - viol-t.

right - ant-c., ***cimic.,*** con., ***ran-s.,*** verat.

tip of - calc., con., olnd.

frostbitten, as if - agar., bor., zinc.

frozen previously - agar., carl., phos.

intermittent - dulc.

joints, of - berb.

nails, roots of - asaf.

nails, under - caust.

night - plat.

paroxysmal - ***tarax.***

second, ball - puls.

burning, toes
under - alum., con.
walking, on - phos.
warm bed agg. - nux-v.
wetting feet, after - nit-ac.

BURNT, as if toe, first - caust.

BURROWING, pain - spig.

CALLOUSES, horny, soles, on - **ANT-C.,** ***ars., calc.,*** plb., ***sil.*** sulph.
tenderness - ***alum.,*** bar-c., lyc., med., ***nat-s., sil.***

callouses, toes, on - **ANT-C.,** ***graph.,*** sil.

CHILBLAINS - abrot., **AGAR.,** ***alumn.,*** am-c., ***anac.,*** ant-c., aur., bad., ***bell.,*** berb., bor., bry., bufo, cadm-s., ***carb-an.,*** carb-v., ***cham., chin.,*** colch., ***croc.,*** crot-h., cycl., hep., hyos., ign., kali-chl., kali-n., ***lyc., merc.,*** mur-ac., naja, ***nit-ac.,*** nux-m., ***nux-v., op.,*** **PETR.,** ph-ac., ***phos.,*** **PULS.,** ran-b., rhus-t., sep., stann., staph., ***sulph.,*** sul-ac., ***thuj.,*** **ZINC.**
cracked - merc., nux-v., petr.
inflammation - ***lach.,*** merc., nit-ac., **PETR.**
purple - ***lach., merc., puls., sulph.***
suppurating - ***lach., sil., sulph.***
swollen - ***merc.***

chilblains, heels, swollen and red - petr.

chilblains, toes - **AGAR.,** ***alum.,*** aur., bor., ***carb-an., croc.,*** kali-c., nit-ac., ***nux-v.,*** **PETR.,** phos., **PULS.,** rhod.

CHILLINESS - **AGAR.,** ant-c., arg-m., ars., bry., ***calc.,*** cedr., ***dros., nit-ac.,*** petr., ***phos., rhus-t., sulph.,*** thuj.
left - stann.
motion, after - calc.
summer - ant-c.

chilliness, toes - **AGAR.,** asar., bor., ***carb-an., carb-v.,*** cast-eq., ***croc.,*** cycl., op., **PETR.,** phos., ***puls.,*** sulph., thuj., **ZINC.**
ball of right big toe - ars-h.
first toe - nit-ac.

CLUCKING, extending to head - calc.

COLDNESS - abrot., absin., acet-ac., ***acon.,*** agar., aloe, alum., alumn., ***am-br.,*** ambr., ***am-c.,*** am-m., ***anac.,*** ang., anth., **ANT-C., ANT-T.,** aphis., **APIS,** apoc., ***arg-n., arn.,*** **ARS., ARS-I.,** asaf., ***asar.,*** asc-t., **AUR.,** bapt., ***bar-c.,*** bar-m., **BELL.,** benz-ac., berb., ***bov.,*** brach., **BROM.,** bry., bufo, ***cact.,*** calad., **CALC.,** calc-p., calc-s., ***camph.,*** cann-i., cann-s., ***canth., caps., carb-an., carb-ac.,*** carb-o., **CARB-S.,** ***carb-v., caul.,*** **CAUST.,** cedr., ***cham., chel.,*** **CHIN.,** ***chin-a.,*** cic., cimic., ***cimx., cina,*** cinnb., ***cist., cocc.,*** coff., ***colch.,*** **CON.,** ***crot-c.,*** crot-h., ***crot-t.,*** **CUPR.,** cupr-ar., daph., **DIG.,** dor., **DROS.,** ***elaps,*** eup-per., fago., **FERR.,** ferr-ar., **FERR-I.,** ***ferr-p.,*** form., ***gels., glon.,*** **GRAPH.,** ***hell.,*** hipp., hura, hydrc., hyos., hyper., iber., ign., ind., **IOD., IP.,** iris, **KALI-AR.,** kali-bi., **KALI-C.,** kali-chl., kali-i., **KALI-N., KALI-P., KALI-S., KREOS.,** lac-ac., lac-d., **LACH.,** lact., laur., led., lil-t., **LYC.,** ***lycps.,*** mag-c., mag-m., mag-s., manc., ***mang., med.,*** **MENY., MERC.,** ***merc-c.,*** mez.,

COLDNESS - morph., ***mur-ac.,*** **NAJA, NAT-C., NAT-M.,** ***nat-p., nat-s.,*** **NIT-AC.,** ***nux-m., nux-v.,*** oena., ol-an., olnd., ol-j., op., ***ox-ac.,*** pall., **PAR., PETR., PH-AC., PHOS.,** ***phyt., pic-ac.,*** pip-m., plan., plat., ***plb., podo., psor.,*** ptel., **PULS.,** raph., **RHOD.,** ***rhus-t.,*** rob., rumx., **RUTA.,** sabad., ***sabin., samb.,*** sang., ***sars.,*** **SEP., SIL.,** spong., **SQUIL.,** ***stann.,*** staph., **STRAM.,** ***stront-c.,*** stry., **SULPH.,** sul-ac., sumb., tab., ***tarent.,*** tell., **THUJ.,** ***verat., verat-v.,*** verb., vesp., ***zinc.***
afternoon - bar-c., chel., chin-s., coca, colch., ***gels.,*** mez., nux-v., sang., ***sep.,*** squil., ***sulph.,*** zinc.
1 p.m. - chel.
2 p.m. - chel., sars., lyc.
3 p.m. - eup-pur., lyc.
4 p.m. - coff., sang.
4 p.m, in open air amel. - coff.
hot face, with - hura.
alternating, with cold hands - aloe, sep., zing.
alternating, with heat - alum.
alternating, with pain in limbs - rhus-t.
anxiety, during - cupr., graph., puls., sulph.
bed, in - alum., ***ferr.,*** kali-c., lach., naja, phos., raph., rhod., thuj.
bones, of - chin.
daytime - **HEP.,** mag-s., nit-ac., phos., ***sep., sil.,*** sulph.
menses, during - nat-p.
diarrhea, with - dig., ***lyc.,*** nit-ac.
dinner, after - cann-i., carb-v., ***sulph.***
dinner, during - sulph.
dysentery, cold feet to knee, in - aloe.
eating, while - ign., sulph.
eating, after - aloe, calc., ***camph.,*** caps.
emission, after - aloe, nux-v.
evening - **ACON.,** aloe, am-br., ***am-c.,*** ars., bar-c., bell., **CALC.,** carb-an., carb-s., ***carb-v.,*** cham., chel., chin., con., graph., hell., kali-s., lyc., mag-c., mang., nat-c., nat-n., nux-v., ox-ac., petr., ph-ac., plan., puls., rhod., rhus-t., sars., **SEP., SIL.,** stront-c., sulph., til., verat., ***zinc.***
5 p.m. - alum., graph.
6 p.m. - cedr.
8 p.m. - bar-c., hep.
9 p.m. - aloe, kreos.
11 p.m. - fago.
air, in the open - mang.
bed, in - aloe, **AM-C.,** ***am-m.,*** aur., **CALC.,** carb-an., carb-s., ***carb-v.,*** carl., chel., ***ferr.,*** ferr-p., **GRAPH.,** kali-ar., ***kali-c.,*** kali-s., lyc., meny., merc., nat-c., nit-ac., nux-v., par., petr., ph-ac., ***phos.,*** raph., rhod., **SEP., SIL.,** staph., sulph., thuj., ***zinc.***
bed, in, amel. - sulph.
excitement, during - mag-c.
extending to, calves - aloe, crot-t.
to, knees - aeth., chel., ign., mang., ***meny.,*** nat-m.

COLDNESS,
fever, during - am-c., ***arn.,*** ars., bar-c., bell., bufo, calad., calc., caps., carb-an., carb-v., chin., hell., ign., ip., ***iris,*** kali-c., kali-s., ***lach.,*** meny., nux-v., petr., ptel., puls., ran-b., rhod., samb., squil., stann., ***stram., sulph., zinc.***
forenoon - ***carb-an.,*** chin-s., cop., fago., hura, mez., petr., sep.
3 p.m.,until - petr.
8 a.m. - ferr., hura, meny.
9 a.m. until 3 p.m. - ***carb-an.***
10 a.m. - fago., med.
11 a.m., lying down amel. - ***sep.***
headache, during - ***arg-n.,*** ars., aur., ***bell.,*** bufo, cact., ***calc.,*** camph., carb-s., ***carb-v.,*** chin., chr-ac., coca, dirc., ***ferr.,*** ferr-p., **GELS.,** lac-d., lach., laur., **MELI.,** ***meny., naja,*** nat-m., phos., plat., ***psor.,*** sars., **SEP.,** stram., ***sulph.,*** verat-v.
headache, after - cupr.
headache, after menses - ***ferr.***
heat, of body during sleep, with - **SAMB.**
heat, of one side of body - ran-b.
heat, of thighs, with - cocc., thuj.
hot, bath amel. - glon.
hot, face, with - acon., ***asaf.,*** cocc., gels., graph., ign., kali-c., nat-c., ruta., samb., ***sep.,*** sil., **STRAM.**
hot, hands with - acon., calad., com., ***nux-m.,*** sep.
hot, head, with - alum., am-c., anac., ***arn.,*** ars., aur., bar-c., ***bell., cact., calc.,*** com., ***ferr.,*** gels., laur., ***nat-c.,*** nit-ac., ***ph-ac.,*** sep., squil., thuj.
hottest weather, in - ***asar.***
house, in, amel. - mang.
icy, cold - agar., alum., anac., ant-c., ***apis,*** ars., aur., cact., calad., **CAMPH., CARB-V.,** cedr., chin., **CROT-C.,** ***cupr.,*** dor., **ELAPS,** ***eup-per., gels.,*** graph., ***hep.,*** ip., kali-i., **LACH.,** ***lyc.,*** manc., mang., meny., ***merc., merc-c.,*** mez., nat-c., nat-p., ***nux-m.,*** par., **PHOS.,** ***psor.,*** rhus-t., samb., sars., **SEP., SIL.,** squil., ***sulph.,*** **VERAT.,** zinc.
burning soles, with - ***cupr.***
chill, during - ant-c., aur., ***ferr.,*** **MENY.,** ***phos.,*** sep., **VERAT.,** ***zinc.***
cold air amel. - camph., led.
left - aeth., carb-v., euph., hydrc., nat-n., psor., pip-m., rhus-t., sulph., sumb., ***tub.***
lying, while - tell.
lying, while, amel. - phos.
menses, during - ***arg-n., calc.,*** cop., ***crot-h., graph.,*** nat-p., ***nux-m., phos.,*** sabin., **SIL.**
menses, after - ***carb-v., chin-s.***
menses, before - calc., hyper., ***lyc., nux-m.***
mental, exertion - agar., ambr., ***am-c., anac.,*** **AUR.,** bell., **CALC.,** calc-p., ***carb-v., caust.,*** chin., cocc., ***cupr.,*** gels., kali-c., ***lach., lyc.,*** **NAT-C.,** ***nat-m.,*** nit-ac., **NUX-V.,** petr., ***ph-ac.,*** **PHOS.,**

COLDNESS,
mental, exertion - psor., **PULS., SEP., SIL.**
midnight - calad.
morning - anac., caps., chel., chin., coc-c., graph., hura, lyc., mag-m., mang., merc., nat-c., nux-v., **SEP.,** ***spig.,*** stram., sumb.
5 a.m. - hura.
7:30 a.m. - ferr.
breakfast, after - verat.
breakfast, after, during headache - **SEP.**
motion, after - ***cocc.***
night - aloe, am-c., am-m., ant-c., ***aur.,*** bov., bry., calad., **CALC.,** ***carb-s., carb-v.,*** chel., com., cop., ***ferr.,*** ferr-i., iod., kali-ar., nit-ac., par., petr., ***phos.,*** psor., raph., rhod., sars., sep., ***sil.,*** sulph., thuj., verat., ***zinc.***
bed, in - am-m., ***aur.,*** **CALC.,** carb-v., chel., ***ferr.,*** nit-ac., petr., phos., raph., rhod., sil., sulph., thuj., zinc.
waking, and on - ***nit-ac.,*** zinc.
noon - chin-s., kali-c., nit-ac., zing.
heat and redness of the face, during - sep.
while the other foot burns - hura.
one cold the other hot - chel., chin., con., dig., ip., **LYC.,** ***puls.***
pregnancy, during - ***lyc.,*** **VERAT.**
right - ambr., bar-c., ***chel.,*** con., ***lyc.,*** puls., sabin., ***sulph.***
walking - bar-c.
sensation of, though warm to touch - ***sulph.***
sitting, while - ars., mez., puls., ***sep.***
amel. - mang.
sleep, during - samb., zinc.
heat of body, with - samb.
stool, after - sulph.
supper, during - ign.
after - lyc.
suppressed, sweat - con., ***sil.***
takes cold through - con., ***sil.***
talking, while - am-c.
urination, during - dig.
vertigo, during - sep.
vomiting, after - sin-a.
waking, on - ***chel.,*** puls., ***samb.,*** verat., zinc.
walking, while - ***anac., aran.,*** asaf., carb-an., ***chin.,*** mang., mez., sil.
after - nit-ac.
air, in open - ***anac.,*** bar-c., mang., plan., plb.
air, in open, fast - ***phos.***
amel. - aloe
sun, in the - ***lach.***
warm room, in - kali-br., mez.
cannot be warmed - ars.
water, as though in - gels., mag-c., meny., merc., **SEP.**
as if cold, running in foot - verat.
wine, after - lyc.
writing, while - chin-s., sep.
coldness, back of feet - graph.
walking, while - graph.
coldness, heels - sep.

coldness, soles - acon., ars., caust., chel., chin-s., colch., ***coloc.,*** dig., hyper., laur., lith., merc., ***nit-ac.,*** nux-v., ***sulph.***
evening, in bed - ***aur.,*** verat.
icy cold - ***nit-ac.***
menses, during - ***calc., graph., nux-m., phos., sil.,*** verat.
morning - chin-s.
5 a.m. with hot face - con.
night - nit-ac.
open air - laur.
painful - caust.
sensation of, although not cold - coloc.

coldness, toes - **ACON.,** agar., ***carl.,*** card-m., chel., chin-s., cinnb., coff., con., daph., dig., ***ferr.,*** gels., lyc., ***med.,*** meny., nux-v., ol-an., ***sec., sulph.***
first toe - ant-t., brom., iod., ran-b.
icy - ***ferr.***
morning - chin-s.
sitting, while - bry.
sitting, after - ***carl.***
tips - aloe.
touched - ant-t.
walking, while, amel. - bry.

COMPRESSION, sensation, feet - ang., cimic.
compression, heels - alum.
compression, toes, first toe - plat.

CONSTRICTION - anac., graph., nat-m., nit-ac., ***petr.,*** stront.
constriction, toes, big toe - ***plat.***
ball, of - graph.

CONTRACTION, of muscles and tendons - acon., alum., ***cann-s.,*** carb-an., ***caust.,*** ferr-s., guare., ind., merc-c., nat-c., nat-m., plat., ***sec.,*** sep., zinc.
bones - staph.
cramp-like - ***nat-m.,*** phos.
left - cycl.
spasmodic - acon., bism.

contraction, heels - am-m., ***colch.,*** led., sep.
convulsive, evening in bed - am-m.

contraction, soles - berb., cham., nux-v., rhus-t., spig., sulph., ***syph.,*** verat., zinc.

contraction, toes - ars., asaf., crot-c., ***ferr.,*** ferr-ar., gamb., gels., guare., jatr., kali-n., mag-s., merc., paeon., phyt., plat., ***sec.***
cramp-like - cham., nux-v., rhus-t.
drawn, down - ***ars.,*** chel., phyt.
drawn, up - apis, ***camph.,*** ferr-s., ***lach.,*** sec.
night - merc.
sitting, while - kali-n.
sitting, while - kali-n.
walking - hyos.
yawning, while - nux-v.

CONVULSION - bar-m., ***calc.,*** camph., ***cupr.,*** iod., ***merc-c., nat-m., nux-v.,*** op., phos., ***sec.,*** stram., ***zinc.***
extending to knees - stram.
menses, during - hyos.
night - iod.
tetanic - ***camph., nux-v.***
tonic - phos.

CONVULSION,
touch - ***nux-v.***

convulsion, toes - **CHEL.,** ***cupr., sec.***
first - apis.

CORNS - ***acet-ac., agar., am-c.,*** **ANT-C.,** ***arn., bar-c., bor.,*** bov., ***bry., calc., calc-s., carb-an., caust.,*** chin., coloc., ***cur., graph., hep., ign.,*** **LYC.,** lyss., nat-c., ***nat-m.,*** nit-ac., ***nux-v.,*** petr., **PH-AC., PHOS., PSOR.,** ran-s., rhod., ***rhus-t.,*** **SEP., SIL.,** staph., ***sulph.,*** ter.
aching - ant-c., lyc., sep., sil., sul-ac., sulph.
boring - bor., calc., caust., nat-c., ***nat-m.,*** phos., ***ran-s., sep., sil.,*** thuj.
burning - ***agar., alum.,*** am-c., ***ant-c., arg-m.,*** bar-c., ***bry., calc., calc-s.,*** carb-v., caust., graph., ***hep.,*** **IGN.,** lith., ***lyc.,*** meph., ***nat-m.,*** nit-ac., ***nux-v., petr., ph-ac.,*** phos., ***ran-b., ran-s., rhus-t.,*** **SEP.,** sil., ***sulph.,*** thuj.
burning, night - nat-m.
drawing - lyc., nat-c., sep.
drawing, night - sep.
horny - ***ant-c.,*** graph., ran-b., sulph.
inflamed - ***ant-c.,*** calc., ***lyc., puls., sep.,*** **SIL.,** ***staph.,*** **SULPH.**
jerks - cocc., dios., phos., **SEP.,** ***sulph.,*** sul-ac.
painful - ***agar.,*** alum., ambr., ***ant-c.,*** arn., aster., ***bar-c.,*** bov., bry., calc., ***calc-s.,*** calad., caust., ***hep.,*** ign., ***iod.,*** kali-c., lach., lith., ***lyc.,*** meph., nat-m., ***nit-ac.,*** nux-v., phos., puls., ran-s., rhus-t., sep., sil., spig., **SULPH.**
painful, touched, when - bry., kali-c.
painful, ulcerated, as if - am-c., bor.
pinching - bar-c.
pressing - agar., ***ant-c.,*** bov., ***bry.,*** calc., ***calc-s.,*** carb-v., ***caust.,*** graph., iod., **LYC.,** ph-ac., phos., ***sep.,*** sil., **SULPH.**
pulsating - calc., kali-c., ***lyc.,*** sep., sil., sulph.
shooting - ***bov.,*** **NAT-M.**
sore - aesc., ***agar.,*** ambr., ant-c., ***arn., bar-c., bry., calc., calc-s., camph.,*** **CARB-AN.,** fl-ac., ***graph., hep.,*** **IGN.,** lith., **LYC.,** med., nat-c., nat-p., ***nux-v.,*** petr., phos., ***puls., ran-b.,*** ran-s., ***rhus-t., sep.,*** **SIL.,** ***spig., sulph.,*** thuj., verat.
stinging - ***agar.,*** **ALUM.,** am-c., ant-c., ars., ***bar-c.,*** bor., ***bov.,*** **BRY.,** calad., **CALC., CALC-S.,** carb-an., carb-v., caust., hep., ign., kali-c., ***lyc.,*** mag-m., **NAT-C., NAT-M.,** nat-p., ***petr.,*** ph-ac., ***phos.,*** ptel., ***puls., ran-s., rhod.,*** **RHUS-T.,** rumx., ***sep., sil.,*** staph., **SULPH.,** sul-ac., ***thuj.,*** verat.
stinging, night - ars., nat-m., sulph.
stinging, rainy weather, in - bor.
stinging, walking - phos.
tearing - am-c., arn., ***bry.,*** calc., calc-s., cocc., kali-c., **LYC.,** ***sep.,*** **SIL., SULPH.,** sul-ac., thuj.
tearing, night - ars.

corns, heel - ***phos.***

corns, soles, horny - **ANT-C.,** ***ars.,*** ***calc.,*** kali-ar., sil.

CRACKED, skin - ***aur-m.,*** carb-an., com., eug., **GRAPH.,** ***hep.,*** hydr., ***lach.,*** ***nat-m.,*** ***petr.,*** sabad., **SARS., SIL.,** sulph.

cracked, heels - ***lyc.***

cracked, soles - ars.

cracked, toes, between - aur-m., carb-an., eug., **GRAPH.,** hydr., ***lach.,*** **NAT-M., PETR.,** ***sars.,*** sabad., **SIL.**

deep - ***hydr.***

under - sabad.

violent itching - ***nat-m.***

CRACKING, joints, in - caust., petr., ph-ac., sars., sulph., thuj.

first, toe - ant-c.

CRAMPS - ***acon.,*** ***agar.,*** am-c., ***ang.,*** arg-c., arg-m., ars., ***asc-t.,*** **BELL.,** berb., bism., bry., **CALC.,** calc-p., ***camph.,*** **CARB-S., CAUST.,** ***colch.,*** ***coloc.,*** **CUPR.,** dig., euph., ferr., ferr-ar., ferr-i., ferr-p., form., gels., gnaph., graph., hep., hyper., iod., ***jatr.,*** ***lac-c.,*** lach., lachn., lil-t., ***lyc.,*** mag-m., **MAG-P.,** manc., meph., ***nat-c.,*** ***nat-m.,*** nat-p., nux-m., nux-v., olnd., ox-ac., ***petr.,*** ***ph-ac.,*** phos., phys., plat., plb., ran-b., ***rhus-t.,*** sanic., ***sec.,*** ***sep.,*** ***sil.,*** spig., ***stram.,*** stry., ***sulph.,*** sul-ac., til., verat., verat-v., verb., zinc.

alternating with dim vision - bell.

bed, in - bry., gnaph., sanic.

chill, during - ***cupr.,*** elat., nux-v.

cholera, in - **CUPR.,** sec., **VERAT.**

daytime - ox-ac., ***petr.,*** ***sep.***

evening, 9 p.m. - lyc.

drawing up limbs, on - ferr.

walking, while - verat.

inner border, of foot, bending foot inward - nat-c., sep.

inside of - crot-t.

left - nat-m.

menses, during - lachn., sulph.

morning, 9 a.m. - lachn.

motion, on - calc., ph-ac.

first motion, after resting - plb.

night - form., lachn., lyc., nat-c., sanic.

outside of - nicc.

sitting during menses - nicc.

sex, on attempting - ***cupr.***

sitting, on - euph.

sleep, on going to - hyper.

standing when - euph.

stretching, on - caust., verat.

walking, while - sil.

cramps, back of feet - com., plb., ran-b., rhus-v.

walking, while - ran-b.

cramps, heels - ***anac.,*** bry., cann-s., crot-c., eug., led., mag-c., sel., sep.

morning, in bed - mag-c.

cramps, soles - acon., ***agar.,*** ***alumn.,*** ***am-c.,*** anac., ang., ***apoc.,*** apoc-a., ars., bar-c., bell., berb., bry., cact., calad., **CALC., CARB-S., CARB-V.,** card-m., **CAUST.,** cham., chel., coff., ***colch.,*** com., crot-t., ***elat.,*** eug., ***ferr.,*** ferr-ar., form., gent-c., ***hep.,*** hipp., kali-c.,

cramps, soles - kali-p., med., mur-ac., nat-a., nat-m., ***nit-ac.,*** nux-v., olnd., ***petr.,*** ***phos.,*** plb., rhus-t., ruta., sang., sec., sel., sep., **SIL.,** stann., staph., ***stront-c.,*** ***stry.,*** **SULPH.,** ***syph.,*** tarent., til., thuj., ***verat.,*** ***verb.,*** zing.

bed, in - ***calc.,*** bell., carb-v., sep., thuj.

bed, putting out of, agg. - chel.

colic, preceding - plb.

dancing, when - bar-c.

daytime - nux-v.

daytime, on trying to rise - nux-v.

drawing on boot - ***calc.***

evening - hipp., nat-m., zing.

7 p.m. - nat-a.

lying down, after - ***carb-v.***

flexing, thigh - bell.

hanging, down, on - berb.

intermittent fever, in - elat.

lain on, on the side - staph.

menses, during - sulph.

morning, 3 a.m. - ferr., form.

moving, on - eug., petr.

night - ***agar.,*** calad., **CALC.,** med., ***nit-ac.,*** ***nux-v.,*** ***petr.,*** **SULPH.**

cholera, in - **SULPH.**

drawing up limbs - kali-c., nux-v.

lying down, when - bry.

lying down, while - sel.

rising, when - plat.

pregnancy, during - **CALC.**

putting out, on - chel., coff.

riding in a carriage, while - thuj.

sitting, while - bry., hipp., stann.

smoking, from - calad.

standing - verb.

stepping, on - chel., sulph.

stretching on - caust.

walking, while - ***bar-c.,*** petr., ***sil.,*** ***sulph.,*** vib.

after - calc.

air, in open, while - carb-v.

amel. - calc., ***verb.***

cramps, toes - ***am-c.,*** arn., ***ars.,*** ***asaf.,*** bar-c., ***bar-m.,*** **CALC.,** cann-s., carb-an., carb-h., carb-s., **CAUST.,** ***cham.,*** ***chel.,*** coc-c., ***crot-h.,*** **CUPR.,** ***cupr-ar.,*** dig., ***ferr.,*** ferr-p., gels., ***hep.,*** hura, ***kali-c.,*** lil-t., ***lyc.,*** mosch., nat-c., nicc., ***nux-v.,*** ol-an., petr., ***ph-ac.,*** phos., phyt., plat., plb., psor., rhus-t., sang., ***sec.,*** sep., sil., stry., sulph., tab., tarent., verat-v.

alternating with spasm of glottis - ***asaf.***

evening - petr.

bed, in - ars.

bed, in, 5 p.m. - lil-t.

fifth, toe, - coc-c.

night - coc-c.

night, on lying - coc-c.

first, toe - calc-p., coloc., gamb., kali-c., nux-v., psor., sil., tarent.

bed, in - gamb.

stretching foot, on - psor.

walking, while - gamb., ***sil.***

flexor tendons - dios.

cramps, toes
fourth, toe - coc-c.
night - coc-c.
night, on lying - coc-c.
labor, during - cupr.
menses, during - sulph.
midnight, bed, in - nux-v.
morning, in bed - nicc.
night - calc., coc-c.
bed, in - ***ars.,*** merc-i-f.
pregnancy, during - ***calc.***
second toe - sep.
stretching out, foot - bar-c., psor., sulph.
third, toe - coc-c., iod.
night - coc-c.
night, on lying - coc-c.

CUTTING, pain - alum., ambr., ars., calc., ***chin-s.,*** coloc., dulc., lyc., mag-m., mur-ac., ***nat-c.,*** osm., plat., thuj.
chill, during - ***chin-s.***
transversely across - plat.
walking, while - thuj.

cutting, heels - am-c., eup-per., mag-m., nat-s., puls., sulph.

cutting, soles - alum., ars., calc., coloc., dios., dulc., elaps, mur-ac., ol-an., sil., sulph.
extending to thighs - ars.
hollow of - mur-ac.
night - sulph.
sitting, while - elaps

cutting, toes - aur-m., calc., carb-an., cina, coloc., dios., led., paeon., ph-ac., puls., sep., ***sil.***
first - alum., ant-c., aur-m-n., con., ph-ac., sang., stry., sulph.
extending into heel - alum.
jerking - ph-ac.
morning - alum., sulph.
rhythmical - ant-c.
walking - alum., aur-m.
night, back, on the, lying - sep.
sleep, during - led.
stepping - alum.
touch, on - ph-ac.
under nail - sil.
walking, when - aur-m.

DECAY, bones, of feet - asaf., calc., ***hecla., merc.,*** **SIL.**

decay, heels - ***calc-p.,*** plat-m., ***sil.***

decay, toes, of left big toe - **SIL.**

DISCOLORATION, of feet
ball of, redness - rhus-t.
blackness - crot-h., sol-n., vip.
blueness - ***arg-n.,*** arn., bor., dros., elaps, kali-br., ***kali-c.,*** lach., led., ***mur-ac.,*** oena., phos., puls., rhus-t., sep., stram., verat., vip.
spots, in - kreos., sulph.
livid - merc-c., ox-ac., stram.
pale - **APIS,** chin., ph-ac.
purple - op., sec.
spots, in - apis.

DISCOLORATION, of feet
redness - agar., apis, calc., ***carb-s.,*** carb-v., graph., hyos., lach., nat-c., phos., ***puls.,*** rhus-t., sars., sep., ***sil.,*** stann., thuj., vesp., vip., zinc.
evening - apis
spots, in - apis, ars., bry., chin., elaps, ***lach.,*** led., lyc., mang., phyt., thuj.
spots, in, burning - ars.
joints - lyc., mang., stann.
spots - phos.
white - apis.
yellow-grayish - vip.

discoloration, back of feet, blue - vip.
marbled - ***caust.,*** thuj.
redness - ***rhus-t.,*** thuj.
8 a.m. - ***rhus-t.***
spots - carb-o., puls., thuj.

discoloration, heels, purplish - puls.
purplish, redness - ant-c., ***petr.***

discoloration, soles, of, blue spots - kali-p.
redness - bry., kali-c., phos., ***puls.***
spots, in - ***ars.***
white spots - nat-m.
as if bleached - bar-c., plb.

discoloration, toes - ***sec.***
blackness - crot-h., phos., sol-n., ***sec.***
fifth, redness, in morning - lyc.
redness, in spots - staph.
first, blackness - iod.
redness - alum., ***am-c.,*** arn., aster., ***benz-ac.,*** bry., coc-c., eup-per., ***nat-m., nit-ac.,*** sabin.
redness, in spots - nat-c.
redness - ***agar., alum., am-c.,*** apis, aster., aur., ***aur-m.,*** berb., bor., ***carb-v.,*** nat-m., nit-ac., ***nux-v.,*** phos., sep., thuj., zinc.
shining - thuj.
wetting feet, after - nit-ac.
tips, blueness - op.
redness - mur-ac., sep., thuj.
violet-colored - stry.
white, bleached between the toes - bar-c., plb.

DISLOCATION, as if, feeling - arum-t., bell.
joints - ang., bufo, calc.

dislocation, toes, as if, feeling - syph.

DRAWING, pain - agar., alum., am-c., ammc., ***anac.,*** ang., arn., ***ars.,*** asaf., ***aur.,*** aur-m-n., bapt., bar-c., bell., bor., bov., bry., calc., camph., cann-s., canth., carb-s., carb-v., ***caul., caust.,*** **CHEL.,** chin., chin-a., chin-s., clem., cocc., coc-c., ***coloc.,*** con., cupr., dig., dios., dros., ferr., ferr-i., fl-ac., ham., hep., hyper., indg., kali-ar., kali-bi., kali-c., lach., led., ***lyc., mag-c.,*** mang., merc., ***mez.,*** mur-ac., naja, nat-c., nat-m., nat-p., nat-s., nit-ac., nux-v., olnd., ***ol-an.,*** petr., ph-ac., plb., **PULS.,** ran-b., rat., ***rhod.,*** **RHUS-T.,** rhus-v., sars., sec., sil., sol-n., spong., stann., ***stront-c., sulph.,*** tarax., thuj., verat., vinc., zinc.
afternoon - com.
air, open, agg. - **CAUST.**
arthritic - arg-n.
burning - tarax.

DRAWING, pain
cramp-like - arg-m., chin., hyper., nat-m., ph-ac.
cutting - bell.
evening - caust., nat-c., ph-ac.
bed, in - ars., hep.
walking - agar.
extending, to back - nit-ac.
to calves - dros.
to hips - sulph.
to knees - nit-ac., sil.
to shoulders - bell.
upward - dros., led., nit-ac., ***sil., spong.,*** sulph.
fatigue, as from - kali-c.
joints - am-c., ***anac.,*** ang., ars., bov., caust., dulc., merc., mosch., stront-c., thuj.
left - ars., nat-m.
motion agg. - nit-ac.
morning - ang., ars., kali-bi., ph-ac.
night - agar., calc.
11 p.m., lying on the other side - com.
paralytic - acon., aur., **RHUS-T.**
paroxysmal - coc-c., nat-m., ph-ac.
pinching - kali-c.
right - ***chel.***
rising, after - bry.
sitting, while - aur-m-n., carb-v., coloc., **RHUS-T.**
amel. - tarax.
spots, in - arn.
standing, while - chin., tarax.
dragging - ars., bov.
walk caustiously, must - ars.
walking, while - bar-c., clem., coloc., crot-h., nit-ac., petr.
warmth of bed amel. - **CAUST., RHUS-T.**

drawing, back of feet - arg-m., asaf., aster., ***bry.,*** camph., ***caust.,*** chel., chin., coloc., con., dig., ferr., gins., ham., indg., jatr., kali-bi., led., mang., mur-ac., nat-c., nat-s., nux-v., ran-b., rhus-v., sars., tarax., zing.
afternoon - com.
cramp-like - arg-m.
evening - nat-c.
motion amel. - mang.
motion, on - camph.
outer part of - ang., arn.
pulsating - arg-m.
rubbing amel. - nat-c.
sitting, while - cycl., mur-ac.
standing - chin., mur-ac., nat-c., tarax.
walking, while - coloc.
amel. - arg-m.

drawing, heels - anac., ang., ***ant-c.,*** aur., aur-m-n., berb., cann-s., carb-an., chin., con., led., lyc., merc., par., ***plat.,*** ptel., rhus-t., sep., sulph., thuj.
cramp-like - plat.
evening in bed - acon., lyc., sulph.
sitting, while - cann-s., chin., indg.
sleep, on going to - aur.
standing, after - berb.
walking, while - berb., led.

drawing, soles - ***alumn.,*** ammc., ***anac.,*** aphis., asc-t., aster., aur-m-n., bar-c., ***bell.,*** cact., cham., caust., cic., colch., coloc., com., con., crot-h., cupr., ***hep.,*** hyos., ign., ***kali-p.,*** led., mag-c., nux-v., sars., sil., sulph.
cramp-like - cact.
evening - com.
extending to, thigh - spong.
extending to, toes - aur-m-n., jatr.
morning, bed, in - sulph.
rheumatic - jatr.
stepping, on, while - mez.
walking - cupr.

drawing, toes - agar., anac., ang., arg-n., asaf., asc-t., aster., ***aur., aur-m-n.,*** bar-c., berb., cact., ***camph., caul.,*** caust., chel., cic., clem., cocc., colch., coloc., con., dig., ham., hell., indg., led., mag-m., mez., nat-c., nat-s., ol-an., plat., rat., rhus-v., ruta., sars., ***sep.,*** sil., stront-c., ***thuj.,*** vinc.
cramp-like - ***anac.,*** plat., vinc.
evening - nat-s.
bed, in - asar., con.
extending upwards - anac., caust., dig., ***thuj.***
fifth - cycl.
first - agar., ***ant-c.,*** aur., bry., caust., chel., colch., coloc., com., con., cycl., jatr., kali-bi., nat-m., plat., plb., rhus-t., sars., sep., sulph., ***thuj.***
ball of first toe - am-c., petr.
cramp-like - plat.
evening - com., thuj.
extending upward - bry.
joints - led., nat-s., ***sulph.***
joints, afternoon - sulph.
motion, on - caust.
motion, on, amel. - plb.
paralytic - aur.
sitting - agar.
sudden - coc-c.
tip - bar-c.
fourth - colch., tarax.
joints, of - aur., berb., sabin., sil., verat.
motion, amel. - lyc.
paralytic - aur.
second - caust., colch., plb.
shifting - arg-n.
sitting - ***aur-m-n.***
tearing - carb-an., clem., sulph., zinc.
third - colch.
walking, while - aur-m-n.

DRYNESS - ars., chel., manc., phos., ptel., sep., sil.
dryness, soles - bism., manc., phos.

ECZEMA, feet, back of feet - merc., ***psor.***

ELECTRICAL, current, sensation of - gels.

EMACIATION - ***ars.,*** **CAUST.,** chin., iod., nat-m., plb.

ENLARGEMENT, sensation of - **APIS,** ***coloc.,*** daph., mang.
walking in open, air, after - mang.
enlargement, toes - ***laur.***
sensation of, toes - apis.

ERUPTIONS - ***anan., ars.,*** aster., bar-c., bov., ***calc.,*** carb-o., ***caust.,*** chin-s., con., croc., crot-c., elaps, genist., lach., med., ***mez.,*** phos., ***rhus-t.,*** rhus-v., sec., sep., stram., sulph.
ball, nodule - zinc.
biting - ***calc.***
black - ***ars., sec.***
bleeding - ***calc.***
blotches - ant-c., jug-r., kreos., lyc., sep., sulph.
burning - bov., ***mez.***
confluent - cop., rhus-v.
coppery spots - ***graph.***
desquamation - chin-s., dulc., **MEZ.**
dry - ***mez.***
elevations - cop.
flea bite, like - sec.
hard - bov., ***lach.***
itching - aster., bov., calc., con., ***mez.,*** sep., sil.
miliary - ars.
nodes - ***ang.***
painful - lyc., phos., spig., sulph.
pimples - ars., bar-c., bov., bry., ***carb-s.,*** con., crot-c., cupr., led., mosch., sel., sep., sulph., zinc.
pustules - ***calc., con., merc., rhus-t.,*** sep.
red - bov., crot-c.
scabs - ***calc.,*** rhus-v., ***sil.***
scaly - rhus-v.
scurf - ***sil.***

eruptions, back of feet - aster., bov., carb-o., ***caust.,*** lach., led., med., merc., petr., ***psor.,*** puls., sars., tarax., thuj., zinc.
elevation - petr., puls., thuj.
itching - aster., ***calc.,*** carb-an., lach., led., ***psor.,*** sep., tarax.
nodules - carb-an., petr.
painful - bov., psor.
pimples - ***caust.,*** led., mosch.
pustules - calc., con., sars., sep.
scaly - psor.

eruptions, heels, boils - calc., lach.
blisters - calc., caust., graph., lach., led., nat-c., petr., phos., sep., sil.
desquamating - elaps
itching - caust., sil.
pustules - ***nat-c.***
ulcerated, of - nat-c.

eruptions, soles, of - anan., ars., bell., bry., bufo, chin-s., con., elaps, kali-bi., manc., nat-m., pip-m., sulph.
desquamating - ars., chin-s., elaps, ***manc.,*** sulph.
pimples - con.
psoriasis - ***phos.***
pustules - ***nat-c.***
scales - pip-m.

eruptions, toes - am-c., crot-c., cupr., cupr-ar., graph., kali-bi., lach., led., nat-c., nit-ac., ph-ac., rhus-v., ruta., ***sil., sulph.,*** zinc.
between - alum., ***petr.***
painful - sulph.
pimples - mosch., sulph.

eruptions, toes
between, soreness - berb., carb-an., ***graph.,*** lyc., merc-i-r., mez., nat-c., ph-ac., ran-b.
white - sulph.
blotches - ant-c., lach., sulph., zinc.
pimples - am-c., bor., sulph., zinc.
pustules - crot-c., cupr-ar., cycl., graph., kali-br., ph-ac.
scabs - **SIL.**
sore to touch - zinc.

ERYSIPELAS, - ***apis, arn.,*** bor., ***bry.,*** dulc., nux-v., puls., ***rhus-t.,*** sil., sulph.
dancing, after - berb., bor.
desquamating - dulc.
spots, in - apis

EXCORIATION, foot, soles - sil.

excoriation, toes, between - aur-m., berb., carb-an., clem., ***fl-ac., graph.,*** lach., lyc., mang., merc-i-f., mez., ***nat-c.,*** nat-m., nit-ac., ph-ac., ran-b., ***sep.,*** **SIL.,** syph., zinc.

EXCRESCENCES, soles, on - **ANT-C.,** ***graph.,*** thuj.

EXTENSION - phyt., plat.

FELON, general
bone, decay - asaf., aur., fl-ac., ***lach.,*** lyc., merc., mez., ph-ac., **SIL.,** sulph.
deep-seated pain agg. in warm bed - sep.
pus, with offensive - fl-ac.
cold application amel. - ***apis, fl-ac., led.,*** **NAT-S., PULS.**
gangrenous - ***ars., lach.***
hangnails, from - lyc., ***nat-m.,*** sulph.
injury, from - ***led.***
itching - **APIS.**
lymphatic inflamed - all-c., ***bufo, hep., lach.,*** rhus-t.
malignant with burning - ***anthr., ars.,*** **TARENT-C.**
maltreated - ***hep.,*** phos., ***sil.,*** stram., ***sulph.***
nail, beginning in - par., petr., ***phyt.,*** plb., puls., ***rhus-t.,*** sep., **SIL.,** ***sulph.***
root of - caust., graph.
under - alum., caust., coc-c., sulph.
panaritium - ***all-c.,*** alum., **AM-C.,** ***am-m., anac.,*** **ANTHR., APIS,** arn., asaf., bar-c., ***benz-ac.,*** berb., bov., ***bufo, calc., caust.,*** chin., ***cist.,*** con., cur., **DIOS.,** eug., ferr., **FL-AC.,** gins., **HEP.,** ***hyper., iod., iris,*** kali-c., kalm., ***lach.,*** led., ***lyc., merc., nat-c., nat-h., nat-m., nat-s.,*** **NIT-AC.,** par., petr., ***phyt.,*** plb., puls., ***rhus-t., sang., sep.,*** **SIL.,** ***sulph.,*** **TARENT-C.,** teucr.
burning - **ANTHR.**
deep-seated - bry., hep., lyc., rhus-t.
periosteum - ***am-c.,*** asaf., calc., calc-p., canth., dios., ***fl-ac.,*** mez., phos., sep., **SIL.,** sulph.
prick with a needle under the nail, from - all-c., bov., ***led.,*** sulph.
purple - ***lach.***

FELON, general
run-around - all-c., alum., ***apis***, bufo, bov., ***caust.,*** con., crot-t., dios., eug., ferr., ***fl-ac., hep.,*** graph., lach., ***merc., nat-h., nat-m., nat-s.,*** par., phos., plb., puls., ran-b., rhus-t., ruta., ***sang.,*** sep., ***sil.,*** sulph., syph.
lymphatics inflamed - all-c., hep., lach., op., rhus-t., sin-n.
vaccination, after - **THUJ.**
sloughing, with - **ANTHR., *ars., carb-ac., euph., lach.***
splinters, from - ***bar-c., hep.,*** iod., lach., ***led.,*** nit-ac., petr., **SIL.,** sulph.
sensation of - nit-ac.
stinging pain - **APIS, LACH.,** sep., **SIL.**
sulphur, after abuse of - apis
suppurative stage - ***calc.,*** **HEP., SIL.**
tendons, affected - graph., ***hep.,*** lach., ***led., merc.,*** nat-s., ***nit-ac.,*** ran-b., rhus-t., **SIL.,** sulph.
winter, every - **HEP.**

FLEXED, toes - ***ars.,*** colch., ***hyos.***

FORMICATION - acon., aeth., **AGAR.,** alum., am-c., ang., ant-c., apis, arn., ars., ars-h., ars-i., arund., bell., bor., canth., caps., carb-an., carb-s., carl., ***caust.,*** chel., cic., clem., coloc., con., croc., ***crot-c.,*** dulc., euph., graph., guai., hep., hyper., ign., jatr., kali-c., kali-n., kreos., lyc., mag-c., manc., mang., mez., ***nat-c., nat-m.,*** nat-p., nux-v., op., par., phos., plb., ***rhod., rhus-t.,*** rhus-v., sars., **sec., *sep.,*** spong., ***stann.,*** stram., stront-c., ***sulph.,*** tarax., tax., zinc.
chill, during - canth.
extending over body - caps., nat-m.
upward - bell., stann.
heat, after - ***sulph.***
morning - carb-an., ***hyper.,*** nat-c.
bed, in - ***rhus-t.***
stepping, on - puls.
night - phos., sulph.
raising foot - sars.
sitting agg. - carl.
standing, while - mang., sep.
stepping - sars.
walking in open air amel. - bor., zinc.
formication, back of feet - mag-c., zinc.
formication, heels - agar., am-c., bell., caust., ferr-ma., ***graph.,*** nat-c., par., phos., stront-c., ***sulph.,*** zing.
evening in bed - nat-c.
extending to toes - bell.
morning, in bed - ***graph.***
sticking - ***sulph.***
formication, soles, of - agar., am-c., bell., berb., calc-p., **CAUST.,** clem., ***coloc.,*** cic., con., fl-ac., hep., hura, kali-c., laur., mag-m., nat-m., pic-ac., plb., raph., sep., spig., spong., staph., sulph., thuj., vip., zing.
evening - zing.
sitting, while - zing.
rest agg. - sep.
rubbing amel. - sulph.
sitting, while - mag-m., staph.
formication, soles, of
standing, while - plb., zing.
stepping - con.
walking, while - plb., spong.
formication, toes - **AGAR.,** alum., am-c., ***am-m.,*** ars., berb., caust., chel., cic., colch., con., euph., euphr., guai., hep., jatr., kali-c., lach., lyc., mag-c., mag-m., nat-c., nat-m., nicc., ***phos.,*** plat., plb., ran-s., ***rhod., sec.,*** sep., stram., sulph., thuj., zinc., zing.
evening - ars., lyc., puls.
fifth - crot-t., phos.
first - alum., ars., brom., ***caust.,*** chin., gins., jatr., phos., plat., plb.
ball of - caust.
evening - nit-ac.
evening, 5 p.m. - cast.
freezing, as after - ***agar.,*** alum., zinc.
night - brom., mez.
waking, on - brom.
twitching, with - crot-t.
freezing, after - caust.
night - hep., nicc.
planter - mag-c., phos., staph.
second - nat-c.
tips - acon., agar., **AM-M.,** colch., spig., sulph.
walking, while - lyc.

FROZEN, sensation - pic-ac., puls.

FULLNESS - aesc., rhus-v., sumb.
veins of - ***ant-t.,*** ars., ***carb-v.,*** sul-ac., sumb.
fullness, soles, of, veins, network as if marbled - caust., lyc., thuj.

FUZZINESS, sensation of - ars., hyper.
sensation of, morning - ***hyper.***

GANGLION, instep, on the - ferr-m.
instep, on the - ferr-m.
ganglion, soles, of right - buf-s.

GANGRENE - ant-c., ant-t., ***ars.,*** calen., ***lach.,*** merc., **SEC.,** vip.
cold - ***sec.***
burning, tearing pains, with - **SEC.**
gangrene, toes - crot-h., cupr., iod., lach., **SEC.**
senile - ***ars., carb-an., carb-v.,*** cupr., ***ph-ac.,*** **SEC.**

GNAWING, pain., ball of - ran-s.
gnawing, toes - benz-ac., hyper., kali-c.
first - kali-c., ***ran-s.***

HARDNESS, soles, skin of - **ARS.**
without sensation - ars.

HEAT - acon., agar., ang., ***apis,*** arn., ars., ars-h., arund., aster., bell., brom., bufo, calad., calc., camph., carb-an., carb-s., carb-v., ***caust.,*** **CHAM.,** cimic., ***cocc.,*** coff., coloc., crot-h., cub., ***glon.,*** hyos., ign., kali-ar., ***kali-bi.,*** kali-chl., kali-i., lach., laur., led., ***lyc.,*** merc., mez., mill., morph., nat-c., nat-m., nat-p., ***nat-s.,*** nit-ac., ***nux-v.,*** par., ***petr.,*** ph-ac., phos., phyt., ***psor.,*** ptel., **PULS.,** rheum, rhus-t., rhus-v., ***ruta., sec., sep., sil.,*** spig., spong., stann., staph., **SULPH.,** sumb., til., vip., zinc.
afternoon - gels., hura
alternately hot and cold - ***gels.,*** graph., sec.

HEAT,
bed, in - calc., fago., hep., hura, merc., mez., ***sang., sil.,*** stront-c., **SULPH.**
burning - ***agar.,*** apoc-a., ars., aster., calc., cham., cocc., fl-ac., ***graph.,*** kali-ar., kali-c., ***lyc.,*** **MED.,** ***nat-s.,*** **PH-AC.,** phyt., plan., **PULS.,** ***sang.,*** sanic., **SEC.,** ***sep.,*** stann., **SULPH.,** ***zinc.***
uncovers them - agar., apoc-a., ***cham.,*** mag-c., **MED.,** ***phos.,*** **PULS.,** ***sang., sanic.,*** **SULPH.**
chill, during - agar., cann-s., nit-ac., rat., ***spong.***
cold, body - ***calad.***
hands, with - ***aloe, calc.,*** coloc., ph-ac., ***sep.***
sweat of hands - hura
dinner, after - calen., phos.
dry heat - bell., phos.
eating, after - calen.
evening - alum., bell., bry., carb-s., caust., kali-c., ***led.,*** mag-m., ***nat-s.,*** nit-ac., nux-m., ***sil.***
8 p.m. - nicc.
after lying down - stront.
cold hands, with - aloe
fire, as if, were forcing to head - zinc.
flushes - colch., stann., **SULPH.**
freezing, as after - agar., kali-c.
lying on back, while - ign.
morning - apis, nat-s., ***nux-v.,*** ptel.
night - calc., ***ign., nat-s.,*** ph-ac., ***sep., sil.,*** staph., **SULPH.**
after walking in open air - ***alum.***
bed, in - ***sil.***
lying on back - ign.
midnight, 3 a.m. - clem.
midnight, 3 to 5 p.m. - hyper.
midnight, after - calad.
midnight, before - mag-m.
one, coldness of the other - chel., dig., ip., **LYC.,** ***puls.***
perspiration, cold, after - hura.
pricking - rhus-v.
sleep, when going to - alum.
tingling - berb., merc., sumb.
uncovers foot - mang., ***sulph.***
walking, after - carl., puls.

heat, back of feet - calc., coloc., cupr-s., plb., ***puls.,*** rhus-t., thuj.
sudden - calc.

heat, heels - kali-bi., spong.

heat, soles - am-m., apoc., ars-s-f., bell., berb., ***calc.,*** carb-s., carb-v., ***carl., cham.,*** clem., ***cocc.,*** coc-c., cub., dulc., eup-per., ***ferr.,*** ferr-p., fl-ac., ***graph.,*** kali-n., ***lach., lil-t.,*** lith., **LYC.,** ***manc.,*** mang., ***med.,*** mur-ac., ***nat-c.,*** nat-m., nit-ac., nux-m., ***nux-v.,*** ox-ac., ***petr., ph-ac., phos.,*** plb., psor., ***puls.,*** samb., ***sang., sanic.,*** sars., ***sep., sil.,*** spig., stann., stram., **SULPH.,** ***thyr.,*** verat., zinc.
afternoon, while sitting - lyc.
chill, after - sulph.
evening - **LACH.,** ***phos., sang.,*** zinc.
lying down, after - am-m., nux-v., ***sulph.***

heat, soles
evening, wine, after - psor.
fever, during - aesc., canth., cupr., ***ferr.,*** graph., ***lach.,*** **SULPH.**
flushes, in - cub.
forenoon - nat-c.
menses, during - carb-v., cham., ***petr., sulph.***
morning - eup-per.
bed, in - nux-v.
motion, amel. - sars.
night - bar-c., fl-ac., **LACH.,** petr., thyr.
sitting, after - cocc.
uncovers them - ***calc.,*** **CHAM.,** cur., fl-ac., med., ***petr., phos.,*** **PULS.,** ***sang., sanic.,*** **SULPH.**

heat, toes - apis, asaf., aster., berb., bor., coc-c., cycl., hura, kali-bi., lach., mag-m., zinc.
afternoon - asaf.
burning - bor.
cold feet, with - apis
crawling - berb.
first - am-c., aster., ***nit-ac.,*** rhus-t.
ball of - am-c., carb-an.
night - coc-c.
tips, heat, shooting, to head like electric sparks - sep.

HEAVINESS - acon., ***agar., agn.,*** **ALUM.,** am-c., anac., ant-c., apis, aran., ***arn.,*** **ARS.,** ***ars-i., aur.,*** bar-c., ***bell.,*** berb., bor., ***bov.,*** bry., cadm-s., ***calc.,*** calc-ar., cann-i., cann-s., canth., carb-ac., carb-s., ***carb-v.,*** carl., caust., cham., chin., clem., coca, ***cocc.,*** colch., coloc., croc., crot-h., ***cycl.,*** eup-per., ferr., ferr-ar., ferr-i., gamb., ***graph.,*** hell., ***ign.,*** ind., iod., ***kali-ar., kali-c.,*** kali-p., kali-n., kreos., lach., ***led.,*** lyc., **MAG-C.,** mag-m., mang., merc., ***nat-c.,*** **NAT-M.,** nat-p., nat-s., nicc., nit-ac., nux-v., ***ol-an.,*** op., ***petr.,*** **PHOS., PIC-AC.,** ***plat.,*** plb., **PULS.,** rhus-v., ***sabad.,*** sabin., ***sars.,*** **SEP.,** ***sil.,*** spong., stann., stram., **SULPH.,** sul-ac., tab., tep., thuj., verat., verb., xan., zinc.
afternoon - lyc., nux-v.
sitting, while - lyc.
walking, while - lyc.
ascending stairs - bor., cann-s., lyc., mag-c.
bending them - led.
bones - staph.
chilliness, during - hell.
dinner, after - ***carb-v.***
eating, after - bry., cann-s., op.
evening - am-c., apis, bor., mag-c., mang., nat-m., plat., thuj.
6 p.m. - mang.
undressing, when - ***apis.***
walking, while - lyc.
forenoon - bry., coloc.
lying, while - led.
menses, during - colch., nat-m., sars., ***sulph.,*** zinc.
amel., during - **CYCL.**
before - bar-c., cycl., lyc., zinc.
morning - apis, carl.
bed, in - mag-m., ***nat-m.,*** sep., sulph.
waking, on - nat-s.
motion, amel. - nicc., zinc.

HEAVINESS, sensation
night - apis, carb-an., caust., nit-ac.
bed, in - caust.
right - ***agn.***
rising after a meal when - bry.
sitting, while - alum., anac., led., **MAG-C.**, ***plat.***, **RHUS-T.**
standing, while - kali-n., ***nat-m.***, phos.
stepping - nit-ac.
vexation, after - nat-m.
walking, while - cann-i., kali-n., kreos., lyc., manc., phos., plb., ***sep.***, ***sulph.***, verat.
after - alum., ***arn.***, cann-s., caust., ***con.***, murx., ***rhus-t.***, ruta.
amel. - ars-i., led., **MAG-C.**, ***nat-m.***, ***sulph.***
heaviness, soles - ph-ac., thuj.

HERPES - **ALUM.**, ***mez.***, ***nat-m.***, ***petr.***, **SULPH.**
herpes, toes - alum.
between - alum., graph.

IMPETIGO, back of feet - ***carb-s.***

INDURATION, heels, muscles - aur., lyc.
induration, soles - **ARS.**

INFLAMMATION - acon., arn., ***ars.***, bor., **BRY.**, calc., calen., ***carb-an.***, ***com.***, dulc., kali-bi., ***merc.***, mygal., ***phos.***, ***puls.***, ***rhus-v.***, sil., **SULPH.**, zinc.
bone - sarr.
dark red - rhus-v., sil.
periosteum - ***aur-m.***, guai.
inflammation, back of feet - calc., mag-c., puls., thuj.
inflammation, heels - ant-c., sabin.
rheumatic - sabin.
inflammation, soles - ***puls.***
inflammation, toes - am-c., berb., carb-an., caust., lach., ***nit-ac.***, ph-ac., phos., ***puls.***, sep., sulph., tarent., teucr., ***thuj.***, zinc.
erysipelatous - **APIS.**
first toe - ***am-c.***, sulph.
ball - phos.
frost-bitten - ***agar.***
as if - agar., bor.
wet, after getting feet - nit-ac.

INSENSIBILITY, to touch and stitches - ant-c.

INVERSION - nux-v., sec.

ITCHING - ***agar.***, alum., am-c., anac., apis, ***ars.***, arum-t., aur., ***bell.***, ***berb.***, bism., ***bov.***, bry., ***calc.***, cann-s., canth., ***caust.***, cham., ***chel.***, ***cocc.***, coloc., con., corn., crot-c., dios., dulc., fago., hura, ***ign.***, jug-r., kali-ar., kali-c., ***lach.***, **LED.**, lyc., mag-c., merc-i-f., mur-ac., nat-m., nat-p., nit-ac., nux-v., ol-an., phyt., psor., puls., ran-s., ***rhus-t.***, rhus-v., sabad., sars., ***sel.***, **SEP.**, spong., stram., **SULPH.**, sul-i., tarent., ***tell.***, thuj., verat., verat-v., ***zinc.***
afternoon - fago.
bed, in - ***apis***, **LED.**, merc-i-f., ***sulph.***, zinc.
biting - bell., berb., spong.
burning - berb., stram.
cold, from - tarent.
evening - kali-c., nux-v., sel., zinc.
frozen, as if - **AGAR.**, kali-c.
it had been - agar., caust., kali-c.

ITCHING,
inner side of - ***ambr.***, bov., bufo, laur.
joints - aur., calc., dig., kali-c., ***mez.***, mur-ac., ph-ac., stann.
midnight, before - puls.
motion amel. - psor., rhus-v., spig.
night - ***apis***, canth., **LED.**, ***lith.***, puls., ***rhus-t.***, sabad.
outer side of - grat., merc-i-f., sars.
stinging - merc-i-f.
rubbing agg. - corn.
scratching, agg. - bism., corn., ***led.***
amel. - cann-i.
sticking - berb., lach., puls., zinc.
tickling - bry.
walking, after - alum.
becoming warm from - alum.
warming up agg. - rhus-v.
itching, back of feet - agar., alum., anac., apis, asaf., bell., berb., ***bism.***, calc., **CAUST.**, chel., coloc., dig., hep., lach., **LED.**, mag-m., nat-m., nat-s., nit-ac., puls., ran-s., ***rhus-t.***, sars., spig., stann., ***tarax.***, thuj.
biting - berb.
burning - berb.
corrosive - agar.
evening - nat-s.
undressing - apis, ***nat-s.***
morning, bed in - ***puls.***
night - dig.
scratching, agg. - berb., ***bism.***, ***led.***
amel. - mag-m., nat-s., tarax.
sticking - berb., mur-ac.
warmth of bed - apis, **LED.**, merc-i-f., sulph., zinc.
itching, heels - berb., bov., calc., card-m., ***caust.***, cham., fl-ac., lach., lob., lyc., mur-ac., nat-c., nicc., olnd., ***ph-ac.***, ***phos.***, puls., rat., sabin., staph., verat.
left - nicc.
rubbing, amel. - mur-ac.
scratching, amel. - caust.
warmth of bed - caust.
itching, soles, of - ***agar.***, ***alum.***, ***ambr.***, ***am-c.***, am-m., ammc., anth., aur., ***berb.***, bov., brach., ***calc-s.***, cann-i., caust., cham., ***chel.***, con., crot-c., cupr., elaps, euph., ferr-ma., gins., graph., ***hep.***, ***hydrc.***, kali-n., ***kali-p.***, kreos., lith., med., merc-i-f., mur-ac., nat-c., nat-m., ol-an., phos., psor., ran-s., rat., sars., sel., ***sil.***, stry., ***sulph.***, ***zinc.***
afternoon, 2 p.m. - ol-an.
biting - berb.
burning - berb., kali-n.
scratching, after - am-c.
evening - am-c., am-m., phos., sel.
motion amel. - mur-ac., olnd., sars.
night - sars., ***zinc.***
prickling - crot-t.
scratching amel. - chin.
sitting - chin.
sticking - berb.
tickling - alum., euph., kali-n.
voluptuous - rat.
scratching, after - sil.

itching, soles, of
walking, while - chin., mur-ac., **SULPH.**
wine, after - psor.

itching, toes - ***agar., alum., ambr.,*** am-c., ***arg-m.,*** arn., ars., ***berb.,*** bry., ***carb-an.,*** caust., chel., ***clem., colch., cycl.,*** euphr., ***graph., hep.,*** ind., iod., jatr., lach., lact., ***mag-c.,*** mag-s., ***merc., mez.,*** mur-ac., nat-c., nat-m., nat-s., nit-ac., nux-v., paeon., ph-ac., phos., plat., ***puls.,*** rhod., rhus-v., ruta., sep., sil., ***staph., stront-c.,*** **SULPH.,** thuj., verat., ***zinc.***
air, cold, after - alum.
air, in open - alum.
between - cycl., graph., jatr., mang., med., merc., mosch., ***nat-m., nat-s.,*** thuj.
biting - berb.
burning - berb., hep., ind., mur-ac., nat-c., paeon., staph.
daytime - ind.
dinner, after - mag-c.
evening - ***alum.,*** ind., merc., nat-s., nit-ac., phos., zinc.
lying down, after - ***clem.***
scratching, agg, after - ***alum.***
undressing - nat-s.
fifth - bor., nicc., rheum, staph.
ball of - bor., puls.
evening - staph.
evening, 4 p.m. - ol-an.
scratching amel. - nicc.
first - alum., am-c., ant-c., ars., cycl., graph., ***kali-c.,*** merc-i-f., nat-c., nit-ac., plat., ruta., staph., verat., zinc.
ball - am-c., mur-ac., ***nat-s.,*** rhus-t., zinc.
burning - nat-c.
creeping - ars.
distal joints - caust., sep.
evening - nit-ac., zinc.
freezing after - am-c., zinc.
sticking - graph., plat., rhus-t., staph., zinc.
tip of - ambr., am-m., kali-c., sep.
fourth - nicc., tarax.
fourth, scratching amel. - nicc.
frozen, toes that had been - **AGAR., ALUM.,** carb-an., nat-c., nux-v., paeon., ***puls., sil.,*** staph., sulph., zinc.
heat, agg. - rhus-v.
morning, falling asleep - mur-ac.
waking, on - spong.
night - hep., puls.
scratch until they bleed, must - ***arg-m.***
scratching agg. - ***alum., arg-m., zinc.***
second, ball - puls.
sticking - berb., graph., plat., puls., staph.
third - nicc.
scratching amel. - nicc.
under - kali-c., phos.
under, nails - sil.
undressing - ***nat-s.***
voluptuous - spong., thuj.
walking, after - alum.
becoming warm from - alum.

JERKING - anac., ars., ***bar-c.,*** bar-m., ***cic.,*** cina, ***graph.,*** hyos., ip., ***kali-bi.,*** lyc., nat-c., nat-s., nux-v., phos., puls., ***sep.,*** **STRAM.,** sil., sul-ac.
sleep, in - nat-c., phos., sep.
on going to - ***bell., kali-c.,*** phos., ***zinc.***
spasm, in - ***cina.***

jerking, back of feet - anac.

jerking, soles, of - crot-t., ferr-ma.

jerking, toes - **AGAR.,** anac., berb., ***calc.,*** calc-p., ***merc.***

KNOCKED, together, feet - ***cann-s.***

knocked, together, toes - ***asaf.,*** plat.

LAMENESS - abrot., am-br., ***aur.,*** bell., ***colch.,*** com., fl-ac., hyper., merc-i-f., nat-m., ***rhus-t.,*** sil., thuj., tub.
afternoon - thuj.
pregnancy, during - sil.

lameness, soles - cupr., kali-p.

lameness, toes - ***aur.***

LOOSE, left - arg-m.

MOTION, constant motion - ***lach.***
convulsive - op., plb., ***zinc.***
difficult - nat-m.
downward, as if stamping - cina.
nervous, in bed - ***zinc.***

motion, toes - fl-ac.
involuntary - op.
restricted - ars.

NAILS, general, toes

brittle - cast-eq., ***sil., thuj.***

burning, nails - alumn., ant-c., calc., caust., **GRAPH.,** hep., merc., nat-m., nux-v., puls., ***sep.,*** sulph.
around - con.
under - calc., ***caust.,*** elaps, kali-c., merc., nit-ac., ***sars.***
roots of - ***asaf.,***

chapped, skin, about the nails - **NAT-M.**

corrugated, nails - ars., fl-ac., sabad., **SIL.,** ***thuj.***
transversely - ars.

cracked, nails - **ANT-C.,** ars., ***nat-m., sil.***

crippled - ars., ***caust.,*** **GRAPH.,** ***nat-a., nit-ac.,*** sabad., sep., **SIL.,** ***thuj.***

crumbling - ars., sep., ***sil., thuj.***

discoloration, nails - ant-c., ars., graph., nit-ac., thuj.
black - ***ars., graph., lept., nat-m.***
around - **NAT-M.**
blood, settles under nails - apis
blueness - acon., aesc., agar., apis, apoc., ***arg-n.,*** arn., ***ars.,*** asaf., aur., cact., ***camph.,*** carb-s., ***carb-v., chel., chin.,*** chin-a., ***chin-s.,*** chlf., cic., cocc., colch., con., ***cupr., dig., dros.,*** eup-pur., ***ferr.,*** ferr-ar., ferr-p., gels., gins., ***graph.,*** ip., manc., merc., merc-sul., ***mez.,*** mur-ac., ***nat-m., nit-ac.,*** **NUX-V.,** op., ***ox-ac., petr.,*** ph-ac., ***phos.,*** plb., rhus-t., sang., sars., sep., ***sil., sulph.,*** sumb., tarent., ***thuj.,*** **VERAT.,** ***verat-v.***

NAILS, general, toes
discoloration, nails
blueness, chill, during - apis, arn., **ARS.,** ***asaf.,*** carb-s., ***carb-v., chel., chin., chin-s., cocc.,*** con., ***dros., eup-pur.,*** ip., kali-ar., mez., **NAT-M., NUX-V.,** petr., ph-ac., **RHUS-T.,** sulph., thuj., verat.
menses, during - ***arg-n., thuj.***
dark - morph., ox-ac.
gray - merc-c., ***sil.***
livid - ars., ***colch.,*** op., ***ox-ac.,*** sul-ac.
purple - apis, ars., op., samb., sec., stram.
red - ars., crot-c., lith.
then black - ***ars.***
white - cupr., nit-ac.
spots - alum., ars., ***nit-ac.,*** sep., **SIL.,** sulph.
yellow - ambr., am-c., aur., bell., bry., canth., carb-v., cham., chin., **CON.,** ferr., ign., lyc., ***merc., nit-ac., nux-v.,*** op., plb., **SEP., SIL.,** spig., ***sulph.***
discoloration, toenails - apis, ***ars.,*** camph., dig., ***graph., nit-ac., ox-ac., sil.***
black - ***lept., nat-m.***
around - **NAT-M.**
blueness - apis
distorted, nails - alum., anan., calc., ***fl-ac.,*** **GRAPH.,** merc., sabad., ***sep.,*** **SIL.,** sulph., ***thuj.***
distorted, toenails - anan., **GRAPH.,** merc., sep., thuj.
drawing, pain, under - nat-m.
dryness - ***sil., thuj.***
dryness, about - nat-m., ***sil.***
eruptions, nails, about - eug., merc., sel.
exfoliation, nails, of - alum., ant-c., apis, ars., cast-eq., chlor., crot-h., form., **GRAPH.,** ***hell., merc.,*** rhus-t., sabin., ***sec.,*** sep., ***sil.,*** squil., sulph., thuj., ***ust.***
grow, nails, do not - ***ant-c.,*** calc., sil.
grow, rapid - fl-ac.
hangnail, nails - ***calc.,*** lyc., ***merc.,*** **NAT-M.,** ***rhus-t.,*** sabad., sep., ***sil., stann.,*** **SULPH.,** ***thuj.***
inflamed - kali-chl.
painful - sel., stann.
horny, nails, growth under - **ANT-C.,** graph.
ingrowing, nails - alum., ***caust.,*** colch., **GRAPH.,** kali-c., kali-chl., **MAG-AUST.,** ***nat-m., nit-ac., ph-ac.,*** plb., **SIL.,** ***sulph.,*** **TEUCR.,** ***thuj.,*** tub.
ulceration, with - ***nit-ac.,*** **SIL.,** ***teucr.***
unhealthy granulation, with - ***lach.,*** sang.
injuries, toenails - **ARN., HYPER.,** ***led.***
lacerations, from - **HYPER.**
splinter of glass, from - calen., hyper., ***sil.***
pain, nails - am-m., ant-c., bell., ***caust., graph., hep.,*** kali-c., ***merc.,*** nat-m., ***nit-ac., nux-v.,*** par., ***petr.,*** puls., ran-b., rhus-t., sabad., sep., ***sil., squil.,*** stann., sulph., zinc.
splinter, as of - ars-h., coc-c., ***nit-ac., sil., sulph.***

NAILS, general, toes
pain, nails, under - caust., eup-per., hep., merc., ***sil.,*** thuj.
in intermittent fever - eup-per.
walking, while - camph.
pain, toenails - caust., ***graph.,*** hura, merc-sul., ***teucr.***
first, as from a splinter - agar., **NIT-AC.**
as from inflammation - lyc., ***sil.***
as if nail would be torn out - thuj.
as if nail would enter flesh - colch., ***graph.,*** kali-c., teucr.
under - ***agar.,*** **NIT-AC.,** ***sil., sulph.***
panaritium, nails - ***all-c.,*** alum., **AM-C.,** ***am-m., anac.,*** **ANTHR., APIS,** arn., asaf., bar-c., ***benz-ac.,*** berb., bov., ***bufo, calc., caust.,*** chin., ***cist.,*** con., cur., **DIOS.,** eug., ferr., **FL-AC.,** gins., **HEP.,** ***hyper., iod., iris,*** kali-c., kalm., ***lach.,*** led., ***lyc., merc., nat-c., nat-h., nat-m., nat-s.,*** **NIT-AC.,** par., petr., ***phyt.,*** plb., puls., ***rhus-t., sang., sep.,*** **SIL.,** ***sulph.,*** **TARENT-C.,** teucr.
burning - **ANTHR.**
deep-seated - bry., hep., lyc., rhus-t.
roughness, toenails - ***graph.,*** SIL.
ribbed - thuj.
ridges, longitudinal - fl-ac.
sensitive, toenails - berb., ***nat-m.,*** nux-v., petr., ***sil.,*** squil., sulph.
sharp, pain, nails - alum., ***calc.,*** caust., ***graph.,*** mosch., ***nat-m.,*** nit-ac., nux-v., ***puls.,*** rhus-t., sep., sil., sulph.
sharp, toenails, first - coc-c., ***sil.,*** sulph., ***thuj.***
under, first - cahin., caust., coc-c.
shooting, pain, toenails, first - hyper., sulph.
night in bed - sulph.
spilt, nails - **ANT-C., SIL.,** ***squil.,*** sulph.
splinters, nails, as from, under the - bell., carb-v., ***fl-ac.,*** hep., **NIT-AC.,** petr., plat., ran-b., ***sil., sulph.***
spotted, nails - alum., ars., ***nit-ac.,*** ph-ac., sep., **SIL.,** sulph., tub.
suppuration, nails, around - con., ph-ac.
under - form.
nail of left great toe - caust.
vaccination, after - **THUJ.**
tearing, pain, nails - colch., ***fl-ac.,*** hep., ***nit-ac.,*** petr., plat., ran-b., ***sil., sulph.***
tearing, toenails - ***camph., carb-v.,*** caust., graph., hep., hura, thuj.
tearing, walking, while - ***camph.***
thick, nails - alum., ***ant-c.,*** calc., **GRAPH.,** merc., sabad., sep., **SIL.,** sulph., ***ust.***
thick, toenails - ***graph.,*** sec.
thin, nails - ars., op.
ulcers, nails - alum., ant-c., **ARS.,** aur., bar-c., bor., bov., calc., caust., con., crot-h., ***fl-ac.,*** **GRAPH.,** ***hep., lach.,*** lyc., ***merc., nit-ac., puls.,*** ran-b., ***sang.,*** sec., sep., **SIL.,** squil., **SULPH.,** thuj.
ulcers, toenails - ***caust.,*** graph., hep., ***mag-aust.,*** merc., ***sep.,*** **SIL., SULPH.**

NUMBNESS - abrot., acet-ac., ***acon.,*** agar., ***alum.,*** alumn., ambr., am-c., am-m., ang., ant-c., ant-t., ***apis, arg-m.,*** **ARG-N.,** arn., **ARS.,** ars-h., ars-i., arund., asar., asaf., ***bapt.,*** bell., bry., cact., ***calc.,*** calc-p., calc-s., ***camph.,*** cann-i., ***carb-an., carb-s., carb-v.,*** carb-o., ***caust.,*** cham., cinnb., coca, **COCC.,** colch., ***coloc.,*** **CON.,** croc., cub., cupr., dig., dios., euph., euphr., fago., ferr., ferr-ar., ferr-i., ferr-p., glon., **GRAPH.,** grat., hell., helon., hyper., ign., iod., ***kali-ar.,*** kali-c., kali-n., kali-p., kali-s., lach., laur., **LYC.,** mag-m., mag-s., mang., merc-c., mez., mill., nat-a., nat-c., nat-m., nat-p., ***nit-ac.,*** **NUX-V.,** op., **PH-AC., PHOS.,** phys., pic-ac., ***plat., plb.,*** psor., ***puls.,*** rhod., rhus-t., sabad., ***sec.,*** sep., sil., spig., stram., sulph., sul-ac., sumb., ***thuj.,*** upa., verat-v., vip., zinc.
afternoon - fago., mang., mez., phos.
2 p.m. - mang.
4 to 8 p.m. with chill - lyc.
alternating with hands - **COCC.**
ascending steps, on - nat-m.
bed, in - carb-an.
chill, with - cedr., ***cimx.,*** ferr., ***lyc.,*** nux-m., **PULS.,** sep., stann., stram.
crossing limbs - laur., ***phos.***
daytime - ***carb-an.***
dinner, during - kali-c.
after - ***kali-c.,*** mill.
eating, after - **KALI-C.**
evening - ***calc.,*** graph., phos., puls., sil., sul-ac., zinc.
excitement, during - sulph.
forenoon - am-m., nat-c.
hollow of - bry., merc-sul.
joints of - cann-i.
left - coloc., ***glon.,*** graph., kali-c., mag-s., med., nat-c., ***nat-m.,*** ph-ac., phos., phys., psor., sul-ac., ***thuj.***
then right - mill.
walking, only while - ph-ac.
lying, while - caust., sulph.
menses, before - hyper.
morning - alum., dios., nux-v., sep., sil.
bed, in - alum., calc-p., mag-s.
motion, on - bapt.
amel. - am-c., puls.
night - am-m., bry., ***ferr.,*** lyc., mag-m., phos., zinc.
night, bed, in - alumn., ***calc.***
outer side of - ang.
painful - mag-m., puls.
pressing on the spine, when - ***phos.***
riding, while - ***calc-p.***
cold wind, in - ham.
right - alum., am-c., ant-c., ars., carb-an., camph., ***kali-bi.,*** mang., rhus-t., sep., zinc.
right, then left - coloc., mill.
sitting - am-c., ***ant-t., calc.,*** calc-p., cann-s., caust., cham., coloc., euph., graph., grat., helon., jug-c., laur., lyc., mill., nat-c., ***phos., plat., puls.,*** rhod., sep., sul-ac.
standing - mang., merc., ***sec.***
stooping - coloc.
stretching - cham.

NUMBNESS, sensation
walking, while - ant-c., graph., ph-ac., ***sec.***
after - rhod.
air, in open amel. - ***thuj.***
numbness, back of feet - graph., thuj.
walking, while, in open air - graph.
numbness, heels - ***alum.,*** arg-m., caust., chel., con., graph., ign., lyc., nux-v., rhus-t., sep., ***stram.,*** thuj.
morning, rising, on - stram., thuj.
sitting, while - ***con.***
stepping - ***alum.,*** arg-m., caust., rhus-t.
numbness, soles, of - ***alum.,*** alumn., ***ars.,*** bry., ***cann-i.,*** cham., chel., **COCC.,** cupr., eupi., fl-ac., laur., merc-sul., nat-c., ***nux-v.,*** olnd., plb., puls., raph., ***sec.,*** sep., sulph., syph., thuj., zinc.
evening - sulph.
extending to thighs - ars.
left - cann-i., sulph.
night - cham.
rubbing amel. - sulph.
sitting - **COCC.,** thuj.
standing - puls., ***sec.***
walking, while - cham., olnd., ***sec.***
amel. - puls., zinc.
numbness, toes - ***acon.,*** apis, ***ars.,*** benz-ac., ***calc.,*** camph., ***caust., cham., chel., con.,*** crot-h., cub., cycl., fago., glon., **GRAPH.,** lyc., ph-ac., ***phos.,*** plb., puls., **SEC.,** thuj.
ball of - puls.
extending upward - ***ars.***
first - cham., nat-c., nat-s., nux-v.
afternoon - nat-c.
morning - nat-s.
morning, while sitting - nat-s.
hot pickles - acon.
morning - lyc.
tips - acon., phos., tab.
beginning in - tab.
walking - ***acon., caust.,*** cycl., ph-ac.

ODOR, offensive without perspiration - ***graph.,*** sep., **SIL.**

PAIN, feet - abrot., agar., ail., aloe, ***alum.,*** alumn., ambr., am-m., ***anac.,*** anag., ant-c., ant-t., ***apis, arn., ars.,*** ars-h., ars-i., arum-t., arund., asaf., asc-t., aster., ***aur., aur-m.,*** bell., berb., bism., blatta, ***calc.,*** calc-s., ***cann-s.,*** carb-ac., carb-o., ***carb-v., caul., caust., chin.,*** cob., cocc., coff., colch., ***coloc.,*** con., crot-c., crot-h., crot-t., ***cupr., dig.,*** dios., dirc., ***dulc.,*** eup-per., fago., ferr., ferr-ar., ferr-i., gels., ***guai.,*** hell., hura, hyos., iod., jatr., kalm., ***lach., led., lith., lyc., merc.,*** merc-c., merc-i-f., ***mez.,*** mill., mosch., mur-ac., nat-a., nat-c., ***nat-m., nat-s.,*** nit-ac., nux-m., ***nux-v.,*** osm., ***petr.,*** phos., ***phyt.,*** pip-m., plan., plat., plb., podo., polyg., psor., puls., ***rhod.,*** **RHUS-T.,** rhus-v., rumx., ***ruta.,*** sabin., sang., sars., sec., sel., ***sil.,*** sol-n., spig., spong., stann., ***staph.,*** stram., stry., sulph., ***syph.,*** tarent., ter., teucr., ***thuj.,*** ust., ***verat.,*** verat-v., wies., zinc.
afternoon - lith., mez., phos., rhus-v., sars.
alternately in each - ***lac-c.,*** nat-p.
ascending - **LED.,** mag-c.

PAIN, feet
ball of - lyc., sil.
begining to walk - lyc.
ulcerative - lyc.
bending, when - coff., sel.
bones - acon., agar., ***alum.,*** ars., ***asaf.,*** aur., bell., bism., ***carb-v., chin.,*** cocc., ***cupr.,*** lach., led., ***merc.,*** mez., nit-ac., plat., ***ruta., sabin.,*** spig., stann., ***staph.,*** teucr., verat., zinc.
chilblains, as from - berb., bor., caust., cham., nux-v.
chill, during - cupr.
coffee, after, amel. - calo.
dinner, after - carb-s.
evening - acon., all-c., ars-h., ferr-m., fl-ac., led., lyc., mag-c., phos., puls., sil., sulph.
exertion, from - bar-c., caust., phos., **RHUS-T.**
extending to, body - ***plb.***
to, calves - dros.
to, hips - ***nux-v.***
to, knees - dirc.
to, tibia - nat-m.
to, toes - chel.
to, upwards - dirc., dros., ferr-i., **LED.,** nat-m., nit-ac., nux-v., ***plb., sil.,*** sulph.
gouty - ***led., nat-s.***
heat - ran-b.
jerking - kali-n., rat.
joints of - ambr., aster., bell., ***bry., calc.,*** caust., cedr., clem., coloc., con., graph., ***guai.,*** hell., ***kali-c.,*** mez., nat-m., nat-s., osm., ph-ac., ***phos., staph.,*** stront-c., tarent., verat.
wandering - coloc.
left - ail., crot-h., hyper., mur-ac., murx., sang.
lifting - berb.
menses, during - am-m., ars., mag-c.
morning - dios., **RHUS-T.,** sulph.
8 a.m. until afternoon - coloc.
11 a.m. - hura.
rising, on - **RHUS-T.**
waking, on - ***sulph.,*** tarent.
motion, on - acon., ars., bry., bufo, caust., coff., ***guai., led.,*** puls., sel., thuj.
motion, on, amel. - abrot., calo., cur., dios., psor., ***rhod.,*** **RHUS-T.,** ***verat.***
night - bar-ac., caul., cham., kali-c., lyc., ***mez.,*** phos., sep., sil., spong., stront-c., ***syph.,*** verat.
noon - arund.
paralytic - acon., ang., cham., ***chin.,*** eug., kalm., led., nat-m., olnd., ol-an., par., ***plb.,*** **RHUS-T.,** tab.
paralytic, left - hyper.
paralyzed - am-m.
paroxysmal - sec.
pressure, on - caust.
rheumatic - ant-c., ***aur.,*** calc., ***caust.,*** colch., ferr-i., ***guai.,*** **HEP.,** ***lach.,*** **LED.,** lith., mag-m., ***merc.,*** merc-i-r., nat-s., ***nit-ac.,*** phos., ***phyt.,*** plb., ***rhod., ruta.,*** sars., stram., stry., zinc.
right - kalm., lith.
sides - arg-m.
outer - caust., zinc.
sitting while - alum., aur-m-n., dig., nat-c., **RHUS-T.,** stann., tarax., valer.
sleep, disturbing - sep.
standing while - chin., eup-per., ***puls.,*** rhus-v., tarax.
stepping, when - ang., bry., caust., **RUTA.,** thuj.
touching agg. - acon., bor., bry., chin., ferr-ma.
ulcerative - am-m., bry., caust., hep., lyc., ***mag-c.,*** **NAT-M.,** nat-s.
uncovering, when - stront.
waking, on - abrot., sep.
walking, while - agn., ambr., am-m., ang., ant-t., ars-h., bar-c., carb-s., caust., clem., coloc., crot-h., ferr., ***guai.,*** lith., mag-c., nat-c., nat-m., nit-ac., petr., phyt., plb., puls., rhus-v., sabad., stry., sulph., tax.
air, in open, after - ***rhus-t.***
amel. - bar-ac., dig., ***puls.,*** **RHUS-T.,** ***verat.***
wandering - ars-h., coloc., iris, ***puls.***
warm bed, in - ***mag-c.,*** verat.
amel. - **CAUST.**
warmth agg. - ***guai.***
weight on, on bearing - calo.
wet weather - ***dulc., rhod., rhus-t.***

pain, back of feet - aesc., agar., alum., asaf., aur., card-m., caust., chel., coloc., ***cop.,*** eup-per., ferr., ferr-i., guai., hell., lach., lil-t., merc-i-f., mez., nat-s., nux-m., ***phyt.,*** plan., plb., puls., sang., sil., syph., ***tarax.,*** xan.
evening - agar., ferr., led.
walking, while - agar.
extending to, pelvis - ferr-i.
to, toes - syph.
menses, during - lyss.
motion, on - cop.
rheumatic - chin., ferr., ferr-i., ol-j., rhus-t., syph., vesp.
sitting while - asaf., ***tarax.***
stepping agg. - nux-m.
stretching out, on - bry.
touch, on - alum., puls.
walking, while - agar., bry., calc., caust., coloc.
warmth of bed amel. - **CAUST.**

pain, heels - acon., agar., alum., am-c., ***am-m.,*** anag., aran., ars., ars-h., aur., bapt., berb., bor., ***calc.,*** calc-p., caps., ***carb-an.,*** cast-eq., cedr., cham., ***chel.,*** cinnb., clem., ***coloc.,*** crot-h., dios., eup-per., euph., ***ferr., ferr-ar.,*** fl-ac., graph., hell., ign., iod., kali-c., ***kali-i.,*** led., lyc., lyss., mang., meph., merc-i-f., ***nat-c.,*** nat-m., nat-s., osm., ***petr.,*** phos., phyt., **PULS.,** ran-b., ran-s., raph., **RHOD.,** ***rhus-t.,*** rhus-v., ruta., sang., sep., spong., sulph., thuj., upa., ***valer.,*** verat., xan., ***zinc.,*** zing.
afternoon - clem.
ascending steps - carb-s.

pain, heels
bone - berb., caps., coloc., crot-h., ign.
elevating the feet amel. - phys.
evening - am-m., ***nat-c.,*** **PULS.,** zinc.
frozen, formerly - phos.
gouty - calc., kali-i., lyc., meph., sabin.
left - bry., xan.
morning - am-c.
first step - rhus-t.
waking, on - am-c., ars.
nails, like, under skin - ***rhus-t.***
night - ***am-m.,*** zinc.
3 a.m. - ***am-m.***
bed, in - ***am-m.***
paralytic - caust., puls.
pulsating - ***nat-c.***
resting, with boot off, amel. - raph., valer.
rheumatic - anan., bapt., mang., meph., phyt., **RHOD.,** sabin.
right - ***am-m.,*** ars-h., lyss., valer.
rising from a seat - graph., puls.
rubbing, amel. - ***am-m.***
sharp - iod.
sitting - **VALER.**
splinter, as if - ***petr., rhus-t.,*** sulph.
standing - agar., am-c., berb., cham.
stepping - am-m., lyc., phos.
stone, as from a small - lyc.
tendons of foot after walking - sulph.
ulcerative - am-c., ***am-m.,*** aur., berb., carb-an., ***caust.,*** graph., ***kali-i.,*** laur., ***nat-s., zinc.***
walk, on beginning to - puls.
walking - acon., agar., ambr., am-c., ***ars.,*** berb., ***caust.,*** cinnb., euph., jatr., kali-bi., lyc., nit-ac., phos., raph., spong., ***zinc.***
amel. - laur., **VALER.**
warmth, amel. - stram.
wine, after - **ZINC.**

pain, soles - agar., alum., am-c., anac., anag., ***ars.,*** bar-c., berb., bov., bry., cact., calc., ***canth.,*** carb-v., **CAUST.,** croc., ***crot-t.,*** cupr., dios., gels., graph., hyos., ***led.,*** lith., ***lyc.,*** lyss., merc., merc-i-f., merc-i-r., mez., nat-p., nit-ac., pareir., ***petr., phos.,*** pip-m., plat., plb., puls., ran-s., sec., ***sil., stann.,*** sulph., ***still.,*** zinc.
afternoon - crot-t.
afternoon, 4 p.m. - plan.
convulsions - ars.
convulsive - bar-c.
evening - berb., mag-m., sil.
extending to, first toe - ***crot-t.,*** merc-i-f.
to, knees - kali-p.
to, lumbar region - plb.
to, toes - sep.
hollow of the - anag., cham., lith., mur-ac., myric., rhus-t., sanic.
lightning-like - daph.
morning - bar-c., dios., zinc.
motion amel. - aloe, coloc., puls.
night - sil., sulph.
paralytic - par.
rheumatic - aphis., calc., med.

pain, soles
rising, on - sulph.
seat, from a, on - graph.
sitting, on - asaf., lyc.
spikes, as if stepping on - ***cann-i.***
splinter, as if - agar.
standing, while - anac., berb., croc., sul-i., syph.
amel. - euph.
stepping, when - ***alum.,*** ars-h., bar-c., berb., brom., bry., ***cann-i., canth.,*** lyc., nat-c., puls., sulph., ***zinc.***
touch agg. - crot-t., puls.
ulcerative - ambr., bar-c., calc., ***canth.,*** graph., kali-n., kreos., lyc., ***nat-s.,*** phos., ***puls.,*** sulph., thuj., zinc.
walking, while - aloe, alum., ambr., ant-c., ***ars.,*** ars-h., bar-c., berb., bry., cact., calc., ***cann-i.,*** canth., carb-v., caust., coc-c., gels., hydrc., ign., kali-c., ***led.,*** lyc., med., merc., nat-c., olnd., par., phos., plb., puls., rhus-t., sil., sulph., viol-t., ***zinc.***
stones, on uneven - hep.
wandering - psor.

pain, toes - am-m., aster., ***aur., benz-ac.,*** berb., brom., ***calc.,*** calc-p., ***caul., caust.,*** chel., cocc., ***coloc.,*** crot-h., dig., dulc., ferr., hell., hura, iod., kali-bi., kali-i., kali-p., lach., lact., lil-t., ***lith., lyc.,*** merc., mez., naja, nat-m., nit-ac., nux-v., ***phos., phyt.,*** pip-m., ***plat.,*** plb., puls., **RHOD.,** rhus-t., rumx., sabad., sang., sec., sel., sep., ***sil., stict.,*** stry., ***sulph., syph.,*** tarent., tell., thuj., ***zinc.***
annually - tarent.
ball of - am-c., tab.
ball of, bone - mez., sep.
ball of, walking, while - am-c.
corrosive - sep.
evening - cist.
extending into hip - ***nux-v., pall.***
fifth - aloe, anag., asar., asc-t., blatta, chel., con., fl-ac., hura, lith., merc-i-f., rumx., staph., ther.
as from chilblains - aloe.
ball of - nit-ac.
ball of, walking, while - nit-ac.
morning - anag.
touch on - lyc.
first - ***all-c., am-c.,*** ammc., anag., asaf., aster., ***aur.,*** bapt., ***berb., benz-ac.,*** both., bry., calc-p., carb-ac., carb-v., chin., ***cimic., colch.,*** coloc., dios., ***dulc.,*** elat., ***eup-per.,*** gnaph., ***graph.,*** hell., hura, ind., ***iod.,*** lac-ac., **LED.,** ***lyc.,*** mang., meph., merc-i-f., merc-i-r., mez., nat-p., nat-s., ph-ac., phos., phys., ***phyt., pip-m.,*** plat., ***plb.,*** puls., ***ran-s., rhod.,*** sabin., ***sil.,*** sulph., tarent., ***zinc.***
alternating with pain, in heart - nat-p.
ball of - ambr., am-c., ***bry.,*** carb-an., ***colch.,*** **LED.,** sep., sulph., tab.
ball of, frozen, as if it had been - carb-an.
ball of, ulcerative - carb-an.
cold applications amel. - sabin.
damp weather - am-c.

pain, toes, first
evening - nat-s., stry., zinc.
evening, bed, in - ***am-c.***
evening, bed, in, amel. - puls.
frozen, as if - bry., phos.
hiccoughs, from - ph-ac.
jerking - agar.
joints - ***apoc.***, aster., ***benz-ac., cann-i.,*** carb-v., ***caust.,*** coff., dulc., ***eup-per.,*** ind., ***iris,*** **LED.,** nat-s., phos., prun., sabin., sang., sil., upa.
joints, gouty - ambr., ammc., ***arn.,*** ars., asaf., aster., ***benz-ac., bry.,*** calc., ***calc-p., caust., cimic., dulc.,*** elat., ***gnaph.,*** kalm., **LED., LYC.,** phos., plat., ***sabin., sil.,*** sulph., zinc.
joints, gouty, left - ammc.
left - ***am-c., eup-per.,*** phos.
lightning, like - daph.
lying amel. - puls.
morning - anag., **LED.,** lyc., merc-i-r.
morning, walking, while - ***led.***
motion, agg. - aster., chin., sabin.
motion, amel. - ind.
nail, as if would enter flesh - colch., ***graph.,*** hep., kali-c., teucr.
nail, as from inflammation - caust., lyc., ***sil.***
nail, as from a splinter - agar., **NIT-AC.**
nail, as if nail would be torn out - thuj.
nail, under - ***agar.,*** carb-v., **NIT-AC.,** ***sil., sulph.***
neuralgic - phyt.
night - ***benz-ac.,*** mang., ***plb.***
noon - pip-m.
pressure, on - alum.
pulsative - asaf.
rheumatic - apoc., cinnb., crot-t., ***led.,*** ol-an., sabin.
rheumatic, left - agn., ***led.***
rheumatic, right - ***benz-ac.,*** bry., cist., lac-c.
right, then left - ***dulc., pip-m., ran-s.***
sudden - bry.
swallowing agg. - ph-ac.
tip - asaf., berb., calc.
tip, pulsating - asaf.
touch agg. - chin., kali-c., mang., ph-ac., sabin.
ulcerative - am-c., caust., nat-c., ol-an., zinc.
ulcerative, stepping, when - sil.
walking, while - aur., bry., calc-p., chin., **LED.,** pip-m., **SIL.**
warm bed - ***am-c.***
fourth - asc-t., brom., calc-s., chel., dios., fl-ac., form., merc-i-f., mur-ac.
fourth, pulsating - mur-ac.
frozen, as if - asar.
formerly - phos.
jerking - ***am-m.,*** mez., par., ran-s.
joints, of - ambr., ***arn., colch.,*** con., graph., ***led.,*** plb., ***sabin.,*** sang., ***sulph.,*** upa.
gouty - arn., asaf., ***caust., dulc.,*** graph., ran-s., ***sabin.,*** thuj.

pain, toes, fourth
joints, of
small joints - caul.
stepping, on - bor.
motion, on - am-c., thuj.
night - ***am-c.,*** coc-c., kali-c., led., merc., merc-i-f., nat-c., plat., ***syph.***
paralytic - aur., ***chin.***
rheumatic - arg-m., **AUR.,** kali-c., stict., stront-c., ***teucr.***
second - berb., bry., coloc., fl-ac., mur-ac., nat-s.
sitting, while - dig.
sleep, during - led.
standing, while - ars., calc., nat-m., sil.
stepping, when - bor., bry., led., sil., thuj.
third - aloe, berb., chel., fl-ac., form., mag-m., mur-ac., thuj.
morning - mag-m.
nail, under, as from splinter - ars-h.
pulsating - mur-ac.
ulcerative - berb.
tendons, extensor, while walking - verat.
touch, on - ***chin.,*** ph-ac., staph.
ulcerative - berb., carb-an., carb-v., caust., ***kali-i.,*** nat-c., ph-ac., sil., valer., zinc.
walking, while - agn., am-c., ant-c., ars., bry., camph., caust., ***kali-c.,*** lyc., mez., nat-m., phos., sil., thuj.
wandering - clem.

PARALYSIS - ang., apis, arn., ***ars.,*** bar-m., ***bell.,*** carb-o., ***chin., cocc.,*** colch., ***con.,*** crot-h., hydr-ac., laur., ***lyc.,*** nux-v., ***olnd., phos., plb.,*** rhus-t., stram., sulph., vip., ***zinc.***
flexors - ***bar-c.***
fright, from - ***stann.***
heel - graph.
partial - plb.
sudden - ***cham.***

paralysis, toes - ars.
extensors of - crot-h., plb.
turn under while walking - ***bad.***

PARALYSIS, sensation of - asaf., asar., ***cham., chel.,*** eug., kali-bi., led., mur-ac., nat-m., phos., sil., tab., zinc.
alternating with tearing - hyper.
morning, after rising - ***phos.***
bed, in - nat-m.
stepping, on - asaf.

PERSPIRATION - acon., am-c., am-m., ang., apis, arn., ***ars., ars-i.,*** **BAR-C.,** ***bar-m., bell.,*** benz-ac., brom., bry., **CALC., CALC-S.,** camph., cann-s., ***canth.,*** carb-an., **CARB-S., CARB-V.,** ***caust.,*** cham., chel., **COCC.,** coc-c., coff., **COLOC.,** croc., ***cupr.,*** cycl., dros., euph., fago., ***fl-ac.,*** **GRAPH.,** hell., hep., hura, hyper., ind., **IOD.,** ip., jab., kali-ar., ***kali-bi., kali-c.,*** kali-p., kali-s., kalm., kreos., ***lac-ac.,*** lach., lact., led., **LYC.,** ***mag-m.,*** mang., med., **MERC.,** mez., mur-ac., naja, nat-a., nat-c., ***nat-m.,*** nat-p., ***nit-ac.,*** ox-ac., ***petr.,*** ph-ac., ***phos.,*** phyt., pic-ac., plb., ***psor.,*** **PULS.,** rhus-t., sabad., sabin., sanic., sec., sel., **SEP., SIL.,** ***squil., staph.,*** **SULPH.,** tarent., **THUJ.,** ***verat.,*** **ZINC.**

PERSPIRATION,
afternoon - graph., lac-ac., plect.
burning, with - ***calc., lyc.,*** mur-ac., petr., sep., ***sulph.,*** thuj.
chill, during - cann-s.
clammy - acon., cann-i., pic-ac., sep., sulph.
cold - acon., ars., **BAR-C.,** bell., benz-ac., **CALC.,** ***calc-s., canth.,*** **CARB-S., CARB-V.,** ***caust.,*** cimic., ***cocc., cupr., dig., dros.,*** fago., graph., ***hep.,*** hura, ind., ***ip., kali-c., kali-p., kali-s.,*** laur., ***lil-t.,*** **LYC.,** ***mag-m.,*** med., ***merc.,*** mez., **MUR-AC.,** nit-ac., ox-ac., phos., pic-ac., plb., ***psor.,*** **PULS.,** ***sanic.,*** sec., ***sep., sil.,*** squil., **STAPH.,** stram., ***sulph.,*** thuj., **VERAT.**
constant - **SIL.,** ***thuj.***
daytime - pic-ac.
diarrhea, during - sulph.
except, feet - chin., phos.
evening - **CALC.,** coc-c., cocc., graph., ***mur-ac.,*** pic-ac., podo.
bed, in - calc., clem., ***mur-ac.***
excoriating - ***bar-c., calc., carb-v.,*** coff., **FL-AC.,** graph., hell., ***iod., lyc., nit-ac.,*** ran-b., ***sanic., sec., sep., sil.,*** squil., zinc.
forenoon - fago.
heat, during ars.
injuries of spine, in - **NIT-AC.**
left - cham., nit-ac.
menses during, from severity of pain - verat.
after - ***calc.,*** lil-t., ***sep., sil.***
before and during - ***calc.***
morning - am-m., bry., coc-c., euphr., lyc., merc., ***sulph.***
bed, in - bry., hell., lach., merc., phos., ***puls., sabin.***
rising, after - am-m.
night - coloc., mang., ***nit-ac.,*** staph., ***sulph.,*** thuj.
2 a.m. - ***ars.***
11 p.m. - hura.
waking, on - mang.
offensive - am-c., am-m., anan., arg-n., ars., ars-i., arund., **BAR-C.,** bufo, ***calc., calc-s.,*** carb-ac., ***carb-s.,*** cob., coloc., cycl., ***fl-ac.,*** **GRAPH., KALI-C.,** kalm., **LYC.,** nat-m., **NIT-AC.,** ***petr., phos., plb., psor.,*** **PULS.,** ***rhus-t., sanic., sec., sep.,*** **SIL.,** staph., ***sulph.,*** **TELL., THUJ.,** ***zinc.***
carrion - sil.
rotten eggs - staph.
sole-leather, like - cob.
sour - ***calc.,*** cob., nat-m., ***nit-ac.,*** sil.
sour, evening - ***sil.***
urine, like - canth., coloc.
profuse - ars., arund., carb-an., ***carb-s.,*** carb-v., cham., coloc., fl-ac., ***graph.,*** ind., ***ip., kali-c.,*** kreos., ***lac-ac.,*** lach., **LYC.,** merc., **NIT-AC.,** petr., phyt., ***psor.,*** puls., sabad., sal-ac., ***sanic.,*** sec., ***sep.,*** **SIL.,** staph., sulph., ***thuj., zinc.***
right - plect., sulph.
sitting, while - bell.

PERSPIRATION,
stool, after - sulph.
suppressed - am-c., apis, ars., bad., **BAR-C.,** ***bar-m.,*** cham., coch., colch., ***cupr., form.,*** graph., haem., ***kali-c.,*** lyc., merc., nat-c., ***nat-m.,*** nit-ac., ph-ac., phos., plb., ***puls.,*** rhus-t., sel., **SEP., SIL.,** sulph., ***thuj.,*** **ZINC.**
swelling of with - graph., iod., kali-c., kreos., ***lyc.,*** petr., ph-ac., plb., sabad.
waking, on - mang.
walking, while - carb-v., graph., nat-c.
warm - ***led.***
winter, worse during - arg-n., ***med.***

perspiration, heel - thuj.

perspiration, soles - acon., **AM-M.,** arn., ***calc.,*** chel., fago., hell., kali-c., ***merc., nat-m.,*** **NIT-AC.,** ***nux-m.,*** petr., ***plb., puls.,*** sabad., **SIL.,** ***sulph.***
cold - acon., ***sulph.***
itching - **SIL.,** ***sulph.***
making sole raw - ***calc.,*** nit-ac., ***sil.***
offensive - ***petr., plb.,*** **SIL.**

perspiration, toes - acon., arn., clem., kali-c., lach., ***phyt., puls.,*** sep., **SIL.,** squil., tell., ***thuj.,*** zinc.
between - acon., anac., arn., ***bar-c.,*** carb-v., ***clem.,*** cob., cupr., cycl., ferr., ***fl-ac., kali-c., lyc., nit-ac., puls.,*** sep., **SIL.,** squil., tarax., thuj., ***zinc.***
evening - clem.
offensive - ***bar-c.,*** cob., cycl., ***kali-c.,*** lyc., nit-ac., ***puls., sep.,*** **SIL.,** ***thuj., zinc.***
rawness, causing - **BAR-C.,** ***carb-v., graph., nit-ac., sanic., sep., sil.,*** **ZINC.**
morning, in bed - lach.
under toes - phyt., tarax.
walking, while - graph.

PINCHING, pain - chin., hyos., ip., sulph.

pinching, back of feet - ***camph.,*** par., sulph., thuj.
extending to thigh - ***camph.***
motion agg. - ***camph.,*** sulph.

pinching, heels - alum., ***chel.,*** nat-c.

pinching, soles - bry., upa.

pinching, toes - bar-c., puls., sul-ac.
fifth - mosch., ph-ac.
first - meph.
fourth - ph-ac.
stretching out foot, on - bar-c.
twitching - sul-ac.

PRESSING, pain - ***alum.,*** anac., ang., arg-n., asaf., aur., aur-m-n., ***bell.,*** brom., caust., cinnb., dig., fl-ac., graph., kali-n., lach., ***led.,*** lil-t., lyc., ***mang-m.,*** mez., mur-ac., naja, nat-s., olnd., petr., ***ph-ac., plat., sars.,*** spig., ***stann.,*** stront-c., ***sul-ac.,*** thuj., verb.
blunt body, as from - ang.
bones - bism., cupr., dig., mez., staph.
drawing - bry., staph.
eating, after - graph.
evening - fl-ac., lach., led.

PRESSING, pain
inner side of - ***led.***
inward - lach.
joints of - ***agar.,*** ang., asaf., aur., coloc., graph., hell., kali-c., led., lyss., merc., ***mez.,*** nat-m., nat-s., sep., stront.
motion agg. - led.
motion amel. - kali-c.
jumping to knee - asaf.
motion agg. - bry., staph.
outer side - ang., bism.
outward - lil-t.
sitting, while - aur-m-n., tarax.
tensive - stront.
walking - ang.
amel. - ***coloc.***
writing, while - coloc.

pressing, back of feet - ang., arg-n., aur-m-n., brom., cahin., caust., ferr-m., hell., jatr., ***led.,*** mur-ac., ***nat-c.,*** plat., sul-ac., tarax., thuj.
drawing - bry.
evening - led.
10 p.m. - arg-n.
pinching - thuj.
sitting, while - cycl., ***tarax.***
tearing - camph.
tremulous - plat.
walking in open air - acon.
amel. - coloc.
writing, while - coloc.

pressing, heels - alum., anac., ang., carb-s., eup-pur., graph., hell., hep., kali-c., petr., ruta, spong., stann.
as if in vise - alum.
stepping - stann.
tearing - stann.
vise, as if in - alum.

pressing, soles - anac., aur., bell., camph., graph., jatr., led., nux-m., olnd., ph-ac., plat., rhus-t., ruta, sabad., sars., tarax.
extending, great toe - ph-ac.
to thigh - led.
inner side - cupr., mur-ac.
motion, on - led.
paroxysmal - ph-ac.
pinching - ph-ac.
sitting, while - plat.
standing, while - sabad.
stepping - kali-c.
walking, while - kali-c., led.
amel. - ***verb.***

pressing, toes - ang., brom., camph., caust., chel., clem., coloc., ***colch.,*** cupr., gins., graph., guare., hell., mez., nat-s., olnd., ph-ac.
afternoon - coloc.
alternating with drawing - gins.
crushed, as if - olnd.
fifth - cycl., ferr-ma., ***led.,*** nat-s., olnd., paeon., ph-ac., ther.
first - arg-m., bor., carb-ac., coloc., cycl., gins., graph., jatr., **LED.,** ***nat-s., plat.,*** rhus-t., sep., sulph.
as if tightly enveloped - ***plat.***
ball of - bor., ***caust.,*** lyc., petr.

pressing, toes
first, joints - asaf., ***caust., coloc.,*** **LED.,** nat-s., rhod.
nail, under - calc.
stepping - bor.
tip - bism.
fourth - ph-ac.
frozen, formerly - phos.
joints - coloc., con., led., nat-s.
motion amel. - coloc.
nails - sars.
stepping - bor.
tips - mosch., led.
walking - mez., phos., sil.

PSORIASIS, soles - ***phos.***

PULSATION - am-m., ang., arg-m., asaf., caust., cann-s., carb-s., eup-per., gels., kali-i., lil-t., mygal., nat-m., nux-m., plb., rhus-v.
dinner, after - plb.
evening - carb-s.
joints of - arg-m.
lying, while - gels.
outer side of - sulph.
right - eup-per.

pulsation, back of - cann-s., rhus-t.

pulsation, heels - ars-m., ***nat-c.,*** nat-s., phos., ran-b.
evening - nat-c.
night - phos.

pulsation, soles - arund., kali-n., petr., sars., sulph.
evening - sulph.
hollow of - sulph.
rest, during - petr.
sitting, while - sars.

pulsation, toes - am-m., asaf., cycl., gamb., kali-bi., ph-ac., plat., zinc.
fifth - agar., plat.
first - ***asaf.,*** ars., meph., ph-ac., plat., rhus-t.
tip of - asaf.
fourth - gamb., mur-ac.
second - gamb., mur-ac.
third - gamb., mur-ac.

RAISED, difficult to raise - tab., zinc.
breathing, deeply, when - carb-v.
forenoon - mang.
impossible to raise - ars., nux-v.

RASH - bov., bry.

rash, toes, between - rhus-t.

RELAXATION - ars., ***gels.,*** nat-c.
lying, when - ars.

RESTLESSNESS - agar., ***alum.,*** arn., ***ars.,*** bar-c., calc., carb-s., carb-v., caust., ***cham.,*** chin., chin-a., cimic., croc., ferr-i., fl-ac., glon., kali-p., ***lil-t.,*** mag-m., **MED.,** ***meph.,*** nat-c., ***nat-m.,*** nat-s., ox-ac., plat., prun., ***puls.,*** **RHUS-T.,** sil., still., ***stram., sulph., tarent.,*** thuj., **ZINC.**
beer, after - nat-m., **SULPH.**
evening - arn., mag-m., nat-m.
bed, in - sulph., **ZINC.**
beer, after - nat-m.
heat, after - **SULPH.**

RESTLESSNESS,
lying, while - alum., **SULPH.**
menses, during - thuj., ***zinc.***
night - ***cham.,*** lyc., nat-c., puls., sulph., thuj., ***zinc.***
sitting, while - alum., bar-c., ***puls.,*** **ZINC.**
spasmodic - cina.
trembling - plat.
waking, on - ferr-i.
walking amel. - ***nat-m.***
restlessness, soles - croc.

SENSITIVE - agar., aloe, anac., ant-c., apis, calc., calc-s., ***kali-c.,*** lac-f., ***lach.,*** led., **LYC.,** med., ***mez., merc-i-r., petr.,*** rumx., ***sil.,*** stann., ***staph.,*** sulph.
cold, to - alum., am-c., zinc.
walking, while - alum.
warmth, to, left on walking - arg-m.
sensitive, heels - jatr., med.
sensitive, soles - aloe, ***alum.,*** ant-c., carb-v., hep., **KALI-C., LYC., MED.,** mez., sabad., sars., ***staph.,*** sulph., zinc.
sensitive, toes - ***calc., carb-an.***
ball of - sil.
first - ars-h., eup-per.
walking, while - calc.

SHAKING - kali-c., tab.

SHARP, pain - acon., agar., agn., ail., ***alum.,*** ambr., am-c., ***anac.,*** ant-c., apis, arg-m., arg-n., arn., ars., arum-d., asaf., aster., aur., bar-c., ***bell.,*** berb., ***bov.,*** bry., calc., ***calc-p., canth.,*** carb-an., carb-s., ***carb-v.,*** caust., cham., chel., chin., chin-a., cina, coloc., cupr., dig., dor., euph., eup-per., fago., ***ferr-p., fl-ac., graph., guai., hell.,*** hep., hura, hyos., hyper., iris, kali-ar., **KALI-C., KALI-S.,** ***kalm.,*** lyc., mag-c., mag-m., manc., mang., meli., meph., ***merc.,*** mez., **MUR-AC.,** ***nat-c.,*** nat-m., nat-s., ***nit-ac., nux-v.,*** ol-an., olnd., par., petr., ***phel.,*** ph-ac., phos., pic-ac., puls., ran-b., ran-s., raph., rhod., rhus-t., rhus-v., ruta., samb., ***sars.,*** senec., ***sep., sil.,*** spig., stann., stront-c., stry., ***sulph.,*** sul-ac., tarax., tarent., ***thuj.,*** verb., viol-t., vip., xan., zinc., zing.
afternoon - mez.
asleep, as if - lyc.
ball, of - lyc., mez., plat., sulph., zinc.
burning - bufo, coloc., rhus-t., ***sulph.,*** zinc.
chill, during - ***eup-per.***
cramp-like - cina.
eating, after - graph.
excoriation, in - phos.
extending, to knee - bell., xan.
upward - bar-c., ***plb.,*** ruta., xan.
morning on waking - thuj.
waking at, 10 a.m. - sil.
motion, on - bar-c., bufo, calc., chin., sulph.
amel. - guai., ***kali-c., kali-s., lyc., rhus-t.***
night - phos., sulph.
numbness, terminating in - ***berb.***
placing, on floor - tarent.
pressure, like - ***cina.***
rhythmical - nat-m.

SHARP, pain
riding in a carriage, when, stitches from inside outward - ***berb.***
shocks, ending in - daph.
sitting, while - asaf., manc.
standing, on - agn., nat-m., ***puls.,*** sil.
stepping, on - ars., bell., ***berb.,*** calc-p., ***nat-m.,*** tarent.
tearing - guai., sil.
twitching - carb-s., ***cina.***
walking, while - nat-m., tarent.
after - kali-c.
air, in open, amel. - nat-m.
air, in open, while - bell., lyc.
weather, on change of - vip.
sharp, back of feet - agar., ***anac.,*** ang., aur., chin., coloc., guai., hep., kali-c., lyc., ***puls.,*** rheum, rhus-t., ruta., spig., sulph., tarax., zinc.
motion agg. - sulph.
sitting - bell.
sleep, during - asar.
standing and sitting - mur-ac.
walking on pavement - sep.
sharp, heels - aeth., agar., ambr., am-c., am-m., ang., ars., arund., bad., bar-c., berb., bry., calc., carl., chel., chin., con., cic., cina, euphr., eupi., eup-per., ferr-ma., ***graph.,*** hep., ign., kali-ar., kali-c., kali-n., kreos., lyc., mag-c., ***manc.,*** meny., merc., nat-c., nat-m., nat-p., ***nat-s.,*** nit-ac., nux-v., ol-an., olnd., ***petr.,*** ph-ac., ***puls., ran-b.,*** rhod., ***rhus-t.,*** ruta., ***sabin.,*** sang., sars., ***sep., sil.,*** stry., spong., sulph., thuj., trom., **VALER.,** zinc.
afternoon - nat-m., ***ran-b.***
sitting, while - nat-s.
boring - ***puls.***
burning - agar., puls., sep., sul-ac.
cutting - berb., eupi., lyc.
darting - rhod.
evening - ang., merc., sep., thuj.
in bed - mag-c., nit-ac.
extending, to, back of feet - sars.
ball of foot - aeth.
thigh - ars.
upward - agar., spong.
itching - berb., nat-m.
left - nicc., thuj.
morning - eupi., ign., ***rhus-t.***
bed, in - bry., puls., sang.
moving, amel. - spong.
moving, on - kreos.
night - am-m., calc., euphr., sep.
bed, in - am-m.
paroxysmal - sep., spong.
prickling - carl.
pulsating - ***ran-b.***
putting it down, when - graph.
rhythmical - carl.
right - agar., chel., sulph.
rising amel. - bry., puls.
rubbing amel. - am-m., nat-s.
scratching, while - sars.
shooting - eupi.

sharp, heels
  sitting, while - agar., ang., berb., cic., cina, ***rhus-t.,*** ruta., sep., sil., spong., **VALER.**
  splinter - mang., nat-c., nit-ac., ***petr.,*** ph-ac., sulph.
  standing, while - berb., con., ran-b., sil., ***rhus-t.,*** spong.
  stepping upon it, when - ars., ***nit-ac.,*** ***rhus-t.,*** sep.
  stinging - bad., berb., sep.
  tearing - sil.
  tingling - berb.
  walking, while - berb., con., nat-s., thuj.
    walking, after - berb., spong.

sharp, soles - aeth., ***agar.,*** agn., ail., alum., ang., ant-c., arn., ars., arum-t., asar., bell., berb., **BOR.,** bry., calc., calc-caust., calc-p., camph., carb-an., chin., cic., clem., cocc., coc-c., coloc., con., crot-h., cub., daph., dig., dros., elaps, eupi., eup-per., ***fl-ac.,*** gamb., gent-l., graph., hura, ***ign.,*** ir-foe., jatr., kali-n., ***kalm.,*** led., lob-s., lyc., mag-m., mag-s., meny., ***nat-c.,*** nat-m., nat-p., nat-s., nicc., nit-ac., nux-v., ol-an., olnd., par., ph-ac., phos., plb., ***puls.,*** raph., rheum, ***rhus-t.,*** rhus-v., sabin., sars., sep., sil., spig., stry., sulph., tarax., thuj.
  afternoon - ***nat-c.***
  ball, on the - am-c., aur-m-n.
  burning - alum., berb., ***fl-ac.,*** ph-ac.
  crawling - arn., berb., mag-m.
  corrosive - plat.
  evening - alum., dig., ph-ac., ***rhus-t.,*** sulph.
    10:30 p.m. - hura.
    in bed - ant-c.
  extending, outward - ***tarax.,*** thuj.
    to hip - plb.
  itching - dros., spig., tarax.
  jerking - ph-ac.
  menses, during - raph.
  morning - alum., fl-ac., nicc.
    on rising from bed - fl-ac., nicc.
  motion, amel. - olnd.
  motion, during - spig.
  outer margin - ars.
  perspiration - **NIT-AC.**
  prickling - ant-c., bell., sep.
  pulsating - berb., clem., con.
  rubbing amel. - alum., ant-c., gamb., kali-n.
  sitting, while - dros., jatr., sars., sep., spig., tarax.
  splinter, like - agar.
  standing while - berb.
  stepping, on - berb., bry., nat-c., nicc., nit-ac., spig., staph., sulph.
  tearing - chin., phos.
  touch, from - sep.
  twitching - dig., nat-s., ph-ac.
  walking, while - agar., bell., cocc., con., eupi., gent-l., meny., plb., ***rhus-t.,*** sep.
    after - ant-c.
    as if walking on needles - ***rhus-t.***

sharp, toes - ***acon., agar.,*** ail., ***alum.,*** am-c., ***am-m.,*** ang., ant-t., apis, arg-n., arn., arum-d., arund., aster., aur., ***aur-m-n.,*** bar-c., ***berb.,*** bov., bry., buf-s., cadm-s., ***calc.,*** calc-p., cann-i., ***carb-s., carb-v., caust.,*** chel., cina, cist., cocc., ***coloc.,*** crot-t., cycl., dulc., elat., fago., ferr-ma., graph., ***hell., hep.,*** hyper., kali-bi., kali-c., ***kalm.,*** lach., led., ***lyc.,*** mag-c., mag-s., med., merc., merl., mez., nat-m., nat-s., **NIT-AC.,** ***nux-v.,*** olnd., ***pall.,*** par., petr., ph-ac., phos., plat., plb., ***puls.,*** ran-b., ***ran-s.,*** rhus-t., sabad., sabin., ***sil., stict.,*** stry., ***sulph.,*** sul-ac., tarax., tarent., thuj., ***verat.,*** verb., zinc.
  afternoon - mez.
  ball - alum., calc-p., daph., dros., spig.
  bed in - agar.
  bending body to left - thuj.
  biting - ***hyper.***
  burning - arund., chel.
  chill, during - lyc.
  cold amel. - aster.
  coming slowly - am-m.
  cramp-like - calc., cina, sil.
  evening - cist., lyc., nat-s.
    on falling asleep - merl.
  extending, to hip - ***nux-v.,*** pall.
  extending, upward - lach., ***nux-v.,*** pall.
  fifth - agar., am-m., apis, asaf., calc., cann-s., chel., con., hep., hura, lyc., ph-ac., rheum, ruta., thuj.
    ball - puls.
    cramp-like - ruta.
    frozen, as if - lyc.
    morning - lyc.
    pulsating - con.
    standing - am-m.
    walking - am-m.
  first - agar., agn., alum., alumn., am-c., am-m., ammc., arn., ars., ***asaf.,*** aster., ***aur-m.,*** bar-c., ***benz-ac., berb.,*** bov., bry., calc., ***cann-i.,*** caps., carb-v., carl., cast., ***caust.,*** chel., ***cist.,*** coloc., crot-t., daph., euphr., ferr-ma., form., gamb., gins., graph., ***hep.,*** hura, hyper., jatr., ***kali-c.,*** kali-n., ***kalm.,*** lach., laur., ***led., lyc.,*** mag-c., mag-s., merl., nat-m., nat-s., nit-ac., ph-ac., phos., pip-m., puls., ***ran-s.,*** rat., rhus-t., sabin., sang., sep., ***sil.,*** sulph., sul-ac., tarax., tarent., thuj., verat., zinc.
    alternating with thumb - sulph.
    ball - alum., am-c., ***cann-i., caust., kali-c.,*** mag-m., mur-ac., mag-c., ph-ac., phos., rhus-t., zinc.
    boring - sabin.
    burning - alum., ambr., berb., ***caust.,*** plat., tarax.
    crawling - berb., plat.
    cutting - sil.
    dinner, after - mag-s.
    drawing - bry.
    evening - alumn., ***cist.,*** euphr., lyc., mag-c., nat-m., phos.
    extending, to ankles - bov.
    extending, to chest - rhus-t.

sharp, toes
first, extending, to hip - ***hep.***
extending, upward - benz-ac., ***hep.***
fine - caust., kali-c., led., mag-s., rhus-t., sulph.
freezing, as after - agar., ***nit-ac.,*** zinc.
hot - thuj.
increasing and decreasing slowly - am-m.
joints - berb., ***benz-ac.,*** calc., ***cann-i.,*** kali-bi., ***led.,*** nat-m., nat-s., sep., sil., stann.
left - agn., alum., coc-c., kalm., led., phos.
long - arn., caust.
morning, in bed - ars.
motion, agg. - phos.
night - alum., form., kali-n.
night, in bed - thuj.
paroxysmal sudden - lyc.
pressure, on - ***hep.,*** nat-s.
prickling - sul-ac., zinc.
pulse-like - berb., hep.
rheumatic - hyper.
right - alumn., benz-ac., ***cist.,*** lyc., phos., ***ran-s.***
sitting, while - ***con.,*** graph., nat-m., sabin., sil.
splinters, like - agar., coc-c.
stamping amel. - caps.
standing, while - am-m., nat-m., rhus-t., sil.
stepping, when - asaf., ***aur-m.,*** berb.
sudden - lyc., nat-m., nat-s.
tearing - am-c.
tickling like electric shocks - sabin.
tips of - aur-m-n., bar-c., bry., carl., coc-c., colch., ***con.,*** kali-c., ***led.,*** mez., nat-s., olnd., par., ***ran-s.,*** sep., stann., staph., sulph., zinc.
tips of, burning - sep.
tips of, pulsating - mez., zinc.
tips of, sitting, while - ***con.***
twitching - berb., hell., kali-n.
walking, while - alumn., am-m., euphr., nat-m., phos., tarax.
fourth - agar., berb., chel., dros., mez., nat-s., ran-b., rhus-t., thuj.
twinging, drawing - berb.
going slowly - am-m.
hot - ***acon.***
itching - ran-s., spig.
jerking - carb-s.
joints - asaf., berb., cann-i.
motion - nux-v.
amel. - agar., cocc.
needle-like - calc., petr.
night - ***nux-v.***
noon, on bending body to left - thuj.
paroxysmal - calc.
second - canth., cham., dros., kali-n., ***led.,*** spig.
ball of - puls.
sitting, while - aur-m-n., calc.
smarting - nat-m.

sharp, toes
sprained - crot-t.
standing, while - ***agar.,*** calc., ***verat.***
stinging - ***verat.***
stool, during - nux-v.
tearing - tarax.
third - agar., asaf., chel., dros., ***led.,*** nat-s., sep., sulph.
tips of - am-c., am-m., aur-m-n., berb., caps., chin., dig., fl-ac., kali-c., merc., mez., nat-s., puls., stry., sulph.
boring - chin.
evening - am-m., puls., ran-b.
falling asleep, on - merl.
lying, while - sulph.
outward - caps.
sitting, while - aur-m-n., sulph.
walking in open air - am-m.
twitching - berb., carb-s., ***cina,*** merl.
walking, amel. - calc.
walking, while - arn., carb-s., crot-t., dros., ***lyc.,*** ran-b.

SHOCKS - agar., all-s., cadm-s., ***phos.,*** spig., stann.
asleep, before falling - ***phos.***
sleep, during - all-s., cadm.
shocks, heels - mag-m.

SHOOTING, pain - arg-m., aster., bell., daph., ferr., iris, **KALI-C.,** tarent., xan.
extending to knees - xan.
sticking ending in electric shocks - daph.
walking, while - bell., tarent.
shooting, heels - trom.
shooting, soles - agar., alum., bell., calc-p., daph., plb., sulph.
extending to hips - plb.
night before going to bed - sulph.
splinters, like - ***agar.***
walking, while - agar., bell., plb.
shooting, toes - ***acon.,*** agar., apis, aster., calc-p., daph., dulc., ***elat.,*** med.
ball of - alum., calc-p., daph.
extending to hips - nux-v., ***pall.***
first - alum., daph., pip-m., sulph., tarent.
joints - ***cann-i.,*** kali-bi., ***stann.***
tip - stann.
joints - ***cann-i.***
tips - ***am-m.***
evening - am-m.

SHRIVELLED - ars., merc-c., verat.

SMALL, seems too - kali-c., raph.

SMARTING, pain - ph-ac.

SOFT, soles, sensation of - ***alum.,*** sulph.

SORE, pain - alumn., ant-t., ***arg-m.,*** arn., arund., bar-c., bell., berb., bry., calc., calc-s., carb-ac., carb-an., carb-v., cham., chin., ***cina,*** clem., com., ferr., ***graph.,*** hyos., kali-ar., kali-bi., kali-n., laur., lil-t., **LYC.,** mag-c., mag-m., merc., ***mez.,*** nat-c., nat-m., nat-s., ol-j., op., ph-ac., phos., plb., puls., ran-b., rumx., **RUTA.,** sars., sep., **SIL.,** sulph., thuj., zinc.
afternoon - phos.
ascending - mag-c.

SORE, pain
ball of - nat-c.
eating, after - graph.
evening - ***arn.,*** mag-c.
morning, lying, amel. - mag-c.
stepping, on - puls.
waking, on - mag-c., nat-s.
night - plb., ***sulph.***
outer side - hep.
paralyzed, as if - ph-ac.
perspiration, from - graph., **lyc.**
pressure, on - cina
sitting, while - ***arg-m.***
standing - ang., **RUTA.**
walking, while - alumn., cham., **RUTA., SIL.**
amel. - arg-m., sep.

sore, back of feet - carb-an., chin., cocc., com., eup-per., indg., kali-i., laur., mag-m., sil.
left - kali-i.

sore, heels - agar., am-m., arg-m., bell., berb., bor., calc-p., caps., carl., caust., ***cimic.,*** cocc., ***cycl.,*** fago., jatr., kali-bi., **LED.,** mag-m., ***mang.,*** nux-m., nux-v., ph-ac., ran-b., sep., teucr., zinc.
left - puls.
paroxysmal - caps.
right - euph.
standing, while - agar., berb., mang.
stepping on it, when - agar., arg-m., bell., ph-ac.
walking, while - am-m., bell., caust., ***cycl.,*** euph., fago., jatr., ***kali-bi., led.,*** lyss., mang., nux-v., ph-ac., puls., sep.

sore, soles - **ALUM.,** alumn., ambr., **ANT-C.,** ***arg-m.,*** arum-t., aster., **BAR-C.,** berb., brach., calc., canth., ***carb-s.,*** caust., cham., ***coloc.,*** crot-h., graph., hep., ***ign.,*** kali-c., ***lac-c.,*** lact., **LED.,** lil-t., lyc., **MED.,** merc., **NAT-C.,** ***nux-m.,*** nux-v., phos., plb., psor., ***puls.,*** rhus-v., sabad., sars., ***sil.,*** stann., sulph., sul-ac., sul-i., syph., thuj.
exercise, amel. - plb.
inflamed, as if - nit-ac.
jerking - sul-ac.
morning, in bed - psor.
bed, in, rising, after - plb.
bed, in, stepping - spig.
night - bar-c.
sitting - thuj.
standing, while - sul-i.
stone pavements agg. - ***ant-c.***
walking, while - ***aloe,*** **ALUM.,** alumn., ambr., **ANT-C.,** ***arg-m., ars.,*** arum-t., ***bar-c.,*** calc., ***canth.,*** carb-s., carb-v., cham., chr-ac., ***con.,*** eup-per., graph., **HEP.,** lac-c., **LED., LYC., MED.,** ***mez., nat-c., nit-ac.,*** nux-v., phos., ***puls.,*** **RUTA.,** sabad., ***sil., staph.,*** squil., sulph., thuj., ***zinc.***
amel. - bar-c.
warmth, amel. - plb.

sore, toes - ***ars.,*** aster., aur., berb., calc., ***canth.,*** caust., ***cina,*** coff., ***coloc.,*** cycl., daph., graph., lyc., nat-c., ***nat-m.,*** **NIT-AC.,** ph-ac., plat., ran-b., ruta., sep., sulph., thuj., zinc.
balls - ph-ac., plat., sil.
formerly frozen - plat.
walking, on - ***ars.,*** caust., ph-ac., sil.
bending foot - hipp.
between - berb., carb-an., ***fl-ac., graph.,*** lyc., merc-i-r., mez., ***nat-c., nat-m.,*** ph-ac., ran-b., **ZINC.**
burning - lyc.
fifth - agar., bry., mur-ac., staph.
first - alum., ***arn., bry.,*** clem., ***nat-c., sulph.***
ball - **LED.,** lyc., pic-ac.
joints - aur., bry., lob-s., nat-m.
tip - zinc.
walking, while -lyc.
fourth - dios.
joints - ***camph.,*** puls.
jumping - cycl.
perspiration, from - graph., sep.
pressure, on - ***cina***
spots - ph-ac.
third - mez.
tips - con.
evening - ran-b.
ulcerated, as if - ph-ac.
walking, while - cycl., lyc., zinc.

SPRAINED, as if - ang., **ARN.,** ars., bar-c., berb., ***bry.,*** calc., ***camph.,*** carb-s., carb-v., caust., cop., crot-t., ***cycl.,*** dros., ferr-ma., ***hep.,*** hyper., ***kalm.,*** kreos., merc., nat-m., nux-v., phos., prun., puls., **RHUS-T.,** sanic., sil., sulph., til., valer., zinc.
left - hyper., sanic.
morning - **RHUS-T.**
touch amel. - cycl.
walking - ars., cycl.
amel. - cycl.

sprained, back of feet - bar-c.

sprained, heels - euph.

sprained, soles, as if - cham., cupr., ***cycl.,*** mur-ac.

sprained, as if, toes - am-c., berb., coloc., zinc.
ascending steps - coloc.
evening - coloc.
first - aloe, ***arn.,*** jug-r., lyc., mez., mosch., sil.
joints - ***arn.,*** aur., kali-c., prun., rat.
morning - jug-r.
morning, bed, in - jug-r.
motion agg. - mosch.
night - aloe, am-c.
night, bed, in - aloe, am-c., jug-r.
sudden - lyc.
fourth - berb.
joints - all-s., bry., carb-an., petr.

STAMPING, feet in sleep - kali-c., sep.

STIFFNESS - alum., all-s., ambr., ang., ant-t., **APIS,** ars., ars-m., asaf., bry., calc-s., caps., caust., cham., chel., cic., ***coloc.,*** dios., dros., ***ferr.,*** ferr-ar., ferr-p., graph., ign., kali-ar., kali-bi., ***kali-c.,*** kali-s., kreos., laur., ***led.,*** merc., mosch., nat-m., nux-v., ***op., petr.,*** phos., ran-b., **RHUS-T.,** sanic., ***sec., sep., stict.,*** stry., ***sulph.,*** sul-ac., tep., thuj., ***zinc.***

air open - nux-v.
alternating with tearing pain - ars.
cold from - cham.
eating, after - graph.
evening - calc-s., kali-s.
sitting - plat.
undressing, when - apis.
morning - apis, ign., ***led.***
morning, on waking - alum.
night - **APIS,** sulph.
rising, after sitting - bry., laur.
amel. - alum.
sitting - plat.
tearing, in, after - sulph.
waking, on - alum.
walking, while - ign.
amel. - alum., laur.

stiffness, toes - **APIS,** ars., brom., ***carl., coloc.,*** dios., ferr., ***graph., led.,*** nux-v., ***sil.,*** stry., ***sulph.***

first - **ATRO,** coloc., sulph.
afternoon - sulph.
morning - dios.
second - colch.
sitting, after - carl.

STRETCHED, out - phos.

convulsively - cina.
inclination to - am-c., op., puls.
morning in bed - ***rhus-t.***
sitting, while - ***puls.***
sole, painful - aster.

SUPPURATION - rhus-v., ***sec.,*** vip.

scurf - ***sil.***

suppuration, soles - berb., bor., fago.

sensation of - calc., kali-n., lyc., prun., spig.

suppuration, toes, under nail of left big toe - caust.

SWELLING - acet-ac., acon., aesc., alum., ambr., am-c., ant-c., **APIS,** apoc., arg-m., ***arn.,*** **ARS.,** ***ars-i.,*** arund., asaf., ***aur.,*** aur-m., bar-c., bar-m., ***bell.,*** berb., bov., **BRY.,** ***cact., calc., calc-ar.,*** calc-s., cann-s., ***canth., carb-an., carb-s.,*** carb-v., **CAUST.,** cedr., ***cench.,*** cham., ***chel., chin.,*** chin-s., ***cocc., colch.,*** coloc., con., cop., corn., crot-h., ***dig.,*** dor., ***elaps,*** eup-per., ***ferr.,*** ferr-ar., ***ferr-m.,*** ferr-p., fl-ac., ***glon., graph.,*** hep., ***hyos.,*** hyper., iod., kali-ar., ***kali-c.,*** kali-i., kali-n., kali-p., kali-s., kreos., lac-c., ***lach.,*** **LED., LYC.,** mang., **MED.,** ***merc., nat-a., nat-c., nat-m.,*** nat-p., ***nit-ac.,*** nux-v., op., pareir., ***petr.,*** ph-ac., ***phos., phyt.,*** plb., prun., **PULS.,** ***rhod., rhus-t.,*** rhus-v., ruta., sabad., ***samb.,*** sars., ***sec., sep.,*** **SIL.,** sol-n., stann., staph., ***stict.,*** stram., ***stront-c.,*** sulph., sul-ac., ter., ther., thuj., verat., vesp., vip., zinc.

SWELLING,

ascending steps, while - ***nat-m.***
bed, out of, when, amel. - sulph.
blue with red spots - elaps, ***lach.***
bones - staph.
burning - canth., con., puls.
chlorosis, in - ***ferr.***
cold - ***apis, calc.,*** kreos.
cramp, after - graph.
dancing, after - bov.
daytime - dig.
edematous - acet-ac., ***anthr.,*** **APIS,** ***apoc., arg-m., arg-n.,*** **ARS.,** arund., asaf., ***aur., aur-m.,*** bov., ***bry., cact.,*** cahin., ***calc., calc-ar.,*** calc-s., ***camph., canth.,*** carb-ac., card-m., ***cench.,*** **CHEL.,** ***chin.,*** chin-a., ***cocc., colch., dig., eup-per., ferr., ferr-i., ferr-m.,*** **GRAPH.,** ***hell., hydr., iod., kali-c.,*** kali-i., ***lach.,*** **LYC.,** ***lycps.,*** mag-c., ***mag-m.,*** **MED.,** ***merc.,*** **MERC-C.,** ***nat-a., nat-m., nat-s., nit-ac., nux-m.,*** petr., ***phos., plb.,*** puls., pyrog., rhus-t., rhod., **SAMB.,** sars., senec., sin-n., stann., ***stront-c., ter.,*** thuj., vesp., ***zinc.***
one only foot - ***kali-c.,*** phos., puls.
evening - ***apis,*** bell., **BRY.,** carb-s., caust., chin-s., cocc., crot-h., ***phos.,*** puls., ***rhus-t.,*** sang., sars., stann., thuj.
amel. - dig., sil.
bed, in - am-c.
walking, while - mang.
exertion, unusual - rhod.
extending to calf - am-c., puls.
hard - ***ars.,*** chin., graph., vip.
hot - ***ars.,*** **BRY.,** chin., ***lyc.,*** puls., rhus-t.
hydrothorax - ***apis,*** merc-sul.
inflamed - calc., carb-an., zinc.
itching - ars., sol-n.
joints - ars., ***calc.,*** hep., lyc., mang., merc., phos., ***rhod.,*** stann., sulph.
left - ***apis,*** com., ***elaps,*** lach., lyc., sang., sil.
left, to right - ***kali-c.***
menses, during - ***calc., graph., lyc., merc.,*** sulph.
before - bar-c., ***lyc.***
morning - ***apis, aur., manc.,*** phyt., sabad., sil.
night - **APIS,** ***carb-v.***
painful - apis, ars., aur., chin., con., ***led., merc.,*** ph-ac., phos., rhus-t., sabad., sars., sil., ***sulph.,*** thuj.
pregnancy - ***merc-c., zinc.***
red - ars., bry., ***carb-v.,*** chin., con., graph., hep., kali-c., merc., mur-ac., nit-ac., ***puls.,*** rhus-t., sil., stann., thuj.
reddish-blue - ars.
rheumatic - ***chel.***
right - lyc., sec., spig., sulph.
shining - alum., **ARS.,** ***sabin., sulph.***
sitting, while - carb-an., lach.
stinging - ***carb-v.,*** lyc., merc., ***phos.,*** **PULS.**
sudden - am-c., arn., cham., verat.
tingling - puls.
tuberculosis - acet-ac., ***stann.***

SWELLING,
walking, while - sil.
after - aesc., ***lach., phos.,*** sep.
air, in open - nit-ac., sulph.
air, in open, after - mang.
warmth of bed - sulph.
washing, after - aesc.
yellowish green - ars.
swelling, back of feet - ars., **BRY.,** calc., carb-an., lyc., ***merc.,*** nux-v., ***puls.,*** rhus-t., staph., ***thuj.***
swelling, heels - ant-c., berb., con., hyper., kali-i., merc., petr., plb., raph.
red - con.
swelling, soles - arund., ***bry., calc.,*** cham., ***chin., coloc.,*** kali-c., **LYC.,** med., ***nat-c., petr., puls.***
evening - petr.
morning - nux-v.
sensation of - ***alum., coloc.,*** zinc.
soft - chin.
stepping - kali-c.
sudden - cham.
swelling, toes - ammc., am-c., ***apis, arn., aur-m.,*** bar-c., ***carb-an., carb-v.,*** chin., coc-c., ***coloc.,*** crot-h., ***daph.,*** **GRAPH.,** hyper., ***led., merc.,*** mur-ac., ***nat-c., nit-ac., paeon., ph-ac., phos.,*** plat., pyrus, ***sabin., sulph.,*** syph., tarent., ***thuj.,*** vip., zinc.
balls of - graph., plat.
evening - am-c.
fifth - phos.
sensation of - mur-ac.
first - ***am-c., apis,*** aster., bar-c., ***benz-ac.,*** bry., chin., coc-c., ***led., mang.,*** med., nat-c., plb., ruta., sabin., sulph., tep.
ball - carb-an.
evening, in bed, agg. - ***am-c.***
gout-like - aster., ***benz-ac.,*** eup-per., plb., ***rhod.,*** sabin.
joints - apis, benz-ac., ph-ac., sang.
left - eup-per.
night - chin.
painful - am-c., bar-c.
right - ***benz-ac.***
joints, of - plb.
night - coc-c.
red - am-c., ***aur-m.,*** carb-v., thuj.
third - crot-c.
tips of - chin., mur-ac., thuj.
sensation of - **APIS.**
wetting feet, after - nit-ac.

SWELLING, sensation of - **APIS,** ars-m., mang., merc., nat-m., ox-ac., phos., sars., sep., til.
swelling, toes, sensation of - **APIS,** sars.

TEARING, pain - ***agar.,*** agn., all-s., alum., ambr., am-c., am-m., ammc., ant-c., ***arg-m.,*** arn., **ARS.,** bar-c., ***bell.,*** berb., ***bism.,*** bor., bov., bry., ***calc.,*** cahin., ***camph.,*** carb-s., carb-v., **CAUST.,** ***cham., chin.,*** chin-a., chin-s., cocc., ***colch., coloc.,*** crot-t., ***dulc., graph.,*** hep., hyper., kali-ar., kali-bi., ***kali-c., kali-n.,*** kali-p., ***kalm.,*** lach., ***lyc., merc., merc-i-r.,*** merl., ***mez.,*** nat-a., ***nat-c., nat-m.,*** nat-p., **NAT-S.,** nit-ac., ol-an., ***phos., puls., rat., rhod.,*** sars., sec., sep., ***sil.,*** spig., spong., ***stann., stront-c., sulph.,*** sul-ac., tep., ***ter.,*** thuj., trom., verat., ***zinc.***
afternoon - kali-bi.
air, open, agg. - ***caust.***
alternating with a paralyzed feeling - hyper.
ball of - hell., kali-n., lyc.
night - plat.
bones - arg-m., carb-v., chin., spig., staph.
chill, after - ***cham.***
covered in bed, in being, agg. - cham.
dinner, after - cahin.
drawing - ars., bov., kali-c., stann., zinc.
evening - graph., lach.
extending to, knee - bar-c., bry.
to, thighs - caust.
to, toes - graph., kali-bi., kali-c.
gouty - graph.
inner side - caust., cina, colch., **KALI-C.**
jerking - chin.
left - ars., nat-m., puls.
menses, during - am-m.
morning - ars., nit-ac.
motion agg. - bar-c., ***cham.***
night - ***ars.,*** hep., ***merc.,*** phos., rhod., ***sulph.***
outer side - ambr., am-m., bism., graph., stann., ***zinc.***
pregnancy, during - phos.
rheumatic - crot-t., ***graph.,*** puls.
right - nit-ac., ***rat.,*** sep., sulph.
rubbing amel. - zinc.
stepping - carb-v.
stitch-like - bry.
storm, during - caust.
touch - ***chin.***
walking, agg. - agn., ***sil.***
amel. - am-m., ***bell.***
wandering - merl.
warmth of bed amel. - ***am-c., caust., cham.***
weather, on change of - vip.
wet, after getting - ***dulc.***
tearing, back of feet - aeth., ang., ***arg-m., arn.,*** ars., berb., bry., ***camph.,*** canth., caust., colch., coloc., ***con.,*** cupr., graph., ign., jatr., kali-bi., kali-c., kali-n., led., lyc., mag-m., merc., merl., mez., nat-c., ***nat-s.,*** plat., plb., ***puls.,*** rat., rheum, sabin., sil., sol-n., spig., sulph., tab., thuj., zinc.
arthritic - sil.
cramp-like - nat-c.
drawing - berb., merl.
evening - con., kali-n., nat-s.
bed, in - con., nat-s.
extending to, buttocks - merc..
to, heels - puls.
to, thighs - ***camph.***
to, toes - kali-c., mag-m., merl.
to, upwards - ***camph.***
forenoon - ars.
lying, while - ars.
motion agg. - ang., plb.
paroxysmal - plb.
periosteum - coloc.
right - rat.
sitting, while - nat-s.

tearing, back of feet
sticking - berb.
touch agg. - sabin.
twitching - cupr., spig., tab.
walking - mag-m., plb.
amel. - zinc.
warmth of bed - plb.

tearing, heels - aeth., am-c., **AM-M.,** anac., ***arg-m., arg-n.,*** arn., ***ars.,*** bapt., berb., bism., calc-caust., caps., carb-an., caust., cina, ***colch.,*** graph., kali-i., kreos., led., ***lyc.,*** merl., mez., mur-ac., nat-s., par., petr., phyt., sep., ***sil.,*** staph., sulph., sul-ac., ***ter.,*** zinc.
afternoon, when standing - nat-s.
bed, in - anac.
cramp-like, when limbs are crossed - ang.
evening, 9 p.m., while spinning - nat-s.
evening, in bed - mag-c., stann.
evening, while sitting - stront.
extending upward - plb., sulph.
morning - petr., sul-ac.
3 a.m. - am-m.
in bed - am-m., anac.
waking, on - petr., sul-ac.
motion, on - dros.
night - am-m.
bed, in - am-m.
paroxysmal - caps.
rubbing amel. - am-m., nat-s.
sitting, while - cina, kali-i., mur-ac.
spinning - mur-ac.
standing, while - berb., kali-i.
stepping, on - berb., sep.
sticking - merl., staph.
sudden - caust.
torn out, as if - stann.
treading agg. - sep.
twitching - am-c., mag-c., merl.
walking, while - berb., dros., nat-s.
amel. - sulph.

tearing, soles - agar., ***alumn.,*** am-c., ammc., ang., ***arg-m., ars.,*** aur., aur-m-n., bell., berb., calc., cic., ***colch.,*** coloc., con., crot-t., cupr., graph., hep., hyos., **KALI-C.,** kali-n., mag-m., ***merc-i-r.,*** merl., mez., mur-ac., nat-c., ***nat-s.,*** olnd., par., phos., plb., psor., puls., sep., sil., ***ter.,*** valer., zinc.
afternoon - kali-n., nux-v.
lying, while - nux-v.
burning - sabin.
constriction - stront.
drawing - colch.
evening - mag-m., sil., sulph.
lasting till 6 p.m. - sil.
extending, above knees - puls., sil.
to back - puls.
forenoon - nat-c.
lightning-like - phel.
menses, during - kali-n.
midnight - sars.
motion, agg. - plb.
amel. - coloc., hyos., psor., sabin.
night - kali-n.
paroxysmal - plb.

tearing, soles
pressure, agg. - plb.
amel. - plb.
rubbing amel. - plb., sulph.
sitting, while - agar., ang., merl., nat-s., phos.
spinning - mur-ac.
sticking - zinc.
sudden - ang., cic.
twitching - cupr., kali-n.
walking, while - agar., bell., berb., con., graph., merl.
warmth of bed - plb.

tearing, toes - ***acon.,*** agar., ***agn.,*** am-c., ***am-m., anac.,*** asaf., ***arg-m.,*** aur., ***benz-ac.,*** berb., bism., bry., calc., camph., carb-an., carb-s., ***carb-v., caust., chin.,*** cic., cocc., ***colch., coloc.,*** con., croc., crot-t., dios., ***graph.,*** hell., indg., jatr., **KALI-C.,** laur., ***led.,*** lyc., mag-m., mag-s., merl., mez., ***nat-c.,*** nat-m., nat-p., nat-s., nicc., ol-an., par., phos., ***plat.,*** plb., psor., ***rat.,*** sep., sil., ***stront-c.,*** sulph., tarent., tep., teucr., thuj., valer., zinc.
balls of - plat.
bed amel. - am-m.
cramp-like - ***anac.***
drawing - carb-an., clem., sulph., zinc.
evening - **AM-M.,** lyc.
6 p.m. - arg-m.
8 p.m. - am-m.
extending upward - anac., stann.
fifth - arn., caust., graph., kali-bi., lyss., mag-c., mag-m., mez., nat-s., sep., thuj., zinc.
evening - zinc.
first - agar., am-c., ***am-m.,*** anac., ***ant-c.,*** arg-m., aur-m., bar-c., ***benz-ac.,*** calc., carb-an., carb-s., caust., cic., cocc., coc-c., con., crot-t., dulc., graph., hep., indg., kali-bi., ***kali-c.,*** kali-i., kali-n., lachn., lyc., mag-c., mag-m., mag-s., merc., merl., mez., mur-ac., nat-c., nat-m., ol-an., par., plat., plb., rat., ruta., sang., sars., ***sil., sulph.,*** tarent., tep., thuj., ***zinc.***
afternoon - am-m.
afternoon, 2 p.m. - ol-an.
ball of - agar., con., caust., dros., petr., ph-ac.
burning - con., rat., ruta.
drawing - agar., kali-bi., mez., sars.
evening - sars., sil.
evening, bed, in - mag-m.
evening, before lying down - mag-s.
extending to, heel - nat-c.
extending to, knee - merc.
forenoon - nat-c.
forenoon, 11 a.m. - sil.
gouty - ant-c., benz-ac.
joint, proximal - con.
left - coc-c., rat.
motion amel. - cocc., dros., plb.
nail - colch., hep., ***thuj.***
nail, under - iod., zinc.
nail, under, left - coloc.
night - kali-i.

tearing, toes
first, paroxysmal - merc.
pressure agg. - ruta.
pulsating - dulc.
rheumatic - crot-t.
right - cic., mag-c., mag-m., mur-ac., sil., ***zinc.***
rubbing amel. - nat-c.
sitting, while - agar., ***am-m.,*** con., mag-m., par.
standing, while - ***am-m.,*** con., nat-m.
sticking - berb., zinc.
spinning - mur-ac.
tendon, extensor - nat-c
tip of - arn., bar-c., bism., caust., **KALI-C.,** sars., zinc.
touch agg. - arg-m.
twitching - am-m., brom.
ulcerative - ol-an., plat.
walking, while - con., hep., mag-m., nat-m.
fourth - carb-v., gamb., mag-c.
gouty - ***benz-ac., graph.***
jerking - chin.
left - ***agn.,*** mag-c., spig.
motion agg. - nat-c., plb.
amel. - anac., cocc., psor.
night - plat., sulph.
amel. - nicc.
paroxysmal - plb.
rheumatic - ***graph.***
rising, after - asaf.
rubbing amel. - laur., nicc., phos.
second - canth., carb-v., dulc., kali-i., lyc., plb., rat.
joints - berb., stront.
right - zinc.
right, pulsating - dulc.
sitting, while - ***am-m.,*** berb., phos.
smarting - merl.
sprained - crot-t.
standing - am-m., anac., stann.
sticking - zinc.
third - ambr., bry., carb-v., lyc., mez., rat.
tips - **AM-M.,** ***camph.***
touch - ***chin.***
twitching - chin.
waking, on - nat-s.
walking, while - ***agn., camph.,*** carb-v., crot-t., mag-c., nat-s., plb.
warmth of bed agg. - plb.

TENSION - agar., ail., ***alum.,*** ambr., ant-t., bell., bor., bry., cann-s., carb-an., ***caust.,*** cham., clem., eupi., kali-c., ***lyc.,*** mag-m., mez., nat-m., petr., ph-ac., phos., plat., puls., rhus-t., sabad., sars., ***seneg., sep.,*** stront-c., ***sulph.,*** thuj., zinc.
afternoon - nat-m.
burning - alum.
dinner, after - ***sulph.***
evening - ***bry.,*** plat., thuj.
morning - sars., ***sulph.***
hearty breakfast, after - puls.
motion, on - thuj.
amel. - mag-m.
moving toes - ***sulph.***

TENSION,
night - agar.
noon - ambr.
outer side - ***zinc.***
sitting, while - **BRY.,** mag-m., plat., **RHUS-T.**
stepping, on - **BRY.,** thuj.
tendons, after walking - sulph.
walking, on - ail., ant-t., bell., clem., petr., ph-ac., thuj.
pavement agg. - sep.

tension, back of feet - alum., ant-t., bor., ***bry.,*** carb-an., caust., lyc., mag-m., nat-c., sec., sep., thuj.

tension, heels - berb., ***caust.,*** led., nicc., phos., thuj.
morning, in bed - phos.
rising, after long sitting - thuj.
standing - berb.
sticking, agg. putting foot down after rising from bed - nicc.
walking, while - berb., led., thuj.

tension, soles - ***alum.,*** bell., berb., ***caust.,*** hyper., lyc., plat., rhus-t., sil., spig., sulph., ***zinc.***
afternoon - lyc.
evening - zinc.
forenoon - alum.
near the heel - bell.
noon - sulph.
walking, while - sulph.
pressure amel. - bell.
sitting, while - lyc.
stepping, when - berb., bry., ***caust.,*** spig., sulph., zinc.
stooping - plat.

tension, toes - mez., nat-s., ph-ac., phos., plat., prun., sars., sulph., thuj.
first - plat., sulph.
morning - sars.
motion, on - sulph., thuj.
stepping - thuj.
walking, while - ph-ac., sulph.

THICK, soles, skin of - **ARS.**

THRILLING, sensation - bapt.
thrilling, toes, first - benz-ac.

TINGLING, prickling, asleep - **ACON.,** ail., all-s., ***alum.,*** ambr., ammc., am-c., am-m., arn., ars., arum-d., bapt., bar-c., berb., ***calc.,*** calc-p., ***carb-s.,*** caust., chel., **COCC.,** ***colch., coloc.,*** con., croc., dig., dulc., euph., ham., hell., hyos., hyper., ***kali-c.,*** lachn., lyc., mag-m., manc., merc-i-f., mez., naja, nat-c., nat-m., ***nit-ac.,*** onos., ***ph-ac., phos., puls.,*** ran-s., ***rhod., sec., sep.,*** sil., stann., stry., sulph., sul-ac., sumb., thuj., zing.
alternating with hands - **COCC.**
eating, after - kali-c.
evening, in bed - carb-an.
extending upwards - **ACON.**
heat agg. - lachn.
left - crot-h., grat.
lying in bed, while - carb-an., ***hyper.***

TINGLING, prickling, asleep
morning - calc-p.
bed, in - nat-c.
night - am-m., mag-m., phos.
painful - mag-m.
right - alum., carb-an.
rising after sitting - ***puls.***
sitting - euph., grat., nat-c.
standing, while - naja, ***puls., sec.***
walking, while - ant-c., berb., ***sec.***
amel. - am-c., ***puls.***
tingling, back of feet - am-c., chin., ran-s.
tingling, heels - alum., am-c., caust., ferr-ma., ***nux-m.,*** rhod.
evening, in bed - nit-ac.
sitting, while - alum., con.
tingling, soles - am-c., alum., arg-n., ars., bell., ***berb.,*** bry., cahin., **CAUST.,** cic., ***cocc.,*** coloc., cub., ferr., ***hep.,*** lyc., nat-c., ***nux-m., nux-v., olnd., rhus-t.,*** ruta., ***sec.,*** sep., ***sil.,*** staph., stry., zing.
evening - rhus-t., zing.
in one spot - ol-an.
rising, from bed, when - lyc.
rising, from sitting - ***puls.***
scratching, after - sil.
sitting, while - arg-n., cic., **COCC.,** staph., zing.
voluptuous - ***sil.***
walking, while - berb., bry., ***olnd., rhus-t., sec.,*** zing.
tingling, toes - ail., ars., arum-d., berb., cic., ***colch.,*** con., hell., ***hep., lach.,*** merc., merc-i-f., ***nux-m.,*** sabad., sec., stry., verat., vip.
first - berb., buf-s., camph., carb-ac., chin., cic., nat-c., ran-s.
tips - mez.
fourth, outer side of - onos.
nails, under - elaps
second - crot-t.
tips - acon-c., **AM-M.,** ***nat-m.***

TREMBLING - am-c., apis, ars., ***bar-c.,*** bell., bor., bov., calc., camph., canth., carb-s., chin-s., coff., coloc., crot-t., ***cupr.,*** cycl., ***hyos.,*** ip., kali-c., kali-n., kali-s., lyc., mag-c., mag-m., **MERC.,** mur-ac., nat-c., ***nat-m.,*** nicc., nux-m., ol-an., op., ox-ac., ***plat., psor.,*** **PULS.,** sars., sec., ***stram., sulph.,*** sumb., ***tab., thuj.,*** verat., zinc.
ball of - mur-ac.
chill, during - canth.
convulsive - hyos., kali-cy.
descending stairs - thuj.
dinner, after - mag-m.
evening, in bed - canth., nat-m.
standing - nux-v.
falling asleep - croc.
forenoon - nat-m., sars.
11 a.m., on rising from bed - nat-m.
fright, as from - coloc.
left - puls.
menses, during - ***hyos.,*** zinc.
as from - coloc.
if menses doesn't come - puls.

TREMBLING,
morning - ars., nat-m.
rising, on - con., crot-t., merc-c.
motion, during - ***camph.,*** puls.
amel. - mag-m.
music, from - thuj.
raising it - zinc.
sitting, while - mag-m., plat., zinc.
amel. - ol-an.
standing, on - ***bar-c.,*** ol-an.
suppression of menses, with - ***puls.***
vomiting - sulph.
walking, while - merc., par., puls.
air, in open, amel. - bor.
trembling, back, of - kali-c.

TUBERCLES - carb-an., rhus-t.

TUMORS, toes, endochondroma - sil.

TWITCHING - ***alum.,*** arg-m., arn., asaf., bar-c., bar-m., canth., carb-an., carb-s., cedr., chel., cimic., cina, crot-t., cupr., dulc., ***graph.,*** **HYOS.,** iod., ***ip.,*** laur., led., mag-c., merc., mur-ac., ***nat-c.,*** nat-s., nux-v., petr., phos., ruta., sant., ***sep.,*** sil., **STRAM.,** stry., sulph., ***thuj.,*** verat.
afternoon, during sleep - ruta., sep.
bed, in - arg-m., cimic., nat-c.
bending them - led.
crawling - thuj.
daytime - sulph.
evening - alum., arg-m., sulph.
sleep, on going to - carb-an.
lying on, back, while - nux-v.
painless side, amel. - nux-v.
midnight - nat-c.
after, during sleep - nat-s.
morning, rising, after - mag-c.
night - canth., lyc., mag-c., nat-s.
sitting, while - crot-t., sulph.
sleep, during - hyos., nat-s., sulph.
on going to - carb-an.
standing, while - sulph., verat.
sticking - nux-v.
stitches in tibia, from - arg-m.
upward - mag-c., thuj.
twitching, back, of - sars.
twitching, heels - all-c., am-c., eupi., kalm., lith., mag-c., mag-m., nat-c.
twitching, soles - crot-t., cupr., graph., plat., sul-ac., sulph., thuj.
motion amel. - sulph.
sitting - jatr., plat.
twitching, toes - acon., agar., anac., calc-p., cic., ***cimic., cupr.,*** hyper., jatr., ***merc.,*** merl., nat-c., ph-ac., phos., stram.
drawing - cic.
evening - merc.
first - agar., am-c., anac., ars., asaf., calc., calc-p., carl., ferr-ma., hell., mez., nat-c., par., phos., puls., ran-s., tep.
afternoon - nat-c.
ball of - am-c.
evening - calc.
evening, bed, in - calc.
evening, sitting - par.

twitching, toes
first, intermittent - anac.
morning - ars., mez.
morning, bed, in - ars., mez.
shooting - tep.
sitting, while - par., phos.
sticking - hell.
tearing - ars., puls.
walking, while - carl.
night - hyper.
on going to sleep - hyper.
second - ir-foe.
third - sul-ac.
tips - ***am-m.,*** thuj.
evening - ***am-m.***
touching big toe - ph-ac.
visible - merc.

ULCERS - ***anan.,*** **ARS.,** bar-c., canth., carb-s., caust., cham., clem., ***carb-ac., con.,*** crot-h., ***fl-ac., graph.,*** ip., ***kali-bi.,*** kali-c., lyc., merc., nat-c., nit-ac., petr., ***phos., psor., puls.,*** sel., sep., sil., sol-n., ***sulph.,*** sul-ac., vip., ***zinc.***
bleeding - ***ars.***
blisters, from - **SULPH.,** zinc.
ulcers, back of feet - ***psor., sep., sulph.***
ulcers, heels - am-c., anac., aran., ***ars., caust.,*** laur., ***nat-c., sep.,*** **SIL.**
bloody, pus with - ars.
blister, spreading from a - ***caust., nat-c., sep.***
left - aran.
shoe, rubbing of the, from - all-c., bor.
ulcers, soles - anan., ***ars.,*** calc., caust., lach., phyt., pip-m., ruta., sec., **SEP.,** sulph.
blisters, from - **ARS.**
ulcers, toes - ***ars., bry.,*** carb-v., caust., cupr-ar., ***graph., nit-ac., petr.,*** plat., ***sep., sil., sulph.,*** thuj.
blisters, originating in - ars., ***graph., petr.***
boring - caust.
burning - caust.
fifth - ant-t.
first - ***paeon., sil.***
border of - graph.
gangrenous - ***lach.***
joint of - ***ars., bor.,*** nat-c., ***sep.***
phagedenic - ***bor.***
leprous - ***graph.***
tips - ant-t., ***carb-v.***

UNCOVER, inclination to - agar., **CHAM.,** ***cur.,*** fl-ac., ***mag-c.,*** **MED.,** ***petr.,*** **PULS.,** ***sang., sanic.,*** sep., **SULPH.**
toward morning - cur.

UNSTEADINESS - agar., camph., merc., sumb.

URTICARIA - ***calc.,*** sulph.

VARICOSE, feet - ant-t., ***ferr.,*** lac-c., lach., **PULS.,** sulph., sul-ac., ***thuj.***

VESICLES - ***ars.,*** aster., carb-o., ***caust., con.,*** elaps, ***graph.,*** lach., ***manc.,*** nit-ac., ***phos.,*** rhus-v., ***sec.,*** sel., sep., sulph., tarax., vip., vinc.
back - aster., bov., carb-o., lach., zinc.
black - **ARS.,** nat-m.

VESICLES,
phagedenic - ***con., sel., sulph., zinc.***
rubbing, from - caust.
suppurating - ***con., graph., nat-c., sil.***
watery - rhus-v.
white - ***cycl., graph., lach.,*** sulph.
vesicles, back of feet - aster., bov., carb-o., lach., zinc.
itching - aster.
ulcerative - zinc.
vesicles, soles - ***ars.,*** bell., ***bufo, calc.,*** kali-bi., ***kali-c., manc.,*** nat-m., sulph.
bloody serum - nat-m.
corroding, eating - ***ars.,*** sulph.
fetid water, with - ***ars.***
spreading - **ARS.,** ***calc.***
ulcerating - **ARS.,** ***calc.,*** psor., sulph.
yellow fluid, with - ***ars., bufo.***
vesicles, toes - ***caust.,*** cupr., graph., ***lach., nat-c.,*** nit-ac., ***petr.,*** ph-ac., rhus-v., ***sel., sulph.,*** zinc.
between - hell., sil.
walking, from - sil.
spreading - graph., ***nit-ac.***
watery - rhus-v.
white - graph.

VIBRATION, sensation, soles - olnd.

WALKS, on outer side of foot - cic.

WARTS, toes - ant-c., spig., ***thuj.***

WATER, sensation as if, cold feet had been put in hot water - raph.
cold water were poured on them - verat.
dipped into cold water - carb-v.
sole - merc.

WEAKNESS, feet - agar., ambr., am-c., **ARS.,** bell., bor., ***bov., calc.,*** canth., carb-ac., carb-o., carb-s., ***cham., chin.,*** chin-s., chlf., clem., coca, coff., colch., croc., crot-t., cycl., eup-pur., ferr., gamb., gels., gins., glon., graph., grat., ***hell.,*** hyos., ign., indg., ip., ***lach.,*** lath., laur., ***lyc.,*** mag-c., mag-s., merc., ***mez.,*** nat-a., nat-c., ***nat-m.,*** nicc., nit-ac., nux-v., ***ol-an., olnd.,*** petr., phel., ***phos.,*** phys., ***plat.,*** plb., ***puls.,*** ran-s., ***rhus-t.,*** ruta., sabad., sars., sec., seneg., ***sil.,*** stann., stram., stront-c., ***sulph.,*** sumb., ***tab.,*** tep., thuj., verat., xan., zinc.
afternoon - alum., bov., hydr-ac., lith., lyc., nux-v.
4 p.m. - **LYC.**
5 p.m. - cham.
walking, while - lyc.
ascending stairs - acon., bor., bry., lyc., mag-c., nux-v.
bending, on - led.
chilliness, during - hell.
dinner, after - mag-m.
eating, after - cahin., ferr., nat-c.,
evening - agar., ign., merc-c., pic-ac., puls.
7 p.m. - ant-c.
walking, after - coc-c.
walking, while - mag-m.
fever, after - nat-s.
forenoon - seneg.

WEAKNESS, feet
headache, during - ol-an.
lying amel. - mag-c., ***nat-m.***
menses, during - ant-t., cast., ***graph.,*** mang., ol-an., zinc.
morning - caust., lyc., mag-m.
4 a.m. - plb.
bed, in - zinc.
rising, on - nat-m.
walking, while - lyc., mag-c., mag-m.
night - ***carb-an.,*** cham., mag-s., nit-ac.
menses, before - mang.
noon - kali-bi.
paralytic - cham., nat-m., olnd., tab.
raise, trying to - merc.
riding, while, amel. - ***nat-m.***
sex, after - calc-p.
sitting - anac., coc-c., ***led.,*** plat., ***rhus-t.,*** thuj.
amel. - ***nat-m.***
standing, while - kali-n., ***nat-m.,*** sars.
trembling - caps.
walk, begining to - mag-m.
waking, on - nat-m.
walking, while - camph., chin., clem., croc., ***graph.,*** ham., kali-n., par.
air, in open - agar., arn., olnd., thuj.
amel. - laur., nat-m., zinc.

weakness, soles - cahin., carb-s., croc., kreos., led., nux-v., olnd., plb., sumb., tep., thuj.
dinner, after - carb-s.
sitting, while - plb., thuj.
walking, while - nux-v., olnd., thuj.

weakness, toes - ars., crot-h., glon.

WET, getting, agg. - agn., ***all-c.,*** cham., ***dulc.,*** merc., nat-c., nat-m., ***nux-m., phos.,*** **PULS.,** ***rhus-t., sep.,*** **SIL.,** xan.

WOODEN, sensation - carl.

wooden, sensation, soles - ars.

WRINKLED - ars.

Female

GENITALIA, female, affections of - acon., agar., agn., am-m., ambr., ang., ant-t., apis, arn., ars., asaf., **BELL.**, berb., bor., ***bry.***, calad., **CALC.**, camph., canth., **CAPS.**, **CAUL.**, ***caust.***, **CHAM.**, ***chin.***, cic., ***cimic.***, clem., **COCC.**, coff., **CON.**, **CROC.**, cupr., dig., erig., euph., ferr., fl-ac., gels., graph., hell., ***helon.***, ***hyos.***, **IGN.**, iod., ip., kali-c., ***lac-c.***, ***lach.***, laur., led., mag-c., mag-m., mang., merc., merc-br., ***mosch.***, mur-ac., nat-c., ***nat-m.***, nit-ac., ***nux-m.***, nux-v., op., perh., phos., **PLAT.**, plb., **PULS.**, rheum, ***rhus-t.***, sabad., sabal., **SABIN.**, ***sec.***, ***sel.***, seneg., **SEP.**, sil., spig., spong., stram., sul-ac., sulph., thuj., ***valer.***, verat., vib., viol-o.
alternating between both sides - ***cimic.***, coloc., **LAC-C.**, lycps., ol-an., onos., rhod.
left - ***lac-c.***, ***lach.***, naja, ***puls.***, rhod., ***thuj.***
right - apis, calc., caust., ***clem.***, hep., ***lyc.***, merc., nux-v., pall., spong., sul-ac., verat.

ABSCESS, genitalia - ***hep.***, kali-p., ***merc.***, nit-ac., ***sep.***, ***sulph.***
abscess, ovaries - bell., chin., ***crot-h.***, ***hep.***, ***lach.***, ***merc.***, ph-ac., plat., psor., pyrog., ***sil.***
left - ***lach.***
menses, during - merc.
abscess, vagina, vulva, labia - ***apis***, ***bell.***, bor., ***hep.***, iod., kreos., lach., ***merc.***, ***puls.***, rhus-t., ***sep.***, ***sil.***, sulph.

ABORTION, spontaneous, (see Pregnancy, chapter, Miscarriage)

ACHING, pain, genitalia - calc-p., ***lil-t.***
aching, pain, ovaries - apis, brom., con., iod., ***kreos.***, lac-ac., lil-t., med., onos., pic-ac., podo., sep., sulph., syph.
left - brom., med., pic-ac., podo., syph.
right - ***lac-ac.***, ***pall.***
walking, rapidly - apis, lac-ac.
aching, uterus - bell., ***calc-p.***, ***con.***, ferr., lach., merc., senec., sep., ust.
morning - ***calc-p.***
sex, during - merc-c.
aching, vagina - **CALC.**, calc-p., elaps.
menses, during - calc.
before - elaps.
nosebleed, after - calc-p.

ANESTHESIA, vagina, during sex (see Insensitivity) - phos.

ANTEVERSION, of uterus - graph., lil-t., nux-v., phos.

APHTHAE, genitalia - agar., ***bor.***, ***carb-v.***, ***helon.***, iod., ***kreos.***, ***merc.***, sulph., ***sul-ac.***, thuj.
aphthae, vagina - alumn., ***arg-n.***, carb-v., ***caul.***, ***graph.***, ***helon.***, ***hydr.***, ign., kreos., lyc., lyss., merc., nat-m., ***nit-ac.***, rhus-t., rob., ***sep.***, thuj.
vulva - helon.

ASCARIDES, genitalia - ferr., ***sil.***, ***sulph.***

ATONY, of uterus - abies-c., alet., aloe, alst., alum., ambr., bell-p., ***carb-v.***, **CAUL.**, ***chin.***, cimic., ***ferr.***, ferr-i., goss., **HELON.**, kali-c., lapa., ***lil-t.***, plb., psor., **PULS.**, rhus-a., ***sabin.***, ***sec.***, ***senec.***, **SEP.**, sulph., ***tril.***, ***ust.***
causing delayed menses - ***thlaspi.***
childbirth, during - am-m., caul., op., plb., puls., sec.
metrorrhagia, in - ***carb-v.***

ATROPHY, ovaries - apis, ***bar-m.***, ***carb-s.***, ***con.***, helon., **IOD.**, orch., ov., plb.

BALL, ovaries, feels like a heavy, in right - carb-an.
ball, uterus, in, sensation of a - ust.
hot, ascending to throat - raph.
ball, vagina, in, sensation like cotton - pulx.

BARTHOLINITIS, genitalia - hep., lach., merc., morg., nit-ac., sep., ***sil.***, tarent-c., thuj.

BEARING down, pain, genitalia and uterus - **AGAR.**, alet., aloe, alum., ***ant-c.***, ***ant-t.***, ***apis***, arg-m., asaf., asc-t., aur., aur-m-n., **BELL.**, bor., bov., bry., ***calc.***, calc-p., canth., ***carb-an.***, **CHAM.**, ***chin.***, ***cimic.***, cocc., ***con.***, cop., croc., cur., der., elaps, ***ferr.***, ***ferr-i.***, frax., ***graph.***, helon., ign., inul., ***iod.***, ip., kali-c., ***kali-fer.***, kali-s., ***kreos.***, ***lac-c.***, **LIL-T.**, lob., lyc., lyss., mag-c., mag-m., ***mang.***, ***merc.***, mosch., **MURX.**, mur-ac., ***nat-c.***, **NAT-H.**, **NAT-M.**, ***nit-ac.***, ***nux-v.***, onos., ***pall.***, **PLAT.**, ***podo.***, ***puls.***, rhus-t., **SABIN.**, **SEC.**, **SEP.**, ***sil.***, **STANN.**, ***sulph.***, tarent., thuj., til., ust., xan., zinc.
afternoon - mag-m., **SEP.**
ascending, steps - ***plat.***
bleeding, with uterine - mag-c.
colds agg. - hyos.
come out, as if everything would - **BELL.**, ***con.***, **KREOS.**, ***lac-c.***, **LIL-T.**, ***nat-c.***, **NAT-H.**, ***nat-m.***, ***nit-ac.***, ***plat.***, ***podo.***, **SEP.**
pregnancy, during - ***kali-c.***
stool, during - ***podo.***
stool, before - ***nat-c.***
crossing, limbs amel. - **LIL-T.**, murx., **SEP.**, zinc.
drinking, after - nux-v.
eating, amel. - sep.
forenoon - sep.
labor, after, colicky, amel. by gush of blood - cycl.
lifting, after - ***agar.***
lying, agg. - ***puls.***
amel. - ***agar.***, cimic., onos., pall., ***sep.***
on left side amel. - pall.
menopause, after - agar.
menses, during - acon., ***agar.***, alet., aloe, am-c., am-m., ant-c., arg-n., ***asaf.***, ***aur.***, **BELL.**, berb., bor., bov., calc., ***calc-p.***, calc-s., caul., caust., ***cham.***, ***chin.***, chin-s., ***cimic.***, cina, ***con.***, ***ferr.***, ***gels.***, graph., hyos., ign., ***kali-c.***, kali-i., ***kali-p.***, kreos., ***lach.***, **LIL-T.**, lob., mag-c., med., mosch., murx., ***nat-c.***, ***nat-m.***, ***nit-ac.***, nux-m., nux-v., pall., ***plat.***, ***podo.***, **PULS.**, rhus-t., ***sec.***, **SEP.**, ***sulph.***, thuj., ***vib.***, xan., zinc.

BEARING down, pain, genitalia and uterus
menses, after - ***agar., con.***, pall., tarent.
before - alum., ***apis***, aur., ***bell.***, bov., ***calc-p., chin.***, chin-s., ***cina, con.***, croc., elaps, ***kali-c.***, mosch., nux-m., ***phos., plat.***, rhus-t., sabad., sec., ***sep.***, sul-ac., tarent., ust., ***vib.***, zinc.
metrorrhagia, with - mag-c.
midnight, after - ***bov.***
morning - **BELL., NAT-M.**, ***nux-v.***, **SEP.**
night, in bed - **SULPH.**
noise aggr - cimic.
nursing of child, while - ust.
perspiration, with hot - til.
pregnancy, during - ***kali-c.***
come out, as if everything would, during - ***kali-c.***
pressing on vulva amel. - ***bell.***, **LIL-T., MURX.**, sanic., **SEP.**
pressure amel. - mag-c.
riding, in a carriage agg. - ***asaf.***
rubbing, amel. - pall.
for itching, after - con.
sitting, bent, agg. - ***bell.***
erect amel. - ***bell.***
she feels as if pushing something up, while - ***ferr-i.***
standing, agg. - ***con.***, dict., ***murx.***, nat-m., ***pall.***, rheum, rhus-t., **SEP.**
amel. - ***bell.***
stool, during - arg-n., ***bell.***, iod., ***lil-t., podo., stann.***
before - nat-c., nit-ac.
urging, with - ***con., corn.***, **NUX-V.**, plat.
stooping, amel. - mag-c.
when - ***lyc.***
supports, abdomen with hands - ***bell., lil-t., murx., sep.***
urging, to urinate, on - nux-v., ***pall.***, **SEP.**
walking, agg. - ***bell., chin.***, coff., ***con.***, kreos., ***lil-t.***, **NAT-H.**, phos., ***plat., rhus-t.***, **SEP.**
in open air amel. - ***puls.***

bearing down, ovaries - ***apis***, canth., ferr-i., ham., lac-d., ***lach., lil-t.***, mag-m., med., plat., ***podo.***
left - lac-d., ***lach.***
right - **APIS.**
standing, while - **LIL-T.**
walking, while - ***lil-t.***, med.

BITING, pain, genitalia - berb., calc., ***caust.***, eupi., graph., kali-c., ***kali-i.***, kali-n., **KREOS.**, ***merc., rhus-t., sil.***, staph., sulph., thuj., zinc.
menses, during - ***rhus-t.***, zinc.
urination, during - ***caust.***, hep., nat-m., thuj.

biting, vagina - cham., ***graph.***, thuj.
between labia - **KREOS.**

BLEEDING, uterus, metrorrhagia - abrot., ***acet-ac., acon.***, agar., ***agn.***, alet., alumn., am-br., am-m., ***ambr.***, ant-c., ***apis, apoc.***, aran., arg-m., ***arg-n.***, arg-o., ***arn., ars., ars-i.***, asar., asc-t., aur., aur-m-n., aur-m-k., aza., bapt., **BELL.**, bell-p., bor., **BOTH.**, ***bov., bry.***, bufo, ***cact.***, **CALC.**, calc-ac., calc-ar., calc-f., calc-i., calc-s., cann-i., ***canth.***, caps., ***carb-an., carb-s., carb-v., card-m., caul., cean., cham.***, **CHIN.**, chin-a., ***chin-s., cimic.***, cina, ***cinnam.***, cit-v., cob-n., ***coc-c., cocc., coff.***, coff-t., ***colch.***, coll., ***coloc.***, cop., **CROC.**, crot-c., **CROT-H.**, cupr., cycl., dict., dig., ***elaps***, erech., ***erig.***, eupi., **FERR.**, ***ferr-ac.***, ferr-ar., ***ferr-i., ferr-m., ferr-p., ferr-s.***, fic., fl-ac., fuli., gall-ac., gels., **HAM.**, ***helon., hep.***, hydr., hydrin-s., ***hyos., ign., iod.***, **IP.**, iris, joan., juni., kali-ar., ***kali-br., kali-c., kali-chl.***, **KALI-FER.**, ***kali-m., kali-n.***, kali-p., kali-s., ***kreos., lac-c.***, **LACH.**, laur., ***led.***, lil-t., ***lyc.***, lycps., mag-aust., mag-c., mag-m., mag-s., mangi., ***med., meli., merc.***, **MILL.**, mit., **MURX.**, nat-a., ***nat-c.***, nat-m., **NIT-AC.**, ***nux-m.***, **NUX-V.**, ***oci-s.***, op., petr., **PHOS.**, ***phyt.***, **PLAT.**, plb., podo., **PSOR.**, prun., **PULS.**, pyrog., **RAT.**, ***rhus-a., rhus-t.***, rob., rosm., ruta, **SABIN.**, samb., ***sang.***, **SEC.**, ***senec., sep., sil.***, squil., staph., ***stram.***, sul-ac., sul-i., ***sulph., tarent.***, tep., ter., ***thlaspi***, thiop., **TRIL.**, ***tub.***, urt-u., **UST.**, verat., **VIB.**, ***vinc., visc.***, x-ray, ***xan.***, yohim, zinc., zinc-s.

acrid - ***sul-ac.***, sulph.

active - ***acon.***, apis, arn., **BELL.**, calc., cham., chin., ***cinnam., coff.***, **CROC.**, ferr., ***ham.***, hyos., ign., **IP.**, mill., **PHOS.**, plat., **SABIN.**, **SEC.**, thlaspi, tril., ***ust.***

alternating, with dyspnea - fl-ac.
mania, with - ***crot-c.***
vagina discharge, with - oci-s., tarent.

anemia, with - calen., ***chin., ferr.***, ferr-m., ferr-p., helon., ***hydr.***, kali-c., kali-fer., **PULS.**, ***thlaspi.***

anger, after - **CHAM.**, kali-c., rhus-t., staph.

atony, from uterine - ***carb-v., chin., ham.***, psor., visc.
malarial - chin.

backache, with, amel. by pressure and sitting - kali-c.

between, the menstrual periods - ***ambr., arn., bell., bov.***, bry., **CALC.**, canth., carb-v., **CHAM.**, chin., ***cimic., cocc.***, coff., ***croc.***, elaps, ferr., ***ham.***, hep., **IP.**, kali-c., lach., lyc., mag-c., mag-s., mang., merc., murx., nit-ac., nux-v., **PHOS.**, puls., **RHUS-T.**, **SABIN.**, ***sec., sep.***, **SIL.**, stram., sulph., zinc.

black - alet., am-c., arn., asar., bell., ***carb-v.***, caul., ***cham.***, chin., coff., **CROC.**, ***elaps, ferr., helon.***, ign., ***kreos.***, lach., lyc., mag-c., nat-m., **PLAT.**, ***puls.***, sabin., ***sec.***, stram., sulph., ***sul-ac.***
liquid - ***am-c., crot-h., elaps, sec., sul-ac.***

breast-feeding, the child, when - calc., phos., rhus-t., ***sil.***

BLEEDING, uterus

bright, red - acal., acon., aran., ***arn.,*** **BELL.,** bov., ***calc.,*** cham., chin., ***cinnam.,*** **ERIG.,** ferr-p., ***ham.,*** hyos., **IP.,** lac-c., ***led.,*** lyc., med., ***mill.,*** mit., **PHOS.,** psor., rhus-t., **SABIN.,** ***sang.,*** sec., ***tril.,*** ust., vib., visc., xan.

clots, with - ***arn.,*** **BELL.,** ***ip.,*** lac-c., **SABIN.,** ***ust.***

copious - ***erig.***

fluid - ham., ust.

painless, and, after labor - mill.

gushing from least motion - acal., ***bell.,*** bov., cham., erig., ***ip.,*** med., ***mill.,*** mit., ***phos., sec., tril.,*** ust., visc.

hot, profuse after labor, collapsing symptoms, with - ip.

profuse after labor, gushes - bell.

miscarriage, after - hyos.

profuse - acal., bell., bov., cham., erig., ***ip.,*** med., mill., mit., ***phos., sec., tril.,*** ust., visc.

cachectic females, in - sec.

cancerous affections, in - kreos., med., phos., thlaspi, ust.

cervix, bleeding easily - ***aln.,*** alum., arg-n., dict., ***hydr.,*** hydrc., ***kali-bi., ust.***

chamomile, tea, from - ***chin.,*** ign.

changeable in color and flow - **PULS.**

chronic - ***card-m., ust.***

coagulated - acal., ***alet., alum., apoc.,*** arg-m., ***arn.,*** **BELL.,** ***cact.,*** **CHAM.,** chin., cocc., coc-c., ***coff., croc.,*** cycl., elaps, erig., ***ferr.,*** ham., helon., ip., kali-c., kreos., lach., laur., lyc., ***merc., murx.,*** nux-v., phos., ***plat.,*** plb., ***puls., rhus-t., sabin., sang.,*** sec., stram., ***thlaspi,*** tril., **UST.,** visc.

coagula escape when quit or during urination - ***coc-c.***

night - coch.

paroxysms - cham., ***ferr., puls., ust.***

confinement after - phos.

expelled in paroxysms - ***ferr., puls., ust.***

mixed with, dark liquid blood - **BELL.,** carb-v., elaps, ***sabin., sec.***

pale watery blood - chin., ferr.

coldness of body, with - ***camph.,*** **CARB-V.,** ***sil., verat.***

comes, suddenly and ceases suddenly - ***bell.***

continuous - apoc., arn., carb-v., caul., ***erig., ham., hydr., hyos.,*** iod., ***ip.,*** kali-c., ***kreos.,*** mill., ***nit-ac.,*** **PHOS.,** ***sec.,*** sulph., ust., vinc.

but slow - carb-v., ham., psor., sec., sulph., ust.

convulsions, with - ***bell., chin., hyos.,*** **SEC.**

curettage, from - calen., nit-ac.

daytime, only - caust.

dark, blood - ars., ***bell., bry., cact.,*** canth., carb-v., ***cham.,*** **CHIN.,** coff., ***croc., crot-h., elaps, ferr., ham.,*** helon., ***kreos.,*** lach., laur., lyc., lyss., mangi., ***nux-m., plat.,*** plb., ***puls.,*** sabin., ***sec.,*** sep., ***sulph.,*** sul-ac., tril., ust.

BLEEDING, uterus

dark, clots, mixed with - **BELL.,** ***cham.,*** chin., ***croc., ferr.,*** kreos., lyc., ***puls., sabin., sec.,*** ust.

daily a little dark blood - lyss.

fluid - bry., crot-t., plat., sabin., sec.

fluid, and thick - nux-m., ***plat.***

thick, paroxysmal flow, debility, after labor - chin.

displaced, uterus, from - trill.

elderly, women, in - ***calc.,*** cham., hydr., ***ign.,*** lach., ***mag-m., mang., merc.,*** phos., sep.

emotions, excitement, etc. - acon., bell., bry., ***calc., cham.,*** cocc., croc., ***helon.,*** hyos., nat-m., ***phos.,*** plat., puls., sep., ***sil.,*** stram., sulph.

exertion, after - **AMBR.,** ***aur., bov.,*** **CALC.,** ***croc.,*** **ERIG.,** mill., ***nit-ac.,*** rhus-t., ***sabin., tril.***

fainting, with - apis, ***chin.,*** ferr., ferr-p., ***ip., kreos.,*** **TRIL.**

fibroids, from - ***calc.,*** calc-f., calc-p., ***ham., hydr., kali-i.,*** lap-a., led., lyc., merc., nit-ac., **PHOS.,** ***plat., sabin.,*** sec., sil., stip., ***sulph.,*** sul-ac., ***thlaspi., tril.,*** **UST.,** ***vinc.***

fluid - ***apis,*** apoc., ars., ***both., carb-v.,*** chin., **CROT-H.,** ***elaps, erig.,*** ferr., **LACH.,** ***mill.,*** nat-m., **NIT-AC., PHOS.,** prun., **SABIN.,** ***sec., sul-ac., ust.***

alternating with clots - ***plb.***

clotted, or, paroxysmal or continual flow, nausea, vomiting, palpitation, pulse quick, feeble when moved, vital depression, fainting on raising head from pillow - apoc.

partly - puls., ***ust.***

menses, between - ham.

fright, after - acon., bell., ***calc.,*** nux-v.

girls, little - ***cina, hydr.,*** xan.

gushing - acal., ***bell.,*** bov., ***cham.,*** chin., ***cinnam., croc., erig., ham.,*** **IP.,** ***lac-c.,*** med., ***mill.,*** mit., **PHOS.,** ***puls.,*** **SABIN.,** ***sec.,*** tril., ***ust.,*** visc.

hard, stool, from passing - **AMBR.,** ***lyc.***

headache, with congestive - bell., glon., lach.

hot blood - **BELL.,** bry., cham., coff., ***hydr., lac-c.,*** puls.

infertile, women - ***arg-n.***

injuries - ***ambr., arn., bell-p., cinnam.,*** ham., ***mill.,*** ruta, ***sec.***

concussions, from - ***arn., bell-p.,*** cinnam., ***mill.,*** phos., puls., ***rhus-t.,*** ruta., ***sec.,*** sulph.

intermittent, flow - ambr., apoc., ***bell., cham.,*** chin., erig., ***ip., kreos.,*** nux-v., **PHOS.,** ***psor., puls.,*** rhus-t., ***sabin.,*** sec., sulph., ust.

iron, after abuse of - ferr., ferr-p., puls.

BLEEDING, uterus

labor, during and after - ***acet-ac.,*** acon., adren., alet., alum., am-m., aml-n., apis, ***arn.,*** ars., ***bell.,*** bry., ***cann-i.,*** cann-s., carb-v., caul., ***cham., chin., cinnam.,*** cocc., coff., ***croc.,*** crot-h., cycl., **ERIG.,** ***ferr., gels.,*** ger., **HAM.,** ***hydr., hyos., ign.,*** **IP.,** kali-c., kalm., kreos., lach., lyc., merc., ***mill.,*** nit-ac., nux-m., nux-v., op., ph-ac., ***phos., plat.,*** plb., puls., ***rhus-t.,*** **SABIN., SEC.,** senec., sep., ***thlaspi,*** tril., ***ust.***

8 days after - ***sabin.***

bright red - bell., ***hyos., ip.,*** mill., phos., ***ust.***

fluid and painless - mill.

clotted - phos., sabin., tril.

constant - ***ip.,*** **NUX-M.,** ***sabal., ust.***

dark - bell., caul., chin., ***gels., ip., sabin.,*** sec., tril., ***ust.***

fluid - sec.

hot - bell., ip.

profuse, collapsic symptoms, with - ip.

profuse, gushes - bell.

inertia uteri, with - am-m., caul., puls., sec., ***ust.***

motion agg., slightest - **CROC.,** sec.

offensive - ***nit-ac., ust.***

putrid - ***ust.***

one week after - ***kali-c.***

paroxysmal flow - chin.

prevents hemorrhage - ***arn.***

profuse - **APIS,** bell., ***ip., plat., sabin.,*** tril.

some days after - **CINNAM.**

thick - chin.

two weeks after - ***ust.***

lying on back agg. - ***cham.***

amel. - ***ip.***

menopausal period, during - ***alet., aloe,*** am-m., aml-n., apoc., arg-m., ***arg-n.,*** aur-m., ***bell.,*** buni-o., **CALC.,** caps., ***carb-v.,*** chin., ***cimic., croc., ferr., gels.,*** **GRAPH.,** hydrin-s., kali-br., kali-c., **LACH.,** ***laur.,*** lyc., ***med., murx.,*** nit-ac., ***nux-v.,*** phos., ***plb., psor., puls., sabin.,*** **SANG.,** sanguiso., sarr., ***sec., sed-ac.,*** **SEP.,** sul-ac., **SULPH.,** ***thlaspi, tril.,*** **UST.,** vinc., zinc-valer.

after - **ARG-N.,** ***arn., ars.,*** calc., ferr., ***hydr.,*** **KREOS.,** mang., ***merc., sep., tarent., vinc.***

before - arg-m., staph.

menses, between - **AMBR.,** arg-n., ***arn., bell., bov.,*** bry., **CALC.,** canth., carb-v., caust., **CHAM.,** chin., ***cimic., cocc.,*** coff., ***croc.,*** elaps, ferr., flav., foll., guare., ***ham.,*** hep., hydr., iod., **IP.,** kali-c., kali-sil., kreos., lach., lap-a., lup., mag-c., mag-s., mang., merc., murx., nat-hchls., nit-ac., nux-v., op., **PHOS.,** puls., **RHUS-T.,** rob., **SABIN.,** ***sec., sep.,*** **SIL.,** stram., sulph., ust., vinc., visc., zinc.

sexual excitement, with - ***sulph.***

after - lyc., merc., rat.

before - calc., mag-m., merc., sil.

return of long suppressed menses, after - ***sulph.***

BLEEDING, uterus

miscarriage, during - anac., ***apis,*** arn., bry., caul., cham., ***chin.,*** **CROC.,** ***erig.,*** hyos., ***ip.,*** **KALI-C.,** ***lyc.,*** mill., ***nit-ac.,*** **PLAT.,** ruta, **SABIN.,** ***sec., sil., thlaspi,*** **VIB.**

after - alet., ***bell.,*** caul., ***cham., chin.,*** croc., ***ferr.,*** hyos., ***ip.,*** kali-c., ***lyc., mill., plat.,*** psor., ***sabin., thlaspi, ust.***

night, 3 a.m. agg. - ***nux-v.***

before - ***lyc.***

excitement, mental or sexual - sil.

threatening miscarriage, in - ***calc.,*** cimic., ***croc.,*** erig., goss., ***ham.,*** **IP., KREOS.,** ***lyc.,*** **PHOS.,** ***puls.,*** ruta, ***sabin.,*** sec., ***tril., ust.***

moon, at full - ***croc.,*** kali-bi.

full and new moon, at - ***croc.,*** kali-bi.

3 days before, at - mang-m.

new moon, at - rhus-t., sil.

motion, agg. - acal., ambr., arg-n., bell., bov., ***bry.,*** cact., calc., cham., ***coff., croc.,*** **ERIG.,** ***helon.,*** **IP.,** lil-t., med., ***mill.,*** mit., phos., psor., ***sabin., sec.,*** sulph., tril., ust., visc.

walking amel. - ***sabin.***

night, agg. - alet., ***mag-m.,*** nat-m., ***rhus-t.,*** sabin.

night-watching, after - ***puls.***

offensive - ***bell., cham.,*** croc., crot-h., ***helon., kreos.,*** lach., ***nit-ac.,*** phos., sabin., ***sec., ust.***

pungent - kreos.

putrid - **ARS.,** carb-v., cham.

painless - bov., calc., carb-an., chin., croc., ***ham.,*** **KALI-FER.,** mag-c., mangi., ***mill.,*** nit-ac., nux-m., plat., sabin., ***sec.,*** ust.

pale, blood - bell., carb-v., chin., ***ferr.,*** hyos., merc., mill., prun., sabin., sec., tarent., ust.

pale, and waxy women, in - acet-ac., kali-c.

paroxysms, in - apoc., bell., ***cham.,*** chin., nux-v., **PULS.,** rhus-t., **SABIN.,** ust.

paroxysms, in, bright red, joint pains - sabin.

thin, light blood, firm coagula, severe labor-like pains - cham.

passive - alet., carb-s., **CARB-V.,** caul., ***chin., chin-s.,*** cimic., cinnam., croc., **ERIG.,** ***ferr., helon.,*** ham., **KALI-FER.,** ***kreos., lyc.,*** plb., ***sec.,*** sul-ac., thlaspi, **TRIL., UST.,** vinc.

persisting - caul., cinnam., nit-ac., thlaspi.

perspiration, with cold - **CARB-V.,** ***sec., verat.***

placenta, preavia, from - ***ip., nux-v., sabin., sep., verat-v.***

retained placenta, from - ***bell., canth., carb-v.,*** caul., ***ip., kali-c.,*** mit., ***puls., sabin.,*** sec., sep., stram.

plethoric, women, in - **ACON.,** arn., ***bell.,*** bry., calc., **CHAM.,** coff., ***croc., erig., ferr.,*** ferr-m., hyos., ign., ***plat., sabin.,*** sil., sulph.

polyps, from - bell., ***calc., con.,*** lyc., phos., ***sabin.,*** sang., thuj.

BLEEDING, uterus
pregnancy, during - ***apis,*** bell., ***cann-i.,*** caul., ***cham.,*** chin., cimic., ***cinnam., cocc.,*** croc., ***erig.,*** ham., **IP.,** kali-c., **KREOS.,** ***nit-ac.,*** **PHOS.,** ***plat., puls., rhus-t., sabin.,*** sec., ***sep., tril.***
fifth and seventh month - **SEP.**
first part, in - nit-ac.
fright, after - ***ign.***
lying amel. - ***ign.***
overexertion, from - arn., ***cinnam., erig., nit-ac.***
sixth month - ***cann-i.,*** erig.
third month - **KREOS.,** sabin.
profuse - acal., acon., alet., am-m., ambr., apis, apoc., arg-n., ***arn., ars.,*** **BELL.,** bov., brom., bry., ***cact.,*** **CALC.,** caul., ***cham., chin.,*** cinnam., ***con.,*** croc., erig., ferr., glon., ham., helon., hyos., iod., **IP.,** kali-c., ***kreos.,*** lyc., mangi., med., mill., mit., murx., nit-ac., ***nux-v.,*** **PHOS.,** plat., plb., puls., **SABIN.,** ***sec., sul-ac.,*** thlaspi, tril., ust., vib., vinc., visc., xan.
puberty, at - helon.
before - ***cina.***
recurrent - ***arg-n., croc., kreos., nux-v., phos.,*** psor., ***sulph.***
riding, from - ***ham.***
rising from, bed - psor.
ropy blood - arg-n., **CROC.,** lac-c., **UST.**
scanty - carb-v., coc-c., lyss., phos.
sleep, during - ***mag-m.***
scrawny, women, in - ***sec.***
sex, during - arg-n.
after - **ARG-N.,** ***arn., ars., hydr.,*** **KREOS.,** nit-ac., ***sep., tarent.***
coitus interruptus, from - ***cocc.***
standing, while - ***mag-m.***
stool, during - ambr., murx.
after every - **AMBR.,** am-m., ind., ***lyc.***
hard stool, from passing - **AMBR.,** ***lyc.***
straining, from - podo.
stringy, blood - arg-n., **CROC.,** lac-c., **UST.**
subinvolution - ***kali-i.,*** lil-t., psor., sec., sulph., ust.
sudden - ***ars.,*** **BELL.,** cinnam., ***ip.***
swelling of glands, with - carb-an.
tall, women - ***phos.***
tarry - plat.
thick, blood - carb-v., ***nux-m.,*** plat., puls., sec., sulph., tril.
thin, fluid - apoc., bry., carb-an., ***carb-v.,*** chin., ***crot-h., elaps, erig.,*** ferr., kreos., **LACH.,** laur., lyc., ***phos.,*** plat., prun., puls., **SABIN.,** ***sec., sul-ac.,*** ust.
mixed with clots - ***chin., elaps, ferr.,*** kreos., ***sabin., sec.***
foul smelling - kreos., ***sec.***
touch agg. - ust.
urination, during - coch.
painful, during - erig., mit.
uterus, from displaced - tril.

BLEEDING, uterus
vagina discharge, with - ***calc.,*** kreos.
after - ***mag-m.***
vexation, after - ***ip.,*** kali-c.
voluptuous itching, with - ***coff.***
walking, after - ambr.
agg. - **AMBR.,** ***mag-m.,*** nat-s., sep.
amel. - ***sabin.***
warm, bath, after - thuj.
watery - ant-t., berb., bov., ***calc.,*** dulc., laur., mang., phos., prun., puls.
instead of menses - ***sil.***
weakly, women - asaf., ***carb-an.,*** **CHIN.,** cocc., croc., ferr., ***ip.,*** nux-v., phos., psor., ***puls.,*** sec., sep., sulph., verat.
widows, in young - kali-c.

BLOTCHES, genitalia - staph.

BORING, pain, ovaries - brom., ***coloc.,*** lach., **LYC.,** sumb., thuj., **ZINC.**
bending up amel. - ***coloc.***
left - brom., sumb., thuj., **ZINC.**
menses, during - thuj.
menses, amel. - zinc.
menses, during, amel. - lach., zinc.
pressure amel. - zinc.
right - **LYC.**
boring, uterus - merc.

BURNING, pain, genitalia - acon., agar., alum., ***ambr., am-c.,*** anan., ***ars.,*** aur., ***aur-m.,*** bar-c., ***bell.,*** berb., bov., bry., bufo, ***calc.,*** calc-ar., calc-p., calc-s., ***canth., carb-an., carb-s., carb-v.,*** cast., ***caust.,*** cham., chel., coc-c., con., cop., cur., dulc., ***eupi., ferr.,*** ferr-ar., ferr-p., ***graph., helon.,*** hep., kali-ar., ***kali-bi., kali-c., kali-i.,*** kali-p., kali-s., ***kreos.,*** lac-c., lach., lap-a., ***lil-t.,*** lyc., mag-s., ***merc., merc-c.,*** murx., **NIT-AC.,** ***nux-v.,*** ox-ac., pall., ***petr., phos., puls., sabin.,*** sec., sep., ***sil.,*** staph., ***sulph., ter.,*** thuj., til., xan., zinc.
bleeding, with - petr.
hemorrhage, with - petr.
lying, amel. - berb.
menses, during - ***am-c., carb-v.,*** kali-br., ***kali-c., kreos., sil.,*** thuj.
before - calc., carb-v., ***sep.***
motion, agg. - ars.
night, in bed - anan.
sitting, while - berb., sep.
touch, on - thuj.
urinating, while - ***ambr.,*** calc., ***caust., eupi.,*** **KREOS.,** ***lac-c.,*** nat-m., plat., sulph.
after - ***caust.,*** **KREOS.,** ***lac-c.,*** merc., ruta.
walking, agg. - berb., thuj.
burning, ovaries - abrot., anan., **APIS, ARS.,** ***bell., bufo, canth.,*** carb-an., coloc., con., ***eupi., fago.,*** goss., ***kali-i.,*** kali-n., ***lac-c.,*** **LACH.,** ***lil-t.,*** lyc., med., merc., nat-m., ***plat., sep., thuj.,*** tub., ***ust.,*** zinc., zinc-valer.
left - abrot., ***lach.,*** med., thuj.
motion, on, before menses - croc., ***thuj.,*** ust.

burning, ovaries
menses, during - bufo, canth.
after - zinc.
miscarriage, during - **APIS.**
moving feet, amel. - **ARS.**
paroxysmal - ***plat.***
riding, while - thuj.
right - ***apis, bell.,*** coloc., kali-n., ust.
sex, after - **APIS,** thuj.
urinating, when - nat-m.
walking, while - thuj.

burning, uterus - anan., ***arg-n., ars., bell., bry.,*** bufo, ***calc-p.,*** carb-an., ***carb-v., con.,*** cur., ***hep., kreos.,*** lac-c., ***lach.,*** lap-a., ***lyc., nux-v.,*** pip-n., ran-b., raph., rhod., ***sec.,*** sep., sul-ac., tarent., ter., thuj., xan.
alternating with pain in limbs - rhod.
cervix - con., ***kreos.,*** sep.
chilbirth, after - rhod.
extending, kidneys, to - anan.
pit of stomach, to - ***raph.***
thighs, to - carb-an.
fibroids, with - lap-a.
menses, during - ars., bry., ***calc-p.,*** canth., carb-v., caust., merc., nat-m., nux-v., ph-ac., phos., rhus-t., sep., sulph., tarent.
after - canth., ***kreos.***
before - bufo, carb-an., con., cur., ***nat-m.***

burning, vagina - ***acon.,*** all-s., alum., antipyrin., aur., aur-m., ***bell.,*** **BERB.,** bov., bufo, calc., ***calc-p., canth.,*** carb-an., carb-v., card-m., ***cham., chel.,*** cop., ferr-p., ***graph.,*** helon., ***hydrc., kali-bi.,*** kali-br., kali-c., kali-p., ***kreos.,*** lyc., lyss., ***merc., merc-c., nat-m.,*** **NIT-AC.,** ***petr.,*** pop-c., ***puls.,*** pulx., sabin., ***sep.,*** spira., **SULPH.,** tarent., ***thuj.***
extending to chest - calc-p.
hour, every day at same - ***chel.***
introitus - hyos.
labia - acon., am-c., aur., bov., ***canth.,*** carb-v., ***graph.,*** helon., ***kreos.,*** lyc., ***merc.,*** puls., ***rhus-t.,*** sep., sil., ***sulph.,*** thuj.
menses, before - calc.
lying on left side agg. - merc.
menses, during - all-s., berb., ***graph.,*** nux-v., sulph.
after - berb., graph., kreos., lyc., ***sulph.***
before - bufo, ***ign.,*** nat-m., ***sulph.***
pregnancy, during - bor.
sex, during - kali-bi., ***kreos., lyc.,*** nat-m., spira., ***sulph.***
after - ***kreos.,*** lyc., lyss.
sitting, while - ***thuj.***
urinating, after - nat-m.
walking, while - ***thuj.***

BURSTING, pain, ovaries - graph., med.
bursting, uterus, as if something had burst - elaps.

CANCER, genitalia - ***arg-m., ars., ars-i., aur-m-n.,*** bell., bov., calc-ar., calc-o-t., calc-s., ***calth., carb-an.,*** carc., cham., chin., ***con., graph., hydr.,*** iod., irid., ***kali-bi.,*** kali-p., kali-s., ***kreos.,*** lach., ***lap-a.,*** mag-p., med., murx., ***phos.,*** phyt., rhus-t., ***sec.,*** sep., ***sil.,*** staph., sulph., tarent., thlaspi, ***thuj.,*** tril., zinc.
bleeding, with - bell., crot-h., kreos., lach., sabin., ***thlaspi,*** ust.
cancer, cervix - carb-an., carc., **CON.,** iod., kreos., thuj.
cancer, ovaries - ars., **CON.,** graph., kreos., ***lach.,*** med., psor., thuj.
cancer, uterus - alum., alumn., anan., apis, ***arg-m., arg-n.,*** **ARS., ARS-I.,** aur., aur-m-n., bell., bov., brom., ***bufo, calc.,*** carb-ac., ***carb-an.,*** carb-s., ***carb-v., carc.,*** chin., cic., clem., **CON.,** ***crot-h.,*** cund., elaps, fuli., **GRAPH., HYDR.,** ***iod.,*** kali-ar., kaol., **KREOS., LACH.,** ***lap-a.,*** **LYC.,** mag-m., med., merc., ***merc-i-f.,*** **MURX.,** ***nat-c., nat-m., nit-ac.,*** **PHOS.,** ***phyt.,*** plat., rhus-t., ruta, sabin., sang., sars., ***sec.,*** **SEP., SIL.,** ***staph.,*** sul-ac., sulph., tarent., **THUJ.,** ***zinc.***
scirrhus - ***alumn.,*** anan., ***arg-m., ars.,*** aur., aur-m-n., **CON.,** kreos., lyc., mag-m., phos., ***phyt.,*** rhus-t., sep., staph.
cancer, vagina - ***ars.,*** con., **KREOS.**
labia, vulva, cancerous - ***ars.,*** con., thuj.

CANDIDA albicans, infection - calc., calc-p., chin., helon., lyc., med., nat-p., nit-ac., puls., sep., ***thuj.***
vagina discharge, with - calc., calc-p., helon., ***med.,*** nat-p., nit-ac., puls., sep., thuj.

CERVICITIS, inflammation of cervix - alum., ant-t., arg-n., ***ars., bell.,*** calen., hydr., kali-bi., kreos., lyc., med., merc., ***merc-c., nit-ac.,*** sep., ***thuj.***
bleeding easily - ***aln.,*** alum., arg-n., dict., ***hydr.,*** hydrc., ***kali-bi., ust.***
excoriation, with - alum., arg-m., arg-n, hydr., kali-bi., kreos., merc., nat-p., ***nit-ac.,*** phyt., sul-ac., thuj.

CHEESY, deposits, genitalia - ***helon.***
cheesy deposits, vulva - ***helon.***

CHILDBIRTH, general, (see Pregnancy, chapter)

CHLAMYDIAL, infection - med., sulph., thuj.

CLUTCHING, and relaxing sensation of uterus - sep.

COLDNESS, genitalia - berb., plat., sabal.
menses, during - plat.
coldness, ovaries, sensation of, left - ferr-i.
coldness, uterus - petr.
coldness, vagina - bor-ac., ***graph., nat-m.,*** sec.
icy - bor-ac.

CONCEPTION, easy - ***bor.,*** canth., merc., nat-c., nat-m.
false conception - caul.

CONDYLOMATA, genitalia (see Excrescences) - aur-m., ***calc.,*** cinnb., euphr., ***lyc.,*** med., ***merc.,*** **NAT-S., NIT-AC.,** ***sabin., sars., staph.,*** syph., **THUJ.**
- cauliflower, like - **NIT-AC.,** thuj.
- dry - ***lyc.***
- itching - euphr., ***lyc., sabin.***
- pediculated - ***lyc.***
- soft, red and fleshy - **NAT-S.**

condylomata, cervix - ***calc., calen.,*** cub., graph., ***kreos., merc., nit-ac.,*** sec., tarent., **THUJ.**

condylomata, vagina - ***nit-ac., phos., staph.,*** tarent., **THUJ.**
- bleed easily - ***phos.***
- labia - aur-m., med., ***thuj.***

CONGESTION, genitalia - acon., alet., ***aloe,*** ambr., aur., ***bell.,*** bell-p., bry., ***caul., chin.,*** cimic., ***coll., croc.,*** fl-ac., ***frax.,*** gamb., gels., ***hep.,*** iod., kali-c., lac-c., lach., ***lil-t.,*** mag-p., ***merc.,*** mit., murx., nux-v., ***phos.,*** plat., puls., sabal., sabin., sec., ***sep.,*** stroph., sulph., tarent., ust., ***verat-v.***
- chronic or passive - aesc., ***aur.,*** calc., cimic., ***coll., helon.,*** lach., ***polym., sep.,*** stann., sulph., ***ust.***

congestion, ovaries - ***acon.,*** aesc., alet., aloe, am-br., **APIS,** arg-n., ***bell., bry.,*** canth., ***cimic.,*** colch., con., ***gels., ham., hep., iod., kali-i.,*** lac-c., lach., ***lil-t.,*** meli., ***merc.,*** naja, ***nat-ch.,*** pall., plat., polyg., puls., rhus-t., sabin., sec., ***sep.,*** staph., sulph., ***syph.,*** tarent., ***thuj., vib.,*** ust., ***zinc.***
- continence, from - apis, graph.
- menses, before - lac-c.
  - suppressed - ***apis.***
- motion agg. - lac-c.

congestion, uterus - aloe, anan., arg-n., **BELL.,** caul., cham., ***chin.,*** ferr., ***gels., hep., lac-c.,*** **LACH.,** ***nat-c., nux-v.,*** **PULS.,** ***sec.,*** senec., **SEP.,** sulph., ter., vib.
- bleeding, after - ***chin.***
- menses, during - acon., alet., **BELL.,** caul., cham., ***chin.,*** **LACH.,** nux-v., **PULS.,** sec., senec., ***sep.***
  - before - ***chin.,*** **LACH.**
  - suppressed, with - sabal.
- sensation of - ***caul.***

CONSCIOUS, of the uterus - **HELON.,** ***lyss.,*** med., ***murx.,*** vib.
- jars, very tender to - ***helon.,*** lyc., lyss., ***med,*** murx.

CONSTRICTING, pain, genitalia - ***bell-p., cact.,*** cham., chin., ***gels., mag-p.,*** nux-v., polyg., ***sep.,*** thuj., ust.

constricting, ovaries - ***cact.,*** puls.

constricting, uterus - **BELL.,** ***cact.,*** chin-s., cocc., lil-t., lyc., plb., ***puls.,*** sabin., sep., staph., tarent.
- extending upwards - cact.
- menses, during - ***agar., bell.,*** **CACT.,** staph.

constricting, vagina - **CACT.,** ***plat., puls.***

CONSTRICTION, ovaries - ***cact.***

constriction, uterus - bell., cact., cham., ***gels.,*** ign., kali-i., murx., mygal., nux-v., plat., sec., sep., tarent.
- band, like a - cact., sec.

constriction, vagina - **CACT.,** kreos., plat., ***puls.***
- sex, during - **CACT.**
- touch, from - **CACT.**

CONTRACTIONS, genitalia - ***lac-c.,*** thuj.

contractions, cervix os, spasmodic, during labor - acon., aml-n., **BELL.,** cact., **CAUL., CIMIC.,** con., **GELS.,** hyos., lach., lyc., sec., vib., xan.

contractions, uterus - ***bell.,*** cact., ***calc-p.,*** chin-s., cimic., cocc., ign., lac-c., murx., nat-m., nux-v., ***puls.,*** sabin., sep., staph., thuj.
- hour-glass - **BELL.,** ***cham., cocc.,*** con., cupr., hyos., ***kali-c.,*** nux-v., ***plat.,*** puls., rhus-t., ***sec., sep.,*** sulph.
- menses, before - caul., cimic., cur.
- menses, during - ***bell.,*** **CACT.,** ***puls., staph.***

contractions, vagina - aur-m-n., ***cact.,*** ham., ***kreos., sep.***
- rising from sitting - kreos.
- spasmodic during vagina discharge - aur-m-n.

CONTUSION, ovaries (see Injuries)

COWPERITIS, inflammation of cowper's glands - acon., cann-s., fab., gels., hep., merc-c., petros., sabal., sil.

CRACKS, genitalia - carb-v., graph., ***nit-ac.,*** urt-u.

CRAMPING, pain, genitalia - con., staph., thuj.
- extending to abdomen - thuj.
- rising from a seat - thuj.

cramping, ovaries - ***bufo,*** cocc., ***coloc.,*** cub., ***naja,*** phos., plat.
- left - ***coloc., naja.***
- menses, during - ***cocc.***

cramping, uterus - agar., aloe, anan., ***bell.,*** bry., bufo, ***cact., calad., calc-p.,*** **CAUL.,** caust., **CHAM.,** chin., ***cocc., con.,*** cop., ***gels., hyos., ign.,*** kali-c., lyc., ***mag-m.,*** **MAG-P.,** nat-m., **NUX-V.,** onos., ***plat., puls.,*** rob., **SABIN.,** ***sep., tarent.,*** **UST.,** ***vib.***
- anger, after - **CHAM.**
- broad ligaments - **CIMIC.,** gels.
- cold damp weather - ***calc-p.***
- double up, compelling her to - ***cact.,*** **COLOC.,** ***cimic.,*** **NUX-V.**
- extending, down thighs - ***kali-i., mag-m.***
  - to stomach - ***cact.***
  - up the back - gels.
- humiliation, from - ***cocc.***
- menses, during (see Dysmenorrhea) - acon., ***bell.,*** **CACT.,** ***calc-p.,*** caul., ***caust.,*** **CHAM.,** ***cimic.,*** **COCC.,** ***coff.,*** **COLOC.,** ***con.,*** der., **GRAPH.,** ***ign., ip., kali-c.,*** kali-i., ***lach.,*** **MAG-P.,** ***nit-ac.,*** **NUX-V.,** onos., ***plat., puls.,*** sec., sep., stann., ***tub.***
  - after - ***cocc.,*** iod., plat., puls.

cramping, uterus
menses, before - **CALC-P.,** ***caust.,*** **CHAM.,** ***mag-p., vib.***
should appear but do not, when - ***cocc., kali-c.***
midnight, after - ***calad.***
motion, from - **COCC.**
night, 11 p.m. - ***cact.***
nursing - cham.
pregnancy, during - ***cupr-ar.***
reaching up - ***rhus-t.***
stool, after - lyc.
touching parts agg. - ***ign.***
vagina discharge, followed by - ***con., mag-m.***
walking, while - tarent.
warmth amel. - caust., nux-m., nux-v.

CUTTING, pain, genitalia - asaf., bor., cann-s., carb-v., caust., con., ip.
left to right - ip.
motion, on - caust., ip.
urinating, when - con.
walking, while - caust.

cutting, fallopian tubes, along - polyg.

cutting, ovaries - absin., acon., ***apis, arg-n.,*** arum-t., atro., ***bell., bor., bry.,*** canth., caps., cocc., coll., ***coloc., con.,*** croc., cub., eup-pur., graph., ham., ***lil-t., lyc.,*** merc., naja, nat-m., nux-m., onos., puls., ***sabad.,*** stram., syph., ***thuj.,*** ust., xan.
extending down thighs - ***apis,*** arg-n., bry., ***cimic.,*** croc., lil-t., phos., podo., wye., ***xan.,*** zinc-valer.
right - xan.
left - graph., phos., puls., ***thuj.,*** ust.
then right - apis.
menses, during - ***apis, bor.,*** cocc., ***lyc., phos.***
right - ***apis, arg-n.,*** xan.
right to left - ***lyc.***
sex, during - syph.
stretching in bed - apis
urinating, when - nat-m.

cutting, uterus - asaf., bufo, ***calc., calc-p.,*** **COCC.,** con., crot-c., cur., ign., ***lac-c., murx.,*** pall., **PULS.,** sep., tarent., thuj.
breath, every - **COCC.**
extending, to sacrum - **CALC-P.**
upwards - lac-c.
menses, during - apis, ***asaf.,*** bell., ***calc.,*** canth., carb-v., ***caust.,*** **COCC.,** ***coloc.,*** ferr., ign., ***kali-c.,*** kreos., lach., merc., murx., nat-c., nat-m., phos., rhus-t., sec., sep., sil., zinc.
before - caust., mag-c., murx., nat-c.
motion, during - **COCC.**
sex, during - **PULS.**
stool, after, amel. - pall.
washing in cold water - crot-c.

cutting, vagina - sil.
sex, during - ***berb., ferr-m.***
urination agg. - sil.

CYSTS, genitalia - ***sabin., sil., thuj.***

cysts, ovarian - **APIS,** apoc., arn., ars., aur., ***aur-i.,*** aur-m-n., bell., ***bov.,*** bry., ***bufo,*** canth., carb-an., chin., ***colch., coloc.,*** con., ferr-i., form., graph., ***iod., kali-br.,*** kali-fer., ***lach.,*** lil-t., ***lyc.,*** med., merc., murx., ***ov., plat.,*** prun., rhod., ***rhus-t.,*** sabin., sep., syc-co., syph., ter., **THUJ.,** zinc.
left - apis, coloc., ***kali-bi.,*** **LACH.,** ***podo.,*** **THUJ.**
right - **APIS,** fl-ac., ***iod.,*** **LYC.,** ***podo.***

cysts, vagina - ***lyc., puls., rhod.,*** **SIL.,** teucr., **THUJ.**
serous - rhod.

DIGGING, pain, genitalia - con.

digging, uterus - bufo, cur.
menses, during - ***nux-v.***

DIPTHTERIA, exudations, genitalia - apis, ***kali-bi., lac-c.,*** merc-cy., sep.

DISCHARGE, vagina, (see Vaginitis) - ***aesc.,*** agar., ***agn., alet.,*** **ALUM.,** alumn., ***ambr., am-c., am-m.,*** anac., ant-c., ***ant-t.,*** apis, ***arg-n.,*** **ARS., ARS-I.,** asaf., aur., ***aur-m., aur-m-n.,*** bad., ***bar-c., bar-m.,*** bell., bell-p., berb., ***bor., bov.,*** bry., **CALC.,** ***calc-f., calc-p.,*** **CALC-S.,** cann-s., ***canth.,*** caps., **CARB-AN., CARB-S.,** ***carb-v.,*** card-m., ***caul.,*** **CAUST.,** cedr., cham., chel., ***chin.,*** chin-a., ***cimic., cinnb., cocc.,*** coff., ***con.,*** crot-c., cub., cur., cycl., dig., dros., dulc., ***eupi., ferr.,*** ferr-ar., ferr-p., ***frax.,*** **GELS., GRAPH.,** guai., ham., ***helon., hep.,*** hura, ***hydr.,*** **IOD.,** ***ip.,*** iris, **KALI-AR.,** ***kali-bi.,*** **KALI-C.,** ***kali-chl., kali-i.,*** kali-m., ***kali-p., kali-s.,*** **KREOS.,** ***lac-ac., lac-c.,*** lac-d., ***lach.,*** laur., ***lil-t., lyc.,*** mag-c., ***mag-m.,*** mag-s., mang., **MED., MERC.,** ***merc-c.,*** merc-i-f., merc-i-r., meli., mez., murx., **MUR-AC.,** naja, ***nat-a., nat-c.,*** nat-h., **NAT-M., NAT-P.,** nat-s., **NIT-AC.,** ***nux-m.,*** nux-v., ***op., orig., pall.,*** penic., ***petr., ph-ac., phos., phys., phyt.,*** pic-ac., **PLAT.,** plb., ***podo.,*** prun., ***psor.,*** pulx., **PULS.,** ran-b., rat., rhus-t., ruta., ***sabin.,*** sanic., sang., sarr., ***sars.,*** sec., senec., seneg., **SEP., SIL.,** squil., **STANN.,** stront-c., **SULPH.,** ***sul-ac.,*** syph., ***tarent.,*** thlaspi, **THUJ.,** ***thymol.,*** til., tril., ***tub.,*** ust., vib., viol-t., ***xan., zinc.***

acids, foods, after - ***nat-p.,*** sil.

acrid, excoriating - aesc., ***agar.,*** **ALUM.,** alum-p., alumn., ***am-c.,*** am-m., amor-r., anac., ange-s., ant-c., apis, aral., ***arg-m., arg-n.,*** **ARS.,** ***ars-i., ars-s-f.,*** aur., aur-i., ***aur-m.,*** aur-m-n., bapt., bar-s., ***bell-p.,*** berb., **BOR.,** ***bov., calc.,*** calc-ar., calc-i., ***calc-s.,*** calc-sil., cann-s., canth., carb-ac., ***carb-an.,*** **CARB-S.,** ***carb-v.,*** **CAUL.,** ***caust.,*** **CHAM.,** ***chel., chin.,*** chin-a., ***clem., con.,*** cop., cub., ***dig.,*** eucal., **FERR., FERR-AR.,** ferr-br., ***ferr-i., ferr-p.,*** **FL-AC., GRAPH.,** ***hed., hep.,*** helon., hydr., ign., ***iod.,*** kali-ar., kali-bi., ***kali-c.,*** hyper., kali-chl., ***kali-i., kali-m., kali-p.,*** kali-s., ***kali-sil.,*** **KREOS.,** ***lac-c., lach., lam.,*** laur., ***lil-t., lob.,*** **LYC.,** ***mag-c.,*** mag-m., mag-s., med., **MERC.,** ***merc-c.,*** merc-i-f., mez., ***murx., myric., nat-m., nat-p.,*** nat-s.,

DISCHARGE, vagina

acrid, excoriating - **NIT-AC.,** nux-m., ***onos., petr.,*** ph-ac., **PHOS.,** phyt., ***polyg.,*** prun., ***psor.,*** **PULS.,** ran-b., rhus-t., rob., ruta., ***sabin.,*** sang., ***sec.,*** **SEP., SIL.,** ***sulph., sul-ac.,*** sul-i., ***syph.,*** thlaspi, thuj., ***tub.,*** urt-u.,vib., zinc., zinc-p., ziz.
- at first acrid, not afterwards - ***ferr.***
  - at first mild, acrid afterwards - ***ran-b.***
- childbirth, after - ***nat-s.***
- children, in - cub.
- dinner, after - ***cham.***
- eats holes in linen - ***iod.***
- food, after acid - **SIL.**
- menopause, during - sang.
- menorrhagia, in chronic - ***iod.***
- menses, during - lach., ***phos.,*** sep.
  - menses, after - **GRAPH.,** kreos., ***lach.,*** mag-c., mez., ***nit-ac.,*** ruta, ziz.
  - menses, before - **GRAPH.,** lach., ***sep., sil., ust.***
  - menses, suppressed, after - ruta
- night, agg. - ***syph.***
- thighs and linen - iod.

afternoon - alum., calc-p., lil-t., mag-c., naja.

albuminous - aesc., agn., ***alum.,*** am-c., ***am-m., ambr.,*** arist-cl., aur., bell., berb., **BOR.,** ***bov.,*** but-ac., calc., ***calc-p.,*** carb-v., elaps, ferr-i., graph., haem., **HYDR.,** inul., iod., kali-m., ***kali-s.,*** kreos., lil-t., mag-c., med., ***mez.,*** **NAT-M.,** pall., ***petr., plat., podo., puls., senec.,*** **SEP.,** ***stann.,*** stram., ***sul-ac., thuj.,*** til., ust.
- hot - ***bor.***
- menses agg, before - ust.
- pregnancy, during - petr.
- walking agg. - aesc.

alternating, with bloody discharge - ambr., oci-s., tarent.
- cough - ***iod.***
- mental states - hydr., murx.
- nasal catarrh - kali-c.
- uterine bleeding, with - ambr.

amber-colored - nat-p., sep.

amenorrhea, in - ***graph.***

anemia, with - **CALC.,** ***cycl.,*** **FERR.,** ***graph., helon., hep., ph-ac., phos., sil.***

atony, from - ***alet., caul.,*** cimic., ***helon.,*** sec., sep., tril., ust.

black - ***chin.,*** croc., kreos., ***rhus-t., sec.,*** thlaspi.

bland - allox., ***alum., am-m.,*** bor., ***brom.,*** calc., calc-p., carb-v., ***caul.,*** cycl., eupi., fago., ferr., ***frax.,*** kali-c., kali-chl., kali-fer., ***kali-m., kali-s.,*** kreos., laur., lil-t., ***merc.,*** nat-m., nux-v., penic., ph-ac., plat., **PULS.,** puls-n, ran-b., ruta, sep., sil., stann., staph., ***sulph., thuj.,*** ziz.
- menses, before and after - ***puls.***
- morning - phyt.
- painless - ***am-m., nux-v.,*** **PULS.**
- rest, agg. - fago.
- urination, before - ***kreos.***

blistering - am-c., canth., kreos., med., ***phos.***

bloody - acon., agar., aloe, ***alum.,*** alum-p., alum-sil., am-m., ***ant-t., arg-m., arg-n.,*** arist-cl., ***ars., ars-i., ars-s-f., bar-c.,*** bar-i., ***bell.,*** bufo, calc., calc-ar., calc-i., **CALC-S.,** calc-sil., canth., carb-s., ***carb-v.,*** caust., **CHIN.,** chin-a., chin-s., ***chlor.,*** chr-ac., cinnb., **COCC.,** coff., ***con.,*** cop., crot-h., dict., foll., graph., ham., hep., hydroph., ***iod.,*** kali-i., ***kreos., lac-c., lach., lyc.,*** mag-m., ***merc., merc-c.,*** murx., **NIT-AC.,** nux-m., petr., ph-ac., ***phos.,*** phys., podo., prot., raph., rob., sabin., **SEP.,** ***sil., spira., sul-ac.,*** sul-i., tarent., ***ter., thlaspi,*** thymol., ***tril.,*** zinc., zinc-p.
- elderly women, in - arist-cl., ***phos.***
- forenoon - sep.
- menses, after - ars., canth., caust., ***chin., lac-c.,*** pyrog., sil., ***tarent., zinc.***
  - appear, with sensation as if menses would - ***sul-ac.***
  - before - aran-ix.
  - instead of - chin.
- morning - kreos.
- night - raph.
- nursing, during - sil.
- pregnancy, during - erig., kali-c., ***nux-m.,*** phos., rhus-t., sep.
- stool, during - murx., ***vib.***
- water - calc., kreos., mang., nit-ac.
- weakness, with - tril.

bluish - ambr.

breasts, sore, with - dulc.

briny - sanic.

brown - aesc., ***am-m.,*** arg-m., arist-cl., berb., cocc., dict., foll., hir., iod., kreos., **LIL-T.,** man., **NIT-AC.,** prot., ***sec., sep., sil.,*** spig., ***thymol.,*** ust.
- menses, during - pic-ac.
  - after - ***lac-c., nit-ac.***
  - before - arist-cl., hir.
- stains linen - ***lil-t.,*** **NIT-AC.**
  - yellow - lac-d.
- urination, after - ***am-m.***

burning - alum., alum-p., ***am-c.,*** ant-c., ***ars.,*** ars-i., ars-s-f., bar-c., **BOR., CALC., CALC-S.,** canth., carb-ac., ***carb-an.,*** carb-s., ***carb-v.,*** cast., cham., ***con.,*** ferr-i., ***fl-ac.,*** hep., hydr., iod., kali-ar., kali-c., ***kali-p.,*** kali-s., **KREOS.,** ***lach.,*** lept., lil-t., mag-c., mag-s., meph., ***merc., nit-ac., phos.,*** **PULS., SEP., SULPH.,** ***sul-ac.,*** sul-i., tarent., thuj.
- abdominal pain, after - calc-p.
- hot - ***bor.,*** calc., calc-s., hep., ***kreos.,*** lept., lil-t., puls., sep., sulph.
- menses, after - ***phos.***
- motion agg. - ***mag-s.***
- watery - hydr.

candida, albicans - calc., calc-p., helon., lyc., med., ***nat-p., puls.,*** nit-ac., sep., ***thuj.***

cervical, excoriation, with - alum., arg-n., kali-bi., merc., nit-ac.

childbed, in - bell-p.

DISCHARGE, vagina
chilliness, with - ***cycl., puls.***
night - lach.
cold, agg. - ***nit-ac.***
colic, after - am-m., calc-p., con., lyc., mag-c., mag-m., sil., ***sulph.,*** zinc.
constant - ***aesc.,*** alum., ***am-m.,*** aur., bell-p., ***bor.,*** calc., erig., **GRAPH.,** ***ign.,*** iod., ***kali-i., kali-m., kreos., lach., mag-m., mez., myric.,*** nat-c., ***nit-ac., nux-v.,*** plat., podo., ***rat.,*** sec., ***senec., sil., sulph.,*** thuj., ziz.
amenorrhea, with - ***plat.***
menses agg. - **IOD.**
after - ***nux-v.***
oozing from vulva - aur.
sexual desire, with increased - ***ign.***
cough, after - con.
alternating with - ***iod.***
during - nat-m.
cramp, after every - mag-m.
cream-like - alum., bufo, calc., ***calc-p., kali-fer.,*** **NAT-P., PULS.,** ***sec.,*** sep., ***staph., tril.***
acid foods, from - nat-p.
afternoon - calc-p.
menses, before and after - tril.
painless - **PULS.**
weakness, from - ***sec.***
dark - ***aesc.,*** agar., croc., ***kreos.,*** nux-m., sec.
daytime, agg. - murx., ***sep.***
agg., after menses - ***kali-fer.***
only, daytime - ***alum., lac-c.,*** plat., sep.
diarrhea, with - puls.
dirty - sec.
dreams, with amorous - ***petr.***
dropping - ars.
eating, after - cham.
evening - bufo, echi., eupi., lil-t., merc., phys., sil., tarent., ***zinc.***
excitement, agg. - calc.
exercising, while - mag-m., mag-s., ***sars.***
agg. - helon., tong.
exertion, agg. - erig., helon.
exhausting - cocc., frax., senec., visc.
flatus, after - caust.
emission of, during - ars.
flesh-colored - ***alum.,*** bar-c., bufo, canth., chin., cocc., kali-i., kreos., lyc., ***nit-ac.,*** phos., sabin., sep., ***tab.***
afternoon, in open air - alum.
menses, after - ***nit-ac.***
non-offensive, like washing of meat - ***nit-ac.***
flocculent - ambr., apis, helon., merc., sep.
flowing down, thighs - alum., ***graph.,*** lept., lyc., lyss., onos., ***senec.,*** syph., tub.
imperceptibly - agn.
warm water - lept.
fright, before the menarche, from - **PULS.**
frothy - but-ac.

DISCHARGE, vagina
girls, in little - ***asper.,*** bar-c., bufol, ***calc.,*** calc-p., ***cann-s.,*** carb-ac., carb-v., ***caul.,*** caust., ***cina, cub.,*** hydr., kali-p., mang., med., **MERC.,** ***merc-i-f., mill., puls.,*** senec., **SEP.,** ***syph.,*** viol-t.
acrid - cub.
infants - cann-i., cann-s.
yellow - merc-i-f.
glairy, like egg white - nat-m., pall.
gonorrheal - ***aur-m., cann-s.,*** cop., *med.,* mez., **NIT-AC.,** ***plat.,*** **PULS.,** sabin., ***sep.,*** **THUJ.**
gray - ***arg-m.,*** berb., helon., kreos., nit-ac., ***sec.***
greenish - amor-r., anan., apis, arg-m., ***arg-n., asaf., bov., carb-ac., carb-an.,*** **CARB-V.,** cop., cub., flor-p., **KALI-BI,** kali-chl., ***kali-i., kali-p., kali-s., lach.,*** **MERC.,** merc-i-r., ***murx., nat-c.,*** **NAT-M., NAT-S., NIT-AC.,** phos., pulx., puls., rob., ***sec.,*** **SEP.,** sulph., ***thuj.,*** x-ray.
acrid - merc-i-r.
greenish-yellow - ***bov., murx., puls.,*** ruta, ***sabin., sep.,*** **SULPH., THUJ.**
menses, after - ***nit-ac.***
morning - murx.
stains, linen - bov., kali-chl., lach., thuj.
walking, agg. - ***nat-m.***
water - ***sep.***
gushing - **CALC.,** ***cocc., eupi., gels.,*** **GRAPH.,** kreos., **LYC.,** mag-c., mag-m., sabin., **SEP., SIL.,** stann., thuj.
cramp, with - mag-m.
menses, after - ***nit-ac.***
squatting, when - cocc.
hair, falling off - alum., graph., ***lyc., nat-m.,*** phos., sulph.
pubes - ***nat-m.***
headache, with - plat.
heat, flushes, with - ***lach.,*** lyc., ***sulph.***
hemorrhoids, suppression, from - am-m.
hepatic derangement, costiveness - hydr.
hoarseness, after - con., ***nat-s.***
honey-colored - ***nat-p.***
hot - bor., ferr-i., ***hydr.***
ichorous - arg-m.
insensibility of vagina, causing - raja-s.
intermittent - carb-v., con., sulph.
itching - ***agar.,*** agn., alum., ***ambr., anac.,*** ars., **CALC.,** ***calc-i.,*** carb-ac., ***caust.,*** cham., ***chin.,*** coff., ***coll.,*** con., cub., ferr., ***fl-ac.,*** hedeo, helin., helon., hoit., ***hydr., kali-bi.,*** kali-c., **KREOS.,** lach., ***merc., nat-m., nit-ac.,*** ph-ac., phos., plat., puls., ***sabin.,*** **SEP.,** sil., staph., sulph., syph., ***zinc.***
menopause, in - ***murx.***
menses, after - kreos., ***ph-ac.***
jelly-like - coc-c., ***graph.,*** pall., ***sabin.,*** sec., sep.
menses, agg. before and after - ***pall.***
labor-like pains, with - dros.
lochia, after - lyss.
loss, of fluids, from - ***alet.***

DISCHARGE, vagina

lumpy - ambr., ***ant-c.,*** ars-m., bor., ***bov.,*** chin., cur., helon., hep., hydr., ***merc., psor.,*** rad-br., ***sep.,*** sil., tarent., ust.

clear - tarent.

menses, after - ***chin.***

offensive - ***chin., psor.***

lying, while - **PULS.**

masturbation, from - ***canth.,*** orig., orig-v., ***plat.,*** **PULS.**

meat water, like - kali-i.

membranous - ***bor.,*** bov., hep., hydr., kali-bi., nit-ac., phyt., vib.

menopause - **GRAPH.,** ***sabin., sang.,*** sars., **SEP.**

continues, after menses cease - ***sang.***

menses, during - alum., am-c., ars., ars-i., bor., bov., calc., carb-ac., carb-an., carb-v., caust., chin., chin-s., ***cocc.,*** con., graph., hura, ***iod.,*** kali-ar., kali-c., ***kreos.,*** lach., ***mag-m.,*** merc., mez., mur-ac., nat-m., nit-ac., phos., psor., puls., sabin., sep., sil., sulph., zinc.

after - aesc., ***alum.,*** alum-p., alum-sil., ars., ***ars-i., bor.,*** **BOV.,** bufo, bry., **CALC., CALC-P.,** calc-sil., calc-s., canth., carb-ac., carb-an., carb-s., ***carb-v.,*** carl., caust., ***cham.,*** chel., chin., chin-a., cocc., ***coloc., con.,*** cop., cub., ***eupi.,*** ferr-i., ***graph.,*** guare., ***hydr.,*** iod., kali-ar., kali-bi., kali-c., kali-n., kali-p., kalm., ***kreos.,*** lac-c., lac-d., lach., lil-t., ***lyc.,*** lyss., ***mag-c., mag-m.,*** merc., ***mez., murx.,*** nat-m., ***nat-p.,*** nat-s., ***nicc., nit-ac.,*** nux-v., pall., ***ph-ac., phos., plat.,*** psor., ***puls., ruta.,*** sabin., **SEP.,** ***sil.,*** spig., ***sulph.,*** sul-ac., sul-i., tab., tarent., thlaspi thuj., tril., vib., ***xan.,*** zinc.

a week - ***kalm.***

some days - ***thlaspi.***

ten days - ***con., hydr.***

two weeks - bar-c., ***bor.,*** calc-p., con., mag-m., sulph.

day-time, usually in - ***kali-fer.***

before - ***alum.,*** alum-p., allox., alum-sil., ang., aran-ix., arist-cl., aur-m., ***bar-c.,*** bar-i., bar-s., berb., bor., **BOV.,** ***bufo,*** **CALC.,** ***calc-p., calc-s.,*** calc-sil., carb-s., ***carb-v.,*** caust., ***cedr.,*** chin., ***cocc.,*** con., cub., ferr., ferr-i., ferr-p., **GRAPH.,** ***hed.,*** hir., iod., kali-m., kali-n., **KREOS.,** lac-c., lac-d., ***lach.,*** mag-m., man., nat-c., ***nat-m.,*** nat-sil., ***nux-v., pall., ph-ac., phos.,*** pic-ac., plat., prot., ***puls.,*** ruta, sabin., **SEP.,** ***sil.,*** sul-i., ***sulph.,*** tarent., thlaspi, vib., ***zinc.***

and after - graph., pall., sul-i.

vicarious - ***dig.***

between - ange-s., **BOR., CALC.,** ***cocc., coloc.,*** foll., hypoth., ***ip., kreos.,*** prot., rob., **SEP.,** sulph., ***xan.***

instead of menses - alum., **ARS.,** berb., bov., calc-p., ***cedr., chen-a., chin., cocc., ferr., graph., iod.,*** lac-c., ***nux-m., phos.,*** psor., puls., senec., ***sep., sil., xan., zinc.***

DISCHARGE, vagina

menses, like the menses - ***alum., caust., kreos.,*** mag-s., zinc.

retarded menses, with - ziz.

scanty, with - calc-p., ***caust., mez.***

smelling like - ***caust.***

suppressed, with - sabin., ziz.

mental symptoms, with - murx.

mercury, after - **NIT-AC.**

milky - ***am-c.,*** anan., ang., ange-s., aur., bar-c., bell., ***bor.,*** **CALC.,** calc-f., ***calc-i., calc-p.,*** calc-sil., canth., carb-s., ***carb-v.,*** chel., coff., ***con.,*** cop., ***euph., ferr.,*** ferr-m., ferr-p., ***graph.,*** haem., ***ign.,*** iod., ***kali-chl.,*** kali-i., **KALI-M.,** ***kreos., lach.,*** lyc., naja, nat-m., ***ovi-g-p.,*** paraf., ***phos., phys.,*** psor., **PULS.,** sabin., sarr., **SEP.,** ***sil., stann., sulph., sul-ac., sumb.,*** xan.

coccygodynia, in - **KREOS.**

day-time - **SEP.**

forenoon - sep.

girls, in little - hyper.

lying down agg. - **PULS.**

menses, during - phos.

morning, when walking - ***phos.***

urination, during - ***calc.***

miscarriage, with history of - alet., ***caul., sabin.,*** sep.

tendency to - caul., ***plb.,*** sep.

moon, at full - **LYC.**

morning - ***aur., aur-m.,*** aur-s., ***bell., calc-p., carb-v., graph., kreos., mag-m.,*** murx., nat-m., phos., plat., **SEP.,** ***sulph.,*** zinc.

girls, in - ***puls.***

rising, on - calc-p., carb-v., graph., kreos., ***sulph.***

urinating, after - ***mag-m.***

walking, when - phos.

motion agg. - ***bov.,*** calc., carb-an., euph-pi., graph., helin., mag-c., ***mag-m.,*** mag-s., ***phys., sep.,*** til.

downward - ***bor.***

mucous - alum., calc., kali-c., mez., phos., sars., sep., sulph., sul-c., zinc.

night - alum., ambr., ***carb-v., caust., con.,*** **MERC.,** ***nat-m.,*** nit-ac., ruta, ***sulph., syph.***

only at - ***carb-v., caust., nat-m.***

offensive - am-m., amor-r., anan., ***aral., arg-m., ars.,*** asaf., bapt., bufo, calc., calc-ar., calc-p., cann-s., caps., **CARB-AC.,** carb-an., ***carb-v.,*** caust., ***chin.,*** chin-a., ***coloc., con.,*** cop., crot-h., cub., cur., ***eucal.,*** graph., ***guare., helon., hep.,*** hydr., **KALI-AR.,** kali-i., **KALI-P., KREOS.,** lach., lam., ***lil-t.,*** lyss., mag-c., man., med., ***merc.,*** merc-c., ***myric., nat-a., nat-c.,*** **NIT-AC., NUX-V.,** oci-s., onos., ***op.,*** **PSOR.,** pulx., ***pyrog., rhus-t.,*** rob., ***sabin., sang., sanic.,*** sarr., ***sec.,*** **SEP.,** ***sil., sulph., syph.,*** ter., thlaspi, ***thymol.,*** tril., tub., ***ust.***

ammonia, like - am-c.

blackish water - rhus-t.

burnt blood, as - hist.

cheese, like old - **HEP.,** sanic.

DISCHARGE, vagina

offensive, evening - sep.

fish-brine, like - hep., med., ***sanic.,*** thuj.

decayed - ***med.***

forceps, delivery, after - calen.

green corn, like - ***kreos.***

horse's urine, like - but-ac.

menopause, in - ***sabin.***

menses, after - ars., coloc., ***guare.,*** kreos., nit-ac., tarent.

before - man.

between - ***coloc.***

like the menses - caust.

suppressed - sabin.

pungent - kreos.

putrid - **CARB-AC.,** colch., ***kali-ar., kali-i.,*** **KALI-P., KREOS.,** lach., mur-ac., ***nat-c.,*** nit-ac., ph-ac., **PSOR.,** sabin., sarr., ***sec., sep.***

sour - hep., ***nat-p.***

sweetish - calc-p., merc-c.

urinous - ol-an.

yeasty - but-ac.

orange, fluid - kali-p.

painful - mag-m., sil., sulph.

painless - ***am-m., kreos., plat.,*** **PULS.**

pains, flowing after abdominal - am-m., bell., caust., cham., con., ferr., ign., kali-c., lyc., mag-c., ***mag-m., merc.,*** naja, nat-c., ***nat-m., sil.,*** sulph., ***zinc.***

paroxysmal - allox., eupi., lyc.

periodical - lyc.

pregnancy, during - **ALUM.,** bor., caul., cimic., ***cocc.,*** con., kali-c., **KREOS.,** med., ***murx.,*** nat-p., petr., **PULS.,** sabin., **SEP.,** ***thuj.***

miscarriage, with tendency to - caul., ***plb.,*** sep.

profuse - acon., aesc., ***agar.,*** agn., ***alum.,*** alum-p., alum-sil., alumn., ambr., ***am-c., ant-c.,*** apis, ***arg-n., ars., ars-i., ars-s-f., asaf., aur.,*** aur-m., bapt., ***bar-c.,*** bell., bor., bov., bufo, bry., cact., **CALC.,** calc-f., calc-p., calc-s., ***calen., carb-ac.,*** carb-s., carb-v., ***caul., caust., cean.,*** chin., chin-a., cinnb., ***cocc.,*** coff., ***con.,*** cub., ***cur., dig., erig., eupi.,*** ferr., ferr-i., ***fl-ac.,*** **GRAPH.,** ***ham., helon.,*** hydr., ***hydrc.,*** iod., kali-p., ***kreos.,*** lac-c., ***lac-d., lach., led., lil-t.,*** lyss., ***lob.,*** lyc., mag-c., mag-m., mag-s., ***med., merc., merc-c., merc-i-f.,*** merc-i-r., ***nat-a., nat-c., nat-m., nat-p., nat-s.,*** nicc., nit-ac., ***onos., petr., ph-ac., phos., phys., phyt.,*** puls., pulx., ***sabin., sec.,*** **SEP., SIL., STANN.,** ***still.,*** **SUL-I.,** ***sulph., syph.,*** thlaspi, ***thuj.,*** til., tril., ***tub.,*** ust., ziz.

day-time - ***alumn.***

menses, after - ***lac-c., mag-s., nux-v.***

before - alum., ***lach.,*** **NUX-V.**

between - plat.

like the menses - ***alum., caust., kreos.,*** mag-s.

serum-like discharge from anus and vagina - ***lob.***

morning - phyt.

DISCHARGE, vagina

profuse, serum like discharge from anus and vagina - **LOB.**

urination, after - sep.

vomit, after efforts to - **SEP.**

walking agg. - phos.

washing am, cold - ***alum.***

puberty, at - ferr., **SEP.**

before - calc., merc., ***puls.,*** sep., thuj.

purulent - aesc., ***agn., alum.,*** alum-sil., alumn., amor-r., anan., ***arg-m.,*** arg-n., ***ars.,*** aur-m., ***bov.,*** bufo, **CALC.,** calc-s., calc-sil., ***cann-s.,*** carb-an., cean., cham., ***chin.,*** cinnb., ***cocc.,*** con., cop., cur., eupi., ***fago.,*** helin., ***hep., hydr., ign.,*** iod., ***kali-bi., kali-fer.,*** kali-p., ***kali-s.,*** kreos., lach., lil-t., lyc., ***merc., merc-c., merc-i-f., nat-s.,*** nit-ac., prun., ***puls.,*** pulx., rob., ***sabin.,*** sec., **SEP.,** sil., ***stann., still., sulph., syph.,*** tril., ust.

menses, during agg. - ***merc.***

after - ***bov.***

rest, from - fago.

rising, from sitting - plat.

ropy, stringy, tenacious - ***acon.,*** acon-l., ***aesc., alum.,*** am-m., ant-t., aran., arg-m., ***asar.,*** bell-p., ***bor., bov., caust.,*** chel., ***coc-c., croc.,*** dict., ferr-br., goss., ***graph.,*** **HYDR.,** iris, **KALI-BI.,** ***kali-br., kali-m., mag-m., merc.,*** mez., ***nat-c.,*** **NIT-AC.,** ***pall.,*** ph-ac., phos., ***phys., phyt.,*** raja-s., **SABIN.,** ***sil.,*** stann., sulph., tarent., tril.

menses, after - chel., phos.

before - ferr.

morning - phyt.

walking, when - bov.

running down, limbs - alum., ant-c., onos., senec.

scanty - but-ac., cur., graph., mag-c., murx., phys., puls., ***sars., sulph.,*** thymol.

serous, fluid - tab.

sex, after - cann-s., mag-c., nat-c., ***sep.***

amel. - merc.

sexual excitement, from - ***canth.,*** hydr., orig., orig-v., plat., ***puls.,*** senec.

sexual excitement, with - ign.

sitting, while - ***ant-t., fago.,*** mag-c., sumb.

walking amel. - cact., ***cocc.,*** cycl.

sleeplessness, after - senec.

slimy - ambr.

squatting, agg. - cocc.

staining, linen - agn., bov., ***carb-an.,*** chel., eupi., fago., graph., ***kreos., lach., lil-t., nux-v., prun.,*** sep., ***thuj.***

stains, indelibly - mag-c., med., ***pulx.,*** sil., vib.

standing, from - aesc., ***ars.,*** carb-an., kreos., lac-c., sep.

amel. - fago.

starch, boiled, like - **BOR.,** ferr-i., **NAT-M., SABIN.,** tep.

sticky, stringy - ***hydr., kali-bi.,*** nit-ac., sabin., tarent.

stiffening, the linen - ***alum.,*** alumn., bell., ***kali-bi.,*** kali-n., ***kreos., lach., sabin.***

DISCHARGE, vagina

stool, during - ferr-i., mag-c., sanic., thuj., zinc.
agg. - calc-p.
after - ***mag-m.,*** vib., zinc.
every stool, with - ***mag-m.***

stooping, agg. - cocc.

stubborn - mez.

suddenly, coming and going - ***carb-v.***

suppressed - ***am-m.,*** asaf., carc., graph., lac-c., lach., med., nat-s., phos., ***sabin.,*** senec., thlaspi., thuj.

sycotic - ***mag-s.,*** **MED.,** ***nat-s.,*** **THUJ.**

syphilitic - ***kali-bi., merc., merc-c.,*** **NIT-AC.,** viol-t.

thick - ***acal.,*** aesc., alum., ambr., amor-r., anac., anan., **ARS.,** ***ars-i.,*** ars-s-f., ***asar., aur., aur-i.,*** aur-s., bar-c., ***bor., bov.,*** bufo, **CALC.,** calc-s., carb-ac., ***carb-v.,*** canth., cast., ***cean., chlol.,*** coc-c., ***coloc., con.,*** cop., cur., goss., **HYDR.,** ***iod.,*** **KALI-BI.,** kali-m., kali-s., kreos., lach., lup., ***mag-m.,*** mag-s., med., mez., murx., myric., ***nat-a., nat-c.,*** nat-m., nit-ac., ***phyt., podo., puls.,*** rob., ***sabin.,*** sarr., ***sec., senec., sep.,*** stann., staph., sulph., syph., ***thuj.,*** tong., vib., ***zinc.***
acrid - bov., hydr.
creamy - calc-p., ***nat-p., puls.,*** sec.
menses, after - ***coloc., nit-ac., pall., sep., tril., zinc.***
before and after - ***zinc.***
between - ***coloc.,*** tril.
profuse, as menses - mag-s.
morning - aur-s.
night, on waking - zinc.
stool, during - ***vib.***
stringy - ***hydr., kali-bi.***
urination, during - **CALC.**
walking, when - ***bov.***
white paste, as - ***bor.***

thin, watery - ***acal.,*** alum., alum-p., alum-sil., ambr., ***am-c.,*** anan., ***ant-c., ant-t., arg-m.,*** arist-cl., ***ars., ars-i., asaf.,*** bapt., bell., bond., ***bufo,*** but-ac., ***calc., calen., carb-an.,*** carb-s., ***carb-v.,*** cast., cham., chin., chin-a., ***cocc., ferr.,*** ferr-ar., ferr-i., ferr-p., fl-ac., frax., gels., **GRAPH.,** helon., ***hydr.,*** iod., ***kali-i.,*** kali-n., kali-s., ***kreos., lac-c.,*** lept., ***lil-t., lob., lyc., mag-c., mag-m.,*** med., merc., ***merc-c.,*** mez., ***murx.,*** naja, nat-c., ***nat-m., nat-p.,*** nicc., **NIT-AC.,** ***ol-an., ph-ac., phos.,*** plat., prun., **PULS.,** ***rhus-t.,*** sabin., sarr., ***sec., sep., sil.,*** stann., ***sulph.,*** sul-ac., syph., tab., ***tarent.,*** thymol., sul-i., ***syph.,*** vib.
afternoon - ***naja.***
dinner, after - cham.
forenoon - mag-c.
menses, after - ars., ***mag-c., nit-ac.,*** tab., ***vib.***
before - sapin.
between - alet.
morning - carb-v.
rising - ***carb-v.,*** sulph.
pregnancy, during - ***cocc.***
scrofulous women, in - ***iod.***

DISCHARGE, vagina

thin, watery, urination, after - nicc.

transparent - agn., allox., ***alum.,*** alumn., am-c., ***am-m., aur.,*** aur-s., **BOR.,** ***bov.,*** bufo, calc., ***calc-p., caust.,*** chlorpr., ***mez.,*** nabal., **NAT-M.,** ***nit-ac.,*** pall., ***petr., plat., podo.,*** **SEP.,** ***stann.,*** stram., ***sul-ac.,*** til., ust.
menses, after - ***pall.***
rising from seat, after - plat.
walking, when - ***bov.***

urinary, symptoms, with - berb., erig.

urinating, while - calc., coff., nat-c., sil.
after - ***am-m.,*** carb-v., con., cur., ***kreos.,*** mag-m., ***nat-c.,*** nicc., plat., **SEP., SIL.**
before - kreos.
ceasing after - ***nat-c.***

urine, from contact of - kreos., ***merc.,*** sulph.

urinous - ol-an.

vagina, pressure, in, with - cinnb.

vaginismus, in - ***ign., plat.***

walking, agg. - ***aesc.,*** alum., anan., ***aur.,*** **BOV.,** calc., ***carb-an., graph.,*** kreos., ***lac-c., mag-c.,*** mag-m., ***nat-m.,*** onos., ***phos., sars., sep.,*** stront-c., ***sulph.,*** til., tong., ***tub.***
amel. - cact., ***cocc.,*** cycl., fago.

warm, bed, agg. - syph.

water flowing down, sensation of - ***bor.***

washing, amel. - alum., kali-c.
cold amel. - ***alum.***

weakness, with - ***aesc., alet., alum., arg-n.,*** bar-c., berb., **CALC.,** calc-p., ***calen.,*** carb-an., **CAUL.,** ***caust.,*** **CHIN.,** ***cocc.,*** coll., con., ***frax.,*** **GRAPH.,** gua., ***ham.,*** helin., ***helon.,*** hydr., ***iod., kali-bi., kali-c.,*** **KREOS.,** ***lyc.,*** lyss., nabal., **NAT-M.,** nicc., onos., ***petr., ph-ac.,*** phos., ***phys., psor.,*** puls., rob., ***senec.,*** sep., **STANN.,** sul-ac., tarent., tril., ***vinc.,*** zinc.
lumbar region, in - con., **GRAPH.**

white - aloe, ***alum.,*** alum-sil., ambr., am-c., ***am-m.,*** anac., anan., ***ant-t., arg-m.,*** arist-cl., ***ars., aur., aur-s.,*** bar-c., ***bell., berb.,*** **BOR.,** ***bov.,*** bufo, ***calc.,*** calc-f., ***calc-p.,*** calc-s., canth., carb-s., ***carb-v.,*** cent., chel., coc-c., ***con.,*** dict., elaps, ***ferr.,*** ferr-ar., ferr-p., ***gels.,*** goss., **GRAPH.,** haem., hydr., kali-c., ***kali-chl., kali-i., kali-m.,*** kali-n., ***kreos.,*** lac-c., lapa., lil-t., lyc., ***lyss., mag-c.,*** mag-s., man., ***merc.,*** merc-c., ***mez.,*** mom-b., nabal., ***naja,*** **NAT-M.,** ***nux-v.,*** oci-s., ol-an., pall., penic., ***petr.,*** phos., ***plat., podo.,*** prun., ***psor., puls.,*** rob., sabin., sarr., sars., **SEP.,** sil., ***stann.,*** stram., sulph., ***sul-ac.,*** sumb., syph., ***tarent.,*** ust., vib., ***zinc.,*** zinc-p.
afternoon - naja.
evening - phos.
menses, after - vib.
morning, on rising agg. - **GRAPH.**
sitting agg. - ***sumb.***
stains, linen yellow - chel.
stool, during - ***vib.***
turn, green - nat-m.

DISCHARGE, vagina
women, type of
blond and phlegmatic - ***cycl., puls.***
cachectic - ***helon.,*** **NIT-AC.**
chilly - ars., calc., lach.
elderly - ars., ***gels., helon.,*** nit-ac., ***phos.,*** sec.
elderly and weak - ars., ***helon.,*** nit-ac., sec., **STANN.**
hysterical - ***am-c., gels.,*** **PULS.**
scrofulous - **CALC.,** carb-an., ***iod.***
students - ***gels.***
thin - phos., ***sec., sep.***
tuberculous - ferr.
yellow - acon., ***aesc.,*** alet., ***alum.,*** alum-p., alum-sil., ***alumn.,*** anan., apis, ***arg-m., arg-n.,*** **ARS.,** ***ars-i., ars-s-f., asar., aur.,*** **AUR-I.,** ***aur-m., aur-s.,*** bell., ***bufo,*** bov., **CALC.,** calc-f., calc-i., ***calc-s.,*** calc-sil., ***carb-an., carb-v.,*** cean., cench., **CHAM.,** ***chel.,*** chin., ***chlor.,*** cinnb., ***coloc.,*** con., cub., cycl., ***eupi.,*** fago., fl-ac., foll., gels., ***gran., graph.,*** **HYDR.,** ign., ***inul., iod., kali-ar., kali-bi.,*** kali-c., ***kali-fer., kali-i.,*** kali-m., ***kali-p., kali-s., kali-sil., kalm.,*** **KREOS.,** lac-c., ***lac-d.,*** lach., ***lac-ac., lil-t., lyc.,*** mag-c., man., ***med., merc.,*** merc-c., ***merc-i-f.,*** merc-i-r., ***murx.,*** myric., ***nat-a., nat-c.,*** nat-m., ***nat-p., nat-s.,*** nit-ac., ***nux-v.,*** oci-s., ***ol-j.,*** onos., ***pall.,*** penic., ***ph-ac.,*** phos., prun., psor., **PULS.,** rob., ***sabin., sec.,*** senec., **SEP.,** sil., spira., ***stann., sul-i.,*** **SULPH.,** sul-ac., ***syph., thuj., tril.,*** ust., ***zinc., zinc-p.***
children, in - ***merc-i-f., syph.***
menopause, at - ***sabin.***
menses, during - calc., ***puls.***
after - ars., lac-d., ph-ac., ***sep.,*** **TARENT.**
before - ang., ars., lac-d., ***nat-m., puls., sep., tarent.***
between - calc., ***coloc.,*** tril.
morning - ***aur-m.,*** kalm., **SEP.**
motion agg. - ***sep.***
night agg. - ***syph.***
scrophulous women, in - ***iod.***
stains linen yellow - ***agn., carb-an.,*** chel., **KREOS.,** nit-ac., ***nux-v.,*** prun.
urination, before - ***kreos.***
yellow-green - arg-m., ***bov.,*** calc-sil., ***kali-bi.,*** merc., ***murx., nat-s., puls.,*** ruta, ***sabin., sep.,*** **SULPH.,** syph., ***thuj.***

DISPLACEMENT, of uterus, (see Prolapsus) - ***abies-c.,*** aesc., ***am-m.,*** aur-m., **BELL., CALC.,** ***calc-p.,*** carb-ac., ***caul., cimic., eupi.,*** ferr., ***ferr-i., frax.,*** graph., helio., ***helon.,*** kali-c., **LACH.,** lappa-a., led., **LIL-T.,** ***mag-m., merc.,*** mel-c-s., ***murx.,*** **NAT-M.,** ***nit-ac., nux-m., nux-v.,*** pall., phos., ***plat., podo., puls.,*** sabal., senec., sec., **SEP.,** ***stann.,*** sulph., ***tarent., thuj.,*** tub., ***ust.***
anterior - graph., lil-t., phos.

DISTENDED, uterus, as if, filled with wind - ph-ac.

DRAWING, pain, genitalia - ***aur.,*** bar-c., mosch.
stool, before - carb-an.
drawing, ovaries - apis, ***ars.,*** atro., bell., ***chin.,*** coloc., goss., lach., lil-t., ***pall., plat.,*** podo.
extending into thighs - ars.
left - coloc.
menses, before - coloc.
motion agg. - **ARS.**
raising arms - ***apis.***
right - ***apis,*** med., pall.
rubbing amel. - ***pall.***
sex, after - ***plat.***
sitting bent, from - **ARS.**
drawing, uterus - **BELL.,** calc-p., ***cham.,*** cop., plat., plb., ***puls.,*** sabin.
menses, before - jug-r.
would appear, as if - calc-p.
sex, after - ***plat.***
drawing, vagina - card-m., cop.

DROPSY, (see Edema)

DRYNESS, genitalia - ***nat-m.,*** **SEP.,** tarent.
dryness, vagina - ***acon., ars.,*** apis, ***bell., berb., ferr.,*** ferr-p., ***graph.,*** **LYC.,** lycps., lyss., **NAT-M.,** puls., **SEP.,** spira., tarent., zinc-chr.
menopause, during - ***nat-m., sep.***
menses, during - ***graph.***
after - berb., ***lyc.,*** nat-m., ***sep.***
uneasy sensation, with - zinc-chr.
dryness, vulva - ***acon., bell.,*** calc., lyc., sep., tarent.
menses, after - sep.

DULL, pain, genitalia, constant - aur-br., hydrc., nicc., sep.
numb, aching - podo.
dull, uterus, wedge-like - iod.

DYSMENORRHEA, painful, menses, (see Menses) - abrot., acetan., ***acon.,*** aesc., agar., agn., alet., alum., alum-p., alum-sil., alumn., am-a., **AM-C.,** am-m., ammc., amor-r., ***anac.,*** anan., ant-c., ***ant-t.,*** ap-g., ***apiol.,*** apis, aquileg., arg-n., arist-cl., arn., ***ars.,*** ars-i., ***ars-m.,*** asar., asc-c., atro., aur., aven., bar-c., bar-i., bar-m., **BELL.,** bell-p., ***berb., bor.,*** bov., brom., bry., bufo, buni-o., **CACT.,** ***calc.,*** calc-ac., calc-i., **CALC-P.,** calc-s., calc-sil., cann-i., canth., carb-an., carb-s., carb-v., cast., ***caul., caust.,*** **CHAM.,** chin., chin-a., chin-s., ***chol., cic.,*** **CIMIC.,** cinnb., ***cit-v.,*** **COCC.,** ***coff., colch.,*** coll., ***coloc., con., croc.,*** crot-c., cupr., cur., ***cycl.,*** der., ***dios., dulc.,*** epip., ergot., **ERIG.,** eup-pur., euphr., ferr., ferr-ar., ferr-i., ***ferr-m.,*** ferr-p., ***gels.,*** glon., ***gnaph.,*** goss., ***graph.,*** grat., ***guai., ham., helon.,*** hir., ***hoit., hydr.,*** hyos., hyper., ***ign.,*** inul., iod., ip., ***kali-ar.,*** kali-bi., **KALI-C.,** kali-fer., ***kali-i.,*** kali-m., kali-n., ***kali-p., kali-per., kali-s.,*** kali-sil., kalm., kreos., ***lac-c., lach., lap-a.,*** laur., led., ***lil-t.,*** lob., ***lyc., macro., mag-c.,*** mag-m., **MAG-P.,** mag-s., mang., ***med., meli.,*** meph., ***merc., merl.,*** **MILL.,** ***mit.,*** morph., mosch., murx., mur-ac., ***nat-c.,*** nat-m., nat-p., nat-s., nicc., nit-ac., nux-m., ***nux-v.,*** ol-an., ***ol-j.,*** onop., op., pall., palo., passi., petr., ph-ac., ***phos.,*** phyt., pic-ac., ***pituin., plat.,*** plb., podo., **PSOR., PULS.,** rauw., ***rhod., rhus-t.,***

DYSMENORRHEA, painful, menses - sabal., ***sabin.,*** sang., sant., sars., ***sec.,*** sel., ***senec., sep.,*** sil., spong., staph., stram., sul-i., **SULPH.,** sul-ac., ***syph., tanac., tarent.,*** tell., ther., thuj., thyr., thyreotr., trio., ***tub.,*** **UST.,** uza., ven-m., ***verat.,*** **VERAT-V.,** vesp., **VIB.,** vib-p., wye., **XAN.,** ***zinc., zinc-valer.***

anger, from - **CHAM.,** ***coloc.***
beginning at - cact., ***calc.,*** calc-p., ***crot-h.,*** foll., gels., ***lach., pituin.,*** sel.
belching, with - vib.
bending back amel. - ***dios.,*** lac-c.
double, must - ***coloc., mag-p.,*** op.
blood, black, with - ***croc.,*** elaps.
blotches, all over, body, with - dulc.
chill, with - ***kali-c., verat.***
cold, after becoming - ***acon., caj.***
coldness, with - **VERAT.**
colic, after - cham., coloc., ***kali-c.***
convulsions, with - aran., caul., ***nat-m., tarent.***
dinner or supper, after - ***phyt.***
discharge of clots amel. - ***vib.***
emotions, from - cham., ign.
end, of menses - buth-a.
excitement, from - **CALC.**
fainting, with - kali-s., ***lap-a.,*** lyc., nux-m.
feet pressing, against support, amel. - med.
feet wet, from getting - acon., dulc., merc., nat-c., nat-m., ***phos.,*** **PULS.,** ***rhus-t.,*** sep., sil.
few drops of blood, with - cast.
first day - gnaph., lach.
flatulence, with - vib.
flow, amel. - kali-fer., ***lach.,*** mag-p., mosch., zinc., ***zinc-valer.***
amel., with scanty - caul., gnaph., graph.
only in the absence of pain - ***cocc.,*** mag-c., plb.
the more the flow, the more the pain - cann-i., cann-s., ***cimic.,*** phos., tarax., tarent., tub.
the smaller the flow, the greater the pain - ***lach.***
fright, from - ***acon.***
frightful - tub.
horrible pain, crying and screaming - ***cact.,*** **CHAM.,** ***coff.,*** **COLOC.,** ***cupr.,*** ign., ***mag-p.,*** plat., sep.
infantilism, with - calc-p.
infertility, in - nat-m., ***phyt.,*** sep.
jerks, with - plat.
lying amel. - ven-m.
back on, with legs stretched - mag-m.
menopausal, period - **PSOR.**
miscarriage, after - senec.
nausea and vomiting, with - **IP.,** kreos., sars., ***sep.,*** verat-v.
no relief in any position - xanth.
perspiration, from checked - ***caj.***
premature - am-c., ***calc.,*** caust., cocc., con., cycl., ign., ***kali-c.,*** lam., lil-t., ***mag-p.,*** nat-m., ***nux-v.,*** ol-an., phos., sabin., sep., sil., sin-n., ***sulph., xan.***
prolapsus, with - ***sep.,*** verat-v.

DYSMENORRHEA, painful, menses
puberty, at - ***phyt., puls., sep.***
rheumatic - caul., caust., ***cimic.,*** cocc., guai., rham-cath.
screams, with - cham., coloc., plat.
sexual desire, with - cham.
spasmodic, neuralgic - acon., agar., **BELL.,** ***caul.,*** cham., ***cimic.,*** coff., coll., **COLOC.,** ***gels.,*** glon., gnaph., mag-m., **MAG-P.,** ***nux-v., puls.,*** sabin., sant., ***sec.,*** senec., sep., verat-v., ***vib., xan.***
uterine congestion, with - acon., ***bell.,*** cimic., coll., gels., puls., ***sabin.,*** sep., verat-v.
strangury, with - verat-v.
sweat, cold, after - cast.
thighs down - cham., chel., ***cimic.,*** kali-c., rhus-t., sep., zinc-valer.
urination, frequent, with - med.
walking, agg. - ***sabin.***
amel. - cortiso.
warmth amel. - ***ars.,*** cast., caust., **MAG-P.,** ***nux-m., sabin.,*** ven-m.
washing, amel. - kali-c.
wet, after getting - puls., sil., ***zinc.***

ECZEMA, vagina, vulva, labia - rhus-t.

EDEMA, ovaries, (see Swelling) - **APIS,** arn., **ARS.,** aur-m-n., bell., bry., **CALC.,** carb-an., chin., ***coloc.,*** con., ***ferr-i.,*** graph., ***iod.,*** kali-br., kali-c., kreos., ***lach., lil-t.,*** **LYC.,** med., merc., nat-s., phos., plat., ***plb.,*** podo., prun., rhod., rhus-t., sabin., ter., zinc.

edema, uterus - aesc., ***apis,*** ars., ***bell.,*** brom., ***bry.,*** calc., ***camph.,*** canth., ***chin., colch.,*** con., ***dig.,*** dulc., ***ferr.,*** ham., **HELL.,** iod., kali-c., lach., lact., led., ***lob.,*** **LYC.,** merc., phos., puls., rhus-t., ruta., sabad., ***sep., sulph.***
piercing, with, in limbs - hell.
daytime - ***bry.***

ENDOMETRIOSIS, acute - ***acon.,*** ant-i., ***apis,*** arn., ***ars., bell., bry.,*** canth., cham., ***cimic.,*** chin., con., ***gels.,*** hep., hyos., ***iod.,*** kali-c., kali-i., lach., lil-t., med., ***mel-c-s., merc-c.,*** nux-v., op., ph-ac., plat., ***puls.,*** rhus-t., ***sabin., sec., sep., sil.,*** stram., sulph., ter., til., verat-v.
chronic - alet., aloe, ***ars., aur-m., aur-m-n.,*** bell., bor., ***calc., carb-ac.,*** caul., chin-a., ***cimic., con.,*** graph., ***helon., hydr.,*** hydrc., inul., ***iod., kali-a.,*** kali-c., kali-s., kreos., lac-c., ***lach.,*** lyc., ***mag-m.,*** med., ***mel-c-s., merc.,*** nat-m., nit-ac., ***nux-v., ph-ac.,*** phos., plb., ***puls.,*** rhus-t., ***sabin., sec., sep.,*** sil., stram., ***sulph.***

ENLARGED, ovaries, (see Swollen) - **APIS,** aur-m-n., **BELL.,** ***carb-an.,*** coloc., **CON.,** ***graph.,*** hep., ***iod.,*** kali-br., lac-c., lach., lil-t., ***lyc., med.,*** meli., spong., ***ust., thuj.***
every cold agg. - ***graph.***
left - ***apis,*** coloc., graph., lac-c., ***lil-t., med., thuj.***
right - **APIS,** ***bell.,*** **LYC.,** mag-m., ***pall.***

enlarged, ovaries, sensation as if - arg-m., arg-n., cur., med., ***sep., sil.***
left - arg-m.
menses, before - ***sil.***
right - arg-n.
enlarged, uterus - aesc., ***am-m.,*** apis, ***aur., aur-m., bell.,*** calc-i., ***carb-an.,*** **CON.,** helon., ***hep.,*** kali-br., ***kali-i., lach.,*** lyc., lyss., mag-m., merc-i-r., ***nat-c.,*** nux-v., ***phyt.,*** plat., plb., sabin., **SEP.,** ***ust.***
sensation, before menses - ***sep.***
enlarged, vagina, as if - sanic.

EPILEPTIC aura, extending from uterus to stomach - bufo.
uterus to throat - lach.

ERECT, vagina, clitoris, after urination, with sexual desire - calc-p.

ERUPTIONS, genitalia - aeth., agar., alum., ***anan., ant-t., apis,*** ars., aur-m., aur-m-n., bry., bufo, calad., ***calc.,*** canth., carb-s., carb-v., caust., ***coff.,*** con., cop., crot-t., ***dulc.,*** ferr., ***graph.,*** ham., helon., kali-c., ***kali-i.,*** kreos., ***lil-t., lyc., merc.,*** nat-m., nat-s., nit-ac., ***nux-v.,*** **PETR.,** plat., rad-br., rob., **RHUS-T.,** ***rhus-v.,*** sarr., ***sep.,*** sil., staph., sulph., ***thuj.,*** viol-t., zinc.
chancres - merc.
erysipelatous - **RHUS-T.**
labia, vulva, with edema - ***apis.***
itching - ambr., graph., lach., ***nit-ac.,*** nux-v., ***sep.,*** sil., ***sulph., urt-u.***
warm, when - aeth.
menses, before - aur-m., ***dulc.,*** verat.
menses, during - agar., aur-m., bry., calc., caust., con., ***dulc., graph.,*** kali-c., ***merc.,*** nux-v., petr., ***sep.,*** staph.
moist - sep.
night - ***merc.***
nodosities - merc.
painful - sil., viol-t.
pimples - aeth., agar., alum., ambr., ant-c., aur-m., ***calad.,*** calc., con., ***graph.,*** kali-c., lach., ***merc.,*** nat-m., nit-ac., ph-ac., sil., ***sulph., thuj.,*** verat., zinc.
burning - alum., calc., cub., kali-c.
burning, small - cub.
menses, before - aur-m., verat.
menses, during - all-s., ant-t., caust., con., hep., kali-c., lyc., merc., nat-m., petr.
nymphae, on - graph.
painful - sil., ***thuj.***
pustules - ***anan.,*** ant-t., aur-m., bry., carb-ac., merc., nit-ac.
black - bry.
hard, black - bry.
labia - ***carb-ac.,*** graph., ***sep.,*** sulph.
menses, before - aur-m.
menses, during - all-s.
rash - ***anan.***
scabby - kali-i., maland., sars.

EXCITEMENT of genitals, easy - foll., lac-c., manc., med., orig., phos., plat., sumb., thlaspi, zinc.
difficult - ign.
erection of clitoris after urination with sexual desire - calc-p.
menses, during - kali-br.

EXCORIATION, genitalia - ***alum., ambr.,*** am-c., berb., ***bov., calc.,*** calc-s., carb-s., ***carb-v., caust., graph., hep., kali-c.,*** kali-s., ***kreos.,*** lac-c., lil-t., lyc., meph., ***merc.,*** nat-c., ***nit-ac., petr.,*** ph-ac., sabin., ***sep.,*** sil., sulph., **THUJ.,** til.
elderly, women - merc.
menses, during - all-c., ***am-c.,*** bov., carb-v., ***caust., graph.,*** hep., ***kali-c.,*** nat-s., ***sars.,*** sil., ***sulph.***
before - kali-c.
mons veneris - sil.
excoriation, cervix - alum., arg-m., arg-n, hydr., kali-bi., kreos., merc., ***nit-ac.,*** phyt., sul-ac., thuj.
excoriation, perineum, of - alum., arum-t., aur-m., ***calc.,*** carb-an., ***carb-v., caust., cham., graph., hep.,*** ign., **LYC.,** ***merc.,*** petr., puls., rhod., sep., ***sulph.,*** thuj.
female - ***calc., carb-v., caust.,*** **GRAPH.,** hep., **LYC.,** ***merc., petr., sep., sulph.,*** thuj.
excoriation, vagina - alum., ars., ***kali-bi.,*** kali-c., merc., nit-ac.

EXCRESCENCES, genitalia - cinnb., crot-h., cub., graph., ***kreos.,*** lac-c., merc., **NIT-AC.,** sec., staph., **THUJ.**
genito-anal surface - nit-ac., thuj.
excrescences, cervix - cub., ***kreos.,*** merc., **NIT-AC.,** sec., tarent., **THUJ.**
bleeding - merc., thuj.
cauliflower - crot-h., ***graph.,*** kali-ar., ***kreos.,*** lac-c., ***phos.,*** **THUJ.**
wart-shaped - ***thuj.***
watery - sec., thuj.

FETUS, (see Pregnancy, chapter)

FIBROIDS, ovaries - apis, calc., coloc., fl-ac., hep., iod., kali-br., lach., merc., plat., ***podo., sep.,*** staph., ***thuj.,*** xan.
fibroids, uterus - ***apis, aur-i., aur-m., aur-m-n.,*** bell., brom., bufo, **CALC., CALC-F.,** ***calc-i., calc-p., calc-s., calen.,*** carc., chin., ***con.,*** erod., ferr., ***frax.,*** goss., graph., ham., hydr., ***hydrc., iod.,*** ip., kali-br., ***kali-c., kali-i., lach., led., lil-t., lyc.,*** med., merc., ***merc-c., merc-i-r.,*** morg., **NAT-M.,** ***nit-ac.,*** nux-v., **PHOS.,** plat., plb., puls., sabal., ***sabin.,*** sang., sec., **SEP.,** ***sil.,*** solid., staph., sul-ac., sulph., ***ter., thlaspi, thuj.,*** **THYR.,** tril., tub., **UST.,** vinc.
bleeding, from - ***calc.,*** calc-f., calc-p., ***hydr.,*** lyc., merc., nit-ac., **PHOS.,** ***sabin.,*** sil., stip., ***sulph.,*** sul-ac., ***thlaspi.,*** **UST.**
hard, stony - con., merc-i-r.

FISTULA, vagina - ***asar.,*** **CALC.,** ***carb-v.,*** caust., ***lach., lyc., nit-ac., puls.,*** **SIL.**
recto-vaginal - thuj.

FLATUS, vagina, from - apis, ***bell.,*** **BROM.,** ***calc.,*** carc., chin., hyos., ***lac-c.,*** **LYC.,** lyss., ***mag-c., nat-c., nux-m., nux-v.,*** orig., **PH-AC.,** ***phos., sang., sep.,*** sulph., tarent.
distended abdomen, with - sang.
menses, during - brom., kreos., nicc.

FORMICATION, genitalia, (see Tingling) - calc-p., elaps, ***plat.***
formication, uterus - elaps, ***plat.***

FULLNESS, uterus - alet., aloe, apis, ***bell.,*** helon.
standing agg. - aloe.
walking agg. - chin., merc.
fullness, vagina - ham., lil-t.
sensation of, during menses - ***puls.***

GANGRENE, genitalia - ars., ***sec.***
gangrene, uterus - apis, ***ars.,*** bell., carb-ac., carb-an., carb-v., chin., cur., ***kreos.,*** **SEC.**
gangrene, vagina - apis, ***ars.,*** bell., calc., chin., kreos., lach., ***sec.,*** sul-ac.
prolapse, after - sul-ac.

GNAWING, pain, genitalia - kali-c., ***lyc.***
gnawing, ovaries - coloc., ***lil-t.,*** plat., podo.
left - coloc.
right - ***lil-t.,*** podo.
walking, agg. - lil-t., podo.
gnawing, uterus - anan.
gnawing, vagina - lyc.

GONORRHEA, (see Bladder) - ***acon.,*** alumn., apis, arg-n., **CANN-S.,** ***canth., cop., cub.,*** jac., kreos., **MED.,** ***merc.,*** merc-c., ***ol-sant.,*** petros., ***puls., sep.,*** sulph., **THUJ.**

GRASPING, pain, ovaries - lil-t.

GRANULATION, vagina - ***alum., nit-ac.,*** staph., tarent.

GRINDING, pain, genitalia - ***con.***
grinding, ovaries - fl-ac., graph.

GRIPING, pain, ovaries - cact., cur., lil-t.
griping, uterus - cham., con.

HANDLES genitals, during cough or spasms - zinc.
fever, during - hyos.

HAIR falling out, genitalia - hell., merc., **NAT-M.,** ***nit-ac.,*** rhus-t., ***sel.,*** sulph., thuj., ***zinc.***
hair falling out, vagina, labia, vulva - merc., nit-ac.

HARDNESS, genitalia, (see Induration) - ***con.,*** **KREOS.,** ***merc.***
hardness, ovaries (see Induration) - ***apis, brom.,*** con., graph., lach., ust.
left - ***brom., graph.,*** lach., ***ust.***
right - **APIS.**

HEAT, genitalia - aur., calc-p., carb-v., chin., ***cimx.,*** coff., ***dulc., helon.,*** hydrc., kali-br., ***kreos.,*** lil-t., merc., merc-c., nux-v., puls., sarr., sec., sep., tarent., tub.
eating agg. - tub.
flushes - sep., sul-ac.
menses, during - chin., kreos.
heat, ovaries - **BUFO,** lac-c., med.
heat, uterus - apis, ars-m., bell., bufo, camph., lac-c., ***lach., nux-v.,*** ped., raph., sarr., sec.
flushes from uterus to head - raph.
menses, during - lac-c.
heat, vagina - ***acon.,*** ars-m., aur., aur-m., ***bell.,*** berb., coloc., ferr-p., ***graph.,*** ham., hydrc., lycps., sec., tarent.
menses, before - ***ign.***
menses, during - aur.
sex, after - lyc., lyss.
vulva - carb-v., tarent.

HEAVINESS, sensation, genitalia - lob., murx., pall., ***plat.***
menses during - lob., murx., ***plat., sep.***
heaviness, ovaries - **APIS,** carb-an., cimic., con., eup-pur., helon., kali-c., lil-t., meli., onos., ***plat., sep.,*** vib.
left - ***lac-c.,*** lach.
right - carb-an.
heaviness, uterus - ***alet.,*** aloe, alumn., ***apis, bell., calc.,*** calc-p., ***caul.,*** **CHIN.,** cimic., con., elaps, ***gels.,*** helon., hydrc., lac-c., ***murx., nux-v.,*** pall., puls., sabin., senec., **SEP.,** sil.
hysteria, after - elaps.
menses, during - chin., nux-v.
standing - aloe.
vagina discharge, with - cimic.
walking, while - ***chin.***
heaviness, vagina, after hysteria - elaps.

HEMORRHAGE, uterus (see Bleeding, uterus)

HERPES, genitalia - ars., bufo, carb-v., caust., cench., ***dulc.,*** graph., kali-c., kreos., ***med.,*** merc., **NAT-M.,** nit-ac., nux-v., **PETR., SEP.,** sulph., ***rhus-t., thuj.,*** urt-u.
cold, from every - ***dulc.***
menses, during - dulc.
herpes, vulva - nat-m., nat-s.
follicular, herpetic - ars., crot-t., ***dulc.,*** merc., nat-m., rob., ***sep.,*** spira., thuj., ***xero.***

HOLDS, vagina, vulva - hyos., lil-t., plat., sabad., sep., zinc.

INDURATION, genitalia - aml-n., ***con.,*** **KREOS.,** ***merc.,*** sep.
injuries, from - ***con.***
induration, cervix, of - alumn., anan., **AUR.,** ***aur-m., aur-m-n., bell., carb-ac.,*** **CARB-AN.,** chin., **CON.,** hydr., ***iod., kreos.,*** lac-c., ***mag-m., nat-c., plat.,*** **SEP.,** ***sil.,*** staph., tarent., verat.
cervix, os, of - ***aur., carb-an.,*** **CON.,** hydr., nux-v., plat., ***podo., ust.***
pessary, after use of - hyper.
induration, cervix and uterus - alumn., ***aur., aur-m.,*** aur-m-n., ***carb-an.,*** **CON.,** helon., hydr., ***iod., kali-fer.,*** kalm., mang., nat-c., nux-v., ***plat., podo.,*** sep., ***ust.***
induration, ovaries - alum., alumn., am-br., ***apis, arg-m.,*** ars., ***ars-i., aur.,*** aur-m-n., ***bar-i., bar-m.,*** bell., ***brom.,*** carb-an., **CON., GRAPH.,** ***iod.,*** kreos., **LACH.,** ***pall.,*** plat., ***psor., sep.,*** spong., tarent., ust., zinc.
left - ***brom., graph.,*** **LACH.,** psor., ust.

induration, ovaries
right - ***apis, carb-an., pall., podo.***
induration, uterus - ***alum., alumn.,*** **AUR.,** ***aur-m., bell., carb-an.,*** cham., ***chin.,*** **CON.,** helon., ***iod., kali-br.,*** lyss., pall., ***plat.,*** sep., tarent.
miscarriages, after repeated - aur.
pessary, after use of - hyper.
induration, vagina - bell., calc., ***chin.,*** clem., ***con., ferr., lyc.,*** mag-m., merc., petr., ***puls.,*** sep., ***sil.,*** sulph.
painful - chin.

INFANTILISMUS, genitalis - ***bar-c.,*** calc-hp., calc-p., chim., con., ferr., helon., iod., ***ov.,*** phos., senec., thyr.

INFERTILITY - ***agn., alet.,*** alum., ***am-c.,*** anag., anan., apis, **AUR.,** ***aur-i.,*** aur-m., aur-m-n., bar-c., ***bar-m.,*** **BOR.,** brom., ***calc.,*** calc-i., cann-i., cann-s., ***canth.,*** caps., carb-s., ***caul.,*** caust., cic., cocc., ***coff., con.,*** croc., dam., dulc., ***eup-pur., ferr., ferr-p., fil.,*** form., ***goss., graph.,*** helon., ***hyos., iod., kali-br.,*** kali-c., ***kreos., lach.,*** lappa-a., lec., lil-t., man., ***med., merc.,*** mill., mit., **NAT-C., NAT-M.,** nat-p., ***nux-m.,*** nux-v., ***orig., ov., phos.,*** phyt., pituin., ***plat.,*** plb., ***puls.,*** ruta, ***sabal., sabin.,*** sec., ***senec.,*** **SEP.,** ***sil.,*** sulph., ***sul-ac., syph.,*** ther., vib., wies., x-ray, ***zinc.***
atrophy of breasts and ovaries - iod.
non retention of semen, from - nat-c.
ovarian atony, from - eup-pur.
profuse, menstrual flow, from - ***calc.,*** merc., mill., ***nat-m.,*** phos., ***sulph.,*** sul-ac.
and too early- sulph.
and too early or too late - ***phos.***
sexual desire, excesses, with - cann-i., ***kali-br., orig., phos., plat.***
without - agn.
sycotic - med., thuj.
vagina discharge, with - caul., ***kreos., nat-c.***
acid, from - ***nat-p.***
weakness, from - caul., merc., sil.

INFLAMMATION, genitalia - ***acon.,*** ambr., anan., ***apis,*** **ARS.,** ***asaf., bell.,*** bry., ***calc.,*** carb-v., ***coc-c.,*** coll., con., ferr., ferr-ar., ***ferr-p.,*** ign., ***kali-c.,*** **KREOS.,** ***lyc.,*** med., **MERC.,** ***merc-c., nat-m.,*** nat-s., ***nit-ac.,*** nux-v., ***petr.,*** **RHUS-T.,** ***sep.,*** staph., sulph., tarent., ***thuj.***
erysipelatous - ***apis,*** **RHUS-T.**
menses, during - acon., bell., calc., merc., nit-ac., nux-v., sep., sulph.
inflammation, (see Cervicitis)
inflammation, fallopian tubes, (see Salpingitis)
inflammation, ovaries, of, (see Oophoritis)
inflammation, uterus, (see Pelvic Inflammatory Disease)
inflammation, vagina, (see Vaginitis)

INJURIES, to genitalia - **ARN., BELL-P.,** ***calen.,*** con., ***hyper.,*** mill., ***rhus-t., staph.***
pelvic organs, to - ***bell-p.***
injuries, ovaries, contusions - arn., ***bell-p.,*** con., ***ham.,*** psor.

INSENSITIVITY, vagina - alum., ***berb., brom.,*** cann-s., ***ferr., ferr-m.,*** kali-br., nat-m., ***phos., sep.***
sex, during - ***berb.,*** brom., ***ferr., ferr-ma., ign., phos., plat.,*** **SEP.,** ***thuj.***

INSUFFICIENCY, of ovaries - lec., ov., ***sep.***

IRRITATION, genitalia - ***agar., am-c.,*** bry., ***calc., canth., carb-v., con.,*** dulc., ***graph.,*** hep., kali-br., kreos., lyc., merc., nat-m., nit-ac., nux-v., ***orig.,*** phos., plat., puls., ***sep., sil.,*** sulph.
irritation, clitoris - ***am-c.***
irritation, ovaries - am-br., ***apis,*** ars., carb-ac., cimic., ***gels.,*** ham., hep., kali-br., lil-t., nux-v., phyt., plat., rhus-t., thuj., **UST., VIB.**
irritation, uterus - ars., ***bell., caul., cimic.,*** ign., ***lil-t., mag-m.,*** murx., ph-ac., ***senec.,*** tarent.
irritation, vagina - caul., cypr., helon.

ITCHING, genitalia - ***agar.,*** alum., alumn., **AMBR., AM-C.,** ***anac.,*** anan., ant-c., ***ant-t., apis,*** ars., ars-i., aspar., aur., ***aur-m., aur-s.,*** bell., berb., bor., bufo, **CALAD., CALC.,** calc-s., ***canth.,*** carb-ac., ***carb-s., carb-v., caust., chin.,*** chin-a., ***coff.,*** colch., ***coll., con., cop., crot-t.,*** dol., ***dulc.,*** elaps, euph., eupi., fago., ***ferr.,*** ferr-ar., ***ferr-i., fl-ac.,*** fuli., ***graph.,*** grin., ***guano,*** guare., ham., **HELON.,** hydr., ign., kali-ar., ***kali-bi., kali-br., kali-c.,*** kali-i., ***kali-s.,*** **KREOS.,** ***lac-c.,*** lach., lac-ac., ***lap-a.,*** lil-t., ***lyc., mag-c., med.,*** menthol, **MERC.,** mez., murx., mur-ac., ***nat-h.,*** **NAT-M.,** nat-s., nicc., **NIT-AC.,** ***nux-v., onos., orig.,*** **PETR.,** ph-ac., **PLAT.,** rad-br., raph., **RHUS-T.,** rhus-v., sabin., **SEP., SIL.,** sol-t-ae., ***spira., staph.,*** **SULPH.,** ***sul-ac.,*** syph., tarax., **TARENT.,** tarent-c., ***thuj., urt-u., zinc.***
afternoon - sol-t-ae.
burning - **AM-C.,** anan., ***aur-m.,*** berb., **CALC.,** ***kali-i.,*** nat-m., nit-ac., ***urt-u.***
clitoris - sulph.
cold, becoming, from - ***nit-ac.***
water amel. - calad.
weather - dulc.
evening - calc., eupi., ***nit-ac.***
flatus from vagina, during - tarent.
intolerable - ***agar.,*** **AMBR.,** ***am-c., calc.***
lying amel. - berb.
menses, during - agar., ***ambr., am-c.,*** calc., calc-s., ***carb-v., caust., coff., con.,*** hep., ***kali-br., kali-c., kreos.,*** lac-ac., lac-c., lach., ***lyc.,*** merc., nat-m., ***petr.,*** plat., sep., ***sil.,*** sul-ac., ***zinc.***
amel. - syph.
after - calc., calc-s., colch., ***con.,*** cur., elaps, ***ferr.,*** graph., kali-br., kali-c., kreos., lyc., ***mag-c., nat-m.,*** **NIT-AC.,** ***ph-ac., sil.,*** sulph., **TARENT.,** ***zinc.***
amel. - ov.
before - bufo, ***calc.,*** carb-v., caust., colch., **GRAPH.,** ***kali-c.,*** lac-c., ***lil-t., merc., sulph.,*** tarent., zinc.
mons veneris - eup-per.
morning - syph.

ITCHING, genitalia
night - ***lac-c., nit-ac.,*** tarent.
bed, in - ***calc.,*** raph.
pregnancy, during - ambr., ***calad.,*** calc., chlol., ***fl-ac., helon., merc.,*** sabin., **SEP.,** urt-u.
pubis - ambr.
scratching, agg. - am-c., onos.
amel. - crot-t., sep.
strong desire for - urt-u.
sex agg. - nit-ac.
sitting agg. - berb.
stinging - urt-u.
urination, during - ambr., carb-v., sil., ***thuj.***
urine, contact of, agg. - **MERC.,** urt-u.
vagina, discharge, from - agar., alum., ***anac.,*** ars., **CALC.,** calc-s., carb-ac., ***carb-v., caust.,*** chin., ***coll.,*** cub., cur., ***fago., fl-ac.,*** hydr., ***kali-bi.,*** kali-c., kali-p., **KREOS.,** med., ***merc., nat-m.,*** **NIT-AC.,** ***onos.,*** ph-ac., puls., ***sabin.,*** **SEP.,** ***sulph.,*** syph., zinc.
voluptuous - ***agar.,*** arund., bov., ***bufo, calad., calc., canth., coff.,*** dulc., elaps, ***kali-br.,*** kreos., ***lach., lil-t.,*** **ORIG., PLAT.,** ***zinc.***
walking agg. - berb., colch., **NIT-AC.,** ***thuj.***

itching, uterus - bell-p.

itching, vagina - agar., alum., alumn., antipyrin., apis, arund., ***aur-m., brom.,*** **CALAD.,** ***calc., calc-s., canth.,*** carb-ac., caust., coff., ***con.,*** cop., cub., elaps, ***ferr-i., helon., hydr., hydrc.,*** **KREOS.,** ***lil-t., lyc., med., merc.,*** **NIT-AC.,** plat., rhus-t., scroph-n., **SEP.,** sil., staph., ***sulph., tarent.,*** thlaspi, ***thuj.,*** zinc.
deep in - con.
evening - ***kreos.***
menses, during - ***con.,*** elaps, helon., kreos.
after - canth., ***caust.,*** con., elaps, ***kreos.,*** lyc., mez., sulph.
before - elaps, ***graph.***
pregnancy, during - acon., ***ambr.,*** ant-c., bor., **CALAD.,** ***coll.,*** ichth., sabin., ***sep.,*** tab.
scratching until it bleeds - sec.
sex, after - agar., **NIT-AC.**
sexual excitement, with - canth.
urinating, when - kreos.
voluptuous - ***calad.,*** **KREOS.,** ***lil-t.***
warm bathing amel. - med.

itching, vagina, labia, between - agar., ***ambr.,*** apis, ***ars.,*** arund., berb., bov., ***calad., calc., canth.,*** carb-ac., ***carb-v.,*** caust., coff., ***coll., con.,*** conv., cop., crot-t., dulc., ***fago.,*** ferr-i., ***graph.,*** grin., gua., ***helon.,*** hydr., kali-bi., kali-c., **KREOS.,** lil-t., ***lyc., merc.,*** mez., nat-m., nit-ac., ***orig.,*** ped., petr., pic-ac., ***plat., rad.,*** rhus-d., ***rhus-t.,*** rhus-v., scroph-n., ***sep.,*** spira., staph., ***sulph., tarent.,*** tarent-c., thuj., ***urt-u.,*** xero, zinc.

itching, vagina, vulva - ambr., ***calad.,*** carb-v., coll., helon., morg., senec., sil., staph., sulph., syc-co., tarent., urt-u.
burning - calad., kali-i., senec., sulph., urt-u.
pin worms, from - calad., cina.
pregnancy, during - acon., ***ambr.,*** ant-c., bor., ***calad., coll.,*** ichth., ***sep.,*** tab.
sexual excitement, with - kali-bi.
urinating, when - ambr., kreos.
vagina discharge, during - agar., alum., ***ambr., anac.,*** calc., ***fago., helon.,*** hydr., kreos., merc., ***sep.,*** sulph.

JARS, uterus, very tender to motion - bell., ***helon.,*** lyc., lyss., ***med,*** murx.

JERKING, uterus - aster.
jerking, vagina, upwards, morning - sep.

KNOTTED, uterus, as if - ust.

LABOR, uterus, (see Pregnancy, chapter)

LABOR-like, pain, genitalia - acon., ***agar., aloe, apis,*** arg-m., ***arn., asaf.,*** aur., **BELL.,** bor., bov., ***bry.,*** calad., calc., camph., ***cann-i.,*** canth., carb-an., carb-v., ***caul.,*** caust., **CHAM.,** chin., ***cimic., cina,*** cocc., ***coff., coloc., con.,*** croc., ***cupr.,*** dios., dros., ***ferr.,*** ferr-i., **GELS.,** ***goss.,*** graph., hedeo, ***hyos., ign.,*** inul., iod., ***ip.,*** **KALI-C.,** kali-p., ***kreos., lach., lil-t.,*** lyc., mag-c., mag-m., mag-p., med., merc., ***mosch.,*** mur-ac., murx., nat-c., nat-m., nit-ac., nux-m., ***nux-v.,*** onos., ***op.,*** ph-ac., phos., **PLAT.,** podo., **PULS.,** ***rhus-t.,*** ruta, ***sabin.,*** **SEC., SEP.,** ***sil.,*** stann., ***sulph.,*** sul-ac., tarent., ther., thlaspi, thuj., til., ***ust., vib., xan.,*** zinc.
alternating with eye symptoms - kreos.
back, in - ***gels.,*** petr.
downward - nux-v.
belching, with - bor.
bend double, must - puls.
cold, from taking - hyos.
easing - caul., cimic., vib.
excessive, labourious, violent - ***cham.,*** puls., sec., ***sep.***
extending to, back and hips - **GELS.,** sul-ac.
to, bladder - carb-v.
to, rectum - ***aloe, nux-v.***
to, right to left - ***lyc.***
to, sacrum - carb-v.
to, thighs - ***aloe,*** apis, ***cham.,*** con., kali-c., nat-m., nux-v., stram., ust., vib.
fainting, causing - cimic., ***nux-v.,*** puls.
fear of death, with - coff.
left sided - puls.
menses, during - ***acon.,*** agar., ***alet.,*** aloe, ***am-c.,*** am-m., ant-c., apis, arg-n., ***asaf., bell.,*** berb., bor., bov., ***calc., calc-p., carb-an.,*** caul., ***caust.,*** **CHAM.,** chin., ***cimic.,*** cina, coff., ***con., cycl.,*** ferr., ***gels., graph.,*** hyos., ***ign., kali-c.,*** kali-s., kreos., ***lac-c., lach., lil-t.,*** lyc., ***mag-p.,*** med., mosch., ***nat-c., nit-ac., nux-m.,*** nux-v., ***plat., puls., rhus-t., sec., sep.,*** sulph., ust.

LABOR-like, pain, genitalia
menses, after - ***cham.,*** iod., kreos., plat., puls.
before - ***alet.,*** aloe, alum., ***am-c.,*** am-m., ***apis,*** aur., ***bell.,*** bor., ***bov.,*** brom., calc., ***calc-p., caul., cham.,*** chin., ***cimic., cina, cocc., coff., colch.,*** cupr., ***cycl., dig.,*** ferr., ferr-p., ***gels., graph., haem.,*** helon., ***hyos.,*** ign., joan., ***kali-c.,*** kreos., lil-t., ***mag-c., mag-m., mag-p.,*** med., meli., nat-m., nit-ac., nux-m., ***nux-v.,*** plat., ***puls.,*** rhus-t., ***sabin.,*** sanic., ***sec., sep.,*** stann., thlaspi, thuj., ust., ***verat.,*** verat-v., vesp., ***vib., xan.,*** zinc.
standing agg., during - ***rhus-t.***
suppressed - cham.
metrorrhagia, during - ***caul., cham., cimic.,*** ham., sabin., sec., thlaspi, visc.
night - carb-v., nat-m.
pregnancy, during - ***caul., cham., cimic.,*** gels., ***puls., sec.***
pressure, amel. - ign.
spasms, with - caul., caust., ***cham.,*** gels., **HYOS.,** ign., ***puls.***
standing, while - ***rhus-t.***
stool, during - ***nat-m., nux-v.***
upward, going - calc., cham., gels., lach.
vagina discharge, with - con.

LANCINATING, pain, genitalia - aeth., clem., meli.
breathing agg. - clem.
urination, during - clem.
lancinating, ovaries - **APIS,** bell., bor., coll., con., cub., goss., **LIL-T.**
menses, after - ***bor.***
menses, during - ***bor.,*** coll.
lancinating, uterus - anan., ***ars.,*** bufo, ***con.,*** crot-c., graph., hura, ign., lac-c., murx., sep., tarent.
extending upward - lac-c., sep.
touch agg. - ign.
washing in cold water, while - crot-c.
lancinating, vagina - berb., hura
walking agg. - berb.

LEUCORRHEA, vagina, (see Discharge, vagina)

LOCHIA, (see Pregnancy, chapter)

LYING, agg. of uterine symptoms - ambr.

MASTURBATION, (see Sex)

MENOPAUSE, general - acon., ***agar.,*** alet., aloe, ***aml-n., apis,*** aquileg., ***arg-n.,*** arist-cl., aur., bar-c., ***bell., bell-p.,*** bor-ac., bov., ***bry., cact.,*** calc., ***calc-ar.,*** camph., caps., carb-v., carc., ***caul., chin., cimic., cocc.,*** coff., ***con., croc.,*** **CROT-C.,*****crot-h., cycl.,*** ferr., ferr-p., ***gels., glon.,*** **GRAPH.,** ***helon.,*** hir., ***hydr., ign., jab., kali-bi.,*** kali-br., ***kali-c., kali-s., kreos.,*** **LACH.,** laur., lyc., mag-c., mag-p-a., magn-gl., man., ***manc.,*** **MANG.,** meli., merc-sul., mosch., ***murx.,*** nat-m., nit-ac., ***nux-m., nux-v.,*** ol-an., orch., ***ov., ph-ac., phos.,*** phys., piloc., plat., plb., **PSOR., PULS.,** rhus-t., ***sabin.,*** sal-ac., ***sang.,*** sars., ***sec., sel.,*** sem-t., **SEP.,** ***stront-c.,*** **SULPH.,**

MENOPAUSE, general - ***sul-ac.,*** sumb., ***tab., ter., ther.,*** tril., ***ust.,*** valer., ***verat.,*** vip., visc., xan., zinc., ***zinc-valer.***
agg. - acon., aml-n., arg-n., ars., ***cimic.,*** coff., glon., ign., kali-br., **LACH.,** lil-t., ***puls.,*** **SEP.,** tab., ther., valer., verat., zinc.
ailments since - lach., sep.
cough, burning in chest and periodic neuralgia, with - sang.
fatigue, causeless, muscular weakness and chilliness, with - calc.
persistent tiredness and fagged womb, with - bell-p.
headache, with - ***carb-v.,*** croc., glon., **LACH.,** ***sang., sep., ther.,*** ust.
heat, with, in vertex of head - carb-an., cimic., croc., **LACH.,** ***sulph.***
hot flashes, with, perspiration - acet-ac., am-m., ant-c., aur., bell., ***carb-v., fl-ac., hep.,*** kali-bi., ***lach.,*** op., phos., ***puls.,*** **SEP.,** ***sulph., sul-ac.,*** **TUB.,** ***xan.***
hypertrophy of one side - lyc.
obesity, with - calc-ar., calc.
premature - absin.
ulcers, superficial, sores, on lower limbs, with - polyg.

MENSES, general, agg. during - acon., agar., aloe, alum., ambr., **AM-C.,** ***am-m., ant-c.,*** **ARG-N.,** ars., ars-i., asar., bar-c., bar-m., bell., bor., **BOV.,** bry., ***bufo, calc.,*** calc-p., cann-s., canth., caps., carb-an., **CARB-S.,** carb-v., ***caust.,*** **CHAM.,** chel., chin., ***cimic., cocc., coff.,*** con., croc., crot-h., cupr., ferr., ferr-i., ferr-p., gels., **GRAPH.,** hep., **HYOS.,** ***ign.,*** iod., **KALI-C.,** kali-n., ***kreos.,*** lach., laur., ***lyc.,*** **MAG-C.,** ***mag-m.,*** merc., mosch., ***mur-ac.,*** nat-c., ***nat-m.,*** nat-p., nit-ac., ***nux-m.,*** **NUX-V.,** oena., op., petr., ph-ac., ***phos.,*** plat., **PULS.,** rhod., rhus-t., sabin., sars., sec., sel., **SEP.,** ***sil.,*** spong., stann., stram., stront-c., **SULPH.,** sul-ac., thea., ***verat., vib.,*** **ZINC.**
acrid, excoriating - all-s., ***am-c.,*** amor-r., ant-t., ars., ars-s-f., aur., aur-m., bar-c., bov., calc-sil., canth., carb-ac., carb-s., ***carb-v., caust.,*** cham., ferr., ***graph.,*** hep., ***kali-ar.,*** kali-bi., **KALI-C.,** kali-m., ***kali-n.,*** kreos., ***lac-c.,*** **LACH.,** mag-c., merc., nat-c., ***nat-s., nit-ac.,*** petr., phos., prun., puls., raja-s., ***rhus-t.,*** sabin., sang., ***sars.,*** sep., **SIL.,** ***stram., sulph.,*** sul-ac., tere-ch., zinc.
after, agg. - alum., am-c., **BOR.,** ***bov.,*** bry., calc., canth., carb-an., ***carb-s.,*** carb-v., chel., chin., ***con.,*** cupr., ***ferr.,*** ferr-i., **GRAPH.,** iod., ***kali-c.,*** **KREOS., LACH.,** ***lil-t., lyc.,*** mag-c., merc., ***nat-m.,*** nat-p., **NUX-V.,** ***nit-ac., ph-ac., phos.,*** plat., puls., rhus-t., ruta, sabin., **SEP.,** sil., ***stram.,*** sulph., sul-ac., verat., ***zinc.*****afternoon** - ferr., lyc., mag-c.
ceases in - ***mag-c.***
while walking only - nat-s.

MENSES, general

ailments, of menses - acon., **BELL.,** calc., ***cham.,*** cimic.., cocc., ferr., ***graph.,*** ip., ***kali-c.,*** kreos., lach., mag-c., nat-m., nux-m., nux-v., phos., ***plat.,*** **PULS.,** ***sabin.,*** sec., ***sep., sulph.,*** verat.

bath, from - nux-m.

amel. - kali-c.

breast, with scirrhus of - brom., con.

careworn, tired women, in - ars.

cause, without - ust.

chagrin, from - coloc.

childbed, after - ***sep.,*** tub.

dancing, from excessive - cycl.

deafness, with - nat-c.

diabetes, in - uran-n.

dropsy, with - apis, apoc., kali-c., senec.

emotions, from - cimic., ign.

footsweat, suppression of, from - cupr.

fright, from - op.

functional - senec.

grief, from - ***ign.***

hands putting in cold water, from - lac-d.

jaundice, with - chion.

liver affections, with - lept.

love, from disappointed - hell., ***ign.***

milk in breast, with - phos., rhus-t.

months, for - lyc., sil.

neuralgic pain in body, with - kalm.

rheumatism, with - bry., caul., cimic., lach., rhus-t.

running, from excessive - cycl.

tuberculosis, in - solid., ust.

weaning, after - puls., sep.

wet, from getting feet - ***puls.,*** rhus-t., sil.

alternating with bloody discharge - tarent.

amelioration, during - alum., apis, aran., bell., calc., calc-f., cimic., cycl., kali-bi., ***kali-c.,*** kali-p., lac-c., **LACH.,** ***mosch.,*** phos., puls., rhus-t., senec., sep., ***stann.,*** sulph., ust., verat., ***zinc.***

of all complaints during - **LACH.,** ***zinc.***

amenorrhea, menses absent (see Suppressed) - ***acon.,*** aesc., agar., agn., alet., all-c., aln., ***am-c.,*** am-m., ammc., ***anac., ant-c., apis, apoc.,*** arg-n., ***arist-cl., ars., ars-i.,*** asar., **AUR.,** aur-i., aven., ***bar-c., bell.,*** bell-p., benz-ac., berb., ***bor.,*** brom., ***bry., calc.,*** calc-i., calc-p., calc-s., calc-sil., cann-s., canth., **CARB-S.,** carb-v., card-m., ***caul., caust., cham.,*** chel., ***chin.,*** chin-a., chlorpr., cic., ***cimic.,*** cina, ***coca, cocc., coch.,*** colch., ***coll., coloc.,*** **CON.,** cortiso., cortico., croc., crot-t., ***cupr., cycl., cypr.,*** dam., dig., ***dros.,*** **DULC.,** euph., eupi., **FERR.,** ***ferr-ar.,*** **FERR-I.,** ***ferr-m., ferr-p.,*** gast., gels., ***glon., goss.,*** **GRAPH.,** ***guai., ham.,*** hedeo, ***hell., helon.,*** hyper., ***hyos.,*** ictod., **IGN.,** indg., ***iod., kali-ar.,*** **KALI-C.,** kali-i., ***kali-n., kali-p., kali-per.,*** kali-s., kreos., lac-d., ***lach.,*** lil-t., linu-c., lob., **LYC.,** ***mag-c., mag-m.,*** mag-s., man., mang., ***merc., merl.,*** mill., ***mit.,*** nat-c., ***nat-m.,*** nat-p., nat-sil., nat-s., nep., ***nux-m., nux-v.,*** ol-an., ***ol-j.,*** op., ovi-g-p., parth., ph-ac., ***phos., phyt.,*** pin-l., pituin., ***plat.,*** plb., podo., ***polyg.,*** **PULS.,** ***rhus-t., sabad.,*** sabin., sang., sanic., sec., **SENEC., SEP.,** sieg., **SIL.,** ***sin-n.,*** spong., ***staph.,*** stram., **SULPH.,** sul-i., symph., tanac., tep., thiop., ***thuj.,*** thyr., **TUB.,** urt-u., ust., ***valer.,*** verat., verat-v., ***vib.,*** wies., wye., x-ray, xan., ***zinc.,*** zinc-p.

girls, in - ***ign.,*** x-ray.

milk in breasts, with - puls., ***rhus-t.***

molimen only - ***ant-c., calc., con., cur.,*** senec.

sexual desire absent - ***helon., sep.***

strain, after psychical and physical - hypoth., ign.

women, in, feeble - ***ars.,*** **SEP.**

hysterical - ***cypr., ign., sil.***

plethoric - **CALC.,** ***petros.***

psoric - ***psor.***

scrofulous - ***bar-c.,*** sulph.

ammoniacal - lac-c.

anger, brings on the flow - cham., nat-m.

appear, as if would - act-sp., ***aloe,*** ambr., am-m., ***apis,*** aur., bry., ***calc-p.,*** canth., carb-v., cina, cocc., ***croc.,*** ferr., hyos., inul., kali-c., kreos., laur., lil-t., lyc., ***mag-c.,*** mag-p., mosch., ***murx.,*** mur-ac., ***nat-c.,*** nat-m., ***onos.,*** phos., phys., phyt., ***plat., puls.,*** sang., ***senec., sep.,*** stann., staph., sul-ac., til., vib.

appears, afternoon, amel. in evening - pall.

cold, after a - ***puls.***

shock, from a - op.

suddenly - ***nat-m., phos.***

before, agg. - alum., ***am-c.,*** am-m., arg-n., asaf., asar., ***bar-c.,*** bar-m., bell., bor., **BOV.,** bry., **CALC., CALC-P.,** canth., carb- an., carb- s., ***carb-v.,*** caust., cham., chin., cina, cocc., coff., ***con.,*** croc., **CUPR.,** dulc., ***ferr.,*** ferr-i., gels., graph., hep., ***hyos.,*** ign., iod., ip., ***kali- c.,*** kali-n., ***kreos.,*** lac-c., **LACH., LYC.,** mag-c., mag-m., ***mang., merc.,*** mez., mosch., mur-ac., nat-c., **NAT-M.,** ***nat- p.,*** nux-m., nux-v., petr., ***ph-ac., phos., plat.,*** **PULS.,** rhus-t., rob., ruta., sabad., sars., **SEP.,** sil., spig., spong., stann., staph., **SULPH.,** sul-ac., thuj., valer., **VERAT.,** ***vib.,*** **ZINC.**

before and after, agg. - calc.

breasts, agg. - bry., ***calc., con., kali-c.,*** **KALI-M., LAC-C.,** lyc., ol-an., ***phyt.,*** puls.

beginning of, at, agg. - ***acon.,*** asar., bell., bry., ***cact.,*** **CALC-P.,** ***caust., cham.,*** cocc., coff., graph., **HYOS.,** ign., iod., ip., **KALI-C.,** ***lyc.,*** mag-c., mag-m., merc., mosch., nat-m., nit-ac., ***phos., plat., puls.,*** ruta., sars., ***sep., sil.,*** staph.**between,** periods, menses appear - ambr., bov., calc., cham., ***ham.,*** helo., hydr., ip., lyc., phos., puls., rhus-t., sabin., sep., sil.

daytime, only - ham.

sexual excitement, with - ambr., sabin.

MENSES, general

black - ***am-c., am-m.,*** ant-c., ant-t., apis, arn., arund., asar., ***bell.,*** berb., bism., calc-p., canth., ***carb-an.,*** carb-s., ***carb-v., cham., chin., cocc.,*** coc-c., ***croc.,*** **CYCL.,** ***elaps, ferr.,*** graph., ham., helon., ***ign.,*** jug-r., kali-m., **KALI-N.,** kali-p., kreos., **LACH.,** ***lyc., mag-c., mag-m.,*** mag-p., ***mag-s.,*** mang., ***nat-h.,*** nat-m., nat-s., nux-m., ***nux-v., ol-an.,*** phos., ***plat.,*** **PULS.,** raja-s., rob., ***sang., sec., stram.,*** sol-t-ae., ***sulph.,*** tep., thal., thuj., ust., xan.

clots, with - alet., arist-cl., ***croc.,*** hoit.

inky - ***kali-n.***

morning, only in - carb-an.

pitch-like - bism., ***cact., cocc.,*** croc., ***graph.,*** kali-m., kali-n., ***mag-c., mag-m.,*** mag-p., med., nux-v., ***plat.,*** sang.

sticky - coc-c.

stringy, and - ***croc.***

bladder symptoms, with - canth., erig., sabal., ***thlaspi.***

bloody, fluid, containing clots - alet., aloe, ant-c., apoc., arn., **BELL.,** bufo, caust., ***cham., chin., ferr.,*** ham., ign., ip., lyc., nat-s., nux-v., plat., plb., puls., **SABIN.,** sang., **SEC.,** stram., ust., vib.

bloody, mucus - alum., apis, bar-c., berb., ***cocc., croc.,*** lachn., nat-s., nux-m., **PULS.,** ***sep.,*** sul-ac., wies.

last day - ***apis.***

morning - nat-s.

breast-feeding, menses during - bor., ***calc., calc-p.,*** chin., ***pall.,*** rhus-t., ***sil.***

nursing agg. - pall., phos., ***sil.,*** vip.

breast, scirrhus of, with - brom.

bright-red - acon., aloe, alum., am-c., anan., ant-t., aran., ***arn.,*** ars., atro., bar-c., **BELL.,** bor., bov., brom., bry., calc., ***calc-p.,*** calc-sil., canth., carb-an., carb-v., ***caust.,*** cench., chin., ***cinnam.,*** coloc., croc., dig., dros., **DULC.,** ergot., **ERIG.,** eupi., ***ferr.,*** ferr-ar., ferr-p., fic., foll., form., glyc., graph., ***ham.,*** **HYOS., IP.,** kali-ar., ***kali-c.,*** kali-chl., kali-m., kali-n., kali-s., kreos., ***lac-c.,*** lachn., laur., led., lil-t., lyc., mag-m., manc., med., meli., merc., **MILL.,** nat-c., nit-ac., nux-m., pall., **PHOS.,** plat., puls., ***rhus-t.,*** sabad., **SABIN.,** ***sang.,*** sapin., ***sec.,*** sep., sil., spig., stram., stront-c., sulph., syph., thuj., ***tril., ust.,*** vib., visc., xan., zinc., zinc-p.

clotted - ***arn., bell.,*** caust., lil-t., ***puls., sabin.***

partly - ust.

dark, then - ***calc-p.***

foul, and - sang.

girls, in - ***calc-p.***

mingled with dark clots - **BELL.,** ***lyc., sabin., sec.***

morning, 9 a.m. - sol-t-ae.

brown - bapt., berb., **BRY.,** calc., ***carb-v., con.,*** goss., mag-c., ***nit-ac.,*** puls., rhus-t., ***sec.,*** sep., thuj., vesp.

coffee-ground, as - ***nit-ac.***

MENSES, general

ceases, suddenly - cocc.

and headache comes on - bell., lith.

lying, on - cact.

walking, after - ***lil-t.***

changeable, in appearance - **PULS.,** sep.

clotted - alet., aloe, ***am-c., am-m.,*** ant-c., ***apis,*** apoc., arg-n., arist-cl., ***arn.,*** bart., **BELL.,** bell-p., berb., bor., bov., bry., bufo, buni-o., cact., **CALC., CALC-P.,** canth., carb-an., carl., ***caust.,*** **CHAM., CHIN.,** ***cimic.,*** cina, ***cocc.,*** **COC-C.,** ***coff.,*** con., ***croc.,*** **CYCL.,** ***ferr.,*** ferr-p., fl-ac., foll., glyc., ***graph.,*** ham., helon., hoit., ***hyos.,*** hypoth., ***ign.,*** inul., **IP.,** jug-r., kali-c., kali-chl., ***kali-m.,*** kali-n., kreos., ***lac-c.,*** **LACH.,** lepi., ***lil-t., lyc.,*** macro., mag-c., ***mag-m.,*** mag-s., man., ***med.,*** merc., **MURX.,** ***nat-h., nat-m.,*** nat-s., nit-ac., nux-m., nux-v., ov., ph-ac., phos., **PLAT.,** plb., prot., psor., **PULS.,** raph., **RHUS-T.,** rhus-v., ***sabad.,*** **SABIN.,** sang., sanic., ***sec.,*** sep., sol-t-ae., spig., staph., ***stram.,*** stront-c., ***sulph.,*** tep., ***thlaspi,*** thuj., til., tril., ***tub., ust.,*** vib., vip-a., visc., xan., ***zinc.,*** zinc-p., zing.

clots and serum - lyc., ust.

dark - aloe, am-c., ambr., apis, arund., **BELL.,** bov., calc-p., cench., ***cham., chin.,*** cimic., ***cocc.,*** coc-c., coff., **CROC.,** culx., ***cycl., ferr.,*** ham., ign., kali-chl., kali-m., kali-n., ***lyc., mag-m.,*** med., nux-m., ***plat., puls.,*** **SABIN.,** ***sec.,*** staph., ***ust.,*** vip., vip-a., zing.

motion agg, slightest - **CROC.**

vaginismus, in - ***ign.***

first day - plb.

gelatinous, bright blood, with - laur.

large - ***apoc., ip., stram.***

last days - ***nat-s.***

offensive - ***bell.,*** berb., cham., ***croc.,*** helon., kreos., plat., sang., ***sec.***

partly fluid - apoc., bell., ***ferr.,*** graph., ham., plb., **SABIN.,** ***sec.,*** ust., vip.

serum, and - lyc., ust.

urinating, while - coc-c.

cramps, during (see Menses, painful) - acon., ***bell.,*** **CACT.,** ***calc-p.,*** caul., ***caust.,*** **CHAM.,** ***cimic.,*** **COCC.,** ***coff.,*** **COLOC.,** ***con.,*** der., **GRAPH.,** ***ign., kali-c.,*** kali-i., ***lach.,*** **MAG-P.,** ***nit-ac.,*** **NUX-V.,** onos., ***plat., puls.,*** sec., **SEP.,** stann., ***tub.***

labor-like pains - ***acon.,*** agar., ***alet.,*** aloe, ***am-c.,*** am-m., ant-c., apis, arg-n., ***asaf., bell.,*** berb., bor., bov., ***calc., calc-p., carb-an.,*** caul., ***caust.,*** **CHAM.,** chin., ***cimic.,*** cina, coff., ***con., cycl.,*** ferr., ***gels., graph.,*** hyos., ***ign., kali-c.,*** kali-s., kreos., ***lac-c., lach., lil-t.,*** lyc., ***mag-p.,*** med., mosch., ***nat-c., nit-ac., nux-m.,*** nux-v., ***plat., puls., rhus-t., sec., sep.,*** sulph., ust.

MENSES, general

dark - acon., alet., aloe, ***am-c., am-m.,*** ambr., anan., ***ant-c., ant-t.,*** apis, arn., ***ars.,*** ars-m., ars-s-f., arum-t., arund., ***asar., bell.,*** berb., ***bism.,*** bor., ***bov., bry., cact., calc.,*** **CALC-P.,** calc-s., cann-i., canth., carb-ac., ***carb-an., carb-s.,*** carb-v., carl., caul., **CHAM.,** ***chin., chin-a., cimic., coc-c., cocc.,*** coff., ***coloc.,*** con., cop., **CROC.,** ***crot-h.,*** cupr., ***cycl.,*** dig., dros., elaps, ***ferr.,*** ferr-ar., ferr-p., ***fl-ac.,*** form., gamb., ***graph.,*** **HAM.,** helon., hypoth., ***ign.,*** jug-r., ***kali-m., kali-n., kali-p., kreos.,*** lac-d., ***lach., aur.,*** led., ***lil-t.,*** lyc., macro., ***mag-c.,*** mag-m., mag-p., mag-s., man., ***med.,*** merc., nat-m., ***nit-ac., nux-m.,*** **NUX-V.,** ol-an., ***ph-ac.,*** phos., **PLAT.,** plb., **PULS.,** ***sabin., sang.,*** **SEC.,** sel., ***sep.,*** spig., ***staph., stram., sulph.,*** sul-ac., ***thlaspi, thuj.,*** tril., **UST.,** wies., ***xan.,*** zinc.
- clots, with - buni-o., hypoth.
- motion, agg. - ***croc.***
- rheumatic patients, in - **CALC-P.**
- wash out, difficult to - ***med.***
- watery, then - thuj.

daytime, only - **ABIES-N.,** cact., ***caust.,*** coff., cycl., ham., kali-c., **PULS.**
- mostly on walking - **PULS.**

delayed, (see first menses)

dysmenorrhea, (see Menses, painful)

evening, only - coc-c., coff., phel.
- lying, while - berb., bov., coc-c.

excitement, returns with the least - **CALC.,** sulph., tub.

exertion, brings on the flow - ***ambr., bov., calc., erig.,*** kreos., nit-ac., rhus-t., tril.

fearsome - nat-m.

feels, like coming - carb-an., lil-t., mosch., onos., phos., puls., senec., vib., zinc-chr.
- diarrhea, with - kali-i.
- frequently - plat.
- uterine spasms, with - kali-c.

flatus, during - mag-c.

flesh colored - apoc., nat-c., ***sabin., stront-c.***

foamy - arn., dros., ferr., ip.

forenoon, only - lycps., nat-s.

frequent, too early, too soon - acon., adlu., ***agar., alet.,*** all-c., all-s., aloe, alum., alum-p., alum-sil., ***am-c.,*** **AMBR.,** ***am-m., anac.,*** anan., ant-c., ***ant-t.,*** apis, ***apoc., aran.,*** aran-ix., ***arg-n., arist-cl.,*** arn., **ARS.,** ars-i., **ARS-M.,** ars-s-f., arund., asaf., asar., aur., aur-a., aur-m., aur-s., bapt., bar-c., bar-i., bar-m., bar-s., **BELL.,** benz-ac., ***bor.,*** **BOV.,** brom., **BRY.,** ***bufo,*** buth-a., ***cact.,*** **CALC.,** calc-ar., calc-i., ***calc-p., calc-s.,*** calc-sil., ***cann-i.,*** cann-s., ***canth.,*** **CARB-AN., CARB-V.,** cast., caul., ***caust.,*** cean., **CHAM.,** chel., ***chin., chin-a., chin-s., cimic., cina, cinnam., clem.,*** **COCC.,** coc-c., ***coff., colch.,*** coll., ***coloc., con., cop., croc.,*** crot-h., cub., culx., cur., **CYCL.,** cyna., daph., dicha., dig., digin., dirc., dulc., elaps, ***erig.,*** eupi., fago., **FERR.,** ferr-ac., ferr-ar., ferr-i., ***ferr-p., fl-ac.,***

MENSES, general

frequent, too early - flav., form., ***gamb.,*** gent-c., ***ger.,*** gink-b., glyc., goss., ***graph.,*** grat., ham., hell., ***helon.,*** hipp., hir., hist., hura, hydr., hydrc., hyos., hyper., ***ign.,*** ind., indg., inul., iod., **IP.,** joan., **KALI-AR.,** ***kali-bi.,*** **KALI-C.,** ***kali-fer.,*** kali-i., ***kali-m.,*** kali-n., ***kali-p., kali-s., kali-sil., kalm., kreos.,*** **LAC-C.,** lach., lachn., ***lam., laur., led.,*** lept., lil-t., lipp., lob., lyc., ***lyss.,*** mag-aust., ***mag-c.,*** **MAG-M.,** mag-p., ***mag-s.,*** man., **MANG.,** merc., merc-ac., ***merc-c., mez., mill., mosch., murx., mur-ac.,*** naja, nat-a., ***nat-c., nat-h.,*** **NAT-M.,** nat-p., nat-sil., nep., nicc., ***nit-ac.,*** **NUX-M., NUX-V.,** ol-an., ***ol-j.,*** onos., op., ***ov.,*** pall., palo., par., paraf., ***petr., phel., ph-ac.,*** **PHOS.,** phyt., pic-ac., **PLAT.,** ***plb.,*** pneu., prun., puls., raph., **RAT.,** rauw., ***rhod.,*** **RHUS-T.,** rhus-v., rosm., ***ruta,*** **SABIN.,** sang., sanguiso., sars., ***sec.,*** sed-ac., ***senec.,*** seneg., ***sep.,*** sieg., ***sil.,*** sin-n., sol-t-ae., spig., ***spong., stann., staph.,*** stram., stront-c., sul-i., ***sulph., sul-ac., sumb.,*** tarent., tell., **THLASPI,** ***thuj.,*** thyr., tong., ***tril., tub., ust.,*** vac., ***verat.,*** verb., visc., voes., wies., wild., ***xan., zinc.,*** zinc-p., zing.
- 2 days too early - lac-c.
- 3 days - asar., ***thlaspi.***
- 4 days - am-c., bov., ***lyc.***
- 5 days - nep.
- 6 days - ***am-c., mang.***
  - or 8 days, every - ***lyc.***
- 7 days - aran-ix., berb., **COCC.,** ***ferr-p., kali-s., lac-c., lach., manc.,*** **NAT-M.,** ***puls., senec., stram., ust., verat., xan.***
  - to 14 days - ***elaps.***
- 8 days - aran., ***cocc.,*** form., lyc.
- 10 days, every - ***phos.***
  - to 14 days - ***ign.***
- 12 to 16 days, every - ***sulph.***
- 14 days, every - bov., brom., calc., calc-p., ***cann-i.,*** cean., ***cocc.,*** ferr-p., ind., ***ip., lac-c., lil-t.,*** lyc., lyss., mag-c., ***merc., murx., nux-v., ph-ac.,*** phos., ***plat., puls.,*** sang., syph., ***thuj.,*** tril.
  - last, 2 weeks - ***calc.***
  - last, 7 to 9 days - ***sec.***
  - menopause, at - ***tril.***
- 15 to 20 days, every - coch.
- 21 days, every - berb., ***bufo,*** ferr-p., ***murx.***
  - intermittent, second day - pneu.
- anemic persons, in - ***mang.***
- chill, after - sulph.
- drive in cold air, after - am-c.
- infertility, in - ***canth., sulph.***
- menopause, in - tell.
- motion agg. - ***croc.***
- overheating, from - ***croc.***
- profuse, and - kali-c., sep., stann.
- scanty, and - alum., lept., nat-m.

fright, from - op.

first menses, (see menarche)

functional - senec.

MENSES, general

girls, in young - ***calc.,*** calc-p., carb-v., chin., ***cocc.,*** sil., verat.

green - graph., ***lac-c.,*** manc., med., psor., puls., pulx., ***sep.,*** tub., x-ray.

grey - thuj.

serum, like - berb.

grief, brings on - coloc., ***ign.***

gushes, in - ***bell.,*** cham., coca, cocc., erig., ***ip.,*** lac-c., phos., puls., ***sabin.,*** sars., ***tril.,*** zinc.

rising, when - ***cocc.***

tip toe, standing, on - cocc.

waking, when - coca.

heart, symptoms, with - cact.

hot - arn., ***bell.,*** bry., kali-c., kreos., lac-c., puls., sabin., sil., sulph.

like fire - lac-c.

lying, cease, when - sil., squil.

hot, applications amel. - ***mag-p.***

indelible - culx., mag-c., mag-p., med., pulx., thlaspi.

injuries, after - **CROC.**

inky - kali-n.

intermittent - acon., alum., alum-sil., am-c., ambr., apis, apoc., arg-n., ***berb.,*** bor., bov., bry., calc., canth., cast., ***caust., cham.,*** chin., ***cimic.,*** clem., coc-c., cocc., colch., con., cop., des-ac., ***cycl.,*** eupi., ***ferr.,*** ferr-ac., ferr-m., ferr-p., glon., ham., iod., kali-i., ***kali-s., kali-sil.,*** **KREOS.,** ***lac-c., lach., lil-t.,*** lyc., lycps., mag-c., mag-m., mag-s., mang., ***meli.,*** merc., mosch., murx., nat-c., nat-s., nicc., ***nit-ac.,*** nux-m., ***nux-v.,*** ph-ac., ***phel., phos., plb., psor.,*** **PULS.,** rat., rhod., rhus-t., ***sabad.,*** sabin., ***sec.,*** senec., ***sep.,*** sil., sol-t-ae., stram., ***sulph.,*** tril., ust., verat., vesp., ***vib.,*** xan., ***zinc.***

alternating with bronchial trouble - ***phos.***

blood, black - elaps.

ceases every, 2 days - mag-s.

2 or 3 days - ferr.

10 or 12 days - ***lyc.***

childbirth, after - acet-ac.

daytime, only - ham.

every other day - ***apis,*** ovi-g-p., ***xan.***

girls, young, in - polyg.

miscarriage, after - plat.

old maids, in - mag-m.

sexual excitement, with - ambr., sabin.

sometimes stronger, sometimes weaker - sabad.

women, childless or young widows, in - arg-n.

irregular - alum-p., am-c., ***ambr.,*** ammc., ***apis,*** apoc., aran., **ARG-N.,** ***art-v.,*** aur-m-n., aur-s., ***bell., benz-ac.,*** bry., buni-o., ***calc.,*** calc-i., calc-p., calc-s., calc-sil., ***carb-ac.,*** carb-s., caul., ***caust.,*** chel., ***chlol., cimic., cinnb., cocc., con.,*** cortico., cortiso., crot-h., cur., ***cycl., dig.,*** eupi., ferr., ferr-p., flav., ***graph.,*** guai., ham., hyos., hypoth., ***ign.,*** inul., ***iod., ip., iris,*** joan., ***kali-ar.,*** kali-bi., kali-p., ***kreos., lach., lac-d.,*** lil-t., ***lyc.,*** mag-c., mag-m., mag-s., ***manc.,*** merc., mosch., ***murx., nat-c., nat-m.,*** nicc., ***nit-ac.,*** **NUX-M.,**

MENSES, general

irregular - ***nux-v.,*** oena., ***ol-j.,*** op., ovi-g-p., phos., ***phys.,*** pip-n., pisc., plat., plb., **PULS.,** rad., rad-br., ruta, sabad., **SEC.,** ***senec.,*** **SEP.,** ***sil., staph., sulph.,*** tab., ***ter.,*** thuj., trio., ***tub.,*** ust., verat., vesp., xan.

between periods - ***bell., bov., calc., caust., cham., cocc., coff., elaps,*** eupi.

epilepsy, in - **ART-V.**

long and variable intervals, in - ***sulph.***

painful - am-c., ***bell.,*** bry., ***calc., caul., cimic.,*** cocc., ***cycl.,*** guai., inul., mag-s., murx., ***nat-m., nux-v.,*** phys., ***puls.,*** sec., ***senec., sep.***

every two weeks or so - ***bov., calc.,*** calc-p., croc., ferr-p., ***helon.,*** ign., mag-s., mez., murx., nit-ac., nux-v., ph-ac., ***phos.,*** phyt., sabin., sec., thlaspi, ***tril.,*** ust.

girls, in, since the first period - puls., sep.

girls, young, in - apis, calc-p., graph., ***mill., puls., sep.,*** xan.

puberty, at - ***puls.,*** sep.

time and amount, in - cimic., coc-c., ign., nux-m., plat.

vagina discharge, before - ***sep.***

itching, causing - petr., sulph., tarent.

jaundice, with - chion.

joints, pain, with - sabin.

jolting, from - ham.

late, too - absin., ***acon., agn.,*** alet., alum., alum-p., alum-sil., am-c., ang., ange-s., ***apis,*** arg-n., arist-cl., arn., ars., ars-i., aster., ***aur.,*** aur-i., aur-s., ***bell.,*** benz-ac., bor., bov., bry., calc., ***calc-p.,*** calc-s., canth., ***carb-ac.,*** carb-an., **CARB-S.,** carb-v., cast., caul., **CAUST.,** cench., cham., ***chel.,*** chin., cic., ***cimic.,*** cinnb., coca, ***cocc.,*** colch., coloc., **CON.,** croc., ***crot-h.,*** cub., **CUPR.,** cur., des-ac., ***cycl.,*** daph., dig., ***dros.,*** **DULC.,** euphr., ***ferr.,*** ferr-i., ***ferr-p.,*** flor-p., gast., ***gels.,*** glon., goss., **GRAPH.,** guai., ham., hell., ***hep.,*** hir., hist., ***hydr.,*** hyos., hyper., ***ign., iod.,*** joan., **KALI-C.,** kali-chl., ***kali-fer., kali-i.,*** kali-m., kali-n., ***kali-p., kali-s., kali-sil.,*** kalm., ***lac-c.,*** lac-d., **LACH.,** lec., ***lept.,*** lil-t., lith., lol., **LYC., MAG-C.,** mag-m., mag-s., manc., man., mang., ***merc.,*** merl., ***mit.,*** nat-c., **NAT-M.,** ***nat-p., nat-s.,*** nicc., nit-ac., **NUX-M.,** nux-v., ***oci-s., ov.,*** penic., ***petr., ph-ac., phos., pituin., plat.,*** pneu., ***podo., polyg., psor.,*** pulm-a., **PULS.,** pulx., rad., rad-br., rhus-t., rob., ruta, sabad., ***sabin.,*** sang., sapin., saroth., **SARS.,** sec., ***sel., senec.,*** **SEP., SIL.,** ***staph.,*** stram., stront-c., **SULPH.,** ***sul-ac.,*** tab., tarent., ter., ***thlaspi,*** thuj., til., tub., ***valer.,*** verat., verat-v., ***vib.,*** voes., xan., ***zinc.,*** zinc-p., ziz.

2 days - ***sulph., ter.***

2 or 3 months - **LACH.,** ***sil.***

5 days - flor-p., **SEP.**

5 months - ***graph.***

6 days - ***polyg.,*** tell.

MENSES, general
late, too, 6 to 8 weeks - ***crot-h.***
6 weeks - ***glon.***
7 days - ***lac-d., polyg.,*** tell.
8 days - aster., ***calc., iod.***
10 days - vib.
14 days - hyper., ***mag-m.***
17 days - ***lac-ac.***
21 days - ***puls.***
alternate months - syph., thlaspi.
alternating with bronchial trouble - ***phos.***
anxiety, with - ***graph., sulph.***
chill, with - **NAT-M.**
infertility, in - ***phos.***
profuse - bell., ***carb-ac., caust.,*** chel., cur., dulc., ferr., ***kali-c., kali-i.,*** lach., nit-ac., ***phos., sil.,*** staph., vib.
puberty, at - ***caust., dros., graph., kali-c., lach., lyc., nat-m.,*** phos., ***puls.,*** sep., sil., ***sulph.***
scanty - ***acon.,*** bov., ***calc.,*** con., ***graph.,*** kali-c., ***merc.,*** sep., vib.
several months - ***kali-c.***
vagina discharge, with - hyper., ziz.
wet feet, from getting - ***graph.***
lifting, agg. - kreos.
liver, affections, with - lept.
lochia-like - amor-r.
lying, agg. - ***am-c.,*** am-m., ***bov.,*** cycl., ***kreos.,*** **MAG-C.,** puls., ***zinc.***
back, on, agg. - cham.
cease while - ***cact., caust.,*** ham., **LIL-T.,** ***puls.,*** sabin., sil., squil.
more, on - kreos., mag-c., puls.
only when - kreos., ***mag-c.,*** sabin., sep.
maroon, colored - kali-fer.
meat, putrid, like - lachn., syph.
washings, like - brom., ***cycl.,*** ferr., nat-c., ***nit-ac.,*** stront-c.
membranous - acet-ac., apoc., ***ars.,*** bell., **BOR.,** brom., ***bry.,*** bufo, ***calc., calc-ac., calc-p., canth.,*** **CHAM.,** cimic., ***coll.,*** con., ***cycl.,*** ferr-m., guai., helio., ***hep., kali-bi.,*** kali-c., kali-chl., kali-m., kiss., lach., **LAC-C.,** ***mag-p.,*** merc., nat-c., nat-m., ***nit-ac., phos.,*** ph-ac., phyt., ***rhus-t.,*** sabin., sep., ***sulph., tril.,*** tub., ust., ***vib.***
puberty, at - cham.
menarche, first menses, appears before the proper age - ambr., ***ant-c.,*** bell., ***calc., calc-p.,*** canth., carb-v., ***caust., cham.,*** chin., cocc., coc-c., ferr., goss., hyos., ip., kali-c., lyc., merc., nit-ac., ***phos., puls.,*** rhus-t., ***sabin.,*** sec., ***sil.,*** sulph., verat.
delayed - acon., agn., alet., am-c., ant-c., apis, ***aur.,*** aur-s., ***bar-c.,*** bry., dam., ***calc., calc-p.,*** calc-s., ***carb-s.,*** cast., caul., **CAUST.,** chel., cic., cimic., cocc., ***con.,*** croc., cupr., dig., dros., dulc., ***ferr.,*** **GRAPH.,** guai., ***ham.,*** helon., hyos., **KALI-C.,** ***kali-p.,*** kali-per., lac-d, lach., ***lyc., mag-c.,*** mag-m., ***mang.,*** merc., **NAT-M.,** ***petr.,*** phos., polyg., **PULS.,** sabad., ***sabin.,*** sang., sars., **SENEC.,**

MENSES, general
menarche, delayed - ***sep.,*** sil., spig., staph., stram., stront-c., ***sulph., tub.,*** valer., verat., vib., ***zinc.***
feels disturbed, if slightly - fl-ac.
breasts, with undeveloped - lyc.
milk, from drinking much - lac-d.
menopause, during - **LACH.,** ***plat., plb.,*** **SABIN.,** ***sec.,*** **SEP.**
mental excitement agg. menses - **CALC.,** ***sulph.,*** tub.
mental symptoms, menses, during - acon., am-c., ars., bell., berb., calc., caust., ***cham., cimic.,*** coff., hydr-ac., ***hyos.,*** lyc., mag-c., mag-m., merc., mur-ac., ***nat-m.,*** ol-an., phos., plat., ***sep.,*** sil., stann., ***stram., verat.,*** zinc.
copious flow amel. - cycl.
after, agg. - alum., aur., nat-m., stram.
amel. - ***lach.***
suppressed menses - ***ferr., ign.,*** nux-m., plat., puls.
before - am-c., calc., caust., cocc., con., cupr., hyos., kali-c., **LACH.,** lyc., mag-m., mang., **NAT-M.,** nit-ac., phos., **PULS., SEP.,** ***stann.***
amel. - cimic.
beginning of, at - acon., cham., ferr., lyc., ***nat-m.***
milk, in breast, with - phos., puls., rhus-t.
milky - ***puls.***
molasses, like - mag-c.
month, alternate - syph., thlaspi.
months, for - lyc., sil.
moon, full, at - ***nux-v.,*** petr., ph-ac., puls., sep.
at full instead of new moon, appeared later - pall.
full or new moon, during - ***croc.***
new moon, at - lam., merc-ac., rhus-t., sil., staph., verat.
morning - am-m., ***bor., bov.,*** sulph.
less during day - am-m.
morning and daytime agg. - bor., cact., carb-an., ***caust.,*** cycl., ***lil-t., puls.,*** sep.
and evening only - ***phel.***
only - bor., ***bov.,*** carb-an., **SEP.**
rising, on - mag-c.
rising, on - plat.
walking, on - glon.
motion, agg. - bov., **BRY.,** canth., caust., croc., erig., ***ferr.,*** helon., ip., ***lil-t.,*** mag-p., sabin., ***sec.,*** thlaspi, ***tril.,*** zinc.
amel. - am-m., bov., ***cycl.,*** kreos., ***mag-c., sabin.***
downward agg. - ***bor.***
only on motion - cact., caust., ***lil-t.,*** manc., nat-s., sec.
mucus, the last day - ***apis.***
neuralgic, pain, in body, with - kalm.
nursing, agg. (see breast-feeding)
night, more at - ***am-c., am-m., bov., coca,*** coc-c., glon., ferr., **MAG-C.,** mag-m., ***nat-m.,*** puls., sep., sulph., ***zinc.***

MENSES, general

night, 11 p.m., flow commences - lac-ac.
more at - ***am-c., am-m.,*** bad., ***bov., coca,*** coc-c., cycl., ferr., glon., kreos., **MAG-C.,** mag-m., ***nat-m.,*** puls., sep., sulph., ***zinc.***
only at - am-c., am-m., bor., **BOV.,** coc-c., coff., cycl., mag-c., mag-p., nat-m.
sleep only during - mag-c.

noon - coca.

offensive - acon-l., alum., alum-sil., aral., ars., bapt., bart., **BELL., BRY.,** calc-p., ***carb-an.,*** carb-s., **CARB-V.,** carl., ***caust., cham.,*** chin., chin-a., cimic., ***coloc.,*** cop., ***croc., crot-h.,*** helon., hist., ***ign., kali-ar., kali-c.,*** **KALI-P.,** kali-s., ***kali-sil.,*** **KREOS.,** lach., lac-c., **LIL-T.,** lyss., mag-c., ***manc., med.,*** merc., nit-ac., nux-v., petr., phos., ***plat., psor.,*** puls., pyrog., raja-s., rheum, **SABIN.,** ***sang.,*** **SEC.,** sep., ***sil.,*** sol-t-ae., spig., ***stram.,*** sulph., syph., ust., vib.
acrid - ***bell., carb-v.,*** raja-s.
ammonia, like - aran., lac-c.
carrion-like - ***psor.***
fish, like spoiled - sol-t-ae., syph.
lochia, like - **LIL-T.**
pungent - kali-c., kreos.
putrid - **ALUM-SIL., ARS.,** cham., hoit., ign., kali-ar., lachn., med., ***psor., sulph.,*** syph.
semen, like - stram., ***sulph.***
sour - carb-v., cimic., sulph.
spoiled fish, like - syph.
strong - **CARB-V.,** cop., ***sil.,*** stram.

onset, trouble at - **PHYS.**

pain, flow, only after the - ***mag-c.***
ceases during pain - ***cycl.***
only in the absence of - ***cocc.,*** mag-c., plb.

painful, menses, (see Dysmenorrhea)

pale - ***alum.,*** alum-p., alumn., am-c., ant-t., apoc., arn., ars., ***atro., bell., berb.,*** bor., ***bov.,*** bry., bufo, calc., calc-s., canth., carb-an., ***carb-v., caul.,*** cench., chin., chin-a., cop., dig., dros., ***dulc.,*** eupi., **FERR.,** ***ferr-ar., ferr-p.,*** form., goss., **GRAPH.,** hyos., ip., ***kali-ar., kali-c., kali-i.,*** kali-n., kali-p., kali-sil., kreos., ***lac-ac., lac-d.,*** laur., led., lyc., mag-m., manc., ***mang.,*** merc., nat-c., **NAT-M.,** nat-p., nit-ac., ***phos.,*** prun., ***puls., rhus-t.,*** sabad., ***sabin.,*** sac-l., ***sec., sep.,*** sil., ***staph.,*** stram., stront-c., ***sulph., tarent.,*** til., tril., ***ust.,*** vib., zinc.
clots, with dark - cench.
then dark and clotted - ***staph.***
epilepsy, in - ***atro.***

pitch-like - bism., **CACT.,** ***cocc., croc., graph.,*** kali-m., kali-n., ***mag-c.,*** mag-m., med., nux-v., ***plat.,*** sang.

pregnancy, during - asar., cham., cocc., ***croc.,*** ip., kali-c., kreos., lyc., ***nux-m.,*** phos., plat., rhus-t., sabin., sec.
first month, during - ***calc.***

MENSES, general

profuse - acet-ac., ***acon., agar.,*** ail., ***alet.,*** all-s., aloe, alum., alumn., am-caust., ***ambr., am-c., am-m.,*** anan., ant-c., ant-t., ***apis,*** **APOC.,** ***aran.,*** arg-mur., arg-n., arist-cl., ***arn.,*** **ARS.,** ***ars-i.,*** ars-m., ars-s-f., arum-m., arund., asar., asc-t., aur., aur-a., aur-i., aur-s., bapt., bar-c., bar-i., bar-m., bart., **BELL.,** bell-p., benz-ac., ***bor.,*** **BOV.,** brom., ***bry.,*** bufo, buni-o., cact., **CALC.,** calc-ac., ***calc-i.,*** **CALC-P.,** ***calc-s.,*** calc-sil., ***calen.,*** camph., ***cann-i.,*** cann-s., ***canth.,*** caps., ***carb-ac., carb-an.,*** carb-s., ***carb-v., card-m., cast., caul., caust.,*** cean., cench., ***cham., chel.,*** **CHIN.,** ***chin-a., chin-s., cimic., cina, cinnam., cit-v.,*** clem., **COCC.,** coc-c., ***coff., coll., coloc., con.,*** cop., cortiso., ***croc., crot-h.,*** culx., cupr., cupr-ar., cur., **CYCL.,** ***dig.,*** digin., dulc., elaps, **ERIG.,** ***eupi.,*** fago., **FERR.,** ***ferr-ar., ferr-i.,*** ferr-m., ferr-p., ferr-r., ferr-s., fic., ***fl-ac.,*** flor-p., frax., ***gamb., gels., ger.,*** glon., glyc., ***goss.,*** grat., guare., hall, ***ham.,*** **HELON.,** ***hep.,*** hir., hoit., hura, ***hydr.,*** hydrc., hydroph., hyper., ***hyos., ign., iod.,*** **IP.,** iris, joan., jug-r., kali-ar., ***kali-bi., kali-br., kali-c.,*** kali-fer., ***kali-fer., kali-i., kali-m., kali-n., kali-p., kali-s.,*** kali-sil., kiss., ***kreos.,*** lac-ac., ***lac-c.,*** lac-v-f., ***lach.,*** lachn., ***laur., led.,*** lil-t., lipp., lob., ***lyc., lyss.,*** mag-arct., mag-aust., ***mag-c., mag-m.,*** mag-s., ***manc.,*** man., ***mang., med.,*** **MERC.,** ***merc-c.,*** mez., **MILL.,** ***mit.,*** mom-b., mosch., **MURX.,** mur-ac., ***nat-a.,*** nat-c., **NAT-M.,** nat-p., nat-s., nat-sil., nep., nicc., ***nit-ac.,*** **NUX-M., NUX-V.,** oci-s., ***ol-j.,*** onos., op., ***ov.,*** pall., paraf., penic., ***petr.,*** ph-ac., phel., **PHOS.,** ***phyt.,*** **PLAT.,** plb., ***prun., puls.,*** raph., **RAT.,** rhod., **RHUS-T.,** rhus-v., ***ruta,*** sabad., **SABIN.,** ***samb.,*** sang., ***sanguiso.,*** **SEC.,** sed-ac., sel., **SENEC.,** ***sep.,*** sieg., ***sil.,*** solid., spong., ***stann.,*** staph., **STRAM.,** stront-c., sul-ac., ***sul-i., sulph., sul-ac.,*** syph., tab., tanac., ***tarent.,*** tep., ter., tere-ch., thiop., ***thlaspi, thuj., tril., tub., urt-u., ust., vac., verat., vib.,*** vib-p., vinc., visc., voes., wies., x-ray, ***xan., zinc.,*** zinc-p., zing., ziz.
afternoon - mag-c., nat-s.
walking, while - nat-s.
alternate period absent, every - ***lach.***
less copious - ***thlaspi.***
alternating with gout - sabin.
breast-feeding, during - ***calc., phos.***
chilliness, after - sulph.
clots, large, with - apoc., coc-c., murx., zinc.
cold, air agg. - am-c.
baths agg. - ant-c.
taking cold, after - ip.
coldness of body, with - coff.
cold limbs, followed by - ***gels.***
icy with - sil.
convulsions, after - ***op.***
dancing, from - ***croc.,*** cycl., erig., sec.
daytime - ***caust.,*** coff., cycl., ham., nat-m., puls.
elderly women - crot-h., lach., ***plat., sars.***

MENSES, general

profuse, erotic, spasms, with - tarent.

evening - merc., murx.

only - ***coc-c.***

excitement, after - **CALC.**

exertion agg. - **AMBR.,** bell-p., ***bov.,*** **CALC.,** ***calc-p.,*** croc., **ERIG.,** ***helon.,*** mill., ***nit-ac.,*** rhus-t., ***sec.,*** tril.

faintness, with - acon., apis, chin., cocc., helon., **IP.,** lach., sulph., tril.

forceps, delivery, after - calen.

infectious disease, after - ergot.

infertility, in - ***canth., mill., phos., sulph.***

intemperate women - crot-h., lach., ***nux-v.***

labor, hasty, after - caul.

lean women, in - ***phos., sec.***

lying, agg. - ***kreos.,*** mag-c.

amel. - hypoth.

down, after - coc-c.

mania, with - ***sep.***

menopause, during - apoc., bov., calc., cimic., croc., helon., ***kali-br., lach., laur., nux-v.,*** paro-i., plb., ***sabin.,*** sec., ***sep.,*** sulph., tril., ***ust.,*** vinc.

long, after - vinc.

miscarriage or childbirth, after - **APIS,** chin., ***cimic.,*** helon., kali-c., ***nit-ac., plat., sabin.,*** sep., sulph., thlaspi, ***ust.,*** vib.

moon, new and full, agg. - croc.

morning - bor., ***bov.,*** carb-an., sep.

motion, from - ***croc.,*** **ERIG.,** ***ferr., helon., sabin., sec.***

only during - lil-t.

nausea, with - apoc., caps., ***ip.***

night - ail., ***am-c., am-m.,*** bov., ***coca,*** cycl., **MAG-C.,** mag-m., nat-m., ruta, ***zinc.***

nymphomania with - ***phos.,*** plat., sec., stram.

obstinate, continuous - nux-m., vinc.

onset, trouble at - **PHYS.**

rheumatic constitutions - ***ars., cimic.***

riding, from - am-c.

in cold air - ***am-c.***

sensation of copious menses - allox.

shocks, from - arn., ip.

short duration, and - am-c., ant-c., bor., kali-c., ***lach.,*** nat-m., phos., ***plat., sil., thuj.***

sitting, while - ***am-c.***

agg. - am-c., mag-m.

sleepiness, with - **NUX-M.**

standing agg. - am-c., **COCC.,** mag-c.

stomach troubles, with - calc., lyc.

tall women - ***phos.***

tenesmus of bladder and rectum, with - erig.

thunderstorm, from - nat-c., phos.

tubercular - ***calc., kali-c., phos.,*** sang., ***senec., stann.***

urination, hot, with - ferr.

painful, with - ***mit.***

vagina discharge, after - ***ferr.***

before - ***thuj.,*** **ZIZ.**

lying agg. - ***kreos.,*** mag-c.

vexation, after - nux-v., rhus-t.

virgins, in - ergot.

MENSES, general

profuse, walking, agg. - ***am-c.,*** **COCC.,** ***croc.,*** erig., ***lil-t.,*** mag-c., nat-s., ***pall.,*** puls., ***sabin.,*** ust., zinc.

amel. - kreos., mag-m.

women, cachectic - **CARB-AN.**

emaciated, in - arg-n., carb-an., phos., ***sec.***

hysterical - ***nux-v.***

intemperate - crot-h., lach., ***nux-v.***

lean - ***iod., phos., sec.***

nervous - ***kali-p.***

pale - ***helon.***

plethoric - ***acon.***

young - kali-br.

young, sedentary habits, of - coloc.

protracted - ***acon.,*** agar., agn., ***aloe,*** am-c., amor-r., apoc., aran., ***arg-n., ars.,*** ars-s-f., arund., asar., aspar., bar-ac., ***bar-c.,*** bell., bor., bov., ***bry.,*** **CALC.,** calc-ar., calc-i., ***calc-s.,*** calc-sil., cann-i., ***canth.,*** **CARB-AN., CARB-V.,** carl., caust., chel., ***chin.,*** chin-a., cina, cinnam., coc-c., ***cocc., coff., coloc., con., croc., crot-h.,*** **CUPR.,** cur., cycl., daph., ***dig.,*** dulc., ***erig.,*** **FERR.,** ferr-ac., ***ferr-ar.,*** ferr-m., ***ferr-p., fl-ac.,*** foll., glyc., graph., grat., ham., hip-ac., hyos., ***ign.,*** ind., iod., ip., ***kali-ar.,*** **KALI-C.,** kali-chl., kali-m., kali-n., kali-p., kali-s., ***kreos., lach.,*** laur., led., **LYC.,** ***lyss.,*** mag-aust., mag-c., ***mag-m.,*** mag-s., ***merc.,*** merc-c., ***mez.,*** **MILL.,** ***murx., nat-a., nat-c.,*** **NAT-M.,** ***nat-p., nat-s., nux-m.,*** **NUX-V.,** onos., ***ph-ac., phos.,*** **PLAT.,** prot., psor., **PULS.,** rad., raph., **RAT., RHUS-T.,** ruta, ***sabad.,*** **SABIN.,** sang., sanguiso., saroth., **SEC., SENEC.,** ***sep., sil.,*** stann., ***staph., stram., sulph.,*** sul-ac., tarent., ***thlaspi,*** thuj., thymol., ***tril., tub., ust.,*** verat-n., vinc., vip., visc., ***xan.,*** zinc., zinc-p.

1 day - aspar.

7 days - ***sabin.***

7 to 14 days - ***thuj.***

8 to 9 days - ***lach.,*** **SENEC.**

8 to 10 days - ***plat.,*** **SEP.**

8 to 18 days - ***thlaspi.***

10 to 12 days - ***murx.***

10 to 14 days - ***ust.***

12 to 18 days - ***tarent.***

12 to 18 days - agn.

14 days - ***coloc., xan.***

18 days - cann-i., ***thuj.***

labor, hasty, after - caul.

not ceasing entirely until the next period - ***ust.***

almost until - carb-v., nux-v., sabin., sec.

replaced by smarting vagina discharge - phos.

scarcely recovers from one, when another begins - thlaspi.

sexual desire, with - kali-br.

puberty, before - calc., cina, sabin., sil.

purple - ***puls.***

rectum, symptoms, with - erig.

MENSES, general

rest, agg. - am-c., ***ferr.,*** mag-m.
ceasing, when at rest, flows only when walking - squil.

return, after having ceased, the periods - alum., ambr., ***bor., calc.,*** carb-v., ***cocc.,*** cycl., ferr., ***kali-c.,*** kali-i., ***kreos., lach.,*** **LYC.,** mag-c., mag-m., mosch., murx., nat-m., ***nux-v.,*** ph-ac., phos., plat., puls., rhod., ***rhus-t.,*** sep., sil., ***staph.,*** stram., thuj., tril., ust., verat., zinc.
childbirth, soon after - tub.
elderly woman, in an - ***calc.,*** lach., mag-c., mag-m., ***phos., plat.,*** sep., staph.
excitement, from - ***calc.***
menopause, after - carl., lyss., mag-c., phos., thea.
overexertion, from - tril.

rheumatism, with - bry., caul., cimic., lach., rhus-t.

ropy, tenacious, stringy - cact., canth., **CROC.,** ***cupr., ign.,*** kali-chl., kali-m., ***lac-c.,*** lach., ***mag-c.,*** mag-m., mag-p., mang., phos., ***plat., puls.,*** sec., ***sep.,*** ust., ***xan.***

scanty - acet-ac., agav-t., agn., alet., ***alum.,*** alum-p., alum-sil., alumn., **AM-C.,** anac., ange-s., ant-t., ***apis,*** **ARG-N.,** arn., ***ars.,*** **ARS-M.,** ***art-v., asaf., atro., aur.,*** aur-a., aur-s., ***bar-c., berb., bor., bov.,*** bry., ***bufo,*** buni-o., ***buth-a., cact.,*** cael., calc., ***calc-ar.,*** calc-f., calc-p., calc-s., calc-sil., cann-i., canth., ***carb-an.,*** **CARB-S.,** ***carb-v.,*** carl., ***caul., caust.,*** chel., cic., ***cimic., cocc.,*** colch., ***coloc.,*** **CON.,** croc., crot-h., crot-t., cub., cupr., cur., **CYCL.,** des-ox., dig., dros., **DULC.,** ***elaps,*** erig., ***euphr.,*** eupi., ***ferr., ferr-ar., ferr-p.,*** form., ***gels.,*** goss., **GRAPH.,** guai., hed., helon., ***hep.,*** hip-ac., hir., hist., hura, hyos., ***ign.,*** iod., iris, ***kali-ar., kali-bi.,*** kali-br., **KALI-C.,** ***kali-i.,*** kali-n., ***kali-p.,*** **KALI-S.,** kali-sil., kalm., lac-ac., lac-c., lac-d., **LACH.,** lam., laur., lept., ***lil-t.,*** lob., ***lyc.,*** mag-arct., ***mag-c.,*** mag-m., mag-s., **MANG.,** ***meli., merc.,*** merc-i-f., merl., mez., mill., mosch., naja, ***nat-a., nat-c.,*** **NAT-M.,** nat-s., nat-sil., nicc., ***nit-ac.,*** nit-s-d., ***nux-m., nux-v.,*** oena., ***ol-an., petr.,*** phel., **PHOS.,** pip-n., pituin., ***plat., plb.,*** pneu., psor., **PULS.,** rat., rhod., rhus-t., ruta, ***sabad.,*** sabin., sac-l., sang., ***sars.,*** sel., **SENEC., SENEG., SEP.,** ***sil., stann., staph.,*** stram., stront-c., stront-nit., **SULPH.,** ***syph.,*** tarent., tell., ter., thuj., thymol., thyreotr., tong., trio., ust., valer., verat., verat-v., ***vib.,*** visc., wye., ***xan., zinc.,*** zinc-p.
acne, with - sang.
ceases when lying down - ***cact.***
chill, with - **NAT-M.**
clotted - cocc.
cold, from a - **NUX-M.**
consisting mostly of vagina discharge - cub.
convulsions with - ***glon.***
copious, then - ***nat-m.***
days, first three - mag-m.
daytime - ***bov.,*** **MAG-C.**
decreasing until they disappear - cocc.

MENSES, general

scanty, dyspnea, with - arg-n.
epilepsy, in - **ART-V.,** ***bufo, caust., kali-bi.***
evening - mag-c.
exertion, from - **NUX-M.**
agg., physical and mental - ***glon.***
first three days - mag-m.
fright, from - **NUX-M.**
infertility, in - ***canth.***
morning, flowing only in - carb-an., ***sep.***
motion agg. - ***sep.***
sexual desire lost - ***lach.***
sleepiness, with - ***helon.***
stomach troubles, with - cocc., puls.
vagina discharge, with - ***mez.***
after - ***sep.***
weakness, from - **NUX-M.**
women, fleshy - ***kali-br., kali-i***
hysterical - **NUX-M.**
plethoric - ***petros.***

short, duration - ***alum.,*** alum-p., **AM-C.,** ***ant-t.,*** arg-n., arist-cl., ars., ars-i., ***asaf.,*** aur-m., ***bar-c.,*** bar-i., ***berb.,*** bov., carb-an., carb-o., ***carb-s.,*** clem., ***cocc.,*** colch., ***con.,*** dirc., ***dulc.,*** euphr., fl-ac., gast., glon., gran., hed., ***graph.,*** iod., ***ip.,*** kali-c., kali-p., kali-sil., ***kreos.,*** **LACH.,** lyc., mag-c., mag-m., mag-s., ***mang., merc.,*** merl., mosch., ***nat-m.,*** nat-s., nicc., ***nux-v.,*** oena., ***ov.,*** phel., ***phos., plat.,*** pneu., ***psor.,*** **PULS.,** rhod., ruta, sabad., sars., ***sep.,*** sil., stront-c., sul-i., **SULPH.,** sumb., ***thuj.,*** til., vib., vip-a., zinc., ziz.
1 to 6 hours only - ***lycps.***
2 days - ant-t., **APIS,** ***mang.,*** pneu., ***verat.***
2 or 3 days - ***sep.***
3 or 4 days - ***lach.***
12 hours - ziz.
alternating days, on - ovi-g-p.
few hours - ***coc-c.,*** vib.
one day only - ***alum., apis, arg-n.,*** bar-c., bor., euphr., lepi., mang., nux-v., psor., pyrog., rad., **SEP.,** thuj.
day only, appear, at the interval, of - apis.
hour only - euphr., psor.
vagina discharge, bloody, followed, by - rad.

shreddy - phyt.

sitting, increased, while - cycl., mag-m.
amel. - kreos.

skin, symptoms, with - bor., carb-v., ***dulc., graph.,*** kali-c., mag-m., ***nat-m.,*** sang., sars., sep., stram., verat.

sleep, gushes during - ***coca.***
only during - mag-c.

spotting, of menses, between the periods - ***bov.,*** caust., eupi., ***ham.***

staining, fast - carb-ac., culx., lach., ***mag-c.,*** med., merc., pulx., sil., thlaspi, thuj.
linen - med.

standing - ***am-c.,*** cocc., mag-c., psor.
cease while - kreos.
increased, while - ***am-c.,*** mag-c.
tiptoe, on, agg. - cocc.

MENSES, general

stomach troubles, with - calc., cham., ***cocc.,*** lyc., nux-v., **PULS.**

stool, increased during - hep., iod., lyc., murx.

hard, from - ambr., lyc.

stooping, amel. - mag-c.

stringy, ropy, tenacious - cact., canth., **CROC.,** ***cupr., ign.,*** kali-chl., kali-m., ***lac-c.,*** lach., ***mag-c.,*** mag-m., mag-p., mang., phos., ***plat., puls.,*** sec., ***sep.,*** ust., ***xan.***

suddenly - acon.

suppressed, (see Amenorrhea) - ***abrot., acon.,*** aeth., ***agn.,*** alet., alum., alum-sil., alumn., ***am-c.,*** ambr., anan., ***ant-c., apis, arg-n.,*** arn., ***ars.,*** ars-h., ars-i., arum-t., ***asc-c.,*** aur., aur-a., aur-i., ***aur-m.,*** aur-m-n., aur-s., ***bar-c.,*** bar-i., **BELL.,** berb., bor., ***brom., bry.,*** bufo, cahin., ***calc.,*** calc-i., ***calc-p.,*** calc-s., calc-sil., ***camph., carb-an., carb-s.,*** carb-v., card-m., caul., ***caust.,*** cean., ***cham.,*** chel., ***chen-a.,*** chin., chin-a., chion., chlol., ***cimic., cocc., coc-c.,*** coch., cod., coff., ***colch., coll.,*** coloc., **CON.,** ***croc., cupr.,*** **CYCL.,** ***dig.,*** dros., **DULC.,** euphr., ***ferr., ferr-ar.,*** **FERR-I.,** ***ferr-p.,*** gast., ***gels., glon.,*** goss., **GRAPH.,** guai., hedeo, ***hell.,*** helon., hep., ***hyos.,*** ign., iod., **IP.,** ***kali-ar.,*** **KALI-C.,** kali-i., ***kali-m., kali-n.,*** kali-p., ***kali-s., kalm., kreos.,*** lac-d., **LACH.,** leon., ***lept.,*** lil-t., lob., **LYC.,** macro., mag-arct., mag-c., ***mag-m.,*** mang., merc., merc-c., mez., mill., morph., mosch., ***nat-m., nat-s., nicc., nit-ac., nux-m.,*** nux-v., ***op.,*** ox-ac., ***par.,*** petr., ph-ac., ***phos., phyt.,*** plat., plb., podo., ***prun.,*** **PULS.,** ***puls-n, rhod., rhus-t.,*** ruta, ***sabad.,*** sabin., sang., sars., sec., sem-t., **SENEC.,** ***sep.,*** **SIL.,** spong., stann., ***staph., stram.,*** stront-c., sul-i., **SULPH.,** symph., ***tanac.,*** tax., ther., thuj., tub., ***uran-n., ust., valer.,*** **VERAT., VERAT-V.,** visc., xan., ***zinc.,*** zinc-p., ziz.

anemia, in - ars., ars-i., caust., ferr-ar., ferr-r., graph., ***kali-c.,*** kali-p., kali-per., mag-ac., nat-m., ovi-g-p., ***puls., senec.***

anger, from - cham., ***coloc.,*** staph.

indignation, with - cham., cod., ***staph.***

asthma, with - **PULS.,** spong.

bathing, from - ***aeth., ant-c., calc-p.,*** cupr., ***nux-m.***

from cold - ***acon.,*** ant-c., kali-m., mosch.

from warm - ***aeth.***

cancer, from - kreos., ***lyc.***

chagrin, from - acon., ***chin.,*** **COLOC.,** puls., ***staph.***

chill, from - bell., dulc., nux-m., puls., sep., ***sulph.***

cold, from - ***acon., act-sp.,*** aral., bell., bell-p., bry., ***caj.,*** calc., ***cimic., coc-c., con., dulc.,*** graph., hell., nux-m., nux-v., ***plat.,*** podo., ***puls., rhus-t.,*** senec., ***sep.,*** sulph.

cold, hands, from - lac-d.

cold, water, from - ***acon., ant-c.,*** bell., calc., cham., cimic., ***con., dulc.,*** graph., lac-c., ***lac-d.,*** phos., ***puls., rhus-t.,*** sulph., ***verat-v.,*** xan.

MENSES, general

suppressed, cold, water, putting feet in - ***nat-m.***

putting hands in - ***con., lac-d.***

congestion, with, cerebral - ***acon.,*** apis, ***bell.,*** bry., calc., cimic., ***gels., glon.,*** lach., psor., sep., sulph., ***verat-v.***

chest, to - acon., calc., sep.

uterine, transient, localized, followed by chronic anemic state - sabal.

convulsions, with - ***bufo,*** **CALC-P.,** ***cocc., cupr.,*** gels., ***glon., mill.,*** **PULS., VERAT.**

dampness, from - calc., ***dulc.,*** graph., ***rhus-t.***

dancing, after excessive - cycl., ***sabin.***

delirium, with - stram.

diabetic attack, during - uran-n.

dropsy, with - apis, apoc., kali-c.

emigrants, in - bry., ***plat.***

emotions, from - ***cham., cimic.,*** kali-m., ***lach.,*** mosch.

exertion, from - bry., ***cycl., nux-m.***

falling, from - coloc.

fever, from - cimic.

fright, from - ***acon.,*** act-sp., bry., calc., cimic., coff., coll., gels., **IGN.,** ***kali-c., lyc.,*** **NUX-M.,** nux-v., ***op., rhus-t.,*** verat.

girls, in young - senec.

grief, from - **IGN.,** nat-m.

heated, after being - ***bry., cycl.***

ironing, by - bry., sep.

injuries, from - ***coloc.***

jaundice, with - chion.

love, from disappointed - hell., **IGN.,** nat-m., ph-ac.

milk, from drinking - lac-d., phos.

nurse, after ceasing to - sep.

pains, with, neuralgic around head and face - ***gels.***

rheumatic - bry., cimic., rhus-t.

perspiration of feet, from suppression of - ***cupr.***

plethoric women, in - ***acon.,*** arn., ***bell.,*** bry., calc., glon., nux-v., op., plat., sulph., verat., **VERAT-V.**

shock, from mental - ***ign., nux-v.***

stool, with urging for - podo.

suddenly - acon.

thunderstorm from - nat-c.

tuberculosis, in - ***lob., lyc., senec.,*** solid., ust.

vexations, from - ***acon.,*** act-sp., ***cham., chin.,*** cimic., coll., **COLOC.,** lyc., op., puls., ***staph.,*** verat.

walking, on - **KREOS.**

water, putting hands in cold - ***lac-d.***

working in - calc.

weakness, from - **NUX-M.**

wet, from becoming - acon., ***calc., dulc.,*** graph., ***hell.,*** nux-v., ***puls., rhus-t., senec.***

getting feet - ***acon., dulc., graph., hell., nat-m.,*** nux-m., **PULS., RHUS-T.,** ***senec., xan.***

MENSES, general

suppressed, women, hysterical - cypr., **NUX-M.,** ol-an., ***sil.***

feeble, in - **SEP.**

plethoric - ***acon.,*** arn., ***bell.,*** bry., calc., glon., nux-v., op., plat., sulph., verat., **VERAT-V.**

psoric - psor.

scrofulous - ***bar-c., sulph.***

tenacious - cact., **CROC.,** ***cupr.,*** kali-chl., lac-c., lach., ***mag-c.,*** mag-m., mang., phos., ***plat., puls.,*** sec.

thick - ant-c., ***arg-n.,*** arn., ***bell., cact., carb-v., cocc.,*** coc-c., cortiso., ***croc.,*** cupr., ferul., ***fl-ac., graph., kali-m.,*** kali-n., ***kali-p.,*** kreos., lac-c., ***lil-t., mag-c.,*** mag-p., mag-s., man., mang., ***nit-ac., nux-m.,*** nux-v., ***plat.,*** **PULS.,** ***sulph.,*** thymol., ***tril., ust., xan.***

thin - acet-ac., aeth., ***alum.,*** alumn., ant-t., ars., ars-m., ***bell., berb., bov., bry., calc.,*** **CARB-V.,** cocc., com., ***dulc., erig.,*** eupi., **FERR.,** ferr-ac., ***ferr-m., ferr-p.,*** ferul., gast., goss., ***graph.,*** haem., hell., kali-c., kali-p., lac-d., lach., ***laur.,*** mag-aust., ***mag-m.,*** mang., mill., nat-c., **NAT-M.,** nat-p., nat-s., ***nit-ac.,*** nux-m., ***nux-v., phos.,*** plb., prun., **PULS.,** ***sabin., sec.,*** sep., spig., stram., stront-c., sulph., sul-ac., tub., ***ust.,*** vib.

clots, with - ***cham., chin., ferr.,*** sec., ***ust.***

coagulating, not - ***kali-p.***

first thin - mag-m.

then clotted - stront-c.

meat water, like - stront-c.

throat, agg. - bar-c., calc., gels., lac-c., mag-c., sulph.

tuberculosis, in - solid., ust.

urinary, symptoms, with - berb., thlaspi.

urinating, only when - mag-aust.

vagina discharge, with - kreos., ***sep.***

vexation, after - acon., coloc., puls., staph.

vicarious - acon., ars., bapt., bell., ***brom.,*** **BRY.,** cact., ***calc.,*** chin., cimic., coll., ***crot-h.,*** cupr., ***dig.,*** dulc., erig., eupi., ***ferr.,*** graph., ***ham.,*** ip., kali-c., **LACH.,** mill., nat-s., nux-v., **PHOS.,** ***puls.,*** sabad., ***sang.,*** sec., ***senec., senec.,*** sep., sil., sulph., tril., ust., zinc.

walking, agg. - mag-c., **PULS.,** sabin.

ceases while - coc-c., sabin., sec.

increased while walking - mag-c., zinc.

less while - cycl., sabin.

only while - ***lil-t.,*** nat-s., sec., squil.

wash, off, difficult to - carb-ac., croc., culx., ***mag-c., med.,*** merc., puls., ***sil.,*** vib.

watery - ***alum.,*** ars., ***carb-v., ferr., graph., kali-c.,*** nat-p., ***puls.,*** sulph.

weakness, during - ***agar., aloe, alum., am-c.,*** am-m., ***ars.,*** ars-i., bar-c., bell., berb., bor., bov., bufo, cact., calc., calc-p., ***calc-s.,*** **CARB-AN.,** ***carb-s., carb-v.,*** caul., ***caust.,*** cimic., ***cinnb., cocc.,*** eupi., ferr., ferr-i., ***graph., helon.,*** ign., ***iod.,*** ip., ***kali-c.,*** kali-n., ***kali-s., lach., lil-t.,*** lyc., ***mag-c., mag-m.,*** mosch., ***murx.,*** nat-a., nat-c., nat-m., ***nicc.,***

MENSES, general

weakness, during - ***nit-ac.,*** nux-m., ***nux-v., petr.,*** phel., ***phos., sabin., sec.,*** senec., **SEP.,** stann., ***sulph.,*** tarent., thuj., tril., tub., ***uran., verat.,*** vinc.

amel. - ***sep.***

breathe, can scarcely, must lie down - ***nit-ac.***

desire to lie down, with - bell., ip., ***nit-ac.***

end of - bov., iod.

going up stairs, when - ***iod.***

painful - bell., bufo.

stool, after - nux-v.

talk, can scarcely - ***carb-an., stann.***

after - ***alum.,*** berb., benz-ac., calc-p., ***carb-an.,*** caul., **CHIN.,** ***cimic.,*** iod., **IP.,** nat-m., ***phos.,*** plat., sec., sulph., thuj.

disproportionate to loss of blood - ***ip.***

appearance of, amel. - cycl., mag-m.

at beginning - phel.

before - alum., aur-s., ***bell.,*** brom., carb-ac., cimic., ***cocc.,*** ferr., iod., ***mag-c., nat-m.,*** nux-m., phel., zinc.

wet, getting feet, from - puls., rhus-t.

white, of egg, like, morning agg. - calc-p.

METRORRHAGIA, (see Bleeding, uterine)

MISCARRIAGE, (see Pregnancy, chapter)

MOISTURE, genitalia - ***petr., thuj.***

sensation of - eup-pur.

vulva and thigh, between - calc.

moisture, vulva and thigh, between - calc.

MOLES, uterus - canth., chin., ***kali-c.,*** merc., ***nat-c., puls.,*** sabin., ***sil.,*** sulph.

promotes expulsion of - canth., sabin.

NEURALGIC pain, genitalia - acon., ***agar.,*** am-br., ap-g., ***apis, aran., atro., bell.,*** berb., bry., bufo, ***cact.,*** calc., canth., ***caul., chin., cimic., coloc., con.,*** crot-c., cupr-ar., ***dios.,*** ferr., ferr-p., ***gels.,*** goss., graph., ham., hyper., kali-br., kali-p., ***lach., lil-t.,*** mag-m., ***mag-p.,*** meli., merc., merc-c., ***murx., naja,*** op., phyt., ***plat.,*** podo., puls., ***sabal.,*** sal-n., sec., ***staph.,*** sumb., tarent., thea., ***ust., vib.,*** visc., ***xan., zinc-valer.***

back, coming from, circumferentially - plan., sep.

to abdomen - sep., visc.

to pubes - bell., ***sabin.***

to thights, to, legs - bufo, carb-ac., cham., ***cimic.,*** puls., ***sabin.***

chest, radiating, to - lach., murx., vesp.

hip to hip - ***bell.,*** calc., chin., ***cimic., coloc.,*** lac-c., pall.

intermittent - ***goss.,*** thlaspi, ziz.

side, right, upwards across body, thence to left breast - murx.

umbilicus to uterus - ip.

NODULES, genitalia - calc., ***lac-c.,*** merc., phos., syph., thuj.

nodules, vagina, in - ***agar.***

labia, borders of - phos.

NUMBNESS, genitalia - bar-c., eup-pur., mosch., ***plat.***
washing in cold water, after - eupi.
numbness, ovaries - apis, ***podo.***
beginning in right, extending to hip and ribs and over thigh, lying on it amel. - apis
painful, extending to limb - podo.
numbness, uterus - phys.
numbness, vagina - berb., brom., phos., plat., sep.
sex, during - ferr., kali-br., phos., plat.

NYMPHOMANIA, (See Sex)

OOPHORITIS, inflammation of ovaries - **ACON.,** aesc., am-br., ambr., ***ant-c.,*** **APIS,** arg-m., arn., ars., ars-i., aur., **BELL.,** brom., ***bry., cact., canth.,*** caps., ***chin.,*** cimic., **COLOC.,** con., crot-h., cub., dulc., euph., graph., ***guai.,*** ham., hep., ign., ***iod., lac-c., lach., lil-t.,*** **LYC.,** mag-p., ***med.,*** **MERC.,** nit-ac., ***nux-v., pall., ph-ac.,*** **PHOS.,** ***phyt., plat.,*** **PODO.,** ***puls.,*** rhus-t., sabad., **SABIN.,** staph., ***syph., thuj.,*** ust., ***verat-v.,*** zinc.
acute - ***acon.,*** am-br., ***apis, bell., bry.,*** cact., ***canth., cimic., coloc.,*** con., ferr-p., guai., ***ham., iod., lach.,*** lil-t., merc., ***merc-c.,*** ph-ac., plat., ***puls.,*** sabin., thuj., visc.
peritoneal involvement, with - ***acon.,*** apis, ars., ***bell.,*** bry., canth., chin., chin-s., coloc., ***hep., merc-c.,*** sil.
feet wet, after getting - ***puls.***
gonorrhea, suppressed, after - ***canth.,*** **MED.,** ***thuj.***
hemorrhage, after - ***chin., plat.***
left - arg-m., caps., graph., ***lach.,*** lil-t., ***thuj.,*** vesp., zinc.
menses, suppressed - ***acon.,*** cimic.
menstrual flow suddenly checked - **ACON.,** ***puls.***
miscarriage, after - sabin.
right - aesc., ***apis, arg-m., bell., bry.,*** iod., **LYC.,** ***pall.,*** **PODO.**
sexual excesses, from - ***chin., ham., plat., staph.***

OPEN feels, uterus - lach., sanic.
opens and shuts, as if - nat-h.
open, vagina, vulva feels - bov., sabal., sec., sep.

OVARIES, complaints following surgery - ars., ***bell., bry., calen.,*** chin., coff., ***colch.,*** hyper., ip., lyc., naja, nat-m., nux-v., orch., ***ov.,*** **SEP.,** ***staph.***

PAIN, genitalia - aloe, ambr., apis, asaf., aur., bar-c., **BELL.,** berb., brom., ***calc., calc-p., carb-an.,*** caust., cham., ***cimic.,*** coc-c., ***con.,*** eupi., ***graph., kali-c.,*** kreos., ***lac-c., lach., lil-t., lyc., merc-c.,*** nat-m., ***nux-m.,*** nux-v., onos., ***phos., plat.,*** **PULS.,** ***sabin.,*** sec., senec., **SEP.,** ***staph., sulph., thuj.,*** til., tril., ***urt-u.,*** ust., ***vib.,*** visc., ***zinc.***
breathing deep - bry.
cough agg. - thlaspi.
labor, after - sabin.

PAIN, genitalia
lying, agg. - ambr., ferr., kreos., murx., ***puls.***
doubled up, amel. - cact., cimic., nux-v.
on back, amel. - onos., sabin.
menses, before - chin., ***croc.,*** lyc., plat., sulph.
between - ***bry.,*** ham., iod., kreos., ***sep.***
motion, on - berb.
night in bed - coc-c.
paroxysmal - ***staph.***
pulsating - ***aesc.,*** bell., brach., bran., ***cact.,*** calc-p., hep., murx.
rising from a seat, on - thuj.
sitting, while - ***lac-c.,*** staph., thuj.
up in bed amel. - coc-c.
spasmodic - ign., kreos., nux-v., thuj., ***xan.***
splinter-like when walking or sitting - cycl.

PAIN, ovaries - acon., aesc., am-m., anan., **APIS,** ***arg-m., arg-n.,*** arn., ars., ars-i., ***atro.,*** aur., **BELL.,** brom., ***bry., bufo, cact.,*** calc., ***canth.,*** carb-ac., ***cench.,*** cham., cimic., cocc., coll., **COLOC.,** cop., con., crot-h., gels., graph., guai., ***ham., helon.,*** hydrc., ***ign., iod., kali-br.,*** kali-p., kreos., lac-ac., ***lac-c.,*** lac-d., **LACH.,** ***lil-t.,*** **LYC.,** lyss., **MAG-P.,** med., ***merc.,*** murx., ***naja,*** onos., ***pall., phos., phyt., plat.,*** plb., **PODO.,** ***puls., ran-b., rhod.,*** sabad., sabal., sarr., sec., senec., ***sep.,*** stann., ***staph.,*** sulph., syph., tarent., ter., ther., **THUJ.,** tub., urt-u., ***ust.,*** vesp., vib., ***xan.,*** wye., zinc., zinc-valer.
alternating, pain in eye, with - sulph.
sides - cimic., coloc., **LAC-C.,** lil-t., onos., ust.
animated, conversation - **PALL.**
bending, backward, amel. - ***lac-c.***
double amel. - ***coloc.,*** kali-p., op.
breast, with pain in - sabal.
breathing agg. - bry., graph., ***lac-c.***
celibacy, from - ***apis,*** kali-br.
changes, in the weather, from - ***ran-b., rhod., rhus-t.,*** thuj.
childbirth, after - lach.
company, amel. - ***pall.***
continence, from - ***apis,*** kali-br.
drawing up leg amel. - ap-g., coloc.
eating amel. - iod.
extending, limbs, amel. - ***plb.***
extending to
abdomen - con., ham.
back, to - abrot., aesc., ***am-c.,*** am-m., asar., bell., ***bor.,*** calc., ***calc-p.,*** caust., ***cham.,*** cic., ***cimic.,*** cupr., cycl., ***gels.,*** graph., ***helon.,*** kali-c., mag-m., merc., nit-ac., ***nux-v.,*** phos., plat., podo., ***puls.,*** rad., sabin., ***senec., sep.,*** spong., ***sulph.,*** syph., vib., ***xan.***
right - rumx.
up the - arg-m.
backward - bell., carb-ac., con., lil-t., sep.
breast, to - lil-t., murx., senec.
chest, to - apis, caul., cham., cimic., ***cupr.,*** lach.
to left - apis.

PAIN, ovaries
extending, to, crural region, down - podo., staph., xan.
diagonally upward - apis, med., ***murx.***
downwards - med.
and forwards - arg-m.
genitals, to - lach.
genito-crural nerve - xan.
groin, to - am-c., bor., ***bufo, caul., cub.,*** kali-c., lil-t., plat., tanac., ***ust.***
to hypogastrium, and - xan.
to left - lil-t., ust.
to through toward left leg - plat.
heart, to - naja.
hips, to - apis, berb., brom., con., lil-t., merc., ust., xan.
knee, to - lac-c., wye.
limbs, down - ***apis, calc.,*** ferr-i., goss., lac-c., ***lil-t., pall.,*** podo., thuj., ust., xan.
left - apis, cham., lil-t., phos., thuj., ust.
right - apis, podo.
liver, to - lach., med., ph-ac.
loins, to - staph.
one to the other - coloc., **LAC-C.,** med., onos., ust.
outward - sep.
pubes - aln., bov., colch., cycl., ***rad.,*** sep., vib.
rectum - ***aloe,*** xero
sacrum, to - arg-n.
shoulder - podo.
shoulder blade, to - bor.
stomach, to - coloc.
thighs, to - ***apis,*** arg-m., ***arg-n., ars.,*** berb., ***bry., cact., calc.,*** carb-an., cham., coloc., graph., ***lac-c., lil-t.,*** nat-m., pall., ***phos., podo.,*** staph., ***thuj.,*** ust., xan., wye., zinc-valer.
to anterior surface - lil-t., nat-m., xan.
to hip, over, region of - xan.
to inner surface - arg-n., ars., ***lil-t., phos.***
to inner surface, and down knee - podo.
to outer surface - lil-t.
upward - cimic., con., lach., lil-t.
uterus, to - ham., ***iod.,*** lach., sep., ust.
vagina, to - sep.
flexing, thigh, amel. - ***coloc., pall.***
gonorrhea, chronic, with - ***plat.***
hawking - graph.
head, with pain in - sabal.
hemorrhagic, subjects, in - crot-h.
intermittent - bell., cham., lac-c., lach., thuj.
jarring, agg. - arg-n., ***bell.,*** lil-t., pall.
labor, after - **LACH.**
left - aesc., abrot., am-br., ap-g., apis, **ARG-M.,** arg-n., ***brom.,*** caps., ***carb-ac.,*** caul., ***cimic., coloc.,*** erig., eup-pur., frax., graph., ***ham.,*** iod., kali-br., kali-c., ***kali-p.,*** **LACH.,** ***lac-c.,*** **LIL-T.,** lyss., magn-gr., med., ***merc.,*** murx., **NAJA,** ovi-g-p., ***phos.,*** pic-ac., ***plat.,*** sulph., ***tarent.,*** thea., ***ther.,*** thlaspi, ***thuj.,*** **UST.,** ***vesp.,*** visc., wye., ***xan., zinc.***
coughing - naja.

PAIN, ovaries
left, lying, on, back amel. - kali-p.
left side agg. - thuj.
left side amel. - kali-p., pall.
walking in open air - carb-ac.
left, extending, to abdomen - ham., lil-t.
to heart - brom., cimic., lac-c., lach., lil-t., ***naja,*** sulph., tarent., vib.
to, right - apis, lac-c., **LACH.,** lil-t., naja, syph., ust.
to, small of back - ***aesc.,*** merc., plat., podo., syph.
thigh, down - lil-t., thuj.
uterus - naja, ust.
lifting, from - rhus-t.
love-sick girls, in - ant-c.
lying, agg. - ambr., murx.
amel. - pall., podo., thuj.
back, on amel. - kali-p., rhus-t.
hard board or floor, on - rhus-t.
left side agg. - thuj.
amel. - kali-p., ***pall.***
painful side amel. - ***bry.***
right side amel. - apis.
menses, during - ***apis,*** arg-m., ***bell.,*** bry., cench., cocc., con., gels., iod., kali-p., lac-c., **LACH.,** lyc., lil-t., merc., ***pall., phos., plat.,*** podo., ther., ***thuj.,*** tub., ust., xan.
after - apis, bor., cupr., goss., graph., iod., **LACH.,** ***pall.,*** ust., zinc.
and during - zinc-valer.
amel., during - ***lac-c., lach.,*** mosch., ust., ***zinc.***
before - ***apis, bell.,*** bry., cact., canth., ***cench., cimic., coloc.,*** graph., ham., iod., joan., kali-n., lac-c., **LACH.,** ***lil-t.,*** pic-ac., podo., sal-n., tarent., ***thuj.,*** ust., vib., ***zinc.***
mental, exertion - calc.
motion, agg. - ***ars.,*** **BELL., BRY.,** ***cench., lac-c., pall.,*** podo., ther.
amel. - iod.
moving, feet amel. - ***ars.***
music, and excitement - pall.
night - kali-p., ***merc.,*** podo., ***syph.***
numbness, with, and shifting gases in ascending colon - podo.
ovulation, at - cocc., ham., puls., sep.
paroxysmal - ***ham.***
pregnancy, during - kali-p., podo., xan.
pressure, agg. - staph.
amel. - coloc., pall., podo., zinc.
pulsating - cop., onos.
raising, arms - ***apis,*** sulph.
the leg - lyc.
restlessness, with, physical - kali-br., vib., ***zinc.***
riding agg. - thuj.
right - absin., alum., ***apis, arg-n.,*** ars., ars-i., aur-m-n., **BELL.,** bran., ***bry.,*** calc., coloc., croc., cub., eupi., fago., graph., ***iod.,*** lach., lil-t., **LYC.,** med., murx., ***pall.,*** phyt., **PODO.,** sarr., syph., ust., xan.
lying on right side amel. - ***apis.***

PAIN, ovaries
right, to left - graph., **LYC.,** xan.
to uterus - iod., podo.
right, extending to, back - xan.
to, hip - xan.
to, point under scapula - aur-m-n.
to, shoulder blade - aur-m-n.
to, thigh - xan.
rubbing, amel. - pall.
sex, after - ***apis,*** lac-c., ***plat., staph.,*** syph., thuj.
sexual desire, during - ***kali-br.***
sitting, bent agg. - ***ars.***
sleep, on going to - kali-p.
society, from - **PALL.**
standing, on - apis, pall.
stepping, agg. - arg-n., ***bell.,*** lil-t., pall.
stooping - apis.
storm, before - ***rhod.,*** rhus-t.
stretching, bed, in - apis
legs, agg. - podo.
amel. - plb.
touch - bry., graph.
turning, in bed - lyc.
urging, to urinate, when - ***thuj.***
urination, during - thuj.
frequent, with - vesp.
walking - ***apis,*** arg-n., ***bry.,*** lil-t., med., merc., pall., podo., thuj.
lying down amel. - carb-ac., podo., sep., ***thuj.,*** ust.
open air, in the, while - ***carb-ac.***
rapidly - lac-ac.
warm, bed agg. - ***apis, merc.***

PAIN, uterus - absin., ***acon.,*** all-c., anan., ant-c., arn., ars., aster., ***aur.,*** bar-m., **BELL.,** ***bry.,*** bufo, cact., calad., ***calc., calc-p.,*** calc-s., carb-an., carb-s., cast., ***caul., caust., cham.,*** chin., ***cimic.,*** cinnam., ***cocc., coff.,*** coloc., ***con.,*** croc., crot-c., cub., cur., ***ferr.,*** ferr-ar., ferr-p., fl-ac., ***gels.,*** graph., ham., helon., hyos., ign., iris, kali-ar., ***kali-c.,*** kali-p., kreos., ***lac-c.,*** **LACH.,** ***lil-t., lyc.,*** lyss., mag-m., med., merc., merc-c., mosch., ***murx.,*** nat-a., ***nat-c., nat-m.,*** **NUX-V.,** onos., op., pall., ***plat.,*** **PODO., PULS.,** ***rhus-t.,*** rob., ***sabin., sec., sep.,*** sulph., tarent., ***ter.,*** ust., verat-v., vib.
after pains, of childbirth - acon., **ARN.,** asaf., aur., ***bell.,*** bor., ***bry., calc.,*** carb-an., carb-v., **CHAM.,** chin., cic., ***cimic.,*** cina, cocc., ***coff., con.,*** croc., **CUPR.,** ***ferr., gels.,*** graph., hyos., **HYPER.,** ***ign.,*** iod., ip., **KALI-C.,** kreos., lach., lyc., nat-c., ***nat-m.,*** nux-m., ***nux-v.,*** op., par., plat., ***podo.,*** **PULS., RHUS-T.,** ***ruta.,*** **SABIN., SEC.,** ***sep.,*** sul-ac., ***sulph., vib., xan.,*** zinc.
child nurses, when - ***arn., cham.,*** con., puls., **SIL.**
childbirth, after - **CAST-EQ.**
alternating, with pain in heart - ***lil-t.***
anger, after - **CHAM.**
ascending agg. - plat.

PAIN, uterus
bath, after a - crot-c.
bending, double amel. - ***acon., cimic.,*** **COLOC.,** ***nux-v.***
cold damp weather - ***calc-p.***
coughing, on - thlaspi.
curettage, after - kali-c., nit-ac., thlaspi
eating, after - ***caust.***
evening - cact., pall., ped.
exertion, after - pall.
extending to
back - ***am-c.,*** am-m., asar., ***bell., bor.,*** calc., ***calc-p.,*** caust., ***cham.,*** cic., ***cimic.,*** cupr., cycl., ***gels.,*** graph., ***helon., kali-c.,*** kreos., mag-m., nit-ac., ***nux-v.,*** phos., plat., podo., ***puls.,*** rad., sabin., ***senec., sep.,*** spong., vib., ***xan.***
to groin - **SABIN.**
body, over whole - xan.
breasts - lyss., murx.
and right side of abdomen - lyss.
left - murx.
chest - caul., cham., cimic., ***cupr., lach., murx.***
coccyx and toes - sec.
diagonally upwards - ***murx.***
down the thighs - ***am-m.,*** apis, ars., berb., bry., bufo, cact., ***calc.,*** cast., ***caul.,*** cham., chel., cimic., coff., colch., con., ***gels.,*** graph., ham., ***kali-c.,*** kali-i., kreos., ***lac-c.,*** lil-t., mag-c., mag-m., nat-m., nit-ac., nux-v., ox-ac., plat., rhus-t., sabin., sep., staph., tril., ust., ***vib.,*** xan.
reading or writing, from - nat-m.
downward - aesc., ***apis,*** ars., ***cact.,*** calc., calc-p., con., ***graph.,*** ham., ip., kali-i., ***kreos.,*** lac-c., mag-m., nat-m., nit-ac., nux-v., sec., ***sep.,*** ust.
epigastrium - iris.
groins - bor., ***caul.,*** kali-c., lil-t., plat., tanac., ***ust.***
heart - xan.
labia, into - lyss.
liver - ph-ac.
pelvis, through, antero-posteriorly or laterally - bell.
pubes - aln., bov., colch., cycl., rad., ***sabin.,*** sep., vib.
rectum - ***aloe,*** xero
sacrum, to - calc-p.
stomach - cact., elaps, ran-b., raph.
throat - gels.
umbilicus - nux-v., sep.
upward - **LACH.,** lyc., lyss., ***murx.,*** phos., ***sep.***
to right side of abdomen - lyss.
flow of blood amel. - arg-n., bell., kali-c., **LACH.,** mosch., sep., sulph., ust., ***vib.***
gradually, comes and goes - ***plat.,*** stann.
humiliation, from - ***cocc.***
jar, agg. - **BELL.,** ***lach., lil-t.***
leaning on it - ped.

PAIN, uterus
lying down - ***ambr., ferr.***
on back amel. - ***onos.***
on right side amel. - sep.
maddening - acon., ***bell., cact.,*** cimic., ***plat.***
menopause period, during - agar., ***cimic.,*** cocc., lach., puls., ***sep.***
menses, during (see Dysmenorrhea) - ***acon., agar.,*** agn., alum., ***am-c.,*** ars-m., **BELL., CACT., CALC.,** ***calc-p.,*** calc-s., caul., ***cham., cimic., cocc.,*** dam., ***gels., ham., ign., kali-c.,*** kali-s., ***kreos., lac-c., lach., lil-t., lyc., mag-m.,*** med., merc., **NUX-V.,** phyt., ***plat.,*** **PULS.,** sars., sep., ***stann., sulph., tarent., tub., ust.,*** xan.
amel., during - bell., ***lach.,*** mosch., sep., sulph., ***zinc.***
at beginning - ***calc., calc-p., caust.,*** graph., ***kali-c., lach.,*** **LAP-A.,** lyc., ***vib.***
before - alum., ***arund., bell.,*** bry., bufo, **CALC., CALC-P., CAUL.,** ***caust., cham.,*** coloc., **KALI-C.,** ***lach., lyc., mag-p.,*** mosch., nat-m., ***nux-v., phos.,*** **PULS.,** sec., **SEP.,** ***sil.,*** ust., ***vib., zinc.***
between - cocc., ham., sep.
cry out, compels her to, during - ***acon., cact., cham.,*** **COLOC.,** ***mag-m.,*** nux-m., ***nux-v.,*** **PULS.,** senec., xan.
suppressed - ***cocc., kali-c.,*** **PULS.**
morning - bufo, ***calc-p.,*** puls.
motion, agg. - **BELL., BRY.,** ***cimic.,*** **COCC.,** con., lil-t.
night - kali-p.
11 p.m. - ***cact.***
menses before - ***calc.***
midnight, after - ***calad.***
nurses, while child - ***arn., cham.,*** puls., **SIL.**
paroxysmal - asaf., **BELL.,** ***caul.,*** caust., **CHAM.,** ***cimic.,*** coloc., con., ign., lac-c., mag-m., nux-m., ***nux-v.,*** **PLAT., PULS., SABIN.,** ***sec.,*** sep., sulph., ***vib.***
periodically, same time each day - cact.
pessaries, after agg. - ter.
pregnancy, during - bry., kali-p., lyss., plat.
pressure, agg. - caul.
amel. - ign., lil-t., ***mag-p.,*** sep.
on back amel. - ***mag-m.***
pulsating - ars., ***bell., cact.,*** cur., ***hep.,*** murx., ***sep.***
reaching up with arms - aur., ***graph.***
reflex symptoms, from - bell., cimic., goss., helon., kali-c., lil-t., plat.
rheumatic - ***bry.***
sex, during - ***ferr-p., hep.,*** merc-c.
after - ***plat.***
shifting - ped.
sitting long - ***bufo.***
stool, during - calc-p., carb-v.
after - lyc.
straining, from - podo.
suddenly, comes and goes - **BELL.,** vib.
touch of cloth - lil-t.

PAIN, uterus
undressing amel. - onos.
urging, to urinate - con., tarent.
walking agg. - **BELL., BRY.,** bufo, med., merc.
wandering - arn., bell., lach., nux-m., **PULS.,** rhus-t., sulph.

PAIN, vagina - bell., ***berb., calc., calc-p.,*** canth., card-m., cham., chin., ferr., ***graph.,*** ham., ***kali-c., kreos.,*** lil-t., ***lyc.,*** merc., nux-v., puls., rhus-t., ***sec., sep., staph.,*** sulph., thuj.
centers, in, from other parts - ***calc-p.***
clitoris - am-c., coll.
extending, chest, to - alum.
meatus, to - berb.
upward - lyss., nit-ac., sabin., sep., sil.
labia - apis, ars., ***bell., berb., calc., cann-s.,*** con., ferr., kali-c., ***kreos.,*** lyc., ***meli., merc-c., phos.,*** plat., ***sep.,*** sulph.
menses, during - ***ars-m.,*** calc.
before - berb., elaps
nosebleed, after - calc-p.
paroxysmal - ***staph.***
pulsating - alum.
scratching agg. - tarent.
sex, during - alumn., **ARG-N.,** bell., ***berb., calc-p.,*** coff., ***ferr., ferr-m., ferr-p.,*** ham., ***hep.,*** hydr., ign., ***kali-bi., kali-c., kreos.,*** **LYSS., NAT-M.,** ***plat., rhus-t.,*** sabin., **SEP.,** sil., ***staph., sulph., thuj.***
sitting agg. - staph.
urination agg. - sil.
vulva, menses, during - rhus-t.
sitting agg. - berb., kreos., staph., sulph.

PELVIC inflammatory disease, infection of uterus - ***acon., agn.,*** alum., **APIS,** ***arn.,*** **ARS.,** ***aur., aur-m.,*** **BELL.,** ***bry.,*** bufo, ***cact.,*** calc., **CANTH.,** ***carb-an.,*** carb-s., caul., ***cham.,*** chin., cocc., ***coff.,*** coloc., con., croc., ferr., ferr-ar., graph., ***ham., hep.,*** hydr., ***hyos.,*** hyper., ign., ***iod.,*** ip., iris, kali-c., kali-p., kreos., **LAC-C., LACH., LYC.,** ***lyss.,*** mag-m., **MED.,** ***merc., nux-v.,*** op., ph-ac., ***phos.,*** **PULS.,** ***rhus-t., sabad.,*** **SABIN., SEC.,** ***sep., sil., stram., sulph.,*** **TER.,** thuj., ***verat., verat-v.,*** vib., visc..
acute - ***acon.,*** ant-i., ***apis,*** arn., ***ars., bell., bry.,*** canth., cham., chin., ***cimic.,*** con., ***gels.,*** hep., hyos., ***iod.,*** kali-c., kali-i., lach., lil-t., ***mel-c-s., merc-c.,*** nux-v., op., ph-ac., plat., ***puls.,*** rhus-t., ***sabin., sec., sep., sil.,*** stram., sulph., ter., til., ***verat-v.***
anger, after - ***cham.***
bleeding, after - ars., ***chin.,*** ham., led., phos., ***sec., thlaspi.***
chronic - alet., aloe, ***ars., aur-m., aur-m-n.,*** bor., ***calc.,*** carb-ac., caul., chin-a., ***cimic., con.,*** graph., ***helon., hydr.,*** hydrc., inul., ***iod., kali-bi.,*** kali-c., kali-s., kreos., lach., ***mag-m., mel-c-s.,*** merc., ***murx.,*** nat-m., nit-ac., ***nux-v., ph-ac.,*** phos., plb., ***puls.,*** rhus-t., ***sabin., sec., sep.,*** sil., stram., ***sulph.,*** visc.
congestion, with arterial - bell., lil-t., ***sabin.***
follicular - ***hydr.,*** hydrc., iod., merc.

PELVIC inflammatory disease
emotional excitement, from - ***hyos.***
indignation, from - ***coloc.***
joy, excessive - ***coff.***
labor, after - bell., ***canth.***, lach., ***nux-v.***, ***sabin.***, ***sec.***, til.
menses, after suppressed - cham., coloc., puls.
miscarriage, after - sabin.
perimetritis, parametritis - acon., ***bell.***, canth., coloc., hep., ***merc-c.***, sil.
puerperal - til.
sexual excesses, after - ***chin.***

PERITONITIS, pelvic - ***acon.***, ***apis***, arn., ars., ***bell.***, ***bry.***, ***canth.***, chin., chin-s., cimic., ***coll.***, gels., ***hep.***, hyos., ***lach.***, **MED.**, ***merc-c.***, op., pall., rhus-t., sabin., sec., ***sil.***, ter., verat-v.
uterine bleeding, with - ars., ham., sabin., thlaspi.

PERSPIRATION, genitalia - dios., ***lyc.***, ***merc.***, ***petr.***, sars., sel., ***sep.***, sil., ***sulph.***, **THUJ.**
offensive - ***calc.***, fago., lyc., ***merc.***, ***nit-ac.***, sil., ***thuj.***
coughing agg. - thuj.

PINCHING, pain, genitalia - kali-c., mur-ac., plat.
menses would appear, as if - mur-ac.
pinching, ovaries - anan., canth., cham., ***plat.***
pinching, uterus - anan., bell., bry., cact., canth., ***cham.***, con.
menses, before - ***alum.***, bry.

POLYPS, genitalia - calc., lyc., ***thuj.***
polyps, cervix - ***ars.***, ***aur.***, **BELL.**, ***bufo***, **CALC.**, **CALC-P.**, caust., ***con.***, hydr., led., ***lyc.***, merc., mez., nit-ac., petr., **PHOS.**, ***ph-ac.***, ***plat.***, puls., rhus-t., ***sang.***, sec., ***sep.***, ***sil.***, ***staph.***, **TEUCR.**, **THUJ.**
soft - ***kali-s.***
polyps, vagina - **CALC.**, merc., petr., ph-ac., psor., ***puls.***, staph., ***teucr.***, **THUJ.**
labia - bell., calc., ***phos.***, teucr., ***thuj.***

PREGNANCY, (see Pregnancy, chapter)

PRE-menstrual syndrome (PMS) - alum., ***am-c.***, am-m., arg-n., asaf., asar., ***bar-c.***, bar-m., bell., bor., **BOV.**, bry., **CALC.**, **CALC-P.**, canth., carb-an., carb-s., ***carb-v.***, caust., cham., chin., cina, cocc., coff., ***con.***, croc., **CUPR.**, dulc., ***ferr.***, ferr-i., ***follic.***, gels., graph., hep., ***hyos.***, ign., iod., ip., ***kali-c.***, kali-n., ***kreos.***, ***lac-c.***, **LACH.**, **LYC.**, mag-c., mag-m., ***mang.***, ***merc.***, mez., mosch., mur-ac., nat-c., **NAT-M.**, ***nat-p.***, nux-m., nux-v., petr., ***ph-ac.***, ***phos.***, ***plat.***, **PULS.**, rhus-t., ruta., sabad., sars., **SEP.**, sil., spig., spong., stann., staph., **SULPH.**, sul-ac., valer., **VERAT.**, ***vib.***, **ZINC.**
before and after, agg. - calc.
breasts, agg. - bry., ***calc.***, ***con.***, ***kali-c.***, **KALI-M.**, **LAC-C.**, lyc., ol-an., ***phyt.***, puls.

PRESSING, pain, genitalia - agar., alet., ***aloe***, ant-c., ***aur-m-n.***, bar-c., ***bell.***, calc., calc-p., calen., carb-ac., chin., ***cimic.***, ***cocc.***, ***coll.***, con., ferr-br., frax., glyc., gnaph., ***goss.***, graph., ***helon.***, kali-bi., lappa-a., ***lil-t.***, mag-c., ***mag-m.***, mang., merc., murx., nat-c., nat-ch., ***nux-v.***, ***plat.***, plb., ***podo.***, polyg., ***sep.***, sulph., thuj., tril., wye., zinc., zinc-valer.
downward, during urination - con.
menses, during - am-c., ant-c., asaf., **BELL.**, berb., bov., calc., ***cham.***, chin., con., ip., mag-c., mag-s., mosch., nat-m., nit-ac., nux-m., nux-v., ***plat.***, puls., ***sep.***, sil., sulph., zinc.
before - chin., ***croc.***
sitting, while - thuj.
stool, during - kali-c.
urination, downward during - con.
pressing, ovaries - ang., ***ars.***, ***coloc.***, ***iod.***, lac-d., **LACH.**, ***lil-t.***, plat., ***sep.***
left - ***lach.***, ***med.***
menses, suppressed - ant-c., bell.
would reappear, as though - ***plat.***
right - ang., ***ars.***, ***iod.***
stool, with urging to, after menses - ***plat.***
pressing, uterus - ***acon.***, anac., anan., ***ant-c.***, **BELL.**, cact., calad., calc., calc-p., canth., cham., chin., ***cocc.***, ***gels.***, ***lil-t.***, ***nat-c.***, ***nit-ac.***, nux-v., ***plat.***, podo., ***puls.***, ***sec.***, **SEP.**, sul-ac., tarent., ust.
menses, before - jug-r.
would appear, as if - ***mur-ac.***, plat.
morning - puls.
stool, during - ***carb-v.***
viscera would protrude from vagina, as if - sep., xan.
pressing, vagina - alum., ant-c., ***bell.***, ***calc.***, chim., cinnb., ***ferr-i.***, graph., ***lil-t.***, lyc., nat-c., ***nit-ac.***, ***nux-v.***, podo., ***sep.***, sil., stann., ***ust.***
menses, during - ant-c., ***bell.***, con., ***lach.***, ***lil-t.***, ***nat-c.***, ***nit-ac.***, plat., ***sep.***, ust.
before - alum., bell., con.
morning - puls.
stool, during - podo.
stooping, when - lyc.
upward, on sitting - ferr-i.

PROLAPSUS, uterus (see Displacement) - abies-c., acon., ***aesc.***, agar., agn., ***alet.***, ***aloe***, ***alum.***, ***alumn.***, am-m., anan., ***apis***, **ARG-M.**, **ARG-N.**, ***ars.***, ars-i., ***arn.***, asper., **AUR.**, aur-m., ***aur-m-n.***, ***bell.***, ***benz-ac.***, berb., ***bry.***, **BOR.**, ***bry.***, bufo, **CALC.**, calc-ar., ***calc-p.***, calc-s., calc-sil., canth., ***carb-an.***, carb-v., caul., ***cham.***, chel., ***chin.***, chin-a., cimic., ***cina***, cocc., coll., ***coloc.***, ***con.***, croc., crot-h., crot-t., ***dulc.***, erig., ***ferr.***, ferr-ar., ferr-br., ***ferr-i.***, ferr-p., ***frax.***, gels., ***graph.***, ***helon.***, hydr., hydrc., ***ign.***, iod., ***ip.***, kali-ar., ***kali-bi.***, kali-br., ***kali-c.***, kali-cy., kali-p., kali-s., kreos., lac-c., ***lach.***, lappa-a., **LIL-T.**, lyc., ***lyss.***, ***mag-c.***, mang., merc., mill., ***mur-ac.***, ***murx.***, nat-c., nat-ch., **NAT-H.**, ***nat-m.***, **NAT-P.**, ***nit-ac.***, ***nux-m.***, ***nux-v.***, onos., op., **PALL.**, ***petr.***, phel., ***ph-ac.***, phos., phyt., **PLAT.**, ***podo.***, psor., **PULS.**, rheum, ***rhus-t.***, ***sabin.***, samb., sang., ***sec.***, sel.,

PROLAPSUS, uterus - senec., **SEP.**, ***sil.***, spig., ***squil.***, ***stann.***, ***staph.***, stram., sul-ac., ***sulph.***, teucr., ***thuj.***, ***til.***, ***tub.***, ***ust.***, zinc., zinc-valer.
afternoon - **SEP.**
alternate days, on - alum.
cervix, low in vagina - calen.
concussion, after - arn.
confinement, after - bell., ***helon.***, ***podo.***, puls., ***rhus-t.***, sec., ***sep.***
crossing legs amel. - lil-t., murx., **SEP.**
diarrhea, from - petr.
electric shocks down the thighs, with - ***graph.***
forceps delivery, after - sec.
fright, after - gels., **OP.**
head, holding and straining, amel. - pyrog.
hot weather, in - ***kali-bi.***
lifting, from - agar., ***aur.***, **CALC.**, nux-v., ***podo.***, ***rhus-t.***
lumbar, with backache - nat-m.
lying down, agg. - puls.
amel. - ***nat-m.***, ***sep.***
on back, amel. - nat-m., onos.
menopause, during - lach., sep.
menses, during - ***aur.***, ***calc-p.***, ***cimic.***, kreos., ***lach.***, ***lil-t.***, nat-c., **PULS.**, **SEP.**
after - agar., aur., ip., kreos.
morning - bell., **NAT-M.**, sep.
nursing, during - podo.8
reaching up, from - ***aur.***, ***calc.***, nux-v., ***sulph.***
sex, agg. - nat-c.
amel. - merc.
standing, agg. - lappa-a.
amel. - bell.
stool, during - ***calc-p.***, con., dirc., nux-v., **PODO.**, psor., puls., ***stann.***
after - ***stann.***
urging to, constant - inul., nux-v., podo.
storm, before a - rhus-t.
straining, from - ***aur.***
urination, during - ***calc-p.***
dribbling, with - ferr-i.
foul, with - benz-ac.
walking agg. - lappa-a.
walks bent - ***am-m.***, ***arn.***
weakness, from - sul-ac.

prolapus, vagina - alum., ***bell.***, calc-ar., chim., ***ferr.***, gran., ***kreos.***, ***lach.***, ***lappa-a.***, ***merc.***, ***nux-m.***, ***nux-v.***, oci., op., plat., plb., podo., psor., **SEP.**, ***stann.***, staph., ***sulph.***, sul-ac., thlaspi, thuj., verat.
lifting, from - ***nux-v.***
pregnancy, during - calc-ar., ***ferr.***
stool during - stann.
weakness, from - sul-ac.

PULSATING, genitalia - alum., apis, ***bell.***, ***calc-p.***, ***coc-c.***, ***lac-c.***, ***merc.***, nat-c., prun.
constant behind pubes - aesc.
lying on the right side - apis
sex, after - ***nat-c.***

pulsating, ovaries - ***bell.***, ***cact.***, calc., con., cop., ***lach.***, ***onos.***, podo.
menses, during - lac-c.

pulsating, ovaries
right - podo.
standing, while - apis, cop.
walking, while - apis.
menses, during - lac-c.
right - podo.
standing, while - apis, cop.
walking, while - apis.

pulsating, uterus - aesc., ars., ***bell.***, ***cact.***, calc-p., con., cur., murx., sabin., sarr.

pulsating, vagina - ***alum.***, ***merc.***
lying amel. - merc.

PUSHES, uterus, up when she sits down - ferr-i., **NAT-H.**

PYOMETRA, retained pus in uterus - lach., merc., ***puls.***, pyrog., ***sep.***

RASH, genitalia - ***anan.***

RAWNESS, genitalia - tarent.

REDNESS, genitalia - ars., aur-m., ***bell.***, calc., ***carb-v.***, ***helon.***, hydrc., kali-bi., led., merc., ***sep.***, ***sulph.***, til.

redness, cervix - hydrc., mit.

RELAXATION, of genitals, during vagina discharge - agn., ***caul.***, sec., sep.

relaxation, vagina, sphincter, of - ***agar.***, ***ambr.***, ars., ***calad.***, ***calc.***, croc., ***ferr.***, ***kali-c.***, ***lyc.***, mag-c., merc., mur-ac., ***nat-c.***, nat-m., ***sep.***, sil., staph., ***sulph.***, ***tub.***

RETROVERSION, of uterus - lil-t., puls., sep., tarent., ust.

SALPINGITIS, inflammation of fallopian tubes - acon., apis, ***ars.***, bell., bry., canth., chin-s., coll., ***coloc.***, eupi., hep., lach., ***med.***, merc., ***merc-c.***, ***puls.***, sabal., ***sep.***, sil., staph., thuj.
accumulation, with, of pus or serum, which escape from uterus from time to time - sil.

SENSITIVE, genitalia - ***aur-m.***, **BELL.**, ***canth.***, chin., ***coc-c.***, ***coff.***, con., merc., ***mur-ac.***, nux-v., **PLAT.**, ***sep.***, **STAPH.**, sulph., tarent., ust., ***zinc.***
menses, before - am-c., cocc., kali-c., ***lach.***, ***plat.***

sensitive, cervix, spot near os uteri - med.

sensitive, vagina - ***acon.***, alumn., aur., ***bell.***, ***berb.***, bry., ***cact.***, calc., carb-v., ***caul.***, caust., ***cimic.***, ***cocc.***, ***coff.***, con., ***ferr.***, ferr-i., ferr-p., ***gels.***, graph., ham., **IGN.**, ***kreos.***, lac-c., **LYSS.**, ***mag-p.***, merc., mur-ac., ***murx.***, ***nat-m.***, nit-ac., nux-v., orig., **PLAT.**, ***plb.***, sec., ***sep.***, ***sil.***, **STAPH.**, sulph., tarent., ***thuj.***
sex agg. - hydr., ***plat.***, ***staph.***, sulph., thuj.
urination agg. - coc-c.

SEX, general

aversion to - agar., ***agn.***, alum., alum-p., am-c., anac., arg-m., arund., **ASAR.**, bar-c., berb., bor., ***brom.***, calad., calc., cann-i., cann-s., carb-an., carb-s., ***caust.***, chlor., ***clem.***, coff., cub., ***dam.***, ether, ***ferr.***, ***ferr-m.***, ferr-ma., ferr-p., fl-ac., franz., ***graph.***, hell., ***hydr.***, ign., ***kali-br.***, kali-c., kali-n., kali-p., kali-s., ***lach.***, ***lyc.***, lyss., mag-c., ***med.***, **NAT-M.**, nep., nit-ac., onos., op., ***petr.***, ***phos.***, plat., plb.,

SEX, general

aversion to - podo., polyg., ***psor.,*** puls., ran-s., ***rhod.,*** rhodi., sabad., sabin., **SEP.,** spirae., stann., staph., stram., sul-ac., ***sulph.,*** tarent., teucr., thal., ther., thuj.

anemic women, in - ***nat-m.***

childbirth, since last - ***lyss.,*** **SEP.**

menopause, during - ***con., sep.***

menses, after - arund., bart., berb., ***caust.,*** kali-c., nat-m., ***phos.,*** sep., sul-ac.

orgasms, painful, from - nat-m.

vagina discharge, with - ***caust.***

vaginitis, in - ***cur.***

coitus interruptus, ailments from - bell-p.

desire, sexual, (Sexual, desire)

enjoyment absent - agn., alum., alum-p., anac., arg-m., ***berb., brom.,*** cael., calad., calc., cann-i., cann-s., **CAUST.,** ***ferr., ferr-m., graph., kali-br., lyc.,*** lyss., ***med.,*** **NAT-M.,** nep., nit-ac., onos., ***phos.,*** plat., pneu., psor., puls., rhodi., **SEP.,** ***sulph.,*** thala., thiop.

diminished - bart., ferr-p., plat., **SEP.,** tarent.

increased - agn., ambr., cann-s., lach., nat-m., ***plat.,*** stann., sulph.

excesses, agg. - acon., **AGAR., AGN.,** alum., anac., ant-c., arn., ***ars.,*** asaf., aur., bar-c., bell., bor., ***bov.,*** bry., ***calad.,*** **CALC.,** ***calc-s.,*** cann-s., canth., caps., carb-an., ***carb-v.,*** caust., cham., **CHIN.,** ***chin-a.,*** cina, cocc., coff., **CON.,** ***dig.,*** dulc., ferr., ***gels.,*** graph., ign., ***iod., ip., kali-br., kali-c.,*** kali-n., **KALI-P.,** led., ***lil-t.,*** **LYC.,** mag-m., ***merc.,*** mez., ***mosch., nat-c.,*** **NAT-M., NAT-P.,** ***nit-ac.,*** **NUX-V.,** op., petr., **PH-AC., PHOS.,** plat., plb., ***puls.,*** ran-b., rhod., rhus-t., ruta., sabad., samb., sec., **SEL., SEP., SIL.,** ***spig.,*** squil., stann., **STAPH., SULPH., THUJ.,** valer., zinc.

headache, after - **AGAR.,** arn., ***bov.,*** **CALC.,** carb-v., ***chin.,*** con., kali-c., lach., merc., ***nat-c.,*** nat-m., nat-p., ***nux-v.,*** ph-ac., phos., pip-m., ***puls.,*** **SEP., SIL.,** spig., ***staph., sulph., thuj.***

mental, symptoms, from - agar., alum., ars., asaf., aur., ***bov.,*** calad., **CALC.,** ***carb-v., chin.,*** chin-a., cocc., ***con., iod., kali-c.,*** kali-p., kali-s., lil-t., **LYC.,** mag-m., med., ***merc., nat-c.,*** nat-m., nit-ac., **NUX-V.,** petr., **PH-AC., PHOS.,** ***plat., puls.,*** sel., **SEP.,** ***sil.,*** spig., **STAPH.,** sulph., thuj., zinc.

excitement, agg. - ***bufo,*** **LIL-T.,** sars.

headache, from - agar., arg-n., arn., ***bov.,*** calad., **CALC.,** ***calc-p.,*** chin., dig., graph., **KALI-C.,** ***lyc., nat-c.,*** nat-m., ***petr., phos.,*** puls., **SEP., SIL.,** staph.

masturbation, disposition to - ambr., ***anac.,*** anan., ***apis,*** bell-p., bufo, ***calad.,*** calc., ***calc-p.,*** carc., caust., ***chin.,*** coff., dys-co., ***gels., grat., kali-br., lach.,*** lil-t., med., ***nat-m., nux-v.,*** op., **ORIG.,** ***orig-v., ph-ac., phos.,*** pic-ac., ***plat.,*** puls., raph., sal-n., **STAPH.,** ***sulph.,*** tarent., thuj., ***tub.,*** ust., ***zinc.***

SEX, general

masturbation, ailments from - agar., alum., ***ambr.,*** anac., ant-c., ***arg-m.,*** ars., bov., ***bufo,*** calad., **CALC.,** calc-s., ***carb-v.,*** **CHIN., COCC., CON.,** ***dig.,*** ferr., **GELS.,** ***hyos., iod.,*** kali-c., ***kali-p., lyc.,*** mag-p., ***merc.,*** merc-c., mosch., nat-c., ***nat-m.,*** **NAT-P.,** nux-m., ***nux-v.,*** **ORIG.,** petr., **PH-AC.,** ***phos.,*** plb., ***puls.,*** **SEL., SEP.,** sil., ***spig.,*** squil., **STAPH., SULPH.**

children, in - ***med.,*** orig., plat.

due to itching of vulva - ***calad., orig.,*** plat., zinc.

headache after - ***calc.,*** carb-v., ***chin., con.,*** lyc., merc., nat-m., nux-v., phos., puls., ***sep.,*** spig., ***staph.,*** sulph.

menses, during - zinc.

sexual desire strong, driving her to - ***gels., grat., nux-v.,*** **ORIG.,** phos., ***plat.,*** raph., **ZINC.**

nymphomania - ambr., agar., ant-c., apis, ***bar-m., bell.,*** calad., calc., ***calc-p.,*** camph., ***cann-i., cann-s., canth., carb-v., cedr., chin., coff., dig.,*** dulc., ***fl-ac.,*** graph., **GRAT., HYOS.,** ***kali-br.,*** **LACH.,** ***lil-t., lyc.,*** **MED.,** ***merc.,*** mosch., ***murx.,*** nat-c., nat-m., ***nux-v.,*** op., **ORIG.,** ***phos.,*** **PLAT.,** plb., ***puls., raph.,*** rob., ***sabad.,*** sabin., sil., ***staph.,*** **STRAM.,** sulph., ***tarent.,*** thuj., ***verat., zinc.***

menses during - ***hyos.,*** kali-br., ***plat., sec., verat.***

before - calc-p., ***phos.,*** stram., ***verat.***

suppressed - ant-c., canth., chin., cocc., hyos., ***murx.,*** phos., ***plat.,*** stram., sil., sulph., verat., zinc.

puerperal - ***chin.,*** kali-br., ***plat.,*** verat.

uterine bleeding, during - mosch., murx., plat., sec.

orgasm delayed - ***berb.,*** brom., caust., ***nat-m.,*** **SEP.**

delayed and painful - ign., nat-m., staph.

easy - ***plat.,*** stann.

involuntary with violent desire - ang., ***arg-n., ars., calc., lil-t.,*** nat-m., ***nux-v., op.,*** **PLAT.,** sul-ac.

lacking - ***brom.,*** calad., ***nat-m.,*** **SEP.**

painful - nat-m., plat., staph.

painful - alumn., ange-s., apis, **ARG-N.,** bell., ***berb.,*** bor., ***cact.,*** calc., ***calc-p.,*** coff., ***ferr.,*** ferr-m., ferr-p., ham., ***hep., hydr.,*** ign., ***kali-bi., kali-c., kreos., lyc.,*** **LYSS.,** merc., **NAT-M., PLAT.,** ***rhus-t.,*** sabin., **SEP.,** sil., **STAPH.,** ***sulph., thuj.***

vagina, in, during - alumn., **ARG-N.,** bell., ***berb., calc-p.,*** coff., ***ferr., ferr-m., ferr-p.,*** ham., ***hep.,*** hydr., ign., ***kali-bi., kali-c., kreos.,*** **LYSS., NAT-M.,** ***plat., rhus-t.,*** sabin., **SEP.,** sil., ***staph., sulph., thuj.***

dryness, from - ferr., ***nat-m., sep.***

sore, tenderness - bell., ***berb.,*** coff., ***ferr.,*** ferr-m., ham., ign., ***kali-bi., kali-c., kreos.,*** **LYSS.,** ***naja, plat., rhus-t., sep.,*** staph., ***sulph., thuj.***

SEX, general

refuses to have conjugal sex - con., ign., lyc., nat-m., ***sep.***

sensation, as after sex - lach., lyc., kreos.

midnight, after - lyc.

sleeping and waking, between - kreos.

voluptuous sensation, tingling, coitus-like - ***alum.,*** am-m., apis, ***bov.,*** bufo, cadm-s., calc., ***calc-p.,*** cann-i., canth., cer-s., coff., elaps, fl-ac., ***kali-br.,*** kreos., lach., lil-t., lyc., mosch., ***nit-ac., nux-v.,*** **ORIG.,** par., phos., **PLAT.,** raph., ***stann.,*** staph., sul-ac., tarent.

anxiety and palpitation, with - plat.

dream, in - sul-ac.

extending into abdomen - plat.

menses, before and during - calc., kali-c.

morning - kreos.

orgasm, with - plat., sul-ac.

scratching the arm, while - ***stann.***

unconsciousness, during partial - meth-ae-ae.

waking, on - am-m., kali-c.

walking, while, amel. - nat-m.

weakness, after - ***agar.,*** berb., **CALC.,** chin., clem., ***con., dig., graph., kali-c., kali-p.,*** lil-t., lyc., mosch., ***nat-m.,*** nit-ac., petr., ***ph-ac., phos.,*** **SEL.,** ***sep., sil.,*** staph., tarent.

SEXUAL, desire

diminished - ***agn.,*** alum., am-c., ambr., anh., ***bar-c.,*** bart., bell., berb., bor., brom., camph., cann-s., carb-an., **CAUST.,** dam., des-ac., ***ferr., ferr-m.,*** ferr-p., ***graph., helon., hep., ign., kali-br., kali-chl.,*** kali-i., kali-m., kreos., ***lyc., lyss., mag-c.,*** man., mur-ac., ***nat-m.,*** oci-s., ***onos., ph-ac.,*** phos., plb., rauw., ***rhod.,*** sabal., saroth., **SEP.,** sil., sulph., tub., visc

evening - ***dios.***

morning - bell.

night - coca.

sex, during - ***kali-br.***

sexual excitement, with - cann-s.

increased - ***agar.,*** **AGN.,** am-c., ***ambr., ant-c., apis,*** arg-n., ***ars., ars-i.,*** arund., ***asaf., aster.,*** aur., aur-a., aur-i., aur-s., bar-c., bar-i., ***bar-m., bell.,*** bov., ***bufo,*** cact., ***calad.,*** **CALC.,** calc-i., **CALC-P.,** calc-sil., **CAMPH.,** cann-i., cann-s., **CANTH.,** ***carb-v., caust.,*** cedr., cench., cham., chin., cimic., coca, ***coff.,*** **CON.,** ***croc.,*** cub., cur., des-ac., ***dig.,*** dulc., ***ferul.,*** **FL-AC.,** form., ***gels.,*** gran., **GRAT., HYOS.,** ***ign.,*** iod., ***kali-bi., kali-br.,*** kali-c., kali-fer., ***kali-p., kreos., lac-c.,*** **LACH.,** ***lil-t., lyc.,*** lyss., man., manc., **MED.,** ***merc., mosch., murx.,*** mygal., ***nat-a., nat-c.,*** nat-m., nat-p., nat-sil., nit-ac., **NUX-V.,** oci-s., ***op., orig.,*** ph-ac., **PHOS.,** ***pic-ac.,*** **PLAT.,** plb., podo., **PULS.,** ***raph., rob.,*** sabad., ***sabin., sal-n.,*** saroth., sars., sel., ***sep., sil., stann., staph., stram.,*** stry., sul-ac., sul-i., ***sulph., tarent.,*** thlaspi, ***thuj.,*** tub., ***ust.,*** valer., **VERAT.,** visc., ***xero, zinc., zinc-p.***

afternoon - calc.

busy, must keep, to repress it - lil-t.

SEXUAL, desire

increased, childbirth, during - ***verat.***

contact of parts, by least - lac-c., ***murx.,*** plat.

dreams, sexual, with - ***op.***

without - zinc.

dysmenorrhea, with - cann-i.

elderly women - apis, ***mosch.***

excitement of fancy, without - ***hyos.***

of sexual parts, with extreme - plat., ***stram.***

girls, in young - plat.

headache, during - sep.

infertile women, in - cann-i.

itching, with - calad., ***canth., hydr.***

lochia, with suppressed - ***verat.***

love disappointment, after - ***verat.***

lying-in women - bell., camph., ***chin., grat., hyos., kali-br., mosch., plat.,*** tarent., verat., zinc.

married, with obsession of being - bell., ***caust.,*** plat., verat.

masturbation, with - zinc.

menopause, at - lach., manc., ***murx.***

menses, during - agar., ars., bell., bufo, camph., ***canth.,*** chin., cina, coff., dulc., ***hyos.,*** kali-br., kreos., ***lach.,*** **LYC.,** ***mosch.,*** nux-v., ***orig., plat.,*** **PULS.,** ***sep.,*** sul-ac., tarent., verat.

after - ars., berb., calc-p., cann-s., caust., ***kali-br.,*** kali-c., ***kali-p., med., nat-m.,*** phos., plat., sep., ***sul-ac.***

before - ars., bell., ***calc-p.,*** cann-i., croc., cub., dulc., kali-c., nux-v., ***phos.,*** plat., stann., stram., ***verat.***

suppressed, from - ant-c.

metrorrhagia, during - ambr., coff., plat., ***sabin.***

morning in bed - aster., cedr., kali-c., kreos.

mucus flow, from - senec.

night - bell., psil., ***syph., zinc.***

rousing - ***med.***

nursing child, when - calc-p., phos.

paralytic affections, in - ***sil.***

pregnancy, during - bell., lach., merc., phos., plat., puls., stram., verat., ***zinc.***

nymphomania, during - zinc.

scratching distant parts, from - ***stann.***

sex, from - ***tarent.***

sleep, disturbing - ***aur.***

spinal affection, in - ***sil.***

unsatisfied passion, in - ***verat.***

urination with erection of clitoris, after - calc-p.

vagina discharge, with - ***ign., orig-v.***

virgins, in - con., med., ***plat.***

widows, in - **APIS, LYC., ORIG.,** phos., ***staph.***

unsatisfied - staph.

worms, from - ***sabad.***

insatiable - aster., ***calc-p.,*** canth., ***lach.,*** med., ***plat., sabin.,*** stram., ***zinc.***

perverted - med., ***plat.,*** sabal., thuj.

SEXUAL, desire
suppression of, agg. - **APIS,** berb., calc., **CAMPH.,** ***carb-o.*** carc., **CON.,** ***hell., lil-t., ph-ac.,*** pic-ac., nat-m., plat., **PULS., STAPH.,** ***thuj.***
amel. - calad.
headache, after - ***con., puls.***
unsatisfied sexual desire, from - verat.
violent - **AGN.,** ***ars.,*** arund., aster., bar-m., **CALC.,** ***calc-p.,*** canth., ***gels.,*** grat., ***hyos., kali-br., lach.,*** lyss., **MED.,** ***mosch.,*** **MURX.,** ***op.,*** **ORIG.,** ***phos.,*** **PLAT.,** ***sabin., sil.,*** stann., ***staph., stram.,*** sumb., ***tarent.,*** thuj., ***tub., verat., zinc.***
involuntary, orgasms, with - ang., ***arg-n., ars., calc., lil-t.,*** nat-m., ***nux-v., op.,*** **PLAT.,** sul-ac.
masturbation, driving her to - ***gels., grat., nux-v.,*** **ORIG.,** phos., ***plat.,*** raph., **ZINC.**
scratching the arm, from - ***stann.***
virgins, in - ***con.,*** **PLAT.**
widows, in - **APIS,** lyc., **ORIG.,** staph.

SHARP, pain, genitalia - aeth., alum., ***ars., aur., bell., bor., calc., calc-p.,*** caust., clem., coc-c., ***con.,*** croc., ***glon.,*** **GRAPH.,** ign., ***kali-c.,*** kali-n., lac-c., lyc., meli., merc., murx., nat-s., nit-ac., pall., **PHOS.,** rhus-t., sep., staph., sul-ac., tarent., thuj.
extending, outward - caust.
to chest - alum., calc-p.
to liver - med.
to vagina - lil-t., puls.
jar, on - bell.
menses, during - lyc., sul-ac., zinc.
before - con.
stool, during - kali-n.
urinating - carb-v.
walking, while - thuj.
sharp, ovaries - abrot., absin., ***ambr., apis, ars., bell.,*** bor., brom., ***bry., bufo, canth.,*** carb-an., cench., ***coloc.,*** con., cur., goss., graph., kali-ar., kali-c., kali-p., ***lac-c., lach.,*** **LIL-T.,** ***lyc., mag-p.,*** med., merc., phos., pic-ac., ***plat., podo., sep., staph.,*** syph., thuj., ust., ***vib.,*** xan.
alternating sides - ***lac-c.***
breathing, on - ***bry.,*** graph.
arresting - ***canth.***
drawing in abdomen - ambr.
extending, left - lac-c.
right - med.
to knee - lac-c., wye.
to thighs - phos., staph., ust.
up side - cimic., lac-c., ***sep.***
hawking - graph.
left - abrot., graph., **LACH.,** thuj.
lying on back amel. - kali-p.
menses, during - kali-p., ***lac-c.,*** phos., ***podo.***
before - ***podo.,*** vib.
motion agg. - ***ars.,*** **BRY.,** cench.
right - **ARS.,** apis, ***bell.,*** lac-c., lec., ***lyc., plat., podo.***
to left - ***lyc.***
standing, while - lil-t.
sharp, ovaries
touch - graph.
sharp, uterus - **ACON.,** anan., **APIS,** ***arg-n.,*** ars., aur., **BELL.,** bor., bufo, calc., coloc., **CON.,** cur., ***ferr.,*** fl-ac., gels., graph., hura, ign., inul., ***kali-c.,*** kali-p., ***lac-c., lil-t.,*** lyss., ***merc., murx.,*** nux-v., phos., plat., sabin., **SEP.,** tarent.
extending, to right side of chest - con.
up back - ***gels.***
upward - **LAC-C.,** murx., ***sep.***
menses, during - bor.
after - tarent.
before - bor.
nursing, while - **SIL.**
riding, while - arg-n.
side to side - **CIMIC.**
walking, while - arg-n., **BELL.**
sharp, vagina - ***alum., ambr.,*** am-c., ars., ***bell., berb.,*** chin., con., ***graph.,*** hydrc., ***kreos.,*** lyss., mur-ac., nat-s., ***nit-ac.,*** phos., puls., ***rhus-t., sabin., sep.,*** stry., tarent.
abdomen from - ***kreos.***
clitoris, night - bor.
discharge, before - ambr.
extending, to chest - alum.
upward - alum., am-c., berb., ***lyss., nit-ac., phos.,*** sabin., ***sep.***
labia - lyc.
between - eupi.
left, through uterus to right ovary - bell., lac-c., phos., thuj.
menses, during - bell., ***berb., con., graph.,*** kreos., rhus-t., sabin., sul-ac.
morning, on waking - ***sep.***
outward - berb.
sex, during - ***berb.***
standing, on - ***nit-ac.***
walking, while - ***nit-ac.***

SHOCKS, uterus, in, on falling asleep - stry.
shocks, vagina, in - kreos.

SOFT, uterus - op.
feels as if - abies-c.

SORE, pain, genitalia - ambr., am-c., arn., ars., ***ars-i.,*** bov., ***calc.,*** calc-p., canth., ***carb-s.,*** **CARB-V.,** ***caust., coc-c.,*** coff., con., ferr-i., ***graph., hep.,*** iod., kali-bi., ***kali-c.,*** **KREOS.,** ***lac-c.,*** lyc., meph., nit-ac., petr., phos., **PLAT.,** puls., rhus-t., sec., ***sep., sil.,*** **STAPH.,** ***sulph., thuj.,*** til., ***zinc.***
menses, during - bov., ***kali-c., nat-m.,*** sil.
after - ***kali-c.***
before - con., ***kali-c.,*** lach., **SEP.**
urination, during - thuj.
after - calc.
walking, agg. - ***lac-c.***
washing, in cold water, after - eupi.

sore, ovaries - alum., ***ant-c., apis,*** arg-m., arg-n., arn., ***ars-i.,*** atro., **BRY.,** ***bufo, canth., chin.,*** cimic., coloc., con., cupr-ar., graph., guai., ham., helon., hep., ***iod.,*** kali-br., kali-c., kreos., ***lac-c.,*** **LACH., LIL-T.,** med., ***nux-m.,*** ol-j., onos., ***pall., plat.,*** psor., puls., rhus-t., sep., ***staph.,*** syph., tarent., ter., ther., thuj., ust., vesp.
extending down the limbs - bry.
left - ***arg-m.,*** atro., coloc., kali-br., **LACH.,** med., ovi-g-p., plat., syph., ust., vesp.
menses, during - ***apis,*** canth., ***iod., kali-c.,*** plat.
after - ant-c., ***iod.,*** kali-c.
before - ***kali-c., lac-c.***
suppressed, from - ant-c., bell.
motion - ther.
pressure agg. - ther.
rectum, with pain in - onos.
right - ***apis, bry., iod.,*** mag-m., murx., ***pall.,*** plat., psor., sec.
uterus, with pain in - ust.
walking agg. - ***apis,*** **ARN., BRY.**

sore, uterus - abies-c., acon., ***aesc.,*** am-c., ant-c., ***apis,*** arg-m., arg-n., **ARN.,** ***ars-i.,*** **AUR., BELL.,** ***bell-p.,*** bov., **BRY.,** ***bufo, calc.,*** calc-p., canth., caul., cham., chin., ***cimic., cocc., con.,*** conv., ***gels.,*** ham., ***helon., hydr.,*** kali-c., kreos., ***lac-c.,*** **LACH.,** lappa-a., ***lil-t.,*** lyss., mag-m., ***mel-c-s.,*** merc., **MURX.,** nux-m., nux-v., ***onos.,*** plat., ***puls.,*** rhus-t., sanic., sec., ***sep.,*** tarent., ***thlaspi, til.,*** tril., ust., **VERAT-V.**
contact of clothing agg. - **LACH.,** lil-t.
jarring, sensitive to - ***arg-m.,*** **BELL.,** ***lach.,*** lappa-a., **LIL-T.**
menses, during - am-c., arg-n., arn., bov., ***bry.,*** carb-v., canth., ***caust., cocc.,*** coff., ***con., ham.,*** ign., kreos., nat-m., ***nux-m.,*** nux-v., ruta., sil.
after - bov., kreos.
before - bov.
motion - **BELL., BRY.**
pregnancy, during - ***bell-p.,*** ham., puls., ***sil.***
riding in a carriage - ***arg-m.***
sex, during - **PULS.,** sep.
standing - lappa-a.

sore, vagina - acon., alum., aur., **BERB.,** brom., calc-p., cimic., coc-c., ***coff.,*** ferr., ferr-i., graph., ***ham.,*** ign., ***kali-bi.,*** kali-c., **KREOS., LYSS.,** merc., nit-ac., ***plat., puls., rhus-t.,*** sep., ***sil.,*** staph., ***sulph.,*** tarent., thuj.
between labia, when urinating - eupi.
evening - rhus-t.
introitus - hyos.
labia, vulva - acon., ambr., ***bell.,*** caust., ***cimic.,*** cocc., ***coff.,*** conv., ferr-i., ***gels., graph., helon.,*** hep., ***ign.,*** kali-br., ***kreos.,*** mag-p., ***merc., murx., nit-ac.,*** nux-v., ovi-g-p., petr., ***plat., sep.,*** sulph., tarent., ***thuj.,*** til., urt-u., zinc.
between labia, when urinating - eupi.
menses, during - kali-c.

sore, vagina
sex, during - bell., ***berb.,*** coff., ***ferr.,*** ferr-m., ham., ign., ***kali-bi., kali-c., kreos.,*** **LYSS.,** ***naja, plat., rhus-t., sep., sulph., thuj.***
preventing - coff., ***plat.,*** rhus-t., sep., ***thuj.***
sitting agg. - sulph.
vulva - carb-v., coc-c., plat., staph., sulph., tarent.

SPONGY, cervix - arg-m., thuj., ust.

SQUEEZED, uterus, sensation of, by a hand - ***cact.,*** gels.

SQUEEZING, ovaries - coloc., ***thuj.***

squeezing, uterus - bell-p., ***cact.,*** gels., kali-i.
menses, during - kali-i.

STIFFNESS, painful of uterus - sep.

STINGING, pain, genitalia - **APIS,** ***ars.,*** berb., calc-p., carb-v., eupi., ***kali-c.,*** kreos., lil-t., lyc., phos., puls., sabin., sep., ***staph.,*** urt-u., zinc.
menses, during - kali-c., kreos., lyc., phos., puls., sabin., sep., sul-ac.
before - zinc.
walking, while - zinc.

stinging, ovaries - **APIS,** bor., bry., canth., con., goss., graph., **LIL-T.,** merc., ***sep.,*** vesp.
cold amel. - apis, vesp.
left - lil-t.
menses during - ***apis.***
right - apis
sex, after - ***apis.***

stinging, uterus - ***apis,*** arg-m., ars., ***calc., con.,*** sabin.

stinging, vagina - ***apis,*** berb., cimic., cimx., coloc., ham., kreos., puls., ***rhus-t.,*** sabin., ***sep.,*** staph.
clitoris, in - apis., bor.
night - bor.

SUBINVOLUTION, genitalia - ***arn., bell.,*** bry., ***calc., carb-v., caul.,*** chin., **CIMIC.,** cycl., frax., ham., helon., ***hydr., kali-bi.,*** **KALI-BR.,** kali-c., ***kali-i., lil-t.,*** mill., ***nat-h.,*** nat-s., ***op.,*** plat., podo., psor., **PULS.,** ***sabin., sec.,*** **SEP.,** staph., **SULPH.,** ter., ***ust.***
breast-feeding, during - ***aur-m-n.,*** calc., caul., cimic., crot-h., ***epip.,*** ferr-i., ***frax., helon.,*** hydr., ***kali-br., lil-t.,*** mel-c-s., podo., ***sec., sep.,*** ust.
miscarriage, after - psor.

SWELLING, genitalia - ***ambr., am-c.,*** **APIS,** arn., **ARS.,** ars-i., ***asaf.,*** aur., aur-m., aur-s., bell., bry., ***calc.,*** calc-p., calc-s., cann-s., ***canth.,*** carb-an., ***carb-v.,*** coc-c., ***coll.,*** coloc., con., dig., ***ferr-i.,*** goss., ***graph., helon.,*** kali-bi., **KREOS.,** ***lac-c.,*** lach., ***lil-t.,*** meph., ***merc., nat-s.,*** **NIT-AC.,** nux-v., ***phos., podo.,*** **PULS., RHUS-T.,** sec., ***sep.,*** sulph., tarent., ***thuj., urt-u.***
edematous - apis, ***graph., merc., nit-ac., phos., urt-u.***
menses, during - chin., graph., lyc., sep., staph., sulph., zinc.
before - lyc., sep.

SWELLING, genitalia
one-sided - nit-ac.
phlegmonous - ***merc.***
pregnancy, during - ***merc., podo.***
swelling, cervix - arg-m., calc., ***calc-p.,*** canth., hydr., ***iod., kreos., nat-m.,*** sarr.
scirrhus-like - anan.
urinary symptoms, with - canth.
swelling, ovaries (see Edema) - ***alum., am-br.,*** **APIS,** ***ars.,*** atro., ***bell., brom., bufo, carb-ac.,*** coll., ***coloc.,*** con., cub., goss., ***graph.,*** ham., ***iod., kali-br., kali-i.,*** **LACH., LIL-T.,** ***med.,*** nat-h., nux-m., ***pall.,*** podo., staph., syph., ***tarent.,*** thea., thuj., ust., zinc-valer.
left - ***brom.,*** carb-ac., graph., kali-br., **LACH.,** lil-t., ***nat-h.***
menses, during - apis, brom., nat-h.
after - ***graph.***
before - brom.
right - ***apis,*** lyc., ***pall.***
swelling, uterus, (see Edema) - ***agn.,*** anan., aur., calc-i., con., cub., ***iod., lach.,*** lap-a., ***lil-t.,*** lyc., ***lyss.,*** meph., plat., sabin., sec., sep., ***tarent.,*** ust.
menses, during - kali-bi., ust.
before - nux-m., ph-ac.
swelling, vagina - ***agar.,*** alumn., calc-p., cann-s., coc-c., ***cur.,*** ferr., ***ferr-i., iod., kreos.,*** merc., **NIT-AC.,** ***nux-v.,*** puls.
clitoris, as if - colch., coll.
labia minora - ***apis,*** chin-s., merc., nit-ac., podo.
pregnancy, during - podo.
between - eupi.
vulva - carb-v., hep., puls., senec., sep.
as if - colch., coll.
pregnancy, during - podo.

TEARING, pain, genitalia - anac., ***bar-c.,*** berb., ***carb-an.,*** carb-v., con., ***kali-c.,*** lyc., nat-c., ***phos.,*** sil., ter.
cry out, making her - ***bar-c.***
evening - bar-c.
extending to anus - ***carb-an.***
to chest - kali-c.
meatus, about the - berb.
menses, during - am-c.
sitting, while - ***con.***
stool, during - carb-an.
walking in open air - phos.
in open air, after - phos.
tearing, ovaries - abrot., graph., ham., kali-i., lil-t., merc., ***plat.***
left - plat.
menses, during - plat.
right - graph., kali-i.
tearing, uterus - ***arg-n., cham.,*** lap-a., lyss., nat-m., plb., stry., tarent.
menses, during - ***agar., am-c.,*** ars., ***bell.,*** calc., ***caust.,*** chin., lyc., merc., nat-c., nit-ac., podo., ***puls.,*** rhus-t., ***sep.,*** sil., staph., sulph., zinc.
before - nat-m.
tearing, vagina - ***am-c.,*** chin., plb.

TEARS, of vagina - **CALEN.,** sec.

TIGHTNESS, in ovarian region, on raising arms - ***apis.***

TINGLING, genitalia, voluptuous - agar., ***alum.,*** apis, bov., bufo, calc., ***calc-p.,*** canth., coff., elaps, ***kali-br.,*** kreos., lach., lil-t., lyc., mosch., ***nux-v.,*** **ORIG.,** petr., ***phos.,*** **PLAT.,** raph., staph., tarent.
anxiety, during - ***plat.***

TUBERCLES, genitalia - ***calc., carb-ac., merc.,*** phos.
stinging burning - ***calc.***

TUMORS, genitalia (see Cancer, Cysts, Fibroids) - ***calc.,*** coc-c., **LYC.,** ***nit-ac., sil.,*** **THUJ.**
encysted - apis, bar-c., calc., carb-s., ***graph., kali-br.,*** kali-c., lyc., nit-ac., rhod., ***sabin.,*** sep., ***sil.,*** sulph., thuj.
erectile - ars., ***carb-an., carb-v.,*** kreos., ***lach.,*** lyc., ***nit-ac., phos.,*** plat., sep., sil., sulph., ***thuj.***
bleeding - arn., coc-c., kreos., lach., ***phos.,*** puls., thuj.
blue - ***carb-v.***
burning - calc., ***carb-an., thuj.***
hard - ***carb-v.***
itching - ***nit-ac.***
pricking - ***carb-v.***
sticking - ***nit-ac.***
hard - ***carb-v.***
tumors, ovaries (see Cancer, Cysts, Fibroids) - **APIS.,** apoc., ***ars.,*** ars-i., aur-m-n., ***bar-m.,*** bov., ***calc., coloc.,*** con., ferr-i., fl-ac., graph., hep., ***iod., kali-br.,*** lach., lyc., med., ov., ***pall., plat., podo., sec.,*** staph., stram., syph., ***thuj.,*** zinc.
left - apis, ***kali-bi.,*** **LACH.,** ***podo., thuj.***
right - ***apis,*** fl-ac., kali-fer., ***iod.,*** **LYC.,** pall., ***podo.,*** xan.
tumors, uterus, (see Cancer, Cysts, Fibroids) - ***aur-m-n., calc.,*** carc., con., ***crot-h.,*** lyc., nat-m., sep., **TER.,** ***thuj.***

TOXEMIA, (see Pregnancy)

TWITCHING, genitalia - sep.

ULCERS, genitalia - alum., **ALUMN.,** am-c., anan., ***arg-n.,*** arg-m., ars., ***asaf.,*** bell., bry., bufo, calc., calc-s., calen., carb-ac., carb-v., con., graph., ***hep.,*** kali-i., lac-c., ***lach., lyc.,*** med., **MERC.,** ***merc-c.,*** merc-i-f., merc-i-r., ***mur-ac.,*** **NIT-AC.,** ph-ac., phos., ***psor., puls.,*** rhus-t., rob., sec., ***sep.,*** **SIL.,** staph., sulph., syph., ***thuj.,*** vesp., zinc.
itching - carb-v.
ulcers, cervix - aln., ***arg-m., ars., aur-m-n.,*** bufo, ***carb-ac.,*** carb-an., fl-ac., ***hydr., hydrc.,*** kali-ar., ***kreos.,*** lyc., med., merc., ***merc-c.,*** methys., murx., phyt., sep., sul-ac., thuj., ***ust., vesp.***
miscarriage, from - aur.
bleeding easily - aln., arg-n., carb-an., kreos.
deep - merc-c.
discharge, with, fetid, acrid - ars., carb-ac.
ichorous, bloody - carb-an., kreos.
elderly, women - sul-ac.

ALTERNATING, with chills -***ph-ac., phos.,*** plat., ***psor.,*** puls., **RHUS-T.,** rheum, rhod., sabad., samb., ***sang., sec., sel., sep., sil.,*** sol-n., spig., stram., sulph., sul-ac., ***tarent.,*** thuj., ***verat., zinc.***
afternoon - calc., ***chin.,*** chin-s., lob., kali-n., myric., rhus-t., sep., sulph.
eating, after - sep.
in open air - ***chin.***
evening - all-c., all-s., alum., ant-s., am-c., ***bar-c.,*** cocc., kali-c., kali-n., lyc., merc., nat-m., ph-ac., puls., sep., sulph.
8 p.m. - elaps
bed, in - am-c.
forenoon - ***calc.,*** chin., elaps, thuj.
fright - lyc.
hot, twitches, with - ***nat-m.***
menses, during - am-c., thuj.
motion, on - ant-t.
night - **ACON.,** ang., ***bar-c.,*** hura, ip., mag-s., ***merc.,*** phos., sabad., sep., sulph.
with perspiration - ***ip.***
noon - kali-n.
alternating, chilliness, with dry, burning heat - ***bell.,*** sang.
alternating, perspiration, with - apis, ars., bell., calad., calc., ***euph.,*** kali-bi., kali-c., kali-i., ***led.,*** lyc., nux-v., phos., puls., sabad., sac-alb., sulph., thuj., ***verat.***
alternating, shivering, with - agar., ars., bov., caust., chin., cycl., ***elaps,*** hep., lach., lob., merc., mosch., nicc., ph-ac., podo., sabad., sang.
alternating, shuddering, with - ars., mag-s., mosch.

ANGER, paroxysms, brought on by - acon., ***cocc.,*** coloc., **CHAM.,** ign., nat-m., nux-v., ***petr.,*** **SEP., STAPH.**

ANTHRAX, intestinal - anthr.

ANTICIPATING - NUX-V.

ANXIOUS, heat, (see Mind, Anxiety)

ASCENDING - ***acon.,*** agar., alum., am-m., ang., ant-t., arund., bell., calad., canth., carb-an., ***cina,*** colch., crot-t., dig., glon., ***hyos.,*** kali-c., ***lach.,*** led., lyc., mang., ***nat-m.,*** **PHOS.,** plb., sabad., sars., **SEP., SULPH.,** sumb., ***verat.***

AUTUMN, fever - absin., **AESC.,** ***ars.,*** bapt., **BRY.,** ***calc., carb-ac.,*** carb-v., chin., **COLCH.,** ***eup-per.,*** lach., **NAT-M.,** ***nux-v.,*** puls., ***rhus-t.,*** **SEP.,** ***verat.***
liver and spleen swollen - absin.

BACTERIAL, infections - ***ars.,*** bapt., echi., nit-ac., pyrog., sil., thuj.

BED, in (see Night and Warmth) - ***acon.,*** agar., agn., am-c., am-m., ant-c., ant-t., ***apis,*** arg-m., ***arn.,*** asar., bapt., bor., ***bry., calc.,*** calen., carb-an., ***carb-v.,*** cham., chel., chin-s., clem., coc-c., **COFF.,** con., eug., hell., hep., ***kali-c.,*** kali-chl., kali-p., ***led.,*** mag-c., **MAG-M.,** mag-s., **MERC.,** ***mez.,*** mosch., nicc., nit-ac., nux-v., ph-ac., phos., **PULS.,** ***rhus-t.,*** samb., sars., sil., spong., squil., **SUL-AC.,** ***sulph.,*** thuj.

BED, in,
amel. - agar., bell., canth., ***caust.,*** cic., cocc., con., hyos., lach., ***laur., nux-v.,*** sil., squil., staph., stram.
driving him out of bed at night - graph., ***merc.***
feeling of heat in bed, yet aversion to uncovering - ***coff.,*** merc.
bed, after getting out of - acon., agn., ambr., am-c., ant-t., ars., asar., bell., calc., carb-an., carb-v., chel., chin., coloc., dros., ***hell.,*** ign., iod., kali-c., mang., ***merc.,*** mez., petr., plat., sel., sep., spig., stront-c., sulph., sul-ac., valer., ***verat.***
bed, heat, on rising from - ***thuj.***
and walking about - nicc.

BILIOUS - acon., ant-c., ***ant-t.,*** ars., ***bell., bry., cham., chel.,*** chin., cocc., coloc., corn., ***elaps, eup-per.,*** gels., ***hep., ip., iris,*** lept., ***merc., mur-ac., nux-v.,*** phos., ***podo.,*** polyp-p, ***puls.,*** stram., sulph., ***verat., verat-v.***
abdomen, cutting pain in - ***elat.***
anger, after - ***cham.***
cold and numb - lept.
debility - ***hydr.***
evacuations, watery - ***elat.***
miasmatic influences, not dependent upon - ***verat-v.***
nausea and vomiting - ***elat.***
plethoric individuals or in those suffering from portal stasis, occurring in hot weather, or on warm wet days - ***nux-v.***
remittent - ***crot-h.***
caused by atmospheric changes in spring, or due to miasmatic influences in autumn - ***gels.***
characteristic gastric and intestinal symptoms - corn.
low type, tendency to hemorrhage - ***crot-h.***
or intermittent - ***podo.***
paroxysm, nausea and vomiting of a bilious substance, accompanied by first a yellow, then a greenish diarrhea - podo.
skin dry, hot, stupor, black down center of tongue - lept.
tympanites - ***nat-s.***
vomiting of bile - ***ip., podo.***

BLEEDING symptoms, or tendency to putrescence - ***anthr., ars., carb-v., crot-h., lach.,*** pyrog., sec.

BLOOD, heat in, sensation, night - nit-ac.

BODY, general
anterior part (see Sides) - canth., caps., ***cham.,*** cina, croc., **IGN.,** iod., led., mez., **RHUS-T.,** sec., sel.
head, but less of the - ***arg-m.***
lower, part - caust., hep., lyc., nat-c., nat-m., ***op.,*** stann.
posterior, part - carb-an., carb-v., **CHAM.,** lyc., mur-ac., nat-c., nat-m., sep., sulph., thuj.

BODY, general
upper, part - **AGAR.,** ***anac., arn.,*** bry., carb-an., cina, dros., euph., meny., nux-v., ***par.,*** plat., ***puls.,*** rhus-t., sel.
with icy-cold feet - lact.

BUBONIC plague - alum., ***ars.,*** ars-i., aur., aur-m., aur-m-n., bad., ***bapt.,*** bar-m., bell., **BUFO,** ***carb-an., carc.,*** chel., chin., chin-a., **CINNB.,** clem., crot-h., **HEP.,** ***hippoz.,*** ign., iod., kali-chl., ***kali-i.,*** lac-c., ***lach.,*** lyc., ***merc., nit-ac.,*** phyt., phos., psor., pyrog., rhus-t., sec., ***sil.,*** sulph., sul-ac., tarent-c., verat., zinc.
burning bubo, with - ars., ars-i., bell., ***carb-an., tarent-c.***
suppurating bubo, with - ***aur.,*** bufo, ***carb-an.,*** chel., **HEP.,** ***iod.,*** kali-chl., ***kali-i.,*** **LACH.,** ***merc., merc-i-r.,*** nit-ac., ***sil., sulph.,*** tarent-c.
refuses to heal, old - ***carb-an., sulph.***

BURNING, heat - **ACON.,** agar., ant-t., **APIS,** arn., **ARS.,** arund., bapt., bar-c., bar-m., **BELL.,** bism., ***bry.,*** bufo, cact., canth., caps., carb-s., ***carb-v., cham.,*** chin., chin-a., chel., ***chlor., cina, con.,*** crot-h., cur., dig., ***dulc., elaps,*** **GELS.,** hell., ***hep.,*** ign., ip., ***kali-ar.,*** lach., ***lyc.,*** mag-c., manc., ***med.,*** merc., ***merc-c.,*** mosch., mur-ac., nat-m., nit-ac., ***nux-v.,*** **OP.,** petr., **PHOS.,** plb., **PULS.,** ***rhus-t.,*** sabin., ***samb.,*** sarr., ***sec.,*** sep., sil., ***spong.,*** stann., staph., stram., sulph., ***tarent.,*** thuj., **TUB.,** verat.
afternoon - **APIS,** ***ars.,*** **BELL.,** berb., ***bry., hep.,*** hyos., ign., lyc., nat-m., nit-ac., nux-v., **PHOS.,** ***puls.,*** rhus-t., stram., sulph.
4 p.m. lasting all night - ***hep.***
4 p.m. lasting several hours - **LYC.**
with transient chills - cur.
alternating, with chill - ***laur.***
with chilliness - **BELL.**
chills, after, passing down back - ***hydr.***
croup, in - spong.
day, in middle of, heat intense, with sensation as if burning up - syph.
distended blood vessels, with - aloe, ***bell.,*** **CHIN.,** chin-s., cycl., dig., ferr., ***hyos., led.,*** **MERL.,** ***puls.,*** sars.
dry, burning, extending from head and face, with thirst for cold drinks - ***acon.***
evening - ***acon.,*** agar., apis, ***ars.,*** **BELL.,** berb., ***bry., carb-v., cham.,*** cina, hell., hep., ***hyos.,*** ign., ip., **LYC.,** ***merc-c.,*** mosch., nat-m., nit-ac., nux-v., **PHOS., PULS., RHUS-T.,** staph., sulph., thuj., verat.
except head and face, which are covered with sweat - stram.
feel, which he does not - canth.
forenoon - bry., lyc., **NAT-M.,** ***nux-v., phos.,*** rhus-t., sulph., thuj., verat.
9 to 12 - **CHAM.**
furious delirium, with - **BELL.,** canth., **STRAM.,** verat.
heat outside, cold inside - **ARS.**
increased by walking in open air - chin.

BURNING, heat
intense, radiating heat, burning hot to touch - vario.
then sweat with relief, then fever with exacerbation of symptoms - ***sal-ac.***
internal, mostly, blood seems to burn in the veins - **ARS.,** ***bry., med.,*** **RHUS-T.**
internal, parts - mez.
interrupted with shaking chills, then internal burning heat with great thirst - sec.
lasting all day - chin., thuj.
midnight - **ARS.,** lyc., ***rhus-t.,*** stram., sulph., verat.
3 a.m. - ***thuj.***
after - **ARS.,** ign., lyc., merc., nat-m., ***phos.,*** sulph., thuj.
before - agar., ars., **BRY.,** ***cham.,*** laur., puls., sep., verat.
morning - ars., ***bry., cham.,*** ign., nat-m., nux-v., rhus-t., sep., sulph., thuj.
night - **ACON.,** agar., apis, **ARS.,** arund., ***bapt., berb.,*** **BELL.,** ***bry.,*** **CACT.,** cann-s., canth., carb-s., ***carb-v., cham.,*** cina, con., ***hep.,*** ign., lyc., merc., nat-m., nit-ac., nux-v., ***op.,*** petr., **PHOS., PULS.,** ***rhus-t.,*** staph., ***stram.,*** sulph., thuj., verat.
9 to 12 p.m. - ***bry.***
bed, in, intolerable heat - **PULS.**
parts lain on - lyss., manc.
pricking over the whole body, with - **CHIN.,** gels.
sleep, during - gins., **SAMB.,** thuj.
sparks - alum., ant-c., led., lyc., mez., sec., ***sulph.***
spot, in one, which is cold to the touch - ***arn.***
spots, in single - sel., zinc.
spreading from the hands over the whole body - **CHEL.**
stinging sensations, with - ***apis,*** merc-c.
stroke, in - ***crot-h.***
sweat, even when bathed in, with red face - op.
thirst, and desire to be covered - manc.
for cold drinks, with - ***acon.,*** bry., **PHOS.,** ***verat.***
with unquenchable - **ARS.,** bell., colch., hep., **PHOS.,** ***verat.***
within and without, body turning hot - **BELL.**

CANDIDA albicans, infection - calc., calc-p., chin., helon., lyc., med., puls., nat-p., nit-ac., sep., thuj.

CATARRHAL, fever - **ACON.,** ***apis, ars., asc-c., asc-t., bad.,*** bapt., bar-m., **BELL., BRY.,** ***cact.,*** carb-v., ***con., cupr-m., dros., dulc., eug., gels., ferr-p.,*** **HEP.,** ***kali-c., kali-i.,*** lach., med., **MERC.,** ***nux-v.,*** op., ph-ac., ***puls.,*** pyrog., ***rhus-t.,*** ruta, ***sabad.,*** senec., sep., sil., ***spig.***
atmosphere, from cold damp, or sudden change from hot and dry to damp air - ***gels.***
change of weather, from every - ***myrt-c.***
chilliness and coldness predominate - ***euph.***
hay catarrh, in - stict.

CATARRHAL, fever
hoarseness, with - aur-m.
menses, during - ***graph.***
pain in stomach - ***card-m.***

CATHETER, fever, after - acon

CEREBRO-spinal, fever - acon., aeth., agar., am-c., ant-t., **APIS,** ***arg-n.,*** arn., ars., bapt., **BELL.,** bry., cact., camph., canth., ***cic., cimic.,*** cocc., crot-h., cupr., dig., **GELS.,** glon., hell., hydr-ac., hyos., ***ign.,*** lyc., ***nat-m.,*** **NAT-S.,** ***nux-v.,*** **OP.,** ***phos.,*** plb., ***rhus-t.,*** sol-n., tarent., verat., **VERAT-V.,** ***zinc.***

CHANGING, paroxysms - ***elat.,*** eupi., **IGN.,** meny., ***psor.,*** **PULS.,** sep.
frequently - ***elat.,*** ign., ***psor., puls.***
homeopathic potencies, after - **SEP.**
no two paroxysms alike - **PULS.**
quinine, after abuse of - arn., ars., ***elat., eup-per.,*** ferr., ign., ***ip.,*** nux-v., **PULS.**

CHICKENPOX infection - acon., **ANT-C.,** ***ant-t.,*** ars., asaf., ***bell.,*** canth., ***carb-v.,*** caust., coff., con., cycl., hyos., ip., ***led., merc.,*** nat-c., nat-m., **PULS., RHUS-T.,** ***sep.,*** sil., **SULPH.,** ***thuj.***

CHILDBIRTH, fever, after (see Puerperal) - ***apis, arg-n.,*** arn., ars., ***bapt.,*** bell., ***bry.,*** **CARB-S.,** cham., cimic., coff., coloc., **ECHI.,** ***ferr.,*** gels., ***hyos.,*** ign., ip., kali-c., **LACH., LYC.,** mill., ***mur-ac.,*** nux-v., op., phos., plat., **PULS., PYROG., RHUS-R., RHUS-T.,** sec., sil., **SULPH.,** verat., verat-v.
lochia, suppressed, from - ***lyc.,*** mill., puls., **SULPH.**

CHILDREN, in - **ACON., BELL.,** ***cham., coff., ferr-p., stram.***
all night, in nursing infants - ***cina.***
dentition, during, with irritation of brain, and convulsions of tendency to them - ***verat-v.***
growth and in young people, during - ***sil.***
newborn, in, with startings - **CAMPH.**

CHILLS, general (see Alternating or Chills, chapt.)
fever with chill - **ACON.,** ambr., anac., ant-c., asar., **ARS.,** ars-i., **BELL.,** benz-ac., ***bry.,*** bufo, calc., caps., carb-v., **CHAM.,** ***chel.,*** chin., ***chin-s., cocc.,*** coff., coloc., ***dig., dros., ferr.,*** ferr-ar., ***graph.,*** **HELL., IGN.,** iod., ip., kali-ar., kreos., ***led.,*** lyc., ***merc., mez.,*** nat-c., nat-m., nat-s., nicc., **NIT-AC., NUX-V.,** ***olnd.,*** petr., phos., ***plb., podo., puls., pyrog.,*** ran-b., **RHUS-T.,** sabad., sabin., ***samb., sang., sep.,*** sil., spig., staph., ***stram.,*** **SULPH.,** ***tarent., thuj., verat., zinc.***
heat and perspiration - ***jab., mez., nux-v.***
perspiration, without subsequent - ***graph.***
shaking - ***sec.***
fever without chill - acon., acet-ac., alum., ambr., ***anac., ang.,*** ant-c., apis, ***arn.,*** **ARS.,** ***bapt.,*** **BELL.,** ben-ac., bov., **BRY.,** cact., ***calc.,*** carb-ac., caust., **CHAM.,** ***chin.,*** chin-a., ***cina,*** clem., coff., con., cur., elaps., eup-per., ***ferr., ferr-ar., ferr-p.,*** **GELS.,** graph., hep., ***ip.,*** kali-ar., kali-bi., kali-c., lach., ***lyc.,*** lyss., mang., merl., nat-m., nicc., nux-m., ***nux-v.,*** petr., podo., puls., **RHUS-T.,** stann., spig., ***stram.,*** sulph., ***thuj.***
afternoon - aesc., anac., ang., apis, **ARS., BELL.,** ***bry.,*** calc., caust., chin., chin-a., clem., coff., con., cur., eup-per., ferr., ferr-ar., ***gels.,*** graph., ip., kali-ar., kali-bi., kali-c., lyc., nat-m., nux-v., puls., rhus-t., ***sang., sil.,*** sulph.
1 p.m. to 2 p.m. - **ARS.**
2 p.m. - **PULS.**
2 p.m. to 3 p.m. - cur., kali-c.
3 p.m. - ars., coff., cur., ferr., lyc., lyc., nicc.
3 p.m. to 4 p.m. - **APIS,** clem., lyc., ***sang.***
4 p.m. - **ANAC.,** ***apis,*** ars., graph., hep., ***ip.,*** kali-bi., **LYC.**
4 p.m. to 8 p.m. - ***lyc.***
5 p.m. - con., kali-bi., kali-c., petr., sabin., stann.
5 p.m. to 6 p.m. - con., petr.
5 p.m. to 6 p.m., very ill humored - con.
5:30 p.m. with pricking in tongue - cedr.
12 p.m. to 1 p.m. - sil.
lasting all night - ars., ***hep.,*** puls., stann.
evening - acon., aesc., alum., ambr., anac., ang., ant-t., apis, arn., ars., ***bapt.,*** **BELL.,** bor., **BRY.,** calc., carb-v., caust., ***cham.,*** chin., chin-a., ***cina,*** coff., coloc., eup-per., ferr., ferr-ar., ferr-p., hep., ip., kali-ar., kali-c., lach., lyc., nat-m., nicc., nux-m., nux-v., ***petr.,*** plat., podo., **PULS., RHUS-T.,** stann., sulph., thuj.
6 p.m. - calc., carb-v., caust., caust., kali-c., **NUX-V.,** petr.
6 p.m. lasting all night - cham., lyc., ***nux-v., rhus-t.***
6 p.m. to 7 p.m. - ***calc.,*** nux-v.
6 p.m. to 8 p.m. - ant-t., caust.
6 p.m. to 12 p.m. - lachn.
7 p.m. - aesc., bov., ***calc.,*** lyc., ***nux-v.,*** petr., rhus-t.
7 p.m. to 8 p.m. - ambr.
7 p.m. to 12 p.m. - aesc.
8 p.m. - coff., ferr., hep., sulph.
daily fever at the same hour, with shortness of breath - cina.
forenoon - ars., bapt., cact., calc., ***cham.,*** **GELS.,** lyc., nat-m., nux-m., rhus-t., sulph., thuj.
9 a.m. to 12 a.m. - **CHAM.**
10 a.m. - **GELS., NAT-M.,** ***rhus-t.,*** thuj.
10 a.m. to 11 a.m. - gels., **NAT-M.,** thuj.
11 a.m. - ***bapt.,*** cact., ***calc.,*** med., **NAT-M.,** thuj.
midnight - **ARS.,** nux-v., stram., sulph.
after - ars., bor., ferr., kali-c., lyc., nat-m., sulph., tax., thuj.
before - acon., ant-c., ars., **BRY.,** ***carb-v.,*** cham., elaps., lyc., mag-m., mag-s., nat-m., petr., puls., sabad.

CHILLS, general
fever without chill,
morning - arn., ars., bry., calc., caust., eup-per., hep., kali-bi., kali-c., nat-m., petr., podo., rhus-t., sulph., thuj.
6 to 10 a.m. - rhus-t.
7 a.m. - podo.
9 a.m. - kali-c.
night - acon., ang., ant-t., apis, **ARS., BAPT., BELL., BRY.,** ***calc., carb-v.,*** caust., cham., ***cina,*** coff., ferr., ***ferr-ar.,*** gels., hep., ip., ***kali-bi.,*** lachn., lyc., nat-m., nicc., nux-v., petr., ***phos.,*** podo., ***puls.,*** **RHUS-T.,** stram., sulph., thuj.
10 p.m. - ars., elaps, ***hydr.,*** lach., petr., sabad.
11 p.m. - cact., ***calc.,*** mag-m.
12 a.m. to 2 a.m. - **ARS.**
12 a.m. to 3 a.m. - **ARS.,** kali-c., med.
1 a.m. to 2 a.m. - **ARS.**
2 a.m. - **ARS.,** benz-ac.
2 a.m. to 4 a.m. - kali-c.
3 a.m. - ang., thuj.
4 a.m. - arn.
noon - ars., spig., stram., sulph.
fever with chilliness - acon., agar., ***anac.,*** apis, ***arn., ars.,*** bapt., bar-m., ***bell.,*** bor., calc., camph., carb-v., ***caust., cham., colch.,*** coff., cur., dros., ***elaps,*** hep., kali-ar., kali-bi., ***kali-c.,*** kali-i., ***kali-s.,*** led., lach., lachn., merc., nat-m., phos., ***podo.,*** puls., ***pyrog.,*** sabin., sec., ***sep.,*** sil., ***spig., squil., sulph., tarent.,*** thuj., ***tub.,*** verat., ***zinc.***

CHLAMYDIAL, infection - med., sulph., thuj.

COLDNESS, external, with - arn., ***ars.,*** bell., bry., calc., ***carb-v.,*** chin., euph., hell., iod., merc., mez., mosch., ph-ac., phos., puls., rhus-t., sabad., spong., stann., verat.

CONTINUED fever, (see Typhoid)

CONVERSATION, from - sep.

CONVULSIONS, after - calc.

COUGHING, increases the heat - ambr., am-c., ant-t., ***arn., ars.,*** bell., carb-v., hep., hyos., iod., ip., kreos., lach., led., lyc., mag-m., nat-c., nux-v., phos., puls., sabad., sep., squil., sulph.

COVERED, parts - arg-m., cham., ***thuj.***

COWPOX, vaccinia - ***acon.,*** ant-t., apis, ***bell.,*** merc., phos., ***sil.,*** sulph., ***thuj.,*** vac.

DAY, febrile heat, only during the - ail., ant-t., bell., berb., carb-v., ***eup-per.,*** ox-ac., sep., sulph., thuj.
periodically, during the - sil.

DEHYDRATION, (see Generals)

DENGUE, fever - ***acon.,*** ars., bell., ***bry.,*** chin., coloc., **EUP-PER.,** ferr., ham., ip., merc., nux-v., podo., ***rhus-t.,*** sec., sul-ac.

DENTITION, during - ***acon.,*** **BELL., CHAM.,** ***ferr-p., gels.,*** phyt., ***rheum, sil., verat-v.***
night - cham., phyt.

DESCENDING - acon., agar., ***alum.,*** bar-c., ***bell.,*** calc-p., canth., ***caust.,*** chel., cic., coff., colch., croc., euphr., laur., mag-c., mez., mosch., nat-c., op., par., ruta., sabin., staph., stront-c., sul-ac., thuj., valer., verat., zinc.

DIARRHEA, after - ars.

DIPHTHERIA (see Throat) - ***chin-a., ign., kali-br., kali-i., kreos.,*** **PHYT.,** ***sal-ac.***
afternoon, returning every - lac-c.
flushed face and sore throat, in alternation with bella - ***kaol.***
high, fever - ***apis, kali-per., merc-c., merc-i-f.***
following violent chill - **PHYT.**
low, fever - ***carb-ac., merc-cy., mur-ac., rhus-t.***
moderate - lac-c.
night, at - ***bapt.***
putrid - ***chin-a., mur-ac.***

DRINKING, agg. - bar-c., calc., cham., cocc.
beer - ***bell., ferr.,*** rhus-t., sulph.
coffee - canth., cham., rhus-t.
coffee, amel. - ars.
cold water, amel. - bism., **CAUST.,** cupr., fl-ac., lob., op., ***phos.,*** sep.
shivering from - ***bell.,*** calen., **CAPS.,** eup-per., ***nux-v.***
water - canth., calc., ign., ***rhus-t.,*** sep.
wine - ars., ***carb-v.,*** fl-ac., gins., iod., nat-m., nux-v., sil.

DRINKS, warm, agg. - sumb.
warm, amel. - ars.

DRY, heat - acet-ac., **ACON.,** aesc., ail., am-c., aml-n., anac., ant-t., ***apis, arn.,*** **ARS.,** ars-i., arum-t., bar-c., bapt., bar-m., **BELL.,** bism., bol., **BRY.,** cact., ***calc.,*** calc-p., camph., carb-an., carb-s., carb-v., caust., ***cedr., cham.,*** chel., chlor., ***chin.,*** chin-a., cimx., cina, clem., cocc., coff., ***colch.,*** coloc., con., cor-r., crot-h., **DULC.,** elaps, ***ferr., ferr-ar.,*** ferr-i., ***ferr-p.,*** hell., hep., hyos., hyper., ign., ***iod.,*** ip., ***kali-ar., kali-c.,*** kali-cy., kali-n., kali-p., kali-s., lach., lact., led., ***lyc.,*** mag-s., meny., ***merc., mur-ac.,*** nat-a., nat-m., nat-s., nit-ac., **NUX-V.,** ***op., petr.,*** plb., ***ph-ac.,*** **PHOS.,** phys., ptel., ***puls.,*** ran-s., ***rhus-t., samb., sec.,*** sep., sil., spig., squil., ***spong., stram.,*** stann., staph., stront-c., ***sulph., sumb., tarent.,*** thuj.
afternoon - alum., ***ars.,*** elaps, gels., ferr., nat-s.
2 p.m. alternating with chill, as if dashed with cold water - chel.
chilliness, with - arg-n.
sleep during - alum.
covered parts, of - **THUJ.**
daytime - bar-m.
evening - aesc., apis, ars., bapt., bell., ***calc-p.,*** carb-v., coff., **CHIN.,** coloc., elaps, graph., ***kali-c., plb.,*** **PULS.,** sul-ac.
7 to 9 p.m., followed by chill until 10 p.m. - elaps
bed, in, with chilliness in back - coff.
distended veins and burning hands that seek out cool places - **PULS.**

DRY, heat
evening,
sleep, on going to - ph-ac.
morning - ***arn.,*** ail., ***bry.,*** calc., cocc., nit-ac., petr., sulph.
morning, on waking - ***arn.***
night - **ACON.,** anac., ant-t., arn., **ARS.,** bapt., ***bar-c., bar-m.,*** **BELL.,** ***bry.,*** calc., carb-an., ***carb-s.,*** carb-v., ***caust., cedr.,*** chel., chin-a., chin-s., cina, ***clem., cocc.,*** coff., ***colch.,*** coloc., con., dulc., ***ferr.,*** hep., graph., kali-n., ***lach.,*** lyc., mur-ac., ***nit-ac.,*** nux-m., ***nux-v.,*** ph-ac., **PHOS.,** ***puls.,*** ran-s., raph., **RHUS-T.,** ***rhus-v.,*** spig., ***sumb., tarent.,*** thea., thuj.
delirium, with - **ARS., BELL.,** ***bry., chin-s., coff., lach., lyc., phos.,*** **RHUS-T.**
driving him out of bed - ant-t.
hot vapors rise up to the brain, is if - ant-t., sarr., sulph.
menses, during - con.
motion, on - ***bry.***
noise, from - bry.
pricking as from needles, with - bol., chin., gels., nit-ac.
rising heat and glowing redness of cheeks, without thirst, after sleep - cina
sleep, during - bov., bry., gins., ph-ac., **SAMB.,** thuj., viol-t.
sleep, going to, on - **SAMB.**
spasmodic gagging, with - **CIMX.**
sweaty hands agg., when put out of bed, with - ***hep.***
swollen veins of arms and hands without thirst - **CHIN.,** sumb.
sex, after - ***nux-v.***
walking in open air - arg-m., nat-m., ***sumb.***

EATING, while - am-c., ***bar-c.,*** cham., chlor., mag-m., nux-v., psor., sil., spig., sul-ac., thuj., valer., viol-t.
amel. - **ANAC.,** ign., lach., mez., zinc.
after - alum., ***ang.,*** arg-n., asaf., bar-c., bell., bor., ***bry.,*** calc., ***caust.,*** cham., chlor., cycl., dig., fl-ac., graph., ign., ind., ***lach.,*** lact., lachn., ***lyc.,*** mag-c., mag-m., nat-m., ***nit-ac., nux-v.,*** petr., **PHOS.,** psor., pyrog., raph., ***sep.,*** sil., sulph., sul-ac., viol-t.
amel. - **ANAC.,** ars., **CHIN.,** cur., ferr., ign., iod., nat-c., phos., rhus-t., stront.
breakfast, after - bar-c., calc., croc., ign., iod., sabad., sulph.
dinner, while - mag-m., sul-ac., thuj., valer.
after - bar-c., bell., ***dig.,*** nit-ac., phos., plan., ptel., sabin., sep., sul-ac., til.

EMACIATION, with hectic fever, and night sweats - ***cocc.***
intermittent - ***aran.***
particularly of face - tarent.
typhoid, in - ***ter.***

ENCEPHALITIS, (see Meningitis) - ***acon.,*** aeth., apis, apoc., arn., ars., bapt., **BELL.,** ***bry.,*** cadm-s., calc., calc-p., ***camph.,*** canth., carb-ac., cham., chin., chin-s., chr-ox., cic., cina, ***con.,*** crot-h., ***cupr., cupr-ar.,*** dig., gels., glon., ***hell.,*** hydr-ac., ***hyos.,*** hyper., iod., iodof., kali-i., kreos., lach., ***merc.,*** merc-c., merc-d., mosch., nux-v., ***op.,*** ox-ac., par., ***phos.,*** phys., plb., puls., rhus-t., ***sil.,*** sol-n., stram., sulph., ***tub.,*** verat-v., vip., zinc.
basilar - ***cupr-cy.,*** dig., hell., iod., tub., ***verat-v.***
cerebro-spinal - ***agar.,*** ail., ***apis,*** arg-n., atro., ***bell.,*** bry., ***cic., cimic., cocc., cupr-ac.,*** cyt-l., echi., ***gels.,*** glon., ***hell.,*** hyos., ip., kali-i., nat-s., op., oreo., phys., sil., stram., sulph., verat-v., zinc-cy., zinc-m.
sopor, with - bor.
traumatic - acon., ***arn.,*** bell., ***hyper.,*** nat-s., sil.
tubercular - ***apis, bac.,*** bell., bry., ***calc., calc-p.,*** cocc., dig., glon., ***hell.,*** hyos., ***iod., iodof.,*** kali-i., ***lyc., merc.,*** nat-m., op., ***sil.,*** stram., ***sulph., tub., verat-v., zinc.,*** zinc-oc.

EVENING - **ACON.,** ***agar.,*** aesc., alum., am-c., anac., ang., anthr., ant-t., apis, aran., arg-m., arn., ***ars.,*** ars-h., aster., bapt., bar-c., bar-m., **BELL.,** ***berb.,*** bor., bov., bry., calad., ***calc., calc-s.,*** calen., caps., carb-s., ***carb-v.,*** caust., ***cham., chel.,*** **CHIN.,** chin-s., ***cina,*** clem., coc-c., coff., con., coloc., cocc., croc., cycl., dros., elaps, euphr., ferr., ferr-ar., ferr-i., graph., hell., ***hep., hyos.,*** ign., ip., kali-ar., ***kali-c.,*** kali-i., kali-n., kali-p., kali-s., **LACH.,** lec., led., **LYC.,** ***merc.,*** mag-m., meny., ***mez.,*** mosch., mur-ac., nat-m., nicc., nit-ac., nux-m., nux-v., petr., ***ph-ac.,*** **PHOS.,** plat., plb., ***psor.,*** **PULS.,** ran-b., rhod., **RHUS-T.,** ruta, ***sars.,*** sabad., sabin., ***sep.,*** **SIL.,** spig., spong., squil., stann., staph., stram., ***sulph.,*** sul-ac., ***thuj.,*** verat., vip., zinc.
5 p.m. - con., kali-c., kali-n., nat-c., nit-ac., phos., rhus-t., sulph., thuj.
6 p.m. - ant-t., arg-n., berb., bor., caust., chin., cocc., hep., kali-c., lac-ac., nux-v., rhod., ***rhus-t.***
6 p.m. to 7 p.m. - calc., phos.
6 p.m. to 8 p.m. - calc., caust., **LYC.**
7 p.m. - ambr., bov., elaps, ***lyc.,*** mag-s., petr., puls., rhus-t.
8 p.m. - ant-t., coff., ferr., hep., lachn., mur-ac., naja, nicc., ***phos.,*** sol-n., sulph.
8 p.m. to 9 p.m. - ars., sulph.
bed, in - ***acon.,*** agn., anac., arg-m., bor., calc., calen., coc-c., coff., hep., kali-c., kali-n., mosch., sars., sulph., thuj.
after lying down - ***acon.,*** asar., bar-c., **BRY.,** carb-ac., chel., coff., hell., mag-m., samb., sul-ac., sulph., zinc.
sweat, with - bor., bov., calc., verat.
chill, after - acon., apis, ars., berb., graph., guai., petr., sulph.

EVENING,
chilliness, with - ***acon.,*** apis, anac., arn., ars., bapt., bor., carb-v., caust., coff., ***cham., elaps,*** ferr-i., hep., kali-c., kali-i., nat-m., sabin., ***sil.,*** sulph., thuj.
delirium, with - ***psor.***
eating, after - anac., ang., raph.
lasting, all night - acon., bol., cocc., graph., hep., lach., lyc., puls., ***rhus-t.,*** sarr., sil.
all night followed by shuddering - cocc.
from 7 to 12 p.m., following 4 p.m. chill - ***aesc.***
morning and - ***hep.***
room, on entering the - ang., nicc., **PULS.,** sul-ac., sulph., zinc.

EXANTEMATIC, fevers, (see Mealses, Scarlet fever) - **ACON.,** ***am-c., ant-c.,*** **APIS,** ***arn., ars., bell.,*** **BRY.,** camph., ***carb-s., carb-v.,*** cham., ***chel.,*** chin., ***chlor., coff., cop., crot-h., dros.,*** **EUPHR.,** ***ferr-p., gels.,*** hyos., ign., ***ip., kali-bi.,*** kali-m., kali-s., mag-c., **MORBILL.,** nux-v., ***phos.,*** phyt., **PULS.,** ***rhus-t., squil.,*** stict., ***stram.,*** **SULPH.,** verat., zinc.

EXERTION, from - acon., alum., ***ant-c.,*** ant-t., arg-m., ars., ***camph., chin.,*** ferr., merc., nit-ac., nux-v., olnd., ox-ac., ***rhus-t.,*** samb., ***sep.,*** spig., spong., stann., stram., ***sumb.,*** valer.
after - am-m., brom., fl-ac., pyrog., rhus-t., sep.
amel. - ign., ***sep.,*** stann.

EXTERNAL, heat - **ACON.,** aeth., ail., alum., am-c., ***anac., ant-t.,*** apis, ***arn.,*** **ARS.,** ***ars-i.,*** asaf., bapt., **BELL.,** bism., **BRY.,** ***calc.,*** **CANTH.,** ***caps.,*** carb-s., ***carb-v.,*** cedr., **CHAM.,** chel., ***chin., chin-s.,*** chlor., cic., cimic., coc-c., ***cocc.,*** coff., colch., coloc., con., cor-r., crot-h., cupr., dig., dulc., hell., hep., ***hyos.,*** **IGN.,** iod., ip., jatr., kali-ar., kali-bi., kali-c., kali-chl., kali-i., kali-n., ***lach., lyc.,*** mag-c., ***merc., merc-c.,*** nit-ac., ***nux-v., op., phos.,*** phyt., plb., **PULS.,** ruta., **RHUS-T.,** sec., sel., sep., **SIL.,** spig., **STRAM.,** ***sulph.,*** sul-ac., ***tarent.,*** verat., zinc.
afternoon, 4 p.m. - coff., ptel.
with chilliness - ars.
with chilliness, and redness without internal heat - **IGN.**
chilliness, with - ***acon.,*** agn., ***anac.,*** alum., ***arn.,*** **ARS.,** asar., atro., ***bell.,*** berb., ***bry.,*** **CALC.,** ***calc-ar.,*** cann-i., ***cocc., coff.,*** coloc., dig., dros., gamb., hep., ***hell.,*** **IGN.,** ***kali-n.,*** lac-c., ***lach., laur., lyc., meny.,*** merc., mur-ac., nat-m., **NUX-V.,** par., ***phos.,*** plb., **PYROG.,** ran-b., raph., rat., rheum, **SEP.,** ***sil., squil., sulph.,*** tab., **THUJ.,** ***verat.***
desire to be fanned in place of thirst during the heat - **CARB-V.**
evening - anac., iod., plb., rhus-t., sulph.
8 p.m. - coff., nat-a.
9 p.m. - elaps
10 p.m. - ars.
11 p.m. - nat-m.
lying down, after - coff., squil.

EXTERNAL, heat
morning - bell.
10 a.m. to 3 p.m. - canth.
night - ***bry., colch.,*** kali-bi., phos., rhus-t.
2 a.m., on waking - hep.
dinner, after - ptel.
sensation, of coldness of the whole body - bar-c.
external heat, without heat - **CHAM.,** ign.
yellow skin, with - merc-c.

FAINTNESS, and languor - gels., ptel.

FORENOON - alum., ***am-c.,*** am-m., arg-m., ars., ***bapt.,*** berb., bry., cact., calc., caps., cedr., **CHAM.,** ***eup-per.,*** gels., ham., kali-c., lyc., ***mag-c.,*** **NAT-M.,** nux-m., ***nux-v., phos., rhus-t.,*** sars., sep., sil., sol-n., spig., sulph., thuj., verat., zinc.
9 a.m. - am-c., **CHAM.**
9 a.m. and 5 p.m. - ***kali-c.***
10 a.m. and 8 p.m. - sil.
10 a.m. as if dashed with hot water, or hot water running through the blood vessels - **RHUS-T.**
11 a.m., with thirst and chilliness - sil.
11 a.m. to 1 p.m. - arg-m.
11 a.m. to 12 a.m. - calc.
alternating with chill - calc., cham., thuj.
before - am-c.
chilliness, with - ars., ***bapt.,*** **CHAM.,** kali-c., sil., sulph., thuj.
heat, of the whole body except the head - arg-m.

GANGRENE, (see Generals)

GASTRIC, fever - ***acon.,*** **ANT-C., ANT-T.,** ***arg-n., arn.,*** **ARS.,** bapt., ***bell.,*** **BRY.,** canth., carb-v., ***cham., chel., chin., colch., coloc.,*** cupr., dig., dulc., eup-per., ***gels., hydr.,*** ign., **IP.,** ***iris,*** mag-m., mag-s., **MERC.,** mur-ac., nat-s., **NUX-V.,** ***phos., podo.,*** **PULS.,** rheum, ***rhus-t., sec.,*** sep., ***sulph.,*** tarax., ***verat.***
anger, after - ***acon., bry.,*** **CHAM.,** ***coloc., nux-v., staph.***
debility - ***hydr.***
hot weather, in, from abuse of ice water and summer beverages - **CARB-V.**
jerking of arms and fingers - ***stram.***
low, nervous, bilious, lingering - ***cocc.***
nervous - daph., ***lach.***
pain in stomach and liver - ***card-m.***
plethoric, or suffering from portal stasis, in hot weather or warm wet days - ***nux-v.***
typhoid form - auran.

GONORRHEA, (see Generals)

HAT, putting on - agar.

HEAD, except - ang., sulph.

HEAT, absent - am-m., agar., **ARAN.,** benz., ***bov.,*** camph., canth., ***caps., caust., cimx.,*** cocc., gamb., graph., ***hep.,*** kali-c., kali-n., led., ***lyc.,*** mag-c., ***mez.,*** mur-ac., nat-c., ph-ac., ran-b., rhus-t., ***sabad.,*** **STAPH., SULPH.,** sul-ac., ***thuj., verat.***

HECTIC fever - abrot., **ACET-AC.**, am-c., arg-m., ***arn.***, **ARS.**, **ARS-I.**, ***asar.***, aur-m., bapt., bry., bol., **CALC.**, ***calc-p.***, ***calc-s.***, **CAPS.**, ***carb-an.***, ***carb-v.***, ***chin.***, ***chin-a.***, chin-s., ***chlor.***, cocc., ***crot-h.***, ***cupr.***, ***ferr.***, ferr-p., guai., hep., ***hydr.***, ***hyos.***, **IOD.**, ***ip.***, **KALI-AR.**, ***kali-c.***, ***kali-p.***, ***kali-s.***, ***lach.***, ***lac-d.***, **LYC.**, med., ***merc.***, mez., mill., ***nat-a.***, nit-ac., nux-v., ***ph-ac.***, **PHOS.**, ***plb.***, ***puls.***, ***pyrog.***, **SANG.**, ***senec.***, **SEP.**, **SIL.**, ***stann.***, ***sulph.***, sul-ac., ***tarent.***, thuj., **TUB.**
- afternoon, or towards evening - ***ph-ac.***
  - every - med.
- anguish, with, red cheeks - **CALC.**
- children, especially in - ***merc.***
- chills, alternate, and heat - **CALC.**
  - shaking, then heat and drenching sweat - ***gels.***
- cough, in whooping, with debility - verat.
- cough, with - ***acet-ac.***
  - night - ***caps.***
- cystitis, in - ***eup-pur.***
- cystitis, or kidney disease - chim.
- daily, forenoon, 11 to 12 or 1 p.m. - arg-m.
- debilitated persons, in, worse after meals - ***sil.***
- disease, after exhausting, loss of fluids, etc. - **CALC.**, **CHIN.**
- dyscrasia - ***iod.***
- edema, in - ***aur-m.***
- emaciation and night sweats - ***cocc.***
  - and tubercular condition - merc-c.
- emotions, after depressing - **CAPS.**, ***lach.***, ***ph-ac.***, staph.
- evening, with sharply circumscribed redness of cheeks, especially left - ***sulph.***
- expectoration, sweetish, purulent, slight mucous rhonchus and sibilant rale - ptel.
- flushes, frequent - **CALC.**
- gonarthrocace - ***ars.***
- hemoptysis, with - mill.
- hepatitis, suppuration - ***phos.***
- hip disease, in - ***calc.***, ***caust.***, phos., ***sil.***
- influenza, after - ***abrot.***
- intermittent paroxysms - ***hep.***
- jaundice - ***sulph.***
- laryngeal and bronchial troubles, eleven a.m. to twelve or one p.m. - ***arg-m.***
- lipoma on neck - ***phos.***
- lungs, chronic bleeding, from - senec.
- lungs, suppuration of - ***lyc.***
- measles, in - ***lach.***
- night, at, preventing sleep - ***ol-j.***
- nostalgia, from - **CAPS.**
- pleurisy, in - ***carb-v.***
- pleuropneumonia, in - ***hep.***
- pneumonia, in - ***sulph.***
- pus, enormous quantities of - ***iod.***
- scarlatina, after - ***aur-m.***
- scrofulosis and rachitis, with, protracted ill-treated cases - petr.
- scurvy - ***am-c.***
- shuddering, constant, in evening - **CALC.**
- skin dry, withered - **CALC.**

HECTIC fever,
- slow progress, in third stage of croupous pneumonia - ***iod.***
  - spinal abscess, in - ***ph-ac.***
- stomach, after a blow on - ***arn.***
- suppurative process, during - ***ars.***, ***carb-v.***, ***chin.***, ***hep.***, ***lyc.***, ***merc.***, **SIL.**, sulph.
- sweat and diarrhea, with - phos.
  - sour, emaciation, and great debility - fl-ac.
- sweats easily - **CALC.**
  - clammy night, after pneumonia - ***lyc.***
  - night, with - ***eup-pur.***, ***lyc.***, ***phos.***, rob.
- syphilis, in secondary - ***aur-m.***
- thirst, no - ars-s-f.
- throat, swelling and redness in, dryness, soreness, as in scarlet fever - sang.
- trachea is implicated - ***iod.***
- tubercles of lungs develop - ***phos.***
- tuberculosis, in - **CALC.**, eucal., ***kreos.***, **PLB.**, polyp-p, ***samb.***, stann., ***tril.***, ***tub.***
  - with appearance similar to chronic - hippoz.
- ulceration, chronic, of mucous membrane - kali-bi.
- urine, with red - calc., sulph.
- weakening - ***abrot.***

HERPES, (see Generals)

HICCOUGH, in place of fever - ***ars.***

HIGH, fever - abrot., **ACON.**, ant-t., ***apis***, **ARN.**, **ARS.**, ***arum-t.***, ***aur.***, **BELL.**, ***bry.***, cact., canth., caps., chel., chin., ***chin-s.***, cina, coff., ***colch.***, **CON.**, croc., crot-h., cupr., dig., dulc., ferr-ar., **GELS.**, hep., hyos., ***kali-ar.***, kali-i., ***lach.***, ***lyc.***, mag-c., meny., merc-c., **MEZ.**, **NAT-M.**, nat-s., nit-ac., nux-m., ***nux-v.***, ***op.***, ph-ac., ***phos.***, **PULS.**, **PYROG.**, **RHUS-T.**, samb., sang., **SEC.**, ***sil.***, staph., ***stram.***, thuj., ***tub.***
- convulsions, with - **BELL.**, ***cic.***, ***hyos.***, op., **STRAM.**
- delirium, with - ant-t., ***apis***, **ARS.**, **BELL.**, ***bry.***, carb-v., chin., ***chin-s.***, ***chlor.***, coff., hep., hyos., iod., **NAT-M.**, nux-v., **OP.**, **PULS.**, sarr., sec., **STRAM.**
- head and face hot, body cold - **ARN.**, ***bell.***, ***op.***, ***stram.***
- sleep, during - ***ant-t.***, apis, caps., chin., gels., ***lach.***, lyc., **MEZ.**, ***nat-m.***, ***nux-m.***, **OP.**, rhus-t., stram.
  - after - cina, op.
- stupefaction and unconsciousness, with - ***bell.***, ***cact.***, **NAT-M.**, **OP.**, ***phos.***

INFLAMMATORY, fever - ***acet-ac.***, **ACON.**, apis, arn., ars., **BELL.**, **BRY.**, ***cact.***, canth., ***cham.***, chin., ***calc.***, con., dig., dulc., ***gels.***, hep., hyos., ip., kali-c., ***lach.***, lyc., **MERC.**, nit-ac., nux-v., ***phos.***, **PULS.**, **RHUS-T.**, sep., sil., ***sin-n.***, ***sulph.***, sul-ac., verat.
- children, in, with excitability - ***coff-t.***
- croup, in - ***spong.***
- does not reach a high grade - ***hydr.***
- lung affections, in - ***kali-n.***
- pulmonary, hepatic, or gastric - ***sang.***

INFLUENZA, infection - ***acon.,*** all-c., arn., **ARS.,** ars-i., **BAPT., BRY.,** calc., camph., ***carc., caust., chel.,*** dulc., ***euph.,*** **EUP-PER.,** ferr-p., **GELS.,** med., ***merc., merc-i-r.,*** naja., ***nux-v.,*** ph-ac., **PHOS.,** ***pyrog.,*** **RHUS-T.,** sabad.
ailments, from - abrot., ars., bry., cadm-m., calc-p., **GELS.,** ***ph-ac.,*** psor., scut., tub.
pain, in limbs, during - ***acon.,*** arn., **BRY.,** ***caust., chel., euph.,*** **EUP-PER.,** ***gels., merc.,*** naja., ***pyrog.,*** rhus-t.
remaining after - calc., lycps.
stomach, flu - ***acon.,*** **ANT-C., ANT-T., ARS.,** bapt., ***bell.,*** **BRY.,** canth., carb-v., ***cham., chel.,*** chin., colch., coloc., cupr., eup-per., ***gels.,*** ign., **IP.,** iris, mag-m., mag-s., med., ***merc.,*** mur-ac., nat-s., ***nux-v., phos., podo.,*** **PULS.,** rheum, ***rhus-t., sec., sulph.,*** tarax., ***verat.***
tendency to get influenza - carc.
weakness, after - abrot., ***carc.,*** con., chin., cypr., ***gels.,*** kali-p., ***ph-ac.,*** scut., x-ray.

INJURIES, after - ***acon.,*** apis, ***arn., calen., coff.***

INSIDIOUS, fever - acet-ac., ***ars., chin.,*** cocc., con., colch., ***sec., sulph., tub.***

INTENSE, (see High, fever)

INTERMITTENT fever - absin., acon., ***cimic., aesc.,*** agar., ***agn., alum.,*** am-m., ***ambr., ang.,*** **ANT-C., ANT-T.,** apis, arg-n., ***arn.,*** **ARS.,** art-v., aur-m., ***bapt.,*** bar-c., ***bell.,*** berb., bov., ***bry., casc., calad., calc.,*** calc-s., camph., ***canth.,*** **CAPS.,** ***carb-v.,*** carb-ac., ***cact.,*** caust., **CEDR.,** cetr., **CHAM.,** ***chel.,*** chim., ***chin-a.,*** **CHIN-S.,** cic., ***cimx., cina,*** **CHIN.,** chin-b., cist., **CIMX.,** ***cocc.,*** coch., ***coff.,*** coff-t., **COLCH.,** ***corn.,*** cur., ***cycl., aran., dros., elaps,*** **ELAT.,** ***eucal.,*** **EUP-PER.,** ***eup-pur., ferr., ferr-m., ferr-p.,*** fl-ac., ***gamb., gels., glon.,*** hell., ***hep.,*** hydr., ***hyos., ign., iod.,*** **IP.,** kali-bi., ***kali-br., kali-c., kali-i., kali-m.,*** kali-p., lach., lachn., led., ***lob., lyc., lyss.,*** mag-c., mag-m., ***mag-p.,*** mag-s., **MENY.,** ***merc., merl., mez.,*** mur-ac., nat-a., **NAT-M.,** ***nat-s.,*** nit-ac., **NUX-M.,** ***nux-v., op., petr., phos., ph-ac.,*** plan., plb., ***podo.,*** polyp-p, psor., **PULS.,** ***rhus-t.,*** rob., ***sabad., samb., sec., sep., sil.,*** spig., stann., staph., ***stram., sulph., sul-ac., tab., tarax., tarent.,*** thuj., valer., ***verat.***
abdominal affections, with - ***petr.***
chilliness, in - ***meny.***
afternoon, in - ***apis.***
2 p.m., worse - ***lach.***
lasting till three or four o'clock next morning - rob.
paroxysm coming every - ***chel.***
anticipating - ant-t., ars., bell., bry., chin., eup-per., gamb., ign., nat-m., nux-v.
each time two hours - chin-s.
apathy, great, and night sweats - ***ph-ac.***
apoplectic - **NUX-V.**
apyrexia - ***ars.***
abdomen bloated - chin.
abdominal viscera, pains in, especially liver, with great lassitude - ***polyp-p***
anemic appearance - ***chin.***

INTERMITTENT fever,
apyrexia,
apathy - ign.
appetite, loss of - chin., ip., ***nat-m., polyp-p, puls.,*** sabad.
quotidian, in - ***ip.***
back, pain in - ign.
in small of - ***ip.***
belching, rancid, sour - sabad.
breathing, oppressed - sabad.
bruised feeling in limbs - ip.
cachectic appearance - chin.
chest, oppression of - sabad.
pain in - sabad.
pain in, in quotidian - puls.
chilly - sabad.
colic - ign.
cough - ***sabad.***
irritation to, in larynx - ign.
loose - eup-per.
with expectoration of bitter taste - puls.
crusty, lips - ***ars.***
debility and painful diarrhea - ***corn.***
debility, in tertian - ***ip.***
delirium - ***nat-m.***
despondent - ***ip.***
diarrhea, mucous - ***puls.***
stools grayish-yellow - ***ip.***
dyspepsia, flatulent, with heat and twitching in epigastric region, eructation, nausea, vomiting and colic, in men - ***petros.***
epigastrium, aching in - ign.
face bloated - ***ars.***
pale - ign., ip., sep.
yellow - ***arn.***
gastric symptoms - **ANT-C.,** ***dros., ip., nux-v.***
head burning in, with cold hands and feet - ign.
dulness in, with loss of appetite - nux-v.
heaviness in - ign.
were smaller, sensation as if - ign.
headache - ***arn., nat-m., polyp-p, puls.***
heaviness of whole body, with chilliness and sleepiness during day - puls.
herpes labialis - ip.
hungry about eleven a.m. - ign.
hypochondria, sensitiveness in - chin.
stitching in left - puls.
itching, of whole body - ***elat.***
kidneys, pain in region of - ***nat-m.***
knees, giving away of, languor - ign.
larynx, sensation of a foreign body lying over - ign.
lassitude - puls.
lassitude, in quotidian - ***ip.***
legs, pain in - puls.
lemon juice with coffee - cit-l., ***hyos., mez.,*** **NAT-M.,** tarax.
limbs, pain in - ign., ***ip.***
lips cracked - ***ars.,*** ign.
pale or swollen - ***ars.***
liver region, continual stitches in - ***nat-m.***
pressure in, sometimes alternating with pain in spleen - ***nat-m.***

INTERMITTENT fever,
apyrexia,
meat, aversion to - ***arn.***
nausea - ***puls.***
sadness - ip.
salivation - ip.
sclerotica, burning and redness of - rhus-t.
sleep continues from heat through sweating stage - ign.
restless - ***ip.***
sound, with snoring - ign.
starting in - ign.
stomach bloated - sabad.
disturbance of digestive organs - ***ferr.***
emptiness, pressure, or weakness in - ***ip.***
stool hard - ign.
frequent watery, with pain in abdomen - ***elat.***
ineffectual urging to - ign.
loose - ip.
taste, loss of - ***nat-m.***
bitter - ***elat.***
insipid water, of - ip.
bitter - ***arn., polyp-p.***
earthy - ***ip.***
pappy - ign.
temples, throbbing in - ign.
thirst - ***cimx., nat-m.***
thoughts, difficulty in collecting - ip.
tongue dry, white - ***nat-m.***
white or yellow - ***polyp-p***
white, in quotidian, with icterus - ***elat.***
urine dark - ***elat.***
scanty - chin.
scanty red - ***ip.***
urticaria, better by rubbing - elat.
vertigo - ***ign., ip.***
vomiting of bile and bitter mucus - sabad.
wanting, or very short - ***gels.***
weakness - ***ars., gels., hep., ip.,*** sabad.
limbs, of - chin., sabad.
whole muscular system, of - ***gels.***
asthma, with, for a year - tab.
attacks, twelve to eighteen, during twenty-four hours - sabad.
autumnal - bapt., bry., chin., nat-m., nux-v., rhus-t., sin-n., verat.
back, pain in small of - **LACH.**
and neck, pains in, before - gels.
bilious - ***puls.***
belching, with - sabad.
breathing, oppression of, constriction of chest, pain in region of liver, thirst worse during chill - ***kali-c.***
broncho-pneumonia, after - chin-m.
cachectic persons - **CALC.,** ***hydr.***
after loss of blood, or from continued and long prostration - chin., chin-s.
calves, with cramps in - ***mag-p.***
change of type, frequent - elat., ***ferr.***
changing, type continually, especially after abuse of quinine - ign.

INTERMITTENT fever,
chest, in, oppression - ***crot-h.***
children, in - ***gels., nux-v., op.***
cholera, during - ***verat.***
chronic - agar., alum., apis, **ARS.,** ***ars-i.,*** **CALC.,** ***calc-p.,*** calc-s., ***carb-ac., carb-v.,*** **CHIN.,** ***chin-a.,*** **FERR.,** ferr-ar., ***ferr-i.,*** graph., ***hep., iod.,*** kali-ar., kali-c., **KALI-S.,** lach., **LYC., NAT-M., NAT-S., NIT-AC.,** nux-v., ***phos.,*** **PSOR., PYROG.,** ***sep., sil.,*** **SULPH., TARENT., TUB.**
abuse of quinine, after - ***plan.***
afternoon and evening, agg. - ars-s-f.
partially recovers, then relapses - ***sulph.***
stomach, pain, with - ***abies-n.***
colic, with - aran.
and lameness in small of back - cocc.
confinement, fifth day after - ***lach.***
congestive - nux-v.
convalescence, in - eucal.
convulsions, in children, with - ***gels.***
tonic - ***nat-m.***
delirium - ***sabad.***
diarrhea, during - ars., chin-a., **CINA,** cocc., con., gels., puls., ***rhus-t.,*** thuj.
dropsy, with - **AUR-M.,** sin-n.
after - ***hell.,*** **LAC-D.**
suppression of, after - cor-r.
dyscrasia - aran.
dysentery, with - polyp-p
elderly people, with coma - alum., ***op.,*** nux-m.
head and body, pain in, when he has no chill, tongue not much coated - ***gels.***
epidemic - ***lyc.***
eruptions, after suppressed - **CALC.**
feet, after, have become wet and cold - nux-v.
food and nausea, regurgitation of - sabad.
sensitiveness to smell of - ***colch.***
gastric - ***arg-n., ip.***
and bilious symptoms, or consequent upon abuse of chinona or quinine, with bitter taste of food, and constipation - ***puls.***
rheumatic - ***ant-t.***
gonorrheal contamination, with - ***thuj.***
gout, with - ferr., led.
head, congestion to - ***cact.***
headache, with - ***cina,*** cist., ***kali-c., polyp-p.***
coming on early in morning, after suppressed - ***nat-m.***
hot days, cool nights - acon., colch., merc.
hunger, ravenous - ***staph.***
ice house, after staying in - eup-per.
incomplete - ***ars.***
consisting only of heat and sweat, with moderate thirst - mang.
irregular, cases, in beginning of - ***ip.***
chiefly cold stage, incompletely developed, hands or ends of fingers and toes, or feet and end of nose alone becoming very cold - ***meny.***
paroxysms - ***ang.,*** hippoz., ***ign., ip.,*** mill., ***nux-v.,*** samb., sulph., sul-ac.

INTERMITTENT fever,
irregular,
periodicity and evolution of stages, in - ign.
liver, complaint, after - **LACH.**
enlarged, with - ferr-ar., ferr-i., ***lyc.,*** nat-m., **NIT-AC.**
functional disease of - ***hydr.***
long-lasting fever, with - **ANT-T.,** cact., canth., colch., ***ferr.,*** hep., ip., sec., sil., ***tarent.***
lungs, hemorrhage, with - ***arg-n.***
malarial - **ARN.**
quotidian - ***gels.***
malignant - ***crot-h.***
marsh fever - ***ang.,*** arn., **ARS.,** ***asc-t.,*** carb-v., **CHIN.,** cina, aran., ferr., **IP., NAT-M.,** ***rhus-t., sang.,*** sin-n., verat.
marshy regions in warm seasons and tropical countries - **CEDR.**
masked - ***ars.,*** ip., nux-v., ***sep.,*** spig., ***tarent., tub.***
choreic or neuralgic manifestations - ***gels.***
menses, after - **NUX-V.**
miscarriage, pains threatening, in early months of pregnancy, during febrile stage - ***puls.***
monthly attacks - **NUX-V.**
morning, worse early in - ***verat.***
nausea and vomiting during paroxysm - ***gels.***
and regurgitation - sabad.
nervous symptoms predominate - ***gels.***
night, midnight, worse after - ran-b., raph.
noon, principally before - ***guare.***
obstinate cases, hot flushes and hot soles at night - sulph.
worse by exposure and neglect or abuse of quinine - ***polyp-p***
occiput, pain in, before - gels.
opium, suppression by - ***calc-ar.***
paralysis follows - **RHUS-T.**
periodicity strongly marked - cedr., gels., ***petros.***
periosteal pains, with - mur-ac.
pernicious - ***apis, arn.,*** camph., cur., nux-v., op., ***verat.***
postponing - chin., cina, gamb., ign., ip.
prevailing, icterus, eyes yellow, stool white, urine dark yellow - ***sang.***
prodromal stage - ***gels.***
prosopalgia, suppressed by quinine - **STANN.**
quartan - acon., anac., ant-c., arn., ***ars.,*** bell., bry., **BUFO,** carb-v., ***chin-s.,*** **CIMX.,** cina, chin., clem., ***coff.,*** cor-r., elat., ***eup-per., hyos., ign.,*** iod., ***ip.,*** lach., lyc., meny., mill., ***nat-m.,*** **NUX-V.,** ***phel.,*** plan., podo., ***puls.,*** rhus-t., ***sabad., sin-n.,*** verat.
diarrhea on days free from fever - ***iod.***
double - ars., chin., dulc., eup-per., eup-pur., gamb., lyc., nux-m., puls., rhus-t.
paroxysm between three and four a.m. - sep.
paroxysm in evening, chill predominating - rhus-t.
since two years - ***nat-m.***

INTERMITTENT fever,
quartan,
six weeks, paroxysm twelve m., then attack like cholera morbus - ***elat.***
two years, resisting many remedies - ***ptel.***
quinine, after abuse of - ***arn.,*** **CALC.,** ***elat., ferr., gels., hep.,*** **IP.,** ***nat-m.,*** **PULS.,** rhus-t., sulph., ***verat.***
relapse into bilious with burning and rending pain - ***lach.***
spleen swollen - ***ran-s.***
quotidian - acon., aesc., anac., ant-c., ant-t., apis, **ARS.,** bapt., bar-c., bell., bry., cact., calc., calc-s., ***caps.,*** carb-v., ***cedr.,*** cham., ***chin-s.,*** cic., cina, cur., ***aran.,*** elaps, elat., eucal., ***eup-per., eup-pur.,*** gamb., gels., graph., ***hep., ign., ip., kali-br.,*** kali-c., lach., ***lob.,*** lyc., mag-c., ***nat-m.,*** nit-ac., nux-v., ***petros.,*** phos., plan., podo., polyp-p, ***puls., rhus-t.,*** sabad., ***samb., sep.,*** spig., stann., staph., ***stram.,*** sulph., ***tarax., verat.***
1 to 3 p.m. - ***nat-m.***
4:45 p.m. to 6.30 p.m. - ***lyc.***
5 p.m., preceded by yawning and pain in maxillary joint, as if dislocated - rhus-t.
8 to 10 p.m. - elaps.
9 a.m. - meny.
11 a.m. - **CACT.**
afternoon - sep.
anthrax, with on back of neck - tarent., sulph.
double - ant-c., ***apis,*** bapt., bell., chin., dulc., elat., graph., led., stram., sulph.
at sunrise and five p.m. - ***aran.***
hour, at same - anac., ang., ***cact.,*** **CEDR.,** ***aran.,*** gels., sabad., stann., spig.
icterus, with - ***elaps.***
marsh fever - ***aran.***
midnight, before - arund.
pressure and swelling at epigastrium and anxious palpitation during day - rhus-t.
scrofula, profuse saliva with, chronic - **CALC.**
scrofulous children, in, chronic - calc-p.
suppressed, became tertian - ***elat.***
regular, at same period every day - aesc., ang., cact., caps., **CEDR.,** ***chin-s.,*** cina, ***chin., aran.,*** gels., hep., kali-c., podo., spig., verat.
chill, without - gels.
relapsing - ***ars.,*** ust.
quinine, after - **ARS.**
remittent, apt to become usually quotidian - ***phos.***
becomes, postponing oftener than anticipating - gamb.
or typhoid, apt to become - ***phos.***
restless, during paroxysm - ***cocc.***
rheumatism, with - led.
or gout - ***led.***
right side, commencing on, first arm then leg gets cold - rhus-t.
sequelae - ***cean.,*** chin., ***gels.***
seven days, every - ***lyc.***

INTERMITTENT fever,
shoulders, pains in neck and, before and after - gels.
simple, uncomplicated - gels.
skin hot, dry, in reactive stage - ***gels.***
parchment like, dry heat after chill - ip.
sleeping, from, on cold floor - ***aran.***
slowly, comes on - stram.
soporous - ant-t.
spasmodic symptoms - calc.
spleen, enlargement of - ***ars., carb-ac., cean., chin-s., chin., aran.,*** ferr-ar., ferr-i., ***kali-i., nat-m., ran-s.,*** rhus-t., ***sul-ac.***
spoiled - ars., ***calc., ferr., ip.,*** nat-m., nux-v., **SEP.,** sulph., ***tarent.***
spring, in - ***cham.,*** gels., sabad.
after suppression, in summer or fall by quinine - ***lach.***
every - carb-v., ***lach.,*** nux-v., sep., sulph.
for several years, annually - ***ign.***
stages distinct - **CHIN-S.,** ***petros.***
indistinct, adynamic condition - ***gels.***
severe chill, little shaking then fever - ***gels.***
stiffness - ***nat-m.***
stomach, derangement of - **CACT.**
chill begins in, agonizing weight - calc.
summer, in beginning of - ***lach.***
suppressed - ***elat.,*** spig.
aching and soreness, with general weakness - ***gels.***
earache, toothache, headache, pain in limbs, etc. - ***puls.***
sweat, without - rhus-v.
swellings, edematous, after - cahin.
tertian - aesc., alum., anac., **ANT-C.,** ***ant-t., apis,*** arn., ***ars., bar-m.,*** bell., bry., calc., calc-s., canth., caps., carb-v., ***cedr., cham.,*** cic., cina, ***chin-s., cimx., chin.,*** cor-r., ***aran., dig.,*** dros., dulc., elat., eucal., **EUP-PER.,** ferr., gamb., gels., ***hep.,*** hyos., ***ign.,*** iod., ***ip., lach.,*** lyc., mez., mill., ***nat-m.,*** nux-m., **NUX-V.,** plan., podo., polyp-p, ***puls.,*** rhus-t., sabad., sulph., verat.
afternoon - bapt.
anteponing - ***nat-m.***
half an hour - ***ip.***
bilious fever, after - sulph.
body drawn up in a heap - ***lach.***
double - aesc., ars., chin., dulc., elat., eucal., eup-pur., gamb., lyc., nux-v., rhus-t.
evening - ***calc.***
evening, 9 p.m. - sabad.
gout of knee follows with tophi and lameness in joints - nux-v.
had been treated with chinona - sabad.
morning chill, evening fever - ferr.
nettle rash, with, disappearing after attack - rhus-t.
nightly at same hour - sabad.
profuse vomiting of bilious matter - ptel.
sometimes morning, sometimes evening - sep.
stages well marked - ***ph-ac.***

INTERMITTENT fever,
tertian,
symptoms of scurvy - ***staph.***
throat, sore, and nausea - ***dros.***
tongue, slimy coated, yellow - kali-s.
tuberculosis, incipient - ***bry.***
typhoid, tendency to run into - **ARS.,** ***bapt.,*** gels., ***mez., sec.***
after - ***gels.***
urethra, traumatic or chronic inflammation of, even stricture - ***petros.***
vomiting, food - ***ferr-p.***
acid, sour masses - nat-p.
bilious, agg. by damp weather or seashore - nat-s.
water, working in cold - **CALC.**
week, once a - am-m., canth., chin., lyc., meny., plan.
every four - nux-m., nux-v., puls., sep.
every three - chin., mag-c., sulph.
every two - am-m., ars., calc., chin-s., chin., lach., plan., puls.
whooping cough, with - ***kali-c., nat-m.***
winter, in - ant-t., ***nat-m.,*** polyp-p, psor.
women, nervous hysterical - ***tarent.***
yearly - ars., carb-v., ***aran.,*** lach., nat-m., psor., sulph., thuj.
young persons, recent cases in - ip.

INTERNAL, heat - **ACON.,** aloe, alum., am-m., anac., **ARN., ARS.,** ars-i., **BELL., BRY.,** berb., calad., ***calc., canth.,*** caps., ***carb-v., caust., cham.,*** chel., chin., ***cic.,*** coloc., ***con.,*** croc., ***ferr.,*** ferr-ar., ferr-i., ***ferr-p., fl-ac., hell.,*** hyos., ign., ***iod.,*** ip., ***kali-ar., kali-c.,*** kali-p., lach., **LAUR.,** ***lyc.,*** **MAG-C.,** mag-m., ***med.,*** **MERC.,** ***mez.,*** nat-m., ***nit-ac.,*** **NUX-V., PETR., PH-AC., PHOS.,** ***puls.,*** **RHUS-T.,** ***sabad., sec., sep., sil., spig.,*** squil., ***stann.,*** **SULPH.,** ***verat., zinc.***
afternoon - graph.
burning - ***ars., bell.,*** brom., caps., bell., hyos., mez., ***mosch.,*** **SEC.**
at 9 a.m. - brom.
in the blood vessels - agar., **ARS.,** ***aur., bry., calc., hyos., med.,*** nat-m., nit-ac., op., **RHUS-T.,** ***sulph.,*** verat.
chill, with external - **ACON.,** ***arn.,*** **ARS.,** ars-i., ***bell.,*** bry., ***calc.,*** **CAMPH.,** caps., ***cham., chel., ferr.,*** ferr-ar., ***ferr-i., ign., iod., ip., kali-ar., kali-c., mez.,*** **MOSCH.,** nat-c., nit-ac., ***ph-ac., phos., puls., rhus-t.,*** sabad., sang., ***sec., sil.,*** squil., sulph., sul-ac., **VERAT.,** ***zinc.***
chillness, with - graph.
cold perspiration, with - anac.
cold to the touch, while the body feels - ***carb-v., ferr.,*** sars.
coldness of single parts, with - chin., ign., ***nux-v., rhus-t.***
evening - anac., calc., ***puls.,*** spig., zinc.
menses, during - nat-m.
morning - alum., carb-v., petr.
8 a.m. - caust.

INTERNAL, heat

night - calc., clem., mag-c., mag-m., mang., petr., spig.

must uncover, which causes chilliness - **MAG-C.**

IRREGULAR, (see Intermittent, Stages)

IRRITATIVE, fever - acon., arn., **ARS.,** bapt., bell., ***bry., camph.,*** canth., ***carb-v.,*** cham., ***chin., cocc.,*** crot-t., cupr., dig., ***gels., graph.,*** hell., hyos., **LACH.,** ***lyc.,*** merc., ***mur-ac., nat-m., nux-v.,*** op., ***ph-ac., podo., puls., rhus-t., sec.,*** sulph., verat.

cerebral congestion, with, causing convulsions, in children - ***verat-v.***

physical irritation, from dentition, or indigestible foreign bodies in intestines - ***cham.***

sharp, with swelling of face, head and hands - rhus-v.

slow - ***acet-ac.,*** **ARS.,** ***bry.,*** calc-s., ***camph.,*** canth., ***chin.,*** cocc., hell., lach., ***lyc., mur-ac., ph-ac., phos.,*** plb., ***sec.,*** sil., sulph., thuj.

ulceration, suppuration, abscess, presence of foreign body, etc. - ***gels.***

LONG, lasting heat - acon., ***ant-t.,*** apis, ***arn., ars.,*** aster., bar-m., ***bell.,*** bol., ***cact.,*** calc-f., ***caps., carc.,*** **CHAM.,** chin., colch., elaps, eup-per., ***ferr.,*** **GELS.,** graph., ***hep.,*** hyos., lach., laur., lyc., nat-m., ***nux-v., sec.,*** sil., ***sulph., tarent.***

followed by chill - apis.

sleep, with - ***chin.***

LOW, fever - **ARS.,** ***bapt., cact.,*** carb-ac., chim., coca, ***crot-h.,*** eucal., nit-s-d., sabin.

debility during convalescence - **COCA.**

diphtheria, in - **ARS.,** ***kali-bi.***

hot weather, in, from abuse of ice water or cold drinks - **CARB-V.**

insomnia, with - ***stram.***

morning, remission slight each - ***lach.***

pneumonia, in - ***seneg.***

pulse slow and accelerated by lifting or turning patient - ***gels.***

typhus, succeeding - ***sumb.***

MALARIA - abies-n., ***arg-n.,*** **ARN.,** carb-ac., **CEDR., CHIN.,** chin-a., ***chin-s., eucal.,*** **EUP-PER.,** ***ferr.,*** ip., ***nat-m., nat-s., nux-v.,*** **PSOR.,** ***sulph.,*** **TER.,** verat-v.

appetite, loss of - ***nat-s.***

ataxy - ***arg-n.***

breath, offensive - ***nat-s.***

chronic - eucal., polyp-p

creeps and fever, alternate - ***nat-s.***

headache, dull - ***nat-s.***

jaundice, with - ***nat-s.***

metastasis of miasmatic - ***bry.***

old, broken-down cases - **LYC.**

periodicity, marked - **CHIN.**

relapsing, obstinate, spleen affected early in disease - eucal.

scrotum, inflammation and sloughing of, followed - op.

weak and languid - ***nat-s.***

MARSH fever - ***ang.,*** arn., **ARS.,** ***asc-t.,*** carb-v., **CHIN.,** cina, aran., ferr., **IP., NAT-M.,** ***rhus-t., sang.,*** sin-n., verat.

bilious, on rice plantations - ***asc-t.***

marshy regions in warm seasons and tropical countries - **CEDR.**

MEASLES, infection - **ACON.,** ***am-c., ant-c.,*** **APIS,** ***arn., ars., bell.,*** **BRY.,** camph., ***carb-s., carb-v.,*** cham., ***chel.,*** chin., ***chlor., coff., cop., crot-h., dros., euph.,*** **EUPHR.,** ***ferr-p., gels.,*** hyos., ign., ***ip., kali-bi.,*** kali-m., kali-s., ***lach.,*** mag-c., **MORBILL.,** nux-v., ***phos.,*** phyt., **PULS.,** ***rhus-t., squil.,*** stict., ***stram.,*** **SULPH.,** verat., zinc.

ailments after - acon., am-c., ant-c., ***ant-t., arg-m., ars., bell.,*** bry., ***calc.,*** **CAMPH.,** ***carb-s.,*** **CARB-V.,** ***caust.,*** cham., chin., cina, coff., cupr-ac., ***dros., dulc.,*** euphr., ***hell., hyos.,*** ign., iod., ***ip., kali-c., kali-m.,*** lob., **MORBILL.,** mosch., nux-m., nux-v., ***phos.,*** **PULS.,** ***rhus-t., sep., stict.,*** stram., ***sulph.,*** zinc.

before eruption - ***bry., puls., stram.***

conjunctivitis, with - euphr., puls.

eruptions-like, limbs - cop., rhus-t.

exanthema repelled, receding - ***bry., phos., puls.,*** rhus-t.

headache, after - bell., ***carb-v.,*** dulc., hell., hyos., ***puls.,*** rhus-t., ***sulph.***

hemorrhagic - ***crot-h.,*** ferr-p.

prophylactic - ***acon.,*** ars., morbill., ***puls.***

respiration, difficult from suppressed - **CHAM., PULS.,** ***zinc.***

MENINGITIS, infection - acon., aeth., ***agar.,*** ail., **APIS,** apoc., arg-n., ***arn.,*** ars., atro., bapt., **BELL.,** ***bry., calc.,*** calc-br., ***calc-p.,*** camph., canth., carb-ac., chin., chin-s., chr-ox., ***cic.,*** cimic., ***cina, cocc.,*** crot-c., crot-h., ***cupr., cupr-ac., cupr-m.,*** dig., echi., ***gels., glon.,*** **HELL.,** ***hippoz., hydr-ac., hyos.,*** hyper., iod., iodof., ip., ***kali-br.,*** kali-i., kreos., ***lach.,*** med., ***merc.,*** merc-c., merc-d., mosch., ***nat-m.,*** nat-s., ***op.,*** oreo., ox-ac., ***phos.,*** phys., ***plb., rhus-t., sil.,*** sol-n., **STRAM.,** ***sulph., tub.,*** verat-v., vip., **ZINC.,** ***zinc-c., zinc-m.***

cerbro-spinal - acon., aeth., agar., am-c., ant-t., **APIS,** ***arg-n.,*** arn., ars., bapt., **BELL.,** bry., cact., camph., canth., ***cic., cimic.,*** cocc., crot-h., cupr., dig., **GELS.,** glon., hell., hydr-ac., hyos., ***ign.,*** lyc., ***nat-m.,*** **NAT-S.,** ***nux-v.,*** **OP.,** ***phos.,*** plb., ***rhus-t.,*** sol-n., tarent., verat., **VERAT-V.,** ***zinc.***

suppressed ear discharge, from - stram.

urine, with pale, clear - bell., hyos., lach., phos.

meningitis, spinal - ***acon.,*** **APIS, BELL.,** ***bry., calc., cic., cimic.,*** cocc., crot-h., cupr., dulc., **GELS.,** ***hyos.,*** hyper., kali-i., ***ip.,*** merc., ***nat-m., nat-s.,*** nux-v., ***op.,*** ox-ac., ***plb., rhus-t.,*** sec., verat-v., ***zinc.***

MENSES, during - ***acon.,*** aesc., ***bell.,*** bry., ***calc.,*** carb-an., ***coc-c.,*** gels., ***graph.,*** helon., kali-bi., kreos., mag-c., mag-m., merc., nat-m., nit-ac., nux-v., ***phos.,*** rhod., **SEP.,** ***sulph.***
absent, amenorrhea - ***cina.***
before - am-c., carb-an., calc., con., cupr., iod., kali-c., lyc., nit-ac., puls., sep., thuj.
menorrhagia - ***coc-c.***
nightly - ***nat-m.***
soon, too - ***kali-bi.***
suppressed - mill.

MENTAL, exertion after - ambr., bell., nux-v., olnd., phos., sep., sil.
amel. - ferr., nat-m.

MIDNIGHT - **ARS.,** coc-c., elaps, lyc., mag-m., mag-s., nux-v., petr., ***rhus-t.,*** sep., ***stram.,*** sulph., verat.
after - ang., ant-c., **ARS.,** bor., caust., chin., cic., cimic., dros., elaps, ferr., ***ferr-ar.,*** ign., ***kali-c., lyc.,*** mag-c., mag-m., merc., nat-m., nit-ac., phos., ran-b., ***ran-s.,*** sabad., sars., sulph., thuj.
before - acon., agar., ant-c., ars., alum., **BRY.,** cadm-s., **CALAD.,** ***carb-v.,*** cham., ***chin-s.,*** elaps, eug., ***graph.,*** hydr., ***laur.,*** lyc., ***mag-m.,*** mag-s., nit-ac., petr., ph-ac., phos., puls., rhus-t., sabad., sep., sulph., sul-ac., verat.
menses, before the - lyc.
noon, and - ars., ***elaps,*** spig., stram., sulph.
perspiration, with, when lying on the back - ***cham.***
sleep, during passing away on waking - ***calad.***
until 8 a.m. - sil.

MONONUCLEOSIS, infection - acon., ail., alumn., anan., ***apis,*** ars-i., ***ars.,*** bapt., bar-c., bar-i., ***bar-m., bell., bism.,*** **CALC., CARC.,** ***cist.,*** clem., ***dulc.,*** **GELS.,** graph., ***hep.,*** iod., ***iodof., kali-i.,*** **MERC.,** ***merc-i-r., phos.,*** ph-ac., ***phyt.,*** rhus-t., sil., ***sil-mar.,*** sulph.
acute adenitis - acon., ail., alumn., anan., ***apis,*** ars-i., bar-c., bar-i., ***bell., bism., carc.,*** clem., ***dulc.,*** graph., ***hep.,*** iod., ***iodof., kali-i., merc., merc-i-r., phyt.,*** rhus-t., sil., ***sil-mar.***
ailments, from - bapt., ***carc.,*** gels.
chronic fatigue, from - ***bapt., calc.,*** **CARC.,** ***gels., merc., ph-ac.,*** sil., thuj.

MORNING - aeth., am-c., ail., ***ang.,*** **APIS,** ***arn.,*** ars., bell., bor., bry., ***calc., caust.,*** carb-an., ***cham.,*** chel., chin., cimic., coff., cycl., dros., eup-per., fl-ac., glon., ***hep.,*** ign., kali-bi., kali-c., ***kali-i.,*** lach., mag-c., nicc., ***nat-m.,*** nux-m., nux-v., ox-ac., petr., phyt., podo., ***rhus-t.,*** sabad., sang., sarr., spong., ***sulph.,*** teucr., thuj., vip.
bed, in - ars., ign., kali-c., nicc., nux-v., petr., **PULS.,** sulph.
5 a.m. followed by shaking chill - ***apis.***
breakfast, after - bar-c., calc., croc., ign., iod., mag-m., phos., sabad., sars., staph.
chilliness, with - **APIS,** arn., **ARS.,** caust., cham., coff., kali-bi., kali-c., kali-i., sulph., thuj.

MORNING,
coffee, after - cham.
morning, 4 to 5 a.m. - sep.
rising, after - am-m., calc., carb-an., coloc., lach., mag-c., rhus-t., sabad.
and walking about - aeth., camph., chel., petr., sep., sulph.
seminal emissions, after - petr.
sleep, during - sulph.
waking, on - acon-c., aeth., camph., chel., eup-per., lac-c., petr., sep., sulph.
amel. - sulph.
walking in open air, after - nux-v.

MOTION, agg. - agar., alum., am-m., ant-c., ant-t., ars., bell., ***bry., camph.,*** canth., **CHIN.,** chin-s., con., cur., ***nux-v., sep.,*** spig., spong., stann., stram., sul-ac.
amel. - agar., apis, **CAPS.,** cycl., ferr., ***lyc.,*** merc-c., puls., rhus-t., sabad., samb., sel., tarax., valer.
brings on chilliness - ant-t., ***apis, arn., chin-s., merc.,*** **NUX-V.,** ***podo.,*** **RHUS-T.,** ***stram.***
wants to be quiet in any stage - **BRY.,** gels.

MUMPS, infection - ***acon.,*** ail., ***am-c.,*** ant-t., anthr., ***ars., arum-t., aur.,*** aur-m., **BAR-C.,** ***bar-m.,*** **BELL.,** ***brom., calc., carb-an.,*** **CARB-V.,** ***cham.,*** **CIST.,** cocc., ***con., crot-h.,*** dor., dulc., euphr., ***ferr-p., hep.,*** hippoz., **JAB.,** kali-ar., ***kali-bi., kali-c.,*** kali-m., kali-p., ***lach., lyc.,*** mag-p., **MERC.,** merc-i-f., merc-i-r., ***nat-m.,*** petr., ***phos.,*** phyt., piloc., **PULS.,** ***rhus-t.,*** sars., ***sil.,*** sul-i., sulph., trif-p., trif-r.
gangrenous - anthr.
left - **BROM.,** ***lach.,*** **RHUS-T.**
metastasis to, brain - apis, bell., hyos.
breasts - carb-v., con., piloc., **PULS.**
testes - ***ars., carb-v., clem., ham.,*** jab., nat-m., **PULS.,** rhus-t.
persistent - bar-ac., bar-c., ***con., iod.,*** sil.
prophylactic - trif-r.
right - ***bar-m., calc., kali-bi., kali-c.,*** **MERC.**
then left - **LYC.**
scarlatina, in - ***calc.***
suppuration with - **ARS., BROM.,** ***bry.,*** **CALC.,** ***con.,*** **HEP.,** ***lach.,*** **MERC.,** ***nat-m., phos.,*** **RHUS-T., SIL.,** sul-ac.

NAUSEA - alum., arund., eup-pur., ***ip., nat-m.***
eating, after - ind.
ephemeral - ***verat.***
peritonitis, in - ***lyc.***
prodroma - ***samb.***

NERVOUS - ***calc., camph.,*** cinnam., ***cham.,*** cocc., ***manc.***
insidious, produced by fits of anger, or accompanied by disposition to anger - **COCC.**
limbs, with pain in - **BRY.**
nausea, with - ***ip.***
stupidity - cic.

NIGHT - ***acon., agar., alum.,*** am-c., am-m., ang., anac., ant-c., ant-t., ***apis, ars.,*** ars-h., ***ars-i.,*** arum-t., arund., ***bar-c., bar-m.,*** **BAPT., BELL.,** berb., bol., bor., **BRY.,** cact., cadm-s., calad., ***calc.,*** calc-s., ***canth.,*** caps., carb-an., **CARB-S.,** ***carb-v.,*** caust., cedr., ***cham.,*** cic., ***cimic.,*** **CINA,** ***cinnb.,*** **COLCH.,** coca, cocc., coff., con., cur., cycl., dig., ***dros.,*** dulc., elaps, ferr., ***ferr-ar., gels.,*** glon., **GRAPH.,** ***hep.,*** hura, hydr., ign., ***kali-bi.,*** kali-c., kali-n., kali-p., kali-s., **LACH.,** lil-t., ***lyc.,*** mag-c., mag-m., mag-s., **MERC.,** ***merc-cy., morph., mur-ac., nat-a.,*** nat-c., nat-m., ***nat-s.,*** nicc., ***nit-ac., nux-v., op.,*** paeon., ***petr., ph-ac.,*** **PHOS.,** plb., psor., **PULS.,** raph., **RHUS-T.,** ***sabad.,*** sarr., ***sep.,*** **SIL.,** spong., staph., ***stram.,*** **SULPH.,** ***tarent.,*** thuj., ***tub.,*** verat., ust., zinc.

anxiety and sweat, with - alum., calc.

chilliness, with - acon., ***agar.,*** apis, ***ars.,*** bapt., carb-s., carb-v., caust., cham., coca, coff., ***colch.,*** cur., ***elaps, graph., kali-bi., rhus-t., sil.,*** **SULPH.,** thuj., tub.

chilly during day, heat at night - dros.

dry burning heat - **ACON.,** anac., arn., **ARS.,** ***bar-c.,*** **BELL., BRY.,** calc., carb-v., caust., cedr., chel., chin-s., ***cina,*** coc-c., coff., ***colch.,*** coloc., ***con.,*** dulc., hep., ***graph.,*** kali-n., ***lach.,*** lyc., ***nit-ac.,*** nux-m., ***nux-v.,*** **PHOS.,** ***puls.,*** ran-s., rhod., **RHUS-T.,** rhus-v., spig., thuj., ***tub.***

with anxiety - acon., ***apis,*** **ARS.,** bar-c., bry., rhus-t.

with sleeplessness - bar-c., ***cham.,*** graph., hyos., ***phos.***

without thirst - ***apis,*** **ARS.**

night, 2 a m - ***ars.,*** bor., tax.

3 a.m. - ang., thuj.

9 p.m. - **BRY.,** lyc., mag-s., nit-ac.

10 p.m. - ars., elaps, hydr., lach., petr.

11 p.m. - mag-m.

perspiration, with - agar., alum., am-m., ***ant-c.,*** **BELL.,** bor., bry., calc., caps., carb-an., cedr., cina, ***colch., con.,*** ferr., glon., ign., mag-c., mag-m., **MERC.,** nat-m., nit-ac., nux-v., op., **PHOS.,** ***psor.,*** **PULS., RHUS-T.,** sabad., ***sep.,*** spig., staph., stram., **SULPH.,** thuj., verat.

clammy sweat and quick pulse - cimic.

waking, on - **BAR-C.,** benz-ac., carb-v., coloc., mag-m., sil., **SULPH.,** tarax., zinc.

amel. - ***calad.***

water, as if hot water were poured over one - ars.

NOISE, from - bry.

NOON - ars., ars-h., bell., ferr-i., mag-c., merc., spig., ***stram.,*** sulph.

NOSE, coryza - **ACON.,** bar-m., calad., ***iod.,*** jab., **MERC.,** sang., spong., ***stict.***

secretion, thick plugs of nasal, especially in old people and children - ***merc-i-f.***

stopped up - spong.

swells - ***guai.***

PAIN, from fever - arn., ars., bell., carb-v., cham., pyrog., sec.

pain in stomach - sec.

PAROXYSMAL, fever - am-m., arund., ***bry., calc.,*** camph., cham., ***chin.,*** cocc., eup-per., hep., lyc., ***merc.,*** nit-ac., op., zinc.

afternoon - agar., calc., sil.

3 p.m. - lyc.

evening - calc., lyc.

7 p.m. - lyc.

forenoon, 11 a.m. - calc.

morning - eup-per., kali-bi.

night - kali-bi., **MERC.**

PAROXYSMS, increasing in severity - ars., ***bry.,*** eup-per., ***nat-m.,*** nux-v., ***psor.,*** **PULS.**

paroxysms, irregular - **ARS.,** carb-v., ***eup-per.,*** ign., ***ip., meny.,*** **NUX-V., PSOR., PULS.,** samb., **SEP.**

long chill, little heat, no thirst - **PULS.**

one stage wanting - ***apis,*** aran., **ARS.,** bov., camph., dros., led., lyc., meny., mez., verat.

short chill, long heat, no thirst - **IP.**

paroxysms, regular - ***chin.,*** **CHIN-S.,** cina.

PERIODICITY (see Intermittent fever) - aran., ars., ***chin.,*** **CHIN-S.,** cedr., cina., eup-per., gels., ham., ip., lyc., lyss., ***nat-m.,*** nux-v., stram., syph.

3 p.m., daily, into night - cur.

and 4 p.m., every 2 or 3 weeks, in afternoon, between - stram.

daily, at 4 p.m., since second day after childbirth, eleven weeks ago - ***lyc.***

11 to 1 p.m., sweats when she begins to get over fever - syph.

at same hour - cedr., ***cina.***

day, each, at 4 p.m., in pulmonary diseases - ***lyc.***

evening, every, after supper, gradually worse, went off by morning - ***gels.***

commencing at dusk and lasting until bedtime - lyss.

hour, every other - symph.

spells, by - ***ham.***

PERSPIRATION, general

absent - acon., alum., am-c., anac., ***apis, aran.,*** arg-n., arn., **ARS.,** ars-i., **BELL.,** bism., ***bov.,*** **BRY., CACT.,** calc., caps., carb-s., ***cham.,*** chin., coff., colch., corn., cor-r., crot-h., dulc., ***eup-per.,*** **GELS.,** ***graph., hyos.,*** ign., iod., ***ip.,*** kali-ar., kali-bi., ***kali-c.,*** kali-p., ***kali-s.,*** lach., led., ***lyc.,*** mag-c., merl., nat-a., nat-c., nat-m., nit-ac., **NUX-M.,** nux-v., olnd., op., phel., ***ph-ac., phos., plat., plb., psor.,*** puls., ran-b., ***rhus-t.,*** sabad., sec., sang., sil., spong., squil., staph., ***sulph.,*** tub., verb.

heat, with - agar., **ALUM.,** am-m., anac., ***ant-c.,*** ant-t., apis, asc-t., ***bell.,*** berb., bor., bry., ***calc.,*** camph., canth., **CAPS.,** carb-an., carb-v., cedr., ***cham.,*** chel., chin., cina, cob., colch., **CON.,** cor-r., ***dig.,*** euph., eup-per., ***ferr.,*** gamb., glon., guare.,

PERSPIRATION, general
heat, with - **HELL.,** hep., hydr-ac., ign., ***ip.,*** kali-bi., ***kali-i.,*** kali-n., lac-c., laur., mag-c., mag-m., ***merc.,*** **MEZ., NAT-C.,** nat-m., nat-p., ***nat-s.,*** nit-ac., ***nux-v.,*** **OP.,** ox-ac., ***par.,*** ph-ac., **PHOS.,** ***podo.,*** **PSOR., PULS., PYROG.,** ***rhus-t.,*** raph., ***sabad.,*** samb., ***sep.,*** sol-t-ae., spig., **STANN.,** ***staph.,*** **STRAM.,** stront-c., **SULPH., SUL-AC.,** ***sumb.,*** thuj., **TUB.,** valer., ***verat.***

PLAGUE, (see Generals, Bubonic)

POLIOMYELITIS, (see Nerves, Chapter)

PUERPERAL, fever - ***acon.,*** cimic., ail., apis, ***arn.,*** **ARS.,** ***bapt.,*** **BELL., BRY.,** ***calc., canth., carb-ac.,*** cham., cocc., coff., ***colch., coloc.,*** **CROT-H.,** ***hyos., kali-c., kreos., lach., lyc., merc., mur-ac.,*** nux-v., op., plat., ***puls., rhus-t., sec.,*** sulph., ter., verat., **VERAT-V.,** zinc.
chill, follows sudden, after four days' confinement - ***phyt.***
intense fever mingles with and follows severe - verat-v.
chills, alternating with often recurring, of short duration, followed by profuse sweat, with restlessness - carb-ac.
constant, after miscarriage - ust.
irritability, with - ***cham.***
lochia, cessation of - sec.
mental excitement, from - coff.
milk, lack of, in breast - ***cham.***
red rash, increased before, seventh day after confinement - ***calc.***
restlessness, with - ***cham.***
stools, frequent watery - ***sec.***
tympanitis - **LYC.,** ***verat-v.***
weeks, six, after confinement, hydrogenoid constitution - nat-s.

PUTRID, (see Zymotic)

RABIES, hydrophobia (see Generals)

RELAPSING, fever - ars., **CALC., FERR., PSOR., SULPH.,** ***tub.***
errors in diet, from - ***ip.***
typhus, in - crot-h.

REMITTENT, fever - **ACON.,** ant-c., ***ant-t., apis,*** arg-n., ***arn.,*** **ARS.,** ***bapt.,*** **BELL.,** bol., **BRY., CHAM.,** chin., ***cocc.,*** coff., coloc., ***crot-h., eucal., eup-per.,*** ferr., ***gels., hyos.,*** ign., ***ip., lach.,*** lept., ***lyc.,*** mag-c., mag-s., **MERC.,** mur-ac., ***nat-s., nux-v.,*** ph-ac., phos., ***podo.,*** polyp-p, puls., ***rhus-t.,*** sep., stram., ***sulph.,*** tarax., verat.
afternoon - **ARS., BELL.,** ***bry.,*** chin., ign., **GELS., LACH.,** ***lyc.,*** nux-v.
autumn, in - ***carb-ac.***
and winter - ***sulph.***
every - carb-ac.
bilious - ***nat-s., podo.***
and malarial, gastric intestinal irritation - eup-per.
constipation, with - ***hydr.***
convalescence, in - eucal.
cough, with - ***podo.***
dullness of mind - ***sulph.***

REMITTENT, fever,
evening - ***acon.,*** arn., **BELL.,** ***bry.,*** chin., lach., **LYC.,** mag-c., merc., mur-ac., nux-v., ph-ac., ***phos.,*** puls., **RHUS-T.,** ***sulph.***
exacerbations, with - sep.
worse every other - verat.
headache - ***polyp-p.***
infantile - **ACON.,** am-m., ant-c., apis, ars., **BELL.,** bor., ***bry.,*** **CHAM.,** cina, coff., ***ferr-p.,*** **GELS.,** ign., ***ip.,*** kali-br., mag-c., merc., ***mur-ac.,*** nux-v., ***podo., puls., rhus-t.,*** sulph.
due to irritation of teething, intestinal troubles, worms or malarial influences - ***gels.***
low type - ***mur-ac.***
intermittent type, taking on, or vice versa - gels.
morning - ***arn.,*** bry., mag-c., podo., ***rhus-t.,*** sulph.
night - acon., ant-t., **ARS.,** bapt., cham., coff., lyc., mag-c., mag-s., **MERC.,** nux-v., ph-ac., ***phos., puls.,*** **RHUS-T.,** ***sulph.***
pleurisy, with - bry., crot-h.
redness of one cheek, with paleness, of the other - ***acon.,*** **CHAM.**
stages, last, diarrhea profuse, sweat, exhaustion - ***corn.***
typhoid fever, prone to become - ant-t., **ARS.,** ***bapt.,*** **BRY.,** carb-ac., colch., ***gels., mur-ac.,*** ph-ac., phos., **PSOR., RHUS-T.,** sec., ter., tub.
from the abuse of quinine - arn., **ARS.,** ***ip.,*** puls., **RHUS-T.**

RESTLESSNESS - **ACON., ARN., ARS.,** bapt., ip., lac-c., ***rhus-t.***
intermittent, in - ***ip.***
nervous, from 12 to 3 a.m. - med.
tossing about - **ACON., ARS.,** bapt., pyrog., vac.
up and down every few hours - lac-c.

RHEUMATIC, fever, pain in joints, with - abrot., ***acon.,*** act-sp., agn., all-c., ***ant-t.,*** apoc., arg-m., ***arn.,*** ars., ars-i., ***ars-s-f.,*** asc-t., **AUR., BELL.,** ***benz-ac.,*** berb., **BRY.,** ***cact., calc.,*** **CALC-P.,** ***calc-s.,*** cann-s., caul., **CAUST.,** cedr., ***cham., chel., chim., chin-s.,*** chlf., ***cimic.,*** clem., ***cocc.,*** **COLCH.,** ***coloc., dulc., ferr.,*** ferr-i., **FERR-P., FORM.,** gels., ***guai.,*** ham., ***hep.,*** ign., indg., **IOD., KALI-BI.,** kali-c., ***kali-chl., kali-i., kali-s.,*** **KALM.,** kreos., ***lac-ac., lac-c., lach., led.,*** **LYC.,** ***mang., merc., nat-m.,*** nat-p., ***nat-s., nux-v.,*** ol-j., ox-ac., ***phos., phyt.,*** pic-ac., ***puls.,*** ran-b., rheum, ***rhod.,*** **RHUS-T.,** ***ruta.,*** sabin., ***sal-ac., sang.,*** sec., senec., sep., **SPIG.,** spong., ***staph.,*** stict., stront-c., ***sulph., ter.,*** teucr., thuj., ***verat-v.,*** viol-t.
articular, overheated, while, violent, after being chilled - ***kali-s.***
cardiac complications, severe - ***lyc.***
cold, after catching - ***merc.***
chilliness - ***nat-m.***
cold, after catching, neuralgic - puls.

RHEUMATIC, fever,
constipation after - **HYDR.**
evening, worse in, and forepart of night - puls.
gastric complaints, followed by, after taking cold - ***cham.***
heart, leaves joints and attacks - ***aur-m.***
inflammatory articular, acute - ***sal-ac.***
follows aching in bones - verat-v.
liver, pain in - ***card-m.***
muscular, especially - ***gels.***
nerves and joints, with rheumatic and gouty affections of, slight - indg.
pains, changing places, persistently return - ***camph.***
prevalent, drawing tearing in limbs, worse at night, constant change of position, worse lying on back - ***rhus-t.***
stomach, with pain in - ***card-m.***
sweats, clammy fetid, or gout, with sour - fl-ac.
wet, from getting - ***nat-s.***

RIDING, in a carriage, while - graph., ***psor.***
amel. - kali-n., ***nit-ac.***
wind, in the after - nit-ac.

RINGWORM, (see Generals)

SCARLET, fever, scarlatina - acon., **AIL., AM-C., APIS,** ***arg-n.,*** arn., ***ars., arum-t.,*** bar-c., **BELL.,** ***bry., calc.,*** canth., ***carb-ac., carb-v., cham.,*** chin., ***crot-c., crot-h., cupr.,*** **ECHI.,** ***gels.,*** hep., hyos., ip., **LACH., LYC., MERC.,** mur-ac., **NIT-AC.,** nux-m., ***ph-ac., phos.,*** **RHUS-T.,** sec., ***stram., sulph.,*** **TER.,** ***zinc.***
ailments after - **AM-C., AM-M.,** aur., bar-c., **BELL.,** ***bry., calc., carb-ac., carb-v.,*** **CHAM.,** dulc., euph., ***hep.,*** hyos., ***lach.,*** lyc., ***merc.,*** nit-ac., petros., phos., rhus-t., ***sulph.***
headache, after - am-c., bell., ***bry.,*** carb-v., cham., dulc., hell., hep., lach., ***merc.,*** rhus-t.
scarlet rash - **ACON., AM-C.,** ars., **BELL., BRY.,** calc., carb-v., caust., ***chlol., coff.,*** con., dulc., hyos., iod., ***ip., kali-bi.,*** lach., ***merc.,*** ph-ac., phos., rhus-t., sulph., zinc.

SEPTIC, fever, (Blood, Septicemia) - acet-ac., **ANTHR.,** ***apis,*** **ARN., ARS.,** ***bell.,*** berb., **BAPT., BRY.,** ***cadm-s., carb-v.,*** **CROT-C., CROT-H.,** ***cur.,*** **ECHI., KALI-P., LACH., LYC.,** ***merc.,*** **MUR-AC.,** op., ***ph-ac.,*** **PHOS.,** ***puls.,*** **PYROG.,** ***rhus-t., rhus-v.,*** **SULPH., TARENT-C.**

SEX, after - graph., nux-v.

SHIVERING, with fever - acon., anac., ant-t., ***apis,*** **ARN.,** ***bell.,*** bry., bov., ***calc.,*** camph., carb-s., carb-v., **CAUST.,** ***cham.,*** chin., ***chin-s.,*** cina, cocc., coff., coloc., ***cur.,*** cycl., ***dros., elaps, eup-per.,*** **GELS.,** graph., **HELL.,** ***hep.,*** ign., ***lach.,*** mag-m., ***mag-p.,*** meny., **MERC., NUX-V.,** petr., ph-ac., ***podo.,*** psor., puls., ***rhus-t.,*** sabad., sep., **SULPH.,** ***tarent.,*** verat., ***zinc.***

SHIVERING,
alternating with heat - acon., ars., bell., bov., ***bry.,*** calc., caust., chin., ***cocc.,*** cycl., ***dros., elaps,*** hep., ***ip.,*** kali-bi., lach., lob., merc., mosch., ***nux-v., plat.,*** ph-ac., sabad.
drinking, from - bell., **CAPS.,** ***eup-per.,*** **NUX-V.**
motion, from - apis, ***arn.,*** **NUX-V.,** podo., stram.
perspiration with heat, and - **NUX-V.,** podo., ***rhus-t.,*** sulph.
uncovering, from - apis, **ARN.,** bar-c., ***calc.,*** chin., ***chin-s.,*** lach., **NUX-V.,** ***psor., rhus-t.,*** stram., ***tarent.,*** **TUB.**

SHUDDERING, with fever - acon., ***bell.,*** caps., **CHAM.,** ***hell.,*** ign., ***kali-i.,*** merc., nat-m., ***nux-v.,*** rheum, ***rhus-t.,*** zinc.
alternating with heat - bov.
constant, with one cheek hot and red - coff.

SIDE, of body
lain on - arn., mag-m.
left - anac., ant-c., bell., **LYC.,** merc., ***mez.,*** nat-m., nux-v., ***par.,*** ph-ac., ***plat., ran-b.,*** **RHUS-T.,** ***sulph.,*** **STANN.,** thuj.
with coldness of right - par., **RHUS-T.**
one cheek red and hot, the other pale and cold - **ACON.**
one side of the body, the hand and foot are red and cold, on the other they are hot in evening and at night - ***puls.***
one-sided - **ALUM.,** arn., asaf., ***bell.,*** **BRY.,** carb-v., ***caust.,*** **CHAM.,** chel., ***clem.,*** **DIG.,** ***graph., kali-c.,*** **LYC.,** mang., **MOSCH.,** mur-ac., nat-c., **NUX-V., PAR.,** ***ph-ac., phos.,*** plat., **PULS.,** ***rhus-t.,*** spig., staph., ***sulph.,*** sul-ac., ***tarax.,*** thuj., verat., verb., viol-o., zinc.
right - **ALUM.,** ***bell., bry.,*** carb-v., ***cham.,*** fl-ac., kali-c., ***mag-c.,*** mag-m., mosch., nat-c., ***nux-v.,*** **PHOS.,** ***puls., ran-b.,*** sabad., spig., tub., verb.

SINGLE, parts - cham., cycl., stann., tub., zinc.

SITTING, while, agg. - graph., phos., rhus-t., sep.
amel. - nux-v.

SLEEP, heat comes on during - ***acon., alum.,*** anac., ant-t., apis, ***ars.,*** astac., ***bar-c.,*** bell., ***bor.,*** bov., ***bry., calc.,*** **CALAD.,** caps., cham., chin., chin-a., cic., ***cina,*** con., cycl., ***dulc.,*** gels., gins., ign., ***lach.,*** led., lil-t., ***lyc.,*** merc., **MEZ.,** ***nat-c., nat-m.,*** nat-p., ***nit-ac., nux-m.,*** **OP.,** ***petr.,*** ph-ac., ***phos., puls.,*** ran-b., ***rheum, rhus-t.,*** **SAMB.,** sep., ***sil.,*** stram., tarax., thuj., ***ust.,*** vario., viol-t.
cold feet and sweat on waking - **SAMB.**
dry heat - samb., thuj.
after - agar., anac., arn., ars., ***bell., bor.,*** calad., calc., caust., cic., ***cina,*** cocc., coloc., con., ***ferr.,*** ferr-ar., ferr-p., hep., ip., kreos., lyc., mag-m., merc., ***mosch.,*** nat-m., nit-ac., ***op.,*** petr., ph-ac., ***phos.,*** ptel., puls., ***samb., sep., sil.,*** **SULPH.,**

SLEEP,
after - **TARAX.,** thuj., zinc.
amel. - **CALAD.,** chin., colch., hell., nux-v., ***phos., sep.***
distressing dreams - lachn.
drowsiness, dulness - ***gels.***
restless - ***cimx.***
somnolency - lachn.
sopor bordering upon stupor, absence of complaint - ***op.***
sleepless - eup-per.
colic, with - alum.
osseous growths - ***calc-f.***
stupid slumber - spong.
want of for - coff.
worse after sleep - ***lach.,*** sulph.

SKIN, alternately cold and clammy and hot and burning - dor.
alternately hot and dry, again drenched with sweat, with thirst - ***kali-i.***
dry - bell., ***hydr.***
more cold than hot - ***iod.***
hot and dry - bell., ***calc., hydr.***
itching pricking - ***spong.***
moist - samb.
sensation as if cold wind were blowing out from skin - ***cupr.***
sensitive - eup-per.

SLOW - acal., asar., gels., mur-ac., **RHUS-T.,** sulph.
lingering - ***nux-v.***
night, at, delirious - ***camph.***
obstinate - agar.
sweats, with night - ***acet-ac.***
tabes mesenterica, in - ***iod.***

SPOTTED - **CIMIC.,** ***dig., eup-per., sil.,*** verat-v.
beginning, at - ***am-c.***
clonic spasms, with - ***cupr-ac.***
typhoid state - ***chlor.***

SPRING, during - **BRY., GELS.**

STAGES, of fever, general
chill followed by heat - **ACON.,** ***alum.,*** ambr., am-c., am-m., ang., ant-c., ***ant-t.,*** apis, aran., ***arn.,*** ars., asar., bapt., bar-c., ***bell.,*** berb., bor., bry., cact., calc., camph., canth., **CAPS.,** carb-an., ***carb-v.,*** caust., cham., ***chin., cina,*** coff., ***colch.,*** con., ***corn.,*** croc., **CYCL.,** dig., ***dros.,*** dulc., elaps, ***eup-per., graph.,*** guai., hell., ***hep.,*** **HYOS., IOD., IGN., IP.,** kali-bi., kali-c., kali-n., kreos., lach., laur., **LYC.,** ***mag-c.,*** mag-m., mang., meny., merc., ***merc-c.,*** mez., mur-ac., ***nat-c.,*** **NAT-M.,** ***nat-s.,*** nit-ac., nux-m., **NUX-V.,** ***op., petr.,*** ph-ac., ***phos.,*** plat., psor., **PULS., RHUS-T.,** sabad., **SANG.,** ***sec.,*** seneg., sep., sil., ***spig., spong.,*** squil., staph., ***stram.,*** **SULPH.,** thuj., ***valer., verat.***
then sweat - am-c., am-m., apis, **ARS.,** bell., bor., bov., ***bry.,*** cact., caps., carb-an., carb-v., caust., cedr., cham., cina, **CHIN.,** cocc., corn., dig., dros., ***eup-per., eup-pur.,*** gels., ***graph.,*** hep., ***ign.,*** **IP.,** kali-c., kali-n., ***lach.,*** lyc., mag-m., nat-c.,

STAGES, of fever, general
chill followed by heat
then sweat - ***nat-m., nat-s.,*** nit-ac., **NUX-V.,** op., **PULS.,** ***rhus-t., sabad.,*** sabin., samb., sep., ***spong.,*** staph., ***sulph.,*** thuj., ***verat.***
alternating with thirst - sabad.
internal chill, then heat and sweat - phos.
sour - lyc.
thirst, with - rhus-t.
chill followed by heat with sweat - ***acon.,*** alum., anac., ant-t., **BELL.,** bry., ***caps.,*** carb-v., **CHAM.,** ***chin.,*** cina, eup-per., ***ferr.,*** graph., hell., ***hep.,*** ign., kali-c., mez., nat-m., nit-ac., ***nux-v.,*** **OP.,** phos., ***puls.,*** **RHUS-T.,** ***sabad.,*** sars., spig., sulph.
with sweat, of the face - alum.
without sweat - graph., nat-m.
thirst then sweat - kali-c., thuj.
then heat without thirst - ***hep.,*** kali-n., nat-m.
chill, then sweat, without intervening heat - alum., am-m., arg-m., ars., ***bry.,*** cact., **CAPS.,** ***carb-an.,*** carb-s., carb-v., **CAUST.,** cedr., cham., chel., cimx., ***clem., dig.,*** graph., hell., hyos., **LYC.,** kali-c., kali-n., mag-c., mag-m., merc., merc-c., **MEZ.,** mur-ac., nat-m., nat-s., nux-v., ***op.,*** **PETR.,** ph-ac., phos., ***rhus-t.,*** sabad., sep., spig., sulph., **THUJ.,** ***verat.***
then cold sweat - ars., verat.
then heat - **BELL.**
sweat, without heat or thirst - am-m., bry., caust., ***staph.***
then heat - bell.
heat, alternating with chill, followed by sweat, then heat - verat.
then heat - verat.
finally sweat - bry., kali-c., ***spig.***
heat, followed by chill - ail., alum., am-m., ang., apis, asar., ***bell., bry.,*** calad., **CALC.,** caps., ***caust.,*** chin., coloc., dros., dulc., elaps, eup-pur., ***hell.,*** ign., kali-c., lyc., meny., merc., nat-m., nicc., nit-ac., **NUX-V.,** petr., ***phos.,*** **PULS.,** ***pyrog.,*** **SEP., STANN.,** ***staph., sulph.,*** thuj., ***tub.***
then heat - am-m., stram.
sweat - ***rhus-t.***
heat, followed by chill, then sweat - agar., alum., ***am-m.,*** ant-c., ant-t., **ARS.,** bell., bor., bry., calc., carb-an., ***carb-v.,*** **CHAM.,** ***chin.,*** cina, **COFF.,** corn., graph., hell., hep., ***ign., ip.,*** kali-c., kali-n., kreos., lach., lob., lyc., ***mang.,*** nit-ac., ***nux-v.,*** op., petr., puls., ***ran-s.,*** rhod., **RHUS-T.,** sep., ***sil.,*** spong., staph., stront-c., sulph., **VERAT.**
cold sweat - caps., ***verat.***
heat, followed by chill, with sweat, with external coldness, then chill, then heat with external coldness - ***phos.***
then heat - aloe, am-c., ant-c., ant-t., calad., calc., carb-v., hell., ign., ran-s., sil.
heat, followed by chilliness - ars.

STAGES, of fever, general,
irregular - **ARS., BRY.,** ***ip.,*** **NUX-V.,** op., ***sep.***
perspiration, alternating with chilliness - ant-c., calc., nux-v., sac-alb.
appears long after the heat has subsided, with renewal of the earlier symptoms - ars.
followed by chill - ***carb-v.,*** euphr., ***hep., nux-v.***
followed by chill, then with perspiration - nux-v.
with heat - nux-v.
following, chill, alternated with heat - carb-ac., corn., kali-c., meny., verat.
alternated with heat, and heat alternating, then heat - bry.
following, chill, with heat - calc., caps., sulph.
perspiration, with heat following chill - acon., alum., anac., ant-c., bell., caps., ***cham.,*** chin., cina, graph., hell., hep., ign., kali-c., nat-m., nicc., nit-ac., nux-v., op., phos., puls., rhus-t., sabad., spig., sulph.
during heat, the coldness and heat, irregularly intermingle - cedr.
followed by dry heat - ant-c.

STANDING, agg. - arg-m., con., ***mang.,*** puls., rhus-t.
amel. - bell., cann-s., iod., ip., phos., sel.

STAPHYLOCOCCUS, infections - **ANT-C.,** ***ars.,*** ars-i., calc., carb-ac., carb-v., caust., cic., clem., con., crot-t., ***dulc., echi.,*** graph., ***hep., iris, kali-bi.,*** kreos., lyc., merc., nat-m., ***nit-ac., ph-ac.,*** phos., pyrog., ***rhus-t.,*** sars., sep., ***sil.,*** staph., sulph., viol-t.

STOOL, during - ars., cham., puls., rhus-t., sulph.
after - ars., bry., caust., nux-v., rhus-t., sel.
before - calc., crot-t., cupr., ***mag-c., merc., phos.,*** samb., verat.

STOOPING - bry., ***kali-c.,*** **MERC.,** sep.
coldness when rising - ***merc-c.***

STORM, before and during - rhod., sil.

STREPTOCOCCUS, infections - ail., arn., ***ars., bell.,*** strep., sul-ac., x-ray.

SUMMER, hot season - ***acon.,*** ant-c., ***ars., bell., bry., calc., caps.,*** carb-v., cedr., chin., cina, eup-per., ***gels., ip., lach.,*** nat-m., puls., ***sulph.,*** thuj., verat.

SUN, from exposure to - ***acon.,*** aml-n., ***ant-c., arn.,*** bapt., **BELL.,** ***cact.,*** camph., ***carb-v.,*** **GLON.,** ***lach.,*** lyss., nat-c., ***op.,*** puls., sep., sil., ***ther.,*** thuj., ***verat., verat-v.,*** zinc.
walking in - ant-c.

TEETH, with pains in - ant-c., nat-c.

THIRST, with - alum., ***anac., ang.,*** arund., **ARS., BRY.,** ***calc., cham.,*** chin-s., cina, ***chin.,*** cist., coff., con., croc., cur., elaps, elat., **EUP-PER.,** ***eup-pur., hep., hyos., ip.,*** kali-bi., lach., lyc., mag-c., med., merc., mill., **NAT-M.,** ***nux-v.,*** **PHOS.,** plan., plat., podo., psor., ***puls.,*** rhus-t., sep., staph., ***stram., sulph., ter.,*** thuj., valer., vac., ***verat.,*** ziz.

THIRST, with
absent - acet-ac., apis, calad., **GELS., PULS.,** vario.
afternoon - ars-h.
anthrax - tarent.
appetite, lost - calc-ar.
chill and icy coldness, follows, attacks come on suddenly - ***nat-s.***
little thirst - ars., ***gels., puls.***
peritonitis, in - ***lyc.***
preceded by, fever, cannot raise head - eup-per.
prodromal, during - ***samb.***
stages, during all - sec.
unquenchable, in kidney disease - ***hep.***
with or without - med.

TINEA, (see Generals)

TOBACCO, smoking, from - cic., ign., sep.

TUBERCULOSIS, infection - acal., ***acet-ac.,*** acon., **AGAR.,** agarin., ***all-s.,*** ant-a., ant-t., ***ars., ars-i.,*** atro., aur-a., bac., bals-p., ***bapt., bar-m.,*** bell., blatta, ***brom., bry., bufo,*** **CALC.,** calc-ar., ***calc-i.,*** **CALC-P.,** ***calc-s.,*** calo., cann-s., ***carb-an., carb-s., carb-v.,*** card-m., ***chin-a.,*** chlor., cimic., coc-c., cod., ***con., crot-h.,*** cupr-ar., ***dros., dulc., elaps,*** erio., ferr-ac., ***ferr-ar., ferr-i.,*** ferr-m., ***ferr-p.,*** fl-ac., form., ***gall-ac., graph., guai.,*** ham., **HEP.,** hippoz., hydr., ichth., **IOD.,** iodof., ip., kali-ar., kali-bi., **KALI-C.,** ***kali-n., kali-p.,*** **KALI-S.,** ***kreos.,*** lac-ac., ***lac-d., lach., lachn.,*** laur., lec., led., **LYC.,** mang., ***med., merc.,*** mill., ***myos., myrt-c.,*** naphtin., nat-a., ***nat-m.,*** nat-s., ***nit-ac.,*** nux-v., ***ol-j.,*** ox-ac., petr., ***ph-ac., phel.,*** **PHOS.,** piloc., ***plb., polyg-a.,*** **PSOR., PULS.,** rumx., ruta, salv., samb., ***sang.,*** **SENEC.,** ***seneg., sep.,*** **SIL., SPONG., STANN.,** stict., ***still.,*** succ., **SULPH.,** sul-ac., teucr., thea., **THER., TUB.,** urea, vanad., **ZINC.**
acute - ant-t., ***ars., bry.,*** calc., calc-i., ***chin., cimic.,*** dros., ***dulc.,*** ferr., ferr-ac., ferr-m., **FERR-P.,** ***hep.,*** iod., ***kali-chl.,*** kali-p., ***kreos.,*** lach., laur., ***med.,*** nat-m., ***phos.,*** **PULS.,** ***sang.,*** **SENEC., SIL.,** stann., ***sulph.,*** **THER.,** tub.
exacerbations in all stages of - ***kali-n.***
menses, suppressed, from - **SENEC.**
bleedings, after - ***chin.***
bones, of - ***dros.,*** phos., puls., stann.
cold, damp weather - ***dulc.***
elderly, people - ***nat-s.***
fever, in - bapt., chin-a., ferr-p.
florida - ***ferr.,*** med., nat-p., ***puls., sang.,*** **THER.**
gonorrhea, after suppressed - **SEP.**
incipient - acal., ***acet-ac., agar., ars-i., bry.,*** cact., **CALC.,** calc-i., **CALC-P.,** ***carb-v., dros., dulc., ferr.,*** ferr-p., **HEP., KALI-C.,** kali-i., **KALI-P.,** ***lach.,*** lachn., **LYC.,** ***lycps.,*** mang., **MED.,** myrt-c., ***nat-s.,*** ol-j., petr., **PHOS.,** polyg., **PSOR., PULS.,** ***rumx., sang.,*** sec., **SENEC., SIL., STANN.,** succ., ***sulph., ther.,*** thuj., tril., **TUB.,** vanad.
injury to the after - mill., ***ruta.***

TUBERCULOSIS, infection,
last stage - ars., bry., **CALC.**, **CARB-V.**, ***chin.***, ***dros.***, ***euon.***, kali-n., **LACH.**, led., lob., **LYC.**, ***phel.***, ***phos.***, ***psor.***, **PULS.**, ***pyrog.***, **SANG.**, ***seneg.***, **TARENT.**
lying, on side agg. - calc.
miners, from coal dust - carb-s., sil.
nursing, mothers - ***kali-c.***
pituitous - ***aesc.***, **ANT-C.**, **ANT-T.**, ***bar-m.***, caust., ***coc-c.***, ***dulc.***, **EUON.**, ***ferr.***, **FERR-P.**, **HEP.**, ***kali-c.***, **KALI-I.**, **KALI-CHL.**, ***kreos.***, ***lach.***, **LYC.**, **MED.**, ***merc.***, ***merc-c.***, mill., ***nat-s.***, **PHOS.**, **PSOR.**, ***puls.***, **SANG.**, **SENEC.**, ***seneg.***, ***sil.***, **STANN.**, ***sulph.***, **THER.**
prophylaxis, for - bac., calc-p., phos., sulph., tub.
purulent and ulcerative - ***ars.***, ***ars-i.***, brom., bry., **CALC.**, ***carb-an.***, ***carb-s.***, ***carb-v.***, chin., ***dros.***, guai., ***hep.***, hyos., **IOD.**, **KALI-C.**, ***kali-n.***, ***kali-p.***, ***lach.***, led., **LYC.**, ***merc.***, nat-m., ***nit-ac.***, ***nux-m.***, **PHOS.**, ***plb.***, ***psor.***, ***puls.***, ruta., sep., ***sil.***, stann., ***sulph.***
recurring - ferr-p., kali-n., tub.
stone-cutters - ***calc.***, lyc., puls., ***sil.***
sycotic - ars., **AUR.**, ***aur-m.***, bar-c., bry., **CALC.**, ***carb-an.***, carb-v., ***caust.***, cham., chin., ***ferr-p.***, ***lach.***, **LYC.**, **MED.**, **NAT-S.**, **NIT-AC.**, ***phyt.***, ***puls.***, sep., ***sil.***, staph., sulph., ***ther.***, **THUJ.**
weakness, in - ars-i., chin-a., ***ph-ac.***, phos., ***stann.***

TROPICAL, fever - ars., **CEDR.**, ***chin.***, eup-per., ***gels.***, ip., nat-m., nat-s., **PSOR.**, ***ter.***

TYPHOID, fever - absin., ***acet-ac.***, aesc-g., **AGAR.**, ail., ***alum.***, ***alumin.***, ant-t., am-c., anac., anthr., **APIS**, ***apoc.***, arg-n., **ARN.**, **ARS.**, **ARUM-T.**, ***asar.***, astac., ***atro.***, aur., **BAPT.**, ***bar-c.***, **BELL.**, ***berb.***, bor., **BRY.**, ***calad.***, **CALC.**, ***camph.***, ***canth.***, ***caps.***, ***carb-an.***, **CARB-V.**, carb-ac., cast., ***cham.***, ***chel.***, chim., ***chin-a.***, ***chin-s.***, ***chlor.***, chlf., ***cic.***, **CHIN.**, **CHLOR.**, ***cimic.***, cinnam., cit-l., coca, ***cocc.***, coff., **COLCH.**, con., croc., **CROT-H.**, cupr., dig., dor., dulc., **ECHI.**, erig., ***eucal.***, ***eup-per.***, **FERR.**, ferr-m., ***fl-ac.***, **GELS.**, glon., ***gymn.***, ***ham.***, hep., ***hell.***, ***hippoz.***, hydr., ***hydr-ac.***, **HYOS.**, ***iod.***, ign., ip., ***iris***, ***kali-c.***, ***kali-m.***, ***kali-p.***, ***kreos.***, **LACH.**, lachn., ***laur.***, lept., **LYC.**, ***mag-p.***, ***manc.***, meli., ***merc.***, merc-c., merc-d., **MERC-CY.**, ***mosch.***, **MUR-AC.**, nat-m., **NIT-AC.**, ***nit-s-d.***, ***nux-m.***, ***nux-v.***, **OP.**, ox-ac., petr., **PHOS.**, **PH-AC.**, pic-ac., ***psor.***, puls., ***pyrog.***, ran-s., **RHUS-T.**, ***rhus-v.***, samb., ***sec.***, sel., ***sep.***, ***sil.***, ***sin-n.***, spong., staph., **STRAM.**, **SULPH.**, ***sul-ac.***, ***tarax.***, **TER.**, ***urt-u.***, **VALER.**, **VERAT.**, ***verat-v.***, **ZINC.**, zing.
abscesses, with multiple - ars., hep., sil.
abdomen, fermentation - cham., ***lyc.***
tympanitic - ***arn.***, ***ars.***, ***bry.***, **CARB-V.**, **CHIN.**, ***colch.***, erig., hell., ***lach.***, **LYC.**, ***manc.***, ***mill.***, caj., ***op.***, ***podo.***, ***rhus-t.***, sulph., **TER.**, **VALER.**, **VERAT.**,

TYPHOID, fever,
abdomen, fermentation - cham., ***lyc.***
tympanitic - ***verat-v.***, **ZINC.**, zing.
abdominal - ant-t., apis, arn., ***ars.***, ***bapt.***, **BRY.**, canth., caps., carb-ac., **COLCH.**, ip., ***lyc.***, ***mur-ac.***, ***nit-ac.***, ***ph-ac.***, **PHOS.**, **RHUS-T.**, ***sec.***, ***sulph.***, ***ter.***, verat.
icteric skin, with - cham., chin., ***crot-h.***, lyc., merc., ***nat-c.***, sulph.
aborting - bapt., pyrog.
acute diseases take on a typhoid form - **RHUS-T.**
afternoon - agar., apis, ***ars.***, ***bry.***, ***canth.***, chin., colch., dig., ***gels.***, ***hyos.***, ip., **LACH.**, lyc., ***nit-ac.***, nux-v., ph-ac., **PHOS.**, puls., rhus-t., sulph., sul-ac., stram.
4 p.m. to 8 p.m. - ***lyc.***
till midnight - ***stram.***
5 p.m. - kali-n., rhus-t., sulph.
ailments since - bac., carb-v., mang., phos., psor., pyrog., tub.
anger, after - ***cham.***
answer questions, will not - ***lycps.***
anxiety - ***ars.***, bry., **CALC.**, chin., ***kali-c.***, rhus-t., ***spong.***, verat.
apathy - apis, ***arn.***, ***ars.***, ***carb-v.***, chin., colch., hell., hyos., ***nit-s-d.***, ***op.***, ***ph-ac.***, stram., verat.
arms cool - ***zinc.***
ataxic - agar.
back, lying on - ***zinc.***
thighs flexed on pelvis - ***verat-v.***
bed, sliding down in - ***ars.***, ***bapt.***, ***bell.***, ***hell.***, **MUR-AC.**, ***zinc.***
bedsores - ***arn.***, ***ars.***, bapt., ***carb-v.***, chin., **FL-AC.**, ***lach.***, mosch., mur-ac., nux-v., ph-ac., pyrog., ***sec.***, ***zinc.***
bilious - ***bry.***, caps., ***chel.***, haem., ***lach.***, ***lept.***, lyc., ***merc.***, nux-v., stram.
lies on right side, painful to lie on left - stram.
blood, reduced by loss of, or malarious poison - **CHIN.**
brain alone seems to be involved - ***hell.***
impending paralysis of - ***zinc.***
breathing, stertorous - ***op.***
bronchitis, epidemic - chel.
bronchial symptoms, dangerous - ***ter.***
calomel, after - ***nit-ac.***
carriers, after inoculation with anti-thypoid serum - bapt.
cellulitis, adenitis - bell., chin-s., merc-i-r.
cerebral - ***apis***, arn., ***bapt.***, ***bry.***, canth., cic., ***gels.***, **HYOS.**, ***lach.***, ***lyc.***, nux-m., ***op.***, ***phos.***, ***ph-ac.***, ***rhus-t.***, **STRAM.**, verat., verat-v.
excitement, of - ***samb.***
resulting in paralysis of brain - ***op.***
chest symptoms - ***ant-t.***, bor., bov., ***carb-v.***, ip., **LACH.**, merc., ***phos.***, ***sulph.***
oppression of, and difficult respiration - ***phos.***
children, in - coff., ***gels.***

TYPHOID, fever,
cholera, in - ***op.***
season, in - **VERAT.**
cold, from taking - cham., ***dulc.***
collapse, in stage of - xan.
congestive - arn., ***bry., gels.,*** glon., ***lach.,*** sang., verat.
threatening, cerebral paralysis - hell., ***lach., lyc.,*** **OP.,** ***ph-ac., phos.,*** tarent., zinc.
threatening, collapse - carb-v.
threatening, paralysis of lungs - ***ant-t.,*** ars., carb-v., ***lyc.,*** mosch., ***phos.,*** sulph.
consciousness, lack of - ***phos.***
constipation, with - ***bry.,*** hydr., nux-v., op.
convalescence, stage, in - anac., ars-i., ars-m., ***aur-m.,*** carb-v., ***chin.,*** cocc., hydr., **FL-AC.,** kali-p., ***lyc., nux-v., ph-ac.,*** **PSOR.,** puls., ***sel., sil.,*** sulph., tarax.
retarded - ***hydr.***
cough and chest symptoms supervening and complicating - ***phos.***
and hemoptysis - ***sul-ac.***
cries of pain, utters - ***zinc.***
cry, inclined to, with fear - acon., bry., cocc., rhus-t., verat.
deafness - apis, ***arn.,*** ars., bell., ***bry.,*** carb-v., chlor., ***hyos.,*** lach., lachn., merc., ***nit-s-d.,*** **PHOS.,** ***ph-ac.,*** psor., sec., stram., ***sulph., verat.***
delirium - acet-ac., agar., arn., ars., ***bapt.,*** **BELL.,** ***bry.,*** **CALC.,** cann-i., chlol., ***crot-h.,*** **HYOS., LACH.,** ***lyc.,*** methyl-b., mur-ac., ***op.,*** ph-ac., phos., ***rhus-t.,*** **STRAM.,** ter., valer., ***verat., verat-v., zinc.***
involuntary diarrheic stools - ox-ac.
furious - ***ars.,*** **BELL.,** ***canth.,*** colch., gels., ***hyos.,*** lyc., ***op.,*** puls., rhus-t., sec., spong., ***stram.,*** zinc.
describe symptoms, cannot, though suffering greatly - ***ign.***
diabetes - sul-ac.
diarrhea - arn., ***ars., bapt.,*** **CALC.,** calc-s., crot-h., cupr-ar., dulc., ***hyos., kali-c.,*** lach., ***merc., mur-ac.,*** ph-ac., ***phos.,*** puls., ***rhus-t., stram., sulph.,*** sumb., ***verat.***
involuntary - apis, ***arn.,*** ars., hyos., mur-ac., ***ph-ac.***
last stage, profuse sweat, physical and mental exhaustion, in - ***corn.***
rumbling in bowels - ***ph-ac.***
stool like pale yellow ochre - ***kali-m.***
eat, cannot, feels weak and miserable - ***glon.***
ecchymosis, with - ***arn.,*** ars., carb-v., mur-ac.
enteric, cerebral, exanthematic, or putrid - **APIS.**
epidemic - ***chel., gymn.***
epigastrium, pulsating - ***puls.***
eruption, petechial, on abdomen - ***apis,*** **ARN.,** ***ars., bell.,*** calc., chin-s., cupr-m., lyc., nit-ac., **RHUS-T.**
erythema nodosum, during invasion - rhus-v.

TYPHOID, fever,
escape, desire to - ***bell.,*** bry., ***hyos.,*** nux-v., ***op., stram.,*** zinc.
evening - arn., ***ars.,*** **BRY.,** ***carb-v., cham.,*** chin., hell., ign., ip., ***lach.,*** **LYC.,** ***mur-ac.,*** nit-ac., nux-v., **PH-AC., PHOS., PULS., RHUS-T.,** ***sulph.,*** sul-ac.
7 p.m. to ***lyc., rhus-t.***
8 p.m. - hep., mur-ac., phos., sulph.
9 p.m. to 12 p.m. - ***bry.***
10 p.m. - lach.
exanthematous - ***ail.,*** **APIS,** arn., ars., arum-t., **BELL.,** bry., calc., carb-v., chlor., ***euphr.,*** lach., merc., mur-ac., nux-m., ph-ac., phos., **RHUS-T.,** sec., stann., sulph.
cold, viscous sweat, with - chlor.
exertion, after overheating from, and taking cold, first stage, with sensitiveness to air - ***astac.***
eyes, nightly agglutination of eyelids, injection of conjunctiva, secretion of yellow mucus at inner canthus, dilated pupils, squinting - ***verat-v.***
face hot, body cold - cham.
hippocratic, sunken - ***ars., camph., carb-v., colch., lach., merc., mur-ac.,*** phos., ***zinc.***
red - ***bell.,*** **CALC.,** ***op.***
fainting - cham.
fancies vivid - cham.
fear of death - acon., ***ars., bapt.,*** bry., cocc., rhus-t., verat.
fluids swallowed eagerly, but with difficulty - ***zinc.***
fear - ***bell.,*** bry., cham., ***hyos., stram.***
gastric symptoms, with - ***bry.,*** canth., carb-v., ***hydr.,*** merc., nux-v., puls.
second stage, during - merc-d.
grief, from - cham., ***ign.,*** **PH-AC.**
hands, constant trembling - ***gels., zinc.***
head squeezed, wants - ***glon.***
headache - ***glon.***
hemorrhagic - alum., alumn., ars., bapt., carb-v., chin., **CROT-H.,** elaps, ***ham.,*** ip., kreos., ***lach., mill., mur-ac., nit-ac.,*** nux-m., ph-ac., **PHOS.,** sec., ***sul-ac.,*** ter.
oozing of dark thin blood from capillaries - crot-h., ***sul-ac.***
headache, with - bell., ***bry.,*** gels., hyos., nux-v., rhus-t.
home, wants to go - ***bry.***
hopeless, feels - ***bapt., psor.***
hydrocephalus - art-v.
icteroid, marked, or scorbutic symptoms - ***merc.***
impatience - ***cham.,*** ign., ***nux-v.***
incipient, with pains in head, back and limbs - **BRY.,** ***gels.,*** **RHUS-T.**
indifference - **ARN.,** ***chin.,*** merc., ph-ac., sec., verat.
insomnia, with - bell., coff., gels., hyos., op., rhus-t.

TYPHOID, fever,

intestines, hemorrhages from - alum., ***arn., ars., carb-v.,*** chlol., ***ham., merc., mur-ac.,*** **NIT-AC.,** ***ph-ac.***

irritability, with - bell., ***bry.,*** chin., cocc., nux-v., rhus-t.

jactitation and trembling - cypr.

jaw, dropping of lower - ***ars., bapt., carb-v., lach., lyc., mur-ac.,*** **OP.,** ***ph-ac.,*** sec., ***verat-v.,*** **ZINC.**

trembling - ***arn.***

laryngeal affections, with - apis, merc.

lips, dry and black - ***ars.,*** bell., ***bry., lach., ph-ac., rhus-t.,*** verat.

dry and cracked - ***arn., ars., bry.,*** mur-ac., rhus-t.

sooty - ***zinc.***

loquacity - bell., bry., ***lach.,*** lachn., rhus-t., stram.

lungs, abscess or cancer of, tendency to gangrene - crot-h.

malarial - ***ham., lycps.***

violent pains, particularly in thighs - ***tarax.***

malignant - ***lac-d.***

measles, in - ***chlor., euph.***

memory, loss of - **ANAC.,** arn., hyos., lach., merc., mur-ac., op., puls., rhus-t., verat.

midnight - ***ars.,*** lyc., ***rhus-t., stram., sulph., verat.***

after - **ARS.,** bry., chin., chin-a., lyc., nux-v., **PHOS., RHUS-T.,** ***sulph.***

before - ars., **BRY.,** ***bapt.,*** calad., **CARB-V.,** nux-v., lach., lyc., ***stram.***

mouth, corner of, drawn down on left side - ***verat-v.***

motions, automatic convulsive, of hands and feet as in hydrocephalus - ***zinc.***

move, inability to - ***ars.***

muttering - apis, ***hyos.,*** lach., ***lyc.,*** ph-ac., ***rhus-t., verat-v.***

nervous symptoms, with - agar., ***bell., hyos.,*** lach., op., ph-ac., phos., stram.

adynamia, and - agar., apis, ars., bapt., ***bell.,*** bry., cocc., colch., gels., hell., ***hyos., ign.,*** lach., lyc., ***mur-ac.,*** ph-ac., phos., rhus-t., ***stram.,*** sumb., valer., zinc.

collapse, and - ***ars., camph.,*** carb-v., chin., ***laur.,*** mur-ac., sec., verat.

continually increase, in third or fourth week - ***chlor.***

predominate - ***bapt., gels.***

night - am-c., apis, **ARS.,** arum-t., **BAPT.,** ***bell.,*** **BRY.,** calad., **CARB-V.,** cham., **CHIN., CHIN-A.,** cocc., ***colch.,*** **LACH.,** ***kali-bi.,*** lyc., **MERC.,** ***mur-ac., nux-v., op., ph-ac., phos., puls.,*** **RHUS-T.,** ***stram.,*** **SULPH.,** sul-ac.

temperature running very high - **BELL.,** ***bry., hyos.,*** rhus-t., ***stram.***

noise and jar, worse from least - **BELL.,** ***ign.***

nose, sooty - ***zinc.***

TYPHOID, fever,

nosebleeds, with - ***acon., arn., bry.,*** croc., cupr-m., ***ham.,*** hyos., ***ip., lach.,*** meli., merc., ***phos., ph-ac., rhus-t., sec., sulph., sul-ac.,*** verat.

onset, at - ***bry., calc., rhus-t.***

pains, violent, particularly in thighs - ***tarax.***

parotitis - acon., ***bell., calc., mang., merc., nat-m.***

pectoral - am-c., ***ant-t.,*** **BRY.,** ***carb-v.,*** chel., chin., ***hyos.,*** kali-bi., ***lyc.,*** nit-ac., **PHOS.,** ***rhus-t., sulph.,*** tub.

pemphigus - crot-h.

peritonitis, with - ars., ***bell.,*** carb-v., coloc., merc., rhus-t., ter.

petechial - anthr., ***arn., ars., bapt.,*** camph., caps., ***carb-v., chin.,*** **CHLOR.,** ***lach.,*** **MUR-AC.,** nit-ac., ***phos., rhus-t., sec.,*** sulph.

fetid stool, intestinal haemorrhage, sopor, so weak that he settles down in bed into a heap - **MUR-AC.**

foul breath, says there is nothing matter with him - **ARN.**

putrid, foul, cadaverous smell to stool, brown, dry, leathery-looking tongue, extreme prostration - **ARS.**

phlebitis - ***lach.***

picking at bedclothes - arn., ars., colch., **HYOS.,** lyc., ***op.,*** ph-ac., psor., ***stram.,*** sulph., ***verat-v., zinc.***

pneumonia - **ANT-T.,** ***bad., benz-ac.,*** **BRY.,** ***hyos.,*** lach., lachn., ***laur.,*** **LYC.,** merc-cy., ***nit-ac.,*** op., **PHOS.,** ***rhus-t., sang.,*** **SULPH., TER.**

bronchial symptoms - ***ant-t.,*** ars., bell., ***bry.,*** hyos., ip., lach., ***phos.,*** puls., rhus-t., ***sang.,*** sulph., ter.

psoric individuals, in - ***sulph.***

pupils fixed, do not react to light - ***zinc.***

refuses things - bell., ***nit-s-d.***

remedy, well selected, has no effect - ***sulph.***

remittent - stram.

repeated over and over in a singing tone any question put to him until interrupted by another question which he repeated as the first and so on, after typhoid - zinc.

restless, wants to go from one bed into another - **ARS.,** bell., ***calc., cina, cham.,*** hyos., mez., ***rhus-t.,*** sep., verat.

putrescent - ars., mur-ac.

scarlatina, in - apis, ***ars., arum-t., chlor.***

sequel, cries a great deal, particularly when alone - ***manc.***

diminished appetite - ***psor.***

eating, very little makes her immediately very full - ***manc.***

nervous deafness - ***phos., ph-ac.***

fear of getting crazy - ***manc.***

feels light, as though she could float or hover in air, in nervous affection - ***manc.***

mental dejection and apathy - ***hell.***

progressive emaciation, with cough - ***myos.***

hoarseness - ***phos., spong.***

TYPHOID, fever,

sequel,

legs feel weak, with fear of paralysis, also nervous debility - ***sel.***

paralysis - ***cupr-m., phos.,*** **RHUS-T.**

raw sensation down throat - ***manc.***

constant desire for some dishes, particularly indigestible things, puddings, half baked bread and the like - ***manc.***

debility of spine, fears he will be paralyzed - sel.

sweat - psor.

weakness - ***chin.,*** coca, ***fl-ac.,*** psor., ***sil.***

shipboard, from confinement on, without good care or food - ***bapt.***

silent, taciturn, averse to talking - ***arn.,*** ars., bell., bry., chin., cocc., hyos., merc., nit-s-d., nux-v., op., **PH-AC.,** rhus-t., verat.

singing - ars., bell., hyos., lyc., mur-ac., ***stram.***

sleepless - ***bell.,*** cham., merc., ***op.,*** mur-ac.

slow, protracted cases - **ARS.**

sopor - ***arn., ars., cocc.,*** lach., ***lyc., op., phos., rhus-t.***

sounds, utters inarticulate - ***zinc.***

spasmodic symptoms - cham.

spine, irritated, in beginning - valer.

soreness, muscular, with - ***arn.,*** bapt., bry., gels., ***rhus-t.***

stage, early - ***nux-v., puls.***

first, when patient seems to have taken cold, sudden onset - ***gels.***

symptoms like early - hippoz.

staring - bell., hell., ***hyos., op., ph-ac.,*** sec., ***zinc.***

stupid form - apis, ***arn., ars.,*** arum-t., **BAPT.,** ***bry.,*** **CARB-V.,** ***chin.,*** chin-s., cic., cocc., ***crot-h., gels.,*** **HELL., HYOS.,** ***lach.,*** lyc., **MUR-AC.,** nux-v., **OP., PH-AC.,** ***phos., rhus-t.,*** sec., ***stram.,*** verat., **ZINC.**

stupor, complete - **HELL., HYOS.,** lyc., **OP.,** stram., ***ph-ac.***

subsultus - **CALC.,** ***zinc.***

like galvanic shocks - ***verat-v.***

sweat, clammy, covers arms, cold - ***zinc.***

sweat, one-sided - ***nux-v.***

swung, as if, to and fro in a swing or cradle - ***ign.***

symptoms similar to - bapt., ***iris.***

teeth, champing - ***verat-v.***

temperature nearly normal - ***hell.***

toxemia, with - ***ars., mur-ac.,*** pyrog., rhus-t.

thirstless - ***apis, arn., gels.***

trembling, of limbs - ***lach.***

twitching - cham.

tympanites, with - ***ars., asaf.,*** bapt., ***carb-v.,*** chin., cocc., colch., lyc., methyl-b., mill., mur-ac., nux-m., ***ph-ac.,*** rhus-t., ***ter.***

typhus abdominalis - plb.

typhus with swelled parotid and sensitive bones - ***mang.***

TYPHOID, fever,

unconscious - ***arn.,*** ars., ***bell.,*** canth., colch., ***hell., hyos.,*** lach., lyc., merc., mur-ac., ***op.,*** phos., ***rhus-t., stram., zinc.***

ulcer, corneal, with - apis, ip.

urination, involuntary - apis, ***arn., ars., bell.,*** colch., hell., ***hyos., lyc.,*** merc., ***op., phos., rhus-t., stram., verat., verat-v., zinc.***

profuse, with - gels., mur-ac., ***ph-ac.***

scanty and painful - apis, ars., ***canth.***

urine, albuminous - ***calc-ar., ph-ac., rhus-t.***

dark - ***carb-v., merc., nux-v., verat-v.***

fetid - apis, ***ars.,*** bapt., ***carb-v.,*** phos., sulph., verat-v.

turbid - ***ars., carb-v., phos., verat-v.***

variola, in - ***chlor.***

visions - ***bell., calc.,*** carb-v., chin., ***hyos., mur-ac.,*** puls., ***stram.***

visions, when closing eyes - ars., ***calc.,*** carb-v., samb.

vomiting, after, diarrhea and coldness have ceased - ***hyos.***

weakness - ***arn., ars., bapt., bry.,*** cupr-m., hydr., merc., ***nuph.,*** **OP.,** ***ph-ac., rhus-t.***

week, second - ***calc.***

fifth - ***lach.***

women, in, and young people - ***ign.***

UNCOVERING, general

amel. - acon., ***ars., bov., cham.,*** chin., chin-a., coloc., ferr., ign., ***led.,*** lyc., mur-ac., nux-v., plat., ***puls., staph.,*** verat.

aversion to - acon., ***arg-n.,*** ars., aur., **BELL.,** ***calc., camph.,*** carb-an., ***chin-s.,*** clem., coff., ***colch.,*** con., ***gels., graph., hell., hep.,*** **MAG-C.,** ***mag-m.,*** manc., ***merc.,*** nat-c., nux-m., **NUX-V.,** ph-ac., phos., **PULS., PSOR., PYROG., RHUS-T., SAMB.,** ***sil.,*** **SQUIL., STRAM.,** ***stront-c.,*** sul-ac., ***tarent.,*** **TUB.**

chilliness from - acon., agar., ***apis,*** **ARN.,** bar-c., ***bell., calc.,*** carb-an., cham., **CHIN.,** ***chin-s.,*** **NUX-V.,** ***psor.,*** pyrog., **RHUS-T.,** sarr., ***sep.,*** squil., ***tarent.,*** **TUB.**

and pain - squil.

in any stage of paroxysm - arn., ars., aur., carb-an., ***chin., gels.,*** graph., hell., ***hep.,*** **NUX-V.,** ***pyrog.,*** **RHUS-T., SAMB.,** squil., stram., ***tarent.***

desire for - **ACON., APIS,** ***arn., ars., ars-i.,*** asar., ***bar-c.,*** bor., ***bov.,*** bry., calad., calc., cham., **CHIN.,** ***chin-a., coff.,*** **EUPH., FERR.,** ferr-i., fl-ac., ***hep.,*** **IGN.,** iod., ***lach.,*** led., lyc., ***mag-c.,*** med., **MOSCH., MUR-AC., NAT-M.,** ***nit-ac.,*** **OP., PETR.,** ***phos., plat.,*** **PULS.,** rhus-t., **SEC.,** spig., **STAPH.,** ***sulph.,*** thuj., ***verat.***

pain from uncovering - stram.

VACCINATION, after - **SIL.,** ***thuj.***

VIRAL, infections - acon., ars., bapt., ***carc., gels.,*** nat-m., ph-ac., rhus-t.

VERTIGO, commencing with - ***cocc.***
ephemeral fever - ***verat-v.***
high fever, with dizziness - ***kali-c.***

VEXATION, heat, from - acon., ***cham.,*** nux-v., ***petr.,*** ph-ac., phos., **SEP.,** staph.

VOMITING, during - all-s., ant-c., ***arn., ars., cact.,*** cham., ***cina, crot-h.,*** dor., ***elat.,*** eup-pur., ***ip.,*** lach., **NAT-M.,** nux-v., stram., verat.
amel. - acon., dig., puls., sec.
puffed stomach, with - ferr-p.

WALKING, in open air - am-c., am-m., arg-m., bell., bor., bry., caust., **CAMPH.,** chin., con., cur., hep., hyos., led., meny., ***nux-v.,*** ph-ac., rhus-t., sabad., ***sep.,*** spig., staph., tarax., thuj.
after - ars., calc., caust., meny., ***petr.,*** **RAN-S.,** ***rhus-t.,*** sabin., ***sep.***
amel. - alum., asar., caps., cic., lyc., mag-c., mosch., ***phos., puls.,*** sabin., tarax.

WARM, covering agg. - acon., **APIS,** calc., ***cham.,*** coff., ferr., **IGN.,** ***led.,*** lyc., mur-ac., nux-v., op., ***petr.,*** **PULS.,** rhus-t., staph., ***sulph.,*** verat.
intolerance of both cold and warm air - cocc.
room agg. - ***am-m.,*** ang., **APIS,** ***bry., ip.,*** kali-c., lach., ***lyc.,*** mag-m., nat-m., nicc., plan., **PULS.,** ***sulph.,*** sul-ac., zinc.
heat of the room is intolerable - **APIS.,** lach., puls., sulph.
weather, in - nit-ac.

WARMTH, agg. - **APIS,** bry., ign., lach., **PULS.,** op., staph.

WASHING, agg. - am-c., rhus-t., sep., ***sulph.***
amel. - **APIS,** bapt., **FL-AC., PULS.**

WEAKNESS, during - acon., alum., am-m., ant-t., ***anthr., apis,*** aran., **ARS.,** ***bapt., bry.,*** calc., carb-v., crot-h., ***eup-per.,*** eup-pur., ferr., gels., ***ign.,*** lyc., morph., ***mur-ac.,*** nat-c., ***nat-m.,*** nicc., nit-ac., petr., ***ph-ac.,*** **PHOS.,** ***puls., rob., rhus-t.,*** sarr., sep., sul-ac., sulph., syph., thuj.
after - ***apis, aran.,*** gent-l., med., morph., sal-ac., sulph., syph.
anthrax, in - tarent.
diarrhea, in - sulph.
ephemeral fever - ***verat-v.***
following prolonged fever - ***colch., psor.,*** **SEL.**
inebriety, bilious or remittent, from - eup-per.
languor, muscular weakness, desire for absolute rest and drowsiness - ***gels.***
weariness, extreme - coca

WET, after getting wet - ***calc., puls.,*** **RHUS-T.**

WINTER - calc., carb-v., chin., nux-m., puls., ***rhus-t.,*** sulph., verat.

WORMS, from - cic., **CINA,** fil., ***indg., ip., merc., sabad., spig.,*** stram., ***sulph.***
excitable and restless boy - stann.
intestinal inflammation and diarrhea - ***merc.***
slow, chronic form in scrofulous children, with large bellies, and sweat about head - ***sil.***

YAWNING, disposed to yawn and stretch - aesc., ***rhus-t.***

YELLOW, fever - ***acon., ant-t., arg-n.,*** **ARS.,** ***ars-h., bell., bry.,*** **CADM-S.,** calc., ***camph.,*** **CANTH.,** ***caps.,*** **CARB-V.,** cean., ***all-c., chin.,*** coff., **CROT-H.,** ***cupr-m.,*** daph., ***gels., glon.,*** hep., ip., kali-p., **LACH.,** ***lob.,*** **MERC.,** ***nat-s., nux-v., phos.,*** plat., ***psor., rhus-t., sulph.,*** sul-ac., ***ter., verat., verat-v.***
anxiety about heart - **LACH.**
awaking, worse on - **LACH.**
bilious remittent, assuming form of - ***nat-s.***
belching, sour, with - **LACH.**
bleed much, small wounds - **LACH.**
blood dark, non-coagulable - **LACH.**
conjunctiva, yellow - **LACH.**
delirium - ***crot-h.***
night - **LACH.**
drowsy - **LACH.**
drugging, after, or in persons accustomed to strong liquor - ***nux-v.***
dyspnea - **LACH.**
epigastrium, sensitiveness to pressure about, and neck - **LACH.**
gastro-hepatic type, with thin blackish or yellowish diarrhea - ***verat.***
head, rush of blood to, red face, fainting - **LACH.**
heartburn - **LACH.**
heat, sudden flushes of - **LACH.**
hemorrhagic, petechial spots and hemorrhages at an early stage - ***phos.***
left side, cannot lie on - **LACH.**
loquacious - **LACH.**
lips dry, cracked and bleeding - **LACH.**
meningeal inflammation threatening, especially in children - cor-r.
nausea after drinking - **LACH.**
nourishment, better after - **LACH.**
pregnancy, during - plat.
pulse, irregular weak - **LACH.**
quarrel, disposed to - **LACH.**
reconvalescence - ***calc.***
skin yellow - **LACH.**
skin purplish - **LACH.**
sleeplessness, persistent - **LACH.**
slow, difficult speech - **LACH.**
stage, first - ***acon.,*** arn., ***bell., bry., ip., lach.,*** puls.
first, as an intercurrent, when bones ache as if broken, headache, backache, thirst and vomiting - ***eup-per.***
second - acon., ant-c., ***ant-t., arg-n., ars.,*** bell., bry., ***crot-h.,*** hyos., ***ip.,*** merc-c., ***rhus-t.,*** sin-n.
third - ***ars., cadm-s., carb-ac.,*** **CARB-V.,** chin-a., chin., chin-s., ***crot-h.,*** dig., **LACH.,** ***merc., nit-ac., phos., ph-ac.,*** sec., ***sulph.,*** **SUL-AC.,** ***verat.***
hemorrhages, with great paleness of face - **CARB-V.**

YELLOW, fever,
- **stomach** weak, craves raw onions - ***all-c.***
- **sweat,** is checked from exposure to a draft of air, when - ***cadm.***
  - stains yellow - **LACH.**
- **tip** of tongue red, center brown - **LACH.**
- **trembling** all over - **LACH.**
- **trembling,** tongue heavy, dry and red cracked tip - **LACH.**
- **urine** almost black - **LACH.**
- **vomiting,** with palpitation - **LACH.**
- **wakefulness,** intense nervous - plat.

ZYMOTIC, fever - acet-ac., anthr., apis, **ARN.**, **ARS.**, ***bell.***, berb., **BAPT.**, **BRY.**, ***cadm-s.***, **CARB-S.**, carb-v., ***cur.***, **CROT-H.**, **ECHI.**, hyos., ip., **KALI-P.**, **LACH.**, **LYC.**, merc., **MUR-AC.**, nux-m., nux-v., op., ph-ac., ***phos.***, ***puls.***, **PYROG.**, **RHUS-T.**, rhus-v., **SULPH.**, tarent.

Food

ACIDS, agg. (see Sour) - **OLND.,** ***nat-p.***
amel. - **PTEL.**
aversion, to - abies-c., arund., ***bell.,*** chin., clem., ***cocc., con.,*** dros., elaps, ***ferr.,*** ferr-m., ***fl-ac.,*** ign., kali-bi., lyc., man., nat-m., nat-p., nux-v., ph-ac., ***sabad., sulph.,*** tub.

ALCOHOL, general
abuse of, ailments from - acon., ***agar.,*** alum., alumn., am-m., anac., ***ant-c.,*** apom., ***arg-n.,*** arn., **ARS., ASAR., AUR., BAR-C.,** ***bell.,*** bor., bov., cadm-s., ***calc., calc-ar.,*** carb-an., ***carb-s., carb-v.,*** card-m., caust., ***chel., chin.,*** chlol., coca, cocc., ***coff.,*** colch., ***con., crot-h.,*** dig., eup-per., ***gels.,*** hep., hydr., hyos., ***ign.,*** ip., kali-bi., **LACH.,** laur., ***led., lob., lyc.,*** naja, ***nat-c., nat-m., nux-m.,*** **NUX-V., OP.,** ***petr., puls.,*** querc., **RAN-B.,** ***rhod., rhus-t., ruta.,*** sabad., ***sang.,*** **SEL.,** sep., ***sil., spig., stram.,*** stront-c., stroph., stry., **SULPH., SUL-AC.,** tab., thuj., ***verat.,*** zinc.
agg. - acon., aeth., ***agar.,*** agav-t., aloe, alum., alumn., ***am-c.,*** am-m., anac., ang., ***ant-c.,*** apom., ***arg-n.,*** arn., **ARS., ASAR.,** aur., **BAR-C.,** ***bell.,*** berb., bor., bov., ***calc., calc-ar.,*** calc-f., calc-sil., ***cann-i.,*** caps., ***carb-ac.,*** carb-an., ***carb-s., carb-v.,*** card-m., ***caust., chel., chin.,*** chlol., cimic., ***coca,*** cocc., ***coff.,*** colch., ***con., crot-h., dig.,*** eup-per., ***ferr.,*** ferr-i., fl-ac., gels., ***glon.,*** gran., grat., guare., ***hell.,*** hep., hydr., hyos., ***ign.,*** ip., kali-bi., ***kali-br.,*** **LACH.,** laur., ***led., lob., lyc., merc.,*** naja, ***nat-c., nat-m.,*** **NAT-P.,** ***nux-m.,*** **NUX-V., OP.,** ***petr.,*** **PHOS.,** phyt., ***puls.,*** querc., **RAN-B.,** ***rhod., rhus-t., ruta,*** sabad., ***sang.,*** **SEL.,** sep., ***sil., spig., stram.,*** stront-c., stry., ***sul-ac., sulph., syph.,*** trinit., **ZINC.**
abstaining, after - calc-ar.
easily intoxicated - **CON.,** naja, phos., ***zinc.***
amel. - ***acon.,*** agar., canth., ***con., gels.,*** lach., op., sel., sul-ac.
aversion to, alcoholic stimulants - ail., alco., ang., ant-t., ars., ars-m., bell., bry., calc., calc-ar., carb-v., cham., chin., cocc., ***hyos.,*** ign., lec., man., manc., ***merc., nux-v.,*** ph-ac., phos., phyt., psor., ***rhus-t.,*** sil., spig., spong., stram., stroph., ***sul-ac.,*** sulph., zinc.
desires - acon., agav-t., ail., alco., aloe, am-c., ant-t., arg-m., ***arn.,*** **ARS.,** ***ars-i.,*** **ASAR.,** aster., ***aur.,*** aur-a., aur-i., bov., bry., bufo, ***calc., calc-ar.,*** calc-s., **CAPS.,** ***carb-ac.,*** carb-an., ***carb-v., chin.,*** cic., ***coca,*** cocc., **CROT-H.,** cub., cupr., ferr-p., fl-ac., gins., hell., **HEP.,** iber., ign., ***iod.,*** kali-bi., ***kreos.,*** lac-c., **LACH.,** lec., ***led., lyc., med.,*** merc., mosch., ***mur-ac.,*** naja, nat-m., nat-p., nux-m., **NUX-V.,** olnd., ***op., phos.,*** plb., ***psor., puls.,*** rhus-t., ***sel., sep.,*** sil., sol-t-ae., ***spig., staph.,*** stront-c., stry-n., **SULPH.,** ***sul-ac.,*** sumb., ***syph.,*** tab., ter., ther., ***tub.,*** ziz.

ALCOHOL, general
desire, for, disgust for, but - thiop.
menses, before - **SEL.**

ALCOHOLISM, (see Mind, Alcoholism)

ALE, agg. - gamb., spong., sulph.
aversion to - ferr., **NUX-V.**
desires - ferr-p., ***med., sulph.***

ALMONDS, desires - cub.

APPETITE, general - ant-c., ars., ***calc.,*** **CHIN.,** ***cina,*** graph., iod., ***lyc.,*** merc-cy., ***nat-m.,*** **NUX-V.,** petr., phos., **PULS.,** sil., stroph., **SULPH.,** verat.
capricious - ail., arn., ars., aster., bell., **BRY.,** bufo, calc., carb-s., carc., cham., **CHIN., CINA,** ***coc-c.,*** coca, fago., ferr., graph., ***hep., ign., iod., ip.,*** kali-bi., kreos., lach., mag-c., ***mag-m.,*** meli., merc., merc-i-f., nat-m., petr., ***phos., puls.,*** rheum, ***sang.,*** sil., staph., sulph., sumb., symph., syph., tep., ***ther., tub.,*** zinc.
drinks, desire for but refuses when offered - bell.
changeable - alum., am-m., ***anac.,*** berb., carc., **CINA,** coc-c., cocc., ***cur.,*** cycl., gels., gran., grat., iod., lach., ***mag-m.,*** meph., merc., nat-m., ***nit-ac.,*** op., phos., podo., puls., syph.
constant - bov., fl-ac., gran., ***kali-bi.,*** kali-p., ***merc.,*** myric., ***nat-c., nat-m.,*** rat., tab.
diminished - acet-ac., agar., agn., all-c., aloe, **ALUM.,** alumn., ant-t., aran., ***arg-n.,*** ars., ***aur.,*** aur-m., bad., bar-c., bar-i., ***bar-m.,*** bell., berb., bor., brom., ***cact.,*** calc., canth., carb-s., carb-v., ***caust.,*** cedr., chel., chin., chin-a., ***cina,*** cop., ***coff., coloc., con.,*** crot-t., cupr., ***cycl., dig.,*** dirc., echi., fago., ***ferr.,*** ferr-i., ferr-p., fl-ac., gamb., ***gels.,*** grat., hell., hura, ***hydr.,*** hyos., ign., iod., kali-bi., kali-c., kali-chl., kali-n., kali-s., kreos., lac-ac., ***lac-d., lach., lyc.,*** mag-s., merc., merc-c., merc-i-f., mez., ***murx.,*** myric., nat-c., nat-m., nat-p., naja, nux-v., ol-an., onos., op., plb., petr., phos., **PIC-AC.,** pin-s., pip-m., plan., ***psor.,*** puls., rheum, rhus-t., ruta., rumx., ***sabad.,*** sabin., sang., sant., sars., seneg., sep., sil., spong., stram., sulph., tab., tell., ter., thuj., til., ust., verat., zinc.
eating, when time for - ***chin.,*** ign.
evening - bor., chlor., dig., nux-m.
menses, during - mag-c.
morning - aloe, asc-t., calc-p., cinnb., lyss., mag-m., myric., narcot., sel., sulph.
noon - ant-t., calc., clem., coloc., indg., mez., nat-m., ox-ac., sulph.
perspiration, after - bell.
easy, satiety - agar., ***am-c.,*** ant-t., arg-m., arg-n., arn., ars., bar-c., bry., calad., carb-an., ***carb-s.,*** carb-v., ***caust.,*** **CHIN.,** ***cic., clem.,*** coc-c., ***colch.,*** con., croc., ***cycl., dig.,*** dulc., ***ferr., ferr-i.,*** fl-ac., ***gels.,*** guare., hydr., ***ign.,*** kali-bi., kali-i., kali-s., led., **LYC.,** mag-c., mag-m., mag-s., mang., merc., mez., nat-c., ***nat-m.,*** nit-ac., ***nux-m., nux-v.,*** olnd., ***op.,*** petr., petros., ph-ac., ***phos.,*** plan., **PLAT.,** ***podo.,*** prun., psor., ptel., ***rheum, rhod.,*** rhus-t., ruta., ***sep.,*** serp., ***sil.,*** spong., ***sulph.,***

APPETITE, general

easy, satiety - tarent., thea., ***thuj.,*** vinc.

evening - phos.

morning - cycl.

sadness, from - plat.

eat, with inability to - chin., elaps, ***sulph.,*** tab.

gnawing - abrot., arg-m., chin., colch., iod., kreos., sil.

increased, hunger - **ABIES-C.,** abrot., acal., ***acon., agar.,*** ail., ***all-c.,*** aloe, ***alum., alumn.,*** **AM-C.,** anac., anan., ang., ant-c., ant-t., **ARG-M.,** arn., **ARS.,** ***ars-i.,*** asaf., ***aur., bar-c., bar-i., bar-m., bell., berb.,*** bov., bry., calad., **CALC.,** ***calc-p.,*** **CALC-S.,** camph., **CANN-I.,** canth., caps., carb-ac., ***carb-an.,*** carb-s., carb-v., caul., ***caust.,*** **CHIN.,** ***chin-s.,*** cic., **CINA, CINNB.,** ***cocc.,*** coc-c., coff., colch., coloc., ***con.,*** cop., crot-c., cub., cupr., cycl., dig., dios., dros., dulc., ***elaps,*** equis., eug., euph., ***ferr., ferr-ar., ferr-i., fl-ac.,*** gamb., ***gels.,*** gent-c., gran., **GRAPH.,** grat., ***guai., guare.,*** hell., hep., hura, hydr-ac., hydr., hyos., ***ign.,*** **IOD.,** ind., jug-c., jug-r., kali-ar., kali-bi., kali-c., kali-chl., kali-i., kali-n., kali-p., ***kali-s.,*** kreos., ***lac-ac., lac-c., lach.,*** lact., laur., led., lept., lil-t., **LYC.,** lyss., mag-c., ***mag-m.,*** mag-p., ***merc., merc-c.,*** mez., ***mur-ac., myric., nat-a., nat-c.,*** **NAT-M.,** ***nat-p., nat-s., nit-ac., nux-m.,*** **NUX-V., OLND.,** onos., ***op.,*** ox-ac., **PETR.,** ***ph-ac.,*** **PHOS.,** phys., ***pic-ac.,*** plat., plb., podo., **PSOR., PULS.,** ran-b., raph., ***rat.,*** rheum, rhus-t., ruta, **SABAD.,** sars., sec., sel., seneg., ***sep., sil.,*** spig., spong., squil., ***stann., staph.,*** stram., stront-c., sul-ac., **SULPH.,** sumb., tab., tarent., tep., ter., ***teucr.,*** ther., thuj., ust., valer., **VERAT.,** zinc.

afternoon - arg-m., chin., colch., guai., lyc., nat-c., nux-v., psor., zinc.

2 p.m. - chin-s., clem.

4 p.m. - calc-p.

5 p.m. - myric.

after drinking - nat-m.

air, open amel. - ant-t.

alternating with loss of appetite - am-m., anac., ars., ***berb., calc.,*** caps., chin., cina, dros., **FERR.,** ***iod.,*** nat-m., nux-v., op., ***phos.,*** puls., sil., sulph., ***thuj.,*** tub.

beer, after - nux-v.

chill, during - ail., **ARS.,** ***chin-s., eup-per., lec.,*** nux-v., ***phos.,*** **SIL.,** staph.

after - ***ars.***

before - ***chin.,*** **CINA,** ***eup-per.,*** **STAPH.**

convulsion, before - calc., hyos.

coryza and cough, with - all-c., hep., nux-v., sul-ac.

daytime - murx., nat-m., ***stann.***

diarrhea, with - nux-v., **PETR.,** verat.

digestion weak, with - merc.

eating, after - acon., agar., ***alf.,*** all-c., alum., ***arg-m.,*** asc-c., aur., bov., ***calc.,*** casc., cast-eq., chin-a., ***chin-s., cic.,*** **CINA,** coc-c., corn., dig., fago., gran., grat., hura, indol., **IOD.,** kali-chl., kali-p., lac-c., lach.,

APPETITE, general

increased, hunger

eating, after - **LYC.,** med., ***merc.,*** murx., myric., nat-m., par., **PHOS.,** phyt., plat., plb., ***psor.,*** ran-s., raph., sars., sil., staph., stront-c., sulph., syc-co., syph., zinc.

increases the - **LYC.**

refuses, but - bar-c.

returns only while - anac., calc., carb-an., **CHIN.,** mag-c., nat-m., phos.

evening - agar., aloe, arn., bor., bov., calad., calc., cann-s., carb-an., cham., chin., chin-s., colch., cop., crot-c., cycl., fl-ac., ***guai.,*** iod., ***kali-n.,*** lyc., mag-m., mez., nat-c., ***nat-m.,*** phos., ***pic-ac., psor.,*** puls., sabad., ***sep.,*** sil., teucr., thuj., zinc.

6 p.m. - sumb.

8 p.m. - pip-m.

9 p.m. - form.

fainting, with - iod.

fever, during - ***chin., cina,*** cur., eup-pur., hell., **PHOS.**

after - ***cimx., cina,*** dulc., eup-per., ign., staph.

forenoon - aloe, arg-m., hell., hep., ind., kali-n., nat-c., nat-m., nux-m., sulph.

10 a.m. - iod., kali-n., lyc., ***nat-m.,*** thuj.

11 a.m. - euphr., hep., hura, hydr., ign., ***iod.,*** kali-n., lach., ***nat-m.,*** phos., **SULPH.,** tub., ***zinc.***

gnawing - med.

headache, with - agn., ars., bry., crot-h., dulc., elaps, ign., ***kali-c.,*** kali-p., kali-s., lac-d., lyc., nux-v., **PHOS., PSOR.,** ptel., sang., sel., ***sep.,*** sil., sulph., syph., thuj.

after - iod.

before - ***calc.,*** dulc., epip., ***phos.,*** **PSOR.,** sep., tub.

intermittent, in - ***phos., staph.***

loses flesh, yet - abrot., acet-ac., ***iod., nat-m.,*** sanic., tub., uran-n.

menses, during - kali-p., spong.

before - mag-c., spong.

morning - agar., ant-c., ***arg-m.,*** asar., aur., bor., bry., calad., ***calc.,*** carb-an., chel., chin., cycl., hyper., lyc., lyss., mur-ac., murx., myric., nat-c., nat-m., psor., ran-b., rhus-t., sabad., sang., ***sel.,*** sep., sil., teucr., zinc.

5 a.m. - nat-c.

7 a.m. - aloe.

8 a.m. - chin.

after stool - aloe

breakfast, after - aloe, tax.

nausea, with - arg-m., caust., chin., cycl., petr., rhus-t., valer., verat.

neuralgia, during - dulc., **PSOR.**

night - abies-n., anan., bry., canth., **CHIN.,** ***chin-s., ign.,*** **LYC., PHOS.,** ph-ac., **PSOR.,** puls., sel., sulph., tarent., tell.

11 p.m. - ox-ac.

12 a.m. - ***med.***

APPETITE, general

increased, hunger

noon - abies-n., acon., am-c., clem., coc-c., colch., coloc., dig., hyper., lact., lyc., mag-c., ***mez.,*** nat-c., ***nat-m., nux-m.,*** stront-c., sulph.

pain in stomach, with - **LACH.,** ***lyc.,*** puls., ***sil.***

during - cimx., ***cina,*** sanic.

sickness before attacks - bry., calc., hyos., nux-v., ***phos., psor.,*** sep.

siesta, after - ang., onos.

sitting, after - rhus-t.

spine, from - lil-t.

stomach full, when - staph.

stool, after - aloe, fl-ac., kali-p., **PETR.**

stool, during - aloe, ferr., sec.

sudden - sulph.

tormenting - arg-m., bell., crot-h., ***iod., olnd.,*** seneg.

umbilicus, from - valer.

unusual time - chin., coc-c., **CINA,** gins.

vanishing, at sight of food - caust., ***crot-c.,*** kali-p., merc-i-f., ***phos.,*** **SULPH.**

drinking water, after - kali-m.

on attempting to eat - ***sil.***

quickly satiated, yet - am-c., arn., ars., bar-c., carb-v., ***chin., cycl.,*** ferr., lith., ***lyc.,*** nat-m., nux-v., petros., podo., prun., ***sep., sulph.***

smell or thought of food, pregnancy during - caust.

vomiting, with - caust., chin., hell., verat.

after - cina, ***colch.,*** olnd., podo., tab.

waking, on - arn., bell., chin., dig., ptel.

weakness, with - lach., merc., ***phos.,*** **SULPH.,** zinc.

limbs, in - zinc.

wine, after - nat-m.

worms, with - ***cina.***

insatiable - ant-c., ***arg-m.,*** arg-n., arum-t., asc-t., aur., bar-c., **CINA.,** ***ferr., ferr-i.,*** **IOD., LYC.,** petr., puls-n, ***sec., sep., spong.,*** squil., stann., staph., ***zinc.***

evening - arg-n., zinc.

morning - arg-n.

noon - asc-t., petr., zinc.

loss, of - abrot., absin., acet-ac., ***acon.,*** aesc., aeth., ***agar.,*** ail., ***all-c.,*** aloe, ***alum.,*** ambr., am-c., am-m., ***anac., anthr., ant-c.,*** ant-t., apis, arg-m., ***arg-n., arn.,*** **ARS.,** ars-h., ars-i., arum-t., **ASAR.,** aster., aur., aur-m., ***bapt., bar-c.,*** bar-i., bar-m., bell., ***berb.,*** benz., ***bol., bor., bov.,*** brach., ***bry., cact.,*** calad., **CALC.,** ***calc-ar.,*** calc-p., calc-s., camph., canth., caps., ***carb-ac., carb-an.,*** carb-s., ***carb-v.,*** carc., ***card-m., caust.,*** **CHAM., CHEL., CHIN.,** chin-a., chin-s., ***chlor., cina,*** cinnb., ***cic.,*** cimic., **COCC.,** ***coff., colch.,*** coloc., ***con.,*** cop., cor-r., crot-t., cupr., cupr-ar., **CYCL.,** daph., ***dig.,*** dros., dulc., echi., elat., eup-per., **FERR.,** ***ferr-ar., ferr-i.,*** ferr-p., ***fl-ac.,*** gels., glon., gran., graph., ***guai.,*** gymn., hep., ***hydr.,*** hydrc., hyos., hyper., ***ign.,*** ind., indg., ***iod.,*** **IP.,** ***iris,*** jatr., jug-c., jug-r., kali-ar., **KALI-BI.,** ***kali-br.,*** kali-c., kali-chl., ***kali-i., kali-n.,*** kali-p., ***kali-s.,*** kreos., lach., lact., laur., ***lec.,*** led., lil-t., lob., **LYC.,** lyss., ***mag-c.,*** mag-m., mag-s., manc., ***mang.,*** med., ***meph., merc., merc-c., mez., mur-ac.,*** murx., myric., naja, nat-a., nat-c., **NAT-M.,** nat-p., nat-s., nicc., nit-ac., ***nux-m.,*** **NUX-V.,** olnd., op., osm., ox-ac., ***petr., ph-ac.,*** **PHOS.,** phyt., pic-ac., pip-m., plat., ***plb., podo., psor.,*** ptel., **PULS.,** raph., rat., **RHUS-T.,** sabad., ***sabin., sang., sarr.,*** sars., sec., senec., ***seneg.,*** **SEP., SIL.,** sol-t-ae., ***spig.,*** spong., squil., stann., stram., stront-c., **SULPH.,** ***sul-ac.,*** sumb., ***syph.,*** tab., tarent., tep., ***ter., thuj.,*** trom., upa., urt-u., verat., vip., xan., zinc., zing.

brain trouble, in - hell.

disease, after severe - ant-c., ars., psor.

drinking water, after - kali-m.

evening - aeth., am-m., arn., ars., bor., carb-v., cinnb., clem., coc-c., coloc., cupr., cycl., dig., graph., hyper., mag-m., merc., murx., nat-c., nat-m., ox-ac., ran-s., senec., sil., sulph., zinc.

exertion, after - ***calc.***

foggy weather, in - **CHIN.**

food, sight of, at - alum., caust., ***colch., crot-c.,*** kali-p., merc-i-f., nux-v., ***phos.,*** **SULPH.**

during pregnancy - caust., colch., ip., lyc., sabad., sep.

tasted, until, then ravenous - lyc.

food, smell of, at - caust., carb-an., **COLCH.,** nux-v., ***sep.***

fullness, from sense of - ***chin., lyc.,*** phos., rhus-t., squil.

habitual - kali-m.

hunger, with - act-sp., ***agar., alum., ars., bar-c.,*** bell., bry., carb-s., carb-v., ***chin., chin-s.,*** **COCC.,** dulc., euphr., ***hell., kali-n.,*** **LACH., NAT-M.,** nicc., **NUX-V.,** olnd., op., ***phos.,*** psor., ***rhus-t.,*** sabad., ***sil., sulph., sul-ac.,*** tax., ***tub.,*** verb.

lifting, from - sep.

menses, during - ammc., brom., calc-p., cupr., cycl., goss., ***ign.,*** lyc., mag-c., puls.

before - am-c., bell., calc-p., ign.

months, for - syph.

morning - abies-n., agar., ail., am-c., ant-t., arg-m., arg-n., bell., benz-ac., bov., carb-v., ***caust.,*** chin., chin-a., cic., coc-c., con., cycl., dig., dios., euphr., ***ferr-m.,*** gymn., hydr., ign., ind., lach., lec., meph., myric., nit-ac., phos., ptel., sars., sel., ***seneg., sep.,*** stram., sulph., tab., tub., zinc.

nausea, from - ars., ***ip.***

noon - agar., ang., anac., arg-n., bor., carb-v., chel., chin., clem., cic., cycl., grat., mang., murx., nat-c., ox-ac., phos., pic-ac., rhus-t., ruta., sars., sulph., sumb., zinc.

offered, when desired thing is - ign.

palpitations, with - coca.

returns after eating - cham.

a mouthful - anac., ***calc.,*** **CHIN.,** mag-c., ***sabad.***

APPETITE, general

loss, of, returns, after thinking of food - calc-p.
sadness, from - nat-m., plat.
sex, after - ***agar.***
smoking, from - bell., sep.
suddenly, eating when - bar-c.
thirst, with - am-c., ant-t., ars., bapt., bor., ***calc.,*** calc-ar., ***colch.,*** coloc., dig., dulc., ***kali-n.,*** kreos., lac-d., lec., lyc., mag-c., nux-v., ox-ac., ***phos., psor.,*** rhus-t., sanic., seneg., sep., sil., ***spig.,*** **SULPH.,** zinc.
uterine disorders, with - alet.
vexation, after - nat-m., petr., phos.

nibbling - ***aeth.,*** ars., calc., mag-c., mag-m., nat-c., petr., rhus-t.

ravenous - abies-c., abrot., ***agar., all-c., alum.,*** **AM-C.,** ***anac.,*** anan., **ARG-M.,** arn., **ARS., ARS-I.,** asaf., ***aur.,*** bar-c., ***bar-i.,*** bar-m., bell., ***berb.,*** bov., ***bry.,*** calad., **CALC., CALC-P., CALC-S.,** camph., **CANN-I.,** caps., carb-ac., ***carb-an.,*** **CARB-S.,** carb-v., carc., card-m., caul., ***caust.,*** **CHIN.,** ***chin-a.,*** **CINA,** ***cocc., coc-c., coff., colch., coloc., con.,*** cop., crot-c., cupr., dros., ***elaps,*** equis., ***eup-per.,*** **FERR.,** ***ferr-ar., ferr-i.,*** ferr-p., ***fl-ac.,*** gamb., gels., gran., **GRAPH.,** ***guai.,*** guare., hell., hep., ***hyos.,*** hura, ***ign.,*** **IOD.,** ind., jug-c., kali-ar., kali-bi., kali-c., kali-chl., ***kali-n.,*** kali-p., kali-s., kreos., lac-c., ***lac-ac.,*** lach., lap-a., laur., lil-t., **LYC.,** lyss., mag-c., mag-m., mag-p., meny., ***merc., merc-c., mez., mur-ac.,*** myric., ***nat-a., nat-c.,*** **NAT-M.,** ***nat-p., nat-s., nit-ac., nux-m.,*** **NUX-V.,** ***ol-j.,*** **OLND.,** ***op.,*** ox-ac., **PETR.,** ***ph-ac.,*** **PHOS.,** phys., ***plat., podo.,*** **PSOR.,** ptel., **PULS.,** ***rat., rhus-t.,*** ruta., **SABAD.,** ***sec.,*** seneg., ***sep.,*** **SIL.,** spig., ***spong.,*** squil., ***stann., staph.,*** stront-c., **SULPH.,** sul-ac., tab., tarent., tep., ter., ***thuj.,*** ust., valer., **VERAT.,** zinc.
afternoon - ***guai.,*** lyc., nat-c., nux-v.
2 p.m. - clem.
4 p.m. - ***calc-p.***
5 p.m. - myric.
ague, before - eup-per., ***staph.***
apyrexia, during - **STAPH.**
contempt, during - plat.
convulsions, after - coc-c.
diarrhea, with - aloe, ***asaf., calc.,*** coch., ***fl-ac., iod., lyc., olnd.,*** **PETR.,** ***stram., sulph., verat.,*** zinc.
preceding - psor.
dysentery, in - **NUX-V.**
eating, after, soon - acon., agar., ***arg-m.,*** asc-c., bov., ***calc.,*** **CHIN-S.,** ***cic.,*** **CINA,** coc-c., corn., fago., grat., **IOD.,** kali-p., lach., **LYC.,** ***med., merc.,*** myric., **PHOS.,** phyt., plb., ***psor.,*** sarr., ***staph.,*** stront-c., ***sulph.,*** zinc.
2 hours after - calc-hp., tax.
3 hours after - **IOD.**
increases the hunger - **LYC.**

APPETITE, general

ravenous, emaciation, with - ***abrot.,*** acet-ac., ars-i., bar-c., **CALC.,** chin., con., gran., ign., **IOD.,** ip., ***kali-i.,*** lyc., **NAT-M., PETR.,** ***phos.,*** psor., sac-alb., sanic., sec., sel., sil., ***sulph., thyr., tub.,*** uran-n.
children, in - ***abrot.,*** ars-i., bar-c., bar-i., calc., calc-p., caust., chin., ***cina, iod.,*** lyc., mag-c., nat-m., nux-v., ol-j., petr., sil., sulph., tub.
epilepsy, after - calc.
before - ***calc.,*** **HYOS.**
evening - agar., aloe, calc., cann-s., cham., chin-s., crot-c., fl-ac., gent-c., gent-l., ***guai.,*** guare., iod., lyc., mag-c., ***mez., nat-m.,*** sabad., sil., teucr., zinc.
6 p.m. - sumb.
8 p.m. - pip-m.
forenoon - aloe, kali-n., ***nat-c.,*** sulph.
10 a.m. - iod., kali-n., meli., ***nat-m.***
11 a.m. - ign., ***iod.,*** **SULPH.,** ***zinc.***
gastralgia, in - ***lyc., sil.***
lying amel. - sil.
marasmus, with - ***abrot.,*** ars-i., ***bar-c.,*** bar-i., **CALC.,** ***calc-p., caust., chin.,*** **CINA, IOD.,** ***kali-i., lyc., mag-c.,*** **NAT-M.,** ***nux-v.,*** petr., ***sil., sulph.***
menopause, at - sulph.
morning - ant-c., ***arg-m.,*** bry., ***calc.,*** hyper., myric., nat-c., plat., sabad., sang., sil.
5 a.m. - nat-c.
nausea, after - bry.
before - mag-m.
neuralgia, with - ***dulc.,*** **PSOR.**
night - abies-n., anan., bry., **CHIN.,** ***ign., lyc.,*** petr., ***ph-ac.,*** **PHOS.,** ***psor.,*** sel., sep., sil., sulph., tarent.
11 p.m. - ***nat-c.***
noon - acon., abies-n., coloc., lyc., ***mez., nat-m., nux-m., zinc.***
perspiration, with - agar.
pregnancy, during night - ***psor.***
sadness, with - ign., nat-m.
sleep, prevents - abies-n., ***chin., ign., lyc., phos.,*** sanic., teucr.
stool, after - kali-p., petr.
thirst, with - carb-v.
walking, while - ant-t., hell., lyc., phos.
weakness, with - bry.

relish, without - ***agar.,*** alum., ang., ant-c., ars., ***bar-c.,*** bar-i., bell., bor., ***bry.,*** calad., calc., carb-s., carb-v., caust., cham., ***chin.,*** chin-a., cic., clem., cocc., coff., colch., cycl., dig., ***dulc.,*** euphr., ***ferr.,*** ferr-ar., ferr-i., ferr-p., hell., hep., ign., iod., kali-n., ***kali-s.,*** lach., lyc., mag-c., ***mag-m.,*** merc., mez., nat-c., **NAT-M.,** nicc., nux-v., **OLND., OP.,** phos., plat., ***puls.,*** **RHEUM,** rhod., **RHUS-T.,** ruta., sabad., ***sil.,*** staph., sulph., ***sul-ac.,*** sumb., thuj., valer., verat., verb.
eat, until begins to - chin., **LYC.,** sabad.

thirst, with - **ARG-N.,** graph., ***kali-bi.***
without - **ARG-N.**

APPLES, agg. - alum., ant-t., arg-n., ars., ars-i., bell., bor., chin., con., mang., merc-c., nat-s., ox-ac., phos., puls., rumx., sep., sulph., thuj.
sour - merc-c.
amel. - guai., ust.
aversion to - ant-t., guai., **HELL.,** lyss.
desires - aloe, ant-t., ap-g., fel., ***guai.,*** menth., sulph., tell.

AROMATIC, drinks agg. smell of - agn., puls.
desires - anan.

ARTICHOKES, aversion to - abies-c., acon., ***mag-c.,*** sulph.

ARTIFICIAL agg. - ***alum.,*** calc., mag-c., sulph.

ASHES, desires - tarent.

BACON, amel. - ran-b., ran-s.
aversion to - rad-br.
desires - ars., calc., ***calc-p.,*** carc., cench., ***mez.,*** rad-br., ***sanic.,*** tell., ***tub.***

BAKED, agg. - carb-v., puls.

BANANAS, agg. - rumx.
aversions - bar-c., elaps.
desires - ther., tub.

BEANS, and peas agg. - ars., **BRY.,** ***calc.,*** carb-v., chin., ***coloc.,*** cupr., erig., hell., kali-c., **LYC.,** nat-m., ***petr.,*** phos., puls., sep., sil., sulph., verat.
aversion to - ***kali-a.,*** ***lyc.,*** med., nat-m.

BEEF, aversion to - merc., ptel.
smell of - ptel.

BEER, agg. - acon., act-sp., ***aloe,*** alum., ant-t., ars., asaf., bapt., bell., ***bry.,*** cadm-s., calc-caust., carb-s., card-m., chel., chlol., chin., chlor., coc-c., cocc., coloc., crot-t., euph., ***ferr.,*** fl-ac., ign., ***kali-bi.,*** kali-m., ***led., lyc.,*** merc-c., mez., mur-ac., nux-m., **NUX-V.,** ***puls., rhus-t.,*** sec., sep., ***sil.,*** stann., staph., stram., ***sulph.,*** teucr., ***thuj., verat.***
easily intoxicated - ***chim.,*** coloc., ign., kali-m.
new - ***chin., lyc., puls.***
smell of - ***cham.***
ailments from - kali-bi., rhus-t., thuj.
bad - nux-m.
amel. - aloe, **LOB.,** mur-ac., nat-p., ***verat.***
aversion to - ***alum.,*** alum-p., asaf., atro., **BELL.,** bry., calc., carb-s., ***cham.,*** **CHIN.,** cinch., ***clem.,*** **COCC.,** crot-t., ***cycl., ferr., kali-bi.,*** med., nat-m., ***nat-s.,*** **NUX-V.,** pall., ph-ac., ***phos.,*** puls., ***rhus-t.,*** sang., sep., spig., spong., ***stann., sulph.***
evening - bry., nat-m., sulph.
morning - ***nux-v.***
desires - **ACON.,** agar., aloe, am-c., ant-c., arn., ars., asar., ***bell., bry.,*** calad., calc., camph., carb-s., carc., ***caust.,*** chel., chin., ***cocc.,*** coc-c., ***coloc.,*** cupr., dig., ***graph., kali-bi., lach.,*** mang., ***med., merc.,*** mosch., nat-a., ***nat-c.,*** nat-p., ***nat-m., nat-s.,*** **NUX-V.,** op., ***petr., phel.,*** ph-ac., phos., psor., ***puls., rhus-t., sabad.,*** sep., ***spig.,*** spong., staph., stram., ***stront-c.,*** **SULPH.,** tell., zinc.
afternoon - psor., sulph.

BEER, general
desires, bitter - aloe, cocc., ***kali-bi.,*** nat-m., nux-v., puls.
chill, during - ant-c., ***nux-v.***
colic, after - ph-ac.
evening - coc-c., ***kali-bi.,*** mang., ***med.,*** nux-v., sulph., ***zinc.***
fever, after - puls.
fever, during - acon., nux-v., puls.
forenoon - agar., phos.
morning - ***nux-v.,*** phel., ***puls.***
thirst, with - ***calad.***
thirst, without - ***calad.***

BERI-beri - ars., ***elat.,*** lath., rhus-t.

BERRIES, agg. - ip.

BITTER, drinks, desires - acon., aloe, ***cod.,*** dig., ***nat-m.,*** ter., ther.
bitter, food, ailments from - nat-p.
desires - cod., **DIG.,** graph., ***nat-m.,*** nux-v., sep.

BOILED, aversions - calc.

BRANDY, whisky, agg. - agar., ***ars.,*** ars-m., bell., calc., carb-ac., chel., chin., cocc., fl-ac., hep., hyos., ign., lach., laur., ***led.,*** med., **NUX-V., OP.,** puls., ***ran-b.,*** rhod., ***rhus-t.,*** ruta, spig., ***stram.,*** sul-ac., **SULPH.,** verat., zinc.
ailments from bad - carb-v.
amel. - olnd., sel.
aversion to - ant-t., ***carb-ac.,*** ign., lob., lob-e., ***merc.,*** ph-ac., rhus-t., stram., zinc.
brandy drinkers, in - ***arn.***
desires - acon., ail., arg-n., ars., ars-m., aster., bov., bry., bufo, calc., chin., cic., coca, cub., ferr-p., ***hep.,*** lach., mosch., mur-ac., **NUX-V.,** olnd., **OP.,** ***petr., phos.,*** puls., ***sel., sep., spig., staph.,*** stram., stront-c., ***sulph., sul-ac.,*** ther.

BREAD, agg. - ***ant-c., bar-c.,*** **BRY.,** carb-an., ***caust.,*** chin., cina, clem., coff., crot-h., crot-t., cupr., ***hydr.,*** kali-c., lith., **LYC.,** merc., ***nat-m., nit-ac., nux-v.,*** olnd., ph-ac., phos., **PULS.,** ran-s., ***rhus-t.,*** ruta, ***sars.,*** sec., ***sep.,*** staph., sul-ac., ***sulph.,*** teucr., ***verat., zinc.,*** zinc-p., zing.
black, agg. - bry., ign., ***kali-c., lyc.,*** nat-m., nit-ac., nux-v., ***ph-ac.,*** phos., ***puls.,*** sep., sulph.
butter, and bread, agg., - carb-an., caust., ***chin.,*** crot-t., cycl., meny., nat-m., ***nit-ac.,*** nux-v., phos., plat., **PULS.,** ***sep.,*** sulph.
ailments from - nat-m., zing.
amel. - ***caust.,*** lact., laur., ***nat-c.,*** phos.
aversion to, bread - agar., aphis., calc., chen-a., **CHIN.,** ***con.,*** corn., cur., ***cycl.,*** elaps, ferr-ar., hydr., ign., kali-a., **KALI-C.,** kali-p., kali-s., ***lach.,*** lact., lil-t., ***lyc., mag-c.,*** manc., meny., **NAT-M.,** ***nat-p., nat-s., nit-ac.,*** nux-m., ***nux-v.,*** ol-an., ***ph-ac., phos.,*** **PULS.,** ***rhus-t., sep.,*** **SULPH.,** tarent.
aversion to, during pregnancy - ant-t., ***laur., sep.***
black - nat-m., ph-ac.

BREAD, general
aversion to, bread, brown - ***kali-c., lyc.,*** merc., ***nat-m., nux-v.,*** ph-ac., puls., sulph.
butter and bread - ***cycl.,*** mag-c., meny., nat-p., sang.
rye - lyc., nux-v.
desires - abrot., aloe, am-c., ***ars., aur.,*** bar-m., bell., bov., ***cham.,*** con., ***cina, coloc.,*** cub., ***ferr.,*** ferr-ar., grat., hell., hydr., ign., ***mag-c.,*** merc., nat-a., nat-c., ***nat-m.,*** nit-ac., op., ***plb.,*** puls., sec., sil., staph., ***stront-c.,*** sumb.
boiled, in milk - abrot.
butter, and bread- agar., ***bar-m.,*** bell., ***ferr.,*** grat., hell., hydr., ign., ***mag-c.,*** **MERC.,** ***merc-sul.,*** puls., stront-c.
dry - ***aur., bar-m.***
evening - cast., tell.
only bread - bov., grat.
rye bread - ***ars.,*** carl., ***ign.,*** plb.
white - aur., bar-m.
sensitive to the smell of foul bread - par.

BREAKFAST, agg. - ***agar.,*** ambr., ***am-m.,*** anac., ars., bell., bor., ***bry., calc.,*** carb-an., carb-s., carb-v., ***caust.,*** **CHAM.,** chin., ***con.,*** cycl., ***dig.,*** euph., form., ***graph.,*** hell., ign., ***kali-c., kali-n.,*** laur., lyc., mag-c., mang., ***nat-c., nat-m., nat-s.,*** nit-ac., nux-m., **NUX-V.,** par., petr., ph-ac., **PHOS.,** plb., puls., rhod., rhus-t., sars., ***sep.,*** sil., stront-c., ***sulph., thuj.,*** valer., verat., **ZINC.**
before - alumn., croc.
breakfast, amel. - ***calc., croc.,*** ferr., ***iod.,*** nat-m., ***staph.,*** valer.
after - acon., alum., am-c., ***am-m., ambr.,*** anac., ***bar-c., bov.,*** bry., ***cann-s.,*** canth., ***carb-an.,*** carb-v., caust., ***chel.,*** chin., cina, graph., hell., ***hep., ign., lach., laur., lyc., mez.,*** nat-p., nat-s., **NUX-V.,** ***petr.,*** phos., ***plat., plb., ran-b., rhus-t.,*** zinc-p.

BROTH, bouillon, agg. - graph., mag-c., sil.
aversion to - ***arn., ars.,*** bell., ***cham.,*** **COLCH.,** graph., kali-i., rhus-t., sil.
sensitive to the smell of - **COLCH.**

BUCKWHEAT, agg. - ip., ***phos.,*** **PULS.,** ***sep.,*** verat.

BUTTER, agg. - acon., ant-c., ant-t., ***ars.,*** asaf., bell., carb-an., **CARB-V.,** caust., chin., colch., ***cycl.,*** dros., euph., ***ferr.,*** ferr-ar., hell., hep., ip., mag-m., meny., merc-c., nat-a., nat-c., nat-m., nat-p., nit-ac., nux-v., ***phos., ptel.,*** **PULS.,** ***sep.,*** spong., sulph., ***tarax., tarent.,*** thuj.
ailments from - carb-v.
aversion to - ars., carb-an., carb-v., **CHIN.,** ***cycl.,*** hep., mag-c., meny., ***merc.,*** morg-g., nat-m., petr., ***phos.,*** prot., ***ptel.,*** **PULS.,** sang.
desires - all-s., carc., ferr., ign., mag-c., ***merc.,*** nit-ac., **PULS.**

BUTTERMILK, agg. - bry., puls.
aversion to - ***cina.***
desires - ant-t., chin-s., ***chion.,*** elaps, ***sabad., sabal., thlaspi.***
tastes too sweet - ran-b.

CABBAGE, agg. - ars., **BRY.,** calc., carb-v., ***chin.,*** cupr., erig., hell., kali-c., **LYC.,** ***mag-c.,*** nat-m., ***nat-s.,*** **PETR.,** phos., podo., ***puls.,*** rob., sep., sil., sulph., verat.
ailments from - ***lyc.,*** petr.
aversion to - bry., carb-v., cocc., kali-c., lyc., petr.
desires - acon., ***acon-l.,*** alum., **CIC.,** con.

CAKES, agg. - ant-c., ip., puls.
desires - lyc., plb., puls.
hot agg. - kali-c., puls.

CANDIES, sweets, desires - ***am-c.,*** **ARG-N.,** bar-c., carb-v., **CHIN.,** ***ip.,*** **KALI-C., LYC.,** mag-m., nat-c., ***phos.,*** rheum, rhus-t., sabad., sulph.

CARBONATED, drinks, desires - colch., **PH-AC.,** ***phos.***

CARROTS, agg. - calc., ***lyc.***

CEREALS, aversion to - ars., phos.

CHARCOAL, desires - alum., ***calc., cic.,*** con., ign., nit-ac., nux-v., ***psor.***
desires, in chlorosis - alum.

CHEESE, agg. - arg-n., ars., coloc., nux-v., phos., ptel., sanic., sep., staph.
old, from - ***ars., bry.,*** coloc., hep., nux-v., ph-ac., ***ptel., rhus-t.,*** sanic., ***sep.***
spoiled, from - ars., bry., ph-ac., rhus-t.
ailments from - nit-s-d.
aversion to - ***arg-n., chel.,*** chin., ***cocc.,*** **NIT-AC.,** olnd., ***sil., staph.,*** tub.
gruyere - ***merc.,*** sulph.
old - chin.
roquefort - ***hep.***
strong - ***hep., merc., nit-ac., sulph.***
desires - aeth., ***arg-n.,*** aster., calc., calc-p., caust., ***chel., cist.,*** coll., ign., man., mosch., ***nit-ac., phos.,*** puls., sep.
strong - arg-n., aster., ign.

CHERRIES, agg. - merc-c.
desires - chin.

CHICKEN, agg. - bac., bry.
aversion to - **BAC., NAT-M.,** ***sulph.***
desires - ***ferr-i., graph., phos.***

CHILLI, (green or red) agg. - phos.

CHOCOLATE, agg. - ***arg-n., bor.,*** bry., calad., caust., coca, kali-bi., lil-t., ***lith.,*** **LYC.,** ox-ac., ***puls.***
aversion to - osm., prot., tarent.
desires - **ARG-N.,** ***calc., carc.,*** lepi., ***lyc.,*** lyss., nat-m., **PHOS.,** puls., ***sep., sulph.,*** tarent.

CIDER, agg. - aster., phos.
amel. - bell.
desires - benz., benz-ac., puls., sulph.

CITRIC acid, agg. - nat-p.
desires - puls., verat.

CLOVES, desires - ***alum., chlor.,*** stront-nit.

COAL, desires - ***alum., calc., cic.,*** ign., psor.

COCOA, aversion to - osm., tarent.

COFFEE, agg. - ***aeth.,*** agar., alet., all-c., anac., ars., arum-t., aster., aur-m., bell., bov., bry., ***cact.,*** calc., ***calc-p.,*** cann-i., **CANTH.,** ***caps.,*** carb-v., caul., **CAUST., CHAM.,** chin., cist., clem., ***cocc.,*** coff., colch., coloc., cycl., fl-ac., form., glon., grat., guare., ***hep.,*** **IGN.,** ***ip.,*** kali-bi., kali-c., kali-n., lyc., mag-c., mang., ***merc.,*** nat-m., ***nat-s.,*** nit-ac., **NUX-V.,** ox-ac., ***ph-ac.,*** plat., psor., ***puls.,*** rhus-t., sep., stram., sulph., sul-ac., ***thuj.,*** vinc., xan.

hot - caps.

menopause period, during - **LACH.**

smell of - fl-ac., lach., ***nat-m.,*** osm., sul-ac., tub.

odor of - sul-ac.

ailments from - **CHAM.,** grat., ***ign., nux-v.,*** ox-ac., thuj.

amel. - acon., agar., arg-m., ***ars.,*** brom., cann-i., canth., **CHAM.,** chel., **COLOC.,** eucal., ***euph.,*** euphr., fago., glon., hyos., ***ign.,*** lach., mag-c., mosch., ***nux-v.,*** op., phos., til.

aversion to - ***acon.,*** alum-sil., ***bell., bry.,*** **CALC.,** calc-s., carb-v., ***caust., cham.,*** chel., ***chin.,*** cinnb., coc-c., ***coff.,*** con., ***dulc.,*** fl-ac., kali-bi., kali-br., kali-i., kali-n., lec., lil-t., lol., ***lyc.,*** mag-p., man., ***merc., nat-c., nat-m.,*** **NUX-V.,** osm., ox-ac., ph-ac., ***phos.,*** phys., puls., rheum, rhus-t., sabad., ***spig., sul-ac., sulph.***

morning - lyc.

noon - ox-ac.

smell of - fl-ac., lach., ***nat-m.,*** osm., sul-ac., tub.

sweetened - aur-m.

unsweetened - ***rheum.***

desires - ***alum.,*** **ANG.,** arg-m., arg-n., ***ars.,*** aster., ***aur., bry.,*** calc-p., ***caps., carb-v.,*** carc., cham., chel., ***chin.,*** colch., ***con.,*** gran., lach., lec., lob., ***mez.,*** mosch., nat-m., ***nux-m.,*** **NUX-V.,** ph-ac., sabin., ***sel.,*** sol-t-ae., sulph.

beans of - chin., nux-v., sabin.

dysmenorrhea, in - ***lach.***

nauseates, which - caps.

strong - ***bry.,*** mosch.

COLD, drinks, agg. - ***agar., all-s.,*** allox., ***alum.,*** alum-p., alum-sil., ***alumn.,*** anac., ***ant-c.,*** apis, ***apoc.,*** arg-n., ***ars.,*** ars-s-f., aur-a., ***bell.,*** bell-p., bor., bry., calad., calc., calc-p., calc-sil., camph., **CANTH.,** ***caps.,*** carb-an., ***carb-v.,*** cham., ***chel., chin.,*** clem., ***cocc.,*** coloc., ***con., croc.,*** crot-t., ***dig.,*** dros., dulc., elaps, **FERR.,** ferr-ar., ferr-p., ***graph.,*** grat., hep., hyos., ***ign.,*** kali-ar., kali-c., kali-i., kali-m., kali-p., ***kali-sil., kreos.,*** lach., lept., lob., ***lyc., mag-p.,*** mang., merc., mur-ac., nat-a., ***nat-c.,*** nat-p., ***nux-m., nux-v.,*** op., ***ph-ac.,*** puls., ***rhod.,*** **RHUS-T.,** sabad., sars., **SEP.,** ***sil., spig.,*** spong., squil., staph., stram., ***sulph., sul-ac., tarent., teucr.,*** thuj., verat.

heated, when - bell-p., ***bry., kali-ar., kali-c., nat-c., rhus-t.,*** samb.

hot weather, in - ***bry., kali-c., nat-c.,*** verat.

COLD, drinks, general

amel. - acon., acon-f., all-c., aloe, ***ambr.,*** anac., ***ant-t.,*** apis, arg-n., ars., ***asar.,*** aster., **BISM.,** bor., brom., **BRY.,** calc., cann-s., ***carb-ac.,*** **CAUST.,** cham., ***clem.,*** coc-c., coff., ***cupr., fl-ac.,*** kali-c., laur., meph., ***onos.,*** op., **PHOS.,** phyt., ***puls.,*** sel., **SEP.,** stann., sumb., tab., thuj., trio., verat., xan., zinc., zinc-p.

aversion to - acon., alum-p., ant-t., arn., ***ars.,*** bell., brom., bry., ***calad., calc-ar.,*** canth., carb-an., caust., chel., chin., ***chin-a.,*** dig., elaps, kali-i., lyss., mag-c., ***med.,*** nat-m., ***nat-p.,*** nat-s., nux-v., onos., ***phel.,*** phos., phys., ***stram.,*** tab., ***verat.***

cold water - **BELL.,** brom., bry., ***calad.,*** canth., caust., chel., **CHIN.,** ***chin-a.,*** ham., kali-bi., lyc., ***lyss.,*** nat-m., **NUX-V.,** ox-ac., ***phel.,*** phos., phys., puls., rhus-t., **SABAD.,** ***stram.,*** sulph., tab.

desires - abel., achy., **ACON.,** agar., agar-em., ail., allox., ***alum., alumn.,*** am-c., am-m., ***ang., ant-t.,*** apis, apoc., ***arg-n., arn.,*** **ARS.,** arum-t., asim., asaf., aster., aur., aur-a., aur-s., ***bell., bism.,*** bor., ***bov.,*** **BRY.,** ***calc., calc-ar., calc-s.,*** camph., cann-i., cann-s., ***caps.,*** carb-an., carb-s., **CARC.,** ***caust.,*** cedr., ***cench.,*** **CHAM.,** chel., **CHIN.,** ***chin-a.,*** cimic., **CINA,** cinnb., clem., ***cocc.,*** coc-c., colch., corn., ***croc.,*** cub., ***cupr., cupr-ac.,*** dig., ***dulc., echi.,*** euph., **EUP-PER.,** fl-ac., ***glon., graph., hell., ign.,*** ip., kali-bi., kali-m., kali-n., ***kali-p., kali-s.,*** lap-a., ***led., lyc., lycps.,*** mag-c., mag-p., manc., ***med.,*** **MERC., MERC-C.,** mez., nat-a., ***nat-c., nat-m., nat-p.,*** **NAT-S.,** nux-v., oena., ***olnd.,*** onos., op., ***ph-ac.,*** **PHOS.,** pic-ac., plat., ***plb., podo.,*** polyg., psor., ***puls., rhus-t.,*** ruta, ***sabad.,*** sabin., sac-l., sars., sec., sel., ***sep.,*** sil., spig., spong., squil., stann., sulph., ***tarent.,*** tell., ***thuj.,*** tub., **VERAT.,** vip., zinc.

afternoon - ***croc.***

afternoon, 3 p.m. - caust.

chill, during - bry., carb-v., tub.

evening - oena.

fever, during - bry., phos., tub.

ice, with - med., ***phos., verat.***

night - eup-per.

thirst, without - ars., ***camph.,*** cocc., ***coloc.,*** graph., nux-v., phos.

COLD, food, agg. - acet-ac., acon., agar., alum., alum-p., alum-sil., ***alumn., ant-c., arg-n.,*** **ARS.,** ars-s-f., bar-c., ***bell.,*** bell-p., ***bov.,*** brom., ***bry.,*** calad., calc., calc-f., ***calc-p.,*** calc-sil., canth., caps., ***carb-s., carb-v.,*** caust., cham., chel., chin., ***cocc.,*** coloc., ***con.,*** crot-t., cupr., dig., **DULC.,** elaps, ferr., fl-ac., ***graph.,*** hell., ***hep., hyos.,*** ign., ip., kali-ar., ***kali-bi., kali-c.,*** kali-i., kali-m., ***kali-n.,*** kali-sil., ***kreos.,*** **LACH.,** lept., **LYC.,** mag-c., mag-m., mag-p., manc., ***mang., merc.,*** merc-i-r., mez., mur-ac., nat-a., nat-c., nat-m., nat-p., ***nat-s., nit-ac., nux-m.,*** **NUX-V.,** par., ***ph-ac.,*** plb.,

COLD, food, agg. - ***puls., rhod.,*** **RHUS-T.,** rumx., sabad., samb., ***sep.,*** **SIL.,** ***spig.,*** squil., ***staph.,*** stram., sul-ac., ***sulph., syph.,*** thuj., ***verat.***
amel. - acon., agn., alum., alumn., am-c., ***ambr., anac.,*** ang., ant-t., ***apis,*** arg-n., ars., ***asar., bar-c., bell., bism.,*** bor., brom., **BRY.,** ***calc.,*** cann-s., canth., ***carb-v.,*** **CAUST.,** ***cham.,*** clem., coc-c., ***cupr.,*** dros., ***euph., ferr.,*** graph., hell., ign., ***kali-c.,*** **LACH.,** ***laur.,*** lyc., mag-c., mag-m., ***merc.,*** merc-i-f., ***mez., nat-m., nux-m.,*** nux-v., op., par., ***ph-ac.,*** **PHOS.,** phyt., **PULS.,** pyrog., rad-br., rhod., rhus-t., sang., sars., sel., ***sep.,*** sil., spig., stann., tab., thuj.
aversions - acet-ac., chel., cycl., ***med.***
desires - abel., am-c., ang., ***ant-t.,*** arg-n., ***ars.,*** asaf., bell., bism., ***bry.,*** caust., ***cham.,*** chin., cina, cocc., croc., ***cupr.,*** cupr-ar., euph., ferr-p., fl-ac., ***ign.,*** kali-p., ***kali-s.,*** lach., lept., ***lyc.,*** med., ***merc.,*** merc-c., nat-m., ***nux-v.,*** olnd., **PHOS.,** pic-ac., pip-n., plb., **PULS.,** rhus-t., ruta, sabad., sanic., sars., sec., ***sil., thuj.,*** tub., ven-m., **VERAT.,** zinc.
pregnancy, in - phos., ***verat.***
menses, during, - am-c.

CONDIMENTS, desires (see Spicy) - ant-c., arg-n., ars., calc-p., chel., fl-ac., ***hep.,*** hyper., nat-m., nux-v., phos., puls., sang., staph., sulph., ***zing.***

COOKED, food, agg. - ars., podo.
desires - mag-c.
sensitive to the smell of - ars., chin., **COLCH.,** ***dig., eup-per., sep.,*** stann.

CORN, agg. - chin., kali-c., puls., sulph.

CORNMEAL, agg. - calc-ar.

CUCUMBER, agg. - ***all-c.,*** ars., ***ign., nat-m.,*** puls., ***rhus-t.,*** sul-ac., verat.
aversion to - mag-m., prot.
desires - abies-n., **ANT-C.,** ***phos., sulph., verat.***

DAINTY, foods, agg. - puls.
desires - ***acon-l,*** arg-n., calc.

DELICACIES, desires - aeth., ***aur.,*** bufo, calc., **CHIN.,** cub., cupr., **IP.,** kali-c., mag-c., mag-m., nat-c., petr., psor., ***rhus-t., sabad.,*** sang., ***spong.,*** **TUB.**
aversion to - caust., petr., sang.
desires - acon-l., aeth., ***aur.,*** bufo, calc., **CHIN.,** cub., cupr., cupr-ar., **IP.,** kali-c., mag-c., mag-m., nat-c., paull., petr., psor., ***rhus-t., sabad.,*** sang., ***spong.,*** **TUB.**

DIGESTION, slow - aur-m., berb., ***calc.,*** **CHIN.,** ***corn.,*** corn-f., cycl., eucal., ***lyc.,*** nuph., ***nux-v., op., par., sabin.,*** sanic., ***sep.,*** **SIL., TARENT.**
weak - alst., ***anac., ant-c., arg-n.,*** ars., asaf., bism., ***bry.,*** caps., ***carb-an., carb-v., chin.,*** coch., coff., colch., ***cycl., dios.,*** eucal., gran., ***graph., hydr.,*** ip., kali-bi., **LYC.,** merc., **NAT-C.,** nat-m., **NUX-V.,** prun., ***puls.,*** spong., zing.

DRINKS, aversion to - agar., agn., aloe, ang., ***apis,*** arn., **BELL.,** berb., bor., bov., bry., bufo, calad., calc., camph., **CANTH.,** carb-an., caust., cham., chin., chin-s., chlor., ***cocc.,*** coc-c., coff., colch., coloc., corn., cupr., dros., **FERR.,** graph., ham., hell., **HYOS.,** ***ign., ip.,*** kali-bi., ***lac-c.,*** lach., lyc., ***lyss.,*** mag-aust., merc., ***nat-m., nit-ac.,*** **NUX-V.,** phys., plb., plb-chr., **PULS.,** rat., sabin., samb., sec., staph., **STRAM.,** verat.
children, in - bor., bry.
desires - cob-n., lyc., ***phos.***
but when offered refused - bell.
thirst, without - bell., camph., coloc., wies.

DRY, food agg. - agar., ***alum.,*** bov., calad., **CALC.,** chin., ferr., ign., ip., kali-i., ***lyc., nat-c.,*** nit-ac., nux-v., ox-ac., petr., ph-ac., ***puls.,*** raph., sars., sil., sulph.
aversion to - merc., phos.
desires - ***alum.***
food seems too dry, while eating - calad., chin., ferr., ign., kali-i., ox-ac., raph.

EATING, while, agg. - aloe, alum., ambr., **AM-C.,** am-m., anac., ang., ant-c., ant-t., arg-m., arn., ars., aur., aur-a., aur-s., ***bar-c.,*** bell., bism., ***bor.,*** bov., ***bry., calc.,*** calc-f., calc-sil., cann-s., canth., ***carb-ac.,*** **CARB-AN.,** carb-s., **CARB-V.,** ***caust., cham.,*** chin., ***cic.,*** clem., ***cocc.,*** coff., colch., **CON.,** cycl., dig., dros., dulc., euph., ferr., ***graph.,*** hell., ***hep.,*** ign., iod., kali-bi., **KALI-C.,** kali-n., kali-p., lach., laur., led., ***lyc.,*** mag-c., ***mag-m.,*** mang., merc., mur-ac., ***nat-c., nat-m.,*** **NIT-AC.,** nux-m., nux-v., ***olnd., petr.,*** ph-ac., ***phos.,*** plat., plb., ***puls.,*** ran-b., ran-s., rauw., rhod., rhus-t., ***rumx.,*** ruta, sabin., samb., sars., sec., ***sep.,*** sil., spig., spong., squil., staph., stram., **SULPH.,** sul-ac., tarax., teucr., thuj., valer., verat., verb., zinc.
amel. - aloe, ***alum., alumn., ambr.,*** am-m., **ANAC.,** aq-mar., arn., aur., bar-c., bell., buth-a., cadm-m., cadm-s., calc-p., cann-i., ***caps.,*** carb-an., carb-v., cham., ***chel.,*** chin., cimic., cocc., ***croc.,*** cur., cyn-d., dig., dros., ferr., fl-ac., graph., **IGN.,** iod., **LACH.,** laur., led., lyc., mag-c., mang., med., merc., methys., ***mez.,*** nat-c., nit-ac., nux-v., par., perh., ph-ac., phos., phyt., plat., prot., puls., rheum, rhod., rhus-t., sabad., sabin., ***sep.,*** sil., ***spig.,*** spong., squil., stann., staph., sulph., sul-ac., tarax., ***thlaspi,*** thymol., **ZINC.**
after agg. - abies-n., acon., ***agar.,*** agn., all-c., **ALOE,** alum., ambr., am-c., ***am-m.,*** **ANAC.,** ant-c., ant-t., ***apis,*** apoc., ***arg-n.,*** arn., **ARS.,** ***asaf.,*** asar., aur., ***bar-c., bell., bism.,*** bor., bov., **BRY.,** bufo, cahin., calad., **CALC., CALC-P.,** camph., cann-s., canth., caps., ***carb-an., carb-s., carb-v.,*** **CAUST.,** ***cham., chel., chin.,*** cic., cina, clem., ***cocc., coc-c., cod.,*** colch., **COLOC., CON.,** croc., ***crot-t., cycl.,*** dig., dros., dulc., eup-per., euph., euphr., ***ferr.,*** ferr-ar., ***ferr-i.,*** ferr-p., ***gran., graph.,*** grat., hell., hep., ***hyos.,*** ign., ***indg.,*** iod., ip., ***jug-r.,*** kali-ar., **KALI-BI., KALI-C.,** kali-n.,

EATING, general

after agg. - kali-p., kali-s., kreos., **LACH.,** laur., led., **LYC.,** mag-c., mag-m., mang., merc., ***mez.,*** mosch., mur-ac., nat-a., ***nat-c.,*** **NAT-M.,** nat-s., ***nit-ac.,*** nux-m., **NUX-V.,** olnd., op., ***ox-ac.,*** par., ***petr., ph-ac.,*** **PHOS.,** phyt., plat., plb., ***podo., psor., ptel.,*** **PULS.,** ***ran-b.,*** ran-s., ***rheum,*** rhod., ***rhus-t.,*** **RUMX.,** ruta., sabad., sabin., samb., sang., sars., sec., ***sel., seneg.,*** **SEP., SIL.,** spig., spong., squil., stann., staph., stront-c., **SULPH.,** sul-ac., ***tarax.,*** teucr., ***thuj.,*** tril., ***trom.,*** valer., verat., verb., viol-t., **ZINC.**

after, eating a little, aversions - bar-c., bry., cham., cina, cycl., ign., **LYC.,** nux-v., prun., rheum, rhus-t., ruta., sil., sulph.

breakfast, agg. - ***agar.,*** ambr., ***am-m.,*** anac., ars., bell., bor., ***bry., calc.,*** carb-an., carb-s., carb-v., ***caust.,*** **CHAM.,** chin., ***con.,*** cycl., ***dig.,*** euph., form., ***graph.,*** hell., ign., ***kali-c., kali-n.,*** laur., lyc., mag-c., mang., ***nat-c., nat-m.,*** nit-ac., nux-m., **NUX-V.,** par., petr., ph-ac., **PHOS.,** plb., puls., rhod., rhus-t., sars., ***sep.,*** sil., stront-c., ***sulph., thuj.,*** valer., verat., **ZINC.**

breakfast, amel. - ***calc., croc.,*** ferr., ***iod.,*** nat-m., ***staph.,*** valer.

long after eating - grat., kali-i., kreos., murx., ***phos.,*** **PULS.**

amel. - acet-ac., acon., agar., aloe, alum., alumn., ambr., am-c., am-m., amor-r., ***anac.,*** ang., arn., ars., ars-i., ***aster.,*** bar-c., bar-i., bell-p., ***bov.,*** brom., ***bry.,*** buth-a., cadm-m., cadm-s., calc., calc-i., ***calc-s.,*** cann-i., ***cann-s.,*** caps., carb-an., carb-s., ***caust.,*** cham., **CHEL.,** chin., cimic., cist., con., ***cupr.,*** dicha., dios., euphr., ***ferr.,*** ferr-ac., fl-ac., gamb., ***gels.,*** goss., ***graph.,*** guat., hed., hell., ***hep.,*** hom., ***ign.,*** **IOD.,** kali-bi., kali-br., kali-c., ***kali-p., kali-s.,*** kalm., kreos., lac-ac., lach., ***laur.,*** lith., mag-c., mag-m., mang., meny., merc., mez., mosch., **NAT-C.,** nat-m., ***nat-p.,*** nicc., nux-v., ***onos.,*** ox-ac., paeon., petr., **PHOS.,** pip-n., plan., plat., plb., ***psor., puls.,*** ran-b., rhod., rhus-t., ***sabad.,*** sars., **SEP.,** sil., spig., **SPONG.,** squil., stann., ***stront-c.,*** sul-i., sulph., ***thlaspi,*** verat., zinc., zinc-p.

before, agg. - acon., alum., ***ambr.,*** am-c., am-m., anac., ang., arn., ars., ***ars-i.,*** ars-s-f., bar-c., bell., ***bov.,*** bry., ***calc., cann-s.,*** carb-an., carb-s., carb-v., caust., cham., ***chel., chin., cina,*** colch., ***croc.,*** dulc., euphr., ***ferr.,*** **FL-AC.,** ***graph.,*** hell., hep., ***ign.,*** **IOD.,** kali-c., ***lach.,*** **LAUR.,** mag-c., mang., meny., merc., mez., mosch., **NAT-C.,** ***nat-p.,*** nit-ac., nux-v., olnd., petr., **PHOS.,** ***plb., puls.,*** ran-b., ***rhus-t., sabad.,*** sabin., sars., seneg., sep., sil., spig., squil., stann., staph., ***stront-c., sulph., tarax.,*** teucr., valer., verat., verb.

fast - ars., cina, iod., ***ip.,*** led., ***nux-v.,*** sulph.

EATING, general

overeating, agg. - acon., aeth., alum., **ANT-C.,** ***ant-t.,*** arg-n., ***arn.,*** ars., asaf., bry., calc., carb-v., caust., chin., ***coff.,*** hep., ign., **IP., LYC.,** mag-c., nat-c., nat-p., nux-m., **NUX-V., PULS.,** staph., sulph., tub.

ailments from - all-s., ant-c., bry., dios., nux-m.

children, in - aeth., calc., ***cina,*** iod., nat-p.

refuses, to eat - ars., bell., caust., cocc., croc., grat., **HYOS.,** ***ign.,*** **KALI-CHL.,** kali-p., op., **PH-AC.,** ***phyt.,*** plat., puls., sep., **TARENT., VERAT., VIOL-O.**

amel. mental symptoms - **GOSS.**

satiety, to - bar-c., bar-s., ***calc.,*** carb-v., chin., **LYC.,** nat-c., nat-m., nux-v., phos., **PULS.,** sep., sil., ***sulph.,*** zinc.

amel. - ars., ***iod.,*** med., phos.

small quantity agg., of a - alet., am-c., arg-n., bar-c., bell., **BRY.,** canth., carb-an., ***carb-v., chin., con.,*** crot-t., cycl., ferr., hep., ***ign.,*** kali-bi., ***kali-c.,*** kali-s., led., lil-t., **LYC.,** merc., nat-m., nat-p., **NUX-V.,** petr., **PHOS.,** puls.

amel., of a - guat.

EEL, desires - ***med.***

EGGPLANT, aversions - ***med.,*** sep.

desires - med.

EGGS, agg. - anthr., ***calc.,*** calc-f., chin-a., ***cocc.,*** colch., ***ferr.,*** ferr-m., led., lyc., merc-c., **PULS.,** ***sulph.***

from odor of eggs - anthr., ***colch.***

ailments from bad - carb-v.

aversion to - anthr., bell., calc-f., carc., **COLCH.,** ***ferr.,*** ferr-m., kali-s., morg., nit-ac., ol-an., phos., prot., **PULS.,** saroth., **SULPH.,** syc-co., tub., upa.

boiled- bry.

children, in - phos.

hard boiled - bry., prot.

odor of - ***colch.***

desires - agar., **CALC.,** calc-p., ***carc.,*** caust., hydr., morg., nat-p., ol-an., olnd., prot., ***puls.,*** sanic., sil.

boiled - **CALC.**

boiled, soft - **CALC.,** nat-p., ol-an., olnd., ***puls.***

fried - nat-p., sil.

EVERYTHING, aversion to - acon-l., alum., am-m., bov., caps., cupr., grat., hyos., ***ip.,*** kali-c., lyc., merc., mez., mur-ac., nit-ac., nux-v., plat., ***puls.,*** rheum, rhod., sars., sep., sulph., thea., ther., thuj.

afternoon, 1 p.m. - grat.

daytime - sep.

forenoon - sars.

morning - lyc., plb.

FARINACEOUS, (see Starchy and Wheat)

aversion to - ars., kali-ar., nat-m., ph-ac., phos., plan., ptel.

desires - aeth., ***alum., calc.,*** calc-p., ***ferr-ac.,*** **LACH.,** ***nat-m., sabad., sulph.,*** sumb.

FASTING, while - acon., aloe, alum., am-m., ***ambr.,*** am-c., am-m., anac., ars., ***bar-c.,*** bar-i., bov., ***bry.,*** cact., **CALC.,** calc-i., cann-i., canth., ***carb-ac., carb-an.,*** carb-v., caust., ***chel.,*** chin., cina, ***coc-c.,*** **CROC.,** dios., ferr., ferr-p., ***graph.,*** hell., ***hep.,*** ign., **IOD.,** ***kali-c.,*** kreos., **LACH.,** laur., lyc., mag-c., mag-m., merc., ***mez.,*** nat-c., nat-p., nit-ac., ***nux-v.,*** petr., ***phos.,*** **PLAT., PLB.,** puls., **RAN-B.,** rhus-t., ***rumx., sabad.,*** **SEP.,** ***spig.,*** **STAPH.,** ***sulph.,*** **TAB.,** ***tarax.,*** teucr., ***valer.,*** verat., ***verb.***

agg. - acon., aloe, alum., am-c., am-m., ambr., anac., ars., ***bar-c.,*** bov., bry., cact., **CALC.,** cann-s., canth., carb-ac., carb-an., carb-v., cast., caust., ***chel.,*** chin., cina, coc-c., **CROC.,** dios., ferr., ferr-p., ***fl-ac.,*** gran., graph., hell., hep., ***ign.,*** **IOD.,** ***kali-c.,*** kreos., ***lach., laur.,*** lyc., mag-c., mag-m., merc., mez., ***nat-c.,*** nit-ac., nux-v., petr., ***phos., plat.,*** plb., puls., ***ran-b.,*** ran-s., rhod., rhus-t., ***sabad., sep., spig.,*** **STAPH.,** stront-c., sulph., tab., ***tarax.,*** teucr., valer., verat., ***verb.***

amel. - agar., alum., alum-sil., am-m., ambr., anac., ant-c., arn., ars., asaf., bar-c., bell., bor., ***bry.,*** calc., calc-sil., caps., carb-an., carb-v., ***caust.,*** **CHAM.,** ***chin.,*** cocc., **CON.,** cycl., ***dig.,*** euph., ferr., hell., hep., hyos., ign., iod., ***kali-c.,*** kali-n., kali-p., kali-pic., lach., laur., lyc., mag-c., mang., nat-c., **NAT-M.,** nig-s., ***nux-m.,*** nux-v., par., petr., ***ph-ac.,*** phos., plb., puls., rhod., rhus-t., sabin., sars., sel., sep., ***sil.,*** stann., stront-c., sul-ac., sulph., thuj., valer., verat., ***zinc.***

headache, from - ars-i., caust., ***cist.,*** elaps, ind., iod., ***kali-c.,*** kali-s., ***lyc.,*** nux-v., ***phos.,*** ptel., ran-b., ***sang., sil.,*** spig., ***sulph.,*** thuj., uran.

if hunger is not appeased at once - cact., cist., elaps, ***lyc.,*** phos., ***sang., sulph.***

FAT, agg. - acon., agn., alet., ant-c., ant-t., arg-n., ***ars.,*** ars-s-f., ***asaf.,*** bell., bry., calc., calc-f., carb-an., carb-s., **CARB-V.,** carc., ***caust.,*** chin., ***colch.,*** cupr., **CYCL.,** ***dros.,*** erig., euph., **FERR.,** ***ferr-ar., ferr-m.,*** **GRAPH.,** ham., ***hell.,*** hep., ***ip.,*** jug-r., kali-ar., kali-c., ***kali-chl., kali-m.,*** kali-n., kali-sil., ***lept., lyc.,*** mag-c., ***mag-m.,*** mag-s., meny., merc., merc-c., merc-cy., ***nat-a., nat-c.,*** nat-m., ***nat-p., nit-ac.,*** nux-v., phos., podo., psor., ***ptel.,*** **PULS.,** rob., ruta, ***sep.,*** sil., ***spong.,*** staph., ***sulph.,*** **TARAX., TARENT.,** ***thuj.,*** verat.

infants, in - but-ac., ***puls.***

rancid - ars., carb-v.

amel. - nux-v.

ailments from - ars., carb-v.

aversion to fats and rich food - acon-l., **ANG.,** ***ars.,*** ars-s-f., ***bell., bry., calc., calc-f., carb-an.,*** carb-s., ***carb-v., carc.,*** **CHIN.,** chin-a., ***colch.,*** croc., **CYCL.,** dros., erig., ferr., grat., guare., hell., ***hep., ip.,*** kali-m., lyc., lyss., mag-s., man., meny., ***merc.,*** nat-a., nat-c., ***nat-m.,*** nit-ac., nux-v., **PETR.,** phos., **PTEL., PULS.,** rheum,

FAT, aversion to fats and rich food - rhus-t., sang., sec., ***sep., sulph.,*** tarent., thyr.

desires, fat - arg-n., ars., calc., ***calc-p., carc.,*** hep., ***kali-n., med.,*** **MEZ.,** nat-c., nat-m., **NIT-AC.,** ***nux-v.,*** phos., prot., rad-br., sanic., sil., ***sulph., tub.***

fat and salt - arg-n., med., nit-ac., phos., sulph., tub.

fat and sweets - ***arg-n.,*** ars., ***med.,*** nat-c., nux-v., phos., **SULPH.,** tub.

FISH, agg. - ars., calad., carb-an., carb-v., chin., chin-a., ***fl-ac.,*** kali-c., ***kali-s.,*** lach., lyc., ***medus.,*** nat-s., ***plb., puls., sep.,*** thuj., urt-u.

fried - kali-c.

pickled - calad.

sensitive to the smell of - ***colch.***

shellfish - ***aloe, brom.,*** bry., carb-v., fl-ac., **LYC.,** ***podo., sul-ac., urt-u.***

spoiled - ***all-c.,*** ars., bell., **BERB.,** ***carb-an., carb-v.,*** chin., **COP.,** euph., ***kali-c., lach.,*** lyc., ***plb., puls., pyrog.,*** rhus-t., ter.

amel. - lac-c.

aversion to - carb-v., ***colch.,*** **GRAPH.,** grat., guare., kali-i., nat-m., ***phos.,*** sulph., ***zinc.***

salty - ***phos.***

desires - calc-p., caust., ***kali-i.,*** man., ***med., meny., nat-m.,*** nat-p., ***nit-ac.,*** phos., sul-ac.

fried - nat-p.

salty - ferr-i., nat-m., nat-s.

FLATULENT, food agg. - ars., **BRY.,** calc., carb-v., ***chin.,*** cupr., hell., kali-c., **LYC.,** nat-m., **PETR.,** puls., sep., sil., verat.

FLOUR, aversions - ars., ph-ac., ***phos.***

desires - ***calc.,*** lach., sabad.

FOOD, aversion, to - acet-ac., ***acon.,*** agar., ail., all-c., ***alum.,*** anac., ***ang., ant-c.,*** ant-t., apis, arg-m., ***arg-n.,*** **ARN., ARS.,** ***ars-i., asaf.,*** asar., aur., bapt., ***bar-c., bar-i., bar-m.,*** **BELL.,** bor., **BRY.,** bufo, ***cact.,*** calc., ***canth.,*** caps, ***carb-an.,*** carb-s., cast-eq., caust., cham., chel., **CHIN.,** ***chin-a., chin-s.,*** cimic., cina, cinnb., **COCC.,** coc-c., coff., **COLCH.,** ***coloc.,*** con., crot-c., ***cycl.,*** cupr., ***dig.,*** dios., ***dulc.,*** elaps, eup-per., **FERR.,** ***ferr-ar.,*** ferr-i., ferr-m., ferr-p., gamb., ***glon.,*** graph., ***grat., guai., hell.,*** hep., ***hydr.,*** hyper., ***ign., iod.,*** **IP.,** kali-ar., kali-bi., ***kali-c.,*** kali-i., kali-p., kali-s., lach., ***laur.,*** lepi., **LIL-T.,** lyc., ***mag-c., mag-s.,*** mang., ***merc.,*** merc-c., ***merc-i-f.,*** mez., mosch., ***mur-ac.,*** **NAT-M.,** nat-p., nat-s., **NUX-V.,** ol-an., olnd., ***op.,*** ph-ac., phos., ***pic-ac., plat.,*** plb., ***podo.,*** prun., ptel., **PULS.,** raph., rat., rheum, ***rhus-t., ruta., sabad.,*** sec., senec., **SEP.,** sil., stann., ***staph.,*** stront-c., sul-ac., sulph., ***tarent.,*** thea., thuj., til., ***tub.,*** upa., verat., zinc.

attempting to eat - ant-t., petros., ***sil.***

breakfast - con., lyc., mag-s.

cold - acet-ac., alum-p.1, chel., cycl., kali-i., ***med.,*** phos.

cooked, food - am-c., asar., bell., bov., calc., chel., cupr., ***graph.,*** guare., ign., ***kreos.,*** lach., ***lyc.,*** mag-c., merc., petr., phos., psor., ***sil.,*** verat., zinc., zinc-p.

FOOD, aversion, to
daytime - mag-s.
diarrhea, in chronic - ant-c., ars., chin., nux-m., phos., puls.
dinner, during - carb-an., coc-c., ol-an., verat.
eating a little, after - am-c., ***bar-c.,*** bry., caust., cham., cina, ign., ***lyc., nux-v.,*** prun., ***rheum,*** rhus-t., ruta, sil., ***sulph.***
evening - ars., mag-c., sil.
hot - calc., **CHIN.,** ferr., kali-s., ***merc-c.,*** petr., ***phos.,*** pyrog., sil., verat.
hunger, with - act-sp., ***agar., alum., ars., bar-c.,*** bry., ***carb-s.,*** carb-v., ***chin., chin-s.,*** **COCC.,** ***dulc., hell., hydr., kali-n., lach.,*** **NAT-M.,** nicc., **NUX-V.,** olnd., op., ***phos.,*** psor., ***rhus-t.,*** sabad., ***sil., sulph., sul-ac.,*** tax., ***tub.,*** verb.
morning - con., lyc., mag-s.
noon - bor., verat.
pregnancy, in - ant-t., ***colch.,*** ip., ***laur., nat-m., sep.***
seen, if - ptel., ***sil.,*** squil.
sight of - ail., ***arn.,*** **ARS.,** caust., chin., ***colch.,*** dig., lyc., mang., ***merc-i-f.,*** mosch., nux-v., phos., ***sil.,*** squil., stann.
smell of - ant-c., ***ars.,*** bell., caust., **COCC., COLCH.,** dig., **IP.,** lyc., ***nux-v.,*** phos., ***podo.,*** **SEP.,** sil., stann., sym-r.
solid, food - ang., ***ferr.,*** lyc., merc., ***staph.***
sudden, while eating - ***bar-c., ruta.***
supper, during - sulph.
tastes, food, until he tastes it, then he is ravenous - **LYC.**
thinking of eating, when - arg-m., ***ars.,*** carb-v., **CHIN.,** colch., mag-s., mosch., nux-m., sars., ***sep.,*** zinc., zinc-chr.
thought of - arg-m., ip.
pregnancy, during - sep.
warm - ***alum-p., bell.,*** bov., ***calc., cham.,*** chel., **CHIN.,** ***cupr.,*** ferr., **GRAPH.,** guare., ***ign.,*** kali-s., ***lach., lyc.,*** mag-c., mag-s., merc., ***merc-c.,*** merc-cy., ***nux-v.,*** petr., **PHOS.,** psor., **PULS.,** ***sil., verat.,*** zinc.

FOOD, poisoning - ant-c., **ARS.,** bapt., bry., ***carb-v.,*** chin., ***coloc.,*** crot-h., ***ip.,*** lach., lyc., nat-p., ***nux-v.,*** ph-ac., ***podo.,*** psor., ***puls.,*** pyrog., sul-ac., ***urt-u.,*** zing.
bad, water - ***ars.,*** bapt., zing.
fish, spoiled - ars., ***carb-v.,*** chin., ***puls.***
fruit, acid, sour - ***ant-c., ip.,*** ox-ac., **NAT-P.,** ***ph-ac., psor.***
shellfish, agg. - ***aloe,*** ars., ***brom.,*** bry., fl-ac., **LYC.,** ***podo., sul-ac., urt-u.***
spoiled, fatty, rich - ars., ***carb-v.,*** chin., ***ip.,*** nux-v., **PULS.**
meat, agg. - **ARS.,** ***carb-v.,*** chin., ***crot-h., lach., puls., pyrog.***

FRESH food, desires - sul-ac.

FRIED, desires - plb.
aversion to - adel., mag-s., plb., puls.

FROZEN, agg. - arg-n., ***ars.,*** bry., ***calc-p., carb-v.,*** coloc., dulc., ***ip.,*** psor., **PULS.,** rumx.
amel. - phos., xan.

FROZEN, general
desires - arg-m., eup-per., nat-s., phos.

FRUIT, agg. - acon., ***aloe, ant-c.,*** ant-t., **ARS.,** ars-s-f., aster., ***bor.,*** **BRY.,** calc., ***calc-p., carb-v., caust.,*** **CHIN.,** ***chin-a., cist.,*** colch., **COLOC.,** ***crot-t.,*** cub., elaps, ***ferr.,*** glon., ign., iod., ***ip., iris,*** kali-bi., kreos., lach., lith., ***lyc.,*** mag-c., ***mag-m.,*** merc., merc-c., ***mur-ac., nat-a., nat-c.,*** nat-p., **NAT-S.,** ***olnd.,*** ox-ac., ***ph-ac.,*** phos., ***podo., psor.,*** **PULS.,** rheum, ***rhod., rumx.,*** ruta, samb., ***sel., sep.,*** sul-ac., sulph., tarax., tarent., trom., **VERAT.**
acid, sour - ***ant-c., ip.,*** ox-ac., **NAT-P.,** ***ph-ac., psor.***
canned - podo.
juicy - ant-c., calc., iod., puls., sulph.
sour - ***ant-c.,*** ant-t., cist., ferr., ***ip.,*** mag-c., ox-ac., ***ph-ac.,*** podo., ***psor.,*** sul-ac., ther.
spoiled - act-sp.
unripe - ip., rheum, rob., sul-ac.
ailments from - ars., rhod.
unripe - rheum.
amel. - lach.
sour - lach.
aversion to - aeth., aloe, ***ant-t., ars.,*** bar-c., carb-v., ***carc., caust.,*** **CHIN.,** ferr-m., ***hell.,*** **IGN.,** kali-bi., kali-br., mag-c., **PHOS., PULS.,** ***rumx., sul-ac.***
green - mag-c.
sour - ferr.
desires - ***acon-l.,*** aloe, ***alum.,*** alum-p., alumn., ***ant-t.,*** ars., ars-s-f., asar., calc-s., ***carb-v., carc., chin.,*** cist., cub., gran., guai., hep., ***ign.,*** kali-a., lach., lepi., ***mag-c.,*** mag-s., med., nat-m., paull., **PH-AC.,** phos., puls., staph., ***sul-ac.,*** **VERAT.**
acid - adel., ant-t., ***ars.,*** calc., calc-s., chin., ***cist.,*** cub., ign., lach., ***mag-c.,*** ther., thuj., **VERAT.**
green - calc., calc-s., lepi., ***med.***

GARLIC, agg. - **PHOS.**
smell of, from the - sabad.
aversion to - ***phos.,*** prot., **SABAD.,** ***thuj.***
desires - nat-m.

GRAPES, agg. - chin., ox-ac., verat.

GREEN, things, aversion to - mag-c.

GRUEL, agg. - chin., kali-c., puls., sulph.
aversion to - ars., ***calc.***
desires - bell.

GUAVA, agg. - sep.

HAM, aversion to - puls.
desires - ***calc-p.,*** mez., uran-n.
fat - calc-p., ***carc., mez.,*** nit-ac., ***sanic., tub.***
raw - uran-n.
rind - calc-p.

HEARTY food, desires - calc., rhus-t., ust.

HEAVY, food, agg. - bry., calc., ***caust.,*** cupr., **IOD.,** ***lyc.,*** mag-c., nat-c., **PULS.,** sulph.

HERRING, agg. - ferr-p., fl-ac., lyc., nat-m.
aversion to - phos.
desires - cist., **NIT-AC.,** ***puls., verat.***

HONEY, agg. - nat-c., nat-m., phos., ***sil.***
aversion to - nat-c., ***nat-m.***
desires - ***sabad.,*** verat.

HOT, drinks, agg. - am-c., ambr., anac., ant-t., apis, asar., ***bar-c., bell.,*** **BRY.,** calc., ***carb-v.,*** caust., ***cham.,*** chion., cupr., euph., ferr., graph., hell., ill., kali-c., ***lach.,*** laur., ***merc-i-f., mez.,*** oena., ***ph-ac.,*** **PHOS.,** ***phyt.,*** **PULS.,** pyrog., sep., stann., sul-ac.
amel. - ail., ars., chel., lyc., nux-v., sul-ac.
aversion to - caust., cham., chin., ferr., graph., ***kali-s., lyc.,*** mang., oena., ptel., ***puls.***
thirst, with - hell.

HOT, food, agg. - acon., alum-sil., alumn., ***am-c., ambr., anac.,*** ang., ***ant-t.,*** apis, ars., arum-t., ***asar., bar-c., bell.,*** bor., ***bry., calc.,*** canth., caps., carb-v., ***caust., cham.,*** chin., chlol., clem., coff., ***cupr., euph.,*** ferr., graph., ***hell.,*** kali-c., ***lach., laur.,*** mag-c., mag-m., ***merc., mez.,*** nat-m., ***nat-s.,*** phyt., ***puls., sep.,*** tub.
amel. - agar., alumn., ant-c., **ARS.,** bar-c., bell., bov., bry., calc., canth., carb-v., caust., cham., chel., ***con., graph., kreos.,*** **LYC.,** mag-c., mag-m., ***mang., mez., mur-ac., nat-m.,*** nit-ac., ***nux-m.,*** **NUX-V.,** par., ph-ac., ***plb.,*** puls., **RHUS-T.,** sep., ***sil., spig.,*** sul-ac., ***sulph.,*** thuj., ***verat.***
aversion to - **CHIN.,** ferr., kali-s., ***merc-c.,*** petr.
desires - ang., ars., chel., cupr., cycl., ***ferr.,*** **LYC.,** ph-ac., ***sabad.***

HUNGER, ailments from - ***alum., aur., cact.,*** calc-f., canth., ***caust.,*** **CROT-H.,** ***crot-t.,*** ferr., **GRAPH.,** hell., **IOD., KALI-C.,** olnd., ***phos.,*** plat., ***psor.,*** rhus-t., sep., **SIL.,** ***spig.,*** stann., **SULPH.,** tub., valer., verat., ***zinc.***
hunger, agg. - ***anac.,*** ars-i., chel., cina, ***graph.,*** iod., ***kali-c.,*** lyc., olnd., phos., ***sil.,*** spig., staph., ***sulph.***

HYPOGLYCEMIA, hunger, agg. (see Fasting) - ***alum., aur., cact.,*** canth., ***caust., cina., crot-t.,*** ferr., **GRAPH.,** hell., **IOD., KALI-C., LYC.,** olnd., **PHOS.,** plat., ***psor.,*** rhus-t., **SIL.,** ***spig.,*** stann., **SULPH.,** valer., verat., ***zinc.***
headaches, if hunger is not appeased at once - cact., cist., elaps, ***lyc., phos., sang., sulph.***
weakness, from not eating - ***alum.,*** **IOD., PHOS.,** spig., **SULPH.,** ***zinc.***

ICE, agg. - arg-n., **ARS.,** bell., bell-p., ***bry.,*** calc-p., **CARB-V.,** dulc., hep., ip., kali-bi., kali-c., ***nux-v., puls.,*** rhus-t., rob.
ailments from ices - arg-n., ars., bell-p., carb-v., puls.
ice-water, from - ***bell-p.,*** carb-v., rhus-t.
desires - arg-m., arg-n., ***ars., calc., elaps,*** eup-per., lept., **MED.,** merc-c., merc-i-f., nat-s., paro-i., **PHOS.,** sil., **VERAT.**

ICE cream, agg. - arg-n., ars., kali-ar., ***puls.***
ailments from - ***puls.***
aversion to - carc., rad-br.
desires - arg-n., ***calc.,*** carc., ***eup-per., med.,*** **PHOS.,** ***puls., sil.,*** tub., verat.

INDIGESTIBLE, things, agg. - bry., calc., caust., cupr., **IOD.,** ip., lyc., nat-c., ***puls.,*** ruta, sulph.
ailments from - ip.
amel. - ign.
desires - abies-c., ***alum.,*** alumn., ***aur.,*** bell., bry., **CALC.,** ***calc-p.,*** cic., con., cycl., ferr., ign., **LACH.,** nat-m., **NIT-AC.,** ***nux-v.,*** psor., **SIL.,** ***tarent.***

INDISTINCT, knows not what desires - arn., **BRY.,** cham., chin., hep., **IGN.,** ip., kreos., ***lach., mag-m.,*** phos., **PULS.,** sang., sil., ***staph., sulph., ther.***

INVIGORATING things, desires - ph-ac., puls., sulph.

JUICY, things, desires - aloe, ***ant-t.,*** ars., chin., gran., graph., mag-c., med., nat-a., nux-v., phos., **PH-AC.,** puls., sabad., ***sabin.,*** sars., staph., verat.

LARD, desires, (see Fat) - ars., nit-ac.

LEMONADE, agg. - calc., phyt., ***sel.***
ailments from - sel.
amel. - ***bell.,*** cycl., phyt., **PTEL.**
desires - ***am-m.,*** **BELL.,** calc., cycl., eup-per., eup-pur., fl-ac., ***jatr.,*** lach., ***nit-ac.,*** puls., sabad., ***sabin.,*** sec., **SEP.,** sul-ac., ***sul-i.,*** xan.

LEMONS, amel. - bell., stram.
desires - ars., **BELL.,** benz., benz-ac., ***merc.,*** nabal., nat-m., puls., ***sabad.,*** **SEP.,** sul-ac., ***tarent.,*** verat.
peel agg. - ip.

LENTILS, aversions - chel.

LIMES, desires - **ALUM.,** ***alumn., calc.,*** calc-p., chel., cic., con., ferr., hep., hyos., ign., nat-m., **NIT-AC.,** ***nux-v.,*** oci., psor., sil., sulph., ***tarent.***

LIQUIDS, agg. - **ARS.,** ***chin., cocc.,*** coloc., crot-t., ferr., ign., ***lach., nat-m.,*** **PHOS.,** ***rhus-t., sil.,*** verat.
aversion to - bell., graph., hyos., nux-v.
desires - ***ang.,*** bell., bry., ***calc-ac.,*** caps., ***ferr., kali-i., merc.,*** nat-m., ph-ac., ***staph., sulph.,*** verat.

LIQUOR, agg. - ant-c., ars., bell., bov., ***cann-i., carb-v.,*** cimic., led., ***ran-b.,*** rhod., rhus-t., sel., sulph., verat.
desires - med.

LOATHING, of food - absin., acon., act-sp., ***alet.,*** alum., alumn., am-c., anac., **ANT-C.,** ***ant-t.,*** arg-m., ***arg-n., arn.,*** **ARS.,** ***ars-i.,*** asaf., asar., bar-c., bar-i., bar-m., **BELL.,** bor., ***bry.,*** calc., ***canth.,*** carb-s., ***carb-v.,*** caust., ***cham.,*** chel., **CHIN.,** ***chin-s.,*** **COCC., COLCH.,** con., crot-t., cupr., cycl., dig., dios., ***dulc.,*** euph., ***ferr.,*** ferr-i., ***gamb., grat., guai.,*** hell., ***hydr.,*** hyos., ign., iod., **IP., KALI-AR.,** kali-bi., ***kali-br.,*** **KALI-C.,** kali-i., kali-p., kali-s., ***kreos.,*** lach., ***laur.,*** lyc., ***mag-c.,*** mag-m., mag-s., mang., meny., ***merc.,***

LOATHING, of food - merc-i-f., mosch., ***mur-ac.,*** nat-a., nat-c., nat-m., ***nux-v., ol-an.,*** op., petr., phel., ***phos., plat.,*** plb., ***prun.,*** psor., ***puls.,*** rat., rheum, rhod., rhus-t., ruta., ***sabad.,*** sars., ***sec.,*** seneg., **SEP.,** ***sil.,*** spig., stann., stram., ***sulph., sul-ac.,*** sumb., tab., tarent., thuj., valer.
alternating with hunger - berb.
beer, after - mur-ac., nux-v.
bite, first, after - caust., cycl., lyc., plat., prun., rheum
convalescence, during - kreos.
diarrhea, chronic, in - ant-c., ars., chin., nux-m., phos., puls.
eat, on attempting to - ant-t., nux-m., petros., ***sil.***
eating, after - alum., cycl., ***ip.,*** kali-c., ol-an., sars.
emotions, after - ***kali-c.***
evening - alumn., ***hep.,*** raph.
intermittent fever, during - ***kali-c.***
morning on waking - phyt.
night - rat.
noon - pic-ac.
pain, during - aloe.
pregnancy, during - colch., ***ip., laur., sep.***
sadness, from - plat.
sudden, while eating - ***bar-c.***
thought of, at the - carb-v.

MANY, things, desires - ***carc,*** **CINA,** kreos., phos.

MAPLE, sugar agg. - calc-s.

MARINADE, desires - ars., aster., ***cist., fl-ac., hep., lac-c.,*** nat-p., ph-ac., ***sang.***

MEAT, agg. - all-s., arg-n., ***ars.,*** bor., ***bry., calc.,*** carb-an., carb-v., caust., ***chin., colch.,*** cupr., ***ferr.,*** ferr-ac., ferr-i., ferr-p., graph., ***kali-bi., kali-c.,*** kreos., lept., lyc., ***lyss.,*** mag-c., mag-m., med., merc., nat-m., nux-v., ***ptel., puls.,*** ruta, sel., sep., sil., staph., sulph., ter., ther., verat.
fresh - ars., ***caust., chin.,*** kali-c.
odor of cooking - ars., colch., sep.
pickled - carb-v.
spoiled - absin., acet-ac., all-c., **ARS.,** bell., bry., camph., carb-an., ***carb-v.,*** chin., ***crot-h., cupr-ar.,*** kreos., ***lach.,*** ph-ac., ***puls., pyrog.,*** rhus-t., urt-u., ***verat.,*** vip.
amel. - lat-m., ***verat.***
aversion to - abies-c., agar., aloe, ***alum.,*** alumn., am-c., am-m., ***ang.,*** aphis., ***arn., ars.,*** asar., aster., ***aur.,*** bell., bor., ***bry., cact.,*** **CALC.,** calc-f., **CALC-S.,** ***cann-s.,*** **CARB-S.,** ***carb-v.,*** card-m., caust., cham., chel., chen-a., **CHIN.,** ***chin-a.,*** cinch., ***coc-c.,*** **COLCH.,** crot-c., crot-h., ***cycl., elaps, ferr., ferr-ar.,*** ferr-i., ***ferr-m.,*** ferr-p., **GRAPH.,** hell., hydr., ***ign., kali-ar., kali-bi., kali-c.,*** kali-p., kali-s., kreos., lachn., lact., ***lap-a.,*** lepi., ***lyc., mag-c.,*** **MAG-M.,** mag-s., manc., meny., ***merc., mez.,*** morph., **MUR-AC.,** nat-a., nat-c., ***nat-m.,*** nat-p., nat-s., nicc., ***nit-ac.,*** **NUX-V.,** ol-an., olnd., op., **PETR.,** ***phos.,*** plan., ***plat., ptel.,*** **PULS.,** rad-br., ***rhus-t.,*** ruta., ***sabad.,*** sec., **SEP.,** sel., **SIL.,** stront-c., **SULPH.,** sumb., ***syph., tarent.,*** tep., ter., thuj., til.,

MEAT, general
aversion to - ***tub.,*** upa., uran-n., x-ray, ***zinc.***
beef - crot-c., merc.
boiled - ars., calc., chel., nit-ac.
dinner, during - nat-c.
evening - sulph.
fat - ***carb-v.,*** hell., nat-m., phos.
fresh - ***thuj.***
liver - nat-m., sulph.
menses, during - plat.
mutton - calc., mag-c., ov.
noon - ol-an., olnd., sulph.
pickled - carb-v.
pork - ang., **COLCH.,** ***dros., psor.,*** **PULS.,** sep.
roast - ***ptel.,*** tarent.
salted - card-m.
scrap - mag-c.
smell of - ars.
soup - arn., cham., rhus-t.
spicy - mag-c.
thinking of it, while - **GRAPH.**
veal - merc., phel., ***zinc.***
desires - abies-c., aloe, anth., aur., aur-m-n., bell-p., ***bry., calc., calc-p.,*** canth., caust., coca, cocc., cycl., erig., ferr., ***ferr-m.,*** graph., hell., hydr., iod., ***kreos., lil-t.,*** **MAG-C.,** man., med., ***meny.,*** merc., morph., nat-m., nit-ac., ***nux-v.,*** sabad., sanic., ***staph., sulph.,*** thiop., tub., viol-o.
boiled - caust.
children, in - mag-c.
lean - hell.
must have - ***calc., nux-v., staph., sulph.***
pickled - abies-c., ant-c., cori-r., hyper., ***mag-c.***
pork - ***calc-p.,*** **CROT-H.,** ***mez.,*** nit-ac., nux-v., rad-br., ***tub.***
raw - ***phos.***
smoked - ***calc-p.,*** carc., **CAUST.,** kreos., **TUB.**
supper, at - graph.

MELONS, agg. - ars., fl-ac., puls., ***zing.***
ailments from - zing.
aversion to - ***ars., chin.,*** verat., zing.
desires, melons - puls.

MILK, agg. - acon., **AETH.,** ***alum.,*** alum-p., alum-sil., alumn., ***ambr., ang., ant-c.,*** ant-t., ***arg-m., ars.,*** ars-s-f., brom., ***bry.,*** **CALC., CALC-S.,** carb-an., carb-s., ***carb-v., cham., chel.,*** **CHIN.,** ***cic.,*** **CON.,** crot-t., ***cupr.,*** ferr., hell., hom., ign., ***iris,*** kali-ar., kali-bi., ***kali-c., kali-i.,*** kali-n., kali-p., kali-sil., lac-c., lach., **LAC-D.,** lact., ***lyc., mag-c.,*** **MAG-M.,** merc., ***nat-a.,*** **NAT-C.,** ***nat-m., nat-p., nat-s., nicc.,*** **NIT-AC.,** nux-m., ***nux-v., ol-j., phos.,*** podo., ***psor., puls.,*** rheum, rhus-t., sabin., samb., **SEP.,** sil., spong., **STAPH.,** stram., **SULPH.,** sul-ac., valer., ***zinc.,*** zinc-p.
boiled - nux-m., sep.
buttermilk - puls.
cold - calc-sil., carc., kali-i., spong.
hot - bry.
mother's - aeth., ***cina,*** nat-c., **SIL.**

MILK, general
agg., sour - podo.
warm - ***ambr.***
ailments from - ***aeth.,*** hom., lac-d., mag-c., ***nat-c.,*** nat-p., nux-m.
boiled - sep.
cold - calc-sil., kali-i.
amel. - acon., ant-c., ***apis, ars., chel.,*** cina, crot-t., ferr., graph., iod., lact., merc., mez., ***nux-v.,*** ph-ac., rhus-t., ruta, squil., staph., verat.
hot - ***crot-t.***
sweet - ars.
warm - ars., calc., ***chel.,*** crot-t., graph.
aversion to - acon-l., **AETH.,** alum-p., am-c., ammc., ***ant-t., arn.,*** ars., bell., bov., ***bry., cact.,*** calad., ***calc., calc-s.,*** calc-sil., carb-s., ***carb-v., carc.,*** chin., ***cina,*** con., convo-s., elaps, ferr., ferr-p., ***guai.,*** guare., ***ign.,*** iod., kali-i., **LAC-D.,** lach., ***lec.,*** mag-c., ***mag-m.,*** merc., ***mez.,*** **NAT-C.,** ***nat-m.,*** nat-p., ***nat-s.,*** nicot., nit-ac., nux-m., nux-v., ol-j., past., pers., ***phos.,*** podo., ***puls.,*** rheum, rhus-t., ***sep., sil.,*** stann., **STAPH.,** sul-ac., ***sulph.,*** tub.
boiled - ***phos.***
but relishes it - bry.
cold - ph-ac., tub.
morning - puls.
mother's (see Breast, chapter) - ant-c., ant-t., ***bor., calc.,*** **CALC-P.,** cham., ***cina,*** lach., ***merc.,*** nat-c., rheum, **SIL.,** stann., stram.
mother's, child refuses - **CALC-P., SIL.**
smell of - bell.
yogurt, sour milk - ***nat-s.***
desires - anac., ***apis,*** aran., ***ars.,*** asar., ***aur.,*** aur-a., aur-s., bapt., bor., bov., ***bry., calc.,*** calc-sil., ***carc., chel., elaps,*** kali-i., ***lac-c.,*** ach., lact., ***lycps.,*** mag-c., mang., ***merc., nat-m., nux-v., phel., ph-ac., phos.,*** **RHUS-T., SABAD.,** sabal., sabin., sanic., ***sil., staph., stront-c.,*** sulph., **TUB.,** ***verat., vip.***
boiled - abrot., nat-s.
cold - adlu., ***apis,*** calc., calc-p., phel., ***ph-ac., phos., rhus-t.,*** sabad., sanic., staph., **TUB.**
hot - ***calc.,*** chel., graph., hyper.
sour - ant-t., man., mang., nat-s.
warm - calc., chel., ***bry.***
sensitive, to the smell of foul - par.

MIXED, agg. - ant-c., ip., **LYC.,** ***puls.,*** sil.

MUSHROOMS, aversion to - lyc., nat-m., nat-s.
poisoning from - ***absin.,*** agar., ***ars.,*** atro., ***bell.,*** camph., pyrog.

MUSTARD, desires - ars., bac., cic., ***cocc.,*** colch., hep., ***lac-c.,*** mez., mill., nicc.

MUTTON, agg. - bor., lyss., ov.

NUTS, desires - cub.

OIL, agg. - bry., ***canth., meny., nat-m.,*** **PULS.**
aversion to - ***meny., nat-m., puls.***

OLIVE, oil agg. - ***nat-m., sulph.***
aversion to - **ARS.,** nat-m., puls.
desires - **ARS.,** calc., **LYC.,** sulph.

OLIVES, aversion to - **SULPH.**
desires - ars., calc., **LYC.,** sulph.

ONIONS, agg. - alum., alumn., brom., carb-v., ***ign.,*** kali-p., **LYC.,** murx., nat-m., nux-v., ornithog., phos., ***puls.,*** sep., ***sulph.,*** **THUJ.**
ailments from - thuj.
amel. - all-c.
aversion to - brom., **LYC.,** nit-ac., op., ***phos.,*** prot., ***sabad.,*** sep., **THUJ.**
desires, raw - ***all-c.,*** all-s., bell-p., cop., cub., med., ***sabad.,*** staph., ***thuj.***

ORANGES, agg. - nat-p., **OLND.,** ph-ac.
aversion to - elaps.
desires - cub., elaps, **MED.,** olnd., sol-t-ae., ther.

OYSTERS, agg. - ***aloe, brom.,*** bry., carb-v., ***coloc.,*** **LYC.,** ***podo., puls., sul-ac.***
amel. - lach.
aversion to - acon., calc., lyc., med., **NAT-M.,** ***phos.,*** sep.
desires - apis, brom., ***bry., calc.,*** **LACH.,** ***lyc.,*** **LYCPS.,** ***nat-m.,*** phos., ***rhus-t., sulph.***

PANCAKES, agg. - ant-c., ***bry.,*** ip., ***kali-c.,*** **PULS.,** verat.

PAPER, desires - lac-f.

PASTRY, agg. - **ANT-C.,** arg-n., ars., ***bry.,*** carb-v., cycl., ip., ***kali-c., kali-chl.,*** kali-m., ***lyc.,*** nat-s., ***phos.,*** ptel., **PULS.,** sulph., sumb., ***verat.***
ailments from - puls.
aversion to, pastry - ***ars.,*** lyc., ***phos., ptel., puls.,*** sumb.
desires - bufo, ***calc.,*** chin., lyc., mag-m., merc-i-f., plb., ***puls.,*** sabad., sulph.

PEACHES, agg. - all-c., ***fl-ac.,*** glon., psor., verat.
sensitive to the smell of - all-c.

PEANUT butter, desires - ***puls.***

PEARS, agg. - bor., bry., merc-c., nat-c., puls-n, ***verat.***

PEAS, aversion to - med.

PEPPER, agg. - alum., ars., ***chin., cina,*** nat-c., ***nux-v.,*** sep., sil.
agg., cayenne - phos.
desires - **CAPS.,** ***lac-c., nat-m.,*** nux-v.
black - ***lac-c., nat-m.,*** nux-v.
cayenne - merc-c.

PICKLES, agg. - apis, ars., nat-m., sul-ac., verat.
aversion to - abies-c., arund.
desires - abies-c., alum., am-m., ***ant-c.,*** arn., ars., carb-an., chel., cod., ham., hep., hyper., ign., kali-bi., ***lach.,*** lact., mag-c., ***myric.,*** nat-a., sec., **SEP.,** ***sulph., sul-i.,*** verat.

PINEAPPLES, aversion to - tub.

PLANTAINS, agg. - rumx.

PLUMS, agg. - mag-c., ***merc.,*** puls., rheum
ailments from - rheum
aversion to - bar-c., elaps, sul-ac.
desires - sul-ac.
sauce - arg-n.

PORK, agg. - acon., acon-l., ***ant-c.,*** ant-t., ars., asaf., bell., **CARB-V.,** caust., clem., ***colch.,*** **CYCL.,** dros., **GRAPH.,** ham., ***ip., nat-a., nat-c., nat-m.,*** **PULS., SEP.,** tarax., tarent., thuj.
smell of - ***colch.***
ailments from - puls., sep.
amel. - mag-c., nat-m., ran-b., ran-s.
aversion to - ang., ***colch., dros.,*** prot., ***psor.,*** **PULS.,** sep.
desires - ***crot-h.,*** rad-br., ***tub.***

POTATOES, agg. - **ALUM.,** alum-p., ***alumn.,*** am-c., am-m., ***bry.,*** calc., ***coloc.,*** gran., mag-c., mag-s., merc-c., merc-cy., ***nat-c.,*** nat-s., ***puls., sep., sil., sulph., verat.***
sweet - calc-ar.
amel. - acet-ac.
aversion to - alum., alum-p., camph., ***phos.,*** sep., thuj.
desires - alum., calc-p., carc., hep., med., nat-c., ol-an., olnd., tub.
raw - calc., carc., cic.

POULTRY, ailments from - carb-v.

POULET - ***bac.***

PUDDINGS, agg. - ptel.
aversion to - ars., calc., ***phos., ptel.***
desires - puls., sabad.

PUNGENT, things aversion to - ***fl-ac.,*** sang.
desires - acon., ars., aster., caps., caust., chin., ***cist., fl-ac., hep., lac-c.,*** nat-p., nit-ac., nux-v., ph-ac., phos., puls., ***sang.,*** sep., stry., sulph.

RADISHES, desires - abies-c., sabad.

RAGS, clean, desires - alum., alumn.

RAISINS, agg. - ip.

RAW, food, agg. - ars., bry., chin., lyc., ***puls.,*** **RUTA,** sulph., ***verat.***
amel. - ign.
aversion to, raw food or salads - lyc., ***mag-c.,*** prot.
desires - ***abies-c.,*** ail., all-c., alum., ant-c., calc., cub., ign., ***lycps.,*** **SIL., SULPH.,** tarent.
ham - ***uran.***
potatoes - ***calc.***

REFRESHING things, aversion to - ***fl-ac.,*** phos., rheum, sang.
desires - allox., aloe, ant-t., ***ars., calc.,*** calc-f., ***calc-p.,*** calc-s., carb-an., ***caust., chin., cist., cocc., fl-ac.,*** hep., iod., mag-s., nat-a., **PH-AC.,** ***phos., puls.,*** rheum, ***sabin.,*** sang., sars., sel., thuj., til., ***tub., valer.,*** **VERAT.**

RICE agg. - all-c., ars., bry., ***calc.,*** caps., carb-v., ip., kali-m., lach., lyc., nat-s., nit-ac., nux-v., ***puls.,*** sep., sulph.
ailments from - kali-m.

RICE, desires - phos., ***staph.***
desires, dry - ***alum.,*** man., ***phos., staph.,*** ter., ter., ther.

RICH, agg. - ant-c., arg-n., ***bry.,*** carb-an., **CARB-V.,** cycl., dros., ferr., **IP.,** kali-chl., nat-m., ***nat-s., nit-ac.,*** phos., **PULS.,** ***sep.,*** staph., tarax., thuj.

ROLLS, stale - aur.
desires, sweet - aur., lyc., puls.

SALAD, agg. - all-c., ars., bry., ***calc.,*** caps., carb-v., ip., lach., lyc., nux-v., ***puls.,*** sulph.
desires - elaps, lepi., lycps., mag-s.

SALMON, agg. - fl-ac.

SALT, agg. - ***alumn.,*** ars., bell., calc., ***carb-v.,*** coca, ***dros.,*** lyc., mag-m., **NAT-M.,** nit-s-d., nux-v., **PHOS.,** puls., ***sel.,*** sil.
ailments from - carb-v., nat-m., nit-s-d., phos., sel.
sight of - sil.
amel. - mag-c., nat-m.
aversion to - acet-ac., allox., arund., bufo, ***carb-v., carc.,*** card-m., chin., clem., ***con.,*** **COR-R.,** cortico., dros., elaps, ***fl-ac.,*** **GRAPH.,** lyc., lyss., ***merc., nat-m.,*** nit-ac., phos., puls., ***sel., sep.,*** sil.
desires - acet-ac., aeth., ***aloe,*** aq-mar., **ARG-N.,** atro., aur-m-n., ***bac., calc.,*** calc-f., ***calc-p.,*** calc-s., **CARB-V.,** ***carc., caust., chin.,*** cocc., ***con., cor-r.,*** dys-co., **LAC-C.,** ***lycps., lyss., manc., med., meph.,*** merc., merc-i-f., merc-i-r., morg., **NAT-M., NIT-AC.,** ***ph-ac.,*** **PHOS.,** ***plb.,*** prot., ***sanic.,*** scarl., sel., sil., staph., sulph., ***tarent.,*** teucr., ***thuj., tub.,*** uva., **VERAT.**
pregnancy, during - ***nat-m., verat.***
salt and sweets - **ARG-N.,** ***calc.,*** calc-p., calc-s., carb-v., ***med.,*** nat-m., ***phos.,*** plb., sulph., tub.

SAND, desires - sil., **TARENT.**

SARDINES, agg. - fl-ac., ***lyc.***
desires - ***cycl., verat.***

SAUCES, with the food, desires - arg-n., nux-v.

SAUERKRAUT, agg. - ars., **BRY.,** ***calc.,*** carb-v., ***chin.,*** cupr., hell., **LYC.,** nat-m., **PETR.,** ***phos., puls.,*** sep., verat.
aversion to - hell., sulph.
desires - carb-an., cham., ***lycps., nat-m.***

SAUSAGES, agg. - acet-ac., ***ars.,*** bell., bry., puls.
ailments from - bell.
aversion to - ***ars.,*** puls.
desires, sausages - acet-ac., calc-p.
spoiled, agg. - **ARS., BELL.,** ***bry.,*** ph-ac., rhus-t.

SHELL-fish agg. - bell., carb-v., ***coloc.,*** cop., euph., levo., ***lyc.,*** phenob., rhus-t., ter., ***urt-u.***

SIGHT of food, agg. - ant-t., **COLCH.,** ***kali-bi.,*** kali-c., ***lyc.,*** merc-i-f., mosch., ph-ac., sabad., ***sil.,*** spig., squil., **SULPH.,** xan.

SLIMY food, aversion to - ***calc.,*** med., **NAT-M.**

SMELL of food, agg. - ***ars.,*** bell., ***cocc.,*** **COLCH.,** ***dig.,*** dros., eup-per., **IP.,** lach., merc-i-f., nat-m., nux-m., nux-v., osm., ph-ac., phos., podo., ptel., sang., **SEP.,** ***sil.,*** stann., sul-ac., sulph., ***thuj.,*** xan.
sensitive to smell, of - arg-n., **ARS.,** ***cocc.,*** **COLCH.,** eup-per., ***ip.,*** lach., **SEP.,** stann.

SMOKED, food agg. - ***calc., sil.***
desires, things - calc-p., carc., **CAUST.,** ***kreos.,*** puls.

SNOW, desires - crot-c.

SNUFF, aversion to - spig.
desires - ***bell.***

SOFT, food desires - alumn., pyrus, sulph.

SOLID food, aversion to - ether, ang., bell., bry., coca, ***ferr.,*** lyc., merc., ***staph.,*** sulph.

SOUP, agg. - alum., alumn., chin., kali-c., staph.
aversion to - ***arn.,*** ars., bell., carb-v., cham., chin., ***graph.,*** kali-c., kali-chl., kali-i., lyc., merc-cy., nat-m., ol-an., puls., ***rhus-t.,*** staph.
desires - ang., ars., bry., ***calc-ar., carc., ferr.,*** kali-chl., merc., nat-m., ol-an., ***staph., sulph.***

SOUR, acids, agg. - **ACON.,** aloe, **ANT-C.,** ant-t., apis, ***arg-n., ars.,*** ars-s-f., aster., ***bell.,*** bor., brom., calad., calc., **CARB-V.,** caust., chin., cimic., cub., dros., ***ferr.,*** ferr-ar., ferr-m., ferr-p., fl-ac., ip., ***kali-bi.,*** kreos., lach., merc-c., merc-cy., merc-d., nat-c., nat-m., **NAT-P.,** nux-v., ox-ac., ph-ac., phos., podo., ***psor., puls.,*** ran-b., ***rhus-t.,*** sel., ***sep., staph.,*** sul-ac., ***sulph.,*** thuj.
and amel. - ***merc., ptel.***
odors - dros.
ailments, from - nat-m., ***nat-p.***
amel. - arg-m., arg-n., ign., lach., ***merc.,*** naja, **PTEL.,** puls., sang.
aversion to - abies-c., arund., ***bell.,*** chin., clem., ***cocc., con.,*** dros., elaps, ***ferr.,*** ferr-m., ***fl-ac.,*** ign., kali-bi., lyc., man., nat-m., nat-p., nux-v., ph-ac., ***sabad., sulph.***
desires - ***abies-c.,*** alum., alum-p., alumn., am-c., am-m., ***ant-c., ant-t., apis, arg-n.,*** **ARN.,** ***ars.,*** ars-s-f., arund., bell., bism., bol., ***bor., brom., bry., calc.,*** calc-s., calc-sil., carb-an., carb-s., **CARB-V.,** ***cham.,*** chel., ***chin.,*** chin-a., ***cist.,*** cod., ***con.,*** conv., **COR-R.,** corn., crot-h., cub., cupr., cupr-ar., der., dig., dor., elaps, erig., eup-per., ***ferr.,*** ferr-ar., ***ferr-m.,*** ferr-p., ***fl-ac.,*** gran., **HEP.,** hipp., ***ign.,*** joan., ***kali-ar.,*** kali-bi., ***kali-c.,*** kali-i., kali-p., kali-s., kreos., ***lach.,*** lact., lyc., ***mag-c.,*** mang., ***med.,*** merc-i-f., ***myric., nat-m., ph-ac.,*** phel., ***phos.,*** plb., ***podo.,*** psor., ptel., ***puls.,*** rhus-t., ***sabad., sabin., sec.,*** **SEP.,** spirae., ***squil.,*** staph., ***stram.,*** stry-p., sul-ac., **SULPH.,** ***sul-i.,*** thea., ther., thuj., ust., uva., **VERAT.,** ziz.
bad effects from sweet and sour foods - acon., cham., ferr., ign., sulph.

SOUR, acids, general
desires, drinks - arn., ars., bor., dig., kali-bi., mag-c., mang., phel., sep.
headache, after - nat-s.
pregnancy, during - sep., ***verat.***
salt, and sour - ***arg-n., calc., calc-s.,*** **CARB-V.,** ***con.,*** **COR-R.,** ***med., merc-i-f.,*** **NAT-M., PHOS.,** ***plb., sulph., thuj.,*** **VERAT.**
sweets, and sour - ***bry., calc., carb-v., kali-c., med., sabad., sec., sep.,*** **SULPH.**

SPICY, food, (condiments, highly seasoned)
agg. - bism., ign., kali-m., naja, **NUX-V.,** phos., sel., sep., zinc.
amel. - hep., nux-m.
ailments from - ***nux-v.***
aversion to - fl-ac., mag-s., phos., puls., ***sang.,*** tarent.
desires - abies-c., alum., ant-c., arg-n., ***ars.,*** aster., calc-f., calc-p., caps., ***carc.,*** chel., **CHIN.,** cic., ***fl-ac., hep.,*** hyper., ***lac-c.,*** mag-s., man., meph., nat-m., nux-m., **NUX-V., PHOS.,** puls., ***sang.,*** sep., staph., stry-p., **SULPH.,** ***tarent.,*** tub., ***zing.***

SPINACH, aversions - ***chel.***

STARCHY, agg. - ***all-c.,*** ars., bell., **BERB.,** bry., ***carb-an., carb-v.,*** caust., chin., **COP.,** euph., ***kali-c., lach., lyc.,*** nat-c., **NAT-M., NAT-S.,** ***plb., puls., pyrog.,*** rhus-t.
amel., in children - nat-c.
aversion to - ars., chin., kali-ar., lyc., nat-a., ***nat-c.,*** nat-s., phos., ***sulph.***
desires - ***alum., calc.,*** calc-p., cic., ***ferr-ac.,*** **LACH., LYC.,** ***nat-m.,*** nit-ac., nux-v., sabad., ***sulph.,*** sumb.

STIMULANTS, agg. - agar., ant-c., chion., fl-ac., ***glon.,*** ign., lach., led., naja, ***nux-v.,*** op., thuj., ***zinc.***
amel. - gels., glon.
desires - alco., aloe, ant-t., ars-s-f., aster., aur., aur-s., calc-i., caps., caust., chin., crot-h., ***fl-ac.,*** gins., hep., iber., iod., kali-i., mur-ac., naja, nat-p., **NUX-V.,** ***puls.,*** sol-t-ae., staph., sul-i., ***sulph.,*** sumb., tab., ziz.

STRANGE things, desires - ***bry., calc., calc-p., chel., cycl., hep., lyss., manc.,*** puls., ter.
pregnancy, during - ***alum.,*** calc., carb-v., ***chel.,*** **LYSS.,** ***mag-c., puls., sep.***

STRAWBERRIES, agg. - ant-c., ***apis, ox-ac.,*** sep., thlaspi., urt-u.
aversion to - chin., ox-ac., ***sulph.***

SUGAR, agg. (see Sweets) - **ARG-N.,** bell., ***calc.,*** **LYC.,** ***merc.,*** nat-p., ox-ac., ***phos.,*** sang., ***sel.,*** **SULPH.,** thuj., zinc.
aversion to - ars., caust., chloram., ***graph.,*** merc., phos., rauw., sin-n., ***zinc.***
desires - am-c., am-m., **ARG-N.,** ***calc.,*** cann-i., carc., dys-co., ***kali-c.,*** **LYC.,** op., ***phos.,*** prot., ***sec.,*** sulph.

SUGAR, general
desires, can only digest if eats large amounts of sugar - nux-v., **STAPH.**
evening - ***arg-n.***
sugared water - bufo, sulph.

SUGARCANE, juice agg. - ars.

SWEETS, agg. (see Sugar) - acon., am-c., anac., ***ant-c.,*** **ARG-N.,** ars., aster., bad., bell., calc., calc-f., ***cham.,*** cina, cycl., ferr., fl-ac., ***graph.,*** hep., **IGN.,** ***ip.,*** lach., **LYC.,** med., ***merc.,*** nat-c., ***nat-p.,*** nux-v., ox-ac., phos., ***puls.,*** sang., ***sel.,*** spig., spong., ***sulph.,*** thuj., zinc., zinc-p.
agg, and amel. - ***arg-n., lyc., phos.***
sensitive to the smell of - aur., nit-ac., sil.
ailments from - **ARG-N.,** phos., thuj.
amel. - am-c., ***arg-n.,*** bell., ***lyc., phos.***
aversion to - ***arg-n., ars.,*** bar-c., beryl., brom., cadm-s., calc-p., carc., card-m., **CAUST.,** chloram., erig., **GRAPH.,** hipp., hippoz., ***kali-c.,*** lac-c., lol., ***lyc.,*** med., ***merc.,*** nit-ac., nux-v., petr., ***phos.,*** puls., rad., rad-br., rauw., rheum, senec., ***sin-n., sul-ac., sulph., zinc.,*** zinc-p.
sweets, or sour, or - bell.
desires - alf., ***am-c.,*** arg-m., **ARG-N.,** ***ars., aur-m-n.,*** bar-c., ***bry.,*** bufo, ***cact., calc., calc-f.,*** calc-p., ***calc-s.,*** **CANN-I.,** cann-s., ***carb-v., carc.,*** **CHIN.,** chin-a., **CHIN-S.,** ***cina,*** coca, ***cocaine,*** dys-co., ***elaps, euphr., ferr., ip.,*** kali-ar., ***kali-c.,*** kali-p., ***kali-s.,*** lil-t., **LYC.,** ***mag-m., med., meny.,*** meph., merc., merc-d., morg., nat-a., ***nat-c.,*** nat-m., ***nit-ac.,*** nux-v., op., petr., ***phos.,*** plat., ***plb.,*** prot., ***puls., rheum, rhus-t., sabad., sec., sep.,*** **STAPH.,** ***sul-ac.,*** **SULPH.,** ***thyr., tub.,*** x-ray.
candies - ***am-c.,*** **ARG-N.,** bar-c., carb-v., **CHIN.,** ***ip.,*** **KALI-C., LYC.,** mag-m., nat-c., ***phos.,*** rheum, rhus-t., sabad., sulph.
dainties - ***acon-l.,*** arg-n., calc.
headache, during - **CALC.**
menses before - lyc., **SULPH.**
only sweets - kali-p.
salt, and sweets - **ARG-N.,** ***calc.,*** carb-v., carc., ***med., plb.***
sour, and sweets - ***bry., calc., carb-v., kali-c., med., sabad., sec., sep.,*** **SULPH.**

TAMARIND, water agg. - sel.

TEA, agg. - abies-c., ***abies-n., aesc.,*** agar., ars., aur-m., calad., cham., ***chin.,*** cocc., coff., dios., ***ferr.,*** fl-ac., hep., kali-bi., lach., lob., ***nux-v.,*** ph-ac., puls., ***rhus-t.,*** rumx., **SEL., SEP.,** ***spig.,*** stroph., ***thuj.,*** verat.
ailments from - abies-n., ***chin.,*** cocc., dios., lob., ***nux-v.,*** sel., thuj.
amel. - aloe, carb-ac., dig., ferr., glon., kali-bi., pyrus.
aversion to - carb-ac., carb-an., chin., dios., ferr-m., kali-p., ***phos., sel.,*** thea., thuj., trinit.

TEA, general
desires - alum., aster., calc-s., ***chin.,*** hep., hydr., lepi., nux-v., ***puls.,*** pyrus, sel., thuj., uran-n.
tea grounds - ***alum.***

THINKING of food, agg. - arg-n., bor., cann-s., carb-v., dros., graph., lach., lil-t., nat-m., ***puls.,*** sars., ***sep.,*** thuj.

THIRST, general - **ACET-AC., ACON.,** aesc., aeth., agar., agn., ail., ***all-c.,*** all-s., aloe, alum., alumn., am-c., ***am-m., anac.,*** anan., ang., ***ant-c.,*** ant-t., anthr., apis, ***apoc.,*** **ARG-N.,** ***arn.,*** **ARS.,** ars-h., ***ars-i.,*** aur., aur-m., ***bapt., bar-c.,*** bar-i., ***bar-m., bell., berb.,*** bism., ***bor., bol.,*** bov., brom., **BRY.,** cact., cadm-s., cahin., caj., **CALC.,** ***calc-ar.,*** **CALC-CAUST.,** ***camph.,*** cann-i., ***canth.,*** **CAPS.,** ***carb-ac.,*** carb-an., carb-s., ***carb-v.,*** carl., cast., caul., **CAUST.,** cedr., **CHAM.,** ***chel.,*** **CHIN.,** ***chin-a., chin-s., cic., cimic., cina,*** cinnb., clem., ***cocc., coc-c., colch., coloc., con.,*** cop., cor-r., ***croc., crot-c., crot-h., cupr.,*** cycl., daph., **DIG.,** dor., ***dros., dulc.,*** elaps, eug., **EUP-PER.,** euph., eupi., fago., ferr-ar., ferr-i., ***ferr-p., fl-ac.,*** form., gamb., gent-c., gins., glon., graph., grat., guai., ham., **HELL.,** ***hep.,*** hydr-ac., ***hyos.,*** **IOD.,** ind., ip., jug-r., kali-ar., ***kali-bi., kali-c.,*** kali-chl., ***kali-i.,*** kali-n., ***kali-p., kali-s., kalm.,*** kreos., ***lach.,*** lachn., lact., ***laur., led.,*** lil-t., lyc., ***mag-c.,*** mag-m., mag-s., manc., mang., **MERC.,** ***merc-c., merc-i-f.,*** merl., ***mez.,*** mill., mur-ac., naja, ***nat-a., nat-c.,*** **NAT-M.,** ***nat-p.,*** nat-s., nicc., ***nit-ac.,*** nux-m., ***nux-v.,*** ol-j., olnd., **OP.,** ox-ac., paeon., petr., ph-ac., **PHOS.,** phys., pic-ac., plan., plat., ***plb., podo.,*** psor., ptel., puls., ***ran-b., raph., rat.,*** rhod., **RHUS-T.,** rob., ruta., sabad., samb., sang., sant., sars., **SEC.,** sel., seneg., sep., **SIL.,** sol-n., sol-t-ae., spig., stann., staph., **STRAM.,** stront-c., **SULPH.,** sul-ac., tab., **TARENT.,** tax., tep., ter., thea., ***ther., thuj.,*** upa., ust., **VERAT.,** ***verat-v.,*** verb., ***zinc.,*** zing.
afternoon - aloe, am-c., am-m., berb., bor., bov., brom., ***calc.,*** carl., chin., clem., colch., con., ham., ign., kali-n., mag-c., mag-m., mag-s., ***nat-c.,*** nat-m., nat-s., nicc., nux-v., petr., ph-ac., phos., phys., ***ran-b.,*** rhus-t., ruta., sars., senec., sil., sulph., verat., ***zinc.***
1 p.m. to 2 p.m. - phos.
1 p.m. to 6 p.m. - ***phos.***
2 p.m. - **PULS.**
3 p.m. - ferr., lyc., nicc., staph.
4 p.m. - chel., ***lyc.,*** sulph.
chill, during - sulph.
6 p.m. - bar-c., ham., tab.
sleep, after - **STAPH.**
alternating, with aversion to drink - berb.
anger, after - bry., nux-v.
anxious - bell.
apyrexia, during - ***cimx., ip.***

THIRST, general

aversions, drinks - agar., agn., aloe, ang., ***apis,*** arn., ***bell.,*** berb., bufo, ***canth.,*** carb-an., chin., cocc., coc-c., coff., corn., cupr., **FERR., HYOS.,** ign., kali-bi., ***lac-c.,*** lach., ***lyss.,*** merc., ***nit-ac.,*** **NUX-V.,** phys., plb., ***puls.,*** rat., samb., sec., ***stram.***

fever, during - con.

headache, during - **FERR.**

beer, agg., after - bry.

burning, vehement - **ACET-AC.,** ***acon.,*** aeth., ***agar., anac.,*** anan., apis, ***ars., aur., bell.,*** **BRY.,** bufo, ***calc., camph.,*** **CANN-I.,** canth., carb-s., ***carb-v., cast.,*** caust., cham., chin., colch., ***coloc., crot-c., crot-h.,*** cub., cupr., elaps, ferr., graph., hep., hyos., iod., jatr., kali-bi., ***kali-n.,*** kali-s., ***laur.,*** lyc., ***lycps.,*** mag-m., **MERC.,** merc-c., merc-i-f., mur-ac., nat-a., nat-c., nicc., nit-ac., op., ph-ac., **PHOS.,** ***plb.,*** puls., raph., ***rhus-t., sec., sil.,*** spong., squil., stann., ***stram., sulph.,*** sul-ac., **TARENT.,** thuj., verat., verb., vip., zinc.

burning, without desire to drink - ***ars.***

chill, during - ***acon.,*** alum., am-m., ant-c., **APIS,** aran., **ARN.,** ars., asar., bar-c., bar-m., bor., bov., ***bry.,*** calad., ***calc.,*** camph., cann-s., canth., **CAPS.,** carb-s., ***carb-v.,*** cham., ***chin-s.,*** cimx., **CINA,** croc., eupi., **EUP-PER.,** ***eup-pur., ferr.,*** gamb., hep., **IGN.,** kali-ar., ***kali-c.,*** kali-i., ***lach., lec., led.,*** mag-m., med., mez., mur-ac., nat-c., **NAT-M.,** nat-s., **NUX-V.,** ol-j., ***op.,*** psor., **PYROG.,** ran-s., ***rhus-t.,*** ruta, sabad., ***sec.,*** **SEP., SIL.,** spong., squil., staph., ***sulph.,*** tarent., thuj., **TUB., VERAT.**

after - all-c., **ARS.,** canth., **CHIN.,** ***cimx.,*** **DROS.,** ferr., hep., kali-bi., kreos., mag-s., mang., ***nat-m.,*** nat-s., psor., **PULS.,** ***sabad.,*** sars., ***sep.,*** sulph., thuj.

yet cannot drink, makes headache unbearable - cimx.

before - am-c., am-m., arn., **ARS.,** bor., ***caps.,*** **CHIN., EUP-PER.,** ***eup-pur., hep.,*** lach., mag-c., nat-m., ***nux-v.,*** ol-j., **PULS.,** sep., sulph.

choking, sensation when drinking, with - squil.

constant, amel. by drinking cold water - alum.

convulsions, during - cic.

after - bell., ign.

coryza, during - mag-m., nat-c.

daytime - hep., kali-n., sulph.

diarrhea, with - acet-ac.

dinner, after - aloe, anac., canth., ***cast.,*** cycl., ferr., gamb., mag-c., mag-m., ***nat-c.,*** nat-m., plb., psor., thuj., zinc.

dread, of liquids, with - agn., am-c., arn., ars., ***bell.,*** cann-i., ***canth., caust., cocc., hell., hyos.,*** lac-c., ***lach., lyc.,*** lyss., merc., nat-m., ***nux-v.,*** rhus-t., samb., sel., ***stram.,*** tarent.

dropsy, with - acet-ac.

eating, while - ail., aloe, ***am-c.,*** bufo, ***cocc.,*** coc-c., ***lach., nat-c.,*** nit-ac., psor., puls.

THIRST, general

eating, after - aloe, anac., bell., ***bry.,*** calad., caust., cocc., coc-c., cycl., elaps, graph., guare., lyc., nat-c., nit-ac., phel., phos., sil.

evening - acon., ***all-c.,*** am-c., am-m., anac., ***ant-c.,*** arg-m., ars., ars-i., bar-c., bell., benz-ac., bism., bor., bov., bry., carl., cham., chin., chin-a., chin-s., clem., coc-c., ***croc.,*** cur., **CYCL.,** elaps, euphr., fago., ferr., ferr-i., ***gamb.,*** gran., graph., grat., ham., ***iod.,*** jatr., kali-bi., kali-c., kreos., laur., lyc., ***mag-c., mag-m.,*** mag-s., merc-i-f., mez., nat-a., nat-c., ***nat-m., nat-s., nicc.,*** ol-an., phos., phys., plb., podo., rat., rumx., seneg., sel., sep., sin-a., spig., spong., squil., sulph., tab., ***thuj., zinc.,*** zing.

8 p.m. - phos.

extreme - **ACET-AC., ACON.,** ***aesc.,*** aeth., agar., ***all-c.,*** all-s., alum., ***am-m.,*** anac., anan., ***ant-c., ant-t.,*** anthr., ***apis,*** **ARG-N.,** ***arn.,*** **ARS.,** ***ars-h.,*** ars-i., asar., aspar., aur., aur-m., bar-c., bar-i., bar-m., ***bell.,*** bism., ***bor., bov.,*** **BRY.,** bufo, ***cadm-s.,*** calad., **CALC., CALC-S.,** ***camph.,*** cann-s., canth., caps., ***carb-ac.,*** carb-an., carb-s., ***carb-v.,*** **CAUST.,** ***cedr.,*** **CHAM.,** ***chel.,*** chlor., **CHIN.,** cic., cina, cocc., coc-c., coff., ***colch., coloc.,*** con., ***cop., croc., crot-c., crot-h., crot-t.,*** cub., ***cupr., cupr-ar.,*** cur., ***cycl.,*** **DIG.,** dros., ***dulc., elaps,*** **EUP-PER.,** ***eup-pur., ferr.,*** ferr-ar., ferr-i., ferr-m., gamb., ***graph.,*** grat., guai., ham., **HELL.,** helon., ***hep.,*** hydr-ac., hyos., hyper., ign., ***iod., ip.,*** jab., jatr., kali-ar., kali-bi., ***kali-br., kali-c.,*** kali-chl., ***kali-i.,*** kali-n., ***kali-p., kalm., kreos., lac-ac.,*** lac-d., lach., lachn., ***laur., led.,*** lil-t., ***lyc., lycps., lyss., mag-c., mag-m.,*** manc., ***med.,*** **MERC., MERC-C.,** merc-i-f., mez., mill., mosch., mur-ac., mygal., nat-a., ***nat-c.,*** **NAT-M.,** ***nat-p., nat-s., nit-ac.,*** nux-m., ***nux-v., olnd., op.,*** ox-ac., par., ***petr., ph-ac.,*** **PHOS.,** ***phyt.,*** plan., plat., plb., ***podo.,*** ptel., puls., **PYROG.,** ran-b., ran-s., ***raph.,*** rheum, rhod., ***rhus-t.,*** **ROB.,** ruta., sabad., samb., ***sang.,*** sec., sel., seneg., ***sep.,*** **SIL.,** spig., ***spong.,*** squil., stann., staph., **STRAM.,** stront-c., stry., **SULPH.,** ***sul-ac.,*** syph., tarent., tarax., tell., ***ter.,*** ther., thuj., **THYR.,** uran., valer., **VERAT.,** verb., ***zinc.***

drinks more than she should - ars.

fever, with - alum., phos.

fever, heat, during - **ACON.,** ***all-c., aloe,*** am-m., ***anac., ang.,*** anthr., ant-c., arn., **ARS.,** arum-t., **BELL.,** berb., **BRY.,** cact., ***calc.,*** calad., ***canth., caps.,*** carb-an., carb-s., carb-v., ***cedr., cham., chin.,*** chin-a., ***chin-s., cina,*** cist., clem., ***cocc., coff.,*** colch., ***coloc., con.,*** cop., cor-r., ***croc.,*** crot-h., cur., dros., dulc., ***elat.,*** **EUP-PER.,** ferr., ***gels.,*** graph., ***hep., hyos.,*** ign., ***ip., kali-ar., kali-c.,*** kali-p., ***lach.,*** lyc., mag-c., mag-m., mang., med., **NAT-M.,** nit-ac., **NUX-V.,** op., petr., ph-ac., ***phos., podo., psor., puls., pyrog., ran-s.,*** rhod., ***rhus-t.,*** sars., ***sec.,*** sep., ***sil.,*** spig., spong., stann., staph., ***stram., sulph.,*** tax.,

THIRST, general
fever, heat, during - ***thuj.,*** **TUB.,** valer., verat.
after - anac., am-m., cact., ***chin.,*** coff., cycl., malar., nux-v., op., puls., pyrog., sep., stann., stram., tub.
stages, during all - acon., bry., eup-per., nat-m.
forenoon - agar., ang., apis, calc-s., chin., elaps, kali-c., kali-n., mag-c., mag-m., mag-s., nat-c., nat-s., zinc.
10 a.m. - nat-a., ***nat-m.***
headache, with - aeth., agar., **BRY.,** cadm-s., camph., chin-s., ***lac-d.,*** **MAG-M.,** ***nat-m.,*** plat., stram., ***ter., verat.,*** zing.
heart attack, after - xan.
labor, during - ***caul.***
large, quantities, for - ***acet-ac., acon.,*** **ARS.,** bad., **BRY.,** calen., camph., carb-s., ***chin., cocc.,*** coc-c., cop., ***eup-per., ferr-p.,*** ham., ***jatr.,*** lac-c., ***lac-d.,*** lil-t., ***lycps., merc-c.,*** **NAT-M.,** ph-ac., **PHOS.,** pic-ac., ***podo.,*** sol-n., ***stram.,*** **SULPH.,** ***thyr.,*** tub., **VERAT.,** vip., xan.
long intervals, at - **BRY.,** hell., podo., ***sulph.,*** verat.
menses, during - nat-m., ***sulph.***
before - sulph.
often - ***acon.,*** arn., ars., ***bell.,*** **BRY.,** cop., ***eup-per.,*** lac-c., ***lac-d.,*** lil-t., ***nat-m.,*** **PHOS.,** ruta, samb., syph., ***tarent., thyr.***
menses, during - am-c., ***bell.,*** cast., ***cedr., cham., coc-c.,*** dig., kali-n., mag-s., nat-m., sep., sul-ac., sulph., verat., ***zinc.***
before - kali-c., mag-c., mang., nat-m., sil., sulph.
morning - am-c., am-m., ant-c., apoc., ars., arund., bell., bor., bry., calc., carb-an., carb-s., caust., chin., chin-s., coc-c., dros., eug., fago., glon., ***graph.,*** grat., hyper., jab., kali-c., kreos., mag-m., mag-s., nat-a., nat-c., nat-m., nat-s., **NIT-AC.,** nux-m., ***nux-v.,*** ox-ac., ph-ac., phos., phyt., plb., puls., rhus-t., sabad., sars., sep., spong., ***stram.,*** sulph., tab., thuj., ***verat.,*** vip.
breakfast, after - mag-s.
milk, after - nat-m.
waking, on - am-c., arund., hyper., jab., mag-s., nit-ac., sel., thuj., zing.
after - sep.
night - ***acon.,*** aloe, ambr., ***ant-c.,*** ant-t., apis, arn., ***ars.,*** bell., bor., bry., ***calc.,*** cadm-s., canth., carb-an., carb-v., cedr., cham., chin-s., cinnb., ***coff.,*** cur., ***cycl.,*** dros., elaps, ***eup-per.,*** fago., fl-ac., gamb., glon., graph., ***hep., kali-c., lach.,*** led., ***lyc., mag-c.,*** mag-m., mang., ***merc.,*** mez., mur-ac., nat-a., nat-c., nat-m., nat-s., nicc., nit-ac., nux-v., op., ***phos.,*** plan., puls., ***rhus-t.,*** sep., **SIL.,** ***spong., sulph.,*** tab., ***thuj.,*** zing.
3 a.m. - mag-m.
midnight - cann-i., mag-m., merc., plat., puls., sulph., sul-ac.
midnight, after - bell., mag-m., mang.

THIRST, general
night, waking, on - aloe, ***apoc.,*** berb., calad., carb-ac., ***coff., nat-s., stram.***
noon - bell., **LYC.,** mag-c., mag-m., nat-c., phos.
pains, with the - acon., aran., **CHAM.,** ***nat-c.***
pains, abdominal, with - chin.
perspiration, during - ***acon.,*** anac., **ARS.,** ars-i., ***bry.,*** cact., calc., cedr., **CHIN.,** ***chin-a., chin-s., coff.,*** gels., ***iod., ip.,*** kali-n., mag-m., nat-c., **NAT-M.,** op., ***ph-ac.,*** puls., ***rhus-t.,*** sec., ***sep.,*** **STRAM.,** tarax., ***thuj.,*** **VERAT.**
perspiration, after - ***ant-c., ant-t.,*** bell., bor., bov., **LYC.,** ***nux-v.,*** sabad.
pregnancy, during - phos., ***verat.***
sex, after - eug.
seldom, but much - ***bry.,*** hell., podo., ***sulph.,*** verat.
sleep, after - ambr., apoc., bell., bor., ther.
after, midday - ther.
afternoon - **STAPH.**
small, quantities, for - anac., ant-t., apis, **ARS.,** arum-t., bell., bry., cact., calc., caps., carb-v., ***chin.,*** cimic., cupr., cupr-ar., gast., ham., ***hell.,*** hep., hyos., kali-n., lac-c., ***lach.,*** laur., **LYC.,** merc-i-r., nat-m., nux-v., phos., ***rhus-t.,*** sanic., squil., ***sulph.,*** tab., tub.
often - acon., ant-t., apis, arum-t., **ARS.,** ***bell.,*** cact., ***chin., coloc., corn.,*** eup-per., hyos., lac-c., lyc., ***nat-a.,*** puls., rhus-t., ***sulph.,*** verat.
smoking, after - spong.
stool, during - ars., bry., cham., chin., dulc., hell., lil-t., mag-c., sulph.
after - alum., ant-t., **CAPS.,** chin., dulc., lyc., ox-ac., sulph., trom.
before - ***ars.,*** bry., cham., chin., dulc., hell., mag-c., podo., sulph.
supper, after - aloe, carb-an., phos., plat.
swallow, inability to, with - bell., cic., hyos., ign., lyss.
thirstless - acet-ac., ***aesc.,*** aeth., agar., ***agn.,*** all-c., ambr., am-c., ***am-m., ant-c.,*** **ANT-T., APIS,** ***arg-n., ars., asaf., bell.,*** berb., ***bov.,*** brom., bry., bufo, calad., ***calen., camph.,*** canth., caps., caust., chel., **CHIN.,** cimic., cocc., coff., **COLCH.,** cor-r., ***con.,*** crot-t., ***cycl.,*** dios., euph., ***ferr.,*** ferr-ar., ferr-m., gamb., **GELS.,** ham., **HELL.,** hep., ***hydr-ac.,*** hyos., ign., indg., ***ip.,*** iris, kali-ar., ***kali-c.,*** kali-n., kali-p., led., ***lyc.,*** mag-c., ***mang.,*** **MENY.,** merc-c., mez., mur-ac., nat-a., nat-c., nat-m., nat-s., nit-ac., **NUX-M.,** nux-v., ***olnd.,*** onos., ***op.,*** ox-ac., petr., **PH-AC.,** phos., plat., ptel., **PULS.,** rhod., **SABAD.,** ***samb.,*** sars., ***sep.,*** spig., ***staph., stram.,*** sulph., tab., ***tarent.,*** thuj., valer., verat.
desire to drink, with - aeth., ***ars., calad., camph., cimx.,*** cocc., coloc., graph., nux-m., phos.

THIRST, general
thirstless, fever, heat, during - acet-ac., ***aeth.,*** agar., ***alum., ant-c., ant-t.,*** **APIS,** arg-m., ars., ars-h., asaf., bar-c., bell., bov., ***calc.,*** camph., ***caps.,*** carb-an., ***carb-v., caust.,*** cham., chin., ***cimx.,*** **CINA,** cocc., con., cycl., dig., ***dros.,*** euph., ***ferr.,*** **GELS.,** guai., hell., hep., ***ign., ip., kali-c.,*** kali-n., lec., ***led.,*** lyc., med., meny., ***mur-ac., nit-ac., nux-m.,*** op., ***ph-ac.,*** phos., ***puls.,*** rheum., rhus-t., ruta, **SABAD.,** ***samb.,*** **SEP.,** sil., spig., spong., squil., stann., staph., stram., ***sulph.,*** tarax., verat.
unquenchable, thirst - ***acet-ac., acon.,*** aeth., agar., aloe, am-c., anac., anan., ***apis,*** **ARS.,** ars-i., ***bar-c.,*** bar-i., ***bell., bry., calc., camph., carb-s.,*** cham., ***crot-h.,*** cupr-ac., cycl., dig., ***dulc.,*** **EUP-PER.,** ***ferr., hyos.,*** iod., kali-n., ***kali-p., lach., merc.,*** merc-c., merc-i-r., nat-a., nat-c., ***nat-m.,*** nicc., ***op.,*** petr., ph-ac., **PHOS.,** ***rhus-t.,*** ruta., sec., stram., sol-n., ***sulph., tarent., verat.,*** zing.
constant sipping of cold water - ***acon.,*** ant-t., ***ars.,*** hyos., onos., sanic.
disgust for drink, with - ***lach.***
vomiting, with - ars.
after - olnd., ***sul-ac.***
before - **EUP-PER.**
waking, on - ***apoc.,*** camph., dros., ferr., hyper., mag-c., ***mag-m.,*** nat-m., rat., stram.
walking, after - ***ferr-m.,*** nat-c., nat-m.
wine, after - sil.
without, desire to drink - ang., cocc., merc-c., mez., nat-m., ***nux-v.***

TOBACCO, (see Toxicity, Tobacco)

TOMATOES, agg. - lith., ox-ac., phos.
aversion to - ***phos., psor.***
desires - ***ferr.,*** ign.

TONICS, agg. - carb-ac.
aversion to - sul-ac.
desires - aloe, caps., carb-ac., carb-an., caust., ***cocc.,*** gels., med., ***nux-v., rhus-t., ph-ac.,*** phos., ***puls.,*** rheum, sul-ac., sulph., ***valer.***

TURNIPS, agg. - ***bry.,*** calc-ar., ***lyc., puls.,*** rob., sulph.
aversion to - bry., puls., sulph.

VEAL, agg. - ars., ***calc., caust.,*** chin., **IP., KALI-N.,** nux-v., ***sep.,*** sulph., verat., ***zinc.***
ailments from - kali-n.
aversion to - merc., phel., ***zinc.***

VEGETABLES, agg. - ***alum.,*** ars., ***bry.,*** calc., caps., cupr., ***hell.,*** hydr., ***kali-c.,*** lept., ***lyc., mag-c., nat-c.,*** **NAT-S.,** petr., verat.
decayed - ***carb-an.,*** **CARB-V.**
green - ***alum.,*** ars., ***bry.,*** cupr., ***hell.,*** lyc., ***nat-c.,*** **NAT-S.,** verat.
aversion to - bell., caust., **HELL.,** hydr., lyc., lyss., **MAG-C.,** ***mag-m., nat-m., phos.,*** ruta.
desires - abies-c., adel., all-c., ***alum.,*** alumn., ars., asar., calc-s., carb-an., cham., ***kali-i., lycps., mag-c., mag-m.,*** onos., ***sulph.***

VINEGAR, agg. - ***acon.,*** aloe, alum., **ANT-C.,** ***ars., bell.,*** bor., calad., ***carb-v.,*** caust., dros., ***ferr.,*** ferr-ar., ***graph.,*** hep., kreos., lach., merc-c., nat-a., nat-c., nat-m., ***nat-p.,*** nux-v., ph-ac., phos., ***puls.,*** ran-b., ***sep.,*** staph., sul-ac., ***sulph.***
sensitive to the smell of - agar.
amel. - ***asar.,*** bry., hell., ign., meny., op., ***puls.,*** sang., stram., tab., tong.
desires - apis, arn., ars., asar., ***bac.,*** bell-p., chel., **HEP.,** ***kali-m.,*** kali-p., lepi., ***nat-m.,*** puls., ***sep.,*** sulph.

WARM, drinks, agg. - ambr., apis, bry., chel., fl-ac., graph., ign., ***lach., phos.,*** phyt., ***puls.,*** pyrog., **RHUS-T.,** sars., sep., sil., stann., ***sulph.,*** verat., zinc-p.
amel. - ***alum.,*** apoc., arg-n., **ARS.,** ***bry.,*** calc-f., ***carb-s., cedr., chel.,*** cupr., ***graph.,*** guare., ***lyc., mang., nux-m.,*** **NUX-V.,** pyrus, **RHUS-T.,** sabad., spong., ***sulph.,*** verat.
aversion to - bry., caust., ***cham., cupr.,*** graph., kali-s., **PHOS., PULS.,** pyrog., rib-ac., ***verat.,*** zinc-p.
desires - ang., **ARS.,** ars-s-f., bell., **BRY.,** ***calad.,*** carb-v., casc., cast-v., cedr., ***chel.,*** chin-a., cocc., cupr., eup-per., eup-pur., ferr-p., graph., hep., ***hyper.,*** kali-ar., kali-c., kali-i., kreos., **LAC-C.,** ***lyc.,*** med., merc-c., pyrus, ***sabad.,*** spig., ***sulph.,*** tub.
angina pectoris, in - spig.
chill, during - **ARS.,** ***cedr., eup-per.***
fever, during - ars., ***casc.,*** cedr., ***eup-per., lyc.***
warm, food, agg. - acon., agn., all-c., alum., ***alum-p.,*** alum-sil., ***ambr.,*** am-c., ***anac.,*** ang., ant-t., ars., asar., ***bar-c., bell.,*** bism., bor., **BRY.,** calc., canth., carb-s., ***carb-v.,*** caust., ***cham.,*** clem., ***coc-c., cupr.,*** dros., ***euph.,*** ferr., gran., hell., ***kali-c.,*** **LACH.,** laur., ***mag-c.,*** mag-m., merc., ***mez.,*** nat-m., ***nit-ac.,*** nux-m., nux-v., par., ***ph-ac.,*** **PHOS.,** phyt., **PULS.,** rhod., ***rhus-t.,*** sars., sep., sil., spig., squil., stann., sul-i., sulph., sul-ac., thuj., verat., zinc.
amel. - ars., asar., chel., kreos., ***laur.,*** lyc., sabad.
aversion to - ***bell., calc., chin.,*** cupr., **GRAPH.,** guare., ***ign., lach., lyc.,*** mag-c., mag-s., merc., ***merc-c.,*** petr., **PHOS.,** psor., **PULS.,** ***sil., verat.,*** zinc.
desires - ang., **ARS.,** ars-s-f., ***bry.,*** cast., cedr., ***chel.,*** chin-a., cocc., cupr., cycl., ***ferr.,*** kali-i., ***lyc., lyc.,*** med., ***ph-ac., sabad.,*** sil.
soups - ars., bry., ***calc-ar.,*** ferr., lyc., nat-m., phel.

WATER, agg. - arg-n., ars., bry., calc., canth., chin-a., ***cocc., crot-t.,*** dros., ferr-m., lach., lob., lyc., nux-m., puls., sabad., sep., spong., stann., sulph.
drinking too much - grat.
seeing or hearing of - lyss.
amel. - ars., **BRY.**

WATER, general
aversion to - am-c., ***apis***, ars., ***bell.,*** berb, brom., ***bry., calad.,*** cann-i., ***canth.,*** carl., caust., cedr., chel., ***chin.,*** chin-a., coc-c., coloc., elaps, ham., hell., **HYOS.,** ***kali-bi., lach.,*** lyc., ***lyss.,*** manc., merc., merc-c., ***nat-m.,*** **NUX-V.,** onos., ox-ac., phel., ***phys., puls.,*** **STAPH., STRAM.,** sul-ac., ***tab.,*** thea., zinc., zing.
cold water - **BELL.,** brom., bry., ***calad.,*** canth., caust., chel., **CHIN.,** ***chin-a.,*** ham., kali-bi., lyc., ***lyss.,*** nat-m., **NUX-V.,** ox-ac., ***phel.,*** phos., phys., puls., rhus-t., **SABAD.,** ***stram.,*** sulph., tab.
pregnancy, during - phos.
thinking of, agg. - ham.
thirst, with - hell.
touch of - am-c.

WHEAT, agg. - ***all-c.,*** ars., bell., **BERB.,** bry., ***carb-an., carb-v., caust.,*** chin., coloc., **COP.,** euph., ***iris, kali-a., kali-c., lach.,*** **LYC.,** nat-c., **NAT-M., NAT-S.,** nux-v., ***plb.,*** psor., ***puls., pyrog.,*** rhus-t., sulph.
amel., in children - nat-c.
aversion to - ars., kali-ar., phos.
desires - ***alum., calc.,*** calc-p., cic., ***ferr-ac.,*** **LACH.,** ***lyc., nat-m.,*** nit-ac., nux-v., sabad., ***sulph.,*** sumb.

WHISKEY, aversion to - ant-t., ***ign.,*** merc., ph-ac., rhus-t., zinc.
desires - acon., ***arn., ars.,*** calc., carb-ac., ***carb-an.,*** chin., cub., fl-ac., hep., **LAC-C.,** ***lach.,*** merc., nux-v., op., ***phos.,*** puls., ***sel., spig.,*** staph., **SULPH.,** ther.

WINE, agg. (see Alcohol) - acon., acon-l., aeth., agar., alum., am-m., ***ant-c., arn.,*** **ARS.,** aur., aur-m., bell., benz-ac., ***bor.,*** bov., bry., cact., ***calc.,*** calc-sil., carb-an., carb-s., carb-v., **CHIN.,** chlol., coc-c., **COFF.,** coloc., ***con.,*** cor-r., eup-per., ign., ***fl-ac., gels., glon.,*** hyos., ign., kali-chl., ***lach., led.,*** **LYC.,** mag-m., ***merc., naja, nat-a., nat-c., nat-m., nux-m.,*** **NUX-V., OP.,** ox-ac., petr., phos., puls., **RAN-B.,** ***rhod.,*** rhus-t., ruta., ***sabad.,*** sars., ***sel.,*** **SIL.,** staph., stront-c., sul-ac., ***sulph.,*** thuj., verat., **ZINC.**
champagne - calc.
red - fl-ac.
sour agg. - **ANT-C.,** ant-t., ***ars.,*** ferr., sep., sulph.
sour, white - **ANT-C.,** ant-t., ***ars.,*** ferr., sep., sulph.
sulphureted - ***ars.,*** chin., ***merc.,*** **PULS.,** ***sep.***
ailments from - carb-v., coff., lyc., nat-m., ***zinc.***
bad, from - carb-v.,
amel. - ***acon.,*** agar., ars., bell., brom., bry., ***canth., carb-ac.,*** chel., chen-v., coca, cocc., ***con.,*** gels., glon., graph., lach., mez., nat-m., nux-v., onos., ***op.,*** osm., phos., ran-b., sel., sul-ac., sulph., thea.
sour, white - ferr.

WINE, general
aversion to - **ACON.,** agar., alum., ars-m., carb-s., carb-v., coff., fl-ac., glon., hyper., ***ign.,*** jatr., jug-r., **LACH.,** lact., man., manc., ***merc.,*** nat-m., nux-v., ph-ac., puls., ***rhus-t.,*** **SABAD.,** sil., ***sulph.,*** tub., ***zinc.,*** zinc-p.
desires - ***acon., aeth.,*** arg-m., arg-mur., ***ars.,*** asaf., bov., ***bry.,*** **CALC.,** calc-ar., calc-s., **CANTH.,** chel., chin., chin-a., chlor., ***cic.,*** colch., cub., eup-per., fl-ac., ***hep.,*** hyper., iod., kali-bi., kali-br., kali-i., ***lach., lec.,*** **LYCPS.,** merc., ***mez.,*** nat-m., nux-v., op., **PHOS.,** puls., sec., sel., ***sep., spig., staph.,*** sul-i., **SULPH.,** ***sumb.,*** syph., ther., thiop., verat., vichy-g.
claret - calc-s., staph., ***sulph.,*** ther.
sensitive to the smell of - tab.
sour agg. - **ANT-C.,** ant-t., ***ars.,*** ferr., sep., sulph.

Generals

ABSCESS, suppurations - all-c., ***anan.,*** **ANTHR.,** ant-c., ant-t., ***apis,*** **ARN.,** ars., ***ars-i.,*** ars-s-f., ***asaf., bar-c.,*** bar-m., ***bell., bell-p.,*** both., ***bry.,*** bufo, calc., calc-f., ***calc-hp.,*** **CALC-I., CALC-S.,** calc-sil., **CALEN.,** ***canth.,*** caps., ***carb-ac.,*** carb-an., ***carb-v., caust., cench., cham., chin.,*** chin-a., chin-s., cic., ***cist.,*** cocc., con., conch., ***croc.,*** crot-h., cupr., digox., ***dulc., echi.,*** elat., ***fl-ac., guai., gunp.,*** **HEP.,** ***hippoz.,*** kali-c., kali-chl., kali-s., ***kreos.,*** **LACH.,** ***lap-a.,*** led., ***lyc.,*** mag-c., ***mang.,*** matth., **MERC.,** merc-d., methyl-b., mez., ***myris.,*** nat-c., nat-m., nat-sal., nat-sil., ***nit-ac.,*** nux-v., ***olnd., ol-j.,*** paeon., petr., ph-ac., **PHOS.,** ***phyt.,*** plb., psor., ptel., puls., ***pyrog.,*** raja-s., ***rhus-t., sec.,*** sep., sieg., **SIL.,** sil-mar., staph., ***stram., sul-ac.,*** sul-i., ***sulph.,*** symph., syph., tarent., ***tarent-c..*** thyr., tub., vesp., ***vip.,*** wies.

- **abort,** remedies to - apis, arn., bell., bry., calc., ***calc-s.,*** guai., ***hep., merc.,*** phyt., sil.
- **absorption,** of pus - ***calc-s.,*** iod., **LACH.,** ***phos., sil.***
- **acute** - acon., ***anan.,*** anthr., apis, ***arn.,*** ars., ***bell.,*** calc-hp., ***calc-s.,*** calen., ***carb-ac.,*** chin-s., crot-h., fl-ac., **HEP.,** hippoz., ***lach.,*** lap-a., lyc., **MERC.,** ***merc-sul., myris., nit-ac.,*** ph-ac., phos., ***rhus-t.,*** **SIL.,** sil-mar., ***sulph.,*** syph., ***tarent-c.,*** vesp.
- **ailments,** from - abrot., ***chin.,*** chin-a., ferr., kali-c., nat-m., ph-ac., ***phos.***
- **blind** - lyc.
- **bluish** - lach., tarent-c.
- **burning** - **ANTHR., ARS.,** merc., ***pyrog.,*** **TARENT-C.**
- **chilly,** within - merc.
- **chronic** - arg-m., arn., ***asaf.,*** aur., calc., ***calc-f.,*** calc-i., calc-p., ***calc-s., carb-v.,*** cham., chin., con., fl-ac., graph., **HEP.,** ***iod.,*** iodof., kali-bi., kali-i., laur., lyc., mag-f., mang., ***merc.,*** merc-c., merc-i-r., ***merc-sul., nit-ac.,*** ol-j., phos., ***pyrog.,*** sars., sep., ***sil.,*** stram., ***sulph.***
- **cold** - ol-j.
- **deep** - calc., ***calc-s.,*** caps., tarent.
- **discharge,** from abscess
  - acrid - ail., **ARS.,** ***asaf.,*** bell-p., brom., ***carb-v.,*** **CAUST.,** ***cham., clem.,*** echi., euphr., fl-ac., gels., ***hep., kali-ox.,*** lach., ***lyc., merc.,*** mez., ***nat-c.,*** nat-m., ***petr.,*** sabad., sanic., sars.
  - black - bry., chin., lyc., ***sulph.***
  - bland - bell., ***calc., hep., lach.,*** mang., ***merc.,*** phos., **PULS.,** rhus-t., ***sil.,*** staph., ***sulph.***
  - bloody - arg-n., arn., ***ars.,*** **ASAF.,** bell., calc-s., ***carb-v., caust.,*** con., croc., crot-h., dros., **HEP.,** iod., kali-c., kreos., lach., ***lyc., phyt.***
  - brown - anac., calc., con., lycps., puls.
  - excoriating - am-c., anac., bell., calc., chel., con., cupr., graph., ign., iod., kreos.

ABSCESS, suppurations

- **discharge,** from abscess,
  - fetid - am-c., ant-t., ***anthr.,*** arn., ***ars.,*** **ASAF.,** aur., bapt., bar-m., ***bell.,*** bov., bry., ***calc., carb-an.,*** **CARB-V.,** ***caust.,*** chel., ***chin.,*** chin-s., cic., clem., con., cycl., dros., fl-ac., ***graph.,*** **HEP.,** kali-c., ***kali-p.,*** **KREOS.,** ***lach.,*** led., ***lyc.,*** mang., ***merc.,*** mez., mur-ac., nat-c., ***nit-ac.,*** nux-m., ***nux-v.,*** paeon., petr., ***ph-ac.,*** phos., ***phyt.,*** plb., ***psor.,*** pyrog., syph., thuj., vip., vip-r.
  - gelatinous - arg-m., arn., bar-c., cham., ferr., merc., sep., ***sil.***
  - gray - ***ambr., ars.,*** carb-an., ***caust.,*** chin., lyc., merc., sep., ***sil.,*** thuj.
  - greenish - ars., ***asaf., aur.,*** carb-v., ***caust.,*** kreos., **MERC.,** nat-c., nux-v., phos., ***puls.,*** rhus-t., sec., sep., sil., staph., syph., tub.
  - sour, smelling - calc., graph., ***hep.,*** kalm., ***merc.,*** nat-c., sep., sulph.
  - suppressed - ***bry., calc.,*** cham., dulc., **HEP.,** ***lach., merc.,*** puls., ***sil.,*** stram., ***sulph.***
  - tenacious - arg-n., ars., asaf., bor., bov., ***calc-sil.,*** cham., coc-c., ***con.,*** euphr., hep., hydr., kali-bi., kali-s., merc., mez., ph-ac., phos., ***puls.,*** sanic., sep., sil., sulph.
  - thick - arg-n., ***calc-sil.,*** euphr., hep., kali-bi., kali-s., ***puls.,*** sanic.
  - thin - ars., ***asaf.,*** carb-v., ***caust.,*** dros., fl-ac., iod., kali-c., ***lyc., merc.,*** nit-ac., phos., plb., puls., ran-b., ran-s., rhus-t., ruta, ***sil.,*** staph., ***sulph.,*** thuj.
  - watery - ***ars.,*** **ASAF.,** calc., ***carb-v., caust.,*** cench., cham., clem., con., dros., fl-ac., ***graph., iod.,*** kali-c., lach., ***lyc., merc., nit-ac.,*** nux-v., ***phyt.,*** plb., puls., ran-b., ***ran-s.,*** rhus-t.
  - whitish - am-c., ars., ***calc.,*** carb-v., hell., ***lyc.,*** nat-m., puls., sep., sil., sulph.
  - yellow - acon., am-c., ambr., anac., ang., arg-m., ars., aur., bov., ***bry., calc.,*** **CALC-S.,** caps., ***carb-v., caust.,*** cench., ***cic., clem.,*** con., croc., dulc., euphr., graph., **HEP.,** iod., kali-n., kreos., lyc., mag-c., mang., ***merc., nat-c.,*** nat-m., ***nit-ac., nux-v., phos.,*** **PULS.,** ***rhus-t.,*** ruta, sec., sel., ***sep., sil.,*** spig., ***staph.,*** sul-ac., ***sulph.,*** thuj., viol-t.
  - yellow-green - ars-i., ***calc-sil.,*** kali-bi., kali-s., merc., ***puls.,*** sil.
- **exertion,** on physical - carb-ac.
- **fever,** after - ph-ac.
  - typhoid - ph-ac.
- **fibrinous,** parts, of - mez.
- **foreign** bodies, to promote elimination of - arn., ***hep., lob.,*** **MYRIS., SIL.**
- **gangrenous** - ***ars., asaf., carb-v., chin.,*** chin-s., ***hep., kreos.,*** **LACH.,** ***merc., nit-ac.,*** phos., ***sil., sul-ac.***
- **hasten,** suppuration, remedies to - ars., bell., guai., **HEP.,** lach., ***merc.,*** nat-sil., oper., phos., phyt., puls., **SIL.,** sulph.

ABSCESS, suppurations,

incipient - am-c., anac., apis, ***arn.,*** ars., aur., ***bar-c., bell.,*** calc., ***carb-an.,*** chel., con., cupr., graph., guai., ***hep.,*** ign., iod., kreos., ***lach., merc.,*** rhus-t.

menses, during - merc.

organs, of internal - calc-s., ***canth.,*** **LACH.,** ***pyrog.,*** sil.

recurrent - anthr., ***arn.,*** ars., berb., calc., calc-mur., calc-p., calc-s., crot-h., echi., hep., ***pyrog., sulph., syph.,*** tub.

slow, developing - hep., ***merc.,*** sil.

ACID, diseases of children suffering from excess of lactic, resulting from overfeeding of milk or sugar - ***nat-p.***

ACIDITY, ailments from excess of - ***nat-p.***

ACQUIRED, immune deficiency syndrome, (see Fevers, AIDS)

ACROMEGALY - ***bar-c.,*** carc., pituit., thyr.

ACTINOMYCOSIS - hecla., hippoz., kali-i., ***nit-ac.***

ACTIVITY, general

amel. - cycl., helon., iod., kali-bi., lil-t., mur-ac., ***sep., rhus-t.***

desire for - ***acon.,*** ars., aur., eucal., rhus-t.

increased - ***bor.,*** brom., ***carc.,*** cic., ***iris,*** lyc., ***med., nat-m.,*** nep., ***sul-ac., tub.***

physical - ars., coca, fl-ac., lycps., nat-s., nep., ***op.,*** phos.

afternoon - rhus-t.

evening - lycps.

midnight, until - **COFF.**

ADIPOSE tissue, increased - agar., ambr., ***am-br.,*** am-m., ang., ant-t., arn., ***ars., asaf., aur.,*** bar-c., bell., bor., bry., **CALC.,** ***calc-ar.,*** camph., canth., **CAPS.,** cham., chin., clem., coc-c., coloc., con., croc., ***cupr-m.,*** dig., euph., **FERR., GRAPH.,** guai., hell., hyos., iod., ip., ***kali-c., lac-d.,*** lach., laur., ***lyc.,*** mag-c., merc., mur-ac., nat-c., nux-m., op., **PHYT.,** plat., plb., ***puls.,*** rheum, sabad., sars., seneg., sep., sil., spig., spong., stram., ***sulph., thuj.,*** verat., viol-o.

children and young people, especially in - ***ant-c.,*** **CALC.**

gout, with - ***lith.***

heart, with fatty degeneration of - ***aur.***

palpitation, causes - crot-h.

pathological deposits, removes, of fatty matter, where the iodide removes normal adipose matter - kali-br.

people, of young - ***ant-c.***

AGILITY - apis, calc-p., coca, coff., form., lach., luna, mang., nux-v., op., rhus-t., stram., tarent., valer.

AFTERNOON, (see Time, general)

AIDS, (see Fevers)

ALCOHOL, general, (see Toxicity)

ALLERGIC, reactions

anaphylaxis, allergic attack - acon., **APIS.,** ***ars.,*** ars-i., ***carb-ac.,*** caust., ***hist.,*** led., ***nat-m.,*** psor., ***rhus-t.,*** sulph., **URT-U.**

ALLERGIC, reactions,

allergy shots, ailments from - carc., ***thuj.***

asthma - ambro., **ALL-C., ARS.,** ***ars-i., bad., carb-v.,*** chin-a., ***dulc., euphr.,*** **IOD.,** kali-i., lach., linu-u, ***naja,*** nat-c., ***nat-s., nux-v.,*** op., ***sabad.,*** sang., ***sin-n.,*** sil., stict., sulph., **THUJ.**

sneezing, with - ***ars., carb-v., dulc., euphr.,*** lach., ***naja, nat-s., nux-v.,*** sin-n., stict.

hives and swelling, with - ***acon.,*** agar., all-c., ***ant-c.,*** **APIS,** arn., **ARS., ASTAC.,** bell., ***bov., calad.,*** **CARB-AC.,** chlor., ***graph.,*** **HIST., LED.,** ***lyc., mez.,*** **NAT-M.,** ***nat-p.,*** nit-ac., ***psor., puls.,*** **RHUS-T.,** ***sal-ac.,*** **SULPH.,** ***sul-ac.,*** **URT-U.,** vesp.

rhinitis - **ALL-C., ARS.,** ars-i., carb-v., **EUPHR.,** iod., kali-i., ***nat-m.,*** **NUX-V.,** puls., ***sabad.,*** sang., sil., wye.

ALTITUDE, sickness - ***acon., arn., ars.,*** aur., bell., **CALC., CARB-V.,** caust., **COCA.,** con., conv., cupr., gels., kola., ***lach.,*** lyc., nat-m., olnd., ***op.,*** puls., **SIL.,** spig., verat.

ascending high, agg. - acon., bry., ***calc.,*** carb-v., **COCA,** ***conv., olnd., sil., spig.,*** sulph.

ANCYLOSTOMIASIS - carb-tcl., chen-a., ***thymol.***

ANXIETY, physical, (see Mind)

ARMS holding away from body amel. - psor., spig., sulph.

ASCARIDES - abrot., acet-ac., acon., aesc., agn., ant-c., ant-t., ***ars.,*** asar., asc-t., **BAR-C.,** bar-m., ***calc.,*** carb-s., carb-v., ***chelo.,*** chin., ***cina,*** crot-t., cupr., dig., dol., ***ferr.,*** ferr-m., gran., graph., grat., hyos., ***ign.,*** indg., kali-chl., lyc., mag-c., ***mag-s.,*** merc., merc-d., naphtin., **NAT-M.,** ***nat-p.,*** nux-v., petr., phos., pin-s., plat., ***ptel., rat.,*** **SABAD.,** ***sant., scirr., sep.,*** sil., ***sin-n., spig., spong.,*** squil., stann., ***sulph.,*** tell., **TER.,** ***teucr.,*** thuj., urt-u., ***valer.,*** viol-o.

female genitalia - ferr., ***sil., sulph.***

ASCENDING, agg. (see Altitude sickness) - acet-ac., acon., aloe, alum., ***am-c.,*** anac., ant-c., arg-m., arg-n., arn., **ARS.,** asar., aur., ***bar-c.,*** bar-m., bell., ***bor.,*** **BRY.,** cadm-s., **CALC.,** ***calc-p.,*** cann-i., cann-s., canth., ***carb-v., carb-s.,*** caust., chin., **COCA,** coff., conv., ***cupr.,*** dig., dios., dros., euph., gels., ***glon.,*** graph., hell., hep., hyos., ign., kali-ar., kali-c., ***kali-i.,*** kali-n., kali-p., ***kalm.,*** kreos., lach., led., lyc., mag-c., mag-m., meny., ***merc.,*** mosch., mur-ac., nat-a., nat-c., ***nat-m.,*** nat-p., nit-ac., nux-m., ***nux-v., ox-ac.,*** par., petr., ph-ac., ***phos.,*** plat., plb., ran-b., rhus-t., ***ruta.,*** sabad., ***seneg., sep.,*** sil., ***spig.,*** **SPONG.,** squil., ***stann.,*** staph., ***sulph.,*** sul-ac., ***tab., tarax.,*** thuj., verb., ***zinc.***

amel. - allox., am-m., arg-m., bar-c., bell., bry., canth., coff., ***con.,*** ferr., lyc., meny., nit-ac., plb., ***rhod.,*** rhus-t., ruta, sabin., stann., sulph., ***valer.,*** verb.

ASCENDING, agg.
high agg. - acon., bry., **CALC.**, carb-v., **COCA,** ***conv., olnd., sil., spig.,*** sulph.
amel. - prot., syph.
steps, agg. - stann.

ATHETOSIS, hammond's disease - lath., stry., verat-v.

ATONY, of body - gels., op.

ATROPHY, of tissues - ars., bar-c., chin., cupr., hep., kali-c., nux-v., phos., ***plb.,*** sec.

AUTO-immune, disorders - ars., ars-i., calen., carc., cortiso., graph., kali-ar., lach., med., merc., nit-ac., psor., rhus-t., syph., thuj.

AVIATOR'S, disease - ars., bell., bor., ***coca, cocc.,*** psor.

AWKWARDNESS, physical, (see Mind) - aeth., **AGAR.,** ambr., anac., **APIS,** ars., asaf., asar., bell., **BOV.,** bry., **CALC.,** calc-s., camph., ***caps., caust.,*** cocc., ***con.,*** dig., **HELL.,** hep., ***ign.,*** **IP., LACH.,** mez., ***nat-c., nat-m., nux-v.,*** op., ph-ac., phos., plb., ***puls.,*** sabin., sars., sep., sil., spong., stann., staph., stram., sulph., thuj., vip.
awkwardness, legs - **AGAR.,** ***alum.,*** **CAUST.,** ***con.,*** gels., ***nux-m.,*** sabad., ***sil., verat.***
knocks against things. - caps., ***colch.,*** ip., kali-n., nat-m., nux-v., op., vip.
stumbling when walking - **AGAR.,** ***calc.,*** caps., **CAUST.,** ***colch., con.,*** gels., ***hyos., ign.,*** iod., **IP.,** ***lach.,*** lil-t., mag-c., ***mag-p., nat-m.,*** nux-v., op., ***ph-ac., phos.,*** sabad., sil., verat.

BACTERIAL, infections (see Fevers)

BANDAGING, amel. (see Binding) - ***arg-n.,*** bry., lac-d., ***mag-m.,*** pic-ac., tril.

BATHING, washing, general
agg. - ***aesc.,*** aeth., **AM-C.,** am-m., **ANT-C.,** ant-t., ***apis, aran.,*** ars., ***ars-i.,*** ars-s-f., ***bar-c.,*** bar-s., ***bell.,*** bell-p., bor., bov., bry., **CALC., CALC-S.,** calc-sil., ***canth.,*** caps., ***carb-s., carb-v., caust., cham.,*** **CLEM.,** con., crot-c., ***dulc.,*** ferr., ***form., graph., hep., ign., kali-c.,*** kali-m., ***kali-n.,*** kali-s., kali-sil., kreos., ***lac-d.,*** lach., laur., lil-t., ***lyc.,*** lyss., mag-c., ***mag-p., mang., merc.,*** merc-c., ***mez.,*** mur-ac., nat-c., nat-m., ***nat-s., nit-ac.,*** nux-m., nux-v., ***op., petr., phos.,*** phys., psor., puls., rad-br., **RHUS-T.,** ***rumx., sars.,*** **SEP.,** sil., ***spig.,*** stann., staph., ***stront-c.,*** **SULPH.,** sul-ac., thuj., urt-c., urt-u., zinc., zinc-p.
face - fl-ac., plan.
cold - acon., **AM-C.,** am-m., ***ant-c.,*** **ANT-T.,** apoc., ars., bell-p., ***bor.,*** bov., ***bry.,*** bufo, **CALC.,** calc-sil., ***canth., carb-v., cham.,*** chim., cimic., **CLEM.,** ***con., dulc.,*** glon., **IGN.,** ***kali-c., kali-m.,*** lach., mag-p., mez., mosch., nux-m., psor., ***rhus-t.,*** ruta, ***sil., spig.,*** stann., ***staph., stront-c.,*** sul-ac., ***sulph.,*** thyr., ***tub.,*** urt-u., ***zinc.***
hot bathing - **APIS,** ***arg-n., bell.,*** bell-p., ***bry., carb-v.,*** **GELS., IOD., KALI-I., LACH., NAT-M.,** op., ***puls., sec.,*** sulph.
lukewarm - acon., ***ang.,*** phos.

BATHING, washing, general
agg.,
rivers, in summer - caust.
sea - ***ars.,*** brom., carc., lim., ***mag-m.,*** med., nat-m., ***rhus-t.,*** sep., zinc.
steam - lyss.
warm - acon., ant-c., ***apis,*** ars-i., bell., caust., iod., ***lach., op.,*** phos., ***stront-c.,*** sulph.
amel. - acon., agar., all-c., ***alum., alumn., am-m.,*** ant-t., ***apis,*** arg-n., ***ars.,*** **ASAR.,** aur., ***bor.,*** bry., bufol, calc., calc-s., cann-i., ***caust.,*** cham., ***chel., euphr., fl-ac.,*** form., hell., hyper., kali-chl., kali-i., ***lac-c.,*** laur., **LED.,** mag-c., mez., mur-ac., nat-m., nux-v., phos., phyt., ***pic-ac., psor.,*** **PULS.,** rhod., sabad., sep., ***spig.,*** staph., thlaspi, thuj., zinc.
affected part, of - alum., ***am-m.,*** ant-t., ars., **ASAR.,** bor., bry., ***caust.,*** cham., ***chel.,*** clem., cycl., ***euphr.,*** laur., mag-c., mez., mur-ac., nux-v., **PULS.,** rhod., sabad., sep., ***spig.,*** staph., zinc.
cold - agar., aloe, alum., ambr., ***apis, arg-n., arn.,*** asar., aster., aur., ***aur-m.,*** bell-p., berb-a., bism., ***bry.,*** bufo, calc-f., ***calc-s.,*** camph., cann-i., cann-s., caust., coc-c., cupr., fago., ***fl-ac.,*** hed., hyper., ind., iod., ***led.,*** mag-s., ***meph., nat-m., phos.,*** phyt., ***psor., puls.,*** rat., sec., sep., spig., sulph., syph.
face - asar., calc-s., cann-i., phos.
hot bathing - anac., **ARS.,** chel., ***hep.,*** lyss., ***mag-p.,*** mez., pyrog., rad-br., rat., ***rhus-a., rhus-t., sil.,*** stroph.
sea - ***med.***
warm - ant-c., bufo, flav., lat-m., mim-p., sec., ***stront-c.,*** thea.
warm bath, head, of - **PHOS.**
feet, of - pneu.
face, of - ***lac-d.,*** lyc., ***phos.***
ailments from - nux-m., phys., rhus-t.
aversion to, (see dread of) - aq-mar., bell-p., calc-sil., caust., coloc., ***hep.,*** kali-m., kali-sil., lyss., mag-p., mang., meny., nat-p., ol-an., ***phys., puls.,*** **SULPH.,** thuj.
cold, agg. - **ANT-C.,** ***bar-c., bell., caps.,*** carb-s., ***caust., colch.,*** elaps, ***form., kreos., lac-d., mag-p., mez.,*** mur-ac., ***nit-ac.,*** phos., ***phys.,*** **RHUS-T.,** sars., ***sep.,*** **TUB.**
ailments from - bell-p., mag-p., phys.
amel. - ***arg-n., arn., asar., aur-m.,*** bism., ***calc-s., fl-ac.,*** ind., iod., kali-i., **LED.,** meph., ***nat-m.***
desire for - aster., meph., phyt., nat-m.
desire for - tarent.
cold - aloe, ***apis,*** asar., caust., chel., fl-ac., ***hyper.,*** iod., ***led.,*** puls., sep.
dread, of (see aversion to) - **AM-C.,** am-m., **ANT-C.,** bar-c., bar-m., ***bell., bor.,*** bov., ***bry., calc., canth., carb-v., cham.,*** **CLEM.,** ***con.,*** dulc., kali-c., ***kali-n., laur.,*** lyc., mag-c., merc., ***mez.,*** mur-ac., nat-c., nat-p., nit-ac., nux-m., nux-v., phos., phys., **PSOR.,** ***puls.,*** **RHUS-T.,** ***sars.,*** **SEP.,** sil., **SPIG.,** stann., ***staph., stront-c.,*** **SULPH.,** sul-ac., ***zinc.***

BATHING, washing, general
face, amel. - ***asar., calc-s.,*** mez., sabad.
hot, bathing agg. - **APIS, KALI-I.,** ***lach., puls. sulph.***
parts, affected amel. - alum., ***am-m.,*** ant-t., ars., **ASAR.,** bor., bry., ***caust.,*** cham., ***chel., euphr.,*** laur., mag-c., mez., mur-ac., nux-v., **PULS.,** rhod., sabad., sep., ***spig.,*** staph., zinc.
sea, bathing agg. - ***ars.,*** carc., ***mag-m.,*** nat-m., ***rhus-t.,*** sep.
ailments from - ars., mag-m., rhus-t.
warm, bath of head amel. - **PHOS.**

BED, in general
getting out of bed, agg. - am-m., ***bry.,*** calc., **CARB-V.,** cimic., cocc., ***con.,*** ign., ***lach., phos., puls., rhus-t.,*** sulph.
amel. - ***aur.,*** dulc., ign., ***puls.,*** sep.
hard, sensation of, see Sensations, general)

BEDSORES - ***agar.,*** ambr., am-c., am-m., ant-c., ***arg-n.,*** **ARN.,** ars., bapt., bar-c., bell., bov., ***calc.,*** calc-p., canth., carb-an., ***carb-v.,*** caust., cham., **CHIN.,** coff., colch., crot-h., dros., euph., fl-ac., **GRAPH.,** ***ham., hep.,*** hippoz., ***hydr.,*** **HYPER.,** ***ign.,*** kali-ar., kali-c., kreos., **LACH., LED.,** ***lyc.,*** mag-m., mang., ***merc.,*** mez., ***nat-c.,*** nat-m., nit-ac., nux-v., olnd., op., paeon., **PETR.,** ph-ac., phos., ***plb., puls.,*** rhus-t., ruta., sel., **SEP., SIL.,** spig., squil., ***sulph., sul-ac.,*** ter., zinc.
black edges, with - **LACH.**
gangrenous sores, turn to - ***sulph.***
gnawing pain - ***sulph.***
putrid - hippoz.

BENDING, turning
agg. - ***am-m.,*** anac., ang., ant-t., arn., ***bell.,*** bov., ***bry.,*** calc., camph., caps., carb-an., carb-v., cham., ***chin., cic.,*** cocc., coloc., ***con.,*** cycl., dros., dulc., nux-v., puls., ***samb.,*** spig., ***spong., stann.,*** staph., thuj., upa., verat., visc., zinc.
affected part - acon., am-c., ***am-m.,*** anac., ang., ***ant-c.,*** ant-t., arg-m., ***arn.,*** asaf., aur., bar-c., ***bell.,*** bor., bov., ***bry.,*** **CALC.,** camph., caps., carb-an., carb-v., ip., ***kali-c.,*** lach., laur., led., ***lyc., mag-c.,*** merc., mur-ac., ***nat-m.,*** nit-ac., ***nux-v.,*** olnd., par., petr., ph-ac., plat., ***puls.,*** ran-b., rhod., ***rhus-t.,*** ruta, sabad., sabin., samb., ***sel., sep., spig., spong.,*** stann., staph., sulph., tarax., teucr., thuj., valer., verat., zinc.
backward - acon., am-c., ***anac.,*** ant-c., aran-ix., asaf., aur., ***bar-c., calc.,*** caps., carb-v., caust., **CHAM.,** chel., cina, cinnb., coff., **COLCH.,** ***con.,*** cupr., dig., dros., dulc., ***ign.,*** iod., ***kali-c.,*** kali-i., kalm., kreos., lach., mag-c., mang., merc-c., nat-m., nat-s., ***nit-ac.,*** nux-v., ph-ac., **PLAT.,** plb., **PULS.,** rad-br., ***ran-b.,*** **RHEUM,** rhod., **RHUS-T.,** ruta, samb., **SEP.,** stann., **STAPH.,** ***sulph.,*** teucr., ***thuj.,*** tong., valer., zinc.
forward, and - asaf., ***chel.,*** coff., nux-v., thuj.

BENDING, turning
agg.,
bed, turning in - ***acon.,*** agar., am-m., anac., ***ars.,*** asar., ***bor.,*** **BRY.,** calc., cann-s., ***caps., carb-v., caust.,*** chin., cina, cocc., ***con.,*** cupr., dros., ***euph., ferr.,*** graph., ***hep.,*** kali-c., lach., led., ***lyc.,*** mag-c., merc., ***nat-m.,*** nit-ac., ***nux-v.,*** petr., ***phos.,*** plat., plb., **PULS.,** ran-b., ***rhod., rhus-t.,*** **RUTA.**
double - dios.
forward - aesc., asaf., ***bell.,*** chel., ***coff.,*** kalm., mag-m., mang., nux-v., thiop., thuj.
inward - am-m., ***ign.,*** staph., verat.
right, to - spig.
sideways - ***bell.,*** bor., ***calc.,*** canth., chel., chin., cocc., ***kali-c.,*** lyc., ***nat-m.,*** plb., stann., staph.
amel., backward - acon., alet., ***alum.,*** ant-c., **ANT-T.,** ***bell.,*** bism., bry., ***calc.,*** calen., cann-s., ***cham.,*** chel., chin., cimic., cocc., ***dios.,*** **DROS.,** fl-ac., ***guai.,*** hep., hyper., ***ign.,*** iod., kali-c., kreos., lac-c., ***lach.,*** lyc., lyss., mag-m., med., merc., nux-v., plb., ***puls.,*** rhus-t., sabad., sabin., sec., seneg., sep., spong., squil., ***thuj.,*** verat., zinc., zinc-oc.
double - acon., arg-n., bov., ***calc.,*** caps., caust., cham., chin., cimic., colch., **COLOC.,** graph., ***kali-c.,*** lil-t., lyc., mag-c., mag-m., ***mag-p.,*** man., merc-c., pareir., plat., plb., puls., ***rheum, rhus-t.,*** sec., ***sep., sulph.,*** thuj., tril.
forward - apis, ***aur., coloc.,*** gels., ***kali-c., teucr.***
inward - am-m., ***bell.***
prolonged - puls., rhus-t., squil.
sideways - meny., ***puls.***

BENT, holding the part, agg. - hyos., lyc., ***spong.,*** teucr., valer.
amel. - bov., bry., ***coloc.,*** nat-m., puls., rhus-t., squil., sulph., verat.

BERI-beri - ars., ***elat.,*** lath., rhus-t.

BESNIER-boek-schaumann, morbus - aq-mar., asar., beryl., hip-ac., hist., man., parathyr., thiop.

BILHARZIASIS, (see Schistosomiasis)

BINDING up, amel. (see Bandaging) - apis, arg-n., bry., chin., gels., mag-m., mang., mim-p., puls., rhod., sil., tril.

BLACKNESS of tissues,
external parts - ***acon.,*** agar., alum., am-c., ang., ant-t., ***anthr., ant-c.,*** apis, ***arg-n.,*** arn., **ARS.,** ars-i., asaf., asar., aur., bapt., bar-c., bell., bism., both., brass., brom., bry., calc., ***calc-ar.,*** camph., canth., ***caps.,*** carb-ac., ***carb-an.,*** carb-o., ***carb-v.,*** caust., cham., ***chin.,*** chin-a., chr-ac., chr-ox., cic., cina, cocc., com., ***con., crot-h.,*** **CUPR.,** cycl., ***dig.,*** dros., ***echi.,*** elaps, euph-c., ferr., gels., ***ham.,*** hell., hep., hyos., ign., iod., ip., ***kali-p.,*** kreos., ***lach.,*** lyc., mag-m., **MERC.,** ***merc-c., merc-cy.,*** mur-ac., nat-m., nit-ac., ***nux-v.,*** **OP.,** ***ph-ac., phos.,*** phyt., ***plb.,*** puls.,

BLACKNESS of tissues,
external parts - ran-a., ran-b., ran-s., sabad., ***sabin.***, ***samb.***, sars., **SEC.**, sep., sil., solid., spig., spong., squil., stann., staph., stram., sul-ac., sulph., ***tarent.***, ter., thuj., **VERAT.**, ***vip.***, ***vip-r.***
cold - ant-t., **ARS.**, ***asaf.***, bell., ***canth.***, caps., ***carb-v.***, chin., merc., **PLB.**, ran-b., **SEC.**, sil., squil., sul-ac., sulph., tarent-c., ***ter.***
diabetic - ***ars.***, con., ***kreos.***, kres., lach., ***sec.***, solid.
hot - acon., ars., bell., mur-ac., op., ***sabin.***, ***sec.***
moist - brom., ***carb-v.***, **CHIN.**, ***hell.***, lach., ph-ac., phos., tarent., ***vip.***
senile - adren., all-c., am-c., ***ars.***, ***carb-v.***, chin., con., crot-h., cupr., echi., ergot., euph., ***kreos.***, **LACH.**, ***ph-ac.***, ***plb.***, **SEC.**, sul-ac., vip.
spots - ars., crot-h., lach., vip.
trauma, from - am-m., ***arn.***, ***calen.***, ham., ***hyper.***, **LACH.**, led., ***sul-ac.***

BLOWING the nose, agg. - arn., ***aur.***, calc., **CHEL.**, graph., **HEP.**, iod., kali-bi., lach., ***merc.***, ph-ac., phos., ***puls.***, spig., **SULPH.**, zinc.

BUBONIC plague, (see Fevers)

BURSITIS - ant-c., ***apis.***, ars., bell., ***bell-p.***, ***bry.***, graph., hep., iod., ***lycpr.***, puls., rhus-t., **RUTA.**, **SIL.**, ***stict.***, ***sulph.***

CACHEXIA, (see Emaciation)

CANCER, general - acet-ac., alum., alumn., anan., anil., ***ant-chl.***, ***ant-m.***, ***apis***, ***ambr.***, apoc., arg-m., arg-n., **ARS.**, ars-br., ***ars-i.***, ***aster.***, ***aur.***, aur-a., aur-i., ***aur-m.***, aur-m-n., aur-s., ***bapt.***, bar-c., bar-i., bell., bell-p., bism., **BROM.**, ***bufo***, **CADM-S.**, ***cadm-i.***, ***cadm-m.***, ***calc.***, ***calc-i.***, ***calc-s.***, ***calen.***, ***carb-ac.***, **CARB-AN.**, ***carb-s.***, ***carb-v.***, **CARC.**, caust., chel., chol., ***cic.***, cinnam., ***cist.***, ***cit-ac.***, clem., croc., crot-h., **CON.**, ***cund.***, cupr., dulc., elaps, eucal., euph., ferr-p., form., ***gali.***, ***graph.***, ***ham.***, hep., ***hippoz.***, **HYDR.**, ***iod.***, ***kali-ar.***, ***kali-bi.***, kali-chl., ***kali-cy.***, ***kali-i.***, ***kali-p.***, ***kali-s.***, ***kreos.***, ***lach.***, ***lap-a.***, **LYC.**, maland., med., ***merc.***, ***merc-i-f.***, methyl-b., ***mill.***, morg-g., ***morph.***, nat-m., **NIT-AC.**, ***ol-an.***, ***op.***, ornithog., ozone, petr., ph-ac., **PHOS.**, **PHYT.**, pic-ac., psor., rad-br., ***sang.***, ***scirr.***, ***sec.***, sed-r., ***semp.***, sep., **SIL.**, squil., ***sol.***, ***sulph.***, sul-ac., symph., syph., tarax., tax., ***ter.***, ***thuj.***, viol-o., visc., ***x-ray***, zinc.
abdomen, omentum, of - lob-e.
bladder - con., crot-h.
bones - aur-i., aur-m., cadm-m., calc-f., con., hecla., ***phos.***, ***symph.***
brain - acet-ac., arn., ***ars.***, ***ars-i.***, art-v., ***bar-c.***, bell., ***calc.***, carb-ac., ***carb-an.***, caust., **CON.**, ***croc.***, gels., glon., graph., hydr., hyper., ***kali-i.***, ***kreos.***, ***lach.***, merc., nit-ac., nux-v., **PHOS.**, ***plb.***, sep., ***sil.***, stram., sulph., ***thuj.***, ***tub.***

CANCER, general
breast - alum., alumn., anag., ***apis***, ***arg-n.***, arn., ***ars.***, ***ars-i.***, **ASTER.**, ***aur-a.***, ***aur-m-n.***, ***bad.***, bapt., bar-i., ***bell.***, ***bell-p.***, ***brom.***, bry., **BUFO,** calc., calc-i., ***calen.***, ***carb-ac.***, ***carb-an.***, carb-s., carb-v., ***carc.***, caust., cham., ***chim.***, cic., cist., ***clem.***, coloc., **CON.**, ***cund.***, dulc., ferr-i., form-ac., ***gali.***, **GRAPH.**, ***hep.***, ho., ***hydr.***, kali-c., ***kali-i.***, kreos., ***lach.***, lap-a., ***lyc.***, **MERC.**, ***merc-i-f.***, nat-cac., ***nit-ac.***, ol-an., ***ox-ac.***, ***phos.***, **PHYT.**, plb-i., ***psor.***, puls., ***sang.***, ***scirr.***, sem-t., ***sep.***, **SIL.**, ***sulph.***, tarent-c., ***thuj.***, tub.
axilla - ***aster.***, con., phyt.
axillary glands indurated - ***carb-an.***
bleeding - ho., kreos., lach., ***phos.***, sang., thuj.
burning, of edges, smells like old cheese - ***hep.***
open tumor - **APIS.**, ***hydr.***
pains, better from external warmth - **ARS.**
towards axilla - ***carb-an.***
contusion, from - ***bell-p.***, **CON.**, phyt.
discharge of blood and fetid ichor from livid red spot on tumor - ***aster.***
drawing pain toward axilla - ***carb-an.***
epithelioma - ***arg-n.***, ***ars.***, ***ars-i.***, brom., **BUFO,** calc., calc-p., ***clem.***, **CON.**, ***hydr.***, ***kreos.***, ***lach.***, merc., ***merc-i-f.***, ***phos.***, ***phyt.***, ***sep.***, ***sil.***, sulph., thuj.
epithelioma - ***hydr.***
face gray, earthy, oldish - **BROM.**
hen's egg in, size of - phyt.
indurations inflamed, very painful, worse by exposure to air - ***phos.***
itching, with - sil.
lancinating - **ASTER.**, ***lach.***
bleeding easily - ***phos.***
large as a small egg, as - ***hydr.***
left feels drawn in - aster.
open - ***hydr.***
nightly, pains - ***aster.***
occult - **BUFO**.
pains, with - ***hydr.***
red spots on skin - ***carb-an.***
right - ***apis.***
open, with burning pain - ***hydr.***
scars, in old - **GRAPH.**, sil.
which had remained, after repeated abscesses - **GRAPH.**
sharp pains, in shoulders and uterus, with - clem.
sleep from pain, cannot - ***aster.***
sore pain, a sort of raw feeling - **MERC.**
stinging of edges, smells like old cheese - ***hep.***
stony hard, large as tea cup - **CON.**
ulceration - ***calc.***, ***hep.***, ***phos.***, **PHYT.**, **SIL.**, sulph.
breast, scirrhus - ***arg-n.***, ars., ***aster.***, ***brom.***, **BUFO,** ***carb-an.***, **CON,** cund., hydr., kreos., lap-a., phyt., sars., ***scirr.***, ***sil.***, sulph.
burning - ***sep.***

CANCER, general

breast, scirrhus,

discharge, ulceration with fetid sanious, and sloughing - cund.

emaciated and cachectic - cund.

hard as cartilage and uneven, which has grown to size of a hen's egg, during menopause - ***con.***

heaviness - ***con.***

injury, caused by - ***con.***, hyper.

left, of - ***carb-ac.***

occasionally twitching in affected part, the mass is immovable - ***con.***

very painful, worse in cold weather and during night - ***clem.***

painful of right, about an inch in diameter, hard but movable, nipples drawn in - ***chim.***

purple, skin, in spots and wrinkled - cund.

right, in - cund.

adhering by entire base to thoracic walls - ***aster.***

with itching - sil.

sharp shooting pain - ***con.***

skin and axillary glands involved - cund.

cervix, of uterus - carb-an., carc., **CON.,** iod., kreos., thuj.

chemotherapy, treatment, side effects - ars., **CADM-S.,** chin., ***ip.,*** nux-v.

clavicles, fungus haematodes - sep.

colloid, cancer - ***lach., phos.***

contusions, after - bell-p., ***con.,*** phyt., symph.

delusion, that, he has a cancer - verat.

deposits, removal of, after - kali-p., maland.

emaciation, with cancer - acon., ***alfa., ars., carc.,*** graph., ***hydr.,*** pic-ac., thuj.

epithelioma, (see skin)

eyes - aur-m-n., **CALC.,** con., ***lyc.,*** **PHOS.,** ***sep., sil.,*** thuj.

epithelioma - cund., ***lach.***

cornea - hep.

eyelids - hydr., lach., phyt., ran-b., thuj.

eyelids, lower - apis, cund., thuj.

fungus - bell., **CALC.,** ***lyc.,*** **PHOS.,** ***sep., sil.,*** thuj.

medullaris - bell., **CALC.,** ***lyc., sil.***

lachrymal glands - ***carb-an.***

face - **ARS.,** ***aur., carb-an., con., kali-ar.,*** kali-c., kali-i., lach., nit-ac., ***phos.,*** sil., sulph., zinc.

antrum - aur., symph.

epithelioma - **ARS.,** cic., con., hydr., kali-ar., **KALI-S.,** ***lach.,*** lap-a., ***phos., sep.,*** sil.

lower - ***dulc.***

lupoid - ***hep.,*** syph.

lupus - alumn., ***arg-n.,*** **ARS.,** aur-m., carb-ac., ***carb-v.,*** cist., **HYDRC.,** kali-ar., ***kali-bi.,*** kali-chl., kreos., lach., psor., ***sep., sil.***

near wing of nose - ***aur.***

open, bleeding - cist.

scirrhus - ***carb-an.,*** sil.

CANCER, general

fear, of cancer - agar., **ARS., CALC.,** calc-f., calc-p., **CARC.,** chin-a., ign., ***kali-ar., med., nit-ac.,*** **PHOS., PSOR.,** ruta.

fungus, haematodes - ant-t., **ARS.,** bell., ***calc.,*** **CARB-AN.,** ***carb-v.,*** clem., ***kreos.,*** **LACH.,** ***lyc., merc., nat-m., nit-ac.,*** **PHOS.,** ***puls.,*** sep., **SIL.,** staph., ***sulph.,*** **THUJ.**

genitalia, female - ***arg-m., ars., ars-i., aur-m-n.,*** bell., bov., calc-ar., calc-o-t., calc-s., ***calth., carb-an.,*** carc., cham., chin., ***con., graph., hydr.,*** iod., irid., ***kali-bi.,*** kali-p., kali-s., ***kreos.,*** lach., ***lap-a.,*** mag-p., med., murx., ***phos.,*** phyt., rhus-t., ***sec.,*** sep., ***sil.,*** staph., sulph., tarent., thlaspi, ***thuj.,*** tril., zinc.

bleeding, with - bell., crot-h., kreos., lach., sabin., ***thlaspi,*** ust.

genitalia, male - ars., bell., ***carb-an.,*** **CON.,** phos., phyt., sil., spong., thuj.

glands - ***ars-i., aster., aur-m.,*** brom., bufo., **CARB-AN., CARC.,** ***cist.,*** **CON.,** ***iod.,*** **PHYT.,** ***scroph-n.,*** sul-i., syph.

adenocarcinoma - ars., aur-m., bufo., carb-an., carc., ***con., phyt.***

hodgkin's disease - ***acon.,*** acon-l., ***ars., ars-i., bar-i.,*** buni-o., ***calc-f., carc.,*** cist., con., cund., ferr-pic., ***iod., kali-m., nat-m.,*** ph-ac., ***phos.,*** **PHYT.,** saroth., **SCROPH-N.,** syph., ***thuj., tub.***

intestines, colon - ***alum., ars.,*** carb-v., graph., **HYDR.,** ***kali-c.,*** lyc., mur-ac., ***nit-ac.,*** ruta., sep., spig..

jaws - ***ant-c.,*** arg-n., ***ars.,*** aur., calc., fl-ac., graph., ***hecla.,*** merc., phos., rhus-t., sil., symph.

bones - ***hecla.,*** symph.

left - ***ars., hecla.,*** merc., phos., sil.

right - ***ant-c.,*** arg-n., ars., aur., calc., fl-ac., graph., hecla., rhus-t.

larynx - ***ars.,*** ars-i., bell., carb-an., clem., ***con.,*** hydr., iod., kreos., lach., morph., nit-ac., phos., ***phyt.,*** sang., thuj.

leukemia - acet-ac., acon., ***aran.,*** **ARS.,** ***ars-i.,*** bar-i., bar-m., bry., ***calc., calc-p., carb-s.,*** carb-v., **CARC.,** ***cean., chin.,*** chin-s., con., cortiso., crot-h., ***ferr-pic.,*** ip., ***kali-p.,*** merc., **NAT-A.,** ***nat-m., nat-p.,*** **NAT-S.,** nux-v., op., phos., ***pic-ac.,*** sulfa., sulph., syph., thuj., tub., ***x-ray.***

acute - ***ars.,*** lach., merc., merc-c., ***nat-m.,*** nit-ac., phos.

children, in - **ARS.**

lymphoid - **ARS.,** ***ars-i.,*** carb-s., carb-v., **CEAN.,** kali-s., mur-ac., nat-a., nat-m., **PHYT.,** pic-ac., thuj.

spleen, involvement - ***cean.,*** nat-m., nat-s., querc., succ.

lips - acet-ac., ***ars.,*** ars-i., aur., ***aur-m.,*** camph., ***carb-an.,*** caust., ***cic., cist.,*** clem., com., **CON., CUND.,** hydr., kali-chl., kali-s., ***kreos., lach., lyc.,*** phos., phyt., ***sep., sil.,*** sulph., tab., thuj.

CANCER, general

lips,

epithelioma - ***cic., con., hydr.,*** lap-a., sep.

lower - ***ars.,*** clem., ***merc-i-f., phos., sep., sil.***

lower - ant-chl., ***ars., cist., clem., con.,*** dulc., ***lyc., phos.,*** **SEP.**, ***sil.***

pressure of pipe - ***con.,*** sep.

ulcers - ***ars., aur-m.,*** carb-an., ***clem.,*** **CON.**, ***kali-bi.,*** lyc., ***phos.,*** phyt.

liver - ars., ***carc.,*** chel., ***chlol., chlor.,*** cholest., con., echi., ***hydr.,*** lach., myric., nat-s., nit-ac., phos., ther.

early - carc., senec.

jaundice, with - myric.

lupus, carcinomatous - agar., alum., alumn., ant-c., arg-n., **ARS.**, ***ars-i.,*** aur-m., ***bar-c., calc., carb-ac., carb-s., carb-v.,*** caust., ***cist., graph.,*** hep., ***hydrc.,*** kali-ar., ***kali-bi.,*** kali-c., ***kali-chl.,*** kali-s., ***kreos.,*** lach., **LYC.**, merc., nat-m., ***nit-ac., phyt., psor.,*** rhus-t., sep., ***sil.,*** spong., staph., sulph., **THUJ.**

hypertrophicus - ars., ***graph.***

rings, in - sep.

vorax - ars., sep., sil., ***staph.,*** sulph.

lungs - ars., calad., con., phos.

melanoma - ***arg-n.,*** card-m., ***lach.,*** ph-ac., sol.

miasm, cancer - ars., **CARC.**, ***cadm-s., con.,*** hydr.

mouth, palate - aur., hydr.

hardness, with - hydr.

noma - alum., alumn., ***ars.,*** calc., carb-v., ***con.,*** elat., kali-chl., ***kali-p.,*** merc., sil., sulph., tarent-c.

nose - alumn., ***ars.,*** **AUR.**, ***aur-m., calc.,*** carb-ac., ***carb-an.,*** cund., ***kreos.,*** merc., ***phyt., sep.,*** sulph.

epithelioma - ***ars.,*** ars-i., ***carb-ac.,*** cund., ***hydr.,*** **KALI-S.**, ***kreos.***

nose wing - med.

flat, on right side - euphr.

noli me tangere on - cist., jug-c., phyt., thuj.

ovaries - ars., **CON.**, graph., kreos., ***lach.,*** med., psor., thuj.

pain, to relieve - acon., anthr., ***apis,*** **ARS.**, aster., aur., bry., bufo., calc., ***calc-ar., cadm-s.,*** carb-an., **CARC.**, cedr., cinnam., cit-ac., ***coloc., con.,*** cund., echi., ***euph., hydr.,*** mag-p., merc., morph., op., ph-ac., sil.

penis, glans, epithelioma on excrescences - arg-n., ***ars.,*** con., thuj.

prostate - carc., **CON.**, crot-h., ***cop., iod.,*** plb., ***psor., sel.,*** senec., ***sil., sulph.,*** **THUJ.**

pain, with - carc., crot-h.

radiation, sickness, for side effects, of - ars., **CADM-S.**, calc-f., chin., fl-ac., ***ip.,*** nux-v., phos., rad-br., **SOL.**, x-ray.

burns, from - calc-f., fl-ac., phos., rad-br., ***sol.,*** x-ray.

rectum - ***alum., ars.,*** carb-v., graph., **HYDR.**, ***kali-c.,*** laur., lyc., mur-ac., nat-s., ***nit-ac.,*** phyt., ***ruta,*** sang., ***sep.,*** spig., tub.

CANCER, general

sarcoma, cutis - ars., bar-c., calc-f., calc-p., carb-ac., carb-an., ***crot-h., cund.,*** cupr-s., graph., hecla., ***kali-m.,*** lach., ***lap-a.,*** nit-ac., phos., sil., symph., thuj.

lymphoid - ars., ars-i.

scars, in old - graph.

scirrhus - alumn., ***anac.,*** arg-m., arn., ***ars.,*** ars-s-f., ***aster.,*** bell-p., ***calc-s.,*** calen., **CARB-AN.**, ***carb-s., carb-v.,*** clem., **CON.**, ***graph., hydr., lap-a.,*** med., nux-v., ***petr., phos., phyt.,*** sep., **SIL.**, squil., staph., ***sulph.***

scrotum - ars., carb-an., fuli., ph-ac., thuj.

epithelioma, of - carb-an., ph-ac.

scirrhus - carb-an.

skin, epithelioma - acet-ac., alum., alumn., arb., arg-m., arg-n., ***ars.,*** **ARS-I.**, ars-s-f., aur., aur-a., ***bell.,*** brom., calc., calc-p., calc-sil., carb-ac., carb-an., ***carc.,*** chr-ac., cic., clem., **CON.**, ***cund.,*** euph., fuli., ho., ***hydr., hydrc.,*** kali-ar., kali-chl., kali-m., ***kali-s., kreos., lap-a.,*** **LYC.**, mag-m., mag-s., merc., merc-c., methyl-b., nat-m., nectrin., nit-ac., phos., ***phyt.,*** puls., rad., rad-br., raja-s., ***ran-b.,*** ran-s., scroph-n., sep., ***sil., sol.,*** sulph., ***thuj.,*** uran-n.

flat - cund.

melanoma - ***arg-n.,*** ars., ***carc.,*** card-m., ***lach., sol,*** ph-ac.

sunlight, from - carc., sol.

smoking, from - ars., calad., con., phos.

sternum - sulph.

stomach - ***acet-ac.,*** am-m., arg-n., **ARS.**, ***ars-i.,*** bar-c., bell., **BISM.**, **CADM-S.**, calc-f., ***caps.,*** **CARB-AC.**, **CARB-AN.**, ***carb-v.,*** **CON.**, ***crot-h.,*** **CUND.**, form-ac., graph., **HYDR.**, ***iris,*** kali-bi., kali-c., ***kreos., lach.,*** **LYC.**, mag-p., ***merc-c., mez.,*** nux-v., ***ornithog.,*** **PHOS.**, plat., plb., sec., ***sep., sil., staph., sulph.***

hiccough, with - carb-an.

pylorus - acet-ac., graph.

vomiting, from - cadm-s., carb-ac., kreos.

submaxillary glands - ***anthr.,*** calc-s., carb-an., ferr-i.

surgery, after - ***calen., carc.***

testes - aur., ***carb-an.,*** clem., **CON.**, phyt., sil., ***spong.,*** thuj.

throat - ***carb-an.,*** led., tarent.

tongue - ***alumn., apis, ars., aur., aur-m.,*** benz-ac., calc., ***carb-an.,*** caust., ***con.,*** crot-h., cund., ***hydr.,*** kali-chl., **KALI-CY.**, ***kali-i., lach., mur-ac., nit-ac., phos., phyt.,*** sep., ***sil.,*** sulph., thuj.

epithelioma - ars., carb-ac., chr-ac., ***hydr., kali-cy.,*** mur-ac., ***thuj.***

ulcers - ***ambr., anthr.,*** ant-c., apis, **ARN.**, **ARS.**, ***ars-i.,*** **ARS-S-F.**, ***aster.,*** aur., aur-a., aur-i., **AUR-S.**, ***bell.,*** **BUFO**, calc., ***calc-s., carb-ac., carb-an., carb-s., carb-v.,*** caust., chel., chim., chin-s., clem., **CON.**, ***crot-c.,*** cund., dor., dulc., ***ferr.,*** fl-ac., fuli., ***gali., graph.,*** **HEP.**, ***hippoz.,*** hydr., kali-ar., kali-c.,

CANCER, general
ulcers - ***kali-i., kreos., lach.,*** **LYC.,** ***lyss.,*** mang., ***merc.,*** merc-i-f., ***mill.,*** mur-ac., ***nit-ac., petr., ph-ac., phos., phyt., rhus-t.,*** rumx., sars., ***sep.,*** **SIL.,** spong., squil., ***staph.,*** **SULPH.,** sul-ac., sul-i., syph., tarent-c., ***thuj., zinc.***
uterus - alum., alumn., anan., apis, ***arg-m., arg-n.,*** **ARS., ARS-I.,** aur., aur-m-n., bell., bov., brom., ***bufo, calc.,*** carb-ac., ***carb-an.,*** carb-s., ***carb-v., carc.,*** chin., cic., clem., **CON.,** ***crot-h.,*** cund., elaps, fuli., **GRAPH., HYDR.,** ***iod.,*** kali-ar., kaol., **KREOS., LACH.,** ***lap-a.,*** **LYC.,** mag-m., med., merc., ***merc-i-f.,*** **MURX.,** ***nat-c., nat-m., nit-ac.,*** **PHOS.,** ***phyt.,*** plat., rhus-t., ruta, sabin., sang., sars., ***sec.,*** **SEP., SIL.,** ***staph.,*** sul-ac., sulph., tarent., **THUJ.,** ***zinc.***
bleeding, with - kreos., med., phos., thlaspi, ust.
menses suppressed, from - kreos., ***lyc.***
scirrhus - ***alumn.,*** anan., ***arg-m., ars.,*** aur., aur-m-n., **CON.,** kreos., lyc., mag-m., phos., ***phyt.,*** rhus-t., sep., staph.
vagina - ***ars.,*** con., **KREOS.**
labia, vulva, cancerous - ***ars.,*** con., thuj.

CANDIDA albicans, infection - calc., calc-p., chin., helon., lyc., med., puls., nat-p., nit-ac., sep., thuj.

CARRYING, ailments from - carb-ac., caust., ruta.
agg. - cadm-s., ruta.
back, on the - alum.. rhus-t., ruta.
head, on the - calc., ruta, tarent.
amel. - ant-c., ant-t., ars., ***ham.,*** coloc., ferr., ip., kali-c., nat-c., nat-m., ph-ac., sep.

CARTILAGES, affections of - **ARG-M.,** cimic., guai., led., merc., nat-m., olnd., plb., ruta, sil.
inflammation of, chondritis, perichondritis - **ARG-M.,** asaf., ***bell.,*** cham., ***cimic.,*** led., lob-s., merc., ***nat-m.,*** olnd., ***plb., ruta,*** sil., syph.
necrosis, in syphilis - crot-h.
pains, of - arg-m., calc-p., lob-s., nat-m., ruta, sulph., symph.
sensitive - **ARG-M.**
sore - **ARG-M.,** ***rhod., rhus-t.***
swelling - **ARG-M.**
tumors - ***calc., sil.***
ulcers of - merc-c.

CELIAC, disease - carc., chin., lyc.

CELLARS, vaults, agg. - aran., **ARS.,** ***bry.,*** calc., ***carb-an.,*** carc., caust., dulc., ***kali-c.,*** lyc., merc-i-f., **NAT-S., PULS.,** ***sep., stram.***

CHICKENPOX, infection (see Fevers)

CHLAMYDIAL, infection (see Fevers)

CHILBLAINS, hands - ***agar.,*** aloe, ***croc., kali-chl., nit-ac.,*** op., **PETR., PULS.,** ***stann., sulph.,*** sul-ac., ***zinc.***
itching - **PULS.,** ***zinc.***
mild weather - stann.
swelling - ***zinc.***
chilblains, fingers - berb., carb-an., lyc., nit-ac., ***nux-v., petr., puls., sulph.,*** sul-ac.
chilblains, fingers
itching - sulph.
painful - sul-ac.
chilblains, feet - abrot., **AGAR.,** ***alumn.,*** am-c., ***anac.,*** ant-c., aur., bad., ***bell.,*** berb., bor., bry., bufo, cadm-s., ***carb-an.,*** carb-v., ***cham., chin.,*** colch., ***croc.,*** crot-h., cycl., hep., hyos., ign., kali-chl., kali-n., ***lyc., merc.,*** mur-ac., naja, ***nit-ac.,*** nux-m., ***nux-v., op.,*** **PETR.,** ph-ac., ***phos.,*** **PULS.,** ran-b., rhus-t., sep., stann., staph., ***sulph.,*** sul-ac., ***thuj.,*** **ZINC.**
cracked - merc., nux-v., petr.
inflammation - ***lach.,*** merc., nit-ac., **PETR.**
purple - ***lach., merc., puls., sulph.***
suppurating - ***lach., sil., sulph.***
swollen - ***merc.***
chilblains, heels, swollen and red - petr.
chilblains, toes - **AGAR.,** ***alum.,*** aur., bor., ***carb-an., croc.,*** kali-c., nit-ac., ***nux-v.,*** **PETR.,** phos., **PULS.,** rhod.

CHILDREN, (see Children, chapter)

CHILLINESS, general, (see Environment, Cold or Chills, Chilliness)

CHRONIC fatigue syndrome (see Generals, Weakness) - **ALUM.,** ***ambr.,*** **AM-C.,** apoc., ***ars., ars-i., aur.,*** bar-c., ***bapt.,*** **CALAD., CALC.,** cann-s., ***carb-v.,*** **CARC.,** ***caust., chel.,*** **CHIN.,** ***chin-s., cocc.,*** **CON.,** ***dig.,*** **FERR.,** ferr-ar., ferr-p., **GELS., GRAPH.,** helon., hyos., ***kali-c.,*** kali-n., ***kali-p.,*** **LACH.,** ***laur., lyc.,*** mag-m., ***mang., merc.,*** mur-ac., nat-a., ***nat-c., nat-m.,*** nit-ac., ***nux-m.,*** **NUX-V.,** ***op.,*** **PH-AC.,** ***phos.,*** **PIC-AC.,** ***psor.,*** puls., sel., ***seneg., sep.,*** **SIL.,** ***stann.,*** staph., ***stram.,*** stront-c., ***sulph.,*** **SUL-AC.,** ***thuj., valer.,*** verat.
acute diseases, after - abrot., aeth., ail., alet., ***alst., anac.,*** ant-t., apis, **ARS.,** aven., calc-p., carb-an., ***carb-v.,*** **CARC.,** ***chin., chin-a.,*** coca, ***cocc.,*** colch., cupr., cur., dig., fl-ac., **GELS.,** guare., ***helon., irid.,*** kali-fer., kali-m., ***kali-p.,*** lath., lob-p., merc-cy., mur-ac., nat-sal., nux-v., **PH-AC.,** ***phos.,*** pic-ac., ***psor.,*** sel., sil., staph., stroph., stry-p., sul-ac., ***tarent-c.,*** verat., zinc-ar.
alternating with activity - ***aur.,*** **CARC., MED.**
exertion, agg. - ***arn.,*** ars., ***calc.,*** cann-s., chin., gels., helon., nux-v., ***ph-ac., rhus-t.,*** **SIL.,** verat.
influenza, from - ***carc., gels.,*** kali-p., ***ph-ac., sil.,*** thuj.
mononucleosis, from - ***bapt., calc.,*** **CARC.,** ***gels., merc., ph-ac.,*** sil., thuj.

CHRONICITY, of complaints - ***alum.,*** arg-n., ***ars., calc.,*** carc., ***caust., con.,*** kali-bi., kali-i., ***lyc.,*** mang., phos., plb., psor., ***sep., sulph.,*** syph., tub.
stubborn - carc., kali-i.

CLOSING eyes, ailments on - ther.

CLOTHING, general
cold, as if - ars-i.
damp, as if - calc., guai., lac-d., lyc., phos., ran-b., sanic., sep., tub., verat-v.
fire, as if on - ars-i.
fit, as if would not - verat-v.
heavy, too - con., euph.
intolerance of - agar., ***am-c.***, aml-n., ***apis***, **ARG-N.**, arn., asaf., asar., ***bov.***, ***bry.***, **CALC.**, ***caps.***, ***carb-s.***, ***carb-v.***, ***caust.***, cench., chel., chin., clem., coc-c., coff., con., **CROT-C.**, ***crot-h.***, dios., euph., glon., ***graph.***, ***hep.***, ign., kali-bi., kali-c., kali-i., kali-m., kali-n., kreos., **LACH.**, lept., lil-t., **LYC.**, mag-m., merc., merc-c., ***nat-m.***, ***nat-s.***, nit-ac., nux-m., **NUX-V.**, olnd., **ONOS.**, op., ***phos.***, polyg., psor., ***puls.***, ***ran-b.***, ***sanic.***, ***sars.***, sec., ***sep.***, ***spig.***, **SPONG.**, ***stann.***, sulph., ***tarent.***, tub., verat-v., vip.
large, as if too - psor., thuj.
looseness of, amel. - am-c., arn., asar., ***bry.***, **CALC.**, ***cann-i.***, ***caps.***, ***carb-v.***, ***caust.***, ***chel.***, chin., coff., ***hep.***, **LACH.**, **LYC.**, mag-m., **NIT-AC.**, **NUX-V.**, olnd., op., ***puls.***, ran-b., ***sanic.***, ***sars.***, ***sep.***, ***spig.***, ***spong.***, ***stann.***, ***sulph.***
pressure of, agg. - arg-n., bov., bry., ***calc.***, carb-v., caust., con., glon., hep., **LACH.**, lil-t., **LYC.**, nit-ac., ***nux-v.***, onos., psor., sec., sep., spong., sulph., ***tub.***
amel. - fl-ac., nat-m., psor., sabad.
tight, as if too - arg-m., caust., chel., glon., nux-v., rumx.
abdomen, about - lach., lyc., mosch.
chest, about - meli.
neck, about - lach.
uncomfortable - spong.
wears his best - con.
wool clothing agg. - hep., morg., phos., ***psor.***, puls., ***sulph.***, tub.

COLD, body temperature (see Chills, Chiliness) - acon., ***aesc.***, aeth., ***agar.***, agn., ail., alst., ***alum.***, ***ambr.***, am-c., am-m., ***anac.***, ***anthr.***, ***ant-c.***, **ANT-T.**, **APIS**, **ARAN.**, arg-m., **ARN.**, **ARS.**, ars-i., arum-t., asaf., asar., aur., aur-m., bapt., bar-c., ***bell.***, berb., bol., bor., bov., brom., ***bry.***, bufo, cadm-s., cact., calad., ***calc.***, ***calc-ar.***, ***calc-p.***, ***camph.***, cann-i., **CANTH.**, ***caps.***, ***carb-an.***, **CARB-S.**, **CARB-V.**, cast., caust., **CEDR.**, ***cham.***, **CHEL.**, **CHIN.**, **CHIN-S.**, ***cic.***, cimic., ***cimx.***, cina, coca, cocc., coff., ***colch.***, coloc., corn., con., cop., croc., crot-h., crot-t., cupr., cupr-ar., ***cycl.***, daph., ***dig.***, dios., dros., dulc., elat., ***elaps***, euon., **EUP-PER.**, ***eup-pur.***, eupi., ***ferr.***, gamb., **GELS.**, ***graph.***, grat., guai., hell., **HELO.**, ***hep.***, ***hyos.***, **IGN.**, ***iod.***, **IP.**, kali-bi., ***kali-c.***, ***kali-i.***, kreos., ***lach.***, ***lachn.***, lac-c., laur., **LED.**, lil-t., lith., lob., **LYC.**, lyss., mag-c., mag-m., mag-s., mang., **MENY.**, merc., merc-c., **MEZ.**, mosch., ***mur-ac.***, naja, ***nat-a.***, nat-c., **NAT-M.**, nat-p., nicc., **NIT-AC.**, **NUX-M.**, **NUX-V.**, ***op.***, par., ***petr.***, phel., ***ph-ac.***, ***phos.***, phyt., plat., plan., plb., ***podo.***, ***psor.***, **PULS.**, ran-b., **RHUS-T.**, ***rob.***, ***ruta.***, **SABAD.**, sabin., ***samb.***, sang., sarr., sars., sel., **SEC.**, senec., seneg., **SEP.**, ***sil.***, spig., spong., stann., **STAPH.**, ***stram.***, sulph., ***sul-ac.***, ***sumb.***, ***tarent.***, ***tarax.***, teucr., ther., **THUJ.**, valer., verb., **VERAT.**, **VERAT-V.**, vip.
affected parts, of - ars., bry., calc., cocc., colch., lach., ***led.***, meny., mez., mez., rhus-t., sec., sil.
onesided, other, other side hot, in septic fevers - meny., puls., rhus-t.
side lain on, morning in bed arn.
afternoon, after siesta - con.
ailments from, (see Environment, Cold)
vital heat, lacking, (see Chills, chapter) - ***aesc.***, ***agar.***, ***alum.***, **ALUMN.**, ***am-c.***, ***am-m.***, ang., ***ant-c.***, **ARAN.**, ***arg-m.***, ***arg-n.***, **ARS.**, ***ars-i.***, ***asar.***, ***aur.***, **BAR-C.**, ***bar-m.***, bor., ***brom.***, ***bufo***, cact., cadm-s., **CALC.**, **CALC-AR.**, ***calc-f.***, **CALC-P.**, ***calc-s.***, **CAMPH.**, caps., **CARB-AN.**, ***carb-s.***, ***carb-v.***, ***caul.***, **CAUST.**, ***chel.***, ***chin.***, ***cimic.***, ***cinnb.***, **CIST.**, ***cocc.***, ***con.***, **CROT-C.**, cycl., ***dig.***, **DULC.**, ***elaps***, euph., **FERR.**, ***ferr-ar.***, **GRAPH.**, ***guai.***, **HELO.**, **HEP.**, ***ip.***, **KALI-AR.**, **KALI-BI.**, **KALI-C.**, **KALI-P.**, ***kalm.***, ***kreos.***, ***lach.***, ***lac-d.***, lac-ac., laur., **LED.**, ***lyc.***, ***mag-c.***, mag-m., **MAG-P.**, ***mang.***, ***med.***, ***merc.***, ***mez.***, ***mosch.***, ***naja***, ***nat-a.***, nat-c., ***nat-m.***, ***nat-p.***, **NIT-AC.**, ***nux-m.***, **NUX-V.**, ***ol-j.***, ***petr.***, **PH-AC.**, **PHOS.**, ***plb.***, **PSOR.**, **PYROG.**, ***ran-b.***, ***rhod.***, **RHUS-T.**, ***rumx.***, ***sabad.***, sars., ***senec.***, ***sep.***, **SIL.**, ***spig.***, ***stann.***, ***staph.***, ***stront-c.***, ***sulph.***, ***sul-ac.***, ***sumb.***, ***tarent.***, ***ther.***, ***thuj.***, ***tub.***, zinc.
afternoon, after siesta - con.

COLD, temperature, (see Environment, Cold)

COLDS, tendency to take - **ACON.**, aesc., agar., all-c., **ALUM.**, alum-p., alum-sil., alumn., am-c., am-m., anac., ***ant-c.***, ant-t., aral., aran., ***arg-n.***, arn., ***ars.***, ***ars-i.***, ars-s-f., **BAC.**, **BAR-C.**, bar-i., bar-m., bar-s., ***bell.***, benz-ac., bor., **BRY.**, calad., **CALC.**, calc-i., **CALC-P.**, ***calc-s.***, calc-sil., ***calen.***, camph., caps., carb-an., ***carb-s.***, ***carb-v.***, carc., caust., **CHAM.**, chin., chin-a., cimic., cinnb., cist., clem., cocc., coc-c., coff., colch., coloc., ***con.***, croc., cupr., cycl., dig., dros., **DULC.**, dys-co., elaps, eup-per., euphr., ***ferr.***, ferr-ar., ferr-i., ferr-p., ***form.***, gast., ***gels.***, goss., ***graph.***, ham., hed., **HEP.**, hyos., hyper., ign., iod., ip., kali-ar., ***kali-bi.***, **KALI-C.**, **KALI-I.**, **KALI-P.**, kali-s., kali-sil., ***lac-d.***, lach., led., **LYC.**, mag-arct., mag-aust., mag-c., mag-m., **MED.**, **MERC.**, mez., naja, **NAT-A.**, ***nat-c.***, **NAT-M.**, nat-p., nat-sil., **NIT-AC.**, ***nux-m.***, **NUX-V.**, ol-j., op., osm., ***petr.***, ***ph-ac.***, **PHOS.**, plat., **PSOR.**, ***puls.***, rhod., ***rhus-t.***, **RUMX.**, ruta, sabad., sabin., samb., sang., sars., sel., senec., **SEP.**, **SIL.**, solid., spig., stann., staph., sul-i., ***sulph.***, ***sul-ac.***, syph., **THUJ.**, **TUB.**, valer., verat., verb., zinc.
chilled, easy - acon., ars., bry., hep., ***merc.***, nat-m., nux-v., phos., puls.
cold, air agg. - acon., all-c., ars., dulc., hep., merc., nux-v., phos.

COLDS, tendency to take
cold, dry weather agg. - acon., bry., caust., hep., nux-v.
feet, from - con., ***sil.***
wet weather agg. - calc., ***dulc.,*** rhus-t., nat-s.
colds, go to the chest - ant-t., ars., ***bac.,*** carb-v., ip., ***phos., tub.***
drafts, from - kali-c., nux-v., ph-ac.
chest on, from - ph-ac.
menses, during - bar-c., graph., mag-c., senec.
first, agg. - calc-p.
overheated, from - kali-c.
sneezing, with alot of - ***all-c.,*** dulc., hep., ip., kali-i., merc., ***nat-m.,*** phos., rhus-t., sulph.
sweating, after - nit-ac.

COMPLEXIONS, general (see Constitutions, Hair)
dark, brunette - ***acon.,*** alum., anac., arn., ars., aur., brom., ***bry., calc.,*** calc-i., caps., **CAUST.,** cham., ***chin.,*** cina, coff., con., graph., **IGN.,** iod., **KALI-C.,** kreos., lac-c., lach., lyc., lycpr., mag-p., mur-ac., nat-m., **NIT-AC.,** ***nux-v.,*** **PHOS.,** pic-ac., **RHUS-T.,** sang., sec., sep., staph., sulph., thuj., viol-o.
brown, olive, disposed to constipation, sad, gloomy, taciturn - aur.
excitable - alum.
eyes - aur., graph., iod., lach., lycpr., mur-ac., nit-ac.
ophthalmia - ***apis***
rigid fibre, with - ***acon., anac.,*** arn., ***ars., bry., caust.,*** kalm., nat-m., ***nit-ac.,*** **NUX-V.,** ***plat.,*** puls., ***sep.,*** staph., sulph.
slight, lean - kreos.
spare and seven were, from eight patients, the eighth blonde - lac-c.
spare habit, yellow - ***calc.***
swarthy - ***chin.,*** **NIT-AC.**
eyes blue and dark hair - lyc., nat-m., sep.
black - **CAUST.,** ***mur-ac., nit-ac.***
blue - ***brom.,*** **CALC.,** caps., ***lob.,*** **PULS.**
dark - ***acon.,*** aur., ***guai.,*** **IOD., LACH.**
baby, nosebleeds - lac-ac.
disposed to sluggishness and indolence - ***lach.***
sycosis - sars.
fair - bell., brom., caps., lob., puls., spong.
gray - med.
eyelashes, delicate - **PHOS.**
fair, blonde, light - agar., ***apis,*** aur., bell., bor., ***brom.,*** bry., **CALC.,** ***caps.,*** cham., chel., clem., cocc., coloc., con., cupr., cycl., dig., ***graph., hep.,*** hyos., ip., ***kali-bi.,*** kreos., lob., lycps., merc., mez., nat-c., op., **PETR., PHOS., PULS.,** ***rhus-t.,*** sabad., sel., sep., ***sil.,*** spig., **SPONG.,** sul-ac., ***sulph.,*** thuj., vario., viol-o.
fibre, with lax - ***bell.,*** **BROM., CALC.,** ***caps., cham.,*** clem., cocc., con., dig., **GRAPH.,** hyos., ***kali-bi.,*** lach., lyc., merc., ***rhus-t.,*** sil., **SULPH.**
grows too rapidly - ***calc.***
hair, sandy, sanguine - arn.

COMPLEXIONS, general
fair, blonde, light
lymphatic ascites, ophthalmia - ***apis***
skin, delicate, thin, white, light hair and eyebrows - ***brom.***
skin fine - ***sil.***
spare and thin - ***apis***
women, graceful - ***phos.***
florid - ***acon., chin-s.***
blotchy, red, thick skin - kali-bi.
lax fibre, with - agar., ***bell.,*** **BROM., CALC.,** ***caps., cham.,*** clem., cocc., con., dig., **GRAPH.,** hyos., ***kali-bi.,*** lach., ***lyc., merc., rhus-t.,*** sil., **SULPH.**
pale - ***calc.,*** kali-p., spig.
delicate - led.
livid - kreos.
disposition sad, irritable - kreos.
sciatica, nervous affections, neuralgia, lumbago, with deficiency of animal heat - ***ol-j.***
scrofulous, flabby - ***merc-d.***
diseases of joints - ***ol-j.***
sensitive, irritable - kali-p.
sickly - ***lach.***
very white, light hair, and more or less tendency to scrofula, post-scarlatinal dropsy - dig.
sallow - fl-ac.
bilious - ***hep.***
cold extremities - ***lyc.***
jaundice - ***podo.***
pale, lupus, recent cases, shallow ulceration - **LYC.**
yellow, dirty, greasy skin - ***psor.***

CONSTANTLY, changing symptoms - **CARC.,** cimic., kali-bi., ***lac-c.,*** **MED.,** mosch., **PULS.,** sanic., tub.

CONSTITUTIONS, temperaments, general - bar-c., **CALC.,** ***calc-p.,*** calc-s., ***lyc.,*** **PHOS., SIL.,** ***sulph.***
anemic - ***ars., calc.,*** **CALC-P.,** cycl., **FERR.,** ***lach.,*** **NAT-M.,** ***phos., sil.,*** spig., ***sulph.,*** verat.
debilitated, rheumatic, scrofulous children, afflicted with ascarides and lumbrici - ***spig.***
face ache - ***chin.***
fluids or vitality, after loss of - **CHIN., KALI-C.**
headache, with congestion, indurated glands - ferr-i.
laryngeal catarrh - ***mang.***
nervous affections, neuralgia, sciatica, lumbago, with deficiency of animal heat - ***ol-j.***
palpitation - ***ferr., verat.***
asthmatic - ***ambr., arg-n., ars.,*** asaf., ***aur., colch.,*** eucal., ill., ***ip., kali-c., kali-i.,*** kali-n., ***mosch.,*** nat-s., phos., ***puls., sulph.***
affected by odor of blossoms - ail.

CONSTITUTIONS, temperaments

bilious - acon., ***aesc.***, ail., ambr., ant-c., ant-t., ***bell.***, berb., **BRY.**, cann-i., **CHAM.**, ***chin.***, ***cocc.***, ***ip.***, ***lach.***, ***merc.***, **NUX-V.**, plat., **PODO.**, ***puls.***, ***sulph.***
- asthma - ***phos.***
- constipation, tendency to - cub., **NUX-V.**
- dry subjects, ague, where disease degenerates into a slow fever - ***tarax.***
- headache, sick - ***iris.***
- hepatic affections - ***merc.***, ***nux-v.***
- lymphatic - ***bell.***
- mercurialization, especially after - ***podo.***
- nervous - ambr., ***apis.***
- stout and robust - ail.

cachexia - **ARS.**, bad., caps., chim., clem., coc-c., cund., ***form.***, ***iod.***, ***kali-bi.***, nat-m., **NIT-AC.**, seneg.
- africana - caps.
- bronchial catarrh of old people - ***hydr.***
- bronchitis, subacute attacks - ***phos.***
- catarrhal, or nerve deafness - ***syph.***
- chronic disease, deep-seated progressive - **LYC.**
- condylomata, of long standing - ***kali-i.***
- cough, with - **NIT-AC.**
- debility and emaciation - **IOD.**
- deep-seated, child weak and exhausted, with no other symptoms - ***sul-ac.***
- dry habit - ***nux-v.***
- dysentery, or gout - ***colch.***
- edema, with - ***ol-j.***
- fever, long-lasting cases of intermittent, when liver is involved and blood is anemic - **NIT-AC.**
- gastric and hepatic functions, disturbance of - hydr.
- glands enlarged and tender - ***kali-m.***
- helminthiasis - cina
- low state - ***iod.***
- mercurial - **AUR.**, ferr-i., ***iod.***, ***kali-m.***
- nosebleed - ***sul-ac.***
- nutrition, from faulty, and assimilation - ***ferr.***
- palpitation, nervous - ***nat-m.***
- phosphatic - **CALC-P.**
- purpura, rheumatism - sec.
- quinine - eucal., ***ferr.***, nat-m., phos.
- salt-eaters seldom have male issue - ***phos.***
- stomach, with, and liver troubles - hydr.
- strength, loss of - arg-n.
- suppression of habitual secretions, caused by a, and excretions - ***graph.***
- syphilitic eruption, pustular, or squamous - ***kali-i.***
- vomiting - ***sul-ac.***
- weakened by loss of blood - **CHIN-S.**
- wounds and ulcers, ordinary, tend to take on a bad appearance - ***cund.***
  - remains long impressed by slight mechanical injuries - ***arn.***

cancerous - ars., **CADM-S.**, **CON.**, ***hydr.***, mez., sep.
- ulcer of cervix os uteri - ***cur.***

CONSTITUTIONS, temperaments

carbo-nitrogenoid - aur., aur-m-n., cupr-ac., cupr-m.

catarrhal - **HEP.**, **KALI-BI.**, **NAT-M.**, ***sep.***, ***sulph.***, ***thuj.***

choleric - acon., ars., aur., **BRY.**, carb-v., ***caust.***, **CHAM.**, coff., **FERR.**, ***hep.***, **HYOS.**, kali-p., ***kalm.***, ***lach.***, ***lyc.***, nat-m., ***nit-ac.***, **NUX-V.**, ***phos.***, ***plat.***, sec., ***sil.***, sulph.
- ardent, disposed to anger, spite or deception, always irritable and impatient - **NUX-V.**
- bilious, dark hair and complexion, with firm fibre - ***bry.***
- dissatisfied with everything - ***apis***
- especially children - **MAG-C.**
- fever, in intermittent, without reaction - phel.
- foxy, mischievous, destructive - tarent.
- haughty - ***lyc.***, ***plat.***
- irascible - ***nux-v.***
- mistrustful, when sick - ***lyc.***
- particular, very, zealous persons, in clined to get angry or excited, or of a spiteful, malicious disposition - **NUX-V.**
- peevish - ***ign.***
- plethoric - sec.
- sedentary - **NUX-V.**
- vigorous persons of dry habit, tense fibre, ardent, irascible, tenacious - ***nux-v.***

dwarfish, cretinism - **BAR-C.**, ***lap-a.***
- mentally and physically - ***bar-c.***

fibre, lax - agar., bor., ***calc.***, ***caps.***, cinnam., hep., **KALI-C.**, **MAG-C.**, ***op.***, sabad., ***sil.***, ***spong.***
- blonde persons, in - bell., ***brom.***, ***calc.***, ***caps.***, cham., clem., con., cocc., dig., ***graph.***, hyos., ***kali-bi.***, lach., ***lyc.***, ***merc.***, rhus-t., sil., ***sulph.***
- flooding, with fainting - ***tril.***
- hemorrhages - ***merc.***
- hepatitis - ***merc.***
- indolent enlargement of tonsils - ***kali-bi.***
- light-haired children - thuj.
- miscarriage - ***ust.***
- too frequent and copious menses - ***thla***spi
- women - sec.

fibre, rigid - **ACON.**, coff-t., **NIT-AC.**, **NUX-V.**, **SEP.**
- cancerous and scrofulous people - con.
- dark persons, in - acon., anac., arn., ars., ***bry.***, ***caust.***, kalm., nat-m., ***nit-ac.***, ***nux-v.***, ***plat.***, ***sep.***, staph., sulph.

gouty - ***apis***, aspar., **BENZ-AC.**, ***calc.***, ***calc-p.***, ***caps.***, ***carb-s.***, ***cham.***, ***colch.***, crot-h., ***guai.***, **LED.**, **LITH.**, **LYC.**, ***mag-c.***, ***meny.***, sabin., ***urt-u.***
- alcoholics - **NUX-V.**
- bladder irritability - ***colch.***
- bronchitis, chronic - ***sulph.***
- deafness, paralytic - ***petr.***
- headache, intermittent, pains semi-lateral, tearing, drawing, crampy - ***coloc.***
- hemorrhage, protracted uterine - ***sabin.***

CONSTITUTIONS, temperaments
gouty,
indigestion, flatulent - **LYC.**
iritis - **RHUS-T.**
kidney colic - pareir.
neck, hard lumps on, extend to left side - sil.
neuralgia - ***coloc.***
ophthalmia, after catching cold - bell.
serous effusion in chest in arthritic pleurisy - ***colch.***
ulcers, mercurial - **LYC.**
uric acid diathesis - **COLCH., LITH., LYC.**
urine, fetid - ***benz-ac.***
glycosuria - ***phos.***
viscous, fetid - form.
hemorrhagic - chlol., ***crot-h.,*** aran., **FERR.,** ***ham.,*** **LACH., PHOS.,** ter.
atonic - mill.
fluidity and dissolution, from, of red blood corpuscles - am-c.
hemorrhoids - crot-h., ***nux-v., sulph.***
nervi-sanguine temperament - ***ham.***
ovaritis - crot-h.
slight wounds bleed much - **PHOS.**
slightest wound causes bleeding for weeks - ***sec.***
stroke - ***crot-h.***
hemorrhoidal - ***aesc.,*** **CALC.,** ***caps., caust.,*** crot-h., ***graph., ham., mur-ac.,*** plat.
constipation, with - ***aesc., hydr., nat-m., nit-ac.,*** **NUX-V.,** ***sulph.***
deafness - sil.
hemoptysis - **MILL.**
herpetic - bov., ***calc.,*** **GRAPH.,** ***lyc.***
chronic bronchitis - ***sulph.***
tumors, with - ***sil.***
hydrogenoid - ant-c., ant-t., arn., ars., caust., ***aran., dulc.,*** nat-m., **NAT-S.,** nit-ac., ***rhus-t.,*** thuj.
attacks at regular hours - aran.
feels every change from dry to wet, cannot tolerate sea air, nor eat plants that thrive near the water, feels best on a dry day, a constitution in which the gonorrheal poison is most pernicious - **NAT-S.**
hysterical - arg-n., cast., plat., **GELS., IGN.,** viol-o.
asthma, palpitation, dyspnoea, prostration, and digestive troubles - **MOSCH.**
headache - ***coff.***
from mental causes, dulness of head - arg-n.
hemorrhoidal patients, perhaps such as suffer from gout or worms, especially those of mournful or alternately sad and gay, who cry easily, are pale, easily fatigued, suffer from wandering pains, are inclined to spasms - ***plat.***
inclined to taking cold - ***bar-c.***
neuralgic headaches - ***plat.***
not - atro.
palpitation - ***sumb.***
sensation of great coldness in head - valer.

CONSTITUTIONS, temperaments
hysterical,
spasmodic asthma, caused by anxious dreams, sensation as if clothing were too tight - ***nux-v.***
dysuria - ***vib.***
wind colic - mill.
lymphatic - am-c., ***apis,*** arn., ars., aster., aur-m., bapt., ***bar-c., bar-m.,*** **BELL., CALC.,** calc-ar., ***cann-i., carb-v., chin., dulc.,*** **FERR., GRAPH.,** ***hep.,*** kalm., ***lyc., merc.,*** murx., ***nat-m.,*** nit-ac., ***petr.,*** phos., ***puls., rhus-t., sep., sil., sulph.,*** thuj.
agalactia - agn.
bronchitis - ***caust.***
exudations, tendency to mucous and serous - seneg.
flabby - ***aster.***
glandular swellings, liable to - bell.
light hair and complexion, slow to act, muscles soft and flabby - ***hep.***
reaction, weak and defective - phel.
scrofulous and tuberculous - calc-ar.
skin, light, blue eyes, feeble - ***apis***
stroke, prophylactic in - ***merc.***
melancholic - ***acon.,*** anac., **AUR.,** ***aur-m.,*** bell., ***bry., calc.,*** chin., cocc., ***colch., graph.,*** **IGN.,** ***lach., lil-t., lyc.,*** murx., **NAT-M.,** ***plat.,*** **PULS.,** ***rhus-t.,*** stram., ***sulph.,*** verat.
asthma, spasmodic, caused by anxious dreams, sensation as if clothing were too tight - ***nux-v.***
bilious, choleric - chel.
colic, wind - mill.
constipation - ***sulph.***
grief, inclined to - **IGN., NAT-M., PULS.**
phlegmatic, dark eyes, indolent - ***lach.***
pneumonia - ***nux-v.***
sanguine, lymphatic - murx.
subject to skin diseases - ***lyc.***
timid, fearful - cocc.
mild - ambr., bell., calad., chim-m., cic., cocc., ***ign., ph-ac.,*** **PULS.,** ***sil., sulph.***
easy - **SEP.**
quick to perceive, rapid in execution - **IGN.**
tearful - **PULS.**
anxious - alum.
yielding, submissive - **PULS.**
nervous - ***acon.,*** agar., alum., ambr., **ANAC.,** arg-n., **ARS.,** bar-c., ***bell.,*** **CALC.,** cann-i., ***carb-v.,*** **CHAM.,** ***chin-s.,*** chin., ***con.,*** cupr-m., dig., graph., ***hep.,*** **HYOS., IGN.,** ***lach.,*** laur., **LYC., MAG-C., MAG-P.,** teucr., ***merc.,*** nat-c., ***nat-m.,*** **NUX-M., NUX-V., PHOS.,** ***ph-ac., plat., puls., rhus-t.,*** sabin., sec., ***sep., sil., stann.,*** stram., ***sulph., valer.,*** viol-o., zinc.
ardent - **NUX-V.**
bashful, timid, ill at ease in society - ***coca***
brains, largely developed - bell.
brunettes - **NIT-AC.**
careful - **NUX-V.**
choreic - tarent.
cough, whooping - ***kali-p.***

CONSTITUTIONS, temperaments
nervous,
delicate - ***calc.***
pale, sensitive - kali-p.
dyspepsia, flatulent - ***lyc., nux-m.***
ears, noises and singing in - ***coff.***
excitable - **CHAM., HYOS.,** ***ign.***
attacks from sudden or intense emotions, or smothering passion - kali-p.
melancholic - asar.
violent throbbing, toothache drives to madness - ***verat.***
exhausted, easily, take cold easily - ***nux-v.***
habit, full - ***caps.***
hair, dark, and gray eyes - calc.
intellectual - chim-m.
irritable, excitable, sanguine - **HYOS.**
canine hunger - ***sil.***
dry skin, profuse saliva, diarrhea, night sweats - ***sil.***
hysterical, intellectual faculties predominate, hysterical neuralgia - ***valer.***
lax fibre, sour smell - mag-c.
lymphatic - dig.
lymphatic - ***apis***
melancholic, indigestion, venous constitution, with tendency to hemorrhoids - ***nux-v.***
menses, premature and profuse - kali-p.
mild, amiable, refined, sensitive, intellectual - chim-m.
paraplegia - cocc.
particular - **NUX-V.**
quick motioned, plethoric, skin excessively sensitive to atmospheric changes - **SULPH.**
sanguine - ***cann-i.***
readily affected - ***glon.***
sensitive - ***acon.,*** ail., ant-c., ***ars., calc.,*** canth., chim-m., chin-s., ***chin.,*** **COFF.,** cupr-m., **IGN.,** kali-p., ***lach., lyc.,*** **NUX-V.,** ***pall.,*** **PHOS.,** ***plat.,*** sabad., ***sil.***
amblyopia - ***sil.***
cannot bear pain - ***arn., cham.,*** **COFF.**
disposed to rheumatism and catarrh - ***colch.***
especially hysterical subjects, anomalous functional disorders of heart - sumb.
have taken too much medicine - **TEUCR.**
imperfectly nourished from imperfect assimilation - **SIL.**
neuralgic headaches - ***plat.***
pain, to, querulous or discontented - chin.
peevish, excitable, hysterical, with sanguine nervous is delicate, falls easily in love, is romantic, bears trials meekly, readily falls into clonic spasms after mental agitation - ***ign.***
remains long impressed by even slight mechanical injuries - ***arn.***

CONSTITUTIONS, temperaments
nervous, sensitive,
sluggish circulation - kali-p.
spoiled natures - mosch.
tenacious - ***nux-m.***
timid - ***calc.,*** **PULS.**
anxious, during cholera season - asar.
dread storm and are afraid of thunder - ***rhod.***
weak, desires to be magnetized - **PHOS.**
women of a sensitive, easily excited nature, dark hair and skin, but mild disposition, quick to perceive, rapid in execution - **IGN.**
zealous - **NUX-V.**
phlegmatic - aloe, ***am-m.,*** ant-t., ***bell.,*** calad., **CALC.,** ***caps.,*** cocc., ***chin., clem.,*** cycl., ***dulc.,*** ferr-p., hep., kreos., ***lach., merc.,*** mez., ***nat-c., nat-m.,*** **PULS.,** seneg., ***sep.***
air, dread open - ***caps.***
aversion to open, and dislike to exercise, physical or mental - nat-c.
awkward, easily offended, indolent, melancholic, lack of reaction, gastric troubles - ***caps.***
blennorrhea, malignant - ***thuj.***
bronchitis - ***caust.***
comprehension slow, memory weak - ***lyc.***
cold and chilly, always - led.
constipation - ***op.***
face ache - ***chin.***
fat, unclean, dread of open air - ***caps.***
good natured, timid women, and especially during pregnancy - **PULS.**
hair, light, irresolute - mez.
headache, chronic, with relaxed muscles and general debility - ***sul-ac.***
indolent - ***caps., lach.***
irresolute - mez., **PULS.**
irritability, want of bodily, well chosen remedy makes no impression - ***op.***
lax - calad.
fibre, light hair, great sensitiveness to slightest contact of ulcers, eruptions and parts affected - ***hep.***
mild and sluggish, light hair - cocc.
nourished, ill, prophylactic in stroke - ***merc.***
pale, weakly, timid - ***calc.***
plethoric - seneg.
scrofulous, restless and irritable, take cold in damp cold changes - dulc.
slow, sandy hair, blue eyes, pale face, easily moved to laughter or tears, affectionate, mild, gentle, timid, yielding - **PULS.**
tonsils, enlargement of, indolent - ***kali-bi.***
plethoric - **ACON.,** ***aur.,*** **BELL.,** ***bry., cact., calc., glon.,*** **NUX-V.,** ***op.,*** ruta, seneg., sulph., ***verat-v.***
adults, headaches with congestion, giddiness, flushed face and constipation - ***nux-v.***
apoplectic, subject to paralysis - con.
constipation - ***op.***
ebullitions - ***bell.***
nervous persons, spasms - **KALI-BR.**

CONSTITUTIONS, temperaments
plethoric,
robust - ***nux-v.,*** ruta.
seemingly plethoric - **FERR.,** ***glon.***
strong, sedentary - con., ***nux-v.***
veta - ***coca***
vigorous, gout - **COLCH.**
psoric - ***ars-i.,*** **CALC.,** ***graph., hep.,*** kreos., **LYC., PSOR., SULPH.**
chronic diarrhea - ***mez.***
impetigo, especially after abuse of mercury - ***clem.***
patient emits a disagreeable odor - ***psor.***
remedies fail to impress, lack of reaction after disease - **PSOR.**
rachitic - ***calc.,*** **CALC-P.,** ***rhus-t., sil.***
rheumatic - ***acon.,*** **CIMIC.,** ***act-sp., bad., benz-ac., calc.,*** **CAUST., CHAM., COLCH.,** ***crot-h., form., guai., lac-ac.,*** **LED., LYC.,** ***kali-i., kali-m., kalm., med., phyt., rhod.,*** **RHUS-T.,** sabin., ***sal-ac.,*** spig., ***sulph.,*** ter.
abuse of alcohol - **LED.**
angina pectoris - phyt.
ataxia, progressive locomotor - nux-m.
bronchitis, chronic - ***sulph.***
caries, with tetter - ***rhus-t.***
intermittent headache, semi-lateral, tearing, drawing, crampy - ***coloc.***
neuralgia - ***coloc.***
periosteal and fibrous tissues affected - phyt.
prosopalgia - ***phyt.***
renal colic - pareir.
sclerotitis - ***kalm.***
serous effusion in chest with arthritic pleurisy - ***colch.***
sweats, night, tearing, lancinating, sensation of cold in affected parts worse at night - ***merc.***
syphilitic and mercurial patients, especially in - ***guai.***
or gonorrheal patients - benz-ac.
urinae, ardor - ***sabin.***
women - ***phyt.***
sanguine - ***acon.,*** ars., aur., ***calc., cham., chin-s., coff.,*** **FERR., HYOS.,** ***ign.,*** murx., ***nit-ac., nux-v.,*** **PHOS.,** plat.
affectionate persons - **PULS.**
amiable persons - chim-m.
asthma, in lively subjects - ***phos.***
bilious, injured knee - apis
changes, frequent and great, in sensations, feelings changing suddenly from greatest hilarity to deepest despondency - croc.
choleric - coff.
pettish, quarrelsome, disputative, easily excited, least contradiction angers, women are weak, delicate, chlorotic, yet have a very red face - **FERR.**
good natured - ***puls.***
hemoptysis - ***phos.***
hair, black, dark eyes, lively, restless, anxious - aur.
hysterical, nervous, headache - ***coff.***
imagination vivid - ***lach.***

CONSTITUTIONS, temperaments
sanguine,
laughter or tears, easily moved to - **PULS.**
muscles soft, flabby - ***calc.***
nervous, bilious - ***apis***
plethoric - **ACON.,** ***arn.***
quick perception - **PHOS.**
romantic, falls in love easily - ***ign.***
scorbutic - ***carb-v.,*** aran., ***kali-m., merc., nat-m., nit-ac., sul-ac.***
caries of teeth - ***ph-ac.***
granular vegetations in vagina - ***staph.***
scrofulous - agar., ***alum.,*** alum., ant-t., anthro., ***apis,*** **ARS., ARS-I.,** arum-m., ***asaf., asc-t.,*** **AUR.,** aur-m., ***aur-m-n.,*** **BAD.,** ***bar-c.,*** **BAR-M.,** ***bell., brom.,*** bufo, **CALC.,** calc-ar., ***calc-p.,*** calen., caps., caust., ***chim.,*** **CIST.,** ***coca,*** **CON.,** cor-r., ***corn.,*** cund., ***dulc.,*** ferr., ***ferr-i.,*** ferr-m., ***ferr-p.,*** ferr-s., ***graph.,*** **HEP.,** hippoz., ***hydr.,*** **IOD.,** iris, **KALI-BI.,** ***kali-c., kali-i., kreos., lac-c., lach., lap-a., lith.,*** **LYC.,** mag-c., **MERC.,** ***mez., nat-c., nat-m.,*** nat-p., **NIT-AC.,** nux-m., ***nux-v., phyt., rhus-t.,*** rumx., ***sars., sep.,*** **SIL.,** ***spong., staph., still.,*** **SULPH.,** ***ther., thuj.***
air, sensitiveness to cold - cist., ***hep., merc.***
albuminuria - calc-ar.
bronchitis, chronic - ***sulph.***
chancre, soft - ***nit-ac.***
cough, suffocating - con.
debilitated - ***hep.***
difficult dentition - **SIL.**
discharge, offensive, unhealthy - ***psor.***
dysmenorrhea - ***senec.***
emaciation - **IOD.**
enlarged - **BAD.,** ***bar-c., bar-m.,*** bell., ***brom.,*** **CARB-V., CON.,** dig., ***graph., merc.,*** ther.
excoriation in throat and nose - mez.
eye troubles - ***con.***
face, pale, rather fair complexion and disposition to corpulence - ***calc.***
herpes on face, with dry, croupy cough - ***spong.***
hydrocele - **SIL.**
hypopion - seneg.
joints, diseases of - ***caust.,*** kali-c., ***ol-j., sil.,*** **SULPH.**
light-haired, sanguine temperament, ruddy complexion - ***aur.***
liver complaint - ***sil.***
lymphatic oedema, blonde hair, pale face, low spirits - ***graph.***
nervous, restless, easily startled - ***psor.***
ophthalmia - sec.
palati, ulceration of velum - ***kali-i.***
pale, thin, cachectic - ***ol-j.***
pleurisy, with croupous exudation - ***hep.***
protracted, ill-treated cases with hectic and profuse fetid suppuration - petr.
ruddy complexion - ***aur.***
slender, lean figure, thin, transparent skin, frequent pulse, great excitability of nervous system, urine of high specific gravity - ***ol-j.***

CONSTITUTIONS, temperaments
scrofulus,
suppurating fistula - ***sil.***
sycosis, with - ***cinnb.***
syphilis - ***cinnb.,*** ph-ac.
or mercurialization is added, especially if - **KALI-I.**
secondary - kali-i.
tuberculosis, incipient - ***still.***
varicosis - ***carb-an.***
venous congestions, especially of portal system - **SULPH.**
young persons - carb-an.
sycotic - ***aster.,*** aran., ***med., nat-p.,*** **NAT-S.,** ***nit-ac., sars.,*** **THUJ.**
a kind of phthisis, not true tuberculosis - ***nat-s.***
syphilitic - ***ars., asc-t.,*** **AUR.,** ***benz-ac., clem., cor-r., crot-h.,*** cund., euph., ferr-i., ***fl-ac., guai., kali-bi.,*** **KALI-I., MERC.,** ***merc-c., merc-d., merc***-i-r., ***mez.,*** **NIT-AC.,** ***petr., phos., ph-ac., phyt., sars., sil., still., sulph.,*** **SYPH.,** ***thuj.***
hereditary, in a girl - sulph.
keratitis parenchymatosa - merc.
hypopion, with sloughing ulcer - sil.
mercurial - **AUR-M-N.,** ***daph.,*** **KALI-I.,** ***lach.***
large doses of - ***petr.***
mercurial-scrofulous - ***apis***
mothers, to prevent disease in offspring - aur-m-n.
prosopalgia - ***phyt.***
torpid, cachectic swelling and induration of glandular system - clem.
tubercular - **ACET-AC.,** ***agar., ars., ars-i., arum-t., brom.,*** **CALC.,** calc-ar., ***calc-p., hep., iod., kali-c., kali-i., lach., lyc., mang.,*** merc., nat-m., ***nat-s.,*** **PHOS.,** ***pix., psor.,*** rhus-t., ***sep., sil.,*** **SPONG., STANN.,** stram., ***sulph.,*** **TUB.**
aphonia - ***phos.***
chest, oppression of, with constant irritation to cough and expectoration, causing evening fever, with hot hands and cheeks - ***kali-n.***
cough, chronic - ***nat-m., phos.***
slight hacking - tub.
expectoration, bloody, shortness of breath, no pain in chest, palpitation - ***ferr.***
hemoptysis - myrt-c.
hyperemia - ***kali-i.***
sputa, bloody or purulent, alternately - ***plb.***
venous - ***carb-an., carb-v., ham., lach.,*** nux-v., ***sulph.,*** sul-ac.
weakly - ***ars., calc., calc-p., carb-v., chin-s., chin.,*** cocc., ***colch., ferr.,*** fl-ac., ***hep., lach., merc., nat-m., nux-v., phos.,*** **PH-AC.,** sec., sep., **SIL.,** spig., **SULPH.,** verat.
assimilation imperfect - ***sil.***
asthma - ***carb-v.***
blood, by loss of - ***chin-s., chin.***
bookworms, sensitive romantic girls, onanists, rakes and drunkards - ***cocc.***

CONSTITUTIONS, temperaments
weakly,
broken down - **CROT-H., NIT-AC.**
by continued influence of syphilis and mercury - **AUR.**
caries following syphilitic nodes - ***staph.***
intemperate, abdominal and renal dropsies - chim.
mania-a-potu - ***op.***
with neuralgia - **PHOS.**
cachectic, diarrhoea and colliquative sweats, glandular affections - phos.
profound debility and great emaciation - **IOD.**
chancre, soft - ***nit-ac.***
chorea - ***stram.***
delicate persons - ***ign., nat-m.***
dysmenorrhea - ***graph.***
emaciated - ***alet.***
erysipelas phlegmonous, phlyctenous or œdematous - ***crot-h.***
fever, intermittent - phel.
florid, sanguine and nervous - chin-s.
fluids and excesses, loss of, violent acute diseases, chagrin, or a long succession of emotions - ***ph-ac.***
especially in anemia - **KALI-C.**
headache, with congestion - ***ferr.***
heart, intermittent action of, with obstruction to hepatic circulation - ***verat.***
heat, diminished animal - alumin.
hectic fever, worse after meals - ***sil.***
hernia and prolapsus, abdominal - kali-p.
irritable, lymphatic, weak, and defective reaction - phel.
meagre, melancholy, chlorotic, sickly complexion, hot flushes, burning vertex, headaches, pain in back, or hot flushes by day and cold flushes by night, insomnia - ***lach.***
menopause - ***crot-h.***
mucous discharges, subjects with - hydr.
muscular development feeble, intellect keen - ***lyc.***
nervous cough - ***phos.***
cold sweat - act-sp.
fat, or plethoric persons and such as have disease of heart and lungs, suffer from veta - ***coca***
nourished imperfectly - ***sil.***
poorly - ***merc-c.***
paraplegia - cocc.
sallow, emaciated - ***fl-ac.***
skin, fine, pale face, light complexion, lax muscles - ***sil.***
starving persons - ars., ign.
stomach, pain in, after eating - mang.
uteri, prolapsus - calc-p.
varix, large, from slight cause - ***sulph.***

CONTRACTIONS, inflammation, after - ***agar.,*** alum., ant-c., arg-m., asaf., ***bell., bry.,*** calc., ***camph.,*** canth., caust., chel., ***chin.,*** **CIC.,** ***clem., cocc.,*** con., dig., dros., dulc., euph., lach., led., **MERC.,** ***mez.,*** nat-m., nit-ac., **NUX-V.,** petr., ***phos.,*** plb., ***psor., puls.,*** ran-b., **RHUS-T.,** ruta.,

CONTRACTIONS, inflammation, after - sabad., sep., ***spong.,*** squil., staph., stram., sulph., teucr., thuj., zinc.

CONTRADICTORY, and alternating states (see Symptoms) - ***abrot., aloe,*** ambr., bell., bry., **CARC.,** cimic., croc., dulc., graph., **IGN.,** kali-bi., kali-c., lac-c., ***lyc.,*** mosch., ***nat-m., plat.,*** plb., **PULS.,** rhus-t., sanic., sep., ***staph., thuj.,*** **TUB.**
rapidly - croc.
reaction, want of, with - valer.

CONVALESCENCE, ailments during or since - ail., ***alet.,*** am-c., apoc., aur., bac., cadm-m., caps., **CARC.,** ***cast.,*** **CHIN.,** ***chin-a.,*** coca, cocc., cupr., ***cur.,*** cypr., ***ferr.,*** ferr-ac., ***gels.,*** guare., kali-m., kali-p., laur., lob., mang., med., nat-p., okou., phos., prot., psor., ***scut., sel., sil.,*** sul-i., ***sulph.,*** syph., **TUB.,** tub-a., zinc.
childbirth, after - arn., bell-p., ***caul.,*** chin., ***graph.,*** **SEP.**
diphtheria, after - ***alet., cocaine,*** cocc., fl-ac., ***helon., lac-c.***
fever, ailments from - carc., chin., ***hell.,*** lyc.
infectious diseases, after - **CARC.,** chin., form-ac., ***gels.,*** ph-ac., ***psor.,*** puls., sulph., thuj., tub., vario.
influenza, after - abrot., bry., cadm-m., carc., **GELS.,** ***ph-ac.,*** psor., scut., tub.
meningitis, after - calc., ***hell.,*** sil.
mononucleosis, after - ***carc.***
pneumonia, after - bry., calc., carb-v., ***kali-c.,*** lyc., morg., **PHOS.,** pneu., sang., sil., sulph.
rheumatism, after tonsillitis - echi., guai., lach., phyt.
typhoid, ailments from - carb-v., pyrog., sulph.

COVERS, agg., intolerance of - ign., med., merc., tab.
amel. and desire for - ***ars.,*** aur., bell., clem., colch., ***hep., nux-v., puls.,*** rhus-t., ***samb.,*** sil., ***squil., stront-c.,*** tub.
aversion to - acon., calc-s., camph., iod., led., med., ***puls.,*** sec., ***sulph.***
kicks off - **BRY.,** cact., ***cham.,*** iod., med., ***puls., sulph.***
coldest weather, in - hep., sanic., sulph.

CONVULSIONS, (see Nerves)

COORDINATION disturbed (see Nerves, Incoordination)

CRACKLINGS - acon., cean.

CRAMP - caps.
night on waking - sulph.

CRETINISM - absin., ***aeth., anac.,*** arn., bac., ***bar-c.,*** bar-m., ***bufo,*** calc-p., hell., ign., iod., ***lap-a.,*** lol., nat-c., oxyt., ph-ac., plb., sep., sulph., ***thyr.***

CORYZA, suppressed agg. general symptoms - am-c., ***am-m.,*** ambr., ars., **BRY.,** calad., **CALC.,** carb-v., caust., cham., ***chin.,*** cina, con., ***dulc., fl-ac.,*** graph., hep., ip., **KALI-BI.,** kali-c., kreos., **LACH.,** laur., lyc., mag-c., mag-m., mill., ***nit-ac.,*** nux-m., **NUX-V.,** par.

CORYZA, suppressed
amel. general symptoms - ***thuj.***

COWPOX, vaccinia (see Fevers)

DAYTIME, (see Time, general)

DENGUE, fever (see Fevers)

DESCENDING, agg. - acon., alum., am-m., ***arg-m.,*** bar-c., bell., berg., **BOR.,** bry., canth., carb-v., coff., ***con., ferr.,*** **GELS.,** ***lyc.,*** meny., nit-ac., phys., plb., psor., ***rhod.,*** rhus-t., ***ruta,*** sabin., sanic., sep., ***stann.,*** stram., sulph., ther., ***verat.,*** verb.

DEVELOPEMENT, (see Children)

DEHYDRATION - ***ars.,*** ars-i., ***calad.,*** **CALC., CALC-P.,** ***carb-an.,*** **CARB-V.,** caust., **CHIN.,** ***chin-a.,*** **CHIN-S.,** ***con., crot-h.,*** dig., ***ferr.,*** **GRAPH.,** ***iod.,*** ip., ***kali-c., kali-p.,*** led., lyc., mag-m., ***merc.,*** mez., nat-c., nat-m., ***nat-p.,*** nit-ac., ***nux-m., nux-v.,*** **PH-AC., PHOS.,** plb., **PULS.,** sec., **SEL., SEP.,** ***sil.,*** stann., **STAPH.,** ***sulph.,*** thuj., valer., **VERAT.,** zinc.
ailments from loss of fluids - ***calad.,*** **CALC.,** ***carb-an., carb-v.,*** caust., **CHIN.,** ***ph-ac.***
amblyopia - ***chin.***
dyspepsia - ***ph-ac.***
fainting - chin., ***ph-ac.***
hysterical attacks - cinnam.
locomotor ataxia - ***phos.***
vertigo - ***chin.***
weakness - ***ph-ac., sec.***

DIABETES mellitus - ***acet-ac., adren.,*** alf., all-s., alumn., am-c., aml-n., ant-t., ***arg-m.,*** arg-n., arist-m., arn., ***ars., ars-br.,*** ars-i., ***aur.,*** aur-m., bar-c., bell., ***benz-ac., bor-ac.,*** **BOV.,** ***bry., calc., calc-p.,*** camph., caps., ***carb-ac., carb-v.,*** **CARC.,** cean., ***cham., chel., chim., chin.,*** chin-a., ***chion., coca, cod.,*** coff., ***colch.,*** con., conv., ***crot-h.,*** cupr., cupr-ar., ***cur., elaps,*** eup-pur., fel., ferr-i., ***ferr-m.,*** fl-ac., glon., glyc., grin., ***hell.,*** **HELON.,** ***hep.,*** iod., ***iris,*** kali-a., kali-br., ***kali-chl.,*** kali-n., ***kali-p., kreos., lac-d., lach., lac-ac., lec.,*** lith., **LYC.,** ***lycps.,*** lyss., mag-s., ***med.,*** mosch., morph., mur-ac., murx., nat-m., nat-p., ***nat-s., nit-ac.,*** nux-v., op., petr., **PH-AC.,** phase., **PHOS.,** ***pic-ac.,*** **PLB.,** ***podo., rat., rhus-a.,*** sal-ac., sec., sep., ***sil.,*** squil., ***sulph., sul-ac.,*** tarax., **TARENT., TER.,** ***thuj.,*** thyr., tub., **URAN-N.,** urea, vanad., zinc., ziz.
debility, with - acet-ac., carc., op., ***ph-ac.***
gangrene, boils, carbuncles and diarrhea, with - ars.
gastro-hepatic origin - ars., ***ars-i.,*** bry., calc., cham., chel., kreos., ***lac-ac.,*** lept., lyc., ***nux-v., phos., uran-n.***
gouty symptoms, with - ***lac-ac., nat-s.***
impotency, with - coca, mosch.
melancholia, emaciation, thirst and restlessness, with - helon.
motor paralysis, with - cur.
nervous origin - ars., aur-m., calc., ***ign., ph-ac., phos.***
pancreatic origin - iris, phos.
rapid course, with - cur., morph.

DIABETES mellitus
weakness, in - ***arg-m., ars., lac-ac., ph-ac.***
diabetes, insipidus - apoc., kali-n., squil., ***uran-n.***

DISCHARGES, (see Mucous, secretions)

DOUBLING up the body - acon., aloe, ant-t., ***ars., calc.,*** caps., caust., cham., chin., cimic., ***cocc.,*** **COLOC.,** dros., graph., ***kali-c.,*** lil-t., lyc., mag-c., ***mag-p.,*** merc-c., nux-v., pareir., plb., puls., ***rhus-a.,*** rhus-t., sabin., sec., ***sep.,*** sin-n., sulph., thuj.

DOWN'S, syndrome (see Children, chapter) - **BAR-C.,** calc., carc., pituit., thyr.

DRIVING, in automobile amel. - nit-ac.

DROPSY, (see Edema)

DUPUYTREN'S, contracture - caust., cimx.

DUST, agg. - blatta., ***brom., lyss.,*** poth., ***sil.***
dust, in internal parts, (see Sensations, general)

DWARFISHNESS, (see Children, chapter)

ECCHYMOSIS - aeth., anthr., arg-n., **ARN.,** ars., bad., bar-c., bar-m., bell-p., both., ***bry.,*** calc., ***carb-v.,*** cham., chin., chlol., coca, ***con., crot-h.,*** dulc., euphr., ***ferr.,*** **HAM.,** ***hep.,*** kreos., ***lach.,*** laur., **LED.,** ***nux-v.,*** par., **PH-AC., PHOS.,** plb., ***puls.,*** rhus-t., ruta., **SEC.,** ***sulph.,*** **SUL-AC.,** ***tarent., ter.,*** trinit., uran-n.
returning yearly - crot-h.

EDEMA, (see Generals, Swelling)
albuminuria, with - **APIS, AUR-M.,** ***chin., eup-pur., helon.,*** hep.
alcoholism, from - ***ars.,*** calc-ar., ***card-m., chin.,*** fl-ac., helon., ***led.,*** lyc., ***nux-v.,*** rhus-t., ***sulph.***
allergic reactions, from - ***apis.***
anemia, with - ***ferr., phos., senec.,*** seneg., ***ter.***
angio-neurotic - agar., ***apis,*** ars., hell., hep., ***rhus-t.,*** urt-u.
asthma, with spasmodic, of children - kali-br.
bleeding, after - apoc., ***chin.***
bright's disease, in - ***apis,*** **LAC-D.,** rhus-t., ter.
sequelae of scarlatina - ***hep.***
chlorosis, with, in scrofulous girls - ***senec.***
debility, with - ***chin., helon.***
diabetes mellitus, with - lac-ac.
diarrhea, with - acet-ac., ***hell.***
nephritis, in - ***phos.***
diseases, debilitating chronic, after, cachectic - ***prun.***
eruption, from suppressed - **APIS,** ***apoc.,*** asc-c., dig., dulc., ***hell.,*** sulph.
exanthema, from suppressed - ***apis,*** ars., hell., rhus-t., sulph., zinc.
external - acet-ac., agar., **ANT-C.,** ***ant-t.,*** **APIS, APOC., ARS.,** ars-i., ***asc-c.,*** aur., ***aur-m., bell., bism., bry., cact.,*** calad., ***calc., calc-ar.,*** camph., ***canth., carb-s., card-m.,*** cedr., chel., **CHIN.,** ***chin-a.,*** cinnb., coca,

EDEMA, general
external - **COLCH.,** ***coll.,*** coloc., ***con.,*** conv., cop., ***crot-h.,*** **DIG.,** ***dulc.,*** eup-pur., euph., ***ferr.,*** ferr-ar., ***ferr-i.,*** ferr-p., **GRAPH.,** guai., **HELL.,** hyos., **IOD.,** kali-ar., ***kali-c., kali-i.,*** kali-n., kali-p., kali-s., ***lac-d., lach., led., liatr., lyc.,*** **MED.,** ***merc.,*** mez., mur-ac., nat-a., nat-c., ***nit-ac., nux-m.,*** **OLND., OP.,** phos., pic-ac., plat., ***plb., puls.,*** rhod., rhus-t., ***ruta., sabin., samb.,*** sars., sec., ***seneg., sep.,*** sil., **SQUIL.,** stram., ***sulph.,*** **TER.,** ***teucr., verat., verb.,*** zinc.
bleeding, after - apoc., chin.
elderly people, in - **KALI-C.**
forenoon - apoc., aur., just., kali-chl., phos., sep., sil.
morning - ***apis.,*** apoc., aur., chin., just., kali-chl., ***nat-c., phos.,*** sep., sil.
motion amel. - nat-c.
overexertion agg. - apis.
painful - dulc.
serum oozing, with - ars., ***jab,*** lyc., merc-c., rhus-t., uran-n.
fever, with - ***hell.,*** verat-v.
hectic fever, with - ***aur-m.***
intermittent - **AUR-M.,** carb-v., chin., ferr., hell., **LAC-D.,** sin-n.
after - chim., ***dulc.***
protracted, after, in marshy districts - all-s.
quinine, from abuse of, in intermittent - ***ferr.***
remittent, from - hell.
suppressed, after - ***ars.,*** chim., dulc., ***ferr.,*** merc., ***sulph.***
fluids, from loss of blood or other - acet-ac., apoc., calc-p., **CHIN., FERR.,** ***ferr-p.,*** helon., lyc., merc., sulph.
heart, disease - aml-n., ***apis, apoc.,*** **ARS., AUR-M.,** ***bry., cact.,*** calc-p., chin-a., chlol., ***colch.,*** coll., cop., crot-h., ***dig., fl-ac., hell., kali-m.,*** **LAC-D., LACH., LYC.,** ***nat-m., prun.,*** sep., ***squil.,*** ter.
diseased right heart, from - merc-sul., phos., ph-ac.
hypertrophy, from - ***ars., dig.,*** lyc.
injury, after - arn., bell-p., led.
internal - ang., ambr., am-c., ant-c., ***ant-t.,*** **APIS,** ***apoc.,*** arg-m., arn., **ARS.,** ars-i., aur., ***aur-m.,*** **BELL.,** ***bry., calc.,*** camph., cann-s., canth., caps., carb-v., **CARD-M., CHIN.,** ***chin-a.,*** cina, **COLCH.,** coloc., ***con.,*** **DIG.,** ***dulc.,*** euph., ***ferr.,*** ferr-ar., ***ferr-p.,*** guai., **HELL.,** hep., hyos., iod., ***ip., kali-ar., kali-c.,*** kali-p., kali-s., lach., lact., laur., ***led.,*** lyc., ***merc.,*** mez., mur-ac., nit-ac., ph-ac., phos., puls., ***rhus-t.,*** sabad., samb., sars., ***seneg., sep.,*** sil., spig., spong., ***squil.,*** stann., stram., **SULPH., TER.,** teucr., verat., viol-t.
kidney - ***apis, asc-c.,*** calc-p., chim., **COLCH.,** coloc., crot-h., eup-pur, sal-ac.
affections, with, prostration - ***ter.***
albuminuria, after scarlatina - cop.
congestion of - ***ter.***
pain in region of - ***dulc.***

EDEMA, general
  kidney, disease
    rapid - ter.
  liver, disease of - **AUR-M.,** ***card-m., chim., chin.,*** cupr-m., ***fl-ac.,*** iris, lach., lept., ***lyc.,*** merc., merc-sul.
  meningitis - apis, ars., ***calc., dig., graph.,*** helon., merc., senec.
  menstrual disorder, from puberty or menopause - puls.
  motion amel. - nat-c.
  newborn, in - ***apis,*** carb-v., coffin., dig., lach., sec.
  overexertion agg. - apis.
  painful - apis, dulc.
  part, around affected - crot-h.
  pregnancy, in - **APIS,** ***apoc., ars.,*** aur-m., colch., ***dig.,*** dulc., hell., helon., ***jab.,*** lyc., merc., merc-c., nat-m., sanic., uran-n.
  quinine, abuse of - apoc., chin.
  red - apis, com.
  saccular - apis, ars., kali-c.
  scarlet fever, from - acon., ***apis, apoc.,*** asc-c., colch., dig., dulc., ***hell., hep.,*** juni., lach., piloc., squil., ***ter.***
  scarlatina, after - ***acet-ac.,*** acon., ***ambr.,*** **APIS,** apoc., **ARS.,** ***asc-c.,*** **AUR-M.,** bar-c., ***bar-m., calc., colch.,*** coloc., cop., ***crot-h.,*** dig., ***dulc.,*** **HELL.,** ***hep.,*** juni., juni., **LACH.,** ***merc., nat-m.,*** nat-s., ***phos.,*** piloc., squil., ***stram.,*** **TER.,** verat-v., zinc.
  serum, oozing, with - ars., lyc., rhus-t.
  soreness in uterine region, with - conv.
  spleen disease, from - **AUR-M.,** ***card-m.,*** **CEAN.,** ***chim., chin.,*** cupr-m., ***fl-ac.,*** iris, **LACH.,** lept., liatr., ***lyc.,*** merc., merc-sul., querc., squil.
    enlargement of, with - ***chin-s.***
  sprain, after - arn., bov., bry., led.
  stone cutters, in - ***sil.***
  sudden - apis, kali-n.
  suppressed, exanthema, from - ***apis,*** hell., zinc.
  thirst, with - ***acet-ac.,*** acon., **APIS,** ***apoc.,*** ars.
    without - ***apis,*** hell.
  uremic symptoms, with - **APIS.**
  urine, black - **LACH.**
    turbid - ***rhus-t.***
    suppressed, from - ***apis,*** aral-h., ***hell.***
      fever and debility, with - hell.

EFFICIENCY, increased - agar., ars., coca, coff., kola., lach., nat-p., op., pic-ac., pip-m., stram.

ELDERLY, people - acet-ac., ***acon., agar., agn.,*** all-s., ***aloe, alum.,*** alumn., **AMBR.,** ***am-c.,*** am-m., ***ammc., anac., ant-c.,*** ant-t., apis., ***arg-n., arn., ars.,*** **AUR., BAR-C.,** ***bar-m., bry.,*** **CALC.,** ***calc-p.,*** camph., caps., ***carb-an., carb-v., caust.,*** chin., chin-s., cic., **COCA,** cocc., ***colch., con.,*** crot-h., cupr., dig., ***fl-ac.,*** gamb., gins., ***graph., hydr., hyos., iod., irid., iris.,*** kali-ar., kali-bi., **KALI-C.,** kreos., **LACH., LYC.,**

ELDERLY, people - merc., mill., nat-c., ***nat-m.,*** nat-s., ***nit-ac.,*** nux-m., nux-v., **OP.,** orch., ***ov.,*** ph-ac., **PHOS.,** puls., rhus-t., ruta.., sanic., sars., sabad., **SEC., SEL.,** ***seneg.,*** sep., **SIL.,** sul-ac., ***sulph.,*** sumb., syph., ter., ***teucr., thiosin.,*** thuja., tub., ***verat.,*** zinc.
    asthma - **AMBR.,** am-c., ant-c., ant-t., **ARS.,** aur., ***bar-c.,*** camph., ***carb-v.,*** caust., chin., kali-c., lach., teucr., nat-s., op., sulph.
    brain, atrophy of - alum., con., phos.
    bronchitis - ***am-c.,*** **ANT-T.,** ***carb-v., dros.,*** eucal., hippoz., ***hydr., lyc., nux-v., seneg., verat.***
    cramps in legs - **CALC.,** cupr., ***cupr-ac., mag-p.***
    deafness - ***cic.***
      paralytic - ***petr.***
    depression, in - ***aur.***
    obesity - am-c., **AUR., CALC.,** fl-ac., **KALI-C.,** op., sec.
    vision weak - **AUR., PHOS.**

ELECTRICITY, general
    amel. - sil.
    ailments from - nat-c.
    electroshock, agg. - phos.
      ailments from - morph., phos.
    spark sensation - agar., arg-m., calc., ***calc-p.,*** lyc., nat-m., **SEC.,** sel.

ELEPHANTIASIS - ***anac., ars.,*** calo., card-m., ***elae.,*** graph., ham., hell., hippoz., ***hydr.,*** iod., lyc., ***myris.,*** sil., still.
    arabum - ars., ***hydrc.,*** myris., ***sil.***

EMACIATION, general - **ABROT.,** ***acet-ac., agar., alum.,*** alumn., ***ambr.,*** am-c., am-m., anac., ant-c., ant-t., ***apis, arg-m., arg-n.,*** arn., **ARS., ARS-I.,** asc-t., aur-m., **BAR-C.,** ***bar-m.,*** bor., ***bry., bufo, cact.,*** **CALC., CALC-I.,** ***calc-p., camph., canth., carb-s., carb-v., cham., chel.,*** **CHIN.,** chin-a., ***chlor., chion.,*** cina, ***clem., cocc., colch., coloc.,*** con., cor-r., ***crot-c.,*** crot-t., ***cupr.,*** dig., dros., dulc., **FERR.,** ***ferr-ar., ferr-i., ferr-m., fl-ac.,*** **GRAPH.,** ***guai.,*** **HELL.,** ***helon., hep., hippoz., hydr., ign.,*** **IOD.,** ***ip.,*** kali-ar., kali-bi., ***kali-c., kali-i., kali-p.,*** kali-s., ***kreos., lach.,*** **LYC.,** mag-c., mag-m., ***merc.,*** mez., mur-ac., ***nat-a., nat-c.,*** **NAT-H., NAT-M.,** ***nat-p., nat-s.,*** **NIT-AC.,** nux-m., **NUX-V.,** ***ol-j., op., petr., ph-ac.,*** **PHOS., PLB.,** ***psor., puls.,*** ruta., samb., ***sars., sec.,*** **SEL.,** sep., **SIL.,** spig., spong., **STANN.,** staph., ***stram., stront-c.,*** **SULPH.,** sumb., ***taren***
  abdomen - ***iod.***
    large - **CALC.,** ***sars.,*** **SULPH.**
  abscesses, suppurations, with - cetr., ***chin., hep.,*** **SIL.**
  affected, parts - ars., bry., caust., ***carb-v.,*** cupr., dulc., **GRAPH., LED.,** ***lyc., mez.,*** nat-m., ***nit-ac.,*** nux-v., ***phos.,*** ph-ac., **PLB., PULS., SEC.,** sel., sep., sil.
  anemia, chlorosis - ***ferr.***
    weakness, with - ferr., **PLB.**

EMACIATION, general
appetite, good - ***calc.,*** **IOD., NAT-M.,** ***petr.***
loss of - ***chel.***
ravenous - ***abrot.,*** acet-ac., ars., ars-i., bar-c., bar-i., calc., calc-f., ***chin.,*** **CINA,** con., **IOD.,** luf-op., ***lyc., nat-m.,*** sanic., sil., thyr., tub., uran-n.
ascites, from loss of fluids - chin., **LYC.**
asthma, in - kali-p.
back, of - tab.
lumbago, with - coloc.
bladder, catarrh - ***canth.***
cystitis, with - ***eup-pur.***
brain, affection, with dry, flaccid skin - ***hell.***
hydrocephalus, traumatic - ***calc.***
tubercular meningitis - ***lyc.***
breasts, inflammation - phos., phyt.
bronchitis - ***uran-n.***
cachexia - acet-ac., arg-m., arg-n., arn., **ARS.,** ars-i., bad., bond., calc., caps., carb-ac., chim., chin., clem., ***coc-c.,*** cund., fl-ac., ***form., hydr., iod., kali-bi.,*** mang., merc., merc-n., morph., mur-ac., nat-m., **NIT-AC.,** phos., phyt., pic-ac., plb., sec., seneg., thal., thuj., vip.
catarrh, acute - ***ant-t.***
certain, parts - bry., calc., caps., ***caust.,*** carb-v., con., dulc., graph., ***iod.,*** led., ***mez.,*** nat-m., nit-ac., ph-ac., **PLB.,** ***sel.,*** sil.
children, (see Children, chapter)
childbirth, after - caul.
chorea, in - ***agar.,*** chlol., ***mygal.***
clavicles, about the - ***lyc., nat-m.***
cold, after catching - ***ip.***
coldness, lies as if dead, yet conscious - ***carb-v.***
cough, with - acet-ac., ***ambr., coff., ferr.,*** **NIT-AC.**
bronchial irritation, from - ***lyc.***
chronic - ***aesc., ol-j.***
whooping - ***cor-r.,*** phel.
diabetes, with - **ARG-M.,** ***ars.,*** **PH-AC.,** rat., tarent., ***uran-n.***
appetite, with good - ***coloc.***
diarrhea - **ACET-AC.,** apis, ***arg-n.,*** **ARS.,** ***bor.,*** **CALC.,** ***calc-p.,*** **CHIN., FERR.,** ***ferr-s.,*** gamb., ***iod.,*** kreos., lyc., **NAT-M.,** ***nit-ac., nux-v., op., petr., phos.,*** **SARS.,** sep., ***sil.,*** sulph.
camp - ***lept.***
chronic - ***ang.,*** chin., coloc., ***dulc., gamb.,*** podo., thuj.
chronic, in adults - ***ol-j.***
rapid - **PHOS.**
watery diarrhea, after attacks of - sil.
diphtheria, in - ***merc-cy.***
diseased, limb - ars., bry., ***carb-v.,*** dulc., ***graph.,*** **LED.,** ***mez.,*** nat-m., nit-ac., ph-ac., phos., **PLB., PULS.,** ***sec.,*** sel., ***sep.,*** sil.
downwards, spreads - calc., cench., ***lyc., nat-m.,*** psor., sanic., sars.
dysentery - ***bar-m.,*** chin., ***ham., merc-c., zinc.***
chronic - chin., nux-v.

EMACIATION, general
elderly, people - ***ambr.,*** anac., ars., **BAR-C.,** carb-v., ***carc.,*** chin., chin-s., ***fl-ac., hydr.,*** **IOD.,** kali-p., **LYC.,** nit-ac., op., rhus-t., ***sec., sel., sil.***
elderly, of, people - **BAR-C.,** kali-p.,
edema, in - ***fl-ac.***
eruption, dry, itch like, with - ***sars.***
esophagus, stricture - phos.
feeding and medicines, in spite of - mag-c.
dehydration, from - **CHIN., LYC., SEL.,** ***verat.***
face, bloated - bar-c.
chronic diarrhea, in - ***calc.***
pale - ***cact.,*** graph., ***nat-c., sil.***
suffering expression - **SIL.**
feet, of - ***ars.,*** **CAUST.,** chin.
fever, hectic, and night sweats - ***cocc.***
intermittent - ***aran.***
particularly of face - tarent.
typhoid, in - ***ter.***
gout, in - ***kali-i.***
grief, after - ign., petr., ***ph-ac.***
hands - chin., ***phos.,*** sel.
heat, hot hands and head - ***ol-j.***
heart, disease - ***cact.***
rheumatic disease - ***cact.***
hysteria - sil.
insanity, with - arn., ***ars.,*** calc., chin., graph., hyos., lach., lyc., nat-m., nit-ac., nux-v., phos., puls., sil., sulph., ***verat.***
kidneys, diseased - ***hep.***
bright's disease - ***iod.***
chronic passive hemorrhage - ter.
lactation, milk scanty and watery - ***plb.***
liver, affection - ***mag-m.***
atrophy, chronic - ***merc.***
drying of body - ***merc.***
dropsy, with, affection - ***fl-ac.***
hypertrophied - ***chen-v.***
lungs, hemoptysis, laryngitis, chronic bronchitis - tab.
hectic, accompanied by phthisical condition - merc-c.
scrofulous - ***jug-c.***
measles - stict.
marasmus after - ***hydr.***
menses, after - ***phos.***
irregular - ***dig.***
mucous membrane, chronic ulceration - kali-bi.
muscular, progressive - ars., carb-s., hyper., kali-hp., ***phos.,*** phys., ***plb.,*** sec.
muscles, relaxation - ***lach.***
neck - ***calc-p.,*** **NAT-M.**
beginning - ***nat-m.***
chronic diarrhea, in - ***calc.***
nerves, with loss of sensation of touch - ***kali-p.***
pancreas, diseased, during last weeks - ***atro.***
paralyzed, part - ***kali-p.,*** nux-v., **PLB.,** ***sec., sep.***

EMACIATION, general
paralysis, with - cupr-m., **GRAPH.,** plb., ***sep.***
sclerosis of cerebrospinal system - **PLB.**
rapid - ***sec.***
wrist drop alternating with colic - **PLB.**
pining boys - **AUR., LYC.,** ***nat-m., ph-ac.,*** **TUB.**
pleurisy - ***ferr-m.***
pneumonia, in, hectic - ***arn.***
progressive - ***nit-ac., ph-ac.***
bronchitis, in - ***iod.***
gradual - ***led.***
hemoptysis - ***acal.***
months, for twelve - ***arg-n.***
muscular - ***phys.,*** crot-h.
onanism, after - tarent.
purpura - led.
slowly - ***cupr-m.***
typhus, after - ***myos.***
rapid - ***ars., ars-i.,*** iod., ***mag-c.,*** **PHOS., PLB.,** ***podo.,*** samb., ***sulph., thuj., tub.***
diarrhea, with - **CHIN.,** ferr-m.
fever, in typhus or intermittent - ***ars.***
paralyzed parts, of - ***sec.***
sweat, with cold, and debility - ***ars., tub., verat.***
rectal troubles - paeon.
rheumatism - viol-o.
arthritic - spig.
chronic, of left hip joint - ***phyt.***
complicated with - ***colch.***
sexual, excesses, from - agn., ***samb.***
impotence - agn., mosch., sel.
seminal losses, from - agn., ***dig., samb.***
sciatica, in - ***ferr.***
scrofulous - ***ars.,*** **BAR-C.,** ***bell.,*** cetr., ***ferr-i., iod.***
children - ***ant-t., bell.***
skin disease, with - ***bar-c.***
swelling of cervical glands - ***bar-m.***
shrivelled up look, with - abrot., ***arg-n.,*** fl-ac., kreos., op., sanic., sars., sil., ***sulph.***
single parts - bar-c., bry., calc., caps., carb-v., ***caust.,*** con., dulc., graph., ***iod.,*** led., ***mez.,*** nat-m., nit-ac., ph-ac., ***plb., puls.,*** sec., ***sel.,*** sil., ***sulph.***
stomach, cancer, with - ars., ***cund., hydr.,*** mez.
stomach, blow, after a - ***arn.***
cardialgia - plb., stram.
dyspepsia, in chronic - ***hydr-ac.***
flatulent - sal-ac.
gastric disorder - ***atro., kreos., merc-d.***
hematemesis - nat-m.
mucous membrane, degeneration of - ***kali-i.***
perforating ulcer - ***kali-c.***
suppuration, from excessive - ***ph-ac.***
syphilis, in - ***aur-m., lyc.***
throat, ulcerated sore - ***kali-bi.***
tuberculosis, in - all-s., ars., ***ars-i.,*** calc-p., erio., ***ferr-i., hydr., iod.,*** myos., ***nat-a., nit-ac.,*** phos., ***ph-ac.,*** sil., ***tub.***
colliquative night sweat - ***nit-ac.***

EMACIATION, general
upwards, spreads - abrot., arg-n.
uterus, neuralgia - nux-v.
weakness, too weak to walk alone - ***chel.***
worms, from - ***cina.***

EXERTION, physical agg. (see Mind) - acon., ***agar.,*** **ALUM.,** ***alumn., ambr.,*** am-c., am-m., ***anac.,*** ant-c., ***ant-t.,*** apis, apoc., ***arg-m., arg-n.,*** **ARN., ARS., ARS-I.,** asaf., asar., aur., ***bar-c., benz-ac., bol.,*** bor., bov., **BRY.,** ***cact.,*** **CALC.,** ***calc-p.,*** **CALC-S.,** ***cann-s., carb-v., caust., chel., chin.,*** chin-a., cic., cina, **COCC.,** coff., ***colch.,*** **CON.,** croc., ***crot-h.,*** cycl., **DIG.,** euphr., ***ferr., ferr-ar.,*** **FERR-I.,** ferr-p., **GELS.,** graph., ***guai., ham.,*** hell., ***helon., hep.,*** ign., **IOD.,** ip., ***kali-ar., kali-bi., kali-c.,*** kali-n., ***kali-p.,*** kali-s., ***kalm., kreos., lach.,*** **LAUR.,** led., lil-t., ***lob., lycps., lyc.,*** meny., ***merc., merc-c., mur-ac.,*** murx., naja, **NAT-A., NAT-C., NAT-M.,** ***nat-p.,*** nit-ac., nux-m., ***nux-v.,*** olnd., ***ox-ac., ph-ac., phos.,*** **PIC-AC.,** plat., ***plb., podo., psor., puls., rheum,*** rhod., **RHUS-T.,** ***ruta.,*** sabad., ***sabin., sang.,*** sars., sec., **SEL., SEP.,** sil., sol-n., **SPIG., SPONG.,** squil., **STANN., STAPH., SULPH.,** sul-ac., ***tarent.,*** thuj., ***tub., valer.,*** verat., ***zinc.***
mental symptoms - plb., sil.
ailments from - agar., alum., ***arn.,*** ars., calc., carb-an., carb-v., cimic., cocc., con., epip., kali-c., mill., nat-c., ovi-g-p., rhus-t., ruta, sanic., scut., sel., ***sil.,*** sulph., ter.
amel. - agar., alumn., brom., canth., carc., fl-ac., ***hep., ign.,*** kali-br., kali-c., **LIL-T.,** nat-m., phys., plb., rauw., ***rhus-t., sep.,*** sil., stann., thlaspi, tril.
air, open in - rauw.
mental symptoms - calc., ***iod., rhus-t., sep.,*** tarent.
impossible - calc-i.

FALLING, liability to - arn., ***caust.,*** iod., mag-c., nux-v., ph-ac., phos.
falling to ground, rolls about, and - cic.
suddenly, when walking or standing - mang.
through, as if - benz.
unconscious - cocc.
screams, and - bufo.
falling out, sensation as if (see Sensations, general)

FANNED, being, agg. - mez.
amel. - ant-t., apis, ***arg-n.,*** bapt., **CARB-V.,** ***chin.,*** chlol., crot-h., ferr., kali-n., lach., med., sec., xan.
desire to be - apis, ars., bapt., **CARB-V.,** caust., chin., chlol., chlor., chol., glon., hist., kali-n., lach., lyc., med., nux-m., ***puls., sec.,*** sulph., tab., zinc.

FATTY degeneration, of organs - ***ars.,*** **AUR.,** ***calc-ar., cupr.,*** kali-c., ***lac-d., lyc.,*** merc., **PHOS.,** vanad.

FEATHER-bed, agg. - ***asaf.,*** cocc., ***coloc.,*** led., lyc., **MANG.,** ***merc., psor., sulph.***

FEELS good and bad by turns - alum., carc., ***med.,*** psor.

FISTULA - alum., aur-m., bac., bar-m., ***berb.,*** bry., bufo, cact., **CALC.,** ***calc-f.,*** calc-hp., ***calc-p.,*** calc-s., ***calen.,*** carb-v., **CAUST.,** con., cop., cund., eucal., ***fl-ac., hep.,*** hydr., iris, kali-c., kreos., lach., **LYC.,** maland., ***nat-s., nit-ac.,*** ol-j., petr., ***phos., puls.,*** pyrog., querc., **SIL.,** stram., stront-c., **SULPH.,** thuj., ***tub.,*** tub-k.
alternates with chest disorders - berb., calc-p., ***sil.***
closing, after - kali-c.
glands, of - cist., lyc., merc., ***phos.,*** phyt., ***sil., sulph.***
operation of, after - berb., calc., calc-p., caust., graph., sil., sulph., thuj.
ulcers of skin, with - ***agar.,*** ant-c., ars., ***asaf.,*** aur., bar-c., ***bell.,*** **BRY., CALC.,** calc-mur., ***calc-p.,*** calc-s., carb-ac., carb-s., ***carb-v.,*** **CAUST.,** chel., ***cinnb.,*** clem., ***con., fl-ac., hep., hippoz.,*** kreos., ***lach.,*** led., **LYC.,** ***merc., mill.,*** nat-c., ***nat-m.,*** nat-p., ***nit-ac., petr.,*** **PHOS., PULS.,** rhus-t., ruta, sabin., sel., stann.

FLABBY, feeling (see Sensations, general)

FLATUS passing, agg. - aloe, ars-i., caust., chin., cocc., fl-ac., mur-ac., nat-p., olnd., ph-ac., podo., verat.
amel. - **CARB-V.,** coloc., ***lyc.,*** nat-s., ***nux-v.,*** puls., sang., scop., staph., sulph.

FOREIGN bodies, sensation as if small foreign bodies or grains of sand were under the skin - **COCAINE.**

FORENOON, (see Time, general)

FRICTION, agg. - con., sep., tell.

FROSTBITE, ailments from (see Emergency) - zinc.

FUNGUS, infection (see Tinea)

GAIT reeling, staggering, tottering and wavering - acet-ac., acon., **AGAR.,** agro., ail., ***alum.,*** am-c., anan., ang., ant-c., ***arg-m.,*** arn., ars., ars-s-f., ***asar.,*** aster., astra-m., aur., aur-s., **BELL.,** bov., **BRY.,** calc., calc-p., ***camph.,*** cann-s., canth., ***caps.,*** carb-an., ***carb-s.,*** carb-v., **CAUST.,** cham., chel., chin., cic., **COCC.,** ***coff.,*** colch., ***con.,*** croc., crot-h., cupr-ar., dig., dub., gels., helo., hydr-ac., hydrc., ign., lac-ac., ***lach.,*** lact., ***lath.,*** lil-t., lyc., mag-s., morph., mur-ac., ***mygal.,*** naja, nat-c., nux-v., onos., op., ***oxyt.,*** paeon., phos., phys., phyt., pic-ac., plat., prun., puls., rhod., rhus-t., stram., sulph., tanac., verat., verat-v., zinc.
sex, after - bov.
alcoholics - ran-b.
places one foot over the other - teucr.
unobserved, when - arg-n.

GANGRENE - ***agar.,*** alum., am-c., **ANTHR.,** ant-c., apis, **ARS.,** ***asaf., bell.,*** calc., **CANTH.,** ***carb-an., carb-v.,*** **CAUST.,** ***chin., colch., crot-h.,*** cycl., euph., hep., hell., ***iod.,*** kali-n., ***kali-p., kreos.,*** **LACH.,** mag-c., merc., ph-ac., ***phos., plb.,*** ran-b., ***rhus-t.,*** ruta., ***sabin.,*** **SEC., SIL.,** ***squil., stram.,*** sulph., sul-ac., tarent-c., verat., vip.

GANGRENE,
aphthae - ***ars.,*** carb-ac., cocc., lach., merc-d., plb.
burns, or sores, from - ***agar.,*** alum., am-c., **ANTHR.,** ant-c., apis, **ARS.,** ***asaf.,*** calc., ***canth., carb-v.,*** **CAUST.,** cycl., euph., ***kreos.,*** lach., mag-c., ph-ac., ***rhus-t.,*** ruta., **SEC.,** ***stram.***
cold - ant-t., **ARS.,** ***asaf.,*** bell., ***canth.,*** caps., ***carb-v.,*** con., crot-h., ***euph., lach.,*** merc., **PLB.,** ran-b., **SEC.,** ***sil., squil.,*** sulph., sul-ac., tarent-c.
feet - ant-c., ant-t., ***ars.,*** calen., ***lach.,*** merc., **SEC.,** vip.
cold - ***sec.***
cold, with burning, tearing pains - **SEC.**
fingers - ***sec.***
hands - ***ars., lach., sec.***
hot - acon., ars., bell., mur-ac., ***sabin., sec.***
inflammation, gangrenous - **ARS.,** ***bell.,*** **CANTH.,** ***carb-an., carb-v., chin., colch., crot-h.,*** euph., hep., ***iod.,*** kali-n., ***kali-p.,*** **LACH.,** merc., ***phos., plb., rhus-t.,*** **SEC., SIL.**
moist - ***carb-v.,*** **CHIN.,** ***hell.,*** ph-ac., squil., tarent.
senile - ***ars., carb-an., carb-v.,*** cupr., ***ph-ac.,*** **SEC.,** sul-ac.
spots - crot-h., cycl., ***hyos.,*** sec., vip.
toes - crot-h., cupr., iod., lach., **SEC.**
traumatic - arn., lach., sul-ac.
wounds, gangrenous - acon., am-c., ***anthr.,*** **ARS.,** ***bell., brom.,*** calen., ***carb-v., chin., eucal.,*** euph., **LACH.,** sal-ac., sec., ***sil.,*** sul-ac., trach., vip., vip-a.

GANGLION - am-c., arn., aur-m., calc., calc-f., ***carb-v.,*** ph-ac., ***phos.,*** plb., rhus-t., **RUTA.,** sil., sulph., zinc.

GLANDERS, horse disease - acon., ***ars.,*** calc., chin-s., ***crot-h.,*** hep., hippoz., ***kali-bi., lach., merc.,*** ph-ac., phos., sep., sil., sulph., thuj.

GIARDIA, parasites - ars., chin., cina.

GONORRHEA, infection (see Bladder)

GOOD health before paroxysms - bry., carc., helon., nat-m., phos., ***psor.,*** sep.

GRANULATIONS - ***alum.,*** anac-oc., ant-t., **ARS.,** ***calc.,*** cund., ***kali-m., lach., sabin.,*** **SIL.**

GROWTH in length to fast - ***calc., calc-p.,*** ferr., ferr-ac., iod., irid., kreos., ***ph-ac., phos.***
young people, in - ***calc-p.,*** hippoz., kreos., ***ph-ac.,*** **PHOS.**

GUILLAIN-barre syndrome - carc., con., thuj.

HAIR, general, head and body
auburn - lach., **PHOS., PULS., RHUS-T.**
baldness, (see Hair, loss of)
beard, falling out, of - agar., ambr., anan., aur-m., ***calc.,*** carb-an., ***graph., kali-c., nat-c., nat-m.,*** nit-ac., ***ph-ac.,*** plb., sanic., sil.
grief, after - ***ph-ac.***

HAIR, general
blonde, hair - agar., ***apis.,*** bor., ***brom.,*** bry., **CALC.,** ***caps., graph., hep., kali-bi.,*** lob., merc., **PETR., PHOS., PULS.,** ***rhus-t.,*** sabad., ***sil.,*** **SPONG.,** ***sulph.***
bristling - acet-ac., ***acon.,*** am-c., arn., bar-c., calc., canth., carl., carb-v., ***cham., chel.,*** cina, coc-c., dulc., gran., hep., lachn., laur., lyc., mag-m., mang., meny., meph., merc., mez., ***mur-ac.,*** nit-ac., nux-v., puls., ran-b., seneg., sil., spong., sul-i., sulph., tarent., verat., ***zinc.***
coming in from open air - am-c.
dinner, during - sil.
painful part - sulph.
seem - acon.
sensation of - acon., am-c., ars., bar-c., chel., dulc., ***lach.,*** mez., sil., spig., vinc.
brittleness - ars., bad., bell., bor., fl-ac., graph., ***kali-c.,*** plb., ***psor.,*** sec., ***sep.,*** staph., thuj.
brunettes, hair - ***acon.,*** alum., anac., arn., ars., ***bry., calc.,*** **CAUST.,** cina., **IGN., KALI-C.,** kreos., nat-m., **NIT-AC.,** ***nux-v.,*** phos., **PLAT.,** puls., ***sep.,*** staph., sulph.
brushing back agg. - carb-s., puls., rhus-t.
child's face, growth of - calc., morg., nat-m., ol-j., psor., sulph., tarent., thuj., thyr., tub.
chin, women in, on - ol-j.
color, changes - kali-i.
combing agg. - ***asar.,*** bell., ***bry.,*** chin., ign., kreos., nat-s., ***sel.***
curly, becomes - mez.
cutting of hair, agg. - acon., **BELL.,** cina, ***glon.,*** kali-i., lappa-a., led., ***phos.,*** puls., ***sep.***
ailments after - ***bell.,*** glon., kali-i., led., phos.
child, refuses - ***cina.***
darker, grows - jab., pilo., wies., wild.
distribution masculine in women - cortico., sep.
dryness - aloe, alum., ***ambr.,*** bad., ***calc.,*** chel., ***fl-ac.,*** hipp., ***kali-c., med.,*** **NAT-M.,** ***phos., plb., psor.,*** sec., **SEP.,** ***sulph.,*** **THUJ**.
electrical - med.
falling out, of hair (see Hair, loss of) - ail., ***alum., ambr.,*** am-c., ***am-m.,*** anan., ***ant-c.,*** ant-t., apis, ***ars.,*** ars-i., ***arund.,*** asc-t., **AUR.,** ***aur-m.,*** aur-m-n., aur-s., bac., ***bar-c.,*** bell., bov., bry., bufo, ***calc.,*** calc-i., ***calc-p.,*** calc-s., ***canth., carb-an.,*** **CARB-S., CARB-V.,** carl., caust., ***chel.,*** chlol., chin., colch., ***con.,*** cop., ***elaps, ferr.,*** ferr-ar., ferr-m., ferr-p., **FL-AC.,** ***form.,*** glon., **GRAPH**., hell., ***hep.,*** hyper., ign., iod., kali-ar., ***kali-bi.,*** **KALI-C.,** kali-i., kali-n., kali-p., **KALI-S.**, kreos., **LACH., LYC.,** ***mag-c.,*** manc., ***merc., merc-c., mez.,*** morg., naja, nat-c., **NAT-M.,** nat-p., **NIT-AC.,** nuph., oena., op., osm., ped., ***petr., ph-ac.,*** **PHOS**., piloc., plb., psor., puls., rhus-t., rhus-v., sanic., sars., sec., ***sel.,*** **SEP., SIL.,** ***skook., staph.,*** **SULPH**., sul-ac., ***syph.,*** tab., tep., ***thal.,*** **THUJ**., thyr., tub., ust., vesp., ***zinc.***
all over - sel.

HAIR, general
falling out, of hair
childbirth, after - ***calc., canth., carb-v.,*** hep., **LYC.,** ***nat-m., nit-ac., sep.,*** sil., **SULPH.**
children, in - bar-c.
dandruff, due to - am-m., thuj.
diseases, after - lyc., manc., ***ph-ac.,*** thal.
extending all over body - alum.
forehead - ars., bell., ***hep., merc., nat-m., phos.,*** sil.
grief, from - ***ph-ac.***
handfuls, in - lyc., ***mez.,*** **PHOS**., sulph.
headache, with - ant-c., nat-m., nit-ac., sep., sil.
menopause - ***sep.***
pregnancy, during - **LACH.,** ***sep.***
occiput, on - ***carb-v., chel., petr.,*** sil., staph.
seaside amel. - med.
sides - ars., bov., calc., ***graph.,*** kali-c., merc., ph-ac., phos., ***staph.,*** zinc.
skin, general - ***alum.,*** ars., ***calc.,*** carb-an., ***carb-v., graph.,*** hell., kali-c., lach., ***nat-m.,*** op., phos., sabin., ***sec., sel.,*** sulph., thal.
spots, in - ***apis, ars., calc.,*** calc-p., carb-an., **FL-AC.,** ***hep., phos., psor.***
and comes in white - vinc.
syphilis, from - merc., nit-ac., ust.
temples - calc., ***kali-c.,*** lyc., merc., ***nat-m.,*** par., sabin.
unusual parts, on - med., thuj., tub.
vertex - bar-c., graph., lyc., thuj., zinc.
young people, in - sil., tub.
gray, becomes - ***ars.,*** graph., hipp., ***kali-i.,*** kali-n., kreos., **LYC.,** op., ***ph-ac.,*** sec., ***sil., staph.,*** sul-ac., ***sulph.,*** thuj.
spots, in - psor.
greasy - arund., benz-n., bran., ***bry.,*** calc., ***caust.,*** lac-c., lyss., ***med.,*** merc., ***nat-m., ph-ac.,*** plb., thuj., tub.
hairy - med., thuj.
horripilation, left side - ped.
lifted up, by the hair, as if - ped.
lip, upper, on - ol-j.
loss, hair, of
baldness, head - ***anac., apis,*** **BAR-C.,** ***fl-ac., graph.,*** hep., lyc., med., morg., ***phos.,*** pix., sel., ***sep.,*** **SIL.,** syc-co., ***zinc.***
chilbirth, after - ***calc., canth., carb-v.,*** **LYC**., ***nat-m., nit-ac.,*** **SEP., SULPH**.
patches, in - ***apis, ars., calc.,*** calc-p., carb-an., fl-ac., ***graph., hep.,*** kali-p., lyc., morg., ***phos.,*** psor., sep.
spots, in - ***apis, ars., calc.,*** calc-p., carb-an., **FL-AC.,** ***hep., phos., psor.***
young, people - ***bar-c., sil.,*** tub.
beard, from - agar., ambr., anan., aur-m., ***calc.,*** carb-an., ***graph., kali-c., nat-c., nat-m.,*** nit-ac., ***ph-ac.,*** plb., sanic., sil.
eyebrows, from - agar., ail., alum., ***anan.,*** aur-m., hell., **KALI-C.,** mill., plb., sel., sil., sulph.

HAIR, general
loss, hair, of
eyebrows, white, from - ars-h.
eyelashes, from - alum., ***apis, ars.,*** aur., bufo, ***calc-s., chel.,*** chlol., ***euphr.,*** med., ***merc.,*** ph-ac., psor., **RHUS-T.,** ***sel.,*** sep., sil., ***staph., sulph.***
forehead, from - ars., bell., ***hep., merc., nat-m., phos.,*** sil.
genitalia, female, from - hell., **NAT-M.,** ***nit-ac.,*** rhus-t., ***sel.,*** sulph., ***zinc.***
female, labia, vulva - merc., nit-ac.
genitalia, male, from - bell., nat-c., **NAT-M.,** ***nit-ac., ph-ac.,*** rhus-t., sars., ***sel., zinc.***
offensive sweat, from - **SULPH.**
occiput, from - ***carb-v., chel., petr.,*** sil., staph.
sides, from - bov., ***graph.,*** kali-c., ph-ac., ***staph.,*** zinc.
temples, from - calc., ***kali-c.,*** lyc., merc., ***nat-m.,*** par., sabin.
lustreless - calc., fl-ac., kali-n., ***med., psor., thuj.,*** tub.
moving sensation - stann.
mustache, women, in - cortico., nat-m., ***sep.,*** thuj., thyr.
falling out, of - bar-c., kali-c., plb., sel.
oily - lyss.
painful, when touched - alum., ***am-c.,*** ambr., **APIS,** ***ars.,*** arund., ***asar., bell.,*** calc., carb-s., ***carb-v., carl.,*** chel., **CHIN.,** chin-s., ***cina, cinnb., coloc.,*** dys-co., ***ferr.,*** ferr-p., fl-ac., ***hep., kali-c.,*** lac-c., lach., mez., nat-m., nat-s., nit-ac., ***nux-v.,*** phos., ***puls.,*** **SEL.,** ***sep.,*** spig., spira., stann., ***sulph.,*** thuj., verat., zinc.
plica polonica - tub.
pulled out, sensation - lyc., mag-c.
head, on vertex - ***acon., arg-n.,*** kali-n., lachn., mag-c., ***phos.***
red, hair - calc-p., lach., **PHOS.,** sep., sulph.
sensation of a hair - all-c., ***arg-n., ars.,*** bell., caps., carb-s., caust., coc-c., croc., ***kali-bi.,*** lac-c., laur., lyc., mosch., nat-m., nat-p., nux-v., ptel., ***puls.,*** ran-b., rhus-t., ***sabad.,*** **SIL.,** ***sulph.,*** ther., thuj.
standing on end, as if - lachn.
occiput - lachn.
sticks together - bor., jac., **MEZ.,** ***nat-m., psor.,*** sars., sep., sulph., tub., ust.
ends at - ***bor.***
tangles, easily - ***bor., fl-ac.,*** graph., lyc., med., nat-m., psor., tub., verat., vinc.
toching agg. - ambr., **APIS, ARS.,** ***bell., carb-v.,*** chin., **CINA,** ***ferr., ferr-p.,*** hep., ign., mez., nit-ac., ***nux-v.,*** ph-ac., phos., ***puls.,*** rhus-t., **SEL.,** sep., stann., verat., ***zinc.***

HAND, lying on part amel. - ***bell.,*** bor., ***bry.,*** calc., canth., con., ***croc.,*** cycl., dros., mang., ***meny.,*** mur-ac., nat-c., olnd., par., ***phos., rhus-t.,*** sabad., ***sep.,*** spig., sulph., thuj.
agg. - kali-n.
amel. near part affected - sul-ac.

HANGOVER, (see Toxicity)

HEAT, sensation in body (see Fevers) - agar., agn., ***alum.,*** am-c., ant-t., **APIS,** ***arg-n.,*** ars., ars-i., asaf., ***aur., aur-i., aur-m., bar-c.,*** bov., bry., ***calc., calc-i.,*** **CALC-S.,** ***camph.,*** **CANN-S.,** canth., caps., caust., chel., chin., cina, cocc., **COC-C., COFF.,** colch., com., ***croc.,*** cycl., ***dros.,*** euph., **FL-AC.,** graph., hell., ign., **IOD.,** ***ip.,*** kali-c., ***kali-i.,*** kali-n., **KALI-S.,** kreos., ***lach., laur.,*** **LIL-T., LYC.,** mag-c., ***mag-m., mang., merc.,*** nat-c., **NAT-M., NAT-S.,** ***nux-m., nux-v.,*** ph-ac., ***phos., psor., plat., ptel.,*** **PULS.,** ran-b., rheum, rhod., rhus-t., ***sabad., sabin.,*** samb., sars., **SEC.,** ***seneg., spong.,*** staph., **SULPH., SUL-AC., SUL-I.,** teucr., thuj., tub., valer., ***verat., zinc.***
coughing - sep., squil.
eating warm food - ***carb-v., ferr., kali-c.,*** lach., ***mag-c.,*** **PHOS., PULS.,** sep., ***sul-ac.***
evening, in bed - ***bry.***
exertion, on - alum., squil.
hand has lain, where - hyos.
motion, least - squil.
night - bar-c., cham., con., nat-m., ***phos.,*** puls., rhus-t., sil., zinc.
side, left - rhus-t.
talking - squil.
waking, on - **BAR-C.,** fl-ac., ***graph.,*** nat-m., ***sil.,*** zinc.
walking - samb.
heat, flushes of - acet-ac., acon., aesc., agn., ail., alum., ***alumn.,*** ambr., am-c., am-m., aml-n., ang., ant-t., apis, ***arn.,*** ars., ***ars-i.,*** arum-t., asar., aur., bapt., bar-c., bell., berb., bism., bor., bov., brom., bry., bufo, ***cact.,*** **CALC.,** ***calc-s.,*** carb-an., ***carb-s., carb-v.,*** **CAUST.,** cham., chel., ***chin.,*** chin-s., cimx., **COCC.,** coff., ***colch.,*** coloc., corn., croc., crot-h., crot-t., cupr., dig., dros., ***elaps,*** eup-per., ***ferr.,*** ferr-ar., ferr-i., ferr-p., gamb., **GLON.,** ***graph.,*** hep., helon., hura, hyos., ***ign., iod., kali-s., kreos.,*** lac-ac., **LACH.,** lob., **LYC.,** lyss., mag-m., **MANG.,** ***meny., merc.,*** nat-a., nat-c., nat-m., nat-p., **NAT-S., NIT-AC.,** ***nux-v.,*** olnd., op., ***ox-ac., petr.,*** ph-ac., **PHOS.,** plat., podo., **PSOR., PULS.,** raph., rumx., ***rhus-t.,*** ruta., sabad., sabin., ***sang.,*** seneg., **SEP.,** ***sil.,*** spig., ***spong.,*** stann., **SULPH., SUL-AC., SUMB.,** teucr., **THUJ., TUB.,** valer., ***xan.,*** zinc.
afternoon - ambr., bell., colch., con., laur., meny., nat-p., plb., samb., **SEP.**
dinner, during - calc-s., nux-v.
alternating with chills - acon., ars., asar., calc., chin-s., com., iod., ***kali-bi.,*** med., ***sep.,*** spig.
anger, after - ***phos.***
chilliness, with - agar., apis, ***ars., carb-v., colch.,*** corn., eup-per., kali-bi., lach., lob., ***merc.,*** plat., puls., sep., sulph., ter., thuj.
downward - glon., sang.
head to stomach - ***sang.***
eating, while - ***calc-s.,*** nux-v., psor.
after - alum., arg-n., carb-v., par., sumb.
amel. - chin.

heat, flushes of
emotions, from - lach., ***phos.***
evening - acon., all-c., arum-t., bor., carb-an., carb-v., elaps, ***lyc.,*** merc-c., nat-p., ***nat-s.,*** nit-ac., phos., ***psor.,*** **SEP.,** ***sulph.***
8 p.m., with nausea - ferr.
8:30 p.m - arum-t., cina, sep.
eating, after - carb-v.
falling asleep, before - carb-v.
exertion, from least - alum., ***sep., sumb.***
followed by chill - **CAUST.,** sang.
headache, during - agar.
menses, during - nat-p.
before - alum., iod., kali-c.
mental exertion, after - olnd.
morning - bism., bor.
eating, after - thuj.
motion - helon.
night - bar-c., spig.
3 a.m., feeling as if sweat would break out - bapt.
palpitation, with - calc., **KALI-C.,** lach., sep.
perspiration, with - acet-ac., am-m., ant-c., aur., bell., camph., ***carb-v.,*** **CON.,** ***fl-ac., hep.,*** kali-bi., ***lach.,*** op., petr., **PSOR.,** puls., ***sep., sulph., sul-ac.,*** **TUB.,** ***xan.***
anxiety, and - ang., kali-bi.
face and hands, on - calc.
night, 12 to 1 a.m - ***fl-ac.***
sitting, while - sep.
sleep, during - cham., nat-m., ***phos.,*** sil., zinc.
upwards - alum., alumn., ars., asaf., ***calc.,*** carb-an., carb-v., chin., cinnb., ***ferr.,*** ferr-ar., **GLON.,** ***graph.,*** indg., iris, kali-bi., ***kali-c.,*** laur., ***lyc.,*** mag-m., mang., nat-s., nit-ac., ***phos.,*** plb., ***psor.,*** **SEP.,** ***spong., sulph., sumb.,*** tarent., ***valer.***
hips, from the - alumn.
walking in open air - caust., sep.
warm water were, dashed over one - calc., cann-s., nat-m., phos., ***puls., rhus-t.,*** sep.
dashed over one, when an idea occurs vividly - ***phos.***
poured over one, as if - **ARS.,** bry., ph-ac., phos., **PSOR.,** ***puls., rhus-t.,*** **SEP.**

heat, vital heat, lacking, (see Chills, chapter) - ***aesc., agar., alum.,*** **ALUMN.,** ***am-c., am-m.,*** ang., ***ant-c.,*** **ARAN.,** ***arg-m., arg-n.,*** **ARS.,** ***ars-i., asar., aur.,*** **BAR-C.,** ***bar-m.,*** bor., ***brom., bufo,*** cact., cadm-s., **CALC., CALC-AR.,** ***calc-f.,*** **CALC-P.,** ***calc-s.,*** **CAMPH.,** caps., **CARB-AN.,** ***carb-s., carb-v., caul.,*** **CAUST.,** ***chel., chin., cimic., cinnb.,*** **CIST.,** ***cocc., con.,*** **CROT-C.,** cycl., ***dig.,*** **DULC.,** ***elaps,*** euph., **FERR.,** ***ferr-ar.,*** **GRAPH.,** ***guai.,*** **HELO., HEP.,** ***ip.,*** **KALI-AR., KALI-BI., KALI-C., KALI-P.,** ***kalm., kreos., lach., lac-d.,*** lac-ac., laur., **LED.,** ***lyc., mag-c.,*** mag-m., **MAG-P.,** ***mang., med., merc., mez., mosch., naja, nat-a.,*** nat-c., ***nat-m., nat-p.,*** **NIT-AC.,** ***nux-m.,*** **NUX-V.,** ***ol-j., petr.,*** **PH-AC., PHOS.,** ***plb.,*** -**PSOR., PYROG.,** ***ran-b., rhod.,*** **RHUS-T.,** ***rumx., sabad.,*** sars., ***senec., sep.,*** **SIL.,** ***spig., stann., staph., stront-c., sulph., sul-ac., sumb., tarent., ther., thuj., tub.,*** zinc.
afternoon, after siesta - con.

HEATED, becoming, (see Environment)

HERNIA, general - am-m., aur., cham., lyc., ***nux-v.,*** sul-ac., sulph., verat.
congenital - thuj.
femoral - cub., ***lyc.,*** nux-v.
infantile - ***aur.,*** calc., cham., lyc., mag-m., nit-ac., ***nux-v.,*** sul-ac.
inguinal - aesc., ***all-c., alum.,*** am-c., ***apis, asar., aur.,*** berb., ***calc.,*** calc-ar., caps., ***carb-an., carb-v., cocc., coff.,*** coloc., ***dig.,*** lach., **LYC.,** ***mag-c.,*** mill., ***mur-ac., nit-ac.,*** **NUX-V.,** ***op.,*** petr., phos., prun., psor., ***rhus-t.,*** sars., ***sil., spig.,*** staph., ***sulph., sul-ac.,*** ter., thuj., ***verat., zinc.***
children, in - **AUR.,** ***calc.,*** cina, lyc., ***nit-ac.,*** nux-v., sil., sulph.
left side - nux-v.
right side - aur., lyc.
incarcerated - lob., ***mill.,*** nux-v., ***op.,*** plb.
inflammation - acon., bar-c., iod., nux-v., op., sulph.
vomiting, with - acon., ars., bell., lach., ***tab.,*** verat.
left - nux-v.
painful - aesc., ***alum.,*** aur., cic., cocc., phos., ***sil.***
right - lyc.
sensitive - ***bell.,*** **LACH.,** ***nux-v., sil.***
stitching - sep.
scrotal, congenital - mag-m.
strangulated - acon., ***all-c.,*** alum., alumn., ars., aur., **BELL.,** calc., caps., ***carb-v.,*** cham., ***cocc., coff.,*** coloc., ***dig.,*** lach., lyc., mill., nit-ac., **NUX-V., OP.,** ***plb.,*** rhus-t., sil., ***sulph., sul-ac., tab.,*** verat.
tender - sil.
umbilical - ***calc.,*** cocc., ***lach.,*** lyc., ***nux-m.,*** **NUX-V.,** ***op.,*** **PLB.,** tub.

HERPES, simplex - acet-ac., acon., aethi-a., agar., aln., ***alum.,*** ambr., am-c., anac., ***anan.,*** antho., ***apis,*** arn., **ARS.,** ***ars-i.,*** aster., aur., ***bar-c., bar-m.,*** bell., berb., bor., **BOV.,** ***bry.,*** bufo, cadm-s., calad., **CALC., CALC-S.,** ***canth.,*** caps., ***carb-ac., carb-an.,*** **CARB-S.,** ***carb-v., caust.,*** chel., chrysar., ***cic., cist.,*** **CLEM.,** cocc., com., **CON.,** crot-h., ***crot-t.,*** cupr., cycl., dol., **DULC.,** eucal., **GRAPH.,** grat., hell., ***hep.,*** hyos., iod., iris, ***kali-ar., kali-bi., kali-c., kali-chl., kali-i.,*** kali-n., kali-p., ***kali-s.,*** kalm., ***kreos., lac-c., lach., led.,*** lith., **LYC.,** mag-c., ***mag-m.,*** manc., mang., **MED., MERC.,** mez., mosch., mur-ac., ***nat-a., nat-c.,*** **NAT-M.,** nat-p., ***nat-s.,*** nit-ac., nux-v., ***olnd.,*** par., ***petr.,*** ph-ac., ***phos.,*** plb., ***psor.,*** puls., ***ran-b.,*** ran-s., rhod., **RHUS-T.,** rumx., ruta., sabad., ***sars.,*** **SEP., SIL.,** spig., spong., squil., stann., ***staph.,*** **SULPH.,** sul-ac., tarax., **TELL.,** teucr., **THUJ.,** valer., vario.,

HERPES, simplex - verat., viol-t., xero, zinc.
alternating, with chest affections and dysenteric stools - rhus-t.
back - all-s., ars., lach., nat-c., sep., zinc.
bleeding - anac., dulc., lyc.
body, all over - dulc., ***psor., ran-b.***
burning - agar., alum., ambr., am-c., anac., **ARS.,** aur., bar-c., bell., bov., bry., calad., ***calc.,*** caps., carb-an., carb-v., **CAUST.,** cic., clem., cocc., ***con.,*** dulc., hell., hep., ***kali-c.,*** kali-n., kreos., lach., led., ***lyc., mang.,*** **MERC.,** mez., nat-c., nat-m., nux-v., olnd., par., petr., ph-ac., phos., plb., ***psor.,*** puls., ran-b., **RHUS-T.,** sabad., sars., sep., ***sil.,*** spig., spong., squil., staph., stram., ***sulph.,*** teucr., thuj., verat., viol-t., zinc.
chapping - alum., aur., bry., cadm-s., ***calc.,*** cycl., graph., hep., kali-c., kreos., lach., lyc., mag-c., mang., merc., nat-c., nat-m., nit-ac., petr., ***puls., rhus-t.,*** ruta., sars., **SEP.,** sil., **SULPH.,** viol-t., zinc.
chronic - aln.
clusters, in - dulc.
cold, water agg. - clem., ***dulc., sulph.***
corrosive - alum., am-c., bar-c., ***calc.,*** carb-v., caust., chel., ***clem., con.,*** **GRAPH.,** hell., hep., kali-c., lach., lyc., mag-c., mang., merc., mur-ac., nat-c., nit-ac., nux-v., olnd., par., ***petr.,*** ph-ac., phos., plb., ***rhus-t., sep.,*** **SIL.,** squil., staph., ***sulph.,*** tarax., viol-t.
crusty - alum., ambr., am-c., anac., ***ars., aur., aur-m.,*** bar-c., bell., bov., bry., **CALC.,** caps., carb-an., carb-v., cic., ***clem.,*** **CON.,** cupr., ***dulc.,*** **GRAPH.,** hell., hep., kali-c., kreos., lach., ***led.,*** **LYC.,** mag-c., **MERC.,** ***mez.,*** mur-ac., nat-m., nit-ac., nux-v., olnd., par., petr., ph-ac., phos., plb., puls., ran-b., **RHUS-T.,** sars., ***sep., sil.,*** squil., staph., **SULPH.,** thuj., verat., ***viol-t.,*** zinc.
dry - alum., ars., ***bar-c., bov.,*** bry., cact., ***calc.,*** carb-v., caust., clem., cocc., cupr., dol., ***dulc.,*** graph., ***hep.,*** hyos., kali-i., kreos., **LED.,** lyc., mag-c., med., ***merc.,*** nat-c., nat-m., nit-ac., par., petr., **PHOS.,** ph-ac., psor., rhus-t., sars., **SEP., SIL.,** stann., ***staph.,*** sulph., teucr., thuj., valer., verat., viol-t., ***zinc.***
fevers, in - carb-v., **NAT-M.,** rhus-t.
gastric problems, with - iris.
glands covered with - dulc., graph.
glandular swelling, with - dulc.
gray - ars.
indolent - lyc., mag-c., psor.
itching - agar., alum., ambr., am-c., anac., ***ant-t.,*** **ARS.,** bar-c., bell., ***bov.,*** bry., calad., calc., caps., carb-an., carb-v., ***caust.,*** chel., cic., **CLEM.,** cocc., con., cupr., dulc., ***graph.,*** hep., jug-r., ***kali-c.,*** kreos., lach., ***led.,*** lyc., mag-c., mag-m., mang., ***merc.,*** mez., nat-c., nat-m., ***nit-ac.,*** nux-v., olnd., par., petr., ph-ac., phos., plb., puls., ran-b., ran-s., **RHUS-T.,** sabad., sars., **SEP.,** ***sil.,*** spig., spong., squil., stann., ***staph., sulph.,*** tarax., thuj., valer., verat., viol-t., zinc.

HERPES, simplex
itching,
menses, before - carb-v.
jerking, pain, with - calc., caust., cupr., lyc., puls., **RHUS-T.,** sep., sil., ***staph.***
mealy - am-c., **ARS.,** aur., bov., bry., **CALC.,** cic., ***dulc.,*** graph., kreos., led., lyc., merc., mur-ac., **PHOS.,** ***sep.,*** **SIL.,** sulph., thuj., verat.
menses, during - petr.
mercurial - aur., mosch., ***nit-ac.***
moist - alum., am-c., anac., ars., bar-c., bell., ***bov.,*** bry., cact., cadm-s., **CALC.,** carb-an., ***carb-v.,*** **CAUST.,** cic., cist., ***clem.,*** con., **DULC., GRAPH.,** grat., hell., hep., kali-c., **KREOS.,** lach., led., **LYC., MERC.,** mez., nat-c., nat-m., nit-ac., ***olnd.,*** petr., **PH-AC.,** phos., ***psor.,*** ran-b., **RHUS-t.,** ruta., **SEP.,** ***sil.,*** squil., staph., **SULPH.,** sul-ac., tarax., ***tell.,*** thuj., viol-t.
neuralgic pains after - ***mez.,*** ran-b., still., ***vario.***
patches - ***ant-c.,*** caust., con., crot-h., ***graph.,*** hyos., **LYC., MERC.,** mur-ac., ***nat-c.,*** nat-m., nit-ac., petr., phos., sabad., sars., **SEP.,** sil., **SULPH.,** zinc.
brown - **SEP.**
pregnancy, during - sep.
red - am-c., ars., bry., cic., ***clem., dulc.,*** kreos., ***lach.,*** led., ***lyc., mag-c.,*** mag-s., ***merc.,*** olnd., petr., ph-ac., staph., tax., tell.
right side - iris.
scaly - agar., anac., anan., ars., aur., bell., bov., cact., cadm-s., **CALC.,** cic., ***clem., con.,*** cupr., ***dulc., graph.,*** hep., hyos., kali-c., led., ***lyc.,*** mag-c., **MERC.,** nat-m., olnd., ph-ac., ***phos.,*** plb., ***psor.,*** ran-b., rhus-t., ***sep.,*** sil., staph., ***sulph.,*** teucr., thuj.
scaly, white - anac., ars., graph., lyc., thuj., zinc.
scaly, white, dry - ars., calc., dulc., lyc., sep., sil., thuj.
spread by coalescing, with pimples or pustules surrounding - hep.
spreading - alum., caps., carb-s., clem., dulc., **MERC.**
spring, every - ***sep.***
stinging - alum., **APIS.,** ***ars.,*** bar-c., bell., bov., bry., calc., caps., carb-v., caust., **CLEM.,** cocc., con., cycl., graph., hell., hep., kali-c., kreos., led., lyc., mag-c., ***merc.,*** mez., mur-ac., nat-c., nat-m., ***nit-ac.,*** nux-v., petr., phos., ***puls.,*** ran-b., ran-s., ***rhus-t.,*** sabad., **SEP.,** ***sil.,*** spong., squil., staph., ***sulph.,*** thuj., viol-t., zinc.
suppressed - alum., ambr., ***calc., lach., lyc.,*** nat-c., sep., ***sulph.***
suppurating - ars., bell., cadm-s., cic., clem., cocc., con., cycl., ***dulc.,*** hep., jug-c., led., ***lyc.,*** mag-c., **MERC.,** ***nat-c.,*** nat-m., ***petr.,*** plb., puls., **RHUS-T.,** sars., **SEP.,** sil., spig., staph., sulph., tarax., thuj., verat., viol-t., zinc.

HERPES, simplex
tearing - ars., bell., bry., ***calc.,*** carb-v., caust., clem., cocc., dulc., graph., kali-c., **LYC.,** merc., ***mez.,*** nat-c., nit-ac., nux-v., phos., puls., rhus-t., ***sep., sil.,*** staph., ***sulph., zinc.***
whitish - anac., thuj., zinc.
yellowish - agar., ars., carb-s., cic., cocc., cupr., ***dulc.,*** hell., kreos., led., ***lyc., merc.,*** nat-c., nit-ac., par., sep., ***sulph.***
brown - carb-s., cupr., dulc., lyc., ***nat-c.***

HERPES, zoster, shingles - agar., apis, arg-n., arn., **ARS.,** aster., bry., bufo, ***canth.,*** carb-o., carb-s., ***caust.,*** cedr., cham., ***cist., clem.,*** com., crot-h., crot-t., dol., dulc., euph., ***graph.,*** grin., ***hep.,*** hyper., iod., **IRIS,** kali-ar., ***kali-bi., kali-chl.,*** kali-i., kali-m., ***lach.,*** **MERC., MEZ.,** morph., nat-c., **NAT-M.,** ***petr.,*** pip-m., prun., puls., **RAN-B.,** ran-s., **RHUS-T.,** sal-ac., sel., semp., ***sep., sil.,*** staph., stry., ***sulph., thuj., vario.,*** zinc., zinc-p., zinc-valer.
chronic - ars., mez., ***nat-m., rhus-t.,*** semp.
neuralgic pains, persisting, after herpes zoster - ars., dol., ***mez.,*** ran-b., ***rhus-t.,*** still., zinc-m.

HIVES, urticaria - ***acon.,*** agar., all-c., ***ant-c.,*** **APIS,** arn., **ARS., ASTAC.,** bell., ***bov., calad.,*** **CARB-AC.,** chlor., ***graph.,*** **LED.,** ***lyc., mez.,*** **NAT-M.,** ***nat-p.,*** nit-ac., ***psor., puls.,*** **RHUS-T.,** ***sal-ac.,*** **SULPH.,** ***sul-ac.,*** **URT-U.,** vesp.

HOOK-worm disease - carb-tcl., chen-a., thymol.

HODGKIN'S disease, (see Cancer)

HOT, applications, amel. - anac., ***ars.,*** calc-f., hep., kali-c., **MAG-P.,** nux-v., rad., ***rhus-t., sil.,*** syph.
hot, sensations, (see Senations, general)

HUNGER, ailments from - ***alum., aur., cact.,*** calc-f., canth., ***caust.,*** **CROT-H.,** ***crot-t.,*** ferr., **GRAPH.,** hell., **IOD., KALI-C.,** olnd., ***phos.,*** plat., ***psor.,*** rhus-t., sep., **SIL.,** ***spig.,*** stann., **SULPH.,** tub., valer., verat., ***zinc.***
agg. - ***anac.,*** ars-i., chel., cina, ***graph.,*** iod., ***kali-c.,*** lyc., olnd., phos., ***sil.,*** spig., staph., ***sulph.***

HYPERSENSITIVE, (see Toxicity, Drugs) - apis., ***ars., coff.,*** med., ***merc.*** nat-c., ***nit-ac.,*** nux-v., ***phos.,*** psor., sul-ac., sulph.
drugs, to allopathic - acon., arn., ***ars.,*** cham., carc., coff., lyc., **MED., NIT-AC.,** nux-v., **PULS.,** sep., sil., **SULPH.**
remedies, to homeopathic potencies, - acon., **ARS.,** ars-i., cham., carc., coff., **MED., NIT-AC.,** nux-v., **PHOS.,** sep., ***thuj.***

HYPERTROPHY, of tissues - ***ant-c.,*** ars., calc., ***clem., dulc., graph.,*** lyc., ran-b., rhus-t., sep., ***sil.,*** sulph., thyr.
exertion, excessive, from - thyr.
one side - lyc.

HYPOSTASIS - am-c., carb-v., rhus-t., sep.

IMMOBILE - lycps., mang., stroph.
one side - stroph.

INCONTINENCE in general - ***aloe, arn.,*** ars., **BELL., CAUST.,** chin., con., dios., ***gels., hyos.,*** mur-ac., nat-m., **PH-AC.,** ***phos., podo., puls.,*** sel., ***sep.,*** staph., ***sulph.***
anticipation, from - arg-n., gels., op.
fright, from - acon., op.

INDOLENCE and luxury, ailments from - carb-v., helon., ***nux-v.***

INTERMITTENT, complaints - **ARS.,** calc., **CHIN.,** ip., lach., nat-m., nit-ac., ***nux-v.,*** ph-ac., ***puls.,*** sec., sulph.

INTOXICATION, ailments from (see Toxicity)

IRRITABILITY, excessive physical - absin., acon., agar., ***ambr.,*** anac., ant-c., ***ant-t.,*** **APIS, ARN.,** ***ars., asaf.,*** **ASAR., AUR.,** bar-c., **BELL.,** bor., bov., bry., camph., cann-i., **CANTH.,** carb-s., caust., ***cham.,*** **CHIN.,** ***chin-s., cocc.,*** **COFF.,** croc., cupr., ***ferr., gels.,*** graph., hell., hep., hyos., ***ign.,*** kreos., ***lach.,*** laur., ***lil-t.,*** mag-c., mag-m., mang., **MED., MERC.,** mez., ***mosch.,*** nat-a., nat-c., ***nat-m.,*** nat-p., **NIT-AC., NUX-V.,** par., petr., ***ph-ac., phos.,*** plat., ***puls.,*** rhus-t., sabin., sec., sel., sep., **SIL.,** spig., squil., **STAPH.,** stram., sulph., **TARENT., TEUCR.,** ***valer., verat.***
when too much medicine has produced an hypersensitive state and remedies fail to act - nux-m., op., ***ph-ac.,*** sep., **TEUCR.**
lack of - agn., ***alum., ambr., am-c., anac.,*** ant-c., ant-t., arn., ***ars.,*** asaf., bar-c., bism., brom., bry., **CALC., CALC-I.,** ***camph.,*** cann-s., **CAPS.,** ***carb-an.,*** **CARB-V.,** caust., cic., ***cocc.,*** colch., coloc., **CON.,** croc., cupr., ***dulc.,*** euph., ferr., **GELS.,** graph., ***guai.,*** **HELL.,** hyos., ***iod., ip., kali-bi.,*** kali-c., lach., **LAUR.,** led., ***lyc.,*** mag-c., mag-m., mez., ***mosch.,*** mur-ac., nux-m., **OLND., OP.,** petr., **PH-AC.,** phos., plb., **PSOR.,** ***rhod.,*** rhus-t., sec., seneg., ***sep.,*** spong., stann., ***stram.,*** stront-c., ***sulph.,*** thuj., ***valer.,*** verb., ***zinc.***

ICTERUS, newborn - chel., chion., coll., merc., nux-v.

INDURATIONS, of tissues - ***agn.,*** alum., ***alumn.,*** ambr., ***anthr., apis, arg-m., arg-n.,*** arn., ***ars.,*** ars-i., ars-s-f., asaf., ***aur.,*** aur-a., aur-i., ***aur-m.,*** **AUR-M-N.,** aur-s., **BAD.,** ***bar-c.,*** bar-i., bar-m., **BELL.,** bov., ***bry., calc.,*** **CALC-F.,** calc-i., camph., cann-i., cann-s., caps., **CARB-AN.,** carb-s., **CARB-V.,** caust., cham., chel., **CHIN.,** cina, ***cinnb.,*** cist., **CLEM.,** cocc., coloc., **CON.,** cupr., cycl., dulc., ferr., ferr-ar., fl-ac., **GRAPH.,** ***hep., hydrc.,*** hyos., ign., ***iod., kali-bi.,*** kali-c., ***kali-chl., kali-i., kali-m.,*** kreos., **LACH.,** lap-a., led., ***lyc.,*** mag-c., **MAG-M.,** mang., ***merc.,*** merc-i-r., mez., nat-c., nux-v., op., ***petr.,*** **PHOS.,** ***phyt., plb.,*** plb-i., ***psor., puls.,*** ran-b., ran-s., rhod., **RHUS-T.,** sec., **SEL., SEP., SIL.,** spig., spong., squil., **STAPH.,** ***still.,*** stram., sul-i., ***sulph.,*** syph., tarent., **THIOSIN.,** thuj., valer., verat.

INDURATIONS, of tissues
cellular tissue - anthr., graph., kali-i., merc-i-r., rhus-t., thiosin.
painful - bell.
pressure, from - ***sulph.***

INFECTIOUS diseases, ailments since - carc., gels., ph-ac., psor.

INFILTRATION, of tissues - calc., carb-an., graph., iod., kali-m., rhus-t., sul-i., sulph.

INFLAMMATION, of tissues - ***acon.***, apis, ***ars.***, **BELL.**, **BRY.**, calc., cann-i., cann-s., ***canth.***, cham., echi., ferr-p., **GELS.**, hep., **HYOS.**, ***iod.***, kali-c., ***lach.***, **MERC.**, **NUX-V.**, ***phos.***, plb., **PULS.**, **RHUS-T.**, sec., sep., **SIL.**, ***staph.***, sulph., ter., ***verat-v.***

absorption, to favor - ant-t., apis, ***kali-i.***, kali-m., lyc., phos., sulph.

cellulitis - ***apis***, ***arn.***, ars., bapt., bell., bry., crot-h., gad., ***hep.***, ***lach.***, mang., merc., ***merc-i-r.***, myris., ***rhus-t.***, ***sil.***, sul-i., tarent-c., vesp.
puerperal - hep., ***rhus-t.***, verat-v.
subacute - mang., sil.

externally - ***acon.***, agar., agn., alum., alumn., ambr., am-c., ant-c., ***apis***, arn., **ARS.**, ars-i., asaf., asar., aur., aur-a., bar-c., **BELL.**, bor., bov., ***bry.***, bufo, ***cact.***, ***calc.***, calc-i., calc-sil., camph., cann-s., canth., caps., carb-an., carb-v., caust., ***cham.***, chel., chin., chin-s., cina, clem., cocc., coff., colch., coloc., ***con.***, cortiso., croc., crot-h., crot-t., cupr., cupr-ac., dig., dulc., **ECHI.**, euph., ***euphr.***, ***ferr.***, **FERR-P.**, ***fl-ac.***, ***gels.***, gran., graph., ***gunp.***, hell., ***hep.***, hyos., ign., iod., ip., ***kali-ar.***, kali-c., kali-m., kali-n., kreos., **LACH.**, lact., led., ***lyc.***, ***mag-arct.***, mag-c., mag-m., mang., ***merc.***, ***merc-d.***, mez., mur-ac., myris., nat-a., nat-c., nat-m., nat-sil., ***nit-ac.***, nux-v., op., ***petr.***, ph-ac., ***phos.***, plb., **PULS.**, ran-b., ***rhus-t.***, sabad., sabin., samb., sars., sep., **SIL.**, ***spig.***, spong., squil., stann., **STAPH.**, stram., sul-ac., sul-i., ***sulph.***, tarax., teucr., thuj., valer., verat., **VERAT-V.**, zinc.

gangrenous, (see Gangrene) - **ARS.**, ***bell.***, **CANTH.**, ***carb-an.***, ***carb-v.***, ***chin.***, ***colch.***, ***crot-h.***, euph., hep., ***iod.***, kali-n., ***kali-p.***, **LACH.**, merc., ***phos.***, ***plb.***, ***rhus-t.***, **SEC.**, **SIL.**

internally - abrot., **ACON.**, agar., ***agro.***, aloe, alum., ang., ant-c., ant-t., ***apis***, arg-m., ***arg-n.***, arn., **ARS.**, ars-i., ars-s-f., ***arum-t.***, asaf., ***aur.***, aur-a., aur-i., aur-s., bar-c., bar-i., **BELL.**, bell-p., ***berb.***, bism., **BRY.**, ***cact.***, calad., calc., calc-sil., camph., ***cann-s.***, **CANTH.**, caps., carb-ac., carb-v., ***cham.***, chel., chin., cic., cina, clem., cocc., coc-c., coff., colch., coloc., ***con.***, cortiso., crot-h., ***cub.***, cupr., dig., dros., dulc., **ECHI.**, equis., euph., ***ferr.***, ferr-ar., **FERR-P.**, **GELS.**, graph., guai., ham., hell., hep., hydr-ac., ***hyos.***, ign., **IOD.**, ip., ***kali-ar.***, kali-bi., ***kali-c.***, ***kali-chl.***, ***kali-i.***, kali-m., ***kali-n.***, kali-s., **LACH.**, laur., lil-t., ***lyc.***, mag-m., mang., **MERC.**, **MERC-C.**, mez., nat-a., nat-c., nat-m., ***nat-ns.***, nat-s., nit-ac., nux-m., **NUX-V.**, op., par., pareir., petr., ph-ac., **PHOS.**, phyt., **PLB.**, podo., **PULS.**, ran-b., ran-s., rheum, rhus-t., ruta, sabad., sabin., samb., sang., sang-n., **SEC.**, senec., seneg., sep., sil., spig., ***spira.***, spong., ***squil.***, stann., stram., stront-c., sul-i., ***sulph.***, sul-ac., tab., tarent., **TER.**, thuj., uva., ***verat.***, ***verat-v.***, vib., vip.

nerves, of - **ACON.**, ***alum-sil.***, ***ant-c.***, ***ars.***, **BELL.**, ***cact.***, caust., ***cic.***, ***coca***, **COFF.**, ***gels.***, ***hep.***, **HYPER.**, iod., ***ip.***, kali-i., ***kalm.***, lac-c., ***lec.***, ***led.***, ***merc.***, ***nat-m.***, ***nux-v.***, **PHOS.**, ***puls.***, ***rhus-t.***, ***sil.***, stram., sulph., zinc.

passive - ***dig.***, ***gels.***, puls., sulph.

sudden - bell.

surgery, after - acon., ***anthr.***, arn., ars., ars-i., ***bell.***, bell-p., calc-s., **CALEN.**, echi., gunp., ***hep.***, hyper., iod., merc-c., merc-i-r., myrt-c., ***pyrog.***, rhus-t., ***sil.***

tendency to inflammation - camph.

tendonitis - anac., ant-c., calen., ***rhod.***, ***rhus-t.***

wounds, of - ***acon.***, arn., calc-f., **CALEN.**, ***cham.***, ***con.***, hyper., kali-bi., lach., led., nat-m., plb., ***puls.***, ***rhus-t.***, ***sul-ac.***, ***sulph.***, vip.

INFLUENZA, (see Fevers)

INHERITANCE, bad - bar-c., bufo, **CARC.**, med., psor., syph., tub.

ITCHING, tickling, internally (see Skin) - acon., agar., alum., am-c., am-m., **AMBR.**, anac., ang., ant-t., apis, arn., asar., bar-c., bell., bor., bov., brom., bry., calc., caps., carb-v., caust., cham., chin., cic., ***cina***, ***coca.***, cocc., colch., ***con.***, croc., dig., euph., ***ferr.***, fl-ac., graph., hep., ign., **IOD.**, ip., ***kali-bi.***, kali-c., lach., ***laur.***, led., mag-c., mag-m., meny., merc., mosch., nat-c., nit-ac., nux-m., **NUX-V.**, olnd., petr., ph-ac., **PHOS.**, plb., **PSOR.**, puls., rhod., rhus-t., ruta, sabad., sabin., sang., seneg., sep., sil., spig., spong., squil., ***stann.***, sulph., tarax., teucr., thuj., verat., zinc.
affected parts, of - dig.

JAR, of body, agg. - ***acon.***, aloe, alum., alum-p., alum-sil., ambr., am-c., ***anac.***, ***ang.***, ***ant-c.***, arg-m., ***arg-n.***, **ARN.**, ars., ***asar.***, bapt., bar-c., **BELL.**, berb., bor., **BRY.**, ***cact.***, calad., ***calc.***, calc-p., calc-sil., camph., canth., carb-ac., carb-s., ***caust.***, cham., chel., ***chin.***, **CIC.**, cina, ***cocc.***, coff., **CON.**, crot-h., dros., dulc., euphr., ***ferr.***, ferr-ar., ferr-p., form., glon., ***graph.***, ***ham.***, ***hell.***, ***hep.***, ign., kali-c., ***kali-i.***, kali-n., kali-sil.1, ***lac-c.***, **LACH.**, ***led.***, ***lil-t.***, ***lyc.***, mag-c., ***mag-m.***, meny., merc., nat-a., ***nat-c.***, ***nat-m.***, nat-p., nat-s., nat-sil., **NIT-AC.**, nux-m., ***nux-v.***, ***onos.***, par., petr., ***ph-ac.***, ***phos.***, plat., plb., podo., ***puls.***, rhod., **RHUS-T.**, ruta, ***sabad.***, sabin., sang., ***sanic.***, seneg., ***sep.***, **SIL.**, ***spig.***, spong., stann., staph., ***sulph.***, tab., tarax., **THER.**, ***thuj.***, valer., verb., viol-t.
agg., sudden - vib.
amel. - ars., caps., gels., hell., ***nit-ac.***

JELLY, body were made of - eupi.

JERKING, of body, (see Muscles, chapter)
bones, in - asaf., chin., sil.
convulsions, as in - acon., agar., ***alum.,*** am-c., am-m., **AMBR.,** ant-c., ant-t., arg-m., arn., ***ars.,*** asaf., bar-c., bar-m., bell., bry., ***calc.,*** camph., cann-s., canth., caps., carb-v., **CAUST.,** ***cham.,*** chin., chin-s., chlol., ***cic.,*** cina, cocc., coff., colch., coloc., crot-h., ***cupr.,*** cupr-ac., cupr-c., dig., dros., dulc., graph., hep., ***hyos., ign.,*** ip., kali-c., kali-chl., kreos., lach., lact., laur., led., ***lil-t.,*** lob., lyc., mag-arct., mag-c., mag-m., mang., ***meny., merc.,*** mez., mosch., mur-ac., ***mygal.,*** nat-c., **NAT-M.,** nit-ac., nux-v., op., ***petr.,*** ph-ac., phel., ***phos.,*** plat., **PLB.,** puls., ***ran-b.,*** ran-s., rat., rhod., rhus-t., sabad., ***sec.,*** sep., sil., sol-n., squil., staph., ***stram.,*** stront-c., ***sulph.,*** sul-ac., tarent., teucr., thuj., valer., verat., viol-t., vip., ***zinc.***
convulsions, as in, night - staph.
convulsions, before - ars., bar-m., laur., verat-v.
evening in bed - petr.
internally - ***acon.,*** agar., ambr., anac., ang., aran-ix., arn., ars., ***bell.,*** bov., bry., calad., **CALC., CANN-I.,** ***cann-s.,*** caust., cic., clem., coca, colch., ***con., croc.,*** dig., dulc., **GLON.,** kreos., ***lyc.,*** mag-c., mag-p-a.1, mang., mez., mur-ac., nat-c., nat-m., ***nux-m., nux-v.,*** petr., phos., **PLAT., PULS.,** ran-s., rhod., rhus-t., ruta, samb., sep., ***sil.,*** **SPIG.,** ***spong.,*** **STANN.,** stront-c., sul-ac., sulph., teucr., thuj., ***valer.***
joints, in - alum., bell., bry., bufo, ***coloc.,*** graph., nat-m., puls., sil., spig., spong., ***sul-ac.,*** sulph., ***verat.***
lightning like, head to foot, from - hydr-ac.
paralyzed parts - ***arg-n.,*** merc., ***nux-v.,*** phos., sec., stram., ***stry.***
run through whole body - ign.
side lain on, in - ***cimic.***
side not lain on - onos.
sleep, during - ***acon., aeth.,*** agar., aloe, ***alum.,*** ambr., anac., ant-c., ant-t., ***apis,*** arg-m., ***ars., bell.,*** bor., brom., bry., calc., carb-v., cast., caust., cham., chin., cimic., ***cina,*** cob., colch., ***con.,*** cor-r., ***cupr., cupr-ac.,*** cupr-ar., daph., dig., dulc., hell., hep., hyos., ign., ip., ***kali-c.,*** lyc., merc., morph., nat-c., ***nat-m.,*** nat-s., nit-ac., nux-v., op., passi., phos., puls., ran-s., rheum, rhus-t., samb., sel., sep., sil., stann., staph., ***stram.,*** stront-c., sul-ac., ***sulph.,*** tarent., thuj., tub., valer., viol-t., zinc., ziz.
sleep, on going to - acon., ***agar.,*** all-s., ***aloe, alum.,*** arg-m., **ARS.,** ***bell.,*** bor., calc., cham., cina, cob., ***colch.,*** cupr., hyper., ***ign.,*** iodof., **KALI-C.,** kali-cy., ***lyc.,*** nit-ac., nux-v., op., phys., ***puls.,*** ran-b., ***sel.,*** sep., sil., stram., ***stront-c., stry., sulph., sul-ac.,*** tub., ***zinc.***
air, as if wanting, from - calc-s.
fear, with - sabal.

JUMPING, agg. - agar., ***arg-m.,*** asar., ***aur.,*** bell., cic., ***croc.,*** grat., hyos., lact., nux-v., pip-m., spig., stict., stram., tarent.

KNEADING bread or making similar motion agg. - sanic.

KNEELING, ailments from - calc., ***cocc.,*** mag-c., puls., sep., spig., tarent.
agg. - ***cocc.,*** mag-c., ***sep.***
amel. - euph.

LABOR manual agg. - ***am-m., bov.,*** ferr., kali-c., ***lach.,*** mag-c., merc., **NAT-M.,** nit-ac., phos., ***sil., verat.***
mental agg. - ***arg-n., gels.,*** graph., lyc., nat-c., ***nux-v.,*** ph-ac., sil.

LASSITUDE, (see Chronic Fatigue or Generals, Weakness)

LEAN, thin people - acet-ac., alum., **AMBR.,** ***arg-m., arg-n., ars.,*** ars-i., bar-c., beryl., bry., cadm-m., ***calc.,*** calc-f., **CALC-P.,** caust., ***chin.,*** coff., cupr., ***ferr.,*** fl-ac., flor-p., graph., ***hep.,*** ign., ***iod.,*** ip., ***kreos.,*** lac-c., lach., ***lyc.,*** mag-c., mang., merc., nat-c., ***nat-m., nit-ac.,*** nux-m., ***nux-v.,*** perh., petr., ph-ac., **PHOS.,** ***plb.,*** puls., rat., saroth., **SEC.,** ***sep., sil.,*** spig., **STANN.,** staph., **SULPH., TUB.,** verat.
abdominal plethora - chel.
bilious, complexion, pimply, and subject to erysipelatous inflammation, pallor of face when excited by movement, or very red and flushed - ***hep.***
fibre, rigid, swarthy, black hair and eyes, brunette rather than the blonde nervous temperament - **NIT-AC.**
invalids, subacute attacks of bronchitis - ***phos.***
irritable, choleric, dark hair, make great mental exertion, or lead a sedentary life - **NUX-V.**
legs body fat - ***am-m.***
lung and hepatic affections, predisposed to - ***lyc.***
nervous affections, neuralgia, sciatica, lumbago, with deficiency of animal heat - ***ol-j.***
nervous temperament, delicate organization - xan.
relaxed - acet-ac.
rheumatism and catarrh, disposed to - ***colch.***
scrawny - **SEC.**
scrofulous diseases of joints - ***ol-j.***
spare, dry - alum.
stooped, walk and sit, standing is the most uncomfortable position - phos., **SULPH.**
tubercular disease, incipient - tub.
upper body wasted, lower semi-dropsical - ***lyc.***
weak - ***ferr., sil.***
and melancholy - ***lach.***

LEANING, against anything
- arg-m., arn., bell., cann-s., canth., cimic., coloc., con., cycl., graph., ***hell.,*** hep., mag-m., ***nit-ac.,*** phos., plat., samb., sil., stann., staph., sulph., ther., thuj.

LEANING, against anything, agg.
after - ***coloc.***
backward - nit-ac., staph.
head, sideways - cina.
sharp edge - agar., caust., chin-s., lyc., ran-b., ruta, ***samb.,*** stann., valer.
sideward - meny.
amel. - bell., ***carb-v.,*** dros., **FERR.,** gymn., ***kali-c.,*** kali-p., mang., merc., nat-c., ***nat-m.,*** nux-v., ph-ac., rhod., rhus-t., sabad., seneg., ***sep.,*** spig., staph.
hard - bell., ***rhus-t.***
sharp edge - nat-c., stann.
desire for - gymn., op., tub.

LEECHES agg., application of - sec.

LEUKEMIA, (see Cancer)

LICE - am-c., ars., lach., ***lyc., merc.,*** nit-ac., olnd., ***psor., sabad.,*** staph., ***sulph.,*** vinc.
head, of - am-c., apis, ars., bell-p., ***carb-ac.,*** lach., led., lyc., ***merc.,*** nit-ac., olnd., ***psor.,*** **STAPH.,** sulph., tub., vinc.

LICHEN, planus - agar., anac., ***ant-c.,*** apis, ***ars., ars-i.,*** chin-a., iod., ***jug-c., kali-bi.,*** kali-i., led., merc., sars., staph., ***sul-i.***
lichen, simplex - alum., am-m., ***anan.,*** ant-c., apis, ***ars., bell.,*** bov., bry., ***calad.,*** cast-v., dulc., ***jug-c.,*** kali-ar., ***kreos.,*** lach., ***led., lyc.,*** merc., nabal., nat-c., ***phyt., plan., rumx.,*** sep., sul-i., ***sulph.,*** thuj., til.

LIGAMENTS, pains in those that have been stretched, as in sprains - ruta.
relaxed - calc-f., ***cupr-ac.,*** ferr-s.

LOCKJAW, (see Emergency, Tetanus)

LUMBRICOIDES - acon., all-s., anac., ***ars.,*** asar., bar-c., bell., calc., carb-s., cic., cham., ***chel.,*** **CINA,** ***ferr-s., gran.,*** graph., hyos., kali-c., lyc., mag-c., merc., nat-m., nux-v., rhus-t., ruta., ***sabad.,*** sec., ***sil.,*** **SPIG.,** stann., **SULPH.,** ter.

LUPUS - agar., alum., alumn., ant-c., arg-n., **ARS.,** ars-i., aur-m., ***bar-c.,*** bell., calc., ***carb-ac., carb-v., caust.,*** cic., ***cist.,*** graph., guare., hep., ***hydrc.,*** kali-ar., ***kali-bi.,*** kali-c., ***kali-chl., kali-s., kreos.,*** lach., **LYC.,** mag-arct., merc-i-r., ***nat-m.,*** **NIT-AC.,** ol-j., ***phyt., psor.,*** rhus-t., sabin., sep., ***sil.,*** spong., staph., sulph., **THUJ.**
lupus, erythematosum - apis, cist., guare., ***hydrc., kali-bi.,*** paull., ***phos.,*** sep., ***thyr.***
lupus, face - alumn., ***arg-n.,*** **ARS.,** aur-m., carb-ac., ***carb-v.,*** cist., **HYDRC.,** kali-ar., ***kali-bi.,*** kali-chl., kreos., lach., psor., ***sep., sil.***
lupus, vulgaris - abr., apis, ***ars., ars-i.,*** aur-i., ***aur-m.,*** calc., calc-i., calc-s., ***cist.,*** cund., ferr-pic., form., graph., guare., ***hep., hydr., hydrc.,*** irid., kali-bi., kali-i., lyc., nit-ac., paull., phyt., staph., ***sulph.,*** thiosin., thuj., ***tub.,*** urea, x-ray

LYING, down
agg. - abies-n., ***acon., agar.,*** alum., ***ambr.,*** am-c., ***am-m.,*** anac., ant-c., ***ant-t.,*** **APIS,** ***apoc.,*** aral., ***arg-m.,*** arn., **ARS.,** ars-i., ***asaf.,*** asar., **AUR.,** ***bapt., bell.,*** bism., bor., bov., ***bry.,*** cact., calad., calc., calc-p., camph., cann-i., cann-s., canth., **CAPS.,** carb-an., carb-s., carb-v., caust., **CHAM.,** chel., chin., cic., cina, clem., cocc., coff., colch., coloc., **CON.,** croc., crot-t., cupr., ***cycl.,*** dig., dios., **DROS.,** ***dulc.,*** **EUPH.,** ***euphr.,*** **FERR.,** ferr-ar., ferr-i., ferr-p., fl-ac., gels., ***glon.,*** graph., grin., ***guai., hell.,*** hep., **HYOS.,** ign., iod., ip., kali-bi., **KALI-BR., KALI-C.,** kali-i., ***kali-n.,*** kreos., ***lach.,*** lact., laur., led., ***lil-t.,*** **LYC.,** mag-c., ***mag-m.,*** mang., **MENY.,** merc., mez., ***mosch., mur-ac.,*** murx., naja, nat-a., ***nat-c.,*** nat-m., **NAT-S.,** nit-ac., nux-m., ***nux-v.,*** olnd., ***op.,*** par., petr., phel., ***ph-ac.,*** **PHOS., PLAT.,** plb., **PULS.,** raph., ***ran-b.,*** rheum, ***rhod.,*** **RHUS-T., RUMX.,** ***ruta., sabad.,*** sabin., sal-ac., **SAMB., SANG.,** sars., sec., sel., seneg., ***sep.,*** spig., spong., squil., stann., staph., stict., stram., ***stront-c.,*** sul-ac., ***sulph.,*** **TARAX.,** teucr., thuj., ***valer.,*** verat., ***verb.,*** viol-o., ***viol-t.,*** zinc., ***zing.***
after, agg. - acon., agar., agn., alum., **AMBR.,** ***am-c.,*** am-m., ant-c., ant-t., ***arg-m.,*** arn., **ARS.,** ***asaf.,*** asar., **AUR.,** bar-c., bell., bism., bor., bov., bry., calad., calc., canth., ***caps.,*** carb-an., carb-v., caust., ***cham.,*** chel., chin., ***clem.,*** cocc., coff., colch., coloc., ***con.,*** croc., cupr., ***cycl.,*** dros., **DULC.,** ***euph., euphr., ferr.,*** graph., guai., hell., hep., ***hyos.,*** ign., ip., ***kali-c.,*** kali-n., lach., laur., led., **LYC.,** ***mag-c., mag-m.,*** mang., ***meny.,*** merc., mez., mosch., mur-ac., nat-a., nat-c., nit-ac., nux-m., nux-v., olnd., op., par., petr., ph-ac., phos., **PLAT.,** ***plb.,*** **PULS.,** ran-b., ran-s., rhod., **RHUS-T.,** ruta., ***sabad.,*** sabin., **SAMB.,** sars., sel., seneg., ***sep.,*** sil., spig., stann., staph., **STRONT-C.,** ***sulph.,*** sul-ac., ***tarax.,*** teucr., thuj., valer., verat., verb., viol-o., viol-t., zinc.
amel. - acon., agar., agn., alum., ambr., am-c., **AM-M.,** anac., ant-c., ant-t., arg-m., ***arn.,*** ars., **ASAR.,** ***bar-c.,*** **BELL.,** bor., **BRY.,** calad., **CALC.,** ***calc-p.,*** camph., cann-s., ***canth.,*** caps., carb-ac., ***carb-an.,*** carb-s., ***carb-v., caust.,*** chel., chin., cic., cimic., cina, clem., cocc., coff., ***colch.,*** coloc., con., conv., croc., cupr., dig., dios., dros., dulc., euph., **FERR.,** ***glon., graph.,*** guai., hell., hep., hyos., ***ign.,*** iod., ip., kali-c., kali-n., kalm., kreos., lach., laur., ***led.,*** lyc., mag-c., mag-m., **MANG.,** merc., mez., mur-ac., nat-c., **NAT-M.,** ***nit-ac.,*** nux-m., **NUX-V.,** olnd., op., par., petr., ph-ac., phos., **PIC-AC.,** plb., ***psor.,*** ran-b., rheum, rhus-t., ruta., sabad., sabin., sars., sec., sel., seneg., sep., ***spig., spong.,*** **SQUIL.,** ***sulph.,*** zinc.

LYING, down

amel.

after - acon., agar., agn., ambr., am-m., anac., ant-c., ant-t., arg-m., arn., **ARS.,** asaf., aur., bar-c., ***bell.,*** bov., **BRY.,** caj., calad., **CALC.,** calc-f., camph., cann-s., ***canth.,*** caps., carb-an., ***carb-s., carb-v.,*** caust., chel., chin., cic., ***cina,*** cocc., coff., colch., coloc., con., ***croc.,*** crot-h., cupr., dig., dios., dros., dulc., euphr., ***fl-ac., graph.,*** guai., hell., ***hep.,*** hyos., ign., ***iod.,*** ip., kali-c., kali-n., kreos., ***lach.,*** laur., led., lyc., mag-c., mag-m., meli., ***merc.,*** nat-c., **NAT-M., NIT-AC.,** nux-m., **NUX-V.,** ***olnd.,*** pall., par., petr., ph-ac., ***phos.,*** **PULS.,** ran-b., rheum, rhod., rhus-t., sabin., samb., sars., sec., sel., ***sep.,*** sil., sin-n., ***spig.,*** spong., **SQUIL.,** stann., ***staph., stram., sulph.,*** sul-ac., tarax., thuj., valer., verat., verb.

inclination to lie down - **ACON., ALUM.,** ***ambr., am-c., anac., ant-c.,*** ant-t., ***apis,*** **ARAN.,** arn., **ARS.,** asar., ***aur., bapt.,*** bell., ***bar-c.,*** bar-m., ***bell.,*** bism., bor., bry., **CALAD.,** ***calc.,*** canth., ***caps., carb-an.,*** **CARB-S.,** ***carb-v., casc., caust.,*** **CHAM.,** ***chel.,*** chin., chin-a., cina, ***cocc.,*** coff., ***con.,*** croc., cupr., ***cycl.,*** dig., dros., dulc., **FERR.,** ferr-p., ***gels., graph., guai.,*** hep., hipp., hyos., ***ign.,*** ip., **KALI-AR.,** ***kali-bi.,*** **KALI-C.,** kali-s., ***lach.,*** led., ***lyc.,*** mag-c., mag-m., mang., merc., mur-ac., nat-a., nat-c., ***nat-m.,*** nat-p., ***nit-ac.,*** **NUX-V.,** op., ***petr., ph-ac., phos., phyt., pic-ac., plan., puls.,*** ran-b., ***rhus-t.,*** ruta., sabad., **SEL.,** ***sep.,*** **SIL.,** ***spong., stann.,*** staph., ***stram.,*** stront-c., ***sulph., sumb.,*** tarax., ***tarent.,*** teucr., thuj., verat., ***zinc.***

abdomen in pregnancy, on - ***podo.***

but agg. by - alum., murx.

eating, after - ant-c., caust., chel., ***chin.,*** clem., ***lach.,*** nat-m., nit-ac., ***sel.***

must - apis.

will not lie down, sits up in bed - kali-br.

LYING, down, position

abdomen, on, amel. - acet-ac., aloe, ambr., am-c., ars., bar-c., **BELL.,** bry., calc., ***chel., cina, coloc.,*** crot-t., ***elaps,*** ind., lach., mag-c., ***med., nit-ac., phos.,*** phyt., plb., podo., rhus-t., sel., sep., ***stann.***

pregnancy, in, on - podo.

back, on, agg. - acet-ac., acon., aloe, alum., am-c., ***am-m., arg-m.,*** arn., ***ars.,*** aur-m., bar-c., bell., bor., bry., bufo, calc., canth., carb-v., ***caust., cham.,*** chin., cina, clem., ***coloc., cupr.,*** dulc., eup-per., euph., hyper., ***iod.,*** kali-c., lach., merc., nat-c., nat-m., ***nat-s.,*** **NUX-V.,** ***op.,*** par., **PHOS.,** plat., ran-b., ***rhus-t., sep., sil., spig.,*** spong., stront-c., ***sulph.,*** thuj.

amel. - ***acon.,*** aeth., am-c., **AM-M.,** ***anac., apis,*** arn., bar-c., bell., bor., **BRY.,** cact., calad., **CALC.,** ***canth., carb-an.,*** caust., chin., cimic., cina, clem., ***colch.,*** con.,

LYING, down, position

back, on, amel. - conv., ferr., grat., hell., ***ign.,*** ip., ***kali-c., kalm.,*** kreos., lach., ***lyc., mang.,*** merc., **MERC-C.,** mosch., nat-c., ***nat-m., nat-s.,*** nux-v., ox-ac., par., ***phos.,*** plat., **PULS.,** ran-b., **RHUS-T.,** sabad., ***sang.,*** senec., ***seneg.,*** sep., sil., spig., ***spong., stann.,*** sulph., ***thuj.,*** verat., viol- t.

unable to turn from the back - ***cic.,*** elaps.

bed, in, agg. - acon., ***agar.,*** aloe, alum., **AMBR.,** ***am-c.,*** am-m., anac., ant-c., ***ant-t., arg-m.,*** arn., ***ars.,*** ars-i., asaf., asar., ***aur.,*** bar-c., bell., bism., ***bor.,*** bov., ***bry.,*** calad., calc., camph., cann-s., canth., caps., carb-an., carb-v., caust., cham., chel., chin., cic., cina, ***clem.,*** cocc., coff., colch., ***coloc.,*** con., croc., cycl., dig., dios., ***dros.,*** dulc., ***euph.,*** euphr., **FERR., FERR-I.,** graph., guai., hell., hep., hyos., ign., **IOD.,** ***kali-c.,*** kali-i., kali-n., kali-p., kali-s., ***kalm.,*** kreos., **LACH.,** laur., ***led., lil-t., lith.,*** **LYC.,** ***mag-c., mang.,*** meny., **MERC.,** ***merc-i-f., mez.,*** mosch., mur-ac., nat-c., ***nat-m.,*** nit-ac., nux-m., ***nux-v.,*** olnd., op., ***ox-ac.,*** par., petr., ***ph-ac.,*** **PHOS.,** phyt., ***plat., plb.,*** **PULS.,** ran-b., rheum, ***rhod., rhus-t.,*** **RUMX.,** ruta., sabad., sabin., samb., **SANG.,** ***sars.,*** sec., ***sel.,*** seneg., **SEP., SIL.,** ***spig.,*** spong., squil., stann., staph., stict., stram., ***stront-c.,*** **SULPH.,** sul-ac., tarax., ***tell.,*** teucr., thuj., valer., ***verat.,*** verb., viol- o., viol-t., ***zinc.***

amel. - ***acon.,*** agar., ambr., ***am-m.,*** anac., ant-c., ant-t., arg-m., arn., ***ars.,*** asar., aur., ***bar-c.,*** bell., bov., **BRY.,** calad., calc., camph., cann-s., ***canth.,*** caps., carb-an., carb-v., ***caust.,*** cham., chel., chin., **Cic.,** cina, clem., **COCC.,** ***coc-c.,*** coff., colch., coloc., ***con.,*** croc., cupr., dig., dulc., ferr., graph., guai., hell., **HEP.,** hyos., ign., iod., ip., kali-c., kali-n., kreos., ***lach.,*** laur., led., ***lyc.,*** mag-c., ***mang.,*** merc., mez., mur-ac., nat-c., ***nat-m., nit-ac.,*** nux-m., **NUX-V.,** olnd., par., petr., ph-ac., phos., puls., ran-b., rheum, rhod., ***rhus-t.,*** sabad., sabin., samb., sars., sec., sel., sep., ***sil.,*** spig., spong., **SQUIL., STANN.,** ***staph., stram.,*** stront-c., sulph., sul-ac., tarax., thuj., valer., verat., verb., viol-t.

side, on, agg. - **ACON.,** am-c., am-m., **ANAC.,** ***arg-n.,*** arn., ars., aur., bar-c., bell., bor., **BRY.,** ***calad.,*** **CALC.,** canth., **CARB-AN.,** caust., chin., ***cina,*** clem., colch., ***con., ferr., ign., ip.,*** **KALI-C.,** kali-n., ***kreos.,*** lach., ***lil-t.,*** **LYC.,** ***merc., merc-c.,*** mosch., nat-m., ***nat-s.,*** nux-v., ***par., ph-ac., phos.,*** plat., ***puls.,*** ran-b., **RHUS-T.,** sabad., ***seneg.,*** sep., ***sil.,*** spig., spong., **STANN.,** ***sulph., thuj.,*** verat., viol- t.

amel. - acon., alum., am-c., am-m., arn., ars., bar-c., bell., bor., bry., calc-p., canth., caust., cham., chin., cina, clem., **COCC.,** colch., cupr., dulc., euph., ign., iod., kali-c., lach., nat-m., **NUX-V.,** par., ***phos.,*** plat., ran-b., rhus-t., ***sep.,*** spig., spong.,

LYING, down, position

side, on, agg. - stront-c., sulph., thuj.

left side agg. - ***acon.,*** ail., anac., ant-t., ***arg-n.,*** arn., ***bar-c.,*** bell., bry., ***cact.,*** canth., carb-an., chin., ***colch.,*** con., eup-per., glon., ***iber.,*** ind., ip., kali-ar., kali-c., kalm., kreos., lyc., mag-m., merc., ***naja, nat-c., nat-m.,*** nat-p., ***nat-s.,*** op., ***par.,*** petr., **PHOS.,** plat., **PULS.,** rhus-t., seneg., ***sep.,*** sil., ***sulph.,*** tab., ***thuj.***

painful side, agg. - ***acon.,*** agar., ambr., am-c., am-m., anac., ***ant-c.,*** arg-m., arn., ***ars.,*** ars-i., ***bapt.,*** **BAR-C.,** ***bell.,*** bry., **CALAD.,** calc., calc-f., cann-s., caps., carb-an., carb-v., caust., ***chin.,*** cina, clem., croc., cupr., cycl., dios., ***dros., graph.,*** guai., **HEP.,** hyos., ign., **IOD.,** ***kali-c., kali-i.,*** kali-n., lach., laur., led., ***lyc., mag-c.,*** mang., ***merc.,*** mez., ***mosch.,*** mur-ac., nat-m., ***nit-ac.,*** **NUX-M.,** ***nux-v.,*** olnd., ***par.,*** petr., ***ph-ac., phos.,*** plat., puls., ran-b., ran-s., ***rheum,*** rhod., ***rhus-t., rumx.,*** **RUTA.,** ***sabad.,*** sabin., samb., sars., sel., sep., **SIL.,** ***spong.,*** staph., stram., tarax., teucr., thuj., valer., verat., verb.

amel. - ambr., am-c., arn., bell., **BRY.,** ***calc.,*** cann-s., carb-v., caust., ***cham., coloc.,*** ign., kali-c., lyc., nux-v., ***puls.,*** rhus-t., ***sep.,*** stram., sulph., viol-o., viol-t.

painless, side, agg. - ***ambr., arg-n.,*** arn., bell., **BRY.,** ***calc.,*** cann-s., carb-v., ***caust.,*** **CHAM.,** chel., chin., **COLOC.,** cupr., fl-ac., hyper., ***ign., kali-c.,*** lyc., mer-i-r., naja., nat-c., nux-v., phos., plan., **PULS.,** ***rhus-t.,*** sec., ***sep.,*** stann., sul-ac., vio-o., vio-t.

amel. - acon., agar., ambr., am-c., anac., ant-c., arg-m., arn., ars., ***bapt., bar-c., bell.,*** bry., ***calad.,*** calc-f., cann-s., caps., carb-an., carb-v., caust., chin., cina, clem., croc., cupr., dios., dros., graph., guai., ***hep.,*** hyos., ign., ***iod., kali-c.,*** kali-n., lach., led., lyc., mag-c., mang., merc., mez., mosch., mur-ac., nat-m., nit-ac., ***nux-m., nux-v.,*** olnd., par., petr., ph-ac., plat., puls., ran-b., rheum, rhod., rhus-t., ***ruta.,*** bad., sabin., samb., sars., sel., sep., ***sil., spong.,*** staph., stram., tarax., thuj., valer., verat., verb.

pains, go to side lain on - ars., ***bry.,*** calc., ***kali-c.,*** merc., ***ph-ac.,*** puls., sep., sil.

to side not lain on - bry., cupr., fl-ac., graph., ***ign.,*** kali-bi., ***rhus-t.***

right, side, agg. - acon., ***alum., am-c., am-m.,*** anac., ***benz-ac., bor.,*** bry., bufo, calc., carb-an., cina, clem., con., ip., ***kali-c.,*** kali-i., kreos., lyc., mag-c., **MERC.,** ***mag-m.,*** mur-ac., ***nux-v., phos.,*** prun., psor., ran-b., sang., seneg., ***spong.,*** sulph., sul-ac., thuj.

LYME disease - ars., merc. thuj.

LYMPHOID tissue, ailments of - carc., rad-br.

MAGNETIZED, desires body to be - **CALC.,** ***lach.,*** nat-c., **PHOS., SIL.**

easy to magnetize - caust., crot-c., lach., ***phos.,*** sep.

magnetism, mesmerism, amel. - acon., bar-c., ***bell., calc.,*** calc-p., chin., con., **CUPR.,** graph., ign., iod., nat-c., ***nux-v.,*** **PHOS.,** sabin., sep., ***sil.,*** sulph., ***teucr.,*** viol-o.

MALAISE, (see Weakness)

MANUAL, work (see Work)

MEASLES, (see Fevers)

MENIERE'S disease - alum., arg-m., ***arg-n.,*** arn., ars., asar., bar-m., bell., benz-ac., bry., calc., ***camph.,*** carb-v., carb-s., ***caust.,*** chen-a., chin., **CHIN-S.,** ***chin-sal., cic., cocc.,*** colch., com., con., crot-h., crot-t., ***dig.,*** eucal., ferr-p., gels., ***glon.,*** gran., hell., hydrobr-ac., jab., kali-c., kali-i., kali-m., kali-p., kalm., laur., mag-c., morg., myric., nat-a., nat-c., nat-m., nat-p., nat-s., ***nat-sal.,*** nux-v., onos., op., petr., ph-ac., **PHOS.,** pic-ac., psor., puls., rad-br., ***sal-ac., sang.,*** seneg., sep., ***sil.,*** stann., tab., ***ther.,*** thyr., zinc.

noises, before vertigo - lachn., sep.

seasick, as if - tab.

MIDNIGHT, (see Time, general)

MOLLUSCUM contagiosum - ***brom.,*** bry., calc., ***calc-ar.,*** kali-i., lyc., merc., merc-sul., ***nat-m., sil.,*** sulph., teucr., ***thuj.***

MONONUCLEOSIS, (see Fevers)

MOON, (see Environment)

MORNING, (see Time, general)

MOTION, general

absent - ***bry.,*** cocc., gels., hell., rhus-t.

agg. - abrot., ***acon., agar., agn.,*** aloe, alum., ambr., am-c., am-m., anac., ant-c., ant-t., ***apis,*** apoc., ***arn., ars.,*** ars-h., ***ars-i., asaf., asar., aspar., aur.,*** bapt., ***bar-c.,*** **BELL.,** ***berb.,*** **BISM.,** bor., bov., **BRY.,** bufo, ***cact.,*** cadm-s., ***calad.,*** calc., ***calc-p., calc-s., camph.,*** cann-i., ***cann-s., canth., caps., carb-an., carb-s., carb-v.,*** card-m., caust., cham., **CHEL., CHIN.,** chin-a., ***chion.,*** cic., ***cimic., cimx.,*** cina, ***cinnb.,*** clem., **COCC.,** coc-c., ***coff.,*** **COLCH., COLOC.,** ***con., croc., crot-h.,*** crot-t., cupr-ar., cupr., ***dig.,*** dros., ***eup-per.,*** euph., ***ferr.,*** ferr-i., ***fl-ac.,*** form., ***gels., glon., graph.,*** **GUAI.,** ***hell., hep.,*** hyos., ign., ***iod., ip., iris,*** jac., ***kali-bi., kali-n.,*** kali-p., ***kalm., lach.,*** laur., **LED.,** lycps., mag-c., mag-m., ***mag-p., mang., med., meli.,*** meny., **MERC.,** merc-c., mez., mosch., ***nat-a.,*** nat-c., ***nat-m., nat-p., nat-s., nit-ac.,*** nux-m., **NUX-V.,** olnd., ol-an., ***onos.,*** op., osm., ***ox-ac.,*** pall., par., ***petr.,*** ph-ac., ***phos., phyt.,*** plat., ***plb., psor.,*** ptel., puls., **RAN-B.,** ran-s., ***rheum,*** rumx., sabad., **SABIN.,** samb., ***sang., sanic., sec., sel.,*** senec., seneg., ***sep.,*** **SIL.,** ***spig.,*** spong., ***squil., stann., staph.,***

MOTION, general

agg. - stram., stront-c., **SULPH.,** sul-ac., tarax., teucr., ***ther.,*** thuj., tril., ***verat.,*** verb., viol-o., viol-t., ***visc., zinc.***

after - **AGAR.,** am-c., ***anac.,*** arn., **ARS.,** aspar., calad., camph., **CANN-S.,** ***carb-v.,*** caust., cocc., coff., ***croc.,*** dros., ***hyos.,*** iod., ***kali-c.,*** laur., merc., ***nit-ac.,*** nux-v., olnd., phos., plb., **PULS., RHUS-T.,** ***ruta.,*** sabin., sep., spig., **SPONG., STANN.,** staph., ***stram.,*** sul-ac., **VALER.,** zinc.

distant parts - apis, ***bry.,*** cocc.

downward - **BOR.,** carb-v., **GELS.,** sanic., sep., sulph.

kneading bread or making similar motion - sanic.

slightest - ***bry.,*** bufo, cadm-s., lat-m., lob., ther.

rotation - bry., cocc., coloc., kali-c.

slow - sep.

sudden - cocc., ferr., kali-c.

violent - acon., arn., ***ars., bry.,*** calc., camph., lyc., mag-c., nux-v., rhus-t., ruta, sep., sil., sul-ac., sulph., symph.

wrong - bry., lyc.

amel. - ***acon., agar., aloe, alum.,*** ambr., ***am-c., am-m., anac.,*** ant-t., ***arg-m., arg-n.,*** arn., ***ars.,*** asaf., asar., ***atro.,*** **AUR., AUR-M.,** ***aur-m-n., bar-c.,*** bar-m., benz-ac., ***bism.,*** bor., bov., ***brom.,*** calc., calc-p., canth., **CAPS.,** carb-ac., carb-an., carb-v., ***caust.,*** cham., chin., ***chin-a.,*** cic., ***cina,*** coca, ***cocc., coloc., com.,*** **CON.,** cupr., **CYCL.,** ***dios., dros.,*** **DULC., EUPH.,** euphr., **FERR.,** ferr-ar., ferr-p., ***gamb., gels.,*** guai., hep., hyos., ign., ***indg.,*** **IOD.,** ***kali-c., kali-i., kali-n., kali-p.,*** **KALI-S.,** ***kreos.,*** lach., laur., ***lil-t.,*** lith., lob., **LYC.,** ***mag-c., mag-m.,*** mang., ***meny., med., merc-c., merc-i-f., mosch., mur-ac., nat-c., nat-s.,*** nit-ac., nux-m., olnd., op., par., petr., ***ph-ac., plat.,*** **PYROG., PULS.,** ***rat.,*** **RHOD., RHUS-T.,** ***ruta.,*** **SABAD., SAMB.,** sel., seneg., ***sep.,*** spig., ***stann., stram.,*** **SULPH.,** sul-ac., **TARAX., TARENT.,** teucr., thuj., ***tub.,*** **VALER.,** verat., ***verb., vib., viol-t., zinc.***

affected part, of - abrot., acon., ***agar.,*** agn., ***am-m.,*** ang., apis, arn., ***ars.,*** ars-i., asaf., asar., ***aur.,*** bell., calc., **CAPS.,** cham., ***chin.,*** cina, ***con.,*** croc., **DULC.,** ***euph.,*** **FERR.,** hyos., ***kali-bi.,*** kali-c., lith., ***lyc.,*** mag-c., ***mag-m.,*** meny., ***mosch.,*** mur-ac., nat-c., ***ph-ac.,*** **PULS.,** ***rhod.,*** **RHUS-T.,** ***sabad., samb., sep.,*** squil., stann., stront-c., **SULPH.,** ***tarax.,*** thuj., valer., verb., viol-t.

air, in open - ***alum., arg-n.,*** dios., ***fl-ac., iod., kali-i.,*** kali-s., ***lil-t.,*** lyc., mag-c., mag-m., **PULS.,** ***rhus-t.***

continued - agar., ***ambr., am-m.,*** anac., aran-ix., bell-p., bry., ***cact., calc-f.,*** **CAPS.,** carb-v., caust., chin., ***cina,*** cob., com., **CON.,** ***cycl., dros.,*** **EUPH., FERR., FL-AC.,** gels., graph., ign., ind., iod., iris,

MOTION, general

amel.

kali-c., kalm., ***lyc.,*** mag-c., man., phos., plat., plb., ***ptel.,*** **PULS.,** rad., rauw., ***rhod.,*** **RHUS-T.,** ruta, ***sabad.,*** sabin., **SAMB.,** sep., ***sil.,*** **SYPH.,** tarax., thuj., tub., ***valer., verat.,*** zinc.

gliding - nit-ac.

rapid - am-m., ***ars.,*** aur-m., brom., ***bry., ferr.,*** fl-ac., graph., ign., nit-ac., scop., ***sep.,*** sil., stann., sul-ac., sulph., tarent., thlaspi, tub.

slow - agar., alum., ambr., asaf., ***aur.,*** bell., calc., caust., coloc., **FERR.,** ferr-ac., ferr-ar., glon., kali-bi., ***kali-p., mag-m.,*** plat., **PULS.,** stann., ***sulph.,*** sumb., **SYPH.,** tarent., zinc.

sudden - rhod., sabad.

violent - aesc., **ARS., BROM.,** cham., dulc., phys., **SEP.,** sil., ***sul-ac.***

wrong - am-m.

aversion, to - **ACON.,** alum., ambr., am-c., anac., ant-c., ant-t., arn., **ARS.,** asar., ***bar-c.,*** **BELL.,** bor., **BRY.,** cadm-s., **CALAD., CALC., CALC-S.,** canth., ***caps., carb-an., carb-s., carb-v.,*** caust., cham., ***chel., chin.,*** chin-a., cina, ***cocc.,*** coff., ***con.,*** croc., cupr., ***cycl., dig.,*** dros., dulc., ferr., ferr-i., ***gels., graph.,*** **GUAI.,** hyos., ***ign.,*** ip., kali-ar., ***kali-bi., kali-c.,*** kali-p., **LACH.,** led., ***lyc.,*** mag-c., mag-m., merc., ***mez.,*** mur-ac., ***nat-a.,*** nat-c., ***nat-m.,*** nit-ac., **NUX-V.,** op., petr., ***ph-ac.,*** phos., psor., puls., **RUTA.,** ***sang.,*** sep., **SIL.,** stann., stront-c., **SULPH.,** tarax., teucr., ***thuj.,*** zinc.

seated, after being - kali-p.

beginning, of, agg. - ***agar.,*** ant-t., asar., cact., calc., **CAPS.,** ***carb-v., caust.,*** chin., cina, cocc., **CON.,** cupr., dig., dros., **EUPH., FERR.,** fl-ac., graph., ***kali-p.,*** lach., led., **LYC.,** mag-c., nit-ac., petr., ***ph-ac., phos.,*** plat., plb., ***psor.,*** **PULS.,** rhod., **RHUS-T.,** ruta., ***sabad.,*** sabin., ***samb.,*** sars., ***sil., ther.,*** thuj., valer., verat., ***zinc.***

continued, amel. - agar., ***ambr., am-m.,*** bry., ***cact.,*** **CAPS.,** carb-v., caust., chin., ***cina,*** com., **CON.,** ***cycl., dros.,*** **EUPH., FERR.,** gels., ind., iris, kali-c., ***lyc.,*** plat., plb., ***ptel.,*** **PULS.,** ***rhod.,*** **RHUS-T.,** ruta., ***sabad.,*** sabin., **SAMB.,** sep., ***sil.,*** tarax., thuj., ***valer., verat.***

desire for - acon., agar., alum., am-c., ***ambr.,*** arg-m., arg-n., ***arn.,*** ars., asar., aur., aur-a., ***bell.,*** bell-p., bism., bor., bry., calc., canth., cench., **CHAM., CHIN.,** coff., coloc., con., ***cupr.,*** euphr., **FERR.,** ferr-ar., ferr-i., hyos., ign., iod., ip., kali-i., kreos., lyc., macro., mag-c., mag-m., mang., merc., mosch., mur-ac., nat-c., nit-ac., nux-m., nux-v., op., petr., ph-ac., phos., puls., ran-b., rhod., **RHUS-T.,** ruta, samb., sec., sep., sil., squil., stann., staph., sul-i., sulph., ***teucr.,*** tub., valer.

MOTION, general

difficult - bell., ***bry.,*** caust., lyc., petr., rhus-t., ***sep.***

disorderly - stram.

paralytic part, of - merc.

exaggerated - agar., ign.

erratic - tarent., verat-v.

incessant, but walking agg. - tarent.

irregular - agar.

oscillatory - agar., elaps, stram.

part, affected of, agg. - ***acon.,*** **AESC.,** agar., am-c., anac., ***ant-c.,*** **ARN.,** ***ars.,*** asaf., asar., bar-c., ***bell.,*** **BRY.,** camph., ***cann-s., caps.,*** caust., **CHAM.,** chel., ***chin.,*** cic., cimic., clem., ***cocc.,*** coff., **COLCH.,** ***coloc., com.,*** con., croc., cupr., dig., ferr-ar., form., ***gels., glon.,*** guai., hep., ign., iod., kali-c., ***kalm., lach.,*** **LED.,** mag-c., mang., meny., ***merc., mez.,*** nat-c., nat-m., nux-m., nux-v., olnd., petr., ***phos.,*** phyt., plat., ***puls., ran-b., rheum,*** **RHUS-T.,** ***rhod.,*** rumx., ruta., sabad., ***sabin.,*** samb., ***sang., sars.,*** sel., sep., ***sil.,*** **SPIG.,** ***stann.,*** staph., ***sulph.,*** thuj., zinc.

amel. - abrot., acon., ***agar.,*** agn., ***am-m.,*** arn., ***ars.,*** ars-i., asaf., asar., ***aur.,*** calc., **CAPS.,** cham., ***chin.,*** cina, ***con.,*** croc., **DULC.,** ***euph.,*** **FERR.,** ***kali-bi.,*** kali-c., ***lyc.,*** mag-c., ***mag-m.,*** meny., ***mosch.,*** mur-ac., nat-c., ***ph-ac.,*** **PULS.,** ***rhod.,*** **RHUS-T.,** ***sabad., samb., sep.,*** squil., stann., stront-c., **SULPH.,** ***tarax.,*** thuj., valer., verb., viol- t.

rhythmic - elaps, stram.

side, one only - stront-c.

slow motion, amel. - calc., **FERR., PULS.,** ***sulph.,*** **SYPH.**

tumultuous - acon., ***glon.,*** tab.

MOTION, sickness (see Emergency)

MOUNTAIN, sickness (see Altitude)

MUCUS secretions, general

amel. - apis, arg-m., arist-cl., ars., ***bry.,*** calc., camph., cimic., cupr., dulc., graph., ip., kali-bi., **LACH.,** lyc., mosch., nux-v., ph-ac., psor., ***puls.,*** rhus-t., senec., sep., sil., squil., stann., stict., stram., **SULPH.,** thuj., verat., ***zinc.***

acrid - aesc., ***all-c.,*** all-s., ***alum., am-c., am-m.,*** anac., ant-c., ***ars.,*** ars-i., ***arum-t., bor.,*** bov., ***brom.,*** calc., cann-s., canth., carb-an., ***carb-v., caust., cham.,*** chin., ***con.,*** euph., ***ferr.,*** fl-ac., ***graph.,*** hep., ***ign., iod.,*** kali-c., kali-i., ***kreos., lach., lyc.,*** mag-arct., mag-c., ***mag-m.,*** mang., ***merc., mez.,*** mur-ac., ***nat-m., nit-ac., nux-v.,*** ph-ac., ***phos.,*** prun., ***puls., ran-b., rhus-t.,*** ruta, sang., ***sep., sil., spig., squil., sul-ac., sulph.,*** thuj.

albuminoid - alum., am-m., berb., bor., bov., coc-c., graph., grat., jatr., ***kali-m.,*** mez., **NAT-M.,** pall., petr., plat., sep., stann.

altered and increased - colch.

bitter taste - aloe, cocc., ***kali-bi.,*** nat-m., nux-v., puls.

MUCUS secretions, general

bland - alumn., arg-n., cycl., euphr., ***hep.,*** kali-i., kali-m., kali-s., ***merc.,*** **PULS.,** sil., sulph.

yellowish-green, thick - **PULS.**

blood-streaked mucus - ***ter.***

bloody - acon., ail., aloe, alum., alum-sil., am-c., am-m., aphis., arg-n., arn., ars., ***ars-s-f., asar.,*** bar-m., ***bell.,*** bor., brom., bry., ***calc-s., canth.,*** caps., carb-an., ***carb-v.,*** caust., ***chin.,*** cocc., cop., ***crot-h.,*** daph., dros., euon., ferr., form., graph., ham., hep., iod., kali-ar., kali-c., kali-chl., kali-n., kreos., ***lach.,*** led., lyc., mag-c., mag-m., mang., ***merc.,*** mez., mur-ac., murx., nat-m., ***nit-ac.,*** nux-m., ***nux-v.,*** op., par., petr., ***phos., puls.,*** sabin., sang., ***sep., sil.,*** sul-ac., sulph., ***ter.,*** thuj., verat., vip., zinc., zinc-p.

bluish - ambr., ars., cupr., cupr-ac., lach.

brownish - am-m., ambr., ars., ***bell.,*** bism., bor., carb-v., grat., hydr., ***kreos.,*** nit-ac., sulph.

burning - acon., aesc., ***ail.,*** all-c., alum., alum-p., am-c., am-m., ***ars.,*** ars-i., ars-s-f., arum-t., bad., brom., calad., ***calc.,*** canth., caps., carb-ac., ***carb-an.,*** carb-v., cast., chin., chlor., cina, ***con.,*** crot-h., fl-ac., ***gels.,*** graph., guai., hep., hydr., iod., kali-c., ***kali-i.,*** kreos., lach., lyc., mag-s., ***merc.,*** merc-c., mez., mur-ac., nat-m., ***nit-ac.,*** petr., phos., phyt., puls., ran-s., ***sabad.,*** sang., sep., sil., sin-n., sul-ac., ***sulph.***

cold - verat.

corrosive - **ALUM.,** am-c., ***am-m.,*** ant-c., **ARS.,** ars-i., ***ars-s-f.,*** arum-t., bor., ***bov.,*** carb-v., **CAUST.,** ***cham., con.,*** ferr., **HYDR.,** ign., ***iod.,*** ip., kali-ar., ***kali-bi., kali-i., kreos., lach.,*** lyc., **MERC.,** mez., nat-m., **NIT-AC.,** ***nux-v., phos., puls., rhus-t.,*** ruta, sep., **SIL.,** staph., sul-ac., ***sulph., thuj.***

dirty, yellowish green, not laudable - **NIT-AC.**

fetid - ars., **BAPT.,** ***carb-v.,*** **KREOS.,** ***lach.,*** **NIT-AC.**

fishy, offensive - calc., graph., med., ol-an., sanic., sep., tell., thuj.

flocculent - agar., ambr., kali-bi., kali-c., kreos., mag-c., merc., phos., sabad., sep., sil., sulph., thuj.

frothy - ***aphis.,*** ars., **NAT-M.,** op., sec., sul-ac.

gelatinous - ***aloe,*** arg-m., ***arg-n.,*** bell., berb., caust., cocc., ***colch.,*** coloc., dig., ***hell., kali-bi.,*** laur., podo., ***rhus-t.,*** sabin., sel., sep.

gray - ***ambr.,*** anac., ***arg-m.,*** ars., carb-an., caust., chin., cop., kali-m., kreos., lach., ***lyc.,*** mag-m., merc., ***sil.,*** thuj.

greenish - acon., ***ars.,*** asaf., aur., bor., ***carb-v.,*** caust., cham., colch., con., ***dros.,*** ferr., hyos., ip., ***kali-bi.,*** kali-c., ***kali-i.,*** kali-s., kreos., lach., led., ***lyc.,*** mag-aust., ***mag-c.,*** mang., med., ***merc.,*** murx., nat-c., nat-m., nat-s., nit-ac., nux-v., ***par., phos.,*** **PULS.,** rhus-t., sabad., sec., ***sep.,*** sil., ***stann.,*** sul-ac., ***sulph.,*** thuj., ***verat.***

hard - agar., bry., con., **KALI-BI.,** ***mosch.,*** nat-c., ***phos., sep., sil.,*** stict., ***sulph., thuj.***

MUCUS secretions, general

honey-like - ars-i.

hot - ***acon., bell.***, bor., euphr., ***iod.***, kreos., op., ***puls.***, sabin., ***sulph.***

increased - acet-ac., acon., agar., agn., **ALL-C.**, ***alum.***, ambr., am-c., ***am-m., ammc.***, ang., ***ant-c.***, ant-t., ***arg-m.***, aphis., ***arg-n.***, arn., ***ars.***, ars-i., arum-m., asaf., asar., aur., aur-s., ***bar-c., bar-m., bell., benz-ac.***, bism., bond., ***bor.***, bov., bry., **CALC.**, calc-s., calc-sil., camph., ***cann-s.***, canth., ***caps.***, carb-an., ***carb-s.***, **CARB-V.**, ***caust., cham.***, chel., ***chin.***, chlor., chr-ac., cina, cinnb., cocc., ***coc-c.***, coff., colch., coloc., ***con., cop.***, croc., cupr., dig., dros., **DULC.**, euph., ***euphr., ferr.***, ferr-i., ***graph.***, grat., guai., hell., ***hep.***, **HYDR.**, ***hyos.***, ign., **IOD.**, ***ip., iris,*** jab., kali-ar., **KALI-BI.**, ***kali-c.***, kali-chl., ***kali-i.***, kali-m., kali-n., kreos., **LACH.**, lact., laur., **LYC.**, mag-arct., mag-aust., mag-c., mag-m., mec., **MED.**, **MERC.**, mez., mur-ac., myric., nat-a., ***nat-c., nat-m., nat-s.***, nicc., ***nit-ac.***, ***nux-m.***, **NUX-V.**, ***olnd.***, op., ***par.***, **PETR.**, ph-ac., **PHOS.**, plat., plb., podo., **PULS.**, ran-b., raph., rat., rheum, rhod., ***rhus-t.***, ***rumx.***, ruta., sabad., sabin., ***samb.***, sars., sec., sel., ***seneg., sep., sil.***, sin-n., spig., spong., ***squil., stann.***, staph., stroph., sul-i., **SULPH.**, sul-ac., **TAB.**, tax., teucr., thal., **THUJ.**, tong., valer., verat., zinc.

jelly-like lumps or cakes - aloe.

lumpy - ***calc-s., hep.***, kali-c., kreos., phos., sabad., sabin., sin-n., stann.

metallic taste - calc., cupr., ip., nux-v., rhus-t.

milky - ***calc.***, carb-v., con., ferr., ***kali-m.***, kali-p., lyc., nat-s., ***ph-ac.***, phos., ***puls.***, sabin., sep., ***sil.***, sul-ac.

musty smell - bor., ***carb-v., coloc.***, crot-h., ***merc.***, nux-v., ***phos., puls., rhus-t., stann.***

offensive, fetid - ail., arg-n., arn., ***ars., ars-s-f.***, arum-t., ***asaf., aur-s.***, bals-p., **BAPT.**, bell., ***calc.***, calc-f., calc-sil., caps., carb-ac., carb-an., ***carb-v., chel.***, chin., chlor., cist., con., cop., crot-h., cupr., echi., ferr., fl-ac., ***graph.***, helon., hep., ***hura,*** kali-ar., kali-bi., kali-br., kali-i., kali-p., kali-per., kali-s., **KREOS.**, **LACH.**, lyc., mag-c., ***merc.***, mur-ac., **NIT-AC.**, ***nux-v.***, petr., ***psor., pyrog., rob., sabin.***, sang., sec., ***sep.***, sil., stann., ther., tril., vip.

passive, flux - ***ph-ac.***

purulent - ***aur.***, **CALC.**, **CON.**, cop., ***graph.***, ign., lyc., ***merc.***, nat-c., ***puls.***, sep., ***sil., sulph.***

ropy, tenacious - acon., agn., ***alum.***, alum-p., am-m., anac., ***ant-c.***, ant-s., ant-t., arg-m., arg-n., ***ars.***, asaf., bar-ac., bar-c., bar-m., ***bell.***, ***bov.***, bry., calc., cann-s., canth., carb-an., carb-s., carb-v., caust., ***cham.***, chin., ***chin-s.***, ***cist., coc-c.***, cocc., colch., con., croc., culx., dulc., euphr., form., graph., hep., ***hydr.***, iod., **KALI-BI.**, kali-c., ***kali-m.***, kali-s., lach., lact., lap-a., laur., lob., lyc., mag-arct., mag-aust., ***mag-c.***, mag-m., ***merc., mez.***, myrt-c., nat-c., nat-m., nux-v., ol-an., osm., ***par., ph-ac.***, ***phos.***, phyt., plat., plb., puls., ***ran-b.***, raph., rhus-t., sabad., sabin., ***samb.***, scroph-n., ***seneg.***, sep., sin-n., spig., spong., squil., **STANN.**, staph., sul-ac., ***sulph.***, sumb., ***tab.***, thuj., tong., ust., verat., zinc.

salty, taste - alum., ***ambr., ars., bar-c.***, calc., chin., dros., fl-ac., ***graph., iod., kali-i., lyc.***, mag-c., mag-m., ***merc., nat-c., nat-m.***, nux-v., ***petr., phos.***, puls., samb., ***sep., sil.***, stann., staph., sulph., zinc.

scanty - ***nat-m.***

sour, taste - calc., graph., ***hep.***, kali-c., kali-n., lam., mag-m., merc., nat-c., nat-p., nit-ac., nux-v., ***plb.***, sep., sulph., tarax.

suppressed - abrot., agar., ***ant-c.***, arist-cl., ars., asaf., **ASAR.**, aur-m., ***bar-c., bry.***, bufo, calc., carb-v., cupr., ***dulc., graph., kali-bi.***, ***lach.***, led., ***lob.***, med., merc., mill., ***mosch.***, ***nux-v.***, plb., ***psor., puls.***, sanic., senec., ***sil.***, ***stram., sulph.***, verat., viol-o., zinc.

sweetish, taste - asar., ***calc.***, cham., lach., mag-c., merc-c., phos., stann.

tenacious - bov., hydr., **KALI-BI.**, sin-n.

thick, slimy - acon., agar., ***alum.***, alum-sil., am-m., ant-c., arg-m., ***arg-n., ars.***, ars-i., ars-s-f., ***aur-s.***, bals-p., ***bar-c.***, berb., bor., calc., calc-s., carb-an., carb-s., carb-v., cast., caust., chin., cist., coc-c., con., cop., cycl., graph., helon., ***hep.***, **HYDR.**, iod., ip., **KALI-BI.**, kali-br., ***kali-i., kali-m., kali-s.***, kali-sil., kreos., lac-ac., lam., lith., lyc., mag-arct., mag-c., ***mag-m.***, mag-s., mang., merc., merc-d., mur-ac., murx., ***nat-c.***, nat-m., nat-s., nat-sil., nicc., ol-an., op., par., phos., **PULS.**, ruta, sabad., samb., sars., scroph-n., sec., sel., seneg., sil., staph., ***sulph.***, tong., thuj., tub., zinc., zing.

thin - ambr., ant-t., ***ars., ars-s-f., asaf.***, asar., ***bell.***, bor., bov., ***calc.***, canth., caps., ***carb-v.***, caust., colch., ***con.***, ferr., ***fl-ac.***, gels., ***graph.***, ***kali-i.***, kali-n., laur., lyc., ***mag-c.***, mez., mur-ac., ***nat-m.***, **NIT-AC.**, nux-v., ol-an., ***puls.***, rhus-t., seneg., ***sil.***, stann., staph., sul-ac., ter., thuj.

ichorous, corrosive - ***kali-i.***

transparent - aesc., alum., cast., crot-h., ferr-m., fl-ac., graph., kali-i., mag-s., mang., **NAT-M.**, phos., puls., sabad., ***sep., sil.***, ***stann.***, sul-ac.

watery, coarse, frothy - **NAT-M.**

transudation of watery portions of blood, causing copious diarrhea - crot-t.

urinous, odor - benz-ac., canth., ***coloc.***, nat-m., nit-ac., ol-an., sec., urt-u.

vicarious - ***bry.***, con., dig., ham., ***lach.***, lycps., mill., nux-v., **PHOS.**, ***puls.***, sec., ***senec.***, sulph.

watery - acon., aesc., ***agar.***, **ALL-C.**, alum., ***am-c., am-m.***, ambr., ant-c., arg-m., **ARS.**, ***asaf.***, asar., bell., ***bov.***, brom., calc., cann-s., ***carb-an., carb-v.***, cast., ***caust., cham.***, ***chin.***, chlor., clem., coff., con., crot-h., cupr., elat., gamb., gels., ***graph.***, grat., ign., iod.,

MUCUS secretions, general

watery - iris, ***jug-c.,*** kali-i., kali-n., ***kali-s.,*** kreos., ***lach., mag-arct., mag-c., mag-m.,*** meny., ***merc., mez., mur-ac.,*** murx., **NAT-M.,** nat-s., nicc., ***nux-v.,*** par., phos., ***plb., podo.,*** puls., ran-b., rhus-t., sabin., seneg., ***sep., sil., squil.,*** stann., staph., sul-ac., ***sulph.,*** thuj., verat.

white - bell., ferr., graph., grat., hell., **KALI-M.,** kali-n., kreos., lyc., mag-arct., mag-c., ***merc.,*** **NAT-M.,** nat-s., nux-v., ol-an., ***phos.,*** prun., ***puls.,*** raph., rat., sabin., ***sep., sil.,*** sul-ac., tab.

full of bubbles, color of white of egg or like boiled mucus - **NAT-M.**

thick, livid - ***kali-m.***

yellow - ***acon.,*** agar., agn., alum., alum-p., alum-sil., alumn., am-c., am-m., ambr., anac., ang., ***ant-c.,*** arg-m., ***arg-n., ars.,*** ars-i., ***ars-s-f.,*** aur., aur-a., ***aur-i., aur-s.,*** bar-c., bar-i., bar-s., ***bell., berb.,*** bov., ***bry., calc.,*** calc-s., calc-sil., ***cann-s., canth.,*** caps., ***carb-an., carb-v.,*** cast., caust., cench., ***cham., cic.,*** cist., clem., con., cor-r., croc., cycl., ***daph., dros.,*** dulc., ***eug.,*** form., gran., ***graph., hep.,*** **HYDR.,** ***iod.,*** kali-ar., ***kali-bi., kali-c., kali-m.,*** kali-n., **KALI-S.,** kali-sil., ***kreos.,*** lac-ac., lach., ***lyc.,*** mag-c., mag-m., mag-s., mang., merc., merc-i-f., mez., mur-ac., ***nat-c., nat-m., nat-p.,*** nat-s., ***nat-sil., nit-ac., nux-v.,*** ol-j., ph-ac., ***phos.,*** prun., **PULS.,** rhus-t., ruta, sabad., sabin., sec., ***sel.,*** seneg., ***sep., sil., spig., stann.,*** staph., sul-ac., ***sul-i., sulph.,*** sumb., ***thuj.,*** verat., viol-t., zinc-p.

honey-colored - nat-p.

yellowish - kali-s.

slimy - ***kali-m.***

yellowish-green - ars-i., ***calc-sil.,*** **HYDR., KALI-BI.,** mang., ***med., merc.,*** nat-s., **NIT-AC., PULS.,** sulph., **THUJ.**

MUCOUS membranes, general - **ARS.,** ***bapt.,*** coc-c., coch., dulc., **MERC.,** nat-a., **NAT-M.,** ***puls.,*** seneg.

affinity for outlets of mucous surfaces where skin and mucous membrane join - **NIT-AC.**

burning - ***apis,*** **ARS.,** ***canth., carb-v.,*** caust., ***ter.***

edges, at - ***nat-m.***

rawness - ***am-m., caust.***

raw feeling - **AESC.**

catarrh - ***am-c., am-m.,*** **ANT-T.,** apis, ***arg-n., bad., bar-m.,*** **BENZ-AC.,** ***calc.,*** **HEP.,** ***kali-bi., merc.,*** myris., **NAT-M.,** nicc., ***ol-j.,*** phel., ***puls., senec., sulph.***

atmosphere favoring relaxation, from conditions of - ***gels.***

blennorrhea, chronic, from atony, great pain - mill.

blenorrhagia - cop., ***nat-m.***

chronic - petr.

spasms from suppressed - ***camph.***

suppressed, or undeveloped - ***gels.***

MUCOUS membranes, general

congestion - anthr., chel.

irritated, with sensation of roughness, smarting or pricking - ptel.

passive, or venous stagnation - ***ham.***

cool, chronic passive hemorrhage - sec.

dryness - ***acon.,*** apis, cor-r., ***nat-m., nux-m.,*** **STICT.,** ***ter.***

swollen - ***aesc.***

epithelium, degeneration, with enterocolitis - ***ter.***

inflammation, destruction - chr-ac.

especially affected parts, covered with squamous - merc-i-f.

eruption, erysipelatous - apis

vesicles - ***am-m.***

exudations, fibrous - ***kali-m.***

lymphatic constitution, in - seneg.

plastic - ***kali-bi.***

sticky - ***kali-m.***

yellow, honey-colored - nat-p.

fissures, of outlets, syphilitic subjects who have used too much mercury and iodide of potash, and debilitated persons broken down by excessive use of alcohol - ***hydr.***

follicles, acts upon - nat-m.

hypertrophied in vagina - ***kreos.***

subjects, in scrofulous - ***iod.***

swelling - ***graph.***

infiltrations, serous and sera-hemorrhagic - anthr.

inflammation - **ACON., ANT-T.,** ***apis,*** **ARS.,** arum-m., **BELL.,** ***bry., dulc.,*** **FERR-P.,** ***merc., nit-ac.,*** nux-m., ***nux-v.***

chronic - euph.

red - anthr.

scrofulous subjects, in - ***iod.***

irritation - **APIS,** caps., fl-ac.

chronic - fl-ac.

et morbus medicinalis - ***hydr.***

meningitis, in - ***gels.***

pruritus, of upper outlets - chlol.

pale - ***chin.,*** **FERR., PHOS.**

chronic, passive hemorrhage - sec.

smarting, edges, at - ***nat-m.***

as from pepper - xan.

softening, black with atony and extension of softening, especially to hard oesophagus, in scrofulous and lymphatic patients - ***kreos.***

syphilitic - ***hydrc.,*** **MERC.**

ulceration - ***am-m.,*** ant-chl., ***ars.,*** arum-m., ***bapt., carb-v., carb-ac., lach.,*** **MERC.,** ***nat-m.,*** **NIT-AC.,** ***phyt., sal-ac.***

erosions - hydr., ***nat-m.***

depressed vitality, with - ***kreos.***

MUMPS, (see Fevers)

MYCOSIS - calc., calc-sil., graph., **SIL.**

MYXOEDEMA - ***ars.,*** cortico., dor., penic., prim-o., sulfa., ***thyr.***

NEUROSIS cordis - ***acon.,*** adren., cact., cham., chin., ***coff.,*** ferr., ***gels., iber., ign.,*** lach., ***lil-t.,*** lycps., ***mosch., nux-v.,*** prun., scut., sep., ***spig., tab.,*** verat., zinc-m.
hemorrhoids, suppressed, from - coll.
influenza, from - iber., saroth.
scarlet fever, from - lach.
tea, coffee, from - agarin.
tobacco, from - agarin., ars., calad., ***conv.,*** dig., ***kalm.,*** lyc., nux-v., ***phos., spig.,*** staph., ***stroph.,*** tab., verat.
utero-ovarian disease, with - cimic., lil-t.

NIGHT, (see Time, general)

NIGHT-watching, ailments from - **CARC.,** caust., **COCC.,** cupr., ***nit-ac.,*** sel., zinc.

NOON, (see Time, general)

NURSING, of others, agg. - abrot., acon., agn., ant-t., ars., ***bell., bor.,*** **BRY., CALC.,** ***calc-p.,*** carb-an., carb-v., **CARC.,** cast-eq., ***caust., cham.,*** chel., ***chin.,*** chin-a., cina, **COCC.,** con., crot-h., crot-t., ***dulc.,*** ferr., ign., iod., ip., ***kali-c.,*** lac-c., lach., lyc., ***merc.,*** mill., nat-c., nat-m., ***nit-ac.,*** nux-v., olnd., **PH-AC.,** phel., ***phos.,*** **PHYT., PULS.,** rheum, ***rhus-t.,*** samb., sel., **SEP., SIL.,** spig., squil., stann., ***staph.,*** stram., ***sulph.,*** zinc.
ailments from - **CARC.,** bry., **COCC.,** cycl., frag., puls.
prolonged, with anemia and debility - ***acet-ac.,*** calc-p., carb-an., ***chin.,*** ph-ac.
weakness, from nursing the sick - **CARC.,** ***cimic.,*** **COCC.,** ***nit-ac.,*** olnd., zinc.
sit up with sick person - carb-v., cocc., ***nux-v.,*** puls.

nursing, children, ailments in - acon., agn., ***ars., bell.,*** **BOR.,** ***bry.,*** **CALC., CALC-P.,** carb-an., carb-v., **CHAM.,** chel., ***chin., cina,*** con., crot-t., ***dulc.,*** ferr., graph., ***ign.,*** iod., ***ip.,*** kali-c., lach., lyc., ***mag-c.,*** merc., nat-c., nat-m., **NAT-P.,** ***nux-v.,*** phel., ***ph-ac.,*** phos., phyt., **PULS.,** rheum, ***rhus-t.,*** samb., sec., sel., **SEP.,** sil., spig., ***squil.,*** stann., ***staph.,*** stram., ***sulph.,*** zinc.

nursing, women, weakness in - ***calc., calc-p., carb-an.,*** **CARB-V., CHIN.,** chin-s., kali-c., lyc., olnd., **PH-AC.,** ***phos., phyt.,*** sep., ***sil., sulph.***

OBESITY - ***acon.,*** adon., agar., ail., alco., all-s., ***am-br., am-c.,*** ambr., ***am-m., ang., ant-c.,*** ant-t., apis, aran-ix., arist-cl., arn., ***ars.,*** asaf., ***aur.,*** bac., bar-c., ***bell.,*** blatta, bor., brom., bry., bufo, calad., **CALC.,** calc-ac., ***calc-ar.,*** calc-caust., ***calo.,*** camph., canth., **CAPS.,** carb-v., caust., cham., chin., chlorpr., cic., clem., ***coc-c.,*** coca, cocc., coloc., con., cortiso., ***croc., cupr.,*** dig., euph., euphr., **FERR.,** ***fuc.,*** **GRAPH.,** guai., ***hura, hyos.,*** iod., ip., ***kali-bi.,*** kali-br., ***kali-c., lac-d.,*** lach., laur., lith., lob., ***lyc.,*** lycpr., mag-c., mag-p., mang., merc., merc-d., mur-ac., nat-a., nat-c., nat-m., nux-m., olnd., op., ***phos.,*** **PHYT.,** plat., plb., ***puls.,*** rheum, rhus-t., rumx., sabad., sabal., sars., sel., seneg., sep., sil., spig., spong., stram., stront-c., ***sulph.,*** thuj., ***thyr.,*** tus-f., valer., verat., viol-o.

OBESITY,
body fat, but legs thin - ***am-m.,*** ant-c.. lyc.
children, in - ***ant-c., bad.,*** bar-c., bell., **CALC.,** ***caps., ferr., kali-bi.,*** sac-l., seneg.
elderly people - am-c., **AUR.,** bar-c., **CALC.,** fl-ac., **KALI-C.,** op., sec.
menopause, during - calc-ar., **GRAPH.,** sep.
pregnancy, after - kali-c., ***sep.***
young people, in - ***ant-c.,*** calc., calc-ac., lach.

OLD age, premature, (see Elderly) - ***agn.,*** alco., alum., ***ambr.,*** arg-m., arg-n., ***bar-c.,*** berb., bufo, carb-v., chin-s., coca., ***con.,*** cortico., ***cupr., fl-ac., kali-c., lyc.,*** nux-v., op., psor., sars., **SEL.,** sep., staph., stram., sulph., ***vip.,***

ORIFICES, affections of - ***aesc.,*** aloe, ***bell., caust.,*** graph., ign., kali-c., lach., lyc., ***merc.,*** mur-ac., nat-m., **NIT-AC., NUX-V.,** phos., podo., rat., ***sep., sil.,*** **STAPH., SULPH.**
cracks - nit-ac.
red - aloe, nit-ac., pyrog., sulph.
stretching agg. - staph.
surgery, agg. - calen., staph.
swelling - nit-ac.

OSGOOD-schlatter's disease - ***calc-p., sil.***

OXYURIS, vermicularis - ars., bapt., ***chelo., cina,*** ign., indg., lyc., ***merc-d., merc-sul.,*** nat-p., rat., ***sant.,*** sil., sin-n., spig., teucr., valer.

PAGET'S, disease - calc-p., sil.

PAINLESSNESS, of complaints, usually painful - **ARN.,** ***hell.,*** **OP., STRAM.**

PAINS, general

agg. during the pain - ars., cham., cimic., coloc., ign., lyc., nat-c., onos., rhus-t., sars., sep., thuj., verat.

appear gradually - acon., bry., calc-sil., carb-o., caust., chin., con., ign., lact., lob., rad., rad-br., sars., sul-ac., tell.
and disappear gradually - acon., ***arg-n.,*** arn., ars., bar-c., bufo, cact., cast., chel., coloc., crot-h., epip., euphr., form., ***gels.,*** glon., ***ign.,*** piloc., kali-bi., ***kalm., lach., lam.,*** led., lol., mez., ***nat-m.,*** nit-ac., nux-m., op., pall., ***phos.,*** phyt., pic-ac., **PLAT.,** ictod., psor., puls., sabal., sabin., **SANG.,** sars., sel., ***sep., spig.,*** **STANN.,** staph., stront-c., stroph., sulph., ***sul-ac.,*** **SYPH.,** tell., valer., verb., xan.
and disappear suddenly - ***arg-m., arg-n.,*** bell., caust., ign., ***puls.,*** rad., rhus-t., ***sul-ac.***

appear suddenly - ***acon.,*** agar., am-c., anh., ***arg-m., ars.,*** aster., atro., bar-ac., **BELL.,** berb., camph., ***canth.,*** carb-ac., caust., ***coloc.,*** croc., cimic., ***crot-h., cupr.,*** cupr-ar., ***dios.,*** eup-per., ferr., form., ***glon.,*** kali-bi., lyc., mag-c., mag-p., mez., morph., ***nat-s.,*** **NIT-AC.,** ***nux-v.,*** ox-ac., phys., plb., ***podo., puls.,*** ran-b., ***sabin.,*** sang., sep., sil., ***spig.,*** stann., stry-p., sul-ac., ***tab., tarent.,*** thuj., ***valer., verb.,*** vip., zinc., zinc-valer.

PAINS, general

appear suddenly,

and disappear gradually - asaf., ***bell.,*** buni-o., calc., coloc., fl-ac., ***hyper.,*** ign., ***lach., med., puls.,*** rad-br., ran-s., sabin., sep., sul-ac.

and disappear suddenly - ***arg-n.,*** asaf., aster., **BELL.,** bor., cact., canth., ***carb-ac.,*** carb-s., cham., coff., crot-h., cupr., dios., eup-per., eup-pur., fl-ac., ictod., ign., iris, **KALI-BI.,** kalm., lyc., ***mag-p.,*** med., merc-c., nat-f., **NIT-AC.,** nux-m., ovi-g-p., oxyt., petr., ***phyt.,*** ictod., ictod., puls., ***rhus-t.,*** sabin., spig., ***stry.,*** thal., thuj., tub., valer., verat.

and disappear suddenly, tension acutely increases, leaves with a snap on first motion - puls., rhus-t.

sleep, felt during, disappearing on waking - sul-ac.

anxiety, from the - **ACON., ARS.,** carb-v., caust., kali-ar., ***nat-c.,*** **PHOS.**

belching amel. - jal.

benumbing, pain - ***acon.,*** agar., agn., am-c., anac., ant-c., ant-t., arg-m., arn., asaf., asar., aur., bell., bov., bry., ***calc.,*** cann-s., carb- an., **CHAM.,** chin., cic., ***cina,*** cocc., con., croc., cupr., cycl., dros., dulc., euph., euphr., ***graph.,*** hell., hep., hyos., ign., ***iris,*** kali-n., laur., led., mag c., mag-m., mang., meny., ***mez.,*** mosch., mur-ac., nat-c., nat-m., nux-m., **OLND.,** op., par., ph-ac., phos., **PLAT.,** ***puls., rheum,*** rhus-t., ruta., **SABAD.,** sabin., ***samb.,*** seneg., sep., stann., staph., sulph., sul-ac., tarax., valer., ***verat.,*** **VERB.,** zinc.

biting, pain - acon., agar., agn., alum., ***ambr.,*** am-c., ant-c., ant-t., arg-m., arn., ars., asar., aur., bell., bry., calad., calc., camph., cann-s., ***canth., caps.,*** carb-an., **CARB-V.,** caust., cham., ***chin.,*** clem., cocc., colch., coloc., con., croc., ***dros.,*** dulc., ***euph., euphr.,*** graph., ***hell.,*** hep., hyos., ***ign.,*** iod., ***ip., kali-c.,*** kali-n., ***kreos.,*** lach., laur., led., lyc., mag-c., ***merc., mez.,*** mosch., mur-ac., nat-c., nat-m., ***nit-ac.,*** nux-m., **NUX-V.,** olnd., op., paeon., par., petr., **PETROS.,** ph-ac., phos., ***prun., puls., ran-b.,*** **RAN-S.,** rheum, rhod., ***rhus-t., ruta.,*** sabad., sabin., sars., sel., seneg., ***sep.,*** sil., spig., squil., stann., ***staph.,*** stram., stront-c., **SULPH.,** sul-ac., ***teucr.,*** thuj., valer., verat., viol-t., **ZINC.**

boring, pain - acon., ***agar.,*** aloe, alum., am-c., am-m., anac., ant-c., ant-t., apis, ***arg-m.,*** **ARG-N.,** arn., ars., ***asaf.,*** **AUR.,** bar-c., **BELL., BISM.,** bor., bov., ***calc.,*** cann- i., canth., caps., carb- an., carb-s., carb- v., ***caust.,*** chin., cimic., ***cina,*** clem., cocc., coc- c., colch., coloc., con., cupr., cycl., dig., dios., dros., ***dulc.,*** euph., euphr., ***hell., hep.,*** ign., ip., ***kali-c.,*** kali-n., kreos., ***lach.,*** laur., led., lyc., mag-c., mag- m., mang., meny., ***merc., mez.,*** mur-ac., ***nat-c., nat-m.,*** nit-ac., nux-m., nux-v., olnd., par., petr., ***ph-ac.,*** phos., plat., ***plb.,*** **PULS.,** ran-b., **RAN-S.,** ***rhod.,*** rhus- t., ruta.,

PAINS, general

boring, pain - sabad., sabin., sel., ***seneg., sep., sil.,*** **SPIG.,** spong., stann., staph., stram., stront-c., ***sulph., tarax., thuj.,*** valer., ***zinc.***

inward - alum., bell., calc., cocc., ***kali-c.,*** mang., zinc.

outward - ant-c., asaf., bell., ***bism.,*** bov., calc., dros., ***dulc.,*** ip., puls., sep., ***spig.,*** spong., ***staph.***

burning, pain

externally - ***acon., agar.,*** aloe, alum., ambr., am-c., ***am-m.,*** anac., ***anthr.,*** ant-c., ant-t., **APIS,** arg-m., ***arn.,*** **ARS.,** ars-i., **ARUM-T.,** ***asaf.,*** asar., ***bapt., bar-c.,*** bar-m., bell., ***berb.,*** bism., ***bor.,*** bov., **BRY.,** ***bufo,*** calad., calc., ***calc-p.,*** camph., cann-s., ***canth., caps.,*** carb- an., **CARB-S., CARB-V., CAUST.,** cham., ***chel.,*** chin., cic., ***cimic.,*** cina, ***clem.,*** cocc., coc-c., coff., colch., ***coloc., con., corn.,*** croc., crot-h., crot-t., cupr., ***cycl.,*** dig., ***dros., dulc.,*** euph., **EUPHR.,** ***ferr., graph., grat.,*** guai., hell., helon., hep., ***ign.,*** iod., ip., **IRIS,** kali- ar., ***kali- bi., kali-c.,*** kali-n., kali-s., ***kreos., lach.,*** laur., led., lob., ***lyc.,*** mag-c., mag-m., ***manc.,*** mang., meny., **MERC.,** ***merc-c.,*** mez., mosch., ***mur-ac., nat-a., nat-c.,*** **NAT- M.,** ***nit-ac.,*** nux-m., **NUX-V.,** ***olnd., op.,*** paeon., par., petr., **PH-AC., PHOS.,** phyt., plat., plb., ***prun., psor., puls.,*** ran-s., **RAT.,** ***rheum,*** rhod., **RHUS-T.,** ***rumx.,*** ruta., ***sabad.,*** sabin., sal- ac., samb., sars., **SEC.,** sel., seneg., **SEP., SIL.,** spig., spong., squil., **STANN.,** ***staph.,*** stram., stront-c., **SULPH.,** sul-ac., ***tarax.,*** teucr., ***thuj.,*** valer., viol-t., ***zinc.***

left upper part of body - kreos.

right side - phos.

internally - abies-c., acet-ac., **ACON.,** acon-f., ***agar., alum.,*** alumn., ambr., ***am-br.,*** am-c., ***am-m.,*** ant-c., ant-t., ***apis,*** arg-m., ***arg-n., arn.,*** **ARS.,** ars-i., **ARUM-T.,** ***asaf.,*** asar., ***aur., bapt., bar-c.,*** bar-m., **BELL., BERB.,** ***bism.,*** bor., bov., **BRY.,** ***bufo,*** calad., ***calc., calc-p.,*** camph., **CANN-I.,** cann-s., **CANTH.,** caps., carb-ac., carb- an., **CARB-S.,** ***carb-v., caust.,*** cedr., cham., ***chel., chin., cic.,*** cina, ***clem.,*** cocc., coff., ***colch., coloc., com., con.,*** crot-t., cund., ***cupr.,*** dig., ***dios.,*** dol., ***dros., dulc.,*** equis., eup- pur., ***euph.,*** euphr., ***fl-ac., gamb.,*** **GRAPH.,** hell., hep., hydr., hyos., ign., iod., ip., ***iris,*** kali-ar., **KALI-BI.,** kali-c., ***kali-i.,*** kali-n., kali-s., ***kreos., lach., laur.,*** led., ***lith., lil-t., lob., lyc.,*** mag-c., mag- m., mang., **MERC., MERC-C.,** ***merc-i-f.,*** **MEZ.,** mosch., mur- ac., ***nat-a., nat-c., nat-m.,*** **NIT-AC.,** nux-m., **NUX-V.,** ***op., osm., ox-ac.,*** par., ***petr., ph-ac.,*** **PHOS.,** phyt., plat., plb., **PRUN.,** ***psor.,*** **PULS.,** ***ran-b.,*** ran-s., rat., ***rhod.,*** **RHUS-T.,** rob., ***rumx.,*** ruta., **SABAD.,** ***sabin.,*** **SANG.,** sang- n.,

PAINS, general

burning, pain

internally - ***sars.,*** **SEC.,** ***seneg.,*** **SEP.,** ***sil.,*** sin-n., **SPIG., SPONG.,** ***stann.,*** staph., stram., stront-c., **SULPH.,** sul-ac., tarax., ***tell., ter., thuj.,*** uran., ust., uva., ***verat.,*** verat-v., viol-o., viol-t., wye., **ZINC.**

internally, as from - ***agar.,*** aloe, alum., ambr., ***apis, arum-t., bapt., bar-c.,*** bell., ***berb.,*** bry., cann- s., caust., chin., ***coloc.,*** ferr., hyos., ***ign.,*** **IRIS,** kali-c., ***lil-t., mag-m.,*** merc., mez., mur-ac., nat-c., ***nux-v.,*** op., osm., par., phos., ***phyt., plat., puls., ran-s., sabad., sang., sep.,*** still., sul- ac., tarent., thuj., verat.

glowing coals - ars., carb-v.

hot coals - sabad.

parts, grasped with the hand - bry., **CAUST.**

chill, during - ars., petr.

cold - arn., med., syph.

coldness, from - cist., mez., mosch.

constricting, pain

externally - acon., agar., alum., ambr., ***am-c., anac.,*** arg-m., ***arg-n.,*** arn., bar-c., ***bell.,*** bry., calad., ***calc.,*** camph., cann-s., ***carb-v.,*** caust., cham., chel., cic., ***cina,*** cocc., colch., coloc., croc., cycl., ***dig.,*** dros., dulc., euphr., graph., hyos., iod., kali-c., ***kali-n.,*** kreos., led., lyc., mang., meny., merc., mez., mosch., nat-c., ***nit-ac., nux-v.,*** olnd., petr., ph-ac., ***phos.,*** **PLAT., PULS.,** ran-b., rhod., rhus-t., ruta, sabad., sep., sil., spig., squil., stront-c., sulph., samb., teucr., thuj., valer., verat., verb., viol-t., zinc.

internally - ***acon.,*** agn., **AMBR.,** am-m., anac., ant-t., arg-m., arn., ars., asaf., asar., aur., bar-c., bell., bism., bor., bry., ***calc.,*** camph., canth., caps., carb-an., ***carb-v.,*** cham., chel., chin., cina, ***cocc., colch., coloc.,*** con., croc., cycl., dig., dros., dulc., ferr., graph., hyos., **IGN.,** iod., ***kali-c.,*** lach., led., lyc., mag-c., meny., merc., ***mez.,*** mur-ac., nat-m., ***nux-v.,*** olnd., petr., **PH-AC.,** phos., **PLAT.,** puls., ran-s., rheum, rhod., rhus-t., sabin., sars., sel., seneg., sep., sil., spong., squil., stann., ***staph.,*** stram., stront-c., ***sulph.,*** sul-ac., ***teucr.,*** thuj., valer., verat., ***zinc.***

cutting, pain

externally - acon., ***alum.,*** ambr., anac., ant-c., arg- m., arn., asaf., asar., aur., **BELL.,** bism., bor., brom., bry., **CALC.,** camph., cann-s., canth., carb- s., caust., chin., cimic., clem., colch., ***coloc.,*** **CON.,** conv., dig., **DROS.,** dulc., euph., ***graph.,*** hell., hep., hyos., ***ign.,*** kali-c., kali-s., led., ***lyc.,*** mag- m., mang., meny., ***merc.,*** mez., mosch., ***mur-ac.,*** **NAT-C.,** nat-m., nit-ac., ***nux-v.,*** olnd., osm., oxyt., par., **PETR.,** ***ph-ac.,*** phos., plat., puls., ran-b., rhod., ***rhus-t.,*** ruta., sabad., ***samb.,*** sars., seneg., ***sep., sil.,*** spig., stann., staph., stram., ***sulph., sul-ac.,*** teucr., thuj.,

PAINS, general

cutting, pain

externally - verat., ***viol-t.,*** zinc.

internally - abies-n., acon., aesc., aeth., agar., ang., all-c., alum., ambr., am-c., am-m., anac., ant-c., ant-t., arg-m., arg-n., ***arn.,*** ars., asaf., asar., aur., bar-c., bar-m., **BELL.,** ***berb.,*** bism., bor., bov., bry., ***calad.,*** **CALC.,** calc-p., camph., cann-i., cann-s., **CANTH.,** caps., carb-an., carb-v., caust., cham., ***chel., chin.,*** cic., cina, clem., cocc., coc-c., coff., colch., ***coll.,*** **COLOC., CON.,** conv., croc., crot-h., crot-t., cub., cupr., cycl., dig., **DIOS.,** dros., ***dulc., elat., equis.,*** ferr., **GAMB.,** gels., graph., guai., hell., hep., hydr., **HYOS.,** ign., iod., ***ip.,*** iris, **KALI-C.,** kali-chl., ***kali-n., kali-s.,*** lach., laur., led., **LYC.,** mag-c., mag-m., mang., meny., **MERC.,** merc-c., mez., mosch., ***mur-ac.,*** nat-c., **NAT-M.,** nit-ac., nux-m., **NUX-V.,** ***op., par., petr.,*** ph-ac., ***phos.,*** plat., plb., **PULS.,** ran-b., ran-s., ***rheum,*** rhod., rhus-t., ruta., sabad., sabin., samb., sars., sel., seneg., ***sep.,*** **SIL.,** ***spig.,*** spong., squil., ***stann., staph., stront-c.,*** **SULPH.,** sul-ac., teucr., thuj., valer., **VERAT.,** verb., ***vib.,*** viol-t., **ZINC.,** zing.

digging, pain - ***acon., agar.,*** alum., ambr., am-c., ***am-m.,*** anac., ant-c., ant-t., arg-m., arg-n., ***arn.,*** ars., ***asaf.,*** asar., aur., bar-c., bar-m., ***bell.,*** bism., bor., ***bov., bry., calc.,*** cann-s., caps., canth., carb-an., carb-v., ***caust.,*** cham., chel., chin., ***cina,*** clem., cocc., colch., ***coloc.,*** con., croc., dig., dros., **DULC.,** euph., ferr., graph., hell., hep., ign., ***kali-bi., kali-c.,*** kali-n., kreos., laur., led., lyc., mag-c., mag-m., mang., merc., mez., mur-ac., ***nat-c.,*** nat-m., nux-m., nux-v., olnd., petr., ph-ac., ***phos., plat.,*** puls., rheum, **RHOD.,** ***rhus-t., ruta.,*** sabad., sabin., samb., seneg., ***sep.,*** sil., **SPIG.,** spong., squil., ***stann.,*** staph., stront-c., sulph., sul-ac., thuj., valer., zinc.

despair, with the - acon., **ARS., AUR.,** aur-ar., calc., carb-v., ***cham., chin.,*** chin-ar., ***coff.,*** colch., hyper., lach., lil-t., mag-c., nux-v., stram., ***verat.,*** vip.

directions of pains

backward - bar-c., bell., ***bry.,*** chel., con., crot-t., cupr., gels., ***kali-bi.,*** kali-c., kali-i., lil-t., merc., nat-m., par., phos., phyt., prun., puls., ***sep.,*** spig., **SULPH.**

crosswise - acon., ambr., anac., arg-m., ***bell.,*** berb., bov., bry., calc., canth., caust., cham., ***chel., chin.,*** cocc., hell., kali-bi., kali-c., kali-m., ***lac-c.,*** laur., lyc., mang., merc., phos., rhus-t., ***seneg., sil.,*** spig., sul-ac., ***sulph.,*** tarax., valer., ***verat.,*** zinc.

downward - acon., agar., agn., aloe, alum., alumn., ant-t., apis, arn., asaf., aur., bar-c., bell., benz-ac., ***berb.,*** bor., bry., cact., canth., ***caps., carb-v.,*** caust., chel., chin., cic., cina, **COFF.,** goss., graph., hyper., kali-c., ***kalm.,*** lach., led., **LYC.,** merc., nat-c., nat-m., nux-v., ph-ac., ***puls.,***

PAINS, general

directions of pains

downward - rheum, rhod., rhus-t., ***sanic.,*** sars., sel., seneg., sep., sil., sulph., verat., verb., zinc.

extend from original side - ther.

forward - berb., bry., carb-v., ***gels., lac-c., sabin., sang.,*** sep., sil., **SPIG.**

inward - alum., arg-n., **ARN.,** bell., bov., ***calc.,*** cann-s., **CANTH.,** carb-v., caust., chin., cina, con., hyos., ***ign., laur.,*** meny., merc., mez., petr., phel., phyt., ***plb.,*** ran-b., rhus-t., ***sabin.,*** sep., spig., spong., squil., stann., staph., sul-ac., sulph., valer., verb.

left side, on - benz-ac., brom., chel., cinnb., crot-c., crot-h., daph., ind., kalm., lepi., lil-t., lycps., merc., merc-i-f., oena., ol-j., op., ox-ac., phys., pic-ac., plan., puls-n

outward - alum., am-m., anh., ***arg-m.,*** arg-n., arn., **ASAF.,** bell., berb., calc., canth., carb-v., chel., ***chin.,*** cimic., cocc., **CON.,** dros., dulc., hyos., kali-bi., kali-c., kali-m., kalm., lith., lyc., mang., merc., mur-ac., nat-c., nit-ac., phel., phos., phyt., plat., prun., ran-b., rhod., rhus-t., sabad., ***sep.,*** sil., spig., spong., stann., stann-i., staph., **SULPH.,** tarax., ***valer.,*** viol-t., zinc.

radiating - agar., apis, arg-n., ars., bapt., berb., caust., cham., cimic., ***coloc.,*** cupr., ***dios.,*** hyper., kali-bi., kali-c., kalm., lil-t., mag-m., mag-p., ***merc.,*** mez., nux-v., phyt., plat., plb., sec., sil., spig., xan.

right side, on - arist-m., brach., bry., cedr., oena., pic-ac., sulph., tarent., wye., yuc.

upward - acon., aloe, alum-sil., anac., arn., ars., ***asaf.,*** aur., **BELL.,** calc., canth., caust., cham., chin., cimic., colch., con., croc., cupr., dulc., eup-pur., euphr., gels., ***glon.,*** hyper., **IGN.,** kali-bi., kalm., kreos., **LACH.,** ***led.,*** mag-c., mang., meny., naja, nat-c., nat-m., nit-ac., nux-v., op., **PHOS.,** puls., rhus-t., sabad., samb., **SANG., SEP., SIL.,** spong., stroph., sulph., thuj., valer., zinc.

disappear suddenly - arum-t., **BELL.,** carb-ac., caust., cimic., ***dios.,*** mag-p., puls., stry-p., sul-ac., sulph., thuj.

drawing, pain - acon., aloe, am-c., anac., arg-m., bar-c., ***bry., camph.,*** **CARB-V.,** ***caul.,*** caust., **CHEL.,** chin-a., clem., coc-c., colch., **COLOC.,** ***crot-t.,*** dig., eupi., euon., ferr-ar., ***gamb.,*** goss., **GRAPH.,** guare., hydrc., kali- bi., kali-c., kreos., lach., lact., lyc., ***mang.,*** merc., mez., **NIT-AC.,** ***nux-v., ol-an.,*** plat., phos., ***puls.,*** raph., rhod., sars., sec., sep., sil., stann., staph., sulph., tab., thuj., **VALER.**

alternating with heart symptoms - acon.

chill, during - lyc.

cold, as from a - plat.

cramp-like, drawing - plat.

eating, after - camph.

evening - coc-c., raph.

8 p.m. - rhus-t.

10 p.m. - bry.

PAINS, general

drawing, pain

extending to,

fingers - apis

toes - apis.

increasing and decreases rapidly - nit-ac.

left, night - lyc.

menses, during - phos.

morning, after rising - ***graph.***

after waking - coloc.

motion, on - calc., cycl.

night - coc-c.

paralytic - coc-c., staph.

position, from wrong - staph.

rheumatic - am-c., carb-v., chel., sul-ac.

right - sep.

rising, after - coloc.

sitting while - samb., **VALER.**

upwards - ***ol-an.***

walking agg. - calc., coca

amel. - rhus-t.

weather, bad, agg. - rhod.

dreams, during - ars., cann-i., ***cham.,*** coloc., mag-m., merc., passi., puls., sin-n.

faintness, from - apis, asaf., **CHAM.,** ***cocc.,*** coloc., ***hep.,*** **IGN.,** ***nux-m., nux-v.,*** phyt., ***valer.,*** verat.

fluid forcing its way, as if - coc-c.

gnawing, pain - ***ars.,*** caust., **MERC.,** sil., staph., sulph.

externally - acon., agar., **AGN.,** alum., ambr., am-c., arg-m., arn., aur., ***bar-c.,*** bar-m., bell., bry., calad., calc., ***canth.,*** caps., ***cham., crot-t.,*** cycl., dig., ***dros.,*** dulc., euph., ferr., ***glon.,*** graph., hell., hyos., ign., ***kali-c.,*** kreos., laur., led., lyc., mag-c., mag-m., mang., ***meny.,*** merc., mez., mur-ac., nat-c., nux-v., olnd., op., ***par., ph-ac., phos.,*** **PLAT.,** plb., ***puls.,*** **RAN-S.,** rheum, rhod., rhus-t., ***ruta.,*** samb., sep., sil., spig., **SPONG.,** stann., **STAPH.,** stront-c., sulph., ***tarax.,*** thuj., verat., zinc.

internally - agar., alum., am-m., arg-m., ***ars.,*** bar-c., ***bell.,*** calad., ***calc.,*** cann-s., ***canth., carb-v.,*** **CAUST.,** chel., cocc., ***coloc., con., cupr.,*** dig., dros., dulc., ***gamb.,*** hep., iod., kali-bi., kali-c., ***kreos.,*** lach., ***lyc.,*** merc., mez., nux-v., olnd., ph-ac., phos., ***plat.,*** **PULS.,** ***ran-s.,*** rhod., **RUTA.,** seneg., **SEP.,** sil., stann., sulph., teucr., verat.

half sleep, during - nit-ac.

heat agg. - tab.

itching, alternating with - stroph.

jerking, pain

externally - acon., agar., agn., ***alum.,*** ambr., anac., ant-c., ant-t., arg-m., ***arn.,*** ars., **ASAF.,** asar., ***aur.,*** bar-c., ***bar-m., bell.,*** bism., bor., bov., ***bry.,*** **CALC.,** camph., canth., caps., ***carb-s.,*** carb-v., **CAUST.,** cham., ***chin.,*** cic., ***cina, clem.,*** cocc., coff., colch., coloc., cupr., iod., kali-c., kali-s., kreos., lach., laur., led., ***lyc.,***

PAINS, general

jerking, pain

externally - mag-c., ***mag-p.,*** mang., **MENY.,** ***merc.,*** mez., mosch., mur-ac., ***nat-c.,*** **NAT-M.,** ***nit-ac.,*** **NUX-V.,** olnd., op., par., ***petr.,*** ph-ac., phos., phyt., plat., plb., **PULS.,** ***ran-b.,*** ran-s., rheum, rhod., **RHUS-T.,** ruta., sabad., sabin., sec., ***sep.,*** ***sil.,*** spig., spong., ***squil.,*** ***stann.,*** staph., stront-c., sulph., sul-ac., **TARAX.,** teucr., thuj., **VALER.,** verat., verb., viol-t., zinc.

affected parts - ***merc.***

internally - acon., agar., aloe, ambr., am-m., anac., arn., ars., **BELL.,** bor., bry., ***calc.,*** cann-s., carb-v., caust., cham., **CHIN.,** clem., cocc., colch., con., croc., graph., **IGN., KALI-C.,** lyc., mang., meny., ***merc.,*** mez., nat-m., **NIT-AC.,** nux-v., petr., ph-ac., plat., plb., **PULS.,** ran-b., ran-s., rhus-t., ***sep.,*** **SIL.,** ***spig.,*** ***stann.,*** stront-c., **SULPH.,** sul-ac., teucr., **THUJ.,** ***valer.***

right side - cupr.

rising from bed - mag-c.

many pains - carc., med., mez., naja, rumx.

morning - xan.

nerves, along - ter.

neuralgic, pain - **ACON.,** all-c., **ARS., BELL.,** ***bry.,*** ***caust.,*** ***cham.,*** chin., cimic., coff., **COLOC.,** dios., gels., ***hyper.,*** **IGN.,** ***iris,*** ***kali-bi.,*** lach., ***lyc.,*** ***mag-c.,*** **MAG-P.,** ***merc.,*** nat-m., ***nux-v.,*** phos., ***psor.,*** puls., ran-a., ***rhus-t.,*** rumx., ***sang.,*** **SPIG.,** stann., sul-ac., ***sulph.,*** thuj., ***verat.,*** verb.

herpes, before herpes zoster - staph.

herpes, after - caust., kali-chl., kalm., ***mez.,*** plan., prun., ran-b., still., ***vario.,*** zinc.

injury, from - calen., hyper.

menses, during - aml-n., aran.

suppressed, from - kalm.

operations, after surgical - all-c., calen., hyper.

palpitations, with - lach.

paralytic weakness and trembling, with - kalm.

periodical - cact.

peripheral - arg-n.

prodrome, as a - nux-v.

sepsis, from - crot-h.

stump, of - all-c., am-m., arn., asaf., hyper., ph-ac., staph., symph.

breathing deep amel. - ph-ac.

suppressed, from - stann.

veins, pressure from distended - sec.

night - ***asaf.,*** ***aur.,*** fl-ac., hep., iod., ***kali-i.,*** lach., mang., ***merc.,*** ***mez.,*** ph-ac., phyt., rhod., still., syph.

operations, after - hyper.

paralytic, pain - acon., agar., agn., alum., ambr., am-c., am-m., ant-c., arg-m., ars., ars-i., asaf., asar., ***aur.,*** bar-c., **BELL.,** ***bism.,*** bov., ***bry.,*** calc., cann-s., canth., carb-v., caust., ***cham.,*** chel., ***chin.,*** **CINA, COCC.,** coff., **COLCH.,** coloc., con., croc., crot-h., **CYCL.,**

PAINS, general

paralytic, pain - dig., dros., ***dulc.,*** euph., euphr., ***ferr.,*** ferr-ar., graph., hell., hep., hyos., ign., iod., kali-c., kali-n., kali-p., kreos., ***laur.,*** led., lyc., mag-c., mag-m., mang., meny., merc., ***mez.,*** mosch., mur-ac., nat-c., ***nat-m.,*** **NUX-V.,** olnd., par., petr., ph-ac., phos., plat., plb., puls., ran-s., rhod., ***rhus-t.,*** ruta., sabad., **SABIN.,** sars., sel., seneg., sep., ***sil.,*** spig., stann., ***staph.,*** stram., stront-c., sulph., sul-ac., teucr., thuj., valer., ***verat.,*** verb., zinc.

paralyzed parts - agar., arn., ***ars.,*** bell., calc., ***caust.,*** cina, ***cocc.,*** crot-t., ***kali-n.,*** lat-m., nux-v., phos., ***plb.,*** rhus-t., sil., sulph.

parts, of affected - con., dig.

injured long ago - glon.

lain on - caust., hep., kali-c., phos., sil.

recently lain on - **PULS.**

uncovered, of - bell.

pinching, pain - agar., alum., ambr., anac., **ARN.,** ***ars.,*** ars-i., asar., bar-c., **BELL.,** bov., bry., ***calc.,*** cann-s., canth., ***caps.,*** carb-an., carb-v., caust., ***cham.,*** cina, clem., cocc., ***colch.,*** coloc., con., croc., dros., dulc., ***euph.,*** guai., hell., hep., ign., iod., kali-c., kali-n., kreos., ***laur.,*** lyc., mag-m., mang., meny., ***merc.,*** ***mez.,*** mur-ac., ***nat-c.,*** nat-m., nit-ac., ***nux-m.,*** **NUX-V.,** op., par., petr., ***phos.,*** ***plat.,*** ***puls.,*** ran-b., ran-s., ***rheum,*** rhod., ***rhus-t.,*** ruta., ***sabad.,*** sabin., sars., seneg., sep., sil., spig., ***spong.,*** stann., staph., stront-c., ***sulph.,*** teucr., thuj., valer., verat., verb., zinc.

externally - acon., anac., ant-c., arg-m., arn., bell., bry., ***calc.,*** cann-s., caps., carb-v., caust., chel., chin., cina, ***clem.,*** cocc., con., croc., dig., dros., dulc., euph., euphr., ***hyos.,*** ***ip.,*** kali-c., kreos., led., mang., **MENY.,** ***mur-ac.,*** nat-c., nit-ac., nux-v., olnd., ***osm.,*** par., ph-ac., phos., **RHOD.,** ***rhus-t.,*** ruta., **SABAD.,** sabin., samb., sars., sil., ***spig.,*** **SPONG., STANN.,** staph., ***sulph.,*** sul-ac., thuj., verat., **VERB.,** viol-t., zinc.

internally - acon., ***agar.,*** agn., alum., ***am-c.,*** am-m., anac., ant-c., ant-t., arg-m., arn., ars., ars-i., asaf., asar., aur., bar-c., ***bell.,*** ***bism.,*** bor., bov., ***bry.,*** **CALC.,** camph., ***cann-s.,*** ***canth.,*** ***caps.,*** carb-an., ***carb-v.,*** caust., cham., **CHEL.,** ***chin.,*** cic., ***cina,*** **COCC.,** coc-c., coff., ***colch.,*** **COLOC.,** com., croc., cupr., cycl., dig., dros., ***dulc.,*** euph., euphr., ***gamb.,*** **GRAPH.,** guai., ***hell.,*** hep., hyos., **IGN.,** iod., ***ip.,*** ***kali-c.,*** kreos., **LYC.,** mag-c., mag-m., mang., ***meny.,*** ***merc.,*** mez., mosch., ***mur-ac.,*** ***nat-c.,*** ***nat-m.,*** nit-ac., nux-m., nux-v., olnd., ***par.,*** ***petr.,*** ph-ac., ***phos.,*** plat., ***plb.,*** ***puls.,*** ***ran-b.,*** ran-s., rheum, ***rhod.,*** ***rhus-t.,*** ***ruta.,*** ***sabad.,*** sabin., samb., sars., seneg., ***sep.,*** sil., ***spig.,*** ***spong.,*** squil., ***stann.,*** ***staph.,*** stront-c., ***sulph.,*** sul-ac., tarax., teucr., ***thuj.,*** valer., verat., **VERB.,** viol-t., ***zinc.***

right side - sep.

PAINS, general
pressing, pain
externally - abrot., ***acon., aesc.,*** **AGAR.,** agn., aloe, alum., ambr., ***am-m., ammc., anac.,*** ant-c., ***ant-t.,*** **APOC.,** arg-m., arn., ars., ars-i., ***asaf.,*** asar., ***aspar., aur., bapt.,*** bar-c., bar-m., ***bell.,*** bism., bor., bov., ***bry., calad., calc., calc-p., camph.,*** **CANN-I.,** ***cann-s.,*** canth., caps., ***carb-ac.,*** carb-an., carb-s., **CAUST.,** cedr., ***cham., chel.,*** chen-a., ***chin.,*** **CHIN-S.,** cic., ***cimic.,*** cinnb., cina, clem., cob., ***cocc.,*** coc-c., coff., ***colch., coloc., con.,*** crot-t., cupr., ***cycl.,*** dig., dios., **DROS.,** ***dulc.,*** elaps, **EUP-PER.,** euph., euphr., **FERR.,** ferr-ar., ***gels., glon., graph., guai., hell.,*** hep., ***hyos., ign.,*** iod., ***ip.,*** **KALI-BI.,** kali-c., kali-n., kali-p., ***kalm., kreos.,*** lach., ***laur., led., lil-t., lyc.,*** mag-c., mag-m., mang., meny., merc., ***mez.,*** **MOSCH.,** mur-ac., nat-a., nat-c., ***nat-m.,*** **NIT-AC.,** nux-m., **NUX-V.,** ***olnd., ox-ac.,*** par., pareir., ***petr., ph-ac.,*** **PHOS.,** phyt., plat., plb., **PODO.,** prun., ***psor.,*** **PULS.,** ran-b., ran-s., rheum, **RHOD., RHUS-T., RUTA.,** ***sabad.,*** sabin., ***samb., sang., sars., sec., seneg.,*** **SEP., SIL., SPIG.,** spong., ***squil.,*** **STANN., STAPH.,** ***stict.,*** stront-c., **SULPH.,** sul-ac., tab., ***tarax., teucr.,*** thuj., ust., valer., ***verat.,*** verb., vib., viol-o., ***zinc.***
internally - ***acon.,*** aesc., agar., agn., ***ail., aloe, alum., ambr.,*** am-c., am-m., ***anac.,*** ant-c., ant-t., arg-m., **ARG-N., ARN., ARS.,** ***ars-i., arum-t.,*** **ASAF.,** asar., ***aur.,*** bar-c., **BELL.,** berb., ***bism., bor.,*** bov., **BROM.,** ***bry.,*** cact., calad., **CALC.,** ***camph., cann-i.,*** cann-s., **CANTH.,** caps., ***carb-an.,*** carb-s., **CARB-V.,** ***caust., cedr.,*** cham., chel., chen-a., **CHIN.,** cic., **CIMIC.,** cina, clem., ***cocc., coc-c., cod.,*** coff., ***colch.,*** **COLOC.,** ***con.,*** cor-r., croc., crot-t., **CUPR.,** cycl., ***dig.,*** dios., dros., dulc., elaps, euph., euphr., ***ferr., gamb., gels., glon.,*** goss., ***graph.,*** guai., **HAM.,** ***hell.,*** hep., hydr., ***hydr-ac.,*** hyos., hyper., ***ign.,*** iod., ip., iris, kali-bi., ***kali-c., kali-i.,*** kali-n., ***kalm.,*** kreos., **LACH.,** ***laur.,*** led., ***lept.,*** **LIL-T.,** ***lith.,*** **LYC.,** mag-c., mang., **MENY.,** ***merc., merc-c.,*** merc-i-f., ***mez.,*** mosch., murx., mur-ac., naja, nat-a., nat-c., **NAT-M.,** ***nit-ac.,*** nux-m., **NUX-V.,** olnd., onos., **OP.,** osm., ***ox-ac.,*** par., **PETR.,** ***ph-ac.,*** **PHOS.,** ***phys., phyt., pic-ac., plat., plb., podo., prun.,*** psor., **PULS., RAN-B.,** ran-s., ***rheum, rhod.,*** **RHUS-T.,** ***rumx.,*** **RUTA.,** sabad., ***sabin.,*** samb., **SANG., SANG-N.,** sars., **SEC., SENEG., SEP., SIL., SPIG., SPONG.,** ***squil.,*** **STANN.,** staph., stict., stram., stront-c., **SULPH.,** sul-ac., tab., ***tarax.,*** tarent., ***ter.,*** teucr., thuj., ust., **VALER., VERAT.,** ***verat-v.,*** verb., vesp., vib., viol-o., viol-t., vip., xan., **ZINC.**
inward - acon., agar., alum., **ANAC.,** ant-c., ant-t., asaf., asar., aur., bar-c., bell., bism., bor., bry., ***calc.,*** cann-s., carb-an., caust., ***chel.,*** chin., ***cocc.,*** coff., croc., cycl., ***dulc., hell.,*** hep., ign., kali-c., ***kreos.,*** laur., mez., mosch., ***nit-ac.,*** nux-m., nux-v., ***olnd.,*** ph-ac., **PLAT.,** ran-s., rheum, rhod., rhus-t., ruta., sabad., sabin., sars., sep., sil., ***spig.,*** **STANN.,** ***staph., sulph.,*** sul-ac., tarax., teucr., thuj., valer., verb., viol-t., ***zinc.***
deep inward with instruments -***bov.,*** verat.
load, as from - ***abies-n.,*** **ACON.,** ***aesc.,*** agar., aloe, alum., ***ambr.,*** am-c., ***am-m., ant-t.,*** aran., arg-m., ***arg-n.,*** arn., ***ars.,*** asaf., asar., aur., ***bar-c.,*** **BELL.,** bism., bor., bov., **BROM., BRY.,** ***cact.,*** calad., calc., camph., cann-s., carb-an., carb-v., caust., cham., ***chel.,*** chin., cina, cinnb., cocc., colch., coloc., ***com., con.,*** croc., corn., crot-t., ***cupr.,*** dig., ferr., gels., graph., hell., hep., hyos., ign., iod., **IP.,** kali-c., kali-chl., kali-n., ***kreos.,*** laur., led., **LIL-T.,** lyc., mag-c., mag-m., mang., ***meli.,*** **MENY.,** merc., mosch., ***nat-c.,*** nat-m., nit-ac., nux-m., **NUX-V.,** olnd., ***op.,*** **PAR.,** petr., ***ph-ac.,*** **PHOS.,** plat., plb., ***psor., puls.,*** **RAN-B.,** ***rheum,*** rhod., **RHUS-T.,** sabad., sabin., ***samb.,*** sars., ***sec.,*** seneg., **SEP.,** ***sil., spig.,*** spong., squil., stann., staph., **STICT.,** stront-c., **SULPH.,** sul-ac., thuj., valer., ***verb.,*** viol-o., zinc., zing.
together - acon., agar., **ALUM.,** ambr., am-m., ***anac.,*** ant-c., ant-t., arg-m., ***arn., ars.,*** asaf., **ASAR.,** aur., bar-c., ***bell., bov.,*** bry., calc., camph., ***cann-s., canth.,*** caps., carb-an., carb-v., caust., cham., chel., chin., cic., cina, **COCC.,** coff., coloc., con., cupr., dig., ***dros.,*** dulc., euph., ferr., graph., guai., ***hell.,*** hyos., ign., iod., ***ip.,*** kali-c., kali-n., laur., led., lyc., mag-c., mag-m., meny., merc., mez., ***mosch., nat-m.,*** nit-ac., nux-m., **NUX-V.,** olnd., op., petr., ph-ac., phos., **PLAT.,** plb., puls., ran-s., rhod., rhus-t., ruta., sabad., sabin., ***sars.,*** seneg., sep., sil., spig., ***spong.,*** squil., ***stann.,*** staph., stram., stront-c., **SULPH.,** ***sul-ac.,*** tarax., teucr., thuj., valer., verat., viol-o., zinc.
within, outward from - ***acon., aloe,*** alum., am-c., am-m., anac., ant-c., arg-m., arn., **ASAF.,** asar., ***aur.,*** bar-c., ***bell.,*** berb., bism., bor., **BRY.,** calc., camph., cann-s., canth., caps., carb-v., caust., chel., chin., **CIMIC.,** cina, clem., cocc., colch., coloc., con., ***cor-r.,*** croc., cupr., dig., ***dros.,*** dulc., euph., ***ferr.,*** graph., guai., hell., hep., ***ign.,*** ip., kali-c., ***kali-i.,*** kali-n., kreos., lach., laur., led., ***lil-t.,*** lyc., mag-m., mang., meli., meny., ***merc., merc-c., mez.,***

PAINS, general
  pressing, pain
    within, outward from - ***mur-ac.,*** nat-c., ***nat-m.,*** nit-ac., nux-m., ***nux-v., olnd.,*** op., ***par.,*** petr., ph-ac., ***phos.,*** plat., ***prun.,*** **PULS.,** ran-b., ran-s., rheum, rhod., ***rhus-t.,*** ruta., sabad., ***sabin.,*** samb., seneg., ***sep., sil., spig., spong., squil., stann.,*** staph., stront-c., **SULPH.,** sul-ac., tarax., ***teucr., thuj., valer., verat.,*** viol-t., zinc.
  radiating, pain - ***arg-n.,*** **BERB.,** dios., **HYPER.,** ***mag-p., tell.***
  scraped, pain, as if - ***acon.,*** aesc., alum., ***arg-m.,*** arn., asaf., ***bell.,*** **BROM.,** bry., carb-v., cham., ***chin., coc-c.,*** coloc., ***con.,*** crot-t., dig., **DROS.,** ***kali-bi., kali-chl., lach.,*** led., ***lyc., mez.,*** **NUX-V.,** ***osm., par.,*** ph-ac., ***phos.,*** phyt., **PULS.,** ***rhus-t., rumx., sabad.,*** sel., seneg., spig., ***stann.,*** **SULPH.,** tell., **VERAT.**
  sensitive, to - ***acon., agar., alum., ambr., am-c.,*** anac., ***ant-c.,*** ant-t., ***arn., ars., ars-i., asar.,*** **AUR.,** ***bar-c., bell., bry., cact.,*** calad., calc., calc-p., ***camph.,*** cann-s., ***canth.,*** caps., carb-an., carb-v., **CHAM.,** ***chin.,*** chin-a., cina, ***cocc.,*** **COFF.,** ***colch., con., cupr.,*** dig., ***ferr.,*** ferr-p., graph., hell., **HEP.,** ***hyos.,*** **IGN.,** iod., ip., kali-ar., ***kali-c.,*** kali-p., **LACH.,** laur., led., **LYC.,** ***mag-c.,*** mag-m., **MED.,** merc., mur-ac., ***nat-c.,*** nat-p., **NIT-AC.,** nux-m., **NUX-V.,** olnd., ***petr.,*** ph-ac., **PHOS.,** ***phyt.,*** plb., **PSOR., PULS.,** ***rhus-t.,*** sabad., sabin., sars., sel., seneg., **SEP., SIL.,** ***spig.,*** squil., **STAPH.,** sulph., thuj., ***tub.,*** valer., verat., vesp., viol-o., ***zinc.***
  sharp, pain
    burning - **ARS.,** aur., ***mez., ol-an.,*** spig.
    crawling - lyc.
    cold, needles - agar.
    downward - **ANT-C.,** arn., ***asc-t.,*** bell., bor., canth., caps., **CARB-V.,** ***caust.,*** chel., cimic., cina, coloc., dios., dros., **FERR.,** gels., kreos., lyc., mang., mez., nit-ac., nux-v., pall., petr., ph-ac., ***phyt., puls., ran-s.,*** **RHUS-T.,** sabin., sars., sep., squil., still., ***sulph.,*** tarax., ust., ***valer.,*** zinc.
    externally - abrot., ***acon., agar.,*** agn., ***aloe, alum.,*** ambr., am-c., ***am-m.,*** anac., ant-c., ant-t., apis, arg-m., ***arn.,*** ars., ars-i., **ASAF.,** asar., aur., ***bar-c.,*** bar-m., **BELL.,** ***berb.,*** bism., bor., bov., **BRY.,** calad., **CALC.,** ***calc-p.,*** camph., ***cann-i.,*** cann-s., canth., ***caps.,*** carb-ac., carb-an., **CARB-S.,** carb-v., ***caust.,*** cedr., cham., ***chel., chin.,*** chin-a., **CIC.,** ***cimic.,*** cina, cinnb., ***clem., cocc.,*** colch., ***coloc.,*** **CON.,** croc., crot-h., crot-t., cupr., cycl., dig., ***dios., dros.,*** dulc., euph., euphr., ***ferr.,*** ferr-ar., ferr-p., form., ***gels., graph., guai., hell.,*** hep., hydr., hyos., ***ign., indg.,*** iod., ip., kali-ar., ***kali-bi.,*** **KALI-C.,** ***kali-n.,*** **KALI-P., KALI-S.,**

PAINS, general
  sharp, pain
    externally - kreos., lach., laur., **LED.,** ***lith., lob., lyc.,*** mag-c., mag-m., ***manc.,*** mang., ***med., meny.,*** **MERC.,** ***mez.,*** mosch., ***mur-ac.,*** naja, nat-a., ***nat-c., nat-h., nat-m., nat-p., nat-s.,*** **NIT-AC.,** nux-m., ***nux-v., ol-an.,*** olnd., ***ox-ac., par.,*** petr., ***ph-ac., phos., phyt.,*** plat., ***plb.,*** psor., **PULS., RAN-B.,** ***ran-s., rat.,*** rheum, rhod., **RHUS-T.,** ruta., ***sabad., sabin.,*** samb., sang., sars., sel., seneg., ***sep., sil.,*** **SPIG.,** ***spong.,*** squil., ***stann.,*** **STAPH.,** still., stram., stront-c., **SULPH.,** sul-ac., **TARAX.,** teucr., **THUJ.,** ***valer.,*** verat., verb., viol-o., ***viol-t.,*** **ZINC.**
      ascending - spig.
      crawling - lyc.
      morning in bed - stann.
      night - euphr.
      one sided - stann.
      vexation, after - rhus-t.
    internally - abrot., ***acon., aesc., agar.,*** agn., all-c., aloe, ***alum.,*** ambr., ammc., am-c., am-m., anac., ant-c., ant-t., apis, arg-m., arg-n., arn., ***ars.,*** ars-i., **ASAF.,** ***asar., aspar., aur.,*** bar-c., bar-m., ***bell.,*** **BERB.,** bism., **BOR.,** ***bov.,*** **BRY.,** ***cact.,*** calad., ***calc.,*** calc-p., camph., **CANN-I., CANTH.,** caps., carb-an., **CARB-S.,** carb-v., card-m., ***caust.,*** cham., **CHEL., CHIN.,** chin-a., cic., cimic., ***cina,*** clem., cocc., ***coc-c.,*** coff., ***colch.,*** coll., ***coloc., con., croc.,*** crot-t., cupr., cycl., dig., dios., dol., dros., ***dulc.,*** euph., euphr., ***ferr., gamb.,*** gels., ***glon.,*** graph., ***guai.,*** hell., hep., hydr., hyos., **IGN.,** iod., ip., kali-ar., ***kali-bi.,*** **KALI-C.,** ***kali-i., kali-n.,*** **KALI-S.,** ***kalm., kreos.,*** **LACH.,** ***laur.,*** **LED.,** ***lyc., mag-c., mag-m.,*** mang., meny., **MERC., MERC-C.,** merc-i-r., merc-n., mez., mosch., mur-ac., ***naja,*** nat-a., ***nat-c., nat-m., nat-s.,*** **NIT-AC.,** nux-m., ***nux-v., ol-an.,*** olnd., op., ox-ac., ***par.,*** petr., phel., ***ph-ac.,*** **PHOS.,** phyt., plan., plat., **PLB.,** prun., psor., **PULS., RAN-B.,** ***ran-s.,*** rheum, rhod., ***rhus-t., rumx.,*** ruta., ***sabad.,*** sabin., samb., sang., ***sars.,*** sec., sel., ***seneg.,*** **SEP., SIL., SPIG.,** spong., **SQUIL.,** stann., ***staph.,*** stram., stront-c., ***sulph.,*** sul-ac., tab., ***tarax.,*** teucr., ***thal., ther., thuj.,*** valer., verat., verb., ***viol-t., zinc., ziz.***
      burning - **ARS.,** aur., ***mez., ol-an.,*** spig.
      cold needles, like - **AGAR.**
    inward - acon., alum., am-m., arg-m., **ARN.,** ***asaf.,*** bar-c., bell., bov., ***bry., calc.,*** cann-s., **CANTH.,** caps., carb-v., caust., cina, clem., cocc., coloc., croc., dros., guai., hyos., ***ign.,*** ip., ***laur.,*** mang., meny., mez., nux-v., olnd., par., petr., ph-ac., phos., ***phyt., plb.,*** **RAN-B.,** rhus-t., ***sabin.,*** samb., sel., squil., staph., sul-ac., tarax., thuj., verb.
    night - euphr.

PAINS, general

sharp, pain

outward - ***alum.,*** am-m., ant-c., **ARG-M.,** arn., **ASAF.,** asar., ***bell., bry., calc.,*** cann-s., canth., carb-v., caust., cham., **CHEL., CHIN.,** clem., cocc., coff., colch., **CON.,** dros., ***dulc.,*** hell., hyos., kali-c., ***lach., laur., lith., lob., lyc.,*** mang., meny., **MERC.,** ***mez.,*** mur-ac., ***nat-c.,*** nat-m., nit-ac., ***ol-an.,*** olnd., **PHEL.,** ph-ac., phos., phyt., **PRUN.,** puls., rhod., ***rhus-t., sabad., sabin., sil.,*** **SPIG., SPONG., STANN.,** ***staph.,*** stront-c., **SULPH.,** ***tarax.,*** ther., thuj., **VALER.,** verat., verb., ***viol-o.,*** viol-t.

outward, to tips of fingers -***lob.***

paralytic - sep.

transversely - acon., ambr., anac., arg-m., ***atro., asc-t.,*** **BELL.,** bov., bry., calc., canth., caust., cham., ***chin.,*** cimic., cocc., cupr., dig., ***kali-bi.,*** kali-c., laur., lyc., merc., mur-ac., phos., ***plb., ran-b.,*** rhod., rhus-t., seneg., ***sep., spig., stict.,*** stront-c., ***sulph.,*** sul-ac., tarax.

upward - acon., alum., arn., ars., bar-c., **BELL.,** bry., calc., canth., carb-v., ***caust., cham.,*** chin., cimic., cina, coloc., dios., ***dros.,*** euphr., gels., ***glon., guai.,*** kali-c., ***lach., lith.,*** mang., ***meny.,*** merc., nat-s., petr., **PHYT.,** ***plb.,*** puls., rhus-t., rumx., ruta., **SEP.,** ***spong., stann., sulph., tarax., thuj.***

wandering - euphr.

shifts to, part lain on - arn., ars., ***bry.,*** calc., ***graph., kali-c.,*** merc., mosch., ***nux-v., ph-ac.,*** **PULS.,** sep., sil.

recently - puls.

part not lain on - bry., cupr., fl-ac., graph., ***ign.,*** kali-bi., puls., rhus-t.

sleep, felt in - nit-ac.

waking amel. - sul-ac.

small spots - agar., aloe, ***alum.,*** am-c., am-m., ambr., apis, arg-m., arg-n., **ARN.,** ***ars.,*** asaf., bell., ***berb.,*** bry., bufo, calc., ***calc-p.,*** cann-s., canth., carb-v., caust., cham., chel., ***cist.,*** coff., ***colch., con.,*** croc., cupr., dios., ferr., fl-ac., gels., glon., graph., hep., hist., ***ign.,*** iod., **KALI-BI., LACH.,** led., lil-t., lith., lyc., mag-c., mag-m., mag-p., meny., merc., mosch., ***nat-m.,*** nit-ac., nux-m., nux-v., ol-an., ***onos., ox-ac., phos.,*** plat., psor., puls., ran-b., ran-s., ***rhod.,*** rhus-t., rhus-v., **SABAD.,** sabin., samb., sars., sel., ***sep.,*** sil., spig., squil., sul-ac., **SULPH.,** ***thuj.,*** verat., zinc.

weather changes agg. - rhod.

sore, pain - ***acon., aesc., agar.,*** agn., aloe, ***alum.,*** alumn., ***am-c.,*** ammc., ant-c., ant-t., apis, **ARG-M., ARN.,** arum-t., ***asar., bad., bapt.,*** bar-c., bar-m., berb., bor., bov., ***bry.,*** calc., calen., ***canth.,*** carb-an., ***carb-s.,*** carb-v., ***caust.,*** cedr., cham., chel., chlor., **CIC., CIMIC., CINA,** clem., cob., coloc., con., crot-h., crot-t., cupr., cycl., dig., **DROS.,** dulc., elaps, euph., eupi., fago., ferr-ar., ferr-p., gamb., goss., grat., **HAM.,** hep., hipp., hyos., ign., iod., ip., kali-c., kali-n., kalm., lach., ***lec., led.,*** lil-t., ***lith.,*** lyc., ***mang.,*** mag-m., mag-s., ***med.,*** merc., merc-i-r., mosch., ***nat-a.,*** nat-c., nat-m., nit-ac., ***nux-m.,*** nux-v., ***olnd.,*** par., petr., ***phos., phyt.,*** **PLAT.,** plb., ***puls.,*** **PYROG.,** ***ran-b.,*** raph., ***rhod.,*** **RHUS-T., RUTA.,** sabad., sabin., seneg., sep., **SIL.,** sol-n., spig., spong., sulph., ***sul-ac.,*** tell., teucr., tarent., thuj., ***tub.,*** verat., verb., viol-o., wies., zinc.

air, open, amel. - caust.

chill, during - tarent.

cramp, after - plat.

evening - agar., am-c., caust., lyc.

11 p.m. - fago.

lying down, after - mag-m., mag-s., petr.

sitting - brom.

exertion, as after great - clem.

externally - ***acon., aesc., agar.,*** aloe, ***alum.,*** am-c., am-m., anac., ant-t., ***apis,*** **ARG-M., ARN.,** ars., asaf., ***asar., aur., bad.,*** **BAPT.,** bar-c., **BELL.,** ***berb.,*** bov., ***bry.,*** calad., ***calc.,*** camph., cann-s., canth., caps., carb-an., carb-s., carb-v., ***caust.,*** cedr., ***cham.,*** chel., **CHIN.,** cic., ***cina, clem.,*** **COCC.,** coff., ***colch., coloc.,*** con., ***croc.,*** cupr., cycl., dig., dros., ***dulc.,*** **EUP-PER.,** euph., ***ferr.,*** fl-ac., form., ***gran.,*** graph., guai., **HAM.,** hell., **HEP.,** hyos., ***ign.,*** ip., kali-c., ***kalm., kreos.,*** lach., laur., ***led., lith., lyc., mag-c.,*** mag-m., ***mang.,*** med., meny., merc., mez., mur-ac., ***nat-c.,*** **NAT-M.,** ***nit-ac., nux-m.,*** **NUX-V.,** ***ox-ac.,*** par., petr., ***ph-ac., phos., phyt.,*** plat., plb., ***puls.,*** **PYROG., RAN-B.,** ran-s., rheum, ***rhod.,*** **RHUS-T., RUTA.,** ***sabad.,*** **SABIN.,** samb., sars., seneg., ***sep.,*** **SIL.,** ***spig.,*** **SPONG.,** squil., ***stann.,*** staph., stram., stront-c., **SULPH.,** sul-ac., tarax., ***thuj., valer.,*** **VERAT.,** viol-t., ***zinc.***

forenoon - mag-m., sars.

headache, during - seneg.

heat, during - agar., mang.

heated walk and rapid cooling, after -***bry.,*** **RHUS-T.**

internally - acon., ***aesc.,*** agar., alum., ambr., am-m., anac., ***apis,*** arn., ***ars.,*** ars-i., asaf., ***aur.,*** **BAPT.,** bar-c., bar-m., bov., bry., **CAMPH.,** cann-i., cann-s., carb-ac., carb-an., carb-s., carb-v., caust., cham., **CHIN.,** cina, clem., ***cocc.,*** coff., ***coloc.,*** con., ***cupr., dros.,*** euph., euphr., ferr., **GELS.,** glon., graph., ***hell.,*** hep., ign., iod., ***ip.,*** kali-c., kreos., lach., ***laur.,*** led., lyc., mag-c., mag-m., ***mang.,*** meny., merc., **MERC-C.,** mosch., mur-ac., nat-c., nit-ac., ***nux-v., op.,*** ph-ac., phos., phyt., **PULS., PYROG., RAN-B.,** ran-s., rhod., rhus-t., rumx., ruta., sabin., samb., sars., sep., ***sil.,*** spig., spong., **STANN.,** staph., stram., stront-c., ***sulph.,*** sul-ac., thuj., valer., ***verat.,*** viol-t., ***zinc.***

PAINS, general

sore, pain,

march, as after a long - chel.

menses, during - nat-c., petr., sep.

morning - aesc., bry., carb-an., chin., euphr., form., mag-m., nat-c., lyc., ox-ac., tab., thuj.

bed. in - grat., petr., rhod., nat-m.

insufficient sleep, after - mag-m.

rising, on - nat-a., sulph.

rising, after - am-m., carb-ac., mag-c., phos., sep., sulph.

waking, on - aesc., alum., bar-c., calc., thuj., til., zinc.

after - crot-h.

motion, on - bapt., ***bry.,*** chel., lach., phyt., plb., staph.

amel. - caust., ***pyrog., rhus-t., tub.***

bed - sol-t-ae.

night - carb-an., caust., ferr-i., ***sil.***

midnight, after - caust.

parts, lain on - **ARN.**, ***bapt.,*** caust., graph., ***hep., mosch., nux-m.,*** **PYRUS., RUTA.**, ***sep.,*** sil., thuj.

affected with cramp-like pain - **PLAT.**

pressure, on - **PLAT.**, plb.

red hard nodules - petr.

rising, amel. - bar-ac., grat., mag-c.

sex, after - **SIL.**

siesta, after - bar-c., eug.

siesta, during - graph.

sitting, on - caust.

spots, in - aloe, **ARN.**, calc-p., carb-ac., colch., **KALI-BI.,** ***nux-v., ox-ac.,*** petr., plat., **SABAD.**

stool, after - calc.

stooping, after - berb.

stormy, weather, in - cham.

touch, on - caust., mang.

waking, after - mag-s., sep.

waking, on - hydrc., spong., sulph., thuj.

walking, while - ***staph.***

amel. - coloc.

working amel. - caust.

splinters, pain - ***aesc.,*** **AGAR.,** ***alum.,*** **ARG-N.,** ***bar-c., carb-v.,*** cic., colch., coll., ***dol., fl-ac.,*** **HEP., NIT-AC.,** petr., plat., ran-b., ***sil.,*** sulph.

tearing, pain - act-sp., coloc., dig., hep., **KALI-BI.,** kreos., led., mosch., nux-v., paeon., petr., phos., ***plb.,*** **RHUS-T.,** sep., sulph., thlaspi, thuj., uran., urt-u.

asunder - agar., alum., am-m., anac., arn., ars., asar., calc., carb-an., carb-v., caust., **COFF.,** colch., con., dig., ferr., graph., ign., ***mez.,*** mur-ac., nat-m., **NIT-AC., NUX-V.,** op., puls., rhus-t., sabin., sep., spig., ***staph.,*** sulph., sul-ac., ***teucr.,*** thuj., zinc.

downward - ***acon., agar., agn.,*** alum., anac., ant-c., ant-t., ars., asaf., aur., ***bar-c.,*** bar-m., **BELL.,** bism., ***bry.,*** calc., canth., **CAPS.,** ***carb-s., carb-v.,*** caust., chel., ***chin.,*** cina, colch., ***coloc.,*** con., croc., dulc., euphr., ***ferr.,*** ferr-p., ***graph.,*** ign.,

PAINS, general

tearing, pain,

downward - ***kali-c.,*** kali-n., kali-p., ***kali-s., laur.,*** **LYC.,** mag-c., ***meny., merc.,*** mez., mur-ac., nat-a., ***nat-c.,*** nat-m., nit-ac., ***nux-v.,*** ph-ac., phos., ***puls.,*** rhod., **RHUS-T.,** sabin., sars., seneg., ***sep.,*** sil., ***spig.,*** squil., stann., staph., **SULPH.,** thuj., valer., ***verat.,*** verb., zinc.

externally - **ACON.,** aesc., ***agar.,*** agn., ***alum., ambr., am-c., am-m., anac.,*** ant-c., ant-t., arg-m., **ARN.,** ***ars., asaf.,*** asar., aur., bar-c., bar-m., **BELL., BERB.,** ***bism.,*** bor., bov., brom., **BRY.,** cact., calad., ***calc.,*** calc-p., camph., cann-s., canth., ***caps.,*** carb-an., **CARB-S.,** ***carb-v., caust., cedr., cham., chel.,*** **CHIN.,** chin-a., cic., cina, clem., cocc., coff., **COLCH.,** ***coloc.,*** con., croc., crot-t., cupr., cycl., dig., dros., ***dulc.,*** euph., euphr., ***ferr., ferr-ar.,*** ferr-p., ***gamb., gels.,*** graph., ***guai.,*** hell., hep., hyos., **HYPER.,** ign., ***indg.,*** iod., ip., kali-ar., ***kali-bi.,*** **KALI-C.,** ***kali-i., kali-n.,*** **KALI-P., KALI-S.,** ***kreos.,*** lach., laur., **LED., LYC.,** lyss., ***mag-c.,*** mag-m., mang., meny., ***merc., mez.,*** mosch., mur-ac., nat-a., ***nat-c.,*** **NAT-M.,** nat-p., **NAT-S.,** ***nicc.,*** **NIT-AC.,** nux-m., ***nux-v.,*** olnd., op., par., petr., ph-ac., phyt., plat., plb., **PULS.,** ***ran-b.,*** ran-s., ***rat.,*** rheum, ***rhod., rhus-t.,*** ruta., sabad., sabin., samb., sars., sec., ***sel.,*** seneg., **SEP., SIL.,** ***spig.,*** spong., squil., stann., staph., stram., ***stront-c.,*** **SULPH.,** sul-ac., tarax., teucr., thuj., ***valer.,*** verat., verb., viol-o., viol-t., **ZINC.**

internally - acon., aesc., ***agar.,*** agn., aloe, alum., ***ambr.,*** am-c., am-m., anac., ant-c., ***ant-t.,*** apis, ***arg-m.,*** arn., ars., ars-i., asaf., asar., ***aur.,*** bar-c., **BELL., BERB.,** bism., bor., bov., **BRY.,** calad., calc., camph., cann-s., canth., ***caps.,*** carb-an., ***carb-s.,*** **CARB-V.,** caust., ***cham., chel.,*** chin., chin-a., cic., cina, clem., cocc., coff., colch., ***coloc.,*** **CON.,** croc., crot-h., cupr., cycl., dig., dios., dros., dulc., euph., euphr., ferr., ***gran.,*** graph., guai., hell., hep., hyos., ***ign.,*** iod., ip., kali-ar., kali-c., ***kali-n.,*** **KALI-S.,** ***kalm.,*** kreos., ***lach.,*** laur., **LED., LYC.,** ***mag-c.,*** mag-m., mang., ***meny.,*** **MERC.,** mez., mosch., mur-ac., nat-a., nat-c., ***nat-m.,*** nit-ac., nux-m., **NUX-V.,** olnd., op., par., petr., ph-ac., ***phos.,*** plat., plb., **PULS.,** ran-b., ran-s., ***rhod.,*** rhus-t., ruta., sabad., sabin., samb., sang., sars., sec., sel., seneg., **SEP., SIL., SPIG.,** spong., squil., ***stann.,*** staph., stram., stront-c., **SULPH.,** sul-ac., ***tarax.,*** thuj., uva., valer., verat., ***verat-v.,*** verb., viol-o., viol-t., ***zinc.***

PAINS, general

tearing, pain

outward - all-c., am-c., bell., bov., ***bry., calc.,*** cann-s., caust., ***cocc.,*** cycl., elaps, euph., ip., mang., mez., mur-ac., nat-c., par., ph-ac., **PRUN.,** puls., ***rhus-t., sil., spig.,*** spong., stram.

upward - acon., alum., ***anac.,*** ant-c., arn., ***ars.,*** asaf., aur., **BELL.,** bism., bor., calc., carb-v., caust., chin., clem., colch., ***con., dulc.,*** euphr., mag-c., meny., merc., ***nat-a., nat-c.,*** nat-m., ***nit-ac., nux-v.,*** ph-ac., phos., puls., rhod., rhus-t., samb., sars., **SEP., SIL., SPIG.,** spong., ***stront-c.,*** sulph., thuj., valer.

sympathetic - carc., phos., tarent.

thunderstorm, before or during a - agar., caust., cedr., nat-c., nat-p., phos., **RHOD.,** sep., ***sil.***

trembling and paralytic weakness, with - kalm.

twinging, pain - aloe, alum., **AM-M.,** ant-c., apis, aur., bell., berb., ***bov.,*** canth., carb-an., caust., ***chel.,*** cocc., coloc., ***crot-t.,*** dros., ***ferr.,*** iod., kali-c., **LAUR.,** lyc., ***mag-c.,*** mag-m., merc., **MOSCH.,** mur-ac., nat-p., ph-ac., phos., plan., **PLB.,** ***prun., rhus-t.,*** sabin., sars., seneg., sil., staph., stront-c., sul-ac., ***valer.***

twisting, pain - ***agar.,*** alum., am-m., anac., ant-c., ant-t., ***arg-n.,*** ars., asaf., bar-c., ***bell.,*** berb., bor., ***bry.,*** calad., calc., ***caps.,*** canth., cham., ***cina,*** con., dig., ***dios.,*** dros., dulc., ***ign.,*** ip., kali-c., kali-n., led., ***merc.,*** mez., nat-c., nat-m., nux-m., ***nux-v.,*** olnd., ox-ac., ph-ac., phos., ***plat.,*** plb., podo., ran-b., ran-s., ***rhus-t.,*** ruta., ***sabad.,*** sabin., sars., seneg., sep., **SIL.,** staph., sulph., sul-ac., thlaspi, thuj., valer., **VERAT.**

unbearable - **ACON.,** ***ars.,*** **CHAM., COFF., HEP.,** ign., ***hyper., phyt., pip-m.***

ulcerative, pain

externally - acon., agar., alum., ambr., am-c., **AM-M.,** anac., ant-c., arg-m., arn., ars., aur., bar-c., bell., bov., **BRY.,** camph., cann-s., ***canth.,*** caps., carb-an., carb-v., ***caust.,*** cedr., cham., chin., ***cic.,*** cocc., colch., cycl., dros., dulc., ferr., ***graph.,*** hep., ***ign., kali-c.,*** kali-n., **KALI-S.,** kreos., lach., laur., mag-c., mag-m., ***mang.,*** merc., ***mur-ac.,*** nat-c., ***nat-m.,*** nit-ac., ***nux-v.,*** petr., ph-ac., phos., plat., **PULS., RHUS-T.,** ruta., sars., ***sep.,*** **SIL.,** spig., spong., staph., sulph., sul-ac., teucr., thuj., verat., ***zinc.***

internally - acon., ***am-c., arg-n.,*** ars., bell., bor., bov., ***bry., cann-s.,*** canth., ***caps.,*** carb-an., carb-s., carb-v., ***caust.,*** cham., chel., cocc., ***coloc.,*** cupr., dig., ***gamb.,*** hell., hep., kali-c., kreos., **LACH.,** laur., mag-c., mag-m., mang., ***merc.,*** mur-ac., nit-ac., ***nux-v.,*** ph-ac., phos., ***psor.,*** **PULS., RAN-B.,** ***rhus-t.,*** ruta., sabad., sep., **SIL.,** spig., stann., staph., stront-c., ***sulph.,*** valer., verat.

PAINS, general

undulating, pain - acon., anac., ant-t., arn., asaf., chin., cocc., dulc., mez., olnd., plan., rhod., sep., spig., teucr., viol-t.

wandering, pains - acon., aesc., am-c., ***am-m.,*** apoc., arg-m., ***arn.,*** ars., asaf., ***aur.,*** bar-c., ***bell.,*** benz-ac., bry., ***calc-p.,*** camph., caps., ***carb-s., carb-v., caul., caust.,*** cedr., chel., ***chin.,*** clem., ***colch.,*** croc., ***dios.,*** eup-pur., gels., goss., graph., ign., iod., ***iris,*** **KALI-BI.,** kali-c., ***kali-fer.,*** **KALI-S.,** ***kalm.,*** **LAC-C.,** ***lach.,*** **LED.,** lil-t., lycps., mag-c., ***mag-p., manc., mang.,*** meny., nat-m., nat-s., ***nux-m., phyt.,*** plat., ***plb.,*** polyg., **PULS.,** ***rad., ran-b.,*** rhod., ***rhus-t., rumx., sabin., sal-ac.,*** sang., sars., sep., sil., ***spig.,*** stel., sulph., tarent., thuj., ***tub.,*** valer., zinc.

touch, on - graph.

violent behaviour, from pain - **AUR., CHAM., HEP.**

wakens, him - acon., ars., chin., kali-c., lach., nux-v., sil., sulph.

weakness, from - ***arg-m.,*** **ARS.,** carb-v., hura, kali-p., ***ph-ac.,*** plb., ***rhus-t., sil.***

PARALYSIS, (see Nerves, Chapter)

PARTS single, effects - agar., alum., bar-c., caust., con., dulc., kali-c., ol-an., plb., rhod., sec., sul-i., valer.

white and insensible, turn - sul-i.

PAROXYSMS, repeated - acon., ***agar., ars.,*** bar-c., bar-m., ***bell.,*** calc., ***caust.,*** **CHAM.,** ***chin.,*** **COCC., COLOC.,** cupr., ***dios.,*** gels., hep., ign., kali-i., lach., lyc., **MAG-P.,** mez., nat-m., **NUX-V.,** phos., plat., plb., ***psor.,*** puls., **SEP.,** stann., sulph., tab., tub., valer., verb.

repeated, easy - asaf., cupr.

PELLAGRA - ***ars.,*** ars-s-r., bov., chin., gels., hep., ped., psor., ***sec., sedi.,*** sulph.

cachexia, with - ars., sec.

fissures, desquamation, skin eruptions - graph., ***hep.,*** ign., phos., puls., sep.

PEMPHIGUS - acon., ***anac.,*** antipyrin., ***ars.,*** arum-t., bell., bufo, calc., calth., canth., carb-o., caust., chin., ***crot-h., dulc.,*** hep., hydrc., jug-c., **LACH.,** ***lyc., manc., merc., merc-c.,*** merc-p-r., ***nat-m., nat-s.,*** nat-sal., ***nit-ac.,*** ph-ac., phos., ***psor.,*** ran-b., ran-s., raph., ***rhus-t., sars., sep., sil., sulph.,*** sul-ac., syph., thuj.

PERIODICITY, (see Time, general)

PHLEBITIS - **ACON.,** agar., ***all-c.,*** ant-c., ***ant-t.,*** apis, arist-cl., ***arn., ars., bell.,*** both., **BRY.,** ***bufo,*** **CALC.,** calc-ar., ***calc-f.,*** carb-s., carb-v., ***cham., chin.,*** chlorpr., **CLEM.,** crot-h., graph., ***ham.,*** hecla., hep., hir., ***iod., kali-c.,*** kali-m., kreos., **LACH.,** ***led., lyc., lycps.,*** mag-c., mag-f., merc., merc-cy., merc-i-r., ***nat-s.,*** nux-v., phos., ***puls.,*** rhod., **RHUS-T.,** ruta, ***sep., sil.,*** spig., stront-br., stront-c., sulfa., ***sulph.,*** thiop., thuj., verat., **VIP.,** vip-a., zinc.

injuries, after - rhus-t.

childbirth, after, forceps with - all-c.

contractions, with - ***sil.***

PHTHISIS, (see Tuberculosis)

PIANO, playing, agg. - anac., calc., kali-c., ***nat-c., sep.,*** zinc.

PLAGUE, bubonic, (see Fevers)

PLETHORA, of body - ***acon.,*** alum., ambr., ***am-c.,*** am-m., ant-c., apis, ***arn., ars.,*** **AUR.,** ***bar-c.,*** **BELL.,** bov., **BRY., CALC.,** canth., caps., ***carb-an., carb-s., carb-v.,*** caust., cham., chel., ***chin.,*** clem., cocc., coloc., con., ***croc.,*** cupr., dig., dulc., ***ferr.,*** ferr-ar., ferr-p., ***graph.,*** guai., hep., **HYOS.,** ign., iod., ip., **KALI-BI.,** ***kali-c.,*** kali-n., ***lach.,*** led., **LYC.,** mag-m., ***merc.,*** mosch., nat-c., **NAT-M.,** nit-ac., ***nux-v., op.,*** petr., ***ph-ac.,*** **PHOS.,** ***puls.,*** rhod., ***rhus-t.,*** sabin., sars., sec., sel., seneg., **SEP., SIL.,** spig., spong., stann., staph., ***stram., stront-c.,*** **SULPH.,** ***thuj.,*** valer., verat., zinc.
- pregnancy, during - acon.

POSITION, change of body, agg. - acon., **BRY., CAPS.,** ***carb-v.,*** caust., ***chel., con.,*** **EUPH., FERR.,** ***lach., lyc.,*** petr., ph-ac., ***phos.,*** plat., plb., **PULS.,** ran-b., rhod., rhus-t., sabad., ***samb.,*** sil., syph., thuj.
- bed or chair, seem so hard - ***arn.***
- desire for, continually - **ARS., RHUS-T.**
- frequent - lyss., spong.
- amel. - agar., ars., caust., ***cham., dulc.,*** **IGN.,** ***meli., nat-s., ph-ac., plb.,*** puls., **RHUS-T.,** sep., staph., syph., teucr., valer., zinc.

POTT'S disease, tuberculosis of vertebrae - aur., calc-p., iod., ph-ac., phos., stann., syph., tub.
- lies on, with drawn up knees - merc-c.

POULTICE, rebels against - bor., bry., ***calc.,*** carb-v., ***cham., lyc.,*** merc., mur-ac., nit-ac., nux-v., phos., puls., rhus-t., sep., spig., staph., ***sulph.***

POUNDING, side lain on - clem.

PRESSURE, agg. - acon., **AGAR.,** alum., ambr., am-c., am-m., anac., ant-c., **APIS,** ***arg-m.,*** arn., ***ars., ars-i.,*** asaf., ***bapt.,*** **BAR-C.,** bar-m., bell., bism., bor., bov., ***bry.,*** cact., ***calad.,*** calc., calc-p., camph., ***cann-s., canth., caps.,*** carb-an., carb-s., ***carb-v.,*** card-m., caust., ***chel.,*** chin., **CINA,** cocc., coc-c., coloc., crot-t., cupr., dig., dros., dulc., ***guai.,*** hell., **HEP.,** hyos., ign., **IOD.,** ip., ***kali-bi., kali-c., kali-i.,*** kali-n., kali-p., **LACH.,** laur., led., **LIL-T., LYC.,** ***mag-c.,*** mag-m., mang., meny., ***merc.,*** **MERC-C.,** mez., ***mosch.,*** mur-ac., nat-a., nat-c., ***nat-m., nat-s., nit-ac.,*** nux-m., ***nux-v., olnd., op.,*** ox-ac., ph-ac., phos., ***plat.,*** puls., ***ran-b., ran-s.,*** rhus-t., ***ruta.,*** sabad., ***sabin.,*** samb., sars., ***sel.,*** seneg., sep., **SIL.,** spig., ***spong., stann., staph.,*** stram., stront-c., sulph., sul-ac., ***teucr.,*** thuj., ***valer.,*** verat., ***verb.,*** zinc.
- boots, shoes, of - bor., paeon.
- hard - pip-n., ruta, spig., tell.
- pain goes to side, lain on - cimic., graph., mosch., nat-m., phys., tell.
- opposite side, on - viol-t.

PRESSURE, agg.
- painless side, of - ***ambr.,*** arn., bell., **BRY.,** ***calc.,*** cann-s., carb-an., carb-v., ***caust., cham., coloc., fl-ac.,*** **IGN.,** ***kali-c.,*** lyc., nux-v., **PULS.,** ***rhus-t., sep., stann.,*** viol-o., ***viol-t.***
- sharp - ign.
- slight agg., hard amel. - aloe, bell., bry., ***cast.,*** caust., **CHIN.,** culx., ign., kali-c., lac-c., ***lach., mag-p., nux-v.,*** plb., sulph.

pressure, amel. - abies-c., acon., agar., ***agn.,*** alum., ambr., ***am-c., am-m.,*** anac., ant-c., ***apis,*** arg-m., ***arg-n.,*** arn., ars., ***asaf., aur.,*** bell., bism., ***bor.,*** bov., **BRY.,** cact., calc., calc-f., camph., ***canth.,*** carb-ac., ***carb-s.,*** caust., ***chel.,*** **CHIN.,** cina, cinnb., ***clem.,*** **COLOC., CON.,** ***croc.,*** crot-t., dig., dios., **DROS.,** ***dulc.,*** form., ***glon., graph.,*** guai., hell., ign., ip., ***kali-bi.,*** kali-c., ***kali-i.,*** kali-p., kreos., laur., ***lach.,*** led., **LIL-T.,** mag-c., **MAG-M., MAG-P.,** ***mang.,*** **MENY.,** merc., mez., mosch., ***mur-ac.,*** **NAT-C.,** ***nat-m.,*** nat-p., ***nat-s., nit-ac., nux-m.,*** nux-v., olnd., ***par., ph-ac.,*** phos., **PLB., PULS.,** ***rhus-t.,*** ruta., sabad., sabin., sang., ***sep.,*** **SIL.,** ***spig.,*** stann., sulph., sul-ac., thuj., ***tril.,*** verat., verb., zinc.
- hard pressure - achy., arg-n., arn., ***bry., coloc.,*** culx., ign., mag-m., plb., rauw., sep., stann.
  - amel., slight agg. - aloe, bell., ***cast.,*** caust., **CHIN.,** culx., ign., kali-c., lac-c., ***lach., mag-p., nux-v.,*** plb., psor., sulph.
  - edge, over a - bell., ***chin.,*** **COLOC.,** con., ign., ***lach.,*** mag-m., ***meny.,*** nux-v., psor., samb., sang., stann., zinc.
- steady - bry., nit-ac., spig.

PUBERTY, (see Children, chapter)

PULSATION, general

externally - ***acon., aesc.,*** agar., alum., alumn., ***ambr.,*** am-c., am-m., ammc., anac., ***ant-t., arg-m., arg-n.,*** arn., ***ars., ars-i., asaf.,*** asar., ***bar-c.,*** bar-m., bell., benz., berb., bov., brom., bry., ***cact.,*** calad., **CALC.,** ***calc-p., calc-s.,*** cann-s., canth., caps., carb-an., ***carb-s., carb-v., caust.,*** cham., chel., chin., chin-a., chlol., cina, clem., cocc., coc-c., coff., ***coloc., con.,*** cop., croc., cupr., dig., dros., dulc., euphr., **FERR.,** ferr-ar., **FERR-I.,** ferr-p., ***fl-ac.,*** gamb., gels., **GLON., GRAPH.,** guai., hell., helo., hep., hyos., ***ign., iod.,*** kali-ar., ***kali-bi.,*** **KALI-C.,** kali-n., kali-p., **KALI-S.,** kiss., **KREOS., LACH.,** laur., ***lil-t., lyc., lyss.,*** mag-c., mag-m., manc., mang., med., **MELI.,** ***merc.,*** mez., mosch., mur-ac., nat-a., ***nat-c.,*** **NAT-M.,** ***nat-p., nat-s., nit-ac.,*** nux-m., ***nux-v.,*** **OLND.,** op., par., petr., ph-ac., ***phos.,*** phys., phyt., ***plat.,*** plb., **PULS.,** ran-b., rheum, ***rhod.,*** rhus-t., ***rumx., ruta,*** **SABAD.,** sabin., samb., sang., sars., sec., ***sel.,*** seneg., ***sep., sil.,*** spig., spong., squil., stann., staph., ***still., stram., stront-c.,*** **SULPH.,** sul-ac., ***tarax.,*** teucr., ***thuj.,*** til., ***urt-u.,*** verat., ***zinc.***

PULSATION, general
afternoon, 2:30 p.m - pall.
air, open, amel. - ***aur.***
bed, in - arn., carb-an., caust., nat-m., sep., upa.
cough, during - ***calc.***
eating, after - arg-n., camph., ***clem.,*** lyc., **SEL.**
evening, in - arn., ***carb-an.,*** caust., nat-m., sep.
rest, during - nat- m.
on, falling to sleep - sil.
excitement agg. - ferr., kreos.
exertion - ferr., iod.
headache - lach.
lying, while - calad., ***glon.***
menses, before - cupr., thuj.
morning, on waking - ***bell.***
motion, agg. - ant-t., ***graph., iod.***
motion, amel. - ***kreos., nat-m.***
music, agg. - kreos.
night - am-m., ***bry.,*** cact., nat-m., ***sil.,*** sulph.
coughing, from - ***calc.***
half awake, while - sulph.
midnight - phys.
midnight after 4 a.m - iris.
plaintive music - kreos.
pregnancy, during - ***kali-c.***
sitting, while - eupi., phys., ***sil.***
sleep, during - nat-m., sulph.
speaking in company, while - carb- v.
standing - alum.
touches anything, when body - glon.
tremulous - nat- c.
waking, on - ferr- i.
walking - dig., ferr.
in open air, after - ambr.

internally - **ACON.,** aeth., agar., aloe, **ALUM.,** ambr., am-c., ***am-m., aml-n.,*** anac., ant-c., **ANT-T.,** arg-m., ***arg-n.,*** arn., ***ars., ars-i., asaf.,*** asar., ***aur.,*** bar-c., ***bell., bor.,*** bov., **BRY.,** ***cact.,*** calad., **CALC.,** calc-p., ***camph.,*** **CANN-I.,** ***cann-s.,*** canth., ***caps.,*** carb-an., carb-s., carb-v., caust., cedr., ***cham.,*** chel., chin., chin-a., ***cic.,*** **COCC.,** coff., colch., ***coloc., con.,*** croc., crot-h., crot-t., cycl., ***dig.,*** dros., dulc., **FERR., FERR-I.,** gels., **GLON.,** ***graph.,*** hell., hep., hyos., ***ign., iod.,*** ip., kali-c., kali-n., ***kreos.,*** lach., ***laur.,*** led., lyc., mag-c., mag-m., mang., **MELI.,** ***merc., merc-c.,*** mez., mosch., murx., nat-c., ***nat-m.,*** nat-p., ***nat-s.,*** nit-ac., nux-m., ***nux-v., olnd.,*** op., par., petr., ph-ac., **PHOS.,** phys., pic-ac., ***plan., plat., plb., psor.,*** **PULS.,** ran-b., rheum, rhod., ***rhus-t.,*** ruta., ***sabad.,*** sabin., ***sang.,*** sars., sec., **SEL.,** seneg., **SEP., SIL.,** ***spig., spong.,*** stann., ***stram., sulph.,*** sul-ac., ***thuj.,*** verat., verat-v., verb., ***zinc.***
upper part of body - nit-ac.

PULSE, (see Pulse, chapter)

QUIVERING, general - ***am-c.,*** **BELL.,** berb., bism., ***calc.,*** caps., caust., ***clem.,*** com., **CON.,** dig., hep., hyos., ign., iod., kali-c., kali-n., lyc., mag-c., mosch., ***nit-ac.,*** nux-v., petr., sars., ***sep.,*** sil.,

QUIVERING, general - stann., stront-c., **SULPH.,** verb.
all over, followed by vertigo - ***calc.***
lying, while - ***clem.***

RABIES, hydrophobia (see Emergency)

RAIN, general, (see Environment, Rain)

RAYNAUD'S disease - **AGAR.,** calc., **HEP.,** ***lac-d., merc., nat-m., pyrog.,*** **RHUS-T., SEP., SIL.,** thuj., zinc.

REACTION, general, lack of - agar., ***alum.,*** **AMBR., AM-C.,** ***anac.,*** ant-c., ant-t., arn., ***ars., ars-i., asaf., bar-c.,*** bism., ***brom.,*** bry., **CALC.,** ***calc-i., calc-s., camph.,*** **CAPS.,** ***carb-an.,*** **CARB-V.,** ***cast.,*** caust., cham., ***chin.,*** cic., ***cocc.,*** coff., **CON.,** ***cupr., dulc.,*** euph., ***ferr.,*** ferr-i., ***fl-ac.,*** **GELS.,** ***graph., guai.,*** **HELL., HYDR-AC.,** hyos., ***iod., ip., kali-br., kali-c., kali-s., lach.,*** **LAUR.,** ***lyc.,*** mag-c., mag-m., **MED.,** ***merc.,*** mez., ***mosch., mur-ac.,*** nat c., nat-m., nat-p., ***nux-m.,*** **OLND., OP.,** petr., **PH-AC.,** ***phos., plb.,*** **PSOR.,** ***rhod., sec.,*** seneg., ***sep.,*** spong., ***stann., stram.,*** stront-c., ***syph.,*** **SULPH., TARENT.,** ***thuj., valer., verat., verb.,*** zinc.
acute danger - ambr., ars., camph., lyc.
chill, after - camph., dulc.
convalescence, in - cast., ph-ac.
exanthemas, in - ant-t., ***bry.,*** cupr., dulc., psor., stram., ***sulph.,*** zinc.
loss of fluids, after - ***chin.***
remedies, to - carb-v., laur., op., teucr.
menopause, at - con.
nervous patients, in - ambr., laur., op., **VALER.,** zinc.
old age, in - con.
suppression, after - lach.
eruptions, of - ars-s-f.
suppuration, in - calc-f., hep.

REDNESS, of affected parts (see Skin) - **ACON.,** ***apis, arg-n.,*** ars., **BELL.,** ***bry., cham.,*** chin., ***ferr.,*** piloc., lach., meli., ***merc., nux-v.,*** op., phos., ***rhus-t.,*** sabin., ***sang.,*** sep., **SULPH.**
bluish, dark - bapt., phyt., rhus-t.
body, whole - op.
fiery - bell., cinnb., med., stram., sulph.
rosy - apis, pyrog., sil.
spots - merc., pic-ac., rhus-t., stict., sulph.
bloody - cor-r., phos.
elevated - mang.
fiery - med.
pink - colch.
small, all over body - squil.
wine - cocc., ***sep.***
streaks - bell., bry., bufo, mygal., pyrog.
white, turning - bor., hell., merc., valer.
yellow or green, turning - con.

RELAXATION, of tissues, (see Muscles) - acon., agar., agn., alum., ant-t., arn., ars., asar., aur., bell., bism., bry., camph., caust., cham., chel., chin., cic., cina, cocc., coff., colch., cupr., cycl., dig., dulc., euph., ferr., ***gels.,*** hydr-ac., ***hyos.,*** ign., ip., kali-c., kali-n., lach., linu-c., lyc., meny., merc., ***morph.,*** nat-c., nat-m., nit-ac., nux-m., nux-v., olnd., ***op.,*** par., petr., ph-ac., phos., plat.,

RELAXATION, of tissues - plb., ran-s., rhod., rhus-t., ruta, sabad., sabin., sel., sep., sil., spig., spong., stann., staph., stram., sulph., tarax., verat., viol-o., viol-t., zinc.
connective tissue - calc., calc-br., caps., ferr-i., hep., kali-c., mag-c., merc-i-r., nit-ac., sec., spong.
sex, after - ***agar.,*** sep.

REST, agg. - acon., ***aesc., agar.,*** alum., ***alumn.,*** am-c., ***am-m., ambr.,*** anac., ang., ant-c., ***ant-t.,*** aran-ix., ***arg-m., arn., ars., asaf.,*** asar., **AUR.,** aur-m., bar-c., bell., bell-p., benz-ac., ***bism., bor., bov.,*** bry., calc., calc-f., **CAPS.,** carb-v., caust., ***cham.,*** chin., cic., cimic., ***cina,*** cocc., ***coloc.,*** com., **CON.,** cortiso., cupr., **CYCL.,** ***dros.,*** **DULC., EUPH.,** ***euphr.,*** **FERR.,** ferr-ar., ferr-p., fl-ac., foll., gels., glon., guai., hecla., hep., hyos., ign., indg., ***iod.,*** iris, kali-c., kali-i., ***kali-n.,*** kali-s., ***kreos., lach.,*** laur., lith-lac., **LYC.,** ***mag-c.,*** **MAG-M.,** mang., ***meny., merc., merc-c.,*** merc-i-f., ***mez., mosch., mur-ac., nat-c.,*** nat-f., ***nat-m.,*** nat-s., nit-ac., ***nux-m.,*** olnd., ***op.,*** par., petr., ***ph-ac.,*** phenol., phos., ***plat.,*** plb., pneu., **PULS.,** pyrog., ***rhod.,*** **RHUS-T.,** ***ruta,*** **SABAD.,** sabin., **SAMB.,** sars., sel., seneg., **SEP.,** sil., spig., spong., stann., staph., ***stront-c.,*** sul-ac., sulph., **TARAX.,** tarent., tell., teucr., ***thuj.,*** tub., tub-r., **VALER.,** ***verat., verb., viol-t., zinc.,*** zinc-valer.
as well as motion, during - am-c., bov., calc., carb-an., carb-v., caust., mez., ph-ac., phos., sulph.

amel. - achy., acon., adlu., aesc., agar., ***agn.,*** alum., alum-sil., alumn., ***am-c.,*** am-m., ambr., ***anac., ang.,*** anh., ant-c., ***ant-t.,*** aq-mar., arg-m., ***arn.,*** ars., asaf., ***asar.,*** aur., bar-c., bar-m., **BELL.,** bism., ***bor.,*** bov., **BRY.,** but-ac., cadm-s., ***calad., calc.,*** calc-f., calc-p., ***camph.,*** cann-i., ***cann-s., canth.,*** caps., ***carb-an., carb-v.,*** caust., cham., ***chel.,*** chin., ***cic.,*** cina, coc-c., ***cocc., coff.,*** **COLCH.,** ***coloc.,*** con., crat., ***croc., cupr.,*** cycl., des-ac., dicha., ***dig.,*** dros., dulc., ***echi.,*** euph., ferr., fl-ac., **GELS.,** get., gink-b., ***graph., guai.,*** guat., gymn., ***hell., hep.,*** hydr., hyos., ign., ***iod., ip.,*** kali-bi., kali-c., kali-i., kali-n., kali-p., kalm., kreos., lac-d., lach., laur., **LED.,** lyc., mag-c., mag-m., mag-p., man., ***mang.,*** meny., ***merc.,*** merc-c., ***mez.,*** mosch., mur-ac., nat-c., ***nat-m., nit-ac., nux-m.,*** **NUX-V.,** olnd., onop., op., ***par.,*** penic., ***petr.,*** ph-ac., phenob., ***phos.,*** phyt., plat., ***plb.,*** prot., pulx., ***ran-b., rheum,*** rhod., rhus-t., ruta, sabad., sabin., samb., sang., ***sars., sec., sel.,*** seneg., **SEP.,** sieg., sil., ***spig., spong., squil.,*** stann., ***staph., stram.,*** stront-c., stroph-s., stry-p., ***sul-ac.,*** sulph., teucr., ther., thuj., trio., verat., vib., viol-t., zinc.

must rest - ***aesc.,*** alum., alum-sil., ***anac.,*** arn., brom., ***bry.,*** lach., lyc., nux-v., op., ***ph-ac.,*** sabad., ***stann.***

RIDING, cars, in a wagon or on the street cars, agg. (see Emergency, Motion sickness) - acon., alum-sil., ***arg-m., arg-n., arn.,*** ars., asaf., ***aur.,*** bell., berb., ***bor.,*** bry., calc., calc-p., carb-v., caust., coc-c., **COCC.,** colch., ***con.,*** croc., cycl., dig., ferr., fl-ac., glon., graph., grat., **HELON.,** ***hep.,*** hyos., ***ign.,*** iod., iodof., kali-c., kreos., lac-d., ***lach.,*** lyc., ***lyss.,*** mag-c., mag-s., meph., nat-m., ***nux-m.,*** op., **PETR.,** phos., plat., ***psor.,*** puls., rhus-t., ***rumx., sanic., sel.,*** **SEP.,** ***sil.,*** spig., staph., sul-ac., ***sulph.,*** **TAB.,** ***ther.,*** thuj., tril., valer.
after - graph., kali-n., nat-c., nat-m., ***nit-ac.,*** plat., **SIL.**
railway - kali-i.
stomach, felt in, nausea without - kali-p.
ailments from - lyc., petr.
amel. - arg-n., ***ars.,*** bar-m., brom., bry., des-ac., ***gels.,*** glon., ***graph.,*** kali-n., lyc., merc., merc-c., ***naja,*** nat-m., **NIT-AC.,** nux-m., phos., puls., tarent., thiop.
aversion to - psor.
down hill - **BOR.,** ***psor.***

riding, horseback, agg. - arist-cl., arg-n., ars., ***bell.,*** bor., bry., ***graph., lil-t.,*** mag-m., meph., ***nat-c.,*** nat-m., psor., ***ruta,*** **SEP.,** sil., spig., ***sul-ac.,*** tab., ther., valer.
ailments from - ther.
amel. - brom., calc., kali-c., lyc., tarent.

riding, ship, ailments from riding in a - ars., petr., tab., ther.

RINGWORM - anac., anag., ars-s-f., **BAC.,** ***bar-c., calc.,*** calc-ac., chrysar., clem., dulc., dys-co., equis., ***eup-per., graph.,*** hell., hep., iod., ***lith.,*** mag-c., med., ***nat-c.,*** **NAT-M.,** phos., **PHYT.,** ***sanic.,*** **SEP.,** spong., sulph., syc-co., **TELL., THUJ.,** torula., **TUB.**
rings, in intersecting - tell.
spots, in isolated - sep.
spring, every - **SEP.**

ringworm, beard - ant-t., anthr., ars., aur-m., ***bac., calc.,*** calc-s., chrysar., ***cic.,*** cinnb., cocc., cypr., ***graph., kali-bi.,*** kali-m., lith., ***lyc.,*** mag-p., med., merc-p-r., nat-s., ***nit-ac.,*** petr., phyt., plan., ***plat.,*** rhus-t., sabad., sep., sil., ***staph.,*** stront-c., sul-i., ***sulph.,*** tell., **THUJ.**

ringworm, face - anag., ***bac.,*** bar-c., calc., cinnb., clem., dulc., ***graph.,*** hell., kali-chl., lith., lyc., ***nat-c., nat-m.,*** phos., **SEP.,** sulph., tarent., ***tell., thuj.,*** **TUB.**

ringworm, head - **CALC., DULC.,** ***phyt., sep.,*** tell., thuj., tub.

RISING, up agg. - **ACON.,** alum., ***am-m.,*** anac., ***ant-t.,*** arg-m., ***arn., ars.,*** asar., bar-c., bar-m., **BELL.,** bov., **BRY.,** cact., calad., ***cann-i., cann-s.,*** caps., carb-an., caust., ***cham., chel.,*** chin., ***cic.,*** **COCC.,** colch., coloc., ***con.,*** croc., **DIG.,** dros., ***ferr.,*** hell., hep., ***ign.,*** kali-c., lach., laur., **LYC.,** mag-m., mang., meny., merc., ***mur-ac., nat-c., nat-m., nit-ac.,*** **NUX-V., OP.,** ***osm.,*** ph-ac., ***phos.,*** plat., plb., ***puls.,*** ran-b., **RHUS-T.,** rumx., sabad., ***sang.,*** sars., seneg., sep., **SIL.,** spong., ***squil.,*** stann., staph., stram., sul-ac., **SULPH.,** tarax., verat., verat-v., ***viol-t.,*** zinc.

RISING, up
amel. - acon., alum., **AM-C.**, am-m., ***ant-t.,*** **ARS.**, asaf., aur., bar-c., bell., ***bor.,*** bov., bry., **CALC.**, cann-s., canth., carb-v., caust., ***cham.,*** chel., chin., cic., coloc., con., ***cupr., dig.,*** ferr., hell., hep., ***hyos., ign., kali-c.,*** laur., ***lyc.,*** mag-c., mang., merc., mosch., naja, nat-c., nat-m., nux-m., nux-v., olnd., petr., phos., puls., rhus-t., sabin., **SAMB., SEP.,** ***sil.,*** spig., squil., stann., sul-ac., sulph., teucr.
bed, from, amel. - ph-ac., puls.

ROCKING, agg. mentally - ars., bor., carb-v., ***cocc.,*** thuj.
amel. - acon., calc., carb-an., **CHAM.,** ***cina,*** helia., kali-c., ***merc-c.,*** plb., puls., pyrog., rhus-t., sac-alb., sec.
to and fro - bell., hyos.
desire for being rocked - acon., carb-an., **CHAM.,** cina, kali-c., pyrog., rhus-t.
physically amel. - acon., ***cham., cina,*** puls., rhus-t.

ROLLING, filth, in his own - camph.
floor, on the - acet-ac., ars., ***calc.,*** cic., **OP.,** paeon., prot., ***sulph.,*** tarent.
side to side - am-c., ars., lach., tarent.
turning over, or, as if - am-c., ars., **BELL.,** cact., crot-h., cupr., gels., ***graph.,*** kali-c., **LACH.,** lyc., lycpr., rhus-t., sabad., **SEP.,** tarent.

RUBBING, general
agg. - ***am-m.,*** **ANAC.,** arn., ars., aur., ***bism.,*** bor., ***calad.,*** calc., cann-s., canth., ***caps.,*** carb-an., ***caust.,*** cham., chel., ***coff.,*** **CON.,** cupr., dros., guai., kreos., ***led.,*** mag-c., mang., merc., ***mez.,*** mur-ac., nat-c., par., ph-ac., **PULS.,** seneg., **SEP.,** ***sil.,*** spig., spong., squil., stann., staph., stram., **STRONT-C., SULPH.**
clothes, of - olnd.
gently, stroking - teucr.
but hard amel. - rhus-t.
amel. - acon., agar., agn., ***alum.,*** ambr., am-c., ***am-m.,*** anac., ant-c., ant-t., ***arn., ars., asaf.,*** bell., bor., bov., bry., **CALC.,** camph., cann-s., **CANTH.,** caps., **CARB-AC.,** carb-an., caust., cedr., chel., chin., cic., cina, colch., ***cycl.,*** dios., ***dros., guai.,*** ham., hep., ***ign.,*** kali-c., kali-n., kreos., laur., lil-t., mag-c., mag-m., mang., meny., ***merc.,*** mosch., ***mur-ac.,*** **NAT-C.,** nit-ac., ***nux-v., ol-an.,*** olnd., osm., pall., ph-ac., **PHOS.,** plat., **PLB.,** ran-b., rhus-t., ***ruta.,*** sabad., sabin., samb., sars., sec., sel., seneg., spig., spong., stann., staph., ***sulph.,*** sul-ac., tarax., ***thuj.,*** valer., viol-t., ***zinc.***
hand, with - arn., ***asaf.,*** **CALC.,** ***caps., cina, croc.,*** **CYCL.,** ***dros.,*** guai., ign., mang., meny., ***merc., mur-ac.,*** **NAT-C.,** ***phos., plb., puls., ruta,*** sulph., ***thuj.,*** zinc.
warm - lil-t.
hard - med., rad-br.
soles - chel.

RUNNING, agg. - alum., alumn., ***ang.,*** arg-m., ***arn.,*** **ARS.,** ars-i., ars-s-f., aur., aur-a., aur-i., aur-s., ***bell.,*** bor., **BRY.,** calc., ***cann-s., caust.,*** chel., chin., cina, ***cocc.,*** coff., ***con.,*** croc., ***cupr.,*** dros., ***ferr.,*** ferr-ar., hep., hyos., ***ign.,*** iod., ip., ***kali-c.,*** laur., ***led., lyc., merc.,*** mez., nat-c., ***nat-m.,*** nit-ac., nux-m., ***nux-v., olnd.,*** phos., plb., **PULS.,** rheum, ***rhod., rhus-t.,*** ruta, sabin., ***seneg.,*** sep., ***sil., spig.,*** spong., squil., staph., **SULPH.,** sul-ac., verat., zinc.
amel. - ars., brom., caust., fl-ac., graph., ***ign.,*** nat-m., nit-ac., **SEP.,** sil., stann., sul-ac., tarent., thlaspi.
better than walking - tarent.
headache, causes - ***bry., ign.,*** nat-c., ***nat-m., nux-v.,*** **PULS.,** tarent.

SCARLET, fever (see Fevers)

SCHISTOSOMIASIS, bilharziasis - ant-t.

SCURVY, scorbutus - acet-ac., ***agav-a.,*** agn., all-s., aln., alum., alumn., ***am-c.,*** am-m., ambr., ant-c., arg-m., aran., ***ars.,*** ars-i., arum-m., aur., bell., bor., bov., brass., bry., ***calc.,*** canth., caps., ***carb-an.,*** **CARB-V.,** cary., caust., cetr., chin., chin-s., cic., ***cist.,*** cit-ac., cit-l., cit-v., coca, coch., con., ***dulc.,*** elat., ***ferr-p.,*** gali., graph., ***ham., hep., iod.,*** jug-r., ***kali-c.,*** kali-chl., ***kali-m.,*** kali-n., kali-p., kreos., lach., lyc., mag-m., **MERC., MUR-AC.,** nat-hchls., ***nat-m., nit-ac.,*** nit-m-ac., nux-m., **NUX-V.,** petr., ph-ac., phos., plb., psor., rat., rhus-t., ruta, sabin., sac-alb., sanic., sep., ***sil.,*** sin-n., sol-t-ae., stann., **STAPH.,** sul-ac., ***sulph.,*** tep., zinc.
scorbutic, gums - all-s., alum., ***alumn., am-c., anan., ant-c.,*** ant-t., **ARS.,** ***ars-i.,*** **ASTAC.,** ***aur-m-n., bov., brom., calc., camph.,*** canth., ***carb-an., carb-s.,*** **CARB-V.,** chin-s., chr-ac., ***cist.,*** coch., ***dulc., hep., iod., kali-c.,*** **KALI-CHL.,** ***kali-i., kali-n.,*** **KALI-P., KREOS.,** lac-ac., lach., ***lyc.,*** **MERC., MUR-AC.,** ***nat-m., nit-ac., nux-m., nux-v., ph-ac., phos.,*** phyt., ***psor.,*** sac-alb., sep., ***staph., sulph.,*** sul-ac., ***ter., zinc.***
salt eaters, in - coch.

SEASHORE, general, (see Environment)

SEASICKNESS, (see Emergency)

SEASONS, (see Environment)

SEDENTARY habits - acon., aloe, alum., am-c., anac., arg-n., ars., asar., ***bry., calc.,*** cocc., con., ***lyc.,*** nat-m., **NUX-V.,** petr., ran-b., rhus-t., sep., ***sil.,*** staph., **SULPH.,** ter.

SENSES, (see Brain)

SENSATIONS, general
adhesion of inner parts - arn., bry., coloc., ***dig.,*** euph., hep., kal-n., merc., ***mez.,*** nux-v., par., petr., phos., ***plb.,*** puls., **RHUS-T.,** seneg., **SEP.,** ***sulph.,*** thuj., verb.
alive, of something, in muscles - berb.
ball, internally - acon., ***arg-n., arn.,*** asaf., ***bell.,*** brom., ***bry.,*** calc., ***cann-i.,*** caust., cham., chin., cob., coc-c., coloc., con., crot-t., cupr., gels., graph., **IGN.,** kali-ar., kali-c., kali-m.,

SENSATIONS, general

ball, internally - lac-c., **LACH.,** ***lil-t.,*** lyc., mag-m., merc-d., merc-i-r., mosch., nat-m., nat-s., nit-ac., nux-m., ***nux-v.,*** par., phos., phyt., plan., plat., ***plb., puls.,*** raph., rhus-t., ruta, ***sabad.,*** senec., **SEP.,** sil., spig., staph., stram., sulph., tab., teucr., ust., ***valer.,*** zinc.

cold, running trough bowels - bufo.

hard - nux-m.

hot - carb-ac., lyc., phyt., raph.

alternating with cold - lyc.

bed, feels too hard - acon., agar., **ARN.,** ***ars.,*** **BAPT.,** bar-c., bry., caust., con., dros., ***ferr., ferr-p.,*** graph., ip., kali-c., lyc., mag-c., mag-m., manc., merc., nux-m., nux-v., op., petr., phos., plat., puls., **PYROG.,** ***rhus-t., ruta.,*** sabad., **SIL.,** spong., stann., sulph., tarax., thuj., verat.

biting, as if - acon., aloe, euon., euph., lach., sel., thuj., voes.

bug like - kali-bi., led., syph., tell.

evening, agg. - am-m., carb-an.

fleas, as of - led., mez., staph., syph., tab., visc.

itching - **RHUS-T.**

lying, after - mur-ac.

lying, down - sil.

parts on which he is lying on, in bed, scratching amel. - chin.

spots, in - aloe, cham., cocc., coloc.

stinging - viol-t.

subcutaneous - lact.

board, sensation - bapt., carb-an., dulc., nux-m., rhus-t., tarent-c.

lying, as if, on - bapt., sanic.

boiling, as if - am-m., led., ust.

water, side lain on - mag-m.

breaking, as if parts were broken - ***ang., cham., chel.,*** **COCC.,** ***dros.,*** **IGN., PHOS., RUTA,** ***verat.***

as if body were frail and easily broken - ***thuj.***

bubbling, sensation of - ambr., ant-c., asaf., bell., ***berb.,*** caps., colch., coloc., ip., junc., laur., lyc., mang., nux-v., ***puls., rheum,*** squil., spig., sulph., tarax.

air, with suppuration - sulph.

bursting - sulph.

buzzing - ***caust., kreos.,*** **NUX-M.,** ***nux-v.,*** **OLND.,** op., **PULS.,** ***rhus-t., sep.,*** **SPIG., SULPH.**

caged, body, as if, in wires, twisted tighter and tighter - **CACT.**

clutching, sensation - ***bell.,*** cact., lil-t., thyr.

coat, of skin drawn over inner parts - ant-t., ars., bar-c., brom., bry., calc., caust., ***cina,*** cocc., ***dig.,*** dros., ***hep.,*** merc., nat-m., nux-m., ***ph-ac., phos., pip-m., puls., sulph.***

cobweb, sensation of a - alum., alumn., ***bar-c., bor.,*** brom., ***calc.,*** con., ***graph.,*** mag-c., ph-ac., plb., ***ran-s.,*** sul-ac., sumb.

cold air, as if, were blowing on him - canth., chel., graph., mosch., nux-v., olnd., puls., rhus-t., sabin., spig., squil., stram.

SENSATIONS, general

constriction, sensation

externally - abrot., ***acon., aesc.,*** aeth., ***agar., all-s.,*** alum., am-c., am-m., ***ammc., aml-n., anac.,*** ant-c., ***ant-t., apis,*** aral., arg-m., arg-n., arn., ***ars., ars-i., arum-t.,*** asaf., ***asar.,*** aur., ***bar-c.,*** bell., berb., ***bism.,*** bor., bov., ***bry., cact.,*** calc., ***calc-p.,*** cann-i., cann-s., canth., ***caps.,*** carb-ac., carb-an., ***carb-s.,*** carb-v., caust., cham., ***chel., chin.,*** **CIMIC.,** cina, **COCC.,** coff., colch., ***coloc.,*** con., ***cupr.,*** dig., dios., ***dros.,*** dulc., euphr., ***ferr.,*** gels., ***glon.,*** **GRAPH.,** guai., ***hell.,*** hep., hydr-ac., **HYOS.,** ***iod., ip.,*** kali-c., kali-n., kreos., ***lach.,*** laur., led., lil-t., ***lob., lyc.,*** mag-c., mag-m., ***mag-p.,*** mang., meny., **MERC.,** ***merc-c., merc-i-r., mez.,*** mosch., mur-ac., naja, nat-c., nat-m., **NIT-AC.,** nux-m., **NUX-V.,** olnd., ***op., ox-ac., par.,*** petr., ***phos., plat.,*** **PLB.,** ***puls.,*** ran-b., ran-s., rheum, rhod., **RHUS-T.,** ruta., sabad., sabin., sars., sec., sel., ***sep.,*** sil., spig., ***spong.,*** squil., **STANN.,** staph., **STRAM.,** ***stront-c., sul-ac., sulph., tab.,*** thuj., ***verat.,*** verb., viol-t., zinc.

sensation, as if caged with wires twisted tighter and tighter - **CACT.**

internally, sensation of a band - acon., ***alum.,*** alumn., ***ambr.,*** am-br., **ANAC.,** ant-c., ant-t., ***arg-n.,*** arn., ars., asaf., ***asar., aur., bell.,*** benz-ac., brom., bry., **CACT.,** calc., cann-i., **CARB-AC.,** ***carb-s.,*** carb-v., caust., **CHEL.,** ***chin., cocc.,*** coc-c., colch., coloc., **CON.,** croc., dig., gels., ***graph.,*** hell., hyos., iod., kreos., laur., lyc., mag-m., ***mag-p.,*** manc., ***merc., merc-i-r.,*** mosch., ***nat-m.,*** **NIT-AC.,** nux-m., nux-v., olnd., op., petr., ***phos.,*** **PLAT., PULS.,** sabad., sabin., sang., sars., **SIL.,** ***spig.,*** stann., **SULPH.,** sul-ac., tarent., til., zinc.

orifices, of - ***acon.,*** alum., ars., ars-i., bar-c., **BELL.,** ***brom.,*** **CACT.,** calc., carb-v., ***chel.,*** cic., cocc., colch., con., crot-h., dig., dulc., ferr., form., graph., hep., ***hyos.,*** ign., iod., ip., **LACH.,** ***lyc.,*** **MERC.,** ***merc-c.,*** mez., ***nat-m.,*** **NIT-AC.,** ***nux-v.,*** op., phos., plat., ***plb.,*** rat., rhod., **RHUS-T.,** sabad., sars., sep., **SIL.,** ***staph.,*** **STRAM.,** sulph., sumb., tarax., ***thuj., verat., verat-v.***

crawling - agar., anag., arund., astac., ***sec.,*** zinc.

drinking, after - ***ars.***

horripilations in affected parts - ***guare.***

mouse, like a - **BELL., CALC.,** nit-ac., rhod., ***sep.,*** **SULPH.**

skin and flesh, between - ***sec.***

sleep, as if gone to - ***ign.***

tingling, with a feeling as if asleep, or of heaviness - ter.

crepitation - **ACON., CALC.,** puls., **RHEUM,** ***spig.***

SENSATIONS, general

delicacy, feeling of - ***gels.,*** ign., nat-m., nux-v., sil., ***thuj.***

discomfort - ars., camph., ***card-m.,*** chel., hippoz., ***nux-m.,*** zinc.

awaking, on - ant-t.

dry, in internal parts - ***acon.,*** **ALUM.,** am-m., arg-m., arn., ars., ***asaf., asar.,*** bar-c., ***bell., bry., calad.,*** camph., cann-i., cann-s., canth., caps., carb-v., caust., chin., cic., cina, cinnb., cocc., con., croc., dros., euph., ferr., ign., kali-c.

dust, in internal parts, feeling of - ***am-c.,*** ars., ***bell.,*** **CALC.,** chel., cina, cocc., crot-c., dros., hep., ***ign.,*** ip., op., ***ph-ac.,*** plat., rheum, sulph., teucr., zinc.

emptiness, sensation - ail., alum., am-c., am-m., ant-c., ant-t., apoc., arg-m., arn., astra-m., aur., bar-c., bry., ***calad.,*** calc., caps., carb-an., carb-v., caust., cham., ***chin.,*** chin-s., cina, cob-n., **COCC.,** coff., coloc., croc., cupr., dig., dulc., euph., glon., graph., hell., hep., hydr., hydr-ac., **IGN.,** iod., ip., **KALI-C.,** kali-n., ***lach.,*** laur., **LYC., MERC.,** ***mur-ac.,*** nat-m., ***olnd., phos.,*** **PULS.,** rhus-t., **SARS., SEP., STANN.,** ***sulph.,*** tab., verat., vib., vinc., xanth., ***zing.***

as if whole body where hollow - aur., ***cocc., kali-c.***

grief, after - cocc., ***ign.***

internal - aur.

faintness, of - **SEP.**

ether, feeling as after inhaling - ***glon.***

falling out, sensation as if - ***bell.,*** cocc., laur., ***lil-t.,*** nux-v., podo., sep.

feels, as if she could feel every muscle and fibre of her right side - sep.

festering, as if - bufo.

flabby, feeling - ***acon.,*** agar., ambr., am-m., ant-t., arg-m., arn., **ARS.,** asar., ***bar-c.,*** bell., bov., bry., **CALC.,** ***calc-p.,*** calc-s., canth., **CAPS.,** carb-an., carb-v., **CAUST.,** ***cham., chel.,*** chin., cic., cina, clem., coff., **CROC.,** ***cycl., dig.,*** euph., euphr., ***ferr., fl-ac.,*** graph., hep., **IGN.,** iod., ***ip., kali-ar., kali-c.,*** kali-n., kali-p., kali-s., laur., **LYC.,** mag-c., mag-m., meny., merc., ***mosch.,*** mur-ac., **NAT-C.,** nit-ac., nux-m., ***nux-v.,*** olnd., par., petr., **PHOS.,** ***plat., psor.,*** puls., rhod., rhus-t., ***sabad.,*** sabin., seneg., ***sep.,*** sil., spong., ***staph.,*** stront-c., **SULPH.,** ***tarax.,*** teucr., thuj., **VERAT.,** ***zinc.***

hard parts, in - caust., ***merc.,*** mez., ***nit-ac.,*** nux-m.

internally - ***calc.,*** kreos., **SEP.**

formication, sensation

affected, part - coloc.

angina, during - dig.

anxiety, with - cist.

bad news, after - calc-p.

body, all over - ail., aran., cist., dig., mag-m., med., zinc-p.

cold - ***agar.,*** frax., lac-c.

body, around - helo.

menses, before - ant-t.

SENSATIONS, general

formication, sensation

dyspnea, with - cist.

emissions, after seminal - mez.

external parts - abrot., **ACON.,** acon-c., acon-f., aconin., aesc., aether, **AGAR.,** agn., alco., all-s., aloe, ***alum.,*** alum-p., alum-sil., ***alumn.,*** ambr., am-c., am-m., anac., ang., ant-c., ant-t., ap-g., apis, ***aran.,*** arg-m., **ARG-N., ARN.,** ars., ars-i., ars-s-f., arum-t., arund., asaf., asar., aur., aur-a., aur-s., ***bar-c.,*** bar-i., bar-m., bar-s., bell., bor., bov., brucin., bry., bufo, cadm-s., calad., calc., calc-p., calen., camph., cann-i., cann-s., canth., caps., carb-an., carb-s., carb-v., card-b., ***carl., cast., caust.,*** cedr., cham., ***chel.,*** chin., cic., cina, cist., clem., ***cocaine, cocc.,*** cod., **COLCH.,** coloc., con., coni., ***croc.,*** cupr-s., cur., dros., dulc., euon., euphr., fago., ferr., ferr-ma., fl-ac., ***gran.,*** graph., guai., guare., ham., hep., hist., hydr-ac., hyos., ***hyper.,*** ign., iod., ip., kali-ar., ***kali-br., kali-c.,*** kali-m., kali-n., ***kalm.,*** kreos., lach., lath., laur., led., ***lyc., mag-arct.,*** mag-aust., mag-c., ***mag-m.,*** mang., ***med.,*** medus., ***merc.,*** merc-c., merc-i-r., ***mez., morph.,*** mosch., mur-ac., nat-a., ***nat-c., nat-m.,*** nat-p., nat-sil., nit-ac., nit-s-d., nux-m., **NUX-V.,** oena., ol-an., ol-j., olnd., onos., op., osm., pall., par., petr., ***ph-ac., phos.,*** phys., ***pic-ac.,*** **PLAT.,** plb., ***puls., ran-b.,*** ran-s., rheum, ***rhod.,*** **RHUS-T.,** rumx., ***sabad.,*** sabin., samb., sars., **SEC.,** sel., seneg., **SEP.,** sil., **SPIG.,** spong., ***squil.,*** stann., staph., stram., stront-c., sul-i., ***sulph.,*** sul-ac., tab., tarax., ***tarent.,*** tell., teucr., thuj., tub., urt-u., valer., vario., verat., verb., viol-t., ***visc., zinc.,*** zinc-m., zinc-p.

painful sensation of crawling through whole body if he knocks against any part - spig.

here and there - op.

internally - ***acon.,*** acon-f., agar., agn., aloe, alum., alum-sil., ambr., am-c., am-m., ant-t., apis, arg-m., ***arn.,*** ars., asaf., bar-c., bell., bor., bov., brom., ***bry.,*** cadm-s., calc., ***canth.,*** caps., carb-an., carb-v., caust., chel., ***chin.,*** cic., cina, cocc., **COLCH.,** coloc., con., cupr., dig., dros., dulc., euphr., ferr., graph., guai., hep., hyos., ign., iod., kali-ar., kali-c., kali-n., kres., ***lach.,*** laur., led., mag-c., mag-m., med., meny., merc., mez., mur-ac., nat-a., nat-c., ***nat-m.,*** nat-p., nat-sil., nux-m., nux-v., olnd., ph-ac., phos., **PLAT.,** plb., prun., ***puls.,*** rheum, rhod., **RHUS-T.,** ***sabad.,*** sabin., **SANG.,** ***sec.,*** sel., seneg., sep., sil., spig., spong., stann., staph., sul-i., **SULPH.,** tarax., teucr., thuj., ***verat.,*** viol-o., ***zinc.,*** zinc-p.

pain, after - sec.

with pain - hyper.

paralyzed part - cadm-s., phos., ***zinc.***

SENSATIONS, general

formication, sensation

suffering parts, of - agar., coloc., con., zinc.

frail, as if body were - gels., sars., sil., ***thuj.***

full, feeling

blood vessels, of - ham., sang.

externally - ***aesc.,*** ars., aur., aur-m., caust., kali-n., laur., nux-m., par., phos., verat.

internally - **ACON., AESC.,** agar., alum., am-c., am-m., aml-n., anac., ant-c., ***ant-t., apis, arn.,*** ars., ***asaf., asar.,*** aur., ***bar-c.,*** bar-m., ***bell.,*** bor., bov., ***bry.,*** cact., calc., calc-i., camph., cann-i., cann-s., ***canth., caps., carb-an., carb-s., carb-v.,*** caust., ***cham.,*** chel., **CHIN.,** cic., **CIMIC.,** cocc., coff., ***colch.,*** coloc., com., ***con.,*** croc., ***crot-t., cycl., dig., ferr.,*** **GLON.,** ***graph.,*** guai., ***ham., hell.,*** hyos., ign., iod., ***iris, kali-c., kali-n.,*** kreos., lach., laur., led., ***lyc.,*** mag-c., mag-m., mang., **MELI.,** meny., merc., mez., **MOSCH.,** mur-ac., ***nat-a.,*** nat-c., nat-m., ***nit-ac., nux-m., nux-v.,*** olnd., op., par., petr., ph-ac., **PHOS.,** ***phyt.,*** plat., plb., ***psor., puls., ran-s.,*** rheum, rhod., **RHUS-T.,** ruta., sabad., ***sabin.,*** sars., ***sep.,*** sil., spig., spong., stann., staph., stict., stront-c., **SULPH.,** sul-ac., thuj., ***valer.,*** verat., verat-v., verb., zinc.

piano, after playing - anac.

furry, inwardly - caust., cocc., dros., merc-c., nux-m., ***phos., puls.***

growing, inner parts as if grown together - bry., euph., hep., ***mez.,*** nux-v., phos., ***plb.,*** puls., **RHUS-T.,** ***sep.,*** thuj.

heaviness, sensation

externally - acon., **AESC.,** agar., agn., aloe, ***alum.,*** ambr., am-c., anac., ant-c., ant-t., arn., ***ars., ars-i.,*** asaf., asar., aur., ***bar-c.,*** bar-m., **BELL.,** bor., bov., **BRY.,** cact., calc., camph., cann-i., cann-s., canth., caps., carb-ac., ***carb-s., carb-v.,*** caust., cham., chel., ***chin.,*** cic., clem., cocc., coff., colch., coloc., **CON.,** croc., crot-h., crot-t., cupr., cur., dig., dulc., euph., euphr., ***ferr.,*** **GELS.,** graph., hell., hep., ign., iod., ***ip.,*** kali-c., kali-n., kali-s., ***kreos.,*** laur., ***led.,*** lyc., mag-c., mag-m., ***meli.,*** meny., ***merc., mez.,*** mosch., mur-ac., ***nat-c., nat-m.,*** nit-ac., nux-m., **NUX-V.,** ***onos.,*** op., par., ***petr.,*** ph-ac., **PHOS.,** pic-ac., plat., plb., ***psor.,*** **PULS.,** ran-b., rheum, ***rhod.,*** **RHUS-T.,** ***ruta., sabad.,*** sabin., samb., sars., sec., **SEP.,** ***sil.,*** **SPIG.,** ***spong.,*** squil., **STANN.,** ***staph.,*** stram., stront-c., **SULPH.,** sul-ac., ***thuj.,*** valer., ***verat.,*** verb., viol-o., ***zinc.***

internally - **ACON.,** ***agar.,*** agn., **ALOE,** alum., ambr., ***am-c., am-m.,*** anac., ant-t., arg-n., arn., ars., asaf., asar., aur., ***bar-c.,*** bar-m., ***bell.,*** **BISM.,** ***bor., bov., bry.,*** calad., **CALC.,** camph., ***cann-i.,*** cann-s., canth., carb-ac., ***carb-an.,*** carb-s., ***carb-v.,*** caust., cham., **CHEL.,** ***chin.,*** cic., clem., ***cocc.,*** coff., colch., ***coloc., con., croc., cupr., dig.,*** dros., ***dulc.,*** euphr., ferr., **GELS.,** ***graph., hell.,*** hep., hyos., ign., iod., ***iris, kali-c.,*** kali-n., kreos., ***lach., laur., lob., lyc., mag-c., mag-m.,*** mang., ***meny., merc.,*** mez., mosch., ***mur-ac.,*** nat-c., **NAT-M.,** nit-ac., ***nux-m.,*** **NUX-V.,** ***olnd., onos., op.,*** par., **PETR.,** ph-ac., **PHOS.,** plat., ***plb., prun.,*** **PULS.,** ran-b., ran-s., rheum, rhod., **RHUS-T.,** ruta., ***sabad., sabin.,*** samb., ***sang.,*** sars., sec., sel., ***senec., seneg.,*** **SEP., SIL.,** ***spig.,*** spong., squil., **STANN.,** ***staph.,*** stram., stront-c., **SULPH.,** sul-ac., tarax., thuj., valer., verat., verb., viol-o., viol-t., zinc.

morning - kali-c., lyc., nat-c., zinc.

night - mag-c.

menses, during - kali-c.

sleep, after - rheum.

storm, before and during - sil.

walking in open air - nit-ac.

heat, sensation in body - acon., ***aeth.,*** ant-t., ***ars., bar-m., bor-ac.,*** cadm-met., calc., calc-p., ***camph.,*** camph-br., ***carb-v., chlol.,*** cupr., ***helo., jatr.,*** lachn., ***sec.,*** tab., ***verat.,*** zinc.

blood vessels, in - abies-c., **ACON.,** ant-c., ant-t., **ARS.,** bell., lyc., op., plb., pyrog., **RHUS-T.,** sulph., sul-ac., ***verat.***

bones, in - ***aran., ars., berb., calc.,*** calc-p., elaps, eup-per., kali-i., lyc., merc., per., pyrog., sep., sulph., ***verat.,*** zinc.

inner parts, in - anh., ars., ***calc., hura, laur.,*** lyc., meny., nux-v., par., sep., sulph.

single parts, in - agar., aran., buth-a., elaps, helo.

taking cold, agg. - acon., ***bac.,*** bell., bry., calc., ***camph.,*** carb-an., cham., cist., coloc., dulc., kali-n., merc., phos., sil., ***tub.***

hot, iron, wires, needles, etc. as if - agar., alumn., apis, ***ars.,*** bar-c., lith., mag-c., naja, nit-ac., olnd., rhus-t., spig., vesp.

knotted, internally - ambr., ant-t., arn., ***ars.,*** asaf., bell., bry., carb-an., carb-v., cham., cic., cina, con., cupr., gels., graph., hydr., hydr-ac., ign., kali-p., kreos., **LACH.,** lob., mag-m., mag-p., ***merc-i-r.,*** nux-v., petr., ***phyt.,*** puls., ***rhus-t., sabad.,*** sec., sep., **SPIG.,** staph., stict., **SULPH.,** ust., valer., zinc.

largeness, body, of, or part of it - bell.

affection of vasomotor nerves - ***kali-br.***

single parts feel larger and thicker - cann-i.

lifted up, as if - hyper., phos., stroph.

sleep, during - stroph.

lightness - ***ars.,*** asar., ***coff.,*** hyos., ***mez., op.***

air, as though she could float or hover in, after typhoid fever - ***manc.***

airy - stict., ***stram.***

lifted, as if - acon.

onanism from, or hysterical behaviour - gels.

SENSATIONS, general

lightness,

raised from ground, as if - ***asaf.,*** cann-i., hep., lyc., ***merc.,*** nux-v., ***phos., plat.,*** ran-b., ***spig.,*** sul-ac., valer., ***verat.***

swimming, as if, or flying in air - calc-ar.

walking, when - thuj.

loose, as if - ***am-c.,*** bar-c., bov., carb-an., caust., chin., croc., hyos., ***kali-c.,*** kali-m., laur., med., nat-s., **NUX-M.,** nux-v., psor., **RHUS-T.,** sec., sul-ac., thuj.

open, and - sec.

motion, body, through whole, now a prickling, now a stinging - ang.

feeling of inability to move even a finger - iber.

nervous - agar.

up and down - lach., plb., ***spong.***

peculiar - cann-i., ***brom.,*** iodof., spong.

plug, sensation of - agar., ***anac.,*** ang., arn., bufo, coloc., ***crot-t.,*** hell., hyper., ***kali-bi.,*** lach., plat., ruta

externally - agar., arg-n., arn., bufo, ***crot-t.,*** hell., ***kali-bi.,*** lach., mosch., plat., ruta.

internally - acon., ***agar.,*** **ALOE,** ambr., am-br., am-c., ***anac., ant-c.,*** arg-m., ***arn., asaf.,*** aur., bar-c., bell., bov., calc., caust., cham., chel., cocc., coc-c., coff., con., croc., dros., ferr., graph., hell., ***hep.,*** **IGN.,** iod., kali-c., kreos., lach., led., lyc., merc., mez., mur-ac., nat-m., ***nux-v.,*** olnd., par., plat., plb., ran-s., rhod., ***ruta.,*** sabad., sabin., sang., sep., spig., ***spong.,*** staph., ***sulph.,*** **THUJ.**

rivet - lil-t., sulph.

prickling, sensation, externally - acon., agar., ***ail.,*** alum., ant-c., ant-t., bell., calc., cann-i., cann-s., caps., carb-s., caust., cimic., coloc., con., croc., ***crot-c., dros.,*** glon., hep., kali-br., laur., ***lob.,*** lyc., med., ***mez.,*** mosch., ***nux-m.,*** onos., **PLAT., RAN-S.,** ruta., sabad., ***sec.,*** sep., staph., sulph., sul-ac., zinc.

internally - abrot., acon., ***ail.,*** aur., cann-s., dios., lach., **NIT-AC.,** ***osm.,*** ph-ac., ***phos.,*** plat., ***ran-b., sabad., sang.,*** sec., seneg., ***verb.,*** viol- o.

pulsation, (see Pulsation, general)

roughness, inner parts - ***alum., calc.,*** **CARB-V.,** ***caust., cocc., dig., dros., laur., mag-c.,*** nux-m., **NUX-V.,** ***par.,*** **PHOS.,** ***ph-ac., puls., rhus-t., sars., seneg., stann., stro***nt., **SULPH.,** ***sul-ac., zinc.***

shocks, electric-like, in body - ***acon., agar.,*** ail., alum., ***ambr.,*** anac., ang., apis, **ARG-M.,** ***arg-n.,*** arn., **ARS.,** ***art-v.,*** bar-c., ***bar-m.,*** bell., bufo, calad., calc., ***calc-p., camph.,*** cann-s., carb-ac., carb-v., caust., ***cic.,*** cimic., ***cina, clem., cocc.,*** colch., con., croc., cupr., ***dig.,*** dulc., ***fl-ac.,*** graph., hell., hep., kali-c., kreos., ***laur., lyc.,*** mag-m., manc., mang., mez., mur-ac., nat-a., nat-c., ***nat-m.,*** nat-p., ***nit-ac., nux-m., nux-v.,*** ol-an., olnd., ***phos.,*** plat., puls., ***ran-b., ruta.,*** sep., spig., squil., stram., ***stry.,*** sulph., sul-ac., sumb., ***tab.,***

SENSATIONS, general

shocks, electric-like, in body - ***thal.,*** **VERAT.,** xan., zinc.

agg. - acet-ac., ***acon.,*** am-c., arn., camph., cham., cic., coff., gels., hep., hyos., hyper., mag-c., merc., nat-m., op., ph-ac., phos., puls., sec., stram., stront-c., sulph., verat.

concussion of brain, from - **CIC.**

convulsions, before - ***bar-m., laur.***

interrupted by painful shocks - stry.

epilepsy, before - ars.

evening in bed - sulph.

explosion like, flying into pieces - aeth., ars., ***bell.,*** bry., carb-an., ***coff.,*** dig., glon., ***mur-ac., nit-ac., nux-v.,*** **PULS., RHUS-T.,** sil., ***stann.,*** staph., sulph., verat.

lancinating - mag-arct.

lying, while - ***clem.***

morning - mang.

motion or rest, during - graph.

move, on beginning to - ***arg-n.***

nervous - acon., ambr., ***arn.,*** camph., carb-v., coff., gels., hyos., hyper., ***ign.,*** iod., op., verat.

pain, from - arg-n., cina, lyc., plat., podo., sul-ac.

painful - zinc-chr.

return of the senses, on - cic.

right side of body - agar.

sleep, during - **ARG-M.,** ***ars.,*** kreos., lyc., mez., ***nat-m., nux-m.***

on going to - agar., alum., **ARG-M., ARS.,** ***bell.,*** calc., ***ip.,*** kali-c., nat-a., ***nat-m., nit-ac., phos., stry.,*** thuj.

slow pulse, with - ***dig.***

touching anything - alum.

violent - plat., stront-c.

pain, as from - plat.

waking, while - lyc., ***mag-m.,*** manc.

wide awake, while - mag-m., nat-p.

sick feeling - abrot., **ACON.,** ***alum.,*** ant-c., ***ant-t., ars.,*** bapt., brom., ***bry.,*** carc., ***chel., chin-s.,*** cimic., ***con.,*** **GELS.,** ip., ***lac-d.,*** lach., lob., ***mez.,*** myris., ***nux-m.,*** **NUX-V.,** nit-ac., petr., ***podo.,*** psor., ptel., puls., sabad., sang., ***spong.,*** stront-c., stroph., ***sulph.,*** sumb., ***tab.,*** tarax., thuj., verat., zinc.

awaking, on - ***lach.***

chilled, after being - ***ip.***

day and night - zing.

does not know why - brom.

head, caused by burning in - ***lach.***

hysteria, in - ***mosch.***

menses, during - zing.

pain, from - stront-c.

queer, before menses - brom.

suddenly - carc., con., tab.

tired feeling, with pains over left eye - ind.

walk, during a, feels as if she must lie down and die - ***kali-c.***

sinking, sensation all over, fancied she would sink through bed - ***dulc.***

SENSATIONS, general

smaller, body - acon., agar., ***calc.,*** cact., croc., euphr., ***glon.,*** graph., kreos., naja, nux-m., nux-v., sabad., sulph., tarent., zinc.

smoke, hot, coming through all orifices, as if - fl-ac.

soft, hard parts feel - caust., ***merc.,*** mez., nit-ac., ***nux-m.***

sparks, of - agar., arg-m., calc., ***calc-p.,*** lyc., nat-m., **SEC.,** sel.

splinters, of - ***aesc.,*** **AGAR.,** ***alum.,*** **ARG-N.,** ***bar-c., carb-v.,*** cic., colch., coll., ***dol., fl-ac.,*** **HEP., NIT-AC.,** petr., plat., ran-b., ***sil.,*** sulph.

squeezing - ***ter.***

spots, sensations occur in - agar., ***alum.,*** arg-m., ars., ***berb.,*** bufo, ***calc-p.,*** caust., ***cist.,*** colch., ***con.,*** fl-ac., glon., hep., ign., **KALI-BI., LAC-C.,** lil-t., ***nat-m.,*** nux-m., ol-an., ol-j., ***ox-ac., phos.,*** rhus-t., sars., sel., ***sep.,*** sil., **SULPH.,** thuj., zinc.
- cold - agar., calc-p., petr., sep., tarent., ***verat.***

stinging - **APIS,** ***gels., kali-c.,*** **LED.**
- bee-sting, like - **APIS**
- different parts at same time - ***canth.***
- inner parts - ***sep.***

strangling, sensation - sulph., valer.
- sleep, falling to, on - valer.

streaming, sensation - ***ox-ac.***

strength, of - ***agar.,*** alco., anh., ars., bell., bov., bry., ***bufo,*** calc-f., carb-o., chin-s., clem., cob., ***coca, coff.,*** corn., cot., elae., erech., ferr., ***fl-ac.,*** gast., gels., gins., helon., kola., lach., lil-t., meny., ***nat-p.,*** nep., ol-j., **OP.,** ped., phos., pic-ac., pip-m., plat., psor., sars., stram., vanad., wies., zinc.
- anger, after - carb-s.
- changing, suddenly - tarent.
- sex, after - merc-c.
- decreased - ars-i., carb-an., carb-v., cocc., ferr-p., laur., mag-m., op., ph-ac., phos., sulph., tub., verat., vinc.
- increased during convulsions - agar.
- muscular - agar., alco., anh., ars., camph., coca, cod., ***fl-ac.,*** gels., keroso., kola., ***nat-p.,*** nitro-o., phos., tab., thea., zinc.
- perspiration, during - op., piloc., stach.
- walking, while - bapt., chin.

swimming - ars-h.

swollen, sensation - ***acon.,*** agar., aloe, alum., ambr., am-m., anac., ant-c., ant-t., apis, ***aran.,*** arg-m., ***arg-n.,*** arn., ars., asaf., asar., aur., bapt., bar-c., ***bell., bism.,*** bov., bry., caj., calad., calc., ***calc-p.,*** cann-i., canth., ***caps.,*** carb-ac., carb-s., carb-v., caust., ***cedr.,*** cham., chin., cimic., cina, ***cocc., coc-c.,*** colch., ***coloc., com.,*** con., ***cor-r.,*** crot-h., crot-t., ***cupr.,*** cycl., dig., dulc., euph., ***euphr., glon.,*** **GUAI.,** hell., hep., hyos., ign., ip., kali-c., kali-n., kreos., **LACH.,** ***laur.,*** led., lyc., mag-c., mang., **MERC., MERC-I-F.,** mez., mosch., nit-ac., nux-m., nux-v., olnd., ***op.,*** **PAEON., PAR.,** petr., ph-ac., phos., plat., plb., **PULS.,** ran-b., ran-s., rhod., **RHUS-T.,** sabad., sabin., samb., ***sang.,*** sars., ***seneg.,*** sep., sil., **SPIG.,** spong., stann., staph., stram., ***sulph.,*** sul-ac., tarax., thuj., valer., verat., zinc.

strumming, in intermittent fever - ***ign.***

threads, of - bry., coc-c., ign., lach., ***osm.,*** par., ***plat.,*** **VALER.**

throbbing - **ACON.,** ***agar.,*** **ALUM.,** ***am-m.,*** **ANT-T.,** ***arg-m., arg-n.,*** ars-m., ***asaf.,*** **BELL.,** berb., ***bor., bry.,*** **CALC.,** ***cann-i., caps., caust., cham.,*** **COCC., GLON., HEP.,** ***ign., iod.,*** **KALI-C.,** ***kreos., laur.,*** **LED.,** ***lyc., meli., merc., nat-c., nat-m., nit-ac.,*** **OLND., PHOS.,** ***plat., plb.,*** **PULS.,** ***rhod., rhus-t., ruta,*** **SABAD., SEP., SIL.,** ***spig., spong.,*** **SULPH.,** ***tarax., thuj.,*** zinc.

tingling, (see formication) - **ACON.,** agar., cub., dios., glon., **PHOS.,** zinc.
- as if circulation had stopped, with anxiety - bar-c.
- frostbitten, as if, when weather changes - agar., colch., zinc.
- quivering sensation, with - med.

trickling, like drops - acon., agar., ambr., arg-n., arn., ars-h., bell., berb., **CANN-S.,** caust., chin-s., cot., croc., glon., graph., kali-bi., lyc., mag-m., nat-m., nux-m., petros., phos., rhus-t., sep., spig., stann., tarent., thuj., vario., verat., x-ray.
- hot drops - stann., sulph.

uneasiness - aml-n., ***apis, bry.,*** camph., ***cham., cina,*** chin., cinnb., cop., cub., ***cupr-m., dulc., hep.,*** jal., lact., lyss., mag-c., nat-c., ***petr., plat., plb.,*** ptel., ***sep., spig., stram.***
- abdomen, tearing in - **CHAM.**
- afternoon, late - merc-sul.
- chill, followed by - ***cop.***
  - internal, with - ***calc.***
- dinner, after - agar.
- dreams, from - ***calc.***
- evening, in, in bed - ***phos.***
- head, from pain in - lyss.
  - hot, at night - canth.
- headache, chronic - ***dulc., iod.***
- heart, about, while sitting, must rise and walk - ***caust.***
- heat, from - ***calc.***
  - heat, with - valer.
- influenza - ars., chel., gels.
- nervous vibrations, caused by very fine - meph.
- night, at - ***caust., cycl.,*** **PULS.**
- pain, with, from head to fingers - ***camph.***
- palpitation, especially at night - spong.
- rigors, with, before menses - ***lyc.***
- sitting long, prevents - ***ant-c.***
- sleep, arousing child from, evening - am-c.
  - prevents - caust.
- strangers, in presence of - sep.

vapors, smoke, fumes, etc., of - apis, **ARS.,** bar-c., brom., ***chin.,*** ign., lyc., ***puls., verat.***

vibration, after lying down - ***clem.***
- nervous, causing uneasiness - meph.

SENSATIONS, general
water, sensation
cold water, sensation as if, were running from clavicle down to toes along a narrow line - caust.
dashing against inner parts, sensation of - ars., bell., carb-ac., carb-an., ***chin.,*** cina, ***crot-h.,*** **CROT-T.,** dig., ferr., glon., hell., ***hep., hyos.,*** jatr., kali-c., kali-m., laur., nat-m., ph-ac., ***rhod., rhus-t., spig.***
hot water - chin., hep., sumb.
hot, as if, in - phos.
breast to abdomen - sang.
flowing through part, as if - sumb.
pain, during - ter.
poured on part, as if - verat-v.
trickling, dropping or flowing, sensation of - arg-n., bufo, ***cann-i., cann-s.,*** caust., glon., graph., kali-bi., lappa-a., nat-m., petros., phos., rhus-t., sep., stann., sumb., tarent., ***thuj.,*** vario., verat.
affected part, on - arg-n.
hot - hep., sep., stann., sulph., sumb.
wavelike, sensations - acon., am-c., aml-n., anac., ant-t., arn., asaf., **BELL.,** ***bism.,*** caps., caust., chin., clem., cocc., coff., con., dig., dulc., ferr-p., fl-ac., glon., graph., hyos., iod., kali-c., kali-n., lach., lyc., mag-c., mez., ***nit-ac.,*** nux-v., olnd., par., petr., plat., rhod., sars., senec., ***sep.,*** sil., spig., stann., stict., stront-c., stroph., **SULPH.,** teucr., verb., viol-t., zinc-i.
wind, sensation of, on body - agar., ***camph.,*** canth., ***chel.,*** chin., ***cist.,*** cor-r., croc., graph., lach., **LYSS.,** med., ***mez., mosch.,*** naja, nat-m., ***nux-v.,*** olnd., petr., puls., rhus-t., sabin., sep., spig., squil., stram., syph., ther., ***thuj.,*** thyr.
blowing on covered parts - camph.
cold - camph., ***chel.,*** croc., cor-r., graph., ***lac-d., laur.,*** **LYSS.,** ***mosch., nux-v.,*** olnd., puls., rhus-t., sabin., samb., spig., squil., stram.
worms, sensation, under the skin - **COCA.**

SENSITIVE, physically, (see Mind)
drugs, to allopathic - acon., arn., ***ars.,*** cham., coff., lyc., **MED., NIT-AC.,** nux-v., **PULS.,** sep., sil., **SULPH.**
externally - ***acon., aesc.,*** agar., aloe, ***alum.,*** ambr., am-c., am-m., ant-c., ant-t., **APIS,** arg-m., **ARN.,** ars., asaf., ***aur., bapt., bar-c.,*** **BELL.,** ***bor.,*** bov., bry., calc., calc-p., camph., cann-s., ***canth.,*** caps., carb-an., carb-v., caust., **CHIN., CHIN-S.,** cimic., cina, ***clem.,*** coc-c., ***coff., colch.,*** coloc., con., ***crot-c.,*** cupr., dig., ***ferr.,*** ferr-p., ***gels.,*** hell., ***hep., hyos.,*** ign., ip., ***kali-bi., kali-c.,*** kali-n., kali-p., kali-s., kreos., **LACH.,** led., lyc., mag-c., mag-m., ment., ***merc., mez.,*** mosch., nat-a., ***nat-c., nat-m.,*** **NAT-P.,** nit-ac., nux-m., **NUX-V.,** olnd., ***op.,*** par., petr., ph-ac., **PHOS.,** plb., psor., **PULS., RAN-B.,** ***ran-s., rhus-t.,*** sabad., ***sabin.,*** sal-ac., sars., sec., ***sel., seneg., sep.,*** **SIL., SPIG.,** spong., squil., ***stann.,*** **STAPH.,** stront-c., ***sulph.,*** sul-ac., teucr.,

SENSITIVE, physically
externally - ***thuj.,*** verat., zinc.
internally - acon., agar., ***alum., am-c.,*** ant-c., ant-t., apis, arn., ***ars.,*** ars-i., asaf., ***asar.,*** aur., ***bapt.,*** bar-c., ***bell.,*** bism., ***bor.,*** bov., ***bry.,*** calad., ***calc.,*** cann-s., **CANTH.,** ***carb-an.,*** carb-s., carb-v., caust., ***cham.,*** chin., cic., clem., ***cocc.,*** coc-c., coff., colch., ***coloc.,*** con., croc., crot-h., cub., cupr., cycl., dulc., ***equis.,*** ferr., ***graph.,*** hell., helon., **HEP.,** ***hyos., iod.,*** ip., ***kali-bi., kali-i.,*** kali-p., **LACH.,** laur., led., ***lil-t.,*** mag-c., ***mag-m.,*** mang., meny., merc., ***merc-c., mez.,*** mosch., nat-a., ***nat-c.,*** **NAT-M.,** ***nit-ac., nux-v.,*** olnd., ***osm.,*** par., **PHOS.,** puls., ran-b., rhus-t., ***ruta,*** sars., ***sec.,*** sel., seneg., sep., **SIL.,** spong., ***squil.,*** stann., ***stram.,*** stront-c., sulph., sul-ac., tarax., tarent., teucr., thuj., valer., verat., zinc.
pain, to (see Pain, body)
remedies, to homeopathic potencies - acon., ***ars.,*** ars-i., cham., coff., **MED., NIT-AC.,** nux-v., **PHOS.,** sep., ***thuj.***

SEROUS membranes, general
acted upon by, specifically - ***apis,*** **BRY.,** ***cimic., hell.***
burning - apis.
disease approaching insidiously rather as sequel to some other disease than as natural termination of an inflammation of brain - ***hell.***
effusions - anthr., **APIS,** ***apoc.,*** arg-n., **ARS., BRY.,** ***kali-m., kali-s., lyc., nat-m., sulph.,*** zinc.
brain and spine, in - arn.
debility, with mental and physical - seneg.
fluid, from loss of vital - chin.
joints and closed sacs, in - ***nat-m.***
mattery - ***kali-s.***
peritonitis, in - ***crot-h.***
pleura and lungs, especially of - jab.
and peritoneum, especially from - uran-n.
weakness of vessels, from - ***dig.***
inflammation, of - **ACON.,** am-c., **APIS,** apoc., arg-m., **ARS.,** ars-i., asaf., ***aur., aur-m.,*** bell., **BRY., CALC.,** calc-p., **CANTH.,** ***carb-v.,*** colch., ferr., fl-ac., **HELL.,** indg., ***iod., kali-c.,*** lach., ***led.,*** **LYC.,** mag-m., ***merc., nat-m., ph-ac., phos.,*** plat., ***psor., puls.,*** ran-b., samb., seneg., **SIL.,** ***squil., stram., sulph., ter.,*** zinc.
chronic - **ARS.**
joints, particularly knees, hips and hands - hippoz.
peritoneum, particularly pleura or - ***ran-b.***
peritonitis, in second stage of, pleuritis and pericarditis - ***kali-m.***
stitches - **BRY.**

SEWING, agg. - agar., bov., ***calc.,*** **CAUST.,** ***cham.,*** cimic., cocc., ***cycl., dros.,*** gels., **KALI-C.,** mag-p., **NAT-M.,** phos., pic-ac., plat., **RUTA,** sep., **SIL.,** ***stann.,*** valer., **ZINC.**

SEWING,
amel. - lach., nat-m.

SHAVING, after agg. - ***carb-an.***, ox-ac., phos., ph-ac., **PULS.**, rad-br., stroph-s.
amel. - brom.

SHINING objects, ailments from - bell., canth., glon., hyos., ***lyss.***, ***stram.***

SHIPBOARD, ailments on (see Emergency, Seasickness) - cocc., petr., tab., ther.

SHOCK, (see Emergency, chapter)

SHOCKS, electric-like, (see Sensations, generals)

SHRIVELLING, of body (see Emaciation) - ***abrot.***, alum., am-c., am-m., ambr., ***ant-c.***, ***arg-n.***, arn., ***bar-c.***, bism., ***bor.***, bry., ***calc.***, camph., cham., chin., cupr., fl-ac., hell., graph., kali-br., ***lyc.***, merc., mur-ac., nux-v., op., ph-ac., plb., psor., rheum, rhod., rhus-t., sabad., ***sars.***, ***sec.***, ***sep.***, sil., spig., stram., ***sulph.***, verat., viol-o., vip., zinc.

SICK feeling - acon., ant-t., bapt., brom., carc., chel., cimic., con., ip., lach., lob., nux-v., petr., ***podo.***, psor., puls., sang., stront-c., stroph., ***tab.***, tarax.
does not know why - brom.
pain, from - stront-c.
queer, before menses - brom.
suddenly - con., tab.

SIDES, of body
atypical - mosch.
alternating sides - agar., ant-c., carc., cimic., cina, **COCC.**, iris, **LAC-C.**, ***lach.***, ***lyc.***, mang., merc., onos., phos., plat., puls., rad-br., sep.
crosswise, left lower and right upper - acon., agn., **AMBR.**, am-c., am-m., ***ant-c.***, ant-t., arg-m., ars-i., asar., bism., ***bor.***, ***bov.***, bry., calad., ***calc.***, cann-s., carb-v., ***caust.***, chel., cic., cina, coloc., colch., croc., cupr., dig., dulc., euph., ***euphr.***, ***ferr.***, graph., hell., hyos., ign., iod., ip., **LAC-C.**, ***lyc.***, mag-c., mang., ***merc-i-f.***, mez., mur-ac., ***nat-c.***, nux-v., **PHOS.**, plat., ***plb.***, ran-b., rheum, rhus-t., ruta., sel., ***sil.***, spig., **SUL-AC.**, viol- o.
left upper and right lower - **AGAR.**, ***alum.***, ***anac.***, ***arn.***, ars., bar-c., bell., brom., camph., caps., ***carb-an.***, cham., chel., chin., coff., con., cycl., euphr., ***l-ac.***, hep., hyper., ***kali-c.***, kali-n., lach., laur., **LED.**, mag-m., meny., merc., mill., mur-ac., nat-m., nit-ac., nux-m., nux-v., olnd., op., par., ph-ac., puls., ran-s., rhod., **RHUS-T.**, sabad., sabin., samb., sars., sec., seneg., spong., ***squil.***, ***stann.***, staph., stram., sulph., **TARAX.**, teucr., ***thuj.***, valer., ***verat.***, ***verb.***, ***viol-t.***
left - acon., ***all-c.***, aloe, ***am-br.***, ***anac.***, ***ant-c.***, ***ant-t.***, ***apis***, ***arg-m.***, **ARG-N.**, ***arn.***, arum-t., **ASAF.**, **ASAR.**, ***asc-t.***, ***aster.***, aur- m-n., bar-m., ***berb.***, bism., ***brom.***, ***bry.***, ***calc.***, cann-s., canth., **CAPS.**, caust., ***cham.***, ***chel.***, ***chin.***, ***cimic.***, **CINA**, **CLEM.**, cocc., ***colch.***, ***coloc.***, **CROC.**, ***crot-t.***, ***cupr.***, ***dulc.***, **EUPH.**, ***euphr.***, ***ferr.***, ferr-p., gels., **GRAPH.**, ***guai.***, hep., ign., ip., iris, ***kali-chl.***, **KREOS.**, **LACH.**, ***lith.***, mag-m., mang., meny., ***merc.***, ***merc-c.***, ***merc-i-r.***, **MEZ.**, mosch., ***mur-ac.***, naja, nat-s., ***nit-ac.***, nux-m., **OLND.**, ***onos.***, ***osm.***, ox-ac., ***par.***, **PHOS.**, phys., plb., ran-b., ***ran-s.***, ***rhod.***, ***sabin.***, sal-ac., **SEL.**, **SEP.**, ***sil.***, ***spig.***, **SQUIL.**, **STANN.**, staph., stront-c., **SULPH.**, sul-ac., tab., ***tarax.***, ***teucr.***, ther., ***thuj.***, ust., vesp., ***viol-o.***, ***viol-t.***, xan.
coldness of - bry., carb-v., caust., lyc., rhus-t., sapin., sulph.
heat of - bell., lac-ac., rhus-t.
left then right - acon., all-c., aloe, arg-n., ars., benz-ac., brom., calc., calc-p., ***colch.***, dulc., elaps, ferr., ***form.***, form-ac., hed., ***iod.***, ip., kali-c., kreos., lac-c., **LACH.**, merc-i-r., naja, nit-m-ac., nux-v., phyt., puls., rhus-t., sabad., stann., tarax.
one sided, symptoms, on - ***aesc.***, ***agar.***, agn., **ALUM.**, ***ambr.***, am-c., am-m., **ANAC.**, ant-c., ant-t., apis, ***arg-m.***, ***arg-n.***, arn., ars., **ASAF.**, asar., aur., ***bar-c.***, bar-m., bell., bism., bor., **BRY.**, ***calc.***, camph., cann-s., ***canth.***, caps., carb-an., carb-v., caust., cham., chel., chin., cic., ***cina***, clem., cocc., coff., colch., coloc., con., croc., cupr., ***cycl.***, dig., dros., ***dulc.***, euph., euphr., ferr., graph., ***guai.***, hell., hep., hyos., ign., iod., iris, **KALI-C.**, kali-n., **KALI-P.**, **KREOS.**, **LACH.**, laur., led., **LYC.**, **Lyss.**, mag-c., mag-m., ***mang.***, meny., merc., ***mez.***, mosch., ***mur-ac.***, nat-c., nat-m., ***nit-ac.***, nux-m., nux-v., ***olnd.***, ***par.***, petr., **PH-AC.**, ***phos.***, **PLAT.**, ***plb.***, ***puls.***, ran-b., ran-s., rheum, rhod., rhus-t., ruta., ***sabad.***, ***sabin.***, samb., **SARS.**, sel., seneg., sep., sil., ***spig.***, spong., squil., stann., ***staph.***, ***stront-c.***, sulph., **SUL-AC.**, tarax., teucr., thuj., valer., verat., **VERB.**, viol- o., viol-t., ***zinc.***
pains, go to side lain on - ars., ***bry.***, calc., ***kali-c.***, merc., ***ph-ac.***, **PULS.**, sep., sil.
pains, go to side not lain on - bry., cupr., fl-ac., graph., ***ign.***, kali-bi., ***rhus-t.***
right - abies-c., ***acon.***, ***aesc.***, ***agn.***, ***alum.***, ***am-c.***, **APIS**, **ARG-M.**, ***arn.***, **ARS.**, ars-i., **AUR.**, **BAPT.**, **BELL.**, ***bism.***, **BOR.**, brom., **BRY.**, **CALC.**, ***calc-p.***, cann-i., cann-s., **CANTH.**, caps., ***caust.***, cedr., cham., **CHEL.**, chin., ***cocc.***, ***colch.***, **COLOC.**, **CON.**, **CROT-C.**, **CROT-H.**, ***dros.***, dulc., euphr., form., guai., ***hep.***, ***ign.***, ***ip.***, ***iris***, kalm., kreos., lil-t., ***lith.***, **LYC.**, **LYSS.**, ***mag-m.***, ***mang.***, meny., ***merc.***, ***merc-i-f.***, ***mez.***, ***mosch.***, mur-ac., nat-a., ***nat-c.***, nit-ac., ***nux-m.***, **NUX-V.**, op., ***pall.***, par., ***petr.***, phyt., ***plb.***, ***podo.***, ***prun.***, **PULS.**, ***ran-b.***, **RAN-S.**, **RAT.**, ***rhod.***, ***sabad.***, ***sabin.***, ***sang.***, **SARS.**, **SEC.**, ***sil.***, spig., ***staph.***, ***stront-c.***, ***sulph.***, **SUL-AC.**, tarax., tell., ***teucr.***, thuj., viol-o., viol-t., ***zinc.***
heat of - op.

SIDES, of body

left, then left - acet-ac., acon., am-c., ambr., anac., ***apis,*** ars., ars-m., aspar., bar-c., bell., benz-ac., bry., calc-p., canth., ***caust.,*** chel., cupr., graph., lil-t., **LYC.,** merc-i-f., mez., ox-ac., ***phos.,*** ptel., rheum, rumx., **SABAD.,** sang., saroth., spong., sul-ac., sulph., syph., thiop., ***verat.***

SITS, general

bed, on, will not lie down - kali-br.

bent forward, straightens difficulty with - lath.

down, desire to - puls.

elbow and knee, on - lob.

erect, hands folded across chest, with - ox-ac.

ground looking, at - stram.

hands supporting the body - berb., sulph.

knees drawn up, resting her head and arms on knees - **ARS.**

legs crossed, uncross can not - bell., ther.

suddenly and lies down - hyos.

supports, weight hands on, with - sulph.

SITTING, general

agg., while - acon., **AGAR.,** agn., ***aloe,*** alum., ***ambr.,*** am-c., **AM-M.,** anac., ant-c., ant-t., ***arg-m.,*** arn., **ARS.,** ***asaf.,*** asar., ***aur., aur-m-n., aur-m., bar-c.,*** bar-m., bell., bism., bor., bov., ***bry.,*** cact., calad., calc., camph., cann-s., canth., **CAPS.,** carb-an., carb-v., caust., cham., chel., ***chin.,*** cic., ***cina,*** clem., cob., ***cocc.,*** coff., colch., ***coloc.,*** **CON.,** croc., cupr., **CYCL.,** ***dros.,*** **DULC., EUPH.,** ***euphr., ferr.,*** fl-ac., ***gamb.,*** graph., guai., ***hell.,*** hep., hyos., ign., iod., ip., ***kali-bi.,*** kali-c., kali-n., kali-p., kali-s., kreos., ***lach.,*** laur., ***led.,*** **LYC.,** mag-c., ***mag-m.,*** mang., ***meny., merc.,*** mez., ***mosch., mur-ac., nat-c.,*** nat-m., nat-p., nit-ac., nux-m., nux-v., olnd., op., par., ***petr., ph-ac.,*** **PHOS., PLAT.,** plb., ***prun.,*** **PULS.,** ran-b., ***ran-s.,*** rheum, ***rhod.,*** **RHUS-T.,** ***ruta., sabad.,*** sabin., samb., sars., sec., ***seneg.,*** **SEP.,** sil., ***spig.,*** spong., squil., stann., staph., stram., stront-c., **SULPH.,** sul-ac., ***tarax.,*** teucr., ***thuj.,*** **VALER.,** verat., **VERB.,** viol-o., **VIOL-T., ZINC.**

chair, low - syph.

cold place, on a - bell., cimic., dulc., glon., ***nux-v.,*** rhus-t., sep., sil.

amel. while - ***acon.,*** agar., agn., alum., ***alumn.,*** am-c., am-m., ***anac.,*** ang., ***ant-t.,*** aral., arg-m., arn., ars., asaf., asar., aur., bar-c., bell., bor., **BRY.,** cadm-s., ***calad.,*** calc., camph., cann-s., canth., caps., carb-an., carb-v., caust., cham., chel., chin., chion., cic., cina, clem., cocc., ***coff.,*** **COLCH.,** ***coloc.,*** con., croc., cupr., cycl., **DIG.,** ***dulc.,*** ferr., gels., ***glon., graph.,*** guai., hell., hep., hyos., ign., iod., ip., kali-c., kali-n., kreos., laur., led., mag-c., mag-m., mang., meny., meph., ***merc.,*** mez., mosch., nat-a., nat-c., nat-m., nit-ac., nux-m., **NUX-V.,** op., par., petr., ph-ac., phos., plb., ***puls.,*** ran-b., ran-s., ***rheum, rhod., rhus-t.,*** sabad., sabin., samb., sars., sec., sel., ***sep., sil.,*** spig., spong., ***squil.,*** stann., staph., stram., sulph., sul-ac., sumb., tarax., thuj., valer., verat., verb., zinc.

bed, up in - ***kali-c.,*** samb.

crooked - sulph.

elbows, knees on - kali-c.

aversion, to, mental - ***ars.,*** iod., lach.

physical - iod., lach.

bent, while, agg. - ***acon., agn.,*** alum., ***alumn., am-m.,*** ang., **ANT-T.,** arg-m., ***ars.,*** asaf., bar-c., bor., bov., ***bry.,*** caps., carb-v., caust., cham., chel., ***chin., cic.,*** **DIG.,** ***dulc.,*** ferr., ***hyos.,*** ign., meny., nat-m., ***nux-v., phos.,*** plb., ***puls.,*** ran-b., ***sep.,*** spig., spong., ***squil.,*** stann., ***sulph., verb.,*** viol-t.

amel. - anac., ***ang.,*** ars., bar-c., ***bell.,*** bor., bry., calad., ***carb-v.,*** caust., ***cham., chel.,*** chin., cina, ***colch., coloc., con.,*** dig., ***ign.,*** **KALI-C.,** lach., ***lyc.,*** mang., ***merc., mez.,*** mosch., nux-m., nux-v., op., puls., ***rheum,*** rhus-t., ***sabad.,*** sars., ***spig., spong., stann.,*** sulph., tarax., verat., verb.

down, on first, agg. - ***agn.,*** alum., **AM-M.,** ***ant-t.,*** arg-m., aur., bar-c., bov., bry., caust., ***chel.,*** chin., ***coff.,*** croc., cycl., graph., ***hell., ip.,*** iris, kali-c., lyc., ***mag-c.,*** mang., merc., murx., nit-ac., ph-ac., phos., puls., ruta, sabin., ***samb.,*** sars., **SPIG.,** ***spong.,*** squil., thuj., ***valer.,*** verat., viol-t.

amel. - acon., ambr., anac., ang., ant-c., ant-t., arn., ars., asar., aur., ***bar-c., bell.,*** bov., bry., calc., cann-s., canth., **CAPS.,** carb-an., ***carb-v.,*** caust., cham., chin., cic., cocc., **CON.,** croc., dig., dros., ***euph., ferr.,*** graph., kali-c., kali-n., lach., ***laur., led.,*** lyc., mang., merc., mur-ac., nat-c., nat-m., nit-ac., ***nux-v., olnd., petr.,*** ph-ac., ***phos.,*** plat., puls., ran-b., rhod., ***rhus-t.,*** ruta, sabad., ***sep.,*** sil., ***spig., staph.,*** stram., stront-c., ***sulph.,*** thuj., ***verat.***

erect, while, agg., - anac., ***ang.,*** ars., aur-s., bar-c., bar-s., ***bell.,*** bor., bry., calad., ***carb-v.,*** caust., ***cham., chel.,*** chin., cina, ***colch.,*** **COLOC.,** ***con.,*** dig., ***ign.,*** **KALI-C.,** kreos., ***lyc.,*** mang., ***merc., mez.,*** mosch., nat-m., nux-m., nux-v., op., puls., rheum, rhus-t., ***sabad.,*** sars., ***spig., spong., staph.,*** sulph., tarax., verat., verb., viol-t.

amel. - ***acon., alumn., am-m.,*** ang., **ANT-T.,** apis, aral., arg-m., ***ars.,*** asaf., bar-c., bell., carb-v., caust., cham., chel., ***chin., cic.,*** con., **DIG.,** ***dulc.,*** ferr., gels., ***hyos.,*** kali-bi., kali-n., meny., nat-m., nat-s., ***nux-v., phos.,*** plb., ***puls., rhod., rhus-t., sabin., sep.,*** spig., spong., squil., stann., ***sulph.,*** verb.

impulse to sit - acon., ***agar.,*** alum., am-c., ***am-m.,*** ambr., anac., ant-c., arg-m., arn., ***ars.,*** asar., bar-ac., bar-c., ***bell.,*** bor., bry., calc., camph., ***cann-s.,*** canth., caps., ***carb-v.,*** caust., cham., ***chel.,*** **CHIN.,** ***cocc.,*** cod., colch., **CON.,** croc., cupr., cycl., dulc., ***euphr.,*** **GRAPH.,** ***guai.,*** hell., hep., hyos., ign., ***iod.,***

SITTING, general

impulse, to sit - ip., jac-c., kali-c., lach., lact., laur., led., lil-t., lyc., mag-aust., mag-c., mag-m., ***merc.,*** mez., mur-ac., nat-a., nat-c., ***nat-m.,*** nat-s., nit-ac., **NUX-V.,** olnd., op., petr., ***ph-ac.,*** **PHOS.,** pic-ac., plb., puls., ran-b., ran-s., rheum, rhod., rhus-t., ruta, sabin., ***sec., sep.,*** sil., ***spong.,*** **SQUIL.,** ***stann.,*** staph., stront-c., sulph., ***tarax.,*** teucr., verat., verb., viol-t., ***zinc.***

inability to sit erect - lyc., stram.

must sit up in bed with knees drawn up, rests her head and arms upon knees - **ARS.,** glon.

squatting - calc., ***coloc.,*** graph., syph.

wet ground, ailments from sitting on - ***ars.,*** calc., caust., ***dulc., nux-v.,*** rhod., ***rhus-t.,*** sil.

SLIDING, down in bed - apis, ars., ***bapt.,*** chin., colch., hell., ***hyos., mur-ac.,*** ph-ac., tab., zinc.

SLUGGISHNESS, of the body (see Weakness) - acon., agar., alum., ***alumn., am-m.,*** ammc., anac., ***ant-t.,*** arn., ars., **ASAR.,** bar-c., bell., bor., brucin., bry., cact., calad., calc., calc-p., camph., cann-s., canth., ***caps.,*** carb-an., ***carb-v., carl.,*** casc., ***chel.,*** chin., cinnb., cocc., ***con.,*** croc., cur., cycl., dig., dirc., dulc., ferr-m., ***gels.,*** graph., grat., guai., hell., hep., hera., hyos., ign., indg., iod., ip., kali-c., kali-m., kali-p., kali-s., lach., laur., lil-t., lyc., mag-aust., mag-c., mag-m., merc., mez., mur-ac., nat-c., nat-m., nit-ac., nux-v., ol-an., olnd., ***op.,*** petr., ph-ac., phel., phos., phys., ***plb.,*** puls., rheum, rhod., ruta, sabin., sars., ***sec.,*** sel., ***sep.,*** sil., stann., stram., stront-c., sul-i., ***sulph.,*** thea., thuj., verb., zinc., zinc-p.

forenoon - sars.

morning - carb-an., chel., lyc., ***mag-m.,*** nat-c., nat-m., ***nux-v., ph-ac.,*** verb.

sitting, while - chel.

processes of body - sil.

rising, on - ammc.

torpor - apis, berb., ***cic., crot-h., gels.,*** kali-br., ***lyc.,*** **NAT-M., NUX-M., OP.,** ***plb.,*** sang., ***stram.***

SMALLER, (see Sensations, general)

SMALLPOX - agar., am-m., ***ant-c.,*** **ANT-T.,** ***apis, ars.,*** bapt., ***bell., bry.,*** canth., ***carb-ac.,*** carb-v., cham., clem., cocc., hyos., maland., **MERC.,** ***nat-m.,*** nit-ac., ***puls.,*** **RHUS-T.,** sarr., sep., sil., stram., ***sulph.,*** **THUJ.,** ***vario., zinc.***

black - ant-c., **ARS.,** ***bell.,*** bry., hyos., ***lach., mur-ac.,*** **RHUS-T.,** ***sec.,*** sep., sil., spig.

diarrhea, during - ant-t., ***ars.,*** **CHIN.,** thuj.

prophylactic - maland., vac., vario.

SMOKE, (see Sensations, general)

SMOKING, habit (see Toxicity, Tobacco)

SNEEZING, agg. - ars., bell., bry., kali-c., ***lyc.,*** phos., rhus-t., **SULPH.,** til., verb.

amel. - chlol., lach., mag-m., naja, thuj.

SNOW-air, general, (see Environment, Snow-air)

SPOTS, symptoms occur in - agar., ***alum.,*** arg-m., ars., ***berb.,*** bufo, ***calc-p.,*** caust., ***cist.,*** colch., ***con.,*** fl-ac., glon., hep., ign., **KALI-BI., LAC-C.,** lil-t., ***nat-m.,*** nux-m., ol-an., ol-j., ***ox-ac., phos.,*** rhus-t., sars., sel., ***sep.,*** sil., **SULPH.,** thuj., zinc.

cold - agar., calc-p., petr., sep., tarent., ***verat.***

STANDING, agg. - acon., ***agar.,*** agn., aloe, ***alum.,*** ambr., am-c., ***am-m.,*** arg-m., arn., ars., asaf., asar., ***aur.,*** bar-c., bar-m., ***bell., berb.,*** bism., bor., ***bry.,*** cact., ***calc.,*** calc-s., ***camph.,*** cann-s., ***canth., caps.,*** carb-an., ***carb-s.,*** carb-v., ***caust.,*** cham., chel., ***chin.,*** chin-a., cic., cina, **COCC.,** coff., **CON.,** croc., cupr., **CYCL.,** ***dig.,*** dros., dulc., ***euph., euphr., ferr.,*** ferr-ar., ferr-p., ***fl-ac.,*** graph., guai., hell., hep., ign., ***kali-bi.,*** kali-c., kali-n., kali-p., lach., laur., led., **LIL-T.,** mag-c., mag-m., mang., meny., merc., mez., mosch., mur-ac., ***murx.,*** nat-c., nat-m., ***nit-ac.,*** nux-m., nux-v., olnd., op., par., petr., ***ph-ac.,*** phos., ***plat.,*** plb., **PULS.,** ***ran-b., rheum,*** rhod., ***rhus-t., ruta., sabad., sabin., samb.,*** **SEP.,** ***sil.,*** spig., spong., stann., staph., stram., stront-c., **SULPH.,** sul-ac., ***tarax.,*** teucr., thuj., ***tub.,*** **VALER.,** ***verat., verb.,*** viol-t., ***zinc.***

erect - ars., bell., ***dios.,*** kali-p.

eyes closed with - arg-n., calad., iodof., lath.

tiptoe, on - cocc.

amel. - agar., agn., am-c., anac., ant-t., arn., **ARS.,** ***asar.,*** bar-c., **BELL.,** bor., bry., ***calad.,*** calc., camph., ***cann-s.,*** canth., carb-an., carb-v., chel., chin., cic., cina, cocc., con., ***colch.,*** croc., cupr., dig., dios., euph., graph., guai., hell., hep., ign., ***iod.,*** ip., kreos., ***led.,*** mang., meny., merc., mez., mur-ac., naja, nat-m., nux-m., ***nux-v.,*** par., petr., ***phos.,*** plb., ***ran-b.,*** rheum, ruta., sars., sec., ***sel., spig.,*** spong., ***squil.,*** stann., staph., stram., sul-ac., tarax., tarent., thuj.

erect - ars., bell., cedr., ***dios.,*** kali-p.

legs, keeps, wide apart - phos., pic-ac., ter.

impossible - acon., acon-f., aeth., ant-t., calc-p., canth., chin-s., cocc., con., cupr., cupr-s., dulc., gels., hep., hydrc., hyos., iod., ***kali-br.,*** lach., merc., merc-n., nat-m., nit-ac., nux-v., op., phys., plb., sabad., sec., stann., staph., stram., sul-ac., tarent.

till afternoon - bell.

falls, after - arg-n.

STAPHYLOCOCCUS, (see Fevers)

STARVING, general - ars., ign.

exhaustion, with - ***ign.***

sensation that he must be - kali-m.

STEAM, agg. - kali-bi.

amel. - ars-s-f., lyss.

STEPPING, downstairs, agg. - stram.

high steps, from agg. - phyt.

STIFFENING out of body - ang., camph., cham., ***cina,*** cic., cupr., ***ign., ip.,*** just., phos., stram.

cough, before - cina, led.

touch, from - apis.

STIFFNESS, of body - abrot., absin., acon., aeth., ***agar.***, am-c., am-m., ***aran.***, arg-m., **ARS.**, ars-i., ars-s-f., **ASAF.**, ***bell.***, bov., brom., **BRY.**, ***calc.***, calc-p., calc-s., camph., cann-i., cann-s., canth., ***caps.***, ***carb-ac.***, ***carb-an.***, carb-o., ***carb-s.***, carb-v., carl., **CAUST.**, ***cham.***, **CHEL.**, ***chin.***, chin-a., ***cic.***, ***cimic.***, **COCC.**, ***colch.***, **CUPR.**, cycl., dig., ***dulc.***, eup-per., ferr-ar., graph., ***guai.***, ***hell.***, hydr-ac., ***hyos.***, iod., kali-ar., kali-bi., ***kali-c.***, kali-p., **KALM.**, ***lach.***, lath., ***laur.***, **LED.**, lith., **LYC.**, ***med.***, meny., ***merc.***, ***merc-c.***, merc-i-r., merc-sul., mosch., naja, nat-a., nat-c.1, ***nat-m.***, ***nat-s.***, nit-ac., nux-m., ***nux-v.***, olnd., op., ox-ac., **PETR.**, ph-ac., ***phos.***, ***phyt.***, ***plat.***, plan., plb., psor., ***puls.***, **RHUS-T.**, ***sang.***, sars., ***sec.***, sel., **SEP.**, **SIL.**, ***spong.***, ***stram.***, ***stry.***, **SULPH.**, tab., ***thuj.***, verat., verat-v., ***zinc.***
- exertion, after - arn., calc., **RHUS-T.**, ***tub.***
- morning in bed - calc-p., ***chin.***, ***lach.***, ***led.***, **RHUS-T.**, staph.
- move, on beginning to - ***agar.***, ***caps.***, kali-p., ***lyc.***, ***psor.***, **RHUS-T.**
- paralytic - ***cocc.***, lith., merc-c., nat-m., plb.
- rising, on - agar., op., plan., psor., **RHUS-T.**
- sleep, after - ***lach.***, morph., ox-ac., **RHUS-T.**, ***sep.***

STONES, calculi (see Bladder, Kidneys, Liver)

STOOP, shouldered - am-m., ***arg-n.***, ***calc.***, calc-p., ***carb-v.***, cocc., coff., coloc., con., gels., lath., ***lyc.***, ***mang.***, med., nat-c., nat-m., nux-v., op., **PHOS.**, ***sil.***, **SULPH.**, ***ter.***, ***tub.***, verat.

STOOPING, agg. - aesc., agar., ***am-c.***, bell., **BRY.**, ***calc.***, caust., lyc., ***mang.***, merc., nux-v., puls., ran-b., sep., sil., ***spig.***, ***sulph.***, tell., ther., ***valer.***
- amel. - cina, ***colch.***, con., ***hyos.***, ign., ***iris***, puls., ran-b.
- easy, stretching difficult - nat-m.
- inability to - bor.
- prolonged agg. - asar., bov., caust., hep., plat.

STORMS, (see Environment, Storms)

STREPTOCOCCUS, (see Fevers)

STRETCHING, agg. - acon., ***aesc.***, agar., alum., ambr., ***am-c.***, ang., ant-t., apis, arn., **ARS.**, arum-t., bar-c., ***bell.***, bor., bov., brach., ***brom.***, caj., calad., ***calc.***, calc-p., camph., cann-s., canth., caps., carb-an., ***carb-v.***, **CAUST.**, **CHAM.**, chel., chin., chlf., cimic., cimx., cina, colch., cycl., daph., dig., dios., dros., ferr., form., gins., gran., ***graph.***, guai., haem., hell., hep., hyos., ind., kali-bi., kalm., kreos., lach., laur., led., lil-t., lob., mag-c., meph., ***merc.***, ***merc-c.***, merc-i-r., ***mez.***, nat-c., ***nat-m.***, nat-s., **NUX-V.**, olnd., op., ox-ac., petr., phel., ph-ac., ***phos.***, plan., ***plat.***, plb., prun., **PULS.**, ***ran-b.***, raph., **RHUS-T.**, ***rhus-v.***, ruta., ***sabad.***, sel., ***sep.***, sil., spong., squil., stann., staph., sulph., tarent., ***teucr.***, valer., verb., viol-o., wild., zinc.
- **abdominal** trouble, in - plb.
- **affected,** parts, agg. - ***alum.***, am-c., am-m., anac., ang., ***ant-c.***, arg-m., arn., aur., bar-c., bell., bov., ***bry.***, **CALC.**, cann-s., caps., carb-v., caust., ***cham.***, ***chin.***, cina, clem., ***colch.***,

STRETCHING, general
- **affected,** parts, agg. - **COLOC.**, con., croc., dig., dros., dulc., ferr., fl-ac., graph., guai., ***hep.***, ign., **IOD.**, kali-c., laur., lyc., mag-m., ***mang.***, meny., merc., ***merc-c.***, mur-ac., nat-m., nux-v., petr., phos., ***plat.***, plb., psor., ***puls.***, ***rheum***, ***rhus-t.***, ***ruta***, sabin., sel., **SEP.**, spig., spong., stann., ***staph.***, **SULPH.**, **THUJ.**, valer., verat.
  - amel. - agar., alum., am-m., anac., ***ant-t.***, asar., bell., berb., bor., carb-an., carb-v., cham., chel., chin., coff., cupr., dig., dros., dios., dulc., ferr., guai., hep., ign., kali-c., mag-c., mez., mur-ac., nat-m., nat-s., nux-m., nux-v., olnd., ox-ac., par., petr., phos., plat., puls., rheum, rhod., **RHUS-T.**, sabad., sabin., **SEC.**, stann., staph., thuj., verb., zinc.
- **afternoon** - arum-t., cina, form., jug-r., nux-v., plat., rhus-t.
  - 1 p.m - form.
  - 4 p.m - cina, plan.
  - 5 p.m to 9 p.m - bell.
  - desire to stretch - amln., plb., sec.
  - sleeping, after - verat.
  - stretching, amel. - sec.
- **air,** open, amel. - ol-an.
- **always** - puls., rhod., rhus-t., sabad., staph., tab.
- **amel.** - alet., ***alum.***, aml-n., **ANT-T.**, arn., bell., berb., ***calc.***, carb-v., dios., graph., ***guai.***, halo., hep., ***ign.***, lyc., man., nat-f., ***nux-v.***, perh., phos., plat., plb., podo., **PULS.**, pyrog., rhus-t., sabad., sabin., ***sec.***, teucr., tub-r.
- **anguish** with impending menses - carl.
- **anxiety,** from - nat-c.
- **arms** - spong., squil., stann., tab.
- **backward** - glon., hydr.
  - amel. - bor., ***dios.***
- **breakfast,** after - lach.
- **chill,** during - alum., ars., bry., caps., coff., daph., elat., ***eup-per.***, ip., ***kreos.***, laur., mur-ac., ***nat-s.***, nit-ac., nux-v., petr., rhus-t., ruta., tab., teucr.
  - before - aesc., ant-t., arn., ***ars.***, ***bry.***, ***eup-per.***, ign., ip., ***nat-m.***, nux-v., plan., rhus-t.
- **coldness,** during internal - bol., nat-s.
- **colic,** during - haem.
- **continually** - puls., rhod., sabad., staph., tab.
- **convulsive,** paroxysmal - ang., bell., camph., carb-h., ***chin.***, cic., cimic., cina, hydr-ac., lach., lyc., merc., nux-v., op., sabad., sec., sil., stram., sulph., thuj., verat.
- **cough,** after - merc., sang.
- **daytime** - mang.
- **dinner,** after - mag- c.
- **eating,** after - ip.
- **evening** - bell., cann-s., chin., graph., nat-c., rhus-t., sumb., tab., verat.
  - chill, during - tab.

STRETCHING, general
fever, during - alum., ***ars.,*** bell., ***bor.,*** bry., **CALC.,** ***calc-p.,*** caust., cham., eup-per., nat-m., ***nux-v.,*** **RHUS-T., SABAD.,** sep., spong., sulph., thuj.
forenoon - aloe, ant-t., bov., mag-c., mez., mill., mur-ac., nat- m.
11 a.m - mit.
hours, for - aml-n., plb.
house, in the - ruta.
impossible - acon., phos.
pains, because of - bell.
lying down, after - **COCC.**
menses, during - ***carb- an.***
after - carb-an.
before - **PULS.**
morning - ars., ***calc., carb-v.,*** cedr., ferr., hell., graph., lyc., nux-v., phos., puls., rhod., sep., sulph., tab., tarent., verat.
6 a.m - sep.
7 a.m - cedr.
amel. - **RHUST-T.,** sec.
bed, in - graph., hell., meph., merc., petr., phos., puls., rhod., sep., sulph.
of arms - petr.
stupefied, as if - meph.
waking, on - dulc., sep.
night - **CAUST.,** cocc., nat-c., sulph.
bed, in - ***cocc.***
sleep, in - nat-m.
violently for hours - aml-n., plb.
waking, when - merc.
noon - am-c., menis.
painful - sec.
perspiration, during - alum., bell., **BOR.,** bry., **CALC.,** caust., cham., **NAT-M.,** ***nux-v.,*** **RHUS-T.,** ***sabad., sep.,*** spong., sulph.
shuddering, during - ars., ***puls.***
sitting, while - alum.
reading, while - euphr.
sleep, during - nat-m.
sleepiness with - ant-t., bell., chin., lach., meph., sabad.
sleeplessness, during - dulc.
slept enough, as if he had not - am-c., mill.
supper, after - nit- ac.
tossing about, with - rhod.
unsatisfactory - ***graph.***
urination, before - **PULS.**
waking, on - bell., dulc., hell., ***ign.,*** meph., nit-ac., merc., phos., sulph.
walking, in open air amel. - ox-ac., plan.
yawning, with - acon., aesc., ***agar.,*** all-c., ***alum., am-c.,*** ambr., aml-n., ang., ant-t., arn., **ARS.,** asar., bar-c., ***bell.,*** bor., bov., ***bry.,*** calc., cann-s., canth., caps., ***carb-v.,*** cast., ***caust.,*** **CHAM.,** ***chin.,*** chin-s., cocc., cur., dig., dros., elat., ferr., ***form.,*** gran., graph., ***guai.,*** hell., hep., ***ign., ip.,*** kreos., ***lach.,*** lact., laur., led., mag-c., mang., meph., merc., merc-c., mez., mur-ac., nat-m., nit-ac., **NUX-V.,** ***olnd.,*** onis., petr., ph-ac., phos.,

STRETCHING, general
yawning, with - plat., plb., **RHUS-T.,** ruta, ***sabad.,*** sec., senec., seneg., ***sep.,*** sil., ***spong., squil.,*** stann., ***staph., sulph.,*** tab., tart-ac., tong., valer., verat., verb., viol-o., zinc.
forenoon - ant-t.
sleepiness, without - viol-o.

STRETCHES, twists, turns - alum., ***bell., calc.,*** chel., ***cina,*** coloc., ign., nux-v., plb., rhus-t., sulph., teucr.
convulsion, before - calc.
cough, after - merc.

SUBSULTUS, tendinum (see Muscles, chapter)

SUPPRESSION of, ailments from
condylomata - merc., nit-ac., staph., ***thuj.***
coryza, agg. - am-c., ***am-m.,*** ambr., ars., **BRY.,** calad., **CALC.,** carb-v., caust., cham., ***chin.,*** cina, con., ***dulc., fl-ac.,*** graph., hep., ip., **KALI-BI.,** kali-c., kreos., **LACH.,** laur., lyc., mag-c., mag-m., mill., ***nit-ac.,*** nux-m., **NUX-V.,** par.
eruptions - acon., ail., alum., am-c., ambr., anac., ant-c., ant-t., ***apis,*** **ARS.,** ***ars-i.,*** ars-s-f., asaf., bad., bar-c., ***bell.,*** **BRY.,** calad., calc., ***camph.,*** caps., carb-an., ***carb-v., caust., cham.,*** chin., ***cic.,*** clem., con., ***cupr.,*** cupr-ac., cupr-ar., **DULC.,** ***gels., graph., hell., hep.,*** hyos., iod., **IP., KALI-BI.,** kali-c., ***kali-s., kreos.,*** lach., laur., ***lyc.,*** mag-c., mag-s., merc., ***mez., nat-c.,*** nit-ac., ***nux-m.,*** **NUX-V.,** op., **PETR., PH-AC.,** phos., plb., **PSOR.,** ptel., ***puls., rhus-t.,*** sars., sel., senec., ***sep.,*** sil., ***staph.,*** **STRAM.,** sul-ac., **SULPH.,** thuj., ***tub., tub-k.,*** verat., verat-v., ***viol-t.,*** x-ray, **ZINC.**
fail to break out - ***ail.,*** am-c., ant-t., ***apis., stram., sulph., zinc.***
exanthemata - ***ail., apis,*** hell., verat.
hemorrhoids - aloe, am-m., apis, ars., ***calc., caps.,*** carb-v., ***coll.,*** cupr., ***ign.,*** lycps., ***mill.,*** **NAT-M., NUX-V., OP.,** phos., puls., ran-b., **SULPH.**
mother milk - ***acon.,*** agar., ***agn.,*** aur., aur-i., aur-s., bell., **BRY.,** calc., calc-sil., camph-br., ***carb-v.,*** **CAUST.,** ***cham., chim.,*** cimic., cycl., dulc., frag., ***hyos.,*** ign., ***iod.,*** lac-d., ***lach., merc.,*** mill., phyt., **PULS.,** ***rhus-t., sec.,*** senec., ***sil.,*** sul-i., ***sulph., urt-u.,*** verat., zinc.
anger, from - ***cham.***

SWELLING, general, (see Edema) - ***acon.,*** agar., agn., alum., ambr., am-c., am-m., anac., ant-c., **APIS,** arg-m., ***arn.,*** **ARS.,** ars-i., asaf., aur., ***bar-c.,*** **BELL.,** bism., bor., bov., **BRY.,** bufo, calad., ***calc.,*** camph., cann-s., ***canth.,*** caps., carb-an., ***carb-s.,*** carb-v., caust., ***cham.,*** chel., ***chin.,*** cic., clem., cocc., coff., colch., coloc., com., con., cop., croc., crot-h., cupr., cycl., dig., dros., ***dulc.,*** euph., euphr., ***ferr.,*** graph., guai., hell., ***hep.,*** hyos., ign., iod., ***kali-ar.,*** **KALI-BI.,** ***kali-c.,*** kali-n., kreos., lach., laur., led., ***lyc.,*** mag-c., mag-m., mang., **MERC.,** mez., mosch., mur-ac., naja, ***nat-c.,*** nat-m., ***nit-ac.,*** nux-m., **NUX-V.,**

SWELLING, general - olnd., op., par., petr., ***ph-ac.***, ***phos.***, ***plb.***, **PULS.**, ran-b., rhod., **RHUS-T.**, ruta, sabad., sabin., samb., sars., sec., seneg., ***sep.***, ***sil.***, ***spig.***, spong., squil., stann., staph., ***stram.***, stront-c., ***sulph.***, sul-ac., ***thuj.***, valer., verat., ***vip.***, zinc.

beads, like - aeth., am-c., apis, iod., ***nat-m.***, phos.

cartilages - **ARG-M.**, ***calc.***, ***sil.***

inflammatory - **ACON.**, agn., alum., am-c., ant-c., ***apis***, arn., **ARS.**, ars-i., asaf., bar-c., **BELL.**, ***bry.***, **CALC.**, cann-s., **CANTH.**, carb-an., carb-v., ***caust.***, chin., cocc., colch., ***con.***, cupr., euph., graph., guai., hep., ***iod.***, ***kali-ar.***, **KALI-BI.**, **KALI-C.**, ***kali-i.***, led., ***lyc.***, mag-c., **MERC.**, nat-a., ***nat-m.***, ***nit-ac.***, nux-v., petr., ***phos.***, ***phyt.***, plb., ***puls.***, ***rhus-t.***, sabin., samb., sars., sec., **SEP.**, ***sil.***, spong., stann., **SULPH.**, thuj., zinc.

lymphatic swellings - berb., iod.

mucous membranes - arg-n., ars-i., hydr.

painful - dig.

parts, affected, of - **ACON.**, **ACT-SP.**, agn., alum., ant-c., ant-s., ***apis***, arn., ***ars.***, ***ars-i.***, asaf., aur., bar-c., **BELL.**, bov., **BRY.**, ***calc.***, cann-s., ***canth.***, carb-an., carb-v., ***caust.***, cedr., cham., chin., cic., clem., cocc., colch., coll., con., **CROT-H.**, crot-t., cub., cupr., dig., dulc., euph., **EUPHR.**, ***ferr.***, ferr-p., ***fl-ac.***, **GELS.**, graph., guai., hell., ***hep.***, hydr., ign., ***iod.***, ***kali-bi.***, ***kali-i.***, ***lach.***, ***led.***, ***lyc.***, mag-c., mang., **MERC.**, **MERC-C.**, ***mur-ac.***, ***nat-c.***, ***nat-m.***, ***nit-ac.***, ***nux-v.***, ox-ac., ***petr.***, ph-ac., ***phos.***, ***phyt.***, plb., ***psor.***, **PULS.**, ran-b., **RHOD.**, **RHUS-T.**, ruta, sabin., ***samb.***, sang., sars., sec., **SEP.**, **SIL.**, spig., **SPONG.**, ***stann.***, ***stram.***, **SULPH.**, thuj., ***valer.***, zinc.

puffy - ***acon.***, ***agar.***, am-c., ***am-m.***, **ANT-C.**, **APIS**, ***apoc.***, arn., **ARS.**, ***asaf.***, aur., ***aur-m.***, bar-c., ***bell.***, ***bry.***, **CALC.**, **CAPS.**, ***carb-s.***, cedr., cham., chin., cina, cocc., colch., coloc., con., **CUPR.**, **DIG.**, dros., ***dulc.***, **FERR.**, **GRAPH.**, guai., **HELL.**, hyos., ***iod.***, ip., kali-c., kreos., lach., laur., led., ***lyc.***, mag-c., merc., mez., mosch., nat-c., ***nit-ac.***, nux-m., **OLND.**, op., phos., ***phyt.***, plb., ***puls.***, rheum, ***rhus-t.***, samb., sars., ***seneg.***, ***sep.***, sil., ***spig.***, spong., **SQUIL.**, staph., stram., ***sulph.***, ***teucr.***, verat., ***verb.***, zinc.

SYMPTOMS, and states, nature of

alternating, mental and physical symptoms - ***abrot.***, alum., ***arn.***, astra-e., aur., bell., **CARC.**, ***cimic.***, con., ***croc.***, ferr., **IGN.**, lach., ***lil-t.***, ***murx.***, ***nux-m.***, **PLAT.**, sabad., stram., ***sul-ac.***, tub.

alternating, physical states - abrot., acon., agar., aloe, ***ambr.***, arn., ***ars.***, bell., berb., ***cann-i.***, ***cann-s.***, **CARC.**, ***cimic.***, ***cocc.***, croc., cupr., dulc., ferr-p., glon., ***ign.***, iris, **KALI-BI.**, **LAC-C.**, lach., **LYC.**, onop., ***phos.***, prot., psor., ***puls.***, stram., sul-ac.,

SYMPTOMS, and states, nature of

alternating, physical states - **SULPH.**, valer., xan., zinc.

constantly, changing symptoms - **CARC.**, cimic., kali-bi., ***lac-c.***, **MED.**, mosch., **PULS.**, sanic., tub.

contradictory, and alternating states - ***abrot.***, ***aloe***, ambr., bell., bry., **CARC.**, cimic., croc., dulc., graph., **IGN.**, kali-bi., kali-c., lac-c., ***lyc.***, mosch., ***nat-m.***, ***plat.***, plb., **PULS.**, rhus-t., sanic., sep., ***staph.***, ***thuj.***, **TUB.**

rapidly - croc.

reaction, want of, with - valer.

many, symptoms - agar., **CARC.**, med., tub.

metastasis - **ABROT.**, agar., ***ant-c.***, apis, ***ars.***, asaf., cact., calc., ***calc-f.***, ***carb-v.***, **CARC.**, ***caul.***, ***cimic.***, colch., ***crot-t.***, ***cupr.***, dig., ***dulc.***, graph., hep., kali-bi., ***kalm.***, kreos., lac-c., ***lach.***, lith., lyc., mag-c., mang., med., merc., mez., ***nat-m.***, nat-p., ***nux-v.***, ***plat.***, ***puls.***, sang., ***senec.***, ***sep.***, sil., sulph., zinc.

sudden, manifestations of - **ACON.**, apis, ars., **BELL.**, coloc., con., cupr., hydr-ac., lyc., ***mag-ac.***, mag-c., mag-p., nat-s., phos., rad-br., tab., tarent., tarent-c., valer., verat.

changing about - ambr., bell., berb., cimic., dios., valer.

SYPHILIS, general - aethi-a., agn., ail., am-c., anac., anag., ***anan.***, ***ang.***, ant-c., ***ant-t.***, ***apis***, arg-i., arg-m., arg-n., arn., ***ars.***, ars-br., **ARS-I.**, ***ars-m.***, ***ars-s-f.***, ***asaf.***, asar., ***asc-t.***, astra-e., **AUR.**, ***aur-a.***, aur-i., **AUR-M.**, **AUR-M-N.**, aur-s., bad., bapt., bell., benz-ac., berb., ***berb-a.***, buni-o., cadm-met., ***calc-f.***, ***alc-i.***, ***calc-s.***, ***calo.***, ***carb-an.***, carb-v., ***caust.***, ***cean.***, ***chim.***, chin-a., chr-ox., ***cinnb.***, clem., cob-n., ***colch.***, ***con.***, convo-s., cop., cor-r., ***cory.***, crot-h., cund., cupr., cupr-s., dam., echi., ery-a., eryth., eucal., euph., ferr., ferr-i., ***fl-ac.***, franc., gels., ***graph.***, ***gua.***, guai., ham., hecla., ***hep.***, hip-ac., ***hippoz.***, hir., hydr., hydrc., iber., ***iod.***, ***iris***, ***jac.***, jac-c., jatr., jug-r., ***kali-ar.***, ***kali-bi.***, kali-br., kali-c., ***kali-chl.***, **KALI-I.**, ***kali-m.***, **KALI-S.**, ***kalm.***, ***kreos.***, ***lac-c.***, lac-d., ***lach.***, **LAUR.**, ***led.***, lith., ***lyc.***, maland., **MERC.**, **MERC-C.**, ***merc-d.***, **MERC-I-F.**, **MERC-I-R.**, ***merc-sul.***, ***mez.***, mill., nep., **NIT-AC.**, nux-v., osm., penic., petr., petros., ***ph-ac.***, ***phos.***, **PHYT.**, piloc., pituit., plat., ***plat-m.***, psor., reser., rhod., rhus-g., ***sabad.***, ***sang.***, ***sars.***, sec., sel., ***sep.***, **SIL.**, spong., ***staph.***, stict., **STILL.**, ***sul-i.***, ***sulph.***, **SYPH.**, ter., thala., thiop., ***thuj.***, thymol., ***thyr.***, vac., ***viol-t.***, xan.

congenital - ars-i., ars-m., ***aur.***, calc-f., ***calc-i.***, cor-r., kali-i., kreos., **MERC.**, ***merc-d.***, ***nit-ac.***, piloc., psor., syph.

TABES, mesenterica - ***ars.***, ars-i., ***aur.***, aur-m., ***bar-c.***, ***bar-i.***, ***bar-m.***, **CALC.**, ***calc-p.***, ***calc-s.***, ***carb-an.***, ***carb-s.***, caust., ***con.***, ***hep.***, ***iod.***, ***kreos.***, ***lyc.***, merc., merc-i-f., ***nat-s.***, ol-j., sulph., ***tub.***

TEMPERATURE, change of, (see Environment)

TENIAE - ***ail.***, arg-n., **CALC.**, ***carb-an.***, carb-s., ***carb-v.***, chin., cina, cupr., cupr-ac., cur., ***fil.***, ***form.***, frag-v., ***gran.***, ***graph.***, grat., kali-c., kali-i., mag-m., merc., ***nat-c.***, nat-s., nux-v., petr., phos., ***plat.***, ***puls.***, ***sabad.***, sant., ***sep.***, ***sil.***, ***stann.***, sulph., ter., thuj., valer.

TENSION, physical

externally - acon., agar., agn., aloe, ***alum.***, ambr., am-c., ***am-m.***, anac., ant-c., ant-t., arg-m., ***arg-n.***, ***arn.***, ars., ***asaf.***, asar., ***aur.***, **BAR-C.**, bar-m., ***bell.***, berb., bism., bor., bov., **BRY.**, calc., camph., cann-s., canth., caps., ***carb-an.***, carb-v., **CAUST.**, cham., ***chel.***, chin., cic., clem., cocc., colch., **COLOC.**, **CON.**, croc., crot-h., ***cupr.***, dig., dros., dulc., euph., euphr., ***ferr.***, glon., graph., guai., hell., hep., hyos., ign., iod., ip., kali-ar., ***kali-c.***, kali-n., kreos., lach., laur., ***led.***, lyc., mag-c., mag-m., mang., meny., ***merc.***, ***mez.***, ***mosch.***, mur-ac., ***nat-c.***, nat-m., nat-p., nit-ac., nux-m., ***nux-v.***, ***olnd.***, op., par., ***petr.***, ph-ac., **PHOS.**, **PLAT.**, plb., **PULS.**, ran-b., ***rheum***, rhod., **RHUS-T.**, ruta, sabad., ***sabin.***, samb., sars., ***sec.***, seneg., ***sep.***, sil., ***spig.***, ***spong.***, squil., stann., ***staph.***, stram., **STRONT-C.**, **SULPH.**, sul-ac., tarax., teucr., ***thuj.***, valer., verat., **VERB.**, ***viol-o.***, viol-t., ***zinc.***

internally - acon., aesc., agar., agn., alum., ambr., am-m., anac., ant-c., ***ant-t.***, arg-m., arn., ***ars.***, **ASAF.**, asar., ***aur.***, bar-c., **BELL.**, ***berb.***, bov., bry., ***calc.***, camph., cann-s., ***caps.***, ***carb-ac.***, carb-an., carb-v., ***caust.***, cham., chel., chin., ***cic.***, ***clem.***, cocc., coc-c., coff., colch., ***coloc.***, com., con., croc., crot-t., cupr., cycl., dig., dros., ***dulc.***, euph., euphr., ferr., gels., ***glon.***, ***graph.***, guai., hell., hep., hydr-ac., ***hyper.***, hyos., ign., iod., ip., kali-c., ***kali-n.***, kreos., lach., laur., led., lob., **LYC.**, mag-c., mag-m., mang., meny., ***merc.***, mez., ***mosch.***, mur-ac., naja, nat-c., nat-m., ***nit-ac.***, nux-m., **NUX-V.**, olnd., ***op.***, osm., **PAR.**, petr., ph-ac., **PHOS.**, plat., plb., **PULS.**, **RAN-B.**, ran-s., ***rheum***, rhod., ***rhus-t.***, ruta, sabad., sabin., samb., sec., seneg., **SEP.**, sil., ***spig.***, spong., squil., ***stann.***, ***staph.***, ***stram.***, **STRONT-C.**, **SULPH.**, sul-ac., tab., tarax., teucr., thuj., valer., ***verat.***, verb., ***zinc.***

tremulous - petr.

TETANUS, lockjaw, (see Emergency)

THROMBOSIS, (see Blood)

THUNDERSTORM, (see Environment, Storms)

TIME, general

afternoon - acon., aeth., ***agar.***, all-c., ***aloe***, ***alum.***, **ALUM-P.**, alum-sil., ***ambr.***, ***am-c.***, ***am-m.***, anac., ***ang.***, ***ant-c.***, ant-t., ***apis***, ***arg-m.***, ***arg-n.***, arn., ***ars.***, ars-i., ***ars-s-f.***, ***asaf.***, ***asar.***, aur., aur-a., aur-i., aur-s., aza., bar-c., bar-i., ***bar-m.***, bar-s., **BELL.**, ***bism.***, bor., ***bov.***, ***bry.***, buth-a., cact., calad., calc., calc-i., ***calc-p.***, calc-sil., camph., cann-s., ***canth.***, caps., carb-an., carb-s., carb-v., caust., cedr., ***cench.***, cham., ***chel.***, chin., ***cic.***, ***cimic.***, cina, cocc., coc-c., coff., colch., ***coloc.***, con., croc., cycl., cyn-d., cyt-l., ***dig.***, dios., dros., ***dulc.***, ***euphr.***, eys., fago., ferr., ferr-ar., ferr-i., ferr-m., ferr-p., ***fl-ac.***, gels., graph., grat., guai., hell., hep., hip-ac., hyos., ***ign.***, iod., ip., kali-ar., ***kali-bi.***, kali-c., kali-cy., kali-m., **KALI-N.**, kali-p., kali-sil., kreos., lach., ***laur.***, ***led.***, lil-t., lob., **LYC.**, mag-c., mag-m., ***mang.***, meli., meny., ***merc.***, mez., ***mosch.***, ***mur-ac.***, nat-a., ***nat-c.***, ***nat-m.***, nicc., ***nit-ac.***, nux-m., ***nux-v.***, ***ol-an.***, op., par., petr., ***ph-ac.***, ***phys.***, phyt., plan., plat., plb., ***ptel.***, **PULS.**, ***ran-b.***, ran-s., rheum, rhod., **RHUS-T.**, ***rumx.***, ruta, sabad., sabin., sal-ac., ***sang.***, ***sars.***, ***sel.***, ***seneg.***, **SEP.**, **SIL.**, **SIN-N.**, spig., ***spong.***, squil., stann., ***staph.***, ***still.***, sul-i., ***sulph.***, sul-ac., tarax., ***teucr.***, thiop., **THUJ.**, til., upa., ***valer.***, ***ven-m.***, verat., verb., ***viol-t.***, wye., x-ray, xero, **ZINC.**, **ZINC-P.**

1 p.m. - arg-m., ***ars.***, cact., chel., cina, grat., kali-c., ***lach.***, mag-c., phos., ***puls.***

1 p.m. to 2 p.m. - ars.

1 p.m. to 9 p.m. - chel.

2 p.m. - ars., calc., chel., cur., ***eup-per.***, ferr., gels., hell., lach., lob., mag-p., nit-ac., ol-an., puls., sang.

2 p.m., 3 p.m. or 4 p.m. till morning - syph.

3 p.m. - ***ang.***, ant-t., ***apis***, ars., asaf., asar., **BELL.**, bry., cedr., cench., chel., ***chin-s.***, clem., con., nat-m., samb., sang., sil., staph., sulph., ***thuj.***

3 p.m. to 5 p.m. - sep., thuj.

3 p.m. to 6 p.m. - apis.

3 p.m. to 3 a.m. - bell.

4 p.m. - ***aesc.***, alum., anac., ***apis***, ars., arum-t., cact., calc-p., carb-v., ***caust.***, ***cedr.***, chel., ***chin-s.***, cob., ***coloc.***, gels., ***hell.***, hep., ip., kali-c., lachn., **LYC.**, mag-m., mang., merc-sul., mur-ac., nat-m., nat-s., nit-ac., ***nux-v.***, puls., rhus-t., stront-c., sulph., verb.

4 p.m. to 5 p.m. - allox., merc-sul.

4 p.m. to 6 p.m. - alum., eys., gels., lyc., **SEP.**

4 p.m. to 7 p.m. - coloc., ***lyc.***

4 p.m. to 8 p.m. - alum., bov., buth-a., chin-s., coloc., ***hell.***, **LYC.**, mag-m., nux-m., sabad., sulph., zinc.

4 p.m. to 10 p.m. - alum., chel., plat.

4 p.m. to 4 a.m. - thuj.

5 p.m. - alum., bov., caust., cedr., ***chin.***, cimic., ***coloc.***, con., ***gels.***, ***hep.***, hyper., kali-c., ***lyc.***, nat-m., ***nux-v.***, **PULS.**, ***rhus-t.***, sulph., **THUJ.**, tub., valer.

5 p.m. to 6 p.m. - ange-s., methys., scirr.

5 p.m. to 8 p.m. - ***lil-t.***

amel. - cinnb., hecla., kali-c., ***nat-s.***, phyt., rhus-t., ***sep.***

evening, and afternoon - kali-c.

TIME, general

daytime - ***agar.***, ***alum.***, am-c., am-m., arg-m., arg-n., calc., caust., cimic., ***euphr.***, ***ferr.***, guai., lac-d., lach., ***med.***, ***nat-a.***, nat-c., ***nat-m.***, ***nit-ac.***, nux-v., phos., ***puls.***, ***rhus-t.***, ***sang.***, **SEP.**, **STANN.**, **SULPH.**

amel. - acon., ***agar.***, arn., bry., cham., cob-n., ***cycl.***, helon., ***jal.***, kali-c., ***mag-p.***, merc., nat-p., nat-s., ***petr.***, sep., syph.

sunrise till sunset - ***med.***

evening - abrot., ***acon.***, aeth., agar., agn., alf., ***all-c.***, aloe, **ALUM.**, alum-sil., alumn., am-br., **AMBR.**, **AM-C.**, ***am-m.***, ***anac.***, ***ang.***, **ANT-C.**, **ANT-T.**, apis, ***arg-m.***, ***arg-n.***, **ARN.**, ***ars.***, ***ars-i.***, ars-s-f., ***asaf.***, ***asar.***, aur., aur-a., aur-i., ***aur-s.***, ***bapt.***, ***bar-c.***, bar-i., bar-m., bar-s., **BELL.**, berb., berb-a., bism., ***bor.***, ***bov.***, ***brom.***, **BRY.**, bufo, buth-a., caj., ***calad.***, **CALC.**, calc-ar., ***calc-i.***, calc-p., ***calc-s.***, **CALC-SIL.**, camph., cann-s., canth., **CAPS.**, **CARB-AN.**, **CARB-V.**, **CARB-S.**, carc., **CAUST.**, cedr., ***cench.***, **CHAM.**, chel., chin., chlorpr., cic., ***cimic.***, cina, clem., ***cocc.***, coff., **COLCH.**, ***coloc.***, com., ***con.***, ***croc.***, crot-h., cupr., ***cupr-s.***, **CYCL.**, cyn-d., cyt-l., dig., dios., dirc., dros., ***dulc.***, euon-a., **EUPHR.**, eys., ***ferr.***, ***ferr-ar.***, ***ferr-i.***, ***ferr-p.***, ***fl-ac.***, flor-p., form., ***gamb.***, ***graph.***, ***guai.***, hecla., **HELL.**, ***hep.***, **HYOS.**, ***ign.***, ***iod.***, ***ip.***, iris, jatr., ***kali-ar.***, ***kali-bi.***, ***kali-c.***, ***kali-i.***, kali-m., **KALI-N.**, ***kali-p.***, ***kali-s.***, kali-sil., ***kalm.***, kreos., **LACH.**, ***laur.***, ***led.***, ***lil-t.***, **LYC.**, **MAG-C.**, ***mag-m.***, ***mang.***, **MENY.**, meph., **MERC.**, merc-c., ***merc-i-r.***, **MEZ.**, mosch., mur-ac., ***nat-a.***, ***nat-c.***, ***nat-m.***, **NAT-P.**, ***nat-sil.***, nep., nicc., **NIT-AC.**, ***nux-m.***, ***nux-v.***, olnd., op., osm., ***ox-ac.***, ***par.***, penic., ***petr.***, **PH-AC.**, **PHOS.**, phyt., pic-ac., pituin., plan., **PLAT.**, **PLB.**, ***psor.***, ***ptel.***, **PULS.**, ***ran-b.***, **RAN-S.**, rheum, ***rhod.***, ***rhus-t.***, **RUMX.**, **RUTA**, sabad., ***sabin.***, sal-ac., ***samb.***, ***sang.***, ***sars.***, sel., ***seneg.***, **SEP.**, **SIL.**, **SIN-N.**, spig., ***spong.***, squil., **STANN.**, staph., stict., **STRONT-C.**, ***sul-i.***, **SULPH.**, **SUL-AC.**, ***sumb.***, ***syph.***, ***tab.***, tarax., tarent., teucr., thiop., ***thuj.***, trio., upa., **VALER.**, verat., verb., vib., viol-o., viol-t., x-ray, **ZINC.**, **ZINC-P.**

6 p.m. - alum., ang., ant-t., arg-m., bapt., calc., calc-p., caust., ***cedr.***, cupr-ac., dig., hep., hyper., ***kali-c.***, kali-i., lachn., laur., nat-m., **NUX-V.**, petr., ***puls.***, ***rhus-t.***, ***sep.***, ***sil.***, ***sumb.***

6 p.m. to 7 p.m. - carc., culx., ***hep.***

6 p.m. to 8 p.m. - rauw.

6 p.m. to 10 p.m. - kali-c.

6 p.m. to 4 a.m. - guai.

6 p.m. to 6 a.m. - kreos., lil-t., ***syph.***

7 p.m. - alum., ant-c., bov., cedr., chin-s., culx., ferr., gamb., gels., ***hep.***, ip., ***lyc.***, nat-m., ***nat-s.***, ***nux-v.***, petr., puls., pyrog., rhus-t., ***sep.***, sulph., tarent.

8 p.m. - alum., ***bov.***, caust., coff., elaps, hep., mag-c., merc., merc-i-r., phos., ***rhus-t.***, **SULPH.**, tarax.

TIME, general

evening,

8 p.m. to 3 a.m. - syph.

9 p.m. - ars., ***bov.***, **BRY.**, calc., ***gels.***, merc., mur-ac., sulph.

9 p.m., amel. - med.

amel. in general - ***agar.***, ***alum.***, aran-ix., arn., arg-m., asaf., **AUR.**, bor., brucin., cast., chel., cob-n., cortiso., halo., hed., kali-n., lob., lyc., mag-c., ***med.***, nat-m., nicc., nux-v., podo., ***puls.***, ***sep.***, stel., thyr., visc.

4 p.m. till going to bed - alum.

eating, after - indg., petr.

eating, amel. - ***sep.***, upa.

every other evening - ***puls.***

lying down after, agg. - ars., graph., hep., ***ign.***, ***led.***, ***merc.***, ***phos.***, puls., sel., stront-c., ***sulph.***, thuj.

amel. - kali-n.

night, and - cench., lil-t., mag-c.

open air agg. - ***am-c.***, carb-an., carb-v., ***merc.***, nit-ac., sulph.

sleep, before going to - ***plat.***

sunset, agg. - aur., kreos., ***merc.***, phyt., ***syph.***

after - ang., bry., ign., lycps., merc., phyt., ***puls.***, rhus-t., syph.

after, amel. - coca, lil-t., med., sel.

amel. - coca, lil-t., med., sel.

till sunrise - ***aur.***, cimic., colch., ***merc.***, phyt., **SYPH.**

twilight, agg. - ***am-m.***, ang., arg-n., ***ars.***, ars-s-f., berb., ***calc.***, ***caust.***, cham., dig., graph., mang., nat-m., nat-s., ***phos.***, plat., plb., **PULS.**, rhus-t., staph., sul-ac., valer.

amel. - alum., bry., meny., ***phos.***, tab., tub.

forenoon - aloe, alum., alum-p., ***alumn.***, ambr., am-c., am-m., anac., ang., ant-c., ant-t., aran., ***arg-m.***, arg-n., ars., ars-s-f., asaf., aur., aur-a., aur-s., bar-c., bar-m., ***bar-s.***, bell., bor., bov., ***bry.***, cact., calc., calc-sil., **CANN-I.**, **CANN-S.**, canth., carb-an., carb-s., ***carb-v.***, caust., cedr., cham., chel., chin., cocc., coloc., con., cupr., cycl., dros., dulc., euph., euphr., ferr., ***fl-ac.***, graph., ***guai.***, halo., hell., ***hep.***, ign., ip., kali-ar., kali-c., kali-m., kali-n., kali-p., kali-sil., kreos., lach., ***laur.***, lyc., mag-c., mag-m., ***mang.***, merc., mez., mosch., mur-ac., ***nat-a.***, **NAT-C.**, **NAT-M.**, nat-p., ***nat-sil.***, nit-ac., ***nux-m.***, nux-v., par., ***pareir.***, petr., ph-ac., plat., plb., **PODO.**, puls., ***ran-b.***, rhod., ***rhus-t.***, rumx., **SABAD.**, ***sars.***, ***sec.***, sel., seneg., **SEP.**, ***sil.***, ***spig.***, spong., **STANN.**, ***staph.***, ***stram.***, stront-c., **SULPH.**, **SUL-AC.**, ***tarax.***, ***teucr.***, valer., verat., verb., ***viol-t.***, zinc., zinc-p.

9 a.m. - bry., ***cham.***, ***eup-per.***, kali-bi., kali-c., lac-c., nat-m., nux-v., podo., sep., sumb., ***verb.***

9 a.m. to 11 a.m. - stann.

9 a.m. to 2 p.m. - nat-m.

TIME, general

forenoon,

10 a.m. - ***ars.,*** bor., chin., chin-s., cimic., eup-per., gels., ***iod.,*** meli., **NAT-M.,** nux-v., petr., ***phos., rhus-t.,*** sep., sil., ***stann., sulph.,*** thuj.

10 a.m. to 11 a.m. agg. - gels., ***nat-m., sep.,*** sulph.

10 a.m. to 3 p.m. agg. - tub.

11 a.m. - arg-m., arg-n., ars., arum-t., asaf., asar., bapt., berb., cact., ***chin-s.,*** cimic., cob., cocc., ***gels.,*** hydr., hyos., ind., ip., lach., mag-p., nat-c., **NAT-M.,** nat-p., ***nux-v., phos.,*** phyt., puls., ***rhus-t., sep., stann.,*** **SULPH.,** ***zinc.***

amel. - ***alum.,*** lil-t., **LYC.,** nat-sil.

midnight - **ACON.,** aran., arg-n., ***ars.,*** ars-i., brom., calad., calc., canth., ***caust.,*** chin., dig., ***dros., ferr.,*** hed., kali-ar., kali-c., lach., lyc., ***mag-m.,*** mez., ***mur-ac.,*** nat-m., nux-m., nux-v., op., phos., puls., ***rhus-t., samb.,*** spong., stram., sulph., verat., zinc.

after - acon., alum., alum-p., alum-sil., ambr., am-m., ***ang.,*** ant-c., ant-t., apis, arist-cl., **ARS.,** ***ars-i.,*** asaf., aur., bar-c., bar-i., bar-m., bar-s., bell., bor., ***bry.,*** calad., ***calc., calc-i., calc-sil., cann-s.,*** canth., caps., ***carb-an.,*** carb-v., caust., cham., ***chel.,*** chin., cocc., coc-c., coff., con., croc., ***cupr.,*** **DROS.,** dulc., euph., euphr., ***ferr., ferr-ar.,*** ferr-i., ferr-p., ***gels.,*** graph., hed., hell., hep., ***ign.,*** iod., **KALI-C.,** kali-m., **KALI-N.,** kali-p., ***kali-sil.,*** lyc., ***mag-c.,*** man., ***mang., merc., mez.,*** mur-ac., **NAT-A.,** nat-c., nat-m., nat-p., nat-s., nat-sil., nit-ac., **NUX-V.,** par., ***ph-ac.,*** **PHOS.,** phyt., plat., **PODO.,** ***puls.,*** ran-b., ***ran-s.,*** rhod., **RHUS-T.,** rumx., sabad., sabin., ***samb.,*** sars., seneg., sep., **SIL.,** spig., ***spong., squil.,*** staph., stram., sul-i., ***sulph.,*** sul-ac., tarax., **THUJ.,** viol-o.

after, amel. - **LYC.,** man., nat-p., nat-s.

before - alum., alum-p., ambr., am-m., anac., ***ang., ant-t.,*** apis, **ARG-N.,** arn., **ARS.,** ars-s-f., asar., ***bell.,*** brom., ***bry., calad.,*** cann-s., caps., **CARB-V.,** ***carb-s., caust.,*** **CHAM.,** chel., chin., **COFF.,** colch., ***cupr.,*** cycl., dulc., ferr., ferr-ar., ***fl-ac., graph., hep.,*** ign., **KALI-AR.,** kali-c., kali-m., ***lach.,*** **LED., LYC.,** mag-c., ***mang., merc., mez.,*** mosch., ***mur-ac.,*** nat-m., nat-p., nat-s., ***nit-ac.,*** nux-v., osm., petr., **PHOS.,** phyt., plat., ***psor.,*** **PULS.,** ***ran-b.,*** **RAN-S.,** rhod., ***rhus-t.,*** **RUMX.,** ***ruta,*** **SABAD.,** samb., ***sep., spig., spong.,*** **STANN.,** ***staph., stront-c.,*** sulph., teucr., thuj., ***valer.,*** verat., viol-t.

until, 4 a.m. - thuj.

until, noon - ***ars.,*** cist., puls.

TIME, general

morning - ***abies-n.,*** abrot., absin., ***acal., acon.,*** aesc., **AGAR.,** agn., all-c., ***aloe, alum.,*** **ALUM-P.,** alumn., ***ambr.,*** am-c., **AM-M.,** ***anac., ang., ant-c., ant-t., apis,*** aran., aran-ix., **ARG-M.,** ***arg-n.,*** arist-cl., ***arn., ars.,*** **ARS-I.,** ***ars-s-f.,*** asaf., asar., **AUR.,** aur-a., aur-i., **AUR-S.,** ***bapt., bar-c., bar-i., bar-m., bar-s.,*** bell., benz-ac., ***berb.,*** bism., ***bor., bov.,*** **BRY.,** bufo, cadm-m., calad., **CALC.,** calc-i., **CALC-P.,** ***calc-sil.,*** cann-i., cann-s., ***canth., caps.,*** **CARB-AN., CARB-S., CARB-V.,** ***cast., caust.,*** **CHAM., CHEL.,** chin., ***chr-ac.,*** cic., cimic., **CINA,** ***cinnb., cist.,*** clem., cob., cob-n., ***coca, cocc.,*** coc-c., cod., ***coff.,*** colch., coloc., ***con.,*** convo-s., corn., cortico., cortiso., **CROC.,** crot-h., crot-t., cupr., cycl., ***dig., dios., dros., dulc.,*** echi., elaps, erig., ***eup-per.,*** euph., ***euphr., ferr., ferr-ar.,*** ferr-i., ***ferr-p., fl-ac.,*** form., ***gamb., gels.,*** gran., ***graph.,*** grat., ***guai.,*** harp., hed., hell., ***hep., hydr.,*** hydroph., hyos., ***ign.,*** iod., ip., iris, ***kali-ar.,*** **KALI-BI.,** ***kali-c., kali-i.,*** kali-m., **KALI-N.,** ***kali-p.,*** kali-sil., ***kalm., kreos.,*** lac-c., **LACH.,** laur., led., lept., lil-t., lith., lob., lyc., mag-arct., ***mag-c.,*** mag-f., ***mag-m.,*** mag-s., magn-gr., mang., med., meny., meph., ***merc.,*** merc-c., ***merc-i-f.,*** mez., mosch., mur-ac., ***naja,*** **NAT-A.,** ***nat-c.,*** **NAT-M.,** ***nat-n., nat-p.,*** **NAT-S.,** nat-sil., nicc., **NIT-AC.,** nuph., ***nux-m.,*** **NUX-V.,** oci-s., olnd., **ONOS.,** ***op.,*** ox-ac., par., pareir., perh., **PETR., PH-AC., PHOS.,** ***phyt.,*** pic-ac., ***plan., plat.,*** plb., **PODO.,** ***psor.,*** ptel., **PULS.,** ***ran-b.,*** ran-s., ***rheum,*** **RHOD., RHUS-T., RUMX.,** ruta, sabad., ***sabin., sal-ac.,*** samb., ***sang., sars.,*** sec., ***sel., senec., seneg.,*** **SEP.,** ***sil.,*** **SPIG.,** spong., **SQUIL.,** ***stann., staph.,*** stel., ***stram.,*** stront-c., stry., **SUL-AC.,** sul-i., **SULPH.,** tab., ***tarax.,*** tell., teucr., ***thuj.,*** **TUB.,** upa., **VALER.,** ***verat., verat-v.,*** ven-m., verb., viol-o., viol-t., visc., ***zinc., zinc-p.***

5 a.m. - aloe, apis, bov., ***chin.,*** cob., dros., helon., ***kali-c.,*** kali-i., nat-c., ***nat-m.,*** nat-p., ph-ac., ***podo.,*** rumx., sep., sil., ***sulph.***

6 a.m. - aloe, ***alum.,*** arn., bov., calc-p., ferr., ***hep.,*** lyc., ***nux-v.,*** ox-ac., sep., sil., sulph., verat.

7 a.m. - eup-per., ***hep.,*** nat-c., ***nux-v.,*** podo., sep.

8 a.m. - ***eup-per.,*** nux-v.

9 a.m. - bry., ***cham., eup-per.,*** kali-bi., kali-c., lac-c., nat-m., nux-v., podo., sep., sumb., ***verb.***

9 a.m. to 11 a.m. - stann.

9 a.m. to 2 p.m. - nat-m.

afternoon, and - sars.

amel. - acon., am-m., ambr., cench., jug-c., merc., phos., sang., still., xero, zinc.

bed, in - aloe, ***am-m., ambr.,*** bry., con., ***kali-c., lyc., nux-v.,*** phos., sep., ***sulph.***

daybreak amel. - colch., syph.

TIME, general

morning,

evening, and - alum., bov., ***calc.,*** caust., coc-c., ***graph.,*** guai., ***kali-c.,*** lach., ***lyc., phos.,*** psor., ***rhus-t.,*** sang., **SEP.,** ***stram., stront-c., thuj.,*** verat., zinc.

morning of one day and afternoon of next - eup-per., lac-c.

night, and - iod., nat-c.

sunrise agg., after - cham., ***nux-v.,*** puls., syph.

sunrise agg., before - lyc.

night - abel., abrot., acet-ac., **ACON.,** agar., agn., agre., aloe, alum., **ALUM-P.,** alum-sil., alumn., ambr., ***am-br.,*** am-c., ***am-m., ammc.,*** anac., ***ang., ant-c., ant-t.,*** apis, apoc., ***aral.,*** aran., arg-m., **ARG-N.,** arist-cl., **ARN., ARS., ARS-I., ARS-S-F.,** ***asaf.,*** asar., aster., ***aur.,*** aur-a., aur-i., aur-m., **AUR-S.,** bac., ***bar-c.,*** bar-i., ***bar-m., bar-s., bell.,*** benz-ac., berb-a., bism., bor., ***bov., brom., bry.,*** bufo, buni-o., but-ac., cact., caj., calad., **CALC., CALC-I., CALC-P., CALC-S., CALC-SIL.,** ***camph., cann-i., cann-s., canth., caps.,*** carb-ac., **CARB-AN., CARB-S.,** ***carb-v., caust.,*** cedr., ***cench.,*** **CHAM.,** ***chel.,*** **CHIN.,** chin-a., chion., cic., cimic., cina, **CINNB.,** clem., ***cocc.,*** coc-c., ***cod.,*** **COFF., COLCH.,** ***coloc.,*** com., **CON.,** convo-s., ***croc.,*** crot-c., ***crot-h.,*** crot-t., ***cupr.,*** **CYCL.,** cyt-l., ***dig.,*** dios., dol., ***dros.,*** **DULC.,** elaps, erig., eucal., ***euphr., equis.,*** **FERR., FERR-AR.,** ***ferr-p.,*** **FERR-I.,** ***fl-ac.,*** flav., ***gamb.,*** **GRAPH.,** grat., guai., hed., ***hell.,*** **HEP., HYOS.,** ***ign.,*** **IOD., IP.,** iris, jal., **KALI-AR., KALI-BI.,** ***kali-br.,*** **KALI-C., KALI-I.,** ***kali-m.,*** kali-n., ***kali-p., kali-sil.,*** kalm., kreos., **LACH.,** laur., ***led.,*** **LIL-T.,** lob., ***lyc.,*** **MAG-C., MAG-M.,** mag-p., man., **MANG.,** meny., meph., **MERC.,** ***merc-c., merc-i-f., mez.,*** mosch., ***mur-ac., nat-a., nat-c., nat-m., nat-p., nat-s., nat-sil.,*** nep., **NIT-AC.,** ***nux-m., nux-v., olnd., op., ox-ac.,*** par., pareir., ***per., ph-ac.,*** phenob., **PHOS.,** ***phyt., pic-ac.,*** plat., **PLB., PSOR., PULS.,** pyrog., ran-b., ran-s., rat., ***rheum,*** rhod., **RHUS-T., RUMX.,** ruta, ***sabad.,*** sabin., sal-ac., ***samb.,*** sang., sarcol-ac., ***sars., sec., sel.,*** senec., seneg., **SEP.,** sieg., **SIL.,** sin-n., ***spig., spong.,*** squil., ***stann., staph.,*** stict., still., stram., **STRONT-C., SUL-I., SULPH.,** ***sul-ac.,*** syph., tarax., tarent., **TELL.,** ter., teucr., thal., thea., ther., ***thuj.,*** trio., valer., verat., vib., ***viol-t.,*** vip., visc., x-ray, **ZINC., ZINC-P.**

10 p.m. - ***ars., bov.,*** cham., **CHIN-S.,** ***graph.,*** ign., lach., petr., podo., puls.

11 p.m. - aral., ars., bell., ***cact.,*** calc., carb-an., lach., rumx., sil., sulph.

1 a.m. - **ARS.,** carb-v., caul., cocc., lachn., mag-m., mur-ac., psor.

1 a.m. to 2 a.m. - ***ars.***

1 a.m. to 3 a.m. - ***kali-ar.***

TIME, general

night,

2 a.m. - all-c., aur-m., benz-ac., ***caust.,*** com., cur., dros., ferr., graph., ***hep., kali-bi., kali-br.,*** **KALI-C.,** kali-p., lach., lachn., lyc., mag-c., mez., nat-m., nat-s., ***nit-ac.,*** ptel., ***puls.,*** ric., rumx., sars., ***sil.,*** spig., sulph.

2 a.m. to 3 a.m. - gink-b., kali-bi.

2 a.m. to 4 a.m. - arist-cl., **KALI-C.,** med.

2 a.m. to 5 a.m. - aesc., aeth., ***aloe,*** am-c., bac., bell., bell-p., chel., cina, coc-c., cur., hed., ***kali-bi., kali-c.,*** kali-cy., kali-p., nat-s., ***nux-v.,*** ox-ac., ***podo.,*** ptel., rhod., ***rumx.,*** sulph., thuj., tub.

3 a.m. - ***am-c., am-m.,*** ant-c., ant-t., ***ars.,*** bapt., bor., ***bry.,*** calc., canth., ***cedr.,*** chin., con., euphr., dulc., ferr., hed., iris, ***kali-ar.,*** kali-bi., **KALI-C.,** kali-n., kali-p., ***mag-c.,*** mag-f., mag-m., ***nat-m.,*** nux-v., podo., ***rhus-t.,*** sec., ***sel.,*** sep., sil., staph., ***sulph., thuj.,*** zinc.

3 a.m. to 4 a.m. - aeth., am-m., arist-cl., caust., kali-bi., kali-c., med., nux-v.

3 a.m. to 5 a.m. - bor., calc-f., mag-c., man., syph.

4 a.m. - ***alum.,*** alumn., ***am-m.,*** anac., ***apis, arn., bor., caust.,*** **CEDR.,** chel., coloc., ***con.,*** cycl., ferr., mag-c., ***mur-ac., nat-s.,*** nit-ac., **NUX-V.,** penic., podo., ***puls.,*** rad-br., sep., sil., stann., ***sulph.,*** verat.

4 a.m. to 4 p.m. - kali-cy., **MED.,** nux-v.

5 a.m. - bov., cob., helon., kali-i., ***podo.***

6 a.m. - aloe, calc-p., ox-ac., sep., sil., sulph., verat.

amel. - alum., ang., arg-m., caust., cupr-ac., laur., man., med., petr.

every other night - ***puls.***

night air agg. - am-c., carb-v., merc., nat-s., nit-ac., ***sulph.***

noon - alum., ant-c., apis, **ARG-M.,** arg-n., ars., bol., brucin., carb-v., cham., chel., chin., cic., coloc., elaps, ***eup-per.,*** gels., kali-bi., kali-c., lach., mag-c., ***nat-m., nux-m., nux-v.,*** paeon., phos., sang., ***sel.,*** sep., ***sil.,*** spig., ***stram.,*** sulph., ***valer.,*** verb., ***zinc.***

noon till midnight - lach.

eating, after - grat., halo., ***mag-m., nat-c.,*** nux-m., valer.

symptoms increasing till noon, then decreasing - acon., ***arg-n.,*** bry., echi., gels., glon., kali-bi., ***kalm.,*** nat-m., nux-v., ***sang.,*** sanic., spig., stann., stram., stront-c., sulph.

periodicity, of symptoms or complaints - acon., ***agar.,*** aloe, **ALUM.,** alum-sil., **ALUMN.,** am-br., ambr., ***anac., ant-c.,*** ant-t., aran., **ARG-M.,** aran., ***arn.,*** **ARS.,** ars-m., ars-s-f., ***asar., bar-c.,*** bell., benz-ac., bov., bry., bufo, ***cact., calc.,*** calc-sil., cann-s., ***canth., caps., carb-v.,*** **CARB-S.,** carl., **CEDR.,** cent., chel., **CHIN., CHIN-A., CHIN-S.,** chr-ac., cina, clem., cocc., colch., croc., crot-h., cupr., dros.,

TIME, general

periodicity, of symptoms or complaints - ***eucal., eup-per.,*** ferr., ferr-ar., ***gels.,*** graph., hep., ***ign.,*** **IP.,** ***kali-ar.,*** kali-bi., kali-c., kali-n., lac-d., ***lach.,*** lact., lil-t., ***lyc., mag-c.,*** mag-s., meny., merc., nat-a., **NAT-M.,** nat-n., ***nat-s.,*** nicc., nicc-s., **NIT-AC.,** ***nux-v.,*** petr., ***phos., plb.,*** prim-o., ***puls.,*** ran-s., ***rhod., rhus-t.,*** rhus-v., ***sabad.,*** samb., ***sang.,*** sec., senec., **SEP., SIL.,** ***spig., stann., staph.,*** sul-ac., ***sulph.,*** tarent., ***tela,*** thal., ***tub.,*** urt-u., valer., ***verat.,*** vip., zinc.

alternate days - alum., chin., lyc., nat-c., nat-m., nux-v., puls.

annually - am-c., ***ant-t.,*** **ARS.,** buth-a., carb-v., carc., cench., crot-h., echi., elaps, gels., kali-bi., ***lach.,*** lyc., naja, nat-m., nicc., psor., rhus-r., ***rhus-t.,*** rhus-v., sulph., tarent., thuj., ***urt-u.,*** vip.

complaints return at same hour - ant-c., ***aran.,*** ars., bov., ***cact.,*** **CEDR.,** cench., chin., ***chin-s.,*** cina, cocc., ign., ip., kali-bi., kali-br., lyc., nat-m., ***sabad.,*** sel., tarent., tub., verb.

neuralgia every day at same hour - cedr., **KALI-BI.,** sulph.

daily - ***aran.,*** ars., caps., ip., nux-v., puls.

every other day - ***alum.,*** anac., ars., calc., cham., ***chin.,*** chin-s., crot-h., fl-ac., ***ip.,*** lyc., lycps., nat-c., nat-m., nit-ac., nux-v., oxyt., psor., puls.

evening - ***puls.***

morning - ***alumn.***

exact - aran., ars., cedr., chin-s., nat-m., tarent.

forty-two days - ***mag-m.***

fourteenth day - am-m., **ARS.,** ars-m., bufo, ***calc.,*** canth., chel., ***chin.,*** chin-s., ***con., ign.,*** kali-br., **LACH.,** nicc., phyt., plan., psor., ***puls.,*** sang., sulph.

fourth day - ars., aur., eup-per., kali-br., lyc., puls., sabad.

half year, every - lach., sep.

regular intervals, complaints return at - **CARB-S.**

seventh day - am-m., ars., ars-h., aur-m., canth., cedr., ***chin.,*** croc., eup-per., gels., ***iris,*** lac-d., lyc., nux-m., phos., plan., rhus-t., sabad., sang., sil., **SULPH.,** tell., tub.

tenth day - kali-p., lach., phos.

third day - anac., aur., chin-s., kali-ar., kali-br.

pregnancy, in - ***lyc., mag-c.***

twenty-eighth day - mag-c., ***nux-m.,*** **NUX-V.,** puls., **SEP.,** tub.

twenty-first day - ant-c., ars., ars-m., ***aur., chin-s., mag-c.,*** psor., sulph., ***tarent., tub.***

TINEA, general

tinea, capitis, favosa - aethi-a., agar., ars., ars-i., ***brom.,*** calc., calc-i., ***calc-mur.,*** calc-s., ***dulc.,*** ferr-i., graph., ***hep.,*** jug-r., ***kali-c.,*** kali-s., lappa-a., ***lyc.,*** med., ***mez.,*** nit-ac., olnd.,

TINEA, general

tinea, capitis, favosa - phos., ***sep., sil.,*** sul-ac., sulph., ust., vinc., ***viol-t.***

tinea, circinate - aesc., ant-c., calc., graph., hep., lyc., merc., mez., psor., rhus-t., sep., sulph., thuj.,

tinea tonsurans - ant-c., ant-t., ***ars., bac.,*** calc., calc-i., ***chrysar.,*** graph., hep., jug-c., jug-r., kali-s., lyc., mez., nat-m., petr., psor., puls., rhus-t., semp., ***sep.,*** sulph., ***tell.,*** thuj., tub., viol-t.

tinea, versicolor - ars., ars-i., bac., calc., carb-an., carb-v., chrysar., kali-s., mez., ***nat-a.,*** nit-ac., phos., phyt., psor., ***sep.,*** sil., sulph., tell., **THUJ.**

TORPOR - ammc., apis, asaf., berb., ***cic., crot-h.,*** cupr., dros., ***gels., hyos., iod.,*** kali-bi., kali-br., kali-s., led., lepi., lob., ***lyc., mag-m., merc-c.,*** **NAT-M., NUX-M., OP.,** ***plb.,*** polyg., ***puls.,*** sang., sil., ***stram.,*** vip.

TOUCH, general

agg. - ***acon., aesc.,*** **AGAR.,** ***agn.,*** aloe, ambr., am-c., am-m., anac., ***ant-c., ant-t.,*** **APIS, ARG-M.,** ***arn., ars.,*** **ASAF.,** asar., aur., bar-c., **BELL.,** bor., bov., **BRY.,** ***cact.,*** calad., calc., calc-p., camph., ***cann-s., canth., caps.,*** carb-an., ***carb-v.,*** caust., **CHAM.,** ***chel.,*** **CHIN.,** ***chin-a.,*** **CHIN-S.,** cic., ***cina, cinnb.,*** clem., **COCC., COFF., COLCH.,** ***coloc.,*** con., croc., **CROT-C.,** crot-h., **CUPR.,** cycl., dig., dros., dulc., ***euph.,*** euphr., ferr., ferr-i., graph., **GUAI., HAM.,** hell., **HEP., HYOS.,** ign., ***iod.,*** ip., **KALI-AR.,** ***kali-bi.,*** **KALI-C.,** ***kali-i., kali-n., kali-p.,*** kali-s., ***kreos.,*** **LACH.,** laur., ***led.,*** **LYC.,** ***mag-c., mag-m.,*** **MAG-P., MANG.,** ***med.,*** meny., ***merc., merc-c., mez.,*** mosch., mur-ac., nat-c., ***nat-m.,*** **NIT-AC.,** nux-m., **NUX-V.,** olnd., ***op.,*** osm., ***par.,*** petr., ***ph-ac., phos.,*** plat., plb., ***puls.,*** **RAN-B.,** ran-s., **RHOD., RHUS-T.,** ruta, sabad., **SABIN.,** sal-ac., ***sang.,*** sars., ***sec., seneg.,*** **SEP., SIL.,** ***spong.,*** squil., stann., **STAPH.,** ***stram., stront-c.,*** **SULPH.,** sul-ac., ***tarax., tell., thuj.,*** valer., ***verat.,*** verb., viol-o., viol-t., ***zinc.***

cannot bear limbs touch each other at night - ***psor.***

children, in - ant-t., apis, ***cina.***

each others - lac-c., psor., sanic.

feet, of - **KALI-C.,** nux-v.

hair, even of a - apis

slight - **ACON., APIS,** ars., **BELL., CHIN.,** coff., ***colch.,*** ham., **HEP.,** ***ign.,*** **KALI-C., LACH.,** lyss., mag-m., **MERC.,** merc-c., ***mez., nit-ac.,*** **NUX-V.,** ph-ac., ***phos.,*** sep., sil., spig., ***stann.***

hard pressure amel. - bell., ***cast., chin.,*** ign., ***lach., nux-v.,*** plb., psor.

throat agg., of - bell., **LACH.**

amel. - agar., alum., ***alumn.,*** am-c., am-m., anac., ant-c., arn., ***ars.,*** **ASAF.,** bell., bell-p., ***bism., bry.,*** **CALC.,** ***calc-ar.,*** canth., ***cast.,*** caust., chel., chin., ***coloc.,*** con., **CYCL.,** dros., euph., euphr., graph., ***grat.,*** hep., kali-c.,

TOUCH, general
amel. - **MUR-AC.,** pall., petr., ph-ac., ***phos.,*** plb., sang., sep., spig., spong., staph., sulph., tarax., **THUJ.,** viol-t., zinc.
aversion to being, touched - ***acon., agar.,*** **ANT-C.,** ***ant-t., arn.,*** ars., ***bell., bry.,*** calc., camph., **CHAM.,** ***chin., cina,*** cocc., ***coff.,*** colch., cupr., iod., **KALI-C.,** ***kali-i., lach.,*** mag-c., mag-m., ***med.,*** merc., mez., nux-v., plb., sanic., ***sil.,*** stram., **TARENT.,** ***thuj.,*** verat.
caressed, to being - ***cina.***
illusions, of - acon., ***alum.,*** anac., ant-t., arn., ars., ***asaf.,*** asar., bar-c., ***bell.,*** bism., bor., bov., bry., ***calc.,*** cann-s., canth., caps., caust., chel., cocc., coc-c., coloc., con., ***croc.,*** dros., dulc., glon., graph., guai., hell., hep., hyos., ***ign.,*** indg., iod., kali-c., kali-n., kreos., ***lach.,*** laur., lyc., mag-c., mag-m., meny., merc., mosch., nat-c., nat-m., nux-v., olnd., op., ***par.,*** ph-ac., phos., plat., ***plb., puls.,*** ran-b., ran-s., rheum, rhod., **RHUS-T.,** ruta., sabad., samb., seneg., sep., sil., ***spig.,*** spong., squil., staph., ***stram.,*** sulph., sul-ac., tarax., thuj., valer., verat., verb.
pain vanishes on touch and appears elsewhere - ant-t., asaf., sang., staph.
slight, agg. - ars., **BELL., CHIN.,** coff., ***colch., ign.,*** **LACH.,** mag-m., **MERC.,** ***mez.,*** **NUX-V.,** ph-ac., ***phos., stann.***
things, impelled to - lycps.

TOUCHING, anything agg. - acon., am-c., am-m., arg-m., arn., bell., bor., ***bry., calc., cann-s., carb-v.,*** caust., **CHAM.,** chin., dros., kali-c., kali-n., led., lyc., merc., nat-c., phos., plat., ***puls.,*** sec., ***sil.,*** spig., verat.
amel. - spig.
cold, things agg. - **AGAR.,** calc., **HEP.,** ***lac-d., merc., nat-m., pyrog.,*** **RHUS-T.,** ***sep.,*** **SIL.,** thuj., zinc.
warm, things agg. - ***sulph.***

TREMBLING, (see Nerves)

TRICHINOSIS - ars., bapt., cina.

TRICHOPHYTOSIS, (see Ringworm) - ant-c., ant-t., ***ars., bac.,*** calc., calc-i., ***chrysar., graph.,*** hep., jug-c., jug-r., kali-s., lyc., mez., psor., rhus-t., semp., ***sep.,*** sulph., ***tell.,*** tub., viol-t.
all over body - psor., ran-b.
intersecting rings over great portion of body, with fever and great constitutional disturbances - tell.
isolated spots on upper part of body, in - sep.

TUBERCLES, (see Skin)

TUBERCULOSIS, (see Fevers)

TUMORS, general (see Cancer)
ascites, with - ***apis.***
angioma, fungus hematodes, hemangioma - abrot., ant-t., **ARS.,** bell., ***calc.,*** **CARB-AN.,** ***carb-v.,*** clem., ***kreos.,*** **LACH.,** ***lyc.,*** manc., ***merc., nat-m., nit-ac.,*** nux-v., **PHOS.,** ***puls., rhus-t.,*** sep., **SIL.,** staph., ***sulph.,*** **THUJ.**

TUMORS, general
atheroma, steatoma - agar., ant-c., anthr., ***bar-c., bell.,*** benz-ac., brom., ***calc.,*** caust., clem., ***con.,*** daph., **GRAPH.,** ***guare., hep.,*** kali-br., ***kali-c.,*** kali-i., lac-ac., lach., ***lob.,*** lyc., mag-arct., mez., nat-c., ***nit-ac., ph-ac., phyt.,*** rhus-t., ***sabin.,*** sil., spong., staph., ***sulph.,*** thuj., vanad.
reappearing every weeks - ***calc.***
suppurating - ***calc., carb-v., sulph.***
bone-like, protuberances - ***calc-f., hecla.,*** lap-a., maland., ruta, sil.
bones, of - mez.
brain, encephaloma - acet-ac., arn., ***ars., ars-i.,*** art-v., ***bar-c.,*** bell., ***calc.,*** carb-ac., ***carb-an.,*** caust., **CON.,** ***croc.,*** gels., glon., graph., hydr., hyper., ***kali-i., kreos., lach.,*** merc., nit-ac., nux-v., **PHOS.,** ***plb.,*** sep., ***sil.,*** stram., sulph., ***thuj., tub.***
burning - ***apis, ars., con.***
colloid - carb-ac., hydr., phos.
conical, acuminate - ant-c., ant-t., hydr., puls., ***sil.,*** syph.
cystic - agar., ***apis,*** apoc., ars., ***aur.,*** **BAR-C.,** benz-ac., bov., ***brom.,*** **CALC.,** calc-f., calc-p., ***calc-s.,*** caust., ***con.,*** form-ac., **GRAPH.,** ***hep.,*** hydr., ***iod., kali-br.,*** kali-c., ***lyc., med.,*** merc-d., nit-ac., **PHOS.,** platan., ***sabin.,*** sil., spong., staph., sulph., ***thuj.***
cystic - ***apis,*** apoc., ars., **BAR-C.,** ***brom.,*** **CALC.,** calc-s., graph., ***hep.,*** sil.
pus, discharging - ***calc.***
enchondroma - ***calc.,*** calc-f., conch., lap-a., ***sil.***
epithelioma - acet-ac., ferr-pic.
epulis - ***calc.,*** plb-a., ***thuj.***
erectile - ***lyc., nit-ac., phos.,*** staph.
fibroid - arb., bell., bry., ***calc.,*** **CALC-F.,** ***calc-i., calc-s.,*** chol., chr-s., ***con.,*** fl-ac., frax., graph., hydr., ***hydrin-m., kali-br., kali-i., lap-a.,*** led., lil-t., lyc., **PHOS.,** phyt., ***sec.,*** **SIL.,** tarent., ter., teucr., thiosin., thlaspi, thyr., tril., ust., xan.
bleeding, with - calc., lap-a., nit-ac., ***phos., sabin.,*** sul-ac., thlaspi, ***tril.,*** ust.
fungus, like - calen., clem., manc., phos., sang., ***thuj.***
hematodes - ars., ***calc.,*** carb-v., **LACH.,** ***nat-m.,*** nit-ac., **PHOS.,** ***puls.,*** sep., ***sil.,*** staph., **THUJ.**
medullaris - ***calc.,*** carb-an., nit-ac., ***phos., sil.,*** thuj.
idiopathic, of dura mater - ***calc-p.***
particularly if syphilitic - ***manc.***
ganglion - am-c., arn., aur-m., ***benz-ac.,*** bov., calc-f., ***carb-v.,*** ferr-ma., iod., kali-m., ph-ac., ***phos.,*** plb., rhus-t., ***ruta,*** sil., sulph., thuj., zinc.
lipoma, fatty - agar., ***am-m.,*** **BAR-C., BELL.,** ***calc.,*** calc-ar., croc., graph., ***kali-br., lap-a.,*** phos., ***phyt., thuj.,*** ur-ac.
liquors, from abuse of - ***calc.***
neck, on - **BAR-C.,** ***phos.***

TUMORS, general
lipoma, fatty
scalp, on - ***croc.***
scrofulous - ***calc.***
nevus - abrot., **ACET-AC.,** arn., ars., bell-p., ***calc.,*** calc-f., carb-an., ***carb-v.,*** con., cund., ***ferr-p.,*** **FL-AC.,** ***graph.,*** ham., lach., ***lyc.,*** med., nit-ac., nux-v., ***petr., ph-ac.,*** **PHOS.,** rad., rad-br., rumx., ***sep., sil.,*** sul-ac., ***sulph., thuj.,*** ust., vac.
neuroma - all-c., calc., calen., ***ruta,*** staph.
noma - alum., alumn., ***ars.,*** bapt., calc., carb-v., ***con.,*** elat., ***guare.,*** hydr., ***kali-chl., kali-p., kreos., lach.,*** merc., ***merc-c., mur-ac.,*** sec., sil., sol-t-ae., sul-ac., sulph., tarent-c.
osteoma - ***mez.***
papillomata - ant-c., ***calc.,*** nit-ac., staph., ***thuj.***
sarcoma, cutis - ars., bar-c., calc-f., calc-p., carb-ac., carb-an., ***crot-h., cund.,*** cupr-s., graph., hecla., ***kali-m.,*** lach., ***lap-a.,*** nit-ac., phos., sil., symph., thuj.
burning - ***bar-c.***
lymphoid - ars., ars-i.
malignant - ***crot-h.,*** lap-a.
neck, in, burning - ***bar-c.***
open - kali-m.
osteo - carb-ac., graph., hecla.

TURNING, general (see Bending)
affected part amel. - bell.
around agg. - agar., aloe., calc., cham., ***ip.,*** kali-c., merc., nat-m., par., ***phos.,*** sil.
bed, in, amel. - nat-m.
must rise for turning - bry., **NUX-V.**
head agg. - am-m., anac., ant-c., ***arn.,*** asar., bar-c., ***bell.,*** bov., ***bry.,*** **CALC.,** camph., cann-s., canth., carb-an., carb-v., caust., cham., chin., **CIC.,** cocc., coff., coloc., ***con.,*** cupr., dros., dulc., glon., ***hep.,*** hyos., ***ign.,*** ip., kali-c., lach., ***lyc.,*** mag-c., mez., ***nat-c., nat-m.,*** nit-ac., ***nux-v.,*** par., petr., ph-ac., ***phos.,*** plat., ***puls., rhus-t.,*** sabad., sabin., samb., ***sang.,*** sars., ***sel., sep.,*** spig., **SPONG.,** stann., staph., sulph., thuj., verat., vio-t., zinc.
left to right amel., from - lach., phos.
over in bed agg. - ***acon.,*** agar., am-m., anac., ars., asar., ***bor., bry.,*** calc., ***cann-s., caps., carb-v.,*** caust., chin., cina., cocc., **CON.,** cupr., dros., ***euph., ferr.,*** graph., ***hep.,*** kali-c., kreos., lach., led., ***lyc.,*** mag-c., merc., ***nat-m.,*** nit-ac., nux-v., petr., phos., plat., plb., **PULS.,** ran-b., rhod., rhus-t., ruta., sabad., sabin., samb., sars., sel., ***sil., staph., sulph.,*** thuj., valer.
rapidly, as if - mosch.
right, to, agg. - carb-v., spig.
rise, before he can - kali-c.
to left agg. - scop., sulph.
walking, when - helo.
sideways agg. - bell., calc., kali-c., nat-m.
something by limbs amel. - ***sep.***
turning and twisting involuntarily - lyc.

TYPHOID, fever, (see Fevers)

TWITCHING, of body - acon., **AGAR.,** agn., alum., ***ambr.,*** am-c., am-m., ant-c., ***ant-t.,*** apis, ***arg-m., arg-n., ars., ars-i.,*** **ASAF.,** aster., atro., ***bar-c.,*** bar-m., ***bell.,*** bor., brom., ***bry.,*** bufo, **CACT.,** ***calc., calc-s., camph.,*** cann-i., ***canth.,*** caps., carb-ac., ***carb-s.,*** carb-v., ***caust.,*** cham., ***chel., chin., chin-s.,*** chlor., ***cic., cimic., cina, clem., cocc., cod.,*** colch., coloc., ***con.,*** croc., crot-h., ***cupr.,*** dig., dros., ***graph.,*** guai., ***hell.,*** **HYOS., IGN., IOD.,** ip., ***kali-ar.,*** kali-br., **KALI-C.,** kali-p., kali-s., kreos., ***lach.,*** laur., ***lyc., lyss.,*** mag-m., mag-p., meny., ***merc., merc-c.,*** **MEZ.,** ***mur-ac.,*** mygal., ***nat-a.,*** **NAT-C.,** ***nat-m., nat-p., nit-ac., nux-v.,*** olnd., ***op.,*** ox-ac., ***par.,*** petr., ***ph-ac., phos.,*** plat., ***plb.,*** psor., puls., rhod., ***rhus-t.,*** ruta, sabin., ***sec.,*** sel., seneg., ***sep., sil., spig.,*** spong., ***stann.,*** **STRAM.,** stront-c., ***stry., sulph.,*** sul-ac., tanac., tarax., thuj., valer., viol-t., ***visc.,*** **ZINC.**
fright, after - ign., ***op., stram.***
here and there - agar., alum., ***cocc.,*** colch., ***kali-c.,*** kali-n., lyc., mez., nat-c., nat-m., ph-ac., phos., rhod., sep., ***stry.,*** sulph., **ZINC.**
internally - atro., bov., ***cann-s.,*** seneg.
morning - rheum.
onesided - apis.
right - caust.
sleep, during - alum., anac., ***ars.,*** bell., caust., cinnb., con., ***cupr.,*** dulc., graph., ***kali-c.,*** lyc., mag-c., mez., nat-c., nat-m., petr., ph-ac., phos., seneg., sil., stann., ***stront-c., sulph.,*** sul-ac., thuj., **ZINC.**
on going to - acon., ***agar., alum.,*** arg-m., **ARS.,** cob., hyper., ***ign.,*** **KALI-C.,** phys., ***sel., stront-c., stry., sulph., sul-ac., zinc.***
subsultus, tendinum - ***agar.,*** ambr., am-c., ***ars., asaf.,*** bell., ***calc., camph., canth., chel., chlor.,*** **HYOS., IOD.,** ***kali-i., lyc., mez., mur-ac., ph-ac., phos.,*** rhus-t., ***sec., stry.,*** sul-ac., **ZINC.**
touch, agg. - ***stry.***
upper, part of body, lying down - nat-m.
wandering - cast., cocc., coloc., graph., ***merc.,*** nat-s., plat.

UNCLEANLINESS, agg. - all-c., **CAPS.,** ***chin., psor.,*** puls., ***sulph.***

UNCOVERING, general
agg. - ***acon.,*** acon-f., ***agar., am-c.,*** ant-c., arg-m., ***arg-n.,*** arn., **ARS.,** asar., ***atro., aur., bell., benz-ac.,*** bor., ***bry.,*** camph., canth., ***caps., carb-an., cham., chin., cic., clem., cocc., coff., colch., con.,*** dios., ***dulc., graph.,*** hell., **HEP.,** hyos., ***ign.,*** **KALI-AR.,** ***kali-bi.,*** **KALI-C.,** kali-i., kreos., ***lach., lycps.,*** **LYC.,** ***mag-c., mag-m.,*** **MAG-P.,** meny., ***merc.,*** mur-ac., ***nat-c., nat-m.,*** **NUX-M., NUX-V.,** ***ph-ac., phos.,*** puls., rheum, **RHOD., RHUS-T., RUMX.,** sabad., **SAMB.,** sep., **SIL., SQUIL.,** staph., stram., **STRONT-C.,** thuj., **ZINC.**
ailments from - kalm., sang-n.

UNCOVERING, general
agg.
least - hep., nux-v., rhus-t., ***sil.***
single part agg. - ***bry.,*** **HEP.,** ***nat-m.,*** **RHUS-T., RUMX., SIL.,** squil., stront-c., ***thuj.***
feet, of - ***calc.,*** cupr., nux-m., sil.
amel. - ***acon.,*** alum., apis, ars., asar., aur., ***bor.,*** bry., ***calc.,*** camph., cann-s., carb-v., cham., chin., coff., ***ferr.,*** ign., **IOD.,** kali-i., kali-s., ***lach.,*** led., **LYC.,** med., merc., mosch., mur-ac., nit-ac., nux-v., onos., op., phos., plat., **PULS.,** rhus-t., ***sec.,*** seneg., sep., ***spig.,*** staph., **SULPH.,** ***tab., verat.***
aversion to - arg-n., ***ars.,*** aur., ***bell.,*** calc-s., clem., colch., hep., mag-c., nat-m., nux-m., ***nux-v.,*** samb., sil., ***squil., stront-c.***
desire for - ***acon., aloe, apis,*** ars-i., asar., calc., calc-s., ***camph.,*** ferr., ***iod.,*** kali-i., led., manc., merc., mosch., op., **PULS.,** ***sec.,*** spig., stram., **SULPH.**
morning - fl-ac.
sleep, going to, on - ***op.***
sleep, in - plat.
waking, on - ***plat.***
kicks the covers of - **BRY.,** camph., ***cham.,*** iod., ***puls.,*** sulph.
coldest weather, in - hep., sanic., sulph.

UNDRESSING, after, agg. - am-m., **ARS.,** calc., ***cocc.,*** **DROS.,** hep., mag-c., mez., mur-ac., nat-s., **NUX-V.,** ***olnd.,*** plat., ***puls.,*** **RHUS-T.,** sep., ***sil., spong.,*** stann.
agg., in the open air - phos.

UREMIA - ***am-c., apis,*** apoc., ars., asc-c., bapt., ***bell., canth., carb-ac.,*** cic., ***cupr.,*** cupr-ac., dig., gels., ***glon., hell.,*** hydr-ac., ***hyos.,*** kali-br., ***kali-s., morph.,*** mosch., ***op.,*** phos., pic-ac., piloc., ***plb.,*** queb., ser-ang., ***stram., ter.,*** urea, **URT-U.,** verat-v.
convulsions, with - apoc., cic., crot-h., ***cupr.,*** cupr-ar., ***dig.,*** hydr-ac., ***kali-s.,*** merc-c., ***mosch., plb., ter.***
head, congestion, with - am-c., apis, ***bell.,*** con., ***cupr., gels., glon.,*** merc-c., ***stram.,*** tab., ter., verat-v.

VACCINATIONS, ailments, from (see Toxicity, chapter)

VACCINIA, (see Cowpox)

VARICELLA, (see Chickenpox)

VARICOSE veins, (See Blood)

VARIOLA, (see Smallpox)

VEINS, (See Blood)

VENESECTION, ailments from - chin., ***led.,*** senec., squil.

VIOLENT, illnesses - ***acon.,*** alum., anac., ***ars.,*** **BELL.,** bry., canth., carb-v., **CARC., CHAM.,** cupr., glon., hep., ***hyos.,*** ign., iod., ***lach.,*** merc., **NUX-V., STRAM.,** sulph., ***tarent., verat.***

VIRAL, infections (see Fevers)

WALK, desire to - calc., ***rhus-t.***
inability to, fall, after a - arg-m.
pregnancy, during - bell-p.
late learning to - ***agar., bar-c.,*** bell., **CALC., CALC-P., CAUST.,** lyc., merc., **NAT-M.,** nux-v., ***ph-ac., phos.,*** pin-s., ***sanic., sil.,*** sulph.
must walk - ars., aur., calc., dig., dios., iod., murx., op., paeon., ruta, stront-c., tarent.
night, at - merc.
tardy development of bones - ***calc.,*** calc-f., ***calc-p.,*** sil.

WALKING, general
agg. - ***acon.,*** **AESC.,** ***agar., agn.,*** aloe, ***alum., ambr.,*** am-c., am-m., anac., ant-c., ***ant-t.,*** apis, arg-m., ***arn., ars.,*** ars-i., asaf., ***asar., atro.,*** aur., ***bapt.,*** bar-c., **BELL.,** ***berb., bov.,*** **BRY.,** ***cact.,*** cadm-s., ***calad.,*** **CALC., CALC-S.,** ***camph., cann-s.,*** canth., caps., ***carb-ac., carb-an., carb-s.,*** carb-v., **CAUST.,** cham., ***chel.,*** **CHIN.,** ***chion.,*** cic., cina, clem., **COCC.,** ***coff.,*** **COLCH.,** ***coloc.,*** **CON.,** conv., ***croc.,*** cupr., cycl., ***dig.,*** dros., dulc., euph., euphr., ***ferr.,*** ferr-i., form., gels., ***glon., gran., graph.,*** guai., ***hell., hep.,*** hyos., ign., ***iod., ip., kali-c.,*** kali-n., kali-p., kreos., ***lach.,*** laur., **LED.,** ***lil-t.,*** lyc., mag-c., mag-m., ***mag-p.,*** mang., meny., ***merc., mez.,*** mosch., mur-ac., ***murx.,*** nat-c., ***nat-m., nat-p., nat-s.,*** **NIT-AC.,** nux-m., **NUX-V.,** olnd., op., paeon., par., ***petr., ph-ac.,*** **PHOS.,** ***phyt.,*** plat., plb., ***psor.,*** puls., ***ran-b.,*** ran-s., ***rheum,*** rhod., **RHUS-T.,** ***ruta,*** sabad., ***sabin.,*** samb., ***sars.,*** sec., ***sel.,*** seneg., **SEP.,** ***sil.,*** **SPIG.,** ***spong., squil.,*** **STANN.,** ***staph.,*** stram., stront-c., **SULPH.,** sul-ac., ***tarax., tarent.,*** teucr., thuj., tub., valer., verat., ***verat-v.,*** verb., viol-o., viol-t., ***zinc.***
backward - mang.
bent - ***bry.***
bridge, on a narrow - ang., ***bar-c.,*** ferr., sulph.
canal, by the side of a - ang.
closed eyes, with - alum., arg-n., calad., iodof., zinc.
dark, in - zinc.
distant parts, in - apis, ***bry.,*** cocc.
downstairs - bor., stram.
fast - ***alum.,*** alum-sil., ***ang.,*** arg-m., ***apis, arn.,*** **ARS.,** ars-i., ars-s-f., ***aur.,*** aur-a., aur-i., ***aur-m.,*** aur-s., **BELL.,** bor., **BRY.,** ***cact., calc., calc-s.,*** calc-sil., ***cann-s., caust.,*** chel., chin., cina, cocc., coff., **CON.,** croc., ***cupr.,*** dros., ***ferr.,*** ferr-ar., hep., hyos., ***ign., iod.,*** ip., ***kali-ar., kali-c.,*** kali-p., kali-sil., laur., ***led., lyc., merc.,*** mez., nat-a., nat-c., ***nat-m.,*** nit-ac., nux-m., ***nux-v., olnd.,*** **PHOS.,** ***plb.,*** **PULS.,** rheum, ***rhod., rhus-t.,*** ruta, sabin., ***seneg.,*** sep., **SIL.,** ***spig.,*** spong., squil., staph., sul-ac., **SULPH.,** verat., zinc.
level, on a - ran-b., verat.
rough ground, over - clem., hyos., lil-t., phos., podo.

WALKING, general

agg.,

running water, over - ang., bar-c., brom., ***ferr.,*** hyos., ***sulph.***

side, to one - aml-n., verat-v.

sideways - caust., kali-c.

stone pavement, on - aloe, ant-c., ars., ***con.,*** ***hep.,*** nux-v., sep.

wind, in - acon., ***agar., ars., asar.,*** aur., aur-a., **BELL.,** ***calc.,*** carb-v., ***cham.,*** chin., con., euphr., ***graph.,*** lach., ***lyc.,*** mur-ac., nat-c., nux-m., **NUX-V.,** ***phos.,*** plat., ***puls.,*** rhus-t., **SEP.,** spig., ***stann.,*** thuj.

ailments from - sel.

air, in open air agg. - acon., ***agar.,*** agn., alum., ambr., ***am-c.,*** am-m., anac., ant-c., arg-m., arn., **ARS.,** asar., aur., bar-c., ***bell.,*** bor., bov., ***bry.,*** calad., ***calc., camph.,*** cann-s., canth., caps., ***carb-ac., carb-an., carb-v.,*** **CAUST.,** cham., ***chel.,*** chin., chin-a., cic., ***cina,*** clem., **COCC.,** ***coff., colch.,*** coloc., ***con.,*** croc., dig., dros., dulc., euph., ***euphr.,*** ferr., graph., ***guai.,*** hell., ***hep.,*** hyos., ign., iod., ip., ***kali-c.,*** kali-n., ***kali-p.,*** kreos., lach., laur., ***led.,*** lyc., mag-c., mag-m., **MAG-P.,** mang., meny., ***merc.,*** merc-c., mez., mosch., mur-ac., nat-a., nat-c., nat-m., nit-ac., ***nux-m.,*** **NUX-V.,** olnd., op., par., petr., ph-ac., ***phos., plan.,*** plat., plb., ***psor., puls.,*** ran-b., ***ran-s.,*** rheum, rhod., ***rhus-t.,*** ruta, sabad., sabin., sars., **SEL.,** ***seneg., sep., sil.,*** **SPIG.,** ***spong., stann.,*** staph., ***stram.,*** stront-c., **SULPH.,** sul-ac., tarax., teucr., thuj., valer., verat., ***verb., viol-t.,*** zinc.

amel. - acon., agar., aloe, **ALUM.,** ambr., am-m., anac., ant-c., arg-m., **ARG-N.,** arn., asaf., ***asar., aur.,*** bapt., bar-c., bell., bism., bor., bov., ***brom., bry.,*** calc., calc-s., caps., carb-ac., carb-s., carb-v., caust., cic., cina, ***con., dulc.,*** **FL-AC.,** gamb., ***graph.,*** hyos., ign., kali-c., **KALI-I.,** kali-n., **KALI-S.,** laur., ***lil-t.,*** **LYC.,** ***mag-c., mag-m.,*** mang., meny., merc., merc-c., ***merc-i-r.,*** mez., mosch., mur-ac., ***naja,*** nat-a., nat-c., nat-m., nit-ac., op., ox-ac., par., petr., ***ph-ac.,*** phos., plat., plb., **PULS.,** rhod., **RHUS-T.,** ***sabin., sang.,*** sars., sel., ***seneg., sep.,*** spig., ***stann.,*** staph., stront-c., ***sulph.,*** sul-ac., ***tarax., teucr., thuj.,*** verat., verb., viol-t., zinc.

amel. - ***acon.,*** agar., agn., alum., alumn., am-c., ***am-m.,*** ambr., anac., ang., ant-c., ant-t., apis, apoc., aran-ix., arg-m., arg-n., arn., ***ars.,*** ars-s-f., asaf., asar., **AUR.,** aur-m., aur-s., bar-c., bell., bism., bov., ***brom., bry.,*** buni-o., calc., calen., canth., **CAPS.,** carb-v., caust., cham., chin., cic., cina, cocc., coloc., **CON.,** cortiso., crot-h., cupr., **CYCL.,** ***dios., dros.,*** **DULC., EUPH.,** euphr., **FERR.,** ferr-ar., ***fl-ac.,*** glon., graph., guai., halo., hep., hyos., ign., indg., iod., kali-bi., kali-c., **KALI-I.,** kali-n., kali-p., ***kali-s.,*** kreos., lach., laur., ***lyc.,*** lycps., ***mag-c., mag-m.,*** mag-p., mang.,

WALKING, general

amel. - aml-n., verat-v.***meli., meny.,*** meph., ***merc.,*** mez., ***mosch.,*** mur-ac., nat-c., ***nat-m.,*** nat-s., nid., nit-ac., nux-m., olnd., op., palo., par., petr., ***ph-ac.,*** phos., ***plat.,*** plb., **PULS.,** pyrog., ***ran-b.,*** raph., ***rhod.,*** **RHUS-T.,** ***ruta,*** **SABAD.,** sabin., **SAMB.,** sars., sel., seneg., ***sep.,*** sil., spig., spong., stann., staph., stront-c., sul-ac., **SULPH., TARAX.,** tere-ch., teucr., thal., thuj., tub., **VALER.,** ***verat., verb., viol-t.,*** vip-a., ***zinc.***

bare feet, on - psor., puls.

bent - am-m., arn., **CON.,** ***hyos., lyc.,*** nux-v., phos., rhus-t., sabin., sulph., ***viol-t.***

closed eyes, with - con.

crooked - am-m.

fast - ant-t., ***arg-n.,*** ars., aur-m., brom., canth., carb-ac., ***ign., mag-c.,*** nat-m., petr., ***rhus-t., sabin.,*** **SEP.,** sil., ***stann., sul-ac.,*** **TUB.**

gliding - nit-ac.

slowly - agar., **AUR.,** aur-i., **AUR-M.,** cact., calc-s., **FERR.,** ferr-ar., iris, ***kali-p.,*** lyc., **PULS.,** sep., ***tarent.***

aversion to - agar., aza., cham., clem., fago., kali-bi., nit-ac.

backward impossible - cocc., mang.

beginning of agg. - acon., ***agar.,*** ambr., am-c., anac., ant-c., ant-t., arn., ars., asar., aur., bar-c., bell., bov., ***bry., cact., calc.,*** cann-s., canth., **CAPS.,** carb-an., ***carb-v., caust.,*** cham., chin., cic., cina, cocc., **CON.,** croc., cupr., cycl., dig., dros., **EUPH., FERR.,** graph., kali-i., kali-n., lach., laur., led., **LYC.,** mag-c., mang., merc., mur-ac., nat-c., nat-m., nit-ac., nux-v., olnd., petr., ph-ac., ***phos.,*** plat., plb., **PULS.,** ran-b., rhod., **RHUS-T.,** ***ruta, sabad.,*** sabin., ***samb.,*** sars., sep., ***sil.,*** spig., staph., stram., stront-c., sulph., ***thuj.,*** valer., verat., ***zinc.***

bones of legs, on, sensation of - cham.

circle, in a - bell., thuj.

cotton, as if on - onos.

desire for - acon., arg-m., arg-n., ***ars., aur.,*** bism., caj., calc., chlor., cod., ferr., fl-ac., gins., ***iod.,*** kali-i., lepi., lil-t., lyc., mag-c., merc., mosch., naja, ***op.,*** paeon., paull., phos., ***rhus-t.,*** ruta, sep., spirae., ***stront-c.,*** tarent., ***thlaspi,*** thuj., valer., zinc-ar.

air, in open - asaf., clem., crot-t., fl-ac., lach., lact., lyc., mez., phos., ***puls.,*** teucr.

night - ars., ***iod.,*** merc., ***op.***

difficult - aur., chin., olnd., ter.

easily - thuj., zinc.

fast, agg. - ***alum.,*** arg-m., ***apis, arn.,*** **ARS.,** ars-i., ***aur., aur-m.,*** **BELL., BRY.,** ***cact., calc., calc-s., cann-s., caust.,*** chel., chin., cina, cocc., coff., **CON.,** croc., ***cupr.,*** dros., ***ferr.,*** ferr-ar., hep., hyos., ***ign., iod.,*** ip., ***kali-ar., kali-c.,*** kali-p., laur., ***led., lyc., merc.,*** mez., nat-a., nat-c., ***nat-m.,*** nit-ac., nux-m., ***nux-v., olnd.,*** **PHOS.,** ***plb.,*** **PULS.,** rheum, ***rhod., rhus-t.,*** ruta, sabin., ***seneg.,*** sep., **SIL.,** ***spig.,*** spong., squil., staph.,

WALKING, general
  fast, agg. - **SULPH.,** sul-ac., verat., zinc.
    amel. - ***arg-n.,*** canth., carb-ac., ***ign.,*** nat-m., petr., **SEP.,** sil., ***stann., sul-ac.,*** **TUB.**
  gressus, gallinaceus - ***aur., ign.,*** **LACH.,** mag-p., **SIL.**
    gressus vaccinus - calc., ***iod.,*** sec.
  hard pavement, on - con.
  infirm - caust., kali-c., mag-c., ***mag-p.,*** nat-c., ol-an., phos., sulph.
  involuntary, with quick steps - coca.
  late learning to walk, children - ***agar., bar-c.,*** bell., **CALC., CALC-P., CAUST., NAT-M.,** nux-v., ***sanic., sil.,*** sulph.
  limping - abrot., acon., ant-c., ***bell., calc.,*** **CAUST.,** ***dros.,*** hep., kali-bi., ***kali-c.,*** lyc., ***merc.,*** nit-ac., phos., **RUTA.,** sabin., sep., sulph.
    pain in knee - spig.
    spontaneous - **APIS.,** bell., ***coloc.,*** lyc., ruta., zinc.
  needles, on, as if - eupi., rhus-t.
  peas, on hard, as if - nux-m.
  rapidly, from anxiety - arg-n., fl-ac., ***sep.***
  rough, ground, on hyos., lil-t.
  slowly, amel. - agar., **AUR., AUR-M.,** cact., calc-s., **FERR.,** ferr-ar., iris, ***kali-p.,*** **PULS.,** sep., ***tarent.***
    slowly and dignified - caj.
  toes, on - crot-h., lath.
  turns right on - helo.
  velvet, on, as if - sec.
  wind, in the, agg. - acon., ***agar., ars., asar.,*** aur., **BELL.,** ***calc.,*** carb-v., ***cham.,*** chin., con., euphr., ***graph.,*** lach., ***lyc.,*** mur-ac., nat-c., nux-m., **NUX-V.,** ***phos.,*** plat., ***puls.,*** rhus-t., **SEP.,** spig., ***stann.,*** thuj.
  wool, on, as if - xan.

WALKS, on outer side of foot - cic.

WARM, temperature, (see Environment)

WARMBLOODED, (see Heat)

WARMTH, desire for - alum., am-br., arg-m., ***ars.,*** bar-c., calc., caps., ***caust., colch.,*** con., ***hep., kali-c.,*** moly-met., ph-ac., psor., ***sabad., sil.,*** thuj., tub.
    warm stove - bar-c., cic., ptel., ***sil.,*** tub.
    warm clothing - alum., ars., ***bar-c.,*** bell., calc., caul., graph., hep., kali-c., nat-c., nat-s., plb., psor., ***sabad.,*** sil.
      afternoon - nux-v.
      in spite of sensation of heat - achy.
    warm bed - ars., spig.

WASHING, clothes, laundry - phos., sep., ***ther.***
    floor - caust., merc-i-r.

WATER, (see Environment, Water)

WEAKNESS, general, (see Chronic fatigue) - abies-c., abies-n., abrot., absin., ***acet-ac.,*** acon., aesc., ***aeth.,*** agar., ***agn.,*** ail., all-c., all-s., ***aloe, alum.,*** alumn., ***ambr.,*** **AM-C.,** am-m., **ANAC.,** anthr., ***ant-c.,*** **ANT-T., APIS,** apoc., ***aran.,*** **ARG-M.,** ***arg-n.,*** **ARN., ARS.,** ars-h., **ARS-I.,**

WEAKNESS, general - ***ars-m.,*** ars-s-f., arum-m., arum-t., asaf., asar., asc-t., aster., ***aur.,*** **BAPT., BAR-C.,** ***bar-m.,*** bell., benz., ***benz-ac.,*** berb., ***bism., bol.,*** bor., bov., brach., **BROM.,** bry., bufo, ***cact.,*** cahin., calad., **CALC.,** calc-i., ***calc-p.,*** calc-s., ***camph.,*** cann-i., cann-s., ***canth.,*** caps., **CARB-AC.,** ***carb-an.,*** carb-h., ***carb-s., carb-v.,*** card-m., cast-v., ***caul., caust.,*** cedr., ***cham.,*** chel., ***chim.,*** **CHIN.,** chin-a., **CHIN-S.,** chion., chlf., chlol., ***cic.,*** cimic., cimx., ***cina,*** cinnb., ***clem.,*** cob., ***cocc.,*** coc-c., ***coff.,*** **COLCH.,** coloc., com., **CON.,** cop., croc., ***crot-c., crot-h., crot-t.,*** cub., ***cupr., cupr-ar.,*** cupr-s., cur., ***cycl.,*** **DIG.,** dios., dor., ***dros., dulc.,*** elat., eug., eup- per., eup-pur., euph., euphr., fago., **FERR.,** ferr-ar., **FERR-I., FERR-M.,** ferr-p., ***fl-ac., form.,*** **GELS.,** gent-l., glon., goss., **GRAPH.,** gran., grat., guai., guare., ***ham., hell.,*** helon., **HEP.,** ***hipp., hydr., hydr-ac.,*** **HYOS.,** ***hyper.,*** hura, ***ign.,*** ind., indg., **IOD.,** ***ip.,*** iris, jab., jatr., jug- r., **KALI-AR.,** ***kali-bi.,*** kali-br., **KALI-C.,** kali- chl., **KALI-FER.,** ***kali-i.,*** kali-n., **KALI-P.,** kali-s., **KALM.,** kreos., lac-ac., ***lac-c.,*** **LACH.,** lachn., **LAUR., LEC.,** led., lepi., lept., lil-t., lob., lob-s., ***lyc.,*** lycps., lyss., mag-c., mag-m., mag-s., manc., **MED.,** meli., meny., meph., **MERC., MERC-C., MERC-CY.,** merc-i-f., merc-i-r., mez., mill., morph., mosch., murx., **MUR-AC.,** mygal., naja, nat-a., nat-c., nat-h., nat-m., nat-n., nat-p., nat-s., nicc., **NIT-AC.,** nuph., ***nux-m., nux-v.,*** oena., **OLND.,** ol-an., ***ol-j., op.,*** osm., ***ox-ac.,*** paeon., pall., par., ped., ***petr.,*** phel., **PH-AC., PHOS.,** ***phys., phyt.,*** **PIC-AC.,** plan., ***plat.,*** **PLB.,** podo., polyg., **PSOR.,** ptel., ***puls.,*** **RAN-B.,** ran-s., ***raph.,*** rat., rheum, rhod., **RHUS-T.,** ***rumx.,*** ruta., ***sabad.,*** sabin., samb., ***sanic., sang.,*** sarr., ***sars.,*** **SEC., SEL.,** senec., ***seneg.,*** **SEP., SIL.,** sin-n., sol-n., sol-t-ae., spig., ***spong.,*** **SQUIL., STANN., STAPH.,** ***stict.,*** still., ***stram.,*** stront-c., stry., **SULPH., SUL-AC.,** sul-i., sumb., syph., **TAB.,** tarax., **TARENT.,** ***tell.,*** **TER.,** teucr., ***ther., thuj.,*** til., tril., trom., **TUB.,** ust., valer., **VERAT.,** verat-v., verb., vesp., vinc., viol-t., vip., xan., ***zinc.,*** zing.
  abortion, weakness, from - ***alet.,*** caul., chin., chin-s., ***helon.,*** ruta, sec., ***sep.,*** sil.
  acute diseases, during or after - abrot., aeth., ail., alet., ***alst., anac.,*** ant-t., apis, **ARS.,** aven., calc-p., carb-an., ***carb-v., chin., chin-a.,*** coca, ***cocc.,*** colch., cupr., cur., dig., fl-ac., **GELS.,** guare., ***helon., irid.,*** kali-fer., kali-m., ***kali-p.,*** lath., lob-p., merc-cy., mur-ac., nat-sal., nux-v., **PH-AC.,** ***phos.,*** pic-ac., ***psor.,*** sel., sil., staph., stroph., stry-p., sul-ac., ***tarent-c.,*** verat., zinc-ar.
  addison's disease, in - ***calc., iod.***
  afebrile - ars., bapt., carb-v., chin.
  afternoon - acon., aeth., ***alet.,*** am-c., amyg., anac., apis, aq-pet., arg-n., aur., bar-c., bell., bor., brom., ***bry.,*** cast., carb-an., carbn., chin-s., coc-c., coca, colch., con., coloc., com., digin., erig., fago., ferr., ***gels.,*** glon., ham., helon., hydr-ac., hyos., ign., iod., iris, ***kali-c.,*** kali-n., lyc., lycps., mag-c., merl., mez., mur-ac., nat-c., nat-m., nat-p., nat-s., nit-ac.,

WEAKNESS, general
afternoon - nux-v., ol-an., phys., phyt., plb., ptel., ran-b., rhus-t., ruta, sang., sep., ***sil.,*** spirae., staph., stram., stry., **SULPH.,** thuj., zinc., zing.
12:00 p.m. - gels., sol-t-ae.
1 p.m. - astac., ferr-p., lyc., phys., pic-ac., verat-v.
2 p.m. - chel., gels., nux-v., sulph.
2 p.m. to 3 p.m. - guano, plb-chr., sulph.
2 p.m. to 4 p.m. - ign.
3 p.m. - ***ham.,*** lyss., mag-c., nat-s., nep.
3 p.m. to 4 p.m. - reser.
4 p.m. - caust., gad., hydr., iris, lyc., mang., merc-i-f., phys.
5 p.m. - coff., coloc., ***lac-d.,*** lyc., merc., stram.
5 p.m. or 6 p.m. - merc.
5 p.m. to 5 a.m. - tarent.
5 p.m. to 11 p.m. - perh.
sleep, after - bor., chin-s., ferr., gels., kali-c., nat-m.
walking, while - caust., lyc., mag-c., pic-ac., ran-b.
after - ery-a., euph., hyper.
amel. - nat-s.
air, open, in - ambr., am-c., am-m., ***atro.,*** bry., calc., chin., clem., coff., coloc., con., ferr., grat., kali-c., mag-c., merc., merc-c., mur-ac., nux-v., ***plat.,*** sang., ***spig.,*** verat.
amel. - chel., colch., **CON.,** croc., gels., grat., hed., naja, nat-m., pic-ac., sabad.
fresh air - calc.
for want of - meli.
fresh air amel. - calc.
albuminuria, in - ***ars., calc-ar., dig., iod., merc-c., nat-c., ter.***
alcoholic drinks amel. - ***canth.,*** nit-s-d., nux-v., thea.
alcoholism, in - ***ars., carb-s., kali-br., nat-s., phos., ran-b., sel., sulph.***
alternating with, activity - aloe, aur.
sensation of strength - ars., chin., colch.
trembling - ferr., plb.
anemia, in - ***chin.,*** **FERR.,** ferr-p., **KALI-C.,** ***nat-c., nat-m.,*** **PHOS.**
anesthetics, from - acet-ac., hyper., ***phos.***
anger, after - mur-ac., staph., zinc.
anxiety, with - am-c., ars., aur., calc., caust., rhus-t.
appetite, with increased - ail., iod.
ascending stairs, from - alum-sil., ***anac.,*** ars., ars-i., ars-s-f., bar-m., blatta-a., **CALC.,** ***calc-p.,*** calc-sil., carb-s., coff., colch., croc., fago., **IOD.,** kali-a., ***lyc.,*** mag-arct., mag-c., nat-m., nat-n., nux-v., ox-ac., ph-ac., phys., pic-ac., puls., sarcol-ac., ***sil.,*** spig., ***stann.,*** sulph., zinc-ar.
ascites, from - ***apis.,*** chin., **LYC.**
bed, on going to - arn., cinnb., lycps., mur-ac., rumx., ter.
beer, after - coc-c., nux-v.
amel. - thea.

WEAKNESS, general
bleeding, in - ***carb-v.,*** **CHIN.,** ***chin-a., chin-s.,*** **FERR.,** ferr-p., ***hyper., ign., ph-ac., phos., rat.,*** stront-c.
severe - chin., stront-c.
breakfast time, about - sep.
after - arg-n., brom., carb-v., cham., con., dig., lach., nux-v., ***ph-ac.,*** sil., still., thea., verat.
amel. - ***calc., con.,*** nat-m., nux-v., ***staph.***
businessman, worn out - ***calc.,*** carc., clem., lyc., **NUX-V.,** sil.
causeless - psor.
chest, as if starts in - seneg.
childbirth, during - ***arn.,*** ars., asaf., **BELL.,** bor., bry., calc., camph., carb-an., carb-v., **CAUL.,** caust., ***cham.,*** chin., cimic., cocc., coff., ***con.,*** **KALI-C., KALI-P.,** kreos., lyc., mag-c., mag-m., merc., mosch., nat-c., ***nat-m.,*** nux-m., ***nux-v.,*** **OP.,** phos., plat., **PULS.,** rhus-t., ruta, sabad., **SEC., SEP.,** stann., sul-ac., sulph., thuj., zinc.
after - ***arn., bell-p.,*** calen., **CAUL.,** ***chin.,*** kali-c., puls., **SEP.**
children, in - ars., bar-c., bell., calc., calc-p., carb-v., ***carc.,*** cham., cina, kali-c., lach., ***lyc.,*** med., nux-v., **SIL.,** ***sulph.,*** tub.
without cause - carc., sul-ac.
chill, during - agar., aran., ars., asar., astac., ***chin.,*** coc-c., ip., lach., ***nat-m.,*** petr., ***phos.,*** psor.
after - apis, sulph.
before - ***ars., chin.,*** nat-m., thuj.
chilliness, with - sep.
cloudy, damp weather, in - sang.
coffee, amel. - eug.
from odor of - sul-ac.
cold weather, in - apis, lach.
after exposure to - ars.
coldness, during - apis, atha., aeth., con., guare., nat-m., thuj.
from - ***ars.,*** **CARB-V., VERAT.**
colic with - cast., tab.
company, in - sep.
conversation, from - ambr., sil.
convulsions, after - acon., agar., ars., art-v., carbn., ***cupr., ip.,*** merc-c., ***oena.,*** sec., stram., stry., sulph., tab., upa.
epileptic - ***aster.,*** camph., ***plb., sulph.***
hysterical - ars.
coryza, during - calc., graph.
cough, from - ars.
after - cor-r., verat.
dampness, from exposure to - ars.
daytime - agar., ***am-c.,*** cench., cob-n., corn., graph., iod., indg., lyc., lyss., mag-c., mosch., nat-a., nat-c., ***nat-m.,*** nit-ac., op., ph-ac., phos., phys., pip-m., plan., ***stann., sulph.,*** tarent., ter., uran-n.
death, as of approaching - ***ars.,*** carc., con., dig., mag-m., nat-c., olnd., op., sec., spig., ***vinc.***

WEAKNESS, general

dentition, in - ***calc.,*** calc-p., cham., ***ip.***

descending steps - stann.

diabetes mellitus, in - ***arg-m., ars.,*** carc., ***lac-ac.,*** **PH-AC.**

diarrhea, from - ***alum.,*** ambr., ***apis,*** **ARS.,** ***bor.,*** both., bry., carb-v., **CHIN.,** coloc., con., ***dulc., ferr.,*** gnaph., ***graph.,*** hura, hydr., ***iod., ip.,*** iris, kali-c., kali-chl., lil-t., mag-c., merc., merc-cy., **NAT-S., NIT-AC.,** ***nux-v.,*** **OLND.,** op., ox-ac., petr., **PHOS.,** phyt., **PIC-AC., PODO.,** ***sec.,*** senec., sep., **SIL.,** ***sul-ac., tab., tarent.,*** **VERAT.,** ***zinc.***

does not weaken - ph-ac.

dinner, during - am-c., bov., nat-a., nat-s., teucr.

after - alum., am-c., am-m., ant-c., ars., ars-h., asar., bapt., bov., cahin., calc., carb-v., cast., chel., ***chin.,*** cob., cycl., dig., euph-a., graph., grat., ign., indg., iod., ***lach.,*** lyc., mag-c., mur-ac., nat-m., nat-p., nit-ac., ol-an., ox-ac., perh., phel., ***ph-ac.,*** phos., plat., plect., sars., sep., ***sil.,*** squil., ***sulph., thuj.,*** zinc.

amel. - ambr., sars.

before - mez., nat-m., sabin., sil., thuj.

diphtheria, in - ***ail., alum-sil., apis, brom., canth., chin-a., crot-h.,*** diph., ***ign., kali-bi., kali-per.,*** lac-c., **LACH., MERC-CY.,** ***merc-i-f., mur-ac., nat-a., nux-v.,*** **PHYT.,** ***sal-ac., sec., sulph.***

stupor, cold limbs, low temperature, pulse rapid, weak - diph.

disease, out of proportion to - ars., sul-ac.

drawing and jerking in limbs, after - sulph.

dream, after a - ***calc-s.***

drinking, after - nat-m.

drugging, from - aven., carb-v., helon., ***nux-v.***

dyscrasia, from some deep-seated - abrot., ***carc.,*** eup-per., hydr., iod., nat-m., nit-ac., ***psor.,*** sul-ac., ***sulph.,*** tub., ***zinc.***

easy - cycl., nat-m., pic-ac., sil.

eat, cannot even - bar-c., stann.

eating, while - am-c., bufo, ***kali-c.,*** mag-c., ptel., sulph.

after - act-sp., alum., ***anac., ant-c.,*** **ARS.,** ars-s-f., asar., bar-ac., **BAR-C.,** bar-s., brom., calc., calc-p., cann-s., carb-an., card-m., ***chin.,*** cina, clem., ***con., croc.,*** crot-c., cycl., dig., ferr., ferr-ma., hep., hyper., kali-c., kali-sil., ***lach.,*** lyc., mag-c., mag-m., meph., merc-c., mur-ac., ***nat-c., nux-m.,*** ox-ac., **PH-AC.,** phos., rhod., rhus-t., ruta, sang., sars., sel., sep., ***sil., staph.,*** sul-ac., sulph., tell., teucr., thea., thuj., uran-n., zinc.

amel. - aster., ***hep.,*** **IOD.,** nat-c., petr., sapin., sep., sil.

before - cinnb.

edema, with - **APIS,** ***ars., eup-per., hell.,*** seneg.

WEAKNESS, general

elderly people - ***ambr.,*** ars., aur., **BAR-C.,** ***calc-p.,*** carb-v., ***carc., con., cur.,*** eup-per., glyc., nit-ac., ***nux-m.,*** op., ***phos.,*** sec., ***sel.,*** **SIL.,** ***sul-ac.***

emissions, after - acet-ac., agar., anac., aur., ***bar-c., calad., calc.,*** calc-p., canth., carb-an., carl., ***chin.,*** chin-b., ***cob., coff., con.,*** cupr., ***cypr.,*** dam., dig., ***dios.,*** ery-a., ferr., form., ***gels.,*** ham., ***hydr.,*** iod., **KALI-BR.,** ***kali-c.,*** kali-p., lach., **LYC.,** med., naja, ***nat-m.,*** nat-p., ***nuph.,*** **NUX-V.,** ***op.,*** **PH-AC., PHOS.,** ***pic-ac.,*** plb., puls., ***sabad., sars., sel., sep.,*** **SIL.,** ***stann.,*** **STAPH.,** sul-ac., ***sulph.,*** ust., zinc.

emotions, from depressing - calc-p., ign., ***ph-ac.***

erections, from - aur., aur-m., carb-s.

erethism, with - ars., chin., sil.

erethism, without - ph-ac.

evening - acon., aloe, alum., ***am-c.,*** am-m., aphis., apis, apoc., ars., asaf., asar., bapt., bell., berb., bor., bov., brom., brucin., bry., calc., calc-p., ***calc-s.,*** carb-v., carl., ***caust.,*** chin., clem., cob., coc-c., coca, coloc., con., ***croc.,*** cycl., dios., dirc., erig., ery-m., euphr., eupi., fago., ferr., ferr-ar., form., ***graph.,*** grat., haem., helon., hep., hydr., hydr-ac., ***ign.,*** indg., iris, jac., jac-c., ***kali-bi.,*** kali-c., kali-m., kali-n., kali-sil., kalm., ***lach.,*** laur., lim., lob., lyc., lycps., mag-c., merc., merl., mez., mur-ac., murx., naja, **NAT-M.,** nat-n., nicc., nit-ac., nux-v., ox-ac., pall., ***petr.,*** phos., plat., plb., psor., puls-n, rat., rhus-g., rhus-t., rumx., ruta, senec., ***sep.,*** sil., spig., stront-c., sulfonam., ***sulph.,*** sumb., tab., ***tart-ac.,*** thuj., tub., upa., valer., zinc., zinc-p.

6 p.m. - helon., lyc., merc.

7 p.m. - gins., mag-c., nat-m., phys., pic-ac., sep., verat., verat-v.

8 p.m. - astac., bar-c., mang., pana., phys., sep.

8:30 p.m. - pip-m.

9 p.m. - dirc., mag-s., op., phys., pic-ac.

9 p.m., amel. - phos.

9:30 p.m. - lyc., sep.

amel. - asc-t., calc-s., colch., nit-ac.

air, in open - chel., **CON.,** grat., naja, nat-m., pic-ac., sabad.

bed, in - lyc.

eating, after - bov., ***croc.***

excess, after any - agar., ***anac., calc-p., carb-v.,*** caust., ***chin.,*** chin-a., corn-f., cur., gins., kali-c., nat-m., ***ph-ac., phos.,*** plb., sel., stroph.

excessive - ars., bapt., chin., ferr., ***ferr-pic., gels.,*** ph-ac., tab.

excitement, after - ***con.,*** phos., stry., thea.

exertion, from - acon., ***alum-p.,*** ambr., ***arn., ars.,*** ars-s-f., aur-a., aur-m., bry., calc., caust., chin., cocc., coff., cycl., ferr., ferr-ac., ferr-i., kali-a., kalm., lac-d., macro., mag-c., merc., nat-c., nit-m-ac., nit-s-d., nux-m., ph-ac., phos., ***pic-ac.,*** rhod., rhus-d., rhus-t., sarcol-ac., sep., sil., ***stann.,*** sul-i., thea., verat.

WEAKNESS, general
exertion, from
slight, from - acon., ***agar.,*** ail., apis, **ARS.,** ***ars-i.,*** ars-s-f., alum., ***am-c.,*** anac., bapt., berb., **BRY., CALC.,** calc-sil., ***carb-v.,*** carb-s., cham., clem., ***cocc., colch.,*** **CON., CROT-H.,** dor., ***ferr.,*** ferr-i., ***gels.,*** ham., ign., jatr., kali-c., kali-n., kalm., lac-d., **LACH.,** ***lyc., mag-m., merc., merc-c., nat-a.,*** **NAT-C.,** ***nat-m., nat-p.,*** nux-m., petr., **PH-AC., PHOS., PIC-AC.,** plb., prot., ***psor.,*** ptel., **RHUS-T., SEL.,** ***sep.,*** sol-n., ***spig.,*** **SPONG.,** ***stann., staph.,*** stram., sul-i., ***sulph.,*** sumb., ther., thuj., **TUB.,** verat., ziz.
amel. - ferr., kali-n.
exhilaration, as after - cinnb.
feet, while washing - merc.
faint-like - ant-t., ***ars.,*** bar-c., berb., ***carb-v.,*** **CAUST.,** cham., ***coca,*** cocc., croc., cupr-c., ***dig.,*** digin., dulc., **EUP-PER.,** ferr., gels., ***goss.,*** ign., kali-c., kali-i., lyc., mez., mosch., **NUX-V.,** olnd., ***petr., tab., verat.,*** zing.
frequent spells during day - murx., nux-m., sep., ***sulph.,*** zinc.
fever, during - acon., alum., am-m., ant-t., ***anthr., apis,*** aran., **ARS.,** ***bapt., bry.,*** calc., carb-v., crot-h., ***eup-per.,*** eup-pur., ferr., **GELS.,** ***ign.,*** lyc., morph., ***mur-ac.,*** nat-c., ***nat-m.,*** nicc., nit-ac., op., petr., ***ph-ac.,*** **PHOS.,** ***puls., pygrog., rob., rhus-t.,*** sarr., sep., sul-ac., sulph., syph., thuj.
after - ***apis, aran.,*** carc., chin., gels., gent-l., med., morph., sal-ac., sulph., syph.
following prolonged fever - ***colch., psor.,*** **SEL.**
inebriety, bilious or remittent, from - eup-per.
food, from sour - aloe.
forenoon - abrot., acon., alum., am-c., ambr., ang., ant-t., bart., brucin., **BRY.,** calc., carb-an., carb-v., corn., fago., fl-ac., graph., grat., hell., indg., kali-cy., kali-n., lach., ***lyc.,*** mag-m., mang., nat-m., nux-m., ox-ac., ***ph-ac.,*** phel., phys., ***plat.,*** ptel., ran-b., sabad., sars., scroph-n., sep., staph., tab., tarent.
9 a.m. - chin-s., cocc., merl., nat-s., ox-ac., ped., perh., peti., phys., ptel., sep.
9 a.m., amel. - tarent.
9 a.m. to 11 a.m. - tarent.
10 a.m. - aq-mar., bor., cast., cench., equis., gels., lycps., merc-d., phys.
10 a.m., amel. - ***gels.***
10 a.m. to 12 a.m. - calc-s.
11 a m - arg-m., ***lach.,*** nat-c., phos., ptel., sep., ***sulph.,*** thuj., zinc.
agg. - ***acal.,*** bar-m., bry., calc., con., corn., lac-c., lach., lyc., ***nat-m., nit-ac.,*** phos., psor., sep., stann., sulph., tub.
fright, from - coff., ***gels.,*** merc., op.
grief, from - ***carc., caust., ign.,*** nat-m., **PH-AC.,** ***pic-ac.***
growing fast, after - calc-p., hipp., ph-ac.

WEAKNESS, general
headache, during - **ANT-C.,** aran., ars-h., bism., bufo, calc-ar., carb-v., chin., chin-s., cob., fago., glon., lil-s., naja, ***sil., thuj.,*** thymol., ***verat.***
headache, from - ars-h., bufo, calc., cob., fago., glon., kali-c., lac-d., naja, sil.
heartburn, from - carb-v., chin., lyc.
heat, from - aster., ***carb-s.,*** coc-c., ***lach., nat-c.,*** nat-p., ***puls., puls-n,*** rhod., **SEL.,** ***sulph.,*** tab., vesp.
bed, of - aster.
flushes of, after - dig., nat-c., **SEP., SULPH.,** ***xan.***
heat of day, during - sel.
walking, amel. - ph-ac.
hot room, in - cinnb., ***puls.***
entering, from bed - aloe.
summer, of - alum., ***ant-c., ars., carb-s., corn.,*** **GELS., IOD.,** ***lach.,*** **NAT-C.,** nat-m., **SEL.**
sun, of - ***ars.,*** **GELS., NAT-C., SEL.**
thrills of heat, from - cocc.
walk, heated, and rapid cooling, after - bry., ***rhus-t.***
humiliation, after - carc., ign., ***staph.***
hunger, from - ***alum., crot-h.,*** **IOD.,** lach., ***lyc.,*** merc., nat-c., **PHOS.,** sep., ***spig.,*** sul-i., spig., **SULPH.,** ter., ***zinc.***
hysterical - nat-m., phos.
impressions, from unpleasant - phos.
indolency and luxury, from - helon.
influenza, after - abrot., ***carc.,*** con., chin., cypr., ***gels.,*** kali-p., ***ph-ac.,*** scut., x-ray.
injuries, from - ***acet-ac.,*** arn., calen., ***camph.,*** carb-v., dig., hyper., ***sul-ac.,*** verat.
intermittent - ***apis,*** nat-a., nat-s.
irritability, with - gall-ac.
jaundice, from - ferr-pic., pic-ac., tarax.
leaning towards left during menses amel. - phel.
left, side, of - ***arg-n., lach.***
lifting, from - **CARB-AN.,** kali-sil., nat-c.
looking down, on - kali-c.
loss of fluids, from - ***calc.,*** **CHIN.,** ***cur.,*** ferr., ferr-ac., ham., hydr., lachn., ***nat-m., nuph.,*** **PH-AC.,** ***phos., psor.,*** sec., ***sep.***
loss of sleep - **COCC.,** colch., cupr., glon., ***hydr., ip., nat-m.,*** nux-v., osm., ***puls.***
love, from unfortunate - ***ph-ac.***
lying, agg. - agar., alum., bar-c., bry., carl., carb-v., coca, cycl., gels., nat-c., nat-m., nit-ac., nux-v., petr., phys., pip-m., ***puls.,*** rhus-g., spig., zinc-m.
amel. - acon-f., ars., bry., hedeo, lach., mag-c., nat-m., nit-ac., ph-ac., ***psor.,*** sabad., ***sep.***
amel., on back - cast.
shower, before - gels.
masturbation, from - aven., bell-p., ***nat-m., phos.***
meeting amel., in interesting - pip-m.

WEAKNESS, general

menopause, during - **CHIN.**, chin-a., ***cocc.***, ***con.***, ***crot-h.***, dig., helon., ***kali-p.***, ***lach.***, magn-gl., phos., sabin., ***sep.***, sul-ac., tab.

menses, during - ***agar.***, ***aloe***, ***alum.***, alum-p., ***am-c.***, am-m., ***ars.***, ars-i., ars-s-f., bar-c., bar-i., bar-s., bell., berb., bor., bov., brom., bufo, cact., calc., calc-i., calc-p., ***calc-s.***, cann-s., **CARB-AN.**, ***carb-v.***, ***carb-s.***, caul., ***caust.***, cimic., ***cinnb.***, ***cocc.***, eupi., ferr., ferr-i., ***graph.***, ***helon.***, ign., ***iod.***, ip., ***kali-c.***, kali-n., ***kali-s.***, ***lach.***, ***lil-t.***, lyc., ***mag-c.***, ***mag-m.***, mag-s., mosch., ***murx.***, nat-a., nat-c., nat-m., ***nicc.***, ***nit-ac.***, nux-m., ***nux-v.***, ol-an., ***petr.***, phel., ***phos.***, pic-ac., ***sabin.***, ***sec.***, senec., **SEP.**, stann., ***sulph.***, tarent., thuj., tril., ***tub.***, uran-n., ***verat.***, vinc., wies., zinc., zinc-p.

amel. - **SEP.**

breath, can scarcely, must lie down - ***nit-ac.***

desire to lie down, with - bell., ip., ***nit-ac.***

end of - bov., iod.

going up stairs, when - ***iod.***

painful - bell., bufo

stand, can scarcely - cocc.

stool, after - nux-v.

talk, can scarcely - alum., ***carb-an.***, ***cocc.***, ***stann.***

after - agar., ***alum.***, ***alumn.***, am-c., am-m., aran., ***ars.***, bell., benz-ac., berb., cact., calc., calc-p., carb-ac., ***carb-an.***, carb-v., cast., ***chin.***, ***chin-s.***, ***cimic.***, ***cocc.***, ferr., ferr-pic., glyc., graph., ***helon.***, iod., **IP.**, kali-c., kali-p., mag-c., nat-m., nit-ac., nux-v., ***phos.***, pic-ac., plat., sapin., sec., sep., stann., sulph., thlaspi, thuj., ***tril.***, tub., ***verat.***, vinc.

disproportionate to loss of blood - alum., ham., ***ip.***

profound weakness - ***alum.***, am-c., am-m., ***ars.***, calc., ***carb-an.***, carb-v., ***chin.***, cimic., ***cocc.***, ferr., glyc., graph., iod., ip., kali-c., mag-c., phos., thlaspi, ***tril.***, ***verat.***, vinc.

appearance of, amel. - cycl., mag-m.

at beginning - brom., cocc., ferr., mag-m., phel.

before - ***alum.***, ***am-c.***, aur-s., ***bell.***, ***alum.***, ***am-c.***, brom., calc., carb-ac., carb-an., carb-v., ***chin.***, cimic., cinnb., ***cocc.***, ferr., glyc., graph., ***haem.***, ***helon.***, ign., iod., kali-p., lyc., ***mag-c.***, merc., ***nat-m.***, ***nicc.***, nux-m., phel., phos., puls., sec., ***verat.***, zinc.

mental, after (see Mind, Exertion)

midnight - ambr., op., ***rhus-t.***

2 a.m. - sep.

3 a.m. - nat-m., ***sec.***, zing.

4 a.m. - sulph.

after - nat-m., rhus-t.

milk, after - sul-ac.

miscarriage, weakness, from - ***alet.***, caul., chin., chin-s., ***helon.***, ruta, sec., ***sep.***, sil.

WEAKNESS, general

mononucleosis, after - abrot., **CARC.**, con., chin., cypr., ***gels.***, kali-p., ***ph-ac.***, scut., x-ray.

morning - ***acal.***, acon-l., agar., alum., am-c., am-m., ***ambr.***, amph., ant-c., ant-s., apoc., aran., ***arg-m.***, **ARS.**, ***ars-i.***, ars-s-f., asc-t., atra-r., atro., aur., aur-a., aur-i., bar-m., bell., bism., bor., brucin., ***bry.***, bufo, caj., ***calc.***, calc-i., ***calc-s.***, canth., caps., carb-an., ***carb-v.***, carb-s., celt., cham., chel., chin-s., cimic., cinnb., clem., coc-c., colch., ***con.***, corn., ***croc.***, crot-h., cycl., dig., digin., dios., dros., erig., euphr., eupi., fago., flor-p., form., ***gels.***, gnaph., ***graph.***, ham., hyper., hom., ***iod.***, jal., kali-bi., kali-c., kali-m., kali-n., kali-p., lac-c., lac-ac., **LACH.**, lact., levo., **LYC.**, ***mag-c.***, ***mag-m.***, meli., ***merc.***, merc-c., merl., morph., mur-ac., naja, ***nat-a.***, ***nat-c.***, ***nat-m.***, ***nat-p.***, ***nat-s.***, nat-sil., ***nit-ac.***, ***nux-v.***, op., osm., ox-ac., ped., perh., ***petr.***, **PH-AC.**, ***phos.***, pic-ac., plat., prun., psor., pulm-a., ***puls.***, ran-b., ***rhus-v.***, rob., ruta, sabad., sang., **SEP.**, ***sil.***, ***spig.***, stach., ***stann.***, ***staph.***, ***stront-c.***, stry., sul-ac., ***sulph.***, sumb., syph., tab., ther., thuj., til., tub., valer., ***verat.***, viol-t., zinc., ***zinc-p.***

5 a.m. - napht.

6 a.m. - pic-ac.

6:30 a.m. - ham.

7 a.m. - cham., elat., graph.

8 a.m. - dios., phys.

8:30 a.m. - fago.

9 a.m. - chin-s., cocc., merl., nat-s., ox-ac., ped., peti., phys., ptel., sep.

amel. - tarent.

10 a.m., until - nit-ac.

bed, in - ***ambr.***, arn., ***carb-v.***, caust., chin., chin-b., ***con.***, ham., hell., hep., hom., lach., mag-c., ***nat-m.***, phos., **PULS.**, ***sil.***, ***staph.***, stront-c.

bed, while sitting up in - nat-m.

fasting - con.

ideas, after copious flow of, at night - tab.

lying - **PULS.**

rising, on - alum., asc-t., aur-m-n., bov., **BRY.**, calc-caust., carbn., caust., chin., cina, colch., com., crot-t., dig., dios., ***dulc.***, eupi., ***ferr.***, ham., hep., ign., iris, **LACH.**, lac-ac., ***lyc.***, mez., nat-m., nux-v., op., petr., **PH-AC.**, phos., plb., puls., puls-n, rhus-v., scut., ***sep.***, ***sil.***, ***stann.***, sulph., thuj., ust.

amel. - acon., carb-v., caust., con., kali-c., mag-c., nat-c., nat-m., phos., ***puls.***

rising, after - alumn., ***arg-m.***, ***arg-n.***, bry., carb-an., hep., kali-n., ***lach.***, ***nit-ac.***, ***nux-v.***, peti., **PH-AC.**, rhod., til.

waking, on - acon., agar., alum., alum-p., am-c., ambr., ant-c., ***arg-m.***, arn., aur., bell., berb., ***bry.***, ***calc.***, calc-sil., cann-s., carb-an., carb-v., cast., cast-v., cham., chel., chin., clem., coca, colch., coloc., con., corn., crot-t., cycl., dros., ***dulc.***, euph., fago., gels., gnaph., graph., grat., hep., hyper., ign., iod., piloc., kali-c., kali-sil.,

WEAKNESS, general
morning,
waking, on - ***lach., lyc.,*** mag-c., mag-s., mang., nat-m., ***nux-v., phos.,*** pic-ac., plb., podo., rhus-t., sabad., ***sang., sep., sil., spig., staph.,*** stram., ***syph.,*** tab., ter., thuj., verat., xan., zinc.
motion, from - agar., ammc., apoc., ***arg-m.,*** **ARS.,** asaf., bry., cann-s., cocc., hydr-ac., kali-bi., kali-n., lach., mang-o., merc., merl., mur-ac., narcin., nat-m., nit-ac., nux-v., phel., ***phos.,*** plb., sep., spig., **SPONG.,** stann., staph., sulph., tab.
amel. - cham., colch., coloc., cycl., gels., kreos., ***lyc.,*** mosch., pip-m., ***plat.,*** plb., ***rhod.,*** stann.
gentle - ferr., kali-n., puls.
least motion, on - anac., lyc., nux-m., spig., verat.
when moved from horizontal position - rob.
moving arms, on - nat-m.
music, from - lyc.
nausea, with - aeth., ***agar.,*** alumn., ang., ant-t., ***ars., calc., camph.,*** cimic., cob., crot-t., gran., hell., ***ip.,*** sabad., sang., sep., stront-c., ***tab., verat.***
nervous, (see Nerves, Weakness)
night - acon-l., am-c., ambr., ant-c., anthr., anthro., calc., canth., carb-an., carb-v., chel., coca, crot-t., ferr-i., graph., hell., hyper., kreos., mur-ac., naja, nat-m., nux-v., rhus-t., sep., ***sil.,*** sulph., tab., thuj.
10 p.m. - elat., fago., phys.
11 p.m. - nat-m.
noon - bov., carb-v., caust., clem., con., cycl., fago., helon., hyper., nat-m., nit-ac., phos., phyt., ptel., sil., sulph., teucr., thuj.
3 p.m. until - hyos.
6 p.m. until - ptel.
12:30 p.m - gels., sol-t-ae.
amel. - hyper.
nursing, the sick, from - **CARC.,** ***cimic.,*** **COCC.,** ***nit-ac.,*** olnd., zinc.
sit up with sick person - carb-v., cocc., ***nux-v.,*** puls.
nursing, breast-feeding, from - ***calc., calc-p., carb-an.,*** **CARB-V., CHIN.,** chin-s., kali-c., lyc., olnd., **PH-AC.,** ***phos., phyt.,*** sep., ***sil., sulph.***
pain, from - ***arg-m.,*** **ARS.,** carb-v., cham., hep., hura, kali-p., kalm., pic-ac., plb., podo., ***rhus-t.,*** verat.
sacrum, in - ***sep.***
palpitation, with - aur., caust., sang., sul-i.
after - kali-c.
paralytic - agar., ***alum.,*** alum-p., ***alumn.,*** am-m., ambr., anac., ang., ***arg-m.,*** **ARS.,** ***art-v.,*** bapt., ***bar-c., bar-m.,*** bell., ***bism.,*** bry., ***calc.,*** calc-ar., camph., cann-i., canth., caps., carb-v., ***caust., cham.,*** chel., ***chin.,*** cimic., cina, **COCC.,** ***colch.,*** con., crot-h., cupr., dig., dros., euph., ***ferr.,*** ferr-ar., ferr-ma., **GELS., HELL.,** hyos., ign., ind., kali-c., kali-n., kali-p., kalm., lach., laur.,

WEAKNESS, general
paralytic - ***merc.,*** mez., mosch., **MUR-AC.,** nat-c., nat-m., nat-p., ***nit-ac.,*** nux-m., nux-v., ***olnd.,*** **PH-AC., PHOS.,** plat., plb., psor., ***puls., rhod., rhus-t.,*** sabad., sarcol-ac., sil., ***stann.,*** stront-c., sulph., valer., **VERAT.,** zinc.
heat, with - ferr.
morning after rising - phos.
motion, on - aeth., arg-m.
pain, with - ***arg-m., verat.***
painful parts, in - cham., ***verat.***
pleurisy, with - sabad.
sense of - stront-c.
sliding down in bed - ***ant-t., apis,*** arn., ***ars.,*** arum-t., ***bapt., bell.,*** carb-v., chin., colch., crot-h., ***hell.,*** hyos., ***lyc., lach.,*** **MUR-AC.,** mosch., nux-m., ***nit-ac.,*** **PH-AC., PHOS.,** ***rhus-t.,*** zinc.
stiffness, with - lith.
periodical - **ARG-N.**
every other morning - nit-ac.
perspiration, during - **ALOE,** ***calc., chin., chin-m.,*** dig., ***piloc., lyc., ph-ac.,*** sal-ac., sul-ac., ***tarent.***
agg., from - acon., agar., am-c., ambr., aml-n., ant-c., ***ant-t.,*** ant-ox., anthr., apis, **ARN.,** ***ars.,*** ars-i., ars-s-f., bar-c., benz., **BRY.,** bov., caj., ***calad., calc.,*** **CAMPH.,** canth., **CARB-AN.,** carb-v., carl., cast., **CAUST., CHIN.,** ***chin-a.,*** **CHIN-S.,** coca, cocc., croc., dig., **FERR.,** ***ferr-ar., ferr-i.,*** ferr-p., gels., graph., hep., hist., hura, hyos., ign., **IOD.,** jatr., kali-bi., kali-n., lac-c., lyc., mag-c., **MERC.,** morph., nat-c., ***nat-m., nit-ac., nux-v.,*** op., ***ph-ac.,*** **PHOS., PSOR.,** puls., ***pyrog.,*** ran-s., rhod., ***samb., sec.,*** senec., **SEP.,** ***sil., stann., sulph., tarax.,*** tarent., **TUB.,** ***verat., verat., verat-v.***
childbirth, after - ***samb.***
cold, during - ***camph., carb-v.,*** cupr., ***merc., ph-ac., ter.,*** **VERAT.**
night - ars., bar-c., bry., ***carb-an., chin.,*** eupi., ferr., ***merc.,*** nat-c., ph-ac., ***phos., samb.,*** stann., tarax., **TUB.**
suppressed foot sweat, from - ***sil.***
sleeping, while, burning heat, dry while awake - **SAMB.**
playing piano, from - anac.
pleasant - cann-s., morph.
pleasure, from - crot-c.
pregnancy, during - alet., alum., alumn., calc-p., caul., ***helon.,*** murx., ***sep., sulph., verat.***
progressive - acon., ars., caust., cupr-ar., ***dig.,*** kreos., ***ol-j., phos., plb.,*** verat.
prolapsus, from - alet., ***helon.***
quinine, from abuse of - ars-s-f., chin., chin-s.
rapid, onset - **ARS.,** bapt., laur., lyc., ***sep.,*** tub., **VERAT.**
early, and - ***merc-cy.***

WEAKNESS, general
reaction, with lack of - ***am-c., carc., laur., OP., sulph., valer.***
obese people, in - **CAPS.**
reading, from - anac., ***aur.,*** ph-ac., plb., ***sumb.***
aloud, from - stann.
rest, during - coloc., con., kreos., lyc., rhod.
amel. - bry.
resting head on something and closing eyes amel. - anac.
restlessness, with - **ARS.,** ***bism.,*** chin-a., ***colch.,*** lycps., lyss., ***ph-ac.,*** **RHUS-T.,** zinc.
riding, from - card-m., cer-b., cocc., petr., ***psor.,*** sep., sulph., tet.
amel., in open air - cinnb.
rising, on - acon-c., ammc., arn., **ARS.,** atro., **BRY.,** clem., coca, fago., ham., hydr., hyper., piloc., lyc., mag-c., nat-a., ***nat-m.,*** olnd., osm., phyt., pic-ac., ptel., rhus-g., rhus-t., sol-t-ae., teucr., thuj., uran-n.
after - am-c., coc-c., hydr., mag-c.
seat, from a -***chin.***
room, in - asar.
agg. from closed - asar.
sadness, from - aur., calc-p., ign., nat-m., ph-ac.
sea, bathing, after - ***mag-m.***
sedentary habit, from - nux-v., sulph.
sensitive, and - ter.
sex, after - ***agar.,*** ambr., berb., **CALC.,** ***carb-an., chin.,*** clem., ***con., dig., graph., kali-c., kali-p.,*** lil-t., lyc., mosch., nat-c., ***nat-m.,*** nit-ac., ***nuph.,*** petr., ***ph-ac., phos.,*** plat., **SEL.,** ***sep., sil.,*** staph., tarent., tax., thlaspi, vichy-g., ***ziz.***
shuddering, with - kali-c.
women, in - berb., sep.
sexual, excesses, after - ***agn., ars.,*** aven., calad., ***chin.,*** coca, con., ***dig.,*** gins., graph., kali-c., lil-t., ***lyc.,*** med., ***nat-m.,*** nat-p., nux-v., onos., ***ph-ac., phos.,*** sec., ***sel., sep.,*** staph., sulph., symph., thuj., ***ust.***
sexual, weakness - agn., calad., kali-br., lyc., nuph., onos., sabal., sel., staph., yohim.
unmarried persons, in - agn.
single parts, in - valer.
sinking, readily - ***merc.***
sit down, desire to - alum., ambr., anac., ars., bry., calc., caust., cham., chin., ***cocc.,*** colch., croc., dulc., kali-n., led., ***lil-t.,*** mag-aust., ***merc.,*** mur-ac., nat-m., nat-s., nux-v., ol-an., olnd., ph-ac., rhus-t., sabin., ***stann.,*** staph., stront-c., sulph., tarax., verat.
sitting - agar., anac., arg-m., ***ars.,*** aur., bry., carl., caust., chel., chin., cocc., colch., fago., graph., kali-n., led., ***lyc.,*** mag-aust., ***mag-c.,*** mang., merc., merc-i-f., mur-ac., ***nat-m.,*** nit-ac., nux-v., phos., ***plat.,*** plb., ptel., ran-b., **RHUS-T.,** ruta, sabad., staph., stront-c., ***sulph.,*** thuj.
amel. - bry., euph-a., glon., nux-v., sapin.
walk, after a - **RUTA**

WEAKNESS, general
sleep, after - agar., ambr., bor., bor-ac., camph., carl., chel., chin-s., coca, colch., con., cycl., dor., ferr., gels., gent-l., ***kali-n., lach.,*** lyc., mez., nat-n., sec., sep., sil., sin-n., zinc.
amel. - alum., mez., ***ph-ac., phos.***
during - bufo.
loss of, from - **CARC., COCC.,** colch., cupr., ***cypr.,*** glon., ***hydr., ip., kreos., nat-m.,*** nux-v., osm., ***puls.***
as from - plat.
sleepiness, from - chlol., ***coff., chlol.,*** gran., hep., nit-ac., rhus-t.
afternoon, walking amel. - ruta
as from - ***aeth.,*** chen-v., cimic., dig., kali-n., merc-sul., peti., petr., phel., plat., ***rhus-t.,*** thuj.
morning - verat.
sleeplessness, from - **CARC., COCC.,** ***cypr., kreos.***
smoking, from - asc-t., calad., clem., ***hep.***
somnambulism after - sulph.
speak, cannot, from - cocc.
sports, after - ***arn.,*** ars., coca, fl-ac., rhus-t.
spring, in - apis, **BRY.**
standing - ***acon.,*** acon-c., agn., ***apis,*** asaf., aster., berb., ***cic.,*** cocc., crot-h., cupr., cur., ham., hep., ***kali-c.,*** kali-n., lach., led., merc., **MERC-CY.,** mur-ac., nat-m., nit-ac., nux-v., ol-an., ped., plat., ran-b., spig., staph., sul-ac., **SULPH.,** ther., zing.
stimulants amel. - phos.
stomach, in - ***calc-p., calc-s., crot-t.,*** **HYDR.,** ***podo.***
as from - mag-c.
pain in, from - ***nux-v., podo.***
and back - sep.
stool, during - aesc., apis, atro., bell., ***bor.,*** carb-s., cob., colch., crot-h., crot-t., ***cupr-ar.,*** kali-i., lact., ***nit-ac.,*** pic-ac., plan., **PLAT.,** sec., ***verat.***
after - acet-ac., aeth., ***ail., aloe,*** ant-t., apis, apoc., ***arg-n.,*** arn., ***ars.,*** **ARS-M.,** ars-s-f., bapt., bism., bov., ***calc., camph.,*** carb-an., ***carb-v., carb-s.,*** cast-v., caust., ***chin., chin-s.,*** clem., cocc., coch., ***colch.,*** coloc., com., ***con.,*** cop., crot-h., crot-t., cupr., dios., ***dulc.,*** elat., eupi., ferr-m., ferr-ma., ***graph.,*** ign., ***iod.,*** ip., iris, ***jatr., kali-p., lach.,*** lil-t., lipp., ***lyc.,*** mag-c., mag-m., ***med.,*** **MERC.,** mez., nat-m., **NAT-S., NIT-AC.,** ***nux-m., nux-v., petr., phos.,*** phys., **PIC-AC.,** plan., ***podo.,*** pyre-p., rham-f., ***rhus-t.,*** sabad., sac-alb., ***sec., sep., sil.,*** sul-ac., ***sulph., tab., ter.,*** thuj., trio., trom., tub., upa., **VERAT.,** vinc.
mucus - bor.
before - hydr., mez., nat-h., ***rhus-t., verat.***
stooping, on - graph.

WEAKNESS, general

storm, before and during a - psor., sang., sil., tub.

thunderstorm, during - caust., nat-c., nat-p., nit-ac., petr., rhod., sil.

stroke, from - ***bar-c.***

suckling, after - carb-v.

sudden - ***acon.,*** act-sp., ***aeth.,*** ail., ***am-c.,*** am-m., ambr., ***ant-a.,*** ant-c., ***ant-t., apis,*** apoc., ***arg-m.,*** arg-n., arn., **ARS.,** ars-h., ***ars-i., bapt.,*** bell., bry., calc., camph., cann-s., carb-ac., ***carb-v., caust.,*** cham., colch., con., **CROT-H.,** ***cupr.,*** cupr-ac., dig., dulc., fl-ac., ***gels.,*** glon., **GRAPH.,** ***hell., hep., hydr-ac., ip.,*** jatr., kali-br., kali-c., kali-cy., kalm., lach., laur., lith., lyc., mag-c., merc-c., merc-cy., naja, nit-ac., ***nux-v.,*** petr., ***phos.,*** ran-b., rhus-t., sabad., sec., ***sel.,*** **SEP.,** sil., spong., stann., stram., ***sulph., tab.,*** tarent., tax., thuj., tub., ***verat., verat-v.,*** vip., zinc.

afternoon - lyc., ran-b.

1:30 p.m. - iodof.

walking, after - graph.

chilliness, during - sep.

daily - ***hep.***

diarrhea, with - crot-t.

dressing, while, after rising - ***stann.***

elderly people, in - kali-cy.

eruption comes out, after the - ars.

evening - fl-ac.

sitting, while - cham., lyc., ran-b.

vanish, as if senses would - ran-b.

vision, with illusion of - sep.

walking, from - carb-v., con., sabad., wild.

sunstroke, from - ***glon., verat-v.***

supper, after - alum., bov., chin., lach., mag-c., sil.

suppressed eruptions, from - ars., ars-s-f.

surgery, from - acet-ac., arn., ***calen.,*** carb-v., hyper., phos., stront-c.

symptoms, with very few - carc., op., syph.

syphilis, in - ***ars., aur.,*** calo., carb-an., carb-v., ferr-i., ferr-lac., ***iod., kali-i., lyc., merc.,*** sars., ***staph.***

talking, from - act-sp., **ALUM.,** am-c., am-caust., ambr., arn., ***calc., cocc.,*** dor., ***ferr.,*** hydrc., ***hyos.,*** iod., jac-c., ***nat-m., ph-ac., psor.,*** sep., sil., **STANN., SULPH.,** ***ust.,*** wies.

other people, from the talking of - alum., am-c., ars., verat.

tea, amel. - dig.

tobacco, from - calad., clem., hep.

toothache, with - mang., mag-p.

after - nat-c.

tremulous - ***agar., alum., anac.,*** anag., ant-c., ant-t., ***apis,*** **ARG-N.,** ***ars., bapt.,*** bell., berb., bor., brom., bry., calc-ar., caps., carb-v., caul., caust., ***chin.,*** chin-s., clem., ***cocc.,*** **CON.,** ***crot-h.,*** cupr., **GELS.,** graph., hep., hyos., kali-c., kali-n., ***kalm.,*** **LACH.,** lyc., lycps., mang., med., ***nat-m., nit-ac.,*** ol-an., olnd., ox-ac., petr., ***phos., plat.,*** plb., ***puls.,*** rhus-t., ***sep.,*** spig., **STANN.,** ther., thuj., tub., verat., vip., zinc.

alternation between tremulous and trembling - ferr.

dinner, after - ant-c.

night, on waking - brom.

smoking, after - hep.

stool, after - **ARS.,** carb-v., caust., **CON.**

trifles, from - am-c., ars.

upper part, with trembling of lower - ambr.

urination, after - ***ars.,*** caust., cimic., ferr., ***gels., lyss.,*** nux-v., ***phos., pic-ac.,*** sep., syph., tub.

urination, after, after copious - caust., gels., med.

vaginal, discharge, from - chin., con.

vertigo, with - ***acet-ac., cocc.,*** crot-t., cupr-s., dulc., graph., hell., ***sil.,*** uran-n.

vexation, after - ***ars., calc-p.,*** lyc., ***nat-m.,*** nux-v., petr., sep., ***staph.,*** verat.

voice away, takes - canth., stann.

vomiting, with - aeth., ars., bol-s., ***calc.,*** chin., crot-t., gran., ip., kali-c., phos., **SANG.,** sulph., tab.

after - aloe, ant-c., ant-t., apom., ars., bar-c., cadm-s., ***colch.,*** der., gran., guai., mag-c., nat-s., op., phyt., sel., ***verat.,*** zinc.

waking, on - aeth., alco., aloe, ambr., aq-pet., arg-m., ars-h., bell., bism., bry., carb-s., card-m., cham., chel., chin., clem., ***cycl.,*** dig., dios., ***dulc., echi.,*** equis., erig., erio., euphr., ferr., ferr-p., form., hipp., hura, ign., lac-ac., **LYC.,** mang., myric., nabal., nat-a., nat-m., nat-p., nux-m., **NUX-V.,** op., **PH-AC.,** podo., ptel., **PULS.,** rhod., rhus-t., sang., sec., sel., ***sep.,*** sulph., sumb., syph., tab., teucr., thuj., upa., xan.

after - arg-m., calc-s., cedr., cycl., iod., wild.

morning - mag-c.

from a dream - ***calc-s.,*** op., teucr.

walking, from - acon., acon-f., aesc., agar., **ALUM., ALUM-P.,** alum-sil., am-c., ambr., ***anac.,*** ang., arg-m., arn., **ARS.,** ***ars-i.,*** aur-a., aur-m., aur-s., bar-c., bar-i., bar-m., bar-s., ***berb.,*** bov., brom., **BRY., CALC., CANN-I.,** carb-ac., ***carb-an., carb-v.,*** carb-s., caust., cench., cham., chel., ***chin.,*** chin-a., clem., coca, cocc., ***coloc.,*** **CON.,** cupr., ***cupr-ar.,*** cycl., digin., ery-a., ery-m., euph., euph-a., fago., **FERR.,** ferr-ar., ferr-i., ferr-ma., ***fl-ac.,*** franz., gins., graph., ham., helon., hep., hyper., ind., indg., ***iod.,*** kali-ar., ***kali-c.,*** kali-m., kali-p., kali-sil., ***lac-d.,*** **LACH.,** led., ***lyc.,*** lyss., mag-c., mag-m., mag-s., ***med.,*** meny., merc., merl., mez., morph., **MUR-AC.,** narcin., ***nat-a., nat-c.,*** nat-hchls., ***nat-m.,*** nat-n., ***nat-s.,*** nat-sil., nicot., **NIT-AC.,** nux-m., nux-v., pall., petr., **PH-AC., PHOS.,** phys., phyt., **PIC-AC.,** ***plb.,*** polyg., **PSOR.,** ***puls.,*** puls-n, ran-b., rheum, rhod., rhus-d., **RHUS-T.,** ruta, sabin., sarcol-ac., **SEP.,** ***sil., spig.,*** **SQUIL.,** stann., ***staph.,*** stram., stront-c., sul-i., **SULPH.,** sumb., tarent., tell., thea., thuj., til., tril., tub., ***verat.,*** wies., wild.,

WEAKNESS, general
walking, from - ***zinc.,*** zinc-p.
air, open, in - act-sp., agar., **ALUM.,** alumn., ***am-c.,*** ambr., ang., arg-m., ars-s-f., berb., bry., ***calc.,*** calc-sil., carb-v., caust., chin., coff., chel., ***cocc., coll.,*** coloc., ***con.,*** euph., ferr., graph., grat., hep., hyos., kali-bi., kali-c., lact., lyc., mag-arct., mag-aust., mag-c., mag-m., merc., nat-m., ***nux-v.,*** ph-ac., puls., rhod., **RHUS-T.,** sang., sep., ***sil., spig.,*** sulph., ***zinc.***
after - graph., sil., spong.
amel. - agar., alum., am-c., asar., caust., chin-s., croc., ***fl-ac.,*** grat., ***kali-i.,*** ox-ac., sapin., ***sulph.***
amel. - ambr., anac., bry., calc., coloc., merc., nat-m., **RHUS-T.,** ***ruta,*** **SULPH.**
breakfast, after, amel. - coca.
commencing to walk, on - ***carb-v.***
cough and expectoration, from - nux-v.
dinner, before - hyper.
eating, after - hep.
heat of the sun, in - ***lach., nat-c.***
house, in - agar., ferr-ma., sapin., sec., sumb.
menses, during - ***murx.,*** phel.
rapidly - agar., coc-c., olnd.
amel. - ***stann.***
riding, after - petr.
short walk, from - ***calc.,*** cann-i., ***con.***
short walk, from, after a - ***nat-c.,*** ruta, ***sulph., ter.,*** tub.
slowly amel. - ***ferr.***
smoking, after - sulph.
storm, before and during a - sil.
warm, room - aloe, ambr., croc., ***iod.,*** merl., **PULS.**
weather agg. - **ANT-C.,** camph., ***iod.,*** lach., ***nat-a.,*** nat-c., nat-m., nat-p., nat-s., podo., puls., ***sel.,*** **SULPH.,** vip.
wine agg. - ars., lyc., phos., ***thuj., zinc.***
amel. - ars., ***thuj.,*** visc.
women, worn out from hard work - calc., helon., ***sep.***
indolence and luxury, from - helon., ***sep.***
working hard, as from - apis.
worms, with - carc., ***cic., cina, merc.***
writing, from - cann-s., ran-b., sil.
yawning, after - eug., ***nux-v.***

WEARINESS, general (see Weakness) - acon., aesc., agar., **ALUM.,** ambr., ***am-c., anac., ant-c., ant-t.,*** arg-m., ***arg-n., arn., ars., ars-i.,*** asaf., asar., aur., aur-m., ***bapt.,*** bar-c., bar-m., bell., **BENZ-AC.,** berb., bism., bov., ***bry.,*** calc., **CALC-P.,** camph., **CANN-S.,** canth., caps., ***carb-ac.,*** carb-an., **CARB-S.,** ***carb-v.,*** caust., cham., **CHEL.,** chin., cic., cimic., cimx., cina, clem., cocc., ***coc-c.,*** coff., colch., coloc., ***con.,*** **CROC.,** ***crot-c., cupr.,*** cycl., dig., dros., dulc., euph., euphr., **FERR.,** ferr-p., **GELS., GRAPH.,** ***ham.,*** hell., helon., ***hep., hyos.,*** ign., ***ip.,*** kali-c., kali-n., **KALI-P.,** kali-s., ***kreos.,*** **LACH.,** lac-ac., ***laur.,*** led., **LYC.,** ***mag-c.,*** mag-m., mang., meny., **MERC.,** mez., mosch., ***mur-ac., nat-c.,*** **NAT-M.,** ***nat-s.,*** nit-ac., ***nux-m.,*** **NUX-V.,** olnd., op., ***par.,*** ***petr.,*** **PH-AC., PHOS., PIC-AC.,** ***plat.,*** plb., ***psor.,*** **PULS.,** ran-b., ***rheum, rhod., rhus-t.,*** **RUTA,** sabad., sabin., samb., sars., sec., senec., seneg., **SEP., SIL.,** spig., spong., squil., ***stann.,*** **STAPH.,** ***stram.,*** stront-c., **SULPH.,** sumb., ***sul-ac., tab.,*** teucr., thuj., **TUB.,** valer., ***verat.,*** verb., viol-o., **ZINC.**
conversation, from - ambr.
eating, after - ant-c., **ARS.,** ***bar-c., carb-an.,*** card-m., chin., kali-c., ***lach.,*** mur-ac., ***nat-m., nux-m., rhus-t.,*** ruta., sang.
eating, while - ***kali-c.***
evening - berb., carb-v., ign., pall., ***mur-ac., sulph.***
in open air - ***carb-v.***
menses, during - ***am-c.,*** bor., calc-p., ***caust., ign.,*** iod., kali-c., mag-c., ***nit-ac., nux-m., petr.,*** thuj.
after - thuj.
before - alum., ***bell., nat-m.***
mental exertion - alum., ***aur., lach.,*** **LEC., PIC-AC.,** ***puls., thuj.***
morning - ambr., am-c., ***ars.,*** bry., calad., carb-s., ***carb-v., cham., kali-chl.,*** lac-ac., **LACH.,** mag-c., mag-m., ***nat-m.,*** **NUX-V.,** petr., **SEP.,** staph., ***sulph.,*** zinc.
playing piano - anac.
reading, from - ***aur.***
sitting, while - ***merc.***
standing, when - ***mur- ac.***
talking, after - **ALUM.,** ***calc-p., sulph.***
too, much - kali-c.
walking, after - ***mur- ac.***

WEATHER, change of (see Environment, Weather)

WET, in general, (see Environment, Wet)

WHITENESS, of parts usually red - ambr., ant-t., ***ars.,*** anac., ang., **BOR.,** ***calc.,*** canth., carb-v., caust., chel., ***chin.,*** cina, coloc., dig., ***ferr., graph.,*** **HELL.,** ***kali-c., kali-m.,*** **LAC-C.,** lac-d., lyc., **MERC.,** ***merc-c.,*** nat-c., ***nat-m., nit-ac., nux-v., olnd.,*** op., petr., ph-ac., ***phos., plb., puls.,*** sabin., ***sec.,*** sep., ***staph., sul-ac.,*** sulph., valer., verat., viol-t., ***zinc.***

WIND, general, (see Environment, Wind)

WORK, manual, fine, agg. - graph., iod., kali-p., ***sil.***

Glands

ABSCESS, suppurations - ***aur., aur-m-n.,*** bad., ***bar-c.,*** bar-m., ***bell.,*** brom., **CALC.,** calc-f., ***calc-hp.,*** calc-i., calc-p., **CALC-S.,** ***carb-an.,*** carb-v., canth., cinnb., cist., clem., coloc., crot-h., ***dulc.,*** echi., fl-ac., ***form., guai.,*** guare., **HEP.,** hyos., ign., jug-r., **KALI-I.,** kreos., ***lach.,*** lap-a., ***lyc.,*** **MERC.,** myris., ***nit-ac.,*** petr., ***phos., phyt., pyrog., rhus-t., sars.,*** sec., ***sep.,*** **SIL.,** sil-mar., spig., squil., sul-ac., **SULPH.,** ***stram., syph.,*** teucr-s., ***tub.,*** zinc.

ABSORBENTS, red lines along - vesp.

ADENITIS, inflammation of - ***acon., alumn., anan.,*** apis, arn., ars., ars-i., ***aur., aur-m., bad., bar-c.,*** **BAR-M., BELL.,** ***bry., brom.,*** bufo, **CALC.,** ***camph.,*** canth., ***carb-an.,*** carb-v., **CARC.,** ***cham., cist.,*** clem., ***con., dulc.,*** ferr-ar., ***hep.,*** kali-ar., ***kali-c., kali-i.,*** kali-p., lach., laur., ***lyc.,*** **MERC.,** ***nit-ac., nux-v.,*** petr., ph-ac., **PHOS., PHYT.,** plb., ***psor., puls., rhus-t.,*** samb., sars., ***sil.,*** spig., squil., staph., **SULPH.,** sul-ac., thuj., verat., zinc.

- acute adenitis - acon., ail., alumn., anan., ***apis,*** ars-i., bar-c., bar-i., ***bell., bism., carc.,*** clem., ***dulc.,*** graph., ***hep.,*** iod., ***iodof., kali-i., merc., merc-i-r.,*** oper., ***phyt.,*** rhus-t., sil., ***sil-mar.***
- chronic adenitis - acon-l., ***ail., aln.,*** apis, ars., ars-br., ***ars-i.,*** arum-d., astac., aur-m., ***bad., bar-c., bar-i.,*** bar-m., ***brom., calc., calc-f., calc-i.,*** calc-p., calen., ***carb-an.,*** **CARC.,** ***cist., clem., con.,*** cory., crot-h., dulc., ferr-i., fil., graph., hep., ***iod., kali-i.,*** lach., ***lap-a.,*** lyc., med., merc., merc-cy., merc-i-f., ***merc-i-r.,*** nit-ac., **PHYT.,** psor., rhus-t., ***rumx.,*** scirr., **SCROPH-N.,** ***sil.,*** sil-mar., ***spong., sulph.,*** tax., thiosin., thuj., tub.
- breasts, particularly of - plan.
- children, in - ***bell.***
- lymphatic - crot-h., ***hep.,*** hippoz., kali-m., ***sil.***
  - with heat and shining redness, hardness and pain - nux-v.
- sebaceous, glands of - chel., **SIL.**
- scirrhus, in - ***carb-an.***
- obscure, infiltration - ***clem.***

ADENOIDS, problems with - agra., ***bar-c., bar-m., calc.,*** calc-f., calc-i., calc-p., ***carc.,*** chr-ac., iod., kali-s., lob-s., merc., mez., phyt., psor., sang-n., sulph., ***thuj., tub.***

- post nasal - mez.
- removal, after - carc., kali-s.

ATROPHY - anan., ars., ***aur.,*** bar-c., carb-an., ***cham.,*** chim., chin., **CON., IOD.,** kali-ar., kali-c., **KALI-I.,** kali-p., kreos., lac-d., ***nit-ac.,*** nux-m., ph-ac., plb., sars., ***sec.,*** sil., ***staph.,*** sul-i., verat.

BORING, pain - ***bell.,*** puls., sabad.

BURNING, pain - alum., ant-c., arn., **ARS.,** ***bell.,*** brom., bry., calc., ***cann-s.,*** carb-v., caust., cic., clem., ***cocc., con.,*** graph., ***hep., ign.,*** kali- c.,

BURNING, pain - laur., merc., mez., nat-m., nux-v., ***phos.,*** phyt., plat., **PULS.,** rhus-t., ***sep., sil.,*** staph., sul-ac., sulph., teucr., ***zinc.***

- scirrhus, in - ***carb-an.***
- lymphatic - ***carb-v.***

CANCER - ***ars-i., aster., aur-m.,*** brom., bufo., **CARB-AN., CARC.,** ***cist.,*** **CON.,** ***iod.,*** **PHYT.,** ***scroph-n.,*** sul-i., syph.

- adenocarcinoma - ars., aur-m., bufo., carb-an., carc., ***con., phyt.***

COLD - ***cocc.***

CONSTRICTING, pain - am-c., anac., bell., ***calc.,*** carb-v., caust., chin., ign., iod., kali-c., lyc., nat-c., nux-v., ph-ac., ***plat., puls.,*** sabad., sep., sil., spong.

CUTTING, pain - arg-m., ***bell.,*** calc., con., graph., ign., ***lyc.,*** nat-c., ph-ac., ***sep.,*** sil., staph., sulph.

- around, glands - con.
- scirrhus, in - ***carb-an.***

DIGGING, up, pain - acon., am-m., arn., asaf., bell., bov., bry., calc., ***dulc.,*** kali-c., nat-c., phos., plat., ***rhod.,*** rhus-t., ruta., sep., spig., stann.

DRAWING, pain - phos.

FISTULA, of - ***phos., sil., sulph.***

FOLLICULAR, disturbed action causes pimples on face, neck, etc. - ***kali-m.***

FORMICATION - acon., ***arn.,*** bell., calc., cann-s., canth., **CON.,** ign., laur., mag-aust., merc., nat-c., ph-ac., ***plat.,*** puls., rhod., ***rhus-t.,*** sabin., ***sep., spong.,*** sulph., zinc.

- suffering parts - con.

GNAWING, pain - bar-c., cham., mez., ph- ac., ***plat.,*** ran-s., ***spong.,*** staph.

HERPES, glands, covered with - dulc., graph.

HODGKIN'S disease - ***acon.,*** acon-l., ***ars., ars-i., bar-i.,*** buni-o., ***calc-f., carc.,*** cist., con., cund., ferr-pic., ***iod., kali-m., nat-m.,*** ph-ac., ***phos.,*** **PHYT.,** saroth., **SCROPH-N.,** syph., ***thuj., tub.***

HOT - ***asaf.,*** chin., **PULS., RHUS-T.**

INDOLENT, with syphilis - **KALI-I.**

INDURATIONS, of - acon., agar., agn., ***alum.,*** alumn., ***am-m.,*** ambr., am-c., ant-c., ***anthr., apis, arg-n.,*** arn., ars., ars-br., ars-i., ***asaf., astac., aster., aur.,*** aur-a., aur-i., ***aur-m., aur-m-n.,*** aur-s., **BAD., BAR-C.,** ***bar-i.,*** **BAR-M., BELL.,** bov., **BROM.,** ***bry.,*** bufo, **CALC., CALC-F.,** ***calc-i., calc-s.,*** calc-sil., camph., cann-s., canth., caps., **CARB-AN.,** carb-s., ***carb-v.,*** caust., **CHAM.,** ***chin., cinnb., cist.,*** **CLEM.,** ***cocc.,*** coloc., **CON.,** cupr., cycl., ***dig., dulc.,*** ferr., ***ferr-i., graph., hecla.,*** hep., hydr., hyos., ign., **IOD.,** kali-c., ***kali-chl., kali-i.,*** kali-n., ***lap-a.,*** lyc., ***mag-m.,*** mang., **MERC.,** ***merc-c.,*** merc-d., ***merc-i-f.,*** merc-i-r., merc-sul., nat-a., ***nat-c.,*** nat-m., nit-ac., nux-v., oper., petr., phos., **PHYT.,** plb., ***psor., puls.,*** raph., rhod., **RHUS-T.,** ***sars.,*** sep., ***sil.,*** spig., **SPONG.,** squil., staph., **SUL-I., SULPH.,** syph., thuj., thyr., tub., verat., viol-t.

- cancerous - **CON.**

INDURATIONS, of
conjunctivitis, with scrofulous - ***iod.***
everywhere - tub.
injuries, after - arn., bell-p., **CON.,** phyt.
knotty like ropes - aeth., **BAR-M.,** berb., ***calc., cist.,*** con., ***dulc.,*** hep., ***iod.,*** lyc., nit-ac., rhus-t., ***sil.,*** sul-i., ***tub.***
lymphatics - am-c., ***carb-s.***
felt like hard cords under skin, painful - ***apis***
if cut across, red, harder or softer, infiltrated with hemorrhagic or bloody, serous matter - anthr.
maxilla, under - anthr.
neck, especially - **BAR-C.**
nodes, under the skin, like - bry., ***calc.,*** caust., mag-c., nit-ac., ***still.***
parotid - brom., ***carb-an.***
scirrhus - ***carb-an.***
scrofula and syphilitic buboes - **BAD.**
scrofulous - **BAR-M.**
secondary deposit - con.
stony hard - ***calc-f.***
syphilis - ***merc***-i-f.
throat, in - anthr., con.
tingling and stitches, with, after contusions and bruises - **CON.**

INFILTRATION, interstitial - **KALI-I.**
acute, lymphatic - kali-m.
hemorrhagic, lymphatic - anthr.

INFLAMMATION, (see Adenitis)

INJURIES, to - ***arn.,*** aster., cann-s., **BELL-P.,** cic., ***cist.,*** **CON.,** ***dulc.,*** glon., ***hep., iod.,*** kali-c., kalm., ***iod.,*** merc., ***petr., phos.,*** phyt., puls., rhus-t., ***sil., sul-ac., sulph.***
indurations, after - arn., bell-p., **CON.,** phyt.

IRRITATION - ***iod.***

ITCHING - am-c., ***anac.,*** ant-c., anth., carb- an., carb-v., ***caust.,*** cocc., **CON.,** ***kali-c.,*** mag-c., merc., nit-ac., ***phos.,*** ran-s., rheum, rhus-t., sabin., sep., ***sil., spong.***

JERKING, pain - arn., asaf., aur., bell., bry., ***calc.,*** caps., caust., chin., ***clem.,*** graph., lyc., meny., merc., nat-c., ***nat-m.,*** nit-ac., nux-v., petr., ***puls.,*** rhus-t., sep., sil., sulph.

LANCINATING, pain - ***carb-an.***

LYMPH, effusion, after inflammation - ***kali-m.***

LYMPHATIC affections - ***lap-a., sulph.***
affections, in scrofula - **BAR-M.**
intense redness in streaks, following course of, from calf upward to body, with great anxiety - mygal.
palpable - tub.
red lines and stripes in course of - anthr.
streaks - ***lach.***
redness and swelling along course, after wounds - ***bufo***
vessels, inflamed, swollen, from hand to shoulder - cupr-m.

NUMBNESS, sensation of, in - anac., asaf., bell., cocc., con., lyc., ***plat.,*** puls., rhus-t., sep., sil., spong.

PAIN, glands - acon., ***alum.,*** ambr., ***am-c.,*** ant-c., ant-t., **ARN.,** ars., ***ars-i., aur., bar-c.,*** bar-m., **BELL.,** ***bry.,*** calc., ***cann-s.,*** canth., ***carb-an., carb-s., carb-v., caust.,*** cham., chin., cic., clem., ***coloc.,*** con., dulc., graph., hell., hep., ign., ***iod.,*** kali-c., kali-s., **LYC.,** mag-c., **MERC.,** ***nat-m., nit-ac.,*** nux-v., petr., ***ph-ac.,*** **PHOS., PULS.,** rheum, **RHUS-T.,** sel., sep., sil., ***spig.,*** spong., squil., stann., staph., stram., ***sulph., sul-ac.,*** **THUJ.,** verat.

PANCREAS, ailments of - ars., ***atro.,*** bar-m., bell., calc-ar., carb-an., carb-v., chion., ***con.,*** hydr., iod., ***iris,*** piloc., kali-i., ***merc.,*** nux-v., ***phos.,*** piloc., puls., ***spong.***
acute affections - con., ***iris.***
burning, pain - ars., calc-ar., ***iris,*** phos.
distress, with sweetish vomiting, diarrhoea and prostration - ***iris.***
cancer - ars., ***calc-ars.,*** **CON., HYDR.,** phos.
diabetes mellitus, (see Generals)
diseased - atro., phos.
duct, catarrh - ***merc.***
catarrh in girls - ***puls.***
enlarged, chronic inflammation - ***iod.***
excites secretion of - iris.
fatty degeneration - ***phos.***
heavy, painful feeling - merc-i-r.
induration, of - bar-m., ***carb-an., con.***
with paroxysms of lack of breath - ***bar-m.***
with vomiting after eating - ***carb-an.***
infarct - ammc.
kidneys, disease of, preceding or accompanying diabetes mellitus, or bright's disease - ***phos.***
pancreatitis - ars., **BELL.,** coloc., ***con., iod., iris, phos.,*** **SPONG.**
acute - ***con., iris.***
chronic - ***iod.,*** **SPONG.**

PAROTID, gland
abscess - **ARS.,** ***lach.,*** lyc., ***phos.,*** phyt., ***rhus-t.,*** **SIL.**
boring, pain - sabad.
burning, pain - apis, merc., phos.
cold air amel. - merc.
clawing, pain - sabad.
cutting, pain - arg-m.
chewing, when - arg-m.
digging, pain - sulph.
dinner, after - sulph.
drawing, pain - agn., ***arg-m.,*** mang.
left - agn.
enlarged - ***ail., kali-bi.,*** nit-ac., rhus-t., ***sil.***
left - ***rhus-t.***
right - nit-ac.
induration - am-c., bar-m., **BROM.,** calc., carb-an., cist., clem., ***con.,*** cupr., ign., kali-c., merc., merc-i-f., nat-m., phyt., **RHUS-T., SIL.**
right - ign., kali-c.
inflamation, (see mumps)

PAROTID, gland

mumps, parotid gland, inflamation of - ***acon.,*** ail., ***am-c.,*** ant-t., anthr., ***ars., arum-t., aur.,*** aur-m., **BAR-C.,** ***bar-m.,*** **BELL.,** ***brom., calc., carb-an.,*** CARB-V., ***cham.,*** **CIST.,** cocc., ***con., crot-h.,*** dor., dulc., euphr., ***ferr-p., hep.,*** hippoz., **JAB.,** kali-ar., ***kali-bi., kali-c.,*** kali-m., kali-p., ***lach., lyc.,*** mag-p., **MERC.,** merc-i-f., merc-i-r., ***nat-m.,*** petr., ***phos.,*** phyt., piloc., **PULS.,** ***rhus-t.,*** sars., ***sil.,*** sul-i., sulph., trif-p., trif-r.

gangrenous - anthr.

left - **BROM.,** ***lach.,*** **RHUS-T.**

metastasis to, brain - apis, bell., hyos.

to, breasts - carb-v., con., piloc., **PULS.**

to, testes - ***ars., carb-v., clem., ham.,*** jab., nat-m., **PULS.,** rhus-t.

persistent - bar-ac., bar-c., ***con., iod.,*** sil.

prophylactic - trif-r.

right - ***bar-m., calc., kali-bi., kali-c.,*** **MERC.**

then left - **LYC.**

scarlatina, in - ***calc.***

suppuration with - **ARS., BROM.,** ***bry.,*** **CALC.,** ***con.,*** **HEP.,** ***lach.,*** **MERC.,** ***nat-m., phos.,*** **RHUS-T., SIL.,** sul-ac.

lancinating, pain - carb-an.

pain - apis, aran., arg-m., ***aur.,*** aur-s., bapt., ***bell.,*** calc-p., cham., coc-c., dios., elaps, fago., ferr-p., lac-ac., lycps., mang., ***merc., merc-i-r.,*** nat-m., phyt., plb., ***rhus-t.,*** sabad., sulph.

afternoon - dios.

lunch, after - sulph.

cold, air - kali-c.

applications amel. - merc.

evening, 8:30 p.m. - merc-i-r.

extending to eye - coloc.

left - coloc., rhus-t.

night,10 p.m. - dios.

right - bell., cocc., merc.

swallowing, when - ***chin.***

touch - ***aur.,*** phos.

pinching, pain, in - aran., nat-m.

sharp, pain - asaf., **BELL.,** bry., calc., cham., chin., ***dulc.,*** ign., ***kali-bi.,*** kali-c., kalm., lyc., merc., nat-c., phos., puls., ***sep.,*** sil., spong., sulph.

sharp, swallowing, when - ign., spig.

sore, pain - ail., arum-t., aur., ***aur-m.,*** bry., calc-p., calc-s., cop., dros., kali-n., merc-i-r., nat-c., phos.

sore, left - arum-t.

sore, right - calc-s.

stinging, pain - apis, merc.

swelling, of - ail., ***am-c.,*** anth., apis, ***arn., ars.,*** **ARUM-T.,** ***aur., aur-m.,*** **BAR-C.,** ***bar-m.,*** **BELL., BROM.,** ***bry.,*** bufo, ***calc., calc-s., carb-an., carb-s., carb-v.,*** **CHAM., CHIN.,** ***chin-a.,*** chlol., ***cinnb., cist., cocc.,*** coc-c., ***con., crot-h.,*** dig., ***dulc.,*** fago., ***ferr-p., graph., hep.,*** hippoz., hyos., ***ign., iris,*** kali-ar., ***kali-bi., kali-c., kali-i.,*** kali-p., ***lach.,*** lac-c., ***lyc.,*** mang., **MERC.,** ***merc-cy., merc-i-r., mur-ac.,*** nat-a., nat-c., **NIT-AC.,**

PAROTID, gland

swelling - nux-v., ***phos., phyt.,*** plb., ***psor.,*** puls., **RHUS-T.,** sarr., ***sep.,*** **SIL.,** staph., stram., sulph., ***sul-ac.,*** sumb., vip.

cold air amel. - ***merc.***

exanthemata, after - anthr., ***arn., bar-c.,*** **BROM.,** ***carb-v.,*** dulc., iod., kali-bi., mag-c., sulph.

hard - am-c., **BAR-M., BROM.,** ***merc.,*** sil., sul-ac.

left - **BROM.,** con., ***lach.,*** **RHUS-T.,** ***sul-ac.***

menses, during - kali-c.

right - am-c., **BAR-C.,** ***bar-m.,*** **BELL.,** carb-an., graph., ***kali-bi.,*** kali-c., ***merc.,*** nit-ac., plb., sep., stram.

right, then left - **LYC.**

tearing, pain - bell.

drinking, when - nat-m.

tingling - phos.

tumor, cystic on, right - calc.

ulcers - bar-c., calc-p., rhus-t., sars., sil.

PINCHING, pain - bry., ***calc.,*** meny., mur-ac., ***rhod.,*** rhus-t., sabad., stann., sulph., verat.

PRESSING, pain - arg- m., ars., asar., aur., ***bell., calc.,*** carb-v., caust., chin., cina, cocc., cycl., hyos., ign., kali-c., ***lyc.,*** mang., meny., **MERC.,** mur-ac., osm., par., ph- ac., puls., rheum, rhus-t., sabin., ***spong.,*** stann., ***staph.,*** stram., ***sulph.,*** verat., zinc.

inward - aur., ***calc.,*** cocc., cycl., rheum, ***staph.,*** zinc.

from without - ***cocc.***

outward - arg- m., cina, ign., lyc., mang., meny., ***merc.,*** par., puls., rhus-t., ***spong.,*** sulph.

PRICKING - arund.

PULSATION - ***am-m.,*** arn., asaf., bell., bov., bry., ***calc.,*** caust., cham., clem., ***kali-c.,*** lyc., **MERC.,** nat-c., nit-ac., ***phos.,*** rhod., ***sabad.,*** sep., ***sil., sulph.,*** thuj.

QUIVERING - bell., calc., kali-c., mez., nat-c., sil.

RELAXED - nux-m.

SCROFULOUS - ***bar-m., carb-an.,*** iod., ***merc-i-f.***

lymphatic - ***merc-i-f.***

SEBACEOUS, secrete in excess - **PSOR.**

SECRETION, profuse - ***jab.***

SENSITIVE - arn., ***aur.,*** **BAR-C.,** bell., ***cham.,*** chin., clem., cocc., **CON.,** crot-h., cupr., graph., hep., ign., kali- c., laur., ***lyc.,*** mag-c., nat-c., nit-ac., nux-v., petr., ph-ac., **PHOS.,** puls., ***sep.,*** sil., spig., squil., sul-ac., zinc.

painful - sul-ac.

SHARP, pain - acon., agn., alum., ***am-m.,*** arg-m., arn., ***asaf.,*** bar-c., bar-m., **BELL.,** bor., ***bry., calc.,*** carb-an., caust., chin., ***cocc., con.,*** cupr., cycl., euph., graph., hell., hep., ***ign., iod.,*** kali-c., kreos., lach., lyc., **MERC.,** ***mez.,*** mur-ac., ***nat-c., nat-m.,*** **NIT-AC.,** ***nux-v.,*** ph-ac., ***phos.,*** plb., **PULS.,** ***ran-s.,*** rheum, ***rhus-t.,*** sabad., ***sep.,*** sil., spig., ***spong.,*** stann., staph., ***sulph.,*** sul-ac., thuj., verat., zinc.

SHARP, pain
around glands - con.

SORE, pain - alum., ant-c., arg-m., ***arn.,*** ars., bry., calc., ***carb-an.,*** caust., ***cic.,*** **CON.,** cupr., ***graph., hep.,*** iod., kali- c., merc., mez., nat- m., phos., plat., ***psor.,*** puls., rhod., rhus-t., ***ruta.,*** ***sep.,*** staph., sulph., sul- ac., teucr., zinc.

SPLEEN, general - abies-c., abrot., ***agar.,*** alum., ***am-c.,*** am-m., anac., arn., **ARS.,** ***ars-i.,*** **ASAF.,** ***bor., bry.,*** calc-p., camph., ***cann-s., canth.,*** caps., carb-an., carb-v., caust., **CEAN.,** cedr., cham., chel., **CHIN.,** coc-c., colch., con., ***dios., dulc., ferr., ferr-m.,*** fl-ac., gran., grin., helia., **IGN.,** ***iod.,*** iris, jug-r., kali-bi., kali-n., ***laur.,*** mag-c., mag-m., mang., merc., mez., ***mur-ac.,*** naja, ***nat-a., nat-m., nat-s.,*** nit-ac., ***nux-v.,*** ph-ac., phos., ***plat., plb.,*** psor., **RAN-B.,** rhod., rhus-t., ***ruta.,*** sars., sil., squil., ***stann.,*** sulph., **SUL-AC.,** ther., thuj., ***urt-u.,*** valer., verat., verb., ***zinc.***
abscess - ***hippoz.***
aching - asar., bor., cean., chin.
dull pain, when touched - ran-b.
extending to, chest - bor.
walking slowly, when, pains extends in direction of long axis - **CHIN.**
atrophy - agn., ***ars.,*** eucal., ***ign., iod.,*** phos., psor.
breathing, deep agg. - card-m., cob., sulph.
burning, pain - anan., bell., carb-an., ***coc-c.,*** ign., sec.
distress, with- ***lept.***
congested - anthr., bar-m., cean., **CHIN-S., CHIN.,** hippoz.,
cutting, pain - cahin., ***cean.,*** chin., crot-h., ***hydr.,*** ptel., tarent., verb.
cold weather agg. - ***cean.***
cough, during - ***puls.***
edema, spleen disease, from - ***cean.,*** chin., **LACH.,** liatr., querc., squil.
ascites, causes - ***chin.***
enlarged - agar., agn., ***anthr., aran., ars., ars-i., aur-m.,*** bell-p., berb., ***calc., calc-ar., caps.,*** carb-v., card-m., **CEAN.,** cedr., **CHIN.,** chin-a., ***chin-s.,*** chion., ***cit-v., cocc., con.,*** dros., ***ferr.,*** ferr-ac., ferr-ar., ferr-i., ***ferr-m.,*** ferr-p., grin., ***helia., hippoz.,*** hydr., ***ign.,*** **IOD.,** kali-br., ***lach.,*** laur., mag-m., malar., merc-i-r., ***nat-m., nit-ac.,*** nux-m., ***nux-v.,*** op., per., ***ph-ac., phos.,*** plb., ***querc., ran-s.,*** ruta., squil., succ., ***sulph., sul-ac.,*** tab., tub., ***urt-u.***
abdominal cavity, fills one-fourth of - ***ars-i.***
ague, in a man subject to, constantly chilly, worse when it rained - ***aran.***
albuminuria, in - ***aur-m.***
asthma, in - tab.
bulging out - tub.
chronic - ***cean.,*** plat.
intermittent fever, in - ***cean.***
splenitis, in - ***cean.***
torpid action of bowels, with - con.
coughing, hurts when - ***sul-ac.***

SPLEEN, general
enlarged,
crepitation, with, on motion of legs - ***ars.,*** bry., ***calc.,*** **CHIN.,** aran., eucal., ***ferr-m.,*** **IOD.,** kali-br., ***kali-i.,*** merc-i-r., ***nat-m., nux-m.,*** petr., puls., ***sul-ac.,*** verat.
edema, with, intermittent fever, in - ***ars.,*** **CHIN-S.**
elderly man, in an - bry.
fever, quotidian, in - rhus-t.
typhoid fever, in - ***apis, cocc.,*** ph-ac.
ilium, to within crest of - ***cean.***
indurated - ***agn.***
maltreated gonorrhea, in - ***brom.***
intermittent, after, and abuse of quinine - aran., ***ran-s.***
checked with quinine, worse in damp weather and exposure to damp walls - ***aran.***
melancholia, with - ***con.***
pain, pressive - ***mez.***
painful - ***caps.,*** ruta, ***sul-ac.***
feels swollen - absin.
edema, in - ***lyc.***
intermittent fever, in - ***caps.***
quinine, after abuse of - aran., ***caps., ran-s.***
sore on pressure - ***ferr.***
tuberculosis, in incipient - tub.
yellow fever, after - ***nit-ac.***
fatty degeneration - eucal., ***phos.***
fullness, sensation of - apoc., kali-i., lec.
grasping pain - ***med.***
gurgling, sensation - verb.
region, of - helo.
hard - ***agn., ars.,*** brom., caps., **CHIN.,** ***ign.,*** iod., ***mez., psor., ran-b.,*** sulph., ***sul-ac.***
heat, in - **ASAF.**
heaviness, as from a load - kali-i., sulph.
painful feeling - merc-i-r.
walking, when - mag-m.
induration - agn., ***ars.,*** eucal., ***ign., iod.,*** phos., psor.
chronic - ***psor.***
intermittent fever, in - **CHIN.**
miasmatic fever, in - eucal.
pressive pain, with - ***mez.***
inflammation - acon., ***apis, arn.,*** ars., ars-i., asaf., bell., bufo, ***bry.,*** **CEAN., CHIN.,** chin-s., con., cupr., ign., iod., nat-a., nat-c., ***nat-m., nit-ac., nux-v.,*** sulph.
injuries - arn., bell-p., ***cean.***
lancinating, pain - anan., bufo, cahin., nat-m.
leucocythemia - bell., con., iod., lyc., merc., nit-ac., phos., rhus-t., sulph.
lump, sensation of, abdomen - sulph.
neuralgic, pain - ***zinc.***
pain, spleen - aesc., ***agar.,*** ambr., am-m., anac., anan., arn., ars., ars-i., asar., bapt., berb., bor., brom., ***carb-v.,*** **CEAN.,** ***chel.,*** **CHIN., *chin-s.,*** cob., ***cocc., coc-c.,*** colch., con., cupr., ferr., ferr-i., ***fl-ac.,*** form., helon., ***hydr., ign.,*** iod., kali-bi., kali-p., kreos., ***lach., lyss.,*** merc-i-r., ***merl., mez., nat-m.,*** nat-s., nit-ac.,

SPLEEN, general

pain, spleen - pall., petr., phos., phyt., plb., rhod., sang., sep., ***stann., sulph., sul-ac., zinc.***

abdomen swollen and tender - ptel.
afternoon, 2 p.m. - cedr., sep.
bending, on, taking deep breath, or coughing - ***chin-s.***
breathing, agg. - agar., am-m.
deep agg. - card-m., cob., sulph.
chill, during - ***bry.,*** caps., **CHIN-S.,** eup-per., nux-v., **PODO.,** rhus-t., ***sep.,*** sulph.
coughing, on - bor., ***chin., chin-s.,*** sul-ac.
distended, as if, causing dull ache - ***helon.***
eating, amel. - rhod.
evening - agar., mag-s.
exercising on - kali-bi., ran-b.
fever, during - anac., ars., bor., **CARB-V.,** ***nat-m., nux-v.***
groin, to, in evening - ars-m.
gravel, with - dol.
inspiration agg. - cob., mez.
intermittent, in - **CHIN.,** petr., tarax.
lying, amel. - phyt., squil.
first worse then better by, on that side - ***cocc.***
left side on, while - agar., cean., ***cocc.,*** colch.
menses, during - apis, pall.
at return of - pall.
walking or coughing, agg. - ***apis***
metrorrhagia, with - ***cean.***
morning - am-m., sang.
motion - ***kali-bi.,*** kali-p.
neurosis, with, of chest - sil.
night - agar.
occiput, pain in, commencing with chill - petr.
ovaritis, in chronic - pall.
posterior, in, aspect - ***lob-c.***
pressing amel. - chin-s.
pressure of clothing agg. - calad., fl-ac., kali-bi., nat-m., puls.
pulsating - ***lyss.***
riding in a carriage - bor., lach.
stool, during - kali-bi.
turning to right side amel. - agar.
vertigo, with - urt-u.
walking while - ***arn.,*** hep., ign., lach., rhod., sel.
amel. - agar.

pinching, pain - ***carb-v., fl-ac.***

extending, hip, to - fl-ac.

pressing, pain - agar., ***ars.,*** bor., ***carb-v.,*** chin., chin-s., crot-t., ***fl-ac.,*** graph., ***ign., kreos.,*** lyss., ***merl.,*** nat-c., ***nat-m., nit-ac.,*** ol-an., polyg., rheum., stann., sulph., zinc.

belching, before - sulph.
lying on left side - agar.

pressure, agg. - zinc.

pressure, feeling of - astac., calad., ***carb-v.,*** kreos., ***nat-m.***

painful - ***fl-ac.,*** kali-m.
intermittent, in - ***ars.***

SPLEEN, general

pressure, feeling of

sticking, with, region of - ol-an.
supper, after - lyss.
walking, when, fast - lyss.

pricking, sensation - arum-m.

pulsation - anan., crot-t., grat., lyss., ran-b., ruta.

rheumatic pains, continuous, pressing, after taking cold by getting wet, better by eating - rhod.

sensitive - arn., ***caps., cean.,*** eucal., kreos., lach., ptel.

intermittent fever, in - **CHIN.**
pressure, agg. - ***arn., ferr-m., lach.***
miasmatic fever, in - eucal.
pressure, on - kreos., ptel.
typhoid, fever, in - **RHUS-T.**

sharp, pain - acon., agar., aloe, alum., am-m., anac., arg-n., arn., **ARS.,** bell., berb., bry., cahin., calad., calc-p., camph., carb-an., ***carb-v., card-m.,*** **CEAN.,** cedr., chel., ***chin.,*** clem., cob., ***cocc., coc-c., con.,*** euphr., hep., ***hydr., kali-bi.,*** kali-n., kali-p., ***lach.,*** lec., led., lith., lyc., mag-c., ***mag-s.,*** nat-a., ***nat-c., nat-m.,*** nat-s., nit-ac., ***nux-m.,*** ol-an., ph-ac., phos., ***psor.,*** puls., ran-s., rhod., ruta., sang., sars., sel., sep., sil., spig., squil., stann., ***sulph., sul-ac.,*** tab., verat., verb., ***zinc.***

backwards, worse on quick walking - camph.
bend double, must - ***nux-m.***
breathing deeply, on - bry., ***card-m.,*** chin., ***cob.,*** mosch., nat-c., ***ran-s.,*** sabad., ***sulph.***
worse when taking deep inspiration and when walking - ***sulph.***
coughing, on - bell., carb-v., con., sulph., zinc.
with expectoration of blood-streaked mucus - sep.
dull - coc-c.
during chills, in intermittent - ***bry.***
eating, while - thuj.
after - verat.
evening - arg-n., colch., crot-t., ***sulph.***
extending, chest, into - aloe
headache, with dull - urt-u.
hematemesis, in - **ARS.**
hepatitis, in chronic - ***nat-c.***
inspiration, worse on deep - ***carb-v.***
intermittent fever, with splenitis - ***arn.***
lightning-like - ***carb-v.***
lumbar region, into, worse on motion or pressure - ***kali-bi.***
worse during sleep and on inspiration - ran-s.
lying, while - ***all-c.,sulph.***
menses, during - bufo.
morning - psor.
motion - kali-p., nit-ac.
pain, especially on inspiration and stooping - card-m.
when walking slowly, in direction of long axis of spleen - ***chin.***

SPLEEN, general
sharp, pain
pityriasis versicolor, in - ***mez.***
pressure agg. - kali-bi., zinc.
sitting - am-m.
in morning on awaking, difficult breathing, must rise - ***am-m.***
standing - mag-c.
better, worse moving - psor.
stitches - ***ars.,*** berb., bry., calad., carb-an., ***carb-v.,*** cean., cedr., chel., chin-s., ***chin., con.,*** jug-c., nat-c., ***nat-m.,*** puls., ran-s., ruta, sang., ***sul-ac.,*** vac., zing.
stooping, on - card-m.
sudden - daph.
upper part, in, while walking - chen-v.
walking, while - acon., arn., chin., ***hep., lach., nat-c.,*** nat-m., psor., rhod., sel., verat.
shooting, pain - alum., ***sulph.***
exercise by walking, agg. - ***lach.***
extending, to breast on left side of neck - ***lach.***
soft - ***anthr.,*** ars-h.
liquefied - hippoz.
sore, pain - ***agn.,*** arn., ***ars.,*** asar., calc., ***caps.,*** **CHIN.,** ***ferr.,*** ferr-m., kali-i., kreos., lec., ***phos., ptel.,*** **RHUS-T.,** sars., stann.
painful - ***calc.***
pressure, on - ***ferr.***
touch to, in quotidian fever - ***ars.***
typhoid fever, in - ***phos.***
unbearable, cannot lie still a moment, like acute rheumatism - grin.
sticking, dull sensation - zinc.
stinging, pain - psor.
swelling - agn., anan., aran., ars., brom., ***bry.,*** caps., **CEAN.,** cedr., **CHIN.,** chin-s., cocc., dros., ***ferr., ferr-ar.,*** grin., ign., ***iod.,*** kali-i., mag-m., nat-m., nit-ac., nux-v., phos., plb., ***ran-s.,*** ruta., sul-ac., tub.
fever, during - ***carb-v., nat-m.***
painful - ***cean.,*** ruta.
quinine, after - ***aran.***
tearing, pain - ambr., con.
as if something were torn away - ambr.
tension - nit-ac., rhod., sulph.
fever, during - ***ars.***
painful, in intermittent - ***ars.***
stooping, from - rhod.
throbbing, painful, as if an abscess were forming, very deep - ***lyss.***
twisting, pain, at night, leaving soreness, when going off, gradually worse and better, leaving feeling as if there were a hole in side - stann.

STINGING, pain - apis, ***cocc.***

SUPPURATING - calc-s., guare., **RHUS-T.**
chronic - ***aur-m-n.***
discharge curdy, or thin, corrosive - **KALI-I.**
especially cervical - ***bar-c.***
indolent, with hard edges - **KALI-I.**
lymphatics - ***carb-v.***
scarlatina, in - ***iod.***

SUPPURATING,
sebaceous, of - **SIL.**

SWELLING, of - acon., ***aesc.,*** agn., alum., ambr., am-c., ***am-m., anthr.,*** ant-c., ant-t., apis, arg-m., arn., ars., **ARS-I.,** ***arum-t., asaf., aur., aur-m., bad., bapt.,*** **BAR-C., BAR-I., BAR-M., BELL.,** bor., bov., **BROM.,** ***bry., bufo,*** calad., ***calc.,*** **CALC-I.,** calc-p., **CALC-S.,** camph., cann-s., ***canth.,*** caps., **CARB-AN.,** ***carb-s.,*** **CARB-V.,** caust., ***cham.,*** chin., cic., **CIST., CLEM.,** cocc., coloc., **CON.,** croc., crot-h., cupr., cycl., dig., **DULC.,** eucal., euph., **FERR.,** ferr-ar., ferr-i., **GRAPH.,** hell., **HEP.,** ***hecla.,*** hippoz., hyos., ign., **IOD.,** iris, ***kali-ar., kali-bi., kali-c., kali-chl.,*** **KALI-I.,** lach., led., **LYC.,** mag-c., mag-m., mang., med., **MERC., MERC-C.,** merc-d., ***merc-i-f., merc-i-r.,*** mez., ***mur-ac., nat-c.,*** nat-m., **NIT-AC.,** ***nux-v.,*** petr., ***ph-ac.,*** **PHOS.,** ***phyt.,*** plb., psor., **PULS.,** ran-b., ran-s., rhod., **RHUS-T.,** ruta., sabad., sabin., samb., sars., ***sep.,*** **SIL.,** spig., **SPONG.,** squil., ***stann.,*** staph., stram., stront-c., sec., **SULPH.,** ***sul-ac., syph.,*** teucr., **THUJ.,** ***uran-n., verat.,*** viol-o., viol-t., zinc.
acute - **BELL.**
bluish - arn., ars., aur., ***carb-an.,*** carb-v., con., ferr-i., hep., ***lach.,*** mang., merc., merc-i-f., puls., sil., sul-ac.
bronchitis, in chronic - ***inul.***
cachectic people - ***kali-m.***
chronic - calc-p., ***hep.***
cold - ***ars.,*** asaf., bell., ***cocc.,*** **CON.,** cycl., ***dulc.,*** lach., rhod., spig.
deafness, with - kali-m.
painless - thuj.
contusions and bruises, after, tingling and stitches - **CON.**
especially after - ***phos.***
diphtheria, in - ***kreos., merc-i-r.***
earache, with - kali-m., merc.
edema, pressure, causing - ***kali-i.***
eggs, size of, hard - ***bar-m.***
emaciation, with - ***ars., ars-i., bar-c., calc., calc-i., calc-p.,*** carb-v., caust., ***cist., con., graph.,*** **IOD.,** ***mag-c.,*** mag-m., nat-m., nit-ac., ***ol-j.,*** petr., phos., ph-ac., psor., ***sil.,*** staph., sulph., sul-ac.
eruptions, with - dulc.
gleet, with, disposition to - ***kali-m.***
hard - agn., ant-c., arn., ars., asaf., ***brom., bry., carb-an.,*** caust., chin., **CON.,** dig., graph., **IOD.,** ***kali-i.,*** lach., led., merc., mez., nux-v., ***phos.,*** phyt., ***puls.,*** **RHUS-T.,** sabin., samb., ***spong.,*** stront-c., ***sulph.***
head eruption on, with - ***psor.***
hip disease, in - **CALC.**
hodgkin's disease - ***syph.***
hot - ***acon.,*** am-c., ant-c., arn., asaf., **BELL., BRY.,** bufo, ***calc.,*** canth., ***carb-an.,*** carb-v., chin., clem., ***cocc.,*** euph., ***hep.,*** kali-c., led., **MERC.,** nux-v., petr., **PHOS.,** ***phyt.,*** puls., rhus-t., sars., sil., ***sulph.***

SWELLING, of
hot,
painful and hot - ***acon., bell., cham., clem.***
induration, and - ***graph.***
infants, in - ***cham.***
inflammatory - ***acon.,*** agn., am-c., ant-c., ***arn.,*** ars., asaf., ***bad., bar-c.,*** **BELL.,** bor., ***bry.,*** calc., ***carb-an., carb-v.,*** caust., ***cham.,*** cinnb., ***clem.,*** cocc., **CON.,** ***hep.,*** hyos., ***kali-i., lyc.,*** mang., **MERC.,** mez., mur-ac., nat-c., petr., ***phos., phyt.,*** puls., ***rhus-t.,*** sars., **SIL.,** sulph., ***thuj.***
itching - sil.
jerking, pain - ***asaf.***
knotted cords, like - **BAR-M.,** ***calc., cist.,*** con., ***dulc.,*** hep., ***iod.,*** lyc., rhus-t., ***sil.,*** tub.
lymphatic - am-c., anthr., astac., berb., **CALC.,** ***carb-s., carb-v., con.,*** kali-br., nat-p.
alternate side - ***lac-c.***
cancer uteri - ***graph.***
chronic - ***nat-m.***
dark red, brittle, or softened as if filled with extravasations - anthr.
diphtheria - ***nat-m.***
heat and soreness - med.
painless - ***sep.***
scarlatina - am-c.
scrofulous - chim., con.
menses, during - kali-c., lac-c.
before - bar-c.
nodes, like - bry., nit-ac.
ophthalmia, strumous - ***merc-d.***
painful - acon., am-c., anan., ***anthr.,*** ant-c., ***arn.,*** ars., ***aur., bar-c.,*** **BAR-M., BELL., CALC.,** ***calc-p.,*** canth., ***caps., carb-an.,*** carb-v., caust., ***chin.,*** clem., **CON.,** cop., cor-r., crot-t., cupr-m., ***hep.,*** ign., ***iod.,*** kali-c., ***kali-i., merc.,*** nat-m., ***nit-ac.,*** nux-v., phyt., psor., ***puls., rhus-t., sil.,*** spig., stann., ***staph.,*** sulph.
rending, tearing - ***ferr.***
scrofulous - **BAR-M.**
under chin - ***anthr.,*** staph.
painless - ars., asaf., **CALC.,** ***cocc., con.,*** cycl., dulc., ***ign.,*** lach., ***nit-ac., ph-ac.,*** plb., ***sep.,*** sil., staph., sulph., thuj.
scabies, in - ***sulph.***
scarlet fever, epidemic - ***merc***-i-r.
after - am-c., bar-c., ***lac-c., lyc., merc.***
sebaceous - **SIL.**
chronic - ***nat-m.***
scrofulous - **CARB-V.,** dig., ther.
scrofula, or syphilitic buboes - **BAD.**
children, worse after slight cold - ***bar-c.***
suppuration - **BROM.**
shooting, pain - ***asaf.***
subcutaneous - ***iod.***
suppurating - ***ars-i., aur-m-n., bad., bell.,*** **CALC.,** ***calc-s., cist.,*** **HEP., KALI-I.,** ***lyc., merc., merc***-i-r., nat-s., ***nit-ac.,*** rhus-t., sep., ***sil.,*** sulph.

SWELLING, of
suppuration, with or without, but especially if suppuration is profuse - **MERC.**
swelling before hardening - nat-p.
syphilis, in - **CARB-V., KALI-I.,** ***merc***-i-f.
secondary - ***merc.***
tabes mesenterica, with, in fleshy, flabby subjects - ***kreos.***

SWOLLEN, sensation - ant-c., aur., ***bell.,*** bry., carb-v., chin., clem., con., dulc., hep., ign., kali-n., lach., merc., nit-ac., nux-m., nux-v., **PULS.,** ***rhus-t.,*** sabin., spig., ***spong.,*** staph., zinc.

TEARING, away, pain - agn., ***ambr.,*** am-c., ***arn.,*** bar-c., ***bell.,*** bov., ***bry., calc.,*** cann-s., ***caps., carb-an., carb-v.,*** caust., ***cham.,*** **CHIN.,** cocc., con., cycl., ***dulc.,*** ferr., graph., ign., ***kali-c.,*** kali-s., kreos., ***lyc.,*** **MERC.,** mez., nat-c., nit-ac., nux-v., phos., **PULS.,** ***rhod., rhus-t.,*** sel., seneg., sep., ***sil., sulph.,*** thuj., ***zinc.***

TENDER, in cachectic people - ***kali-m.***

TENSION - alum., ambr., arg- m., arn., aur., ***bar-c.,*** bell., bov., ***bry.,*** calc., carb- an., ***caust.,*** clem., coloc., ***con.,*** dulc., graph., kali- c., lyc., merc., mur-ac., nux-v., **PHOS.,** ***puls., rhus-t.,*** sabad., sabin., sep., sil., ***spong.,*** staph., stront-c., ***sulph.,*** thuj.

THROBBING - asaf.

THYROID, gland - aloe, ambr., bad., bell., ***brom.,*** **CALC.,** calc-f., ***calc-i.,*** calc-s., caust., cist., con., ferr-i., fl-ac., form., graph., **IOD.,** kali-c., **KALI-I.,** ***lach.,*** lycps., ***lyc.,*** nat-c., **NAT-M.,** nat-p., nat-s., phos., ***sep.,*** sil., **SPONG.,** ***thyr.***
air, blowing through throat glands and thyroid on breathing - spong.
coldness, in region of - nat-a.
constriction, in - ***calc-s.,*** **CROT-C.,** elaps, ***iod.,*** spong.
finger, as from a - nat-a.
cretinism - absin., ***aeth., anac.,*** arn., bac., ***bar-c.,*** bar-m., ***bufo,*** calc-p., hell., ign., iod., ***lap-a.,*** lol., nat-c., oxyt., ph-ac., plb., sep., sulph., ***thyr.***
enlargement of, due to hypertrophy - kali-i.
menses, after suppressed - ***ferr-i.***
tender - ail.
formication, sensation - ambr.
goitre - adren., ***ail.,*** aloe, am-c., am-m., ***ambr.,*** am-c., ***apis,*** ars-i., arum-t., ***aur., aur-i.,*** aur-s., ***bad.,*** bar-i., ***bell., brom.,*** **CALC.,** ***calc-f., calc-i., calc-s., carb-an., carb-s., caust.,*** chr-s., ***cist.,*** cob., con., ***crot-c.,*** dys-co., ferr., ***ferr-i., fl-ac.,*** form., ***fuc.,*** glon., ***graph., hep., hydr.,*** hydr-ac., **IOD.,** ***iris,*** kali-c., ***kali-i., lach., lap-a., lycps., lyc.,*** mag-c., mag-p., mang., merc., ***merc-i-f., merc-i-r.,*** morg., ***nat-c.,*** **NAT-M.,** ***nat-p., nat-s., phos.,*** phyt., pineal., plat., podo., puls., ***sep., sil.,*** **SPONG.,** stram., sulph., syc-co., tab., ***tarent., thyr., tub.,*** urt-u.
asthma, causes - **SPONG.**
constriction, with - ***calc-s.,*** **CROT-C.,** ***iod., lyc., spong.***

THYROID, gland

goitre,

cough, from - psor.

diarrhea, with - ***cist.***

distension, sensation like - spong.

egg, size of a hen's - ***brom.,*** cist.

exophthalmic goitre - adren., aml-n., anh., aq-mar., aran-ix., ars., ars-i., atra-r., ***aur., aur-i.,*** bad., bar-c., ***bell.,*** brom., ***cact., calc.,*** calc-f., cann-i., chin., chin-a., chr-s., cimic., colch., con., crot-h., cupr., cyt-l., echi., ***ferr., ferr-i.,*** ferr-p., ***fl-ac.,*** flor-p., fuc., ***glon.,*** **IOD.,** kali-c., mag-c., mag-f., nux-v., op., phos., ***piloc., lycps., nat-m., phos., piloc.,*** saroth., scut., sec., sel., ***spong.,*** stram., thal., thala., ***thyr.,*** verat.

grief, from - aml-n.

menses, after suppression of - **FERR.**

tuberculosis history, with - dros.

hard - ***iod.,*** spong.

indurated - aeth., berb., iod., nit-ac., ***spong.***

large, irregular, knotty - spong.

right side - ***lyc.***

left, side - chel., ***lach.***

lumpy - spong.

menses, before agg. - cimic.

moving sensation on swallowing - ***spong.***

obese people, in - calc., fuc.

painful - **IOD.,** ***plat.,*** spong.

menses, during - iod.

swallowing, on - ***spong.***

painless, well-marked - ***iod.***

pregnancy, in - hydr.

pressing, pain - ***nat-c.***

puberty, in - calc-i., hydr.

pulsation - iod., lyc.

otorrhoea, with - ***calc.***

right, side - caust., hep., iod., ***lyc.,*** mag-c., merc-i-f., nat-c., ***phos., sep.,*** sil., spong.

sensitive, to contact - ***kali-i.***

tender - spong.

tickling - plat.

twitching - lyc.

vascular - ***apis, calc.***

vertigo, with - ***iod.***

hypertrophy, in basedow's disease - spong.

indurated, region of - ***spong.***

itching - ambr.

myxoedema - ***ars.,*** cortico., dor., penic., prim-o., sulfa., ***thyr.***

pain - am-c., ***bar-c.,*** calc-s., carb-v., cupr., **IOD.,** elaps, ***plat.,*** spig., ***spong.***

moving head, on - iod.

parathyroid - calc-p.

pressing, pain - ***bar-c.***

round, hard swelling on upper right part - ***nat-c.***

sharp, pain - am-c., iod., nat-c., ***spong.,*** sulph.

swallowing, on - spong.

soreness, pain - ail., ***kali-i.,*** nicc.

swelling - ail., ars., aur-s., ***carb-an.,*** caust., clem., con., ***kali-i.,*** nat-c., nit-ac., ol-j., thuj.

increasing rapidly - ***kali-i.***

middle lobe, of - ***nat-c.***

THYROID, gland

swelling,

right - merc.

sensation of swelling - benz-ac.

right - mag-c., xan.

sensitive to touch and pressure - ***kali-i., spong.***

swollen, with suffocating spells at night, barking cough, with stinging in throat - ***spong.***

painful on touching neck and on pressure - ***spong.***

tension - agar.

tumors - ***calc-i.,*** thuj.

TUBERCULOSIS, in, affected - ***iod.***

ULCERATIVE, pain - am-c., ***am-m.,*** aur., bell., bry., calc., canth., caust., cham., chin., cic., cocc., graph., hep., ign., kali-c., **MERC.,** mur-ac., nat-c., nat-m., ***nit-ac.,*** petr., **PHOS.,** ***puls., rhus-t.,*** ruta., **SIL.,** staph., sul-ac., teucr., ***zinc.***

ULCERATION, of - ***ol-j.***

lymphatics, of - ***rhus-v.***

sebaceous - dig.

ULCERS - ***ambr.,*** ant-c., arn., **ARS.,** asaf., aur., ***bell.,*** calc., ***canth.,*** carb-an., carb-v., caust., clem., coloc., ***con.,*** cupr., dulc., ***hep.,*** hyos., ign., kali-c., kali-p., kreos., ***lach.,*** lyc., merc., nit-ac., ph-ac., **PHOS.,** ***phyt.,*** rhus-t., sars., sep., **SIL.,** spong., squil., ***sulph.,*** sul-ac., thuj., zinc.

fistulous, especially on neck - bar-c.

Hands

ABDUCTED, fingers, spasmodically - ***glon.,*** kali-cy., lac-c., lyc., **SEC.**

ABSCESS, (see Felon) - anan., hep., lach., merc., sil.

back - plb.

splinters, from - ***bar-c., hep.,*** iod., lach., ***led.,*** nit-ac., petr., **SIL.,** sulph.

abscess, fingers - fl-ac., hep., lach., mang.

abscess, palm - ars., cupr., fl-ac., sulph.

ACHING, pain - aesc., ang., asaf., calc-p., croc., dios., euphr., ham., kalm., led., mez., nit-ac., ptel.

afternoon, 1 p.m., sitting, while - lycps.

evening - led.

exercise amel. - dios.

extending to, elbow - cer-s.

to, fingers - elat.

joints of - clem., ***kali-c.,*** phys.

morning - dios.

night - dios.

aching, back of - arg-n., carb-v., hep., kali-c., merc., verb.

midnight, after - hep.

aching, fingers - abrot., ang., apis, bry., cic., dios., euphr., gymn., ham., hell., kalm., lob-s., mez., rhus-t.

first - abrot., carb-ac., com., fl-ac., rhus-v., sabad., stann.

ball of - calc-p.

evening - dios., rhus-v.

joints - phys., spong., sumb.

metacarpal - am-m., nat-m.

metacarpal, last - sumb.

metacarpal, middle - zinc.

motion, on - sabad.

tip - teucr.

fourth - arn.

joints - arn., gamb.

joints of - bry., cann-i., coloc., com., led., kali-bi., tax.

first joint - tax.

morning - merc-i-r.

nails, under - caust.

second - phos., pip-m., rhus-t.

morning, in bed - rhus-t.

third - ***arn.,*** led., naja, pip-m.

tips - com., phyt.

writing, while - fago.

aching, palm - merc-i-f., nat-s.

aching, thumbs - calc-p., chel., chin., laur., sang.

evening, 9 p.m. - dios.

ball of right - sang.

joints - asaf., berb., osm.

using it - phos.

AMPUTATED, fingers, stump painful - all-c., ***calen.,*** **HYPER.,** phos., ***staph.***

ANCHYLOSIS, fingers, first joint of - crot-h.

first joint of, last joint - fl-ac.

ARTHRITIC, nosodities - ant-c., ***benz-ac., calc.,*** carb-s., ***hep., led.,*** plb.

arthritic, nosodities, finger joints - ***aesc.,*** agn., ***ant-c.,*** **APIS, BENZ-AC., CALC.,** ***calc-f., calc-p.,*** **CAUST.,** ***clem., colch., dig.,*** **GRAPH.,** hep., **LED., LITH., LYC.,** ox-ac., ran-s., ***rhod., sil., staph., sulph., urt-u.***

stiffness, with - ***carb-an., graph.,*** **LYC.**

AWKWARDNESS - ***agar., apis,*** **BOV.,** carb-s., ***con.,*** graph., kali-n., ***lach., manc., phos.,*** plb., ptel., rhus-v., sep., sil.

diverted or talking, when. - **HELL.,** nit-ac.

drops things, (see Weakness, fingers) - abrot., alumn., **APIS,** bell., **BOV.,** bry., ***con.,*** cycl., hell., hyos., gins., kali-bi., ***lach., nat-m.,*** nux-v., sep., sil., ***stram., sulph.***

reins, when driving carriage - abrot., lyc.

menses, during. - alumn.

awkwardness, fingers - agar., ***apis,*** asaf., **BOV.,** ***calc.,*** calc-s., carb-s., graph., ***hell.,*** hyos., nat-m., ***nux-v.,*** **PHOS.,** plb., ptel., sep., ***sil.***

as if were thumbs. - **PHOS.**

BLISTERS, fingers, phagedenic - calc., ***graph.,*** hep., kali-c., ***mag-c.,*** nit-ac., ran-b., sil., sulph.

tips of - alum., cupr.

blisters, palm - bufo, ran-b.

blisters, thumbs - hep.

BLOOD, rush of to - elaps, nat-s., ***nux-m.,*** ph-ac., phos.

afternoon - nat-s.

arm hanging down - ph-ac., phos., sul-ac.

stomach, from - phos.

blood, fingers, rush of to - phos.

hang down, on letting arm - phos.

tips - rhus-t.

BOILS - ***calc.,*** coloc., iris, lach., led., ***lyc., psor.***

back of - calc.

small - iris.

boils, fingers - calc., ***lach.,*** sil.

boils, thumbs - hep., kali-n.

BORING, pain - bism., daph., ***nat-c.,*** pall., ran-s.

joints - coloc.

boring, back of - hep.

boring, fingers - carb-v., cocc., daph., hell., lach., mag-c., mez., ran-s.

back of - lach.

ball of - kali-n.

bones - aur-m-n., ran-s.

first, joints - nat-s.

metacarpal - aur-m-n.

middle - carb-v.

joints - aur., aur-m-n., carb-v., coloc., daph., hell., mez., nat-s.

nails - colch.

pisiforme, bone - nat-c.

second, last joint of - carb-v.

middle point of - hell.

third phalanx of - mez.

tips - sulph.

boring, palm - mez., spig.

boring, thumbs - ***led.,*** mag-c.

BROKEN, sensation as if, fingers, index - cham.

broken, thumbs, as if - cham.

BURNING, pain - **AGAR.,** am-c., anac., ant-t., apis, arg-m., arg-n., ***ars.,*** ars-h., arund., aur-m., berb., bry., ***calc., calc-s.,*** canth., cann-s., ***carb-s.,*** carb-v., ***caps.,*** cedr., cham., chel., con., corn., daph., elaps, fago., ***fl-ac.,*** graph., hep., hyos., hura, jug-r., kali-ar., kali-bi., kali-c., ***kali-s.,*** lach., laur., led., lil-t., lyc., mag-c., **MED.,** merc., mez., nat-c., nat-m., nat-p., nat-s., nit-ac., nux-m., nux-v., ox-ac., ***petr.,*** ph-ac., ***phos.,*** plat., ***puls.,*** ran-s., rhod., ***rhus-t.,*** rhus-v., sars., sel., ***sep.,*** sol-t-ae., ***spong., stann.,*** stront-c., thuj., **SULPH.,** zinc.

afternoon - cham., fago., phos.
2 p.m. - laur.
ball, of - zinc.
between fingers - alum., rhus-v.
index finger and thumb - alum., berb., iod., rhus-t., sulph.
chill, during - ***spong.***
cold and numb, or - ***lyc.***
and wet, after getting feet - phos.
eating, after - phos., sulph.
eczema, in - ***merc.***
evening - cedr., phos., **PULS., SULPH.**
fever, during - hura
forenoon - fago., nat-s.
while the other is cold - fago.
frost-bitten, as if - lyc.
internal - ph-ac.
itching - nat-m.
joints - nat-c.
evening - nat-c.
menses, during - carb-v., sec.
morning - petr., sulph.
waking, on - petr.
nettles, as from - carl., nat-m.
night - lac-c., pall.
noon - am-c., mag-c.
one hot and pale, the other cold and red - mosch.
radial side of hand - phos.
spots, in - cop., fl-ac., mang., zinc.
steam, from - kali-bi.
ulnar side of hand - anac., sep., stann., zinc.
warm from fast walking - dulc.
washing in cold water agg. - ***caps.***

burning, back of - agar., alum., apis, aur-m., berb., bry., ***calc.,*** carl., cop., dulc., fl-ac., laur., nat-s., nux-v., rhus-v., ***sulph.***

afternoon - nat-s.
evening - **SULPH.**
morning - sulph.
nettles, as from - carl.
spots - cop., fl-ac.
warm from walking - dulc.

burning, fingers - ***agar.,*** alum., anan., apis, ars., asaf., ***berb.,*** bor., calc., carl., carb-v., caust., coff., coloc., con., croc., dig., fago., fl-ac., gamb., gran., graph., kali-ar., ***kali-c.,*** lyc., merc., mez., mosch., ***nat-c.,*** nicc., nit-ac., nux-v., ***olnd.,*** petr., plat., rhod., rhus-v., sec., ***sil.,*** staph., ***sulph.,*** sul-ac., tep., teucr., ther., vip.

back of - brom., cocc., ran-s., sil.
ball of - ***sulph.***
cold, burning - carb-v.
evening - alum.
external - ars., fl-ac.
first - acon., ***agar.,*** alum., arund., berb., card-m., chel., ferr-ma., hura, ***kali-c.,*** mez., olnd., sil.
and crawling - ***agar.***
back of - acon., berb.
external - chel.
joints, metacarpal - berb., fl-ac.
last - berb., nat-c.
middle - berb.
tip - kali-c., olnd.
volar - con.
forenoon - fago.
fourth - spig., stann., tarax., zinc.
inner side of - fl-ac., mill.
joints, metacarpal - sabad.
outer side of - apis, prun.
tip - apis, aur-m-n., fl-ac., kali-c., sul-ac.
frostbitten, as if - agar., bor., lyc.
inner surface - zinc.
joints - apis, bufo, cann-i., carb-v., caust., vinc.
second - apis, carb-v., coloc., ***kali-c.,*** mez., sul-ac.
back of - nat-c.
joints, metacarpal - berb., carb-v.
nail - kali-c.
outer side of - berb.
spots - sul-ac.
sides of - sars.
third - carb-v., osm., tarax.
back of - sulph.
joints, metacarpal - berb., carb-v.
middle - nat-p., sil.
middle, 9 a.m. - sil.
nail, on inner border of - osm.
tips - am-m., anthr., apis, bell., caust., con., croc., crot-c., gins., mang-m., mur-ac., nat-s., sabad., ***sars., sil., sulph.,*** tab.

burning, palm - aesc., ail., all-s., apis, ars., ***calc., calc-s., canth.,*** carb-s., ***carb-v.,*** chel., cop., fl-ac., form., graph., ham., ***ip.,*** lac-c., ***lach., lachn.,*** lil-t., ***lyc.,*** mag-c., ***med.,*** merc., mez., mur-ac., nat-c., nat-m., ox-ac., ***petr., phos.,*** phys., rhus-t., rumx., sabad., ***sang.,*** sanic., sars., sec., ***sep.,*** **STANN., SULPH.,** tarent., tep., upa.

bath, warm, after - nat-c.
eating, after - phos.
evening - **LACH.,** rumx., upa.
in bed - graph.
menses, during - carb-v., petr.
midnight - rhus-t.

burning, palm
night - **LACH.**
palms and soles - ***lach.***
radial side of hand - phos.
rubbing, after - **SULPH.**
stinging - bor., sulph.
ulnar side of hand - anac., sep., stann., zinc.
burning, thumbs - agar., arum-t., arund., berb., chel., gran., graph., ***hep.,*** lach., laur., mag-arct., mag-aust., merc., nux-v., olnd., ol-an., sars., staph., vesp., zinc.
afternoon - agar.
ball of - laur., lith., nux-v.
evening, in bed - graph.
joints - spig.
morning, in bed - ars.
night - sars.
spots - lach.
tearing - agar.
tip - con., croc., gymn., lach., olnd., mur-ac., sil., sulph., teucr.

CALLOUSES, horny, on - ***am-c., ant-c.,*** bor., **GRAPH.,** kali-ar., rhus-v., sil., **SULPH.**
cracks, deep, with - cist., graph.

CHAPPED, (see Roughness) - ***alum., aesc.,*** apis, am-c., ***anan., arn.,*** aur., **CALC., CALEN.,** carb-ac., **GRAPH.,** ham., **HEP.,** hydr., ***kali-c.,*** kreos., ***lyc., mag-c., merc., nat-c., nat-m.,*** **PETR.,** puls., **RHUS-T., SARS., SEP.,** ***sil.,*** **SULPH.,** ***zinc.***
working in water, from - alum., ant-c., **CALC.,** cham., hep., merc., ***rhus-t.,*** sars., ***sep.,*** **SULPH.**
chapped, fingers - **NAT-M.**
about the nails - **NAT-M.**
tips - bar-c.

CHILBLAINS - ***agar.,*** aloe, ***croc., kali-chl., nit-ac.,*** op., **PETR., PULS.,** ***stann., sulph.,*** sul-ac., ***zinc.***
itching - **PULS.,** ***zinc.***
mild weather - nit-ac., stann.
swelling - ***zinc.***
chilblains, fingers - berb., carb-an., lyc., nit-ac., ***nux-v., petr., puls., sulph.,*** sul-ac.
itching - lyc., sulph.
painful - sul-ac.

CLENCHING, fingers - am-c., ***apis,*** arg-n., ***ars., bell., chin.,*** chin-a., ***cic., coloc.,*** **CUPR.,** ***glon., hydr-ac., hyos., ip.,*** lach., ***laur.,*** lyc., ***med.,*** meny., ***merc., nux-m., nux-v., oena.,*** op., par., phos., ***plat.,*** sang., stram., ***stry.,*** ter.
chill, at beginning of - ***cimx.***
convulsive - glon., mag-p., nux-m., ***nux-v.***
epileptic convulsion - **CUPR.,** ***lach.,*** lyc., ***mag-p., oena.***
headache, after - coloc.
noon - am-c.
seizing something, when - arg-m., arg-n., ***dros.,*** stry.
stretching out arms - stry.

clenching, thumbs - ***aeth., apis,*** ars., art-v., arum-t., bell., brach., ***bufo, camph., caust., cham., cic., cocc.,*** **CUPR.,** ***glon.,*** hell., hyos., ign., ***lach.,*** mag-p., **MERC.,** oena., phyt., ***sec.,*** sep., staph., stram., sulph., viol-t.
falling on head - ***cupr.***
epilepsy, in - ***bufo, caust., cic., cupr., lach., stann.,*** staph., sulph.
epilepsy, in after fright - ***ign.***
rheumatism, in - kali-i.
sleep, during - viol-t.

CLOSED, fingers - lyc., stry.
sleep, during - hyos., sul-ac.
closed, thumbs - cocc., hyos.

CLUCKING, thumb - rhus-t.

COBWEB, sensation of, on hands - bor.

COLDNESS - abies-c., acet-ac., ***acon., agar.,*** aloe, alum., alumn., ambr., am-c., amyg., anac., ang., anth., ***ant-t., apis,*** apoc., ***arg-n., arn.,*** **ARS., ARS-I.,** asaf., asar., atro., **AUR.,** aur-m-n., ***bar-c., bar-m., bell.,*** benz-ac., berb., ***bov.,*** brach., ***brom.,*** bry., ***cact., calc.,*** **CALC-AR., CALC-P.,** calc-s., **CAMPH.,** cann-i., cann-s., ***carb-ac., carb-an., carb-s.,*** **CARB-V.,** ***caust., cedr.,*** cham., **CHEL., CHIN.,** ***chin-a., chin-s.,*** cimic., ***cina,*** cinnb., cocc., coff., colch., coloc., com., con., cop., ***croc., crot-c.,*** crot-h., crot-t., ***cupr.,*** cupr-s., **CYCL.,** ***dig.,*** dor., ***dros.,*** elaps, ***eup-per.,*** eup-pur., euph., euphr., fago., **FERR.,** ferr-ar., **FERR-I., FERR-P.,** ***gels.,*** gins., glon., **GRAPH.,** grat., ***hell.,*** hep., hura, hydrc., hyos., ***ign.,*** ind., indg., inul., **IOD., IP.,** iris, jatr., **KALI-AR.,** kali-bi., **KALI-C.,** kali-i., kali-n., **KALI-P.,** kali-s., kreos., lac-ac., lac-d., **LACH.,** lact., laur., ***led.,*** lil-t., lob-s., **LYC., LYCPS.,** mag-s., manc., ***mang., med.,*** **MENY., MERC.,** merc-c., merc-i-r., merc-sul., ***mez.,*** morph., mosch., **MUR-AC.,** naja, **NAT-C., NAT-M., NAT-P.,** nat-s., ***nit-ac.,*** **NUX-M.,** ***nux-v.,*** oena., ol-an., **OLND.,** ***op., ox-ac., pall.,*** **PETR., PH-AC.,** ***phos., phyt.,*** **PULS.,** ***pyrog.,*** ran-b., raph., ***rob., rhus-t.,*** rumx., **RUTA., SABIN., SAMB.,** ***sang.,*** sars., **SEC., SEP.,** sil., spig., spong., squil., stann., staph., ***stram.,*** stry., **SULPH.,** sul-ac., ***sumb., tab.,*** tarax., tep., ther., ***thuj.,*** verb., **VERAT.,** ***verat-v.,*** vip., ***zinc.***
afternoon - alumn., chin-s., gels., nux-v., sulph.
1 p.m. - chel.
2 to 3 p.m. - chel.
4 p.m. - petr.
4:30 p.m. - mez.
5 p.m. - ***rhus-t.***
after 3 p.m. - eup-pur.
alternating hands - cocc.
alternating with, cold feet - aloe, sep., zing.
with, head - nit-ac.
with, heat - bell., bor., chin., cimic., cocc., fago., par.
blue - ***arg-n.,*** benz-n., bor., ***cact., camph.,*** cocc., con., ***crot-h.,*** crot-t., elaps, inul., morph., ***nux-v.,*** oena., plb., stram., stry., zinc.
breakfast, after - verat.

COLDNESS, general
chill, during - asar., ars., aur., bell., cact., ***camph.,*** canth., ***carb-v.,*** cedr., chel., colch., con., dros., hep., hyos., ip., led., lyc., mang., ***meny.,*** **MEZ.,** mur-ac., nat-c., ***nat-m.,*** **NUX-V.,** ***op.,*** petr., **PHOS.,** plb., samb., **SEC.,** sep., spong., staph., stann., stram., sulph., thuj., **VERAT.**
cough, during - rumx., ***sulph.***
cutting and tearing in abdomen, with - ***ars.***
daytime - ars-m., phos.
diarrhea - apis, brom., dig., **PHOS.**
dinner, after - cann-i.
eating, after - aloe, camph., caps., con.
elderly people - bar-c.
emission, after - ***merc.***
evening - ***acon.,*** agar., aloe, alumn., ambr., ars., aur., carb-an., ***carb-v.,*** carl., chel., chin., colch., coloc., graph., hep., nat-c., ox-ac., phos., sulph., thuj., verat.
7 p.m. - ***lyc.,*** phos.
8 p.m. - hep., tarax.
air, open - mang.
bed, in - aur., carb-an., colch.
heat, after - thuj.
heat, during - agar., sabad.
excitement, from - lil-t.
fever, during - arn., asaf., canth., cycl., dros., euphr., hell., ip., nit-ac., puls., ran-b., sabad., sul-ac.
forenoon - calc., chin., grat., mez., nat-m.
9 a.m. - dros., mez.
10 a.m. - con., fago., led.
headache, during - ambr., carb-v.
after - cupr.
heat, internal - ***arn.***
of body, with - ars-m.
of one side of body, with - ***ran-b.***
of thighs, with - thuj.
hot face, with - agar., **ARN.,** ars., asaf., camph., chin., con., cycl., euph., graph., hyos., ign., ruta., sabin., sil., spig., **STRAM.,** sumb., ***thuj.***
feet, with - ***aloe, calc.,*** coloc., ph-ac., ***sep.***
fingers, with - thuj.
forehead, with - ars., asaf., asar.
head, with - **ARN.,** asaf., ***aur.,*** **BELL., GLON.,** hell., iod., ***nat-c.,*** petr., sumb.
hottest weather, in - ***asar.***
icy - ***acon.,*** agar., ***ambr.,*** anac., ***arg-n.,*** ars., asar., aur., bell., ***cact., camph., carb-v., caust.,*** cedr., chin., coloc., ***eup-per.,*** hep., ip., lach., lyc., ***manc., meny., mez., nat-c.,*** **NUX-M.,** ***nux-v., ph-ac.,*** phos., ***plb.,*** sanic., sep., sil., squil., thuj., **VERAT.**
left - ambr., chin., kali-m., thyr.
lying down - kali-c.
amel. - phos.
menses, during - aesc., ***arg-n.,*** ferr., ***graph.,*** kali-i., ***phos.,*** sabin., sec., sulph., verat.
mental exertion - lach., ***ph-ac.***

COLDNESS, general
morning - bell., chel., chin., cina, coloc., cycl., fago., gels., lyc., mang., spong., stram., sumb.
7:30 a.m. - ferr.
8 a.m. - ferr.
8:30 a.m. - mez.
after rising - coloc.
motion, after - alumn., ***cocc.***
nausea, during - gran.
night - ***aur.,*** bry., ***phos.,*** sep., thuj.
noon - kali-c., zing.
numb and cold - chel., ***lach., ox-ac.***
one hand - ***chin.,*** dig., ferr., lyc., ***mosch., puls.,*** rhust-t., sulph.
fingers of other hot - thuj.
hot and pale, the other cold and red - mosch.
one hot, other cold - ***chin.,*** cocc., ***dig., ip., mosch., puls., tab.***
sweat of the other - ip., mez., mosch.
painful - caust.
perspiration, during - chin., dig., fago., ***lil-t.,*** merc-c., nit-ac.
reading, while - lyc.
right - ant-t., cann-i., chel., ferr., ***gels.,*** med., pall., sec.
cold, numbness of left - ferr.
cold, warmth of left - lac-ac., mez., mosch.
then left - med.
rising, after - fago.
sacrum, pain in, during - hura
sensation cold, yet warm to touch - phos.
sleep, during - ign., merc., samb.
talking, while - am-c., ph-ac.
urination, during copious - dig.
vertigo, with - merc., sep.
vexation, after - phos.
waking, on - dig.
walking, while - asaf., camph., chin.
in open air - mang., phos., plb.
warm room - mez., ***nux-v.,*** plan.
to touch, sensation - phos.
wine after - verat.
with pain - ***calc., graph., sabin.***
wraps, them up - petr.
writing, while - chin-s., mez.
after - agar.

coldness, back of hands - anac., chin-s., naja, phos., rhus-t.
afternoon - chin-s.
heat of palms, with - anac., coff.

coldness, fingers - ***acon.,*** act-sp., ang., apis, calad., ***calc., calc-p.,*** caust., ***carb-s., cham.,*** **CHEL.,** cic., cocc., colch., coloc., con., crot-h., ***dig.,*** gels., gins., **GRAPH.,** ***hell.,*** hydr-ac., **KALI-C.,** ***lac-c., lac-d.,*** lyc., med., ***meny.,*** merc., mosch., mur-ac., par., plan., ***ph-ac.,*** plb., ptel., rat., rhod., ***rhus-t.,*** rumx., sars., sec., ***sep.,*** sulph., sumb., **TARAX., THUJ.,** verat., vip.
afternoon, 2 p.m. - plan.
alternating with headache - ***cupr.***

coldness, fingers
chill - ***apis, cact.,*** dig., meny., ***nat-m.,*** nux-v., par., ph-ac., ***rhus-t., sep.,*** verat.
evening - sulph., thuj.
extending, to middle of upper arms - graph.
to nape of neck - coff.
to palms and soles - dig.
first - rhod.
fourth - lyc.
joints - chel.
left - thuj.
morning - chin-s., rat.
nails, under - cann-s.
night - ***mur-ac.***
right - ang.
second - mur-ac., phos., rhod.
joints of - agar.
sitting, while - cham.
third - rhod., sulph.
evening - sulph.
tips - abrot., ***ant-t., arn.,*** brom., ***caps.,*** carb-v., ***carl.,*** **CHEL.,** coloc., cist., hell., jatr., lac-d., lob., meny., merc., mur-ac., ph-ac., ran-b., sal-ac., sars., spig., sulph., sumb., ***tarax., thuj., zinc.***
chill, during - mur-ac., ran-b.
fever, during - ***caps.***
morning, after rising - coloc.
open air - ph-ac.
rest of body is hot - thuj.
sensitive to cold - sec.
writing, after - carl.

coldness, palm - ***acon.,*** dig., hyos., jatr.

coldness, thumb, tip of - mang.

CONSTRICTION - cocc., ***cupr.,*** nux-v., prun.

constriction, fingers - aeth., carb-an., croc., dros., elaps, lach., nux-v., phos., sep., spong.
periodical - ***phos.***
under nails, cramp-like - elaps

CONTRACTION, (see Dupuytren's) muscles and tendons - ***anac.,*** ars., aur., bell., bism., calc., cann-s., carb-s., carb-v., ***caust.,*** cimx., cina, cinnb., colch., coloc., euphr., ferr-s., hydr-ac., kali-bi., lyc., mag-p., mag-s., merc., merc-c., mur-ac., ***nux-v.,*** op., ph-ac., phos., ***sec., sil.,*** sol-n., ***stann.,*** sulph., tab., zinc.
alternating with feet - stram.
extending over forearm - coloc.
grasping involuntarily things taken hold of - ambr., dros., sulph.
paroxysmal - cann-s., cina, phos.
tearing - sulph.
tendons of - carb-v., ***caust.,*** lach., sulph.
flexor - ***benz-ac., plb.,*** sulph.

contraction, fingers - aeth., alum., ambr., am-c., anac., ***ant-t., apis,*** arg-m., ***arg-n., ars.,*** bell., benz-ac., ***calc.,*** cann-s., carb-s., carb-v., **CAUST.,** chel., chin., cina, cocc., coff., colch., crot-t., ***cupr.,*** cycl., ***dros., ferr.,*** ferr-ar., ferr-p., gins., ***graph.,*** hyos., kali-cy., kali-i., lyc., **MAG-P.,** mag-s., mang., med., ***merc.,*** morph., ***nat-c.,*** nux-v., oena., op., ox-ac., par., ph-ac., phos., ***plat.,*** plb., rhod., rhus-t., ruta., sabad., sabin., ***sec.,*** sel., sep., ***sil.,*** spig., stann.,

contraction, fingers - sulph., tarent., tell.
adductors - arg-n.
afternoon - morph.
chill, before - ***cimx.***
cholera - cupr.
convulsions, during intervals of - sec.
cramp-like - calc.
epilepsy - ***lach., mag-p., merc.***
first - alum., caps., cycl., graph.
flexors - ***ars., caust.,*** cimx., ***sil.,*** spig.
fourth - sabad., sulph.
grasping - arg-n., ***dros.,*** stry.
after - graph.
lying on that side while - crot-t.
morning - phos.
periodical - ***phos.***
second - cina, sil.
spasmodic - ***anac., bell., calc.,*** caust., ***cic., cina,*** colch., ***dros., glon., hydr-ac., ip.,*** kali-c., ***lach., laur.,*** **MAG-P.,** med., meny., mosch., phos., phyt., ***sec.,*** ter.
third - sabad.
flexor - ***benz-ac.***
vomiting blood, after - ars.
yawning when - crot-t., nux-v.

contraction, palm, of - anac., carb-an., ***caust.,*** nux-v., sabad., stann., stry., ***verat.***

contraction, thumb - colch., ***hell.,*** sec., staph.
right - cycl.

CONVULSION - acon., ambr., anac., arum-t., bar-m., ***bell.,*** bism., calc., ***camph.,*** cann-s., carb-s., carb-v., caust., coloc., dros., graph., ***iod.,*** kali-bi., kali-i., ***merc.,*** mosch., nat-m., paeon., plat., plb., ***sec., stram., stry.,*** sul-ac., tab., ***zinc.***
clonic - ***stry.***
menses, during - hyos.
taking hold of something - ambr., ***dros.,*** stry., sulph.
tetanic - camph., zinc.

convulsion, fingers, (see Clenching) - am-c., arn., ars., ***bell., calc.,*** cann-s., cham., **CHEL.,** ***cic.,*** clem., cocc., coff., ***cupr.,*** dros., ferr., hell., ***ign.,*** iod., ip., kali-n., lach., lyc., merc-c., mosch., nat-m., nux-v., phos., plb., ***sec.,*** sant., stann., staph., sulph., tab., verat.
first - cycl.
stretching them - staph.
tonic - ars.

convulsion, thumbs - aesc., arum-t., ***bell., cocc., cupr.,*** cycl., nat-m.

COVERED, hands wants - ign.

CRACKED, skin (see Chapping) - ***aesc.,*** **ALUM.,** ***am-c.,*** anan., ant-c., arn., ***aur., aur-m.,*** bar-c., **CALC.,** ***carb-s.,*** cench., ***cist.,*** cycl., **GRAPH.,** ***hep.,*** kali-c., kali-s., kreos., ***lach., lyc., mag-c.,*** maland., ***merc., nat-c., nat-m.,*** **NIT-AC., PETR.,** phos., ***psor., puls., rhus-t.,*** rhus-v., ruta., sanic., **SARS.,** sec., ***sep.,*** **SIL., SULPH., ZINC.**
ball of - hep.
burning - ***petr.,*** sars., zinc.
cold, from - sanic., zinc.
deep and bleeding - alum., ***merc.,*** **NIT-AC., PETR.,** sanic., ***sars.***

CRACKED, skin
itching - merc., ***petr.***
wetting, from - alum., ant-c., **CALC.,** ***cist.,*** kali-c., nit-ac., ***puls., rhus-t.,*** rhus-v., sars., **SEP., SULPH.,** zinc.
winter in - alum., **CALC.,** ***cist., merc.,*** **PETR.,** ***psor., sanic.,*** **SEP., SULPH.**
cracked, back of - ***merc.,*** mur-ac., nat-c., petr., ***rhus-t., sanic.,*** **SEP.**
cracked, fingers - am-m., bar-c., **CALC.,** ***cist., hep.,*** kali-c., mag-c., ***merc.,*** **PETR.,** phos., **SARS.,** sil., zinc.
base, of - sulph.
between - ***aur-m., ars., graph.,*** sulph., zinc.
first - sil.
joints of - ***graph.,*** mang., merc., phos., ***sanic., sulph.***
that ulcerate - ***merc.***
nails, on - **ANT-C.,** ars., lach., ***nat-m., sil.***
tips of - ***aur-m.,*** bar-c., **GRAPH., PETR.**
cracked, palms of - ***cist., merc-i-r., petr.,*** sulph.
cracked, thumbs - sars.
bend, of thumb joint - mang.

CRACKING, fingers, joints, in - ars-m., bar-c., caps., ***carb-an.,*** kali-n., merc., rhus-t., sulph.
closing the hand - ars-m.
feels impelled to make them crack - meph.
third joint - hydr., phos.
cracking, thumb, joints, in - ant-c., bar-c., kali-n., nux-v.

CRAMPS - acon., aeth., ***agar.,*** ambr., anac., ars., **BELL.,** bism., **CALC.,** calc-s., carb-v., caust., cina, cocc., ***coloc., cupr.,*** dios., dulc., euphr., ferr-ar., ferr-ma., ***graph.,*** jatr., hep., ***kali-bi., kali-c.,*** lact., lyc., ***mag-p.,*** mang., merc., merc-c., merc-i-f., mur-ac., naja, ***nat-m.,*** nat-p., nit-ac., olnd., ***phys.,*** plat., plb., puls., ruta., sabad., sec., sil., spig., stram., stry., sul-ac., sulph., tab.
afternoon - calc-s., dios.
3 p.m. - dios.
alternating, with dim vision - bell.
with feet - stram.
ball of - plat.
bones, metatarsal - aur.
cholera - **CUPR.,** ***sec.***
closing hand, on - chin.
evening - lyc.
9 p.m. - lyc.
exertion - plat., sec., ***sil.***
extending agg. - plb.
flexing, after - merc.
grasping - ambr., **DROS.,** graph., lyc., nit-ac., plat., stann.
grasping, a cold stone - nat-m.
left - calc., euphr., nat-p., sulph.
morning - ***calc.***
motion - ars., merc., sec.
amel. - acon.
night - ***calc.***
bed in - plb.
resting, after - plb.
right - acon., merc-i-r., plb., sabad.

CRAMPS, general
transversely across - ruta.
ulnar side of - anac., cocc., puls.
writing - ***alum-sil., anac., cycl.,*** euph., gels., **MAG-P.,** ***nat-p.,*** phos., pic-ac., plat., sil.
cramps, back of, at night in bed - anac.
cramps, fingers - am-c., anac., ***arn.,*** ars., calc., ***carb-v.,*** card-m., **CHEL.,** com., con., ***cupr., cupr-ar.,*** cycl., der., dulc., euph., euphr., ferr., graph., hyper., ign., kali-c., lil-t., lyc., mag-c., mag-p., **MERC.,** ***nat-m.,*** nux-v., plb., sabad., ***stann.,*** staph., ***sulph.,*** tab., tril., verat.
childbirth, during - **CUPR., DIOS.**
cholera, with - ***colch.,*** **CUPR.,** sec., **VERAT.**
cold, air in - am-c.
cutting with shears - con.
evening - ars.
first - anac., cycl., graph., kali-chl., nat-p., sulph.
writing, while - ***cycl.***
fourth - calc., cocc., com., sulph.
writing, while - cocc.
joints - euphr., mag-c., plat.
metacarpo-phalangeal - anac.
proximal - ars., calc.
midnight, in bed - nux-v.
morning - tab.
moving, on - merc.
night in bed - ars.
periodical - ***phos.***
pick up a small object, on attempting to - ***stann.***
playing piano or violin - ***mag-p.***
second - am-m., caust., hura, lil-t., plb., ***sulph.***
sewing, while - kali-c.
shoemaking - ***stann.***
stretching them, when - ars.
third - hura, sep., ***sulph.***
evening - sep., ***sulph.***
extending to elbow - sep., sulph.
tips - ars.
writing, while - brach., cupr., cycl., **MAG-P., STANN.,** ruta, tril.
cramps, palms - coloc., mur-ac., naja, spig., stann., stry., zing.
cramps, thumbs - agar., aml-n., anac., anag., asaf., mang., nat-m., plat., valer.
holding objects - graph.
playing piano - zinc.
muscles, adductor - merc.
extensor - zinc.
twitching, with - valer.
writing, while - agar., aml-n., bell., brach., ***cycl.,*** mur-ac.

CUTTING, pain - mur-ac., ***nat-c.,*** stann., stry., ust.
bones - anac.
cutting, fingers,first - mang.
fourth - bell., ball of - stann.
joints - bapt., mur-ac., ph-ac.
second, joint - caul.

cutting, fingers
tips - hyper., petr.
cutting, thumbs - con., merc-i-f., stry.
DECAY, of bone, metacarpal bone - sil.
decay, fingers, bone, of - ***sil.***
DISCOLORATION, of hands
black - sol-n., sul-ac., tarent., vip.
dots, in - petr.
spots, in - sol-n.
blotches - ars., sep.
itching - sep.
blueness - acon., aesc., agar., am-c., ***ant-t., apis, arg-n.,*** **ARN.,** ***ars.,*** bar-c., benz-n., bor., ***brom., cact., camph., carb-an., carb-v., chin-a., cocc.,*** con., ***crot-h.,*** crot-t., cupr., ***dig.,*** dros., elaps, helo., inul., ***kali-c.,*** **LACH.,** ***laur.,*** morph., **NUX-V.,** oena., ***plb.,*** ph-ac., phos., puls., rhus-t., samb., ***spong., stram.,*** stry., tab., ***verat., verat-v., zinc.***
chill, during - ***camph.,*** dros., nux-v., ph-ac., ***spong.,*** stram., **VERAT.**
coldness, with - ***nux-v.,*** sep.
convulsion, with - ***aesc.***
hanging down, when - sep.
marbled - cupr.
morning - spong.
night - phos., samb.
night, waking, after - samb.
spots - nit-ac.
spots, in elderly, people - bar-c.
washing in cold water, after - am-c.
winter, in - cupr.
brownish-red - arg-n., sulph., sul-ac.
afternoon - sulph.
spots - arg-n., nat-m.
streaks - sul-ac.
copper, colored spots - nat-ac.
greenish - crot-h.
lividity - **ARS.,** merc., morph., naja, nux-v., op., ox-ac., plb., stram., stry.
lividity, spots - lyc.
mottled - **LACH.,** naja.
paleness - ***ars.,*** bell., ***calc., camph.,*** cedr., con., ign., ***ip., sang., sec.,*** zinc.
purple - apis, kali-p., ***lach.,*** naja, op., ***phos.,*** rhus-t., sec., thuj., vip.
chilliness, during - thuj.
spots - ***kali-c.***
redness - **AGAR., APIS,** bar-c., ***bell.,*** berb., bry., carb-an., ***fl-ac.,*** hep., mez., nat-s., nux-v., phos., plan., puls., rhus-t., seneg., sep., staph., stram., sulph., sumb., vesp.
left - cocc., right - staph.
spots - all-s., alum., ***bell.,*** berb., ***cor-r.,*** elaps, kali-i., lach., mag-m., mang., merc., nat-c., nat-m., ***ph-ac.,*** puls., sabad., sep., stann., tab., zinc.
yellowness - canth., ***chel.,*** cupr-ar., elaps, ign., ***lyc., sil.,*** spig.
dark - aran.
greenish - cupr-ar.
spots, in - elaps, med.

discoloration, back of hands
blotches - apis, arg-n.
itching - cit-v.
red - arg-n., cit-v.
stinging - apis
blueness - carb-o., plb.
spots - sars., sec.
brown - iod., thuj.
as if bruised - ***nat-m.***
spots - cop., ***lach.,*** lyc., ***nat-m.,*** petr., sep., sulph.
brownish - ***iod., thuj.***
petechiae - berb.
purpura hemorrhagica - ***lach., phos.***
redness - aur-s., berb., brom., cic., cimic., ***crot-h.,*** dulc., ferr., mur-ac., sulph., sul-ac., sumb., vip.
afternoon - cimic.
evening - cimic., sulph.
evening, in open air - dulc.
morning - sulph.
nettles, as from - nat-s.
streaks in - vip.
warm, from walking, when - dulc.
redness, in spots - ***agar.,*** bell., calc., cic., cop., hura, nat-c., osm., stann., sulph.
dusky - berb.
itching - brom., dros.
white - ***berb., calc.,*** nat-c., nit-ac.
yellow, in spots - cop., crot-c.
discoloration, fingers - act-sp.
black - sec., vip.
blue - benz-n., caust., ***cocc.,*** corn., ***crot-h., cupr.,*** nat-m., nux-m., nux-v., op., ox-ac., ***petr., sil.,*** vip.
blue, morning - petr.
brown, spots - ant-t.
ecchymoses - coca.
first, finger, black - phos.
redness, blotches - arg-n.
redness, blotches, back of - arg-n.
spots - apis, rhus-t.
fourth, finger, redness - lyc.
freckles - ferr.
greenish - colch.
joints - cann-s., ***cham.,*** cinnb., chel., ***lyc.,*** pall., spong., sulph.
livid - chin-s., ox-ac.
pale - verat.
redness - ***agar.,*** apis, apoc., arg-n., arum-i., benz-ac., berb., ***bor.,*** cann-i., ***cit-v.,*** fl-ac., graph., kali-bi., lach., ***lyc., nux-v.,*** plb., sil., sulph., ther., ***thuj.,*** zinc.
blotches - arg-n.
evening - sulph.
frost-bitten, as if - lyc.
points - lach.
spots - benz-ac., cor-r., plb., zinc.
stripes - apis
second, finger, second point of - ars-h.
spots - ***con.,*** corn., lyc., mang., ***nat-m., ph-ac., plb.***
tips, black - sol-n.

discoloration, fingers
tips, blue - agar., bor., colch., crot-c., op., phos.
blue, evening - phos.
redness - berb., calc., fago., mur-ac.
redness, after chilblains - berb.
white - alum., der., fl-ac.
yellow in spots - elaps
violet - stry.
white - gins., lach., vip.
coldness, during - gins.
yellow - ant-t., ***chel.,*** con., elaps, ph-ac., sabad.
spots, in - ant-t., bism., con., elaps, sabad.

discoloration, palm
brown spots - iod., nat-c., thuj.
red spots - apis, sep.
between index finger and thumb - iod.
redness - fl-ac.
yellow - ***chel.***

discoloration, thumbs
black - vip.
brownish - sulph.
dark - cic.
redness - cimic., lach., vesp.
white - vip.
in spots - sulph.
yellow - sulph.

DISLOCATION, fingers, joints, easy - bell., hep., teucr.
pain, as if, joints - mag-c., phos.

dislocation, thumbs, as if, feeling, joint - calc-p., cupr., puls.

DRAWING, pain - aesc., agar., agn., aloe, am-c., anac., ang., arg-m., arg-n., asaf., aur., bry., calc., cann-s., canth., carb-an., carb-s., carb-v., card-m., **CAUST.,** cham., chel., chin., chin-s., ***cina,*** cist., ***clem.,*** coloc., dios., euph., ***euphr.,*** grat., ham., kali-bi., kali-c., led., lyc., mag-c., mag-m., merc., mez., mur-ac., nat-c., nat-p., nat-s., ***nit-ac.,*** ol-an., petr., ph-ac., phos., plat., ptel., ***rhod.,*** **RHUS-T.,** sec., ***sil.,*** spig., stann., staph., ***stront-c., sulph.,*** tell., thuj., zinc.
asleep, falling - nit-ac.
ball of - aur-m., nat-c.
while writing - nat-c.
between index finger and thumb - agar.
bones - agar., ars., carb-v., mang., nat-c.
closing hand, on - chin.
cold, as from taking - cham.
cramp-like - anac., ang., arg-m., aur., cann-s., chin., ***cina,*** euphr., grat., lact., lyc., mosch., ph-ac., ***plat., sil.***
dinner, after - kali-bi.
evening - nat-s., nit-ac., ph-ac., ptel.
extending to, arm - nat-s.
to, elbow - phyt., sep., tab.
to, fingers - canth., colch., nat-s.
to, ring fingers - elaps
to, upward - nux-v.
extensors - ferr-i., led., nat-c.
grasping - chin.
inward - mag-c., mag-s., nux-v., sec.

DRAWING, pain
jerk-like - plat.
joints of - **ANAC.,** ang., ars., aur-m-n., chel., clem., coloc., ***mang.,*** nat-p., nat-s., phos., thuj.
rest, during - aur-m-n.
morning - ars., dios., kali-bi., lyc., ph-ac.
motion, on - caps., meny.
outward, while playing piano - merl.
paralytic - cham., mez., nit-ac., sil.
paroxysmal - cann-s., lyc.
rheumatic - ant-t., euphr., puls., **RHUS-T.,** zing.
shocks - phyt.
spots, in - arn.
sprained - nit-ac.
tendons - spig.
ulnar side - anac., arn., carb-an., sep.
waking, on - nit-ac.
wetting with warm water, after - ***phos.***
writing, while - euph., meny., ***sil.***
after - thuj.

drawing, back of - ***anac.,*** arg-m., asaf., chel., chin., ***ferr-i.,*** jatr., kali-bi., lyc., staph., viol-o., zing.
crampy - anac., arg-m.
motion, on - staph.
rheumatic - zinc.

drawing, fingers - acon., agar., ambr., am-c., ang., **ANT-C.,** ant-t., arn., ars., asar., aur., aur-m-n., bar-c., ***bell.,*** bry., ***camph.,*** carb-an., carb-s., ***carb-v., caul., caust.,*** cact., cina, ***cit-v.,*** clem., ***coloc.,*** com., con., dig., dios., ham., hell., hep., indg., kali-c., lyc., mag-s., mang., merc., mez., mosch., mur-ac., nat-c., nat-s., nit-ac., nux-m., nux-v., ***petr.,*** plat., plb., puls-n, **RHUS-T.,** rhus-v., sep., ***sil.,*** stann., staph., ***stront-c.,*** sulph., thuj., zinc.
afternoon - sulph.
cramp like - zinc.
evening - lyc., sulph.
bed, in - asar.
extending to, elbow - eupi., nat-m., plat.
to, shoulder - nux-m.
extensors, muscles - hep.
first - acon., agar., alum., anac., bar-c., calc., carb-v., caust., chel., chin., dig., kali-bi., mang., par., petr., plat., sabad., sulph., thuj., verb.
cramp like - plat.
distal - stann.
evening - anac., sabad., verb.
evening, bed, in - kali-bi.
extending upward - chin.
extensor tendon - nit-ac.
forenoon - thuj.
forenoon, 11 a.m. - thuj.
joints of - ruta.
jerk like - plat.
joints of, metacarpal - arg-m., euon.
middle - arg-n., berb., calc., camph., lyc., staph., ust.
paralytic - agar., bar-c., sabad., verb.
forenoon - thuj.

drawing, fingers
fourth - arn., bry., calad., chel., com., kali-n., nat-s., ph-ac., phos., sil., sulph., thuj.
bones - sars.
cramp like - phos.
evening - arn.
flexing amel. - ph-ac.
joints - caust., ruta.
joints, night - ruta.
morning, rising, on - kali-bi.
motion amel. - thuj.
tip - kali-c.
jerking - sulph.
joints - aloe, aml-n., **ANT-C.,** asaf., aur., ***bar-c.,*** carb-v., **CAUST.,** cist., ***coloc.,*** euon., hyos., nat-s., ph-ac., phos., plan., plat., rhod., ***rhus-t.,*** seneg., sep., sil., stann., staph., sulph., tep., ust.
evening - staph.
first - card-m., com., croc., kali-c., ph-ac., ol-an., staph.
first, motion, agg. - staph.
first, motion, amel. - com.
first, rheumatic - card-m.
middle - ruta.
motion, agg. - com.
motion, amel. - coloc., **RHUS-T.**
paralytic - staph.
morning - kali-c.
motion, on - hyos.
night - ***merc.,*** phos., puls.
paralytic - bell., ***sil.***
paroxysmal - lyc.
second - am-m., ars., calc., carb-v., chel., chin., cocc., crot-t., mang., par., stann., sulph., thuj., zinc.
afternoon - sulph.
crampy - stann.
evening, bed, in - ars.
jerky - stann.
joints - arg-m., bell., upa.
joints, distal - carb-v.
sitting, while - aur-m-n., **RHUS-T.**
sleep, during - rheum
tearing - carb-an.
third - ***calc.,*** cina, kali-bi., kreos., rat., stann., sulph., zinc.
during rest - cina, rat.
joints of - arg-m., mur-ac., ruta, upa.
joints of, night - ruta.
tips - am-c., ***ars.,*** kreos., petr., zinc.
extending, hand to - am-c.
extending, up arm - ***ars.,*** zinc.
wetting with warm water, after - phos.

drawing, palm - aloe, aur-m., ***caust.,*** chin., ***coloc.,*** led., nat-s., ***rhus-t.,*** sabin., zinc., zing.
evening - nat-s.
extending to fingers - ***caust.,*** sabin.

drawing, thumbs - acon., alum., ambr., anac., ***arn.,*** bry., chin., ***coloc.,*** con., indg., kali-bi., nat-m., nat-s., par., puls., rhus-v., spong., stann., sulph., thuj.
afternoon - sulph.
alternating with drawing, to occiput - arg-m.
ball - cupr., dulc., ***spong.***

drawing, thumbs
cramp-like - anac., meny.
evening - thuj.
exertion agg. - sulph.
extending up arms - ars., chin., colch., spong., zinc.
to wrists - ars.,
jerking of arms - cocc.
joints - aloe, ang., chel., nat-s.
first - coloc., colch., nit-ac., spig., thuj.
second - bar-c.
waking - nit-ac.
motion - ***coloc.***
amel. - nat-c., thuj.
paralytic - mosch., nit-ac., sabad.
paroxysmal - ferr-ma., thuj.
sudden - coc-c., ol-an.
tip - zinc.
writing, while - thuj.

DRAWN, outward, the left hand, while playing the piano - merc.

drawn, thumbs, inward - ***aeth., apis,*** ars., art-v., arum-t., ***bell.,*** brach., ***bufo, camph., caust., cham., cic., cocc.,*** **CUPR.,** ***glon.,*** hell., hyos., ign., ***lach.,*** mag-m., mag-p., merc., oena., phyt., ***sec.,*** stann., staph., stram., sulph., viol-t.

DROPPED, reins, often unconsciously, while driving - ***abrot.,*** con.

DRYNESS - acet-ac., aesc., aeth., all-c., **ANAC.,** anag., ***ars.,*** atro., **BAR-C.,** bell., ***calc-p.,*** cann-s., chel., cimic., clem., crot-h., fago., ham., ***hep.,*** iris, lach., lob., **LYC.,** ***nat-c., nat-m.,*** ol-j., op., ***ph-ac.,*** phos., plb., ptel., puls., ***rhus-t.,*** rhus-v., rob., sabad., **SULPH.,** ***sul-ac.,*** sumb., ***thuj., ust., zinc.***
afternoon - fago., gels.
forenoon - sabad.
10 a.m. - gels.
morning - zinc.
night - til.
parchment like, skin of - ***anac.,*** **BAR-C.,** crot-h., ***sulph.***

dryness, fingers - anac., anag., nat-m., puls., ***sil.***
afternoon - ***sil.***
evening - puls.
nails about - nat-m., ***sil.***
tips - ant-t., ***sil.***

dryness, palm - bad., bell., bism., haem., laur., ***lyc.,*** pip-m., rhus-v., sabad., tax.

DUPUYTREN'S, contracture, (see Contractures) - caust., cimx.

ECZEMA - ars., calc., ***canth.,*** clem., **GRAPH.,** ***jug-c.,*** lyc., ***merc., mez., nit-ac.,*** phos., ***sil.***
back of - ***graph., jug-c., merc.,*** **MEZ.,** nat-c., phos., ***sep.***

eczema, fingers - ***calc., lyc.,*** sil., staph.
painful - arn.

ELECTRICAL, current, sensation of - gels.

electrical, current, sensation of, fingers, on touching things - ***alum.***

EMACIATION - ars., chin., cupr., graph., ***phos.***, **PLB., SEL.**
emaciation, fingers - lach., ***sil.***, thuj.
index - lach., thuj.
tips - ars.
emaciation, thumbs - thuj.
ball, of - **PLB.**

ENLARGEMENT, sensation of - aran., bapt., cann-i., clem., ***cupr.***, kali-n., nux-m., ptel.
enlargement, fingers - benz-ac., calad.
osteoarthropathy, hypertrophic - thuj.
touching something, when - ***caust.***

ERUPTIONS - alum., am-m., anag., ant-t., ars., bar-m., **CARB-V.**, ***cic.***, cist., ***clem.***, cocc., com., con., cop., dulc., **GRAPH.**, ***hep.***, ***kali-s.***, kalm., kreos., ***lach.***, **LYC.**, med., ***merc.***, ***mez.***, ***mur-ac.***, nat-c., ***nat-m.***, ***nat-s.***, ***nit-ac.***, oena., ***petr.***, phos., psor., puls., ***rhus-t.***, rhus-v., ruta., sanic., ***sars.***, sel., sep., ***staph.***, still., ***sulph.***, ***sul-ac.***, zinc.
black - ***sec.***
bleeding - ***alum.***, ***lyc.***, ***merc.***, ***petr.***
blotches - ars., arg-n., carb-an., indg., kali-chl., merc., rhus-t., rhus-v., sep., spig., stann., sulph., urt-u.
brown - nat-m.
burning - bufo, nit-ac., rhus-t.
scratching, after - ***mez.***, **STAPH.**
touch, on - canth., **CIC.**
cold, weather - sep.
confluent - cic., cop., genist., phos.
cracked - ***alum.***, ***lyc.***, ***merc.***, ***petr.***
crusty, and full of cracks - ***anthr.***, **GRAPH.**, ***petr.***, ***sanic.***
desquamation - all-s., alum., am-c., am-m., bar-c., ferr., ***graph.***, laur., merc., mez., nat-m., ***ph-ac.***, phos., rhus-t., ***sep.***, sulph.
discharge, thin watery, palm - crot-h., ***nat-s.***
dry - anag., bov., lyc., merc., ***psor.***
elevated - bar-m., **CIC.**, kali-c., lach., merc., nat-m., nit-ac., rhus-v., sul-ac., urt-u.
exudation, yellow - ***rhus-v.***
fine - **CARB-V.**
furfuraceous - ***alum.***
hard - am-m., bov., led., ph-ac., rhus-t., spig.
itch-like - ***anan.***, ***psor.***, ***sep.***
itching - ars., **CARB-V.**, daph., ***graph.***, jug-r., ***mez.***, mur-ac., nit-ac., phos., psor., sanic., sep., staph., urt-u., zinc.
midnight, after - sul-ac.
millet, seed-like - bar-m.
moist - ***clem.***, kali-c., kali-s., mang., merc., ***mez.***, ***petr.***, ran-s., rhus-t.
nodules - ***petr.***, sep.
pimples - acon., ***agar.***, am-c., anac., ant-c., arg-n., ars., bell., ***bov.***, bry., ***canth.***, carb-s., ***carb-v.***, chin-s., ***cic.***, cupr-ar., dig., elaps, hep., iod., kali-ar., kali-chl., ***kreos.***, lac-ac., ***lyc.***, merc., mur-ac., nit-ac., ol-an., op., psor., ***rhus-t.***, rhus-v., sarr., ***sel.***, ***sulph.***, ***tarax.***, ***zinc.***
burning - bov., rhus-t.
greenish - cupr-ar.
hard - bov., ***rhus-t.***, rhus-v.

ERUPTIONS, general
pimples, itching - acon., am-c., bov., hep., kreos., ***lyc.***, sel., sulph., tarax.
itching, periodically - sulph.
red - acon., ars., anac., bov., sulph., til.
scurfs forming - mur-ac.
stinging - acon.
suppurating - anac., elaps
warm in bed, when becoming - mur-ac.
purple - ***petr.***
purulent - anac., sars.
red, evening - **SULPH.**
swelling - ***rhus-t.***
watery - rhus-t.
pustules - ***anac.***, asc-t., ***carb-s.***, chel., cic., fl-ac., ***kali-bi.***, ***merc.***, nat-m., phos., ***psor.***, rhus-t., rhus-v., ruta., sanic., sars., ***sep.***, sil., squil., staph., **SULPH.**
confluent - anac., rhus-v.
itch, resembling - ruta., ***sulph.***
itching - asc-t., squil., **SULPH.**
rawness - ***petr.***, ***sulph.***
red - bell., berb., bov., canth., carb-an., cic., cycl., jug-r., lyc., ***merc.***, ***ran-s.***, spig., spong., sulph., sul-ac., verat.
scales - anac., ***anthr.***, arn., ***clem.***, ***graph.***, hep., ***merc.***, mur-ac., ***petr.***, ***psor.***, sars., sec., ***sep.***
white - ***graph.***, ***sep.***
worse, in winter - ***petr.***, ***sep.***
scurfy - sars., sep.
sloughing - ***ars.***, kali-bi.
ulnar, side of, boils - coloc.
vesicles - ant-c., lach., sel.
eruptions, back of - berb., bov., chel., cupr., jug-r., kali-chl., ***kali-s.***, kreos., ***merc.***, ***mez.***, mur-ac., nat-c., phos., pix., puls., sanic., ***sep.***, **SULPH.**
cold - ***sep.***
confluent - cop.
copper-colored, spots - psor.
cracked - ***merc.***
crusts, yellow - ***merc.***, ***mez.***
desquamating - am-m., bar-c., calc., ***graph.***, merc.
elevated - anac., dros., plb., sul-ac.
excrescences, wart-like - **THUJ.**
itching - am-m., ***merc.***, ***mez.***, sanic., **SULPH.**
night - ***merc.***
measles, back of, like - cop.
moist - bov., kreos., ***mez.***
pemphigus - sep.
petechiae - berb.
pimples - acon., **AGAR.**, am-m., calc-p., canth., ***carb-s.***, carb-v., cic., kali-chl., mur-ac., tarax., zinc.
itching - am-m., zinc.
psoriasis, syphilitic - aur., ***ars.***, phos., ***merc.***
pustules - anac., cimic., sanic., ***sil.***, sulph.
rash - ***dig.***
red - jug-r., sul-ac.
patches - calc.
spots - bell.
scabs - mur-ac., plb., ***sep.***, sulph., sul-ac.

eruptions, back of
spots, red - bell.
tetter - lyc., sars., ***sep.,*** sulph.

eruptions, fingers - arn., ars., bor., canth., caust., ***cist.,*** cupr., cycl., fl-ac., graph., hep., ***kali-s., lach.,*** mez., mur-ac., ph-ac., ran-b., rhus-t., rhus-v., sars., sep., sil., spig., sulph., tab., tarax., thuj.
back of - mur-ac.
blotches - ant-c., arg-n., ars., berb., caust., cocc., con., lach., led., nat-c., rhus-t., verat.
burning - caust., ran-b.
copper-colored spots - cor-r.
desquamation - agar., bar-c., elaps, ***graph.,*** merc., ***mez., rhus-v.,*** sabad., ***sep.,*** still., ***sulph.***
desquamation, tips of - bar-c., elaps, ph-ac., phos.
dry - anag., psor.
elevated spots - syph.
excrescences - ars., thuj.
greenish - ars.
wart-like - thuj.
first - agar., ***calc.,*** kali-c., mag-c., nat-c., sil.
pimples - anac., sulph.
pustules - anac.
tubercles - lyc.
wart-like - lyc.
fourth - cycl.
itching - caust., ran-b.
joints - cycl., hydr., ***mez.,*** **PSOR.**
dry - **PSOR.**
nails, about - eug., merc., sel.
crusts - ***ars.***
desquamation - chlol.
pustules - bell.
pustules spreading over hand to wrist - ***kali-bi.***
ulcers - ***ars.***
vesicles - ail., ***nat-c.***
painful nodules - ***calc.***
phagedenic blisters - calc., ***graph.,*** hep., kali-c., ***mag-c.,*** nit-ac., ran-b., sil., sulph.
pimples - anac., ant-c., arn., ars., bar-c., berb., canth., carb-ac., cycl., elaps, graph., ***kali-c., lyc.,*** mez., mur-ac., ***ph-ac.,*** sars., ***spig.,*** tab., tarax., ***ther., zinc.***
red - ph-ac.
tips of - elaps
pustules - anac., bar-c., bor., cinnb., cocc., cupr., kali-bi., rhus-t., sars., sang., spig., zinc.
tips of - ***psor.***
scabs - anag., cit-v., kali-bi., lyc., mur-ac., rhus-v., thuj.
scales, white - lyc., ***sep.***
sides, of - ***mez.,*** sabad., tarax., tax.
third - cycl.
tips, of - ars., bar-c., ***cist.,*** cupr., elaps, ***nat-c.,*** psor.

eruptions, fingers, between the - ***canth.,*** carb-s., ***graph.,*** hell., lach., lyc., nit-ac., olnd., phos., ***psor.,*** puls., rhus-v., sep., ***sulph.,*** sul-ac.
burning - nit-ac.

eruptions, fingers, between the
desquamation - am-m.
between index finger and thumb, - am-m.
first and second fingers - cic.
itching - ars., canth., lyc., mag-c., nit-ac., **PSOR., SULPH.**
after midnight - sul-ac.
moist - ***graph.***
pimples - ars., lyc., mag-c., ph-ac., puls.
index and thumb, burning on touch - canth.
index finger and thumb - agar., bry., canth., ham., sulph., thuj.
index, and thumb, itching - ars., sulph.
third and fourth - canth.
pustules - caps., rhus-t.
scaly - laur.
second and third - ***sulph.***
third and fourth - mag-c.
urticaria - hyper., merc.
washing, worse from, itching agg. in warmth of bed, palm - ***rhus-v.***

eruptions, palm - anag., arn., aur., crot-h., ***graph.,*** kali-c., ***nat-s., sep., sulph.***
ball of - ant-c., mez.
copper-colored, spots - cor-r.
desquamation - am-c., arn., chin-s., elaps, graph., hydr., rhus-t., ***sep.,*** sabad., ***sulph.***
dry, tetter - ***caust., nat-s., sel., sulph.***
elevated, red blotches - ***fl-ac.***
pimples - nat-s., psor., spig., thuj.
hard itching, discharging stony concretion - thuj.
pustules - ***lach.***
raw - ***nat-s.***
red, spots - apis.
scales - hep., ***lyc., nat-s.,*** petr., pip-m., rhus-t., sabad., sars., ***sel.,*** sep., ***sulph.***
scurfy, tetters - cinnb., ***lyc., nat-s.,*** sulph.
smooth, spots - cor-r.

eruptions, thumbs - hep., sanic.
between and index finger - bruc., iod.
dry - verat.
pimples - arn., bry., canth.
tubercle - ***ars.***
pimples - ant-c., berb., ***kali-c., lyc., ther.***
beside the ball of - berb., ther.
itching - kali-c.
pustules - cic., sanic.
tip of - ail.
vesicles - ail., nit-ac.

EXCRESCENCES, on hands - ant-c., lach., thuj.
horny, on - ant-c., thuj.

EXOSTOSES, fingers - ***calc-f.***

EXTENSION, fingers, difficult - arn., ***ars., camph.,*** carb-s., ***coloc.,*** cupr., ***cupr-ar.,*** hyos., merc., mosch., plat., plb., stram., syph., tab.

FELON, general
bone, decay - asaf., aur., fl-ac., ***lach.,*** lyc., merc., mez., ph-ac., **SIL.,** sulph.
pain, deep-seated agg. in warm bed - sep.
pus, with offensive - fl-ac.
cold application amel. - ***apis, fl-ac., led.,*** **NAT-S., PULS.**
gangrenous - ***ars., lach.***
hangnails, from - lyc., ***nat-m.,*** sulph.
injury, from - ***led.***
itching - **APIS.**
lymphatic inflamed - all-c., ***bufo, hep., lach.,*** rhus-t.
malignant with burning - ***anthr., ars.,*** **TARENT-C.**
maltreated - ***hep.,*** phos., ***sil.,*** stram., ***sulph.***
nail, beginning in - par., petr., ***phyt.,*** plb., puls., ***rhus-t.,*** sep., **SIL.,** ***sulph.***
nail, root of - caust., graph.
nail, under - alum., caust., coc-c., sulph.
palm of - lach., ***sil.,*** sulph.
periosteum - ***am-c.,*** asaf., calc., calc-p., canth., dios., ***fl-ac.,*** mez., phos., sep., **SIL.,** sulph.
prick with a needle under the nail, from - all-c., bov., ***led.,*** sulph.
purple - ***lach.***
run-around - all-c., alum., ***apis,*** bufo, bov., ***caust.,*** con., crot-t., dios., eug., ferr., ***fl-ac., hep.,*** graph., lach., ***merc., nat-h., nat-m., nat-s.,*** par., phos., plb., puls., ran-b., rhus-t., ruta., ***sang.,*** sep., ***sil.,*** sulph., syph.
lymphatics inflamed - all-c., hep., lach., op., rhus-t., sin-n.
vaccination, after - **THUJ.**
sloughing, with - **ANTHR.,** ***ars., carb-ac., euph., lach.***
splinters, from - ***bar-c., hep.,*** iod., lach., ***led.,*** nit-ac., petr., **SIL.,** sulph.
sensation of - nit-ac.
stinging pain - **APIS, LACH.,** sep., **SIL.**
sulphur, after abuse of - apis
suppurative stage - ***calc.,*** **HEP., SIL.**
tendons, affected - graph., ***hep.,*** lach., ***led., merc.,*** nat-s., ***nit-ac.,*** ran-b., rhus-t., **SIL.,** sulph.
thumbs - all-c., am-m., bor., ***bufo,*** eug., fl-ac., gran., ***hep.,*** kali-c., kali-i., nux-v., op., sep., ***sil., sulph.,*** sul-ac.
palmer surface of - hep.
winter, every - **HEP.**

FISTULOUS, openings, palm - ars.

FLEXED, fingers - ambr., ***ars.,*** caust., chin., colch., **CUPR.,** ***hyos.,*** **MERC.,** nux-m., nux-v., ***phos., plat.,*** **PLB.,** sec., ***stram.***
extending, arm - plat.
extension, and flexion alternately, jerking - kali-c.
index flexed - sep.

FORMICATION - ACON., agn., arn., ars., ars-h., arund., atro., bar-c., bry., canth., carb-s., caust., chel., cupr., dulc., ***graph.,*** guare., ***hyos., hyper.,*** kali-n., kreos., lac-ac., lach., lyc., mez., nux-v., op., ph-ac., phos., ***plat., rhod.,*** **SEC.,** seneg., spig., ***sulph.,*** thuj., verat.
chill, during - canth.
evening - lac-ac., nat-c., ph-ac.
menses, during - ***graph.***
morning - ***hyper.,*** nat-c.
night - ars.
pressing them - spig.
right - nat-c.
ulnar side of - agar.
writing, after - agar.
water, after putting them in - ***sulph.***
yawning in open air, while - ***phos.***

formication, back of - bar-ac.

formication, fingers - **ACON.,** aeth., agar., alum., ars., brom., ***calc., caust.,*** colch., gins., graph., hep., kali-c., kreos., lach., **LYC.,** ***mag-c., mag-s.,*** mez., mur-ac., ***nat-c., nat-m.,*** nit-ac., op., paeon., phos., plat., plb., psor., ran-b., ***rhod., rhus-t.,*** samb., sep., ***sil.,*** staph., sul-ac., ***thuj.,*** verat.
anxiety, from - verat.
back of - bar-ac., ran-b.
evening - alum., ars., colch.
first - croc., phos., mag-s., tab.
tip of - graph., nat-m., thuj.
fourth - agar., ***aran.,*** mag-s., phos., rhod.
tip - sep., sul-ac.
morning, in bed - psor.
second - acon., caust., mag-s., mez., sul-ac., tab.
tip - kali-c., thuj.
third - ***aran.,*** caust., mag-s., sulph., tab.
tip - thuj.
tips - **AM-M.,** cann-s., cupr., glon., graph., hep., mag-m., mag-s., morph., **NAT-M.,** ***nat-s.,*** plat., **SEC.,** sep., spig., stry., sulph., tep., ***thuj.***
afternoon - ***am-m.***
evening - nat-c.
writing, while - ***acon.***

formication, palm - bar-c., berb., ol-an., par., seneg., spig., vip.

formication, thumbs - alum., chel., phos., mez., plb., rhod., zinc.
flexor, side of - plat.
proximal joint - cina.
tip - am-m., cina, nat-m.

FULLNESS - brom., ***caust.,*** fl-ac., nat-s., ***nux-m.,*** puls., sumb.
afternoon, knitting, while - nat-s.
evening - nux-m.
palm, at night - ars.
taking hold of anything - ***caust.***

fullness, palm - ars.

fullness, veins of hand - alum., alumn., am-c., arn., bar-c., calc., cast., **CHEL.,** ***chin., cic.,*** ind., laur., nux-v., olnd., op., ***phos.,*** **PULS.,** rheum, rhod., rhus-t., ruta., sulph., sul-ac., sumb., ***thuj.,*** **VIP.**

fullness, veins of hand
afternoon - alum.
chill, during - **CHEL.,** ***meny.***
evening - alum.
fever, during - chin., hyos., ***led.,*** meny.
washing in cold water, after - ***am-c.***

FUNGUS, fingers, hematodes - ***phos.***

FUZZINESS, sensation of - hell., ***hyper.,*** merc.
morning - hyper.
fuzziness, fingers, sensation of - ars., colch.

GANGLION, back of hands - am-c., ***ph-ac.,*** plb., **RUTA.,** ***sil.,*** zinc.
ganglion, palm - **RUTA.**

GANGRENE - ***ars., lach., sec.***
gangrene, fingers - ***sec.***

GNAWING, pain - bar-c., berb., cadm-s., gran., laur., merc., plat.
ball - kali-n.
ulnar side of extending to index finger. - sulph.
gnawing, fingers - berb., cina, mag-c., olnd., ph-ac., sant., stront.
bones of - ran-s.
convulsions, during - sant.
first - kali-bi., phos., ran-s.
bones - ran-s.
joints, first joint - kalm.
nails, under - **ALUM.**
tips of - fago.
gnawing, palm - kalm., ***ran-s.***
evening - ran-s.
gnawing, thumbs - kali-bi., mag-c., olnd.
scratching, from - olnd.
tip - nat-m.

HARDNESS, of skin, (see Callosities) - am-c., **GRAPH.,** rhus-v., **SULPH.**

HEAT - acon., aesc., **AGAR.,** aloe, alum., alumn., anac., ***ant-t.,*** apis, arg-n., ars-i., arum-d., arund., asaf., ***bar-c.,*** bar-m., **BELL.,** berb., bol., bor., brom., bufo, cadm-s., calad., calc., calc-s., camph., cann-s., caps., carb-an., carb-s., ***carb-v.,*** cast., ***cham.,*** chin., chin-a., chin-s., **CHEL.,** chlor., cina, clem., cocc., coff., colch., com., corn., croc., crot-t., cub., cur., ***cycl.,*** daph., dig., dros., dulc., eup-per., euphr., fago., ferr., ferr-i., ferr-ma., ferr-p., ***fl-ac.,*** form., gad., gamb., gels., ***glon.,*** gran., ***graph.,*** grat., ***guai.,*** ham., hep., hydr., hyos., hura, ign., ***iod.,*** iris, ***kali-bi., kali-c., kali-p.,*** kali-n., kali-s., kreos., lac-ac., **LACH.,** lact., laur., **LED.,** ***lil-t.,*** **LYC.,** ***mag-c.,*** mang., merc., merl., mez., mill., morph., mur-ac., murx., **NAT-C.,** nat-m., nat-p., nat-s., nicc., **NIT-AC., NUX-M.,** ***nux-v.,*** ol-an., **OP.,** ox-ac., ***petr., ph-ac.,*** **PHOS.,** phel., phys., pip-m., ***plan., psor.,*** ptel., **PULS.,** raph., rat., rheum, **RHOD.,** rhus-t., rhus-v., ruta., ***sabad.,*** sang., sarr., sars., **SEP.,** sil., sol-t-ae., ***spig.,*** spong., ***stann.,*** **STAPH.,** stront-c., **SULPH.,** sumb., tab., **TARAX.,** til., verat., zinc.
afternoon - ***apis,*** berb., fago., gels.
2 p.m. - lyc.
3 p.m. during cold sweat - hura

HEAT, general
afternoon, 3 to 5 p.m. - sulph.
4 p.m. - fago.
5 p.m. - petr.
air, open, amel. - phos., verat.
alternating with shivering - phos.
anxiety, with - carb-v., lyc., phos.
ball of - carb-v.
chill, during - agar., alum., ***apis, chin., cina,*** kali-c., mez., ***nat-c.,*** nux-v., ph-ac., phos., puls., spong.
after - sulph.
cold, during - apis, cadm-s., nat-s., puls., rat.
after - sep.
and pale, the other hot - mosch.
internal, during - alum., coff.
coldness, alternating with - cocc., sec.
of face, during - cina, nat-c.
of feet, during - acon., calad., com., mur-ac., ***nux-m., sep.***
of feet, during, or hot feet and cold hands - **SEP.**
of left arm, during - sep.
dry - bell.
eating, after, hot and burning - lyc., phos., sulph.
evening - aloe, alum., asaf., bell., cann-s., carb-an., dros., euphr., ferr., kali-c., lac-ac., ***led.,*** lyc., murx., nat-m., nux-m., nux-v., petr., rhus-t., sars., sep., ***stann.,*** sulph.
6 p.m. - asaf.
7 p.m. - cocc.
8 p.m. - nicc.
9 p.m. - sarr.
air, open - carb-an.
bed, in - kali-c.
burning - petr.
chilliness, during - asaf.
lying, after - carb-v.
lying, while - asar., sulph.
reading, while - ferr-p.
shivering, during - ***sulph.***
excitement, from - graph., phos., sep.
fever, during - zinc.
flushes, in - calc., colch., hydr., pip-m., **SULPH.**
beginning in hands - ***phos.***
forenoon, 10 a.m. - fago., gels., pip-m.
fright, after - calc.
internal - spig.
left - stann.
lying on the back, while - ign.
menses, during - carb-v., petr., sec.
morning - alumn., calc., chin-s., cycl., fago., hura, kali-c., nux-m., ***nux-v.,*** sulph.
8 a.m. - fago.
coldness, during - calc., fago., nux-m., nux-v., sulph.
writing, while - chin-s.
night - arg-n., ***calc.,*** com., ***ign.,*** nit-ac., sil., staph., sulph., til.
1:30 a.m. - chin-s.
2 to 5 a.m. - ign.
3 a.m. - clem.

HEAT, general
night, bed, in - ***sil.***
bed, in, after walking in open air - alum.
bed, in, with cold feet - ***sulph.***
cold legs and feet, with - com.
noon - mag-c.
one hand, coldness of the other - chin., cocc., ***dig.***, ***ip.***, mosch., ***puls.***, tab.
onesided - lyc., mez.
perspiration, cold, during - hura
right - staph.
shivering, during - ign.
sitting, while - calc.
sleep, when going to - alum.
stitching pain, during - gamb.
stool, during - hep.
sudden - ferr-m., glon.
talking, from - graph.
vomiting, after - verat.
writing, while - chin-s., mez.
heat, back of - all-s., ang., ***apis,*** chel., cycl., **NAT-C.,** nux-v., **RHUS-T.,** sep., sulph., thuj.
heat, fingers - apis, bor., fago., lact., mag-c., mang., par., rhus-t., thuj.
alternately hot and cold as if dead - par.
nails - hura.
sensation - lyc.
tips - daph., fago., hura, nat-c., rhod.
heat, palm - **ACON.,** alum., am-m., anac., arg-n., ars., ars-m., **ASAR.,** bad., berb., ***bor.,*** **BRY.,** ***calc.,*** carb-an., carb-o., carb-s., carb-v., chin-a., coff., colch., com., crot-h., cub., ***eup-per., ferr.,*** ferr-p., ***fl-ac., gels.,*** ham., hep., hydr., ind., **IP.,** iris, kreos., lac-c., **LACH.,** laur., ***lil-t., lyc.,*** mag-m., ***med.,*** merc., **MUR-AC.,** naja, nat-c., nit-ac., ***nux-v.,*** ol-an., ol-j., ***petr.,*** ph-ac., **PHOS.,** raph., rheum, rhus-v., ***samb., sep.,*** sil., ***stann.,*** **SULPH.,** sumb., tab., tarent., tax., til., verat., zinc., zing.
afternoon - arg-n., gels., stann., ***sulph., zinc.***
5 p.m. - chel., lil-t., til.
chill, after - sulph.
coldness, after - asar., merc., sulph.
of the backs of, with - anac., coff.
dry heat - ars-m., chin-a., ferr-p., gad., gels., ptel.
evening - acon., iod., mag-m.
after lying down - am-m., nux-v.
flushes - cub.
forenoon - calc., fl-ac.
menses, during - carb-v., ***petr.***
morning - carb-an., sil.
in bed - nux-v.
night - **LACH.,** nit-ac., ***ol-j.***
sitting, while - ferr-p.
spreads from - chel.
ulnar side of hand - laur.
walking in open air, after - lyc.
heat, thumbs - phos., zinc.

HEAVINESS - acon., acet-ac., aesc., ang., ***alum.,*** am-c., ***ars., bar-c.,*** **BELL.,** ***bov.,*** bry., cann-s., ***caust.,*** chel., cycl., iris, ***kali-n., lyc.,*** manc., nat-m., nicc., ol-an., ox-ac., ***ph-ac.,*** **PHOS.,** phyt., pic-ac., plb., puls., rhod., sars., sil., spong., stann., sul-ac., teucr., ***zinc.***
evening - lyc.
hanging arm, down - sul-ac.
menses, during - zinc.
before - bar-c., kreos., zinc.
motion amel. - cann-s., nicc.
night - kali-n.
right - bov., cann-s., sulph.
warmth of bed agg. - goss.
writing, while - caps., ***caust., chel.,*** lyc.
heaviness, fingers - berb., par., phos., ***plb.,*** rhus-v.

HERPES - ***bor., bov., calc.,*** cist., ***con.,*** **DULC.,** ***graph.,*** kreos., merc., ***mez., nat-c.,*** nat-m., ran-b., sars., sep., ***staph.,*** verat., **ZINC.**
herpes, back of - carb-s., graph., lyc., nat-c., petr., sep., thuj.
herpes, palm - ***aur., kreos.,*** psor., ran-b., ***sep.***
herpes, fingers - ambr., caust., ***cist.,*** **GRAPH.,** ***kreos.,*** merc., nit-ac., psor., ran-b., thuj., zinc.
between the - ambr., graph., merc., ***nit-ac.***
herpes, fingers, between - ambr., graph., merc., ***nit-ac.***
fingers, between, index and thumb - ambr.

HORNY, excrescences on hand cracked, at base - thuj.

INDURATION, muscles - ars., ***sulph.***
induration, fingers, muscles - caust., crot-h., graph., med., phyt., ***ruta.***
tendons - carb-an., **CAUST.,** ***ruta.***
induration, palm - ***cist., lyc.***
tendons - sulph.

INFLAMMATION - anac., ***anthr.,*** arn., ars., ***bry.,*** bufo, cocc., ***crot-h.,*** cupr., ferr., hep., ***kalm., lach., lyc.,*** manc., ***rhus-t., sil.,*** sulph., vesp.
callosities - ***phos.***
dark red - anthr., ***lyc.,*** rhus-t.
erysipelatous - graph., ***lach., rhus-t.***
inflammation, fingers - **AM-C.,** apis, calc-s., con., ***cupr., hep.,*** kali-c., lyc., ***mag-c.,*** mang., nat-m., nit-ac., puls., ran-b., ***sil.,*** tarent.
bone - ***staph.***
periosteum - **LED.**
erysipelatous - rhus-t., rhod., sulph., thuj.
joints - ***lyc.***
joints, middle - lyc.
bursitis - ***ruta.***
nails, around - con., hell., ***nat-m., nat-s.,*** ph-ac.
root of - hep., kali-c., stict.
tips - ***thuj.***
inflammation, palm - bry.

INJURIES, hands, contusion - ***arn., ruta.***
dissecting wounds - ***apis,*** **ARS., CALEN., LACH.,** ***pyrog.,***
fracture, with laceration - ***hyper.***
sprain - **ARN.,** ***calc., rhus-t., ruta.***

injuries, fingers, amputated stump painful - ***calen.,*** **HYPER.,** phos., ph-ac., ***staph.***
lacerations - **CALEN.**, hyper.
splinter of glass - myris., sil.
injuries, thumbs, cat bite - calen., hyper., lach., led.

INSENSIBILITY - stram.
burning, to - ***plb.***
pain, to - kreos., plb.
pricking, to - plb.
insensibility, fingers, heat of stove - ***plb.,*** thuj.

ITCHING - **AGAR.,** aloe, ***alum.,*** ambr., **ANAC.,** ***anthr.,*** ant-s., apis, arg-m., ars., asc-t., aur., bar-c., ***berb., bov.,*** bry., calc., ***camph.,*** cann-s., canth., ***carb-an.,*** carb-s., ***carb-v., caust.,*** chin-s., ***cit-v.,*** colch., dios., fago., fl-ac., glon., gran., graph., ham., ***hep.,*** jug-r., kali-ar., kali-bi., ***kali-c., kali-s.,*** kreos., ***lach., lyc.,*** med., ***merc.,*** mur-ac., ***nit-ac.,*** ol-an., osm., ***petr., ph-ac., phos.,*** phyt., plan., plat., ***psor.,*** ran-b., ***rhus-t.,*** rhus-v., ruta., sabad., sars., sel., ***sep.,*** sil., stann., **SULPH.,** tarax., zinc.
ball of - con., graph., ***sep.***
spots, in - ***sep.***
biting - berb.
burning - **AGAR.,** apis, arg-m., ***kali-bi.,*** kali-c.
chilblains, as of - **AGAR.,** arg-m., ***cit-v., puls.***
crawling - berb.
evening - ***sulph.***
10 a.m. - mag-c.
bed, in - phos.
lying down, after - ph-ac.
hot water amel. - ***rhus-t.,*** rhus-v.
midnight - rhus-t.
lying down, after - kali-bi.
morning, rising, on - rhus-v., sulph.
waking, on - ham., ***sulph.***
motion amel. - sars.
nettles, as from - nit-ac., urt-u.
night - canth., ***lith.,*** ruta., sabad.
rising from bed - rhus-t., sulph.
rubbing, after - ***nat-m.***
amel. - berb., ham., nit-ac.
scratching, agg. - ars., ham., ***ph-ac.,*** **SULPH.**
amel. - alum., anac., camph., merc., ol-an.
sticking - berb., lach., merc-i-f.
touch, on - psor.
water, on immersing in - rhus-v.
itching, back of - **AGAR.,** alum., anag., apis, ars-i., bor., calc., ***camph.,*** carb-an., caust., ***cimic.,*** cina, com., ***dig., euph.,*** eupi., fago., gran., indg., jug-r., merc., merc-i-r., mez., nat-c., nat-s., ol-an., ***ph-ac.,*** phos., plat., ptel., ***puls.,*** rhus-v., rumx., stann., **SULPH.**
afternoon - cimic.
burning - stann.
corroding - merc.
evening - cimic., merl., **SULPH.**
flea bites, as from - bor., nat-c.
forenoon - ***sulph.***

itching, back of
night - dig., phos., sulph.
rubbing, after - rhus-v.
scratching, agg. - ph-ac.
amel. - alum., camph., ol-an., merc.
spots - sulph.
stinging - ars-i., camph., phos.
warmth agg. - ***sulph.***
itching, fingers - ***agar., alum.,*** am-c., **ANAC.,** apis, ars., ars-h., arum-d., asc-t., aur., berb., calad., calc., cann-s., carb-an., carb-v., ***caust.,*** cit-v., coc-c., ***con.,*** euph., hep., jatr., jug-r., lach., lact., lyc., mag-c., mang., merc., mez., nat-c., nat-m., nux-v., ox-ac., petr., phos., plan., plat., prun., puls., ran-b., ***rhod.,*** rhus-v., sel., sil., stry., **SULPH.,** ***sul-ac.,*** tarent., thuj., **URT-U.,** zinc.
afternoon - coc-c., jug-r.
back of - ars., berb., carb-an., caust., **CON.,** merc-i-r., nat-m., sars., sulph.
bed, on going to - nux-v.
burning - euph.cool, when - thuj.
evening - calad., sulph.
bed, in - nat-m.
first finger - agar., anac., calc., carb-an., caust., crot-h., fl-ac., hell., hura, lach., lyc., nat-m., plat., sil., teucr.
evening - fl-ac.
joints, last - petr.
joints, metacarpal - berb., fl-ac., verat.
joints, middle - euph., manc., nat-m.
tip - am-m., nat-m.
tip, morning - am-m.
tip, scratching does not amel. - am-m.
fourth finger - anac., asc-t., con., lach., lyc., ol-an.
night - sulph.
frozen, as if they had been - ***agar.,*** spig.
formerly - lyc.
joints - alum., apis, ***bor.,*** bry., ***camph.,*** hydr., nux-v., petr.
back of - ***bor.***
lying, while - calad.
nails, round - ***hep.,*** merc.
under - sep.
phalanx, middle and last - lyc.
scratching agg. - alum., ars., arum-d., arum-i., arum-m., arum-t.
second finger - ars., ars-h., chel., crot-h., crot-t., gran., kali-n., lith., nat-m., olnd., ph-ac., rhod., teucr., verat., verb.
smoking, from - calad.
third finger - asc-t., crot-h., crot-t., lith., ***rhod.,*** teucr., ther.
tips - ambr., plat., prun., spig., ***sul-ac.***
warm room agg. - nux-v.
itching, fingers, between - alum., anac., aur., brom., camph., carb-s., carb-v., caust., cycl., grat., mag-c., nat-s., ***ph-ac., puls., psor.,*** rhod., rhus-v., sel., **SULPH.**
evening - ran-s.
morning - **SULPH.**
waking, on - rhus-v., sulph.
night - anac.

itching, fingers, between
thumb and index finger - ***agar.***, ambr., aur., grat., hura, iod., jatr., kreos., plb., sumb.
thumb and index finger, night - ***agar.***
itching, palm - agar., alum., ambr., **ANAC.**, apis, arg-m., arg-n., ars., aur., ***benz-ac.***, berb., calc., ***camph.***, carb-v., ***caust.***, chel., cinnb., com., con., crot-h., dios., form., graph., ***gran.***, grat., ***hep.***, hydr., ind., jatr., ***kali-c.***, ***kali-p.***, lyc., mag-c., mag-s., mang., merc., ***mur-ac.***, nat-m., ol-an., petr., phys., ran-b., ***rhus-t.***, ***rhus-v.***, ***sel.***, sil., spig., staph., stram., stry., **SULPH.**, ther.
afternoon - form., nat-m.
burning - agar., aur-m., ran-b., spig.
burning, rubbing, after - **SULPH.**
evening - dios., mag-c., mang., ol-an., sulph., ther.
intervals of 10 or 12 hours - rhus-v.
licking amel. - mang.
midnight - rhus-t.
morning - mag-c., ol-an.
moving about amel. - com.
night - **ACON.**, carb-v., hydr.
root of fingers, near - kali-c., lyc.
rubbing, amel. - **ANAG.**, mag-s.
scratching, agg. - mang.
amel. - chel., graph., mag-c., mang., ol-an.
stinging - ran-b., ruta.
washing, after - rhus-v.
itching, thumbs - aur-m., carb-v., chel., cimic., con., kali-n., lach., mez., olnd., sep., vesp.
ball of - ***agar.***, aloe, gamb., manc., spong., verat.
burning - aur-m., mang.
evening - cimic.
nails, under - sep.
nettles, like - lach.
scratching amel. - chel., olnd.
tickling - kali-n.
tip - ant-c.

JERKING - bar-m., brom., ***cina***, ***cocc.***, ***coff.***, ***cupr.***, ***graph.***, hyos., jug-r., ***merc.***, nat-c., ***nat-m.***, nux-v., pall., ran-b., sec., **STRAM.**
convulsive - bar-m., merc.
electric shocks - jug-r.
exertion, on - ***merc.***
going to sleep, on - nat-c.
grasping, on - nat-c.
jerking, fingers - ***calc.***, cadm-s., **CIC.**, **CINA**, ***cocc.***, ***merc.***, ***merc-c.***, mez., ***nat-c.***, nit-ac., ***op.***, stram.
epilepsy - **CIC.**
extending, into shoulder - ***ars.***
to both arms in chorea - ***cupr.***
fourth - com., meny.
gastric fever - stram.
joints - carb-s.
rheumatic - carb-s.
painful - cocc.
second - stann.
writing, while - stann.

KNOBBY, finger ends - ***laur.***

LAMENESS - abrot., acet-ac., agar., ars., ***cupr.***, fl-ac., ***kali-bi.***, nat-m., nat-s., phos., rhus-t., ***sil.***, stront-c., ***sulph.***, tab., ***zinc.***
exertion, after - ***sil.***
morning,10 a.m. - abrot.
spasms, before - kali-bi.
sudden - cann-s.
writing, while - ***sil.***
lameness, fingers - bor., ***calc.***, carb-v., hyper., kali-c., ***sep.***
second - cimic., rhus-t.
third - bry.
writing, after - bry.
lameness, thumbs - calc-s., kali-c.

LONGER, fingers - kali-n., phos.

LYING, hand on part, amel. - ***bell.***, bor., calc., canth., con., ***croc.***, cycl., dros., mang., ***meny.***, mur-ac., nat-c., olnd., par., ***phos.***, rhus-t., sabad., sep., sil., spig., sulph., thuj.
agg. - kali-n.
near part amel. - sul-ac.

MOTION, hands, of
automatic - ***acon.***, cann-i., coca, ***kali-i.***, nux-v., zinc.
he strikes his face - acon.
to head - plb.
clutching - ***hyos.***
convulsive - apis, bell., ***kali-c.***, ***nat-m.***, ***op.***, plb., ***zinc.***
diminished power of - carb-s., con., ***plb.***
face, toward - stry.
hasty - ***bell.***
inco-ordination - ***bell.***, ***cupr.***, ***gels.***, merc., plb., puls.
playing, with - ***mur-ac.***
sleep, during - ars.
write, when trying to, power of direction impaired - aesc., ter.
motion, fingers, of - agar., fl-ac., ***lach.***, ox-ac., ***stram.***, tarent.
automatic - zinc.
constant - kali-br., ***stram.***, sulph.
counting, as if he were, with - mosch.
difficult - plb., rob., tarent., vip.
afternoon - mag-s.
first, spasmodic - con., ign.
irregular - ***cupr.***
sleep, during - ars.
motion, thumbs, of, convulsive - calc., calc-p., coc-c., con., crot-c.

NAILS, general, fingers
biting, fingernails, habit of - acon., am-br., ***ant-t.***, arn., ***ars.***, arum-t., bar-c., brom., calc., **CINA.**, hura., hyos., ign., lyc., med., ***nat-m.***, nit-ac., phos., plb., sanic., senec., sil., stram., sulph.
blood, fingernails, oozing from - ***crot-h.***
rush of to - ***op.***
brittle, nails - cast-eq., ***sil.***, ***thuj.***
brittle, fingernails - ***alum.***, ***ambr.***, ant-c., ars., calc., cast-eq., ***cupr.***, ***dios.***, ***fl-ac.***, **GRAPH.**, ***lyc.***, med., merc., ***nit-ac.***, ***phos.***, **PSOR.**, sep., ***sil.***, squil., ***sulph.***, ***thuj.***

NAILS, general, fingers

burning, nails - alumn., ant-c., calc., caust., **GRAPH.,** hep., merc., nat-m., nux-v., puls., ***sep.,*** sulph.
around - con.
under - calc., ***caust.,*** elaps, kali-c., merc., nit-ac., ***sars.***
roots of - ***asaf.,***

chapped, skin, about the nails - **NAT-M.**

claw-like, fingernails - ars.

corrugated, nails - ars., fl-ac., sabad., **SIL.,** ***thuj.***
transversely - ars.

cracked, nails - **ANT-C.,** ars., ***nat-m., sil.***

crippled - ars., ***caust.,*** **GRAPH.,** ***nat-a., nit-ac.,*** sabad., sep., **SIL.,** ***thuj.***

crippled, fingernails - alum., ***caust.,*** **GRAPH.,** ***nit-ac., sabad., sep.,*** **SIL.,** sulph., ***thuj.***

crumbling - ars., sep., ***sil., thuj.***

curved, fingernails - ***nit-ac.***
tuberculosis, in - med., tub.

discoloration, nails - ant-c., ars., graph., nit-ac., thuj.
black - ***ars., graph., lept., nat-m.***
around - **NAT-M.**
blood, settles under nails - apis
blueness - acon., aesc., agar., apis, apoc., ***arg-n.,*** arn., ***ars.,*** asaf., aur., cact., ***camph.,*** carb-s., ***carb-v., chel., chin.,*** chin-a., ***chin-s.,*** chlf., cic., cocc., colch., con., ***cupr., dig., dros.,*** eup-pur., ***ferr.,*** ferr-ar., ferr-p., gels., gins., ***graph.,*** ip., manc., merc., merc-sul., ***mez.,*** mur-ac., ***nat-m., nit-ac.,*** **NUX-V.,** op., ***ox-ac., petr.,*** ph-ac., ***phos.,*** plb., rhus-t., sang., sars., sep., ***sil., sulph.,*** sumb., tarent., ***thuj.,*** **VERAT.,** ***verat-v.***
chill, during - apis, arn., **ARS.,** ***asaf.,*** carb-s., ***carb-v., chel., chin., chin-s., cocc.,*** con., ***dros., eup-pur.,*** ip., kali-ar., mez., **NAT-M., NUX-V.,** petr., ph-ac., **RHUS-T.,** sulph., thuj., verat.
menses, during - ***arg-n., thuj.***
dark - morph., ox-ac.
gray - merc-c., ***sil.***
livid - ars., ***colch.,*** op., ***ox-ac.,*** sul-ac.
purple - apis, ars., op., samb., sec., stram.
red - ars., crot-c., lith.
then black - ***ars.***
white - cupr., nit-ac.
spots - alum., ars., ***nit-ac.,*** sep., **SIL.,** sulph.
yellow - ambr., am-c., aur., bell., bry., canth., carb-v., cham., chin., **CON.,** ferr., ign., lyc., ***merc., nit-ac., nux-v.,*** op., plb., **SEP., SIL.,** spig., ***sulph.***

distorted, nails - alum., anan., calc., ***fl-ac.,*** **GRAPH.,** merc., sabad., ***sep.,*** **SIL.,** sulph., ***thuj.***

drawing, pain, under nails - nat-m.

dryness - ***sil., thuj.***
about - nat-m., ***sil.***

NAILS, general, fingers

eruptions, nails, about - eug., merc., sel.

exfoliation, nails, of - alum., ant-c., apis, ars., cast-eq., chlor., crot-h., form., **GRAPH.,** ***hell., merc.,*** rhus-t., sabin., ***sec.,*** sep., ***sil.,*** squil., sulph., thuj., ***ust.***

grow, nails, do not - ***ant-c.,*** calc., sil.
grow, rapid - fl-ac.
slow, fingernails - ***ant-c.***

hangnail, nails - ***calc.,*** lyc., ***merc.,*** **NAT-M.,** ***rhus-t.,*** sabad., sep., ***sil., stann.,*** **SULPH.,** ***thuj.***
inflamed - kali-chl.
painful - sel., stann.

hardness, fingernails - ars.

horny, nails, growth under - **ANT-C.,** graph.

inflammation, fingernails - kali-c.
root of - ***hep.,*** stict.

ingrowing, nails - alum., ***caust.,*** colch., **GRAPH.,** kali-c., kali-chl., **MAG-AUST.,** ***nat-m., nit-ac., ph-ac.,*** plb., **SIL.,** ***sulph.,*** **TEUCR.,** ***thuj.,*** tub.
ulceration, with - ***nit-ac.,*** **SIL.,** ***teucr.***
unhealthy granulation, with - ***lach.,*** sang.

injuries, fingernails - **ARN., HYPER.,** ***led.***
lacerations, from - **HYPER.**
splinter of glass, from - calen., hyper., ***sil.***

pain, nails - am-m., ant-c., bell., ***caust., graph., hep.,*** kali-c., ***merc.,*** nat-m., ***nit-ac., nux-v.,*** par., ***petr.,*** puls., ran-b., rhus-t., sabad., sep., ***sil., squil.,*** stann., sulph., zinc.
splinter, as of - ars-h., coc-c., ***nit-ac., sil., sulph.***
under - caust., eup-per., hep., merc., ***sil.,*** thuj.
in intermittent fever - eup-per.
walking, while - camph.

pain, fingernails - alum., ant-c., ***calc-p., caust.,*** colch., ***graph.,*** hep., merc., myric., naja, nat-m., ***nit-ac.,*** nux-v., ***petr.,*** puls., raph., **SIL.,** squil., sulph., teucr.
around the nails - lith.
root of - calc., ***calc-p.,*** sang.
touched, when - caust., petr.
ulcerative - ***calc-p.,*** nat-s., puls.
under - **ALUM.,** ant-c., berb., bism., calc-p., caust., elaps, naja, ***nat-s., nit-ac.,*** ran-b., raph., sars., ***sil., sulph.***
horny growths, from - ***ant-c., graph.***
pressure, on - sars.
splinters, as from - bell., carb-v., ***fl-ac.,*** hep., **NIT-AC.,** petr., plat., ran-b., ***sil., sulph.***
touched, when - caust.

panaritium, nails - ***all-c.,*** alum., **AM-C.,** ***am-m., anac.,*** **ANTHR., APIS,** arn., asaf., bar-c., ***benz-ac.,*** berb., bov., ***bufo, calc., caust.,*** chin., ***cist.,*** con., cur., **DIOS.,** eug., ferr., **FL-AC.,** gins., **HEP.,** ***hyper., iod., iris,*** kali-c., kalm., ***lach.,*** led., ***lyc., merc., nat-c., nat-h., nat-m., nat-s.,*** **NIT-AC.,** par., petr., ***phyt.,*** plb., puls., ***rhus-t., sang., sep.,*** **SIL.,** ***sulph.,*** **TARENT-C.,** teucr.

NAILS, general, fingers
panaritium, burning - **ANTHR.**
deep-seated - bry., hep., lyc., rhus-t.
roughness, fingernails - ***graph.,*** SIL.
ribbed - thuj.
ridges, longitudinal - fl-ac.
sensitive, fingernails - berb., ***nat-m.,*** nux-v., petr., ***sil.,*** squil., sulph.
sharp, pain, nails - alum., ***calc.,*** caust., ***graph., hyper.,*** mosch., ***nat-m.,*** nit-ac., nux-v., ***puls.,*** rhus-t., sep., sil., sulph.
sharp, thumbnails, under - am-m., bapt., coc-c., ***graph.,*** kali-n., ***thuj., zinc.***
root of - fl-ac.
shooting, pain, fingernails - ***hyper.***
first - hyper., sulph.
night in bed - sulph.
spilt, nails - **ANT-C., SIL.,** ***squil.,*** sulph.
splinters, nails, as from, under the - bell., carb-v., ***fl-ac.,*** hep., **NIT-AC.,** petr., plat., ran-b., ***sil., sulph.***
spotted, nails - alum., ars., ***nit-ac.,*** ph-ac., sep., **SIL.,** sulph., tub.
suppuration, nails, around - con., ph-ac.
under - form.
nail of left great toe - caust.
vaccination, after - **THUJ.**
suppuration, fingernails, first - calc., nat-s.
tearing, pain, nails - colch., ***fl-ac.,*** hep., ***nit-ac.,*** petr., plat., ran-b., ***sil., sulph.***
tearing, thumbnails, under - carb-v., fl-ac., kali-c., zinc.
extending upward - berb.
night, in bed - sulph.
thick, nails - alum., ***ant-c.,*** calc., **GRAPH.,** merc., sabad., sep., **SIL.,** sulph., ***ust.***
thick, fingernails - alum., **GRAPH.,** sabad.
thin, nails - ars., op.
tough, fingernails - chin-s.
ulcerative, pain, thumbnails - am-m., nat-s.,
ulcers, nails - alum., ant-c., **ARS.,** aur., bar-c., bor., bov., calc., caust., con., crot-h., ***fl-ac.,*** **GRAPH.,** ***hep., lach.,*** lyc., ***merc., nit-ac., puls.,*** ran-b., ***sang.,*** sec., sep., **SIL.,** squil., **SULPH.,** thuj.
ulcers, fingernails - alum., bar-c., ***bov.,*** caust., con., ***hep.,*** iod., kali-c., lach., lyc., ***merc., nat-m.,*** plat., puls., sang., sep., **SIL., SULPH.,** sul-ac., ***thuj.***
around - **CARB-S.,** chlol., con., hell., ***nat-s.,*** phos., ***rhus-t., sang.,*** **SIL.,** ***sulph.***
under - **ARS.**
ulcers, thumbnails, under - kali-bi.

NODULES, first finger, volar - con.

NUMBNESS - abrot., ***acon.,*** aesc., agar., aloe, alum., ambr., am-c., ***apis,*** arg-n., ***ars.,*** ars-h., asaf., asc-t., aster., atro., bapt., bar-c., bell., bor., bry., bufo, cact., ***calc.,*** calc-i., calc-p., calc-s., ***camph.,*** cann-s., carb-ac., **CARB-AN.,** carb-o., ***carb-s., carb-v., caust.,*** cedr., chel., cimic., ***coca,*** **COCC.,** ***colch.,*** com., ***con.,*** croc., **CROT-C.,** cub., ***cupr.,*** cycl., dios., ***dulc.,*** elaps, eupi., euphr., ***ferr.,*** ferr-ar., ferr-p., ***fl-ac., gels.,*** gins., **GRAPH.,** guare., hell., helo., hep., hydrc., ***hyos., hyper., kali-ar.,*** **KALI-C., KALI-N.,** kali-p., ***kali-s., lach.,*** **LYC.,** lyss., manc., med., merc., merc-c., merc-i-f., merc-sul., ***mez.,*** naja, ***nat-m., nit-ac.,*** nux-m., ***nux-v., onos., op.,*** ox-ac., **PHOS.,** phys., pic-ac., ***plb., psor.,*** ptel., ***puls.,*** pyrog., raph., sarr., ***sec.,*** sep., ***sil., spig.,*** stram., stry., stront-c., sulph., sumb., ***thuj.,*** verat-v., vip., ***zinc.***
afternoon - mez.
air, cold - lyc.
alternating hands - **COCC.**
back of - caj., laur., med., phos.
carrying anything - ambr., sep.
chill, during - ***apis, cimx.,*** ferr., guare., ***lyc.,*** nux-m., nux-v., ph-ac., **PULS.,** sec., **SEP.,** stann.
daytime - apis, ***zinc.***
eating, after - con., lyc.
evening - bor., nux-m.
excitement, during - ***sulph.***
exercise - ruta.
extending to arm - agar., aster., dios., fl-ac.
grasping anything - ***calc., cham.,*** sep.
anything, amel. - spig.
heat in stomach, with - con.
lain on - ambr., am-c., graph., ***kali-c.,*** petr.
left - acon., aloe, aster., cact., carb-an., con., ***crot-h.,*** dig., dios., euphr., ferr., fl-ac., ***glon., graph., lac-c., lach., lat-m.,*** med., merc-sul., mez., naja, nat-c., ***nit-ac.,*** phyt., ***rhus-t.,*** stry.
during menses - ***graph.***
right hand, cold - ***ferr.***
lying, on - ambr., mag-c., nat-m., puls.
on hard substance - nat-m.
menses, during - ***graph.,*** kali-n., sec.
morning - ***carb-an.,*** fl-ac., ***kali-c.,*** mag-c., ***nit-ac., phos.,*** sil., ***spig., thuj.***
4 a.m. - nat-c.
5 a.m. - fl-ac.
7 a.m. - dios.
bed, in - ***carb-an.,*** fl-ac., lyc., nat-c., nit-ac., ***phos.***
waking, on - alum., calc-p., ***ferr., kali-c., phos., zinc.***
washing, on - ***carb-v.***
motion, on - bapt.
amel. - am-c., ***apis,*** cann-s., carb-an., ***ferr.,*** nat-m., puls., spig., stront.
night - agar., ambr., bry., carb-v., lyc., kali-n., mag-m., pall., sep., **SIL.**
grasping anything - sep.
lain on - am-c., petr.
sleep, in - croc.
one hand numb, the other asleep - ***phos.***
painful - euphr., mag-m.
paralytic - nit-ac.
pocket, on putting hand into - nat-m.
prosopalgia, side of - cocc.
radial nerve, distribution of - ph-ac.
resting, hand on anything - nit-ac.
head on hand - squil.
riding in a carriage - form.

NUMBNESS, general
right - am-c., asc-t., cann-s., cycl., elaps, ***gels.,*** graph., ***hep.,*** kali-p., lil-t., lyss., merc., nat-m., nit-ac., phos., sil., spig., thuj.
right, then left - ***cocc.***
sewing, while - ***crot-h.***
sitting - am-c., graph., merc.
talking - lyc.
ulnar side - dig., plb.
ulnar side, after writing - agar.
using, after - graph.
waking, on - alum., calc-p., form., manc., mez.
walking, while - rhod.
water, after emersion in - carb-v., sulph.
wetting, on - ***rhus-t.***
wetting, on, amel. - spig.
writing, on - agar., ***zinc.***

numbness, fingers - abrot., ***acon.,*** act-sp., agar., ail., alum., am-c., am-m., ***aml-n.,*** anac., ant-t., ***apis, ars., ars-i.,*** aster., atro., ***bar-c.,*** bar-m., bell., bry., bufo, **CALC.,** calc-i., ***carb-an.,*** carb-o., ***carb-s., carl., caust.,*** cham., ***cic., cimic., cimx.,*** coff., colch., ***con.,*** crot-h., cub., ***cupr.,*** **DIG.,** dios., euph., euphr., ***ferr.,*** ferr-ar., ***ferr-i.,*** ferr-p., fl-ac., gins., **GRAPH.,** ***hep.,*** hydrc., ***iod., kali-ar.,*** kali-c., ***kali-chl.,*** kali-n., ***kreos.,*** lach., lil-t., **LYC.,** mag-m., merc., merc-c., merc-i-f., morph., mosch., ***mur-ac.,*** nat-m., nat-p., nit-ac., nux-m., nux-v., ol-an., olnd., paeon., ***par.,*** ph-ac., **PHOS., PLAT.,** ***plb.,*** podo., ptel., puls., rhod., **RHUS-T.,** sarr., sars., **SEC.,** ***sep., sil.,*** spong., stann., staph., stram., stront-c., ***sulph.,*** ter., ***thuj.,*** verat., zinc.
air, cold - nit-ac.
carrying load on arm - carl.
chest affections - ***carb-an.***
chill, during - cedr., ***cimx.,*** ferr., ph-ac., **SEP.,** stann., thuj.
convulsion, between - ***sec.***
eating after - ***con.***
epileptic, during - cupr.
evening - sep., ter.
on lying down - mag-m.
extending upwards - ***ars.***
fever, during - thuj.
before an attack of intermittent - puls.
first - agar., apis, bar-c., calc., ***caust.,*** euphr., hura, kreos., lyc., nat-m., ***par.,*** phos., rhod., ***rhus-t.***
chill, during - ph-ac.
left hand - anac., nat-m., rhus-t., thuj.
morning - lyc., nat-m., ***rhus-t.***
side of - ph-ac.
tip of - graph., spong., thuj.
up radial side of arm - anac., carb-an., phos.
forenoon - fl-ac., sulph.
fourth - alum., anac., arg-n., ***aran.,*** calad., calc-s., coca, com., dig., dios., eupi., inul., lyc., med., nat-c., nat-m., op., ***plat.,*** sars., sulph., sumb., thuj.
afternoon - calc-s., nicc.

numbness, fingers
fourth, evening - sulph.
evening, bed, in - sulph.
left - dios., sumb., thuj.
morning - calc-s., lyc.
morning, on waking - lyc.
night - nat-c.
right - inul.
rising amel. - nat-c.
rubbing amel. - nat-c.
sitting, after - alum.
tip of - plb.
waking, on - coca, lyc.
writing, while - com.
grasping anything - acon., am-c., calc.
headache, during - podo.
joints - euphr.
morning - am-c., caust., cham., dios., ***ferr.,*** kreos., lyc., merc., phos., puls., rhus-t., ***sulph.***
morning, bed, in - puls.
rising, on - stram., zinc.
night - am-c., kali-n., ***mur-ac.,*** puls.
one sided - cact., ph-ac.
perspiration, during - nux-v.
playing piano, while - sulph.
right - hydrc., nat-p., sep.
second - calc., carb-o., dig., euphr., gamb., lyc., mur-ac., nat-m., phos., rat., rhus-t.
cool air - phos.
morning - lyc., nat-m., rhus-t.
night - mur-ac.
tip, left - thuj.
sitting, while - ***cham.***
third - alum., anac., ang., ***aran.,*** arg-n., calc., carb-o., com., dig., eupi., lyc., nat-m., nicc., op., phys., rat., sabad., sars., sulph., sumb., thuj.
afternoon - nicc.
evening, 7 p.m. - phys.
evening, in bed - sulph.
left - sumb., thuj.
morning - lyc.
morning, waking, on - lyc.
night - nat-c.
rising, amel. - nat-c.
right - rat.
writing - com.
tip, of - thuj.
tips of - ant-t., ***apis,*** arg-n., ars., cann-s., carb-an., carb-s., ***caust.,*** chel., graph., kali-c., kali-p., ***lach.,*** mag-m., mez., mur-ac., ph-ac., **PHOS.,** ***sec., spong.,*** stann., ***staph.,*** sumb., tab., tell., thuj.
chill, during - mur-ac., stann.
morning - kali-c., ***lach.***
rubbing amel. - mag-m.
stretching hands, on - tell.
wetting, after a - rhus-t.
whooping cough, during - ***spong.***
writing, after - carl.

numbness, palm - acon., bry., con., lob-s., op., phos., psor., stram., syph.
morning - psor.

numbness, thumbs - alum., calad., cann-i., ***caust.,*** euphr., hura, kali-c., nat-m., op., plat., plb., stront-c., stry., verb.
afternoon - alum.
ball of - gamb.
left - alum., calad., nat-m.
morning - kali-c., plat., nat-m.
painful - ***caust.***
proximal joint - cina.
right - ox-ac., plb.
tip of - cina, phos., zinc.

PAIN, hands - abrot., acon., ***act-sp.,*** aesc., agar., alumn., am-m., anac., anag., apis, ars., arum-d., bar-c., bell., benz-ac., bol., brom., ***calc.,*** carb-s., carb-v., caul., cham., cic., cist., clem., cocc., ***colch.,*** com., crot-c., crot-h., cupr., ***dig.,*** dios., ery-a., euphr., fago., ferr., ferr-ar., fl-ac., gels., gent-l., grat., ***guai.,*** gymn., ***hep.,*** hura, iodof., kali-bi., kalm., kreos., lach., led., lil-t., lith., lyc., ***merc-i-f.,*** merc-i-r., ***mez.,*** mosch., naja, nat-c., nat-s., phos., phys., phyt., plb., ptel., puls., ran-s., **RHUS-T.,** rhus-v., rumx., ruta., sabin., sang., sars., sol-n., ***staph.,*** stry., ***sulph.,*** tab., tarent., tell., ust., vesp.
afternoon - cist., rumx.
alternating with head symptoms - hell.
ball of - aur., cupr., nat-c.
writing, while - nat-c.
bed, in - iodof., merc-i-f.
bone, metacarpal - agar.
bones, between - anac.
jerking - anac., chin.
chill, during - nux-v.
closing hand, on - caul, dios., med., merc.
cold amel. - guai., lac-c., ***led., puls.***
epileptic fit, before (left) - ***calc-ar.***
evening - abrot., acon., cist., dios., led., nat-s., nit-ac., ph-ac., ptel.
extending to shoulder - fl-ac., ham., lat-m., vesp.
forenoon - dios., fago., hura
writing on a cold table, from - fago.
gouty - ***carb-s.,*** gins., lyc.
grasping anything - get., kali-c., ***nat-s.***
holding, anything - coff., guai., nat-c., phos., sep., sil.
jerking - chin., mez., nat-c., nat-n., puls.
joints of - **ANAC.,** bell., clem., coloc., con., kali-c., kalm., ***lac-c.,*** lach., nat-s., phos., phys., plb., ***puls.,*** thuj.
gouty - pin-s., plb.
waking, on - lach.
morning - calc., dios., kali-bi., lyc., nat-c., ph-ac., sang.
waking, on - agar.
motion, on - bapt., caps., form., gent-l., ***guai.,*** laur., meny., plb., puls., sep.
amel. - bar-c., com., dios.
night - am-c., dios., merc-i-f., phos., sel., sulph.
paralytic - ***act-sp.,*** agar., bar-c., cham., mez., nit-ac., sel., tab.

PAIN, hands
paroxysmal - ang., arg-n., calc., cina, coloc., euph., ***euphr.,*** ferr-m., lyc., mang., ***meny.,*** merc., ph-ac., plat., ruta., sec., sil., tab., verb.
playing piano - merc.
pulsating - am-m., carb-v., gels., rhus-t., sulph.
running agg. - agar.
touch, on - myric., nit-ac., ***sulph.***
ulnar side of - arum-d., nicc., rhus-t., sep.
jerking - arn.
night - nicc.
uncovering, during fever, from - ***nux-v.,*** stram.
waking, on - nit-ac.
wandering - ars-h., ***iris,*** tell.
warmth, external, agg. - bry., caust., ***guai.,*** lac-c., led., ***puls.***
washing, on - alum., iod., merc., sulph.
wet weather - ***rhus-t.***
writing, while - acon., agar., ant-c., ars-i., bar-c., cinnb., euph., fl-ac., kali-c., **MAG-P.,** meny., ***merc-i-f.,*** sabin., samb., ***sil.,*** sul-ac., thuj., valer., zinc.

pain, back of - am-c., arg-m., arg-n., arn., asar., bar-c., berb., carb-v., cycl., ferr., ham., hep., kali-bi., kali-c., merc., merc-i-f., nat-c., phys., tarent., verb., zing.
extending to shoulder - ham.
night - am-c., anac.

pain, fingers - ***acon.,*** agar., alum., alumn., am-c., ant-c., apis, ars., arund., bar-c., benz-ac., bol., bry., cact., ***calc.,*** calc-p., calc-s., ***carb-an.,*** **CAUL.,** caust., chin-s., cist., clem., ***colch.,*** crot-h., ***dios.,*** elat., grat., ***guai., hep.,*** hydr., iodof., iris, kali-bi., kali-c., kalm., lach., lact., laur., lil-t., lyc., mang., mez., mosch., ***nat-a.,*** nat-s., nicc., ***nit-ac.,*** nux-m., olnd., ox-ac., petr., ***phyt.,*** plat., ***plb.,*** raph., **RHOD.,** ***rhus-t., sars.,*** sep., spig., ***sil., stry.,*** sulph., tarent., tell., thuj., upa., urt-u., verat., vip.
between, evening - ***rhus-t.***
bones of - alum., apis, ars., crot-h., dios., mez., **SIL.,** verat.
grasping, when - verat.
chill, during - nux-v.
closed, when - nat-s., verat.
cold air - agar.
agg. - stram.
amel. - caust., ***lac-c.***
cramp-like - lil-t.
creeping - acon.
evening - lyc., sulph.
writing, while - calc-p.
exertion, on - bry.
extending, to elbow - nat-m., plat., ***plb.***
to shoulder - nux-m., ***plb.***
first - acon., ammc., cham., chel., chin., cocc., con., crot-h., ***fl-ac.,*** hura, hydr., ind., iris, jug-r., kali-n., kalm., lil-t., lyc., lyss., mag-m., mang., med., merc-i-f., nat-a., nat-p., pall., plan., **SIL.,** spig., thuj.
ball of - calc-p., kreos.
evening - kalm., mang.

pain, fingers
first phalanx - osm., plat.
forenoon - thuj.
joints of - acon., **ACT-SP.,** arg-n., berb., caul., ***coloc.,*** nat-m., nat-p., nat-s., phys., rhus-t., spong., verat-v., viol-o., zinc.
joints of, metacarpal - bry., calc., ham., jatr., mang., puls., rhus-t.
joints of, middle - berb., rhod., rhus-t.
nail - berb., con., kali-c., puls., ran-b., **SIL.**
paralytic - agar., ***caust.,*** crot-h., plan., sabad., spig., verb.
rheumatic - ***hydr.***
second phalanx - staph.
third phalanx - mosch.
tip of - berb., nat-m., teucr., zinc.
ulcerative - plat., **SIL.**
forenoon - thuj.
fourth - all-c., aloe, canth., chel., cinnb., coca, coloc., con., dios., gels., hyos., kalm., lith., naja, nat-p., phyt., rhod., rhus-t., stry., tarent.
afternoon - calc-p., chin-s.
frozen, as if - verat.
joints - aeth., aloe, ant-c., aur., arg-m., calc., colch., crot-h., kalm., lach., lyc., mur-ac., nat-p., rhod., sabad., teucr.
joints, last - aloe, hyper.
joints, metacarpal - calc., lach., teucr.
joints, middle - rhod.
joints, on bending fingers - mur-ac.
joints, rheumatic - hyper., ***lach.***
morning - nat-a., nux-m.
rheumatic - tell.
sitting, reading - com.
tip - ambr., carb-v., kali-c., myric., nat-a., nat-c., spig., zinc.
using fingers - tarent.
grasping amel. - lith.
jerking - ***am-c.,*** ars., ***chin.,*** meny., mez., ph-ac., ran-s., rheum, staph.
joints - **ANT-C.,** ars., arund., aur., benz-ac., bry., ***calc.,*** calc-p., carb-v., **CAUL., CAUST.,** cist., ***colch.,*** coloc., fl-ac., ***guai.,*** hydr-ac., iris, kali-bi., kali-n., lac-ac., led., lith., manc., mez., nat-s., onos., ox-ac., phos., polyg., pyrus, rhod., sep., sil., staph., still., sulph., ***tarent.,*** upa.
evening - ***calc.,*** staph.
extending upward - brom.
first - arund., iris, upa., verb.
first, dislocation, as of - alum., ruta.
first, evening - iris
first, pulsative - polyg.
first, rheumatic - arg-n., ferr., plan.
first, wandering - polyg.
gouty - ***calc., hep.,*** **LYC.,** ***sulph.***
jerking - anac., nat-m., rhus-t.
moved, when - ang., ars., sep.
paralytic - arg-m.
paroxysmal - anac., kali-n., mag-c.
pressure, on - iod., lyc., sil.
pulsative - polyg.

pain, fingers
joints, second - carb-an., jac., lil-t.
short, as if tendons were too - nux-v.
third - ang., sep.
third, motion, on - ang., sep.
waking, on - ***calc.***
wandering - coloc., polyg., psor., sulph.
menses after, amel. - ***caul.***
morning - crot-h., coloc., kali-c., merc-i-r.
move, on beginning to - ***rhus-t.***
rising, after - coloc.
moving, when - ***guai.,*** hep., kali-c., nit-ac., rhus-t.
moving, amel. - lith.
night - bor., kali-n., ***mag-s., merc.,*** puls., sulph.
paralytic - benz-ac., sil., verb.
paroxysmal - agar., ang., calc., ***euphr., meny.,*** mur-ac., olnd., ph-ac., plat., rat., ruta., sil., verb.
pressure amel. - lith.
pulsative - anag.
rheumatic - alumn., bapt., ***calc., caul.,*** clem., **COLCH.,** grat., nicc., ***phyt.,*** ust.
second - all-c., alum., bapt., carb-s., cinnb., crot-h., hura, iris, lact., lith., lyc., med., myric., nat-c., nat-p., nux-m., osm., ran-s., rhus-v., sil., sulph., verat., upa.
joints - carb-ac., iris, nat-a., nat-m., puls-n, stann., verat-v.
joints, last - ant-t., bell., crot-h., iris
joints, metacarpal - nat-m., puls.
joints, middle - carb-ac., stann., stict., verat.
joints, tip - lyc., merl., par., zinc.
motion, during - alum., verat.
stretching them apart - am-c.
syphilitic - ***nit-ac.***
tendons, flexor - aster.
third - all-c., ***arn.,*** colch., crot-h., ***gymn.,*** led., lil-t., naja, pip-m., thuj.
coldness, during - crot-h.
inner side - glon.
joints - ***calc.,*** merc-c., op., rhus-t., stann., tarent., thuj., verat-v.
joints, rheumatic - sang., thuj.
metacarpal - lyss., verat-v.
middle - rhus-t., stann.
middle, last - plan.
nail - nat-m.
phalanx, first - ***arn.***
phalanx, second - chel.
rheumatic - thuj.
tip - cham., nat-a.
tips of - berb., caust., cist., colch., hyper., merc-i-f., paeon., ***sars.,*** sec., stry., ***sil.,*** sulph.
evening - caust., merc-i-f.
extending to shoulder - gels.
morning - sulph.
playing piano - ***gels.***
squeezed, as if - bell.
tendons, extensors - sil.
ulcerative - graph., kali-c., **SIL.**

pain, fingers
ulcerative - am-m., berb., sars., **SIL.,** ***sulph.***
variola, in - ***thuj.***
vibrating - berb.
waking from sleep - sabad.
walking, after - croc.
wandering - ars-h., iris, nat-a.
warm water, putting hands in - ***caust.,*** ***phos.***
warmth amel. - agar., ***ars.,*** ***bry.,*** ***calc.,*** **HEP.,** lyc., rhus-t., stram.
writing - acon., bry., calc-p., cist., iris, mur-ac.

pain, palm - anac., asc-t., aur-m., berb., calc., crot-c., crot-h., ill., led., merc-i-f., mez., ***nat-a.,*** nat-s., phyt., ***rhus-t.,*** sabin., stry., tarent.
cutting bread - ***calc.***
evening - nat-s.
extending to fingers - sabin.
motion, on - anac.
pulsating - berb., merc-i-f.

pain, thumbs - agar., am-c., anag., aster., bry., calc-p., calc-s., cham., chel., chin., chin-s., cinnb., coc-c., con., dios., dulc., ferr., jac-c., kali-bi., **KREOS.,** laur., led., mag-m., mang-m., merc., merc-i-f., nat-c., pall., phos., rumx., sang., ***spong.,*** stry., tarent., vip.
abduction, on - con.
afternoon - calc-s., sulph.
ball of - arn., bry., calc-p., lach., ox-ac., sang., ***spong.,*** xan.
evening - chin-s.
extending to, back of head and neck - plb.
extending to, forearm - spong.
bones - mez.
evening - dios., stry., tarent., thuj.
extending, to elbow - calc-s.
extending, to shoulder - aster.
joints - ambr., asaf., berb., dios., erig., kali-c., kali-i., kali-n., mang-m., nat-m., osm., petr., sul-ac., ***sulph.,*** verat.
extending to shoulder - aster.
gouty - carb-v., lyc.
motion, on - kali-n.
pulsating - caust., nat-m.
rheumatic - ambr., caul., ***graph.***
splinter, as from - colch.
ulcerative - kali-c.
left - anag., **KREOS.,** merc-i-f.
lifting, on - ruta.
morning, rising, after - mag-m.
motion, on - cham., coc-c., ferr., kali-bi., phos.
amel. - jac.
paralytic - acon., ***caust.,*** laur., mez., prun., rhod.
paroxysmal - agar., prun.
pressure amel. - tarent.
pulsating - fl-ac., merc-i-f.
right - ol-an., ***spong.***
tip - carb-v., lyc., nat-m., sulph., zinc.
pulsating - bor.
twitching - acon.
writing, while - thuj.

PANARITIUM, (See Nails, general, felon) - ***all-c.,*** alum., **AM-C.,** ***am-m.,*** ***anac.,*** **ANTHR., APIS,** arn., asaf., bar-c., ***benz-ac.,*** berb., bov., ***bufo,*** ***calc.,*** ***caust.,*** chin., ***cist.,*** con., cur., **DIOS.,** eug., ferr., **FL-AC.,** gins., **HEP.,** ***hyper.,*** ***iod.,*** ***iris,*** kali-c., kalm., ***lach.,*** led., ***lyc.,*** ***merc.,*** ***nat-c.,*** ***nat-h.,*** ***nat-m.,*** ***nat-s.,*** **NIT-AC.,** par., petr., ***phyt.,*** plb., puls., ***rhus-t.,*** ***sang.,*** ***sep.,*** **SIL.,** ***sulph.,*** **TARENT-C.,** teucr.
burning - **ANTHR.**
deep-seated - bry., hep., lyc., rhus-t.

PARALYSIS, hands - act-sp., agar., ambr., ***apis,*** ars., bar-c., bar-m., calc., calc-caust., calc-p., cann-s., carb-o., **CAUST.,** ***cocc.,*** colch., cupr., ferr., ***gels.,*** hydr-ac., kali-c., lach., laur., merc., nat-m., nux-v., phos., ***plb.,*** ***rhus-t.,*** ruta., ***sil.,*** tab., ***zinc.***
left - bar-c., calc-p.
palm - plb.
right - **CAUST.,** elaps, **PLB.**

paralysis, fingers - ***calc.,*** calc-p., ***caust.,*** ***cocc.,*** ***mez.,*** ***phos.,*** ***plb.***
extensors - ***ars.,*** ***caust.,*** ***cocc.,*** ***lach.,*** **PLB.**
first - mag-c.
cramps, with - carb-s.
partially - mag-c.
flexors - ***mez.***
fourth - plb.
sensation of - hell., lact., nat-m.
sensation of, rest, amel. - hell.

paralysis, thumbs - kali-c., mag-c.
evening - mag-c.
knitting - kali-c.

PARALYSIS, sensation of, hands - acon., ambr., am-m., bism., ***carb-an.,*** **CAUST.,** chel., ***chin.,*** elaps, ***kalm.,*** kali-n., lob., meny., nat-s., nit-ac., nux-v., phos., pip-m., prun., sil., staph., stront-c., sulph., ***tab.***
knitting, while - am-m.
morning, after, rising - phos.
after, rising, 3 a.m. - plb.
motion amel. - acon.
piano playing - carb-an., cur., plb., rhus-t., zinc.
pressure, on - nit-ac.
rubbing amel. - chel.
sleep, during - plat.
writing, while - acon., agar., ***caust.,*** chel., ***cocc.***

paralysis, fingers, sensation of - acon., ars., asar., aur., bry., ***carb-v.,*** ***chin.,*** cycl., dig., euon., gran., kreos., lact., lil-t., meny., ***mez.,*** phos., plb., staph.
extending over whole side - both.
grasping, when - carb-v., ***mez.***
joints - ***aur.,*** calc-p., par., ptel., verb.
third - plb.
sensation of - nat-m.

paralysis, thumbs, sensation of, - lachn., merc-i-f.
on extending and grasping - sulph.
right - lachn.

PEMPHIGUS, fingers - lyc.

pemphigus, thumbs - lyc.

PERSPIRATION - acon., **AGN.,** ambr., aml-n., anac., ***ant-t.,*** **ARS.,** ars-i., bar-c., bell., brom., **CALC.,** ***calc-s.,*** camph., canth., caps., carb-o., carb-s., carb-v., ***caust.,*** cham., chel., ***cina, cit-v.,*** cocc., coff., ***con., coloc.,*** cupr., dig., dirc., dulc., ***fago., fl-ac.,*** glon., graph., guare., hell., ***hep.,*** hura, ***ign.,*** iod., ***ip., kali-bi.,*** kreos., lac-ac., laur., ***led.,*** lith., ***lyc., merc., merc-c.,*** nat-a., nat-c., ***nat-m.,*** nat-p., **NIT-AC.,** ***nux-v.,*** oena., ol-an., op., ox-ac., ***petr.,*** phel., ph-ac., **PHOS.,** phys., pic-ac., puls., pyrus, rhod., ***rhus-t.,*** sars., **SEP., SIL.,** spig., stict., **SULPH.,** tab., **THUJ.,** verat., ***zinc.***

afternoon - bar-c.
air, open - agn.
alternately in one or the other - cocc.
between the fingers - sulph.
chill, during - eup-per., ***ip., puls.***
clammy - anac., ***ars.,*** carb-ac., ind., merc., nux-v., **PHOS.,** pic-ac., plan., pyrog., spig., sulph., zinc.
cold - acon., ant-c., ant-t., ***ars.,*** ars-i., ambr., ***atro.,*** bell., ***brom., calc-s.,*** **CANTH.,** caps., carb-ac., cham., ***cimic., cina,*** cocc., ***hep.,*** iod., ***ip., kali-bi.,*** kali-cy., ***lach., lil-t., lyc.,*** merc-c., morph., **NIT-AC.,** nux-v., ***ox-ac., ph-ac., phos.,*** phyt., pic-ac., plb., ***psor.,*** rheum, ***rhus-t.,*** sanic., sars., ***sec.,*** **SEP.,** ***spig., sulph., tab., thuj.,*** **TUB.,** ***verat., verat-v.,*** zinc.
nose, with - ***nux-v.***
warm room, in - ambr.
coldness, during internal - tab.
copious - ***ip., nit-ac.,*** **SIL.**
coughing, on - ant-t.
daytime - nit-ac., ol-an., pic-ac.
dysmenorrhea - tarent.
evening - ign., glon., sulph.
before lying down - sulph.
exhausting - nat-c.
forenoon - fago.
noon until evening, daily - lac-ac.
heat, with - nit-ac.
injuries of the spine - **NIT-AC.**
itching, with - sulph.
migrain, in - ***calc.***
morning - lyc., phos., puls., sulph.
bed, in - phos.
rising, after - puls.
night - coloc.
offensive - calc-s., coloc., hep., nit-ac.
only, on - agn., verat.
ophthalmia - brom., cadm-s., ***calc., con., dulc.,*** **FL-AC.,** gymn., ind., ***iod., led., petr.,*** **SULPH.**
prolapsus uteri - ***lil-t.***
rising, on - am-m., fago.
sitting, while - calc.
sleep, on going to - ars.
stool, after - ***sulph.***
sulphur, odor of - sulph.
urine, odor of - coloc.
walking in open air - agn.
writing, while - coff.

perspiration, back of - lil-t., lith.
cold - lil-t.
exercising, while - thuj.

perspiration, fingers - agn., ant-c., bar-c., carb-v., ign., rhod., sulph.
between - sulph.
tips - carb-an., carb-v., sep.

perspiration, palm - ***acon.,*** agar., ***all-c.,*** all-s., aml-n., am-m., anac., ant-t., bar-c., brom., bry., cadm-s., ***calc.,*** calc-p., camph., cann-i., caps., carb-v., caust., ***cham.,*** chel., coff., ***con.,*** dig., **DULC.,** fago., ***fl-ac.,*** glon., gymn., hell., hep., hyos., **IGN.,** ind., ***iod.,*** jatr., ***kali-c.,*** kali-s., kreos., laur., ***led.,*** lil-t., lob., lyc., manc., ***merc.,*** naja, nat-m., nit-ac., **NUX-V.,** petr., ***phos., psor.,*** rheum, rhus-t., **SEP., SIL.,** spig., **SULPH.,** tab., tarent., ***tub.***
afternoon - bar-c.
clammy - anac., coff., spig.
cold - ***acon., cham.,*** coff., nux-v., rheum, spig.
coldness, during - gran.
back of hand, with - hell.
on back, during - all-c.
daytime - dulc.
evening - tab.
exertion, on - ***calc., psor.***
morning - am-m.
night - ***psor.***
midnight, after - merc.
pressed together, when - rheum
room, in - caust.
soup, after - phos.
walking in open air - nux-v., rhus-t.

PINCHING, pain - bar-c., euphr., ol-an.
back of - euphr., ol-an.

pinching, fingers - am-c., caust., colch., euphr., stront.
evening - colch.

pinching, palm - mang.

pinching, thumbs - bry., kali-i., mang.

PRESSING, pain - anac., ang., arg-m., arg-n., arn., asaf., aur., bell., bry., carb-v., clem., coloc., cupr., cycl., dulc., fl-ac., hell., hep., kali-c., ***lach., led.,*** lil-t., ***mang., merc., mez.,*** mur-ac., nat-m., nat-s., olnd., ph-ac., ***plat.,*** plb., puls., rhod., ruta., sars., sil., stann., staph., thuj., verb., zinc.
asunder - ***led.***
ball of - cupr., zinc.
bones - arg-m., aur., sars., staph.
closing hand - merc.
inward - lach.
joints of - ang., asaf., coloc., hell., kali-c.
motion amel. - kali-c.
waking, on - asaf.
motion, agg. - led., staph., verb.
outward - lil-t.
palm - asaf., olnd., plb.
touch, agg. - cupr., staph.
ulnar side of - led., nat-s., stann.
walking, while - nat-s.

pressing, back of - anac., ang., arg-m., arn., asaf., berb., carb-an., cycl., kali-c., staph., verb.
evening - ang.
rheumatic - ang.
pressing, fingers - ***agar.***, ***anac.***, ang., arg-m., asaf., bell., bry., coloc., con., cycl., dig., euph., euphr., hell., ***led.***, **LYC.**, merc., ***mez.***, mur-ac., ***nat-s.***, nux-v., olnd., ph-ac., phos., ***plat.***, rhod., ruta., sabin., ***sars.***, sep., stann., staph., sulph., tarax., verb., zinc.
as if bones were crushed - olnd.
between fingers - led., puls., thuj.
first - chel., nat-s., tarax., zinc.
joints - nat-s.
joints, distal - bell.
fourth - arg-n., aur., led., nat-s., ph-ac., ruta, tarax., thuj.
ball - staph., sulph.
bending, amel. - ph-ac.
joints - ruta.
moving, hand - spig.
rest, during - aur.
sitting, while - arg-n.
walking, while - nat-s.
tips - spig.
joints - arg-m., arn., asaf., coloc., con., hell., mez., nat-s., ***sars.***, spong., stann.
joints, metacarpal-phalangeal - ruta.
joints, motion, amel. - coloc.
middle - ruta.
motion, on - hyos.
nails, under - caust.
second - nat-s., tarax.
joints - nat-s., spong.
third, outer side - thuj.
pressing, thumbs - arg-m., hell., nat-s., phos., verb.
ball of - ang., euph., meny.
inner side - asaf.
joints - asaf., aur., graph., indg., ***led.***, mez., nat-s.
evening - nat-s.
morning - mez.
rest, during - aur.

PSORIASIS, diffusa - ***ars.***, ***calc.***, ***clem.***, ***graph.***, ***kali-bi.***, ***lyc.***, mez., **PETR.**, ***rhus-t.***, ***sulph.***
psoriasis, back, of, chronic - ***ars.***, aur., bar-c., **GRAPH.**, hep., ***lyc.***, ***maland.***, **PETR.**, ***phos.***, phyt., ***rhus-t.***, sars., ***sulph.***
syphilitic - aur., ***ars.***, phos., ***merc.***
psoriasis, fingers - lyc., teucr.
first - anag., teucr.
second - anag.
psoriasis, palm - aur., calc., ***clem.***, crot-h., graph., hep., kali-s., ***lyc.***, ***merc.***, ***mur-ac.***, ***nat-s.***, petr., **PHOS.**, ***psor.***, sars., ***sel.***, sil., ***sulph.***, sul-ac., x-ray.
syphilitic - ***ars.***, ***ars-i.***, aur., phos., ***merc.***, ***sel.***

PULSATION - am-m., bry., carb-v., cic., coc-c., fago., glon., phys., plb., rhus-t., sumb., thuj.
burning - phys.
dinner, after - plb.

PULSATION, general
forenoon - nicc.
heat, in - sumb.
morning - fago.
bed, in - thuj.
motion, amel. - am-m.
sticking - thuj.
stool, straining at - cic.
touching anything - glon.
writing amel. - nicc.
pulsation, back of - dros., nat-s.
motion amel. - nat-s.
pulsation, fingers - ***am-m.***, anan., apis, bar-c., bor., fago., ferr-ma., fl-ac., glon., hura, kali-bi., lith., plat., ***sulph.***, teucr., xan.
evening - fl-ac.
first - gymn., hura, mag-s., sulph., til.
tip of - hura, nat-m.
tip of, evening - nat-m.
fourth - hura, zinc.
tip of - nat-s., sep.
joints - bufo, ***hep.***
nails, around - con.
under - am-m., ***graph.***, sep.
second - bar-c., dios., hura, sabad.
third - crot-h., sol-t-ae.
tips of - aml-n., bell., crot-h., carb-v., gels., glon., phyt.
noon - gels.
pulsation, thumbs - bor., carb-v., ***hep.***, hura, nat-m., sars., stront-c., zinc.
eating, after - nat-m.
nail, under - **AM-M.**
night - sars.
sitting, while - nat-m.
tip of - bor., chin-s., ferr-ma., mag-c., zinc.

RASH - ***agar.***, bry., ***carb-v.***, cupr., dig., kali-ar., led., **LYC.**, phyt., rhus-t., stram., verat.
palm - form.
rash, fingers - hydr., sil.

RELAXATION - gels., nat-c.

RESTLESSNESS - acet-ac., ***alum.***, arg-n., ***ars.***, bell., calc., calc-ar., calc-s., camph., fago., fl-ac., glon., ***hyos.***, **KALI-BR.**, kali-c., lac-c., nat-m., phos., plb., rhus-t., stram., **TARENT.**
daytime - rhus-t.
delirium, during - stram., sulph.
night - arg-n., kali-c.
in bed - lac-c.
sleep, during - rhus-t.
sleep, during - acet-ac., ars., calc., rhus-t.

RHEUMATIC, pain, hands - act-sp., aesc., alumn., ammc., asc-t., bapt., bor., **CAUL.**, ***clem.***, **COLCH.**, com., ery-a., euphr., ***guai.***, ***lac-c.***, lach., lyc., med., ***merc-i-f.***, phyt., ptel., ***puls.***, **RHUS-T.**, sang., ***stry.***, ***viol-o.***, ust., zinc.
rheumatic, fingers, joints - ***act-sp.***, ***aesc.***, alumn., ***calc.***, **CAUL.**, ***colch.***, ***coloc.***, ferr., ***glon.***, ***gran.***, ***guai.***, ***kali-bi.***, lac-ac., lach., lith., ***manc.***, plan., ***podo.***, tell., teucr.
afternoon - chin-s.
goes to heart - nat-p.
rheumatic, thumbs - jac.

ROLLING, in - op., ph-ac.

ROUGHNESS, (see Chapped) - alum., bar-c., ***graph.,*** **HEP.,** kali-c., laur., med., nat-c., nit-ac., ***petr.,*** ph-ac., phos., ***rhus-t.,*** rhus-v., sabad., ***sulph.,*** sul-ac., ***zinc.***
back of - ***nat-c.***
cold weather - ***zinc.***
dead skin - mez.
evening - sulph.
palm - tab.
spots - zinc.
roughness, fingers - ph-ac., zinc.
tips - **PETR.**

SCARS, cicatrices, deep, stinging on - kali-bi.

SEBACEOUS cysts, on - ph-ac., plb., **SIL.**

SENSITIVE, back of - con.
sensitive, palm - merc-c., nat-c.
sensitive, fingers - ***lac-c.,*** lach., ***led., sec.***
cold, to - agar., sec.
skin at nails - ant-c.
tips - cist.
separated, must keep fingers - lac-c., lach.
tips - nat-c., ***staph.***

SHAKING - atro., cann-i., kali-c., lyc., **PLB.**

SHARP, pain - acon., aesc., ambr., am-c., am-m., anac., ang., apis, arn., ars., arund-d., asaf., bapt., bar-c., ***bell.,*** berb., bov., bry., cahin., calc-s., camph., caps., carb-ac., ***carb-an.,*** carb-s., carb-v., ***caust.,*** cham., chel., chin., ***cina, coloc.,*** con., cycl., dios., euphr., ferr., form., gins., glon., graph., guai., hell., hyper., ign., ***kali-c., kalm.,*** lac-ac., lach., led., lil-t., lyc., mag-c., ***mag-m.,*** mag-s., manc., mez., mosch., mur-ac., nat-m., ***nat-s.,*** nit-ac., nux-v., ol-an., par., petr., ph-ac., phos., pic-ac., plat., puls., ***plb., ran-b., rhus-t.,*** sabad., samb., ***sars.,*** seneg., sep., sil., ***spong.,*** stann., staph., ***sulph.,*** tab., thuj., ***verb.,*** vip., ***zinc.***
acute - merc-i-f.
ball of - anac., carb-an., cham., cupr., kali-n., mag-m., mang., ran-s., sil., sulph., zinc.
evening, in bed - mag-m.
bones - ars., chel., chin., mang., ph-ac., sars.
breath, with each - am-c.
burning - gamb., plat., rhod., sulph.
cold water amel. - apis
evening - lac-ac., mag-m., rhod.
bed in - mag-m., plat.
extending to, elbow - ang., ***caust.***
to, fingers - cina, euphr., gels., petr.
to, upper arm - canth.
fine - arn., arund., clem., led., nat-m.
forenoon - thuj.
hollow of - acon., cann-s.
pulsating - acon.
itching - nat-m.
joints - bry., sars., ***sep., spig.,*** squil.
morning, in bed - petr.
on waking - thuj.
motion, on - am-m., vip.
amel. - acon., ***rhus-t.***
of arms - caust.
night 10 p.m. - cham.
pricking - plat.

SHARP, pain
radial side of - cham., phos.
shifting - euphr.
to larynx and back to hand - euphr.
shocks in heart, during - glon.
splinters, as of, on touching hair on hand - ign.
stinging - aesc., ambr., led., merc., squil., sulph.
subcutaneous - par.
tearing - bell., chel., zinc.
touched, when - lyc.
twitching - caust., ***cina,*** lyc., mez.
ulnar side of - anac., berb., carb-an., merc-i-f., mill., stann., tarent.
walking in open air - am-m.
wandering - con., plat.
washing - clem.
after - aesc.
water, from - clem.
writing, while - ***coloc.***
sharp, back of - anac., berb., caust., ferr., lyc., sulph., zinc.
sharp, fingers - aesc., agar., agn., ambr., am-c., ***am-m., anac., apis,*** arn., ars., arund., bapt., bar-c., berb., bov., brom., bry., ***calc.,*** cann-i., carb-an., carb-s., ***carb-v., caust.,*** **CIC.,** con., daph., ***dig.,*** dios., dros., elaps, fl-ac., graph., hep., ind., jug-r., **KALI-C.,** kalm., lil-t., lyc., ***mag-m.,*** mag-s., mang., merc., ***mez.,*** mur-ac., ***nat-m.,*** nat-p., ***nat-s.,*** nit-ac., pall., par., petr., ph-ac., phos., phyt., plat., plb., ran-s., ***rhod., rhus-t.,*** sabad., sabin., ***sars.,*** sep., sil., spig., ***stann.,*** staph., sulph., ***sul-ac.,*** tab., tarent., tep., ***thuj.,*** trom., verb., viol-t., vip., xan., zinc.
afternoon - thuj.
back of - caust., nat-m., sabad.
between fingers - carb-s., cycl., puls.
first and second - ran-s.
index finger and thumb - aur., ol-an.
bones - ph-ac.
breath, with each - am-c.
burning - alum., caust., iod.
cold air, when in - am-c.
coldness, during - gins.
evening - alum., ang., thuj.
extending to elbows - caust.
extending to tips - berb., dros.
first - aeth., agar., ambr., bapt., berb., calc., camph., carb-v., cham., chel., croc., dig., hura, kali-c., kalm., lyss., lyc., meny., merc., nat-m., nat-p., par., phos., rhod., sabad., ***sil.,*** stann., staph., tarent., thuj., verb.
as from a thistle - aeth.
back of - grat., nat-m., par., rhus-t.
bending arm - carb-v.
between, first and thumb - verb.
evening, in bed - rhod.
evening, in bed, 5 p.m. - thuj.
evening, in bed, 8 p.m. - hura
extending finger agg. - kali-c.
extending outward - meny.
joints of - bov., calc., nat-m., nat-s.

sharp, fingers
first, joints of, evening - nat-m.
joints of, last - agn., cham., gamb., hura, lyc., petr., stann., sulph.
joints of, metacarpal - agar., bapt., bar-ac., berb., carb-ac., mag-c.
joints of, middle - arn., carb-v., indg., kali-c., nat-m., verb.
joints of, working - bov.
morning - lyc.
motion, on - verb.
nail - coc-c., kali-c., sep., thuj.
skin - berb., camph., carb-v., nat-m.
tip - carb-an., berb., kali-c., nat-c., nat-s., sulph., zinc.
tip, on touch - mur-ac.
tip, when grasping anything - ***rhus-t.***
forenoon - trom.
fourth - ars., asaf., berb., brom., cact., caps., carb-s., ***caust.,*** cham., kali-c., laur., led., merc-i-f., nat-c., nat-m., phyt., sang., sil., tarax., thuj., verb., zinc.
ball - berb., caps., sulph.
joints - aloe, bry., sars.
joints, metacarpal - aloe, anac., merc-i-f.
joints, middle - brom., bufo
distal phalanx - carb-v.
tip - am-m., arg-n., aur-m-n., bar-c., fl-ac., kali-c., merl., sul-ac.
frozen - lyc.
jerking - ***carb-s.***
joints - ***acon.,*** aloe, am-m., asaf., aur-m-n., bar-c., calc., camph., carb-s., ***carb-v.,*** cham., con., ferr-ma., ***hell.,*** hyper., indg., iod., mang., meny., mosch., nat-m., nit-ac., paeon., ph-ac., phyt., plat., sars., ***sep.,*** spig., stann., stict., ***sulph.,*** sul-ac., tep., thuj., trom., zinc.
first - aloe, calc., com., kali-bi., sul-ac.
middle - carb-v., con.
morning - dios., mez.
7 a.m. - dios.
motion amel. - am-m.
nails, around - lith., merc.
under - calc., caust., con., graph., nat-m., nat-s., puls., sil., sulph.
palmar surface of - **RHUS-T.**
paroxysmal - ust., verb.
rising from sitting - carb-v.
second - arn., calc., carb-an., caust., chel., cinnb., cupr., dios., euphr., gamb., kali-bi., kali-c., kali-n., lach., lyc., merc., nat-p., olnd., ox-ac., sil., sul-ac., sulph., sumb., thuj., verat.
afternoon, 5 p.m. - thuj.
evening - lyc.
joints, metacarpal - carb-v., mang.
joints, metacarpal, last - ant-t., arn., carb-v.
joints, metacarpal, middle - sep., thuj.
nail, under - kali-c., lyc.
proximal phalanx - ph-ac.
tip - arn., bell., cast., kali-c., lyc., mag-m., mez., stann., viol-o.
tip, 9 p.m. - cast.

sharp, fingers
splinter, as from - **ARN.,** ***bell.,*** carb-v., colch., hep., lach., **NIT-AC.,** petr., puls., ran-s., sil., sulph.
stinging - ambr., ***apis,*** arund., sil.
third - ant-c., arg-n., cann-s., carb-s., caust., crot-h., hura, kali-c., kali-n., nat-c., phyt., sil., thuj., trom., viol-t.
joints - mang., sil.
joints, 9 a.m. - sil.
motion amel. - viol-t.
nail, behind - sulph.
tips of - abrot., alum., ambr., am-c., **AM-M.,** arund., aur-m-n., bell., berb., buf-s., carb-an., chin., coc-c., con., elat., graph., hyos., ***lach.,*** led., lept., mag-m., merc., mez., mur-ac., nicc., osm., **PETR.,** puls., **RHUS-T.,** sec., spig., ***stann.,*** **SULPH.,** ***thuj.,*** vip.
chill, during - bell.
evening - ***am-m.***
extending up arm - fago.
frozen, as if they had been - spig.
grasping anything, when - **RHUS-T.**
hang down agg. - sulph.
night - ***sulph.***
rubbing, amel. - mag-m.
walking in open air - ***am-m.***
writing, while - bapt., ***bry.***

sharp, palm - apis, berb., bor., calad., carb-an., caust., clem., ***con.,*** eupi., gamb., hell., kali-a., lyc., mag-c., mang., mur-ac., nat-m., nat-s., nicc., nit-ac., par., ph-ac., phos., rhus-t., sel., seneg., sep., staph., **SULPH.,** thuj., verb., zinc.
acute - gamb.
cold water amel. - apis
crawling - ill.
drawing - ph-ac.
evening - bor., calad., lyc., thuj.
10 p.m. - sulph.
in bed - graph.
extending to, back of forearm - gamb.
to, elbow - eupi.
midnight - rhus-t.
morning, in bed - calc.
tearing - verb.
tingling - staph.

sharp, thumbs - agar., ambr., anac., ars., asaf., bapt., bell., berb., bry., carb-s., cham., colch., dulc., elat., graph., ***guai.,*** hura, lith., lob-s., lyc., lycps., mag-c., mang., meny., merc., nat-m., nat-s., pall., ran-b., rheum, sabad., sang., sars., sil., ***staph.,*** stram., sulph., tab., tarent., thuj., verb., ***zinc.***
afternoon - lyc.
alternating with stitches in great toe - sulph.
back of - ph-ac.
ball of - am-m., anac., berb., carb-an., carb-v., dig., gamb., graph., hura, lith., manc., ox-ac., petr., ph-ac., ***sil.,*** tarent., verat.
as if stung - hura
evening while writing - ox-ac.
burning - dig., staph., stram.
drawing - bry.

sharp, thumbs
evening in bed - graph.
extending to back of hand - asaf.
intermitting - berb.
itching - ***staph.***
jerking - ***carb-s.***
joints - clem., con., thuj.
first - agn., bry., cham., grat., ign., led., nat-m., sars., thuj., til.
metacarpal - verb.
second - am-m., bar-c., gran., ign., laur., nat-c., spong., thuj., zinc.
left - lith., ox-ac.
morning - ars.
bed, in - ars., stram.
motion amel. - anac.
nail, root of - fl-ac.
under - am-m., bapt., coc-c., ***graph.,*** kali-c., ***thuj., zinc.***
needle-like - zinc.
pressure agg. - dig.
pressure amel. - mag-c., tarent.
right - guai.
tingling, when writing - sabad.
tip - agar., ambr., am-m., bar-c., berb., calc-p., graph., mag-s., mez., nat-c., nat-m., nat-s., phyt., sabad., sep., staph., vip., ***zinc.***
dinner, after - mag-s.
evening, sitting, while - am-m.
evening, walking, while - merc-c.
taking hold of anything, agg. - mez.
waking, on - nat-m.
touch, amel. - anac.
twitching - nat-s.
writing, while - ox-ac., sabad.

SHOCKS - ***agar.,*** stann., sul-ac., valer., zinc.
shocks, fingers, if he touch anything - ***alum.***
shocks, thumbs, proximal joint - con.

SHOOTING, pain - acon., apis, calc-s., form., nicc-s., pic-ac., sulph.
ball of - sulph.
motion amel. - acon.
shooting, back of - berb., ferr.
shooting, fingers - agar., ind., nicc-s., phyt., tep., trom.
first - nat-p., stann., tarent.
joints - ***acon.,*** caust., phyt., tep., trom.
forenoon - trom.
nails, around - lith., merc.
under - caust.
second - cinnb., nat-p., sumb.
joints - sumb.
third - crot-h., trom.
tips - ***am-m.,*** bell., berb., elat., lept., ***sulph.***
chill, during - bell.
evening - ***am-m.***
night - ***sulph.***
shooting, palm - sulph.
night, 10 p.m. - sulph.
shooting, thumbs - arum-d., dulc., sang.
ball of - tarent.
tip of - phyt.

SHRIVELLED - abies-c., ang., ***ars.,*** bism., camph., hep., ***lach., lyc.,*** merc-c., ***ph-ac.,*** **PHOS., VERAT.**
skin of - aeth., mez.
shrivelled, back of - mur-ac.
shrivelled, fingers - ambr., ant-c., crot-t., cupr., merc., ph-ac., ***phos.,*** sec., ***verat.***
cholera, in - ***camph.,*** **VERAT.**
perspiration, during - ant-c., canth., **MERC.,** ph-ac., pyrog., **VERAT.**
tips of - ambr., sulph.
morning, on waking - ambr.

SHUDDERING - chel., kali-i., laur., nicc., ran-b.

SORE, pain - abrot., ***arn.,*** ars., bell., bism., calc-p., carb-v., crot-h., cupr-ar., dros., ferr., ***hep., kali-bi.,*** lil-t., mag-c., mez., nat-c., nat-m., nicc., olnd., ph-ac., phos., rhus-v., ***ruta.,*** sars., sil., sulph., vip.
extending into arm on moving it - hep.
to elbow - dros.
joints, of - alumn., ***arg-m.,*** asaf.
metacarpal I (bones) - iod.
metacarpal IV - verb.
morning, lying amel. - mag-c.
on waking - mag-c.
moving it - sil.
paralyzed, as if - ph-ac.
ulnar side - carb-an.
sore, back of - carb-v., graph., hep., hura, ***ruta.***
sore, fingers - alum., am-c., apis, brach., bry., camph., com., croc., **LED.,** mez., nat-m., nit-ac., petr., ruta., rhus-t., sec., sep., sulph.
between fingers - ***ars.,*** graph.
end phalanges - nat-m.
fourth - chin-s., verb.
fourth, joints - chin-s.
joints - alum., bry., caul., iod., lac-ac., lyc., nat-m., sep., sulph.
of, first - caust., crot-h., lac-ac.
of, first metacarpophalangeal - spig.
third - alum., sep.
left, morning - merc-i-r.
motion amel. - ruta.
nails - ***petr.***
under - caust., sulph.
periosteum - **LED.**
second - cann-s., dios., kali-c.
joints - agar., carb-an.
third - ruta.
middle joint - sulph.
tips - calc-p., nat-c., ***sars.***
sore, palm - am-m., ars., nat-c.
sore, thumbs - am-c., brach., coc-c., cupr., kreos., vip.
ball of - arn., hura, ran-b.
distal, joint - spong.
left - am-c., kreos.
cold, becoming - am-c.
root of - phos.
metacarpophalangeal joint - spig.
nail, under - mez.
tip - calc-p., vip.

SPRAINED, as if - acon., ambr., ***am-c.,*** anac., ***arn.,*** bar-c., bov., ***bry.,*** **CALC.,** ***carb-an.,*** carb-v., ***caust.,*** dios., hep., kali-n., kalm., nit-ac., phos., prun., puls., rhod., ***rhus-t., ruta.***, sabin., seneg., sil., sulph., thuj., verb., zinc.

sprained, back of - am-m., bar-c.

sprained, fingers, as if - aloe, graph., kali-n., nat-m., phos., puls., sulph.
first - alum., cham., spig., stann.
fourth - lyc., nux-m., phos.
joints, first - nat-m.
second - mag-c.
third - phos.

sprained, thumbs, as if - calc-p., cham., kali-n., **KREOS.,** lachn., nat-m., phos., prun., rhod.
grasping, while - phos.
joints - ang., calc-p., camph., con., cupr., graph., kali-n., nat-m., petr., phos., rhod., spig., sulph., verat.
carpometacarpal - verb.
left - ***kreos.***
motion, on - phos.
writing, while - prun.

STIFFNESS - ***agar.,*** alum., ***ars.,*** ars-m., arum-t., arund., asaf., aster., aur., aur-m., bell., bov., bry., ***calc., calc-s.,*** carb-ac., ***carb-an.,*** carb-s., cham., chin-a., cocc., ***coloc., cupr.,*** cur., dios., ***ferr.,*** ferr-ar., ham., hyos., kali-ar., kreos., lil-t., ***lyss.,*** merc., mosch., nit-ac., ***nux-v.,*** phos., plb., plat., ptel., sanic., sars., sep., sil., ***stict., stry.,*** thuj., vip., wye., zinc.
afternoon - calc-s.
chilliness - kali-chl.
cold, from - cham., phos.
covered, from being - sep.
cramp-like - plat., stann.
evening - calc-s.
forenoon - calc-s.
grasping - nit-ac.
holding anything - mosch.
morning, on waking - alum., ***ars., ferr., lach., led.,*** sanic.
paralytic - cham.
playing piano - ***zinc.***
rheumatic - ***agar., ars.,*** bell., chel., ***ferr., kali-c., lyc., merc.,*** nat-c., ph-ac., puls., **RHUS-T.,** ***ruta.,*** sabin., sanic., sep., staph., ***sulph.,*** thuj., viol-o.
waking, on - alum., lach., led.
walking amel. - alum.
work, at - merc.
writing, while - cocc.

stiffness, fingers - ***agar.,*** am-c., aml-n., ant-t., ***apis, ars.,*** ars-i., aur-m., ***bell.,*** berb., bov., bry., ***calc., calc-s.,*** camph., cann-i., ***carb-an., carb-s., caul., caust.,*** chin., chin-a., coloc., con., ***cupr.,*** dig., dios., ***dros.,*** dulc., eup-per., ***ferr.,*** ferr-ar., fl-ac., graph., ham., hell., hep., hydr-ac., iod., kali-n., **LED.,** lil-t., **LYC.,** lyss., ***manc., merc.,*** merc-i-f., nat-m., nat-s., olnd., ox-ac., ***petr.,*** plb., ptel., puls., **RHUS-T.,** rhus-v., sang., sec., ***sil.,*** sol-n., spong., stann., stry., sulph., verat., vinc.
chill, during - eup-per., ferr., ***rhus-t.***

stiffness, fingers
cutting with shears - con.
evening - petr.
exertion, after - **RHUS-T.,** ***stann.***
extending them, with - carb-s.
first - acon., am-m., arg-n., ***calc., kali-c.,*** sabad.
writing, while - ***kali-c.***
forenoon - fl-ac.
fourth - aloe, ***calc-s.,*** con., hell., mur-ac., ***sil.***
morning - calc-s.
night - mur-ac., sil.
rest amel. - hell.
gouty - **AGAR.,** ***carb-an., lyc.,*** petr., sulph.
grasping, anything, when - am-c., ***carb-an., dros.***
after - graph.
holding a book, while - lyc.
lying, while - hep.
morning - am-c., ***ars., calc.,*** calc-s., ***ferr., lach., led., rhus-t.,*** thuj.
painful - manc.
second - bor., calc-s., carb-an., dros., ***phos.,*** **SIL.**
last joint - bell.
spinal, affections - apis
stretching, out arm - dulc.
third - mur-ac., sulph., til.
evening - sulph.
night - mur-ac.
work, at - merc., lyc.
writing, while - aesc., cocc., stann.

stiffness, thumbs - aeth., ***calc-s.,*** cann-i., ferr., ***kali-c.,*** **KREOS.,** ***led.,*** puls., sabad.
afternoon - calc-s.
painful - ferr., kreos., sabad.
sewing, while - aeth.
writing, while - ***kali-c.***

STRETCHED, out - bell., dulc.
as if to grasp something - dulc., phos.

stretched, fingers, out, spasmodic - sec.

SUPPURATION, fingers - bor., mang.
nails, around - con., ph-ac.
under - form.
under, of first finger - calc., nat-s.
vaccination, after - **THUJ.**

SWELLING - acon., aesc., ***agar.,*** am-c., anac., ang., **APIS,** aran., arn., ***ars.,*** ars-i., arum-d., arum-t., arund., atro., ***aur.,*** bar-m., ***bell., bry., bufo, cact., calc.,*** carb-ac., carb-s., caust., cham., chel., chin., chin-a., chin-s., clem., ***cocc.,*** **COLCH.,** com., corn., crot-h., crot-t., cub., cupr., ***dig.,*** elaps, euphr., ***ferr.,*** ferr-ar., ferr-p., fl-ac., grat., guare., ***hep.,*** hyos., iod., kali-ar., kali-c., kali-p., lac-c., ***lach., lyc.,*** manc., ***merc.,*** mez., ***mosch.,*** mur-ac., naja, nat-c., nat-m., ***nit-ac.,*** nux-v., op., ***phel.,*** ph-ac., ***phos.,*** plan., plb., ***psor.,*** rhod., ***rhus-t., rhus-v.,*** ruta., ***samb.,*** sanic., ***sec.,*** sil., sol-n., spong., ***stann., stict.,*** stram., ***sulph.,*** sul-ac., tep., thuj., vesp., vip.
afternoon - ***nat-c.***
behind the thumb - am-m.
bones - ***aur.***
dark - ***bell.,*** **LACH.,** ***vip.***

SWELLING, general
daytime - nat-m.
eczema, with - psor.
edematous - **APIS,** ***aur., cact., calc-ar., canth.,*** chin-a., crot-h., ***lyc., phos.***
endocarditis - ***aur-m., cact.***
erysipelatous - **RHUS-T.,** ***rhus-v.***
evening - aloe, lyc., rhus-t., ***stann.,*** sulph.
extending to, elbow - crot-c., crot-h., ruta.
to, pectoral muscles - crot-h.
feeling, as if - ***aran., cocc.,*** mang.
gangrenous - **ARS., LACH., SEC.**
hard - graph.
hot - ***bell., bry.,*** chel., ***cist., rhus-t.***
inflammatory - aur., cupr.
intermittent, in - ***lyc.***
itching - sol-n., ***urt-u.***
left, with heart symptoms - ***cact.***
menses, during - ***graph., merc.***
morning - nat-m.
on waking - sanic.
motion, amel. - nat-c.
night - aran., ars., caust., dig., kali-n.
after waking - samb.
nodular swellings - ars., nat-m., nit-ac., sul-ac.
painful - ars., ***cur.,*** dig., **LACH.,** vesp.
pale - bell., lyc., nux-v.
phlegmonous - plb.
phthisis, in - ***stann.***
red - lyc.
reddish - graph.
right - ***dig.,*** hep., lyc., nat-m., phos.
room, when entering - aeth.
sensation of - aesc., aeth., aran., chel., chin-s., laur., mang., mez., ***op.,*** raph.
grasping anything, when - **CAUST.**
walking in open air, after - mang.
shining - bell., vip.
tendons - plb.
walking, in open air - mang.
washing - aesc.

swelling, back of - am-m., calc., chin., mez., mur-ac.
left hand - am-m., ***calc-ar.,*** chin.

swelling, fingers - act-sp., aeth., agar., alum., am-c., ammc., ant-c., ***apis, ars.,*** benz-ac., bor., ***bry.,*** bufo, calc-s., carb-an., carb-s., carb-v., ***cit-v.,*** cupr., ***dig.,*** euphr., ***graph.,*** hep., ***kali-bi., kali-n.,*** lach., ***lyc., mag-c., merc.,*** mur-ac., nat-c., nat-p., nat-s., ***nit-ac.,*** nux-v., olnd., ***phos., phyt.,*** plb., psor., ran-s., **RHUS-T.,** rhus-v., sec., sil., spong., ***sulph.,*** sumb., tab., tep., ***thuj.,*** verat-v., vip.
afternoon - calc-s.
bones of - ***carb-an.***
burning, with - olnd.
constipated, while - mag-c.
cramp, after - graph.
dissecting wound, from - **ARS.,** ***lach.***
eruptions, with - psor.
evening - stront-c., sulph.
first - chin-s., ***fl-ac.,*** lac-ac., ***lach., lyc.,*** mag-c., phos., staph., sulph., thuj.
forenoon - calc-s.

swelling, fingers
fourth - bry., hyos., ***mang.,*** rhus-t.
middle joint - sulph.
hanging down arm, when - am-c., phos.
hard - ars.
joints - ang., am-c., anag., apis, ***ars.,*** berb., ***bry.,*** bufo, ***calc., caul.,*** caust., ***cham.,*** chin., colch., euphr., ***hep.,*** hyos., iod., ***lac-ac., lyc.,*** med., ***merc., nit-ac., phyt.,*** rhod., ***rhus-t.,*** spong., sulph.
burning and pulsating - bufo
first joint - merc., vinc.
gouty - anag., ***kali-i.,*** **LYC.,** ***sulph.***
hot - bry., ***hep.***
middle - lyc.
left, in heart disease - lycps.
midnight - carb-an.
morning - ***ars.,*** calc-s., nat-c., nit-ac., ran-s., sec., sulph.
night - carb-an., dig.
nodular swellings - anac., ***lyc.,*** mag-c.
red - mag-c.
second - apis, bor., calc-s., iris, mag-c., phos., sulph., syph., thuj.
5 p.m. - thuj.
afternoon - calc-s.
joints - lyc.
joints, distal - carb-v.
joints, middle - graph.
sensation, on grasping - bry.
third - bry., calc., olnd., sulph., thuj.
middle joint - sulph.
tips - fl-ac., kreos., mur-ac., ***rhus-t.,*** tab., ***thuj.***
walking, after - act-sp.

swelling, palm - cham., ***lyc.***
night - ars.
sensation of - ars.

swelling, thumbs - berb., coc-c., cupr., hep., naja, nux-v., rhus-t., sang., spig., sulph., vesp., vip.
containing pus - sulph.
joints, of - nux-v., phos., spig., sulph.
sensation of - berb., plb.

swelling, veins - alum., ***arn.,*** ars-h., bar-c., calc., cast., ***chel., chin., cic.,*** crot-t., cycl., ***fl-ac., ham., laur., led.,*** manc., meny., merc., ***nux-v.,*** olnd., ***op.,*** ph-ac., ***phos.,*** plan., plb., **PULS.,** rheum, rhod., ***rhus-t.,*** sars., staph., stront-c., sumb., sulph., thuj.
afternoon - alum., mez.
5 p.m. - chel.
eating, after - ruta.
hanging, down - phos.
forenoon - indg.
washing in cold water, after - am-c.

TEARING, pain - ***acon., agar.,*** alum., ***ambr.,*** am-c., am-m., ammc., anac., arg-m., arn., ars., ***aur.,*** bapt., bar-c., berb., ***bell., bism.,*** bor., brom., calc., ***calc-p.,*** canth., carb-an., carb-s., ***carb-v.,*** **CAUST.,** chel., ***chin.,*** chin-a., chin-s., ***cina, colch.,*** coll., ***coloc.,*** cupr., dig., dulc., euph., ***graph.,*** indg., kali-ar., kali-bi., **KALI-C.,** ***kali-n.,*** kali-p., kalm., kreos., lach., laur., led., ***lyc., mag-m.,*** mag-s., ***mang.,*** meny., merc., merl., ***mez.,*** mur-ac., nat-c., nat-m., **NAT-S.,** ***nit-ac., ol-an., petr.,*** ph-ac., ***phos.,*** plat., plb., puls., rheum, ***rhod., rat.,*** rhus-t., ruta., sars., sec., ***sel.,*** sep., ***sil., stann.,*** staph., stront-c., ***sulph.,*** tab., tep., teucr., thuj., verb., ***zinc.***

afternoon - kali-bi.
2 p.m. - laur.
alternating in each - caust.
ball of - anac., kali-n., mag-m., mang., sil.
evening, bed in - mag-m.
bed, only while in - ***lyc.***
bones - arg-m., ars., aur., bism., caust., chel., chin., cupr., dig., graph., kali-c., nat-c., phos., ph-ac., stann., zinc.
bones, metacarpal, first finger - iod.
burning - merl.
evening - ***alum.,*** brom., graph., kali-n., led., lyc., nat-c., rhod., ***sel.,*** thuj.
bed, in - mag-m.
extending, into back - caust.
to fingers - kali-c., lyc.
to shoulder - lat-m.
to upper arm - ***ars.,*** lach., lat-m.
extensor tendons - merl.
feather covering, under - lyc.
forenoon - thuj.
hang down, letting arm, amel. - arn.
jerking - chin.
joints - cadm-s., ***coloc.,*** indg., lach., spig., sulph.
evening - sulph.
motion, on - sulph.
night - ***phos.***
pulsating - spig.
left - nit-ac., ph-ac., phos.
lying on left side - ***phos.***
morning - ars., carb-v.
night - lyc., merc., ***sel.***
bed, in - phos.
noon - thuj.
paroxysmal - rhod., thuj.
pressive - stann.
pressure, agg. - chel.
radial side of - canth., caust., kali-bi., ol-an., sulph.
as if flesh would be torn from bone - ol-an.
as if in bone - caust.
rheumatic - ammc., chel., ***graph.,*** puls.
riding in a carriage - zinc.
right - canth., rat.
rubbing amel. - kali-n., laur.
sitting, while - nat-s.
sticking - zinc.
touch, agg. - ***chin.,*** nit-ac.
twitching - cupr., rat., stann.

TEARING, pain
ulnar side - arn., berb., bism., cast., lyc., mur-ac., nat-m., nicc., rhod., sep.
extending to, elbow - sep.
extending to, little finger - rhod.
extending to, wrist - lyc.
motion, amel. - nicc.
paroxysmal - rhod.
writing, while - nicc.
uncovering - lyc.
undulating, amel. - mez.
wandering - berb., stann.

tearing, back of - anac., caust., chel., kali-c., kali-n., mez., sulph., verb., zinc.

tearing, fingers - ***acon., agar.,*** agn., alum., ***ambr.,*** am-c., ***am-m.,*** anac., apis, ***arg-m.,*** arn., ***ars.,*** ars-i., asaf., ***aur.,*** bar-c., ***bell.,*** berb., bism., brom., bry., cact., calc., calc-p., carb-an., ***carb-s.,*** **CARB-V., CAUST.,** chel., ***chin., chin-a.,*** clem., coff., ***colch., coloc.,*** crot-t., cupr., daph., ***dig.,*** dios., gran., graph., guai., hell., ign., iod., kali-ar., kali-bi., ***kali-c., kali-n.,*** kali-p., kreos., ***led., lyc., mag-c.,*** mag-m., ***mag-s.,*** manc., ***mang.,*** meny., ***merc.,*** merc-c., ***mez.,*** mur-ac., nat-c., nat-m., nat-p., ***nat-s.,*** nicc., ol-an., olnd., ***ph-ac.,*** **PHOS.,** plb., psor., puls., rhod., ***rhus-t.,*** ruta., sabad., samb., sabin., ***sars.,*** sep., ***sil., stann., staph., stront-c.,*** **SULPH.,** sul-ac., tep., teucr., thuj., verb., ***zinc.***
back of - berb., carb-an., hell., nat-c., sars., zinc.
between fingers - alum., cycl.
index finger and thumb - agar., ***kali-c.,*** lyc., ran-b., rat.
index finger and thumb, while writing - ***ran-b.***
second and third fingers - phel., nat-s.
third and fourth fingers - aeth.
wrist and knuckle of thumb - lyc.
bones - ph-ac.
cold, amel. - led., puls.
washing - ol-an.
evening - brom., carb-v., lyc., stront-c., zinc.
6 p.m. - lyc.
8 p.m. when spinning - am-m.
bed, in - lyc.
moving them, when - sulph.
sleep, before going to - sulph.
extending to, arm - alum., merc.
to, chest, elbow, shoulder and wrist - vip.
to, wrist - mag-c., vip.
extensor, tendons - hep., puls.
first - agar., ambr., am-m., bell., ***bism.,*** calc., caust., chel., dig., gamb., iod., kali-bi., kali-c., kali-i., kali-n., lyc., mang., nat-c., nat-m., nicc., par., ran-b., rhod., sabad., sep., til.
afternoon, while spinning - nat-s.
back of - grat.
evening - agar., mag-c.
evening, bed, in - mez.
extending it - am-m.
extending to elbow - kalm.

tearing, fingers
first, extending to forearm - nat-m.
joints of - ambr., **BELL.,** berb., calc., carb-v., caust., kali-c., nat-m., nux-v.
joints of, afternoon - lyc.
joints of, afternoon, in rough weather - rhod.
joints of, evening - agar., am-m.
joints of, last - am-m., ambr., bell., nux-v.
joints of, metacarpal - berb., calc., carb-v., chel., lyc., mag-m., merc-c., spig., stann.
joints of, metacarpal, motion amel. - stann.
joints of, metacarpal, pressure amel. - mag-m.
joints of, middle - agar., **BELL.,** calc., carb-v., kali-c., nat-m.
joints of, paralytic - bell., chel.
nail - am-m., colch., con., kali-c., sep.
nail, afternoon - am-m.
nail, under, cold water agg. - sul-ac..
night - kali-n.
outer side - merc.
paralytic - dig.
side - berb., plb.
side, inner - mez.
splinter, as from - agar.
tendons - nat-m.
tip - kali-c., nat-m., zinc.
twitching - dig., mag-m.
writing, while - ran-b.
forenoon - ars., sulph.
fourth - agar., am-m., anac., arg-m., ars., bar-c., bell., bism., brom., canth., carb-v., chel., coc-c., colch., cycl., inul., kali-c., laur., mag-c., merc., mez., nat-c., nit-ac., phos., sulph., tab., thuj.
afternoon - canth., indg.
back of - mag-c.
ball of - mur-ac.
bones of - sars.
evening - ambr., arn.
forenoon - sulph.
jerking - agar.
joints - agar., arg-m., aur., calc., carb-v., kalm., lyc., nat-s., sabin., teucr.
joints, last - aeth., arg-m., aur., kalm., lyc., sabin., teucr.
joints, metacarpal - agar., ***benz-ac.,*** calc., lyc., sabin.
joints, middle - agar., calc., iod., mur-ac., sabin.
motion, agg. - carb-v., sars.
motion, amel. - kali-c.
night - nat-c.
night, rising amel. - nat-c.
paralytic - hell.
rheumatic - hell.
tip - ambr., anthr., arn., carb-v., kali-c., nat-c., spig., zinc.
jerking - chin., dig., zinc.

tearing, fingers
joints of - ***acon., agar.,*** agn., am-c., am-m., arg-m., asaf., **AUR.,** berb., bry., calc., carb-s., carb-v., cist., clem., colch., ***coloc.,*** dig., hell., kali-bi., kali-c., kali-n., lachn., led., **LYC.,** mag-c., merc., merc-c., ph-ac., phos., psor., puls., rheum, ***rhus-t.,*** sabin., samb., sars., **SIL.,** stann., stront-c., ***sulph.,*** teucr., thuj., zinc.
cramp-like - kali-n.
evening - lyc., stront.
extending, into wrist - mag-c.
extending, to shoulder - ***ars.***
first, distal - brom., kali-i.
first, evening - kali-i.
forenoon - ars., mag-c., sulph.
gouty nodes in - agn.
motion, on - ***led.***
night, bed, in - ***phos.***
paralytic - dig.
pressive - stann.
rising after - asaf.
second - carb-v., sabin., staph.
sleep, before going to - sulph.
third, proximal - agar., aur., bism., carb-v., lyc., mag-c., ***zinc.***
twitching - ph-ac.
lying on left side - ***phos.***
morning - hell., mez., nat-s.
motion, during - led., stann.
nails, under - ***bism.,*** calc-p., fl-ac., kali-c., kali-n., naja.
night, bed in - mag-s., phos., puls.
paralytic - dig., meny.
pressive - stann.
pulsating - spig.
right - ***bism.,*** chel.
second - agar., am-m., ang., aur-m., ***bism.,*** calc., calc-p., carb-v., caust., cycl., form., hell., iod., kali-i., kali-n., lyc., mag-m., mang., merc., nat-s., plb., sabad., ***sil.,*** sulph., til.
afternoon - nat-s.
afternoon, 3 p.m - caust.
afternoon, while spinning - nat-s.
dinner, after - aur-m.
evening - kali-i.
feather covering, under - lyc.
joints - agar., berb., brom., laur., lyc., mag-m., merl., par., sil.
joints, last - am-m., arg-m.
joints, metacarpal - berb., laur., lyc., merl.
joints, middle - berb., brom., hell., kali-c., mag-m., ruta, sil.
nail - ambr., teucr.
nail, under - lyc.
night - lyc.
outside - merl.
phalanx, first - ph-ac.
phalanx, second - nicc., ph-ac., ruta.
phalanx, last - mez., zinc.
phalanx, tendons - merl., sil.
phalanx, tendons, on bending - sil.
phalanx, tip - lyc., merl., zinc.

tearing, fingers
second, side, inner - mez.
twitching - mag-m.
uncovering amel. - lyc.
third - agar., aloe, ***bism.,*** brom., calc., camph., carb-v., cycl., kali-i., mag-m., merl., ol-an., sabad., ***sulph.,*** til.
evening - ambr., kali-i.
forenoon - sulph.
jerking - agar.
joints - calc., carb-v., merc-c., op., teucr., thuj.
joints, last - teucr.
joints, metacarpal - ***benz-ac.***
joints, middle - calc., op., thuj.
joints, middle to metacarpal joint - mur-ac.
nail, behind - sulph.
night - nat-c.
night, rising amel. - nat-c.
phalanx, first - arn.
phalanx, first, third - colch., zinc.
tip - arn.
tips of - ambr., **AM-M.,** arn., ***ars.,*** berb., ***bism.,*** calc., caust., chel., cupr., mag-c., mag-s., ***staph.,*** zinc.
evening - **AM-M.**
extending to shoulder - ***ars.***
morning, after rising - mag-c.
night - mag-s.
pressure agg. - chel.
touch - ***chin.***
twitching - am-m., staph.
writing, while - nat-s.

tearing, palm - bapt., bell., berb., calc., carb-v., caust., ill., inul., lyc., mang., spig., stront-c., sulph., thuj., zinc.
between index finger and thumb - zinc.
evening - stront.
extending to finger - sulph.
to forearm - stront.

tearing, thumbs - agar., ambr., am-c., am-m., anac., arg-m., arg-mur., astac., aur., berb., bov., brom., calc., carb-v., clem., hyper., indg., kali-bi., kali-c., kali-i., kali-n., laur., lyc., mag-c., mag-m., mang., nat-m., nat-s., nicc., par., phel., phos., plb., rat., rhod., sil., spig., ***staph.,*** sulph., sul-ac., zinc.
alternating sides - rat.
ball of - am-m., anac., berb., bism., dros., gamb., kali-c., lyc., merl., ph-ac., ran-b., ***sil.,*** staph., teucr.
motion amel. - staph.
between first finger and thumb - agar., rat.
bones - carb-v., chel., sul-ac.
burning - agar.
drawing - anac., clem., mag-m., zinc.
evening - hyper., mag-c.
extending, to chest - sul-ac.
to elbow - anac.
toward tip while sitting - nat-s.

tearing, thumbs
joints - am-c., am-m., aur., aur-m., aur-m-n., benz-ac., calc., cast., chel., chin., cupr., graph., iod., kali-bi., ***led., lyc.,*** merc., merc-c., nat-m., nat-s., **SIL.,** sulph., sul-ac., tell., thuj., zinc.
bending, impossible - lyc.
motion, amel. - led.
paralytic - chel.
paroxysmal - lyc.
second - bar-c., zinc.
writing, while - grat.
left - bov., kali-c., lyc.
margin - mang.
inner - kali-i.
outer - mang.
nail, under - bar-c., carb-v., fl-ac., kali-c., zinc.
extending upward - berb.
night in bed - sulph.
night - kali-n.
paroxysmal - nat-m.
phalanx, distal - aur.
proximal - sep.
sudden - ran-b.
tip - ambr., carb-v., lyc., phel., ***staph.,*** zinc.
burning - carb-v.
torn, out, as if would be - kali-i.
twitching - brom., rat., staph.
sul-ac.
writing, while - ran-b.

TENSION - alum., am-c., apis, arg-m., bell., canth., carb-v., caust., chin., clem., ferr-ma., hyper., kali-c., lach., laur., lyc., mang., meny., merc., nat-c., nat-p., plb., prun., psor., sep., stront-c., sulph., sul-ac., thuj., zinc.
bones, of - mang.
convulsive - lyc., ***zinc.***
evening - sulph.
hanging, arm down - sul-ac.
joints, of - mang.
stretching, on - laur.
amel. - nat-c.

tension, back, of - alum.

tension, fingers - aeth., alum., ambr., aml-n., apis, arg-m., benz-ac., carb-an., caust., coc-c., ***crot-h.,*** hep., hyos., iod., kali-c., lach., mag-c., mang., nat-m., nat-s., nit-ac., ph-ac., ***phos.,*** psor., ***puls.,*** rhod., sulph., thuj.
bending, when - caust., sep., thuj.
eruptions, with - psor.
evening - sulph.
first - nat-m., sep.
fourth - canth., hyper., phos.
joints - carb-an., ***caust.,*** croc., iod., kali-c., kali-n., mag-c., ***nat-m.,*** nit-ac., phos., puls., sep., spong., sulph.
left - phos.
motion, during - hep., ph-ac.
impeded - ***coloc.***
pressed, when - phos.
third - mang., phos.

tension, thumbs - ***coloc.,*** prun., sulph., thuj.
ball, of - cupr.

THRILLING, sensation - bapt., **CANN-I.**
thrilling, fingers, tips of - ail.

THROWS, hands about in sleep - nat-c.

TINGLING, prickling, asleep - acet-ac., **ACON.,** aesc., agar., ail., ***alum.,*** am-c., ***apis,*** arn., ars., arum-d., bapt., bar-c., bell., ***calc.,*** calc-p., ***carb-an., carb-s.,*** **COCC.,** colch., croc., crot-h., eupi., form., graph., hell., hyos., ***kali-c., kali-n.,*** lac-c., ***lach.,*** lil-t., ***lyc.,*** mag-c., meny., ***mez.,*** mur-ac., nat-c., nat-m., nat-s., ***nit-ac., nux-v., ph-ac., phos.,*** ptel., ***rhod.,*** rhus-t., ruta., sep., ***sel.,*** stram., stry., ust., ***verat.***
alternating with feet - carb-an., cocc.
grasping anything - cham., rhus-t.
lain on - ambr., am-c., ars., ***chin.,*** kali-c., petr.
left - cact., ***crot-h., lach.***
midnight - rhus-t.
morning - calc-p., form., kali-c., nit-ac., ***phos.***
motion, agg. - bapt.
amel. - am-c., carb-an., sep.
night - mag-m., sep., ***sil.***
painful - mag-m.
palm - apis, calad., cupr., ***rhus-t.,*** ruta., seneg., stry., sumb.
playing piano - sulph.
riding, while - form.
right - carb-an.
standing, while - agar.
waking, on - croc., ***phos.***
washing, after - aesc., ars.
writing, while - agar.
tingling, back of - apis, jatr., plat.
tingling, fingers - **ACON.,** ail., ***alum.,*** ambr., ***am-m.,*** apis, ***ars., bar-c.,*** bell., ***calc.,*** calc-s., ***carb-s.,*** con., croc., cupr-ar., ***dig.,*** form., ***glon.,*** kali-c., lac-c., lact., lil-t., lob., ***lyc.,*** mag-c., ***mag-m.,*** mag-s., merc., nat-c., **NAT-M.,** ol-an., ox-ac., paeon., ***par.,*** ph-ac., ptel., ***puls., ran-b.,*** rat., rhod., ***rhus-t., sec.,*** sep., **SIL.,** spig., stry., sulph., sul-ac., tab., ***thuj., verat.***
first - plat.
fourth - alum., carb-an.
sitting - alum.
joints - verat.
morning - dios.
waking, on - ail.
nail, under - cann-s., colch., ***nat-s.***
night, on waking - bar-c.
second - apis
sitting, while - alum.
third - alum., sil.
tips - acon., acon-c., acon-f., **AM-M.,** cact., cann-s., ***colch.,*** croc., fl-ac., ***hep.,*** **KALI-C.,** lach., nat-m., ***nat-s.,*** rhod., ***rhus-t., sec.,*** sep., sulph., ***thuj.***
grasping, when - ***rhus-t.***
hanging down the arm - sulph.
morning - ***kali-c.***
tingling, thumbs, prickling, asleep - alum., ambr., fl-ac.
tip of - ambr., am-m.

TOUCH, fingers, cannot bear, to have them touch each other - ***lac-c., lach.,*** sec.

TREMBLING - ***acon.,*** **AGAR.,** all-c., alum., alumn., am-c., ***aml-n., anac., ant-c.,*** **ANT-T.,** ***apis, arg-n.,*** arn., ***ars., ars-i.,*** atro., aur-m., bapt., bar-c., ***bell.,*** bism., bov., bry., cahin., **CALC., CALC-P.,** ***calc-s.,*** camph., cann-i., carb-ac., ***carb-an., carb-h., carb-s.,*** **CAUST.,** chel., ***chin.,*** chin-a., ***cic.,*** cimic., cist., coca, ***cocc., coff.,*** colch., ***cop., crot-c., crot-h.,*** crot-t., cupr., cycl., dios., dig., dulc., elaps, ***ferr., gels., glon.,*** guare., helo., hydr-ac., ***hyos., ign.,*** ind., ***iod.,*** kali-ar., kali-br., ***kali-c.,*** kali-i., kali-n., ***kali-p.,*** kali-s., ***lac-c.,*** lac-d., ***lach.,*** lact., laur., led., lil-t., lyc., lyss., mag-c., mag-m., ***mag-p.,*** mag-s., manc., med., **MERC.,** mez., morph., nat-a., nat-c., **NAT-M.,** nat-p., nat-s., nicc., **NIT-AC.,** ***nux-m.,*** **NUX-V.,** ***onos., op.,*** ox-ac., par., ph-ac., **PHOS.,** phys., ***phyt., plat.,*** **PLB.,** ***psor., puls.,*** rheum, rhod., rhus-t., sabad., samb., sars., sep., ***sil.,*** spig., spong., **STANN.,** ***stram.,*** stry., **SULPH.,** tab., ter., thea., ***thuj.,*** tub., valer., **ZINC.**
afternoon - ***calc.,*** lyc., lycps., mez., nat-c.
anger, after - sep.
anxiety, with - am-c., bov., cic., ***plat.,*** puls.
bright's disease - lycps.
chill, during - canth., chin.
contradiction, after - cop., ***nit-ac.***
convulsive - colch., ***hyos., plb.***
delirium tremens - ***coff., kali-br., lach.,*** **NUX-V.,** ***stram.***
dinner, during - grat., tab.
after - ant-c., mag-m.
eating, while - bism., **COCC.,** olnd., stram.
emotions, from - nat-m., plb.
evening - ***all-c.,*** caust., ferr., mez., plan., ***plb.***
bed, in - nat-m.
exercise after - ferr-ma., hyos.
fine work at - sulph.
forenoon - sars., sulph., valer.
fright, after - op., samb.
grasping amel. - stann.
hanging down, while - phos.
headache, with - calc-p., carb-v.
holding objects, on - ***agar.,*** bism., cann-s., con., **MERC., PLB.,** sabad., ***sil.,*** spig., ***staph.,*** stram.
hand free - cocc., **MERC.,** plat.
hand still - ***coff.***
taking hold of, on - cann-s., ***led.,*** lyss., **MERC.,** ***sil.,*** stram., verat.
them, out - caust., ***cocc., coff., gels.,*** ign., **MERC.,** ***merc-c., phos.,*** plat., **PLB.,** ***puls.,*** tab.
hunger, with - olnd.
intermittent - ***calc.***
left - calc., ***glon.,*** lac-c., puls., stann.
manual labor - plb., **MERC.,** ***sil.***
menses, during - agar., ***hyos., zinc.***
mental, exertion, on - bor.
worry agg. - plb.
morning - ars., aur-m., ***kali-c.,*** lyc., ***nat-c., nat-m.,*** phos., sulph.
breakfast, at - ***carb-an.***
rising, on - crot-t.
motion amel. - ***crot-h.,*** zinc.

TREMBLING, general
mouth, carrying something to, when - kali-br., **MERC., PLB.**
moving them, on - agar., ant-c., ***camph.,*** iod., ***kali-br., led., plb.,*** puls.
in typhoid - ***gels.***
news, after unpleasant - nat-m.
night - am-c., bufo, carb-v.
noon - cic., sulph.
pain, with - **CAUST.**
paralytic - ant-c., ***cocc.,*** **MERC., PLB.**
raising them high - **COCC., MERC.**
resting them on table, when - stann., ***zinc.***
right - all-c., anac., caust., mez., sep., sulph.
rising, after - nux-v.
rubbing amel. - ***nat-m.***
sitting, while - ***led.,*** sil.
sleeping, after - morph.
threading needle, while - ran-b., ***sil.***
tobacco, from - ***nux-v.***
typesetting from - plb.
typhoid, in - ***arg-n., zinc.***
using them, from - ***phos., sil.***
vertigo, after - ***zinc.***
from - gran.
vomiting, while - calc., calc-p., ***sulph.***
waking, on - ant-c., ***nat-s.***
walking, while - ***led.***
after - sulph., ust.
weakness - ***led.,*** **MERC.,** plb., ***stann.***
weather, cold, moist, in - ***dulc.***
writing, while - agar., ***all-c.,*** alum., ***ant-c.,*** bar-c., bism., camph., caps., ***carb-ac.,*** **CAUST.,** chel., ***chin., cimic., colch.,*** ferr., hep., hyos., ***ign.,*** kali-br., ***kali-c.,*** lycps., ***lyss.,*** **MERC.,** morph., ***nat-m., nat-p., nat-s.,*** olnd., ***phos., ph-ac.,*** **PLB.,** ***puls.,*** sabad., samb., ***sil.,*** stann., **SULPH.,** thuj., ***zinc.***
after - thuj.
trembling, fingers - ars., bry., cic., cupr-ar., ***glon.,*** hyper., iod., ***merc.,*** morph., nat-m., nit-ac., olnd., phos., plat., plb., rhus-t., sep., stront.
first - ***calc.***
convulsive - ***calc.***
motion, on - plb.
night - olnd.
second - stann.
writing, while - ***cimic.***
trembling, thumbs - ambr., plat.

TUBERCLES - ars., carb-an., hydrc., kali-chl., ***merc.,*** nit-ac., rhus-t., rhus-v., sep., spig., stram.
tubercles, fingers - berb., caust., ***con.,*** hydrc., ***lach., led.,*** lyc., nat-c., rhus-t., verat., zinc.
tubercle, thumbs - ***ars.,*** caust.

TUMORS, hands, metacarpal bones, between - ph-ac., tarent.
enchondroma, fingers - sil.

TWINGING, fingers - rhus-t.
back of - rhus-t.

TWITCHING - aloe, alumn., ant-t., ***asaf.,*** bar-m., ***bell.,*** brom., canth., caust., ***cina, cocc., coff.,*** colch., con., ***cupr.,*** dulc., ***graph.,*** **HYOS.,** ign., iod., kreos., ***lach.,*** lact., lyss., mag-s., manc., mang., meph., merc., mez., ***nat-c.,*** nat-m., nat-s., nit-ac., nux-m., ***nux-v.,*** oena., ***op.,*** ph-ac., phyt., ***plat.,*** plb., ran-b., rheum, rhod., sabad., sant., sec., sep., ***stann., stram.,*** stry., sulph., ***sul-ac.,*** thuj., valer., viol-t., zinc.
afternoon, sitting, while - lach.
between index finger and thumb - mag-s., stann.
chill, during - nux-m., nux-v.
convulsive - brom., colch., nux-v., phyt.
coughing, when - ***cina.***
daytime - sulph.
exertion agg. - ***merc.***
fright, after - op.
hollow of - caps.
lying, while - merc.
midnight, after - nat-c.
after, during sleep - nat-s.
before - nat-c.
morning - cupr., nat-c., rheum.
rising, after - cupr.
night - canth., con., nat-c., nat-s.
sleep, during - con., nat-s.
waking, on - stann.
paroxysmal - rhod.
rising, on - cupr., nat-m.
sitting, while - lach.
sleep, during - con., cupr., ign., nat-s., ph-ac., viol-t.
spasm, at beginning - sulph.
taking hold of anything - nat-c.
tremulous - sec.
ulnar side of - fago., ox-ac.
twitching, back of - nat-c.
twitching, fingers - ***acon., agar., alum.,*** am-c., ***anac.,*** ars., bism., bry., cadm-s., ***caust.,*** cham., chel., ***chin., cic., cimic., cina, cocc.,*** crot-t., **CUPR.,** dig., dulc., ign., iod., kali-bi., kali-br., kali-c., lach., lith., lyc., mag-c., mang., ***merc., nat-c.,*** nux-v., op., ***osm.,*** ox-ac., ph-ac., **PHOS.,** plat., plb., puls., rhod., rhus-t., sabad., spig., ***stann.,*** stront-c., sulph., ***sul-ac.,*** tab.
bones - mez.
cramp-like - anac.
daytime - phos.
evening - lyc., puls., sulph.
lying down, after - puls.
first - am-m., dig., lyc., mang., nat-s., pall., rhod., sil.
evening - am-m., mang.
sitting, while - pall.
fourth - chin., com., kali-bi., meny., nat-c., phos.
hand, palm - chel., sep.
joints - nat-c.
morning - pall.
rising, after - mag-c.
motion, during - bry.
night - mag-c., nat-c.
sleep, during - nat-c.
pulse, synchronous with - anac.

twitching, fingers
second - arn., chin., dulc., fl-ac., kali-n., nat-a., sil., stann., thuj.
sewing, when - kali-c.
sleep, during - anac., cupr., lyc., nat-c., puls., rheum, sulph.
third - chin., kali-n., mang., nat-c.
afternoon - mang.
tips - am-m., **ARS.,** merc., phos., staph., sul-ac., thuj.
toothache, with - mag-c.
writing, while - caust.

twitching, palm - caps., chel., sep.

twitching, thumbs - aeth., agar., alum., am-c., anag., apis, arg-m., ars., asaf., calc., fl-ac., hell., lach., mosch., nat-c., phos., plb., rhus-t., sul-ac.
afternoon - arg-m.
writing, while - arg-m.
between thumb and index finger - stann.
first, joint - zinc.
morning, bed in - ars.
paralytic - mosch.
visible - am-c.
writing while - arg-m., phos.

ULCERS - ***anan., ars.,*** caust., kali-bi., naja, psor., rhus-v., sep., sil., stront-c., sul-ac.
back of - dros., ***hydr.,*** psor., syph.
cracked - ***merc.***
palm - ***lyc.,*** pip-m., psor.

ulcers, fingers - alum., ***ars., bor., bov., bry., calc.,*** carb-an., carb-v., caust., cupr-ar., ***kali-bi.,*** kreos., lyc., mag-c., mang., nat-m., petr., plat., ***ran-b., sep.,*** sil., ***sulph.***
first - ***calc.,*** kali-bi., lyc.
nail of - iod., nat-s.
joints - ***bor.,*** mez., ***sep.***
itching - ***mez.***
painful - lyc.
second - aloe
tips - alum., ant-t., **ARS.,** carb-v., fl-ac., ***nat-c., petr.,*** plat., sars., ***sec., sep.***
burning - **ARS.,** ***sep.***
offensive - ***petr.***

ulcers, thumbs - caust., kali-bi., nat-c.
tip of - caust., kali-i.

UNSTEADINESS - bell., chlf., elaps, lyc.
writing, while - agar., hep., morph.

URTICARIA - apis, berb., bufo, ***carb-v., hep.,*** hyper., nat-c., ***nat-m.,*** nat-s., ***sars.,*** **SULPH.,** ***urt-u.***
morning - chin.
red, after rubbing - nat-m.
spots, in - ***apis.***
whitish - nat-m.

urticaria, back of - acon., apis, berb., cop., hyper., indg., ***sulph.,*** thuj.
when hands become cool - thuj.

urticaria, fingers - hep., thuj., urt-u.
cold, on becoming - thuj.

urticaria, palm - rhus-v., stram.

VESICLES - ***anag.,*** ant-c., aran., arn., ars., bor., bov., chin., **CARB-AC.,** carb-s., caust., clem., cocc., com., hell., hep., kali-ar., kali-bi., kali-c., kali-i., ***kali-s.,*** lac-ac., ***lach.,*** mag-c., mag-m., ***merc.,*** merl., mez., ***nat-m., nat-s., petr.,*** phos., plan., ***psor.,*** ptel., ***ran-b., rhus-t., rhus-v.,*** ruta., sanic., sars., sec., ***sel., sep.,*** spig., ***sil., squil., sulph.,*** ter., vip.
areola, red - bov., ruta.
black - ***sec.***
ball, of - ant-c., mez.
burning - ***canth.,*** rhus-v.
confluent - ruta.
corroding - clem., ***graph.,*** kali-c., mag-c., nit-ac., sil.
crops, in - ***anag.***
denuded spots, on - nat-m.
elevated base - kali-bi.
hard - lach.
healing, new vesicles appear after - ***anag.***
inflamed - ***rhus-t.***
itching - **CARB-AC.,** nat-m., sep.
patches - rhus-t.
phagedenic - graph., kali-c., ***mag-c., nit-ac.,*** sil.
spots, in - cic.
stinging - mag-c.
watery - anag., ***ars., nat-c., psor.,*** rhus-t., ruta.
white, with red areola - sanic., uran.
yellowish - rhus-v., ***sulph.***

vesicles, back of - anac., arg-n., brom., ***calc., canth.,*** cic., ***graph.,*** indg., kali-chl., ***kali-s., mez.,*** phos., pix., psor., puls., **RHUS-T.,** rhus-v., sol-n., **SULPH.,** zinc.
burning - mez.
cold, from taking - zinc.
discharging acid fluid - sol-n.
itching - cic., kali-chl., **MEZ.,** phos., sulph.
agg. - phos.
moist - mez.
red - psor.
spots, in - rhus-t.
watery - calc., rhus-v.
yellow - arg-n.
yellowish fluid, discharging acid fluid - sol-n.

vesicles, fingers - bell., bor., calc., ***cit-v., clem.,*** cupr., cupr-ar., cycl., fl-ac., ***graph.,*** hep., ***kali-c., kali-s.,*** lach., mag-c., mang., ***mez., nat-c., nat-m.,*** nat-s., ***nit-ac., ph-ac.,*** phos., ***plb., puls., ran-b., rhus-t.,*** rhus-v., ***sars., sel., sep., sil., sulph.***
becoming ulcers - calc., graph., kali-c., mag-c., nit-ac., ran-b., sil.
bluish - ***ran-b.***
burning - ran-b.
between - canth.
first - ***calc.,*** kali-c., mag-c., nat-c., sil., sulph.
cold, after washing - nat-c.
discharging water - kali-c.
phagedenic - ***calc.***
fourth - graph.
itching - ran-b.
tips of - ail., ***ars., cupr., nat-c.***
filled with blood - **ARS.**

vesicles, fingers, between - anag., ***apis, calc., canth., hell.,*** iod., laur., ***nat-m.,*** olnd., phos., **PSOR.,** ***puls.,*** rhus-t., rhus-v., ruta., ***sel.,*** **SULPH.**
burning - nit-ac.
index, and thumb - grat., ***nat-s.,*** **SULPH.**
itching, - ars., canth., mag-c., nit-ac., ***psor.,*** **SULPH.**between,
itching, after midnight - sul-ac.
second and third - ***sulph.*****vesicles,** palm - ***anthr.,*** bufo, canth., caust., ***kali-c.,*** mag-c., ***merc.,*** ran-b., rhus-t., rhus-v., ruta.
itching - caust., ***kali-c.,*** rhus-t.
large - anthr.
scratching after - mag-c.
third and fourth - mag-c.
transparent- merc.
yellow - anthr., bufo, rhus-t., rhus-v.
watery - bell.

vesicles, thumbs - ***hep., lach.,*** mang., mez., ***nat-c.,*** nat-s., nit-ac., ***ph-ac., sep.***
ball, of - ph-ac.
between, thumb, and index, desquamation - am-m.
dry - verat.
pimples - arn., bry., canth.

VIBRATION, sensation - berb., carb-s.

WARTS - anac., ***ant-c.,*** **BAR-C.,** berb., bov., bufo, **CALC., CAUST., DULC.,** ***ferr.,*** ferr-ma., ferr-pic., ***fl-ac.,*** kali-c., kali-chl., ***lach., lyc., nat-c., nat-m.,*** **NIT-AC.,** ***ph-ac.,*** phos., ***psor., rhus-t., sep.,*** sil., **SULPH., THUJ.**
flat - berb., **DULC.,** lach., ruta., ***sep.***
horny - ***ant-c., caust., sep., thuj.***
itching - ***sep.***
knuckles - pall.
large - dulc.
sensitive - nat-c.
sore - ambr., fl-ac., ruta.

warts, fingers - ambr., ***bar-c.,*** berb., ***calc.,*** carb-an., ***caust., dulc., ferr., fl-ac.,*** **LAC-C.,** lach., lyc., ***nat-m., nit-ac.,*** petr., psor., ran-b., ***rhus-t.,*** sang., sars., ***sep.,*** sulph., **THUJ.**
first - ***caust.,*** thuj.
horny - ***caust.***
joints - sars.
nails, close to - **CAUST.,** dulc., fl-ac., graph., lyc., sep.
second - berb., lach.
third - ***nat-s.***
tips - **CAUST.,** dulc., thuj.

warts, palm - ***anac.,*** berb., bor., ***dulc.,*** nat-c., ***nat-m.,*** ruta.
flat - dulc., nat-m., ruta.
painful on pressure - nat-m.

warts, thumbs - berb., lach., ran-b., ***thuj.***

WASHES, dry hot hands frequently - ***phos.***
always washing her hands - plat., psor., ***syph.***

WEAKNESS - acon., alumn., ang., arn., ars., bell., bism., ***bov.,*** bufo, canth., caps., carb-v., caust., cham., chin., chin-s., cimic., ***cina,*** colch., com., croc., cupr., cur., dios., ***fl-ac.,*** gels., glon., hell., hep., hipp., jug-r., ***kali-bi.,*** kali-c., ***kali-n.,*** kreos., lach., lyc., ***merc.,*** merc-i-f., **MEZ.,** nat-a., nat-c., nat-m., nat-p., ***nat-s., nit-ac.,*** nux-m., nux-v., phos., phys., plb., rhod., rhus-t., ***ruta.,*** sabin., sec., sep., sil., ***stann.,*** sulph., sumb., tab., verat., zinc.
afternoon - bov.
5 p.m. - cham.
after sleep - nux-v.
chill, during - laur.
cramp-like - caust.
dinner, after - mag-m.
eating, after - bar-c., nat-c.
evening - dios.
grasping objects, on - nat-m., ***nat-s.***
headache, during - ol-an.
laughing - carb-v.
lying, amel. - mag-c.
hard substance - nat-m.
on table, when - stann.
menses - alumn., ol-an., zinc.
morning - calc., caust., dios., lyc., nat-m.
bed, in - nat-m.
motion, on - plb., thuj.
night - kali-n.
after fever - nat-s.
on waking - mez.
numb as from electric shocks - fl-ac.
paralytic - act-sp., **ALUMN.,** ang., **ARS.,** bism., ***bov.,*** crot-h., nat-m., ***sil., stann.***
pressure, on - mez., nit-ac.
rising, on - nat-m., plb., sulph.
after - nux-m., plb.
sprained, as if - indg.
supper, after - nat-m.
trembling - lycps., ***stann.***
waking, on - mez.
walking, while - grat., plb.
warm room, in - ***caust.***
writing, while - ***aesc.,*** aml-n., bism., brach., caps., carb-v., chel., **MEZ.,** sabin., ***stann., zinc.***
writing, after - plb.

weakness, fingers - ambr., **ARS.,** ***bov.,*** carb-an., ***carb-v.,*** cic., crot-h., cur., fago., hipp., hura, ***kali-n.,*** lact., led., lyc., ***nat-m.,*** par., phos., **RHUS-T.,** sil., zinc.
daytime - phos.
drops things, (see Awkwardness) - ***ars.,*** carb-an., ***nat-m., sil., stann.***
first - kali-c., nat-m.
writing, while - kali-c.
grasping, when - **ARS.,** carb-an., carb-v., kali-br., ***sil.***
night - ambr.
paralytic - **ARS.,** carb-v.
playing the piano - ***cur., stann., zinc.***
second - nat-m.
third - plb.
tips - ***mez.***
writing, while - fago., kali-c.

weakness, thumbs - kali-c., nat-m., sil., sulph.
writing, while - kali-c.

WENS, (see Sebaceous cysts)

WITHERED, skin of hands - **LYC.,** nat-c., nat-m., ph-ac.

WOODEN, sensation - **KALI-N.**

WOUNDS, fingers, dissecting - ***apis,*** **ARS., CALEN., LACH.,** ***hyper., pyrog.,***

WRINKLED, back of - mur-ac., ***ph-ac.***
wrinkled, fingers - ambr., cupr., ***ph-ac.,*** sol-n.

WRITING, difficult and slow after breakfast - carb-v.

Head

ABSCESS - ***calc., hep.,*** lyc., ***merc., sil.***

ACNE, forehead - ant-c., ***ars.,*** aur., bar-c., bell., ***calc., caps.,*** **CARB-AN., CARB-S., CARB-V., CAUST.,** ***cic.,*** clem., **HEP.,** ***kreos.,*** led., ***nat-m., nit-ac.,*** **NUX-V.,** ***ph-ac.,*** **PSOR., RHUS-T., SEP., SIL., SULPH.,** viol-t.

ACHING, pain, (Headaches, general)
aching, brain, (see Brain, chapter)

ACROMEGALY - ***bar-c.,*** carc., pituit., thyr.

ADHESION, scalp to the skull, as if - mag-arct.
skin, of forehead - sabin.

AIR or wind, sensation of, in head - benz-ac., lyss.
above the eyes, a current of - bor.
extending to abdomen - aloe.
passing through sensation as of - anan., aur., benz-ac., colch., ***cor-r.,*** meny., mill., nat-m., petr., puls., sabin., sanic.
and on head, sensation of - ***aur.***
rocking, on - **COR-R.**
vertex, in - ***carb-an.***

AIR, sensitive to a draft (see Cold) - ***acon., ars.,*** **BELL.,** benz-ac., bor., cadm-s., ***calc., calc-ar., calc-p., caps.,*** **CHIN.,** coloc., gels., ***hep.,*** kali-ar., ***kali-c.,*** kali-n., kali-s., lac-c., ***merc., nux-m., nux-v.,*** phos., ***sanic., sel.,*** **SIL.,** stront-c., ***sulph.,*** valer., verb.
agg. - am-m., ***aur., bell.,*** nit-ac., nux-m., nux-v., ***sil.,*** verat., zinc.

ALIVE, sensation as if something, were in head - ant-t., asar., croc., crot-c., hyper., ***petr., sil.,*** sulph.
pressing, crawling pain, spreading out from centre, as of something alive - tarax.
everything in head were, as if - petr.
night - hyper.
in bed - hyper.
walking, while - sil.
alive, sensation as if something, were in crawling in forehead as of a worm - alum.

ANXIETY, in head - nat-c., nat-m., sars.

ASLEEP, sensation as if - alum., apis, calad., carb-an., con., cupr., merc., mur-ac., nat-m., nit-ac., op., sep.
debauch, after a - ***op.***
eating, after - con.
left side - calad.
lying, while - merc.
asleep, sensation as if forehead in - mur-ac.
left half of - calad.

AURA, epileptic, starting in head - caust., lach., stram., sulph.

BALANCING, difficult to keep the head erect - glon.
motion, on - crot-h., fl-ac., lyc., rhus-t.
pendulum-like - cann-i.
sensation in - aesc., bell., ***glon.,*** lyc.

BALL, sensation of a, beating against skull on beginning to walk - plat.
fast in brain - staph.
lying on right side - anan.
rising up - acon., cimic., lach., plat., plb., sep., staph.
rolling in brain - anan., bufo, hura, lyss.
ball, sensation of a, in forehead - ant-t., carb-ac., caust., kali-c., lac-d., ***staph.***

BAND, (see Constriction)

BEATS, head against the bed (see Head, Striking) - ***apis,*** ars., con., hyos., mill., prot., rhus-t., scut., stram., tarent., ***tub.***
against wall in sleep - mag-c.
feels as if he could beat head to pieces - nit-ac.

BENDS, head backward must (see Drawn back) - arn., ***cham.,*** kali-n.
walks with head thrown backward - ***arn.***

BITING, pain - arg-m., bar-c., carb-v., cham., grat., kali-bi., kali-i., lyc., mez., phel., ran-s., rhod., sec.
forehead - spig.
occiput - iod.
right, side - thuj.
rubbing agg. - staph.
scratching amel. - grat.

BLEEDING, internal (see Nerves, Stroke)

BLOCK solid, sensation as of a, forehead - kali-bi., kreos.

BLOOD-vessels, distension of, head - acet-ac., ***ars.,*** cact., **CHIN.,** ***chin-s., ferr., glon.,*** ph-ac., sang., stry., thuj., xan.
menses, during - ***croc.***
sensation, as if - guai.
veins, in - am-m., bell., stict.
blood-vessels, of temples, distended - amyl-n., ars., ***aur.,*** cedr., **BELL., CHIN.,** cub., cupr., ***glon.,*** jab., ph-ac., ***sang.,*** sulph., tab., thuj.

BLOWS, sensation, as from (see Injuries) - aeth., alum., ant-t., arn., bov., caust., chel., hell., indg., led., mang., med., nat-m., nux-v., olnd., ph-ac., plat., ran-b., ruta., sabad., sol-n., spig., sul-ac., valer., zinc.
back of head and neck, on - cann-i.
blows, forehead, on, awakens at 1 a.m. - psor.
frontal eminence, left - squil.
morning on waking - sol-n.
right, side - sul-ac.
blows, periosteum - ruta.
blows, occiput, on - dig., hell., **NAJA,** ***lyss.***
sub-occipital - apis.
blows, temples - ***sul-ac.***
blows, vertex, stupefying pain - valer.

BOARD, or bar, before, sensation as if - acon., aesc., calc., ***carb-an.,*** cocc., ***dulc.,*** eug., helon., kreos., lyc., olnd., op., plat., plb., ***rhus-t., sulph.,*** zinc.
morning, 11 a.m. - zinc.

BODY, hot in forehead - kali-c.

BOILING, sensation (see Bubbling) - **ACON.,** alum., cann-i., caust., chin., coff., dig., graph., grat., hell., kali-c., kali-s., laur., lyc., mag-m., mang., med., merc., sars., sil., sulph.
water, as if - acon., indg., rob.
side lain on - mag-m.
boiling, sensation seething in left side of vertex - lach.

BOILS - anac., ***ant-t., arn., ars.,*** aur., bar-c., bell., ***calc., calc-mur.,*** calc-s., dulc., ***hep.,*** jug-r., kali-bi., ***kali-c.,*** **KALI-I.,** led., mag-m., mez., mur-ac., nit-ac., ***psor.,*** rhus-t., scroph-n., ***sil., sulph.***
boils, forehead - am-c., led., mag-c., phos., sep.
above the eyes - calc-s., nat-m.
boils, occiput - ***kali-bi., lyc., nat-c.***
boils, temples - mur-ac.
right - mur-ac.

BORES, head in pillow - **APIS,** ***arn.,*** arum-t., **BELL.,** ***bry.,*** camph., **CINA.,** crot-t., dig., ***hell.,*** helo., hyper., ***med.,*** podo., ***stram.,*** sulph., tarent., **TUB.,** zinc.
sleep, during - hyper.

BORING, pain, digging - act-sp., agar., am-c., am-m., anac., ang., ant-c., ant-t., ***arg-n.,*** ars., aur., bar-c., bar-m., ***bell.,*** bism., bor., bov., bry., cadm-s., calc., camph., cann-s., canth., carb-an., carb-s., **CAUST.,** cham., chin., chin-a., chin-s., cimic., clem., ***cocc.,*** colch., ***coloc.,*** dros., dulc., graph., hell., ***hep.,*** hipp., hyper., ***ign.,*** indg., ip., kali-c., kali-i., kali-p., ***kali-s.,*** lach., laur., led., lyc., mag-c., mag-m., mag-s., mang., merc., ***mez.,*** mosch., mur-ac., nat-m., ***nat-s.,*** nit-ac., nux-v., olnd., ol-an., op., paeon., petr., phel., ph-ac., phos., ***plat.,*** puls., ran-s., rhod., rhus-t., ruta., sabad., sabin., samb., seneg., ***sep.,*** sil., ***spig.,*** squil., stann., staph., stram., sulph., ***tab.,*** thuj., valer., zinc.
afternoon - aloe, mag-s., nicc., sang., sep.
air, cold, amel. - phos., thuj.
bed, in warm - arg-n., puls.
bending back - aur., mang.
chilliness, during - ***sang.***
closing eyes amel. - sep.
coffee, after - nux-v.
cooling of head agg. - carb-an.
coughing agg. - aur., bell., bry., ***nux-v.***
dinner, during - am-c.
after - zinc.
eating, after - nux-v.
evening - aloe, anac., arg-n., coloc., hipp., mag-c., mag-m., nat-s., plan., puls., sep., zinc.
amel. - nux-v.
bed, in - mag-s.
extending from within out - dulc., puls., sep., zinc.
to ears - sep.
to nose - phos.
to teeth - sep.
to temples - sep.
heat and cold agg, of the face, with - puls.
heat and cold agg. - grat.
laying head on table amel. - ang.

BORING, pain
light agg. - nux-v.
menses, during - calc., mag-c., sep.
mental exertion - nux-v.
morning - arg-n., camph., cham., dios., hep., hyper., lyss., nicc., nux-v.
waking, after - apis, arg-m., arum-t., aur., mez.
motion, on - hep., ***sep.***
amel. - calc.
even of talking - dulc.
night - am-c., arg-n., carb-v., clem., dulc., lyc., sep., sulph.
midnight, before - dulc.
noise agg. - nux-v.
opening mouth - spig.
pressure - bell.
amel. - hell., ip., sep.
rising up - mang.
rubbing amel. - ol-an.
sitting, while - agar.
sleep amel. - sep.
stooping, on - hep., merc., ***sep.***
stooping, on, amel., rising up or bending backward agg. - mang.
twisting, screwing pain from right side to both temples, after going to bed, spreading over whole returns daily, after a walk on entering a room - sabad.
waking, on - cham.
amel. by sleep when sufficient - sep.
walking, while - bufo, coloc.
writing, while - dros.

boring, forehead - agar., am-m., anac., ant-c., ant-t., apis, arg-m., ***arg-n., ars.,*** aur., aur-m-n., bar-c., ***bell., bism.,*** bov., brom., bry., calad., calc., carb-s., carb-v., chel., chin., chin-s., cimic., colch., ***coloc.,*** cycl., dios., ***dulc.,*** hell., hep., hydr-ac., ign., ip., iris, kali-c., laur., led., mag-m., mang., ***merc.,*** mez., mosch., ***nat-m., nat-s.,*** nicc., ol-an., phel., phos., ***plat.,*** psor., puls., ruta., sabad., sabin., ***sang.,*** sep., ***sil., spig., spong.,*** squil., staph., sul-ac., sulph., zinc.
above - zinc.
afternoon - bism.
air, open - calc.
chilliness, during - sang.
cold application amel. - colch.
eating, after - bism.
evening - calc., nat-s.
extending to nose - bism., mang.
eyes, over - agar., arg-n., ***ars.,*** asaf., aster., aur-m-n., **BELL.,** calc-caust., cimic., colch., cupr-ar., dulc., ip., laur., led., lyc., mag-s., ol-an., sep., spig., sulph.
afternoon - sang.
closing eyes amel. - ip.
cold air, in - sep.
evening in bed - mag-s.
forenoon, 10 a.m. - cimic.
forenoon, 11 a.m. - ***spig.***
left - ***arg-n.,*** cimic., cupr-ar., kali-c., lyc., nux-m., spig.
morning - sulph.

boring, forehead
eyes, over, pressure, amel. - ip.
right - ***aur.,*** colch., sulph.
thunderstorm, in - sep.
walking amel. - ars.
walking, while - aur-m-n.
forenoon until evening - sep.
frontal eminence - am-c., arg-m., ***bell.,*** led., mang., ol-an., ***plan.,*** sabad., thuj.
left - **ARG-N.,** ol-an., thuj.
right - bell., colch.
touch amel. - thuj.
intermittent - arg-m.
inward - bell., calc., cocc., kali-c.
morning - ***bell.,*** calc., dios., sulph.
waking, on - ***bell., bry.***
motion, on - dulc., sep.
amel. - bism.
night - carb-v., sulph.
nose, above - bism., coloc., **HEP.,** mang., nat-m., sulph.
outward - ant-c., bell., bism., bov., dros., ***dulc.,*** ip., sep., spig., spong., ***staph.***
pressure agg. - calc.
amel. - anac., colch.
reading, while - led.
sides - arg-m., ***arg-n.,*** aur., aur-m-n., ***bell.,*** brom., calc., cimic., colch., ***coloc.,*** led., mez., nat-s., ***puls.,*** spong., staph.
8 a.m. - bor.
evening - arg-m.
extending to nape - arg-n.
left - arg-m., arg-n., aur., brom., spong.
morning - ***bell.,*** staph.
motion - arg-n.
right - coloc., puls., ruta.
walking in open air, during - spong.
walking in open air, after - calc.
stooping agg. - calc.
walking, while - arg-n., coloc.
after - calc.
in open air - sul-ac.
writing, while - dros.

boring, occiput - agar., ***arg-n.,*** gels., hell., merc., ***mez.,*** mosch., nat-m., ***nat-s.,*** nicc., ol-an., ph-ac., plan., ran-s., ***rhus-t.,*** sabin., spig., stann., stront-c., zinc.
afternoon - nicc.
evening - zinc.
intense pain as if a bolt had been driven from neck to vertex, agg. each throb of heart - cimic.
sides - arg-m., aur-m-n., ol-an., sabin., stront.
night - stront.
spot - stront.

boring, sides - agar., ang., arg-n., arum-t., aur., aur-m-n., bell., bov., bry., chin., clem., coloc., cop., eup-pur., hep., iris, kali-i., laur., led., mag-c., mag-m., mag-s., mang-m., mez., nat-m., nat-s., phos., puls., stann., staph., zinc.
afternoon - mag-s.
bending backward - aur.
coughing agg. - aur.
dinner, after - zinc.

boring, sides
evening - mag-m., zinc.
changing to stitching - bell.
extending to occiput - mag-c.
left - aur., chin., cop., mag-c., mag-s., nat-m., nat-s., staph., zinc.
morning - arum-t., aur., mag-c.
8 a.m - arg-n.
waking - staph.
motion agg. - bell.
outward - bell.
right - anac., ***arg-n.,*** arum-t., bov., bry., clem., coloc., stann., ***zinc.***
sitting - phos.
spots, in - hep.
standing - zinc.
violent - ***arg-n.***

boring, temples - acon., agar., aloe, alum., alumn., ang., ant-c., apis, ***arg-n., ars.,*** aur-m-n., bar-c., bar-m., bell., bov., bufo, calad., calc., ***camph.,*** carb-an., carb-s., carb-v., cham., clem., ***coloc.,*** cycl., dios., dulc., ***ferr., ferr-ar.,*** ferr-p., grat., ***hep.,*** ip., ***kali-i.,*** led., mag-m., ***mang.,*** mez., mur-ac., nat-a., nat-s., ol-an., paeon., ph-ac., ***phos.,*** psor., ptel., rhod., sep., sil., stann., stram., sulph., ***thuj.***
afternoon - aloe, nat-s.
5 p.m. - nat-s.
bending backward agg. - mang.
closing eyes amel. - ip.
cold agg. - grat.
coughing, on - kali-bi.
daytime - stann.
evening - aloe, alum., coloc., plan.
10 p.m. - arg-n.
extending, to head - hep.
to malar bone - carb-an.
forenoon - alum.
heat agg. - grat.
inward - hep.
left - alum., ***arg-n.,*** calc., ***clem.,*** ph-ac., rhod.
menses, before - ***ant-c.***
morning - apis, camph., cham., hep., lyss., mez.
waking, on - apis
noon - ***arg-n.***
outward - ant-c., ***dulc.***
pressure amel. - calad., ip., stann.
pulsating - ***ferr.***
rest, during - dulc.
right - bell., coloc., ***hep.,*** nat-s., ptel.
to left - nat-a.
sitting upright - mang.
stooping amel. - mang.
tearing - ***rhod.***
touch amel. - ***coloc.***

boring, vertex - agar., ang., ***arg-n.,*** bar-c., bell., caust., chel., chin., cimic., colch., cycl., dros., ***lach.,*** led., mag-s., mosch., mur-ac., nit-ac., olnd., ph-ac., phos., puls., samb., spig., ***sulph.***
outward - spig., staph.
spots, in - bor., colch., sulph.

BRAIN, general (see Brain, chapter)

BRITTLE, sensation - chel., cupr., fl-ac., nat-m., par., rad-br., thuj.

BUBBLING, sensation in - acon., asaf., bell., berb., bry., indg., kali-c., kreos., nux-v., par., ***puls.,*** rob., ***spig., sulph.***
leaning back while sitting amel. - spig.
night - par., puls.
walking, while - nux-v., spig.

bubbling, sensation in, forehead, as if bubble bursting in - ***form.***

bubbling, sensation in, occiput - indg., sumb.

BURNING, pain - **ACON.,** agar., ail., alum., am-c., anan., ant-t., ***apis,*** arg-m., ***arg-n., arn., ars.,*** arum-t., aur., aur-m., aur-s., ***bar-c.,*** bar-m., bell., berb., bism., bov., ***bry., calc.,*** calc-ar., ***calc-p., canth.,*** carb-ac., carb-an., carb-s., ***carb-v., caust.,*** chel., chin., cocc., coff., coloc., crot-c., crot-t., cupr., dig., ***dros.,*** dulc., ***eug., form., glon.,*** graph., ***hell.,*** helon., ***ip., kali-ar., kali-bi.,*** kali-c., kali-p., kali-s., ***kreos.,*** lachn., lact., lil-t., lith., mag-m., manc., mang., med., **MERC.,** ***merc-c.,*** merl., **MEZ.,** mur-ac., nat-c., nat-m., nat-s., nit-ac., nux-v., par., ***petr.,*** phel., ph-ac., **PHOS.,** phys., plat., plb., psor., rhod., rhus-t., rob., ruta, sabad., sang., sec., sep., ***sil.,*** spig., stann., staph., stront-c., sulph., sul-ac., tab., tarax., tarent., tax., verat., verat-v., zinc-s.
afternoon - canth., fago.
air, open, in, amel. - ***apis,*** mang., myric., **PHOS.**
alternating with pain - brom.
body cold - **ARN.**
brain were on fire, as if - ***canth.,*** hydr-ac., ***phos.***
chilliness, with - ant-t., kali-c., sil.
cold bathing agg. - form.
contracting - bism.
dinner, after - ***alum.,*** grat.
ears, burning along - rhus-t.
evening - am-c., carb-ac., jug-r., merc-i-r., phys.
bed in - carb-v., ***merc.,*** nat-c.
hot iron around as from, or hot water in - acon., coc-c.
light agg. - ***glon.***
lying on back, while - agar.
amel. - canth.
in bed agg. - ***merc.***
menopause, during the - ***lach.***
menses, during - nat-m.
mental, employment amel. - helon.
exertion - ***sil.***
morning - arn., canth., glon., mur-ac., ***nux-v.,*** phos., phys.
waking, on - chin., coc-c.
motion, agg. - ***apis,*** arn.
amel. - helon.
night - arn., lyc., ***merc., sil.***
noon - ***sulph.***
pressing - mang.
pressure of hand amel. - apis
room, on entering from air - ***caust.***
rubbing amel. - phos.

BURNING, pain
scratching, after - cob., kali-n., lach., merc., ol-an., par.
sitting, while - canth., phos.
upright amel. - merc.
sneezing amel. - lil-t.
sparks, like - nit-ac.
spine, burning along, with - pic-ac.
spots, in - ars., glon., graph., nit-ac., raph.
standing, while - canth.
stooping agg. - ***apis.,*** mur-ac.
talking, from - sil.
tearing - merc.
touched, when - ip., nat-m.
vomiting, after - eug., nat-s.
walking, while - rhus-t.
amel. - canth.
warm room - apis, **PHOS.**
wrapping up warmly amel. - aur., **SIL.**

burning, forehead - acon., ***alum.,*** am-c., ant-t., ***ars.,*** aur., aur-m., bell., bism., bry., carb-ac., carb-an., carb-v., ***caust.,*** cham., chel., ***chin.,*** coloc., conv., crot-t., cupr., dulc., eup-per., glon., grat., hyos., ip., kali-c., **KALI-I.,** kali-p., lil-t., ***lyc.,*** lyss., mag-m., mang., meny., merc., merc-i-r., mez., mur-ac., ***nat-c.,*** nat-m., nux-m., ***nux-v.,*** ox-ac., **PHOS.,** phys., podo., psor., rhus-t., rhus-v., sabad., sec., sep., ***spig.,*** stann., staph., stront-c., sul-ac., tarent., teucr., ther., zinc.
air, open, amel. - alum., **PHOS.,** stann.
cold hand amel. - carb-ac., ***phos.***
dinner, after - ***alum.,*** grat.
eating, after - ***nux-v.***
evening - nat-c.
bed, in - nat-c.
extending to eyes - ***spig.***
eyes, over - acon., agar., **ARS.,** chel., coloc., dig., dros., meny., merc., nux-m., rhus-t., sil., sulph.
afternoon - sulph.
evening - chel.
night - **ARS.**
left - merc., spig.
morning - mur-ac., nux-v., phos., phys.
morning, on rising amel. - nux-v.
night - lyc., ***merc.***
day and night - ***lyc.***
right - coloc., ***mang.,*** **SPIG.**
room, on entering - ***caust.***
scratching, after - laur.
sides - aur., caust., clem., coloc., fl-ac., merc., ph-ac., **SPIG.**
sitting, while - alum.
spot - mang.
standing, while - ***alum.***
stool, during - kali-p.
stooping - mur-ac.
touched, when - ip., nat-m.
waking, on- ***nux-v.***
walking, when - rhus-t.

burning, occiput - aesc., agar., ***apis,*** aur., aur-m., chin-a., cupr., ***gels.,*** indg., kali-c., kali-n., lyc., mag-m., med., nat-c., **PHOS.,** pic-ac., rhus-t., sep., ***spong.,*** staph., sulph.
covering head agg. - gels.
extending down neck in morning - chin-a.
evening, in bed - kali-n.
left - chin-a.
lying, on occiput - sulph.
scratching, after - sulph.

burning, sides - bapt., bar-c., bell., calc., canth., coloc., dros., mang., ph-ac., **PHOS.**
left, morning on waking - lyss.
right - spong.

burning, temples - alum., am-m., apis, aur., bar-c., calc., cann-i., carb-ac., carb-an., caust., chel., cimic., cinnb., ***coloc.,*** con., crot-t., cupr., ***merc.,*** nit-ac., phel., **PHOS.,** phyt., plat., rhus-t., sabad., sars., spig., staph., sul-ac., verb., viol-t.
above - mur-ac.
blow, as from - sul-ac.
extending to cheek - mez.
left - am-m., chel., cupr., merc., nit-ac., plat., sabad., sars., ***spig.,*** staph., verb.
right - alum., aur., bar-c., carb-an., caust., cimic., con., mang., rhus-t., viol-t.
wave, like - sul-ac.

burning, vertex - agar., alumn., arn., ars., ***aur.,*** bapt., ***bry.,*** **CALC.,** ***calc-p.,*** carb-ac., carb-s., ***carb-v.,*** caust., chin-s., coc-c., ***con., crot-c.,*** cupr., dros., dulc., ***glon.,*** **GRAPH.,** helon., hyper., ***lach.,*** merl., ***nat-m.,*** nat-s., ***ph-ac., phos.,*** podo., ran-s., raph., sabad., sep., stann., **SULPH.,** viol-t., zinc.
biting - dros.
chilly, when - caust.
extending to temples - phos.
grief, after - ***calc., ph-ac.***
menopause, during - **LACH.**
menses, during - ***lach., nat-m., phos., sulph.***
morning - coc-c.
waking, on - coc-c.
noon - sulph.
rubbing amel. - phos.
spots, in - ***arn.,*** ars., ***graph.,*** raph.
transient - nat-c.

BURROWING, pain - agar., ant-t., aur., bar-ac., calc., cham., clem., coc-c., colch., eupi., ***hep., mag-m.,*** phos., rat., samb., sep., ***spig.,*** squil., til.
afternoon - ant-t.
air, in open - agar., rat.
cold amel. - phos.
bending head backwards, amel. - hep.
binding up amel. - hep.
dinner, after - agar., kali-c.
extending to cheeks - calc.
to eyes - calc.
to nose - calc., ***phos.***
to teeth - calc.
lying amel. - junc., ***spig.***
morning - agar., hep.
rising, after - bar-ac., junc., squil.

BURROWING, pain
motion, agg. - ***spig.***
of upper lids agg. - coloc.
night - agar.
noise - ***spig.***
opening mouth - ***spig.***
talking loud - spig.
walking in open air - agar.

burrowing, forehead - agar., bar-c., cham., coc-c., dulc., eupi., kali-c., mag-m., mez., plat., sep., spig.
extending to mouth - eupi.
eyes, over - dulc., kali-c., plat.
while walking - plat.
left - agar.
morning, rising, on - bar-c., squil.
sides - agar., clem., ol-an.

burrowing, occiput - agar., ph-ac., ***spig.***
left - agar.
lying amel. - ***spig.***

burrowing, sides - agar., carl., clem., phos., rat.
air, open - rat.
extending to occiput - clem.
forenoon - agar.
walking - clem.
in open air - agar.

burrowing, temples - agar., bar-c., cham., clem., coloc., mang.
dinner, after - agar.
midnight - agar.

BURSTING, pain - aesc., alum., am-c., ***am-m.,*** ant-c., apis, arg-n., ars., ars-m., asaf., asar., aster., bapt., bar-c., **BELL.,** berb., bov., brom., **BRY.,** cact., calad., **CALC.,** cann-s., ***caps.,*** carb-an., ***caust.,*** cham., chel., **CHIN.,** chin-a., cimic., clem., cob., coc-c., coff., **CON.,** cupr., dig., dios., dol., euph., ***euphr., ferr.,*** ferr-ar., ferr-p., **GLON.,** ***graph.,*** gymn., ham., ***hep.,*** hydr., ign., ***ip.,*** kali-ar., kali-bi., kali-c., kali-n., kali-p., kali-s., kalm., kreos., **LACH.,** lachn., lac-ac., ***lyc.,*** **LYSS.,** mag-m., **MERC.,** mez., mill., mosch., naja, nat-a., nat-c., **NAT-M.,** nat-p., nat-s., nicc., ***nit-ac., nux-m., olnd.,*** op., ***petr.,*** ph-ac., **PHOS.,** phys., pic-ac., prun., psor., ptel., ***puls., rat.,*** rhus-t., sabad., sang., **SEP.,** ***sil.,*** sol-n., ***spig., spong.,*** stann., stront-c., ***sulph.,*** sul-ac., thuj., verat., zinc.
air, open in - **BELL.,** glon.
air, open in, amel. - kali-bi.
binding up head amel. - lac-d., mag-m., sil.
calvarium were being lifted, as if - **CANN-I.**
closing eyes, on - ***chin.***
contraction of muscles of the face, at - spig.
coughing, on - **BELL., BRY.,** cact., calc., **CAPS.,** ***chin.,*** coc-c., dios., hep., hydr., kali-bi., ***lach.,*** lac-ac., merc., **NAT-M.,** nux-v., ol-j., ***ph-ac., phos.,*** puls., rumx., sep., sil., spig., ***spong.,*** staph., **SULPH.**
day, every - ***sulph.***
daytime - ***sulph.***
eating, after - ***graph.,*** nat-s., nux-v.
dinner, after - kali-bi.
evening - caps., clem., ham., rat.

BURSTING, pain
fever, with - aesc., bell.
fly to pieces, as if would - arg-n., asaf., bar-c., carb-an., caust., graph., hep.
increasing and decreasing gradually - mez., stront.
influenza, during - ***bry., eup-per.,*** naja.
jar, from any - bell., ***chin.,*** sil.
lying down amel. - ***ferr.,*** kali-bi., ***lach.,*** mag-m., sang.
menses, during - berb., ***bry.,*** calc., ***glon.,*** kreos., lyc., nat-m., nat-s., sang., sep.
before - brom., calc., cham., ham., nat-m.
instead of - nux-m.
mental exertion - arg-n., ptel.
mental exertion, reading or writing amel. - ign.
morning - am-m., dios., ham., lach., lac-c., phos.
first opening the eyes on - ***bry.***
gradually increasing till evening - bry., sang., sep.
waking, on - cham., ***con.,*** hydr., nux-v.
motion, from - ***bry.,*** caps., ***chin., coff., ferr.,*** kali-bi., ***lach.,*** lyss., mag-m., rhus-t., sep., sil., sol-n., spig.
continued hard motion amel. - sep.
of the eyes - chin., ptel., ***puls.***
night - cact., carb-an., cedr., ***hep.***
waking him - ***hep.***
opening eyes amel. - ***chin.***
press with hands, must - carb-an., ***glon., mag-m.***
resting head amel. - kali-bi.
rubbing amel. - **PHOS.**
sitting, while - phos.
bent over, while - rat.
sleep amel. - ***sang.,*** sep.
sneezing - nat-m.
split open with a wedge, as if - lachn.
stool, after - rat.
straining at - ind.
stooping, while - ***ham.,*** hep., hydr., kali-bi., lyss., nat-m., ptel., sep., stry.
talking aloud, while - ign., ***spig.***
turning after - lyss.
waking, on - cham., chin., con., ham., hydr., ***lach.,*** nux-v.
walking, while - caps., carb-an., kali-bi., stront.
in open air amel. - ***sang.***
weather, wet, agg. - carb-an.
weeks, every six - **MAG-M.**
wrapping up amel. - ***mag-m.***

bursting, forehead - ***am-c.,*** ant-c., ***ars.,*** bar-c., ***bell.,*** **BRY.,** calad., ***calc.,*** caps., chin-s., crot-c., dulc., ***ferr., gels., glon., graph.,*** hell., hydr., indg., ***kali-c.,*** kali-n., kali-p., lac-c., lac-d., lyc., ***mag-m.,*** **MERC.,** nat-a., ***nat-c.,*** **NAT-M.,** nat-s., ***nux-v., olnd.,*** **PULS.,** rat., ruta., ***sang.,*** sep., sil., sol-n., spig., spong., staph., stry., sulph., thuj., ust., **ZINC.**
bandaging amel. - lac-d.
coughing, on - ***nat-m.,*** ol-j., staph., stict.
eating, after - am-c., ***graph.***

bursting, forehead
evening - ruta.
exercise, after - nat-c.
extending to nose - ***dulc.***
eyes, over - crot-c., kali-bi., mag-m., nit-ac.
lying, while - ***gels.***
menses, during - lyc., nat-m.
morning - sulph.
7 a.m. to 5 p.m. - nat-c.
10 a.m. - ***gels.***
motion, on - nat-c.
night - ***crot-c.***
paroxysmal - kali-c.

bursting, occiput - aloe, ***calc., carb-v.,*** ferr., ***gels., ip., lach.,*** nux-m., ***nux-v., op.,*** spig., spong., staph., zinc.
excitement - ***ferr.***
extending, over head, beginning in upper cervical region, causing bursting pain in forehead and eyeballs agg. 10 a.m. while lying, nausea, cold sweat and cold feet - ***gels.***
extending, to top of head, is so severe she thinks head will burst and she will go crazy - **CALC.**

bursting, sides - asar., brom., ***glon.,*** nicc., nit-ac., ***puls.,*** zinc.
eating, after - nit-ac.
evening - zinc.
menses, during - glon., lach.
standing, while - zinc.

bursting, temples - apis, ***bell.,*** brom., cact., chin-s., cimic., ***cina,*** glon., hell., ign., ind., ip., kalm., ***lach.,*** lil-t., merc-i-f., ***sang.,*** sol-n., staph.
afternoon - sang.
coughing, on - cina
right - ***bell.,*** sang.
walking in open air amel. - ***sang.***

bursting, vertex - alum., ***am-c.,*** am-m., bapt., calc., **CARB-AN.,** ***cimic., ferr.,*** graph., ***hyper.,*** lac-ac., ***nat-s.,*** nit-ac., **SIL.,** spig., spong., stront-c., xan.
afternoon, while walking - stront.
binding up head amel. - **SIL.**
blown off, as if - cham.
coughing, on - sanic.
fly off as if would - cimic.
forced, asunder, as if - kali-i., lac-d., nux-v., ***sil.***
morning - am-m.
night - carb-an.
split open, as if - zinc.
walking, while - stront.
wet weather - carb-an.

CARBUNCLES - ***anthr., ars., hep., lach., sil., sulph.***

CEREBELLAR disease - helo., sulfon.

CEREBRAL hemorrhage (see Brain, Strokes) - **ACON.,** ***arn., aur., bar-c.,*** **BELL., BOTH.,** ***camph.,*** carb-v., ***chin.,*** **COCC., COLCH.,** coff., con., ***cupr., crot-h., ferr.,*** ferr-p., **GELS.,** glon., helon., ***hyos.,*** **IP., LACH.,** laur., ***lyc.,*** merc., ***nat-m.,*** nit-ac., ***nux-m., nux-v.,*** **OP.,** ***phos.,*** plb., ***puls.,*** stram.

CEREBRO-spinal axis, ailments of - agar., arg-n., chin., cocc., ***gels.,*** ign., ***nux-v.,*** phos.

CEPHALAHEMATOMA - ***calc-f., merc.,*** **SIL.**

CHILLINESS, (see Coldness)

CHIRPING - bry.

CLUCKING, in - sulph.

clucking in, occiput - spig.

clucking in, temples, in - bry.

COLD, air, head sensitive to - ant-c., ***ars., bar-c., bell.,*** benz-ac., bor., brom., ***carb-an., carb-v.,*** card-m., **CHIN.,** eup-per., ferr-p., ***graph.,*** grat., **HEP.,** hyos., kali-ar., ***kali-c.,*** kali-p., ***lach., lyc.,*** mag.c., ***mag-m., merc., mez., nat-m.,*** nux-m., **NUX-V.,** ***phos., psor., rhus-t.,*** sanic., ***sep.,*** **SIL.,** squil., ***stront-c.,*** thuj., zinc.

evening - ant-c.

morning - carb-v.

night - ***phos.***

walking in cold air - **CARB-V.**

COLDNESS, chilliness - acon., abrot., **AGAR.,** agn., alum., alumn., ambr., am-c., anan., ant-c., apis, ***arn., ars.,*** ars-i., asaf., asar., ***aur.,*** bar-c., **BELL.,** benz-ac., bor., **CALC.,** calc-p., calc-s., ***cann-s.,*** caps., carb-an., carb-s., ***carb-v.,*** chel., chin-a., chlor., cimic., cist., coca, cocc., ***colch., con., croc.,*** cupr., dios., dulc., eup-per., ferr., ferr-ar., ferr-i., ferr-p., gels., gins., glon., ***graph.,*** grat., ham., hura, ind., iod., kali-ar., ***kali-c.,*** kali-p., kali-s., kreos., ***lach.,*** lachn., lact., ***laur., lyc.,*** mag-m., mag-s., mang., ***meny., merc.,*** **MERC-C.,** merc-i-r., morph., mosch., naja, ***nat-m., nit-ac.,*** nux-v., olnd., phel., ph-ac., ***phos.,*** phyt., raph., **RHUS-T.,** rhus-v., rumx., ***ruta.,*** sabad., ***sanic., sep.,*** sil., **STANN.,** staph., **STRONT-C.,** stry., ***sulph.,*** sumb., ***tarent.,*** thea., til., valer., ***verat.,*** verb., vip., zing.

afternoon - ars., ***arum-t.,*** gamb., gels., ol-an., valer.

air, as from cold - acon., arg-n., ***laur.,*** nat-m., petr.

in open - ***ars.,*** phos.

in open, amel. - ***laur.,*** sep.

alternating with heat - bell., calc., kali-n., merc., ***phos.,*** verat.

begins in - ***bar-c.,*** nat-m., stann.

begins in spreads from the - mosch., valer.

breakfast, after - arn.

burning, after - sulph.

congestion of, with - glon.

covered, amel. - ***aur.,*** grat., kali-i., nat-m., sanic.

even when - mang.

evening - alum., ars-i., dulc., hyper., kreos., merc., stry., ***sulph.,*** zinc.

headache, during - ***ars.,*** sulph.

COLDNESS, chilliness

heat, with - chin., puls., verat.

heated, from being - **CARB-V.**

icy - ***agar., ars.,*** bar-c., **CALC.,** calc-p., ind., laur., phos., nux-v., ***sep.,*** valer.

internally - arn., bell., **CALC.,** staph.

lying, while, amel. - calc.

menses, during - ant-t., calc., mag-s., sep., sulph., ***verat.***

morning - cedr., dios., lact., sumb., ***tarent.***

motion, on - chel., sep.

night - cimic., lyc., mang., ***phos., sep.,*** stront.

pain, with - ***gels., phos.***

painful parts - ***kali-i.***

perspiration, with - merc-c.

of body - phos.

pressure of hat., from - valer.

riding, after - lyc.

scratching, after - ***agar.***

sitting, while - mez.

spot, as of a cold - sulph.

spreads from - mosch., valer.

stool, during - staph.

after - plat.

before - carb-an.

stooping, agg. - alum., sep.

walking amel. - gins.

warm room - ***laur.,*** merc-i-r., tarent.

water, as from cold - ***cann-s.,*** carb-an., croc., cupr., glon., sabad., ***tarent.***

coldness, forehead - acon., ***agar.,*** anac., arn., ***ars.,*** bell., ***camph.,*** carb-s., cedr., cham., chin., chin-a., cimic., cinnb., cist., coff., colch., gels., glon., ***graph., hep.,*** hydr-ac., hyper., ***lach., laur.,*** lyc., mag-m., merc., mez., mosch., oena., phel., ph-ac., puls., ran-s., staph., sulph., sul-ac., tarent., verat., ***zinc.***

afternoon - nat-a.

air, from, as from a draft - ***laur.,*** staph.

cold, penetrates painfully - zinc.

alternating with heat - spig., staph.

evening - hyper., sulph., zinc.

externally - cist., cinnb., gels., laur., sulph.

fever, during - chin., puls., zinc.

with external heat - agar.

ice, as from - agar., glon., laur.

menses, during - sulph.

morning - cedr.

night - lyc.

one-sided - spig.

spots, in small, as of cold finger - ***arn.***

warm room, in - cist., ***laur.***

coldness, occiput - acon., agar., aloe, alum., berb., ***calc.,*** **CALC-P.,** cann-i., **CHEL.,** chin-s., coc-c., ***dulc.,*** echi., gels., gins., ***kali-n.,*** nux-m., ***phos.,*** plat., podo., ***sep.,*** sil., tarent., thea., verat.

air, like cool - acon.

as if frozen - gels., nux-v., ***sep.***

cold damp weather - ***dulc.***

evening - alum., ***dulc.***

left side - cocc.

right side - ***form.***

rising from neck like cold air - **CHEL.,** sep.

coldness, sides - ***asar.,*** bar-c., ***calc.,*** cann-s., ***con.,*** croc., kali-bi., lach., lob., phos., tarent., verat.
left - lach., phos.
one-sided - ***calc.,*** con., lach., ruta.
right - am-m., bar-c., ***calc.,*** verat.
evening - alum., ***dulc.***
evening, but feels burning hot - bar-c., ***calc.***
spots in - croc.
above the ear - asar.
warmth amel. - lach.

coldness, temples - bell., ***berb.,*** gamb., merc-c., ol-an., ph-ac., plat., rhod., tarent.
right - berb., tarent.

coldness, vertex - agar., am-c., arn., ***arum-t.,*** aur-m., ***bry.,*** calc., **CALC-P.,** calc-s., ferr-p., grat., kali-c., kali-i., kali-s., ***laur.,*** mang., myric., ***nat-m.,*** plat., psor., ***sep., sil.,*** sulph., tarent., valer., **VERAT.**
afternoon - ***arum-t.***
as if without covering upper part - arum-t.
covered, even when - mang.
extending to sacrum - acon.
icy - agar., arn., ***laur.,*** valer., ***verat.***
when covered - valer.
menses during - ***sep.,*** sulph., ***verat.***
motion, during - sep.
spots, in - mang., ***sulph.***
a small - mang.
stooping, on - sep.
warm room - ***laur.***
water, as from cold - tarent.

COMMOTION, painless, in - caust.

CONCUSSION of brain (commotion) - ***acon.,*** **ARN.,** bell., bry., **CIC.,** con., ham., ***hell.,*** hep., ***hyos.,*** **HYPER.,** kali-i., kali-p., led., merc., nat-s., op., ph-ac., ***rhus-t.,*** sep., sul-ac., sulph., zinc.
knocking foot against any, when - bar-c.
misstep, from - led.

CONGESTION, hyperemia (see Fullness, Pulsation) - acet-ac., ***acon.,*** aesc., aeth., agar., aloe, alum., alumn., ***ambr.,*** am-c., am-m., aml-n., ***anac., ant-c.,*** **APIS,** arg-m., ***arg-n.,*** **ARN.,** ***ars.,*** ars-h., ars-i., asaf., aster., ***aur.,*** aur-s., bar-c., **BELL.,** ***bor.,*** bov., brom., **BRY.,** ***bufo,*** **CACT., CALC.,** ***calc-p., calc-s., camph.,*** cann-i., ***cann-s., canth.,*** carb-ac., ***carb-an.,*** **CARB-S., CARB-V.,** caust., ***cedr., cham.,*** chel., ***chin.,*** chin-a., chlor., cic., ***cimic., cinnb.,*** clem., ***cocc.,*** coc-c., ***coff.,*** colch., coloc., ***con.,*** cop., cor-r., corn., ***croc.,*** crot-h., crot-t., **CUPR.,** cur., ***cycl.,*** dig., ***dulc.,*** elaps, eug., eup-per., **FERR.,** ferr-ar., ferr-i., ***ferr-p., fl-ac.,*** form., gamb., **GELS., GLON.,** gran., ***graph., grat.,*** **HELL.,** hura, hydr., hydr-ac., ***hyos.,*** ign., indg., ***iod.,*** jatr., kali-ar., ***kali-bi., kali-br., kali-c.,*** kali-chl., ***kali-i.,*** kali-p., kali-s., kali-n., kalm., kreos., ***lac-d.,*** **LACH.,** lac-ac., lact., ***laur.,*** lil-t., **LYC.,** lyss., ***mag-c.,*** mag-m., ***mag-s., mang.,*** **MELI.,** ***merc.,*** merc-c., merc-i-f., ***mill.,*** mosch., naja, nat-a.1, ***nat-c., nat-m.,*** nat-p., ***nat-s., nit-ac.,*** nux-m., ***nux-v.,*** ol-an., ***op.,*** paeon., ***par.,*** petr., phel., ***ph-ac.,*** **PHOS.,** ***pic-ac., plb.,*** plat., ***psor.,***

CONGESTION, hyperemia - ***puls., ran-b., rhus-t.,*** sabin., sal-ac., **SANG.,** sec., seneg., ***sep., sil., spong.,*** staph., ***stram., stry.,*** **SULPH.,** ***sul-ac., tab.,*** tarax., tarent., tell., thea., thuj., urt-u., valer., ***verat., verat-v.,*** viol-o., ***zinc.,*** zing., ziz.
afternoon - am-c., cham., chin-s., graph., lach., nat-m., paeon., ran-b., sil.
5 p.m. to midnight - glon.
air, in open - lil-t., nat-c., ran-b., ***sulph.***
amel. - **APIS,** ***ars.,*** camph., caust., ***coc-c.,*** grat., hell., mag-m., mosch., nat-c.
alcoholic liquors agg. - ***calc.,*** calc-s., ***glon., lach., zinc.***
alternating, with congestion to heart - ***glon.***
icy cold sensation - ***calc.***
anger, after - ***bry., cham.,*** staph.
anxiety, with - ***acon., aur.,*** cycl.
bed, while in - anac., kali-c., lyc., mill., ***sulph.***
amel. - nat-c.
bending on, backward - bell.
forward - lac-c.
blowing nose, on - nit-ac.
chest, during shocks in - tab.
coffee, from - am-c., ***cact.,*** mill., ***rumx.***
constipation, during - aster., crot-h., ***nux-v.***
convulsions, during - **BELL.,** canth., crot-h., **GELS.**
before - **GLON.**
coughing, on - acon., ambr., anac., bell., calc., calc-s., carb-v., caust., cham., chin., dulc., ferr., hyos., iod., kali-c., kali-p., kali-s., lach., laur., lyc., mag-c., mag-m., merc., mosch., nit-ac., nux-v., phos., rhus-t., samb., seneg., sep., sil., spong., stram., sulph.
dinner, after - cycl., nux-m., psor.
eating, after - bor., calc., cinnb., cop., cycl., glon., nux-m., petr., sulph.
before - uran.
high living, from - verat-v.
epilepsy, before - calc-ar.
evening - calc., caust., chin-s., croc., fl-ac., hyos., indg., mag-m., mill., nat-c., nat-p., nux-v., phos., puls., rhus-t., sulph., trom.
excitement, during - asaf., ***phos.***
after a pleasant surprise - **COFF.**
exercise, on taking - sulph.
extending to from abdomen - crot-t.
to from back - ***phos.***
to from chest - ***glon.,*** lyss., mill., sulph.
forenoon - mag-c., mag-s.
fright or grief, from - ***ph-ac.***
headache, before - lyc.
heart, as if blood rushed from heart to head - nux-m.
at every throb of - cimic., ***glon.***
heat of face, with - acon., asaf., canth., cham., chin-s., coff., cop., ferr., ***ferr-p.,*** hell., kalm., mang., phos., rhus-t., sil., ***sulph.,*** valer.

CONGESTION, hyperemia
lifting, after - nat-c.
lochia, from suppressed - acon., bell., bry., cimic.
lying, while - cycl., lac-c., lyss., mang., naja
amel. - nat-c.
on temple - mur-ac.
on the back - ***sulph.***
menses, during - acon., **APIS,** ***bell., bry.,*** cact., ***calc.,*** calc-p., calc-s., caust., cham., ***chin.,*** cinnb., con., elaps, ***ferr-p.,*** gels., ***glon.,*** iod., mag-c., mag-m., manc., merc., mosch., nat-m., ***nux-m., nux-v., phos.,*** sang., **SULPH.,** verat., verat-v.
after - chin., ign., ***nat-m.,*** sulph., thuj.
before - ***acon.,*** **APIS,** ***bell.,*** bry., cupr., gels., ***glon.,*** hep., hyper., iod., ***kali-c.,*** lyc., manc., ***meli., merc.,*** tril.
suppressed, from - ***acon., apis,*** arn., **BELL.,** ***bry., calc.,*** calc-s., cham., ***chin.,*** **CIMIC.,** cocc., coc-c., **FERR., GELS., GLON.,** ***graph.,*** **LACH.,** merc., op., stram., sulph.
mental exertion, from - agar., ***aur.,*** **CACT.,** ***calc.,*** cham., nux-v., ***phos.,*** psor.
morning - calc., cham., chin-s., glon., lach., lac-ac., ***lyc.,*** mag-c., mag-s., naja, raph., tell.
rising, on - eug., lyc.
waking, on - ***calc., lyc., ph-ac.***
motion, from - glon., grat., kali-chl., mang., nux-v., petr., sulph.
rapid, from - ***petr.***
music, from - ***ambr.***
night - am-c., anac., ***aster.,*** berb., ***calc., calc-s.,*** carb-v., cycl., kali-c., mill., **PSOR.,** puls., sil., ***sulph.***
a stream from chest to head like a gust of wind with nosebleed - ***mill.***
noon - cham., naja.
agg. toward, gradually ceasing toward evening, with terrible pain, presses head against wall and fears going mad - stram.
nosebleeds, with - ant-c., bell., bry., carb-v., croc., lach., lil-t., meli., nux-v., pic-ac., ***psor.***
feels as if, were coming on - ign., lac-ac.
painful - sil.
pains, when, suddenly cease - cimic.
pale face, with - ***ferr., glon.***
periodical - ***cycl.,*** ferr.
perspiration, during - thuj.
where perspiration fails in ague - **CACT.**
rage, during - acon., **BELL.,** hyos., lach., nux-v., ***op.,*** phos., ***stram.,*** verat.
raising the head - lyc.
redness of face, with - acon., **BELL.,** canth., cop., cor-r., coff., ***glon., graph.,*** meli., merc-c., phos., sil., sol-n.
riding, from - grat., sulph.
rising, on - eug., mag-s., nat-c., sil., sulph.
rising, on, amel. - aur., mill.
room, on entering - ol-an.
shaking the on - nit-ac., nux-v.

CONGESTION, hyperemia
sitting, while - lac-ac., mag-c., mang., nat-c., ***phos.,*** thuj.
must sit up - aloe
sleep, during - glon., sil.
amel. after - grat.
smoking, from - ***bell., mag-c.***
speaking, when - coff., sulph.
spoken to harshly, when - ign.
standing, from - kali-c., mang.
stepping heavily, from - bar-c.
stool, during - aloe, ***bry., nux-v., sulph.***
after - lach., sulph.
before - aloe
stooping, when - acon., am-c., aur., ***bell., calc-p.,*** canth., ***cor-r.,*** elaps, lach., lyc., mill., myric., nat-c., nit-ac., ***puls.,*** rhus-t., seneg., sep., ***sulph.,*** tell., ***verat.***
streamed, as if blood from below upwards or within outwards - ox-ac.
sun, from exposure to - ***acon., bell., cact., gels., glon.,*** verat-v.
suppressed, from - **VERAT-V.**
discharges or suddenly ceasing pains - cimic.
talking - coff.
uremic poison, from - am-c., apis, ***bell.,*** con., ***cupr., gels., glon.,*** merc-c., ***stram.,*** tab., ter., verat-v.
waking - am-c., bell., ***calc.,*** carb-v., sil.
walking, while - caust., lach., mang., ran-b.
fast - ***phos.***
fast, amel. - cham.
in open air - caust., ran-b.
warm room - **APIS,** calc-s., ***carb-v., coc-c., kali-s.,*** **PULS., SULPH.**
wet, from getting the feet - dulc.
wine, after - sil.
writing, while - cann-s.

congestion, forehead - aloe, bad., bell., cimic., ***cinnb., fl-ac.,*** glon., lac-ac., mag-s., nat-c., ran-b., ***sil.,*** spong., stann., viol-t.

congestion, occiput - aloe, bor., ***chel., dulc., gels., glon.,*** ol-an., pip-m., staph., ***sulph.,*** thuj., ***verat-v.***
stooping, after - lyc.

congestion, temples - chel., glon., sil., zing.

congestion, vertex - absin., cann-i., **CINNB.,** nat-c., phos., ran-b., sil.

CONSTRICTION, tension (see Drawing, Pressing) - ***acon.,*** aesc., ***aeth.,*** agar., agn., aloe, alum., am-br., am-c., ***anac.,*** ang., ***ant-t.,*** antipyrin., **APIS,** arg-m., ***arg-n., arn.,*** ars., ***asaf., asar.,*** bapt., bar-c., bar-m., bell., berb., bov., ***bry.,*** bufo, calc., calc-s., ***camph.,*** cann-i., cann-s., carb-ac., carb-an., ***carb-s.,*** **CARB-V.,** card-m., **CAUST.,** cham., ***chel.,*** chin., chin-a., ***chin-s.,*** cimic., cic., cina, clem., ***cocc.,*** coc-c., coff., colch., coloc., ***con.,*** croc., ***crot-c.,*** crot-h., ***cycl.,*** daph., dig., dios., dulc., eug., ferr., ferr-ar., ferr-p., fl-ac., gamb., **GELS.,** gent-c., glon., ***graph., grat.,*** guare., ***hell.,*** helon., hep., hydrc., hyos., hyper., ign., indg., ***ip.,*** iris, kali-ar., kali-bi., ***kali-br.,*** kali-c., kali-i., kali-n., kali-p., kali-s., kreos., lach., lac-c.,

CONSTRICTION, tension - laur., lob., ***lyc., lyss.,*** mag-c., mag-m., mag-s., manc., mang., med., ***meny., merc.,*** merc-i-f., merl., ***mosch.,*** mur-ac., nat-c., ***nat-m.,*** nat-p., nat-s., **NIT-AC.,** nux-m., ***nux-v.,*** olnd., op., ***par., petr.,*** phel., ph-ac., ***phos.,*** phys., pip-m., ***plat.,*** plb., prun., psor., puls., ran-b., rhod., rhus-t., ruta., sabad., sabin., samb., sel., sep., ***sil.,*** spig., spong., stann., staph., ***stront-c.,*** **SULPH.,** sul-ac., tab., tarax., tarent., ther., thuj., valer., verat., verb., viol-o., vip., ***zinc.***

afternoon - graph., mag-c., naja, nit-ac., phos.
air, open, agg. - mang., merc., nat-m., valer.
amel. - berb., coloc., kali-i., lach., lyc.
alternating with relaxation - bism., calc., lac-c.
armor, as if in - apis, ***arg-n.,*** cann-i., **CARB-V.,** clem., coc-c., ***crot-c., graph.,*** nat-m.
band or hoop - ***acon.,*** aeth., all-c., ***am-br.,*** anac., ant-t., arg-m., ***arg-n.,*** asaf., bapt., bell., brom., camph., cann-s., **CARB-AC.,** carb-an., carb-s., ***carb-v.,*** card-m., ***chel.,*** clem., ***cocc.,*** crot-h., ***cycl.,*** dios., **GELS.,** glon., ***graph.,*** guai., ***hep.,*** hyos., indg., ***iod.,*** ip., iris, kali-c., kali-s., laur., med., ***merc.,*** nat-m., **NIT-AC.,** op., osm., petr., phys., plat., rhus-v., sabin., sang., sars., ***spig.,*** stann., **SULPH.,** sul-ac., ***ter.,*** teucr., ther., verat., ziz.
after dinner - kali-c.
hot - acon., coc-c.
bending backward amel. - thuj.
brain, was compressed, as if whole - asaf.
breakfast amel. - bov.
chill, during - tarent.
closing eyes amel. - ***chel.,*** sulph.
coughing, on - ferr., iris, petr.
dinner, after - bar-c., kali-c., kali-n., lyc.
drinking agg. - merc.
eating, after - con., dios., kali-c., lyc., nat-m., sep.
emotion, after - nat-m.
evening - anac., asaf., camph., hyper., kali-bi., merc., murx., mur-ac., phos., ***rhus-t.,*** sep., stront-c., sulph., tab., tarent., valer.
amel. - anac.
in bed - asaf., merc., ol-an.
extending to eyes and nose - nit-ac.
hat, as of a tight - phys.
pressure of, agg. - **CARB-V.**
heat of sun amel. - stront.
heated, when - **CARB-V.**
laughing, when - iris
lean, forward on a table, must - con.
light from candle - cann-i.
looking, sideways - dig.
steadily agg. - par., ***puls.***
lying amel. - nat-m.
back, on, while - mez.
menses, during - gels., helon., iod., lyc., merc., plat., sulph.
before - hep., nat-c., sil.
mental exertion, from - iris, par., ***sulph.***

CONSTRICTION, tension
morning - agar., bry., cham., con., gamb., graph., kali-bi., nat-m., nux-m., sulph., sumb., tarax.
amel. - glon.
rising, after - lyc.
motion, from - asar., ***bry.,*** carb-v., hipp., iris, ir-foe., mez., par., valer.
amel. - op., sulph., valer.
in open air amel. - acon.
net, as if in a - apis, nat-m.
night - merc., mez., nux-v.
paroxysmal - crot-c.
periodic - phos.
pressure amel. - aeth., anac., lach., meny., thuj.
reading, while - agn.
rising amel. - dig., laur., merc.
room, on entering - bov.
amel. - hep., valer., verb.
sitting, agg. - fl-ac.
amel. - asar., nat-m.
bent forward agg. - asaf.
sleeping agg. - graph., merc.
sleeping agg, on affected side - caust.
sneezing, on - kali-chl.
standing agg. - mag-c.
stool, during - coloc.
stooping agg. - berb., coloc., dig., med., thuj.
string, as if by - anac., asaf., bell., chin., cycl., **GELS.,** graph., hell., iod., lach., merc., merc-i-r., mosch., nat-c., ***nat-m.,*** nit-ac., plat., psor., **SULPH.**
from nape to ears - anac.
supper, after - ***carb-v.***
swallowing on - mag-c.
talking - nat-m.
thread were stretched from nape to eyes, as if - lach.
uncovering head amel. - ***carb-v.***
vomiting amel. - stann.
waking, on - anac., ***ant-t.,*** bry., graph., naja, nux-v., tarent.
walking, while - ang., ***asar., chin.,*** hipp., thea.
in open air amel. - ox-ac.
warm room - acon., ***bry.,*** cann-i., ***carb-v.,*** plat.
warmth amel. - stront.
washing, after - ***ant-t.***
wet weather agg. - sulph.
writing, while - gent-l., ***lyc.***

constriction, forehead - ***acon., aesc.,*** aeth., agn., ail., aloe, alum., ***ambr., anac., ant-t.,*** apis, arg-n., arn., ars., asaf., ***bar-c.,*** bapt., bell., berb., bism., bry., calc., ***calc-p.,*** calc-s., camph., cann-s., ***carb-ac.,*** carb-an., carb-s., carb-v., card-m., caust., ***cham.,*** chel., chin., clem., coff., cocc., colch., coloc., crot-t., ***cycl., dig.,*** dros., dulc., elat., euph., fl-ac., gels., glon., ***graph., grat.,*** haem., ham., hell., helon., hep., hyos., ign., ip., iris, kali-ar., kali-c., kali-n., kali-p., kali-s., lac-c., lac-ac., laur., lepi., mag-m., manc., mang., med., meny., **MERC.,** mosch., ***naja, nat-c., nat-m.,***

constriction, forehead - nat-p., ***nit-ac.,*** nux-m., nux-v., olnd., osm., par., ***phos.,*** phys., phyt., ***plat.,*** plb., psor., ***puls.,*** rheum, ***rhod.,*** rhus-t., ruta., sabad., sabin., sep., ***sil.,*** spig., stann., staph., ***sulph.,*** ***sul-ac.,*** sul-i., tarax., ther., valer., verat., verb., zinc.
above - con., sumb.
across - arn., bar-c., cann-i., iris, laur., lepi., naja, op., par., phys., sabin., sep., verat.
alternating with expansion - tarax.
band, as from - aeth., ant-t., bar-c., ***cact.,*** **CARB-AC.,** ***carb-v.,*** cedr., ***chel.,*** ***coca,*** gels., ***graph.,*** helon., indg., iod., iris, lil-t., manc., med., **MERC.,** ***merc-c.,*** merc-i-r., mill., phos., sang., sulph., sul-i., tarent.
closing eyes amel. - ***chel.***
laughing, from - iod.
noon - ***chel.***
coughing, on - iris, mosch., verb.
eating, after - bar-c., rhus-t.
eyes, over the - aeth., anag., apis, ars., asaf., bell., bor., bry., ***card-m.,*** chel., colch., dulc., euphr., ***glon.,*** iod., ip., meny., merl., nux-m., plat., ***puls.,*** sang., sil., sul-i.
left - bor.
looking intently - ***puls.***
right - nat-c.
touch amel. - meny.
hand, on part amel. - con.
intermittent - arn., hyos., plat.
margin of orbits to temples, from - cann-s.
pressure amel. - aeth., ***anac.***
morning - naja
rising, on - sumb.
narrow, as if too - gels.
stooping, amel. - con.
string, as by - merc-i-r., nat-c.

constriction, nerves - graph.

constriction, occiput - agar., alum., anac., ***asaf.,*** bar-c., berb., calc., calc-s., cann-s., **CARB-S.,** carb-v., ***chel.,*** chin., ***cimic.,*** coloc., dulc., euph., glon., **GRAPH.,** hell., hyos., ip., kali-i., lach., lact., laur., lob., lyc., mag-c., manc., merc., ***mez.,*** mosch., mur-ac., murx., nat-c., nat-m., par., psor., ruta., stann., staph., ***sulph.,*** sumb., thuj., verat., viol-o., ziz.
alternating with tension of face - ***viol-o.***
coughing, on - mag-c., mosch.
evening - mur-ac., murx., sumb.
extending, into nape of neck - graph., nat-c.
to finger joints - plect.
to forehead - mur-ac.
upward, downward and toward ears - **GLON.**
forenoon - agar., alum.
night, lying on back - mez.
side - staph.
standing, on - mag-c.
swallowing - mag-c.
waking, on - anac., graph.
writing, while - lyc.

constriction, sides - ant-t., apis, asaf., bar-c., calc., caust., chin-s., clem., coloc., dig., fl-ac., mur-ac., ruta, spig., ***stront.***

constriction, sides,
extending, into orbits and teeth - crot-h.
to left upper teeth, stitch-like in spots, on stooping, amel. on rising - dig.

constriction, temples - acon., ail., alum., ambr., ***anac.,*** ant-t., arn., ars., bar-c., berb., bov., calc., ***cann-s.,*** carb-v., caust., ***carb-an.,*** cinnb., clem., coloc., elaps, elat., glon., hell., hyper., ip., lith., lyc., mag-m., mang., merl., mur-ac., naja, nat-m., ol-an., pall., ph-ac., ***plat.,*** plb., ***puls.,*** rheum, ***squil.,*** tab., thuj., verat., verb., zinc.
band from temple to like a - carb-ac.
cough, during - lach., mag-c., merc., mosch., verb.
morning - sulph.
opening mouth - ang.
pressure amel. - alum.

constriction, vertex - ant-t., apis, cact., calc., carb-an., chel., con., gent-c., kali-i., kali-n., lyc., meny., mosch., naja, nat-m., phos., plat., rheum, sep., stann., staph., stront-c., verat., verb.
afternoon and night - kali-n.
evening - phos.
exertion of vision - gent-c.
extending to jaw - stront.
menses, during - lyc., nat-m., phos.
mental exertion - gent-c.
morning - kali-n., staph.

CONTRACTION, sensation of, of scalp - aeth., ***carb-v.,*** lyc., lyss., merc., par., plat., ran-s., rhus-t., sanic., stann., spig.

contraction, sensation of, forehead - bell., ***cycl.,*** lyc., ***sanic.***

CONVULSIONS, of the right side of head - mygal.

COVERS, head (see Coldness, uncovering)

CRACKING, sensation in - acon., ars., calc., carb-v., cham., con., dig., glon., kalm., puls., sep., spig.
as if something broke - sep.
blowing nose, after - hep.
evening - acon.
forehead - acon., spig.
motion agg. - acon.
shivering, with - kalm.
siesta, during - dig.
sitting, while - carb-v., coff.
amel. - acon.
turning the when - sep.

CRACKING, occiput - ***calc.,*** carb-v., ***sep.***

cracking, side - acon., arn., ars., calc., cham., coff., ***hep.***

cracking, vertex - ***coff.,*** con.

CRAMPING, pain - ***acon.,*** alum., ***ambr.,*** am-m., anac., ang., ***ant-t.,*** ars., asaf., calc., carb-v., cina, colch., ***coloc.,*** croc., eug., gels., ***ign.,*** kali-c., mag-m., mez., nit-ac., nux-v., olnd., petr., ***ph-ac.,*** ***plat.,*** psor., ran-s., rheum, sep., squil., stann., teucr., thuj., verb., zinc.
evening - alum.
extending to malar-bone - bell.
morning, early, after rising - mag-c.

CRAMPING, pain
rubbing forehead amel. - thuj.
study and exertion from, after ague - gels.
suppressed catarrh, from - ***acon.***
vexation, after - mag-c.
cramping, forehead - aeth., bell., calc., croc., ign., nat-c., ***plat.***
above root of nose - arn., bell., spong.
as if would lose senses - ***acon.,*** ign.
extending to eyes - nat-c.
to lower jaw - bell.
to nose - nat-c.
to vertex - calc.
cramping, occiput - am-m., ***camph.,*** dios.
small spot, in - am-m.
stooping - camph.
cramping, sides - bell., phos., sars., thuj.
left - phos., thuj.
cold, crampy - phos.
right - bell.
cramping, temples - agar., ***calc.,*** cann-s., cina, indg., ***kali-c.,*** nat-m., ***petr.,*** plat., sil., verb., zinc.
afternoon - ***plat.***
extending into teeth - nat-m.
left - agar., indg., kali-c., sil.
muscle - cocc.
right - nat-m.
tickling, with - cann-s.
cramping, vertex - chin., coloc., phos.

CRAWLING, sensation (see Formication)

CRUSHED, pain, as if shattered, beated to pieces - acon., aeth., alum., anan., **ARG-M.,** ars., aur., bar-c., bell., bov., calc., camph., caul., caust., cham., ***chin., cocc.,*** coff., ***con.,*** euph., graph., hell., hyos., **IGN.,** iod., ***ip.,*** kali-c., ***lach.,*** lyss., mang., merc., mur-ac., nat-m., nat-s., nux-v., ph-ac., **PHOS.,** puls., rhus-t., **RUTA,** ***sep., sil.,*** stann., stront-c., sul-ac., verat., verb., vib.
morning - sul-ac.
crushed, vertex - ip.

CUTTING, pain - acon., aesc., agar., ail., alum., ambr., am-c., ***apis,*** arg-m., ***arg-n., arn., ars., aur.,*** bell., bism., cadm-s., **CALC.,** camph., cann-s., canth., caps., carb-ac., ***carb-an.,*** carb-s., carb-v., caust., chel., chin., cina, cinnb., cocc., con., croc., cupr., dig., dros., ferr., glon., graph., hell., hep., hura, ip., **IRIS,** ***kali-bi.,*** kali-chl., ***kali-i.,*** kreos., ***lach.,*** lyc., mag-c., manc., merc., mosch., mur-ac., nat-m., nit-ac., par., petr., psor., puls., sang., sars., sep., ***sil.,*** spig., squil., staph., tarent., til., verat.
afternoon - nat-p., ptel.
air, agg. - nat-m.
amel. - am-c.
binding up head amel. - carb-ac.
blowing nose - sep.
brain were cut to pieces, on stopping, as if - nicc.
closing eyes amel. - til.
cold air agg. - kali-i., ***spig.***
applications amel. - til.
coughing, when - asim., bell., ziz.

CUTTING, pain
evening - ***bell.,*** kali-i.
exertion, on - ambr., til.
heat agg. - kali-i.
amel. - ***lach.***
knife, as with a - alum., ***arg-n., arn., bell.,*** calc., cocc., ***con.,*** kali-bi., lach., mag-c., mag-s., nat-m.
followed by sensation of coldness - arn.
light - carb-ac.
lying amel. - ambr.
menses, after - ***nat-m.***
morning - coloc., mag-c.
motion, agg. - chin., til.
amel. - kali-i.
of arms - caust.
of eyes - dros.
night - dig.
noise - carb-ac.
rest, agg. - caps.
amel. - til.
sleep, amel. - stram.
sleep, during - dig.
split by a wedge, as if, body icy cold, thirst - lachn.
standing, while - agar., calc.
stepping agg. - alum., ambr.
stooping, on - arn., caust., chin., dros., ferr-p., nicc.
storm, before - ***sil.***
supporting head on hands amel. - dros., hydr.
thinking of it amel. - cic.
turning head - cupr.
vexation, after - ***mag-c.***
walking, agg. - calc.
amel. - ***caps.,*** hep.
wind, in cold - lyc.
cutting, forehead - acon., aesc., agar., am-c., ***arg-n., bell.,*** bism., calc., camph., carb-ac., ***caust., chel.,*** cinnb., coc-c., coloc., con., ***cupr.,*** cycl., dios., dros., ferr., jug-r., kali-bi., ***lach.,*** lyc., lyss., mag-c., mang., nat-m., podo., sabin., seneg., sep., stann., staph., tarent., ter., **VALER.**
air, open agg. - kali-bi.
blowing nose, on - sep.
coughing, on - hyos., ziz.
extending, right to left - ***aesc.***
to occiput - ***bell.,*** bism.
eyes above - ***hydr.***
right - bism., ***chel.,*** nat-a.
knife, as with - ***lach.,*** mang., nat-m., sabin., ter.
left, side - caust.
lying down - camph.
menses, during - apis
morning - coloc., viol-t.
motion, on - acon., arn., lach.
of arms violently - caust.
nose, above root of - led.
pressure agg. - calc., ***cupr.***
pulsating - acon.
standing, while - agar.
stooping, when - caust.

cutting, forehead
walking agg. - calc.
cutting, occiput - aesc., ail., ***arg-n.,*** aster., ***aur-s., bell., bufo, calc.,*** canth., ***caps.,*** carb-an., chin., ***con., cupr.,*** dig., glon., med., mur-ac., nat-m., sang., sars., **SULPH.**
extending, to eyes - chin.
to forehead - arg-n., camph.
knife, as with a - ***con.,*** nat-m.
motion agg. - chin.
night - **SYPH.**
pressure agg. - calc.
pulsation, with every - ***con.***
stooping agg. - chin.
walking - calc.
cutting, sides - arg-n., ***arn.,*** aur., ***bell., calc., chel.,*** cic., cocc., hura, iris, kali-bi., ***lach.,*** mang., nat-m., nat-p., rumx., spig., tarent.
ascending - lach.
coughing, on - mang.
knife, as with a - ***arn.***
left - ***arg-n.,*** cupr.
morning - tarent.
pressure, on - aesc.
right - ***bell.***
warm applications amel. - lach.
cutting, temples - acon., agar., ail., alum., apoc., arg-m., ***arg-n.,*** arum-t., aster., bapt., bar-c., **BELL.,** calc., camph., canth., carb-ac., carb-s., ***chel.,*** chin., cimic., coc-c., ***coloc., croc.,*** crot-c., cupr-ar., cycl., dios., eup-per., euphr., form., genist., glon., graph., guai., ***ham.,*** hura, ***hydr.,*** iris, kali-bi., **KALI-I.,** lac-c., lach., ***lyc.,*** mag-c., manc., med., nat-p., ***nit-ac.,*** onos., ph-ac., phos., plb., ptel., ***puls.,*** rhus-t., sang., senec., stram., stront-c., sulph., tarent., verb., xan.
extending to eyes - berb., chin.
to eyes, jaw - glôn.
to eyes, temple to temple - **BELL.,** ***chin., sulph.***
knife, as with a - cycl., ferr., lach., stram.
knife, as with a, during difficult stool - ***lyc.***
left - bar-c., ***coloc.,*** genist., guai., ***kali-i.,*** onos.
when chewing - am-c.
lying down, after - camph.
motion, agg. - chin.
pressure agg. - verb.
rhythmical - calc.
right - apoc., ***chel.,*** ptel., stram., verb.
stool, straining at - ***lyc.***
stooping, agg. - chin.
cutting, vertex - acon., aur., ***bell.,*** calc., ***carb-an.,*** con., ***lach.,*** nat-m., senec., **THUJ.,** verat.
walking, while - ***carb-an.***

DANDRUFF - all-s., alum., ***am-m., ars.,*** bad., ***bar-c.,*** bran., ***bry., calc., calc-s.,*** **CANTH., CARB-S.,** carc., ***dulc.,*** fl-ac., **GRAPH.,** hep., hera., iod., kali-c., kali-chl., kali-p., ***kali-s.,*** lac-c., ***lyc.,*** mag-c., ***med., mez.,*** **NAT-M.,** ***olnd.,*** **PHOS.,** ***psor.,*** sanic., ***sep., staph.,*** sul-i., **SULPH.,** ***thuj.***

DANDRUFF, scalp
white - alum., ***kali-chl., mez.,*** **NAT-M.,** ***phos.,*** **THUJ.**
yellow - **KALI-S.**

DECAY, of bones - arg-m., asaf., **AUR.,** caps., ***fl-ac., hep.,*** hippoz., ***nat-m.,*** **NIT-AC.,** ***ph-ac.,*** **PHOS., SIL.,** ***staph.***

DIGGING, pain (see Boring)

DISTENTION, (see Bloodvessels)

DRAGGING, sensation in - ant-t., calc., canth., crot-h., gels., laur., merl., nat-m., rhus-t.
extending to shoulders - gels.
sitting and leaning against high pillow amel. - gels.

DRAWING, pain - ***acon.,*** aeth., ***agar.,*** ail., ang., alum., ambr., am-c., ant-t., apis, aran., arg-m., arg-n., ***ars.,*** asar., aur., aur-m., bapt., bar-c., bell., berb., bism., bor., bov., ***bry., calc., calc-p.,*** camph., canth., caps., carb-an., ***carb-s., carb-v., caust., cham.,*** **CHIN.,** cimx., cimic., cina, coff., coloc., ***con.,*** croc., cupr., cycl., dulc., eug., eupi., ferr., ferr-ar., ***gels., glon.,*** gran., ***graph.,*** guai., hell., hipp., hydr., ip., kali-c., ***kali-i.,*** kali-p., kali-s., kalm., ***kreos.,*** lach., lil-t., lyc., ***mag-c.,*** mang., meny., **MERC.,** merc-c., mez., ***mosch.,*** nat-a., nat-c., ***nat-m.,*** nat-p., nit-ac., **NUX-V.,** ol-an., petr., ***phos., plat., plb., puls.,*** ran-s., rheum, ***rhod., rhus-t.,*** ruta., sabad., sabin., sars., seneg., ***sep., sil.,*** squil., stann., ***staph.,*** stront-c., stry., **SULPH.,** ***sul-ac.,*** thuj., til., valer., verat., zinc., zing.
afternoon - agar., ant-t., dulc., gins., verat-v., zing.
air, cold, agg. - ***caust.***
open, in - ***con.,*** grat., kalm., mang., plect.
open, in amel. - asar., hell., olnd.
bed, in - agar., hell., hipp.
warm amel. - caust.
breath, when holding - agar.
chewing, while - sulph.
chilliness, during - eupi., ***glon.***
church, while in - zinc.
closing eyes - sabad.
amel. - til.
cold applications amel. - til.
cough, during - iris
damp weather, during - ***rhod., rhus-t.***
amel. - caust.
dinner, after - bell., nat-c., phos.
dinner, during - kali-c.
draught of air from - til., valer.
eating, after - ant-t., bell., chin., crot-h., mill., nat-c., phos.
amel. - con., sulph.
eating, during - dulc.
evening - all-c., aloe, ang., bov., cast., crot-h., dulc., graph., hipp., kali-n., kalm., ol-an., phos., ran-b., stront-c., sul-ac., valer., zinc.
amel. in - coloc.
extending, ears, to - mag-m., sep.
eyes, to - **NIT-AC.**

DRAWING, pain
extending, face, to - ant-t., aran., graph., mag-m., seneg.
forward - carb-v., nat-m.
here and there - ambr., ip., mosch., nux-v.
neck, to - graph.
nose, to - ant-t.
occiput, to - ***ars.,*** glon.
spine, to - kali-n., ***mosch.,*** thuj.
teeth, to - mag-m., sep.
temples, to - asar., sep.
forenoon - kali-c.
hat, pressure of - carb-v.
heat of sun amel. - stront.
heated, when - carb-v.
house, on entering, amel. - mang., plect.
lying down amel. - asar.
with head high amel. - gels.
menses, during - berb., mag-c., sang.
mental exertion, from - bor., calc-caust., cina, coff., gins., nat-m., sulph.
morning - agar., ang., dros., hell., kali-bi., mag-c., mez., petr., rhod., sulph., zinc.
rising, on - nat-m.
waking, on, passes off on rising - am-c.
motion, on - arg-n., bism., tab., til.
amel. - arg-m., bell., eupi., ***rhod., rhus-t.***
moving on - cact., staph.
nausea, during - croc.
night - agar., ***kali-c.,*** nat-m., phos., rhus-t., sep.
noon - phos.
amel. - **BRY.**
paroxysms - carb-v., thuj.
periosteum, as if in - ***merc., merc-c.***
preceded by drawing in arm - petr.
pressure, agg. - agar., cina
amel. - chin.
pulsating - ars.
rising, when - bry., coloc., nat-m.
round the head - bov., carb-v.
sitting, while - arg-m., chin., meny., ***mur-ac.,*** squil.
sneezing, amel. - mag-m.
frequent, amel. - lil-t.
standing, while - agar., mag-c.
amel. - ***tarax.***
stooping low, on - ***ign.***
stretching agg. - agar.
stripes, as if, in - arg-n.
swallowing, on - mag-c.
thunderstorm, during - ***rhod.***
tightening - asaf., bar-c., cann-i., carb-v., ***caust.,*** clem., coloc., dig., ***graph.,*** gymn., hep., kali-chl., lyc., mag-c., mag-m., mang., meny., ***mosch.,*** nat-c., nat-m., nit-ac., nux-v., olnd., op., par., petr., rhod., sabad., samb., stram., sulph., ther., verb.
to and fro - ambr.
touch, on - con., **STAPH.**
waking, when - agar.
walking while - chel., coloc.
warmth, amel. - stront.
of bed amel. - caust.

drawing, forehead - acon., **AGAR.,** all-c., am-c., anac., ang., ant-c., ant-t., ***arg-n., ars.,*** asaf., asar., aur-m., aur-m-n., bad., bar-c., ***bell.,*** benz-ac., bor., bry., calc., cann-i., cann-s., canth., ***caps.,*** carb-an., carb-s., carb-v., cast., caust., chel., chin., cic., ***cimic.,*** cina, clem., cocc., colch., ***coloc.,*** con., ***croc.,*** cycl., dulc., eupi., ferr., gins., ***graph., guai.,*** hell., hipp., ***ign.,*** **KALI-C.,** kali-n., kali-p., lact., laur., led., lil-t., ***lyc., mag-c., mang.,*** meny., **MERC.,** mez., mosch., ***nat-a., nat-c., nat-m.,*** nat-s., nit-ac., **NUX-V.,** petr., phos., ***plat.,*** psor., ***puls.,*** ran-b., rat., rheum, ***rhod.,*** ruta., sabad., sabin., sel., seneg., ***sep.,*** sil., squil., ***stann.,*** staph., ***stront-c., sulph.,*** tarax., ter., thuj., valer., verb., viol-o., ***zinc.,*** zing.
afternoon, 2 p.m. - verat.
alternating with pains in the wrist - sulph.
chill, during - petr.
dinner, after - phos.
evening - ang., bar-c., graph., kali-c., kali-n.
exertion, during - ***zinc.***
extending to, ears - mang.
eyes - agar., cann-i., glon., hep., ***kali-c.,*** lil-t.
to, lower jaw - nat-m., rhus-t.
to, neck - bor., kali-n., ***mosch.,*** viol-t.
to, nose - **AGAR.,** dulc., glon., guai., ***kali-c.,*** nux-v.
to, occiput - dros., graph., ***sep.***
to, teeth - rhus-t.
to, upward - nit-ac
to, vertex - sep.
eyes, above - ***agar.,*** asaf., bry., calc., ***cann-i.,*** carb-an., ***chel.,*** colch., con., ***ign.,*** lyss., nat-m., nit-ac., ***puls.,*** seneg., sil., spig., stann., sulph., thuj., zinc.
blowing, nose agg. - mag-c.
extending, upwards - staph.
feel as if projecting, with sensation as if a thread were tightly drawn through eyeball and backward into middle of brain, sight weak - **PAR.**
left - chel., mag-c., nat-m., thuj., spig.
mental exertion - calc.
right - aur., carb-v., dulc., ign., lyss.
forenoon - ***kali-c.,*** mag-c., sulph., thuj.
forenoon, 10 a.m. - thuj.
intermittent - agar., thuj.
left - asaf., bar-c., cina, clem., colch., ***coloc.,*** cycl., dulc., ***rhod.,*** thuj., verb., viol-o.
lying, while - nat-m.
menses, during - mag-c.
mental exertion - asar., ***calc.,*** sulph.
morning - agar., am-c., mez., nat-m., ***nux-v.***
waking, on - agar., am-c., ***nux-v.,*** thuj.
night - nat-m.
night, midnight - ***kali-c.***
noon - petr., zing.
nose, above root of - acon., agar., asar., ***carb-v.,*** caust., ***hep.,*** meny., merc., nat-m., rheum, spong., zing.
above root of, mental exertion, on - nat-m.
opening eyes agg. - ars.

drawing, forehead
paroxysmal - zinc.
pressure amel. - mang.
raising the eyes - puls.
reading - bor.
right - caps., meny., nit-ac., rat., ruta., sabin., stann.
rising, after - coloc.
side of forehead - stann.
right, side - ars.
to left and back to left - cycl.
to left and to left temple - cycl.
left to temple - plat.
sitting, while - ***aur-m-n.***
standing, while - agar., tarax.
stooping - bor., dulc., mang.
touch amel. - cycl.
turning eyes to side - dig.
walking, while - arg-n., mang., rat.
wandering - chel.
wine agg. - rhod.
worm, as if a, crept through - sulph.
writing - bor.

drawing, occiput - ***agar.,*** ambr., anac., ant-t., ***arg-m.,*** arg-n., **ARN.,** asaf., aur-m-n., bell., **BRY.,** cact., calad., calc., ***calc-p.,*** camph., cann-s., carb-s., ***carb-v.,*** caust., ***chel.,*** chin., cocc., coc-c., coloc., corn., cycl., dros., ***ferr., gels.,*** gins., glon., graph., guai., hyper., ip., kali-bi., kali-c., ***kali-n.,*** laur., mag-c., mang., meny., merc., mill., mosch., ***mur-ac.,*** nat-c., nat-p., nat-s., ***nux-v.,*** ph-ac., phos., plat., plect., puls., ran-b., raph., rhod., rhus-t., sabin., sel., ***sep.,*** spig., squil., staph., sulph., valer., ***zinc.***
afternoon - agar.
bed, in - agar., graph.
bend head backward, must - chin.
bending head backward amel. - cact.
forward, on - staph.
bones of occiput - chin., ph-ac.
chewing, while - sulph.
eating, after - agar., ant-t.
evening in bed - graph.
extending, ears, to - bar-c., cann-s.
forehead, to - arg-m., chel., chin., nat-c., sars.
neck, to, before going to sleep - ***bry.***
neck, to, nape of - merc., mur-ac., nat-c., plect., sulph.
nose, to - corn.
upper neck region and shoulders, to, amel. resting head high on pillow, with eyes half shut, sleepy - gels.
upward from nape of neck - ambr., carb-v., ferr., sep., staph.
forenoon - sulph.
mental exertion - ***calc.,*** chin.
morning - kali-bi.
motion, agg. - ph-ac.
amel. - arg-m.
of head - ***cact.,*** staph.
noon amel. - **BRY.**
occipital protuberance, extending to eye - mur-ac.

drawing, occiput
pressure amel. - chin., mang.
side, as he turns head to side - calc.
sides - alum., aur-m-n., ***carb-v., chel.,*** chin., ***fl-ac.,*** kali-n., kali-s., laur., meny., mez., nat-s., phos., sep., thuj., zinc.
alternating with similar sensation in the ball of thumb - arg-m.
bending head backward amel. - chin.
cramp-like - kali-n., plat., ***sulph.***
drawn back, as if head would be - nat-c.
extending from left to right - ***squil.***
extending to forward - cycl.
forenoon - alum., sulph.
left - calc., ***carb-v., chel.,*** cycl., zinc.
left to lower jaw- plat.
paroxysmal - rhod.
pressive - ***chin., spig.***
rheumatic - coff.
right - alum., caust., nat-c., rhod., zinc.
sneezing - calc.
warm room - zing.
sitting, while - chin., meny., squil.
standing, while - chin., mag-c.
stooping - mang.
swallowing - mag-c.
touch, on - chin.
walking amel. - chin.
wandering - mez.

drawing, sides - ***acon.,*** alum., anac., ang., ant-t., apis, ***arg-m.,*** arg-n., arn., asaf., bar-c., bar-ac., bell., brom., bry., calc., camph., canth., caps., carb-v., caust., ***cham.,*** chin., cimx., cina, clem., cocc., colch., coloc., dig., dros., fl-ac., gran., guai., hell., indg., iod., ip., ***kali-c.,*** kali-n., kali-p., lach., led., lyc., meny., nat-s., nit-ac., nux-v., ph-ac., phos., plat., rhus-t., ruta, sars., sep., spong., sul-ac., thuj., valer.
air, open - grat.
dinner, after - phos., zinc.
draft of cold air - caust.
evening - phos.
extending to, behind ears - caust.
to, clavicle - ind.
to, face - cupr.
to, forehead - bry., phos., sul-ac.
to, neck - ***chel.,*** cupr-ac., lyc.
to, orbits - crot-h., stann.
to, teeth - crot-h., iod., nat-m.
to, temple - iod.
forward - hell.
increases gradually and ceases suddenly, feeling as if a nerve had been torn - arg-m.
left - anac., ant-t., apis, arg-m., arn., bar-c., brom., caps., cinnb., colch., hell., iod., **KALI-C., NIT-AC.,** rhus-t., sars., sep.
extending to, frontal eminence - guai.
motion agg. - arg-n.
night - phos.
rheumatic - sep.
right - alum., arg-n., asaf., ***bell.,*** calc., camph., cocc., fl-ac., lach., lyc., ***ph-ac.,*** phos., sars., spong., sul-ac., thuj., valer.
side lain on - ph-ac.

drawing, sides
spots - phos.
tearing - phos., thuj.
twitching - plat.
warm bed amel. - caust.

drawing, temples - acon., ***agar.,*** ambr., ang., ant-c., ***ant-t., arg-m.,*** asar., aur-m., bar-c., ***bell., bry.,*** cact., ***calc.,*** cann-i., canth., carb-s., casc., caust., chel., chin-s., ***cina,*** coc-c., coff., colch., ***coloc., con.,*** croc., cupr., cycl., dulc., eupi., guai., hep., hipp., indg., kali-bi., kreos., ***lach.,*** laur., lyc., mang., merc., mez., mosch., nit-ac., ***nux-v.,*** ol-an., olnd., ***petr.,*** ph-ac., phos., phyt., plat., ran-b., raph., rhod., rhus-t., ruta., sabad., sabin., sars., seneg., spig., squil., stann., stront-c., sulph., sul-ac., tab., tarax., thuj., til., zinc., zing.
afternoon - dulc.
air, open, amel. - olnd.
ceasing suddenly - caust.
chewing agg. - thuj.
chilliness, during - eupi.
closing eyes - sabin.
coughing - ***cina.***
eating, after - calc.
eating, while - calc.
evening - alum., alumn., calc., dig., ran-b., zinc.
extending, to ear - hell.
to eye - aloe.
to face - ant-t., arg-m., ***bry.,*** seneg.
to forehead, across - bell., chin-s., lach., lact., lyc., sabin.
to head - ambr., dulc.
to jaw, upper - arg-n.
to malar bone - **BRY.**
to vertex - aur-m., cycl.
increasing gradually - caust.
left - ant-c., ***arg-m.,*** colch., caps., cycl., dulc., ***lach., petr.,*** ph-ac., plat., ***spig.,*** staph., sul-ac., ***tarax.,*** thuj., zinc.
motion, on - tab.
one-sided - cham.
periodical, every two days - cact.
pressure agg. - cina.
amel. - ant-c.
pulsating - staph.
right - ***bell., calc.,*** caust., ***cina,*** coff., ***merc., nit-ac.,*** sabad., ***sars.,*** squil.
sitting, while - arg-m., ***tarax.***
spots - sul-ac.
standing amel. - ***tarax.***
touch, on - con.
walking - con.
amel. - ***tarax.***
worm creeping sensation - sulph.

drawing, vertex - anac., ant-t., arg-m., ***arn.,*** ars., bov., ***calc., calc-p.,*** caust., ***chel.,*** cinnb., crot-h., dulc., grat., hell., indg., iod., ***kali-c.,*** kali-p., led., nux-m., nux-v., ol-an., ph-ac., phos., ran-b., ran-s., ruta., sars., sil., spig., spong., stann., thuj., til., zinc.
before going to bed - cinnb.
cramp-like - phos.
evening - bor., crot-h., dulc., ol-an.

drawing, vertex
extending, to eyes - nux-m.
to forehead - led.
to neck - chel.
to nose while eating - dulc.
to temple - bor., chel.
morning - hell.
motion agg. - ph-ac.
paroxysmal - zinc.
pressure amel. - ph-ac.
walking, while - chel.

DRAWN, backward (see Falling) - ***acon.,*** acet-ac., ***ant-t., apis, bell.,*** camph., cann-i., ***carb-ac.,*** cedr., ***cham., chin.,*** **CIC.,** ***cimic., cina, cupr.,*** cur., dig., ***eup-per., gels., glon., hell., hep., ign., ip.,*** kreos., ***lyc., mag-c., med.,*** mur-ac., nat-c., ***nat-m.,*** nit-ac., ***nux-v., op., phel.,*** samb., ***stram.,*** stry., verat-v., viol-t., zinc.
convulsions, in - **CIC.,** ***ign.,*** mosch., ***nux-v., op.,*** tab.
menses, during - zinc.
sleep during - alum., ***hep.***
downwards - sulph.
forwards - bar-m., hydr-ac., merc., mur-ac., par., plb., sang.
headache in occiput and vertex, with - spig.
sideways - ars., ***bar-c.,*** bell., calc., camph., caul., ***caust.,*** chel., chin., cic., cina, colch., cupr., dulc., eup-pur., gels., hura, kali-ar., lac-c., ***lach., lachn.,*** **LYC.,** merc., ***nux-v.,*** plb., puls., ***rhus-t.,*** sabad., sil., stram., sulph., tax.
epilepsy, before - bufo, ***caust.,*** **LYC.**
first left then right - ***stram.***
first right then left - ang., ***nux-m.***
right, to - ***caust., ferr.,*** **LYC.,** ***nux-m.***
upon shoulders - ***agar.,*** hydr-ac.

DRYNESS, scalp - skook.
dryness, vertex - ars., frax.

DULL, pain, (see Headaches, general) - ***aesc., agar.,*** ail., ***all-c.,*** alum., ***anac.,*** ant-c., ***apis,*** arg-m., ***arg-n.,*** arum-t., ***bapt.,*** bar-c., bism., bov., bry., calc., camph., cann-i., canth., carb-an., ***carb-s.,*** carb-v., caust., cham., chel., ***chin., cimic.,*** cina, ***clem., cocc., coll.,*** coff., croc., crot-h., crot-t., cupr., ***dios., dulc., echi.,*** eup-pur., ferr., **GELS.,** glon., ***graph.,*** ham., hell., hep., hyos., ***hyper.,*** ign., ***ind., kalm., lach.,*** lachn., lact., laur., led., ***lyc.,*** mag-m., mang., meny., meph., ***merc.,*** mosch., ***nat-c.,*** nat-m., nat-s., ***nit-ac.,*** **NUX-V.,** ***op.,*** petr., ***ph-ac.,*** phos., plat., ***podo.,*** **PULS.,** ran-s., rheum, rhod., ***rhus-t.,*** sabad., ***sang.,*** sars., sec., ***seneg.,*** sep., sil., spig., spong., squil., ***stry.,*** sulph., sul-ac., teucr., ter., thuj., urt-u., verat., verb., viol-o., viol-t.
afternoon - bapt.
brain, base of - gels., hyos.
chill, during - petr.
dinner, after - mag-m., nat-c.
eating amel. - ind.
evening - carb-s., ind., pall., rhus-t.
hemorrhage, during - kali-c.
heat, during - agar.
menses, during - lyc.

DULL, pain
morning - agar., chin., hep., ind., kali-c., lach., nit-ac.
after rising - sep., squil.
morning, waking - ars.
move must, and close eyes - agar.
night - nat-c.
pressure amel. - ***apis,*** cimic.
rising amel. - ars.
smoking - ant-c.

dull, forehead - ***aesc., agar.,*** aloe, ant-c., ant-t., arn., asar., bapt., calc., camph., cann-i., **CARB-AC.,** ***chel.,*** cimic., ***cinnb.,*** cocc., coff., ***coll.,*** coloc., **CUPR.,** cupr-ar., ***dulc.,*** euph., ***euphr.,*** fl-ac., form., ***glon.,*** graph., hell., hydr., hyos., ign., ind., iris, laur., lept., mygal., nat-c., nat-m., ph-ac., phos., ***plat.,*** plb., puls., rheum, sabad., sars., ***sep.,*** verat., zinc.
chill, during - cham.
eye, over - apis, cann-i., nat-a., ***sep.,*** urt-u., zinc.
right frontal eminence, in, then in left - acet-ac.

dull, occiput - ***aesc.,*** alum., ambr., asar., bry., calc., **CARB-V.,** chin., cic., cimic., ***crot-h.,*** cycl., ***echi.,*** fl-ac., **GELS.,** indg., ***ip., lach.,*** med., nat-c., ***nat-s.,*** ran-s., ***rhod.,*** rumx., samb., ***sec.,*** stram., stront-c., thuj., urt-u.
extending to vertex - ***cimic.***
headache coming once a week and spreading over head, amel. by binding head tightly, followed by blindness and sore eyeball - arg-n.

dull, sides - canth., croc., dros., laur., spong., thuj., zinc.
left - ***cinnb.,*** mez., phos., spong., thuj., zinc.
pressure amel. - mez.

dull, temples - aesc., ***agar.,*** calc., **CARB-AC.,** chin., cupr-ar., echi., ind., laur., ph-ac., stront-c., verat.
from temple to temple - lob.

dull, vertex - aeth., ang., ant-c., cimic., gels., graph., lach., mez., phos.

EBULLITIONS, night - bor.

ECZEMA - ***agar., ant-t., arum-t.,*** **ARS.,** astac., ***aur., bar-c., bar-m.,*** berb-a., brom., **CALC.,** calc-s., **CARB-S.,** ***caust.,*** clem., ***cocc., cic., dulc., fl-ac.,*** **GRAPH., HEP.,** hydr., iris, kali-ar., ***kali-bi.,*** kali-m., ***kali-s., kreos., lappa-a.,*** **LYC.,** merc., ***mez.,*** nat-m., nat-p., ***olnd.,*** **PETR.,** ***phyt.,*** **PSOR.,** ***rhus-t., sars.,*** sel., sep., staph., ***sil.,*** **SULPH.,** tell., tub., ust., viol-o., ***viol-t., vinc.***
about the ears - ***ars.,*** arund., bov., chrysar., clem., crot-t., ***graph.,*** hep., kali-n., ***mez.,*** olnd., petr., psor., ***rhus-t.,*** sanic., tell.
behind ears - ars., arund., bov., **CALC.,** ***chrysar.,*** **GRAPH.,** ***hep.,*** jug-r., kali-m., **LYC.,** ***mez., olnd., petr.,*** **PSOR.,** rhus-t., sanic., ***scroph-n.,*** sep., staph., sulph., tell., tub.
margin of hair from ear to ear posteriorly - ***nat-m.,*** nit-ac., petr., **SULPH.**

eczema, occiput - **CAUST.,** ***lyc., petr.,*** **SIL.,** ***staph.,*** sulph.

EDEMA, glabella - kali-c.
scalp, of - ***apis, ars.***

ELONGATED, sensation - ***hyper.,*** lachn.
vertigo, with, and urging to urinate - hyper.

EMPTY - alum., am-c., anac., ant-c., ***arg-m.,*** arn., ***ars.,*** asaf., aster., bar-c., bell., berb., bov., cact., calc., camph., caps., carb-s., ***carb-v.,*** caust., chin-s., ***cina,*** clem., ***cocc., cor-r., cupr.,*** cycl., dulc., euphr., ferr., ferr-ar., ferr-p., glon., gran., ***graph.,*** hipp., hyos., ign., jab., lyc., ***manc.,*** mang., myric., naja, nat-a., nat-c., nat-m., nat-p., nux-v., ox-ac., ***phel.,*** **PHOS.,** pic-ac., plan., ***puls., sec., seneg.,*** sep., spig., staph., stram., ***sulph.,*** zing.
afternoon - nux-m.
air, in open - cocc., sulph.
bed, amel. on getting warm in - cocc.
eating, after - cocc., graph., meny.
headache, during - calc.
intoxication, as after - acon., agar., ambr., spig.
morning - anac., bov., chin-s., euphr., sulph., verat.
night agg. lying on occiput, amel. by pressure of hand - sep.
pressure of hand amel. - mang., sep.
riding amel. - euphr.
sitting, while - spig.
sleep, after restless - hipp.
talking, while - lyc., spig., ***sulph.***
warm bed amel. - cocc.

empty, in, forehead - alum., **CAUST.,** croc., spig., sulph., sul-ac.
as if between forehead and brain - caust.

empty, occiput - mang., nat-c., sep., ***staph., sulph.***
empty, while brain in front seems too large - hell.

empty, sides - stann.

empty, temples - cycl.

ENLARGED, sensation (see Expanded, Swollen) - **AGAR.,** ant-c., apis, apoc., **ARG-N., ARN.,** ars., ars-m., bapt., **BELL.,** ***berb.,*** **BOV.,** cact., caj., ***caps., cimic.,*** cob., coll., com., ***cor-r.,*** daph., ***dulc., echi., gels.,*** gent-l., gins., **GLON.,** hell., ***hyper.,*** indg., kali-ar., kali-i., ***lac-d.,*** lach., lachn., lac-ac., lact., laur., lith., ***mang.,*** meph., merc., merc-c., nat-c., ***nat-m.,*** **NUX-M., NUX-V.,** ***par.,*** phel., ***plat.,*** **RAN-B.,** ran-s., rhus-t., ***sil., spig.,*** sulph., tarax., ther., til., verat., zing.
afternoon, 4 p.m. - ***mang.***
bandaging amel. - ***arg-n.***
elongated - hyper.
extended upward, the vertex seems - lachn.
the vertex seems, and as if split open by a wedge from the outside - lach.
fever, with intermittent - ***cimic.***
headache, with - gels.
lying, while, rising agg. - rhus-r.
rising amel. - dulc.
menses, during - arg-n., ***glon.***
pregnancy, during - **ARG-N.**
pulling on boots, agg. - coll.
stool, during - cob.
weather, in cold, damp - dulc.

ENLARGED, sensation,
widened, sensation as if - aloe.
enlarged, occiput - dulc., med.

ERUPTIONS - ***agar.,*** **ARS.,** ars-i., arund., ***bar-c., bar-m., bov.,*** cadm-s., **CALC.,** ***calc-s., carb-an.,*** **CARB-S.,** ***carb-v., caust.,*** cic., ***clem.,*** crot-t., cupr., cycl., dulc., **GRAPH.,** ***hep., jug-c.,*** kali-ar., ***kali-bi.,*** kali-br., kali-c., kali-n., kali-p., ***kali-s., lyc., mag-c.,*** **MERC., MEZ.,** naja, ***nat-m.,*** nat-p., ***nit-ac.,*** **OLND.,** ***petr., phos.,*** phyt., plan., ***psor., rhus-v.,*** **RHUS-T.,** ***ruta.,*** **SEP.,** sil., **STAPH., SULPH., SAL-AC.,** tell., zinc.
bleeding after scratching - alum., ***ars., bov., calc.,*** cupr-ar., ***dulc.,*** lach., ***lyc., merc., nat-a.,*** petr., ***psor.,*** staph., **SULPH**.
blotches - ***apis,*** arg-n., sep.
moist - ***psor.***
boils, (see Head, Boils)
burning - ***ars., bar-c.,*** cic., ***graph.,*** kali-bi., ***nit-ac.,*** petr., phos., ***sars.,*** **SULPH**., tarax.
copper-colored - ***carb-an.,*** lyc., sulph.
cracks - ***graph., petr.***
crusts - acet-ac., agar., alum., anan., ant-c., ***ant-t.,*** **ARS**., ***ars-i.,*** arum-t., astac., ***aur., bar-c.,*** bar-m., brom., ***calc., calc-s., caps.,*** carb-ac., ***carb-s.,*** carb-v., ***caust., chel.,*** chin., ***cic.,*** **CLEM., CROT-T., DULC.,** ***eup-per., fl-ac.,*** **GRAPH**., hell., ***hep., hydr.,*** iod., ***iris, kali-ar.,*** kali-bi., kali-c., kali-chl., kali-p., ***kali-s., kreos.,*** lith., ***lyc.,*** **MERC**., ***merc-i-f.,*** **MEZ**., mur-ac., **NAT-M**., nat-p., ***nat-s., nit-ac., olnd.,*** ol-j., ***petr.,*** phos., ***phyt.,*** **PSOR**., ***rhus-t.,*** ruta., ***sars., sep., sil., staph.,*** **SULPH**., sul-ac., ust., ***vinc., viol-t.***
bloody - ***calc.***
brown - **DULC.**
greenish - ***kali-bi.,*** petr., sulph.
malignant - ***brom., phos.***
moist - ***anan., bar-c., calc., graph.,*** **PSOR**., ruta., staph.
serpiginous - ***psor., sars.***
ulcerated - ars., ***mez.,*** **PSOR.**
vermin, with - carb-ac., lyc., ***mez.,*** staph., vinc.
white - alum., calc., ***mez.,*** **NAT-M.,** tell., ***thuj.***
white, with thick white pus beneath - **MEZ.**
yellow - calc., ***calc-s.,*** dulc., ***kali-bi.,*** **KALI-S.,** merc., nat-p., ***petr., psor., spong., staph.,*** sulph., viol-t.
desquamating - ***calc.,*** lach., merc., merc-c., mez., nat-m., **OLND**., phos., staph.
dirty - ***psor.,*** sulph., thuj.
dry - ars., ***calc., fl-ac.,*** kali-ar., merc., ***mez.,*** **PSOR**., sep., ***sil.,*** **SULPH**.
offensive - merc., ***sep., sulph.***
eczema, (see Head, Eczema)
excoriating - ***calc.,*** **GRAPH., HEP., MERC**., ***nat-m., nit-ac.,*** **PETR**., ***ph-ac., psor., rhus-t., sep.,*** **SULPH**., ***viol-t.***
hard - ant-c., carb-an., nat-m.
herpes, (see Head, Herpes)

ERUPTIONS, general
impetigo, (see Head, Impetigo)
itching - am-m., ars., ***bar-c., carb-s., cic.,*** ferr-m., fl-ac., ***graph., hep.,*** hipp., led., ***lyc.,*** mag-c., **MERC.,** ***mez.,*** nat-c., nat-m., ***nit-ac., olnd.,*** phos., ***phyt., psor.,*** rhus-t., ***sep., sil.,*** staph., **SULPH**., zinc.
menses, before - ***mag-m.***
moist, when - ***psor.***
morning - ***hep.***
night agg. - ***mag-m.,*** merc-i-f., rhus-t., vinc.
rainy, weather, in - ***mag-c.***
warm, covering agg. - ***lyc.,*** **SULPH.**
warm, room agg. - ***clem., mag-m.***
margin of hair - calc., ***nat-m.,*** nit-ac., petr., sep., **SULPH**., tell.
miliary, menses, before - sep.
milk crust - ars., ***calc.,*** dulc., euph., ***graph., lyc.,*** nat-p., ol-j., psor., rhus-t., sep., ***sulph.,*** tub., ust.
eroding - staph.
foul - staph.
moist - alum., ***anan., ars.,*** **BAR-C**., ***bar-m., calc.,*** **CARB-S.,** ***cham., cic.,*** **GRAPH., HEP.,** ***hydr.,*** kali-ar., ***kali-bi.,*** kali-s., ***lyc., merc., mez., nat-m., nit-ac., petr., phyt.,*** **PSOR**., ***rhus-t., sars.,*** sep., ***sil., staph.,*** **SULPH**., ***thuj.,*** ust., vinc., ***viol-t.***
glutinous moisture - **GRAPH**., ***nat-m., sulph.***
hair, that eats the - ars., ***kali-bi., merc., nat-m., rhus-t.***
yellow - ***clem., iris,*** **KALI-S.,** ***psor.,*** staph., ***viol-t.***
nodes - asaf., ***caust., chin.,*** con., ***hep., kali-i.,*** mag-c., nat-c., nat-s., nit-ac., ***phyt.,*** rhus-t., **SIL**., thuj.
offensive - bar-m., brom., calc., graph., ***hep.,*** lyc., merc., mez., nit-ac., psor., rhus-t., sep., sil., staph., sulph., vinc.
painful - arg-m., bar-c., cann-s., clem., ferr-ma., **GRAPH., HEP.,** kali-c., lyc., mag-c., merc., par., sulph.
pimples - act-sp., agar., alum., ***ambr.,*** anac., arg-m., **ARS**., aur., bar-c., bar-m., ***bov.,*** calc., calc-s., carb-s., ***con.,*** crot-c., cund., cycl., **HEP**., kali-bi., kali-c., kali-p., ***kali-s.,*** **LED**., merc-i-r., mez., ***mur-ac.,*** nat-c., ***nat-m.,*** nux-v., olnd., petr., ***phos.,*** sec., ***sil.,*** spig., staph., **SULPH**., tarax., tarent., ***zinc.***
came out all over scalp like small-pox, shot like feeling under them - am-c.
margin of hair in front - nit-ac.
pustules - ammc., ***ars.,*** arund., bov., ***calc., hep., iris,*** kali-br., ***merc.,*** merc-i-r., mur-ac., ***psor.,*** puls., rhus-t., sep., ***sil.,*** **SULPH**.
rash, (see Head, Rash)
scales - alum., ***ars.,*** arund., bell., ***calc.,*** carb-s., ***cic., fl-ac.,*** **GRAPH**., ***kali-bi.,*** kali-n., ***kali-s., kreos., lyc.,*** merc., mez., naja, nat-m., **OLND**., phos., phyt., ***sep., sil., staph.,*** sulph., ***thuj.***

ERUPTIONS, general
scales, bleeding after scratching - lyc.
dry - ars., ***calc.***, mez., ***ph-ac.***, ***sil.***, staph.
fine - clem., par.
fish like - mez.
offensive - ***nit-ac.***
patches - graph., kali-n., lyc., phos., ***sil.***
washing amel. - **GRAPH.**
white - alum., calc., ***mez.***, **NAT-M.**, tell., ***thuj.***
winter agg. - ***sil.***
working amel. - **GRAPH.**
scurfy - alum., ars., ars-i., ***bar-c.***, ***calc.***, com., con., **GRAPH.**, hep., iod., ***merc.***, nat-m., **OLND.**, ***psor.***, sep., sil., ***staph.***, ***viol-t.***
black - ***calc-p.***
dry - ***bar-c.***
moist - alum., ***anan.***, ***bar-c.***, ***calc.***, ***graph.***, nit-ac.
white - nat-m.
sensitive, extremely - **HEP.**, ***nit-ac.***, **STAPH.**
serpiginous - ***calc.***, ***clem.***, ***psor.***, ***sars.***
sore - ***hep.***, nat-m.
touch, on - phos.
spots - ars., kali-c., mosch., zinc.
suppurating - ars., ***bar-m.***, ***calc-s.***, cic., clem., graph., hep., lyc., ***mez.***, ***psor.***, ***rhus-t.***, ***sep.***, staph., **SULPH.**, vinc.
tubercles, (see Head, Tubercles)
vesicles, (see Head, Vesicles)

eruptions, forehead - agar., alum., ambr., am-c., am-m., **ANT-C.**, arg-m., ars., aur., bad., bar-c., bar-m., bell., ***bov.***, bry., cadm-s., ***calc.***, ***calc-p.***, caps., carb-an., carb-v., caul., ***caust.***, cham., chin., cic., clem., cycl., dulc., ferr-ma., ***hep.***, hura, **KREOS.**, **LED.**, ***lyc.***, mag-m., mur-ac., nat-a., nat-c., **NAT-M.**, nat-p., nit-ac., **NUX-V.**, ***par.***, ***ph-ac.***, ***phos.***, ***psor.***, **RHUS-T.**, rhus-v., ***sars.***, **SEP.**, sil., staph., **SULPH.**, sul-ac., viol-t.
menses, before - mag-m., sars.
moist, menses, before - sep.
pimples - agar., alum., ***ambr.***, am-c., am-m., anac., ars., aur., bell., ***bov.***, bry., calc., calc-p., canth., carb-v., chel., chin., ***clem.***, con., cycl., ferr-m., gran., hep., hura, indg., kali-bi., kali-br., kali-chl., kreos., lach., ***led.***, mag-m., meph., mez., ***mur-ac.***, nat-c., nat-m., ***nat-p.***, nit-ac., olnd., par., ***ph-ac.***, phos., ***psor.***, puls., ***rhod.***, rhus-v., ***sep.***, sol-n., ***sulph.***, tab., tarent., zinc., ziz.
burning - ars., bell., canth.
itching - alum., calc., mag-m., ***sulph.***, ziz.
itching, rubbing agg. - mag-m.
painful - ambr., clem., indg., sep., staph.
red - ambr., anac., bell., carb-v., nat-c., sep., nat-m., sol-n.
sore to touch - ambr., hell., ph-ac., zinc.
stinging, on rubbing - sulph.
washed smarting when - nux-v.

eruptions, forehead
pimples, white - carb-v., kali-br., sulph., zinc.
wine, after - zinc.
scurfy - calc., dulc., mag-c., mur-ac.
scurfy, forehead and temples - dulc., mur-ac.

eruptions, occiput - arg-n., bufo, **CAUST.**, ***clem.***, cycl., ***graph.***, kali-bi., kali-n., ***lyc.***, merc., nat-c., nat-m., olnd., ***petr.***, ***psor.***, puls., **SIL.**, ***staph.***, **SULPH.**
crusts - **CAUST.**, ***clem.***, ***lyc.***, ***nat-m.***, ***sil.***
moist - ***clem.***, olnd., ***petr.***, **SIL.**, ***staph.***, ***thuj.***
nodes - ***mag-m.***
pimples, on - am-m., buf-s., clem., cycl., kali-bi., kali-n., lyc., merc., **SULPH.**
pustules - ammc., puls., **SIL.**

eruptions, temples - ***alum.***, ***ant-c.***, arg-m., bell., bry., calc., carb-v., caust., ***dulc.***, lach., lyc., ***mur-ac.***, ***nat-m.***, nit-ac., sabin., spig., sulph., thuj.
crusts - ***dulc.***, ***mur-ac.***
itching - zinc.
pimples - arg-m., carb-v., ***mur-ac.***, nit-ac.

ERYSIPELAS - ***anthr.***, ant-t., **APIS**, apoc., ***ars.***, bell., carb-s., ***chel.***, ***chin.***, cupr., dor., ***euph.***, **GRAPH.**, ***lach.***, ***ph-ac.***, ***phyt.***, ***rhus-t.***, ***ruta***, sulph., ter., verat-v.
extending to face - ***apis.***
left - samb.
to right - ***rhus-t.***

erysipelas, forehead - apis, kali-i., ruta., sulph.
spots - kali-i., sulph.

erysipelas, occiput - ***ph-ac.***, rhus-t.

EXOSTOSES - anan., **ARG-M.**, **AUR.**, ***calc.***, **CALC-F.**, ***fl-ac.***, ***hecla.***, ***kali-i.***, **MERC.**, ***mez.***, **PHOS.**, ***phyt.***, sil., still., syph.
painful - ***aur.***, ***kali-i.***, **MERC.**

EXPANDED, sensation (see Enlarged, Swollen) - ***arg-n.***, bell., cann-i., carb-ac., dulc., euph., nux-m., sol-n., stront.
inflated, feels - kali-i.
ring-like - merc.
shaking head agg. - carb-ac.
stool, during - cob.

expanded, forehead - ***nux-m.***
relaxed and, alternately - ***lac-c.***

FALLING, of head (see Heaviness)
backward - aeth., ***agar.***, ant-t., bov., camph., cham., chin., cic., ***colch.***, ***dig.***, dios., glon., ***ign.***, kali-c., laur., ***led.***, mur-ac., oena., ***op.***, ***phel.***, samb., ***spig.***, tarent.
sitting, while - chin., ***dig.***, oena., op.
vertigo, during - led., ph-ac., ***spig.***
walking, while - ***chin.***, ***dig.***, phel.
forward - agn., calc., cham., clem., ***cupr.***, elaps, gels., glon., hipp., hydr-ac., hyos., ***ign.***, kali-c., kali-p., laur., lyc., ***merc.***, ***nat-m.***, nux-m., ***op.***, par., phos., phys., pic-ac., plat., plb., ***puls.***, ran-b., sars., sec., ***sil.***, staph., sulph., verat.
and to left - calc-ac.

FALLING, of head
forward, looking at anything, when sinking of head forward - ***cic.***
rising, on - hipp.
sitting, while - ***nux-m.,*** oena., staph.
stooping, when - cist., ***puls.***
vertigo, during - calc-ac., ph-ac., sars.
walking, while - carb-s., hipp., mez.
wrinkling of forehead and open air amel. - phos.
hither and thither - bar-c., bell., ***cupr., nux-m.,*** phel.
pieces, sensation as if head would fall in, when stooping - glon.
side, to side, in brain - nicc., sul-ac.
to, left temple on stooping - nat-s.
to side, to which stoops - am-c.
walking in the open air - sul-ac.
sideways, of head - am-c., ang., arn., ars., cann-s., ***cina,*** dios., eup-per., ferr., fl-ac., hyos., kali-i., ***mygal.,*** nux-m., op., prun., stram., sulph., tarax.
child leans, all time - cina.
left side, to - nux-m., sil.
right side, to - am-c., ferr.
vertigo, with - sil., spong.
waking, on - sulph.
walking, while - dios., ferr.
falling, forward, sensation
brain, in - ***alum.,*** am-c., ant-t., bar-c., berb., bry., carb-an., cham., coff., ***dig.***, grat., hipp., kali-c., kreos., laur., mag-s., nux-v., ***rhus-t.,*** sabad., sul-ac.
pain, as if fell forward and came up again - sul-ac.
raising head amel. - alum.
stooping, on - alum., ant-t., bar-c., ***carb-an.,*** chel., coff., dig., kali-c., laur., mag-s., nat-m., ***nat-s., nux-v.,*** rhus-t.
forehead, in, as if everything would fall out - ***acon.,*** all-c., bar-c., bell., brom., bry., canth., carb-an., caust., cham., chel., colch., coloc., hell., hep., kali-c., kreos., mag-m., mag-s., mez., nux-v., phos., plat., puls., rat., rhod., sabad., sep., spig., spong., stann., staph., stront-c., tab., ***thuj.,*** verb.
coughing, while - hep.
moving the eyes, on - puls.
stool, during - rat.
stooping, on - bar-c., hell., mag-s., nat-c., spig., staph.

FLATTENED, sensation in, forehead - cor-r.
as if pressed flat - verat.

FLY off, as if, vertex - acon., ***bapt., cann-i.,*** cann-s., ***cimic.,*** iris, passi., ***syph.,*** thlaspi, visc., xan., yuc.
fly off, as if, vertex, air, cold, letting in - cimic.

FONTANELLES, open - ***apis,*** apoc., **CALC., CALC-P.,** ***ip., merc., puls., sep.,*** **SIL.,** ***syph., sulph.,*** tub., zinc.
close and reopen - calc-p.

FONTANELLES, open
posterior - calc-p., sil.
sinking - mag-c.
reopening - calc-p.
sunken - ***apis,*** calc.

FOREIGN body in head, sensation of - arg-n., ars., cina, merc., phos., phys.

FORMICATING, pain, forehead - puls.

FORMICATION, sensation - ***acon.,*** aesc., ***agar.,*** alum., am-c., am-m., ***ant-c.,*** **ARG-N.,** ars., arund., bar-c., ***calc., calc-p.,*** calc-s., cann-s., carb-v., cast-eq., chel., coca, coc-c., colch., cupr., ***cycl.,*** dulc., fago., ***ferr.,*** hyos., kali-bi., lach., laur., mez., nat-s., nit-ac., nux-v., ***pic-ac.,*** psor., puls., ran-b., rhod., ***rhus-t.,*** sep., sil., ***sulph.,*** thuj.
evening - bar-c., calc.
in bed - ran-b.
heat amel. - ***acon.***
morning - arg-n., thuj.
scratching until parts bleed - alum.
walking, on - ***coc-c.***
in open air - lyc., rhus-t.
formication, forehead - apis, arn., arund., benz-ac., chel., chin., cic., ***colch.,*** glon., kali-c., laur., manc., nux-v., ph-ac., phos., puls., rhus-t., rhus-v., tarax., ***zinc.***
above the - kali-c.
formication, occiput - ars., brom., carb-v., ***sep.,*** thuj.
formication, side, left - spig.
right - nit-ac.
formication, vertex - arn., calc-p., cann-i., caust., ***cupr.,*** lil-t., ***nat-s.***

FROZEN, head and brain, as if - ***indg.***

FULLNESS, (see Enlarged) - abrot., **ACON.,** ***aesc.,*** agar., ail., all-c., am-c., ***am-m.,*** ang., **APIS,** ***arg-n.,*** arn., arum-t., asaf., ***aster.,*** aur., bapt., ***bell.,*** berb., ***bor.,*** bov., ***bry.,*** **CACT.,** ***calc., calc-p.,*** calc-s., cann-i., canth., caps., carb-ac., carb-an., carb-s., ***carb-v., card-m., carl.,*** cast., cham., chin., ***chin-a., chin-s.,*** chr-ac., cimic., ***cinnb.,*** clem., cob., cocc., coff., ***con.,*** corn., crot-h., crot-t., cupr., cupr-ar., cycl., daph., ***dig., dios.,*** dulc., echi., elaps, ***ferr.,*** ferr-ar., ferr-p., fl-ac., form., ***gels., gent-c.,*** **GENT-L., GINS., GLON.,** graph., grat., guai., gymn., ***ham., hell.,*** helo., hydr., ***hyos.,*** hyper., ign., iris, jac., jug-c., kali-ar., kali-c., kali-i., kali-p., kali-s., kalm., kreos., lac-ac., ***lac-d.,*** **LACH.,** lact., laur., lil-t., lyc., meph., ***merc.,*** merc-i-r., mill., naja, nat-a., nat-c., nat-m., nat-p., ***nicc., nit-ac., nux-m.,*** nux-v., onos., op., osm., ***paeon., petr.,*** phel., ***phos.,*** phys., phyt., pic-ac., plan., ***psor.,*** puls., ***ran-b., ran-s.,*** raph., ***rhus-t.,*** rumx., samb., ***sang.,*** senec., ***sel.,*** sep., sil., sol-n., ***spong.,*** stram., ***stry.,*** **SULPH.,** ***sul-ac.,*** tab., tanac., tell., ***ter.,*** thuj., til., urt-u., ust., valer., verat-v., ***xan.,*** ziz.
afternoon - arg-n., coca, ferr., gels., guare., lac-ac., lact., lith., mill., nat-p., osm., phys., sang., stry., ***sulph.***
to night - sil.
waking, on - carb-v.

FULLNESS, sensation
air, in open amel. - cinnb., carl., grat., jac.
ascending, on - bor.
bending head backwards - osm.
breakfast, after - con., hydr.
burst, as if would - am-c., aster., cann-i., daph., **GLON.,** ip., lil-t., merc., nit-ac.
descending, on - **BOR.**
dinner, after - gins.
eating, during - con.
after - bor., con., gins., hydr., ***hyos.***
after, amel. - onos.
before - uran.
evening - arg-n., cimic., ferr., guare., ham., naja, nat-m., nat-p., thuj.
fever, during - **GLON.,** lach.
intermittent - asaf.
leaning head to left - chin-s.
lying, while - naja
menses, before - brom.
menses, during - ***apis,*** arg-n., ***bell., calc.,*** eupi., gent-c., ***glon.,*** puls., ***xan.***
on appearance of - ***glon.***
mental exertion, from - **CACT.,** cinnb., helon., ind., meph., ***nat-p.,*** phos., ***psor.***
amel. when mind is employed - helon.
morning - am-m., arg-n., arn., bor., carl., cann-i., chin-s., chr-ac., cinnb., cob., ***con.,*** cop., dulc., hydr., indg., ***lach.,*** mag-m., nat-p., nicc., petr., pic-ac., rhus-t., sul-ac., tell.
10 a.m. to 10 p.m. - lac-ac.
waking, on - arg-n., con., glon., kalm., lil-t., til.
motion agg. - calc-p.
night - arg-n., ***aster.,*** chr-ac.
noon to 2 p.m. - pic-ac.
pressure of hat, agg. - calc-p.
amel. - agar., arg-n., cop., hydr.
raising, on - sulph.
reading, while - cop., helon., indg.
rising, on - am-m., cinnb., glon., sil.
sewing agg. - petr.
sex, after - phos.
shaking, on - carl., glon.
siesta, after - mill.
sitting, while - bor., glon.
up agg. - calc-p.
sleep, after, agg. - hep., sulph.
amel. - onos.
sneezing, on - hydr.
stool, amel. after - corn.
when straining at - ham.
stooping, when - acon., lac-ac., merl., nicc., petr., pic-ac., rhus-t., spong.
talking, after - sulph.
urine, copious flow amel. - gels.
vertigo, during - am-m., bor., bry., chr-ac., con., crot-t., cycl., gymn., helon., lac-ac., lact., merc., nat-m., nat-p., podo., sol-n., til., urt-u.
waking, on - agar., asaf., carb-v., guare.
walking in open air amel. - ***apis, bor.,*** hydr., ***lyc.,*** **PULS.**
warm room - ***apis,*** hydr., lact.

FULLNESS, sensation
wine, after - ail.
writing, while - chin-s.

fullness, forehead - acon., aesc., agar., ***am-c.,*** am-m., ang., ***apis,*** apoc., arg-n., bapt., ***bell.,*** berb., bor., ***bry.,*** cahin., calc., calc-s., cann-i., carb-an., **CARB-S.,** chr-ac., cimic., **CINNB.,** clem., coca, con., cop., euph., eupi., gels., ***glon.,*** gymn., ***ham.,*** hell., ***helon.,*** hydr., hyos., indg., ind., lac-ac., laur., lil-t., mag-s., meph., naja, ***nat-a.,*** nat-p., nicc., ox-ac., pall., ***phos.,*** phys., phyt., pip-m., podo., psor., ran-s., rhus-t., rumx., sang., sep., staph., stict., ***sulph.,*** sul-ac., thea., til.
afternoon - phys., sang.
closing eyes amel. - ***bry.***
eating amel. - psor.
evening - ***bry.,*** naja, nat-m., sumb.
eyes, over - hydr., lil-t., nat-p., ox-ac.
with vertigo - podo.
forenoon - rhus-t., sul-ac.
morning - arg-n., bor., carl., fago., glon., nat-p., til.
nose, over, evening - naja
reading, while - indg.
sex, after - phos.
stool amel. - fago.
stooping, on - acon.
walking, while - dig.
washing amel. - psor.

fullness, occiput - ***acon.,*** agar., all-c., apis, bapt., caj., coca, cann-i., cham., cinnb., con., glon., helon., kreos., osm., puls., sulph., sumb., ther., thuj.
coughing on - all-c.
evening, in - sumb.
walking in open air - thuj.
lying on face amel. - ***coca.***

fullness, sides - arg-n., asaf., cimic., cycl., fl-ac., glon.

fullness, temples - apis, bell., cic., cinnb., cob., ***echi.,*** glon., gnaph., jac., lil-t., lith., nat-m., plan., rumx., sep., sumb.
first right, then left, then to nape where it disappears - jac.

fullness, vertex - aesc., ***am-c.,*** apis, calc-p., chin-s., chr-ac., cimic., **CINNB.,** eup-per., **GLON.,** gymn., ham., helon., hyper., kali-bi., lac-ac., meph., osm., pic-ac., psor.
eating, after - ***cinnb.***
evening - cimic.
reading, while - hell.
sitting up agg. - calc-p.
stooping - pic-ac.

FUNGUS, (see Tinea) - ***apis,*** bac., calc-i., ***calc-p., phos., thuj.***

GLANDS, swollen, of, glabella - kali-c.

GNAWING, pain - calc., canth., ***coloc.,*** led., lyc., nat-m., paeon., par., phos., ran-s., zinc.
ear pain, with - ran-s.
night - merc-i-r.
when stepping heavily - lyc.
pulsating - par.

gnawing, forehead - con., dros., merc-i-r., nat-s., ruta, sulph., zinc.
eye, above right, morning - dros.
frontal eminence - bell.
nose, above - calc-ac., merc., ph-ac., phos., raph.
gnawing, occiput - calc., cycl., dros., glon., led., ***nat-s.,*** nicc., ol-an., raph., zinc.
erosive - thuj.
gnawing, sides - bell., phos., ***thuj.***
gnawing, temples - led., ran-s., sol-n.
right - sol-n.
gnawing, vertex - ***ant-c.,*** dros., meny., ran-s., spong.

GRASPING, pain - arg-n., ars., chin., con., hell., mag-m., nat-s.
grasping, forehead - ***ant-c.,*** meny., ran-s.
cold feet, bath amel. - nat-s.
eating amel. - anac.
frontal eminence, left - agar.

GRINDING, pain - agar., anac., aur., myric.
coughing agg. - aur.
evening - anac.
pressure amel. - anac.

GRIPING, pain - alum., con., mag-m., mag-s., sep.

GRUMBLING - hep., indg., sul-ac.

GURGLING - asaf., bry., sep.
gurgling, temples - bry.

HACKING, pain - am-c., ars., aur., kali-n., lyc., ph-ac.

HAIR, (see Generals, Hair)

HAMMERING, pain - ***am-c., ars.,*** aur., **BELL.,** cadm-s., calc., chel., ***chin.,*** chin-a., ***chin-s.,*** cic., cimic., clem., ***cocc., coff., cur.,*** dros., **FERR., FERR-AR.,** ferr-p., **GLON.,** ***hep.,*** indg., iris, kali-i., ***lach.,*** mag-s., manc., mez., **NAT-M.,** nicc., nit-ac., ph-ac., ***psor.,*** puls., rhus-t., rheum, **SIL., SULPH.,** ***tarent.,*** verb.
evening, while lying - clem.
morning - **NAT-M.**
vivacious talking, from - **SULPH.**
hammering, forehead - am-m., cham., cic., **FERR.,** kali-i., kreos., mez., nicc., **LYC.,** olnd., rheum, verb.
middle, of - **LYC.**
hammering, occiput - act-sp., camph., ferr-p., nat-m., psor.
sides, of - ign.
hammering, sides - iris.
hammering, temples - ars., benz-ac., chel., chin., ***ferr.,*** hep., nat-m., psor.
hammering, vertex - hyper., phos.

HANDS, holds head with - glon., hyos.
coughing, on - **BRY.,** nicc., **NUX-V.,** sulph.
grasps forehead - sulph.
leans, on - iod.
rubs, with - verat.

HAT, aversion to - calc-p., carb-an., carb-v., crot-c., ***iod., led., lyc.,*** mez., nit-ac., sil.

HAT, sensation of - calc., calc-s., ***carb-v.,*** cycl., ***graph.,*** lach.

HEADACHES, general - abrot., absin., acet-ac., acon., act-sp., aesc., aeth., agar., ail., all-c., aloe, ***alum., alumn.,*** ambr., ***am-c.,*** am-m., ammc., anac., ang., **ANTHR.,** ***ant-c.,*** ant-t., **APIS,** ap-g., apoc., **ARG-M.,** ***arg-n., arn.,*** **ARS.,** ars-i., arum-t., asaf., asar., ***aur.,*** bad., ***bapt.,*** bar-c., bar-m., **BELL.,** berb., benz-ac., berb., bism., ***bor.,*** bov., brom., **BRY.,** bufo, ***cact.,*** calad., **CALC.,** calc-p., **CALC-S.,** camph., cann-i., cann-s., canth., carb-an., carb-s., ***carb-v.,*** cast., caul., ***caust.,*** **CEDR.,** ***cham.,*** chel., **CHIN.,** chin-a., **CHIN-S.,** ***cimic.,*** cina, ***cinnb.,*** clem., cob., coca, **COCC.,** coc-c., ***coff.,*** colch., ***coloc.,*** com., con., conv., corn., croc., **CROT-C.,** ***crot-h., crot-t.,*** cund., ***cupr.,*** cupr-ar., cur., cycl., daph., ***dig., dios., dros., dulc.,*** elaps, elat., eug., eup-per., euph., euphr., eupi., ***ferr., ferr-ar., ferr-i., ferr-p.,*** fl-ac., gamb., **GELS.,** gent-c., gins., **GLON.,** gran., ***graph.,*** grat., guai., gymn., ham., ***hell., hep.,*** hipp., hura, hydr., hydr-ac., ***hyos.,*** hyper., ictod., ***ign.,*** indg., ind., ***iod.,*** ip., **IRIS,** jal., jatr., jug-r., ***kali-ar., kali-bi., kali-c.,*** kali-chl., **KALI-I.,** ***kali-n., kali-p., kali-s., kalm., kreos., lac-d.,*** **LACH.,** lachn., lac-ac., lact., laur., ***lec., led.,*** lil-t., lob., ***lyc.,*** lyss., mag-c., ***mag-m.,*** **MAG-P.,** mag-s., ***manc.,*** mang., ***med., meli.,*** meph., **MERC.,** merc-c., merc-i-f., merl., ***mez.,*** mill., morph., mosch., murx., mur-ac., naja, ***nat-a., nat-c.,*** **NAT-M.,** nat-p., ***nat-s.,*** nicc., **NIT-AC.,** ***nux-m.,*** **NUX-V.,** oena., ol-j., osm., ox-ac., pall., ***par., petr.,*** phel., ***ph-ac.,*** **PHOS.,** phys., phyt., pic-ac., plan., plat., ***plb., podo.,*** prun., **PSOR.,** ptel., **PULS.,** ran-b., ran-s., raph., rheum, rhod., ***rhus-t.,*** rhus-v., rumx., sabad., sang., sec., sel., seneg., **SEP., SIL.,** sol-n., ***spig.,*** spong., stann., ***staph.,*** stram., stry., **SULPH.,** sul-ac., tab., tanac., tarax., tarent., tax., tell., ***ter.,*** thea., ***ther., thuj.,*** til., tril., trom., urt-u., ust., valer., verat., viol-o., viol-t., vip., xan., ***zinc.,*** zinc-s., zing., ziz.
acids, from - bell., morph., ***nat-p., sel.***
afternoon - ***acon.,*** aeth., ***agar., alum.,*** ambr., ***am-c.,*** am-m., anac., ant-t., arn., ars., ars-i., asar., aur., ***bad.,*** bar-c., bar-m., **BELL.,** berb., bov., bry., bufo, calad., calc., calc-ar., calc-f., calc-p., calc-s., canth., carb-an., carb-s., ***carb-v.,*** caust., chel., chin., chin-a., chin-s., cic., cimic., cob., coca, cocc., colch., coloc., con., ***cupr.,*** cycl., dig., dios., dros., equis., euphr., fago., ferr., ferr-ar., ferr-i., ferr-p., form., gamb., gels., genist., glon., ***graph.,*** grat., ham., hell., iber., ign., ind., indg., iod., iris, kali-ar., kali-c., ***kali-n.,*** kali-p., kali-s., kalm., kreos., ***lac-c.,*** lach., lact., laur., ***lyc.,*** lycps., lyss., mag-c., mag-m., mag-s., ***mang.,*** merc-i-r., ***mez., mur-ac.,*** nat-a., ***nat-c.,*** nat-m., nat-p., ***nit-ac.,*** nux-m., nux-v., op., pall., petr., ***ph-ac.,*** phos., phyt., pic-ac., ***plat.,*** plb., polyg., ptel., puls., ran-b., rhus-r., ruta., sabin., ***sars.,*** sec., **SEL.,** seneg., sep., ***sil.,*** spong., stram., ***stront-c., sulph.,*** sul-ac., tab., tell., valer., ***verat., zinc.***

HEADACHES, general

afternoon, 1 p.m - ail., coca, lyc., mag-c., phys., pic-ac., ptel.

1 to 3 p.m - chin-s., plan.

1 to 5 p.m - lac-ac., mag-c.

1 to 10 p.m - mag-c., plat., sil., spig.

2 p.m - ***ars., chel.,*** grat., iod., laur., lyss., phys., ptel.

2 p.m. until late in the evening - bad., chel.

2 p.m. to 7 a.m - ***bad.***

3 p.m - apis, **BELL.,** fago., ***fl-ac.,*** guai., hura, iber., lycps., lyss., nat-a., sep., sil., thuj., verat-v.

3 to 4 p.m - brom., clem.

3 to 9 p.m - arn., lyss., nat-a., tarent.

4 p.m - arg-mur., arg-n., bar-c., caust., chin-s., dios., helon., meli., nat-m., phys., pic-ac., stry., ***sulph.,*** verat-v.

4 p.m. to 3 a.m - **BELL.**

4 to 8 p m - caust., hell., **LYC.**

5 p.m - bufo, equis., helon., iod., nat-m., paeon., pic-ac., ptel., ***puls.,*** sulph.

5 to 6 p.m - chin-s., lil-t., sep.

5 to 9 p.m - plat.

5 to 10 p.m - ***puls.***

amel - ip., ol-an.

evening, until next - cist., kali-n.

night, lasting all - colch., cupr., verat.

air, cold, from - am-c., **ARS., AUR., BELL.,** bov., ***bry., calc., camph.,*** carb-an., ***carb-v.,*** **CAUST., CHIN.,** ***chin-a., cocc., coff.,*** **DULC.,** ferr., ferr-ar., grat., ***hep.,*** ign., ***iris, kali-ar., kali-bi.,*** **KALI-C.,** kali-chl., kali-p., ***lac-c., lach., lyc., mag-m., mang.,*** nat-m., ***nit-ac.,*** **NUX-M., NUX-V.,** ***phos.,*** plat., ***psor., puls.,*** **RHOD., RHUS-T.,** ruta., ***sep.,*** **SIL.,** ***sulph., verat.***

amel - aloe, arg-n., ars., bufo, caust., cimic., croc., dros., euphr., ferr-p., ***glon.,*** iod., kali-s., ***lyc.,*** lyss., **PHOS.,** ***puls., seneg.,*** sin-n.

draft of, from - ***acon., ars., bell.,*** benz-ac., cadm-s., ***calc.,*** caps., caust., ***chin.,*** coloc., eup-pur., ferr-p., gels., ***hep.,*** ichth., ign., iris, kali-ar., ***kali-c.,*** kali-p., kali-s., lac-c., ***merc.,*** nux-m., ***nux-v.,*** phos., ***psor.,*** rhod., ***rhus-t., sanic., sel.,*** **SIL.,** stront-c., sul-ac., ***sulph.,*** valer., verb.

walking, in, while - caps.

air, open, (see Walking, in open air) - alum., ang., ***arg-m.,*** bar-c., bar-m., ***bell.,*** bov., bry., cadm-s., ***calc.,*** calc-ar., calc-p., ***carb-an., caust.,*** cedr., cham., ***chel.,*** **CHIN.,** cimic., cina, ***cocc.,*** coff., colch., ***con.,*** cycl., eup-per., euphr., ferr., glon., grat., ***hep.,*** hipp., ign., iod., ip., ***kali-c.,*** kalm., lach., laur., ***lil-t.,*** lyc., ***mang.,*** meny., **MERC.,** ***mez.,*** mur-ac., nat-m., ***nux-v.,*** petr., phos., ran-b., rhus-t., spig., staph., sulph., valer., zinc.

amel. - acon., ***all-c.,*** aloe, ***alum.,*** ambr., am-c., ang., ***ant-c.,*** ap-g., ***apis, aran.,*** arg-n., arn., ***ars.,*** ars-i., asar., aur., bar-c., bell., berb., bov., calc., calc-s., camph., cann-i., cann-s., ***carb-ac.,*** carb-s.,

HEADACHES, general

air, open, amel. - ***carb-v.,*** caust., ***cimic.,*** clem., cob., coc-c., ***coff.,*** coloc., com., con., croc., dulc., fago., ***ferr.,*** ferr-ar., ferr-i., ***glon.,*** grat., ham., ***hell.,*** hydr., hydr-ac., hyos., iod., jatr., ***kali-bi.,*** kali-c., ***kali-i.,*** kali-n., ***kali-p., kali-s.,*** lac-c., lach., laur., ***led.,*** lith., **LYC.,** lyss., ***mag-m.,*** mag-s., **MANG.,** meny., merc-i-f., mez., mosch., nat-a., nat-c., ***nat-m.,*** nat-p., ***nicc.,*** nux-v., olnd., op., petr., phel., ph-ac., **PHOS.,** pic-ac., plat., **PULS.,** ran-b., rhod., sang., sars., sel., **SENEG., SEP.,** sin-n., sol-n., spong., stann., sulph., sul-ac., ***tab.,*** tarent., thuj., viol-t., **ZINC.**

alcohol, spirituous liquors, from - acet-ac., **AGAR.,** alum., ***ant-c., ars.,*** asaf., ***bell.,*** bry., bufo, ***calc.,*** calc-s., cann-i., carb-v., ***chel., chin.,*** chlor., cimic., ***coff.,*** coloc., con., ***gels.,*** hell., hydr., ***ign.,*** ip., **LACH.,** ***led.,*** lob., ***lyc.,*** merc., ***nat-m.,*** nit-ac., ***nux-m.,*** **NUX-V.,** ***op., phos., puls.,*** **RAN-B.,** ***rhod., rhus-t., ruta.,*** sabad., ***sel., sil., spig.,*** spong., ***stram., sulph., verat., zinc.***

amel. - arg-n., bufo, cast., hell., ***ign., kreos.,*** naja, phos., sep.

alternating, with

abdominal and uterine symptoms - aloe.

asthma - ang., glon., kali-br.

cough - lach., psor.

diarrhea - ***podo.,*** sec.

frightful dreams - chin.

heartburn - rob.

hemorrhoids - abrot., aloe.

lumbago - aloe, lycps., meli.

lumbo-sacral region - meli.

nausea - squil.

oppression of chest - glon.

pain in

abdomen - aesc., ***ars.,*** cina, ***gels., iris,*** plb., rhus-r.

back - aloe, brom., meli.

chest - lachn.

joints - ***lyc.,*** sulph.

limbs - sulph.

loins - aloe, lycps.

nape of neck - hyos.

pelvis - ***gels.***

stomach - ars., bism., ox-ac., plb., verat.

teeth - ***lycps.,*** psor.

prolapsus ani - ***arn.***

red sand in urine - ***lyc.***

somnolence and many dreams - ars.

stitches in hypochondrium - aesc.

altitudes, in high - ***coca.***

anemic - ars., calc-p., ***chin.,*** cycl., ferr., ***ferr-p.,*** ferr-r., kalm., ***nat-hchls.,*** nat-m., zinc.

anger, from - acon., arg-n., ***bry.,*** cast., ***cham.,*** coff., coloc., dulc., ***ign.,*** kali-c., ***lyc.,*** mag-c., mez., ***nat-m., nux-v., petr., phos., plat.,*** ran-b., rhus-t., sep., **STAPH.**

anxiety, with - acon., ars., lyss., plat.

after - aeth.

agg. lying down - ***sep.***

HEADACHES, general

arterial excitement, tension, with - acon., ***bell.,*** ***glon.,*** glyc., meli., ictod., usn., ***verat-v.***
arteries, painful, pulsating - caust.
ascending, steps, on - alum., ant-c., arn., aster., **BELL., BRY.,** cadm-s., **CALC.,** carb-s., ***carb-v.,*** cimic., crot-h., ***cupr.,*** ferr., ferr-ar., ***gels., glon.,*** hydr., ign., ***kalm.,*** lac-c., ***lach.,*** lob., ***lyc.,*** meny., meph., ***mosch.,*** nat-a., ***nux-v.,*** par., ***ph-ac., phos., psor.,*** ptel., ***rhus-t.,*** sang., ***sep.,*** **SIL., SPONG.,** staph., ***sulph., tab.,*** thuj., zinc.
attention, from too eager - anac., ***ign.,*** nux-v., sabad.
autumn agg. - aloe.
awake, when trying to keep - phys.
back, pain in, headaches, with - ail., benz-ac., cina, cob., daph., fl-ac., graph., hydr., menis., merc., myric., ol-an., op., sabad., sabin., ***sil.,*** verat., ziz.
pain, in small of back - apoc., cob., lac-c., sil.
back, pressing up against something hard, amel - sang.
ball, were beating against the skull on beginning to walk, as if - plat.
bandaging, (see Binding)
bathing, after (see Washing) - **ANT-C.,** ***bell., calc.,*** canth., caust., kreos., ***nit-ac., rhus-t.,*** puls., sep., sil.
amel. - lac-ac.
feet, of - asc-t.
after, cold - **ANT-C.,** ***bell., caps., nit-ac.,*** phos., ***rhus-t.,*** sars., sep.
sea bathing, after - ***ars.,*** mag-m., ***rhus-t.,*** sep.
bed, on going to - alum., ars., ***lyc.,*** mag-m., ***merc.,*** puls., sabad., sep., sulph., zinc.
amel. - ***alum.,*** colch., mag-c., rhus-t., sep.
must leave the bed - coloc., rhus-t., sep., ***thuj.***
beef, after - ***staph.***
beer, from - all-c., bell., calc., caust., ***coc-c.,*** coloc., ferr., kali-chl., merc., ***nux-v., rhus-t.,*** verat.
and bread, agg. from - crot-t.
belching, amel. - bry., cann-i., carb-v., cinnb., gent-c., hep., ign., lach., sang.
bending, head
backward, while - anac., aur., ***bell.,*** bry., carb-ac., ***carb-v.,*** caust., chin., ***clem.,*** cic., cob., colch., cupr., cycl., dig., dros., elaps, glon., ign., kali-c., kali-s., lyc., mang., osm., ***puls.,*** sep., spig., spong., stann., valer., viol-o.
amel. - apis, arg-n., bell., ***cact., cham.,*** cocc., gels., ***hep., glon.,*** lec., ph-ac., rhus-t., thuj., verat.
walks with head bent backwards - ***arn., ars.***
forward, (see Stooping) - bell., carb-an., cimic., ***cob.,*** rat., ***rhus-t.,*** viol-o.
amel. - carb-ac., cimic., hyos., ign.

HEADACHES, general

bending, head, side, to one - chin., kali-s., meny., spong.
to one, amel - meny., ***puls.,*** sep., stram.
to painful, while - mez., tab.
bilious - am-pic., anac., ***arg-n.,*** bapt., ***bry.,*** cham., chel., ***chion.,*** cycl., eup-per., ***ip.,*** iris, lob., merc-sul., ***nux-v.,*** podo., ***puls.,*** rob., ***sang.,*** stry., tarax.
binding, from the head (see Pressure) - calc., cham., lach., rhus-t., thuj.
amel. - agar., apis, ***arg-m.,*** **ARG-N.,** arn., bell., bry., ***calc.,*** carb-ac., glon., ***hep.,*** ign., iod., lac-d., ***mag-m.,*** merc., nux-v., ***pic-ac.,*** psor., **PULS.,** rhod., **SIL.,** spig., stront-c.
hair, up the agg. - acon., alum., ambr., am-c., ***arg-m.,*** arn., ars., aur., bar-c., bar-m., **BELL.,** bry., calc., canth., carb-an., carb-s., ***carb-v.,*** carl., chel., ***chin.,*** chin-a., ***cina,*** cinnb., coloc., ***glon., hep.,*** indg., iod., kali-c., ***kali-n.,*** kali-p., kreos., lach., laur., lyc., mag-c., mag-m., ***mez.,*** mosch., mur-ac., nat-c., nat-p., ***nit-ac., nux-v.,*** petr., ph-ac., ***phos.,*** psor., ***puls.,*** rhus-t., sep., ***sil.,*** stann., ***sulph.,*** zinc.
belching, amel - bry., carb-v., cinnb., gent-c., lach., sang.
biting, teeth agg. - am-c.
blinding, (see Vision, Blindness) - asar., aster., ***bell., caust.,*** **CYCL.,** ferr-p., ***gels.,*** **IRIS KALI-BI.,** lac-d., ***lil-t., nat-m., petr., phos., psor., sil., stram., sulph.,*** zinc.
blindness, or visual disturbances, precede or attend - bell., ***cycl.,*** epip., ***gels.,*** ign., ***iris, kali-bi.,*** kali-c., lac-c., ***lac-d., nat-m.,*** nicc., nux-v., pic-ac., podo., psor., ***sang.,*** sil., spig., ***ther.,*** zinc-s.
enlarged feeling - arg-n.
followed by violent headache, sight returns as headache becomes worse - ***iris, kali-bi.,*** lac-d., nat-m.
heaviness, eyes and lids, of - bell., gels.
injection - ***bell.,*** meli., nux-v.
lachrymation - chel., phel., rhus-t., spig., tax.
soreness, with - aloe, cedr., ***cimic., eup-per.,*** gels., hom., menthol, nat-m., phel., ***scut.,*** sil., ***spig.***
vision returns as headache comes on - ***iris,*** lac-d., nat-m.
blowing, nose agg - alum., ambr., aster., **AUR.,** ***bell.,*** calc., ***chel.,*** euphr., ferr., **HEP.,** mur-ac., nit-ac., **PULS., SULPH.**
boat, from riding in a - ***cocc.,*** colch., ferr., ***tab.***
bones, in - ***ant-c., arg-m.,*** **AUR.,** bar-c., ***bell.,*** bry., ***calc.,*** canth., carb-v., caust., cham., **CHIN.,** cocc., cupr., graph., guai., **HEP.,** ign., ip., ***lyc.,*** mang., **MERC.,** ***mez.,*** nat-c., **NIT-AC.,** nux-v., ***ph-ac., phos.,*** puls., rhod., rhus-t., ***ruta.,*** sabad., sabin., samb., **SEP.,** ***sil.,*** spig., staph., sulph., verat., viol-t., zinc.
bread, from eating - manc., zing.
bread, and beer agg - crot-t.

HEADACHES, general

breakfast, after - agar., bufo, ***carb-s.,*** cham., hydr., hyper., indg., ***iris, lyc., naja,*** nat-m., nit-ac., nux-m., ***nux-v.,*** par., ph-ac., phos., plb., sul-ac.
amel. - am-m., ap-g., arum-t., bov., caj., canth., carb-ac., cimic., cinnb., con., croc., eup-per., fl-ac., ind., nat-p., petr.
before - calc., cimic., ind., rumx.
missing - calc., phos.

breath, holding, when - agar.

breathing, deeply, on - anac., cact., crot-h., mang., rat.

bright objects, agg. - ***bell.,*** oreo., ph-ac., ***sil.,*** spig.

bruised, feeling of scalp, with headaches (see Sore, pain) - aesc., ***chin.,*** coloc., sil.

business man, in - arg-m., bry., ***nux-v.,*** pic-ac.

candy, after - ant-c., arg-n.

catarrhal, (see Sinus, catarrhal)

changes in, temperature - ran-b.

chewing, while - am-c., ambr., ind., am-m., kali-c., olnd., phos., ptel., sulph., thuj., verb.

chill, during - acon., agar., am-c., anac., ang., ant-t., ***aran., arg-m.,*** arn., ***ars.,*** bapt., **BELL.,** bor., ***bry.,*** **CACT.,** ***calc.,*** camph., caps., carb-an., ***carb-s.,*** carb-v., cham., ***chin.,*** chin-a., chin-s., cimic., cina, coca, coff., coloc., con., cor-r., crot-h., ***cupr.,*** daph., dros., dulc., elat., ***eup-per., eup-pur.,*** eupi., ferr., ferr-ar., ferr-p., gels., ***graph.,*** hell., hep., hipp., ign., ip., kali-ar., kali-c., kali-n., ***kali-s.,*** kreos., lach., lact., led., lyc., mag-c., mang., mez., **NAT-M., NUX-V.,** ***petr.,*** phos., podo., puls., rhod., rhus-t., ruta., sang., seneg., **SEP.,** spig., ***spong.,*** stram., ***sulph.,*** tarax., thuj., verat.
after - acon., alum., ant-t., arn., berb., bor., bov., caust., cedr., ***cimx.,*** cob., dros., mang., **NAT-M.,** phos.
before the - aesc., ***ars.,*** bell., ***bry.,*** calc., carb-v., cedr., chin., corn-f., elat., ***eup-per., eup-pur.,*** ip., kali-n., lach., nat-c., ***nat-m.,*** plan., puls., rhus-t., spong., ***thuj.***

chilliness, with - ***arg-n.,*** camph., ign., mang., ***puls., sang., sil.***
coldness in, back and occiput - berb.
hands and feet - bell., ***calc.,*** ferr., lach., meli., ***meny.,*** naja, sep., sulph., verat.
head - calc., calc-ac., sep., verat.

choreic, persons, in - ***agar.***

chronic - am-c., ***arg-n., ars., bry., caust.,*** chin-s., cocc., con., lach., lyc., lyss., ***nat-m.,*** phos., plb., ***psor.,*** sep., ***sil., sulph.,*** thuj., tub., zinc.
elderly, people, of - bar-c., calc-p., iod., phos.
lasting seven days - ***caust.***
sedentary persons - anac., ***arg-n.,*** bry., nux-v.

clamped together - am-c., ant-t., berb.

HEADACHES, general

cold, weather, in - acon., ***agar., am-c., ars., aur., bell.,*** **BRY.,** ***calc.,*** calc-s., ***camph., caps.,*** carb-v., ***caust.,*** cocc., ***colch.,*** con., **DULC.,** ***hell.,*** **HEP.,** hyos., ign., kali-c., ***kali-i.,*** lyc., ***merc., mosch.,*** nat-m., ***nux-m.,*** **NUX-V.,** ***ph-ac.,*** phos., rhod., **RHUS-T.,** ***sabad.,*** sep., ***spig., stront-c., sulph.,*** verat.
damp - ***am-c.,*** ars., brom., **BRY., CALC.,** carb-an., ***carb-v.,*** cimic., colch., **DULC., GLON.,** ***lach., lyc., mang.,*** **MERC.,** ***mez.,*** mosch., nat-c., **NUX-M., NUX-V.,** phyt., **RHOD., RHUS-T., SIL.,** ***spig.,*** stront-c., **SULPH.,** tub., ***verat.,*** zing.
dry - acon., ***asar.,*** bry., ***caust.,*** **HEP.,** ***nux-v.,*** sabad., ***spong.***

close, eyes, compelled to - ***agar.,*** aloe, arn., ***bell.,*** calc., ***carb-v.,*** chin-s., euph., mez., nat-m., ***sil.***

closed, eyes, as if something - ***cocc.,*** sulph.

closing, eyes, on - **ALL-C.,** aloe, alumn., ant-t., apis, ars., ***chin.,*** ferr., ferr-p., grat., hep., ip., lac-c., lach., nux-v., op., ph-ac., sabin., ***sil., ther.,*** thuj.
amel. - ***acon., agar.,*** aloe, ant-t., **BELL.,** brom., ***bry., calc., carb-v., chel., chin.,*** chin-s., ***cocc.,*** coff., con., euph., ferr-p., ***hell.,*** hyos., ***ign.,*** iod., ip., kali-p., ***lac-d.,*** mez., ***nat-m.,*** **NAT-S.,** ***nux-v.,*** phys., plan., plat., podo., rhus-t., sang., ***sep.,*** **SIL.,** ***spig., sulph.,*** til., zinc.
partially - ***aloe,*** cocc-s., oreo.

clothing, about the neck agg - arg-n., ***bell.,*** crot-c., ***glon., lach.,*** sep.

cloudy, weather, in - bry., ***calc., cham., chin., dulc., mang.,*** merc., ***nux-m.,*** **RHUS-T.,** ***sep.,*** sulph.

coffee, from - acet-ac., am-c., arg-n., arn., arum-t., ***bell., bry.,*** calc-p., caust., **CHAM.,** ***cocc.,*** form., glon., ***guar.,*** hep., ***ign.,*** kali-n., lach., lyc., merc., mill., nat-s., **NUX-V.,** pall., ***puls.***
amel. - cann-i., chin., coloc., glon., hyos., til.
smell of, from - lach.

cold, amel. in general - ***all-c.,*** aloe, ars., bism., cycl., ferr-p., lyc., phos., ictod., ***puls.,*** spig., ***tab.***
applications, amel. - ***acon.,*** **ALOE,** alumn., ***am-c., ant-c.,*** ant-t., ***ars.,*** asar., aur-m., ***bell.,*** bism., ***bry.,*** bufo, ***calc., calc-p.,*** caust., cedr., cham., chin-s., cinnb., cycl., ***euph.,*** euphr., ferr., ferr-ar., ferr-p., ***glon.,*** ind., iod., kali-bi., kalm., lac-c., ***lac-d., lach., led.,*** meny., merc-c., merl., mosch., myric., ***nat-m., phos.,*** plan., ***psor., puls.,*** seneg., ***spig., stram., sulph., zinc.***

cold, becoming, from agg. - acon., agar., ant-c., ***ars.,*** **BELL., BRY.,** cadm-s., ***calc.,*** carb-an., ***carb-v.,*** **CHAM.,** ***chim.,*** chin-a., clem., colch., ***con.,*** **DULC.,** grat., ***hep.,*** lach., ***lyc.,*** **MAG-P.,** ***merc., mez.,*** mosch., ***nat-m., nit-ac.,*** **NUX-V.,** petr., **PHOS.,** ***puls., rhus-t.,*** **SIL.,** ***spig., stram., stront-c., sulph.,*** sul-ac., ***verat.,*** verb.

HEADACHES, general

cold, becoming, from agg.

feet - ***bar-c.,*** cham., kali-c., phos., ***puls.,*** **SIL.**

feet, amel. - sulph.

head getting cold, on - ***aur.,*** **BELL.,** ***calc.,*** ***carb-v.,*** hep., hyos., kali-c., ***led.,*** nat-m., ***nux-v.,*** puls., **SEP., SIL.**

cold, taking cold, from agg. - ***acon.,*** ant-c., arn., ***bell.,*** ***bry.,*** ***calc.,*** carb-s., ***carb-v.,*** caust., ***cham.,*** chin., coff., coloc., con., dulc., graph., hep., hyos., ***kali-bi.,*** ***kali-c.,*** ***kali-p.,*** kali-s., lach., merc., ***nit-ac.,*** nit-m-ac., ***nux-v.,*** petr., ***phos.,*** ***puls.,*** rhus-t., samb., sep., ***sil.,*** ***sulph.,*** verat.

coldness, with, in - calc., calc-ac., sep., verat.

hands and feet, of - bell., ***calc.,*** ferr., meli., ***meny.,*** naja, sep., sulph., verat.

colic, with - aloe, cocc.

combing, the hair - ars., ***bry.,*** carb-v., chin., chin-a., ***cina,*** hell., ign., kreos., lac-c., ***mez.,*** sel., sep.

amel. - form.

backward - puls., rhus-t.

come off, as if, top of head would - alum., bapt., cact., ***cann-s.,*** cham., ***cimic.,*** cob., cupr-s., lith., merc., sang., ther.

jar, at every - cob., merc.

straining at stool - ind.

company, or crowd, while in - mag-c., plat., ***plb.,*** staph.

concussion, from (see Injuries)

confusion, mental, with - agar., ***aur.,*** glon., nat-a., petr., stram., tarax.

lose senses or go mad, as if would - ***acon.,*** agar., chin., med., stram., tarent., verat.

unable to collect one's senses - carb-v., chin., crot-h., cycl., kreos., ***mang.,*** mez., nit-ac., rhus-t., sars., sil., stann., sulph.

congestion, pain, as from - guai., nit-ac.

congestion, of head, (see Head, Congestion)

congestive - ***acon.,*** aml-n., arg-n., **BELL.,** ***bry.,*** ***cact.,*** chin-s., ***ferr-p.,*** ***gels.,*** **GLON.,** glyc., joan., **LACH.,** ***meli.,*** nat-m., nux-v., op., phase., ***sang.,*** sil., sol-n., sulph., usn., ***verat-v.***

menses, before and during - aster., ***bell.,*** bry., cimic., cocc., croc., ***cycl.,*** ferr., ***gels.,*** ***glon.,*** graph., kali-p., kreos., lac-c., ***lach.,*** nat-c., ***nat-m.,*** ***nux-v.,*** puls., ***sang.,*** ***sep.,*** ***sulph.,*** ***ust.,*** verat-v., xan.

metrorrhagia, during - bell., glon.

passive - ***chin-s.,*** ferr-p., ***ferr-py.,*** gels., op., sil.

constant, continued - arg-m., cann-s., carb-v., ***chin-s.,*** ***cimic.,*** cupr., dulc., **FERR.,** ***gels.,*** ***glon.,*** hep., hydr., hyos., indg., lob., lept., nat-m., ph-ac., phos., rhod., rhus-r., sep., still., ter.

fixed, lasts for weeks, months, even years, with rare intermissions - ter.

two or three days - croc., **FERR.**

HEADACHES, general

constipated, while - ***aloe,*** alum., am-c., **BRY.,** ***calc-p.,*** coff., ***coll.,*** con., crot-h., euon., hydr., ign., iris, ***lac-d.,*** lach., mag-c., merc., ***nat-m.,*** ***nat-s.,*** nicc., nit-ac., ***nux-v.,*** op., ***plb.,*** petr., ***podo.,*** ***puls.,*** rat., torula., verat., zinc.

contracting, pain - chin., dig., bism., hep., lyc., mang., nat-c., nit-ac., petr., sep.

contradiction, after - ***aur.,*** ***bry.,*** ***coff.,*** lyc., mag-c., nat-m., petr., phos., rhus-t.

copper, abuse of - hep.

corrosive, pain - alum.

coryza, with - **ACON.,** ***aesc.,*** ***agar.,*** **ALL-C.,** alum., anan., ant-c., ***arg-n.,*** arn., ***ars.,*** ars-i., ***aur.,*** bad., **BELL.,** bov., **BRY.,** ***calc.,*** carb-v., caust., cham., ***chim.,*** ***chin-a.,*** **CHLOR.,** cic., cimic., cina, coff., coloc., con., cor-r., croc., dios., dulc., euphr., ***ferr.,*** ferr-ar., ferr-i., ferr-p., ***gels.,*** graph., hell., hep., hyos., ign., ***iod.,*** jac., kali-ar., ***kali-bi.,*** ***kali-c.,*** ***kali-i.,*** kali-p., kali-s., kalm., ***lach.,*** **LYC.,** mag-m., **MERC.,** ***merc-i-r.,*** naja, nat-a., nat-c., nit-ac., **NUX-V.,** petr., ***phos.,*** phyt., psor., ***puls.,*** rhod., rhus-t., rumx., sabad., samb., ***sang.,*** senec., ***sep.,*** ***sil.,*** ***spig.,*** stann., ***sulph.,*** ***thuj.,*** verat.

as from - nit-ac., phos., sulph.

in begining - sep., sil.

dry, with - croc., ***sep.***

preceded by - ant-c.

suppressed, from having a - ***acon.,*** am-c., ars., bell., bry., ***calc.,*** carb-v., cham., chin., cina, ***kali-bi.,*** kali-c., lach., lyc., ***nux-v.,*** puls., sep., sil.

coughing, on - acon., aeth., alum., ambr., am-c., ***anac.,*** ang., ant-t., apis, ***arn.,*** ars., asim., aur., bad., bar-c., **BELL.,** brom., **BRY.,** cact., ***calc.,*** ***calc-s.,*** **CAPS.,** ***carb-v.,*** caust., ***chel.,*** ***chin.,*** chin-a., chion., cimx., ***cina,*** coc-c., ***coloc.,*** **CON.,** ***cupr.,*** dios., eup-per., ferr., ferr-ar., ferr-i., ferr-p., ham., hep., hydr., hyos., ign., ***ip.,*** ***iris,*** ***kali-ar.,*** kali-bi., ***kali-c.,*** kali-n., kali-p., kali-s., **LAC-D.,** ***lach.,*** lac-ac., led., ***lob.,*** ***lyc.,*** mag-s., mang., med., ***merc.,*** mez., mur-ac., naja, **NAT-M.,** ***nicc.,*** ***nit-ac.,*** ***nux-v.,*** oena., ol-an., ol-j., ***petr.,*** ***ph-ac.,*** **PHOS., PSOR.,** ***puls.,*** rhus-t., rumx., ruta., ***sabad.,*** ***sang.,*** sars., seneg., ***sep.,*** sil., ***spig.,*** ***spong.,*** **SQUIL.,** ***stann.,*** staph., stict., **SULPH.,** sul-ac., tarent., tax., tril., verat., zinc., ziz.

amel. - arg-mur.

cry out, pains compel one to - anac., ***ars.,*** bov., ***bry.,*** cact., camph., ***coloc.,*** cupr., kali-c., lyss., mag-m., petr., ***sep.,*** sil., stann., stram., tarent.

crying, suppressing - ***nat-m.,*** ***uva.***

damp, houses, living in, from - ***ars.,*** calc., ***carb-v.,*** ***dulc.,*** nat-s., phys., puls., rhod., ***rhus-t.,*** ***sil.,*** ***verat.***

dancing - ***arg-n.***

dark spots, before eyes, with - aspar.

darkness, agg. - aloe, carb-an., ***carb-v.,*** lac-c., onos., ***sil.***

HEADACHES, general

darkness, amel. - acon., arn., ***bell.,*** brom., **BRY.,** chin., hipp., lac-d., mag-p., mez., ***sang.,*** sep., ***sil., stram.,*** zinc.

daytime - agar., am-c., aur., bry., calc., cann-s., caust., chel., chin-s., cina, cist., cob., coca, crot-t., eup-per., ferr., fl-ac., ham., jac., kali-c., lyc., lyss., merc-i-r., ***nat-m.,*** nicc., petr., phos., rumx., sep., stann., staph., zinc.

deafness, with - chin-s., verb.

delirium, with - agar., bell., chin-s., sil., stram., syph., verat.

dentition, during - ***acon.,*** bell., ***cocc.,*** calc-p., ***cham.,*** coff., hep., hyos., ign., merc., nit-ac., nux-v., rhus-t., sil.

dehydration, from loss of fluids - ars., ***calc., carb-v.,*** **CHIN.,** cina, cocc., con., kali-c., lach., merc., ***nat-m., nux-v.,*** phos., ***ph-ac., puls., sep., sil., staph., sulph.,*** verat.

profuse uterine hemorrhages, after - chin., ***glon.***

descending, on - **BELL.,** ***ferr.,*** meny., merc-i-f., ***rhus-t.***

diarrhea, with - aeth., agar., aloe, ambr., apis, calc-p., cham., con., glon., graph., ind., jatr., kali-n., podo., stram., verat.

alternating - ***aloe,*** podo.

amel. - agar., alum., apis, lachn.

dinner, after - am-c., alum., bell., ***calc-p., calc-s.,*** carb-s., cast., chin-s., cimic., con., dios., gent-c., gins., glon., hyper., jug-r., kali-bi., kali-c., kali-n., lob-s., mag-m., merc-i-f., ***nat-m.,*** nat-p., nux-v., phel., phos., phyt., raph., stram., ***sulph.,*** thuj., valer., zinc.

amel., after - arg-n., arum-t., genist., phos., ptel., uran-n., zing.

before - indg., nux-v.

delayed, from - cact., cist., lyc.

dogs, after bites of - bell., lyss.

dreams, after unpleasant - cob., sulph.

drinking, from - acon., bry., ***cimx., cocc.,*** crot-t., lyc., merc., sep.

aversion for - **FERR.**

cold drinks, from - con., dig., kali-c.

amel. - alumn., bism.

heated, when - bry.

quickly after - nat-m.

drowsiness, with - ***ail.,*** ant-t., bran., chel., dub., ***gels., ind.,*** lept., myric., stel.

drugs, after abuse of - ***aven.,*** bell., cham., coff., dig., graph., hyos., lach., lyc., **NUX-V.,** op., puls., sep., valer.

eating, during - am-c., arn., ***ars.,*** atro., ***bry.,*** cact., chel., ***cocc.,*** coff., con., dulc., gels., ***graph.,*** ign., ind., lach., ***lyc.,*** mag-m., manc., nat-m., nit-ac., nux-v., ***ph-ac.,*** puls., ran-b., rhus-t., sabin., sec., sul-ac., tab., verb., zinc.

amel., during - alum., ***anac.,*** ap-g., bov., cadm-met., carl., ***chel., chin.,*** coca, ign., iod., kali-p., ***lach., lith., lyc.,*** phel., phos., ***psor.,*** sep., sil., sin-n., sulph., zinc.

HEADACHES, general

eating, after - agar., **ALUM.,** ambr., am-c., ant-c., arn., ars., bar-c., bar-m., bell., bov., ***bry.,*** bufo, ***calc., calc-p., calc-s.,*** canth., caps., carb-an., carb-s., ***carb-v.,*** cast., caust., ***cham.,*** chel., chin., chin-a., chin-s., cina, cinnb., ***cocc., coff., com.,*** crot-t., dios., euon., ferr., ferr-ar., ferr-p., gels., glon., ***graph.,*** grat., ***hyos.,*** ign., ind., kali-ar., kali-c., kali-n., kali-s., lach., ***lith.,*** lob., ***lyc.,*** mag-c., mag-m., meny., merc., merc-i-f., mur-ac., ***nat-a.,*** **NAT-C., NAT-M.,** nat-p., nat-s., nit-ac., nux-m., **NUX-V.,** paeon., ***petr.,*** phel., ***ph-ac.,*** **PHOS.,** plat., prun., **PULS.,** ran-b., ***rhus-t.,*** rumx., ruta., sars., seneg., sep., ***sil.,*** staph., **SULPH.,** valer., verat., ***zinc.***

amel. - aloe, ***anac.,*** arg-n., ars-i., arum-t., caj., carb-ac., carb-an., card-m., caust., chel., chin., cist., coca, con., gels., genist., ind., iod., ***kali-bi.,*** kali-p., lachn., laur., lyc., mag-c., mez., petr., phos., phyt., phys., psor., rhus-t., sabad., scut., **SEP.,** spig., tell., thuj.

overeating, after - coff., **NUX-M., NUX-V., PULS.**

eating, before - am-m., cann-s., carb-an., nux-v., ran-b., sabad., ***sil.***

eating, impossible - kali-n.

epileptic attacks, after - bufo, ***calc., caust.,*** cina, cupr., kali-br.

before - cina.

elderly, people, of - ambr., am-c., cypr., iod.

onanism, from - bry., calc., sulph.

emotional disturbances, from (see Excitement) - arg-n., cham., coff., epip., ***gels., ign.,*** mez., ph-ac., ***pic-ac.,*** plat., rhus-t., sil.

emissions, after - sel.

empty feeling in stomach, with - ***ign.,*** kali-p., ***sep.***

erosive, pain - plat., sulph.

eruptions, suppressed - ant-c., bry., lyc., **MEZ.,** nux-m., **PSOR.,** ***sulph.***

evening - acon., agar., **ALL-C.,** alum., ***ambr.,*** am-c., ***anac.,*** ang., ant-c., ant-t., apis, arg-m., ars., asaf., aur., bad., bar-c., bar-m., **BELL.,** bor., bov., brom., bry., calc., ***calc-s.,*** camph., canth., caps., ***carb-an., carb-s., carb-v., caust.,*** cedr., cham., chel., chin., chin-s., cic., cimic., cina, cist., clem., cob., cocc., coc-c., colch., coloc., croc., crot-t., cycl., cupr., cupr-ar., ***dig.,*** dios., ***dulc.,*** echi., elaps, elat., eug., euphr., ferr., ferr-ar., ferr-p., form., glon., graph., hell., hep., hipp., hydr., hyper., indg., ind., iris, jug-c., jug-r., kali-ar., ***kali-bi., kali-c.,*** kali-chl., kali-i., ***kali-n.,*** kali-p., **KALI-S.,** kalm., lach., lachn., lac-ac., laur., led., lept., lil-t., lob., ***lyc.,*** lycps., lyss., ***mag-c., mag-m.,*** mag-s., mang., meny., meph., ***merc.,*** merc-i-f., merc-i-r., **MEZ.,** mosch., murx., ***mur-ac., nat-a., nat-c., nat-m.,*** nat-p., ***nit-ac.,*** nux-v., par., petr., ***ph-ac., phos.,*** phys., plan., ***plat.,*** plb., psor., **PULS.,** ran-b., rat., rhod., rhus-t., ruta., sabad., sabin., sang., sars., sel., ***seneg., sep., sil.,*** spig., ***stann.,***

HEADACHES, general

evening - staph., stram., ***stront-c.,*** **SULPH.,** ***sul-ac.,*** tell., ter., teucr., ther., thuj., til., valer., ***zinc.***

6 p.m - cob., gels., nat-s., paeon., ptel., puls., rhus-t., sep.

7 p.m. - bad., ***cedr.,*** chin-s., cocc., elaps, lyc., mag-c., nat-m., rhod., rhus-t., sep., ***sulph.,*** verat-v.

8 p.m - gymn., lac-ac., merc-i-r., phys., sol-n., stry., sulph.

8 to 9 p.m - helon., indg.

9 p.m - coca, dios., eupi., gels., lyss., osm., pic-ac., ptel.

9 p.m. to1 a.m. - crot-h.

10 p.m - carb-s., dios., ham., laur., mag-p., myric., phys.

11 p.m - **CACT.,** cast., dios., indg., merc-i-r., pip-m., stram., valer.

amel. - am-c., ***bry.,*** calc-f., ham., kali-bi., lach., mang., nat-a., ***nat-m.,*** phys., pic-ac., spig., ter.

bed., in - arg-m., ars., carb-v., cycl., hipp., laur., lyc., nat-m., phos., ***puls.,*** sep., **SULPH.,** zinc.

amel - mag-c., **NUX-V.,** sulph.

lasting all night - alum.

and following day - kali-n.

twilight, at - ang., caj., puls.

walking, when - ther.

excitement, emotional, after - ***acon.,*** arg-m., ***arg-n., arn., aur., bell.,*** benz-ac., bry., ***cact.,*** cham., chin., ***chin-a.,*** chin-s., ***cocc., coff.,*** con., cycl., ery-a., ***ferr-p., gels.,*** ign., kali-p., kreos., ***lach., lyc., lyss.,*** **NAT-M., NUX-V.,** ***op.,*** par., petr., **PH-AC., PHOS.,** ***pic-ac.,*** **PULS.,** rhus-t., scut., **STAPH.,** sulph., tub., ***verat.***

depressing or sad news, after - calc., cocc., ***gels.,*** ign., nux-v., op., staph.

exertion, of body, agg. - acet-ac., aloe, ambr., anac., arg-n., arn., berb., ***cact.,*** **CALC.,** ***calc-p.,*** cocc., **EPIP.,** gels., gins., glon., kali-p., lact., med., merc., mez., nat-c., ***nat-m., nux-v.,*** ph-ac., phos., pic-ac., rhus-r., rhus-t., sep., sil., spong., tub., ***valer.,*** zing.

amel. - agar., apis, mag-m., merc-i-f., ***rhod.,*** rhus-g., ***sep.***

exertion, mental, from agg. - acon., agar., agn., ambr., am-c., ***anac.,*** apis, aran., arg-m., ***arg-n.,*** arn., ars-i., asaf., asar., aster., **AUR.,** bell., benz-ac., bor., ***bry.,*** **CACT.,** cadm-s., **CALC.,** calc-ar., **CALC-P.,** calc-s., cahin., ***carb-ac.,*** carb-an., carb-s., ***carb-v., cham., chin.,*** chin-a., chion., cimic., cina, cinnb., ***cist.,*** cob., ***cocc.,*** coc-c., coff., ***colch.,*** coloc., ***con.,*** crot-h., cupr., daph., ***dig.,*** elaps, ***epip.,*** fago., ferr-i., ***ferr-pic., gels.,*** gent-c., gins., **GLON.,** graph., hell., helon., hipp., hydr., hyper., hydr., ***ign.,*** ind., ***iris,*** kali-ar., kali-c., kali-n., ***kali-p.,*** kalm., ***lac-c., lach.,*** lact., lob., **LYC.,** ***lyss., mag-c., mag-m.,*** mag-p., manc., med., meli., meph., merc., mez., morph., naja, ***nat-a.,*** **NAT-C., NAT-M., NAT-P.,** ***nat-s.,*** nicc., ***nit-ac., nux-m.,***

HEADACHES, general

exertion, mental, from agg. - **NUX-V.,** olnd., ol-an., op., ox-ac., ***par., petr.,*** **PH-AC.,** phase., ***phos.,*** **PIC-AC.,** pimp., ***pip-n.,*** plat., plb., prun., ***psor.,*** ptel., **PULS.,** ran-b., rhus-t., rhus-v., rob., ***sabad.,*** scut., sel., ***sep.,*** **SIL.,** ***spig., staph.,*** stram., ***sulph.,*** ter., ther., tub., zinc.

amel. - am-c., ars., calc-ac., calc-p., ham., helon., ign., merc-i-f., nat-m., nit-ac., par., phos., phys., pip-m., psor., sabad.

exhaustion, asthenia, with - ***ars., chin., gels.,*** ign., ind., lac-c., lob., ***pic-ac.,*** sang., sulph.

extending to, head pain

around the head - calc-s.

back - aloe, anac., bell., calc., caust., dig., kali-n., lyc., mag-c., mosch., nat-m., nit-ac., petr., phos., prun., ***puls.,*** rhod., rhus-t., samb., sep., sil., spig., spong., stann., stront-c., sul-ac., thuj.

base of brain - ambr., cina, laur., mang., phos., senn.

cheek - hep., ***hyper.,*** indg., rhus-t.

chest - con., nat-m.

chin - hyper.

ears - agar., lach., merc., nux-v., puls., rhus-t.

elbows - kali-n.

epigastrium - thuj.

eyes - ***arg-n.,*** asaf., brom., ***calc.,*** caust., croc., ***crot-h.,*** ign., ***kali-c.,*** kali-s., ***lach., lyss.,*** mag-m., merc., nat-m., nicc., **NIT-AC., PULS.,** rhus-t., ***seneg., spig.,*** **SULPH.**

left - ign.

face - am-m., anac., ant-t., aran., arg-m., ***bry.,*** graph., guai., indg., lyc., mag-m., nat-m., phos., puls., rhus-t., sars., seneg., sil., spig., tarent., thuj.

finger tips - camph.

forehead - aloe, bar-c., **BELL.,** bor., ***bry.,*** carb-v., chin., cupr., dios., ferr., gran., kali-c., kali-s., lact., olnd., ph-ac., prun., stann., staph., sulph., til., viol-t.

jaws - ***arg-n.,*** bell., calc-p., kali-chl., mez., spig.

upper malar bone - nux-v.

left side - camph., cann-s., ***spig.,*** staph.

limbs, through - acet-ac.

neck - anac., bar-c., berb., ***bry.,*** chel., chin., cocc., guai., jac., kali-c., kali-n., kalm., ***lach.,*** lil-t., lyc., merc., mosch., nat-m., nux-m., onos., phel., sabin., viol-t., ziz.

nose - agar., ant-t., ars., bism., bor., calc., cimic., colch., ***glon.,*** guai., **LACH.,** lachn., lyc., lyss., nat-c., nux-v., ph-ac., phos.

root of nose - agar., ***bism.,*** kali-c., kali-n., ***lach.,*** nux-v.

occiput - bell., calc., carb-v., chel., glon., helon., nat-c., op., pip-m., puls., **PRUN.,** ***sep.,*** **THUJ.,** til.

left side - calc-ac.

right side - phos., **PRUN.**

right side - anac., asaf., cast., eupi., hell.

scapula - puls.

right - chel.

HEADACHES, general

extending to, head pain

shoulder - glon., graph., podo.

spine, down - ***cocc.,*** dirc., nux-v., syph.

teeth - **CHIN.,** crot-h., ferr., graph., ign., kalm., kreos., lach., lyc., lycps., lyss., mag-c., merc., mez., psor., puls., rhus-t., sep., sil., staph.

roots of - ip.

temples - asar.

throat - anac., merc., psor., tarent.

tongue - ***ip.***

vertex - glon., par., sep., spig., staph.

zygoma - ***hyper.,*** kali-chl.

eyebrows, as if pressing down - carb-an.

eyes, as would be forced out - ruta.

as if would fall out - sep.

eyestrain, headaches, from - ***agar.,*** arg-n., ***aur.,*** bell., ***bor., cact., calc., carb-v., caust., cimic., cina,*** gels., ***ham.,*** jab., **KALI-C.,** kali-p., kali-s., **LYC.,** mag-p., mur-ac., ***nat-c.,*** **NAT-M.,** ***nat-p., onos.,*** par., **PH-AC.,** ***phos.,*** phys., **RHOD.,** ***rhus-t.,*** **RUTA.,** sep., **SIL.,** ***spong.,*** staph., sulph., ***tub.,*** valer., zinc.

face, flushed, hot - ***acon., bell.,*** cham., ferr-p., gels., ***glon.,*** mag-p., ***meli.,*** naja, nat-m., nux-v., podo., ***sang.,*** sep.

on moving the face - apis, spig.

pale - acon., ***calc.,*** chin., ign., ***lach.,*** lob., meli., nat-m., sil., spig., tab., ***verat.***

fainting, after - mosch.

faintness, with - ars., ***calc.,*** carb-v., ***gels.,*** glon., graph., hippoz., lyc., mosch., nat-m., nux-v., ***sil.,*** stram., ***sulph.,*** verat., zing.

fall, after a - ***arn.,*** hyper., ***nat-s.,*** rhus-t.

fasting, from - ars-i., caust., ***cist.,*** elaps, ind., iod., ***kali-c.,*** kali-s., ***lyc.,*** nux-v., ***phos.,*** ptel., ran-b., ***sang., sil.,*** spig., ***sulph.,*** thuj., uran.

empty feeling in stomach, with - ***ign.,*** kali-p., ***sep.***

if hunger is not appeased at once - cact., cist., elaps, ***lyc., phos., sang., sulph.***

fatty food, from - ***carb-v.,*** colch., cycl., ***ip.,*** nat-c., nat-m., **PULS.,** sang., sep., thuj.

fever, during the - acon., aesc., agar., am-c., ***ang.,*** ant-t., **APIS, ARN.,** ***ars.,*** asaf., **BELL.,** berb., bor., bry., cact., calc., camph., caps., carb-s., carb-v., **CHIN.,** chin-a., chin-s., cina, ***cocc.,*** coloc., corn-f., ***crot-h.,*** cupr., dros., dulc., elat., **EUP-PER.,** graph., ***hep.,*** hipp., hyos., ***ign.,*** kali-ar., kali-bi., kali-c., ***lach.,*** lob., lyc., **NAT-M.,** ***nux-v., op.,*** plan., ***podo., puls., rhus-t.,*** ruta., ***sabad.,*** sep., **SIL.,** spig., sulph., ***thuj.,*** valer., verat.

after the - ***ars.,*** calc., ***carb-v.,*** **EUP-PER., NAT-M.,** sil.

before the - bry., chin., puls., rhus-t., sil., spong.

flatulence, with - asc-t., calc-ac., calc-p., cann-i., ***carb-v.,*** xan.

as if from - carb-v., chin-s., mag-c., nit-ac., sulph.

flatus, emission of, amel. - aeth., cic., sang.

HEADACHES, general

footsteps - **COFF., NUX-V.,** ***sil.***

foreign body, as if - ***con.,*** fl-ac., rhod.

forehead, headaches (see Headaches, forehead)

forenoon - aeth., alum., alumn., ant-c., ***aur., bar-c.,*** bry., ***calc.,*** canth., carb-s., caust., chel., chin-s., cimic., cinnb., clem., cob., cocc., coc-c., ***con.,*** cop., cupr-ar., gamb., genist., ham., hydr., ind., indg., iod., jab., jac., ***kali-c.,*** kali-s., kalm., lach., lachn., lact., merc-i-f., ***nat-c., nat-m.,*** nicc., phel., phyt., polyg., ptel., ran-b., rhod., rhus-t., rumx., ***sars., sep.,*** sol-n., sulph., sul-ac., trom.

8 a.m - bov.

9 a.m. to 1 p.m - cedr., mur-ac.

to 4 p.m - caust., cedr.

to 12 - cedr., ***meli.***

10 a.m - apis, ***aran.,*** ars., **BOR.,** cimic., ***gels.,*** **NAT-M.,** ***sil.,*** thuj.

to 2 p.m - alum.

to 3 p.m - **NAT-M.**

to 4 p.m - ***stann.***

to 6 p.m - apis

11 a.m. - cann-i., ip., spig., sol-n., sulph.

fright, after - **ACON.,** ***arg-n.,*** calc., ***chin-a., coff., cupr.,*** hipp., hyos., **IGN.,** ***nux-v., op.,*** ph-ac., ***plat.,*** **PULS.,** samb.

frowning, from - ars., mang., nat-m.

amel. - calc-caust., caust., phos., sulph.

gastralgia, attending or following - bism.

gastric, headache - acet-ac., acon., aesc., agar., ail., aloe, alum., am-c., ***anac.,*** **ANT-C.,** apis, ***arg-m.,*** arg-n., ***arn.,*** ars., asar., atro., bell., berb., bism., **BRY.,** ***calc., calc-p.,*** calc-s., cann-i., caps., caul., ***caust., carb-v.,*** cham., ***chin.,*** cic., cina, cocc., ***coff., coll.,*** euph., ***eup-per.,*** form., gamb., gels., glon., ***hydr.,*** ign., indg., **IP., IRIS,** kali-ar., kali-bi., kali-c., kali-p., kali-s., lach., lept., ***lyc.,*** naja, nux-m., **NUX-V.,** op., par., ***phos.,*** phyt., plat., podo., **PULS.,** rham-cal., rob., **SANG.,** ***sep., sil.,*** stict., **SULPH.,** ***tab.,*** tarent., verat.

anxiety, with - ***caust.***

bilious - am-pic., anac., ***arg-n.,*** bapt., ***bry.,*** cham., chel., ***chion.,*** cycl., eup-per., ***ip.,*** iris, lob., merc-sul., ***nux-v.,*** podo., ***puls.,*** rob., ***sang.,*** stry., tarax.

gouty - guai.

nodules on scalp, with - sil.

grief, from - ***calc.,*** **IGN., NAT-M.,** op., ***ph-ac., puls.,*** **STAPH.**

hair, cutting, after - **BELL.,** glon., led., puls., sabad., ***sep.***

letting down amel. - bell., cina, dirc., ferr., phos.

hammering - ***am-c., ars.,*** aur., **BELL.,** cadm-s., calc., chel., ***chin.,*** chin-a., ***chin-s.,*** cic., cimic., clem., ***cocc., coff., cur.,*** dros., **FERR., FERR-AR.,** ferr-p., **GLON.,** ***hep.,*** indg., iris, kali-i., ***lach.,*** mag-s., manc., mez., **NAT-M.,** nicc., nit-ac., ph-ac., ***psor.,*** puls., rhus-t., rheum, **SIL., SULPH.,** ***tarent.,*** verb.

evening, while lying - clem.

morning - **NAT-M.**

HEADACHES, general

hammering, vivacious talking, from - **SULPH.**

hang down, letting feet - ***puls.***

hat, from pressure of - agar., alum., arg-m., ***calc-p.,*** carb-an., **CARB-V.,** caust., ***crot-t.,*** ferr-i., ***glon.,*** hep., kali-n., ***lach.,*** laur., led., lil-t., lob., lyc., mez., nat-m., **NIT-AC.,** petr., phys., sel., sep., ***sil.,*** staph., sulph., ***valer.***

hawking, agg. - conv.

hearts, action labored, with - lycps.

heat, amel. - ***arg-n.,*** ars., ***aur., bell., bry.,*** caps., ***caust., chim.,*** cinnb., cocc., colch., ***coloc., gels.,*** hyos., ***ign.,*** iris, ***kali-c.,*** kali-i., lach., ***mag-m.,*** **MAG-P.,** ***nit-ac., nux-m., nux-v., psor.,*** rhod., ***rhus-t.,*** **SIL.,** stann., staph., ***stram.,*** stront-c., sulph., sumb.

hot applications, amel. - ***arg-n.,*** ars., ***aur., bry.,*** chim., cinnb., colch., coloc., ***gels.,*** glon., iris, ***kali-c.,*** kali-i., lach., mag-m., **MAG-P.,** nux-m., **SIL.**

of hand - cinnb., iris.

heated, from becoming - ***acon., aloe,*** am-c., ***arum-t.,*** **ANT-C.,** ***apis,*** arg-n., arn., bar-c., **BELL.,** ***bry.,*** calc., calc-s., camph., caps., ***carb-s.,*** **CARB-V.,** con., dig., dros., form., **GLON.,** grat., ign., ***ip., kali-c.,*** kali-p., ***kali-s., kalm.,*** lach., **LYC.,** nat-a., ***nat-m.,*** nux-m., op., phos., ptel., puls., ***sep., sil.,*** staph., ***stram., sulph., thuj.,*** zinc.

by a fire or stove - **ANT-C.,** ***apis, arn., arum-t., bar-c.,*** bry., cimic., com., euph., **GLON.,** lac-d., ***manc.,*** merc., nux-v., ***phos., puls.,*** rhus-t., ***sanic., zinc.***

bed, from - ***lyc.,*** nux-m.

walking, agg. head, but amel. pain limbs - lyc.

hemorrhage, excesses or vital losses (see Dehydration) - carb-v., ***chin.,*** ferr., ph-ac., sil.

hemorrhoids - coll., nux-v.

high, altitudes, in - ***coca.***

hold must, head - glon.

head and eyes down, must - apis

holding, hands near head amel. - carb-an., glon., petr., ***sul-ac.***

head erect, while - bar-c.

hot, drinks agg - ***arum-t.,*** **PHOS., PULS.,** ***sulph.***

soup amel - kali-bi.

humiliation, from - carc., lyc., op., staph.

humming, pain - aur., hep., squil., staph., sulph.

hunger, with - anac., cact., ***epip.,*** ign., ***lyc., psor.***

hysterical, headache - ***arg-n.,*** arn., **ASAF.,** ***aur.,*** bell., bry., cann-s., caps., cham., cimic., ***cocc., coff.,*** gels., hell., hep., hyos., **IGN.,** iris, kali-bi., lach., lact., mag-c., mag-m., ***mosch.,*** nat-m., nit-ac., ***nux-m.,*** nux-v., ph-ac., phos., ***plat.,*** rhus-t., ruta., scut., ***sep.,*** stict., stram., tarent., valer., verat.

ice cream, after - ***ars.,*** **PULS.**

increasing, gradually - acon., bry., carb-v., caust., con., lact., lob., sars.

and decreasing gradually - arn., ars., bar-c., bufo, crot-h., glon., jab., mez., nat-m., op., pic-ac., ***plat.,*** psor., sabin., sars., spig., **STANN.,** staph., stront-c., sulph., verb.

and decreasing rapidly - ***arg-n.,*** **BELL.,** coca, merc-c., ***spig., sulph.***

but ceasing suddenly - arg-m., caust., ***ign., sul-ac.***

influenza, with - ***bry.,*** camph., ***eup-per.,*** gels., lob-p.

injuries, mechanical, after (see Head, Injuries) - **ARN.,** ***bell.,*** calc., carc., ***cic.,*** con., dulc., ***glon., hep., hyper.,*** lach., merc., ***nat-m.,*** **NAT-S.,** nit-ac., petr., ***phos.,*** puls., ***rhus-t., staph.,*** sulph., sul-ac.

headache, from blows - **ARN.,** ***calc-s., hell., hyper., nat-m.,*** **NAT-S.**

from concussion - **ARN.,** ***bell.,*** calc-s., carc., cocc., ferr-p., hep., lac-c., merc., **NAT-S.,** phos.

inspiration, during an - ***anac.,*** brom., carb-v., rat.

deep - ***cact.***

intermittent pains - agar., alumn., anac., arg-m., ***ars.,*** cann-i., caul., cina, cupr., ferr., ***gels.,*** ign., iod., iris, kalm., mill., nit-ac., plan., plat., psor., sang., sep., stann., ter., valer., verat.

intoxication, after - ***ant-c.,*** bell., ***bry., carb-v.,*** cocc., coff., glon., laur., **NUX-V.,** ***puls.,*** spong., stram., sulph., tarax.

as if - ambr.

iron, from abuse of - ferr., puls., ***zinc.***

ironing, from - **BRY.,** sep.

itching, pain - chin., sep., sil.

jar, from any - am-c., am-m., arn., bar-c., **BELL., BRY.,** ***calc.,*** calc-s., ***carb-s., carb-v.,*** chel., ***chin.,*** chin-a., cina, cob., cocc., con., crot-h., ***ferr-p., gels.,*** **GLON.,** grat., ***hep.,*** ind., ***kali-c.,*** kali-p., ***kali-s.,*** lac-c., lac-d., lach., **LED.,** ***lyc., mag-m.,*** mang., merc., nat-a., ***nat-m.,*** **NIT-AC.,** ***nux-v.,*** onos., petr., ***ph-ac., phos.,*** phyt., ***psor., rhus-t.,*** sabad., sang., ***sep.,*** **SIL.,** ***spig., sulph., ther., thuj.,*** vib.

as from - sep.

joy, from excessive - ***coff.,*** cycl., op., ***phos.,*** puls., scut.

lain, with head to low, as if - phos.

laughing, from - ars., chion., cocc., ip., iris, mang., ***nat-m.,*** phos., ther., zinc., zing.

leaning, against something, while - ang., bell., cycl., nat-m.

amel. - anac., aral., aran., arn., **BELL.,** brom., cann-s., con., dros., gels., gymn., kali-bi., meny., merc., nux-v., rhod., sabad., sabin., sang., seneg., spig., sulph.

HEADACHES, general

left, sided headaches - aloe, alum., ***ambr., ant-c.,*** apis, ***ars., ars-i., asaf., asar., bell.,*** bism., ***bov.,*** **BROM.,** bry., calad., ***calc.,*** calc-p., cann-s., canth., carb-s., carb-v., caust., ***cham., chin.,*** chin-a., chin-s., cimic., cina, ***coloc.,*** con., conv., ***croc.,*** crot-h., cupr., ***cycl.,*** eup-pur., ***euph., ferr., ferr-i.,*** fl-ac., ***graph., guai.,*** gymn., ham., hydr., ign., ***iod., kali-c.,*** lac-c., ***lach.,*** lac-ac., lil-t., lith., ***lob.,*** lyc., ***mag-c.,*** med., ***merc.,*** merc-i-f., merc-i-r., murx., nat-m., ***nit-ac., nux-m., olnd.,*** pall., ***par.,*** phel., ***phos.,*** plan., ***plat.,*** plb., ptel., ran-b., ran-s., ***rhod., rhus-t.,*** sabad., ***samb.,*** sec., ***sel.,*** **SEP., SPIG.,** ***sulph.,*** tab., ***tarax., thuj.,*** trom., verat-v., viol-o., viol-t., xan., ***zinc.,*** zing., ziz.

and face, of, extending to neck - guai.

lying, on left side agg. - ars., calad., kali-bi., phos.

on right side amel. - brom.

then right - arn., eup-per., glon., ***lac-c.,*** lach., ***nux-m.,*** squil., sulph.

with redness and bloated swelling of the cheek with nausea and vomiting - apis.

lemonade, from - ***sel.***

lie down, must - alum., am-c., anac., bell., ***bry., calc.,*** calc-p., calc-s., chin., ***con.,*** croc., crot-h., euphr., **FERR.,** ferr-ac., ferr-i., gels., graph., iod., kali-bi., kali-c., kali-p., kali-s., lach., lyc., mag-m., mosch., nat-c., ***nat-m.,*** nat-p., nit-ac., ***nux-v.,*** olnd., op., petr., ph-ac., phos., psor., puls., ***rhus-t.,*** sang., sars., ***sel., sep.,*** sil., stann., stict., sulph., zinc.

prone with head hanging over side of bed - zinc.

with head high - arg-m., **ARS.,** bry., carb-v., ***com., gels.,*** nat-m., ***phos.,*** **PULS.,** ***spig.,*** stront.

with head low - absin., arn., cadm-s., ***hell.,*** ign., mosch., ***nux-v.,*** phys., ***spong.,*** thuj.

lifting, from - ambr., ***arn.,*** bar-c., ***bry., calc.,*** cocc., ***graph., lyc., nat-c.,*** nux-v., ***ph-ac.,*** **RHUS-T.,** ***sil.,*** sulph., valer.

light, agg. in general - acon., agar., aloe, anan., ***ant-t.,*** arg-n., arn., ***ars.,*** **BELL.,** ***bov., bry.,*** bufo, cact., **CALC.,** caul., ***chin., cocc., coff.,*** euphr., ferr., ***ferr-p., gels., glon., ign.,*** kali-bi., kali-c., kali-p., lac-c., ***lac-d., lyc.,*** lyss., med., nat-a., ***nat-c.,*** **NAT-M.,** nat-p., nux-v., oreo., ***ph-ac.,*** phel., ***phos.,*** podo., ***sang.,*** sanic., scut., ***sep., sil.,*** sol-n., stict., ***stram., sulph.,*** syph., tab., ***tarent.,*** ziz.

amel. - lac-c., sil.

artificial, from - bufo, croc., ***glon.,*** mang., nat-c., phos., ***sang.,*** **SEP.,** ***sil., stram.,*** zinc.

daylight - ***calc., hep.,*** nat-m., **PHOS.,** sep., **SIL.**

gas, working under - bell., **GLON.,** nat-c., nat-s.

limbs crossing, agg. - bell.

listening, to reading and talking - ***mag-m.***

HEADACHES, general

liver derangements, with - chel., jug-c., lept., ***nux-v.,*** ptel., ***sang.***

looking, downward, from - alum., kalm., nat-m., olnd., phyt., spig., sulph.

downward, from, out of window causes vertigo, anxiety, headache and sweat - ox-ac.

fixedly at anything, from - anac., ***aur.,*** cadm-s., calc., caust., cina, gent-c., glon., helon., ***ign.,*** lac-c., lith., mur-ac., ***nat-m.,*** nux-v., olnd., **ONOS.,** par., ***puls., ruta.,*** sabad., sars., ***spig., spong.,*** sulph., tarent.

fixedly at anything, from, amel - agn., sabad., sars.

sideways, from - acon., dig., sil.

amel - olnd.

upward, from - acon., aeth., arn., arum-t., bapt., bell., ***calc.,*** calc-s., caps., caust., coca, colch., cupr., glon., gran., graph., ***ign.,*** lach., ***lac-c.,*** plat., plb., **PULS.,** sep., sil., stram., ***sulph., thuj.***

amel - thuj.

lying, while - agar., ambr., ***am-c.,*** anac., ant-t., ars., asaf., ***aur.,*** bar-c., bar-m., ***bell.,*** bov., cadm-s., calc., camph., **CARB-V.,** cham., chel., cimic., clem., ***coloc., con.,*** cupr., dios., ***dulc.,*** euph., euphr., eupi., ***gels., glon.,*** hep., ign., kali-ar., kali-c., lac-c., lach., led., lith., ***lyc.,*** mag-c., mag-m., mang., ***meny., merc.,*** mez., mur-ac., nat-p., nat-s., nit-ac., nux-v., onos., ***op.,*** ox-ac., petr., ***ph-ac., phos.,*** phys., ***plat.,*** puls., ran-b., rhod., ***rhus-t.,*** sanic., sep., spig., stann., staph., stront-c., sulph., ther., thuj., zinc.

abdomen, on, amel., occipital pain - grat.

amel. - ***alum.,*** ambr., am-m., anac., arn., asar., ***bell.,*** benz-ac., ***bry.,*** bufo, ***cact., calc.,*** calc-p., calc-s., camph., canth., chel., ***chin., chion.,*** chin-s., coc-c., colch., con., dig., ***dulc.,*** epip., ferr., ferr-i., ferr-p., fl-ac., gels., ham., ***hell.,*** hipp., ign., kali-bi., ***kali-c.,*** kali-s., lach., ***lac-d., lyc., mag-c.,*** merc., mosch., mur-ac., nat-c., ***nat-m., nit-ac., nux-v.,*** olnd., petr., ***ph-ac., phos.,*** sabad., sang., ***sil.,*** spig., spong., sulph., tab., zinc., ziz.

back, on, while - ail., bry., cact., cinnb., ***cocc.,*** coloc., ign., lac-c., nux-v., petr., phos., plect., ***sep.,*** spig.

amel - bry., cast-v., ign., kali-p., nux-v., par., petr., puls., spong., verat.

occiput, on - cocc., coloc., nat-m.

room, in a dark, amel - acon., **BELL.,** brom., **BRY.,** ***lac-d.,*** podo., ***sang.,*** sep., **SIL.**

agg. - onos.

stones, as if, lying on hard - plat.

lying, while on side - bell., calad., graph., ign., ***kreos.,*** nux-v., psor., puls., stann.

amel. - cact., ***cocc.,*** ign., meny., merc., sep.

left - cinnb., cycl., nux-v.

amel - nux-v.

HEADACHES, general

lying, painful side, on - ***ars.,*** calad., calc., carb-v., chel., chin., graph., ***kali-bi.,*** mag-c., ***nux-v.,*** petr., ph-ac., puls., rhus-t., ***spong.,*** stann., staph.

lying, painful side, on amel. - anac., arn., bry., calc-ar., hipp., ign., nux-v., plan., puls., sep.

head high, with - ***bell.,*** gels.

low, with - absin., aeth.

lying, painless side, amel - mag-c., ***nux-v.***

lying, right - alum., brom., carb-v., mang., merc., nux-v., phos., staph.

amel - brom., cinnb., nux-v.

maddening, pains - ***acon.,*** ambr., ***ars.,*** **BELL.,** bry., cact., ***calc.,*** cham., ***chin.,*** coloc., cupr., **GELS.,** ign., ind., iod., ***ip., lyss.,*** mag-c., med., meli., ***nat-m., nit-ac.,*** psor., puls., sep., ***stram., tarent.***

feeling in brain - plan.

malaria, in - ***ars.,*** caps., cedr., chin., ***chin-s.,*** cupr-ac., ***eup-per.,*** gels., ***nat-m.***

measles, after - bell., ***carb-v.,*** dulc., hell., hyos., ***puls.,*** rhus-t., ***sulph.***

meat, after - caust., ***puls.,*** staph.

menopause, during - aml-n., cact., ***carb-v., chin., cimic.,*** croc., ***cycl., cypr.,*** ferr., ***glon.,*** ign., **LACH.,** ***sang.,*** **SEP.,** stront-c., sulph., ***ther.,*** ust.

menses, during - acon., agar., aloe, alum., am-c., am-m., ant-c., apis, ***arg-n.,*** ars., asar., **BELL.,** berb., bor., ***bov.,*** brom., ***bry.,*** bufo, cact., ***calc.,*** calc-p., calc-s., canth., carb-an., ***carb-v.,*** cast., ***caust.,*** cham., chim., chin-a., cic., cimic., ***cocc.,*** coff., coloc., con., cub., cupr., cur., cycl., dulc., eupi., ferr., ferr-ar., ferr-p., ***gels.,*** gent-c., **GLON., GRAPH.,** hep., ***hyos.,*** hyper., ***ign.,*** kali-ar., kali-bi., ***kali-c.,*** kali-n., kali-p., kali-s., kalm., **KREOS.,** ***lac-d., lach., laur.,*** **LYC.,** ***mag-c.,*** mag-m., mag-s., med., ***murx.,*** nat-a., ***nat-c.,*** **NAT-M.,** nat-p., ***nit-ac., nux-m., nux-v., phos., plat., puls.,*** rat., rhod., ***sang.,*** **SEP.,** sil., stann., ***sulph., verat.,*** xan., zinc.

amel., during - all-c., bell., glyc., joan., lach., lil-t., meli., ***verat., zinc.***

after - agar., asar., ***bry., calc.,*** calc-p., carb-ac., carb-an., ***chin.,*** eupi., ***ferr.,*** ferr-p., glon., kali-br., ***lach., lith.,*** lyc., mosch., naja, ***nat-m., nat-p.,*** ol-an., plat., ***puls., sep.,*** thuj.

cessation, on - bry., ***carb-v.,*** glon., naja, nit-ac., **PULS.**

morning, on awaking, after sudden cessation of - ***lith.***

top would fly off., as if - ust.

before - ***acon.,*** agn., alum., ***am-c.,*** arg-n., ars., ***asar., bell., bor., bov., brom.,*** **BRY.,** bufo, ***calc.,*** calc-p., calc-s., carb-an., ***carb-v.,*** caust., ***cimic., cinnb.,*** cupr., ferr., ferr-ar., ferr-i., ***gels., glon.,*** graph., hep., hyper., iod., kali-p., **KREOS.,** ***lac-c.,*** lac-d., ***lach.,*** laur., lil-t., ***lyc.,*** manc., ***meli.,*** merc., nat-a., ***nat-c., nat-m.,*** nit-ac., ***nux-m.,*** nux-v., ol-an., petr., ***plat.,*** phos.,

HEADACHES, general

menses, before - ***puls., sep.,*** sil., stann., ***sulph.,*** thuj., ***verat.,*** vib., ***xan.,*** zinc.

amel. when flow begins - all-s., alum., kali-p., ***lach., meli.,*** verat., zinc.

begining of, at - ant-t., berb., brom., carb-an., graph., hyos., iod., ***kali-c.,*** lach., laur., ***nat-m.,*** nit-ac., plat., rhod.

suppressed, from - acon., alum., bell., ***bry., carb-s.,*** **PULS.,** sep.

mental, exertion (see exertion)

mercury, from - arg-n., ***asaf., aur.,*** carb-v., chin., clem., fl-ac., **HEP.,** ***iod., kali-i.,*** led., merc., mez., **NIT-AC.,** podo., puls., ***sars.,*** staph., still., sulph.

metallic substances, from abuse of - merc., sulph.

migraine, headaches (see gastric, periodic) - acon., **AGAR.,** ***anac.,*** **ANT-C.,** apis, ***arg-m.,*** arn., ***ars.,*** **ASAF.,** ***asar.,*** aur., bell., **BRY.,** ***cact.,*** calad., ***calc., calc-p.,*** caust., cedr., ***cham.,*** chel., **CHIN.,** cic., cimic., cina, cocc., **COFF.,** coloc., ***eup-per.,*** **GELS.,** glon., graph., **IGN., IP., IRIS,** kali-bi., ***kali-p.,*** lac-c., lach., lyc., **NAT-M.,** ***nat-s.,*** **NUX-V.,** op., **PHOS., PULS., SANG.,** scut., ***sep.,*** **SIL.,** spig., ***stram., sulph., tab.,*** tarent., ***ther.,*** **THUJ.,** ***valer.,*** **ZINC.**

milk, after drinking - brom., lac-d., phys.

morning - acon., **AGAR.,** alet., all-s., ***alum.,*** alumn., ambr., am-c., am-m., ***anac.,*** ang., ant-t., arg-m., arg-n., ***arn.,*** ars., ars-i., asaf., asar., ***aur., bar-c.,*** bar-m., ***bell.,*** benz-ac., berb., bor., ***bov., bry., cact.,*** cadm-s., ***calc., calc-p.,*** calc-s., camph., cann-s., canth., ***carb-an., carb-s., carb-v.,*** cast-eq., caust., cham., ***chel.,*** chin., chin-a., chin-s., cic., cina, clem., cob., coca, coc-c., coff., ***coloc., con.,*** croc., ***crot-t.,*** cund., cupr., cycl., dios., dulc., euphr., ***eup-per.,*** ferr., ferr-ar., ferr-i., ferr-p., ***fl-ac.,*** form., glon., ***graph.,*** grat., guai., hell., ***hep.,*** hipp., ***ign.,*** ind., iod., ip., iris, jatr., ***jug-c.,*** jug-r., kali-bi., ***kali-c.,*** kali-i., ***kali-n.,*** kali-p., ***kali-s.,*** kalm., kreos., lac-c., lac-d., ***lach.,*** lachn., lact., led., lil-t., lith., mag-c., mag-m., manc., ***mang.,*** merc., merc-i-f., merc-sul., ***mez., murx.,*** mur-ac., nat-a., nat-c., ***nat-m.,*** nat-p., nicc., ***nit-ac.,*** nux-m., **NUX-V.,** ol-an., paeon., pall., ***petr., ph-ac., phos.,*** phyt., ***podo., psor.,*** puls., ran-b., rheum, ***rhod., rhus-t.,*** rumx., ruta., sabad., samb., sang., sars., scut., ***seneg., sep., sil., spig., squil., stann., staph.,*** stram., stront-c., stry., ***sulph.,*** sul-ac., tab., ***thuj.,*** verat., zinc.

5 a.m - calc., kali-bi., **KALI-I.,** stann.

6 a.m. until evening - crot-t.

9 a.m.to1 p.m. - cedr.

to 4 p.m. - cedr.

to 12 noon - cedr.

10 a.m. - ***aran., nat-m., sil.***

until, 10 a.m. - ***arn.,*** lachn., mag-c., ***nat-m.***

amel. - bov., caust., kreos., nat-m., verat.

HEADACHES, general
morning,
bed, in - ***agar.,*** alum., am-c., anac., ant-t., aur., bar-c., ***bell.,*** berb., bov., ***bry.,*** calc., calc-p., carb-an., ***carb-s., cham.,*** chin., chin-s., cic., coc-c., coff., con., dig., dulc., ferr., ferr-p., ***graph.,*** hell., ***hep.,*** ign., ip., jug-c., ***kali-c.,*** kali-i., ***kali-p.,*** kali-s., kreos., ***lac-d., lach.,*** lact., laur., lyc., mag-c., mag-m., mag-s., mang., merc., mez., murx., ***nat-m., nit-ac.,*** **NUX-V.,** petr., ***phos., psor.,*** ptel., ran-b., rheum, ***rhod.,*** rhus-t., ruta., squil., staph., sulph., sul-ac., thuj., verat., zinc.
first motion, on - **BRY.**
nausea, with - calc., cob., ***eup-per.,*** graph., nat-m., nux-v., sep., sil., sulph.
breakfast is delayed, if - calc.
ceases toward evening - ***bry.,*** calc., ***kali-bi.,*** kalm., ***nat-m.,*** plat., sang., spig., sulph.
comes and goes with the sun - cact., kali-bi., ***kalm.,*** lac-d., ***nat-m., sang., spig.,*** sulph., tab.
increases and decreases with the sun - acon., **GLON.,** ***kalm.,*** nat-c., ***nat-m., phos., sang., spig., stann.,*** stram., tab.
until noon, or a little later, then gradually decreases - phos., sulph.
during day - cact., ther.
rising, on - ***agar.,*** am-c., am-m., apis, arg-n., asc-t., aur-m., bar-c., bar-m., **BRY.,** camph., chel., chin-s., cob., colch., crot-t., **CYCL.,** dig., dulc., fago., glon., ham., hep., hydr., ind., iod., ip., jug-c., ***kali-p.,*** kalm., lac-d., ***lach.,*** lyc., mag-c., mag-m., merc., mur-ac., nicc., nux-v., petr., phos., ***psor.,*** ptel., puls., rhus-t., rumx., ruta., ***sep.,*** squil., staph., stront-c., **SULPH.,** tarent.
rising, on, amel - ***alum.,*** ars., cham., coc-c., crot-h., ***graph., hep.,*** ign., jug-c., **KALI-I.,** merc-i-r., murx., nat-m., ***nit-ac.,*** **NUX-V.,** ph-ac., phos., **RHOD.**
same hour, at - kali-bi.
until noon - ars., conv., ip., ***nat-m.,*** nicc., phos., sep., ***tab.***
3 p.m - aur.
5 p.m - mang.
10 a.m - ***arn.,*** lachn., mag-c., ***nat-m.***
10 p.m - phys.
waking, on - agar., ail., ***alum., alumn., arg-n., arn.,*** ars., benz-ac., bov., **BRY.,** bufo, calc., calc-p., calc-s., cann-i., carb-an., carb-s., caust., cham., ***chel.,*** chin., chin-a., cic., cimic., cob., coc-c., coff., colch., con., ***croc.,*** crot-h., crot-t., cupr-ar., dig., elaps, erig., euphr., ***eup-per.,*** fago., form., **GRAPH.,** hell., ***hep.,*** hipp., ign., ind., jug-c., ***kali-bi., kali-c., kali-i.,*** kali-n., kali-p., kali-s., ***kalm.,*** kreos., ***lac-c.,*** **LACH.,** lil-t., lob., ***lyc.,*** mag-c., merc-i-f., morph., murx., mur-ac., myric., ***naja,*** **NAT-M.,** nicc., **NIT-AC., NUX-V.,** ol-an., op., peti., ***ph-ac., phos.,*** phys., pip-m., plan., plat., ***psor.,*** puls., rhus-r., rumx., ***sep.,*** squil., stann., staph., ***sulph.,*** sul-ac., **TARENT.,** ***thuj., thyr.***
waking, and on, opening the eyes, on first - bov., ***bry.,*** graph., ign., kalm., ***nat-m., nux-v.,*** onos., stry., tab.
preceded by disagreeable dreams - murx.
until 10 a.m - ***arn.***

motion, from - acon., agn., aloe, ambr., am-c., am-m., ***anac.,*** anan., ***ant-c.,*** ant-t., ***apis,*** arg-m., ***arg-n.,*** arn., ars-i., ***aur.,*** bapt., **BELL.,** benz-ac., berb., bism., bov., **BRY.,** bufo, cact., calc., ***calc-p.,*** calc-s., camph., cann-s., canth., ***caps., carb-s.,*** **CARB-V.,** caust., cham., chel., ***chin.,*** chin-s., chion., chlor., cic., ***cimic.,*** cinnb., cob., ***cocc., coff.,*** colch., coloc., ***con.,*** croc., ***crot-h., crot-t.,*** cupr., cycl., dulc., eupi., fago., ***ferr-p.,*** fl-ac., ***gels.,*** gent-c., ***glon.,*** graph., grat., hell., ***hep.,*** hipp., ign., iod., kali-ar., kali-bi., kali-c., kali-n., kali-s., kalm., ***kreos.,*** lac-c., lac-d., ***lach.,*** laur., **LED.,** lob., ***lyc.,*** lyss., ***mag-c.,*** mag-m., ***mag-p., mang., meli.,*** merc., **MEZ.,** ***mosch.,*** naja, nat-a., nat-c., ***nat-m.,*** nat-p., nicc., **NIT-AC.,** ***nux-m., nux-v.,*** olnd., petr., ***ph-ac., phos.,*** phys., pic-ac., plat., podo., ***psor.,*** ptel., rat., rheum, rhod., rumx., sabad., samb., ***sang.,*** sanic., ***sars., sep., sil.,*** sol-n., ***spig.,*** spong., squil., ***stann., staph.,*** sulph., thea., ***ther.,*** thuj., verat., verat-v., zing.
amel. - ***agar.,*** am-m., ant-t., arg-m., ***ars.,*** asaf., asar., benz-ac., calc., ***caps.,*** cedr., cham., cic., cina, coff., coloc., com., con., dros., euph., ferr., guai., hipp., hyos., ign., indg., iod., ***iris,*** kali-i., kali-n., kali-p., ***lyc.,*** mag-c., mag-m., mang., meny., merc-i-f., mosch., ***mur-ac.,*** nat-c., ***nux-m.,*** op., petr., phos., psor., ***puls., rhod.,*** **RHUS-T.,** ruta., samb., seneg., stann., staph., sulph., tarax., ***valer.,*** verb.
eyes, of, agg. - bell., ***bry.,*** cimic., coloc., cupr., gels., ichth., ign., ***nux-v., phys.,*** puls., rhus-t., spig.
gentle, amel. - chin., glon., helon., iris, kali-p., ***puls.***
quick, from - cor-r., iod., mez., nat-c., nat-m., ***petr.***
up and down amel. - ***chin.***
violent, from - calc., cocc., dros., ***iris,*** mez.
amel. - ind., rhus-t., ***sep.***

move, on beginning to - iris, ***sep.,*** ther.
amel - valer.
pains compel one to - chin., ph-ac.

moving, arms on - bar-c., berb., caust., coc-c., lept., nat-s., ptel., rhus-t., spong.

moving, eyelids - **BELL.,** ***bry., chin., coff.,*** coloc., ***ign., nux-v.,*** rhus-t.

HEADACHES, general

moving, eyes - acon., agn., am-c., arn., bad., bapt., bar-c., bar-m., **BELL., BRY.,** ***caps.,*** chel., ***chin.,*** chin-s., cimic., cinnb., ***colch., coloc.,*** con., crot-t., cupr., dig., dros., gels., hell., ***hep.,*** ign., ind., jug-r., kali-c., mag-s., mur-ac., ***nat-m.,*** **NUX-V.,** ***op.,*** plat., puls., rhus-t., sang., ***sep., sil., spig.,*** sulph., valer.

moving, head, on - acon., alum., ***am-c., arn., ars., asar.,*** bar-c., **BELL.,** berb., ***bry., calc.,*** calc-s., camph., cann-s., canth., ***caps., carb-s., carb-v.,*** caust., ***chin., cimic.,*** cic., clem., cocc., coc-c., colch., con., cor-r., com., cupr., dros., euph., **FERR.,** ***ferr-ar.,*** ferr-i., ferr-p., fl-ac., **GELS.,** genist., gent-c., ***glon.,*** graph., ***hell.,*** hep., ind., iod., ip., kali-ar., kali-c., kali-s., lach., lact., lac-c., lyc., mag-c., mang., **MEZ.,** ***mosch.,*** nat-a., nat-c., ***nat-m.,*** nat-p., ***nux-m., nux-v.,*** ph-ac., plat., puls., rhod., samb., sang., sars., sec., sep., ***sil.,*** sol-n., ***spig.,*** spong., staph., sulph., ther., verat., vib., viol-o.

amel - ***agar., chin.,*** cina, con., gels., kali-p., plan., sulph.

nodding - lam., sep., ***sulph.***

muscular soreness, with - gels., rhus-t.

music, from - acon., ambr., cact., **COFF.,** ***nat-c.,*** nux-v., ***ph-ac., phos.,*** podo., viol-o.

narcotics, after abuse of - ***aven.,*** bell., cham., coff., dig., graph., hyos., lach., lyc., **NUX-V.,** op., puls., sep., valer.

nausea, during - acon., aesc., ail., ***alum.,*** alumn., ambr., ***am-c.,*** **ANT-C.,** ant-t., apis, arg-m., arg-n., arn., ***ars.,*** asar., aur., benz-ac., ***bor., bry.,*** calc., ***calc-p.,*** calc-s., camph., cann-s., ***caps., carb-ac., carb-s., carb-v.,*** **CAUST.,** ***cedr.,*** chel., chin., chin-a., chin-s., cic., cimic., cob., **COCC.,** ***coloc.,*** **CON.,** cor-r., croc., crot-h., ***cupr.,*** cycl., dros., ***dulc.,*** epiph., ***eug.,*** eup-per., eup-pur., ferr., fl-ac., form., gels., ***glon., graph.,*** grat., hep., hipp., ign., ind., **IP., IRIS,** kali-ar., ***kali-bi., kali-c.,*** kali-p., ***kali-s.,*** kalm., kreos., ***lac-c., lac-d., lach., lept.,*** lith., ***lob.,*** lyc., mag-c., ***merc.,*** mez., mill., ***mosch.,*** nat-a., nat-c., ***nat-m.,*** nat-p., nat-s., ***nit-ac., nux-m.,*** **NUX-V.,** ***op.,*** petr., ***phos.,*** phyt., plat., ***puls.,*** ran-b., rhus-t., ruta., **SANG.,** ***sars.,*** seneg., ***sep.,*** sil., spig., ***stann.,*** stram., stront-c., ***sulph., tab.,*** tarax., tep., ter., ther., thuj., verat., zinc., zing.

trembling of body, with - bor.

neck, pain in, with headaches - acon., ail., ***alum.,*** anac., arg-n., arn., asar., bar-c., ***bell.,*** bor., bry., bufo, ***calc-p.,*** cann-i., cann-s., canth., ***carb-s., carb-v.,*** caust., chel., chin., clem., con., elaps, euph., fago., gall-ac., **GELS.,** ***glon.,*** graph., ***hell.,*** hura, hydr-ac., hyos., jac., kali-c., kali-i., ***kalm.,*** lach., laur., lil-t., lyc., lyss., mag-c., mag-s., manc., merc., merc-i-f., mosch., myric., ***nat-m.,*** peti., ***pic-ac.,*** plb., psor., ptel., ran-b., rhus-r., sars., serp., spong., sulph., stry., tep., ziz.

HEADACHES, general

neck, nape of - aeth., alum., ambr., am-c., anac., asar., bar-c., ***bell.,*** berb., bor., bry., ***calc., calc-p.,*** cann-s., carb-an., carb-v., caust., chel., cinnb., clem., **COCC.,** con., corn., crot-t., **GELS.,** ***glon.,*** graph., ***hell.,*** hyos., hydr-ac., iod., ip., kali-c., kali-n., ***kalm.,*** lac-c., lil-t., lyc., mag-c., manc., merc., mez., mosch., mur-ac., nat-c., ***nat-m.,*** op., paeon., par., **PH-AC.,** ***phyt.,*** **PIC-AC.,** plect., plb., ***puls.,*** ran-b., rhus-t., sabin., sars., sil., spong., ***stry.,*** sulph., tarax., tarent., verat.

nervous - acet-ac., acon., **AGAR.,** agn., ail., anac., apis, ***arg-m.,*** **ARG-N.,** arn., ***ars.,*** **ASAF.,** ***asar.,*** asc-t., atro., aur., bell., bry., ***cact.,*** calad., ***calc.,*** camph., cann-s., caul., caust., cedr., ***cham.,*** **CHIN.,** chin-a., chlor., cic., cimic., cina, coca, cocc., **COFF.,** coloc., croc., crot-t., form., **GELS.,** glon., graph., hydr., **IGN.,** ***ip.,*** iris, ***kali-p.,*** lact., **NAT-M., NUX-V.,** op., ***petr., ph-ac.,*** **PHOS.,** ***plat.,*** **PULS.,** rhus-r., rhus-t., sang., scut., ***sep.,*** sil., spig., stict., ***stram.,*** sulph., tarent., ter., ***ther.,*** **THUJ.,** ***ust., valer., verat.,*** verat-v., **ZINC.**

night - act-sp., ***alum.,*** alumn., ambr., am-c., am-m., anac., ang., ***ant-t.,*** arg-n., arn., ***ars.,*** arum-t., aster., ***aur., bell.,*** berb., bor., bov., bufo, cact., ***calc., calc-p., calc-s.,*** camph., canth., ***carb-an.,*** carb-s., carb-v., ***caust., cedr.,*** cham., chel., ***chim., chin-a.,*** chin-s., cic., clem., ***cocc.,*** colch., con., ***crot-c.,*** cupr-ar., cycl., dig., dulc., elaps, eug., glon., graph., grat., guai., ham., ***hep.,*** hydr-ac., hyos., ign., ind., ***kali-c., kali-i.,*** kali-n., ***kali-p., kali-s.,*** kreos., lach., lac-c., lact., lac-ac., ***laur.,*** led., lob., **LYC.,** ***mag-c.,*** mag-m., **MERC.,** ***merc-c.,*** merc-d., ***mez.,*** mill., nat-a., nat-c., nat-m., nat-p., **NIT-AC.,** nux-m., nux-v., op., par., ph-ac., ***phos., phyt.,*** plat., ptel., puls., raph., rhus-r., rhus-t., sars., sep., ***sil.,*** sol-n., spig., stram., stront-c., stry., ***sulph.,*** **SYPH.,** tarent., ***thuj.,*** verat., zinc.

1 a.m - pall.

1 a.m. to 10 a.m - chin., elaps.

2 a.m - ars., cimic., sulph.

3 a.m - ***agar.,*** bov., chin-s., nat-m., thuj.

4 a.m - chel., con., raph., stram.

5 a.m - dios., **KALI-I.**

amel. - bufo, ham., mag-c., sol-t-ae., spira.

bed, in - aloe, ***alum.,*** alumn., fago., hipp., hyper., merc-i-f., ***sulph., thuj.***

drives him out of - ***thuj.***

lighting the gas amel - ***lac-c.,*** sil.

lighting the gas amel. - ***lac-c.,*** sil.

midnight, about - agar., all-s., arn., ars., elaps, hep., ***kali-c.,*** mag-s., myric., plat., puls., sep.

till morning - hep.

midnight, after - agar., ***ars.,*** bufo, carb-an., cham., ferr., hep., ign., kali-ar., kali-c., nat-s., ph-ac., psor., rhus-t., sep., ***sil.,*** spig., ***thuj.***

before - am-m., anac., caust., chin., dulc., ***lach.,*** puls., rhus-t., sep.

HEADACHES, general

night,

sleep, amel - agar.

preventing - kali-n., sulph.

waking, on - ***agar.,*** alumn., ambr., ant-t., aster., bufo, canth., cinnb., coloc., ferr., gels., gins., glon., hyper., lac-ac., mag-c., mang., merc-i-f., mez., nat-a., nit-ac., nux-v., ph-ac., ***psor.,*** rumx.

night-watching, (see sleep, loss of)

nodding, the head, on - lam., sep., ***sulph.***

noise, from - acon., agar., anac., anan., ang., arg-n., arn., ***ars.,*** ars-i., bapt., bar-c., bar-m., **BELL.,** bor., ***bry.,*** bufo, ***cact.,*** calad., **CALC.,** ***calc-s.,*** cann-s., caps., carb-an., carb-v., caust., ***chim., chin-a.,*** cic., ***cocc., coff.,*** colch., ***com., ferr-p.,*** gels., graph., hell., hyos., ign., iod., kali-ar., kali-bi., kali-s., ***lac-c., lac-d., lach.,*** lyc., ***lyss.,*** mag-m., manc., merc., merc-i-f., mur-ac., **NAT-A.,** ***nat-c.,*** nat-p., **NIT-AC.,** ***nux-v., ph-ac., phos.,*** ptel., sang., sanic., ***sil., sol-n., spig., stann.,*** stict., tab., **THER.,** yuc., zinc.

distant talking, of - mur-ac.

ear, in, roaring - aur., ***chin., chin-s.,*** ferr., sang., sulfon.

falling water, of - **LYSS.,** nit-ac.

footsteps - bell., bry., **COFF.,** gels., **NUX-V.,** ther.

hammer on anvil, of - manc.

rattling of vehicles - **NIT-AC.,** ***ther.***

voices, especially - bar-c., lyss.

noon - aeth., agar., alum., ant-c., arg-m., arg-n., asar., bell., bov., calc-ar., calc-p., cann-i., carb-v., ***cedr.,*** cham., chel., chin-s., cic., cob., graph., gymn., ign., indg., jab., kali-bi., kali-n., kalm., lyc., lycps., lyss., mag-c., mang., merc., mur-ac., ***naja,*** nat-c., ***nat-m.,*** phos., puls., rhus-t., spong., ***sulph.,*** zinc., zing.

until evening - sil.

until midnight - ***caul., sulph.***

nosebleeds, after - aml-n., ***bor.***

agg. - aml-n., ant-c.

amel. - ant-c., brom., bry., bufo, carb-an., cham., chin., dig., ferr-p., ham., hyos., kali-bi., ***lach.,*** mag-s., ***meli.,*** mill., ***petr., psor.,*** raph., rhus-t., tab., tarent., tub.

numbness, with - chel., indol., plat.

lips, tongue and nose, of - nat-m.

nursing, infant, after - bell., bry., ***calc.,*** cham., chin., dulc., phos., ***puls., sep.,*** sil., staph.

occiput, headaches, (see Headaches, occiput)

odors, from, strong - acon., anac., arg-n., ***aur., bell.,*** cham., chin., ***coff., colch.,*** graph., **IGN.,** ***lyc.,*** nux-v., **PHOS.,** sel., ***sep., sil., sulph.***

alcohol, of - sol-t-ae.

coffee, of - lach.

dirty clothes, of - carb-an.

eggs, strong odor from - colch., **SULPH.**

oversensitiveness to, from - sabad.

strong and agreeable - arg-n.

tobacco - ***ign.***

HEADACHES, general

one-sided, headaches - acon., aesc., aeth., ***agar.,*** agn., **ALUM.,** ambr., am-c., am-m., ***anac.,*** ang., ant-c., ant-t., ***apis, arg-m.,*** **ARG-N.,** ***arn., ars.,*** ars-i., arund., ***asaf., asar.,*** aur., ***bar-c.,*** bar-m., ***bell., bism.,*** bor., ***bov., bry., bufo, cact., calc.,*** calc-p., camph., cann-i., cann-s., ***canth., caps.,*** carb-an., carb-s., carb-v., caust., ***cham., chel., chin.,*** chin-a., chin-s., ***cic.,*** cina, cinnb., clem., cocc., **COFF.,** colch., ***coloc.,*** con., cop., ***corn.,*** croc., crot-h., cupr., cycl., dig., dios., dros., dulc., elat., elaps, eug., euph., euphr., eup-per., ***ferr.,*** ferr-ar., ferr-i., ferr-p., ***gels., glon., graph., guai.,*** hell., hyos., ***ign.,*** iod., ind., ip., iris, ***kali-ar., kali-bi., kali-br.,*** **KALI-C., KALI-I.,** kali-n., **KALI-P.,** ***kali-s.,*** kalm., kreos., ***lac-d., lach.,*** lact., ***laur.,*** led., ***lyc.,*** mag-c., mag-m., manc., mang., meny., ***merc., mez.,*** mill., mosch., murx., mur-ac., nat-a., nat-c., nat-m., nat-p., nicc., nit-ac., nux-m., ***nux-v.,*** olnd., par., petr., **PH-AC.,** ***phos., phyt.,*** **PLAT.,** plb., ***psor.,*** **PULS.,** ran-b., ran-s., rheum, rhod., ***rhus-t.,*** ruta., ***rob.,*** sabad., sabin., samb., ***sang.,*** **SARS.,** sel., seneg., ***sep., sil.,*** **SPIG.,** spong., squil., stann., staph., stict., stram., stront-c., ***sulph.,*** **SUL-AC.,** ***syph.,*** tab., tarax., tarent., teucr., ***thuj.,*** ust., valer., ***verat.,*** **VERB.,** viol-o., viol-t., **ZINC.,** zing.

alternating from one side to the other - agar., bell., calc., calc-ar., cedr., chin., colch., cupr., dros., euon., hell., hydr., hyper., ***iris,*** kali-bi., **LAC-C.,** lil-t., lyc., nat-m., nat-p., nicc., ***nux-v.,*** plan., phos., sep., sil., valer.

alternating from one to the other, with pain in left arm - ptel.

both, (see Sides, both)

ceases on one side, becomes more violent on the other - ***lac-c., nat-m.***

coffee, from excessive use of - ***cham.,*** nux-v.

ears, behind the - asar., calc-p., caust., chel., onos., sang.

air, open - kali-p.

behind the left - ambr., kali-p., sang.

motion - kali-p.

extending, arm, to - cimx., fago.

eye, to - ars., ***asaf.,*** brom., calc., caust., crot-h., mag-m., nat-m.

neck - guai., ***lach.,*** lyc., merc.

neck and shoulders, neck stiff - lach.

side to side, from, through temples - alum., chin., phos., plan., sang.

waist - lyss.

itching - dig.

left, side, (see Left sided, Headaches)

lying, amel. - dig.

painful side, on amel. - anac., arn., bry., hipp., ign., sep.

painless side, on amel. - mag-c., ***nux-v.***

right side, on with hands over, amel. - brom.

HEADACHES, general
one-sided, headaches
lying, side lain on - ***ars.,*** calad., calc., carb-v., chel., ***chin.,*** mag-c., nit-ac., ***nux-m.,*** nux-v., ph-ac., puls., ***spong.,*** stann., staph.
side not lain on - calc-ar., ***graph.,*** puls.
while - carb-v., petr., rhod., sep., spong.
right, side, (see Right sided, Headaches)
spot, in - kali-bi., kalm.
opening, mouth - fago., spig.
opium, from abuse of - acet-ac., aven., cham., nux-v.
overheated, (see Heated)
pains in, with headache
abdomen - cina, coloc., verat.
back, amel. - kali-p.
sciatica, during - petr.
back, lumbar region - rad-br.
limbs - sang.
palpitations, with - aeth., bell., cact., lith., spig.
reverberation in head - aur., bell., ***glon.,*** spig., spong.
paroxysmal - acon., agar., ambr., ant-t., arn., ***ars.,*** asaf., **BELL.,** bufo, calc., carb-v., ***cedr., cham.,*** chin., chin-a., cocc., colch., ***coloc.,*** crot-t., cupr., dig., ferr., ferr-ar., ferr-p., ign., ***kali-ar.,*** kali-c., kali-n., kali-p., ***kalm.,*** **LACH.,** lyc., ***mag-p.,*** mosch., mur-ac., murx., nat-a., nat-c., nat-p., nicc., nit-ac., nux-m., petr., ph-ac., plat., psor., ran-b., **SANG.,** sars., sep., ***sil., spig.,*** spong., squil., stann., ***stram.,*** stront-c., thuj., valer., ***verat.,*** viol-t., zinc.
periodic, headache - act-sp., ***aeth.,*** aloe, **ALUM.,** ambr., ammc., ***anac., apis,*** aran., arn., **ARS.,** ***ars-i.,*** asaf., bell., benz-ac., ***cact., calc.,*** calc-s., ***carb-v.,*** **CEDR.,** cham., **CHIN.,** ***chin-a.,*** **CHIN-S., COLOC.,** cupr., eup-per., ***ferr., ferr-ar., ign., kali-ar.,*** kali-bi., ***kreos.,*** lac-d., ***lach.,*** laur., lob., ***lyc.,*** mur-ac., ***nat-a.,*** nat-c., **NAT-M.,** nat-p., nat-s., nicc., **NIT-AC.,** ***nux-v., phos.,*** plat., prun., ***puls., rhus-t.,*** **SANG.,** sel., **SEP., SIL.,** ***spig., stram., sulph.,*** tab., ***tub.,*** zinc.
afternoon, 2 p.m. to bed time - sep.
4 p.m.-3 a.m - bell.
increasing until midnight, every third attack alternately more or less violent - ***lob.***
certain hours, at - nat-c.
day and night - bor., caust., kreos., led., rhus-t., sul-ac., viol-t.
every, day - ***ars., bell.,*** calc., cedr., coloc., con., eup-per., form., hep., lach., lyc., mag-c., mag-m., mang., merc-i-r., mur-ac., ***nat-m., nux-m., nux-v.,*** petr., phos., sabad., seneg., sep., ***sil.,*** spig., stann., sulph., zinc.
day, at same hour - aran., ars., cedr., cimic., gels., **KALI-BI.,** mur-ac., spig.
day, continues two or three days - croc.
day, earlier each day - form.
eight days - iris

HEADACHES, general
periodic, headache
fourteen days - ***ars.,*** calc., ***chel.,*** chin., chin-a., ign., nicc., phyt., psor., puls., sang., ***sulph., tub.***
fourteen days, lasting two or three days - **FERR.**
other day - alum., ambr., ars., cact., ***cedr.,*** chin., cimic., eup-per., merc-c., nat-m., nux-v., ***phos.,*** psor., sang., sulph.
seven days - ars., calc., calc-ar., dys-co., epip., eup-per., gels., ***iris, lac-d.,*** lyc., morg., nux-m., ***phos.,*** phyt., psor., rhus-t., sabad., ***sang.,*** sep., ***sil., sulph.,*** syc-co., ***tub.***
six weeks - ***mag-m.***
sunday - tub.
ten days - ***lach.***
three or four days - aur., eup-per., sang.
three days-seven days - eup-per.
twenty one days - aur.
two-three weeks - ferr.
year, before winter - aloe.
lasting several days - tab.
morning, 7 a.m - ***ars.***
9 a.m. to 1 p.m - ***cedr.,*** mur-ac.
every - ***chin.,*** hep.
every other, on awaking - ***chin.,*** eup-per., per.
on awaking, with vertigo and nausea, also in evening, often amel. by pressure, in open air, or by eating - kali-bi.
noon to 10 p.m - form.
perspiration, during - ant-c., apis, arg-m., arn., ***ars., bry.,*** canth., carb-v., caust., chin-s., eup-per., glon., graph., hyos., kali-n., lachn., lyc., mag-s., ***merc.,*** nat-m., nat-s., op., ox-ac., plat., puls., rhus-t., ***sulph.,*** tarent., thuj.
after - calc., ***chim.,*** merc., puls., ***sep.,*** staph., sulph.
amel. - bov., carb-s., chin-a., clem., graph., mag-m., ***nat-m.,*** nat-s., nux-v., psor., spong., ***sulph.,*** tarent., thuj.
cold - **GELS.,** graph., **VERAT.**
preceded by headache - ferr., lyc.
profuse - lob., tab.
suppressed, from - ***ars., bell.,*** bry., ***calc.,*** **CARB-V.,** ***cham., chin.,*** lyc., merc., ***nux-v.,*** phos., ***puls.,*** rhus-t., sep., **SIL.,** ***sulph.***
position, as from wrong - lyc.
pregnancy, during - ***bell.,*** bry., calc., caps., caust., ***cham.,*** cocc., hyos., nux-m., plat., ***puls.,*** rhus-t., ***sep.,*** sulph.
pressure, external, agg. - ***agar.,*** am-c., ant-c., ***arg-m., bar-c.,*** bar-m., bell., bism., bov., calc., camph., cast., chin., ***cina,*** cinnb., ***cupr.,*** glon., ***kali-c.,*** kali-p., kali-s., lach., lact., lyc., ***mag-c.,*** mag-m., merc-i-f., mez., mur-ac., nat-a., nat-c., ph-ac., ***prun.,*** sabin., sars., sulph., teucr., valer., verb.
abdomen, on, causes headache - **ARS.**
back of neck agg - sec.

HEADACHES, general

pressure, external

amel. - agar., alum., ***alumn.,*** **AM-C.,** ***anac.,*** ant-c., ***apis,*** aran., ***arg-m., arg-n.,*** **BELL., BRY.,** cact., ***calc.,*** calc-s., camph., carb-ac., carb-an., carb-v., chel., ***chim.,*** chion., cimic., ***cinnb.,*** clem., ***coloc.,*** con., dros., **FERR.,** ***ferr-i.,*** ferr-p., ***glon.,*** guai., hell., hep., hydr., ind., ip., ***kali-bi.,*** kali-n., kalm., ***lac-d.,*** **LACH.,** laur., lil-t., ***lyc.,*** mag-c., **MAG-M., MAG-P.,** meny., merc., merc-i-f., mez., mur-ac., nat-c., **NAT-M.,** nat-p., ***nat-s.,*** nicc., ***nux-v.,*** olnd., par., phos., ***pic-ac.,*** podo., **PULS.,** ***pyrog.,*** ran-s., rhus-t., sabad., sabin., ***sang., sep., sil., spig.,*** **STANN.,** staph., ***sulph.,*** sul-ac., tarent., thuj., verat., ***zinc.***

cannot bear pressure though it does not agg - seneg.

cold hand amel - ***calc.***

hard, amel - anac., arg-n., ***bell.,*** bry., carb-an., **CHIN.,** ***mag-m.,*** **MAG-P.,** meny., nux-m., ***sang., zinc.***

rain, agg. - phyt.

amel - cham.

raising, amel. - ang., carb-v., ign., kali-c., mag-c., nat-m., rhus-t., spig.

arms to head - sulph.

head - ang., ars., bar-c., bov., cact., calc., caps., chin-s., cinnb., coca, dros., ign., lach., ***nux-m.,*** seneg., spong., squil., sulph., tarax., ***thuj.,*** verat., viol-t.

reading, agg. - agn., apis, arg-m., arn., asaf., aur., bor., bov., bry., ***calc.,*** calc-s., carb-s., carb-v., caust., cham., chel., chin-s., cimic., cina, cinnb., clem., coca, cocc., coff., crot-t., ery-a., ferr-i., glon., helon., ign., lach., lyc., lyss., merc., mez., **NAT-M.,** nat-s., nux-v., olnd., op., par., ph-ac., ***plat.,*** ptel., ***ruta.,*** sabad., ***sep.,*** sil., sulph., ***tub.***

amel - ham., ign.

respiratory affections, with - lact.

rest, agg. (see Motion)

amel. - ***bry.,*** cocc., ***gels.,*** lith., meny., nux-v., oreo., puls., ***sang., sil.,*** spig.

resting, on arm, while - nat-m.

on arm, while, amel - dros., seneg., staph.

on hand, while - bell., chin.

on a cushion quietly amel. - alum.

riding, in a carriage - asaf., ars., chin., **COCC.,** colch., ferr., ferr-ar., ferr-p., ***graph., hep., ign.,*** iod., ***kali-c.,*** kali-p., lach., ***lyc.,*** meph., naja, ***nux-m.,*** phos., phyt., raph., **SEP.,** ***sil.,*** sulph., thuj.

after - nat-m., ***nit-ac.,*** plat., **SIL.**

amel. - brom., graph., kali-n., merc., ***nit-ac., sanic.***

noise and jarring of, agg. - **NIT-AC.**

riding, cars, in - arg-n., **COCC.,** coloc., graph., kali-c., ***med., nit-ac.,*** petr., sulph.

amel. - ***nit-ac.***

riding, horseback amel - calc.

HEADACHES, general

right, sided headaches - ***alum.,*** arg-m., ars., asaf., **BELL.,** ***bism.,*** bov., ***bry.,*** bufo, ***cact.,*** **CALC.,** carb-an., **CARB-V.,** ***caust.,*** cham., ***chel.,*** cimic., ***cina,*** cist., coca, coc-c., coff., ***con.,*** croc., ***crot-c.,*** crot-h., cycl., euph., ferr-ar., gels., gins., gran., graph., grat., guai., ***hep.,*** **IGN.,** iod., **IRIS,** jac., kali-c., lach., ***lyc.,*** mag-c., meny., merc., merc-i-r., ***mez.,*** mill., ***mosch., nat-m.,*** nit-ac., nux-m., ol-an., plat., ***plb., ran-b., rat.,*** rheum, rhod., ***rhus-t., ruta.,*** **SABAD.,** ***sang.,*** **SEP.,** sil., spong., sulph., tarax., tarent., thuj., urt-u., verat., zinc.

blurred vision before the attack - **IRIS.**

dimness of left eye, with - arg-n.

evening in bed - con.

foreign body, as of a - ***con.***

lying, on painful side amel. - hipp.

on right side agg. - mag-c.

morning, left side, evening - bov.

periodic - ***cact.***

stroke of an anvil, as of - manc.

then left - arn., bry., colch., cupr., dig., merc-i-r., staph., tax.

warm room, entering - ***spig.***

rising, after - arn., glon., laur., nat-m., ox-ac., phos., stram., tarent.

amel. - asaf., hep., ign., kali-i., merc., nat-c., nat-s., nit-ac., rhus-r.

lying, from - aesc., am-m., anac., ang., apis, arn., ars., asar., aur-m., bapt., **BELL.,** bov., bry., ***calc.,*** calc-s., camph., caps., carb-an., cham., chel., cinnb., clem., coca, coloc., con., cor-r., ***dulc.,*** fago., glon., graph., hep., iod., ip., kali-n., mur-ac., nat-c., ***nat-p.,*** nux-v., olnd., **PH-AC.,** ***phos.,*** puls., rhod., ruta., sep., **SIL.,** squil., sulph., staph., ust.

amel. - aloe, ambr., am-c., ars., aur., **BELL.,** calad., carb-an., carb-v., cham., chin., cic., cupr., ferr., gels., hep., ign., ***kali-c.,*** kali-n., laur., lith., mag-c., nat-m., nit-ac., nux-v., ph-ac., **PHOS.,** phys., plb., puls., ran-b., rhod., rhus-t., sabin., spig., verat.

sitting, from - aesc., apis, ***bell.,*** chin., cob., ferr., grat., lam., laur., lyc., mang., mur-ac., ox-ac., puls., sil., spong., verat.

amel - arg-m., phys., spig., spong.

standing position to, amel. - ***alum.,*** ang., aur., bar-c., bry., calc., canth., carb-v., chin., con., dig., ***kali-c.,*** laur., mag-c., nat-c., olnd., puls., rhus-t., spig., stann., teucr.

stooping, from - acon., asar., colch., cor-r., daph., hep., ***kali-c.,*** laur., lyc., mag-m., mag-s., mang., mur-ac., nux-v., sul-ac., viol-t.

amel - calc-ac., con., ign., indg.

upright, erect - acon., ang., arn., ars., asar., bell., bov., bry., caps., caust., cham., cic., dros., hell., hep., ign., ***kali-c.,*** lac-d., laur., lyc., mag-m., ***mang., mur-ac.,*** spong., sul-ac., tarax., verat., viol-t.

HEADACHES, general

rising, from

upright, erect, amel. - ant-t., cic., mag-c., rhus-t., sabin.

roaring in ears, with - aur., ***chin-s.,*** ferr., sang., sulfon.

rolling, head from side to side amel - ***agar.,*** kali-i., med., ph-ac.

room, in - hyos.

crowded, in - ***lyc.,*** mag-c., **PLAT.,** plb.

entering a, on - caust., chel., laur., mez., nat-m., ***nicc., ran-b.,*** ran-s., rhus-t., sabad., spong.

from cold air - colch., con., puls.

pains coming on in room are amel. outdoors and vice versa - mang., ran-b.

rubbing, agg. - alum., calc-p., caust., dios., nit-ac.

amel. - ars., canth., carb-ac., chin-a., form., ham., indg., laur., ol-an., op., ***phos.,*** phys.

running, from - arn., ***bry., ign.,*** nat-c., ***nat-m., nux-v.,*** **PULS.,** tarent.

salivation, with - fagu., iris, merc.

scarlatina, after - am-c., bell., ***bry.,*** carb-v., cham., dulc., hell., hep., lach., ***merc.,*** rhus-t.

school girl, headache - acon., bell., ***calc.,*** **CALC-P.,** kali-p., ***lac-c.,*** mag-p., ***nat-m.,*** **PH-AC.,** ***pic-ac.,*** psor., ***puls.,*** tub., zinc.

scratching, amel - mang.

sewing - cina, lac-c.

sex, after - agar., arg-n., arn., ***bov.,*** calad., **CALC.,** ***calc-p.,*** chin., dig., graph., **KALI-C.,** ***lyc., nat-c.,*** nat-m., ***petr., phos.,*** puls., sel., **SEP., SIL.,** staph.

desires - sep.

excesses, after - **AGAR.,** arn., ***bov.,*** **CALC.,** carb-v., ***chin.,*** con., kali-c., lach., merc., ***nat-c.,*** nat-m., nat-p., ***nux-v.,*** ph-ac., phos., pip-m., ***puls.,*** **SEP., SIL.,** spig., ***staph., sulph., thuj.***

onanism, after - ***calc.,*** carb-v., ***chin., con.,*** lyc., merc., nat-m., nux-v., phos., puls., ***sep.,*** spig., ***staph.,*** sulph.

repression of desire, after - ***con., puls.***

sexual desire, after excessive pollutions - alum., bov., ***calc.,*** caust., cob., con., ham., kali-c., lach., lyc., nat-c., ***nux-v.,*** sel., sep., staph., viol-o.

sexual, excitement, with - apis, plat-m.

shaking, head - acon., ***arn.,*** ars., bar-c., **BELL.,** bor., ***bry.,*** calad., ***calc.,*** calc-s., carb-an., ***carb-s., carb-v., caust.,*** chin., ***colch., coloc.,*** con., ***cor-r., ferr.,*** ferr-ar., ferr-p., **GLON.,** ***hep.,*** kali-n., kali-s., lact., ***led.,*** lyc., mang., merc., ***mosch., nat-m., nit-ac., nux-m.,*** **NUX-V.,** petr., ***ph-ac., phos., rhus-t.,*** ruta., ***sep., sil., spig.,*** sang., sol-n., squil., stann., staph., stram., sulph., sul-ac.

amel. - cina, gels., hyos., phos.

shopping, from - epip., ***sep.***

sides, (see One-sided headaches, see Aching, pain, sides)

HEADACHES, general

sides, both - all-c., ***alum.,*** asar., bov., ***calc-p.,*** calc-s., carb-an., chin., cor-r., cupr., cycl., dig., dios., euphr., glon., kali-bi., **KALI-I.,** lyc., mag-c., mag-m., ***merc-c.,*** merc-i-f., mez., ol-an., phos., plat., squil., til.

singing, from - alum., ptel.

sinus, headaches, from catarrhal - acon., aesc., ***all-c., alum.,*** ambr., am-m., ***ars., ars-i., aur.,*** bell., ***bry., calc.,*** **CALC-S.,** camph., carb-s., ***carb-v.,*** caul., cham., chin., chin-a., ***chlor.,*** cic., cimic., cina, **DULC., EUPHR.,** ***ferr., ferr-ar.,*** ferr-p., ***gels.,*** **GRAPH.,** gymn., hell., **HEP.,** ***hydr.,*** ign., ***iod., kali-ar.,*** **KALI-BI.,** ***kali-c.,*** **KALI-I.,** ***kali-s.,*** kalm., ***lach.,*** laur., ***lyc., mang.,*** **MERC.,** merc-i-f., mez., nat-a., ***nat-m.,*** **NUX-V.,** ***phos., puls.,*** ran-b., rumx., sabad., samb., sang., sil., staph., ***stict.,*** still., ***sulph.,*** teucr., **THUJ.**

sitting - ***agar.,*** alum., am-m., ang., aral., arn., ars., asaf., asar., bism., bor., bry., bufo, ***calc.,*** canth., carb-an., ***caust.,*** cham., ***chin.,*** cic., coff., con., cycl., dros., euph., ferr., ferr-ar., ferr-p., gent-c., grat., guai., indg., lac-d., lach., led., lyc., mag-c., meny., merc., merc-i-r., mez., ***mosch.,*** mur-ac., nat-a., ***nat-c., phos.,*** plat., puls., ran-b., rat., rhod., rhus-t., ruta., sabad., seneg., sil., spong., squil., ***staph.,*** sulph., ***sul-ac.,*** tarax., verat., zing.

amel. - ant-t., arn., ars., asar., ***bell.,*** calc., calad., cic., cocc., coff., ***con.,*** gels., glon., ***guai.,*** hipp., ign., kali-ar., kali-c., ***kreos.,*** lam., lith., mag-c., mag-m., mang., merc., nat-m., nux-v., phos., rhus-t., sep., sulph., verat.

up, agg. - mang.

up or erect, amel. - ant-t., ***cic., gels.,*** kali-c., merc., phos.

sleep, during - agn., ars., camph., cham., colch., dig., ferr., graph., hyos., led., mag-c., petr., thuj.

morning, second agg - ham.

after - aesc., aeth., ***agar.,*** ail., alum., ambr., ***anac., ant-t.,*** arg-n., arn., ars., ***aur.,*** bad., bar-c., ***bell., bov., bry.,*** cadm-s., calad., ***calc.,*** calc-s., carb-an., **CARB-S.,** ***carb-v.,*** caust., cham., chin., chin-s., chion., cic., cimic., cina, cinnb., clem., ***cocc.,*** coff., ***con.,*** croc., crot-h., dig., dros., erig., euphr., eup-per., gels., ***graph.,*** ham., hell., hep., ign., ip., kali-ar., ***kali-bi., kali-c.,*** kali-n., kali-p., kali-s., **LACH.,** lact., ***lyc., mag-c.,*** mag-m., meny., merc., mill., morph., ***naja,*** nat-a., nat-c., **NAT-M.,** nat-p., nat-s., nit-ac., nux-m., ***nux-v.,*** op., ox-ac., pall., par., peti., petr., ph-ac., ***phos.,*** plb., psor., ptel., puls., raph., rheum, rhus-r., rhus-t., rumx., ruta., sabad., sel., sep., ***sil.,*** squil., staph., stram., ***sulph.,*** sul-ac., ***tarent., thuj.***

afternoon nap - calc-p.

HEADACHES, general

sleep, after, amel. - bell., camph., chel., colch., ferr., ***gels.***, ***glon.***, graph., ham., hyos., kali-n., lac-c., laur., ***pall.***, **PHOS.**, pic-ac., puls., ***sang.***, ***sep.***, thuj.
good sleep, amel. by - epip., ***phos.***, ***sep.***
restless sleep - crot-c., stram.
afternoon - calc-p.
amel. - acon., bad., cocc-s., gels., glon., hell., ign., nat-m., pall., ***sang.***, scut., sep., sil.
before going to - agar., nux-m.
damp room, in - bry.
disturbed, with - ars.
falling asleep on, amel. - anac., ang., nit-ac.
loss of, from late hours - ant-c., arg-m., ***carb-v.***, carc., **COCC.**, coff., colch., ***laur.***, ***nux-v.***, rhus-t., sulph.
from night watching - ambr., bry., carb-v., **COCC.**, colch., **NUX-V.**, ***puls.***, sulph.
roused, on being, from - ***arn.***, ***cocc.***, phos.
siesta, after a - bov., calad., calc-s., carb-v., chel., coff., ign., merc-i-r., nux-m., rhus-t., sep., sulph.
amel. - kali-n., pall.

sleepiness, with - ***ail.***, ant-t., chel., dub., ***gels.***, ind., lept., stel.

sneezing, agg. - am-m., apis, arn., bor., ***bell.***, benz-ac., ***bry.***, ***carb-v.***, cina, grat., hydr., ***kali-c.***, kali-p., kali-s., ***nat-m.***, ***nit-ac.***, nux-v., **PHOS.**, sabad., ***spig.***, **SULPH.**
amel. - calc., lil-t., lyc., mag-m., mur-ac.

spinal - alum.
complaints agg. - caul.

spinning, from - carb-an.

spirituous liquors, from (see Alcohol)

spitting, with - epip.

spot, pain in small - alum., bor., carb-v., caust., colch., dulc., eupi., ferr-ma., graph., helon., hep., hydr-ac., ***kali-bi.***, ***kalm.***, lach., lact., lith., nux-m., ox-ac., phos., plan., psor., ran-s., rat., sang., sol-n., spig., sulph., sul-ac., tell., thuj., vinc., zinc.

sprained, sensation - carb-an.
back of head - psor.

standing, while - agar., alum., arg-m., arn., ars., calc., calc-s., canth., chin., dig., guai., ip., kali-ar., kali-c., kali-s., ***mag-c.***, mang., ***nat-m.***, **PULS.**, ran-b., rheum, rhus-t., spong., staph., ***sulph.***, tarax., verat., zinc.
amel. - calc., camph., ran-b., tarax.

stepping, (see Walking) false step - anac., bar-c., bry., cob., hep., led., puls., **SIL.**, sol-n., spig., thuj., vib.
heavily agg. - aloe, alum., ambr., am-c., ***ant-c.***, bar-c., **BELL.**, **BRY.**, ***calc.***, calc-p., ***carb-s.***, ***caust.***, chel., ***chin.***, cocc., coc-c., coloc., **CON.**, dros., **GLON.**, hell., hydr., ign., kali-c., kali-p., kali-s., ***lach.***, ***led.***, ***lyc.***, ***mag-m.***, meny., mez., nat-a., ***nat-m.***, **NIT-AC.**, nuph., ***nux-v.***, ph-ac., ***phos.***, ***phyt.***, ***psor.***, **RHUS-T.**, ***sep.***, **SIL.**, ***spig.***, spong., sulph., thuj.

stimulants, (see Alcohol)

HEADACHES, general

stomach, as from - alum., carb-v., con., mag-m.

stool, after - aloe., ambr., am-c., apoc., bell., bufo, carb-an., ***carb-s.***, caust., chel., cupr., ign., lach., lyc., nat-c., ox-ac., petr., phos., podo., sabad., sep., sil., spig., ther., zinc.
after, amel - aeth., agar., aloe, apis, asaf., bor., corn., cupr., lachn., ox-ac., ptel., thuj., verat-v.
before - aloe, ox-ac., merc., ***puls.***
pressing, at, from - bell., ***bry.***, calc-p., cob., coloc., ***con.***, glon., ham., hell., ign., ***ind.***, iod., ***lyc.***, mang., nat-m., ***nux-v.***, ox-ac., phos., psor., ***puls.***, rat., ***sil.***, spig., ***sulph.***, thuj., vib.

stooping, from - acet-ac., acon., aesc., aloe, ***alum.***, am-m., ang., ant-t., ***apis***, arg-mur., arn., asar., bapt., ***bar-c.***, bar-m., **BELL.**, berb., bor., bov., **BRY.**, ***calc.***, calc-p., calc-s., camph., canth., caps., carb-ac., carb-v., caust., cham., ***chel.***, chin., chin-s., cic., cob., ***cocc.***, ***coff.***, colch., ***coloc.***, com., con., corn., cupr., cycl., ***dig.***, dros., ***dulc.***, ***ferr.***, ferr-i., ferr-ma., ferr-p., form., gels., ***glon.***, ham., ***hell.***, ***helon.***, ***hep.***, hydr., hydr-ac., hyos., ***ign.***, kali-bi., ***kali-c.***, ***kali-n.***, kali-p., ***kali-s.***, kreos., lach., laur., ***led.***, lyc., lyss., mag-m., manc., **MANG.**, med., meny., **MERC.**, merc-i-r., mill., mur-ac., nat-a., nat-c., ***nat-m.***, nat-p., nat-s., nicc., ***nit-ac.***, ***nux-m.***, ***nux-v.***, par., ***petr.***, ***phos.***, phys., phyt., pic-ac., plat., plect., ptel., **PULS.**, rheum, rhus-r., ***rhus-t.***, samb., ***sang.***, ***seneg.***, senn., **SEP.**, ***sil.***, sol-n., **SPIG.**, spong., ***stann.***, staph., stry., **SULPH.**, sul-ac., teucr., ***thuj.***, **VALER.**, ***verat.***, vib., zing.
amel - ang., bar-c., caust., ***cina***, con., dig., elaps, fago., ***hyos.***, ign., indg., laur., mang., mez., nux-v., phos., tarax., verat., verb., viol-t.

stove, heat of (see heat)

straining eyes, from (see eyestrain)

sudden, pains - agar., ***arg-m.***, aster., **BELL.**, berb., camph., cimic., croc., ferr., ***gels.***, mez., morph., phys., ***sabin.***, ***tab.***, valer.
come and go suddenly - asaf., aster., ***bell.***, ***cedr.***, fl-ac., ***ign.***, kali-bi., mag-p., med., merc-c., ***sulph.***
decreasing gradually - asaf., calc., fl-ac., puls., ran-s., sabin.
urination, during - tab.

summer - ***ant-c.***, bar-c., **BELL.**, ***bry.***, **CARB-V.**, **GLON.**, graph., lyc., **NAT-C.**, ***nat-m.***, ***nat-s.***, **PULS.**, sulph., thuj.

sun, from exposure to - ***acon.***, act-sp., ***agar.***, aloe, **ANT-C.**, ***arum-t.***, ***bar-c.***, **BELL.**, brom., brucin., **BRY.**, cact., cadm-s., ***calc.***, calc-s., ***camph.***, cann-i., ***carb-v.***, cast-v., ***chim.***, chin-s., ***cocc.***, euphr., ferr-p., ***gels.***, genist., **GLON.**, hipp., hyos., ign., kali-bi., kalm., **LACH.**, manc., nat-a., **NAT-C.**, ***nat-m.***, ***nux-v.***, **PULS.**, sang., ***sel.***, spig., ***stram.***, syph., ***sulph.***, ***ther.***, valer., verat-v., zinc.
amel. - graph., stront.

supper, amel. (see eating) - am-c., colch., lachn.

HEADACHES, general

suppressed eruptions - ***ant-c.,*** bry., lyc., ***mez.,*** nux-m., ***psor.,*** sulph., zinc.

sutures, pain follows - **CALC-P., FL-AC.**

swallowing, when - gels., kali-c., mag-c.

sweets, from - ant-c., **ARG-N.,** lyc., phos.

syphilitic - ars., asaf., ***aur.,*** aur-a., fl-ac., hep., ***kali-i.,*** led., ***merc.,*** mez., ***nit-ac.,*** phyt., sars., still., ***syph.,*** **THUJ.**

talking, while - ***acon.,*** agar., ***aran.,*** arg-n., ***aur., bell.,*** bry., cact., ***calc., calc-s.,*** canth., chin., cic., ***cocc.,*** coff., con., dros., dulc., euphr., fl-ac., ***gels.,*** glon., hyos., ***ign.,*** iod., jug-r., ***lac-c.,*** lac-d., led., ***mag-m.,*** meli., merc., ***mez.,*** **NAT-M.,** nux-v., par., ph-ac., phos., psor., puls., rhus-t., sang., sars., ***sil.,*** spig., spong., **SULPH.,** zinc.

amel. - dulc., eup-per., ham., lac-d., sil.

distant - mur-ac.

others, of - aran., bar-c., cact., ign., mag-m., merc., syph.

while, aloud - spig.

tapping, on spine - cina.

tea, from - chin., lach., nux-v., paull., sel., sep., ***thuj.,*** verat.

amel. - carb-ac., cimic., ferr-p., kali-bi.

strong - ***carb-ac.,*** glon.

temples, headaches, (see Headaches, temples)

thinking, of pain agg. - ant-c., arn., calc-p., cham., chin., con., euph., ferr-p., ***hell.,*** helon., hydr., ign., nat-s., ol-an., ***ox-ac.,*** pip-m., sabad., sin-n., staph.

amel. - agar., camph., ***cic.,*** helon., ***ox-ac.,*** pall., prun.

thunderstorms, during - morg., ***nat-p.***

before - bry., carc., lach., ***nat-c.,*** **PHOS., RHOD.,** ***sep., sil.***

tobacco, smoking, from - acet-ac., acon., alum., ant-c., ***ant-t., bell.,*** brom., ***calad.,*** calc., carb-ac., caust., clem., cocc., coc-c., ferr., ferr-i., ***gels.,*** glon., hep., ***ign., lob.,*** mag-c., **NAT-A.,** nat-m., nux-v., op., par., petr., plan., ***puls.,*** sil., spig., thuj., zinc.

amel. - am-c., ***aran.,*** calc-p., ***carb-ac.,*** naja.

toothache, with - ail., ***cham.,*** **HECLA.,** ***ign., kali-c.,*** lac-d., **LACH.,** lyss., plan., ***sang.,*** sil., verat.

touch - ***acon., agar.,*** agn., all-c., alum., ***arg-m.,*** bar-c., ***bell.,*** bor., bov., bry., calc., camph., casc., cast., carb-an., carb-v., chel., ***chim.,*** chin-a., cinnb., con., cupr., daph., ***gels.,*** grat., hep., ***ign.,*** ip., kali-bi., ***kali-c.,*** kali-n., kali-p., ***kalm.,*** lact., laur., led., lyc., lyss., mag-m., mag-s., ***merc.,*** **MEZ.,** mur-ac., nat-m., nit-ac., nux-m., ***nux-v.,*** par., ***ph-ac.,*** phos., rhod., sabin., ***sars.,*** sep., ***sil.,*** spig., staph., ***sul-ac.,*** tarent.

amel. - ars., asaf., bell., bry., ***calc.,*** coloc., con., cycl., kali-n., ***mang.,*** meny., ***mur-ac., phos.,*** sars., thuj., viol-t.

vertex, on, from - sabin.

touching the hair, from - agar., carb-v.

trauma, from - ***arn.,*** hyper., ***nat-s.***

HEADACHES, general

trembling, with, all over - ***arg-n.,*** bor., ***gels.***

hands, of - calc-p.

turning, body - cham., glon., graph., lyc., merc-i-f., nat-c., nat-m., plan., ***sil.***

body, in bed - crot-h., meph.

forward amel. - ign.

head - ars., canth., chin-s., clem., cocc., coloc., gels., genist., glon., graph., hyos., ign., kali-n., lyc., nat-c., nat-m., ph-ac., phos., phys., pic-ac., rhod., sil., spong.

quickly - genist., ign., nat-c.

twanging, as from breaking a piano string - lyc.

unconsciousness, with headache - acon., aeth., agar., ambr., arg-n., arn., aur., bell., ***bov.,*** cann-i., carb-v., cast., cocc., ***crot-h.,*** cycl., ferr., glon., hep., iod., kali-c., laur., mag-c., mang., ***mosch.,*** **NAT-M.,** nux-m., ***nux-v., petr.,*** phos., prun., puls., rhus-t., sabin., ***sil.,*** stann., stram., tarax., ***verat.***

pain with, and after - bov.

on moving - calc., carb-an., rhus-t.

uncovering body, from - benz-ac.

amel. - cor-r.

uncovering, head amel. - glon., lyc.

uremia, in - anac., arn., cann-i., carb-ac., cupr-ar., ***glon.,*** hyper., ***sang.***

urination, during - acon., coloc., nux-v., ***tab.,*** vib.

after - caust.

amel. - agar., fl-ac, **GELS.**

before, if the call be not attended to - fl-ac., sep.

profuse, with - acon., asc-t., ***gels., ign.,*** lac-d., ***sang.,*** scut., sil.

amel. - ***acon.,*** agar., ferr-p., **GELS.,** ***ign., kalm., meli., ph-ac.,*** sang., ***sil.,*** ter., verat.

uterine complaints, agg. - bell., caul.

utero-ovarian - bell., ***cimic., gels.,*** helon., ign., joan., lil-t., plat., ***puls., sep.,*** zinc.

vaccination, after - sil., thuj.

vascular, headaches (see congestive) - aml-n., ***bell.,*** meli., **GLON.,** ***lach.,*** sec.

vaults, cellars, etc. - **ARS.,** bry., carb-an., **PULS.,** ***sep., stram.***

veal, eating, from - kali-n.

vertex, headaches, (see Headaches, vertex)

vertigo, with - acon., agro., bry., calc-ar., ***chin.,*** chin-s., ***cocc., eup-pur., gels.,*** glon., ign., lept., lob-p., ***nux-v.,*** podo., sep., xan.

after - ***calc.,*** kali-bi., phos., plat., plb., ran-b., sep., til., upa.

vexation, after - acon., ***bry.,*** cast., ***cham.,*** cocc., ***coff.,*** ign., ip., lyc., ***mag-c.,*** **MEZ.,** ***nat-m.,*** nux-v., ***petr.,*** phos., ran-b., rhus-t., **STAPH.,** verat.

vinegar, agg. - teucr.

applying, amel. - meli., op.

HEADACHES, general

violent, pains - acon., aeth., agar., am-c., am-m., aml-n., ***anac.,*** ant-c., ***apis, arg-m.,*** arg-n., ***ars.,*** aur., ***bar-c.,*** **BELL., BRY., CACT.,** cadm-met., cann-s., canth., **CARB-S., *chin., cimic.,*** cimx., cina, cinnb., ***cocc.,*** coc-c., ***coff.,*** colch., coloc., croc., ***crot-h.,*** cupr., euphr., ***gels.,*** **GLON.,** grat., ***hell., hyos., ip.,*** kali-ar., kali-bi., ***kali-br.,*** kali-c., ***kali-i.,*** kali-p., kali-s., ***lac-d.,*** **LACH.,** laur., led., **LIL-T., *lyc.,*** lyss., mag-c., manc., **MELI.,** meph., ***merc., mez., morph.,*** mosch., ***nat-m., op.,*** oreo., passi., ***phos.,*** plat-m., plb., ***rhus-t., sang.,*** scut., ***sep.,*** **SIL., *sol-n., spig., stram.,*** stry., ***sulph.,*** syph., tarax., ther., thuj., zinc-valer.

menopause, during - ther.

red face, with, and diarrhea - **BELL.**

visual disturbances, (see blindness)

vomiting, with headaches - arg-n., ars., asar., bar-m., ***bry.,*** calc-ac., cham., chin., cocc., con., eug., ferr-p., glon., **IP., IRIS,** lac-c., ***lac-d.,*** lach., lob., lyc., meli., mez., nat-m., ***nux-v.,*** phyt., puls., rob., ***sang.,*** sec., sep., sil., tab., verat., zinc-s.

after - cham., cocc., ferr., nat-c., nux-v.

amel. - arg-n., asar., calc., cycl., gels., glon., kali-bi., lach., lac-d., manc., morg., op., raph., ***sang.,*** sep., sil., stann., sul-ac., sulo-ac., tab., tub.

walking, while - acon., act-sp., aloe, ***alum.,*** anac., ang., ant-t., arn., ars., ars-i., asar., aster., bar-c., bar-m., **BELL., BRY.,** cadm-s., calc., calc-s., ***caps.,*** carb-an., ***carb-s., carb-v.,*** caust., ***chin.,*** chin-a., chion., cic., clem., cob., ***cocc.,*** coloc., con., corn., dig., dros., ferr., ferr-i., ferr-p., **GLON.,** gran., guai., hell., hipp., hyos., hura, ign., iod., ***kali-c., kali-m.,*** kali-p., ***lach.,*** laur., ***led.,*** **LYC.,** mag-c., mang., meny., merc., merc-i-f., mur-ac., nat-a., nat-c., nat-p., ***nat-s., nit-ac.,*** nux-v., olnd., par., ***petr., ph-ac., phos.,*** phyt., plat., ptel., ***puls.,*** ran-b., raph., rheum, rhod., ***rhus-t.,*** sabad., ***sars., sep., sil.,*** spig., spong., staph., stront-c., sulph., tab., tarax., tarent., thea., ***ther.,*** ust., verat., verb., viol-t., zinc.

amel. - am-c., ant-c., aran., asar., bor., calc., canth., caps., carb-ac., cham., chin., coca, coloc., ***cycl.,*** dros., fago., gels., glon., ***guai.,*** ham., ***hyos.,*** **LYC.,** mag-c., mang., ***mur-ac.,*** nat-c., nat-m., **PHOS.,** puls., ran-b., **RHOD., RHUS-T.,** seneg., sep., sin-n., spig., staph., sulph., ***tarax., thuj.***

compelled to stand or walk - chin.

walking, air, in open, while - acon., alum., am-c., ant-c., ***arn.,*** atro., ***bell.,*** bor., bov., bry., ***calc.,*** caust., ***chin.,*** chin-s., ***cina,*** coff., ***com.,*** dulc., euphr., ferr., grat., hell., ***hep.,*** ign., kali-c., lam., laur., lil-t., ***lyc.,*** mang., merc., ***mur-ac.,*** nat-c., nat-m., nicc., nit-ac., nux-m., ***nux-v.,*** par., petr., plat., puls., ran-b., ***rhus-t.,*** sabad., ***sars.,*** sel., sep., spig., ***spong.,*** staph., stront-c., ***sulph.,*** sul-ac., tarax., thuj., zinc.

HEADACHES, general

walking, air, in open, after - ***am-c.,*** bar-c., bell., ***bov.,*** calc., caust., chel., chin., coca, coff., con., ferr., ***hep.,*** kali-bi., mez., mur-ac., nicc., nit-ac., nux-v., pall., petr., puls., ran-b., ran-s., rhus-t., ***sabad.,*** spig., spong., **SULPH.,** zinc.

amel. - aeth., ***agar.,*** ambr., am-c., ang., **ANT-C., APIS,** aral., aran., **ARS.,** asar., bar-c., bor., bov., canth., carb-an., caust., chin-s., cimic., cina, coff., coloc., cor-r., ***croc.,*** crot-t., eup-pur., fago., genist., glon., ***hyos., iris,*** **KALI-S., *lach.,*** laur., lith., **LYC.,** mag-c., ***mag-m.,*** mang., merc-i-f., mosch., ***nat-m.,*** olnd., phel., **PHOS., *plat.,* PULS.,** ran-b., **RHOD., *rhus-t.,*** sang., sars., ***seneg., sep.,*** sol-n., **SULPH.,** viol-t., ***thuj.***

head erect, with, amel. - ***nux-m.***

rapidly, while - **BELL., BRY., *calc.,*** chel., ferr-i., ***iod.,*** mang., nat-c., **PULS.,** tab.

in the wind, from - chin., mur-ac., nux-v.

slowly, while - hipp.

amel. - agar., coc-c., eup-per., ferr., lyc., **PULS.,** sep., visc.

wandering, pains - alumn., am-c., arg-n., calc., carb-v., chin., colch., ign., kali-bi., led., lyc., mag-p., mang., nat-s., phos., plan., podo., ***puls., sang., spig.,*** sulph.

mist before eyes, then fleeting pains agg. at occipital protuberance, down neck and shoulders, amel. lying in a dark, quiet place, and from sleep - podo.

warm, general

bed - **BELL., *carb-v.,* LYC., *mez.***

food, agg. - arum-t., mez., phos., puls., sulph.

room, agg. - acon., aeth., **ALL-C.,** aloe, alum., am-m., ant-c., **APIS,** arn., ars., ars-i., asaf., arum-t., bar-c., bell., bov., bry., bufo, calc., cann-i., carb-s., **CARB-V.,** caust., cham., chel., cimic., cob., coca, coc-c., coff., colch., com., croc., euph., ferr-i., ham., hydr., hyos., iod., ip., kali-i., kali-n., **KALI-S.,** lact., laur., led., lil-t., lyc., lyss., mag-c., mag-m., mang., mez., mosch., nat-a., nat-c., nat-m., nat-p., nicc., ph-ac., **PHOS., PLAT.,** plb., **PULS.,** ran-s., rhod., sang., sel., **SENEG.,** sep., sin-n., sol-n., spong., stram., sulph., tab., til., verat., verb., zinc.

amel. - am-c., aur., bell., bry., bov., cham., chel., **CHIN.,** cocc., coff., eup-per., ferr., hep., kali-c., lac-c., mag-c., **MANG.,** merc., nux-m., nux-v., rhus-t., spig., sil., staph., **SULPH.,** sul-ac., thuj., valer., zing.

weather amel. - calc.

begins with the warm weather - glon., **NAT-C.,** nat-s.

warmth, agg. - all-c., aloe, bry., euphr., glon., hyper., ***led.,*** nicc., phos., ***puls.,*** sep.

alternating with cold - carb-v., ran-b., verb.

amel. - am-c., chin., coloc., ichth., ***mag-p.,*** nux-v., ***phos.,*** rhus-t., ***sil.***

HEADACHES, general

washing, cold water, amel. - acon., aloe, ant-t., ***ars.,*** asar., aur-m., ***bry.,*** calc., calc-p., caust., cham., cinnb., cycl., euph., ***glon.,*** ind., iod., kalm., lac-c., myric., nat-s., ***phos.,*** plan., psor., zinc.

feet, amel. - nat-s.

hands, from - rhus-r.

head, from - ***am-c., ant-c.,*** bar-c., bell., bry., ***calc.,*** calc-s., canth., carb-v., cham., glon., lyc., merc., nit-ac., ***nux-m.,*** phos., puls., ***rhus-t., sep.,*** spig., stront-c., ***sulph.***

water, on hearing running - ***lyss.***

waves of pain (see Paroxsmal) - ant-t., asaf., bell., chin., cocc., ferr., plat., **SEP.,** spig., viol-t., zinc.

weather, changes of, headaches from - ***ars., bry., calc., calc-p., carb-v.,*** dulc., guai., lach., mez., nat-c., ***nux-m., ph-ac., phos.,*** phyt., ***psor., ran-b., rhod.,*** **RHUS-T.,** ***sil.,*** spig., verb., vip.

weight on the shoulders, from carrying - mag-s.

wet, from getting - ars., ***bell.,*** bry., **CALC.,** ***colch., dulc.,*** hep., kali-c., ***led.,*** lyc., ***nat-m.,*** nux-m., phos., ***puls.,*** **RHUS-T.,** ***sep.***

feet, wetting - gels., phos., ***puls., rhus-t.,*** sep., ***sil.***

head, wetting - bar-c., ***bell.,*** led., phos., puls., sep.

sweating, while - acon., calc., ***colch.,*** dulc., ***rhus-t.,*** sep.

wind, exposure to - ***acon., ars-i.,*** asar., ***aur.,*** bry., ***calc-i., carb-v.,*** **CAUST.,** cham., chin., glon., ham., **HEP.,** ign., ***kali-c., kali-i., lac-c.,*** lach., lyc., ***mez., mur-ac.,*** nat-s., ***nux-m.,*** **NUX-V.,** ***phos.,*** puls., ***rhod.,*** **RHUS-T.,** ***sanic., sep.,*** **SIL.,** ***spig.***

cold - ***acon.,*** anag., ***aur.,*** **CAUST.,** ***bry.,*** **HEP.,** ***ign., lac-c., mez., mur-ac.,*** **NUX-V.,** ***psor.,*** **RHUS-T.,** ***sanic., sep.***

riding in - ***ars-i.,*** bry., ***calc-i., carb-v.,*** **CAUST.,** glon., ***kali-c., kali-i.,*** lyc., **RHUS-T.,** ***sanic.***

windy, stormy, weather, headaches from - asar., ***aur.,*** bry., cham., chin., lach., mur-ac., ***nux-m.,*** nux-v., phos., puls., ***rhod., rhus-t., spig.***

wine, from - ant-c., arn., ***ars.,*** bell., cact., ***calc., carb-an., carb-v.,*** coff., con., **GELS.,** glon., ign., kali-chl., lach., ***led.,*** lyc., nat-a., ***nat-c.,*** nat-m., nux-m., ***nux-v., ox-ac.,*** petr., ***ran-b., rhod.,*** rhus-t., sabad., ***sel., sil.,*** stront-c., ter., verat., **ZINC.**

amel. - arg-n., calc., coca.

sour - ***ant-c.,*** ars., ferr., sulph.

winking - ***all-c.***

winter, headaches - aloe, ***aur-m-n., bism.,*** carb-v., nux-v., sabad., ***sil.,*** **SULPH.**

work, from - anac., bufo., calc., nux-v.

amel. - merc-i-f.

while doing some disagreeable - chin.

HEADACHES, general

worm, as if creeping - alum.

worms, complaints - ***calc.,*** chin., **CINA,** graph., nux-v., plat., sabad., ***sil.,*** spig., ***sulph.***

wrapping, up head - ***acon., apis, arum-t., bor.,*** bry., ***calc., carb-v.,*** cham., ***cob.,*** ferr., ***ferr-i.,*** ferr-p., gels., ***glon.,*** ign., **IOD.,** lach., ***led.,*** **LYC.,** merc., nit-ac., op., **PHOS.,** plat., **PULS.,** sec., seneg., sep., ***spig.,*** staph., ***sulph.,*** thuj., ***verat.***

amel. - agar., apis, arg-m., ***arg-n., ars., aur., bell.,*** benz-ac., ***bry., colch., con., cupr., gels.,*** **HEP.,** hyos., kali-ar., kali-c., kali-i., kali-p., ***lach.,*** mag-c., ***mag-m., mag-p.,*** meny., mez., mur-ac., nat-m., ***nit-ac., nux-m.,*** **NUX-V.,** ph-ac., ***phos.,*** pic-ac., ***psor.,*** **RHOD., RHUS-T.,** ***sanic., sep.,*** **SIL.,** ***squil., stront-c., thuj.***

wrinkling, forehead agg. - nat-m.

writing, from - aran., arg-n., ars., asaf., ***aur.,*** bor., ***calc.,*** carb-an., caust., cimic., clem., dros., ***ferr.,*** ferr-i., gent-c., glon., ign., ***kali-c.,*** kali-p., lyc., ***lyss.,*** manc., meph., **NAT-M.,** phos., ran-b., rhus-r., ***rhus-t., sil.***

yawning, when - agar., bar-c., chin., cycl., mag-c., nux-v., phyt.

amel. - mur-ac., nat-m., staph.

ends, with - ign., staph.

HEADACHES, forehead - acet-ac., **ACON.,** ***aesc., aeth., agar., ail., all-c., aloe, alum.,*** alumn., **AM-C., AM-M.,** ammc., anac., ang., ***ant-c., ant-t., apis,*** apoc., aran., ***arg-m., arg-n.,*** **ARN., ARS.,** ars-i., arum-t., arund., ***asaf., asar.,*** aster., ***aur., bapt.,*** bar-c., bar-m., **BELL.,** berb., **BISM.,** bor., bov., brom., **BRY.,** bufo, cact., caj., calad., ***calc., calc-p., calc-s., camph.,*** cann-s., canth., **CAPS.,** ***carb-ac.,*** carb-an., ***carb-s., carb-v.,*** card-m., caul., ***caust., cedr., cham., chel.,*** chim., ***chin.,*** chin-a., ***chin-s.,*** chlol., ***cic.,*** cimic., cina, ***cinnb.,*** cist., clem., cob., coca, **COCC.,** coc-c., colch., ***coll., coloc.,*** con., com., croc., ***crot-c.,*** crot-h., crot-t., ***cupr.,*** cupr-ar., ***cur., cycl., dig., dios.,*** **DROS.,** ***dulc.,*** echi., ***elaps,*** elat., euph., ***euphr., ferr., ferr-ar.,*** ferr-i., ***ferr-p.,*** fl-ac., form., ***gels.,*** gins., ***glon.,*** gran., ***graph.,*** grat., gymn., guai., ***ham.,*** hell., helon., **HEP.,** hipp., hura, ***hydr.,*** hydr-ac., **HYOS., IGN.,** ind., iod., ***ip., iris,*** jug-c., kali-ar., kali-bi., ***kali-c.,*** kali-chl., ***kali-i.,*** kali-n., kali-p., **KALI-S.,** ***kalm., kreos.,*** **LAC-C.,** ***lac-d., lach.,*** lachn., lac-ac., lact., **LAUR.,** lec., led., ***lept.,*** lil-t., lith., ***lyc.,*** lycps., lyss., ***mag-c., mag-m.,*** mag-s., manc., mang., ***med., meli., meny.,*** **MERC.,** merc-c., ***merc-i-f.,*** merc-i-r., merl., mez., mosch., ***mur-ac., mygal., naja,*** **NAT-A., NAT-C., NAT-M.,** nat-p., nat-s., ***nit-ac., nux-m.,*** **NUX-V.,** ***olnd.,*** ol-j., op., osm., ***ox-ac., par., petr.,*** phal., ph-ac., **PHOS.,** phys., ***phyt.,*** pic-ac., pip-m., plan., ***plat., plb.,*** podo., ***psor.,*** ptel., **PULS.,** ***ran-b.,*** raph., rheum, rhod., ***rhus-t., rhus-v., rumx.,*** ruta., samb., ***sang., sars.,*** sec., ***sel.,*** seneg., ***sep.,*** **SIL., SPIG.,** ***spong.,*** **STANN.,** ***staph., sol-n.,*** stict., stram., stront-c., stry., **SULPH.,** sul-ac., ***syph.,*** tab., tarax., ***tarent.,*** tell., teucr., thea., ***ther., thuj.,*** til., tril., trom., uran., ust., ***valer.,***

HEADACHES, forehead - verat., verat-v., verb., vib., viol-t., xan., zinc., zing.

above the forehead - acon., calc-p., kalm., lyc., merc-i-f., naja, ***olnd.,*** psor., sep., thuj.

above the, mental exertion, on - psor.

afternoon - ail., ***aloe,*** alum., ambr., anac., arg-n., bad., bor., bov., bry., bufo, calc-s., cann-i., cast., caust., chin., chin-s., cic., cimic., coca, colch., con., cycl., dios., dirc., fago., form., gels., glon., graph., hipp., ign., ind., ir-foe., jab., ***kali-c.,*** kali-cy., kali-n., kali-s., kreos., lac-c., lact., laur., lil-t., lyc., lyss., mag-c., mag-s., mang., merc-i-r., mur-ac., myric., naja, nat-a., nat-m., nit-ac., op., peti., ph-ac., phos., pip-m., puls., ran-b., rhus-t., sang., senec., serp., sil., sol-t-ae., stront-c., sulph., tab., tarent., valer.

3 p.m. - hura, lyc., lycps., sep., verat-v.

3-7 p.m. - tarent.

3-8 p.m. - arn.

4 p.m. - arg-mur., chin-s., phys., pic-ac., ***sulph.***

5 p.m. - paeon., stram.

riding in a carriage, while - lyc.

waking, on - sulph.

walking, while - ***kali-c.***

air, cold - ***bell.,*** calc., carb-an., caust., ferr., ***iris,*** kali-bi., ***nux-v.,*** rhus-t., sep., sil., zing.

cold amel. - lyc., **PHOS.,** pip-m.

air, open - agar., ***bell.,*** calc., carb-an., chel., euphr., kali-bi., kalm., lac-c., lachn., lil-t., ***mang., nux-v.,*** rumx., sil., staph.

amel. - acon., alum., ang., ***apis,*** arg-m., aur., aur-m., berb., calc., camph., carb-ac., cast., cimic., colch., coloc., cor-r., crot-t., euphr., ***ferr., ferr-i., ferr-p.,*** ham., hell., hydr-ac., jac., jug-r., kali-bi., lach., ***mag-m.,*** mag-s., merc., nuph., ***phos.,*** pic-ac., pip-m., sanic., sars., seneg., sep., sulph., sul-ac., tab., tarax., viol-t.

alternating with pain in small of back - brom.

crampy pain in chest at last tearing in nose and shoulders - lachn.

from side to side - ***iris,*** **LAC-C.,** lil-t.

gouty pain in joints - sulph.

pain in occiput - acon., agn., mosch., sulph.

anger, after - ign., petr., ***staph.***

ascending steps - alum., ***ant-c.,*** arn., cimic., ign., meny., sulph.

bending the head, backward - chin., stann.

backward, amel. - bell., sanic., thuj., verat.

forward - tarent.

binding up, amel. - lac-d.

blowing nose - alum.

business men - ***arg-m.***

chill, during - eup-pur., **NAT-M.**

after - mang.

closed, eyes forcibly - ***cocc.***

closing eyes amel. - ***agar.,*** aloe, **BELL.,** ***bry.,*** calc., nat-m.

cold, with - cimic., ***cinnb.***

HEADACHES, forehead

cold, applications amel. - chel., ***cycl.,*** merl., ***phos.,*** **SULPH.**

hand amel. - carb-ac.

wet weather - ***calc., dulc., rhus-t., spig.***

company agg. - ***plb.***

coughing - acon., anac., ant-t., ***apis,*** arn., ***asc-t.,*** asim., **BELL.,** brom., **BRY.,** ***calc.,*** chel., coca, ferr., ferr-i., ferr-p., form., hep., hyos., iod., iris, kali-bi., kreos., lyc., mez., mosch., **NAT-M.,** ***ol-j., phos.,*** rumx., ruta., seneg., sep., spong., staph., stict., sulph., verb.

coughing, amel. - arg-mur.

daytime - ***calc.,*** caust., chel., con., cund., kali-c., lach., lil-t., lyc., mag-c., nat-m., nuph., petr., phos., ptel., ran-b., sep., sil., sol-t-ae., tarent., zinc.

descending - ***bell., ferr.***

dinner, after - am-c., calc-s., chin-s., cimic., con., phyt., sulph., thuj.

diversion, amel. - ***pip-m.***

eating - alum., am-c., aran., bov., brom., ***bry.,*** calc-s., calen., ***carb-v.,*** cham., chel., ***chin.,*** chin-s., clem., ***cocc.,*** colch., con., graph., hydr., inul., kali-bi., kali-br., ***kali-c.,*** kali-n., kali-s., lyc., mag-c., ***nat-m.,*** nat-s., op., ***phos.,*** phyt., plat., sars., sulph., tab., valer., zinc.

amel. - carb-an., chel., ***cist.,*** genist., phyt., psor., **SEP.,** ***thuj.***

evening - acon., agar., alum., alumn., anac., ang., ant-t., aran., arg-m., arg-n., ars., ars-i., arum-t., bad., bapt., bar-c., bism., bor., bov., brom., bry., cact., calc-s., camph., cast., caust., chel., chin., chin-s., cimic., cina, cinnb., cocc., crot-h., ***cycl.,*** dig., dios., dulc., erig., fago., ferr., ferr-ar., ferr-i., ferr-p., fl-ac., graph., ham., hell., hipp., hura, iber., indg., ind., iod., ***iris,*** ir-foe., jug-r., kali-c., kali-i., kali-n., ***kali-s., kalm.,*** lach., lac-ac., lepi., lil-t., lyc., lycpr., lyss., mag-c., mag-m., mag-s., merc., merc-i-f., merc-i-r., myric., nat-m., nit-ac., nuph., ol-an., osm., paeon., ped., peti., ph-ac., phos., phys., pic-ac., plat., plb., podo., psor., ***puls.,*** ran-b., ran-s., rat., rhus-r., rumx., sars., sel., seneg., sep., sil., sin-n., staph., ***sulph.,*** sul-ac., tab., thuj., uran., ust., valer., zinc.

7 p.m. - chin-s., nat-m., ***sulph.,*** verat.

7-8 p.m. - sep.

7-9 p.m. - cocc.

8 p.m. - sol-n.

amel. - chin., clem., coca, kali-bi., naja, op.

bed, in - fl-ac., mag-s., sep.

singing, after - rumx.

exercise, from slight - ***epip., sang.***

exertion, mental agg. - anac., ***arg-m.,*** arg-n., arn., asar., bor., ***calc.,*** coff., cop., dig., fago., hydr., ***iris,*** kalm., lact., lyss., manc., meli., mez., ***nat-c., nat-m.,*** **NAT-P.,** nat-s., ***nux-v.,*** ol-an., ox-ac., petr., ***ph-ac., pic-ac.,*** pip-m., plb., psor., puls., rhus-r., rob., ***sil.,*** sep., ter.

HEADACHES, forehead

extending, backward - agar., arn., bry., ***crot-c.,*** cupr., eup-per., kali-bi., ***lach.,*** lil-t., mur-ac., onos., ***phyt.,*** **PRUN.,** ran-s., spong., tab., ther., **THUJ.**

backward, over whole head - anac., lach., mur-ac., sel., valer.

cheeks, to - brom., lachn., mosch., puls., sang.

ears, to - aur-m., glon., osm., squil., ter.

eye teeth, to - kalm.

eyes, to - agar., ant-t., apis, asar., ***bad.,*** calc-p., cann-i., cham., chel., ***crot-h.,*** gins., glon., grat., hep., ign., kali-bi., ***kali-c.,*** lac-c., lach., lact., lil-t., mur-ac., nit-ac., nux-m., ***phos.,*** puls., sabin., seneg., ***spig.,*** thuj.

face, to - brom., chin., lachn., meny., merc., mosch., puls., sang., sep., tab.

lower jaw, to - nat-m.

molars, upper - ***kalm.***

neck, to - chel., kali-n., kalm., lil-t., lyc., mosch., onos., viol-t.

nose, to - ***agar., calc.,*** calc-p., cina, croc., dios., dulc., glon., kali-bi., ***kali-c.,*** **LACH.,** mang., mosch., nat-c., nux-v., op., phos., ph-ac., psor., sep.

nose, to, root of - acon., aloe, bapt., glon., kali-bi., ***kali-c., lach.,*** nux-v., phos., ptel., ***puls.***

occiput, to - ars., **BELL.,** bism., ***bry.,*** calc., camph., ***cann-s.,*** canth., carb-ac., ***cham.,*** chel., chin-s., chlol., **CIMIC.,** coc-c., colch., con., cupr., dios., eup-per., ***form., kali-bi.,*** kali-n., kali-p., kalm., kreos., ***lac-d., lil-t.,*** lycps., merc-i-r., naja, nat-c., nat-m., ***nux-v.,*** par., phos., phys., pic-ac., plat., **PRUN.,** sabad., sabin., ***sep.,*** sulph., ther., **THUJ.,** zing.

orbits, to - chel., gins.

outward - bar-c., olnd.

parietal bone, to - chel.

shoulder, to - ***kalm.***

temples, to - arn., bor., canth., cimic., dios., hell., hydr., ign., kali-p., phys., thuj.

vertex - cimic., glon., hell., ip., kreos., merc., ruta., sep., sil., valer.

eyes, above - acon., aesc., aeth., agar., ail., all-c., aloe, alum., ambr., am-c., ang., ant-c., ***apis,*** arg-m., ***arg-n., arn., ars.,*** ars-i., asaf., aspar., aur-m., bapt., bar-c., ***bell.,*** berb., bor., bov., brom., ***bry.,*** cadm-s., ***calc., calc-p.,*** calc-s., cann-i., canth., caps., carb-ac., carb-an., carb-v., caust., **CEDR.,** chim-m., ***chel., chin., chin-s.,*** chlol., cimic., cina, cinnb., cist., coca, colch., con., cop., ***croc.,*** crot-h., cupr., dig., dios., dros., echi., elaps, ferr., ferr-ar., ferr-i., ferr-p., fl-ac., ***gels., glon.,*** gymn., ham., hell., ***hep.,*** hipp., hura, hydr., hydrc., hyos., hyper., ign., ind., iod., ip., ***iris,*** jug-r., kali-ar., ***kali-bi.,*** **KALI-C.,** kali-n., kali-p., ***kali-s.,*** kalm., **LAC-C.,** ***lac-d.,*** **LACH.,** lac-ac., lact., laur., lil-t., lith., lob., ***lyc.,*** lyss., mag-c., mag-p., mang., med., ***meph.,*** merc., merc-i-r., merl., mez., mosch., naja, nat-a., nat-c., ***nat-m.,*** ***nat-p.,*** nit-ac., nux-m., **NUX-V.,** ol-an., onos., op., osm., ox-ac., ***petr.,*** ph-ac., ***phos., phys., phyt.,*** pic-ac., plan., plat., plb., ***psor.,*** ptel., **PULS.,** ran-b., raph., rheum, rhus-r., rhus-t., sabad., ***sang., sanic., sel., seneg., sep.,*** **SIL.,** ***sol-n.,*** **SPIG.,** spong., ***stann.,*** staph., sulph., sul-i., tab., tarent., tax., tell., ter., teucr., ther., thuj., urt-u., ***valer.,*** verat., viol-t., ***zinc.,*** zing.

afternoon - carb-v., cinnb., com., kali-bi., ***lac-c.,*** lyss., puls., sang., sulph.

1 p.m. - chin-s., dios., phys.

3 p.m. - hura, pip-m.

4 p.m. - com.

motion - cinnb.

air, cold, in - kali-bi.

open, in - calc., chel., colch., ham.

open, in, amel. - echi., kali-bi., pip-m., phos., ***sep.***

alternating sides - ***iris,*** **LAC-C.,** ***lil-t.***

bed, on going to - ferr.

breakfast, after - hyper., ***lyc.***

close the eyes, compels him to - ***bell.***

cold applications amel. - agn., cedr., chel., kali-bi., lac-d., ***lach., spig.***

damp weather - ***sil., spig.***

dry wind - **ACON.**

contraction, of brow - ***arn.***

coryza, as from - sulph.

coughing, after - ***ol-j., spig.***

dark, in the - onos.

daytime - phos., pic-ac., sulph.

eating, after - bry., colch., nit-ac., sulph.

amel. - chin.

evening - ars., chel., ferr., iod., kalm., lyss., nat-m., plan., ***puls.,*** ran-b., ***sep.,*** stry.

6 p.m. - colch., dios., lil-t.

8 p.m. - chin-s.

9 p.m. - lyss.

reading, while - ***chel.,*** lyss.

extending, outward - nat-c., sec.

temples - ***arn.,*** bor., dios., hell., nat-a., phys.

to ear - aur-m., glon., lac-c., osm.

to eyes - con., lil-t.

to face - ***mag-p.***

to head - gymn.

to nose - all-c., bov., ***calc.,*** **LACH.,** phys., ran-b.

to occiput - bism., chel., cimic., dios., kali-p., kalm., kreos., ***lach.,*** lyc., naja, sep., zing.

to root of nose - **LACH.**

vertex - arg-n., gymn., phos., phys.

forenoon - cinnb., glon., ***mez.,*** rhus-t., sulph., thuj.

8 a.m. - hydr.

9 a.m. - lyss., petr., pip-m.

9 a.m. until 3 p.m. - ***caust.***

10 a.m. - crot-c., petr., stram., tell.

10 a.m. to 4 p.m. - ***stann.***

11 a.m. - mag-p., merc-i-r., myric., verat.

walking, while - thuj.

glasses, from wearing - ruta, sil.

HEADACHES, forehead
eyes, above
heat of stove agg. - ***arn.***
left - acon., ***aesc.,*** aeth., ambr., ant-t., arn., ***ars.,*** arum-t., asaf., bar-c., berb., brom., **BRY.,** caj., calc-p., camph., cann-i., cedr., ***chel., colch.,*** cupr., echi., euph., ferr., glon., ham., hell., helo., hydr., ign., ***ip.,*** iris, ***kali-bi., kali-c.,*** kalm., lac-c., ***lach.,*** lil-t., lob., lyss., mag-c., mag-s., meny., merc-c., merc-i-r., mosch., mur-ac., naja, nat-p., nit-ac., ***nux-v.,*** onos., ox-ac., ***ph-ac., phos.,*** pip-m., psor., puls., ptel., rhus-r., ***sep.,*** **SPIG.,** stann., stram., sul-ac., tell., ter., uran., verat., verat-v., verb.
extending, over whole increasing and decreasing gradually - ***stann.***
extending, to occiput and finally over whole body - ***bry.***
extending, vertex, to - ferr-i.
lying on left side amel. - ***bry.***
periodical - sep.
sex, after - cast., cedr.
then right - kali-bi., ***lac-c., lach.,*** nit-m-ac., ***psor.,*** zing.
light, from - chel., chin-s., mez., nat-m., nux-v., pic-ac., spig.
looking, at bright objects - sol-n.
down - ***nat-m.***
intently at anything - puls.
lying down, after - chim-m., ***ran-b., sang.,*** tell.
amel. - cupr., kali-bi.
menses, during - cimic., graph., ***lach., lyc.,*** nat-p., sang.
after - mag-m.
amel. - kali-bi.
before - bell., graph., hyper., nat-p., sil., xan.
mental exertion, during - ph-ac., **PIC-AC.,** ***puls.,*** sep., ***spig.***
morning - agar., alum., alumn., ***arg-n., chin.,*** chin-s., coc-c., dios., dros., ***kali-bi., lac-c., lach., mez.,*** nat-a., nux-m., **NUX-V.,** petr., phys., sol-n., ***stann.,*** sulph.
4 a.m. - spig.
6 to 12 a.m. - ***glon.***
in bed - coc-c., ***nux-v.,*** sol-n., spig.
until 4 p.m. - ***mez.***
waking - bell., phos.
motion, during - ***bry.,*** cinnb., cupr., mag-m., onos., ***nux-v.,*** plb., ***sang.,*** sol-n., ***spig.,*** ther.
amel. - dios., ***puls.***
narrow line, in a - bry.
night - ars., ***chel., glon.,*** hyper., ***kali-bi.,*** lyss., ***mez.***
midnight after - ambr.
noise - chin-s.
noon - form., ham.
numbness, followed by - ***mez.***
periodical - ***chin-s., tub.***
pressure amel. - chin-s.

HEADACHES, forehead
eyes, above
pulsating - ***bry.,*** caust., chel., dig., ***glon.,*** ham., ***kali-bi., lach., lyss.,*** mag-m., nat-m., ***pic-ac.,*** plat., ptel., **PULS.,** sep., ***spig.,*** ther.
reading - calc., chel., ph-ac.
right - acon., aesc., agar., am-m., anac., aran., arg-n., ars., aur-m., bapt., ***bar-ac., bell.,*** bism., bry., **CARB-AC.,** carb-an., **CHEL.,** ***chin.,*** cinnb., cist., coca, cocc., coc-c., com., cycl., daph., dig., dros., dulc., euon., ferr., fl-ac., ***gels.,*** gins., glon., graph., ham., hyos., ***ign.,*** iris, kali-n., lac-c., lach., ***lyc., mag-p.,*** mang., merc-i-f., mez., mur-ac., ***nat-m., nux-m., ol-an.,*** op., phys., phyt., **RAN-B.,** rhus-t., rumx., **SANG.,** ***spig.,*** staph., stront-c., tab., tarent., viol-t., xan., ziz.
then left - calc., ***lac-c., nat-m.,*** ptel., sep., sin-n.
sewing, while - **LAC-C.**
sex, after - cast., cedr.
sitting, while - ter.
sleep amel. - kali-bi.
sneezing, when - echi.
standing amel. - ***ran-b.***
stooping, when - dros., kali-bi., ***ign.,*** lyss., nat-m., petr., ***puls.,*** sin-n., sol-n., ***spig.***
sudden - ***mez.***
supper, during - chlor.
waking, on - bry., ***lac-c.,*** nat-a., sol-n., ***spig.***
walking, while - agar., chin., puls., thuj.
amel. - dros., ***ran-b.***
in open air, amel. - bor., chel., hydr., nux-v., ***sep.***
warm applications amel. - ***arg-m.,*** **ARS.,** ***aur-m., mag-p.,*** sang., ***thuj.***
warm room agg. - mez., ***puls.***
warmth - chel., mez.
eyes, behind - acon., asc-t., bad., ***bell.,*** berb., bism., cann-s., chel., cimic., cob., cop., daph., dig., fago., ***fl-ac.,*** gels., glon., kali-n., ictod., lach., led., merc-c., pall., phos., ***podo.,*** rhus-t., ***sel.,*** seneg., sep., ***ther.,*** ziz.
eyes, between - **CUPR.,** ***hep.,*** ictod., lach., lyc., phos.
eyes, extending to upper jaw - ***fl-ac.***
eyes, using agg. - ***plat.***
fire, near a - nux-v.
footsteps - **NUX-V., SIL.**
forenoon - arn., ars-i., brom., bry., calc-s., chin., clem., cocc., coloc., con., dig., euphr., fl-ac., gamb., gels., ign., kali-c., lach., lyc., mag-c., mag-s., meli., merc-i-r., myric., nat-a., peti., rhus-t., sars., sel., seneg., sep., sol-n., ***sulph.,*** ust., zinc.
10 a.m. - ***gels.,*** **NAT-M.**
amel. - ind., lact.

HEADACHES, forehead
frontal eminence - acon., agar., ambr., am-c., arg-m., ***arg-n.,*** bar-c., bell., berb., ***caust., cina,*** clem., cocc., colch., croc., dulc., ***ferr.,*** gran., grat., hell., hyos., kali-bi., kali-c., ***lach.,*** laur., lycps., merc-c., mez., naja, nat-c., nit-ac., nux-m., onos., op., pip-m., plan., polyg., puls-n, sin-a., spong., squil., stann., ***thuj.,*** verat., verb., xan., zinc.
afternoon - mag-s., nat-m.
4 p.m. - ferr.
air, draft of, in - verb.
open amel. - ***ferr.***
alternating with pain in cervical region - thuj.
blow, as from - sul-ac.
catarrhal - kali-bi.
descending steps - ***ferr.***
dinner, after - kali-bi., zinc.
evening - fl-ac., lycps., sin-a.
7 p.m. - thuj.
8 p.m. - thuj.
extending, ears,to - bov., nat-c., zinc.
eyes, to - calc-ac., thuj.
jaw, to - bell.
nose, to - cina, croc., dulc., op., squil.
occiput, to - coc-c., nat-c.
outward - verb.
supra-orbital foramen - aur-m.
temple, to - thuj.
vertex, to - ***ferr.***
left - agar., ambr., ***arg-n.,*** aur-m., ***cina,*** dulc., gran., ***lach., lycps.,*** nat-c., onos., puls-n, squil., **THUJ.,** zinc.
looking steadily - spong.
morning - agar.
3:30 a.m. - thuj.
10 a.m. - thuj.
waking, on - agar.
pressure amel. - ***ferr.,*** lycps.
pulsating - ***arg-n.,*** nit-ac.
rest, during - thuj.
right - acon., am-c., ***arg-m., caust.,*** cocc., colch., hell., kali-br., merc-c., mez., sin-a., xan., zinc.
shaking head, on - sul-ac.
sitting, while - hell.
stooping, on - dulc.
waking on - thuj.
walking in open air - thuj.
warm bed agg. - arg-n.
room agg. - spong.
hammering in - am-m., cham., cic., **FERR.,** kali-i., kreos., mez., nicc., **LYC.,** olnd., rheum, verb.
hat, from the - hep.
heat during - apis, ferr-i., sep., sulph.
amel. - cinnb., mag-m., **SIL.,** stann., ***sulph.***
increase gradually - erech.
intermittent - ant-c., stann.
laughing - iris, ***nat-m.***
leaning forward sewing - ***bor.***

HEADACHES, forehead
left side - acet-ac., acon., aeth., agar., ant-c., ant-t., apis, arg-m., ***arg-n.,*** arn., asaf., ***asar.,*** aur., aur-m., bell., bov., bry., cact., camph., carb-an., caust., chel., chin., chin-s., cic., cina, clem., coca, cocc., colch., coloc., cund., cupr., dulc., euph., euon., fl-ac., glon., gran., grat., haem., ham., hipp., hyos., iod., ip., kali-bi., kali-n., kalm., kreos., ***lac-c.,*** laur., lil-t., lith., lyc., lyss., mag-c., mag-m., meny., merc., mez., mur-ac., nat-c., nat-m., nat-s., ol-an., op., par., phel., ph-ac., phys., pip-m., plan., plat., prun., psor., ptel., rhod., rhus-t., sabin., sars., seneg., sel., sep., sil., spig., spong., stann., staph., sulph., sul-ac., tab., tarax., **THUJ.,** valer., verb., zinc.
extending to, occiput - nat-c.
to, right side - agar., chin., haem., ***iris,*** lycps., rhus-r., squil.
looking steadily - glon.
lying, while - alum., arg-m., bov., bry., camph., cham., chim-m., cinnb., coloc., fl-ac., ***gels.,*** lachn., mag-s., merc., nat-s., ran-b.
amel. - anac., ***bell.,*** calc., con., cupr., glon., ham., kali-bi., ***lac-d.,*** meli., nat-p., pip-m., rhus-t., sep., spig., tab., ***thuj.***
head low, with amel. - ***spong.***
on back - cinnb., ***coloc.***
on back, amel. - dig., nux-v., spong.
on side, amel - nat-m.
on side, left agg. - ***cinnb.***
on side, right amel. - cinnb.
meninges - hyos.
menses, during - aesc., alum., am-c., am-m., apis, bell., brom., ***bry.,*** cact., carb-an., cahin., cast., cinnb., cycl., euph., ***gels.,*** graph., helon., iod., kali-bi., lac-d., lyc., mag-c., merc., nat-c., nat-m., nat-p., nux-v., phos., plat., rat., sang., sep., sil., sulph.
after - ferr.
at close of - crot-h.
before - acon., bell., brom., ***calc.,*** cimic., cinnb., kali-p., lac-c., sil.
middle, of forehead - agar., ail., ***ars.,*** atro., calc., ***carb-an.,*** colch., crot-c., ***cupr.,*** fl-ac., kali-bi., **KALI-I.,** ***lyc.,*** **MERC.,** mez., phys., pic-ac., psor., ***puls.,*** rat., sabad., sang., sel., **SIL.,** ***staph.,*** verb.
football, during - nat-s.
frontal sinuses from chronic coryza - ***ars.,*** **KALI-BI.,** ***sang.,*** **SIL.,** ***thuj.***
hammering - **LYC.**
hat agg. - sel.
menses, before - ***calc.***
straining at stool - rat.
walking, while - sil.
in open air - tarax.
morning - agar., alum., am-m., arn., aster., aur-m., bapt., bell., bov., brom., bry., ***calc., calc-s.,*** canth., carb-s., chel., chin-s., cimic., coca, crot-h., crot-t., cycl., dios., equis., euphr., ferr., form., hydr., ***kali-bi.,*** kali-c., ***kali-s.,*** kreos., ***lac-c.,*** **LACH.,** lact., lil-t., lyc., lyss., mag-c., mag-s., med., merl., mez., murx., naja,

HEADACHES, forehead

morning - nat-a., nat-c., nicc., nit-ac., nux-m., ***nux-v.,*** ol-an., ox-ac., paeon., phos., psor., raph., rhus-r., rhod., scut., seneg., sep., sil., stram., stry., **SULPH.,** tarent., thuj., ust., zinc.

6 a.m. - sulph.

10 am to 3 pm - ***nat-m., tub.***

amel. - mag-s., ox-ac., petr.

bed, in - anac., dulc., graph., inul., mez., nux-v., ran-b., rhod.

every other morning lasting all day - ***calc.***

rising, on - am-m., asar., bar-c., bry., carb-an., cob., con., dulc., ferr., ham., iber., kali-bi., kali-n., kalm., lac-d., ***lach.,*** lil-t., lyc., mag-c., nat-c., nat-m., psor., raph., sep., sil.

amel. - anac., graph., hep., **NUX-V.,** phos., ran-b., rhod., ***sulph.***

waking, on - acon., agar., alum., alumn., anac., ant-t., arg-m., arg-n., arn., bell., berb., ***bry.,*** calc., calc-s., carb-ac., carb-an., carb-s., chin-s., cina, cinnb., coc-c., coff., colch., coloc., ***crot-h.,*** dig., erig., euphr., fago., ferr., ferr-p., fl-ac., gels., glon., graph., hep., hydr., ign., ind., ***kali-bi.,*** kalm., kreos., lac-ac., lac-c., lact., lyc., lyss., mag-c., mag-m., morph., myric., naja, nat-a., **NUX-V.,** ol-an., ox-ac., petr., ph-ac., phos., raph., rhus-t., rumx., ruta., sang., sol-n., staph., ***sulph.,*** tell., ther., thuj.

motion on - acon., agn., ang., ant-t., ***ars.,*** atro., aur., aur-m., **BELL.,** bism., bov., **BRY.,** ***calc.,*** canth., ***chel.,*** cimic., cinnb., cupr., cupr-ar., cycl., dig., dulc., fago., ferr-i., **GLON.,** graph., ign., iod., kali-bi., ***kali-c., lac-d., lach.,*** lyc., mag-c., meli., meny., mosch., nat-c., nat-p., ***nux-v.,*** ph-ac., phys., rhod., rob., rumx., sabad., ***sang.,*** sep., ***sil.,*** sol-n., ***spig.,*** staph., **SULPH.,** tab., ***ther.***

amel. - ***agar.,*** hydr., ***iris,*** petr., pip-m., ***puls., rhod.***

eyelids, of - ***bry.,*** coloc.

eyes of the - ***bad.,*** bapt., bell., **BRY.,** chel., chin-s., cimic., dros., gels., ***hep.,*** ign., jug-r., kali-c., mur-ac., ***pic-ac.,*** puls., rhus-t., sil., spig., valer.

hands of - coc-c.

must move the head to and fro - ***agar.***

rapid - dros., nat-m.

night - ***acon.,*** anac., arg-n., ars., camph., caust., chin-s., cinnb., croc., crot-h., cycl., fago., ham., hep., hura, kali-c., lachn., lac-ac., lyc., mag-s., merc., merc-i-r., naja, pip-m., ptel., puls., puls-n, raph., sang., sil., sin-n., spig., tarent., ***thuj.,*** til.

after 2 a.m. - cimic.

3 a.m. until evening - lyc.

amel. - clem., phys.

midnight - hep., mag-s., petr.

after - **LAC-C.**

until morning - hep.

waking, on - cinnb., merc-i-f., puls-n.

HEADACHES, forehead

noise - acon., agar., ***bell.,*** cact., ***chin-s.,*** cit-v., colch., con., ***iod.,*** lac-c., lac-d., ***sil., spig.***

noon - chel., dirc., fago., ign., puls-n, **SULPH.,** verat., zinc.

nose, above root of - ***acon.,*** agar., am-m., ant-t., arn., ***ars., ars-i.,*** aster., ***bapt.,*** bar-c., ***bell., bism.,*** bor., brom., ***calc.,*** calc-p., camph., canth., ***caps.,*** chel., coc-c., coloc., **CUPR.,** dig., dulc., ferr., ***glon.,*** guai., ham., ***hep., ign.,*** **KALI-BI.,** ***kali-c.,*** kali-chl., **KALI-I.,** kreos., ***lach.,*** merc., ***merc-i-f.,*** mosch., nux-v., plat., ***prun.,*** puls., raph., ***rhus-v.,*** **STAPH.,** stict., ***ther.,*** viol-t., xan.

evening - ferr.

left half - mur-ac.

menses, during - arn., hep., ***ign.,*** kali-bi., ***lach.***

night - rhus-v.

pulsating - **ARS.**

at root begins and extends gradually over the head, with delirium and vomiting - cimic.

odors, strong - sel.

paroxysmal - aesc., ant-t., ars., berb., ***psor.,*** **SEP.,** ***spig.***

periodic - lac-d., laur., mag-m., merc-c., nat-s., nux-v., ***sil.,*** sulph., teucr., ***tub.***

on alternate days - merc-c.

pressure - calc., camph., dios., mag-m., mur-ac., ph-ac., teucr.

amel. - ail., am-m., anac., apis, aral., **BELL., BRY.,** ***calc.,*** carb-ac., cast., ***chel., chin.,*** cimic., clem., colch., croc., ***ferr.,*** gels., ***glon.,*** ham., hell., hydr., ip., kali-i., kalm., ***lac-d.,*** lil-t., mang., meny., merc., merl., mur-ac., nat-c., **NAT-M.,** nat-s., ***nux-v.,*** olnd., op., phys., **PULS.,** sabad., spig., stann., sulph., sul-ac., tarent.

pulsating - alum., ***am-c., am-m., ars.,*** asar., **BELL.,** ***bry., calc.,*** cann-i., ***caps.,*** carb-v., ***caust.,*** cic., cimic., cocc., coloc., cupr-ar., ***dig.,*** **FERR., GLON.,** ***ign., iris,*** kali-i., ***kalm.,*** kreos., **LAC-C., LAC-D.,** laur., **LYC.,** lyss., mag-c., meli., merc-i-f., mez., naja, ***nat-m.,*** nicc., nux-m., olnd., petr., phos., **PULS.,** ruta., sec., sep., **SIL.,** sol-n., spong., ***stram.,*** ther., verb., zinc.

reading, while - arn., bor., bry., ***calc.,*** caust., chin-s., cocc., coff., ferr-i., lob-s., lyc., lyss., op., phys., pip-m., rob., tarax.

by candle light - ***spig.***

riding in a carriage - acon., ***cocc.,*** glon., ***lyc.,*** nux-m.

amel. - kali-n.

in cold wind - ars-i., calc-i., ***cocc.,*** glon., lyc.

right side - acet-ac., ***acon.,*** agar., aloe, anac., ant-t., apis, arg-n., arn., ***ars.,*** arum-t., asaf., bar-c., ***bell.,*** berb., bov., brom., bufo, canth., ***carb-ac.,*** cast., ***chel.,*** chin., chin-a., cimx., cinnb., cocc., coc-c., colch., crot-h., cupr-ar., cycl., dig., dios., dros., euphr., ferr., ferr-ar., ferr-i., ferr-p., fl-ac., glon., grat., hell., ***hep., ign.,*** indg., iod., ***iris,*** kali-bi., kalm., kreos.,

HEADACHES, forehead
right side - lach., ***laur., lyc.,*** lyss., meny., merc., merc-i-f., ***mez.,*** mosch., nat-m., nat-s., nicc., ol-an., op., osm., phel., phos., pic-ac., ***phyt.,*** **PRUN.,** psor., ***ran-b.,*** rat., rhod., rhus-r., rumx., ruta., sabad., sabin., ***sang.,*** sars., seneg., sep., sil., spig., spong., squil., stann., staph., stram., sulph., sul-ac., tarent., teucr., thuj., urt-u., valer., verb., zinc.
afternoon - agar., stram.
evening - ant-t., apis, nat-m., sang., merc-i-r.
extending to, cheek - lachn.
to, left side - acet-ac., aesc., aeth., cycl., ign., iris, nat-m., **SABAD.,** sanic.
to, occiput, through head - **PRUN.**
forenoon - dig., fl-ac.
morning on waking - colch., phyt.
night - sulph.
rising, after - cob., dulc., glon., iber., kalm., mur-ac., phys., ***sang.,*** verat.
amel. - chin-s., ***cinnb.,*** spong., sulph.
stooping, from - asar., ***bell.,*** mag-s.
room, in a - acon., bry., cact., caust., coca, colch., con., jug-r., lach., plat., ran-b., rhod., rhus-t., sep.
amel. - bell., mang.
warm - acon., **APIS,** bov., carb-ac., caust., ferr-i., lac-ac., lil-t., merc., mez., ***phos.,*** plat., **PULS.,** ran-b., sel., ***sanic., seneg.,*** sin-n., verb.
amel - lac-c., sil., sulph.
rubbing amel. - ars., ham., ol-an., op., ***phos.,*** phys.
sewing, from - iris, lac-c.
shaking the head - ***carb-s.,*** coc-c., con., ***glon.,*** merc-c., sep.
sitting, while - aeth., agar., ***alum.,*** aur-m-n., bism., calc., cast., caust., ***chin.,*** con., glon., ***iris,*** ham., ***lac-d.,*** lach., merc., mez., phos., ruta., seneg., spig., spong., staph., tarax., ter., verat.
amel - acon., ars., ***bell.***
sleep, after - ant-c., ant-t., calc., cham., cinnb., con., erig., euphr., fago., hell., lyc., myric., nat-a., sol-n., stram., thuj.
amel. - kali-bi., **PHOS.,** ***sep.***
smoking, from - calad., caust., ferr-i.
sneezing - apis, arn., echi., ***nat-m.,*** sabad.
spot - alum.
standing, while - agar., ***alum.,*** ars., calc-ac., canth., chin., ham., kali-c., mag-c., merc., phel., **PULS.,** ran-b., rheum, sang., spig., spong., staph., tab., tarax.
amel. - calc., iris, teucr.
stepping - alum., **BELL.,** ph-ac., sep., ***sil.***
stool, during - apis, ***sil.***
after - bufo, chel., podo., sep.

HEADACHES, forehead
stooping, from - acon., am-c., am-m., ang., arg-mur., arg-n., arn., asar., atro., aur-m., bar-c., **BELL.,** berb., bor., bov., brom., **BRY.,** ***calc., calc-s.,*** camph., canth., carb-an., carb-v., caust., chel., cob., coff., ***coloc.,*** cupr., cycl., dros., dulc., elaps, fago., fl-ac., ***gels.,*** gran., guai., haem., ***hep.,*** hyos., ign., ind., ip., junc., kali-bi., kali-i., kali-n., kreos., lact., laur., lyc., lyss., mag-m., manc., **MANG., MERC.,** merc-c., murx., mur-ac., myric., ***nat-m., nux-v.,*** phos., pic-ac., plat., ptel., **PULS.,** rat., ***rhus-v.,*** sanic., ***sil.,*** sol-n., **SPIG.,** stann., staph., **SULPH.,** tarent., teucr., **VALER.,** verat., zing.
stooping, from, amel. - bar-c., bell., caust., con., verb.
sunlight - ign., nat-m.
talking - cocc., iod., nat-m., ***sil.***
touch - alum., am-m., chin., cupr., ip., ***kali-c.,*** lepi., lyc., mur-ac., nat-m., sil., spong.
amel. - **BELL.,** calc-ac., chin., cycl., mur-ac., viol-t.
turning, eyes upward - ***lac-c.***
turning, head - canth., chin-s., coc-c., gels., glon., ***nat-m.,*** phos., ph-ac., rhod.
quickly - bry., ign., **NAT-C.,** ph-ac.
to right - aeth.
walking, while - acon., anac., ***arn.,*** ars., **BELL., BRY.,** ***calc.,*** calc-s., chin., clem., coca, cocc., coloc., dros., euphr., gran., ind., kali-bi., ***kali-c.,*** kali-n., lac-d., lept., mag-c., naja, peti., ph-ac., phys., ***puls.,*** rat., rhus-v., sabad., sars., ***sil.,*** spong., sulph., ust., viol-t.
air, in open, while - acon., ant-c., arg-n., asim., **BELL.,** calc., carb-ac., ***caust., chin., cina,*** coca, coff., hell., hyos., kali-cy., lyss., merc., nat-m., plat., sars., spong., tarax., ***thuj.***
amel. - bor., camph., chel., cor-r., crot-h., ham., hydr., hyos., ***iris, lyc.,*** mag-m., phys., ***plat.,*** scut., sep., sulph., thuj.
amel. - calc-ac., chin., coca, dros., ***iris,*** puls., ran-b., rhod., sang., staph.
wandering - aesc.
warm applications amel. - ***ars.,*** cinnb., kali-c., mag-m., mag-p., ***sil.,*** sulph., ***thuj.***
warmth, in - calc.
waves, of pain - **SEP.**
weight of the hat - hep.
wet feet, from - ***spig.***
wind, cold - aur., ***carb-v.,*** lac-c., nux-v., rhus-t.
wine, after - ran-b., rhod.
wrinkling - nat-m.
amel. - phos.
writing, while - aran., bor., calc., dros., ferr-i., gent-l., kali-c., lyc., op., ran-b., sanic., sil., zinc.

HEADACHES, occiput - ***acon., aesc., aeth., agar.,*** ail., ***all-s.,*** aloe, alum., alumn., ***ambr., am-c.,*** ammc., am-m., ***anac.,*** ant-t., **APIS,** ***arg-n.,*** **ARN.,** ***ars., ars-i.,*** arund., asaf., asar., aur., aur-m-n., bapt., bar-c., bar-m., **BELL.,** ***benz-ac.,*** berb., bism., bor., bov., ***brom.,*** **BRY.,** cact., calad., ***calc., calc-p.,*** calc-s., camph., cann-i., cann-s., canth., caps., ***carb-ac., carb-an.,*** **CARB-S., CARB-V.,** card-m., **CAUST.,** cedr., cham., ***chel.,*** **CHIN.,** ***chin-a.,*** chin-s., ***cic.,*** **CIMIC.,** ***cinnb.,*** clem., cob., coca, **COCC.,** coc-c., ***colch.,*** coloc., con., conv., ***cop.,*** corn., croc., ***crot-c., crot-h.,*** crot-t., cupr-ar., cycl., daph., dig., dios., ***dulc., echi., elaps,*** euph., ***eup-per.,*** ferr., ferr-ar., ferr-i., ferr-p., **FL-AC.,** form., **GELS., GLON.,** gnaph., ***graph.,*** grat., guai., ham., ***hell., helon.,*** hep., hydr., hydr-ac., hyos., ***hyper.,*** hura, ***ign.,*** indg., ind., ***iod., ip., iris,*** jatr., **JUG-C.,** kali-ar., ***kali-bi., kali-br., kali-c., kali-chl., kali-i., kali-n.,*** kali-p., ***kali-s., kreos.,*** **LAC-C.,** ***lach.,*** lachn., lac-ac., lact., laur., ***lec.,*** led., ***lil-t.,*** lith., lob., ***lyc., lycps.,*** lyss., mag-c., ***mag-m.,*** mag-s., manc., mang., ***med.,*** meph., merc., merc-i-f., ***merc-i-r., mez.,*** mill., ***morph., mosch.,*** murx., ***mur-ac.,*** myric., ***naja, nat-a., nat-c.,*** nat-m., ***nat-p., nat-s.,*** nicc., ***nit-ac.,*** nux-m., **NUX-V.,** ol-j., **ONOS.,** ***op.,*** ox-ac., osm., pall., paeon., par., **PETR., PH-AC.,** ***phos.,*** phys., ***phyt.,*** **PIC-AC.,** pip-m., plan., plat., ***plb.,*** prun., psor., ptel., ***puls., pyrog.,*** ran-b., ran-s., raph., rhod., ***rhus-r., rhus-t.,*** rumx., sabad., ***sabin.,*** sang., sanic., ***sars.,*** sec., ***seneg.,*** **SEP., SIL.,** ***spig., spong.,*** squil., stann., ***staph.,*** stram., stront-c., ***stry., sulph.,*** sul-ac., ***tab.,*** tarax., ***tarent.,*** teucr., ***thuj.,*** til., trom., urt-u., valer., verat., ***verat-v.,*** verb., xan., ***zinc.,*** zinc-m., zing.

- **afternoon** - aeth., agar., ang., bov., canth., cast., chel., chin-s., cimic., clem., coca, dios., dirc., fago., hydr., ind., iod., iris, kali-n., mang., ol-an., osm., ph-ac., phos., rhus-r., rhus-t., rumx., sars., sep., sulph.
  - 1 p.m. - ptel.
  - 3-6 p.m. - phos.
  - 4 p.m. - gels.
- **air,** open - bov., cob., hydr-ac., iod., lob., nux-m.
  - amel. - all-c., alum., ***apis,*** carb-an., ***cimic.,*** hydr., ***kali-c.,*** mag-m., mag-s., glon., mosch., pic-ac., sep.
- **alternating,** with, pain, in forehead - mosch.
  - in joints - sulph.
  - in sacrum - alum., carb-v., ***nit-ac.***
  - in temples - zinc.
- **anger,** from - ip., petr., ***staph.***
- **ascending,** steps - ***bell., carb-v.,*** carl., ip., mosch., pic-ac.
- **bandaging,** the head - calc., gels.
  - amel. - plb.
- **bending** head backward - ***anac., carb-v.,*** colch., ip., osm., staph., tarent.
  - amel. - aeth., bar-c., cact., chin., fago., murx., raph., ***rhus-t.,*** spig.
- **binding,** up hair - alum., bell., ***carb-v., kali-n., nit-ac.***
  - amel. - kali-n.

HEADACHES, occiput

- **blindness,** with - ***petr.***
- **breakfast,** after - aster., gels.
- **chagrin,** after - petr., ran-b.
- **chill,** during - petr.
- **closing,** eyes - ***calc.,*** ip., ***lach.,*** op., ***stram.***
  - amel. - ***hell., sep.***
- **cold,** air, amel. - ***carb-v.,*** euph., ***lac-c.***
  - application amel. - ***acon.,*** aloe, alumn., ant-t., ***ars.,*** asar., ***bell.,*** bism., ***bry., calc., calc-p., caust.,*** cham., chin-s., cinnb., euph., ferr., ***glon.,*** ind., iod., ***lac-c., lach.,*** mag-s., ***mosch.,*** myric., ***nat-m., phos.,*** psor., ***puls., seneg., spig., stram., sulph.,*** zinc.
- **coryza,** with - sep.
- **coughing,** on - alum., anac., carb-an., carb-v., ***coca,*** coloc., ***ferr., ferr-m., ferr-p., glon., lach.,*** mag-c., merc., mosch., nat-m., nit-ac., pyrog., sang., sep., sil., ***sulph.,*** tarent.
- **damp,** weather - ***bar-c.,*** brom., **CALC.,** ***calc-p.,*** **DULC.,** ***rhus-t.***
- **dark,** agg. - carb-an., ***carb-v.,*** lac-c., onos.
  - amel. - mag-p., ***sep., stram.***
- **daytime** - carb-v., ign., mag-c., petr., ph-ac., plan., seneg., stry.
- **drawing,** the eyes together - nat-m.
- **eating,** after - agar., alum., canth., carb-v., dios., gels., ***kali-bi.,*** mill., nat-m., ol-an., pip-m.
- **emotions,** from - benz-ac., petr.
- **evening** - all-c., alum., ambr., bar-c., bell., bov., brom., canth., carb-an., carb-s., chin-s., cimic., colch., dios., form., gels., graph., hyper., indg., jab., kali-br., kali-chl., kali-n., lob., lyc., mag-c., mez., mur-ac., nit-ac., ol-an., op., ptel., ran-b., ran-s., rhus-r., seneg., sep., stann., staph., stront-c., sulph., thuj., uran., zinc.
  - amel. - coca, sep.
  - bed, in - dulc., kali-n., sarr.
  - gas light - zinc.
- **exercise,** amel. - cact.
- **exertion,** after - ***gels.,*** nit-ac., ***ox-ac.***
- **extending,** chest, to - graph.
  - down back - ***aeth.,*** cimic., ***cocc.,*** crot-h., graph., lil-t., lyss., nat-m., pic-ac., podo., sang., sep., ***stry.,*** thuj.
  - ears, to - aesc., bar-c., cann-s., chel., colch., plan., plb., puls., stry.
  - eyes, to - atro., chin., ery-a., gels., ***glon.,*** **LACH.,** nat-s., ***petr.,*** pic-ac., **SANG.,** sanic., sars., ***sep., sil.,*** **SPIG.,** stry., ***verat.,*** zinc.
  - forehead, to - ambr., ***arg-n.,*** aur., bov., brom., ***calc., carb-v., chel.,*** chin., clem., con., dios., dirc., ferr., fl-ac., **GELS.,** ***glon., kali-bi.,*** kali-c., **LAC-C.,** ***lach.,*** mang., merc., mez., mosch., mur-ac., ***nat-m.,*** nat-s., ol-j., op., ***petr., ph-ac.,*** plb., ptel., ***rhus-t.,*** sanic., ***sars.,*** **SANG.,** ***sil.,*** sulph., tarent., ter.
    - in waves - ***sil.***

HEADACHES, occiput
extending,forward - aeth., ambr., anac., aur., chin., mag-m., merc., ***ph-ac.,*** rat., sanic., ***sil.***
head, to - canth., carb-v., caust., **CHIN., GELS.,** ***glon.,*** kalm., mag-p., merc., ***mez.,*** pic-ac., ***puls.,*** sabad., sang., ***sil.,*** **STRAM.**
over whole head - chin.
jaw, to - bar-c., kali-chl., nit-ac.
lower, to - cham.
neck, to - ambr., ***bell., bry., carb-v.,*** **COCC.,** glon., hell., hep., kali-c., laur., ***lil-t.,*** phyt., podo., sulph.
down back of neck - arg-n., bell., berb., ***bry.,*** cimic., ***cocc.,*** com., ***graph.,*** hell., ***hep.,*** hydr-ac., kali-c., kali-n., laur., lil-t., lob., mang., merc., mur-ac., nat-c., **NUX-M., NUX-V.,** pic-ac., podo., ran-b., sabin., sep., sulph., tarent.
nose, to - corn.
right to left - dig., mez., staph.
shoulders, to - ***bry.,*** caust., dios., ***gels.,*** hep., ***ip.,*** kali-c., kali-n., podo.
while lying on back - ***bry.***
temples, to - anac., arn., cann-i., coca, ***glon.,*** plb., seneg., ***spig.***
throat, to - laur.
upward - all-c., berb., **CALC.,** caust., **GELS.,** glon., ol-an., ph-ac., ***puls., sang.,*** sars., sep., **SIL.**
vertex, to - ambr., bov., ***calc.,*** cann-i., ***caust.,*** **CIMIC.,** dig., ***dulc.,*** glon., hell., hura, lac-c., lac-ac., lyc., mag-m., nat-c., phel., rat., sep., **SIL.**
fanning, amel. - ***carb-v.***
fever, during - **NUX-V.,** ***verat-v.***
foreign, body, as if - arg-m.
forenoon - agar., all-c., alum., ***bry.,*** chel., ***chin., cob.,*** cop., dios., gels., indg., lact., lyc., nat-c., op., phys., phyt., psor., rhus-t., ***sep.,*** spong., sulph.
11 a.m. - gels.
mental exertion, after - rhus-t.
shaking head - cann-i.
sitting while - rhod.
grief, after - **PH-AC.**
hammering - act-sp., camph., ferr-p., nat-m., psor.
heat, during - graph., lyc.
agg. - ***euph., gels.,*** ip., ***phos., puls.***
stove, of - ***carb-v.,*** puls.
heated, from becoming - ***carb-v.,*** ip., kali-c., lac-c., ***stram.***
hot, applications amel. - ***gels., ign.***
indigestion, after - cann-s., ***ip.,*** petr., ran-b., ***staph.***
jarring, agg. - anac., **BELL.,** ***bry., carb-v., calc.,*** ferr-p., ***gels.,*** **GLON.,** ***ip.,*** kali-n., **LED.,** ***mag-m.,*** mag-s., **NIT-AC.,** staph., ***stram.,*** ther.
laughing, agg. - zinc.
leaning, head back - tarent.
amel. - spig.

HEADACHES, occiput
light, amel. - lac-c.
looking, at bright objects - plb., ***stram.***
lying, while - agar., camph., canth., chel., **CHIN.,** euph., ***eup-per., gels.,*** ip., lachn., lyss., mag-s., nux-v., ***onos., op.,*** pip-m., puls., sep., spig., spong., staph.
abdomen, on, amel. - grat.
amel. - alum., ***graph., hell.,*** iod., ***kali-s.,*** nit-ac., ph-ac., spig., tab.
back of head, on - agar., cact., ***petr., sep.,*** sulph.
amel. - ***kali-p.,*** ph-ac.
head high, with amel. - ***gels., spig.***
low amel. - ***mosch.***
lying, side of head, on amel. - cact., ***sep.***
lying, side, either side agg. - ***carb-v.***
left amel. - ars.
right - ***carb-v.,*** petr., staph.
menses, during - ***bell., bry., calc., carb-an., carb-v., kali-n., lac-c.,*** mag-c., mag-m., nit-ac., nux-v., ***phos.***
after - ***carb-v.***
before - calc., nat-c., nit-ac.
contracting the eyes, during - ***carb-v.***
scanty flow, with - alum., ***carb-v.***
mental, labor - anac., aster., calc., ***carb-ac.,*** carb-an., ***carb-v., cimic., coc-c., colch., elaps, gels.,*** ign., kali-n., lob., ***nat-c.,*** nat-s., nit-ac., ***par., pic-ac.,*** psor., rhus-r., rhus-t.
amel. - cact., calc.
morning - agar., ***all-s.,*** arum-t., bov., ***bry.,*** cedr., chin-s., cob., colch., cop., dios., euph., gels., ***helon., jug-c.,*** junc., **LAC-C.,** ***lach.,*** lob., lyc., mag-c., mag-s., morph., ***nat-m.,*** nit-ac., nux-m., ***nux-v.,*** op., petr., ***ph-ac.,*** puls., ***ran-b.,*** raph., rhod., rhus-r., rhus-t., sabin., sanic., ***sep., sil.,*** spig., sulph.
bed, in - agar., eupi., ***jug-c., nux-v., ph-ac.,*** sep.
lying on back - ***all-s., bry.,*** sep.
rising, on - cimic., cinnb., gels., kali-bi., mag-m., merc-i-f., ***nux-v.***
amel. - jug-c., kali-p., spig.
room, in, amel. - bov.
waking, on - arn., arg-m., ***bry.,*** con., fl-ac., grat., hell., kali-bi., **LAC-C.,** ***lach.,*** mill., ***morph., nat-m.,*** op., ox-ac., ***petr., ph-ac.,*** rhus-t., sanic., ***sulph.,*** uran.
3 p.m. - cob.
5 p.m. - rhus-t.
amel. at noon - ***bry.***
until 2 p.m. - clem.
motion, agg. - am-c., aur., ***bell.,*** bism., ***bry.,*** calc., ***carb-v.,*** chin., chin-a., coc-c., cupr., elaps, eup-per., ***ferr., gels.,*** glon., ***hell., hyper.,*** iod., ***ip.,*** kali-c., kali-n., lac-c., ***lach.,*** lac-ac., lyc., mag-p., manc., mang., ***mez.,*** mosch., nit-ac., ***nux-v., ox-ac.,*** petr., ph-ac., ***sep., sel.,*** spig., spong., staph., ***stram.,*** thuj.
amel. - ***agar.,*** carl., euph., pip-m., ***rhus-t.,*** stann.
eyelids - bry., ***carb-v.***

HEADACHES, occiput

motion, head, of - ***bry.***, cact., ***carb-v., gels.***, ip., petr., staph., ***stram.***

neuralgic - aesc.

night - bor., carb-s., carb-v., cedr., ***chel.***, clem., hipp., kali-n., ***kali-p.***, lyc., ***mez.***, osm., sep., stront-c., ***sulph., thuj.***

1 a.m. - bry., rhus-t.

2 a.m. - sulph.

3 a.m. - chin-s.

3-4 a.m. - spig.

midnight - sep.

noise, agg. - anac., ***bry.***, calc., ***carb-v.***, cimic., ***gels.***, ign., ip., ***nit-ac., ph-ac.***, plb., spig., ***stram.***

noon - cob., murx., nat-c., sulph.

occipital protuberance - **BRY.,** ***calc-p.***, colch., dig., mur-ac., ***rhus-t., sil.***, uran.

afternoon - chin-s.

heat, from - ***sil.***

motion agg. - **BRY.**

pressure of hat agg. - ***sil.***

touch, on - nat-c.

walking in wind - mur-ac.

occiput, and forehead - aeth., ***alum.***, ambr., anac., aphis., arn., asaf., aur., bell., bry., calc., camph., cann-i., canth., caps., carb-v., chel., chin., chin-s., cimic., cina, clem., colch., con., corn., dig., dios., eup-per., ferr., gels., glon., graph., grat., guai., hydr-ac., hyos., ign., iod., iris, kali-bi., kali-c., kali-n., lach., lachn., laur., lyc., mag-c., mag-m., mang., merc., mez., mosch., mur-ac., nat-m., ol-j., onos., op., petr., ph-ac., prun., ptel., raph., rhus-t., sabad., sabin., sars., seneg., sep., serp., spig., spong., squil., stry., sulph., sul-ac., tab., thuj.

morning, on waking - kali-bi., ***lach.***, **ONOS.**

paroxysmal - ***aesc., bell.***, chen-v., cimic., ***gels.***, **LACH.,** ***stram.***

perspiration, amel. - clem.

pressure, agg. - am-c., calc., camph., dios., ph-ac., spig., sulph.

amel. - ***bry.***, calc., ***carb-v., cast.***, colch., dios., gels., grat., hydr., hyos., kali-n., mag-c., ***mag-m., mag-p.***, mang., ***nux-m.***, **NUX-V.,** ***plb.***, sabin., sep., spig., tarent., ***zinc.***

hat of, agg. - **CARB-V.,** ***kali-n.***, lob., ***nit-ac.***, petr., sil.

pulsating - act-sp., agn., alum., am-c., asar., **BELL.,** bor., ***calc.***, camph., ***carb-v.***, caust., ***chel.***, cimic., con., ***crot-h.***, dros., **EUP-PER.,** ***ferr., gels., glon., ign.***, kali-br., ***kali-n., kali-s.***, **LACH.,** ***led.***, lyss., mag-m., mang., ***nat-m.***, nit-ac., ***petr., phos.***, psor., puls., ***sep., stram.***, valer.

rheumatic - bar-c., staph.

riding, agg. - petr., phyt.

rising, after - gels., mur-ac., lyss.

after, amel. - chin., eup-per., grat., jug-c., kali-p., puls.

bed, from, agg. - ***mur-ac.***

HEADACHES, occiput

rubbing, amel. - canth., carb-v., laur., ol-an., ph-ac., tarent.

screwed, together, as if - grat., mag-c., merc.

sex, after - agar., bov., calad., calc., chin., graph., kali-c., nat-m., petr., sep., sil., staph.

neurasthenia, in - gels.

sexual excesses, after - ***calc.***, **CHIN., PHOS.**

shaking, head - apis, calc., cann-i., **CARB-V.,** con., ***glon., ip., kali-br.***, mosch., ***nit-ac., petr.***, staph.

head, amel. - gels.

sides - aesc., all-c., aster., cann-s., cham., ***chel.***, colch., elaps, **FL-AC.,** glon., guai., hyos., ign., ind., kali-bi., kali-n., led., mag-c., mag-s., meph., mez., ol-an., ph-ac., phys., ptel., sep., ***sil.***, **STRAM.,** sulph.

bending backward - colch.

blood, stagnated as if - sulph.

daytime - ph-ac.

evening, 8 p.m. - stram.

forenoon - all-c., dios.

hammering - ign.

left - agar., am-c., cham., ***chel.***, guai., led., ol-an., nuph., phys., ptel., puls., thuj.

sitting, while - ***agar.***

to right - squil.

morning - dios., puls.

pressure amel. - hyos.

right - aesc., aster., cann-s., colch., hep., ign., ***iris***, ind., kali-bi., myric., sep., stram.

to left - dig., ***mez.***, staph.

to left eye - iod.

shaking head - glon.

touch, on - thuj.

waking, after - ***sulph.***

walking, on - aster.

sitting, while - ***agar.***, cast., caust., chin., euph., indg., ***kali-br., kali-s.***, meny., ***mosch.***, ph-ac., ran-b., rhod., spig., squil., zinc.

amel. - asar., gels., ign., mag-c., mag-m., nux-m.

sleep, after - aesc., aeth., agar., ail., alum., ambr., ***ars.***, bov., bry., ***calc., carb-v.***, caust., ***chel.***, chin., chin-a., ***cimic.***, cinnb., cocc., ***con.***, eup-per., ***gels., graph.***, hep., ***ip., kali-bi., kali-c., kali-n.***, **LACH.,** ***lyc.***, mang., ***nat-s.***, nit-ac., ***nux-v., op.***, ox-ac., ***pall.***, petr., ph-ac., ***phos.***, prun., ptel., puls., ***rhus-t.***, sep., ***sil.***

amel. - nit-ac.

sneezing - grat., lach.

standing, while - ***carb-v.***, cast., ***hell., ip.***, kali-c., kali-n., lac-c., mag-c., mosch., ph-ac., staph., tab.

amel. - ***chin.***, nux-v., plb., tarax.

position, in one - cham.

stool, while pressing at - ***ign.***

stooping - acon., aesc., aloe, alum., ant-t., ***calc.***, camph., carb-ac., ***carb-v.***, chin., cob., colch., con., cupr., elaps, fago., ***ferr., gels., hell.***, helon., kali-c., ***kali-n.***, lyc., mag-s., mang., nit-ac., nux-m., ph-ac., ***phos.***, prun., rhus-r., ***spig.***, staph., sulph.

HEADACHES, occiput
stooping, amel. - ign., ol-an., verat.
changes to forehead, on - carb-an.
sun, heat of - **ACON., BELL.,** brom., **BRY.,** camph., carb-v., ***gels.,*** **GLON.,** ***nat-c., nat-m.,*** sol., ***ther.***
suppurating, as if - bor., mang.
swallowing, agg. - gels., kali-c.
thinking, agg. - ign., nit-ac.
touch, agg. - cupr., gels., ***kali-n.,*** mang., ***nit-ac.,*** op.
amel. - mang.
hair, the agg. - ***carb-v., kali-n., nit-ac.***
turning, eyes, agg, upward - **LAC-C.**
eyes, agg. - sep.
head - ***carb-v.,*** mang., ***op.***
urinate, if desire to, be delayed - sep.
copious flow of, amel. - ***gels.***
vexation, after - alum., ip., petr., ***ran-b.,*** staph.
walking - asar., bell., ***bry., calc., carb-v., chin.,*** con., ***glon., graph., ip.,*** kali-br., kali-c., **LED.,** mur-ac., nit-ac., phys., ***spig.,*** sulph., staph., ***stram.,*** tarax.
walking, air, in open - bov., ***calc., caust.,*** cina, ferr-p., mang., spig., staph., zinc.
amel. - cimic., mang., rhus-t., ***seneg.,*** sulph., tab.
slowly amel. - plb.
wandering - nat-s.
warm, wrapping up amel. - ***gels.,*** ign., ***nux-v.,*** **RHUS-T., SIL.**
clothing agg. - ip., nit-ac., staph., ***stram.***
food - ip., mez., puls., sulph.
warm, room - ***all-c., apis,*** bov., ***bry.,*** carb-v., ***cimic., mag-m., mez.,*** mosch., ***puls., seneg., stram.,*** sulph.
amel. - bov.
wet, weather - lyss.
wine, agg. - zinc.
amel. - gels.
writing, from - carb-an., cocc., gels.
yawning, agg. - cocc.
amel. - staph.

HEADACHES, sides - acon., aesc., aeth., ***agar.,*** agn., **ALUM.,** ambr., am-c., am-m., ***anac.,*** ang., ant-c., ant-t., ***apis, arg-m.,*** **ARG-N.,** ***arn., ars.,*** ars-i., arund., ***asaf., asar.,*** aur., ***bar-c.,*** bar-m., ***bell., bism.,*** bor., ***bov., bry., bufo, cact., calc.,*** calc-p., camph., cann-i., cann-s., ***canth., caps.,*** carb-an., carb-s., carb-v., caust., ***cham., chel., chin.,*** chin-a., chin-s., ***cic.,*** cina, cinnb., clem., cocc., **COFF.,** colch., ***coloc.,*** con., cop., ***corn.,*** croc., crot-h., cupr., cycl., dig., dios., dros., dulc., elat., elaps, eug., euph., euphr., eup-per., ***ferr.,*** ferr-ar., ferr-i., ferr-p., ***gels., glon., graph., guai.,*** hell., hyos., ***ign.,*** iod., ind., ip., iris, ***kali-ar., kali-bi., kali-br.,*** **KALI-C., KALI-I.,** kali-n., **KALI-P.,** ***kali-s.,*** kalm., kreos., ***lac-d., lach.,*** lact., ***laur.,*** led., ***lyc.,*** mag-c., mag-m., manc., mang., meny., ***merc., mez.,*** mill., mosch., murx., mur-ac., nat-a., nat-c., nat-m., nat-p., nicc., nit-ac., nux-m., ***nux-v.,*** olnd., par., petr., **PH-AC.,** ***phos., phyt.,*** **PLAT.,** plb., ***psor.,*** **PULS.,** ran-b., ran-s., rheum, rhod., ***rhus-t.,*** ruta., ***rob.,*** sabad., sabin., samb., ***sang.,*** **SARS.,** sel., seneg., ***sep., sil.,*** **SPIG.,** spong., squil., stann., staph., stict., stram., stront-c., ***sulph.,*** **SUL-AC.,** ***syph.,*** tab., tarax., tarent., teucr., ***thuj.,*** ust., valer., ***verat.,*** **VERB.,** viol-o., viol-t., **ZINC.,** zing.
afternoon - aeth., alum., bry., canth., cast., chin-s., coca, colch., ferr., graph., indg., lach., laur., mag-s., merc-i-r., nat-m., nicc., nit-ac., nux-v., ol-an., ***sep.,*** valer., zinc.
air, open, in - fago., fl-ac., mang., mez., **SEP.,** trom.
amel. - am-c., carb-an., fago., kali-c., mang., nat-m., phos., rat., ***sep.,*** sulph.
alternating from one side to the other - agar., bell., calc., calc-ar., cedr., chin., colch., cupr., dros., euon., hell., hydr., hyper., ***iris,*** kali-bi., **LAC-C.,** lil-t., lyc., nat-m., nat-p., nicc., ***nux-v.,*** plan., phos., sep., sil., valer.
with pain in left arm - ptel.
appearing, gradually - con.
ascending, steps - hydr.
bed, in - ars., iod.
amel. - tab.
breakfast, at - gels.
ceases on one side, becomes more violent on the other - ***lac-c., nat-m.***
coffee, from excessive use of - ***cham.,*** nux-v.
cold, after taking - kali-c.
applications amel. - acon., caust.
combing, hair - merc-i-f.
coughing, on - apis, aur., cimic., dirc., mang., vib.
daytime - cact., ferr., hydr., mag-m.
dinner, after - ***form.,*** nit-ac., paeon.
ears, behind the - asar., calc-p., caust., chel., onos., sang.
air, open - kali-p.
behind the left - ambr., kali-p., sang.
motion - kali-p.
eating, after - ***ars.,*** bar-c., bell., calc-s., coc-c., form., ham., kali-c., lach., mag-c., nux-v., paeon., phos., zinc.
amel. - calc-p., colch., form., nat-m.
evening - aloe, arg-m., ***ars.,*** bar-c., calc-s., canth., caust., chin., chin-a., dios., elaps, fl-ac., graph., ham., indg., ind., kali-c., kali-n., lyc., lyss., mag-c., mag-m., merc-i-r., mez., nicc., nux-v., pall., phos., ***puls., sep.,*** sil., spig., sulph., tab., zinc., zing.
amel. - phos., ptel., sep.
bed, in - arg-m., ars., con., plat., sep.
exertion, mental - hyper., ign., phos.
extending, arm, to - cimx., fago.
backward - mag-c., mag-s., verat-v.
brow, to - chin-s.
ear, to - ars-m., chin-s., grat., lyc., ***merc.***
ear, to, behind - pic-ac.
eye, to - ars., ***asaf.,*** brom., calc., caust., crot-h., mag-m., nat-m.
face, to - kali-bi.
forehead, to - iod., sil.

HEADACHES, sides
extending, forward - ant-c., con., guai., kali-c., mang.
nape, to - elaps, sars.
neck, to - chel., cupr., guai., ***lach.,*** lyc., ***merc.***
and shoulders, neck stiff - lach.
occiput, to - lach., nux-m., phos., tab.
one side to the other - carb-v., clem., ***nat-m.,*** plan., rhus-t.
scapula, to - ***chel.***
shoulders, to - caust., ***lach.***
side to side, from, through temples - alum., chin., phos., plan., sang.
teeth, to - crot-h., graph., lyc., ***merc.***
temples, to - bell., kali-bi.
to eye - ***asaf.,*** brom., caust., croc., mag-m., nat-m.
waist, to - lyss.
foreign body, as of - ***con.***
forenoon - alum., cact., carb-an., cast., euphr., fl-ac., hydr., indg., jug-c., jug-r., kalm., lach., nat-m., peti., plb., sars., stront-c., verat.
hammering - iris.
jarring - **BELL.,** ***lyc.,*** **SPIG.**
leaning on the affected side - ***ars.,*** chin.
left, side, (see Left sided, Headaches)
light, bright - cact.
looking intently - thuj.
lying, amel. - dig.
painful side, on amel. - anac., arn., bry., hipp., ign., sep.
painless side, on amel. - mag-c., ***nux-v.***
right side, on with hands over, amel. - brom.
side lain on - ***ars.,*** calad., calc., carb-v., chel., ***chin.,*** mag-c., nit-ac., ***nux-m.,*** nux-v., ph-ac., puls., ***spong.,*** stann., staph.
not lain on - calc-ar., ***graph.,*** puls.
while - carb-v., petr., rhod., sep., spong.
menses, during - am-m., ars., berb., calc., calc-p., cast., chin., cic., colch., cycl., lob., lyc., mag-c., mag-m., nat-c., nux-v., puls., ***sang.,*** sep., verat.
after - ***ferr.***
before - calc-p., cinnb., puls.
milk, after - ***brom.***
morning - aloe, alum., ***ars.,*** bell., bov., chin-s., chr-ac., dios., euphr., fl-ac., gels., ***graph.,*** ham., hipp., hydr., jug-c., mag-c., mang., sars., **SPIG.,** tab.
bed, in - graph., nicc., nux-v., scut., **SPIG.**
rising, on - ars., cact., calc., gels., mag-s., puls., spig.
amel. - graph., merc-i-r.
waking, on - arum-t., aur., cina, merc-i-r., mur-ac., phos., puls., tab.
7 a.m. till 5 p.m. - ***puls.***
motion, on - agn., arg-n., ars., bell., calc-p., chin., dirc., glon., hipp., mang., ***nux-v.,*** phos., ph-ac., prun., sabad., sil., **SPIG.**
amel. - ***agar., iris.***

HEADACHES, sides
night - acon., cact., ***caust., graph.,*** kali-n., mag-c., mez., nat-m., nicc., ol-an., plb., staph., tarent.
amel. - mag-c.
midnight, after - ***thuj.***
noise, from - cact., manc., phys.
noon - calc-p.
paroxysmal - acon., ***ars.,*** kali-c., puls., ***sep.***
periodic - ***graph.,*** kali-bi.
pressure, on - agar., kali-c., stram.
amel. - mez., sulph.
pressure of glasses on temples - lyc.
pulsating - arg-n., ***ars.,*** aur., bell., ***brom., cact.,*** calc-p., carb-ac., con., hura, kali-c., laur., nat-c., ***nit-ac.,*** puls., sec., zinc.
raising - cact.
reading - lyc.
riding, while - naja.
right, side, (see Right sided, heaches)
rising, after - chin., graph., ***spig.***
amel. - carb-v., dig., graph., indg., ol-an., rhod., tab.
from stooping, amel. - kali-c., mang., sul-ac.
room, agg. - am-m., ***bov.,*** euphr., ***fl-ac.,*** **PHOS.,** sabad.
amel. - mag-s.
rubbing, amel. - chin-a.
shaking, the head - trom.
sitting - am-m., canth., chin-s., fago., indg., mag-c., nicc., phos., rat., rhod., sulph.
amel. - ars., calad., con.
sneezing agg. - am-m., arn., **BELL.,** grat., ***spig.***
sound of talking - cact.
spot, in - kali-bi., kalm.
small - ***kali-bi.***
standing, while - calc., canth., dig., kali-c., mag-c., mang., plb., zinc.
stepping on - calc-p., ***lyc.,*** **SPIG.**
stool, during - **SPIG.**
stooping, agg. - alum., ang., calc-ac., caps., chin-s., cor-r., dig., euphr., glon., hep., hipp., indg., laur., phos., puls.
amel. - dig., iris
supper, after, amel. - sulph.
talking - ign.
touch, agg. - agar., agn., bor., cupr., dirc., laur., merc-i-f., nit-ac.
amel. - bry., thuj.
turning, eye outward - raph.
eyes to affected side - con.
walking - arg-m., arg-n., ars., bell., calc., clem., con., kali-c., ***lyc.,*** mez., nat-m., plb., **SPIG.,** trom.
fast - sep.
walking, air, in open - alum., chin-s., grat., ign., mag-s., **SPIG.**
amel. - ***iris,*** mang., merc-i-r., **PHOS.**
wandering - nat-s.

HEADACHES, sides

warm, applications amel. - lach., ***nux-v.***

room, on entering, from open air - spong.

writing, while - gels., lyc.

with, inclined to left - chin-s.

HEADACHES, sutures, pain follows the - bell., **CALC-P.,** coloc., fl-ac.

HEADACHES, temples - acon., act-sp., aesc., aeth., agar., ail., aloe, ***all-c., alum.,*** ambr., anan., ***apis,*** apoc., **ARG-M.,** arg-n., **ANAC.,** ***arn.,*** arum-t., ars., ***ars-i.,*** asar., aspar., aster., ***atro.,*** aur., ***bad., bapt.,*** bar-c., bar-m., **BELL.,** benz-ac., berb., bor., brom., bry., calc., calc-p., camph., cann-i., cann-s., caps., **CARB-AC.,** carb-an., carb-s., caust., cedr., ***cham., chel.,*** **CHIN.,** chin-s., chlol., cic., cina, ***cinnb.,*** clem., cob., ***cocc.,*** coc-c., coff., colch., coloc., con., corn., cor-r., crot-h., crot-t., cupr., cupr-ar., **CYCL.,** ***daph.,*** dios., dros., echi., elaps, elat., euphr., eup-per., eupi., ***ferr.,*** ferr-ar., ferr-i., ***ferr-m.,*** ferr-p., ***fl-ac.,*** form., ***gels.,*** gent-c., gent-l., glon., graph., gymn., ham., hell., hep., ***hipp.,*** hura, hydr., hydr-ac., hyos., hyper., ign., ***ind.,*** iod., ***ip., iris, jatr., jug-c., kali-bi.,*** **KALI-C.,** kali-chl., kali-p., kali-s., kalm., **KREOS., LAC-C.,** lac-d., ***lach.,*** lachn., laur., lec., led., lept., lith., lob., **LYC.,** lycps., ***lyss., mag-c., mag-m.,*** manc., ***mang.,*** med., meli., ***merc.,*** merc-c., merc-i-f., merl., ***mez.,*** mosch., murx., mur-ac., myric., ***naja,*** nat-a., nat-c., nat-m., nat-p., nat-s., nit-ac., nuph., **NUX-M.,** ***nux-v.,*** ol-j., onos., ***op.,*** osm., ox-ac., pall., **PAR.,** ***petr., ph-ac.,*** phos., phys., phyt., pic-ac., plan., **PLAT.,** ***plb.,*** podo., psor., ptel., **PULS.,** ran-b., raph., rheum, rhod., ***rhus-t.,*** rob., rumx., ***ruta., sabad.,*** **SABIN.,** ***sang.,*** sec., sel., ***sep.,*** sil., sol-n., spig., ***stann.,*** staph., stram., stry., sulph., ***sul-ac.,*** sumb., tab., **TARAX.,** ***tarent.,*** **THUJ.,** uran., verat-v., **VERB.,** viol-t., xan., ***zinc.***

afternoon - aloe, alum., bell., bov., bry., canth., carb-s., caust., chin-s., coca, cod., coloc., corn., dios., dirc., dulc., equis., fago., gamb., grat., guai., hipp., iber., iod., kali-bi., lac-c., laur., lyc., mag-s., myric., nat-a., nat-ac., ol-an., peti., plat., ptel., rumx., sang., sil., stront-c., sulph., zing.

5 p.m. - bry., nat-a.

air, cold - hyos., kali-bi., ***spig.***

open - aur., ***chin.,*** coff., coloc., equis., hyos., jac., kali-bi., mang., naja, ol-an.

amel. - asar., atro., camph., cast., coloc., com., crot-t., glon., hell., hydr., hyos., jatr., lith., nuph., olnd., phos., **PULS.**

alternating, heat of face, with - coc-c.

sides - hyper., **LAC-C.**

ascending steps - ***glon.,*** kalm., sulph.

bending head, backwards, on - ***anac., chin.,*** mang., thuj.

forwards (see stooping)

chill, after - bor.

cold water amel. - aur-m., coc-c., kalm.

coughing, on - alum., ambr., ant-t., ***bry.,*** caust., ***chin.,*** cina, coca, kali-c., kreos., **LYC.,** mang., ***puls.,*** rhus-t., sulph., tarent., tax., verb.

HEADACHES, temples

damp cold weather - nux-m.

dark, in the - onos.

daytime - ars., calc., hell., hep., hydr., jatr., kali-n., lyss., mez., stann.

dinner, after - dios., kali-bi., pall., sulph.

getting dinner too late - ***cact.***

driving or riding in a carriage - lith., lyc.

eating after - alum., aran., canth., cast., clem., con., dios., hydr., hyos., indg., kali-bi., kali-n., mag-c., ol-an., phos., zing.

evening - acon., aloe, alum., am-c., ang., apis, aran., calc-s., camph., cast., caust., chin., cinnb., colch., cop., crot-h., dig., dios., equis., fl-ac., hydr., hyper., inul., jac., kali-c., kali-i., kali-n., kreos., lach., lac-ac., lith., ***mag-m.,*** mez., nat-m., nit-ac., nux-m., nux-v., ph-ac., psor., **PULS.,** ran-b., rhus-r., sep., stram., stront-c., sulph., sul-ac., tab., tarent., thuj., zing.

bed, in - chel., glon., ***mag-m.,*** ol-an., ph-ac., rhus-t.

exertion, after - cact., hell., psor.

exertion, mental - anac., ***chin.,*** dig., gent-c., hell., kalm., manc., mez., nat-c., nat-m., nux-v., ph-ac., pip-m., ***psor., puls., sulph.***

amel. - calc-ac.

extending, backward over ears - arg-m., cedr., gymn., nat-p.

centre of head - dirc.

ear - aur., bov., gels., puls.

eye - aloe, ant-c., asim., berb., cedr., coc-c., gels., nat-p., phos., pip-m.

eyebrows - pic-ac.

face - am-m., ant-t., arg-n., ***bry.,*** kali-c., lachn., puls., rhus-t., seneg.

jaw - arg-n., calc-p., glon., kali-c., lob., rhod., stann.

neck - bry., kali-i., pic-ac., puls.

nose - glon.

occiput - cham., cinnb., coff., iris, iod., kali-bi., kalm., lil-t., lycps., pic-ac., puls., rhus-v.

over forehead - ***all-c.,*** anac., berb., bor., ferr., glon., hep., lil-t., lyc., mez., ph-ac., phos., sil., squil., tab.

shoulder, face distorted - graph.

teeth - bry., carb-v., lachn., sars., sulph., ***verb.***

last molar - hydr.

temple to temple - alumn., asc-c., **BELL.,** ***cedr.,*** chel., ***chin.,*** con., glon., ham., hydr., ***lac-c.,*** lil-t., lob., lyss., manc., mez., naja, nat-n., ***phos.,*** plan., rhod., sep., ***sulph.***

temple to and back again - hydr., ***lac-c.,*** lil-t.

upwards - am-m., laur., rhus-v.

vertex - am-m., coc-c., cycl., kali-bi., laur., phos.

zygoma - coc-c., kali-c., phos.

HEADACHES, temples

forenoon - alum., ars., asar., ***caust., cham.,*** clem., cob., dios., fago., genist., hipp., hydr., indg., ***jug-c.,*** kali-c., lach., lil-t., lycps., mag-s., nat-a., peti., phyt., podo., rhus-t., seneg., sulph.

hammering - ars., benz-ac., chel., chin., ***ferr.,*** hep., nat-m., psor.

heat, amel. - mur-ac., nux-m., ***syph.***

intermitting - atro., bad., clem., iod., murx., nat-m., nat-p., pic-ac., ***stann.,*** stict., sulph.

left side - aesc., agar., ***arn.,*** asar., aspar., aur-m., bar-ac., ***cimic.,*** dig., ***kali-chl.,*** kali-n., ***merc.,*** mur-ac., nuph., nux-m., onos., ox-ac., rhod., sang., sil., ***spig., staph.,*** sumb., viol-t.

alternating with pain, in right knee - meli.

periodical. - spig.

pulsating. - spig.

to right - aur-m., calc., hipp., merc-i-f., ol-j., ptel., sulph.

lying, while - camph., clem., graph., lith., ***mag-m.,*** spong.

amel. - asar., benz-ac., chel., chin-s., colch., ferr., gels., ***lach.,*** mag-c., nux-v.

menses, during - am-m., berb., calc., cast., lac-c., **LYC.,** nat-c., nat-s., sang.

before - lach.

morning - all-c., am-c., apis, bar-c., cact., camph., carb-s., clem., cob., coloc., cop., cund., dios., dirc., equis., ***gels.,*** graph., ham., ign., jac., kali-n., lith., lil-t., lyss., nat-a., nat-p., phos., podo., psor., rhus-r., rhus-t., rumx., sang., sep., sulph., tarent., thuj.

amel. - mag-s.

rising, on - aur-m., coca, ***lach.,*** lil-t., nat-a., nit-ac., sulph.

waking, on - ail., anac., asim., atro., calad., calc., camph., carb-s., cast-eq., coff., graph., ind., ***lach.,*** lith., med., naja, nat-a., nat-p., nit-ac., tab., zinc.

motion - agn., cact., caust., **CHIN.,** cinnb., cob., cupr., dirc., ***echi.,*** gels., glon., hipp., hydr., kali-bi., ***mez.,*** ph-ac., phos., phys., rhod., thuj., zinc.

amel. - carl., com., lil-t., ***mez.***

moving the eyes - ***bad.,*** chin., coloc., sulph.

night - arn., ars., arum-t., bry., cact., cop., dig., ferr., grat., kali-c., lyc., mag-s., merc-i-f., mur-ac., rhus-r., sang., tarent., thuj.

noise agg. - cact., cann-s., cimic.

noon - ars., dios., dirc., fago., pall., ptel., sulph.

opening, mouth - ang.

opera, from attending - cact.

paroxysmal - aesc., cact., lil-t.

pressure, agg. - aspar., bism., cast., cina, cop., daph., kali-n., lil-t., mur-ac., nat-a., nat-m., ***prun.,*** sulph., verb.

pressure, amel. - aeth., alum., ant-c., aral., ***cact.,*** calad., calc-ac., ***chin.,*** coc-c., cop., dios., dirc., echi., ***glon.,*** guai., hydr., iod., kali-i., kalm., lil-t., mag-c., **MAG-M.,** meny., nat-c., par., phos., plan., podo., stann., thuj., verat.

on opposite side amel. - jac.

HEADACHES, temples

pulsating - alum., am-c., anan., apis, ***arg-n.,*** arn., aur-m., ***bell.,*** benz-ac., bor., camph., ***caps., carb-s.,*** caust., cedr., chel., ***chin., chin-s.,*** coc-c., coloc., corn., ***echi.,*** ferr., **GLON.,** hep., jug-r., kali-n., lac-c., lac-d., **LACH.,** merc-i-f., nat-s., nit-ac., ***phos., podo., puls.,*** sep., sol-n., spig., ***stann., stram.,*** sulph., thuj.

mastoid process - iris.

reading, while - calc-ac., carb-ac., clem., coca, mez., nat-m., phys., pip-m., sulph.

right side - aloe, apis, ars., ars-i., bell., cact., ***caust., chel., coloc.,*** dros., ferr-ar., ***ferr-m., gels., jug-c.,*** meli., mosch., ***nat-a., nux-v.,*** pall., puls., rhus-t., ***tarax.,*** thuj., trom., verb., ziz.

alternating with pain, in right knee - meli.

lying upon in while - stann.

to left - glon., lil-t., pall., plat., ptel., sep.

rising, after - fago., lycps., verat.

amel. - calc-ac., rhus-t., stann.

room, in - jatr., laur., phos., ran-b., rhod., sabad.

amel. - ***chin.,*** coff., hyos., ol-an., zing.

rubbing amel. - canth., ol-an., phos., plat.

shaking the head - carb-s., glon.

side, lain on - puls., stann.

not lain on - graph.

sitting, while - am-m., arg-m., chin., lil-t., mang., mez., nicc., phos., staph., sul-ac., tarax., verat.

amel. - ars., asar., calc-ac., coff., coloc., lith., mang.

sleep, during - mag-c.

sneezing - am-c., cina

standing, while - ars., cast., chin., coloc., glon., guai., staph., verat.

amel. - tarax., zing.

stepping, on - carb-s., coloc., hell., lyc., sol-n.

stool, straining at - ***bell.,*** nux-v., ***puls.,*** thuj.

stooping from - am-m., bov., ***brom.,*** calc-ac., carb-ac., chin., coff., coloc., cycl., dios., dros., fago., fl-ac., glon., guai., hep., kali-bi., kali-c., lach., lyss., mur-ac., nat-a., nat-s., phos., plat., ***puls.,*** sol-n., sulph., thuj., verat.

amel. - ang., mang., verat.

sun, exposure to - nat-a.

talking - mez.

temple and forehead - agar., agn., ant-c., ant-t., aran., arn., ***ars.,*** arum-t., atro., aur., bar-c., ***bell.,*** berb., bov., bry., ***camph.,*** canth., cedr., chel., chin., chin-a., chin-s., clem., coloc., cor-r., crot-t., cycl., dig., dios., dulc., elat., ferr., ferr-ar., fl-ac., gels., glon., gran., hell., hipp., hura, hydr-ac., ind., iris, kali-bi., kalm., lachn., lil-t., lyc., lycps., mag-m., mag-s., mang., merc-i-f., merl., mez., mur-ac., myric., naja, nat-a., nat-m., nat-p., op., ph-ac., phos., phys., phyt., pip-m., psor., rhod., sabad., sabin., sel., seneg., **SEP.,** spig., stann., sulph., tab., tanac., verat., zinc.

temple and occiput - acon., aesc., ***alum.,*** bov., cann-s., nux-v., rhus-r., spig.

HEADACHES, temples

toothache, with - mur-ac.

touch, agg. - aur., berb., cast., chel., ***chin.,*** con., cupr., daph., led., ***mez.,*** nux-m., peti., staph.

amel. - ars., calc-ac., cycl.

turning, eyes out - raph.

eyes up - puls.

walking, from - agn., alum., ant-t., ars., asar., bufo, bry., cast., chin., cocc., coloc., con., cupr., dios., genist., glon., hell., kali-bi., lil-t., lyss., mang., mez., nat-m., nat-s., phos., ran-b., rhod., spig., sulph.

amel. - chin., guai., staph., tarax.

walking, air, open, in - arn., bry., coff., hyos., mang., nat-m., rhod., spig., tarax., zing.

amel. - psor., rhod.

wandering - acon., ***aesc.,*** carb-s., ***cham.,*** merl., plan., spig., verat-v.

wind, riding against the - calc-i.

wine, from - ***cact.,*** zinc.

winking, agg. - all-c.

wrapping, up amel. - mur-ac.

HEADACHES, vertex - acet-ac., acon., aeth., agar., agn., ***alum., alumn.,*** ambr., am-c., ***anac.,*** ant-c., ant-t., **APIS,** arn., ars., ars-i., arum-t., aur-m-n., bad., bell., ***benz-ac.,*** bor., bov., **BROM.,** bry., ***bufo,*** **CACT.,** cadm-s., calc., ***calc-p.,*** calc-s., ***cann-s.,*** **CARB-AN.,** ***carb-s., carb-v.,*** cast., ***caust.,*** cedr., cham., ***chel.,*** chen-a., ***chin.,*** chin-a., **CIMIC.,** ***cinnb.,*** cob., coca, cocc., coc-c., coff., colch., ***con.,*** conv., ***corn.,*** crot-c., ***crot-h., cupr., cur.,*** daph., dig., dios., dros., dulc., echi., ***elaps,*** euph., ***eup-per., ferr., ferr-ar.,*** ferr-i., ***ferr-p., form., gels.,*** gent-c., glon., gran., graph., hell., ***hep.,*** hura, ***hydr., hyper., ind.,*** iod., iris, kali-bi., kalm., kreos., lac-c., lac-d., ***lach.,*** lac-ac., lact., laur., ***lil-t.,*** lith., ***lyc.,*** lyss., ***meny., merc., merc-i-f.,*** merc-c., ***merc-i-r., mez.,*** mosch., mur-ac., naja, nat-ac., ***nat-c.,*** nat-m., nat-p., ***nit-ac., nux-m., nux-v.,*** ol-j., ox-ac., pall., par., ***ph-ac., phos.,*** phys., ***phyt.,*** pic-ac., podo., ptel., puls., ***ran-b.,*** **RAN-S.,** rheum, rhod., rumx., sabad., sang., sanic., ***sep., sil.,*** sol-n., ***spig.,*** spong., squil., stann., staph., stram., **SULPH.,** sul-i., syph., tab., tell., ther., ***thuj.,*** ust., valer., **VERAT.,** verb., xan., ***zinc.***

afternoon - alum., alumn., ambr., ars., bufo, calc-s., carb-v., ***cimic.,*** crot-h., graph., helon., hura, hyper., indg., ir-foe., kali-n., lac-ac., lyc., lyss., mang., merc-i-r., mur-ac., nat-a., nit-ac., osm., phel., phos., phys., sulph.

air, cold, amel. - ind.

open - ferr., iris, sulph.

amel. - carb-an., cimic., ferr., gamb., glon., ind., kali-n., puls., rat., tarent.

alternate days - hydr.

ascending steps - ant-c., cimic., ferr., lob., meny.

blowing, nose - sulph.

chewing - sulph.

cold applications amel. - ***acon., alumn.***

coldness, during - kali-n.

HEADACHES, vertex

coughing, on - alum., ***anac.,*** apis, caust., con., cupr., kali-c., sabad., squil., sulph.

daytime - sep., sulph., tab.

deep inspiration, on - ***anac.***

dinner, after - con., nat-c., nat-m., thuj.

driving or riding in a carriage - lyc.

eating, after - bad., calc-s., cast., dirc., kali-bi., lyc., mag-c., nat-c., phel., rhus-t., sulph., tab.

evening - acon., ambr., apis, bor., canth., carb-an., cimic., crot-h., cycl., dulc., fago., form., glon., ***hep.,*** hyper., kali-c., kali-i., lach., lith., lyc., merc., mur-ac., nit-ac., ol-an., petr., ***ran-b.,*** rhus-t., sep., sil., stann., stront-c., ***sulph.,*** thuj., zinc.

bed, in - carb-v., stann.

exertion, mental - aster., carb-v., con., ***ferr-pic.,*** gent-c., nat-m., ***nux-v.,*** ph-ac., ***pic-ac.,*** ran-b., ***sep.***

extending, backward - chel., kali-bi., kali-n.

downward - kali-n.

ear - agar., phos.

from one to other - pall.

eyes - ign., nux-m.

forehead - caps., ***caust.,*** cham., ***cocc.,*** led., mez., nicc., nux-m.

malar-bones - tarent.

neck - calc-p., ***chel.,*** glon., kalm.

nose, while eating - dulc.

occiput - calc-p., ***chel.,*** gels., indg.

palate - nat-m.

shoulder - lyc.

temples - carb-v., caust., cham., chel., hipp., kalm., phos.

throat - cham.

zygoma - phos.

forenoon - ***alum.,*** bar-c., bov., bry., calc., fl-ac., gamb., glon., kali-cy., mag-s., nat-a., nicc., nux-m., pic-ac., rhus-t., sulph.

10 a.m. - lac-ac.

10:30 a.m. - hydr.

11 a.m. - hydr.

hammering - hyper., phos.

fever, during - graph.

jarring agg. - bell., cob.

lying, while - carb-v., chel., hipp., stann.

amel. - calc-p., phos., spig.

on left side - ***cinnb.***

meditating, while - ***lyss.***

menses, during - calc., carb-an., cast., ferr-p., lach., laur., lyc., mag-c., nat-m., nat-s., nux-v., ol-an., phos., rat., sulph.

morning - agar., ambr., aster., bar-c., bov., carb-ac., graph., hydr., hyper., iris, lac-c., merc., nat-c., nat-p., ox-ac., pall., ran-b., staph., **SULPH.,** thuj.

amel. - laur.

bed, in - carb-v., hell.

rising, on - bar-ac., carb-v., caust., cimic., kali-n., nicc., podo., ***sep., sulph.***

amel. - ol-an.

HEADACHES, vertex

morning, waking, on - alum., bar-ac., ***bry.,*** bufo, calc., carb-an., caust., cedr., croc., hyper., ***kali-bi.,*** nat-p., puls., ***sulph.,*** tab., verat.
5 a.m. - calc.

motion, on - alum., alumn., aur., ***bell.,*** calc-p., canth., ***chin.,*** echi., ***ferr.,*** glon., ip., iris, lach., lob., lyss., mez., ***ox-ac.,*** ph-ac., phyt., sep., spig., thuj., verat.

moving, the eyes, on - sep.
the head - alum.

night - acon., agar., aster., carb-an., ferr., glon., hipp., ir-foe., kali-n., laur., lyc., mez., mur-ac., ol-an., rat., sulph.
amel. - mag-c.
on going to sleep, amel. - phyt.

noise, from - ***cact.,*** calc., ferr-p., ***ferr-pic.,*** iod., spig.

noon - ***puls-n, sulph.,*** thuj.

paroxysmal - chel., ***chin.,*** cimic., hydr.

periodic - ***sil.***

pressure, agg. - ant-c., bell., cast., caust., ***chin.,*** cina, kali-c., kali-n., ***lach.,*** nat-c.
amel. - alum., alumn., ***arg-n., cact.,*** dirc., eup-per., ferr., ***meny.,*** ph-ac., phys., stann., ***verat.***

pulsating - agar., alum., ars., bell., ***bry.,*** canth., carb-an., ***ferr., glon.,*** hyper., kreos., ***lach., lyc.,*** lyss., nat-c., ***nux-v.,*** phos., ***sep., sil., stram.,*** sulph., ***verat.***

reading, while - carb-v., helon., lyc., lyss., nat-m.

rising, from a seat - cob.

room, on entering - ***ran-b.***

rubbing, amel. - carb-ac., phos.

sitting, while - cast., lyc., peti., phos., verat., viol-t.
amel. - con., gels.

sleep, amel. - calc.

sneezing, on - apis, bar-c., nux-v., sulph.

spots, in - nux-v., psor., sol-n., spig.

standing, while - alum., mang., ran-b., sul-ac., verat.

stool, during - ind., lyc.

stooping, from - acon., alum., alumn., am-m., berb., calc., calc-p., coloc., elaps, glon., helon., iris, kreos., lyc., lyss., meny., nux-m.
amel. - laur., verat.

touch, agg. - bov., caust., chel., cinnb., kali-bi., mez., peti., phos., sulph.
by laying hand on it, amel. - kali-n.

touching, the hair agg. - ***carb-v.,*** nit-ac.

urinating, after - caust.

vertex and forehead - acet-ac., acon., all-c., aloe, ambr., anac., ant-c., ant-t., arg-n., bar-c., bell., berb., bor., bry., bufo, calc., cann-i., carb-an., cast., caust., cinnb., corn., crot-t., dig., dios., glon., graph., grat., helon., hura, hydr-ac., ign., indg., kali-bi., laur., lyss., mag-c., mang., meny., merc., mez., mosch., mur-ac., myric., naja, nat-c., nat-m., nat-p., nux-v., ol-an., ol-j., ox-ac., phel., ptel., puls., rhus-r., ***sep.,*** sil., sol-n., stann., valer., zinc.

HEADACHES, vertex

voices, agg. - ***ferr-pic., lyc.***

waking, on - kali-bi., thuj.

walking, from - carb-an., calc., cedr., con., glon., hura, peti., phyt., spong., sulph.
amel. - peti., sang.
air, in open - calc.
amel. - acon., aster., thuj.
sun, in the - bar-c.
rapidly, agg. - chel.

wet, weather - ***carb-an.***

writing, from - gels., nat-m., ran-b.

HEADLESS, sensation of being - asar., calc-i., nit-ac.

HEAT, in- abies-n., acet-ac., **ACON.,** aesc., aeth., agar., ***all-c., aloe, alum., alumn., ambr.,*** am-c., am-m., anac., ang., ant-c., ***ant-t.,*** **APIS,** arg-m., arg-n., arn., ars., ars-i., asaf., asar., aster., ***aur., aur-m.,*** bad., bapt., bar-c., **BELL.,** benz-ac., berb., bism., **BOR.,** brom., ***bry.,*** **CACT.,** calad., **CALC.,** calc-ar., ***calc-p., calc-s.,*** camph., cann-i., cann-s., canth., carb-ac., carb-an., ***carb-s., carb-v.,*** caust., cham., ***chel.,*** chin., chin-a., chin-s., cimic., ***cina,*** cinnb., clem., ***cocc.,*** coff., colch., ***coloc., con.,*** corn., croc., ***crot-t.,*** cupr., ***cur., cycl.,*** daph., dig., dios., dros., dulc., euph., euphr., eupi., ***ferr., ferr-ar.,*** ferr-i., ferr-p., ***fl-ac., form., gamb., gels.,*** gins., **GLON.,** gran., **GRAPH.,** grat., gymn., haem., ***hell.,*** helo., hura, hydr., hydr-ac., hyos., hyper., ***ign.,*** ind., indg., iod., ***ip.,*** iris, jatr., kali-ar., kali-bi., kali-br., kali-c., ***kali-chl.,*** kali-i., kali-n., kali-p., kali-s., kalm., ***lac-d.,*** **LACH.,** lact., ***laur.,*** led., lyc., lyss., ***mag-c., mag-m.,*** mag-s., manc., ***mang.,*** meny., merc., merc-c., merl., ***mez.,*** morph., ***mosch.,*** naja, nat-a., ***nat-c., nat-m.,*** nat-p., nicc., ***nit-ac., nux-m., nux-v.,*** ol-an., ***op.,*** paeon., petr., phel., ph-ac., **PHOS.,** phys., ***phyt.,*** pic-ac., plat., ***plb., podo.,*** psor., puls., ran-b., ran-s., rat., rheum, rhus-t., ruta., sabad., sabin., samb., sarr., sec., senec., ***sep., sil.,*** spig., spong., squil., ***stann.,*** staph., ***stram., stront-c., sulph.,*** tab., tarent., tax., ther., tell., thuj., til., valer., ***verat.,*** verb., vinc., viol-o., ***xan.,*** zinc.
abdomen, from pain in - grat.
afternoon - anac., arg-n., ***arum-t.,*** bad., berb., bry., cann-s., ***carb-an.,*** carb-s., chin-s., dios., fago., graph., ***hyper.,*** ip., kali-n., lyc., mag-c., mag-m., mag-s., mang., nat-a., nat-c., nat-m., nicc., ol-an., phos., phys., ***puls.,*** sant., sep., spong., stront-c., sulph.
4 p m - ***mang.***
agreeable - camph., cann-s., nicc., thuj.
air, in open agg. - verat.
amel., in open - **APIS,** ***ars.,*** clem., con., grat., kali-i., kali-s., laur., mag-m., mang., mosch., nat-c., phel., **PHOS.,** sulph.
surrounded by hot air, as if - aster.
alternating, with chilliness - asaf., phos., sep.
with diarrhea - ***bell.***
with rigor in back - spong.

HEAT, in
anxiety, with - canth., coff., phos., sil., stront-c., sulph.
back, with coldness of - thuj.
bed, in - ang., arg-n., carb-an., carb-v., cycl., lyc., nat-c., ***nux-v.,*** staph.
amel. - kali-c., nat-c.
beer, after - chel., sulph.
boiling, in brain - acon.
breakfast, after - laur.
breathing, deep - bor.
burning - ail., ***apis,*** aster., aur-s., camph., hell., kali-c., mur-ac., ***phos.,*** plan., sil., verat.
chill, during - acon., alum., ***apis,*** **ARN.**, ***ars.,*** asar., ***bell.,*** berb., ***bry.,*** cedr., cina, chin., eup-per., gels., lachn., nat-s., nux-v., **OP.**, rhod., stram., verat.
after - berb., caust., dros., mez., phos.
before - stram.
chilliness, after - **SANG., SIL.**
after, extending from head to stomach - ***sang.***
before - zinc.
during - ant-c., asaf., asar., ***bor.,*** **BRY.**, ***cocc.,*** colch., dig., hell., mag-m., ***merc.***
cold, bath, amel. - euphr., ind., mez., nat-m., sep.
head, cold to touch, though - hydr.
water, cold amel. - ***apis, con.***
coldness of body, with heat in head - ***acon.,*** agar., **ARN.**, ***ars.,*** asaf., ***bufo, cact.,*** calc., chin., chin-s., clem., gels., hell., hipp., hyos., ip., ***lachn.,*** mag-s., mang., mez., nux-v., ran-b., plb., phyt., stram., sulph., verat.
of abdomen, with - camph.
of, face, with - thuj.
of, feet, with - alum., am-c., anac., ***arn.,*** ars., bar-c., ***bell., cact., calc.,*** carb-an., con., ***ferr.,*** ferr-ar., ***gels.,*** hell., ***ip.,*** laur., mur-ac., ***nat-c.,*** ph-ac., sep., squil., ***sulph.,*** thuj.
of, fingers, with - hell.
of, hands, with - asaf., asar., bar-c., bell., calo., hell., iod., ***ip.,*** lact., lyc., nat-c., petr., ph-ac., sep., sumb.
of, limbs, with - ***arn.,*** aur., **BELL.**, bufo, ***cact.,*** cadm-s., camph., cann-i., cann-s., chel., com., ***ferr.,*** glon., jug-c., led., stram.
constipation, with - verat.
contradiction, from - cop.
coryza, during - anac., **ARUM-T.**, calc., graph., jatr., lach., mag-m., phos.
cough, during - am-c., ant-t., arn., ***ars.,*** carb-v., ip., ***sulph.***
descending, to toes - ***calc-p.***
diarrhea, during - ***apis, arn.,*** **BELL.**, bor., ***bry.,*** hell., kali-br., ox-ac., rhus-t.
dinner, during - grat., nat-c., nux-v., sars.
after - alum., bell., berb., caust., cycl., graph., mag-m., phel.

HEAT, in
eating, after - alum., bell., berb., canth., carb-v., caust., clem., cycl., graph., ***hyos., kali-c.,*** laur., ***lyc.,*** mag-m., ***petr.,*** phel., phos.
hot food, after - mag-c.
epilepsy, before - ***caust.***
evening - ***acon.,*** alum., am-m., bar-c., bor., calc., calc-s., canth., carb-v., chel., coc-c., cycl., grat., indg., ip., kali-c., laur., lil-t., lob., lyc., mag-c., mag-m., merc-i-r., nat-c., nat-p., nux-v., ol-an., ph-ac., phys., puls., ran-b., ***rhus-t., sep., sil.,*** sulph., thuj., zinc.
lying - ars.
exertion, from - berb., con.
extending, to toes - ***calc-p.***
flashes of - aesc., aeth., alumn., am-m., ant-t., arn., ars., aur., bar-c., calc-p., calc-s., cic., cocc., colch., corn., dig., ***ferr., ferr-ar.,*** ferr-p., ***glon., graph.,*** hell., hep., ***kali-c.,*** kali-p., kali-s., lact., laur., led., mag-c., mag-m., mag-s., mang., nat-m., nat-p., oena., phos., ptel., ***sep.,*** sil., ***sulph.,*** tab., xan., zinc., ziz.
forenoon - bry., lyc.
fright, after - ***ph-ac.***
grief, after - ***ph-ac.***
headache, with - nat-m., sep.
after - nat-c.
heart, during oppression of - glon.
with palpitation of - coloc., iod.
heat, of head, with face - aeth., arg-n., berb., bry., calc-p., cann-s., canth., clem., corn., glon., hura, jatr., iris, kali-c., kali-i., kali-n., nat-m., op., phos., sabad., sep., stront-c., sulph.
with hands - canth., lach., laur., mag-c., ol-an., phel., phos.
with palms - bor., tarent.
hot, body, as if, fell forwards - kali-c.
iron around, as if from a - ***acon.***
water - all-c., indg.
water thrown on scalp and penetrating to brain, as from - peti.
laughing agg. - ther.
lying down, while - arn., ars., jug-r.
amel. - kali-c., nat-c., ***phos.,*** rhus-t.
menopause, at - ***sulph.***
menses, during - ***apis, arn., bell.,*** **CALC.**, carb-an., caust., cham., ***ferr-p., ign.,*** ip., ***kali-i.,*** lach., lyc., mag-c., mag-m., mag-s., nat-m., nat-s., nux-m., petr., sulph.
after - ferr-i., iod.
before - apis, bell., ***calc., con., crot-h., ign., iod.,*** ip., ***lyc.,*** petr., ***thuj.***
mental, exertion, from - anac., aur., berb., **CACT.**, ***con., sil.***
midnight - aur-m., lyc., sil.
after - nit-ac.

HEAT, in
morning - alum., am-m., ang., ant-c., ant-t., ***bry.,*** calc., calc-s., carb-an., carb-v., chin., clem., cycl., dios., euphr., hipp., hyper., indg., ***kalm.,*** kali-n., lyc., ***merc-i-r., mez.,*** nat-a., ***nat-c.,*** **NUX-V.,** petr., phos., ***podo.,*** sep., ***sulph.,*** til., zinc., zing.
bed, in - staph.
rising on - agar., am-m., bar-c., calc., corn., cycl., dulc.
rising on, amel. - sulph.
waking, on - berb., calc., lyc., nat-m., sil., stann., **SULPH**.
motion, agg. - calc.
music, from - **AMBR.**
night - ambr., am-m., ang., arg-n., arn., camph., cann-s., lyc., meph., nat-c., nat-m., nit-ac., rhus-r., ruta., ***sil.,*** staph., til.
bed, in - carb-an., lyc., nat-m., **SULPH**.
waking, on - arn., til.
noon - ant-c., bell., jatr., mag-m., nat-m.
nosebleed, amel. - bufo, lach., ***psor.***
painful - sep.
pale face, with - ambr., puls., thuj.
periodical - calad.
pressure, amel. - arg-n., hydr., nux-v.
hands of, amel. - nux-v.
raising, head, agg. - calc.
reading, while - nat-s.
redness of face, with - aeth., aster., ***bell.,*** bry., cact., cann-s., kali-i., mag-c., mag-m., mag-s., merl., nat-c., phel., plb., stront-c., sulph., tarent., zinc.
riding, while - lyc.
rising, on - bar-c., calc., mag-s.
amel. - carb-an., kali-c., sulph.
stooping, from - grat., nat-c.
rising, up - aeth., calad., canth., cycl., gamb., kali-c., ***lil-t., mang.,*** nat-s., plb., rheum, rhus-t.
abdomen, from - alum., indg., kali-c., mag-m., nat-s., plb.
back, from - phos.
chest, from - acon., glon., ***lil-t.,*** lyss., mill., ***phos.,*** sulph.
room entering - am-m., mag-m.
sewing, while - petr.
scratch, must - mez.
siesta, after - clem., cycl., rhus-t.
sitting, while - canth., merc., nat-c., ph-ac., spong.
sleep, before - alum., coc-c., sulph.
amel. - laur.
sleepiness, with - kreos., stann., stront.
sneezing, amel. - lil-t.
soup, on taking - phos.
speaking, by - ph-ac., phos.
spot, in small - carb-v., mez.
standing, agg. - alum., canth.
amel. - phos.
stool, during urging to - clem., mag-m., ox-ac.
after - bell., lyc., nat-c.
stooping, when - kali-c., petr., valer.
storm, on approach of - nat-c.

HEAT, in
stove agg. - bar-c., ***glon., phos.***
thinking, of it agg. - hell.
toothache, one-sided - am-c., sil.
transient - agar., arn., cann-i., mag-m., sulph., tab., valer.
urinating, while - ***sep.***
vapor, as from warm - ol-an.
waking, on - calc., chel., lyc., nat-m., phos., sil., stann., **SULPH**., tarent., til.
before - hyper.
walking, while - bor., glon., indg., mez., nit-ac., ***phos.,*** sep., stront.
in open air amel. - ***phos., sulph.***
warm, room - **APIS,** ***ars., calc-s., carb-v.,*** caust., ***coc-c.,*** indg., ***kali-s.,*** lyss., mag-m., nat-c., nicc., ***phos.,*** **PULS**., ran-s., **SULPH**.
washing, hands in cold water amel. - rhus-v.
wine, after - lyc., nux-v., petr.
as from - rhus-r., sabad.
writing, on - aran., bor., kali-c., ran-b.

heat, forehead - ***acon.,*** aeth., ***alum.,*** am-m., ang., ant-t., **APIS,** ***ars.,*** asaf., asar., bad., bapt., **BELL.,** brom., calc., calc-s., camph., canth., carb-an., carb-s., ***carb-v.,*** caust., cham., chel., chin., chin-a., cimic., cinnb., clem., coc-c., cocc., colch., coloc., croc., crot-h., cupr., cycl., euph., euphr., eupi., fl-ac., gels., gins., ***glon.,*** gran., graph., grat., gymn., hell., hep., hydr., hyos., indg., ind., jatr., kali-ar., kali-bi., kali-c., kali-n., kali-p., ***kali-s.,*** kreos., ***lach.,*** lact., laur., led., lyc., mag-m., mag-s., manc., merc., merc-c., ***mez.,*** nat-a., ***nat-c.,*** nat-m., nat-p., nicc., ***nux-m.,*** **NUX-V.,** ol-an., op., petr., phel., ph-ac., ***phos.,*** phys., pic-ac., ***puls.,*** ran-b., rat., rhus-r., ***sabad.,*** senec., sep., sil., spong., ***stann.,*** staph., ***stram.,*** ***sulph.,*** tarax., tarent., tax., tell., thuj., til., verat., viol-o., zinc.
afternoon - chin-s., ip., nicc., sep., spong.
air, cool, amel. - alum., **APIS,** ***phos.***
alternately in either protuberance - lact.
alternating with coldness - staph.
chill, during - ars.
after - caust.
chilliness, during - asaf., asar., sep.
cold to touch, but - mag-m.
coldness, of hands and feet - camph.
of limbs - chin.
dinner, after - alum., caust.
evening - canth., gran., ip., lyc., mag-m., nat-c., ran-b., sep.
while writing - ***ran-b.***
forenoon - calc., carb-an., nat-c., thuj.
headache, with - sil.
morning - am-m., ant-c., cycl., indg., kali-n., nat-c.
night - ang., ph-ac., staph., til.
noon - zinc.
side of - ph-ac.
walking, while - mez.
warm, water trickled down inside, as if - glon.
wind, as from - staph.

heat, forehead
warmth, in middle of, feeling of, then coolness as from draught of air - laur.
writing, while - kali-c.
heat, occiput - aesc., aur-m-n., bell., brom., camph., cann-i., cann-s., cic., cinnb., coc-c., ***con.,*** dig., fl-ac., glon., indg., jatr., kalm., lob., manc., med., merc-i-f., ***nat-m.,*** nat-s., nux-m., ph-ac., puls., rhus-r., ***sulph.,*** sumb., tarent., thuj., verat-v., ***zinc.***
diarrhea, during - bell., ***zinc.***
evening - sumb.
excitement agg. - ***con.***
flashes of - aesc., lach., sumb.
morning - sulph.
walking in open air, amel. - sulph.
warm room, in - sulph.
heat, sides - am-m., calc., caust., cinnb., cycl., kali-bi., petr., phel., pic-ac., tarent., til.
in flashes - kali-bi.
right, evening - am-m.
heat, temples - berb., euph., glon., hura, ign., lyc., merl., ol-an., phel., podo.
cold cheeks, with - berb.
heat, vertex - ***acon., aur., benz-ac., calc.,*** calc-s., camph., carb-an., carb-s., cham., chel., coc-c., ***con.,*** corn., ***crot-c., daph.,*** eupi., ***eup-per., ferr-p., glon.,*** **GRAPH.,** grat., helo., hep., ***hyper.,*** **LACH.,** laur., lepi., mag-s., ***med., merc-i-r., mez., mur-ac.,*** nat-c., nat-m., nat-p., ***nat-s., nux-m., ph-ac., phos.,*** podo., rhus-r., **SULPH.,** tarent., thea.
grief, after - ***calc., ph-ac., phos.***
menopause, during - carb-an., cimic., croc., **LACH.,** ***sulph.***
prolapse uterus, with - ***lach., sep.***
menses, during - ***nat-s., sulph.***
morning - podo.
night,11 p.m. - **MERC-I-R.**
pressure amel. - eup-per.
spots, in - ***arn., graph., mez.***
thinking, while - ***nat-s.***
warm applications amel. - ***kali-i.***

HEAVINESS, sensation, (see Pressing) - acet-ac., ***acon.,*** aesc., aeth., ***agar.,*** agn., ail., all-c., aloe, ***alum.,*** ambr., am-c., ***am-m.,*** anac., anan., ang., ant-t., **APIS,** apoc., ***arg-n., arn., ars.,*** ars-i., arum-t., asaf., asar., asc-t., aur., aur-m-n., bapt., bar-c., bar-m., ***bell.,*** berb., bism., bor., bov., brom., ***bry.,*** bufo, ***cact., calc.,*** calc-ar., ***calc-s., camph., cann-i., canth., carb-ac., carb-an.,*** **CARB-S., CARB-V.,** ***card-m.,*** cast., caust., cedr., ***cham., chel.,*** **CHIN.,** chin-a., ***chin-s.,*** cic., cimic., cinnb., ***clem.,*** coca, coc-c., cocc., coff., ***colch.,*** coloc., ***con., corn.,*** cop., croc., ***crot-c., crot-h., crot-t., cupr.,*** cycl., ***dig.,*** dios., ***dros., dulc., elaps,*** euphr., eupi., ferr., ferr-ar., ferr-i., ferr-p., fl-ac., form., ***gamb.,*** **GELS.,** gins., ***glon.,*** gran., graph., grat., guare., gymn., haem., ***hell.,*** hep., hipp., hura, hydr., hydr-ac., ***hyos.,*** hyper., ***ign.,*** indg., iod., ***ip.,*** iris, jatr., kali-ar., ***kali-bi.,*** kali-c., ***kali-i., kali-n., kali-p.,*** kali-s., kreos., lac-c., **LACH.,** lachn., ***lact., laur.,*** led., lil-t., lob., ***lyc., mag-c., mag-m., mag-s.,*** manc., ***mang.,*** med., ***meny.,*** meph., ***merc.,*** merc-c., merc-i-f., merc-i-r., ***merl.,*** mez., morph., mosch., murx., **MUR-AC.,** naja, ***nat-a., nat-c.,*** **NAT-M.,** ***nat-p.,*** nat-s., ***nicc.,*** **NIT-AC.,** nux-m., **NUX-V.,** ***olnd.,*** ol-an., onos., ***op.,*** osm., paeon., par., **PETR.,** ***phel., ph-ac., phos.,*** phys., phyt., **PIC-AC.,** pip-m., plan., plat., ***plb.,*** prun., ptel., ***puls.,*** ran-b., ran-s., rat., ***rheum, rhus-t.,*** ruta., ***sabad., sabin.,*** sang., ***sars., sec., seneg., sep., sil.,*** sol-n., spig., ***spong.,*** squil., ***stann.,*** stram., ***stront-c., staph.,*** **SULPH.,** ***sul-ac., tab., tarax., tarent.,*** tell., ter., thea., ther., ***thuj.,*** til., ust., valer., verat., verat-v., verb., viol-o., ***viol-t.,*** vip., ***zinc.,*** zing.
afternoon - all-c., alum., am-c., ***arg-n.,*** bry., bufo, cham., chel., chin-s., ferr., gamb., gels., hyper., indg., jug-r., kali-i., kali-n., lact., mag-c., mag-m., mang., murx., nat-c., nicc., pall., puls., sil.
4 p.m. - ***mang.***
air, in cold - carb-an.
in open - laur., lil-t.
in open, amel. - ant-t., **APIS, ARS.,** caust., clem., ferr-i., gamb., hell., hydr., mang., mosch., nicc., phos., ***puls.,*** tab., zinc.
alternating with clearness of mind - murx.
ascending, on - meny., rhus-v.
back, and limbs, with drowsiness and pain in - gamb.
with pain in - apoc.
bed, while lying in - am-c.
beer, after - chel.
bending, back amel. - ***cocc.,*** ph-ac.
forward, on - nat-m., ph-ac.
blood, as if too full of - ***glon.,*** ign., lil-t.
breakfast, after - carb-s.
candle-light, from - bov.
chill, during - dros., kali-n., sulph.
after - dros.
coffee, strong, amel. - corn.
cold, after taking - dulc.
amel. - chin-s.
congestion, as from - dig.
coughing, on - euphr., tax.
daily - nat-m., sil.
darkness, agg. - sil.
amel. - brom.
descending, on - meny.
dinner, after - am-c., nat-c.
amel. - carb-an.
drinking, as if had been - acon., agar., bell., cocc., dulc., kali-n., lach., laur., sabin.
dull - apoc., caj., calc., fl-ac., glon., nat-s., phys., rumx., verb.
eating, while - aeth.
after - am-c., bry., cast., cedr., euphr., gins., graph., grat., jug-r., kali-i., mag-c., mag-s., nat-c., ***nat-m.,*** op., ***phos.,*** tab.
erect, on becoming - con.

HEAVINESS, sensation
evening - ambr., apoc., arg-n., ars., bar-c., bov., bufo, cedr., chin-s., coloc., ferr., fl-ac., hydr-ac., kali-i., kali-n., kalm., laur., lith., lyc., phos., plan., rumx., sep., ***stann.,*** sulph., tarent., zinc.
exercise, on - calc.
eyestrain, from- mur-ac.
falls, backward, head - ant-t., bor., camph., chin., kali-c., laur., mur-ac., op., phel.
forward, as if head would - agn., alum., bar-c., berb., chel., hipp., kali-c., nat-m., ip., par., phos., plb., rhus-t., sulph., sul-ac., tab., viol-t., zinc.
side, to - arn.
side, to one, as if head would - bry., fl-ac., phel.
fever, during the - calc., dig., sep., thuj.
forenoon, until night - sil.
headache, from - lyc.
heat, from - com., hell.
after the - tarent.
of sun - brom., nat-c.
holding, head, erect, on - dros., tarax.
lean, on something, desires to - ***bell.,*** gymn., staph.
light, from strong - cact.
looking, sideways, while - agn.
steadily, agg. - mur-ac.
steadily, amel. - sabad.
lying, while - am-c., bov., ***glon.,*** mag-c., merc., nicc., nux-m., puls., sep., ***sulph., tarax.***
amel. - manc., ***nat-m.,*** olnd., rhus-t., tell.
back, on - cact., mez.
head high amel. - sulph.
head too low, as if had been - ***phos.***
side, on - meny.
side, on, amel. - cact.
side, on, right on - anan.
menses, during - calc., carb-an., ferr-p., ***ign., kali-c., mag-c.,*** mag-m., ***mag-s.,*** nat-m., nux-v., zinc.
after - all-s., nat-m.
before - cimic., crot-h., ign.
menstrual pain, colic - ant-t.
mental, exertion, from - ***calc.,*** crot-h., ferr-i., lyc., **NAT-C.,** nat-m., **PH-AC., PHOS.**
morning - acon., agar., alum., am-m., ars., arum-t., berb., bov., bry., calc., ***carb-an.,*** cast., chel., chin., chin-a., cimic., clem., coca, com., con., croc., eupi., gamb., hell., hydr., hyper., indg., kali-c., kali-i., kali-n., kali-p., kali-s., kalm., ***lach.,*** lyc., mag-m., mang., mez., nat-m., nat-s., nicc., **NUX-V.,** op., ox-ac., paeon., pall., ***petr.,*** phos., phys., phyt., pic-ac., plb., ruta, sabin., sars., sep., sil., spig., sulph., sul-ac., tarent., verat., zinc.
morning, rising, on and after - am-m., anac., ang., ars., aur., bell., clem., coc-c., coff., hell., hipp., hura, kali-bi., kali-i., kali-p., mag-c., mag-m., mur-ac., nat-m., nicc., phos., rhod., sep., stront-c., sulph.

HEAVINESS, sensation
morning, rising, on, and after amel. - kali-i., mag-s., ***nat-m.,*** nicc.
waking, on - ant-t., bar-c., bell., bry., calc., calc-p., cann-i., cham., chin., croc., crot-t., euphr., ferr., fl-ac., ip., lach., lil-t., lyc., mag-s., mang., nat-m., nicc., nit-ac., phos., rhus-t., sol-n., squil., ***tarent.,*** uran., verat.
motion, from - acon., arg-n., bism., bov., ***calc.,*** canth., colch., fl-ac., lyc., phys., plat., ***sars., stann., sulph.,*** thuj.
amel. - mag-c., mosch., stann.
eyes of, on - bry., chin., nux-v., ***rhus-t.***
head, of - calc., indg., sars., spig.
night - arg-n., carb-an., kali-i., kali-n., lil-t., mez., nit-ac., sil., tarent., til.
waking, on - chel., cic., mez., nat-c., til.
nosebleed, amel. - dig.
painful - cic., gran., hell., nicc., olnd., sabad., verb.
paroxysmal - nat-m.
perspiration, during - ***ars.,*** caust., eup-per.
amel. - nat-m.
pressed, brain feels compressed - hyper.
forward, as if brain were - bry., canth., laur., thuj.
weight on brain, like a - chel., nux-v., sil.
weight on head, like a - cocc., phel.
pressure, amel. - ail., **CACT.,** camph., cop., mur-ac., nat-m., sabin.
raising, on - calc., dros., ign., op., spong., sulph.
raising, on, amel. - bry.
reading, while - bry., ***calc.,*** crot-t.
riding, while - phyt.
rising, on - am-m., ang., aur., bapt., calc., hura, iod., olnd., sulph., tarax., viol-t.
amel. - calc., con., laur., nicc.
from stooping - grat., mag-s., sulph., viol-t.
sewing, while - petr.
shaking, head amel. - gels.
siesta, after a - bov., bry., mag-c., rhus-t.
sitting, while - aeth., alum., ang., ars., bism., caust., chin., cic., manc., merc., olnd., squil., ***sulph.***
amel. - sulph.
bent over, while - ***con.***
erect - alum.
sleep, amel. - laur.
smoking, agg. - ferr-i., gels.
sneezing, on - seneg.
standing, on - alum., ars., bov., calc., caust., kali-c., mag-c., manc., nicc., plb.
stool, after - apoc.
stooping, on - acon., alum., bell., ***berb.,*** bov., bry., camph., ***carb-an.,*** colch., con., fl-ac., grat., hell., hyos., indg., kali-bi., kali-i., laur., nat-m., nicc., nit-ac., ***nux-v.,*** petr., ***ph-ac.,*** phos., plat., **PULS.,** rhus-t., senn., spong., ***sulph.,*** sul-ac., tab.
after - calc.
amel. - dros., ign., tarax., viol-t.

HEAVINESS, sensation
swallowing, agg. - kali-c.
talking, from - ***ambr.,*** cact., nat-m., sulph.
thinking, of it agg. - ***hell.***
urine, profuse discharge, amel. - fl-ac., **GELS.**
vexation, after - mag-c.
waking, on - bar-c., bell., bry., calc., calc-p., cann-i., cham., chel., chin., cic., con., crot-t., euphr., ferr., fl-ac., ign., lach., lil-t., mag-s., nat-c., nat-m., nicc., nit-ac., rhus-t., sep., sol-n., squil., sulph., tarent., til., verat.
walking, while - hell., hipp., kali-bi., laur., puls., rheum, rhus-t., spong., sulph., thea.
amel. - kali-bi., mag-c.
open air amel. - hydr.
open air, after - bov.
warm, room - **APIS, ARS.,** chin-s., ferr-i., hydr., laur., merc., paeon., ***phos.,*** rhus-t.
washing, amel. - mag-c., phos.
wine, after - rhus-t.
wrinkling, forehead, amel. - phos.
writing, while - ***calc.,*** ferr-i., gent-l., lyc.

heaviness, forehead - ***acon., aesc.,*** aeth., agar., ail., all-c., ***am-c., am-m.,*** ang., ***ant-c.,*** ant-t., apis, apoc., arg-m., arg-n., arn., ars., arum-t., asaf., asar., aspar., bapt., bar-c., bar-m., ***bell.,*** berb., ***bism., bov.,*** brom., **BRY.,** bufo, ***calc.,*** calc-s., camph., cann-i., canth., ***carb-an.,*** carb-v., ***cham.,*** chel., chin-s., ***cic.,*** cinnb., cist., clem., ***coloc.,*** con., conv., crot-h., crot-t., dulc., elaps, ferr., ferr-ar., ferr-i., ferr-p., fl-ac., gamb., ***gels.,*** gins., glon., gran., grat., haem., ham., hell., hep., hipp., hura, hydr., hyos., indg., ip., jac., jatr., kali-bi., kali-c., ***kali-i.,*** kali-n., kali-p., kali-s., kreos., lac-c., lach., laur., led., lil-t., lith., lyc., ***mag-c., mag-m.,*** mag-s., mang., merc., merc-i-r., mur-ac., naja, nat-a., nat-c., ***nat-m.,*** nat-p., nicc., nit-ac., nux-m., ***nux-v.,*** olnd., op., ***ox-ac.,*** pall., phos., phyt., plb., ***puls.,*** rhod., ***rhus-t.,*** ruta., sabin., sars., sep., **SIL.,** sol-n., ***stann.,*** staph., stront-c., ***sulph.,*** tarent., tax., tell., thea., verat., zinc.
afternoon - am-c., chel., chin-s., kali-i., mang., nicc., pall., sil.
4 p.m. - ***mang.***
air, in open, amel. - mang.
all would come out, as if - acon., kreos., mag-s.
dinner, after - sars.
eating, after - aeth., am-c., mag-c.
evening - coloc., lith., mag-m., nat-m., sulph.
menses, during - zinc.
forenoon - carb-an., gamb., ***mang.,*** nicc., sarr., sars.
frontal sinuses - puls.
heat of sun - ***brom.,*** nat-c.
menses, during - zinc.
mental exertion - calc.
morning - arum-t., chin., nat-m., nicc., ox-ac., pall., sulph., verat.
rising, after - ang.
waking, on - bell., calc., nat-m.

heaviness, forehead
motion, on - ***bism.,*** fl-ac.
noon - sulph.
pressure, amel. - mur-ac.
reading, agg. - calc.
standing, while - mag-c.
stone, lay there, as if - bell., ruta.
stooping, when - acon., ***carb-an.,*** rhus-t., tell.
waking, on - bell., sulph.
walking, while - camph., con., sulph.
weight pressed forward in, as if a, must hold head upright - ***acon., rhus-t.***
sank down in it - nux-v.
writing, while - ***calc.***

heaviness, occiput - ***aesc.,*** aeth., ***agar.,*** alumn., ant-t., apis, aur., aur-m-n., bapt., bar-c., bar-m., ***bell.,*** bism., bov., ***bry.,*** cact., cahin., caj., ***calc., calc-ar.,*** calc-s., ***cann-i.,*** cann-s., ***canth., carb-an.,*** **CARB-V.,** ***carl.,*** cham., **CHEL.,** chin., clem., colch., ***con.,*** cop., ***crot-h., dulc., eup-per., ferr.,*** ferr-p., graph., gels., gins., hell., ***ign.,*** indg., kali-c., kali-i., kali-n., kali-p., kali-s., kreos., ***lach.,*** lac-ac., lact., laur., ***lyc.,*** mag-m., mang., ***meph., mez., mur-ac.,*** myric., **NAT-M.,** nat-s., nicc., nit-ac., nux-v., ***op.,*** paeon., **PETR.,** ph-ac., phos., pic-ac., ***plb.,*** prun., psor., ptel., ruta., sabin., sec., sel., sep., spig., spong., stann., ***sulph.,*** sumb., tarax., thuj., til., tril., zinc.
afternoon - ferr., lact., spong.
bending head forward - colch., con., ph-ac.
chill, during - cann-i.
draws eyelids together - **NAT-M**.
evening - bov., kali-i.
extending, down arms - nit-ac.
downward - nit-ac., sep., sulph.
ear to ear - ferr.
nape, into - sulph.
shoulders, to - bry.
forenoon - indg.
heat of sun - ***brom.***
lead, as if full of - kali-c., ***lach.,*** mur-ac., op., ***petr.,*** spong.
lying down, after - ***tarax.***
back on, while agg. - bry., cact.
side, on, amel. - cact.
morning - cham., **LACH.,** sep., sulph.
menses, during - mag-m.
motion agg. - bar-c., bism., colch., lyc., thuj.
night - chel., mez.
could not be raised from pillow, as if - ***chel.***
lying on back - mez.
raise, difficult to - ***chel., lach.,*** op., sep.
raise, pain in occiput like a weight, must raise head with hands - ***eup-per.,*** op.
rising, on - aur.
sink, as if head would, backward - ign., kali-c., mur-ac., op.
sitting bent, while - ***con.***
step, at every, a jolt as if a weight were on occiput - bell.
stooping, amel. - tarax.
swallowing agg. - kali-c.

heaviness, occiput
waking, on - bry., cham., hell., **LACH.**
walking, while - spong.
in open air - staph.
heaviness, sides - aeth., am-c., arg-n., bov., ***cact.,*** cedr., elaps, eug., grat., hydr., kalm., kali-c., kali-i., lyc., mag-m., sabad., sabin., stann., sul-ac., tarent.
left - sul-ac.
right - am-c., bov., sars.
heaviness, temples - agar., bell., bism., bov., cact., carb-an., cimic., cinnb., clem., ferr., glon., kali-i., led., nit-ac., phyt., rhus-t., sabad., sars., sep., stann., tell.
as if a weight hung at both sides - agar., rhus-t.

HEAVING, up and down sensation - bell., con., lyc.

HEMATOMA - ***arn.,*** calc-f., merc., sil.

HERPES - agar., ***anan.,*** bad., bar-c., ***caps.,*** chrysar., cupr., kali-c., ***lyc., mag-c.,*** nat-m., olnd., ***petr., psor.,*** ran-b., **RHUS-T.,** ***thuj.***
herpes, forehead - bad., bar-c., bor., caps., dulc., tarent.
herpes, occiput - ***arg-n., petr.***
herpes, temples - ***alum.,*** cadm-s., ***psor.***

HOLD, head up, unable to - ***abrot., aeth.,*** ant-t., atro., bapt., ***calc-p.,*** cham., cocc., con., croc., cupr., fago., **GELS.,** glon., hipp., ign., lil-t., lyc., ***mang.,*** mez., nat-m., nux-m., nux-v., olnd., ***op.,*** petr., phel., ph-ac., ***puls.,*** rhus-t., sabad., ***sil.,*** tab., ***verat.,*** zinc.
headache, with - petr.
steady, unable to - squil.

HOLLOW, (see Empty)

HOT body, in forehead, sensation - kali-c.

HUMMING, pain - aur., hep., squil., staph., sulph.

HYDROCEPHALUS - acon., am-c., **APIS,** apoc., ***arg-n.,*** arn., ***ars., aur., bac.,*** bar-c., bell., ***bry.,*** **CALC.,** ***calc-p.,*** canth., carb-ac., chin., chin-s., ***con.,*** cupr-ac., cypr., ***dig., ferr.,*** ferr-i., gels., ***hell., hyos.,*** indg., ***iod., iodof.,*** ip., kali-br., ***kali-i.,*** kali-p., lach., ***lyc.,*** mag-m., ***merc., nat-m., op.,*** ph-ac., ***phos.,*** plat., podo., ***puls.,*** samb., **SIL.,** sol-n., ***stram., sulph.,*** **TUB.,** verat., zinc., zinc-m.
coldness, with, of face - agar., arg-n., **CAMPH.,** hell., ***verat.***
diarrhea, after - zinc.
headache, with - petr.
lies, with head low - apis, merc., sulph., zinc.
sweat, with - merc.
vision, with loss of - apoc.
hydrocephalus, brain - ***apis,*** apoc., ***calc.,*** calc-p., hell., iodof., merc., ***sil.,*** sulph., tub., ***zinc.***
diarrhea, after - zinc.
vision, loss of, with - apoc.

IMPETIGO - ***ant-c.,*** bar-c., calc-p., ***caust.,*** con., ***iris,*** **MERC.,** ***petr.,*** rhus-t., rhus-v., sil., sulph., ***viol-t.***
margin of the hair - ***nat-m.***
impetigo, forehead - ant-c., kreos., led., ***merc., rhus-t.,*** sep., sulph., ***viol-t.***

INFLAMMATION, (see Brain, chapter)
inflammation, of, periosteum - ***aur., aur-m.,*** **FL-AC.,** ***kali-i.,*** led., ***mang., merc., merc-c.,*** **MEZ.,** ***nit-ac.,*** **PH-AC.,** ***phos.,*** puls., ***rhod., rhus-t., ruta., sil., staph.***

INJURIES, blows, concussions etc. - acet-ac., acon., am-c., ***anac.,*** **ARN.,** aur., **BAD.,** ***bell.,*** bell-p., both., bry., ***calc., calc-p.,*** calc-s., calen., camph., cann-s., ***carc.,*** caust., chin., ***cic.,*** cina, ***cocc., con.,*** cupr., echi., euphr., ***glon., ham.,*** **HELL.,** ***hyos.,*** **HYPER.,** ***iod., kali-p.,*** kreos., lac-c., ***lach.,*** laur., ***led.,*** lyc., mag-arct., mag-m., ***mang.,*** merc., mez., nat-m., **NAT-S.,** nux-m., ***nux-v.,*** op., ph-ac., ***puls., rhus-t., ruta,*** seneg., ***sep., sil., spig.,*** staph., stram., stry., sul-ac., sulph., ***symph., teucr.,*** valer., ***verat.,*** verb., viol-t., zinc.
ailments, after - acon., **ARN.,** bell., bell-p., both., calc., calc-p., calc-s., calen., ***carc.,*** chin., ***cic., cocc.,*** con., cupr., dulc., ferr-p., glon., **HELL.,** hep., ***hyos.,*** hyper., ***kali-p.,*** lac-c., lach., ***led., lob.,*** mang., merc., ***nat-m.,*** **NAT-S.,** nit-ac., nux-v., op., petr., ph-ac., phos., puls., pyrar., rhus-t., sep., staph., sul-ac., sulph., tell., ***teucr.,*** verat., zinc.
scalp, of - calen.
concussion, brain, after - **ARN.,** bell., calen., chin., **CIC.,** ***cocc.,*** **HELL.,** hep., ***hyos., hell.,*** **HYPER.,** ***kali-p., led., lob.,*** mang., merc., **NAT-S.,** ***nat-m.,*** **OP.,** ph-ac., rhus-t., sep., stram., sul-ac., ***teucr.,*** zinc.
amel. - hell.
commotion of the brains, ailments from - sul-ac., teucr.
epilepsy, after - ***arn., cic.,*** hell., hyper., ***nat-s.,*** zinc.
headache, blows, from - **ARN.,** ***calc-s., hell., hyper., nat-m.,*** **NAT-S.**
concussion, from - **ARN.,** ***bell.,*** calc-s., cocc., ferr-p., hep., lac-c., merc., **NAT-S.,** phos.
injuries, after - **ARN.,** ***bell.,*** calc., ***cic.,*** con., dulc., ***glon., hep., hyper.,*** lach., merc., ***nat-m.,*** **NAT-S.,** nit-ac., petr., ***phos.,*** puls., ***rhus-t., staph.,*** sulph., sul-ac.
mental, functionings altered - carc., ***hell.,*** kali-p., ***nat-s.,*** op., stram.
scalp, of - ***calen.***
vertigo, after injuries - cic., **NAT-S.**

INTOXICATION, as from - ***absin.,*** acon., aesc., ***agar., ail.,*** aloe, am-c., anac., ***apis,*** aran., arn., ars., asc-t., ***bapt.,*** bell., berb., ***bry.,*** cann-i., carb-an., ***carb-v.,*** caust., chel., chin., ***cocc.,*** croc., crot-t., cycl., euphr., eupi., ***gels., glon.,*** graph., ***hell.,*** hydr-ac., iod., kali-n., kreos., laur., mag-m., menthol, mez., nat-c., ***nat-m.,*** nit-ac., nux-m., **NUX-V.,** ***op.,*** par., ***ph-ac., phos.,*** ptel., ***puls., querc.,*** rhod., ***rhus-t.,*** samb., sep., spig., ***sulph.,*** tanac., tarax., sul-ac., valer., xero, zinc.

ITCHING, scalp - abrot., acon., ***agar.***, agn., ***alum.***, ***am-c.***, ***am-m.***, anac., anag., anan., ***ant-c.***, ***apis***, ***arg-n.***, ars., ars-i., arund., asar., aur., aur-s., bad., **BAR-C.**, benz-ac., berb., ***bov.***, bry., **CALC.**, **CALC-S.**, caps., ***carb-ac.***, ***carb-an.***, **CARB-S.**, ***carb-v.***, ***caust.***, chin., ***clem.***, cob., coff., coloc., com., con., corn., ***crot-h.***, cupr-ar., ***cycl.***, daph., dig., ***dros.***, elaps, eup-pur., fago., ferr., ferr-ar., ferr-i., ferr-p., ***fl-ac.***, ***form.***, **GRAPH.**, ***hep.***, hura, ind., iod., jug-c., jug-r., ***kali-ar.***, kali-bi., kali-c., kali-chl., kali-i., kali-n., kali-p., ***kali-s.***, lach., ***laur.***, led., **LYC.**, mag-c., mag-m., manc., ***med.***, meph., ***merc.***, merc-c., ***merc-i-f.***, merc-sul., **MEZ.**, **NAT-M.**, nit-ac., nux-v., ***olnd.***, paeon., par., ***petr.***, ph-ac., ***phos.***, ran-s., rat., rhod., rhus-t., ***ruta.***, ***sabad.***, sarr., ***sars.***, sel., ***sep.***, ***sil.***, ***spong.***, ***staph.***, stry., **SULPH.**, ***sul-ac.***, tab., tarax., ***tarent.***, ***tell.***, thuj., til., verat., vinc., zinc.

- afternoon - sep.
  - 2 p.m. - chel.
- biting - agar., agn., ***mez.***, puls., rhus-t., staph., thuj., verat., vinc.
- bleeds, must scratch until - alum., bov., carb-an., mur-ac., ***sabad.***
- burning - ars., berb., ***calc.***, dros., ***hep.***, kali-c., ***mez.***, ***ruta.***, sabad., ***sil.***, vinc.
- cold, when becoming - ars.
- corrosive - ars., caps., con., ruta, sep., staph.
- crawling - ***arg-n.***, lach., led., sil.
- damp, weather - ***mag-c.***
- daytime - hydr., **OLND.**
- evening - arg-n., calc., calc-p., ***carb-v.***, chin-s., ***cycl.***, mag-c., mez., ph-ac., rhod., ***sel.***, staph., ***sulph.***, ther.
- forenoon - mag-c., sabad.
- headache, after - sep.
- internal - tarax.
- lying, while - mez.
- morning - ***agar.***, bov., ***kali-c.***, kali-p., kali-s., lyc., lyss., mag-c., meph., ol-an., plan., seneg., staph., ***sulph.***, zinc.
- night - agar., ars., aur-s., ***calc.***, cob., cupr-ar., hyper., kali-p., ***mez.***, **OLND.**
  - 3 to 5 p.m. - kali-p.
- painful - ars.
- rainy weather - ***mag-c.***
- rubbing agg. - ***dros.***, nat-m.
  - amel. - ***dros.***, nat-m.
- scratching, agg. - ***calc.***, ***lyc.***, **PHOS.**, ***sil.***
  - amel. - agar., bar-c., caps., caust., mag-c., mez., nat-m., ol-an., ***olnd.***, ph-ac., ran-s., ruta, sabad., sars., thuj.
  - changes place, after - ***cycl.***, ***mez.***, sars., staph.
  - not amel., after - bov., calc., carb-an., mur-ac., sars.
- sleep, when going to - agn.
- sore - zinc.
  - after scratching - petr., sil.
- spots - sil., zinc.
- stinging - caust., mez., sars.
- sudden - ph-ac.
- undressing, when - ars.
- walking in open air - calc.

ITCHING, scalp

- wandering. - bar-c., mag-c., mosch.
- warm, from exercise, when - **LYC.**, sabad.
  - when head becomes - ***bov.***, mez., sabad., ***sanic.***, staph.
- warmth of bed agg. - bov., ***calc.***, ***carb-v.***, lyc., ***mez.***, ***sil.***, staph., ***sulph.***

itching, forehead - agar., alum., ambr., am-m., anac., ars., aur-m., bell., berb., bov., canth., caps., carb-an., carb-v., caust., cham., chel., clem., con., fl-ac., gamb., gran., hura, hyper., kali-bi., lach., laur., led., lyc., mag-c., merc., nat-m., olnd., ol-an., pall., petr., phos., ***rhus-t.***, samb., sars., sil., spig., squil., ***sulph.***, tab., verat.

- air, in open, amel. - gamb.
- burning - ***kali-bi.***
- corrosive - con., ph-ac.
- dinner, during - hep., mag-c., sulph.
- evening - ***sulph.***, zinc.
- menses, before, itching, eruption on - sars.
- rubbing amel. - ol-an., samb., tab.
- scratching amel. - bov., mag-c., squil.

itching, occiput scalp - ***am-c.***, ars., bor., calc., ***chel.***, cinnb., fago., kali-c., mez., sars., ***sep.***, **SIL.**, ***staph.***, **SULPH.**, tell., thuj.

- evening - sep., ***staph.***, stront.
- morning - ***sulph.***
- scratching agg. - ***staph.***
  - amel. - chel., ruta.
- warm room agg. - fago., sulph.

itching, side, right - mang., sars.

- left - sil., spig.

itching, temple, right - graph.

itching, vertex - sep.

JERKING, of head - ***agar.***, alum., ant-t., ars., ***bell.***, cann-i., caust., cham., ***cic.***, cina, ***hyos.***, ign., lam., mygal., ***nat-m.***, ***nux-m.***, op., ***sep.***, ***stram.***, stry., sumb., verat-v., zinc.

- backwards - alum., atro., bov., ***cic.***, cina, hyper., kali-c., merc., nux-v., sep., stry.
  - and forwards - ars., nux-m., sep., stry.
- behind forward, from - kali-c., ***nux-m.***, ph-ac., sep., spong., ***stram.***, stry.
- daytime - ***sep.***
- head forward and knees upward - bell.
  - during cough - ther.
- here and there - chel., stram., stront.
- involuntary, back and forward, while sitting - sep.
- left - aeth., spig.
- lying on the back, while - ***cic.***, ***hyper.***
  - the head jerks clear of the pillow - **STRAM.**
- one side to another, from - kali-c., nat-s., nux-m., plb., samb.
- right, to - ***nat-s.***
- sitting, while - sep.
- sleep, during - ***arn.***
  - head jerks backwards, during - ***hyper.***
  - on falling asleep - puls.
- talking, while - ***cic.***
- walking quickly or ascending stairs, on - **BELL.**

JERKING, pain - acon., aeth., agar., ambr., am-c., anac., ant-t., apis, ***arn.,*** asaf., bar-c., **BELL.,** bism., bor., ***bry.,*** calc., cann-i., canth., ***carb-ac.,*** carb-an., ***carb-s.,*** carb-v., caust., ***chin.,*** crot-t., cycl., dig., dulc., eupi., glon., graph., ***ign.,*** indg., kali-c., kali-p., ***kali-s.,*** kreos., lach., lyc., mag-c., mag-m., meny., merc., mill., ***mur-ac.,*** nat-c., ***nat-m.,*** nit-ac., nux-v., paeon., ***petr.,*** ph-ac., phos., plb., prun., ***puls.,*** rat., sabad., samb., ***sep.,*** sil., ***spig.,*** spong., squil., ***stann.,*** **SULPH.,** teucr., thuj.
afternoon - mag-c.
alternating sides - samb.
ascending steps, on - **BELL.,** ***ign.***
behind forwards - ph-ac.
drinking cold water amel. - kali-c.
extending, forward - arg-n.
to nape - calc.
light agg. - carb-ac.
lying amel. - chin.
menses, during - eupi.
motion, on - ***chin.***
amel. - stann.
noise agg. - carb-ac.
raising the eyes - ***ign.***
turning suddenly, on - sil.
walking, while - **BELL.,** ***chin.***
in open air - ***chin., spig.***
wandering - chel., stront.

jerking, forehead - apis, arn., bor., cann-i., caust., cham., ***chin.,*** lyc., mang., op., ***prun., sep., sil., stann.,*** sulph., ***sul-ac., thuj.***
across - sabad.
alternating with dull aching - stann.
coughing - sul-ac.
evening - alumn.
extending backward - ***prun.***
outward - lyc.
left - alum., caps.
night - sil.
stool, after - spig.
stooping, on - sil.

jerking, occiput - acon., ***bell.,*** cedr., fl-ac., glon., kali-c., prun., rhus-t., ***spig.,*** stann., sulph., thuj.
intermitting - canth.
walking in open air - ***spig.***

jerking, sides - aeth., alum., calc., caust., ***chin.,*** graph., kreos., nat-m., nicc., nit-ac., sabin., spig., spong.
left - aeth., cupr., spig.
right - graph., kreos., ***prun.,*** sabin.

jerking, temples - acon., apis, arg-m., arn., calc., carb-ac., cast., ***chin.,*** dig., glon., kali-c., lact., lil-t., mang., ox-ac., plb., rhus-t., ***spig.,*** stann., sulph., valer.
extending, downward - anac.
lower jaw to - rhus-t.
teeth, to - rhus-t.
upper jaw to - ***chin.***
upward - am-m., spong.
jerking pain, with arms, on - spig.
left - cupr., stann.
right - sul-ac.
stepping on - ***spig.***

jerking, vertex - anac., ***calc.,*** gent-c., kali-i., meny., mur-ac., ran-s., sil., spig., spong.
here and there - kali-i.
paroxysmal - sil.

KNOCKING, in head (see Pulsation) - am-c., ang.
ball striking skull, like a - plat.

KNOCKS, head against things - apis, ars., **BELL.,** con., hyos., mag-c., **MILL.,** rhus-t., **TUB.**
pain as if knocked in the head - mosch.

LANCINATING, pain (see Cutting) - acon., aesc., alum., ambr., am-c., anan., arn., ***ars., bell.,*** cadm-s., calc., ***cupr.,*** dros., gins., graph., hep., hura, ip., kali-i., mag-c., manc., sang., spig., squil., tarent.
air, cold, agg. - kali-i., ***spig.***
open amel. - am-c.
cold applications amel. - ***ars.***
evening - ***bell.,*** kali-i.
exertion, on - ambr.
heat agg. - kali-i.
lying amel. - ambr.
morning - mag-c.
rising, after - mag-c., coloc.
motion amel. - kali-i.
night - tarent.
stepping - ambr.
stooping, on - arn.
turning head agg. - cupr.
vertigo, with - nat-m.
waking, on - tarent.
walking fast - ***calc.***
in open air amel. - hep.

lancinating, forehead - ***am-c., bell., calc.,*** coloc., ***cupr., dros.,*** ferr., gins., jug-r., lyc., tarent.
afternoon - sol-t-ae.
extending to occiput - ***bell.***
frontal eminence - thuj.
left - thuj.
morning - viol-t.
rising, on - coloc.
moving eyes - ***dros.***
pressure agg. - ***cupr.***

lancinating, occiput - aesc., aster., aur-s., ***bufo,*** canth., ***con., cupr., sang.,*** sec., syph.
night - syph.
pulsation, with every - ***con.***

lancinating, sides - bell., ***calc.,*** cocc., hura, kali-bi., spig., tarent.
extending to eye, ear, temples and lower jaw - hura
morning - tarent.

lancinating, temples - ail., anan., aster., ***bell.,*** blatta, crot-c., ***cupr.,*** form., ***ham.,*** hura, **KALI-I.,** manc., plb., senec., tarent.
left when chewing - am-c.
temple to temple - **BELL.**

LARGE, sensation, (see Enlarged) - **BAR-C.,** caj., ***calc., calc-p.,*** cor-r., merc., ***sil.***

LEAN, on something, desire to - ***bell.,*** carb-v., gymn.

LICE, head - am-c., apis, ars., bac., bell-p., ***carb-ac.,*** cocc., graph., lach., ***lyc., merc.,*** nit-ac., olnd., ***psor.,*** **STAPH.,** sulph., tub., vinc.

LIFTING, up of the skull, sensation of - cann-i., ***lac-d.***

LIGHTNESS, sense of - abies-c., hyos., ***jug-c.,*** manc., nat-a., nat-ch.
nausea, after - lyss.

LIGHTNESS, occiput, in - sec.

LOOSENESS, (see Brain, chapter)

LUMP, sensation as of - ant-t., arn., cham., chel., ***con.,*** staph.
lump, sensation as of, forehead, in - cham., pip-m., staph.

LUPUS - calc., lyc.

LYING, in an uncomfortable position, as if - cimx., clem., lyc.
hard, as if on something - ***manc.,*** ph-ac.
too low, as if from - phos.

MADDENING, pains - ***acon.,*** ambr., ***ars.,*** **BELL.,** bry., cact., ***calc.,*** cham., ***chin.,*** coloc., cupr., **GELS.,** ign., ind., iod., ***ip., lyss.,*** mag-c., med., meli., ***nat-m., nit-ac.,*** psor., puls., sep., ***stram., tarent.***
feeling in brain - plan.

MASTOID process, abscess, threatened of - **AUR., CAPS.,** carb-an., ***fl-ac., hep., lach., nit-ac.,*** **SIL.**

MOTIONS, of head - aloe, ars., aur., aur-m., bell., benz-ac., bry., bufo, ***calc-p.,*** cann-i., caust., ***cic.,*** crot-h., mez., nux-m., sec., sep., stram., tarent.
backward and forward - agar., aur., ***cham., cina,*** lam., lyc., ***nux-m., ph-ac.,*** sep., ***verat-v.***
constant - ***agar.,*** ant-t., ars., ***bell.,*** cann-i., cham., cocc., ***hyos.,*** lam., mygal., nux-m., op., ***stram.,*** stry., verat-v., zinc.
left side, to - cocc.
convulsive - **AGAR.,** ***calc., camph., caust., cocc., cupr., nux-m.,*** stram., tarent.
hiccough, after - bell.
talking and swallowing are impossible - nux-m.
with convulsive motions of arms - cic.
difficult - colch., hipp., kali-i., stann.
forward - merc., nat-m., sep., stry.
hither and thither - ars., nit-ac., op., ***stram.***
impossible - spig., tarent., zinc.
involuntary - alum., agar., ***cann-i.,*** caust., hell., lyc., merc., nat-m., zinc.
nodding of - aur-m., aur-s., calc., caust., cham., kali-bi., lyc., ***mosch., nat-m.,*** ph-ac., ***verat-v.***
pains, moves head to relieve - chin., ***kali-i.,*** sec.
pendulum-like - cann-i., sec.
rising from the pillow, spasmodic - bell., stram.

MOTIONS, of head
rolling head - ***agar., apis, arn.,*** ars., **BELL.,** ***bry.,*** caust., ***cic., cina,*** clem., colch., cor-r., ***crot-t., cupr.,*** cyt-l., dig., ***hell., hyos.,*** kali-br., kali-i., ***lyc., med., merc.,*** naja, ***nux-m.,*** oena., ***op.,*** ph-ac., phos., ***podo.,*** pyrog., sec., ***sil.,*** spong., ***stram.,*** sulph., ***tarent.,*** **TUB.,** verat., verat-v., zinc.
day and night, with moaning - ***hell., lyc.***
paroxysms, in - merc.
sitting, while - ***nux-m.***
too weak to move body, when - ***ars.***
rubs against something - tarent.
shaking the head, involuntarily, which makes him dizzy - **LYC.**
sideways - aur., bell., caust., clem., hell., lyc., ***med.,*** nat-s., nux-m., tarent.
rocks head from side to side to relieve pain - kali-i., ***med.,*** tarent.
throwing head about - ***bell.,*** caust., merc., phos., ***tarent.***
talking, while - puls.
throwing head about, backward - acet-ac., camph., cina, ***glon.,*** hell., kali-n., lob., merc., mygal., phyt., ***stram.,*** tab., tanac.
throwing head about, epilepsy, in - lach.
tosses - ***acon., cocc., cupr.,*** ign., ph-ac., ***tarent.***
turning, of, backward - laur.
side, to - op.
side, to, right - plb.
side, to, left - lyc., tarent.
side, to, wrong side, when spoken to - ***atro.***
wagging - bell., cham.
wavering - kali-c.
motions, of scalp - caust., nat-c., nat-m., sep., sulph.

MOVE, up and down, sensation - zinc.
head seems to - sep.

MOVEMENTS, in head - ***acon.,*** aloe, alum., am-c., anan., ang., ant-t., ***ars., bar-c.,*** bar-m., **BELL.,** ***bry.,*** calc., carb-an., carb-s., caust., **CHIN.,** chin-a., cic., cob., cocc., con., croc., ***crot-c.,*** crot-h., cycl., dig., elaps, eug., **GLON.,** graph., guai., ***hep., hyos.,*** indg., ***kali-c.,*** kali-n., kali-p., kali-s., kalm., lach., lact., ***laur., lyc.,*** mag-s., mez., mosch., mur-ac., nat-m., nat-s., nicc., ***nux-m., nux-v.,*** phel., phos., plat., rheum, ***rhus-t.,*** **SEP.,** ***sil.,*** sol-n., spig., stann., staph., stront-c., ***sulph.,*** sul-ac., tab., tell., verat., xan.
afternoon - graph., mag-m., mez., nat-m., sulph.
amel. in - bar-c.
air, in open - laur.
in open, amel. - indg., mag-m.
ascending stairs, while - bell., crot-h., lyc., nat-m., par.
bending the by - asar., dig.
amel. - spig.
carrying a weight - lyc.
coughing, when - acon., ***bry.,*** carb-an., lact., mag-s., sep., sul-ac.

MOVEMENTS, in head
drawing load, while - mur-ac.
drinking, when - acon., bry.
eating, after - alum., mag-s.
amel. after - aloe
evening - eug., mag-m., nat-m., plat., stront-c., sulph.
leaning, when - cycl.
lying on right side - anan.
menses, during - mag-m.
morning - cic., grat., guai., hyos., indg., lact., nat-s., spig., tab.
rising, on - bar-c.
waking, on - cic.
motion, from - acon., ***ars.***, bry., calc., carb-an., ***caust.***, cic., cob., croc., led., lyc., mag-c., mag-s., mang., nat-m., nux-m., nux-v., spig., staph., ***sulph.***, tab., tell.
amel. - lach., petr., staph.
moved, as if something, from back of neck up to head - glon.
moving the by head - am-c., ***ars.***, bar-c., calc., chin-s., cocc., con., croc., glon., kali-c., kali-s., lach., lact., mang., mez., nat-m., ***nux-m., rhus-t.***, sep., sol-n., spig., squil., stann., ***sulph.***, sul-ac., thuj., xan.
night - anan., hyper., puls.
waking, on - par.
nodding the on - ***sulph.***
pressure amel. - bell.
rising up, when - cham., indg., lyc., phos.
amel. - alum., laur., mill.
room, while in - indg., mag-m.
in warm - lact.
shaking, head - sep.
sitting, while - grat., sil.
amel. - spig.
speaking, while - acon., cocc., zinc.
standing, while - cycl., mang.
step, making a - bar-c., guai., led., lyc., **RHUS-T.**, sep., ***sil., spig.***, thuj.
stool, while at - spig.
stooping, on - alum., am-c., ant-t., berb., bry., carb-an., coff., dig., hydr-ac., kali-c., laur., mag-s., mill., nat-s., nux-v., rheum, rhus-t.
stumbling, from - bar-c., led., sep., sil., thuj.
thinking about it amel. - cic.
turning when - cham., ***glon.***, kali-c., kalm., spig.
turning, when, quickly, when - nat-a.
waking, on - cic., par., phos.
walking, while - acon., bar-c., bell., carb-an., cic., cob., cocc., crot-h., guai., hyos., indg., led., lyc., mag-c., mag-s., nuph., nux-m., nux-v., rhod., ***rhus-t.***, sep., ***sil., spig.***, staph., ***sulph.***, verat., verb., viol-t.
in open air, while - aloe, caust., plat., ***rhus-t.***, sul-ac.

NAIL, pain, as if from a - ***agar.***, arn., ***asaf.***, carb-v., caust., **COFF.**, dulc., euon., ***graph.***, hell., ***hep., ign.***, lach., nat-m., ***nux-v.***, olnd., ptel., ***puls.***, ruta., sang., ***sep.***, staph., thea., **THUJ.**
air, open, in - coff.

NAIL, pain, as if
alcoholics, after - ruta.
menses, during - arn., ***ign., nux-v.***
morning, rising, on - ptel.
walking about amel. - ***agar.***
in open air - ***thuj.***
nail, forehead, as if, in - caust., hell., ***ign.***, iris., lyc., sabin., **THUJ.**
extending from occiput to - mosch.
frontal eminence, left - **THUJ.**
left side - thuj.
nail, occiput, as if, in - ***cimic., hep., mosch.***, puls., tarent.
extending to vertex - ***cimic.***
one-sided - puls.
nail, sides, as if, in - acon., ***agar.***, chel., ***coff.***, **HEP.**, ***ign., nat-m., nux-v.***, ruta., staph., **THUJ.**
dinner after - **THUJ.**
driven outward, were, amel. lying on it - **IGN.**
pressure, amel. - **THUJ.**
right - ***agar.***
nail, temples, as if, in - ***am-br., arn.***, cocc., dulc., ham., ***hep., ign.***, kali-i., sang., spira.
morning - sang.
right - spira.
temple to - ham.
nail, vertex, as if, in - euon., form., hell., hura, manc., nicc., ***nux-v.***, staph., **THUJ.**
night, 3 to 4 a.m. - ***thuj.***
walking in open air, amel. - ***thuj.***

NAUSEA, in - cocc.

NEURALGIC, pain - ***acon., aconin.***, aesc., all-c., arg-n., ***ars., bell.***, bism., ***cedr.***, chel., ***chin-s.***, cimic., coll., der., ***gels., mag-p.***, meli., menthol, oreo., pall., phos., ***spig.***, tarent., zinc-valer.
scalp, of - ***acon., cimic.***, hydr., phyt.

NODDING, (see Motions, of Head)

NODES, headache, during (see Eruptions, Exostoses, Swollen glands) - kali-i., phos., sil.
nodes, scalp, in - caust., coloc., kali-i.

NODULES, in scalp - ***coloc., kali-i.***

NOISES, in, head (see Hearing, Noises) - chin-s., dig., kali-i., nat-s., phos.
buzzing - caust.
chronic - ***kali-i.***
cracking - aloe, kalm.
deafness, with - carb-s., graph.
eustachian tube, inflammation, with - **HYDR., MERC.**
explosion-like, during sleep - cann-i.
humming or roaring - calc., ***carb-v.***, caust., chin-s., ***dig.***, graph., kali-i., mag-c., ***nat-s.***, nux-v., ph-ac., ***phos.***, sars., sulph., thuj., verat., zinc.
coughing, on - hep.
stool, during and after - zinc.
walking - verb.
roaring - caust., graph., phos.
coryza, during - sep.
singing locusts - bry.

noises, occiput, in - phos.

NODOSITIES, forehead - still.

NUMBNESS, sensation of (see Asleep) - ***acon.,*** all-c., aloe, alum., ambr., am-c., anac., ant-t., apis, ars., arund., asaf., asar., aur., aur-m., aur-m-n., bapt., bell., bor., ***bry.,*** bufo, calc., calc-ar., calc-p., carb-ac., carb-an., carb-v., chel., cocc., coff., colch., coloc., con., dig., dios., ferr-br., ***fl-ac.,*** glon., **GRAPH.,** ham., hura, jatr., ***kali-br., lach.,*** lil-t., lyc., lyss., mag-m., meny., meph., merc., merc-i-f., ***merl.,*** mez., mur-ac., nat-m., **NIT-AC.,** nux-v., olnd., ol-an., op., par., ***petr.,*** phos., phys., ***plat.,*** sep., sil., stram., sulph., thuj., upa., zinc.

dinner, after - carb-v.
lying, while - merc., sulph.
menses, during - plat.
morning - carb-v.
soreness then numbness extending to body - ambr.
resting head on arm - nat-m.
walking in open air, amel. - mang., ***plat.***

numbness, forehead - bapt., bar-c., brom., coll., dig., ***fl-ac.,*** ham., ***mag-m.,*** merc., ***mur-ac.,*** nat-a., ***phos.,*** **PLAT.,** sil., valer.
blow, as if from a - plat.
board lay there, as if a - acon.
evening - nat-a.
extending to nasal bone - ***plat.***
morning, on waking and while lying, amel. exercise and wrapping head warmly - mag-m.
warm room - plat.

numbness, occiput - ***agar.,*** ammc., bry., ***calc-p.,*** carb-v., caust., fl-ac., gels., kali-c., ***lach.,*** merc-i-f., merl., nat-c., plat., raph., tell.
too tightly bound, as if - ***carb-v., plat.***

numbness, sides - ***aur., calc., chel.,*** cina, ***con.,*** hura, ***lach.,*** lyss., ol-an., tarax., thuj.
left - lyss., ol-an., stram.
right - ***chel.***
then left - anac.

numbness, temples - ang., aur., myric., phos., phys., **PLAT.,** zing.

numbness, vertex - carb-s., ***mez.,*** pall., phos., ***plat.***
preceded by feeling as if scalp and brain were contracted, amel. on motion and open air - plat.

OILY, forehead - ***hydr., psor.***

OPEN, as if - ***carb-an., cimic.,*** guano, sil.

open, fontanelles (see Head, Fontanelles)

OPENING, and shutting - **CANN-I.,** ***cann-s., cimic., cocc.,*** lyc.
moving head or turning eyes, on - ***cimic.***
as if opened and let in cold air - ***cimic.***

opening, and shutting, occiput - ***cocc.,*** sep.
air, open, amel. - sep.
cold application, amel. - sep.

PAIN, head, general (see Headaches)

PARALYSIS, sensation of, after emissions - sil.
forehead - sep.
muscles of occiput - dulc.
talking, while - calc.

PECKING, pain - carb-an., mosch., nux-v., rhus-t., ruta.

pecking, forehead - carb-an., nat-m.

pecking, temple, left - nit-ac.

PERSPIRATION, of scalp - aesc., ***agar.,*** **ANAC.,** ***ant-t., apis,*** ars-i., bar-c., ***bar-m., bell.,*** benz-ac., bor., bov., bufo, **CALC.,** ***calc-p., calc-s.,*** camph., carb-s., ***carb-v., caust.,*** **CHAM., CHIN.,** cimx., clem., cycl., dig., eup-pur., gamb., glon., ***graph.,*** grat., **GUAI.,** ***hep.,*** iod., ip., ***kali-c., kali-p.,*** kali-s., laur., led., ***lyc.,*** mag-c., ***mag-m.,*** **MERC.,** ***mez.,*** mosch., **MUR-AC.,** nat-m., ***nit-ac.,*** nux-v., ol-an., olnd., op., ***petr.,*** phel., ph-ac., **PHOS.,** plb., psor., **PULS.,** ***pyrog.,*** **RHEUM,** sabad., ***sep.,*** **SIL.,** spig., staph., ***stram.,*** stry., sulph., tab., tarent., thuj., tub., valer., verat-v., zinc.

bed, in - bry.
breakfast, after - par.
chill, after - sulph.
clammy - cham., merc., nux-v.
cold - acon., ant-t., benz-ac., bry., bufo, ***calc.,*** camph., cina, cocc., con., dig., ***hep., lob.,*** merc., merc-c., ***nux-v., op.,*** petr., ***phos.,*** podo., ***verat.***
air, in - ***calc.***
coughing, on - ant-t., calc., ip., merc., sil., tarent.
daytime - ol-an., stram.
and night - sulph.
eating, while - nux-v., petr.
epilepsy, before - ***caust.***
evening - anac., bar-c., ***calc.,*** mag-m., mur-ac., sep., sil.
after lying down - petr.
except the head - ***bell.,*** merc., mur-ac., nux-v., **RHUS-T., SAMB.,** ***sec., sep.,*** **THUJ.**
fetid - ***calc., merc.,*** puls., ***staph.***
forenoon - mag-c.
headache, with - mez., **SULPH.**
heat, during - sep.
hot - ***cham., cimic., glon., op.,*** podo.
menses, during - cham., merc., phos., verat.
mental exertion - kali-c., kali-p., ph-ac., ran-b.
midnight - ph-ac., rhus-t.
morning - ***calc.,*** cann-s., dulc., hep., ***mez.,*** nat-m., nux-v., ***sep.***
rising, on - nat-m.
musk-like odor - ***apis, sulph.***
musty - nat-m.
night - ars., bov., bry., **CALC.,** calc-p., carb-an., cham., chin., cic., coloc., hep., kali-c., lyc., ***merc.,*** nat-m., nit-ac., podo., rhus-t., sanic., sep., ***sil.,*** sulph., syc-co.
oily - ***bry., merc.***
one-sided - ambr., bar-c., nit-ac., ***nux-v.,*** **PULS., SULPH.**
painless side - aur-m-n.

PERSPIRATION, of scalp
only on the head - acon., am-m., ***calc.,*** cham., kali-m., phos., ***puls.,*** rheum, sabad., sanic., sep., ***sil.,*** spig., stann.
reading, while - nat-s.
sleep, during - bov., bry., ***bry.,*** **CALC.,** ***calc-p.,*** carb-an., ***cham., chin., cic.,*** dys-co., ***lyc., merc.,*** nat-m., ***podo.,*** rhus-t., sanic., ***sep., sil.,*** syc-co.
on falling a - graph., sep., ***sil.***
soup, after - phos., rheum
sour - ***bry., cham., hep., merc.,*** rheum, ***sep.,*** **SIL.**
stool, during - ptel.
uncovered parts - thuj.
waking, on - ph-ac.
walking, after - ***calc.,*** carb-v., merc.
in open air - bor., ***calc.,*** **CHIN.,** ***graph.,*** guai., phos., thuj.
washing, after - **GRAPH.**

perspiration, forehead - acet-ac., ***acon.,*** aeth., agar., aml-n., anag., ant-t., ***ars.,*** ars-i., asaf., bapt., bell., ***brom.,*** bry., ***cact., calc.,*** camph., **CANN-I.,** caps., carb-o., carb-s., ***carb-v.,*** cham., chel., ***chin.,*** chin-a., cic., cina, colch., con., croc., crot-t., cupr., dig., dros., elaps, eup-pur., glon., ***guai.,*** hell., ***hep.,*** iod., ***ip.,*** jab., kali-ar., ***kali-bi., kali-c.,*** kali-p., lachn., ***laur.,*** **LED.,** lyc., **MERC-C.,** mosch., ***nat-a.,*** **NAT-C.,** nat-m., nat-p., ***nit-ac.,*** nux-v., **OP., PHOS.,** ph-ac., phyt., ran-a., sabad., **SARS.,** sil., sin-n., ***stann.,*** staph., stram., sulph., ***tab.,*** **VERAT.,** vesp., ***zinc.***
afternoon - ferr-i.
anxiety, as from - nux-v., ***verat.***
burning - nat-c.
chill, during - ***acon.,*** bry., ***calc., chin.,*** cina, dig., ***led., nat-s., cic.***
clammy - acet-ac., carb-an., cina, colch., ***hep., op.***
cold - ***acon.,*** acet-ac., ant-t., ***ars.,*** asaf., bapt., bell., bry., bufo, ***cact., calc.,*** camph., caps., carb-s., **CARB-V.,** ***chin., cina,*** cocc., ***colch.,*** croc., cupr., ***dros., gels.,*** glon., ***hell., hep., ip., kali-bi.,*** kali-c., kali-p., ***lach., laur., merc.,*** merc-c., nat-m., **OP.,** ox-ac., petr., phos., ***phyt., plb.,*** sabad., ***sec.,*** sep., ***staph.,*** sul-ac., sulph., ***tab.,*** **VERAT.,** vip., zinc.
chill, during - chin., cina
heat, during - dig.
trembling with anxiety - sep.
warm room, in - ambr.
cough, during - ant-t., chlor., ip., verat.
diarrhea, during - sulph.
dinner, during - lyc.
after - nat-s., par., sars., sulph.
dream, frightful - bell.
easy - rheum
eating, while - carb-v., nit-ac., nux-v., sulph., sul-ac.
evening - anac., carb-v., chin., ol-an., puls., ran-b., ***sars.,*** senec.
6:30 p.m. - ol-an.
lying, after - carb-v.

perspiration, forehead
evening, walking, while - chin.
writing - ran-b.
fever, during - ant-t., dig., ip., mag-s., sars., staph., **VERAT.**
greasy - coloc., hydr., ***psor.***
hat, from pressure of - nat-c.
headache, during - glon., ***kali-c.,*** ph-ac., ***phyt.,*** sulph.
hot - cham., chin.
menses, during - phos., verat.
morning - ambr., ang., dios., ***kali-c.,*** nux-v., phys., stann., staph.
4 a.m. - stann.
6 a.m. - nux-v.
8 a.m. - dios.
bed, in - staph.
stool, during - phys.
motion, during - valer.
night - bry., cann-s., chin., crot-t.
pain in abdomen, during - crot-t.
noon - nat-m., valer.
offensive - led., sil.
rising from a seat - ***verat.***
up in bed, when - mag-s.
sitting, while - camph., ir-fl.
sleep, during - cham.
sour - led.
sticky - cham., cocc.
stool, during - crot-t., **VERAT.**
after - crot-t., ip., merc., nat-c., **VERAT.**
storm, during approach of - nat-c.
vomiting - ant-c., mag-c., phos.
walking in open air, while - guai., led., merc., nux-v.
warm - acon., act-sp., anac., camph., cham., glon., phys., puls.

perspiration, occiput - anac., ars., **CALC.,** chin., ferr., mag-c., mosch., nit-ac., nux-v., **PH-AC.,** ***sanic., sep., sil.,*** spig., stann., **SULPH.**
sleep, during - **CALC.,** ***sanic.***
walking, while - sulph.

perspiration, vertex - ruta.

PINCHING, pain - alum., bar-c., caust., colch., kali-c., lyc., mez., nux-v., ***petr.,*** phos., sil., teucr., verb.
evening - alum.
sleep, after - rheum
stooping - alum.
walking, on - sil.

pinching, forehead - acon., anac., calc., eug., mez., nit-ac., nux-m., petr., psor., rheum, staph., verat.
above eyes - ars.
extending to root of nose - op.

pinching, occiput - am-m., carb-v., chel., hipp., mag-m., meny., ***petr.,*** ph-ac.

pinching sides - calc., crot-h., lyc., mez., petr., sep., squil.

pinching, temples - **ARG-M.,** calc., carb-an., crot-h., ***kali-c.,*** lec., merc., mez., olnd., petr., ph-ac., ***sulph.,*** **VERB.,** zinc.

pinching, temples
extending to ear - nat-p.
to forehead - mez.
to nose - mez.
forceps, as with - calc., ph-ac., verb.
left - kali-c., nat-p., ph-ac., zinc.
right - crot-h., merc., olnd.
pinching, vertex - mag-m., ph-ac., rheum, sep.

PLUG, peg or wedge, as from a (see Nail) - ***anac.,*** arg-m., asaf., bov., caust., cocc., con., dulc., hep., jac., kreos., olnd., plat., prun., ran-s., rhod., rhus-t., ruta., ***sul-ac.***
plug were thrust suddenly in by increasingly severe blows - sul-ac.
split wide open by a wedge, body cold, head burns, cannot get warm, whines - lachn.
plug, peg or wedge, forehead - anac., asaf., caust., jac., sul-ac.
plug, peg or wedge, occiput - ***arg-m.,*** bov., canth., con., hep., puls., rhod., tarent.
plug, peg or wedge, sides - ***asaf.,*** dulc., **HEP.,** ***plat.***
plug, peg, or wedge, temples - ***anac., asaf.,*** cocc., dulc., hep., sul-ac., ***thuj.***
mental exertion, on - ***anac.***
plug, peg, or wedge, vertex, intense pain as if a bolt were driven from neck to agg. each throb of heart - ***cimic.***

PRESSING, pain (see Bursting, Drawing) - ***acon., aesc., aeth., agar.,*** agn., all-c., aloe, alum., ***alumn.,*** ambr., ***am-br., am-c., am-m., anac.,*** ang., ***ant-t.,*** apis, aran., arg-m., ***arg-n., arn.,*** ars., ars-i., arum-t., ***asaf., asar.,*** aster., aur., ***bapt.,*** bar-c., bar-m., **BELL.,** benz-ac., berb., ***bism.,*** bor., bov., brom., ***bry.,*** cadm-s., calad., ***calc.,*** calc-p., ***calc-s., camph.,*** cann-i., cann-s., canth., ***caps.,*** carb-ac., ***carb-an.,*** **CARB-S., CARB-V.,** ***caust.,*** cham., chel., **CHIN.,** chin-a., ***chin-s., chlol., cic.,*** cimic., cina, cinnb., clem., ***cocc.,*** coc-c., ***coff., coloc., con.,*** cor-r., crot-c., croc., crot-h., cub., cupr., cycl., daph., ***dig., dros.,*** dulc., eug., ***euph.,*** euphr., ***euon.,*** eupi., ferr., ferr-ar., ferr-i., ferr-p., fl-ac., gamb., gels., **GLON.,** ***graph.,*** grat., guai., ***hell.,*** helon., ***hep.,*** hipp., hydr-ac., ***hyos.,*** hyper., ***ign.,*** indg., iod., ***ip.,*** iris, kali-ar., kali-bi., ***kali-c., kali-i., kali-n.,*** kali-p., ***kali-s.,*** kalm., ***kreos.,*** **LAC-C., LACH.,** lam., lact., laur., led., ***lil-t.,*** lob., ***lyc., lycps., lyss., mag-c., mag-m.,*** mag-s., mang., meli., ***meny.,*** **MERC.,** merc-c., merc-i-f., merc-i-r., merl., ***mez.,*** mosch., ***mur-ac.,*** myric., nat-a., nat-c., **NAT-M.,** nat-p., nat-s., nicc., **NIT-AC.,** ***nux-m.,*** **NUX-V.,** ***olnd.,*** ol-an., ***op.,*** osm., par., ***petr., ph-ac., phos.,*** pip-m., ***plat., plb.,*** prun., **PSOR., PULS.,** ***ran-b., ran-s.,*** rheum, ***rhod., rhus-t.,*** rhus-v., ***ruta., sabad.,*** sabin., ***samb.,*** sars., ***seneg., sep.,*** serp., ***sil., spig., spong.,*** squil., ***stann., staph., stront-c.,*** **SULPH., SUL-AC., TAB., TANAC.,** ***tarax., tarent.,*** ter., ther., ***thuj.,*** valer., verat., verb., viol-t., xan., zinc., zing.
afternoon - alum., ang., cann-i., carb-an., carb-v., cham., coloc., graph., hell., kali-c., kali-n., lyc., mag-c., naja, nat-c., nit-ac., op., phos., ph-ac., senec., sep., stram.

PRESSING, pain
afternoon, 2 p.m. - alum.
air, cold, agg. - ferr., ***sil.***
in open - agar., caust., chel., ***chin.,*** ferr., glon., hep., laur., meny., ***merc.,*** nux-v., rhus-t.
in open, amel. - alum., ***arg-m.,*** bov., cinnb., coloc., ***hell.,*** hydr-ac., jatr., lach., lyc., mag-m., mang., ***phos.,*** sabin., seneg.
amel. - bell., **LACH.,** nit-ac., spig.
armor, as if in - apis, ***arg-n.,*** asaf., ***berb.,*** cann-i., ***carb-v.,*** clem., ***cocc., crot-c., cycl., graph.,*** hell., ***ip., lil-t.,*** **NIT-AC.,** peti., pyrog., ***spig.,*** stry., sulph., zinc.
ascending, steps, on - arn., lyc., **MENY.,** ***ph-ac.***
asunder - acon., aesc., aloe, ant-c., ***arg-n.,*** arn., ars., bar-c., ***bell.,*** bov., ***bry.,*** calc-p., caps., ***carb-an.,*** chel., **CHIN.,** cocc., con., daph., euph., gels., hell., hyper., ign., kali-bi., kali-i., kali-n., lach., lil-t., ***lyc., merc., mez.,*** nat-m., nux-m., ***nux-v.,*** par., ***prun.,*** puls., ran-b., rhus-t., sabad., sabin., samb., ***sep., sil.,*** spig., ***stann., staph.,*** stront-c., tarax., ***thuj.,*** zinc.
band, as if by - ***carb-ac.,*** clem., cocc., ***gels.,*** glon., iod., ip., ***merc., mosch., nit-ac.,*** op., osm., ***spig., stann.,*** **SULPH.**
bed, while in - kalm., nat-s., ol-an., pip-m., ran-b., rhus-t., sulph.
bending, backward, agg. - mang.
backward, amel. - ***bell.,*** ph-ac., thuj.
head forward, on - bell., ferr-p., nat-m., ph-ac.
binding, up the head amel - ***arg-n.***
blowing, nose agg. - chel.
boards, as if compressed by two - ip.
breakfast, after - chel., hydr., sars.
amel. - bov., ***psor.***
burning - aloe, alum., lact., mang., nux-m., sep., sul-ac., tarax.
cap, like a - apis, ***arg-n.,*** asaf., berb., ***carb-v., cocc.,*** coc-c., crot-c., ***cycl., graph.,*** hell., ip., ***lil-t.,*** peti., pyrog., stry., sulph., zinc.
changeable - bell., gins., ***ign.***
chill, during - sep., tarent.
with coldness all over - camph., stann.
closing, eyes amel. - chel.
coffee, after - arum-t., nat-s.
cold, application amel. - ***phos.***
company, while in - lyc., mag-c.
congestion, as from - apis, chin., dig., merl., nux-m., rhus-v.
constipation, during - jatr.
constricting - ***cocc.,*** graph.
coughing, while - acon., alumn., ambr., anac., ***arn.,*** brom., **BRY.,** chel., coc-c., con., hep., kreos., nit-ac., petr., phos., ruta, sars., sep., spig., verb.
covered, pressing with distress, while - ***led.***
cramp-like - ars., colch., ph-ac., ***plat.,*** ran-s., zinc.
darkness, in - sil.

PRESSING, pain
deep-seated - agar., ***arg-n., bell.,*** caust., cic., con., gins., indg., lach., nat-m., nat-s.
descending, on - meny.
digging - bry., clem.
dinner, during - pall.
after - agar., alum., alumn., calc., carb-an., chin., ol-an., ruta., seneg., tab., thuj., ***zinc.***
downward - agar., ambr., ant-t., asar., cic., ***cina,*** cocc., con., ***cupr.,*** hura, laur., mang., meny., merc., merc-i-f., mur-ac., nit-ac., nux-v., ***ph-ac., phos.,*** plat., rhus-t., senn., sil., spig., spong., ***sulph.,*** verat.
drawing - agar., ang., ant-c., ant-t., arg-m., ars., asaf., aur., carb-v., caust., coff., hell., hep., ign., iod., kali-c., mosch., nat-c., nit-ac., olnd., ran-b., ran-s., ***rhod.,*** rhus-t., sabad., sars., spig., stann., staph., tarax., thuj.
drinking, agg. - cocc., merc.
dull - aloe, apis, canth., cimic., con., ferr., hydr-ac., lith., op., phys.
eating, while - graph.
after - alumn., calc., carb-an., carb-v., clem., ***cocc.,*** con., graph., hydr., hyos., kali-c., lyc., nat-m., nat-s., ol-an., pip-m., ran-b., ruta., sep., tab., thuj., zinc.
amel. - psor.
evening - acon., agar., alum., ambr., ***anac.,*** arg-n., ars., cast., cham., chel., coc-c., colch., coloc., dig., dios., dulc., ferr., fl-ac., hell., hydr-ac., hyper., kali-bi., kali-n., kalm., ***lyss.,*** mag-m., mag-s., mang., nat-c., nat-m., nat-s., ol-an., phos., plat., rhod., ***rhus-t.,*** ruta, sep., staph., **SULPH.,** tab., tarent., thuj., valer., ***zinc.***
amel. - ran-b.
in bed - carb-v.
lying down, after - stann.
sunset, after - nat-s.
walking, while - dulc.
excitement, after - chin-s.
exertion, agg. - **BELL.,** ***hell., nat-c.***
extending, to eyes - sil.
to forehead, left - ph-ac.
to neck, nape of - kali-c., lyc.
eyes, from using - gent-c., helon.
fever, during - ruta, sep.
forward - asar., ***bry.,*** nit-ac., sil., sulph.
gnawing - ***ran-s.***
scalp - hyos.
hat, as from a tight hat - sulph.
pressure of - ***calc-p., carb-v.,*** **NIT-AC.,** phys., sep., sulph.
hay-fever, with - sabad.
head, high amel. - ***spig.***
heated, when - am-c.
hiccough, during - ***bry.***
hot, things, from - ***arum-t.***
increasing and decreasing slowly - ***stann.***
intermittent - ph-ac., sulph.

PRESSING, pain
inward - ***alum., anac.,*** asar., bov., calc., cham., ***cocc.,*** coff., ***dulc.,*** graph., ***hell.,*** ign., merc., nit-ac., olnd., petr., ph-ac., ***plat., ran-s.,*** sabad., sep., sil., spig., stann., staph., zing.
sharp corners, as if by - cham.
jerk-like, pressing - dig.
knots, as from - phos.
light, agg. - cann-i.
looking, steadily - helon., ***puls.***
lying, while - glon., lach., ***lyc.,*** merc., nat-s., nux-v., **TARAX.**
side, on - bar-c., calad.
menses, during - acon., bell., berb., ***bry.,*** cast., ***cimic.,*** cycl., eupi., ***gels., graph.,*** iod., **KREOS.,** lyc., merc., ***nat-m.,*** nat-s., nux-m., nux-v., plat., ***sep.,*** sil., stann., ***sulph.***
after - ust.
before - bell., cimic., hep., ***nat-m.,*** nux-v., petr., sep., sil.
mental, exertion, from - anac., ***arg-n.,*** arn., asar., ***cact., calc.,*** calc-s., ***carb-an.,*** cham., ***cocc.,*** coff., colch., dig., helon., ign., kali-c., ***lyc., mag-c.,*** mez., **NAT-C.,** nat-s., ***nux-v.,*** ol-an., par., ***ph-ac.,*** **PIC-AC.,** ***sep.,*** sil., ***sulph.,*** ter.
attention is concentrated, while - helon.
reading, while - **BELL.,** ***cocc.,*** helon., ***lyc.***
morning - ***acon.,*** agar., alumn., ambr., arg-n., asaf., benz-ac., bor., bov., ***bry.,*** cann-s., caust., cedr., ***cham.,*** chin., cimic., coloc., ***con.,*** croc., cycl., dig., gamb., glon., ***graph.,*** kali-bi., kali-n., **LACH.,** lyc., mez., myric., nat-c., nat-m., nat-s., nicc., ***nux-v.,*** paeon., ***petr.,*** ph-ac., phos., pip-m., psor., puls., rhus-t., ***sil.,*** sulph., thuj.
3-4 a.m. - thuj.
rising, after - calc., ruta.
rising, on - cinnb., graph., **LACH.,** lyc., mag-c., ox-ac., psor., sabin., squil., **SULPH.**
waking, on - agar., alumn., anac., arg-n., bell., coc-c., ***con.,*** ferr., gels., ***graph.,*** hep., mez., **NAT-M.,** ol-an., ph-ac., zinc.
motion, on - acon., agn., ***arg-n.,*** **BELL.,** bism., **BRY.,** ***calc.,*** carb-v., cocc., cupr., dulc., ferr-p., glon., ***hell.,*** hyper., lach., mang., mez., nat-s., ph-ac., phos., pic-ac., rhod., ***spig.,*** sulph., thuj.
amel. - ***agar., ferr.,*** op., pip-m., sulph., ***valer.***
arms, of - rhus-t.
eyes of - ***bell., chel.,*** hep., ***puls.***
head, of the - coloc., ***glon.,*** nat-s., staph.
head, of the - while walking - ars.
muscles of face - ***spig.***
open air, in, amel. - acon.
night - ambr., guai., hep., lyc., mang., nit-ac., nux-v., ***sil.,*** sulph.
2 a.m. - ars.

PRESSING, pain
night, waking, on - canth., mang., nat-c., plat., ***psor.***
noise, agg. - ***nit-ac.,*** ph-ac., spig.
noon - agar., cedr., kali-n., manc., sil., ***sulph.,*** zinc.
sleep, after - calad.
toward, amel. - bry., nat-m.
nosebleed, before - ***carb-an.***
opening eyes, after sleep - rhus-t.
outward - ***acon.,*** agar., ***am-c.,*** anac., arg-n., ***arn.,*** ars., **ASAF.,** asar., ***bell.,*** berb., ***bry.,*** calc., camph., carb-ac., ***carb-an.,*** chel., cimic., cob., coloc., con., ***cor-r.,*** dros., dulc., euph., ferr., ferr-ar., ferr-p., fl-ac., glon., ***hell.,*** hep., hyper., ign., indg., kali-ar., kali-c., ***kreos.,*** **LACH.,** laur., lil-t., lyc., meny., ***merc.,*** **NAT-M.,** nux-m., ***olnd.,*** par., ***ph-ac.,*** phys., phyt., pic-ac., ***prun.,*** psor., ptel., ran-s., rhod., sabad., sabin., samb., ***sep., sil.,*** spig., spong., stann., staph., sulph., tarax., thuj., zinc.
contents would be forced out, as if - lil-t.
sharp instrument, as if by a - prun.
paralytic - nat-c.
paroxysmal - agar., carb-v., cham., ign., **LACH.,** ter.
part, lain on - ph-ac.
perspiration, amel. - thuj.
pressure, amel. - alum., alumn., ***arg-n.,*** asaf., ***cact.,*** chin., dios., ***hell.,*** lach., ***meny.,*** merc., nat-m., nat-s., ***nux-v.,*** op., ***puls.,*** pyrog., sang., stann., thuj.
upon the floor, desires - sang.
pulsating - arn., ***bry., chin.,*** **PULS.,** ***ruta.,*** verat.
pulse, synchronous, with - hell.
raising eyes - ***bry.***
reading, while - agn., bell., ***cocc.,*** hell., lyc.
rhythmical - ruta.
riding in a carriage - cocc., ***nit-ac.***
rising, on - apis, asaf., bell., cinnb., glon., mag-s., nit-ac., ***spig.***
after, amel. - laur., ran-b., stann.
stooping, from - lyc.
room, in - am-m., coc-c., laur., **LYC.,** mag-c., ***nat-m., nat-s., phos.,*** **PULS.,** sulph.
amel. - ***chin., hep.,*** merc., valer.
crowded - mag-c.
entering, on - bov.
warm - acon., **APIS,** cann-i., ***coc-c.,*** **PULS.**
rubbing, amel. - op., ph-ac., phos.
running, amel. - hipp.
shaking, on - **BELL., BRY.,** ***chin.,*** coloc., ferr-p., **GLON.**
sitting, while - agar., alum., ***bry.,*** benz-ac., fl-ac., **LACH.**
amel. - asar., **BELL.,** calad., pic-ac.
erect, while - mang.
up in bed amel. - **BELL.,** canth.

PRESSING, pain
sleep, agg. - ***arg-n., bry.,*** calad., cocc., **LACH.,** merc., nat-m., rhus-t., thuj., tarent., ***verat.***
amel. - thuj.
siesta, after, agg. - calad.
sleeping, on the affected left side while - caust.
smoking, from - ***calad.,*** mag-c.
sneezing, after - apis, cina.
spots, in - asar., acon., ***bell.,*** cic., con., dig., dulc., ign., glon., meph., nit-ac., nux-v., ox-ac., ph-ac., psor., thuj., zinc.
standing - alum., staph.
stepping, agg. - **BELL.,** ***bry.,*** coc-c., ***glon.,*** hell., lyc.
stool, during - coloc., gran., merc.
after - ***lyc.,*** sil., spig.
before - merc.
stooping, on - ***bell., bry., calc.,*** canth., carb-v., cham., chel., coloc., fl-ac., hep., lyc., mag-m., merc., merc-c., par., petr., phos., ***puls.,*** sil., ***spig.,*** stann., thuj., zing.
amel. - caust., mang.
compelled to stoop - cann-i., ign.
sun, in, passes off in shade - brom.
supper, after - carb-v., ran-b.
talking, loudly, from - spig.
tea, after warm, amel. - glon.
thinking, of it - cham., cocc., dig., ***helon.***
turning, eyes sideways - ***sil.***
toward affected side - con.
upward - fl-ac., guai., meph., ph-ac., spig.
vise, as if in a - aeth., agar., ***alum.,*** am-c., am-m., ant-t., ***arg-n.,*** aster., atro., ***bar-c.,*** bov., bry., ***cact.,*** cadm-s., carb-v., caust., chel., chin., cina, clem., ***cocc.,*** daph., euph., ***glon.,*** graph., grat., hell., lyc., mag-c., mag-s., **MERC.,** ***nat-m.,*** nicc., **NIT-AC.,** olnd., op., petr., **PLAT.,** ***puls.,*** ran-b., ran-s., rat., rhus-t., sabad., sars., spig., stann., sulph., sul-ac., ***tarent.***
open air, amel. - caust.
vomiting, amel. - stann.
walking, while - alum., arn., ars., ***asar., bell., bry.,*** calc., caust., ***chin.,*** clem., cocc., kali-c., **LACH.,** lyc., nat-m.
in open air, while - agar., **BELL.,** chin., con., dulc., ferr., glon., hell., lil-t., staph., thuj.
wandering - graph., ***ign.***
washing, after amel. - ferr., phos., ***psor.***
cold amel. - euphr.
weight, as from - agar., alum., alumn., ars., bell., ***bism.,*** cact., cann-s., carb-v., ***cina,*** cupr., laur., led., **MENY.,** merc-i-r., ***mosch., nit-ac., nux-v.,*** ph-ac., plat., ***rhus-t.,*** sars., sil., ***spig.,*** sulph., squil., ***thuj.,*** verat.
wet, weather agg. - sulph.
wrapping, up head amel. - kali-c.
writing, while - bor., carb-an., ferr-i., gent-l., ign., kali-c., nat-c.

pressing, forehead - **ACON.,** ***aesc., aeth., agar.,*** agn., **ALOE,** alum., alumn., ambr., ***am-c.,*** am-m., ammc., ***anac.,*** ang., ant-c., ***ant-t.,*** **APIS,** ***arg-m., arg-n., arn., ars., ars-i.,*** **ASAF.,** asar., aster., ***aur.,*** bapt., ***bar-c.,*** bar-m., **BELL.,** ***berb., bism.,*** bor., bov., ***brom.,*** **BRY.,** cact., calad., ***calc.,*** camph., cann-i., cann-s., canth., caps., carb-an., carb-s., carb-v., cast., ***caust., cedr., cham., chel.,*** chim-m., ***chin.,*** chin-a., cic., cimic., cina, ***cinnb.,*** clem., ***cocc., coc-c.,*** coff., colch., ***coloc.,*** con., cop., ***cor-r.,*** croc., crot-t., cupr., ***cycl., dig., dros.,*** dulc., elaps, ***euph.,*** euphr., eupi., ***ferr., ferr-ar., ferr-i., ferr-p.,*** fl-ac., gels., gent-l., gent-c., gins., ***glon.,*** gran., graph., grat., guai., ham., hell., hydr-ac., ***hyos.,*** hura, ***ign.,*** indg., ***iod.,*** ip., iris, jatr., kali-ar., kali-bi., ***kali-c.,*** kali-i., ***kali-n., kali-p., kalm., kreos.,*** lac-c., **LACH.,** lachn., lact., laur., led., lept., lil-t., ***lyc.,*** lycps., lyss., ***mag-c., mag-m.,*** manc., mang., meny., ***merc., mez.,*** mosch., ***mur-ac.,*** naja, ***nat-a., nat-c., nat-m., nat-p., nat-s., nit-ac.,*** nux-m., **NUX-V.,** ***ol-an., olnd., op.,*** osm., ***ox-ac., par.,*** petr., ***ph-ac.,*** **PHOS., PHYT.,** pip-m., ***plat.,*** plb., plect., prun., ***psor.,*** ptel., ***puls., ran-b.,*** raph., rheum, ***rhod.,*** rhus-t., ruta., sabad., ***sabin.,*** samb., ***sang., sars., seneg., sep., sil., sol-n., spig., spong.,*** squil., ***stann., staph., stict.,*** stram., stront-c., **SULPH.,** sul-ac., tarax., tarent., teucr., thea., ***ther.,*** thuj., til., ust., ***valer.,*** verat., verb., vinc., viol-t., ***zinc.***

above - ***aloe,*** arg-n., chin., coloc., con., dig., dulc., ***iod.,*** nat-m., ***olnd., par.,*** sep., ***sil.***

afternoon - ***aloe,*** carb-v., chin., ***kali-c.,*** nit-ac., ran-b., senec., sulph.

1 p.m. - fl-ac.

air, open - ***bell.,*** calc., caust., ***glon.,*** laur., mang., rhus-t., valer.

amel. - ***alum.,*** **APIS,** brom., ferr-i., ***nat-c., phos., sabin.,*** seneg., sep., tarax.

alternating, with expansion - tarax.

alternating, with stitching - **VALER.**

ascending, steps - ang., arn., **BELL.,** meny.

backward - dios., spong., tab.

ball, as from - **BELL.,** con., mag-s., **STAPH.**

band, as from - ***aeth., ant-t., carb-ac.,*** carb-v., cedr., **CHEL.,** coca, con., helon., indg., iod., iris, kali-p., ***lac-c.,*** lil-t., ***merc.,*** mill., **SULPH.,** tarent.

closing eyes amel. - ***chel.***

laughing, when - iris.

bed, in - ran-b.

bending head, backward - chin., stann.

backward, amel. - ***bell., ign.***

down, on - nat-m., ***coloc.***

chill, during - ***ars.,*** cham., sep.

close, the eyes, compelled to - **BELL.,** calc., carb-v., ***nat-m.,*** nux-v., plat.

closing, eyes amel - ***chel., nat-m.***

cold, air agg. - ***nux-v.***

cold applications amel. - ***ant-t., apis, ars.,*** calc., **PHOS.**

pressing, forehead

company, agg. - ***plb.***

coughing, on - acon., alum., arn., bell., brom., bry., chel., con., hep., kreos., nit-ac., phos., ruta., sars., sep., spong., verb.

cramp-like - **PLAT.**

crowded, room - ***mag-c., plat.***

daytime - mag-c., op., ***phos.,*** sil., **STICT.**

descending, steps - ***ferr.,*** meny.

dinner, after - ***alum.,*** calc., con., kali-bi., plat., sars., seneg., zinc.

downward - ***aloe,*** ambr., am-m., ant-t., ***asar.,*** bell., bry., cina, cocc., ***glon.,*** mur-ac., ***par.,*** **PHOS.,** ph-ac., rhus-t., sabin.

dull, point, as with a - caust.

eating, after - ***am-c.,*** carl., clem., ***cocc.,*** con., graph., nat-m., nat-s.

eating, after, amel. - chel., kali-p., psor.

eating, while - lyc.

evening - ***acon.,*** alum., anac., ang., cast., coff., coloc., dig., dulc., kalm., kali-c., mag-m., mang., nat-m., ***nat-s., ph-ac.,*** phos., **PULS.,** ran-b., sep., ***sulph.,*** tab., thuj., valer., ***zinc.***

excitement - par.

exercise, after - nat-c.

extending, downward - ***bry.,*** chin-s., merc.

eyes, to - asar., bell., carb-s., carb-v., caust., ***chel.,*** ign., kali-bi., kali-c., kali-n., laur., mur-ac., nux-m., op., ***phos.,*** samb.

inward - agar., graph., laur.

neck, to - bor., chel., spong.

nose, to - agar., aloe, am-m., ***calc.,*** kali-c., lyc., mez., ph-ac., ***phos.***

occiput, to - anac., bry., ***cann-s.,*** chel., coc-c., lyc., par., spong., thuj.

outward - aloe, anac., asaf., bar-c., eupi., hell., lact., prun., psor., ***spig., stann.,*** staph.

side of head - indg.

temples, to - ***carb-s.,*** chel., gran., sep.

temples, to, on bending backwards - chin.

vertex, to - glon., kreos., lyc., puls.

eyes, over - ***acon.,*** aeth., agar., **ALOE,** alum., alumn., am-c., ***anac.,*** ang., ant-c., apis, arg-m., arg-n., arn., ars., ars-i., asaf., aster., bar-c., ***bell., bism.,*** bor., bov., brom., **BRY.,** calc., ***calc-p.,*** cann-i., carb-an., carb-s., ***carb-v., card-m.,*** caust., ***chel.,*** chin., chin-a., cist., con., ***crot-h.,*** dig., dros., dulc., euph., eupi., euon., fl-ac., ***glon.,*** grat., gymn., haem., hep., ***ign.,*** indg., iod., ***kali-ar., kali-c.,*** kali-n., kali-p., kalm., kreos., lach., lil-t., lith., lyc., lyss., mag-c., merc., merc-c., merc-i-r., merl., mez., morph., **NAT-M.,** ***nat-p.,*** nat-s., nit-ac., ***nux-m., nux-v.,*** op., paeon., petr., ph-ac., ***phos.,*** phyt., pic-ac., plan., plect., **PULS.,** rheum, ***rhus-t.,*** ruta., sabad., sant., seneg., sep., ***sil.,*** sol-t-ae., spig., spong., stann., staph., stront-c., ***sulph.,*** tab., teucr., ther., thuj.,

pressing, forehead

eyes, over - urt-u., ***valer.,*** zinc., zing.

afternoon - ***acon.,*** cann-i., carb-v., ph-ac., sulph.

air, in open - staph.

close the eyes, compelled to - nux-v.

closing the eyes, amel. - ip.

daytime - sep.

dinner, after - phos.

evening - camph., iod.

extending, eyes, into - con.

extending, nose, to - bov.

extending, outward - sec.

eyes would be forced out, as if - cocc., gymn., ign., lachn., nat-m., phos., sabin., seneg., sep., sil., tarent.

left - ***acon.,*** arg-m., bry., camph., cupr., mur-ac., ***nux-v.,*** phos., ***sep.,*** sulph., ***ther., thuj.,*** verb.

left, extending to right - thuj.

light by - sep.

margin of orbits to temples, from - cann-s.

menses, before - sep.

menses, during - lac-c.

morning - alumn., kali-n., lach., mag-c., petr., sulph.

morning, waking, on - alumn.

motion agg. - **BRY.,** ***sep.***

opening eyes agg. - sil.

outward - ang., bell., ip., kali-c., lyc., phos.

pressing down upon the eyes - arg-m., bell., hell., ***hep., phos.,*** plat., sabin., spig., zinc.

pressive pain above left eye, followed by a dull, pressive pain in occipital protuberances, thence spreading over whole body, on quick motion and after eating, pain so severe that it seemed a distinct pulsation in head - ***bry.***

pressure amel. - apis., ip.

pressure so severe, when rising, could only half open eyes, could not look up - stram.

raising, eyebrow agg. - nat-m.

right - am-m., ant-c., caust., ***chel.,*** con., dulc., ***ign.,*** nat-m., plat., rhus-t., ***sang.,*** sil., spig., spong., staph., thuj., urt-u., zinc.

right, upward and inward - bism.

stooping agg. - merc-c., spong., teucr.

stunning - plat.

walking after - con.

walking in open air - ***sep.***

wavelike - plat.

fever, during - ars., glon., thuj.

fingers, as from a - ol-an., stront.

forenoon - cocc., mag-c., mag-m., nat-c., nat-m., nat-s., nicc., sars., sulph., zinc.

10 a.m. - nat-m.

menses, during - sulph.

forward - hydr., laur., mag-s., nux-m., rhus-t.

pressing, forehead

frontal eminence - agar., ambr., anac., arg-m., ***arg-n.,*** asaf., bar-c., bell., brom., calc., ***caust.,*** cham., chin., cimx., croc., cupr., dulc., ***ferr.,*** ferr-p., gins., gran., guai., nit-ac., olnd., op., osm., par., ph-ac., plat., raph., sabad., ***sabin.,*** sars., ***spig.,*** spong., stann., sumb., thuj., verb., zinc.

afternoon, 3 p.m. - bry.

air, open, in - ran-b.

air, open, in, amel. - ***ferr.***

close the eyes, compelled to - calc.

descending steps agg. - ***ferr.***

dinner, after - zinc.

evening - dulc.

extending, eye, to - thuj.

extending, occiput, to - spig.

extending, outward - anac., ph-ac., prun., spig., spong., staph.

extending, right eye, to - calc.

extending, vertex - ***ferr.***

left - agar., ambr., gran., ***nux-m.,*** squil., staph., thuj.

morning - ***ferr.***

morning, rising, after - ***ferr.***

night - anac., calc., ***caust.,*** ph-ac., spong., zinc.

night, midnight - sulph.

pressure amel. - ***ferr.,*** op.

right - ***caust.,*** hell., mez., ph-ac., ***sabin.,*** spong., zinc.

rubbing amel. - op.

sitting, while - spong.

studying agg. - cham.

touch agg. - ***chin.***

walking in open air - dulc., hell.

warm room, on entering - spong., verb.

frontal, sinus - mag-m.

hand, lying on part amel. - meny.

hat, as from a tight - ***alum.***

hiccough, from - ***bry.***

house, in, agg. - ***apis,*** cact.

intermittent - arn., hyos., plat.

inward - agar., aloe, alum., anac., ant-c., bapt., bell., brom., calc., cocc., croc., ferr., hell., hep., ***kali-c.,*** laur., mosch., ***nux-v.,*** olnd., ***plat.,*** ran-s., rhod., rhus-t., sep., spig., **STANN.,** staph., sulph., verb., zinc.

jarring, agg. - acon., ***bry., bell.,*** glon., ***spig., sulph.***

left, sides - agn., ambr., ant-c., ant-t., arg-m., asaf., ***aur.,*** camph., cann-s., caust., cic., cina, coloc., crot-t., euph., ign., ***iod.,*** kali-n., mag-c., merc., mur-ac., nat-c., nat-m., nux-m., ***nux-v., ph-ac.,*** plat., ran-b., ***rhod.,*** sabin., **SARS.,** seneg., spong., squil., staph., teucr.

light, agg. - cact.

looking, intently - puls., spong.

lying, amel. - ***bell.,*** nat-m., nat-s.

back, on - ***coloc.***

back, on, amel. - ***nux-v., spong.***

menses, during - cast., lac-c., lyc., nux-v., ***sep., sil., sulph.***

after - ***ferr.***

pressing, forehead
menses, before - ign., ***sil.***
mental exertion, from - anac., arn., asar., bor., cocc., ***dig.***, ***mag-c.***, mez., ***nat-c.***, ***nat-s.***, petr., ph-ac., ***psor.***, sabad., ***sil.***
morning - agar., ambr., am-m., ant-t., bor., brom., calc., caust., lyc., mez., nat-c., ***nat-m.***, ***nat-s.***, nit-ac., ***nux-v.***, pic-ac., ***psor.***, ran-b., ***sabin.***, ***sil.***, **SULPH.**, ***ther.***, zinc.
rising, after, amel. - ***ran-b.***
rising, on and after - calc-ac., graph., nat-c., sil., spig., sulph.
waking on - agar., anac., ant-t., arg-n., gels., mag-c., mag-m., mez., ***nat-m.***, ol-an., ***ph-ac.***, ***spig.***, ***sulph.***, zinc.
motion, on - ant-t., **BELL.**, ***bism.***, ***bry.***, carb-v., cocc., cupr., dulc., graph., kali-c., nat-s., par., ph-ac., sep., ***spig.***, spong., staph., sulph., ***ther.***
amel. - ***cic.***, psor., valer.
arms, of, violent - rhus-t.
eyelids, of - coloc.
eyes, of - ***chel.***, dulc., ph-ac., ***puls.***
head, of - lyss., plat., staph.
muscles - bell.
narrow, as if too - gels.
night, waking, on - canth., ***sil.***
noise, agg. - **BELL.**, cact.
noon - gent-l., ***sulph.***, zinc.
nose, above - ***acon.***, aesc., aeth., ambr., am-m., ant-t., arn., asar., ***bapt.***, bar-c., ***bell.***, bism., bov., brom., camph., cann-s., **CARB-AC.**, carb-v., chel., chin., ***cimic.***, ***cist.***, ***coloc.***, euphr., glon., ham., helon., hep., hydr., ***ign.***, iod., kali-n., manc., meny., merc., mez., mosch., ph-ac., raph., ruta, sil., spong., ***stict.***, tarax., til., verb., viol-t., zinc., zing.
cold, amel. - euphr.
morning - sil.
pressing upon eyelids - chel.
opening the eyes - ***ars.***, ph-ac.
opening the eyes, hindering - bell.
orbits, margin of - anac., hyos., spig.
to temple from - cann-s., chin.
outward - **ACON.**, aloe, alum., all-c., ***am-c.***, anac., ang., arg-n., ***arn.***, **ASAF.**, ***bar-c.***, bar-m., ***bell.***, benz-ac., ***berb.***, brom., ***bry.***, calc., ***camph.***, cann-i., cann-s., canth., ***caps.***, carb-v., cast., caust., chel., ***chin.***, cic., cimx., cina, colch., ***coloc.***, con., ***cor-r.***, cupr., ***dros.***, dulc., ***ferr.***, graph., hell., hep., ip., ***kali-c.***, ***kali-p.***, ***kreos.***, **LACH.**, lact., ***lil-t.***, lyc., lyss., mag-m., mag-s., mang., med., meny., merc., mez., mur-ac., nat-c., nat-m., nat-p., ***nux-m.***, nux-v., ***olnd.***, op., ph-ac., ***phos.***, plat., prun., ***psor.***, ptel., ***puls.***, ran-b., rat., rhod., rhus-t., sabad., senec., ***sep.***, ***sil.***, **SPIG.**, ***spong.***, ***stann.***, staph., ***stront-c.***, ***sulph.***, sul-ac., tarax., teucr., thea., thuj., ***verb.***, viol-t.

pressing, forehead
outward, brain would come out, as though - acon., all-c., am-c., ang., arn., **BELL.**, brom., ***bry.***, canth., carb-v., caust., chel., colch., coloc., ***kali-c.***, kreos., **LACH.**, mag-m., mag-s., mang., med., mez., nat-c., nux-v., ***phos.***, plat., puls., rat., rhod., sabad., sep., ***sil.***, spig., spong., stann., staph., stront-c., sul-ac., thuj., verb.
eyes would spring out, as if - kali-n.
paroxysmal - mur-ac., plat., sep., verat., zinc.
pressure, amel - am-c., ***arg-n.***, calc., chin., mur-ac., ***nat-m.***, ***nat-s.***, ***spig.***, stann.
on temple, from - calc.
raising, the head - bar-ac.
reading, while - arn., bor., ***calc.***, carb-s., cocc., ***nat-m.***
riding - **COCC.**
right, sides - anac., arg-n., arn., ***ars.***, asaf., ***bell.***, ***caust.***, **CHEL.**, ***chin.***, coc-c., crot-h., euph., ferr-i., guai., hell., ign., iod., ***kali-c.***, kali-n., meny., merc., mez., mosch., nat-s., ***nux-v.***, par., phos., ***plat.***, rhus-t., ruta., sabin., ***sars.***, ***spig.***, stann., ***staph.***, sul-ac., teucr., thuj., valer., verb., viol-t.
then left - colch.
to left temple - cycl.
to left and back to right - cycl.
to occiput - kali-n.
rising, on - asaf., ***bell.***, mag-s., ***spig.***, ***stram.***
amel. - spong.
room, in - ***acon.***, brom., nat-c.
shaking, the head - sep.
sides - agar., alum., ang., chel., chin., cina, ign., lyc., spig., ruta, verb.
extending to back - spong.
sitting, while - agar., alum., ***spong.***
amel. - ***bell.***
smoking - calad., coloc., ***mag-c.***
sneezing, after - apis
spots - **NUX-M.**, psor., ***zinc.***
standing, while - **ALUM.**, sang., staph.
stool, during - ***bry.***, coloc., ***nux-v.***, rat., ***spig.***
after - sep., spig.
stooping, while - acon., arg-n., ***bell.***, bor., **BRY.**, calc., canth., carb-s., carb-v., caust., chel., ***coloc.***, cupr., fl-ac., kreos., kali-n., lyss., mag-m., merc., nat-c., ***par.***, plat., sep., sil., ***spig.***, spong., stann., staph.
after - hyos.
amel. - bar-c., bell., caust., con., verb.
sudden - ther.
supper, after - nat-m., ran-b.
talking, after - sil., ther., thuj.
thinking, of it - nat-s.
touch, amel. - cycl., mur-ac.
uncovering, body amel. - cor-r.
upward - glon., nit-ac., valer.
waking, on - agar., anac., ant-t., arg-n., cina, gels., mez., ***nat-m.***, ol-an., ***ph-ac.***, rhus-t., sulph., thuj., zinc.

pressing, forehead
walking, while - anac., arg-n., ***arn., bry.,*** calc., caust., clem., ***chin.,*** cocc., ***kali-c.,*** nat-m., ***spig.***
air, in open - am-c., arg-n., **BELL.,** calc., caust., ***chin., cocc.,*** dulc., nat-m., plat.
air, in open, amel. - bor., calc., cor-r., ***sang., sep.***
rapidly - caust.
warm, room - acon., **APIS,** ferr-i., ***plat.,*** ran-b.
room, amel. - am-c.
stove agg. - ***apis, arn.***
weight, of hat - carb-v.
weight or stone, as if - acon., am-m., aur., bell., cham., con., dig., ***glon.,*** kali-c., ***nat-m., par.,*** rhus-t., sep., spig., tarax.
sinking weight, as a - thuj.
writing, while - bor., kali-c., lyc.

pressing, occiput - acon., ***agar.,*** all-c., ***aloe, alum.,*** ambr., ammc., am-m., anac., ant-t., apis, ***arg-m.,*** arn., ***ars., ars-i.,*** asaf., asar., aur., bapt., bar-c., ***bell.,*** berb., ***bism.,*** bor., ***bov., bry.,*** cact., ***calc.,*** calc-p., camph., cann-i., cann-s., canth., carb-ac., carb-an., **CARB-S., CARB-V.,** card-m., caust., cedr., cham., ***chel., chin.,*** chin-a., cic., cinnb., cocc., coc-c., ***colch.,*** coloc., con., cop., croc., ***crot-c.,*** cupr., dig., ***dulc., euph.,*** fl-ac., ***gels.,*** gent-l., gins., glon., **GRAPH.,** grat., guai., ***hell., hep.,*** hydr-ac., ***hyper., ign., iod., ip.,*** jatr., kali-bi., ***kali-c.,*** kali-n., kali-p., lach., laur., lec., lob., ***lyc.,*** mag-c., ***mag-m.,*** mag-s., manc., mang., meny., meph., ***merc., mez.,*** mosch., ***nat-a., nat-m., nat-p., nat-s., nit-ac.,*** nux-m., **NUX-V.,** ol-an., ***onos., op.,*** ox-ac., paeon., par., **PETR.,** phel., ph-ac., ***phos.,*** pip-m., plb., puls., ran-b., ran-s., rhod., ***rhus-t.,*** ruta., sabad., sabin., sars., **SEC.,** sel., seneg., ***sep.,*** **SIL.,** ***spig., spong.,*** squil., ***stann., staph.,*** stram., stront-c., ***sulph.,*** sul-ac., tab., ***tarax., tarent.,*** teucr., ***thuj.,*** til., valer., verb., zinc., zing.
afternoon - ang., gent-l., iod.
1 p.m. - mang.
air, open, agg. - iod., nux-m., plect.
amel. - ***all-c.,*** carb-an., ***carb-v.,*** kali-c., mag-m., mag-s., mez., puls.
anger, after - ***petr., staph.***
asunder - aloe, ***calc.,*** nux-v., staph.
band, as from - anac., psor., sulph.
bending head, backward amel. - ph-ac.
forward - staph.
burning - mang.
closing eyes agg. - ip.
coughing - alum.
dinner, after - agar., con.
downward - hydr-ac., merl.
eating, after - carb-v.
amel. - kali-p.
evening - anac., coc-c., mez., rhod., sep., stann., staph., thuj.
until midnight - sep.
walking in open air - thuj.
warm room - coc-c.

pressing, occiput
exercise, mental or physical, amel. - cact.
extending, downward - hep., hydr-ac., laur., nat-c.
eyes, to - ***carb-v.***
forehead, to - ambr., aur., ***calc.,*** camph., carb-v., fl-ac., mang., mez., mur-ac.
forward - ant-t., bov., ***chel.,*** hydr-ac., mang., nat-c., ph-ac., sabad.
into back and chest at noon - ***graph.***
neck, to - calc., ***graph.,*** hep., laur., nat-c., nux-v.
outward - mez., ph-ac.
shoulders, to - hep., ip.
side, to - asar.
teeth, to - ferr.
upward - all-c., ambr., onos., puls., staph.
vertex, to - bov., carb-an., dig., glon.
fever, during - rhus-t.
forenoon - bov., caust., iod., kali-bi., nat-c.
forward - chel., mang., nux-v., ol-an., ph-ac., plb., sabad.
hand, laying on part, amel. - mang.
hard, as if lying on something - ph-ac.
hat, as from a tight hat - ***alum.***
holding head erect amel. - spong.
intermittent - carb-an., phel.
inward - bar-c., calc., ign., mag-c., meph., olnd., ox-ac., ph-ac., sep., spig., stann., ***staph.,*** stront-c., thuj.
between vertex and occiput - ox-ac.
looking up - ***graph.***
laying, as if, on something hard - ph-ac.
left, sides - calc., ***chel.,*** dulc., lyc., mez., sep., stann., sulph., sul-ac., zinc.
lying, down, after - **TARAX.**
on back - plect.
menses, during - ***nux-v.***
mental exertion - ***carb-ac., colch.,*** nat-c.
morning - caust., cedr., ***graph.,*** hell., kali-bi., mag-s., nux-m., ***nux-v.,*** paeon., ***petr.,*** sil., ***sulph.***
waking, on - coc-c., kali-bi., ***sulph.***
motion - ***bism.,*** **BRY.,** colch., cupr., ***hyper.,*** iod., ip., nat-s., ph-ac., spong.
of head - mez.
night - ***sulph.***
noise agg. - ***carb-v., nit-ac.,*** ph-ac., ***spig.***
outward - bell., berb., bry., ***calc.,*** carb-v., chin., ***gels.,*** mez., ph-ac., prun., stann., ***staph.,*** stront-c., til.
paroxysmal - zinc.
pressure amel. - **NUX-V.**
pulsating - kali-n., mosch., peti., sulph., zinc.
reading - carb-ac.
right, sides - anac., aur., ***calc.,*** carb-v., caust., dig., hep., lyc., nat-c., ph-ac., ***rhod.,*** seneg., sep., ***spig.,*** verb.
extending to left - dig.
extending to scapula - hep.
rising from bed - cinnb.
rubbing amel. - ph-ac., ***phos.***

pressing, occiput
sides - anac., asar., aur., bov., bry., calc., camph., carb-an., carb-v., cast., caust., ***chel.,*** colch., con., crot-t., dig., **FL-AC.,** glon., ign., hydr-ac., ***laur.,*** mag-s., mez., nat-c., nat-p., ***nat-s.,*** nux-v., ph-ac., psor., ruta, sabin., sep., ***sil.,*** spig., spong., stann., sulph., sul-ac., zinc.
asunder - zinc.
as from a blow - dig.
evening - mez., nat-s., zing.
extending, neck, to - calc., ***chel., laur.***
extending, outward - ph-ac., stann.
hands, layng on amel. - sul-ac.
lying down amel. - mag-s.
pressure agg. - ph-ac.
pressure amel. - spig.
pulsating - bell., zing.
sitting, while - fl-ac.
spot - spig.
stooping agg. - spig.
sub-occipital region - ***carb-v.***
turning the head - ph-ac.
walking in open air - caust.
sitting, while - fl-ac.
amel. - nux-m.
spots, in - carb-an., glon., olnd., ol-an., sep.
as with a button - acon., ***lyc.,*** thuj., zinc.
standing, on - ***ip.,*** kali-c., sel.
amel. - plb.
stool, during - gran.
stooping, on - carb-v., ***colch.,*** nux-m., ph-ac.
sub-occipital region - ambr., ***carb-v.,*** iod.
supper, after - ***carb-v.***
talking, from - spig.
tight hat, as from - ***alum.***
touch agg. - cupr., kali-n.
vise, as in a - am-m., grat., mag-c., merc.
walking, while - ***chin.***
after - zinc.
amel. - nux-m.
in open air - staph.
in open air amel. - mang.
warm room agg. - ***all-c., carb-v.,*** coc-c., mag-m., ***mez.***
weight or stone - anac., asar., ***bell.,*** cann-s., ***carb-v.,*** caust., ***chel.,*** cina, cocc., cupr., graph., hell., kali-n., laur., led., meny., nux-v., **PETR.,** ph-ac., plat., sulph.
wrapping up head amel. - **SIL.**
writing, while - carb-an.

pressing, sides - acon., aeth., agar., agn., alum., am-m., anac., ang., arg-m., arn., arum-t., ***asaf., asar.,*** aur., ***bar-c.,*** **BELL.,** bov., bry., ***cact., calc.,*** cann-s., ***caps.,*** carb-an., caust., cedr., ***chel.,*** chin., cic., clem., coca, coloc., com., con., cor-r., crot-h., cupr., dig., dios., dros., euph., fl-ac., ***glon.,*** grat., guai., hydr-ac., ***hell.,*** **HEP.,** ign., iod., kali-bi., ***kali-i.,*** kali-n., kalm., kreos., laur., lil-t., lyc., lyss., mag-c., mag-m., mang., meny., mez., mur-ac., **NAT-M.,** nat-s., nux-m., olnd., paeon., ph-ac., phos., pip-m., ***psor.,*** rheum, rhus-t., sabad., ***sabin.,*** samb., ***sars.,*** sep., **SPIG.,** spong., squil., stann., staph., stront-c., sulph., tab.,

pressing, sides - ***thuj.,*** verat., verb., viol-t., zinc.
air, open amel. - ***kali-i.***
all sides, from - ***acon.,*** tarax.
alternating with stitches - anac.
asunder - ***cor-r., spig.***
band tied around like a - dios.
behind and before, from - nux-m., spong.
bending head forward - ang.
blunt instrument as from - calc.
board, like a heavy - eug.
both sides - acon., aeth., alum., arg-m., asar., bar-c., bell., bov., bry., camph., ***chin.,*** cic., com., gamb., glon., hell., lam., mag-c., mag-m., mag-s., meny., nat-m., prun., sabad., sil., tarax.
brain, as if something were lying on the - grat.
against the bone - mez.
burning, pressing - mang., staph.
chewing warm food - phos.
dinner, after - zinc.
downward - calc., con.
entering warm room - phos.
evening - zinc.
extending, to eyes - ***lyss.***
to forehead - hydr-ac.
to orbita - stann.
to temple, toward - iod., kali-n.
foreign body, as of - con.
forenoon - alum.
forward - bar-c., hell., verb.
hoop, like a - ther.
internal, while leaning against wall - cann-s.
inward - asaf., bar-c., bell., ***bov.,*** calc., croc., dulc., kali-c., lyss., mag-c., nat-s., olnd., plat., sars., staph., sulph., sul-ac., zinc.
jerk-like - dig.
left - ***asaf.,*** bov., crot-h., hell., iod., mez., nit-ac., ph-ac., rhus-t., sars., ***stront-c.,*** sul-ac., sulph., ***thuj.***
left, lying, on, while - caust.
looking up - caps.
lying - spong.
morning - carb-v., sars.
outward - ***asaf.,*** asar., bell., cina, dros., kreos., merc., ph-ac., spig., spong., stann., verb., viol-t.
left - asaf., bell., calc.
right - cina, dros., ph-ac., spig., spong., stann., verb., viol-t.
right - agar., agn., anac., arg-m., arg-n., asar., bar-c., bry., caust., ***chel., clem.,*** dros., grat., ***hep.,*** ign., kalm., lil-t., ***mez.,*** olnd., plat., sabad., spong., tab., thuj., verb., zinc.
then left - cupr.
to left - alum.
rising from bed, amel. - carb-v.
stooping, after - kali-c.
room, in - am-m.
screw behind each ear, as from - ox-ac.
screwed in, as if, amel. in open air - bar-c., ***kali-i.***

pressing, sides
screwed, together as if - am-m., bar-c., bell., mag-c., zinc.
side, lain on - carb-v., ph-ac.
towards he bends - chin.
skull feels smaller - grat.
stooping - caps., cor-r.
stupefying, as with blunt instrument - dulc., olnd., ruta.
sudden, as from blunt tool, pressed in - asaf.
supper, after - sulph.
talking, from - fl-ac., ign., thuj.
tool, as from a blunt - asaf., dulc., hep., olnd., ruta.
toothache, on same side, with - staph.
turning eyes to painful side agg. - con.
walking - clem.
walking, in open air, amel. - ***kali-i.,*** mang., phos.

pressing, temples - acon., aesc., ***agar.,*** agn., aloe, ***alum.,*** ambr., ***am-br., anac.,*** ang., ***ant-t.,*** apis, ***arg-m., arg-n.,*** arn., ***ars.,*** ars-i., ***asaf., asar.,*** aur., bar-c., ***bell.,*** benz-ac., berb., ***bism.,*** bor., bov., brom., ***bry.,*** bufo, calad., ***calc.,*** camph., cann-i., ***cann-s.,*** canth., ***caps.,*** carb-ac., carb-an., carb-s., **CARB-V.,** cast-eq., caust., cedr., ***cham., chel., chin.,*** chin-a., cimic., cina, cinnb., cob., clem., coca, ***cocc.,*** coc-c., coff., colch., ***coloc.,*** con., ***crot-c.,*** cupr., ***cycl., dig.,*** dios., dros., dulc., echi., elaps, elat., euon., euph., ferr., ferr-ar., ferr-i., ***ferr-p.,*** fl-ac., gent-c., gent-l., gins., **GLON.,** gran., graph., ***guai.,*** hell., hep., hipp., hura, hydr-ac., hyos., hyper., ign., ind., iod., ip., jatr., kali-bi., ***kali-c., kali-i.,*** kali-n., kali-p., kalm., kreos., **LACH.,** lachn., lac-c., laur., lec., led., lith., lob., **LYC.,** ***mang.,*** meny., ***merc.,*** merl., ***mez.,*** mosch., naja, ***nat-a.,*** nat-c., **NAT-M.,** nat-p., nat-s., ***nux-m.,*** nux-v., olnd., ol-an., ***op.,*** osm., ***par.,*** petr., ph-ac., ***phos.,*** phys., **PLAT.,** plb., podo., ***prun.,*** psor., ptel., ***puls.,*** ran-b., ran-s., rheum, ***rhod.,*** rhus-t., ***sabad., sabin.,*** samb., sars., sil., spig., spong., ***squil., stann., staph.,*** stront-c., ***sulph.,*** sul-ac., tab., tarax., tax., teucr., ther., thuj., verat., ***verb.,*** viol-t., ***zinc.***
above temple, rising from sitting - mang.
afternoon - alum., ***coloc.,*** dulc., nat-c., nat-m., sil.
air, open, amel. - phos.
alternating with drawing, in occiput - bry.
in vertex - phos.
bending backwards agg. - mang.
breakfast, after - hyper.
coughing, when - verb.
crushed, as if - caul.
cutting - bell.
daytime - carl., hep., ***stann.***
closing eyes amel. - ip.
digital - ambr., ant-t., arn., asaf., cham., cocc., dulc., hell., nit-ac., rhus-t., sep., staph.
dinner, after - agar., alum., ol-an., thuj.
eating, while - calc.
after - calc., con., hyos.

pressing, temples
evening - alum., ang., calc., ***cham.,*** chel., colch., dig., dios., hell., nat-s., ph-ac., rhus-t., thuj.
amel. - anac.
excitement - par.
exertion, during - nat-c.
extending, brain, to - glon.
downward - sabad.
ears, to - lach.
eyes, above, to - alum.
eyes, to - anac.
forehead, across - alum., bry., seneg., sol-n.
forward - verb.
head, to - ambr., psor.
malar, to - **BRY.**
neck, to - bov., chel.
occiput, to - lil-t., ph-ac., sabad.
temple to temple - sulph.
upward - rhus-t.
vertex, to - carb-s., chel., kali-bi.
eyes in, as from strabismus - podo.
faintness, with - petr.
fever - sep.
forenoon - ***cham.,*** kali-c., podo., thuj.
forward - verb.
house, in - phos.
increasing and decreasing gradually - **STANN.**
inwards - ***acon., alum., anac.,*** ant-c., ant-t., ***asaf.,*** asar., bell., bor., bov., ***calc.,*** cocc., con., dulc., fl-ac., hell., jatr., kali-c., ***kali-i.,*** lith., ***lyc.,*** mez., nat-c., **NAT-M.,** nit-ac., ol-an., ***ph-ac., plat., ran-s.,*** rhod., sabad., sabin., seneg., sol-n., ***spig.,*** **STANN.,** staph., ***sul-ac., ther., thuj.,*** valer., zinc.
left - asaf.
intermittent - bor., ph-ac., sep.
jerk-like - dig.
leaning forward on a table amel. - con.
left - ***asar.,*** aur., brom., ***chin., coloc.,*** dulc., lith., **MEZ.,** mur-ac., ph-ac., ***puls., rhod.,*** sars., sulph., ***zinc.***
lying, on back amel. - ign.
on side, when - ign.
with head high amel. - ***spig.***
meditating, while - ***cham.,*** ph-ac., psor., ***sulph.***
menses, during - ***bry.,*** **LYC.**
mental exertion - dig., ph-ac.
morning - apis, bov., chin., cycl., mez., ***phos.,*** ruta., **SULPH.**
bed, in - graph.
rising, after - nit-ac., **SULPH.**
morning, waking, on - apis, calc., ferr., ***nux-v.,*** ph-ac.
motion, on - cupr., **LACH.,** par., ph-ac., phos., ***spig.***
amel. - ferr., mez., psor.
night - alum., sep.
noise - ***spig.***
noon - agar., sil.

pressing, temples

outward - acon., aloe, anac., asaf., berb., bism., bry., calc., canth., carb-v., cast-eq., caust., chin., dros., ***fl-ac.,*** **GLON.,** ign., indg., ip., kali-c., kreos., **LACH.,** lact., lil-t., lob., ***mez.,*** mur-ac., nat-c., nat-m., nux-m., op., par., ph-ac., phys., phyt., ***prun.,*** ran-s., rhod., ***sabad.,*** sabin., samb., senec., ***spig.,*** spong., stann., stront-c., sulph., teucr., valer., verb., viol-t.

heat of face and flickering before eyes, with - aloe

left - asaf., carb-v., mez., mur-ac., sabin., verb.

right - caust., dros., kali-c., mur-ac., nat-c., nux-m., ph-ac., sabad., spong., stann., stront.

paroxysmal - ***kali-c.***

pressure, on - bism., nat-m., ph-ac.

amel. - dios., ip., meny., par., ***stann.***

pulsating - camph., ***cocc., glon.,*** grat., nux-v.

reading - carb-an., mez., **NAT-M.,** par.

right - ***alum., bell.,*** bor., caust., cedr., ***cham., chel., guai.,*** hell., ***kali-c.,*** kali-n., nit-ac., par., ***ph-ac.,*** phos., rhus-t., sil., ***spig., stann.,*** tarax., verb.

lying on it - stann.

noon until evening - sil.

to left - apis, lyc.

rising, after - nit-ac.

after, up amel. - stann.

from seat - mang.

screws, as with - acon., arg-n., **LYC.,** sabad.

shaking head - ***asar.,*** chin.

sharp - mang.

side, lain on - stann.

not lain on - graph.

sleep, after - hep., rhus-t.

sneezing, after - cina.

speaking, from - mez.

spots, in - helon., ox-ac., psor.

stool, during - merc.

after - sil.

before - merc.

stooping, on - phos., ***lach.,*** samb., ***spig.***

amel. - mang.

thinking of the pain, agg. - **CHAM.**

touch agg. - arg-m., aur., cupr., led., sars.

touching the hair agg. - agar.

urinate, if the desire be not soon attended to - ***fl-ac.***

vise, as if in - anac., cocc., con., dios., ham., ***lyc., nat-m., nux-m.,*** plat.

waking, on - calad., ***calc.,*** ferr., ***nux-v.***

walking, while - asar., chin., hell., **LACH.,** mang., nat-m.

wavelike - plat.

wedge, as if - ***thuj.***

writing, while - **NAT-M.**

pressing, vertex - **ACON.,** act-sp., aesc., ***agar.,*** agn., all-c., ***aloe,*** alum., ***alumn., ambr., am-c., anac.,*** ant-t., apis, ***arg-n.,*** arn., ***ars.,*** asaf., aur., bar-c., **BELL.,** benz-ac., bov., brom., bry., bufo, **CACT.,** ***calc., calc-ar., calc-p.,*** camph., ***cann-s.,*** canth., **CARB-S., CARB-V.,** cast., ***caust.,*** cedr., cham., ***chel., chen-a.,*** chin., chin-s., cic., cimx., **CIMIC.,** ***cina,*** cinnb., clem., cocc., coc-c., colch., coloc., con., croc., crot-h., cupr., ***cycl., dig.,*** dulc., dros., eug., euphr., eup-per., ***ferr., ferr-ar.,*** ferr-i., ***ferr-p.,*** fl-ac., gels., **GLON.,** ***graph.,*** hell., helon., hep., hipp., hydr., hydr-ac., hyos., ***hyper.,*** ign., indg., ***iod.,*** ip., jac-c., ***kali-bi., kali-c., kali-i.,*** kali-n., ***kali-p.,*** kalm., kreos., **LACH.,** laur., led., lil-t., lith., **LYC.,** ***lyss.,*** lac-c., mag-c., mag-m., manc., mang., med., ***meny.,*** merc-i-r., ***mez.,*** mosch., ***naja,*** nat-a., nat-c., nat-m., ***nat-p.,*** nat-s., ***nicc.,*** nit-ac., ***nux-m., nux-v.,*** olnd., ol-an., op., ***ox-ac.,*** pall., ***petr., phel.,*** **PH-AC.,** ***phos., phys., phyt.,*** pic-ac., plat., puls., ***ran-b.,*** ran-s., rheum, rhod., rhus-t., rumx., sabad., sabin., ***sars., sep.,*** **SIL.,** spig., spong., squil., **STANN.,** ***staph.,*** stram., **SULPH.,** sul-ac., syph., tab., ***thuj.,*** valer., ***verat.,*** verb., viol-t., xan., zinc.

afternoon - alum., carb-v., graph., op.

4 to 8 p.m. - **LYC.**

air, open, amel. - acon.

ascending steps - **MENY.**

asunder - carb-an., hyper., nux-v., ran-b.

band drawn tightly over, from ear to ear - ip.

binding head up amel. - **SIL.**

bound, as if - acon., cycl., kalm.

cold air, from - ***ferr.***

coughing, on - ***anac.***

dark, in, while - sil.

daytime - carb-s., ***crot-h.***

dinner, after - calc., con., mag-c.

draw eyes together, must - ***sulph.***

eating, after - ***cinnb.***

evening - acon., ambr., carb-v., chin-s., coloc., dig., hep., kali-c., petr., sil., stann., ***sulph.***

5 p.m. - stram.

6 p.m. - hyper.

extending, brain, to - sulph.

eye, to - calc., sil.

forehead, to - cham., hydr-ac., ign., nat-m., sulph.

head, to - dig.

occiput, to - bar-c., ***ph-ac.***

shoulder, to - gels.

spine, to, no pain - benz-ac.

finger, as from - nit-ac., thuj.

forenoon - ***acon.,*** glon.

11 a.m. - kali-bi.

grief, after - ***ph-ac.***

hands, laying on parts agg. - kali-n.

hard body, as from - ***ign.,*** nux-v., thuj.

ice amel. - alumn.

increasing and decreasing slowly - sars., **STANN.**

inspiration, deep, on - ***anac.***

intermitting - chel., ***cina,*** ph-ac., stann.

inward - ***anac.,*** asaf., caust., ***dulc.,*** ferr., glon., hell., nit-ac., nux-v., ox-ac., **PH-AC.,** plat., ran-s., sep., sil., stann., staph., ***sulph.,*** zinc.

jerking - sil.

pressing, vertex
lying, while - ***lyc.***
menses, during - cast., ***calc.,*** ferr-p., ***nat-s., nux-v.***
mental exertion, after - ***cham., lyc.,*** nat-s., ***nux-v., sep.***
morning - agar., ***alumn.,*** ambr., chel., coc-c., ox-ac., rhus-t., squil., **SULPH.**
5 a.m. - calc.
waking - calc.
waking, after - verat.
waking, on - ***alumn.,*** coc-c.
motion agg. - aur., ph-ac.
night - ***acon.,*** agar., lyc., sulph.
4 a.m. - ***alumn.***
noise agg. - ***bell., cact.***
noon - manc.
outward - ***am-c.,*** calc., calc-p., **CARB-AN.,** cham., **CIMIC.,** ***ferr.,*** glon., ***lach.,*** op., ph-ac., phys., **SIL.,** spig.
paroxysmal - chel., sil., zinc.
plug, as if - **ANAC.**
pressure, agg. - ***bell.,*** cina, kali-n.
amel. - ***alumn.,*** **CACT.,** ***cina, meny.,*** nat-m., stann., ***verat.***
pressure, hard, amel. - alumn.
riding in a carriage, while - lyc.
screwed up in a vise, as if - daph.
small spot - spig.
standing, while - alum., sul-ac.
stooping, when - calc., cham., indg., ***lyc.,*** lyss.
sun, while standing in - ***bar-c.***
talking, from - iod., mez., peti., spig.
talking, hearing - ***cact.***
thinking about it agg. - **CHAM.**
touching the hair, on - ***carb-v.***
turning, head - hyos.
in a circle, as if, after - calc.
upward - **CIMIC.,** ***ferr.,*** helon.
urinate, if the desire to, be not soon attended to - ***fl-ac.***
walking, while - ***hep.***
in open air, while - calc.
rapidly - chel.
wrinkling forehead, compels - ***sulph.***

PRICKLING, sensation - alum., am-m., apis, arg-n., aur., bar-c., calad., carb-an., cham., chin-s., con., cupr., hydr-ac., lachn., merc., mur-ac., nat-m., nit-ac., op., ph-ac., sabad., sep., tarent., thuj., verb., viol-o.
above root of nose - kali-bi.
debauch, after a - ***op.***
eating, after - con.
forenoon - ph-ac.
intermittent - verb.
left-side - calad.
like needles - agar., all-c., am-c., asaf., caul., hep., kali-c., mang., nat-m., sep.
lying, while - merc.
needles, as from - con., eug., rhus-t., thuj.
spots, in - apis

prickling, forehead - apis, aur., chin-s., ferr., lil-t., ***mur-ac.,*** sabad., sep., thuj., verat., ***viol-o.***
left side - calad.

prickling, temples - ail., ant-c., apis, cupr., cocc., euphr., rhus-r., tarax., tarent., thuj., verb.
evening - lachn.
needles, as with - nicc., zinc.

prickling, vertex - carb-ac.

PULLED, pain, sensation as if hair were - ***acon., aeth., alum.,*** ambr., ***arg-n.,*** arn., aur., bar-c., canth., carb-an., **CHIN.,** ferr., indg., iod., ***kali-c.,*** kali-n., ***laur.,*** lyc., mag-c., mag-m., mur-ac., petr., ph-ac., ***phos.,*** psor., ***rhus-t.,*** sel., sil., stann., ***sulph.***
out - ars., bell., ***sulph.***
skin were - sep.

pulled, occiput - arn., kali-p., ***nux-v.***

pulled, side - phos.

pulled, temple - bry.

pulled, vertex, from the - ***acon.,*** alum., ferr., indg., kali-n., ***mag-c.,*** mag-m., ***sulph.***

PULLING, pain, like - canth., ***lach.,*** petr.
extending into teeth - staph.

pulling, forehead, like - plb.

PULSATING, throbbing - ***acon.,*** aeth., agar., ail., aloe, alum., am-c., am-m., ***aml-n.,*** anac., anan., ant-t., apis, ***arn., ars., ars-i., asaf.,*** asar., aster., aur., bar-c., bar-m., **BELL.,** ***bor.,*** bov., brach., ***bry., cact.,*** cadm-s., calc., calc-ar., calc-p., calc-s., ***camph., cann-i.,*** cann-s., canth., ***caps.,*** carb-an., carb-s., ***carb-v., cast., caust.,*** cedr., ***cham.,*** chel., **CHIN., CHIN-S.,** cimic., cinnb., clem., cob., cocc., coff., colch., con., ***croc., crot-h.,*** crot-t., cupr., cur., cycl., daph., dig., dros., eug., ***eup-per.,*** euphr., eupi., ***ferr., ferr-ar.,*** ferr-i., ferr-p., ***gels.,*** **GLON.,** graph., grat., guai., hell., hep., hipp., hyos., ***ign.,*** indg., ind., ***iod., ip., kali-ar.,*** kali-bi., ***kali-c.,*** kali-i., ***kali-n.,*** kali-p., ***kali-s., kalm., kreos.,*** **LACH.,** lachn., lact., lam., ***laur.,*** led., ***lith.,*** **LYC.,** mag-c., mag-m., mag-s., manc., mang., merc., mez., mill., mur-ac., myric., nat-a., nat-c., nat-m., nat-p., nicc., ***nit-ac., nux-m.,*** nux-v., olnd., ol-an., ***op.,*** par., ***petr.,*** ph-ac., phel., ***phos.,*** pic-ac., plb., psor., ***puls., pyrog., rheum,*** rhod., ***rhus-t.,*** ruta, sabad., sabin., **SANG.,** ***sars.,*** sec., ***seneg., sep.,*** **SIL.,** sol-n., ***spong.,*** squil., stann., ***stram.,*** **SULPH.,** tab., ter., ther., thuj., til., verat., ***verat-v.,*** zinc.
afternoon - aeth., alum., cast., caust., coca, glon., graph., grat., hura, ind., lyc., mag-s., mang., ***merc-i-r.,*** nat-m., phel., phys., sil.
air, in open, agg. - carb-an., cocc., eup-pur., iris
amel. - kali-bi., kali-i., mang., nicc., phos., ***pic-ac.***
alternating between head and chest - bell.
ascending on - alum., aster., ***bry.,*** glon., nat-p., ***sep.***
fast - glon.

PULSATING, throbbing
bathing, after - cast.
cold, amel. - ars., ind., phos.
bed, while in - chel., con., cycl., graph., sep.
bending backward - aur., glon., **LYC.**
amel. - ***bell., nat-m., sil.***
binding up head amel. - pic-ac., sil.
blood, after loss of - ***chin.***
blowing nose - aster.
breakfast, amel. - nat-m., nit-ac.
burning - apis, coff., ***rhus-t.***
chewing, while - phos.
chill, during - cann-i., eup-per.
after - bor.
with chilliness - sil.
closing eyes agg. - sep.
cold, preceding a - lach.
coughing, from - arn., aur., dirc., ferr., hep., hipp., ***ip.,*** iris, kali-c., led., **LYC.,** ***nat-m.,*** nit-ac., ph-ac., phos., seneg., sep., sil., spong., sulph.
darkness amel. - sep.
dinner after - alum., ***am-c.,*** carb-an., kali-bi., mag-c., nat-c., ol-an., plb., zinc.
drawing - ars.
drinking, agg. while - acon.
agg. - ars.
eating, after - am-c., ars., carb-v., clem., cocc., sel.
before - cocc.
ending in shooting - **BELL.**
evening - acon., am-m., bar-c., bov., calc., canth., carb-v., cast., cic., clem., ***cocc.,*** con., cycl., fl-ac., glon., indg., ***iris,*** kali-i., lac-ac., lyc., mag-s., ***nat-m.,*** nit-ac., ox-ac., ***puls.,*** ruta., stram., zinc.
agg., until gets to sleep - cast.
asleep, on falling - sil.
bed, in - cycl., lyc., sep.
excitement, during - ***sulph.***
exertion, from - gins., glon.
extending, neck or chest to - nat-m.
teeth, to - mez.
fever, during the - ***bell., eup-per.***
forenoon - alum.
gnawing - par.
hammers, as if from little, awakens every morning - ***nat-m.,*** psor.
heat, during - eup-per., glon., rhus-t.
of body - nat-m.
here and there - acon., aeth., indg.
inspiration, during - ***carb-v.***
intermittent - ferr-ma., verat.
jar, from any - ***bell.,*** glon., ***ther.***
jerking - bry., ign., phos.
laughing, from - lyc., phos.
leaning head backward, on - **LYC.**
lies senseless with closed eyes - arg-n.
lying, while - aloe, calc-ar., glon., lachn., naja, phos.
amel. - anac., calc., kali-bi.
back, on - sep.
head high, amel. - nat-m., ***spig.***
must lie down - ***bell.,*** sang.
part, on the - ***petr.***

PULSATING, throbbing
lying, side, lain, on - sep.
side, on, amel. - nat-m., sep.
menses, during - acon., bell., ***chin.,*** croc., ***glon.,*** ign., lac-d., ***lach.,*** mag-c., ***nat-c.,*** nux-m., puls., sang., verat-v.
after - calc-p., carb-an., ferr., glon., nat-m.
before - ***bell., bor.,*** chin., ***crot-h.,*** gels., ***glon., lach.,*** nat-m., ***petr.,*** sulph.
painless throbbing, during - eupi.
suppressed - ***puls.***
mental exertion, from - agar., ***nat-m., pic-ac.,*** psor., ***puls., raph.,*** sil., vib.
milk, from - brom.
morning - alum., asar., aur., bov., ***calc.,*** canth., cedr., ***cob.,*** gamb., glon., graph., grat., indg., kali-bi., lact., lyc., nat-c., ***nat-m.,*** nicc., ***nit-ac., nux-v.,*** plb., podo., sars., sep., sil., spig., ***sulph.***
comes on gradually and goes off about breakfast - ***nit-ac.***
every, lasts all day - ***calc.***
increases until evening - eup-pur., sang., sep.
rising, on - ***asar.,*** caust., nat-m.
waking, on - alum., ***bry.,*** kreos., lach., ***nat-m.,*** phos., ruta., ***sulph.***
motion, agg. - acon., ***anac., apis,*** ars., ***bell., bry.,*** calc-p., caust., chin., cimic., ***cocc.,*** colch., dirc., eupi., ferr., ferr-p., ***gels., glon.,*** grat., ***iod.,*** kali-bi., ***lach., lyc., nat-m.,*** nit-ac., nux-m., ***sep., stram., sulph.***
amel. - aloe, lact.
moderate, amel. - iris, vib.
sudden, from - calc-p., ferr.
moving head agg. - ***sulph.***
night - aloe, arg-n., ars., ***cact.,*** carb-v., chel., ferr., glon., hura, hyos., lyc., nat-m., sars., sil., ***sulph.***
agg., after 12 p.m. - **FERR.**
bed, in, before sleep - chel.
comes on during the, with nausea and vomiting - **SIL.**
driving out of bed - arg-n.
waking - carb-v., sulph.
nosebleed, after - bor.
painless, with fear of going to sleep - ***nux-m.***
paroxysmal - caust., glon.
periodic - ars., ferr.
perspiration amel. - ***nat-m.***
pressure, amel. - aeth., ***am-c.,*** bell., bry., ferr., glon., kali-bi., kali-n., nat-m., ***puls.,*** pyrog.
upon forehead causes beating - mag-m.
with hands amel. - apis, carb-an., guai.
raising head suddenly agg. - nat-p., squil.
reading, while sitting - lyc., ***nat-m.***
respiration, during difficult - ***carb-v.,*** glon.
resting head amel. - kali-bi.
riding, while - cocc., ***glon.,*** phos.
rising, on - chin-s., dirc., glon., phos.
amel. - nat-c.
from stooping - mag-m.

PULSATING, throbbing
rising, up in bed - ars.
room on entering - aeth., mag-m., mang.
rubbing amel. - aeth.
shaking head agg. - ***glon.***
sitting, while - am-m., cast., guai., indg., lyc., ol-an.
amel. - mag-m.
sleep amel. - sang.
spots, in - nux-m.
standing, while - cast., guai., plb.
amel. - camph.
stool, while straining at - ign.
stooping, on - alum., ***apis,*** asar., bar-c., **BELL.,** colch., ferr., ferr-p., ***glon.,*** hydr-ac., kali-bi., lach., ***laur.,*** mag-m., nat-c., nat-m., ***nux-v.,*** phos., puls., sulph.
after - hyos.
stretching limbs out, on - phos.
sunlight agg. - acon., sulph.
talking agg. - acon., aur., ***cocc., nat-m.,*** sil., ***sulph.***
tea, warm, amel. - glon.
thinking of it amel. - ant-c.
transient, in one-half of - cham.
turning, around agg. - glon.
eyes agg. - sep.
ulcerative - am-c., bov., cast., mang.
vertigo, during - glon., sec.
waking, on - aur., carb-v., cinnb., lach., lyc., nat-m., phos., podo., ruta., sulph.
walking, open air, in - ***am-c.,*** mag-s.
open air, in, amel. - ars., eup-pur., ***guai.***
quickly, while - calc., ferr., nux-v., ***puls.***
walking, while - alum., aster., ***bell.,*** calc., ***glon.,*** kali-bi., ***nat-m.,*** nat-s., nux-v., plb., sars., sil., ***sulph.***
stepping, when - alum., ***phos.***
warm, food agg. - sulph.
room, agg. - iod., ***puls.,*** sulph.
room, amel. - am-c., cocc.
wine, after - ox-ac.
wrapping, head up warmly amel. - sil.
writing, while - kali-c., manc.
yawning, after - calc.

pulsating, forehead - acon., aeth., aloe, alum., ***am-c.,*** am-m., ang., ant-t., apis, apoc., arg-m., ars., ***ars-i.,*** asaf., asar., aur., aur-m., bapt., bar-c., **BELL.,** bor., brach., bry., ***calc.,*** calc-p., ***camph., cann-i.,*** cann-s., canth., ***caps.,*** carb-v., cast., ***caust.,*** cic., cinnb., clem., cocc., con., corn., croc., ***dig.,*** dulc., euph., eupi., ***ferr., ferr-ar., ferr-p.,*** gamb., **GLON.,** graph., grat., hell., ign., iod., **IRIS,** kali-ar., kali-c., ***kali-i.,*** kali-n., kali-p., ***kalm., kreos.,*** **LAC-D.,** laur., ***lyc.,*** lyss., mag-c., ***mag-m.,*** mag-s., ***merc., merc-i-f.,*** mez., meli., nat-c., nat-m., nat-p., nit-ac., ***nux-m.,*** olnd., op., ox-ac., par., ***petr.,*** phos., **PULS.,** ran-b., rheum, rhod., rhus-t., ruta., sabad., sars., seneg., sep., ***sil.,*** spig., ***spong.,*** stann., ***stram.,*** ther., thuj., verb., vib., zinc.
afternoon - alum., alumn., caust., lyc., mag-s., sil.
2 p.m. - nat-m.

pulsating, forehead
afternoon, 3 p.m. - lyc.
air, open, amel. - aeth., ***arn., am-c.,*** kali-i., **PULS.**
ascending stairs - nat-p., par.
bending head forward - nat-m.
cough during - hep., phos., spong.
dinner, after - ***am-c.,*** kali-c., zinc.
eating, after - ***am-c.,*** cocc.
evening - am-m., cic., cocc., lyc., mag-s., ruta., stram.
9 p.m. - calc., caust.
extending occiput, to - bry., ***con.,*** ther.
eyes, over - ***bell., gels.,*** glon., gymn., ign., ***kali-bi., lac-c., lach.,*** lyss., ***nat-m., nux-m.,*** ptel., ***sep.,*** spig., stram., ther., vib.
arteries - caust.
forenoon - gamb., lyc.
frontal eminence - aesc., ***arg-n.,*** calc., cocc., hyos., iris, lyc., mez., nit-ac., ran-b.
afternoon, 4 p.m. - nit-ac.
evening - ***iris,*** lyc.
evening, 6 p.m. - lyc.
evening, 8 p.m. - ir-fl.
left - ***arg-n.,*** cocc., verb.
right - aesc., calc., lyc., mez.
slow - verb.
left - acon., ***arg-n.,*** cimic., cocc., kali-c., ***kreos.,*** nux-m., par., spig., verat.
menses, during - acon., ***bell.,*** bor., bry., cact., calc., calc-p., ***chin., glon., ign., lach.,*** mag-c., ***nat-c.,*** **PULS.,** sang., ***tarent.***
morning - asar., ***canth.,*** grat., ***nat-m.,*** sil.
rising, on - asar., ***nat-m.***
waking, on - ***nat-m.,*** ruta.
motion, during - ars., ***gels., glon.,*** merc., pic-ac.
amel. - ***puls.***
night - fago., hura, ***merc.,*** nat-m.
noon - lyc.
one-sided - aur., kali-bi., ptel.
pressure, on - mag-m.
amel - aeth., am-c., nat-m.
reading, while - lyc.
riding, while - ***glon.,*** grat.
in cold air - ***am-c.,*** cocc.
right - ***ant-t.,*** sars., ***sep.***
rising up in bed - ars., glon.
root of nose, above - ***ars.,*** camph., gamb., mez., puls.
forenoon - gamb.
walking amel. - puls.
standing while - kali-c.
stooping, on - asar., bar-c.
talking agg. - cocc.
walking, on - ***aeth.,*** kali-c., sars.
in open air - am-c., sars.
warm room amel. - ***am-c.,*** cocc.

pulsating, occiput - aeth., agar., ail., aloe, ***alum.,*** am-c., anac., asar., bar-c., **BELL.,** berb., bor., **BRY.,** ***calc., camph., cann-i.,*** cann-s., ***carb-an.,*** carb-s., ***carb-v.,*** caust., ***chel.,*** con., cop., ***crot-h., dros.,*** eup-per., ***eup-pur., ferr., ferr-ar.,*** ferr-p., ***gels., glon.,*** hep., hura, ign., indg., kali-bi., kali-br., ***kali-c., kali-n.,*** kali-s., lac-c., ***lach.,*** laur., lyc., lyss., ***mag-m.,*** mang., mez., ***nat-m., nit-ac., petr.,*** **PHOS.,** phys., pic-ac., plb., ***psor., puls.,*** ran-b., rhus-t., ruta., **SEP.,** spig., ***stram., sulph.***
afternoon - nat-m.
cough, during - ***ferr.,*** ferr-p., sep.
daytime - petr.
evening - bar-c., kali-n., puls.
extending, forward - bar-c., lac-c., op., sulph.
sides and forehead, to - ferr.
to forehead - carb-v., sil., ***spig.***
to frontal eminence - bar-c.
to vertex - hura
whole head, over - mag-m.
hammer, like beats of - camph., ***nat-m.,*** psor.
lying on back, while - ***petr.***
morning, after rising during menses - mag-m.
moving, on - **BELL., BRY.,** ***eup-per., ferr., ip., lach.,*** **STRAM.**
amel. - aloe
night - aloe, lyc.
paroxysmal - ***glon.***
pressure, amel. - alum., cast., kali-n.
rising, on - gels., phos.
from stooping - mag-m.
rubbing, amel. - caust.
shaking head - kali-br.
sides - ***alum.,*** am-c., cast., caust., ***eup-pur.,*** indg., kali-n., laur., plb., ran-b., stram., ***sulph.***
evening, in bed - kali-n.
sides, rising, on - gels.
sitting, while - kali-br., ran-b.
amel. - mag-m.
standing amel. - **CAMPH.**
stool, during - ***ign.***
stooping, on - ***ferr.,*** mag-m.
walking agg. - kali-br.
in open air amel. - dig.
warm room - mag-m.

pulsating, sides - aeth., agar., alum., am-c., ant-t., arg-n., ars., aur., bar-c., bell., bov., bry., calc., calc-p., canth., ***cham.,*** chin., coca, con., croc., dirc., eup-per., glon., ***graph.,*** hura, indg., iris, kali-c., kali-i., kali-s., kalm., laur., lyc., mag-c., mag-m., mag-s., nat-c., nit-ac., ol-an., petr., ***phos.,*** plb., rhod., rhus-t., sars., sep., spong., sul-ac., verat., zinc.
afternoon - alum., graph., lyc.
3 p.m. - hura
bending backward - aur.
coughing agg. - aur., dirc.
deep-seated - sars.
dinner, after - kali-c., mag-c., ol-an.
evening - canth., con., phos.
forenoon - plb., sars.

pulsating, occiput
house, in, amel. - mag-s.
left - am-c., bar-c., calc., hura, mag-m., nat-c., ***nit-ac.,*** phos.
to right - nux-m.
lying on side, while - sep.
menses, during - nat-c.
morning - aur., bov., ***nit-ac.***
motion, agg. - bell., ***calc-p.***
right - aeth., agar., alum., aur., con., graph., kali-c., mag-c., ***phos.,*** rhod., sul-ac., zinc.
right, to left - bov.
rising, after - glon.
shaking - glon.
side on which he lies - sep.
sitting - phos.
standing, while - kali-c.
stooping, on - glon., laur.
walking, while - kali-c.
in open air - mag-s.

pulsating, temples - acon., aesc., aeth., agar., all-s., ***alum.,*** am-c., am-m., ant-c., ant-t., arg-n., ***ars., ars-i., asaf.,*** aur-m-n., bar-c., **BELL.,** bor., ***bry.,*** cact., cadm-s., calc., calc-p., calc-s., camph., ***caps.,*** carb-s., carb-v., cast., ***cedr.,*** cham., ***chel.,*** chin., chin-s., cic., cocc., coloc., cupr-ar., daph., ferr., ***ferr-ar.,*** ferr-p., fl-ac., ***gels.,*** gins., **GLON.,** gymn., ***grat.,*** hell., hep., hyper., hura, ***iod.,*** kali-c., kali-i., kali-n., kali-p., kali-s., kreos., ***lac-c.,*** lac-d., ***lach.,*** lac-ac., laur., lyss., med., nat-a., nat-c., nat-m., nat-p., nat-s., ***nit-ac., phos.,*** phys., plb., podo., rhus-t., sabad., ***sang.,*** sars., ***spig.,*** spong., ***staph., stann.,*** stram., ***sulph.,*** sul-i., tab., thea., thuj., verat., verat-v.
afternoon - alum., glon.
ascending stairs - glon.
blood-vessels - bell., chin., chion., mur-ac., tab.
chill, before - carb-v.
cough, during - hep.
evening - am-m., bry., fl-ac., glon., kali-i., lac-ac.
sitting, on - am-m.
walking - glon.
forenoon - carl.
fever, during - glon.
left - chin-s., ***coloc.,*** nit-ac., ***phos.***
lying, while - naja
menses, before - ***lach.***
midnight - sars.
morning - bov., lach., ***podo.,*** stry.
waking on - lach.
motion, on - caust., **CHIN.,** ***gels., glon.***
night - ***cact.,*** chel.
noon - ars., thuj.
paroxysmal - glon.
right - aesc., alum., chel., ***cupr-ar., hep.***
stooping, while - sul-i.
waking on - carb-v.
walking, while - aeth., bar-c., ***glon.,*** nat-s., sulph.

pulsating, vertex - aeth., agar., ***alum.,*** anac., ars., bry., calc., cann-i., carb-an., ***caust., cham., chel., chin-s.,*** cinnb., cocc., corn., ***ferr., ferr-ar.,*** ferr-p., ***glon.,*** grat., ham., hura, ***hyper.,*** kali-c., kali-s., kreos., ***lac-d.,*** lach., ***lyc.,*** lyss., manc., ***merc-i-r.,*** nat-a., ***nat-c., nat-m.,*** nat-p., ***nux-v.,*** petr., phel., phos., pic-ac., plan., puls., sars., ***sep., sil., stram., sulph., ter.,*** thea., verat.
afternoon - ***hyper.***
ascending steps agg. - carl., ferr.
attention, from fixing - nux-v.
bending head back amel. - **SIL.**
dinner, after - nat-c.
forenoon - alum., glon.
menses, after - ferr., ***lach.***
mental exertion - nux-v.
morning - alum., bry., caust., nat-c., ***sep.***
motion, on - ***bry., calc., cocc.,*** ferr., glon., lach., sep., ***verat.***
of the eyes - cocc.
waking, on - bry., ***lyc.***
walking, while - carb-an., ***sars.***
rapidly, while - ferr., puls.

PULSATING, pain (see Head, Pulsating)
drinking cold water, when heated, after - bry.
menses, after, with sore eyes - nat-m.
pain, with, external - lach.
with, stomach, in - ***kali-c.***

PUSHED, forward, as if - ***canth.,*** ferr-p., grat., nit-ac., nux-m., nux-v., rhus-t., staph.
pushed, to forehead from occiput, sensation as if a load were - pall.

PUSHES, sensation, (see Pressure) - croc., ***nat-m.,*** ph-ac., phos.
pressure, amel. - ***arg-n.***

QUIVERING, sensation - bov., cann-s., lact.
running and walking, while - nux-v.
shaking on - xan.

RAISE, the head, difficult to, night - chel.
frequently from pillow - stram.
unable to - bell., carb-v., chel., ***lach.,*** laur., nux-v., ***op., puls.***
lying on back, while - chel., nux-v.
morning on waking - ***lach.***
stooping, after - bell., rhus-t.

rash, forehead - ail., arn., indg., lil-t., rheum, teucr.
itching - rheum.

REMOVED, as if calvarium - arum-t., cann-i.

RESTLESSNESS - ambr., bell., caust., jab., merc., phos., pip-m., ruta., sec., sil.
forenoon - phos., sil.
weak, when too to move body, will roll head from side to side - ***ars.***

RESTLESSNESS, occiput - ambr.

RHEUMATIC, pain - acon., act-sp., am-m., ***ars., asar.,*** asc-t., ***aur., bell.,*** benz-ac., berb., **BRY.,** cact., calc., ***calc-p., caps., carb-s.,*** caul., ***caust.,*** cham., chin., ***cimic.,*** colch., coll., **COLOC.,** cycl., der., **DULC.,** ***eug.,*** graph., ***guai.,*** hep., ign., ip., kali-ar., kali-bi., kali-s., ***kalm., lach.,*** led., lyc., mag-m., mang., **MERC.,** ***nat-m., nit-ac.,*** nux-v., petr., ***phos., phyt.,*** plat., podo., ***puls., ran-b.,*** **RHUS-R., RHUS-T.,** ***sang.,*** **SEP.,** ***sil.,*** spig., stict., stram., sulph., ***verat.***

RIGID, feeling - ***caust.,*** phos., rheum

RINGWORM - bac., **CALC., DULC.,** ***phyt., sep.,*** tell., thuj., tub.

RISING, sensation, in - glon., lac-d., nat-c., nux-v., rhus-t., thuj.
drinking beer, while - rhus-t.
sinking, and - **BELL.,** cob.
walking rapidly, while - nux-v.

rising, sensation of something in, from vertex to forehead - glon.

ROLLING, in head - cupr-ar., eug., graph., hura, phys., sep.
brain, were rolled into small bulk, as if - ***arn., coc-c.***
lead, ball rolled about, as if - lyss.
study, after - cupr-ar.
vertigo, during - sep.
vomiting, agg. - eug.

rolling, of the head, (see Motions, of head)

RUBBING - camph., con., hyos., tarent.
against something - tarent.
hand, with the - verat.

rubbing, inclination to rub forehead - glon.

SCRAPED, feeling, amel., on motion, while lying the pain shifts to side lain on - ***ph-ac.***

SCRATCHING, head - nat-m.
waking, on - calc.

SEBACEOUS cysts, wens - agar., ***bar-c., calc.,*** **GRAPH.,** ***hep., kali-c., lob.,*** lyc., nat-c., nit-ac., **SIL.,** sulph.

SEBORRHEA - ***am-m., ars.,*** bry., bufo, calc., chin., graph., ***iod.,*** kali-br., kali-c., kali-s., lyc., merc., mez., nat-m., phos., ***plb.,*** psor., raph., rhus-t., sars., sel., sep., staph., sulph., thuj., ***vinc.***

SENSITIVENESS of, external - ***agar.,*** am-c., bell., bor., bov., ***carb-an.,*** chin., chin-s., grat., lach., lyc., mag-c., merc., nat-m., nux-v., phos., sabin., tong.

sensitiveness of, scalp - cinnb., ***mag-m.***
motion, to - hell.
touch, to - **CHIN.,** hell., kali-n.

sensitiveness of, vertex - alum., kali-n., mag-c., mag-m., phos., squil., sulph., zinc.

SEPARATED, as if, head from body, were - alum., ant-t., cann-i., **COCC.,** ***daph.,*** nat-c., nat-m., nux-m., **PSOR.,** ther.
night - ***daph.***
bones, were, as if - ther.

separated, vertex were, as if - ***ther.***

SHAKING, sensation (see Looseness, Motion, Waving) - acon., aloe, ant-c., ant-t., ***am-c.,*** anac., arn., ***ars.,*** asar., aur., bar-c., bell., benz-ac., bufo, ***calc.,*** cann-i., carb-v., caust., chel., cic., cinnb., cocc., cop., crot-h., cub., elaps, eupi., fl-ac., glon., grat., graph., ***hyos.,*** ign., indg., kali-c., kali-p., lact., led., lith., ***lyc., mag-c.,*** mag-p., mag-s., ***mang.,*** merc., mez., nit-ac., nux-m., nux-v., op., pall., petr., ph-ac., phos., plat., plb., rhod., sars., sep., ***sil.,*** sol-n., ***spig.,*** stann., stront-c., sulph., tab., verat., verb., viol-t., zinc.

against frontal bone - aur.
air, agg. - aloe
ascending steps, when - lyc.
chills, during - ars.
cold agg. - nux-m.
cough, during - ant-t., calc., chin., hep., ***lact.,*** mag-s., rhus-t.
eating, agg. after - nux-m.
heat, except that of bed, amel. - nux-m.
menses during - ant-c., cic., cinnb., cub.
motion, on - calc., mang.
of head, on - arn., ars., cic., cocc., lact., lyc., mag-c., mez., nux-v., sol-n., ***spig.***
of head, on laying head down - aloe
rising, from stooping - lyc.
shaking, head - calc., mang.
shuddering, with - mez.
speaking, on - cocc.
stamping, on - bar-c.
steel spring, as of a - grat.
step, at every - calc.
stepping heavily, when - led., ***lyc.,*** nux-v., ***sil., spig.***
striking foot against anything - bar-c., sep., sil.
stooping, on - berb.
talking, while - phos., verat.
walking, while - anac., ***ars.,*** caust., cic., cocc., hyos., led., ***lyc.,*** mang., nux-v., sep., sil., spig., verb., viol-t.
begining, to - plat.
open air, in - caust., ***nux-v.***
warm, room amel. - nux-m., nux-v.
wrapping, up warmly amel. - nux-v.

shaking, forehead - aur., ***merc.***
shaking, occiput - calc., sulph.
shaking, temples - cocc., kali-c., stront.

SHARP, pain - ***acon.,*** aeth., ***agar.,*** agn., aloe, ***alum.,*** ambr., ***am-c.,*** am-m., anac., anan., ant-c., ***ant-t.,*** apis, arg-m., arg-n., ***arn.,*** ars., ***ars-i.,*** asaf., ***aur.,*** bapt., ***bar-c., bar-m., bell., berb., bor., bov., bry., calc., calc-s.,*** camph., cann-i., cann-s., canth., ***caps.,*** carb-ac., carb-an., carb-s., carb-v., cast., ***caust.,*** cham., ***chel.,*** **CHIN.,** chin-a., ***cic.,*** cina, cocc., coc-c., ***con.,*** cop., croc., crot-t., cupr., cycl., daph., dig., dirc., dulc., elaps, eug., ***euphr.,*** eupi., ***euon.,*** ferr., ferr-ar., ferr-i., ferr-p., gels., glon., grat., guai., hell., ***hep.,*** hipp., hydr-ac., ***hyos., ign.,*** indg., iod., ***ip.,*** kali-ar., kali-bi., **KALI-C.,** ***kali-i., kali-n.,*** **KALI-P., KALI-S.,** lach., lachn., lact., lam., ***laur.,*** lob., ***lyc., mag-c., mag-m.,*** mag-p., ***mag-s.,*** manc., ***mang., merc.,*** merc-c., merc-i-f., merl., mez., mill., mosch., ***mur-ac.,*** nat-a., ***nat-c., nat-m., nat-p.,*** nat-s., nicc., ***nit-ac.,*** nux-m., ***nux-v.,*** ol-an., op., ***par., petr., ph-ac., phos.,*** plan., plat., plb., **PULS.,** raph., rat., rhod., ***rhus-t.,*** ruta, sabad., ***sabin., sars.,*** sel., seneg., ***sep.,*** serp., ***sil., spig.,*** spong., ***squil.,*** stann., staph., ***stront-c.,*** stry., **SULPH.,** ***sul-ac.,*** tab., tarax., tarent., teucr., ***thuj.,*** til., ***valer.,*** verat., verb., viol-t., zinc.

afternoon - aeth., alum., bov., canth., cham., grat., indg., ***lyc.,*** mag-c., nat-c., nicc., ol-an., phel., puls., sars., sep., sil., stront.
4 p.m. - asaf., laur.
4 p.m. every day, with coldness and trembling - asaf.
air, in open - ***mang.,*** sil.
amel. - am-c., nicc., sars., ***sep.,*** tab.
bed, while in - nat-c., plat., thuj.
blowing, nose, on - mur-ac.
boring, stitching - am-c., ruta.
breakfast, after - ***bry.***
burning - arg-m., ph-ac., phos., rhod.
chilliness, during - eupi., sil.
cold hand, touch of, amel. - euphr.
coryza, during - coc-c., kali-c., lyc.
stopped - croc.
coughing, when - alum., anac., ant-t., arn., ***ars., bry.,*** calc., calc-s., ***carb-v.,*** caust., chel., cimic., cina, coloc., con., hep., hyos., kali-ar., ***kali-c.,*** mez., nit-ac., ph-ac., phos., ruta., sabad., stann., sulph., sul-ac., thuj., verb., zinc.
deep-seated - all-c., lach., tab.
descending, on - merc-i-f.
dinner, during - zinc.
after - ant-t., bar-c., mag-c., mur-ac., phos., ***puls., zinc.***
drawing - kreos., ***mang.,*** sil., squil.
dull - kali-c., mag-m., sep., sil.
eating, after - alum., ant-t., bar-c., lyc., mag-c., phel., phos., sep., sulph., ***zinc.***
evening - ambr., bar-c., bell., bov., calc., canth., carb-an., carb-v., caust., chel., dig., dulc., graph., hyper., indg., kali-i., lyc., mag-c., mang., mur-ac., nat-c., nat-m., nit-ac., petr., phos., plat., puls., rat., sel., sep., ***sil.,*** staph., stram., stront-c., sulph., thuj., valer.
in bed - carb-v.
exertion, during - ambr., nat-c.
extending, backwards - ***bry.***
chest, or neck, to - ***nat-m.***
ears - rhus-t.
eyes, to - ***calc., kali-c., lach., spig.,*** **SULPH.**
eyes, out of - sep., sil.
face, to - rhus-t., sars.
frontal eminence - guai.
malar bone, to - indg., rhus-t.
occiput, to - carb-v., ***lyc.,*** mag-c., puls.
outward - alum., sil.
root of nose, to - ***kali-c., lyc.,*** rhus-t.
teeth, ears and neck, to - ***merc.***
temples - carb-v.

SHARP, pain
extending, upward - thuj.
fever, during the - asaf., gels., ***nux-v.,*** puls.
fright, from least - cic.
heat, amel. - kali-c.
of stove, from - bar-c.
intermittent - ph-ac.
jerking - calc., ***nat-m.,*** nux-v., puls., thuj.
lying, while - canth., nat-c., puls., sep.
amel. - ambr., calc., dulc., nat-m., nit-ac., ***sep.***
side, on affected amel. - arn., chel., sep.
side, on well amel. - mag-c.
menses, during - acon., berb., calc., lyc., mang., rat.
after - berb., ***lyc., nat-m.,*** ol-an., plat.
appearance of, amel. - cycl.
before - calc-p., ***ferr.***
mental exertion, after - lyc., pimp.
morning - agar., alum., am-m., arg-m., bry., canth., caust., cham., cic., con., glon., grat., hep., indg., lyc., mag-c., mag-s., mang., nicc., petr., plb., sars., sil., stront-c., thuj., til., verat.
3 a.m. - ferr.
rising, on and after - bar-c., ***mag-c.,*** plb., stront.
waking, on - caust., petr.
motion, on - agn., ant-t., calc., caps., cham., chin., hep., hyper., kali-c., kali-n., mag-p., nat-m., rat., ***sep.,*** sil., spong.
amel. - caps., sulph.
continued amel. - calc-ac.
sudden - petr.
moving, arms - nat-s.
eyes, on - caps., hyper., kali-c.
head - caps., hyper., kali-c., nat-m.
jaw, the, agg. - kali-c.
night - am-c., arum-t., dig., hep., ***lyc.,*** mag-c., nat-m., sep., sil., spig., ***sulph.***
waking, on - hep.
noon - con., elaps
until goes to sleep - mur-ac.
odors, from strong - sel.
periodic - calc., mur-ac.
pressure, amel. - aeth., calad., guai., mur-ac., sil., sulph.
pulsating - calc., ferr., kali-n., ***spig.***
raising, head amel. - kali-c.
reading, while - carb-v., caust., lyc.
respiration, on deep - rat.
rising, on - agar., calc.
amel. - ol-an., puls.
lying, from - calc.
seat, from - mur-ac.
stooping, from - calc., hep., mur-ac.
room, in - am-m., bar-c., bov., con., nat-m., nicc., sel., sep.
amel. in - mang.
rubbing, amel. - canth., phos.
scratching, amel. - plat.
sitting while - caust., chin., indg., mag-c., nit-ac., phos., rat., squil., ***tarax.***
standing, while - mag-c., nit-ac., plb.
still, amel. while - mang.

SHARP, pain
stepping - aloe, alum., alumn., ambr., **BRY.,** sep.
stooping, when - alum., am-m., berb., bry., calc., caps., cycl., ferr-p., glon., ***hep.,*** kali-c., mag-m., mur-ac., nicc., ***par.,*** puls., staph., sulph., thuj.
after - aloe, calc., rhus-t.
sun, from exposure to - bar-c., sel.
talking, after - agar., nat-m.
loudly - sulph.
tearing - berb., coloc., hyos., kali-bi., merc., mur-ac., nat-m., phos.
touch, from - hep., ip., spig., staph.
amel. - ars., ***coloc.***
vexation, after - mag-c.
waking, on - canth., hep., petr., thuj.
walking, while - alum., bry., calc., carb-an., crot-t., merc., nit-ac., plb., sep., staph., sulph., thuj.
about, amel. - canth., hep.
after - bry., hep., tarax., tell.
air, in open - sul-ac.
air, in open, amel. - hep.
warmth, of bed - thuj.
stove, of - bar-c.
washing, face, on - cop.
amel. during, but agg. after - spig.
weather, on change of - vip.

sharp, forehead - acon., aesc., agar., ***agn., alum.,*** am-c., am-m., anac., anan., ang., ant-t., apis, arg-n., ***arn., asaf.,*** aur., bar-c., bar-m., **BELL.,** ***berb., bov.,*** bry., ***calc., calc-s.,*** camph., canth., caps., carb-v., caust., cham., chel., ***chin.,*** cic., cina, cocc., coc-c., ***coloc., con.,*** cupr., cycl., dig., dros., ***dulc., elaps,*** euph., euphr., ferr., ferr-p., gels., gins., gran., grat., guai., hell., ***hep.,*** hyos., ign., ip., ***kali-c., kali-n.,*** kali-p., ***lach.,*** lact., laur., led., ***lil-t., lyc.,*** mag-c., ***mag-m., mang.,*** meny., ***merc., merc-c., mez.,*** mosch., ***mur-ac.,*** nat-c., nat-m., nat-p., ***nit-ac.,*** nux-v., op., ***petr.,*** ph-ac., phos., plan., ***plat.,*** plb., podo., ***puls.,*** rat., rhod., rhus-t., ***ruta.,*** sabad., sabin., ***sars.,*** sel., senec., ***sep., sil., spig.,*** spong., squil., ***stann., staph.,*** stram., ***stront-c., sulph., sul-ac.,*** tarax., ter., til., valer., verat., verb., viol-t., ***zinc.***
above - aloe, chin., mez., nat-m., ol-an., ruta., sulph.
burning - chin.
dull - mez.
morning, in bed - mez.
afternoon - aeth., alum., grat., mag-c., mur-ac., nat-c.
afternoon, 2 p.m. - alum.
air, open - ***mang.,*** sil.
amel. - sars., ***sep.,*** tab.
behind, eyes - phos.
burning - cupr., meny., phos., staph., thuj.
chill, during - arn.
with - mang.
cough, during - anac., arn., hep., hyos., mez., sulph.
daytime - sulph.

sharp, forehead
dinner, after - ant-t.
drawing - aur., chel., mang., ruta, squil.
eating, during - lyc.
after - alum., sulph.
evening - alum., bov., dig., mag-c., mag-m., mang., nat-c., nat-m., sil., sulph.
6 p.m. - mag-c.
8 to11 p.m. - ***sil.***
bed, in - nat-c.
extending, chest to - cham.
ear, to - mang., rhus-t., squil.
eye, to - ***ant-t.,*** mang.
lower jaw, to - brom.
nape - anan.
nose, to - coloc., psor.
occiput, to - ***bell., cedr., cham.,*** nat-m., petr., phos.
outward - colch., con., lyc., sep., sulph.
temple - mur-ac., ruta.
vertex - caust., meny., sep.
externally - ang., dig., hell., hep., staph., ***tarax.***
eyes, over - agar., aloe, alum., am-c., anac., ang., arum-t., bell., berb., bor., ***bov.,*** bry., calc., caps., ***cedr.,*** **CHEL.,** coc-c., colch., ***ferr.,*** ferr-p., kali-c., **KALI-I.,** kali-p., lach., ***lyc.,*** mag-p., mag-s., manc., mang., mez., nat-m., ol-an., paeon., petr., ph-ac., ***phos.,*** pip-m., rhus-t., sel., ***sep.,*** sil., ***spig.,*** sulph., tarent., valer.
blowing nose - mag-c.
coughing - hyos.
dinner - arn., am-c., bor.
eating, after - am-c.
evening - hep., inul., kali-bi., pip-m.
left - caust., ***lac-f.,*** **KALI-I.,** mag-c., ph-ac., ptel., **SEL.,** ***sep.,*** thuj., zinc.
left, extending to right - thuj.
morning - alum., nit-ac., sep.
night - lyc.
night, 3 a.m. - pip-m.
right - anac., ***bov.,*** carb-v., ***cur., lyc., mag-p.,*** mang., tarent.
stooping - ip.
walking in open air amel. - ***phos.,*** sep.
forenoon - mang., sars.
frontal eminence - agar., aloe, am-c., arg-n., arn., ***asaf.,*** bar-c., bell., bov., calc., canth., cham., chel., chin., cocc., croc., euon., grat., guai., lact., laur., led., lyc., mag-m., meny., mez., mur-ac., nat-c., nit-ac., plb., raph., ruta., sabad., sars., **SPIG.,** stann., staph., sul-ac., ***thuj.,*** verb.
above - zinc.
afternoon - arg-n.
afternoon, 2 p.m. - laur.
afternoon, 4 p.m. - nit-ac.
dinner, during - am-c.
evening - alum., lyc., nit-ac., sars.
evening, 6 p.m. - lyc.
evening, 7 p.m. - sars.
extending, ear, into - nat-c.
extending, brain, into - sul-ac.
extending, nose, to - squil.

sharp, forehead
frontal eminence,
extending, outward - bar-c., bell., verb.
left - arn., ***arg-n.,*** asaf., croc., mang., nat-c., sars.
motion amel. - pip-m.
motion on - staph.
noise, from - agar.
open air amel. - pip-m.
outward - bar-c., bell.
pulsating - ***spig.***
right - bell., bov., kali-p., pip-m., squil.
standing, while - canth.
stooping, when - bar-c., lact.
tearing - chel., mez.
waking, on - thuj.
washing, when - bar-c.
itching - ang.
jerking - lyc., mang.
light, from - bov.
lying, agg. - cham.
lying, amel. - calc., ***lyc., sep.***
mediation, on - lyc.
menses, during - phos.
after - plat.
middle, of - aur., chel., gels., indg., sars., stann., valer.
afternoon - gels.
eating, after - nit-ac.
evening - bov., mag-m.
extending outward - kali-c., ph-ac., phos.
motion, agg. - sep.
noon - gels.
pulsating - petr.
stooping, when - gels., rat.
walking, amel. - sep.
walking, in open air - laur.
morning - arg-n., con., grat., hell., kali-c., lyc., petr., sars., sil.
rising, after - coloc., con.
waking, on - arn., petr.
motion, on - ***bov., kali-c.,*** lyc., mag-c., ***sep.,*** spong., staph.
moving, eyes - ***dros.***
night - cham., nat-m., spig.
midnight, on coughing - hep.
noon - con., mur-ac., zinc.
nose, over - agar., berb., camph., chin., kali-bi., kali-c., nat-m., nit-ac., psor., ran-b., rhus-t., sars., sep., sil.
pressing - mang., nat-m.
pressure, agg. - mur-ac.
pulsating - sars.
raising, head amel. - kali-c.
raising, the eyes - arn.
reading - lyc., ***ruta.***
rhythmical - kali-n.
rising, after - agar.
room, in - con.
amel. - mang.
sides - agar., am-m., anac., asaf., ant-c., berb., bov., bry., calc., calc-ar., canth., cocc., cycl., dig., dros., euphr., grat., hyos., kali-n., kali-s., kreos., lach., mag-m., mang., nat-m., nat-s., ***sars.,*** staph., sides

sharp, forehead
sides - sul-ac., tarax., thuj., verat., verb., zinc.
afternoon - am-m., phos.
air, open, amel. - carb-an.
coryza, with - stann.
dinner, after - nat-m.
evening - chel., lyc., nat-m., phos., sul-ac., sulph.
extending, brain, into - sul-ac.
extending, eye, into - psor.
extending, face, to - cycl.
extending, jaw, to - all-c.
extending, left to right - squil.
extending, outward - mag-c., spong.
extending, teeth, to - all-c.
laughing, on - glon.
left - ***arg-n., bar-c., calc.,*** caust., chin., coloc., ***euph., lyc.,*** mang., phos., spong., ***stann.,*** **STAPH.,** tarax.
left, to right - cocc., squil.
morning - carb-an., mez., nicc., sars.
morning, 9 a.m. - sil.
morning, 10 a.m. - nat-s.
morning, 11 a.m. - calc.
morning, rising, after - carb-an.
opening eyes - ***sil.***
pressing - dig.
pressure, amel. - sul-ac.
right - ***alum.,*** bell., ***cocc., lyc.,*** mag-c., nux-v., ***phos.,*** ruta, sil., sul-ac.
right, to left - aesc.
sitting, while - calc., merc., ruta.
stooping - kali-n.
touch, amel. - chin.
sitting, while - chin.
sleep, on going to - alum.
standing, while - alum.
still amel. - mang.
stooping, on - berb., bry., ***dros., kali-c.,*** mag-m., mur-ac., rat., staph., sulph.
sunlight - bov.
talking, loud - sulph.
tearing - cham.
touch, on - ip.
transversal - chel., spong.
twitching - mag-m., mang., mez., spong.
walking, while - crot-t., kali-n., mang., merc., sep., spong., sulph.
air, in open - merc., sars., spong.
air, in open, amel. - ***sep.***
warm, applications amel. - kali-c.

sharp, occiput - acon., aesc., aeth., aloe, ambr., ammc., ant-t., arn., ***bar-c.,*** bar-m., ***bell.,*** bov., bry., ***bufo,*** calc., canth., ***carb-an.,*** carb-v., caust., cham., ***chel.,*** cimic., coc-c., ***con.,*** dig., dulc., euphr., ferr-p., gels., glon., grat., hell., ***hep., hyper.,*** ign., indg., iod., iris, kali-bi., ***kali-c.,*** kali-i., kali-n., kali-p., ***lac-c.,*** laur., ***lyc.,*** mag-c., ***mag-m.,*** mang., meny., ***merc., mur-ac.,*** nat-c., ***nat-m.,*** nit-ac., nux-m., petr., **PHOS.,** puls., ran-b., rhus-t., samb., sars., sec., ***sep.,*** sil., spig., spong., squil., staph., stront-c., stry., sulph., sul-ac., ***tarax.,*** teucr., thuj., verat., verb., viol-t., zinc.

sharp, occiput
burning - carb-v., staph.
coughing, on - coloc., sulph.
deep-seated - canth., cop.
dinner, after - ant-t.
eating, after - alum.
evening - alum., ambr., carb-v., hyper., lyc., mag-c., mur-ac., sep., thuj.
extending, across - agar.
back of chest - eupi.
ears, through - puls.
eye, to - sanic.
forehead to - bov., chel., ferr-p., **LAC-C., NAT-M.,** sanic., sars., thuj.
forward - nat-m., sars.
frontal eminence, to - bar-c.
nape of neck, to - mang., mur-ac., stry.
upper jaw, left side - cham.
vertex, to - sep.
forenoon - lyc.
lying down, on - puls.
menses, during - kali-n.
morning - agar., kali-c., mang., petr., verat.
waking, on - arn., mang.
motion, on - ***kali-c.,*** kali-n., spong.
night - lyc.
occipital protuberance - nit-ac.
pulsating - ***carb-an., con.,*** cop., hep., kali-n.
room, on entering - nat-m.
sides - acon., bov., calc., ***chel.,*** grat., guai., indg., kali-bi., kali-n., laur., lyc., mag-m., nat-c., nat-m., phos., sars., spig., sulph., sul-ac., verb., viol-t.
afternoon - euphr., petr.
breakfast, during - nit-ac.
dinner, after - canth., ol-an.
drawing - chel.
evening - carb-an., nat-c., nit-ac.
evening, sleep amel. - nit-ac.
extending, forehead, to - ***chel.***
extending, neck, to nape - mur-ac.
extending, side to side - agar.
extending, upward - staph.
left - alum., bell., ***chel.,*** nit-ac., petr., samb., sars., sul-ac.
morning - agar., bov., eupi.
morning, 7 a.m. - bov.
pinching - chel.
pressing - chel.
right - ***calc.,*** mang., ***nat-c.,*** nit-ac., ***sanic.,*** sulph.
right, extending to forehead - chel., sanic.
right, extending to left forehead - staph.
spot - spig.
tearing - euphr., samb.
twitching - cham., mag-m.
sitting, while - indg., squil.
sleep amel. - nit-ac.
stepping agg. - con., kali-c., sep.
stooping, after - aloe, kali-c., rhus-t.
tearing - aeth., thuj.
touch, agg. - kali-n.
turning the head - mang., ***spong.***
warm room - bov.

sharp, sides - aeth., alum., am-c., am-m., anac., asaf., aur., bar-c., bar-m., bell., ***berb.,*** bor., bov., brom., bry., calc., calc-p., camph., cann-s., canth., caps., carb-ac., carb-v., cast., caust., cham., chel., chin., cic., cinnb., cocc., coc-c., con., crot-h., cupr., cycl., dig., eup-pur., euph., euphr., eupi., ferr., ferr-p., gamb., graph., grat., guai., hyos., hyper., indg., iod., ***kali-bi.,*** kali-c., kali-p., **KALI-S.,** lach., laur., ***mag-c., mag-m.,*** mag-s., mang., meny., merc-c., mez., mill., mur-ac., nat-c., ***nat-m.,*** nat-p., nat-s., nicc., nit-ac., ***nux-v.,*** ol-an., petr., ph-ac., phos., plat., plb., puls., rat., rhod., sars., sep., sil., spig., staph., sulph., tarax., ***tarent.,*** thuj., verb., ***zinc.***
 afternoon - alum., canth., nicc., sep.
  3 p.m. - mag-c.
 alternating sides - agar.
 bending body to right - mag-m.
 bowing, on - thuj.
 burning - phos., staph.
 coughing, on - anac., ***bry.,*** cimx., mang., sulph.
 daytime - nicc.
 dinner, after - bar-c., mag-c., zinc.
 evening - bar-c., canth., carb-v., caust., mag-c., nat-m., plat.
 exerting arms - nat-s.
  eyes and - hyper.
 extending, backward - mag-c.
  deep into brain - anac., indg.
  down arm - cimx.
  eye, to - calc., mag-m.
  face, to - kali-bi.
  forehead - con., mur-ac., sil.
  forward - kali-c., mag-c., mag-m., mang., thuj., verb.
  frontal bone, to - con., guai.
  neck, to - sars.
  occiput, to - cic., mag-c., phos., tab.
  outward - mag-c.
  orbit - mur-ac.
  outward - mag-c.
  side to side, from - carb-v., mag-c.
  vertex - meny.
 forenoon - alum., am-m., nicc., plb.
  standing - plb.
  walking - plb.
 fright, from - cic.
 heat, during - cham.
 intermittent - plat., spig.
 left - aeth., ***bar-c.,*** berb., calc., calc-p., cann-s., cham., con., crot-h., cycl., kali-c., lach., ***mang.,*** mez., nat-c., nat-m., ***plat.,*** rhod., sars., sil., staph., sulph., tab.
  extending to frontal eminence - bar-c., guai.
 looking up - caps.
 lying on painless side amel. - mag-c.
 menses, during - ***calc-p.,*** mag-m.
  before - calc-p.
 morning - alum., mag-c., mag-s., nat-m., nicc., ***nux-v.,*** sars.
  until evening - nat-m.
  waking - staph.

sharp, sides
 motion agg. - sil.
 nail, as from a - carb-v.
 night - nat-m.
  menses, after - ol-an.
 outward - mag-m., staph.
 pressure on - kali-c.
 pulsating - aeth., calc., petr.
 reading, while - lyc.
 right - alum., anac., bor., brom., caust., cic., cupr., grat., iod., kali-bi., ***mag-c., mur-ac.,*** nit-ac., ph-ac., plb., rat., sars., tarent., thuj.
 room, in - am-m.
 sit, down, must - con.
 sitting, while - mag-c.
  down, on - rat.
 spot, in - spig.
 standing, while - mag-c.
 stooping, on - alum., caps., hep., mang.
 talking - canth.
 tearing - carb-v., con., sars., spig., thuj.
 turning to right - mag-s.
 waking, on - thuj.
 wandering - ***kali-bi.,*** tarent.

sharp, temples - acon., aesc., aeth., agar., aloe, ***alum.,*** ambr., am-c., am-m., anac., ang., ant-c., ant-t., **APIS,** apoc., arg-m., ***arn.,*** ars., ars-i., arum-t., asaf., asar., bapt., bar-c., bar-m., ***bell.,*** berb., bor., bov., bry., cadm-s., calad., ***calc.,*** calc-s., camph., ***cann-i.,*** canth., ***carb-an.,*** carb-s., carb-v., **CAUST.,** ***cham.,*** chel., **CHIN.,** cimic., cina, cocc., coc-c., coff., ***coloc.,*** cop., crot-h., ***cupr., cycl.,*** daph., dig., dulc., euph., euphr., eupi., ***ferr.,*** ferr-ar., ferr-i., ferr-p., gamb., ***glon.,*** gran., graph., grat., ***guai.,*** hell., hep., hydr., hyper., ign., iod., iris, kali-bi., ***kali-c.,*** **KALI-I.,** kali-n., kali-p., kreos., laur., lec., **LYC.,** ***lyss.,*** mag-c., mag-m., mag-s., manc., ***mang.,*** meny., ***merc.,*** merc-i-f., merl., mez., mur-ac., nat-c., ***nat-m.,*** nat-p., ***nit-ac.,*** nux-m., ***nux-v.,*** ol-an., ***par.,*** ph-ac., ***phos.,*** plat., plb., psor., ***puls.,*** ran-b., ran-s., rheum, rhod., rhus-t., ruta., sabad., sal-ac., sang., ***sars.,*** sel., sep., ***sil.,*** sol-n., ***spig.,*** spong., squil., ***stann., staph.,*** stram., stront-c., stry., ***sulph.,*** sul-ac., tab., tarax., tarent., ther., thuj., verb., viol-t., zinc.
 afternoon - canth., cham., nit-ac., stront.
  1 p.m. - sars., sep.
  3 p.m. - ***pip-m.***
 air open, in - ***mang.***
 alternating, with heat and coldness - bor.
  with pressure - meny., tab.
 bending head backward, amel. - thuj.
  head forward - thuj.
 boring, amel. on touch - calc., coloc.
 breathing, when - anac.
 burning - ars., bar-c., cupr., phos., plat., sars., staph.
 chewing, on - am-c., am-m.
 chill, during - graph., stann.
 cold amel. - ***apis.***
 cough, during - alum., caust., cina, kali-c.
 descending stairs - merc-i-f.

sharp, temples
dinner, after - kali-n., mag-c.
drawing - cycl.
dull - bor., caust., cycl., sars., staph., zinc.
evening - ***caust.,*** dig., graph., hyper., nat-c., nit-ac., phos., sep., sil., stront.
6 p.m. - kali-i., sep.
8 p.m. - stram.
bed, in - nat-c., sep.
extending, brain, into - aloe, croc., ph-ac.
brain, through - dig.
downward - ang.
eyes, to - ant-c., berb., graph., lec., ph-ac.
forehead, to and across - anac., berb., bor., ***ferr.,*** sil., squil., tab.
inward - acon., arg-m., arn., lach., rhus-t., til.
occiput, to - carb-s., ***cham., pip-m.***
outward - bar-ac., berb., calc., dulc., lyc., nux-m., rhus-t., sil., sulph.
teeth, to - sars.
temple to temple - **CHIN.**
zygoma, to - kali-c.
forenoon - am-m., hep., indg., lyc., mag-c.
10 a.m. - hep.
11 a.m. - lyc.
intermittent - bor., calc., stann.
itching - ang.
jerking - cycl., mang., rhus-t., squil.
left - aeth., ambr., asaf., calc., carb-s., ***chel.,*** cocc., coc-c., crot-h., gent-c., mag-c., pip-m., plat., ***sep., spig., staph.,*** tarax.
to right - calc., cocc.
light, looking at a bright - **NAT-M.**
looking at sun, white or red color - graph.
lying on the painful part amel. - chel.
mental exertion - lyc., sil., sulph.
morning - cham.
motion, during - agn., calc., kali-c., stann.
moving the jaw - calc., kali-c.
needles like - zinc.
burning - ars., staph.
night - dig., ferr., lyc.
3 a.m. - ***ferr.***
sleep, during - dig.
paroxysmal - berb.
pressure, agg. - coc-c., verb.
amel. - aesc., aeth., guai., thuj.
pulsating - stann., staph.
raising head amel. - kali-c.
reading - ***caust.***
rheumatic - lyc.
rhythmical - bor., stann.
right - agar., ***alum.,*** bor., ***caust.,*** coff., coloc., crot-c., grat., ***lyc., ph-ac., phos., sars.,*** squil., stront.
to left - aesc.
scratching, amel. - plat.
shaking head - nat-m., ***nux-v.***
singing, while - alum.
sitting, while - ***caust.,*** guai., nit-ac., ***tarax.***
standing agg. - guai.
amel. - mur-ac., tarax.
stepping agg. - aloe.
stool, during - lyc.

sharp, temples
stooping - kali-c., mang., ***par.***
talking, after - agar.
tearing - ars., dig., kali-c., viol-t.
touch, agg. - sars., staph.
touch, amel. - ars., ***coloc.,*** cycl., mur-ac.
walking, while - ptel., sep.
after - bry., tarax., tell.
amel. - guai., staph.
in open air - tarax.
warm applications amel. - kali-c.
warm room, in - sel.
yawning amel. - mur-ac.

sharp, vertex - acon., aesc., aeth., alum., alumn., am-m., anac., ***bar-c.,*** bell., bor., bov., ***bry., calc.,*** caps., carb-an., carb-v., ***caust.,*** chel., chin., cimx., cimic., ***con.,*** cop., cupr., cycl., dig., eupi., ferr., ferr-i., ferr-p., graph., hell., hyper., guai., indg., iod., ip., kali-i., kali-n., lach., laur., lith., ***lyc., mag-c.,*** mag-m., meny., ***mez.,*** mill., nat-c., ***nat-m.,*** nicc., nit-ac., olnd., ol-an., petr., phel., ***ph-ac., phos.,*** puls., raph., rat., ruta., sabad., sars., sep., sil., ***spig., stann.,*** staph., stront-c., stry., sulph., tab., thuj., valer., verb., zinc.
afternoon - alum., bov., indg., mur-ac., nit-ac.
3 to 6 p.m. - am-m.
burning - cupr., phos., stann., staph., zinc.
coughing, on - alum., con., ***sabad.***
evening - ***calc.,*** carb-an., nit-ac., petr.
extending, brain, to - spig., staph.
forehead, to - caps., mez., nicc.
head, to - lach.
head, to, through whole - bar-c.
inward - petr.
occiput - mag-c.
outward - staph.
palate, into - nat-m.
pharynx, to - cham.
temples, to - carb-v., phos.
within outward - spig.
forenoon - nicc.
10:30 a.m. - mag-c.
intermittent - ph-ac.
leaning head on something amel. - nat-m.
menses, after - ol-an.
morning - am-m., phos.
until afternoon - graph.
needles, like - staph.
night - chel., lyc., nit-ac.
noon - mur-ac.
paroxysmal - ***caust.,*** chel.
perspiration, amel. - graph.
pressure, amel. - ph-ac.
pulsating - aeth.
reading, while - carb-v., lyc.
rubbing amel. - aeth.
spots - chel., kali-bi.
stooping, on - alumn., am-m.
sun, exposure to - ***bar-c.***
trembling - anac.
touch, agg. - ph-ac.
walking, while - carb-an.
rapidly - chel.
washing amel. - spig.

sharp, vertex
wet weather - ***calc.***

SHATTERING, pain - kali-c.

SHOCKS, in head - acon., aeth., agar., ***all-c.,*** alum., ars., asaf., aster., bapt., bar-c., bar-m., ***bell.,*** benz-ac., bov., calc., camph., **CANN-I.,** carb-s., carb-v., caust., ***cic.,*** clem., ***coca, croc., crot-c.,*** ferr., ferr-ar., ferr-p., fl-ac., ***glon.,*** graph., ***hell.,*** hydr-ac., indg., ip., ***kali-ar.,*** kali-c., kali-p., ***kali-s.,*** lach., laur., led., lob., ***lyc.,*** lyss., mag-s., ***mang.,*** merc., mill., mur-ac., nat-c., ***nat-m.,*** nat-p., nat-s., nit-ac., nux-v., olnd., ph-ac., phos., plb., psor., puls., ran-b., raph., rhus-t., sabad., samb., sang., seneg., ***sep., sil., spig.,*** stann., sulph., ***sul-ac.,*** tarent., thea., thuj., valer., verat-v., zinc.
ascending, on - ant-c., arn., bell., meny., par., ph-ac.
cold, air - ***cic.***
consciousness, on regaining - cann-i.
coughing when - ars., ***calc., ip., lach.,*** lyc., mag-s., mang., ***nat-m.,*** rhus-t., seneg., spig., sul-ac., sulph.
drinking cold water, on - thea.
eating, after - lyc.
electric, like - agar., ail., ***all-c., alum.,*** arn., carb-v., ***cic.,*** hipp., lob., nat-s., nux-m., op., ***phos.***
falling asleep, while sitting - alum.
evening - nit-ac., sul-ac.
falling asleep, on - sil.
in bed - sil.
extending, cheek, to - puls.
from elbow to head - agar.
here and there - zinc.
limbs, to - ***ail.,*** **CIC.,** nux-m.
hawking, on - **RAPH.**
here and there - zinc.
lying, while - nit-ac.
menses, during - bor.
mental, exertion, after - phos.
morning - phos.
bed, in - nux-v., sul-ac.
bed, in, rising, on - sep., tarent.
bed, in, rising, on, amel. - nux-v.
motion, from - ***am-c., cic., lyc.,*** merc., prun.
night, 1 a.m., waking him - psor.
noise, from - nit-ac.
outward - clem.
pinching - sep.
pressure amel. - bell., thuj.
pulse, at each beat of - ***cimic.,*** **GLON.**
reading, from - carb-v.
regaining consciousness, on - cann-i.
running, while - nat-m.
shaking when - mang.
siesta, after a - sep.
while sitting - alum.
sitting after a full meal, while - lyc.
sleep, on going to - nat-c., phos.
sneezing, when - bar-c.
stitching - petr.
stool, during - phos.
stooping, on - merc., nit-ac., petr., thuj.

SHOCKS, in head
sudden - ***cic., kali-i.***
talking, while - nat-m.
waking, him - psor.
walking, while - bell., mang., petr.
open, air, in - spig.
rapidly - ant-c., arn., **BELL.,** nat-m., par., ph-ac.
writing, while - raph.

shocks, forehead - acon., am-c., ang., camph., caust., croc., glon., hipp., kali-c., laur., mag-s., nat-m., olnd., phos., plat., psor., rhus-t., sang., seneg., sep., spig., stann., sul-ac., thuj., zinc.
axe, as with an - nux-v.
finger, as with a - nat-m.
motion, on - mag-c.
painful - sul-ac.
sleep, during - dig.
stool, after - spig.
walking - mag-c.
wavelike - sep.

shocks, occiput - arn., cann-i., hell., lyc., mang., ***phos.,*** plb., ran-b., sabad.
dull, heavy, throbbing pain through head, with sensation like a heavy blow on back of head and neck - cann-i.
extending, forehead, to - clem., sabad.
just as he was losing himself in sleep, like a loud report - phos.
mental exertion - ***phos.***

shocks, sides - alum., am-c., bov., chel., graph., kali-c., kali-s., laur., mag-m., nat-s., phos., plat., plb., puls., sars., spig., sulph.
right - graph., puls.

shocks, temples - agn., am-c., bar-c., camph., croc., ***iris,*** lach., **LYC.,** olnd., ph-ac., ***plat.,*** spig., sul-ac., thuj.
cough, during - **LYC.**
painful - sul-ac.
peg were struck in deep, as if - sul-ac.
stool, during - lyc.
sudden, deep in, causes starting - croc.

shocks, vertex - calc., lyc., lyss., mang., nat-c., phos.
bolt, as from a, from neck to agg. at each throb of heart - cimic.
electric like - carb-ac., nat-s.
extending to forehead - nat-m.
sleep, on going to - nat-c.

SHOOTING, pain - acet-ac., ***acon.,*** aeth., agar., ***alum.,*** ambr., am-c., ant-t., apis, arg-m., bar-c., ***bell.,*** berb., bry., calc., caps., carb-v., caust., cham., cimic., colch., ***con.,*** corn., dulc., ***eup-per., ferr.,*** gels., gran., ***hell.,*** hep., hura, hyos., ign., indg., iod., ip., ***kali-bi.,*** **KALI-C.,** kali-n., lach., lact., laur., ***mag-c.,*** mag-m., mag-p., manc., mang., merc., mur-ac., naja, nat-c., ***nat-m., nit-ac.,*** nux-v., petr., plan., ptel., puls., rhus-r., ***rhus-t., sep.,*** sil., staph., sulph., ***ter.,*** teucr., thuj., valer.
afternoon - ***ferr.,*** plan., sulph., tarent.
air, cold - iris
open, in, amel. - naja
bending head backward - anac.

SHOOTING, pain
blowing nose, on - kali-c.
coughing, on - arn., bry., calc., carb-v., con., mang.
cramps, during - hell.
cries, extorting - sep.
eating agg. - sulph.
evening - bell., tarent.
amel. toward - kali-bi.
exercise, during - nat-c.
extending, downward into teeth - ***kalm.,*** sep.
from behind forward - nat-m.
from within outward - alum., cinnb., nat-c., rhus-t., sulph.
here and there - am-c., bapt., calc., hydr-ac., mag-c., mag-s., nicc., plb., rat., sul-ac.
here and there, flying - asar., calc., stront.
upward - guai., sep., sil.
vertex, to - sep.
increasing and declining - bar-c.
lying down - cimic., kali-bi., ***rhus-t.***
with head low - ***rhus-t.***
menses, during - apis
after - berb.
before - calc-p., ferr., nat-m., ol-an.
morning - arum-t., caust., ptel.
begins, in, increases till noon and ceases toward evening - kali-bi.
rising, after - mag-c.
rising, before, agg. - ***nat-h.***
waking, on - caust.
moving head amel. - mag-p., sulph.
night - tarent.
noon - calc-p., sep.
pressure amel. - bell., cupr-s., mag-p.
pulsating - aeth., **BELL.,** ferr., nux-v.
rising agg. - phys.
singing, while - alum., ptel.
sitting up, while - ***lyc.***
amel. - acon.
sneezing, on - am-m., cina
step, at every - sep.
stooping, on - bell., indg., kreos., nit-ac., sulph., sul-i.
talking, from - nat-m., thuj.
teeth, clenching, amel. - sulph.
turning eyes up - arum-t.
vexation, after - mag-c.
walking, while - bell., phys.
yawning, from - bar-c.

shooting, forehead - ***acon.,*** aesc., agar., ant-t., apis, arn., ***bell.,*** berb., chin., cinnb., ***coloc.,*** **CON.,** cycl., dig., dulc., euph., ferr., fl-ac., ***iris,*** kali-bi., ***kali-c.,*** kali-n., kreos., mag-c., mag-m., mang., merc., merc-i-f., mosch., naja, nat-c., plb., **PRUN.,** puls., rhod., rhus-t., rumx., sabad., senec., ***sep.,*** sil., **SPIG.,** stram., sulph., tarent., til.
air, open, in - mang.
diagonally - chel.
eating amel. - **SEP.**
evening - mag-m.

shooting, forehead
extending, occiput, to - **BELL.,** cinnb., nat-c., **PRUN., SEP.**
flying - asar., jatr., sep.
intermittent - mag-c.
inward - canth., coloc., gels., lach.
left - ***merl.,*** **SEP.**
menses, during - ***rat.***
morning - iris
motion - ***lach.***
quick - iris
night in bed - sulph.
noon - con.
outward - con., lyc., senec.
over eyes - ***acon.,*** agar., am-c., ant-c., berb., bov., bry., caust., **CEDR.,** ***kali-bi.,*** kali-p., lyss., nat-a., nat-m., nit-ac., ph-ac., ***prun., sep.,*** sulph., zinc.
4 p.m. - sol-n.
4 p.m, extending occiput, to - **PRUN.,** sol-n.
afternoon - sulph.
left - ***acon.,*** agar., **CEDR.,** nat-a., pip-m., ***sep.,*** sulph.
left, 3 p.m. - pip-m.
left, extending, occiput, to - **SEP.**
left, extending, vertex, to - phyt.
morning on waking - agar.
outward - bar-ac., bell., con., ferr., glon., gran., lyc., ph-ac., puls., senec., sep., sulph., verb.
pressure amel. - kali-p.
right - bry., nat-a., **PRUN.**
rubbing amel. - kali-p.
upward - ph-ac., scut.
violent shooting pains from root of nose along left orbital arch to external angle of eye, with dim sight, begins in morning, increases till noon, and ceases toward evening - kali-bi.
rhythmical - kali-n.
right - **BELL., PRUN., SPIG.**
stooping, on - kreos.
walking, while - kali-bi., kali-n.

shooting, occiput - acon., aeth., agar., ail., alum., anac., arum-t., asaf., bell., bov., calc., caps., cedr., ***chel., cimic.,*** cinnb., con., dig., glon., grat., hep., ***hyper.,*** indg., iod., **JUG-C.,** kali-c., kali-n., lac-c., laur., lyc., mag-c., mag-m., meny., mur-ac., naja, nat-m., nit-ac., ol-an., phos., ***sang.,*** sec., ***sil., sulph.,*** teucr., zinc.
diagonally across - agar.
evening - mag-c.
extending, back, down - cimic.
eye, to - cimic., ***sulph.***
forehead - ***cinnb.,*** lac-c.
spine and arms, down - ***crot-h.***
temples, to - ***cann-i.***
vertex, to, like a bolt - ***cimic., cann-i., sil.***
forward - chel., ***cinnb.***
pulsation, with every - ***con.***
turning eyes upward - arum-t.
upward - ambr., sep., sil.

shooting, sides - acon., aesc., aeth., agar., aloe, alum., am-c., am-m., anac., arg-n., bar-c., calc., camph., canth., caust., cham., ***chel.,*** cocc., con., ***ferr.,*** fl-ac., iris, kali-c., lach., lil-t., mag-c., mag-m., mang., meny., nat-m., phos., phys., plan., ***prun.,*** rumx., sabin., sars., stann., tarent.
cough, during - mang.
extending, eye - ***prun.***
half of right hand, to - phos.
root of nose - phos.
lain on - mag-c.
left - canth., ***cinnb., ferr.,*** tarent.
left, talking, while - canth.
left, then right - aesc.
night - tarent.
periodical - ***chel.***
right - lil-t., mag-c., plan., stann.

shooting, temples - acet-ac., acon., aesc., aeth., agar., alumn., anac., apis, arum-t., bapt., ***bell.,*** calc-p., caust., chel., cimic., coca, com., cupr-s., dig., echi., ***form., gels.,*** glon., ***iris,*** kali-bi., **KALI-C.,** kalm., lil-t., lyc., merc-i-f., naja, ***nit-ac.,*** phos., phys., phyt., pic-ac., pip-m., ptel., rhus-t., sang., sep., ***spig., stram.,*** sulph., sul-i., ***tarent.,*** thea.
afternoon - sep., sulph.
air open, amel. - naja
bending head backward agg. - anac.
cold air agg. - ***spig.***
cough, during - mang.
evening - nit-ac., tarent.
extending, from temple to from - alumn., asc-c., **BELL.,** chel., ***chin.,*** phos., plat., sang.
inward - arn., berb., canth., dirc., **KALI-C.,** rhus-t.
occiput, to - kalm., ***spig., stram.***
outward - bell., dulc., kali-bi., rhus-t.
outward, out and in - staph.
upward - chin-s.
upward, up and down - ang.
zygoma, to - ***phos.***
forenoon, 10:30 a.m. - kalm.
heat agg. - rhus-t.
left - aeth., anac., cimic., ***merl., nit-ac.,*** rhus-t., sep., spig.
lying agg. - kali-bi.
morning on waking - ***alumn.***
night - sang., ***tarent.***
noon - calc-p., sep.
pressure amel. - ***calc.***
pulsating - acon.
right - ***bell.,*** calc-p., ***iris,*** sulph., tarent.
right, extending to left side of occiput - ***iris.***
spreading out in a circle - ***caust.***
stool, during - lyc.
transient - iris, tarent.

shooting, vertex - acon., aeth., agar., alum., am-m., bar-c., bell., berb., bov., bry., calc., caps., carb-an., carb-v., caust., cham., chel., chin., cimic., con., cupr., dig., hura, iod., ip., iris, kali-bi., kalm., lach., laur., lyc., mag-c., mez., mill., nat-m., nit-ac., phel., ph-ac., phos., phyt., spig., stram., sulph., tab., ter., valer., zinc.
across - lac-ac.
air, cold - iris
boring through - sil.
coughing, on - alum.
deep - caps., indg., lyc., staph., tab.
drawing, head backward - phel.
extending, forward, to - cham., nicc.
temples, to - kalm.
inward - aloe, lach., lyc.
transient - indg., mill.

SINKING, sensation - glon.
something were sinking, from occiput, on stooping, as if - kali-c.

SKULL-cap, sensation of - acon., apis, ***arg-n.,*** asaf., ***berb.,*** cann-i., **CARB-V.,** chin-a., coc-c., con., ***crot-c.,*** **CYCL., GRAPH.,** hell., helo., ip., kali-s., ***lil-t., lyss.,*** petr., pyrog., stry., sulph., zinc.
afternoon, 4 p.m. - calc-s.

SMALLER, head, feels - acon., coff., ***grat.,*** pic-ac.

SMARTING, pain (see Sore) - bapt., camph., canth., chin., euphr., glon., ham., rhus-t., sabin.

smarting, forehead - bapt., canth., carb-an., gels., graph., hydr., lach.
on touch - graph.

SNAPPING, in vertex, at every step - con.

SORE, pain, bruised - abrot., acon., aesc., agar., aloe, alum., alumn., am-c., am-m., anac., ***apis, arg-m., arn., ars., ars-i., aur.,*** bad., ***bapt.,*** bar-c., bar-m., **BELL.,** benz-ac., bor., ***bov.,*** bry., ***calc., calc-p.,*** camph., cann-i., ***canth., caps., carb-ac., carb-s., carb-v.,*** caust., cham., chel., **CHIN.,** chin-a., ***chin-s.,*** cimic., ***cinnb.,*** cob., coff., con., cop., corn., ***cupr.,*** cupr-ar., daph., ***eup-per.,*** eup-pur., ***euph.,*** euphr., ***ferr., ferr-ar.,*** ferr-p., fl-ac., **GELS.,** ***glon., graph.,*** gymn., ham., ***hell.,*** **HEP.,** hipp., ***ign.,*** ind., iod., **IP.,** kali-bi., kali-n., kali-p., ***kreos.,*** lac-c., ***lac-d., lach.,*** lachn., lac-ac., lact., led., ***lyc.,*** lyss., mag-c., ***mag-m.,*** manc., mang., med., **MERC., MEZ.,** mosch., mur-ac., naja, nat-a., nat-c., nat-m., ***nat-s.,*** nicc., **NIT-AC.,** ***nux-m.,*** **NUX-V.,** olnd., op., ***par., petr.,*** ph-ac., ***phos., phyt.,*** pic-ac., plan., plat., prun., ***puls.,*** raph., rat., rhod., ***rhus-t., ruta.,*** sabad., sang., sars., sec., ***sep.,*** **SIL.,** sol-n., sol-t-ae., ***spig.,*** stann., ***staph.,*** stram., ***sulph., sul-ac., sul-i., syph., tarent.,*** tep., ter., ***thuj., verat.,*** zinc., zing.
afternoon - alum., bufo, nicc., phos., sang.
air, open - calc., eup-per.
amel. - ang., ***ip.***
breakfast, after - merc.
closing eyes amel. - ***chin.,*** plan., sil.
cold air - ***chin.,*** ind., thuj.
applications amel. - euph.
combing hair - alum., ***ars.,*** asar., carb-s., ***chin., hep.,*** lac-c., mang., nat-s., ***rhus-t.,*** sars., ***sil., sulph.***
conversation amel. - eup-per.
dinner, after - mag-m.
amel. - rumx.

SORE, pain
evening - acon., bov., ***calc.,*** cast., chel., ***euphr.,*** graph., mag-c., nit-ac., phos., ***puls., zinc.***
in bed - plan.
forenoon - sep.
heated, on becoming - petr.
jarring agg. - bar-c., **BELL.,** calc., hell., ***led.,*** nit-ac., nux-v., phyt., sil.
leaning head to right amel. - stram.
lying agg. - aur., crot-h., euphr., nux-m.
on part agg. - **NIT-AC.,** nux-m., plan., spig.
menses, during - ***gels.,*** mag-c., nux-v.
mental exertion, after - anac., ***aur.,*** **CHIN.,** daph., ***phos.,*** prun.
morning - aur., bov., caust., cob., con., gymn., hep., hyper., ind., merc., mez., nicc., **NUX-V.,** petr., plan., sul-ac.
rising - ars.
rising, amel. - aur.
waking, on - ambr., anac., con., ***cupr-ar., ign., plan.,*** tarent.
motion, on - caps., carb-s., ***chin.,*** **CIMIC.,** cupr-ar., glon., iod., mang., merc., nat-a., nux-v., rumx., ***tell.***
amel. - aur., mur-ac., ***ph-ac., puls.***
night - cob., coca, phos.
painful part - ***spig.***
paroxysmal - ***verat.***
pressure, from - arg-m.
of hat - carb-v., **NIT-AC.,** ***sil.***
on pillow - cupr-ar., **NIT-AC.**
reading agg. - aur.
riding on cars agg. - glon.
rubbing amel. - ars., thuj.
shaking, head - ***bell., glon.,*** mang., nit-ac.
sneezing - arn., bell., bry., grat.
speaking, while - aur., ***chin.,*** spig.
spots - ambr., ***ox-ac., sil.***
stooping, on - bapt., ***coloc.,*** hell., lyc., nicc., rumx.
sun, from exposure to - manc., nit-ac.
touch, on - ars., nit-ac., phos., ph-ac., sul-ac.
turning eyes - cupr., hep., mur-ac.
vexation, after - **MEZ.**
waking, on - ind., plan., tarent.
walking, while - **CAPS.,** hyos., nit-ac., nux-v., ph-ac., phos., raph., stram.
in open air - ***chin.,*** coff.
in open air, amel. - ***puls.***
in wind - chin.
warm, bed agg. - ***calc., carb-v.***
room - ***coff., puls.***
room, amel. - eup-per.
warmth amel. - ***nux-m.***
wet weather, during - **CALC.,** ***nat-s.,*** phyt.
writing - aur.

sore, forehead - acon., ang., ant-t., apis, ***arn.,*** ars., bapt., bufo, canth., carb-an., cob., coff., ***coloc.,*** cupr-ar., dros., ***euph.,*** gels., glon., ***hep.,*** hipp., hydr., indg., iod., lach., lil-t., lyc., mag-s., merc., merc-i-f., mur-ac., nat-a., nat-c., nat-m., ***par.,*** ph-ac., plan., plat., podo., prun., **PULS.,** ran-b., ***rumx.,*** sang., sarr., **SIL.,** sol-n., spig., spong., stann., sulph., sul-ac., tell., teucr., thuj., zinc., ziz.
breaking sensation after dinner - nat-s.
daytime - sil.
evening - ph-ac.
eyes, above - cann-i., gels., ***kali-c.,*** plan., plat., ***sil.***
opening eyes agg. - ***sil.***
forenoon - mag-s.
frontal, eminence, in - arn., dros., lach., plan., plat., sul-ac.
mental exertion - ph-ac., ***sil.***
midnight, till morning - hep.
morning - cob., hep., sil.
9 a.m. to 1 p.m. - mur-ac.
waking, on - hep., sol-n.
motion agg. - cupr-ar., hep.
moving eyes - hep.
nose, above - ars., carb-an.
orbital arch, margin of - spig.
rubbing, amel. - ars.
sleep amel. - thuj.
spots, in - par.
stooping - lyc.
surface of brain, as if on - ph-ac.
touch, on - nat-m.
violent blow, as after - arn., chel., sol-n., sul-ac.
waking, on - hep., thuj.

sore, occiput - ***aesc.,*** agar., alum., ars., aur., bapt., ***bry., calc.,*** cann-i., carb-ac., carb-an., chel., cic., **CIMIC.,** coff., crot-c., crot-h., dirc., **EUP-PER.,** ***euph.,*** ferr., ferr-p., **GELS.,** ***glon.,*** grat., ***hell.,*** hyos., indg., ***ip.,*** kali-p., mag-s., merc-i-f., mez., ***mur-ac.,*** nat-m., nat-s., nicc., nit-ac., **NUX-V.,** ***ph-ac.,*** phyt., pip-m., plan., rhus-t., sabad., sep., spig., **STAPH.,** sulph., tab., tarent., zinc.
broken loose from rest of skull, as if - chel.
chill, during - hell.
cold applications amel. - euphr.
coughing, on - tarent.
looking up - graph.
lying amel. - alum., hell.
on occiput - sep.
on the sore side amel. - ***bry.,*** plan.
motion, on - **CIMIC.,** ***crot-h., nux-v.***
amel. - euph., ***rhus-t.***
night - agg. - sep.
pressure, on - sanic., tab.
amel. - sep.
pulsating - ***eup-per.***
sides - caust., euph., grat., iod.
stooping - hell.
touch, on - calc., sep.
wound were pressed, as if - sabad.

sore, sides - ambr., ars., benz-ac., bov., ***chin.,*** con., crot-h., dros., eup-per., grat., ip., kali-i., laur., lil-t., mag-c., merc-i-f., mez., nat-m., nit-ac., **NUX-V.,** petr., phyt., plan., plat., rat., ***rhus-t.,*** **RUTA.**, sil., staph., sulph.
extending to ears - grat.
to eyes - crot-h.
to teeth - crot-h., rhus-t.
forenoon - bov., mag-c.
lain on - bar-c., **NIT-AC.**
not - ***rhus-t.***
left - carb-an., cupr-ar., laur., lil-t., par., sulph.
lying, impossible on painful side - staph.
on painful side amel. - plan.
on painless side amel. - nux-v.
morning - ars.
motion agg. - ***chin.***
pressure, on - ang.
right - aesc., ambr., dros., merc-i-f., mez., nit-ac., plat., staph., zinc.
spots, in - agar., ambr., ang., ant-c., plat., sulph., zinc.
touch agg. - petr.
amel. - dros.
turning eyes, toward painful side - con.
wandering - ind.

sore, temples - aesc., atro., calc-p., cast., cham., cob., coca, cupr-ar., daph., dirc., glon., grat., gymn., haem., meny., merl., ***mez.,*** nicc., nux-m., ph-ac., phys., plan., plb., ***puls.,*** ***rhus-t.,*** sang., tarent., **VERB.**
coughing, on - tarent.
daytime - phys.
evening - ph-ac., ***puls.,*** rhus-t.
forenoon - nicc.
left - cham., gymn.
mental exertion, on - ph-ac.
morning - cob., plan.
night - cop.
right - calc-p., cop., dros., nicc.
touch, on - meny.

sore, vertex - agar., ***alum.,*** ant-c., apis, arg-m., bov., bry., bufo, cast., caust., chel., cimic., cinnb., ferr., ferr-p., glon., hyper., ind., iod., kali-bi., kali-c., kali-n., ***lach.,*** lac-ac., ***mag-c.,*** mag-m., nat-m., nicc., nux-v., olnd., petr., ph-ac., phos., phyt., rhod., rhus-t., sabin., sep., sil., spig., squil., **SULPH.,** sul-i., thuj., ***zinc.***
afternoon - nicc.
air, cold, amel. - ant-c., thuj.
air, open amel. - gamb.
chill, during - hell.
cough, during - kali-c.
evening - mag-c., sulph., ***zinc.***
forenoon - nicc.
lying on painful side agg. - nux-m.
menses during - mag-c.
mental exertion - ph-ac.
morning - bov., hyper., squil.
pressure amel. - hell.
pulsating - caust.
spots, in - ***caust.,*** vinc.
touch, on - zinc.

SPLASHING - asaf., bell., ***carb-an.,*** hep., hyos., nux-v., rhus-t., spig., squil.
walking rapidly, while - carb-an.

SPRAINED, sensation - carb-an.
back of head - psor.

STAGNATION, of blood, sensation - bar-c.
stagnation, temple in - chel.

STIFFNESS, sensation of - canth., ferr., glon., nat-m., nat-s.
evening, bed, in - sil.
motion, on - nat-s.
motion, on, of head agg. - colch.
must bend head back - kali-n.
waking, on - anac.
stiffness, sensation of, occiput, in - anac., calc., ferr., gins., kali-n., phos., sil.
extending, nose, to - lach.

STOMACH, as if rising from - alum., carb-v., con., mag-m.

STONE, as if from, (see Heaviness)

STOPPED, sensation - nat-c.

STRIKES, the head against the wall or bed with twitching of eyelids and frontal muscles - mill.
strikes, the head with fists, from pain - ars.

STUNNING, pain, stupefying - acon., aeth., agar., alum., am-c., anac., ant-c., ant-t., arg-m., ***arg-n.,*** ***arn., ars.,*** ars-i., asaf., asar., aur., bapt., bar-c., bar-m., ***bell.,*** bov., bry., ***bufo,*** **CALC.,** calc-ar., ***carb-an.,*** **CARB-V.,** caust., chin., chin-s., cic., cimx., cina, cinnb., con., crot-t., cupr., cycl., dros., ***dulc.,*** fl-ac., glon., gran., **GRAPH.,** ***hell., hyos.,*** iod., ***iris,*** kali-bi., kali-c., ***kali-n.,*** kali-p., kali-s., lac-c., ***lach., laur., led., lyc., mag-c.,*** mang., meny., ***mez.,*** mosch., ***mur-ac., naja, nat-a.,*** ***nat-c., nat-m.,*** nat-p., nit-ac., ***nux-m.,*** **NUX-V.,** ***olnd.,*** op., petr., ph-ac., ***phos.,*** **PSOR.,** ***puls.,*** rheum, rhod., ***rhus-t.,*** ruta, sabad., sabin., samb., sep., **SIL.,** ***stann., staph.,*** sulph., tarax., ***tarent.,*** thuj., valer., verb., ***zinc.***
afternoon - cham., hell.
cold, agg. - puls., ***rhus-t.***
amel. - ***puls.***
chilliness, with - ***puls.***
compressing - ***mosch.***
coughing, on - aeth., kali-n.
drawing - asar.
eating, after - **NUX-V.**
evening - ***puls.***
morning - agar., arn., **NAT-M., NUX-V.,** ***rhus-t., tarent.,*** zinc.
rising, after - calc.
waking, on, as from liquor - chin., kali-n., **NAT-M., NUX-V.,** ***tarent.***
motion, agg. - rheum.
amel. - ***meny., puls.,*** **RHUS-T.**
and rest, during - **CALC.**
of head - staph.
night - arg-n., kali-n.
periodical - ***ars.***

STUNNING, pain
pressing - ***ant-t.,*** arg-m., arn., ars., ***asar.,*** calc., cic., cina, ***crot-t.,*** cupr., ***dros.,*** dulc., ***euon.,*** hell., ***hyos., mez., ruta., sabad., stann.,*** sulph., verb.
pressure amel. - iod., podo.
reading while - **CALC.,** caust.
sitting - caust., cina.
smoking, while - ant-c.
standing - staph.
stinging - verb.
stooping agg. - rheum.
sunshine, from - nux-v.
throbbing - nat-m., sabin.
tightening - asaf., olnd.
warm room agg. - nat-c., nat-m., ***phos., puls.***

stunning, forehead - agar., anac., ***ant-c.,*** arg-m., arn., ***ars.,*** asaf., asar., bapt., ***bell.,*** **CALC.,** cann-s., carb-an., caust., cic., cina, con., cycl., dros., ***euph.,*** fl-ac., gran., ***hyos., kali-n.,*** laur., led., ***mag-c.,*** mang., meny., ***mur-ac., nat-c.,*** nat-p., olnd., par., ***ph-ac.,*** phos., plat., ruta., sabad., sep., ***stann., staph.,*** tarax., thuj., valer., ***verb., zinc.***
air, open amel. - tarax.
eyes, over - ars., euon., stann.
right - ars.
morning, waking - ph-ac.
motion, agg. - ph-ac.
nose, above - ***acon.,*** ant-t., asar., mosch.
standing - staph.
stooping agg. - calc-ac.
violent, sweats from anxiety, while walking in open air - ant-c.

stunning, occiput - ***cann-i.,*** cina, ***dulc., hell.,*** mang., ***naja,*** seneg., sulph., tarent., zinc.
forehead, to - mez.

stunning, sides - asaf., daph., dulc., euph., hell., ***mez.,*** olnd., stann., sul-ac., verb.
right - euph., ***mez.,*** sul-ac.

stunning, temples - acon., ars., asar., cina, iod., podo., rheum, sabad., ***verb.***

stunning, vertex - bov., cycl., dulc., phos., rheum, valer.

SUNSTROKE - ***acon.,*** agar., **AML-N.,** ***ant-c.,*** apis, arg-m., ***arn., ars.,*** **BELL.,** bry., ***cact., cadm-met., camph., carb-v.,*** crot-h., cyt-l., euph-pi., ***gels.,*** **GLON.,** hydr-ac., hyos., kalm., **LACH.,** lyc., lyss., **NAT-C.,** nat-m., nux-v., ***op.,*** pop-c., rhus-t., **SOL.,** stram., syph., ***ther.,*** thuj., usn., valer., **VERAT.,** ***verat-v.***
chronic effects - nat-c.
sleeping in sun, from - acon., ***bell.***

SURGING, sensation - ***acon.,*** aur., ***bell.,*** canth., ***chin.,*** chin-s., cimic., ***glon.,*** hep., hyos., ind., lach., mag-p., ***meli.,*** nux-v., pall., rhus-t., senec., sulph.
becoming erect amel. - alum.
lying, while - ox-ac.

surging, forehead like waves rolling up and down - ***sep.***

surging, occiput extending to forehead - cann-i., lach.

SWASHING, sensation - acon., apis, ***ars.,*** asaf., ***bell.,*** carb-ac., ***carb-an.,*** chin., cimic., dig., ***hep., hyos.,*** indg., lyc., mag-m., nux-v., ph-ac., ***rhus-t.,*** samb., ***spig.,*** squil., sul-ac., viol-t.
shaking, on - ***spig.,*** squil.
walking, while - nux-v., ***spig.***

SWELLING, of - apis, bell., cupr., dig.

swelling, forehead, shining swelling - phos.
frontal eminence, hard swelling - ars.
glabella - fl-ac., kali-c., sel.

swelling, glands of - ***bar-c., calc., merc., psor.,*** **SIL.,** ***sulph.***

swelling, occiput - bar-c., mag-m.

SWELLINGS - petr.
forehead, sore - hell.
tumor - anac., arg-n., ars., ***calc.,*** caust., daph., hell., kali-c., nux-v., petr., ph-ac., puls., rhus-t., ruta, sep., sil.

SWOLLEN, distended, feeling - aeth., agar., am-c., aml-n., anac., ant-t., **APIS,** ***arg-n.,*** arn., ars., bapt., bar-c., ***bell.,*** berb., bism., bov., cann-i., caps., **CEDR.,** chin-s., cimic., cina, cob., coc-c., coll., cor-r., cupr-ac., daph., dig., dulc., gels., gins., **GLON.,** guai., indg., kali-i., lach., lachn., lact., laur., lil-t., lith., mang., meph., merc., merl., nat-m., nux-m., **NUX-V.,** op., par., plan., ***ran-b.,*** ran-s., rhus-t., samb., sep., spig., stront-c., sulph., tarax., ther.
waking, on - ars., samb.
walking, open air, in - aeth., mang.
washing, after - aeth.

swollen, forehead - acon., agar., ars., cic., dulc., hep., indg., lyc., merc., mez., nux-v., phos., pip-m., rhus-v., ruta., sep., spong.
expanding, alternating with contracting - tarax.
feels broad and high - cund.

swollen, occiput - bry., dulc., pip-m., puls.
glands, occiput - **BAR-C.,** mag-m.

swollen, sides - caust., nux-m., par.

swollen, temples - bufo, calc., cham., euph., par.
above - sep.
left - cham., euph.
right - bufo, calc., par.

swollen, distended, feeling, vertex - all-c.

TEARING, pain - aesc., aeth., agar., ***agn.,*** ail., alum., ambr., am-c., ***am-m., anac.,*** ant-c., ***arg-m., ars.,*** ars-i., asar., **AUR.,** aur-m., bell., ***berb.,*** bor., bov., ***bry.,*** calad., ***calc.,*** calc-p., ***calc-s.,*** camph., cann-s., ***canth.,*** caps., carb-an., ***carb-v.,*** cast., caust., ***cham., chel., chin.,*** chin-a., cina, cinnb., ***cocc.,*** coff., colch., ***coloc., con.,*** croc., crot-t., cupr., ***cycl.,*** dig., dros., eupi., ferr., ferr-ar., ferr-i., **FERR-P.,** graph., ***guai.,*** hell., hyos., hyper., ***ign.,*** indg., iod., ***ip.,*** kali-ar., kali-bi., ***kali-c.,*** kali-n., kali-p., ***kali-s., kalm., kreos.,*** lach., laur., led., lil-t., **LYC.,** ***mag-c., mag-m.,*** mag-p., mag-s., manc., ***mang.,*** **MERC.,** ***merc-c.,*** mez., mill., ***mur-ac.,*** nat-a., nat-c., **NAT-M.,** nat-p., nat-s., nicc., ***nux-v., ol-an.,*** petr., ***ph-ac.,*** phos., plat., plb., psor., ***puls.,*** ran-b., rat., rheum, rhod., ***rhus-t.,*** ruta., samb., sars., sel., ***sep., sil.,***

TEARING, pain - **SPIG.**, squil., ***stann., staph.,*** stram., stront-c., **SULPH.**, sul-ac., tarax., ter., teucr., thuj., til., viol-t., vip., zinc.
aching, jerking - phos.
afternoon - aeth., calc., cast., caust., chel., graph., grat., guai., kali-i., kreos., laur., ***lyc.,*** mag-c., mag-s., nat-c., nicc., ol-an., sil., sulph., zinc.
3 to 10 p.m. - calc.
until evening - lyc.
air, amel. - alum., ant-c., ***arg-m.,*** aur., carb-s., mag-s., sulph.
from cold - bov., caust., grat., ign., rhus-t., stram.
in open - calc., mang., ol-an.
around - calc-p., calc-s.
asunder, (see Bursting) - agar., am-m., coff., ***mur-ac.,*** nat-s., op., ***puls.,*** staph., sul-ac., ***verat.***
bed, amel. - aur-m., caust.
bending, back agg. - anac.
forward amel, burning, tearing in, on - cupr.
forward amel. - ign.
binding, up amel. - sil.
breakfast, during - sul-ac.
bruised, tearing - bov., merc.
chill, during - eupi., hyper., kali-n.
chill, with - anac.
cough, during - alum., arn., calc., cupr., mur-ac., puls., sep., verat.
crazy feeling runs up back - lil-t.
cutting - bell.
daily, every day, at, pressure, agg., open air, amel. - ***arg-m.***
damp, cold weather - **CALC.**, ***rhod., rhus-t.***
amel. - caust.
digging - coloc., spig.
dinner, during - zinc.
after - carb-an., mag-c., ol-an., zinc.
drawing - am-c., calad., canth., caps., cina, guai., ***kali-c.,*** lach., ***mang.,*** nux-v., ol-an., rhus-t., sil.
boring, drawing - carb-an.
eating, while - con., sul-ac., zinc.
after - carb-an., mag-c., ***nux-v.,*** ol-an., phel., sep., zinc.
evening - ail., alum., ambr., am-c., calc-p., cocc., coloc., grat., hyper., kali-n., lachn., ***lyc.,*** mag-c., mag-m., merc., nat-c., nicc., olnd., petr., ***puls.,*** sars., sil., ***spig.,*** staph., sulph., sul-ac.
bed, in - laur., sil., thuj.
midnight, until - laur.
exertion, physical - ***anac.***
extending, ear, to - nux-v., sulph.
eye, left, in paroxysms - nicc.
eye, out, of - sil.
face, to - am-m., anac., bry., guai., lyc., sil., squil., ***staph.,*** thuj.
neck, to - anac., ***chin., kalm., merc.***
nose, to - lyc., nat-c., nux-v.
occiput, to - rheum.
right temple - carb-v.
scapula, to - puls.

TEARING, pain
extending, teeth, to - chin., lyc., ***merc., staph.***
throat, to - anac., merc.
upwards - am-c.
fever, during the - puls.
forenoon - alum., ant-c., ***ip.,*** kali-n.
heat, amel. - mag-p., ***rhod., rhus-t.,*** staph., stram.
intermittent - ***coloc.,*** ferr., hyos., nicc., rheum, ***stann.,*** sulph.
jerking - agar., arn., ***chin.,*** kali-c., mag-c., mur-ac., paeon., puls., rat., teucr., thuj.
knitting, while - mag-s.
leaning, head on hands amel. - dros.
leaning, on table amel. - sulph.
lying, amel. - ***calc., calc-p., calc-s., chin., lyc.,*** spig.
back, on, amel. - ign.
must lie down - colch., ***con., nat-m.***
quietly, towards morning, amel. - merc.
while - mag-c., thuj., zinc.
maddening - mag-c.
menses, during - am-m., calc., cast., lyc., mag-c., ***nat-c.,*** rat.
after - berb.
before - ars., cinnb., glon., laur.
mental exertion, from - ***acon.,*** ran-b.
amel. - calc-ac.
morning - alum., arg-n., bor., bov., cic., ***coloc.,*** con., hyper., indg., mez., nicc., nux-v., phos., ran-s., rhod., sars., sil., staph., verat.
bed, in - arg-n.
rising, on - ip., staph., stram., stront.
until evening - ant-c., zinc.
until noon - ip.
waking, on - graph., ***phos.,*** puls., staph., verat.
motion, agg. - ***agn., aur.,*** calc., canth., ***carb-v.,*** carb-s., ***chin.,*** chin-a., ***cocc.,*** coff., ***coloc.,*** lith., phos., rat., sars., sil., **SPIG.**, staph., verat.
amel. - caps., mur-ac., ***rhod., rhus-t.,*** sulph.
moving, eyes agg. - dros., ***mur-ac.***
head agg. - ***coloc.***
upper eyelids - ***coloc.***
night - agar., ***caust.,*** cham., hep., laur., ***lyc.,*** mag-c., merc., ***sil.,*** sulph., thuj.
waking, on - arg-n.
noise agg. - coff., **SPIG.**
noon - cham., graph., zinc.
opening, mouth - spig.
overheated, after being - ***kali-c.***
paralytic - nat-c.
paroxysmal - carb-v., caust., ***coloc.,*** nicc.
periodic - anac., mur-ac.
pressive - aur., camph., chel., sars., squil.
pressure, agg. - agar., ***arg-m.,*** bism., ***sil.***
amel. - ***calc.,*** camph., carb-an., mag-c., mag-m., mag-p., nat-c., sulph.
pulsating - ars., carb-an., ***cocc.,*** mag-m., nat-c., rhus-t., sil., spong., zinc.
respiration, on deep - rat.

TEARING, pain
rising on - am-m., kalm.
stooping. from - mang.
up in bed agg. - cham., ***lyc.,*** mur-ac.
room, amel. in - ol-an.
entering, on - mag-m.
rubbing amel. - calc., laur., phos.
saw, as if with a - ***sulph.***
shooting - arg-m., berb., caust., chel., chin., cic., hyos., hyper., phos., sil., sulph., vip., zinc.
sitting, while - indg., lith., mag-c., mez., nicc., phos., ***spig.***
amel. - ***carb-v.,*** mag-m.
upright agg. - ign., mur-ac.
spots, in - aloe, ***colch.,*** lyc., ph-ac.
standing, while - lith., ran-b., **SPIG.**
still, amel. - ***tarax.***
step, a false, agg. - **SPIG.**
stinging - caps., cocc., hyper., ***ign.,*** mag-m., ***nat-m.,*** nicc., ph-ac., puls., sulph., zinc.
stooping, on - arn., asar., bov., canth., carb-an., ***coloc.,*** ip., rhus-t., sil.
talking, on - cocc., sars.
thunderstorm, during - **RHOD.**
to and fro - ambr.
touch, agg. - arg-m., chel., ip., staph.
amel. - mur-ac.
turning, on - canth., coloc.
in bed - cham.
twitching - ***chin.,*** kali-c., sil.
vertigo, after - plat.
vomiting, after - thuj.
waking, on - arg-n., graph., phos., thuj., verat.
walking, while - cast., ***chin.,*** con., sars., **SPIG.,** tarax.
amel. - ant-c.
in air - lyc.
in air, amel. - ant-t., coloc., ***thuj.***
wandering - ambr., ant-c., berb., colch., con., nat-s., rhus-t., sel.
warmth, of bed amel. - aur-m., caust.
of bed agg. - lyc., merc., sulph., thuj.
room amel. - ***carb-v.***
water, cold, agg. - sulph.
waves, in - caust.
wrapping head up amel. - ***phos.,*** rhod., ***rhus-t.,*** sil.
writing, while - ran-b.
yawning, passes off with much - mur-ac., staph.

tearing, forehead - act-sp., aeth., agar., ***agn.,*** alum., ambr., am-c., am-m., ***anac.,*** ant-c., ant-t., arg-m., arg-n., arum-t., ars., asaf., asar., ***aur.,*** aur-m-n., ***bell., berb.,*** bism., bov., brom., ***bry.,*** cact., calc., calc-p., camph., canth., ***caps.,*** carb-an., ***carb-s., carb-v.,*** cast., caust., ***cham.,*** chel., chin., cina, ***cinnb.,*** cocc., coc-c., colch., ***coloc., con.,*** cupr., cycl., dros., euphr., gran., ***graph.,*** grat., ***guai.,*** hell., ***hep.,*** hyos., ***ign.,*** indg., ip., kali-ar., kali-bi., ***kali-c.,*** kali-n., kali-p., kalm., kreos., ***lach.,*** lachn., laur., led., **LYC.,** mag-c., mag-m., mag-s., ***mang.,*** **MERC.,** merc-i-r., merl., ***mez.,***

tearing, forehead - mur-ac., nat-a., nat-c., nat-m., nat-s., nit-ac., nux-v., op., phel., phos., ***plb.,*** puls., rat., rhod., sabad., samb., ***sars., sep.,*** **SIL., SPIG.,** ***stann.,*** staph., stront-c., ***sulph.,*** sul-ac., thuj., til., zinc.
above forehead - iod., lyc., zinc.
across - bry., kalm., lachn.
afternoon - alum., chel., graph., laur., lyc., sep., sulph.
2 p.m. - laur., sep.
2 p.m. till 3 a.m. - ant-t.
2-4 p.m. - mag-s.
air, open - mang.
amel. - alum., aur., mag-s.
alternating with pain in arms - sil.
coffee, agg. - cham., kali-n.
dinner, after - mag-c., zinc.
eating, after - sep., sulph.
amel. - chel.
evening - agn., alum., coloc., hell., lyc., mag-m., ***merc., puls.,*** sars., sil., staph.
6 p.m. - brom.
sitting while - staph.
extending, chest, to - cham.
eyes, to - ***kali-c.,*** mur-ac., nat-c., nat-m., samb., spig.
nape, to - berb.
neck muscles, to, then to right arm - bry.
neck, down, into face and teeth - lyc.
nose, to - lyc., nat-c.
nose, to, root - bov., ***kali-c.***
nose, to, wing - sep.
occiput, to - bov., kali-n.
temple, to - caust., gran.
vertex, to - alum., merc., sil.
eyes, behind - bism., squil.
eyes, over - agar., agn., ***ars.,*** aur., aur-m., calc., chel., ***chin.,*** ferr-i., iod., kali-ar., kali-c., kali-i., lach., laur., lyc., mag-p., mang., merc., mez., phos., sang., sep., sil.
afternoon - sang., sep.
air, open, amel. - aur-m., merc.
evening - agn.
intermitting - ***ars.***
left - aeth., arg-m., ***iod.,*** laur., merc., ***merc-c.,*** stann., verb., zinc.
morning - ***chin.,*** lyc.
motion agg. - agn.
night - ***lyc.***
opening eyes on - euph.
pressing the eye, when - arg-m., lyc.
pressure amel. - ***anac.***
right - agn., anac., bism., **CARB-AC.,** mag-p., mang.
walking about amel. - ***ars.***
fever, during - ***ars.***
flying pain - rat., seneg.
forenoon - alum., sars.
frontal eminence - agn., alum., ambr., arg-m., arg-mur., bell., bov., calc., chel., chin., cina, cocc., hell., kali-c., lyc., mang., mill., nat-c., sabad., ***sep.,*** sil., **SPIG.,** ***thuj.,*** verb., ***zinc.***
afternoon, 2 p.m. - lyc.

tearing, forehead
frontal eminence, air, open in - verb.
dinner, after - ***zinc.***
evening - alum.
extending, ear, to - bov., nat-c., zinc.
extending, occiput, to - spig.
extending, orbit, to - zinc.
extending, temple, to - arg-m., mang.
left - kali-c., mang., mez., nat-c., sep., ***zinc.***
left, under - **SPIG.**
left, under, extending to eyes - **SPIG.**
right - ambr., ***arg-m.,*** sep., **SPIG.**
speaking, while - mang.
intermittent - agar.
lying, amel. - kali-p., ***lyc.***
menses, during - cast., ***cinnb.***
before - ***cinnb.,*** kali-p.
before, amel. when flow begins - kali-p.
mental exertion - anac.
middle of forehead - bov., caust., glon., laur., stront-c., sul-ac.
afternoon - mag-c.
dinner, after - chel.
extending, to left side - sul-ac..
morning - bov.
morning - ***coloc.,*** graph., mez.
sitting, while - mez.
waking, on - graph.
motion, during - agn., aur., mag-m., sil.
night - ambr., caust., hep., lyc., ***merc.,*** plb., thuj.
noon - graph., zinc.
nose, above - aeth., agar., ambr., chel., lyc., nat-c., nat-m.
pressing upon eyelids - chel.
paroxysmal - cham., mur-ac., ***stann.,*** zinc.
periodic - ***cham.,*** plb.
pulsating - mag-c.
radiating - lyc.
riding in a carriage amel. - kali-n.
rising, on - kalm., lyc.
sides - ***agn.,*** arg-n., arum-t., aur., bov., camph., ***carb-an.,*** caust., coloc., euph., grat., guai., kali-i., lachn., ***lyc.,*** lyss., ***mag-m.,*** mang., ***meny., merc.,*** mez., nat-s., nuph., ol-an., ***puls.,*** seneg., ***stann.,*** staph., til., zinc.
evening - sul-ac.
evening, 4 p.m. - mag-c.
extending, cheek, to - guai., lachn.
extending, eyebrow, to - ***lyc.***
extending, root of nose, to - ***lyc.***
extending, temples, to - kalm., mez.
extending, vertex, to - sep.
intermittent - stann.
left - aur., euph., kali-c., mang., ***merc.,*** tarax., ***zinc.***
menses, during - nat-c.
morning - ol-an.
motion agg. - aur., euph.
motion of muscles, on - mang.
pressure amel. - nat-c., sul-ac.

tearing, forehead
sides, right - ***carb-an.,*** kali-n., ***lyc., meny.,*** nux-v., puls., ***stann.,*** sul-ac., thuj., zinc.
right, to occiput - kali-n.
stitch, like - meny.
sitting, while - aeth., cast.
stooping - stann.
sitting, while - am-m., merc., **SPIG.,** staph.
standing, while - merc., **SPIG.**
stooping, when - asar., bov., dros., ip., mag-m., ***stann.,*** staph., ***sulph.***
supper, during - zinc.
touch, on - ip.
waking, on - puls., thuj.
warm room, in - caust.

tearing, occiput - acon., aeth., ***agar.,*** ail., ambr., am-m., ***anac.,*** arg-m., ***ars.,*** asaf., ***aur.,*** bar-c., bar-m., bell., berb., bism., bov., calc., camph., canth., carb-an., carb-s., **CARB-V., CAUST.,** chel., colch., ***con., cupr.,*** form., grat., ***guai.,*** hyos., ***hyper.,*** ign., indg., kali-bi., kali-c., kali-n., kali-p., laur., led., ***lyc., lyss.,*** mag-c., ***mag-m.,*** mang., ***merc., merc-c.,*** merl., mur-ac., nat-s., nit-ac., **NUX-M., NUX-V.,** phel., ***ph-ac.,*** puls., ran-b., sabad., ***sep.,*** **SIL.,** ***spig.,*** squil., stann., stront-c., sulph., ***tarax., thuj.,*** verat., ***zinc.***
afternoon - mang.
2 p.m. - grat.
bending head backward - anac.
amel. - bar-c.
burning - cupr.
coughing - cupr.
evening - ambr., carb-an., hyper., ran-b., sil.
extending, forehead, to - ambr., ***aur.,*** carb-v., chin., merc.
forward - aeth., anac., ***aur.,*** chin., merc., **SIL.**
nape of neck, to - berb., **NUX-M., NUX-V.,** ran-b.
temple, to - anac., arn.
throat, to - laur.
upward - ambr., berb., ol-an., sars., **SIL.**
upward, and forward - ambr., **CAUST.,** mag-m., rat.
vertex, to - ambr., ***caust.,*** mag-m., rat., sep.
fever, during - puls.
house, on entering - mag-m.
jerking - anac., mag-c.
laughing, from - zinc.
lying, while - ambr.
mental exertion amel. - calc-ar.
morning - agar., verat.
on rising - ***lyss.***
waking, on - verat.
motion agg. - ***aur., carb-v.,*** ph-ac., sil., ***spig.***
moving head forward, on - cupr.
night - lyc., thuj.
noise agg. - ph-ac., ***spig.***
paroxysmal - **CAUST.**
pulsating - kali-c., mag-m., mez.
room, on entering - mag-m.
rubbing, amel. - laur.

tearing, occiput
sides - agar., aur., bar-c., berb., bov., camph., carb-an., ***carb-v., carl.,*** caust., colch., con., guai., kali-bi., kali-c., led., mag-c., mag-m., mur-ac., ***nat-s.,*** puls., ran-b., rhus-v., sabad., ***sil., stann., stront-c.,*** zinc.
bending head backward amel. - bar-c.
cold draft - caust.
damp weather, amel. - caust.
evening - carb-an., nat-s.
extending - caust.
extending, forehead, to - aur., mur-ac.
extending, head, to - canth., sabad., ***sil.***
extending, neck, to - ambr.
intermittent - sep.
laughing, when - zinc.
left - con., lyc., samb., sep., ***stann.***
morning - anac., puls., ***sil.***
motion agg. - ***aur.***
moving head to left - mag-c.
paroxysmal - mur-ac.
pressing - lyc., zinc.
pulsating - kali-c.
rest, during - nat-s.
right - ***aur.,*** bism., chel., guai., kali-c., mag-c., mag-m., ***stront.***
shooting back and forth - carb-an.
twitching - bism., mag-m.
walking, while - con.
sitting, while, amel. - ***carb-v.,*** mag-m.
erect agg. - ign.
spots, in - ***colch.***
standing still amel. - ***tarax.***
touch agg. - mang.
vomiting - thuj.
walking, while - con., tarax.
warm room amel. - ***carb-v.***
wrapping up head amel. - **SIL.**

tearing, sides - aesc., aeth., agar., alum., ambr., ammc., am-c., am-m., ***anac., arg-m.,*** arg-n., ars., aur., aur-m-n., bar-c., bar-m., bor., bov., brom., bry., ***canth.,*** caps., ***carb-an.,*** carb-s., ***carb-v.,*** cast., caust., ***cham., chel.,*** chin., cic., cina, coc-c., colch., ***coloc.,*** con., croc., dig., ***gran., graph.,*** grat., ***guai.,*** hell., ign., indg., ***kali-c.,*** kali-p., laur., led., lith., ***lyc.,*** mag-c., mag-m., ***mang., merc.,*** merl., mez., mill., ***mur-ac.,*** nat-a., nat-c., nat-s., nicc., nux-v., ol-an., ptel., phos., plb., ***puls.,*** rat., rhod., ruta., sars., ***sel.,*** sep., ***sil., spig.,*** stann., stront-c., sulph., sul-ac., teucr., thuj., til., verb., **ZINC.**
afternoon - alum., nicc., ol-an., zinc.
2 p.m. - grat., laur.
bed, in - thuj.
cold water agg. - sulph.
damp weather amel. - caust.
dinner, after - mag-c., mag-s., ol-an., zinc.
drawing - bov., ***caps.,*** mang., phos., ***zinc.***
evening - graph., lyc., nicc., phos., thuj.
amel. - ruta.
sitting, while - phos.
extending, down neck into face and teeth - lyc.

tearing, sides
extending, ear, to - lyc., ***merc.***
eye, to - ***mag-m.***
face, to - kreos.
forward - indg.
inward - mag-c.
side to side - clem., rhus-t.
teeth and glands of throat - graph., merc.
upward - phos.
vertex - ***mang.***
forenoon - alum.
glowing - sulph.
intermittent - ant-t., spig.
left - ars., aur., ***caps., chin-a.,*** cina, ***coloc.,*** graph., ***guai.,*** **KALI-C.,** laur., led., ***sars., sel., spig.,*** staph., tell., thuj.
lie down, must - ***con.***
lying, amel. - lyc.
menses, during - mag-c., nat-c.
morning - mang., thuj.
motion, on - **SPIG.**
night - arg-n., phos.
night, air, cold - bov., caust., ign.
pulsating - ars.
reading while - aesc.
right - alum., anac., arg-m., bov., ***carb-an., chel., con.,*** mag-c., mang., ***mur-ac., puls.,*** sulph., sul-ac., thuj., verb.
rising, on - lyc.
from stooping - mang.
sitting, while - am-m., mag-c., phos.
spots, in - bar-c., spig.
standing - mang.
stepping - **SPIG.**
stinging - mang., sars.
stooping, on - mang., sil.
touch, agg. - bar-c.
twitching - teucr.
walking, while - cast., **SPIG.**
in open air - kali-c.

tearing, temples - acon., aeth., agar., ***agn.,*** ail., alum., ambr., am-c., ***am-m., anac.,*** ant-c., ***arg-m., arg-n., arn.,*** arum-t., asaf., ***asar.,*** aur., aur-m., ***bell., berb.,*** bism., bov., bry., calc., calc-p., camph., canth., carb-s., carb-v., cast., caust., ***cham., chel.,*** chin., chin-a., chin-s., cic., cina, cocc., colch., coloc., con., cop., cupr., cycl., dig., dulc., gran., grat., guai., ham., hell., hyper., indg., iod., kali-bi., ***kali-c., kali-i.,*** kali-n., kali-p., kalm., kreos., lach., lachn., lact., laur., led., lyc., lyss., mag-c., ***mag-m.,*** mag-s., ***mang.,*** merc., merl., mez., mur-ac., nat-c., ***nat-m.,*** nat-s., nicc., ***nux-m.,*** nux-v., olnd., ol-an., par., petr., ph-ac., phos., plb., ***puls.,*** ran-b., rat., rhod., rhus-t., ruta., sabad., sabin., samb., seneg., ***sep.,*** sil., ***spig.,*** spong., stann., staph., sulph., sul-ac., thuj., til., verb., viol-t., **ZINC.**
above, temples - zinc.
afternoon - aeth., cast., guai., mag-c., mag-s., sil., sulph.
1 p.m. - sil.
4 p.m. - caust., lyc.

tearing, temples
air, open, in - ***mang.,*** ol-an.
amel. - aur., ***puls.***
alternating with pressing - bell.
bending, head backward - anac.
breakfast, during - sul-ac.
burning - chin-a., lyc.
chill, during - hyper.
cold agg. - grat.
cough, during - alum., puls.
dinner, during - am-c., zinc.
after - zinc.
eating, while - con.
after - con.
evening - am-c., kali-c., kali-n., lachn., led., mag-c., olnd., ***puls.,*** sil., sulph., sul-ac.
6 p.m. - kali-i.
lying down, on - mag-c.
until morning - kali-n.
downward - bry., laur.
extending, brain, into - ambr., anac.
ear, to - aur-m., bov.
eye, to - gran.
face, to - am-m., arg-n., bry., kali-c., lachn., seneg.
forehead, across - cast., lyc., mez., ph-ac.
jaw, to - arg-n., kali-c.
neck, to - bry., kali-i.
occiput, to - kali-bi., rhus-v.
teeth, to - bry., carb-v., lachn., ***verb.***
upward - alum., am-m., laur., mag-c., rhus-v., ***sep.***
vertex, to - laur., ***mang.***
zygoma, to - coc-c.
forenoon - alum., am-m., arg-n., indg., nicc.
sitting, while - nicc.
heat, agg. - grat.
intermittent - dulc., samb.
jerking - anac., lyc., mag-c., puls.
laid on, in side - puls.
left - acon., agn., ***anac., arg-m.,*** arn., ***asar.,*** carb-s., gran., grat., guai., kali-bi., **KALI-C.,** mag-c., mag-m., ***merc., ph-ac., rhod.,*** **SEP.,** ***spig.,*** staph., sulph.
to right - aur-m., iod.
to side of head - **SEP.**
menses, during - am-m., nat-c.
morning - am-c., con.
motion, during - ***agn., chel.,*** chin-a., ph-ac., sang., sil.
night, agg. - lyc., thuj.
paroxysmal - carb-v., ***kali-c.***
pressure - bism.
amel. - kali-n., mag-c., nat-c.
pulsating - ***sang.,*** staph.
raising eyes, on - puls.
right - agar., alum., am-m., arum-t., asaf., bov., camph., ***chel.,*** chin-a., dig., lact., laur., mur-ac., nat-s., ran-b., rhus-t., sang.
shaking head - ***sang.***
spots, in - carb-v., rat.
standing - mur-ac.
stitching - lyc., mur-ac., zinc.
stooping, when - carb-s., samb.

tearing, temples
touch - ***arg-m.,*** chel., cupr.
amel. - mur-ac.
twitching, tearing, in, temple lain on, moves to the other side on turning - puls.
walking, while - cast., sulph.
in open air - arn., mang.
warmth of bed agg. - puls.
yawning amel. - mur-ac.

tearing, vertex - act-sp., agar., agn., alum., ***ambr.,*** am-c., anac., ant-c., arg-m., **AUR.,** bar-c., bar-m., ***bell.,*** benz-ac., bor., bov., ***canth.,*** cast., carb-v., caust., chel., colch., con., dulc., hyper., indg., iod., ***kali-c.,*** kali-n., kali-p., kalm., kreos., ***lach.,*** lachn., laur., ***lyc., mag-c.,*** mag-s., mang., merc., mez., ***mur-ac.,*** naja, nat-c., nit-ac., nux-v., phel., ph-ac., phos., ran-b., ran-s., rat., rhus-t., ruta., ***sars.,*** sil., spig., ***stann.,*** thuj., vinc., ***zinc.***
afternoon - kreos., phos.
cough, during - alum.
dinner, after - mag-c.
eating, after - inul., phel.
evening - ***calc.,*** hyper., lyc.
7 p.m. - lyc.
extending, brain, to middle of - thuj.
ear, to - agar., phos.
occiput, to - indg.
over temples - ang.
shoulder, to - ***lyc.***
zygoma, to - phos.
forenoon - bor.
jerking - mag-c.
lying, while, amel. - ***lyc.***
menses, during - ***laur.,*** mag-c., rat.
morning - bov., ran-b.
motion agg. - aur., bell.
night - laur., ***merc.,*** thuj.
10:30 p.m. - alum.
paroxysmal - carb-v., zinc.
pressure agg. - ***bell.***
sitting, while - phos.
standing, while - ran-b.
writing, while - ran-b.

TENSION, (see Constriction) drawing upward of skin of forehead - carb-an.

tension, occiput - lyc.

tension, scalp, of - ***acon.,*** arn., asar., ***bapt.,*** canch., caust., iris, med., ***merc., par.,*** rat., sel., stict., ***viol-o.***

tension, vertex - lob.

THIN, cranium seemed thin - ***bell., calc-p.,*** puls.

THROBBING, (see Pulsating)

THROWING, head about (see Motions of head)

TICKLING, in - ferr., phos.

tickling, in forehead - brom., ferr., mag-c.

tickling, in temples - sep.

TIED, feels as though - colch.

TIGHTNESS, (see Constriction)

TINEA, favosa, (see Fungus) - aethi-a., agar., ars., ars-i., ***brom.,*** calc., calc-i., ***calc-mur.,*** calc-s., ***dulc.,*** ferr-i., graph., ***hep.,*** jug-r., ***kali-c.,*** kali-s., lappa-a., ***lyc.,*** med., ***mez.,*** nit-ac., olnd., phos., ***sep., sil.,*** sul-ac., sulph., ust., vinc., ***viol-t.***
tinea tonsurans - ant-c., ant-t., ***ars., bac.,*** calc., calc-i., ***chrysar.,*** graph., hep., jug-c., jug-r., kali-s., lyc., mez., psor., rhus-t., semp., ***sep.,*** sulph., ***tell.,*** tub., viol-t.
tinea, versicolor - bac., chrysar., mez., ***nat-a., sep.,*** sulph., tell., thuj.

TINGLING, sensation - acet-ac., acon., am-c., apis, arg-m., arn., bar-c., cadm-s., caust., chel., cic., cocc., ***colch., cupr.,*** hyos., laur., nux-m., phos., ph-ac., plat., puls., rheum, ***rhus-t.,*** sec., sulph., tarax., thuj., verb.
large bell were struck, as though a - sars.
speaking aloud, on - zinc.
walking, while - verb.

tingling, forehead - **ARN., AUR., CHEL., CIC.,** ***colch.,*** indg., ph-ac., puls., sabad., stram., tarax., verat., viol-o., viol-t., zinc.

tingling, occiput - rhus-t.
stupefying, on stepping - sulph.

tingling, temples - bor., plat., rheum, stront-c., sulph.
coldness of spot, with - plat.

tingling, vertex - aesc., calc., colch., ***cupr.,*** hyos., lac-c., sulph.
coughing - sulph.
menses, omiting - cupr.

TIRED, feeling - apis, arn., chin-a., con., ferr-p., iris, lach., nat-m., nux-m., **PHOS.,** ***psor.,*** sil., zinc-valer.

TORN, pain, as if, (see Sore or Tearing) - agar., alum., am-m., ang., arg-m., ars., aur., bell., bov., camph., **CARB-AN.,** caust., cham., ***chin., coff.,*** con., euphr., ferr., graph., hell., hep., ***hyper.,*** ign., ip., iod., kali-n., lach., mag-c., merc., mosch., ***mur-ac., nicc.,*** nit-ac., ***nux-v.,*** op., ph-ac., phos., plat., puls., ***rhus-t.,*** sep., stann., ***staph.,*** stront-c., sulph., thuj., verat., zinc.
clasped by a hand and were being torn and twisted - mur-ac.
morning on waking - con.
moving the eyes - ***rhus-t.***
agg. or sitting up in bed, amel. moderate exercise - mur-ac.

torn, forehead - am-m., asar., coff., graph., hep., mez., nux-v., ***puls.,*** thuj.
forenoon - graph.

torn, occiput - con.

torn, sides - nux-v., sulph.

torn, temples - mur-ac.

torn, vertex - **CARB-AN.,** caust., mur-ac., thuj., zinc.

TREMBLING, sensation - ambr., anan., ant-c., ***ant-t.,*** bell., bufo, calc., carb-v., caust., ***chel., cic.,*** cinnb., ***cocc.,*** cop., cub., graph., ***ign.,*** indg., kali-c., ***lith., mag-p.,*** merc., ***op.,*** petr., plat., ***plb.,*** sulph., tab.
conversation, from - ambr.
convulsive - cocc.

TREMBLING, sensation
cough, during - ant-t.
epilepsy, before - ***caust.***
extending pit of stomach, to - phys.
exertion, after - ant-t.
menses, during - ant-c., cic., cinnb., cub.
moving, agg. - ant-t., cic.
noises in ear, with - kali-c.
paroxysmal - carb-v.
talking, after - ambr.

TUBERCLES, on scalp - anac., ant-c., bar-c., **CALC.,** carb-an., kali-c., ***lyc.,*** nat-m., ph-ac., phos., ***phyt., psor.,*** sil.
itching - phos.

TUMORS - anan., apom., arn., aur., ***bar-c.,*** bell., calc., ***calc-f., con.,*** cupr., fl-ac., glon., graph., ***hecla.,*** hydr., ***kali-i.,*** merc., merc-p., phos., ***plb.,*** sep., sil., still.
nevus on right temple, flat, in children - fl-ac.

TURNED, to left in convulsions - mygal., plb.
to right in convulsions - stram.

TURNING, and twisting, sensation of - aeth., bell., bry., calc., indg., iris, **KALI-C.,** petr., rhus-t., sabad., sil.

TWANGING, as from, breaking, a piano, string - lyc.

TWISTING, head - nat-m.

TWITCHING, muscles of the head - ***agar.,*** aloe, ambr., apis, arn., bar-c., ***bell.,*** bry., calc., cann-s., carb-v., caust., cham., chel., chin., ***cic.,*** crot-t., cycl., eupi., glon., graph., ign., kali-c., laur., lyc., mag-c., merc., mygal., nat-c., nat-p., nat-s., nit-ac., nux-v., ***op.,*** petr., ***ph-ac.,*** phos., rat., rhus-t., sabad., ***sep.,*** sil., stann., staph., stram.
afternoon - aeth., bor., rhus-t.
ascending steps, on - glon., hell.
blowing, nose - aster.
cough, during - lyc., puls.
eating, after - cham.
evening - fl-ac., mur-ac., rhus-t., sil.
jerking, the arms, when - spong.
lain, on part - rhus-t.
lying down, while - nit-ac.
morning - cham., glon., nux-v., phos., sep.
motion, agg. - eupi., hell., phos.
of the arms - chel.
night - chel., rhus-t., sil.
noon - glon.
pressure, amel. - hell.
pulsating - ph-ac.
sensation - hell.
standing, after - fl-ac.
stepping, when - spong.
stool, during, agg. - phos.
stooping, on - berb., hell., nit-ac., petr.
touch, agg. - chel.

twitching, forehead - acon., ***agar.,*** alumn., ant-t., arn., berb., bor., bry., caust., cham., chin., kali-chl., lach., mag-m., mez., phos., ***prun.,*** rhod., sabad., ***sep.,*** sil., spong., stann., sulph., thuj.
afternoon - bor.
lying down - hep.
evening - alumn., fl-ac.
extending, brain, into - camph.
rising, amel. - hep.
stooping - berb.

twitching, occiput - acon., bism., canth., mag-c., ***mag-m.,*** merc., ph-ac., rhus-t., sars., ***spig.,*** sulph., thuj.
extending to forehead - anac., ph-ac.

twitching, sides - aeth., agar., anac., ang., bar-c., calc., cann-i., caust., cupr., glon., graph., ***nit-ac.,*** ox-ac., plb., valer., verb.
extending, from side to side - merc.
throat, to - chin.
vertex, to, when jerking, arms and on stepping - spong.
left - anac., calc., cann-i., cupr., ***nit-ac.,*** verb.
right - aeth., agar., bar-c., caust., ox-ac., plb., valer.
touch, agg. - bar-c.

twitching, temples - acon., agar., am-c., am-m., anac., apis, arg-m., bar-c., berb., bov., bry., calc., carb-an., chel., ***chin.,*** crot-h., cycl., glon., kali-c., lil-t., merc., ox-ac., phos., plb., ***spig.,*** squil., stann., sul-ac., valer., verb.
dinner, after - phos.
extending, brain, into - camph.
jaws or teeth, to - rhus-t.
vertex, to - cycl.
left - am-m., anac., bar-c., bov., chel., kali-c., phos., stann.
right - merc., squil., sul-ac., valer.
spots, in - rat.
tearing, in temple lain on, moves to other side on turning, agg. on raising eyes - puls.
walking, while - ***spig.***

twitching, vertex - chel., gent-l., mag-c., meny., mur-ac., petr., phos., ran-s., sil.

TWITCHING, pain - arn., **BELL.,** bry., carb-v., chin., ign., kali-c., lyc., sil., **SULPH.**
afternoon, 1 p.m. - mag-c.
stooping - arn.
walking - **BELL.**

twitching, occiput - kali-n.

twitching, temple, above - zinc.

ULCERATIVE, pain - acon., **AM-C.,** ant-t., bor., ***bov.,*** bufo, carb-v., cast., caust., ***hep.,*** kali-c., kreos., mag-c., mang., merc., nux-v., petr., puls., rhod., sep., stann., stront-c., sulph., ***sul-ac.***

ulcerative, forehead - graph., hep., mur-ac., nux-v.
periodical, with constipation - nux-v.
touch - graph.

ulcerative, occiput - am-c., kreos., mang., nux-v., sep.
coughing - sulph.

ulcerative, occiput
gland - am-c.
left - mag-c.

ulcerative, vertex - cast., kreos., zinc.

ulcerative, temples - mur-ac., ***puls.***

ULCERS - ***anan., ars., bar-m., calc-p.,*** chel., nit-ac., ***phos.,*** ruta., ***sil.,*** tarent., thuj.

ulcers, on occiput - sep., **SIL.**

UNCOVERING, agg. - acon., agar., ant-c., arg-m., arn., ***ars., aur., bar-c.,*** **BELL.,** benz-ac., bor., ***calc.,*** camph., canth., ***carb-v.,*** cham., chin., chin-a., cic., clem., cocc., coff., ***colch., con., graph.,*** **HEP.,** ***hyos.,*** ign., kali-ar., ***kali-c.,*** kali-p., kreos., ***lach.,*** led., mag-c., mag-m., ***merc., mez.,*** naja, nat-c., ***nat-m.,*** nat-p., ***nit-ac., nux-m.,*** **NUX-V.,** ph-ac., ***phos., psor.,*** puls., rhod., **RHUS-T.,** ***rumx.,*** sabad., samb., ***sep.,*** **SIL.,** ***squil.,*** staph., stram., ***stront-c., thuj.,*** til.

UNSTEADY, feeling - bell., clem., phos., rhus-t., sep., ***sulph.***
study, after, agg. - cupr-ar.

URTICARIA - ***agar.***

VACANT, feeling - sec., sulph.

vacant, feeling, forehead, morning, waking, after - sulph.

VESICLES - ***ars.,*** bov., clem., crot-h., kali-bi., olnd., psor., sep., ***sulph.,*** tell., tep.

VIBRATING, (see Shaking)

VIOLENT, pains - acon., aeth., agar., am-c., am-m., aml-n., ***anac.,*** ant-c., ***apis, arg-m.,*** arg-n., ***ars.,*** aur., ***bar-c.,*** **BELL., BRY., CACT.,** cadm-met., cann-s., canth., **CARB-S.,** ***chin., cimic.,*** cimx., cina, cinnb., ***cocc.,*** coc-c., ***coff.,*** colch., coloc., croc., ***crot-h.,*** cupr., euphr., ***gels.,*** **GLON.,** grat., ***hell., hyos., ip.,*** kali-ar., kali-bi., ***kali-br.,*** kali-c., ***kali-i.,*** kali-p., kali-s., ***lac-d.,*** **LACH.,** laur., led., **LIL-T.,** ***lyc.,*** lyss., mag-c., manc., **MELI.,** meph., ***merc., mez., morph.,*** mosch., ***nat-m., op.,*** oreo., passi., ***phos.,*** plat-m., plb., ***rhus-t., sang.,*** scut., ***sep.,*** **SIL.,** ***sol-n., spig., stram.,*** stry., ***sulph.,*** syph., tarax., ther., thuj., zinc-valer.
menopause, during - ther.
red face, with, and diarrhea - **BELL.**

WALKING, while - petr., ***spig.***

WANDERING, pains - alumn., am-c., arg-n., calc., carb-v., chin., colch., ign., kali-bi., led., lyc., mag-p., mang., nat-s., phos., plan., podo., ***puls., sang., spig.,*** sulph.
mist before eyes, then fleeting pains agg. at occipital protuberance, down neck and shoulders, amel. lying in a dark, quiet place, and from sleep - podo.

WARM, coverings on, agg. - ***acon., apis,*** asar., aur., ***bor.,*** bry., ***calc.,*** carb-an., ***carb-v.,*** cham., chin., ***ferr.,*** ign., **IOD.,** lach., ***led.,*** **LYC.,** merc., mur-ac., nit-ac., ***op.,*** **PHOS.,** plat., **PULS.,** ***sec.,*** seneg., sep., ***spig.,*** staph., sulph., thuj., ***verat.***

WASHING, agg. - ***am-c., ant-c., bar-c., bell.,*** bry., ***calc., calc-p., calc-s.,*** canth., carb-v., cham., ***glon.,*** led., lyc., merc., nit-ac., ***nux-m.,*** phos., ***puls., rhus-t., sep.,*** spig., stront-c., sulph.

WATER, sensation of - am-c., anan., asaf., bell., cina, dig., ferr., ***hep.,*** mag-m., ph-ac., plat., samb.
cold, poured on head - ***cupr.,*** tarent.
dripping on head - cann-s.
drop running, temple - verat.
in the head - bufo, plat.
warm water, in - am-c., peti., sant.
wrapped up in - all-c.

WAVES of pain (see Paroxsmal) - ant-t., asaf., bell., chin., cocc., ferr., plat., **SEP.,** spig., viol-t., zinc.

WAVING, sensation, (see Shaking) - ***acon.,*** alum., apis, aur., ***bell.,*** canth., caust., chel., ***chin.,*** chin-s., ***cimic.,*** cina, coff., cupr-s., dig., dulc., ferr., fl-ac., gels., **GLON.,** graph., ***hep., hyos.,*** ind., indg., ***lach.,*** laur., ***lyc.,*** lyss., ***mag-m.,*** mag-p., mang., ***meli.,*** merc., mill., nux-v., pall., par., petr., rhus-t., sars., sel., senec., seneg., **SEP.,** sulph., thuj.
bending backward - dig.
confusion, with - mang.
convulsions, before - cimic.
motion, amel. - petr.
open, air amel. - mag-m.
rising from stooping - lyc.
standing agg. - dig.
stooping, after - hyos., lyc.
turning head agg. - ***glon.***
water in, as from - asaf., bell., cina, dig., ferr., mag-m.
wave-like motion upward - ***glon., lach.***
waving, forehead - asaf., **BELL.,** merc., petr., **SEP.**
like a heavy body swaying back and forth - op.
right to left, from - glon.
waving, occiput - gels., sil.
to forehead - mang.

WEAKNESS, sensation - alum., ***ambr.,*** ant-c., ant-t., asaf., aur., bell., bry., canth., carb-v., caust., cham., chin., cinnb., graph., hep., hyper., kali-c., kreos., ***merc.,*** nat-m., nit-ac., nux-m., op., ph-ac., phos., plan., psor., ran-b., raph., rhus-t., sars., sep., spong., squil., stann., stram., sulph., sul-ac., tab., tanac., tarent., thuj., zinc.
afternoon - sep.
breathing, on deep - carb-v.
coffee, after - ***cham.***
cough, after - bar-c., hep.
dinner, during - sulph.
after - rhus-t.
exertion, after - hydr-ac.
extending to lower limbs, as if paralyzed - phys.
throat, to - graph.
headache, after - nat-m.
were coming on, as though - ambr., iod., lac-c., phos., stram., thuj.
heat, after - sep.

WEAKNESS, sensation
lying on back, while - puls.
mental exertion, after - cinnb.
causes mental weakness - spong.
morning - cham., phos., ran-b.
rising, after - ph-ac.
noon - ars.
noon, evening - plan., raph.
pain, from - ars.
after - thea.
piano, music unbearable - nat-c., phos.
side, lain on - mag-m.
standing, while - rhus-t.
stomach, during weakness in - ars.
turning, as after much - nat-m.
walking, while - sulph.
in the sun - nat-m.
working in hot room, as from - glon.

WENS, (see Sebaceous cysts)

WEIGHT, (see Heaviness, Pressing)

WET, getting - bar- c., **BELL.,** led., ***puls.***

WHARBLING - sep.

WRAPPED, (see Uncovering, warm covering)

WRINKLED, forehead - acet-ac., alum., brom., ***caust., cham., cycl., graph.,*** grat., ***hell., lyc.,*** mang., merc., nat-m., ox-ac., phos., rheum, rhus-t., ***sep., stram., syph.,*** zinc.
brain symptoms, in - ***hell.,*** **STRAM.**
chest symptoms, with - **LYC.**
headache in - aster., ***caust.,*** grat., hyos., nat-m., phos., **STRAM.,** sulph., viol-o.
sensation of - ***graph.,*** thuj.

Hearing

ACUTE, (see Sensitive) - **ACON.,** agar., aloe, alum., am-c., ***anac.,*** ang., apis, arn., ars., ars-i., ***asar.,*** atro., ***aur.,*** **BELL.,** bor., bry., cact., calad., calc., ***cann-i.,*** carb-s., carb-v., cham., **CHIN.,** chin-a., ***cic.,*** cimic., ***cocc.,*** **COFF.,** coff-t., ***colch.,*** **CON.,** cop., cupr., ***graph., hep., iod., kali-c., kali-p., kali-s.,*** **LACH.,** ***lyc.,*** lyss., mag-c., merc., mur-ac., ***nat-a.,*** **NAT-C.,** ***nat-m., nat-p., nux-m.,*** **NUX-V., OP.,** petr., ***ph-ac., phos.,*** phys., phyt., ***plan.,*** plb., ptel., ***puls.,*** sang., sec., seneg., ***sep.,*** **SIL.,** ***spig.,*** stram., ***stry., sulph.,*** **TAB.,** ***ther.,*** thuj., ***verat.,*** viol-o., zing.

bed, in - kali-c.
deafness, precedes - **SULPH.**
dull, then - ***iod.***
cracking in ears, preceded by - graph., mur-ac.
discharge of moisture, after - spig.
evening - coca, rhod.
asleep, on falling - calc., calad.
bed, in - ***kali-c.***
fever, during - acon., bell., calc., **CAPS., CON.,** ip., lyc., nux-v.
headache, during - acon., bry., coff., phyt.
labor pains, during - cimic.
menses, during - ***hyper.,*** mag-c., nux-v.
morning - ***fl-ac.***
music, to - **ACON.,** aloe, ambr., bufo, ***cact., cham., coff., lyc., nat-c.,*** **NUX-V.,** ph-ac., ***sep.,*** sulph., ***tab.,*** viol-o.
amel. - **AUR.,** ***aur-m.***
menses, during - ***nat-c.***
organ - lyc.
piano - phos., sabin., sulph.
violin - viol-o.
night - atro.
noises, to - **ACON.,** aloe, am-c., apis, arn., ***ars.,*** **AUR.,** bar-c., **BELL.,** bor., bry., bufo, calad., ***calc.,*** caust., caps., chen-a., ***chin., cic., cocc., coff.,*** **CON.,** crot-h., ***ferr.,*** ferr-p., fl-ac., ***gels., ign., iod., ip., kali-c., kali-p.,*** lac-c., **LACH., LYC.,** mag-c., mag-m., mill., **MUR-AC.,** ***nat-a., nat-c., nat-p., nat-s.,*** **NIT-AC.,** nux-m., **NUX-V.,** ol-an., **OP.,** ***phos., ph-ac.,*** plb., ***sang.,*** sec., ***sep., sil., spig.,*** stann., ***sulph.,*** tab., **THER.,** ***tub.,*** **ZINC.**
cause nausea - ***cocc., ther.***
high-pitched - chen-a.
perspiration, during - **CAPS.**
rumpling of paper - bor., calad., ferr., ***nat-c., nat-s.,*** tarax., zinc.
scratching on linen and silk - **ASAR.**
vertigo, during - spig.
perspiration, during - acon., bell., calc., **CHAM.,** ***coff.,*** **CON.,** ip., lyc., nat-c., **NUX-V.,** zinc.
roaring, with - ***lyc.***
sensation, with singular, of deafness from one ear to the other, as if a tube went through head - med.
sight, with loss of - stram.

ACUTE, hearing
sleep, during - alumn., ***calad.***
sleeplessness, with, clock striking and cocks crowing at a distance keep her awake - **OP.**
sound of, affect the teeth - ***lach., ther.***
hammer, a - sang.
long retained - lyc., phos.
vehicles, while deaf to voices - ***chen-a.***
step, every - **COFF.,** ***nux-v.***
typhoid fever, in - ***lyc.***
voices and talking - ***agar.,*** am-c., ars., cact., carb-v., ***cocc., coff.,*** con., ign., ***kali-c.,*** kali-p., ***mur-ac., op.,*** ph-ac., ptel., verat., **ZINC.**
her own - op.
waking, on - carb-v., puls.
water running - **LYSS.**
worry agg. - ign.

CONFUSED - **CARB-AN.**
chorea, after - sec.
listens attentively to conversation and at the end knows nothing about it - plat.
tones become commingled - **CARB-AN.**

DEAFNESS, general - acon., ***agar.,*** agn., ***all-c.,*** alum., ***ambr., am-c., anac.,*** ant-c., ant-t., ***arg-n.,*** arn., ars., ***ars-i.,*** asaf., ***asar.,*** aur., ***aur-m.,*** bar-c., ***bar-m.,*** **BELL.,** bor., bry., ***calc.,*** caj., cann-s., caps., ***carb-s., carb-v.,*** carl., **CAUST.,** cham., chel., **CHIN.,** chin-s., chlf., chlor., ***cic.,*** coca, cocc., con., croc., crot-h., ***crot-t.,*** cupr., dros., dulc., ***elaps, fl-ac., form., gels., glon.,*** **GRAPH.,** hell., **HEP.,** ***hydr.,*** hydr-ac., **HYOS.,** jatr., kali-ar., ***kali-bi., kali-br.,*** kali-c., ***kali-n.,*** kali-p., kreos., lach., lachn., laur., led., **LYC.,** ***lyss., mag-c.,*** mag-m., mang., med., meny., meph., ***merc.,*** merc-c., ***merc-d.,*** mosch., nat-c., ***nat-m.,*** nat-p., nat-s., nicc., nit-ac., ol-an., olnd., petr., ph-ac., ***phos., plat.,*** plb., psor., ***puls.,*** raph., rheum, rhod., rhus-t., sabad., sarac., ***sec.,*** sep., sil., **SPIG.,** spong., stann., ***stram., sul-ac.,*** **SULPH.,** syph., thuj., vario., verat., vip., zinc.

acute diseases, almost complete, during - lachn.
afternoon - sil.
air, worse in open - calc.
alternating with abnormal - cadm-s.
amblyopia, with - ***puls.***
blowing, nose - spig.
blurred, with - ***glon.***
boring finger, amel. - spig.
brief, sudden attack - sep.
catarrhal - ***asar.,*** bell., ***caps., caust., gels., merc.,*** **PULS., SULPH.**
marked cachexia, with - ***syph.***
pain from throat into middle ear, with - ***gels.***
scrofulous subjects, in - ***iod.***
chorea, after - sec.
cold, from, after cutting hair - ***led.,*** **PULS.**
congestion, from - cact.
congestive, after typhoid - phos.
convulsions, after - sec.

DEAFNESS, general

coryza, in, after changeable weather - ***gels.***
changeable weather from, after suppression of, or otorrhea - ***led.***
cough, with - chel.
delirium, with, almost complete - **BAPT.**
dinner, during - sulph.
discharge, with, from ear - am-m., bor., ***caust.,*** **HEP.,** ***lyc., merc.,*** **PULS.**
profuse fetid, from right - ***merc.***
purulent fetid - tell.
yellow, green - ***elaps.***
watery - ***elaps.***
dryness, with - ***calc., lach.***
eating, after - **SULPH.**
elderly, people, in - ***cic., merc-d., petr.***
eustachian, catarrhal - **CALC.,** ***kali-s.,*** **PULS.**
scrofulous subjects, in - ***iod.***
eustachian, swelling of tube and tympanic cavity, from - kali-m.
chronic disease of larynx, with - ***mang.***
noises, with - **PETR.**
evening, agg. - anan.
9 p.m., on lying down agg. - merc-c.
exanthema, after acute - ***carb-v.***
suppressed by cold - ***ph-ac.***
fever, in catarrhal - ***euph.***
febris nervosa stupida - meli.
intermittent fever, after suppression of by quinine - ***calc.***
typhus, in - ***apis, arg-n., ars.,*** **BELL.,** ***chlor.,*** dig., ***nit-ac., nit-s-d., nux-m.***
after - ***arn.***
yellow fever, in - ***verat.***
fullness, with, and cracking when blowing nose or swallowing - ***mang.***
glands, with swelling of - kali-m.
head, injury, from - **ARN.**
region of auditory nerve - chin-s.
headache, with - bar-m., chin-s., ***stram.,*** verb.
bending, back, amel. - fl-ac.
congestion to, with - ***chin.***
rheumatic pain in, from - am-m.
liver, disorder, with - ***chel.***
hydrocephalus, in acute - hell.
increasing, after arthritic affection of head - rhod.
gradually - syph.
typhus, in - ***agar.***
inflammation, with, of left - ***merc-sol.***
influenza, in - ***gels.***
leaflet before, sensation of - ant-c.
left, in - all-s., arg-n., chin-b., ol-j., puls., **SULPH.,** thlaspi
catarrhal - ***all-s.***
buzzing in head, with - acon.
otorrhea, with - phos.
shaking head, on, singing and roaring - **CALC.**
loud sounds, followed by - sep.
measles, after suppressed - **PULS.,** ***sulph.***
meatus, external, dry, with - ***graph.***

DEAFNESS, general

melancholy, in, after mortification - ***ign.***
meningitis, in - ***glon.***
cerebrospinal - ***cic., hydr-ac.***
infantum, sequel - ***arn., hell.***
menses, during - ***calc.,*** lyc.
mental, in, derangement - stram., verat.
mercury, after abuse of - ***carb-v., nit-ac.***
momentary, produced by sudden sound on tympanum - polyg.
morning, after rising - stann.
moving, on, quickly, with faintness - verat-v.
nerve, from paralyzed auditory - ***caust., glon., hyos., kali-p.,*** verat-v.
weakness of auditory, fibres, from - mag-p.
nervous - mosch., ***petr., plat.,*** sal-ac., ***sil.,*** tab.
cachexia, with marked - ***syph.***
typhoid, after - ***ph-ac.***
night, at - ***cedr.***
noise, with, better when in a - **GRAPH.**
buzzing - cact.
left, in, like a swarm of bees - ***coff.***
ears, noises in, with - bor., ***petr., psor., sal-ac.***
disappearing on blowing nose and coughing - ***sil.***
follows loud sounds and humming - ***sep.***
head, in - ***coca***
hissing and humming, with - sulph.
preceded by subjective - ***petr.***
ringing, with, and roaring - ***aur-m.***
erysipelas, in - rhus-t.
which went off when at rest, but reappeared when she moved - ***nux-v.***
roaring, with - ***chen-a.,*** **PH-AC.**
thunderous - tell.
singing, and other noises - ***nux-v.***
rumbling, with, in left - ***elaps.***
rushing, with, as of water - ***cocc.***
isochronous with pulse - **PULS.**
very little, of both ears, had to use a trumpet, with - med.
nose, with, cracking on blowing - kali-m.
blowing, agg. - **SULPH.**
otitis, after - ***merc.***
palsy, complicating motor - plb.
paralysis, with - ***sil.***
paralytic, in old people, or in arthritic subjects - ***petr.***
partial, or transitory - ***med.***
with dry wax in left ear - ***lach.***
periodical - ***spig.***
pneumonia, in typhoid - lachn.
oversensitiveness of hearing, preceded by - **SULPH.**
progressive - ***petr.***
rheumatism, with - ***fl-ac.***
humming, consequent upon a chill, with - ***petr.***
riding, in a carriage or train, amel. - **GRAPH., NIT-AC., PULS.**
wagon, in a, amel. - ***graph.***

DEAFNESS, general
  right, in - ***arn., calc., kali-s., led.***
    as if a leaflet were lying before tympanum - ant-c.
    catarrhal - sulph.
    passes off by noon - ***ham.***
    seven or eight months, for - nat-c.
  scarlatina, after - ***crot-h., graph., hep., lach.,*** **LYC.,** ***puls.,*** **SULPH.**
  scarlet fever, after - **LYC.**
  multiple sclerosis, in - ***phos.***
  scrofulous, in, subjects - ***calc., iod., sulph.***
  sensitiveness, after painful, of hearing - ***con.***
  sexual, in those addicted to, excess or drunkenness - ***petr.***
  sopor, with, in scarlatina - ***phos.***
  speech, with loss of, from massive doses of quinine - ***gels.***
    produced by massive doses of quinine - ***gels.***
  stooping, after - mang.
  stopped up, sensation, as if - calad., ***lach., mang., merc-d., nat-c., nit-ac.,*** **PULS.,** ***sep.,*** spig., verat.
    a skin were drawn over - bell.
    something lay in front of membrana tympani - ***calc.***
    something were lying before ear - ***mag-m.***
  stupefaction, with, dizziness and vacancy in head - kreos.
  stupefied, as if, especially after stroke - ***hyos.***
  sudden - ***plb.***
    faint, after a - ***sil.***
    painless, at night, with constant roaring and cracking in ears - ***elaps***
    right ear, after taking cold - ***elaps.***
    roaring and humming, with - nicc.
    temporary - ***gels.***
  sweating, better by - calc.
  swellings, from - ***kali-m.***
  syphilis, from hereditary - lac-c.
    decay of left molars, with - ***nat-c.***
    left, in, in a subject treated with large doses of mercury for - ***petr.***
  syphilitic - ***kreos., nit-ac.***
  throat, caused by, affections - ***sang.***
  tonsils, with enlarged - ***kali-bi., merc., nit-ac., staph.***
  transient, caused by swelling of tonsils and glands of the throat, extending into ears - med.
  tympanitic, from swelling of, cavity with watery condition of tongue - nat-m.
  vertigo, with - ***chin-s., cic.,*** coloc., colch., crot-h., ***sal-ac., sil.***
    heavy food, mostly after fat - ***sin-n.***
    stooping, when - ***merc-c.***
    typhoid, in - ***cic.***
  voice, especially to human - **PHOS.,** rhus-t., sil., **SULPH.**
    sounds unnatural, especially in right ear - ter.
  waking, on - oena.

DEAFNESS, general
  walking, when - chin-s.
  warm, better in a, room and worse in cold, damp weather - ***puls.***
  washing, worse from, and changing linen, better by electricity - sil.
  water, caused by, filling ears - verb.
  wax, from hardening of earwax - ***con.,*** sel.
    hard black cerumen, with - **PULS.**
  weather, worse in damp, with tinnitus - anan.
  words, especially for - bufo.
  years, for several - rhod.

DIFFICULT - aur., bar-c., ***calc-p., caust.,*** **CUPR-M.,** ***form.,*** **PHOS.,** sabad.
  as if ears closed, as if something had fallen before ear - ***verb.***
  human voice and during full moon - ***sil.***
    also after typhus, with cold extremities - ***phos.***
    heard with - ***fl-ac.***
  humming before ears, with increased - ***dros.***
  left ear, in - bor.
  menses, during - kreos.
    before - ***kreos.***
  overexertion, after - sil.
  roaring in ears, with - ***sal-ac.***
  typhus, in - cupr-m.

DISTANT, sounds seem - all-c., cann-i., cham., coca, eupi., **LAC-C.,** nux-m., peti., sol-n.
    voices seem - cann-i., coca, nitro-o., sabal.
      his own - arn., cann-i.

DULL - agar., am-c., ***all-c.,*** iber., polyg.
  acute disease, after severe - ***ph-ac.***
  blowing nose amel., worse during cold and rainy weather - ***mang.***
  burning in ear, after - ***caps.***
  buzzing, with - ***elaps***
  catarrhal fever, in - ***dulc.***
  cotton were in ear, or something lying before right, as if - ***cycl.***
  diphtheria, after - **PHYT.**
  distant sounds, from mental or bodily exhaustion - ***ph-ac.***
  evenings, amel. - merc-i-r.
  feet, worse getting wet - ***dulc.***
  must be spoken to loudly - iodof.
  rheumatism, in - ***kali-c.***
  right side, worse - aster.
  roaring and humming in ears, worse stooping, caused by - ***croc.***
  swelling and catarrh of eustachian tubes and tympanitic cavity, with - ***sil.***
  typhus, in - arg-n., ***bapt.***
  warmth from walking, amel. - ***merc-i-r.***

ILLUSIONS, of (see Noises, in ear) - absin., agar., am-c., ***anac., antipyrin.,*** ars., atro., bell., ***cann-i.,*** carb-o., carb-s., carb-v., ***cham.,*** cocaine, ***coff.,*** con., crot-h., elaps, eup-pur., hyos., kali-ar., lyss., med., merc., naja, nat-p., puls., rhodi., ***stram., sulph.,*** thea.

ILLUSIONS, of
as if tone came from another world - **CARB-AN.**
his own voiced seems to have changed - alum.
sounds, appear to come from left side when they really come from the right - ***nat-c.***
remained longer - ptel.
seem double, whistling - med.

IMPAIRED - aeth., agar., agn., alet., ***all-c., ambr., am-c., am-m., anac., ang.,*** ant-c., ***apis,*** arg-m., arg-n., ***arn., ars.,*** asaf., ***asar.,*** aster., ***aur.,*** aur-m., aur-s., ***bapt.,*** **BAR-C.,** ***bar-m.,*** **BELL.,** bor., ***bov.,*** bufo, ***bry.,*** cact., calad., **CALC.,** ***calc-p.,*** cann-i., caps., **CARB-AN.,** carb-o., **CARB-S., CARB-V., CAUST.,** cedr., cham., ***chel.,*** **CHIN.,** chin-a., chin-s., chlf., cist., clem., ***cic., cocc.,*** coc-c., coff., colch., coloc., com., ***con.,*** cor-r., croc., crot-c., crot-h., ***crot-t.,*** **CUPR.,** ***cycl.,*** dig., ***dros.,*** dulc., ***elaps, ferr.,*** ferr-ar., ***ferr-i.,*** ferr-p., ***fl-ac., form.,*** gamb., ***gels., glon.,*** **GRAPH.,** grat., guare., guai., ***hep., hydr.,*** hydr-ac., **HYOS.,** ign., ***iod., ip.,*** jatr., ***kali-bi., kali-br., kali-c.,*** kali-chl., kali-i., kali-n., kali-p., kali-s., kalm., ***kreos., lach.,*** lachn., ***lact., laur., led.,*** **LYC.,** ***mag-c., mag-m.,*** mag-p., ***mang.,*** med., meny., meph., ***merc.,*** merc-i-r., merl., mez., mosch., ***mur-ac.,*** nat-a., ***nat-c.,*** **NAT-M.,** ***nat-p.,*** nicc., **NIT-AC.,** nux-m., ***nux-v.,*** olnd., onos., op., par., **PETR., PH-AC., PHOS.,** phys., plat., ***plb., psor.,*** **PULS.,** rheum, rhod., ***rhus-t., ruta., sabad., sabin., sal-ac.,*** sars., **SEC.,** sel., ***sep.,*** **SIL.,** ***spig., spong.,*** squil., stann., ***staph., stram.,*** **SULPH.,** ***sul-ac.,*** tab., tarax., tarent., ***tell.,*** tep., ther., thuj., valer., ***verat.,*** **VERB.,** viol-o., zinc.
adenoids, from - agra., calc-i., sul-i.
hypertrophied adenoids and tonsils - ***agra.,*** aur., bar-c., calc-p., merc., nit-ac., staph.
afternoon - elaps, sil.
pain in the ear, with - ign.
air, amel. - mag-c., merc.
open, agg. - calc.
alcoholism, in - ***kali-br.***
alternating with, obscuration of sight - cic.
otorrhea - puls.
eye symptoms - guare.
band, as if caused by a band over the ears - mag-arct.
belching, during - petr.
bending, backward, amel. - ***fl-ac.***
birth, from - meph., tub.
blowing, nose amel. - hep., ***mang.,*** merc., ***sil.,*** stann.
burning, and stinging, after - caps.
catarrh of eustachian tube - ars-i., **ASAR., CALC.,** caps., caust., dulc., gels., graph., ***hep.,*** hydr., ***iod.,*** kali-bi., **KALI-M., KALI-S.,** lach., ***mang.,*** menthol, ***merc-d.,*** merc-sul., mez., morg., nit-ac., **PETR.,** ***phos.,*** **PULS.,** rhus-t., ros-d., ***sang.,*** sep., ***sil.,*** thiosin.
change, of clothing - ***sil.***
change of, weather agg. - mang., sabin.
clock, near - ph-ac.

IMPAIRED, hearing
cold, after a - ars., bell., ***elaps,*** lach., ***led.,*** mag-c., merc., **PULS.,** sil.
wet weather, agg. - acon., dulc., kali-m., ***mang., merc., puls., sil.,*** visc.
cold, sensation in abdomen, with - ***ambr.***
concussions, from - **ARN.,** chin-s., croc., hell., nat-s.
confusion, of sounds - **CARB-AN.,** plat., sec.
cough, during - chel., puls.
cough, amel. - ***sil.***
damp, weather agg. - anan., calen., calen., ***mang.,*** puls., sabin., sil.
decreased, with hallucination - ***hyos.***
deficient, in meniere's disease - ***sal-ac.***
diminished - tell.
frequent pain in head and toothache, with - petr.
left, in - asar., ***calc.***
roaring in head, from - ***sil.***
diminution, rapid - phos.
dinner, after - sulph.
direction, of sound, cannot tell - ***carb-an.***
distance, when at a - ph-ac.
amel. - gamb., ph-ac.
all sounds seem far off - cann-i., lac-c., nux-m.
disturbed, when given in large doses for rheumatism - sal-ac.
earwax, after removal of, amel. - ***con.***
eating, agg. - sil., spig., **SULPH.**
elderly, people - bar-c., ***cic.,*** kali-m., merc-d., ***petr.***
evening - anan., ant-c., cham., kali-c., merc-c., nicc., plb., tarax.
9 p.m. - phys.
forenoon - asaf., clem., ***ham.,*** mag-c., phys.
11 a.m. - mag-c.
lasting till 8 p.m. - phys.
fright, after - mag-c.
fever, during - rhus-t.
grief, from continued, overexertion, sexual excesses, or drain on system,
headache, in occiput, with - ign.
hiccough, after - bell.
humiliation, after - ign.
hydrocephalus, acute, in - ***dig.***
increasing, and decreasing slowly - kali-c.
intermittent - mag-m., sil.
leaf or membrane, like, before the ear - acon., agar., alum., am-c., ant-c., ***arg-n.,*** asaf., ***asar.,*** bell., calad., ***calc.,*** cann-s., chel., ***chin.,*** cocc., ***cycl., graph.,*** kali-i., led., ***mag-m.,*** mang., med., nit-ac., par., ***phos.,*** sabad., sel., ***sul-ac.,*** tab., verat., **VERB.**
shaking, head, and boring in ear amel. - sel.
left - anac., ***arg-n.,*** bor., bry., chel., coc-c., jac-c., mag-m., nat-c., op.
then right - sulph.
lessening - anac.

IMPAIRED, hearing
- **measles,** after - arg-n., asar., ***carb-v., merc.,*** **PULS.,** ***sil.,*** spig., ***sulph.,*** ter.
- **membrane** retracted and thickened - mez.
- **menses,** during - ***calc.,*** mag-m., ***kreos.***
  - before - ferr., ***kreos.***
  - suppressed, agg. - ***cub.***
- **mercury,** abuse of - ***asaf., carb-v., nit-ac., petr., staph., sulph.***
- **moon,** full agg. - sil.
- **morning** - calc., clem., gamb., merc-i-r., sil., stann.
- **night** - ***cedr.,*** elaps
- **nitric** acid, abuse of - petr.
- **noises,** with - caust., cocc., con., dig., lyc., mag-c., merc., nit-ac., petr., ph-ac., sep., sil., sulph., ther.
  - amel. - calen., chen-a., **GRAPH.,** nit-ac., piloc.
- **obtuse** - ***dulc.***
- **overheated,** from becoming - merc., merc-i-f.
- **pain,** in ear, with - cham., cycl.
- **paralysis,** of the auditory nerve, from - ***bar-c., bell.,*** calc., ***caust.,*** chel., dulc., ***glon.,*** graph., ***hyos.,*** kali-p., lyc., merc., nit-ac., nux-v., ***op.,*** petr., ***ph-ac., puls.,*** sec., ***sil.***
- **periodic** - caps., sec., ***spig.***
- **plug,** as from a - sep.
- **pregnancy,** during periodic - caps.
- **pressing,** on ear amel. - ***phos.***
- **quinine,** after abuse of - ***calc., chin-s.***
- **reading,** aloud, while - verb.
- **report,** loud, followed by deafness - sep.
  - relieved after - graph., hep., mur-ac., ***sil.,*** tarent.
- **rheumatic**-gouty diathesis - ***ferr-pic.,*** ham., kali-i., led., sil., sulph., visc.
- **riding,** in a carriage amel. - ***graph.,*** **NIT-AC.,** ***puls.***
- **right** - ***arn., calc.,*** cocc., cycl., ***ham., kali-s., led.,*** merc., phys.
  - right, then left - elaps
- **room,** in a - mag-c.
- **rubbing,** amel. - ***phos.***
- **scarlet** fever, after - bell., **CARB-V.,** ***crot-h., graph., hep., lach.,*** **LYC.,** ***nit-ac., puls., sil.,*** **SULPH.**
- **sexual,** excesses - ***petr.***
- **singing,** after - apoc.
- **stooping,** agg. - ***croc.,*** merc.
- **storm,** before - nux-m.
- **sudden** - dig., ***elaps, gels.,*** nicc., nit-ac., ***plb., sec.,*** sep., ***sil.***
- **suppressed,** coryza or otorrhea, after - led.
  - discharges, after - lob.
  - eczema, after - lob.
  - eruptions about the - ***mez.***
  - intermittents - ***calc., chin-s.***
- **swallowing,** on - ars., aur., phos.
  - amel. - alum., merc.
- **tired,** when - sabin.

IMPAIRED, hearing
- **tonsils,** enlarged, with - agra., aur., ***bar-c.,*** calc-s., ***hep., kali-bi.,*** lyc., med., ***merc., nit-ac.,*** plb., psor., ***staph.***
  - hypertrophied tonsils and adenoids - ***agra.,*** aur., bar-c., calc-p., merc., nit-ac., staph.
- **transient** - sep., sulph.
- **typhoid,** after - ***apis, arg-n., ars., nit-ac., ph-ac.***
- **voice,** the human - ***ars.,*** bov., bufo, calc., ***carb-an., chen-a., fl-ac.,*** ign., iod., kali-p., mur-ac., onos., **PHOS.,** rhus-t., ***sil., still.,*** **SULPH.**
  - except, for - ign.
- **walking,** while - chin-s.
  - wind, in the - phos.
- **warm,** from walking, on becoming - merc.
  - becoming, amel. - merc-i-r.
- **warm,** room, agg. - kali-s.
  - amel. - ***puls.***
- **washing,** agg. - sil.
- **working,** in water - ***calc.***
- **yawning,** amel. - sil.

IMPRESSION of sounds last heard continue for a long time - ptel.

INDISTINCT - am-c., chlf.
- misunderstands - bov.

LOST, (see Hearing, deafness)

NOISES, in ears, (see Illusions, Tinnitus) - acon., act-sp., ***aesc.,*** agar., ***agn.,*** ail., all-c., aloe, alum., ***ambr.,*** am-c., am-m., anac., anag., ang., ant-c., ant-t., ***arg-n., arn., ars., ars-i.,*** arund., ***asar.,*** asaf., aster., atro., ***aur., bar-c., bar-m.,*** **BELL.,** berb., bism., ***bor.,*** bov., brom., ***bry.,*** **CACT.,** cadm-s., cahin., calad., **CALC.,** calc-p., ***calc-s.,*** camph., **CANN-I.,** cann-s., canth., carb-ac., carb-an., carb-h., carb-o., ***carb-s., carb-v., carl.,*** cast., **CAUST.,** ***cedr.,*** cham., ***chel.,*** **CHIN.,** chin-a., **CHIN-S.,** chlf., ***cic.,*** cimic., clem., coca, cocc., ***coc-c.,*** coff., colch., coloc., com., ***con.,*** cop., croc., crot-t., ***cupr.,*** cupr-ac., cur., cycl., daph., ***dig.,*** dios., dirc., dros., dulc., elaps, ery-a., euon., eup-per., ***eup-pur.,*** ferr., ferr-ar., ferr-i., ferr-p., fl-ac., form., gamb., ***glon.,*** **GRAPH.,** guare., hell., hep., hura, hydr., hydr-ac., hyos., hyper., ***ign.,*** ill., indg., ***iod.,*** jatr., kali-a., kali-bi., kali-br., ***kali-c.,*** kali-chl., **KALI-I.,** kali-n., ***kali-p., kali-s.,*** kalm., ***kreos., lac-c., lach.,*** lachn., lact., lac-ac., laur., led., lepi., **LYC.,** ***lyss.,*** mag-c., mag-m., mag-s., manc., mang., meny., ***merc.,*** merc-c., mez., morph., mosch., mur-ac., myric., naja, nat-a., nat-c., ***nat-m., nat-p., nat-s.,*** nicc., ***nit-ac.,*** nux-m., ***nux-v.,*** olnd., ***op.,*** osm., paeon., ***par.,*** **PETR.,** phel., **PH-AC.,** ***phos.,*** pic-ac., pin-s., plan., ***plat., plb.,*** **PSOR.,** ptel., **PULS.,** rheum, ***rhod.,*** rhus-t., ruta., sabad., sabin., ***sal-ac.,*** **SANG.,** sarr., sars., ***sec.,*** seneg., ***sep., sil.,*** **SPIG.,** spong., stann., ***staph.,*** stram., stront-c., stry., **SULPH.,** sul-ac., ***tab.,*** tarax., tarent., tep., teucr., thea., ther., thuj., til., **TUB.,** valer., verat., xan., zinc.

NOISES, in ears
afternoon - all-c., ***ambr., ant-c.,*** carb-v., cham., dios., elaps, gamb., hydrc., kalm., mag-c., ptel., puls., rhus-t., spig., sulph., thuj., verat., verat-v.
2 p.m. - hydr., verat., verat-v.
3 p.m. - elaps, fago., mag-c.
4 p.m. - dios., ***lyc.,*** puls.
5 p.m. - ol-an., sulph.
6 p.m. - ol-an.
air, in open - agar., carb-an., graph., tab.
amel. - ars., cic., puls., thuj.
anxiety, agg. - act-sp.
bagpipe, as from distant - nat-c.
bat, sounds as from - mill.
night - ph-ac.
beating, someone beating a door - ant-c.
distant, amel. on rising - mez.
bed, driving out of - sil.
bell, of a clock - mang.
bells, ringing - auran., ars., chin., ***chin-s., clem.,*** crot-h., led., mang., ***nat-s.,*** **PETR.,** ph-ac., sars., ***spig.,*** sul-ac., valer.
constant clear, bell. sound - ***petr.***
large bell, as of - alum.
left ear, in - chin-b.
morning - mang.
noise as of little - arund.
like that following tolling of a, interrupted by cracking sound - rhod.
spinal irritation, in - ***chin-s.***
whistling, or running of trains, first left, then right, worse by lying on right side, like - merc.
blowing - hydr-ac., ox-ac., ***phos., sel.***
blowing, nose, when - bar-c., ***calc., carb-an., hep.,*** kali-chl., lyc., mang., meny., ph-ac., stann., teucr.
boiling, water, like - cann-i., ***dig.***
oil, like - thuj.
boring, into ear amel. - aeth., lach., meny., nicc.
breakfast, during - carb-v., nit-ac., zinc.
breathing, when - bar-c., ***iod.,*** nat-s.
bubbling - bell., con., dulc., euphr., graph., hura, kali-c., kali-n., lyc., ***nat-c.,*** nat-m., rheum, sil., thuj.
bursting of a bubble - ***nat-c.,*** sulph.
buzzing - abrot., acon., agar., all-c., ant-c., aloe, alum., ambr., ***am-c., arg-m.,*** **ARG-N.,** ***arn., ars., ars-i., aur., aur-m., bar-c., bar-m., bell., berb.,*** bor., ***cact.,*** cahin., calad., ***calc.,*** calc-s., ***camph.,*** **CANN-I.,** carb-an., carb-s., ***carb-v.,*** carl., cast., ***caust.,*** cedr., chel., **CHIN.,** chin-a., **CHIN-S.,** chlf., cimic., cocc., coc-c., ***coff., con.,*** cop., croc., crot-c., dig., dios., dros., ***dulc., elaps, eup-per.,*** euph., ***ferr-p.,*** ferr-pic., ***form.,*** gamb., glon., ***ham.,*** hep., hydr-ac., ***hyos., iod.,*** kali-ar., **KALI-C.,** kali-i., kali-p., kali-s., kalm., ***kreos., lac-c., lach.,*** lact., ***laur.,*** **LYC.,** lyss., ***mag-c.,*** mag-m., merl., merc., ***mur-ac., nat-m.,*** nicc., nit-ac., ***nux-m.,*** **NUX-V.,** olnd., ***op., petr.,***

NOISES, in ears
buzzing - ***pic-ac., phos.,*** **PLAT.,** plb., ***psor.,*** puls., rhod., sabad., sabin., sal-ac., sec., sel., ***sep., spig.,*** stront-c., ***sulph.,*** sul-ac., ***sul-i., tarent.,*** ther., thuj., zinc.
afternoon - gamb.
alternating with whistling - mag-c.
awaking, on - ***ars.***
bee, like a - rhod.
swarm of, left, in, with deafness - ***coff.***
bright's, in disease - ***ars.***
chill, with - ***glon.***
constant - ***elaps, phos.***
deafness, in - am-c., ***kreos., psor.***
descending stairs, while - crot-c.
dinner, after eating - agar.
epilepsy, after - ***caust.***
evening - ***bar-c.,*** gamb., murx., sel., ***spig.,*** sul-ac.
bed, in - lact.
forenoon - ant-c., rhod.
fly, as if a, were enclosed - ***elaps***
head, from rush of blood to - ferr-p.
piercing in, with - ***sulph.***
headache, with - dios.
heart palpitation, in - ***arg-m.***
hysteria, in - ***aur.***
intermittent fever, in - ***ars.***
lameness of legs, morning, agg. - sil.
leaning on head amel. - kali-c.
left - ***berb., coff.***
sensitiveness, with - ***aur-m.***
meningitis, in, infantum, sequel - ***arn.***
menses, during - ***kreos.***
before - ***kreos.***
mental exertion, after - ferr-pic.
morning - dios., mag-m.
waking, on - nat-m.
night - am-m., **DULC.,** ***euph.,*** lac-c.
noon - cedr., fago.
obstruction, with, of nose - ***lach.***
one ear and then the other - ***sulph.***
otitis media, in - ***cact.***
outside, as if - alum.
perspiration, during - **ARS.**
puerperal fever, in - cimic.
right ear - elaps, lac-c., lyss., mag-m., ***mur-ac.,*** sulph.
neuralgia, with - sul-ac.
sleepless at night - ***euph.***
side lain on - mag-m.
sitting, while - am-m.
stool, during - lyc.
after - ***calc-p.***
stroke, in - **NUX-V.**
sunstroke, in - ***verat-v.***
swallowing, when - rhod.
sweat, with, intermittent - **ARS.**
vertigo, with - ***arg-n., ars.,*** bell., **CHIN-S., *cic., glon.,*** laur., nat-s., zinc.
typhoid, in - ***cic.***
whistling, agg. - rhod.
work, with inability to, read or think - ***nat-m.***

NOISES, in ears
cannonading - bad., chel., chen-a., mosch.
distant - chel., plat.
cat, like a spitting - calc., nit-ac., plat., sil.
afternoon - nit-ac.
synchronous with pulse - ***sep.***
chewing, when - aloe, alum., bar-c., bar-m., ***calc.,*** carb-v., ***graph., iod.,*** **KALI-S.,** mang., meny., nat-m., **NIT-AC.,** nux-v., ***petr.,*** sil., sulph.
chill, during - cedr., chin-s., glon., nat-m., rhus-t., puls., ***tub.***
chirping - agar., bry., calad., ***carb-s.,*** carb-v., ***caust.,*** cedr., euph., ferr., kali-s., lach., ***lyc.,*** meny., mur-ac., ***nat-s.,*** nicc., ***nux-v., puls.,*** rat., ***rhus-t., sil.,*** sulph., tarax., ***tub.***
evening - ***carb-s.,*** lyc., nat-s.
intermittent, during - ***lyc., nat-s.,*** nux-v., ***puls., rhus-t.,*** tub.
morning in bed - puls.
night - carb-v., mur-ac., nux-v., rhus-t.
right - rat.
clashing - ***mang.,*** sabad., sil.
closing, eyes - chel.
clucking - agar., ***bar-c.,*** cadm-s., ***elaps, graph.,*** kali-c., lyc., petr., rheum, sep., sil.
left, while lying on it - bar-c.
rising from stooping, when - graph., sep.
stooping on - graph.
cold, drinks after - kali-c.
convulsions, after - ***ars., caust.***
coughing, on - nux-v., sil.
covering, eyes with hands amel. - spig.
cracking - agar., ambr., ***bar-c., bar-m., calc.,*** carb-s., cocc., coc-c., ***coff., com.,*** dulc., ery-a., ***form.,*** gels., glon., ***graph.,*** hep., **KALI-C.,** kali-chl., ***kali-m.,*** kali-s., kalm., ***lach.,*** mang., meny., mosch., mur-ac., nat-c., ***nat-m.,*** **NIT-AC.,** ol-an., ped., **PETR.,** ***psor., puls.,*** rhod., ***rhus-t.,*** sil., stry., sulph., tarent., thuj., zinc.
blowing nose - ***hep.,*** kali-c., kali-chl., mang.
breakfast, after - zinc.
burst, as if drum had, during sleep - ***lach.***
chewing, when - aloe, alum., bar-c., ***calc., graph., kali-s.,*** meny., ***nat-m.,*** **NIT-AC.,** ***petr.,*** sil., sulph.
coughing, while - nux-v.
deafness, with - ***psor.***
eustachian tubes, caused by problem in - **PETR.**
eating, when, in evening - ***graph.***
evening - petr.
eating, while - ***graph.,*** petr.
intermittent - petr.
jaw, on moving, only in morning, while lying in bed - ***graph.***
left, in - ***com., form.***
headache, with - ***form.***
loud, during night - ***mur-ac.***
lying, amel. - bar-c.
morning - nat-c.
bed, in - ***graph.***
breakfast, after - zinc.

NOISES, in ears
morning,
breakfast, during - **NIT-AC.**
moving jaw - ***graph.***
moving, body - puls.
head - graph., ***puls.***
the jaw - aloe, ***graph.***
night - ***mur-ac.***
opening the mouth - dulc.
painful, now and then, in right - ***kali-c.***
painful, chewing, when - ***nat-m.***
reading aloud - aloe
right - hep.
sleep, during - dig., ***lach.***
sneezing, on - ***bar-c.,*** bry., ***graph.***
swallowing, when, with earache - kali-m.
stroking cheek - sang.
swallowing, when - agar., alum., ***bar-c., calc.,*** cic., coca, coc-c., der., ***elaps,*** kali-chl., mang., nat-m., sil., thuj.
turning head - ***caust.***
walking fast - ***bar-c.***
yawning, when - cocc.
crackling - acon., agar., alum., ambr., ars., aur., ***bar-c.,*** bor., calc., cann-i., carb-v., coc-c., con., dulc., ***elaps,*** eup-pur., glon., ***graph.,*** hep., kali-ar., kali-c., kali-i., kali-s., lach., meny., mosch., nit-ac., puls., rheum, sabad., sep., spig., sulph., teucr., thuj.
blowing nose - hep., teucr.
burning of birch bark, very much worse upon swallowing, like - eup-pur.
chewing, when - alum., carb-v.
evening - acon., bor.
left, worse in - bor., coc-c.
lying upon ear - bar-c.
morning, during breakfast - carb-v.
motion of jaws - carb-v.
opening the mouth, on - dulc.
right, in, with sensation as if external auditory passage were closed - coc-c.
sneezing, on - bar-c.
swallowing, when - alum., bar-c., elaps, eup-pur., graph., hep., kali-i.
or chewing - alum.
synchronous with pulse - coff., puls.
walking, while - bar-c., meny.
winding a watch, in left, like - ambr.
crash, a, as from breaking a pane of glass, on falling asleep - zinc.
crashing - aloe, bar-c., con., dig., ***graph.,*** zinc.
as from breaking of a pane of glass - aloe, dig., zinc.
night - bar-c.
asleep, on falling - ***dig.,*** zinc.
creaking - agar., ambr., graph., mosch., stann., thuj.
as from a wooden screw, at each attempt to swallow - agar.
bed, in - graph.
evening - stann.
left, in, when swallowing saliva - thuj.
morning in bed on moving jaws - graph.
swallowing, when - agar., graph., ***thuj.***

NOISES, in ears
croaking, like frogs, while sitting - mag-s.
walking, while - mang.
cymbals, and drums - lob., lol.
daytime - ph-ac., sulph.
dancing - stram.
din, when stepping hard - ***lyc.***
double, the sound is, when whistling, or when two persons whistle thirds - med.
drumming - bell., bor., canth., ***cupr., cupr-ac., dros.,*** dulc., ***lach.,*** manc.
distant - ***cupr.,*** dros., mez.
in ear on which he lies, in morning, disappears on rising - ***cupr.***
dull - bor.
left ear, as if over subterranean vault - bor.
lain on, the ear, amel. rising up - ***cupr.***
morning - lach.
waking, on - lach.
walking, while - manc.
ears, as if he heard with, not his own - alum., psor.
eating, while - con., ***graph.,*** nat-m., petr., sil., sulph., zinc.
eating, after - agar., canth., cinnb., con., mag-c., op., sil.
epilepsy, after - ***caust.***
before - hyos.
evening - acon., alum., bar-c., bor., calc., canth., ***carb-s., caust.,*** cinnb., croc., gamb., glon., ***graph.,*** hydrc., kali-n., lach., lact., ***lyc.,*** mag-c., ***merc., merc-i-r.,*** murx., nat-a., nat-m., nicc., ***nux-v.,*** op., petr., ph-ac., plat., plb., ptel., ***puls.,*** rhod., sel., sep., ***sil.,*** spig., stann., ***sulph.,*** sumb., tab., thuj., valer., zinc.
7 p.m. - mag-c., phys.
8 p.m. - ham.
9 p.m. - hydr.
10 p.m. - nat-a.
bed, in - croc., ***graph.,*** lact., ***merc.,*** phos., rhod., sel., **SULPH.,** valer.
excited, when - sulph.
explosion, like an - cann-i., dig., graph., nat-c., phos.
as from breaking glass - aloe, dig., zinc.
blowing nose, on - hep.
sleep, during - dig., mag-c., stann.
falling, asleep, when - dig., zinc.
far, sounds seem, off - all-c., lac-c.
as if tones came from another world - **CARB-AN.**
fever, during - lach., ***tub.***
finger, noise as of the breaking of a, nail at every step in walking - con.
flapping - ***calc.***
as of wings - jac-c.
fluttering, sounds - acon., agar., alum., ars., ars-i., aur., ***bar-c., bell.,*** berb., bor., ***calc.,*** carl., ***carb-s.,*** caust., cham., chin., cocc., con., cupr., dros., dulc., ***graph.,*** hep., iod., kali-c., kali-i., ***kali-p., kali-s.,*** lach., laur., ***lyc.,***

NOISES, in ears
fluttering, sounds - mag-c., ***mag-m.,*** mang., meny., ***merc.,*** mosch., nat-m., nat-s., nit-ac., olnd., petr., ***ph-ac.,*** phos., **PLAT.,** ***psor., puls.,*** rheum, rhod., sabad., sel., sep., sil., **SPIG.,** spong., stann., staph., ***sulph.,*** zinc.
belching, with - caust., graph.
bird, as of a - ant-t., cham., mag-c., mang., ***ph-ac.***
large bird, before left ear - ant-t.
breathing, when - ***bar-c.***
butterfly, as of - jac., nat-m.
dinner, during - nat-m.
evening - mag-c., mang., tab.
5 p.m. - sulph.
lying amel. - ***bar-c., ph-ac.***
morning - bell.
waking, after - bell.
rhythmical - sil.
right - mag-c., mag-m., nat-s.
swallowing, when - ars.
forenoon - carb-v., chin-s., fl-ac., hura, mag-c., ***nat-m.,*** rhod.
9 a.m. - euphr., hura
11 a.m. - mag-c., ***nat-m.***
gong, like, while lying - sars.
guns, sound of - am-c., cann-i., graph., spong.
as if a battery of, were discharged at night - spong.
night - spong.
swallowing, when - graph.
gurgling, in ears as of air bubbles - ***lyc.***
hammering, sounds of - spig.
headache, during - acon-c., carb-s., **CHIN.,** cycl., dios., euphr., gels., ***naja, puls., sil.***
heart, as if coming from the, sleep amel. - ***glon.***
pulsating sound, with - spong.
hell, has the sounds of, constantly in ears - plb.
hissing - acon., aeth., agar., alum., bar-c., benz-ac., bry., cahin., ***calc., cann-i.,*** caust., chin., **DIG.,** dros., ferr-pic., glon., ***graph.,*** hep., ill., kali-n., kreos., ***lach.,*** lyc., mag-m., med., mur-ac., nat-s., ***nux-v., pic-ac.,*** sil., sulph., sumb., teucr., thuj., valer.
boiling water, as from - ***bar-c.,*** bry., ***cann-i., dig.,*** lyc., mag-m., sulph., thuj.
morning, side lain on - mag-m.
clock, near - ph-ac.
deafness, in - ***dig., dros.,*** sulph.
epilepsy, after - ***caust.***
evening - calc., hep.
hand, when passing, over ear, when talking, or forcing inspiring through nose - teucr.
heart, synchronous with beats of - benz-ac.
mastoid, seemingly in, cells - med.
nervous, with, affections - valer.
morning with snuffing and belching - teucr.
synchronous with pulse - benz-ac.
talking, while - teucr.
horn, of blowing a - ***kalm.***
cracking in head, after - ***kalm.***
howling - sep.

NOISES, in ears

humming - abrot., ***acon.,*** act-sp., agar., all-c., all-s., aloe, ***alum., am-c.,*** am-m., aml-n., ***anac.,*** anag., ant-c., ***arg-n., arn., ars.,*** ars-i., ***aur., bell.,*** bry., calc., calc-s., ***canth.,*** carb-ac., carb-an., ***carb-s.,*** carb-v., card-m., ***carl.,*** casc., cast., ***caust.,*** cham., chel., **CHIN.,** chin-a., ***chin-s.,*** cob., ***con.,*** cop., ***croc.,*** crot-t., ***cycl.,*** daph., dirc., ***dros.,*** dulc., ***ferr.,*** ferr-ar., ferr-i., ferr-p., gels., glon., ***graph.,*** hep., hyos., iod., kali-ar., kali-c., kali-m., kali-p., kali-s., kalm., kreos., lact., laur., **LYC.,** mag-m., meny., merc., merc-c., mez., mosch., ***mur-ac.,*** nat-a., nat-c., ***nat-m.,*** nat-p., nicc., ***nit-ac.,*** nux-m., ***nux-v., op., petr.,*** **PHOS.,** ***psor., puls.,*** rhod., sabad., sang., sec., seneg., **SEP.,** sil., ***spig.,*** stann., ***stry., sulph.,*** tab., ter., verat., verat-v., zing.

air, open, agg. - tab.

amel. - ***ars.***

worse on entering room - ***ars.***

alternating, sides - sulph.

ataxia, in locomotor - ***arg-n.***

bees, as of, in left - chin-b.

bells, as from - alum.

chewing - ***iod.***

chill, during - ***ars.,*** puls.

congestion, with - sang.

deafness, with - ***psor.,*** sulph.

followed by - ***sep.***

rheumatic, consequent upon a chill, with - ***petr.***

evening - alum., nicc., sep., spig.

supper, after - canth.

fever, during - ***ars., nux-v.***

head, on moving, or body - ***puls.***

hysteria, in - ***aur.***

impairment of, worse stooping, causing - ***croc.***

leaning head on table amel. - ferr.

left, in - cob.

lying - all-c.

down, on - all-c.

ear, on the - mez.

meningitis, in infants, after - ***arn.***

menses, during - ***kreos.***

before - bor., bry., ***kreos.***

mental anxiety agg. - act-sp.

morning - ***alum.,*** carb-s.

11 a.m. - zing.

rising, after - alum., ars., sil.

waking, on - nat-m., rhod.

motion, on - ***puls.***

night - agar., ***nux-v.***

noises, loud, agg. - ol-an., tab.

right, in - am-m.

room, in, agg. - tab.

sea, like a, chill - ter.

sitting, while, agg. - bell.

sleep, after - act-sp.

synchronous with pulse - carl., puls.

talking, while - op.

valvular, in, heart disease - chel.

vertigo, with - bell., sep.

veta, in - ***coca***

NOISES, in ears

humming,

warm room agg. - ***ars.***

inspiration, during - bar-c., ***iod.***

landslide, sudden sounds as of a far-off - chin-b.

left - agar., anac., ***berb.,*** bov., bry., carb-s., chel., cic., cob., coc-c., coff., ery-a., graph., mag-s., myric., nat-c., nat-m., sars., stann., staph., zinc.

sounds seem to come from, side when they really come from right - ***nat-c.***

loose, as if - ***calc., graph.***

loud sounds, followed by deafness - ***sep.***

lying, while - agar., all-c., cann-i., con., ***cupr.,*** lil-t., ***mag-c.,*** merc., nat-c., nat-m., phos., plat., puls., sil., ***sulph., tarent.***

amel. - ***bar-c.,*** bell., nat-c., nat-s., **PH-AC.**

upon the ear - am-c., bar-c., cupr., mag-m., mez., rhus-r., sep., spong.

machinery, sound of - hydr.

afternoon, 2 p.m. - hydr.

menses, during - ars., ***bor.,*** chin., ***ferr.,*** kreos., mosch., ***petr., verat.***

after - chin., ferr., kreos.

before - ***bor.,*** bry., ***ferr., kreos.,*** phys.

suppressed, from - calc., graph., puls.

mental, exertion - ***caust.,*** con., ferr-pic.

mice, sound of - rhus-t.

midnight - am-c., rat.

2 a.m. - chin-s.

lying on the ear - am-c.

waking, on - rat.

mill, sound of - bry., cit-v., iod., mez., naja, nux-v.

morning on waking - naja

distance, at a - bry., mez.

morning - alum., ant-c., arg-n., ars., aur., bell., calc., carb-s., carb-v., caust., clem., dios., dros., dulc., ***graph., lach.,*** mag-c., merc., mez., naja, nat-a., nat-c., nat-m., ***nat-s.,*** phel., ph-ac., plat., puls., rhod., sil., sulph., tab., teucr., zinc.

after - alum., ars., calc., nux-v., sil.

bed, in - arg-n., aur., graph., mag-c., nat-m., puls., sulph.

on moving the jaw - graph.

rising, on - mez.

waking, on - hyper., **LACH.,** ***naja,*** nat-m., rhod., tarent.

motion, during - nat-c., nux-v., ***puls.,*** staph., sulph.

moving, head - ***graph.,*** puls., staph.

jaw - ant-c., ***carb-v.,*** dulc., ***graph.***

murmuring - ***bell.***

sleep, after - act-sp.

music, amel. - aur., ***aur-m.***

music, he seems to hear - ail., bell., calc., ***cann-i.,*** kalm., lyc., ***merc.,*** nat-c., phos., plb., puls., sal-ac., sarr., stram., sulph.

delirium, with frightful - plb.

evening - lyc., puls.

on lying down - puls.

NOISES, in ears
music, he seems to hear
organ melody in head and after a few turns were snapped off - ***merc.***
piping - ***bor.***
rest, during - nat-c.
shrill - coff.
whimpering tune - ant-c.
nails, driven into a board at a distance, sound of - agar.
night - agar., am-c., am-m., bar-c., carb-an., cham., chin., chin-s., coc-c., con., cycl., ***dulc.,*** elaps, euph., ***graph.,*** lil-t., lyss., mur-ac., nicc., ***nux-v.,*** ph-ac., rat., sep., ***sil.,*** spong., sulph., ther., tub., zinc.
headache, with agg. - cycl.
waking, on - con., hydr.
noise, agg. - coloc., ol-an., kali-p., plat., phos., tab.
noon - cedr., fago., glon.
pain, with every attack of - ***ars.,*** lach.
palpitations, with - coca.
perspiration, with - **ARS.,** ign.
piping, worse in left - bor.
rain, sound of - kali-i., rhod., rhus-r.
as of a gentle, worse towards evening - rhod.
vertigo, in - coff-t.
rattling - bar-c., ***rhus-t., sep.***
reports, in - aloe, am-c., aster., ***bad., bar-c.,*** **CALC.,** cann-i., ***chin.,*** chel., cic., dig., eup-pur., graph., hep., kali-c., mosch., nat-c., nit-ac., phos., plat., rhus-t., sabad., sil., staph., zinc.
afternoon on going to sleep - rhus-t.
blowing the nose - hep., mang.
breaking of glass, like the - aloe, dig., zinc.
distant shots, as of - am-c., bad., chel., ***dig.,*** plat.
drops of blood, with - mosch.
menses, during - mosch.
morning - nat-c., zinc.
breakfast, after - zinc.
night - bar-c., ***spong.***
sleep, during - dig.
sleep, on going to - dig., rhus-t., zinc.
swallowing, when - ***cic.,*** mang.
violent in ears - aster.
right - aesc., ail., ang., bor., brom., calc-p., cast., cham., chlor., colch., con., ferr., ***hep.,*** lyc., meny., merc., merc-c., mez., mill., mur-ac., ***nat-s.,*** phos., rheum, rhod., rhus-v., sep., spong., stront-c., tub., xan.
opening the mouth - ***glon.***
ringing - **ACON.,** ***aesc., agar.,*** agn., ail., ***all-c.,*** aloe, alum., alumn., ambr., am-c., am-m., ang., anan., anac., ant-c., apis, ***arg-n.,*** arn., ***ars.,*** ars-i., arund., asaf., atro., ***aur.,*** aur-m., ***bar-c.,*** bar-m., **BELL.,** berb., ***bor.,*** brom., bry., **CACT., CALC.,** calc-i., **CALC-S.,** ***camph.,*** **CANN-I.,** cann-s., ***canth.,*** carb-an., ***carb-o., carb-s.,*** **CARB-V.,** ***carl.,*** chen-a., **CAUST.,** ***cham., chel.,*** **CHIN.,** chin-a., **CHIN-S.,** chlf., chlol., chlor., cic., ***cit-v., clem.,***

NOISES, in ears
ringing - ***cocc.,*** coc-c., coca, coff., colch., coloc., com., ***con.,*** croc., crot-h., cupr., ***cycl., dig.,*** dios., ***dulc.,*** elaps, ery-a., ***euph.,*** euphr., ***ferr.,*** ferr-ar., ferr-i., ferr-p., ***fl-ac., form.,*** gamb., ***glon., gran., graph.,*** guare., ***ham.,*** hep., ***hell.,*** hura, ***hydr.,*** hydr-ac., hydrc., hyos., ***ign.,*** ill., iod., ***ip.,*** kali-ar., kali-bi., **KALI-C.,** kali-cy., **KALI-I.,** kali-n., kali-p., **KALI-S.,** kalm., kreos., lac-c., lach., lachn., lec., led., **LYC.,** ***mag-c.,*** mag-s., manc., mang., ***meny., merc.,*** merc-cy., ***mez.,*** mill., morph., mur-ac., myric., nat-a., nat-c., ***nat-m.,*** nat-p., ***nat-s.,*** nit-ac., ***nux-m., nux-v.,*** olnd., op., ***osm.,*** paeon., ***par.,*** phel., **PETR.,** ***ph-ac., phos.,*** plan., **PLAT.,** plb., **PSOR.,** ***ptel.,*** **PULS.,** rat., ***rhod.,*** rhus-v., rumx., ruta., sabad., sal-ac., ***sang.,*** sars., **SEP.,** sel., ***sil.,*** sol-t-ae., ***spig.,*** spong., ***stann.,*** stram., staph., **SULPH.,** sul-ac., tab., tarent., ter., teucr., thuj., til., valer., verat., vinc., viol-o., xan., zinc.
afternoon - carb-v., kali-n., kalm.
2 p.m. - verat-v.
3 p.m. - fago.
4 p.m. - dios.
6 p.m. - ol-an.
air, open - carb-an.
angina, in - ***dig.***
anthrax, in - anthr.
blowing nose - ***carb-an.,*** teucr.
boring, with finger in - chel.
amel. - meny., nicc.
chill, during - cedr., chin., **CHIN-S.,** graph., rhus-t., ***sep.***
closing eyes - chel.
cold water amel. - euphr.
coldness, during - graph.
confused, in left - ery-a.
congestion, with, to - ***sang.***
cough, with - sil.
daytime - sulph.
agg., as day advances, so that he can scarcely hear in evening, after catching cold - rhod.
deafness, with - ***aur-m.,*** **CHEN-A.,** ***psor.***
erysipelas, in - rhus-t.
dinner during - ***sulph.***
after - cinnb., mag-c.
amel. after, and from wine, worse from coffee - arg-n.
evening, late in - cinnb.
disagreeable, constant - ***fl-ac.***
distant - all-c., arg-n., coca, ***spig.***
sensation as if ear were stopped, with - spig.
dull - spong.
epileptic fit, before - **HYOS.**
evening - bar-c., caust., croc., kali-n., ***merc.,*** rhod., sil., valer.
7 p.m. - phys.
8 p.m. - ham.
bed, in - croc., ***merc.,*** phos., rhod., valer.
excitement, from - mag-c.
eyes, after using, right, in - puls.

NOISES, in ears
ringing,
falls, and roaring till he, asleep - ***nat-m.***
fine, in right, when blowing nose, squeaking as if air were forced through mucus - teucr.
forehead, with pain in, and eyes - cact.
forenoon - carb-v., fl-ac.
9 a.m. - euphr.
11 a.m. - nat-m.
hardness, with buzzing - ferr-p., ***psor.***
head, after arthritic affection of, with deafness - rhod.
headache, during - acon-c., aur., carb-s., caust., **CHIN.,** cycl., dios., euphr., ***naja, puls.***
nervous, in - ***naja.***
temples, in - **CHIN.**
heart, disease, with - ***dig.,*** tub.
hemicrania, in - ***chin-a.***
hemorrhage, in postpartum - ***cham.***
left - agar., arn., bor., caust., **CHIN-S.,** cic., coc-c., ery-a., ***gamb.,*** graph., mag-s., myric., myris., ***nux-v.,*** par., sars., stann., staph.
walking, when - chel.
low, with headache - coca
lying, after - croc.
lying, down agg. - sulph.
meningitis, in - ***arg-n., glon.***
menorrhagia, in - ***ferr-s.***
menses, during - **FERR.**, verat.
before - ***ferr., ign.***
midnight, on waking - rat.
2 a.m. - chin-s.
morning - clem., mang., nux-v., phel., sulph.
bed, in - arg-n., mag-c., sulph.
clothing, after - mez.
rising, on - alum., mez., ***nux-v.***
motion, during - ***nux-v.***
moving, on - staph.
head agg. - staph.
nervous, with, affections - valer.
night - carb-an., cycl., ph-ac., sulph., zinc.
forcing him to rise and walk about - sil.
noon - glon.
nose, when blowing - ***carb-an.***
one, burning in the other - kali-c.
pain, with, in rectum during stool - ***lyc.***
palpitation, with - ***phos.***
paralysis, with - ***sil.***
rest, amel. - nux-v., staph.
went off when at, but reappeared when she moved - ***nux-v.***
right - ***aesc.,*** ail., ang., bor., brom., cham., chlor., colch., coloc., con., ***ferr., lac-c.,*** lyc., meny., mill., nat-s., osm., ***rhod.,*** rhus-v., spong., thuj., xan.
headache, with dull - erig.
night - zinc.
rising, amel. - tarent.
rubbing amel. - meny.
sex, after - ***dig.***
and roaring - ***dig.***
sitting, while - ars., merc-cy., ***sulph.***

NOISES, in ears
ringing,
sleep, followed by - ill.
sneezing, on - euph.
stitches, with, in one side of, generally in one temple or in back part - ***puls.***
stool, during - ***lyc.***
after - apoc.
stopping up ear with finger does not amel. - croc.
suffocating, caused by, weight in stomach after eating - sulph.
talking, while - spig.
toothache, with - ***cocc.***
turning head - nat-c.
typhoid fever, in - ***cocc.***
vertigo, with - alum., carb-v., cocc., coff-t., com., ***dig.,*** myric., nat-m.
slight, also pressure about head - myris.
waking, on - arg-n., mag-c., rat., sulph., tarent.
walking, while - chel., manc., nicc., rhus-t.
air, in open - agar., carb-an.
wind, with feeling of cold, especially in left ear - vinc.
rising, on - acon., mez., ***phos.***
amel. - nat-c., tarent.
seat, from, a - lac-ac., ***verat.***
stooping, from - mang., sep.
roaring - ***acon.,*** agar., ***agn.,*** all-c., alum., ***ambr.,*** am-c., am-m., ***anac.,*** ant-c., ant-t., arg-n., arn., ***ars., ars-i., asar.,*** atro., ***aur., aur-m.,*** bapt., **BAR-C.,** ***bar-m.,*** **BELL.,** berb., bism., **BOR.,** bov., brom., ***bry.,*** cact., cahin., calad., ***calc., calc-s., camph.,*** cann-s., ***canth.,*** carb-ac., carb-an., ***carb-h.,*** **CARB-S., CARB-V.,** ***carl.,*** cast., **CAUST.,** cedr., ***cham.,*** chel., chen-a., **CHIN.,** ***chin-a.,*** **CHIN-S.,** chlf., cic., ***cinnb.,*** cimic., clem., coca, ***cocc.,*** coc-c., coff., ***colch., coloc., con.,*** cop., croc., crot-t., cupr., ***cycl.,*** daph., dig., dirc., ***dros.,*** dulc., ***elaps,*** euph., euon., ferr., ferr-ar., ***ferr-i.,*** ferr-p., ***gels.,*** **GRAPH.,** ***hell., hep.,*** hydr., hydr-ac., hyos., ign., ill., indg., ***iod.,*** jatr., kali-ar., kali-br., ***kali-c.,*** kali-chl., kali-i., kali-n., kali-p., ***kali-s., kreos.,*** lac-c., ***lach.,*** lac-ac., lact., ***laur., led.,*** **LYC.,** ***mag-c., mag-m.,*** manc., mang., merl., meny., ***merc., merc-c.,*** mez., morph., mosch., mur-ac., nat-a., nat-c., ***nat-m., nat-p., nat-s.,*** nicc., ***nit-ac.,*** **NUX-V.,** olnd., ol-an., ***op.,*** paeon., ***petr.,*** **PH-AC.,** ***phos., plat.,*** plb., psor., ptel., **PULS.,** rheum, ***rhod.,*** rhus-t., rumx., ***sal-ac.,*** sang., ***sec.,*** seneg., ***sep.,*** **SIL., SPIG.,** spong., ***staph.,*** stram., stront-c., stry., ***sul-ac.,*** **SULPH.,** tab., tep., ter., teucr., thea., ***ther.,*** thuj., til., verat., ***verat-v.,*** viol-o., zinc.
afternoon - all-c., ***ambr., ant-c.,*** cham.
3 p.m. - elaps, mag-c.
4 p.m. - **LYC.**
coming from open air - thuj.
rising, on - lac-c.
air, open, amel. - ***cic.,*** puls., thuj.
alive, as if something, were in them - sil.
bed, driving out of - mag-c.

NOISES, in ears
roaring,
blowing nose - meny.
boring finger in ear, amel. - cast., lach.
cataract, in - sec.
cattle - thuj.
cerebral congestion, in - ***aur.,*** ferr-p., ***op., sulph., verat-v.***
chill, after - cahin.
cholera, in, fourth day - ***ph-ac.***
cold, after taking, in a draft of air and becoming heated - ***kali-c.***
feet becoming, from - ***sil.***
colic, in flatulent - ***lyc.***
constant - ***petr.***
coryza, with - **ACON.,** sep.
day, worse as, advances, so that he can scarcely hear, in evening, after catching cold - rhod.
daytime - ph-ac., sulph.
deafness, in - ammc., ***aur-m., nux-v.,*** **PH-AC.**
eustachian tubes, caused by affection of - **PETR.**
sudden, with - nicc.
dinner, after - cinnb., con.
eating, while - con., sil.
after - cinnb., op., sil.
before - sil.
epilepsy, after - ***caust.***
eating, after - ***cinnb.***
evening - alum., calc., ***carb-s.,*** caust., cinnb., graph., hydr., mag-c., op., petr., plat., plb., ptel., ph-ac., spig., **SULPH.,** sul-ac., thuj.
7 p.m. - mag-c.
9 p.m. - hydr.
bed, in - hep., sulph.
begins in, lasts through night and disturbs sleep - ***coc-c.***
waking, on - hydr.
fainting spells, with - uran-n.
fall, with inclination to - ***calc.***
fever, during - ***ars.,*** lach., ***nux-v.***
forehead, constant, with pressing stitching pain in, extending over whole head, particularly in vertex and occiput, with heaviness and confusion of head - ***lyc.***
frequent, during day - calad.
head, after arthritic affection of - rhod.
congestion to, in young people, with - graph.
heaviness of, with - phos.
headache, with - ***aur.,*** gels., ***sil.,*** staph.
impairment of hearing, stooping agg. - ***croc.***
hemicrania, in - ***chen-a.***
holding hand over eyes, amel. - spig.
hour in right, for an, worse lying on left side, better lying on right, with headache - phos.
hysteria, in - ***lyc.,*** coc-c., ***nux-v.***
inspiration, during - bar-c.
jerking - staph.

NOISES, in ears
roaring,
left - agar., bor., bov., bry., coc-c., ***coloc.,*** graph., nat-c., nat-m., thuj.
afternoon, on rising - lac-ac.
decay of left molar teeth, with - ***nat-c.***
severe cold, as after - all-c.
lying, while - con., graph., ***mag-c.,*** merc., plat., **SULPH.**
amel. - ***ph-ac.***
on the ear - mag-m., spong.
on the ear, amel. - phos.
machinery, as from - ***hydr.***
measles, after suppression of - ***sulph.***
meningitis, in cerebrospinal - ***hydr-ac.***
menses, during - ***ars.,*** bor., kreos., ***petr., verat.***
at time for return of - phys.
before - bor.
suppressed - graph.
mental confusion, with - bapt.
exertion agg. - con.
morning - alum., calc., carb-s., mag-m., merc., nat-s., ph-ac., plat., tab.
11 a.m. - mag-c.
bed, in - ***aur.,*** nat-m.
rising, after - alum., calc., nat-s., ***nux-v.***
waking, on - hyper.
motion agg. - nat-c.
music amel. - ign.
nausea, with - ***calc.***
nervous - ***kali-p.***
night - am-c., chin., coc-c., con., elaps, euph., ***hydr.,*** **GRAPH.,** ***kali-br.,*** nicc., nux-v., sep., ***sil.,*** zinc.
synchronous with pulse - ***kali-br.***
waking, on - con., hydr.
pain, in ear - petr.
every attack of, with - ***ars.,*** lach.
right, in paroxysms, with - stront.
painful - lach.
palpitation, with - iber.
paroxysms, in, with headache as if brain were compressed, mostly in forehead - ***staph.***
of pain, with each - ***ars.***
perspiration, during - ars., ign.
pertussis, in - ***caust.***
pouring, like water, over a dam - bry.
pulsating - merc.
in ear upon which she lies - spong.
reading, agg. - acon.
rhythmical - ***coloc., kali-br.,*** sep., ***sul-ac.***
right - am-m., bar-c., cast., caust., con., mag-c., merc-c., mur-ac., nat-s., phos., rheum, ***sil.,*** stront.
like the sea, at each inspiration - ***bar-c.***
rising, on - acon., ***phos.***
from a seat - verat.
room, in, agg. - cic., mag-c.
sex, during - graph.
after - carb-v., dig.
sitting, while - con., nat-m., phos., sulph.
up amel. - mag-c., op.
sneezing, on - mag-c.

NOISES, in ears
roaring,
sound, at every - coloc., ol-an.
stool, straining at - lyc.
stooping, when - croc.
after - mang.
supper, after - canth.
swallowing, amel. - rheum
talking, agg. - nat-c.
thunderous, with deafness - tell.
tornado, in left, like distant - asar.
typhoid fever, in - ***cocc., lyc.***
vertigo, with - ***bell.,*** calc., carb-v., cocc., crot-t., gran., hell., nat-c., ***op.,*** petr., ***phos., psor.,*** stry.
rising, on - **PHOS.**
violent - zinc.
vomiting, with bilious - ***crot-h.***
walking, while - colch., cycl., ferr., nat-m.
water, as from rushing - **CHAM.**
waterfall, as from on opening mouth during dinner - sul-ac.
wind, as of - **PETR.**
distant storm of - ***chel.***
work, with inability to, read or think - ***nat-m.***
yawning, when - verat.
rolling, sound - ***graph., plat.***
morning - ***plat.***
rubbing, amel. - meny.
rumbling - apis, ***asar.,*** bry., ***elaps,*** equis., ***plat.,*** sel., sep.
evening, in bed - sel.
left, in, as of thunder, with impairment of hearing - ***elaps***
noise, like, of cars or striking of clocks - chlf.
otalgia, with - ***plat.***
tornado, like a distant - ***asar.***
rushing - abrot., agar., am-c., ***arn.,*** ars., aster., ***aur.,*** bar-c., bor., bov., brom., calc., caust., ***chel., chin-s.,*** cinnb., ***cocc., coloc.,*** con., dulc., euphr., ***gels.,*** glon., ***graph.,*** hep., hydr-ac., ***hyos.,*** kali-ar., **KALI-C.,** kali-cy., kali-n., ***kali-p., kali-s., lach., led.,*** lil-t., **LYC.,** lyss., mag-c., mag-s., mang., merc., mez., mosch., nat-a., nat-c., **NAT-M.,** nat-p., **NIT-AC.,** nux-v., ox-ac., **PETR., PHOS.,** phyt., plat., ***puls.,*** rhus-t., ***sel.,*** sep., sil., spig., stann., staph., ***sulph., sul-ac.,*** tab., ther., verat., viol-o.
belches, from - caust.
distant - brom.
evening - bar-c., caust., mag-c., petr., sep.
headache, during - tub.
hysteria, in - aur.
lying, while - agar., con., lil-t., merc., nat-m.
lying, while, on the ear - am-c.
menses, during - bor., ***kreos.***
before - bor.
mental exertion - con.
midnight, after, when lying on the ear - am-c.
morning - dulc., merc.
night - am-c., caust., con., euph., lil-t., nux-v., ther.

NOISES, in ears
rushing,
pulse, isochronous with, with deafness - **PULS.**
right - ***mag-c.,*** nat-a.
rising from a seat - verat.
room, in - mag-c.
sex, during - graph.
steam escaping, like - glon., sil.
synchronous with pulse - **PULS.,** sil.
water, as of - aster., **CHAM.,** ***cocc.,*** kali-n., mag-c., mag-s., petr., ***puls.***
after 4 p.m. - ***puls.***
waterfall, like a - ars., aster., aur., bry., caust., cann-i., chel., chin-s., con., lyss., mag-c., nat-p., petr., rhus-t., sul-ac., ther.
waterfall, like a, opening the mouth, on - sal-ac.
rustling - aloe, ***bell.,*** bor., brom., carb-v., caust., mang., merc., phos., puls., sil., ther., viol-o.
bird, like a - cham.
blowing nose - sil.
distant, like - brom.
moving jaws, on - aloe, carb-v.
straw, as of, when jaws are moved - carb-v.
sex, after - carb-v., dig.
sex, during - graph.
scratching like a bird - cham.
shrieking, on blowing nose - ph-ac., stann.
noise when blowing nose - stann.
shrill sound, bell ringing out of tune, singing like a - petr.
shrill sound, blowing nose, on - ph-ac.
simmering, better resting head on table - ferr.
singing - acon., am-m., arg-m., arn., ars., asar., atro., bell., bry., cact., ***calc.,*** calc-p., calc-s., ***camph.,*** cann-i., cann-s., carb-o., ***carb-s., caust.,*** cedr., chel., **CHIN.,** ***chin-a.,*** chlf., chlor., cimic., coff., coloc., ***con.,*** croc., cupr-ac., ery-a., ferr., ferr-ar., ferr-m., ferr-p., fl-ac., glon., ***graph., hyos.,*** kali-bi., **KALI-C.,** kali-i., ***kali-p.,*** lac-ac., ***lach.,*** lachn., ***lyc.,*** merc-i-r., mur-ac., nat-a., ***nat-c.,*** nat-m., nat-p., ***nux-v.,*** olnd., ol-an., onos., op., petr., phel., ph-ac., phos., phys., ***psor.,*** rhus-t., ***sang.,*** sec., sep., ***stram.,*** sul-i., sumb., ter., verb.
afternoon, while walking in open air - lachn.
5 p.m. - ol-an.
awaking, on - ***ars.***
closing eyes, on - chel.
cracking sound, with, in left - ery-a.
deafness, with - ***nux-v., psor.***
debility, with - **CHIN.**
drowsiness, with - calc-p.
earache, with - ***sang.***
evening - merc-i-r., sumb.
giddiness, with - ***stram.***
head, better resting, on table - ferr.
intermittent fever, in - ***ars.***
left - bry., tarent.
snapping in - lac-ac.
locusts, like - nux-v., rhus-t.
lying, while - cann-i., ph-ac., ***phos.***

NOISES, in ears
singing,
menses, during - ***petr.***
after - ***chin., ferr.***
before - ferr.
morning - phel.
nervous people - ***coff.***
night - mur-ac., nux-v.
lying down, after - ***phys.***
periodic - ***cann-i.***
dreamy spells, ceasing when coming to himself, during - cann-i.
resting, head on table amel. - ferr.
right - asar., calc-p., lachn., ***nat-c.***
walking in open air, when - lachn.
sitting, while - ars.
steam, escaping - phys.
tea-kettle, like a - ***lach.,*** tarent.
left, in - tarent.
vertigo, with - ***camph., sang.,*** stram.
walking, in open air, while - lachn.
water, as from boiling - **LYC.**
sitting, while - am-m., ars., bell., con., mag-s., merc-cy., nat-c., nat-m., op., sulph.
smacking, as if opened and closed while it contained a thick paste - bor.
snapping - ambr., bar-c., bor., ***dulc., graph.,*** hep., ***kali-c.,*** lac-ac., puls., tarent.
belching, after every - ***graph.***
electric sparks, like - ambr., ***calc.,*** dulc., ***hep.,*** rheum, sabad.
evening - tarent.
blowing nose, on - hep.
opening the mouth on - dulc.
swallowing, when - bar-c.
synchronous with the pulse - ars-s-r.
turning the head, on - ***caust.***
sneezing, on - bar-c., euph., graph., mag-c.
squashing, on swallowing - **CALC.**
yawning - mang.
squeaking - eup-pur.
snapping - ***hep.***
belches, after every, as if air penetrated eustachian tube - ***graph.***
head, on turning - ***caust.***
pulsations, corresponds to, of temporal artery - ars-s-r.
sparks, as of, from an electric machine - ***calc.***
standing, amel. - bell.
steam, escaping, like - caust., glon., lach., phys., tarent.
stool, during - lyc.
after - apoc., calc-p.
stooping, when - croc., ***graph., mang.***
striking, sensation as of, of a clock - ter.
stupefying - bar-c.
surging - sarac.
right, in, worse from excitement, or moving - sulph.

NOISES, in ears
swallowing, when - agar., alum., ars., ***bar-c.,*** bar-m., benz-ac., ***calc., cic.,*** coca, coc-c., ***elaps, eup-per.,*** graph., hep., kali-chl., kali-i., lepi., mag-c., mang., nat-m., rhod., sil., thuj.
amel. - rheum.
swashing - sarr., spig., **SULPH.**
jaws, on moving - ant-c.
synchronous with pulse - am-m., ars., benz-ac., ***bufo,*** chen-a., coff., coloc., hydrobr-ac., kali-br., med., merc., ***nux-v., puls.,*** rhus-t., sep., sil., sul-ac.
talking, while - nat-c., op., spig., teucr.
teething, while - aloe, caust., ***mang., nit-ac.,*** phos., ***thlaspi.***
thundering - am-m., ***calc.,*** carb-o., caust., chel., ***graph., lach.,*** ol-an., petr., ***plat.,*** rhod., sil.
morning - ***plat.***
night - am-m.
sitting - am-m.
tick-tack, sound - calad., gad.
ticking, sound - ***chin., graph.,*** mag-s., nat-m., petr., ter.
as of a distant watch - ***chin.***
evening - nat-m.
tinkling - agn., ***aloe,*** am-c., am-m., atro., bar-c., bell., berb., carb-v., ***caust.,*** cham., chin., ***con.,*** ferr., graph., hippoz., kali-c., lyc., mag-c., meny., mur-ac., nat-m., nat-s., nux-v., olnd., ol-an., op., par., petr., ***puls.,*** sars., stann., staph., sulph., ter., valer., viol-o.
head, on moving, or body - ***puls.***
trumpets, din like - bell.
sound as the blowing of a, in left, at night - chin-b.
turning, head - ***caust.,*** nat-c.
twanging, a harp string - lyc., sulph.
wire, a loose - phel.
twittering - calad.
valve, opening and shutting, as if - ***graph.,*** xan.
vertigo, with noises in ear - alum., arg-m., ***arg-n.,*** arn., ars., asar., bar-m., bell., benz-ac., bry., calc., ***camph.,*** carb-v., carb-s., ***caust.,*** chen-a., chin., **CHIN-S.,** ***chin-sal., cic., cocc.,*** colch., com., con., crot-h., crot-t., ***dig.,*** eucal., ferr-p., gels., ***glon.,*** gran., hell., hydrobr-ac., jab., kali-c., kali-i., kali-m., kali-p., kalm., laur., mag-c., morg., myric., nat-a., nat-c., nat-m., nat-p., nat-s., ***nat-sal.,*** nux-v., onos., op., petr., ph-ac., **PHOS.,** pic-ac., psor., puls., rad-br., ***sal-ac., sang.,*** seneg., sep., ***sil.,*** stann., tab., ***ther.,*** thyr., zinc.
before - lachn., sep.
seasick, as if - tab.
voices, hears - phos., ***stram.***
confused, worse swallowing, or walking in open air - benz-ac.
persons, of absent, at night - ***cham.***
waking, on - bell., con., hydr., lach., naja, nat-m., puls., rat., rhod., tarent.
start, with a - dig., zinc.

NOISES, in ears

walking, while - bar-c., chel., colch., cycl., ferr., manc., mang., meny., nat-m., nicc., rhus-t., spig.

air, in the open - agar., carb-an., lachn.

amel. - bell., cop.

fast - bar-c.

warbling, of birds - bell., bry.

warm, room agg. - ars., cic., mag-c., thuj.

watch, as of, when winding - ambr.

water, as if, boiling, sound - bry., cann-i., dig., sulph., thuj.

were in ear - nit-ac.

dropping, as if, from a height into a long, narrow vessel, while lying down - nat-p.

running, like - cact.

rushing, like - aster., petr.

afternoon, 4 p.m., after - ***puls.***

deafness, with - ***cocc.***

left, in - lyss.

tearing pains, as of murmuring, with, at night - ***petr.***

water-fall, like a - ther.

waves, like - aster.

whirring - kali-c., lyc., merc-c., nux-v., puls.

evening, in bed - lact.

mill, like a - ***nux-v.***

rhythmical - merc.

whispering - am-c., anac., dulc., rhod.

evening - rhod.

morning - dulc.

whistling - aeth., alum., ***ambr.,*** aur., bell., bor., carb-an., caust., chel., cur., elaps, ferr., graph., hep., hura, kreos., lyc., mag-c., manc., merc., mur-ac., ***nux-v.,*** puls., sars., sep., sil., teucr., verat., zinc.

afternoon, in - ***ambr.***

alternating with roaring - mag-c.

blowing the nose - carb-an., hep., lyc., ph-ac.

evening - lyc., sep.

forenoon - hura.

9 a.m. - hura.

left - caust.

right, in, at night - chin-b.

walking, while - manc.

wind, with feeling of cold, especially in left ear - vinc.

writing, while - sep.

whizzing - agar., alum., am-c., ***arg-n.,*** bell., berb., brom., calc., ***caust.,*** chel., ***cupr-ac., hep.,*** hura, kali-c., kali-p., kali-s., ***lach.,*** laur., led., **LYC.,** ***mag-c., mang.,*** merc., ***mur-ac.,*** naja, nat-c., nat-p., nicc., nit-ac., olnd., **PETR.,** ph-ac., phos., ***plat.,*** plb., rhus-t., sang., sep., sil., ***sulph.,*** sul-ac., tab., tarent., thuj., zinc.

blowing nose, on - hep.

daytime - ph-ac.

deafness, with, caused by affection of eustachian tubes - ***mang.,*** **PETR.**

dull - zinc.

evening - ph-ac., sul-ac., zinc.

lying down, after - plat.

writing, while - sep.

forenoon, 11 a.m. - mag-c.

NOISES, in ears

whizzing, sound

insects, as from - ***lach.***

left, in - arg-n.

morning - plat.

night - am-c.

bed in, amel. - phos., plat.

right, in - ***mag-c.,*** zinc.

whistling, when - ped.

wind, sound of - abrot., am-c., calc., carb-s., ***chel.,*** ign., ***led.,*** mag-c., mosch., **PETR.,** ***phos.,*** plat., ***puls., sep.,*** spig., sulph., vinc.

afternoon - mag-c., puls.

4 p.m., after - ***puls.***

night - sep.

noise, agg. - plat.

storm - caust., con., mag-c.

storm, noises as from a - led.

strong wind, rushing, as from a, or as from wings of a bird - mosch.

whirlwind - croc.

windmill, like, left - xan.

writing, while - carl., sep.

yawning, when - acon., cocc., mang., mez., verat.

REVERBERATING, noises - ***bar-c.,*** cadm-s., ***carb-s.,*** **CAUST.,** ***cic.,*** cop., ***graph.,*** hep., hydr-ac., kali-br., kali-c., ***kali-p.,*** lac-c., ***lach.,*** **LYC.,** merc., mosch., mur-ac., nat-c., nat-s., ***nit-ac., nux-v., ph-ac.,*** **PHOS.,** plat., ***puls., rhod., sars.,*** sec., **SEP.,** sil., spig., stann., sulph., zinc.

afternoon, 4 p.m. - ***lyc.***

blowing nose - ***bar-c.,*** hep.

every sound - ***caust., lyc.,*** phos.

difficult hearing, with - **CAUST.,** ***lyc.,*** merc.

forenoon - ***nux-v.***

morning - ***caust., nux-v.,*** phos.

morning, before breakfast - ant-c.

painful - cop., nit-ac.

sounds - cadm-s., ***caust., kali-br.,*** ph-ac.

of loud, for a long time - rhod.

re-echo in head, and make her shudder - sec.

speech, of one's - nit-ac.

step, of every word and - ***graph.***

steps, of - **CAUST.**

strong - ***nux-v.***

swallowing, when - ***cic.***

vibrate, sounds, in pregnancy - merc.

voice - caust., phos.

his, own - ***caust.,*** lac-c., nat-s., ***nit-ac.,*** nux-v., ph-ac., ***phos.,*** sars., ***spig.,*** zinc.

waking, on - puls.

walking, amel. - cop.

words, of - **CAUST.,** ***sars.***

and sounds, especially music - ***phos.***

his, own, sound very loud - ***caust.***

SENSITIVE to sounds - **ACON.**, apis, ***ars.***, **BELL.**, bry., bufo, chlol., ***cic.***, chin-b., ***chin.***, ***cocc.***, **COFF.**, crot-h., ***ferr.***, ferr-p., ***gels.***, ***ign.***, ***iod.***, ***ip.***, ***kali-c.***, kali-p., **LACH.**, ***lachn.***, lac-ac., ***lyc.***, mag-c., med., mur-ac., ***nat-c.***, ***nux-m.***, **NUX-V.**, **OP.**, **PHOS.**, ptel., sec., ***sep.***, ***sil.***, stann., ***ther.***, **ZINC.**

amenorrhea, in - xan.

anxiety, causes - sil.

apples, cannot bear to hear others eat, hawk or blow their noses - lyss.

bells, church, ringing makes him anxious and causes a sharp salty taste, with stitches in throat - lyss.

brain sensitive - con.

to loud or shrill noises - ***calc.***

to male voices - bar-c.

chill, during - caps.

convulsions, in puerperal - ***bell.***, ***phos.***

noises or shock shorten attack of - ***hell.***

day, during - zing.

door latch, fall of a, rumpling paper, etc. - ***bor.***

dysmenorrhea, in - xan.

faintness, of crowded street causes - asaf.

fatigues, annoys and, her - ***med.***

headache, agg. - ***bell.***, ***coff.***, sep., ***sil.***

excruciating nervous, during menses - ***kali-p.***

neuralgic - ***spig.***

head, on account of sensitiveness of, fear of - con.

intermittent fever, in - ***caps.***

labor, in spasmodic, pains - cimic.

with difficult - zinc.

left, in, ear, with buzzing - ***aur-m.***

linen, scratching of, or silk is insupportable - **ASAR.**

morbidly with symptoms akin to early stages of meningitis - atro.

morning, in - ***fl-ac.***, ***nux-v.***

music, cannot endure - **ACON.**, ***cham.***, ***coff.***, ***lyc.***, ***nat-c.***, **NUX-V.**, ph-ac., ***sep.***

agg. - viol-o.

amel. - **AUR.**

cry, makes her - ***graph.***

menses, during - ***nat-c.***

shrill sound, has a - ***coff.***

sounds and noises set her in a tremor - aloe

noise, to - chin-s.

agg. from least - ***bell.***, ***ther.***

crackling of a newspaper drives him to despair - ferr.

nausea, excites - ***cocc.***

palpitation, causes - agar.

painful - am-c., arn., ***coff.***, seneg., ***sil.***, ***spig.***

sudden sounds - ***sang.***

noise startles, deafness follows - ***con.***

seasickness, noise excites - ***cocc.***

shrill, every, sound and reverberation penetrates her whole body, especially teeth, makes vertigo worse and causes nausea - ***ther.***

SENSITIVE to sounds,

sing, cannot bear to hear others - lyss.

sleep, on going to - ***calc.***

especially when wanting to - ***calad.***

frightens from - apis

hears every little noise in - alum.

slightest startles him from, in typhus - ***calad.***

soreness, with general sensation of - mag-m.

starting, causes - **ACON.**, ant-c., **BELL.**, ***con.***, lyss., **PHOS.**, sabad., stram.

noise in left, with fright - mill.

sudden, dreads, noise - ***cocc.***

sunstroke, in - ***verat-v.***

talking, to - agar., am-c., cact., ***cocc.***, ***coff.***, con., ***ign.***, **ZINC.**

temper, disturbs - ***colch.***

trembling, causes, in intermittent - ***cocc.***

voice, intolerance of human - ***kali-c.***, mur-ac.

walking, to, of persons over heavy carpet - ***lachn.***

water, running, aggravates dysentery and nervous headache, and causes return of convulsions - ***lyss.***

SLEEP, heard everything while seemingly in profound, could not speak - eup-per.

TINNITUS, (see Noises, in ears) - ***bell.***, bism., ***caust.***, cedr., all-c., ***chin.***, **CHIN-S.**, ***coc-c.***, ***iod.***, kali-br., lac-c., merc-sol., ***nat-s.***, ***phos.***, plat., ***plb.***, ***puls.***, ***sil.***, **THIOSIN.**

catarrh, from, of inner ear - ***hydr.***

deafness, with - bor., ***petr.***, ***sal-ac.***

disappearing on blowing nose and coughing - ***sil.***

epilepsy, in menstrual - ***cedr.***

headache, after a cold drink, with - ***kali-c.***

head, caused by rush of blood to - ***arn.***

heart, in dilated - ***tab.***

hectic fever, in - phos.

hyperaemia, dependent upon - ***sal-ac.***

ideas, with tumult of - camph.

nervous exhaustion, from - ***kali-p.***

night, in the - lyss.

continuous during - zinc.

right, worse in - rhod.

scar tissue, from -calen., sil., **THIOSIN.**

sitting up, when, synchronous with heartbeats - ***nux-v.***

swallowing, when blowing nose or - ***calc.***

vessels, with injection of, along handle of malleus - chin-s.

whooping cough, in - ***all-c.***

yellow fever, in - ***sulph.***

VANISHING, intoxication, with, or drunkenness of previous day, worse after dinner, and in sun - **NUX-V.**

vertigo, with - **NUX-V.**

VOMITING, listening produces - aran.

WEAK - **CARB-AN.**

at times, at times acute - ***anac.***

Heart

HEART, affections of the, general - **ACON.,** ***am-c.,*** apoc., ***ars., ars-i.,*** **AUR., AUR-M.,** ***bad., brom.,*** **CACT.,** ***calc., caust., cench., coll.,*** **CRAT.,** ***crot-h., cupr.,*** ferr., gels., glon., ***hydr.,*** hyos., ***iod., kalm.,*** **LACH.,** lat-m., ***laur., lil-t.,*** **LITH., LOB.,** ***lycps., mosch.,*** **NAJA,** ***nat-m.,*** op., **PHOS.,** ***psor.,*** **PULS.,** seneg., **SPIG., SPONG.**
neuralgia, with - spig.
overlifting agg. - arn., calc., ***caust.***
streptococcal infection, after - led., lyc., med.

ACHING, pain - adon., aesc., ail., ambr., aml-n., aur-m., aur-s., ***cact.,*** calc., con., crot-h., cupr-ar., ***dig.,*** glon., kali-bi., ***lach.,*** lith., ***lycps., merc.,*** merc-i-r., naja, **NAT-M.,** ***nat-p., nux-v., phos.,*** pyrus, rumx., seneg., spong., stroph., tab., tarent., ***verat-v.,*** vesp.
dysmenorrhea, with - crot-h.
evening - kali-bi.
in bed - kali-bi.
headache, with - crot-h.
noon - agar.

ADHESION, sensation of, pericardium - ***graph.***

ANEMIA, from heart disease - ars., crat., stroph.

ANEURISM, of, (see Blood) - **CACT.,** calen., ***carb-v.***
capillary - ***calc-f.,*** fl-ac., tub.

ANGINA, pectoris, (see Chest, pains) - acet-ac., ***acon.,*** adren., agar., **AM-C.,** ***aml-n.,*** anac., ang., **APIS,** arg-c., **ARG-N., ARN., ARS.,** ars-i., **AUR., AUR-M.,** bism., **CACT.,** camph., caust., cer-b., ***chel.,*** **CHIN-A.,** ***chin-s.,*** chlol., chr-ac., ***cimic.,*** coca, ***cocaine,*** conv., ***crat.,*** crot-h., ***cupr., cupr-ac., cupr-ar., dig., dios., glon., haem., hep., hydr-ac.,*** ip., ***jug-c., kali-c.,*** kali-i., kali-p., ***kalm.,*** **LACH.,** lact., **LAT-M.,** ***laur.,*** lil-t., lith., lob., ***lyc., mag-p.,*** magn-gr., morph., ***mosch.,*** **NAJA,** ***nat-i.,*** nat-n., ***nux-v.,*** olnd., **OX-AC.,** petr., **PHOS.,** phyt., pip-n., prun., **RHUS-T.,** ***samb.,*** saroth., sep., **SPIG., SPONG.,** staph., stict., ***stram.,*** stront-c., stront-i., stry., ***tab., tarent., ther.,*** thyr., ***verat.,*** verat-v., zinc-valer.
abuse of, coffee, from - coff.
stimulants, from - nux-v., spig.
drinking, water agg. - ars.
heart disease, from organic - ***ars-i., cact.,*** calc-f., crat., kalm., nat-i., tab.
hot drinks, amel. - spig.
lies, on knees, body bent backwards - nux-v.
muscular origin - cupr., hydr-ac.
pain, excessive - agar.
pseudo angina pectoris - aconin., cact., ***lil-t., mosch.,*** nux-v., tarent.
rheumatism, from - cimic., lith.
standing, amel. - ars.
straining, overlifting, from - ***arn.,*** carb-an., caust.
tobacco, from - calad., kalm., lil-t., nux-v., spig., staph., tab.

ANXIETY, region of - **ACON.,** ***aeth.,*** agar., alum., ***ambr.,*** am-c., ***aml-n.,*** anac., **ANT-T.,** apis, ***arg-n.,*** arn., **ARS.,** ***ars-i.,*** aster., **AUR.,** ***aur-m.,*** **BELL.,** bov., ***brom., cact., calc.,*** **CAMPH.,** cann-s., ***canth., carb-o., carb-s.,*** **CARB-V.,** carl., ***caust.,*** **CENCH.,** ***cham.,*** chel., chin., chin-a., chin-s., cic., cina, ***cocc., coff.,*** colch., ***con.,*** croc., ***crot-c., cupr.,*** cycl., ***dig.,*** echi., elaps, ***euon., ferr., ferr-i.,*** ferr-p., ***gels., glon.,*** gran., graph., hell., hydr., hydr-ac., hyos., **IGN.,** ***iod.,*** **IP., KALM.,** ***kreos., lach., lact.,*** lob., ***lyc.,*** **MENY.,** ***merc., merc-c.,*** mez., mosch., ***naja,*** nat-s., nit-ac., ***nux-v.,*** olnd., op., ox-ac., petr., **PHOS.,** ***plb., plat., prun., psor., puls.,*** ran-b., ***rhus-t.,*** sabad., sal-n., sec., sep., sil., ***spig., spong.,*** stann., stict., stram., sulph., ***tab., tarent.,*** **THER.,** thuj., ***verat.,*** viol-t., vip.
afternoon - canth., rhus-t.
dinner, after - arg-n., bell.
when leaning back in chair - glon.
epilepsy, with - ***lyc.***
evening - bell., brom., ***puls.***
expectoration, copious, amel. - ***ip.***
headache, after - sep.
before - plat.
lying on left side agg. - bell., glon., ***nat-m., phos., spig.***
menses, during - bell.
morning - alum., aster.
2 a.m. - ***kali-c.***
4 to 5 a.m. - ***alum.***
rising, after, amel. - alum.
moving about, agg. - ***dig.***
amel. - ***aur.,*** caust., op.
night - alum., **ARS.,** aster., calc., lyc., rhus-t.
4 a.m. - alum.
11 p.m., after lying down - kali-bi.
bed, in - cann-s., thuj., viol-t.
nausea, during - plb.
pain in heart, with - acon., cact., kali-ar., mill., ***op., phos.***
paroxysmal - arg-n., **KALM.,** lach., verat.
rising and walking amel. - glon.
sight of decisive colors - ***tarent.***
sitting, while - agar., ***caust.,*** kali-c.
stretching out body after physical exertion - lyc.
supper, after - bell.
thinking of it agg. - bar-c., ox-ac.
vexation, after - lyc.
walking amel. - ***caust.,*** glon.
air, in open - cina, spong.

AORTA, (see Blood)

APPREHENSION, region of - acon., ant-t., ***aur.,*** carl., ***kali-ar.,*** meny., mez., phos., plb., plat., ***rhus-t.***

ARTERIOSCLEROSIS, (see Blood, chapter)

ARTERITIS, (see Blood, chapter)

BORING, pain - aur-m., ***cupr.,*** rhod., ***seneg.***
pressure amel. - aur-m.

BLOOD pressure, (see Blood, chapter)

BLOOD vessels, (see Blood, chapter)

BUBBLE, starts from and passes through the arteries - nat-p.

BURNING, pain - arn., aur-m., carb-v., hydr., kali-c., kali-i., lyss., med., ***op., puls.,*** rumx., tarent., ust.
- as if - kali-c., op., tarent.
- noon, at - agar.
- palpitations, with - kali-c.

burning, region of - acon., aesc., ***agar.,*** arg-n., ***ars.,*** bell., ***carb-v., carl., caust., cic., kali-c.,*** plat., ***puls.,*** verat., ***verat-v.***
- coughing agg. - agar.
- extending to left scapula - agar.
- hiccoughs agg. - agar.
- sneezing agg. - agar.

BURSTING, pain - am-c., asaf., lyss., med.

bursting, sensation of being too full - ***aesc.,*** aml-n., aur-m., ***bell.,*** buf-s., ***cact.,*** cench., coll., conv., ***glon.,*** glyc., iber., lact., ***lil-t.,*** pyrog., ***spig.,*** **SPONG.,** stroph., ***sulph.,*** vanad.
- at night when lying on the back amel. by sitting up - asaf.

CEASE, fears heart will, unless constantly on the move - **GELS.,** trif-p.
- sitting up, or - trif-r.

cease, sensation as if, had ceased - antipyrin., ***arg-m., arg-n.,*** arn., aster., ***aur., cact.,*** chin-a., **CIC.,** cimic., conv., crat., **DIG.,** ***lach., lil-t.,*** lob., ***lycps.,*** magn-gr., ***phase., rumx., sep.,*** spig., tarent., trif-p., zinc.
  - pregnancy, during - arg-m.
- then started suddenly - ***aur.,*** conv., lil-t., sep.

cease, sensation as if, would cease - aur., ***calc.,*** chin-a., cimic., conv., lil-t., **LOB.,** nux-m., onos., sep., trif-p., vib.
  - dinner, after - sep.

CIRCULATION, (see Blood)

COLDNESS, region of - arn., ***carb-an.,*** graph., ***helo., kali-bi., kali-chl., kali-n.,*** lil-t., ***nat-m., petr.,*** pyrog.
- as if the heart were cold - calc., ***carb-an.,*** graph., ***helo.,*** kali-bi., ***kali-m.,*** kali-n., lil-t., ***nat-m.,*** petr.
- icy coldness during chill - arn., camph., kali-c., **NAT-M.,** olnd., petr.
- mental exertion, during - ***nat-m.***

CONGESTION, of - **ACON.,** ***asaf., apoc.,*** cham., cycl., **GLON.,** hyper., ***lil-t., nux-m.,*** phos., ***puls.,*** sulph.
- convulsions, in - ***glon.***
- menses, after - ***ign.***
- night - nit-ac., ***puls.***
- walking rapidly - nux-m.

CONGESTIVE, heart failure - **ACON.,** apis., ***asaf.,*** **APOC.,** cham., **CRAT.,** cycl., dig., **GLON.,** hyper., lach., ***lil-t., nux-m.,*** phos., ***puls.,*** sulph.

CONSTRICTION, sensation - aeth., agar., ***ail.,*** alum., aml-n., ang., ***anth.,*** apis, ***arn.,*** **ARS., ARS-I.,** asaf., asc-t., aur., berb., bufo, **CACT.,** cadm-s., calc., ***calc-ar.,*** cann-i., cann-s., chlor., cocc., cund., ***dig.,*** ferr., ferr-ar., ferr-i., ferr-p., graph., hydr., ***ign.,*** **IOD.,** ***kali-ar.,*** kali-bi., ***kali-c.,*** kali-chl., kali-p., lac-ac., ***lach., laur.,*** **LIL-T.,** lyc., ***lycps.,*** lyss., merl., mur-ac., ***naja, nat-m.,*** nit-ac., ***nux-m.,*** nux-v., phos., phyt., ***plb.,*** rad-br., rhus-t., samb., ***spig., spong.,*** tarent., verat., zinc.
- bending chest forward amel. - lac-ac., lil-t.
- drinking water amel. - ***phos.***
- eating, agg. - alum.
  - a little - lil-t.
- epilepsy, before - ***calc-ar., lach.***
- exertion - asaf., bry.
- extending to back - ***lil-t.***
- grasping sensation - ***acon.,*** adon., aml-n., arn., ars., **CACT.,** calc-ar., coc-c., colch., **IOD.,** iodof., kali-c., ***lach., laur.,*** **LIL-T.,** lycps., mag-p., magn-gr., ***nux-m.,*** ptel., rhus-t., ***spig.,*** spong., ***sulph., tarent.,*** thyr., vanad., visc.
  - in heart and on right side - bor.
- grief, after - ***ign.***
- heartbeat amel. - nit-ac.
- night - ***lil-t.***
- nosebleed, with - verat.
- urging to stool, with - calc-ar.
- walk erect, inability to - ***lil-t.***

CONSCIOUS, heart's action - iber.

CRACKING, in region of - mag-c., ***nat-c.***

CRAMP - anan., ***ars.,*** bry., cupr., kali-bi., ***kali-c.,*** **LACH.,** mez., myric., sep., tarent., thuj., zinc.
- music, from soft - thuj.

CRAMPY, pain in - ars., ***bry.,*** **LACH.,** laur., ptel.
- exertion - bry.
- raising arm - bry.

CROUP, cardiac - ***spong.***

CUTTING, pain - abies-n., abrot., ***acon., aesc.,*** anac., apis, apoc., ***arg-n.,*** **ARS.,** ***ars-i.,*** ars-m., asc-t., aur., aur-m., bell., ***bry., cact.,*** calc., cann-i., caust., cer-b., chel., cimic., ***colch., con., croc.,*** daph., dig., ***glon., iber., iod.,*** jac-c., ***kali-c.,*** kali-i., kali-n., ***kalm.,*** lac-ac., ***lac-d., lat-m.,*** lil-t., lith., magn-gr., med., menthol, ***naja, ox-ac.,*** paeon., phyt., sabin., sep., ***spig.,*** syph., **SULPH.,** tab., tarent., ther.
- afternoon, 4 p.m. - ars-m.
- evening - cinnb.
- menses, during - ***con.***
- morning - cund.
- motion, on - ***cact.***
- region of - anac., aur-m., ***brom., calc-p.,*** cinnb., ***dios.,*** myric., ***phos.,*** spig., verat.
  - interrupting breathing - ***calc., calc-p., dios.***

DILATATION, of - adon., ***alum.,*** am-c., ***ant-t., apis, ars.,*** ars-i., ***bar-c.,*** **CACT.,** cimic., coff., conv., ***crat.,*** cupr., ***dig.,*** gels., hydr-ac., iber., ***iod., kali-i., lach., laur.,*** lil-t., ***lyc., lycps., naja, nat-m., nux-v.,*** ph-ac., ***phase., phos.,*** phys., plb., prun., ***psor., puls., spig.,*** stroph., tab., verat-v.

DRAWING, pain, in - agar., aur-m., ***canth.,*** card-m., cod., ***ferr.,*** ferr-m., lyss., nat-m., olnd., **SPIG.**

as if heart and ovary were drawn together - ***naja.***

region of - calc., meny.

DRAWN, downwards, the heart - thuj.

EDEMA, dropsy, from heart disease - aml-n., ***apis,*** **APOC.,** arn., **ARS.,** ***ars-i.,*** asc-c., **AUR-M.,** ***bry., cact., calc-p.,*** chin-a., ***chlol.,*** coff., ***coffin., colch.,*** **COLL.,** ***conv.,*** cop., **CRAT.,** crot-h., ***dig., digin., fl-ac., hell.,*** iod., kali-c., ***kali-m.,*** kalm., **LAC-D., LACH.,** liatr., **LYC.,** lycps., merc-d., merc-sul., ***nat-m.,*** ph-ac., phos., ***prun.,*** rauw., ***sep., squil., stroph.***

pericardium - ant-a., ***apis.,*** **APOC., ARS., COLCH., DIG.,** iod., ***lach.,*** **LYC.,** ***sulph., zinc.***

EMPTINESS, sensation of - cocc., med., sulph.

region of - con., graph., naja, sulph.

ENDOCARDITIS - ***abrot., acet-ac.,*** **ACON., ARS.,** ars-i., **AUR.,** ***aur-m.,*** bism., ***bry., cact., calc.,*** cocc., coc-c., ***colch.,*** dig., ferr., ***iod.,*** kali-ar., ***kali-c., kali-i.,*** **KALM.,** ***lach.,*** led., nat-m., ***naja,*** ox-ac., ***phos.,*** phyt., plat., plb., ***sep.,*** **SPIG.,** ***spong.,*** tarent., ***verat-v.***

acute - ***acon.,*** ars., bell., ***cact., colch.,*** conv., dig., ***lach.,*** magn-gr., ***naja,*** phos., ***spig.,*** spong., tab., verat-v.

malignant - acon., ars., ***chin-s.,*** crot-h., lach., vip.

pain and great anxiety - ***aur., kalm.***

rheumatic - acon., adon., ***ars.,*** **AUR.,** ***aur-m.,*** aven., bell., ***bry., cact., colch.,*** dig., ***hyos.,*** kali-c., ***kali-n.,*** **KALM., LACH.,** ***phos.,*** plat., ***rhus-t., spig., spong., sumb.,*** verat.

scanty menses, with - nat-m.

EXUDATION, in valves of - ***spong.***

FALLING, drops were, from the - cann-s.

FAT, about the heart with nervous irritability - **AUR.**

FATTY, degeneration, of - adon., **ARN., ARS.,** ***ars-i.,*** **AUR., AUR-M.,** ***bar-c.,*** **CACT.,** ***calc.,*** caps., cimic., crat., crot-h., cupr., cupr-ac., ***ferr.,*** fuc., ***iod.,*** **KALI-C.,** kali-fer., kali-p., ***kalm., naja,*** ph-ac., **PHOS.,** phys., ***phyt.,*** stroph., stry-p., vanad.

FLUTTERING, of (see Chest) - acon., ***alumn., ambr.,*** apoc., ***arg-n., arn.,*** ars-i., ***asaf.,*** aur., ***aur-m., bry., cact.,*** calad., ***calc.,*** calc-s., carb-v., ***cench.,*** cupr-ar., daph., ***dig.,*** eup-pur., form., gels., hydr-ac., ***kali-bi., kali-br., kali-i., kali-p., kalm.,*** lac-c., ***lach., laur.,*** **LIL-T.,** lec., ***lith.,*** lyss., ***med.,*** mosch., **NAJA, NAT-M., NAT-S., NUX-M.,** nux-v., ***ox-ac.,*** **PH-AC.,** ***pic-ac.,*** rat., ***rhus-t., samb., sep., spig.,*** stry., ***sulph.,*** sumb., thea., verat-v., zing.

afternoon, after quick exertion - sumb.

during headache - form., sumb.

air open, amel. - **NAT-M., NAT-S.**

alternating with soreness - aur-m.

ascending steps - ***bry.,*** **CALC.**

dinner, after - ***sep.***

evening - pic-ac.

excitement after slight - ***aml-n.,*** **LIL-T.,** ***lith.***

faintness, after - asaf., ***calc., gels., lil-t., mosch.,*** **NAT-M., NAT-S.,** ph-ac., stry.

grief, after - ***nat-m.***

lying, while - **NAT-M.**

on left side - ***daph., dig., gels., nat-m.,*** spig.

on right side - ***alumn.***

menses, after - spig.

morning - naja, stry.

night - naja

wakens her - ***lil-t.***

raising arms, on - dig., ***sulph.***

rest, during - **LIL-T.**

sitting - ***asaf.***

thinking of it - ***arg-n.***

waking, on - ***kali-i.,*** naja

writing, while - naja

fluttering, sensation, as if - absin., ***acon.,*** aml-n., apoc., asaf., ***cact., cimic.,*** conv., crot-h., ferr., glon., ***iber., kalm.,*** lach., ***lil-t.,*** lith., ***mosch.,*** naja, ***nat-m.,*** nux-m., ph-ac., ***phase., phys.,*** pyrog., ***spig.,*** sul-ac., thea.

FULLNESS - ***acon., aesc.,*** arg-m., arg-n., ***asaf.,*** **AUR., AUR-M.,** ***bov.,*** bufo, caust., ***cench.,*** colch., ***glon.,*** **LACH.,** ***lil-t., lycps.,*** med., pyrog., ***puls.,*** sep., ***spong.,*** **SULPH.**

as if too full - ***aesc.,*** aml-n., aur., ***bell.,*** bufo, ***cact.,*** cench., coll., conv., ***glon.,*** glyc., iber., lact., ***lil-t.,*** pyrog., ***spig., spong.,*** stroph., ***sulph.,*** vanad.

ascending stairs - **AUR.,** aur-m.

evening - **PULS.**

menses, during - ***puls.***

night - colch.

while lying on left side - colch.

GOUTY - aur., ***benz-ac., calc., carb-v., caust., colch., kalm., led.,*** **LYC.,** ***puls., spong.***

GRASPING sensation, in - ***acon.,*** adon., aml-n., arn., ars., **CACT.,** calc-ar., coc-c., colch., **IOD.,** iodof., kali-c., ***lach., laur.,*** **LIL-T.,** lycps., mag-p., magn-gr., ***nux-m.,*** ptel., rhus-t., ***spig.,*** spong., ***sulph., tarent.,*** thyr., vanad., visc.

in heart and on right side - bor.

GRIPING, pain, in - ***cact.,*** visc.

GURGLING - bell., ***psor.,*** rhus-t.

when lying - ***psor.***

HANGING, by a thread, as if heart were - kali-c., lach., lil-t., lyc.

HARD, body, the heart - nat-c.

HEART, attack, angina pectoris - **ACON.**, apis, arg-n., **ARN.**, ars., aur., **CACT.**, carb-v., ***dig., glon.***, iod., ***kalm.***, **LACH., LAT-M.**, ***laur., naja***, nux-v., phos., rhus-t., ***spig.***, verat., ***tarent.***
fear of death, during - **ACON.**, ars., asaf., cact., cench., **DIG.**, kali-ars., ***naja, phos., plat.***, psor.
drinking, water agg. - ars.
standing, amel.
stopped, sensation as if heart had, with acute anxiety - ***arg-m., arg-n.***, aster., ***aur., cact.***, chin-a., **CIC., DIG.**, ***lach., lil-t., lycps., rumx., sep.***, spig., tarent., zinc.

HEART is on right side, sensation as if - ***bor., lil-t.***

HEAT, region of - ***ant-t., cann-s.***, croc., **GLON.**, lachn., lyss., med., op., plan., sabad., ***spong.***, sul-i.
evening - naja
extending, over body - ars., ***nux-m.***
to head - **GLON.**
flushes of - ars., carb-v., **GLON.**, lyc., merl., nit-ac., ***nux-m.***, **PHOS.**, plb., sep., sil., ***sulph.***
waking, on - benz-ac.

HIGH blood pressure, (see Blood)

HYPERTROPHY, of - **ACON.**, ***aml-n., arn., ars.***, aspar., **AUR., AUR-I.**, ***aur-m.***, bell., ***brom.***, **CACT.**, ***caust.***, cer-b., chlol., ***conv., crat., dig., ferr., glon., graph., hep., iber., iod.***, kali-bi., **KALI-C., KALM.**, ***lach.***, lil-t., **LITH.**, ***lyc., lycps., naja, nat-m.***, nux-v., ***phos.***, phyt., plb., ***puls., rhus-t., spig.***, **SPONG.**, staph., stroph., ***verat-v.***, visc.
athletes, of, uncomplicated - ***arn.***, brom., caust., ***rhus-t.***
numbness and tingling of left arm and fingers, with - **ACON., RHUS-T.**
over-exertion, from - ***arn.***, brom., ***calc., caust., kali-c.***, **RHUS-T.**
sensation, of - acon.

INFLAMMATION, of - ***acon.***, apis, ars., **AUR.**, ***bry., cact., cann-s., carb-s., carb-v., caust.***, cocc., ***colch., dig.***, kali-i., ***kalm., lach., led., naja, phos., psor., puls.***, rhus-t., **SPIG.**, sulph., sumb., ***verat-v.***
bright's disease, with - ***apis***, apoc., ***ars.***, asc-t., cann-s., colch., ***dig.***, kali-n., phos.
compelled to lie on the back with head, raised - ***acon.***
lying on side impossible - ***cact.***
inflammation, (see Endocarditis)
inflammation, (see Myocarditis)
inflammation, (see Pericarditis)

JERKING, pain, in - calc-ar., carb-v., con., fl-ac.

JERKS, in - agar., arg-n., ***calc.***, fl-ac., nat-m., **NUX-V.**, sumb., tarent.
evening - sumb.

LOOSE, sensation as if - aur., crot-h.

MOVEMENT, region of - sulph.

MURMURS - agar., ***aml-n., apis, ars., ars-i.***, aspar., ***aur., aur-m.***, bar-c., **CACT.**, ***calc.***, carb-ac., ***chel.***, chin-a., ***cocc., colch.***, **COLL.**, ***crot-h.***, cupr-s., **DIG., FERR.**, ferr-ar., ferr-i., ***glon.***, hep., hydr-ac., ***hydr.***, iber., ***iod.***, ip., kali-ar., kali-br., ***kali-c.***, **KALM.**, ***lach., lith.***, lob., ***lyc., lycps., merc.***, **NAJA**, nat-a., nat-c., ***nat-m., nit-ac., phos.***, plb., ***psor.***, puls., **RHUS-T., SPIG., SPONG.**, stann., stram., ***sumb.***, tab., tarent., tub.
valvular disease, with - acon., ***adon.***, apoc., ***ars.***, ars-i., aur., aur-br., aur-i., ***bar-c., cact.***, calc., calc-f., camph., ***conv., crat., dig.***, ferr., gala., ***glon.***, iod., ***kali-c.***, kalm., lach., laur., lith., ***lycps.***, **NAJA**, ox-ac., phos., plb., ***puls.***, rhus-t., sang., ser-ang., ***spig., spong.***, stigm., ***stroph., tarent.***, thyr., visc., zinc-i.
incompetent - cact., crat., kali-c., spong.
mitral and tricuspidal regurgitation - apoc., cact., laur., psor., stroph.

MYOCARDITIS - acon., adon., ***ars-i.***, aur-m., cact., chin-a., crat., ***dig.***, gala., iod., lach., phos., stroph., ***vip.***

OPPRESSION - ***acon., adon., adren., aesc., agar., ambr.***, am-c., ***aml-n.***, anac., ant-t., ***apis***, **ARS.**, ***ars-i.***, arund., aspar., **AUR., AUR-M.**, bapt., bell., ***brom.***, bry., bufo, **CACT.**, calc., ***calc-ar., camph.***, cann-i., cann-s., ***carb-v.***, card-m., ***caust.***, cer-b., cham., ***chin.***, chlor., cimic., clem., colch., coll., cot., ***crat.***, croc., cupr., ***dig.***, dios., eup-per., fago., ferr., ***gels., glon.***, graph., haem., hell., helo., ***hydr-ac.***, hyos., ***iber.***, ign., ***iod.***, **IP.**, kali-ar., ***kali-c.***, kali-i., kalm., ***lach.***, lat-m., ***laur., lil-t., lycps.***, mag-m., magn-gr., med., meny., ***merc.***, merc-c., mez., ***naja, nat-a.***, nat-c., ***nat-s., nux-m., nux-v.***, ol-j., op., ox-ac., **PHOS.**, plb., prim-v., **PULS.**, sapo., sarr., sil., sin-n., **SPIG.**, ***spong.***, stict., stram., sumb., ***tab., tarent.***, ter., ***thea.***, thuj., thyr., tub., vanad., verat-v., viol-t., vip., visc.
afternoon - bapt.
ascending stairs - **AUR., AUR-M.**
drawn downwards - thuj.
eating, after - bufo
evening - brom., bufo, cact., kalm., **PULS.**
exertion, on least - ***brom., laur., nat-a.***
flatulence, with - alum.
left side, on - ***colch., lach., naja***, **SPIG.**
lying amel. - ***laur., psor.***
with head, low - colch., **SPONG.**
melancholy - aur., caust.
morning - graph., kalm., nat-s., ***tarent.***
motion, on - bufo, coll., eup-per.
night - ***aur.***, colch., kali-c.
palpitations, with - ambr., coca, grat., hyos., kali-n., phos., sep., spig.
respiration, deep - aur-m., nat-a., rumx.
sitting - agar., **NAT-S.**
standing - prun.
thinking of it agg. - ***gels.***
walking amel. - colch.

PAIN, heart - abies-n., ***abrot.,*** **ACON.,** ***adon.,*** aesc., **AGAR.,** ail., ambr., ***aml-n.,*** **APIS, ARG-N.,** ***arn.,*** **ARS.,** ***ars-i., asaf.,*** asc-t., aspar., aster., **AUR.,** ***aur-m.,*** bell., ***benz-ac., brom., bry.,*** bufo, **CACT.,** ***calc., calc-ar.,*** calc-f., ***camph., cann-i.,*** canth., carb-s., ***carb-v.,*** card-m., caust., **CENCH., CER-B.,** cer-s., ***cham.,*** chin., chlor., **CIMIC.,** ***cina,*** clem., coff., ***colch.,*** con., conv., corn., crat., ***crot-h., cupr., daph., dig.,*** dios., fago., ferr., ferr-i., ferr-m., ferr-p., ***ferr-t., glon., graph., haem., hydr-ac.,*** iber., ***iod., lil-t.,*** lith., lob., **LYCPS.,** piloc., **KALI-AR.,** ***kali-bi., kali-c., kali-chl.,*** kali-i., kali-p., **KALM.,** lac-d., **LACH.,** ***lat-m., laur.,*** lepi., ***lil-t.,*** **LITH.,** ***lob., lycps., lyss.,*** magn-gr., med., ***merc.,*** merc-c., merc-i-f., merc-i-r., ***naja,*** nat-a., ***nat-m.,*** nat-p., nux-v., oena., olnd., onos., ovi-g-p., ***ox-ac., paeon., phos.,*** phyt., pip-n., prun., ***psor.,*** ptel., **PULS.,** ran-s., rhod., **RHUS-T.,** rumx., ***samb., sang.,*** seneg., sep., sin-n., **SPIG.,** ***spong.,*** squil., ***staph.,*** stront-c., ***stroph.,*** **SULPH.,** syph., ***tab.,*** tarax., ***tarent.,*** tell., ***ther.,*** thuj., thyr., verat., ***verat-v.,*** vesp., viol-o., vip., zinc., zinc-i., zinc-valer.

- afternoon - euphr.
  - 4 p.m. - trom.
- alternating, with pain in great toe - nat-p.
  - with pain in uterus - ***lil-t.***
  - with rheumatism - ***benz-ac., kalm.***
- aneurism, with - cact.
- aorta - adren., stry.
- apex, at - lil-t.
  - to base - med., merc., thuj.
  - to base, and back, at night - syph.
- ascending agg. - ***crot-h.***
- base, at - lob.
- bending forward agg. - ***lil-t.,*** **LITH.**
- bladder, after pain in - lith.
- breathing almost impossible - arg-n.
  - short, with - stroph., thyr.
- childbirth - ***cimic.***
- chill, during - ***calc.***
- coughing, on - tarent.
- eating, after - ***kali-bi.,*** lil-t., lyc., manc., nat-m., stront.
- epilepsy, before - ***calc-ar., lyc.***
- evening - ph-ac., **PULS.,** raph., sulph., thuj.
- excitement from - ***cupr., dig.***
- exertion - cer-s., ***dig., lil-t.***
- expiration, during - phyt.
- extending to,
  - arm, left - ***lat-m.,*** visc.
  - arm, right - ***lil-t.,*** phyt., spig.
  - arms, both - lat-m., sec.
  - axilla - ferr-i., lat-m.
  - back - aloe, ***ars-i.,*** **CENCH.,** ***crot-t.,*** glon., ***kali-c., lil-t., naja, spig.,*** **SULPH.**
  - hand, left - ***acon.,*** am-m., ***aster., aur., cact., cimic., crot-h., dig.,*** iber., **KALM.,** ***lat-m., naja, nux-v., rhus-t., spig., tab.,*** ther.
  - leg, right - alumn.
  - nape of neck and shoulder - ***naja.,*** scop.
  - nape of neck, left shoulder and left arm - fago.

PAIN, heart

- extending to, occiput - ars.
  - scapula, left shoulder, down left arm to fingers - ***acon.,*** arn., bism., ***cact.,*** cimic., crot-h., ***kalm., lat-m.,*** lepi., naja, ***ox-ac., rhus-t., spig.,*** tab.
  - scapula, left - aloe, ***lil-t., naja, spig., sulph.***
  - scapula, right - spig.
  - shoulder - ***verat.***
  - shoulder, neck and - naja, scop.
  - shoulder, left arm, and - fago.
  - sternum - ***spig.***
- fainting, with - arn.
- forenoon - thuj.
- itching, with - magn-gr.
- loudly spoken to, when - ***camph.***
- lying down, after - agar.
  - agg. - agar., ***aur.,*** kali-n., lil-t., merc., nux-v., ox-ac., **PULS.,** rumx., **SPONG.,** ***sulph.,*** thyr.
  - back, on - asaf., merc-i-f., rumx.
  - back, on, amel. - ***cact.,*** kalm., lil-t., ***psor.***
- lying down, left side, on, agg. - bar-c., brom., ***cact.,*** colch., ***crot-h.,*** dig., dios., iber., ***kali-ar., lach., naja, nat-m.,*** **PHOS.,** ***psor.,*** puls., sep., **SPIG.,** tell., zinc-i.
  - could lie only on left - ***ars-m.,*** rumx.
  - with head, low - **SPONG.**
- lying down, right side, on - arg-n., lil-t., rumx.
  - agg. - alum., arg-n., bad., kali-n., kalm., lach., lil-t., plat., rumx.
  - amel. - lach., nat-c., ***phos., psor.,*** tab.
  - could lie only on - ***naja,*** **SPIG.**
- menses, during - ***arg-n., cact., con.,*** lith., ***puls.***
  - after - ***lach., lith.***
  - before - ***cact.,*** crot-h., eupi., lach., ***lith.,*** sep., spong.
  - painful, during - **CON.**
- morning - calc-p., dig.
  - bending over the bed, on - ***lith.***
  - chocolate, after - raph.
  - rising, on - con.
  - waking, on - ***tarent.***
- moving, agg. - bry., ***cact.,*** kali-i., lil-t., phyt., spig.
  - amel. - ***mag-m.***
- night - ***arg-n.,*** cann-i., coc-c., ***naja,*** nat-m.
- noise, from - agar.
- palpitation, during - plb.
- paroxysmal - ***laur.***
- plug, at - ran-s.
- pressure of hand amel. - ***nat-m.***
- pseudo angina pectoris - aconin., cact., ***lil-t., mosch.,*** nux-v., tarent.
- pulsating - arg-n., camph., clem., ***glon.,*** graph., ***kali-c., lycps., nux-v.,*** rumx., sil., spig., tarent.
- radiating - ***glon.***
- reflex, from - asaf., naja
- respiration agg. - crot-h., rumx.
- riding in a carriage - naja, raph.

PAIN, heart
right side, as if, on - bor., ox-ac., ***phyt.***
rising, from a recumbent position - ***laur.***
from a seat - ***gels.***
rubbing, amel. - lil-t.
sex, after - ***dig.***
sitting, while - ***mag-m.***
erect - acon.
smoking, from - conv.
sneezing, agg. - agar., bor., dros., merc.
spine, touching, agg. - tarent.
standing - aur-m-n.
stairs, going up and down, agg. - lac-c.
stooling, agg. - con.
stooping, on - ***lil-t.,*** olnd.
symptoms, few, with -
symptoms, vary - lycps.
tobacco, agg. - cact., scop.
touching spine - tarent.
urination, during - aspar., ***lith.***
after, amel. - ***lith., nat-m.***
before - ***lith.***
waking, after - fago., ***tarent.***
walking - arg-n., ***cact., nat-m.,*** ox-ac., ph-ac., ***ran-b.,*** rhus-t., seneg., spig., sulph.
amel. - colch., ***puls.***
wandering - ***aur., kalm., puls.***
from joint to joint and then locates in - ***aur.***
wine, agg. - glon.
yawning - merc-i-f.

pain, region of heart, (see Chest) - aeth., am-caust., aml-n., arg-n., ars., ars-m., **ARUM-T.,** asaf., ***benz-ac.,*** brach., calc-p., cann-i., cann-s., carb-o., ***cimic.,*** dios., ***graph.,*** hydr-ac., jab., kali-bi., kali-s., **LAT-M.,** lac-ac., laur., lob-s., merc-c., merc-i-f., ***naja, nat-m.,*** onos., plb., phos., phyt., sec., sin-n., sol-n., sol-t-ae., ***spong.,*** stann., sulph., sul-ac., tab., tell., thea., thuj., verat., xan., zinc., zinc-m.
acute - aml-n., bov., calc-p., dios., ***iod.,*** mez.
afternoon - fago.
drinking after - nat-m.
evening - fago., sulph., thuj.
in bed - ***nat-m.***
extending to left arm - **LAT-M.**
forenoon - fago.
inspiration, deep - calc-p.
morning - dios., fago., nat-m.
respiration - stry.
deep - rumx.
quick and difficult - nux-v.
waking, on - kali-bi.

PALPITATIONS - ***abies-c.,*** **ACON.,** ***adon.,*** aesc., ***aeth.,*** **AGAR.,** agarin., aloe, ***alum.,*** alumn., ***ambr., am-c., am-m.,*** **AML-N.,** anac., ant-c., ***ant-t., apis,*** apoc., ***arg-m.,*** **ARG-N.,** ***arn.,*** **ARS., ARS-I.,** art-v., ***asaf.,*** asc-t., aspar., aster., **AUR.,** ***aur-m.,*** aur-m-n., aven., ***bad., bar-c., bar-m., bell.,*** benz-ac., berb., ***bism.,*** bor., ***bov., brom., bry.,*** bufo, **CACT., CADM-S., CALC.,** calc-ar., ***calc-p.,*** calc-s., ***camph., cann-i., cann-s.,*** canth., ***carb-an., carb-s., carb-v.,*** carl., ***caust., cedr., cham., chel.,*** **CHIN.,** ***chin-a., chin-s.,*** cimic., ***coca, cocc.,*** coc-c., coff., **COLCH.,** ***coll.,*** coloc., **CON.,** cop., com., ***conv.,*** crat., ***crot-c., crot-h.,*** crot-t., ***cupr.,*** cupr-ar., ***cycl.,*** **DIG.,** digin., ***dios.,*** dulc., ***elaps, eup-per.,*** eupi., fago., ***ferr., ferr-ar., ferr-i., ferr-p.,*** form., ***gels.,*** **GLON.,** ***graph.,*** grat., ***guai.,*** ham., hell., ***hep., hydr.,*** hydr-ac., ***hyos.,*** hyper., ***iber., ign.,*** **IOD.,** ip., ***kali-ar., kali-bi.,*** **KALI-C.,** ***kali-chl., kali-fer., kali-i., kali-n., kali-p., kali-s.,*** **KALM.,** kreos., ***lac-d.,*** **LACH.,** lact., ***laur., lec.,*** led., ***lil-t., lob.,*** **LYC.,** ***lycps.,*** lyss., mag-aust., ***mag-c., mag-m., manc., mang., med., meli.,*** **MERC.,** ***merc-c., merl.,*** mez., ***mill., mosch.,*** murx., mur-ac., mygal., **NAJA, NAT-A., NAT-C., NAT-M., NAT-P.,** ***nit-ac., nux-m.,*** **NUX-V.,** ***olnd.,*** ol-j., ***op.,*** osm., ***ox-ac.,*** par., petr., pic-ac., ***phase.,*** **PH-AC., PHOS.,** ***phys., plat., plb., podo., prun., psor.,*** **PULS.,** ***pyrog.,*** rhus-r., ***rhus-t.,*** rumx., sabin., sang., ***sars., sec.,*** seneg., **SEP.,** ***sil.,*** **SPIG., SPONG.,** squil., stann., staph., ***stram., stront-c.,*** stry., sulo-ac., sumb., **SULPH.,** ***sul-ac.,*** sul-i., **TAB.,** tarax., tarent., tell., tep., ter., thea., ***ther., thuj., thyr.,*** tril., trinit., upa., ust., valer., **VERAT.,** ***verat-v., viol-t.,*** vesp., yohim, ***zinc.***
afternoon - arg-n., bell., chel., chin-s., colch., crot-t., dig., euphr., form., gels., ***lyc.,*** lyss., phos.
1 p.m. - chel.
2 p.m. to 6 p.m. - carc.
3 to 5 p.m. - agar.
air, in open - ambr., caust.
alternating, with, aphonia - ox-ac.
cheerfulness - spig.
hemorrhoids - coll.
pain in lower limbs - benz-ac.
suppressed menses - coll.
anemia, with - ferr., puls., nat-m.
from anemia - ars., ***chin.,*** dig., kali-c., kali-fer., nat-m., ***ph-ac.,*** phos., ***puls.,*** spig., verat.
anger - arn., ***phos.,*** sep., staph.
anticipation, during - ***arg-n.,*** dys-co.
anxiety - **ACON.,** aesc., agar., alum., ***am-c.,*** ant-t., ***apis, arg-m., arg-n.,*** **ARS.,** aspar., **AUR.,** ***aur-m.,*** bar-c., bor., ***bry., cact.,*** **CALC.,** ***calc-p.,*** calc-s., ***camph.,*** cann-s., carb-s., carb-v., ***caust., chel.,*** **CHIN.,** ***chin-a., cocc., coff., colch., croc.,*** cupr., **DIG.,** elaps, ***ferr.,*** ferr-ar., ferr-p., ***graph., hep., hyos., iod.,*** ip., **KALI-AR.,** ***kali-c., kali-n., kali-p.,*** kali-s., ***kalm., lach., laur., lil-t.,*** lith., ***lyc., merc.,*** mez., ***mosch., nat-a., nat-c.,*** **NAT-M.,** ***nat-p., nit-ac.,*** nux-v., ***olnd., op.,*** osm., **PH-AC., PHOS.,** ***plat., plb., psor.,*** **PULS.,** ***rhus-t.,*** ruta., ***samb.,*** sars., ***sec., sep.,*** sil., **SPIG.,** ***spong., stram.,*** **SULPH.,** thuj., ***verat., viol-t., zinc.***
children, in - ***calc-p., phos.***
cramplike pain in precordial region, with - ***lach.***
dropsy, hydropericardium - ***colch.***
evening and morning - **PHOS.**
excitement, after - ***plat.***
falling asleep, prevents - ***sulph.***

PALPITATIONS, general

anxiety, mental exertion agg. - aur-m.
sudden - ***chel.***
tremulous, caused by quick motion or excitement - ***cocc.***
weakness, with - ***calc-p.***

ascending, steps - ang., arg-n., **ARS.**, aspar., ***aur-m.,*** aur-s., bell., berb., bov., ***bry.,*** bufo, ***cact.,*** CALC., calc-s., crot-t., ***croc.,*** dig., ***ferr-i.,*** helon., ***iod., kali-p., lyc., lycps., naja, nat-a., nat-c.,*** **NAT-M., NIT-AC.**, ***ph-ac.,*** **PHOS.**, plb., plat., ***puls.,*** sabin., spong., **SULPH.**, tab., ter., thea., ***thuj.,*** verat.

attention, is directed to anything, when - nat-c.

audible - aesc., agar., am-c., apis, ***ars.,*** bell., ***calc.,*** camph., colch., ***dig.***, glon., ***iod.,*** lyc., nat-m., sep., spig., thuj.
at night - am-c., ***ars.,*** colch.

bathing, agg. - am-c.

beats, for six to ten - nat-m.

bed, on going to - fago., sol-t-ae., upa.

beer, after - sumb.

belching, from - coloc.
amel. - aur., bar-c., ***carb-v.,*** morg-g., mosch.

bending, forward chest - kalm., **SPIG.**

breath, holding - cact., spig.
takes away - chin.

breathing, deep, amel. - carb-v.

bubbling - bell.

burning at heart, with - kali-c.

children, growing too fast - ph-ac.

chill, during - gels., lil-t., ph-ac., phos., ***merc.,*** sep., sulph.
before - **CHIN.**

chilled, from becoming - ***acon.***

choking in throat, with - iber., lach., naja.

coffee, after - bart., **NUX-V.**

cold bathing, amel. - ***iod.***
washing hands in cold water - ***tarent.***

colic, with - plb.

company, in - plat.

convulsions, after - kali-p.
before - ***cupr., glon.,*** lach.

convulsive - ***nux-v.***

coryza, during - anac.

cough, during - agar., aml-n., ***calc.,*** calc-p., cupr., kali-n., ***nat-m.,*** psor., ***puls.,*** stram., ***sulph.,*** tub.

daytime - **ACON.**, ***iod.,*** rhus-t.

digestion, during - **LYC.**, morg-g., ***sep.***

dinner, after - calc., chin., crot-t., hep., ign., phos., ***puls.,*** sil., stram., sulph.

drawing, up chest and throwing back right arm - ferr-ma.

dreams, during - acon., alum., am-c., ***cact., iod.,*** lil-t., lycps., rhus-t., sep.

drinking, after - benz-ac., **CON.**, senec.
cold water - thuj.

dyspepsia, with - abies-c., ***abies-n.,*** arg-n., cact., ***carb-v., chin.,*** coca, coff., coll., dios., hydr-ac., lyc., ***nux-v., puls.,*** sep., spig., tab.

PALPITATIONS, general

eating, after - ***abies-c., acon.,*** alum., am-m., ***arg-n.,*** aspar., bad., ***bov.,*** bufo, **CALC.**, ***camph., carb-an., carb-v.,*** coc-c., cop., crot-t., cupr., hep., ***ign., iod.,*** kali-c., lil-t., **LYC.**, manc., merc., ***nat-c., nat-m.,*** nat-p., ***nit-ac., nux-v.,*** phos., plb., psor., **PULS.**, rhus-t., ***sep.,*** sil., sulph., thuj.

emissions, after - ***asaf.***

emotional causes - ***acon.,*** am-val., ambr., anac., cact., ***calc-ar.,*** cham., ***coff.,*** gels., hydr-ac., ***ign.,*** iod., lach., lith., ***mosch.,*** nux-m., nux-v., op., plat., sep., tarent.

emptiness of, with - olnd.

epilepsy, before - ars., ***calc., calc-ar.,*** cupr., ***lach.***

evening - ***agar.,*** alum., arg-n., brom., bufo, cact., canth., ***carb-an., carb-s.,*** carb-v., ***caust.,*** chel., cycl., dig., dulc., ***graph., hep., kalm., lec., lyc., lycps., manc.,*** mez., murx., ***nat-m.,*** par., **PHOS.**, sep., sil., ***sulph.,*** tab., thuj.
8 p.m. - ***calc.***
bed, in - ***arg-n.,*** calc., kali-n., **LYC.**, ***nat-m., nit-ac.,*** ox-ac., petr., ***phos.,*** sars., ***sep., sulph.***
lying down - nat-c.
sitting - petr.

exaltation, after - ***coff.***

excitement, after - alum., ***ambr.,*** aml-n., **ARG-N.**, ***ars., ars-i., asaf., aur., aur-m., bad., bell., cact.,*** calc., ***calc-ar., chim.,*** chin-a., ***cocc.,*** **COFF.**, ***crot-h., dig.***, dys-co., ferr., ***kali-p.,*** **LIL-T.**, ***lycps., naja,*** nat-m., ***nit-ac., nux-v., ph-ac.,*** **PHOS.**, ***plat., podo.,*** prot., ***puls.,*** seneg., ***sep.***
sudden, after - acon., alumn., ***cact.,*** **COFF.**, ***lach., nux-v.***

exertion, physical - am-c., ***apoc.,*** **ARG-M., ARG-N., ARN., ARS.**, ***ars-i.,*** **ASAF., AUR.**, ***aur-m., bar-c., bov.,*** **CACT., CALC.**, ***calc-ar., carb-an.,*** carb-s., carb-v., **CHIN.**, chin-a., **CHIN-S.**, cimic., **DIG.**, ferr-i., ferr-p., gran., ***graph.,*** **IOD.**, ***kali-c.,*** kali-i., ***kali-m.,*** **LACH.**, ***laur.,*** **LYCPS.**, ***med.,*** meny., ***merc.,*** **NAJA**, ***nat-a.,*** **NAT-M.**, ***nat-p., nit-ac., ph-ac.,*** **PHOS.**, ***podo.,*** **PSOR.**, ***puls., rhus-t.,*** sil., **SPIG.**, ***spong., stann.,*** **STAPH.**, ***stram., sulph.,*** sumb., vesp.
amel. - mag-m.
dinner, after - nit-ac.
heart-strain - ***arn.,*** bor., ***caust.,*** coca.
mental - ***ambr., cact., calc-ar.,*** coca, cocc., cod., ***ign., iod.,*** kalm., nat-c., ***nux-v., plat., podo., staph., sulph.***
slightest, even - bell., brom., cimic., coca, conv., ***dig., iber., iod.,*** nat-m., sarcol-ac., ***thyr.***
sudden - ***arg-m., arg-n., arn.***
unusual - ***arg-n.,*** arn., ***cact.,*** chel.

expanding, chest - lach.

extending to, occiput - sep.

PALPITATIONS, general
fear, with - ***acon.,*** alum., aur-m., ferr., ***kali-ar.,*** merc., nat-m., nit-ac., op., ***phos.,*** puls., spong.
fever, during - ***acon.,*** aesc., **ARS.,** bar-c., **CALC.,** ***cocc.,*** crot-h., merc., **NIT-AC.,** phos., **PULS.,** ***sars., sep.,*** sulph.
flatulence, with - carb-v., coca, coll., ham., lycps., nux-v.
from - nat-m.
flatus amel. - abies-c., carb-v., morg-g.
footsweat, after - ***ars., sil.***
forenoon - kali-c., ***lach.,*** nat-m., sulph.
9 a.m. - chin.
fright, after - **ACON.,** ***aur-m.,*** cact., ***coff., nat-m., nux-m., op., puls.,*** stram., verat.
grief, from - ***dig., ign.,*** nux-m., ***op., ph-ac.***
gurgling - bell.
hands, washing in cold water - tarent.
headache, during - aeth., arg-n., bell., brom., bufo, cact., carb-o., hep., lith., plb., sil., ***spig.***
after - cimic.
heart-labored, with, reverberated in head - aur., bell., ***glon.,*** spig., spong.
holds right arm - aur.
hot feeling, with, uncomfortable - ant-t., calc., kali-c., petr.
hunger, during - ***kali-c.,*** phos.
hysteria, in - bar-c., ***cedr., gels., mosch., nat-m., nux-m.***
indigestion, with - nat-c., nux-v., puls.
inspiration, deep, during - asaf., cact., kalm., **SPIG.**
irregular - alum., **ARS.,** ***chel., cocc., lyc., mang.,*** merc., nat-m., nit-ac., ***ox-ac., sang.***
joy, after - ***bad., coff.,*** puls.
kneeling, when - ***sep.***
labor, pains, during - puls.
leaning, back, when - ***chin-a., lach.***
forward and resting on arms, when - sul-ac.
lying, while - ***ars.,*** asaf., ***benz-ac., cact.,*** chel., coc-c., crot-t., cur., ***ferr., glon.,*** grat., kali-c., kali-n., ***lach.,*** lil-t., lyc., lycps., nat-c., **NAT-M., NUX-V.,** ***ox-ac.,*** ph-ac., **PULS.,** ***rhus-t.,*** sep., ***spig.,*** spong., **SULPH.,** thyr., viol-t.
amel. - arg-n., ***colch., lach., laur., phos., psor.***
back, on - ammc., ***arg-m., ars.,*** asaf., aur., ***cact., lach., kali-n.***
amel. - ***kalm., lil-t.***
dinner, after - crot-t., **NUX-V.**
one position, long - alumn.
lying, side, on - ang., bar-c., brom., daph., ***hydr., lil-t., nat-c.,*** nat-m., ***phos.,*** puls., tub., viol-t.
left - ammc., ang., ***bar-c.,*** brom., bry., **CACT., CAUST.,** chin., chin-s., cinnb., clem., daph., dig., graph., glon., ***kali-ar.,*** kali-c., ***kalm., lac-c., lach., lil-t., lyc.,*** myric., ***naja, nat-c.,*** **NAT-M.,** nat-p., **PHOS.,** phys., plb., **PSOR., PULS.,** rhus-t., ***sarr.,*** sep., ***spig., tab.,*** thea.

PALPITATIONS, general
lying, side, on
left, amel. - mag-m.
right agg. - ***alumn., arg-n.,*** bad., kali-n., ***lil-t.,*** plat., spong.
amel. - glon., ***lach.,*** **PHOS., PSOR.,** ***tab.***
maids, in old - bov.
menopause period - ***aml-n., calc-ar., crot-h.,*** ferr., glon., kali-br., **LACH.,** sep., ***tab.,*** tril., valer.
menses, during - agar., alum., ***arg-m.,*** aur., ***bov.,*** bufo, ***cact., croc.,*** crot-h., cupr., ***ign.,*** iod., kali-n., merl., ***nat-m.,*** nat-p., ***nit-ac., phos.,*** phys., rhus-t., sep., ***sil., spig., sulph., tab.,*** thuj.
after - agar., iod., ***nat-m.,*** nit-ac., seneg.
amel., during - eupi.
before - alum., ***cact.,*** crot-h., ***cupr.,*** eupi., ign., ***iod.,*** lach., ***lith., nat-m., sep.,*** **SPONG.,** zinc.
suppressed - ***acon.,*** bell., ***cact.,*** calc., chin., coff., cycl., ***lil-t., lyc.,*** merc., nat-m., nux-v., phos., ***puls.,*** rhus-t., sep., ***verat.***
metastasis, from - abrot., aur., cact., colch., dig., iod., kalm., lach., naja, ***phos.,*** spig., spong., sulph.
midnight - kali-n.
1 to 2 a.m. - **SPONG.**
2 a.m. - benz-ac., iber., ***kali-bi.***
3 a.m. - **ARS.,** chin., nit-ac.
4 to 5 am. - lyc.
after - spig.
wakes up - bad., benz-ac., calc., **SPONG.**
morning - agar., alum., bar-c., ***carb-an.,*** caust., chel., chin-s., ***hydr.,*** kali-c., ***kali-m.,*** **LACH.,** lyc., ***lycps., nat-m.,*** nux-v., **PHOS.,** podo., ***rhus-t., sarr.,*** sep., **SPIG.,** sulph., thuj.
7 a.m. - sol-t-ae.
bed, in - ***ign.,*** kali-c., ***rhus-t.***
breakfast, after - phos.
amel. - ***kali-c.***
waking, on - agar., alum., ***carb-an.,*** chin-s., hep., kali-c., **LACH.,** ***nat-m.,*** nux-v., phos., rhus-t., ***sep.,*** thuj.
must lie still with closed eyes - carb-an.
suddenly, after - ***kali-bi.***
motion - acon., agar., ***am-c., apoc., arg-n., arn.,*** aspar., ***aur.,*** aur-s., bell., bov., brom., cact., ***calc.,*** **CANN-S.,** ***carb-s., carb-v.,*** chin., ***cimic., cocc., con.,*** **DIG.,** ***ferr.,*** ferr-i., ferr-p., ***graph., hyos.,*** iod., jatr., kali-n., kali-p., kalm., ***lach.,*** merc., ***naja, nat-m., nit-ac.,*** **PHOS.,** ***prun.,*** **PSOR.,** sabin., ***sil.,*** sol-t-ae., **SPIG.,** ***staph., stram.,*** sulph., verat., zinc-s.
amel. - ***arg-m., arg-n.,*** glon., mag-m., par., phos., ***rhus-t.***
arms, of, agg. - ***acon.,*** am-m., bor., bry., camph., chel., ***dig.,*** ferr., led., ***naja, puls., rhus-t.,*** seneg., ***spig.,*** spong., **SULPH.,** thuj.
arms, of left, agg. - phos.
beginning to move - cact.
compelled to move - ferr.

PALPITATIONS, general

motion, every agg. - chin.

from the first movements of the child - ***sulph.***

slightest - acon., bell., ***cact., calc-ar., carb-v.,*** cimic., ***con.,*** dig., ferr., iber., ***lil-t.,*** med., ***merc.,*** nat-m., ***nit-ac.,*** **PHOS., SPIG.**

slow amel. - ferr., puls.

violent or quick, after - ***cocc., sil., spig.***

mouth, with foul odor from - spig.

music, when listening to - ***ambr.,*** carb-v., ***staph.,*** sulph.

nausea, with - arg-n., brom., olnd.

faintness with, causing her to become sick - ***arg-n.***

nervous, causes - atro., cact., ***coff.,*** glon., hydr-ac., hyos., ign., kali-c., kali-p., lil-t., ***lycps.,*** mag-p., ***mosch., naja, phos.,*** sep., spig., ***sumb.***

palpitation, with small pulse from supression of discharge in women - **ASAF.**

night - agar., alum., am-c., ***arg-m.,*** **ARG-N.,** ***ars.,*** asaf., ***aur.,*** bar-c., ***benz-ac., cact.,*** **CALC.,** ***calc-s.,*** carb-ac., coc-c., colch., dig., ***dulc.,*** ferr., ferr-ar., **FERR-I.,** ferr-p., iber., ign., ***iod.,*** kali-n., lil-t., ***lyc., merc.,*** merc-c., morg., mur-ac., nat-a., nat-c., nat-m., nit-ac., ***ox-ac.,*** petr., ***phos.,*** **PULS.,** sep., sil., sol-t-ae., ***spig., sulph., tab.,*** thea., tub., ***verat.***

11 to 3 a.m. - ***colch.***

bed, in - cact., ***ox-ac.,*** ferr., ***iod., ph-ac.,*** **PULS.,** ***rhus-t., spig.,*** **SULPH.**

pressure in pit of stomach - sulph.

waking - nat-c.

waking every half hour - ***lyc.***

noise, from every strange - agar., ***nat-c.,*** **NAT-M.,** nat-p., nat-s., phos.

noon - dig., mez., sol-t-ae., staph., sulph.

eating, before - mez.

nosebleeds, with - ***graph.***

onanism, after - ***dig., ferr., ph-ac.***

opening, eyes, on - carb-an.

painful - agar., mag-m., spong., zinc.

pains, during - acon., bov., bufo, cimic., glon., hep., ign., kali-bi., lach., nux-v., spig.

changing locality - lach.

precordial - ***acon., ars., cact.,*** caust., cham., ***coff., hydr-ac.,*** laur., mag-m., naja, ***spig.,*** spong.

shoulder, left - acon., crat.

paroxysmal - ***acon., aur., lach., lyc., mag-p.,*** merc-i-f., nat-m., nit-ac., ***nux-v., plb.,*** phos., ***puls.***

periodic - aesc., chel., colch., thuj.

perspiration, during - jab., merc., spong., tab., verat.

cold, with - am-c.

preaching, agg. - naja.

pregnancy, during - ***arg-m., con., laur.,*** **LIL-T.,** ***nat-m., sep.,*** sulph.

pressure, with the hand amel. - ***arg-n.***

puberty agg. - aur.

PALPITATIONS, general

pulsations through the body, with - sabad.

pulse, very frequent, with (see Pulse) - olnd., thyr.

irregular, with - cact., dig.

slow, with - lyc., verat.

soft, with - iber.

raising, arms, on - dig., ***spig., sulph.***

red face, with - agar., aur., bell., glon.

relaxation, with yawning, after - lyc.

rest, during - lil-t., ***mag-m.***

riding in a wagon - ***arg-n.,*** aur., cact.

amel. - ***nit-ac., rhus-t.***

rising, on - ***bry.,*** cact., con., ***dig.,*** ferr-i., kali-n., sulph.

bed, from - ars., colch., ***con., lach.,*** **PHOS.**

seat - brom., ***cact.,*** ferr-i., ***lach.,*** mag-m., **PHOS.**

roused, on being suddenly - chin-s.

sex, during - ***calc.,*** crot-t., ***lyc., ph-ac.,*** **PHOS.,** ***visc.***

after - am-c., ***dig., sep.***

sexual, excesses, after - coca, sec.

excitement - ***ph-ac.***

sighing, amel. - **ARG-M.**

singing, in church, while - carb-an.

sitting, while - agar., ***ang.,*** **ASAF.,** ***aspar.,*** benz-ac., ***carb-v.,*** coloc., ***ferr.,*** ferr-p., gins., ***lach., mag-m.,*** nat-c., phos., ***rhus-t., sil.,*** **SPIG.**

amel. - ars., cact., ***lach.***

bent - ang., dig., kalm., ***rhus-t.,*** spig.

forward - kalm.

eating, after - ***phos.***

erect amel. - kalm.

up, agg. - ***colch., phos.***

up, amel. - asaf., ***cact., lach.***

sleep, during - alst., am-c., ***aur., calc., cann-i.,*** ferr-i., iber., kali-bi., kalm., ***merc., merc-c.,*** morg-g., ***nat-c.,*** ph-ac., phos., ***sep.,*** spong., sulph., zinc.

nap, during - calc.

on going to - ***calc., carb-v.,*** colch., ***lach., nat-m.,*** phos., sil., **SULPH.**

sleepiness, with - cimic.

sleeplessness, with - cimic., coca, ***ign.,*** spig.

smokers, in - calad., lycps.

soreness of uterus, with - conv.

speak, unable to - **NAJA.**

spoken to off his loss, when - gels.

standing, while - agar., aur-m-n., cact., dig., ***ferr.,*** kali-n., ***lach., nat-m.,*** sil.

a long time - alumn.

stiff, as if - aur-m.

stool, during - ***ant-t.,*** cycl., nit-ac., petr., ***sulph.***

after - ***agar.,*** **ARS.,** caust., **CON.,** grat.

loose, with - ant-t.

stooping - ang., cact., ***nat-c., cann-s., spig., sul-ac.,*** thyr.

startles, from sleep - petr., ph-ac., phos.

stretching - phos.

upper limbs - cocc.

PALPITATIONS, general
sudden - ***bar-c.,*** lyc., ***mang.,*** mosch., ***stry.***
sun, heat of, agg. - coff., glon., spig.
supper, after - cupr., ***lyc., ph-ac.,*** **PULS.**, rumx.
suppressed, eruptions, after - ***ars., calc.***
surprise, after - ***coff.***
swallowing - sol-t-ae.
talking - **NAJA,** plat., ***puls.,*** rumx.
before, in public - acon., gels., lyc., plat.
impossible - naja.
tea drinking, from - arg-n., chin.
thinking, of it - alum., alumn., ***arg-n., aur-m.,*** bad., ***bar-c.,*** cact., ***gels.,*** ign., ***lycps., ox-ac.,*** sumb.
about his wrongs - iod.
throat, extending to - graph., ***nat-m., spong.***
thunderstorm - ***nat-p., phos.***
thyroid, toxicosis, in - dys-co.
tobacco, from - acon., agar., ars., cact., ***calad., gels.,*** ign., ***nux-v.,*** phos., spong., stroph., thuj.
tremulous - ***ars., calc., cocc.,*** lyc., ***mang., plb.,*** staph.
trembling, with - acon., ars., asaf., benz-ac., cact., calc-ar., gels., lach., nat-m., rhus-t., sulph.
tumultuous, violent, vehement - abies-c., absin., acon., aesc., ***aeth., agar.,*** alum., alumn., ambr., ***am-c., aml-n.,*** ammc., ***ang., ant-c., apis,*** **ARG-N.**, ***ars.,*** ars-i., ***aur., aur-m.,*** bapt., bar-c., bell., ***bism.,*** bry., ***cact.,*** **CALC.**, ***calc-ar.,*** cann-i., carb-ac., ***carb-s., carb-v.,*** carc., ***chel., chin., chin-a.,*** cimic., ***coca,*** coc-c., coff., ***colch., con.,*** conv., cop., ***crot-t.,*** cupr., cupr-s., ***cycl.,*** **DIG.**, ***ferr-m.,*** gels., grat., ***guai.,*** **GLON.**, helo., hep., hell., hyos., iber., **IOD.,** kali-ar., **KALI-C.**, kali-chl., ***kali-i., kali-n., kali-p.,*** kali-s., ***kalm., lach.,*** lachn., ***lil-t., lob., lycps., lyss.,*** mag-aust., morph., ***naja,*** nat-a., nat-c., **NAT-M.,** ***nux-m., olnd.,*** ox-ac., ***phos.,*** phys., ***plb.,*** prun., ***plat.,*** **PULS.**, pyrog., rhus-t., rumx., sec., seneg., **SEP.**, ***spig., spong., staph.,*** stram., stry., ***sulph.,*** tab., ***tarent.,*** tell., thuj., upa., ***verat., verat-v.,*** viol-o., vesp., yohim.
and excitement of mind - asaf.
turning, in bed - cact., ***dig., ferr-i., lach., lyc., manc., naja, phos.,*** **SULPH.**
in bed to right side - alum.
unrequited, affections, from - ***cact., ign.,*** **NAT-M.**, ***ph-ac.***
urina, spastica - coff.
urination, with copious - coff.
affections, of heart, with - laur.
uterine disease, with - conv., lil-t.
uterus, with soreness of - conv.
vertigo, with - adon., aeth., cact., cocc., conv., cori-r., ***iber.,*** sil., spig., tub.
throat, choking, with - iber.

PALPITATIONS, general
vexation, from - acon., agar., arg-n., ***aur-m.,*** **CHAM.,** coloc., ***ign.,*** iod., lyc., ***nat-m., nux-v.,*** petr., ***phos.,*** **SEP.**, staph., verat.
violent - arg-n., calc., ***crat.,*** dig., **GLON.,** iod., kali-c., ***lycps.,*** mur-ac., nat-m., ***puls.,*** sep.
visible - ant-t., ***ars., aur.,*** bov., cann-s., ***carb-s.,*** **CARB-V.**, chel., com., con., dulc., glon., ***graph., iod., kalm., lach.,*** naja, petr., ***puls.,*** sep., **SPIG.**, ***staph., sulph.,*** thuj., ***verat.***
apex beat through clothing - mag-p.
vision, with dim - puls.
vomiting, with - olnd.
waking, on - acon., agar., ***alum.,*** aran-s., ***ars., benz-ac., bufo, calc., cann-i., carb-an.,*** chin-s., colch., con., eupi., hep., ign., kali-bi., kali-c., kali-i., kali-n., **LACH.**, **NAJA,** nat-c., ***nat-m.,*** nit-ac., ***ox-ac.,*** petr., **PHOS.**, plat., rhus-t., ***sep., sil.,*** spong., staph., thuj., zinc.
lying on, left side, from - chin-s., ***phos.***
menses, before - alum.
startled, from a dream - ***acon.,*** dig., eupi., merc., rad., rhus-t., sil., ***sulph.,*** zinc.
suddenly - acon., anan., chin-s., con., dios., ***kali-bi., merc.,*** sec.
walking - acon., ***apoc.,*** arg-n., aur., **AUR-M.**, brom., ***cact.,*** calc., chel., chin., dig., ***iod., kali-i.,*** lyc., merc., **NAJA,** nit-ac., phos., psor., seneg., ***sep.,*** spig., ***staph.***
air, in open - ambr., chel., lyc., ***nux-v.,*** plat., ***sep.,*** sulph., thuj.
long, distances amel. - ***sep.***
amel. - ***arg-n., ferr.,*** gels., glon., ***mag-m., nux-m., rhus-t.***
eating, after - phos.
rapidly - **AUR-M.,** bufo, euphr., ferr., ferr-p., **IOD.**, kalm., ***nat-m., ph-ac., phos., puls.,*** **SEP.**, thuj.
amel. - ***arg-n., sep.***
slowly - ***nit-ac.***
walking, slowly, amel. - ***ferr., puls.***
warm, bath agg. - ***iod., lach.***
drinks amel. - nux-m.
room - ***lach.,*** puls.
soup - ***lach., phos., puls.***
water, in, as if - bov., sumb.
weakness, with - hydr.
empty feeling in - olnd.
heart, of - coca, ***crat.,*** dig., phos.
wine - ***naja, nux-v.***
woman, on seeing a - ***puls.***
worms, from - spig.
writing - ferr-p., nat-c., upa.
yawning, with - calc.

PARALYSIS - acon., ***ant-t.,*** ars., ars-i., ***bell., bufo,*** cann-i., **CARB-V.**, cimic., chlor., ***crot-h., cupr., dig., gels., hydr-ac., iod.,*** **LACH.**, **NAJA**, **OP.**, ox-ac., ***phos., plb.,*** sang., sumb., verat., verat-v.

PERICARDITIS - **ACON.,** adon., anac., ant-a., ***ant-t., apis,*** apoc., **ARS.,** ***ars-i., asc-t.,*** bell., ***bry., cact.,*** cann-s., ***canth.,*** chlor., ***cimic., colch., dig., iod.,*** kali-ar., ***kali-c.,*** kali-chl., ***kali-i., kalm., lach.,*** magn-gr., ***merc.,*** merc-c., naja, nat-m., ox-ac., phase., plat., **PSOR., SPIG.,** ***spong.,*** squil., **SULPH.,** ***verat., verat-v.***
  chronic - apis, ***aur-i.,*** calc-f., kali-c., spig., squil., sulph.
  lying amel. - ***psor.***
  rheumatic - acon., anac., bry., colch., colchin., crat., kalm., rhus-t., ***spig.***

PLUG, sensation of, at - ran-s.

PRESSING, pain - acon., agar., ambr., ant-t., ***arg-n., arn.,*** **ARS.,** ***asaf.,*** **AUR., AUR-M.,** bell., bov., ***bry.,*** **CACT.,** ***calc.,*** cann-i., carb-an., card-m., ***cench.,*** cham., chin-s., coc-c., colch., coll., con., cycl., ***eup-per., glon., graph.,*** grat., ***hydr-ac.,*** hyos., hyper., iod., kali-bi., kali-c., ***kalm., lac-d.,*** **LACH.,** ***lil-t.,*** lith., lyc., ***lycps.,*** lyss., manc., nat-c., ***nat-m.,*** nat-s., ***nux-v.,*** olnd., ol-an., pall., petr., ***phos.,*** plb., ***puls., rhus-t.,*** sang., sec., ***seneg.,*** sep., sil., ***spig., spong.,*** stram., stront-c., ***tarent.,*** thuj., verat., vip., zinc., zing.
  ascending stairs - **AUR., AUR-M.**
  breathing - graph.
  below heart - lyc.
  eating, after - ***kali-bi., lil-t.,*** lyc.
  evening - **PULS.,** sulph., thuj.
    in bed - ***nat-m.***
  forenoon - thuj.
  lying, when - kali-bi.
  menses, during - ***arg-n.***
    instead of - cham.
  morning - ***lith.,*** nat-m.
  night - ***arg-n.,*** cann-i., coc-c.
  pressure of hand amel. - ***nat-m.***
  standing - aur-m-n.
  urination, during - lith.
    after, amel. - ***nat-m.***
  walking - arg-n., seneg.
    amel. - colch., puls.

PULSATION - lyc., sulph.
  morning in bed - graph.

PURRING, feeling in region of - caust., glon., iod., pyrog., ***spig.***

RHEUMATIC, pain in - ***abrot.,*** acon., am-c., anac., ant-t., apis, ***arg-n.,*** ars., **AUR.,** aur-m., ***benz-ac., cact., cimic.,*** cocc., ***colch., crot-h.,*** dig., gels., guai., ***kali-ar., kali-c., kalm., lach., led.,*** **LITH.,** ***lycps.,*** **NAJA,** phyt., ***puls., rhus-t.,*** sac-alb., ***sang., sep.,*** **SPIG.,** ***spong.***

SHARP, pain - abies-n., ***abrot., acon.,*** aesc., agar., alumn., am-c., ***anac.,*** anan., **APIS,** ***arg-m., arn.,*** ars., ars-m., asc-t., aur., aur-m., bell., berb., brach., **BRY.,** bufo, ***cact., calc.,*** calc-ar., ***calc-p.,*** camph., cann-i., ***canth.,*** caps., carb-ac., carb-s., carb-v., card-m., **CAUST.,** cer-b., ***cham., chel.,*** chin., chin-a., ***cimic., clem.,*** coc-c., ***colch., coloc.,*** crot-t., ***cupr., cycl.,*** daph., dig., dios., euphr., gels., ***glon.,*** graph., ***ham.,*** helo., ***hep., hydr.,*** hyos., iber., ign., iodof., jac-c., kali-bi., ***kali-c., kali-i.,*** kali-n., kali-p., kali-s., **KALM.,** ***kreos.,***

SHARP, pain - **LACH.,** lachn., ***laur.,*** lith., ***lyc.,*** lycps., ***lyss.,*** mag-c., **MAG-M.,** manc., med., meny., merc-i-f., merc-i-r., ***mur-ac.,*** myric., **NAJA,** nat-c., nat-m., nit-ac., ox-ac., par., paeon., **PETR.,** ph-ac., phos., plat., plb., podo., **PSOR.,** ***puls., ran-b., ran-s., rhus-t.,*** rhus-v., sabin., sang., sep., sin-n., **SPIG., SPONG., STAPH., SULPH.,** sul-ac., tarent., thuj., trom., valer., verb., viol-t., vip., ***zinc.***
  afternoon - sep.
  apex to base, from - med.
  back to clavicle and shoulder, from - spig.
  base to apex, at night - syph.
  bending, double - anac.
    forward while sitting - viol-t.
  burning - anan., ***mur-ac.***
  coughing, from - agar., mez., nat-m.
  drinking, after - chin.
  eating, after - aspar.
  evening - dios., lyss., mur-ac., nat-c., rhus-t., verb.
    sleep, on going to - mez.
  expiration - crot-t., ign., zinc.
  extending to
    axilla - mur-ac.
    back - agar., am-c., ***anac., glon., kali-c.,*** mur-ac.
    right lower lung - alumn.
    scapula, left - agar., ***kali-c., kalm.,*** paeon., rumx., **SULPH.**
    shoulder, down left, into arm and fingers - ***acon.,*** arn., asper., bism., ***cact.,*** cimic., crot-h., ***kalm., lat-m.,*** lepi., naja, ***ox-ac., rhus-t., spig.,*** tab.
    stomach - lyc.
    within-out - clem.
  fainting, with - arn.
  forenoon - acon.
  inspiration, on - aesc., anac., ***calc-p., chel.,*** crot-t., laur., mag-m., nat-c., plb.
    deep, agg. - ***acon.,*** aesc., agar., aur-m., ***calc.,*** con., mez., ***mur-ac., ran-b., sulph.***
    deep, amel. - cann-i.
  lying, while - rumx., verb.
    amel. - ***psor.***
    left side - camph., kali-c., lyc.
    on back - ***sulph.***
    only on the right side, can lie - **SPIG.**
    only on the right side, can lie, with the head high - **SPIG.**
  menses, during - ***con.***
  morning, rising, after - nux-v., zinc.
    waking, after - mez.
  motion agg. - aur-m., cham., con., ***ran-b.,*** **SPIG.,** ***sulph.***
  night - aur-m., mag-m., ***mez.,*** nit-ac., ***sulph.***
  noon - verat-v.
  numbness and lameness of left arm - ***rhus-t.***
  periodical - ***spig.***
  pressure of hand amel. - aur-m., ***puls.***
  reading aloud, while - ***calc.,*** nat-m.
  respiration, during - anac., ***calc.,*** mag-m., ***spig., staph.***
  ringing of a church bell - lyss.

SHARP, pain
rubbing amel. - mur-ac.
sitting, while - rhus-t.
sleep, during - aur-m.
sneezing - mez.
stooping - glon.
straightening up difficult - mur-ac.
synchronous with beat of heart - dig., iber., ***rhus-t.,*** **SPIG.,** zinc.
talking - carb-an.
waking, on - fago.
walking - acon., ***kali-i., lyss.,*** nat-m.
air, in open - nat-m.
amel. - puls., rhus-t.
wiping arms agg. - apis.

SHOCKS, region of the, belching agg. - agar.
coughing agg. - agar.
noise, from, sudden - agar.

SMOTHERED, heart as if - stroph., thyr.

SORE, pain - acon., **APIS, ARN.,** bapt., **BAR-C.,** calc-ar., ***cact.,*** camph., cann-i., ***cench., cimic., crot-h., fl-ac., gels.,*** haem., hyos., kali-bi., lach., laur., lept., lil-t., ***lith., lycps., mag-c.,*** med., ***naja, nat-m.,*** ox-ac., puls., sec., ***spig.,*** sul-ac., tab.
foot sweat, suppressed, agg. - aur., bar-c.

SPACE, as if in too small a - eup-per.

SQUEEZING sensation - ***acon.,*** adon., aml-n., arn., ars., bor., **CACT.,** cadm-s., calc-ar., coc-c., colch., ***iod.,*** iodof., kali-c., lach., laur., ***lil-t.,*** lycps., lyss., mag-p., magn-gr., nux-m., ptel., spong., ***thyr.***

STAGNATION, as if - lyc., sabad., zinc.

STRAIN of the heart from violent exertion, as if heart had been strained - ant-t., arn.

SUSPENDED, feels, thread, by a - kali-c., lach.

SWELLING, as if - ang., asaf., cimic., ***glon., lach.,*** pyrog., sep., ***spong.,*** sulph., thlaspi.

SYSTOLE, extra - dys-co.

TEARING, pain, region of - am-m., ars., bell., ***cact.,*** cer-b., cimic., clem., colch., crot-t., daph., elaps, glon., hyos., ***iber., kalm.,*** lach., **LAT-M.,** lil-t., lith., ***lyc.,*** mag-c., magn-gr., menthol, ***ox-ac.,*** paeon., phyt., ***spig.,*** syph., tab., ***ther.,*** thuj.

THREAD, torn loose and swinging by, heart - dig.

TREMBLING, from excitement - lith.
sadness, as from - nux-m.

UNDULATION of, sense of, warm - rhod.

UNSTEADINESS of - tab.

VACUUM, as if beating in a - nux-m.

VALVULAR disease, with murmurs - acon., ***adon.,*** apoc., ***ars.,*** ars-i., aur., aur-br., aur-i., ***bar-c., cact.,*** calc., calc-f., camph., ***conv., crat., dig.,*** ferr., gala., ***glon.,*** iod., ***kali-c.,*** kalm., lach., laur., lith., ***lycps.,*** **NAJA,** ox-ac., phos., plb., ***puls.,*** rhus-t., sang., ser-ang., ***spig., spong.,*** stigm., ***stroph., tarent.,*** thyr., visc., zinc-i.

VALVULAR disease, with murmurs
incompetent - cact., crat., kali-c., spong.
mitral and tricuspidal regurgitation - apoc., cact., laur., psor., stroph.

WEAKNESS, of - adon., adren., aether, agarin., ***alco.,*** aml-n., ant-t., ***apoc.,*** atro., camph., ***cocaine, coffin.,*** conv., **CRAT.,** ***dig., digin., glon.,*** sac-alb., saroth., ser-ang., stroph., ***stry-s.,*** thyr., verat.
metrorrhagia, during - am-m., dig.
smoking, from - scut.

weakness, sensation, about the heart - am-c., ant-c., ant-t., arn., ***ars-i., aur., aur-m.,*** calc., carb-v., colch., ***crat.,*** crot-h., gels., graph., hell., kali-bi., kali-c., kali-fer., lach., lil-t., lob., ***merc.,*** **NAJA, NUX-V.,** op., ***ph-ac.,*** phos., pyrog., ***rhus-t.,*** sang., stroph., sumb., thuj., verat., zinc-i.
lung troubles, chronic, after - ars-i.
sinking, cold and dyspnea at 3 a.m. - ***am-c.***

Hips

ACHING, pain - **AESC.,** ail., bapt., bry., carb-ac., carb-an., ***caust.,*** dios., eup-per., gamb., ham., lyss., med., merc-i-f., mosch., ***phos., phyt.,*** puls., ***rhus-t.,*** staph., still., tab., tarent.
- dinner, after - kali-bi.
- evening - dios.
- extending, along sciatic nerve - carb-an.
  - to ankle - aesc., merc-i-r., plan.
- menses, before - lach.
- morning - aesc.
  - rising amel. - phos.
- night, waking, on - puls-n
- sitting, while - eup-per., ***rhus-t.,*** sabad., staph., verat.
- stooping - gent-l.
- waking, on - hep.
- walking, while - ham., staph.

BOILS - alum., am-c., bar-c., graph., hep., jug-r., lyc., ***nit-ac., ph-ac.,*** rat., sabin.

BORING, pain - arn., ***coloc.,*** kali-i., ***kreos.,*** lil-t., ***mez.,*** rhod.
- gluteal muscles - merc., staph.
- night - ***kali-i.***
  - 4 a.m. - ***coloc.***

BROKEN, sensation as if - ph-ac., zing.

BUBBLING, sensation - ***led.***

BURNING, pain - ***ars.,*** arund., arum-m., bell., berb., ***carb-v.,*** caust., cur., ***euph.,*** gels., hell., iod., ***kali-c.,*** kali-n., kreos., lith., mag-m., nicc., rhus-t., tarent., valer., ***zinc.***
- afternoon - mag-m.
- bending, to painful side agg. - mag-c.
- evening - mag-m., nicc.
  - after lying down - mag-m.
  - scratching - mag-m., nicc.
- extending to shoulder - mag-c.
  - to heel - arund.
- external - aur-m-n., carb-v.
- gluteal muscles - agar., euphr.
  - right - euphr.
- itching - lith.
- joints - iris, kali-n., nux-v.
  - tearing - kali-n.
- menses, during - med.
  - before - ***kali-c.***
- motion, amel. - kali-c.
- night - bell., ***euph.,*** mag-m.
- noon - nicc.
  - after scratching - nicc.
- prickling - caust.
- rest, during - kali-n.
- spots - rhus-t.

CHILLINESS - calc-p., ham.

COLDNESS - agar., bell., bry., carb-v., caust., gad., gran., ham., hura, kali-bi., merc., merl., mez., morph., rhus-t., tax., ther., thuj., valer.
- morning, 9 a.m. - ham.
- left - carb-v., caust., thuj.
- right - bell., bry., kali-bi., merl., rhus-t.

COMPRESSION, sensation - tarent.

CONSTRICTION - anac., ang., ***coloc.,*** eug., lyc.

CONTRACTION, of muscles and tendons - am-m., carb-v., coloc., euph., meny.

CONVULSION - phos.

CRACKING, joints, in - aloe, anac., calc., ***camph., cocc., croc.,*** glon., nat-m., rhus-t.
- morning on rising - aloe.

CRAMPS - ***ang.,*** arg-m., aur., bell., cann-s., carb-an., carb-v., caust., cimic., coloc., cop., cur., jug-c., nat-m., ***ph-ac., phos.,*** ruta., ***sep.,*** sul-ac., valer.
- eating, while - ph-ac.
- gluteal muscles - agar., bell., gels., hyos., ***hyper.***
- labor, during - ***cimic.***
- left - jug-c.
- menses, during - form.
- night - jug-c., sep.
- right - sul-ac.
- sitting, while - ph-ac.
- walking - carb-an., sep.

CUTTING, pain - agn., alum., berb., ***bry.,*** calc., dig., gamb., gins., graph., ***ign.,*** kali-bi., lyc., mur-ac., nat-s., ***phyt.,*** tell.
- extending into abdomen - gins.
- left - kali-i.
- motion, on - lyc.
- right - agn.
- sitting, while - calc.mur-ac.

DISCOLORATION, hips
- blackness - crot-h.
- redness - lac-ac., ph-ac., rhus-t., vip.
  - in spots - lac-ac., rhus-t.
  - in spots, hot - rhus-t.
  - stripes, extending to umbilicus - ph-ac.

DISLOCATION, feeling - agar., am-c., ang., bry., ***caust.,*** chel., con., dulc., fl-ac., hura, ***ign.,*** ip., kreos. laur., mag-m., merc., mosch., osm., pall., psor., **PULS.,** sanic., sulph., thuj., zinc.
- left - chel., dulc., hura, ***kreos.,*** laur., pall., sulph.
- right - agar., con., thuj.
- sitting, while - ***ip.***
- stepping - ***caust.,*** psor., sulph.

dislocation, spontaneous - ***aesc.,*** bell., bry., **CALC., CALC-F.,** ***caust., coloc.,*** lyc., puls., ***rhus-t., ruta,*** sulph., ***thuj.,*** zinc.
- pain, from - aesc., bry., carb-an., dros., kali-i., nit-ac.
- sitting down, on - ip.

DRAWING, pain - acon., aeth., am-c., am-m., ***ant-c.,*** arg-m., ***arg-n., arn., ars.,*** asar., aster., aur., bapt., benz-ac., bry., ***calc.,*** calc-p., ***caps., carb-an., carb-s., carb-v.,*** caust., cham., **CHEL.,** chin., cinnb., ***cocc.,*** coc-c., colch., ***coloc., con.,*** crot-h., ***dig., dulc.,*** ferr-ma., gels., hell., ***hep., kali-bi., led.,*** lil-t., lyc., mang., meph., naja, nat-c., ***nat-m.,*** nat-p., ***nit-ac.,*** par., petr., ph-ac., ***phyt.,*** plat., plb., **PULS.,** ran-b., rhod., ***rhus-t.,*** ruta., ***sep.,*** sil., spig., stann., ***stront-c., sulph.,*** ter., ther., ***thuj.,*** til., verat., **ZINC.**
- afternoon - chel., sulph.

DRAWING, pain
bending, body backward - ***caps.***
leg back - ant-c.
burning - til.
coryza, during - sep.
cramp-like - aur., ***coloc.,*** plat., verat.
drawing back the leg - ferr-ma.
evening - ***ant-c.,*** ran-b., ther.
walking, while - ant-c., calc., crot-h., ran-b.
extending, downward - aeth., am-c., cann-s., ***carb-an.,*** carb-s., ***carb-v.,*** cinnb., crot-h., kali-bi., lil-t., nat-m., ***puls., rhus-t.,*** sep., ther., thuj.
inward - thuj.
to foot - thuj.
to knee - rhus-t.
to sacrum - ant-c., stann.
to right side - stann.
forenoon - sulph.
gluteal muscles - camph., cycl., gels., mosch., ***sulph.,*** verat.
left - ***acon.,*** aeth., ***am-m.,*** **ANT-C.,** stann., ***sulph.***
lying, on painful side, amel. - ferr-ma.
with leg flexed, amel. - ***coloc.***
menses, during - nit-ac.
morning - ars., colch., stront.
motion, on - ***acon.,*** gels., sep.
amel. - ***arg-m.,*** lil-t., **RHUS-T.,** ther.
preventing - sil.
move, on beginning to - nit-ac.
night - ***coloc.***
paroxysmal - arg-m., cocc., coloc., zing.
pressure, amel. - ***bry.***
rheumatic - lyc., meph., ***rhod., rhus-t.***
right - ***chel.,*** kali-bi., lil-t., nit-ac., sep., ther.
rising from a seat - nit-ac.
sitting, while - caust., chin., **RHUS-T.,** ther.
with thigh extended - ***arn.***
spots, in - til.
standing, while - verat.
amel. - chin.
sticking - arg-m., clem.
touch agg. - ***caps.***
twitching - colch., sil.
walking, while - ***am-m., ant-c.,*** asar., bry., calc., ***carb-v.,*** caust., coloc., ***hep.,*** ran-b., ***sulph.***
amel. - chin., cinnb., ***rhus-t.,*** ther.
wandering - bry.

EMACIATION - calc.

ERUPTIONS - ***nat-c.,*** nicc., osm.
pimples - hyper.
vesicular - calc.

FISTULOUS, hips, openings - ***calc., carb-v., caust.,*** **LACH.,** ***ph-ac.,*** **PHOS.,** ***sil.***

GNAWING, pain - am-c., ***am-m.,*** benz-ac., ***elat.,*** **EUP-PUR.,** ***kali-i.,*** pall.
night - ***kali-i.***
sitting, when - am-m.

GURGLING, left - sep.
near the - sep.

HEAT - ***chel.,*** phos., rhus-t., zinc.

HEAVINESS - agar., all-c., ***alum.,*** ant-t., ars-m., ***con.,*** kali-c., kreos., mag-m., mag-s., nat-a., ph-ac., sars.
walking amel. - ph-ac.

HERPES - ***nat-c.,*** nicc., ***sep.***

HIP-joint, disease, (see Suppuration) - acon., **AESC.,** am-c., anac., ***ang.,*** apis, ***arg-m.,*** arn., ***ars.,*** ars-i., ***asaf.,*** asar., ***aur., bell., bry.,*** **CALC., CALC-P.,** ***calc-s., canth., caps.,*** carb-ac., carb-s., ***carb-v.,*** **CARD-M.,** ***caust., cham.,*** **CHIN.,** chin-a., cist., colch., **COLOC.,** dig., ***fl-ac.,*** graph., hecla., ***hep.,*** hippoz., hydr., iod., iris, **KALI-C.,** ***kali-i., kali-p.,*** **KALI-S.,** lac-c., ***lach., lyc., merc., nat-m.,*** nat-s., ***nit-ac., nux-v., ol-j., petr.,*** **PH-AC.,** ***phos., phyt., puls., rhus-t.,*** sep., **SIL., STRAM.,** staph., ***sulph.,*** **TUB.**
left - ***stram.***
right - **LED.,** ***phyt.***

INFLAMMATION, of joints - aesc., apis., rhus-t., ruta.

INJURIES - **AESC., ARN.,** ***bry., calc-p.,*** con., ***rhus-t.,*** ruta, sil., tarent.

ITCHING - agar., alum., aur., ***bov.,*** bry., caust., chel., dig., dios., lach., led., mag-c., mag-m., merc., nat-c., nat-m., nat-p., nicc., osm., ph-ac., phos., puls., sars., ***sep.,*** sulph., zinc.
burning - chel.
after scratching - mag-c.
corrosive - led.
evening - mag-m., nicc., zinc.
evening, before lying down - mag-m.
gluteal region - coloc., fl-ac., mur-ac., ph-ac., tarax.
morning - alumn.
becoming cool agg. - dios.
noon - nicc.
region of - mag-c.
spots, in - osm.
standing - mag-c.
stinging - dios., led.
tuber ischiadicum - agar.
walking, while - chel.
warm in bed - ***sulph.***

JERKING, pain - ***ars.,*** cann-s., graph., mag-c., ***pall., puls.,*** valer.
joint, in - bell., nux-v., puls., sulph.
hips - sulph.
sciatica, in - ***kali-bi.***

LAMENESS - abrot., aesc., am-m., ammc., ars-m., bry., calc-p., cocc., dios., euph., fl-ac., rhus-t., ***ruta,*** sars., zing.
afternoon, 2 p.m. - dios.
bathing, while - ars-m.
left - am-m., ***fl-ac.***
rising from a seat, after - ars-m.

LAMENESS, of
stepping - euph.
walking, amel. - ars-m.
walking, while - dios., euph.

NUMBNESS - agar., ***apis,*** ars-m., bapt., calc., rhus-t., staph.
extending to abdomen, while standing - sulph.

PAIN, hips - abrot., ***acon.,*** act-sp., adeps., ***aesc., agar.,*** ail., alum., am-c., am-m., ammc., anac., ***anag.,*** ant-t., apis, ***arg-m., arn.,*** **ARS.,** ***ars-i.,*** arum-t., asar., asc-t., aster., ***aur.,*** bad., bapt., ***bar-c., bell.,*** benz-ac., ***berb.,*** bov., brom., ***bry.,*** **CALC.,** ***calc-p., calc-s.,*** cann-i., ***canth.,*** carb-ac., ***carb-an.,*** carb-s., **CARD-M.,** ***caust.,*** cham., **CHEL.,** cimx., ***cimic.,*** cinnb., clem., cocc., coff., **COLCH., COLOC.,** con., cop., ***crot-t.,*** cupr., dig., dios., dros., euon., ***euph.,*** fago., ***ferr., ferr-i., fl-ac.,*** form., gels., grat., gran., ham., helon., **HEP.,** hura, ***hydr.,*** hyper., ***indg., iod.,*** jug-c., ***kali-ar., kali-bi., kali-c., kali-i.,*** kali-n., ***kali-p., kali-s., kalm., kreos.,*** lac-c., ***lac-d., lach.,*** **LED.,** ***lil-t.,*** lith., lob-s., ***lyc., lyss.,*** mag-c., mag-s., ***med., merc.,*** merc-i-f., merc-i-r., mez., ***murx.,*** nat-a., ***nat-h.,*** nat-m., ***nat-s.,*** nux-m., ox-ac., pall., ***ph-ac., phos.,*** phys., ***phyt.,*** plat., plb., plumbg., podo., prun., psor., ptel., **PULS.,** rhod., **RHUS-T.,** rhus-v., ruta., sabad., sabin., sang., ***sars.,*** seneg., ***sep.,*** **SIL.,** sin-n., stann., staph., **STRAM.,** ***sulph.,*** tarent., tax., tell., ter., ***thuj.,*** til., trom., ust., ***valer., verat.,*** verat-v., xan., zing.
after-pains - ***sil.***
afternoon - abrot., agar., chel., naja, sulph.
1 p.m. - hura.
3 p.m. - ***lach.***
alternating, from hip to hip - **LAC-C.,** verat.
ascending, steps - bry., nat-s., ***plb.,*** podo., rhus-t., thuj., verb.
bed, going to - fl-ac.
bending, trunk, backwards - caps., ***puls.***
right, to - ***rhus-t.***
blow, as from - kali-c.
childbirth, during - ***cimic.***
chill, during - arn., calc., lyc., nux-v., rhus-t., sep.
confinement, after - **HYPER.**
coughing, on - arg-m., bell., **CAUST.,** rhus-t., sulph., ***valer.***
crossing, limbs - all-s.
daytime - kali-bi., lyss.
eating, while - ph-ac.
after - ***indg.***
evening - agar., ant-c., aster., dios., fago., ***ferr., kali-bi.,*** merc-i-r., phos., ***tarent.,*** ther., valer.
9 p.m. - erig.
walking, while - ant-c., con., crot-h., erig., ran-b.
exertion, after - **CALC., RHUS-T.**
extending to, back - fago., rhus-t.
to, downward - am-c., bar-c., ***indg.,*** **KALM.,** ***med.,*** merc-i-r., plan., rhus-t.
extending to, feet - berb., cact., fago., lach., lyc., mag-p.
to, groin - anac., phys.
to, heel - ars-m., ***kali-i.***
to, hepatic region - grat.

PAIN, hips
extending to, hip to hip - thuj., ust.
to, knees - arg-n., bar-c., caps., carb-ac., coloc., ***hydr., kali-bi., kali-c., kalm.,*** lach., ***med., nat-s.,*** nux-m., nux-v., ***ph-ac.,*** puls., rhus-t., rhus-v., ***sep.,*** xan.
to, leg, in front of - dios., ***phyt.***
to, sacrum - ant-c., lyss.
to, testes - staph.
to, thigh - am-m., kreos., lil-t.
to, toes - ***kalm.,*** nat-a.
fall, as from a - arg-m.
flexing, leg - stann.
flexing leg amel. - kali-bi.
forenoon - equis., kali-n., prun.
gluteal, region (see Pelvis, Pain, buttocks) - am-m., eup-per., euphr., hura, kalm., laur., lepi., med., nit-ac., puls., rhus-t., sol-t-ae., spig., tab.
sitting, while - am-m., sulph.
after - laur., puls.
sleep, during - am-m.
walking - spig., tab.
gouty - bell., graph., ***led., nit-ac.,*** petr.
instrumental delivery, from - hyper.
jerking - kali-bi., ***lyc.,*** mag-m., **MEZ.,** ***puls.,*** sil., ***sulph.***
of limbs - ***lyc.***
laughing - arg-m.
left - ***acon.,*** agn., ***am-m.,*** ant-c., arg-n., ars-m., benz-ac., brom., **CAUST.,** cocc., eup-per., laur., lyc., ***nat-s.,*** onos., pall., sang., ***sanic., stram.,*** sulph., xan., zinc.
lying on right side, when - bell., ***cham.***
lying - coloc., kali-i., murx., plb., ***valer.***
after - acon.
down - lyc.
on hip - ars-m., bapt., caust., kali-bi., rhod., **RHUS-T.,** verat-v.
on opposite side - bell., cham.
on painful side amel. - bell., ***coloc.,*** ferr-ma.
on side - **RHUS-T.,** prun.
menses, during - ***calc.,*** cop., ***graph.,*** sep., tarent.
before - calc., ***cimic.,*** lach., sars., thuj., ust.
morning - aesc., agar., am-c., aster., coloc., dios., ferr-ma., fl-ac., lyc., **RHUS-T.,** sabin., staph., stront.
5 a.m. - verat.
in bed - ***puls.***
rising, amel. - phos.
waking, on - am-c., kali-n., ***med.***
motion, on - acon., agar., agn., all-s., arg-m., ***carb-s., coloc.,*** euph., fl-ac., gels., helon., kali-bi., ***kalm., lac-c., led.,*** mag-c., merc., ***nat-s., nux-v.,*** sanic., sep., ***sulph.,*** zinc.
amel. - arg-m., ferr., ***gels.,*** lil-t., ***lyc.,*** nat-a., ***puls., rhus-t., valer.***
motion, on bed, in - ***agar.,*** nat-s., sulph., valer.
move, beginning to - ***caust.,*** con., ***ferr., lyc., ph-ac., puls., rhus-t.,*** sabin.

PAIN, hips

night - am-m., bell., cham., ***coloc.,*** euph., ferr., ferr-ma., kali-bi., ***kali-c., kali-i.,*** lach., merc., nat-s., petr., prun., ***rhus-t.,*** sin-n., ***sulph.,*** syph., tarent.

bed, in - hyper., ***phos.***

midnight, before - ***ferr.,*** prun.

ovarian, complaints - ***nat-h.***

paralytic - acon., am-m., arg-m., ***aur., bell.,*** cham., chel., cocc., dros., euon., led., lyc., nux-v., phos., plb., sol-n., stann.

paroxysmal - ***bell.,*** bov., caust., cocc., coloc., zing.

pressure, agg. - lyc.

pulsating - polyg., ptel.

rheumatic - abrot., ***acon., aesc.,*** all-s., ant-t., arn., cact., ***carb-ac., carb-s.,*** **COLCH.,** form., hydr., ***kali-bi., kalm., lac-c., led., lyc.,*** mag-s., ***med.,*** meph., merc-i-f., merc-i-r., nat-m., ***nit-ac.,*** ph-ac., ***phos., phyt.,*** plb., podo., ***puls.,*** **RHUS-T.,** sabad., sang., sin-n., stann., sulph., stram., tarent., ***valer.,*** verat-v., zinc.

left - ***acon.,*** lyc., nat-m., sang., ***sanic., stram.***

and right shoulder - ***ferr.***

right - calad., carb-ac., erig., nux-m., ***sep.***

and left shoulder - **LED.**

right - aesc., ***agar.,*** alum., ant-c., bar-c., carb-an., corn., daph., indg., kali-bi., ***kali-c.,*** lac-c., **LED.,** lil-t., **LYSS.,** merc-i-r., mez., ***murx.,*** pall., phos., sep.

to left - lith.

to thigh - lil-t.

rising, on - **AESC.,** kali-n., sarr.

from a seat - agar., **AESC.,** ***aur.,*** card-m., chel., con., kali-n., led., lyc., nat-c., ***nat-s.,*** ph-ac., ***rhus-t.***

rotating the leg, inwards, on - ***coloc.***

sitting, while - arn., asar., caust., chin., eup-per., petr., ph-ac., ***rhus-t.,*** staph., sulph., ther.

amel. - aur., tarent., zinc.

down - lyc., nat-s.

sleep, after - acon., ***lach.***

preventing - sep.

sneezing, when - arg-m.

standing - kali-c., ***led., valer.,*** zinc.

amel. - staph.

stepping, when - arg-n., asar., ***caust.,*** kali-c., phos., **RHUS-T.,** sabin., sulph.

stool, during - pall.

stooping, on - agar., card-m., coloc., gent-l., lyc., ***nat-s.,*** sil.

stretching out limb., on - ruta.

sudden - lyc.

thinking, about the pains - ***ox-ac.***

touch, on - asar., ***bell.,*** kali-c., nat-m., ph-ac., ruta., ***sulph.***

turning, in bed - am-c., ***nat-s.***

ulcerative - calc.

urinating, while - ***berb.***

vexation, from - ***coloc.***

PAIN, hips

walking, on - agar., am-c., ammc., ***am-m.,*** ant-c., arg-m., arg-n., ars-h., asar., ***aur.,*** calc., carb-an., carb-v., ***coloc.,*** con., dros., euph., ham., ***hep., hydr.,*** iris, lac-c., ***led.,*** lyc., mag-c., ***med.,*** mez., nat-s., pall., ***ph-ac.,*** psor., rhod., rumx., sep., stann., staph., ***sulph.,*** zinc.

after - tell.

amel. - am-c.

amel. - am-c., ***ferr.,*** kali-bi., **KALI-S., LYC., PULS.,** ***rhus-t., valer.***

in open air - bar-c.

amel. - ***acon.,*** lyc.

wandering - ***colch.,*** med., ***iris.***

warmth, amel. - ***rhus-t.,*** staph.

wet, weather - ***phyt., rhus-t., sil.***

yawning - arg-m.

PARALYSIS, sensation of - brom., nat-m., phos., plb., ***verat.***

alternates from hip to hip - verat.

evening - phos.

lying amel. - phos.

sitting amel. - phos.

walking, while - verat.

amel. - ph-ac.

PARALYTIC, pain - acon., am-m., arg-m., ***aur., bell.,*** cham., chel., cocc., dros., euon., led., lyc., nux-v., phos., plb., sol-n., stann.

PINCHING, pain - caust., dulc., kali-c., led., mag-c., zinc.

only during rest - nat-s.

only during sitting - mur-ac.

PRESSING, pain - acon., agar., arg-m., asar., aur-m-n., berb., carb-v., caust., ***cimic., coloc.,*** crot-t., ***euph.,*** ferr-ma., hell., hep., kali-bi., ***led.,*** lyc., mez., mosch., nat-c., nat-s., nit-ac., petr., ***puls.,*** **RHUS-T.,** sabad., ***sep., stann., zinc.***

above hip - con., sep.

coughing, on - ***caust.***

extending to ankles - led.

to sacrum - carb-v.

forenoon - puls.

gluteal region - cact., cimic., iod., mez.

increasing and decreasing slowly - sep.

labor, during - ***cimic.***

left - acon., cocc., coloc., hell., lyc., puls.

as from a ball - ***con.***

lying, on right side - sabad.

morning, in bed - agar.

motion, agg. - ***led.***

amel. - puls.

paralytic - cocc.

paroxysmal - cocc., coloc.

right - arg-m., ***asar., kali-bi., led.,*** **LYSS.,** nit-ac., sabad., ***sep.***

stepping with left leg - arg-m.

rising, from seat - nit-ac.

rubbing, amel. - nat-s.

sitting, while - arn., aur-m-n., caust., petr., staph.

stepping, on - arg-m., **RHUS-T.**

stool, during - pall.

PRESSING, pain
tearing - led.
from before backwards - sep.
walking, while - acon., asar., caust., coloc.
begining to walk - nit-ac.

PULSATION - am-c., ars., ars-h., ***coloc.,*** crot-h., hep., ***ign.,*** mag-m., merc., rhod., staph., sil., til.
evening - am-c.
morning - ars-m.

RELAXATION, of joint - apis, ***calc., thuj.***
standing - thuj.

RESTLESSNESS, while sitting - form.

RHEUMATIC, pain - abrot., ***acon.,*** **AESC.,** all-s., ant-t., arn., cact., ***carb-ac., carb-s.,*** **COLCH.,** form., hydr., ***kali-bi., kalm., lac-c., led., lyc.,*** mag-s., ***med.,*** meph., merc-i-f., merc-i-r., nat-m., ***nit-ac.,*** ph-ac., ***phos., phyt.,*** plb., podo., ***puls.,*** **RHUS-T.,** sabad., sang., sin-n., stann., sulph., stram., tarent., ***valer.,*** verat-v., zinc.
left - ***acon.,*** lyc., nat-m., sang., ***sanic., stram.***
left, and right shoulder - ***ferr.***
right - calad., carb-ac., erig., nux-m., ***sep.***
right, and left shoulder - **LED.**

SENSITIVE - bapt., ***coloc.,*** mag-m., zinc.

SHARP, pain - acon., aeth., ***agar.,*** agn., ail., **ALUM.,** am-m., ammc., anan., ant-t., ***apis,*** apoc., arg-m., **ARS.,** aster., bar-c., ***bell., berb., bry., calc.,*** calc-p., canth., caps., **CARB-AN.,** ***carb-s.,*** cast., ***caust.,*** cham., ***chel.,*** chin., ***chin-a.,*** cic., ***cina,*** cinnb., clem., coca, cocc., colch., ***coloc.,*** con., crot-h., cupr., dulc., euon., euph., euphr., ***ferr.,*** ferr-ar., ferr-p., ***fl-ac.,*** form., gran., graph., grat., ham., ***hell.,*** hyos., ign., ***kali-bi., kali-c., kali-i.,*** kali-n., ***kalm.,*** kreos., lac-c., laur., led., lil-t., ***lyc., mag-c.,*** mag-m., manc., mang., meny., ***merc., merc-c.,*** mez., nat-a., nat-c., ***nat-m.,*** nat-p., ***nat-s., nit-ac.,*** nux-v., ox-ac., par., ph-ac., phos., phyt., **PLB.,** ptel., raph., ***rhus-t.,*** sabad., sabin., ***sep., sil.,*** sol-n., sulph., tab., tell., teucr., thuj., verat-v., ***zinc.***
acute - caust.
afternoon - canth., merc-c.
4 p.m. - ptel.
on moving right arm toward left - plb.
ascending steps, on - ph-ac.
bending to painful side agg. - mag-c.
burning - cic., mag-c.
carrying, when - caps.
chill, during - ail.
coughing, on - bell., caps., sulph.
cramp-like - cina.
dinner, after - phos.
drawing - dulc.
evening - sulph., tab.
bed, in - ant-t., ***sep.***
extending to, abdomen - caust., chel., coca.
back, small of, on coughing -sulph.
backwards - laur.
chest - phos.
downward - aeth., aster., ***bry.,*** calc-p., calc-caust., caust., cinnb., colch., ferr., ***kalm.,*** **PLB.,** ***sil., sulph.***

SHARP, pain
extending to,
foot - bry., ***caps.,*** sulph.
genitals - eupi.
groin - dulc.
heel - ***kali-i.***
ilium to ilium - lil-t.
knee - ***bry.,*** caps., colch., ***coloc., kali-c., kali-i.,*** mez., nat-a., **PLB.**
outward - merc-c.
shoulder - mag-c.
small of back - alum.
tibia - ferr.
gluteal muscles - asaf., aur., cham., chin-s., con., hyos., meny., mur-ac., staph., tab., viol-t.
jerking - meny.
inspiration, on - alum.
itching - led., mag-c.
agg. by scratching - led.
amel. by scratching - mag-c.
left - am-m., **CARB-AN.,** cic., cocc., nat-s., sep., stram.
morning, rising, on - mang., nat-m., ***sulph.***
motion, on - agn., calc., ***coloc., merc.,*** merc-c., nat-a., ***sulph.***
amel. - caust., kali-n., laur., ***meny., merc-c.,*** nat-c., sabad., stel.
night - ***am-m.,*** **LYC.,** ***merc., sep.,*** sulph.
paroxysmal - alum., cast., nat-c., par.
periodic - ***merc.***
pressure amel. - ***am-m.,*** sulph.
pulsating - arg-m.
rheumatic - chel., ***lyc.***
right - chel., ***coloc.,*** fl-ac., lil-t., ***lyc.,*** merc-c., sabad., sep., sulph., zinc.
rising from a seat - chel.
rising from a seat - chel.
rubbing amel. - phos.
sitting, while - **CARB-AN.,** con., euph., kali-c., ***kali-i.,*** laur.
standing, while - kali-c., ***kali-i.,*** kali-n., laur., meny.
stepping - arg-m., calc., dulc., mang.
stool, during - cinnb.
stooping, on - calc., ***thuj.***
stretching leg amel. - dulc.
sudden - bar-c.
tearing - colch., ph-ac.
touch agg. - bry.
twitching - cina.
walk, on beginning to - calc., ph-ac.
walking, amel. - ***ferr., kali-i.,*** plb.
bent - ***bry.***
walking, while - arg-m., berb., calc., cocc., ***coloc.,*** dulc., euphr., gran., ham., meny., merc., nat-c., nat-m., ***nat-s.,*** sol-m.
slowly amel. - ***sep.***
warmth, agg. - still.
amel. - ***coloc.***

SHOCKS - agar., aloe, arg-m., arn., bell., nat-m., verat.
left, then right - ***arg-m.***

SHOOTING, pain - ail., **ARS.**, bell., bry., ***calc.***, calc-p., ***chel.***, cinnb., ***ferr.***, form., ***hyper.***, lach., sabad., ***sulph.***, thuj.
coughing - caps.
evening - ***ferr.***, ***sulph.***
7 p.m. - form.
extending to,
abdomen - chel.
calf, to - thuj.
down femur - ***sulph.***
foot - ***caps.***, lach., sulph.
knee - ***caps.***, ***nux-v.***
joint - colch., ***ferr.***, sulph.
daytime - sulph.
evening in bed - ***ferr.***
morning - ***sulph.***
night - sulph.
motion amel. - sulph.
night, before falling asleep - ***sulph.***
right - chel., sabad., sulph.
rising from a seat, when - chel.
tearing extending to leg - colch.
walking amel. - ***ferr.***

SHUDDERING - gran., lyc., ptel.

SORE, pain - abrot., ***acon.***, aesc., agar., all-c., alum., am-c., am-m., anac., apis, ***arg-m.***, ***arn.***, ars., bov., bry., carb-ac., carb-an., ***caust.***, ***cina***, cob., cop., croc., crot-h., dulc., ***ferr.***, fl-ac., form., gins., hura, kali-bi., ***kali-c.***, kreos., ***laur.***, lil-t., mag-m., manc., mang., ***nat-c.***, nat-m., **PH-AC.**, phyt., puls., **RUTA.**, sars., **SEP.**, ***sil.***, ***staph.***, ***sulph.***, tarent., tell., thuj., zinc., zing.
ascending steps - ph-ac.
bending to painful side agg. - mag-c.
chill, during - **ARN.**
extending to,
ankles - manc.
downward - aesc.
gluteal muscles - arg-m., euph., hura, ***puls.***, seneg., zinc.
knees - abrot.
shoulder - mag-c..
forenoon - am-m., equis.
during menses - nat-c.
left - nat-m.
lying, while - staph.
on it - ***caust.***, cop., kali-bi., nat-m., sep.
menses, during - ***mag-m.***, ***nat-c.***
before - calc., ***lach.***
morning - agar., alum., ars., bry., fl-ac., rat.
rising, after - agar., fl-ac.
walking - mag-m.
motion, on - ***arg-m.***, cob., croc., fl-ac., ***kali-c.***, ph-ac., sulph.
move, on beginning to - ***sep.***
moving, body to one side - sulph.
while sitting - euph.
night - ars., nat-m.
bed, in - form., phos.
lying on it - ***caust.***, kali-bi.
pressure, on - alum., caust., ***cina.***
right - lil-t., nat-c., ***sep.***
rising from seat - ***aesc.***, anac., kali-bi., nat-c., sep., tarent.

SORE, pain
sitting, while - kali-bi., mang., sang., sulph.
amel. - tarent.
sneezing, when - ***kali-c.***
standing, while - tarent.
stooping, when - ***sil.***
touch, on - ruta.
walk, on beginning to - ph-ac.
walking, on - alum., bry., caust., cop., kali-bi., mag-m., tarent., tell.
amel. - agar., nat-c., sep.

SPRAINED, as if - aesc., am-m., ***arg-m.***, ***arn.***, ars., bar-c., ***calc.***, ***caust.***, cham., chin., con., ***euph.***, hep., ***ign.***, ip., kali-n., laur., lyc., merc-i-r., mez., ***nat-m.***, nit-ac., nux-v., petr., ***phos.***, psor., ***puls.***, ***rhod.***, **RHUS-T.**, rhus-v., seneg., sol-t-ae., stann., ***sulph.***, tell.
breathing deep - nat-m.
evening - cham., con., merc-i-r.
extending to small of back - lyc.
left - laur., lyc., nat-m.
morning - ars., kali-n., lyc.
motion - ang., ***euph.***, lyc., petr., sulph.
night - ars.
paroxysmal - caust.
right - pall., rhod.
rising, from seat - aesc., anac.
sneezing, when - arg-m.
stepping, on - arg-n.
sudden - lyc.
tuber ischiadica - hep.
walking, while - arg-m., calc., con., lyc., mez., rhod., stann.
after - tell.
in open air - cham., hep., mez.

STIFFNESS, of - acon., agar., ang., arg-m., ars., aur., ***bapt.***, bar-c., ***bell.***, chin-s., euphr., ***ham.***, hell., ***lyc.***, med., nat-m., ***ph-ac.***, phys., rheum, **RHUS-T.**, ***sep.***, **SIL.**, ***staph.***, ***stry.***, sulph., ***zinc.***
morning - arg-m., ars., chin-s., **RHUS-T.**, ***staph.***
move, on beginning to - ***ph-ac.***, **RHUS-T.**, staph.
rising, from a seat - agar.
turning, over, on - ***sulph.***
walking, amel. - ***ph-ac.***

SUPPURATION, (see Hip-joint disease) - ***ars.***, asaf., asar., ***aur.***, ***calc.***, ***calc-p.***, calc-s., calc-sil., **CHIN.**, graph., ***hep.***, ***merc.***, ***ph-ac.***, ***puls.***, rhus-t., ***sep.***, **SIL.**, staph., ***stram.***, sulph.

SWELLING - plb.
sensation of - lil-t.

TEARING, pain - ***acon.***, aesc., agar., all-s., alum., ambr., am-m., ***arn.***, ***ars.***, aur-m., bar-c., ***berb.***, bry., ***calc.***, calc-p., cann-s., ***canth.***, ***caps.***, ***carb-v.***, ***caust.***, cina, clem., ***coloc.***, colch., dios., dulc., ***euph.***, ***ferr.***, ferr-i., ferr-p., gamb., graph., hep., ***iod.***, iris, ***kali-ar.***, kali-bi., **KALI-C.**, ***kali-n.***, ***kali-p.***, ***kalm.***, lach., led., ***lyc.***, mag-c., **MAG-M.**, mag-s., merc., merc-c., merc-i-f., ***mez.***, ***nat-c.***, nat-p., nicc., ol-an., par., ph-ac., ***rat.***, rhod., ***rhus-t.***, sabin., ***sep.***, ***sil.***, stann., stram., ***syph.***, tab., tax., ter., thuj., ***zinc.***

TEARING, pain
above hip - sep.
afternoon - kali-n., mag-m.
4 p.m., lasting all night - mag-c.
alternating with right upper arm - bry.
breathing, when - alum.
coughing agg. - ***caps.***
drawing - acon., ars., aur-m., dulc., kali-bi., kreos., ter., zinc.
evening - kali-n., mag-m., mag-s., sulph.
after going to bed - ***ferr.,*** lyc., ***mag-m.,*** nat-c.
extending to,
downward - ***alum.,*** am-m., caust., ***coloc., kalm.,*** led., lyc., mag-m., mag-s., ***rat.,*** tep.
ankles - calc.
foot - caps., ***kalm.,*** lyc., mag-s., sep.
hypogastrium - zinc
knee - canth., ***caps.,*** colch., ***coloc., kali-c., lyc., mag-m., rat., rhus-t.,*** sil.
knee, when coughing - ***caps.***
lumbar region - alum.
sacrum - ***carb-v.***
sciatic nerve, down to - calc., ***coloc.,*** lyc.
stomach - bry.
toes - nicc.
forenoon - nat-c.
gluteal muscles - agar., coc-c.
left - acon., lyc., mag-c.
lying - ferr., mag-m., nat-c.
on the sound side, amel. - mag-m.
menses, during - nat-c.
morning - ***ars., mag-m.,*** stront.
motion, during - acon., ***calc., coloc., iod., merc.,*** sil.
amel. - agn., alum., ***ferr., euph.,*** kali-n., nat-c., **RHUS-T.**
night - agar., arn., mag-c., mag-m., ***merc.,*** sep.
paroxysms - ***alum.,*** carb-v., ***coloc.***
pressive - ambr., zinc.
amel. - ***merc-i-f.***
pulsating, pains - ***merc.***
rheumatic - ***acon., calc.,*** graph., ***kalm., rhus-t.***
right - agar., agn., coc-c., daph., lachn., ***mag-m., nat-c.,*** ter.
rubbing amel. - ol-an.
sitting, while - am-m., caust., euph., kali-c., par., ph-ac.
standing, while - ***coloc., rhus-t.***
walking, while - ***aesc.,*** caust., ***coloc.,*** mag-m., ***rhus-t.,*** samb., ***sil.,*** sulph.
amel. - ***ferr.,*** stront.
warmth of bed - **MERC.**

TENSION - aeth., agar., ***bell.,*** berb., bry., calc., ***carb-v.,*** coc-c., ***coloc.,*** con., crot-t., euph., ferr-ma., ***lyc.,*** mez., ***nat-m.,*** nit-ac., ph-ac., ***rhus-t.,*** sep., stront-c., sulph., thuj.
afternoon - aeth.
evening, amel. - coc-c.
extending, downwards - berb., sulph., thuj.
to groin - thuj.

TENSION, in
left - ***lyc., rhus-t.,*** sulph.
morning, waking - carb-v.
motion agg. - ph-ac.
rheumatic - lyc.
right - nit-ac.
sitting, while - ***rhus-t.***
standing, while - lyc.
walking, while - bell., calc., carb-v., lyc., nit-ac., sep., ***sulph.,*** thuj.

TINGLING, prickling, asleep - bar-c., rhus-t.
asleep, night - bar-c.

TUBERCLES - rat., rhus-t.

TWITCHING - ***ars., calc.,*** cocc., ***coloc.,*** mag-c., ***mag-m.,*** mez., ph-ac., sep., sil., stann., sulph., valer.
evening, in bed - mag-m., sil.
motion amel. - sulph.

UNSTEADINESS - aesc., calc-p., nat-m., ruta.

WATER, cold, running down to toes - bell.
warm, seems bathed in - coc-c.

WEAKNESS, of - adeps., **AESC.,** agar., ***all-c.,*** apis, arg-m., brach., calc., **CALC-P.,** carb-v., chin., cinnb., ham., ign., ***kali-c.,*** mang., murx., ***ox-ac., pic-ac.,*** podo., rhus-t., **RUTA,** sars., sep., syph., tarent., thuj., ***verat.,*** zing.
ascending stairs - podo.
evening - tarent.
before going to bed - chin-s.
morning - chin., mang.
waking, on - arg-m.
motion amel. - chin.
paralytic - arg-m., ***kali-c.,*** mang.
right - ***arg-m.***
then left - ***verat.***
rising, from seat agg. - sep.
sex, preventing finishing - all-c.
standing - zing.
walking, while - arg-m., chin-s., coca, ***verat.***
continued, amel. - sep.

Intestines

ACHING, dull, pain, the whole length of the - *ferr-m.*
were seized one by one, as if - mez.

ANTIPERISTALTIC, (see Peristalsis, reversed)

APPENDICITIS, (see Inflammation) - **BELL., BRY.,** cadm-s., ***calc-s., chin.,*** chel., ***cocc., coloc.,*** con., ***crot-c.,*** dulc., ***echi.,*** graph., ***hep.,*** ign., **IRIS-T.,** ***lach., lyc., merc.,*** **MERC-C.,** ***nit-ac.,*** **PHOS.,** ***plb.,*** **SIL.,** ter.

BLEEDING, hemorrhage - ***acon.,*** agar., ***ambr.,*** anthr., ***ars.,*** bapt., bar-m., ***cact., canth.,*** **CHIN.,** colch., **COLCH.,** ***coll., crot-h., erig., eucal., ferr-p.,*** **HAM., IP.,** ***kali-bi., kali-i., kali-p., merc., nit-ac., nux-v.,*** **PHOS.,** ***psor.,*** sars., ***sec., senec., sil., tril.,*** tub., ***urt-u.,*** verat.
anus, prolapsus, with - **APIS.**
bilious fever, in - ***chel.***
black, blood - ***rhus-t.***
bright, blood - caust.
bright red, in streams - ***acon.***
chronic, with hemorrhoids - ***anac., sulph.***
clotted masses, large, followed by shivering - med.
coagula - ***alum.***
colon pain, after - ***ham.***
congestion, from portal - **HAM.**
dark, fluid, fetid - ***ham.***
and tough, enveloped in viscid mucus - coll.
liquid - **MUR-AC.**
offensive - ***ars.***
venous, about a quart, better pain in abdomen - ***arn.***
decomposed - **LACH.**
tar like, in large quantities - ***ham.***
edema, in, following intermittent - cit-l.
epithelial, with, degeneration - **TER.**
exertion, after much, lifting or internal injuries - **ARN.,** ***ham., mill., rhus-t.***
exertion, after physical, blood bright and clear - cinnb.
hypochondriasis, with - ***psor.***
infiltrations - anthr.
involuntary, with, spasmodic twitching of lower jaw - **ALUM.**
menses, during - lyss.
vicarious - phos., ust.
metrorrhagia, after checked - acet-ac.
nasal catarrh, with - ***calc.***
painless, in large quantities - ***bism.***
passive - ham., **TER.**
bright red, after stool, with faintness when profuse - ***ign.***
cirrhosis of liver, in - ***sulph.***
secondary, after removal of hemorrhoid - ***nit-ac.***
standing, blood oozing on, or walking, with dark fluid hemorrhage during stool - ***crot-h.***
stitching, with sharp, pains in rectum - ***graph.***

BLEEDING, hemorrhage
stool, during - ***nat-m., puls.***
and immediately after - vib.
purpura hemorrhagica, in - phos.
soft, during - ***hep.***
with or without - ***rat.***
typhus, or typhoid - ***alum., arg-n., ars., bapt.,*** chlor., **LACH.,** ***mill.,*** **MUR-AC., NIT-AC.,** ***nux-m.***
syncope, in, with - nux-v., ph-ac., ***rhus-t., ter.***
ulceration, with - ***ham.,*** **TER.**
urinating, after - ***merc.***
urine, with flow of - **ALUM.**
weather, in autumnal cold damp - ***colch.***
women, elderly, large quantities of blood discharged at once with constipation - psor.
yellow fever, in - **CANTH., LACH.**

BREAKING, as if, on bending - adon.

BURNING, pain - ars., manc.. phos., sulph.

CANCER, colon - ***alum., ars.,*** carb-v., graph., **HYDR.,** ***kali-c.,*** lyc., mur-ac., ***nit-ac.,*** ruta., sep., spig..

CATARRH, of - **ARS.,** ***arund., bad., bry., calc., cham.,*** **CHEL.,** ***colch., coloc., cop., dulc.,*** eucal., ***ferr.,*** ferr-p., ind., ***ip., mag-c.,*** senec., **VERAT.**
blennorrhea, with - hydr.
depression and apathy - grat.
cholera epidemic, in - rhus-t.
chronic - ***ars., hydr., lach.,*** nat-m., ptel., ***sin-n.***
after great straining discharges a mass of exudation - ***lach.***
morning, agg. - ***nit-ac.***
diseases, in eruptive - ***apis***
liver, with affection of, and bladder - cham.
nephritis, in - ter.
pneumonia, before - ***chel.***
ulceration, followed by - ***hydr.***

CECUM, general
cutting, pain - ***hydr.***
distended, hard - plb.
gurgling, on pressure - chin-s.
dull, pain, worse turning to right side - ammc.
gurgling, region of, typhoid pneumonia, in - ***phos.***
on pressure - ***apis.***
region of, ague, in - puls.
inflamed, (see Typhlitis) - **BELL.,** ***calad., card-m.,*** **COLCH.,** ***crot-h., lach., merc., nat-s.,*** **OP.,** ***plb.,*** **RHUS-T.,** ***samb.,*** **THUJ.**
appendix also painful, with frequent paroxysmal aggravations - ***crot-h.***
deep circumscribed swelling, lies on back with right knee drawn up - hep.
painful, with swelling, tenderness, fecal accumulation and vomiting - ***lac-d.***
peritonitis, with - ***bell.,*** **LACH.,** ***lyc.***
region, painful - ***colch.***
swollen, hard, hot and red, painful to touch - ***merc.***

CECUM, general
jerking, worse turning to right side - ammc.
pain - chel., jal., ***lac-d., stram.***
cannot bear pressure of bed cover - ***bell.***
intense, in typhoid - ***iod.,*** phos.
radiating to chest, back and extremities - ***kali-c.***
rumbling - chel., elat.
sensitive, in chronic intestinal catarrh - ***lach.***
typhoid pneumonia, in - ***phos.***
typhus, in - **APIS,** colch., lach.
tenderness - ***colch.***
tenderness, with pain and swelling - ***lach.***
sharp, pain - ***hydr.***
shooting, pain, turning, agg., to right side - ammc.
sore, pain - ***nit-ac.***
stitches, with sneezing - agar.
swelling large, hard, painful to touch and motion - ***plb.***
ulcers, in - ***nit-ac.***

CELIAC, disease - chin., lyc.
celiac plexus, neuralgia - phos.
pressive pain causing anxiety and sweat - camph.

CHOLERA - acon., agar-ph., ***ars.,*** aven., bell., bry., **CAMPH.,** ***canth., carb-v.,*** chin-s., cic., colch., **CUPR.,** ***cupr-ac., cupr-ar.,*** dig., euph-c., ***grat.,*** gua., ***hydr-ac., ip.,*** iris, jatr., kali-bi., lach., ***laur.,*** merc-c., mur-ac., naja, nux-m., nux-v., ***op.,*** ph-ac., ***phos., podo., psor.,*** quas., rhus-t., ***sec.,*** sul-ac., sulph., ***tab.,*** ter., thuj., **VERAT.,** xan., zinc-m.
infantum - acon., **AETH.,** ant-c., ant-t., ***apis,*** arg-n., ***ars., bell., bism.,*** bry., cadm-s., ***calc.,*** calc-ac., ***calc-p.,*** camph., camph-br., canth., carb-v., cham., chin., colch., coloc., colos., corn., ***crot-t.,*** cuph., cupr., cupr-ac., ***cupr-ar., dulc.,*** elat., ***euph-c., ferr.,*** ferr-p., graph., grat., **GUAI.,** hydr-ac., indol., ***iodof., ip., iris,*** jatr., kali-bi., kali-br., ***kreos., laur., mag-c., med.,*** merc., nat-m., ***op.,*** ox-ac., passi., ***phos.,*** phyt., podo., ***psor., puls.,*** raph., ***rhus-t.,*** sars., ***sec.,*** sep., ***sil., stram.,*** sulph., ***tab.,*** thuj., ***verat., zinc-m.***
body remains warm - bism.
opisthotonos, with - med.
epidemic diarrhea - ars., ***ip.,*** phos.
morbus - acon., ant-c., ant-t., **ARS.,** bism., camph., caul., cedr., chlor., ***colch.,*** coloc., crot-h., ***crot-t., cupr., cupr-ar.,*** dios., elat., ***ferr., grat.,*** **GUAI.,** hydr-ac., ***ip., iris, jatr.,*** kali-bi., op., oper., ph-ac., ***phos.,*** **PODO.,** ***psor.,*** raph., ***sec., tab.,*** thuj., **VERAT.**
prophylactic - ars., ***camph., cupr.,*** cupr-ac., ***verat.***
symptoms like, during menses - ***am-c.,*** bov., verat.

COLD, as if - plan.
balls, running through, as if - bufo.
water, flowing through, rectum, anus, to - mill.
menses, during - kali-c.

COLDS, agg. - dulc.

CONTENTS, fluid as if were - polyg.

CORD, bound and loosened, as if - chion.
cord, extending from anus to navel - ferr-i.

CRAMP-like pain, sigmoid flexure, to back, with vomiting - ***dios.***

CRAMPING, pain - ***abrot.,*** acet-ac., ***acon.,*** aesc., aeth., **AGAR.,** ail., all-c., **ALOE,** ***alum., alumn.,*** ambr., ***am-c.,*** **AM-M.,** ***anac.,*** anan., ang., ***ant-c., ant-t., apis,*** aran., arg-m., ***arg-n.,*** arn., ***ars.,*** ars-i., ***asaf., asar., aur.,*** aur-m., bar-c., bar-i., ***bar-m.,*** **BELL.,** ***berb., bism., bor., bov.,*** brom., ***bry.,*** bufo, cact., calad., **CALC.,** ***calc-p.,*** calc-s., camph., cann-s., canth., caps., ***carb-ac., carb-an.,*** **CARB-S., CARB-V.,** card-m., carl., caul., ***caust.,*** cedr., **CHAM., CHEL.,** ***chin.,*** chin-a., ***cic., cina,*** cinnb., clem., cob., coc-c., **COCC.,** ***coff., colch.,*** **COLOC.,** ***con., cop.,*** corn., croc., ***crot-t.,*** cub., **CUPR.,** ***cupr-ar., cycl., dig.,*** **DIOS.,** dros., **DULC.,** echi., elaps, ***elat.,*** erig., ***eup-per., euph., euphr.,*** eupi., ***ferr.,*** ferr-ar., ferr-p., gamb., ***gels.,*** gent-c., glon., gnaph., ***gran.,*** **GRAPH.,** ***grat.,*** guai., ***ham., hell., hep., hydr.,*** hydrc., ***hyos.,*** hyper., **IGN.,** iod., **IP.,** ***iris,*** jab., jatr., jug-r., kali-ar., ***kali-bi., kali-br., kali-c.,*** kali-i., kali-n., kali-p., ***kali-s., kreos., lac-c., lach.,*** lact., ***laur.,*** lec., ***led., lil-t.,*** lob., **LYC.,** lycps., lyss., ***mag-c.,*** **MAG-M., MAG-P.,** mag-s., manc., mang., meny., ***merc.,*** merc-c., merl., ***mez., mosch., mur-ac.,*** naja, ***nat-a., nat-c., nat-m.,*** nat-p., ***nat-s., nit-ac., nux-m.,*** **NUX-V.,** olnd., ol-j., onos., **OP.,** ox-ac., paeon., pall., ***par., petr.,*** phel., **PH-AC.,** phos., ***phyt., pic-ac.,*** plan., ***plat.,*** **PLB., PODO.,** prun., psor., ptel., **PULS.,** ***ran-b.,*** ran-s., ***raph.,*** rat., ***rheum,*** rhod., ***rhus-t.,*** rhus-v., ***rumx.,*** ruta, sabad., sabin., samb., sars., ***sec.,*** senec., seneg., **SENN.,** ***sep.,*** **SIL.,** ***spig.,*** **SPONG.,** squil., **STANN.,** ***staph., stram., stront-c.,*** **STRY., SULPH.,** ***sul-ac.,*** sumb., tab., tarax., ***tarent.,*** tell., ***ter.,*** teucr., ***thuj.,*** trom., ***valer.,*** **VERAT.,** verb., vib., viol-t., vip., ***zinc.,*** **ZING.**
afternoon - agar., alum., bism., bry., carb-s., carb-v., coloc., corn., grat., kali-n., laur., lyc., mag-c., nat-c., nat-m., nat-s., nicc., op., par., phyt., sil., senec., sulph., ***verat.***
1 p.m. - mag-m.
3 to 10 pm - lyc.
4 p.m. - caust., coloc., hell., **LYC.**
4 to 9 p.m. - ***coloc.***
5 p.m. - aran., tell.
air, cold in - ***am-c.,*** lyc.
open, in - ign.
amel. - nat-c.
alternating, pain in chest, with - ***ran-b.***
vertigo, with - verat.
ascending steps - hell.

CRAMPING, pain
bed, in - alum., dig., dios., kali-c., lact., nat-m., nux-v., psor., rhus-t., sabin., valer.
belching, amel. - carb-v., kali-c., sep., ***sulph.***
bending, backward amel. - bell., ***dios.,*** nux-v., onos.
forward amel. - ***acon.,*** am-c., ***caust., chin.,*** coff., ***colch.,*** **COLOC.,** ***kali-c., lach., mag-p.,*** phos., ***plb.,*** prun., ***rhus-t.,*** sars., senec., ***stann.,*** stram., zinc.
breakfast, after - agar., eupi., grat., ham., kali-bi., lyc., nux-m., stront-c., **ZINC.**
chill, during - **COCC.,** led.
before - ars., ***spong.***
chilliness, during - rhus-t., sep.
coffee, from - ***cham.,*** ign., nat-m., ***nux-v.***
cold, after taking - ***all-c.,*** alum., alumn., ***dulc.,*** nat-c., nit-ac.
as after taking - hep., petr., stann.
constipation, during - merc., ***op., plb., podo.,*** sil.
convulsions, with - ***cic.***
coughing, when - chel., plb., tarent.
diarrhea, with - ars., petr., phos., sep., zinc.
before - ars., kali-n., mag-c., mag-m., phos., sulph.
dinner, during - am-c., kali-c., mag-s., zinc.
after - agar., alumn., caps., cocc., crot-t., gent-c., kali-c., **MAG-C.,** naja, phos., ***ran-b.,*** thuj., trom., valer., **ZING.**
drinking, water, after - cham., **COLOC.,** ***crot-c., manc.,*** nat-m., nit-ac., ***nux-v., puls.,*** raph., ***rhus-t.***
eating, while - carb-v., caust., dulc., kali-p., ***nux-v.***
after - ***all-c., ant-t.,*** bell., carb-v., caps., caust., chin., cic., cocc., coc-c., ***colch., coloc.,*** con., cupr., gamb., ***graph.,*** grat., hell., kali-c., kali-p., lyc., ***nat-c.,*** nux-m., ***puls., rhus-t.,*** sars., ***sulph., verat.,*** zinc.
2 hours - sil.
amel. - ***bov.,*** psor.
extending, to
left chest - kali-n.
lumbar region - alum., guai., kali-n., nat-m.
stomach - kali-n.
upward - mag-m.
evening - alum., am-c., bism., calad., **CALC.,** carb-v., cast., chin., cycl., grat., ***iris,*** kali-n., led., mag-c., mag-m., mag-s., merc., nat-m., petr., ph-ac., plan., plb., ***puls.,*** sars., senec., stann., sulph., sul-ac., tarent., thuj., ***valer.,*** zinc.
bed, in - alum., ars., hyos., ***valer.***
fever, during - caps., carb-v., elat., rhus-t., rob.
flatus, from - euph., graph., kali-c., mang., phos., sulph.
before passing flatus - ars., graph., guai., mez., mur-ac., rheum., sil., spig., tarax.
passing, from - aur., canth., ***chin.,*** mur-ac., nit-ac., spig., ***squil.,*** staph.

CRAMPING, pain
flatus, from
passing, from, amel. - ***acon., am-c.,*** cimx., ***coloc., con., echi., graph., hydr.,*** lyc., mag-c., merc-c., nat-a., ***nat-m.,*** nux-m., ol-an., psor., rumx., sil., spong., squil., sulph.
forenoon - agar., am-c., am-m., coloc., **DIOS.,** kali-bi., kali-n., lyc., mag-c., ***nat-c.,*** paeon., sars., sulph., tell., xan.
9 a.m. - mag-c.
10 a.m. - carb-s.
11 a.m. - corn.
fruit, after - calc-p., ***chin., coloc., puls.***
holding, abdomen amel. - coloc., mang.
hot milk, amel. - ***crot-t.***
humiliation, from - ***coloc., staph.***
hysterical - ars., bell., bry., ***cocc., ip., mag-m., mosch.,*** nux-v., ***stann., stram., valer.***
ice cream, after - **ARS.,** ***calc-p., ip., puls.***
indignation, after - **STAPH.**
inspiration, on - aesc., am-m., brom., guai., ***sulph.***
jerking - graph., mur-ac., plat.
kneading abdomen, amel. - ***nat-s.***
leaning, on a sharp edge - ran-b., samb.
lying, while - ***phos., spig.***
abdomen on, amel. - am-c., chion., ***coloc.,*** der.
amel., while - cupr., ferr.
back, on, from - phys.
with limbs drawn up amel. - ***rhus-t.***
right side, on, amel. - phys.
side, on - coloc., ign.
amel. - nat-s.
melons, from - **ZING.**
menses, during - acon., alum., ***am-c.,*** anac., ars., bar-c., ***bell., bor.,*** brom., calc., ***caul., caust., cham.,*** chel., ***chin., chin-s., cimic., cinnb.,*** clem., **COCC.,** ***coff., coloc., con., cupr.,*** form., gran., ***graph.,*** ign., ***kali-c.,*** kali-n., kali-s., mag-m., ***mag-p.,*** mosch., nat-c., ***nat-m.,*** nat-s., nicc., ***nit-ac., nux-v., plat., puls.,*** sabin., sars., ***sep.,*** stront-c., **SULPH.,** vib., zinc.
after - ***am-c.,*** cocc., kreos., merl., puls.
before - aloe, alum., ***am-c.,*** bar-c., ***bell.,*** brom., ***calc-p.,*** carb-v., ***caust., cham.,*** chin., ***cinnb., cocc., coloc., croc., cupr.,*** cycl., hyper., ***ign.,*** **KALI-C.,** ***lach.,*** mag-c., ***mag-p.,*** manc., nux-v., ph-ac., ***plat., puls., sep.,*** spong.
from hip to hip - thuj.
milk, after - bufo., cupr., ***lac-d.,*** mag-s., raph.
morning - agar., am-c., calc., carb-s., **CAUST.,** coc-c., coloc., colch., con., cupr., **DIOS.,** dulc., euphr., graph., hep., kali-bi., kali-c., kali-n., lact., lob., ***lyc.,*** mag-m., mang., nat-c., nat-m., nit-ac., **NUX-V.,** phos., plan., psor., ***puls.,*** rat., ruta, sabin., sars., sep., staph., sulph., tarent., xan., zinc.
bed, in - agar., euph., kali-c., lact., mag-c., nat-m., **NUX-V.,** psor., ***puls.,*** sabin.

CRAMPING, pain
morning,
fasting, from - dulc.
rising, on - nat-m., ruta.
after - am-m., ars., mag-m., nit-ac.
amel. - nat-m.
uncovering, on - rheum.
waking, on - agar., cob., colch., lyc., mang., nat-m., rheum., xan.
5 a.m. - cob.
6 a.m. - ***coloc.***
motion, on - alum., brom., **COCC.,** corn-f., **IP.,** mag-p., ***mur-ac., nit-ac., nux-v.,*** phys., ran-b., raph., rhus-t., ***zinc.***
motion, amel. - bov., ***gels.,*** rhus-t.
night - alum., arg-n., bry., **CALC.,** calc-s., carb-s., ***chin.,*** cupr., ***cycl.,*** dig., euphr., graph., ign., ***iris,*** kali-c., kali-s., mez., myric., nat-c., ***nat-s., nit-ac.,*** osm., ***podo., rhus-t.,*** senec., sep., stront-c., ***sulph.,*** sul-ac., ***valer.***
1 a.m. - ***mag-m.***
2 a.m. - nat-s., phos.
3 a.m. - carb-v.
bed, in - dig., rhus-t.
midnight - alum., **COCC.,** coloc., lyc., **NIT-AC.,** petr., rhus-t., ***zinc.***
after - am-m., aur., sulph.
uncovering, on - bry.
noon - alumn., carb-v., kali-c., mag-c., sulph.
pressure, amel. - am-c., brom., **COLOC.,** ***mag-p.,*** mang., ***podo., stann.***
riding, while - psor.
rising, from a seat - kali-c.
amel. - chin., spong.
rubbing, from - sulph.
sex, during - graph.
sitting, while - chin., dig., elaps, ferr., par., rhus-t., spong.
amel. - bell., mur-ac.
bent, while - carb-v., dulc.
head on knees, with amel. - euph.
sleep, during - kali-n.
amel. - alum., mag-m.
smoking, after - bufo., brom.
soup, after - zinc.
standing, while - bell., gent-c., mur-ac., zinc.
amel. - chin.
bent, amel. - spong.
stool, during - ***agar., aloe, am-c.,*** anac., ***apis,*** asc-c., aur., bapt., ***bor.,*** canth., caust., coc-c., colch., con., corn., crot-t., cupr-ar., cycl., dig., dulc., ferr., grat., hep., hydr., iris, kali-bi., kali-c., ***lil-t., mag-c.,*** mang., ***merc., nux-v.,*** op., phel., phos., plan., podo., puls., ***rheum,*** rhus-t., sec., senn., sep., **SULPH.,** sul-ac., zinc.
after - agar., ***aloe,*** **AM-C.,** ***ars.,*** carb-an., carb-s., ***carb-v., coloc.,*** con., cupr., eup-per., glon., graph., grat., kali-bi., kali-c., lil-t., lyc., mag-m., nat-c., ***nat-m.,*** nit-ac., ***op.,*** plb., rheum., rhod., **SULPH.,** sul-ac.

CRAMPING, pain
stool, during
amel. - agar., aloe., carb-s., cinnb., coc-c., **COLOC.,** ferr., ***gamb., gels.,*** indg., ***mag-c.,*** naja, nat-a., **NAT-S., NUX-V.,** puls., seneg., sulph., ***verat.***
before - aesc., ***agar.,*** **ALOE,** alum., **AM-C.,** ***am-m.,*** ang., **ARG-N.,** ***ars.,*** arum-d., arum-i., arum-m., aur., bell., ***bry.,*** calc., ***calc-p.,*** camph., cann-s., canth., carb-an., carb-s., **CHIN.,** ***chin-s.,*** cina, coc-c., ***colch., coll.,*** **COLOC.,** ***crot-t.,*** cupr., cupr-s., cycl., dig., ferr., ferr-ar., ferr-i., ***gamb.,*** gels., glon., gran., grat., guai., hep., hyper., ign., ***jatr.,*** kali-ar., kali-bi., kali-c., kali-n., kali-s., lact., ***lil-t.,*** lycps., **MAG-C.,** mag-m., ***mag-p.,*** mang., meny., ***merc.,*** merc-i-r., ***mez.,*** mur-ac., nat-a., nat-c., nat-m., nat-p., nit-ac., ***nux-v.,*** **OP.,** petr., phel., ***phos.,*** phys., **PODO.,** puls., rat., rhod., rhus-t., rhus-v., sep., spig., stram., **SULPH.,** ***thuj., trom., verat.,*** zinc.
hard - meny., ***op.***
stooping, agg. - am-c., dulc., nux-v., ***sulph.***
supper, after - alum., calc., coff., gels., grat., ol-an., ***zinc.***
suppressed, hemorrhoidal flow - **NUX-V.**
tea, after - hyper.
tranverse colon, in - guai., staph.
turning, amel. - euph., mag-c.
urination, on - bar-c., ***cham., merc.,*** sul-ac.
amel. - tarent.
vaginal discharge, with - zinc.
before - con., mag-c., mag-m., sulph.
vegetables, after - cupr.
vexation, after - cham., **COLOC.,** ***staph.***
waking, on - alum., coc-c., colch., euphr., ferr., lyc., mez., nat-m., stann., ***stront-c.,*** xan., ***zinc.***
walking, while - ang., bell., chin., ***coloc.,*** cupr., gent-c., graph., kali-bi., mur-ac., nat-p., phos., ph-ac., prun., ***ran-b.,*** stann., ***zinc.***
amel. - chin., cycl., dig., elaps, ferr., par., puls., ***sulph.***
in open air - agar., am-c., bry., ph-ac., rhus-t., sil., sulph.
wandering - mur-ac., spig., staph.
warm, milk amel. - ***crot-t.,*** op.
room, amel. - am-c.
warmth, amel. - alum., am-c., cupr-s.
wet, getting feet - ***all-c.***
wine, after - lyc.
yawning - zinc.

CRAMPING, hypochondria, region - aesc., aloe, am-m., arg-m., bar-c., bell., bry., bufo, calc., ***calc-s.,*** camph., caust., cupr., dios., ign., iod., ***ip.,*** kali-bi., ***kali-c.,*** kali-i., ***lact., lyc.,*** mag-c., ***mur-ac.,*** nat-m., nit-ac., ph-ac., phos., plat., sep., sil., stann., sulph., ***zinc.***
alternating, with oppression of chest - zinc.
belching, amel. - sep.

CRAMPING, hypochondria
bending forward, agg. - dig.
coughing, on - lyc.
evening - calc-s., dios.
extending, to,
back, across the - **SIL.**
downward - hell.
hips, to - sil.
lumbar vertebrae, to - camph.
umbilicus, to - ph-ac.
upward - mag-c.
flatus amel. - mur-ac., sep.
intermittent - mag-c.
left - plat., zinc.
extending to stomach - phos.
menses, before - sulph.
morning - teucr.
motion agg. - zinc.
night - calc-s.
paroxysmal - nit-ac., sep., sil.
periodic - ph-ac.
respiration, deep - croc.
right - carb-an., iod., kali-c., mag-c., nat-m., ph-ac., phos., rhus-t., samb., staph., sulph., verb., zinc.
rubbing amel. - phos.
sitting - carb-an., rhus-t.
stepping - caust.
stool, during - sul-ac.
after - caust.
stooping, on - lyc.
turning the body - lyc.
walking, while - sulph.
after - ph-ac.

CRAMPING, hypogastrium, region - ***acon., agar.,*** aloe, am-c., am-m., ***ars.,*** aur., ***bell.,*** bism., ***bry.,*** calc., carb-an., carb-s., ***carb-v., chel.,*** chin., cimic., ***cocc., coll.,*** coloc., ***con., cupr-ar.,*** cycl., dig., ***dios., gels.,*** guai., helon., kali-c., kreos., lil-t., lyc., mag-c., mez., meny., ***nat-c.,*** nit-ac., ***nux-v., prun.,*** psor., ran-b., rhus-t., ruta., sep., ***sil.,*** spig., spong., squil., stann., ***stry.,*** **SULPH.,** sul-ac., thuj., zinc.
bending double, compelling - ***prun.***
to left agg. - bell.
daytime - stram.
diarrhea, with - ars.
eating, after - con., ran-b.
evening - dulc., lyc.
flatus amel. - kali-c., mez., squil.
forenoon - agar.
left - lyc.
lying agg. - sulph.
on back - ambr.
menses, during - ***agar.,*** **AM-C.,** ***ars.,*** **COCC.,** ***con.,*** **GRAPH.,** ***mag-p.,*** nat-m., sulph.
after - kreos.
before - cimic., ***cocc.,*** **KALI-C.,** ***mag-p.,*** manc., ***nat-m., nit-ac.,*** sars., **SULPH.,** ***vib.,*** zinc.
metrorrhagia, with - mag-c.
morning - ambr., ars., dios., fago., hyos.

CRAMPING, hypogastrium
night - chel.
1 a.m.- mang.
menses, before - mang.
paroxysmal - chin., sep.
pressure amel. - fago.
retracting abdomen agg. - bell., kali-c.
right - ambr.
sit upright, must - sulph.
sitting - chin.
upright, amel. - sulph.
standing - chin.
stepping - calc.
stool, during - ***ars.***
after - agar., lyc.
before - agar., anac., ***ars., coll., gels.,*** meny., stram.
stooping, on - am-c.
supper, after - ran-b.
touch, on - cycl.
urination, during - bar-c., sul-ac.
after - sul-ac.
before - ***chel.,*** sul-ac.
vaginal, discharge, before - sulph.
walking - sulph., zinc.
in open air - agar., calc.
wandering - chin.
warmth, amel. - ***ars.***

CRAMPING, inguinal, region - ***aloe,*** am-c., am-m., bov., ***bry.,*** calc., carb-v., ***chel.,*** cimic., ***gamb.,*** indg., kali-c., kali-i., ***kreos.,*** mag-c., nat-s., petr., phos., rat., stann., sulph., sul-ac., zinc.
afternoon, 3 p.m. - mag-c.
4 p.m. - nicc.
ascending stairs - alum.
dinner, after - nat-c.
extending to knee - aloe.
face, causing face to flush - cimic.
forenoon, 11 a.m. - mag-c.
inspiration, on - sulph.
intermittent - nat-c.
left - chel., kali-n., sars., stann.
menses, during - kali-c.
after - bor., kreos., plan.
morning - rat.
paroxysmal - nat-m.
right - aloe, bov., carb-v., dig., gamb., indg., mag-c., nat-c., sul-ac., zinc.
rising, from sitting - zinc.
rubbing, on - ***sulph.***
amel. - mag-c.
sitting, while - kali-c., petr., spong.
stool, during - nicc.
stooping - sulph.
stretching, on - am-c.
talking - calc.
walking, while - kali-n., mag-c., ***sulph.***

CRAMPING, sides (see Abdomen)

CRAMPING, umbilical, region - acon., agar., ***aloe,*** alum., am-m., anac., ant-c., ant-t., arn., aspar., bar-c., ***bell.,*** berb., ***bry.,*** calc., ***camph., carb-an.,*** carb-s., caul., caust., ***chel.,*** cham., ***chin.,*** cimic., ***cocc.,*** coc-c., **COLOC.,** ***crot-t.,*** cycl., **DIOS.,** dulc., euphr., fl-ac., ***gamb.,*** gent-c., gran., graph., grat.,

CRAMPING, umbilical, region - guai., ham., hyos., ign., ***iod.,*** **IP.,** jug-c., kali-bi., kali-i., kali-n., kreos., ***laur.,*** lec., led., lyc., mag-c., mag-m., mang., meny., merc-c., ***mez., mur-ac.,*** myric., naja, ***nat-c.,*** nat-m., nicc., nit-ac., nux-m., ***nux-v.,*** ox-ac., petr., ***ph-ac.,*** phos., ***phyt., plat., plb., podo., ptel., raph.,*** rheum, rhus-t., sabad., samb., sang., senec., sil., spig., squil., stann., staph., stront-c., ***sulph.,*** tab., tarent., thuj., ***verat.,*** verb., ***zinc.***

afternoon - euphr., nat-c., plb., **SULPH.**
4 p.m. - sulph.
5 p.m. - mag-c., sang.
below, umbilicus - kali-c., kali-n., mag-c., mag-m., nat-c., nat-m., phos., zinc.
supper, after - calc.
bend, body, must - lyc.
bending, body - nit-ac.
forward - con.
forward amel. - ***aloe,*** **COLOC.,** senec.
breakfast, during - alum.
after - agar., kali-bi.
cold, after taking - ***bry.***
as after taking - stann.
diarrhea, with - kali-n.
before - coloc., mag-c., plat.
dinner, during and after - ant-t., bry., calc., **COLOC.,** ham.
eating, after - bell., carb-v., graph., kali-n., mag-m., ***nux-v.,*** plat., sulph.
evening - alum., caust., phos., plat., **SULPH.**
bed, in - nux-m.
stool, during - inul.
extending, abdomen, to - calc.
anus, to - nat-m.
back, to - plat.
chest, to - kali-n.
downward - plat.
groin, to - thuj.
hip, to - mag-c.
sacrum, to - mag-c.
stomach, to - carb-v., mag-c., sulph.
throat, to - kreos.
flatus, amel. - bar-c., carb-v., mag-m., mez., sulph.
as from - plat., zinc.
forenoon - agar., lyc., nat-c.
fruit, after - **COLOC.**
inspiration, on - anac.
menses, before - ***kreos.***
morning - aeth., bor., bov., lyc., mag-c., nat-m.
bed, in - caust., lyc.
rising, after - aeth.
waking, on - bov.
motion - bar-c., nit-ac.
night - bry., cycl., lyc., nux-m., ***podo.***
bed, in - nux-m.
waking, on - cycl.
noon - mag-m., ***sulph.***
periodical - ph-ac.
rising, from stooping - chin.
sitting, while - ***all-c.,*** chin., ph-ac., sulph.
bent - ant-t.
soup, after - kali-n.
sour food, after - asaf.

CRAMPING, umbilical
standing - bry., gent-c.
stool, during - cocc., ***corn.,*** indg., iod., phos.
before - ***coloc.,*** graph., ***ham.,*** kali-n., lec., mag-m., mur-ac., phos., plb., psor.
amel. - meny.
stooping - am-m., phos.
supper, after - gels.
urination, after - mag-c.
vaginal, discharge, with - mag-c.
before - sil.
walking, while - ***all-c.,*** gent-c., zinc.
amel. - bar-c.

CROHN'S, disease - ***aloe,*** ars., chin., merc-c.

CUTTING, pain - calc.
tranverse colon - guai., ph-ac., sep., zinc.

DIARRHEA, (see Rectum)

DISTENTION, from flatus, (see Flatus, Abdomen, Distention) - acon., ***agar.,*** agar-ph., ail., all-c., am-caust., ant-c., ***ant-t.,*** anthr., arn., ars., ars-m., atro., aur-s., bell., bol-lu., bov., brass., ***brom.,*** bry., cahin., calc-p., ***canth.,*** card-m., cedr., chel., chin., cit-v., coca, colchin., ***coloc.,*** corn., cot., crot-t., cupr-ac., cupr-ar., cycl., cyt-l., der., dirc., euph., fago., ferr., ferul., ***gamb.,*** gins., guare., ign., iod., jatr., jug-r., kali-bi., kali-s., laur., lob., **LYC.,** mang., ***merc., merc-c.,*** morph., nat-c., ol-an., ***onis.,*** ox-ac., petr., ph-ac., ***phos.,*** plb., podo., rham-cath., rhod., rob., sant., ***sec., sil.,*** sol-n., sol-t-ae., spira., ***stram.,*** sul-ac., ***sulph.,*** tarent., **TER.,** teucr., ***thuj.,*** til., trom., verb., vichy-g., vip.

afternoon - ***carb-v.,*** cham., fago., mill., rat., stront-c., vichy-g.
4 p.m. - sep.
alternating with tension in chest, evening - lyc.
ascending colon, of - plb.
ascites, at night, agg. after involuntary discharge of offensive water from rectum - prun.
belching, amel. - sep., thuj.
dinner, after - anac., corn., lyc., nicc., sep.
drinking, after - ***nux-v.***
eating, after - aloe, ambr., asaf., ign., nux-v., plb., ***puls.,*** spira., zinc.
eating, as after, too much - nat-m., tax.
evening - con., hyper.
7 p.m. - caust.
8 p.m. - ol-an.
9 p.m. - dirc.
agg. - ant-c., vichy-g.
flatus, emission of, amel. - gins., **LYC.,** mang., ph-ac., rhod.
forenoon - tong.
griping, eating, after, on standing, amel. sitting quietly, agg. on walking - ign.
stool, before - hyper.
hard - hep., lach., ***sil.***
hysterical - raph.
inflammatory - bell., kali-i.
menses, during - aloe, nicc.
before - arum-t.

DISTENTION, from flatus
milk, after - con.
morning - aloe, cist.
soup, after - ol-an.
movable - aloe, plb.
night - valer.
10 p.m. and 11 p.m. - ***sulph.,*** trom.
noon, when walking - coloc.
painful - ***bar-c.,*** bry., caust., coff-t., hell., ***lach.,*** plb., rhod., stann.
morning, after waking - nat-c.
evening - mez., nat-m.
night - alum.
night, dinner, before - spig.
eating, after - rhus-t.
menses, at beginning of - berb.
riding in a carriage - sep.
passing, from - petr., phos.
amel. - all-c., am-m., ant-t., bov., bry., calc., ***carb-v., kali-i.,*** **LYC.,** ***mag-c.,*** mang., mur-ac., nat-c., nat-m., ***ph-ac., sulph.***
amel., rising, after - mur-ac.
as from - con., graph., hep.
does not amel. - phos.
periodic, agg. after eating - aloe
pressive - ***nux-v.***
night, emission of flatus, with - arg-m.
motion amel. - op.
sac-like - cann-s.
pressive, sitting, on - op.
soft - mag-s.
spots, in - grat., nat-c., tarent.
stool, agg. after - graph., **LYC.,** petr.
amel. - calc-p., corn.
supper, after - arn.
water, by - ***nat-m.***
distention, sensation of (see Abdomen) - morg.
splenic flexure of - mom-b.
transverse colon - bell.

DIVERTICULOSIS - aloe, ars.

DRAWING, pain - calc.

DRYNESS, of - alum., ***op., plb.***

DUODENUM, general
aching, with colic - ***caps.***
catarrh - ***puls.***
chill, from - kali-m.
jaundice, in - ***hydr.,*** **MERC.,** ***nat-m.***
yellow-coated tongue, with - ***kali-s.***
congested - bar-m.
inflamed - ars-s-f., bar-m., lyc., ***podo.,*** uran-n.
chronic - ***lyc.***
pain - astac.
awoke at 1 a.m., into umbilical region - merc-sul.
sitting bent, agg. - lyc.
red, dark - bar-m.
sensitive, with colic - ***caps.***
ulcers, duodenal - aloe, alum., ***arg-n.,*** calen., dys-co., ger., ***kali-bi.,*** symph., ***uran-n.***

DYSENTERY - ***acon., aeth.,*** **ALOE,** alst., alumn., ambro., ant-t., ***apis, arg-n., arn.,*** **ARS.,** ars-i., asc-t., ***bapt.,*** bar-m., ***bell., bry.,*** **BUFO, CANTH., CAPS.,** ***carb-ac.,*** **CARB-S., CARB-V.,** caust., ***cham.,*** chap., **CHIN.,** chin-a., ***cinnb.,*** cist., clem., **COLCH., COLL., COLOC.,** ***con.,*** cop., ***corn., crot-c., crot-h.,*** crot-t., cub., cuph., cupr., ***cupr-ar., dirc., dulc.,*** elat., ***erig., eucal.,*** ferr-p., gamb., **GELS., HAM.,** ***hep., ign., iod.,*** **IP.,** ***iris, kali-bi., kali-chl.,*** kali-m., kali-p., ***lach.,*** lept., ***lil-t., lyc.,*** **LYSS., MAG-C.,** mag-m., ***mag-p.,*** manc., **MERC., MERC-C.,** ***merc-cy., merc-d.,*** merc-sul., ***mill.,*** mur-ac., ***nit-ac., nux-m.,*** **NUX-V.,** ***op., ox-ac., petr.,*** **PHOS.,** ***phyt.,*** plb., ***psor., puls.,*** raph., rheum, rhod., **RHUS-T.,** sec., ***silphu.,*** staph., **SULPH.,** ***sul-ac., tanac., ter.,*** tril., ***trom.,*** vac., verat., xan., xanth., zinc., zinc-s., ***zing.***
abuse of local treatment - chin., lil-t.
anxiety, with - ***ars., carb-v.***
autumn, agg. - acon., ***colch.,*** dulc., ***ip.,*** merc-c., sulph.
chronic, intractable cases - aloe, arg-n., ***ars., chin.,*** cop., ***dulc.,*** hep., ***merc-c., nit-ac., nux-v.,*** ph-ac., podo., rhus-a., ***sulph.***
cold feet to knees in dysentery - aloe
elderly people - bapt.
emaciated, undersized children - ***bar-m.***
hemorrhoidal form - aloe, coll., ham.
long intervals between - ***arn.,*** chin.
nausea from straining pains, little thirst - ip.
night - ***merc.,*** sulph., trom.
periodic recurrence in spring or early summer - kali-bi.
plethoric, nervous, climacterial females - lil-t.
rheumatic pains all over - asc-t.
septic origin, of - crot-h.
tearing down thighs - rhus-t.
thirst, with great - acon.

EMPTINESS, knotted feeling, with - cham.

FERMENTATION, in - agar., ambr., ang., aran., brom., ***bry.,*** calc., carb-ac., carb-an., carb-v., **CHIN.,** coff., croc., ***gran.,*** hell., ***hep.,*** inul., lup., **LYC.,** mag-m., merl., mur-ac., ***nat-m.,*** nat-s., ***phos.,*** plb., rhus-t., ***sars.,*** seneg., sep., stram., sulph., wies.
contents were in motion, as if - corn.
diarrhea, during - sars.
before - gran.
drinking, agg. - wies.
eating, after - nat-s.
amel. - rhus-t.
fluid were poured from one intestine into another, as if - arg-m.
forenoon - cast-eq.
fruit, after - **CHIN.**
grumbling - acon.
menses, during - lachn., **LYC.,** ***phos.***
sensation of - agar., rhus-t.
stool, during and after - mez.
before - sulph.
vomiting, before - coff.

FALLS, to side lain on - merc.

FISTULA, discharge of pus, gases, and pale matter - sil.

GANGRENE - plb.

GURGLING, in descending, worse after eating - aloe

FLATUS, intestinal, (see Distension, flatus, from) - aesc., aeth., ***agar.,*** agn., all-c., **ALOE,** alum., alumn., ambr., am-c., **AM-M.,** ammc., ***ant-c.,*** ant-t., ***apis,*** apoc., **ARG-N.,** arn., **ARS.,** ***ars-i.,*** asaf., asar., ***aur.,*** bapt., bar-c., bar-i., bar-m., bell., bor., bov., brom., bufo, cahin., **CALC.,** calc-f., ***calc-p.,*** **CALC-S.,** ***caps.,*** ***carb-ac.,*** **CARB-AN., CARB-S., CARB-V.,** ***caust.,*** **CHAM.,** ***chel.,*** **CHIN.,** ***chin-a.,*** ***chin-s.,*** cic., cinnb., clem., ***coca, cocc.,*** coff., **COLCH.,** coll., ***coloc., con., cop., crot-c., crot-t.,*** cycl., dig., ***dios.,*** dirc., ***elaps,*** eup-per., euph., fago., ferr., ferr-ar., ferr-i., ferr-p., ***fl-ac., form., gels.,*** gins., glon., **GRAPH.,** gran., ***guai.,*** hell., helon., hep., **HYDR.,** hyper., ***ign., iod.,*** indg., jug-r., kali-bi., ***kali-c.,*** kali-chl., kali-i., ***kali-n.,*** kali-p., kali-s., kalm., ***lac-c., lac-d., lach.,*** lil-t., **LYC., MAG-C.,** mag-m., ***mag-p.,*** mang., meny., meph., ***merc.,*** mez., mosch., ***mur-ac.,*** myric., ***nat-a., nat-c., nat-m.,*** nat-p., **NAT-S., NIT-AC.,** naja, **NUX-M.,** ***nux-v.,*** **OLND., OP.,** ornithog., ox-ac., petr., phel., ***ph-ac., phos.,*** **PIC-AC.,** ***plat.,*** plb., ***podo.,*** prun., ***psor., puls., raph.,*** rheum, rhod., rhus-t., rumx., sabad., sang., sars., ***sel., seneg.,*** **SENN.,** ***sep.,*** **SIL.,** squil., stann., staph., stront-c., **SULPH.,** ***syph.,*** tab., **TARENT.,** teucr., ***thuj.,*** til., **VERAT.,** verat-v., vesp., vinc., xan., ***zinc., zing.***
- **acids,** after - ph-ac.
- **afternoon** - aur-m., ***calc-s.,*** carb-v., kali-n., lyc., op.
  - 4 p.m - ***lyc.***
  - eating, after - fago.
  - stool, during - fago.
- **back,** felt in - rhod.
- **bath,** after - calc-s.
- **bed,** rising from - zinc.
- **breakfast,** after - caust., nat-p., **NAT-S.**
  - before - agar.
- **cecal** region - carb-s., nat-s.
- **children** - arg-n., lyc.
- **croaking** - arg-m., coloc., lyc., sabad.
- **dinner,** during - ant-c.
  - after - agar., calc-s., myric., naja, nit-ac., verat.
- **drinking,** after, with distention of abdomen - ambr.
- **eating,** after - ambr., ant-c., **ARG-N.,** aster., ***aur.,*** bor., bufo, calc., carb-an., ***carb-v.,*** caust., coc-c., con., ***dios.,*** ferr-m., kali-n., **LYC.,** ***mag-m.,*** nat-p., **NUX-V.,** puls., rumx., thuj., ***zinc.***
  - distention of abdomen, with - ambr., chin., ***lyc.***
- **elderly** people - ***carb-ac.,*** carb-v., chin., lyc., ***phos.***

FLATUS, intestinal
- **evening** - aloe, alum., ***am-c.,*** apoc., calc-f., cist., glon., ham., hyper., ***lyc.,*** merc., nat-m., ***nit-ac., nux-v.,*** pic-ac., plan., ***puls.,*** sang., ***sep.,*** sol-t-ae., verat., zinc.
- **fermenting,** as if - ***chin.,*** lyc., rhus-t.
- **food,** all, turns to gas - carb-v., chin., kali-c., ***lyc.,*** nux-m., nux-v., teucr.
- **forenoon** - guai., hipp., nat-m., ***puls.,*** zinc.
- **fruit,** from - **CHIN.**
- **here** and there - ***carb-v.,*** cham., chin., cocc., cycl., **LYC.,** nat-m., nat-s., spig., verat.
- **hypochondria,** region - acon., ***aur.,*** **CARB-V.,** ***cham., chin.,*** cist., ***cycl.,*** euph., hyos., **LYC.,** ***phos.,*** podo., sil., sulph., sul-ac., tarent., verat.
  - left - mez., nat-m., sulph.
- **hypogastrium,** region - mag-m., phos., zinc.
  - obstructed, in - graph., staph.
- **hysterical** - alet., ***ambr.,*** arg-n., ***asaf.,*** caj., cham., cocc., ***ign.,*** kali-p., ***nux-m.,*** plat., puls., raph., ***sumb.,*** tarax., thea., ***valer.***
- **incarcerated** in flexures (see obstructed) - am-c., aur., bell., calc., calc-p., carb-ac., ***carb-v., cham., chin.,*** colch., ***coloc., graph.,*** hep., ign., kali-c., lim., ***lyc., nux-v.,*** pall., phos., plb., puls., ***raph.,*** rhus-g., rob., staph., sulph., thuj.
- **inguinal** rings - cham.
- **left,** side - am-m., ***aur., carb-v.,*** **CON.,** crot-t., dios., euph., lyc., nat-m., ph-ac., seneg., staph., **SULPH.**
- **menses,** during - kali-c., kali-p., nux-m., podo., vesp., vib.
  - before - zinc.
- **milk,** after - carb-v., merc., ***nat-c., nat-m., nat-s., phos.,*** sul-ac.
- **morning** - ***arg-n.,*** calc., cann-i., cedr., cist., con., hep., kali-c., kalm., lach., lyc., merc., nit-ac., nux-v., petr., ***plat., podo., puls.,*** senec., squil., ***sulph., verat.,*** tarent.
  - bed, in - euph., nux-v.
  - rising, on - cann-i.
  - waking, on - ***arg-n., calc.,*** cist., con., rumx.
- **night** - agar., ambr., ammc., arn., ***aur.,*** calc., ***carb-v.,*** calc-s., cocc., com., cist., ferr., hyper., ign., op., ***kali-ar.,*** kali-c., lyc., merc., nat-m., ***nat-s.,*** nux-m., puls., stry., thuj., zinc.
  - midnight - aur., **COCC.**
  - midnight, after, with distention of abdomen - ambr.
- **noon** - nat-s.
- **numbness,** with - med.
- **obstructed,** intestinal - agar., aloe, ***alum.,*** ambr., anac., ang., ant-c., ant-t., **ARG-N.,** arn., ***ars., ars-i.,*** asar., **AUR.,** ***calc.,*** camph., canth., caps., ***carb-an.,*** carb-v., carb-s., ***caust., cham.,*** **CHIN.,** ***cocc.,*** coff., **COLCH.,** ***coloc., con.,*** dulc., euph., ***graph.,*** guai., hep., ign., ***iod., kali-ar., kali-c., kali-n., kali-p.,*** kali-s., kalm., ***lach., lyc.,*** meny., mez., mosch., nat-c., ***nat-m.,*** nat-p., ***nat-s.,*** **NIT-AC.,** nux-v., ox-ac., phel., ***ph-ac., phos., plat.,*** plb., prun., **PULS., RAPH.,** rheum, rhod.,

FLATUS, intestinal
obstructed, intestinal - rhus-t., sars., sep., **SIL.,** spig., squil., stann., staph., stry., ***sulph.,*** **TARENT.,** teucr., til., **VERAT.,** ***zinc.***
afternoon - kali-n.
descending colon, with constipation - ***aur., iod., lyc.,*** rhod., ***sulph.***
evening - nit-ac.
hard stool, with - caust.
midnight - coloc.
morning - mang., nit-ac., sulph., zinc.
night - nat-m., sil., sulph.
sitting, from long - lyc.
stool, after - lyc., pic-ac.
before - lyc.
surgery, after - arn., chin., op., raph.
waking - sil.
offensive - ***aloe,*** arn., bry., ***carb-v.,*** ferr-ma., graph., olnd., sil., sulph.
painful - asc-t., carb-v., ***cham.,*** chin., coll., iris, lyc., mag-p., nat-s., ***nux-v.,*** ox-ac., puls., rhod., staph., verat., zinc-valer.
hot drinks, amel. - phos.
palpitations, with - ***arg-n.,*** cact., carb-v., ***nux-v.***
pressing, bladder, on - ***carb-v.,*** ign., kali-c.
rectum, on - calc., ign., nat-s.
upward - arg-n., asaf., carb-v., graph., thuj.
pushing - nat-s.
upward - asaf.
riding, in a carriage, while - calc-f., ferr.
right, side - bism., **CALC.,** graph., lil-t., ***nat-s.,*** ox-ac., ***phos.,*** thuj., zinc.
rolling - thyr.
sides - phos.
siesta, after a - cycl.
sitting, while - phos.
from long - lyc.
sleep, during - kali-n.
sour food, from - ***ph-ac.***
stool, during - acon., apoc., arg-n., arum-d., asaf., ***crot-t.,*** dig., fago., nat-m., ***nat-s.,*** petr., phel., podo., staph., thuj.
after - calc-s., **LYC., PIC-AC.,** plb.
before - apoc., cast., ***fl-ac.,*** gels., hep., **LYC.,** ***op.,*** phel., sumb., viol-t.
supper after - coc-c., hyos., psor., zinc.
tea drinking - ***chin.***
urination, during - merc.
vegetables, after - caps., ***lyc.***
walking, while - lyc.
air, in open - sep.
amel. - phos., sil.
wandering - ***carb-v.,*** chin., **LYC.,** nat-m., puls., sil.
wine, from - chin.

FLUID, as if full of - polyg.

GIARDIA - ars., chin., cina.

GNAWING, pain, transverse - gels.

HANGING, down, as if - ***agn.,*** alum., **IGN.,** ***psor.,*** **STAPH.**
afternoon when walking - alum.
bed, when turning in - bar-c., merc., merc-c.

HARDNESS, of ascending colon - **PLB.**

HEAT, in - ***canth.***
at lower end of - ***calc.***

HEAVINESS, as from a load, etc., intestines would sink down, as if - pimp.

HOOK-worm, disease - carb-tcl., chen-a., cina, thymol.

ILEO-cecal, region (see Cecum)
aching, dull, pain - **BRY.,** ***carb-s., card-m.,*** chel., **CHIN.,** ***cocc.,*** colch., con., cop., ***crot-h.,*** dulc., ***echi.,*** gnaph., ***hydr., lach.,*** **MERC-C.,** ***nit-ac.,*** **PHOS.,** ***plb., ter., thuj.,*** verat.
turning on right side agg - ammc.
burning - ***calad.***
distension - ***colch.,*** fago., mag-m.
rumbling - **PLB.**
sharp - agar., ammc., carb-s., ***card-m.,*** hura.
stool, after - carb-s.
walking - hura.
sore, bruised, tenderness, etc - **APIS,** ***ars., bapt.,*** **BELL., BRY.,** ***calad., carb-ac., cocc., colch.,*** cop., ***gamb., kali-bi.,*** kali-c., ***lach., lyc., merc., merc-c., nit-ac., phos.,*** plb., ter.

ILEUM, inflamed - ***podo.,*** ars-s-f.

ILEUS, complaints of - ars., bell., bry., cham., cocc., coloc., lyc., nit-ac., nux-v., ***op.,*** plat., plb., ***rhus-t.,*** sil., sulph., tarent., ***thuj.,*** verat., zinc.
paralytic ileus of colon transversum - stront.

IMPACTION, of - alum., **BELL.,** ***caust.,*** gels., lac-d., ***lach.,*** **OP., PLB.**

INACTIVITY, of - aeth., **ALUM.,** ***op.,*** phys.

INFLAMMATION, of (see Appendicitis, Peritonitis, Typhlitis) - **ACET-AC., ACON., ANT-T., APIS, BELL., BRY.,** ***cact., cham., colch.,*** cop., cupr-s., grat., jal., ***lach.,*** lycps., ***merc., ox-ac.,*** plb., rhus-t., sulph., **TER.,** verat-v.
acute catarrhal, during damp weather, warm or cold - ***gels.***
children, in, from milk and farinaceous diet - ***lyc.***
followed by dysentery - jug-c.
chronic - ***hydr.,*** phyt., ***ox-ac.,*** sulph.
catarrhal - ***hydr.***
dyspepsia, with - ***hydr-ac.***
croupous - ***hydr., merc-c.***
diarrhea and constipation, alternate - ***ign.***
distension, with, of abdomen - sal-ac.
ascites, in - ***apis.***
eating, probably caused by, baked beans - tarent.
enterocolitis - ***nuph., ter.***
colicky pains in rectum and characteristic stools - ***nuph.***
fever, with high - pyrog., ***verat-v.***
follicular - podo.
foreign, from a, body - ***calen.***

INFLAMMATION, of
gastro-enteritis - **BRY., CACT.,** cupr-m., ***phyt.,*** **RHUS-T.**
hiccough, with - **HYOS.**
ileo-cecal, with - lac-d.
lancinating pain, with - ***merc.***
meteorism, with - ***uran-n.***
mucous - asar., colch., cop., kali-p., rhus-t., zinc-valer.
acute - iris.
nutrition, with faulty, followed by affection of nervous centers - lac-d.
pseudo-membranous - merc-c.
stools, with, of mucus and blood - ***urt-u.***
subacute, mucous - ***asc-t.***
typhlitis, after - ***ang.***
typhoid, with - **BRY.,** ***hyos.,*** **RHUS-T.**
worm fever, with - ***merc.***

INTUSSUSCEPTION - ***acon., arn.,*** **ARS.,** ***bell., bry., colch.,*** **COLOC.,** ***cupr., kali-bi.,*** kreos., ***lach., lob., lyc., merc., nux-v.,*** **OP.,** ***phos.,*** **PLB.,** ***rhus-t., samb.,*** sulph., tab., tarent., thuj., **VERAT.**
colic, with agonizing - **COLOC.,** ***cupr.***
and fecal vomiting - ***plb.***
violent and convulsions, with - ***op.***
motion, agg. - ***ars., bry.***
rushes about, bent double, pressing great anguish - ***coloc., verat.***
pressure, agg., sensitive to - ***ars.***
singultus, with - ***cupr.***
threatening sloughing - ***lach.***

IRRITATION - cina, cham., chin., coloc., cypr., lyc., ***nux-v., podo.***
alternates to chest - ***seneg.***
brain, affecting, and other organs - cina.
dentition, during - cypr.
dysentery, followed by - jug-c.
eczema, after suppressed - ***cupr-ac.***
inflammatory, subacute, from mouth to anus - ***nat-c.***
mental, after extreme, exertion - ***nux-m.***
mastitis, in - phos.
phlegm, with constant accumulation of, in bronchial tubes - ***seneg.***
strabismus, with, in helminthiasis - nat-p., ***spig.***

JEJUNUM - ***podo.***
pale hypertrophied follicles - ant-t.
pustular eruption - **ANT-T.**

KNOTTED - asaf., elaps, sabad., sulph., ust., verat.

LIQUID, flows from stomach, to - mill.

LOOSE, as if intestines, were - ail., cann-i., cann-s., coloc., cycl., ***lach.,*** mag-m., mang., merc., mez., nat-m., nux-v., phys., rhus-t.
afternoon, 3 p.m. - phys.
diarrhea were about to set in, as if, 5 p.m. - coca.
lost their hold - mag-m.
shaking, and loose - mang.
walking, while - mang.

MARBLE, dropped down at stool, as if - nat-p.

MUCOUS membrane
anthrax - anthr.
ecchymoses - sal-ac.
edematous, discolored, cloudy red - anthr.
epithelial degeneration, with hemorrhages - **TER.**
false membranous form actions in small, produced by gradual exudations of plastic lymph - ***lept.***
pale - ant-t.
pustular foci - anthr.
pustules, small conical, filled with serum - ant-t.
reddish swollen, edematous, hemorrhagic prominent infiltrations, grayish or greenish yellow, discolored surface, sloughing center - anthr.
secretion, increased, of - ***mag-c.***

NEURALGIA, of - **CUPR-AR.**

OBSTRUCTED, sensation, as if - ***op.***

OBSTRUCTION, fecal impaction - alum., ***caust.,*** gels., lac-d., ***lach.,*** **OP.,** ***plb.***
obstructions, filled with hard feces - plb.

PAIN, intestines, (see Abdomen)
along course of - ***crot-h.,*** dios., ***lac-c.***
whole length, worse on pressure or movement - ferr-i.
ascending - rhus-t.
awakens, better on rising - chr-ac.
descending - ***asar.,*** berb., ipom.
just below ribs - all-s.
severe, in intussusception - verat.
pain and distension, especially of transverse - ***merc-c.***
region of left superior flexure - jal.
right and left, in - arund.
sigmoid flexure, about - ***colch.,*** jal.
stool looking like pea soup, and consisting of yellowish-greenish and bloody mucus of offensive odor - ***podo.***
transverse, at 3 a.m., followed by diarrhea - podo.
deranged liver, with - ***lept.***

PARALYSIS, of - **ALUM.,** bry., caust., con., lyc., mag-m., nux-v., **OP.,** ***phos.,*** **PLB.,** ***rhus-t., sec.,*** tab., thuj.
surgery, laparotomy, after - acon., ***arn.,*** bell., **CALEN.,** merc-c., ***op.***

PARALYZED, inactive feeling in transverse colon - acon.

PERISTALSIS, general
decreased - alum., hep., op.
increased - aloe, chin.
inertia, feeling of - aloe, alum., cadm-s.
constipation, causing - ***plat.***
congestive, of lower - ***coll.***
of lower, hemorrhoids and constipation, especially during pregnancy - ***coll.***
lost contractility, in constipation of infants - alum., ***lyc., op.***

PERISTALSIS, general
paralysis, of - alum., caps., carb-v., cocc., ***op.,*** phos., ***plb.***
lead poisoning, from - ***alum., op.,*** plb.
lower portions are affected, when - ***phos.***
paralytic, half, half crampy condition - plb.
paralyzed, action almost, in spinal irritation - rhus-t.
inactive feeling - acon., alum., op.
reversed - ***asaf.,*** cocc., elaps, ign., ***nux-v.,*** op., rhus-t., verat.
as if, feeling - asaf.
sluggish - ***card-m.***
stool, disposition to, but peristaltic motion in upper is wanting - cocc.

PERITONITIS, (see Inflammation) - ***acet-ac.,*** **ACON.,** aloe, alumn., **ANT-T., APIS,** ***arn.,*** **ARS.,** ars-i., atro., ***bapt.,*** **BELL., BRY.,** bufo, ***cact., calc., canth., carb-v.,*** card-m., ***cham.,*** cocc., coff., **COLCH.,** ***coloc., crot-c., crot-h.,*** cupr., ***echi., ferr.,*** ferr-ar., ferr-p., gamb., ***gels.,*** **HYOS.,** iod., ***ip., kali-c., kali-chl.,*** kali-i., ***kali-n.,*** kali-p., **LACH., LAUR., LYC.,** ***merc., merc-c., mez., nux-v., op., ox-ac.,*** **PHOS.,** plb., ***puls.,*** **PYROG., RHUS-T.,** sabin., ***sec., sil.,*** spong., squil., ***sulph.,*** **TER.,** thuj., ***uran.,*** urt-u., ***verat., verat-v.***
chronic - apis, ***lyc.,*** merc-d., sulph.
puerperal - acon., ***bell.,*** bry., ***merc-c.,*** pyrog., sulph., ter.
pseudo-peritonitis, hysterical - bell., coloc., verat.
spots, in - rhus-t.
tubercular - ***abrot.,*** ars., ars-i., calc., carb-v., ***chin.,*** iod., psor., sulph., ***tub.***

PHLEGMASIA - ***kali-i.***

PLUG, sensation of, pressed in - anac.
sides - sep.

PRESSURE, transverse colon, in, forenoon - all-s.

PRESSIVE pain, in middle of ascending - cahin.

PRICKING, in - arund.

RUMBLING, in (see Flatus) - acet-ac., ***acon.,*** acon-c., acon-f., aconin., aesc., **AGAR.,** ail., alco., all-c., ***aloe, alum.,*** alumn., am-caust., am-m., ambr., aml-n., ammc., am-c., am-m., **ANAC.,** ang., ant-c., ***ant-t.,*** anthr., aphis., apis, apoc., ***arg-m., arg-n.,*** arist-m., ***arn., ars.,*** ars-i., arum-d., asaf., asar., arund., asaf., asc-t., atha., aur., aur-m., bapt., bar-ac., bar-c., bar-i., bar-m., bapt., ***bell.,*** berb., berbin., ***bism.,*** bol., bor., bov., brom., ***bry.,*** bufo, cact., cahin., ***calc.,*** calc-ac., calc-caust., calc-i., calc-p., calc-s., cann-s., ***canth.,*** caps., ***carb-ac., carb-an.,*** carb-s., ***carb-v.,*** card-m., carl., casc., cass., cast., ***cast-v.,*** **CAUST.,** cedr., ***cham., chel.,*** **CHIN.,** ***chin-a.,*** chin-s., chlor., chr-ox., ***cic.,*** cimic., cinnb., clem., cob., coca, ***cocc.,*** coc-c., coff., ***colch.,*** colchin., coll., ***coloc.,*** con., coni., cop., cori-r., ***corn.,*** cot., croc., ***crot-c., crot-t.,*** cupr-ar., ***cycl.,*** delphin., dig., digin., **DIOS.,** ***dirc.,*** dor., dros., ***dulc.,*** echi., elaps, elat., erig., erio., eup-pur., euph., euphr., eupi., fel., ***ferr.,*** ferr-ar., ferr-i., ferr-ma., ferr-p., fl-ac., form., **GAMB.,** ***gels.,*** gent-l., gins., ***glon.,*** gnaph., ***graph.,*** grat., guai., gymn., haem.,

RUMBLING, in - **HELL., HEP.,** hipp., **HYDR.,** hydr-ac., hydrc., hyos., ***ign.,*** ill., ind., indg., iod., ip., ***iris,*** **JATR.,** jug-r., junc., ***kali-bi.,*** kali-br., kali-c., kali-i., kali-n., kali-p., kali-s., kiss., lach., lachn., lact., laur., led., lepi., lil-s., lina., linu-c., lipp., lob., lil-t., **LYC.,** lyss., ***mag-c., mag-m.,*** mag-s., ***manc.,*** mang., mate, mela., meny., ***merc.,*** merc-br., merc-c., merc-i-f., merc-i-r., merl., ***mez.,*** mill., mim-h., mit., mosch., mur-ac., musa, naja, nat-a., nat-c., ***nat-m.,*** nat-n., ***nat-p.,*** **NAT-S.,** ***nit-ac.,*** nit-s-d., ***nux-m.,*** **NUX-V.,** ol-an., ***olnd.,*** ol-an., onos., ***op.,*** osm., ost., ox-ac., paeon., par., pen., ***petr.,*** phel., **PH-AC., PHOS.,** phys., ***phyt.,*** pic-ac., pimp., plan., plat., plat-m., ***plb.,*** plect., ***podo.,*** polyg., polyp-p, ***psor.,*** ptel., **PULS.,** puls-n, ***ran-b., ran-s.,*** raph., rham-cath., rham-f., rheum, rhod., rhus-t., rhus-v., ric., rob., ***rumx.,*** ruta, ***sabad.,*** sabin., samb., sang., sant., sarr., ***sars.,*** schin., sec., senec., ***seneg., sep.,*** serp., **SIL.,** sin-a., sin-n., sol-t-ae., solin., ***spig.,*** spira., spong., ***squil.,*** stann., ***staph.,*** still., stram., stront-c., stry., sul-ac., **SULPH.,** sumb., sul-ac., tab., tanac., tarax., ***tarent.,*** tax., tep., ter., teucr., thea., ***thuj.,*** til., tong., torula., tril., upa., uran-n., valer., verat., verb., ***verat.,*** vichy-g., vinc., viol-t., vip., wies., xan., ***zinc.,*** zinc-s., zing.
afternoon - agar., am-c., am-m., ammc., carb-v., grat., ign., iris, lyc., mag-s., naja, ***nat-s.,*** nux-v., ox-ac., ***sulph.,*** tab.
1 p.m. - glon., mag-c., ptel.
2 p.m.- ptel.
4 p.m. - dirc., ir-foe., phys.
5 p.m. - fago., ir-foe.
till midnight - sars.
riding, while - nat-s.
standing, amel. - ir-foe.
walking, while - tab.
air, in open, amel. - nat-c.
alternating with, yawning and belching - ant-t.
annoying, women, in - rumx.
ascending colon, in - ***podo.***
palpitation from mental emotion or exertion, with - ***podo.***
bed, in - bry., glon., grat.
belching amel. - bor., sars.
breakfast, during - nat-m., plan.
after - all-c., cycl., grat., sulph., thuj.
amel. - mag-m.
before - eaux
burning - asc-t., vichy-g.
bursting bubbles, as from - ant-c., coloc.
coffee, after - nat-m., ox-ac.
amel. - adel., carl., phos.
colic, after - ars.
convulsions, during - ars., cupr.
cramps, as in, morning and evening, after eating amel. - mag-c.
croaking of frogs, like - caust., ***coloc.,*** graph., nux-v., sabad., spig.
daytime - nit-ac., ptel., vichy-g.

RUMBLING, in

diarrhea, during - calc., crot-t., glon., hyos., iris, kali-c., sars.
amel. - apoc.
after - cahin., mag-m., nat-c.
before - ant-t., ars., bry., ***crot-t.,*** cycl., iris, kali-n., mag-m., mag-s., nat-m., ***sulph.***
sensation, as if, would come on - **ALOE,** apis, ***cham.,*** cob., colch., ***dulc.,*** ferr., graph., **HYDR.,** kali-bi., kali-c., mag-s., myric., naja, nat-a., phos., ptel., sars., stann., ***stry.***

dinner, after - alum., ant-c., bor., coloc., grat., naja, nat-m., ox-ac., staph., ***sulph.,*** ter.
after, agg. - nat-m.
before - kali-c.
stool, before - colch.

drink, of - hydr-ac.

drinking, after - cham., graph., merc., rhod.

eating, while - calc., ferr-ma., graph., sin-a.
after - abies-c., acon., alum., ant-t., bry., calc., ***carb-v.,*** caust., ***chin.,*** coc-c., ***cycl.,*** grat., ign., meny., mez., mur-ac., naja, nat-m., nat-s., nit-ac., phos., plan., ***puls.,*** rhod., sars., sep., stann., ***sulph.***
amel. - graph., mag-c., mosch., squil., sul-ac.
before - mag-m., sel.

emptiness, as from - ant-c., arn., caust., clem., sabad.
hunger, and - euphr.

empty feeling, with - sars.

evening - agar., bov., chin., ferr., ferr-i., kali-n., lyc., mag-c., merc., mez., nat-c., nat-m., ***nat-s.,*** ox-ac., petr., plb., plan., **PULS.,** rumx., sabin., sars., sep., sulph., sul-ac., ***tarent.,*** zinc.
6 p.m. - nat-c.
7 p.m. - dirc., mag-c., nicc., stry.
8 p.m. - phys.
agg. - tarent., zinc.
bed, in - bry., grat.
eating, after - naja, phos.
lying, while - ran-b.
stool, during - zinc.

expiration, on - calc.

extending, sacral region, towards - phos.
stomach, to - kali-cy.
upwards and downwards - caps.

fasting, while - tax.

flatus, passing, amel. - acon., ant-t., ars., bor., bov., **CARB-V.,** caust., coc-c., hell., ***iris,*** **LYC.,** nat-c., **NAT-S.,** ol-an.
after - sul-ac.

food, when food enters cardia - stann.

forenoon - agar., am-c., ant-c., bry., cast-eq., coloc., fl-ac., nat-m., plect., stry., tarent.
9 a.m. - coloc., com., euphr., dirc., mag-c.
to 11 a.m. - tarent.

hypogastrium - aesc., aloe, ang., ant-c., carb-v., card-m., carl., chin., coloc., con., iris, mur-ac., rhus-t., spig., squil., stann., staph., tax.
morning - ambr.
night - com.
4 a.m. - iris.

RUMBLING, in

iliac region - plect.
fossa - plb.
morning, on pressure - dios.

inguinal - phos.

inspiration, on - calc., mag-c., mag-m., manc., tab.

left side - arg-m., bell., con., euph., lyc., ph-ac., sep., sulph., tarax., thuj., zinc.
upper - staph.

liquid, as of - ***jatr.***
emptied from a bottle - **JATR.**
mixed with air - osm.

lying, on - cann-i., coloc., ph-ac., plan., sep., stann.
amel. - am-c., sil.
left side, on, while - glon.
right side, on, while - coc-c.

menses, during - aloe, kali-c., ***kreos.,*** lyc., puls., sep.
before - aloe, bell., bry., calc-p., ferr., kali-c., lac-c., lyc., staph., tarent., ***zinc.***

midnight - alum.
after - rhus-t.

milk, after - ang., carb-an.

morning - agar., all-c., all-s., am-m., apis, arg-n., ars., arum-t., bov., bufo, coloc., dios., graph., haem., mag-c., mag-m., myric., nat-a., nat-m., ***nux-v.,*** plan., plat., plb., stront-c., samb., ter., ***zinc.***
6 a.m. to 3 p.m. - ptel.
9 a.m. - com., euphr., dirc., mag-c.
9 a.m. to 11 a.m. - corn., euphr., nat-m.
bed, in - coloc., croc., ***nux-v.,*** peti.
diarrhea, before - nux-v.
flatus amel., emission of - bov., chr-ac., coloc.
stool, before - ferr-i., hell., nux-v.

motion, on - lyc., mag-c., ***manc.,*** sil.

night - acon., arg-m., bor., cann-i., coc-c., euphr., jatr., kali-n., merc., raph., **SULPH.,** tarent.
10 p.m. - corn., phys., ptel.
1 a.m. - caul., ferr.
3 a.m. - asc-t., carb-v.
4 a.m. - ferr.
5 a.m. - ferr-i., petr., sulph.
flatus amel., emission of - bor., euphr.
stool, during - glon.
before - **SULPH.**

noon - graph., ox-ac., phos.
eating, while - graph.
eating, while, after - phos.

painful - lob., phos.

peas, rolled about, as if - agar.

pressure, agg. - agar.
amel. - tarent.

quaking, as frogs - arg-m., graph.

right, side - bism., zinc.

rising, on - ***bry.,*** crot-t., ferr.
after - plb.

sensation, of - agar.

short, abrupt - agar.

sitting, while - canth., caust., mur-ac.

RUMBLING, in
sleep, during - ***agn.,*** cupr., puls.
smoking, amel. - still.
splenic flexure, in - ***agar.,*** **LYC.**
stomach - mag-c., ph-ac., sep.
stool, during - arn., chel., cycl., elaps, form., gamb., hep., ***iris,*** kali-bi., mez., ptel., rat., seneg., sul-ac., thuj.
after - agar., coloc., ***crot-t.,*** dulc., ferr-ma., **JATR.,** kali-bi., ***lyc.,*** mez., nat-c., nat-m., ox-ac., plb., ptel., sulph., sul-ac., thuj.
amel. - ferr.
as before - hall
before - ars., ***asc-t.,*** brom., cact., carb-s., card-m., colch., dulc., ferr-i., form., gnaph., grat., hell., indg., ***iris, jatr.,*** kali-ar., kali-c., kali-n., kali-s., **MAG-C.,** mag-m., merc., ***mur-ac., nat-m., nat-s.,*** nux-v., olnd., ox-ac., ***phos.,*** rat., rhod., sabad., spig., spong., stront-c., sulph., tax.
stretching, on - stann.
supper, after - ***aloe,*** ol-an., phos.
swallowing, after - arn., am-c.
thunder, like distant - agar.
umbilical region - sul-ac.
below - mag-c., phos.
urination, during - stram.
waking, on - all-s., am-m., arg-n., ars., ferr., form.
6 a.m. - asc-t., mez.
7 a.m. - dios., nat-m., zing.
walking, on - ***lyc.***
open air, in - am-c., gamb., ***lyc.,*** ptel.
warm clothes amel. - am-c.
water is poured from a bottle, as when, after stool - ferr-ma.
yawning - croc.
yeast, as if full of - stict.

RUNNING, something alive, sensation in - cycl., thuj.

SCHISTOSOMIASIS, bilharziasis - ant-t.

SHIVERING, in - arg-n.

SHORTENING, sensation - anac.

SORE, pain - manc.

SWELLING, size of a fist in transverse, with long continued diarrhea - ***merc.***

TORPID - all-s., asim., phys., ***card-m.,*** chin., cocc., ***coloc., kali-c., nat-m., nux-v.,*** **OP.,** phos., ***plat.,*** sumb., sep., sin-n.

TUBERCULOSIS, of - ***carb-s.,*** chin-s., tub.

TYPHLITIS, (see Inflammation) - **APIS,** ***ars.,*** **BELL., BRY.,** ***calad., card-m., chin., colch., crot-h.,*** gins., **LACH.,** ***lyc.,*** **MERC.,** ***nat-s.,*** **OP.,** ***phos., plb.,*** **RHUS-T.,** ***samb., sep., sil., stram.,*** sulph., **THUJ.**

TYPHOID, fever, typhus (see Fevers)

ULCERS and ulceration - ***arg-n.,*** **ARS.,** bapt., ***calc.,*** **CARB-V.,** ***coloc., kali-bi.,*** merc., lept., ***lyc.,*** nat-p., **NIT-AC.,** phos., plb., sal-ac., sin-n., sulph., ***ter.,*** uran-n.
bleeding, with - **TER.**
chronic, with liver disorder - ***lept.***
vomiting of ingesta, hectic fever and emaciation - kali-bi.
corroding, with, stinging pain - cupr-m.
diarrhea, causes - ***sil.***
chronic, hectic fever, with - phos.
tuberculosis, in - olnd.
duodenal - aloe, alum., ***arg-n.,*** calen., dys-co., ger., ***kali-bi.,*** symph., ***uran-n.***
enterocolitis, with - ***ter.***
peyer's gland, of - ***ter.***
remittent fever, in infantile - ***mur-ac.***
round, with blackish fundus, in small intestines - ars-s-r.
tuberculosis, with - phos.
typhoid fever, in - agar., ***bapt.,*** **NIT-AC.,** ***ter.***
upper part of, diphtheria, in - phyt.

UPTURNING, sensation of, as if intestines lost their hold - mag-m.

WEAKNESS, of - ***aloe,*** merc.

WORM, sensation, writhing along in - calad.

WORMS, general - acon., aesc., all-c., all-s., ***ambro.,*** apoc., apoc-a., arg-n., ***ars.,*** art-v., bapt., bell., calad., ***calc.,*** carb-v., carc., ***chelo.,*** chin., cupr-ac., cupr-o., ***cic.,*** **CINA,** dol., ***ferr., ferr-m.,*** ferr-s., fil., ***gran.,*** graph., helm., ign., indg., ip., kali-m., lyc., med., merc., merc-c., morg., ***naphtin.,*** **NAT-M., NAT-P.,** ***nux-m.,*** nux-v., passi., petr., podo., puls., quas., ***rat., ruta, sabad., sant.,*** sec., ***sil., sin-n.,*** **SPIG.,** spong., squil., ***stann.,*** **SULPH.,** sumb., ***ter.,*** teucr., tub., ***valer.,*** verat., ***viol-o., viol-t.***
ancylostomiasis - carb-tcl., chen-a., ***thymol.***
ascarides - abrot., acet-ac., acon., aesc., agn., ant-c., ant-t., ***ars.,*** asar., asc-t., **BAR-C.,** bar-m., ***calc.,*** carb-s., carb-v., ***chelo.,*** chin., ***cina,*** crot-t., cupr., dig., dol., ***ferr.,*** ferr-m., gran., graph., grat., hyos., ***ign.,*** indg., kali-chl., lyc., mag-c., ***mag-s.,*** merc., merc-d., naphtin., **NAT-M.,** ***nat-p.,*** nux-v., petr., phos., pin-s., plat., ***ptel., rat.,*** **SABAD.,** ***sant., scirr., sep.,*** sil., ***sin-n., spig., spong.,*** squil., stann., ***sulph.,*** tell., **TER.,** ***teucr.,*** thuj., urt-u., ***valer.,*** viol-o.
female genitalia - ferr., ***sil., sulph.***
children, in - **CALC.,** cic., **CINA,** ***gaert., ign.,*** **NAT-P.,** ***nux-m., ruta,*** **SPIG.**
dentition, with constipation - ***dol.***
difficult - **SIL.**
masturbation, with - calad.
convulsions, with - indg.
headache, causes - ***calc.,*** chin., ***cina,*** graph., nux-v., plat., sabad., ***sil.,*** spig., ***sulph.***
hookworm - card-m., chen-a., thymol.
itching, from - ***calc.,*** calc-f., chin., ***cina,*** ferr., ign., ***nat-p., sabad.,*** sin-a., ***teucr., urt-u.***

WORMS, general

lumbricoides - acon., all-s., anac., ***ars.,*** asar., bar-c., bell., calc., carb-s., cic., cham., ***chel.,*** **CINA,** ***ferr-s., gran.,*** graph., hyos., kali-c., lyc., mag-c., merc., nat-m., nux-v., rhus-t., ruta., ***sabad.,*** sec., ***sil.,*** **SPIG.,** stann., **SULPH.,** ter.

nerves and eyes, complaints - art-v., cina.

oxyuris vermicularis - ars., bapt., ***chelo., cina,*** ign., indg., lyc., ***merc-d., merc-sul.,*** nat-p., rat., ***sant.,*** sil., sin-n., spig., teucr., valer.

teniae - ***ail.,*** arg-n., **CALC.,** ***carb-an.,*** carb-s., ***carb-v.,*** chin., cina, cupr., cupr-ac., cur., ***fil., form.,*** frag-v., ***gran., graph.,*** grat., kali-c., kali-i., mag-m., merc., ***nat-c.,*** nat-s., nux-v., petr., phos., ***plat., puls., sabad.,*** sant., ***sep., sil., stann.,*** sulph., ter., thuj., valer.

trichinae - ars., bapt., cina.

Joints

ABSCESS - ***ang.***, ars-i., bac., calc., calc-f., ***calc-hp.***, ***calc-p.***, calc-s., conch., fl-ac., guai., ***hep.***, kali-c., kali-i., ***merc.***, myris., nit-ac., ph-ac., ***phos.***, ***psor.***, puls., ***sil.***, ter., ***teucr.***, thuj., tub.
 about the - calc-hp., merc., phos., psor., sil.

ACHING, pain - aesc., all-c., arn., bell-p., bol., bry., carb-an., ***carl.***, ***chin-s.***, clem., erig., ***gels.***, kali-c., ***kalm.***, led., merc., mosch., phos., ptel., pyrus, rhod., rhus-t., ***ruta.***
 chill, during - cann-i.

ARTHRITIC, nodosities - abrot., agn., ***ant-c.***, **APIS**, arn., ***aur.***, **BENZ-AC.**, berb., ***bry.***, **CALC.**, **CALC-F.**, ***calc-p.***, ***calc-s.***, carb-an., caul., ***caust.***, ***cic.***, cimic., ***clem.***, ***colch.***, ***dig.***, ***elaps***, elat., eucal., eup-per., fago., ***form.***, **GRAPH.**, ***guai.***, ***hecla.***, hep., iod., kali-ar., ***kali-i.***, kali-s., **LED.**, **LITH.**, **LYC.**, mang., med., ***meny.***, ***merc.***, nat-m., nux-v., plb., ***puls.***, ran-b., ***rhod.***, ***rhus-t.***, ruta, ***sabin.***, ***sil.***, ***staph.***, sul-ac., sulph., urea, ***urt-u.***
 chill, during - cann-i.
 condyles, on - ***calc-p.***
 painful - **LED.**, nit-ac.
 pinching and cracking on motion - **LED.**
 skin, in, over joints - **LED.**

ARTHRITIS, inflammation - **ACON.**, ***ang.***, **APIS**, ***arn.***, ***aur.***, **BELL.**, **BRY.**, ***calc.***, ***caust.***, ***ferr-p.***, ***guai.***, hyper., ***iod.***, ***kali-c.***, ***kali-i.***, ***kalm.***, ***kreos.***, ***lac-ac.***, lach., **LED.**, lith., ***lyc.***, ***mang.***, meny., ***merc.***, ***nat-m.***, ***nat-s.***, ***phyt.***, ***psor.***, ***puls.***, ***rhod.***, ***rhus-t.***, ***ruta.***, sabin., ***sars.***, ***sep.***, **SIL.**, ***sulph.***, verat-v.
 erysipelatous - ***bry.***, rhod.
 evening - acon.
 heat agg. - guai., led.
 night - acon., **IOD.**, mang., ***rhod.***
 serous membranes - **ACON.**, am-c., **APIS**, apoc., arg-m., **ARS.**, ars-i., asaf., ***aur.***, ***aur-m.***, bell., **BRY.**, **CALC.**, calc-p., ***carb-v.***, colch., ferr., fl-ac., **HELL.**, indg., ***iod.***, ***kali-c.***, lach., ***led.***, **LYC.**, mag-m., ***merc.***, ***nat-m.***, ***ph-ac.***, ***phos.***, plat., ***psor.***, ***puls.***, samb., seneg., **SIL.**, ***squil.***, ***stram.***, ***sulph.***, ***ter.***, zinc.
 synovitis - ***apis***, bell., ***bry.***, calc., caust., ferr-p., iod., kali-c., kali-i., led., lyc., merc., phyt., puls., rhus-t., sep., sil., sulph., verat-v.

BORING, pain - arg-m., clem., coloc., mang., ***rhod.***, thuj.
 decay, of - aur-m.

BROKEN, sensation, as if - carb-an., par.
 motion, on - par.

BURNING, pain - abrot., ant-t., ***carb-v.***, guare., kali-c., ***mang.***, ***nat-c.***, nat-n., ***nit-ac.***, ***plat.***, thuj., zinc.

BURSAE - **ARN.**, calc-p., cann-s., kali-m., **NAT-M.**, **SIL.**, stann., **STICT.**
 cysts - cann-s., caust., ***graph.***, iod., kali-br., ***sil.***, ***sulph.***

BURSITIS - ant-c., ***apis.***, ars., bell., ***bell-p.***, ***bry.***, graph., hep., iod., ***lycpr.***, puls., rhus-t., **RUTA..**, **SIL.**, ***stict.***, ***sulph.***

COLDNESS, sensation - ***camph.***, cinnb., ***nat-m.***, petr., rhus-t., sumb.
 air, in open - nat-m.
 morning - sumb.
  bed, in - sumb.

COMPRESSION, sensation - coloc., merc.

CONTRACTION, of muscles and tendons, of - ***anac.***, ***aur.***, ***caust.***, cimx., ***colch.***, ***form.***, ***graph.***, ***merc.***, ***nat-m.***, ***nit-ac.***, petr., sec., stront.

CONSTRICTION - ***anac.***, ***aur.***, calc., carb-an., ***coloc.***, ferr., **GRAPH.**, ***lyc.***, **NAT-M.**, **NIT-AC.**, ***petr.***, sil., ***stront.***

CRACKED, skin, bends of - hippoz., **GRAPH.**

CRACKING, of - acon., agar., am-c., anac., ***ang.***, ***ant-c.***, brom., calad., ***calc.***, ***camph.***, **CAPS.**, carb-an., carb-s., carl., caul., ***cham.***, chin., chlf., clem., ***cocc.***, croc., ***ferr.***, gins., guare., ***kali-bi.***, ***kali-c.***, ***kali-s.***, **LED.**, ***lyc.***, lyss., ***merc.***, ***nat-c.***, ***nat-m.***, nat-p., ***nat-s.***, **NIT-AC.**, ***nux-v.***, **PETR.**, ***phos.***, plb., raph., **RHUS-T.**, ***sabad.***, ***sep.***, ***sulph.***, ***thuj.***
 bending, on - lyc.
 convulsions during - acon.
 morning - brom.
  after rising - brom.
 turning when - caul.
 walking, while - am-c., bry., caul., cocc.

CRAMPS - ***anac.***, ang., aur., ***bell.***, ***bry.***, **CALC.**, camph., canth., caust., cic., cocc., ***hyos.***, ***ign.***, lach., laur., merc., op., ***par.***, ph-ac., **PLAT.**, plb., rhus-t., ***sec.***, ***stram.***, ***sulph.***, verat.

CUTTING, pain - cadm-s., guare., hyos., ***sabad.***, vesp.

DECAY, of - ***nit-ac.***

DISCOLORATION, redness - **BELL.**, ***cocc.***, colch., ***kalm.***, ***merc.***, **PULS.**, **RHUS-T.**, ***verat-v.***

DISLOCATION, as if - agar., anac., ***arn.***, bry., caps., kali-i., merc., nit-ac., phos., ***ruta***, stram., sulph.

DISTENSION, sensation - mang.

DRAWING, pain - acon., am-c., ant-s., ant-t., arg-m., bar-ac., ***bry.***, calc., ***carl.***, cham., ***cimx.***, ***cist.***, clem., coc-c., coloc., hyos., kali-bi., ***led.***, lyc., mez., nat-c., nat-m., nat-s., nit-ac., ***nux-m.***, ***par.***, phos., plat., ***puls.***, rhod., sec., sulph., tep.
 chill, during - **CIMX.**
  before - calc.
 cramp-like - ***par.***, ***plat.***
 evening - nat-c., nat-s., ***puls.***
 holding them long, in the wrong position - staph.
 morning - cham.
  after rising - phos.
 motion amel. - coloc., phos.
 muscles, near - hyos.
 paralytic - cham., nat-m., staph.
 sitting, while - coloc.

DRAWING, pain
- sticking - calc.
- tearing - coloc.
- waking, after - nat-c.
- walking, while - ang.
- wandering - acon., cham.
- wine, after - ***led.***

DRYNESS - canth., croc., lyc., **NUX-V.,** ph-ac., **PULS.**

ECZEMA - am-c., **GRAPH.,** led., merc., phos., ***sep., sulph***
- bends, of - am-c., **GRAPH.,** led., merc., ***sep., sulph.***

EDEMA, dropsy, of - ***apis,*** arn., ***bry.,*** canth., cedr., chin., chin-s., iod., kali-m., ***ran-b.,*** samb.
- fractures, after - bov., bry.

ERUPTIONS - aeth., ant-c., ***apis,*** calc-p., hura, ***merc., nat-m.,*** nat-p., phos., **PSOR., RHUS-T.,** sep., ust.
- bends of - caust., **GRAPH.,** ***hep.,*** led., ***nat-c., nat-m., psor.,*** sep., staph.
  - itching - sep.
  - pimples - sep.
- desquamation - phos.
- itching - phos.
- pimples - ***calc-p.,*** sep.
- scabs - ***staph.***
- winter - ***merc., psor., rhus-t.***

EXCORIATION, bends of - bell., ***caust.,*** **GRAPH.,** lyc., ***mang., ol-an., petr., sep.,*** squil., ***sulph.***

FISTULA, of - ***calc.,*** hep., ol-j., **PHOS., SIL.,** ***sulph.***

FORMICATION, sensation, of - arn., carl., ip., sec.

FULLNESS - cinnb., ham.

GNAWING, pain - ***dros.,*** mag-c., mang., **RAN-S.,** zinc.
- caries in - ***aur-m.***

GOUTY, pain - ***abrot.,*** agar., **AGN.,** ***alum.,*** ambr., am-c., am-m., anac., anag., ant-c., ***apis,*** **ARG-M., ARN.,** ***ars.,*** ars-h., ***ars-i., asaf.,*** asar., aur., ***bapt., bar-c.,*** **BELL.,** ***benz-ac.,*** bism., bor., bov., **BRY.,** ***bufo,*** **CALC., CALC-P., CALC-S.,** canth., carb-an., ***carb-s.,*** carb-v., **CAUST.,** cham., ***chel., chim., chin., chin-a., cinnb., cocc.,*** **COLCH.,** ***coloc.,*** dros., ***dulc.,*** eup-per., ***ferr.,*** ferr-ar., ferr-i., ferr-p., ***form., graph., guai.,*** hell., ***hep., hyos., ign., iod., kali-ar.,*** **KALI-C.,** ***kali-i.,*** kali-n., kali-p., ***kalm., laur.,*** **LED., LYC., MAG-C.,** mag-m., ***mang.,*** meny., **MERC.,** ***mez., nat-a., nat-c., nat-m.,*** nat-p., ***nat-s.,*** nit-ac., nux-m., **NUX-V.,** ol-j., petr., ***ph-ac., phos., phyt., plb.,*** **PSOR.,** ***puls., ran-b.,*** ran-s., ***rhod.,*** **RHUS-T.,** ruta., **SABIN.,** ***sal-ac.,*** samb., ***sang., sars.,*** sec., **SEP.,** ***sil.,*** spig., **SPONG.,** squil., ***stann.,*** **STAPH.,** stram., ***stront-c.,*** **SULPH.,** sul-ac., tarax., ***thuj.,*** valer., verat., verb., viol-o., viol-t., zinc.
- alternates with, asthma - sulph.
  - with, pain in forehead - sulph.
- debilitated men, in - ***staph.***
- extending left to right - ***colch.***

GOUTY, pain
- gastric symptoms, with - ***ant-c.***
- increase as cough diminishes - coloc.

HEAT - ***cimic.,*** guai., guare., **LED.,** ***kalm., stict.***

HEAVINESS - ***cham., chin., mez.,*** nit-ac., ***ph-ac.,*** plb., ***staph.***

HERPES - dulc., ***kreos.,*** staph.

INFLAMMATION, of, (see Arthritis)

INJURIES, to - arn., bell-p., ***bry., rhus-t., ruta.***

ITCHING - apis, clem., merc., nat-p., nux-v., sep., ***spig.,*** zinc.
- bends of - nit-ac., ***ph-ac.,*** sel., sep., zinc.

LAMENESS - abrot., brom., cinnb., **RHUS-T., RUTA.,** ***sil.***
- chill, during - ***rhus-t., tub.***
- fever, during - ***rhus-t., tub.***
- sprain, after - calc., **RHUS-T., RUTA.**
- waking, after - nat-c.

LOOSENESS, sense of, in - croc., **STRAM.,** wild.

LYME disease - ars., merc. thuj.

NUMBNESS, sensations - alum., con., ip., ***led., lyc.,*** plat., puls.
- cold wet, after exposure to - ***rhus-t.***
- rheumatism, in - puls.

PAIN, joints - acon., aesc., agar., all-c., ***alum., apis, apoc.,*** aran., **ARG-M., ARN.,** ***ars., ars-i.,*** asaf., asc-t., aster., aur., bar-c., ***bell., bol.,*** **BRY.,** caj., ***calc.,*** **CALC-P.,** calc-s., cann-i., ***caps.,*** carb-ac., carb-an., ***carb-s., caust.,*** cedr., ***cham., chin.,*** chin-a., ***cimx., cinnb.,*** cist., ***cocc., colch., coloc.,*** con., cop., croc., crot-t., cycl., daph., dig., dios., ***dulc., ferr., ferr-ar.,*** ferr-i., ***ferr-p.,*** gels., ***guai.,*** hell., hydrc., hydr., ign., ip., ***iod.,*** iris, jac-c., jatr., ***kali-bi., kali-c.,*** kali-n., kali-p., ***kalm., lac-c., lac-ac.,*** **LED.,** ***lyc.,*** lyss., ***mang., merc.,*** mez., morph., ***nat-a.,*** nat-m., ***nat-s.,*** nit-ac., **NUX-V.,** ol-an., par., ***ph-ac., phos., phyt.,*** **PLB., PULS.,** ran-s., raph., ***rheum, rhod.,*** **RHUS-T.,** ***ruta.,*** sabad., ***sabin., sang.,*** sel., senec., ***sil.,*** sol-n., sol-t-ae., ***staph., sulph.,*** sul-ac., ter., thuj., verat-v.
- afternoon - dig.
  - afternoon. sleeping, after - dig.
- air, open - ***phyt., rhus-t.***
- alternating with, colic - plb.
  - with, pain in forehead - sulph.
  - with, pain in limbs - bry.
  - with, pain sides - ***lac-c.,*** mang.
  - with, with uterine hemorrhage - sabin.
- amenorrhea - ***lach.***
- bed, in - calc-p., hell., ***kalm., led.,*** stront-c., ***sulph.***
- bending, on - ***cocc., ran-b., ruta.***
- chill, during - **CIMX.,** ***ferr., hell.***
- cold, after exposure, to - ***calc.,*** **CALC-P.,** con., **DULC.,** ***kalm., ph-ac.,*** **RHUS-T.**
  - from taking - ***calc-p.,*** caps., ***mang., nux-m.,*** **RHUS-T.**
  - weather, in - **CALC., CALC-P., DULC.,** ***ph-ac.***
  - weather, in damp - ant-t., **COLCH.**

PAIN, joints
cough, diminishes when - coloc.
eating, after - ***bry.***
evening - hydr., ***kalm.,*** lac-ac., ***led.,*** nat-c., stront-c., teucr.
exertion, after - ***calc.,*** sabin.
fatigued, as if - con., dig., graph.
forenoon - ars., caust., sabad.
sitting, while - ars.
jerking - mang., nat-c., plat., sul-ac., verat.
lying, while - chin., ruta.
left side - phos.
right side - merc.
side, on - puls.
morning - ***aur.,*** caust., dios., nit-ac., **NUX-V.,** staph., viol-o.
bed, in - **AUR.,** ***chin.,*** **NUX-V., PULS.**
waking, on - sol-n., verat.
motion, agg. - acon., ***ant-t., arn.,*** **BRY.,** caps., ***cham., cocc.,*** **COLCH.,** croc., cycl., ferr-p., ***guai., kali-bi., kalm., lac-ac., lac-c.,*** **LED.,** lyc., ***mang.,*** nux-v., par., phos., ***phyt.,*** plb., rheum, ***ruta.***
amel. - ***arg-m.,*** **AUR.,** caps., cedr., chel., chin., dros., ***ferr.,*** nat-s., ***phos., rhod.,*** **RHUS-T.,** sulph., teucr.
night - ***carb-an.,*** cedr., dios., gels., hell., **IOD.,** kali-c., ***kali-bi.,*** lac-ac., ***led., mang.,*** **MERC.,** nat-c., plb., ***rhod.,*** sil., stront-c., ***sulph.***
10 p.m. - cedr.
10 p.m. until 6 a.m. - ***rhus-t.***
after midnight - nux-v.
amel. - ***ars., mag-p., plb.***
numbness, with - ***lyc.***
position, in wrong - staph.
pressure, amel. - bry., form.
side, not lain on - nux-v.
sleep, during - sul-ac.
small, joints, amel. after menses - ***caul.***
stretch, desire to - puls., rhus-t.
swelling, without - iod.
touch, agg. - cocc., ***mang.***
waking, after amel. - sul-ac.
walking, while - nat-s., ***ran-b.***
after - bry., calc-p., caj., cann-i., caps., carb-ac., carb-s., cedr., cinnb., cist., crot-t., dios., ***ferr.,*** gels., jac-c., kali-bi., lac-ac., ***led.,*** lyss., merc., nat-m., nat-s., ***nux-v.,*** olnd., phys., phyt., plb., raph., rhus-t., ruta., sel., sol-t-ae., sulph.
wandering - anag., ***ant-t., ars.,*** **AUR.,** ***calc-p., camph.,*** cedr., chel., ***cinnb., coca, cocc., colch.,*** form., hell., ***hyper., iris,*** **KALI-BI.,** ***kali-s., kalm.,*** lac-ac., **LAC-C.,** ***lach., mang., merc-c.,*** nat-a., nat-s., phyt., **PULS.,** ***rhod.,*** sabin.
warmth, agg. - caust., cedr., ***guai., lac-c.,*** **LED., PULS.**
bed, of - calc., lac-c., **LED.,** ***plb., sabin., sulph.***
amel. - **ARS.,** ***bry., caust., lyc., nux-v., rhus-t., sulph.***

PAIN, joints
wine, after - ***led.***
sour, after - **ANT-C.**
winter - calc-p., ***kalm.***

PARALYSIS, sensation of - acon., arn., ***caps.,*** cham., croc., graph., ***led.,*** par., plb., rhus-t., sulph.
night - ***led.***

PARALYTIC, pain - am-c., apis, arg-m., **ARN.,** asar., **AUR.,** bov., ***calc.,*** **CAPS.,** ***carb-v., chin.,*** **COLCH.,** ***croc., dros.,*** **EUPH.,** kali-c., ***led., mez.,*** nat-c., ***par., plb., puls., rhus-t., sabin.,*** sars., ***seneg.,*** **STAPH.,** stram., **VALER.**

PERSPIRATION - **AM-C.,** ars., bell., bry., calc., dros., led., ***lyc.,*** mang., nux-v., ph-ac., ***rhus-t.,*** sars., stann., sulph.
bends, of - sep.
morning - lyc.
night - sars.
cold - rhus-t.
morning - am-c., lyc.
painful - am-c., lyc.

PINCHING, pain - kreos., meny.

PRESSING, pain - agn., ***alum.,*** calc., carb-an., chin., clem., coloc., ***kali-c., led.,*** lyc., nat-s., par.
motion, agg. - led.
amel. - ***kali-c.***
tearing - led.

PULSATION - am-m., arg-m., brom., led., ***merc.,*** mill., rhod., rhus-t., ***ruta.,*** sabad., thuj.

RELAXATION - bar-c., laur.

RESTLESSNESS - sil., sulph.

RHEUMATIC, pain - ***abrot., acon.,*** act-sp., ***aesc., agar.,*** alumn., am-m., ***ant-t., apis, arg-m.,*** **ARN., ARS.,** ***ars-i., aur.,*** **AUR-M-N., BAD.,** bapt., ***bell.,*** **BENZ-AC., BRY.,** ***cact., calc., calc-p., calc-s., camph.,*** cann-s., ***caps., carb-ac., carb-s., carb-v.,*** card-m., ***caul.,*** **CAUST.,** cedr., **CHAM., CHEL.,** ***chin., chin-a., cimic.,*** clem., **COLCH.,** ***coloc., corn., crot-c., crot-h., crot-t.,*** cupr., ***dig., dulc.,*** elaps, euph., eup-per., ***ferr., ferr-ar.,*** ferr-p., **FORM.,** ***gels.,*** grat., ***guai., ham.,*** hell., ***hep.,*** hydrc., ***ign., kali-ar., kali-bi., kali-c.,*** kali-chl., **KALI-I.,** kali-p., ***kali-s.,*** **KALM.,** ***lac-ac., lac-c., lach.,*** led., **LYC.,** ***mag-c.,*** mag-p., mag-s., **MED.,** meph., ***merc.,*** merc-i-f., merc-i-r., merc-sul., ***mez.,*** mill., mur-ac., **NAT-A.,** ***nit-ac.,*** nux-m., ***nux-v.,*** ol-an., pall., ***petr., ph-ac., phos.,*** **PHYT.,** plat., ***psor.,*** **PULS.,** ***ran-b.,*** **RHOD., RHUS-T.,** ***ruta., sal-ac.,*** **SANG., SARS.,** sec., ***sep., sil.,*** spig., squil., stann., ***stel.,*** stict., **SULPH.,** ***syph., tarent.,*** ter., thuj., teucr., ***valer., verat.,*** viol-t., zinc.
acute - **ACON.,** ***ant-c., ars.,*** asc-c., ***bell.,*** **BRY.,** calc-s., caul., ***cham., chel.,*** chin., chin-s., cimic., **COLCH.,** ***dulc.,*** glon., ign., ***kali-bi., kalm., lac-c., lach.,*** **MERC.,** ***nux-v., puls., rhod.,*** **RHUS-T.,** sal-ac., sang., verat.
alternating with,
chest problem - led.
diarrhea - cimic., dulc., ***kali-bi.***

RHEUMATIC, pain
alternating, with, dyspnea - guai.
eruptions - crot-t., staph.
gastric, symptoms - **KALI-BI.**
hemorrhoids - abrot.
lung troubles - **KALI-BI.**
pain in heart - benz-ac.
bed, drives him out of - **CHAM.,** ***ferr.,*** lac-c., led., **MERC., RHUS-T.,** sulph., ***verat.***
cold, after a - acon., arn., ***bry.,*** calc., ***calc-p., coloc., dulc.,*** gels., ***guai., merc., nit-ac.,*** ph-ac., ***rhus-t.,*** sulph.
after a, amel. - ***guai., lac-c.,*** **LED., PULS., SEC.**
after becoming - ***ph-ac.,*** **RHUS-T.**
weather, after - ars., **BRY., CALC-P.,** carb-v., ***colch., dulc., kali-bi., kalm.,*** nit-ac., ***nux-v., ph-ac., phos., puls., rhod.,*** **RHUS-T.,** sul-ac., ***tub.***
diarrhea checked - ***abrot.***
chronic, in - ***nat-s.***
following - ***kali-bi.***
eruptions, acute, after - dulc.
extending, to lower limbs - ***kali-c.***
upward - ***kalm.,*** **LED.**
upper to lower limbs - ***kalm.***
flatus, amel. - coloc.
gonorrhea, after suppressed - ***clem.,*** con., ***cop.,*** crot-h., daph., kalm., ***lyc.,*** **MED.,** ***phyt., puls., sars., sep., sulph.,*** **THUJ.**
hemorrhoids, suppressed - ***abrot.***
injured parts - ***caust.***
left to right - **LACH.,** naja, ***rhus-t.***
mercury, abuse of - arg-m., arn., asaf., ***bell.,*** calc., ***carb-v., cham.,*** **CHIN., GUAI., HEP.,** ***kali-i., lach.,*** lyc., mez., ***nit-ac.,*** ph-ac., ***phyt.,*** podo., puls., rhod., **SARS.,** ***sulph.,*** valer.
overheated and exertion from - ***zinc.***
perspiration, with - **FORM., MERC.,** ***sulph., til.***
places least covered by flesh, in - sang.
right to left - **LYC.**
spring - ***colch.***
syphilitic - ***benz., fl-ac.,*** kali-bi., **KALI-I.,** kalm., ***merc., nit-ac., phyt.***
warm weather, in - **COLCH.,** ***kali-bi.***
first warm days - bry.

SCRAPING, as if, in - bry., ***sabad.***

SENSITIVE, morning, in - nit-ac.

SHARP, pain - acon., agar., ***agn.,*** aloe, ***apis, arn., asaf., bar-c., bell., bov.,*** **BRY., CALC.,** ***camph.,*** carl., ***carb-s., caust.,*** cedr., cham., clem., ***cocc., colch., con.,*** dig., ***dros., graph., guai.,*** **HELL.,** ***hep., hyos., ign.,*** ind., **KALI-C.,** ***kali-i., kali-n.,*** kali-p., ***kali-s., kreos.,*** lac-ac., ***led., mag-m.,*** **MANG.,** ***meny.,*** **MERC.,** ***merc-c.,*** mill., ***nat-m.,*** par., ***phos.,*** phys., ***plan., puls., rhod.,*** **RHUS-T., SABIN.,** ***sars., sep.,*** **SIL., SPIG.,** ***spong., stann., staph.,*** stict., ***stront-c.,*** **SULPH.,** ***sul-ac.,*** **TARAX., THUJ.,** trom., verat., **ZINC.**
burning - ign.
chill, during - ***calc.,*** **HELL.**
before - ***calc.***

SHARP, pain
cold, after taking - caust.
drawing - puls.
evening - acon., nat-c., par.
exercise, during - calc.
extending into bones - cham.
fever, during - ***hell.,*** merc., **RHUS-T.,** sil., thuj.
motion, on - ***bry., hyos.,*** sarr.
amel. - dros., ***rhus-t.***
night - cedr., ***kali-i.,*** nat-c., sil.
pressure, on - zinc.
pulsating - led.
rising from a seat - ***rhus-t.***
shocks, like - verat.
tearing - ***calc.,*** camph., sabin.
touch, on - bry.
transversely - **ZINC.**
twitching - carb-s.
wandering - acon., cedr.

SHOOTING, pain - ***camph., hep.,*** plan., tep., trom., verat.
electric shocks, like - verat.

SORE, pain - abrot., ***agar., alum.,*** alumn., ang., anac., ***apis,*** apoc., **ARG-M., ARN., AUR.,** ***bell., bov.,*** bufo, calad., ***calc.,*** carb-an., ***carb-s., carb-v., caust., cham.,*** chel., **CHIN.,** chlf., ***cist.,*** clem., cob., coff., coloc., ***con., crot-h.,*** cupr., ***dig., dros., ferr.,*** hyos., ***hyper.,*** kali-i., ***lac-c., led., lith., mez., mur-ac., nat-m.,*** nat-n., nat-p., ***nit-ac.,*** **NUX-V.,** par., **PH-AC.,** phos., phys., pic-ac., plb., **PULS., RHUS-T.,** ***ruta., sep., spig.,*** squil., ***sulph.,*** tub., ***verat.,*** viol-o., zinc.
bending, after - coff.
cold, from becoming - ***ph-ac.***
descending, on - ***arg-m.***
evening - cham.
7 p.m. - cham.
forenoon - aur.
lying, agg. - aur., ***nux-v.***
on painful side amel. - ***nux-v., rhus-t.***
morning - aur., caps., cob., nit-ac., **PH-AC.,** pyrus, verat.
bed, in - anac., aur., carb-v., chin., coff., **NUX-V.,** ***rhus-t.***
waking, on - abrot.
motion, on - agar., ***arg-m., arn., calc.,*** chin., nux-v.
amel. - caps., ***chin.,*** coloc., **COM., RHUS-T., TUB.**
night - ***con.,*** spig.
nosebleed, after - agar.
paralytic - ***arn., calc.***
rising, on, amel. - aur., coff., ***nux-v.***
sitting, when - coloc.
sleep, nap, after - dig.
touch, on - dulc.

SPRAINED, sensation, as if - agar., agn., alum., ***ambr.,*** am-c., arg-m., ***arg-n.,*** **ARN.,** ars., ***arum-t.,*** bar-c., bell., ***bry., calc., calc-p.,*** caps., ***carb-an.,*** carb-ac., ***caust.,*** cham., chel., chin., cocc., ***con., cor-r.,*** dig., ferr., fl-ac., ***graph., ign.,*** kali-c., ***kali-n., lach.,*** **LED.,** ***lyc.,*** mag-c., ***merc.,*** mez., ***nat-m.,*** nux-v., par., ***petr.,*** **PHOS.,** ***prun.,*** **PULS.,** ran-b., ***rhod.,*** **RHUS-T.,** ***ruta.,*** sabin., sars., ***sep.,*** sil., ***spig.,*** spong., ***stann.,*** staph., **SULPH.,** thuj., valer., verat.

quick, motions, by - phos.

walking, after - nit-ac.

STIFFNESS, of - abrot., aesc., ***agar.,*** ant-s., apis, **ARS.,** ***aur.,*** bapt., ***bell.,*** cact., ***calc.,*** canth., ***caps., carb-an., carb-s.,*** **CAUST.,** ***chin-s.,*** cimic., clem., ***cocc., colch., coloc.,*** ferr-ar., ***form.,*** get., graph., kali-ar., ***kali-bi., kali-c., kali-i.,*** kali-s., lac-ac., ***lac-c.,*** lach., **LED., LYC.,** ***nat-a., nat-m.,*** nat-p., ***nux-v.,*** **PETR.,** ***phos.,*** psor., ***puls.,*** **RHUS-T., SEP., SIL.,** ***staph., stict.,*** **SULPH.,** ***zinc.***

afternoon, sleeping, after - chin.

bath, too warm, after - rhus-t.

chill, during - bry., ***calc.,*** **CAUST.,** led., ***lyc.,*** nux-v., ***op.,*** petr., rhus-t., sep., sulph., thuj.

cold water applied amel. - ***led.***

edema, with - kali-ars.

evening, 9 p.m. - phys.

heat agg. - ***lac-c.***

lying, down, after - caps., caust.

morning - ant-s., caps., cimic., ***kali-bi., led.,*** **RHUS-T.,** staph.

motion, on - cham.

numbness, with - colch.

painful - ***cocc.***

paralytic on rising from sleep - caps., chin.

rheumatic - ***calc., lyc.,*** **RHUS-T.**

rising, on - ***agar., calc., carb-an.,*** **RHUS-T.,** staph.

sitting, while - caust.

sleep, after - chin.

SWELLING, of - **APIS,** ***abrot.,*** acon., **ACT-SP.,** agn., anag., ***ant-t.,*** **APIS,** apoc., ***arn., ars.,*** asc-t., aur., ***aur-m.,*** **BELL.,** berb., **BRY.,** bufo, ***calc.,*** calc-f., chin., ***cimic.,*** clem., ***cocc.,*** **COLCH.,** con., ***ferr-p., guai., ham.,*** **HEP.,** ***kali-chl.,*** kali-i., ***kalm., lach., lac-ac.,*** **LED.,** ***lyc.,*** mang., med., ***merc., nat-m., nux-v., rhod., rhus-t.,*** sabin., ***sal-ac.,*** sil., sol-t-ae., stict., **SULPH.,** tarent., ***ter.,*** thuj., ***verat-v.***

afternoon - chin.

bluish - **LACH.**

dropsical - ant-t., apis, ***caust., nat-m.***

edematous - ***led., thuj.***

exertion, after - act-sp.

sensation, of - caj., caps., ***par.,*** sabin.

white - ***caust.,*** kali-s., ***sulph.***

TEARING, pain - ***acon., agn.,*** aloe, ***ambr.,*** am-c., ant-s., ant-t., apis, **ARG-M.,** ***ars., ars-i., aur.,*** **BELL.,** ***bov., bry.,*** cact., ***calc., camph., carl.,*** **CAUST.,** ***chin.,*** cist., ***colch., coloc., con., dros., graph.,*** grat., **GUAI.,** ***hyos., iod., kali-bi.,*** **KALI-C.,** ***kali-n.,*** kali-s., kreos., ***led.,*** **LYC., MERC.,** nat-c., nat-m., nat-p., ***nat-s., nit-ac., nux-v.,*** petr., ***ph-ac., phos., plat.,*** **PULS.,** rhod., **RHUS-T.,** ***sabin., sars., sep., sil.,*** spig., ***staph., stram.,*** **STRONT-C., SULPH.,** tep., teucr., thuj., ***tub.,*** **ZINC.**

chill, during - ***cimx., hep.,*** led., lyc., nux-v., phos., **RHUS-T.**

downward - ***sulph.***

drawing, on exertion - calc-caust.

evening - ***merc.,*** nat-c., stront.

eruptions, during the - ***merc.***

extending into long bones - ***caust.***

fever, during - ***calc.,*** caust., ***hell.,*** lyc., merc., ph-ac., phos., **RHUS-T.,** ***sulph., tub.***

in limbs not lain on - nux-v.

jerking - con., caust., **CHIN., RHUS-T.,** sulph.

lying on left side - phos.

motion - hyos., led.

amel. - ***coloc.***

night, in bed - hell., ***hep., led.,*** **MERC.**

paralytic - **BELL.,** chin., cocc., dig., **STAPH.**

sticking - **LED.,** ***zinc.***

twitching - led.

wandering - ***camph., kali-bi.***

warm room, agg. - ***sabin.***

warmth, agg. - ***led.***

tearing, joints and muscles - agar., anac., arg-m., arn., asaf., asar., aur., ***bell.,*** bism., calc., ***camph.,*** cann-s., carb- v., chin., colch., cupr., cycl., hyos., led., meny., petr., ph-ac., ruta., sars., sep., spig., spong., stann., sulph., zinc.

TENSION - am-c., ***am-m.,*** anac., apis, arg-m., ***bov., bry., caps., carl., caust.,*** clem., croc., iod., ***iris, kali-c.,*** **LED.,** ***lyc., mag-c., mag-m.,*** manc., ***mang., mez.,*** mur-ac., **NAT-M.,** ***nit-ac., puls.,*** rhod., ***rhus-t., seneg., sep.,*** stann., ***sulph.,*** sul-ac., ***teucr.,*** verat., zinc.

evening - ***iris.***

shifting - iris.

THRILLING, sensation - cinnb.

TREMBLING - cycl., mang., nit-ac.

TWITCHING - alum., bell., bry., graph., nat-c., nat-m., nit-ac., puls., sil., spig., spong., ***sul-ac.,*** sulph., ***verat.***

ULCERS - ***sep.***

UNSTEADINESS - mez.

URTICARIA - clem., verat.

VESICLES - nat-p., phos., **RHUS-T.**

WEAKNESS, of - ***acon.,*** aesc., agar., agn., ***aloe,*** alum., am-c., anac., ang., ***ant-t., arg-m.,*** **ARN.,** ars., asar., aur., bar-c., bell., bor., bov., ***bry.,*** **CALC.,** calc-p., cann-s., canth., ***carb-an.,*** carb-v., carb-s., ***caust.,*** cham., chel., ***chin.,*** chin-a., cimic., clem., cocc., colch., coloc., **CON.,** cupr., cycl., dig., dros., dulc., euph., ***ferr.,*** ferr-ar., ferr-p., graph., hep., hyos., ign., **KALI-C.,** kali-n., ***kali-s.,*** kreos., ***lach., led.,*** **LYC.,** mang., **MERC.,** merc-c., mez., morph., mosch., murx., ***nat-c., nat-m., nit-ac.,*** nux-m., ***nux-v.,*** olnd., par., ***petr., ph-ac., phos.,*** plat., plb., podo., **PSOR.,** ***puls.,*** ran-b., raph., rheum, rhod., **RHUS-T., RUTA,** sabad., sars., **SEP.,** ***sil.,*** spong., stann., ***staph., stront-c.,*** sul-ac., **SULPH.,** tarax., thuj., valer., ***verat.,*** viol-o., zinc., zing.

chill, during - raph.
diarrhea, after - bor.
forenoon - ars.
morning, in bed - carb-v.
  motion, on - cimic.
motion, on - con., chlf.
move, on beginning to - ***euph.***
rising amel. - carb-v.
sitting, while - ars., graph., phos.
stooping, when - graph.
walking, after - bor., zing.
  amel. - bor.

Kidneys

KIDNEYS, general - ***adren., APIS,*** apoc., ***ars.,*** bell., benz-ac., **BERB.,** ***calc.,*** calc-ar., ***cann-i.,*** **CANTH.,** caust., ***chel., chim.,*** chin., coc-c., coloc., **EQUIS.**, helon., ***hep.,*** kali-c., ***lac-ac.,*** **LYC.,** ***merc., merc-c.,*** **NAT-M.,** ***nit-ac.,*** nux-v., oci., pareir., **PHOS.,** ***polyg., puls.,*** rhus-t., samb., ***sars., sec.,*** scop., solid., squil., stront-c., ter., uran-n., ***urt-u.,*** viol-o., zinc.
chlorosis, in - ***puls.***
dwellings, worse from living in damp - ***ter.***
ear and eye symptoms, with - viol-o.
function, derangement - apis, dig., solid.
inactive - ***apis,*** ars., ***berb.,*** benz-ac., helon., solid.
left - ***berb.,*** chin., coloc., lyc., merc., pareir., ***zinc.***
right - ***apis,*** berb., coc-c., ***lyc.,*** nux-v., oci., ***sars.***
sleeplessness, renal affections cause - ***hyos.***

ABSCESS - arn., ***ars.,*** bell., ***canth.,*** cetr., chin., ***hep.,*** hippoz., lyc., ***merc.,*** puls., ***sil.,*** sul-i., ter., verat-v.

ACHING, pain (see Dull, pain) - apoc., benz-ac., **BERB.,** ***calc., cann-i., canth.,*** chel., cinnb., coc-c., ***crot-h.,*** equis., ***eup-pur., helon.,*** kali-bi., ***lyc.,*** med., ***nat-a.,*** scut., tarent., ***ter.,*** zing.
constant, tenderness, with extreme - ***helon.***
keeping awake at night - cann-i.
pain, urination, better by profuse - med.
riding, when - ***calc.***
right, in - ***crot-h.***
urinating, worse evening - ***canth.,*** helon.
night - calc., ***cann-i.***
riding, while - ***calc.***
urination, during - aesc., agn., ant-c., berb.
amel. - **LYC.,** tarent.

aching, region of - acon., agar., all-c., ambr., ant-c., apoc., **BERB.,** brach., calc., carl., caust., coc-c., elat., equis., ham., ***hydr., kali-bi.,*** lyc., merc-c., mit., nat-a., pall., phos., phys., sabad., sep., still., tab.
afternoon - ***chin-s.,*** sang.
constant, almost, dull - ter.
worse in right, where pain shoots through to bowels - kali-bi.
evening - ***canth.***
night, 10 p.m. - ir-fl.
urination, before - tab.
waking, on - still.

ADDISON'S disease - ***adren.,*** ant-c., apom., ***arg-n., ars., ars-i.,*** bac., ***bell.,*** **CALC.,** calc-ar., calc-p., carb-v., caust., chin., cupr., ***ferr., ferr-i.,*** hydr-ac., **IOD.,** kali-ar., ***kali-c.,*** kreos., lyc., mang., ***med.,*** **NAT-M.,** nat-s., ***nit-ac.,*** ol-j., **PHOS.,** pic-ac., psor., sec., **SEP., SIL.,** ***spig., sulph.,*** ther., thuj., ***tub.,*** vanad.
anemia and asthenia - ***ferr.***
vertigo, with - **CALC.**
weakness, in - ***calc., iod.,*** sep.

BLEEDING - canth., merc-c., ***phos.***

BRIGHT'S disease (see Nephritis) - am-be., ant-t., **APIS,** apoc., arg-n., **ARS.,** ars-h., ars-i., atro., **AUR-M., AUR-M-N.,** berb., ***brach.,*** bry., ***calc.,*** calc-ar., calc-p., calc-s., ***cann-s., canth., carb-ac.,*** caul., ***chel.,*** chim., ***chin., coc-c., colch.,*** coloc., con., ***cop., crot-h., cupr., dig.,*** eup-pur., ***ferr., ferr-p.,*** **GLON.,** hell., helon., ***hep., kali-bi., kali-c., kali-i.,*** kali-m., kali-p., ***kalm.,*** kreos., ***lach.,*** **LYC.,** ***lycps.,*** **MERC-C.,** ***merc-cy., merc***-i-r., mez., myris., **NAT-C.,** ***nat-m., nit-ac.,*** ol-j., op., ***phos.,*** **PH-AC.,** ***phyt.,*** **PLB., RHUS-T.,** sars., ***sec., sulph.,*** **TER.,** uran-n.
alcohol, from abuse of - ***ars., berb., carb-v., crot-h., lach., nat-c., nux-v.***
anesthesia, with - **PHOS.**
atheromatous degeneration of arteries - ***calc., lith., ph-ac.,*** **PLB.,** ***sil.***
blows on loins, especially from - ***canth.***
childbed, during - ph-ac.
convulsions, with uremic - **CUPR-M.,** ***dig.,*** **KALI-BR.**
diphtheria - ***apis, merc-c.,*** phyt.
edema, with - ***apis, ars.,*** calc-ar., ***cupr-m., dig., hell.,*** helon., jab., ***lach.***
far advanced with - **LAC-D.**
followed by renal - jab., ***ter.***
exposure, from, to cold and damp - calc., colch., ***dulc.,*** kali-c., merc-c., nux-v., ***rhus-t.,*** sep.
eyeball, protrusion of - ***lycps.***
eyes, amaurosis, with - ***apis, ars.,*** cann-i., colch., ***gels., hep.,*** kalm., ***merc-c.,*** ph-ac., plb.
amblyopia, with - ant-t., ***phos.***
gout, with, and mercurio-syphilis - ***kali-i.***
heart complications, with - ***ars., aur-m.,*** colch., ***crot-h., cupr-m., dig.,*** kali-bi., kali-p., ***kalm., lach., ter.,*** uran-n.
heat, in a man exposed to - rhus-t.
hemorrhages, with - phos.
nervous exhaustion - ***phos.***
preceded or accompanied by disease of pancreas - ***phos.***
pulmonary edema, with, secondary to it - **KALI-I.**
scarlatina, after - ***apis, ars.,*** asc-c., bell., bry., colch., ***hell.,*** kali-c., ***lach.,*** **LYC.,** ***merc-c.,*** rhus-t., ***sec.,*** seneg.
retinitis - ***crot-h.***
standing, difficulty in, and walking - ***kalm.***
weakness, with great - ***ars.,*** ars-i., ferr-s., helon., ***merc-c., phos., ph-ac.***

BRUISED pain - cact., manc., ***pareir.,*** zinc.
as of a great blow, making her cry out - ***cact.***
weakness - manc.

bruised, region of left, while standing and walking - zinc.

BUBBLING, sensation in, region of - **BERB.,** lyc., ***med.***

BURNING, pain - apis, ***ars., ars-h.,*** arund., ***bell., benz-ac., berb.,*** bufo, cann-i., **CANTH.,** ***coloc., helon.,*** hep., ***ip., kali-bi., kali-c., kali-i.,*** kali-n., ***lac-d.,*** nat-m., ***nux-v.,*** ph-ac., ***phos.,*** phyt., pin-s., ***puls.,*** rheum, sep., **TER.,** zinc.

BURNING, pain
extending,to, bladder - bell.
through left ilium to pubis, in women - arund.
left - ***benz-ac.,*** lachn., zing.
ileum, passing through, to pubis - arund.
lying, while - lac-d.
nephritis, in - ***nux-v.***
with hematuria - **TER.**
oppressed breathing and faintness, with - bufo.
outline, can trace their, by the burning - ***helon.***
small spot, in a, near, worse pressing hard, moves downward and forward - berb.
urination, during - rheum
before - rheum, thuj.
burning, region of - ars., ***berb.,*** canth., ***coloc.,*** kali-n., ***lac-d.,*** nat-m., phyt., ***ter.***
burning, ureters - bell., cedr., pin-s., ter.
extending, along - cedr., pin-s.
to bladder - bell., ***ter.***

CALCULI, (see Stones)

CATARRH - canth., coll., petr., sil., sulph.

COLD, affected by a - ***polyg.***
cold, sensation - spira.
region of - cham., coc-c.

COLIC, pain of (see Stones) - ***apis, arg-n., arn., ars.,*** aspar., **BELL.,** benz-ac., **BERB.,** ***calc-ren., cann-s., canth.,*** **CARB-AN.,** ***chlf.,*** coc-c., colch., ***coloc., dios.,*** erig., equis., eup-pur., indg., ***kali-c.,*** **LYC.,** med., ***nux-m., nux-v.,*** oci., ***op.,*** par., **PAREIR.,** polyg., **SARS.,** sil., ***tab.,*** ter., **VERAT.,** zinc.
anodynes, after - ***nux-v.***
chest, with spasmodic difficulties of - coc-c.
constant urging to urinate - ***nux-v.***
cramp in left - agar.
cramp-like, towards bladder - nit-ac.
crampy pains - cur.
glans pressing, amel. - canth.
hematuria, with - oci.
itching, with - ***dios.***
left lumbar region, in - ***pareir.***
lie, inability to, on right side - ***nux-v.***
nausea, with or without - senec.
radiates from left to groin, following course of ureter - ***pareir.***
right ureter to bladder - **LYC.**
sweat, with - ***nux-v.***
urination, profuse, amel. - med.
worse from pressure or motion - coc-c.

CONGESTION - acon., atro., ***bell.,*** bry., ***canth.,*** chel., ***colch., nux-v.,*** pic-ac., ***puls.,*** senec., **TER.**
albuminuria, with, from amenorrhea - ***helon.***
dropsy, causing - ***ter.***
engorged - anthr.
hyperemic state, in organic disease of heart - ***apis***
after cardiac hypertrophy, pressure around waist and increase of urine - aur.

CONGESTION,
hyperemia, in heart disease and morbus brightii - ***aur-m.***
injected, worse in tubular substances - ars-h.
passive - crot-h., ham.
serum, with extensive effusion of, in abdominal cavity and tissues of legs - hell.
uneasiness, as if congested - coch.

CONSTRICTING, extending, down ureters to penis, pressure on glans amel., at times pain goes upward - canth.
extending, to bladder - nit-ac.

CONTRACTED, pain - dig., nit-ac., plb.

CONTRACTING, pain - clem., mang.
down ureters to penis - **CANTH.**

CRAMPING - cadm-s., **CAUST.,** ***chel.,*** cycl., kali-i., ***nit-ac.,*** oci.
afternoon, from 4 to 9 p.m. - ***chel.***
cramping, ureters - nit-ac., polyg.

CRUSHING, pains - anan.

CUTTING, pain - acon., apis, arg-n., ***arn.,*** bad., bell., ***berb.,*** bufo, cadm-s., cann-i., **CANTH.,** clem., coc-c., ***colch.,*** coloc., daph., eup-pur., ***graph.,*** helon., ip., **KALI-BI.,** ***kali-i., merc.,*** mez., ***nux-m.,*** plb., ***polyg., staph.,*** tab., zinc.
downward pressure before urinating - graph.
left into bladder - berb.
paroxysmal, and burning in both - **CANTH.**
urination, before - graph.
yellow fever, in - ***cadm-s.***
cutting, region of - plb., ***staph.,*** zinc.
heat amel., cold, agg. - ***staph.***
lancinations, friction and pressure amel. - plb.
cutting, ureters - aesc., ***apis,*** aspar., ***arg-n., arn., ars.,*** **BELL.,** ***benz-ac.,*** **BERB.,** cann-s., ***canth.,*** **CARB-AN.,** chlol., coc-c., colch., con., ***dios.,*** equis., erig., eup-pur., indg., kali-ar., ***kali-c., lach.,*** **LYC.,** ***med.,*** nat-s., ***nux-m., nux-v., oci., op.,*** **PAREIR.,** ***phos.,*** polyg., psor., **SARS.,** senec., sep., sil., ***tab.,*** ter., **VERAT.,** zinc.
alternating with pain in glans - canth.
urination, after - apis
vomiting, with - **OCI.**

DARTING, pain - berb., ***kali-i.,*** staph.

DIGGING, pain - ***berb.,*** cur., kali-i.
sticking, as if suppurating, worse on deep pressure - ***berb.***
digging, region of, pressure agg. - **BERB.**

DISTENDED - helon., solid.

DRAGGING, ureters, like labour pain with urging to urinate - ***cham.***

DRAWING, pain - **CLEM.,** coc-c., ***nux-m.,*** **TER.,** zinc.
addison's disease, in - ***iod.***
left - ***benz-ac.,*** kali-c.
stooping, when - ***benz-ac.***
right, 5 a.m. - coc-c.
stooping, when - ***benz-ac.***
tensive, riding, while - agar.

DRAWING, pain
transient, in right, extending to right hip - ter.
violent, in nephritis, with hematuria - extending right to hip - *ter.*
drawing, region of - aloe, alumn., benz-ac., berb., ***cann-s.,*** carl., cinnb., ***iod.,*** kali-n., lach., meny., ruta., **TER.,** ***zinc.***
evening, sitting, while - meny., ruta.
extending into, inguinal, region - cann-s.
right hip - ter.
drawing, ureters - berb., cham., ***nat-m.,*** sulph., thuj.
left - calad., coc-c.
right - astac.

DULL pain (see Aching) - ambr., ***benz-ac.,*** berb., ***equis.,*** eup-pur., ham., nat-a., phos., still., ***ter.***
cystitis in - **EUP-PUR.**
evening, late in - ***canth.***
left, in - ***nuph.***
motion, worse from, or - coc-c.
pressure, on - coc-c., ***nat-s.***
right side, most on, with heat - phyt.
stones, with kidney - ***canth.***
uterus, down - ter.
urinate , with frequent desire to - zing.
dull, in region of - ***hydr.,*** mit.
right, with urgent desire to urinate - ***equis.***

EDEMA, dropsy, from kidneys disease - ampe-qu, ant-t., **APIS,** ***apoc., arg-n., ars., asc-c.,*** aspar., aur., ***aur-m., bry., calc-p., chim.,*** coc-c., **COLCH.,** coloc., crot-h., ***dig.,*** digin., ***dulc.,*** eup-pur., ***hell.,*** helon., lac-d., liatr., ***lyc., merc., merc-c.,*** merc-d., ***nat-m.,*** nit-ac., phos., plb., ***prun.,*** rauw., ***sal-ac., senec., solid.,*** **TER.,** ur-ac.
constitutions, in broken-down, and intemperate subjects - ***chim.***
dysuria, and - coloc.
nephritis, after - ***hell.***
prostration, with - ***ter.***
scarlatina, after - ***apis,*** apoc., ***ars.,*** asc-c., bell., ***canth., colch., hell.,*** helon., hep., jab., kali-c., **LYC.,** ph-ac., ***rhus-t.,*** seneg., **TER.**
anasarca, especially with albuminuria - cop.

FATTY degeneration - ars., **PHOS.,** ***ter.***
bright's disease, in - **ARS.,** ter.
cells of both substances granulated - ars-h.
granular degeneration - eucal., ***kali-i., plb.***
with general edema - ***ter.***

FLOATING, kidneys, reflex symptoms, from - apis, bell., berb., ***calc.,*** cham., coloc., gels., ign., lach., puls., ***sep.,*** stry-ar., sulph., zinc.

FLUTTERING sensation, region of - berb., brach., chim.

FORMICATION - hydrc.
region of - dirc.

GNAWING, pain - ***berb., tarent.***
in a small spot near, worse pressing hard, moves downward and forward - berb.
gnawing, region of - berb., brach.

GRIPING, pain - cadm-s.

HEAT - ***ars-h., bell.,*** kali-i., lach., ***nux-v.,*** zing.
extending to bladder - aur.
nephritis, in - bell., ***nux-v.***
heat, region of - berb., cimic., ***helon., nat-m., phos.,*** phyt., plb., ter.
sitting, while - nat-m.

HEAVINESS - ***carl.,*** equis.
morning - sang.
waking. on - aeth.
sitting agg. - ***carl.***
heaviness, region of - cimic., dirc., ***helon.,*** phos., sang., tell., ***ter.***
afternoon - helon., sang.
evening - helon.
night - tell.
motion agg. - cimic.

HOT sensation, with frequent desire to urinate - zing.

INACTIVE - acon., **APIS.,** ***coch., ter., zing.***
atony - ***coch.***
children, especially in - acon., apis., ***stram.***
duration, complete cessation of function up to fifty hours, in reconvalescence from typhus - ***zing.***
peculiar torpid action - apoc.
scanty, with, smoky urine, brain possessed by unexcreted urea - ***ter.***

INFLAMMATION, kidneys, (see Bright's diseases or Nephritis)
inflammation, ureters, acute - acon., arn., ***ars.,*** aur., ***bell., benz-ac.,*** berb., bry., ***cann-s., canth.,*** chin., ***cop., cupr-ar.,*** epig., ***ferr-m.,*** hecla., hep., kali-bi., ***merc-c.,*** nit-ac., ***puls., rhus-t.,*** stigm., ***ter.,*** thuj., ***tritic., uva., verat-v.***
chronic - ars., ***benz-ac.,*** berb., ***chim.,*** chin., chin-s., ***cop.,*** hep., ***juni., kali-bi., ol-sant.,*** pareir., puls., sep., sil., ***stigm.,*** sulph., ***uva.***

LAMENESS, region of - cimic., phys., ***sol-v.***
left, with cramp, extending into thighs - agar.
waking, on - ptel.

LANCINATING, pain, sudden, acute, prolonged, extending from left ureter into bladder - coc-c.

NEPHRITIS, inflammation, kidneys (see Bright's disease) - ***acon., all-c.,*** alum., am-c., **APIS,** ***arg-n.,*** **ARN.,** ars., arund., ***asc-c., aur.,*** **BELL., BENZ-AC., BERB.,** ***bry.,*** cact., calad., calc-s., camph., cann-i., ***cann-s.,*** **CANTH.,** ***caps., carb-ac.,*** caust., ***chel., chim.,*** coc-c., ***colch.,*** coll., cop., crot-c., crot-h., cub., dig., ***ery-a., eup-pur.,*** ferr., ***gels., hell., helon., hep.,*** indg., ***kali-ar., kali-c.,*** **KALI-CHL.,** ***kali-i.,*** kali-p., kali-s., lil-t., lith., **LYC.,** ***lycps.,*** med., ***merc., merc-c.,*** merc-cy., nat-s., nit-ac., ***nux-v.,*** **OCI.,** pareir., ph-ac., ***phos., phyt.,*** pic-ac., plb., ***polyg.,*** prun., ***puls., rhus-t., sabin.,*** samb., ***sars.,*** sec., ***senec.,*** sep., solid., ***stront-c.,*** stroph., **SULPH.,** sul-ac., tarent., **TER.,** ***thuj.,*** tub., uran., zinc.

NEPHRITIS,
acute parenchymatous - ***acon.***, ant-t., **APIS**, apoc., ***ars.***, ***aur-m.***, ***bell.***, **BERB.**, ***cann-s.***, ***canth.***, carb-ac., chel., ***chim.***, ***chin-s.***, ***colch.***, ***con.***, conv., ***cupr-ar.***, dig., dulc., eucal., eup-per., fab., ferr-i., fuch., ***glon.***, guai., ***hell.***, helon., ***hep.***, hydrc., irid., juni., kali-bi., ***kali-chl.***, kali-cit., kali-s., kalm., lach., med., ***merc-sul.***, ***methyl-b.***, **NAT-S.**, nit-ac., ol-sant., ph-ac., ***phos.***, pic-ac., plb-a., polyg., rhus-t., sabal., ***sabin.***, ***samb.***, sec., senec., ser-ang., ***squil.***, ***stram.***, **TER.**, tub., tub-k., uran-n., vac., ***verat.***, ***verat-v.***, zinc.
bloody, ink-like, albuminous urine, with - **COLCH.**
bronchitis, with - ter.
cardiac, and hepatic affections, with - ***aur.***, ***calc-ar.***
chronic, parenchymous nephritis - **APIS**, ***ars.***, ***aur-m.***, benz-ac., berb., ***brach.***, ***calc-ar.***, calc-p., cann-i., ***canth.***, chin-a., conv., dig., ***euon.***, eup-pur., ferr-ar., ***ferr-m.***, ferr-p., form., glon., ***helon.***, hydr-ac., juni., kali-ar., ***kali-chl.***, ***kali-i.***, ***kali-m.***, kalm., lon-x., ***lyc.***, ***merc-c.***, nat-hchls., ***nit-ac.***, ***piloc.***, ***plb.***, senec., ***ter.***, urea
cold, from, or exposure to wet - ***acon.***, ant-t., ***apis***, canth., ***dulc.***, kali-c., rhus-t., ter.
edema, with - acon., adon., ant-t., **APIS**, ***apoc.***, **ARS.**, aur-m., canth., colch., cop., ***dig.***, ***hell.***, merc-c., piloc., ***samb.***, senec., ***squil.***, ter.
exanthema, after - hep.
frequency, of - gels., kali-p.
heart, and hepatic affections, with - adon., ars., ***aur.***, ***calc-ar.***, ***dig.***, glon., stroph., verat-v.
influenza, after - eucal.
injury, from - kali-c.
interstitial nephritis, chronic - apis, ***ars.***, ***aur-m.***, aur-m-n., cact., chin-s., ***colch.***, conv., ***dig.***, ferr., ***ferr-m.***, ***glon.***, ***iod.***, kali-c., ***kali-i.***, lith., ***merc-c.***, merc-d., ***nit-ac.***, nux-v., op., ph-ac., phos., plb., sang.
malaria, from - eup-per., ter.
palpitation, with - kali-ar.
pneumonia, with - chel., phos.
pregnancy, during - apis, apoc., ***cupr-ar.***, helon., kalm., ***merc-c.***, sabin.
pyelo-nephritis - ***apis***, ars., ***berb.***, calc-s., hep., kali-s., merc-c., rhus-t., sul-i., ter.
coma, with - bapt.
rheumatism, with - rad., ter.
scarlet fever, diphtheria, from - acon., ***apis***, ***ars.***, bell., ***canth.***, conv., cop., dig., ferr-i., ***hell.***, ***hep.***, kalm., lach., ***merc-c.***, methyl-b., nat-s., nit-s-d., ***rhus-t.***, sec., ***ter.***
slow - merc-c.

NEPHRITIS,
suppurative - acon., arn., ***ars.***, bell., calc-s., camph., ***cann-s.***, ***canth.***, ***chin-s.***, eucal., hecla., ***hep.***, hippoz., kali-n., lyc., ***merc.***, ***merc-c.***, naphtin., polyg., puls., ***sil.***, sul-i., verat-v.
toxemic - ***crot-h.***, merc.
vomiting, with - hell.

NEPHROTIC, syndrome - ars., ***apis.***

NEURALGIC pain - op., ter.

NUMBNESS, region of - **BERB.**

OPPRESSIVE pain, worse from pressure or motion - coc-c.

PAIN, kidneys - acon., ***aesc.***, aeth., ***agn.***, ***all-c.***, aloe, ***alum.***, ambr., aphis., ***apis***, ***arg-n.***, ***arn.***, ars., arund., aur-m., ***bell.***, bad., ***benz-ac.***, **BERB.**, ***bry.***, cahin., ***calc.***, ***calc-p.***, ***cann-i.***, ***cann-s.***, **CANTH.**, ***caps.***, cedr., ***chel.***, ***chen-a.***, ***chim.***, cimic., ***cinnb.***, ***clem.***, coc-c., cod., **COLCH.**, ***crot-c.***, ***dios.***, ***dulc.***, erig., ***eup-pur.***, ***ferr.***, ferr-ar., ferr-i., ferr-p., gall-ac., gamb., ham., hell., ***helon.***, ***hep.***, hydr., hyper., ***ip.***, ***ipom.***, iris, kali-ar., ***kali-bi.***, kali-br., ***kali-c.***, ***kali-chl.***, kali-i., ***kali-m.***, kali-n., kali-p., lach., lec., lept., ***lith.***, lob., ***lyc.***, lycps., lyss., manc., ***med.***, meph., merc-c., mez., ***mill.***, nat-a., ***nat-m.***, nat-s., ***nit-ac.***, nux-m., ***nux-v.***, ox-ac., ***pareir.***, ***ph-ac.***, ***phos.***, ***phyt.***, ***plb.***, polyg., ptel., ***puls.***, ran-s., rat., rhus-t., samb., **SARS.**, scop., ***sel.***, ***senec.***, ***sep.***, solid., squil., still., stroph., tab., ***tarent.***, ***ter.***, ***thuj.***, uran-n., ***zinc.***, zing.
afternoon - bad., chin-s., sang.
4 p.m. to 8 p.m. - **LYC.**
4 p.m. to 9 p.m. - ***chel.***
albuminuria, with - apis, ars., ***helon.***
pregnancy, during - apis., ***aur-m.***
alternating, with vertigo - alum.
apyrexia, during - bell., chin., hep., lyc., staph.
bending, body, on - chin.
bilious attacks, with - **NUX-V.**
blowing, nose - ***calc-p.***
breathing deeply, when - aeth., arg-n., astac., ***benz-ac.***, sel.
inhaling, worse when - astac.
bright's disease, in - ***apis.***
chest, with spasmodic difficulties of - coc-c.
pains penetrate, on taking a deep breath - ***benz-ac.***
chill, during - ars., canth., kali-c., lyc., nux-v., puls., zinc.
coughing - ***bell.***
dancing, while - alum.
desire, be delayed, if - con., pall., rhus-t.
diabetes, in - ph-ac., phos.
evening - canth., ox-ac., sil., tarent.
extending to,
abdomen - berb., canth., kali-bi., ***nux-v.***
over the - hydr-ac.
bladder, to - arg-n., ars., bell., berb., canth., chel., coc-c., kali-i., ***lyc.***, nit-ac., oci., petr., phyt., ***sars.***, tab.

PAIN, kidneys
extending, to
chest and shoulder, to - glyc.
epigastrium, to - hydr-ac.
left - thuj.
hip, to - arn., berb., lyc., ***nux-m., nux-v.,*** ox-ac., ter.
ilium, to right - sang.
perineum, to - lyc., sep.
sacrum and coccyx, to - graph.
testes, to - ***berb.,*** cahin., dios., equis., erig., ***lyc.,*** nux-v., syph.
thighs, to - ***berb.,*** ip., pareir.
right - ***nux-v.***
uterus, to - nat-m.
vagina, labia, to - eupi.
fever, in apyrexia of intermittent - ***nat-m.***
hematuria, with - ip., phos.
hemorrhage, in chronic passive, from kidneys - ter.
iritis, rheumatic in - ***ter.***
jar, from - aeth., alum., ***bell., berb.,*** calc-p., cann-s.
laughing, when - ***cann-i.,*** cann-s.
left, in - all-c., **BERB.,** chlf., ferr-i., ***lyc.,*** mill.,
chilliness, with - mill.
followed by profuse hematuria, lasting from five to eight days - ***mill.***
mornings, on sitting down - chin-b.
paroxysms of pain running along ureter and in back, with - ***ipom.***
lifting, when - ***calc-p.***
lying, while - aeth., berb., colch., coloc., conv., nux-v., rhus-t.
abdomen, on amel. - chel.
back, on - chel.
amel. - nux-v.
legs (knees) drawn up, with, amel. - colch.
menses, during - berb., cur., verat.
at beginning of - ***berb.,*** raph., ***verat.***
dysmenorrhea, in - ***verat.***
morning - alum., bell., ***cahin.,*** ham., kali-c., tarent.
waking, on - ox-ac.
motion, agg. - aesc., alum., arg-n., ***berb.,*** cahin., ***canth.,*** chel., coc-c., ***colch.,*** dor., ***gels., ham.,*** kali-bi., kali-i., ***nux-v.***
amel. - ter., thuj.
nephritis, in - ***arn., chel.***
night - ars-h., calc., cann-i., chel., cinnb., tarent.
undressing, while - helon.
paroxysmal - aran., ***bell., chel., coc-c.,*** sulph.
penis, alternating with pain in tip of - **CANTH.**
phlebitis, in, worse from motion - ***ham.***
pressure, on - ***berb.,*** canth., colch., dor., ferr., helo., ***solid.***
over - thuj.
prostate gland, with frequent slight pains in - gnaph.
pruritus vulvae, in - tarent.
pulsating - bufo.

PAIN, kidneys
radiating - ***berb.,*** pareir.
riding - alum., berb., ***calc.***
as from, over a rough road, worse from dancing - alum.
right - apis, bell., berb., colch., ***lith., lyc.,*** lyss., ***senec.***
could only lie on back, worse from pressure and motion - ***colch.***
inspiration, worse on - sel.
over, intense, severe during urination - ***senec.***
scarlatina, in - ***lyc.***
septic disease, in - ***tare***nt.
sitting, while - ***berb., pall.,*** ter., valer.
sneezing, agg. - ***aeth.,*** ars., ***bell., calc-p.***
worse on, deep breathing and lying down - aeth.
spine, especially near - ***lyc.***
standing, amel. - berb.
stooping, when - alum., apis, ***berb.,*** chin., ***sulph.***
after long time of - sulph.
straightening, out legs agg. - colch.
swelling, of right knee, with - benz-ac.
thigh, extending to right - ***nux-v.***
tired, when - ter.
touch, worse from - arg-n.
urging, to urinate, during - ***ars-h., canth.,*** coc-c., ***ferr.,*** graph., hep., ***kreos.,*** merc-c., ruta.
urination, during - aesc., ant-c., berb., phos., ***puls.,*** rheum, ***senec.***
after, amel. - **LYC.,** ***med.,*** tarent.
before - graph., ***lyc.***
urinate, with desire to - ***ferr.***
yellow fever, in - ***ars-h.***
urinating, also on - puls.
urine, if, is restrained - con.
walking, while. - alum., carb-an., clem., ham., nit-ac., ***nux-v.,*** zinc.
amel. - ferr.
wine, from - benz-ac., nat-p., zinc.

PAIN, kidneys, region of - abrot., all-s., alum., ars-h., bov., cadm-s., cahin., ***calc., calc-p.,*** chel., ***chin-a.,*** cop., erig., fl-ac., hydr., kali-n., kreos., myric., ox-ac., phys., rhus-t.
bands of clothing, from - chel.
digging, when - calc-p.
extending to,
calves - ***berb.***
chest - benz-ac.
downward - berb., ***sars.***
from genitals, anus and thighs - kreos.
groin - kali-bi., pareir., petr.
groin, anxious nausea, with - cann-s.
prostate gland - graph., sel.
thighs - agar., **BERB.,** hep., ip., kali-bi., nux-v.
ureters - canth., chel., oci., phyt.
lie only on the back, can - colch.
stretching, after - calc.

PAIN, ureters - ***aesc.,*** agar., aloe, ***apis,*** benz-ac., ***berb.,*** calad., ***canth.,*** cann-i., cann-s., ***chel., dios.,*** epig., equis., ***hedeo,*** hydrang., indg., ***ipom.,*** kali-c., lith., **LYC.,** ***nux-v., oci., pareir.,*** phyt., pic-ac., ***sars.,*** tab., tarent., ***ter.,*** uva.
extending to,
bladder - gall-ac.
penis and testes - cann-i., canth., con., ***dios., nux-v.***
right thigh - nux-v.
thighs and feet - pareir.
urethra, into - **BERB.,** canth., coc-c.
urethra, into, and seminal cords - clem., dios.
inter-paroxysmal - ***berb.,*** calc., chin-s., hydrang., ***lyc.,*** nux-v., ***sep.,*** urt-u.
left side - ***aesc.,*** agar., aloe, benz-ac., ***berb.,*** calad., canth., cann-s., epig., ***hedeo,*** hydrang., ***ipom.,*** kali-c., ***lyc., pareir.,*** tab., uva.
radiating from renal region - **BERB.,** ***ipom.,*** pareir.
right side - apis, berb., cann-i., cann-s., canth., ***chel., dios.,*** equis., indg., lith., **LYC.,** ***nux-v., oci.,*** phyt., pic-ac., ***sars.,*** tab., tarent., ***ter.***
vomiting, with - **OCI.**

PIERCING, pain, in both ureters, with urging to urinate - ***berb.,*** nat-s.

PINCHING, pain - zinc.

PRESSING, pain - am-br., aphis., ars-h., ***calc., canth., carl.,*** cimic., clem., coc-c., gels., hyper., ***kali-c., nit-ac., nux-v.,*** pall., ran-s., ter., ***thuj.,*** zinc.
addison's disease, in - ***calc., iod., nit-ac.***
back, extends over, to between shoulders, worse night - ars-h.
distensive pain - ***canth.***
drawing, in right - zinc.
dull pain, with - ***canth.***
left - lyss.
haematuria, with - ***nux-v.***
instrument, as if produced by blunt, as large as end of thumb - ***gels.***
left, in - zinc.
morning - kali-c.
motion, agg. - coc-c.
amel. - ter.
nephritis, in - ***nux-v.***
night - calc.
pressure, worse from, or motion - coc-c.
shoulder blades, extends to - ars-h.
sitting, while - pall., ruta, ***ter.,*** thuj.
better in motion - ter.
urination, before - graph.
pressing, region of - agar., ars-h., ***berb.,*** bor., cimic., ham., hydr., iod., kali-c., lyc., pall., ruta, yhuj., zinc.

PROLAPSE, of - ***bell.,*** cham., coloc., gels., ***ign.,*** lach., puls., sulph., zinc.

PULSATION - act-sp., ***berb.,*** bufo, canth., chel., kali-i., med., pic-ac., sabin., sulph.
extending into abdomen - kali-i.

PULSATION,
restless sensation - puls-n

SENSITIVE, region of - ***acon.,*** **APIS, BERB.,** calc-ar., cann-s., ***canth.,*** equis., ***helon., lyc.,*** phyt., ***solid., sol-v., ter.***
left, to touch - zinc.
colitis, in - ***nuph.***
nervous system, in affection of sympathetic - phos.
pressure, to - sel., tab.
albuminuria, in - ***calc-ar.***
pressure, on deep - vesp.
leaning against cushioned carriage - am-be.
right - ***helon.***
right, worse from touch - ***nux-v.***
touch, to slightest - ***hep.***

SHARP, pain - ***acon.,*** aesc., aeth., agar., anan., ant-t., ***arn., ars.,*** astac., bapt., ***bell.,*** **BERB., BOR.,** bov., calc-f., cann-i., ***canth.,*** carb-an., ***chel.,*** chin., ***coc-c., coloc.,*** crot-t., cycl., dig., erig., gamb., grat., hep., ***ip.,*** kali-ar., **KALI-BI.,** ***kali-c.,*** kali-i., ***kali-n.,*** kali-p., kali-s., ***lach.,*** lob., ***lyc.,*** mag-m., mang., ***mez., nat-m.,*** nat-p., ***nux-v.,*** ph-ac., phos., ***plb.,*** ran-s., sep., stann., ***staph.,*** sulph., ***tarent., ter.,*** upa., valer., vip., zinc.
afternoon - crot-t., ***tarent.***
arms in moving - ant-t.
ascending - aesc., apis.
breathing, on, or sneezing - ***ars.***
arresting - crot-t.
cold, becoming - ***staph.***
deep, penetrating, dull in right, worse during inhalation - cycl.
dinner, after - zinc.
downward, apparently through ureters - ***lach.***
dull, in right - zinc.
eating, after - con.
evening - zinc.
bed, in - coc-c.
expiration - kali-c.
extending to,
bladder - arg-n., bell., **BERB.,** coc-c., cupr-ac., **KALI-BI.,** ***lach.,*** oci.
bladder, and urethra - berb.
chest - zinc.
down ureters - apis, arg-n., bell., **BERB.,** calad., ***chel.,*** coc-c., cupr-ac., **KALI-BI.,** ***lach.,*** **LYC.,** pareir., tab., ter.
down ureters, worse touch or motion, deep inspiration - arg-n.
knee - berb., ip., kali-bi.
urethra - ***berb.,*** coc-c.
uterus - nat-m.
inspiration, on deep - ***ars.,*** astac., crot-t., cycl., laur.
intermittent - zinc.
itching - staph.
needle-like - staph.
knives, as from - ***arn.***

SHARP, pain
left, in - gamb., kali-c., lyc., mang., zinc.
at intervals - zinc.
worse rising from seat and motion, not from touch, cannot lie long in one position - ***nux-v.***
lying on face, amel. - chel.
morning - chel.
4 a.m. - cinnb.
motion - kali-bi.
of arms, on - ant-t.
night - ***tarent.***
pulsating - bufo
radiating - **BERB.**
right, in - agar., astac., bad., bapt.
afternoon - bad.
near spine, down to bladder - berb.
rubbing amel. - kali-c.
stitches - anan., cann-i., ***coloc.,*** ***kali-c.,*** ran-s.
sitting, while - ***berb.,*** dig., valer.
sneezing - ars.
standing, while - zinc.
amel. - berb.
urinating, after - bufo
walking - zinc.
warm bed amel. - ***staph.***

SHOOTING, pain - aesc., apis, bapt., ***berb.,*** ip., pareir.
down left ureter - pareir.
left, in - aesc., bapt.
right, from, down thigh to knee, like cramp - ***ip.***
sixth week of pregnancy, in - ***ip.***

SMARTING, pain - ***kali-c.***

SORE, pain - acon., agar., alum., ***apis,*** ***arg-n.,*** ars., ***asaf.,*** asar., benz-ac., **BERB.,** brach., ***cact.,*** cadm-s., calc., ***calc-ar.,*** ***cann-s.,*** ***canth.,*** ***chel.,*** cinnb., clem., ***coc-c.,*** colch., ferr-i., **GRAPH.,** hell., ***helon.,*** ***hep.,*** kali-c., kali-i., ***manc.,*** meny., merc., merc-c., ***nat-s.,*** ***nux-v.,*** ***pareir.,*** phys., phyt., plb., **PULS.,** ***rat.,*** rhus-t., sel., senec., solid., tab., tarent., tell., ***ter.,*** ***vesp.,*** visc., zinc.
afternoon - kali-c.
diabetes, in - rat.
evening - meny.
exerting the muscles, while - apoc.
jar - aeth., alum., ***bell.,*** ***berb.,*** calc-p., ***cann-i.***
left - benz-ac., zinc.
right - ***helon.,*** ***nux-v.,*** phyt.
heat agg. - phyt.
sitting, while - kali-c., meny.

sore, region of - abrot., benz-ac., **BERB.,** brach., cann-s., ***chel.,*** ***coc-c.,*** equis., hydr., kali-c., mang., merc-c., nat-a., ***nux-v.,*** phos., phys., phyt., ***rhus-t.,*** tell., ter., zinc.
extending to thighs - ***berb.***

sore, ureters - apis, berb., oci.

STABBING, pain, region of - anan., arn., ***berb.,*** erig.

STICKING, pain - ***mez.***
extends straight forward into abdomen - ***berb.***

STICKING, pain
left, in, while standing and walking - zinc.
motion, agg. - coc-c.
pressure, agg. - coc-c., zinc.

STINGING, pain - ***apis,*** astac., bell., berb., erig., kali-bi.
extending, bladder, into - bell., **KALI-BI.**
left, in - erig.
night, at, worse when inhaling - astac.
right, in - ***apis.***
small spot, in a, worse pressing hard, moves downward and forward - berb.

STONES, kidney - act-sp., apoc., arn., bell., **BENZ-AC., BERB., CALC.,** ***calc-ren.,*** ***canth.,*** chin-s., coc-c., ***coloc.,*** equis., eup-pur., hydrang., ***ipom.,*** **LITH., LYC.,** med., mill., morg-g., nat-s., oci., **PAREIR.,** ***phos.,*** **SARS.,** ***sep.,*** ***sil.,*** ***tab.,*** ter., **URT-U.,** uva.
congestive and inflammatory symptoms, with purulent chalky, or sandy sediment - ***phos.***
nephritis, caused - ***berb.,*** ***nux-v.***
colic, pain from stones - ***bell.,*** **BENZ-AC.,** ***berb.,*** **CALC.,** ***calc-ren.,*** ***canth.,*** ***chlf.,*** coc-c., colch., ***coloc.,*** equis., hydrang., **LITH., LYC.,** med., mill., oci., **PAREIR.,** ***phos.,*** polyg., **SARS.,** ***sil.,*** tab., ter.
glans pressing, amel. - canth.
hematuria, with - oci.
passage, with writhing, twitching, crampy pain - ***dios.***
urination, profuse, amel. - med.

SUPPRESSION, of urine, kidney, (see Bladder, Retention of urine) - **ACON.,** ***aeth.,*** ***ail.,*** am-caust., ***anthr.,*** **APIS,** apoc., aran., **ARN., ARS.,** ***ars-h.,*** ***ars-i.,*** ***arum-t.,*** aur., ***bell.,*** bism., bufo, ***cact.,*** calc., ***camph.,*** **CANTH.,** ***carb-ac.,*** carb-s., **CARB-V.,** caust., ***cic.,*** ***colch.,*** con., ***crot-h.,*** ***cupr.,*** cupr-s., ***dig.,*** dulc., elaps, ***elat.,*** ***erig.,*** ***eup-pur.,*** ***hell.,*** hep., ***hydr.,*** ***hyos.,*** iod., ***kali-bi.,*** kali-chl., ***lac-c.,*** **LACH., LAUR.,** lil-t., **LYC.,** merc., ***merc-c.,*** merc-cy., ***morph.,*** nit-ac., nux-v., ***op.,*** osm., petr., ***phos.,*** phyt., ***plb.,*** ***podo.,*** puls., pyrog., ***rob.,*** **SEC.,** sep., ***sil.,*** **STRAM.,** ***stront-c.,*** ***sulph.,*** sul-ac., tab., tarax., ***tarent.,*** ***ter.,*** ***urt-u.,*** **VERAT.,** vip., zinc.
alternating with frequent urging - sep.
cholera, in - **ARS.,** camph., ***carb-v.,*** ***cupr.,*** sec., **VERAT.**
concussion of spinal column, from - ***arn.,*** rhus-t., ***tarent.***
convulsions, with - **CUPR.,** dig., hyos., ***stram.***
dentition, during - ter.
dropsy, and - ***apis,*** aral-h.
fever, with - ***arn.,*** ***ars.,*** ***bell.,*** ***cact.,*** ***canth.,*** colch., crot-h., ***hyos.,*** ***op.,*** ***plb.,*** ***sec.,*** ***stram.***
gonorrhea, from suppressed - **CAMPH., CANTH.**
menses, during - kali-bi.
newborns, in - acon., apis.

SUPPRESSION, of urine
perspiration, with - acon., ***apis,*** arn., ars., bell., camph., ***canth.,*** dulc., hyos., ***lyc.,*** **OP.,** puls., stram., sulph.
stupor, with - dig., plb.
unconsciousness, during - dig., plb.
violent - apis, cic., ***cupr.,*** cycl., sulph.

SWELLING - ***apis.,*** berb., kali-i.

TEARING, pain - aesc., **BERB., CANTH.,** kali-c., ***lyc., mez.,*** raph., ***rhus-t.,*** zinc.
agonizing as from passing calculus, in back and hips - arn.
cutting, in right - zinc.
digging, as if suppurating, worse on deep pressure - ***berb.***
extending, downwards - arg-n., bell., sars.
to thighs, with stiffness - ***berb.***
left, in, sharp intermittent - zinc.
morning, rising, after - ***berb.***
one-sided - berb.
pulsating - ***berb.***
radiating - **BERB.**
right, in - astac., ***berb.,*** zinc.
rising, soon after, in morning, extends to whole back, between pelvis and thorax - berb.
standing, amel. - berb.
stooping, on - berb., raph.
wet weather - ***rhus-t.***
tearing, ureters, extending downwards, touch, motion and inspiration agg. - arg-n., bell.

TENSION, hematuria, in - ***nux-v.***
nephritis, in - ***colch.***
left painful - ***kali-c.***

THROBBING, pain - act-sp., ***bell.,*** berb., sabin.
right - bell., ***berb.***

TUBERCULOSIS - ***ars-i.,*** bac., calc., ***calc-i., chin-a.,*** hecla., kali-i., kreos.

TWISTING, pain - anan.

TWITCHING, region of - canth., mang.

ULCERATIVE, pain - cann-s.

UREMIA - ***am-c., apis,*** apoc., ars., asc-c., bapt., ***bell., canth., carb-ac.,*** cic., ***cupr.,*** cupr-ac., dig., gels., ***glon., hell.,*** hydr-ac., ***hyos.,*** kali-br., ***kali-s., morph.,*** mosch., ***op.,*** phos., pic-ac., piloc., ***plb.,*** queb., ser-ang., ***stram., ter.,*** urea, **URT-U.,** verat-v.
convulsions, with - apoc., cic., crot-h., ***cupr.,*** cupr-ar., ***dig.,*** hydr-ac., ***kali-s.,*** merc-c., ***mosch., plb., ter.***
head, congestion, with - am-c., apis, ***bell.,*** con., ***cupr., gels., glon.,*** merc-c., ***stram.,*** tab., ter., verat-v.

URIC acid diathesis - ***benz-ac.,*** berb., chin-s., coc-c., ***colch., lyc.,*** nat-s., sep., thlaspi., thuj., ***urt-u.***

WEAKNESS, of - **APIS,** ***ars.,*** benz-ac., **BERB., CANTH.,** chin., coc-c., coloc., **EQUIS.,** helon., kali-c., **LYC.,** merc., merc-c., nux-v., oci., pareir., ***phos.,*** polyg., rhus-t., samb., ***sars.,*** scop., solid., squil., stront-c., ter., viol-o., zinc.

WEAKNESS, of
function, defective - apis, solid.
inactive - ***apis,*** ars., ***berb.,*** benz-ac., helon., solid.
kindred to bright's disease - uran-n.,
left - ***berb.,*** chin., coloc., merc., pareir., ***zinc.***
right - ***apis,*** berb., coc-c., ***lyc.,*** nux-v., oci., ***sars.***

WEARINESS, region of - arg-n., benz-ac., ***berb.,*** carb-an., cham., cimic., helon., manc., phyt., tarent.

Knees

ABSCESS - ***bell., calc., guai.,*** hep., hippoz., ***iod., ol-j.,*** **SIL.**
gonarthrocace - ***ars.,*** **CALC.,** ***iod.,*** **SIL.**

ACHING, pain - ***aesc.,*** apoc., asc-t., bell., brom., bry., calc., calc-p., cann-i., carb-ac., chel., cic., clem., cob., com., cop., corn., dios., ***eug.,*** fago., fl-ac., gamb., glon., hell., ***hydr.,*** jatr., lach., led., lil-t., lob-s., lyc., lyss., mang-m., med., ***merc.,*** mez., ***mur-ac.,*** nat-m., nux-v., ***ol-j.,*** op., osm., petr., phys., ptel., ***podo.,*** puls-n, pyrus, **RHUS-T.,** rhus-v., ***stram.,*** stront-c., syph., tab., upa., verat-v., xan., zinc.
afternoon - dios., lycps.
alternating in each - cycl.
chill, during - ***nat-m.,*** nux-v., ***rhus-t.***
evening - cob., cycl., dios., erig., ***led.,*** lycps.
fire, when near - sumb.
lying down after - lil-t.
morning - bry., carb-ac., dios., sumb.
bed, in - sumb.
morning, walking - bry., ***lach.***
motion, agg. - lycps.
motion, amel. - ***agar.,*** bar-c., cycl., dios., ***mur-ac.,*** **RHUS-T.**
night - coc-c., ***kali-bi.***
noon - dios.
sitting while - agar., bar-c., led., **RHUS-T.**
standing agg. - stront.
walking while - ***hydr.,*** nat-m., stront.
in cool air amel. - sumb.
wandering - clem.
aching, hollow of - arg-m., berb., brom., hep., ip., plb., rumx.
standing, while - rumx.
aching, patella - acon., calc., coc-c., tep.

ARTHRITIS, nodosities - ***bufo, calc., led., nux-v.***

BANDAGED, sensation as if - ***anac.,*** ars., **AUR.,** coloc., ***graph.,*** kali-c., mag-m., ***nat-m.,*** nit-ac., nux-m., plat., **SIL.,** sulph., zinc.
right - graph., mag-s.
sitting, while - ***anac.,*** ars., graph.
walking, while - ***aur.,*** coloc., graph.

BENDING, agg. - carb-an., lyc., mag-arct., sulph.

BLOOD, rush of to, - lact., phel.
afternoon, 1 p.m. - phel.
sitting, while - phel.
standing - phel.

BOILS - am-c., ***calc., nat-m., nux-v.***

BORING, pain - agar., alum., am-c., aur., ***aur-m-n.,*** bufo, calc-p., canth., ***caust.,*** chel., coloc., crot-t., grat., ***hell.,*** indg., mag-c., mez., nat-c., nat-p., nat-s., plan., ran-s., sep., zinc.
evening - coloc., mag-c., zinc.
motion, agg. - bufo
amel. - sep.
night - ***calc-i.,*** calc-p.
stretching, when - calc-p.
sitting, while - agar., ***aur-m-n.,*** coloc., grat., indg., mez.
stretching agg. - calc-p.

BORING, pain
walking, while - mez.
wandering - nat-s.
boring, patella - am-c., hell., kreos., led., nat-c.
forenoon - nat-c.

BROKEN, sensation, pain as if - chel., colch., cupr., dros., hep., lyc., merc.
ascending steps, on - colch.
lying - merc.
walking, while - dros.
broken, patella, as if - bry., con.

BUBBLING, sensation - arg-m., bell., berb., nat-m.
popliteus - rheum.
walking, while - dros.
bubbling, as if, in patella - asar.

BURNING, pain - am-c., anac., apis, ***arg-m.,*** arund., asaf., bar-c., bell., berb., brom., bry., cann-s., carb-v., **CHEL.,** fl-ac., kali-n., lachn., lyc., ***mur-ac.,*** nit-ac., petr., ph-ac., phos., plat., plb., ***rhus-t.,*** sabad., stann., stront-c., sulph., sul-ac., tab., tarax., tarent., tep., thuj.
afternoon - lyc.
ascending steps - sulph.
morning - phos.
stinging - bell.
walking, while - stram.
amel. - phos.
burning, hollow of - am-c., ars-h., ***bar-c.,*** berb., cast-eq., ***chel.,*** grat., indg., ***iod.,*** lith., petr., sulph., sul-ac., thuj.
cold hands agg. - am-c.
extending down back of leg - ***bar-c.***
night, in bed - bell., chin., ***sep.***
rising, from sitting, - chin.
sitting, while - bar-c., grat.
soreness - bar-c.
walking amel. - grat.
warm, when - chin.
burning, patella - bar-c., tarax., thuj.

BURSAE - **ARN.,** calc-p., cann-s., kali-m., **NAT-M., SIL.,** stann., **STICT.**
cysts - cann-s., caust., ***graph.,*** iod., kali-br., ***sil., sulph.***

CHILLINESS - card-m., ***coloc.,*** ign.

CLUCKING, hollow of - asar.
outer side of - arg-m.
sitting - bell.

COLDNESS, in - acon., **AGN.,** ambr., ***apis,*** **ARS.,** ***asar.,*** aur., ***benz-ac.,*** camph., cann-s., carb-s., **CARB-V.,** ***card-m., chin., chin-a., chin-s., cimx., colch.,*** coloc., cop., daph., euphr., graph., ***ign., lach., merc., nat-m., nit-ac.,*** petr., **PHOS.,** ***puls.,*** raph., rhod., ***sec., sep.,*** **SIL.,** stann., sulph., ***verat.***
chill, during - **APIS, CARB-V.,** ign., **PHOS.,** sil.
cold, perspiration, with - ars.
evening - agn., euphr.
in, bed - ars., aur.
waking, on - euphr.
forenoon - thuj.
hottest weather, in - ***asar.***

COLDNESS, in
lying, while - ars.
menses, during - cop.
night - **CARB-V.,** cop., euphr., **PHOS.,** raph., sep., ***verat.***
bed in - **PHOS.,** sep.
waking, on - euphr.
outer side - dig.
right - chel.
sensation of, although warm - ***coloc.***
spot - petr.
swollen knee - ***led.***
walking in open air, after - sil.
warmed, cannot be - ars.
water, cold, as if, poured over - verat.
wind, as from - benz-ac., ***cimx.***
coldness, hollow of - agar., ars-h.
coldness, patella - aur., nat-m., verat.

COMPRESSION - aur., led., nat-m., nat-s., plat., spig.
walking while - spig.

CONSTRICTION - ***anac.,*** nat-m., ***nit-ac., plat.,*** sil., sulph., zinc.
afternoon - nit-ac.
evening - sulph.
bend of knee - nit-ac.

CONTRACTION, hollow of, muscles and tendons - ***am-m.,*** ang., ars., bell., berb., calc., carb-an., carb-v., **CAUST.,** ***cimx.,*** coloc., con., euphr., ferr., ***graph.,*** **GUAI.,** kreos., lach., led., med., merc., ***mez., nat-c.,*** **NAT-M.,** nat-s., nit-ac., nux-v., ol-an., ox-ac., petr., phos., ***rhus-t.,*** rhus-v., ruta., samb., sars., ***staph., sulph.,*** syph., ***tell.,*** verat.
bending - rhus-t.
chill, during - ***cimx.***
lying, while - staph.
on back, while - nat-s.
rising from the feet - ruta, staph., sulph.
walking - am-m., carb-an., phos.

CONVULSION- ars., berb.

CRACKING, joints, in - acon., alum., am-c., ***ars.,*** aster., ***benz-ac.,*** bry., calad., ***calc., camph.,*** caps., **CAUST.,** ***cham., cocc., con.,*** cop., ***croc.,*** gins., glon., hura, ign., lach., ***led.,*** mag-s., ***mez.,*** nat-a., nat-m., nit-ac., ***nux-v.,*** petr., podo., ***puls.,*** raph., sel., ***sep.,*** **SULPH.,** tab., tep., thuj., verat.
ascending, stairs - hura.
cartilage, as if slipped - petr.
descending stairs - **CAUST.,** hura
extending, limb - nat-a.
flexing, when - calad., nat-a., sel.
left - aster., calad.
lying down, when - sel.
painless - acon.
right - mez.
stretching, when - con., cop., mag-s., ran-b., rhus-t., thuj.
walking, while - alum., ***ars.,*** bry., calad., ***calc.,*** **CAUST.,** glon., hura, led., mag-s., nat-m., nit-ac., nux-v., tab.
cracking, patella - con., ran-b.

CRAMPS - ang., arg-m., arn., arund., berb., bry., cadm-s., ***calc.,*** carb-an., carb-v., ***coloc.,*** crot-t., dios., hep., hyper., lach., led., petr., plb., sulph., tab., ***zinc.***
above - arg-m.
afternoon 3 p.m. - dios.
alternating with each other - sulph.
drawing on boot - calc.
morning - dios.
motion amel. - arg-m.
night - bry.
10 to 11 p.m. - sulph.
sitting, while - bry., paeon.
long, after - chin.
standing, while - ang.
waking, on - lach.
walking while - ang., carb-an., chin., petr.
cramps, hollow of - bell., berb., ***calc.,*** cann-s., caust., kali-n., lyc., paeon., petr., phys., plb., sulph.
stamping foot, when - berb.
stretching leg - ***calc.***

CUTTING, pain - ***acon.,*** arg-m., bar-c., ***calc.,*** calc-p., form., graph., kali-bi., manc., mez., nat-p., plat., stry., ***sul-ac.,*** tax., verat.
night - form.
walking, when - ***calc-p.***
cutting, hollow of - sep.

DECAY, of bone - sil.

DISCOLORATION
dark brown in spots, posterior portion - phos.
redness - lac-ac., lachn., petr.
anterior part - merc., nat-m.
in spots - lyc., petr.
posterior part - am-c., kreos.
discoloration, patella, on going upstairs - cann-s.
red streaks - ph-ac.

DISLOCATED, feeling - bufo.

DISLOCATION, sensation, as if - ***arg-m., arn.,*** bufo., gels., ***ign.,*** merc., puls., thuj.
dislocation, patella, of - gels.
going upstairs, when - cann-s.

DRAWING, pain - ***acon., agar.,*** aloe, ***alum.,*** ambr., am-c., ammc., ***anac.,*** ang., ant-c., arg-m., arg-n., ars., ars-i., asar., aster., aur., aur-m-n., bapt., benz-ac., **BRY.,** cact., ***calc.,*** camph., cann-i., ***caps.,*** carb-s., carb-v., card-m., ***caul.,*** **CAUST.,** cham., ***chel., chin., chin-a.,*** clem., cist., cocc., coloc., com., croc., crot-h., cupr., cupr-ar., cycl., dig., dios., gran., graph., grat., ***guai.,*** hell., hep., indg., iod., jug-r., kali-ar., kali-bi., kali-c., kali-n., kali-p., kali-s., lach., ***led., lyc.,*** mag-c., mag-m., med., merc-c., mez., mur-ac., naja, nat-a., nat-c., ***nat-m.,*** nat-p., ***nat-s.,*** nit-ac., nux-v., ol-an., olnd., osm., ***ox-ac.,*** par., ph-ac., ***phos.,*** plat., ptel., **PULS.,** rat., ***rhod., rhus-t.,*** rhus-v., sabad., sabin., sec., sep., sil., spig., spong., stann., staph., ***stront-c.,*** sulph., thuj., verat., ***zinc.***

DRAWING, pain
afternoon - ammc., cycl., dios., lyc., ptel., sep., stront-c., sulph.
7 p.m. - lyc.
sleep, after - cycl.
air, open, agg. - **CAUST.**
alternating in each - bry., coloc., puls.
arthritic - sep.
ascending - alum.
bed, in - rhod.
bending, when - anac.
boring - mez.
cramp-like - arg-m., lyc., olnd., phos., sulph.
crossing limbs, when - ang.
ending with a twist - nit-ac.
evening - cham., nat-c., nat-m., sep., sulph.
extending, downward - cham., kali-n., lach., mag-c., nat-s., ph-ac., rhus-v., sec.
to ankles - rhus-t..
to feet - kali-n., nat-c., phos.
to soles - mag-c.
upward - indg., kali-c., nit-ac.
forenoon - coloc.
gouty - ***ant-c.,*** crot-h., sep.
jerking - stann.
left - nat-m., sil.
lying agg. - ***agar.***
menses, during - zinc.
morning - dios., kali-bi., nux-v.
bed, in - nux-v.
rising, after - kali-bi.
motion, on - coloc., iod., staph.
amel. - agar., arg-m., ***rhod., rhus-t.***
night - spong., sulph., zinc.
paralytic - chel., mag-m., nat-m., staph.
paroxysmal - coloc., croc., lyc., phos.
periodic - sec.
rheumatic - iod., mez., ***rhus-t., zinc.***
rising, after - coloc.
from a seat - chin., cocc., sep.
setting foot upon the floor - aur.
sharp - nat-c., nat-m., sil.
sitting, while - ***agar.,*** anac., chin., coloc., cycl., dig., lach., led., mez., ***nat-m.,*** **RHUS-T.,** staph., verat.
amel. - chin., kali-c.
standing, while - ang., ***calc.,*** chin., carb-v., cupr., cycl., stann., verat.
amel. - chin.
stepping - aur.
stretching, agg. - caust.
amel. - anac.
supporting body, knee - ph-ac.
swelling - lach.
tearing - bry., clem., ol-an.
twitching - stann.
waking, on - agar.
walking, while - anac., ang., aur., ***calc.,*** chin., clem., coloc., ***cupr.,*** kali-c., ***led.,*** ph-ac., phos., sep., spig., staph., verat.
after, amel. - grat.
amel. - ***agar.,*** chin., ***lyc.,*** **PULS., RHOD., RHUS-T.**
warmth of bed - **CAUST.,** ***lyc.***
wine, after - benz-ac., zinc.

drawing, hollow of - agn., alum., ***arg-m., bry.,*** calc-p., cann-s., canth., carb-an., carb-s., ***caust.,*** chin., cycl., graph., ***led.,*** lyc., mag-c., meny., mosch., mur-ac., ***nat-m.,*** nat-s., ***nux-v.,*** ol-an., phel., ph-ac., ***phyt.,*** rhod., ***rhus-t.,*** stann., staph., thuj., verat., zinc.
ascending - alum.
bending knee - ***rhus-t.***
evening, in bed - asar.
extending to, calf - mosch., stann.
to, downward - agar., mosch., phel., stann.
to, thigh - verat.
jerking - chin.
lying down, on - staph.
motion, amel. - nat-s., staph.
outer side - tarax.
pressure, amel. - arg-m.
rising from a seat - ***nux-v., rhus-t.***
sitting - meny., mur-ac., nat-s.
with limbs crossed - ***lyc.***
standing, while - cycl., graph., meny., verat.
synchronous with pulse - chin.
tearing - nat-m.
tendons - asar., chin.
trembling - staph.
walking, while - ***caust.,*** graph., mag-c., nat-m., ***nux-v., phyt.,*** rhod., zinc.

drawing, patella - berb., calc., caust., crot-h., cycl.
extending into leg - berb.
gouty - crot-h.
walking - crot-h.

DRYNESS, joint - ars-m., nux-v.
sensation of - benz-ac.

ECZEMA, hollow of - ***graph.***
rubrum - anil., arn., rhus-t.

ENLARGEMENT, sensation of - alum.

ERUPTIONS - anac., ant-c., ars., canth., carb-v., ***dulc.,*** iod., ***lac-c.,*** lach., merc., ***nat-m.,*** nat-p., ***nux-v.,*** ph-ac., phos., ***psor.,*** rhus-t., sabad., samb., sars., sep., ***thuj.***
blebs - ***anthr.***
blotches - ant-c., sulph.
burning - nux-v.
copper-colored - stram.
crusty - sil., ***psor.***
gritty - nat-m.
itching - anac., hep., nat-m., nux-v., ph-ac., thuj., zinc.
painful - arn.
pimples - ant-c., bry., hep., hura, nicc., ph-ac., puls., sars., sep., sulph., ***thuj.,*** zinc.
pustules - ***iris, phos.***
red spot - petr.
scaly - ***hydr.***
varicellae like - thuj.

eruptions, hollow of - **ARS.,** ***bov.,*** bry., calc., ***carb-s.,*** chin., dulc., **GRAPH.,** ***hep.,*** kali-c., led., ***merc., nat-m.,*** petr., phos., ***psor.,*** sars., sep., tep., zinc.
burning - ***merc.***
crusty - ***bov.***

eruptions, hollow of
dry - bry., ***psor.***
moist - ***graph.,*** **MERC., SEP.**
pimples - puls., sep.
pustules - bry., ***carb-s., cinnb.***
rawness - ambr.
red - merc., nat-m.
scabies - ars., bry., merc.
scabs - puls.
sore - merc.
spots - petr.

EXCORIATION, bend of - ***ambr.,*** **SEP.**

EXOSTOSES, patella - calc-f.

FISTULOUS, openings - ***iod.***

FLEXED - lyc., sulph.

FORMICATION - apis, crot-t., cycl., gent-l., kali-c., rat., rhus-t., zinc.

GANGRENE- phos.

GNAWING, pain - benz-ac., kali-i., ***merc., nat-m.,*** ran-s., zinc.
night - ***kali-i., nat-m.***

HEAT - apoc., arund., aur-m., ***bar-m.,*** bry., camph., cina, coc-c., colch., hyos., ign., kali-c., ***lach., lyc.,*** meny., ol-j., phos., ***sars.,*** sulph., verat.
hot air blew through, as if - ***lach.***
morning - sulph.
sitting - sulph.
night - coc-c.
heat, hollow of - dros.

HEAVINESS - act-sp., anac., apis, asar., berb., camph., cann-s., caust., cocc., ***con.,*** euphr., graph., ***hyos.,*** kali-n., lach., ***led.,*** lyc., mag-m., merc., nat-m., nit-ac., **NUX-M.,** ox-ac., phos., ***plat.,*** puls., rhus-t., ruta., sanic., sars., spong., ***stann.,*** staph., sulph., verat.
afternoon - mag-c.
ascending steps - caust., dig., hyos.
left - phos.
menses, during - sars.
morning, in bed - sulph.
rest, worse during - **NUX-M.**
rising, from a seat, after - berb., puls.
sitting - camph., mag-c.
walking, while - mag-c.
after - berb., calc-s.
amel. - kali-n., ruta.

HERPES - ars., carb-v., ***dulc., graph.,*** kreos., merc., nat-c., **NAT-M.,** ***petr.,*** phos., ***sulph.***
herpes, hollow, of - **ARS.,** calc., ***con.,*** **GRAPH.,** kreos., led., nat-c., **NAT-M.,** ***petr.,*** phos., ***psor., sulph.***

HOUSEMAID'S, knee, (see Bursae)

INFLAMMATION - ***apis, arn., bar-m.,*** bell., **BRY.,** ***benz-ac., calc., cocc., fl-ac., guai., iod.,*** lac-ac., ***led.,*** med., ***nux-v., phos.,*** phyt., ***psor.,*** **PULS., RHUS-T.,** ***sars.,*** sil., ***sulph., thuj.,*** tub.
erysipelatous - nux-v., **RHUS-T.,** sulph.
gonorrhea, suppressed - ***med.,*** sil., ***thuj.***

INJURIES - apis., ***arn.,*** bell-p., **BRY.,** calc., **RHUS-T., RUTA.,** thuj.

ITCHING - acon., ambr., ant-c., ars-m., asc-t., aster., aur., berb., bov., bry., calc-i., ***caust.,*** cinnb., cob., ***coloc.,*** fago., hep., hura, ign., kalm., kali-c., kali-n., lach., lachn., lith., lyc., mag-m., ***mang.,*** merc-i-f., ***mez.,*** mur-ac., nat-c., nat-m., nat-p., nit-ac., petr., phos., ***psor.,*** rhus-t., sars., **SULPH.,** thuj., ***zinc.***
burning, after scratching - nat-c.
on falling asleep - mur-ac.
evening - ***mang.,*** zinc.
night - cinnb.
scratching amel. - bov., mag-m.
sitting, while - fago.
stinging - merc-i-f.
tendons - rhus-t.
itching, bend of - ars., bov., caust., chin., coloc., ***con.,*** lyc., mang., ***nat-c.,*** nat-m., nit-ac., phos., ***psor.,*** rat., ***sars., sep.,*** spong., **SULPH., ZINC.**
biting - lyc.
burning - chin., lyc.
after scratching - coloc., rat.
evening - rat., rhus-t., sars., ***zinc.***
night - mang.
painful, after scratching - rhus-t.
itching, patella - aloe, asaf., bufo, caust., hydr., nit-ac., phos., samb., sars.

JERKING - ***arg-n., ars.,*** colch., meny., ***mez.,*** **PULS.,** spig., stram., ***sul-ac.***
first, sleep, in - ars.
sitting - mez.
upward, during cough - ther.
when sitting - ***ars.,*** lyc., ***meny.***

KNOCKED, together - agar., arg-m., ***arg-n.,*** bry., ***caust.,*** chel., clem., coff., ***colch., con., glon.,*** nux-v.
fright, after - cinnb.

LAMENESS - abrot., ***all-c.,*** ars., aur., ***bar-c.,*** berb., bry., ***calc.,*** calc-s., caps., carb-v., cinnb., cocc., com., dios., fl-ac., ***kali-c.,*** merc., rheum, ***rhus-t.,*** **RUTA,** sep., ***spong., sulph.***
descending - sulph.
kneeling, when - ars-h.
left - ***calc.,*** calc-s.
morning - abrot., caps., dios., lyss.
right - com., lyss., spong.
rising from a seat, after - ***berb.***
sitting - kali-c.
walking, while - bry., cinnb., merc.
after - carb-v.

MOTION
difficult - dios.
impossible - bry., ***chel.***
involuntary, to and fro - thuj.

NUMBNESS, of - alum., calc., carb-v., caust., cinnb., ***coloc.,*** fl-ac., graph., kali-c., lach., onos., ***plat.,*** thuj.
evening when stooping - ***coloc.***
morning - caust.
while sitting - sulph.
nap, during - calc.
night - graph.
rising, from sitting - chin.

NUMBNESS, of
sitting, after - alum.
sleep, during - graph.
walking fast, on - kali-c.
numbness, hollow of - onos.
sitting - plat.

PAIN, knees - abrot., ***acon., aesc.,*** agar., ***all-c.,*** aloe, alumn., am-c., anac., anag., ***ang.,*** ant-c., ***ant-t., apis,*** apoc., ***arn., ars., ars-i.,*** asaf., asc-t., aster., **AUR.,** aur-m-n., bad., bapt., ***bar-c., bell.,*** bell-p., **BENZ-AC.,** berb., ***bol.,*** brom., **BRY.,** cact., cahin., caj., calad., **CALC.,** ***calc-p., calc-s.,*** cann-s., ***canth.,*** caps., carb-ac., carb-an., carb-s., carb-v., card-m., cedr., **CAUST.,** cham., **CHEL.,** ***chin.,*** chin-a., ***cimx., cinnb.,*** cist., clem., ***cocc.,*** cod., colch., ***coloc., com., con., cop.,*** crot-c., cupr., daph., dig., dios., erig., elaps, euon., ferr., ferr-ar., fl-ac., form., gamb., ***gels.,*** glon., ***guai.,*** guare., ham., hell., hura, hydr., hyper., indg., ***iod.,*** jac-c., jug-c., kali-ar., kali-bi., **KALI-C.,** kali-chl., kali-i., ***kali-s.,*** kali-p., ***kalm., lac-ac., lac-c., lach.,*** **LED.,** lil-t., lob., ***lyc.,*** lyss., mag-c., ***med.,*** meli., ***merc.,*** merc-i-f., merc-i-r., ***mez.,*** mosch., murx., ***myrt-c.,*** nat-a., ***nat-m.,*** nat-p., ***nat-s.,*** nit-ac., ***nux-v.,*** ol-j., op., ox-ac., petr., ***phos.,*** phys., ***phyt.,*** pic-ac., pip-m., ***plat., plb.,*** podo., ***psor., puls., pyrog., rhod.,*** **RHUS-T.,** ***rhus-v.,*** rumx., ruta., sanic., ***sars.,*** seneg., sep., sil., ***stict., stront-c.,*** stry., ***sulph.,*** sul-ac., sumb., syph., tarent., tax., thuj., valer., **VERAT.,** verat-v., ***verb.,*** xan., zinc.
afternoon - abrot., arund., dios., erig., lycps., mag-c., ***nat-m.,*** phyt., rumx., sep., sulph.
air, open - **CAUST.,** ***phyt.***
air, amel. - pic-ac., sumb.
alternating with, heat and pressure on forehead - hell.
with, pain in elbow - dios.
ascending stairs, on - agar., ***alum.,*** arn., ***bad.,*** bell., cann-s., ***carb-v.,*** colch., dios., lith., nux-m., ***plb.***
bending, on - canth., chin., nit-ac., ***spig.,*** stann.
chill, during - agar., ars-h., chin., ***cimx., cocc., nat-m., nat-s., nux-v.,*** podo., puls., rhus-t., sep., sulph.
cold, when exposed to - ***calc-p., kalm., sep.***
amel. - ***led.,*** plb., ***puls.***
convulsive - nux-v.
cough, during - bry., caps.
cramp-like - bell., chin.
crossing, limbs - anag., petr.
damp, weather - ***calc., phyt., rhus-t.***
descending, steps, when - arg-m., ***bad.,*** cann-s., eupi., merc., nit-ac., ***rhus-t.,*** ruta, verat.
drawing, up limbs amel. - cham.
eruptions, suppressed, after - ***sep.***
evening - carb-an., cast-eq., cist., cob., coloc., cycl., dios., dulc., erig., ***kali-i., led.,*** lyc., lycps., murx., plan., ***rhod.,*** zinc.
bed, in - calad., colch.
exertion, after - caust., con., dulc., graph., ***mag-c.,*** nat-c., zinc.

PAIN, knees
extending to,
downward - kali-p., ***phos.,*** rhus-t.
feet - ***phos., tarent.***
groin - rhus-t.
hip - lach., ***led.,*** sol-n., tarent.
instep - elat.
limb - carb-v., chel., ferr., ***kali-c.,*** lyc.
limb, amel. - ferr.
soles - plb.
tibia - indg.
toes - valer.
up leg - dios., rhus-t.
fatigue, as from - con., dig., dulc., graph., ip., mag-c., ruta, sulph., verat.
fire, when near - sumb.
flexing, limb - phys.
amel. - ferr.
forenoon - coloc., dios., jug-c., merc-i-r., thuj.
9 a.m. - trom.
gouty - **BENZ-AC., CALC.,** con., ***eup-per., guai., lach., led., nux-v.,*** petr., verat.
increasing and decreasing slowly - zinc.
jerking - ***am-c., anac., chin.***
kneeling, when - ***bar-c.***
left - aster., bapt., benz-ac., brom., carb-ac., chin., kalm., pall., ***plat.***
left, then right - ***calc-p.***
lying - carb-an., calad., ***kali-i.,*** lil-t.
amel. - caj., sulph.
on right side - verat-v.
menses, during - cop., mag-c.
morning - abrot., ant-t., asc-t., bry., calc., carb-ac., coloc., dios., hyper., kali-bi., ***lach.,*** mez., nat-a., ***nux-v.,*** phos., sep., sumb., zinc.
rising - kali-bi., led., lyc., ***rhus-t.***
rising, after - agar.
motion - berb., bol., **BRY.,** bufo, cact., ***carb-s., cocc.,*** **CHEL.,** ***guai.,*** ign., iris, kali-bi., ***kalm.,*** lac-ac., lac-c., ***led.,*** lyc., merc., nat-a., petr., ***plb.,*** plan., rheum, staph., verat.
amel. - agar., calc., colch., cycl., dios., indg., ***jac.,*** lob., **LYC.,** mez., nat-s., pic-ac., **PULS.,** ran-b., ***rhod.,*** **RHUS-T.,** sep., ***stict.,*** sulph., ***verat.,*** zinc.
continued, amel. - ***jac., rhus-t.***
move, on beginning to - ***led., puls., rhus-t.,*** verat.
moving foot - staph.
neuralgic - bell., lac-ac., nat-a.
night - cact., caj., calc-p., carb-v., cast., coc-c., dios., gels., ***kali-bi., kali-i.,*** lach., ***lyc., merc.,*** mez., ***nat-m., petr.,*** phyt., ***rhod., sulph.,*** zinc.
11 p.m. until 7 a.m. - ***sulph.***
in sleep - zinc.
noon - arund., cinnb., dios.
paralytic - all-c., anac., arg-m., bar-c., berb., carb-v., chel., ***chin.,*** cocc., colch., coloc., crot-h., ***euon.,*** fago., ***kali-c.,*** mag-m., mosch., phys., plb., puls., ruta., sulph., verat.

PAIN, knees
left - lach.
paroxysmal - bell., nux-v., ***plb.***
pressure, agg. - ol-j., ran-b.
amel. - acon-c., ars.
pulsating - calad., calc., tarent.
raising limb - bar-ac.
right - agar., ***chin.,*** fl-ac., grin., meli., ***puls., sulph., verb.***
alternating with pain in right temple - meli.
and left hand - ***agar.***
hanging down, on - ***psor.***
then left - benz-ac.
rising, from a seat - asc-t., berb., carb-v., chin., fago., kali-c., mez., ***nux-v.,*** **RHUS-T.,** rumx., **SULPH.,** ***verat.***
rising, kneeling, from - ***spig.***
rubbing amel. - cast., cedr., ***phos.,*** tarent.
sitting, while - ***agar.,*** asaf., asc-t., aur-m-n., bell., calc., camph., carb-v., cast-eq., cist., coloc., crot-h., graph., indg., lach., led., mag-c., mez., nat-s., phys., **RHUS-T.,** verb.
after - anac., bell., berb., con., dig., nit-ac., nux-v., **RHUS-T.,** sep., zinc.
squatting, when - calc.
standing, while - alumn., arg-m., calc., carb-an., iod., lach., nux-v., podo., stront-c., ***sulph.,*** valer.
stepping, when - caust., con., nat-c.
stool, after - dios.
stooping, after - anac., croc., graph., plan.
stretching, agg. - ant-c., calc-p., med.
amel. - dros.
tendency - meli.
striking - carb-v.
thinking, of it - ox-ac.
touch, on - acon., calc., ***chin.,*** hyper., lyc.
turning, in bed - carb-v.
on turning the limb - am-c., calc., verat-v.
ulcerative - caust.
waking, on - zinc.
walking, on - ammc., anac., ant-t., arg-n., asaf., asc-t., ***aur.,*** aur-m-n., ***berb., bry., calc-p.,*** caps., caust., **CHEL.,** chin., ***cinnb.,*** cist., clem., ***coloc.,*** crot-h., cycl., dig., dios., dros., euph., form., gels., grat., ***guai.,*** hydr., iris, jac., jatr., kali-bi., ***kali-c., lac-ac., lach.,*** **LED.,** lil-t., ***mag-c., med.,*** merc., merc-i-r., mez., ***mygal.,*** nat-c., nat-m., nat-s., nit-ac., phys., petr., plan., staph., stront-c., thuj., verb., vip.
after - alum., berb., cycl., hydr., kali-n., mosch., phys., ***rhus-t.,*** valer.
amel. - ***agar.,*** grat., ***kali-s.,*** **LYC.,** nat-c., nat-s., ***puls., pyrog., rhod.,*** sulph., ***valer., verat.***
continued, amel. - dios.
open air amel. - sumb.
wandering - clem., dios., iris, kali-bi., ***kalm.,*** lil-t., lycps., nat-s., osm., ***puls.,*** ran-a., tarent.

PAIN, knees
wandering, from one to the other - dios., **LAC-C.**
warm, bed - dios., **LED.,** mosch., ***petr.,*** plb., ***puls., sulph.***
warmth, agg. - ***guai.,*** **LED.**
amel. - ars., canth., rhus-t.

pain, hollow of - agar., ***alum.,*** anag., arg-m., ars., ars-h., berb., brom., calc., calc-p., carb-an., carb-s., card-m., cast-eq., chel., chin., colch., con., cupr., dios., dros., fago., fl-ac., gels., graph., gymn., hep., jatr., ip., kali-bi., kalm., lac-c., mag-c., manc., mang., nat-a., ***nat-c.,*** nat-m., ***nit-ac.,*** olnd., op., ox-ac., par., ph-ac., ***plb.,*** rhus-t., rhus-v., rumx.
bend, must - squil.
bending knee - calc-p., cast-eq., chin., rhus-t.
contracting, pain - squil.
extending, downward - ***alum.,*** merl., mang.
extending, to heel - ***alum.***
to leg - carb-an., ***rhus-t.***
to tendo achillis - kali-bi.
left - ars-h., nat-p.
motion, on - ***nat-c.,*** ph-ac., ***plb.***
night - alum.
paralytic - agar., con.
pulsating - olnd.
right - berb.
rising from a seat - ars-h.
sitting, while - berb.
standing - graph., par., rumx., squil.
as if tendons were too short - graph.
touch agg. - ph-ac.
walk, on beginning to - nit-ac.
walking, on - ars., card-m., ***caust.,*** chel., colch., fago., gels., mag-c., nat-a., ***nux-v.,*** rhod., ***rhus-t.***

pain, patella - am-c., aml-n., ars-h., asaf., bell., berb., bry., cact., calc., ***carb-ac.,*** chel., clem., coc-c., kali-n., kalm., kreos., lac-ac., led., nat-c., ***nit-ac.,*** psor., rhus-t., sarr., sil., stram., valer., zinc.
bending - alum., nit-ac., pyrog.
evening - coc-c., zinc.
extending to back - tarent.
forenoon - nat-c.
motion - aml-n., coc-c., ery-a.
amel. - psor.
night - zinc.
paralytic - kali-n.
pressure, agg. - alum., coc-c.
rheumatic - clem.
rising, from a seat - calc.
sitting, while - bell., calc.
tendon of - ***chel., zinc.***
on walking - ***zinc.***
ulcerative - asaf.
walking - acon., berb., coc-c., led., ***nit-ac.***
wandering - psor.

PARALYSIS - ambr., ars., chel., lath.
sitting, while - chel.

paralysis, sensation of - anac., berb., ***chel.,*** gels., jug-r., kali-c., op., phos.
ascending stairs - plb.

paralysis, sensation of
evening in bed - colch.
forenoon, walking, while - bry.
rising, from a seat - berb., plb.
sitting, while - ***chel.,*** kali-c.
walking, while - berb., brom.
after - aur., berb., ***carb-v.,*** croc., ***hyper.,*** lach.
amel. - lach.

PERSPIRATION - am-c., ars., bry., ***calc.,*** clem., dros., led., ***lyc.,*** plb., sep., spong., ***sulph.***
circumscribed - clem.
cold - ars.
fever, after - plb.
night - ars., carb-an.
popliteus - bufo, ***carb-an.***
swelling, with - lyc.

PINCHING, pain - ang., merc-i-f., sil.
pinching, hollow, of - bell.

PRESSING, pain - alum., ***anac.,*** ang., arg-m., arg-n., asaf., ***aur.,*** aur-m-n., bar-ac., bor., brom., cadm-s., calad., ***calc., camph.,*** carb-v., chel., cic., clem., coloc., com., cop., cupr., cycl., dig., fl-ac., gins., hell., jatr., kali-c., lac-c., **LED.,** ***mag-m.,*** mang-m., mez., mur-ac., nat-m., nat-s., nit-ac., ox-ac., rheum, sars., **SIL.,** spig., stann., stront-c., **SULPH.,** tab., ***thuj.,*** verb.
bending - tarax.
constrictive - ***anac., aur.,*** cann-s., **SIL.**
drawing - camph., nat-s.
evening - coloc., fl-ac., lec., nat-s.
sitting, while - ***led.,*** nat-s.
extending downward - mang-m.
motion, on - hep., lac-c., ***led., sulph.***
amel. - arg-m., aur-m-n., com., cycl., kali-c., mez., tab.
night on waking - led.
paroxysmal - coloc.
pressure amel. - mez.
sitting, while - ***anac.,*** arg-m., asaf., ***aur-m-n.,*** bar-ac., camph., coloc., gins., led., mez., nat-s., ran-s., verb.
standing, while - verb.
sudden - nat-s.
tearing - led.
touch, on - staph.
twisted, as if - clem.
walking, while - anac., arg-n., asaf., cop., cycl., ***led.,*** nat-s.
after - acon.
wavelike - dulc.

pressing, hollow of - alum., arg-m., bell., brom., chin., plat., ***sulph.***
alternating with pressing in axilla - spong.
bending knee - spong.
cramp-like - sulph.
drawing - spong.
extending downward - rheum, ***sulph.***
jerking - spong.
motion, on - hep.
outer tendon - spong.
side of knee - staph., tarax.
sitting - plat., sulph.
walking while - alum., spong.

pressing, patella - alum., bell., calc., coc-c., led., ***sulph.***

PSORIASIS - ***iris, phos.***

PULSATION - ***acon.,*** arg-m., brach., brom., calad., ***kali-c.,*** kali-n., merc., tarent., verat-v., zinc.
evening - calad., kali-c.
lying, while - calad.
morning, on waking - verat-v.
motion amel. - kali-c.
night - kali-n.
painless - merc.
sitting, while - brom., zinc.
standing, when - arg-m.
walking, after - zinc.

pulsation, hollow of - coloc., olnd.

pulsation, patella - coloc., spig.
evening - coloc.

RASH - ***iod., led.,*** nux-v., sep., ter., zinc.
rash, hollow of - ***hep.,*** sep., zinc.

RELAXATION - lith., phos., plb., sulph.
walking, amel. - phos.

RESTLESSNESS - alumn., ***anac.,*** asar., lach., ***lyc.,*** spig., ***rhus-t.,*** staph., thuj.
night, in bed - lyc.

RHEUMATIC, pain - ***acon., agar.,*** ammc., aml-n., apoc., ***ars.,*** ars-h., asc-t., aur., bapt., ***benz-ac., berb.,*** bol., brom., **BRY.,** cact., **CALC.,** ***calc-p., caust.,*** cimic., ***cinnb., clem., cocc.,*** con., cop., ferr-p., form., graph., gels., ***guai.,*** hydr., hyper., iris, ***jac.,*** jug-r., ***kali-bi.,*** **KALI-C.,** ***kalm.,*** lac-ac., ***lac-c., lach., led., lyc.,*** **MED.,** merc-i-r., mez., nat-m., nicc., ***nux-v.,*** ol-j., ***petr., phos., phyt.,*** plb., ptel., puls-n, ***rhod.,*** **RHUS-T.,** ***ruta,*** sal-ac., sanic., sep., ***stict.,*** stry., **THUJ.,** trom., ***verat-v.,*** zinc.
left - bapt., ***berb., glon., phyt.***
right - cinnb., grin., jac., kali-bi., led., lob., nicc., phos., ***phyt.***
on hanging down - ***psor.***

SCRAPING, pain - samb.
scraping, patella - samb.

SENSITIVE - ars., bry., ***lach.,*** rhus-t., ***sars., sep.,*** sulph., verat.

SHARP, pain - acon., aeth., ***agar.,*** aloe, **ALUM.,** am-m., ammc., anac., ant-c., ant-t., ***apis,*** apoc., ***arg-m.,*** arn., ars., ars-i., arund., asaf., asc-t., aur., aur-m., aur-m-n., bapt., ***bar-c.,*** bar-m., **BELL.,** berb., bov., brach., ***bry.,*** bufo, ***calc., calc-s.,*** canth., ***carb-an.,*** carb-s., caust., cedr., cham., chel., chin., chin-a., cina, cinnb., clem., cocc., coc-c., ***coloc.,*** con., ***elaps,*** euph., euphr., ferr-ma., ferr-p., gran., graph., grat., ***guai.,*** gymn., ham., ***hell.,*** hep., hura, hydr., hyper., ign., indg., ***iod.,*** iris, ***kali-ar.,*** **KALI-C.,** kali-chl., kali-n., kali-p., ***kali-s., kalm.,*** lac-ac., lac-c., lach., laur., ***led.,*** lith., lyc., lyss., mag-c., mag-m., manc., mang., med., meny., ***merc.,*** merc-c., mez., mur-ac., myric., nat-a., nat-c., ***nat-m.,*** nat-p., nat-s., **NIT-AC.,** nux-v., ol-an., olnd., ***petr.,*** ph-ac., ***phos.,*** phys., phyt., pip-m., plb., podo., ptel., ***puls.,*** rat., rheum, rhod., ***rhus-t.,*** sabad., sanic.,

SHARP, pain - ***sars., sep., sil.,*** spig., spong., ***stann., staph.,*** stict., stront-c., stry., **SULPH.,** sul-ac., tab., tarax., tep., ***thuj.,*** trom., valer., verat., verb., viol-t., vip., zinc.
afternoon, 4 p.m., while walking - pip-m.
ascending stairs - agar., bar-c., bry., sulph.
bed, in - thuj.
bending, on - cham., mur-ac., tab.
boring - hell.
burning - apis, ***arg-m.,*** lith., mur-ac., ***staph.,*** sul-ac.
coughing, on - nit-ac.
crawling - carb-an.
crossing limbs - mur-ac.
drawing, after - guai., ***staph.***
evening - aeth., ***alum., am-m.,*** ant-t., calc., kali-c., lyc., plb., spong., stront-c., thuj.
9 p.m. - ptel.
bed, in - ant-t.
lying, while - petr., spong.
extending, into leg - ferr-p., mez.
outward - cham.
to hip - ***lach.,*** lyc.
upward - dulc.
forenoon - bov., calc.
itching - meny., viol-t.
kneeling, when - bar-c., ***bar-m.***
morning - calc., ign., lyc., nat-c., ***staph.***
4 to 8 a.m. - ign.
motion, on - ign.
rising, after - phos., rhod., ***staph.***
sitting, on - nat-c.
walking, while - nat-c.
motion, on - ***bry.,*** bufo, cham., coloc., ***elaps,*** ferr-p., led., merc-c., plb., spong., ***staph., sulph.***
amel. - ***calc.,*** camph., ***cham., kali-c.,*** merc-c., phos., viol-t.
sideways agg. - sars.
moving it back and forth amel. - plb.
night - bell., ***calc., camph.,*** carb-an., ***kali-bi.,*** phos.
10 p.m. - chel.
noon, riding, while - calc.
paralytic - bar-ac.
paroxysmal - phos.
rheumatic - acon., asar., chel., **KALI-C.,** ***lach.***
rising from a seat - agar., bov., rhus-t., thuj.
shifting - cham., lyc.
while sitting - asaf.
shooting - berb.
sitting while - alum., ***am-m.,*** asaf., aur-m-n., ***calc.,*** euph., indg., merc., nat-c., ***rhus-t.,*** stann., staph., sul-ac.
amel. - mur-ac., rat., sil.
sleep preventing - caust.
smarting - sep.
sore - bry.
sprained - ***arn.,*** petr.
standing, while - aeth., calc., hell., nit-ac., plb., rat., rhus-t., rumx., sulph.
after sitting - rhus-t.
starting on falling asleep, from - merc.
stepping, on - anac., caust., verb.

SHARP, pain
stretching, on - bov., laur., med.
amel. - mur-ac.
sudden - lyc., mez.
tearing - asar., berb., bry., ***calc.,*** lyc., merc.
thunderstorm, during - med.
touch, on - ant-c., ***arn.,*** tab.
transversely - rhus-t.
twitching - euph.
walking, while - agar., aloe, am-m., aur-m-n., ***bry.,*** bufo, ***calc.,*** calc-caust., caust., cinnb., cocc., coloc., euphr., hell., lach., ***led.,*** lyc., merc., mur-ac., petr., rheum, rhus-t., spig., sulph., thuj., ***valer.***
amel. - alum., ***kali-c.,*** nat-m., phos., ***rhus-t.,*** spig.
begining to walk - thuj.
in open air - dulc., hell., merc., sulph.
in open air, amel. - ***alum.***
warm covering, from - bry., ***elaps.***
weather changes, from - vip.

sharp, hollow of - agar., agn., ammc., bell., berb., ***bry.,*** carb-an., carb-s., chel., coc-c., coloc., cupr-ar., mang., merc-i-f., mill., nat-m., ol-an., plb., rat., sars., sep., stann., sul-ac., sulph., tab., thuj.
afternoon, while walking - bry.
chill, during - ***lyc.***
hot - sulph.
itching - coloc.
motion, on - agn., coloc.
night - lyc., nit-ac.
prickling - sul-ac.
rising from a seat - rat.
sides - guai.
sitting, while - mang., stann., sulph.
standing, while - agn., berb.
walking, while - ang., berb., ***bry.,*** carb-an., mang.

sharp, inner side - bar-c., berb., bry., canth., cham., cinnb., euph., laur., meny., phos., sars., staph., zinc.
dinner, after - grat.
extending to great toe - carb-s.
morning - ammc.
motion amel. - zinc.
nails, as from - nat-m.
pressing - zinc.
sitting, while - euph., plb.
standing, while - thuj.
step, at every - phos.
walking, while - rhus-t.

sharp, outer side - ant-c., cham., nicc., sabad., stann., staph., tarax., thuj.
burning - merl., mur-ac., staph.
sitting - sabad.
standing, while - nicc., stann.
touched, when - staph.
walking, while - cham., cocc., nit-ac., staph.

sharp, patella - ang., ***bar-m.,*** bell., ***camph.,*** carb-v., cham., cina, coc-c., cupr-ar., graph., kreos., lac-ac., lachn., meny., nat-m., nicc., ph-ac., staph., sulph., thuj.
above - verb.
afternoon - nicc.

sharp, patella
ascending stairs - thuj.
behind - sep.
below - bell., meny.
burning - asaf., lachn.
drawing - calc.
electric sparks, like - coc-c.
extending, downward - caust.
to hip - calc.
kneeling, when - ***bar-m.***
motion, agg. - ph-ac., staph.
amel. - viol-t.
right - nicc.
rising from a seat, after - carb-v.
rubbing amel. - manc.
sitting, while - bell., camph., merl., spig.
tearing - arg-m.
tensive - spig.
walking, while - ang., calc., coloc., sep.
continued amel. - coloc.

sharp, tendons - ant-t., berb., con., euphr., merl., nat-m., ph-ac., phos., raph., ***rhus-t.,*** samb.
evening - ant-t.
motion, on - ph-ac., ***rhus-t.***
rising from a seat, when - ***rhus-t.***
standing, while - berb.
touch, on - ***rhus-t.***
walking, while - ant-t., berb., euphr.
in open air - con.

SHOCKS - agar., arg-m., carl., sul-ac., verat.
falling asleep - ***agar., arg-m.***

SHOOTING, pain - ***acon.,*** agar., apis, ***bar-c.,*** brach., bufo, ***coloc., iod., ferr-p., kali-bi.,*** lyss., **NIT-AC.,** podo., rhus-t., sulph., tep., trom.
ascending stairs - agar.
coughing - nit-ac.
kneeling, when - ***bar-c.***
moving agg. - bufo, ***coloc., ferr-p.***
night - ***kali-bi.***
side to side, from - rhus-t.
standing, while - agn.
agg. - nit-ac., sulph.
walking, while - ***coloc.,*** sulph.
in open air - sulph.

shooting, hollow of - agn., bell., cupr-ar., sulph.
hollow of, sitting - sulph.

shooting, patella - bell., cupr-ar.

SHUDDERING - lyc., nat-m.
walking, amel. - nat-m.

SORE, pain - acon., aesc., ambr., ang., ***arg-m.,*** **ARS.,** ars-h., asaf., asar., ***aur.,*** bar-c., berb., brach., ***bry.,*** bufo, calc., calc-p., camph., canth., carb-ac., carb-an., caust., chel., ***chin.,*** chin-s., cic., cist., coloc., ***con.,*** cupr., cycl., elaps, **GRAPH.,** ham., hell., ***hep.,*** hura, hyos., jatr., ***kali-ar.,*** kali-bi., ***kali-c.,*** kali-p., lac-ac., lac-c., lach., **LED.,** lyc., mag-p., ***meph.,*** mez., mur-ac., myric., nat-c., nat-m., nat-p., nat-s., ***nux-v.,*** ol-an., ***ol-j.,*** petr., phos., ***plat.,*** plb., ***puls.,*** rhod., rhus-v., rumx., ruta., sabad., sarr., sep., spig., ***stann.,*** staph., sulph., tarent., tax., tell., thuj., urt-u., verat., zinc.

SORE, pain
alternating in each - cycl.
ascending steps - mur-ac.
bending it, on - aspar., carb-an., hell., spig., sulph.
chill, during - chin-s., phos.
before - chin-s.
descending stairs on - sulph., verat.
evening - abrot., dios., lach.
bed, in - thuj.
left - ***con.,*** phos., plat.
lying on sore side - nat-m.
menses, during - mag-c.
morning - graph., nux-v., zinc.
bed, in - aur., graph., nux-v.
rising, after, amel. - aur., graph.
motion, on - ***arg-m.,*** chin., ***kali-c.,*** puls., verat.
amel. - carb-ac., cycl., ***puls.,*** sulph.
move, on beginning to - nat-a.
night - **GRAPH.,** puls.
paroxysmal - plb.
pressure, on - caust., chel., hell.
raising limb, while sitting, on - phos.
rising after, amel. - aur., graph.
from seat - ars., ***berb.,*** sulph., verat.
from seat, amel. - phos.
sitting, while - ang., arg-m., ars., asaf., bry., coloc., jatr., sabad., sep.
amel. - zinc.
sneezing, on - ***kali-c.***
standing in open air - con.
touch, on - ars., spig.
walking, while - ***arg-m., bry., calc-p.,*** carb-an., cycl., dios., mur-ac., nat-s., thuj., zinc.
after - ***berb.,*** tell.
amel. - ars., ***puls.***
in open air, while - con.

sore, hollow of - ambr., kali-n., manc., mez., plb., stann., zinc.
morning - zinc.
walking - zinc.

sore, patella - acon., alum., ***arg-m.,*** bry., ***carb-ac.,*** chin., ery-a., hell., ***led.,*** nit-ac., petr., sil.
below - calc-ac., zinc.
bending the knee - hell., nit-ac.
descending steps - nit-ac.
side - puls.
sitting amel. - arg-m.
tendons - sep.
walking, while - arg-m., ***led.,*** nit-ac.
on level, amel. - nit-ac.

SPRAINED, pain, as if - agar., am-c., arg-m., ars., calc., ***calc-p.,*** carb-s., caust., chin., cod., con., elaps, gent-l., graph., ***ign.,*** hipp., kali-bi., kreos., ***lach., lyc.,*** meny., nat-m., nit-ac., phos., prun., rhod., **RHUS-T.,** ***ruta,*** sars., spig., sulph., ***thuj.***
above - ambr.
ascending stairs - nux-m.
descending stairs, when - nit-ac.
evening - petr., sulph.
extending to thigh - kali-n.

SPRAINED, pain, as if
fever, during - lach.
forenoon, while walking - nat-c.
left - ars., sulph.
lying - petr.
down amel. - ***sulph.***
morning - cod., sulph.
after rising - arg-m.
moving, on - arg-m., nux-m.
right - arg-m., calc., nat-c., nux-m., sulph.
rising, on - ars., kali-c.
after sitting long - kali-bi.
sitting, while - am-c., calc.
stepping - plat., sulph.
sudden - lyc.
turning leg - am-c.
walking, while - agar., ***calc-p.,*** graph., ip., lyc., nat-c., nat-m., petr., spig., ***sulph.***
after - tell.
on a level, amel. - nit-ac.
sprained, patella - calc., kali-n., nit-ac.

STIFFNESS, of - aesc., alum., ***am-m., anac.,*** ang., ant-c., ***apoc., ars.,*** ars-m., **ATRO.,** aur., aur-m., bell., ***berb.,*** bov., **BRY.,** bufo, ***calc., calc-s., cann-i.,*** carb-s., ***carb-v.,*** card-m., **CAUST.,** ***chel.,*** clem., cocc., ***coloc.,*** con., dig., dios., elaps, euph., ferr-ar., ferr-ma., ***graph.,*** hell., hydr., hyos., ***ign.,*** kali-ar., ***kali-bi.,*** kali-c., lach., lac-ac., lath., **LED.,** lob., **LYC.,** merc., merc-sul., mez., mur-ac., ***nat-m., nat-s., nit-ac., nux-v.,*** ol-an., op., ***petr., phos.,*** phys., phyt., pin-s., pip-m., plan., **PLAT.,** plb., podo., ***psor., puls.,*** rheum, **RHUS-T.,** ***ruta.,*** sang., sars., ***sep.,*** **SIL.,** spig., ***stann., staph.,*** **STRY., SULPH.,** sumb., tarent., tep., ***ter.,*** **THUJ.,** vip., ***zinc.***
alternating, between right and left - coloc., nat-m.
with tearing pains - ***ars.***
ascending steps, after - hydr., ign.
bandaged, as if - ***anac.***
descending stairs - merc.
evening - ***plat.***
kneeling, when - sep.
left - thuj.
morning - calc-s., stry.
rising, on - aesc., caps., ign., ***lyc.***
move, on beginning to - ***carb-v., caust., euph., lyc.,*** puls., **RHUS-T.**
night - ***lyc.***
painful - ant-c., **BRY.,** ***nit-ac.***
paralytic - aur.
rheumatic - **BRY.,** ***lyc.,*** merc., ***phos.,*** **RHUS-T.**
right - lyc.
rising from a seat - aesc., mur-ac., nat-m., **SULPH.**
sitting, while - anac., coloc., stry.
after - ***lach., lyc.,*** **RHUS-T.,** stict., **SULPH.**
sore - stry.
squatting, preventing - ***coloc., graph.***
standing, while - sil.
stretching out, on - bov., ***puls.***
sudden - stann.
tendons - hell.

STIFFNESS, of
walking, while - bell., ***caust.,*** kali-bi., ***led.,*** ol-an., phyt., **PULS.,** sil., sumb.
after - **RHUS-T.**
in open air - hell., hyos.
stiffness, hollow of - ambr., caust., dros., graph., lyc., mez., nit-ac., petr., stann., sulph.

SUPPURATION - hippoz., ***iod.***

SWELLING - acon., ***aesc.,*** ammc., ***anthr.,*** ant-c., ant-t., ***apis, arn., ars., ars-i.,*** arund., aur-m., ***bar-m.,*** benz-ac., **BERB., BRY.,** bufo, **CALC.,** ***calc-p.,*** calc-s., ***chin., cic., clem., cocc.,*** coc-c., ***colch.,*** con., ***cop.,*** ferr., ferr-ar., ***fl-ac.,*** **HEP.,** ***iod.,*** kali-ar., ***kali-c.,*** kali-s., kreos., lac-ac., ***lac-c., lach.,*** **LED., LYC.,** ***med.,*** merc., mur-ac., ***nat-m.,*** nit-ac., ***nux-v., phyt.,*** **PULS.,** pyrus, ***rhod.,*** **RHUS-T.,** ***sal-ac., sars., sep.,*** **SIL.,** ***sulph.***
alternate, and wrist - kreos.
dropsical - ***ant-t., apis, bry., calc., con.,*** dig., ***fl-ac.,*** hyper., ***iod., merc.,*** **RHUS-T.,** ***sil.,*** **SULPH.**
fatty - dig.
gonorrhea, after - ***clem.,*** **MED.**
gouty - ***benz-ac.,*** **CALC.,** ***kali-i.,*** **LED.,** ***lyc.,*** plb.
hot - **BELL.,** ***calc., chin., ferr-p., iod.,*** **PULS., VERAT-V.**
left - ***aesc., cic.***
night - ***calc.***
painful - ***apis,*** aur-m., chin., ***cic., led., mag-c., nit-ac., nux-v.,*** **PULS.,** ***rhus-t.,*** sep., sal-ac., sars.
painless - ***lyc.,*** **PULS.**
purple - aran.
rheumatic - ***acon., apis, ars.,*** berb., **BRY.,** calc-s., clem., **LED.,** ***lyc., rhus-t.,*** sal-ac., verat-v.
cold application, amel. - ***lac-c.,*** **LED.,** ***puls.***
right - ***benz-ac.,*** chin., ***elat.,*** **SULPH.,** tarent., ter., ***tub.***
scrofulous - arn., ***ars.,*** **CALC.,** ***ferr., iod., lyc.,*** **PULS.,** ***sil.,*** **SULPH.**
spongy - ***calc., kali-i.,*** **SIL.**
white, swelling (fungus articulosum) - ***ant-c.,*** arn., ***calc., iod., kali-i., lyc., ol-j., phos., puls., rhus-t., sil., sulph., verat-v.***
swelling, hollow of - ars., ***mag-c., rhus-t.***
sensation of - ***nit-ac.***
swelling, patella - coloc., sep.
swelling, sensation of - alum., am-c., canth., carb-v., dig., ***kali-i., lach.,*** merc., nit-ac.
afternoon - alum.
night - ***kali-i.***
sitting, while - am-c.

TEARING, pain - ***acon., agar.,*** **ALUM.,** ambr., ammc., am-c., am-m., arg-m., ***arg-n., arn.,*** ars-h., asar., asc-t., aur-m., **BAR-C.,** ***berb., bell.,*** bry., ***calc.,*** camph., cann-i., canth., carb-an., carb-s., carb-v., ***caust.,*** cham., ***chin., cist., clem.,*** cocc., coc-c., ***colch.,*** coloc., con., crot-t., dios., dulc., euph., fl-ac., gran., grat., guai., hep., hyper., ign., ***indg.,*** iod., iris, jatr., kali-bi., **KALI-C.,** kali-i.,

TEARING, pain - ***kali-n.,*** kali-p., ***lach.,*** lachn., lact., laur., **LED., LYC.,** lyss., mag-c., ***mag-m.,*** mag-s., mang., ***merc.,*** merl., mez., mill., ***mur-ac., nat-c.,*** nat-m., nat-p., ***nat-s.,*** nicc., nit-ac., op., par., petr., ***phos., plb.,*** psor., **PULS.,** rat., ***rhod.,*** **RHUS-T.,** ***sars., sep., sil., spig., stann., stront-c., sulph.,*** sul-ac., teucr., thuj., til., vip., **ZINC.**

afternoon - alum., carb-s., lyc., nicc.
1 p.m. - sars.
2 p.m. - sars.
3 p.m. - sulph.
4 p.m. - fago.
5 p.m. - chin.
air, open, agg. - **CAUST.,** phos.
alternating with each other - ars., mag-m., puls.
bed, in - **SULPH.**
before going to - ammc.
boring - agar., canth.
cold, on becoming - ***calc., kali-c., lyc., merc.,*** phos., **RHUS-T.,** sep., ***sil.***
crossing limbs - mur-ac.
dinner, after - mag-c., phos., sep.
amel. - phos.
drawing - arg-n., caust., cham., stann., ***sulph.,*** thuj.
eating, after - bry.
evening - alum., ammc., caust., ***cist.,*** coloc., kali-bi., kali-c., kali-n., mag-c., led., **LYC.,** petr., phos., ***puls., sulph.***
lying, after - alum., ***nat-s.***
walking amel. - ***coloc.***
extending, ankle, to - caust., cham., bry., indg., rhus-t.
downward - **ALUM.,** ***bar-c.,*** bry., canth., chin., indg., ***lyc.,*** merl., nat-c., nat-s., op., phos., thuj.
feet, to - lyc., sil., sulph.
hip, to - caust., mur-ac., nit-ac., puls.
hip, to, crest of ilium - sulph.
lumbar region - fago., stront.
thigh - chin., mag-c., nicc.
to toes - ***alum.,*** caust., sulph.
upward - caust., ***chin.,*** dulc., fago., fl-ac., mez., mur-ac., nat-c., nicc., nit-ac., phos., puls., spig., stann., stront-c., sulph., zinc.
inner side - alum., bar-c., calc., ol-an., ran-b., stann.
walking, while - ran-b.
walking, while, amel. - bar-c.
jerking - puls.
left - calad., ***kali-i.,*** lachn., ***psor.,*** sulph., zinc.
lying - con.
down, after, amel. - sulph.
midnight - stront.
morning - lyc., stront-c., zinc.
bed, in - merl.
rising, on - asc-t.
motion, on - ars., asar., ***chin.,*** kali-bi., **LED.,** ***merc.,*** plb.
amel. - ***agar.,*** asar., ***bell.,*** kali-n., psor., ***rat.,*** **RHUS-T.,** ***sil.***

TEARING, pain
night, bed, in - carb-an., ***merc.,*** nat-c., nat-s., nit-ac., ***puls.,*** rhod., **SULPH.**
noon - ***sulph.***
outer side - canth., caust., hep., hyper., iod., kali-i., kali-n., spig.
sitting, while - kali-i.
paralytic - ***chin.***
paroxysmal - cast.
pressure, on - plb., spig.
amel. - plb.
rheumatic - ars-h., asar., hyper., ***lach.,*** **RHUS-T.**
right - agar., ***coloc.,*** kali-n., rat., spig., zinc.
rising from seat, on - calc., caust., mur-ac.
amel. - sil.
rubbing amel. - canth., cast., ol-an., ***phos.,*** plb., sul-ac., ***zinc.***
sitting, while - ***agar., arg-m.,*** bar-c., con., dulc., kali-c., led., mag-m., merl., ***mur-ac.,*** puls., ***rat.,*** sep., ***sil.,*** stann., thuj.
amel. - zinc.
sleep, preventing - caust., lyc.
standing, while - ***agar.,*** berb., mag-c., sars., sulph.
amel. - sil.
stepping - caust.
stitch-like - alum., calc., sil.
stretching - petr.
sudden - lyc., op.
supper, after - sep.
torn, off, as if - phos.
open - calad., mag-c.
touch - ***chin.***
twitching - brom., kali-i., kreos., plb.
walking, while - ***am-m.,*** asc-t., bar-ac., berb., calc., camph., grat., lachn., **LED.,** merc., nit-ac., ***spig.,*** stront-c., ***sulph.,*** zinc.
after - clem., nit-ac.
air, in open, while - dulc.
amel. - ***agar.,*** alum., bar-c., bell., coloc., grat., ***indg.,*** kali-n., mur-ac., **PULS., RHUS-T.,** sulph.
wandering - lact.
warm, wrapping, amel. - nat-c.
warmth, amel. - **CAUST.**
of bed - ***led.,*** **MERC.,** plb.
weather, change of - vip.
yawning, when - sars.

tearing, hollow of - ars., berb., calc., calc-caust., iod., kali-c., kali-n., lyc., mag-c., merl., mez., ***mur-ac.,*** nat-m., ph-ac., phos., plb., sars., ***tarax., valer., zinc.***
drawing - ars.
evening - lyc.
extending, to calf - zinc.
to hip - mur-ac.
to thigh - mag-c., mez., ph-ac.
morning - zinc.
night - mur-ac., phos.
rising, from seat - mur-ac.
sitting, while - mur-ac., tarax.
amel. - ***valer., zinc.***
walking, while - kali-n.
agg. - berb., kali-n., ***zinc.***

tearing, patella - **ALUM.,** arg-m., berb., caust., clem., ***colch.,*** con., kreos., lachn., merl., phos., psor., stront-c., ***sulph.,*** zinc.
behind knee - sep.
dinner, after - phos.
drawing - cocc., merl.
jerking - chin.
motion, on - berb.
amel. - psor.
night - caust.
rubbing amel. - phos.
sitting, while - con., merl.
waking, on - clem.
walking, amel. - sulph.

TENSION - acon., aesc., alum., ant-t., ***arn.,*** ars., ***bar-m.,*** berb., ***bry.,*** calc., canth., caps., carb-v., ***caust.,*** cham., clem., coc-c., coloc., croc., crot-t., dig., euphr., hell., ign., kali-bi., kali-c., lach., laur., ***led.,*** lyc., ***mag-c.,*** merc., mez., mur-ac., **NAT-M.,** ***nit-ac.,*** nux-v., ol-an., pall., par., ***petr., phos.,*** puls., rhod., ***rhus-t., seneg., sep.,*** sil., stann., ***sulph.,*** tab., thuj., zinc.
ascending stairs - nux-v., sep., spig., ***sulph.***
below, knee, squatting - calc.
evening - coloc.
kneeling, when - sep.
morning, waking - carb-v.
motion - berb., kreos., nit-ac.
night - sulph.
rheumatic - mez.
right - sulph., zinc.
rising from a seat - calc., petr., **RHUS-T.,** ***sulph.,*** thuj.
sitting, while - cycl.
after - petr.
sleep, after - carb-v.
standing, while - croc., cycl.
stepping - petr., spig.
impossible - lyc.
stretching agg. - berb., ***ign.***
walking, while - ammc., berb., carb-v., kali-c., ***led.,*** sep., sil., ***sulph.,*** tab., thuj., zinc.

tension, hollow of - aesc., ***am-m.,*** anag., ang., ant-c., ant-t., arg-m., ars., bell., ***berb., bry., calc-p., caps.,*** carb-an., carb-v., carb-s., **CAUST.,** cham., cic., ***cimx.,*** coc-c., coloc., corn., cycl., dig., ***graph.,*** hep., kali-ar., ***lach.,*** lact., ***lyc.,*** lyss., ***mag-c.,*** mag-s., med., meny., ***nat-c.,*** **NAT-M.,** nit-ac., ***nux-v.,*** olnd., pall., petr., ph-ac., phos., ***phyt.,*** plat., ***puls.,*** rheum, **RHUS-T.,** ***ruta.,*** samb., sang., sep., stann., **SULPH.,** ***thuj.,*** valer., verat., vip., zinc.
afternoon - nit-ac.
cramp-like - phos.
daytime - nat-m.
menses, during - nat-p.
morning on rising - caust., ***lyc.***
motion agg. - ph-ac.
rising from a seat - calc-p., lact., nat-m., **NUX-V., RHUS-T.**
room, entering - mag-c.
sitting, while - ars., ***caust.***
standing, while - ars., ***bar-c.,*** graph., nux-v., samb., verat.
stepping - mag-c.

tension, hollow of
stooping, on - ***sulph.***
tendons - sep.
touch agg. - ph-ac.
walk, when beginning to - ***caust.***
walking, while - carb-an., ***caust.,*** cic., coloc., euphr., graph., lact., mag-c., mag-s., merc., nat-m., ***nux-v., phyt.,*** **SULPH.,** verat.
continued walking amel. - ***calc-p.,*** carb-an., ***caust., rhus-t.***
in open air - plat., zinc.

THRILLING, sensation - **CANN-I.**

TINGLING, prickling, asleep - alum., ant-t., aur., hyper., plat., rhus-t.
rising, from sitting - chin.
sitting, while - alum.

TREMBLING - acon., agar., ***alum., anac.,*** ant-t., bell., cadm-s., calc., calad., ***camph.,*** caps., ***chel.,*** chin-s., con., dios., ***glon.,*** hep., iris, kali-c., lach., laur., ***led.,*** lil-t., lyss., mang., merc., mur-ac., nat-m., nicc., nux-v., olnd., op., phos., ***plat.,*** plb., psor., ***puls.,*** rhus-t., ***ruta.,*** sep., sil., stann., staph., stry., tarent., verb.
afternoon - nicc.
ascending steps - dros., nat-m.
descending steps - coff.
emissions, after - nat-p.
evening, lying down after - puls.
standing while - nux-v.
walking, while - mang.
night, on waking - chel.
rising from sitting - chin., nat-p.
sitting, while - bell., ***led.***
amel. - laur.
standing - calad., nux-v., olnd., tarent.
stepping up a step - nat-m.
walking, while - dios., dros., ***ind., led.,*** mang., tarent.
after - zinc.
amel. - chin.
in open air - ***hep.,*** laur.

trembling, patella - mur-ac.

TUMORS - ant-c.

tumors, hollow of - calc-f., phos., sil.

TWISTING, sensation - dios., sep.

TWITCHING - ***agar.,*** aloe, am-c., anac., arg-m., asaf., ***bell.,*** brom., calc., carb-an., caust., chel., chin., eupi., graph., lyc., mag-c., meny., merc., mez., nat-p., nit-ac., ox-ac., phos., prun., puls., rhod., staph., sul-ac., thuj., verat.
afternoon - caust.
below, knee - cycl.
convulsive - lyc.
evening - carb-an., lyc.
sleep, on going to - carb-an.
inside of - agar., ***asaf.,*** brom., canth., sul-ac.
motion amel. - meny.
outer side - arg-m., ***asaf.,*** canth.
intermittent - canth.
sitting, while - arg-m.
sitting, while - anac., arg-m., ***mez.,*** staph.
standing - sul-ac.

twitching, hollow of - agar., am-m., bell., dig., laur., nux-v., spong.
bending knee - spong.
rhythmical, with - dig., puls.
standing - nux-v.
touch amel. - dig.
walking in open air, after - nux-v.

twitching, patella - am-c., caust., mez., spig., thuj.
evening - am-c.
itching - stann.
standing - mez.
under - stann.

ULCERS - anac., ***calc.,*** ph-ac., ***phos.***

UNSTEADINESS - ***acon.,*** ars., ***calc.,*** carb-v., chin., cycl., laur., mang., merc., phys., puls., ***rhus-t.,*** **RUTA,** stry., thuj.

URTICARIA - zinc.

urticaria, hollow of - ***zinc.***

VESICLES - ant-c., arn., carb-v., ***caust.,*** iod., iris, nat-p., phos., rhus-t., sabad., sars., sep.
greenish - iod.
itching - carb-v.
scratching after - sars., sep.
stinging - ***rhus-t.***
varioloid - ant-c.

vesicles, hollow of - chin., iod., phos., puls., sars., sep.

WEAKNESS, of - abrot., acon., act-sp., ***agar.,*** all-s., ***alum., ambr., anac.,*** ang., ant-t., ***arg-m., arg-n.,*** arn., ***ars.,*** ars-h., ars-i., arund., asar., aur., bapt., ***bar-c.,*** bell., ***bol.,*** bor., ***bov., bry.,*** cahin., calad., ***calc.,*** calc-ar., calc-s., caj., ***camph., cann-i., canth.,*** carb-s., carb-v., carl., ***caust.,*** cham., chel., ***chin., chin-a., chin-s.,*** cimic., cinnb., clem., cob., **COCC.,** colch., ***coloc.,*** **CON.,** cor-r., croc., ***cupr.,*** cycl., ***dig., dios., dulc.,*** euphr., fago., ***ferr.,*** ferr-ar., ***ferr-p., gels.,*** gins., ***glon.,*** graph., ***hell.,*** hura, ***hydr.,*** hyos., ***ign.,*** indg., iod., ***ip., iris,*** jac-c., jatr., kali-bi., kali-br., ***kali-c., kali-n.,*** kali-s., kreos., lac-ac., ***lach.,*** lact., ***lec., led.,*** lith., ***lyc.,*** mag-m., mang., med., ***merc.,*** merc-i-r., mez., mosch., **NAT-M., NAT-S.,** ***nit-ac., nux-m., nux-v.,*** ol-an., olnd., op., osm., ox-ac., petr., ***ph-ac., phos.,*** pic-ac., ***plat.,*** **PLB.,** podo., ***psor.,*** puls., ran-b., ***rhus-v.,*** **RUTA.,** sabad., sarr., ***sars.,*** sep., ***sil., stann., staph.,*** stry., sulph., sul-ac., sul-i., syph., tab., tax., tell., thea., **THUJ.,** verat., zinc.
afternoon - caust., chin-s., ham.
walking, while - caust.
ascending stairs - ***bry., canth.,*** caust., **CON.,** dig., dios., hura, hyos., iod., ***kali-c.,*** merc., ox-ac., ***plat.,*** plb., ***ruta., stann., sulph., thuj.***
bath, after a warm - calc.
descending stairs - bell., hura, ***kali-c.,*** lac-ac.
dinner, after - phel., nit-ac., til.
eating, after - anac., ***lach.***
evening - anac., bry., dios., nat-m., sang., sarr.
exercise - cob., equis.
extending and flexing amel. - ferr.

WEAKNESS, of
forenoon - sulph., valer.
fright, after - cinnb., merc.
injury, after - bell-p., rhus-t., ***ruta.***
kneeling, when - ***tarent.***
knock together, as if they would - ***agar.,*** berb., cinnb., ***cocc., colch.,*** **NUX-V.**
left - chel.
mental exertion, on - bor.
morning - chin., ***dios., nat-m.***
in bed - sulph.
rising, after - petr., phos., staph.
motion, on - cycl., phos.
amel. - chin., phos.
night - calc.
paralytic - mosch., stann.
raising leg - colch.
rest amel. - **BRY.**
rising, after - ferr-ma.
from seat - berb., laur., puls.
sex, after - agar., **CALC.,** con., kali-c., lyc., petr., ***sep.,*** sil.
shifting from one to the other - cic.
sitting, while - camph., cic., coloc., mag-c., mosch., phos.
amel. - staph.
standing, while - acon., ***anac.,*** calad., carb-v., chin., ***cic., cupr.,*** iod., merc., ***mosch.,*** plat., prun., sul-ac.
stool, after - trom.
sudden - cham.
touch - chin.
vexation, after - caust.
walk, as after a long - cocc., cor-r., dulc., euph.
walking, while - acon., agar., anac., bell., ***bry.,*** calc., carb-v., caul., chel., ***chin.,*** **COCC., COLOC.,** con., ***cupr.,*** cycl., dig., dios., hyos., kali-c., kali-n., ***lec., led.,*** lil-t., mag-c., nat-n., ***nat-s.,*** petr., plat., puls., spong., staph., zinc.
after - aur., calc-s., caust., clem., ind., phyt., ***rhus-t.,*** ruta.
air, in open - calad., hyos., ***zinc.***
amel. - cham., dios., petr., phos., ruta.

weakness, hollow of - adeps., aur., bov., ferr., plat., rheum, staph., valer., zinc.
morning - valer.
rising from a seat - ferr., staph.
sitting, while - plat.
standing, while - rheum
walking, while - zinc.
after standing - ferr.
cannot walk - adeps..

Larynx

AIR, trachea, hot, from - rhus-t.
as if, in waves, goes through - lyc.

ANESTHESIA - kali-br.

BLOW, as from a - ruta.

BORING, pain - coc-c.

BURNING, pain - **ACON.,** ***aesc., alumn.,*** am-caust., ***am-m.,*** aphis., apis, ***arg-n., ars.,*** ars-i., ***bell.,*** bov., brom., bufo, ***calc-p., canth.,*** carb-s., ***carb-v., caust., cham.,*** chel., ***clem.,*** coc-c., cur., elaps, ferr., ferr-i., ferr-p., ***gels., graph., hydr-ac., iod.,*** ip., ***kali-bi., kali-i.,*** kali-n., lac-ac., ***lob.,*** mag-s., mang., ***merc., mez.,*** myric., ***nat-a.,*** **NIT-AC.,** oena., ***par., ph-ac., phos.,*** phyt., ***puls.,*** pyrog., ***rhus-t., rumx.,*** sang., **SENEG.,** ***spong., stict.,*** tab., ***tarent.,*** thuj., urt-u., zing.
afternoon - am-m.
coryza, during - am-m., ***seneg.***
cough, during - ars., bell., bufo, ***carb-v., caust.,*** cham., ***chel.,*** coc-c., ***dros., gels.,*** iod., mag-m., phos., pyrog., rumx., ***seneg.***
deep, inspiration - ***rumx.***
epiglottis - wye.
extending, to abdomen - ambr.
to nostrils - ***kali-bi.***
hoarseness, with - am-m.
night - ***puls.***
scraping, when - ***canth., kali-bi.***
talking, after - ***ferr., kali-bi.***

burning, larynx and trachea - ***am-m.,*** ant-c., ***ars.,*** bar-c., canth., ***carb-v.,*** caust., cham., cina, cycl., ferr-ar., gels., graph., hydr-ac., iod., lach., lact., ***lob.,*** lyc., mag-m., merc., merc-c., mez., myric., par., phos., ***puls., rumx., seneg.,*** sep., ***spong.,*** staph., sulph., ter., zinc.
cold air amel. - ***puls.***
cough, during - ant-c., carb-v., ***caust.,*** cina, iod., lach., mag-m., pyrog., **SPONG.,** sulph., zinc.
lying, while - ***puls.,*** seneg.

burning, throat pit - ars.

burning, trachea - ***acon., ant-t.,*** ars., ars-i., ***asaf.,*** bov., ***carb-v., caust., cham., coc-c.,*** clem., ***dros.,*** euph., gels., ***iod., kali-bi.,*** kali-n., ***lach.,*** mag-s., mang., ***merc-c.,*** mez., myric., ph-ac., ***phos.,*** phyt., ***sang., seneg., spong.,*** sulph., tep., thuj., zinc.
cough, with - ***caust., ferr.,*** gels., mag-s., phyt., **SPONG.,**
evening, 6 to 8 p.m. - thuj.
motion, on - seneg.

BURSTING, pain - kali-ar.

CANCER - ***ars.,*** ars-i., bell., carb-an., clem., ***con.,*** hydr., iod., kreos., lach., morph., nit-ac., phos., ***phyt.,*** sang., thuj.

CATARRH - ***acon.,*** aesc., ***all-c., alumn.,*** ant-t., apis, arg-m., ***arg-n.,*** ars-i., ***arum-t., bell., brom.,*** bry., **CALC., CALC-P., CALC-S.,** canth., carb-v., ***caust., cham.,*** chin-a., **COC-C.,** ***con.,*** croc., cub., dros., ***dulc.,*** eup-per., ferr-ar., ***ferr-p., ham., hep.,*** iod., ***kali-bi.,*** kali-i., ***kali-s.,*** mang., menthol, merc., ***nat-m.,*** osm., ***ph-ac.,*** phos., rhus-t., **RUMX.,** ***samb.,*** **SANG.,** ***seneg., sil., spong.,*** stict., **SULPH.,** ***tarent.,*** tub.
suffocative - ambr., coff., sang., spong.

catarrh, larynx and trachea - acon., ***all-s.,*** alum., ***am-c., am-m.,*** **ANT-T.,** arn., **ARS.,** ***bad., bar-c.,*** bar-m., bell., ***brom.,*** **CALC.,** ***calc-p.,*** **CALC-S.,** camph., cann-s., canth., carb-an., ***carb-s.,*** **CARB-V.,** ***caust., cham., chim.,*** chin-a., ***coc-c., coff., colch.,*** con., crot-t., dros., ***dulc.,*** ferr., ferr-ar., ***ferr-p.,*** gels., graph., ***hep., hippoz., hydr.,*** hyos., ign., ip., **KALI-AR., KALI-BI.,** ***kali-br.,*** **KALI-C.,** kali-p., ***kali-s.,*** kreos., lob., ***lyc.,*** **MANG.,** meph., **MERC.,** ***nat-a., nat-m.,*** **NUX-M., NUX-V.,** phel., ***ph-ac., phos., rhod., rumx.,*** **SANG., SENEG.,** ***sil.,*** spig., ***spong.,*** **STANN., SULPH.,** verat., verb.
alternating with uterine complaints - ***arg-n.***
change of weather, before - ***kali-bi.***
damp weather - ***calc.,*** dulc., ***kali-bi.***
elderly people, in - ***ammc., ant-t., ars.,*** **BAR-C.,** ***hydr.,*** **SENEG.**
evening - carb-an.
measles, after - ***carb-v.***
morning - nux-v.
night - carb-an., carb-v., spig.
sudden - **ARS.**

catarrh, trachea - alum., ***ammc., ant-t.,*** arg-n., ***ars., bar-c., bry.,*** calc., cann-s., carb-v., ***caust.,*** chin., chin-a., coc-c., conv., cot., ferr-ar., ferr-i., hep., iber., ill., ***kali-bi., mang.,*** merc., naphtin., nat-m., nux-m., nux-v., par., ***ph-ac.,*** **RUMX., SANG., SENEG.,** sil., ***stann.,*** stict., sulph., tab.

CLEARING larynx, scraping - ***aesc., agar.,*** all-s., aloe, alum., ***alumn., ambr., am-c.,*** am-m., anac., **ANT-T.,** aphis., ***apis, arg-m.,*** **ARG-N.,** ***ars.,*** aur-m-n., bar-c., **BELL.,** bor., bov., **BROM.,** ***bry.,*** cahin., ***calc., calc-f., calc-p., calc-s.,*** camph., ***cann-s., carb-s., carb-v., carl.,*** card-m., **CAUST., CHAM.,** chel., chin-s., ***chlor.,*** cimic., cocc., ***coc-c.,*** colch., ***con.,*** crot-t., ***cycl., dig., dros., echi.,*** **EUPHR.,** ferr., ***fl-ac.,*** graph., grat., ***hep.,*** hydr., hydr-ac., ***iod.,*** ip., kali-ar., ***kali-bi., kali-c., kali-i., kali-p., kali-s.,*** kalm., ***kreos., lach.,*** laur., led., lob., ***lyc.,*** mag-c., mag-m., ***mang., merc.,*** mur-ac., ***naja,*** nat-a., nat-c., ***nat-m.,*** nat-s., nit-ac., nux-m., **NUX-V.,** op., paeon., ***par.,*** petr., ***ph-ac.,*** **PHOS.,** phyt., plat., prun., **PULS., RHUS-T., RUMX.,** ***sabad., sang.,*** sanic., ***sel., seneg., sep., sil., spong., stann.,*** **SULPH.,** syph., ***tarent.,*** thuj., ***zinc.***
daytime - ***caust.,*** con., ***stann.***
eating, after - bell., carb-v., ***graph.,*** hep., ***kali-bi.,*** kali-s., ***lyc., nat-s.,*** nit-ac., nux-m., phos., plat., puls., sanic., ***sil.,*** thuj.

CLEARING, larynx
evening - ***arg-m.,*** **BROM.,** ***carb-v.,*** **CAUST.,** chel., cimic., ***coc-c., con., lyc.,*** nat-a., ***rumx.,*** stann., ***tarent., zinc.***
7 p.m. - bry., grat.
ice cream, after - thuj.
incessant - ***phos.***
lying amel. - nat-c.
morning - ***cann-s.,*** **CAUST.,** chin-s., ***cina,*** iod., kali-bi., kali-c., nat-m., ***op., sel., stann., tarent.***
night - am-c., **ANT-T.,** ***cycl.,*** mag-c., ***merc., rumx.***
reading aloud, from - ***arg-m., seneg.***
talking, from - ***mang., stann.***
wind, from - kali-c.

CLOSED, nearly - calc-f.
salivation, with - tarax.

COATED, seems (see Velvety)

COLD, sensation on breathing - arn., **BROM.,** camph., chin., ***cist.,*** cor-r., iod., lith., ***rhus-t.,*** sulph.
expiration, on - rhus-t.
inspiration cold, expiration hot - ***sulph.***
shaving amel. - ***brom.***

CONDYLOMATA, (see Polyps) - ***arg-n.,*** calc., hep., ***merc-c., nit-ac., thuj.***

CONSTRICTION, in - **ACON.,** ***agar., all-c., alum., alumn.,*** am-c., ***ant-c.,*** ant-t., arg-m., ***ars.,*** asar., asc-t., bar-c., **BELL.,** ***brom.,*** bufo, calad., ***calc.,*** camph., ***carb-an.,*** carb-s., caust., ***cedr., cham., chel., chlor., cocc.,*** coc-c., coff., coloc., ***cor-r., crot-c., cupr.,*** dios., ***dros.,*** eug., euphr., ferr., ***gels., glon.,*** hell., hep., ***hyos., ign.,*** **IOD.,** ***ip., kali-c.,*** kali-i., kali-n., ***lach.,*** laur., ***lob.,*** lycps., manc., **MANG.,** med., meny., mez., ***mosch., naja,*** nat-a., ***nat-m.,*** nit-ac., ***nux-v.,*** oena., ol-an., ox-ac., ph-ac., **PHOS.,** ***phyt.,*** plat., ***plb., puls.,*** sang., ***seneg.,*** sep., ***sil., spong.,*** still., ***stram., sulph.,*** sul-ac., ***tarent.,*** thuj., ***verat., zinc.***
air, open, in - ***hep.,*** kali-c.
amel. - coloc.
anger, after - sulph.
auditory canal, scratching, from - sil., sulph., tarent.
cough, during - ***agar., ars., bell., chel.,*** **COR-R., CUPR., DROS.,** euphr., **HYOS.,** ign., ***ip., puls.,*** stram., ***sulph.,*** verat.
amel. - asar.
crumb, sensation of - ***coc-c.,*** lach.
drinking - acon.
after - ***ars.,*** meph.
eating, after - ***puls.***
evening - brom., hep., kali-c., lycps., nux-v., ol-an.
in bed - ferr., naja
on falling asleep - ***kali-c., spong., sulph.***
inhaling, on - ***hep.***
night - acon., ***phos.***
before midnight - ***spong.***

CONSTRICTION, in
scratching auditory canal, from - agar., ***carb-s.,*** kali-c., lach., mang., psor., ***sil., sulph., tarent.***
singing agg. - ***agar.***
sitting, while - ***spong.***
sleep, during - ***agar., cench., coff., crot-h., kali-c., kali-i.,*** **LACH.,** ***naja,*** nit-ac., **NUX-V.,** ***sep., sil.,*** **SPONG.,** ***sulph., valer.***
lying on either side, during - ***kali-c., spong.***
on falling asleep - ***agar., arg-n.,*** **KALI-C., LACH.,** ***phos., spong., sulph., valer.***
on falling asleep while lying on either side - ***arg-n., kali-c., spong.***
spasmodic - dig.
swallowing, on - ***dig.***
talking, while - ***dros., mang.,*** meph.
touch, from - bell.
waking, on - ***lach.,*** manc., ***phos.,*** thuj.
walking amel. - **DROS.**

constriction, larynx and trachea - alum., asar., **BELL.,** ***calad.,*** camph., canth., ***cham., cocc.,*** coloc., dros., ***hell.,*** ictod., ign., ***ip.,*** lach., laur., **MANG.,** meny., ***mosch., nux-m., nux-v.,*** ol-an., ox-ac., ph-ac., ***phos., plb., puls.,*** rhus-t., ***sars.,*** sil., ***spong.,*** verat.
lying, on - ***kali-bi.,*** puls.
night - ***phos.,*** puls., rhus-t.
waking, on - rhus-t.

constriction, throat-pit - ***apis,*** **BROM.,** ***ign.,*** ph-ac., rhus-t., ***staph.,*** valer., zinc.
anger open - ***staph.***
bending neck agg. - ph-ac.
eating amel. - rhus-t.
sleep, on going to - valer.
swallowing, when - staph.

constriction, trachea - alum., **ARS.,** bell., ***brom.,*** cact., ***calad.,*** canth., ***cham.,*** chel., cist., cocc., gua., hydr-ac., ign., ip., ***lach.,*** laur., mag-c., mosch., ***nux-v., phos., puls.,*** sars., ***spong.,*** stann., verat., xero.
evening, lying down, on - ***ars.***

CRAWLING, pain - am-m., ant-t., arn., bov., bry., calc-s., ***caps., carb-v., caust.,*** colch., **CON.,** ***dros.,*** graph., iod., **KALI-C.,** kreos., ***lach.,*** laur., led., lyc., mag-m., meny., **NAT-M.,** nit-ac., prun., ***psor.,*** rhus-t., ***sabin.,*** sang., sep., stann., stram., stront-c., sulph., ***thuj.,*** zinc.
cough, from - kreos.
eating, after - nit-ac.
evening - carb-v.
lying, after - caps.
morning - iod.
night - lyc.
sitting, while - ***psor.***
swallowing, when - staph.

crawling, trachea - anac., arn., ***caps.,*** colch., ***lach.,*** led., lyc., mag-m., nit-ac., nux-m., ruta., ***seneg.,*** spong., stann.
cough, from - colch., mag-m.
evening, lying down, after - caps.

crawling, trachea
night, 2 am, waking - lyc.

CROUP, in (see Coughing, Croupy) - **ACON.**, all-c., alumn., anac., ***ant-t., ars., ars-i.***, arum-t., asaf., ***bell.***, **BROM.**, bry., ***calc., calc-f., calc-i.***, **CALC-S.**, ***canth., carb-ac., carb-v.***, caust., ***cham.***, chin., ***chlor., cupr.***, dros., euph., gels., **HEP.**, ictod., ign., ***iod.***, ip., **KALI-BI.**, kali-br., ***kali-chl., kali-n., kali-p.***, kaol., lac-ac., ***lach., lob.***, lyc., meph., merc-i-f., mosch., naja, ***nat-m., nit-ac.***, petr., **PHOS.**, ***samb., sang.***, **SPONG.**, ***still., verat-v.***
eating, after - anac.
exposure to cold dry air, after - **ACON.**, **HEP.**, kali-bi., **SPONG.**
to, fauces - **BROM.**
to, trachea - ***iod.***, **KALI-BI.**, ***kali-chl., phos.***
gangrenous - ***ars.***
heated, from being - **BROM.**
lying agg. - ***hep.***
membranous - ***acet-ac.***, acon., alumn., am-c., ***am-caust.***, ammc., ant-t., ***apis***, ars., ars-i., ***arum-t.***, bell., **BROM.**, calc-i., ***carb-ac.***, caust., con., dros., ferr-p., ***hep., iod.***, **KALI-BI.**, ***kali-br., kali-chl., kali-m.***, kali-ma., kali-n., ***kaol., lac-c., lach., merc-cy., merc-i-f., naja, nit-ac.***, **PHOS.**, samb., ***sang.***, spong.
night, after - **SPONG.**
before midnight - **SPONG.**
paroxysmal - ***hep., kali-br.***
recurrent - ***calc.***, **CALC-S.**, **HEP.**
sequelae - ***calc., carb-v.***
sleep, after, agg. - **LACH.**, ***spong.***
whooping cough, during - **BROM.**

CRUMB, sensation of, in larynx - ***bry.***, coc-c., **LACH.**, pall., plb.

CUTTING, pain - all-c., ***arg-m.***, canth., kali-n., manc., merc-c., ***merc-cy.***, nit-ac., vinc.
coughing, on - **ALL-C.**, ***staph.***, sulph.
swallowing, on - merc-cy.

DOWNY, feeling (see Velvety)

DRAWING, pain - caust., kali-c., sulph.

DRYNESS, of - ***acon.***, aesc., agar., all-s., ***alum.***, am-c., am-m., ant-t., apis, ***ars.***, ars-i., atro., **BELL.**, ***bry., calc.***, calc-ar., calc-f., carb-an., ***carb-v.***, card-m., carl., ***caust.***, cist., ***clem.***, coc-c., colch., **CON.**, ***cop., crot-h.***, cycl., ***dros.***, ferr-p., fl-ac., gels., hep., hura, hydr-ac., hyos., iod., ip., ***kali-bi., kali-c.***, kali-chl., ***kali-s.***, kalm., lac-ac., **LACH.**, lachn., laur., ***lyc., mag-m., mang.***, med., ***merc.***, merc-c., ***mez.***, nat-a., nat-c., ***nat-m.***, nicc., nux-m., ***nux-v.***, op., osm., ***par.***, petr., ***phos., phyt.***, plan., ***puls., rhus-t.***, rhus-v., sabad., ***sang.***, **SENEG.**, ***sep.***, **SPONG.**, stann., ***stict.***, still., stram., **SULPH.**, sul-ac., tep., ter., thuj., verat., verat-v., verb., ***zinc.***
air, open, in - ***mang.***, nat-c.
aversion to drink - **BELL.**
bronchials - camph.
coughing, on - bell., osm., polyg.

DRYNESS, of
eating, after - zinc.
amel. - zinc.
epiglottis - lach., wye.
evening - carb-v., phyt., ***rhus-t.***, zinc.
forenoon - seneg.
hawking, from - ***spong.***
constant, with - am-m.
fever, during - ***ars.***, hep., nux-v., ***petr.***, phos.
morning - iod., ***nat-m., nux-v.***, phyt., seneg., sep., ***zinc.***
5 a.m. - kali-c.
waking - nat-m., ***par.***, sars.
night - ***bell.***, carb-v., hep., kali-c., lach., nat-m., ***phos., sulph.***
2 to 3 p.m. - ***kali-c.***
singer's, in - sang.
spot - cimic., ***cist.***, **CON.**, crot-h.
waking, on - am-c., ***cist.***, hep., kali-c., lach., nat-m., phos.
winter, in - mez.

dryness, larynx and trachea - agar., alum., ant-c., ***ars.***, calc-s., carb-v., caust., chin., coloc., dros., ferr., gels., hyos., ***kali-ar.***, kali-bi., kali-chl., lact., laur., lob., nat-c., nat-m., nicc., par., rhod., sep., stann., ter., teucr.

dryness, trachea - **ACON.**, ***ars., ars-i.***, bell., brom., calc-ar., carb-an., ***carb-v.***, clem., cycl., dros., fl-ac., ***iod.***, laur., ***lyc., merc.***, mez., nat-m., petr., phos., ***puls.***, rhus-t., ***rumx.***, sang., sep., ***spong.***, stann., tarent., verb.
close room - clem., ***puls.***
morning - phyt., rhod.
waking, on - ***par.***

DUST, as from, in - ***agar., alumn., am-c.***, **ARS.**, aur-m., ***bell., brom., calc.***, calc-s., ***chel., chin.***, cina, ***coc-c.***, crot-c., cycl., **DROS.**, glon., ***hep.***, ictod., ***ign.***, iod., ***ip.***, **LYC.**, meph., nat-a., ***nat-m.***, ph-ac., pic-ac., **PULS.**, **SULPH.**, teucr.

EDEMA, glottidis - **APIS**, ars., arum-t., bell., chin., chin-a., chlor., ***crot-h.***, hippoz., ign., iod., jab., **KALI-I.**, ***lach.***, merc., ***sang.***, staph., ***stram., vip.***
vocal cords - **LACH.**

FISSURES - bufo.

FLAPPING sensation - ***lach.***

FLESH, hanging in sensation of - lach., **PHOS.**, spong.

FOOD, drops into - acon., cann-s., gels., kali-bi., ***kali-c., lach., meph., nat-m.***

FOREIGN object, sensation - ***agar.***, ant-c., ant-t., ***arg-m.***, **BELL.**, brom., ***bry., calc-f., coc-c., dros., hep.***, iod., kali-c., ***lach.***, lob., med., ***nat-m.***, op., ***phos.***, ptel., rumx., ***sang., sil.***, tarent., ***thuj.***
morning - caust.
behind larynx - ***coc-c.***

foreign object, trachea, sensation - hyos., ***kali-c., sang.***, sin-n.

FOREIGN, substances, drop into larynx when drinking or talking - ***meph.***

FULLNESS - cob., naja.
evening - naja.
morning - cob.
singers, in - sang.

FURRY - phos.

HAIR, trachea in, sensation of - naja, sil.

HEAT - all-s., alumn., anan., ant-c., apoc., carb-s., **IOD.,** kali-bi., mag-m., naja, phyt.
heat, trachea - cahin., chel., petr., phyt., rhus-t.

INFLAMMATION, (see Laryngitis)
inflammation, trachea - ***acon., ant-t.,*** ars., ars-i., ***bell., brom.,*** bry., canth., ***carb-v.,*** cham., chin., dig., dros., ***dulc., hep., iod.,*** ip., ***kali-bi.,*** lob., ***mang., nat-m.,*** nux-v., ***puls., rumx., samb., sang., spong.,*** verat.

INSENSIBILITY, of larynx - ***kali-br.***

IRRITATION - acet-ac., **ACON.,** ***aesc.,*** **AGAR.,** ***alum., alumn.,*** ambr., am-c., am-m., anac., anan., ant-c., ant-t., ***aphis., apis,*** **ARG-M., ARG-N.,** ***arn.,*** ars., asar., bar-c., bar-m., **BELL.,** ***brom.,*** bov., **BRY.,** calad., ***calc., calc-p.,*** camph., canth., caps., carb-ac., ***carb-an., carb-s.,*** **CARB-V.,** card-m., ***carl.,*** **CAUST.,** ***cham.,*** chel., chin., ***chlor.,*** cimic., cina, ***cist.,*** coca, **COC-C.,** ***cocc.,*** coff., colch., coloc., **COM.,** ***con.,*** cop., ***cor-r.,*** **CROT-C.,** ***crot-h.,*** crot-t., ***cupr.,*** dig., dios., **DROS.,** echi., ***euphr.,*** ferr., ferr-i., fl-ac., form., ***gels.,*** guai., guare., ***ham.,*** **HEP.,** hydr-ac., ***hyos.,*** hyper., **IOD.,** ***ip.,*** **IGN., KALI-BI., KALI-C., KALI-CHL.,** kali-i., ***kali-p., kali-s.,*** lac-c., **LACH.,** lachn., lac-ac., laur., lith., ***lob.,*** **LYC.,** mag-c., mag-m., manc., **MANG.,** meny., ***merc.,*** merc-c., mez., mur-ac., myric., **NAJA,** nat-c., **NAT-M.,** nat-p., nicc., nit-ac., nux-m., ***nux-v.,*** olnd., osm., ***ph-ac.,*** **PHOS.,** ***phyt.,*** plan., **PULS.,** ***rhus-t., rumx.,*** sabad., sabin., **SANG.,** ***seneg., sep., sil.,*** **SPONG.,** ***squil., stann., staph.,*** stront-c., ***sulph., sul-i.,*** sumb., tab., tarax., ***tarent.,*** teucr., ***thuj.,*** trom., verat., verb., ***zinc.***
afternoon - coca, ferr-i., phos.
2 p.m. - coca.
cold air - **ACON.,** ***ars.,*** **BELL.,** calc-p., **CARB-V.,** cimic., crot-h., fl-ac., ***hep.,*** ip., ***kali-bi.,*** mang., ***naja, nux-m.,*** nux-v., osm., ox-ac., **PHOS., RUMX.,** sil., spong., sulph.
damp weather - ***kali-bi., rhus-t.***
eating, after - nit-ac., ***rumx.,*** staph.
evening, bed, in - cocc., coc-c., ***hyos.***
fever, during - hep.
heated, from becoming - ant-c., ***brom., carb-v., puls.***
lying on either side, on going to sleep - ***kali-c., spong.***
lying, while - ***ign.***
morning on waking - kali-bi., naja
in bed - ***caust.***
night - ambr., ***kali-c.***
before midnight - ***acon., spong.***
recurrent - ***calc.,*** **CARB-V.**
sleep, during - **LACH.,** ***phos., spong.***
suppressing the cough amel. - ***hyos.***
swallowing, empty - lyc., ***nat-m.,*** op.

IRRITATION, of
talking - ***alumn.,*** **ARG-M.,** ***bell.,*** **DROS.,** ***caust., hep., kali-bi., mang., nat-m.,*** **PHOS.,** ***rhus-t., seneg., spong., sulph.***
upper part - ***spong.***
warm damp weather - ***iod.***
room - iod.
irritation, throat pit - ***apis,*** bell., card-m., ***cham.,*** croc., ***hyos.,*** **IGN.,** iod., kreos., lac-c., mang., ph-ac., rhus-r., **RUMX., SANG.,** ***sil.,*** squil.
irritation, trachea - acet-ac., acon., aesc., agar., alum., ambro., ang., ant-t., apis, ***arg-m., arg-n., arn.,*** **ARS.,** asaf., bar-c., bar-m., bell., bov., brom., ***bry., calc.,*** cann-s., carb-an., carb-s., **CARB-V.,** ***caust., cham.,*** chin., cina, ***coc-c.,*** cocc., colch., coloc., con., ***cor-r.,*** croc., dig., **DROS.,** euph., ferr., ferr-i., ferr-p., ***graph.,*** grat., hep., hydr-ac., hyos., ign., ***iod.,*** **IP., KALI-BI., KALI-C.,** ***kali-i.,*** kali-n., ***kali-p.,*** kaol., ***lach.,*** laur., led., **LYC.,** mag-c., ***mang.,*** menth., ***merc-sul.,*** mez., mur-ac., naja, nat-a., ***nat-m.,*** nicc., ***nit-ac.,*** nux-m., **NUX-V.,** ***osm., petr.,*** **PHOS.,** plat., prun., psor., ***puls.,*** rhod., ***rhus-t., rumx.,*** sabin., **SANG.,** seneg., **SEP., SIL.,** spig., **SQUIL., STANN.,** staph., ***stict.,*** still., stront-c., **SULPH.,** syph., teucr., ***thuj.,*** trif-p., verat., xero, zinc.

ITCHING - ambr., am-c., ant-t., ***arg-n.,*** bell., cact., ***calc.,*** calc-f., carb-v., cist., colch., con., dig., fl-ac., lach., laur., lyc., mang., ***nux-v., puls.,*** sil., zinc.
night - ***cist.***
itching, throat-pit - phos.
itching, trachea - ***agar., ambr.,*** cham., ***cist.,*** colch., con., kali-bi., laur., ***nux-v.,*** phos., **PULS.,** rumx.

JERK, in, when drinking - nat-m.

LANCINATING, pain, trachea - ***iod.***

LARYNGISMUS, stridor - ***agar.,*** alum., ***ant-c., ars.,*** ars-i., arum-d., ***asaf.,*** **BELL.,** ***brom., chel., chlor., coff., cor-r.,*** crot-h., ***cupr.,*** dig., **GELS.,** guai., guare., hydr-ac., **IGN.,** ***iod., ip.,*** kali-br., lac-ac., ***lach.,*** laur., ***mag-p., mang., meph.,*** **MOSCH.,** naja, ol-an., ***op., phos.,*** phyt., plat., plb., ***samb.,*** sang., sars., ***sil., spong.,*** stram., sulph., ***tab., tarent., verat.***
alternating with contraction, of fingers and toes - asaf.
cough, before the - ***ip.***
daily - chel.
expiration, on - ***chel., chlor.***
midnight, to 7 a.m. - ***chlor.***
waking out of sound sleep - ***samb.***
night - ***samb.***
sleep, during - ***chlor.,*** lac-ac., ***lach.,*** spong., ***sulph.,*** thuj.
on falling asleep - ***phos.***
swallowing - ***cupr.,*** merc-c.
warm room - ***iod.***

LARYNGITIS, inflammation, of larynx - **ACON.**, ***aesc.***, **ALL-C.**, ***ant-c.***, ***ant-t.***, ***apis***, ***arg-m.***, **ARG-N.**, ***ars.***, ars-i., aur-m., **BELL.**, ***brom.***, bry., ***bufo***, calad., ***calc.***, calc-s., carb-ac., carb-an., carb-s., ***carb-v.***, ***caust.***, ***cham.***, ***chel.***, ***chlor.***, ***crot-c.***, ***crot-h.***, **DROS.**, ***dulc.***, ferr-p., **GELS.**, ***guai.***, **HEP.**, hydr-ac., ***iod.***, ***ip.***, **KALI-BI.**, kali-i., ***lach.***, ***mang.***, ***merc.***, merc-i-r., ***naja***, ***nat-m.***, ***nit-ac.***, ***nux-v.***, ph-ac., **PHOS.**, ***puls.***, ***rhus-t.***, **RUMX.**, ***sang.***, sel., seneg., ***spong.***, ***still.***, ***sulph.***, tab.

- atrophic - am-m., ***kali-bi.***, kali-i., lach., mang., phos., sang.
- catarrhal, chronic - am-br., am-i, ant-s., ant-t., ***arg-m.***, ***arg-n.***, bar-c., bar-m., calc., calc-i., ***carb-v.***, ***caust.***, coc-c., cot., ***dros.***, ***hep.***, iod., irid., **KALI-BI.**, kali-c., kali-i., ***lach.***, ***mang.***, ***merc.***, merc-c., nat-m., nit-ac., ***nux-v.***, ***par.***, ***phos.***, ***puls.***, rhus-t., sang-n., ***sel.***, ***seneg.***, ***stann.***, still., sulph., thuj.
- damp, weather - ***kali-bi.***
- evening, agg. - ***cedr.***, kali-bi., ***rhus-t.***
- follicular - arg-n., hep., ***iod.***, kali-i., sel., sulph.
- gangrenous - ***ars.***, ***bell.***, ***lach.***, ***phos.***
- heated, from getting - **BROM.**, **PULS.**
- recurrent - ***brom.***, ***calc.***
- singers, in - ***ant-c.***, ***arg-m.***, **ARG-N.**, ***mang.***
- speakers, in - **ARUM-T.**, ***carb-v.***, ***still.***
- syphilitic - ***hep.***, ***iod.***, ***merc.***, ***merc-i-r.***, ***nit-ac.***, ***still.***
  - hereditary - ***aur.***, fl-ac., ***hep.***, kreos., merc., merc-i-f., ***merc-i-r.***, ***nit-ac.***, ***phyt.***, sulph., thuj.
  - secondary symptoms, associated with - merc-c., merc-sul., nit-ac.
  - tertiary symptoms, associated with - ***aur.***, cinnb., iod., ***kali-bi.***, ***kali-i.***, lach., ***merc-c.***, merc-i-f., merc-i-r., mez., ***nit-ac.***, sang., thuj.
- urticaria, suppressed - ***ars.***

LEAF, trachea, closing up trachea, like a - ant-t., mang.

LIQUIDS, pass into larynx - ***acon.***, anan., ***lach.***, ***meph.***

LUMP, sensation - ***coc-c.***, ***kali-c.***, ***lob.***, ***med.***, ***nat-m.***

- behind larynx that compels swallowing - ***coc-c.***, ***lach.***, ust.

MEMBRANE, (see Croup) - bufo.

- false - cub.
- seems to move about in - ***kali-c.***
- sensation of, skin - lach., phos., thuj.

MOVEMENT, up and down of - lyc., op., stram., ***sul-ac.***, sul-i.

- cough, with - lach.

MUCUS, in - acon., ***aesc.***, ***all-c.***, alum., ***alumn.***, ***ambr.***, am-br., am-c., am-m., amyg., anan., **ANT-T.**, ***arg-m.***, **ARG-N.**, ***ars.***, ars-i., ***arum-t.***, asaf., asar., ***aur.***, ***bar-c.***, bell., **BROM.**, bufo, calc., ***calc-p.***, ***camph.***, ***canth.***, carb-an., ***carb-v.***, ***caust.***, ***cham.***, chin., chin-s., cina, cist., cocc., **COC-C.**, ***con.***, ***crot-t.***, dig., ***dros.***, echi., ***euphr.***, ***ferr.***, ferr-i., ferr-p., ***form.***, ***graph.***, grat., ***hep.***, hydr-ac., **HYOS.**, **IOD.**, iris, **KALI-BI.**, **KALI-C.**, ***kali-chl.***, kali-i., kali-n., ***kali-p.***, ***kali-s.***, kreos., lac-ac., ***lach.***, laur., **LYC.**, ***mang.***, ***merc.***, mill., ***naja***, nat-a., **NAT-M.**, nat-s., ***nux-v.***, ***olnd.***, ***ol-j.***, osm., ***par.***, phel., ***ph-ac.***, **PHOS.**, psor., ***puls.***, **RUMX.**, **SAMB.**, ***sang.***, ***sel.***, ***seneg.***, sep., ***sil.***, ***stann.***, ***staph.***, ***sulph.***, ***tarent.***, ***thuj.***, verb., ***zinc.***

- air passages, tenacious mucus in the - med.
- ascending stairs - arg-m.
- blood-streaked - am-c., anan., sol-n.
- blue - ***kali-bi.***, nat-a.
- cold air, in - ***rumx.***, seneg.
- copious - alumn., anan., ***carb-v.***, ***coc-c.***, ***nat-m.***, **RUMX.**, ***seneg.***
- cough, after each paroxysmal - ***agar.***, **COC-C.**, kali-bi., ***nat-m.***, ***seneg.***, sulph.
- eating, after - bell., caust., graph., hep., kali-bi., ***lyc.***, ***nat-s.***, nux-m., ***olnd.***, ol-an., ph-ac., phos., puls., sanic., ***sil.***, thuj., tub.
- ejected with difficulty - alum., alumn., ***aur.***, bar-c., bov., ***calc.***, ***canth.***, carl., ***caust.***, ***cham.***, ***cina***, cocc., crot-t., ***form.***, ***kali-bi.***, ***kali-c.***, ***lyc.***, ***mang.***, mosch., naja, nat-a., ***nat-m.***, ***nux-v.***, ***par.***, rumx., sars., ***seneg.***, sep., ***sil.***, staph., ***sulph.***, ***tarent.***
- evening - ***carb-v.***, crot-t., iod., ***puls.***, ***rumx.***, tarent., ***zinc.***
- green - ***hep.***, par.
- laughing - ***arg-m.***, kali-bi.
- morning - ***alumn.***, am-m., dig., ***kali-bi.***, ***ol-j.***, ***mang.***, **NAT-M.**, ***nux-v.***, ***olnd.***, par., ***sel.***, ***seneg.***, ***sil.***, ***sulph.***, tarent., thuj.
  - rising, after - ***cina***, ***olnd.***, sil.
  - waking, on - sars., sulph.
- night - ***puls.***, ***rumx.***, thuj.
  - speaking, on - ox-ac.
- overheated, from being - ***brom.***
- rattling - sul-ac.
  - evening - crot-t.
- saltish - ***am-c.***
- stooping, comes up when - ***arg-m.***
- talking from - kali-bi.

NARROW sensation, trachea - cist.

NECROSIS, of cartilages of - ***calc.***, crot-h., ***kali-bi.***

NODES, vocal cords - sel.

NUMBNESS - kali-br.

- **numbness,** trachea - acon., stict.

PAIN, larynx - ***acon.***, **ALL-C.**, alum., ambr., am-c., ant-t., arg-m., arg-n., ***arum-t.***, asc-t., **BELL.**, ***brom.***, bry., calad., ***calc.***, canth., carb-an., carb-s., ***carb-v.***, caust., ***chel.***, chin-s., ***cist.***, cob., coc-c., colch., crot-c., crot-t., cupr., cycl., der., dirc., dros., euphr., ferr., ferr-i., fl-ac., gels., graph., grat., ***hep.***, hura, ***iod.***, ip., just., ***kali-bi.***, kali-c., kali-chl., kali-ma., kali-n., kreos., **LACH.**, lyc., mag-m., mang., med., merc-c., nat-m., nit-ac., ***nux-v.***, osm., **PHOS.**, ***puls.***, rhus-v., ***rumx.***, ruta., sabad., sang., sarr., sars., sel., sep., spong.,

PAIN, larynx - stann., stram., sulph., sul-ac., tab., tarax., tep., thuj.
air, hot, from trachea - rhus-t.
bending head backward - ***bell.,*** bry., **LACH.,** ***rumx.,*** sil.
amel. - hep.
blowing nose, on - ***caust.***
cold, air - **HEP.,** ***sil.***
cold, drinks - calc., ***hep.***
compressed, as if - acon.
contractive - brom., dros., ign., ***iod.,*** ox-ac., ph-ac., spong., staph., stram., sul-ac., tab., thuj., verat.
speaking, when - dros.
coughing on - ***acon.,*** **ALL-C.,** arg-m., arum-t., **BELL.,** bor., ***brom., bry., calc., carb-v., caust., chel.,*** chin., coc-c., dros., ***hep.,*** iod., ***kali-bi., kali-c.,*** kreos., ***lach.,*** mag-m., med., nat-m., nux-v., ***osm., phos., puls.,*** rumx., sars., ***spong., stann.,*** sulph.
amel. - asar.
grasps the larynx - **ACON., ALL-C.,** ant-t., ***bell., dros.,*** **HEP.,** iod., lach., ***phos.***
coughing on, torn loose, as if something were being - **ALL-C.,** ***calc.***
draft of air - arg-m.
eating, while - rumx.
evening - ***nux-v.,*** spong.
expectoration, where detached - cham., cina, lyc., nux-v.
extending, downward - cham., glon., ip., verat.
to abdomen - crot-c.
to teeth - crot-h.
to, ear, left - zinc-chr.
upward - stann.
fever, during - bell., hep., ***iod.,*** mosch., **NUX-V.,** ***phos.,*** **PULS.**
grasps throat - acon., all-c., ant-t., arum-t., asaf., dros., iod., naja, phos., spong.
drinking, when - acon.
left - caust., ***crot-h., hep., lach.,*** rhus-t.
lifting a weight - sil.
morning - ***nux-v.,*** sep.
waking, on - kali-bi.
motion, on - ***bell.,*** spong.
moving head, on - hura
nail, as if a, in - spong.
pressure, on - ***ars.,*** card-m., chel., ***hep.,*** **PHOS.**
reading, after - euphr., nit-ac., ***spong.,*** stann.
respiration agg. - ***bell., carb-v., hep.,*** kali-n.
right - agar., kali-n., puls., stann., stict.
singing, when - ***acon.,*** **SPONG.**
sneezing, on - aphis., bor., phos.
speaking, on - ***acon.,*** coc-c., **PHOS.**
spot, in a small - ***hep., lach.***
swallowing, on - bapt., ***bell.,*** calc., card-m., chel., hep., ign., kali-bi., kali-ma., kali-cy., lyc., ***merc-c.,*** ph-ac., phos., **SPONG.,** ***sul-ac.***
as if food passed over sore spot - ***kali-bi.***

PAIN, larynx
talking, while - ***acon.,*** all-c., am-c., apis, arg-m., bapt., ***bell.,*** bry., carb-v., card-m., coc-c., ***hep.,*** kali-bi., merc-cy., **NICC.,** nit-ac., osm., **PHOS.,** rumx., sang., **SPONG.,** sulph., sul-ac.
amel. - rhus-t., sel.
tobacco smoking, from - bry.
touch, on - acon., alum., ***ant-t., bell.,*** brom., caust., crot-h., hep., **LACH.,** nat-m., **PHOS., SPONG.**
turning neck, on - ***bell., bry.,*** lach., spong.

pain, throat pit - caust., ***lach.***
extending to root of tongue and into hyoid bone - ***lach.***

pain, trachea - ***acon.,*** aesc., arg-m., **BRY.,** calad., ***cist.,*** hep., ip., lach., mez., sars., spong., stann., thuj.
air, hot, trachea, from - rhus-t.
coughing, on - bell., **BRY.,** camph., **CAUST.,** ***chel., chin.,*** cor-r., ign., **KALI-BI.,** ***kali-i.,*** kali-n., ***kreos.,*** laur., nat-m., ***nux-v.,*** osm., ox-ac., ph-ac., **PHOS.,** ***phyt.,*** psor., ***puls., rumx., sang.,*** spong., staph., ***sulph.,*** thuj.
as after long or much coughing - carb-an.
on, in a streak down - **CAUST.**
expectoration, where detached - cham., cina, lyc., nux-v.
hawking - camph.
inspiration, on - ***bry.,*** caps., ***caust., chel., hep., kali-c.,*** laur., lyc., ***manc.,*** nat-m., psor.
morning - mez.
talking, on - bry.

PARALYSIS - ***alum.,*** am-c., bell., both., canth., **CAUST.,** ***cina,*** cocaine, cocc., ***crot-h., gels.,*** **LACH.,** ***naja,*** ox-ac., ***phos., plb., stram.***
epiglottis - acon., gels.
vocal cords - kali-p., lach., ox-ac., seneg.

PIERCING, pain - brom., cham., kali-c., nit-ac., phos.

piercing, trachea - kali-c., nit-ac.

PLUG, sensation, (see Lump) - ***ant-c.,*** arg-m., bell., ***calc.,*** dros., ***hep.,*** kali-c., ***lach., lob.,*** nat-m., phos., sep., **SPONG.,** sulph.

plug, sensation, trachea - ***lach.***
closing, as if - mang.

POLYPS - ***arg-n.,*** ars., berb., calc., hep., kali-br., nit-ac., psor., ***sang., sang-n., teucr., thuj.***
vocal cords, on - berb., ***thuj.***

PRESSING, pain - acon., agar., anac., bell., ***caust.,*** **CHEL.,** euphr., ***iod.,*** kali-bi., sep., tarax., thuj.
blowing the nose, on - ***caust.***
morning - carb-v., sep.
singing - spong.
supper, after - ***hep.***
swallowing agg. - ***chel.,*** lyc.
amel. - tarax.
talking agg. - ***kali-bi.***

pressing, throat-pit - graph., mag-c., phos.
breathing, deep - caust.

pressing, trachea - ant-c., carb-v.

PRESSURE, in throat-pit - aesc., anac., **BROM.,** ***caust.,*** cic., graph., **LACH.,** ***lob.,*** phos., ***rumx.,*** sarr., staph.
anger, after - staph.
inspiration, on caust.
swallowing agg. - staph.

PRICKLING, in - ***calc.***

PULSATING - ***all-c.***

PURRING on coughing - nat-c.

RATTLING - am-c., ***ant-t., arg-n.,*** **BROM.,** carb-s., ***con.,*** crot-t., ferr-p., hep., hydr., ip., kali-bi., spong., sul-ac.
rattling, trachea, in - acon., am-c., **ANT-T.,** bar-c., bell., carb-ac., carb-an., carb-v., caust., cham., euphr., ferr-p., **HEP.,** hyos., **IP.,** kali-c., ***kali-s., laur.,*** merc., nat-m., nit-ac., oena., op., ox-ac., petr., puls., samb., ***sep.,*** sil., squil., sulph., sul-ac.
lying on left side - anac.
cough, before - kali-c.

RAWNESS, pain - ***acon., aesc., agar., all-c., all-s., alum., alumn., ambr.,*** am-c., anac., anan., apis, **ARG-M., ARG-N., ARS.,** ars-i., asar., ***bell.,*** bov., **BROM.,** ***bry.,*** bufo, ***calc., cann-s., carb-an.,*** carb-s., ***carb-v.,*** carl., ***caust.,*** **CHAM.,** chin., chin-a., ***chlor., cist., coc-c., coff.,*** dulc., ***gels.,*** graph., hydr-ac., ***hydr., iod., kali-bi.,*** kali-c., **KALI-I.,** kali-ma., kali-n., ***kali-s.,*** kreos., **LACH.,** lac-ac., lact., laur., lec., lyc., mag-m., ***mang.,*** med., ***merc.,*** **NAJA,** ***nat-m.,*** **NUX-V.,** ol-an., osm., ox-ac., phel., ***ph-ac.,*** **PHOS.,** ***puls., rhus-t.,*** **RUMX.,** ***samb., sang.,*** sars., ***seneg., sep., sil., stann., staph.,*** stront-c., **SULPH.,** ***tarent., zinc.***
cold air - **ACON.,** calc-p., ***carb-v., nat-m., nux-v., phos.,*** **RUMX.,** sil., ***sulph., tub.***
coughing, from - ***all-c.,*** **ARG-M.,** ***arg-n., ars., bell.,*** **BROM.,** bry., bufo, carb-v., **CAUST.,** cham., chlor., iod., ***kali-c.,*** mag-m., ***naja,*** **NUX-V.,** osm., phos., **PULS.,** ***rumx., seneg.,*** sep., sil., spong., **SULPH.,** ziz.
inspiration, during - **ACON.,** brom., **HEP.,** hipp., **PHOS.,** ***rumx.,*** sil.
evening - ***carb-v.,*** **PHOS.**
morning - calc., ***carb-an.,*** carl., ***caust.,*** cob., ***iod., rhus-t., sil., stann.,*** **SULPH.,** zinc.
waking, on - rhus-t.
night - anac.
scraping, from - agar., ***cann-s., carb-v., rumx.***
singing, when - arg-m., dros., ***stann.***
smoking, from - osm.
swallowing, on - calc.
talking, from - ***alumn.,*** **ARG-M.,** ***arg-n., ars., calc.,*** carl., coc-c., ***kali-bi., nat-m., rumx., stann., staph.,*** **TARENT.**
waking, on - alum.
rawness, throat pit - arg-m.
rawness, trachea - ***acon., agar., ambr., anac.,*** **ARG-M.,** arg-n., arn., ***calc., calc-s., carb-an., carb-s., carb-v.,*** **CAUST.,** ***coc-c.,*** coff., dig., fl-ac., graph., ***iod., ip.,*** kreos., lact., laur., **LYC.,** ***mang., mez.,*** nat-c., ***nat-m.,*** nit-ac., **NUX-V.,** osm., par., ***petr.,*** **PHOS.,** psor., ***puls.,*** **RUMX.,** ***sang., sars., seneg.,*** **STANN.,** staph., ***stram.,*** stront-c., ***sulph.,*** zinc.
coughing, when - ***arg-m.,*** arg-n., arn., ***calc., carb-v., caust., gels., graph.,*** laur., naja, nat-c., nux-v., **PHOS.,** ***rumx.,*** stann., ***staph., sulph.***
coughing, from - carb-an., laur., naja, ***staph.***
inspiration, on - carb-v.
morning - ***carb-an.***
night - calc., sulph.
swallowing - puls.
talking - **ARG-M.**

REMOVED, as if - spong.

ROUGHNESS - ***alum.,*** alumn., apis, calc., ***carb-an.,*** **CARB-V.,** cast., ***caust.,*** chin., cimic., con., dros., ***ferr.,*** ferr-p., graph., ***hep.,*** ip., ***kali-c.,*** kali-i., kreos., ***lach.,*** laur., lyc., mag-m., mag-s., **MANG.,** merc., nat-a., nat-s., nicc., **NUX-V.,** ol-an., ***phos.,*** plb., ***puls.,*** rhod., **RHUS-T.,** sabad., sars., ***seneg., sep., sil.,*** **SPONG.,** ***stann., sulph.,*** sul-ac., tarent., tep.
coughing, from - bar-c., carb-an., ***carb-v., caust.,*** dig., ***hep.,*** **KALI-C.,** kreos., ***mang., nux-v., phos.,*** sabad., ***seneg.,*** spong.
amel. - nicc., stann.
morning - ***calc.,*** coff., kali-bi.
talking, after - arg-m., coc-c., lyc., staph., tarent.
uncovering - kali-c.
roughness, larynx and trachea - ***agar.,*** ambr., am-c., anac., ant-c., apis, ars., ars-i., bor., bov., brom., ***calc.,*** canth., caps., ***carb-an.,*** **CARB-V.,** ***caust.,*** cimic., chin., cist., coc-c., coff., colch., cur., dig., dros., ***ferr.,*** ferr-ar., gels., graph., ***hep.,*** hipp., hydr-ac., iod., kali-ar., ***kali-bi.,*** kali-c., kali-i., kali-n., kreos., lach., lact., ***laur.,*** lyc., mag-m., ***mang.,*** meny., merc., merc-sul., mur-ac., nat-c., nit-ac., nux-m., ol-an., ox-ac., phel., ***ph-ac., phos.,*** plb., prun., puls., rhod., rhus-t., sabad., sang., ***seneg.,*** sep., ***sil., stann.,*** stront-c., ***sulph., sul-ac.,*** verat., zinc.
cough, from - anac.
eating, after - anac., zinc.
amel. - zinc.
evening - cimic.
morning - bor., calc., ***carb-an.,*** zinc.
talking, agg. - am-c., lyc.
walking in open air, after - ***sil.***
wet weather in - phos.
roughness, throat-pit - bor.
roughness, trachea - apis, bar-c., carb-an., dig., dros., hep., kali-c., kreos., laur., led., phos., phyt., rhus-t., sabad., sep., spong., tarent., verb.

SCRAPING, (see Clearing larynx)

SCRATCHING - acon., alum., alumn., am-c., anan., ant-c., arg-n., bov., calc., carb-v., cist., coloc., gamb., ***graph.,*** ign., kali-c., kali-n., ***laur.,*** lyc., mag-c., mag-m., nat-m., nit-ac., nux-v., phos., psor., ***seneg.,*** stann., verat., zinc.
inspiration, agg. - coloc.
night, 2 a.m., wakens him - lyc.
singing, when - agar.
wind from - kali-c.

scratching, trachea - stann.

SENSITIVE - ***acon.,*** **BELL.,** ***calad.,*** carb-s., ***caust.,*** cedr., cor-r., fl-ac., ***graph.,*** hep., lac-c., **LACH., NAJA,** ***phos., spong.,*** sulph., sul-ac., syph.
cold air, to - **ACON.,** ***ars., bell.,*** calc-p., ***carb-v.,*** carl., cimic., crot-h., fl-ac., **HEP.,** ip., ***mang., naja,*** nux-m., nux-v., osm., ox-ac., ***phos.,*** **RUMX.,** sil., spong., stann., sulph.
morning - kali-bi.
pressure, to - ***ars.,*** bell., **PHOS.**
to slightest - bell.
sound of the piano, to - **CALC.**
touch, to - **ACON.,** ***caust., con.,*** crot-h., ***graph., hep.,*** **LACH.,** ***naja,*** **PHOS., SPONG.**

sensitive, trachea, cold air, to - ***rumx.***

SHARP, pain - acon., ang., aphis., ***arg-m.,*** asar., bar-c., bell., bor., ***brom.,*** bufo, ***calc.,*** calc-caust., canth., caps., cham., chin., ***chel., cist.,*** cob., coc-c., croc., cur., dig., dirc., dros., hep., hydr-ac., hyos., ***iod., indg., kali-c., kali-s.,*** laur., led., ***mang.,*** meny., merc-c., mur-ac., naja, ***nit-ac.,*** olnd., ox-ac., ***phos.,*** sars., seneg., spig., spong., stann., sul-ac., ***thuj., til.,*** zinc.
air, open, in - ox-ac.
cough, during - aloe, bufo, dros., kali-c., mur-ac., ***phos.,*** sulph.
evening - indg.
excitement, from - ***cist.***
extending, pharynx, to - dros.
to ear - arg-m., nat-m.
to ear, swallowing, when - **MANG.**
vertex - arg-m.
forced inspiration, on - hep.
night, cough, during - phos.
pressing - sars.
supper, after - ***hep.***
swallowing, when - ***brom.,*** iod., **MANG.**
amel. - spig.
impending - meny.
touch, on - sil.
walking in open air, while - ox-ac.

sharp, throat-pit - bor., phos.

sharp, trachea - ***arg-m.,*** bell., canth., lach., **STANN.,** thuj.
breathing, on - ant-c., thuj.
exertion, slightest, on - manc.
night - canth.
swallowing agg. - thuj.

SHOCKS, larynx, in, on waking - manc.
coughing - sulph.

shocks, trachea, in - bry., cina, spong.
sleep, in- spong.

SKIN, sensation of - ***alum., alumn.,*** caust., kali-c., ***lach., phos., thuj.***

SMOKE, sensation of - **ARS., BAR-C.,** ***brom.***
sleep, before - ***ars.***

SORE, pain - **ACON.,** all-s., alum., ***ambr.,*** ant-c., aphis., apis, **ARG-M.,** ***arg-n., ars.,*** ars-i., bapt., bar-c., **BELL.,** ***brom.,*** bry., calad., ***calc-s., cann-s.,*** carb-an., **CARB-S.,** ***carb-v.,*** cast., ***caust., chin.,*** chin-a., cic., ***con.,*** cop., crot-h., **DROS.,** fl-ac., ***graph., hep., ign.,*** iod., ***kali-bi.,*** kali-c., ***kali-i., kali-s.,*** **LACH.,** lac-c., mag-m., ***med., mez.,*** nat-a., ***nat-m., nicc., nux-m.,*** osm., ox-ac., **PHOS.,** ***rhus-t., rumx., ruta.,*** sang., ***sep., sil.,*** **SPONG., STANN.,** ***still.,*** **SULPH.,** sul-ac., teucr., zinc.
breathing, on - sil.
coughing, on - ambr., **ARG-M., BELL.,** ***brom.,*** carb-an., ***carb-v., caust., caps.,*** chin., ***dros.,*** fl-ac., ign., kali-c., kali-i., nat-m., ***nux-m.,*** **PHOS.,** ***puls.,*** rumx., sep., ***stann.***
evening - kali-bi., ***phos.***
inspiration, on - dros.
morning - ***arg-n.,*** chin-s.
waking, on - kali-bi.
singers - alum., ***arg-n.,*** arn., **ARUM-T.,** caps., cupr., ferr-p., ***lach., rhus-t.,*** sil., ***stann.,*** zinc.
swallowing, on - **BELL.,** calc., chin-s., **DROS.,** fl-ac., gels., mag-m., **SPONG.**
touch - **ACON.,** alum., apis, bapt., bar-c., **BELL.,** brom., bry., ***caust.,*** chin-s., cic., ***con., crot-h., graph.,*** hep., lac-c., **LACH.,** mez., ***nicc.,*** **PHOS.,** rumx., **SPONG.,** sulph., ***sul-ac.,*** teucr., zinc.
turning the head, on - ***carb-v.,*** lach., ***spong.***

sore, larynx and trachea - ambr., alum., am-m., ***arg-m.,*** ars., ars-i., bar-c., ***bell.,*** bov., brom., ***bry.,*** calc., ***calc-s.,*** **CARB-S., CARB-V.,** ***caust.,*** chin., cina, graph., hep., ign., iod., kali-ar., kali-p., lach., lyc., mag-m., merc., nat-c., nux-m., ***nux-v.,*** **PHOS.,** rhus-t., ruta., rumx., seneg., sep., sil., spig., spong., **STANN., SULPH.**

sore, trachea - ***ambr.,*** ant-c., apis, ***bell.,*** brom., ***bry.,*** carb-an., carb-s., carb-v., ***caust.,*** cham., ***chin., hep.,*** kali-c., lyc., nat-c., ***nat-m.,*** nat-p., nux-v., ***phos.,*** **RUMX.,** sep., ***sil.,*** stann., sulph., zinc.
coughing, on - am-c., ***arg-n.,*** **BRY., CAUST.,** chel., cina, iod., iris, kali-i., nux-v., osm., psor., ***rumx.,*** sep., **STANN.,** sulph.

STINGING, pain - ***alumn.,*** am-c., bufo, canth., cham., dirc., ***iod.,*** **NIT-AC.,** ***seneg.***

STOPPAGE, sensation of - aur-m., rhus-t., spong., verb.

STREAK, larynx - caust., olnd.

SUFFOCATIVE, catarrh - ambr., calc., coff., sang., spong.

SULPHUR, vapor, as from - am-c., aml-n., **ARS.,** asaf., ***brom.,*** ***bry.,*** calc., ***carb-v.,*** ***chin.,*** croc., **IGN.,** ip., kali-chl., ***lach.,*** **LYC.,** mosch., par., **PULS.**
cough, during - brom., lyc., ***puls.***

SUPPORTS, on coughing - ***acon.,*** **ALL-C.,** ant-t., ***bell.,*** ***dros.,*** **HEP.,** iod., lach., ***phos.***
on, swallowing - dros.

SWOLLEN - anan., arn., **BELL.,** chel., calad., coc-c., ***hep.,*** ***iod.,*** kali-i., lac-c., ***lach.,*** ox-ac., sil., spong., sulph.
arytenoid cartilage - tub.
evening - coc-c.
swollen, throat-pit - ***lach.***
swollen, sensation of - ***chel.,*** carb-v., hydr-ac., ip., ***kali-bi.,*** ***lach.,*** laur., ox-ac., sang., sulph.

TEARING, pain - anan., bell., bor., caps., ign., lac-ac., seneg.
coughing, on - **ALL-C.,** ***bell.,*** bor., ***calc.,*** ***cist.,*** med., ***phos.,*** ***staph.***
evening - bor.
swallowing agg. - ign.

TENSION - chin., ***cocc.,*** ***iod.,*** kali-n., lach., manc., mez., naja
bed, in - naja.
evening - naja.
menses, during - cop.

TICKLING - ***acon.,*** ***aesc.,*** aeth., ***agar.,*** **ALL-C.,** ***alum.,*** ***alumn.,*** ***ambr.,*** am-br., ***am-c.,*** ***am-m.,*** anac., ang., ant-t., ant-s., aphis., apis, ***arg-m.,*** ***arg-n.,*** ***arn.,*** **ARS.,** asaf., aspar., aur-m., aur-m-n., ***bad.,*** bapt., bar-c., **BELL.,** bor., bov., ***brom.,*** ***bry.,*** bufo, cact., cadm-s., ***calc.,*** calc-ar., ***calc-f.,*** ***calc-p.,*** ***caps.,*** ***carb-ac.,*** ***carb-an.,*** ***carb-s.,*** ***carb-v.,*** ***carl.,*** ***caust.,*** ***cham.,*** ***chel.,*** chin-s., chlor., ***cimic.,*** cina, cinnb., ***cist.,*** clem., coca, **COC-C.,** ***cocc.,*** colch., coloc., com., **CON.,** cop., ***crot-c.,*** ***crot-h.,*** ***cupr.,*** ***cycl.,*** daph., dig., dios., **DROS.,** ***dulc.,*** euph., ***euphr.,*** ferr., ferr-i., fl-ac., glon., graph., gymn., **HEP.,** hipp., hyos., ***ign.,*** ind., inul., **IOD.,** **IP.,** ***iris,*** ***kali-bi.,*** **KALI-C.,** ***kali-i.,*** kali-n., ***kali-p.,*** kalm., kreos., lac-c., **LACH.,** lact., laur., led., **LYC.,** lob., ***mag-c.,*** mag-m., mang., meny., ***merc.,*** merc-c., mez., mur-ac., ***naja,*** nat-c., **NAT-M.,** nat-p., nat-s., nicc., ***nit-ac.,*** **NUX-V.,** oena., ol-an., olnd., onos., **OP.,** ox-ac., par., ***ph-ac.,*** **PHOS.,** phys., phyt., plan., ***prun.,*** ***psor.,*** **PULS.,** rhod., ***rhus-t.,*** **RUMX.,** ***sabin.,*** **SANG.,** ***sars.,*** ***seneg.,*** ***sep.,*** ***sil.,*** sol-n., sol-t-ae., spira., **SPONG.,** ***squil.,*** ***stann.,*** **STAPH.,** ***stict.,*** ***sulph.,*** sumb., tab., tarax., ***tarent.,*** tell., thuj., uva., ***vinc.,*** zinc., zing.
daytime only - nat-m.
eating amel. - carb-an.
fever, during - ***cimx.***
lying amel. - ***euphr.,*** ***mang.***
morning - iod.
tickling, throat-pit - **APIS,** aspar., bell., cann-s., caust., **CHAM.,** cinnb., cocc., coloc., ***con.,*** crot-h., ign., ***iod.,*** kreos., lac-c., lach., lith., mag-m., nat-c., nat-m., ph-ac., phos., ***puls.,*** rhus-r., **RUMX.,** **SANG.,** ***sil.,*** squil., tarax.
tickling, trachea - ***acon.,*** aesc., ***agar.,*** ail., am-m., anac., ang., ant-t., ***arn.,*** ars., arum-t., asaf., aur-m., bar-c., bell., bov., brom., bry., ***calc.,*** ***caps.,*** carb-ac., carb-an., ***carb-s.,*** ***carb-v.,*** casc., caust., ***cham.,*** chin., chin-s., cina, cist., coc-c., coloc., com., ***con.,*** cop., dig., dulc., eupi., ***euphr.,*** ***ferr.,*** ferr-i., gymn., hyos., indg., **IOD.,** ir-foe., iris, ***kali-bi.,*** **KALI-C.,** kali-p., ***kalm.,*** kreos., lac-c., lach., lact., laur., mag-c., mag-m., ***med.,*** mez., nat-a., nat-m., nat-s., nicc., nit-ac., ***nux-v.,*** ol-an., osm., ox-ac., petr., **PH-AC.,** ***phos.,*** plat., prun., ***psor.,*** **PULS.,** rhod., rhus-r., **RHUS-T.,** **RUMX.,** sabin., **SANG.,** sanic., ***seneg.,*** ***sep.,*** sil., spig., ***spong.,*** squil., **STANN.,** staph., ***stict.,*** ***still.,*** sulph., tarent., teucr., thuj., verat., zinc.

TIGHTNESS - bar-c., carb-v., ***cocc.,*** graph., kali-bi., mez., nat-m., phos., teucr., verat., verb.

TINGLING - ***agar.,*** ***caps.,*** ***iod.,*** ***mag-m.,*** sep.

TUBERCULOSIS, (see Lungs) - ***agar.,*** anan., ant-c., ***arg-m.,*** ***arg-n.,*** ars., ars-i., atro., bapt., brom., bufo, ***calc.,*** calc-p., canth., ***carb-an.,*** ***carb-s.,*** ***carb-v.,*** ***caust.,*** chr-ox., cist., ***dros.,*** elaps, ferr-p., ***hep.,*** ***iod.,*** ip., ***jab.,*** ***kali-bi.,*** kali-c., ***kali-i.,*** kali-m., kreos., ***lach.,*** led., lyc., **MANG.,** merc., ***merc-i-r.,*** merc-n., naja, ***nit-ac.,*** ***phos.,*** ***sel.,*** ***seneg.,*** ***sil.,*** **SPONG.,** **STANN.,** sulph., tub.
short hacking cough and loss of voice - **STANN.**
singers and public speakers - ***ant-c.,*** ***arg-m.***
tuberculosis, trachea - ***ars.,*** ***calc.,*** ***carb-an.,*** ***carb-v.,*** caust., chin., coloc., con., ***dros.,*** hep., iod., kali-n., lyc., mang., nit-ac., seneg., spong., ***stann.,*** tub.

TUMORS, benign - caust., kali-bi., sang., thuj.

ULCERATION - bufo, ***calc.,*** ***carb-v.,*** ***caust.,*** ***cinnb.,*** crot-h., ***hippoz.,*** kali-bi., ***nit-ac.,*** ***phos.,*** ***spong.,*** ***syph.***
vocal cords - aur-i., iod., lyc., merc-n.

VELVETY, sensation - brom., calc., chen-a., cina, ***dros.,*** ***hep.,*** ***ph-ac.,*** **PHOS.,** sulph.

VOICE, general
altered - ox-ac.
aphasia, (see Mind)
aponia, (see Voice, lost)
barking - ***bell.,*** brom., ***canth.,*** dros., lyc., nit-ac., spong., stann., stram.
bass - brom., camph., carb-s., ***caust.,*** **DROS.,** laur., mag-s., phos., pop-c., sang-n., stann., sulph., sumb., verb.
bleating - nux-m.
broken - camph., iod., merc., plb., tab.
attempting to sing high, when - phos.
changeable - alumn., ant-c., ***arg-m.,*** ***ars.,*** **ARUM-T.,** bell., carb-v., caust., dros., ferr., lach., mang., rumx., seneg.
changes timbre continually - ant-c., arg-m., arum-t., bell., carb-v., caust., con., dros., graph., lach., rumx., sep., spong., stram.

VOICE, general

changed - bell., carb-s., chlf., lyc., merc., murx., nat-m., ox-ac., tab.

cracked - dros., ***spong.***
- evening - ***spong.***
- singing, when - ***graph.***

croaking - acon., lac-ac., **STRAM.,** sul-ac.

croupy - ***acon., ail., all-c.,*** brom., caust., hep., kali-s., spong., sul-ac.

crowing - ***acon.,*** ars., chin., cina, samb., **SPONG.**

deep - ambr., am-caust., anac., ant-c., arn., ***arum-t.,*** aur-m., bar-c., ***brom.,*** **CARB-V.,** ***chin.,*** chin-s., coc-c., ***colch.,*** dig., **DROS.,** hep., iod., lac-ac., laur., mag-m., mag-s., nux-v., op., par., ***phos.,*** samb., spong., ***stann.,*** sulph., verat., ***verb.***
- eating, after - anac.
- moist cold air, in - sulph.
- open air - coc-c.

finer, than usual - ***stram.***

guttural - ars., gels.

higher - acon., alumn., ars., bell., bry., cann-i., cupr., dros., ***rumx.,*** **STRAM.**
- hawking, after - stram.
- suddenly - stram.

hissing - bell., ***nux-v., phos.***

hoarseness - acet-ac., **ACON.,** ***aesc.,*** agar., **ALL-C.,** aloe, ***alum.,*** alumn., ***ambr., am-caust., am-c., am-m.,*** anac., anan., ang., antipyrin., ***ant-c., ant-t., apis,*** **ARG-M., ARG-N.,** arn., ***ars.,*** ars-i., ars-m., arum-m., **ARUM-T.,** asaf., asc-t., ***asim.,*** atro., aur., aur-m., aur-s., bad., bapt., ***bar-c.,*** bar-m., **BELL.,** benz., benz-ac., berb., bov., **BROM., BRY.,** bufo, ***cact.,*** cahin., caj., **CALC.,** calc-caust., calc-f., ***calc-p., calc-s., camph.,*** cann-i., ***canth.,*** **CAPS.,** ***carl., carb-an., carb-s.,*** **CARB-V.,** cast., **CAUST., CHAM.,** ***chel., chin.,*** chin-a., chin-s., ***chlor.,*** cic., cimic., cina, cinnb., clem., coca, ***coc-c.,*** coch., ***coff., colch., coll., con.,*** cop., ***crot-c., crot-h., crot-t.,*** cub., ***cupr.,*** der., ***dig.,*** **DROS.,** ***dulc.,*** elaps, eup-per., ***euphr., ferr.,*** ferr-ar., ***ferr-i.,*** ferr-p., ***gels.,*** gins., ***graph.,*** grat., ***ham.,*** **HEP.,** ***hippoz.,*** hydr-ac., hydr., ***hyos.,*** hyper., ign., **IOD.,** inul., ***ip.,*** iris, just., kali-ar., **KALI-BI.,** ***kali-c., kali-chl., kali-i.,*** kali-m., kali-n., ***kali-p., kali-s.,*** kreos., **LACH.,** lachn., ***lac-ac.,*** lact., ***laur.,*** led., lob., ***lyc.,*** lyss., mag-c., ***mag-m.,*** mag-p., mag-s., **MANG.,** ***med.,*** meny., meph., **MERC.,** ***merc-c.,*** merc-i-f., ***merc-i-r.,*** merc-sul., merl., ***mez., mur-ac.,*** murx., ***naja,*** nat-a., ***nat-c.,*** **NAT-M.,** nat-p., nat-s., nicc., ***nit-ac., nux-m., nux-v.,*** oena., ol-an., ***op., osm.,*** ox-ac., ***par.,*** pen., ***petr.,*** phel., ***ph-ac.,*** **PHOS.,** ***phyt.,*** pic-ac., plan., plat., plb., **POP.,** prun., psor., ptel., ***puls.,*** raph., ***rhod., rhus-t., rhus-v., rumx.,*** sabad., ***samb., sang.,*** sang-n., sarr., sars., sec., **SEL.,** senec., ***seneg., sep., sil.,*** sol-n., ***spig.,*** **SPONG., STANN.,** ***staph.,*** stict., ***still.,*** **STRAM.,** stront-c., stry., ***sulph., sul-ac.,*** sumb., tab., tarax., **TELL.,** tep., thea.,

VOICE, general

hoarseness, of - ***thuj.,*** til., ***trif-p.,*** trom., ***verat.,*** verat-v., verb., vesp., vinc., viol-o., xan., ***zinc.,*** zing.
- afternoon - alum., ***am-m.,*** brom., ***carb-v.,*** coc-c., kali-bi., petr., phos., ***rumx.,*** sulph.
  - 4 p.m. - chin.
  - 5 p.m. - chel.
- air, cold - ***cupr., hep., nux-m.,*** thuj.
  - draft of - merc.
  - dry - ***cupr.***
  - open in - bry., **MANG.,** ***nux-m.***
  - open in, amel. - calc-s.
- annually at same time - nicc.
- calling aloud, when - am-c.
- changing, once loud, once weak - ars.
- children, in - cham.
- chill, during - hep.
- chronic - ampe-qu, ***arg-n.,*** bar-c., calc., carb-v., ***caust.,*** graph., ***mang., phos.,*** sil., ***sulph.***
- cold bath, after - ***ant-c.***
  - damp weather, from - ***carb-v., dulc., mang., rumx., sil.,*** sulph., tub.
  - worse at end of a cold - ip.
- colds, from - arn., ip., sel.
- coryza, during - acon., all-c., alum., am-c., am-m., ***ars.,*** ars-i., ars-m., bar-c., ***benz-ac., bry.,*** calc., carb-s., **CARB-V., CAUST.,** cham., ***dig.,*** dulc., eup-per., ferr-p., graph., hep., ***kali-bi.,*** kali-c., ***kalm., mag-m.,*** mag-s., **MANG., MERC.,** ***merc-i-r.,*** nat-a., ***nat-c.,*** nat-m., ***nit-ac.,*** osm., ***petr.,*** phel., **PHOS.,** pop-c., puls., ***ran-b., rumx.,*** seneg., ***sep., spig., spong.,*** sulph., sul-ac., ***tell.,*** thuj., trif-p., verb., zinc.
  - preceding - kali-c.
- cough, during, amel. - ***stann.***
- croup, after - ***carb-v., lyc.***
- crying, when - acon., **BELL.,** phos., spong.
- damp weather, in - carb-s., ***carb-v.,*** chlor., ***kali-bi.,*** sulph.
- daytime - ***acon., ars.,*** tarent.
- dinner, after amel. - mag-c.
- diphtheria, after - phyt.
- eating, after - anac.
- evening - alum., alumn., arg-m., brom., calc-p., calc-s., ***carb-an., carb-s.,*** **CARB-V., CAUST.,** cimic., cinnb., coc-c., coloc., crot-t., ***graph., kali-bi.,*** lach., lact., mag-c., ***mang.,*** nicc., **PHOS.,** raph., ***rumx.,*** sep., ***sulph.,*** thuj.
  - bed, in - nux-v.
  - reading, after - calc-f., cupr.
  - sunset, after - stram.
- exertion agg. - arn., ***rhus-t.***
- forenoon - ***arum-t.,*** benz-ac., calc., ***caust.,*** eup-per., hep., lachn., mag-c., ***mang.,*** nit-ac., ***nux-v.,*** sulph., sumb.
- fever, during - ***hep., puls.,*** sep., sulph.
- hay fever, in - all-c., carb-v., ran-b.
- heart complaints, with - coca, hydr-ac., núx-m., ox-ac.
- heated, becoming - brom.

VOICE, general

hoarseness, of

hysterical - cocc., gels., ign., nux-m., plat.
laughing, when - calc-f.
lost on exertion of voice - carb-v.
menses, during - calc., gels., ***graph.,*** lac-c., spong., syph.
after - ***bry., carb-v., dros.,*** maland., sulph.
before - gels., graph., lac-c., mang., syph.
suppressed - senec.
morning - ***acon.,*** alum., ant-t., ***apis,*** arn., ars., arund., asim., benz-ac., ***bov.,*** **CALC., CALC-P.,** ***carb-an.,*** carb-s., carb-v., cast., **CAUST.,** cinnb., coc-c., coca, ***coff.,*** colch., cop., cupr., ***dig.,*** dios., ***euphr., iod., kali-bi.,*** kreos., lach., lyc., mag-m., ***mang.,*** naja, ***nat-m.,*** nicc., ***nit-ac.,*** nux-v., **PHOS.,** plan., ***sil.,*** **SULPH.,** thuj., upa.
menses, during - cop.
rising, after - ***carb-an., ham.,*** ind., iod., mag-m., plan.
waking on - aloe, ***coff.,*** dig., ***ham., par.,*** sars.
motion amel. - lac-c.
mucus, in larynx - ang., aphis., ***bar-c., calc-p.,*** camph., ***caust., cham.,*** chin., ***kali-bi.,*** kali-s., ***mang., phos., psor., rumx.,*** **SAMB., SEL.,** ***stann., sulph.,*** stram., tarax., zinc.
nervous aphonia with heart disorder - coca, hydr-ac., nux-m., ox-ac.
night - alum., arg-n., calc., calc-f., calc-s., carb-an., cimic., lyc., naja, spig., sumb.
noon - carb-s.
overheated, from being - ***ant-c., brom.,*** haem.
overuse of the voice - acon., alum., ***arg-m., arg-n., arn.,*** **ARUM-T., CAPS.,** carb-v., **CAUST.,** ***coca,*** coll., ferr-p., ferr-pic., ***hep.,*** iod., ***kali-p., mang.,*** med., merc-cy., merc-sul., ***nat-m., phos.,*** **RHUS-T.,** ***sel.,*** seneg., spong., ***still.,*** sulph., tab., ter.
painful - ***arg-m.,*** **BELL.,** ***brom., iod., kali-bi.,*** kali-br., **PHOS.,** ***stann.***
talking, when - merc-cy.
painless - ***ant-c.,*** bell., **CALC.,** ***calc-sil.,*** **CARB-V.,** ***caust., dig.,*** ip., ***par., phos.***
paroxysmal - ***gels.,*** par.
periodical - ***nux-v.,*** par.
reading aloud, while - ***calc-f.,*** cupr., med., naja, sel., seneg., verb.
riding in open air - osm.
rising, after - cimic., ham., iod., plan., sol-t-ae., sumb.
from bed amel. - nux-v.
singing, from - **AGAR.,** alum., ***arg-m., arg-n.,*** arn., **ARUM-T.,** ***bry.,*** caps., ***caust.,*** hep., ***mang., nat-m., nit-ac.,*** osm., **SEL.,** sep., spong., ***stann.***
amel. - rhus-t.
high notes causes cough - arg-n.
smallpox, after - maland.
smoking amel. - mang.

VOICE, general

hoarseness, of

sneezing amel. - kreos.
speakers, in - arn., caps., caust., rhus-t.
speech, preventing - ***caust.,*** cupr., ***mag-m.,*** par., **PHOS.**
spring in - all-c.
stooping agg. - caust.
sudden - abrot., ***bell.,*** carb-v., mag-m., seneg., sep., ***spong.***
swallowing amel. - spong.
talking, from - ***alum.,*** alumn., am-c., ant-t., **ARG-M., ARG-N.,** arn., **ARUM-T.,** ***calc.,*** **CAPS.,** ***carb-v.,*** **CAUST.,** ***coc-c., ferr., kali-bi.,*** lach., ***mang.,*** morph., naja, ***nat-m., nit-ac., ph-ac., phos.,*** psor., **RHUS-T.,** sel., ***stann.,*** staph., stram.
a while, improves after - coc-c., ***rhus-t.***
amel. - ant-c., caust., graph., tub.
painful - merc-cy.
vaginal discharge, with - nat-s.
waking, on - aloe, coff., dig., iod., ***par.,*** plan., sars., sol-t-ae., tarent.
walking in open air, after - bry., calc., calc-p., ***nux-m.,*** osm.
against the wind - acon., arum-t., ***euphr.,*** hep., ***nicc.,*** **NUX-M.**
amel. - alum.
warm room - alum., bry., iod., ***kali-s., puls.***
going into open air from warm room - ***coc-c.***
wet weather agg. - ***carb-v.***
after getting - merc-i-r., ***rhus-t.***
whooping cough, in - viol-o.

hollow - ***acon.,*** alum., ant-c., ant-t., ***ars., arum-t.,*** bar-c., bell., cahin., camph., canth., carb-v., ***caust.,*** cham., chin., colch., crot-t., dig., **DROS.,** hep., ign., ***ip., kali-bi.,*** kreos., lach., ***led.,*** lyc., mag-s., op., phos., plb., puls., ***samb.,*** sec., **SPONG.,** ***stann.,*** staph., ***thuj.,*** **VERAT.,** verb.

husky - ***acon.,*** aloe, alum., ***am-m.,*** aur., ***bar-c.,*** bar-m., bell., ***brom.,*** calc., ***calc-sil.,*** camph., ***caust., chin., coc-c.,*** croc., **DROS.,** echi., graph., ***hyos., kali-n., lac-c., lyc.,*** mang., merc., merc-i-r., nat-m., nat-s., onos., **PHOS.,** rumx., sabad., ***sel.,*** sil., ***spong., stann., sulph.***
morning - ***sil.***
waking, on - alum.
open air, in - coc-c.

indistinct - am-caust., **BROM., CAUST.,** lyc.

inflexible - **STRAM.**

interrupted - ***alum., ars.,*** cic., dros., euphr., mag-c., ***spong.***

lost - ***acon.,*** ail., ***alum.,*** **ALUMN.,** am-c., **AM-CAUST.,** am-m., anan., **ANT-C.,** ***ant-t.,*** **ARG-M., ARG-N.,** ***ars.,*** ars-i., ***arum-t.,*** arund., ***bapt., bar-c., bell.,*** **BROM.,** bry., cahin., calc-ar., calad., camph., cann-i., canth., ***carb-ac.,*** carb-an., ***carb-s.,*** **CARB-V., CAUST.,** cedr., chin-s., ***chlor., cina,*** con., ***crot-c.,*** crot-t., ***cupr.,*** dig., ***dros.,*** elaps, ***ferr.,*** ferr-ar., ferr-i., ***ferr-p., gels.,*** graph., ***hep.,***

VOICE, general

lost - ***hyos., ign.,*** iod., ***kali-ar., kali-bi., kali-c., kali-i.,*** kali-n., ***kali-p.,*** kali-s., ***lach., lac-ac., merc., merc-c., merc-i-f., naja,*** nat-a., nat-c., ***nat-m.,*** nat-p., nicc., ***nit-ac., nux-m., nux-v.,*** ol-an., ox-ac., paeon., par., **PHOS.,** ***phyt.,*** plat., plb., ***puls.,*** pyrus, ***rhus-t., rumx., sang., sel., seneg.,*** sep., ***spong., stann.,*** **STRAM.,** stry., ***sulph.,*** sul-ac., tarent., ter., ***verat.,*** vesp., vip., zinc-m.

air, cold - carb-v., ***rumx.,*** sulph.

damp - ***chlor.***

anger, after - staph.

anxiety, with - ***ferr.***

chronic - phyt.

colds, from - alum.

cold, exposure to - ***caust., rumx.,*** xan.

cough, with - mang.

damp weather - ***bar-c.,*** chlor.

drinking cold water when overheated - ***crot-t.***

epilepsy, before - calc-ar.

eruptions, after - kali-ar.

evening - brom., **CARB-V.,** ***phos.***

exertion, on - ant-c., **CARB-V.,** lac-c.

fright, from - ***acon., gels., op.***

grief, from - cham., ign., nat-m.

heart disorder, in - coca, hydr-ac., nux-m., ox-ac.

heated, from being - ***ant-c.,*** haem.

hysterical - ***hyos., ign., nux-m.,*** plat., sep.

intermittent in singers - cupr.

menses, during - ***gels.***

before - gels., graph., syph.

momentarily - alum., dros., spong.

morning - alum., ***brom., carb-v., caust.,*** dig.

waking, on - ***ail.***

motion, on - ant-c.

mucus, in from - ***bar-c.***

night - ***carb-an., carb-v.***

overuse of - arg-m., ***arg-n., arum-t.,*** caps., ***caust., ferr-p., graph., merc.,*** **RHUS-T.,** ***sel., seneg.,*** stann.

painless - ant-c., ***phos.***

paralysis, from - bar-c., bell., both., canth., **CAUST.,** cocaine, cocc., ***gels.,*** kali-p., ***lach.,*** merc., ox-ac., ***plb.***

periodic - gels.

prolonged talking, from - ***phos.***

reading, while - plb.

singers - **ARG-N.,** arum-t., **CAUST.,** graph., mang., rhus-t., sel.

periodically - cupr., rhus-t.

sudden - alum., ***bell.,*** **CAUST.,** seneg.

tongue affections, without - both.

waking, on - nux-m., ptel.

warm, air amel. - seneg.

room, in - ***ant-c.,*** puls.

wind, after exposure to northwest - ***arum-t.***

VOICE, general

loud - bell., cann-i., hyos., lach., mosch., nux-m., sulph.

low - alumn., am-caust., ang., ant-c., ***arn., ars., cact., calc.,*** camph., cann-i., ***canth.,*** cham., chin., crot-t., hep., ***ign.,*** lyc., osm., ox-ac., puls., sec., ***spong.,*** staph., sul-ac., tab., verat.

muffled - gels., lach., lyc., rumx., sumb., sul-ac.

nasal - all-c., alum., aur., bell., bov., bry., ***caust.,*** ferr., ***fl-ac.,*** gels., ***iod.,*** **KALI-BI.,** ***kali-i.,*** kali-n., ***lac-c., lach.,*** lyc., mag-m., mag-s., ***manc.,*** merc., nat-c., nat-m., nux-v., ph-ac., ***phos.,*** plb., rumx., sang., sep., sin-n., spong., ***staph.,*** sulph., sumb., thuj.

catarrhal - kali-i., mag-m., ph-ac.

coryza, with - ip.

evening - sep., sumb.

morning - bov., sulph.

tonsils, enlarged, with - staph.

piping - bell., ***spong.***

powerful - hydr-ac.

rough - acon., ***all-s., alum.,*** ambr., am-c., ant-c., apis, ars., ars-i., ***bar-c.,*** **BELL.,** ***brom.,*** bry., cahin., ***calc.,*** calc-ar., canth., ***carb-s.,*** **CARB-V.,** ***caust., cham., chin.,*** chin-a., ***coc-c., coff.,*** crot-t., cupr., cycl., dig., dros., ***graph.,*** hep., **HYOS.,** ***iod.,*** kali-ar., **KALI-BI.,** kali-c., kali-n., mag-m., mag-s., ***mang., meny., merc.,*** merc-c., merc-i-r., mez., nat-m., nit-ac., ***nux-v.,*** op., ox-ac., **PHOS.,** plb., prun., **PULS.,** ***seneg., sil., spong.,*** stram., ***sulph.,*** sumb., thuj., zinc.

afternoon - alum., coc-c., sulph.

air, draft of, agg. - ***merc.***

on going into open - **MANG.**

bed, before going to - ox-ac.

evening - alum., coloc., kali-bi., sulph.

forenoon - sulph.

morning - ***calc.,*** coc-c., coff., ***mang.***

smoking amel. - ***mang.***

talking, from - am-c., ***coc-c.***

shrieking - alum., **ARUM-T.,** cupr., ***stram.***

shrill - acon., lyss., samb., spong., stram.

speaking through mouthful, as if - nux-v.

squeaking - ars., lac-ac., **STRAM.**

toneless - agn., ambr., ***calad.,*** carb-an., chin., **DROS.,** hep., nat-c., rhod., samb., spong., **STRAM.,** thuj.

tremulous - acon., agar., ***ars., camph.,*** canth., ***cocc.,*** cupr., gels., ***ign.,*** iod., kali-i., laur., **MERC.,** mez., ***nux-m.,*** op., ***phos.,*** psor.

trumpet, like - verb.

unsteady - seneg.

weak - abrot., absin., acon., alum., am-caust., ***ant-c.,*** **ANT-T.,** arg-m., ***arg-n.,*** arn., ars., ars-i., bar-c., bar-m., ***bell., brom., calc., calc-s., camph.,*** **CANTH.,** carb-an., ***carb-v., caust., cham., chin.,*** clem., coc-c., coca, ***coll., crot-h.,*** cupr-ac., ***cycl.,*** daph., dig., dros., dub., ***ferr., ferr-p., gels.,*** **HEP.,** ***ign.,*** iod., kali-i., lach., laur., ***lyc.,*** lyss., ***naja,*** nat-a., nat-c., ***nat-m.,*** nit-ac., ***nux-v.,*** op., osm., ox-ac.,

VOICE, general

weak - par., pen., petr., ***ph-ac., phos.,*** plb., ***pop-c.,*** prim-v., prun., psor., ***puls.,*** **RHUS-T.,** ***sec., spong.,*** **STANN.,** ***staph., stram.,*** stry., ***sulph.,*** sul-ac., tab., thuj., **VERAT.,** zinc.

anger, after - ***staph.***

evening in bed - phos.

fever, during - ***hep.***

headache, after - gels.

menses, during - plb.

talking, after - ***coc-c.,*** daph., ***ph-ac.,*** **STANN.,** ***sulph.,*** sul-ac.

whispering - am-caust., ars., ***calc.,*** camph., cupr., ***ferr.,*** ign., iod., ***merc.,*** nit-ac., ol-an., phos., phyt., rumx., ***stann.,*** stram., sul-ac., tab., zinc-m.

whistling - acon., ars., bell., brom., ***calc., cham.,*** chin., hep., iod., kreos., laur., laur., sabad.,

evening - ***calc.***

inspiration, on - coloc.

lying down, after - ***calc.***

on left side - arg-n.

morning - coloc.

WEAKNESS, of larynx - alumn., bar-c., ***caust.,*** gels., plb., rhus-t., sulph.

Legs

ABDUCTED - colch., nux-v., plat., stry.
abducted, then adducted - lyc.
standing, while - pic-ac.

ABSCESS - ***anan.,*** chin.
psoas - arn., asaf., chin., ***cupr., ph-ac., sil.,*** staph., ***sulph.,*** symph., ***syph.***

abscess, calves - chin.

abscess, lower - sulph.

abscess, thighs - ***hep.,*** lach., **SIL.,** tarent.

ACHING, pain - aesc., aur., ***calc-p., cimic.,*** cob., **EUP-PER., GELS.,** ***med., merc.,*** merc-i-f., nat-a., ptel., pyrog., **RHUS-T.,** rumx., ***tub.***
bones - **EUP-PER.,** lyc., mag-m., ***merc., mez.,*** ph-ac., phos., ***puls.,*** rumx., zinc.
chill, during - eup-per., gels., nux-v., **RHUS-T.**
evening - still.
fever, during - **GELS.,** ***merc., puls.,*** pyrog., **RHUS-T.**
joints, of - ferr-i.
menses, during - calc-p., caul., cimic.
morning, on waking - aur.
motion, after - calc-p.
amel. - ***puls.,*** **RHUS-T.**
night - med.
posterior part - ***helon.,*** **PIC-AC.**
riding, while - rumx.
standing - aesc.
walking, while - merc., nux-m.
amel. - ***tub.***
wet weather, during - calc., ***calc-p.,*** dulc., rhus-t.

aching, calves - ang., ars., berb., chlol., eup-per., fago., ***gels.,*** jatr., ***kali-bi.,*** led., lycps., lyss., merc., mur-ac., ptel., ***puls.,*** sep., sin-n., tarax., teucr.
morning, waking, on - lycps.
motion agg. - rumx.
walking, while - myric.
in open air - fago.

aching, lower - aesc., agar., alum., anac., ***ars.,*** aur., bapt., bol., ***bry., carb-ac., carb-an.,*** chel., chlol., com., dios., ***eup-per.,*** fago., ferr-s., fl-ac., gamb., ham., **IP.,** ***kali-c., kali-i., lac-ac.,*** **LACH.,** laur., ***led.,*** lil-t., med., ***merc.,*** merc-i-f., ***mur-ac.,*** **PH-AC.,** phos., ***phyt.,*** ptel., puls., **PYROG., RHUS-T.,** rumx., sep., sil., sin-n., still., sul-i., sumb., syph., **TUB.,** vac., verat-v., zinc.
afternoon - erig., lycps., ptel., sep.
chill, during - **EUP-PER.,** ***nat-m.,*** nux-v., **RHUS-T.,** ***tub.***
before - ***eup-per.,*** puls.
corns, as from - asc-t.
cough, with - ***carb-an.***
evening - erig., ***still.,*** uran.
10 p.m. - fago.
extending to, heel - kalm.
to, hips - nit-ac.
to, toes - kali-n.
fever, during - puls., ***pyrog.,*** **RHUS-T., TUB.**

aching, lower
forenoon - ptel.
8 a.m. - lach.
lying on left side - com.
maleoli - chin-s., graph.
inner - berb., mez., verat-v.
outer - cic., laur.
menses, during - ambr.
after - calc-p.
morning - agar., aur.
waking, on - aur.
motion - dig., laur., merc-i-r.
amel. - dios., ***mur-ac.,*** puls., **RHUS-T.**
night - caust., med.
noon - com.
sitting, while - agar., brom., led., **RHUS-T.**
walking, while - bry., cupr-ar., phyt.
amel. - kali-n., **RHUS-T.**
wandering - chin-a.

aching, thighs - agar., anac., bol., calc-p., caust., chim., cinnb., cob., daph., ham., hep., ***ip.,*** kali-i., ***lach.,*** merc-i-f., mur-ac., nat-a., nat-p., phyt., ***pyrog.,*** **RHUS-T.,** sabad., sep., spig., still., stry., ***thuj., tub.,*** verat-v.
afternoon - lycps.
anterior part - cupr., dig., hell., nat-a., nat-s., pic-ac.
extending to ankle - nat-a.
lower part - lyc., ***thuj.,*** tub.
ascending stairs - sep.
bone - bry., fl-ac., **IP.,** ***merc-i-r.,*** phos., tep.
evening, 7 p.m. - gels.
sleep, after - cycl.
extending, downward - caps., nat-a., phys.
to knee on coughing - caps.
fever during - ***ip.,*** pyrog., **TUB.**
middle of - asar., chin., cocc., lach.
morning, bed in - sumb.
motion on - dig.
amel. - mur-ac., **RHUS-T.,** tub.
night - cinnb., ***kali-bi.,*** sulph.
outer side - nat-a., still.
extending to foot - still.
paralyzed, as if - verat.
posterior part - carb-ac., dros., ind., led., mez., naja, ptel.
rising - lycps.
walking, while - calc-p., meny., staph.

aching, tibia - agar., anac., berb., bufo, ***carb-ac.,*** chin-a., clem., com., fago., fl-ac., gamb., ign., **LACH.,** mez., nat-m., nit-ac., **PH-AC.,** sep., sil., stry.
afternoon, sitting, while - agar.
daytime - clem.
forenoon - agar.
morning - lycps.
sitting, while - agar., anac.
standing - agn.
walking, while - clem., ign., stry.

ALIVE, sensation of, lower - sil.

alive, sensation, thigh - meny.

ATAXIA - ***agar.***, **ALUM.**, arag., ***arg-n.***, ars., ***calc.***, ***caust.***, ***cocc.***, crot-c., ***fl-ac.***, ***gels.***, ***graph.***, ***hell.***, ***helo.***, ***kali-br.***, ***lach.***, ***lil-t.***, naja, nux-m., ***nux-v.***, ***onos.***, ***phos.***, ***plb.***, ***sil.***, ***stram.***, ***sulph.***, ***zinc.***

AWKWARDNESS, (see Generals) - **AGAR.**, ***alum.***, **CAUST.**, ***con.***, gels., ***nux-m.***, sabad., ***sil.***, ***verat.***
knocks against things. - caps., ***colch.***, ip., kali-n., nat-m., nux-v., op., vip.
stumbling when walking - **AGAR.**, ***calc.***, caps., **CAUST.**, ***colch.***, ***con.***, gels., ***hyos.***, ***ign.***, iod., **IP.**, ***lach.***, lil-t., mag-c., ***mag-p.***, ***nat-m.***, nux-v., op., ***ph-ac.***, ***phos.***, sabad., sil., verat.

BANDAGED, legs, sensation as if - alumn., anac., benz-ac., ***plat.***, til.
joints - nat-m.
walking, while - til.
bandaged, calves - card-m., nat-p., nit-ac.
bandaged, lower - ant-c., chlor., lyc., nat-m., petr., pic-ac., stann., sulph., sul-ac.
evening - ant-c., nat-m.
bandaged, thighs - acon., nit-ac., ***plat.***, sulph.
walking, while - ***acon.***, tarent.

BEND, irresistible desire to, legs - hep., sec.

BLISTERS, lower, black - ***ars.***
blisters, thighs, black - ***anthr.***
scratching, after - lach.

BLOOD, rush of to - **AUR.**, calc., elaps, zinc., lact., phel.
blood, lower, rush of to - lact., meph., nux-m., phos., **SPONG.**, **SULPH.**, ***zinc.***
as if blood stagnated - zinc.
left - nux-m.
night, on waking - meph.

BOILS - all-c., am-c., apoc., ***ars.***, aur-m., bell., carb-s., clem., **HEP.**, hyos., kali-bi., nat-m., nit-ac., nux-v., petr., ph-ac., phos., ***rhus-t.***, rhus-v., sec., sep., sil., stram., ***sulph.***, thuj.
boils, calves - bell., **SIL.**
boils, lower - ***anan.***, ***anthr.***, ***ars.***, ***calc.***, cast-eq., ***mag-c.***, ***nit-ac.***, nux-v., **PETR.**, **RHUS-T.**, ***sil.***
blood - mag-c.
boils, thighs - agar., all-s., alum., am-c., apoc., aur-m., ***bell.***, ***calc.***, carb-s., ***clem.***, ***cocc.***, ***hep.***, ***hyos.***, ***ign.***, kali-bi., ***lach.***, ***lyc.***, mag-c., ***nit-ac.***, ***nux-v.***, ***petr.***, ph-ac., phos., plb., rhus-v., ***sep.***, **SIL.**, thuj.
right - calc., hell., kali-bi., kali-c., rhus-v.

BORING, pain - aeth., act-sp., am-m., apis, aran., cadm-s., canth., coloc., ***ign.***, kali-bi., ***merc.***, ran-b., ran-s., ***rhod.***
bones - ***carb-v.***, coloc., kali-bi., nat-c., rhod.
joints of - alum., coloc., mag-c., ***zinc.***
evening - coloc.
walking, while - coloc.
stretching amel. - act-sp.
boring, calves - coloc., ***cupr.***, mez., sulph.
evening - sulph.
standing - coloc.
boring, lower - aeth., ***anac.***, aran., ars., bov., caust., hell., ***ign.***, merc., merc-i-f., mez., ***nux-m.***, phos., rhod., sil., stann., sulph.
bone, marrow - mag-c.
morning - aran.
boring, lower, maleoli - cic., mez.
inner - led., sulph.
evening in bed - led.
outer, morning bed, in - arg-n.
boring, thighs - act-sp., agar., ang., ***apis,*** asar., caps., carb-an., hell., ign., led., merc., merc-i-f., mez., nat-p., ran-b., rhus-t., sabad., spig., spong., staph., tarax.
bones - carb-an., kali-bi., phos., led., mez.
crural nerves - ***apis.***
motion, amel. - caps.
sitting, when - agar.
boring, tibia - anac., ars., asc-c., **AUR.**, ***aur-m-n.***, brom., chel., cina, ***clem.***, coloc., grat., led., mang., **MERC.**, ***mez.***, nat-c., trom.
evening - grat., nat-c.
forenoon - trom.
left - asc-c., aur-m-n.
morning - clem.
night - **AUR.**, **MERC.**, ***mez.***
sitting, while - agar., ***aur-m-n.***, mez.
walking, while - mez., nat-s.
amel. - ***aur-m-n.***

BROKEN, sensation as if - ars., **RUTA.**
rising after sitting - **RUTA.**
broken, lower - carb-an., graph., thuj., vac., ***verat.***
going upstairs - ***ars.***, thuj.
night - ***merc.***
on waking and turning in bed - carb-an.
stepping - mez., verat.
broken, thighs - bor., cocc., dros., ill., nit-ac., nux-v., plat., puls., ***sulph.***, tep., ***tub.***, valer., verat.
crossing, legs - aur.
sitting, while - ill., verat.
with legs stretched out - plat.
standing, while - valer.
amel. - ill.
walking - dros.

BUBBLING, sensation, downward - bell., olnd., squil.
bubbling, calves - crot-h., rheum, spig.
bubbling, lower - ant-c., arn., berb., con., rheum, rhus-t.
bubbling, thighs - berb., olnd., sil.

BURNING, pain - agar., alum., anac., ***apis,*** ars., bapt., bar-c., bufo, carb-an., carb-v., cast-eq., caust., chin., chin-a., dulc., gels., ***kali-c.***, lach., led., ***lyc.***, mag-c., mag-m., mang., nat-c., nit-ac., ph-ac., ***phos.***, plat., prun., ptel., puls., ***rhus-t.***, ruta., ***sil.***, thuj., ***zinc.***
bones - euph.
joints - bar-c., nat-c., phos., stront.
spots - ***mang.***
night - fago.
bed, in - kali-c.
noon - agar.

BURNING, pain
posterior part - ***helon.,*** **PIC-AC.**
rheumatic - apis
spots - lyc., mag-c., ph-ac.
undressing, when - mez.
burning, calves - agar., alum., am-c., aur., dig., eupi., mang., mez., plb., ran-s., rhus-t., sars., sulph., tarax., tarent., zinc.
evening - alum., sulph.
right - ***agar.***
walking, in open air - mez.
burning, lower - ***agar.,*** alum., anac., ***apis,*** **ARS.,** ***asaf.,*** bapt., bell., berb., bor., bov., calc., cast-eq., caust., chel., coc-c., con., crot-h., dig., hyos., jug-r., ***kali-bi.,*** kali-br., ***kali-c.,*** ***led.,*** lyc., mang., merc-c., merl., mez., nat-c., ***nat-s.,*** pall., ***petr., pic-ac.,*** prun., rhus-t., ***sep.,*** staph., stront-c., ***sulph.,*** tarax., tarent., tep., thuj., ***zinc.***
afternoon, while sitting - sulph.
dinner, after - agar.
evening - agar., ***nat-s.,*** sang., seneg., sulph.
hanging down - graph.
morning - agar., nat-s., sulph.
after exercise - sulph.
night - sep.
right - ***agar.***
rising, when - sulph.
scratching - chel., corn., ir-foe., seneg., sulph.
sparks, as from - anac.
stretching, agg. - berb.
touch agg. - bor., con.
warm bed - sep.
burning, thighs - agar., alum., am-c., ***apis,*** arg-m., ***ars.,*** aur-m-n., arund., ***berb.,*** bov., bor., carb-an., carb-s., carb-v., clem., coloc., con., crot-c., crot-t., dulc., ***euph.,*** eup-per., grat., kali-i., lachn., laur., ***lyc., manc.,*** merc., ***mez.,*** mur-ac., nat-c., olnd., plb., ph-ac., ***phos.,*** psor., rhod., rhus-t., ***sulph.,*** sul-ac., tab., til., ***zinc.***
anterior, part - chin.
band, around - bor.
bend of - bar-c., mag-m., mang., nat-s.
evening - nat-s.
sitting, while - bar-c.
walking, while - nat-s.
cold, yet they are - ph-ac.
coughing, agg. - bor.
extending to the ankles - apis, arund.
inner side of - agar., bry., cocc., ***lachn., lyc.,*** mez., sars., sulph.
evening - agar., bry.
menses, during - sars.
rubbing, after - samb.
rubbing, amel. - sulph.
touch - ***lyc.***
upper, of - ruta.
walking, while - agar., ***lyc.***
near genital organs of, female - bor., kreos., laur., sulph.
male - bar-c., crot-t., ferr-ma., rhus-t.
night, bed, in - carb-v., ***euph.,*** graph.
outer side - zinc.
posterior - agar., mag-m., mez., ph-ac., staph.

burning, thighs
rising from sitting - chin.
rubbing, after - sulph.
amel. - phos.
scratching, after - grat., mag-m., plan.
amel. - alum.
sitting, while - asaf., grat., phos.
standing - ph-ac.
touch, agg. - bor., phos.
walking, while - coloc.
amel. - ph-ac.
burning, tibia - agar., ang., arg-m., arn., bry., ***caust., kali-bi.,*** lach., ***mag-c.,*** ph-ac., rhus-t., sabad., tarax., verat., **ZINC.**
night - ***caust., ph-ac.***
spot - ***mag-c.***

CARBUNCLES, thighs - agar., ***arn.,*** asim., ***hep.***

CHILLINESS - cocc., par., sep.
sneezing - spig.
chilliness, lower - ***ars.,*** cinnb., ***hep.,*** mosch., par., puls., rhod., sep., samb., spong.
sciatica, in - ***nux-v.***
touch, on - chin.
chilliness, thighs - acon., arn., ars-i., bar-c., chin., cic., ***psor.,*** puls., sars., ***spong.***

CHOREA, (see Nerves) - ***cocc.,*** rhod., stict.
chorea, lower - ***cocc.,*** rhod., stict.

CLAWING, pain, calves - mang.
clawing, thighs, posterior part - con.
clawing, sensation, lower, morning, in - stront.
clawing, sensation, thighs - bry.

CLUCKING - bell.

COLDNESS - ***aeth.,*** agar., apis, ***ars., ars-i.,*** asaf., bapt., **BELL., CALAD.,** calc., calc-s., carb-an., carb-s., ***chel.,*** cic., coff., crot-c., crot-t., ***dig.,*** ip., **LAC-C.,** ***led.,*** lyc., ***mez.,*** mosch., mur-ac., nat-c., nat-m., **NIT-AC.,** nux-v., ol-an., **OP.,** ***ox-ac.,*** par., petr., ***phos.,*** plb., **PULS.,** rhod., rhus-t., sars., ***sec.,*** **SEP.,** sil., spong., ***stram.,*** stront-c., stry., ***sulph.,*** tarent., verat.
alternates with heat in head - sep.
daytime - nat-c.
forenoon - rumx.
until bedtime - sep.
icy cold - apis, ***sep.***
in spots - agar., berb.
left - agar., sulph.
menses, during - calc., cham., bufo, lil-t., ***sec., sil.***
morning - con.
nausea, during - arg-n.
night - agar., carb-v., ***lac-c.,*** petr., phos.
on waking - ***nit-ac.***
noon - nit-ac.
in bed - chel., lyc., sars.
when lifting covers - lyc.
painful limb - ***led.,*** merc.
paralyzed limb - ***ars., cocc.,*** dulc., graph., ***nux-v., rhus-t.***
right - echi., nit-ac., petr.

coldness, calves - ars., berb., bufo, chel., hyper., lach., mang., rumx.
evening - mang.
while sitting, amel., rising - mang.
forenoon - berb.

coldness, lower legs - acon., agar., alum., alumn., aloe, ambr., anthr., ant-t., aphis., ***apis, arg-n., ars.,*** ars-i., aur., bar-c., bell., brom., bry., **CALC.,** calc-p., calc-s., ***camph., carb-an., carb-s.,*** **CARB-V.,** ***caust.,*** cedr., ***cham., chel., chin., chin-a., chin-s.,*** cic., cocc., coff., ***colch.,*** com., ***crot-c., cupr.,*** **DIG.,** dios., ***dulc.,*** elaps, euph., euphr., ***ferr.,*** graph., ham., ***hep.,*** hura, hydrc., hyper., ign., iod., kali-ar., kali-i., **LAC-C., LACH.,** ***laur., led.,*** lyc., mang., ***med., meny., merc.,*** mez., mosch., ***naja, nat-c.,*** nat-m., ***nat-p., nit-ac., nux-m., nux-v., op., ox-ac., petr., ph-ac., phos.,*** pic-ac., plat., plb., psor., puls., **RHUS-T.,** samb., sang., ***sec., sep.,*** **SIL.,** spong., **STRAM.,** stront-c., ***sulph.,*** sumb., ***stry., tab.,*** ther., thuj., ***tub.,*** **VERAT.**
afternoon - aloe, alumn., nux-v.
4 p.m. - chel., sang.
6 p.m. - puls.
air in open, when - ham.
burning in thighs, with - tab.
dinner, after - cedr.
dressing, when - anth.
evening - aloe, chel., colch., euphr., mang., puls., sang., ***sil.,*** sulph.
in bed - aur., colch., ph-ac., **SEP.,** sil., tub.
waking - euphr., ***nit-ac.***
fever during - carb-an., ***eup-pur.,*** meph., sep., **STRAM.**
flushed face - ***op.***
heat of body, with - tab.
of face, with - ***arn.***
icy - ***apis,*** aur., **CALC.,** chel., ***sep., sil., tab.***
inner side of leg - ruta.
left - chin., euph., ***hyper.,*** ol-an., sang., tub.
chill, during - carb-v., caust., thuj.
lying, while ,- chin-s.
menses during - arg-n., bufo, ***calc.,*** lil-t., ***sec., sil.***
before - ***lyc.***
morning - hep., hura.
7 a.m. - hura.
night - agar., aloe, com., kali-ar., ***merc.,*** thuj., verat.
as from snow water - verat.
waking, on - nit-ac.
noon - nit-ac.
right - ambr., chel., ***elaps,*** mang., sabin.
chill, during - ***bry.,*** chel., elaps, sabad., ***sep.***
up to knee - ambr.
sex, after - ***graph.***
sitting, while - camph., hyper., led., mang.
snow, as from being in - verat.
standing, while - samb., nat-m.
uncovering, amel. - ***camph., med.,*** **SEC.,** ***tub.***

coldness, lower legs
walking, while - ***nit-ac.,*** plat.
in the sun - ***lach.***
warm room - acon., meny., **SIL.**
warmed, cannot be - ars.
wind, as from - bar-c., samb.

coldness, thighs - aloe, arn., ars., bar-c., berb., bry., ***calc.,*** camph., chin., cimic., coc-c., cop., hura, ign., kali-bi., lyc., ***merc.,*** nit-ac., nux-v., op., phos., puls., ran-b., rhod., sabad., sars., **SPONG.,** ***sulph.,*** tax., tep., ***thuj.***
afternoon - lyc.
chill, during - ***thuj.***
cold air blew on it, as if - camph.
colic, during - ***calc.***
convulsions, with - ***calc.***
daytime - lyc., tax.
evening - bry., ***calc.***
6 p.m. - puls.
rising from sitting - rhod.
heat, during - spong.
icy cold, as if ice water poured down sciatic - acon.
morning - arn., sulph.
night - coc-c., cop., ign., merc., nux-v.
posterior, part - agar.
right - camph.
shaken - ***thuj.***
sitting, while - chin., ran-b.
standing, while - berb.

coldness, tibia - mosch., rhus-t., samb.

COLDNESS, sensation of - agar., berb., carb-v., caust., chin., euph., ***merc.,*** mez., nat-c., petr., rhod., spong.

COMPRESSION, sensation, calves - jatr., led., sol-n.

compression, lower - arg-n., led., nat-s.

compression, thighs - ***plat.,*** sabad., stront.
motion agg. - sabad.
continued amel. - sabad.

CONSTRICTION - alum., alumn., am-br., ***anac.,*** ars., carb-an., carb-s., chin., graph., **LYC.,** mur-ac., petr., ***phos., plat.,*** stront-c., sulph., sul-ac.

constriction, lower - ***anac.,*** ars., benz-ac., **CHIN.,** guai., ***lyc.,*** manc., nit-ac., petr., ***plat.,*** stann., ***sulph.,*** sul-ac.
garter, as with a - alumn., ant-c., card-m., **CHIN.,** ***cocc., manc.,*** raph.
painful - ant-c.

constriction, thighs - acon., anac., carb-v., lyc., manc., mur-ac., nit-ac., **PLAT.,** sulph., sul-ac.
as by a, band - ***coloc.,*** nit-ac., sulph.
by a, string - am-br., lyc., manc.
from a, tightly drawn bandage - acon., **PLAT.**
sitting, while - ***plat.***
walking, while - lyc., olnd.

CONTRACTION, muscles and tendons - aesc., ambr., am-c., **AM-M.,** anac., ***ars.,*** aster., ***bar-c.,*** bism., canth., **CAUST.,** ***coloc., guai.,*** hydr-ac., nat-c., nat-m., nux-v., olnd., ph-ac., ***phos.,*** puls., ***rhus-t.,*** sec., sil., stry., tarent., tell., zinc.
evening - olnd.
menses, during - phos.
rousing, on - olnd.
standing - bar-c.

contraction, calves - agar., agn., arg-n., ars., ***bov.,*** calc-p., caps., ***caust.,*** jatr., led., med., nat-c., nat-m., puls., sil.
cramp-like - ferr.
spasmodic - ars., bart., merc., sil.
walking, while - agar., ***lyc.***

contraction, lower - am-c., **AM-M.,** apoc., ***aster.,*** bad., cann-i., canth., cedr., ***cic.,*** ferr., merc-c., mez., ***nat-m.,*** nux-v., ox-ac., ***phyt.,*** puls., sulph.
evening - cedr.
evening, while walking - ferr.
sciatica, in - ***nux-v.***

contraction, thighs - ambr., asar., berb., carb-v., cham., mag-c., ol-an., plat., puls., ***rhus-t.,*** ruta., sabin.
abscess, after - ***lach.***
as if drawn together - cann-s.
bend of - agar., carb-an., ***caust., rhus-t.***
bend of, while walking - ***rhus-t.,*** thuj.
chill, during - cimx.
hamstrings - ***acon.,*** agar., ***ambr.,*** am-c., ***am-m.,*** ant-c., ant-t., asar., ***bar-c., calc-p.,*** carb-an., **CAUST.,** ***cimx.,*** graph., **GUAI.,** kali-ar., led., ***lyc.,*** lyss., med., nat-c., **NAT-M.,** nat-p., ***nit-ac.,*** **NUX-V.,** phos., ***phyt.,*** puls., ***rhus-t., ruta.,*** samb., sulph.
lower, part of thigh - sul-ac.
menses, after - nat-p.
menses, before - cham.
sitting down, when - sabin.
spasmodic - asar.
walking, while - carb-an., **NUX-V.,** pall., ***rhus-t.***

CONVULSION - ars., cann-i., ***cic., cina,*** cocc., ***crot-c., cupr.,*** gamb., hydr-ac., ***hyos., ign., ip., lach., lyss., merc-c.,*** mosch., nux-v., ***op.,*** phos., ***plb.,*** sec., ***squil.,*** spong., ***stram.,*** **STRY.,** tab.
alternately flexed and extended - ***cic., cupr.,*** lyc., nux-v., tab.
clonic - coc-c., ***plb.,*** sep.
night - plb.
1 to 4 a.m. - tab.
painful - stry.
right - sep.
spasmodically adducted - lyc., ***merc.***
then in upper - phos.
tonic - phos., plb.

convulsion, calves - berb., cupr., ferr-m.

convulsion, lower - acet-ac., ant-t., ars., cann-i., card-m., cupr-s., ***jatr.,*** kali-i., ***merc-c.,*** podo., sep., stram., stry., tab., tarent., tell.
right - acet-ac., podo., stram.

convulsion, thighs - ars., dig., podo.

CRACKED, skin - ***alum., aur., aur-m.,*** bar-c., ***calc.,*** **HEP.,** lach., merc., nat-c., nat-m., petr., ***sulph., zinc.***

CRACKING, joints, of - ***benz-ac.,*** brach., bry., ***camph.,*** caust., ***cham.,*** cocc., con., led., nux-v., petr., puls., ran-b., sel., ***sep.,*** tab., thuj.
stepping - euphr., mag-s.
stooping - croc.
walking - bry.

CRAMPS - ambr., ant-t., ars., bar-c., cahin., ***calc.,*** cedr., cimic., cina, **COLOC.,** crot-h., **CUPR.,** elaps, eup-per., ***ferr., ferr-m.,*** graph., hyos., iod., jatr., kali-bi., kali-s., **MAG-P.,** merc-n., merc-p-r., mur-ac., oena., ph-ac., phos., pic-ac., phyt., plb., sec., sep., sil., tarent., vip., zinc.
bending foot forward - coff.
colic, with - coloc.
crossing limbs - alum.
descending stairs - arg-m.
drawing, on boot - ***calc.***
evening - jatr., sil.
extending leg - bar-c., ***calc.***
lifting legs, when - coff.
morning - bov., bry., nit-ac.
night - ***ambr.,*** ars., bry., calad., carb-v., eug., ***eup-per.,*** iod., ip., lachn., lyc., mag-c., mag-m., nit-ac., nux-v., ***rhus-t.,*** sec., sep., staph., sulph.
pregnancy, during - ***gels.,*** ham., sep., ***vib.***
right - bufo.
sitting, while - olnd., paeon., ***rhus-t.***
walking, while - am-c., carb-v., ***lyc.,*** nit-ac., rhus-t., sep.
after - nit-ac.
standing while - euph., euphr.
stepping out when - alum.

cramps, calves - ***acon., agar., alum.,*** alumn., ***ambr.,*** am-c., ***anac.,*** anag., ant-t., arg-m., **ARG-N.,** ***ars.,*** aspar., bapt., bar-c., bell., berb., bov., bry., bufo, cadm-s., **CALC.,** ***calc-p.,*** calc-s., ***camph.,*** cann-i., carl., carb-ac., carb-an., carb-s., carb-v., card-m., ***caust.,*** **CHAM.,** chel., chin., chin-a., clem., cocc., coff., ***colch.,*** **COLOC.,** ***con., crot-h.,*** **CUPR.,** dig., dulc., elaps, euphr., eupi., ***ferr.,*** ferr-ar., ferr-m., ferr-p., gins., ***gnaph.,*** **GRAPH.,** guai., **HEP.,** hydrc., hyos., ign., ***iris,*** jatr., kali-ar., kali-bi., kali-br., ***kali-c.,*** kali-i., kali-p., lach., lachn., lac-ac., lact., led., lob., **LYC.,** lyss., ***mag-c., mag-m., mag-p.,*** manc., ***med.,*** merc., merc-c., nat-a., ***nat-c., nat-m.,*** nat-p., ***nit-ac.,*** nux-m., ***nux-v.,*** oena., olnd., ***petr., ph-ac., phos.,*** **PLB.,** puls., ***rhus-t.,*** rhus-v., sang., sars., **SEC.,** ***sel., sep.,*** **SIL.,** sin-n., sol-n., spig., stann., staph., stry., **SULPH.,** tab., tarent., ***verat., verat-v., zinc.***
afternoon - alum., ant-t., elaps, hyos.
ascending - berb.
bed, in - ars., bov., **CALC., CARB-S.,** ***caust., eupi., ferr., ferr-m.,*** graph., hep., ign., ***kali-c.,*** lac-ac., lachn., mag-c., nux-v., phys., **RHUS-T.,** sep., sil., **SULPH.**
flexing thigh, on - nux-v.

cramps, calves
bending, knee - cocc., hep., ign.
amel. - calc., cham., rhus-t.
bending, thigh - bell.
carrying a weight - graph.
cholera, in - ***ant-t., camph., colch.,*** **CUPR.,** ***jatr., kali-p., mag-p.,*** **SULPH., VERAT.**
crossing feet, on - alum.
dancing, while - ***sulph.***
daytime - graph., ***petr.***
while sitting bent - ***lyc.***
descending, on - coca
drawing, up knee - coff.
drawing, up leg - kali-c., nit-ac.
evening - kali-n., mag-c., nux-v., sel., sil., sulph.
bed, in - ***ars.,*** bell., mag-c., nit-ac., ***puls.***
sleep, on going to - berb., nux-m.
exertion, after - sil.
flexing leg, on - cocc., coff., kali-c., nux-v.
humiliation, after - ***coloc.***
labor, during - nux-v.
lifting the foot - agar.
lying, while - bry., led., mag-c., sel.
amel. - anac.
upon the one which he was lying - staph.
menses, during - cupr., phos., verat.
before - ***phos.,*** vib.
morning - bry., carb-an., lach., nit-ac.
bed in - bov., ***caust.,*** graph., hep., ign., lac-ac., lach., nat-c., nit-ac., sil., ***sulph.***
stretching, leg, when - nat-c.
forenoon - nat-m., sulph.
rising, on - ferr., lac-ac.
waking, on - lob.
motion, on - bapt., bufo, calc., coca, hyos., ign., lyc., nux-m.
amel. - arg-m., bry., ferr., rhus-t.
of feet - cham.
lying, while - nux-m.
night - ***ambr.,*** anac., arg-n., ars., berb., bry., **CALC.,** carb-an., carb-v., caust., coca, cocc., dig., ***eupi., ferr., ferr-m., graph., kali-c.,*** led., **LYC.,** lyss., ***mag-c., mag-m.,*** mag-p., med., ***nit-ac.,*** nux-m., ***nux-v.,*** petr., plb., rhus-v., sars., sep., stann., **SULPH.,** zinc.
bending foot - chin.
pregnancy, during - ***sep.,*** vib.
pulling on boot - ***calc.,*** nit-ac.
right - agar., kali-c., lyss., trom.
rising from, a seat - alum., ***anac.***
from, bed - ferr., mag-c.
sex, during - cupr., ***graph.***
after - coloc.
on attempting - ***cupr.***
sitting, while - ign., lyc., olnd., plat., **RHUS-T.**
after walking - plat., **RHUS-T.**
sleep, during - ant-t., graph., inul., ***kali-c.,*** nat-m., tep.
before - ***nux-m.***

cramps, calves
standing, on - euphr., ferr., nat-m.
on toes - alum.
long - euphr.
stepping, on - ***sulph.***
stool, after - ox-ac., trom.
stretching, foot, when - chin., nit-ac., thuj.
in bed - **CALC.,** carl., cham., lyss., nat-c., pin-s., ***sulph.***
leg, amel. - bell.
leg, when - bar-c., bufo, **CALC.,** carl., lyc., nat-c., nux-v., sep., ***sulph.***
on waking, when - aspar.
walking, while - phos.
thinking, about it - spong., staph.
turning, foot while sitting - nat-m.
over in bed - mag-c., zinc.
waking, on - graph., lob., staph., verat-v.
walking, on - agar., am-c., **ANAC.,** arg-m., arg-n., ars., berb., **CALC-P.,** cann-s., coca, dulc., ign., kali-c., lact., lyc., mag-m., nat-m., nit-ac., puls., **SULPH.,** sul-ac.
after - carb-an., plat., **RHUS-T.**

cramps, lower - acet-ac., agar., alum., ambr., am-c., anag., ang., ***ars.,*** arum-t., arund., bar-c., bell., blatta, ***bov.,*** bry., bufo, ***calc.,*** camph., ***carb-an., carb-s., carb-v.,*** caust., **CHAM.,** chlor., cina, cit-v., ***colch.,*** **COLOC.,** crot-h., **CUPR.,** dig., dios., eug., ***ferr.,*** ferr-p., gels., glon., graph., iod., ***jatr.,*** kali-bi., **KALI-CHL.,** lach., lact., lil-t., lyc., ***mag-p.,*** manc., merc-c., nat-c., ***nat-m., nit-ac.,*** olnd., petr., ***ph-ac.,*** plat., plb., podo., ***puls., rhus-t.,*** sars., sec., stry., **SULPH.,** tab., verat., verat-v., verb., zinc-s.
bed, in - dios., nux-v., plb., ***puls.,*** rhus-t.
chill, during - cupr., elat., ***nux-v.***
cough, during - dros.
daytime - ***ferr-m.,*** ox-ac.
drawing up leg - zinc.
evening - orig., sep.
9 p.m. - lyc.
after lying down - ***puls.***
exertion, physical - alum.
extension, on - ***calc.,*** plb.
forenoon, while in bed - rhus-t.
labor, during - bell., cupr., mag-p.
lifting, when - calc., iod.
lying, while - am-c.
menses, during - ***gels., graph.***
morning - ars., arum-t., crot-h.
4 to 5 a.m. - bufo
in bed - zinc.
on waking - arum-t.
motion, on - verat-v.
night - ambr., carb-an., carb-v., merc., merc-d., nat-m., pall., ***sulph.***
pressing upon flexors - lyc.
pressing upon flexors, amel. - ox-ac., rhus-t.
sitting - iod.
amel. - cina.
sleep, when going to - hyper.
stool, during - colch., cupr., ***sulph.,*** verat.
stretching out the foot, when - ***sulph.***

cramps, lower legs
urinate, on attempting to - ***pareir.***
walking, while - ***carb-an., carb-v.,*** cina, gels., hep.

cramps, thighs - ***agar.,*** ambr., ***arg-m., ars., asar.,*** brach., bell., cann-s., carb-an., ***carb-s.,*** carb-v., cina, **COLOC.,** crot-h., cycl., dig., ***ferr.,*** ferr-ar., ferr-p., hep., ***hyos.,*** iod., ip., kali-ar., ***kali-bi., kali-c.,*** kali-p., ***lyc.,*** lyss., mang., mur-ac., naja, ol-an., ph-ac., ***plat.,*** plb., ***puls.,*** ran-b., rhus-t., ruta., sabin., ***sec., sep.,*** stry., **SULPH.,** tarent., tep., ter., valer., ***verb.,*** verat.
ascending stairs - carb-v.
bed, in - mur-ac.
daytime, during - petr.
evening - bell.
in bed - ***ars.***
flexing leg - plat.
inner, side - plat., sep.
intermittent - plat.
left - cina, rhus-t.
menses, during - wies.
night - ***ambr.,*** carb-an., hep., ***ip.,*** kali-c.
outer, side - ant-c.
posterior, part - plat.
pulsating - plat.
raising, thigh - carb-v., hep.
right - sulph., tarent.
sitting, while - iod., plat.
sleep, during - ***kali-c.***
on going to - tep.
walking, while - carb-v., ***sep.***
in open air - ***verb.***

cramps, tibia, region of - ***am-c.,*** calc., carb-an., coloc.
extending to toes - sars.

CROSSED, lower, when walking - lath.
crossing, legs impossible - ***lath.***

CURVATURE of bones - am-c., hep.

CURVING, and bowing - ***calc., calc-p.,*** lyc., sil.

CUTTING, pain - alum., bell., calc., dros., dulc., ***graph.,*** ign., lyc., mag-m., mur-ac., ***nat-c.,*** sep., sil., stann., sul-ac.

cutting, calves - alum., ***chel.,*** coloc., dros., ph-ac., stry., ***thuj.***
sitting, while - mur-ac.
walking, while - ***thuj.***

cutting, lower - agar., ***anac.,*** ars-h., bell., calc., coloc., con., gamb., guare., mur-ac., ph-ac., ***plat., rhus-t., thuj.***
motion, on - con.
paroxysmal - thuj.
standing, on - arg-m.

cutting, thighs - ant-t., ***aur-m., bell., calc.,*** dig., dros., gels., stann., ***stry., sul-ac.***
crossing limbs, on - dig.
menses, during - stram.
motion, on - calc.
sitting, while - bell.

cutting, tibia - calc., carb-ac., mag-c.

DECAY, of bones - aur., aur-m., aur-m-n., ***calc., mez., nit-ac., sep.,*** **SIL.**
decay, lower, fibula - **SIL.**
decay, thighs, femur - ***calc.,*** **SIL.,** ***stront.***
decay, tibia - asaf., aur., calc., guai., hecla., kali-i., lach., ph-ac., phos., **SIL.**

DISCOLORATION, general
black and painful spots - nux-v.
blotches - ant-c., crot-t., lach., nat-c., sulph.
bluish - bism., cupr., ***ox-ac.,*** sec., verat.
spots - am-c., ant-c., con., lach., phos., ***sulph.,*** **SUL-AC.**
brownish - arg-n.
ecchymoses - agav-a., phos., sol-v., ***sul-ac.***
greenish - vip.
yellow as from a bruise - con.
livid - kali-a., morph.
marbled - **CAUST.,** lyc., thuj.
purple in spots - bor., ptel.
purpura hemorrhagica - ***lach., phos., sec.,*** ter.
redness - petr., plb., ptel., sep., stram., vip.
redness, in spots - ars., ***calc., caust.,*** con., ***graph.,*** kali-i., ***lach.,*** lyc., merc., mez., petr., ph-ac., sil., ***sulph., sul-ac.***
inner side of - petr.
spots - ant-c., bry., hyos., kali-br., kali-n., nat-c., sulph.
yellow - kali-br., vip.
in stripes - vip.

discoloration, calves
blotches - petr.
blue spots - kali-p.
redness in spots - ***con.,*** graph., kali-br., lach.
spots - con., graph., ***sars.***
yellow spots - kali-br.

discoloration, lower
black - iod., vip.
in spots - vip.
blood specks - phos.
blotches - lac-ac., ***nat-c.,*** phos.
blue - arg-n., ambr., ***anthr., carb-an., carb-s.,*** con., elaps, lyc., kali-br., mur-ac., **NUX-V.,** ox-ac., plb.
left, during menses - ambr.
spots - ***sars., sul-ac.***
spots, indurated - ***sars.***
brown, bluish - ***anthr.,*** vip.
spots - ***petr.,*** thuj.
crusts - mez.
cyanosis - con., elaps
dark, when in depending position - hydr-ac.
ecchymoses - crot-h.
marbled - **CAUST.**
mottled - con., led.
purple - led., vesp.
spots - **APIS,** ***crot-h.***
purpura - kali-i., ***lach.,*** **PHOS.,** ***sec.***
reddish - aeth., am-c., arn., arund., con., cop., elaps, hydr-ac., kali-bi., kali-br., ***lach.,*** lyc., merc., ***nat-c.,*** phos., puls., rhus-t., rhus-v., sulph., thuj.
evening - fago.

discoloration, lower
reddish, spots - ***calc.,*** con., dulc., graph., guare., kali-br., kali-n., lyc., merc., sars., sil., sul-ac., zinc.
spots, become covered with crusts - ***zinc.***
spots, burning - ph-ac.
walking, while - nux-v.
spots - ***calc., chel.,*** con., ***lyc., phos., stann., zinc.***
white spots - calc.
yellow spots - carl., hydrc., stann., vip.
discoloration, thighs
blotches - lac-ac.
blue - anthr., bism., both., kreos.
marks - arn.
spots - ant-c., ***arn.,*** kreos., morph., mosch., vip.
brownish, inside thigh - ***thuj.***
spots - cann-s., nat-s., ***mez.***
cyanosis - ars.
greenish - kali-n.
livid - anthr., arn.
marbled - **CAUST.**
redness - anac., bell., kali-c., rhus-t., nat-m., puls., sil., thuj.
night - rhus-v.
spots - bell., calc., caps., crot-t., cycl., ***graph.,*** med., merc., petr., plan., rhod., rhus-t., sulph.
spots, burning - ph-ac.
spots, itching - graph., nat-m.
spots, itching, when scratched - med.
spots - am-c., ant-c., cann-i., cycl., ***graph.,*** mur-ac., rhod.
white, in spots - calc.
yellow marks - arn.
discoloration, tibia - ambr., ant-c., calc-p., ***caust.,*** kali-n., ***lach.,*** mag-c., ***phos., sil.,*** sul-ac.

DISLOCATION, sensation, as if, feeling - merc., sarr.

DRAGGING, pain, lower - bar-c., con., merc., ***nux-v., op.,*** **PHOS.,** plb., ***sec.***
walking, while - atro., con., merc., ***nux-v., op., plb., sec.,*** ter.

DRAWING, pain - ***acon., agar., alum.,*** am-c., am-m., anac., ***ang.,*** ant-c., ant-t., ***arg-m., arg-n.,*** ars., ars-i., ***bapt.,*** **BAR-C.,** bell., berb., bism., ***bry.,*** calc., calc-p., caps., carb-s., **CARB-V.,** ***caust., cham.,*** **CHEL.,** chin., cina, cinnb., cist., clem., ***con.,*** dig., ***dulc., ferr.,*** ferr-i., ***gels.,*** **GRAPH.,** grat., **HEP.,** ***iod.,*** kali-ar., kali-bi., ***kali-c.,*** kali-n., kreos., lach., led., ***lyc.,*** mag-c., ***merc.,*** mez., nat-a., ***nat-c., nat-m., nit-ac., nux-v.,*** par., petr., ph-ac., ***phos.,*** pic-ac., plat., ***puls.,*** rat., **RHUS-T.,** rhus-v., sars., ***sep., sil.,*** stann., ***stront-c., sulph.,*** thuj., ***tub., valer.,*** verat., ***zinc.***
bones - anac., bar-c., calc., ***chin., con.,*** graph., ***kali-c.,*** mag-c., ***rhod.,*** sabin., sep., **VALER.,** zinc.
cramp-like - ***arg-n.,*** chin., gels., graph., ***hep.,*** iod., merc-i-f., nat-m., phos., ***sulph.***
ending in jerking - ***sil.***

DRAWING, pain
evening - caust., ***nat-m.,*** nit-ac., **PULS.,** sil., stront-c., sulph., zinc.
bed, in - carb-v., ***sulph.***
motion amel. - stront.
exposure to cold - ***calc-p., phos.***
extending, downward - chel., gels., graph., nat-m., nit-ac., ***puls.,*** sil.
to head - thuj.
to shoulder - bell.
to tips of toes - calc.
to upward - sep.
fever, with - kali-n.
joints - chel., lyc., ***rhod.,*** sep., stront.
left - ***bar-c., carb-v.,*** con., nat-m., petr.
menses, during - con., nit-ac., nux-m., rhus-t., sep., ***spong.***
before - phos., sep.
morning, bed, in - ***sulph.***
rising, after - kali-bi.
motion, during - ***gels.***
amel. - ***arg-n.,*** ferr., iod., lyc., merc-i-f., **RHUS-T.,** sep., stront-c., ***tub.,*** **VALER.**
night - phos., ***nat-c.,*** nat-m., ***tub.,*** zinc.
paralytic - **CARB-V.,** ***chel.,*** mez., par.
paroxysmal - nat-m.
periosteum - rhod.
motion amel. - rhod.
night - rhod.
rheumatic - iod., ***zinc.***
right - chel., nit-ac., phos.
sitting - ***arg-n.,*** chin., iod., **VALER.**
storm, during - caust.
walking, while - asaf., coloc., ***gels., hep.***
after - anac.
amel. - ***lyc.,*** **RHUS-T.,** ***tub.,*** **VALER.**
wet weather - rhod.
drawing, calves - acon., agar., agn., ***alum., anac.,*** ang., ant-c., ant-t., ***arg-m., arg-n., ars.,*** asaf., aster., aur-m-n., bapt., berb., bism., bry., cahin., calc., ***calc-p.,*** camph., ***cann-i.,*** caps., **CARB-AN.,** carb-s., cast., caul., caust., chel., ***cic.,*** cist., cocc., coc-c., colch., coloc., con., ***cupr.,*** dios., eupi., fl-ac., gels., gins., graph., ***guai.,*** hell., hyper., ***kali-bi.,*** kali-i., kali-n., ***kali-p., led.,*** lyc., manc., med., meny., ***mez.,*** nat-a., nat-c., nat-s., nit-ac., nux-m., ***nux-v.,*** plat., ***puls.,*** pyrus, rat., ***rhus-t.,*** rhus-v., rumx., sabin., sang., sec., **SIL.,** spig., stann., ***sulph.,*** tab., thuj., upa., verat., viol-t., zinc.
afternoon - agar., cast.
alternating, with pressure - gins.
with sole of foot - sulph.
ascending stairs - arg-n.
chill, during - ***ars.,*** thuj.
cramp-like - **ANAC.,** ang., arg-m., ***carb-an.,*** coloc., graph., manc., plat., ***sil.,*** sulph.
descending stairs - arg-m.
evening - alum., calc., ***puls.,*** rat., verat.
extending, downward - agar., alum., bism., chel., coc-c., fl-ac., sang., thuj., zinc.
to achillis tendon - fl-ac.
to heels - sang.

drawing, calves
extending to knees - chel.
to knees, hollow of - rhus-t.
to thighs - chel.
upwards to back - manc.
griping - sulph.
lying down amel. - nux-m.
middle of - nit-ac.
motion, on - cocc.
night - ars., graph.
paralytic - ***nux-v.***
paroxysmal - ant-t., cist., coc-c., graph., thuj.
pressive - bry., gins., nat-c.
right - ***agar.***
rising, on - graph.
sitting, while - cast., coloc., kali-i., puls., sulph.
down after walking - plat.
standing, while - arn., nat-s., nux-m.
stretching, on - graph.
tearing - calc., kali-n.
twitching - mez.
walking - alum., ***anac.,*** cann-i., **CARB-AN.,** ***lyc.,*** nat-c., ***nux-v., sil.,*** spig., verat-v., viol-t.
amel. - agar., arg-m., sulph.

drawing, lower - acon., ***agar., alum.,*** am-c., ***am-m., anac.,*** ant-c., arg-m., arg-n., ***ars.,*** asaf., ***bapt., bar-c., bell.,*** bor., ***bry., calc.,*** camph., carb-an., carb-s., carb-v., ***caul., caust.,*** cham., **CHEL.,** chin., cic., cina, cist., clem., coloc., con., crot-h., ***cycl.,*** dig., dulc., ***ferr.,*** ferr-m., fl-ac., ***gels.,*** goss., graph., ***guai.,*** ham., hell., ***hep.,*** hyos., iod., kali-bi., ***kali-c.,*** kali-n., kali-p., kali-s., kreos., lach., lact., ***led., lyc., mag-c.,*** mang., ***meny., merc.,*** merc-c., ***mez.,*** mosch., mur-ac., nat-c., ***nat-m., nat-s.,*** nit-ac., ***nux-v.,*** ol-an., olnd., petr., ph-ac., phos., phyt., plat., **PULS.,** rat., ***rhod.,*** **RHUS-T.,** ***rhus-v.,*** sabad., sars., ***sep., sil.,*** sol-t-ae., spong., squil., stann., staph., stront-c., stry., sulph., ***tarax.,*** thuj., til., ***tub.,*** viol-t., zinc.
afternoon - elaps
air, open, agg. - ***caust.,*** graph.
amel. - ***mez.***
bed, in - ign., ***lyc.***
bending, backward - clem.
bones - kali-c., nit-ac., zinc.
burning - rat.
chill, during - ***puls., rhus-t., tub.***
before - ***nux-v.***
cold, becoming - ***phos.***
cramp-like - anac., caust., chin., cina, dulc., graph., hep., ***meny., merc.,*** mosch., nat-c., nat-m., petr., ph-ac., rhod.
crossing, limbs - kali-n.
in bed - ***phos.***
drawing up limbs, amel. - cinnb.
ending in jerking - ***sil.***
evening - ant-c., arg-m., bar-c., caust., cham., cycl., fl-ac., lyc., mag-c., nat-c., phos., **PULS.,** rat., ***sil., sulph.,*** zinc.

drawing, lower
extending, downward - anac., bism., calc., dulc., kali-c., lach., mag-c., mag-m., rhod., sil., spig., thuj.
to knee - nit-ac.
to heel - sep.
to toes - agar., calc., rhod., sep.
upwards - carb-an., lach., lact., meny., nat-m., nit-ac.
jerking - thuj.
lying - am-m.
menses, during - ***con.,*** spong.
morning - ang., ars., indg., ***sulph.***
motion, agg. - ***gels.,*** iod.
amel. - ***iod.,*** ph-ac., **PULS., RHOD., RHUS-T.,** ***tarax.***
night - anac., carb-an., cham., kali-c., ***lyc.,*** phos., ph-ac., thuj., ***tub.,*** verat.
11 p.m. - com., mill.
paralytic - acon., agn., arg-m., bell., chel., hep., hyos., kali-c., meny., nat-m., nit-ac., ***phos.,*** rhus-t., ***rhus-v.***
paroxysmal - merc., ph-ac., thuj.
resting feet on floor while sitting - ***ars.***
rheumatic - ang., carb-v., cimic., elaps, iod., lyc., mez., ***phos.***
riding, while - lyc.
right - ***agar., chel.,*** nat-m.
rise from seat - ph-ac.
rising, after - coloc.
from a seat, on - rat.
sitting, while - agar., am-c., am-m., anac., ant-c., arg-n., ***ars.,*** bar-c., caust., chin., coloc., cycl., dig., iod., led., meny., mez., rhus-t., stann., ***tarax.***
amel. - cina.
letting foot hang down - ***ars.***
standing, while - caust., mez., nat-s., tarax.
amel. - cina.
talking, while - ol-an.
tendons - nat-s., phys., pyrus
walking, amel. - agar., am-m., ***lyc.,*** ph-ac., ***puls.,*** **RHOD., RHUS-T.,** sep., ***tub.***
walking, while - anac., ang., coloc., ***gels.,*** hep., hyos., nat-s., ***nux-v.,*** stront.
bent amel. - am-m.
in open air - cina, ***lyc.***
warmth, of bed, agg. - ***lyc.***
of bed, amel. - **CAUST.**

drawing, thighs - acon., ***agar.,*** agn., ***alum.,*** ambr., am-c., ***anac.,*** ang., ant-c., apis, ***arg-n., arn.,*** ars., ars-i., asaf., asar., asc-t., aster., aur., bar-c., bar-m., ***bell.,*** berb., bry., calc-p., ***camph.,*** canth., carb-ac., carb-an., ***carb-s., carb-v., caul., caust.,*** cham., **CHEL.,** ***chin., chin-a.,*** cinnb., ***clem.,*** cocc., coc-c., colch., ***coloc.,*** con., cupr., ***cycl.,*** dig., ***dulc.,*** euon., eupi., ***ferr.,*** ferr-ar., ferr-i., ***gels.,*** graph., grat., ***guai., hep.,*** hyos., ind., iod., kali-bi., **KALI-C.,** kali-chl., kali-n., kali-p., kreos., lach., led., ***lyc.,*** mag-c., mang-m., meny., ***merc.,*** merc-c., ***mez.,*** mur-ac., nat-a., nat-c., ***nat-m.,*** nat-s., ***nit-ac., nux-m., nux-v., ol-an.,*** phos., ***plat.,*** plb., **PULS.,** ***ran-b.,*** rat., ***rhod.,*** **RHUS-T.,** rhus-v., ruta., sabad.,

drawing, thighs - sabin., samb., sars., ***sep., sil.,*** spig., spong., squil., ***stann.,*** staph., ***stram.,*** **SULPH.,** tab., ter., ***thuj.,*** valer., verb., viol-t., ***zinc.,*** zing.
afternoon - agar., lyc., ***ran-b.,*** sep., sulph.
air, open, agg. - **CAUST.**
alternating, right then left - sulph.
anterior part - agar., ant-c., arg-m., arg-n., bar-c., bry., dig., dulc., kali-bi., lyc., ***meny.,*** rat., samb., staph., stram., ***sulph., vib.***
cramp-like - meny.
evening - sulph.
extending to knee - agar., bar-c.
menses, before - ***vib.***
paralytic - dulc.
walking amel. - bar-c., ***sulph.***
ascending, while - ***bar-c.,*** hyos., kali-bi., kali-c., lyc.
backwards - sulph.
and forth - phos.
bend of - ang., arg-m., chin., gamb., graph., merl., nat-m., thuj.
burning - rat.
chill, during - ferr., ***puls.,*** sep.
before - ***nux-v.***
coryza, during - sep.
cramp-like - anac., arg-n., ars., aur., carb-v., chin., ***cycl.,*** dig., ***gels.,*** iod., kali-n., lyc., ***meny.,*** mur-ac., plat., rhus-v., ruta, ***sep.,*** samb., ***sulph.,*** thuj., valer., verat., ***verb.***
crossing limbs, while - agar., ***rhus-t.***
dinner, during - sulph.
after - sulph.
drawing, up legs amel. - ***caust.,*** cinnb., guai., ***rhus-t.***
evening - colch., kali-c., meny., nit-ac., **PULS.,** rat., ***sulph.,*** thuj., ***zinc.***
bed, in - carb-v., colch., kali-c., ***sulph.***
sleeping, after - cycl.
walking, while - ***sulph.***
extending into penis - clem.
limb, amel. - agar.
downward - ***agar.,*** anac., apis, asaf., bar-c., bell., bry., ***calc-p.,*** carb-v., coc-c., coloc., kreos., merc., mez., mur-ac., nux-v., ***ran-b.,*** sil.
outward - bell.
to feet - asaf., ***sil.***
to hip - bry., ruta.
to knees - ***agar.,*** coloc., grat., guai., nat-m.
to sacral region - ruta.
to sole - kreos.
to toes - apis, ***gels.***
upward - graph., sep.
femur - alumn., asar., bar-c., berb., carb-an., ***chin.,*** cob., colch., coloc., graph., guai., ip., kali-bi., meny., merc-c., mez., nat-m., sabin., sep.
inner side of - am-c., ant-c., asaf., berb., caul., chel., chin., ***coloc.,*** dig., gels., kali-bi., nat-p., nit-ac., par., ran-b., sil., stann., sulph., thuj., zinc.
afternoon - ***coloc.,*** sulph.
evening - kali-bi.

drawing, thighs
inner, side of, forenoon - sulph.
pressing - stann.
sitting, while - dig., ran-b.
tearing - berb.
knee, above the - am-c., caust., kali-n., led., mez., myric., nat-m., plat., thuj.
jerking - plat.
while sitting - nat-m., thuj.
lying on it, amel. - carb-v.
menses, during - ***cham.,*** con., ***puls.,*** spong., ***stram.***
as if, would appear - bry.
before - cham., spong., ***vib.***
middle of - guai., kali-bi., mez., staph., sulph., thuj.
while at rest - thuj.
morning - kali-n., ***sulph.***
motion, agg. - iod., nat-m.
amel. - arg-n., con., ***dulc., ferr.,*** hyos., iod., **PULS., RHOD., RHUS-T.**
night - ars., kali-c., nat-m., **PULS.**
midnight, after - merc.
outer side - agar., anac., ang., arg-mur., aster., berb., carb-v., cic., coloc., led., meny., op., stann., ter., thuj., valer., zinc.
crossing limbs - stann.
pressing - stann.
paralytic - agar., bell., cocc., colch., ***hep.,*** hyos., **KALI-C.,** ***nux-v.,*** staph., ter.
paroxysmal - arg-n., ars., grat., nat-m., ***rhod.,*** sep., squil.
posterior part - ***agar., am-m.,*** ant-c., asar., bry., calc., ***cycl.,*** dig., dulc., led., lyc., ***nat-m.,*** ran-b., zinc.
evening - calc.
lying, while - asar.
motion amel. - caps.
sitting - ***am-m.,*** dig., led.
walking, amel. - dig., zinc.
walking, while - ***agar.,*** am-m., ***ran-b.,*** samb.
rheumatic - agar., ang., carb-v., iod., meph., **RHOD., RHUS-T.,** sep., verat., ***zinc.***
right - ***camph., chel.,*** nat-m.
rising from a seat - ang., chin., graph., rat., rhus-t., thuj.
amel. - aur.
sex, after - nit-ac.
siesta, during - phos.
sitting, while - am-c., anac., arg-n., aur., chin., dig., dulc., iod., led., mang-m., meny., mur-ac., plat., ran-b., **RHOD., RHUS-T.,** spig., squil., ***sulph., thuj.,*** verb.
amel. - aur., kali-bi., nit-ac., rhus-t., sulph.
down - nit-ac.
sprained - carb-v.
standing, on - kali-c., rhus-t., verat., viol-t.
stepping - plat.
sticking - am-c., hyos.
stooping, when - sulph.

drawing, thighs
tearing - ***acon., anac., chin.***, clem., ***coloc., dulc., guai.***, merc., nux-v., **RHUS-T.**, spig., stann., tep., thuj.
upper part - arg-m., carb-an., euphr., mez., mosch., ***plat.***, thuj.
extending upward - euphr.
walking, while - agn., ang., asar., berb., ***carb-s.***, carb-v., **COLOC.**, clem., con., gels., hyos., ind., kali-bi., kreos., nat-m., ***nux-v.***, plan., plat., squil., ***sulph., verb., viol-t.***
after - camph.
after, sitting - agar.
amel. - bar-c., dulc., ***lyc.***, phos., **RHUS-T.**, ***sulph., valer.***
wandering - dulc., mez., nux-m., rhus-v.
warm bed, in - kali-c., ***lyc., merc., nat-m.***, **PULS.**
amel. - **CAUST.**, ***lyc.***
wave-like - mez.

drawing, tibia - acon., ***agar.***, **ANAC.**, ang., ***ant-c.***, ang., ***arg-m.***, ars., asaf., aur-m-n., bar-c., bell., brom., bry., calc., ***calc-p.***, carb-an., carb-v., caust., chel., ***chin.***, clem., ***coloc.***, crot-h., dig., graph., hyper., indg., kali-ar., kali-bi., ***kali-c.***, kali-n., ***led.***, mag-s., ***mang., merc.***, mez., mill., mosch., nat-s., nit-ac., nux-v., petr., ***puls.***, ran-a., ***rhus-t.***, sabin., sars., sil., ***staph.***, sulph., zinc.
afternoon, while sitting - agar.
burning - nat-c.
crampy - nat-c., petr.
descending a mountain - bar-c.
evening - ang., chin., ***sulph.***, thuj.
6 p.m. - arg-m.
7 p.m. - sulph.
9 p.m. - thuj.
extending downwards - nat-c., zinc.
to, ankle - brom.
to, feet - mag-m., sulph.
upwards - sars.
jerking - carb-an.
morning - kali-bi.
motion, amel. - arg-n., **AUR-M-N.**, ***mang.***, **VALER.**
noon - ***agar.***
paralytic - petr.
rheumatic - zinc.
sitting, while - ***agar.***, chin., coloc., cycl., mang., staph., **VALER.**
amel. - cycl., mang.
standing, while - agar., mang.
stretching leg - chin.
walking, while - ang., crot-h., cycl., thuj.
amel. - ***agar., aur-m-n.***, bar-c., chin., cycl., ***mang.***, **VALER.**

DRAWN, backwards, legs - bufo, plb.
sitting, while - spong.
thigh, on the - canth., op., plb.
when attempting to walk - spong.

drawn, inward - acon.

DRYNESS - agar., op.

ECZEMA - ***anil.***, apis, arn., ars., ***bov.***, chel., jug-r., kali-br., merc., ***petr., psor., rhus-t.***

eczema, calves - ***graph.***

eczema, lower - ***apis***, **ARS.**, carb-v., **GRAPH.**, kali-br., ***lach.***, led., ***lyc., merc., nat-m.***, **PETR.**, ***rhus-t., sars.***, **SULPH.**

eczema, thighs - petr., ***rhus-t.***

ELECTRICAL, current, sensation of, lower legs - bol., dor.

EMACIATION - ***abrot.***, am-m., ***apis***, arg-m., ***arg-n., ars.***, berb., ***calc.***, chin., dulc., lath., nat-m., nit-ac., ph-ac., ***plb., sanic.***, sel.
painful, limb - ***ol-j., plb.***

emaciation, calves - sel.

emaciation, lower - ***abrot., apis***, benz-ac., berb., ***bov., calc., caps.***, chin., nit-ac., **NUX-V., RHUS-V.**, sarr., sel., syph., thuj.

emaciation, thighs - bar-m., ***calc., nit-ac.***, plb., sac-alb., ***sel.***

ENLARGEMENT, sensation of, lower - cedr., nux-m., ***plat.***, sep.

ERUPTIONS - agar., am-c., am-m., ***ant-c.***, apis, arn., **ARS.**, arund., ***bar-c.***, bar-m., bell., ***bov.***, bry., **CALC.**, ***calc-p.***, carb-o., ***carb-v.***, **CAUST.**, chel., chin., chin-a., chin-s., chlor., ***clem.***, con., cop., crot-c., ***crot-t.***, cupr., cupr-ar., dulc., elaps, ***euph.***, fago., ***graph.***, iod., jug-r., ***kali-ar.***, kali-bi., kali-br., ***kali-c., kali-s.***, kreos., lach., led., ***lyc.***, mag-c., manc., mang., ***merc.***, murx., nat-c., nat-m., nat-p., nit-ac., nux-v., **PETR.**, ph-ac., phos., phyt., plan., **PSOR.**, ***puls.***, **RHUS-T.**, ***rhus-v.***, rumx., ruta., sabad., sars., sec., sel., **SEP., SIL.**, staph., stram., stront-c., **SULPH.**, tarax., tep., thuj., til.
black - sec.
bleeding after scratching - calc., cupr.
blotches - ant-c., lach., nat-c., sulph.
burning - bov., fago., lac-ac., ***merc.***, nux-v., til.
after scratching - til.
cold bathing amel. - ***lyc.***
confluent - cop., rhus-v.
desquamation - agar., ars., calc-p., chin-s., crot-t., elaps, kreos., mag-c., merc., sulph., thuj.
dry - bry.
eating - nux-v., ***sulph.***
elevations - aur., cop., cupr., kali-br., mag-c., petr., puls., thuj.
flea bites - sec.
gangrenous - hyos.
gritty - nat-m.
groups, in - nat-m.
hard - aur., bov.
hot - chel., fago.
itch-like - ars., bry., chel., sulph.
itching - ***agar.***, anac., arg-n., bov., bry., ***calc.***, caust., daph., dulc., fago., jug-r., ***kali-c.***, lac-ac., lach., led., mang., ***merc.***, mur-ac., ***nat-c.***, **NAT-M.**, nat-p., nicc., ***nux-v.***, petr., puls., rhus-t., rumx., sel., **SEP.**, ***sil.***, **STAPH.**, sulph., tarax., til.
knots, reddish, hard - kali-bi.

ERUPTIONS, general
lumpy - petr., ther., thuj.
miliary - alum., ars., bov., daph., merc., nux-v., sil., sulph.
moist - ***bov.,*** bry., chel., kreos., merc., nat-m.
nodules - petr., ther., thuj.
painful - arn., bov.
papular - lach., lachn., merc., nux-v., ph-ac., rhus-t., sel., sep., thuj.
petechiae - agav-a., am-m., ars., kali-i., sol-v.
phagedenic - ars., nux-v., sulph.
pimples - agar., ant-c., am-c., am-m., arg-n., arn., asc-t., bar-c., bell., berb., bov., bry., calc., calc-p., cann-s., cast., chel., chin-s., clem., con., crot-c., elaps, fago., fl-ac., ***graph.,*** hura, iris, ir-foe., kali-bi., kali-br., kali-c., kali-chl., ***kali-s.,*** mag-c., mang., merc., mez., morph., nat-m., nat-p., nicc., petr., ph-ac., ***puls.,*** rumx., ***sars.,*** sep., sil., stann., staph., stront-c., sulph., thea., thuj., til., verat., zinc.
bleeding - agar., thea.
burning - mang.
burning, when scratched - staph.
flat - ant-c., plan.
hard - plan.
indolent - chel.
itching - asc-t., bell., elaps, ***hep.,*** kali-bi., mang., ***petr., ph-ac.,*** sel., ***sep.,*** stann., staph., sulph.
itching, after scratching - mag-c.
painful - bry., thea.
red - asc-t., chel., clem., graph., kali-c., sars., sulph., thea., til.
white - plan.
yellow - ant-c.
pustules - am-c., ars., bry., crot-c., clem., cupr-ar., dulc., hyos., jug-c., kali-bi., kali-br., lyc., mez., rhus-t., rumx., sars., stram., thuj., verat.
black - ***ars.,*** nat-c., sec.
burn - mez.
groups - hyos.
red - lyc., mez.
red, areola - ant-c.
suppurating - con., thuj.
red - bell., bov., chel., crot-c., kali-bi., mag-c., merc., nat-m., rhus-v.
rough - rhus-v.
scabs - arn., ars., bell., ***bov.,*** calc., ir-foe., ***kali-br., lach.,*** mez., podo., rhus-v., ***sabin., sil.,*** staph., zinc.
elevated, white - mez.
scales - calc-p., clem., kali-ar., ***kali-s.,*** pip-m., rhus-v.
in spots - ***merc.,*** zinc.
scurfs - bar-m., ***merc., petr.***
in spots - ***merc.***
smooth - mag-c.
sore - merc.
spots like a burn - lach.
stinging - ant-c., nux-v., petr., sabin.
ulcerating - ph-ac.
varicella, like - ant-t.
white - agar.

eruptions, calves - apis, bell., caust., kali-ar., mag-c., petr., phyt., sars., sep., ***sil.,*** thuj.
blotches - aur., carb-v., lach., merc., petr., phos., thuj.
desquamation - mag-c.
elevated - mag-c.
itching - carb-v., petr., ph-ac., sars., sep., sil., thuj., zinc.
lumps - nit-ac.
nodes, white - thuj.
pimples - agar., arg-n., asc-t., bov., bry., elaps, hura, kali-bi., lach., nat-c., ph-ac., puls., rumx., sabin., sars., ***sep.,*** staph., zinc.
becoming ulcers - ph-ac.
pustules - kali-bi., kali-br.
red - hyos., mag-c.
spots - ***con., lyc.,*** phyt.
scabs - kali-br.
smooth - mag-c.
stitching - sep.

eruptions, lower - agar., alum., am-m., ars., arund., bov., bry., calc., ***caust.,*** chin-s., chlor., cupr., cupr-ar., daph., fago., kali-ar., kali-bi., kali-br., kali-c., lach., merc., mez., murx., ***nat-c., nat-m.,*** nit-ac., ***petr.,*** ph-ac., ***podo.,*** puls., ***rhus-t.,*** rumx., ***sec.,*** sep., staph., stram., sulph., thuj., zinc.
bleeding after scratching - ***cupr-ar.***
blotches - ant-c., arg-n., aur., carb-v., cocc., hura, jug-r., kreos., lac-ac., merc., nat-c., petr., phos., rhod., thuj.
burning - aur., calc., lac-ac., ***rhus-t.***
copper-colored spots - graph.
denuded spots - calc.
desquamating - agar., ***carb-an.,*** mag-c., merc., ***sulph.,*** thuj.
dry - calc-p., clem., ***dol.***
elevations - aur., cupr., kali-br.
spots - ***syph.***
excoriations - ***graph., tarent-c.***
groups, in - nat-m.
itching - arund., aur., ***calc.,*** carb-v., lac-ac., psor., puls., ***rhus-t.,*** rumx.
corrosive to touch - nat-m.
leprous spots - ***graph., nat-c.***
menses, during, spots painful - ***petr.***
moist - apis, bry., ***calc., graph., merc., petr., rhus-t.,*** tarent-c.
patches, large as the hand - caust.
petechiae - am-m., phos.
pimples - agar., am-c., arg-m., arn., arum-t., bell., bov., chin-s., elaps, fl-ac., hura, ir-foe., kali-bi., kali-chl., merc., morph., ***nat-m.,*** nicc., ***puls.,*** sars., ***sep.,*** staph., stront-c., sul-ac., thuj., verat.
bleeding easily - agar.
burning - arg-m., puls., staph.
itching - asc-t., bell., elaps, kali-bi., sep., stront-c., ziz.
moist - puls.
red - ir-foe., kali-chl., rumx.
scratching, after - agar., nat-c.
white - agar., staph.

eruptions, lower
pustules - arg-n., ars., ***dulc.***, ***kali-bi.***, kali-br., ***lach.***, mez., ***psor.***, rumx., staph., stram., **SULPH.**, ***thuj.***
itching - ***arg-n.***, asc-t.
vaccination, after - sulph., thuj.
red - bell., kali-bi., mag-c., merc., sulph.
patches - ***calc.***, sil., sul-ac.
scabs - arn., calc-p., ir-foe., kali-br., ***lach.***, **NIT-AC.**, ph-ac., podo., ***sep.***, staph., **SULPH.**, zinc.
scales in spots - ***merc.***, zinc.
scurfy - ars., calc., ***kali-bi.***, sabin., sep., staph., zinc.
ulcerate - ***nat-c.***
varicella, like - ant-t.
white - agar.
spots - ***calc.***

eruptions, thighs - agar., ars., aster., bar-m., ***calc.***, chin-s., crot-t., fago., ***graph.***, kali-ar., kali-bi., kali-c., kreos., merc., ***nat-c.***, nat-m., nit-ac., nux-v., osm., petr., phos., plan., ***psor.***, ***rhus-t.***, rhus-v., ***sil.***, staph., sulph., thuj., ***til.***
areola red - nat-m.
between - ***carb-v.***, hep., kali-c., nat-m., nat-s., ***petr.***, puls., sel.
blotches - aur., carb-v., crot-h., merc., rhod., zinc.
blue spots - ***arn.***
burning - fago., til.
after scratching - til.
copper-colored spots - ***mez.***
menses, during - mez.
crusts - anac., ***clem.***, graph., ***ph-ac.***
desquamation - chin-s., crot-t., kreos., sulph.
elevated - plan.
hot - fago.
inside, during menses - kali-c., nux-v., sil.
pimples - sulph.
itching - agar., alum., ***carb-v.***, fago., kali-c., mag-m., merc., nat-m., petr., sep., ***til.***
knots - kali-bi., nat-c.
knots, reddish, hard - kali-bi.
moist - ***crot-t.***, merc., nat-m.
petechiae - ***ars.***
pimples - agar., ant-c., asc-t., bar-m., berb., bov., bry., calc., cann-s., cast., chel., clem., cocc., elaps, fago., fl-ac., graph., ***kali-c.***, ***kali-chl.***, kali-cy., ***lach.***, lyc., mag-c., ***mang.***, meph., ***merc.***, ***mez.***, ***nat-m.***, ***petr.***, ***phos.***, plan., rumx., sars., ***sel.***, ***stann.***, staph., ***sulph.***, thea., ***thuj.***, ***til.***, zinc.
biting - agar.
burning - mang.
burning, morning and evening - mang.
burning, when scratched - agar., ***staph.***, ***til.***
flat - ant-c., plan.
indolent - chel.
itching - asc-t., chel., nat-m., stann., staph., sulph., zinc.
itching, after scratching - mag-c.
itching, evening - mang., sulph.
itching, morning - mang.

eruptions, thighs
painful - bry., thea.
painful, on touch - phos.
red - asc-t., chel., clem., graph., kali-c., sars., sulph., thea., ***til.***
red areola, with - nat-m.
sore, from scratching - mang., nat-m.
white - plan.
pustules - am-c., ***ant-c.***, dulc., grat., ***hyos.***, ***jug-c.***, lach., lyc., mez., staph., stram., ***thuj.***, verat.
burn - mez.
in groups - hyos.
red - lyc., mez.
with points depressed - verat.
yellow - ***ant-c.***
red - mag-m., merc., rhus-v.
patches - calc., cycl.
rough - kreos., rhus-v.
roughness like ham - kreos.
scaly - mez.
scurfs - bar-m., merc., ***mez.***
in spots - ***merc.***

eruptions, tibia, papular - sul-ac.
watery, vesicles - bell.

ERYSIPELAS, legs - ***sulph.***

erysipelas, lower, legs - anan., **APIS**, arn., ars., ***bor.***, ***bufo***, ***calc.***, ***hep.***, ***hydr.***, **LACH.**, lyc., merc., ***nat-c.***, ***puls.***, ***rhus-t.***, ***sil.***, ***sulph.***, ***ter.***, zinc.

EXCORIATION, lower legs - lach.

excoriation, thighs, between - aeth., ***ambr.***, ***am-c.***, anan., ars., bar-c., bufo, ***calc.***, carb-s., **CAUST.**, ***chin.***, chin-a., goss., ***graph.***, **HEP.**, iod., kali-ar., **KALI-C.**, **KREOS.**, ***lyc.***, **MERC.**, ***nat-c.***, nat-m., ***nit-ac.***, ***petr.***, phos., rhod., **SEP.**, squil., ***sul-ac.***, **SULPH.**, zinc.
walking, from - **GRAPH.**, ruta., ***sulph.***, sul-ac.

EXOSTOSES, tibia - ***ang.***, ***aur.***, ***aur-m.***, bad., calc-f., ***calc-f.***, ***calc-p.***, ***cinnb.***, ***dulc.***, ***hecla.***, merc., **NIT-AC.**, phos., ***phyt.***, rhus-t., sars.

EXTENSION, lower difficult - carb-o., dig., pic-ac., stry.
impossible - con., plb.
sitting, while - ***lath.***
necessary - sul-ac.
paroxysm, during - nux-v., stry.
before - bufo.
spasmodic - bufo, cina.
on waking - **BELL.**

FISTULOUS, openings, lower, legs - ruta.
fistulous, thighs - ***calc.***

FLEXED, lower, upon thigh - bufo, ***hyos.***, ***op.***, ***plb.***
cannot allow one leg to be bent in the morning in bed - ***zinc.***
painfully - nux-v.
walk, when he tries to - ***plb.***, spong.
flexed, thighs, abdomen, upon - arg-n., ***ars.***, carb-v., cham., ***cina***, ***cupr.***, hydr-ac., ***hyos.***, ***merc-c.***, ***mur-ac.***, ox-ac., ***plb.***, verat., zinc.
walk, when he tries to - ***plb.***

FLUTTERING, thighs - cench.

FORMICATION - aeth., arn., ***ars.,*** aster., bov., **CALC.,** ***calc-p.,*** caps., caust., euphr., graph., ***helo.,*** hep., lachn., nit-ac., op., ***plat.,*** rhod., rumx., sabad., **SEC.,** ***sep.,*** stry., sulph.
bones - ***guai.***
crossing legs - plat.
evening, in bed - sulph.
menses, during - graph., ***puls.***
night in bed - helo.
paralyzed limb - ***nux-v.***
riding - ***calc-p.,*** rumx.
sitting, while - kali-c., plat.
after - ***calc-p.,*** sep.
standing - hep.
walking - hep.

formication, calves - agar., alum., ant-c., bar-c., cast., caust., ***cham.,*** coloc., ip., lach., nux-v., onos., plb., rhus-v., sang., sol-n., spig., sulph., sul-ac., zinc.
evening - alum.
sitting, while - bar-c.
standing, while - verat.
walking, while - sul-ac.
in open air, after - nux-v.

formication, lower - agar., alum., amyg., apis, arg-m., ***arg-n., arn.,*** ars., aster., bar-c., bell., bov., calc., ***calc-p.,*** caps., carb-o., carb-s., caust., graph., guai., ***hep.,*** jatr., ***kali-c.,*** kreos., lac-ac., lach., lil-t., morph., naja, nicc., **NUX-V.,** op., pall., ***ph-ac.,*** phos., pic-ac., ***plat.,*** puls., ***rhod.,*** **SEC., SEP.,** stann., staph., stram., sulph., sul-ac., ***tab.,*** tarent., tax., verat., ***zinc.***
evening - lac-ac., ***plat.,*** sep.
walking - graph.
extending upwards - bell.
night in bed - ***zinc.***
rising, from seat - sulph.
sitting - guai., ol-an., ***plat.***

formication, thighs - acon., arg-m., ars., caust., euph., ***guai.,*** hydr-ac., ***nat-c.,*** nit-ac., ***pall.,*** phos., **SEC.,** sep., spig., staph., stram., sul-ac.
extending to, abdomen - ars.
to, toes - guai., sep.
numb while sitting - hep.
sitting - guai.

formication, tibia - sul-ac.

FULLNESS, veins of legs - ***calc., carb-v., chin-s.,*** puls., sulph., ***vip.***

fullness, lower, legs - bell., clem., com., ham., mez., nat-c., osm., ph-ac., staph.
fever, during - **CHIN-S.**
hanging down, when - ***carb-v.***
joints - ***ham.***
menses, during - ambr.

FUNGUS, thighs, haematodes - ***phos.,*** sang.

GANGRENE - anthr., ***ars.,*** crot-h., lach., sec.

gangrene, lower - ***anthr.,*** crot-h., iod., ***sec.***

gangrene, thighs - crot-h., ***sec.***

GNAWING, pain - alum., ***ars., bell.,*** lyc., nit-ac., plat., ran-s., ruta.
walking, amel. - **BELL.**

gnawing, calves - euph.

gnawing, lower - alum., ars., ***aur.,*** bell., brom., ***kali-i.,*** nat-c., nit-ac., phys., stront-c., tarax.
bones - dros.
standing, while - tarax.

gnawing, thighs - berb., benz-ac., kali-bi., kreos., par., stront-c., stry.
anterior part - berb.
bone, in - bell., dros., led., nit-ac.
marrow - bell., stront.
middle of, evening, while sitting - kali-i.
outer side - kreos.
while sitting - kreos.
posterior part - berb., par.

gnawing, tibia - ***carb-an., kali-i.,*** nit-ac.

GROWING pains - acon., agar., bell., calc., **CALC-P.,** ***ferr-ac., guai.,*** mang., ol-an., **PH-AC.,** phos., sil.
legs, in - bell., **CALC-P.,** cimic., ***eup-per.,*** **GUAI.,** kali-p., mag-aust., mag-p., mang., nat-p., **PH-AC.**
night, at - calc-p.

GOOSEBUMPS - bapt., chin-a., rhod.

goosebumps, lower - calc., rhod., staph.

goosebumps, thighs - aur., calc., ign., spig., staph.

HEAT - acon., bapt., bor., bry., coloc., eupi., lil-t., mang., ***mez.,*** morph., nat-m., nit-ac., op., phys., plat., sol-t-ae., spig., stram., sulph., verat.
chilliness, after - nit-ac.
internal - staph.
inner side - mang.
joints, of - eupi.
left - cycl.
night - acon., plat.
1 a.m. - mang.
on waking - coloc., spig.
sensation - ***mez.***

heat, lower - acon., apoc., ars., bapt., berb., bov., calc., ***calc-p.,*** cic., ***crot-c.,*** crot-h., crot-t., cycl., graph., guai., ***ham.,*** hyos., iod., kali-br., lil-t., ***lyc.,*** mang., ***meph.,*** mez., ***nat-s.,*** nit-ac., ox-ac., ph-ac., spig., staph., sulph., ***verat.***
afternoon, 3 p.m. - gels.
alternately hot and cold - ***verat.***
dry - sulph.
evening - cycl., ***nat-s.***
8 p.m. - sulph.
flushes - cob.
here and there - graph.
midnight, after - nit-ac.
morning - nat-s., plat.
night - ***meph.***
after going to bed - fago.
sitting agg. - berb.
uncovers them - crot-c.
walking, after - rhus-t.

heat, thighs - all-c., bor., carb-o., clem., coc-c., dros., kali-c., murx., nit-ac., rhus-t., stann., staph., sulph., zinc.

heat, thighs
alternating with coldness - nit-ac.
cold, back, with - ***sulph.***
hands and feet, with - **THUJ.**
creeping - chin.
dry - ***sulph.***
internal - chin., staph.
night - nit-ac.
pregnancy, during - podo.
prickling - osm.
sitting, after, agg. - graph.
stool, after - ***lyc.,*** trom.

HEAVINESS, tired legs - acet-ac., acon., ***agar.,*** aloe, all-s., **ALUM.,** alumn., ambr., am-c., am-m., anac., ang., ant-t., ***aran.,*** **ARG-M.,** ***arg-n., arn., ars.,*** asaf., asar., bar-c., ***bell.,*** **BERB.,** bov., brom., bry., cact., cahin., **CALC.,** calc-ar., calc-p., calc-s., ***camph.,*** **CANN-I.,** caps., ***carb-ac., carb-s.,*** **CARB-V.,** cast., caust., cham., ***chel.,*** chin., chin-a., cic., ***cimx.,*** clem., **COCC.,** coc-c., ***coloc.,*** colch., **CON.,** cor-r., crot-h., dig., dios., ***dulc.,*** eupi., ferr-i., fl-ac., **GELS.,** gins., ***graph.,*** guai., ***ham., hell., hep., ign.,*** ind., indg., iod., ip., ***kali-ar.,*** kali-bi., ***kali-c.,*** kali-n., **KALI-P.,** kali-s., kreos., **LACH.,** laur., ***lec.,*** led., ***lyc.,*** lyss., ***mag-m., med., merc., merc-c., merc-i-f., mez.,*** murx., nat-a., **NAT-C.,** ***nat-m.,*** nat-p., nat-s., ***nit-ac., nux-m., nux-v., onos.,*** op., osm., ***petr., ph-ac., phos.,*** **PIC-AC.,** phyt., ***plat.,*** plb., ptel., ***puls.,*** rhod., rat., **RHUS-T.,** ***ruta., sabad.,*** sanic., sars., sec., senec., ***seneg., sep.,*** **SIL.,** sin-a., spig., spong., ***stann.,*** staph., stram., stry., **SULPH.,** sul-ac., ***tarent., thuj.,*** til., verat., verb., xan., ***zinc.***
afternoon - **ARG-N.,** bry., fago., nux-v., phyt., zinc.
3 p.m. - plan.
4 p.m. - kali-cy.
air, open - graph.
ascending, steps - bry., lyc., ***med.,*** phos., stann., thuj., verb.
bones, sitting - sulph.
constipation - tep.
daytime - ***puls.***
descending, steps - verb.
dinner, after - kali-n., sulph.
evening - alum., am-c., clem., ***coloc.,*** fago., kali-n., nat-m., nicc., op., thuj.
6 p.m. - op.
9 p.m. - pic-ac.
bed, in - indg.
exertion, after - **CON., GELS., LACH., PIC-AC., RHUS-T.**
fatigue, as from - arg-n., calc., chen-a., con., ***gels.,*** kreos., lact., lach., mag-m., merc-i-f., mosch., murx., nat-s., pic-ac., psor., puls., rhus-t., ruta., sulph.
forenoon - ***merc.,*** puls.
11 a.m. - zing.
humiliation, after - puls.
joints - calc., nit-ac., ph-ac.
lying, while - nit-ac.

HEAVINESS, tired legs
menses, during - ***am-c.,*** calc-p., cocc., ***graph.,*** kali-n., nicc., nit-ac., ***sep.,*** sulph., ***zinc.***
after - nat-m.
before - ***carl., con., graph.,*** lach., ***lyc.,*** phel.
suppressed - ***graph.,*** nat-m., nux-v., phos., rhus-t., ruta., verat.
midnight, after - crot-t.
morning - ambr., ars., calc., card-m., kreos., lec., mur-ac., phos., ***sil.,*** sulph., verat.
bed, in - caust., mag-m., sulph., zinc.
waking, on - calc., phos., sumb.
motion - **LACH.**
amel. - mag-c., nat-m., nit-ac.
night - carb-an., carb-v., caust., petr., ***sulph.,*** thuj.
bed, in - sulph.
periodical - ***aran.***
riding, during - rumx.
rising, from sitting - mag-c.
sitting, while - **ALUM.,** croc., mag-c., mag-m., nat-c., nit-ac., plat., sars., spig., stann.
sleep, after - ***sep.***
standing, while - bry., stann., sulph., valer.
stretching, leg amel. - anac.
vexation, after - lyc., nux-v.
walking, while - anac., arn., bell., **BERB.,** bry., ***calc.,*** **CANN-I., CARB-V.,** chin., chin-s., **CON.,** crot-t., **GELS.,** hep., kali-c., **LACH.,** ***lec.,*** lyc., ***mag-m., med.,*** petr., phos., pip-m., puls., rhod., rhus-t., sars., spig., ***stann., sulph.,*** thuj., zinc.
after - anac., **ARG-M.,** kali-bi., kali-m., murx., ruta., sil., stann., ***sulph.***
air, in open - lyc., sil.
amel. - rat., rhod.
begining to - zinc.

heaviness, calves - agar., ***aloe, arg-n.,*** ars-i., berb., cham., euphr., kali-c., lyss., mag-m., plat., rhus-t., sep., stann., staph., sulph.

heaviness, lower - ***aeth., agar.,*** **ALUM.,** ***ambr.,*** am-c., am-m., ang., ant-t., ***arg-n.,*** ars., arum-t., asar., ***bell.,*** berb., ***bry.,*** brach., bufo, cact., cahin., ***calc., calc-p., camph.,*** **CANN-I.,** cann-s., ***carb-ac., carb-s., carb-v., caust., cham., chel., chin., cimx.,*** clem., ***colch., coloc.,*** croc., crot-t., cupr., dig., ***ferr.,*** ferr-p., ***gels., graph.,*** hep., ind., ***kali-bi., kali-c.,*** kali-n., lach., led., lyc., ***lyss., mag-m., med., merc.,*** nat-a., ***nat-c., nat-m.,*** nat-p., nit-ac., **NUX-M.,** ***nux-v., onos., petr., phos., phyt., pic-ac.,*** plat., ***plb., puls.,*** **RHUS-T.,** ruta., sarr., sars., sec., sep., ***sil.,*** spong., stann., stront-c., ***sulph.,*** tarax., ***tarent.,*** thuj., valer., verat., verb., zinc.
afternoon - nat-c.
ascending steps - hep., **NAT-M.,** ***phos.***
chill, before - ***cimx.***
crossing legs - bell., stann., verb.
eating, after - arn., dros.
evening - alum., am-c., ***apis,*** puls., uran.
exertion agg. - **GELS.,** pic-ac.
forenoon - puls.

heaviness, lower
left - thuj.
menses, during - ***calc-p.,*** nicc., ***sars.***
before - ***lyc.***
morning - ars.
night - ***caust.,*** kali-c.
painful - plat.
rest, during - nit-ac.
rising, from sitting - nit-ac.
sitting, while - **ALUM.,** ***mag-m.,*** plat., rhus-t., spig., thuj.
standing - alum., samb.
walking, while - alum., bell., coloc., ***nat-c.,*** rhus-t., stann., ***sulph.***
after - kali-n., nit-ac.
amel. - kali-n., nit-ac., rhus-t., sec.

heaviness, thighs - agar., ***agn.,*** am-c., **ANG.,** aran., ***arn.,*** ars., asar., ***bell., bry., calc.,*** camph., caust., cham., ***chin.,*** croc., crot-t., ***dulc.,*** graph., ***guai.,*** hell., ***ip., kali-c.,*** lach., lyss., ***lyc.,*** mag-c., mag-m., ***merc.,*** murx., nat-s., nux-v., petr., ph-ac., phos., ***puls.,*** rheum, ***rhod., sars., sep.,*** squil., ***stann., thuj.,*** verb., zinc.
ascending, steps - asar.
lying - staph.
menses, during - ***am-c.,*** carb-an., ***cast.,*** cub., ***graph.,*** nit-ac., ***sars.***
before - bell., brom., carb-an., cocc., kali-n., nux-m.
midnight, after - crot-t.
morning - ***calc.,*** kali-c.
night - kali-c., sep.
paralytic - kali-c., kali-n.
paroxysmal - thuj.
right - rat.
sitting, while - kali-c., kali-n., mag-c., rat., sars.
stool, after - lyc.
walking - bell., cic., mag-c., sars., zinc.
after - ang.

heaviness, tibia - dig., kali-n., spong.

HERNIA, thighs, femoral - ***lyc.,*** nux-v.

HERPES - ***alum.,*** **BOV.,** caust., clem., com., **GRAPH.,** kali-c., lach., led., **LYC., MERC.,** mur-ac., **NAT-M.,** nicc., ***petr.,*** sars., ***sep.,*** sil., staph., **TELL.,** zinc.

herpes, calves - cycl., ***lyc.,*** sars.

herpes, lower - ars., calc., calc-p., com., ***graph.,*** kali-c., ***lach.,*** lyc., lyss., mag-c., merc., nat-m., ***petr.,*** sars., ***sep.,*** staph., ***zinc.***

herpes, thighs - ***clem., graph.,*** kali-c., ***lyc.,*** **MERC.,** mur-ac., **NAT-M.,** nit-ac., petr., sars., ***sep.,*** staph., zinc.

HYPERTROPHY, tibia (see Thick) - calc-p., ***sil.***

INCOORDINATION, (see Ataxia) - ***alum.,*** bell., chlol., crot-c., ***nux-m., onos., phos., plb., sil., sulph.***

INDURATION, lower, muscles - graph., ***mag-c.,*** sulph.

INFILTRATION, with bloody serum - dig.

INFLAMMATION, psoas, muscles - ***calc.***
psoitis, if suppuration seems impending, also if pelvic bones are involved - asaf.

inflammation, lower - ***acon., bor.,*** bov., ***calc.,*** com., nat-c., sulph.
dancing, after - bor.
nosebleed, with - bor.
periosteum - ***aur.,*** **ASAF.,** ***kali-bi.,*** **LED.,** ***merc., ph-ac.,*** **PHOS.,** sil., still., ***sulph.***

inflammation, thighs - nat-c., rhus-t., ***sil.***

inflammation, tibia - ***asaf., aur., calc., guai.,*** hecla., kali-i., lach., **PH-AC., PHOS., SIL.,** ***still.,*** stront.
periosteum of femur - ***aur., mez., phyt.***

ITCHING - **AGAR.,** aloe, ***alum.,*** alumn., ***ambr., am-c.,*** am-m., anac., ***ant-c.,*** ant-s., ant-t., **APIS,** arn., **ARS.,** ars-i., arund., asaf., asc-t., aster., aur., ***bar-c.,*** bell., berb., ***bism., bov.,*** brach., bry., bufo, cact., ***calc.,*** calc-i., cann-i., cann-s., canth., carb-ac., carb-s., **CARB-V., CAUST.,** cham., **CHEL.,** chin., chin-a., cinnb., clem., ***cocc.,*** coc-c., coloc., com., con., corn., crot-c., cupr., cycl., dig., dios., dulc., elaps, euphr., fago., gins., **GRAPH.,** gran., grat., hep., hura, ign., iod., ir-foe., jug-c., jug-r., kali-ar., kali-bi., kali-c., kali-i., kali-n., kali-p., kalm., lach., lachn., lact., laur., led., lith., **LYC.,** mag-c., mag-m., mag-s., mang., **MERC.,** merc-i-f., **MEZ.,** mur-ac., nat-a., nat-c., **NAT-M.,** nat-p., ***nat-s.,*** nicc., ***nit-ac.,*** nux-v., ol-an., ***olnd.,*** osm., paeon., pall., ***petr.,*** ph-ac., ***phos.,*** phyt., plat., plb., prun., **PSOR., PULS.,** ran-b., ran-s., **RHUS-T.,** rhus-v., rumx., ruta., sabad., sars., sec., sel., seneg., **SEP., SIL.,** ***spig.,*** **SPONG.,** stann., **STAPH.,** stram., **SULPH.,** stront-c., stry., tab., **TARENT.,** tarax., ***tell.,*** thea., ther., ***thuj.,*** til., verat., ***zinc.***
afternoon - coc-c., fago., nat-c.
2 p.m. - ol-an.
5 p.m. - fago.
air, open, in - alum., aster., rumx., still.
bed, in - cupr-ar., kali-c., lyc., merc-i-f., nux-v., ***puls.,*** sil., staph., tarax., til., zinc.
biting - alum., bell., ***berb.,*** spig., spong.
boil, at the site of a previous - graph.
burning - ***agar.,*** alum., anac., apis, ***berb.,*** calc., dulc., hep., kali-n., led., lith., mez., mur-ac., nat-c., nit-ac., nux-v., paeon., rhus-t., sars.
asleep, on falling - mur-ac.
scratching, after - mag-c.
spots, in - rhus-t.
chilly, on becoming - rhus-t.
cold, on becoming - dios., tarent.
corrosive - ars., bufo, chel., euph., led., tax.
creeping - ars.
daytime - calc., ind.
dinner, after - laur., mag-c.
dressing, while - nux-v.
evening - alum., am-m., aster., clem., cycl., fago., ind., kali-c., kali-n., lyc., mag-c., mag-m., mang., merc., mez., nat-m., ***nat-s.,*** nicc., nit-ac., nux-v., phos., rhus-v., rumx., sars., sel., sep., stront-c., sulph., tarax., tell., thuj., zinc.

ITCHING, general
evening, 6 p.m. - aster., fago.
8 p.m. - con.
10 p.m. - plan.
frozen, as if - kali-c.
heat, after - ***rhus-v.,*** **SULPH.**
menses, during - inul.
midnight - puls.
morning - alumn., ant-c., rumx., sabad., sars., sep., sulph.
motion amel. - mur-ac., olnd., psor., spig.
night - am-m., bar-c., canth., cinnb., cocc., cupr-ar., dig., hep., hura, merc-i-f., ***mez.,*** nat-m., phos., phyt., **RHUS-T.,** rhus-v., rumx., sabad., ***sulph.,*** til., zinc.
noon - nicc.
pain, during - fl-ac.
paroxysms - corn.
prickling - crot-t.
rubbing, agg. - corn.
amel. - cupr., paeon.
scratching, agg. - ***alum., bism.,*** corn., ***led.***
amel. - alum., bov., cann-i., chin., kali-c., laur., led., mag-c., mag-m., nat-c., nat-s., nicc., olnd., pall., tarax., thuj.
sitting - asaf., chin., fago.
sleep, on going to - mag-m., mur-ac., sep.
spots, in - calc., graph., osm., phos., sars.
standing, while - mang., verat.
sticking - ant-c., ***berb.,*** calc., caust., graph., lach., plat., rhus-t., staph., zinc.
spots, in - calc.
stinging - dios., merc-i-f.
tickling - alum., bry., cocc., coloc., euph., ign., kali-n., lach., pall.
tingling - com.
touch agg. - nat-m.
undressing, while - agar., apis, cact., cupr., cupr-ar., dios., fago., ham., jug-r., mag-c., **NAT-S.,** ***rumx.,*** still.
varices - graph.
voluptuous - euphr., rat., ***sulph.***
waking, on - sulph.
walking, while - asaf., chel., chin., cocc., dios., mur-ac., nux-v., sulph.
after - alum.
warm bed agg. - ***agar., alum.,*** led., ***sulph.***
warmth, agg. - rhus-v.
amel. - cocc.
wine, after - psor.

itching, calves - aloe, alum., berb., cact., calc., carb-ac., carb-s., **CAUST.,** chel., cinnb., cocc., crot-c., cycl., euphr., graph., ***hep.,*** hura, ip., kali-bi., laur., lyc., mag-c., mag-m., ***mang.,*** mez., mur-ac., nat-c., nat-m., ***nit-ac.,*** ol-an., paeon., phos., phyt., rhus-t., rumx., sabad., ***sars., sulph.,*** sul-i., tarax., ther., thuj., verat., verat-v., zinc.
bleeding, after scratching - cycl., mez.
burning - berb., mez.
after scratching - cycl., sars.
evening - cycl., daph., euphr., sars.
walking, while - euphr.
lying, down, on - tarax.
morning - cycl., rumx., sars.

itching, calves
night - rumx., ***zinc.***
rubbing, amel. - paeon.
scratching, amel. - laur., mag-c., mag-m., nat-c.
spots, in - graph., sars.
standing - verat.
undressing - cact.
voluptuous - euphr., ***mang.***
walking, while - cocc.

itching, lower - **AGAR.,** aloe, ***alum.,*** anac., ant-t., arund., asc-t., aster., bell., berb., bism., brom., bufo, cact., **CALC., CAUST.,** chel., coc-c., coloc., con., corn., crot-h., cupr-ar., dulc., euph., hura, ir-foe., iod., jug-r., kali-bi., kali-c., kali-n., kali-p., lach., laur., ***lyc.,*** merc., **MEZ.,** nat-c., nat-m., nicc., nux-v., osm., pall., ***petr., phos.,*** phyt., rumx., ***rhus-t.,*** sabad., sars., seneg., **SIL.,** staph., stram., stront-c., **SULPH.,** tarent., thuj., verat., zinc.
afternoon - coc-c., fago.
air, open, in - aster.
atmosphere, exposure to - still.
bed, in - carb-s., ***cupr-ar.,*** sulph.
burning - agar., calc., kali-c.
cold, when - dios.
corrosive - bism., bufo., dig., euph., ph-ac.
evening - agar., fago., kali-c., kali-n., rumx., sulph.
6 p.m. - aster.
8 p.m. - con.
in bed - ambr., staph.
menses, during - inul.
morning - sabad.
walking, after - sulph.
night - cupr-ar., hura, ***mez.,*** nat-m., phyt., rumx., **RHUS-T., SULPH.**
paroxysms - corn.
rubbing, agg. - corn.
amel. - cupr-ar.
scratching, amel. - laur.
spots - calc.
touch, agg. - nat-m.
touching, foot, on - **KALI-C.**
undressing, agg. - agar., cact., cupr-ar., dios., ***rumx.***
waking, on - ***sulph.***

itching, thighs - agar., ***alum.,*** anac., ang., ant-c., ***ars.,*** ars-h., asc-t., aster., **BAR-C.,** ***bar-m.,*** berb., bry., **CALC.,** carb-ac., carb-s., ***carb-v., caust.,*** chin., cinnb., clem., con., corn., crot-c., crot-t., dios., ***euph.,*** fago., gran., ***guai.,*** kali-c., ***kali-i.,*** kali-n., lach., lachn., lith., lyc., lyss., mag-m., merc., mur-ac., nat-m., nit-ac., nux-v., osm., pall., petr., phos., plb., ran-b., rhus-v., ***sars.,*** sep., sil., ***spig.,*** spong., stann., stront-c., **SULPH.,** tab., thea., ***thuj.,*** til., ***zinc.***
afternoon - nat-c.
5 p.m. - dios., fago.
air, open, in - aster.
between - ars., ***carb-v.,*** cinnb., ***kali-c.,*** nat-m., nit-ac., petr., rhod., stann., sulph.
biting - alum., berb., chel., lyc., spig.
boil, at site of a previous - graph.

itching, thighs
burning - agar., ***alum.,*** anac., apis, ***bar-c.,*** berb., calc., cic., dulc., led., mang., nux-v., rhus-t., sars.
scratching, after - mag-m., phos., samb.
spots in - rhus-t.
chilly, becoming - dios.
corrosive - agar., ars., chel., dig., euph., led., ph-ac., tarax.
crawling - sulph.
daytime - calc.
evening - anac., ***ant-c.,*** aster., fago., lyc., stront-c., ***zinc.***
bed, in - nux-v., sil., zinc.
open air - aster.
sleep, before going to - mag-c.
inner side - alum., ***cinnb.,*** mang., samb., sil., sulph.
itch-like - ol-an.
morning dressing while - mag-c., nux-v.
near genital organs - ars., bar-c., ***carb-v.,*** caust., ***graph.,*** kali-c., lyc., mag-m., rhus-t., sabin.
night - ***bar-c.,*** dulc., led., nit-ac., rhus-v., **SULPH.,** til., zinc.
undressing - nux-v.
nodules, scratching, after - mag-m.
outer, side - mag-m., nit-ac., stann., zinc.
pain, during - fl-ac.
painful, scratching, after - euphr.
rubbing amel. - anac., ang.
scratching, agg. - ars., mag-m.
amel. - ***alum.,*** led., pall.
does not amel. - mag-m., nit-ac.
sleep, on going to - sep.
spots - phos.
sticking - ant-c., berb., calc., caust., graph., rhus-t., stann.
spots, in - calc.
tickling - cocc., coloc., kali-n., lach., pall.
walking, while - euphr., nux-v.
warmth of bed - ***alum.,*** bar-c., ***caust., sulph.***

itching, tibia, over - ant-c., aster., bism., cact., ***calc.,*** chel., cocc., crot-t., grat., hep., kali-c., kali-n., lach., mag-m., ***mang., nit-ac., ph-ac.,*** phos., plb., ***rumx.,*** sars., sep., spig., staph., stront.

JERKING, of - ***agar., alum.,*** ambr., am-c., anac., ant-t., apoc., ***arg-m., arg-n., ars.,*** asaf., bar-c., berb., ***carb-s.,*** carb-v., ***calc.,*** chel., chin-s., **CIC., CINA,** cinnb., cocc., coff., crot-h., ***cupr., gels., glon.,*** guare., helo., hep., ***ign., kali-c.,*** kali-i., ***lil-t., lyc.,*** mag-c., ***manc.,*** meny., merc., ***mygal., nat-a., nat-c., nat-m.,*** nit-ac., onos., **NUX-V.,** ***op.,*** ph-ac., ***phos., plat.,*** puls., sep., sil., squil., stann., **STRAM.,** stront-c., **SULPH.,** ***sul-ac., tarent.,*** thuj., ***verat.,*** **ZINC.**
afternoon - ***ars.***
coughing while sitting - ***stram.***
evening - am-c., cinnb., hep., mag-c.
forenoon - sep.
hang down, must, let leg - ***verat.***
left - cod., mag-c., nat-c., nit-ac., sep.

JERKING, of
lying, while - alum., am-c., anac., arg-n., ***verat.***
on back - nat-s.
motion, on - mang.
amel. - hep., ***thuj.,*** valer.
night - ***arg-n., phos.***
pain, in thigh, from - lyc.
painful - hep., ***meny.***
right - meny., mez., sep., zinc.
when a stranger enters the room - zinc.
when falling asleep - ***arg-m.***
sitting, when - ***ars.,*** lyc., ***meny.,*** sep.
sleep, during - ***ant-t., arg-n.,*** cinnb., con., cupr., ***kali-c., lyc.,*** mag-c., nat-c., ***nat-m.,*** nit-ac., ph-ac., ***phos., sulph.,*** **ZINC.**
on going to - ***agar., anac., arg-m.,*** cham., hyper., **KALI-C.,** mag-c., nat-c., ***nat-m., sulph., thuj., zinc.***
on going to, one leg is jerking, up - sulph.
sleeplessness, during - thuj.
standing, while - mygal.
stepping out, on - coff., rhus-t.
stitches, in first toe, from - sil.

jerking, calves - ***graph.,*** **OP.,** tarax.

jerking, lower - ***agar., arg-n.,*** ars., carb-v., dig., hyper., ***kali-i.,*** lyc., ***meny.,*** nat-c., ***phos.,*** plat., sep., sil., sul-ac.
afternoon - ars.
drawing pain, after - phos.
falling asleep - ***ars.,*** hyper., **KALI-C.,** nat-c., sep.
lying on back, while - nat-s.
motion, amel. - carb-v.
sitting, when - ars., carb-v., ***meny.***
sleep, during - cinnb.
walking - phos.

jerking, thighs - ***arg-n.,*** caps., kali-bi., ***kali-c., kali-i.,*** lach., lact., laur., lyc., ***meny.,*** nat-c., nat-m., nux-v., phos., plat., rhus-t., sep., stram.
evening - kali-bi.
posterior part - manc., phos
on walking - phos.
right - lyc., ***meny.***
drawing, up leg or standing amel. - ***meny.***
sitting, while - meny.
walking, when - sep.

LAMENESS - ***aesc.,*** apis, arn., ars., ***bell.,*** berb., calc-p., carb-v., caust., **COLCH.,** dig., fl-ac., iod., lyc., **NAT-M.,** ox-ac., ph-ac., ***phos., plb., rhus-t.,*** sep., sil., stann., **SULPH.,** zinc.
afternoon - myric.
chill, during - ign., ***lyc., rhus-t., tub.***
evening - ***lyc.***
fever, during - ***rhus-t., tub.***
menses, during - mag-m., phos.
before - nit-ac.
morning - nat-m., ***sil.***
suppressed perspiration - **COLCH., RHUS-T.**

LAMENESS, general
walking, while - ammc., bell., calc., carb-an., ***colch.,*** coloc., dros., eup-per., kali-i., lyc., nit-ac., puls., ***rhus-t.,*** zinc.
lameness, lower - carb-v., hep.
lameness, thighs - aloe, ***ars., ars-m.,*** aur., bar-c., ***carb-v.,*** card-m., ***calc.,*** caust., ***chin.,*** cinnb., cocc., dros., hep., hyper., ***iris, kali-c.,*** lyss., ***merc.,*** nux-v., puls., sarr., sil., ***stann.,*** sulph., ***zinc.***
ascending stairs - bar-c.
flatus, from - carb-v.
menses, during - ***carb-an.***
motion amel. - cocc.
involuntary - op.
right - sil.
rising from seat - sil.
walking, on - bar-c., cinnb., zinc.
amel. - sil.
in open air - nux-v.

LIGHTNESS, sensation of - ***ph-ac.,*** stict.
walking, after - valer.

LIMPING - abrot., acon., ant-c., ***bell., calc.,*** **CAUST.,** ***dros.,*** hep., kali-bi., ***kali-c.,*** lyc., ***merc.,*** nit-ac., phos., **RUTA.,** sabin., sep., sulph.
pain in knee - spig.
spontaneous - **APIS.,** bell., ***coloc.,*** lyc., ruta., zinc.

LOCOMOTOR, ataxia (see Ataxia)

LONGER, sensation, lower - ***kali-c.,*** kreos., stram., thuj.
seems at night on lying down - carb-an.

LOOSE, as if flesh were - thigh - nat-c.

LUMPS, in, calves - merc., nit-ac.

MILK, leg (see Phelbitis)

MOTION, chorea like - agar., ***arg-n.,*** coff., ***mygal.***
control, loss of - alum., cann-i., chlor., ***gels.,*** glon., ***plb.,*** stram.
convulsive - ***merc-c., mygal., plb.,*** stram.
difficult - carb-s., ***plb.***
involuntary - merc., stram.
with pain - cocc.
slow - merc.
motion, lower - caust.
automatic - hell.
one, of - hell.
awkward - con.
convulsive - acet-ac., agar., ***caust.,*** merc-c., ***mygal.,*** op., plb., sul-ac.
difficult - camph., chel., kali-n., nat-m., ox-ac., pic-ac., **PLB.**
downward, on sneezing - spig.
dread of - ham.
involuntary - bry., crot-c., stict.
night - ***stict.***
night, in sleep - ***caust.***
wavelike - sep.
motion, thighs, involuntary - op.

MOUSE, sensation of, running up - ***calc., sep.,*** **SULPH.**

NODULES - ***agar.,*** carb-an., carb-v., ***caust.,*** chin., dulc., hep., kali-c., mag-m., mang., merc., mez., petr., rhod., stront-c., thuj.
pressing and tearing - kali-c.
nodules, lower - agar., ***merc.***

NUMBNESS, (see Tingling) - acon., acet-ac., agar., ail., ***alum.,*** alumn., ***ambr.,*** ant-c., ant-t., ***apis, arg-m., arg-n.,*** ars., ars-i., aster., aur., berb., bov., bufo, **CALC.,** ***calc-p.,*** calc-s., cann-i., ***canth., carb-an.,*** carb-s., carb-v., caust., ***chel.,*** chin., chin-a., ***chin-s.,*** cic., cimic., cocc., colch., ***con.,*** croc., cupr., cupr-ar., euph., euphr., ***fl-ac.,*** **GRAPH.,** guare., ign., iod., kali-ar., ***kali-br.,*** **KALI-C.,** kali-n., kali-p., ***kali-s.,*** kreos., lac-c., lact., led., ***lyc.,*** lyss., ***merc.,*** merc-c., mez., morph., mosch., naja, nat-m., nat-s., nux-m., ***nux-v., onos.,*** ox-ac., olnd., op., ***petr.,*** ph-ac., ***phos., pic-ac.,*** plat., **PLB.,** psor., **PULS.,** rheum, ***rhod., rhus-t., sec., sep.,*** sil., ***spong.,*** squil., sulph., sul-ac., **TARENT.,** ter., teucr., thuj., vip.
afternoon, sitting, while - teucr.
ascending stairs - nux-m.
chill, during - con.
crossing the legs, when - agar., ang., ***carb-an., crot-h.,*** fl-ac., laur., plat., rheum, sep., squil.
evening - mez., sil., sulph.
sitting, while - sil.
exertion, during, cramp-like numbness. - alum.
extending to waist-line - ***calc-p.***
gouty limbs - ***acon.***
joints - mosch.
kneeling, after - op.
lain on - alumn., am-c., bufo, ***carb-an., rhus-t.***
left - cupr-ar., kreos., lac-c., ***meny.,*** nat-m., phos., sep., sulph.
lying, while - aur., kali-c., sulph.
meals, after - kali-c.
menses, during - ***kali-n.,*** **PULS.,** ***sec.***
before - ang.
morning - phos.
bed, in - ***aur., sulph.,*** teucr.
night - alum., ***calc-p.,*** graph., ph-ac.
pain after the pain has left - cocc.
resting, after - op.
riding, while - ***calc-p.***
right - alumn., **KALI-C.,** sil., sul-ac., sulph.
and left arm - tarent.
side, affected ovary - apis.
siesta, during - nat-m.
sitting, while - ***ant-c., ant-t.,*** calc., ***calc-p.,*** chin., con., crot-h., euph., euphr., ***graph.,*** kali-c., lyc., lyss., nux-v., ph-ac., plat., sep., sil., sulph., teucr.
after - sep.
standing, while - sep.
stool, after - trio.
walking while - ***alum.,*** graph., **KALI-N.,** lyc., ***plb., rhus-t., sep., thuj.***

numbness, calves - acon., ars., berb., ***bry.,*** cham., ***coloc.,*** dulc., graph., lach., nux-v., phos., sil., verat-v.
afternoon - dulc.
evening - dulc.

numbness, lower - acet-ac., ***acon.,*** agar., ail., aloe, ***alum.,*** alumn., ambr., ***am-c.,*** am-m., anac., anan., ang., ***ant-c.,*** ant-t., ***apis, aran., arg-m., arg-n.,*** arn., ***ars.,*** ars-i., asar., aster., atro., bapt., bell., bor., bov., bufo, cact., ***carc., calc-p.,*** camph., canth., ***carb-an., carb-s.,*** carb-v., ***caust.,*** cedr., cham., chin., chin-s., ***cocc., coloc.,*** **CON.,** ***crot-h.,*** cupr., dios., dulc., euph., eup-per., ***eup-pur.,*** fago., ferr., ferr-ar., ferr-i., ferr-p., glon., **GRAPH.,** ***ham., hyper.,*** ign., iod., ***kali-c.,*** kali-p., lac-c., lach., lact., laur., **LYC.,** mag-m., med., ***merc., merc-c.,*** mez., ***nat-m.,*** nit-ac., nux-m., **NUX-V.,** ***onos., op., ox-ac.,*** petr., ***phos., phys., phyt.,*** pic-ac., **PLAT.,** plb., ***psor., puls.,*** rhod., **RHUS-T.,** rumx., samb., sec., **SIL.,** stram., sulph., tab., ***tarent.,*** thuj., verat-v., vip., zinc.
afternoon - alum., bov., fago., nicc.
during sleep, sitting - alum.
air, open, amel. - pic-ac.
bed, in - plat., zinc.
bones - graph.
chill, during - eup-pur., ***nux-v.***
cold weather agg. - apis
convulsion, before - plb.
crossing, while - ***agar.,*** carb-an., ***crot-h.,*** laur., phos., sep.
daytime - ***carb-an.***
evening - ***calc.,*** hyper., merc-c., ***plat.,*** puls.
in bed - nit-ac.
while lying on it - alum.
while sitting - ***calc.,*** dios., graph., ***plat.***
excitement, during - ***sulph.***
gouty - ***acon.***
lain on - am-c.
left - ***arg-n.,*** asar., bor., cann-i., ***crot-t.,*** dios., fl-ac., ***hyper.,*** lac-c., ***lil-t.,*** med., nicc., onos., ***phos.,*** puls., sep., stram.
lying, on back, while - nicc.
lying, on left side, while - ***phos.***
lying, while - aloe, bell., phos., puls., sumb.
on it while - alumn.
menses, during - **PULS.**
morning - ***ambr.,*** caust., dios., hep., nicc.
bed, in - ***ambr.,*** hep., nicc.
motion, during - laur.
amel. - mag-m., puls.
night - alum., ***am-c.,*** kali-c., nit-ac., phos., merc., zinc.
bed when going to - psor.
noon - spong.
after sleep - spong.
one, pain in the other - sil.
right - alumn., cedron., dios., eup-pur., kali-c., lac-c., lyss., nux-m., sabad., tarent., zinc.
then left - spong.
rising, when - puls., sulph.
from a seat - ***puls.,*** sulph.
rubbing amel. - stram.

numbness, lower
sitting, while - agar., am-c., am-m., ***ant-c.,*** bad., ***calc.,*** con., grat., ign., lyc., nicc., nux-v., ***phos., plat., puls.,*** sul-ac., thuj.
after - **ACON.,** ***graph.,*** lyss.
sleep, after - ***spong.***
standing, while - am-c., nux-v.
stretched, when - cham.
walking, while - ***coloc., rhus-t., sep.,*** thuj.
after sitting - nux-v.

numbness, thighs - acon., agar., ***ars.,*** asar., aster., berb., cadm-s., ***calc.,*** canth., carb-s., carb-v., chel., cic., ***con.,*** dig., dulc., euph., euphr., ***ferr., fl-ac.,*** glon., guai., ***graph.,*** hep., iod., kali-c., ***kreos., lac-d., med.,*** merc., nux-m., nux-v., oci., ox-ac., ***plb.,*** plat., podo., sec., ***spong.,*** tep.
anterior - chel., ***lac-d.,*** plan.
coldness, with - camph.
crossing legs - fl-ac., nux-m., rheum.
evening, when crossing legs - fl-ac.
extending to foot - con.
fever, during - spong.
lain on, one - tell.
left - med., phos.
lying, while - merc.
menses, before - podo.
morning, after, waking - kali-c.
in bed - aur.
night - plb.
outer side - caj., lac-d., ***plb.***
paralytic - acon., merc.
rising from a seat, on - chin., sulph.
sitting, while - graph., merc., puls., sil., thuj.
after - graph.
after eating - ign.
and bending knee - camph.
standing, while - chin.
walking, while - carb-v., sul-ac.

numbness, tibia, about - kalm., samb.

OOZING, lower edematous legs, from - ***graph.,*** **LYC.,** tarent-c.

OSGOOD-schlatter's, disease - ***calc-p., sil.***

OWN, felt as if not his own legs - ***agar., bapt.,*** op., sumb.

PAGET'S, disease - calc-p., sil.

PAIN, legs - abrot., aesc., **AGAR.,** alumn., ***anac.,*** ant-c., ***apis,*** arn., ***arg-m., ars., ars-h.,*** ars-i., ***aur.,*** bad., ***bell.,*** berb., ***bol., bov., bry.,*** cact., ***calc., calc-p., calc-s.,*** carb-ac., carb-s., ***carb-v., caust.,*** cedr., ***cham., chel., chin.,*** chin-a., cimic., ***coloc.,*** con., cupr., dig., echi., elaps, ***ferr.,*** ferr-ar., ***gels.,*** graph., ***guai.,*** ham., hell., ***indg.,*** kali-ar., kali-n., kali-p., ***kalm., lac-c.,*** lach., ***lil-t., lith., lyc.,*** mag-c., ***mag-p., med., merc.,*** merc-c., merc-i-f., merc-i-r., ***mez.,*** myric., nat-a., ***nat-c., nat-m., nit-ac., nux-v., petr.,*** ph-ac., ***phos., phys., phyt.,*** pic-ac., plan., ***plat.,*** **PLB.,** plumbg., prun., psor., ptel., ***puls., ran-b.,*** rhod., **RHUS-T.,** sang., sars., sec., seneg., ***sep., sil.,*** sol-n., **STANN.,** stront-c., ***sulph.,*** tarent., ***tarax.,*** ter., ***valer.,*** vip., xan., ***zinc.***

PAIN, legs
afternoon - bell., sang.
4 p.m. - ***coloc.***
air, open - ***cocc.,*** graph., ***mag-p.***
alternating with eye symptoms - kreos.
bathing - sulph.
bones - **AGAR.,** aran., carb-v., chin., coloc., con., guai., **IP.,** kali-bi., kali-c., lyc., mag-m., ***merc.,*** mez., olnd., petr., ***rhod.,*** sabin., ***sulph.,*** valer., zinc.
as if no marrow - sulph.
walking, while - mag-m.
chill, during - arn., **ARS.,** bry., caps., **CHIN.,** ***ferr.,*** led., lyc., mez., nat-m., **NUX-V.,** phos., **PYROG.,** ***puls., rhus-t.,*** sep., sulph., thuj.
before - ***nux-v.***
cold, amel. - ***apis, coff., guai., lac-c.,*** **LED., PULS., SEC.**
becoming - ***agar., ars.,*** bry., calc., ***dulc.,*** graph., ***kalm.,*** **NUX-V.,** ph-ac., ***phos.,*** **RHUS-T.,** ***tarent., tub.***
crossing limbs, in bed - arn., phos.
dancing amel. - ***sep.***
daytime - phos., plumbg.
eating, after - ***indg.,*** kali-c.
ending in jerking - ***sil.***
evening - ambr., calc., ferr-ma., kali-c., kali-n., **KALI-S.,** ***led., lyc.,*** mez., ***nat-m.,*** nat-s., nit-ac., plan., plumbg., puls., sep., sil., stront-c., zinc.
bed, in - carb-an., ferr-ma., ***kali-s.,*** phos., sulph.
exertion, from and as from - alum., bar-c., **CALC.,** ***caust.,*** ign., phos., **RHUS-T.,** stann.
extending, downward - aeth., aloe, am-c., am-m., ***apis,*** arg-n., ars., bar-c., berb., bry., ***calc.,*** cann-s., caps., carb-an., ***carb-v.,*** card-m., caust., cham., cocc., coloc., crot-h., dios., elat., eup-pur., ferr., gnaph., guai., hyper., ind., iris, kali-ar., kali-bi., kali-c., ***kali-i.,*** kali-p., **KALM.,** lac-c., **LACH.,** lyc., mag-p., mur-ac., nat-m., nit-ac., nux-m., ***nux-v.,*** ph-ac., ***phyt., plb.,*** puls., ***rhus-t.,*** ruta., sep., staph., still., ***sulph.,*** tell., ther., thuj., verat., zinc.
to foot - ***apis, colch.,*** lach., merc-i-f., phyt., sang., zinc.
upwards - acon., agar., cimic., eup-pur., guai., kali-p., lach., **LED.,** ***nux-v., phyt., plb.,*** podo., rhus-t., ruta., thuj., verat., zinc.
fatigue, as from - nat-m., phos., verat.
feather beds - ***asaf.***
flexing limb, on - nux-v.
gouty - ***bry.***
hang down, letting limb, amel. - bell., **CON.,** verat.
inner side of - petr.
jerking - ***valer.***
joints - ambr., arn., ***ars., bar-c.,*** bry., chel., cimic., ***dig., guai., kalm., led., lyc., mang.,*** phos., ***phyt., puls.,*** rhod., ***rhus-t.,*** sabin., ***sep., sil.,*** stront-c., ***sulph.,*** sul-ac.

PAIN, legs
labor-ike - aloe.
lying, while - carb-v.
amel. - am-m., ***dios.,*** ham.
menses, during - ambr., bell., bry., caul., ***cham.,*** con., cycl., graph., ham., kali-n., mosch., nux-m., nux-v., phos., rhus-t., sec., sep., spong., stram., verat.
before - berb., ***caul.,*** lach., nit-ac., nux-v., phos., sep., syph., vib.
midnight, 3 to 5 a.m. - ***kali-c.,*** sep.
4 a.m. - coloc.
after - ***ars.,*** nux-v.
before - **FERR.,** prun.
morning - anac., aur., caust., phos., sang., sil., stann., sulph.
9 a.m. - phys.
amel. - aur., colch., merc., mez., nux-v., syph.
bed, in - ant-t., bov., bry., nit-ac., sulph.
rising, on - phos., **RHUS-T.,** stann.
waking, on - aur., nat-m.
motion, agg. - acon., alum., ***apis,*** berb., **BRY.,** calc-p., carb-s., cocc., ***guai.,*** kali-p., kreos., ***lac-c., led.,*** mang., ***merc.,*** nat-s., ***nux-v., phos., phyt., plb.,*** puls., ***ran-b.,*** sulph.
amel. - ***agar., arg-m., aur-m-n., bell., calc.,*** calc-p., caps., ***coloc.,*** cupr., euph., **FERR.,** gels., ***indg., kali-bi.,*** kali-p., **KALI-S., LYC.,** ***merc.,*** merc-i-r., ***mur-ac., nat-s., ph-ac., plan.,*** **PULS.,** ***rat.,*** **RHOD., RHUS-T.,** ruta., ***sep.,*** stront-c., sulph., ***tarax.,*** **TUB.,** ***valer.,*** verat., ***zinc.***
move, beginning to - calc., carb-v., ***caust., ferr.,*** gels., indg., ***kali-p.,*** **LYC.,** mag-c., nit-ac., ***petr., plat., rhod.,*** **RHUS-T.,** thuj.
neuralgic - cupr., ferr., nat-a., plb., ter.
night - alum., alumn., ambr., arn., ***ars.,*** bar-c., ***bell., bry.,*** carb-an., carb-v., caust., cham., coloc., ery-a., ***ferr.,*** graph., hep., iod., kali-c., ***lac-c., lyc.,*** mag-c., ***mag-p.,*** mag-s., mang., ***med.,*** **MERC.,** ***mez., nat-c., nat-m.,*** **NIT-AC.,** ***nux-v., phos.,*** **PHYT., RHUS-T.,** sang., sep., staph., ***sulph.,*** ter.
10 p.m. - plan.
11 p.m. to 7 a.m. - ***sulph.***
bed, in - **MERC.,** ***mez., sulph., verat.***
paralytic - agar., ***am-m.,*** ang., carb-v., caust., ***cham.,*** chel., chin., cimic., cina, ***cocc.,*** dig., mez., ***nat-m.,*** podo., prun., ***seneg., sep., sil., stann.,*** stront-c., ***sulph.,*** verat.
paroxysmal - ***ars.,*** **BELL.,** ***caust.,*** chin-s., ***coff., coloc., gels., ign., kali-i., lyc., mag-p.,*** nat-m., **PLB., RHUS-T.,** ***tarent., tub.***
periodical - ***ars.,*** lyc., lyss., rhus-t.
perspiration amel. - ***gels.***
pressure, agg. - ***phos.,*** plb.
amel. - ***ars.,*** **MAG-P.**
raising the foot, pain preventing flexion - berb.

PAIN, legs

sitting, while - ***agar.,*** am-m., ant-c., **ARG-M.,** ***aur-m-n.,*** calc., carb-v., cham., chin., cob., croc., ham., ***indg.,*** iod., led., **LYC.,** mag-m., nit-ac., olnd., paeon., ph-ac., plat., ***sep.,*** staph., sulph., ***valer.,*** verat.

standing, while - aesc., ***agar.,*** phyt., ptel., stann., ***valer.***

upright - agar., bry., graph., puls.

upright amel. - bell.

stepping out - berb.

stool, during - coloc., ***nux-v., rhus-t., tell.***

before - bapt.

touch, by - ***bell.,*** berb., ***bry.,*** calc., ***chin.,*** guai., mez., nux-v., plat., puls., ruta., sulph.

ulcerative - benz-ac.

undressing - nat-s.

vexation, after - sep.

walking - ambr., am-m., anac., ant-c., arn., asaf., berb., bry., calc-p., ***coloc.,*** gels., hep., hyos., led., lyc., merc., nit-ac., nux-m., ***nux-v.,*** ol-an., petr., ***phos., phyt.,*** plb., ***ran-b.,*** sep., stann., stram., ***sulph.,*** tab., tarent., thuj., viol-t.

amel. - ***agar.,*** am-c., ***am-m., arg-m., ars., bell.,*** chin., dig., ***dulc.,*** **FERR.,** ***indg., kali-i., kali-s.,*** **LYC.,** ***puls.,*** **PYROG., RHUS-T.,** ***seneg.,*** sep., ***tub., valer., verat.***

in open air, after - phos.

wandering - aesc., ars-h., ***caul., iris, kali-bi., kalm., lac-c., lach.,*** mag-p., ***sang.,*** vib.

warm when - hell., **LAC-C.,** ***led., puls.,*** verat., zinc.

amel. - ***ars., bar-c., caust.,*** graph., ***lyc.,*** nat-c., ph-ac., ***phos.,*** stront-c., sulph.

warmth of bed - coloc., ***ferr., guai.,*** led., **MERC.,** plb., ***sulph.,*** syph., **VERAT.**

amel. - ***agar., ars.,*** bell., caust., ***dulc.,*** **LYC.,** ***mag-p.,*** **NUX-V.,** ***ph-ac., phos.,*** **PYROG., RHUS-T.**

weakness, with - plb.

weather, changing - ***berb., kali-bi.,*** lach., ***ran-b., rhod.***

wet - bor., ***ran-b., rhod., rhus-t.,*** ruta., ***ter.,*** **VERAT.**

windy - lach.

PAIN, calves - agar., ***anac.,*** ant-t., arg-n., ***arn., ars.,*** arund., benz-ac., bor., ***cact.,*** **CALC.,** calc-p., canth., cham., chel., cic., colch., cupr., dig., ***elaps,*** eug., eupi., ***gels.,*** glon., hell., hyper., iod., jug-c., ***kali-bi.,*** kali-br., kalm., lach., lith., lyc., mag-c., merc-c., merc-cy., ***merc-i-r.,*** mez., nat-p., ***nux-v.,*** ox-ac., phos., pic-ac., pip-m., plb., ***puls., rhus-t.,*** sabad., sang., sec., sel., sil., sin-n., stry., sulph., sul-ac., tarent., ***ter.,*** thuj., upa., verat., verat-v., xan.

afternoon - rhus-t.

4 p.m. lying on back with leg flexed - nat-m.

ascending steps - arg-n., rhus-t., sulph.

bathing, after - pip-m.

bending foot, on - calc.

PAIN, calves

blow, as from a - euph.

chill, during - ***ars.,*** thuj.

coughing, on - ***nux-v.***

crossing legs - dig., valer.

deep, in - glon.

descending steps - ***arg-m.,*** puls-n

drawing, up feet amel. - cham.

evening - alum., calc., nux-v., ***puls.,*** staph., verat.

bed, in - staph.

sitting with knees bent - coca

extending down tibia - led.

fatigue, as from - sulph.

flashes of - xan.

menses, during - berb.

morning - calc-p.

stairs, on going down - rhus-t.

walking, on - gels.

motion, on - bry., ***nux-v.,*** rumx.

amel. - agar., am-c., ars-i., cupr., ***rhus-t.***

of feet - cham.

night - anac., arg-n., cham., ***gels.,*** lyc., nux-v., pic-ac., sabad., sulph., vesp.

pressure amel. - eupi.

rheumatic - ant-t., jal., lach., lycps., plb., puls.

rising, on first - nat-p.

sitting, while - agar., puls., sul-ac., sulph.

spasmodic - raph.

standing - arn., arund., euphr., iris, nux-m.

stepping - calc.

tensive - berb., cupr.

touch - ***calc.***

ulcerative - agar.

walking - alum., anac., ***ars.,*** arund., **CALC.,** caps., ***carb-an.,*** gymn., ign., iris, jatr., lyc., mur-ac., ***nux-v.,*** onos., puls., spig., sulph., verat-v., zinc.

after - am-m., cinnb., ***rhus-t.***

warmth of bed amel. - ***nux-v.***

PAIN, lower - abrot., acet-ac., ***aesc.,*** **AGAR.,** ***alum.,*** am-c., am-m., ***anac., apoc., arn., ars.,*** asc-t., bad., bapt., bar-c., **BELL.,** benz-ac., berb., blatta, bov., calc-p., ***caps.,*** carb-s., carb-v., caul., ***caust.,*** cham., ***cimx.,*** cinnb., cina, cocc., coc-c., ***coff.,*** colch., coloc., crot-c., dios., ***dulc., eup-per.,*** fago., fl-ac., form., ***gels.,*** glon., **GUAI.,** gymn., hell., ***hydr.,*** indg., ***iod.,*** jac., kali-ar., ***kali-bi., kali-c., kali-i., kali-n.,*** **KALI-S.,** ***kalm., kreos.,*** **LACH.,** ***led., lyc.,*** lycps., lyss., mag-c., mag-s., manc., ***merc.,*** merc-c., merc-i-f., merl., ***mez.,*** murx., naja, nat-a., nat-c., nat-m., nat-p., nit-ac., ***nux-m., nux-v.,*** op., ***petr.,*** ph-ac., ***phos.,*** phys., ***phyt., plat., plb.,*** podo., ***puls., pyrog.,*** **RHOD., RHUS-T.,** ***rhus-v.,*** rumx., ***sang.,*** sarr., ***sep., stann., staph., stry., sulph., syph.,*** tarent., ter., teucr., thuj., ***tub.,*** valer., ***verat.,*** xan.

afternoon - ***coff.,*** elaps, lycps., nux-m., podo., ptel., rumx., sep.

alternating with,

cold feet - rhus-t.

heaviness of head - hell.

ascending stairs - bad.

PAIN, lower
bones - **AGAR.,** dios., dros., ***dulc., guai., kali-bi., kali-i., led., lyc., merc., mez.,*** nux-v., ***phyt.,*** plat., **SYPH.**
chill, during - ***ars., cimx.,*** lyc., ***nat-m., puls.,*** **PYROG.,** sep., ***spong.,*** tub.
before - ***eup-per.,*** eup-pur., ***puls.***
cold, air agg. - ars., ***kalm., rhus-t.,*** tub.
applications amel. - ***led., puls., syph.,*** thuj.
cold, becoming - agar., dulc., kalm., ph-ac., phos., rhus-t., tub.
from taking - ***iod.***
cough, during - bell., caps., ***nux-v., sulph.***
cramp-like - sul-ac.
crossing limbs - anag., phos., ***rhus-t.,*** stann.
cry out, causes him to - sep.
damp weather - ***dulc., rhus-t.,*** **VERAT.**
daytime - murx.
diarrhea - manc.
dinner, after - sulph.
eating, while - ph-ac.
after - ***kali-c.***
elevating feet amel. - bar-c., dios.
evening - ars., caust., chel., cinnb., crot-h., fl-ac., kali-n., kalm., lyc., merc-c., ***phos.,*** plan., **PULS.,** staph., ***sulph.***
6 p.m. - elaps, ptel.
7 p.m. - nat-a.
bed, in - alum., staph.
exertion, on - lycps.
after - ign., ***nat-m.,*** sul-ac.
extending to,
ankle - kali-bi., ptel.
feet - kalm., pic-ac., ptel., ***rhod.,*** still.
hips - nit-ac., nux-v.
hypogastrium - caust.
toes - kali-n., ***rhod.***
fever, with - ***puls.,*** ran-s., **RHUS-T.,** ***spong.***
flexing, on - plan.
on, foot - bad.
gouty - anan., ***apis, bry.,*** psor., sars.
growing pains - bell., **CALC-P.,** cimic., ***eup-per.,*** **GUAI.,** kali-p., mag-p., mang., nat-p., **PH-AC.**
at night - calc-p.
hanging down - bar-c., hep., ***puls.***
jerking - am-c., anac., cinnb., mez., nit-ac., phos., rat., rhus-t.
labor-like - carb-v.
left - nat-c.
lying, on - calc., carb-v., ***kali-i.***
menses, during - ***ambr., bell.,*** bov., carb-an., con., petr., spong.
after - calc-p.
morning - aesc., agar., aur., dios., ***eup-pur.,*** lach., led., rhod., ***sulph.***
5 a.m. - kali-p.
bed, in - psor.
waking, on - aur., kali-p.
motion - acon., alum., berb., ***carb-s., colch., guai.,*** iod., kali-br., ***kalm.,*** laur., merc., nux-v., op., ***staph., tarax.***

PAIN, lower
motion, amel. - ***agar., coloc.,*** dios., ***dulc., gels.,*** indg., ***kali-p.,*** **KALI-S.,** nit-ac., plan., **PULS.,** ***pyrog., rhod.,*** **RHUS-T.,** ***tub.***
neuralgic - ars., dirc., kalm., nat-a.
night - **AGAR.,** am-m., ***bar-c.,*** caust., ***coff.,*** croc., kali-bi., ***kali-c., kali-i.,*** lyc., **MERC.,** mez., mur-ac., **NIT-AC.,** ***petr., ph-ac., phos.,*** **PHYT.,** ***plb., rhus-t.,*** sec., spong., ***sulph.,*** **SYPH.,** thuj.
amel. - ***puls.***
in bed - ***phos.***
one, numbness in the other - sil.
paralytic - acon., ***agar.,*** am-c., bar-c., cham., chel., chin., cocc., eug., kali-n., mosch., nat-m., ***nit-ac., phos.,*** ruta., stront-c., sul-ac., sulph.
paroxysmal - cocc., ***gels.,*** plb., ***rhod.,*** **RHUS-T.,** sul-ac., thuj.
rest, during - nit-ac.
right - benz-ac., bov.
rising, on - agar., plan., puls.
sitting, while - agar., am-m., arg-m., arg-n., ars., brom., carb-v., caust., clem., crot-h., dios., ***dulc.,*** **KALI-S.,** led., lob., mosch., nat-m., nat-s., ***pyrog., rhod.***
amel. - ***puls.***
sleep, after, amel. - plan.
on going to - kali-c., ***kalm., lach.***
spots - petr.
standing - ***agar.,*** berb., ***kali-bi.,*** mez., nat-s., podo.
stooping - plan.
stretching - ars., dros., plan., ruta.
touch, on - acon., bor., nit-ac., petr., puls.
ulcerative - ***kreos.,*** osm., puls.
undulating - plat.
vexation, after - sep.
waking - abrot., aur., kali-p.
walking - am-m., bar-c., bry., carb-an., chel., cupr-ar., fago., ferr., ***guai.,*** hep., ign., mag-s., nat-p., nux-v., petr., phyt., puls., tab.
amel. - ***agar.,*** am-c., ***dulc., indg.,*** kali-n., **KALI-S., LYC.,** ***puls.,*** **RHUS-T.,** ***tub., valer.,*** **VERAT.**
warmth of bed - ***guai.,*** **MERC.,** mez., petr., plb., psor., staph., ***sulph.,*** **SYPH., VERAT.**
amel. - agar., am-c., ars., ***merc.,*** mez., **NUX-V.,** ***ph-ac., pyrog., tub.***
wave-like downwards - cocc.
wet, getting - ***rhus-t.***

PAIN, thighs - abrot., aesc., ***agar.,*** aloe, ***alum.,*** alumn., am-c., ammc., **ANAC.,** ant-t., apis, arg-m., arn., ***ars.,*** ars-h., ars-i., arum-t., asc-t., aster., aur., ***aur-m.,*** bar-c., bar-m., ***bell.,*** benz-ac., ***berb.,*** brach., ***bry., cact.,*** calc., calc-p., calc-s., camph., cann-i., ***caps.,*** carb-ac., ***carb-s., carb-v.,*** carl., cham., chel., ***chin., chin-s., cimic., cimx., cist.,*** cob., cocc., coff., colch., ***coloc.,*** com., cupr., cupr-ar., daph., dig., dios., dros., ***dulc.,*** echi., eug., euph., euphr., ferr., ferr-i., ferr-ar., ferr-p., fl-ac., form., ***gels., guai.,*** hell., ***hep.,*** hura, hydr., ***hyper.,***

PAIN, thighs - ***indg.,*** iod., iris, jug-c., jal., kali-ar., ***kali-bi., kali-c., kali-i.,*** kali-n., ***kalm.,*** lac-ac., lach., laur., ***led.,*** lil-t., lith., ***lyc.,*** mag-c., mag-m., mag-s., ***med.,*** meny., ***merc.,*** merc-i-f., ***mez.,*** mosch., mur-ac., ***murx.,*** myric., naja, ***nat-a., nat-m., nit-ac.,*** nux-m., op., ***petr., ph-ac.,*** phos., phys., ***phyt.,*** pic-ac., **PYROG., PLB.,** podo., puls., ***rhus-t.,*** sabin., sarr., ***sars., sep.,*** sil., spong., stann., ***staph.,*** stry., ***sulph.,*** sul-ac., stram., stront-c., syph., tarent., ***thuj.,*** trom., verat., ***verb.,*** xan., zinc.

afternoon - agar., coff., lyc., sep., sulph.
air, open - ant-t., **CAUST.**
alternating, with convulsive pain, in arms - sil.
with pain, in lumbar region - am-c.
anterior, part - all-c., ars., ***aur-m.,*** berb., bry., carl., ***coff.,*** cupr., cupr-ar., dig., hell., ***hyper.,*** kalm., led., ***lil-t.,*** lyss., naja, nat-s., pic-ac., ***plb., puls., rhus-t.,*** sanic., staph., sulph., syph., ***thuj.***
lower - agar., anac., ***calc-p., lyc.,*** mag-c., ***thuj., tub.***
morning - ars.
near groin - euph.
walking, while - euph., staph.
arthritic - asc-t.
ascending stairs agg. - bar-c., carb-v., kali-c., sep.
bed, in - iod., iodof.
blow, as from a - bar-c., lyc., sulph., sul-ac.
bone, in - **AGAR.,** am-c., aur., bry., cann-i., dros., ***euph.,*** fl-ac., ***indg.,*** ip., kali-bi., ***led., mez.,*** naja, nat-m., nat-s., nit-ac., phos., puls., sep., thuj., verat., zinc.
crossing limbs, on - aur.
evening, lying down, after - ip., verat.
forenoon - verat.
night - aur., dros., ***mez.***
night, sleep, during - dros.
night, stretching leg, amel. - dros.
sitting, while - sep.
wavelike - sep.
break, as if it would - aur., thuj.
change of weather agg. - berb.
chill, during - ars., **BOR.,** chin., ***cimx., dulc.,*** nat-m., puls., **PYROG.**
coughing, on, extending to knee - ***caps.***
cramp-like - carb-v., chin., sul-ac.
crossing limbs - ***agar.,*** aur., dig.
crural nerves - ***apis,*** ars., coff., **GNAPH.,** ***staph.,*** xan.
damp weather - kali-c.
daytime - kali-c., mag-c.
descending, on - **SABIN.**
dinner, after - carb-s., sulph.
drawing, up legs, amel. - cinnb., rhus-t.
driving - asc-t.
emissions, after - ***agar.***
evening - agar., asc-t., aur., colch., dios., ferr., hyper., kali-c., mag-c., murx., nit-ac., **PULS.,** stry., sulph., thuj., zinc.
4 to 8:30 - rhus-t.
lying down, after - sep.
sitting, while - stront.

PAIN, thighs
exertion, from - am-c., anac., ***caust.,*** kali-c., ***nat-c.***
extending to,
ankles - nat-a.
chest - puls.
down thigh, during effort to urinate - pareir.
down thigh, on coughing - caps.
down thigh, stool, during - ***rhus-t.***
downward - ***aur-m., guai., kali-c., kalm., murx., nit-ac.,*** sars.
downward, during menses - berb., kali-i., ***nit-ac.,*** xan.
downward, to heel - ***lac-d.***
knee - ***aur-m., guai.***
upwards - puls., sabin.
fall, as after a - plat.
flexing knee, amel. - ars.
flying - trom.
forenoon - jug-c.
groin, near - euph., ***rhus-t.***
hamstrings - ***am-m.***
inner side - aloe, am-c., ars-h., calc-p., nat-s., ol-an., sabin., sang., sars., sil., spong., sulph., tarax., verb.
above knee - alumn., ammc., calc-p., cann-i., chel., cina, dig., fl-ac., kalm., kreos., lil-t., puls., stry., sul-ac.
extending to chest - puls.
jerking - ang., cinnb., ***gels.,*** led., mang., mez., nat-c., puls., rat., rhus-t., sil., valer.
knee, above the - anac., lyc., ***ph-ac.,*** thuj., ***tub.***
left - hura, iris, mag-m., ***rhus-t.***
lying - am-c.
menses, during - am-c., ***berb.,*** bov., ***carb-an.,*** carl., cast., ***cham.,*** cimic., con., ***crot-h., kali-i.,*** kali-n., ***kalm.,*** lac-c., ***mag-m., nit-ac.,*** nux-v., petr., ***puls., sars., xan.***
before - cham., crot-h., mag-m., spong., vib.
middle of - aeth., ars., asar., chel., chin., cocc., ***indg.,*** kali-i., lach., mag-m., murx., staph., sulph.
anterior part of - cob., **SABIN.,** sulph.
anterior part of, rest, during - sulph.
anterior part of, walking, while - **SABIN.**
as if tendon would snap on stepping - plb.
evening - ***kali-i.,*** murx.
internal part of - lil-t., ol-an., sulph., verat.
menses, before - mag-m.
morning, in bed - mag-m.
posterior part of - am-br., dios., laur.
pulsating - bry.
sitting - kali-i.
walking agg. - staph.
morning - am-c., aur., caust., dios., sulph., sumb., viol-t.
9 a.m. - trom.
rising, on - ars., ***lac-d.***
waking, on - sulph.

PAIN, thighs
motion, on - ***berb.,*** cocc., coff., colch., dig., gels., ***guai.,*** iod., lyc., merc., nat-m., petr., plb., sanic., sep., sil., spig., ***staph.***
amel. - aeth., ***agar.,*** caps., cham., con., ***dulc.,*** **FERR.,** hyos., ***indg.,*** kreos., ***lyc.,*** merc-i-f., mosch., **PULS.,** ***rhod.,*** **RHUS-T.,** sabin.
neuralgic - ***phyt.,*** plb.
night - am-m., aur., cham., cinnb., coff., dros., euph., ferr., iod., kali-bi., lach., mag-s., ***merc., mez.,*** nux-v., sep., stry., sulph.
sleep, during - sep.
noon - stry.
walking, after - phys.
outer side of - agar., am-m., anag., carb-v., chin-s., com., fl-ac., kreos., lil-t., merc-i-f., ***phyt.***
paralytic - aeth., agar., am-m., ars., bell., bry., carb-v., cham., chel., chin., ***cina,*** cocc., colch., dios., dros., ***ferr.,*** ferr-ar., guai., kali-c., kali-i., laur., nit-ac., ph-ac., nux-v., sil., staph., stront-c., sul-ac., tep., verat., zinc.
paroxysmal - ***anac., aur-m.,*** bell., ***kali-i.,*** nit-ac., ***plb., rhod.,*** sul-ac.
posterior part - ***agar., am-m., ars.,*** bar-ac., camph., caps., carb-ac., cham., dios., dros., ***hep.,*** ind., lach., led., mez., naja, nit-ac., nux-m., sep., ***sulph.***
relaxing the muscles, amel. - ***ars.***
sitting, while - ***am-m.,*** hep., sep., sulph.
stepping, agg. - bar-c., mez.
pulsative - ars., bell., bry., com., ol-an., tarent.
raising, the limb - carb-v., cocc.
riding, as after - mag-m.
right - agar., cist., ***coloc.,*** kali-c., kalm., lith., stram.
rising, on - arn., carb-s., cham., chin., ***ferr.,*** lycps., ***rhus-t.***
from a seat - cham., chin., ***ferr.,*** nit-ac., petr., ph-ac., thuj.
rubbing, amel. - tarent.
scar, in an old - lach.
scratching, after - euphr.
sex, after - agar., nit-ac.
shaking limb - merc-i-f.
sitting, while - ***agar.,*** am-c., anac., arn., cist., coloc., ***ferr., guai., hep.,*** ind., kali-i., ***kali-s., lach.,*** led., lil-t., **LYC.,** mag-m., mill., mur-ac., plat., **PYROG.,** ***rhod.,*** ruta, sep., stront-c., ***sulph.,*** thuj., verb.
amel. - aur., zinc.
from sitting - kali-c.
walking, after - hydr.
sleep, during - bar-c., sep.
after - acon., ***lach.***
amel. - sep.
spots, in - mang.
standing, while - aur., berb., calc., mag-s., syph., valer., verat., zinc.
amel. - euph.
stepping - asar., petr., verb.
stool, during - ***rhus-t.***

PAIN, thighs
straining, at stool, after - sep.
to urinate, during - carb-an., pareir.
stretching limbs - ***ars., caps.,*** cham., cimx., ruta.
amel. - agar., dros., ***ferr.***
and turning from side to side amel. - merc-i-f., **RHOD., RHUS-T.**
touch, on - aur., lyc., nit-ac., nux-v., sep.
twitching - ***coloc.,*** phos.
ulcerative - arg-m., kali-c., sep., staph.
urination, during - berb.
walking - agar., ***am-m., arn., ars.,*** asar., aur., ***berb.,*** brach., calc-p., cham., chin., cist., ***coloc.,*** dios., ***dros.,*** euph., ***guai.,*** kali-c., led., mag-s., ***med.,*** meny., nat-a., nat-m., nux-m., ph-ac., plat., ***pyrog.,*** sabin., ***spig.,*** stann., ***staph.,*** sulph., tarent.
amel. - ***agar., bell., dulc., ferr., indg.,*** **KALI-S., LYC.,** ***merc., puls.,*** **RHOD., RHUS-T.**
wandering - fl-ac., hydr., iris, ***kali-bi.,*** trom.
9 a.m. - trom.
wind, before a heavy - berb.

PAIN, tibia - **AGAR.,** anac., anag., arg-m., ars., ***aur., aur-m-n.,*** bad., bapt., bar-c., berb., calc., ***calc-p.,*** carb-ac., ***carb-an.,*** carb-v., card-m., ***cast-eq.,*** caust., cina, ***clem., dulc.,*** ferr-i., hyper., ***iod.,*** kali-ar., ***kali-bi., kali-i.,*** kalm., **LACH.,** ***led.,*** mang., ***merc., mez.,*** nat-m., ***nit-ac., nux-m., ph-ac., phos., phyt.,*** pic-ac., ***puls.,*** **RHUS-T.,** sarr., sep., sil., stann., staph., tarent., thuj., verat., zinc.
blow, as from a - sep.
crossing, limbs - **RHUS-T.**
damp, weather - ***dulc.,*** mez., ***phyt., verat.***
elevating, leg amel. - aur., bar-c.
evening - ***led.***
extending the leg, when - aur.
fatigue, as from - dig., dulc.
morning - ***agar.***
motion, on - berb.
amel. - ***agar.,*** arg-m., aur-m-n., ***dulc.,*** psor., ***rhus-t.,*** verat.
night - ***aur., kali-i., ph-ac., phyt.,*** **RHUS-T.**
bed, in - ***aur.,*** carb-an., ***merc., mez.,*** psor., **RHUS-T.**
occiput in , with - carb-v.
paralyzing - card-m.
pulsating - arg-m.
rheumatic - rumx.
sitting, while - ***agar.,*** anac., euphr.
spots, painful - ambr.
standing - aur-m-n., rat.
touch, on - lyc., phos., puls.
walking, while - bry., carb-an., clem., coc-c., dig., ign., merc., merl., mez., nat-m., nat-s., ***nux-m.,*** phos., rhod., stry.
amel. - **AGAR.,** aur-m-n., ***dulc., tub.,*** verat.

PARALYSIS, legs, (see Nerves, chapter) - ***abrot.,*** **AGAR.,** ***alum.,*** anac., ang., apis, apoc., **ARG-N.,** arn., **ARS.,** ars-i., bar-c., bar-m., ***bell.,*** berb., bry., ***calc.,*** calc-s., ***camph.,*** **CANN-I.,** canth., ***caps., carb-ac.,*** carb-s., carb-v., caul., chin-s., ***cic., cocc.,*** colch., **CON.,** ***crot-c.,*** crot-t., ***cupr., dulc.,*** form., ***gels.,*** hyos., ***ign.,*** iod., iris, kali-ar., ***kali-c., lach., lath.,*** lith., lyc., lycps., mang., merc., ***merc-c.,*** morph., ***mygal.,*** nat-m., ***nux-m.,*** **NUX-V.,** ol-an., ***olnd., op., ox-ac., phos., pic-ac.,*** **PLB.,** ***psor.,*** **RHUS-T.,** ruta., sars., ***sec.,*** sep., ***sil.,*** stann., ***stram., sulph.,*** tab., ***tarent.,*** ter., ***thal., verat.,*** verat-v., zinc.

anger, after - ***nat-m.***
childbirth, after - ***caust., plb.,*** **RHUS-T.**
cold, from - ***cocc., rhus-t.***
colic, with - ***plb.***
damp weather - lath.
exertion, following - **NUX-V.,** ***rhus-t.***
extending to upper limbs - agar., ***ars., con.,*** hydr-ac., ***kali-c.,*** mang.
fulgurating pains, in abdomen, with - ***thal.***
grief, from - nat-m.
jerking, of eyes, with - alum-m., arg-n.
left - ter.
night - phos.
then right arm and leg - mag-c.
painless - ***alum., arg-n., ars.,*** bar-c., bell., calc., camph., cann-i., ***carb-ac.,*** carb-s., carb-v., cic., **COCC., CON.,** ***cupr., gels.,*** kali-c., ***lath.,*** lyc., ***merc.,*** nat-m., nux-m., nux-v., **OLND.,** ***op., phos.,*** **PLB., RHUS-T.,** ***sec.,*** sil., stram., sulph., zinc.
post diphtheritic - **ARS.,** ***cocc., con.,*** gels., ***lach.,*** nat-m., nux-v., ***phos., plb., sec., sil.***
right - abrot., lac-c., ox-ac., plb.
then left - ***ox-ac.***
sexual excesses - ***nat-m.,*** **NUX-V.,** ***phos.***
sitting, after - sil.
spasms, after - stram.
of the arms - agar.
standing - sep.
stroke, after - caust., lach., **NUX-V.,** ***phos.***
sudden - ***nux-v.***
suppressed eruptions - ***psor.***
tetanus, followed by - nux-v.
vaccination, after - ***thuj.***
wet, becoming - ***nux-v.,*** **RHUS-T.**

paralysis, lower - ars.

paralysis, thighs - ***chel.,*** kali-c., manc., stram., sulph.
extensors - ***calc.***
inside - ***nux-v.***

PARALYSIS, as if, sensation - acon., **AESC.,** ***alum.,*** am-c., **AUR.,** berb., ***calc-p., chel., dig.,*** hyper., lach., phos., rheum, ***rhus-v.,*** stront-c., ***verat.***
night - ***calc-p.,*** phos.
right - phos.
then left - ***verat.***
sitting, while - ***calc-p.***

paralysis, lower, as if - ***acon.,*** **AESC.,** amyg., atro., bell., both., brom., camph., carb-o., ***carb-v.,*** chel., chin., lath., mag-c., manc., med., morph., ***nat-m., nit-ac.,*** olnd., plb., ***rhus-v.,*** sep., tab., vip.
chill, during - ars., ign., stram.
rheumatic - chel., ph-ac.
walking, while - stront.
after - croc.

paralysis, thighs, as if - agar., aur., bar-c., berb., ***chel.,*** cocc., crot-t., lach., nux-v., ***rhus-t.,*** sulph., verat., zinc.
anterior muscles - ang.
extending to knees - ferr-i., thuj.
lying, while - sulph.
posterior muscles - led.
sitting, while - caust., ***chel.***
walking, while - caust., dros.

PERSPIRATION - ars., asaf., bor., calc., coc-c., coloc., con., croc., hep., **HYOS., KALI-N.,** mang., merc., nux-v., ***phos., rhod.,*** sec., ***sep.,*** ter., ***verat., zinc.***
evening, in bed - ter.
except - lyc.
fetid - ***phos.***
menses, during - calc., lil-t.
menstrual colic, during - ant-t.
morning - lyc.
bed, in - rhod.
bed, in, waking, after - con., ***sep.***
night - am-c., ars., coloc., con., kali-n., mang., ***merc.,*** rumx., ter., ***zinc.***
paralyzed limbs - stram.
walking, while - ery-a.

perspiration, lower - agar., am-c., ars., bry., ***calc., calc-p., caps.,*** coc-c., coloc., **EUPH.,** hyos., kali-bi., **MANG.,** merc., mez., nux-v., **PETR., PODO.,** ***psor.,*** rhod., rumx., ***sep., stram., sulph.,*** thuj.
clammy - rumx.
cold - ***caps.,*** euph., ***merc., phos., psor.,*** thuj.
evening, bed, in - agar., ter.
except leg - lyc.
fetid - ***phos.***
inner surface - agar.
morning - ars., euph., sulph.
5 a.m. - sulph.
waking, on - coloc.
night - ***agar.,*** am-c., ***calc.,*** coloc., mang., ***merc., sulph.,*** thuj.
sticky - ***calc.***

perspiration, thighs - acon., **AMBR., ARS.,** ***bor.,*** caps., ***carb-an.,*** coloc., crot-t., dros., euph., eup-pur., ***hep.,*** hyos., ***kali-bi.,*** merc., ***nux-v.,*** rhus-t., ***sep.,*** sulph., **THUJ.**
cold - crot-t., ***merc., sep.***
except - lyc.
inner surface of - ***thuj.***
midnight, after - ars., nux-v.
morning - euph., rhus-t., thuj.
near genitals - thuj.

perspiration, thighs
near, male genitals - crot-t.
offensive - ***crot-t.***
night - ***carb-an.,*** coloc., ***merc., sep.***
sensation, of - caps.
sleep, at beginning of - ars.
spots, in - caps.
walking, in open air - caps.

perspiration, thighs, between - aur., ***cinnb.,*** hep., nux-v.
corrosive - cinnb.
morning - carb-an., nux-v.
night - aur., carb-an.
offensive - ***cinnb.***
walking, while - ambr., ***cinnb.***

PHLEBITIS, milk leg, phlegmasia alba dolens - **ACON.,** agar., ***all-c.,*** ant-c., ***ant-t.,*** apis, arist-cl., ***arn., ars., bell.,*** both., **BRY.,** ***bufo,*** **CALC.,** calc-ar., ***calc-f.,*** carb-s., carb-v., ***cham., chin.,*** chlorpr., **CLEM.,** crot-h., graph., ***ham.,*** hecla., hep., hir., ***iod., kali-c.,*** kali-m., kreos., **LACH.,** ***led., lyc., lycps.,*** mag-c., mag-f., merc., merc-cy., merc-i-r., ***nat-s.,*** nux-v., phos., ***puls.,*** rhod., **RHUS-T.,** ruta, ***sep., sil.,*** spig., stront-br., stront-c., sulfa., ***sulph.,*** thiop., thuj., verat., **VIP.,** vip-a., zinc.
injuries, after - rhus-t.
childbirth, after, forceps with - all-c.
contractions, with - ***sil.***

PINCHING, pain - anac., bell., ***calc.,*** carb-an., carb-v., graph., iod., kali-c., mez., ***nat-c.,*** nit-ac., ph-ac., phos., sep., sil., sulph., zinc.
evening - mez.

pinching, calves - ant-c., dig., hyos., mang., myric., nat-c., ph-ac., stann., thuj.
cramp-like - ph-ac.
lying - berb.
motion, on - nat-c..
rubbing, amel. - ph-ac.
sitting, when - asaf., berb.

pinching, lower - hyos., nux-m., ph-ac., sabad., sil.
stitching - hyos.
walking, while - sabad.

pinching, thighs - anac., colch., dros., dulc., ***led.,*** mag-m., mang., ph-ac., prun., sul-ac., zinc.
inner side - mag-m., mang., meny., sul-ac.

pinching, tibia - mez., sil.

PRESSING, pain - anac., ***arg-m.,*** asaf., cic., cimic., cycl., dros., kalm., led., mez., nat-s., ***olnd.,*** ph-ac., ran-s., ***rhod.,*** ruta., ***sars., stann., staph.,*** sulph., ***verat.,*** zinc.
bones - con., ***guai.,*** kali-c., kali-n.
cramp-like - dros.
drawing - ran-s.
evening - nit-ac.
extending downwards - nit-ac., rhod.
grasping - ***stront.***
joints - bar-c., naja, sep., stront.
left - phos.
night - kali-n.
sitting, while - ***arg-m.***

PRESSING, pain
walking, while - asaf.
after - anac.
amel. - kali-n.

pressing, calves - agar., ***anac.,*** ars., calc., ***led.,*** mur-ac., sep., stann., staph., tarax., verat.
cramp-like - anac., verb., verat.

pressing, lower - ***agar., anac.,*** ang., arg-m., aur., ***bell.,*** camph., carb-an., carb-an., carl., chel., cic., clem., euph., hell., indg., kali-c., kalm., lach., ***led.,*** lil-t., ***mang.,*** nat-c., nat-s., ***ph-ac.,*** ran-s., ruta, sars., ***stann.,*** teucr., thuj., verat., verb., zinc.
below the knee - ***chel., cupr.,*** ph-ac.
drawing - agar., anac.
evening - lach.
sitting, while - nat-s.
menses, during - ambr., carb-an.
morning - led.
rheumatic - anac.
sitting, on - agar., anac., arg-m., nat-s.
spots formerly ulcerated - petr.
walking, while - anac.
amel. - sep.

pressing, thighs - acon., ***agar.,*** all-c., ***aloe, anac.,*** ang., arn., asar., camph., caps., caust., chel., chin., coloc., con., crot-t., cupr., cycl., dros., eupi., ***guai.,*** hell., ign., ind., kali-c., ***kali-i.,*** kali-p., ***led.,*** merc., mez., ***mur-ac.,*** nat-s., nux-v., ***olnd., ph-ac.,*** phyt., prun., ***ruta.,*** sabin., ***sars.,*** sil., ***stann.,*** sul-ac., tarent., thuj., verat.
anterior, part - bell., dig., lyc., mang.
bandaged, as if - tarent.
below the groin - rhus-t.
bend of - am-c., ang., bar-c., dig., rhus-t., ruta.
bones - con., guai., ***led.,*** merc., nat-s.
cramp-like - anac., rhus-t., verat.
cough, during - caps.
deep-seated - ign., merc.
dragging down - con., merc.
drawing up legs amel.- guai.
inner side of - anac., mosch., nit-ac., sars., spong., stann., sul-ac., tarax.
extending backward - spong.
sitting while - calc.
sudden - mosch.
upper - rhus-t.
lower part of - bism., hell., nit-ac., ph-ac., sars., spig., spong., thuj., ***tub.,*** verb.
posterior - asar., petr., sars.
menses, during - ***carb-an.,*** kali-i., lyc., nux-v.
morning - con.
motion, amel. - eupi., ind., spig.
night - ruta., sulph.
outer side of - anac., ang., olnd., ph-ac., ruta, spig., sul-ac.
outward - aloe
paroxysmal - **ACON.**
periosteum - spig.
plug, as with a - ***agar.,*** **ANAC.**

pressing, thighs
posterior part - dros., ind., ***led.,*** zinc.
sitting, while - ind.
stooping - dros.
walking amel. - zinc.
pressure, agg. - spig.
pulsating - stann.
rhythmical - **ANAC.**
rising, from a seat - ang.
shooting - sabin.
sitting, while - coloc., ***guai.,*** ind., led., mang., mur-ac., rhus-t., sars., spig., verb.
amel. - aur.
sticking - olnd., sul-ac.
stool, after - ***lyc.***
stretching leg - ang.
walking - anag., aur., ***led.,*** meny.

pressing, tibia - agar., ang., asaf., aur., bell., brom., calc., carb-an., caust., coloc., cycl., kali-n., kalm., led., meny., ***merc.,*** mez., nat-c., petr., ph-ac., puls., sep., sil., stann., staph., thuj., zinc.
bending knee - rhus-t.
motion, on - cycl.
pulsating - stann.
sitting, while - chin., coloc., con., cycl., staph.
stretching the leg - aur., chin., con.
walking, while - calc., carb-an., cycl.
amel. - asaf., ***ph-ac.***

PSORIASIS, lower - kali-ar., **PHOS.**

PULSATION - ars-m., ***kali-c.,*** nat-m., nux-v., ***sars.,*** sep., ***sulph.***

pulsation, calves - alum., jatr., nat-m., plat.
morning - alum.
outer side - graph.
sitting, while - nat-m., plat.

pulsation, lower - anac., ant-t., arg-m., ars-h., ars-m., brom., kreos., med., merc-i-f., nat-s., ph-ac., pic-ac., plat., rhus-t., sil., stann., still., stront.
evening - still.
rest, during - arg-m., ph-ac.
spots, in - plat.
walking, on - nat-s.

pulsation, thighs - ars., berb., bry., com., dig., murx., nit-ac., plat., ruta., sec., ***sil.,*** spong., stann., tarent.
night - ars.
tendons, of - caust.

PURRING, lower - sep.

PUSHED forward, legs in sleep - lyc.

QUIVERING, (see Trembling)

RAISED, leg, with difficulty - chel., sulph.

raising, affected limb agg., (see Hang down)

RASH - alum., bry., mez., nat-m., nux-v., rhus-t., sep., tep., zinc.
itching - alum.

rash, calves - ***calc.,*** hyos., nat-m., sil.

rash, lower - calc., daph., hyos., ***nat-m.,*** sil.

rash, thighs - bry., caust., cub., merc., mez., nat-m., ***nux-v.,*** ol-an., osm., ***petr.,*** rhus-t., **SULPH.,** ter.

rash, thighs
brownish - mez.
burning, during menses - nux-v.
gnawing, after scratching - mez.
itching, burning, during menses - rhus-v.
worse after scratching - mez.

RAT, lower legs, feels a rat running up the leg - ail., ***calc.***

RELAXATION - ambr., am-m., ang., camph., canth., cic., guai., hell., lach., lyc., nat-c., nit-ac., nux-m., op., phos., plb., puls., stram., verat.

relaxation, lower - carb-v., kali-c.

RESTLESSNESS, legs - ail., am-c., ***anac.,*** **ARS.,** aster., ***bell.,*** calc., ***calc-p.,*** carb-v., ***caust.,*** chin., ***chin-a.,*** con., cop., graph., hep., iod., kali-ar., **KALI-C.,** ***lyc., mez.,*** mosch., mur-ac., nat-a., nat-c., ***nat-m.,*** petr., ***phos., phyt., plat.,*** prun., **RHUS-T.,** ruta, ***sep.,*** stann., ***sulph.,*** tab., **TARENT., ZINC.**
evening - graph., kali-c., lyc., mag-c., ***nit-ac.,*** sec., ***sep.,*** stann., ***sulph.,*** tab., **TARENT.**
bed, in - alum., calc., carb-v., **CAUST.,** hep., ***lyc.,*** mez., ***nat-m.,*** **TARENT.**
bed, in, from pain in the calves - staph.
left, night - nat-c.
uncovers - mag-c.
lying, while - alum., fago., hep., lyc.
amel. - ars.
menses, during - lac-c.
morning, bed, in - **CAUST.**
motion amel. - **RHUS-T., TARENT.**
night - **ARS., CAUST.,** graph., hep., ***lyc.,*** nat-c., nat-m., ***phyt.,*** rhod., **TARENT.,** zinc.
bed, in - **CAUST., RHUS-T., TARENT.**
before midnight - nux-v.
pain, in the calves, from - staph.
room, close - aster.
sitting, while - alum., anac., caust., ***lyc.,*** mosch., nat-m., plat., **RHUS-T.**
sleep, during - coloc.
before going to - **ARS., KALI-C.,** ***lyc., nat-m.***
preventing - nux-v.
standing, while - anac., plat.
warmth of bed - aster., mez., **LACH.**

restlessness, lower - acon., agar., alum., ambr., **AM-C.,** ***anac., arg-n.,*** **ARS.,** aster., ***bell.,*** cact., ***calc., calc-p., camph.,*** carb-s., ***carb-v., caust.,*** chel., ***chin., chin-a.,*** cimic., ***cimx.,*** con., eupi., **FERR.,** ferr-ar., ferr-p., ***glon., graph.,*** hep., hyos., ***kali-c.,*** kali-n., kali-s., ***lach.,*** lac-c., ***lyc., mag-c.,*** **MED.,** ***meph.,*** merc., ***mez., mosch.,*** naja, nat-a., nat-c., ***nat-m.,*** nat-p., ***nit-ac., nux-m.,*** osm., ox-ac., ***phos., plat.,*** prun., ***psor.,*** **RHUS-T.,** ***ruta., sep.,*** spong., squil., stann., ***sulph., tarax.,*** **TARENT., TUB.,** ust., **ZINC.**
daytime, during rest - hep.
evening - alum., carb-v., ***caust.,*** kali-c., lyc., ***merc.,*** nat-c., ***plat., sep.,*** stann., **TARENT., ZINC.**

restlessness, lower
evening, before going to sleep - ***ars., lyc., nat-m., tarent.***
sleep, preventing - stann.
fever, during - bell., bor., **CALC.,** ***nux-v.,*** **RHUS-T., SABAD.,** sep., sulph.
insanity, in - **TARENT.**
morning, in bed - **CAUST.,** hep., ***psor.***
night - ***ars.,*** **CAUST.,** ***cham.,*** con., eupi., mag-c., phos., ***zinc.***
bed, in - ***bell., carb-v., caust., lyc.,*** puls-n, **RHUS-T.,** ***ruta.,*** **TARENT.**
lying, while - ruta.
must put it out of bed to cool it - mag-c., ***sulph.***
rising, after - ***psor.***
sitting, while - alum., anac., ***plat.***
sleep, during - **CAUST.,** ***nat-m.***
before - **ARS.,** ***lyc., nat-m.***
walking, while - anac.

restlessness, thighs - ***anac., camph.,*** carb-v., caust., form., kali-c., ***mag-m.,*** ph-ac., ***plat.,*** puls., squil.
evening in bed - mez.
sitting, while - anac., form., ph-ac., plat.
tremulous - plat.

RHEUMATIC, pain, legs - ang., arg-m., ant-c., ant-t., ***apis,*** cact., cadm-s., calc-s., ***carb-s., carb-v., caust.,*** cimic., ***clem.,*** colch., graph., ***guai., kali-c.,*** kali-n., ***kalm., lac-c.,*** lact., **LED.,** lith., mang., meph., merc-c., nat-m., nit-ac., ***ph-ac., phos., phyt.,*** plb., ***rhod.,*** rhus-r., ***rhus-t.,*** sang., ***sep.,*** stann., stront-c., sul-ac., ***verat., zinc.***
alternating sides - ***lac-c.***
leaves and goes to upper limbs. - ***led.***

rheumatic, lower legs - am-c., aml-n., anac., anan., asaf., ***bell.,*** berb., ***cact., carb-s.,*** carb-v., card-m., cimic., clem., corn., ***dulc., elaps, guai.,*** ham., hyper., iod., ***kali-c.,*** kali-n., ***kalm., lach., led., lith., lyc.,*** lyss., lycps., mag-m., ***med.,*** mez., nat-m., ***nit-ac.,*** pall., petr., ph-ac., phos., ***phyt., rhod., rhus-t.,*** rumx., sep., stront-c., stry., ust., ***verat.,*** zinc.
gonorrhea, after - **MED.,** ***sars.***
left - elaps, mag-s., zinc.
right - ***kalm.,*** lach., ruta., viol-t.

rheumatic, thighs - agar., ant-t., ***arg-n., ars.,*** asc-t., bapt., bell., carb-s., ***carb-v.,*** dulc., ***guai.,*** hydr., iod., kali-bi., ***kali-c.,*** lach., lyc., mag-s., merc., mez., naja, ph-ac., plb., sabin., sang., sanic., sep., ***stann.,*** stry., ***zinc.***
turning in bed agg. - ***nat-s.***
uncovering limb - ***mag-p.***
urination amel. - tell.
vexation - coloc.
walking, agg. - bar-c., berb., ***chin-s.,*** coff., ***coloc.,*** ign., lach., ***led.,*** nat-a., nat-s., psor., ***sulph.,*** zinc.
amel. - agar., am-m., caps., ***coc-c.,*** **FERR.,** indg., ***kali-bi., kali-i.,*** kali-p., **LYC.,** ph-ac., **RHUS-T.,** ruta., sep., syph., ***valer.***
warm room agg. - **PULS.**
warmth agg. - ***guai.,*** **LED.,** verat., zinc.

SCIATICA, pain - acon., agar., ***am-m.,*** anan., ang., ***arg-n., arn., ars.,*** asar., bar-c., ***bell.,*** berb., **BRY., BUFO,** ***calc., calc-p.,*** caps., ***carb-s.,*** card-m., ***caust., cham.,*** chel., chim., chin-s., ***cimic.,*** cist., cocc., coc-c., ***coff.,*** **COLOC.,** cur., ***dios.,*** dros., ***elaps, elat.,*** euph., eup-pur., ***ferr., ferr-ar.,*** ferr-p., fl-ac., ***gels.,*** **GNAPH.,** ***graph., guai.,*** hep., hyper., ***ign., indg.,*** **IRIS,** ***kali-ar., kali-bi.,*** kali-c., **KALI-I.,** ***kali-p.,*** lac-ac., ***lac-c.,*** lac-d., ***lach.,*** lachn., ***led., lyc.,*** lyss., **MAG-P.,** ***meny.,*** merc., mez., nat-a., ***nat-m., nat-s.,*** nit-ac., ***nux-m.,*** **NUX-V.,** ***ol-j.,*** pall., ***petr.,*** ph-ac., ***phos., phyt.,*** plan., ***plb., podo.,*** psor., ***puls., ran-b.,*** **RHUS-T.,** ***ruta.,*** sal-ac., ***sep.,*** sil., ***staph., still.,*** stram., ***sulph.,*** **TELL.,** ter., ***valer., verat.,*** xan., ***zinc.***
afternoon - am-m., bell., bry., chel., coff., indg., kali-bi., nux-v.
air, open, amel. - **KALI-I.,** mez., **PULS.,** thuj.
alternating, side - **LAC-C.**
with numbness - ***gnaph.***
ascending - acon., agar., podo., ruta.
atrophy, with - ***ol-j., plb.***
bed, in - hyper., kali-bi., ***kali-i.,*** lyc., ruta., sep.
beginning, at ankle - ars., cimic., plat.
bending, backward - caps.
forward - thuj.
brown spots, on the skin - ***sep.***
burning, with - ***ars.,*** bufo, coloc., gels., ***gnaph.,*** lach., lyc., ***phos., rhus-t.,*** ruta.
change in weather - ***kali-bi.,*** lach.
cold, agg. - ***ars.,*** asar., caust., coloc., ***mag-p.,*** pall., ***phos., ran-b.,*** **RHUS-t.,** sil.
applications, agg. - ***ars., bry., mag-p., nux-v., phos.,*** **RHUS-T.,** ruta.
coldness, of painful limb - ***led.,*** merc., sil.
coughing, agg. - ***caps.,*** caust., sep., ***tell.***
daytime - coloc., sep.
descending - am-m., ruta.
evening - am-m., bry., chel., coloc., ferr., hyper., indg., iris, kali-bi., ***kali-i.,*** led., meny., mez., pall., ***phos., puls.,*** valer.
flexing leg amel. - ***ars.,*** coloc., graph., guai., ***kali-bi., kali-i.,*** tell., ***valer.***
on the abdomen amel. - ***coloc.***
forenoon - sep.
hang down, agg. - valer.
over sides of bed, letting leg - ***verat.***
heat agg. - ***led.,*** verat., zinc.
heel, becomes localized in - anan., sep.
hip to knee - coloc., elat., ***lach.,*** plan.
hot, weather - kali-bi.
injury, after - ***arn., hyper., ruta.***
jarring, agg. - **BELL.,** ***nux-m., tell.***
laughing, agg. - ***tell.***
left - ***am-m.,*** arag., cimic., elat., eup-pur., iris, ***kali-bi., kali-c.,*** kali-i., lach., phos., tell., thuj.
lifted, when - nux-v.
living, in cold damp house - ***ars., nat-s., rhus-t.***

SCIATICA, pain
lying - coloc., ferr., gnaph., ***kali-i.,*** meny., ***nat-m.,*** ruta., sep., tell., valer.
amel. - **AM-M.,** bar-c., ***bry., dios.,*** lach.
back, on - kali-i., rhus-t.
amel. - ***phos.***
left side, on - kali-c., ***phos.***
painful side, on - dros., ***kali-c.,*** **KALI-I., LYC.,** nux-v., ***phos.,*** **RHUS-T.,** sep., ***tell.***
amel. - **BRY.,** ***coloc.***
right side, on - rhus-t.
amel. - ***phos.***
stretched out, with limb - cham.
mental, exertion - mag-p.
midnight - ferr., ***nux-m.***
4 a.m. - coloc.
after - ***ars.,*** rhus-t.
before - ferr., led.
morning - arg-n., ars., ***bry.,*** kali-bi., nux-v., staph., sulph.
motion, agg. - acon., **BRY.,** calc., chel., ***cocc., coff., coloc., dios.,*** eup-pur., gels., gnaph., ***guai., iris, kali-c.,*** lac-c., lach., led., mag-p., merc., mez., nux-m., nux-v., pall., ***phos., phyt.,*** plb., puls., ***ran-b.,*** sep., ***staph.,*** syph.
amel. - acon., agar., ***arg-m.,*** caps., cham., coc-c., ***dulc., euph.,*** **FERR.,** gels., indg., ***kali-bi., kali-i., kali-p.,*** kreos., lac-c., ***lyc.,*** meny., nat-s., ***puls.,*** rhod., **RHUS-T.,** ***ruta.***, sep., sil., sulph., ter., valer.
continued, agg. - coloc.
slow, amel. - ***ferr.,*** kali-p., ***puls.***
move, on beginning to - ***gels.,*** **RHUS-T.,** ruta., thuj.
night - arg-n., ***ars.,*** bell., cham., coff., ***coloc.,*** ferr., ***ferr-ar.,*** gels., gnaph., hyper., indg., iris, kali-bi., ***kali-i.,*** led., ***merc., mez.,*** nux-v., pall., phyt., plb., ***puls., rhus-t.,*** sep., staph., ***syph.,*** tell., verat., zinc.
amel. - staph.
noon - coloc., nat-m.
numbness, with - cham., ***coloc.,*** **GNAPH.,** nux-v., ***phyt., rhus-t.***
overheated, from being - zinc.
pain, in spine and all over, with - ***petr.***
periodical - ***chin-s., lyc.,*** lyss., ***rhus-t.***
every 4 days - ***lyc.***
pregnancy, during - gels.
pressure, agg. - ***coloc.,*** dros., ***kali-bi.,*** kali-c., ***kali-i., lyc.,*** phyt., plb.
amel. - ars., coff., coloc., **MAG-P.,** meny., phyt., ***rhus-t.***
pulsating - coloc., lac-ac.
regular, intervals - carb-s.
right - carb-s., chel., chin-s., ***coloc., dios., lach., lyc., phyt.,*** plan., sep., ***tell.***
rising, from seat - aesc., cham., coloc., ferr., kali-p., lach., ***lyss., nat-s.,*** rhus-t., ruta., sep., staph., sulph., thuj.

SCIATICA, pain
sitting, agg. - agar., **AM-M.,** berb., ***bry.,*** coloc., dios., ferr., indg., iris, kali-bi., kali-i., lach., **LYC.,** lyss., ***meny.,*** merc., ruta., sep., staph., ***valer.***
amel. - gnaph., guai., kali-i.
sleep, after, agg. - **LACH.,** led.
sneezing - sep., ***tell.***
standing, agg. - ***aesc.,*** agar., bar-c., ferr., kali-bi., kali-i., nux-v., ***sulph., valer.***
amel. - bell., mag-p., meny., staph.
stepping, agg. - asar., bar-c., gnaph., nux-m.
stool, pressing at - ***nux-v., rhus-t., sep., tell.***
stooping, agg. - agar., card-m., dros., nat-s., ***tell.***
stretching, the leg, agg. - arn., berb., ***caps.,*** cham., guai., ***valer.***
amel. - ferr.
suddenly, come and go - **BELL., KALI-BR.,** ***mag-p.,*** sulph.
summer, with cough in winter - staph.
tonic, contractions, chronic - ***nat-m.,*** tell.
touch, agg. - bell., berb., caps., **CHIN-S.,** cocc., ***coloc.,*** ferr., gels., guai., ***kali-c.,*** **LACH.,** ***led., mag-p.,*** mez., sulph., verat.
turn over, on the well side before he can rise from bed - ***kali-c.***
turning in bed agg. - ***nat-s.***
uncovering, limb - ***mag-p.***
urination, amel. - tell.
vexation - coloc.
walking, agg. - bar-c., berb., ***chin-s.,*** coff., ***coloc.,*** ign., lach., ***led.,*** nat-a., nat-s., psor., ***sulph.,*** zinc.
amel. - agar., am-m., caps., ***coc-c.,*** **FERR.,** indg., ***kali-bi., kali-i.,*** kali-p., **LYC.,** ph-ac., **RHUS-T.,** ruta., sep., syph., ***valer.***
warm, room agg. - **PULS.**
warmth, agg. - ***guai.,*** **LED.,** verat., zinc.
agg., bed, of - ***coloc.,*** led., ***merc.***
amel. - **ARS.,** bell., caust., ***coloc.,*** kali-c., ***kali-p.,*** **LYC., MAG-P.,** nat-m., ***nux-v.,*** pall., ***phos.,*** **RHUS-T.,** ***sil.,*** staph., thuj.
bed, of - *ars.,* caust., **LYC.,** ***mag-p., nux-v., phos., sil.***
washing in cold water - ***calc.,*** **RHUS-T.,** sulph.
wet weather - ***phyt.,*** ran-b., **RHUS-T.,** ruta.
amel. - asar.
wind, before a heavy - berb.
winter, in - ign.

SCRAPING, pain, leg bones - am-c., **ARS.,** ***asaf.,*** led., **PH-AC., RHUS-T.**
evening - am-c.
twitch up the legs, must - am-c.
walking amel. - am-c.
scraping, thighs - am-c., ***chin.,*** grat.
evening - am-c.

SCRATCHING, pain, calf - dulc.
scratching, thighs - staph.

SENSITIVE - ***agar.,*** am-m., ars., aur., ***mag-m.,*** ***petr.,*** plb., sep., sil., zinc.
sensitive, calves - ***nat-m.,*** plb., sil.
sensitive, lower - berb., ***calc.,*** calc-s.
cold, to a draft of air - ***zinc.***
sensitive, thighs - ***agar., gels., merc.,*** rhus-t., ruta., sulph.
sensitive, tibia - ***puls.***

SEPARATED, sensation - nux-v., op., stram.
separated, and spasmodic drawing together, lower - lyc., op.
as if severed from his body - op., ***stram.***
standing, on - phos.

SHAKING - ***merc.,*** tarent.
right then left - lyc.
shaking, lower - con., lyc., stry., tarent.

SHARP, pain - aesc., aeth., ***agar.,*** ail., alum., apis, ***arg-m.,*** ars., ars-h., asar., bar-c., **BELL.,** bov., bry., cahin., calc., carb-s., carb-v., cast-eq., caust., chin., chlor., cic., cinnb., ***cocc.,*** coloc., con., dros., dulc., euphr., ***ferr.,*** gels., ***grat.,*** kali-ar., ***kali-c., kali-s.,*** kalm., kreos., led., ***lyc., mag-c., manc.,*** mang., ***merc.,*** merc-c., mur-ac., nat-c., nat-m., ***nat-p.,*** nit-ac., nux-v., op., phos., phyt., **PLB.,** prun., ***puls.,*** **RHUS-T.,** ***sars., sep., sil., stann.,*** staph., ***sulph., tarent., thuj.,*** tub., zinc.
bones - ars., ***bell.,*** carb-v., caust., graph., ***iod.,*** lyc., ***merc.,*** nit-ac., sil., stront-c., zinc.
periosteum, as if in - ars.
burning - thuj.
chill, during - ferr., ***tub.***
evening - ***ars.,*** nat-m.
extending, downward - aesc., anac., ars., ***kali-c., sil.***
upward - bar-c.
ice-cold needles, as of - agar.
inner side - plb.
extending to big toe - ars.
paroxysmal - ***gels.***
resting, after - op.
rising from a seat, on - mag-c.
scratching, from - prun.
amel. - sil.
splinters, as from - ***nit-ac.***
stepping, hard - merc.
stool, during - ***rhus-t.***
touched, when - merc., ***nit-ac.***
walking, amel. - arg-m., ars., **BELL.,** ***cocc.,*** **KALI-C., KALI-S.,** ***lyc.,*** **PULS., RHUS-T.,** ***stel., tub.***
walking, during chilliness - sep.
sharp, calves - ***agar.,*** aloe, ***alum.,*** am-c., am-m., ang., arg-n., asaf., bell., berb., bry., calc., ***calc-p.,*** camph., carb-v., caust., chel., clem., coc-c., coloc., con., cycl., dros., dulc., euph., eupi., gamb., ***graph.,*** grat., ***guai.,*** hell., ***indg.,*** jatr., kali-n., led., ***lyc.,*** meny., merc., nat-p., nux-v., ph-ac., ***plb.,*** puls., ***rhus-t.,*** sars., sil., ***spig.,*** spong., ***staph., sulph.,*** tarax., ***tarent.,*** thuj., upa.
afternoon - grat.
bent, when - chel.

sharp, calves
bones - dros.
dinner, after - grat.
drawing, on boots, when - graph.
evening - sulph.
extending, downward - chel., eupi., ph-ac., ***sulph.***
from within out - berb.
upward - ***guai.,*** xan.
itching - coloc., staph.
lying, on - puls.
motion, on - berb., calc.
paroxysmal - caust., plb.
pressure amel. - plb.
room, in a, amel. - grat.
rubbing, after - thuj.
scratching, agg. - chel.
amel. - staph.
sitting, while - am-m., asaf., clem., ***dros.,*** mang., mur-ac., ***rhus-t.,*** tarax.
amel. - tarax.
stepping, on - sil.
tearing - calc., mang.
twitching - guai.
walk, after a - am-m.
walking, while - arg-n., grat., nat-p., sil., spong., staph.
amel. - ***dros., rhus-t.***
in open air - ***chin.,*** merc., sil.
wandering - berb.
warmth of bed, amel. - plb., upa.
sharp, lower - acon., aesc., aeth., ***agar.,*** agn., ***alum.,*** alumn., am-c., ***anac.,*** ant-c., ***apis,*** arg-m., ars., aster., atro., ***bell.,*** berb., bov., ***bry., calc.,*** cann-i., caps., ***carb-an.,*** carb-s., carb-v., ***caust.,*** cham., chel., ***chin.,*** clem., cob., ***cocc.,*** coc-c., ***coloc., con.,*** dig., dulc., echi., ***euph.,*** euphr., ***ferr., gels.,*** glon., ***graph.,*** grat., ***guai.,*** hell., ***hyper.,*** ind., jug-r., kali-c., ***kali-i.,*** kali-s., ***kalm.,*** lac-ac., lach., led., ***lyc.,*** meny., ***merc.,*** merc-c., ***mez.,*** mosch., ***mur-ac.,*** naja, nat-a., nat-c., nat-m., nit-ac., ***nux-v.,*** pall., petr., ph-ac., phos., pic-ac., ***plat., plb.,*** ran-s., raph., rheum, ***rhus-t.,*** rhus-v., samb., sars., sec., senec., ***sep.,*** **SIL.,** staph., stram., sulph., tarax., tarent., ***thuj., tub.,*** verb., viol-t., vip., zinc.
afternoon - lyc.
sitting, while - alum., alumn.
sitting, and sleeping, while - alum.
blowing, nose when - graph.
chill, during - ferr., lyc.
crossing, legs - nux-v., phos.
eating, amel. - ***nat-c.***
evening - ***ferr.,*** lac-ac., lyc.
in bed - alum., ***ferr.***
extending, downward - chel., ***kalm., sil.***
upward - bell., ***guai.,*** tarax., ***xan.***
falling, asleep, on - ***lach.***
hanging, down leg - graph.
itching - coloc., dulc.
jerking - ***carb-s.***
menses, during - raph.

sharp, lower
motion, during - coloc., merc., sars.
amel. - alum., ***kali-c., kali-s., lyc., rhus-t., tub.***
paroxysmal - ***gels.***
pulsative - coc-c.
riding, in a carriage, while - nat-m.
right - stict.
rising, on - carb-an.
sitting, while - am-m., euph., phos.
standing, while - phos., sil., tarax.
stool, during - rhus-t.
walking, while - anac., ***sulph.***
amel. - agar., ***kali-c., kali-s.,*** lyc., ***rhus-t., tub.***

sharp, thighs - acon., aesc., **AGAR.,** ***alum.,*** ammc., ***anac.,*** agn., apis, ***arg-m.,*** **ARS.,** ars-i., arund., asaf., asar., aster., ***aur-m.,*** bar-c., **BELL.,** berb., ***bov., bry.,*** calc., ***calc-p., carb-an.,*** carb-s., carb-v., caust., cham., chel., chin., chin-a., chin-s., cinnb., coff., ***coloc.,*** con., dig., dros., dulc., eupi., ***ferr.,*** ferr-ar., ferr-ma., form., gels., graph., ***guai.,*** hell., ***ind.,*** inul., ip., iris, ***kali-c., kali-i., kali-s., kalm.,*** kreos., lach., laur., lith., lyc., mag-c., mag-m., manc., ***mang.,*** meph., ***merc.,*** merl., mez., ***mur-ac.,*** myric., naja, nat-a., ***nat-c.,*** nat-m., nat-p., nit-ac., nuph., ***nux-v.,*** olnd., ox-ac., ***pall.,*** ph-ac., ***phos.,*** phyt., plb., ***ptel.,*** rat., rhod., ***rhus-t., sabad., samb., sars., sep., sil., spig.,*** spong., squil., ***stann.,*** staph., stict., stram., stront-c., sulph., tab., ***tarax., tarent., thuj.,*** trom., ***zinc.***
afternoon, walking, on - nat-c.
anterior, part - ang., dros., samb.
ascending - ph-ac.
bed, in - lach., zinc.
bend of - cann-s., caust., dig., gamb., grat., sil., spong.
walking, while - dig., spong.
bone - dros.
walking - cocc., mur-ac.
boring - anac., ph-ac., rhus-t., tarax.
burning - anac., **ARS.,** arund., berb., carb-an., graph., iris, mur-ac., olnd., sulph.
cramp-like - calc.
crural nerves - ***apis,*** ars., ***coff., staph.***
drawing - sabad., samb., spong., thuj.
up leg amel. - mag-m.
electric - agar.
evening - caust., mur-ac.
extending, downward - aesc., apis, ***aur-m., ars., bry.,*** calc-p., carb-v., cinnb., coloc., ***kali-c., kali-i., kalm.,*** mur-ac., ***nux-v.,*** pall., ***sil.,*** staph.
outward - berb., rhus-t.
to chest - caust.
to sole of foot - kreos.
to toes - ***apis.***
upward - ***lach.***
forenoon - bry.

sharp, thighs
inner side - arn., bar-c., calc., carb-s., chel., cocc., lac-ac., laur., nat-m., sabin., spong., stann., ***staph.,*** sulph., tarax., verb.
afternoon - stry.
itching - stann., staph.
pressure agg. - laur.
rubbing, amel. - sulph.
sitting, while - calc., tarax.
stepping, on - berb.
touch, on - cocc.
twitching - sabad.
itching - anac., guai., ***spig., staph.***
knee, above the - anac., arn., asaf., **BELL.,** berb., calc., caust., cham., dig., ferr., grat., guai., kreos., led., mang., meny., nux-v., olnd., phos., ruta., sars., spong., staph., ***zinc.***
burning - meny.
knee, above the, paroxysmal - alum.
pulsating - spong.
rising from sitting - rhus-t.
rubbing amel. - phos.
sitting - **BELL.,** phos., spong.
transverse - **ZINC.**
twitching - mang.
walking in open air - sars.
evening - ***mang.,*** nux-v.
lying, while - puls., zinc.
menses, before - staph.
morning, rising on - nat-m.
sitting, on - nat-c.
motion, on - coff., ***coloc.,*** iris, kreos., merc., nat-a., ph-ac., plb., staph.
amel. - alum., arg-m., ***kali-c., kali-s., rhus-t.***
near male, genitals - nat-m.
night - ars., calc., ***cinnb.,*** coff., ***kali-bi.,*** nat-m., nit-ac.
bed, in - ***ferr.,*** graph., zinc.
bed, in, amel. - ***kali-c., staph.***
noon - form.
outer side - anac., asaf., bar-c., bell., calc., caust., cham., cocc., ir-foe., mang., mur-ac., rhod.
evening - cham.
motion amel. - rhod.
pulsating - cocc.
sitting, amel. - mang.
sitting, while - bell., cocc., mur-ac., spig.
walking, while - mang., mur-ac.
paralytic - sep.
posterior part - canth., con., euphr., iris, ***kali-bi., kali-c., kali-i.,*** laur., meny., merc-i-f., nuph., sil., staph., zinc.
above the knee - dulc., guai.
evening, while yawning - zinc.
motion, amel. - caps.
pulsating - berb.
sitting, while - con., spig.
standing - chin., euphr.
walking in open air - con.
pressure amel. - dulc., nuph., plb.
pulsation, with every - ***anac.***
rheumatic - bapt.

sharp, thighs
rising, from bed - nat-c., ph-ac.
from sitting amel. - mur-ac.
rubbing, amel. - anac., mosch.
scratching, amel. - guai.
sitting, while - **BELL.,** ***con., dulc.,*** kali-c., ***kali-i.,*** mur-ac., nat-c., ph-ac., ***spig.***
down, on - bov., ph-ac.
sleep, after - **LACH.**
before - ***sulph.***
standing, while - calc., carb-an., euphr., rhus-t., stann.
stepping, when - ***calc.,*** lyc.
sudden - chin-s., sep.
tearing - asar., carb-an., hell., kali-c., kali-i., ph-ac., sep., zinc.
touch, on - puls.
transverse - **ZINC.**
twitching - ang., carb-s., mag-m., sabad., stann., stram.
upper part - aeth., carb-v., cham., kali-i., mez., ph-ac., sil., spong., thuj.
extending upwards - cham., euphr.
walking, while - berb., calc., carb-v., caust., coc-c., con., kali-c., ***kali-i.,*** lyc., nat-c., plb., sabad., sep., sil., ***spig.,*** spong., staph., zinc.
amel. - ***agar.,*** alum., ***arg-m., dulc., ferr., kali-c., kali-s.,*** lach., ***rhus-t.,*** sulph.
bent, while - ***bry.***
on beginning to walk agg. - ferr., ph-ac.
rapidly - sulph.
wandering - graph.

sharp, tibia - alum., am-m., ***ant-c.,*** aur., berb., bov., bry., cham., chel., ***chin.,*** coloc., dig., guai., hyper., kali-c., kali-i., led., meny., mez., nat-c., ph-ac., phos., puls., rhus-t., samb., sep., spig., **SULPH.,** thuj., ***zinc.***
boring - euphr., staph.
burning - arg-m.
drawing - guai.
evening in bed - alum., arg-m.
itching - coloc.
left - aur., bov.
motion, amel. - meny.
pulsating - meny.
right - alum., coloc.
sitting, while - nat-c.
tearing - guai., phos., rhus-t.
walking, while - chin., nat-c., zinc.

SHIVERING, legs, (see Shuddering) - ***graph., kali-c.,*** meny., plat.

SHOCKS - agar., ***ars., cic.,*** der., nux-v., op., phos., plat., plb., sulph., thuj., ***verat.,*** zinc.
painful - ars.
right, when falling asleep - ***arg-m.***
sleep, during - ***agar.,*** **ARS.,** zinc.
violent, cause legs to jerk - cic.

shocks, lower - agar., plat., sep.

shocks, thighs - ***agar.,*** dios., euphr., fl-ac., sep.
extending, downward - graph.
upward - agar., euphr.

SHOOTING, pain - aesc., aeth., ***alum.,*** **BELL.,** ***coloc.,*** gels., ***lach.,*** mag-s., ***nux-v.,*** phos., **PLB.**
extending, down sciatic nerve - ***coloc.,*** lach., ***ruta.***
downwards - aesc., anac., **PLB.**
stool during - rhus-t.
walking amel. - **BELL.**
warm bed amel. - ***mag-p.***

shooting, calves - alum., bell., ***calc-p., lyc., plb.,*** sulph., tarent.
evening - sulph.
pulling on boot - graph.

shooting, lower - ***acon.,*** aesc., aeth., anac., bell., cann-i., ***con., ferr., gels.,*** guai., ***hyper.,*** iod., naja, ***rhus-t., sil.***
evening in bed - ***ferr.***
paroxysm - ***gels.***

shooting, lower
periosteum, in - hyper.
right - iod.
upwards - ***guai.,*** xan.

shooting, thighs - acon., aesc., ***alum.,*** anac., ***apis,*** **ARS.,** ars-i., arum-d., aur-m., **BELL.,** ***calc-p.,*** cinnb., form., iris, kali-bi., ***kali-c.,*** lec., myric., naja, sep., sil., stram., sulph., tarent., trom.
back of - ***kali-c.,*** ind.
crural nerves - apis
extending, downward - aesc., apis, aur-m., calc-p., form., kali-bi., ***kali-c.,*** lec., sep.
to foot - anac.
to toes - ***apis,*** sep.
night - kali-bi.
before falling asleep - sulph.
noon - form.
sitting - bell.
sudden - sep.
walking amel. - sulph.

SHORT, sensation as if - ambr.
left - cinnb.
right - merc.

short, calves sensation as if - carl., ***sil.***
descending stairs - arg-m.

SHORTENING, (see Contractions)

SHORTENED, muscles and tendons (see Limbs, chapter)

SHORTER, one than the other leg - caust., cinnb., lycps., mez., nat-m., sulph., til.
right feels shortened - crot-c.

SHUDDERING, lower, shivering - cinnb., con., dig., ***graph.,*** hura, kali-c., meny., mez.

shuddering, thighs - phos., ran-b.
afternoon - lyc.
shivering - ang., arn., bry., cann-s., chin., cina, ign., kali-bi., lyc.

SMALL, lower, seems too - kali-c.

SNAKE, lower, feels as if crawling up leg - ail.

SOFTENING, thighs, femur, of - sil.

softening, tibia, of - calc-f., calc-p., ***guai.***

SORE, pain - aesc., agar., alum., alumn., ant-t., apis, ***arn.,*** asar., aster., ***bell., berb.,*** bufo, ***calc.,*** carb-an., carb-s., ***carb-v.,*** caul., **CAUST.,** ***chel., cocc., con.,*** crot-t., cupr., **EUP-PER.,** ferr-i., form., graph., ham., kali-bi., ***led.,*** lyc., mag-c., mag-m., manc., mang., merc., myric., ***nat-c.,*** nat-m., nat-p., nat-s., ***nit-ac., nux-v., ph-ac., phos.,*** pic-ac., plb., ptel., puls., **RHUS-T.,** ***rhus-v.,*** **RUTA.,** sanic., ***sep.,*** sil., spig., spong., ***stann., sulph.,*** valer., verat., zinc.
afternoon - myric.
ascending, steps, on - nat-m., stann.
bones - calc., ***led., mang., nit-ac.***
dancing amel. - sep.
evening - sulph.
forenoon - nat-s., ptel.
inner side of - petr.
joints - agar., ***arg-m.,*** calc., ***dig.,*** nat-c., ph-ac., sarr., sep.
descending - arg-m.
leg, laid on - graph.
menses, during - caul., mag-m., nit-ac., sep.
before - caul.
morning - carb-an., ***caust., ph-ac.***
on rising - nux-v., stann.
motion, on - calc.
paralytic - calc.
night - phos.
paroxysms, in - plb.
right - ang.
rising to walk, when - cycl., ***eup-per.***
sitting agg. - apis
standing, while - alum., alumn.
walking, while - aesc., ***chel.***
after, agg. - agar., ***berb.,*** **RUTA.**
in open air, after - ***sulph.***

sore, calves - ***aesc.,*** alum., ant-c., ant-t., arn., ars-i., berb., ***bry.,*** caust., ***chel.,*** chim., clem., coca, croc., crot-h., **EUP-PER.,** fago., ***ferr.,*** ferr-i., ***gels.,*** jatr., ***kali-c.,*** lac-ac., mag-m., merc-cy., mez., mosch., nat-m., ***nux-m.,*** nux-v., pic-ac., plb., puls-n, rhus-t., sep., stann.
eating, after - clem.
evening - ferr-i., stann.
in bed - mag-m.
menses, during - mag-m.
night - ***gels.***
paralytic - mag-m.
sitting, while - jatr.
touch, on - ant-c.
walking, while - alum., ***chel.,*** staph.

sore, lower - acon., agar., alum., alumn., am-m., ang., apis, asar., aur-m., bad., **BELL.,** ***berb.,*** brach., bry., ***calc.,*** canth., carb-ac., carb-an., carb-s., card-m., cast-eq., **CAUST.,** chel., chin., chlor., cic., cimic., clem., coff., ***coloc.,*** con., croc., dig., **EUP-PER.,** ferr., ferr-i., gels., graph., ***guai.,*** hura, hyos., iod., **KALI-C.,** kali-n., kali-p., ***led.,*** lyc., lyss., mag-c., mag-m., merc., ***mez.,*** nat-a., ***nat-c.,*** nat-m., nat-p., nat-s., ***nit-ac.,*** nux-m., osm., petr., ***ph-ac.,*** phos., ***phyt.,*** pic-ac., plb., prun., psor., ***puls., rhus-t.,*** **RUTA.,** ***sep.,*** sil., stann., ***sulph.,*** tarent., tep., thuj., valer., zinc.

sore, lower
alternating with bruised sensation arms - cic.
ascending steps - bad., nat-m.
bones - chin.
evening - alum., bry., lyss., mag-m.
in bed - puls.
fatigue, after - clem.
lying down, when - alum., calc.
menses, during - petr.
morning - chlor., prun.
bed, in - **CAUST.,** ferr.
rising, after - plb.
waking, on - kali-n.
motion, on - ***bufo,*** dig., nux-v., ***puls.***
night - gels., ***merc., mez.,*** nux-v., sulph.
numb - bad.
periosteum - chin.
pressing, with hands, amel. - puls.
rising, after, amel. - ferr.
sitting, while - bry., ruta., sep.
spots - sil.
standing, while - alum., dig.
touch, on - con.
urination, during - ***nat-c.***
walking, while - ***aesc.,*** aur-m., berb., canth., carb-an., chlor., coloc., ferr., graph., ph-ac., sol-n.
after - guai., **RUTA.**

sore, thighs - ***acon.,*** all-c., ***am-c.,*** am-m., anac., ang., arg-m., ***arn.,*** ars., asar., aur., bapt., bar-c., **BELL.,** berb., bry., ***calc.,*** calc-p., calo., ***camph.,*** caps., carb-an., carb-s., **CAUST.,** cham., ***chel.,*** chin., clem., ***cocc.,*** coff., crot-h., dig., dulc., ferr-i., fl-ac., gels., graph., grat., ***guai., ham., hep.,*** hyper., iod., kali-bi., kali-c., kali-n., lach., lact., laur., ***led., lyc.,*** lyss., mag-c., ***mag-m.,*** mang., ***meny., merc.,*** merc-i-f., mez., mosch., murx., nat-a., ***nat-c.,*** nat-s., nicc., ***nit-ac., nux-v.,*** ol-an., olnd., ***ph-ac.,*** phos., ***plat.,*** plb., ***puls.,*** **RHUS-T., RUTA.,** sabin., sang., sanic., seneg., ***sep., sil.,*** spig., squil., staph., ***sulph.,*** tab., ***thuj.,*** valer., viol-t., zinc.
afternoon, on walking - hyper., nat-s., valer.
anterior, part of - arg-m., cham., ***hep.,*** laur., ***lyss.,*** nat-c., nux-v., plb., **RUTA.,** sabin., ***sulph.,*** zinc.
evening - ***sulph.***
pressure, on - ***sulph.,*** zinc.
upper part - tarax.
walking, while - olnd., spig.
ascending, steps - calc., ***ph-ac.***
bend of - berb., bov., dig., laur., mang., nat-s., sars.
evening - nat-s.
menses, before - sars.
menses, during - bov.
walking, while - nat-s.
bending knee - ***puls.***
between - am-c., ars., calc., **CAUST.,** graph., kali-c., lyc., ***nat-c., nit-ac.,*** rhod., ***sep.,*** squil., sulph.

sore, thighs
bones - bry., ***calc.,*** graph., mag-c., meny., ***mez.,*** nit-ac., phos., **PULS., RUTA.,** sabin., ***sil.,*** sulph.
chill, during - ***ars.,*** eup-per.
cold damp weather - **CALC-P.**
drawn up, when - sabin.
evening - kali-c., mag-m.
in bed - mag-c.
sitting - meny.
exertion - ol-an.
extending to calves - chel., valer.
to lumbar region - kali-n.
genitals, near - **GRAPH.,** ***merc.,*** rhod.
female - kreos.
male - caust., ***crot-t.,*** nat-m., nit-ac.
grasping it, on - merc.
inner side - bell., ***camph.,*** cocc., fl-ac., mez., nat-p., phel., spig., staph., thuj.
ascending stairs - nat-p.
innner side, evening - sulph.
leaning to left side amel. - phel.
menses, during - phel.
riding horseback, after - spig.
turning, on, in circle to left - cocc.
walking rapidly - mez.
jarring agg. - valer.
lower, part, above knee - cupr., kali-c., lyc., nit-ac., sul-ac.
lying, while - sil., staph.
lying, while, on it - ***caust.,*** kali-bi.
menses, during - ***am-c.,*** bov., ***nit-ac.***
middle of - am-c., bar-c., bry., ***calc.,*** chel., cocc., graph., hep., kali-bi., laur., mag-m., nat-c., nat-s., nicc., ph-ac., phos., plat., ruta, sabin., thuj., valer.
afternoon while sitting - nicc.
ascending stairs - ***calc.***
evening, in bed - mag-m.
menses, during - am-c., indg.
sitting, while - nicc., plat.
standing - valer.
touch, on - kali-c.
walking when beginning to - ph-ac.
walking, in open air - thuj.
morning - lyc., nat-c., ***sulph.,*** viol-t.
after rising - valer.
in bed - **CAUST.**
waking, on - kali-n., ***sulph.***
motion, on - arg-m., dig., lyc., nux-v., phos.
amel. - caps.
night - aur., sep., sulph.
in one lain on - ***caust.***
outer side - anac., aur., meny., sulph., zinc.
paroxysmal - sul-ac.
periosteum - led.
perspiration, amel. - ***gels.***
posterior part - chin., fl-ac., ign., ***indg.,*** mang., mez., phos., **RUTA.,** zinc.
raising leg while sitting - cocc.
right - ***camph.***
rubbing, amel. - am-c.
scratching, after - mang.
sitting, while - chin., ign., kali-c., kreos., meny., sil., sulph.

sore, thighs
skated as if, too much - crot-h.
sleep, during - sep.
after agg. - ph-ac.
standing, while - grat., kali-c.
stepping, forward - nit-ac.
stretching out on - caps., **RUTA.**
touch, amel. - am-c., lyc., mang., nat-c., ruta, sep., sulph., tarax.
turning, in bed - kali-n.
walking, while - am-c., arn., calc., chel., ***guai.,*** mag-c., nat-c., nat-s., olnd., ph-ac., ***sil.,*** spig.
amel. - **BELL.,** caps.
on beginning to walk - ph-ac., **RHUS-T.**
walking, after - ***arn.,*** calc., ***camph.,*** crot-h., mag-c., meny., merc., ph-ac., ***ruta.***
sitting - cocc.
fast - staph.
in open air - guai.

sore, tibia - agar., alum., asaf., ***asar., aur., aur-m., calc.,*** carb-an., caust., coff., con., graph., hyos., iod., ***kali-bi.,*** kali-c., ***kali-s.,*** mag-c., ***mang., mez.,*** nat-m., ***nit-ac.,*** nux-v., petr., **PHOS.,** psor., ***puls., rhus-t.,*** **RUTA.,** sep., ***sil., syph.,*** thuj.
drawing up toes - puls.
evening - alum.
morning, in bed - psor.
motion, on - sep.
sitting agg. - sep.
night - ***mez.,*** nit-ac., nux-v.
in bed - ***merc., mez.***
standing - alum., mag-c., mang.
walking, while - alum., carb-an., mag-c.

SPASM, (see Convulsion)

SPRAINED, as if - ***arn.,*** berb., carb-v., caust., nat-m., olnd., puls., rhus-t.
sitting, on - ip.

sprained, calves - graph.

sprained, lower - agar., am-c., ars.
walking, while - am-c.

sprained, thighs - am-c., caps., led., stann., staph.
abduction, on - caps.
walking - stann.

sprained, tibia, muscles - calc.

STAGGERING, (see Ataxia and Vertigo)

STIFFNESS - ***acon.,*** agar., alum., am-m., aml-n., anac., ang., ant-t., apoc., ***arg-m.,*** arg-n., ars., ars-h., **ATRO.,** aur., ***aur-m.,*** bar-c., ***bell.,*** **BERB.,** brom., ***bry.,*** bufo, ***calc.,*** calc-s., caps., carb-an., carb-o., ***carb-s., carb-v.,*** chel., chin., chin-a., ***cic., cina, cocc., coc-c.,*** con., cupr., dig., dros., **EUP-PER.,** ***ferr.,*** ferr-ar., ferr-p., ***ham., hydr-ac.,*** ign., jatr., kali-c., kali-i., ***lac-c.,*** lact., ***lath., lyc., mag-p., mang., merc.,*** merc-c., ***nat-m., nat-s.,*** nit-ac., **NUX-V.,** ol-an., op., ox-ac., ***petr.,*** phos., phys., **PLAT.,** plb., podo., puls., ran-b., rhod., **RHUS-T.,** sars., sec., **SEP., SIL.,** ***spong.,*** stram., ***stry.,*** sulph., tab., ter., thuj., ***verat., zinc.***
afternoon - brom.

STIFFNESS, legs
bending, on - phos., plan.
chill, during - ***nat-s., tub.***
before - petr., ***phos.,*** psor., rhus-t.
cold damp weather - ***lath.***
descending stairs - ***rhus-t.,*** stry.
epilepsy, before - ***bufo.***
evening - arg-m., calc-s., ***lyc., phos., plat., puls.,*** sil.
nap, after a - ***carb-v.***
rising on amel. - mang.
extending to hip joint - sep.
left - ***arg-n.,*** phos., stram.
morning - bell., ***petr.,*** rhod., **RHUS-T.,** staph., ***verat.***
night - alum., ***lyc.,*** nit-ac.
painful - cic., sec.
with - ***cocc.***
paroxysms - stry.
right - ***coc-c.,*** mang.
rising, on - agar., caps., cycl., **EUP-PER.,** ***hep.,*** psor.
rubbing amel. - stram.
sciatica - cur., ***lyc., nux-v.***
sitting, while - mang., plat.
after - bell., ***calc.,*** carb-an., dig., nux-v., ***puls.,*** **RHUS-T.,** ***sep.,*** zinc.
sleep, after - ***sep.***
standing - verat.
stretching amel. - stram.
walking, while - ol-an., ran-b., thuj.
after - **RHUS-T.**
amel. - ***carb-v.,*** dig.
in open air - **BERB., MANG.,** puls., **RHUS-T.**

stiffness, calves - ***arg-n.,*** con., zinc.

stiffness, lower - bell., mang., nat-m., petr., plat.

stiffness, thighs - am-c., am-m., ars., aur., aur-m., aur-s., bry., ***calc.,*** calc-s., carb-v., cham., cic., cocc., colch., ***coloc.,*** dig., dirc., gins., ***graph.,*** hell., hydr-ac., ign., lac-c., lil-t., merc., ***nat-m.,*** petr., phos., puls., rhod., rhus-t., sars., sec., ***stry.,*** thuj.
afternoon - ***calc-s.***
anterior muscles - ***calc., stry.***
contracted, as if - sars.
cramp, like a - bry.
evening, when rising from a seat - rhod.
morning - bry., ***calc.***
rising, on - ign.
walk, on beginning to - ***calc.***
paralytic - cham., cocc.
standing, while - carb-v.
walking, while - am-c., bell., ***calc.,*** cic., graph., petr., ***stry.***

STRETCHED, out (see Drawing, legs up) - ambr., merc., nat-m., nux-v., ***oena.,*** phos., rhus-t., spong., stry., sul-ac.
must stretch - nat-m., rhus-t.

stretched, out, lower - cham., dig., lach., led., nat-c., ***plat., rhus-t.,*** ruta., spong., stann., sulph.
epilepsy, before - ***bufo.***

stretched, out, lower
evening - nat-c.
morning in bed - ***rhus-t.***
on waking - ***plat.***
night - stann.
noon - am-c.

STRETCHING, (see Generals)

stretching, thigh amel. - cham.

SWAYING, lower, to and fro when standing - cycl.

SWELLING - act-sp., am-c., apis, ***ars.,*** arund., aur-m., ***bar-m., berb.,*** bry., ***calc.,*** carb-s., ***carb-v.,*** caust., ***chel.,*** con., ***dulc., graph.,*** iod., ***kali-ar.,*** kali-bi., ***kali-c., kali-n.,*** lach., ***led., lyc.,*** merc., nat-c., nat-m., nat-p., nit-ac., nux-v., petr., ***phos.,*** plb., polyg., puls., ***rhus-t.,*** rhus-v., ***sep.,*** **SIL.,** sol-t-ae., **SULPH.,** verat.
bluish - lach.
cinchona, after abuse of - **PULS.,** ***sulph.***
cold - asaf.
daytime - dig.
dropsical - acet-ac., aeth., **APIS,** ***apoc.,*** arg-m., **ARS.,** ***ars-i.,*** arund., aur., ***aur-m., cact.,*** cahin., ***calc.,*** calc-ar., calc-s., ***carb-ac., carb-s., cench., chel., chim.,*** **CHIN.,** cocc., ***colch., dig., dulc.,*** eup-per., ***ferr.,*** ferr-i., ***fl-ac., graph., hell., hippoz., hydr.,*** iod., ***kali-c., lach., led.,*** **LYC.,** ***mag-m., med., merc.,*** mur-ac., onos., phos., ***phyt.,*** plb., puls., rhod., ***rhus-t.,*** ruta, **SAMB.,** sanic., sars., ***senec.,*** sulph., ***ter.,*** xan., ***zinc.***
albuminuria, in - ***apis, ars., calc-ar., ferr., lach., sars., ter.***
scarlet fever, after - **APIS,** bar-m., crot-h., ***hell.***
evening - am-c., cocc., hyper., nat-m., phos., puls., rhus-t., stann.
hard - aur., ars., bov., chin., graph., led., mag-c., mez., rhus-t.
hot - acon., am-c., ***arn.,*** ars., ***bry.,*** calc., carb-an., ***chin.,*** cocc., coc-c., colch., graph., iod., kali-c., led., lyc., petr., puls., sars., sec., sep., stann.
inflammatory - acon., calc., iod., puls., rhus-t., sil.
itching - cocc.
large - sulph.
lymphatic - bar-c., berb.
menses, during - apis, apoc., ars., calc., graph., lyc.
morning - sil.
painful - acon., ant-c., arn., ars., carb-an., chin., con., daph., lach., mag-c., merc., nux-v., puls., sep., sil.
burning - ant-c., ***ars.,*** mur-ac., petr., ph-ac., puls.
cutting - ph-ac.
drawing - arn., led., puls.
pressing - led.
pulsating - ph-ac., plat.
sharp - acon., am-c., arn., bry., carb-v., cocc., graph., iod., led., lyc., merc., petr., ***puls.,*** sars.
tearing - colch., led., merc., plat., puls.

SWELLING, legs
painful, tense - bry., chin., led., sars., thuj.
red - acon., am-c., ant-c., arn., bry., calc., carb-v., chin., hep., lach., nat-c., nux-v., petr., puls., sabin., sars., sil., stann., thuj.
bright - iod.
spots - acon., chin.
spots, or blue-black blisters - ars.
rheumatic - hep.
shining - acon., arn., ars., bell., bry., merc., sabin., sulph.
soft - chin., led.
stinging - **APIS,** graph., **LED.,** ***puls.***
transparent - ***apis,*** sulph.
walking, while - phos., rhus-t.
in open air - phos.
waxy - apis.
white - apis, ars., bell., ***calc.,*** graph., iod., kreos., lyc., merc., nux-v., rhus-t., sulph.

swelling, calves - berb., bry., ***calc.,*** carb-v., chin., ***dulc.,*** graph., hyos., ***led.,*** mez., phos., puls., sil., sulph.
veins, of - cycl.

swelling, lower - acet-ac., ***acon.,*** agn., arn., **ARS.,** ars-i., ***aur., aur-m., bad.,*** bor., bov., ***bry.,*** bufo, ***cact., calc.,*** calc-s., carb-s., ***caust., cench.,*** chel., clem., ***chin., colch.,*** coloc., cop., ***crot-c., crot-h., dig.,*** dulc., ***ferr.,*** ferr-i., ***graph., hell.,*** iod., kali-ar., ***kali-bi.,*** kali-c., ***kali-chl.,*** kali-i., kali-n., kali-p., kali-s., ***lach.,*** **LED., LYC.,** manc., ***med., merc.,*** morph., ***nat-c.,*** nat-s., nux-v., plb., ***puls., rhod.,*** rhus-t., rhus-v., ruta., **SAMB.,** sec., ***sep.,*** **SIL.,** ***stann.,*** sulph., ***syph., ter.,*** vip., ***zinc.***
afternoon - chel.
4 p.m. - sang.
bluish - **LACH.,** ***led., puls.***
cold - nux-v.
evening - agn., bufo, dulc., mez., nat-m., sang., stront.
exertion, from - rhod.
hard - aur., bov., graph.
menses, during - sulph.
morning - ***aur.***
painful - dig., **LED.**
red - aur., bov.
sitting, while - sep.
standing, while - merc-cy., mez., sep.
walking amel. - ***aur., sep.***

swelling, thighs - agn., arn., ars., both., calad., carb-o., chin., con., ***ham.,*** kali-c., kali-n., ***lach.,*** led., lyc., merc., puls., ter., vip.
bend of - dig.
evening - agn.
femur - ***mez.,*** **SIL.,** ***stront.***
glands of - ***calc.***
sensation of - prun.

swelling, tibia - ***aur-m., calc-p.,*** graph., lach., ***merc., phos.,*** rhus-t., stann., sulph., thuj.

TEARING, pain - ***acon.,*** aeth., ***agar.,*** agn., **ALUM.,** ambr., anac., ant-c., ant-t., ***arg-m.,*** arn., **ARS.,** ***aur-m.,*** bar-c., ***bell.,*** berb., ***calc., calc-ar.,*** canth., ***caps.,*** carb-s., carb-v., **CAUST.,** ***cham., chin., chin-a., cic.,*** cina, ***colch.,*** **COLOC.,** ***con.,*** dulc., eupi., ***ferr., graph.,*** hep., ***ign., indg.,*** **KALI-AR.,** ***kali-bi.,*** **KALI-C.,** kali-n., kali-p., ***kali-s.,*** **KALM.,** kreos., lach., **LYC.,** mag-c., ***mag-m.,*** mag-s., merc., mez., nat-a., ***nat-c.,*** nat-p., **NAT-S.,** nicc., **NIT-AC.,** nux-m., nux-v., par., ph-ac., phos., **PLB.,** ***puls.,*** rhod., **RHUS-T.,** sars., sep., ***sil.,*** stann., ***stront-c., sulph., tarax.,*** teucr., thuj., ***tub.,*** valer., ***verat.,*** verb., zinc.
air, open, agg. - **CAUST.**
bones - **AGAR.,** am-m., arg-m., ars., aur., bar-c., carb-v., chin., ***kali-c., kali-n.,*** lyc., mag-c., mag-s., ***merc.,*** mez., **NIT-AC.,** phos., ***rhod.,*** stront-c., teucr., thuj., ***zinc.***
chill, during - ***ars.,*** **RHUS-T.**
cold, becoming - ***phos., rhus-t.***
coughing - ***caps.***
eating, while - ph-ac.
evening - alum., mag-s., nat-c.
evening, bed, in - ***ferr., sulph.***
walking, while - sulph.
extending, downwards - ***ars.,*** bar-ac., ***bar-c., cham., cic.,*** eupi., ***kalm.,*** mag-s., ***sulph.,*** valer., verat., verb.
upward - ***bell.,*** nat-c., ***nux-v.,*** sep., stront.
flatulence, from obstructed - carb-v.
hanging over side of bed amel. - verat.
joints - bar-ac., ***bell.,*** calc., kali-c., merc., ***stront-c., teucr.,*** zinc.
left - con., lyc., sil.
to right - ambr.
lying on painful side agg. - **ARS.**
menses, during - ***bell., berb.,*** bry., cham., con., rhus-t., sep., sul-ac.
morning - hep., stront.
motion, during - alum., ars., ***bry., kalm.***
amel. - ***arg-m., ars.,*** euph., ***puls., rhod.,*** **RHUS-T.,** sep., ***tarax., valer.,*** zinc.
night - alum., anac., ***ars., cic.,*** kali-c., lyc., ***merc.,*** **NIT-AC.,** ***rhod., verat.***
4 a.m. - coloc.
when lying upon it - **ARS.**
when putting feet out of bed amel. - sulph.
paralytic - ***cham.***
paroxysmal - sulph.
right - sulph.
rising from a seat, amel. - mag-c.
sitting, while - agar., ***alum.,*** arn., **BELL.,** ph-ac., valer.
low - sulph.
standing, while - sulph.
stool, during - ***rhus-t.***
storm, during - caust.
stretch leg, must - sulph.
touch, agg - ***chin.***
walking, while - nicc., sep., ***sil.,*** stront-c., sulph.
amel. - bar-c., **BELL.,** ***ferr., lyc.,*** **RHUS-T.,** sulph., ***valer.,*** verat.

TEARING, pain
warm applications amel. - ***caust., cham.***
warmth of bed - ***sulph.***
amel. - **CAUST.,** ***coloc., rhus-t.,*** **LYC.**
wet weather - ***dulc., rhod., rhus-t.***
tearing, calves - agar., ***alum.,*** ambr., am-m., arn., ars., aur-m., berb., bry., calc., ***calc-p.,*** canth., carb-s., carb-v., cast., ***caust.,*** chin., cic., cina, colch., ***coloc.,*** croc., euph., ***ign., indg.,*** kali-bi., kali-c., kali-i., kali-n., laur., led., lob., mag-c., mag-m., mang., merc., mez., mur-ac., nat-c., nat-m., **NAT-S.,** olnd., par., phel., plb., ran-b., raph., rat., sabad., sil., staph., sulph., tab., teucr., ***valer., zinc.***
above - sep.
afternoon - mag-c., nat-c., **VALER.**
4 p.m., when laying right limb across the left - ***valer.***
5 p.m. - cast., valer.
bed, in - am-m.
below - lyc., sep.
chill, with - sil.
cramp-like - ran-b.
dinner, after - canth.
drawing - calc., kali-n.
eating, after, agg. - bry.
evening - am-m., mag-m., nat-s., ran-b., sulph.
bed, in - sil.
extending, downward - arn., carb-v., caust., mag-m., phel., sulph., zinc.
to heel - ***coloc.,*** mag-m.
to hollow of knee - nat-s.
to toes - sulph.
upward - arn., mag-m.
lacerating - plb.
lying with limbs crossed - ***valer.***
motion, agg. - berb., plb.
agg., of foot and toes - caust.
amel. - dulc., indg., ***rat.,*** sabad., sulph., ***valer.***
night - mur-ac., sabad.
paroxysmal - ambr., aur-m., plb.
pressive - berb.
amel. - plb.
pulsating - **VALER.**
right - agar., ***caust.,*** rat.
rubbing, amel. - cast., nat-s.
sitting, while - agar., am-m., ars., cina, coloc., euph., indg., mur-ac., rat., sulph., **VALER.**
standing, while - berb., coloc., euph., ***ign.,*** kali-i., mag-m., sulph.
sticking - staph.
twitching - am-m., zinc.
walking, while - canth., ***ign.,*** olnd., plb., ran-b.
VALER.
amel. - agar., kali-i.,
warmth, of bed - plb.
amel. - ars.

tearing, lower - ***acon.,*** agar., agn., **ALUM.,** ***ambr.,*** anac., anag., arg-m., ***arg-n., ars.,*** asaf., aur-m., bar-c., **BELL.,** berb., bor., brom., bry., cadm-s., ***calc.,*** calc-p., camph., caps., ***carb-an.,*** carb-s., ***carb-v.,*** **CAUST.,** ***cham.,*** chel., chin., chin-a., chin-s., ***cic.,*** cina, ***cinnb.,*** colch., ***coloc.,*** con., croc., crot-t., cupr., cycl., ***dulc., euph., ferr., graph., guai.,*** hell., hep., ***hyper., ign., indg.,*** ip., iod., kali-ar., kali-bi., ***kali-c., kali-i., kali-n.,*** kali-p., kali-s., ***kalm.,*** lach., lachn., lact., ***led., lob., lyc.,*** mag-c., ***mag-m., merc.,*** merl., ***mez.,*** mill., nat-a., nat-c., nat-m., nat-p., **NAT-S.,** nicc., ***nit-ac.,*** nux-v., ol-an., op., pall., petr., ph-ac., phos., ***puls.,*** rat., ***rhod.,*** **RHUS-T.,** sabad., samb., ***sars.,*** sel., ***sep., sil.,*** spong., ***stann., staph.,*** **SULPH.,** tab., ***tarax.,*** teucr., thuj., til., verat., verb., ***zinc.***
afternoon - alumn., indg., led., nicc., nux-v., sulph.
2 to 5 p.m. - sil.
walking, while - nicc.
air, open, agg. - **CAUST.,** con.
arthritic - sil.
below knee - cupr.
bones - carb-v., kali-c.
burning - bell.
chill, during - ***ars., ferr.,*** kali-n., ***rhus-t., sulph., tub.***
cramp-like - stann.
eating, while - ph-ac.
evening - alum., caust., kali-bi., kali-i., kali-n., led., ***lyc.,*** nicc., ***sulph.***
extending, downward - agar., agn., ars., aur-m., ***bar-c.,*** calc-p., carb-an., caust., ***cham.,*** chel., ***lyc.,*** nicc., nux-v., thuj., verb., ***zinc.***
to toes - **ALUM.,** nux-v., zinc.
upward - **BELL.,** caust., con., guai., lach., sulph.
forenoon - sil.
jerking - lyc.
lying, while - ***alum.***
menses, during - mag-m.
midnight - lyc.
morning - ambr., dulc., sulph.
bed, in - sulph.
motion, amel. - agar., ***alum.,*** arg-m., **BELL.,** ferr., kalm., ***rat., rhod.,*** **RHUS-T.,** sil., ***tarax., tub.***
night - ***alum.,*** am-m., anag., ***ferr.,*** kali-c., ***lyc., merc.,*** **NIT-AC.,** sulph.
10 p.m. - form.
noon - sulph.
numbness in the other, with - ***sil.***
paralytic - agar., bell., ***cham.,*** til.
paroxysmal - aur-m.
pregnancy during - verat.
pulsating - arg-m.
rheumatic - ambr., ***calc.,*** **CAUST.,** colch., graph., ***kalm., lyc., merc.,*** nit-ac., petr., rhod., **RHUS-T.,** ***zinc.***
right - rat.
rubbing, amel. - phos.

tearing, lower
sitting, while - agar., ***alum.,*** am-c., caust., cina, euph., ***indg.,*** ph-ac., sil., stann., staph., **SULPH., VALER.**
uncovering amel. - ***sulph.***
veins, of - cham.
walking, while - bar-c., ***sil.,*** stann., **SULPH.**
amel. - agar., ***alum.,*** arg-m., asaf., ***bar-c.,*** **BELL.,** ***euph., ferr.,*** grat., ***indg.,*** kali-n., **LYC., RHUS-T., VALER.,** ***tub.***
in open air - euph.
in open air, amel. - cina.
wandering - lact., rhod.
warm, clothing amel. - agar., ars., **LYC.**
warmth of bed - **MERC.,** plb., sil., ***sulph.***
amel. - ***agar.,*** **CAUST.,** ***cham.,*** **LYC.,** ***tub.***

tearing, thighs - ***agar.,*** aloe, **ALUM.,** ***am-c., am-m.,*** anac., ang., **ARS.,** asaf., asar., aur., ***aur-m., bar-c., bell.,*** benz-ac., berb., bor., bry., ***calc., camph.,*** canth., caps., ***carb-an.,*** carb-s., carb-v., ***caust.,*** cham., chel., ***chin., chin-a., cic.,*** cina, cinnb., ***clem.,*** coc-c., coff., ***colch., coloc.,*** con., cycl., ***dulc., euph.,*** ferr., ***ferr-ar., graph.,*** grat., ***guai.,*** hep., hyper., ***kali-ar.,*** kali-bi., ***kali-c., kali-i.,*** kali-s., ***kalm.,*** lach., laur., led., **LYC.,** lyss., mag-c., mag-m., mag-s., mang., ***merc., merl., mez.,*** mur-ac., nat-a., ***nat-c., nat-m.,*** **NAT-S.,** nicc., nit-ac., nux-v., ol-an., par., petr., phel., ***ph-ac.,*** phos., **PLB.,** ***phyt.,*** prun., puls., ***rat.,*** rhod., ***rhus-t.,*** sabad., sabin., ***sars.,*** sec., sep., ***sil., spig., stann., stront-c., sulph.,*** sul-ac., ***syph.,*** tax., tep., ter., thuj., trom., ***valer., zinc.***
afternoon - ***coff.,*** graph., nat-c.
menses, during - nux-v.
sleep, after - nux-v.
air, open agg. - ***caust.***
anterior part - am-m., ars., bar-c., chin., ***coff.,*** con., euph., mag-c., mur-ac., **PLB.**
bend of - ant-t., gamb.
bone - ***am-m.,*** ang., mur-ac., ***nit-ac.,*** stann., thuj., ***zinc.***
burning - merl.
cold air agg. - ***kalm., rhus-t.***
cramp-like - nat-c.
crossing limbs, when - agar.
dining, after - sep., sulph.
drawing - ***acon.,*** agar., ***anac., ars., chin.,*** clem., ***coloc.,*** carb-an., dulc., merc., nux-v., **RHUS-T.,** spig., stann., tep., thuj.
eating, after - dros.
evening - am-m., colch., graph., kali-c., lyc., nat-c., ran-b., stront.
in bed - mag-m.
extending, downward - agar., ***am-m.,*** ant-t., ***aur-m.,*** canth., carb-v., caust., cham., ***cic.,*** kali-i., ***kalm.,*** lach., led., lyc., mag-c., mag-m., nat-c., ph-ac., **PLB.,** rat., ***rhus-t.,*** sec., sil., tep., thuj.
to ankles - ars.
to hip - graph.
to knees - ars., guai., nat-c., sulph.

tearing, thighs
extending, upward - colch., nux-v., ***valer.,*** zinc.
flexed, when knees are - lyc.
inner side - ***am-m.,*** berb., calc., caps., kali-bi., kali-c., merl., plb., sulph., zinc.
intermittent - nat-c.
jerking - chin., mag-c., ***rhus-t.***
knee, above the - aloe, alum., carb-an., cast., colch., hep., kali-c., kali-i., kreos., led., mag-c., mag-m., mang., mez., ***nit-ac.,*** ol-an., puls., ***rhus-t.,*** sars., sil., teucr.
back and forth - sil.
drawing - dulc., kreos.
evening - colch., mag-m., sars.
evening, bed, in - colch., mag-m.
morning, in bed - hep.
night - mag-m., sars., sil.
paroxysmal - alum.
standing, when - plb.
twitching - ***rhus-t.***
walking, while - mez.
left - ***am-m.,*** kali-i., mag-m., sep.
lying while - ***alum.,*** clem.
amel. - ***phyt.***
menses during - carb-an., kali-c., nux-v., ***petr.***
morning - graph., ran-b., rhod., sulph.
rising, after - bar-c.
motion, agg. - aur., berb., bry., calc., coff., ***coloc., kalm., merc., plb.,*** sec.
amel. - ***alum.,*** coc-c., ***dulc., euph.,*** merc-i-f., mur-ac., ***rat., rhod.,*** **RHUS-T.,** sep., ***sulph., valer.,*** zinc.
night, bed, in - ***alum.,*** carb-an., coff., colch., kali-c., puls., sulph., ***syph.***
bed, in, amel. - tax.
numbness, with - agar., hep., rhod.
outer side - anac., ***am-m.,*** bar-c., berb., carb-an., caust., cycl., euph., kali-n., led., lyc., mez., nat-c., ph-ac., ***phyt.,*** ran-b., ***rhus-t.,*** sars., spig., ***valer.,*** zinc.
paralytic - bell., caust., lyc., mez., sep.
paroxysmal - alum., carb-s., carb-v., ***chin.,*** coff., ***coloc.,*** **PLB.**
periosteum - spig.
posterior part - agar., bell., canth., dulc., eupi., graph., hep., kali-bi., kali-c., kali-i., ***lam.,*** mag-m., phos., rat., ***sel.***
crossing limb - rat.
rhythmical, evening after lying - phos.
pressure, amel. - coff.
pulsating - caust., lyc., phos., sec., sil.
riding, after - nat-m.
right - ***am-m.,*** clem., ***phyt.,*** sep.
rising, from seat, on - cic., thuj.
amel. - carb-an., caust., kali-c., mag-c., sil.
rubbing, amel. - sul-ac.
scratching - caust.
sitting, while - agar., ***alum.,*** **AM-M.,** asaf., bell., calc., carb-an., clem., coloc., ***dulc.,*** euph., hep., kali-c., **LYC.,** mag-c., mur-ac., ph-ac., ***phyt., rat., spig.,*** stann., zinc.

tearing, thighs
sitting, amel. - aur., nit-ac.
down - nit-ac.
smarting - graph., lyc.
standing - carb-an., euph., kali-c., mez., nat-c., ***phyt.,*** ran-b.
sticking - coloc., dulc., iod., lyc., mag-c., mur-ac., sep.
stretching the limb amel. - agar.
supper, after - sep.
touch - ***chin.***
twitching - asaf., bell., ***chin.,*** guai., mag-c., nicc., stront.
upper, portion of - arn., colch., kali-c., lyc., mez., puls., thuj.
walking, while - agar., ars., aur., bar-c., cic., ***coff.,*** con., dulc., lyc., mur-ac., ***nit-ac.,*** ran-b., sep.
after - clem.
amel. - ***alum.,*** coc-c., ***dulc.,*** euph., **LYC.,** mur-ac., rat., ***rhod.,*** **RHUS-T.,** sulph., syph., ***valer.***
warmth of bed - kali-c., merc.
amel. - bar-c., ***caust.,*** **LYC.**

tearing, tibia - agar., alum., ambr., am-c., ***arg-m.,*** arg-n., ***ars.,*** bell., berb., ***bry.,*** carb-an., ***caust., colch.,*** con., cycl., dulc., euph., ***ferr.,*** graph., grat., guai., ***kali-bi.,*** **KALI-C.,** ***kali-i.,*** kali-n., lachn., ***led.,*** lyc., merl., mur-ac., nat-c., nat-s., **NIT-AC.,** ***ph-ac., phos., puls.,*** rat., ***rhod.,*** sars., sep., ***sil.,*** spong., staph., ***sulph.,*** thuj., verat., ***zinc.***
cramp-like - con.
evening - kali-i., kali-n., led., ***sulph.***
in bed- con., lyc., mez.
extending downwards - guai., kali-n., sars., verat., zinc.
downwards, to big toe - nat-c.
menses, during - kali-c., ***sep., sil.***
morning - kali-n., phos.
motion, on - cycl.
amel. - arg-m., ***rhod.***
paralytic - mez.
rhythmical - phos.
right - agar., arg-m., rat.
sitting, while - euph., grat., led., mang., mur-ac.
amel. - mur-ac.
twitching - lyc.
walking, while - con., sulph., thuj.

TENSION - ***alum.,*** ambr., ang., ant-t., aur., ***bar-c.,*** berb., calc., ***carb-an.,*** carb-v., caust., clem., ***coloc.,*** hep., mag-c., ***mag-m.,*** mang., merc., mez., mur-ac., ***nat-c., nat-m.,*** nit-ac., ***nux-v.,*** ph-ac., phos., plat., ***puls.,*** rhus-t., sars., ***sep.,*** sil., stann., sulph., ***zinc.***
cramp-like - stram.
night - merc., nat-c., ***puls.***
paralyzed limb - ***nux-v.***
right - hep., mang., phos.
sitting, while - nat-c.
standing - ***bar-c.***
walking, while - mang., nat-c., nat-m.
amel. - bar-c., mag-m.
warmth of bed - ***puls.***

tension, calves - acon., ***alum.,*** am-c., ***anac.,*** ang., ***arg-m.,*** ars., asaf., bar-c., bell., berb., bov., ***bry.,*** calc., canth., caps., carb-an., card-m., cast-eq., caust., ***cham.,*** chel., cic., ***cimx.,*** cocc., colch., con., cupr., dulc., ign., ***kali-bi., kali-c.,*** kali-i., kali-n., kreos., laur., led., lyc., mag-m., mur-ac., nat-c., **NAT-M.,** nat-p., nux-v., ox-ac., pall., ***phos.,*** plat., ***puls., rhus-t.,*** rhus-v., ***sabad.,*** sep., ***sil.,*** staph., sulph., valer., zinc.
afternoon - ox-ac.
5 p.m. - **VALER.**
standing, while - valer.
walking, while - ox-ac.
ascending stairs - ***arg-m.,*** prun., sulph.
bent, when - chel.
burning - asaf.
cold, taking - am-c.
cramp-like - rhus-v., sil.
descending stairs - ***arg-m.***
dinner, after - canth.
drawing - puls.
evening - ***alum.,*** caust., chel., dulc.
forenoon - sulph.
lower, part of - nit-ac.
morning - ferr-ma., sulph.
walking, while - sulph.
motion, of feet - cham.
motion, on - berb., cocc., kali-n., nat-c.
rising from a seat, on - alum., kali-c.
sitting, while - lyc., mur-ac., **NAT-M.,** plat., **VALER.**
standing, while - alum., kali-c., kali-i., stann.
stool, after - ox-ac.
stretching, on - ign.
amel. - chel.
walking, while - ***alum., anac.,*** bar-c., berb., caps., ***carb-an.,*** colch., ign., led., nat-c., ***nat-m.,*** nit-ac., phos., psor., ***rhus-t.,*** sabad., ***sil.,*** spig., zinc.
amel. - alum., kali-i., ***rhus-t.,*** stann.
in open air - bar-c., zinc.

tension, lower - ***agar., alum.,*** am-c., am-m., ***anac.,*** ant-c., ant-t., bar-c., bar-m., bor., bov., ***bry., calc.,*** carb-an., carb-s., caust., cham., chel., cimx., coloc., con., dulc., graph., hep., ign., kali-bi., kali-c., laur., mag-m., mang., mez., mur-ac., **NAT-M.,** nux-v., ph-ac., phos., psor., ***puls.,*** rhod., ***rhus-t., sep.,*** sil., spong., stann., stram., stry., sulph., tab., tarax., ***thuj., zinc.***
afternoon - bry., sulph.
dinner, after - sulph.
evening - ant-c., dulc., kali-bi., led., **PULS.**
left - bor.
lying, while - ***am-m.***
menses, during - spong.
morning - sulph.
night - agar., alum., thuj.
noon - thuj.
rheumatic - mez., puls.
right - ***agar.,*** tarax.
rising, after - agar.
sitting, while - ***am-m.,*** anac., ant-c., carl., rhus-t.

tension, lower
squatting, on - calc.
standing, when - bar-c.
walking, while - graph., kali-c., mang., rhod., ***sulph.,*** tarax., thuj.
amel. - ***am-m.,*** bar-c.
tension, thighs - ***agar., alum.,*** ambr., **AM-M.,** ant-c., ant-t., arn., aur., ***bar-c.,*** bar-m., berb., bry., ***camph., carb-v.,*** **CAUST.,** cham., chel., chin., cic., ***clem., coloc.,*** crot-t., eupi., ***guai.,*** hell., hep., ind., ***kali-bi., kreos., lac-d., lach., lyc., mag-m.,*** mang., meny., ***merc.,*** mez., ***nat-m., nux-v.,*** ol-an., olnd., op., petr., ***plat.,*** prun., **PULS.,** rat., rhod., ***rhus-t.,*** ruta., ***sabin., sep.,*** spig., ***spong.,*** staph., sulph., tab., tarax., ***tarent., thuj.***
afternoon - nat-m.
anterior, part - ang.
ascending steps - hyos., nat-m.
bearing the weight upon the leg, with knee bent - cham.
bend of - agar., arg-m., berb., carb-an., ***caust.,*** zinc.
bending, knee - ang., caust.
bone - lyc.
burning - olnd.
drawing - coloc., **PULS.**
evening - ant-c., lyc., **PULS.,** rat., sulph.
extending downwards - ***alum., nat-m.,*** rhus-t., sep., sulph.
forenoon - sulph.
walking, while - sulph.
hamstrings - agar., ***ambr., am-m.,*** ant-c., ant-t., asar., bar-c., ***calc-p.,*** carb-an., **CAUST.,** cimx., graph., **GUAI.,** kali-ar., led., ***lyc.,*** lyss., med., nat-c., **NAT-M.,** nat-p., ***nit-ac.,*** phos., ***phyt.,*** puls., ***rhus-t., ruta.,*** samb., sulph.
crossing legs - rhus-t.
lying, amel. - bar-c.
menses, during - nat-m., spong.
morning - carb-v.
on rising - caust.
motion, amel. - ***bar-c.,*** mag-m., ***puls.***
of leg amel. - mag-m.
night - ***alum., lyc.,*** sulph.
posterior, part - euph., petr.
rheumatic - mez.
sitting, amel. - aur., guai.
sitting, while - ant-c., ***camph.,*** lyc., meny., merc., ***plat.,*** spig., ***tarent.***
standing, while - ***bar-c.,*** nux-v., rat.
stepping - spong.
walking, while - ambr., aur., berb., chin., ***guai.,*** ind., lyc., meny., nat-m., puls., ***rhus-t.,*** sep., spig., staph., sulph., thuj., til.
warmth, of bed - ***puls.***
tension, tibia - zinc.
descending - bar-c.

THRILLING, sensation, lower - **CANN-I.,** lyss., phys., stry.

THROMBOSIS, legs - ***apis., both.***

TINGLING, prickling, asleep - agar., ***alum.,*** am-c., arn., aur., ***calc-p.,*** carb-ac., carb-an., carb-s., ***carb-v.,*** caust., com., dig., **GRAPH.,** grat., guai., hyper., ign., **KALI-C.,** lachn., **LYC.,** mag-m., ***merc.,*** merc-i-f., nat-m., nit-ac., nux-v., op., **PETR.,** ***ph-ac.,*** rumx., sanic., ***sep., sil., sulph.,*** sul-ac., spig., thuj., til.
kneeling, after - op.
lying, while - ***kali-c., sulph.***
on the limb - carb-an.
menses, during - ***graph., puls.,*** sec.
morning, in bed - ***sulph.***
night, in bed - sanic.
resting, after - op.
right - carb-an., kali-c.
rising, from sitting - caps.
scratching amel. - sil.
sitting, while - ***calc-p.,*** chin., ***graph.,*** guai., ign., kali-c., lyc., mosch., nux-v., ***op., ph-ac.,*** sep., ***sil.***
warm room agg. - com.
tingling, calves - bar-c., berb., caust., cham., lach., onos.
tingling, lower - acet-ac., agar., am-c., arn., asaf., bapt., bar-c., ***calc., calc-p., carb-an., carb-h.,*** carb-s., cic., con., corn., ***crot-h.,*** dig., euph., fl-ac., gels., hyper., ind., iod., ***kali-c.,*** kreos., lachn., lil-t., mag-m., manc., merc., merc-i-f., mez., naja, nux-m., nux-v., petr., puls., ***rhus-t., sec., sulph.,*** thuj., verat.
afternoon - ***gels.***
daytime - ***carb-an.***
evening - ***calc.,*** ign., manc.
excitement, from - calc-p.
rising, after sitting - ***puls.***
sitting - am-c., bar-c., ***calc.,*** camph., cic., crot-h., ign.
with limbs crossed - agar., carb-an., ***crot-h.,*** fl-ac., laur., ***phos.,*** sep.
standing - am-c., naja.
walking, while - asaf.
tingling, thighs - arg-m., canth., caust., cic., coc-c., hep., ***merc.,*** nit-ac., ox-ac., sabad., sec., sil., thuj., verat.
extending to testes - sabad.
menses, during - sec.
painful - caust.
rising, from seat - chin.
sitting, while - cic., sil.

TREMBLING - acon., ***agar., ambr.,*** am-m., anac., apis, ***arg-m.,*** **ARG-N.,** arn., ***ars.,*** ars-i., bell., ***calc.,*** calc-s., canth., caps., carb-s., carb-v., ***caust.,*** chin., chin-a., chin-s., ***cic.,*** cist., ***cimic.,*** cob., cocc., coloc., ***con.,*** corn., ***crot-h.,*** cupr., fl-ac., ***glon.,*** helo., hep., hyos., iod., ip., kali-ar., kali-bi., kali-c., kali-s., **LACH.,** lact., ***lath., led.,*** lyc., manc., ***med., merc.,*** nat-a., nat-c., ***nat-m.,*** **NIT-AC., NUX-V.,** olnd., **OP.,** petr., phos., phys., ***phyt.,*** pip-m., ***plb., puls.,*** ran-b., raph., rhus-t., sars., sec., seneg., sep., sil., sol-n., spig., stram., sulph., ***verat.,*** zinc.
air, in open - caust.
alone, being, amel. - ambr.
anxiety - bor., rhus-t., sars.

TREMBLING, of
ascending stairs - ***caust.,*** corn., nat-m., nux-m.
carrying a weight - graph.
chagrin, from - ran-b.
chill, as from - caust.
evening - lyc., plb., puls.
first lower then upper limbs - spig.
forenoon, 10 a.m. - gels., ptel.
jerking - lyc.
lying, while - plb.
menses, during - agar., caust., graph., hyos., mag-c., nat-c.
morning - ***arg-m., nit-ac.,*** puls.
motion, after - phos.
amel. - **RHUS-T.**
night - hep.
reclining - fl-ac.
rhythmical - ***ign.***
rising, after sitting, on - ***nat-m.,*** nux-m.
sex, after - **CALC.**
sitting, while - plan., plb.
spoken, to, when - merc.
standing - caust.
for some time after - ***led.,*** olnd.
stool, after - ars.
vexation, after - ran-b.
walking, while - caust., ***con.,*** cur., led., merc., nux-m., **NUX-V.**
amel. - ***nat-m.***

trembling, calves - meny., nat-m., sulph.

trembling, lower - ail., am-m., arg-m., ars., bar-c., bell., bufo, canth., carb-s., ***caust.,*** cic., coff., coca, coloc., ***cycl.,*** dig., dios., dor., ferr., ferr-m., fl-ac., gels., kali-c., lact., lyc., manc., med., merc., nat-c., ***nat-m.,*** ol-an., onos., ***phos.,*** pic-ac., ***plat., plb., puls., ruta., sil., stry.,*** sulph., tarent., zinc.
ascending ladder - ***caust.***
evening - plat., puls., sil.
after lying down - plat., ***puls.***
forenoon,11 a.m. - arg-n., nat-m.
left - ***cic.***
menses, before - kali-c.
morning - bufo, phys.
after rising - ***arg-m.***
motion - canth.
night - bufo
room, in amel. - caust.
sex, after - **CALC.**
sitting, while - ***plat.***
sleep, when going to - ***cham.***
standing, while - kali-c.
stool, after - ars.
walking, while - ***led.,*** puls.
in open air - coloc.

trembling, thighs - act-sp., ***anac.,*** apis, ars-h., asaf., bar-c., carb-s., cocc., ***con.,*** kali-c., laur., mag-m., ph-ac., phos., ***plat.,*** rat., sol-n., sep.
evening - rat.
kneeling, on - cocc.
raised, when - act-sp.
right - con., lac-c., rat.
sensation - caust.
sex, after - **CALC.**

trembling, thighs
sitting, while - plat.
walking, while - ***con.***

TUBERCLES, calves - petr.

tubercles, lower legs - ant-c., caust., crot-h., nat-c., petr.

tubercles, thighs - ***nat-c.***

TUMORS, calves - kali-br., ***sulph.***

tumors, lower - tarent.

tumors, thighs - merc., phos.
between thigh and vulva - goss.

tumors, tibia, osteosarcoma - syph.
varicose - arn.

TWINGING, calves, sitting, while - **VALER.**

TWISTING, sensation - graph.

TWITCHING - agar., ***alum., ambr.,*** arg-m., ars., asaf., asar., bar-c., bell., berb., calc., camph., carb-an., ***carb-v.,*** caust., ***chel.,*** cic., ***cina,*** cocc., ***cupr.,*** dig., dulc., glon., graph., ***hell.,*** hep., ign., ip., jatr., kali-c., lach., mag-c., manc., mang., merc., mez., nat-c., nat-m., nit-ac., ***nux-v., op.,*** ph-ac., **PHOS.,** plat., rheum, ***rhus-t.,*** sec., sep.,

TWITCHING - ***sil.,*** spong., ***stront-c., sulph., teucr.,*** thuj., ***verat.,*** viol-t., ***zinc.***
evening - alum., am-c., mez.
after falling asleep - mag-c.
in bed - carb-v.
on falling asleep - sil.
exercising, while - mang.
forenoon, while sitting - sep.
left - sil.
lying, while - merc.
menses, during - cocc.
motion, on - chel., mang.
nap, during - nat-m.
night - thuj.
bed, in - ***ambr.,*** mag-c., nit-ac., ***phos.,*** rhus-t., stront-c., ***verat.***
falling asleep, on - stront.
painful limb - rhus-t.
paralyzed limb - ***nux-v.***
rest, during - ***valer.***
right - sep., sil.
sitting, while - sep.
and letting limbs hang out of bed, amel. - ***verat.***
sleep, on going to - ***agar., arg-m., ars.,*** carb-an., sep.
sleeplessness, during - thuj.
stepping out, when - ***rhus-t.***
stool, during - verat.
waking, on - nat-m.
walking, after - cocc., plat.
amel. - ***valer., verat.***
warmth of bed agg. - ***rhus-t., verat.***

twitching - ***ars., calc.,*** cocc., ***coloc.,*** mag-c., ***mag-m.,*** mez., ph-ac., sep., sil., stann., sulph., valer.
evening, in bed - mag-m., sil.
motion amel. - sulph.

twitching, calves - agar., ant-t., sars., bar-c., chel., coloc., dig., eupi., **GRAPH.,** jatr., kali-bi., laur., mag-m., merc., mez., nat-c., nit-ac., olnd., op., phos., puls., rat., ran-s., rhus-t., tarax., viol-t., zinc.
convulsive - ***op.***
cramp-like - ***jatr.***
forenoon, while sitting - nat-c.
morning - eupi.
bed, in - laur., puls., zinc.
motion, amel. - coloc.
paroxysmal - nit-ac.
sitting - nat-c.
stretching out foot - laur.
synchronous with pulse - dig.
touch - tarax.
amel.- dig.

twitching, lower - agar., agn., ***alum.,*** am-c., **ANAC.,** ant-t., ars., ars-i., asaf., atro., berb., bell., bry., calc., ***camph.,*** carb-an., carb-v., carl., caust., cedr., ***chel.,*** con., crot-t., ***cupr.,*** dig., goss., ***graph.,*** guai., guare., ***hell.,*** hyos., ign., iod., ***ip.,*** kali-n., kreos., ***lach.,*** lyc., lyss., mag-c., mag-m., mang., merc., ***merc-c.,*** mez., morph., ***mosch.,*** mygal., nit-ac., ***op.,*** petr., phos., phyt., plan., plat., ***rhus-t.,*** rumx., sep., sil., squil., stram., stry., sulph., teucr., til.,

twitching, lower - valer., ***verat.***
afternoon, while sitting - ars., lach.
convulsive - ars., bad., phyt., stram.
evening - alum., am-c., dig., lyc., mez.
bed, in - carb-an., carb-v., kali-n.
sitting, while - carb-an.
exertion from - mang.
extending, downward - plat.
to stomach - lyc.
motion amel. - ***valer.***
night - bry., con., ir-foe., mag-c., stry.
painful - bell., petr., ***rhus-t.***
rest, during - calc., meny.
siesta, during - crot-t.
sitting - anac., plat., squil.
sleep, during - ***agar.,*** cinnb., crot-t., lyc., sep., verat.
stepping out, when - ***rhus-t.***
sticking, with - calc.
stitches in sole, from - dig.
touch - agn., ars.
upward - kreos., morph.
walking, while - agn., petr., phos.
after - plat.

twitching, thighs - ***anac.,*** ant-t., arg-m., arn., ars., asaf., aur., bar-c., bar-m., berb., calc., caps., carb-an., carb-v., ***caust.,*** chin., cimic., dig., ***graph.,*** guai., iod., ***kali-ar.,*** kali-bi., **KALI-C.,** ***kali-s.,*** lach., lact., laur., lyc., ***lyss.,*** mag-c., ***mang.,*** meny., merc., ***mez.,*** mur-ac., nat-a., nat-c., ***nat-m.,*** nux-v., petr., ph-ac., phos., plb., puls., rat., rheum, ***rhus-t.,*** sabad., ***sep.,*** sil., squil., stann., stram., stront-c., ***sulph.,*** tarax., tep., verat., zinc., zing.
afternoon - lyc.
bone, as if in - sulph.
chilliness, during - sep.

twitching, thighs
evening - kali-bi., mang., puls., zinc.
bed, in - ***berb.,*** carb-v., puls.
forenoon - merc.
inner side - anac., asaf., chel., mang., mosch., plb., zinc.
afternoon - plb.
intermitting - asaf.
near genitals - arn.
paralytic - mosch.
walking, after - mang.
lower, part - mez.
anterior part - ***berb.***
morning - rat.
motion amel. - kreos., ***rhus-t.,*** squil.
outer side - laur., verat.
posterior part - aur., canth., carb-v., lyc., ol-an., olnd., phos., rheum
crossing limbs, on - aur.
morning, in bed - carb-v.
sitting, while - rheum
walking in open air - phos.
pulsating - ph-ac.
sitting, while - squil.
sleep, during - **KALI-C.**
standing - mez.
sudden - nat-c.
synchronous with pulse - verat.
touched, when - **KALI-C.**

twitching, thighs
upper part - mosch., thuj.
walking, while - sep.

twitching, tibia - mez.

ULCERS - am-c., anac., anan., ***anthr.,*** **ARS.,** ***asaf.,*** bell., ***calc.,*** canth., ***carb-s.,*** **CARB-V.,** card-m., caust., ***cist., com., crot-h., ferr-m., graph., grin., hydr.,*** hydr-ac., ip., jac-c., kali-ar., ***kali-bi., kali-c., kali-i.,*** **KALI-S.,** ***lac-c.,*** **LACH., LYC.,** ***merc., mez.,*** murx., ***mur-ac., nat-c., nat-m.,*** nux-m., paeon., pall., petr., ph-ac., phos., ***phyt.,*** **PSOR.,** ***puls.,*** ran-b., ***rhus-t.,*** ruta., ***sabin.,*** sang., **SEC.,** sel., ***sep.,*** **SIL.,** ***sin-n.,*** still., ***sulph., sul-ac.,*** tep., thuj.
atonic - pall.
black base - ***anthr.,*** **ARS.,** ***asaf.,*** **CARB-V.,** ip., **LACH., LYC., SEC.,** ***sil., sul-ac.***
bleeding easily - carb-v., **MERC.,** ph-ac.
bluish areolae - aesc., **ARS., CARB-V., LACH.,** ***puls.,*** **SIL.**
burning - **ANTHR., ARS.,** carb-ac., **CARB-S., CARB-V.,** ***caust.,*** **LYC.,** mag-c., **MERC., PULS., SIL.,** sulph., zinc.
from touch - ***merc.***
callous edges - kali-chl.
deep - ars., ***aur.,*** **CALC., CALC-S.,** com., **MERC.,** ***nit-ac.,*** **PSOR.,** ***puls.,*** **SIL., SULPH.**
dirty base - lach.
eating vesicles - nat-c., sep.
elevated margins - petr.
elevating limb amel. - ***bell., calc., carb-v.***
fetid - ***bry.,*** **CARB-V., LACH., MERC.,** ***mur-ac.,*** **PSOR., PULS.**

ULCERS, legs
fistulous - calc., ruta.
flat - lach., sel.
gangrenous - **ARN.,** ***carb-v.,*** **LACH., LYC., SEC.**
high edges - hydr.
indolent - ***carb-v., hydr.,*** **LACH.,** ***still.***
irritable - ***hydr., phyt.***
itching - **LYC.,** ***ph-ac., psor.,*** **SIL.**
mottled - **CARB-V., LACH., PULS.**
obstinate - petr., sulph.
painful at night - ***lyc.***
painless - ars., carb-v., graph., plat., sep., sil., sulph.
phagedenic blisters - ***lach.,*** nat-c., sep., rhus-t.
puffy - ***sabin.***
red base - lac-c., petr.
running, oozing - petr.
sanious - ***com.,*** sulph.
serpiginous - paeon.
smooth - sel.
stinging - ars., nat-c., sabin., sil.
superficial - lach., petr.
tearing - lyc.
varicose - ***aesc., carb-v.,*** card-m., ***graph., ham.,*** hydr-ac., kali-s., ***nat-m.,*** syph.
warmth agg. - ***carb-v., sabin.***

ulcers, lower - am-c., anac., anan., ***anthr.,*** **ARS.,** ***asaf., aur.,*** bar-c., bar-m., ***calc., calc-s.,*** canth., **CARB-S., CARB-V.,** caust., ***cist.,*** clem., ***crot-h., ferr-m., graph., grin.,*** hydr., ip., jac-c., ***kali-ar., kali-bi., kali-c., kali-i.,*** **KALI-S.,** ***lac-c.,*** **LACH., LYC., MERC.,** ***mez.,*** murx., ***mur-ac., nit-ac.,*** nux-m., petr., ***ph-ac.,*** phos., ***phyt., psor., puls.,*** ran-b., ***rhus-t.,*** ruta., sel., **SIL.,** ***sin-n.,*** staph., still., ***sulph.,*** syph., tep., vip.
burning - **ANTHR., ARS.,** ***carb-v., lyc., merc., nit-ac.,*** puls., **SIL.,** syph.
carious - asaf.
flat - staph.
gangrenous - **ANTHR., ARS.,** ***carb-v.***
itching - lyc., nat-c.
painful - **ANTHR., ARS.,** sil., staph.
night - ***anthr., carb-v.,*** caust., ***lyc., nit-ac., sil.***
rubbing, from - staph.
rupia - kali-br.
stitching - ars., nat-c.
tearing - lyc.
warmth, agg. - ***carb-v., hydr., merc.,*** mez.

ulcers, thighs - ***calc.,*** crot-h., kali-c., merc., ***mez., nat-s.,*** nit-ac., sil., syph., thuj., ***zinc.***
outer side of - ***nat-s.***
scratching, from - kali-c.

ulcers, tibia, on - ***asaf., cinnb.,*** cist., ***graph.,*** lach., ***mez.,*** nit-ac., ***ph-ac.,*** **PSOR.,** ***sabin.,*** sang., sulph., ***syph.,*** vip.

UNCOVER, inclination to - crot-c., ***plat.,*** sec., ***sulph.,*** zinc.
night - ***plat., sulph.,*** zinc.

uncover, lower, inclination to, morning, on waking - ***plat.***

UNSTEADINESS - acon., caust., lycps., ***nux-v.,*** phos., rhod., stram., ***verb.***

unsteadiness, calves - nat-m.

unsteadiness, lower - agar., bry., merc., ptel., ***sulph.***
afternoon - sulph.

unsteadiness, thighs - calc., ruta.

URTICARIA - ***apis, calc.,*** **CHLOL.,** clem., kali-i., merc., plan., sulph., zinc.
scratching, after - clem., spig., zinc.

urticaria, calves - carb-v.

urticaria, lower - ***calc., chlor.,*** rhus-t., **SULPH.**

urticaria, thighs - all-c., caust., clem., iod., merc., sulph., ***zinc.***
itching - caust., dulc.
scratching, after - clem., ***zinc.***

VARICOSE, veins, legs - ***ambr.,*** arg-n., **ARN.,** ***ars.,*** **CALC.,** calc-f., calc-p., ***carb-s.,*** **CARB-V.,** card-m., ***caust.,*** clem., ***crot-h., ferr.,*** ferr-ar., FL-AC., ***graph.,*** **HAM.,** ***hep., kali-ar., kreos.,*** lac-c., ***lach.,*** **LYC., LYCPS.,** ***nat-m., plb.,*** **PULS.,** sabin., sars., sil., spig., ***sulph.,*** sul-ac., ***thuj.,*** vip., **ZINC**.
cramping - graph.
distended during menses - ambr., lach., puls.
drawing - graph.
painful agg. by warmth - **FL-AC., SULPH.**
pregnancy, during - acon., apis, ***arn., ars.,*** **CARB-V.,** ***caust.,*** **FERR., FL-AC.,** ***graph., ham., lyc., lycps., mill., nux-v., phos.,*** **PULS.,** ***sep., zinc.***

varicose, calf - clem., ***plb.***

varicose, lower - ***calc.,*** **CARB-S., CARB-V., CAUST.,** coloc., ferr., ***fl-ac.,*** graph., **HAM., LYC.,** ***mill., nat-m.,*** **PULS.,** sil., ***sulph.,*** **ZINC.**
bleeding - ***ham., puls.***
inflamed - arn., ***ars., calc., ham.,*** kreos., lyc., lycps., ***puls.,*** sil., spig., sulph., zinc.
itching - ***graph.***
left - fl-ac.
menses, during - ambr.
network in skin - berb., ***calc., carb-v., caust.,*** clem., ***crot-h., lach.,*** lyc., nat-m., ox-ac., plat., sabad., thuj.
painful - brom., ***caust.,*** coloc., ***ham., lyc., mill.,*** **PULS.,** sang., ***zinc.***
menses, during - graph.
pregnancy, during - mill.
painless - calc.
pimples, covered with - ***graph.***
pregnancy, during - acon., apis, ***arn., ars.,*** **CARB-V.,** ***caust.,*** **FERR., FL-AC.,** ***graph., ham., lyc., lycps., mill., nux-v., phos.,*** **PULS.,** ***sep., zinc.***
pulsating - ruta.
sensitive - ***fl-ac.,*** graph., ***ham.,*** lach., puls.
sharp - kali-c., lyc.
soreness - arn., graph., ***ham.,*** puls.
stinging - ***apis,*** graph., ***ham.,*** **PULS.**
swollen - ***apis,*** berb., ***puls.***
tearing - sul-ac.

varicose, lower
tension - graph.
tongue - ***dig.***, ***fl-ac.***, ***ham.***, ***puls.***, ***thuj.***
ulceration - ars., **LACH.,** lyc., puls., sil.
ulcers - ***aesc.***, ***carb-v.***, card-m., ***graph.***, ***ham.***, hydr-ac., kali-s., ***nat-m.***, syph.
varicose, thigh - ***calc.***, ferr., **HAM.,** lac-c., ***puls.***, sep., ***zinc.***

VESICLES - acon., am-c., ***ant-c.***, apis, arn., **ARS.,** aster., bell., ***bov.***, ***bufo***, ***calc.***, cann-s., carb-o., carb-v., **CAUST.,** chin., clem., cupr., elaps, ***graph.***, hyos., iod., kali-ar., kali-bi., lach., lachn., manc., **NAT-C., NAT-M.,** nat-p., **NIT-AC.,** ***petr.***, ph-ac., phos., **RHUS-T.,** rhus-v., sabad., sars., sec., sel., ***sep.***, ***sil.***, **SULPH.,** verat., zinc.
bloody serum - ***nat-m.***
burning - verat.
cold, come out in - dulc.
corroding - bor., caust., graph., sep., sil., sulph.
itching - ***calc.***, carb-v.
red - ***calc.***
borders, with - corn-s.
scratching, after - sars., sep.
spreading - nit-ac.
stinging - ***rhus-t.***
ulcerating - sulph., zinc.
varioloid - ant-c.
water, fetid, with - ars.
white - mez., thuj.
yellow fluid - ars., bufo
vesicles, calves - caust., sars., sep.
vesicles, lower - ***ant-c.***, bov., **CAUST.,** com., dulc., hyos., kali-bi., ***kali-c.***, mang., ***psor.***, **RHUS-T.,** ***sec.***, staph., stram., ***sulph.***, vip.
vesicles, thighs - ant-c., aster., cann-s., caust., clem., ***crot-t.***, ***kali-c.***, lach., nat-c., olnd., sars., sel., sulph., verat., vip.
areola red - sulph.
black - ***anthr.***
burning - verat.
itching - aster., clem.
scratching, after - sars.
ulcers, become - aster.
white with red border - cann-s.
vesicles, tibia, watery - bell.

VEXATION, felt in legs - ***nux-v.***

VIBRATION, sensation, lower - ambr., berb., caust.
vibration, calves - phel.
vibration, thigh - caust.

WALKING, (see Generals, Walking)

WARTS, thighs - med.

WATER, drops of cold water trickled down front of legs - acon.
cold, running down hips to toes - bell.
warm, were running down - bor.
water, lower, oozing from - sac-alb., graph., **LYC.,** tarent-c.

WEAKNESS, of - acet-ac., acon., **AESC.,** aeth., ***agar.***, ail., all-s., aloe, **ALUM.,** alumn., ambr., am-c., ***am-m.***, ***ang.***, ***apis***, **ARG-M., ARG-N., ARS.,** asar., **AUR.,** ***bapt.***, bar-c., bell., benz-ac., berb., bor., brach., ***bry.***, ***bufo***, calad., **CALC.,** calc-i., calc-s., cann-i., cann-s., **CARB-AC.,** ***carb-s.***, ***carb-v.***, cast., **CAUST.,** cham., chel., ***chin.***, ***chin-a.***, ***cic.***, ***cina***, cist., **COCC.,** coc-c., colch., **CON.,** ***corn.***, ***crot-c.***, ***crot-t.***, ***cupr.***, dig., dros., ery-a., euphr., ***ferr-i.***, **GELS., GLON.,** ***graph.***, grat., guai., ham., ***hell.***, hipp., ***hydr.***, ***hyos.***, ind., ip., ***kali-ar.***, kali-bi., ***kali-br.***, ***kali-c.***, ***kali-n.***, ***kali-p.***, lil-t., ***lyc.***, mag-c., ***mag-m.***, mang., ***med.***, merc., ***mez.***, murx., **MUR-AC.,** ***nat-a.***, **NAT-C.,** ***nat-m.***, nat-p., nicc., ***nit-ac.***, ***nux-m.***, **NUX-V.,** olnd., ***op.***, ox-ac., ***petr.***, ***ph-ac.***, **PHOS., PIC-AC.,** ***plat.***, **PLB.,** puls., ***ran-b.***, rhod., **RHUS-T.,** ***ruta.***, sang., ***sars.***, ***sec.***, seneg., ***sep.***, **SIL.,** spong., ***stann.***, stry., ***sulph.***, ***sul-ac.***, ***stront-c.***, tab., tarent., ***thuj.***, til., verat., verb., vip., xan., **ZINC.**
afternoon - ***arg-n.***, carb-v., nag-m., nat-c., nux-v., pip-m., plb., rumx., zinc.
1 p.m. - ham.
ascending steps - agar., ***ars.***, asar., bell., **CALC.,** lyc., nicc., nux-v., phos., pic-ac., ***ruta.***, sars., thuj.
bones, sitting - sulph.
change of temperature - act-sp.
child late learning to walk - **CALC.**
childbirth, after - ***rhus-t.***
descending steps - nux-m., ***ruta.***, sil., stann., sulph.
diarrhea, during - bor.
dinner, after - am-c.
eating, after - mur-ac.
evening - hydr-ac., indg., nit-ac., sulph., zinc.
10 p.m. - plan.
menses, during - kali-n., mag-m.
walking, while - sang., thuj., verat.
exertion, after - ***anac.***, **CALC., GELS., RHUS-T.**
false step, from - ph-ac.
feet wet, getting, after - phos., ***rhus-t.***
fever, catarrhal, during - sep.
forenoon - arg-n., nat-m., ptel., ***ran-b.***
forenoon, 11 a.m. - arg-n., nat-m., zinc.
hunger, during - ***zinc.***
joints - cinnb., nit-ac., rhus-t., stront.
menses, during - arg-n., ***cocc.***, kali-n., mag-m., ***nit-ac.***, nux-m., sulph., ***zinc.***
morning - ambr., ant-t., ***arg-m.***, bar-c., carb-an., iod., mur-ac., ***nat-m.***, **NUX-V.,** ***phos.***, ***rhus-t.***, sep., ***sil.***, sulph.
bed, in - nat-m., plb., sulph., ***zinc.***
waking, on - ***arg-m.***, nat-m., sep.
painful - aloe, nux-m., plan., stann.
paralytic - anac., arg-n., **COCC.,** dig.
right - nat-m., stann., sulph.
rising from a seat, on - ***glon.***, mag-c., nat-m., ruta., zinc.
sex, after - ***calc.***
sitting, while - ars., bar-c., led., mag-c., plat.
smoking, from - calad., ***clem.***

WEAKNESS, of
standing, while - agar., ***anac.***, berb., ***bry.***, dirc., hell., nat-m., **NUX-M.**, plat., stann., zinc.
stool, after - plect.
tremulous - caps., dig.
vexation, after - caust., lyc., nat-m., ***nux-v.***
walking, after and while - **AESC., ARG-M.**, bapt., berb., ***bor.***, **CALC.**, ***calc-s.***, carl., **CON., GELS.**, glon., hell., kali-n., led., **MAG-M.**, mosch., ***mur-ac.***, nux-v., ***plb.***, ***ran-b.***, **RHUS-T.**, ***ruta.***, ***sil.***, stann., sulph., zinc.
amel. - bor., cann-s., dros., nat-m., zinc.
continued, amel. - zinc.
in open air - grat., mag-m., sang., seneg., verat.

weakness, calves - aesc., aloe, ***arg-n.***, calc., calc-i., ***calc-p.***, calc-s., carb-v., cast., cham., chin-s., coc-c., croc., dulc., ferr., ferr-i., kali-c., kali-n., ***kalm.***, kreos., ***nat-m.***, nicc., osm., plb., sil., stront-c., sulph., thuj., valer., zinc.
afternoon - cast., valer.
ascending - bell.
chill, during - thuj.
evening - dulc., eupi.
kneeling, when - ars-i.
motion, on - cast.
night - ***sulph.***
rising from a seat - zinc.
sitting, while - stront.
amel. - nicc.
walking, while - aloe, croc., gran., nicc., osm.
amel. - plb.
amel., after - calc-s.

weakness, lower - acet-ac., acon., act-sp., ***aesc.***, ***agar.***, all-c., aloe, ***alum.***, alumn., ambr., ***am-c.***, am-m., anan., ***arg-m.***, ***arg-n.***, ***ars.***, arund., asaf., aspar., atro., ***bar-c.***, bell., benz-ac., bor., ***bov.***, brom., bufo, ***bry.***, ***cact.***, ***calc.***, ***calc-p.***, ***calc-s.***, camph., ***cann-i.***, ***canth.***, carb-o., carb-s., carb-v., ***caust.***, cham., chin-s., chlor., ***cic.***, cimic., clem., **COCC.**, coloc., **CON.**, cop., corn., ***cupr.***, cycl., dig., dios., dulc., elaps, euph., eup-per., ***ferr.***, ***ferr-m.***, ferr-p., fl-ac., form., gels., gins., ***glon.***, grat., guai., ***ham.***, hell., ***hydr.***, hyos., hura, ind., indg., iris, jab., jatr., kalm., ***kali-bi.***, ***kali-c.***, ***kali-cy.***, ***kali-n.***, kreos., ***lach.***, led., lil-t., ***lyc.***, ***mag-c.***, mag-s., mang., med., ***merc.***, mez., murx., ***nat-a.***, ***nat-c.***, nat-m., nat-p., **NAT-S.**, nit-ac., nuph., **NUX-M., NUX-V.**, ***olnd.***, onos., ***op.***, ox-ac., ***petr.***, **PH-AC.**, ***phos.***, phys., phyt., ***pic-ac.***, ***plat.***, **PLB.**, psor., puls., **RHUS-T.**, rumx., ruta., sabad., sars., seneg., ***sep.***, ***sil.***, staph., stront-c., stry., ***sulph.***, tarent., ***thuj.***, valer., verat., vip., xan., ***zinc.***
afternoon - am-m., hura, nat-c., rat.
walking, while - ***rhus-t.***
ascending, while - ***ruta.***
stairs - acon., ***bry.***, corn., ***hura***, hyos., ruta.
changes of temperature - act-sp.

weakness, lower
childbirth, after - ***caust.***, ***rhus-t.***
crossing legs - verb.
diarrhea, after - bor.
dinner, after - agar.
eating agg. - hyos.
evening - abrot., brach., coc-c., kali-n., merc., onos., phys.
on going up stairs - rhus-t., rumx.
walking, while - onos.
exertion, slight, after - cic., ziz.
forenoon - coloc., ptel., ran-b., rhus-t., sars.
journey, after - pic-ac.
menses, during - bov., sars., sulph., zinc.
morning - acon., ambr., ***arg-m.***, ars., bar-c., brach., chlor., dios., nux-v., sulph.
bed, in - sulph.
rising, on - ***arg-m.***, hura, rat., rhod.
waking, on - ***arg-m.***, caust., sumb.
motion, during - clem., nat-s., pic-ac.
amel. - aur-m-n., cham., dios., nat-s., stront.
night - am-m., sulph.
noon - ***rhus-t.***
painful - calc., cann-i., crot-h., plat.
paralytic - bell., cod., kali-n.
right - tarax.
rising, on - bry.
after amel. - caust.
from seat - atro., puls.
room in a amel. - grat.
sexual excesses after - staph.
sitting, while - acon., alumn., aur-m-n., camph., cic., indg., plat., **RHUS-T.**, sulph., ***thuj.***
amel. - valer.
sleep amel. - tell.
standing, while - aster., chin., nat-p., ol-an., samb., valer.
stepping - plat.
stool, after - con.
waking, on - arg-m.
walk, on beginning to - ***bry.***
walking, while and after - agar., am-c., ***caust.***, chel., chin., ***con.***, ***gran.***, ind., lyc., mez., nit-ac., **NUX-M.**, onos., ph-ac., plat., plb., ***rhus-t.***, stram., ***sulph.***, tarax., tarent., zinc.
after - kali-n.
in open air - grat.

weakness, thighs - acon., agar., all-c., aloe, ***alum.***, am-c., ammc., anac., arg-m., ***ars.***, arund., asar., bor., brach., bry., ***calc.***, caps., carb-an., carb-s., caust., cham., chel., ***chin.***, chin-a., chin-s., clem., **COCC.**, coc-c., coloc., **CON.**, croc., crot-h., cycl., dulc., euph., gins., ***glon.***, graph., ***guai.***, ham., hell., hura, ip., kali-bi., ***kali-c.***, kali-i., lac-ac., lil-t., lyc., mag-s., mang., ***merc.***, ***merc-c.***, mez., **MUR-AC.**, nat-a., nat-c., nat-m., nat-p., **NAT-S.**, nit-ac., ***nux-v.***, ***olnd.***, ph-ac., ***phos.***, pip-m., ***plat.***, ***plb.***, puls., raph., rat., ***rheum***, ***ruta.***, sars., ***seneg.***, sep., sil., sol-n., spig., squil., ***stann.***, staph., stront-c., sulph., tarent., thuj., verb., verat.

weakness, thighs
afternoon - fago., kali-c.
ascending steps, during - ars., ***bry.,*** coloc., mez., sep.
emission, after - ***agar.,*** calc.
evening - chin., fago., mag-c., stront-c., tarent.
left - chel., glon.
menses, during - am-c., am-m., bov., carb-an., cast., nicc., sars.
midnight, after - merc.
morning - brach., ***calc.,*** nat-c.
chill, during - verat.
rising, after - phos., rhod., squil.
walk, on beginning to - ***calc.***
night - ham.
sleep, during - sep.
painful - stann.
paralytic - arg-m., puls.
pregnancy - ***ip.***
right - ***con., kali-c.***
rising, on - thuj.
from a seat, on - ruta.
sex, after - agar., ***calc.***
sitting, after - acon., anac., arg-m., croc., mag-c., mag-s., mang-m., ph-ac., plat., puls.
standing, while - mag-m., plat., stann.
stool, after - lyc.
sudden - cic., hep.
waking, on, amel. - sep.
walking, while - anac., arg-m., aur., bufo, ***calc.,*** caust., chel., chin., con., hep., ***kali-i.,*** lycps., mag-c., mag-s., merc., mez., ***olnd.,*** puls., ***ruta.***
after - ind., nit-ac., sol-t-ae.
amel. - mag-m., rat.
in open air - ang., arg-m., spig.

WEIGHT, sensation, tibia - walking rapidly - spong.

WHIZZING, thigh - bell.

WIND, sensation, as if cool wind - bar-c., calc., lil-t.

WIND, lower - samb.

WOODEN, sensation - ***arg-n., ars.,*** chin-s.
walking while - **KALI-N.,** plb., rhus-t., thuj.

WRINKLED, leg - rhod.

Limbs

ABDUCTED, lies with - **CHAM.,** ***psor.,*** sulph.
convulsion, during - cupr., nux-v.

ACHING, pain - **AGAR.,** am-c., ***ant-c.,*** apoc., ***arn., ars., aur., bapt., bell.,*** bov., ***bry., calc-p.,*** cann-i., ***carb-v., carl., cham., cimic.,*** chin., chin-a., ***cocc.,*** cupr., ***cur.,*** **EUP-PER.,** ferr., ferr-ar., fago., ***gels., glon.,*** ham., hell., ***hydr.,*** hydrc., **IP.,** jug-c., lac-c., lach., led., ***lyc.,*** lyss., ***merc.,*** merc-c., mez., mosch., ***mur-ac.,*** naja, nat-a., ***nat-m.,*** nit-ac., **NUX-V.,** osm., ***phyt.,*** plb., podo., ptel., ***puls., pyrog.,*** **RHUS-T.,** ***samb.,*** staph., still., stram., stront-c., sumb., ***syph., tub., verat.,*** zinc.
afternoon - nit-ac., ptel.
bed, in - carl., **MERC.**
chill, during - aran., arn., ars., **EUP-PER.,** ***ip.,*** nat-m., ***nux-v.,*** **PYROG.,** ***rhus-t.,*** sabad., tub.
cold, as from - nit-ac.
fever, during - puls., ***pyrog., rhus-t., tub.***
forenoon - am-c., nat-a.
left - ***sumb.***
lying upon the, while - dros.
morning, 7 a.m. - myric.
motion, amel. - am-c., ***mur-ac., puls.,*** **RHUS-T.,** ***tub.***
night - am-c., ***aur., merc., nux-v.,*** podo.
sex, after - tub.
waking, on - puls., tell.
walking, while - op.
amel. - nat-a., **PYROG., RHUS-T.,** ***tub.***
aching, bones - **EUP-PER.,** form., **IP.,** ***lyss., mur-ac.,*** nit-ac., ***tub.***
chill, during - ***arn., ars.,*** chin., **EUP-PER.,** ***ferr.,*** **IP.,** mag-c., mur-ac., nat-m., ***puls., pyrog., rhus-t.***
aching, joints - aesc., all-c., bol., carb-an., ***carl., chin-s.,*** clem., erig., ***gels.,*** kali-c., ***kalm.,*** led., merc., mosch., phos., ptel., pyrus, rhod., rhus-t.
chill, during - cann-i.
aching, muscles, extensor - calc-p.
flexors - ptel.

ALIVE, sensation of - ign.

AMPUTATION, pain, from - ***acon., all-c.,*** am-m., ***arn., asaf.,*** bell., **CALEN., COFF.,** cupr., hell., **HYPER.,** kalm., ph-ac., **PHOS.,** rauw., spig., staph., symph., verat.

ANTHRAX - ***anthr., ars., sec.***

ATAXIA - ***agar.,*** **ALUM.,** arag., ***arg-n.,*** ars., ***calc., caust., cocc.,*** crot-c., ***fl-ac., gels., graph., hell., helo., kali-br., lach., lil-t.,*** naja, nux-m., ***nux-v., onos., phos., plb., sil., stram., sulph., zinc.***

AWKWARDNESS, of - aeth., **AGAR.,** ambr., anac., **APIS,** ars., asaf., asar., bell., **BOV.,** bry., **CALC.,** calc-s., camph., ***caps., caust.,*** cocc., ***con.,*** dig., **HELL.,** hep., ***ign.,*** **IP., LACH.,** mez., ***nat-c., nat-m., nux-v.,*** op., ph-ac., phos., plb., ***puls.,*** sabin., sars., sep., sil., spong., stann., staph., stram., sulph., thuj., vip.
awkwardness, legs - **AGAR.,** ***alum.,*** **CAUST.,** ***con.,*** gels., ***nux-m.,*** sabad., ***sil., verat.***
knocks against things. - caps., ***colch.,*** ip., kali-n., nat-m., nux-v., op., vip.
stumbling when walking - **AGAR.,** ***calc.,*** caps., **CAUST.,** ***colch., con.,*** gels., ***hyos., ign.,*** iod., **IP.,** ***lach.,*** lil-t., mag-c., ***mag-p., nat-m.,*** nux-v., op., ***ph-ac., phos.,*** sabad., sil., verat.

BANDAGED, sensation as if - arund., ***chin.,*** nit-ac., **PLAT.**

BLISTERS - ***ars.***
blood, becoming gangrenous - ***sec.***

BOILS - all-c., am-c., apoc., ars., aur-m., ***bell., brom.,*** calc., carb-s., clem., cob., elaps, graph., guare., **HEP.,** hyos., iris, kali-bi., kali-n., ***lyc., merc.,*** mez., nat-m., nit-ac., nux-v., petr., ph-ac., psor., rat., ***rhus-t.,*** rhus-v., sec., sep., stram., **SULPH.,** thuj.

BORING, pain - ***carb-v.,*** coloc., ***mez.,*** plan.
chill, before - ***carb-v.***
rheumatic - plan.
boring, bones - arg-m., ***carb-v.,*** cocc., mang., phos.
boring, flexor muscles - plan.
boring, joints - arg-m., clem., coloc., mang., ***rhod.,*** thuj.
decay, of - aur-m.

BROKEN, sensation as if - aeth., carl., **COCC., EUP-PER.,** ***ip.,*** plb., raph., tril.

BUBBLING, sensation - rheum.

BURNING, pain - abrot., anac., ***ars., bell.,*** cann-i., carb-an., ***carb-v.,*** chin., cocc., coloc., ***kali-ar.,*** kali-br., kali-c., kali-p., kreos., laur., led., nit-ac., ***ph-ac.,*** phos., plan., plat., plb., staph., vip.
afternoon - gels.
bed, in - carb-v., fago., led.
evening, in bed - carb-v.
external - carb-an.
loss of fluids - ***ph-ac.***
menses, during - ***carb-v.***
morning - phos.
night - kali-c.
scratching, after - kreos.
spots - plan.
wandering - plat.

BURSAE - **ARN.,** calc-p., cann-s., kali-m., **NAT-M., SIL.,** stann., **STICT.**
cysts - cann-s., caust., ***graph.,*** iod., kali-br., ***sil., sulph.***

CARBUNCLES - **ANTHR.,** ***arn.,*** **ARS.,** ***hep.,*** **LACH., SIL., SULPH.,** tarent-c.

CHILBLAINS - abrot., **AGAR.,** all-c., aloe, ***alum., alumn., arn., ars.,*** aur., ***bad., bell.,*** bor., bufo, cadm-s., ***carb-an., carb-v., cham.,*** chin., ***cop., croc., cycl.,*** hyos., kali-ar., kali-c., kali-chl., kalm., ***lyc., mur-ac.,*** **NIT-AC.,** ***nux-v.,*** **PETR.,** ph-ac., ***phos.,*** plan., **PULS.,** rhus-t., sep., stann., staph., ***sulph.,*** sul-ac., ***thuj., zinc.***
cutting - kali-c.

CHILBLAINS,
inflamed - ***ars.***, cham., kali-c., lyc., ***nit-ac.***, ***nux-v.***, **PULS.**, staph., ***sulph.***
painful - arn., ***ars.***, aur., hep., ***nit-ac.***, ***petr.***, ph-ac., phos., ***puls.***, sep.
pressing - kali-c.
pulsating - ***nux-v.***
sharp, stitching - kali-c.
vesicular - carb-an., mag-c., ***nit-ac.***, phos., **RHUS-T.**, sep., sulph.

CHILLINESS - agar., ***ars.***, cham., cimic., chlor., coff., ***gels.***, ***hyos.***, lac-ac., ***nat-m.***, ***nux-v.***, plb., ***psor.***, puls., ***rhus-t.***, sec., stram.

CHOREA, (see Nerves, Chorea) - **AGAR.**, apis, ***arg-n.***, ***ars.***, ***asaf.***, ***bell.***, ***calc.***, **CAUST.**, ***cedr.***, ***cham.***, ***chel.***, chin., ***chlol.***, ***cic.***, ***cimic.***, cocc., coff., con., ***croc.***, ***cupr.***, dulc., ***hyos.***, ***ign.***, iod., ip., kali-c., ***lach.***, laur., lyc., merc., mez., **MYGAL.**, ***nat-m.***, nux-v., ***op.***, plat., puls., rhod., rhus-t., sabin., sec., ***sep.***, sil., stann., ***stram.***, stront-c., sulph., tanac., **TARENT.**, verat-v., zinc.
crosswise - agar.
fear, from - ***calc.***, **CAUST.**, ***ign.***, ***kali-br.***, ***laur.***, ***nat-m.***, ***stram.***, zinc.
sex, agg. - ***cedr.***
sleep amel. - ***agar.***, ***mygal.***

COLDNESS - ***acon.***, aeth., ***agar.***, alum., alumn., ***ant-c.***, **ANT-T.**, anthr., ***apis***, ***arg-n.***, **ARS.**, ***ars-h.***, ***ars-i.***, atro., ***aur-m.***, bell., bism., both., bry., bufo, ***cact.***, **CALC.**, ***calc-p.***, calc-s., **CAMPH.**, cann-i., cann-s., ***canth.***, ***caps.***, carb-ac., carb-an., ***carb-h.***, ***carb-s.***, **CARB-V.**, caust., cedr., ***cham.***, ***chel.***, chen-a., chin., chin-a., chin-s., ***cic.***, cocc., ***coff.***, **COLCH.**, ***coloc.***, con., ***croc.***, ***crot-h.***, ***crot-t.***, **CUPR.**, cupr-ar., cycl., **DIG.**, dros., ***dulc.***, echi., ***eup-per.***, ***ferr.***, ferr-ar., ***ferr-p.***, ***gamb.***, ***gels.***, gins., glon., ***ham.***, hell., helon., hep., hydr-ac., ***hyos.***, ***iod.***, ip., ***iris***, jatr., jug-r., ***kali-bi.***, ***kali-br.***, ***kali-c.***, kali-chl., kali-n., ***kali-p.***, kali-s., ***kalm.***, ***lach.***, ***laur.***, ***led.***, ***lept.***, lil-t., ***lyc.***, ***lycps.***, lyss., manc., ***med.***, ***merc.***, ***merc-c.***, ***mez.***, morph., ***mur-ac.***, naja, ***nat-c.***, ***nat-m.***, nat-p., nit-ac., nux-m., ***nux-v.***, olnd., ***op.***, ***ox-ac.***, paeon., pall., petr., ***ph-ac.***, ***phos.***, phys., ***phyt.***, plb., ***pic-ac.***, ***puls.***, raph., ***rhus-t.***, ruta., ***sabad.***, sabin., sarr., **SEC.**, ***sil.***, spig., spong., stann., **STRAM.**, stront-c., stry., sulph., sul-ac., ***tab.***, tarent., ter., **VERAT.**, ***verat-v.***, verb., vip., ***zinc.***
abdomen, pain in, with - ars.
afternoon - ars., chin-s., lyc., thuj.
air, open - chin.
exercising, in - plb.
alternating with heat - bell., ***lyc.***, stram.
company, in - aur.
convulsion, with - aeth., **BELL.**, ***cic.***
daytime - spig.
diarrhea, with - **ARS.**, **CAMPH.**, ***carb-v.***, cop., ***laur.***, nux-m., podo., ***sec.***, ***tab.***, **VERAT.**
evening - ars., chin., jatr., merc-cy., nux-v., phyt., puls., rhus-t., sulph.
stool, during - sulph.
warm room, in - brom.

COLDNESS,
excitement - ***lach.***
fever, during - carb-an., kali-ar., sep., **STRAM.**
forenoon - sulph.
heat of, with, body - chin., ***colch.***, ***rhus-t.***
face - cham., chin., hell.
ice, like ice in spots - **AGAR.**
internal - rhus-t.
left - carb-v., caust., ***elaps.***
menses, during - arn., ***calc.***, cham., ***sec.***, ***sil.***
mental exertion - ***lach.***
morning - anac., bry., calc-p., con., crot-h., hep., ***nux-v.***, lyc., ***sulph.***, thuj.
motion amel. - ***acon.***
night - carb-v., stram.
bed, in - carb-an.
heat of other side, with - ***puls.***
painful parts - led., mez., sil.
paralyzed limb - ***ars.***, caust., cocc., dulc., ***graph.***, ***nux-v.***, **RHUS-T.**, zinc.
sitting, while - kreos.
warm bed unendurable, yet - **CAMPH.**, **LED.**, ***mag-c.***, ***med.***, **SEC.**

COMPRESSION - arg-n., led., nat-s.

CONSTRICTION - alumn., arund., carb-s., ***chin.***, con., ***lyc.***, nit-ac., rhus-t.
constriction, bones - am-m., anac., aur., chin., cocc., ***coloc.***, ***con.***, ***graph.***, kreos., lyc., merc., nat-m., **NIT-AC.**, nux-v., petr., phos., **PULS.**, rhod., ***rhus-t.***, ***ruta.***, sabad., sep., sil., stront-c., **SULPH.**, zinc.

CONTRACTION, muscles and tendons - acon., acon-c., ***ars.***, ***bar-c.***, ***bell.***, bry., **CALC.**, canth., carb-s., carb-v., **CAUST.**, cedr., **COLOC.**, con., ***crot-c.***, ***crot-h.***, ***cupr.***, ferr., ferr-m., **GRAPH.**, ***guai.***, hydr-ac., hydrc., jatr., kali-ar., ***kali-i.***, **LYC.**, ***merc.***, mill., mur-ac., ***nat-c.***, ***nat-m.***, ***nux-v.***, oena., op., ph-ac., ***phos.***, plb., ***ruta.***, **SEC.**, ***sep.***, ***sil.***, still., stram., sulph., syph., vib.
chill, during - **CIMX.**
left - rhus-t.
morning - am-m.
night - plb.
paralysis, of extensors, from - ***ars.***, **PLB.**
periodic - ***sec.***
skin - cupr.
slow - stram.
stiff during exacerbation of pains - guai., ***phos.***
sudden - sec.
contraction, of muscles and tendons, of joints - ***anac.***, ***aur.***, ***caust.***, cimx., ***colch.***, ***form.***, ***graph.***, ***merc.***, ***nat-m.***, ***nit-ac.***, petr., sec., stront.

CONVULSION - absin., ***acon.***, aesc., ***agar.***, ant-c., ant-t., aran., ***ars.***, ***art-v.***, aster., atro., ***bell.***, bism., brom., ***bufo***, ***calc.***, ***camph.***, canth., ***carb-ac.***, carb-h., carb-o., ***caust.***, ***cham.***, ***chlf.***, chin-a., ***chlor.***, **CIC.**, **CINA**, ***cocc.***, ***con.***, ***crot-c.***, **CUPR.**, cupr-ar., ***cupr-s.***, ***dig.***, glon., ***hydr-ac.***, ***hyper.***, **HYOS.**, ***ip.***, jatr., kali-i., ***lach.***, ***lyc.***,

CONVULSION - ***merc-c., merc-cy.,*** morph., ***mosch., nux-m.,*** **NUX-V.,** ***oena.,*** olnd., **OP.,** ox-ac., phos., ***picro., plb., puls.,*** ran-s., sabad., sant., ***sec., sil.,*** **STRAM., STRY.,** tab., tarent., thea., valer., ***verat.,*** verat-v.
alternately extended and flexed - carb-o., ***cic., cupr.,*** lyc., nux-v., ***sec., tab.***
alternating with trembling, of body - nux-v.
of upper and lower - ***hyos.,*** stram.
alternation of single muscles - bell.
chill, during - ***lach.,*** merc., nux-v.
clonic - ***ars.,*** atro., brom., carb-o., coc-c., cupr., cupr-s., ign., nux-m., op., phos., ***picro., plb.,*** **SEC.,** ***stram.,*** **STRY.,** sul-ac.
coffee agg. - stram.
cough, during - ***cupr.***
eating, while - plb.
extensor muscles - **CINA.**
flexor muscles - ***bell.***
hiccough, after - bell.
interrupted by painful shocks - stry.
left - ***ip.***
menses, during - nux-m., tarent.
before - puls.
morning - squil.
motion agg. - cocc., nux-v.
one sided - elaps, plb.
one side, other side paralyzed - apis, ***art-v.,*** hell., ***stram.***
right - chen-a.
right side, left side, paralyzed - ***art-v.***
sex, during - bufo
stretching limb amel. - sec.
tetanic - ***ars., hyper.,*** hydr-ac., mill.
tonic - carb-o., plb., ***sec.***
vertigo after, on rising from a chair - nux-v.
vinegar amel. - stram.

CRAMPS - anan., ***ars.,*** atro., **BELL.,** bufo, ***calc.,*** calc-s., camph., carb-o., carb-s., ***caust.,*** cedr., ***cocc.,*** colch., **COLOC.,** ***con., crot-c.,*** crot-h., **CUPR.,** ***dios., dulc.,*** eup-per., ferr., ***graph., hell., hyos.,*** ign., jatr., kali-bi., ***kali-c.,*** kali-p., kali-s., **LYC., MAG-P., MERC.,** merc-c., merc-sul., ***mur-ac.,*** nat-m., ***nit-ac.,*** nux-v., olnd., op., ox-ac., ***petr.,*** phos., ***phyt.,*** **PLAT.,** ***plb., rob., rhus-t., sec.,*** sel., **SEP.,** ***sil.,*** staph., **SULPH.,** ***tab.,*** tarent., ***verat., zinc.,*** zinc-s.
afternoon - sulph.
chill, during - cupr., ***sil.***
cold air agg. - bufo
discharge of semen - bufo
exertion, after - mag-p.
intermittent - phyt.
morning - sulph.
motion, on - nux-v.
night - merc.
pregnancy - ***cupr., verat.,*** vib.
pressure, agg. - zinc.
right - elaps
stool, during - bell.

CROSSING of limbs, agg. - agar., alum., ang., aquileg., arn., ***asaf.,*** aur., bell., bry., ***dig.,*** kali-n., laur., lyc., mur-ac., nux-v., phos., plat., rad., rheum, rhod., ***rhus-t.,*** valer.
amel. - abrot., ant-t., rhod., **SEP.**
legs impossible - ***lath.***

CURVATURE, of bones - am-c., hep., sil.

CURVING, and bowing of - ***calc., calc-p.,*** lyc., ***sil.***

CUTTING, pain - apis, cina.
coughing - caps.
sneezing, on - caps.

DECAY, bones, of - ***ars.,*** **ASAF.,** aur., ***calc.,*** calc-f., calc-p., ***con., fl-ac.,*** graph., ***guai., hep.,*** **LYC., MERC.,** ***mez.,*** **NIT-AC.,** ***ph-ac., phos., puls.,*** ruta., sec., ***sep.,*** **SIL.,** ***staph., sulph., ther.***
decay, periosteum - ant-c., **ASAF.,** aur., bell., ***chin.,*** cycl., hell., ***merc.,*** mez., **PH-AC.,** puls., rhod., rhus-t., ruta., sabin., ***sil.,*** staph.

DISCOLORATION, of
blackness - ars., tarent., vip.
blotches - berb., cimx., cocc., hura
red - lach., sulph.
blue - agar., apis, bism., bol., **CARB-V.,** ***crot-c., dig.,*** kali-ar., ***lach.,*** lyss., ***merc., op.,*** rob.
dark colored - vip.
ecchymoses - merc-c., ***sec.,*** **SUL-AC.,** ***tarent., vip.***
greenish yellow - vip.
leaden colored - sec.
lividity - agar., bapt., chlol., ox-ac., phos., sul-ac.
spots, in - bapt., vip.
yellowish - vip.
marbled - berb., ***thuj.***
mottled - ***ars.,*** **LACH.**
paleness - hydr-ac., naja, ox-ac., rob., sec.
purple - apis, ***verat-v.,*** zinc.
in spots - apis, ***lach.***
redness - ***bell.,*** carb-o., merc-n., sep., stram., vip.
blotches - lach., sulph.
disappearing on pressure - chin-s., kali-br., verat-v.
redness, spots, in - cadm-s., elaps, lach., vip.
bluish red - vip.
burning - berb., ph-ac., sulph., tab.
itching - berb., euph., zinc.
swollen - plb.
washing, after - sulph.
yellowish - phos.
spots, in - vip.

DISLOCATION, joints, as if - agar., anac., ***arn.,*** bry., caps., kali-i., merc., nit-ac., phos., ***ruta,*** stram., sulph.

DISTENSION, sensation, joints - mang.

DRAGGING, pain - con., naja, ***sulph.***
from hip to groin as if everything would be pressed out - ox-ac.
walking, while - naja.

DRAWING, pain - acon., agar., ***alum., am-c.,*** anac., ang., ant-t., ***arg-m., ars.,*** asaf., aur., aur-m., ***bapt.,*** bar-c., bell., ***bry.,*** calc., calc-p., calc-s., cann-s., canth., caps., carb-an., ***carb-s.,*** **CARB-V.,** carl., ***caul.,*** caust., cham., ***chel., chin.,*** chin-a., cimic., cit-v., ***cocc.,*** colch., ***coloc.,*** con., ***cupr., dulc.,*** ferr., ***graph., hep.,*** hyos., hyper., ip., jatr., kali-ar., ***kali-bi., kali-c.,*** kali-n., kali-p., kali-s., lach., lact., ***led., lyc.,*** mag-m., mag-s., med., ***merc., mez.,*** mill., naja, ***nat-m.,*** nat-p., **NIT-AC.,** nux-m., ***nux-v.,*** petr., ph-ac., phos., ***plat.,*** plb., ***puls., rhod.,*** **RHUS-T.,** rhus-v., sabad., ***sec.,*** sep., sil., spong., stram., **SULPH.,** ***thuj., valer.,*** verat., zinc., zing.
- afternoon - calc., lyc.
- air, open, amel. - sabin.
- beginning with a jerk - ***cocc.***
- chill, during - ***ars.,*** ferr., hell., lyc., ***merc., nux-v.,*** ph-ac., ***puls.,*** **RHUS-T.**
  - after - puls.
- cold, after taking - nit-ac., zing.
- coldness, during - graph., ***puls.***
- convulsions, before - ars.
- cramp-like - asaf., ***graph.,*** kali-n., petr., ***plat.,*** sil.
- evening - calc-p., coloc., led., mag-s., ph-ac., ***puls.,*** rhus-t., **SULPH.**
  - 6 p.m. - **RHUS-T.**
  - 9 p.m. - mag-s.
- extending downward - lyc.
- feather bed agg. - sulph.
- forenoon - merc.
- left - cocc., mez.
- lying, while - **RHUS-T.**
- menses, during - con., **NUX-M.,** ***spong.,*** stram.
- morning - acon., calc-p.
  - when waking - ***aur., hep., nux-v.***
- motion, from - cann-s., caps., ***led.,*** naja, ***nux-v.,*** sabad., thuj., verat.
  - amel. - ***arg-m.,*** ferr., led., ***lyc.,*** nux-m., ***rhod.,*** **RHUS-T.,** thuj., **VALER.**
- night - bell., calc., **CARB-V.,** ***cham.,*** cit-v., graph., hep., ***lyc.,*** merc., ***nux-v., puls., rhod.,*** **RHUS-T.,** sabin.
- paralytic - ***aur., cocc., hep., mag-m.,*** mez., ***nux-v.,*** **RHUS-T.,** sabad.
- paralyzed limbs - ***cocc.***
- paroxysmal - ***cocc.***
- sitting, while - coloc., led., **VALER.**
- stretching amel. - nit-ac.
- walking, while - coloc., verat.
  - amel. - ***lyc.,*** **VALER.,** verat.
- wandering - caust., ***chin., cocc., colch.,*** jatr., kali-n., puls., ***sulph.***
- warm bed - **SULPH.**
- warmth amel. - cham., ***nux-v., rhus-t.***
- wine, after, agg. - ***led.,*** mez.

drawing, bones - cham., ***chin., cocc.,*** gels., graph., kali-c., led., merc., ***mez.,*** petr., sulph., zinc.
- as from a thread through shafts - bry.
- long bones - ***led.***

DRAWING, up, of, agg. - ***agar.,*** alum., am-m., ***anac., ant-t.,*** asar., bell., bor., bry., **CARB-V.,** cham., chel., chin., coff., coloc., dig., dros., dulc., ferr., ***guai.,*** hep., ign., kali-c., mag-c., mez., mur-ac., nat-m., nux-v., olnd., par., petr., plat., **PULS.,** rheum, rhod., **RHUS-T.,** sabad., sabin., **SEC.,** stann., staph., thuj., verb., zinc.
- amel. - acon., agar., ***alum., am-c.,*** am-m., anac., ***ant-c.,*** arg-m., arn., aur., ***bar-c.,*** bar-m., bell., bov., ***bry.,*** **CALC.,** calc-s., cann-s., caps., ***carb-v.,*** caust., cham., ***chin.,*** cina, clem., colch., con., croc., dig., dros., dulc., ferr., graph., guai., ***hell., hep.,*** ign., ***kali-c.,*** kali-i., lac-c., laur., ***mang.,*** meny., ***merc.,*** **MERC-C.,** mur-ac., ***nat-m.,*** nux-v., petr., phos., plat., plb., ***puls.,*** **RAN-B.,** rheum, ***rhus-t., ruta.,*** sabin., sel., **SEP.,** spig., spong., stann., staph., **SULPH., THUJ.,** valer., verat.

DRAWN, together - ars., lyc.
- spasmodically - lyc., merc.

ECZEMA - ***anil.,*** arn., ***ars.,*** kali-br., merc., ***psor.***

ELECTRICAL, current, sensation of. - agar., ail., bol., dor., gels.

EMACIATION - ars., ***calc.,*** carb-s., clem., nit-ac., phyt., **PLB.,** ***sec.,*** stront-c., **SULPH.**
- diseased limb, of - ***ars.,*** bry., ***carb-v.,*** dulc., ***graph.,*** **LED.,** ***mez.,*** nat-m., nit-ac., ph-ac., phos., **PLB., PULS.,** ***sec.,*** sel., ***sep.,*** sil.
- paralyzed limb, of - ***kali-p.,*** nux-v., **PLB.,** ***sec., sep.***

ENLARGEMENT, sensation of - alum., ant-c., sep.

ERUPTIONS - agar., alumn., ***am-c.,*** am-m., anac., ***apis,*** **ARS.,** arund., ***bar-c.,*** bar-m., bell., bov., brom., ***bry.,*** **CALC.,** calc-p., calc-s., canth., carb-o., carb-s., carb-v., **CAUST.,** chel., chin., chin-s., chlor., cimic., cob., con., cop., crot-c., crot-t., cupr., cupr-ar., elaps, euph., fago., fl-ac., ***graph.,*** guare., hep., iod., jug-r., ***kali-ar.,*** kali-bi., kali-br., **KALI-C.,** kali-p., kali-s., ***kreos.,*** lach., led., **LYC.,** mag-s., manc., **MERC., MEZ.,** mur-ac., murx., nat-c., **NAT-M.,** nat-p., ***nit-ac.,*** nux-v., oena., petr., ph-ac., phos., pip-m., plan., podo., ***psor., puls.,*** **RHUS-T.,** rhus-v., ***rumx.,*** ruta., sabad., sars., sec., sel., **SEP., SIL.,** stram., staph., stront-c., **SULPH.,** tab., tarax., tep., ***thuj.,*** til.
- areola red - nat-m.
- black - ***ars., sec.***
- bleeding - ***calc.***
  - after scratching - alum., cupr-ar.
- blotches - ant-c., aur., berb., carb-v., cimx., cocc., hura, lach., merc., mur-ac., nat-c., nat-m., sars., sulph., zinc.
- burning - **ARS.,** bov., fago., lac-ac., **MERC.,** nux-v., **RHUS-T.,** til.
  - after scratching - sulph., til.
- confluent - ***cop.,*** phos., rhus-v.
- cracked - phos.

ERUPTIONS,
desquamating - agar., ***am-c.,*** am-m., arn., ***ars.,*** bar-c., calc., chin-s., ***crot-t.,*** elaps, ferr., hydr., kreos., merc., **MEZ.,** rhus-v., sep., sulph., thuj.
dry - bry., merc.
elevations - alumn., anac., aur., cic., cop., crot-h., crot-t., cupr., cupr-ar., dros., gent-c., gent-l., kali-br., merc., nat-m., nit-ac., petr., plan., plb., puls., sul-ac., thuj., urt-u.
erythematous - ars., thuj.
excrescences - ars., thuj.
exuding - crot-h., cupr., hell., ***kali-s., merc., nat-m.,*** rhus-v., sol-n.
thin water - crot-h., tarent-c.
yellow water - cupr., hell., ***rhus-v.,*** sol-n.
flea bites, like - led., sec.
gritty - nat-m.
groups - nat-m.
hard - bov.
hot - fago.
induration after eruptions - kali-br.
itch-like - ars., bry., ***sulph.***
itching - agar., arg-n., ***bov.,*** bry., calc., fago., gent-c., gent-l., lac-ac., lach., led., mag-s., merc., nat-m., nux-v., phos., puls., ***rhus-t.,*** rumx., sep., sulph., tarax., til., urt-u.
knots, reddish, hard - kali-bi.
measles, like - cop., rhus-t.
moist - bry., ***merc.,*** nat-m.
nodules - petr., sep.
painful - **ARN.,** bov., hep., merc.
patches - ***carb-v.,*** iris, jug-c., phos., ***puls., sars.,*** thuj., viol-t.
petechiae - ***ars.,*** aur-m., berb.
pimples - acon., agar., am-c., am-m., anac., ant-c., ant-t., arg-n., arn., **ARS.,** asc-t., bar-c., bar-m., bell., berb., bov., **BRY.,** bufo, calc., ***calc-p., calc-s.,*** cann-s., carb-an., carb-s., cast., **CAUST.,** chel., chin-s., cit-v., clem., cob., com., ***con.,*** crot-c., cupr-ar., elaps, fago., ***fl-ac., graph.,*** hura, iris, ir-foe., jatr., kali-ar., kali-br., ***kali-c.,*** kali-chl., kali-p., kali-s., kreos., lac-ac., ***lach., lyc.,*** mag-c., mag-m., mang., ***merc.,*** mez., morph., mur-ac., ***nat-m., nat-s.,*** nicc., ol-an., op., osm., ph-ac., plan., plat., psor., puls., rat., **RHUS-T.,** rhus-v., rumx., sabad., sars., sel., **SEP.,** spig., stann., staph., stront-c., ***sulph.,*** tab., tarax., thuj., til., valer., ***verat.,*** zinc.
pustules - am-c., anac., ant-c., arg-n., ars., asc-t., bry., chel., cocc., chlor., cop., crot-c., cupr., cupr-ar., elaps, fl-ac., hyos., iris, jug-c., kali-bi., kali-br., lach., lyc., merc., mez., rhod., ***rhus-t.,*** rhus-v., rumx., ruta., sars., sil., squil., staph., stram., **SULPH.,** tab., tarent., thuj., vac., verat.
rash, itching - alum.
red - bell., bov., chlol., crot-c., gins., jug-r., kali-bi., mag-s., merc., nat-m., rhus-v., valer.
rough - rhus-v.

ERUPTIONS,
scabs - arn., ars., cit-v., ir-foe., kali-br., **KALI-S.,** ***mez.,*** mur-ac., phos., plb., podo., rhus-t., rhus-v., **SIL.,** staph., sul-ac., zinc.
scales - arn., ***ars-i., kali-s., merc., mez.,*** phos., pip-m., rhus-t., rhus-v., sec., sulph., zinc.
scurfs, brownish - am-m., bar-m., cinnb., merc.
varicella, like - ***ant-t.***

ERYSIPELAS - anan., **LACH.,** vip.

EXOSTOSES - aur., aur-m., **CALC-F.,** dulc., **HECLA,** mez., ph-ac., rhus-t., **SIL.,** sulph.

FALL, liability to - ***caust.,*** ign., iod., mag-c., mur-ac., nux-v., ph-ac., phos.

FANNED, wants hands and feet - **MED.**

FLEXED - acon., ars., carb-h., carb-o., colch., sec.
convulsion during - colch., hydr-ac., ***hyos.,*** phos., plb.

FLOATING, in air, as if - nux-v., ***ph-ac.,*** stict.

FORMICATION - ***acon., agar., alum., arg-n.,*** ars., ars-h., ***bar-c.,*** cact., ***camph.,*** caps., carb-ac., carb-s., carl., caust., crot-c., hep., hipp., hydr-ac., ***ign.,*** kali-ar., kali-c., lach., ***laur.,*** **LYC.,** ***mez., nux-v.,*** **PH-AC.,** ***phos.,*** plb., psor., ***puls., rhod.,*** **RHUS-T.,** sabad., **SEC.,** stram., stry., **TARENT.,** teucr., verat., ***zinc.***
after - stry.
evening - graph.
in bed - sulph.
joints - arn., carl., ip., sec.
left - sulph.
menses, during - ***graph.***
morning, in bed - teucr.
paralysed parts - rhus-t.
paralysis, in - **PHOS.**
right - agar., hipp.
sitting, while - kali-c., teucr.
waking, on - ***puls.***
in side lain on - ***puls.***
walking - graph.
weather, rough - rhod.

FREEZING, easily - agar., zinc.

FULLNESS - ***aur.,*** aur-m., nux-m., phos., ***puls.,*** rhus-t.

FUNGUS, haematodes - ***phos.,*** sang.

FUZZINESS, sensation of - hyper., **SEC.**

GANGRENE - **ARS.,** ***carb-an., carb-v., chin., crot-h.,*** **LACH.,** ***phos., plb.,*** **SEC.,** verat., vip.
diabetic - carb-ac., con., lach., solid.
spots, in - vip.
swelling, like - anthr.

GLOW, sensation of, from foot to head - ***visc.***

GNAWING, pain - ***ars.,*** cocc., dros., eup-per., lach., merc., nit-ac.
flexor muscles - merc.
night - nit-ac.

GROWING, pains - bell., **CALC-P.,** cimic., ***eup-per.,*** **GUAI.,** kali-p., mag-p., mang., nat-p., **PH-AC.**
night, at - calc-p.

GROWING too fast - ***calc.,*** **CALC-P.,** ferr., ferr-ac., iod., irid., kreos., **PH-AC., PHOS.**

GOOSEBUMPS - acon., sec.

HANG, down, letting, agg. - ***alum., am-c.,*** berb., **CALC.,** ***carb-v., caust.,*** cina, dig., hep., ign., lyc., nat-m., nux-v., ox-ac., par., ph-ac., phos., phyt., plat., plb., ***puls.,*** ran-s., ruta., ***sabin.,*** stann., sulph., sul-ac., thuj., valer., ***vip.***
amel. - acon., am-m., anac., ant-c., arg-m., arg-n., ***arn.,*** asar., ***bar-c., bell.,*** bor., ***bry.,*** camph., caps., caust., chin., cic., cina, ***cocc.,*** coff., colch., coloc., **CON.,** cupr., dros., euph., ferr., graph., hep., ign., ***iris, kali-c.,*** kreos., ***lach., led.,*** lyc., ***mag-c., mag-m.,*** merc., ***mez.,*** nat-c., nat-m., nit-ac., nux-v., olnd., ***petr.,*** phos., plb., puls., ran-b., ***rhus-t.,*** ruta., ***sil.,*** stann., sulph., sul-ac., teucr., thuj., verat., verb.

HEAT - agar., bapt., brom., bufo, carb-ac., cupr., ***guai.,*** lil-t., nat-m., stann., ***sulph.,*** verat., ***zinc.***
alternating with cold - bell., ***lyc.,*** stram.
chilliness, over back, during - gins.
creeping - op.
eruption, before - nat-m.
night - arn.
night, in bed - fago., ***led.***
paralyzed limb - ***alum.,*** phos.
uncover, must - agar.
warmth of bed intolerable - ***led.***

HEAVINESS, tired - acon., aesc., ***agar.,*** ail., ***aloe, alum.,*** ambr., ammc., am-c., amyg., anac., ant-c., ant-t., ***apis,*** **ARG-M.,** ***arg-n., arn.,*** **ARS.,** ***ars-i.,*** asaf., atro., bar-c., bar-m., **BRY.,** bufo, calad., ***calc.,*** calc-p., camph., cann-i., cann-s., caps., carb-an., ***carb-s., carb-v., caust., cham.,*** **CHEL.,** ***chin.,*** chin-a., cimic., ***clem.,*** coff., ***coloc.,*** **CON.,** cor-r., ***crot-h.,*** crot-t., ***cupr.,*** cycl., dig., dulc., eupi., ferr., ferr-ar., ferr-i., ferr-p., **GELS.,** gins., glon., gran., ***graph.,*** **HELL.,** hep., hipp., hyos., hyper., iod., ip., ***kali-ar.,*** kali-bi., ***kali-c.,*** **KALI-P.,** kalm., kreos., lach., lact., led., ***lyc., lyss.,*** mag-c., manc., **MERC.,** ***merc-c.,*** merc-i-f., ***mez.,*** morph., nat-c., ***nat-m.,*** nit-ac., **NUX-V.,** ***onos.,*** op., osm., paeon., par., petr., **PH-AC., PHOS.,** phys., ***pic-ac.,*** pin-s., plb., ***puls.,*** ruta., ***sabad.,*** sabin., ***sec., sel., sep., sil.,*** spig., stann., stram., ***sulph.,*** tep., ter., ther., thuj., trom., verat., zinc., zing.
afternoon - mag-m.
3 p.m. - plan.
4 p.m. - pic-ac.
ascending stairs - clem., lyc.
breakfast, after - ther.
chill, during - coc-c., sep.
before - ther.
daytime - sulph.
dinner, after - ant-c., sulph.
emissions, after - ph-ac., puls.

HEAVINESS, tired
evening - ammc., am-c., par., phos., ***sabad.***
9 p.m. - cocc.
exertion, on - ***lach.***
fever, during - **CALC., GELS., NUX-V., RHUS-T.,** sulph.
forenoon - caust., cham., grat., phos., ***sabad.,*** stront.
left - anac., carb-v.
lying on left side - merc-i-f.
menses, during - cocc., nat-m.
before - bar-c., com., ***lyc.,*** merc., nit-ac., zinc.
suppressed - graph.
mental exertion, from - ***ph-ac.***
morning - calad., carb-an., caust., iod., nat-m., ***nit-ac.,*** pall., ***zinc.***
6 a.m. - pic-ac.
after, amel. - lyc., nat-m.
bed, in - dulc., nat-m., ***nit-ac.,*** phos., ***zinc.***
breakfast, after - verat.
rising, on - phos.
waking, on - bar-c., clem., lyc., nat-m., phos., ***sulph.,*** verat., ***zinc.***
walking - nux-v., pic-ac.
motion, on - ***lach.,*** mez.
amel. - caps., cham.
night - carb-v., caust., petr., sep.
3 a.m. on waking - mez.
4 a.m. - lyc.
noon, walking, while - dig.
painful - agar.
paralytic - plb.
playing piano, after - anac.
pregnancy, during - ***calc-p.***
rest, during - caps.
rising after sitting - carb-v.
amel. - merc., nat-m.
sex, after - bufo
sexual excesses - ***puls.***
sitting, while - caps., ruta.
storm, during - ***phos.***
waking, on - cham., sep., tep.
walking, while - acon., ***calc.,*** paeon., **PIC-AC.**
amel. - carb-v.
in open air - lyc., sil., zinc.
in open air amel. - carb-v.

HERPES - alum., bor., caust., com., ***con.,*** cupr., ***dulc., graph.,*** led., ***lyc.,*** manc., mang., merc., mur-ac., ***nat-m.,*** nicc., nux-v., petr., psor., sars., sec., sep., staph., thuj., zinc.

INCOORDINATION - ***agar.,*** **ALUM.,** ***arag.,*** arg-n., bell., ***calc.,*** carb-s., caust., chlol., coca, cocc., **CON.,** ***cupr., gels.,*** merc., ***onos., ph-ac., phos., plb.,*** sec., ***stram., sulph.,*** tab., ***zinc.***

INFLAMMATION - ***lach.,*** merc-n., vip.
bones - ***asaf., aur., calc.,*** **FL-AC., MERC.,** ***mez.,*** **PH-AC.,** ***rhus-t.,*** **SIL.**
erysipelatous - anan., **LACH.,** vip.

ITCHING - abrot., **AGAR.**, aloe, ***alum.***, alumn., ambr., am-c., am-m., anac., ant-c., ant-t., apis, arn., ***ars.***, ars-i., asc-t., aster., aur., bar-c., bar-m., bell., berb., ***bism.***, bov., brach., bry., ***calc.***, calc-i., ***calc-s.***, cann-s., canth., carb-ac., carb-s., carb-v., ***caust.***, chel., chin., chin-a., cimic., cinnb., clem., cocc., coc-c., coloc., com., con., corn., cupr., cycl., dig., dios., dulc., fago., gran., graph., grat., ham., hura, ign., indg., iod., jug-c., jug-r., ***kali-ar.***, kali-bi., kali-br., kali-c., kali-i., kali-n., kali-p., kali-s., lac-ac., lach., lachn., laur., led., lyc., mag-c., mag-m., mag-s., mang., merc., merc-i-f., mez., mill., mur-ac., nat-a., nat-c., nat-m., nat-p., **NAT-S.**, nicc., nit-ac., ***nux-v.***, ol-an., olnd., op., osm., paeon., pall., ph-ac., ***phos.***, phyt., plat., ***plb.***, prun., ***psor.***, puls., ran-b., ***rhus-t.***, rhus-v., rumx., ruta., sabad., sars., sel., ***sep.***, ***sil.***, ***spig.***, spong., **SULPH.**, tarent., **TELL.**, thuj., til., verat., zinc.

afternoon - fago.
amel. - alum., ant-t., bov., camph., cann-i., chel., chin., coloc., graph., ***jug-c.***, ***kali-c.***, led., laur., ***mag-c.***, mag-m., ***mang.***, merc., mill., **NAT-C.**, nat-s., nicc., ol-an., olnd., pall., ph-ac., tarax., ***thuj.***
bed, in - fago., lyc., nux-v., rumx.
burning, on scratching - lach., nat-p., phos., rumx., sabad., sabin., **SULPH.**
evening - com., daph.
in bed - sulph.
extensor surface - coc-c.
forenoon - com.
left - sulph.
morning, on rising - ***rumx.***
night, bed in - rumx.
paralyzed limb - phos.
scratching agg. - ***alum.***, ars., ***bism.***, corn., ham., ***led.***, petr., ph-ac., rhus-v., stront-c., **SULPH.**
sex, after - agar.
undressing when - ***nat-s.***, rumx.

JERKING - acon., aesc., ***agar.***, ***alum.***, ***ambr.***, ***am-m.***, ***anac.***, ***apis***, arg-m., ***arg-n.***, ***ars.***, ***bar-m.***, bell., cadm-s., cann-i., ***caust.***, **CHAM.**, chel., ***chin.***, **CIC.**, cimic., **CINA**, colch., crot-h., ***cupr.***, ***glon.***, graph., **HYOS.**, hyper., ***ign.***, iod., ***kali-i.***, ***kali-n.***, kali-s., ***lil-t.***, ***lyc.***, **MERC.**, mur-ac., nat-c., ***nat-m.***, nux-m., onos., op., phos., phyt., **PLB.**, sec., ***sep.***, sil., ***stram.***, sulph., sumb., ***tarent.***, ***valer.***, verat., ***visc.***, ***zinc.***

alternation of flexors and extensors - ***plb.***
evening - graph.
in bed - kali-n.
falling asleep - ***agar.***, ***alum.***, arg-m., **ARS.**, cob., ***gels.***, hyper., **IGN.**, **KALI-C.**, ***nat-a.***, nat-m., ***phys.***, ***sel.***, sil., ***sulph.***, ***thuj.***
left side paralyzed, right side convulsed - art-v.
lying, while - ***anac.***
on back - calc-p.
on side - onos.
motion, on - sep.
amel. - ***merc.***, ***thuj.***, valer., zinc.
night - ***ambr.***, ***kali-i.***, phos., sec., sep., ***visc.***

JERKING,

one leg, and one arm - apis, apoc., hell., stram.
side, other side paralyzed - apis, art-v., bell., ***stram.***
painful - cupr., sec.
paralyzed parts - arg-n., merc., ***phos.***, ***nux-v.***, ***sec.***, ***stry.***
periodical - bar-m.
right - sep.
side, lain on - cimic.
not lain on - onos.
sleep, during - ***ail.***, cann-i., cann-s., colch., ***cupr.***, ***kali-c.***, ***lyc.***, merc-c., nat-c., phos., puls., ***sil.***, **ZINC.**
walking amel. - valer.

JUMPING, sensation of something alive in arms - croc.

KNOCKED, together - agar., ***con.***

LAMENESS - abrot., ***agar.***, aloe, ***apis***, ***ars.***, ***aster.***, bov., bry., cann-i., ***carl.***, ***caust.***, ***cham.***, chel., ***chin.***, **CINNB.**, ***cocc.***, **COLCH.**, ***con.***, cupr., ***dros.***, ***form.***, kali-chl., kali-n., kreos., **MERC.**, nat-c., ***rhus-t.***, ***ruta.***, ***sil.***, ***spong.***, stram., verat., ***zinc.***

evening - sil.
flexor muscles - calc-p.
left arm, and foot after fright - stann.
morning, waking, on - abrot., nat-c., ***zinc.***
night - ***cham.***

LIGHTNESS, sensation of - agar., ***asar.***, cann-i., carl., chin., ***coff.***, dig., gins., hyos., nat-m., nux-m., ***op.***, **PH-AC.**, rhus-t., spig., stict., ***stram.***, thuj.

LOCOMOTOR, ataxia (see Ataxia)

LOOSE, as if flesh were - staph., ***thuj.***

LUPUS, one elbow - hep.

MILK, leg (see Phelbitis)

MISSING, steps when going down stairs - ruta, ***stram.***

MOTION, of limbs

agg. - ***bell.***, nux-v., sars., stram.
agility, great - ***stram.***
constant - ***ars.***, ***bell.***
convulsions, between - ***arg-n.***
sleep, during - **CAUST.**
control of, lost - ***bell.***, chin-s., ***gels.***, merc-c., op., ***stram.***
difficult - acon., anac., ars., atro., aur., ***camph.***, carb-ac., chel., ***con.***, ***cupr.***, cycl., dulc., gels., hydr-ac., lyc., ***pic-ac.***, stront.
difficult, walking, after - gels.
involuntary - agar., alum., bell., calc., ***crot-c.***, ***cupr.***, ***hell.***, ***merc.***, nat-m., op., phos., ***stram.***
one arm and leg - ***apoc.***, ***cocc.***, ***hell.***
one side - ***alum.***, calc.
paralyzed limb - arg-n., merc., phos.
peculiar to daily duties - bell.
stool, after - carb-v.
thinking of movements - aur.

MOTION, of limbs
irregular - ***agar., bell.,*** **HYOS.,** kali-br., lach., ***plb., sec.,*** stram., **TARENT.**
loss of power of - ***apis,*** ars., ***bell.,*** canth., carb-h., cocc., hydr-ac., lath., lyc., naja, oena., op., sars., sec., ***stram.,*** stry., ***tarent.***
irregular, loss of power of, morning, on waking - sil., zinc.
ludicrous - zinc.
oscillatory - acon., zinc.
sleep, during - ***caust.***
slow motion - merc-n., verat.
upward then forcibly thrown downward - **BELL.**
waving motion of left arm and leg with sighing - bry.

MOTIONS, convulsive - absin., acon., **AGAR.,** agar-ph., ***arg-n.,*** aster., aur-m., **BELL.,** calc-p., cann-i., carb-s., ***caust., chlor.,*** cocc., colch., crot-h., ***cupr.,*** kali-c., lyc., ***merc-c.,*** mygal., **OP.,** phos., ***plb.,*** rhus-t., ***sant., sec.,*** **STRAM.,** sul-ac., verat., ***zinc., ziz.***
lying on back, when - calc-p.
on side amel. - calc-p.
morning on waking - rhus-t.
motion on - cocc.
now in upper, now in lower - hyos.
sneezing - phos.
trembling of body, alternating with - arn.
use, on attempting to - cocc., **PIC-AC.**

MOUSE, sensation of, running down - lyss.
running up limbs - ***calc.,*** sep., ***sil., sulph.***

NODES - ***agar., ars.,*** carb-an., caust., lyc., mag-c., ***mez.,*** mur-ac., nat-m., nit-ac., ph-ac., sil., zinc.

NEURALGIC, pain - acon., **ARS.,** cann-s., ***cham.,*** chel., colch., ***coloc., corn., gels., lyc., mag-p.,*** nat-a., ***plb., puls., tarent.***

NUMBNESS, (see Nerves, Numbness) - abrot., ***acon.,*** **AGAR.,** ail., ***alum., ambr., ant-t., apis,*** **ARG-M., ARG-N.,** ***arn., ars.,*** ars-h., aster., atro., ***aur.,*** bar-m., bell., bry., bufo, ***calc., calc-p., calc-s.,*** camph., cann-i., cann-s., canth., ***carb-ac.,*** carb-an., carb-o., **CARB-S., CARB-V.,** ***carl.,*** caust., cedr., ***cham.,*** chel., ***chin., chin-a.,*** chin-s., cic., **COCC.,** ***con., crot-c., crot-h.,*** cupr., cupr-ar., ***dulc.,*** eup-pur., fago., ***fl-ac.,*** **GELS., GRAPH., GUAI.,** ham., hyos., ***hyper.,*** ign., iod., ***kali-ar.,*** kali-c., kali-p., ***kali-s.,*** kalm., ***kreos.,*** lact., laur., ***led.,*** **LYC.,** ***merc.,*** mez., naja, ***nat-m.,*** nat-p., nat-s., nit-ac., **NUX-M.,** ***nux-v.,*** oena., ***onos.,*** **OP., OX-AC.,** paeon., ***petr.,*** **PHOS.,** phys., plat., ***plb., psor., puls., rhod.,*** **RHUS-T.,** sarr., **SEC.,** ***sep., sil., stram., sulph.,*** tab., ***tarent.,*** tax., ter., ther., thuj., valer., verat., vip., xan., ***zinc.***
afternoon - ham.
4 p.m. - puls.
alternating arms and legs - ***phos.***
childbirth, during - cupr.
chill, during - rhus-t.
cold, becoming - sumb.
daytime - lyc.

NUMBNESS, of
evening - dulc., graph.
on remaining in one position - fago.
paralytic - valer.
perspiration, after - tax.
exaltation, with - nat-m.
exertion, during - alum.
fever, during - apis, carb-v., cocc., kali-c., **LYC.,** nat-m., ***nux-v., puls.,*** rhus-t.
left - alum., carb-o., caust., cupr-ar., dios., med., mez., prot., ***sumb.***
arm, and right leg - ***tarent.***
lying, while - aloe, ***aur., carb-v., chin.,*** kali-c., ***sulph., verat.,*** **ZINC.**
after eating - aloe
normal labor, after - ***sep.***
on them - am-c., arn., bar-c., bry., bufo, ***calc.,*** carb-an., **CARB-V.,** ***chin.,*** glon., ***kali-c.,*** lyc., mez., phel., ***puls.,*** rheum, rhod., **RHUS-T.,** ***sil., sumb.***
still agg. - ***graph.***
manual labor - ***sep.***
menses, during - ***graph.***
migratory - ***cocc.***
morning - ***ambr.,*** ox-ac., ***zinc.***
10 a.m. - ant-t.
waking, on - aur., bufo, calc-p., ***zinc.***
motion amel. - am-c., anac., aur.
night - croc., graph., kali-c., lyc., ph-ac.
waking, on - mez., thuj.
one side, the other paralyzed - cocc.
right arm, and left leg - ars., kali-c.
side not lain on - fl-ac.
sitting, while - am-c., cham., cop., ***graph.,*** lact., sulph.
sleep, during - nat-m.
waking, on - ***aur.,*** bry., bufo, erig., mez., puls., thuj.
walking in the open air - alum., ***graph.***
warmth agg. - sec.

OSGOOD-schlatter's, disease - ***calc-p., sil.***

OWN, felt as if not his own legs - ***agar., bapt.,*** op., sumb.

PAGET'S, disease - calc-p., sil.

PAIN, limbs - ***abrot., acon., aesc.,*** aeth., **AGAR.,** all-s., ***alum.,*** alumn., am-c., anac., anthr., ***apis,*** ant-t., apoc., arg-m., ***arn.,*** **ARS.,** ars-h., ars-i., asaf., asc-t., aster., ***aur., bapt.,*** bar-c., **BELL.,** berb., ***bol.,*** both., **BRY.,** cact., ***calc.,*** calc-p., calc-s., cann-i., canth., caps., carb-an., carb-h., carb-o., carb-s., carb-v., ***carl., caul.,*** **CAUST.,** cedr., ***cham.,*** **CHEL.,** ***chin.,*** chin-a., cimic., ***cina,*** cinnb., coca, cocc., coff., **COLCH.,** ***coloc.,*** con., cop., crot-h., crot-t., cupr., dig., dios., ***dros., dulc.,*** elaps, **EUP-PER.,** eup-pur., euph., fago., ***ferr.,*** ferr-ar., form., ***gels., graph.,*** glon., ***guai.,*** ham., ***hell.,*** hep., hydr., hyos., ign., ind., indg., ***ip.,*** iris, jatr., jug-c., **KALI-AR.,** ***kali-bi., kali-c., kali-i.,*** kali-n., kali-p., **KALI-S., KALM.,** ***kreos.,*** lac-ac., lach., lact., led., lith., **LYC.,** lycps., ***lyss.,*** mag-p., **MED.,** meph., **MERC.,** ***merc-c.,*** merc-i-f., merc-i-r., merl., mez., ***mur-ac.,*** naja, ***nat-a., nat-c.,*** nat-m., ***nat-p., nit-ac.,*** **NUX-V.,** op., osm., ox-ac., ***ph-ac., phos.,*** phys., **PHYT.,** plat.,

PAIN, limbs - plan., **PLB.,** podo., psor., ptel., **PULS., RHOD., RHUS-T.,** ***ruta,*** sabad., sabin., ***sang., sars., sec.,*** sel., sep., sil., sol-n., squil., staph., stram., stront-c., ***stry.,*** **SULPH.,** sul-ac., sumb., tab., tarent., tax., tell., thuj., ***valer.,*** **VERAT.,** vip., zinc.
afternoon - calc., cina, glon., kali-c., lyc., lycps., nit-ac., ptel., staph., thuj.
air, cold, from - **ARS.,** daph., kali-ar., ***kalm., sel., tarent.***
cold, from, open, amel. - **KALI-S., PULS.,** sabin.
alternately, in arms and legs - merc-i-r.
alternating sides - **LAC-C.**
with chill and heat - brom.
appear, and disappear gradually - ***stann.***
ascending, stairs - ***calc.,*** phos.
changes of the weather - ***calc-p.,*** **RHOD.,** ***sil.***
childbirth, after - rhod.
chill, during - ang., aran., arn., **ARS.,** asaf., aur., bar-c., **BOV.,** bry., ***calc.,*** calc-s., ***caps.,*** carb-s., caust., ***chin-s., cimx., cina, cocc.,*** **COLOC.,** cycl., **DULC., EUP-PER.,** ***eup-pur., euph., ferr.,*** form., ***gels., graph.,*** hell., ***hep., ign.,*** **IP.,** ***kali-ar., kali-c.,*** **KALI-N.,** ***kali-s.,*** lach., led., **LYC., MEZ.,** mur-ac., ***nat-a.,*** nat-c., nat-m., **NUX-V.,** ***op.,*** petr., ***ph-ac.,*** plb., ***psor.,*** **PULS., PYROG.,** ran-b., **RHUS-T.,** sabad., **SEP.,** sil., squil., stram., sulph., **TUB.,** xan.
chill, before - **ARN.,** ***calc., carb-v., cina,*** **EUP-PER.,** lyc., nux-v., rhus-t.
coffee, amel. - arg-m.
cold, applied, amel. - apis, ***guai., lac-c.,*** **LED., PULS., SEC.,** thuj.
becoming - **ARS.,** bry., ***calc.,*** graph., ***kalm.,*** **NUX-V.,** ***ph-ac., phos., puls., ran-b.,*** **RHUS-T.,** tarent.
water, agg. - ant-c., ***ars., phos., rhus-t., tarent.***
water, amel. - ***puls.***
convulsions, after - plb.
coryza, during - calc., caust., hep., ph-ac.
draft, of air even warm - ***sel.***
drinking, agg. - **CROT-C.**
eating, after - am-m., bry., ***indg.,*** kali-bi., sep.
amel. - nat-c.
evening - am-c., apoc., ***ars., bell.,*** cact., calc., calc-p., colch., ***kalm., kali-s., led.,*** mag-s., sol-n., sulph.
after lying down - ***ars.***
exercise, as after violent - aesc.
exertion, slight, after - ***agar.,*** alum., bar-c., berb., calc., **CAUST.,** cimic., con., gels., ign., kali-c., kali-n., mag-c., nat-c., ***nat-m.,*** phos., ***rhus-t., ruta.,*** sabin., ***sep.,*** sil., stann., sulph., sul-ac., zinc.
fatigue, as from - petr.

PAIN, limbs
fever, during - ***arn.,*** ars., bell., **BRY.,** ***calc., chin.,*** **EUP-PER.,** ***ferr.,*** **GELS.,** ***merc.,*** nat-m., **NUX-V.,** phos., ptel., puls., ***pyrog., rhod., rhus-t.,*** sec., sep., sulph., tub., valer.
flesh, were loose, as if - nat-m., sulph.
forenoon - am-c., mag-m., merc., nat-a., plan.
fright, from - merc.
influenza, during - ***acon.,*** **BRY.,** ***caust., chel., euph.,*** **EUP-PER., GELS.,** merc., naja., rhus-t.
jerking - am-m., **CARB-S.,** ***puls.***
lain, on - dros., ***graph.,*** **KALI-C., NUX-M.,** nux-v., sep.
left - nit-ac.
then right - ***colch.,*** elaps, kali-c., ***kreos.,*** **LACH.,** naja, nit-m-ac., phyt., ***plan.,*** rhus-t.
lying, on - ***ars.,*** bry., iod., lyc., ***merc.,*** nux-v., rhus-t., verat.
menses, during - ***bell.,*** berb., bry., cast., ***cimic.,*** con., ***graph.,*** kali-n., ***kalm.,*** nit-ac., nux-m., nux-v., phos., sep., spong., stram., verat.
mental, exertion - colch.
morning - arg-n., calc-p., cinnb., clem., kali-bi., lyc., phos., sulph.
4 a.m. - gels.
bed, in - ***nux-v.,*** **PULS.,** ***rhus-t.***
toward - ***ars.,*** bov., ***kali-c., nux-v.,*** rhus-t., thuj.
waking, on - aesc., aur., ***hep.,*** op., ***puls.,*** sulph., tell., zinc.
motion, on - aesc., berb., **BRY.,** calc-p., caps., chin., ***cocc.,*** **COLCH.,** ***coloc.,*** dulc., ***euphr., guai., kalm., led.,*** merc-c., naja, ***nat-m., nux-m., nux-v., ox-ac., phyt., plb., ran-b., sil.,*** squil., zinc.
amel. - agar., ***arg-m., aur.,*** cham., chin., ***con.,*** dig., ***dulc., ferr., kali-c.,*** kali-p., **KALI-S.,** lach., ***lyc., med.,*** merc., ***mur-ac., nat-s.,*** psor., **PULS., PYROG.,** ***rat.,*** **RHOD., RHUS-T.,** ***ruta.,*** sep., thuj., ***tub., valer., zinc.***
amel., continued - agar., **CHAM., RHUS-T.**
beginning to - agar., caps., carb-v., ***caust.,*** **FERR.,** fl-ac., graph., ***kali-p.,*** lach., ***led.,*** **LYC.,** ***med.,*** nit-ac., petr., ***ph-ac.,*** **PHOS.,** plb., psor., **PULS.,** pyrog., rhod., **RHUS-T.,** ruta., ***sil.,*** valer.
night - acon., ***agar.,*** alum., am-c., arn., ***ars., asaf., aur.,*** bry., calc., carb-v., **CHAM.,** cinnb., dulc., ***ferr., fl-ac.,*** gels., graph., ***hep.,*** kali-bi., ***kali-c., kali-i.,*** kalm., ***lach.,*** lyc., mag-c., **MERC.,** ***merc-i-f.,*** merc-sul., ***mez.,*** nat-m., ***nit-ac., nux-v.,*** phos., ***phyt.,*** **PLB.,** podo., ***puls., rhod., rhus-t.,*** sabin., ***sars., sulph.,*** syph., thuj.
2 to 3 a.m. - **KALI-C.**
bed, drives out of - **CHAM.,** ***ferr.,*** kali-c., **MERC.**
crampy - phos.

PAIN, limbs
night, midnight - sulph.
midnight, after - **ARS.**, gels., ***merc., sars., sulph., thuj.***
midnight, before - bry.
noise - cocc., **COFF.**, ***nux-v.***
noon - bry., sulph.
until midnight - bell., mag-s., rhus-t.
paralyzed parts - ***agar.***, am-m., arn., ***ars.***, bell., calc., ***caust.***, cina, ***cocc.***, crot-t., ***kali-n., lat-m.***, nux-v., ***phos., plb.***, sil., sulph.
paroxysmal - **CARB-S.**, caul., ***caust., cocc., mag-p.***, **NUX-V.**, phos., **PLB.**, **PULS.**, ***sec.***
perspiration, amel. - ***ars., bry., nux-v.***, thuj.
pressure, agg. - cina, cocc., merc., ***plb.***
amel. - ***ars.***, bry., ***mag-p., plb.***
pulsative - bell., **KALI-C.**
riding, while - bry.
right, then left - bell., **LYC.**, mez., sang., sulph.
sex, after - **SIL.**, tub.
sitting - ***pyrog.***, **VALER.**
sleep, during - ***ars.***
after agg. - ***agar., lach.***, merc-c., op.
from waking - ars.
on going to - ***kali-c.***
thinking, about the pain agg. - ox-ac.
thunderstorm agg. - **MED.**, ***nat-c.***, **RHOD.**
tickling - nat-m.
touch agg. - **CHEL.**, ***chin.***, cocc., lyc., tarax., vip.
changing place, on - ***sang.***
ulcerative - agar.
waking, on, amel. by motion - abrot.
walking, on - coff., lyc., merc., op., ruta.
after - raph., rhod., rhus-t., ***ruta.***, sulph.
amel. - ***agar., arg-m., ars., cham.***, chin., ***ferr.***, kali-i., ***kali-s., lyc., merc.***, nat-a., phos., ***puls., rhod.***, **RHUS-T.**, ruta., seneg., ***valer., verat.***
warmth, agg. - ant-t., apis, ***bry., guai.***, iod., kali-i., ptel., ***puls.***, **SEC.**, sep., stel., ***sulph.***, thuj.
amel. - aesc., agar., am-c., ant-c., arg-m., **ARS.**, ***bry.***, cact., ***caust.***, cham., chin., ***colch., coloc., graph.***, **KALI-BI.**, ***kali-c.***, **KALI-P.**, kalm., ***lyc.***, **MAG-P.**, merc., ***nux-v., ph-ac.***, pyrog., **RHUS-T.**, **SIL.**, ***sulph.***
of bed, agg. - apis, ***lac-c., led.***, **merc.**, phyt., stel., ***sulph., verat.***
of bed, amel. - **ARS.**, ***kali-bi., nux-v., ph-ac., pyrog.***, **RHUS-T.**
wet, weather - am-c., ant-c., ***arg-m.***, bell., bor., bry., **CALC.**, carb-v., caust., **COLCH.**, con., ***dulc.***, hep., lyc., **MERC.**, nat-s., ***nit-ac.***, nux-m., ***phyt.***, **PULS.**, **RHOD.**, **RHUS-T.**, ruta., ***sars., sep., sil.***, sulph., ***tub.***, **VERAT.**
wine - led., mez., zinc.
sour - ***ant-c.***
wrong position in - tarax.

pain, bones - ***arg-m., arn., ars.***, **ASAF.**, ***aur., calc., calc-p.***, carb-v., caust., ***cham.***, chin., cinnb., ***cocc., colch., con., cupr.***, **EUP-PER.**, ***ferr., fl-ac.***, gels., graph., ***guai., hep.***, iod., ***ip.***, kali-c., ***kali-i.***, lach., ***led., lyc.***, mag-s., mang., **MERC.**, ***merc-i-f.***, mez., mur-ac., nat-m., **NIT-AC.**, **NUX-V.**, **PH-AC.**, ***phos.***, **PULS.**, **PYROG.**, ***rhod., rhus-t.***, **RUTA.**, ***sars., sep., sil., staph., sulph.***, ther.
middle of long - bufo, ***phyt.***
periosteum - cham., mang.
touch, on - sulph.
walking, in cold air - sep.

pain, muscles, attachment, of - phyt., rhod.
flexors - anac., arn., carb-s., caust., cic., dros., gels., kalm., merc., mez., op., ***phos.***, plan., plb., rhus-t., sep.
morning - caust.
forenoon - caust.
exertion, from - gels.
motion, agg. - acon., nux-v.
rheumatic - merc-i-f.
waking, on - sep.

pain, periosteum - ant-c., **ASAF.**, aur., bell., bry., ***camph., cham., chin.***, colch., coloc., ***cycl.***, graph., hell., ign., ***kalm.***, led., ***mang., merc., mez.***, **PH-AC.**, ***phyt.***, puls., ***rhod.***, rhus-t., **RUTA.**, sabad., sabin., ***sil.***, spig., staph.

pain, tendons - am-m., arn., benz-ac., berb., ***bry.***, caust., colch., coloc., harp., iod., kali-bi., kalm., prun., **RHUS-T.**, ***ruta,*** sabin., thuj., zinc.

PARALYSIS, (see Nerves) - abrot., **ACON.**, **AGAR.**, ***all-c.***, aloe, **ALUM.**, ambr., ***anac., arg-n., ars., art-v., aur., bapt., bar-c.***, bar-m., ***bell., bry.***, **BUFO,** ***calc.***, calc-s., carb-o., carb-s., carb-v., **CAUST.**, ***chel., cic., chin.***, **COCC.**, coff., ***colch., con., crot-c.***, crot-h., ***cupr., cur., dros., dulc.***, ferr., ***form., gels., guare.***, hydr-ac., hyos., ***kali-ar., kali-c., kali-i.***, kali-n., ***kali-p., kalm., lach.***, laur., lyc., meph., merc., ***merc-c.***, mill., morph., ***naja, nat-m., nit-ac., nux-v., olnd., op.***, ph-ac., ***phos.***, pic-ac., ***plat.***, **PLB.**, puls., rhod., **RHUS-T.**, ***ruta., sec., sep.***, **SIL.**, spong., stann., ***stram.***, stront-c., **SULPH.**, tab., tax., ***tarent.***, thuj., ***verat.***, vip., ***zinc.***
afternoon, 5 to 6 p.m. - ***con.***
anger, after - nat-m., ***nux-v.***, staph.
appearing gradually - **CAUST.**, ***con.***
ascending - agar., ***ars., con.***, hydr-ac., ***kali-c.***, mang.
cholera, after - verat.
cold, after catching - dulc., rhod.
coldness, of parts with - caust., ***cocc.***, dulc., graph., ***nux-v., rhus-t.***
descending - ***bar-c.***, merc.
elderly, people - ***bar-c., con., kali-c.***
evening - cur., sil., stront.
exertion, after - ars., ***caust., gels.***, nux-v., ***rhus-t.***
extensor muscles - alum., ars., calc., ***cocc., crot-h.***, **PLB.**
flexor muscles - caust., ***nat-m.***

PARALYSIS, of
fright, from - stann.
hysterical - cur., **IGN.,** plb., tarent.
mental emotion, after - ***apis,*** **IGN.,** nat-m., nux-v., stann.
morning, bed, in - phos., zinc.
nettlerash, after disappearance of - cop.
pain, from - nat-m.
painless - abies-c., acon., aeth., alum., ambr., ***anac., arg-n.,*** arn., ***ars., aur., bapt.,*** bar-c., bry., cadm-s., **CANN-I., COCC.,** colch., **CON.,** crot-h., ***cupr.,*** cur., **GELS.,** graph., **HYOS.,** kalm., ***laur.,*** **LYC.,** ***merc.,*** nat-m., ***nux-v.,*** **OLND.,** ***op., ph-ac., phos.,*** **PLB.,** ***puls.,*** rhod., **RHUS-T.,** ***sec.,*** sil., stram., sulph., ***verat., zinc.***
partial - ***ars., nux-v.***
post diphtheritic - ant-t., apis, arg-m., arn., ***ars.,*** camph., carb-ac., ***caust., cocc., crot-h.,*** gels., kali-br., kali-p., lac-c., ***lach., nat-m.,*** nux-v., phos., sec., sulph.
rheumatic - bar-c., ***caust., cocc.,*** lyc., rhus-t., sulph.
rising amel. - phos.
river bath in summer - ***caust.***
sex, after - phos.
sexual excesses - ***nat-m., nux-v., rhus-t.***
single, parts - anac., ***ars.***
spastic - ***benz-d-n.,*** gels., ***hyper., lach., nux-v.,*** plect., sec., ***stry.***
stiffness, with - caust., con., lach., lyc., nat-m., rhus-t., sil.
stroke, after - ***alum.,*** anac., apis, ***bar-c.,*** cadm-s., ***caust., cocc., crot-c., crot-h., cupr., gels.,*** **LACH.,** ***laur., nux-v.,*** **OP.,** ***phos., plb.,*** sec., stann., ***stront-c.,*** zinc.
suppressed eruptions - caust., ***dulc.,*** hep., ***psor., sulph.***
intermittent - nat-m., rhus-t.
perspiration - ***colch., rhus-t.***
toxic - ***apis, ars.,*** bapt., gels., lac-c., ***lach.,*** mur-ac., rhus-t.
typhoid, in - ***agar., lach., rhus-t.***
wet, after getting - **CAUST.,** ***rhus-t.***

paralysis, hemiplegia - acon., ***alum., anac., apis,*** arg-n., ***ars.,*** bapt., bar-m., ***both., cadm-s.,*** **CAUST.,** ***cocc.,*** coc-c., cop., elaps, ***graph.,*** hyos., ***kali-c., kali-i.,*** kali-p., ***lach., mur-ac.,*** nat-c., ***ph-ac., phos.,*** plb., **RHUS-T.,** ***sars., stann.,*** staph., stront-c., ***sul-ac.,*** tab., thuj.
anger, after - staph.
left - acon., anac., **APIS,** arg-n., arn., ***bapt.,*** bar-m., bell., brom., caust., ***elaps,*** **LACH.,** lyc., nit-ac., **NUX-V.,** ox-ac., petr., podo., **RHUS-T.,** ***stann.,*** stram., sulph.
mental excitement - stann.
shock, after - apis.
onanism - stann.
one side, numbness, the other - cocc.
pain, caused by - nat-m.

paralysis, hemiplegia
right - ***apis,*** arn., bell., calc., **CAUST.,** colch., **CROT-C.,** ***crot-h.,*** elaps, ***graph.,*** nat-c., op., phos., ***plb., rhus-t.,*** sang., sil., stront-c., sulph.
spasms, after - stann.
twitching of one side, the other is paralyzed - ***apis,*** art-v., ***bell., stram.***

paralysis, sensation of - ***abrot., aesc., alum.,*** apis, ars., bell., ***bry.,*** carb-h., ***chel.,*** cinnb., ***cocc., con.,*** cupr., ***dig.,*** dros., ferr., ***gels.,*** **GRAPH.,** hell., hep., ***kali-i.,*** laur., merc., ***mez., nit-ac., rhus-t.,*** sabad., sil., zinc.
fever, after - sil.
flexors - colch.
headache, with - mez.
joints - acon., arn., ***caps.,*** cham., croc., graph., ***led.,*** par., plb., rhus-t., sulph.
night - ***led.***
morning - dulc., sil., zinc.
motion agg. - plb.
night - ***led.***
pressure, on - nit-ac.
walking, while - **RHUS-T.**

PARALYTIC, pain - ***aur.,*** fl-ac., ***mag-m., merc-c., nux-v., rhus-t.,*** sabad., thuj.

PERSPIRATION - aur., aur-m., ***con., carb-v.,*** cupr., glon., ***lac-ac.,*** ol-j., op., stram.
clammy - ars., calc., ***cact.,*** chin-s., lil-t., merc-c., nux-m., op., phos., plb., ***tab.***
when menses should appear - ***lil-t.***
cold - ***ars., asaf.,*** aur., aur-m., bell., ***cact.,*** canth., dros., ***lach.,*** lachn., ***merc-c., morph.,*** phos., ***sec.,*** spong., stram., ***tab., verat., verat-v.***
menses, during - ars., phos., sec., **VERAT.**
left arm, and left leg - lac-d.
morning - ***carb-v.,*** con.
night - calc., carl., con., kali-n.
paralyzed limb, of - ars., caust., cocc., ***merc., rhus-t.,*** stann.
stool, during - gamb.

PHLEBITIS, (see Legs, chapter)

PINCHING, pain - carb-an., rhod.

PLAYING, agg.
organ, from - lyc.
piano, from - anac., calc., cur., gels., kali-c., mag-p., ***nat-c., sep.,*** sulph., zinc.
sensation of heaviness - anac.
violin, from - calc., ***kali-c.,*** mag-p., viol-o.

PRESSING, pain - agar., arund., ***asaf.,*** bar-c., bell., ***carb-v.,*** chin., dig., dros., ***gels.,*** guare., kali-c., ***led., nat-m.,*** nux-m., olnd., petr., phyt., ruta., spig., thuj.
bones - ***alum.,*** coloc., kali-c.
constrictive - arund., ***chin.***
cramp-like - dros.
drawing - sulph., thuj.
finger, as by a - carb-an.
flexor muscles - arn., cic., ***dros.***
rheumatic - ***merc.***

PRESSING, pain
walking, on - ***bar-c.***
in open air, after - ***chin.***
wandering - agar., kali-c., nux-m.

PULLING - bell.
pregnancy, during - plb.

PULSATION - ant-t., ars., bar-c., berb., chin-a., ***ferr., ign., kali-c., lach.,*** nat-a., ol-an., ***rhus-t.,*** sep., zinc.
chill, during - zinc.
night - ***ferr.,*** sep.
rest, during - ***ferr.***
walking slowly, amel. - ferr.
wrist, motion, agg. - phos.

PURRING - sep.

PUSHED forward, legs in sleep - lyc.

QUIVERING, (see Trembling)

RASH - alum., ant-t., ***apis,*** ars., bell., bry., calad., ***chlol.,*** cop., cupr., daph., ***dig.,*** form., kali-ar., led., mez., nat-m., nux-v., ***petr.,*** phyt., **PULS.,** rheum, ***rhus-t.,*** sep., sil., ***sulph.,*** sul-i., tep., ***vesp.,*** zinc.

RELAXATION - arn., ars., asaf., bar-c., ***carb-h., carb-o., carb-v., chin.,*** cic., clem., con., ferr., grat., hell., lyc., nit-ac., nux-m., nux-v., **OP.,** sep., tab., vip.
dinner, after - nit-ac.
morning, from open air - ***nux-v.,*** sep.
on waking - lyc.
rising, after, amel. - lyc.

RESTLESSNESS - acon., ail., all-c., ***alum.,*** aml-n., **ARS.,** aster., bell., canth., carb-v., ***carl., caust.,*** chel., **CHIN.,** ***chin-a.,*** cic., ***cimic., cimx.,*** colch., coloc., ***cupr., dulc.,*** eupi., fago., **FERR.,** ***ferr-ar., glon.,*** graph., hyos., ***iod.,*** jal., **KALI-BR.,** ***kali-c., kali-p.,*** **LYC.,** mag-c., merc., merc-i-r., nat-a., nat-c., ***nat-m., nit-ac.,*** **NUX-V.,** op., ox-ac., petr., phys., ***phyt., plat.,*** **PULS., RHUS-T.,** ***ruta.,*** sanic., sep., **SIL.,** squil., ***stann.,*** **STRAM.,** stry., sumb., **TARENT., ZINC.**
convulsions, before - bufo
covering agg. - aster.
evening - calc., **CAUST.,** ***kali-c.,*** mag-c., merc-i-r., nat-c., ***nit-ac.***
bed, in - **ARS.,** carb-v., con., **KALI-C.,** ***lyc.***
sitting, after - ***mag-c.***
lying, while - ars., merc.
mental exertion amel. - ***nat-c.***
motion amel. - fago.
music amel. - **TARENT.**
night - ***alum.,*** bell., bufo, **CAUST.,** ***colch.,*** hep., ***lyc., nit-ac.,*** phys., **RHUS-T.,** ***sep.,*** spig., **ZINC.**
bed, before going to - **ARS., KALI-C.,** ***lyc.***
midnight, before - nux-v.
sitting, while - merc.
sleep, during - **CAUST.,** coloc.
walking in open air amel. - sumb.
warm bed agg. - aster., ***lach.***

RHEUMATIC, pain - ***abrot., acon.,*** act-sp., ***aesc., agar.,*** alumn., am-m., ***ant-t., apis, arg-m.,*** **ARN., ARS.,** ***ars-i., aur.,*** **AUR-M-N., BAD.,** bapt., ***bell.,*** **BENZ-AC., BRY.,** ***cact., calc., calc-p., calc-s., camph.,*** cann-s., ***caps., carb-ac., carb-s., carb-v.,*** card-m., ***caul.,*** **CAUST.,** cedr., **CHAM., CHEL.,** ***chin., chin-a., cimic.,*** clem., **COLCH.,** ***coloc., corn., crot-c., crot-h., crot-t.,*** cupr., ***dig., dulc.,*** elaps, euph., eup-per., ***ferr., ferr-ar.,*** ferr-p., **FORM.,** ***gels.,*** grat., ***guai., ham.,*** hell., ***hep.,*** hydrc., ***ign., kali-ar., kali-bi., kali-c.,*** kali-chl., **KALI-I.,** kali-p., ***kali-s.,*** **KALM.,** ***lac-ac., lac-c., lach.,*** led., **LYC.,** ***mag-c.,*** mag-p., mag-s., **MED.,** meph., ***merc.,*** merc-i-f., merc-i-r., merc-sul., ***mez.,*** mill., mur-ac., **NAT-A.,** ***nit-ac.,*** nux-m., ***nux-v.,*** ol-an., pall., ***petr., ph-ac., phos.,*** **PHYT.,** plat., ***psor.,*** **PULS.,** ***ran-b.,*** **RHOD., RHUS-T.,** ***ruta., sal-ac.,*** **SANG., SARS.,** sec., ***sep., sil.,*** spig., squil., stann., ***stel.,*** stict., **SULPH.,** ***syph., tarent.,*** ter., thuj., teucr., ***valer., verat.,*** viol-t., zinc.
acute - **ACON.,** ***ant-c., ars.,*** asc-c., ***bell.,*** **BRY.,** calc-s., caul., ***cham., chel.,*** chin., chin-s., cimic., **COLCH.,** ***dulc.,*** glon., ign., ***kali-bi., kalm., lac-c., lach.,*** **MERC.,** ***nux-v., puls., rhod.,*** **RHUS-T.,** sal-ac., sang., verat.
alternating with, chest problem - led.
diarrhea - cimic., dulc., ***kali-bi.***
dyspnea - guai.
eruptions - crot-t., staph.
gastric, symptoms - **KALI-BI.**
hemorrhoids - abrot.
lung troubles - **KALI-BI.**
pain in heart - benz-ac.
bed, drives him out of - **CHAM.,** ***ferr.,*** lac-c., led., **MERC.,** sulph., ***verat.***
cold, after a - acon., arn., ***bry.,*** calc., ***calc-p., coloc., dulc.,*** gels., ***guai., merc., nit-ac.,*** ph-ac., ***rhus-t.,*** sulph.
after a, amel. - ***guai., lac-c.,*** **LED., PULS., SEC.**
after becoming - ***ph-ac.,*** **RHUS-T.**
weather, after- ars., **BRY., CALC-P.,** carb-v., ***colch., dulc., kali-bi., kalm.,*** nit-ac., ***nux-v., ph-ac., phos., puls., rhod.,*** **RHUS-T.,** sul-ac., ***tub.***
diarrhea checked - ***abrot.***
chronic, in - ***nat-s.***
following - ***kali-bi.***
eruptions, acute, after - dulc.
extending, to lower limbs - ***kali-c.***
upward - ***kalm.,*** **LED.**
upper to lower limbs - ***kalm.***
flatus, amel. - coloc.
gonorrhea, after suppressed - ***clem.,*** con., ***cop.,*** crot-h., daph., kalm., ***lyc.,*** **MED.,** ***phyt., puls., sars., sep., sulph.,*** **THUJ.**
hemorrhoids, suppressed - ***abrot.***
injured parts - ***caust.***
left to right - **LACH.,** naja, ***rhus-t.***

RHEUMATIC, pain
mercury, abuse of - arg-m., arn., asaf., ***bell.,*** calc., ***carb-v., cham.,*** **CHIN., GUAI., HEP.,** ***kali-i., lach.,*** lyc., mez., ***nit-ac.,*** ph-ac., ***phyt.,*** podo., puls., rhod., **SARS.,** ***sulph.,*** valer.
overheated and exertion from - ***zinc.***
perspiration, with - **FORM., MERC.,** ***sulph., til.***
places least covered by flesh, in - sang.
right to left - **LYC.**
spring - ***colch.***
syphilitic - ***benz., fl-ac.,*** kali-bi., **KALI-I.,** kalm., ***merc., nit-ac., phyt.***
warm weather, in - **COLCH.,** ***kali-bi.***
first warm days - bry.

ROSEOLA, after abuse of mercury - ***kali-i.***

SCIATICA, pain, (see Legs, Sciatica)

SCRAPING, pain - bry., **CHIN.,** coloc., **PH-AC., RHUS-T.,** ***sabad.***
bones - **PH-AC.**

SENSITIVE - camph., coff., ***cupr.,*** cycl., ***ferr-p.,*** lath., ***mang.,*** sul-ac., tarax., ter., verat-v., zinc.
side not paralyzed - plb.
cold, to - am-c., ars.
warmth , to - ***sulph.***

SHAKING - kali-br., ***op.***
evening - nux-v.
faintness, after - asaf., arn., colch., ***gels.,*** kali-br., kreos., lyc., merc-c., sec., stry.
night - stram.
noon, after eating - graph.
sleeping, when, after dinner - nux-v.

SHARP, pain - abrot., ***acon., aesc., agar., alum.,*** anan., ant-t., ***apis, arg-m.,*** arn., ***ars.,*** asar., aur., bar-c., bell., benz-ac., ***berb., bry.,*** bov., ***calc.,*** calc-s., cann-i., ***carb-s.,*** carb-v., carl., caust., chin., cimic., cina, cocc., ***colch.,*** coloc., ***con.,*** dros., ***dulc., elat., ferr.,*** ferr-ar., ferr-i., ferr-p., ***gels., guai., hep., iris, kali-ar., kali-bi.,*** **KALI-C.,** ***kali-i.,*** kali-n., kali-p., **KALI-S.,** kalm., ***laur., lyc., merc.,*** merc-c., merl., ***nat-h., nat-p., nat-s., nit-ac.,*** paeon., par., ph-ac., phos., phyt., plan., ***plb., psor., puls.,*** rhod., **RHUS-T.,** sec., senec., ***sep.,*** sil., ***spig.,*** staph., ***stel., sulph., tarent.,*** thea., thuj., **VALER.,** xan., zinc., zing.
afternoon - plan.
4 p.m. - elaps
burning - **ARS.,** aur., spig.
chill, during - ***ars., hep.,*** lyc., psor., ***rhus-t.***
before - calc., ***plb.,*** rhus-t.
cold in paralyzed parts - agar.
condyles - agar.
coughing, on - caps.
cramp-like - cimic., ***cina,*** plat.
drawing - ***puls.***
eruptions, after - ***dulc.***
evening - ***ars.,*** calc., ***dulc., led.,*** par., plan., plb., sil.
sleep, before - sulph.
exercising in open air amel. - plan.
extending inward - phyt.
fever, during - ***dulc.,*** psor., **RHUS-T.,** sulph.

SHARP, pain
heated, after - zinc.
hot, in paralyzed parts - **ARS.**
jerking - **CARB-S.**
left - ***aesc.***
menses, during - ***graph.***
morning - ***kali-bi.,*** phos.
bed, in - ***nat-h.***
motion - bry., ***guai.,*** hyos., ***plb.***
amel. - alum., ***arg-m., ferr., kali-c.,*** **KALI-S.,** ***phos.,*** psor., **RHUS-T.,** ***stel., tub., valer.***
continued, amel. - agar.
night - ***dulc., ferr., hep., sil.***
2 to 3 a.m. - **KALI-C.**
noise agg. - cocc.
paralyzed parts - ars., nux-v.
paroxysmal - gels., ph-ac.
pressure, from - phos., plb.
amel. - ars., plb.
rubbing, amel. - ***plb.***
sitting, while - plan., zinc.
sneezing - caps.
splinters, as from - ***nit-ac.***
spots, in - rhus-t.
tearing - ***ars., carb-s.,*** coloc., ***sec.***
walking amel. - ***alum., ars., kali-c., kali-s., phos.,*** psor., ***rhus-t.***
wandering - arg-m., arn., aur., ferr., kali-n., ***kali-s.,*** kalm., lyc., merl., psor., ***puls., stel.***
warm, bed agg. - ***carb-v., led.,*** stel.
room - plan., stel.

SHOCKS - ***agar.,*** ail., alum., bell., ***cic., cocc.,*** **LYC.,** plat., verat-v.
jarring of the carriage - ***arn.***
lightning-like - plb.
noise, from - bar-c.
pulsating - plat.
sleep, on going to - ***agar.,*** alum., **ARG-M., ARS.,** ip., ***nit-ac.***
waking - lyc.

SHOOTING, pain - ***acon., aesc., agar.,*** aur., bufo, ***calc., con., hep.,*** iris, ***kali-bi., merc.,*** plan., spig., xan.
coughing, on - caps.
cramp-like - plat.
left - aesc.
morning - kali-bi.
motion continued amel. - agar.
move, on beginning to - agar.
noise, from - cocc.
sneezing, on - caps.

SHORTENED, muscles, and tendons (see Contractions) - ambr., am-c., **AM-M.,** anac., ars., aur., ***bar-c.,*** calc., carb-an., carb-v., **CAUST.,** cic., cimic., **CIMX., COLOC.,** con., cupr., dig., dros., **GRAPH.,** ***guai.,*** hell., hep., hyos., kali-c., kreos., lach., led., ***lyc.,*** mag-c., ***merc.,*** mez., mosch., ***nat-c.,*** **NAT-M.,** nit-ac., ***nux-v.,*** ox-ac., petr., ph-ac., phos., plb., puls., ran-b., rheum., ***rhus-t.,*** ruta., samb., ***sep.,*** sil., stann., sul-ac., sulph.

SHRIVELLED - ars., phyt., ***rhod.***

SMUTTINESS- ars., sil.

SORE, pain, bruised - abrot., ***acon.,*** aesc., ***agar., all-c., alum.,*** alumn., am-c., ammc., anac., anthr., ***apis,*** apoc., ***arg-m.,*** arg-n., **ARN.,** ars., aster., ***aur.,*** aur-m-n., ***bad.,*** **BAPT.,** ***bar-c.,*** **BELL.,** bov., ***bry.,*** bufo, ***calc.,*** camph., ***carb-ac., carb-an.,*** **CARB-S., CARB-V.,** ***caust.,*** cham., **CHEL.,** ***chin., chin-s.,*** chlf., **CIMIC.,** ***cist., clem.,*** cob., cocc., ***colch., con.,*** cupr., ***daph., dros.,*** dulc., elaps, elat., **EUP-PER.,** ferr., ferr-ar., ferr-i., ferr-p., ***gels.,*** gins., graph., ***ham.,*** hell., ***hep.,*** hyper., **IP.,** kali-bi., kali-br., kali-c., kali-n., kali-p., ***kalm., kreos., lac-ac., lac-c., lach.,*** lact., ***lec., led.,*** lil-t., ***lyc., lyss.,*** mag-c., mag-s., manc., **MANG.,** ***merc.,*** merc-i-f., mez., nat-a., nat-c., **NAT-M.,** nat-p., **NIT-AC., NUX-V.,** petr., ***ph-ac., phos., phyt., pic-ac.,*** plb., ***puls.,*** ran-s., **RHUS-T.,** rhus-v., **RUTA.,** sars., sec., sel., **SIL.,** sol-n., **SPONG.,** ***stann.,*** **STAPH., SULPH.,** sul-ac., tarax., til., ***thuj., tub.,*** valer., ***zinc.***
- afternoon - cina, cob., kali-c., pall., ***staph.,*** thuj.
- ascending stairs - phos.
- bed, in contact with - **ARN.,** aur., merc-n., ***nux-v., rhus-t.***
- chill, during - ***arn., bapt., nux-v., rhus-t., tub.***
- cold, becoming, from - ***ph-ac.***
- during - gins.
- daytime - sulph.
- dinner, after - nit-ac.
- evening - am-c., ferr-i., petr., sil.
  - lying down, on - petr.
- exertion, after - ***agar.,*** cimic., **RHUS-T.**
- fever, during - arn., ars., bell., **CHIN.,** ***nat-m., nux-v.,*** phos., **PULS.,** ***rhod., tub.***
- forenoon - mag-m.
- fright, during - merc.
- lying, while - lyc., ***nux-v.***
  - in the one on which he lies - **ARN.,** graph., **RUTA.**
  - side not lain on - ***rhus-t.***
- menses, during - nit-ac., phos., sep.
  - before - nit-ac., phos.
  - scanty menses - carb-v.
- morning - aesc., apoc., arg-n., ***aur.,*** clem., **NUX-V.,** sulph.
  - 4 a.m. - ***lyc.***
  - 6 a.m. - ptel.
  - in bed - ***aur., rhus-t., staph., zinc.***
  - rising, after - carb-v., ***nat-m.,*** sulph.
  - rising, after, amel. - ***aur.***
  - waking, on - zinc.
- motion, during - aesc., agar., ***bry.,*** carb-an., chin., croc., graph., ***ham.,*** lach., ***nux-v.***
  - amel. - aur., **RHUS-T.,** ***tub.***
  - continued amel. - nat-a., **RHUS-T.**
- night - nat-m., ***nux-v.***
  - after sleeping - cycl.
- noon - sulph.
- paralyzed parts, in - plb.

SORE, pain
- pressure, on - ***cina.***
- right - caust.
- rising, on - ant-t.
  - after, amel. - naja, ***nux-v.***
- sex, after - **SIL.**
- sitting, while - asaf., bry., sabad.
  - after a walk - ***ruta.***
- sleep, after - ***arg-n.,*** ptel.
- spots here and there - **KALI-BI.**
- standing, on - alum., sulph.
- touch, on - graph.
- ulcer, limb with - graph.
- waking, on - aesc., naja, sulph., ***zinc.***
- walking, while - apoc.
  - after - raph., rhod., **RUTA.**
  - amel. - agar., ***aur.,*** ruta.
  - in open air amel. - clem.
- warmth amel. - ***nux-v.,*** **RHUS-T.**

sore, bones - acon., ***agar.,*** am-m., anac., **ARG-M.,** ***asaf.,*** aur., bar-c., bov., ***calc.,*** cann-s., carb-v., chin., **COCC.,** ***con., cor-r., crot-h., cupr.,*** **EUP-PER., GELS.,** graph., **HEP.,** ***ign.,*** **IP.,** ***kali-bi., led., lith., lyss.,*** mag-c., ***mang., mez.,*** nat-m., ***nit-ac.,*** **NUX-V.,** ***par.,*** petr., ***ph-ac., phos., puls.,*** **RUTA.,** sabad., sep., ***sil., spig.,*** sulph., symph., valer., verat., zinc.
- long bones - agar., ***calc., calc-p.***
- menses, during scanty - carb-v.
- morning in bed - **NUX-V.**
- paralytic - ***calc.***
- sitting - am-m.

SPASM, (see Convulsion)

SPRAINED, as if - carb-v., **RHUS-T.,** rhod.

STAGGERING, (see Ataxia and Vertigo, chapter)

STIFFNESS - abrot., absin., acon., aeth., ***agar.,*** am-c., am-m., ang., ***aran.,*** arg-m., **ARS.,** ars-i., ars-s-f., **ASAF.,** ***bell.,*** bov., brom., **BRY.,** ***calc.,*** calc-p., calc-s., camph., cann-i., cann-s., canth., ***caps., carb-ac., carb-an.,*** carb-o., ***carb-s.,*** carb-v., carl., **CAUST.,** ***cham.,*** **CHEL.,** ***chin.,*** chin-a., ***cic., cimic.,*** **COCC.,** ***colch.,*** con., **CUPR.,** cycl., dig., ***dulc.,*** eup-per., ferr-ar., graph., ***guai., hell.,*** hydr-ac., ***hyos.,*** iod., kali-ar., kali-bi., ***kali-c.,*** kali-p., **KALM.,** ***lach.,*** lath., ***laur.,*** **LED.,** lith., **LYC.,** ***med.,*** meny., ***merc., merc-c.,*** merc-i-r., merc-sul., mosch., naja, nat-a., nat-c.1, ***nat-m., nat-s.,*** nit-ac., nux-m., ***nux-v.,*** olnd., op., ox-ac., **PETR.,** ph-ac., ***phos., phyt., plat.,*** plan., plb., psor., ***puls.,*** **RHUS-T.,** ***sang.,*** sars., ***sec.,*** sel., **SEP., SIL.,** ***spong., stram., stry.,*** **SULPH.,** tab., ***thuj.,*** verat., verat-v., ***zinc.***
- afternoon - thuj.
- air, open - acon.
- chill, during - ***chin-s.,*** eup-per., ***nat-s.,*** op., ***rhus-t.***
  - before - ***chin-s.,*** psor., ***rhus-t.***
- cold air, in - kali-c., rhus-t.
- convulsions, during - acon., alum., am-c., arg-m., ars., ***asaf., bell., camph.,*** canth., caust., cham., chin., ***cic., cina, cocc.,*** coloc., ***dros.,*** hell., hyos., ***ign.,*** **IP.,** kali-c., ***laur.,*** led., ***lyc., merc.,*** **MOSCH.,** nit-ac.,

STIFFNESS, of
nux-m., ***oena.,*** ***op.,*** ***petr.,*** phos., **PLAT.,** plb., sec., sep., sil., stram., sulph., thuj., ***verat.,*** ***zinc.***
after - led.
cough, during - bell., caust., cina, ***cupr.,*** ip., led., mosch.
cough, before - **CINA.**
epilepsy, before - bufo
evening - calc-s., ***puls.,*** ***sil.,*** thuj.
sleep, after - cycl.
exertion, after - arn., calc., **RHUS-T.,** ***tub.***
forenoon, 11 a.m. - brom.
standing, after - verat.
fright, after - ***bry.***
grasping, on - am-c., cham.
headache in occiput - ***petr.***
left - nit-ac., rhus-t.
menses, during - calc-p., ***rhus-t.***
morning - am-c., am-m., cact., calc-p., caps., chlor., cimic., ***kali-bi.,*** ***lach.,*** ***led.,*** ***petr.,*** ***phos.,*** sel., sep.
bed, in - calc-p., ***chin.,*** ***lach.,*** ***led.,*** **RHUS-T.,** staph.
cold bathing amel. - led.
rising, on, and after - mag-c., ***petr.***
waking, on - am-c., ox-ac., ***zinc.***
move, on beginning to - ***agar.,*** ***caps.,*** kali-p., ***lyc.,*** ***psor.,*** **RHUS-T.**
night - ***nux-v.,*** ***sil.***
noon - am-c., bov.
paralytic - ***cocc.,*** lith., merc-c., nat-m., plb.
right - am-m., kali-bi.
rising, on - agar., op., plan., psor., **RHUS-T.**
sitting, after - carb-an., carb-v.
sleep, after - ***lach.,*** morph., ox-ac., **RHUS-T.,** ***sep.***
standing - chin.
swoon., during - bov.
tetanic - absin., ars., hyos., ***phyt.,*** sang., zinc.
walking, while - acon., ter.
after - **RHUS-T.,** verat.
amel. - am-m., calc., carb-v., ***lyc.,*** ***rhus-t.***
warm stove, as approaching a - ***laur.***

STRETCHED, out, limbs (see Drawing, up) - ambr., merc., nat-m., nux-v., ***oena.,*** phos., rhus-t., spong., stry., sul-ac.
must stretch - nat-m., rhus-t.

STRETCHING, out limbs before convulsions, (see Generals) - calc.

SWELLING, of - absin., apis, ***arn.,*** ars., ***bar-c.,*** both., chin., chin-s., crot-h., ***dulc.,*** kali-ar., kali-p., ***kalm.,*** lach., merc., **MERC-SUL.,** nat-a., op., ***petr.,*** plb., rhus-t., ***sec.,*** ***sil.,*** still., vip.
annual, dark red at first, hot weather - vip.
cramp, after - graph.
doughy - vip.
dropsical - ant-c., **APIS,** apoc., **ARS.,** ***ars-i.,*** ***aur.,*** bell., bry., ***cact.,*** chel., ***chin.,*** chin-a., ***colch.,*** **COLL.,** ***crot-h.,*** ***con.,*** ***dig.,*** ***dulc.,*** ***eup-per.,*** ***ferr.,*** ferr-p., ***fl-ac.,*** ***hell.,*** ***iod.,*** kali-ar., kali-c., kali-n., kali-p., ***kalm.,*** led., ***lyc.,*** ***merc.,*** ***merc-sul.,*** mur-ac.,

SWELLING, of
dropsical - ***naja,*** ***nat-a.,*** op., plb., prun., puls., sabin., samb., seneg., ***sep.,*** squil., ***sulph.,*** ***ter.,*** xan.
flabby, livid - both.
sensation of - ant-c., ars-m., chin., ***glon.***

TEARING, pain - **ACON.,** **AGAR.,** alum., ***ambr.,*** ***am-c.,*** ***am-m.,*** anac., ant-c., ant-t., ***arg-m.,*** ***arn.,*** ***ars.,*** asar., **AUR.,** aur-m., ***bar-c.,*** bell., benz-ac., ***berb.,*** bism., bov., ***bry.,*** cact., ***calc.,*** calc-s., canth., ***caps.,*** ***carb-s.,*** ***carb-v.,*** ***carl.,*** ***caust.,*** cedr., ***cham.,*** ***chel.,*** **CHIN.,** ***chin-a.,*** ***cina,*** ***cocc.,*** coc-c., ***colch.,*** ***coloc.,*** ***con.,*** crot-h., ***cupr.,*** ***dulc.,*** ***euph.,*** eupi., ***ferr.,*** form., ***gels.,*** ***graph.,*** ***guai.,*** hell., hyos., iris, kali-ar., kali-bi., ***kali-c.,*** ***kali-i.,*** ***kali-n.,*** kali-p., kali-s., kalm., **LACH.,** lachn., lam., laur., led., ***lyc.,*** ***lyss.,*** ***mag-c.,*** ***mag-m.,*** mag-s., meph., **MERC.,** ***merc-c.,*** merl., mill., mur-ac., naja, nat-a., ***nat-c.,*** nat-p., **NAT-S.,** ***nit-ac.,*** ***nux-v.,*** ***ol-an.,*** osm., paeon., ***ph-ac.,*** ***phos.,*** plb., ***psor.,*** ***puls.,*** **RHOD.,** **RHUS-T.,** ruta., sabin., sars., ***sec.,*** sel., sep., sil., **SPIG.,** squil., sulph., sul-ac., ***tab.,*** thuj., **TUB.,** vinc., ***zinc.***
alternating with pain in teeth - merc.
asunder, as if they would be torn - nat-c.
bed, in putting limb out of - merc.
burning - ***ars.,*** merl.
changes in weather agg. - ***gels.***
chill, during - **ARS.,** **BELL.,** ***caps.,*** ***ferr.,*** graph., hell., ***hep.,*** ***kali-c.,*** kali-s., led., **LYC.,** ***nux-v.,*** ph-ac., phos., ***puls.,*** **RHUS-T.,** ***sabad.,*** sulph., ***tub.***
before - carb-v.
cold, after taking - ***dulc.,*** ***guai.,*** sel.
becoming - ***phos.***
food and drink - ***cocc.***
coryza, with - nit-ac.
cramp-like - nat-c., ruta.
eating, after - ***cocc.***
evening - ***ars.,*** ***dulc.,*** ***ferr.,*** mag-s., ***puls.,*** sulph., sul-ac.
bed, in - con., ***ferr.***
sitting, on - am-m.
exertion, after - zinc.
extending, downward - ***sulph.***
to feet - mag-s.
to head - carb-v.
extensor, muscles sitting - verat.
feather bed agg. - sulph.
fever, during - **CALC.,** **CARB-V.,** **CHIN.,** ***dulc.,*** ***ferr.,*** ***kali-c.,*** **LYC.,** ***nux-v.,*** phos., ***puls.,*** ***rhus-t.,*** ***sep.,*** ***sil.,*** ***sulph.,*** **TUB.**
heated, after being - zinc.
jerking - asar., **CHIN.,** paeon.
left arm, and leg - form.
and right thigh - agar.
lying, on painful side agg. - **ARS.**
lying, amel. - **AM-M.**
menses, during - sul-ac.
before - ***berb.***
suppressed - dig.
morning - hep., lyc., meph.
on waking - carb-v., ***hep.***

TEARING, pain
motion - guai., naja, plb.
amel. - **AGAR.,** ***arg-m., ars., cham., euph., ferr., lyc.,*** mur-ac., psor., ***puls., rhod.,*** **RHUS-T.,** sep., ***sulph.,*** thuj., ***tub.***
slow, amel. - ***ferr.,*** **PULS.**
move, when beginning to - agar.
night - ***calc.,*** carb-v., ***cham., dulc.,*** eupi., ***ferr., hep., lyc.,*** nux-v., ***puls., rhod.,*** **RHUS-T.,** sabin., sars., ***tub.***
bed, driving him out of - ***cham., ferr., merc.***
one side - **ARS.**
paralytic - **CHAM.,** ***chin.,*** **COLCH.,** ***mag-m., phos., plb.***
paralyzed parts - arn., ***ars.,*** bell., calc., caust., **CHAM.,** ***cocc.,*** crot-t., ***kali-n.,*** lat-m., ***nux-v., phos., plb.,*** rhus-t., sil.
paroxysmal - anac., paeon., **PLB.**
periodic - ***gels.,*** lyc.
pressure agg. - merc., plb.
rheumatic - am-m., ***colch., guai., puls.,*** **RHUS-T.,** ***sulph.***
rubbing amel. - canth., ***phos.***
sitting, while - **AGAR., AM-M.,** zinc.
stretching out on - cham., hipp.
sudden - carb-s.
thunderstorm, during - ***nat-c.***
tossing about in bed amel. - cham.
touch agg. - ***chin.***
twitching - ***am-m.,*** cact., chin., ph-ac.
wandering - **AM-M.,** arg-m., ***carb-s., caust.,*** cham., ***colch.,*** con., ***ferr., kali-bi.,*** laur., lyc., ***merc.,*** nat-s., ***puls.,*** rhod.
warm bed, in - sulph.
weather amel. - ***colch.***
warmth amel. - ***lyc.***
wet after getting - ***dulc.,*** **RHUS-T.**
wet weather - ***dulc.,*** lyc., ***rhod., rhus-t.***

tearing, bones - acon., ***agar.,*** alum., ***am-m.,*** anac., ***arg-m.,*** arn., ars., asaf., **AUR.,** ***aur-m., bar-c., bell., berb.,*** bism., bor., bov., bry., calc-p., cann-s., canth., ***caps., carb-v., caust.,*** cham., chel., **CHIN.,** ***cina, cocc.,*** coloc., con., crot-t., ***cupr., cycl.,*** dig., ***dros.,*** dulc., ***ferr.,*** graph., hell., hep., ign., iod., **KALI-C.,** ***kali-n.,*** **LACH.,** laur., ***lyc., mag-c.,*** mag-m., mang., **MERC.,** ***merc-c., mez.,*** nat-c., nat-m., ***nit-ac.,*** nux-v., ***ph-ac., phos.,*** plb., puls., **RHOD.,** rhus-t., ***ruta., sabin.,*** samb., sars., sep., **SPIG.,** spong., stann., ***staph., stront-c.,*** sulph., sul-ac., ***tab., thuj.,*** valer., verat., verb., ***zinc.***
long, in middle of - ***zinc.***
burning - sabin.
cramp-like - aur., olnd., ***valer.***
epiphysis, in arg-m.
jerking - ang., ***bry.,*** **CHIN.,** cupr., mang.
paralytic - **BELL.,** ***bism.,*** chel., chin., ***cocc.,*** dig.
pressive - **ARG-M.,** arn., asaf., bism., bry., coloc., **CYCL.,** staph., teucr.
sticking - bell., cina, mur-ac., sabin.

tearing, periosteum - bry., ***mez.,*** ph-ac., ***rhod.***

TENDONS, (see Musculoskeletal)

TENSION, limbs - bov., ***bry.,*** calc., ***carl., cimx., cupr.,*** hep., iod., mag-m., nux-v., ***plat.,*** plb., ***puls., rhus-t.,*** sec., sulph., ***thuj.***
afternoon - calc.
chill, during - rhus-t.
before - ***rhus-t.***
morning - ***nux-v.***
night - hep., ***puls.,*** rhod., sulph.
rising from a seat - ***rhus-t.***
suddenly, increases gradually and ceases - **PULS.**
walking, after - sulph.

tension, bones - agar., ***asaf.,*** **BELL.,** bry., cimic., cocc., ***con.,*** crot-h., dig., dulc., kali-bi., merc., nit-ac., rhod., ***ruta., sulph., valer.,*** zinc.

THRILLING, sensation - nit-ac., nux-v.
excitement, from - nux-v.

TINGLING, prickling, asleep - **ACON.,** ***alum., alumn., ambr.,*** anac., arg-n., ***arn.,*** ars., atro., bell., camph., ***carb-an.,*** carb-o., ***carb-s., carb-v.,*** con., ***cupr., gels.,*** **GRAPH.,** ***ign.,*** kali-bi., ***kali-c.,*** kreos., lach., ***led.,*** **LYC.,** ***merc.,*** morph., ***nat-m.,*** op., ox-ac., **PETR.,** ***ph-ac.,*** **PHOS.,** plb., psor., **PULS.,** ***rhod.,*** **RHUS-T.,** ***sec., sep., sil., stram.,*** stry., ***sulph.,*** sumb., tanac., tep., teucr., thuj., ***verat.,*** verat-v., zinc.
afternoon - teucr.
morning - kali-bi., teucr.
lying, while - kali-c.
rest, during - anac., carb-an.
night - ***merc.***
lying, while - ***sulph.***

TOTTERING - aesc., ***agar.,*** **ALUM.,** ***ambr., am-m., anac., apis,*** **ARG-M.,** arg-n., ***ars.,*** **AUR., BAR-C.,** ***calc.,*** camph., ***carb-ac.,*** carb-an., ***carb-v.,*** **CAUST.,** ***chin.,*** cic., **COCC., CON.,** ***fl-ac., gels., glon., hell.,*** hyos., ign., ***iod., lath., mag-p., merc., mur-ac., nat-c., nat-m.,*** **NUX-V.,** ***op.,*** ox-ac., ***ph-ac.,*** **PHOS., PIC-AC., PLB.,** rhod., **RHUS-T.,** ***sars.,*** sec., ***sil.,*** stram., ***stry., sulph., tarent.,*** teucr., verb.

TREMBLING, of - ***acon.,*** aeth., ***agar., alum.,*** alumn., ***ambr., anac.,*** ant-c., ***apis,*** **ARG-N.,** arn., **ARS., ARS-I.,** ***asaf.,*** bar-m., bell., bor., bry., bufo, ***calc.,*** camph., ***canth.,*** caps., carb-ac., carb-an., carb-o., ***carb-s., carb-v.,*** carl., cast., **CAUST., CHEL.,** ***chin.,*** chin-a., ***chin-s., cic., cimic.,*** cob., **COCC.,** coff., colch., ***con.,*** cop., ***crot-c.,*** crot-h., cupr., cupr-ar., dig., dor., dulc., euphr., eupi., ferr-i., ferr-ma., **GELS.,** glon., graph., hep., hydr-ac., ***hyos.,*** hyper., ***ign.,*** **IOD.,** kali-ar., kali-c., kali-i., kali-n., kali-p., kali-s., ***kalm., lach.,*** lact., laur., lob., lyc., lyss., mang., ***mag-p.,*** med., meph., **MERC.,** ***merc-c., mez.,*** morph., nat-m., **NIT-AC., NUX-V., OP.,** ox-ac., ***petr., phos.,*** **PLB.,** ***plat., puls.,*** ran-b., raph., rhod., **RHUS-T.,** ***rhus-v.,*** sabad., ***sec., sil.,*** spig., ***spong.,*** squil., **STRAM.,** stront-c., ***sulph., tab.,*** thuj., til., ***verat.,*** viol-o., vip., ***visc.,*** zinc.
afternoon - anac., carb-v., ***gels.***
walking, while - ran-b.

TREMBLING, of
alcoholics, in - **ARS.,** ***bar-c., nux-v.***
anger, after - ***nit-ac.***
anxious - merc., ***puls.***
chagrin - ran-b.
chill, during - ang., anac., ars., bry., chin., chin-s., cina, **COCC.,** con., eup-per., ferr., ***gels.,*** merc., ***par.,*** petr., plat., sabad., sul-ac., zinc.
cigar, after - op.
colic, after - plb.
contradicted, when - nit-ac.
conversation, from - ***ambr.***
convulsive - acon., asaf., carb-h., crot-h., op.
coughing, from - bell., ***cupr., phos.***
crying, while - tarent.
dinner, after - nit-ac.
drawing - lyc.
emission, after - **NAT-P.**
evening - agar., chel., ***cocc.,*** mez.
asleep, on falling - carb-an.
walking, while - dig.
excitement - **MERC.,** phos.
exertion, after - ***merc.,*** nat-m., ***phos.,*** **RHUS-T.,** sec.
fever, during - ***zinc.***
fright, after - **OP.**
frightened, as though - **OP.,** paeon., tarent.
holding them long in the same position - staph.
internal - carb-an., ***chin.,*** gins., staph.
invisible - ***chin.***
meditating, while - bor.
menses, during - ***hyos.,*** nat-m., ***nit-ac.,*** plat., stram.
before - hyos., kali-c., lyc., ***nat-m.***
morning - carb-v., euphr., kali-c., nat-c., nat-m., **NIT-AC.,** ***sil.,*** staph.
walking, while - euphr.
motion, on - **MERC.,** sulph.
night - calc., hep., rhod.
walking, on - nat-m.
one limb - stram.
paralyzed parts - **CAUST.,** plb.
periodic - ***merc.***
resting against anything amel. - plb.
sex, after - ***agar.***
sexual excitement, during - graph.
sleep, starting, from - petr.
something is to be done, when - **KALI-BR.**
standing, on - dirc., ***merc-c., zinc.***
stool, after - ars., carb-v., ***con.***
stretched, out, when - merc-c.
using hands - ferr-i.
vomiting, after - ars., eupi.
walking, while - acon., ars., cupr., ferr-i., **MERC.,** sulph.
after - cupr.
in open air, while - ***nux-v., phos.***

TUBERCLES - ant-c., caust., crot-h., nat-c.

TWITCHING, of - ***agar., alum.,*** alumn., ambr., ***apis,*** arn., ***ars.,*** ars-i., asaf., **BELL.,** calad., calc., cann-i., carb-ac., carb-v., carl., caust., ***cham.,*** **CHEL.,** ***chin., chin-s., cic.,*** cimic., **CINA,** ***cocc., coff.,*** colch., coloc., ***crot-c., cupr.,*** cypr., dros., dulc., graph., ***hell.,*** **HYOS., IGN.,** kali-ar., kali-c., kali-i., kali-n., kali-p., kali-s., kreos., lach., lyc., ***merc., merc-c.,*** morph., mur-ac., ***mygal.,*** nat-a., ***nat-c., nat-m.,*** nat-p., nat-s., nit-ac., ***nux-m., nux-v.,*** **OP.,** paeon., petr., ph-ac., phos., plb., puls., ran-s., **RHUS-T.,** ***rhus-v.,*** sec., ***sep., sil.,*** **STRAM., STRY.,** sulph., **VALER.,** ***visc., zinc.***
afternoon, when trying to sleep - alum.
backward and inward - cupr.
bed, in - merc-n., nux-v., stry.
chill, after - puls.
chill, during - acon., dig., jatr., lyc., nux-m., ***nux-v.,*** op., ox-ac., stram., tab.
convulsions, during - ***op.***
after - nux-v.
cough, during - cupr.
cramp-like - plat.
daytime - carb-v., petr., ***sep.,*** sil.
electric shocks, as from - agar., ***ars.,*** colch., nat-m., plat., ***ter., verat.***
evening - caust., graph.
bed, in - ***carb-v.,*** kali-n., nux-v.
sitting, while - am-m.
fever, during - all-s.
flexor muscles - op.
forenoon - alumn.
lightning-like - stry.
manual labor amel. - agar.
menses, during - ***coff.,*** oena.
morning - phos., sulph.
after rising - alumn.
sleeping - cham.
motion amel. - ***ars.,*** cop., phos., valer.
moving them, when - ***lyc.,*** sep.
night - ambr., calc., mag-c., nat-c., phos., sep., sil., staph., stront.
in bed - **ARS.,** merc-n., stry.
followed by - **RHUS-T.**
one arm and one leg - apis, apoc., hell., stram., tub.
one side, paralysis, of the other - ***apis,*** art-v., ***bell., stram.***
paralytic - cina
paralyzed parts - apis, ***arg-n.,*** merc., nux-v., phos., ***sec.,*** stram., ***stry.***
paroxysmal - stram.
respiration simultaneous, with - hyos.
sitting, while - **VALER.**
sleep, during - acon., alum., ambr., ***ars.,*** bell., cham., cob., ***colch.,*** cupr., ***hell.,*** hep., ***kali-c., lyc.,*** mag-c., morph., nat-c., nat-m., petr., puls., ***sep.,*** sil., ***stront-c.,*** sulph., thuj., ***zinc.***
before - alum.
on falling asleep - alum., **ARS.,** ***cham.,*** mag-c., ***nat-m.,*** puls.
waking - nit-ac.
sudden - arn.
thunderstorm, during - phos.

TWITCHING, of
touched, when - puls.
vexation, after - ign., petr.
vomiting, during - stram.
waking, on - op.
wandering - am-m., cast., cocc., coloc., graph., ***merc.,*** nat-s., plat.
write, on attempting to - nat-m.

ULCERS - merc-c.
varicose - **CARD-M.,** merc-c.

UNCONSCIOUS - ***agar.,*** camph., cann-s., stram.
walking, while - stram.

UNCOVERING, agg. - aur., ***bry.,*** con., **HEP.,** ***nat-m.,*** **RHUS-T., SIL.,** squil., stront-c., **THUJ.**

URTICARIA - acon., ant-c., ***apis, bell.,*** berb., ***calc.,*** chin-s., **CHLOL.,** ***cop.,*** dulc., hydrc., hyper., kali-br., kali-i., indg., ***lach.,*** lyc., merc., ***nat-m., rhus-t., rhus-v., sulph.,*** tarax., ***urt-u.***

VARICOSE, veins (see Blood, Varicose veins) - ***ambr.,*** arg-n., **ARN.,** ***ars.,*** **CALC.,** calc-f., calc-p., ***carb-s.,*** **CARB-V.,** card-m., ***caust.,*** clem., ***crot-h., ferr.,*** ferr-ar., FL-AC., ***graph.,*** **HAM.,** ***hep., kali-ar., kreos.,*** lac-c., ***lach.,*** **LYC., LYCPS.,** ***nat-m., plb.,*** **PULS.,** sabin., sars., sil., spig., ***sulph.,*** sul-ac., ***thuj.,*** vip., **ZINC**.
cramping - graph.
distended during menses - ambr., lach., puls.
drawing - graph.
painful agg. by warmth - **FL-AC., SULPH.**
pregnancy, during - acon., apis, ***arn., ars.,*** **CARB-V.,** ***caust.,*** **FERR., FL-AC.,** ***graph., ham., lyc., lycps., mill., nux-v., phos.,*** **PULS.,** ***sep., zinc.***

VESICLES - acon., am-m., anac., **ANT-C., ANT-T.,** arn., arg-n., **ARS.,** ars-i., bell., bov., brom., bufo, calad., ***calc.,*** calc-p., calc-s., cann-s., canth., ***caust.,*** carb-o., ***carb-v.,*** chin., chlor., cit-v., crot-h., clem., cupr., cupr-ar., daph., ***dulc.,*** elaps, fl-ac., graph., hep., hura, indg., iod., iris, kali-ar., kali-bi., kali-chl., kali-i., kali-s., ***lach.,*** lachn., mag-c., manc., mang., ***merc.,*** mez., nat-c., **NAT-M.,** nat-p., nit-ac., ph-ac., **PHOS., RAN-B.,** rhus-r., **RHUS-T., RHUS-V.,** ruta., sabad., sars., sec., sel., sil., sol-n., spong., ***sulph.,*** verat., vip., zinc.
white - agar.

VEXATION, felt in legs - ***nux-v.***

WALKING, (see Generals, Walking)

WANDERING, shifting, pains - acon., agar., **AM-M.,** ***arn.,*** ars., asaf., bapt., bell., bry., ***calc-p.,*** **CARB-S.,** ***caul., caust.,*** cedr., cham., chin-a., cinnb., colch., coloc., form., ign., ***kali-bi.,*** kali-n., **KALI-S.,** ***kalm.,*** lac-ac., **LAC-C.,** laur., ***lyc., mag-p.,*** merc-i-r., ***merl.,*** mosch., nat-a., nat-s., ***nux-m.,*** nux-v., ***phyt., plb.,*** **PULS.,** ***rhod.,*** sabin., sars., sep., ***sil.,*** sulph., ***tarent., tub.,*** valer., ***verat-v.***

WEAKNESS, of - abrot., acet-ac., acon., ***agar.,*** all-c., ***alum.,*** am-c., am-m., aml-n., ***anac., ant-c., ant-t., apis,*** apoc., **ARG-M., ARG-N., ARS.,** ***ars-h., ars-i.,*** atro., aur., aur-m., bar-c., ***bar-m.,*** bell., berb., bor., bov., brach., **BRY.,** cahin., **CALC.,** ***calc-p.,*** calc-s., cann-i., cann-s., ***canth.,*** caps., carl., carb-h., carb-o., carb-s., ***carb-v.,*** **CAUST.,** ***cham.,*** chel., chin., chin-a., ***chin-s., cic.,*** cimic., cimx., cinnb., clem., cob., cocc., ***coc-c.,*** coff., colch., **CON.,** croc., ***crot-t., cupr.,*** cupr-ar., dig., ***dulc.,*** elaps, eup-pur., euphr., **FERR.,** ferr-ar., ***ferr-i., ferr-m.,*** ferr-p., **GELS.,** gent-l., gins., glon., ***graph.,*** grat., ham., hydr-ac., hell., ***hep.,*** hura, hydr., hyos., hyper., ign., ind., iod., iris, jac-c., jatr., ***kali-ar., kali-bi., kali-br.,*** **KALI-C.,** ***kali-n., kali-p., kali-s., kalm.,*** kreos., ***lach.,*** lact., lob., **LYC.,** mag-c., manc., meny., **MERC.,** ***merc-c.,*** merc-i-f., merl., mez., morph., mur-ac., ***naja,*** nat-a., ***nat-c., nat-m.,*** nat-p., ***nit-ac., nux-v.,*** olnd., op., osm., ox-ac., pall., ***petr., ph-ac.,*** **PHOS.,** phys., pic-ac., plat., **PLB.,** psor., ptel., ***puls., ran-b.,*** raph., **RHUS-T.,** rumx., ruta., ***sabad.,*** sabin., sars., ***sec.,*** sep., **SIL.,** sin-n., spig., spong., squil., ***stann.,*** **STAPH.,** stry., ***sulph.,*** sumb., tab., ***tarent.,*** tep., ter., ***thuj.,*** til., upa., valer., **VERAT.,** verat-v., ***zinc.,*** zing.
afternoon - acon., bar-c., brach., mag-m., til.
4 p.m. - pic-ac., **RHUS-T.**
sitting, while - thuj.
walk, after a short - ol-an.
walking, while - gins.
alternation with dim vision - bell.
bath, in river, after - ant-c.
chill, during - ant-t., cann-i., rhus-t., sep., thuj., verat.
crying, after - con.
daytime - sulph.
dinner, after - nit-ac.
eating, after - ***bar-c.,*** cann-s., ***clem.***
amel. - paeon.
emissions, after - ***ph-ac.***
evening - ***agar.,*** am-c., bar-c., ***calc.,*** dulc., euphr., kali-bi., lyc., mez., naja, ***nuph.,*** paeon., phos., ***rhus-t.,*** sabad.
lying down, on - naja
walk, after short - nat-m.
exertion, least, after - ***anac.,*** **ARS.,** bry., ***calc.,*** **CARB-V.,** cic., ***kali-c., phos.***
extending through back during chill - thuj.
fever, during - bell.
forenoon - ant-t., cham., grat., lach.
lying in bed, while - carl., sulph.
on left side - merc-i-f.
menses, during - calc-p., mag-m.
mental exertion, from - ph-ac.
midnight - pic-ac.
morning - alum., brach., cham., colch., cinnb., dulc., ***nit-ac.,*** ox-ac., pall., phos., sulph., til.
bed, in - canth., nat-m., phos.
rising, on - bov., coc-c., hep., nat-a., ***nat-m.,*** phos., puls.
waking, on - arg-m., bar-c., crot-t., euphr., ***lyc.,*** nat-c., pic-ac., sep., ***zinc.***
motion, during - rumx.
amel. - caps., cham., ***lyc.,*** phos., **RHUS-T.**

WEAKNESS, of
  night - ***cham., merc.,*** til.
    toothache, during - clem.
  noon - gels., zinc.
  paralytic - alum., am-m., ***anac.,*** ars., bell., carb-v., **CAUST.,** ***cham.,*** ferr-ar., ***kali-bi., kali-br., kali-c.,*** merc-c., nux-v., phos., sabad., **VERAT.**
  periodic - ars., ***calc.,*** kreos.
  pregnancy, during - calc-p.
    legs, during - plb.
  pressure, on - nit-ac.
  rheumatic - bov.
  rising from bed - phos., ***puls.***
    after - chel.
    amel. - arg-m., lyc., nat-m.
  seat - caust., dig.
  sitting, while - arg-m., chel., merc., nux-v., ruta., thuj.
    long, after - sars.
  sleep, after - merc-c.
    insufficient after - am-c.
  standing, while - anac., berb., dirc., hell., stann., zinc.
  stiffness, with - caust., con., lach., lyc., nat-m., rhus-t., sil.
  stool, after - ***ars.,*** colch.
  sudden - **CHAM.,** lyc., naja, nat-p.
    with hunger - ***zinc.***
  urination, after, amel. - spira.
  waking, on - chin., kali-n., sol-t-ae., tep.
  walking - ***anac.,*** **ARG-M.,** berb., ***bry.,*** cob., colch., ham., lyc., naja, nat-p., petr.
    amel. - gins., phos., sulph.
    open air, in, while - am-c., colch., euph., ***dig.,*** ferr., mag-m., merl., nux-v., pic-ac., raph., sang., ***zinc.***
      amel. - am-c., cham., clem.

WHIRLING, sensation - glon.

WRINKLED - ars., ***sec.***

Liver

LIVER, general - abies-c., abrot., **ACON.,** ***aesc., agar.,*** all-c., ***aloe, alum., am-m.,*** ant-t., ***apoc., arg-n., arn.,*** **ARS.,** ars-i., asaf., ***aur.,*** aur-m., ***bapt.,*** bar-c., **BELL., BERB., BRY., BUFO CALC.,** ***calc-f.,*** **CALC-P.,** camph., **CARB-S.,** ***carb-v.,*** **CARD-M.,** ***cham.,*** **CHEL., CHIN.,** ***chol., cimx.,*** cinnb., clem., ***cocc., colch., coll., coloc., con.,*** **CORN.,** ***croc., crot-c., crot-h., cupr.,*** dig., dol., dros., dulc., ferr., ***fl-ac.,*** gels., ***graph.,*** grin., ***hep., hydr.,*** **IOD.,** ***iris, kali-bi.,*** **KALI-C.,** kali-s., **LACH.,** ***laur.,*** **LEPT., lyc.,** mag-c., **MAG-M., MERC.,** merc-c., mur-ac., nat-a., nat-c., ***nat-m.,*** **NAT-S., NIT-AC., NUX-M., NUX-V.,** petr., ***ph-ac.,*** **PHOS.,** plat., ***plb.,*** **PODO.,** ***prun., psor.,*** ptel., puls., ran-b., ran-s., rhus-t., ruta., sabad., ***sang.,*** sel., **SEP.,** sil., spig., **SULPH.,** sul-ac., tab., ***tarax.,*** verat., vip., ***zinc.***

ABSCESS - ars., ***bell.,*** bol., bry., chin-a., fl-ac., **HEP.,** ***kali-c., lach., lyc., med.,*** **MERC., MERC-C.,** ***nux-v.,*** phos., puls., raph., rhus-t., ruta, sep., **SIL.,** ***ther.,*** vip.
- as if abscess would burst - ***laur.***
- coughing, when, pain as if ulcerated - ***lach.***
- pain from abscess, to right shoulder and elbow - med.

ACHING, pain (see Pain, liver)

ASCITES, (see Edema)

ATROPHY, of - apoc., ars., ***arg-n.,*** **AUR.,** ***bry.,*** **CALC.,** ***carb-v.,*** **CARD-M.,** ***chel., chin., chion.,*** chlol., ***cupr., hydr.,*** **IOD.,** ***lach.,*** lept., ***lyc.,*** mag-m., ***merc., mur-ac., nat-m.,*** nat-s., nit-ac., ***nux-v.,*** **PHOS.,** ***plb.,*** puls., sel., sep., ***sulph.***
- acute - card-m., crot-h., dig., lept., phos., podo.
  - jaundice, from - ***phos.***
  - yellow - acon., bell., bry., **CALC.,** dig., ip., lept., **PHOS.,** podo.
- chronic, with emaciation and dessication of body - card-m., ***merc.***
- hepatitis, during - ***hep.***
- nodulated, in marasmus - ***hydr.***
- nutmeg or alcoholic variety - ant-t., ars., bry., ***carb-v.,*** ip., **LACH.,** laur., lept., **LYC.,** ***nat-m.,*** **NUX-M.,** ***nux-v., phos.,*** puls., sulph., verat.
- typhus, fever in, with albuminuria - ***calc-ar.***

BALL, as if, in - aesc., bar-c., nux-m.
- below liver - arn., bor., echi., gels., lach., ***nat-s.,*** thuj., verat., zinc.
- hard ball, in - nux-m.

BILE, general
- absence of - ***chion., plb.***
- decreased - **CHEL.,** gels.
- increased - aloe, ars., asc-c., ***bell., bry., cham.,*** chlor., **IP.,** ***merc., nat-s., nux-v., phos.,*** **PODO.,*****puls.,*** sep., ***sulph., verat.***
  - bilious coating on tongue, or bitter taste, with - ***nat-s.***
  - menses, during - ***phyt.***

BILE, general
- increased then deficiency, jaundice, with - ***iris.***
- violet color of bile - ***amyg.***

BILE-ducts, ailments of - am-m., chel., ***chol.,*** gels., merc-d., nat-p., rheum
- catarrh - card-m.
  - inflammation - ***hydr.***
- gangrenous ulcerative inflammation - hippoz.
- neuralgia - dios.
- obstruction, causes edema - ***kali-m.***
- relaxed - ***gels.***
- spasmodic affections - dios.

BILIOUS, liver - ***bry.,*** chion., ***coloc.,*** eup-per., ***hydr.,*** iris, ***lept.,*** nat-s., ***nux-v.,*** podo., ***ptel.,*** sang., tarax.
- fever, bilious - lept.
  - derangement partaking of malarial character - eup-per.
  - symptoms, marked some days before paroxysms of intermittent - ***podo.***
- headache, bilious - berb., ***bry., coloc.,*** corn., ***crot-h.,*** eup-per., ***hydr., ip., lept., merc., nux-v.,*** **PODO.,*****ptel., puls.,*** sang., seneg.
  - attacks, with pains in occiput - **NUX-V.**
- salivation, with general bilious condition - ***iris.***

BRUISED, pain - carb-v.
- fullness, with - ***kreos.***
- stooping, when - ***alum.***
- touched or bending, when - ***clem.***

BUBBLING, sensation, in - laur., lil-t.

BURNING, pain - ***acon., agar.,*** aloe, am-c., anan., bry., carb-s., carb-v., crot-c., ***gamb., kali-c.,*** **LEPT.,** med., ***nit-ac.,*** plb., stann., ***ther.***
- distress, in back part - ***lept.***
- pulsative - anan.
- right, in, lobe, before stool composed of blood, bile and black fecal matter - polyp-p
- spot, in one, in passage of gall stones - ph-ac.
- stool, after - lept., ***stann.***
- tensive - bry.
- touch, worse from - ther.
- vomiting, with - ***aesc.***
- yellow fever, in - ***ars.***

burning, region of liver - am-m., **ARS.,** aur., ***aur-m., bry.,*** chel., ***crot-c., gamb.,*** **KALI-C.,** ***lac-c., lach.,*** laur., mag-c., mag-m., ***med.,*** mur-ac., ***nit-ac.,*** ph-ac., ***phos.,*** plb., sang., stann., sulph., ter., ***ther.,*** thuj., zinc.

CANCER, liver - ars., ***carc.,*** chel., ***chlol., chlor.,*** cholest., con., echi., ***hydr.,*** lach., myric., nat-s., nit-ac., phos., ther.
- burning pain, with - ars., bell., carb-an., con., hydr., lyc., sep., sil., tarent.
- early - carc., senec.
- jaundice, with - myric.

CHOLECYSTITIS, inflammation, of gallbladder - card-m., chel., chion., ***chol., lach.,*** lept., morg-g., myric., ***phos.,*** podo., pyrog.
- septic - bry., bufo, ***lach., phos., pyrog.***

CIRRHOSIS, liver - abies-c., apoc., ars., ***ars-i.,*** aur., ***aur-m.,*** calc-ar., ***card-m.,*** casc., ***chin.,*** crot-h., ***cupr.,*** fel., fl-ac., graph., ***hep., hydr., iod.,*** kali-bi., kali-i., ***lyc., merc.,*** merc-d., ***mur-ac.,*** nat-c., nit-ac., nux-v., ***phos.,*** plb., podo., quas., senec., **SUL-AC.,** ***sulph.,*** urea.
atrophy, with - ant-t., ars., bry., ***carb-v.,*** card-m., ip., **LACH.,** laur., lept., **LYC.,** ***nat-m.,*** **NUX-M.,** ***nux-v., phos.,*** puls., **SUL-AC.,** sulph., verat.
boils, with - nat-p.
hypertrophic - merc-d.

CLAWING, pain, region of liver - bell., ***nat-s.***

COLDNESS, region of liver - bar-c., med.

CONGESTION, (see Engorgement) - ***agar., apoc.,*** ars-h., bry., ***card-m., chel.,*** chin., med., ***phos., podo., ptel.***
acute - ***bell., nux-v., verat.***
ascites, in - ***aur-m.***
asthma, with - ***verat.***
bleeding, with - ***ham.***
blood, full of thick black - bar-m.
bright's disease, in - atro.
catarrh, with bronchial - ***verat.***
cholera-like symptoms, with - ***verat.***
chronic - ***lyc.***
cutting pains, with, and abdominal flatulency - **NAT-S.**
dysmenorrhea, with, in feeble, torpid subjects - sang.
heart, in organic disease of - ***apis***
hemorrhoidal colic, with - merc-c.
jaundice, with - podo., ptel.
pain, from, in back and right side - **LYC.**
passive - ***gels.***
portal system, and - ***aesc.***

CONSTRICTION, region of liver - ***lach.***

CONTRACTION, region of liver - ip., mag-c., mang.
left - bar-c.
right - sulph.

CRAMPING, pain, region of liver - carb-an., iod., kali-c., mag-c., nat-m., ph-ac., phos., rhus-t., samb., staph., sulph., verb., zinc.

CUTTING, pain - ang., aur., ***berb.,*** bufo, calc-f., ***carb-an.,*** colch., crot-c., ***dios., iris, lach.,*** merc-i-r., nux-m., ptel.
deep inspiration, agg. - ptel.
lying down, even while - ***carb-an.***
sudden - merc-i-r.
cutting, region of liver - ang., ***aur.,*** bry., ***carb-ac.,*** crot-c., dulc., iod., kali-c., ptel., stann., stry.

DRAGGING, pain - calc., cham., coc-c., phos., podo., **NUX-V.,** ptel.
caused by turning to left side - ***ptel.***
ligaments, at - agar.
lying on left side, when - ***card-m., mag-m., nat-s., ptel.***
pressure amel. - plat.
painful, after light-colored papescent stool - polyp-p

DRAWING, pain - ***card-m.,*** caul., kali-c., mag-m.
drawing, painful - ptel.
inhaling, worse when - ***camph.***
towards small of back - ***calc.***
drawing, region of liver - agar., alum., aur., bry., calc., cham., con., mag-m., nat-m., sep., stann., sulph., zinc.

DULL pain - ***hyos.,*** plb.
constant - ***carb-v.***
cough, with a little dry - ***sulph.***
grinding, in evening - ***dios.***
jaundice, with - ***merc.***
lying on right side - ***ptel.***
pressure, from - ***ptel.***
worse standing, bends forward - aloe.

EDEMA, general, from liver disease - ***apoc.,*** ars., ars-s-f., asc-c., aur., **AUR-M., CALC., CARD-M.,** cean., chel., ***chim., chin.,*** cop., cupr., ***ferr., fl-ac.,*** iris, kali-ar., ***kali-m.,*** **LAC-D., LACH.,** lept., liatr., **LYC.,** merc., merc-sul., mur-ac., ***nat-m., nux-v.,*** polym., tarax., vip.
ascites - chim., ***chin., merc.,*** seneg.
especially in old persons - ***kali-c.***
feet, of - ***carb-s.***
hydrothorax - crot-h., ***kali-c.***
external warm applications cause pains to move to other places - ***kali-c.***
induration of liver, with - aur., ***card-m.,*** lact., mur-ac.

ENGORGEMENT, (see Congestion) - ***anthr., chin-s., hep.,*** sulph.
chronic - ***hep.***
heart disease, in - cact., dig.
lying on left side, agg. - ***nat-s.***

ENLARGED - aesc., agar., aloe, ant-t., ***ars.,*** ars-i., aur., ***aur-m.,*** bar-m., ***bry.,*** bufo, ***calc., calc-ar., carb-v.,*** carc., ***card-m., chel.,*** **CHIN.,** chin-a., ***chion., cocc.,*** coloc., ***con.,*** crot-h., ***dig., ferr.,*** ferr-ar., ferr-i., ferr-p., ***fl-ac.,*** glyc., graph., ***hep., hippoz.,*** hydr., ***iod., kali-c.,*** kali-s., lach., lact., ***laur.,*** **LYC., MAG-M.,** ***merc., merc-d.,*** merc-i-r., mur-ac., ***nat-m.,*** **NAT-S.,** ***nit-ac., nux-m.,*** **NUX-V.,** ***phos.,*** plb., ***podo.,*** ptel., sec., sel., sep., sil., ***stel., sulph.,*** tab., ***tarax., tub.,*** urt-u., vip., ***zinc.***
abscesses, as if caused by - anan.
alcoholics, in - absin., am-m., ars., fl-ac., lach., **NUX-V.,** sulph.
anger, after - ***cocc.***
appetite, with loss of, particularly in morning - sel.
ascites, with - ***mag-m.***
asthma, in emphysematous, can be felt below ribs, - ***ter.***
cephalalgia, with - 4mag-m.
children, in - calc-ar., ***nux-m.***
in nursing - ***chin.***
who are bottle fed - nat-p.
chronic - con., ***mag-m.,*** plat., ***nux-m.,*** sulph.
after tedious intermittent - ***nux-m.***
with torpid action of bowels - con., ***mag-m.***

ENLARGED,
constipation, inability to lie on right side, with recurring attacks of indigestion, biliousness and constipation - ***mag-m.***
contracted, then - plb.
diabetes, in - ***nat-s.***
downward, about two inches - phos.
edema, causes - ars., ***kali-m.***
in intermittent - ***ars.***
extends two or three inches beyond ribs, after abuse of mercury - ***hep.***
fatty, border extends to navel - ***chel.***
hard - ***con., fl-ac., merc.***
particularly left lobe - ***fl-ac.***
sore to touch, could be felt more to left above navel as a small hard lump - zinc.
swelling, convex, region of right, extending toward precordial region, and nearly to right crest of ileum - con.
heart affections, with - mag-m.
hypertrophy, after - aur.
organic disease, from - ***dig.***
hepatitis, in - ***ars., merc.***
hydrothorax, in - ***lach.***
intermittent fever, in - chin., aran.
chronic - ***nat-m.***
jaundice, in - ***calc.***, dig., sep., ***tarax.***
left lobe - ***hep., mag-c.***, mag-p.
causing respiratory embarrassment and cough, with thick expectoration - ***card-m.***
malarial - merc-i-r.
marasmus, in - hydr.
pain and anger, after - cocc.
goes through from left lobe - dol.
painful - **CHEL.**
anterior and superior aspect, in - ***lach.***
pressure, on - con.
pressure, with - lact.
and stinging, caused by high living, abdominal plethora, and debauchery - **NUX-V.**
projects from under ribs - ***merc.***
sensitive to touch - ***ferr.***
intermittent fever, in - ***eup-per.***
swollen feeling - bar-c.
tense swelling, hot - ***acon.***
typhoid fever, in - ***phos.***

FATTY, degeneration, of - arg-n., aur-m., ***calc.***, carb-v., card-m., ***chel.***, hippoz., kali-bi., kali-c., ***lyc.***, lyss., mag-m., ***merc.***, nat-m., nux-v., **PHOS.**, ***pic-ac.***, sulph., vanad.
conjunctiva, with yellow - ***phos.***
depending upon long-lasting bone disease like caries of vertebrae or hip joint - ***phos.***
heart disease, sequel of - ***phos.***
dilatation of right, caused by cerebral edema - phos.
jaundice, malignant, and a gone, weak sensation in abdomen - ***phos.***
nervous hyperemia - ***lyc.***
stitches - ***phos.***

FULLNESS, sensation of - apoc., ***ferr.***, kreos., ***lach., myris.***, nat-m., **NUX-V.**, ***podo., sep.***, sulph., thuj.
bruised, sensation, with - ***kreos.***
inflammation, in subacute - ***hydr.***
jaundice, with - podo.
pain, with, in left hypochondria - ***lach.***
sharp pains, with, and soreness on moving and coughing - ***eup-per.***
fullness, region of liver - aesc., aloe, ***chel.***, eup-per., kali-c., nat-m., ***podo.***, sang., thuj.

GALLBLADDER, general (see Bile, Cholecystitis) - ars., aur., ***bapt.***, bell., **BERB.**, ***bry., calc.***, **CARD-M.**, ***cham., chel.***, **CHIN.**, ***chion., chlf., chol.***, **COLOC.**, cupr., dig., ***dios.***, euon., fel., ferr-s., gels., ***hydr., ip., iris***, jug-c., kali-ar., ***kali-bi., kali-c., lach.***, laur., ***lept., lith.***, **LYC.**, mag-p., mang., merc., merc-d., morg., myric., **NAT-S.**, ***nux-v.***, op., ***phos.***, podo., ptel., puls., rhus-t., sang., ***sep.***, sulph., tab., tarax., ter., **VERAT.**
catarrhal inflammation of mucous lining - ***hydr.***
dull, aching distress - aesc.
full of pale, yellow watery bile - bar-m.
to bursting - ars-h.
obstruction, with colic - ***chin.***
pain - ferr-s.
dull, hard, at seven a.m. - ***dios.***
extends from right, when at its height, attended with nausea - ***podo.***
extends to spine - bapt.
pressing or shooting - berb.
surgery, after gallbladder removed, agg. - card-m., **CHIN.**, ***lyc.***

GALLSTONE, colic pain from - am-m., alum., ***ars.***, aur., ***bapt.***, **BELL.**, **BERB.**, ***bry.***, **CALC.**, **CARD-M.**, ***cham., chel.***, **CHIN.**, ***chion., chlf.***, **CHOL.**, **COLOC.**, cupr., dig., **DIOS.**, euon., fel., ferr-s., gels., ***hep., hydr., ip., iris***, jug-c., kali-ar., ***kali-bi., kali-c., lach.***, laur., ***lept., lith.***, **LYC.**, mag-p., mang., merc., merc-d., **MORG.**, myric., **NAT-S.**, ***nux-v.***, op., osm., ***phos.***, podo., ptel., puls., rhus-t., sang., ***sep.***, sulph., tab., tarax., ***ter.***, thuj., **VERAT.**
bending, forward amel. - chin., card-m., ***coloc.***, mag-p.
chill, with - ***chel.***
dyspepsia, in chronic - ***hydr-ac.***
fullness, sensation of - myric.
heaviness, stitches, burning, in one spot - ph-ac.
incarcerated, beaten up with yolk of egg, applied inwardly and outwardly - ***nit-s-d.***
indigestion, after - ***staph.***
jaundice, with - **BELL.**, ***card-m.***, chel., **MERC.**, nat-s., **NUX-V.**, ***podo.***
pain from region of stomach to region of gall bladder, with excessive nausea - podo.
mercury or quinine, after - **BELL.**
pain, extending quickly downward across navel into intestines - ***chel.***
periodic - ***chin.***

GALLSTONE, colic
radiating pains, with - ***berb.,*** chel.
spreading over abdomen - ***all-c.***
sticking pains, with - card-m., chel.
stools, with clay colored - ***chel.***
touch, slight agg. - chin.
two weeks, every - sep.
violent pain between ileum and ribs - ***lith.***
vomiting, with - ***chel.***
warmth, amel. - ***mag-p.***

GANGRENE - ars., ***sec.***

GNAWING, pain - bufo, laur., ruta., sil.

HARD, (see Induration) - **ARS.,** ***aur-m., calc.,*** cann-s., ***carb-s., card-m., chel.,*** **CHIN.,** ***chin-a., con.,*** **DIG.,** ***fl-ac.,*** **GRAPH.,** ***hydr.,*** **IOD.,** ***kali-i.,*** lact., ***laur., lyc., mag-c.,*** **MAG-M.,** ***merc., nit-ac., nux-v.,*** **PHOS.,** podo., **RAT.,** ***sil., sulph.,*** zinc.
left lobe - ***card-m.***
small and, as if - abies-c.

hard, region of liver - ***calc-p.***

HEAT, in, sensation of - ***aloe,*** aur., ***kali-c., lach., lept., merc.,*** myric., plb., sabad., stann., ther.
stool, after - stann.

heat, region of liver - aur., ***kali-c.***

HEAVINESS, as from a weight, etc, in - agar., ars., ***bol.,*** bry., ***carb-v.,*** kali-c., ***lach.,*** lact., ***mag-m.,*** nat-s., ***nux-m.,*** nux-v., ph-ac., plb., ***ptel., sep.,*** tab.
aching - phyt.
dyspepsia, in - kali-m.
intermittent fever, in - ***carb-v.***
lying on right side - ***ptel.***
pain, with, in left hypochondrium - ***lach.***
painful - merc-i-r.
spot, of one, in passage of gall stones - ph-ac.

HEPATITIS - **ACON.,** act-sp., anag., anan., apis, **ARS.,** ars-i., aur., bapt., **BELL.,** ***bry., calc., camph., cham., carc.,*** **CARD-M.,** cean., **CHEL., CHIN.,** cocc., corn., cupr., dol., ***hep., hippoz., hydr.,*** ign., iod., ***kali-c.,*** kali-i., kali-p., ***lach.,*** **LYC.,** ***mag-m.,*** mang., ***merc.,*** merc-d., nat-a., nat-c., ***nat-m.,*** **NAT-S.,** ***nit-ac.,*** **NUX-V., PHOS.,** phyt., ***podo., psor., ptel.,*** puls., pyrog., sec., sil., staph., stel., tab., sulph., zing.
abscesses, as if by - anan.
acute - **ACON.,** ***bell., kali-c., podo.,*** sulph.
subacute - cham., ***hydr.***
bad, food or water, after - ars., bapt., zing.
bend, has to, double - ***bell.***
children, of - ***lyc.***
chronic hepatitis - ***arn.,*** aur., ***bell., carc.,*** **CARD-M.,** ***corn.,*** crot-h., ***lach.,*** **LYC.,** ***mag-m.,*** nat-c., ***nat-m.,*** **NAT-S.,** ***nit-ac., nux-v.,*** **PHOS.,** ***psor.,*** ran-s., sel., sil., ***sulph.***
aversion to exercise, with - ***aur.***
enlargement and induration, with - phyt.
cold, after taking - ***cham.***
constipation, with - ***nux-v., podo.***
diffuse - ***phos.***

HEPATITIS,
dirty needles, from - bapt., led., pyrog.
distention of abdomen, with - chin., lyc.
fever, causes - ***sang.***
gastric, with, troubles - ***cham.***
humiliation, after - ***lyc.***
jaundice, with - astac., ***cham., hep.***
mercury, after - ***lyc.***
nausea, with - **CHEL.**
pain spreads to back and kidneys - ***bell.***
peritonitis - ***apis***
pneumonia, with - ***lyc.***
recovery slow - nat-s., phos.
sensitive to pressure and touch - ***lach.***
suppuration, with hectic, night sweats, enlargement and marked soreness - ***phos.***
syphilitic - ***cupr-m.***
vexation, after - ***cham.***

INFLAMMATION, liver (see Hepatitis)

INDURATION, of (see Hard) - abies-c., ammc., anag., **ARS.,** ***aur., chel.,*** **CHIN.,** cinnam., ***con.,*** **DIG., GRAPH.,** ***fl-ac.,*** lact., laur., lyc., **MAG-M.,** merc., nux-v., ***phos.,*** podo., **RAT.,** ***sil., sulph., tarax.,*** zinc.
ascites, with - aur., ***aur-m.,*** lact., mur-ac.
headache, with - **MAG-M.**
chronic - ***mag-m.***
constipation, with chronic - ***graph.***
fever, liver-cake of ague - ***nit-ac.***
hepatitis, with - ***merc.***
jaundice, with - **BELL.,** ***calc., tarax.***
marasmus, in - hydr.
pressure, with, and stinging caused by high living, abdominal plethora, debauchery - **NUX-V.**
sclerosis, especially when there is a succession of boils - ***nat-p.***
stitches, with - ***mag-c.***
syphilis, in - ***kali-i.***

IRRITABILITY, with - ***bry., cham.,*** **NUX-V.,** ***podo.***

ITCHING, liver region - lyc.

JAUNDICE, (see Skin, yellow) - **ACON.,** aesc., agar., agn., ***aloe,*** alum., ***ambr., am-m.,*** ant-c., ***ant-t.,*** arg-n., arn., ***ars.,*** ars-i., ars-s-f., asaf., astac., ***aur., aur-m-n.,*** **BELL.,** ***berb., bry.,*** bufo, ***calc., calc-p.,*** calc-s., calen., cann-s., ***canth.,*** carb-s., ***carb-v.,*** **CARD-M.,** casc., ***caust., cean.,*** cedr., ***cham.,*** **CHEL.,** chen-a., **CHIN.,** ***chin-a.,*** **CHION.,** chol., cina, coca, cocc., **CON.,** ***corn.,*** corn-f., croc., **CROT-H.,** cupr., ***dig., dol.,*** dulc., elat., euph., eup-per., ***ferr.,*** ferr-ar., ***ferr-i.,*** gels., graph., hell., ***hep., hydr., ign.,*** **IOD.,** iris, jug-c., kali-ar., kali-bi., kali-c., kali-p., **LACH.,** laur., ***lept.,*** **LYC.,** mag-m., mang., med., **MERC.,** ***merc-c., merc-d., merc-sul.,*** myric., nat-a., nat-c., ***nat-m.,*** nat-p., **NAT-S., NIT-AC., NUX-V.,** olnd., ***op.,*** ost., petr., ph-ac., **PHOS.,** pic-ac., **PLB., PODO.,** ***ptel., puls.,*** ran-b., rheum, rhus-t., rumx., ruta, sabad., ***sang., sec.,*** **SEP.,** ***sil., spig.,*** still., ***sulph.,*** sul-ac., tab., ***tarax.,*** tarent., thuj., thyr., verat., ***vip., yuc.***

JAUNDICE,

abdomen, itching, with - cham.
acute - ***chel.***
of blood rather than hepatic origin - crot-h.
albuminuria, with - ***dig.***
anemia, with - ***phos.***
brain disease, pregnancy - phos.
anger, after - ***acon., aur-m-n., bry.,*** **CHAM.,** chin., ign., nat-m., ***nat-s.,*** **NUX-V.,** sulph.
arms, with rheumatism of - ***chel.***
atrophy, from acute - **PHOS.**
bile, increase with, then deficiency of - ***iris.***
biting itching, with, over abdomen - ***merc***-sol.
brain disease, with - ***phos.***
catarrh, caused by gastro-duodenal - ***kali-m., kali-s., nat-m.***
children, in - ***astac.,*** podo.
scrofulous, in - ph-ac.
chronic - aur., chel., ***chion., con.,*** iod., ***phos.,*** sulph., ter.
hepatitis, with diarrhea - ***puls.***
relapsing - sulph.
cider, from - chion.
cold, from catching - cham., dulc., merc-sol., nux-v.
from a, with intestinal catarrh - ***acon.***
concomitant as a - phos.
confusion of consciousness, with - ***phos.***
convulsions, with - agar.
after - agar., **NUX-V.**
diarrhea, with - ***merc., nux-v., podo., puls.***
after - chin.
heart, from weakened - ***lycps.***
drowsiness, with - ***nat-m.***
yellow sclera, with - ***phos., sang.***
emotions, from - bry., ***cham.,*** lach., nux-v., vip.
extension of catarrhal process - am-m., ***chel.,*** chion., ***chin.,*** dig., ***hydr.,*** lob., ***merc.,*** nux-v., podo.
fatty degeneration, with - ***phos.***
fever, during - card-m., ***ferr.,*** lach., ***nux-v.,*** vip.
flatulence, with - berb., ***carb-v., cham., chin.,*** ign., ***lyc., nux-v.,*** plb.
food, after too much or rich - ***carb-v.***
fright, from - ***acon.***
fruits, unripe, from - rheum.
diarrhea, with white - ***rheum.***
grief, from - ***ph-ac.***
head congestion, with violent - **MERC.**
headache, with - sep.
hematogenous - phos.
hemorrhagic - chel., ***crot-h., mag-m., phos.***
hepatitis, with - ***hep., lach.,*** mang., ***nat-s.***
high living, after - **NUX-V.**
humiliation, after - bry., ***lyc.***
hyperemia of liver - ptel.
fullness, soreness and pain - podo.

JAUNDICE,

intermittent fever, after - am-c., ***ars., chin-s., con.,*** ferr., nat-c., nat-m., ***nux-v., sang.,*** **SEP.,** ***tub.***
prevailing, during - ***sang.***
quinine after abuse of - ***ars.***
itching - thyr.
loss of vital fluids, from - chin.
lung symptoms, with - card-m., chel., hydr.
malarial symptoms, with - ***nat-s.***
malignant - acon., ***ars.,*** ars-i., chel., ***chin.,*** **CROT-H.,** ***dig.,*** elaps, ***lach.,*** merc., ***pic-ac.,*** **PHOS.**
masturbation, after - chin.
menses, arrested, with - chion.
mercury, after - ***ars.,*** asaf., ***aur., carb-v.,*** **HEP.,** ***iod., nit-ac., sulph.***
nervous excitement, from - ***phos.***
neuralgia, with, of stomach - ran-b.
newborn children, in - **ACON.,** ***bov.,*** bry., cham., ***chel., chin.,*** chion., coll., **ELAT.,** ign., **MERC.,** merc-d., myric., ***nat-s.,*** nit-ac., **NUX-V.,** podo., puls., sep., sulph.
stool, with bilious - elat.
nursing children, in - bov., bry., ***cham., chin., merc., nux-v.,*** sulph.
pregnancy, during - aur., phos.
organic lesion, from - ***iod.***
operation for hemorrhoids, after - ***croc.***
overeating, from - ***ant-c., bry., carb-v.,*** cham., hydr., nat-c., ***nux-v., puls.***
pain, with - ***sep.***
dull, with - ***merc.***
pneumonia, with - ***phos.***
pregnancy, during - aur., **NUX-V.,** ***phos.***
liver atrophied - **ACON.**
psoric persons, in, with or without hardness and swelling of liver - ***sulph.***
quinine, after - ars., bell., chin., ***hep.,*** ip., merc., **NUX-V.,** ***puls.***
quotidian, in, gastric, typhoid or bilious fever - ***hydr.***
returning again and again, after chin and merc. - podo.
rings - ***nat-c.,*** nat-m.
sexual excess, after - chin.
skin, dark, with, walnut color of - tab.
spots - ambr., ant-t., **ARN.,** ars., canth., **CON.,** crot-c., cur., dol., cur., elaps, **FERR.,** hydrc., iod., kali-ar., kali-c., ***lach., lyc., nat-c.,*** nat-p., nux-v., **PETR., PHOS.,** plb., ***psor., ruta.,*** sabad., **SEP.,** stann., **SULPH.,** ***thuj.,*** vip.
turning green - con.
stool, with, clay-colored - ***lept.***
white - ***dig.***
white or green - nat-p.
structural disease, with - ***hydr.***
summer, every - chin-a., ***chion.***
tendency to - pic-ac.
torpid with, and constipation - still.

JAUNDICE,
urinary symptoms, with - carb-v., cham., chin., ign., lyc., nux-v., plb.
urine, with dark yellow - ***sang.***
vexation - ***cham.,*** kali-c., ***nat-s.***

LANCINATING, pain, region of liver - aur-s., aeth., bufo, calc-f., caust.

LUMP, sensation of - arg-n., arn., bar-c., brom., croc., cupr., cycl., hep., lach., mag-c., nat-c., nat-m., nat-s., nux-m., op., plb., tab., thuj., verat.

MENTAL, symptoms, with liver disease
anger, after - **CHAM.,** ign., ***lyc.,*** **NUX-V.,** ***staph.***
crying - ***mag-m.***
depression, with - alum., aur., ***chel.***
disgust for life - aur., podo.
grief, morbid, from - ***ign., ph-ac.***
humiliation, after - **CHAM.,** ign., ***lyc.,*** **NUX-V.,** ***staph.***
hypochondriasis, especially in drunkards - **NUX-V.**
irritability - ***bry., cham.,*** **NUX-V.,** podo.
mania - lach., merc.
nervous, in consequence of excessive hepatic action - ***podo.***
thinks his liver is affected, and he will have to go to bed - ***nux-m.***

PAIN, liver - **ACON., AESC.,** aeth., agar., ***aloe,*** alum., ***ambr.,*** am-c., anan., ***arg-n.,*** arn., ***ars., ars-i.,*** asar., ***bapt.,*** **BELL.,** ***berb.,*** brom., ***bry.,*** bufo, cahin., ***cact., calc.,*** calc-f., ***calc-p., calc-s.,*** camph., ***carb-ac., carb-an., carb-s.,*** carb-v., ***card-m.,*** caust., **CHEL., CHIN.,** ***chin-a., chin-s., cimx.,*** cimic., colch., ***con., crot-t., crot-h.,*** dios., euphr., fago., ferr., ferr-ar., ***ferr-p., form.,*** graph., hell., hyos., ign., ***iod.,*** iris, ***kali-ar., kali-br., kali-c.,*** kali-p., ***kali-s.,*** kalm., kreos., **LACH.,** lact., ***laur., lec., led.,*** **LEPT.,** ***lith.,*** **LYC., MAG-M.,** mang., ***med.,*** **MERC.,** ***merc-c., merc-i-f.,*** merl., mill., ***nat-m.,*** **NAT-S., NIT-AC.,** nux-m., **NUX-V.,** pall., ***phos.,*** phyt., plb., **PODO.,** ***prun.,*** psor., ***ptel.,*** ran-s., ruta., sabad., sec., sel., **SEP.,** ***sil.,*** stram., ***sulph., tarax.,*** tarent., ust.
abdomen, spreading over - ***all-c.***
above - merc.
air, open - ars., carb-v.
anger, after - ***cocc.***
anteriorly, then posteriorly - arum-t.
appetite, with poor - ***ptel.***
ascending, on going up stairs - bapt.
awaking, on - bry.
back, with pain low down in, before menses, thick and black - nux-m.
bed, before going to - ***chin-s.***
bending, on, taking a deep breath, or coughing - ***chin-s.***
forward amel. - ***aloe,*** calc-f., nat-m.
breakfast, after - graph.
breathing, on - **BELL.,** ***bry., calc.,*** lyc., ***nat-s., sel.***
breathing, during - ***calc.***
cheese, after - ptel.

PAIN, liver
chest, through left, and down arm - ***arn.***
chill, during - ***ars.,*** bry., **CHIN.,** ***nux-v.,*** **PODO.,** ***sep.,*** verat.
before - tarent.
chronic - ***chel.,*** nat-m.
cirrhosis, in - ***iod.***
cold food, after - mang.
constant, with hardness and edema - ***con.***
worse before paroxysm of intermittent, with nausea and vomiting - tarent.
constipation, with - verat.
cough, with - bor.
coughing, agg. - bor., brom., ***bry.,*** caps., ***chin-s.,*** cimx., cocc., hep., kali-bi., lach., psor., sulph.
day, all - ***ferr.***
diarrhea, after - vip.
die, as though she would, they were so acute - med.
distension, with, after eating - ***caust.***
drinks, better from warm, or food - ***graph.***
earwax, with accumulation of - ***con.***
eating, after - ambr., mag-m., ***nat-m., ptel.***
amel. - ***chel.***
to satiety - **LYC.**
evening - all-c., caust., ***chel., chin-s.***
exercising, on - ang., iris, merc., nit-ac., nux-v.
extending, to
back, to - ***aesc.,*** **CHEL.,** euphr., ***iod.,*** jug-c., ***kali-c.,*** **LYC., MAG-M.,** ***nat-m.,*** Yuc.
chest, to - chel., dios.
downward - ***chel.,*** ptel.
epigastrium, to - bell., kali-i., ***lach.***
hip to - vip.
right nipple, to - ***dios.***
right to left, from - ***merc-i-f.***
shoulder, left, to - lept., myric.
right, to - crot-h., ***kali-bi., med.,*** merc-c.
faint feeling, with, in epigastrium - ust.
fever, during - ***ars., chin.,*** elat., hyos., nux-v.
flatus, as from incarcerated - ***carb-an.***
flying - ***coloc.***
heaviness, to right shoulder - bry.
humiliation, after - ***lyc.***
inspiration, on - sel.
intermittent fever, in - ***chin., kali-c.***
jarring, agg - **BELL.,** ***bry.,*** chin., ***form.,*** **LACH.,** ***nat-s.,*** nit-ac., sel., **SIL.**
jaundice, in - aur., podo., ***sep.***
fatigue and pain, with - ***polyp-p.***
lodged, as if something had, in right side, with stinging - **LACH.**
laughing - psor.
left lobe - carb-s.
lying, amel. - mag-m., nat-s.
left side, on agg. - arn., ***card-m., mag-m., nat-s., ptel.***
on back agg. - caust.
painful side, on agg. - calc-f., ***lyc., phyt.***
painful side, on, amel. - sulph.
painless side, on, amel. - calc-f.

PAIN, liver
lying, while
right side, on agg. - **BELL.**, calc-f., dios., ***lyc.***, mag-m., ***merc.***, phos., ***phyt.***, psor., sep., sil.
amel. - ambr., **BRY.**, **MAG-M.**, ***nat-s.***, ***ptel.***
menses, during - bufo, ***nux-m.***, ph-ac.
before - con., nux-m., podo., ***puls.***, tarent.
dysmenorrhea, with - ph-ac.
vicarious, in - ***dig.***
mental labor, after - mang., ***merc.***, **NAT-S.**, ***nux-v.***, ***sulph.***
migrated from place to place until they had travelled through whole body - lyc.
morning - agar., bry.
4 to 9 a.m. - ***chel.***
motion, agg. - ***bell.***, ***bry.***, bufo, ***kali-bi.***, phyt., ***sep.***
moving, after - ***sep.***
nausea, with - ***ind.***
and constipation - ***merc-c.***
night - bufo, calc., ind.
ovaritis, in chronic - pall.
paroxysmal - **BELL.**, ***berb.***, ***chel.***, ph-ac., zinc.
pressure, agg - bell., berb., brom., **CHIN.**, clem., psor., sabad., sel., tab.
posterior part, in - ***lact.***
pulsating - anan., bufo., nux-v.
restlessness, with - calc-f.
riding in a carriage - brom., sep.
right lobe, in - carb-v., ust.
right side, pain in, over liver - kali-m.
from ligament to gall bladder, walking, agg. - ***bapt.***
rub, inclination to, with hand - ***podo.***
rubbing, amel. - phos., **PODO.**
sitting, while - calc-f.
for long agg. - **CALC-P.**
smaller, seems to be, than usual - ***kali-c.***
sneezing, on - ***psor.***
standing, while - aloe.
stepping - calc.
stomach complaint, with, - ***kali-bi.***
extends toward - ***lach.***
going to, and spleen, after shivering - sep.
stool, with white - ***calc.***
stooping, on - aloe, alum., calc., clem., cocc., kali-c., lyc.
touched, when - aeth., agar., bry., calc., carb-an., carb-v., **CHIN.**, cimx., clem., hep., **LYC.**, mag-m., **MERC.**, ***nat-s.***, ***nux-v.***, ran-b., **SEP.**, sulph., valer.
turning in bed - arn.
upper, part - ***hydrc.***
urging to urinate, on - ***ferr.***
urinate, with desire to - ***ferr.***
vertigo, with - **CHEL.**, merc-i-f.
vexation, after - bry., ***cocc.***, ***nat-s.***, ***staph.***
vomiting, of bile, with - bufo.

PAIN, liver
walking, while - ***bapt.***, con., hep., kali-c., lec., ***mag-m.***, ***nat-s.***, psor., ***sep.***, thuj.
warm drinks, amel. - ***graph.***
yawning - psor.
yellow fever, in - canth.

PAIN, liver, region of - ***aesc.***, agar., ***aloe***, ***alum.***, ambr., am-c., ***arg-n.***, arn., ***ars.***, arund., ***astac.***, bapt., **BELL.**, bov., brom., ***bry.***, ***bufo***, cahin., calc-f., ***calc-p.***, calc-s., cahin., ***carb-ac.***, carb-an., carb-v., ***card-m.***, cedr., **CHEL.**, chen-a., chim., chin-b., ***chin-s.***, cinnb., clem., ***colch.***, ***con.***, ***crot-c.***, ***crot-h.***, echi., fago., hydr., iber., ***iod.***, ***iris***, ***kali-bi.***, ***kali-c.***, ***kalm.***, ***lept.***, **LYC.**, lyss., ***mag-m.***, ***merc.***, mill., ***nat-c.***, ***nat-m.***, **NAT-S.**, **NIT-AC.**, **NUX-V.**, ***ol-j.***, pall., ***phos.***, phyt., plan., **PODO.**, ptel., rhus-t., ***sang.***, sec., sep., sil., stram., stry., ***sulph.***, tarent., thuj., trom.
bending to left agg. - agar.
coughing, on - bor., caps., chin-s., cimx., cocc., kali-bi., lach., psor., sulph.
eating, amel. - ***chel.***
to satiety, after - **LYC.**
extending, to
back - ***aesc.***, **CHEL.**, euphr., ***iod.***, jug-c., ***kali-c.***, **LYC.**, **MAG-M.**, ***nat-m.***, yuc.
back, sitting for long, while - calc-p.
inguinal region and testes - ars.
left - brom., ***nux-m.***
left scapula - ***lept.***
lying, amel. - ***ambr.***, crot-h., ptel., sep.
can lie only on abdomen - ***lept.***, ***phyt.***
on painful side agg. - **BELL.**, ***lyc.***, ***mag-m.***, ***nat-m.***, phyt., sil.
on painless side amel. - calc-f., ***ptel.***
motion agg. - sep.
sitting for long - **CALC-P.**

PINCHING, pain - aesc., berb., ***kali-c.***
breath, caused him to hold - berb.
griping, in a small spot - zinc.

PORTAL system, congestion - ***carb-v.***, ***card-m.***, mill., ***nux-v.***, ***polyp-p.***
dysmenorrhea and piles, resulting in - **COLL.**
head from - mill.
rumbling, with flatulent - ***coll.***
stool composed of blood, bile, in black fecal matter - polyp-p
constipation caused by stagnation of - ***croc.***
obstruction causes headache - ***nux-v.***
causes hypertrophy of heart - ***nux-v.***
stagnation, signs of - ***nux-v.***
caused by suppression of habitual sanguineous discharge, causes nephritis - ***nux-v.***
stasis - ***led.***, ***nux-v.***, sep.
hemorrhoidal colic, with - merc-c.
vertigo, with - **NUX-V.**
torpidity - ***podo.***
veins, distended - aesc., ***aloe***, ***coll.***, lept., lyc., ***nux-v.***, ***sulph.***

PRESSING, pain - ***acon.,*** aesc., agar., all-c., ***aloe, ambr.,*** am-c., anac., arg-n., arn., ***ars., asaf.,*** berb., ***bry.,*** cahin., ***calc., calc-p.,*** calc-s., ***carb-an.,*** carb-s., carb-v., ***card-m.,*** **CHEL.,** ***chin., cocc., con.,*** dig., ***graph.,*** kali-ar., ***kali-c.,*** kali-s., kreos., lact., ***laur.,*** lith., ***lyc.,*** **MAG-M.,** ***merc.,*** nat-c., ***nat-m.,*** **NAT-S.,** ***nux-m.,*** **NUX-V.,** ol-an., petr., ph-ac., ***phos.,*** plb., ***prun.,*** ran-s., raph., ***ruta.,*** sabad., sabin., **SEP.,** ***sil., stann., sulph.,*** tab., ter., thuj., ***zinc.***
alternating with pain in spleen, during apyrexia - ***nat-m.***
vomiting and diarrhea - ***verat.***
breathing, painful, on - ***lyc.***
cirrhosis, in - ***iod.***
coughing and bending over agg. - ***cocc.***
eating, worse after, vomiting - anac.
extending to,
chest, to, after dinner - asaf.
scapula, to right, after menses - bor.
shoulder, right - sep.
heavy, dull pressure - ***kali-bi.***
hepatitis, painful, in - ***ars., merc.***
indigestion, with chronic - ***sulph.***
indurated livers, in, caused by high living - **NUX-V.**
lying, on, on left side - arn., ***card-m.***
jaundice, painful, in - ***kali-c.***
painful, worse on pressure, corresponding to region of gall bladder in a small spot, spasmodically - ***berb.***
pressure, feeling of - ***all-c., aloe,*** arn., berb., ***carb-an., card-m.,*** lith., **NUX-V.,** sep., tab.
right side, painful, in - elaps
step, with every, when walking - ***calc.***
tension, and pressure, after eating - **LYC.**
walking, while, below liver - thuj.
painful, when, and touching it, worse lying on right side - **MAG-M.**

pressing, region of liver - acon., agar., all-c., aloe, anac., arn., bar-c., bell., brom., ***calc., calc-p.,*** carb-v., ***card-m.,*** **CHEL.,** ***chin., cocc., con.,*** elaps, ferr., hep., iod., ***laur.,*** lil-t., **LYC.,** ***lyss.,*** **MAG-M.,** merc., ***nat-m.,*** nit-ac., ph-ac., plb., rhus-t., sars., sep., ***sil.,*** staph., sul-ac., sulph., ***tarent.,*** thuj., zinc.
lying on painful side - ***mag-m.***

PRESSURE, sensitive to - ***arg-n., arn.,*** act-sp., ars-h., astac., ***card-m., chin., dig., ferr.,*** fl-ac., hydr., ***iod.,*** **MAG-M.,** ***nux-v.,*** plb., ***ptel.,*** tab.
clothing, must loosen - **NUX-V**.
deep pressure - acon.
left lobe - acon.
pneumonia, in - ***chel.***
spots, in - ***lyc.***

PULSATION, region of liver - act-sp., bell., brach., brom., ***calc-p., chel.,*** kali-i., laur., med., nat-s., nux-v., ptel., sarr., sep., sil., sulph.

SENSITIVE, (see Tender) - ***carb-v., lyc., merc.,*** sel.
clothing unendurable - ***carb-v.***
stitches, with, in influenza - ***phos.***

SENSITIVE,
touch, to - ant-t., ***apis, bell., carb-v., chel., chin., iod., merc., nat-s.,*** ol-j., ***phos., sil.***
to a light - ***lach.,*** ptel., tarent.
typhoid fever, in - ***merc.***
yellow fever, in - canth.

SHARP, pain - ***acon., aesc., agar.,*** aloe, ***alum.,*** arg-n., am-c., am-m., ***asaf.,*** asar., ***bell.,*** **BERB.,** ***bov.,*** **BRY.,** bufo, ***cact.,*** **CALC.,** calc-f., ***calc-p., calc-s.,*** camph., canth., carb-s., ***carb-v., card-m., caust.,*** cedr., ***cham.,*** **CHEL.,** ***chin.,*** clem., ***cocc.,*** colch., ***coloc.,*** **CON.,** ***crot-h.,*** cupr., cycl., fago., form., graph., ***hep.,*** hyos., ***kali-bi., kali-c.,*** kali-p., kali-s., kreos., ***lach.,*** lact., ***laur.,*** **LEPT.,** lyc., mag-c., **MAG-M., MERC.,** merc-c., merc-i-f., mosch., ***nat-c., nat-m., nat-p., nat-s., nit-ac.,*** nux-m., **NUX-V.,** ol-an., ***ox-ac.,*** ph-ac., phos., plb., ***podo., ptel.,*** psor., ***puls.,*** **RAN-B.,** ***ran-s.,*** sabad., ***sel.,*** **SEP.,** ***sil., spig.,*** stann., ***sulph., sul-ac., tab., zinc.***
afternoon, sitting - nat-m.
bed, on turning in - ***arn.***
belching, on - merc.
breath, on taking - ***acon.,*** aloe, **BRY.,** ***crot-h.***
amel. by a deep - ***ox-ac.***
caused him to hold - berb.
took away, had to bend over - ***berb.***
breathing, on - ***acon.,*** agar., aloe, ***berb.,*** **BRY.,** ***calc-p.,*** con., ***crot-h., merc., nat-s.,*** **RAN-B.**
cirrhosis, in - ***iod.***
coughing, from - **BRY.,** carb-v., eup-per., kali-c., merc., ***nat-m.***
diabetes, in - sul-ac.
dorsal region, in - ***lyc.***
evening - sep.
sitting - am-c.
expiration, on - chin.
extending, to
back - **CHEL.**
chest and arm - ***dios.***
chest, to, impeding respiration - aloe.
chest, into - calc., ***ran-b.***
navel, to - brom.
nipple - ***dios.***
from right to left - card-m.
right shoulder - **SEP.**
sternum, towards - ars-m.
thigh - cob.
upward - ***ran-b.***
gastritis, in - ***cocc.***
hemicrania, in - ***cham.***
hepatitis, in - ***merc.***
chronic - ***nat-c.***
inspiration, agg. from deep - ptel.
intermittent fever, during apyrexia of - ***nat-m.***
jaundice, in - card-m.
lying, on it amel. - card-m., kali-c.
on left side - ***card-m.***
on right side - merc.
menses, before - con.
morning, 8 a.m. - calc-f.

SHARP, pain
motion, on - clem., kali-c., sel.
and pressure agg. - sel.
worse from, or contact - **NUX-V.**
nausea, with - agar.
needles sharp, as from - agar.
outward - chin.
pregnancy, in - ***caust., kreos.***
pressure, agg. - ***ptel.***
amel., with hand - merc-i-f.
riding in carriage - caust.
rising from stooping - alum.
running - spig.
sitting - calc-f., nat-m.
stooping, during or after - ***calc.***
supper, after - zinc.
touching, agg. - ***bry.***
walking, while - hep., kali-bi., ***nat-s., puls.***
amel. - calc-f.
yellow fever, in - ***ars.***

sharp, region of liver - acon., ***aesc., agar.,*** alum., am-m., anac., brom., ***bry.,*** **CALC.,** ***calc-p.,*** carb-an., carb-v., ***card-m.,*** **CAUST.,** cham., **CHEL.,** chin., ***cob., cocc., coloc.,*** **CON.,** ***crot-h.,*** euphr., fago., form., hyper., iod., ***kali-bi., kali-c., kreos.,*** lact., ***laur.,*** lyc., mag-c., mag-m., ***merc., merc-c.,*** mez., mur-ac., naja, ***nat-c.,*** nat-m., ***nat-s., nit-ac.,*** nux-v., ol-j., ph-ac., phos., podo., psor., ***ptel.,*** **RAN-B.,** ***ran-s.,*** rhus-t., sars., ***sep.,*** spig., spong., staph., sul-ac., ***sulph.,*** sumb., tab., tarent., tep., verb., ***zinc.***
bending to left - agar.
extending, to
back - **CHEL.,** euphr.
chest - mag-c.
heart - zinc.
thigh - cob.
left side - brom.

SHOOTING, pain - ***chin.,*** crot-h., **LEPT., NUX-V.,** ***ox-ac.***
desire, with, to take deep breath - ***calc-p.***
extending to back - ***chel.***
and shoulder - **CHEL.**
inspiration, agg. from deep - ***cob.***
thighs, into - cob.

SORE, pain - acon., aesc., am-c., ant-t., ***apis, arg-n.,*** arn., **BELL.,** ***calc., calc-p., calc-s.,*** carb-an., ***carb-s.,*** **CARB-V.,** ***card-m., chel., chin., chion.,*** clem., ***con.,*** **DIG.,** ***eup-per., ferr., ferr-ar.,*** fl-ac., ***iod.,*** kali-c., **KALI-I.,** ***kali-p.,*** kali-s., ***kreos.,*** **LACH., LEPT., LYC.,** ***mag-m., merc.,*** **NAT-S., NUX-V.,** ***ol-j.,*** pall., ***phos., podo.,*** ptel., raph., sel., ***sep., sil., sulph.,*** tab., ***tarent.,*** zinc.
beating, worse from motion, walking, lying on right side - ***sil.***
bilious fever, in - ***eup-per,***
extending, to, shoulder, to, and spine - ars-m.
hepatitis, with, when suppuration ensues - ***phos.***
inhaling, worse on - ***camph.***
jaundice, in - **MERC.,** podo.
left lobe - ***card-m.***

SORE, pain
rheumatism, like acute, unbearable, cannot lie still a moment - grin.
shoulder, with pain in right - ***nux-v.***
touch, on - kali-c.

sore, region of liver - act-sp., ***aesc., ambr.,*** arn., ars., bapt., **BRY.,** ***calc-p.,*** carb-ac., carb-v., ***card-m., chel., chin.,*** chion., ***clem., con.,*** **DIG.,** eup-per., fago., ***fl-ac., iod., kali-i., kreos.,*** lact., **LYC.,** ***mag-m., mur-ac.,*** **NAT-S., NUX-V.,** ***ol-j., phos., phyt.,*** **RAN-B.,** sec., ***sep., sil.,*** sulph., tarent.
exertion, after - ***kali-i.***
lying on right side - ***sil., mag-m., merc.***

SQUEEZING, sensation - ***dios.***

STICKING, pain - ***kali-c.,*** zinc.
cough, in whooping - ***bry.***
fine worse from motion or contact - **NUX-V.**
needles, as with - cast.
persistent, first anteriorly then posteriorly - plb.
pressure, with - ***laur.***
worse on, corresponding to region of gall bladder in a small spot, spasmodically - berb.
walking, when - hep.

STIFFNESS, sensation - nat-m.
on bending to left - ***nat-m.***

STINGING, pain - ***acon.,*** bry., ***merc.,*** **NUX-V.,** psor., stann.
rubbing, better from - phos., plb.
vexation, after - ***cham.***

SWELLING - acon., ***aesc.,*** ant-t., ***ars.,*** aur., ***bar-m., bell.,*** bufo, bry., calc., cann-s., **CARD-M.,** ***chel.,*** **CHIN.,** chin-s., ***con.,*** cupr., cur., dol., dros., ***ferr.,*** ferr-ar., ***iod., lach.,*** lact., ***laur.,*** **LYC., MERC.,** nat-m., **NAT-S.,** nux-m., **NUX-V.,** ***phos.,*** podo., ***ptel.,*** sep., sil., ***sulph.,*** tarent.
abuse of quinine, after - nux-v.
left lobe - ***card-m.***
mental exertion, after - nat-s.

TEARING, pain - alum., caust., carb-v., clem., ***con., dios.,*** kreos., zinc.
evening - caust.
extending to, hip - alum.
intermittent - zinc.
supper, after - zinc.

tearing, region of liver - alum., ***con.,*** kali-c., mez., ***nux-m.,*** zinc.

TENDER, (see Sensitive) - ail., ***crot-h., iod., podo.,*** tarent., sulph.
along margin - ***lyc.***
bilious colic, in - ***iris.***
diabetes mellitus, in - kali-br.
headache, with - ***iris.***
pain in right shoulder, with - ***nux-v.***
stitches and soreness on moving and coughing, with - ***eup-per.***
subacute inflammation, in - ***hydr.***

TENSION, in - ***aloe,*** ant-t., bry., calc., ***card-m., carb-v., ferr.,*** hyper., lact., ***lyc.,*** mag-m., mur-ac., ***nat-m., nat-s.,*** nit-ac., sep., sulph.

contractive, in nutmeg liver - ***lach.***

lying on left side - ***card-m.,*** mag-m., nat-s., ptel.

painful - bry., ***puls.***

pressing, when, on it - lact.

short, as if too, on awaking from midday nap - ***carb-v.***

THROBBING - chel., ***sil.***

as if an ulcer would form - nux-v.

pulsating, laming pain, like abscess - bufo

TWINGING, pain - nux-v.

TWISTING, pain - ***dios.,*** podo.

painful, with sensation of heat - ***podo.***

TWITCHING, region of liver - acon., mag-c., merc., nat-c., sep., valer.

coughing - lyc.

ULCERATIVE pain - **LACH.,** ***sil.***

subcutaneous ulceration - ***laur.***

worse from touch - ***chin.***

VOMITING, from bilious disorders - ***iris, merc.,*** merc-i-f., ***nux-v., podo.***

WEAKNESS, of liver - ars., ***benz-ac.,*** **CARD-M.,** ***chel.,*** **CHIN.,** chin-a., cinnam., crot-h., ***hydr., lach., led.,*** lept., **LYC.,** mag-m., mill., ***nat-s.,*** **NUX-V.,** ***phos., podo.,*** sang., sulph., tarax.

colic, with - sang., ***sulph.***

constipation, with - ***kali-m., nux-v.***

cough, with - **NIT-AC.**

dysentery, with, and diarrhea - ***corn.***

facial neuralgia, periodic - polyp-p

headache, causing - bry., iris, lyc., **NUX-V.,** ***podo., sang.***

intermittent fever, in - ***hydr.***

jaundice, with, from biliary concretions - ***sang.***

and great depression of mind, with constipation - still.

malarious districts, in - ***chion.***

WRENCHING, on stooping - ***kali-c.***

Lungs

ABSCESS - acon., ars-i., bell., **CALC**., caps., chin., chin-a., ***crot-h***., **HEP**., ***hippoz.***, iod., ***kali-c.***, kali-n., kali-p., ***lach., led., lyc., mang., merc.***, **PHOS**., ***plb.***, ***psor.***, ***puls.***, sep., **SIL**., ***sulph.***, sul-ac., ***tub.***
left - ***calc.***

ADHESION, sensation of, pleura, of - abrot., carb-an., hep., ran-b., sulph.

AIR, entering too much, or forced in - chlor., sabin., ther.
air, bronchial tubes - all-s., ***aral.***, bac., calc-sil., ***cham.***, chin., ***cori-r., dulc., hep.***, iod., kali-c., mang., merc-sul., naja, ***psor., sil., tub.***
air, clavicle - chlor., rumx.

ASPHYXIA, death apparent (see Emergency, Asphyxia or Death apparent)

ASTHMA, general - ***acon., agar.***, all-c., aloe, alum., alumn., **AMBR.**, ***am-c.***, aml-n., anac., ant-a., ant-c., ***ant-t., apis***, aral., **ARG-N.**, arn., **ARS., ARS-I.**, arum-t., ***asaf.***, asar., asc-t., atro., ***aur.***, bac., ***bar-c.***, bar-m., ***bell.***, **BLATTA,** ***bov., brom., bry., cact., calad., calc.***, camph., cann-i., ***cann-s., caps.***, carb-an., carb-s., ***carb-v.***, **CARC.**, card-m., caust., cham., chel., ***chin., chin-a., chlol.***, chlor., ***cic.***, cina, cist., ***coca***, cocaine, cocc., coc-c., ***coff., colch.***, coloc., ***con.***, croc., ***crot-h.***, crot-t., **CUPR.,** ***cupr-ac.***, cupr-ar., daph., ***dig., dros., dulc., euph.***, eup-per., ***ferr., ferr-ar.***, ferr-i., ferr-p., gall-ac., ***gels.***, glon., ***graph.***, grat., grin., ***hep., hippoz.***, hydr-ac., hyos., ictod., ***ign.***, ill., ***iod.***, **IP., KALI-AR.**, ***kali-bi., kali-br.***, **KALI-C.**, ***kali-chl., kali-i.***, **KALI-N.**, ***kali-p., kali-s.***, lac-d., ***lach.***, lact., ***laur., led.***, lem-m., **LOB.,** ***lyc.***, magn-gr., manc., ***med.***, meny., ***meph.***, merc., merc-i-r., mez., morph., ***mosch., naja, naphtin.***, nat-a., nat-c., ***nat-m.***, nat-p., **NAT-S.**, ***nit-ac.***, nux-m., ***nux-v.***, ol-an., ***op.***, par., petr., phel., ***phos., phyt.***, plat., plb., podo., ***psor.***, ptel., **PULS.**, queb., ran-s., raph., rhod., rumx., ***ruta.***, sabad., sabin., **SAMB.**, ***sang.***, sars., scroph-n., sec., sel., ***seneg., sep.***, **SIL.**, sin-n., spig., **SPONG.**, squil., ***stann., ster., still.***, **STRAM.**, stront-c., stry., **SULPH.**, ***sul-ac.***, syph., syc-co., tab., tela, ter., ***thuj.***, tub., vario., ***verat.***, verat-v., viol-o., viol-t., **VISC.**, xan., zinc., zinc-m., ***zing.***
air, draft of, agg. - kali-c., nux-v., rumx., ***sil.***
mountain, air amel. - syph., tub.
open, amel. - ***am-c.***, ip., naphtin., ***puls.***
sea air, amel. - brom.. med.
alcoholics - ***meph., nux-v.***
allergic, hay fever, with - **ALL-C.**, ***ambr.***, apis, aral., **ARS.**, ***ars-i.***, arum-t., ***bad., carb-v.***, **CARC.**, chin-a., chlor., ***dulc., euphr.***, **IOD.**, ***ip., kali-i., lach.***, linn-u., ***lob., med., naja***, naphtin., ***nat-s., nux-v.***, ol-an., ***op.***, phle., ***sabad.***, sang., sep., ***sil., sin-n., stict.***, sul-i., sulph., **THUJ.**, tub.
sneezing, with - **ALL-C.**, ***ars., carb-v., dulc., euphr.***, lach., ***naja, nat-s., nux-v.***, sin-n., stict.

ASTHMA, general
altitude, from - arn., carb-v., ***coca,*** sil.
alternating, with
eruptions - ***ars., calad.***, caust., ***crot-t.***, dulc., graph., ***hep., kalm.***, lach., mez., mut., ***psor.***, rat., rhus-t., ***sulph.***
diarrhea, nocturnal - ***kali-c.***
gout - benz-ac., lyc., ***sulph.***
headache - ang., glon., kali-br.
urticaria - calad.
vomiting, spasmodic - cupr., ip.
anger, after - ***ars.***, carc., **CHAM.**, ign., nux-v., staph.
anxiety, with - ***arg-n.***, **ARS.**, ***dig., kali-ar.***
autumn - ***chin.***
belching, amel. - carb-v., nux-v.
bending, head backwards amel. - cham., **SPONG.**, ***verat.***
forwards, rocking - kali-c.
bronchial catarrh, with - acon., **ANT-T.**, ***ars.***, **BLATTA.**, blatt-a., ***bry.***, calad., caps., cupr-ac., ***erio.***, eucal., ***grin., ip.***, kali-i., ***lob.***, nat-s., onis., sabal., sulph.
burning, in throat and chest, with - aral.
change, of weather - ***ars.***, chel., dulc.
children - ***acon.***, ambr., **ANT-T., ARS.**, calc., **CARC., CHAM., IP.**, kali-br., kali-c., kali-i., **KALI-N., KALI-S.**, lob., **MED.**, ***mosch.***, **NAT-S.**, nux-v., psor., **PHOS., PULS., SAMB.**, sanic., ***sil.***, stram., sulph., ***thuj.***, **TUB.**, vib.
vaccination, after - **ANT-T.**, ***carc., sil.***, **THUJ.**
cold, air agg. - acon., ***lob., nux-v.***, petr., rumx.
amel. - bry., ***carb-v., cham., merc.***
damp, weather - ars., **DULC.,** ***med.***, **NAT-S.**
dry weather - acon., caust., hep.
water, agg. - ***meph.***
amel. - cham.
cold, taking, from - acon., dulc., ip., ***lob.***, phos., ***podo., puls.***, rumx., sil., **SPONG.**, ***stann., tub.***
heated, when - ***sil.***
summer, in - ***ars.***
constitutionally - calc., iod., phos., sil., sulph., tub.
constriction in throat, with - cham., dros., ***hydr-ac.***, lob., ***mosch.***
coryza, with - ***all-c., ars.***, ars-i., calc., ip., nit-ac., phos., sulph.
after, summer in - all-c., ars.
preceded by - ***all-c.***, aral., ***ars.***, just., naja, nux-v.
coughing, asthmatic - ***acon., alum.***, ambr., ***am-c.***, am-m., anac., **ANT-T.**, aral., arg-n., arn., **ARS.,** ***ars-i.***, asaf., aspar., bar-c., bar-m., ***bell., brom.***, bry., calad., calc., calc-s., carb-an., carb-s., ***carb-v.***, caust., cham., ***chin.***, chin-a., chlor., cic., **CINA,** coc-c., cocc., con., cor-r., croc., ***crot-t.***, **CUPR.,** dig., dol., **DROS.**, dulc., ***euph.***, euphr., ferr., ferr-ar., ferr-i., ferr-p., guai., ***hep.***, hyos., ign., iod., **IP.**, ***kali-ar., kali-bi., kali-c.***, kali-chl., kali-n.,

ASTHMA, general

coughing, asthmatic - kali-p., ***kreos.***, ***lach.***, lact., laur., ***led.***, lob., lyc., merc., mez., mosch., mur-ac., nat-m., nat-s., nicc., nit-ac., ***nux-m.***, **NUX-V.**, op., petr., phel., ***phos.***, prun., psor., ***puls.***, rhus-t., sabad., ***samb.***, ***sang.***, ***sep.***, ***sil.***, spig., ***spong.***, squil., stann., ***stram.***, sulph., sul-ac., verat., viol-o., zinc., zing.
agg. - ***meph.***
after - phos.

cramp, muscular spasm of various parts, with - cupr.

cyanosis, with - ars., carb-v., cupr., samb.

dampness, from (see wet, weather) - ars., carc., **DULC.**, ***med.***, **NAT-S.**, ***thuj.***

despondency, thinks she will die, with - ***ars.***, psor.

diarrhea following, with - nat-s.

digestion disturbed, after - arg-n., ***bry.***, carb-v., ***ip.***, kali-m., ***lob.***, lyc., ***nux-v.***, puls., sang., verat-v., zing.

dinner, after - thuj.

dry weather, agg. - caust., cham.

dust, from inhaling - ***blatta.***, brom., ictod., ***ip.***, kali-c., pot-a., poth., ***sil.***

eating, after - ***kali-p.***, ***nux-v.***, ***puls.***
amel. - ambr., ***graph.***
satisfying, agg. - asaf.

elderly, people, in - ***ambr.***, **ANT-T.**, **ARS.**, ***bar-c.***, calc., ***carb-v.***, ***con.***, phel., ***sil.***, sulph.

emotions, after - ***acon.***, ambr., **ARS.**, ***carc.***, cham., ***coff.***, cupr., ***gels.***, **IGN.**, nux-v., pall., verat.

epiglottis, spasms or weakness of - med.

eruptions, after suppressed - ***apis***, ***ars.***, calad., ***carb-v.***, ***dulc.***, ***ferr.***, hep., ***ip.***, ***psor.***, **PULS.**, sec., ***sulph.***

evening - bell., ***cist.***, ferr., nux-v., ***phos.***, **PULS.**, ***sulph.***, stann., ***zinc.***
bed, in - am-c., graph., sep.
lying down, after - aral., ***ars.***, ***cist.***, con., ferr-ac., ***grin.***, lach., ***meph.***, merc-p-r., naja, puls., ***samb.***, sulph.
night, 9 p.m. - bry.

exertion, from - arn., calc., coca, sil.

excitement - acon., ambr., aml-n., ***asaf.***, ***carc.***, cham., chin-s., coff., ***cupr.***, grin., hydrc., ***ip.***, kali-p., ***lob.***, ***mosch.***, nux-m., ***nux-v.***, ***phos.***, sumb., tela, thymu., ***valer.***, verat.

expectoration, amel. - ***ant-t.***, aral., calad., ***erio.***, grin., hyper., ***ip.***, kali-bi., sep., stann., ***zinc.***

faceache, with, after disappearance of tetter on face - dulc.

flatulence, from - **CARB-V.**, ***cham.***, ***chin.***, ***lyc.***, mag-p., ***nux-v.***, op., phos., ***sulph.***, zinc.

fog, agg. - hyper.

formication, preceded by - cist., lob.

fright, after - carc., op., samb.

gastric derangements, with - arg-n., ***bry.***, carb-v., ***ip.***, kali-m., ***lob.***, lyc., ***nux-v.***, puls., sang., verat-v., zing.

ASTHMA, general

goitre, with - spong.

gonorrhea, from suppressed - ***nat-s.***, thuj.

gout, rheumatism, with - led., sulph., ***visc.***

hay, asthma (see allergic)

head, on knee position - kali-c.

heart, problems, with - acon., ***acon-f.***, adon., ***adren.***, am-c., apis, arn., ars., ars-i., aur-m., ***cact.***, ***calc-ar.***, carb-v., ***chin-a.***, cimic., coll., conv., ***dig.***, ***glon.***, grin., ***iber.***, kali-n., kalm., lach., laur., lycps., magn-gr., naja, op., ox-ac., psor., ***queb.***, spig., spong., stroph., sumb., visc.
fatty degeneration of, from - **ARN.**, phos.

heat, agg. - lach., puls.

hemorrhoids, with - junc., nux-v.

hives, from - apis, puls.

horse, coming in contact with - cast-eq.

humid - acon., ***ars.***, bry., ***cann-i.***, coch., cupr., ***dulc.***, eucal., euph-pi., grin., hyper., iod., kali-bi., **NAT-S.**, sabal., ***seneg.***, stann., ***sulph.***, thuj.
children, in - ***nat-s.***, samb., thuj.

hydrothorax, with - colch.

hysterical - ambr., cocc., ign., lob., **MOSCH.**, **NUX-M.**, ***nux-v.***, phos., **PULS.**, stann., stram., sulph.
tears, flow of, ending in - anac.

injury, of spine, after - ***hyper.***, ***nat-s.***

insomnia, with - ***carc.***, chlor.

intermittent, fever, with - mez.

itching, with - calad., cist., lob., psor., sabad.

laughing, agg. - ars.

leaning, backwards - psor.

meal, after every satisfying - asaf.

measles, after - brom., ***carb-v.***

menses, during - kali-c.
scanty - arg-n.
seizures, in, awaking him during sleep - cupr., ***iod.***, ***lach.***, spong.
waking from sleep - cupr., ***iod.***, ***lach.***, spong.
after suppression of - ***puls.***, spong.
before - sulph.

mental, exertion - sep.

mercury, after - aur.

midnight, after - **ARS.**, calc-ar., ***carb-v.***, ***ferr.***, ferr-ar., ***graph.***, ***lach.***, **SAMB.**
must spring out of bed - **ARS.**, ***graph.***, **SAMB.**

miner's asthma, from coal dust (see dust) - ***blatta***, card-m., nat-a., ***sil.***, sulph.

moldy, environment, from - carc., ***med.***, **NAT-S.**, ***thuj.***

morning - ***aur.***, ***calc.***, carb-an., ***carb-v.***, carc., ***coff.***, ***con.***, dig., **KALI-C.**, ***meph.***, phos., ***verat.***, zing.
bed, in - alum., con.
10 a.m. - carc.
10 to 11 a.m. - ***ferr.***
waking, early - am-c., ant-t., ***ars.***, grin., kali-bi., ***kali-c.***, nat-s., nux-v., zing.

ASTHMA, general

morning,

waking, on - alum., ***con.,*** sep.

music, agg. - ambr.

nausea, with - ant-t., ip., lob.

nervous - ***ars.,*** kali-p., mag-p., stram.

night - am-m., ***ant-t.,*** **ARS.,** aur., ***brom.,*** bry., ***carb-v.,*** **CHEL.,** ***chlol.,*** ***cist.,*** coff., coloc., daph., ***dig.,*** ***ferr.,*** ferr-ar., ***ip.,*** kali-ar., ***kali-c.,*** lach., ***meph.,*** nux-v., ***op.,*** phos., **PULS.,** sang., ***sep.,*** ***sulph.,*** ***syph.,*** zinc., ***thuj.***

9 p.m. - bry.

10 p.m. - meph.

11 p.m., when urinating - chel.

11 p.m. to 2 a.m. - **ARS.,** ***ars-i.***

2 a.m. - **ARS.,** ***kali-bi.,*** med., ***rumx.***

2 to 3 a.m. - **KALI-AR., KALI-C.**

2 a.m. to 4 a.m. - ***kali-c.,*** med.

3 a.m. - ***chin.,*** ***cupr.,*** **KALI-C., KALI-N.,** ***nux-v.***

4 to 5 a.m. - kali-s., ***nat-s.,*** stann.

5 a.m. - kali-i., nat-s.

noon - ***lob.***

odors, from - asar., sang.

palpitations, with - ars., cact., eucal., kali-ar., puls.

periodic - all-s., ***alum.,*** ant-t., **ARS.,** ***asaf.,*** ***carb-v.,*** ***chel.,*** ***chin.,*** chin-a., ***hydr-ac.,*** ip., nux-v., ***phos.,*** ***plb.,*** ***seneg.,*** sulph., tab., thuj.

every 8 days - chin., ign., sulph.

rash, after suppression of acute - acon., ***apis,*** ars., ***puls.***

recent, uncomplicated cases - ars., hydrc.

rheumatism, with - benz-ac., kali-c., visc.

rheumatic-gouty complaints, with - visc.

riding, agg. - meph.

rocking, amel. - kali-c.

rose cold, following - ***sang.***

sailors, as soon as they go ashore - **BROM.**

seashore, amel. - ***med.***

sex, during - aeth., ambr.

after - ***asaf.,*** cedr., kali-bi.

sexual excitation, with - nat-c.

sleep, coming on during - ***acon.,*** ***ars.,*** ***carb-v.,*** ***hep.,*** ***kali-c.,*** ***lach.,*** meph., nat-s., op., sep., ***sulph.***

after - aral., grin., ***lach.,*** samb.

falling asleep, after - am-c., ***grin.,*** lac-c., ***lach.,*** merc-p-r., op.

sit up, must, in bed - ars.

skin disease, with - ars., ip.

smoking, from - ars., ***calad.,*** lob., puls.

amel. - merc.

spasmodic - agar., am-c., ambr., ***ant-t.,*** arg-n., **ARS.,** ***asaf.,*** bapt., ***bell.,*** ***cact.,*** cann-i., caust., cham., cic., ***cocc.,*** coff., con., **CUPR.,** ***dros.,*** ***ferr.,*** ferr-p., ***gels.,*** ***graph.,*** guai., ***hydr-ac.,*** ***hyos.,*** ign., **IP.,** ***kali-br.,*** ***kali-c.,*** ***lach.,*** laur., led., lil-t., **LOB.,** ***mag-p.,*** ***meph.,*** merc., ***mez.,*** ***mosch.,*** nat-s., nux-m., **NUX-V.,** ***op.,*** ph-ac., phos., plat., ***plb.,*** ***puls.,*** raph., rumx., samb., ***sars.,*** ***sep.,*** **SPONG.,** ***stram.,*** sulph., ***sumb.,*** ***tab.,*** **VALER., ZINC.**

spring, in - aral.

stool, amel. - ictod.

sudden, attacks - ars., cupr., ip.

suffocative - ***ant-t.,*** ars., cupr., ***ip.,*** ***samb.***

summer, in - arg-n., ars., syph.

amel. - carb-v.

suppressed, foot sweat, from - ol-an., sil.

suppression, from - hep.

sycotic - ***med.,*** **NAT-S.,** sil., ***thuj.***

talking, agg. - ***dros.,*** meph.

amel. - ferr.

tetter recedes with attack - sulph.

thirst, nausea, stitches and burning in chest, with - kali-n.

thunderstorm, during - phos., sep., ***sil.,*** syph.

tuberculosis, with - meph.

uremia, with - solid.

urinating, while - chel.

urination, painful at night, with - solid.

urine supersaturated with solids, with - nat-n.

vaccination, after - **ANT-T., SIL., THUJ.**

vexation, from - ars.

vertigo, with - kali-c.

vomiting, with - ant-t., ip., lob.

amel. - cupr.

warm, food agg. - ***cham.,*** ***lob.***

room agg. - ***am-c.,*** carb-v., kali-s.

room from the open air - ***bry.,*** ***lob.***

weather, change of agg. - carc., **DULC., NAT-S.,** sil., ***thuj.***

wet, weather, in - ***aur.,*** carc., ***chin.,*** con., **DULC., NAT-S.,** sil., ***thuj.,*** verat.

warm, wet weather - ***bell.,*** ***carb-v.,*** ***nat-s.***

wheezing - ail., all-c., aloe, ***alum.,*** ***ambr.,*** am-c., ***ant-t.,*** ***apoc.,*** aral., arg-n., **ARS.,** ***ars-i.,*** ***brom.,*** calad., calc., calc-s., ***cann-s.,*** ***caps.,*** carb-s., **CARB-V.,** card-m., ***cham.,*** ***chin.,*** ***chin-a.,*** chlol., ***cina,*** crot-t., ***cupr.,*** dol., ***dros.,*** erio., ferr., ferr-i., ***fl-ac.,*** graph., ***grin.,*** hep., hydr-ac., ***iod.,*** iodof., **IP.,** just., ***kali-ar.,*** ***kali-bi.,*** **KALI-C.,** ***kali-s.,*** ***lach.,*** **LOB.,** ***lycps.,*** ***lyc.,*** manc., merc., murx., naja, ***nat-m.,*** ***nat-s.,*** ***nux-m.,*** nux-v., ***nit-ac.,*** ox-ac., phos., prun., sabad., ***samb.,*** sang., sanic., seneg., sep., spong., squil., stann., sulph., ***syph.***

afternoon - fl-ac.

daytime - ***lyc.***

evening - lycps., murx.

bed, in - nat-m.

lying down, on - ***ars.***

expectoration amel. - ip.

expiring, when - ***lyc.,*** nat-m., ***sep.***

inspiring, while - ***alum.,*** ***caps.,*** ***chin.,*** ***kali-c.,*** spong.

midnight, after - ***ars.,*** ***samb.***

night - ***ars.,*** kali-bi.

sitting up, while - nat-c.

sleep, during - nux-v.

smoking, on - calad., kali-bi.

warm room - ***kali-s.***

ASTHMA, general
  whooping, cough, from - meph.
  wind, walking against - cupr.
  windy, weather - carc.
  winter, attacks - ***carb-v.,*** nat-m., ***nux-v.,*** phel.

ATELECTASIS, lungs, collapsed - **ANT-T.,** ***hyos.***

BLEEDING, from lungs and chest - ***acal., acet-ac.,*** **ACON.,** ***all-s.,*** aloe, ***alum.,*** am-c., ***anan., ant-t., apoc., aran.,*** arg-n., **ARN., ARS.,** aur-m-n., aspar., ***bell.,*** brom., ***bry.,*** bufo, **CACT.,** ***calc., calc-p.,*** calc-s., canth., carb-an., carb-s., carb-v., ***card-m.,*** casc., caust., cham., **CHEL., CHIN.,** chin-a., chin-s., chlor., cinnam., ***coc-c., colch., coll.,*** con., ***cop., croc.,*** crot-h., cupr., cupr-s., ***dig.,*** dros., dulc., elaps, erech., ***erig.,*** **FERR.,** ***ferr-ac.,*** **FERR-AR.,** ***ferr-i.,*** ferr-m., ferr-p., ***gall-ac., ger.,*** **HAM.,** hyos., **IP.,** kali-ar., kali-bi., ***kali-c., kali-chl., kali-i.,*** kali-n., kali-p., kali-s., ***kreos., lach., lam., led.,*** lyc., ***lycps.,*** mag-c., mag-m., mang., meli., merc., ***merc-c.,*** **MILL.,** ***nat-a.,*** nat-n., **NIT-AC.,** ***nux-m., nux-v.,*** ol-j., op., ***ph-ac.,*** **PHOS.,** ***plb., puls., rhus-t., sabin., sang.,*** sarr., **SEC.,** ***senec.,*** sep., sil., **STANN.,** staph., ***stram.,*** stront-c., stroph., sulph., ***sul-ac.,*** tab., ***ter.,*** tril., tub., ***urt-u.,*** vanad., verat., verat., ***verat-v.***
    alcoholics, in - ars., hyos., led., **NUX-V.,** op.
    alternating with rheumatism - led.
    anger, from - ***nux-v.***
    coagulated - acal., acon., ***arn., bell.,*** brom., bry., canth., carb-an., caust., **CHAM.,** ***chin.,*** coc-c., coll., con., ***croc.,*** crot-h., dros., ***elaps,*** erig., ***ferr.,*** ferr-m., ham., ***hyos., ip.,*** kali-n., kreos., mag-m., ***merc., nit-ac.,*** nux-v., ph-ac., ***puls.,*** **RHUS-T.,** ***sabin.,*** sec., sep., stram., stront-c., sul-ac.
      black - kreos.
      brown - bry., rhus-t.
      dark - arn., coll., ham., mag-c., puls.
    exertion, after - acon., ***arn.,*** ferr., ip., ***mill.,*** puls., ***rhus-t., urt-u.***
    frothy, foaming - acon., ***arn.,*** dros., ferr., ip., ***led.,*** mill., op., ph-ac., ***phos.,*** sec., ***sil.***
    fullmoon, during - kali-n.
    hemorrhoidal flow, after suppression of - acon., ***carb-v., led., lyc.,*** **NUX-V.,** phos., ***sulph.***
    hot blood - acon., ***bell.,*** mill., psor.
    lying-in women, in - ***acon., arn., chin.,*** hyos., ip., lach., ***puls.,*** sulph., tril.
    menses, after suppression of - ***acon.,*** ars., ***bell., bry.,*** con., ***dig.,*** ferr., graph., ham., mill., ***phos.,*** **PULS.,** ***sang., senec.,*** sep., sulph., ust.
      before - ***dig.***
    nursing mothers - ***chin.***
    pneumonia, results of - calc-s., ***sul-ac.***
    puerperal fever - ham.
    walking slowly amel. - ***ferr.***
    whiskey, after - merc., puls.
    whooping cough, in - con., ip.
    wine, after - acon.

BREATH, cold - acon., ant-t., ars., **CAMPH.,** carb-o., **CARB-V.,** ***cedr., chin.,*** chin-s., cist., colch., ***cop.,*** cor-r., ***helo.,*** jatr., merc., ***phos.,*** rhus-t., ***tab.,*** ter., **VERAT.**
    chill, during - **CARB-V.,** verat.
  breath, hot - **ACON.,** aeth., agar., anac., ***ant-c.,*** apis, ***ars.,*** asaf., asar., ***bell.,*** calc., calc-p., cann-s., **CARB-S.,** ***cham.,*** chel., coc-c., coff., ***ferr.,*** kali-br., mag-m., ***mang.,*** med., merl., mez., naja, ***nat-m., phos.,*** ptel., raph., ***rhus-t., rhus-v., sabad.,*** squil., ***stront-c., sulph.,*** sumb., trif-p., zinc.
    afternoon - ***bad., rhus-t.***
    as if - rad-br.
    chill, during - anac., camph., cham., **RHUS-T.**
    cold limbs, with - cham.
    coryza, during - mag-m.
    evening - mang., sumb.
    fever, during - zinc.
    morning, on waking - sulph.

BREATHING, (see Breathing, chapter)

BRONCHITIS, inflammation, bronchial tubes - ***acet-ac., acon.,*** **AESC.,** ***all-c., alum., alumn.,*** am-c., am-i, ***am-m.,*** am-p., ant-a., ***ant-c.,*** **ANT-T.,** ***apis, arn.,*** **ARS.,** ars-i., ***asc-t., aur-m.,*** bar-c., **BAR-M.,** ***bell., benz-ac.,*** blatta, ***brom.,*** **BRY.,** ***cact., calc.,*** calc-f., ***camph., cann-s., carb-s., carb-v.,*** card-m., ***caust., cham., chel.,*** chin., chlol., chlor., ***cina, cist., coc-c.,*** colch., cop., dig., **DROS.,** ***dulc.,*** eup-per., euphr., ***ferr-i.,*** **FERR-P.,** ***gels.,*** grin., ***guai.,*** **HEP.,** ***hippoz., hyos., iod.,*** **IP.,** kali-ar., ***kali-bi., kali-c., kali-chl.,*** kali-p., ***kreos., lach., lob.,*** **LYC.,** mang., ***merc.,*** merc-sul., morg., ***naja,*** nat-a., ***nat-m.,*** **NAT-S.,** ***nit-ac., nux-v., ph-ac.,*** **PHOS.,** piloc., pix., ***plb., psor.,*** **PULS.,** ***rhus-t., rumx.,*** **SANG.,** ***sang-n.,*** **SENEC.,** ***seneg., sep.,*** **SIL.,** solid., **SPONG.,** ***squil.,*** **STANN.,** ***stict.,*** sul-ac., ***sulph., ter.,*** thuj., **TUB.,** uran., ***verat.,*** verat-v., verb., zinc.
    capillary - ***ant-t.,*** bell., carb-v., ***ferr-p., ip.,*** seneg., ter.
    children - am-c., ***ant-t., dulc.,*** ferr-p., **IP., KALI-C.,** nat-a., ***phos.***
    chronic - alum., alumn., ***am-c.,*** am-caust., am-i, am-m., ***ammc.,*** ant-a., ***ant-s.,*** **ANT-T.,** ***ars., ars-i., bac., bals-p.,*** bar-c., ***bar-m., calc.,*** calc-i., calc-sil., ***canth.,*** carb-an., ***carb-v.,*** cean., chel., chin., coc-c., con., ***cop.,*** cub., dig., dros., ***dulc.,*** erio., eucal., grin., ***hep., hydr.,*** hyos., ichth., iod., ***ip., kali-bi.,*** kali-c., ***kali-i.,*** kali-s., kreos., lach., ***lyc.,*** merc-sul., myos., myrt-c., nat-m., nat-s., ***nit-ac.,*** nux-v., phos., pix., ***puls.,*** rumx., sabad., sabal., sang., sec., ***seneg.,*** sep., sil., silphu., spong., squil., ***stann.,*** stry., ***sulph.,*** tax., ter., tub., verat.
    alternates with diarrhea - seneg.
    children - **ANT-T.** ***dulc.,*** **IP., KALI-C.,** phos., sil.
    cold, from every - mang.

BRONCHITIS, inflammation
elderly people - all-c., ***am-c.,*** ammc., ant-c., **ANT-T.,** ars., bac., ***camph., carb-v., dros.,*** **HIPPOZ.,** ***hydr.,*** kali-c., kreos., ***lyc.,*** **PHOS.,** ***nux-v.,*** seneg., ***sil.***
fibrinous - brom., bry., calc-ac., ***kali-bi.,*** phos.
toxemic - am-c., ant-t., bry., colch., diph., ***merc-c.***
winter, each - morg.

BRONCHIECTASIS, chonic dilatation of - acet-ac., all-c., all-s., alumn., am-c., **ANT-T.,** ***ars., bac., bals-p.,*** benz-ac., ***calc.,*** cop., crot-h., eucal., ferr-i., grin., ***hep.,*** ichth., **KALI-BI.,** ***kali-c.,*** kreos., ***lyc.,*** med., myos., myrt-c., phel., ***phos., puls.,*** sang., sil., ***stann.,*** sulph., tub.

BUBBLING, in - ant-t., tell.
in right - tell.

CANCER - ars., calad., cob., con., phos.

CATARRH, (see Expectoration) - ***acon.,*** alum., ***ammc., ant-c.,*** **ANT-T.,** ***apis, arn.,*** **ARS.,** ars-i., ***aur-m.,*** **BAR-C., BAR-M.,** benz-ac., **BRY., CACT., CALC.,** ***calc-s.,*** canth., carb-s., carb-v., ***caust.,*** chel., ***coc-c.,*** cop., ***dros.,*** **DULC.,** ferr., ferr-ar., ferr-i., ***ferr-p., guai.,*** **HEP.,** ***hippoz., hydr., iod., kali-ar.,*** **KALI-BI.,** ***kali-c.,*** **KALI-CHL.,** kali-p., **KALI-S.,** ***kreos.,*** lac-d., ***lach., lact.,*** **LYC., MERC.,** ***nat-m., nat-s.,*** **NUX-V.,** ***petr.,*** phel., **PHOS.,** ***psor.,*** **PULS.,** ***rhus-t., rumx., samb.,*** **SANG.,** ***senec.,*** **SENEG., SIL.,** sin-n., ***spong.,*** **STANN., SULPH.,** ***ter., tub.***
alternating with diarrhea - seneg.
elderly people - ***ammc., ant-t.,*** **BAR-C.,** ***chin., nat-s.,*** phel., **SENEG.,** ***tub.***
morning - aur., sul-ac.

COLD, breath (see Breath, cold)

COLDS, (see Nose, Colds and Coryza)

CONGESTION, hyperemia of chest and lungs - **ACON.,** adren., ***aesc.,*** aloe, alum., ambr., ***aml-n.,*** ammc., ***am-c., apis, arn.,*** ars-i., ***aur.,*** **BELL.,** both., brom., **BRY., CACT.,** ***calc.,*** **CAMPH.,** carb-s., ***carb-v.,*** cent., ***chin.,*** chlor., cimic., ***coc-c.,*** cocc., conv., ***cupr.,*** cycl., **DIG.,** ***ferr.,*** ferr-i., ferr-m., ***ferr-p.,*** gad., ***gels., glon., graph., iod.,*** **IP.,** ***kali-c.,*** kali-chl., kali-i., kali-n., **LACH.,** lact., lil-t., ***lyc.,*** mag-m., ***meli., merc.,*** merl., ***mill.,*** nat-m., ***nit-ac.,*** **NUX-V.,** ol-an., ***op.,*** **PHOS.,** ***puls.,*** rat., rhod., **RHUS-T.,** ***sang.,*** sarr., sec., ***seneg.,*** **SEP.,** ***sil.,*** **SPONG.,** squil., stel., stroph., sulfon., **SULPH., TER.,** ***thuj., verat-v.***
afternoon - seneg.
alternating with congestion of head - ***glon.***
coldness of body, with - carb-v.
desire to urinate, if not obeyed - **LIL-T.**
excitement - ***phos.***
exertion, after - ***spong.***
exposure to cold air - cimic., ***phos.***
lying down impossible - **CACT.**
menopause, at - arg-n., **LACH.**
menses, during - glon.
before - kali-c.
delayed - graph., nux-m., ***puls.***

CONGESTION, hyperemia
menses, suppressed, with - acon., calc., sep.
morning - elaps, pall.
on waking - carb-v., phos., sulph.
motion, after - ***spong.***
night - ***ferr.,*** nit-ac., ***puls.***
pregnancy, during - ***glon., nat-m., sep.***
sea, bathing - ***mag-m.***
sensation as of blood stopping - sabad., ***seneg.***
sleep, during - mill., puls.
urination, desire, if not attended to - lil-t.
uterine hemorrhage, after - **AUR-M.,** ***chin., phos.***
waking, on - **LACH.**
walking in open air - mag-m., ***phos.***
weakness and nausea - ***spong.***
writing, after - am-c.

CONVULSIVE, breathing (see Breathing, paroxymal)

COUGHING, (see Coughing chapter)

CRAMP, in - mosch., zinc.
drinking cold water - thuj.
waking, after - arum-t.

CROUP, (see Coughing chapter) - ***acet-ac.,*** **ACON.,** anac., ant-t., apis, ***ars., ars-i.,*** arum-d., ***bell., brom., calc-s., carb-ac.,*** cham., ***chin., chlor., cina,*** cinnb., cor-r., cub., cupr-s., dros., ***gels.,*** **HEP., IOD.,** ***ip.,*** **KALI-BI.,** ***kali-m.,*** kali-s., ***lac-c.,*** **LACH., PHOS.,** ***phyt., rumx., ruta.,*** **SAMB.,** ***sang.,*** **SPONG.,** staph., stict., **STRAM.**
barking, cough, with - **ACON.,** all-c., ant-t., aur-m., **BELL.,** brom., caps., cimx., clem., ***coc-c.,*** cor-r., cub., **DROS.,** ***dulc.,*** **HEP.,** hipp., ***kali-bi.,*** lac-c., lact., lyc., lyss., merc., mur-ac., ***nit-ac.,*** nux-m., phos., phyt., ***rumx.,*** **SPONG.,** stann., stict., **STRAM.,** sulph., verat.
eating, after - anac.
evening - cinnb.
expiration, on - acon.
face, bluish - brom., ***carb-v.***
morning - ***calc-s.***
night - ars., carb-ac., ***hep., ip.,*** phyt., ***spong.***
midnight, after, agg. - ***ars.***
sopor, stertorous breathing and wheezing, the child starts up, kicks about, suffocating turning black and blue in face, after which cough with rattling breathing sets in again, suffocation and paralysis of lungs appear unavoidable, with - samb.
waking, only after - **CALC-S.**
winter, alternating with sciatica in summer - staph.

CYANOSIS, (see Breathing, cyanosis)

DISCHARGES, from, (see Expectoration)

DISTENSION, lungs, can not - asaf., crot-t.

DRAWN, downwards - am-c.

EDEMA, pulmonary, (see Pulmonary, edema)

EMPHYSEMA - **AM-C., ANT-A., ANT-T.,** arn., ***ars., aur-m., bell., brom.,*** bry., calad., calc., ***calc-p., calc-s., camph.,*** carb-s., ***carb-v.,*** chin., chin-a., ***chlor.,*** cupr., cur., ***dig.,*** dros., echi., eucal., ferr-m., glon., grin., **HEP.,** ***ip.,*** kali-c., lac-d., **LACH., LOB.,** ***lyc., merc.,*** myrt-c., naphtin., ***nat-m.,*** nat-s., nit-ac., nux-v., op., ***phel., phos.,*** puls., sars., seneg., sep., **SIL.,** spong., ***stry.,*** sul-ac., sulph., ter.

smoking, from - am-c., calad.

EMPYEMA - apis, arn., **ARS.,** ***ars-i., calc.,*** **CALC-S.,** ***carb-s., carb-v., chin., chin-a.,*** dig., ferr., ***hep.,*** iod., ***kali-c.,*** **KALI-S.,** ***lach.,*** lyc., **MERC.,** ***nat-a., nit-ac., phos., sep.,*** **SIL., SULPH.,** tub.

pleurisy, after - sil.

EXPECTORATION, general - acon., aeth., aesc., agar., agn., ***all-c.,*** all-s., aloe, alum., ***alumn., ambr.,*** am-c., ***ammc., am-m.,*** anac., ang., ***ant-c.,*** **ANT-T.,** aral., aran., **ARG-M., ARG-N.,** arn., ***arum-t.,*** **ARS.,** atro., asar., aspar., aur., bad., **BAR-C., BAR-M.,** bell., benz-ac., bism., **BLATTA,** ***bor.,*** bov., **BRY.,** bufo, ***cact.,*** calad., **CALC.,** ***calc-s.,*** cann-s., ***canth., caps.,*** carb-ac., carb-an., ***carb-s., carb-v.,*** **CAUST.,** cham., chel., **CHIN., CHIN-A.,** chin-s., cimic., cimx., ***cina,*** cob., coca, cocc., **COC-C.,** cod., con., cop., corn., croc., crot-t., cub., cupr., cycl., der., dig., ***dirc.,*** dor., **DROS., DULC.,** erig., ery-a., eug., **EUPHR.,** eupi., ferr., ferr-ar., ferr-i., ferr-p., fl-ac., gamb., ***graph.,*** guai., ham., **HEP.,** hipp., hydr-ac., **HYDR.,** hyos., hyper., iber., ign., indg., ***iod.,*** ip., iris, kali-ar., **KALI-BI.,** ***kali-c., kali-chl., kali-i.,*** kali-n., kali-p., ***kali-s.,*** kreos., lac-ac., lac-d., **LACH.,** lact., laur., **LOB.,** ***lob-s.,*** **LYC.,** mag-c., mag-m., mag-s., ***mang., med.,*** merc., merc-c., mez., mur-ac., naja, nat-a., ***nat-c.,*** **NAT-M.,** nat-p., ***nat-s.,*** nicc., **NIT-AC.,** nux-m., ***nux-v.,*** oena., ol-j., olnd., op., osm., ox-ac., **PAR.,** ***petr.,*** phel., ***ph-ac.,*** **PHOS.,** phys., plan., plb., **PSOR., PULS.,** raph., rat., rheum, rhod., rhus-r., ***rhus-t.,*** rumx., ruta., sabad., sabin., ***samb.,*** **SANG.,** sec., sel., ***senec., seneg., sep.,*** **SIL.,** sin-n., spig., ***spong.,*** **SQUIL., STANN.,** ***staph.,*** stict., sulph., sul-ac., tab., tarax., ter., ***thuj.,*** uran., ust., verat., vinc., xan., ***zinc.***

acrid - ***alum.,*** am-c., ***am-m.,*** anac., ***ars.,*** carb-v., ***caust.,*** cham., coc-c., con., ferr., ign., iod., kreos., lach., lyc., mag-m., ***merc.,*** mez., nat-m., nit-ac., nux-v., phos., ***puls.,*** rhus-t., sep., ***sil.,*** spig., squil., sulph., sul-ac.

afternoon - alum., am-m., anac., ars., ***bad.,*** caust., chin., chin-s., clem., coc-c., eucal., hydr., lyc., mag-c., mill., naja, nux-v., op., phos.

4 p.m. - op.

5 p.m. - caust., hydr., mag-c.

air, agg. - chin-s., cob., merc., nux-v., plan., sac-alb., sep.

agg, cold - ***lach.,*** plan.

cold, amel. - calc-s.

wind - lycps.

open - chin-s., cob., ***lach.,*** merc., nux-v., ***sac-alb.,*** sep.

amel. - arg-n., calc-s.

EXPECTORATION, mucous

air, walking, in - merc., nux-v., ***sac-alb.***

air passages, mucous in the - acon., aeth., agn., ***alum., ambr., am-c., ammc., ang.,*** **ANT-T.,** ***arg-m., arg-n., ars.,*** ars-i., **ARUM-T.,** asaf., **AUR., BAR-C.,** bell., bov., ***brom., bry.,*** cahin., **CALC., CALC-S.,** ***camph., cann-s.,*** caps., carb-s., carb-v., carl., **CAUST.,** ***cham.,*** chin., ***cina,*** cocc., ***coc-c.,*** croc., crot-t., cupr., dig., dros., ***dulc.,*** euphr., gels., ferr., ferr-ar., ferr-i., ferr-p., **HEP., HYOS., IOD.,** iris, kali-ar., **KALI-BI.,** ***kali-c.,*** kali-p., kali-s., kreos., lach., laur., **LYC.,** mag-m., med., ***merc.,*** merc-sul., naja, **NAT-M.,** ***nat-s., nux-v., olnd.,*** osm., ox-ac., ***par.,*** phel., ***ph-ac.,*** **PHOS.,** plb., ***puls., rumx., samb.,*** **SANG.,** senec., **SENEG.,** ***sil., spong.,*** **SQUIL., STANN.,** staph., sul-ac., ***sulph.,*** teucr., thuj.

ascending and descending - ***coc-c., lach.***

ejected with difficulty - ant-t., ***cann-s., caust.***

evening - crot-t., ***puls.***

forenoon - **STANN.**

morning - ***cann-s.,*** caust., olnd.

night - ***puls.,*** thuj.

ash, colored, spots - arund.

ball, feels like a round, and rushes into mouth - syph.

balls, in shape of - agar., ***arg-n., coc-c.,*** lyc., med., ph-ac., ***sil.,*** squil., **STANN.,** sulph.

bitter, green - med.

little albuminous - ph-ac.

batter, breaks and flies like thin - phos.

bed, in - am-c., ***calc.,*** ferr., ***phos.,*** sep.

sitting up in, on - ***phos.***

bilious, like bile - bar-c., dig., puls., samb.

blackish - arn., aster., bell., ***chin.,*** cur., ***elaps,*** hydr-ac., ***kali-bi.,*** led., lyc., ***nux-v.,*** ox-ac., puls., rhus-t.

grains, with - chin.

lumps in centre - arn., ox-ac.

yellow - hydr-ac.

bloody, spitting up of - ***acal.,*** acet-ac., **ACON.,** aesc., agn., ail., all-s., aloe, alum., ambr., am-br., **AM-C.,** am-m., anac., ***anan.,*** ant-c., ant-s., ***apis, aran., arg-n.,*** **ARN., ARS.,** arum-m., asar., aspar., aur., bad., ***bell.,*** bism., ***bor.,*** brom., ***bry.,*** bufo, ***cact., calc.,*** calc-s., **CANN-S.,** ***canth.,*** caps., carb-an., carb-h., carb-o., ***carb-s., carb-v., card-m.,*** casc., ***cench., cham., chin.,*** chin-a., chlor., cina, cist., cob., coc-c., coll., ***con.,*** cop., ***croc., crot-t.,*** **CROT-H.,** ***cupr.,*** cur., daph., der., ***dig.,*** dios., ***dros., dulc.,*** elaps, erig., eug., euphr., **FERR.,** ***ferr-ar., ferr-i.,*** **FERR-P.,** fl-ac., gamb., gels., graph., guai., ***ham.,*** hell., hep., hippoz., hydr-ac., ***hyos.,*** ill., ind., iod., **IP.,** jug-c., kali-ar., ***kali-bi.,*** kali-c., kali-i., kali-ma., kali-n., kali-p., kali-s., ***kreos.,*** lach., lachn., **LAUR., LED.,** ***lyc.,*** lycps., ***mag-c.,*** mag-m., manc., ***mang., merc.,*** merc-c., ***mez.,*** **MILL.,** mur-ac., ***nat-a.,*** nat-c., ***nat-m.,*** nat-p., **NIT-AC.,** nux-m., nux-v., oena., ***op.,*** ph-ac., **PHOS.,** ***plb.,*** psor., **PULS.,** ***rhus-t.,*** ruta.,

EXPECTORATION, mucous

bloody, spitting up of - sabad., ***sabin.,*** sal-ac., sang., sarr., **SEC.,** sel., ***sep., sil.,*** sol-m., squil., **STANN.,** staph., **SULPH.,** ***sul-ac.,*** tarax., ***ter.,*** thuj., verat., ***zinc.***

acrid - ***am-c., ars., canth.,*** carb-v., hep., **KALI-C.,** ***kali-n.,*** rhus-t., **SIL.,** sulph., sul-ac., zinc.

afternoon - alum., clem., kali-n., lyc., mag-c., mez., mill., nux-v.

1 p.m. - clem.

2 p.m. - nux-v.

4 p.m. - mill.

5 p.m. - mag-c.

alcoholics, in - hyos., ***led.,*** nux-v., ***op.,*** sul-ac.

black - arn., bism., canth., chin., croc., crot-c., dig., dros., **ELAPS**, kali-bi., ***nit-ac.,*** nux-v., ph-ac., puls., zinc.

breastfeeding, during - ***ferr.***

bright-red - acal., **ACON.,** am-c., aran., ***arn.,*** ars., **BELL.,** bry., cact., ***calc.,*** canth., carb-an., ***carb-v.,*** cench., chin., cob., dig., dros., **DULC.,** ferr., ferr-ac., ferr-p., ger., **HYOS.,** ***ip., kali-bi.,*** kali-n., laur., ***led., merc.,*** mill., nit-ac., nux-m., nux-v., **PHOS.,** puls., ***rhus-t.,*** sabad., **SABIN.,** ***sec.,*** sep., sil., tril., ***zinc.***

brown - **BRY.,** ***calc.,*** **CARB-V.,** con., puls., ***rhus-t.,*** sil.

chronic - sul-ac.

clearing the throat, when - am-c.

cough, with - acal., ***acon., ferr-ac.,*** ferr-p., ***ip., led.,*** phos.

without, or effort - ***acon., ham.,*** mill., ***sul-ac.***

dark - acal., acon., ***am-c.,*** am-m., ***ant-c., arn., asar.,*** bell., ***bism., bry., cact., canth.,*** carb-v., cench., **CHAM.,** ***chin.,*** coc-c., coll., con., **CROC.,** crot-t., ***cupr.,*** dig., dros., ***elaps,*** erig., ferr., ferr-m., ferr-p., ham., kali-i., kali-n., ***kreos.,*** led., ***lyc., mag-c.,*** mag-m., merc., mur-ac., ***nit-ac., nux-m.,*** **NUX-V.,** ***ph-ac., phos.,*** plat., ***puls.,*** sec., ***sel., sep.,*** stict., sulph., sul-ac.

drinking, after - calc.

eating, after - sep.

erection, after a violent - nat-m.

evening - cub., nat-c., sep.

coughing, when - nat-c., sep.

lying down, after - sep.

exertion, after - ip., mill.

fall, after a - ***ferr-p., mill.***

hawking, on - cham., ferr., hyper., kali-n., ***nit-ac.***

heart-disease, with valvular - cact., lycps.

liver colored - puls.

lumps - mag-c.

menopause, during - lach.

menses, during - iod., kali-c., nat-m., ***phos.,*** sep., **ZINC.**

before - phos., **ZINC.**

suppressed, during - acon., ***carb-v., dig., led., lyc.,*** **NUX-V.,** ***phos.,*** puls., sulph.

EXPECTORATION, mucous

bloody, spitting up of

moon, full - kali-n.

morning - acal., acon., aesc., ail., alum., ant-c., bell., cupr., ***ferr.,*** indg., ip., laur., mez., nit-ac., ph-ac., sel., sep., sil., sol-t-ae., sul-ac., zinc.

bed, in - nit-ac., **NUX-V.**

coughing, on - bell., sep., sil.

lying down, while - merc.

menses, during - **ZINC.**

rising, on - aesc., ***ferr.***

mucous, bloody - ***acon.,*** ail., alum., **AM-C.,** anac., ant-t., ***apis, arg-n.,*** **ARN., ARS.,** bell., bism., ***bor., bry.,*** cact., ***calc., calc-s.,*** card-m., chin., cina, cob., coll., con., cupr., daph., dig., ***dros., dulc.,*** eug., euphr., **FERR.,** ferr-i., fl-ac., **GELS.,** hep., iod., **IP.,** kali-ar., ***kali-bi.,*** kali-c., ***lach.,*** lachn., **LAUR.,** lyc., mag-m., manc., med., ***merc., merc-c., nat-m.,*** nux-m., ol-j., op., **PHOS.,** sabin., ***sec.,*** sel., senec., sil., spong., squil., stict., sul-ac., zinc.

night - arn., ars., ***ferr.,*** mez., puls., rhus-t., sulph.

noon - sil.

pale - am-c., arn., ars., bell., bor., ***bry.,*** calc., canth., carb-an., carb-v., chin., dig., dros., dulc., ferr., graph., ***hyos.,*** ip., kali-n., kreos., laur., led., mag-m., ***mang.,*** merc., nat-c., nux-m., phos., puls., rhus-t., sabad., sabin., sec., sep., sil., sulph., zinc.

periodical attacks - kreos.

puerperal fevers, in - ham.

purulent - arg-n., chin., sulph.

respiration, from violent effort at - ***sec.***

streaked - ***acon.,*** alum., ***am-c.,*** anac., ant-c., ***arg-n., arn.,*** **ARS.,** bism., ***bor.,*** **BRY.,** ***cact.,*** calc., ***caust., chel., chin.,*** cina, cocc., con., crot-h., cub., cupr., daph., dig., dros., dulc., erig., eug., euphr., **FERR.,** ***ferr-ar.,*** hep., hyos., iod., ***ip.,*** kali-bi., kali-c., kreos., lach., lachn., ***laur., lyc.,*** mag-m., med., merc., ***merc-c.,*** mez., ***nat-m.,*** nit-ac., nux-m., ***op., phos.,*** puls., ***sabin.,*** sang., sec., ***sel.,*** senec., seneg., sep., sil., spong., squil., sul-ac., ter., tub., ***zinc.***

stringy - ***croc.***

taking, after - hura

thick - cupr.

thin - ferr., nux-m., sabin.

threads of blood mixed with white sputa - aur-m.

traumatic - mill.

tubercular - acal., ***acon.,*** all-s., calc-ar., ferr., ***ferr-ac.,*** ferr-p., ***ham., ip.,*** mill., nit-ac., nux-v., ***phos.,*** piloc., tril.

uncoagulated - alum., ant-t., bov., bry., dulc., ph-ac., ***phos.,*** sec., stram., sulph.

valvular disease, with - cact., lycps.

vicarious - bry., ham., phos.

viscid - **CROC.,** ***cupr.,*** mag-c., sec.

walking, while - cham., merc., sul-ac., zinc.

working, while - merc.

EXPECTORATION, mucous
blue, and white alternately - arund.
bluish - arund., brom., ***kali-bi.,*** nat-a., sulph.
gray - coc-c.
breakfast, after - sep.
brick, dust, color - bry., ***phos.,*** rhus-t.
brownish - agar., ***ars.,*** bry., caps., ***carb-an., carb-v.,*** hyos., lyc., mag-c., phos., puls., sil.
frothy - carb-an.
lumps - agar., phos.
yellow - lyc.
burned, when dry on the floor, looks as if - ***phos.***
calcareous, tubercles - sars.
casts, (see membranes) - ip.
cheese, like - chin., fago., lyc., puls., sal-ac., sanic.
cold, weather, from - ***ammc.***
cool, cold - bry., calad., cann-s., ***cor-r.,*** lach., merc., nit-ac., nux-v., ***phos.,*** rhus-t., sac-alb., sin-a., sulph.
constant, almost day and evening - ***arg-m.,*** **SQUIL.**
copious - agar., ail., all-s., alum., ***alumn.,*** am-c., **AMMC.,** ***am-m.,*** ant-a., ant-c., **ANT-T.,** arg-m., **ARS.,** ***ars-i.,*** asc-t., aspar., asar., bals-p., bar-m., ***bism., blatta,*** bry., **CACT., CALC.,** calc-p., **CALC-S.,** calc-sil., canth., carb-ac., carb-s., ***carb-v., caust.,*** cean., ***chel., chin.,*** chin-a., cic., cina, cob., **COC-C.,** cod., cop., cupr., cycl., daph., dig., dios., ***dros., dulc.,*** eucal., euph., **EUPHR.,** eup-per., ***ferr., ferr-ar., ferr-i.,*** ferr-p., gall-ac., graph., grin., guai., **HEP.,** hepat., hippoz., hydr., indg., ***iod.,*** ip., jab., kali-ar., ***kali-bi., kali-c.,*** kali-i., kreos., lach., ***laur.,*** led., lob., **LYC.,** med., merc., merc-i-f., merc-i-r., myos., myric., myrt-c., nat-a., nat-s., oena., petr., ***ph-ac.,*** phel., **PHOS.,** phyt., plb., ***psor.,*** **PULS.,** ***rumx.,*** ruta., ***samb.,*** sang., sanic., sel., ***senec., seneg.,*** **SEP.,** ***sil.,*** silphu., ***squil.,*** **STANN.,** stict., sulo-ac., ***sulph.,*** sul-ac., ter., ***thuj.,*** trif-p., tril., ***uran-n.,*** verat., viol-o., wies., zinc., zing.
daytime - cic., ***sil.***
elderly people - ***ammc., ant-t., ars.,*** **BAR-C.,** ***kreos.***
evening - ***carb-v.,*** graph.
lying down, on - graph.
meals, after - sanic.
morning - agar., ***alum.,*** calc., ***calc-s., carb-v.,*** cob., ***coc-c.,*** dig., euph., euphr., kali-bi., ***ph-ac., phos.,*** psor., sanic., squil., ***stann.***
9 a.m. - cob.
mouthful at a time - **EUPHR.,** lyc., ***phos.,*** rumx.
moving, while - ***ferr.***
night - carb-v., ***kali-bi.***
paroxysmal cough, after each - ***agar., alumn., anan., arg-n.,*** **COC-C.,** kali-bi., sulph.
warm room - ***kali-c.***

EXPECTORATION, mucous
corrosive - iod.
cream, like - ambr.
crumbly - ox-ac.
dark - ***ars.,*** bism., ***carb-an.,*** cupr., kali-bi., med., naja, nux-m., oena.
daytime, only - acon., ail., alum., ***alumn.,*** am-c., anac., ang., ant-t., ***arg-m.,*** arn., **ARS.,** asaf., ***bell.,*** bor., bry., ***calc.,*** calc-s., caps., carb-an., carb-s., ***caust.,*** **CHAM.,** chin., cic., cocc., coc-c., colch., ***con.,*** dig., euphr., ferr., ferr-ar., ferr-p., ***graph.,*** guai., **HEP.,** ***hyos.,*** kali-c., lach., ***lyc.,*** mag-c., mag-m., mag-s., ***mang.,*** **MERC.,** ***nit-ac., nux-v.,*** op., petr., phos., **PULS.,** rhus-t., ***sabad.,*** samb., sanic., **SIL.,** squil., ***stann.,*** staph., ***stront-c.,*** **SULPH.,** verat., zinc.
agg.- ***ars.,*** calc-s., ***caust.,*** mag-s., ***spig.***
difficult - agn., ail., ***all-s.,*** alum., ambr., ***ammc.,*** ang., **ANT-T.,** apis, aral., ***arn., ars.,*** arum-t., arund., asc-t., aspar., atro., aur., ***bar-c.,*** bor., ***bov., brom.,*** bry., ***calc.,*** camph., cann-s., canth., carb-an., **CAUST.,** cham., ***chel.,*** chin., chin-a., chin-s., chlor., cina, coca, ***coc-c.,*** con., cop., cor-r., crot-h., cub., ***cupr.,*** der., dig., dros., ***dulc.,*** euphr., ferr., ferr-ar., ferr-i., ferr-p., ***hep.,*** hydrc., hyos., ign., **IP.,** ***iod.,*** jatr., kali-ar., ***kali-bi., kali-c., kali-s.,*** kreos., ***lach.,*** lob., lyc., mag-c., mag-m., mang., med., nat-a., ***nit-ac.,*** nux-m., nux-v., oena., op., osm., ox-ac., par., ***phos.,*** plan., plb., ***psor.,*** **PULS.,** rat., ***rumx.,*** **SENEG.,** sep., ***squil.,*** staph., stram., sulph., sul-ac., tarent., thyr., zinc.
adhering to throat, teeth and lips - **KALI-BI.**
afternoon - chin., chin-s.
2 p.m. - chin-s.
elderly people - ***ammc.***
tongue, can raise sputa only on to, whence it must be removed by wiping - apis.
dinner, after - alumn.
dirty, looking - calc.
drinking, amel. - am-c.
dust, as if mixed with - phos.
easier, after each cough - aspar.
easy, (see hawked up) - acon., ail., ant-t., **ARG-M.,** arund., aur., bac., carb-v., cimic., ***coc-c.,*** coloc., dig., dol., dulc., erio., euphr., hep., iod., ***ip.,*** kali-bi., kali-s., kalm., kreos., lach., lact., mag-m., mang., meli., ***nat-s.,*** oena., plb., ***puls.,*** ruta., sil., squil., **STANN.,** staph., sulph., tell., tub., verat.
daytime - ail., ***arg-m.,*** coc-c., dig., sil., staph.
evening - ***arg-m.,*** dig.
morning - arund., mang.
profuse, and - arg-m.
motion, on - ip.
night - meli.
waking, on - meli.
eating, after - bell., ***lyc.,*** nux-m., ***phos.,*** sanic., sil., staph., thuj.
elderly people - ***ammc., ant-t.,*** calc.
epithelium, exfoliated - chin-s.

EXPECTORATION, mucous

evening - agn., all-c., alum., ***alumn.,*** ant-c., ***arg-m., arn.,*** ars., aur., bar-c., ***bell.,*** bor., bry., bufo, calc., cann-s., canth., carb-s., ***caust.,*** chin., chin-s., ***cina,*** coc-c., crot-t., cub., dig., ***graph.,*** hydr., hydr-ac., ***ign.,*** iod., kali-ar., kali-c., kali-n., kali-s., ***kalm.,*** kreos., lach., ***lyc.,*** mur-ac., naja, nat-a., nat-c., nat-m., nux-m., nux-v., oena., rhod., rhus-t., ***ruta.,*** sep., sil., stann., staph., sulph., sul-ac., thuj., verat.

bed, in - calc., ***nux-m.,*** sep.

getting warm - ***nux-m.***

lying down, after - graph., kali-n., psor., sep.

flakes - ail., phos.

flies, forcibly out of mouth - ***bad., chel.,*** kali-c., kali-m.

forenoon - bry., calc-s., chin-s., coc-c., iris, lyc., oena., ***sil.,*** **STANN.,** sulph., zinc.

10 a.m. - iris.

frequent - agar., asar., chen-a., cina, daph., ***euphr.,*** hep., iod., lact., laur., lyc., ***puls.,*** ruta., samb., ***seneg.,*** sep., sil., ***stann.,*** sulph., verat.

frothy - ***acon.,*** alet., all-c., am-c., ant-t., ***apis,*** aral., arg-n., ***arn.,*** **ARS.,** asc-t., atro., bufo, calc., canth., cench., chlor., cob., cub., daph., dios., dros., eucal., ***ferr.,*** ferr-p., fl-ac., hep., hura, ***kali-i.,*** kali-p., lach., led., mill., nat-m., nux-v., oena., op., paull., petr., ***phos.,*** plb., ***puls.,*** rumx., sec., sil., stict., stram., sulph., ter., thuj., uran., urt-u., zinc.

blood and mucus, containing - op.

containing, threads like fine twine - croc.

morning - cub., dios., sulph., thuj.

8 a.m. - dios.

9 a.m. - cub.

gelatinous, (see viscid) - agar., ***alumn.,*** **ARG-M.,** ***arg-n.,*** arn., bar-c., bry., ***cact.,*** chin., chin-s., cupr., cur., dig., ***ferr., kali-bi.,*** kreos., laur., med., **SAMB.,** ***sil.,*** sulph., viol-o.

glairy - ***arn.,*** carb-h., **NAT-M.,** ***nat-s.***

globular - agar., ***alumn.,*** am-m., ant-t., arg-m., ***bad.,*** calad., calc., calc-f., ***chel.,*** chin-b., coc-c., ***kali-c.,*** mang., rhus-t., sel., sil., **STANN.,** thuj.

granular - agar., ***bad., calc., chin.,*** hyper., ***kali-bi.,*** lach., lyc., mang., mez., ***phos.,*** sel., sep., ***sil.,*** spong., thuj.

morning 3 to 4 a.m. or 4 to 11 p.m. - lyc.

offensive - ***sil.***

sneezing, while - mez.

grayish - am-p., **AMBR.,** anac., ant-s., **ARG-M.,** ***ars.,*** arum-t., benz-ac., bufo, cahin., ***calc.,*** calc-i., calc-p., calen., cann-s., carb-an., ***carb-v.,*** chel., chin., ***cina,*** coc-c., cop., cur., dig., dros., dulc., eupi., ferr-ac., ham., iod., ***kali-bi.,*** kali-c., ***kali-i.,*** kali-m., kali-s., kalm., kaol., ***kreos.,*** lac-ac., lach., **LYC.,** mag-m., mang., med., merc-c., nat-a., nat-c., nat-m., ***nat-s., nux-v., par.,*** petr., ***phos.,*** psor., ***puls.,*** rhus-t., ***seneg., sep.,*** sol-t-ae., spong., **STANN.,** sulph., syph., tab., tep., ***thuj.***

EXPECTORATION, mucous

greenish - anan., ***arg-m., arn., ars.,*** ars-i., arum-t., asaf., aur., benz-ac., bor., bov., bry., bufo, cahin., ***calc.,*** **CALC-SIL.,** ***calc-s., cann-s., carb-an.,*** **CARB-S., CARB-V.,** coc-c., colch., ***coloc., cop., crot-c.,*** cub., cur., dig., dros., ***dulc.,*** eupi., ***ferr., ferr-ar.,*** ferr-i., ***ferr-p.,*** ham., hyos., iod., kali-ar., **KALI-BI.,** kali-c., **KALI-I.,** kali-p., ***kali-s.,*** kreos., led., **LYC.,** mag-c., ***mang.,*** med., **MERC.,** ***merc-i-f., merc-i-r., nat-c.,*** nat-m., nat-p., **NAT-S.,** nit-ac., nux-v., oena., ol-j., ox-ac., **PAR.,** ***petr.,*** **PHOS.,** plb., **PSOR., PULS.,** raph., rhus-t., ***sep., sil.,*** **STANN., SULPH.,** syph., thuj., ***tub.,*** zinc.

evening, lying down, while - ***psor.***

morning - ars., crot-c., ***ferr., lyc.,*** mang., nat-m., ***nit-ac., par., psor., sil., stann.***

7 to 10 a.m. - sil.

waking, on - ferr., ***psor.***

hard - agar., am-m., ant-c., bry., calad., ***con.,*** dig., fago., iod., kali-bi., kali-c., kreos., lach., mang., **NAT-C.,** nat-s., ox-ac., phos., sep., ***sil., spong., stann.,*** staph., stront-c., sulph., sul-i., thuj.

hawked, up, mucus - agar., all-c., ***alum.,*** am-c., am-m., ant-c., ***ant-t.,*** aphis., bism., calc., caps., carb-an., ***carb-v., caust., cham.,*** cina, con., croc., crot-t., dros., **EUPHR.,** ferr-i., ferr-ma., hep., iod., ***kali-bi.,*** kali-c., lach., lam., laur., ***lyc.,*** meph., naja, ***nat-m., nux-v.,*** ol-an., osm., ox-ac., ***par.,*** petr., ph-ac., ***phos., plat.,*** plb., rhod., rhus-t., **RUMX.,** ***sel., seneg., sep., sil.,*** sulph., ***stann.,*** tarax., thuj.

bloody - am-c., cham., ferr., hyper., kali-n.

morning - ant-t., ***nat-m., sel.***

water - **GELS.**

house, in the - calc-s.

impossible, (see swallow, difficult)

infrequent - acon., alum., arn., bell., caps., ign.

jelly-like, (see gelatinous)

liquids, contact of, at back part of mouth. from - am-caust.

liver, colored like - graph., lyc., puls., sep., stann.

lumpy - acon., agar., ail., aloe, am-m., arg-n., ***arn.,*** ars., bor., bry., calad., **CALC-S.,** carb-ac., carb-v., cet., chel., cob., coca, coc-c., colch., coll., dig., ***hep., hydr.,*** indg., kali-ar., ***kali-bi., kali-c.,*** kreos., lac-d., lach., lyc., mang., nat-a., nat-m., osm., ox-ac., par., phos., puls., ***sel.,*** **SIL.,** sin-n., sol-t-ae., spong., sulph., thuj., verat., wies.

evening - kreos.

lump, like core of boil - ment.

morning - carb-ac., cob., lyc., mang., nat-a.

9 a.m. - cob.

smoke-colored lumps, streaked with blood - kali-c.

masses, in - ars., coc-c., kali-n., sin-n.

membranous - alum-sil., ***brom., calc-ac.,*** chin-s., hep., ip., ***kali-bi.,*** kali-n., ***merc-c.,*** **SPONG.**

EXPECTORATION, mucous

milky - am-c., ***ars.***, aur., carb-v., ferr., **KALI-CHL.**, phos., plb., puls., ***sep.***, ***sil.***, ***sulph.***, zinc.

morning - acal., acon., ***agar.***, ail., ***all-s.***, ***alum.***, ***alumn.***, ambr., ***am-c.***, am-m., ***ang.***, ***ant-c.***, **ANT-T.**, apis, aral., aran., arn., ars., arund., aur., bar-c., bar-m., bell., bor., **BRY.**, bufo, ***calc.***, calc-p., calc-s., caps., carb-ac., carb-an., ***carb-s.***, **CARB-V.**, ***caust.***, chel., cimx., cina, cob., coc-c., colch., crot-t., cub., cupr., ***dig.***, dios., dros., euph., ***euphr.***, ***ferr.***, ferr-ar., ferr-i., ***ferr-p.***, fl-ac., **HEP.**, hipp., hyos., ign., ind., iod., ip., kali-ar., kali-c., ***kali-i.***, kali-p., kali-s., kreos., lac-ac., lach., led., lyc., ***mag-c.***, mag-m., ***mang.***, meph., mez., mur-ac., nat-a., nat-c., ***nat-m.***, ***nat-p.***, nat-s., ***nit-ac.***, nux-v., ol-j., **PAR.**, phel., ***ph-ac.***, **PHOS.**, phyt., psor., **PULS.**, rheum, rhod., ***rhus-t.***, sanic., sel., seneg., **SEP.**, **SIL.**, sol-t-ae., spong., **SQUIL.**, ***stann.***, staph., stront-c., **SULPH.**, **SUL-AC.**, tab., ***thuj.***, verat., zinc., zing.

8 to 9 a.m. - sil.

8:30 a.m. - spong.

9 a.m. - cob., phyt.

after - chin-s., coca, mag-m., ***puls.***, sep., sulph.

bath, after - calc-s.

bed, in - ***calc.***, ferr., nit-ac.

rising, on - calc., ferr., ***phos.***, **PULS.**

rising, after - chin-s., iod., mag-m., sulph.

waking, after - ***agar.***, aur., carb-v., lyc., psor., ***sulph.***, thuj.

mucus, in the air passages (see Expectoration, general)

muddy-like, pus, flies like batter - phos.

night - agar., alum., am-m., arn., ars., bell., calc., calc-s., carb-s., carb-v., ***caust.***, chin-s., coc-c., cycl., dulc., euphr., ferr., ferr-ar., gamb., hep., kali-c., kali-s., led., lyc., mag-aust., meli., mez., op., phos., puls., pyrog., raph., rhod., rhus-t., sabad., **SEP.**, sil., ***staph.***, sulph.

2 a.m., after - phos.

3 a.m. - op.

bed, in - sulph.

midnight, after - ***led.***

before, on getting into bed - ***sep.***

noon - bell., calc-s., sil.

noon to 3 p.m. - calc-s.

odor, general

burnt - cycl., dros., nux-v., puls., ran-b., sabad., squil., sulph.

fetid - arn., ars., bell., bor., bry., ***calc.***, ***caps.***, carb-ac., carb-v., cocc., cop., euphr., ferr., ***guai.***, kali-c., kali-p., led., lyc., mag-c., nat-c., nit-ac., ph-ac., ***phel.***, phos., ***pix.***, psor., puls., sac-alb., ***sang.***, sep., sil., stann., sulph., thuj.

garlic, like - ars.

herbaceous - ph-ac.

milky - aur., dros., phos., sep., spong.

musty - **BOR.**, jug-c.

EXPECTORATION, mucous

odor, general

offensive - alum., all-s., ***arn.***, **ARS.**, asaf., asar., aur., bell., **BOR.**, bry., **CALC.**, ***caps.***, ***carb-an.***, carb-s., carb-v., caust., cham., chin., chin-a., con., cop., ***cupr.***, dig., dirc., dros., euphr., eupi., fago., ferr., ferr-ar., ferr-i., ferr-p., graph., **GUAI.**, hep., hura, ign., iod., kali-c., kali-i., ***kali-p.***, kreos., led., **LYC.**, mag-c., mag-m., merc., **NAT-A.**, **NAT-C.**, nat-m., ***nat-p.***, ***nit-ac.***, nux-v., **PHEL.**, ***ph-ac.***, ***pix.***, ***psor.***, puls., pyrog., ***rhus-t.***, sabin., sac-alb., **SANG.**, seneg., ***sep.***, ***sil.***, squil., **STANN.**, sulph., thuj., zinc.

old catarrh, of an - ***bell.***, ***ign.***, mez., ***puls.***, sabin., ***sulph.***, zinc.

sour - calc., cham., dulc., kali-c., merc., nit-ac., nux-v., sulph., sul-ac.

sweetish - squil.

violets, of - phos., puls.

oleaginous - petr.

opaque - chin-s., **KALI-CHL.**

painful - ars., cub., elaps, merc-c.

as if from heart - elaps.

pale - kali-bi., lycps.

pasty - kali-bi.

phosphorescent - phos.

pieces, in - alum., nit-ac., rhus-t., sep.

prune, juice, like - ***ars.***

purulent - acet-ac., acon., agar., ail., all-s., am-c., ammc., ***anac.***, anan., ***ant-t.***, arg-m., ***arn.***, ***ars.***, ars-i., asaf., asc-t., aur., ***bac.***, ***bals-p.***, bar-c., bell., **BLATTA**, brom., bry., bufo, **CALC.**, calc-p., ***calc-s.***, calc-sil., ***carb-an.***, ***carb-s.***, carb-v., cham., ***chin.***, ***chin-a.***, cic., ***cimx.***, cina, cocc., ***cod.***, **CON.**, cop., cupr., ***dig.***, ***dros.***, dulc., ***ery-a.***, eucal., ***ferr.***, ferr-ar., ferr-i., ferr-p., gels., graph., guai., hep., hepat., ***hydr.***, hyos., ign., ill., iod., ip., kali-ar., kali-bi., **KALI-C.**, kali-i., ***kali-n.***, ***kali-p.***, ***kali-s.***, kalm., ***kreos.***, lach., laur., led., **LYC.**, mag-c., mag-m., ***merc.***, myos., myrt-c., **NAT-A.**, ***nat-c.***, nat-m., nat-p., nat-s., ***nit-ac.***, nux-m., nux-v., oena., op., ***ph-ac.***, **PHOS.**, ***pix.***, ***plb.***, psor., ptel., ***puls.***, ***rhus-t.***, ruta, sabin., samb., sang., sang-n., sec., **SEP.**, **SIL.**, sol-n., squil., ***stann.***, ***staph.***, stront-c., ***sulph.***, syph., ter., tril., tub., verat., zinc., zinc-s.

ropy - all-s., alumn., **ANT-T.**, apis, ***coc-c.***, **HYDR.**, ip., **KALI-BI.**, ***lach.***, lob., med., ***merc.***, ***nat-s.***, rumx., ***seneg.***, stict., viol-o.

rusty - ***acon.***, arn., ***ars.***, atro., **BRY.**, **LYC.**, **PHOS.**, pyrog., ***rhus-t.***, ***sang.***, ***squil.***

saliva, like - ars., astac., eug., med., merc., mez., thuj.

scabs, coughed up every few weeks - ferr.

scanty - acon., ail., alum., alumn., am-m., ***ant-t.***, apis, apoc., ars., asc-t., brom., bry., calc-s., ***caust.***, cham., cimic., clem., cupr., dig., ery-a., ***ferr.***, ferr-p., ign., kali-bi., kali-c., lach., lyc., mez., morph., nit-ac., ***nux-v.***, op., paeon.,

EXPECTORATION, mucous
scanty - **PHOS.,** phyt., ***puls.,*** rumx., samb., sang., sep., sil., spong., squil., **STANN.,** stict., tarent., thyr., zinc.
sea, bathing, after - mag-m.
side, is easier after turning from left to right - ars., kali-c., lyc., ***phos., rumx., sep., thuj.***
sit, up, must, at night to raise - ferr.
sitting, up, in bed, on - ***phos.***
epidemics, like dead - merc-c.
slate, colored - kali-bi., nat-a.
soap, suds, like - kali-i., kali-p.
soap-like - arg-n., ph-ac.
starch, like - ***agar., arg-n.,*** bar-c., cact., coca, dig., laur., nat-a., ***phyt., sel.,*** sulph.
stringy - aesc., agar., alum., **ALUMN.,** ***arg-m.,*** ars-i., arum-t., asaf., calc-s., ***caust.,*** chin-s., cimic., ***coc-c.,*** ery-a., ferr., ***hydr.,*** iber., **KALI-BI.,** ***lach.,*** lob., ***phos.,*** rumx., ruta., **SANG.,** sanic., seneg., stict.
swallow, must, what has been loosened - ambr., ***arn.,*** calad., ***cann-s.,*** **CAUST.,** chr-ac., coca, **CON.,** dig., dros., eug., gels., iod., ***kali-c.,*** **KALI-S.,** lach., lyc., mur-ac., ***nux-m.,*** osm., rumx., seneg., ***sep., spong., staph.,*** zinc., zing.
syrup, like - carb-an.
taste, general
almonds, like - caust., dig.
bad - carb-an., lach., lycps., nat-m., puls., sep.
bilious - puls.
bitter - acon., ail., arn., ***ars.,*** bry., calc., canth., **CHAM.,** chin., chin-a., ***cist.,*** coloc., con., ***dros.,*** ign., kali-ar., kali-bi., kali-c., kali-n., med., ***merc.,*** nat-a., nat-c., nat-m., ***nit-ac., nux-v.,*** **PULS.,** pyrog., sabad., ***sep.,*** stann., sulph., ***verat.***
boiled, cabbage, like - sulph.
burnt - ang., bry., dros., nux-v., ***puls.,*** rhus-t., squil., sulph., zinc.
catarrh, of an old - ***bell., ign.,*** mez., nux-v., phos., **PULS.,** sabin., ***sulph.,*** zinc.
chalk, like - ign., nux-v.
cheese, like old - ***chin., kali-c., lyc.,*** phos., ***thuj.,*** zinc.
putrid cheese - aur., kali-c., phos., zinc.
clay, like - cann-s., chin., phos., puls.
copper, like - cupr., kali-c., lach., nat-m.
earthy - ars., caps., chin., ferr., hep., ign., mang., merc., nux-m., phos., puls., stront.
eggs, like bad - acon., arn., carb-v., con., eupi., graph., hep., merc., mez., mur-ac., ph-ac., phos., sep., stann., sulph.
like yolk of - kali-c., ph-ac., phos., sep., staph., sulph., thuj.
fish, like - acon.
flat - alum., am-m., anac., ***ant-c.,*** ant-t., arg-m., arn., ars., aur., aur-s., bell., ***bry., calc.,*** cann-s., caps., ***chin.,*** chin-a., cop., euphr., ***ign.,*** ip., kali-ar., kali-c., kreos., ***lyc.,*** nat-a., nat-c., nat-m., nat-p., nat-s., op., ***par.,*** petr., ph-ac., phos., puls., rhus-t.,

EXPECTORATION, mucous
taste, general
flat - sabad., sabin., sep., stann., ***staph.,*** stront-c., sulph., thuj.
greasy - alum., ***asaf.,*** **CAUST.,** cham., fl-ac., kali-c., lyc., ***mag-m.,*** mang., merc-c., mur-ac., petr., phos., **PULS.,** rhus-t., sarr., ***sil.,*** thuj.
herbaceous - calad., gels., ***nux-v., ph-ac.,*** puls., sars., stann., verat.
herring, like - anac., nux-m.
leather, like that of russian - arn.
meal, like - lach.
meat, like - ars., bell., bry., carb-v., dulc., kali-c., lach., nit-ac., phos., puls., rhus-t.
broth, like - iod.
metallic - agn., alum., ***calc.,*** cench., cocc., ***cupr., ferr.,*** hep., ***ip.,*** kali-bi., kali-c., kreos., lach., merc., nat-c., nat-m., nux-v., ran-b., ***rhus-t.,*** sars., seneg., sulph., zinc.
milky - phos.
musty - **BOR.,** led., lyc., merc., ph-ac., rhus-t., teucr., thuj.
nauseous - ***ars.,*** asaf., bry., calc., canth., carb-an., chin., cina, cocc., coc-c., cop., dig., ***dros.,*** ferr., ferr-ar., iod., ***ip.,*** kali-ar., kali-c., led., ***merc.,*** nat-m., nit-ac., nux-v., phos., psor., **PULS.,** sabad., samb., sel., sep., sil., squil., ***stann.,*** sulph., tarent., zinc.
onions, like - ars., ***asaf.,*** mag-m., petr., sulph., sul-ac.
oranges, like - phos.
peach, kernels, like - laur.
peas, raw, like - puls., zinc.
pepper, like - acon., ars., mez., sabad., sulph.
putrid - acon., all-s., alum., ***arn., ars.,*** ars-i., bell., bov., bry., ***calc.,*** carb-an., carb-s., ***carb-v.,*** caust., ***cham.,*** cocc., con., cupr., dig., dros., dulc., ferr., ferr-i., ferr-p., ham., hep., iod., ip., ***kali-ar.,*** kali-c., kalm., kreos., lach., led., lyc., merc., ***nat-a., nat-c.,*** nat-p., nit-ac., nux-v., ph-ac., phos., ***puls.,*** rhus-t., samb., sarr., sep., sil., ***stann.,*** staph., sulph., verat., zinc.
rancid - alum., ambr., asaf., bar-c., bry., caust., cham., ip., lach., merc., mur-ac., nux-v., petr., phos., puls., thuj.
salty - acon., agar., alum., ***ambr.,*** am-c., ang., ant-t., aral., **ARS.,** ars-i., bar-c., bell., bov., ***calc., cann-s.,*** carb-s., ***carb-v., chin.,*** chin-a., cocc., coc-c., coloc., con., cop., dros., euph., ***graph.,*** hyos., iod., kali-bi., ***kali-i.,*** kali-p., kalm., lac-ac., lach., lepi., **LYC.,** ***mag-c.,*** mag-m., ***merc., merc-c.,*** mez., ***nat-c., nat-m.,*** nat-p., nit-ac., ***nux-m.,*** nux-v., ***ph-ac.,*** **PHOS.,** plan., psor., **PULS.,** raph., rhus-t., sac-alb., samb., **SEP.,** sil., spong., squil., ***stann.,*** staph., sulph., sul-ac., tarax., tarent., ther., tub., verat., wies.
morning - ***ph-ac.***
sea-weed, like - spong.
smoky - bry., nux-v., puls., rhus-t., sep.
soapy - bar-c., dulc., iod., merc.

EXPECTORATION, mucous
taste, general
sour - ***ambr.,*** ang., ant-t., ars., ***bell.,*** bry., **CALC.,** cann-s., carb-an., carb-v., cham., chin., coc-c., con., crot-t., dros., ferr., graph., hep., hyos., ign., iod., ip., kali-ar., ***kali-c.,*** kali-n., lach., laur., lyc., mag-c., mag-m., mag-s., ***merc.,*** nat-c., nat-m., nit-ac., **NUX-V.,** petr., ph-ac., **PHOS.,** plan., plb., ***puls.,*** rhus-t., sabin., sep., spong., stann., ***sulph.,*** sul-ac., tarax., verat.
sulphur, like - cocc., nux-v., ph-ac., phos., plb., sulph.
sweetish - acon., alum., am-c., anac., ant-s., ant-t., apis, ars., ars-i., asar., astac., aur., **CALC.,** calc-s., cann-s., canth., carb-an., chin., cob., cocc., coc-c., cop., ***dig.,*** dirc., ferr., ferr-ar., hep., hepat., iod., ip., iris, kali-ar., kali-bi., ***kali-c.,*** kali-n., kali-p., kreos., laur., lyc., lycps., mag-c., mag-m., merc., mez., nux-v., **PHOS.,** ***plb.,*** ptel., ***puls.,*** rhus-t., ***sabad.,*** samb., sang-n., ***sanic.,*** sel., senec., sep., ***squil.,*** **STANN.,** sulph., sul-ac., sumb., tub., zinc.
tar, like - con.
tobacco, juice, like - ***puls.***
urine, like - graph., phos., seneg.
wine, like - bell., bry.
wood, like - ars., ign., stram., sulph.
thick - acon., agar., aloe, ***alumn.,*** ambr., am-m., ***ant-t., arg-m.,*** **ARG-N.,** ***ars.,*** atro., aur-m., **BLATTA,** bry., ***cact., calc.,*** calc-s., carb-ac., carb-an., ***caust.,*** chlor., ***cist.,*** cob., ***coc-c., cycl., dulc.,*** ery-a., eucal., eupi., ferr., ferr-ar., ferr-i., ferr-p., glon., ham., **HEP.,** hura, **HYDR.,** iod., ip., **KALI-BI.,** kali-chl., kali-p., kalm., kreos., ***lac-c.,*** laur., ***lyc.,*** mag-m., merc-i-r., naja, nat-p., oena., ol-j., op., ox-ac., phos., ***phyt., puls.,*** pyrog., raph., ruta., sac-alb., sang., senec., seneg., ***sep.,*** **SIL.,** squil., ***stann.,*** stram., sulph., syph., tarent., thuj., **TUB.,** ust., vario., zinc.
afternoon - eucal.
evening - kreos., sulph.
morning - agar., lyc., ***phos., puls., sil.,*** **STANN.,** sulph., tarent., thuj.
rising, after - ***phos.,*** puls., sulph.
waking, after - lyc.
night - calc., ***cycl.,*** lyc., sac-alb.
thin - acon., all-s., am-c., ant-c., bry., colch., cupr., daph., ***ferr.,*** gels., iber., kali-n., mag-c., sac-alb.
tough - aesc., acon., agn., ***all-c., alumn.,*** ambr., anac., ant-c., ***ant-t.,*** atro., ***ars.,*** ars-i., aur., bell., bov., ***bry.,*** **CALC.,** ***cann-s.,*** canth., carl., ***carb-an.,*** carb-v., ***caust.,*** cham., cist., cob., cocc., ***coc-c.,*** cupr., ***dulc.,*** euphr., **HEP.,** indg., ***iod.,*** iris, **KALI-BI.,** kali-c., ***lac-c.,*** mag-c., mag-m., mang., merc-i-r., mez., nux-m., nux-v., par., petr., ph-ac., phos., phyt., puls., ***rumx.,*** ruta., samb., sang., sanic., senec., seneg., ***sep.,*** sil., spong., squil., **STANN.,** staph., tarent., thuj., verat., vinc., ***zinc.***

EXPECTORATION, mucous
tough,
morning - calc., ***cann-s.,*** **KALI-BI.,** petr., ***phos.,*** phyt., sars., ***sil.***
9 a.m. - phyt.
bed, in - calc.
transparent - agar., alum., alumn., am-c., am-m., ant-t., ***apis,*** **ARG-M.,** arn., ***ars.,*** asaf., ***bar-c.,*** bor., bry., calc-s., ***caust.,*** chin., ***ferr., kali-bi.,*** kali-m., kreos., laur., ***med., mez.,*** **NAT-M.,** petr., ***ph-ac.,*** **PHOS.,** puls., ***sel.,*** senec., **SENEG.,** ***sil., stann.,*** sulph.
morning - sel.
tubercles, discharge from - hep., mag-c., ***phos., sil., spong.***
discharge, brown - phos.
offensive - mag-c., phos., sil.
viscid - acet-ac., acon., ***agar.,*** agn., ail., ***all-c.,*** all-s., aloe, alum., **ALUMN.,** ***ambr., am-br.,*** am-m., ammc., anac., ant-c., ant-s., ant-t., aral., **ARG-M., ARG-N.,** ***ars.,*** ars-i., asar., asc-t., aspar., aur., ***bad.,*** bals-p., ***bar-c.,*** bar-m., bell., bor., ***bov., bry.,*** bufo, ***cact., calc.,*** calc-s., ***cann-s.,*** canth., carb-ac., ***carb-s., carb-v., caust., cham.,*** chin., chin-a., cimic., cob., coca, **COC-C.,** colch., ***cupr.,*** dig., ***dulc.,*** eucal., euphr., ferr., ferr-ar., ***ferr-i.,*** ferr-p., graph., grin., hell., **HEP., HYDR.,** hyper., iber., indg., ***iod.,*** jug-c., kali-ar., **KALI-BI.,** ***kali-c.,*** kali-m., kali-p., kali-s., kreos., lac-ac., ***lac-c.,*** lach., laur., lyc., mag-c., mag-m., mang., med., merc., ***merc-c.,*** merc-sul., ***mez.,*** morph., myrt-c., naja, naphtin., ***nat-a.,*** nat-c., nat-m., nat-p., nat-s., ***nit-ac., nux-v.,*** oena., ***olnd.,*** onos., op., osm., ***paeon., par.,*** petr., ph-ac., **PHOS.,** ***phyt.,*** plb., ***psor.,*** **PULS.,** ***pyrog.,*** quillaya, rhus-t., ***rumx.,*** ruta, sabad., sabin., **SAMB.,** sang., sang-n., sec., **SENEG.,** ***sep., sil.,*** silphu., spig., ***spong.,*** squil., **STANN.,** ***staph.,*** sulph., sul-ac., tep., thuj., tub., ust., verat., wies., ***zinc.***
while - cham., merc., nat-m., sul-ac., zinc.
walking, while - cham., merc., nat-m., sul-ac., tub., zinc.
after - ferr.
watery - acon., agar., all-c., am-c., am-m., ang., ***ant-a.,*** arg-m., ***ars.,*** bell., bov., bry., carb-an., ***carb-v.,*** cham., chin., croc., ***daph.,*** euphr., ferr., ferr-p., ***graph.,*** grin., guai., jac-c., ***kali-i., kali-s., lach.,*** lyc., ***mag-c.,*** mag-m., ***merc.,*** mez., mur-ac., nat-c., ***nat-m.,*** nux-v., oena., op., phos., phys., piloc., plb., puls., ran-s., rumx., sac-alb., sep., silphu., squil., ***stann.,*** sulph., sul-ac., tanac., thuj., tub.
white - ***acon.,*** ail., ***agar.,*** alum., ***alumn.,*** ambr., ***am-br.,*** am-c., am-m., **ANT-T.,** ***apis,*** apoc., ***arg-m.,*** arn., ***ars.,*** arund., aur-m., bar-c., ***bor.,*** bov., ***calc.,*** calc-s., caps., carb-ac., carb-an., ***carb-v., caust.,*** cench., chin., chin-a., chin-s., chlor., cina, cob., ***coc-c.,*** crot-t., cupr., cur., dulc., eucal., ferr., ferr-ar., ferr-i., ferr-p., fl-ac., hyper., ***iod.,*** ip., ***kali-bi.,*** **KALI-CHL.,** kali-i., kali-p., ***kreos., lac-c.,***

EXPECTORATION, mucous
white - laur., **LYC.**, manc., ***med.***, merc-i-r., mez., **NAT-M.**, nicc., oena., ol-j., onos., ox-ac., par., petr., ph-ac., **PHOS.**, phys., ***puls.***, puls-n, raph., rhus-t., sac-alb., sang., ***sel.***, senec., **SENEG.**, **SEP.**, sil., ***spong.***, ***squil.***, ***stann.***, stront-c., ***sulph.***, syph., tarent., tell., thuj.
albuminous - ***agar.***, alum., **ALUMN.**, am-c., am-m., ant-t., ***apis***, **ARG-M.**, arn., ***ars.***, asaf., ***bar-c.***, bor., bov., bry., calc-s., ***caust.***, chin., **COC-C.**, cur., ***ferr.***, ip., ***kali-bi.***, ***laur.***, ***med.***, ***mez.***, **NAT-M.**, ***nat-s.***, petr., ***ph-ac.***, **PHOS.**, ***sel.***, **SENEG.**, ***sil.***, ***stann.***, sulph.
daytime - ***arg-m.***, ***stann.***
eating, after - sil.
evening - ***arg-n.***, calc-s., crot-t.
morning - ***agar.***, ***alumn.***, carb-v., **KALI-BI.**, ***nat-m.***, ***phos.***, puls., ***sulph.***
night - sep.
opaque - **KALI-BI.**
yellow - ***acon.***, ail., aloe, alum., ambr., am-c., ***am-m.***, anac., anan., ***ang.***, ant-c., arg-m., ***arg-n.***, ***ars.***, ***ars-i.***, arum-m., arum-t., asc-t., astac., aur., aur-m., aur-s., ***bad.***, bar-c., bar-m., bell., bism., **BLATTA,** bor., bov., brom., ***bry.***, bufo, ***cact.***, **CALC.**, **CALC-P.**, **CALC-S.**, cann-s., ***canth.***, carb-an., carb-s., ***carb-v.***, caust., cench., cham., chlol., cic., cist., coca, ***coc-c.***, coloc., con., cop., cub., cupr., cur., daph., dig., ***dros.***, eug., eupi., ferr., ferr-ar., ferr-i., ***ferr-p.***, graph., ham., **HEP.**, hura, **HYDR.**, hydr-ac., ***ign.***, iod., ip., kali-ar., ***kali-bi.***, ***kali-c.***, ***kali-chl.***, ***kali-p.***, **KALI-S.**, ***kreos.***, lac-ac., lach., linu-c., **LYC.**, mag-c., mag-m., mang., med., ***merc.***, merc-i-f., ***merc-i-r.***, mez., mur-ac., ***nat-a.***, ***nat-c.***, nat-m., ***nat-p.***, ***nit-ac.***, nux-v., oena., ***ol-j.***, op., ox-ac., par., ***petr.***, ***ph-ac.***, **PHOS.**, phyt., plb., ***psor.***, **PULS.**, pyrog., rumx., ***ruta.***, sabad., sac-alb., samb., sang., ***sanic.***, sel., senec., seneg., **SEP.**, **SIL.**, spig., ***spong.***, **STANN.**, ***staph.***, ***sulph.***, sul-ac., syph., tarent., ***thuj.***, **TUB.**, verat., ***zinc.***
afternoon - anac., calc-s.
12 to 3 p.m. - calc-s.
forenoon - staph.
lemon colored - kali-c., lyc., phos., puls.
morning - ail., aur., ***calc.***, ***calc-p.***, cench., ***kali-bi.***, lyc., mag-c., mang., ***phos.***, ***ph-ac.***, **PULS.**, ***sil.***, **STANN.**, tarent.
7 to 10 a.m. - sil.
waking, on - aur.
night - staph.
orange colored - ***kali-c.***, phos., puls.
yellowish-white - ambr.

GANGRENE, of - arn., **ARS.**, ***caps.***, carb-ac., ***carb-an.***, ***carb-v.***, ***chin.***, crot-h., dulc., eucal., hep., **KREOS.**, ***lach.***, lyc., lyss., osm., ***phos.***, ***plb.***, sil., sul-ac., sec., tarent.

HARD body, and small, right, as if - abies-c.

HEPATIZATION - ant-t., ***brom.***, ***cact.***, calc-s., ***camph.***, ***chel.***, ferr., ***iod.***, ***kali-c.***, ***kali-chl.***, ***kali-i.***, kali-p., ***lach.***, ***lob.***, ***lyc.***, merc., ***nux-v.***, op., **PHOS.**, ***sang.***, **SULPH.**, ***ter.***, ***tub.***
left - ***lach.***, ***lyc.***, ***myrt-c.***, phos., ***sulph.***
lying on, back agg. - ***phos.***
left side, agg. - **PHOS.**
right side, agg. - kali-c., ***merc.***
right side, amel. - **PHOS.**
right - ***kali-c.***, **KALI-I.**, ***phos.***
upper right half - ***chel.***

HOT breath, (see Breath, hot)

INFLAMMATION, lungs, (see Pneumonia)
inflammation, bronchials, (see Bronchitis)
inflammation, pleura, (see Pleurisy)

IRRITATION, in air passages - **ACON.**, ***agar.***, agn., all-s., aloe, ***alum.***, am-br., am-c., am-m., aml-n., ***anac.***, ant-t., aspar., bar-c., cahin., ***calc.***, carb-ac., ***carb-s.***, ***carb-v.***, ***caust.***, **CHAM.**, chin-s., ***chlor.***, clem., coc-c., coff., colch., coll., ***con.***, crot-t., dios., ***gels.***, hyos., **IOD.**, **KALI-BI.**, ***kali-c.***, kali-i., **LACH.**, lob., lyc., mag-s., merc-i-r., mez., ***mosch.***, mur-ac., nat-a., nat-s., **NUX-V.**, osm., ox-ac., ***ph-ac.***, **PHOS.**, plan., psor., ***puls.***, raph., **SEP.**, ***stann.***, ***sulph.***, sul-ac.
afternoon - bapt.
cold air - acon., all-c., ***ars.***, ***bell.***, brom., bry., calc-p., ***carb-v.***, caust., cimic., cupr., fl-ac., **HEP.**, ip., ***kali-bi.***, kali-c., kali-p., ***lach.***, ***mang.***, naja, nux-v., osm., ox-ac., **PHOS.**, **RUMX.**, ***sil.***, spong., sulph.
evening - chel., cimic., dios., sulph.
7:30 p.m. - cimic.
bed, in - agn., am-c., coff., hyos., kali-c.
heated, when - **APIS.**
increases the more one coughs - cist., **IGN.**, raph., squil., teucr.
morning, rising after - alum., alumn.
night, on waking - thuj.

MEMBRANE - bufo.
sensation of on skin - lach., phos., thuj.

MOUNTAIN, sickness (see Emergency, Altitude)

MURMURS, lungs (see Chest or Heart) - agar., ***aml-n.***, ***apis***, ***ars.***, ***ars-i.***, aspar., ***aur.***, ***aur-m.***, bar-c., **CACT.**, ***calc.***, carb-ac., ***chel.***, chin-a., ***cocc.***, ***colch.***, **COLL.**, ***crot-h.***, cupr-s., **DIG.**, **FERR.**, ferr-ar., ferr-i., ***glon.***, hep., hydr-ac., ***hydr.***, iber., ***iod.***, ip., kali-ar., kali-br., ***kali-c.***, **KALM.**, ***Lach.***, ***lith.***, lob., ***lyc.***, ***lycps.***, ***merc.***, **NAJA,** nat-a., nat-c., ***nat-m.***, ***nit-ac.***, ***phos.***, plb., ***psor.***, puls., **RHUS-T.**, **SPIG.**, **SPONG.**, stann., stram., ***sumb.***, tab., tarent., tub.

NARROW, sensation of chest - mez., phos.

PAIN, lungs (see Chest, pains) - ***lyc.***, **PHOS.**, rumx., ***sulph.***, ***tub.***
apex - dol., guai., puls., tub.
inspiration agg. - cimic.
left - calc-s., ***con.***, med., myric., ther., tub.
right - **ARS.**, cimic.
right, extending to base of - cimic.

PAIN, lungs
left - **PHOS.**, sulph.
above nipple - **ARUM-T.**, **SULPH.**
apex and middle part - acon., am-c., ***anis.***, ant-s., crot-t., ill., ***lob-c.***, ***myrt-c.***, paeon., phos., ***pix.***, puls., ***ran-b.***, rumx., sil., spig., stann., stict., ***sulph.***, ***ther.***, tub., ust.
centre of - rumx.
evening agg. - ***sulph.***
lower part - agar., ampe-qu, asc-t., calc-p., cimic., ***lob-s.***, lyc., myos., ***nat-s.***, ***ox-ac.***, **PHOS.**, ***rumx.***, sil., squil.
right - bry., ***elaps***, echi., rumx., sulph.
apex and middle part - abies-c., ***ars.***, bor., ***calc.***, com., crot-t., ***elaps***, erio., ***ill.***, ***iodof.***, ***phel.***, sang., upa.
as if lobe were adhering to rib - ***kali-c.***
lower part - am-m., berb., bry., cact., card-m., ***chel.***, dios., kali-c., lyc., ***merc.***, xan.

PARALYSIS - am-c., ***am-m.***, ***ant-a.***, **ANT-T.**, ***arg-n.***, arn., ***ars.***, ars-i., bac., **BAR-C.**, ***calc.***, camph., **CARB-V.**, **CHIN.**, cupr., ***cur.***, diph., dulc., ***gels.***, ***grin.***, hydr-ac., ***iod.***, ip., kali-i., **LACH.**, ***laur.***, ***lob-p.***, **LYC.**, merc-cy., morph., ***mosch.***, op., ***phos.***, senec., ***stann.***
elderly people - ***ant-t.***, ***ars.***, **BAR-C.**, carb-v., **CHIN.**, lyc., op., phos.
left - asc-t.
scarlatina, in - ***calc.***
sensation of - lob.
left - med.

paralysis, diaphragm - arg-n., bell., cact., cimic., con., cupr., mosch., rhus-t., mez., sil.

PLEURISY - abrot., **ACON.**, ant-a., ant-t., ***apis***, ***arn.***, ***arg-n.***, ***ars.***, ars-i., arum-t., asc-t., bad., ***bell.***, ***bor.***, **BRY.**, ***cact.***, ***calc.***, ***cann-s.***, ***canth.***, **CARB-AN.**, ***carb-s.***, ***carb-v.***, card-m., ***chel.***, chin., ***colch.***, ***dig.***, ***dulc.***, erio., ferr-m., ***ferr-p.***, form., ***guai.***, ***hep.***, ***iod.***, ***kali-ar.***, **KALI-C.**, ***kali-chl.***, ***kali-i.***, kali-p., ***kali-s.***, ***laur.***, led., lob-c., ***merc.***, merc-d., ***mur-ac.***, nat-m., nat-s., ***nit-ac.***, op., ***phos.***, ***ran-b.***, rhus-t., sabad., ***sang.***, **SENEG.**, sep., sil., spig., ***squil.***, ***stann.***, **SULPH.**, sul-ac., tub., verat-v.
breathing, deep, agg. - ***bry.***, guai.
bright's disease, with - ars., ***merc-c.***
chronic - ars-i., bry., ***hep.***, ***iod.***, iodof., kali-c.
debility, paralytic, with - sabad.
elderly people - ***bry.***, kali-c., ***nit-ac.***
exudation - abrot., ferr., seneg.
left - ***kali-i.***
neglected - **ARS.**, ***ars-i.***, bry., ***calc.***, camph., canth., ***carb-v.***, chin., ferr., ***hep.***, ***iod.***, lach., lyc., ***nat-m.***, ***seneg.***, ***sep.***, ***sil.***, **SULPH.**
pleura-pneumonia - **ANT-T.**, ***asaf.***, **BRY.**, ***calc.***, ***camph.***, ***caps.***, ***chin.***, ***dulc.***, ***ferr.***, ***hep.***, ***iod.***, ***kali-i.***, ***lach.***, **PHOS.**, ***rhus-t.***, ***seneg.***, ***sulph.***
recurrent - guai.

PLEURISY,
rheumatic - acon., ***ant-t.***, ***arn.***, **BRY.**, ***dulc.***, nux-v., ran-b., rhod., rhus-t., sabad., ***sulph.***
right - bor., ***bry.***
tuberculosis patients, in - ***arg-n.***, ars-i., bry., ***calc.***, hep., ***iod.***, iodof., kali-c., ***seneg.***

PNEUMONIA - **ACON.**, aesc., ***agar.***, ***all-c.***, am-c., am-i, ant-a., ***ant-c.***, ant-s., **ANT-T.**, ***apis***, apom., ***arg-n.***, ***arn.***, **ARS.**, **ARS-I.**, aur-m., ***bad.***, bar-c., ***bell.***, ***benz-ac.***, ***brom.***, **BRY.**, ***cact.***, ***calc.***, camph., ***cann-s.***, canth., caps., carb-ac., ***carb-an.***, ***carb-s.***, **CARB-V.**, **CHEL.**, ***chin.***, ***chlor.***, ***con.***, cop., com., crot-h., ***cupr.***, ***dig.***, dulc., ***elaps***, ***ferr.***, ***ferr-ar.***, ***ferr-i.***, **FERR-P.**, ***gels.***, glyc., **HEP.**, ***hippoz.***, ***hyos.***, ***iod.***, ***ip.***, kali-ar., ***kali-bi.***, ***kali-br.***, ***kali-c.***, ***kali-chl.***, ***kali-i.***, ***kali-n.***, ***kali-p.***, ***kali-s.***, ***kreos.***, ***lach.***, ***lachn.***, ***laur.***, **LOB.**, **LYC.**, lycps., **MERC.**, ***mill.***, myrt-c., ***nat-m.***, ***nat-s.***, ***nit-ac.***, nux-v., op., ox-ac., ***ph-ac.***, **PHOS.**, podo., ***psor.***, **PULS.**, ***pyrog.***, ran-b., **RHUS-T.**, rumx., ***sabad.***, ***sang.***, **SENEG.**, **SEP.**, ***sil.***, spig., spong., ***squil.***, ***stram.***, stry., **SULPH.**, ***ter.***, urt-u., ***verat.***, **VERAT-V.**
aconite, after, abuse of - ***bry.***, sulph.
ailments since - kali-c., phos., tub.
alcoholics - ***hyos.***, ***kali-br.***, ***nux-v.***, ***op.***
bleeding, after - ***chin.***, ***ph-ac.***
catharrhal - ***ant-t.***, ***kali-s.***
cerebral type - acon., arn., bell., bry., cann-i., cann-s., canth., lach., merc., nux-v., phos., puls., rhus-t., stram., sulph.
chronic - carc., phos.
elderly persons - ant-a., ***ant-t.***, ars., ***bry.***, ***dig.***, ***ferr.***, ***hyos.***, ***nat-s.***, ***nit-ac.***, ***nux-v.***, ***op.***, phos., ***seneg.***
grief, after - ign.
infants - ***acon.***, **ANT-T.**, ***bry.***, ***ferr-p.***, **IP.**, ***kali-c.***, ***lob.***, ***lyc.***, ***merc.***, ***nux-v.***, op., **PHOS.**, ***sulph.***
infarcts - tub.
left, lung - ***acon.***, ***calc.***, ***lach.***, ***nat-s.***, ***ox-ac.***, **PHOS.**, ***sang.***, sulph.
lower lobe - ***chel.***, ***nat-s.***, sulph.
upper - ***acon.***
lie on the back, must - acon., ***cact.***, sulph.
lying on, back, amel. - acon., phos., sulph.
back, with head thrown back - phos.
right side agg. - ***kali-c.***
measles, after - ***kali-c.***
menses, before - senec.
suppressed - **PULS.**
neglected - am-c., ant-s., ***ant-t.***, ars-i., bry., ***carb-v.***, chin., hep., kali-i., lach., ***lob.***, **LYC.**, ***phos.***, plb., pyrog., ***sang.***, ***sep.***, **SIL.**, sul-i., **SULPH.**
pleura-pneumonia - **ANT-T.**, ***asaf.***, **BRY.**, ***calc.***, ***camph.***, ***caps.***, ***chin.***, ***dulc.***, ***ferr.***, ***hep.***, ***iod.***, ***kali-i.***, ***lach.***, **PHOS.**, ***rhus-t.***, ***seneg.***, ***sulph.***
right, lung - ars., ***bell.***, **BRY.**, ***brom.***, ***carb-an.***, ***chel.***, elaps, ***kali-c.***, kali-i., ***lyc.***, ***merc.***, ***phos.***, ***sang.***, squil., stram.
lower lobe - ***kali-c.***, ***merc.***, ***phos.***

PNEUMONIA,
right, upper lobe - **CALC.,** ***chel.***
secondary - ferr-p., phos.
stages, congestive - ***acon.,*** aesc., bell., ***ferr-p., iod.,*** sang., ***verat-v.***
consolidation - ant-t., ***bry., iod.,*** kali-i., kali-m., ***phos.,*** sang., sulph.
resolution - ant-s., ***ant-t.,*** ars., ars-i., carb-v., ***hep.,*** iod., kali-i., kali-s., ***lyc.,*** nat-s., ***phos., sang.,*** sil., ***sulph.***
sycotic, pneumonia - **NAT-S.**
typhoid - **ANT-T.,** ***bad., benz-ac.,*** **BRY.,** ***hyos.,*** lach., lachn., ***laur.,*** **LYC.,** merc-cy., ***nit-ac.,*** op., **PHOS.,** ***rhus-t., sang.,*** **SULPH.,** ***ter.***
weakness, from loss of fluids - ***chin.***

PULMONARY, edema - acet-ac., ***am-c.,*** **ANT-T., APIS, APOC., ARS.,** ***asaf., aspar., aur-i., aur-m.,*** **BRY.,** calc., ***canth., carb-s., carb-v.,*** chel., chin., chin-a., coch., **COLCH.,** ***crot-h.,*** crot-t., ***dig., dulc.,*** ferr-m., ***fl-ac.,*** **HELL.,** ***hyos., iod., ip.,*** jab., ***kali-ar.,*** **KALI-C.,** ***kali-i., kali-p.,*** **LACH.,** ***lact.,*** **LYC.,** ***merc.,*** **MERC-SUL.,** mez., mur-ac., ***nat-m.,*** op., ***phos., psor.,*** puls., ***ran-b.,*** rat., ***sang.,*** senec., ***seneg., sil., spig., squil.,*** stann., stroph., ***sulph., ter.,*** tub., uran., verat., ***zinc.***
alcoholics, in - crot-h.
sudden - rhus-t.

RAWNESS, pain, in air passages - ***acon., aesc., agar., all-c., all-s., alum., alumn.,*** am-caust., ***ambr.,*** am-c., anac., anan., apis, **ARG-M., ARG-N.,** arn., **ARS.,** ars-i., ***arum-t.,*** asar., ***bar-c., bell.,*** benz., bov., **BROM.,** ***bry.,*** bufo, ***calc., cann-s., carb-an.,*** carb-s., ***carb-v.,*** carl., ***caust.,*** **CHAM.,** chin., chin-a., ***chlor., cist., coc-c., coff.,*** dirc., dros., dulc., eup-per., ***gels.,*** graph., ***hep.,*** hydr-ac., ***hydr., iod., kali-bi.,*** kali-c., **KALI-I.,** kali-ma., kali-n., kali-per., ***kali-s.,*** kaol., kreos., **LACH.,** lac-ac., lact., laur., lec., lyc., mag-m., ***mag-p., mang.,*** med., ***merc.,*** **NAJA,** ***nat-m.,*** **NUX-V.,** ol-an., osm., ox-ac., phel., ***ph-ac.,*** **PHOS.,** ***puls., rhus-t.,*** **RUMX.,** ***samb., sang.,*** sars., ***seneg., sep., sil.,*** spong., ***stann., staph.,*** stront-c., **SULPH.,** ***tarent., zinc.***
coughing, from - ***coc-c.,*** phos., stann.

RESPIRATION, general, (see Breathing, chapter)

STUFFED up, as if, lungs with cotton, as if - kali-bi., med.

SUFFOCATIVE, (see Breathing, Difficult)

TICKLING, air passages, in - acet-ac., **ACON.,** ***alum., alumn., ambr.,*** am-c., am-m., anac., ang., ant-t., ***arg-m.,*** arg-n., ***arn.,*** ars., arum-t., ***asaf.,*** atro., aur-m., bar-c., bell., bov., ***brom., bry.,*** cahin., ***calc.,*** **CALC-F.,** calc-p., canth., ***carb-an.,*** carb-s., ***carb-v., caust.,*** **CHAM.,** chin., cimic., cina, ***coca,*** cocc., ***coc-c.,*** colch., coloc., **CON.,** ***cupr.,*** dig., ***dros., euphr., ferr.,*** ferr-i., ham., hep., **HYOS.,** ign., inul., ***iod.,*** **IP.,** iris, ***kali-bi.,*** **KALI-C.,** kali-ma., kali-n., kali-s., **LACH.,** lact., laur., led., **LYC.,** mag-c., mag-m., ***merc.,*** mur-ac., ***naja,*** nat-c., **NAT-M.,** nat-p., olnd., ol-an., ol-j., op., petr., ***ph-ac., phos.,*** prun., ***puls., rhus-t.,*** rumx., sabad., ***sabin.,*** **SANG.,** sars., ***seneg.,*** **SEP.,** ***sil., spong., squil., stann.,*** **STAPH.,** sulph., ***tab.,*** teucr., thuj., verat., zinc.
afternoon - naja.
2 p.m. - arg-n., **COC-C.**
3 p.m. - hep., naja
3 to 4 p.m. - calc-f.
air, draft of - merc.
in open - ***lach.,*** ox-ac., **PHOS.**
blood, taste of, with - ham.
daytime - coloc., ***euphr.,*** lyc., nat-m., staph.
daytime, and night - nat-m.
evening - alumn., ***bell.,*** bry., calc-p., ***caps., carb-v.,*** chin., chin-s., cimic., coloc., graph., **LYC.,** merc., nat-m., rhus-t., sulph.
6 p.m., expectoration of mucus, amel. - sulph.
bed, in - ***bell.,*** calc-p., ***caps.,*** graph., **SANG.**
falling asleep, before - merc.
going to sleep, on - ***carb-v.,*** lyc.
midnight, until - rhus-t.
forenoon - calc-f.
inspiring, on - brom., hipp.
lying, while - **HYOS.,** lac-c., ph-ac., seneg.
amel. - ***euphr.,*** **MANG.**
on left side - ***phos.***
morning - ***alumn.,*** cahin., ***carb-v.,*** coloc., **IOD.,** lyc., nat-m., ***op.,*** thuj.
rising, after - alumn., ***arn.***
waking, after - ***carb-v.***
night - am-c., arg-n., ***asaf., bry., calc.,*** coc-c., ***coloc., cycl., dros.,*** kali-bi., kali-c., lyc., mag-m., myric., nat-m., rhus-t., rumx., sanic., zinc.
2 a.m. - nat-m.
3 a.m. - ***am-c., bufo,*** cahin.
11:30 p.m. - **COC-C.**
midnight, after - chin-s.
smoking, from - atro., coloc.
talking, on - ***alum., alumn.,*** atro., ***hep., kali-bi.,*** lac-c., ***phos.***
throat-pit, in, from - **APIS,** aspar., bell., cann-s., caust., **CHAM.,** cinnb., cocc., coloc., ***con.,*** crot-h., ign., ***iod.,*** kreos., lac-c., lach., lith., mag-m., nat-c., nat-m., ph-ac., phos., ***puls.,*** rhus-r., **RUMX., SANG.,** ***sil.,*** squil., tarax.
tobacco - acon.
waking, on - carb-v., ham.
walking in open air - ***ox-ac.***
warm room - all-c., ambr., ***arn., brom., bry.,*** dig., **DROS., IOD.,** ***ip., lyc.,*** mez., ***nat-c.,*** **PULS.,** seneg., spong., sulph.

TUBERCLES - hep., mag-c., ***phos., sil., spong.***
discharge, brown - phos.
offensive - mag-c., phos., sil.

TUBERCULOSIS, lungs - acal., ***acet-ac.,*** acon., **AGAR.,** agarin., ***all-s.,*** ant-a., ant-t., ***ars., ars-i.,*** atro., aur-a., bac., bals-p., ***bapt., bar-m.,*** bell., blatta, ***brom., bry., bufo,*** **CALC.,** calc-ar., ***calc-i.,*** **CALC-P.,** ***calc-s.,*** calo., cann-s., ***carb-an., carb-s., carb-v.,*** card-m., ***chin-a.,*** chlor., cimic., coc-c., cod., ***con., crot-h.,*** cupr-ar., ***dros., dulc., elaps,*** erio., ferr-ac., ***ferr-ar., ferr-i.,*** ferr-m., ***ferr-p.,*** fl-ac., form., ***gall-ac., graph., guai.,*** ham., **HEP.,** hippoz., hydr., ichth., **IOD.,** iodof., ip., kali-ar., kali-bi., **KALI-C.,** ***kali-n., kali-p.,*** **KALI-S.,** ***kreos.,*** lac-ac., ***lac-d., lach., lachn.,*** laur., lec., led., **LYC.,** mang., ***med., merc.,*** mill., ***myos., myrt-c.,*** naphtin., nat-a., ***nat-m.,*** nat-s., ***nit-ac.,*** nux-v., ***ol-j.,*** ox-ac., petr., ***ph-ac., phel.,*** **PHOS.,** piloc., ***plb., polyg-a.,*** **PSOR., PULS.,** rumx., ruta, salv., samb., ***sang.,*** **SENEC.,** ***seneg., sep.,*** **SIL., SPONG., STANN.,** stict., ***still.,*** succ., **SULPH.,** sul-ac., teucr., thea., **THER., TUB.,** urea, vanad., **ZINC.**

- acute - ant-t., ***ars., bry.,*** calc., calc-i., ***chin., cimic.,*** dros., ***dulc.,*** ferr., ferr-ac., ferr-m., **FERR-P.,** ***hep.,*** iod., ***kali-chl.,*** kali-p., ***kreos.,*** lach., laur., ***med.,*** nat-m., ***phos.,*** **PULS.,** ***sang.,*** **SENEC., SIL.,** stann., ***sulph.,*** **THER.,** tub.
  - exacerbations in all stages of - ***kali-n.***
  - menses, suppressed, from - **SENEC.**
- bleedings, after - ***chin.***
- bones, of - ***dros.,*** phos., puls., stann.
- cold, damp weather - ***dulc.***
- elderly, people - ***nat-s.***
- fever, in - bapt., chin-a., ferr-p.
- florida - ***ferr.,*** med., nat-p., ***puls., sang.,*** **THER.**
- gonorrhea, after suppressed - **SEP.**
- incipient - acal., ***acet-ac., agar., ars-i., bry.,*** cact., **CALC.,** calc-i., **CALC-P.,** ***carb-v., dros., dulc., ferr.,*** ferr-p., **HEP., KALI-C.,** kali-i., **KALI-P.,** ***lach.,*** lachn., **LYC.,** ***lycps.,*** mang., **MED.,** myrt-c., ***nat-s.,*** ol-j., petr., **PHOS.,** polyg., **PSOR., PULS.,** ***rumx., sang.,*** sec., **SENEC., SIL., STANN.,** succ., ***sulph., ther.,*** thuj., tril., **TUB.,** vanad.
- injury to the after - mill., ***ruta.***
- last stage - ars., bry., **CALC., CARB-V.,** ***chin., dros., euon.,*** kali-n., **LACH.,** led., lob., **LYC.,** ***phel., phos., psor.,*** **PULS.,** ***pyrog.,*** **SANG.,** ***seneg.,*** **TARENT.**
- lying, on side agg. - calc.
- miners, from coal dust - carb-s., sil.
- nursing, mothers - ***kali-c.***
- pituitous - ***aesc.,*** **ANT-C., ANT-T.,** ***bar-m.,*** caust., ***coc-c., dulc.,*** **EUON.,** ***ferr.,*** **FERR-P., HEP.,** ***kali-c.,*** **KALI-I., KALI-CHL.,** ***kreos., lach.,*** **LYC., MED.,** ***merc., merc-c.,*** mill., ***nat-s.,*** **PHOS., PSOR.,** ***puls.,*** **SANG., SENEC.,** ***seneg., sil.,*** **STANN.,** ***sulph.,*** **THER.**
- prophylaxis, for - bac., calc-p., phos., sulph., tub.

TUBERCULOSIS,

- purulent and ulcerative - ***ars., ars-i.,*** brom., bry., **CALC.,** ***carb-an., carb-s., carb-v.,*** chin., ***dros.,*** guai., ***hep.,*** hyos., **IOD., KALI-C.,** ***kali-n., kali-p., lach.,*** led., **LYC.,** ***merc.,*** nat-m., ***nit-ac., nux-m.,*** **PHOS.,** ***plb., psor., puls.,*** ruta., sep., ***sil.,*** stann., ***sulph.***
- recurring - ferr-p., kali-n., tub.
- stone-cutters - ***calc.,*** lyc., puls., ***sil.***
- sycotic - ars., **AUR.,** ***aur-m.,*** bar-c., bry., **CALC.,** ***carb-an.,*** carb-v., ***caust.,*** cham., chin., ***ferr-p., lach.,*** **LYC., MED., NAT-S., NIT-AC.,** ***phyt., puls.,*** sep., ***sil.,*** staph., sulph., ***ther.,*** **THUJ.**
- weakness, in - ars-i., chin-a., ph-ac., phos., stann.

ULCER, in - **CALC.,** carb-v., chin., **KALI-C.,** kali-n., ***led., lyc., nit-ac.,*** **PHOS.,** puls., ruta., sep., **SIL.,** stann., ***sulph., sul-ac., tub.***

WAVES, moving in lungs, as if - dulc.

WHEEZING, (see Asthma)

Male

GENITALIA, general - ***agn.,*** arn., aur., bar-c., berb., calad., ***clem.,*** coff., erig., gels., hyos., lach., ***lyc., med.,*** merc., nit-ac., ***puls.,*** rhus-t., ***sabal.,*** sel., ***sep., staph.,*** sulph., ***thuj.***
alternating between both sides - cimic., coloc., ***lac-c.,*** lycps., ol-an., onos., rhod.
left - ***lach.,*** naja, ***puls.,*** rhod., ***thuj.***
right - apis, calc., caust., ***clem.,*** hep., ***lyc.,*** merc., nux-v., pall., spong., sul-ac., verat.

ABSCESS, penis - bov., hippoz.
abscess, prostate - sil.
abscess, testes - hep., merc., still.

ABSENT, penis, sensation, as if - ***cocaine.***

ACHING, pain, genitalia - **ARN.,** chin., jatr.
aching, penis, glans, after urination - puls.
aching, prostate - sabal., ***thuj.***
bladder, and prostate, deep in pelvis, morning and forenoon after sex - all-c.
sitting and walking, while - cycl.
aching, scrotum, sides of - lach., meny.
aching, spermatic cord - all-c., chel., chin-s., ***clem.,*** mang., nux-v., ***sars.,*** senec.
erections, after, without sex - mag-m., nux-m., ***sars.***
extending to testes - senec.
morning - sars.
urination, during - stront.
aching, testes - asaf., **AUR.,** berb., bism., ***calc.,*** carl., ***caust.,*** chel., ***clem.,*** con., cop., ***ham.,*** ***iod.,*** jatr., lyss., ***nat-m.,*** nux-v., nuph., **PULS.,** ***staph.,*** still., sumb., thuj., ust.
emission, after - ***ph-ac.***
evening - chin-s.
left - con., jatr., nuph., still., sumb.
morning - sars.
noon - ***caust.,*** ust.
right - ***bism.,*** calc., ***caust.,*** chin-s., nat-m.
sexual excitement, from - ***iod., staph.***
walking, while - ***staph.,*** sumb., thuj.

ADHERE, testes to scrotum - tarent.

ASLEEP, as if - form.
ascending stairs, on - form.

ATROPHY, genitalia - carb-an., cer-s., iod., phos., staph.
atrophy, penis - agar., aloe, amyg., ant-c., arg-m., ***arg-n., berb.,*** caj., ***cann-i.,*** carb-s., **IGN., LYC.,** merc-sul., op., pic-ac., plb., staph.
atrophy, testes - agn., ant-c., ant-ox., ***arg-n., aur.,*** bar-c., bufo, ***caps., carb-an.,*** carb-s., cer-s., chim., ***gels., iod.,*** kali-br., **KALI-I.,** ***lyss.,*** meph., plb., ***rhod., sabal.,*** staph., x-ray, zinc.
sexual excesses, after - **STAPH.**

BALL, prostate, sensation of sitting on a - cann-i., ***chim.,*** **SEP.,** sil.

BEARING, down, genitalia - asaf., coloc.

BITING, pain, genitalia - graph., hep., plat., ***puls.,*** ran-s., staph., thuj.
biting, penis - cocc., ign., nat-c., nat-m., nux-v., phos.
glans - kali-c., nux-v., phos.
prepuce - merc., ***nux-v.,*** puls., thuj.
urination, after - bell., bor., calad., chin-s., cop.
biting, prostate - carb-an., con.
biting, testes, scrotum - plat., ran-s.
between scrotum and thigh - hep.

BLEEDING, penis, prepuce, from - ars-h.
bleeding, scrotum, from - petr.

BLENORRHEA, penis, glans, of - alum., alumn., calad., caust., ***cinnb.,*** cor-r., dig., ***jac-c.,*** lach., ***lyc., merc.,*** mez., nat-c., ***nat-m., nit-ac., nux-v.,*** petr., psor., ***sep., sulph., thuj.***
blue spots, penis - sulph.

BLUE, spots, genitalia - ars.

BLUENESS, penis, glans - ars.
blueness, scrotum - amyg., ***ars.,*** merc-cy., ***mur-ac.,*** puls.
eruptions, after - tep.

BOILS, genitalia, on pupes - apis.

BORING, pain, testes - mur-ac., plb., sil.

BUBBLING, sensation, penis - graph., kali-c.
erection, during - graph., kali-c.
bubbling, sensation, scrotum - staph.

BURNING, pain, genitalia - agar., ambr., anac., arn., bov., **CALC.,** cann-s., **CANTH.,** carb-ac., jac-c., kali-c., ***kreos.,*** mag-m., petr., prun., puls., rhus-t., stann., sumb.
night - agar.
seminal emission, during - calc.
sex, during - ***kreos.***
urination, during - arg-n., caps., carb-s., clem., kali-bi., kali-c., petr., psor., sul-ac., tarax., tarent., thuj.
after - alum., arg-n., kali-c., caust.
before - nat-c., tarax.
walking, after - ambr.
burning, penis - ***all-c.,*** ant-c., ant-ox., ***ars., cann-i.,*** cann-s., canth., caust., chin., ***coch.,*** kali-i., ***merc., mez.,*** mur-ac., naja, rhus-v., sang., spong., stann., sulph., thuj., ***viol-t.***
erection, during - ***mag-m.***
evening after sex - lyc.
morning in bed - mag-m.
root of - ol-an., rat., rhus-t.
scratching, after - carl.
sex, during - clem., jug-r., ***kreos.,*** sep.
walking, while -cann-s.
burning, penis, glans - ***all-c.,*** ant-c., ant-t., arn., ars., berb., calc., cann-s., cinnb., clem., ***coch.,*** crot-t., culx., ***dor.,*** lyss., merc., nux-v., ***pareir.,*** ph-ac., stann., **THUJ.,** ***viol-t.***
behind, during urination - ery-a.
dragging, and, in vesiculae seminales to glans - ***mang.***
ejaculation, during - clem.
itching - cinnb.
tip, of - calc.
urination, during - thuj.

burning, penis, glans
urination, during - anac., ***ars.,*** coch., ***lyc.,*** mez., ***pareir.***
after - anac., coc-c., coch., ***sars.***
before - anac., coch., ***stann.***
on beginning to urinate - psor.

burning, penis, prepuce - ars., berb., bufo, calad., calc., ***merc., nit-ac.,*** nux-v., ***puls.,*** rhus-t., rhus-v., sep., sil., ***sulph., thuj.***
erection, during - ars.
sex, after - lyc.
stool, after - sil.
urination, after - berb., cann-s., canth., clem., coloc., con., grat., kali-bi., kali-c., led., mag-m., ***merc., nat-c.,*** nat-m., nat-s., seneg., teucr., thuj., zinc.**burning,** prostate - all-c., ambr., caps., cop., lyss., ph-ac.

burning, scrotum - ars., ***calc.,*** cann-i., carl., cop., euph., lachn., meny., mez., petr., plat., rhod., rhus-v., sil., spong., sulph.
between, and thighs - bar-c.
itching - cocc.
rubbing, after - rhus-t., rhus-v., thuj.
scratching, after - ***nat-s.,*** thuj.
sides, of - euph., stry., tarent.

burning, spermatic cord - ambr., ***berb.,*** carb-s., clem., mang., staph., thuj.
Left - berb.
right - clem.
walking, while - ***berb.***

burning, testes - apis, bar-c., berb., coff., iod., ***nit-ac.,*** ph-ac., plat., **PULS.,** staph., sumb., tarax., ter.
swelling, without - **PULS.**

CANCER, genitalia - ars., bell., ***carb-an.,*** **CON.,** phos., phyt., sil., spong., thuj.

cancer, penis, glans, epithelioma on excrescences - arg-n., ***ars.,*** con., thuj.

cancer, prostate - carc., **CON.,** crot-h., ***cop., iod.,*** plb., ***psor., sel.,*** senec., ***sil., sulph.,*** **THUJ.**
pain, with - crot-h.

cancer, scrotum - ars., carb-an., fuli., ph-ac., thuj.
epithelioma, of - carb-an., ph-ac.
scirrhus - carb-an.

cancer, testes - aur., ***carb-an., clem.,*** **CON.,** ox-ac., phyt., sil., ***spong.,*** thuj.

CHANCRES, penis, (see Ulcers)

CHLAMYDIAL, infections - med., sulph., thuj.

COLDNESS, genitalia - agar., **AGN.,** aloe, berb., brom., calad., camph., cann-s., caps., carb-s., caust., ***dios., gels.,*** hell., ind., ***iris, lyc.,*** merc., pic-ac., psor., sabal., ***sulph.,*** uran-n.
evening - ***dios.***
morning - sulph.
urination, during - iris.

coldness, penis - agar., **AGN.,** bar-c., berb., caps., dios., helo., indg., **LYC.,** merc., ***onos., sulph.***
glans - berb., merc., ***onos., sulph.***
prepuce - berb., ***sulph.,*** zinc., zing.

coldness, penis
small, and cold - ***agn.,*** lyc.

coldness, scrotum - ***agn.,*** aloe, ***berb.,*** brom., ***calad.,*** calc., ***caps.,*** dios., gels., iris, lyc., ***merc., ph-ac.,*** sep., staph., sulph.
morning, on waking - ***caps.***

coldness, testes - **AGN.,** aloe, berb., brom., camph., caps., cer-s., ***dios.,*** gels., helo., ***merc.,*** sil., zinc.
evening - aloe, ***merc.***
left - brom.
night - ***agn.,*** aloe.

COMPRESSING, pain, testes - am-c., petr., sil., ***spong.,*** squil., staph., thuj., zinc.
right - arg-m., staph.

CONDYLOMATA, genitalia - alumn., apis, ***arg-n.,*** aur., ***aur-m.,*** aur-m-n., ***calc., cinnb.,*** euphr., ***fl-ac.,*** **HEP.,** ***lyc., med., merc., merc-d., mill.,*** **NAT-S., NIT-AC.,** ***ph-ac., phos.,*** psor., ***sabin., sars., sep., staph.,*** **THUJ.**
anus, and genitalia - nit-ac.
bleed easily - ***calc., cinnb.,*** med., ***mill.,*** **NIT-AC.,** sulph., ***thuj.***
bleeding when touched and fetid - ***cinnb.,*** **NIT-AC.,** thuj.
burning - ph-ac.
cheese, smelling, like stale - ***calc., hep., sanic.,*** thuj.
hot - ph-ac.
itching - lyc., psor., ***sabin.,*** staph., thuj.
sensitive - ***staph.***
soft - ***sep.***
sore - ph-ac.
sticking pain - nit-ac.
syphilitic - aur-m., ***cinnb.,*** euphr., kali-i., ***merc.,*** merc-c., merc-cy., merc-d., merc-i-f., merc-i-r., nat-s., ***nit-ac.,*** plat-m., ***sabin.,*** staph., ***thuj.***

condylomata, penis - alumn., ant-t., ***apis,*** aur., aur-m., bell., ***calc.,*** **CINNB.,** euphr., ***hep., kali-i.,*** lac-c., ***lyc., merc.,*** merc-c., ***mill., nat-s.,*** **NIT-AC.,** nux-v., ***ph-ac.,*** **PSOR., SABIN.,** ***sanic.,*** **SEP.,** ***staph., sulph.,*** **THUJ.**
bleeding - ***cinnb.,*** **NIT-AC.,** sulph., ***thuj.***
burning - apis, ***cinnb.,*** **NIT-AC.,** ph-ac., ***psor., sabin., thuj.***
butternut-shaped, hard growth on the dorsum of the penis - **SABIN.**
cauliflower, like - lac-c., **NIT-AC.**
fan shaped - **CINNB.,** ***thuj.***
glans -***ant-t., aur., aur-m., cinnb., kali-chl., kali-i., lac-c.,*** lyc., ***med., nit-ac., ph-ac.,*** psor., ***sabin., sep., staph., sulph.,*** **THUJ.**
itching - staph.
itching - ***psor., sabin.,*** staph.
oozing - aur-m., ***cinnb., lyc., nit-ac., psor., thuj.***
offensive - ***nit-ac.***
prepuce -***aur., aur-m.,*** aur-m-n., caust., **CINNB.,** cub., ***lyc., med.,*** merc., merc-c., ***nit-ac.,*** ph-ac., **PSOR.,** ***sabin.,*** **THUJ.**
edge of, itching and burning - psor.

condylomata, penis
prepuce, fraenum - **CINNB.**
soreness - euphr., **NIT-AC.**, ph-ac., ***sabin.***, ***thuj.***
and itching - ***psor.***, ***sabin.***
condylomata, scrotum - ***aur.***, ***aur-m.***, sil., **THUJ.**

CONGESTION, prostate - ***acon.***, ***aloe***, arn., bell., ***canth.***, con., cop., cub., ferr-p., gels., kali-br., kali-i., lith., ***ol-sant.***, puls., ***sabal.***, thuj.
congestion, scrotum - coloc.

CONSTRICTING, pain, genitalia - puls.
constricting, penis, root of, morning, on waking - ***kali-bi.***
constricting, prostate - canth., ***caust.***, puls., sulph.
constricting, spermatic cord - am-c., berb., nux-v.
standing, while - nux-v.
walking, while - nux-v.
constricting, testes - **AM-C.**, berb., bufo, merc-ac., nux-v., ol-an., ***plb.***, sulph.

CONSTRICTION, genitalia, sensation as if - arn., asar., kali-c., mosch.
constriction, penis - kali-bi.
glans, behind - coloc., plb., puls.
sex, after - calad.
prepuce - merc., nit-ac., rhus-t., sabin., sulph.
string, as if by - plb.
constriction, penis, prepuce - acon., ***apis***, arn., bell., cann-s., ***canth.***, caps., dig., euph-pr., euphr., ***merc.***, ***merc-c.***, ***nit-ac.***, ol-sant., ph-ac., ***rhus-t.***, sabin., sulph., ***thuj.***
constriction, seminal cords, sensation as if - kali-c.

CONSTRINGING, sensation, genitalia - arn., asar., kali-c., mosch.

CONTINENCE agg. - apis, calc., ***con.***, fl-ac., lyc., plat.

CONTRACTING, spermatic cord - alum., berb., calc., **NUX-V.**
contracting, testes - alum., camph., ***chin.***, merc-ac., nux-v., plb.

CONTRACTION, penis - ign.
contraction, scrotum - acon., arn., berb., cann-s., clem., ferr-m., op., plb.
contraction, testes - camph.

CONTUSIONS of genitalia - arn., bell-p., con.

CRAB-lice - cocc., sabad., staph.

COWPERITIS, inflammation of cowper's glands - acon., cann-s., fab., gels., hep., merc-c., petros., sabal., sil.

CRAB-lice, genitalia - cocc., sabad., staph.

CRACKS, penis, glans - ***ars.***, kali-c., mosch., rhus-t.
prepuce - hep., merc., sep., sul-i., sulph.

CRAMPING, spermatic cord - arg-m., kali-c., **NUX-V.**, petr.,
extending, from rectum to testes - sil.
to testes - dios.
cramping, testes - agn., arg-m., am-c., caps., chin., con., ign., lyc., nux-v., petr., phos., plb., spong.
afternoon - chin.
emission, after - caps.
erections, after - con.
evening - con.
extending from rectum to - sil.
rest, during - arg-m.
right- arg-m., phos.

CRUSHED, pain, testes - **ARG-M.**, calc., ***caust.***, con., dig., **RHOD.**, ***spong.***, thuj.
jar, from a - colch.
right, while walking - **ARG-M.**

CUTTING, pain, genitalia - bor., sil.
urinate, when beginning to - iris, ***mang.***, merc., petr., sec.
cutting, penis - alumn., anac., cic., con., crot-h., euon., lyc., nat-c., ol-an., ph-ac., still., thuj.
burning cutting - ph-ac.
glans - con., iod., lyc., ph-ac., thuj.
urination, after - coch.
urination, before - coch.
urination, during - coch., ***lyc.***
prepuce, urination, after - berb., canth., dig., nat-m.
tip - calc.
cutting, scrotum - con., meny.
septum - caust., con.
cutting, spermatic cord - bell., berb.
cutting, testes - aur., bell., berb., cahin., calc., coc-c., ***con.***, lyc., nuph., ph-ac., ***sep.***, ter.
night in bed - coc-c.
sex, during - kali-i.

CYSTS, genitalia - sil., thuj.

DISCHARGES, (see Emissions, Seminal)

DRAGGING, pain, penis, at root of - chel.
burning from vesiculae seminales to glans - mang.
dragging, prostate - nat-a., sil.
dragging, spermatic cord - berb., chin-a., ***iod.***, sars., sec., spong., sumb.
dragging, testes - cann-s., ***gels.***, iod., ***kali-c.***, lach., ***med.***, sumb.
afternoon, extending to groins - gels.
emissions, after - ***ph-ac.***

DRAWING, pain, prostate - clem., ***cycl.***, kali-bi., mez.
sitting or walking - ***cycl.***
drawing, penis - alum., asaf., canth., coc-c., graph., grat., **IOD.**, ***kali-c.***, lact., lyc., merc., mez., ol-an., psor., puls-n, ran-s., rhod., sabad., teucr., valer., ***zinc.***
afternoon - asaf.
evening - puls.
glans - alum., asaf., cic., graph., iod., kali-c., lact., lyc., mez., spong., thuj.
lower, side - cic.
prepuce - coc-c.
root - lact., zinc.
drawing, scrotum - am-c., cahin., clem., meny.

drawing, spermatic cord - ***agar.***, agn., ***all-c.***, alum., ammc., am-c., anag., ang., ant-c., arg-m., aur-m., bell., ***berb.***, bry., cann-s., canth., ***chel.***, cimic., ***clem.***, ***con.***, crot-t., ***ham.***, hydr., ***ind.***, lact., ***mang.***, med., ***merc.***, mez., nat-c., nat-m., nat-p., nit-ac., ***nux-v.***, ol-an., ***ox-ac.***, ph-ac., ***phos.***, plb., psor., ***puls.***, rhod., sec., spong., ***staph.***, sulph., ***tarent.***, tep., ter., ***zinc.***
afternoon, 4 p.m. - arg-m.
evening - ammc.
extending into, abdomen during urination - clem.
into, abdominal ring - ***berb.***, bry.
into, testes - ***berb.***, nux-v., ***puls.***, staph., teucr.
left - agar., ars., tarent.
morning - calc-s., nat-c.
motion amel. - arg-m., rhod.
paroxysmal - merc.
right - arg-m., sabin.
sitting - berb.
spasmodic - agar.
standing, while - ant-c.
upward - clem., ***bell.***, ***ol-an.***
urination during - agar., bell., ***canth.***, caps., clem.
and after - caps.
walking, while - ***berb.***, crot-t.

drawing, testes - acon., aesc., agar., ammc., am-c., apis, **AUR.**, ***aur-m.***, bapt., bell., berb., calc-ac., calc-s., canth., carb-s., card-m., ***chel.***, ***chin.***, ***clem.***, ***cocc.***, coloc., ***con.***, cop., graph., ***ham.***, hipp., hyos., ip., kali-c., kali-n., kali-s., mang., ***merc.***, mur-ac., ***nat-c.***, nat-m., nat-p., nit-ac., ol-an., op., ox-ac., ***nux-v.***, phos., ph-ac., plb., psor., ***puls.***, **RHOD.**, rhus-t., sabad., sep., sil., ***staph.***, ***sulph.***, ter., ***thuj.***, tus-p., verat., ***zinc.***
evening - agar., sulph.
extending, to abdomen - calc., ***iod.***, kali-n., **RHOD.**
to hip - chel.
to inguinal ring - aur-m., bry.
to spermatic cord - aesc., berb., bry., ***clem.***, fl-ac., kali-n., ***zinc.***
to thighs - aur., rhod., sep.
upward - clem.
left - aesc., ang., calc-s., chin., ***con.***, kali-c., ***rhod.***, ter., thuj., ***zinc.***
then right - ***zinc.***
morning - calc-s., nat-c.
motion amel. - ***rhod.***
paroxysmal - aur-m.
right - acon., anag., **AUR.**, bry., **RHOD.**
sexual, excitement, after - kali-n.
sitting, while - ter., zinc.
stooping, while - zinc.
urination, during, agg. - cahin.
walking amel - thuj.

DRYNESS, penis, glans - ***calad.***, lyss.

ECZEMA, genitalia - arg-n., ars., chel., ***crot-t.***, ***graph.***, hep., ***lyc.***, nat-m., nit-ac., petr., rhus-t., sep., sulph., thuj.

eczema, penis, back of - alum., rad-br.

eczema, scrotum - alum., alumn., ant-c., canth., chel., ***crot-t.***, ***graph.***, hep., olnd., petr., ph-ac., ***rhus-t.***, sanic., sulph., ***thuj.***
rubrum - chel.

EJACULATION, (see Seminal Emissions) - agar., mag-aust., sel.

acrid - cop., gels., ***hydr.***, ***merc-c.***, thuj.

bloody - ambr., cann-s., ***canth.***, ***caust.***, cub., fl-ac., led., lyc., **MERC.**, ***merc-c.***, mill., ***petr.***, puls., ***sars.***, sulph., tarent., wies.
night - **MERC.**

burning, during sex - ***calc.***, cann-i.

cold, during sex - ***nat-m.***

copious - agar., bell., carl., carb-s., carb-v., iod., kali-c., merc-i-f., nat-m., par., petr., ph-ac., ***pic-ac.***, sep., sil., staph., sulph., ther., zinc.
dreams, with - kali-c., pip-m., sars.
longer, and - osm.
night - aur., carb-an., ***dig.***, hipp., ign., ol-an.
3 a.m. - pip-m.
sex, after - bar-c.

desire for ejaculation - ign., ***mag-arct.***, nux-v.
erection, without - sulph.
evening and after dinner, without sexual desire - nat-c.
morning, in bed - puls.
rising, after - nux-v.
waking, after - petr., rhus-t.

difficult - anan., carb-s., cimic., lach., lim., lyss., ***zinc.***

excessive - carb-v., iod., sulph., zing.

failing during sex - agn., bar-c., bufo, ***calad.***, calc., carb-s., coff., ***eug.***, **GRAPH.**, hydr., kali-c., kali-i., ***lach.***, lim., ***lyc.***, ***lyss.***, mill., nat-m., nux-v., ph-ac., ***psor.***, zinc.
occurs afterwards during sleep - lyss.
though the orgasm is present - cann-i., graph.

frothy - mur-ac.

hemiplegia, in - mag-aust.

hot - agar., calc., tarent.

incomplete - ***agar.***, agn., aloe, anan., arg-m., bar-c., berb., calad., calc., ***camph.***, canth., carb-s., coff., ***con.***, dig., ***form.***, hydr., ign., ***kali-c.***, lach., ***lyc.***, lyss., nat-m., nux-m., ***phos.***, plb., sel., sep., sul-ac., sulph., ther., zinc., zing.
erection, with - calad., ***form.***
before - ***sulph.***
intromission, before - ***sulph.***

insensible - nat-p., plan.

larger and continues longer - osm.

late, too - ***agar.***, berb., bor., **CALC.**, erig., eug., ***fl-ac.***, hydr., lach., lyc., ***lyss.***, merc-c., ***nat-m.***, petr., ***zinc.***
sexual desire, without - ***nat-m.***
the orgasm subsides several times before it leads to ejaculation - eug.
some time after the orgasm - calc.

lemon-colored - hura.

lump, feeling as a - cer-s.

lumpy - alum.

EJACULATION, general
milky - cann-i., ***cann-s.,*** cop., cupr-ar., graph., ***hydr., kali-bi.,*** lach., ***nat-m., petros.,*** puls., sep.
odor, abnormal - ***sel.***
little odor - agn.
odorless - agn., ***sel.***
stale urine, like - ***nat-p.***
strong - ***lach.***
painful - ***agar.,*** arg-n., ***berb., calc.,*** cann-i., ***cann-s., canth.,*** clem., ***con., kali-c.,*** kali-i., ***kreos.,*** merc., mosch., nat-ac., nat-c., ***nit-ac.,*** ran-s., sabad., ***sabal.,*** sars., ***sep.,*** **SULPH.,** sul-ac., thuj.
painful, cutting - con.
pale - bell.
purulent, yellowish green - agn., alum., ***arg-n.,*** baros., ***cann-s.,*** canth., caps., cob., ***cop., cub.,*** dig., ***hep., hydr.,*** jac., kali-i., ***kali-s., merc., merc-c.,*** nat-m., ***nat-s.,*** ol-sant., ***puls.,*** sabin., sep., sil., sulph., ***thuj.,*** tus-f., zing.
quick, too (see Impotency) - ***agn.,*** aloe, bar-c., ***berb.,*** bor., brom., bufo, ***calad., calc.,*** carb-an., carb-s., ***carb-v., chin., cob., con., ery-a.,*** eug., ***gels.,*** **GRAPH.,** ind., **LYC.,** ***nat-c., nat-m.,*** nux-v., ol-an., onos., petr., ***ph-ac., phos.,*** pic-ac., ***plat., sel., sep.,*** staph., ***sulph., titan.,*** ust., **ZINC.**
dream of sex, during - sumb.
enjoyment, without - bufo, calc., sul-ac.
erection is complete, before - calad., **GRAPH.,** ***sulph.***
shortly after an - ***ph-ac., sulph.***
excitement, almost without - bufo, eug.
intromission, before - ***sulph.***
reddish-brown - fl-ac.
short - sep.
siesta, during - ther.
sticky - ***staph.***
stream, running in a - agn.
sudden - phos.
thick - alum., alumn., med.
threads, with - med.
thin - sel.
voluptuous sensation, without - calc.
watery - bart., bor., ***cann-s.,*** fl-ac., led., med., mez., mill., mur-ac., ***nat-m., nat-p., sel., sep.,*** sulph., thuj.
weak - bell., sep.

ELEPHANTIASIS - ***anac., ars.,*** calo., card-m., ***elae.,*** graph., ham., hell., hippoz., ***hydr.,*** iod., lyc., ***myris.,*** sil., still.
arabum - ars., ***hydrc.,*** myris., ***sil.***

EMISSIONS, genitalia, agg. (see Seminal) - agar., ***alum.,*** ars., ***bar-c.,*** bor., bov., ***calc.,*** cann-s., carb- an., carb-v., caust., ***chin.,*** cob., dig., ***iod.,*** **KALI-C.,** led., ***lyc.,*** merc., mez., nat-c., **NAT-P., NUX-V.,** petr., ***ph-ac., phos., pic-ac.,*** plb., ***psor.,*** puls., ran-b., rhod., sabad., **SEL., SEP.,** ***sil., staph., sulph.,*** thuj.

EMPYOCELE, genitalia - ***ars-i., calc.,*** **CALC-SIL.,** ***sep.,*** **KALI-S.,** ***psor., puls.,*** **SIL., SULPH.**

ENLARGEMENT, prostate - alf., ***aloe,*** alum., ***am-m., apis,*** apoc., ***arg-n.,*** asar., aspar., ***aur-m.,*** **BAR-C.,** ***benz-ac., berb.,*** cact., **CALC.,** calc-f., calc-i., cann-s., canth., chr-s., cic., ***chim., cimic.,*** clem., **CON.,** cop., **DIG.,** ***dulc.,*** eup-pur., ***ferr-m.,*** **FERR-PIC.,** ***gels.,*** graph., hep., ***hydrang., hyos., iod.,*** kali-bi., kali-br., ***kali-i.,*** kali-p., lith., ***lyc., med., merc., nat-c.,*** nat-p., ***nat-s., nit-ac.,*** nux-v., ol-an., ol-sant., oxyd., ***pareir.,*** ph-ac., ***phos.,*** pic-ac., pip-m., ***pop., psor.,*** **PULS.,** rhus-a., ***sabal.,*** sars., ***sec., sel., senec., sil.,*** solid., ***spong., staph., sulph.,*** ther., ***thiosin.,*** **THUJ.,** thyr., trib., tritic., uva.
dribbling, urine after stool and urine - **SEL.,** ***thuj.***
ejaculation, painful, with - sabal.
elderly men, in - aloe, **BAR-C.,** ***benz-ac., con.,*** **DIG.,** ferr-pic., ***iod.,*** nat-c., nux-v., **SABAL., SEL.,** ***staph.,*** sulph., ***thuj.***
gonnorrhea, history, with - med., thuj.
hemorrhoids, with - staph.
high blood pressure, with - dig.
impotency, with - dig., lyc., sel.
pressure, in perineum, with - berb.
enlargement, prostate, sensation of - alum., berb., bry., chim., cycl., nux-v., ***ther.***
enlargement, spermatic cord - fl-ac., kali-i.
enlargement, testes - arg-n., ars., bar-c., bar-m., ***berb.,*** cinnb., con., ***ham., iod., merc.,*** merc-i-r., puls., stigm.
left - ***alum.,*** helo., spong.
left, for two years - spong.
right - arg-n., **AUR.**
walking, while - ***clem.***

ERECTIONS, penis, troublesome - alum., ***am-c.,*** am-m., anac., ant-c., arn., ***aur.,*** aur-m., berb., ***cann-i.,*** **CANTH.,** cham., chin., cocc., coff., dig., ***euph.,*** ferr., ferr-i., ferr-p., ***fl-ac.,*** graph., ham., hyos., ign., ***iod.,*** kali-bi., ***kali-c., kali-i., kreos.,*** laur., led., lith., lyc., mag-m., mag-s., morph., mur-ac., ***nat-c., nat-m.,*** nat-p., nicc., nit-ac., **NUX-V.,** ***op.,*** ox-ac., petr., ***ph-ac.,*** **PHOS., PIC-AC., PLAT.,** ***plb., puls.,*** rhod., rhus-t., seneg., ***sep., sil.,*** stann., ***staph., stram.,*** sul-ac., tab., tarent., ust., verat.
afternoon - alum., caps., carb-s., cham., eug., lyss., ***nux-v.,*** pip-m., thuj., ust.
2 p.m. - alumn., mag-s.
3 p.m. - ***equis.***
urination, after - nat-c.
siesta, after - eug., ***nux-v.,*** sep.
sitting, while - alum.
walking, while - hyper.
bed, in - ant-c., kali-bi., upa.
causeless - ***am-c.,*** carl., ferr., tarax.
causeless, lying down, on - ox-ac.
child, in a - aloe, ***lach.,*** med., ***merc.,*** ph-ac., plat., ***tub.***

ERECTIONS, penis

continued - agar., ***am-c.,*** ambr., apis, arg-n., arn., bell., camph., ***cann-i., cann-s.,*** **CANTH.,** ***caps.,*** carb-s., carb-v., caust., cinnb., clem., ***coloc.,*** dig., ***dios.,*** euph., fl-ac., ***gins., graph.,*** hyos., ign., iod., ***kali-br.,*** kali-c., kali-chl., lach., lat-m., ***laur.,*** led., lyss., ***med.,*** merc., mur-ac., mygal., ***nat-c.,*** nat-hchls., ***nat-m.,*** nat-p., nit-ac., nux-v., oena., op., opun-v., ped., ***petros.,*** ph-ac., ***phos., pic-ac.,*** pip-n., ***plat., puls.,*** raph., rhod., ***rhus-t.,*** sabin., sel., sep., sil., sin-n., spirae., staph., ***stram.,*** tarax., ***thuj.,*** verat., visc., yohim, zinc., zinc-pic., zinc-valer.

curvature of penis, with - canth.
daytime - clem.
dreams, during - ***camph.***
eating, after - hyos.
elderly man, in a - arn.
falls asleep, as soon as he - pic-ac.
morning - asc-t., dig., erech., ***puls.,*** yohim.
nausea, with - kali-bi.
night - carb-v., corn., ***dios., fl-ac., kali-br., lach.,*** nat-m., nit-ac., plat., sep., sin-n., staph., thuj.
pollutions, with - lyss.
after - ars., plb., rhod., sabad.
semipriapism - oena., ***puls.***
sex, after - sep.
spinal disease, with - ***pic-ac.***
trance-like state, with - ***camph.***
urine, with retention of - coloc.

convulsive - nit-ac.
convulsive, child, in a - lach.

coughing, when - cann-s., canth.

day and night - ferr., ***phos.***

daytime - anac., cann-i., cann-s., ***chel., clem.,*** kali-c., lach., lyc., mez., nat-c., ***phos.,*** puls., sabin., sil., sin-n., sul-ac., valer.

delayed - **BAR-C.,** ***calc.,*** canth., carb-s., iod., mag-c., merc-c., nit-ac., osm., par., pic-ac., ***sel.,*** sil.

difficult - pers., tere-ch.

dinner, during - alumn., nicc.

disturbing sleep - alum., ambr., ant-c., aur., carb-v., coloc., hep., kali-c., lach., led., lith., merc., merc-ac., ***nat-c.,*** nat-m., ol-an., op., par., ph-ac., pic-ac., plat., plb., ran-b., sep., ***sil., stann.,*** thuj.

dreams, with amorous - aur., cact., camph., ***cann-i.,*** clem., coloc., kreos., lac-ac., led., merc., mur-ac., ***nat-c.,*** nat-m., par., ***ph-ac.,*** pic-ac., plat., plb., ran-b., rhod., ***sars.,*** sep., sil., sin-n., ***spig.,*** stann., thuj.

easy, too - ***con.,*** ferr., ferr-i., kali-c., lyc., nux-v., ***phos., pic-ac., plb.,*** rhod., sabin., sumb., wild.

eating, after - nicc.

elderly man, in a - arn., fl-ac., phos.

emission, after - aloe, ars., grat., kali-c., mez., nit-ac., **PH-AC.,** rhod., sep.
enjoyment, without - ambr., carb-v., mag-m., nat-c., sel., tab.

ERECTIONS, penis

evening - alum., alumn., bar-c., cact., caps., cinnb., fago., lach., laur., ***lyss.,*** nat-s., phos., sil.
evening, 6 p.m. - equis.
bed, in - cinnb., con., nit-ac.
lying down, after - nit-ac.
shivering and great desire, with - bar-c.

excessive - ***aur-m.,*** **CANTH.,** cop., **FL-AC.,** ***graph.,*** nat-m., ***ph-ac., pic-ac.,*** op., staph.
erotic, lascivious thoughts, during - cop., **PIC-AC.**
night - staph.

exhausting - aur-m.

falling asleep, on - pic-ac.

forenoon - caps., caust., lach., nicc., ol-an., ox-ac., phys.
lying down, when - ox-ac.
riding in a carriage, when - form.

frequent - acon., agar., ***agn.,*** alum., alum-p., alumn., am-m., anth., anthro., apis, arund., aster., ***aur., aur-m.,*** bell., berb., cann-i., cann-s., ***canth., caps.,*** carb-v., caust., ***chel.,*** chin., cic., cimx., clem., ***coc-c.,*** cod., coloc., corn., cyt-l., ***dig., dios.,*** erig., ***ferr.,*** graph., ham., helon., kali-c., kali-n., kalm., lach., lat-m., ***laur.,*** lyc., ***mag-m., med.,*** merc., merc-c., mez., mur-ac., nat-c., ***nat-m.,*** nat-p., nit-ac., nux-v., onis., ph-ac., ***phos.,*** pic-ac., ***puls.,*** ran-b., rhus-t., sabad., sabin., sep., sil., sin-n., ***spig.,*** sumb., ***tab.,*** ther., ust., valer., visc., zinc.
daytime - ***chel.,*** jug-r., lyc., mez., nat-c.
eating, after - hyos.
elderly man, in an - caust.
morning - ***cimx., mag-m.,*** ran-b.
nausea, with - kali-bi.
night - ***alum.,*** corn., helon., jug-r., ***merc.,*** nat-m., ***nit-ac.,*** sin-n.
prostatic fluid, with loss of - ***puls.***
puts hands to penis - ***stram.***
sex, after - kali-bi.

fruitless - con., gins., plat.

impetuous - kali-c.

incomplete - achy., ***agar.,*** agav-t., **AGN.,** aq-mar., aran-ix., arg-n., ars., ars-i., ***bar-c.,*** berb., ***calad., calc., camph.,*** carb-v., caust., chen-v., chin-a., ***cob.,*** coc-c., **CON.,** ferr-p., form., **GRAPH.,** ***hep.,*** ign., ind., iod., kali-ar., kali-i., lach., linu-c., lyss., **LYC.,** mang., merc., merc-cy., moly-met., mur-ac., naja, nat-a., ***nat-c., nat-m., nat-p.,*** nit-ac., ***nuph., nux-m., nux-v.,*** oena., pers., ***petr., ph-ac., phos.,*** pic-ac., plb., rhod., rhodi., sars., ***sel.,*** **SEP.,** stann., sul-i., **SULPH.,** tarent., ther., upa., zinc.
constant - ***kali-i.***
desire, strong, with - ***phos.***
without - agn.
diabetes, with - coca, mosch., ph-ac.
ejaculation too soon - calad.
excitement, during sexual - coc-c., sel.
forenoon - caust.
fright, during sex, from - sin-a.

ERECTIONS, penis
incomplete,
gonorrhea, after - calad.
imaginary - stry-p.
morning - nat-c.
sex, after - caust.
night - calc.
onanism, after - arg-n.
penis becomes relaxed - arg-n., nux-v., ph-ac.
psychical - onos.
sex, during - ***camph., con.,*** cyna., ***form.,*** **GRAPH.,** hep., **LYC.,** lyss., nux-v., ***ph-ac., phos., sep.,*** **SULPH.,** ther.
sexual excess, after - arn.
vertigo, with - tarent.
intolerable - hura.
involuntary - anac., bell., clem., tarax.
lascivious fancies, with - sel.
lying, back, on - onos.
lying, while - alum., ox-ac.
midnight - ambr., nit-ac., osm.
midnight, until 4 a.m. - osm.
midnight, waking, on - ambr.
morning - agar., ***agn.,*** all-c., aloe, ambr., **AM-C.,** ars., ars-h., ars-i., asc-t., aster., bar-c., bond., brom., calad., calc., canth., caps., carb-an., caust., cham., chin-b., ***cimx.,*** coc-c., cop., dig., ***graph.,*** guai., kali-ar., kali-c., kali-n., kali-p., kali-sil., ***lach.,*** lac-ac., lact., mag-arct., ***mag-m.,*** mur-ac., nat-a., nat-c., nat-m., nat-p., nat-s., nicc., nit-ac., ***nux-v.,*** ol-an., osm., pall., ***ph-ac.,*** phos., plat., plb., psor., ***puls.,*** ran-b., ***rhod.,*** rhus-t., ***sel., sil.,*** tab., ther., thuj., valer., viol-t.
bed, in - cann-s., ***nux-v.,*** phos., ***puls.,*** sabad., thuj.
desire, without - am-c., ambr., calad., chin-b., ***nat-m.,*** sel.
dreams, during - colch.
only - ***bar-c.,*** pall.
riding, after - aur., calc.
rising, on - bar-c., calc., canth., caps., dig., osm.
standing, while - ***ph-ac.***
waking, on and after - ambr., anac., arn., bor., ***card-m.,*** nat-c., ox-ac., petr., ph-ac., phos., pic-ac., plat., puls., ***sil.,*** sulph., thuj.
and after, 6 a.m. - guai.
night - agar., aloe, alum., alum-p., alum-sil., ambr., **AUR.,** aur-i., bar-c., bell., brom., bry., calad., calc., **CANTH.,** ***caps.,*** carb-v., ***caust.,*** cent., con., corn., cycl., ***dios.,*** euph., ferr., ferr-i., ferr-p., **FL-AC.,** gins., gymn., helon., hep., ***kali-br.,*** kali-c., kali-p., ***lach., merc.,*** merc-c., mez., ***nat-c.,*** nat-m., nat-p., nicc., **NIT-AC.,** ol-an., osm., ***op.,*** par., petr., ph-ac., **PHOS., PIC-AC.,** pip-m., **PLAT.,** plb., ***puls.,*** rhod., rhus-t., sabin., seneg., sep., ***sil.,*** sin-n., stann., staph., sul-i., sumb., tell., thuj., yuc., zinc., zinc-p.
2 a.m. - aloe.
3 a.m. to 8 a.m. - brom.
4 a.m. - calad., pic-ac., pip-m.

ERECTIONS, penis
night, at
bed, when becoming warm in - ant-c.
pollution, after - nit-ac.
rising, after - caj.
sleep, during - ***fl-ac.,*** op., rhod., ther.
half asleep, cease when fully awake - calad.
urging to urinate, with - ***rhus-t.***
urinating, during - staph.
after - aloe
before - sin-n.
waking, on - dig., guare., ***hep.,*** nit-ac., sil., yuc.
noon - kali-n., ***nux-v.***
after a nap - ***nux-v.,*** sep.
and afternoon - par.
painful - acon., ***agav-a.,*** agn., alum., alum-p., alum-sil., ***anac.,*** ant-c., anthro., **ARG-N.,** aur., bell., berb., bor., bry., cact., ***calad.,*** calc-p., ***camph., camph-br., cann-i.,*** **CANN-S., CANTH., CAPS.,** chin., clem., ***colch.,*** con., cop., crot-t., ***cub.,*** cur., ***dig.,*** erig., ery-a., eug., ferr-i., fl-ac., gels., graph., grat., hep., hyos., ign., jac-c., ***kali-br.,*** kali-c., ***kali-chl.,*** kali-i., kali-p., kali-sil., lact., ***lup.,*** lyc., mag-m., merc., merc-c., mosch., mur-ac., mygal., nat-c., nat-m., nat-p., ***nit-ac., nux-v.,*** oena., ol-sant., ***petros., phos., pic-ac.,*** pip-m., plb., **PULS.,** sabad., sal-n., sel., seneg., sep., ***sil., staph.,*** sulph., sumb., tab., **TER.,** ***thuj.,*** tus-p., yohim, zinc., zing.
children, in - ***tub.***
day and night - ***dig.,*** phos.
desire, without - all-c., ***calad.***
disturbing sleep - cact.
evening - calc-p., cann-s.
sleep, before - con.
fatigue, with - sabad.
morning - agn., all-c., calad., lact., nat-c., ***nux-v.,*** sabad., sep., sil.
sex, after - bry., grat.
sitting, while - sep.
night - alum., ant-c., ***cact., caps.,*** dig., ***hep., merc.,*** nit-ac., nat-m., ***phos., thuj.,*** zinc-p.
dream, during an erotic - chin.
emission, after - grat.
sex, after - bry., calad., grat.
sex, during - hep.
voluptuous dream, during - chin.
pollutions, after, painful - ***kali-c.***
sitting, when - gins.
spasmodic - ***nit-ac.***
swelling of, prepuce, from - jac-c.
scrotum - jac-c.
waking, on - wild.
pollutions, during - agar., anac., aur., ***calc.,*** cann-i., cann-s., ***canth.,*** carb-ac., carb-an., caust., chin., dig., dios., ery-a., form., ***gins., iod., kali-br.,*** kali-chl., kali-p., led., lyc., ***merc.,*** nat-m., ***nux-v.,*** par., phos., pic-ac., pip-m., puls., sil., staph., sulph., ther., viol-t.
after - aloe, ars., grat., kali-c., kali-i., mez., nit-ac., **PH-AC.,** plb., rhod., sabad., sep.

ERECTIONS, penis
pollutions, without - ***aur., gins.,*** plat.
riding, while - ***bar-c., calc-p., cann-i.,*** form.
impotence at all other times, with - bar-c.
rising, after - aur., caj.
rubbing scrotum, by - crot-t.
seldom - achy., ars., carb-s., lyc., merc-c., ***nuph.***
enjoyment, without - sel., tab.
opposite sex, when with - cer-b.
sex, after - agn., aur-s., bry., calad., cann-i., cann-s., caust., graph., grat., nat-c., rhod., sec., ***sep.,*** tarent.
sexual indifference, with - lyss.
sexual desire, without - agn., ambr., ***am-c.,*** anac., arn., asc-t., bor., bry., bufo, ***calad., calc-p., cann-i.,*** cann-s., ***canth., caps.,*** carb-v., caust., chin-b., eug., euph., fl-ac., ***graph.,*** ham., hyos., iod., kali-c., kali-n., kali-p., kalm., lach., ***laur.,*** lyss., mag-m., mag-p-a., mag-s., nat-c., ***nat-m.,*** nat-p., ***nit-ac., nux-v.,*** ol-an., ped., petr., ***ph-ac.,*** phos., ***pic-ac.,*** plat., ***plb.,*** sabad., sabin., ***sel.,*** sil., ***spig.,*** staph., sul-ac., sul-i., sulph., tab., tarent., ther., thiop.
morning - ambr., am-c., calad., chin., ***nat-m.,*** sel.
waking, after - arn.
short, too - ambr., arg-n., berb., calad., calc., camph., carb-v., ***con.,*** fl-ac., ***graph.,*** ign., laur., lyc., ***nat-c., nux-m., nux-v., ph-ac.,*** plb., ***sel.,*** sep., zinc.
sitting, while - alum., ***cann-i.,*** cann-s., euph., gins., sep.
sleep, during - alum., aster., chin., dig., ***fl-ac.,*** kali-c., merc., merc-c., ***nat-c.,*** nat-m., nux-v., ***op.,*** par., ph-ac., plat., rhod., ***ther.,*** thuj.
after - ***lach.***
disturbing - kali-c., sep.
impotence when awake, with - op.
subsiding on urinating - lith.
sleeplessness, during - ant-c., ***canth., plat.,*** sep., ***thuj.***
stool, after - nat-m., phos.
before - kali-bi.
during - carl., ***ign.,*** samb., ***thuj.***
urging, with - thuj.
ineffectual - ***ign.,*** thuj.
strong - ***agn.,*** alum-sil., ars-i., ***aur.,*** calad., **CANTH.,** cedr., cham., cinnb., clem., corn., cyt-l., **FL-AC.,** ***graph.,*** helon., kali-chl., ***lach., laur.,*** mag-m., merc-c., mez., ***nat-m.,*** nux-v., par., **PHOS., PIC-AC.,** ***puls.,*** sabin., sep., sil., tarax., ther., yohim, zinc., zinc-p.
morning - bart., cedr., nux-v.
lasting without increase of desire - yohim.
sitting, while - sep.
waking, on - all-c., bor.
night - aur., cedr., corn., lach.
pain in abdomen, with - zinc.
undressing in a cold room, while - ***lyss.***
sudden - bar-c., nux-v.
supper, during - nicc.

ERECTIONS, penis
thoughts, without erotic - arn., ol-an., petr., ph-ac., phos., sabad., sul-ac.
toothache, with - daph.
urinating, after - aloe, form., lil-t., lith., nat-c., rhus-t.
after, morning - form.
before - rhus-t.
urging to urinate, with - aspar., canth., mosch., rhus-t.
while - cahin., canth., digin., mag-m., staph.
violent - agn., ***alum.,*** alum-p., ambr., am-c., anac., ***anan.,*** arn., aur., bar-c., camph., cann-i., cann-s., ***canth.,*** carb-s., caust., ***cham.,*** chin., cinnb., ***clem.,*** coloc., con., cop., eug., **FL-AC.,** ***gels., graph., hyos.,*** ign., iod., ***kali-br.,*** kali-c., ***kali-chl., kali-m.,*** kali-sil., led., lyss., mag-arct., med., ***merc-c., mez., mygal., nat-c.,*** nat-m., nat-p., ***nit-ac., op.,*** osm., ph-ac., **PHOS., PIC-AC., PLAT.,** ***plb.,*** psor., rhus-t., sabin., sel., sep., ***sil.,*** sin-n., staph., ***stram., thymol.,*** verat., zinc., zinc-p.
day and night - ***canth.,*** merc-c., ***nit-ac., phos.,*** sabin.
daytime - cann-s., canth., caps., ferr., hyos., lach., phos., puls., sabin., sil., ***zinc.***
evening - cinnb., con., led., mez., nat-c., nux-v., ***phos.,*** staph., tarax.
morning - ambr., ***kali-p., nat-c.,*** nat-m., phos., psor., sel.
rising, when - agn.
waking, on - ***nat-c.***
night - ***fl-ac.,*** kali-c., merc-c., nat-c., ***pic-ac., plat.,*** sin-n., zinc-p.
dreams and pollutions, with - sin-n.
elderly man, in a - ***fl-ac.***
frequent - aur., laur.
headache, with - ***pic-ac.***
itching of scrotum, with - ***kali-m.***
siesta, after - eug.
sleep, during - calad., ***dios., fl-ac., merc-c., nat-c., pic-ac.***
thoughts, without sexual - lyss., sil.
urine, before the passage of large quantities of - sin-n.
waking, on and after - ambr., anac., arn., bor., carb-v., ***card-m.,*** ferr., gnaph., ***hep.,*** kali-c., lach., nat-c., nat-m., op., ox-ac., petr., ph-ac., phos., pic-ac., plat., puls., ***sil.,*** stann., ***sulph.,*** tarent., thuj.
walking, while - cann-i.
wanting, (see Male, Impotency)

ERUPTIONS, genitalia - agar., ambr., anan., ant-c., ant-t., apis, arn., calad., calc., carb-v., chel., chin-s., cinnb., clem., crot-h., ***crot-t., dulc., graph., hep.,*** iod., kali-bi., ***lach.,*** lyc., ***merc.,*** nat-c., nat-m., ***nit-ac.,*** **PETR.,** ph-ac., rad-br., **RHUS-T., RHUS-V.,** sabin., sars., ***sep.,*** sil., spong., tell., thuj.
blotches - bell., bov., bry., crot-t., ***merc.,*** nat-c., sep.
burning - calc., kali-c., ***merc.,*** nit-ac., phos., ***rhus-t.,*** spong.
copper colored - calc.

ERUPTIONS, genitalia
crusts - caust., **NIT-AC.,** sars., thuj.
dry - ***petr., sep.***
scaly - calc., merc-i-f., sars.
elevated - lyc., merc.
erosion in spots - bar-c.
hairy parts, on - ***lach.***
hard - bov., kreos.
itching - agar., ambr., arn., bry., calad., crot-t., graph., hep., lach., nat-m., ***nit-ac.,*** **PETR., RHUS-T.,** sabin., ***sep., sil.,*** spong., ***til.***
moist spots, on - ***sil.***
miliary - bry., **RHUS-R.,** ***rhus-t., sars., sil.***
moist - ***carb-v.,*** **GRAPH., HEP.,** merc., nat-m., ***petr.,*** ph-ac., **RHUS-T.,** ***sars.,*** sep., sil.
pimples - ambr., calad., chel., graph., kali-bi., lach., ***merc.,*** nat-m., ***nit-ac.,*** sil., ***thuj.,*** til.
pustules - ant-ox., ant-t., cupr-ar., ***podo.***
painful - ***ars-h.,*** coc-c., ***hep., kali-bi.,*** merc.
red - ant-t.
rash - bry., dulc., rhus-t.
painful - antipyrin., ***bell.,*** bry., calad., cann-s., caust., ***cinnb.,*** gels., lach., ***merc.,*** nat-m., petr., ***rhus-t.,*** sep., ***sulph.,*** thuj.
red - bry., merc., nit-ac., ***petr.,*** ph-ac., rhus-v., sep., ***thuj.,*** zinc.
syphilitic - ***ars-i.,*** merc., **NIT-AC.**
urticaria - clem., cop., merc., nat-c.
vesicular - ant-t., carb-v., chin-s., **CROT-T.,** cupr-ar., ***merc., nat-c.,*** nat-p., **NIT-AC.,** petr., ph-ac., **RHUS-T.,** ***rhus-v.,*** sep.

eruptions, penis - ***crot-t.,*** graph., petr., ph-ac., ***rhus-t.,*** sep., tep.
back of, eczema - alum., rad-br.
copper-colored - calc.
erythematous - petr., samb.
nodules, hard, painful, suppurating - bov.
pimples - anac., bell., jac., lach., ***nit-ac.,*** ph-ac., sulph.
itching - jac-c.
pustules - ant-t., ***ars-h.,*** bov., coc-c., murx.
red rash - bry., ***petr.,*** samb.
scabs - ***kali-bi., nit-ac.***
spots on - caust., cinnb.

eruptions, penis, glans - ***ars-h., bry.,*** calad., ***carb-v., cinnb.,*** cor-r., jac-c., ***kali-bi., lach., lyc., merc., nit-ac., petr., ph-ac., rhus-t.,*** sep., stann.
itching - petr., sep.
pimples - jac., lach., nit-ac., ph-ac.
small, red - cinnb.
reddish - petr., sep.
shining red points - ***cinnb.***
tubercles - sep.

eruptions, penis, prepuce - anan., ***ars-h., calc., caust.,*** cinnb., dulc., ***graph.,*** hep., ***merc.,*** nat-c., **NIT-AC.,** ***petr.,*** ph-ac., ***rhus-t.,*** sang., sars., sep., sil., ***thuj.***
blotches - sep.
burning - caust., ***merc.,*** nit-ac.

eruptions, penis, prepuce
itching - nit-ac., sil.
moist - sil.
pimples - arn., nit-ac., sil.
scurfy, inside - caust.
red, in spots - nit-ac.
tubercles - sep.
under part - carb-v., caust., ***merc.,*** **NIT-AC.,** ***rhus-t.,*** sep., thuj.
scurfy - caust.

eruptions, scrotum - ant-c., ars., ***ars-i., calad.,*** chel., ***crot-t.,*** cupr-ar., **GRAPH., HEP.,** ***kali-c.,*** nat-m., **PETR.,** ph-ac., ***rhus-t., rhus-v.***
blotches - arn.
crusts - anac., chel.
desquamative - ars., crot-t., rhus-v.
dry - calad., chel., ***merc-i-f.***
itching - ars., ***calad., crot-t.,*** **GRAPH.,** nat-m., ***nat-s.,*** **PETR.,** ***rhus-t.***
moist spots - ***sil.***
night - ***calad., crot-t.***
moist - **GRAPH.,** hep., **NAT-M.,** ***petr., rhus-t.,*** sars., ***sil., thuj.***
scrotum and thighs, between - hep., graph., **RHUS-T.,** ***sars.***
pimples - ***calc-p.,*** kali-ar., ph-ac., sars., ***thuj.,*** zinc.
scrotum and thighs, between - ***petr.***
pustules - anac., ant-ox., ant-s., ant-t., ars., crot-t., cupr-ar., podo., tep.
rash - ***petr.,*** puls., ***rhus-t.***
red - chel., petr.
rhagades - ***petr.***
scaly - ***calad.,*** calc., ***merc-i-f.***
scurfy, cracked, dry and red - chel.
thighs, between - hep., nat-m., ***petr.,*** puls., ***rhus-t.***
tubercles - bufo.

ERYSIPELAS, penis, prepuce - ***apis,*** **ARS., LACH.,** ***puls.,*** **RHUS-T.**

erysipelas, scrotum - ***apis, arn., ars.,*** canth., crot-t., graph., merc., nat-m., op., ph-ac., plb., ***puls.,*** **RHUS-T.,** ***rhus-v.***

EXCITABILITY of genitals, sexual desire - agar., aloe, ang., ant-t., ars., aur., aza., cann-i., canth., carb-v., cer-s., chin., cocc., coff., ***dios.,*** erech., gins., ***graph.,*** hep., hyos., ***lyc.,*** meny., naja, ***nat-m.,*** nux-v., op., **PHOS.,** plat., sil., staph., stram., ***sulph.,*** thea., wies.
daybreak at - cedr.
dreams, during erotic - hyos.
loss of excitability - ***agn.***
noon - thuj.

EXCORIATION, genitalia - ***cham.,*** graph., **HEP.,** ***podo.,*** rhod., ***sulph.***

excoriation, penis - cop., kali-i., **NIT-AC.**
glans - anan., cor-r., **MERC.,** merc-i-r., ***nat-c., nat-m., nit-ac.,*** sep., ***sulph.,*** **THUJ.**

excoriation, penis, prepuce - alum., anan., ***ars.,*** calen., cann-s., carb-v., ***caust.,*** cop., ***cor-r., hep.,*** ign., ***mez.,*** **MERC.,** mur-ac., **NIT-AC.,** nux-v., ph-ac., phyt., ***psor.,*** sep., ***sil., thuj.,*** verat.
easy - ***nat-c.***
margin, on the - cann-s., cham., **IGN.,** ***mur-ac.,*** nit-ac., nux-v., rumx.
sex, after - calen.

excoriation, perineum - alum., arum-t., aur-m., ***calc.,*** carb-an., ***carb-v., caust., cham., graph., hep.,*** ign., **LYC.,** ***merc.,*** petr., puls., rhod., sep., ***sulph.,*** thuj.

excoriation, scrotum - **ARS.,** calc., ***calc-p.,*** chel., **HEP.,** kali-c., nit-ac., petr., ph-ac., **SULPH.,** sumb., ***thuj.***
between, and thighs - bar-c., caust., ***graph.,*** hep., **LYC., MERC., NAT-C.,** ***nat-m., nit-ac.,*** nux-v., **PETR.,** rhus-t., ***sulph., thuj.***
sides of - berb., sumb., ***thuj.***

EXCRESCENCES, genito-anal surface - nit-ac., ***thuj.***

excrescences, penis, glans, epithelioma on - arg-n., ***ars.,*** con., thuj.
prepuce - cinnb., ph-ac., sabin., thuj.

excrescences, testes - bar-c., thuj.

FESTERING, prostate, sensation - cycl.

FIRMNESS, testes, increased of - brom.

FISTULOUS, openings, scrotum - ***iod.,*** phyt., spong.

FLACCIDITY, genitalia - **AGN.,** ant-t., asc-t., ***calad.,*** camph., carb-ac., carb-an., carb-s., coff., crot-h., dig., ***dios., gels.,*** hell., lyc., phos., sil., staph., sumb., tab., ust.
relaxed, flabby, cold and weak - absin., **AGN.,** ***calad.,*** caps., ***chin., con., dios., gels.,*** ham., ***lyc.,*** nuph., ***ph-ac.,*** phos., ***sel.,*** sep., staph., sulph., uran-n.
sex, during - nux-v., ph-ac., sulph.
suddenly - graph., lyc., nux-v.

flaccidity, penis - agar., **AGN.,** ant-ox., ***bar-c., calad., cann-i.,*** canth., carb-ac., hell., jac-c., lach., **LYC.,** merc., ***mur-ac., nux-m., nux-v.,*** ph-ac., pic-ac., plb., prun.
glans - mag-m., nat-c.

FLOWING, everything toward - coloc.

FORMICATION, genitalia - acon., berb., calc-p., clem., **PLAT., SEC.,** ***tarent.***
emission, after - ph-ac.

formication, penis - acon., alum., carl., coloc., ph-ac., puls., **SEC.,** tab., valer.
fraenum - ***ph-ac.***
glans - alum., chel., merc., ***nat-m.,*** ph-ac.
after urination -***puls.***

formication, scrotum - carb-v., carl., ***chel.,*** chin., com., merc., nit-ac., ph-ac., plat., rhus-v., **SEC.,** sil., ***staph.,*** thuj.
evening in bed - chim.

formication, testes - agn., berb., carb-v., euphr., hipp., merc., rhod., thuj., zinc.

FRETTING, testes, corrosion, sensation of - ph-ac., plat.

FULLNESS, prostate - alum., ***chim.,*** berb., bry., ***cycl.,*** nux-v.

fullness, spermatic cord, sense of - fl-ac.

GANGRENE, genitalia - ars., ***canth.,*** crot-h., kali-i., laur.

gangrene, penis - ***ars., canth., kali-i., kreos.,*** **LACH.,** ***laur., sec.***
paraphimosis, from - ars., canth., ***lach.,*** merc., ***merc-i-r.,*** sec., tarent.
threatening - ***fl-ac.***

gangrene, scrotum - fl-ac.

GNAWING, pain, testes - ph-ac., plat.

GONORRHEA, (see Bladder) - ***acon.,*** agn., apis, ***arg-n., baros.,*** benz-ac., ***camph.,*** **CANN-S.,** ***canth., caps., clem., cop., cub.,*** dig., ***dor.,*** echi., equis., eucal., euph-pi., fab., ferr., ***gels.,*** hep., ***hydr.,*** ichth., jac., ***kali-bi.,*** kali-s., kreos., **MED.,** ***merc., merc-c.,*** merc-p-r., methyl-b., naphtin., nat-s., ***nit-ac.,*** nux-v., ***ol-sant.,*** pareir., ***petros.,*** pin-c., ***puls.,*** sabal., sabin., sal-n., ***sep.,*** sil., stigm., ***sulph.,*** ter., **THUJ.,** tritic., ***tus-f.,*** zing.
acute, inflammatory - ***acon.,*** arg-n., atro., ***cann-s., canth.,*** caps., ***gels.,*** petros.
adenitis, lymphangitis, with - acon., apis, ***bell.,*** hep., ***merc.***
chordee - acon., ***agav-a., anac.,*** arg-n., bell., berb., ***camph-br., cann-i.,*** cann-s., ***canth.,*** caps., clem., cop., gels., hyos., jac., ***kali-br., lupin.,*** merc., ***oena.,*** ol-sant., phos., ***pic-ac.,*** pip-m., sal-n., ter., tus-f., yohim, zinc-pic.
chronic, subacute stage - arg-n., cann-s., ***cop., cub.,*** erig., ***hep.,*** hydr., ***kali-s.,*** merc., merc-c., merc-i-r., naphtin., ***nat-s., ol-sant.,*** pin-c., psor., ***puls.,*** rhod., ***sabal.,*** sep., sil., stigm., sulph., ***thuj.***
cowperitis - acon., ***cann-s.,*** fab., gels., ***hep.,*** merc-c., petros., ***sabal.,*** sil.

GRASPING, genitals (see Handles)

GRINDING, shooting, pain, morning, spermatic cord - phyt.

GURGLING, sensation, genitalia - phyt.

gurgling, sensation, testes, afternoon, 5 p.m. while sitting - valer.

HAIR, falling off, genitalia - bell., nat-c., **NAT-M.,** ***nit-ac., ph-ac.,*** rhus-t., sars., ***sel.,*** thuj., ***zinc.***
offensive sweat, from - sil., **SULPH.,** thuj.

HANDLES, genitals - ***acon.,*** bell., bufo, canth., colch., ***hyos., merc.,*** plat., ***puls.,*** sep., ***stram.,*** thuj., ust., ***zinc.***
children - ***acon.,*** bufo, ***merc.,*** plat., ***stram., zinc.***
cough, with - ***zinc.***
spasms, with - sec., stram.
constantly - stram.
tearing at genitals - tab.

HARDNESS, prostate (see Induration) - **CON.,** ***cop.,*** iod., med., plb., senec., ***sil., thuj.***
enlargement, without - cop.
hardness, prostate, as if - senec.

HEAT, genitalia - canth., carb-o., coff., dulc., meph., prun., sil., spong., ***sul-ac.,*** sumb., tarent., tub.
eating agg. - tub.
night - meph.
heat, penis - ars., aur., bell., canth., coc-c., euphr., ferr., jac-c., ***mez.,*** phos., plat., rhus-v., sep., ***spong.***
glans - **MERC-C.,** sep.
prepuce - cann-s., merc., plat-m.
heat, prostate - ptel., ***puls.***
heat, scrotum - calc., ***chel.,*** ph-ac., puls., ***spong.,*** sul-ac.
sides, in - sumb.
spots, in - coloc.
heat, spermatic cord - kali-c., ***spong.***
discharge, seminal, with - sabal.
heat, testes - acon., coc-c., ham., kali-c., nat-m., ***nux-v.,*** oci., ***puls.,*** sep., sil., spong., sul-ac., sumb.

HEAVINESS, genitalia - agar., am-c., clem., cupr., elaps, hura, lob., ***nat-c.,*** nux-v., ox-ac., ph-ac., ***psor.,*** tarent., thuj.
urination, during - ph-ac.
heaviness, prostate - cact., caust., ***con.,*** cop., graph., hydrc., ***med.,*** puls., sulph.
lascivious thoughts, during - graph.

HEMATOCELE, genitalia - con., ***ham.,*** ruta.
acute - acon., ***arn.,*** con., erig., ***ham.,*** nux-v., ***puls., sulph.***
chronic - iod., ***kali-i.,*** sulph.

HERNIA, testes - ars., ***bar-c.,*** calc., carb-v., hep., ***merc.,*** nit-ac., ***sil.,*** thuj.

HERPES, genitalia - anan., aur-m., calc., ***caust.,*** crot-h., ***crot-t., dulc., graph., hep.,*** jug-r., ***med., merc.,*** **NAT-M.,** nit-ac., **PETR.,** ph-ac., sars., ***sep.,*** sil., ***tell.,*** ter., ***thuj.***
thighs, between - eup-per., nat-m., ***petr.***
herpes, penis, prepuce - ars., carb-v., caust., ***crot-t., dulc., graph., hep.,*** jug-r., kali-i., med., ***merc.,*** mez., ***nat-c.,*** **NAT-M.,** ***nit-ac., petr., ph-ac., rhus-t., sars., sep., thuj.***
herpes, scrotum - anan., ***calc.,*** cinnb., crot-h., ***crot-t.,*** **DULC.,** ***graph., kali-c.,*** **PETR.,** tell.
scrotum and thighs, between - eup-per., graph., lyc., nat-m., **PETR.**
hydrocele, with - **GRAPH.**

HYDROCELE, scrotum - abrot., ampe-qu, **APIS,** ***arn.,*** ars., ars-i., ***aur.,*** bry., calad., ***calc.,*** calc-f., ***calc-p.,*** canth., ***carb-s.,*** chel., chin., clem., ***con., dig.,*** dulc., ***fl-ac.,*** **GRAPH.,** ***hell., hep.,*** **IOD.,** ***kali-i., lyss.,*** merc., ***merl., nat-m., nux-v.,*** phos., ***psor.,*** **PULS.,** ran-b., **RHOD.,** rhus-t., samb., ***sel.,*** **SIL.,** ***spong.,*** squil., ***sulph.,*** sul-ac., tub.
boys, of - ***abrot., ars., aur., calc., calc-s., graph., kali-chl.,*** **PULS., RHOD., SIL.,** sul-i., ***sulph.***
congenital - rhod.
bruise, caused by a - ***arn.,*** bell-p., con.

HYDROCELE, scrotum
eruptions, suppressed, after - abrot., calc., hell.
gonorrheal orchitis, after - ***phos.***
herpetic, eruptions, with - **GRAPH.**
induration, with - calad., rhus-t.
injury, from - samb.
itching, with - ***ambr.,*** carb-v., caust., ***crot-t.,*** euph., ***graph., hep.,*** nit-ac., nux-v., petr., ph-ac., rhus-t., ***sars.,*** sel., sil., thuj., urt-u.
left side - ***dig.,*** **RHOD.**
multioculair - apis
nodules, with, hard and suppurating - nit-ac.
numbness, with - am-c., ***ambr.,*** sep.
overlifting, from - rhus-t.
painful - am-c., berb., ***clem.,*** iod., kali-c., ***merc.,*** nux-v., ***thuj.***
prurigo, with - ***ant-c.,*** aur., ***graph.,*** mur-ac., nat-s., ***nit-ac.,*** nux-v., ***rhus-t.,*** staph.
retraction, with - plb.
spots, brown, with - con.
suppressed eruption, after - ***abrot., calc.,*** hell.
sweat, with - bell., ***calad.,*** calc., cor-r., cupr-ar., ***dios.,*** fago., nat-m., ***petr.,*** sep., ***sil., sulph.,*** thuj., uran-n.
tubercles, with - con., ***iod.,*** sil., sulph., teucr.

IMPOTENCY, male - ***agar.,*** **AGN.,** alco., alum-p., ***anac., ant-c.,*** ant-ox., ***arn., alum.,*** am-c., arg-m., ***arg-n.,*** ars., ars-i., arum-d., aur., aur-i., aur-s., aven., **BAR-C.,** bar-i., bart., bell-p., berb., bor., ***bufo,*** **CALAD., CALC.,** calc-i., **CALC-S.,** ***camph.,*** cann-i., cann-s., caps., carb-ac., carb-an., carb-s., carb-v., carc., ***caust.,*** cer-s., **CHIN.,** chin-s., chlf., chlol., chlor., cinnam., ***cob., coc-c.,*** coch., cod., ***coff.,*** coloc., **CON.,** corn., cortico., cot., crot-h., crot-t., dam., dig., ***dios.,*** dol., dulc., elaps, ery-a., ery-m., eug., eup-pur., euph., ***ferr.,*** ferr-i., ferr-m., ferr-p., ***fl-ac.,*** gast., ***gels.,*** gins., glyc., ***graph.,*** halo., ***ham., hell.,*** helon., ***hep.,*** hydrc., hyos., ***hyper.,*** ign., ***iod.,*** kali-bi., ***kali-br.,*** kali-c., kali-i., kali-p., kali-s., kreos., ***lach.,*** lappa-a., lath., ***lec.,*** **LYC.,** ***mag-c.,*** **MED.,** meny., ***merc.,*** morph., ***mosch.,*** mur-ac., nat-c., ***nat-m., nat-p., nit-ac., nuph., nux-m.,*** **NUX-V.,** oci-s., ***onos., op.,*** orch., ox-ac., oxyt., pall., perh., petr., ***ph-ac.,*** phase., **PHOS.,** ***phyt., pic-ac.,*** plan., ***plb.,*** polyg., ***psor., puls.,*** rhod., rhodi., rhodi-o-n., ruta, ***sabad., sabal.,*** sabin., ***sal-n.,*** saroth., sec., **SEL., SEP.,** sil., spong., ***stann., staph.,*** stram., ***stry.,*** sul-ac., sul-i., **SULPH.,** sumb., ***syph.,*** tab., teucr., thal., thala., ther., ***thuj.,*** trib., tus-p., ***uran-n.,*** ust., ***yohim,*** zinc., zinc-p.
afternoon - lyss.
amorous caresses, even after - calad.
awake, when - op.
chronic - lyc.
cold, from a - mosch.
constant erection, after - carb-s.
continence, from - **CON.,** ***phos.***
desire, after - **PHOS.**
suppression of desire, from - ***phos.***
diabetes, with - ***helon.,*** mosch.
disappearing during sex - ambr., ***camph.,*** fl-ac., mag-aust., nux-v., ***ph-ac.***

IMPOTENCY, male
elderly men, in - **LYC.**
enlarged, prostate, with - dig., lyc., sel.
evening and night - ***agar.,*** kali-p., pall.
excitement, from excessive - phos.
fright during sex, from - ***sin-a., sin-n.***
gonorrhea, after - ***agn., calad.,*** cob., cub., hydr., med., sulph., ***thuj.***
suppressed from - calad., med., thuj.
lascivious fancies, with - sel.
masturbation, from - arg-n., ***gels.,*** graph., kali-c., kali-p., phos., sal-n., stram.
memory, with loss of - **KALI-BR.**
morning - ***agn.,*** carb-an., crot-t., eug., graph., lact.
nervous prostration, from - dam.
penis relaxed when excited - **CALAD.,** ***ham.***
small and cold - **AGN.,** ***bar-c.,*** berb., caps., **LYC.,** ***sulph.***
perspiration, after - **LYC., PHOS.,** stram.
pollutions, after - ***phos.***
sadness, with - ***aur., calad., gels.,*** **KALI-BR.,** ***spong.***
sexual excesses, after - ***agn.,*** alum., aven., **CHIN.,** ***eup-pur.,*** graph., ***kali-br.,*** kali-c., kali-p., **LYC., PHOS.,** ***staph.***
small and cold - **AGN.,** ***bar-c.,*** berb., caps., **LYC.,** ***sulph.***
stultified by sudden laxness of penis - arg-n., camph.
suddenly - chlor., ***fl-ac.***
syphilis, from - merc.
tobacco, from abuse of - calad., lyc.
waking, on - ***card-m.,*** op.
white urethral discharge, chronic with - ***agn., calad.,*** cob.
work, with aversion to - onis.

INDURATION, penis - con., sep.
elderly man, in an - ***berb.,*** con.
prepuce - ***lach.,*** merc-i-r., sep., ***sulph.***
leather-like - sulph.

induration, prostate (see Hardness) - **CON.,** ***cop., iod.,*** plb., ***psor., sel.,*** senec., ***sil., sulph.,*** **THUJ.**

induration, scrotum - con., **RHUS-T., SULPH.**

induration, spermatic cord - ph-ac., ***syph.***

induration, testes - acon., ***agn.,*** alum., ***arg-m.,*** arg-n., arn., ars., ars-i., ***aur., bar-c.,*** bar-m., bell., ***brom., calc., calc-f.,*** calc-p., ***carb-an.,*** carb-v., ***cinnb.,*** **CLEM., CON.,** ***cop., graph., iod.,*** kali-ar., kali-c., kali-chl., ***kali-i.,*** kali-s., lach., lyc., **MED.,** ***merc., merc-i-r.,*** merl., nit-ac., ***nux-v.,*** ox-ac., phos., ***phyt.,*** plb., ***puls.,*** **RHOD., SIL., SPONG.,** ***staph.,*** stry., ***sulph.,*** thuj., ust., ***viol-t.***
chronic - ***aur.,*** bar-c., ***rhod.***
epididymis - ars., ***aur., med.,*** merc., nit-ac., **RHOD., SPONG.**
gonorrhea, after - ***alum., clem.,*** cop., ***med.,*** **RHOD.,** sulph.
left - ***brom.,*** con., kali-chl., mez., oci., ***rhod., thuj.***

induration, testes
right - arg-n., arn., ***aur., clem., con.,*** lach., merc., ***nit-ac., ox-ac.,*** ph-ac., **RHOD.,** sil.
swollen - ***merc.***

INFLAMMATION, genitalia - ***acon.,*** **APIS, ARS.,** calc., cann-s., **CANTH.,** carb-s., cast., con., ***merc.,*** mur-ac., nat-c., nat-m., nit-ac., nux-v., ph-ac., plb., puls., ***rhus-t.,*** sep., ***spong.,*** staph., thuj.
lymphatic glands - merc.
otorrhea, from suppressed - zinc.

inflammation, of penis - ***arn., ars.,*** cann-s., canth., crot-t., cub., iris, jac-c., ***kali-i.,*** led., merc., nat-c., plb., ***psor.,*** sars., sep., ***sulph.***
warmth of bed agg. - jac-c.
fraenum - ***calc., nit-ac.,*** sumb.

inflammation, penis, glans - alum., ***alumn., apis,*** arn., ars., ***aur.,*** bry., ***calad., calc.,*** cann-s., canth., carb-s., caust., **CINNB.,** ***cor-r.,*** cupr., ***dig.,*** graph., ***jac-c.,*** **KALI-CHL.,** kali-p., ***kali-s.,*** lach., led., ***lyc.,*** lyss., ***merc., merc-c.,*** mez., nat-a., nat-c., ***nat-m., nit-ac.,*** nux-v., petr., ph-ac., ***psor., rhod.,*** rhus-t., sars., sep., sil., ***sulph., thuj.***

inflammation, penis, prepuce - ***acon., apis, ars.,*** calad., ***calc., cann-s., canth.,*** **CINNB.,** coc-c., con., cor-r., crot-t., dig., elaps, ***gels.,*** hep., ***jac., jac-c.,*** lach., lyc., **MERC.,** merc-c., mez., mur-ac., nat-a., ***nat-c., nit-ac.,*** ol-sant., ***rhus-t.,*** sabin., sep., sil., ***sulph., sumb., thuj.,*** viol-t.
erysipelatous - ***apis,*** **ARS., LACH.,** ***puls.,*** **RHUS-T.**
inner surface - crot-t., ***nit-ac.***

inflammation, prostatitis, (see Prostatitis)

inflammation, scrotum - anac., ***ars.,*** crot-t., jac-c., mur-ac., nat-m., plb., ph-ac., podo., ***rhus-t., rhus-v.***
erysipelatous - ***apis, arn., ars.,*** canth., crot-t., graph., merc., nat-m., op., ph-ac., plb., ***puls.,*** **RHUS-T.,** ***rhus-v.***

inflammation, spermatic cord - arn., ***berb.,*** calc., ham., kali-c., nux-v., psor., **PULS.,** ***rhod.,*** **SPONG.,** ***syph.***

inflammation, testes, (see Orchitis)

INJURIES, to genitalia - **ARN., BELL-P.,** ***calen.,*** con., ***hyper.,*** mill., ***rhus-t., staph.***

injuries, to penis - arn., bell-p., calen., hyper., mill., rhus-t., staph.

IRRITATION, in prostate - cact., ***dig.,*** gnaph.

ITCHING, genitalia - agar., agn., ***alum., ambr.,*** am-c., anac., ***ang.,*** ars., benz-ac., berb., ***calad.,*** **CALC.,** canth., carb-ac., carb-an., carb-s., ***carb-v.,*** carl., **CAUST.,** ***chel.,*** chin-s., cinnb., clem., coff., com., con., crot-t., dulc., ***eup-per.,*** euphr., ***fago., graph.,*** ictod., ***ign., iris, kali-bi.,*** kali-c., kali-i., kali-s., lyc., ***mag-m., merc.,*** nat-a., nat-c., nat-m., ***nat-s., nit-ac., petr.,*** plan., **PLAT.,** ***podo.,*** rad-br., rhus-d., ***rhus-t.,*** rhus-v., ***sars.,*** scroph-n., sel., ***sep.,*** sil., sumb., ***sulph.,*** tarax., tarent-c.
burning, and - **CALC.,** carb-ac., nat-c., nat-m., urt-u.

ITCHING, genitalia
emission, after - ph-ac.
hairy parts - kali-bi., lyss.
hot applications amel. - rhus-v.
morning, on waking - sulph.
in a red raw spot - graph.
night - agar., rhus-v.
bed, in - ign., ***merc.***
painful - ictod.
rubbing, agg. - con.
scratching, agg. - iris, tril.
amel. - ign.
spots, in - bar-c.
stitching as from vermin - nat-c.
thighs, between - carb-v., nat-m., ***petr.***
genitalia and scrotum - ***nat-m.,*** viol-t.
urinatiall over, especially on genitals, on, during - arg-n., sil.
voluptuous - berb., **PLAT.,** sumb.

itching, penis - ***acon.,*** agar., agn., alum., ambr., ang., ***ant-c.,*** ars., ars-i., aur-m., bell., benz-ac., berb., ***calad.,*** calc., cann-i., ***canth.,*** caps., carl., carb-ac., **CAUST.,** cham., chin., cinnb., coc-c., com., ***con.,*** cop., cor-r., ***crot-t.,*** cupr., der., dig., graph., ham., ***hep., ign.,*** indg., iod., kali-ar., kali-bi., kali-c., kali-n., lach., lachn., led., ***lyc.,*** mag-m., merc., ***mez.,*** nat-c., nat-m., ***nat-s.,*** nit-ac., nux-v., petr., ph-ac., phos., **PLAT.,** ***puls.,*** rhus-v., sabad., sel., sep., spong., staph., ***sulph.,*** sumb., thuj., ***viol-t.***
alternating with stitching in anus - ***thuj.***
evening, in bed - chin., ***ign.,*** mag-m., nux-v., phos., sumb.
root of - ars., lyss., ***rhus-t.***
rubbing without effect - con.
sex, during - sep.
voluptuous - caust., mang., sep., spong.
increases the excitement during sex - sep.

itching, penis, fraenum - caust., ***hep.,*** lyc., ***ph-ac.***

itching, penis, glans - agn., alum., ***ambr.,*** ant-c., arn., ***ars.,*** ars-i., ***aur-m.,*** bell., ***benz-ac.,*** calc., cann-i., cann-s., caps., carb-ac., ***carb-v.,*** caust., ***chel.,*** chin., **CINNB.,** colch., con., **CROT-T.,** dros., euphr., ferr-ma., gymn., hell., hep., ictod., ind., indg., ip., iod., ***kali-bi.,*** kali-c., led., ***lyc.,*** lyss., mag-m., mang., merc., ***mez.,*** nat-c., nat-m., ***nat-s.,*** **NIT-AC.,** ***nux-v.,*** petr., ***ph-ac.,*** psor., senec., sep., ***sil.,*** spong., **SULPH.,** ***thuj.***
increasing the excitement during sex - sep.
tip of - ant-c., nat-m.
urination, during - thuj.
walking, air, in open - ang.

itching, penis, prepuce - agar., aloe, ang., ars., berb., calc., cann-s., ***canth., caps.,*** carb-v., **CAUST.,** ***cham.,*** **CINNB.,** colch., **CON.,** euph., graph., gymn., ***hep.,*** **IGN.,** jac-c., ***lyc., merc.,*** mez., nat-a., nat-c., nat-m., nat-p., **NIT-AC.,** nux-v., **PETR.,** phos., ***puls.,*** **RHUS-T.,** ***sep., sil., sulph.,*** sumb., tarax., ***thuj., viol-t.,*** zinc., zing.
herpes, with - sars.
stool, after - aloe.

itching, penis, prepuce
raphe - euphr.
tip - ars.
underside - camph., caust., **LYC.,** ***nit-ac., nux-v., puls., rhus-t.,*** sil., ***thuj.***

itching, scrotum - acon., agar., alum., alumn., am-c., ***ambr.,*** anac., ang., ant-c., ant-t., ant-s., ***apis,*** arg-m., ars-m., ***arum-d.,*** **AUR.,** ***bar-c.,*** berb., calad., ***calc.,*** calc-ac., ***calc-p.,*** cann-i., ***carb-ac.,*** **CARB-S.,** carl., **CAUST.,** cham., ***chel.,*** chin., ***cist., cocc.,*** coc-c., com., con., **CROT-T.,** ferr., ferr-ma., form., **GRAPH.,** hep., hipp., indg., jatr., **KALI-C.,** ***kali-chl., kali-s.,*** lachn., lac-ac., ***lyc., mag-m.,*** manc., ***mang.,*** meph., ***merc., mur-ac.,*** nat-a., nat-c., **NAT-M.,** nat-p., nat-s., **NIT-AC.,** ***nuph., nux-v.,*** **PETR.,** ph-ac., plat., prun., puls., rat., ***rhod.,*** **RHUS-T.,** rhus-v., ***sars., sel., sil.,*** spong., ***staph.,*** **SULPH.,** thuj., **URT-U.,** ***viol-t., zinc.***
afternoon - tell.
burning - carb-ac., cocc., gran.
corrosion, painful - **CROT-T.**
evening - alum., sulph., thuj., ***zinc.***
bed, in - calc.
extending to perineum - rhus-t., ***sars.***
to, septum - caust.
to, sides of - agar., ant-c., coff., croc., petr., thuj.
friction amel. - junc., mag-m., rhus-v., staph.
morning - coc-c., puls.
scratching, after - ***nat-s.***
night - calad., com., crot-t., kali-c., lyc., ***nat-m.***
noon - com., ***sulph.***
preventing sleep - kali-c.
scratching, agg. - rhus-v.
amel. - alum., carb-ac., ***crot-t.,*** viol-t.
not relieved by - ***mur-ac., zinc.***
septum - caust.
sides of - agar., ant-c., coff., croc., petr., thuj.
sleep, preventing - kali-c.
spots, in - nicc., sil.
voluptuous - ***ambr., anac.,*** cocc., ***crot-t.,*** euphr., mur-ac., spong., ***staph.***
rubbing agg. - staph.
sexual excesses, after - **STAPH.**
walking agg. - ***crot-t.***
warm agg., when - rhus-v.

itching, spermatic cord - mang., ox-ac.

itching, testes - iod.

JERKING, in penis - cinnb., form., mez., ***thuj.,*** zinc.
glans, in - bar-c.
sleep, during - cinnb.

jerking, in prostaate, region of - form.

jerking, pain, spermatic cord - ang., mang., ox-ac., plb.

KRYPTORCHISM, genitalia - aur., psor., syph., tub.

LANCINATING, pain - croc.

LICE, crab, genitalia - cocc., sabad., staph.

LONG, as if - calad.

MASTURBATION, (see Sex)

METASTASIS, genitalia - ***abrot., carb-v., puls.***

MOISTURE, penis, glans - nit-ac., sep.
corona glandis - nat-m., staph.
odor, saltish - sep.
sour - sep.

moisture, scrotum - ***calc-p.,*** chel., cop., nat-c., **PETR.,** ***sil.,*** **SULPH., THUJ.,** zinc.
acrid - bar-c., cop.
between, and thighs - ***bar-c.,*** carb-v., **HEP.,** lyc., merc., nat-c., nat-m., petr., rhod., ***sulph., thuj.***
purulent - jac.
serum, running with - bell., ***calc-p.,*** hep., kali-i., rhus-t.
spots, on - sil.

MOTION, in testes, sensation as if - sabad., thuj., valer.

MUCUS, penis, glans - graph., nit-ac.

NEURALGIC, pain, testes - arg-n., ***aur.,*** bell., ***berb., clem., coll.,*** con., euphr., ***ham.,*** ign., ***mag-p.,*** merc., nux-v., ol-an., ***ox-ac.,*** oxyt., ***puls.,*** spong., verat-v., zinc-m.

NODES, penis, glans - bell.
spermatic cords - syph.

NODULES, prostate, on- ***bar-c.,*** thuj.

nodules, scrotum, hard, brown on- ***nit-ac.,*** syph.

nodules, testes, hard, brown on - ***psor.***

NUMBNESS, genitalia - ambr., bar-c., dig., form., ***graph.***
ascending stairs, on - form.

numbness, penis - ***merc.,*** plat.
glans, and prepuce - berb.
morning, erections, with violent - ambr.

numbness, scrotum, knees up to - bar-c.

numbness, testes - caps., carb-s., nat-c.

ODOR, genitalia, offensive - ***nat-m., sars., sulph.,*** **THUJ.**
briny, odor, sex, after - sanic.
semen, of - kali-c.

ONANISM, from (see Sex)

ORCHITIS, inflammation of testes - **ACON.,** am-c., anan., ant-t., ***arg-n.,*** **ARN.,** ***ars., aur.,*** **BAPT.,** bar-m., ***bell., berb.,*** chel., ***chin.,*** **CLEM., CON.,** cub., der., ***euph.,*** gels., ***ham.,*** hippoz., kali-ar., kali-c., ***kali-i., lyc., merc.,*** mez., nat-a., nat-c., ***nat-m., nit-ac., nux-v.,*** **PAROT.,** phos., ***phyt., plb.,*** podo., **PULS., RHOD., RHUS-T., SPONG.,** ***staph.,*** sul-ac., verat-v., zinc.
acute - ***acon.,*** ant-t., arg-m., arg-n., ***bell.,*** brom., cham., chin., chin-s., ***clem.,*** cub., gels., ***ham.,*** kali-s., ***merc.,*** nit-ac., nux-v., phyt., polyg., ***puls., rhod., spong.,*** teucr-s., verat-v.
chronic - agn., ***aur.,*** bar-c., ***calc-i.,*** chin., ***clem., con.,*** gels., ***hep.,*** hyper., iod., ***kali-i.,*** lyc., merc., nit-ac., phyt., ***puls.,*** **RHOD.,** rhus-t., ***spong.,*** sulph., ust.

ORCHITIS, general
contusion, from - **ARN.,** bar-m., ***con., ham., puls.,*** zinc.
epididymis - ***acon.,*** apis, arg-n., ars., ***aur., bell.,*** berb., cann-s., ***chin., clem., gels., ham.,*** kali-n., ***med., merc.,*** nit-ac., phyt., **PULS., RHOD.,** sabal., **SPONG.,** sulph., teucr-s., thuj., vib.
extending right to left - spong.
gonorrhea, from suppressed - **AGN.,** ant-t., arg-n., aur., bar-m., bell., brom., canth., chel., **CLEM.,** ***con., ham.,*** kali-chl., ***kali-s.,*** **MED.,** ***merc., mez.,*** nat-c., nat-m., ***nit-ac.,*** **PULS.,** ***rhod.,*** rhus-t., sel., ***spong.,*** **THUJ.**
left - brom., mez., oci., **PULS.,** ***rhod.***
metastatic - ***puls.,*** staph.
night - **CLEM.**
right - ***arg-n.,*** chel., **CLEM.,** ***puls.,*** **RHOD.**
syphilitic - aur., ***kali-i.,*** merc-i-r.
warmth of bed agg. - **CLEM.**

PAIN, genitalia - ***acon.,*** agn., ***apis,*** arg-m., **ARG-N.,** asim., ***aur., bell.,*** berb., ***brom.,*** cahin., ***cann-s.,*** caps., cer-b., cham., chin., ***clem., con.,*** eupi., gins., ***ham.,*** hydr., ign., iod., jatr., kali-c., lyc., ***lycpr.,*** merc., merc-i-r., nit-ac., nux-v., ***ox-ac., oxyt.,*** ph-ac., pic-ac., plat., ***puls., rhod.,*** sal-n., sep., ***spong.,*** staph., sulph., tarent., ***thuj.***
sex, during - arg-n.

PAIN, penis - arn., ***ars., cann-i., cann-s.,*** canth., caul., chel., clem., coc-c., cycl., dig., dulc., ***ign.,*** jac-c., lac-c., kali-bi., kali-c., lith., ***merc.,*** mez., naja, nat-c., osm., phos., plb., prun., rhod., rhus-t., rhus-v., sabad., stry., sumb., tarax., thuj.
cough, during - ign.
motion agg. - berb.
needles, like - asaf.
root - equis., hydr., ign., ***petros.***
spasmodic - nux-m.
stool, during - hydr.
swelled prepuce, from - ***rhus-t.***
tip - camph., hipp., nuph., osm., phos., psor.
urination, at beginning - psor.
touch, on - sumb.
urination, during - ferr-i., nat-m., petr., phos., sulph.
walking when - cann-s., ign., puls-n, thuj.

pain, penis, glans - all-c., asaf., asar., berb., calc., **CANTH.,** ***chel.,*** cic., colch., ***cop.,*** cycl., ***ferr-p.,*** kali-bi., med., mez., ***merc.,*** nat-c., nat-m., osm., ox-ac., **PAREIR.,** ph-ac., viol-t.
behind during erections after sex - nat-c.
urging to urinate, on - aran., aur., ferr-p., lyc., pareir., thuj.
urination, during - acon., act-sp., anac., casc., lyc., ox-ac., prun.
after - anac., lyc., phos., ***puls.***
before - ***canth.,*** lyc.
behind glans during erection after sex - nat-c.

pain, penis, prepuce - ***acon.,*** apis, bell., ***berb.,*** calad., ***cann-s., canth.,*** cinnb., coc-c., con., ***cop.,*** cor-r., cycl., ign., ***lyc., merc.,*** merc-c., ***nit-ac.,*** nux-v., osm., ***rhus-t.,*** sabin., sep., sulph., ***thuj.,*** verat.
rubbing, slight, agg. - cycl.
urination, during - phos.

PAIN, prostate - acon., ***all-c., alum.,*** apis, asaf., bar-c., ***bell.,*** berb., bov., brom., cact., calc-p., ***caps., caust., chim.,*** **CON.,** cop., crot-h., ***cub.,*** cupr-ar., ***cycl.,*** dig., gnaph., graph., laur., ***lyc.,*** lyss., med., merc., ol-an., pareir., ***phos.,*** podo., polyg., **PULS.,** ***rhus-t.,*** **SABAL.,** ***sel.,*** sep., solid., ***staph.,*** sulph., sul-i., tarent., **THUJ.**
blowing nose, on - alum.
cancer, in - carc., crot-h.
erection, during - alum.
extending to urethra - staph.
gonorrhea, during - ***caps.,*** cub., med.
jarring agg. - **BELL.**
riding agg. - staph.
sex, after - ***all-c.,*** alum., caps., ***psor.,*** sel.
sitting, while - ***chim., cycl.,*** dig., rhus-t.
standing - cycl.
stool, after - phos.
urging to stool - ***cycl.,*** rhus-t.
urinate, urging to - ***cycl., rhus-t.***
urination, during - ***apis,*** cop., lyc., med., pareir.
after - lyc., polyg., **PULS.**
at close of - coca.
walking, agg. - all-c., brom., ***cycl.,*** kali-bi., sulph.
amel. - ***rhus-t.***

PAIN, spermatic cords - all-c., ammc., am-c., anth., apis, ***arg-n.,*** arn., arund., aur., ***bell., berb.,*** cahin., ***calc.,*** calc-ar., camph., ***cann-s.,*** caps., chel., chin., chin-s., cimic., ***clem.,*** coloc., con., ***dios.,*** echi., grat., **HAM.,** ind., kali-c., lith., mang., meny., ***merc., merc-i-r.,*** morph., nat-p., ***nit-ac.,*** nux-v., ***ol-an., ox-ac.,*** osm., oxyt., ***phos., phyt.,*** pic-ac., plb., polyg., ***puls., sars., senec.,*** sil., ***spong.,*** staph., stry., sulph., tarent., ***thlaspi, thuj.,*** tub., tus-f., verat-v.
cough, during - ***nat-m.***
emission, after - ***nat-p.***
erection, after - mag-m., nux-m., ***sars.***
exertion, after - calc-ar., ox-ac.
extending, abdomen - rhod.
down - sars.
epididymis, into - ***berb.,*** senec.
testes, into - all-c., ***berb.,*** dios., **HAM.,** lith., merc., osm., plb., puls., senec.
thighs, to - rhod.
upward - osm.
left - berb., calc., grat., nat-p., plb., stry., tub.
sitting and standing - berb.
then right - calc.
urination, after - lith.
morning - clem., sars.
motion agg. - ox-ac.
neuralgic - ***arg-n.,*** aur., ***bell., berb.,*** clem., ham., menth., nit-ac., nux-v., ***ox-ac.,*** phyt., ***spong.***

PAIN, spermatic cords
riding carriage amel. - tarent.
right - cimic., ***clem.,*** echi., morph., ox-ac.
sex, after - arund., mag-m., nat-p., sars., ther.
sitting, while - berb.
stool, during - coca, phos.
urination, during - ***apis,*** bell., canth., clem., polyg., stront-c.
wine, after - calc-ar.

PAIN, testes - abrot., alum., alumn., am-c., ant-ox., **ARG-M.,** ***arn.,*** asaf., **AUR.,** bapt., ***bell., berb.,*** bism., ***calc.,*** cann-s., carb-s., ***caust.,*** chel., cimic., **CLEM.,** cocc., ***coloc., con.,*** der., dig., dios., equis., ***ham.,*** ign., ind., ***iod.,*** kali-br., kali-i., kali-n., kalm., ***lith.,*** lycps., lyss., ***merc.,*** nat-c., ***nat-m.,*** nat-p., nit-ac., nux-v., ol-an., op., osm., ox-ac., ***plb.,*** ph-ac., phos., pip-m., polyg., **PULS., RHOD., SPONG.,** sabad., sel., **SEP.,** sil., **STAPH.,** tarax., tarent., thuj., tub., ust., verat-v., ***zinc.***
afternoon - dios., kalm.
2 p.m. - ery-a.
coughing, on - am-c., nat-m., osm., zinc.
emission, during - caps.
after - caps., mag-m., ox-ac., ***ph-ac.***
erections, after - con., mag-m., ox-ac.
evening - chin-s., lycps., sel., ust., verat-v.
bed, in - ***arg-m.***
urination, before - equis.
extending, abdomen, through - fago.
abdomen, to - iod.
spermatic cord, into - arum-t., plb., polyg., staph.
spermatic cord, into, suddenly shifting to bowels causing nausea - ham.
stomach, to - ham.
left - alum., con., der., dios., kali-br., lycps., nat-c., polyg., ***staph.,*** sumb., tub., verat-v.
lying agg. - sil.
morning - ***clem.,*** kalm., sars., verat-v.
motion, agg. - asaf., berb., ery-a., mag-m., ox-ac.
amel. - arg-m., carb-s., ***rhod.***
night - cer-s., osm., sil.
noon - ***caust.,*** ust.
paroxysmal - spong.
pressure of clothing agg. - **ARG-M.**
right - alum., **ARG-M.,** arg-n., **AUR.,** ***caust.,*** bism., chel., cob., coloc., dig., ind., jac-c., morph., nat-a., nat-m., nat-p., osm., **RHOD.**
thigh, to - sep.
to left - kalm.
urination, after, amel. - cob.
rising, after - mag-m.
sexual excitement, after - ***iod.,*** kali-n., lyss., staph.
sickening as from a blow - nat-a.
sitting, while - **PULS.,** rhod.
standing agg. - rhod.
stepping heavily - colch., coloc.
stool, during - coca, phos.
touch, on - alum., mag-m., nit-ac., ph-ac., spong., staph., zinc.

PAIN, testes
urination, during - polyg.
walking, while - **ARG-M.,** clem., coloc., jac-c., ***lyc.,*** ox-ac., ***staph.,*** sumb., thuj., zinc.
wine agg. - thuj.

PERSPIRATION, genitalia - acet-ac., agn., alum., am-c., ars., ars-i., asc-t., **AUR.,** bar-c., ***bell., calad., calc., canth.,*** carb-an., carb-s., ***carb-v.,*** carl., con., ***cor-r.,*** dios., **FL-AC.,** ***gels.,*** hep., ***hydr.,*** ign., iod., lachn., lyc., mag-m., ***merc.,*** merc-i-f., mez., ***petr.,*** ph-ac., ***puls.,*** sars., **SEL., SEP.,** ***sil.,*** staph., ***sulph.,*** **THUJ.**
cold - ***carb-v.***
coughing agg. - thuj.
evening - carb-s.
exertion, after - sep.
fish, brine, like - sanic., med., thuj.
sex, after - sanic.
morning - ***aur.***
musty - thuj.
night - bell., staph.
offensive - aloe, ars-m., fago., ***fl-ac., hydr., iod.,*** merc-d., ***nat-m.,*** psor., ***sars., sep.,*** sil., **SULPH.,** ***thuj.***
pungent - ***dios., fl-ac.***
sweetish - ***thuj.***
walking, air, in open - ph-ac.

perspiration, penis - lachn., nat-m., nit-ac., thuj.

perspiration, scrotum - acon., agn., am-c., ***aur.,*** bar-c., bell., calad., ***calc., calc-p.,*** carb-an., carb-s., carb-v., caust., ***con.,*** cupr-ar., daph., ***dios.,*** gels., ***ham.,*** hep., hydr., ***ign., iod.,*** lachn., ***lyc., mag-m., merc.,*** mez., ***nat-s., petr., psor., rhod., sel., sep.,*** **SIL.,** staph., **SULPH., THUJ.,** ust.
cold - plan.
evening - nat-s., sil.
morning - thuj., ust.
night - ham., mag-m.
one side of - thuj.
strong smelling - ***dios., thuj.***
sweetish smelling - ***thuj.***
thighs, between - cinnb.

PHIMOSIS, penis - acon., apis, ***arn.,*** bell., calad., ***calc., cann-s., canth., cinnb.,*** coloc., cycl., ***dig.,*** euphr., ***ham., hep.,*** jac., ***lyc.,*** **MERC.,** nat-m., **NIT-AC.,** ol-sant., ph-ac., ***rhus-t.,*** sabad., sabin., sep., ***sulph.,*** sumb., thuj.
friction, from - arn., calen.
gangrene, threatening, with - ***ars.,*** canth., ***cinnb., lach., merc-i-r.***
paraphimosis - bell., ***coloc.,*** kali-i., ***lach.,*** **MERC.,** ***merc-c.,*** nat-m., **NIT-AC.,** ***rhus-t.,*** sep., thuj.
suppuration, with - ***caps., cinnb., hep., merc., nit-ac.***
swelling, extensive, of glans - ***kali-i.***

PINCHING, pain, penis - acon., alum., brom., chel., graph., osm.
glans - kali-bi., mez., ph-ac.
prepuce - jac-c.

pinching, scrotum - **CLEM.,** mez.

pinching, testes - caps., ***clem.,*** con., kali-c., nat-m., sep., **SPONG.**
afternoon - caps.
urinating, while - caps.
after - caps.

PRESSING, pain, genitalia - alum., asaf., benz-ac., cocc., kali-c., kali-n., mag-m., merc., ***plat.***
alternating with contraction of anus - ***bell.***
cramp-like morning in bed - phos.
downwards - bell., cinnb., lil-t., ***plat.***
outwards, morning in bed - nux-v.
stool, during - ***kali-c.***
stool, before - nat-c.

pressing, penis - iod.
glans - alum., caps., lyc., nit-ac., puls., seneg.
urination, before - chin.
tip, after urination - coloc.

pressing, prostate - all-c., ***alum.,*** apis, asaf., berb., brom., cact., ***caust.,*** chim., ***con., cycl.,*** laur., ***lyc.,*** merc., ol-an., ***phos., puls., sel.,*** sulph., thuj.
erection, at beginning of - ***alum.***
nose, on blowing - alum.
sex, during - ***alum.***
standing - cycl.
urination, during - ***lyc.***
after - lyc., **PULS.**
walking, while - all-c., brom., ***cycl.***

pressing, spermatic cord - anth., berb., brom., ***clem.,*** kali-n., mang., meny., nat-c., ***puls.,*** sil., spong., sulph., thuj.
downward - ***iod.,*** nux-m.

pressing, testes - am-c., ***aur.,*** berb., ***bism.,*** calc., ***cann-s.,*** carb-v., **CAUST.,** ***con.,*** clem., gins., ign., kali-n., lach., mang., merc., nat-c., nat-m., nat-p., ph-ac., **PULS.,** ***rhod.,*** sabad., ***sil.,*** spong., squil., ***staph., sulph.,*** thuj., **ZINC.**
extending from lumbar region on coughing - osm.
to spermatic cord - zinc.
to spermatic cord and abdomen - kali-n.
left - ***con.,*** sabad., zinc.
noon - caust.
right - ***aur.,*** bism., ***caust., staph.***
sexual, excitement, after - kali-n.
sitting - thuj.
standing, while - ***cann-s.,*** puls.
touch, agg. - bism., ph-ac., staph.
walking, agg. - ph-ac., staph.

PRIAPISMUS, penis, painful erections (see Erections) - lyss.

PRICKING, genitalia - ***nit-ac.***

PROSTATE gland, general - aesc., aloe, apis, bar-c., baros., caust., chim., **CON.,** crot-h., dam., ***dig.,*** fab., ***ferr-pic.,*** hep., ***hydrang., iod., kali-i.,*** lyc., med., ***mela.,*** merc., pareir., phos., phyt., pic-ac., polyg., pop., **PULS., SABAL.,** ***sel.,*** sep., ***solid., staph.,*** sul-i., sulph., **THUJ.**
rectal troubles, with - podo.

PROSTATIC fluid, emissions - agar., ***agn.,*** alum., am-c., ***anac., apis, aur.,*** bell., calad., ***calc.,*** cann-s., canth., casc., chim., ***con.,*** daph., dig., ***elaps, ery-a., euph.,*** gels., ***hep., lyc.,*** lyss., ***mag-c.,*** mang., ***nat-c., nat-m., nit-ac.,*** nux-m., ***petr.,*** **PH-AC.,** ***phos.,*** pic-ac., plat., plb., ***psor., puls.,*** sabal., **SEL., SEP.,** ***sil., spig.,*** **STAPH.,** ***sulph.,*** tab., tarent., ***thuj.,*** thymol., ***zinc.***

causeless - zinc.

dribbling - ***phos.,*** **SEL.**

easily discharged, so, that even an emission of flatus causes - mag-c.

emotion, with every - **CON.,** hep., puls., sel., zinc.

erections, during - nit-ac., **PH-AC.,** ***puls.***

without - aur., bell., cann-s., con., euph., ***lyc.,*** lyss., ***nat-m., phos.,*** **SEL.,** thuj.

flatus, while passing - con., ***mag-c.***

fondling, women, while - agn., **CON.**

involuntary - sel.

night - sel.

lascivious thoughts, during - **CON.,** ***lyc., nat-m.,*** **NIT-AC.,** ***ph-ac., phos.,*** pic-ac.

morning - ran-b.

sitting, while - ***sel.***

sleep, during - sel.

stool, with - agar., ***agn.,*** alum., am-c., anac., ars., aur-m., ***calc.,*** carb-v., carl., ***caust.,*** **CON.,** cor-r., elaps, ***hep., ign., iod., kali-bi., nat-c., nat-m.,*** nat-p., ***nit-ac.,*** **NUX-V.,** ***petr.,*** **PH-AC.,** ***phos.,*** **SEL., SEP.,** ***sil.,*** staph., sulph., zinc.

after - am-c., anac., ***calc., caust.,*** cur., ***hep., iod., kali-c.,*** lyss., ***nat-c., nit-ac.,*** phos., ***sel., sep., sil.,*** **SULPH.,** zinc.

difficult, with - anac., ***agn.,*** alum., am-c., arn., cann-i., ***carb-v.,*** con., gels., ***hep., nat-c.,*** **NIT-AC., PH-AC.,** ***phos.,*** psor., ***sep.,*** **SIL.,** ***staph.,*** **SULPH.,** zinc.

soft, diarrheic, during - ars.

soft, with - anac., ***sel.***

talking to a young woman, while - ***nat-m., phos.***

thinking of it - nat-m.

tobacco agg. - daph.

urination, during - anac., hep., nat-c., nit-ac., sep., sulph.

after - anac., calc., cur., ***daph., hep.,*** hipp., ***kali-c.,*** lyc., lyss., ***nat-c.,*** nat-m., sel., sep., ***sil.,*** **SULPH.**

before - psor.

walking, while - agn., **SEL.,** sil.

PROSTATITIS, inflammation of - acon., aesc., agn., alum., **APIS,** arn., bell., bov., cact., cann-i., canth., ***caps., caust.,*** **CHIM.,** ***con., cop., cub.,*** cycl., ***dig., dulc.,*** ferr-pic., ***hep.,*** hipp., hydrang., ***kali-bi.,*** lach., lil-t., lith., ***lyc.,*** med., ***merc.,*** merc-d., nit-ac., ***nux-v.,*** pareir., ***petr., ph-ac.,*** polyg-s., **PULS., SABAL.,** sec., ***sel.,*** senec., ***sep., sil.,*** solid., ***staph., sulph.,*** sul-ac., **THUJ.,** zinc.

acute - acon., aesc., aloe, ***apis, bell.,*** bry., canth., **CHIM.,** colch., ***cop.,*** cub., dig., ***fab.,*** ferr-p., ***gels., hep., iod.,*** kali-br.,

PROSTATITIS, general

acute - kali-i., merc-c., ***merc-d., nit-ac.,*** ol-sant., pic-ac., ***puls.,*** sabad., **SABAL.,** sal-n., sel., ***sil.,*** solid., ***staph., thuj.,*** tritic., ***verat-v.,*** vesi.

chronic - alum., ***aur.,*** bar-c., calad., carb-s., caust., clem., ***con., ferr-pic.,*** graph., hep., hydrc., iod., ***lyc., merc., merc-c., nit-ac.,*** nux-v., phyt., ***puls.,*** sabad., ***sabal., sel., sep.,*** sil., solid., ***staph.,*** sulph., **THUJ.,** ***trib.***

gonorrhea, suppressed, from - bell., ***cop.,*** cupr., ***dig., med., merc.,*** **NIT-AC.,** ***nux-v., petr., puls., sep.,*** staph., ***sulph.,*** **THUJ.**

yellow discharge, with thick - cub.

PSORIASIS, penis, prepuce - graph., ***sep.***

psoriasis, scrotum - ***nit-ac., petr.,*** thuj.

PULLING, genitalia, with gravel - canth.

PULSATING, prostate - caust., polyg.

pulsating, region of - bov.

straining to urinate, while - dig.

PULSATION, genitalia - berb.

sex, after - nat-c.

pulsation, penis - berb., brach., ***cop.,*** ham., nit-ac., rhod.

glans - coc-c., ham., nat-m., nit-ac., prun., ptel., rhod.

urination, during - ferr.

left side - osm.

root -thuj.

pulsation, scrotum - hep., nat-c.

sex, after - kali-i.

pulsation, spermatic cord - ***am-m.,*** sumb.

walking, while - sumb.

QUIVERING, prostate, nervous - form.

quivering, scrotum - spig.

RASH, genitalia - bry., dulc., rhus-t.

rash, scrotum - ***petr.,*** puls., ***rhus-t.***

REDNESS, spots, penis - caust.

redness, glans - ***ars.,*** calad., cann-s., ***cor-r.,*** crot-t., ***dor.,*** iris, merc., nat-m., rhus-t., sabin., sars.

spots, in - nat-m., petr., sep., sil.

tip - nat-m.

redness, penis, prepuce - calc., cann-s., **CINNB.,** ***cor-r.,*** lach., lyc., ***merc.,*** prun., rhus-t., rhus-v., rumx., sil., ***sulph.,*** sumb.

prepuce, spots - aloe.

redness, scrotum - anac., ant-s., apis, ***chel.,*** cop., **CROT-T.,** ***merc.,*** **PETR.,** puls., rhus-t., rhus-v., sulph.

bluish - ***mur-ac.***

sides of - agar., ars., petr.

spots, in - lac-ac.

thighs, between - petr.

and scrotum - ambr., cop., nat-m., **PETR.,** thuj.

REITER syndrome - jac., med.

RELAXED, scrotum - acet-ac., ***agn.,*** aloe, am-c., arn., astac., bell., cahin., ***calad., calc.,*** calc-p., camph., caps., carb-ac., carb-an., carb-s., chin., chin-s., **CLEM.,** ***coff., dios., ferr.,*** ferr-i., ***gels., hell.,*** hep., hydrc., iod., iris, lach., ***lec.,*** **LYC.,** mag-c., ***mag-m.,*** merc., ***nat-m.,*** nit-ac., ***nuph.,*** ol-an., op., ***ph-ac.,*** pic-ac., ***psor.,*** **PULS.,** ***rhus-t.,*** sel., sep., ***sil.,*** **STAPH., SULPH.,** sul-ac., sumb., **TAB.,** tarent., thuj., ***tub., uran-n.,*** ust.
erection, during - lyc., sil.
evening in bed - ***sulph.***
right - clem.

RETRACTION, penis - berb., euphr., **IGN.,** mosch., ***nuph.,*** plb., puls.
retraction, penis, prepuce - bell., ***calad.,*** cocc., coloc., ign., nat-c., **NAT-M.,** nux-v., prun., sulph.
difficult - sabin.
morning - nat-c.
night - cocc.
sex, after - ***calad.***
retraction, scrotum - acon., lyss., petr.
retraction, testes - agar., alum., alumn., arg-n., ***aur., bar-c.,*** bell., ***berb.,*** brom., ***calc.,*** calc-p., camph., ***canth.,*** chin., cic., **CLEM.,** coll., coloc., crot-t., euphr., iod., meny., nit-ac., ***nux-v., ol-an.,*** op., pareir., phos., plat., ***plb.,*** psor., puls., ***rhod.,*** sec., sil., ***stram.,*** sulph., syph., thuj., thyr., tub., ***zinc.***
left - calc., crot-t., pareir., thuj.
painful - mag-aust.
night - mag-aust.
right - alum., clem., puls.
walking, while - ***rhod.***

SARCOCELE, genitalia - **AUR.,** calc., iod., ***merc-i-r., puls.,*** rhod., spong.
indolent - tarent.

SCURF, penis, on inside of prepuce - caust.
scurf, spots, red, on corona - cor-r., nit-ac.

SEMEN, genitalia, dribbling - ***calad.,*** canth., dam., gels., pic-ac., ***sel., thuj.***
sleep, in - plb., ***sel.,*** sil., tax.
unnoticed - sel.

SEMINAL discharge, (see Ejaculation or Seminal Emissions)

SEMINAL, emissions, (see Ejaculation) - abr., abrot., absin., acet-ac., acon., acon-c., aesc., ***agar., agn.,*** aloe, ***alum.,*** alumn., ***am-c.,*** ambr., ***anac.,*** anan., ang., anis., ant-c., aphis., aq-mar., ***arg-m., arg-n.,*** arn., ars., ars-i., ars-s-f., ***art-v., aur.,*** aur-s., ***aven.,*** **BAR-C.,** bar-i., ***bar-m., bell., berb., bism.,*** **BOR.,** ***bov.,*** brom., bry., ***bufo,*** cadm-s., ***calad.,*** **CALC.,** calc-ac., calc-ar., calc-caust., calc-i., ***calc-p.,*** calc-s., calc-sil., calen., camph., camph-br., cann-i., cann-s., canth., caps., carb-ac., ***carb-an.,*** carb-s., ***carb-v., carl.,*** casc., ***cast., caust.,*** cer-s., ***cham.,*** **CHIN.,** chin-a., chin-s., chlol., chlor., ***cic.,*** cimic., ***cimx.,*** clem., ***cob.,*** coc-c., coca, ***cocc.,*** cod., coff., coff-t., coll., coloc., colocin., ***con.,*** cop., ***cor-r.,*** crot-t., ***cupr., cycl.,*** **CYPR.,** dam., **DIG.,** ***digin.,*** **DIOS.,** dros., erech., erig., ***ery-a., eug.,*** euph., **EUPH-A.,** ***ferr.,***

SEMINAL, emissions - ferr-ar., ferr-br., ferr-i., ferr-p., ***form., gels., gins., graph.,*** grat., guai., ham., ***hep.,*** hera., hura, ***hydr.,*** hydr-ac., hyper., ign., ind., iod., iris, jac-c., kali-ar., ***kali-br., kali-c.,*** kali-chl., kali-i., kali-m., **KALI-P.,** kali-sil., kiss., ***lach.,*** lac-ac., ***lact.,*** lath., led., lil-t., linu-c., ***lup.,*** **LYC.,** lyss., ***mag-arct.,*** mag-c., ***mag-m.,*** mag-p., ***med., merc., merc-c.,*** merc-i-f., merc-i-r., merc-sul., ***mill., mosch.,*** mur-ac., naja, ***nat-a.,*** **NAT-C., NAT-M., NAT-P.,** nat-sil., ***nit-ac., nuph., nux-m.,*** **NUX-V.,** ol-an., ***onos.,*** op., opun-v., orch., ***orig.,*** osm., ox-ac., paeon., par., ped., petr., petros., **PH-AC., PHOS.,** phys., ***pic-ac.,*** pip-m., plan., ***plat.,*** plb., plb-p., ***psor., puls.,*** puls-n, ran-b., ran-s., rheum, rhod., rhus-t., ruta, ***sabad.,*** sabal., sac-alb., ***sal-n.,*** samb., sang., ***sars.,*** scut., **SEL., SEP.,** ***sil.,*** sin-n., ***sol-o.,*** spirae., stann., **STAPH.,** stict., ***stram., stry.,*** sul-ac., sul-i., **SULPH.,** sumb., tab., tarax., ***tarent.,*** tax., ***ter.,*** ther., ***thuj., thymol.,*** titan., trib., ***tub.,*** upa., uran-n., ***ust.,*** verb., vib., viol-o., ***viol-t.,*** visc., voes., wies., ***yohim,*** zinc., ***zinc-p., zinc-pic.,*** zinc-valer., zing., ziz.
afternoon - carb-an.
4 p.m. - carb-an.
catalepsy, after - grat.
relaxed penis, with - cor-r.
siesta, during - aloe, ***alum.,*** carb-an., caust., clem., cor-r., merc., par., phos., staph., stict., sulph., ther.
agg. in general - alum., cob.
agg. in general, old symptoms - alum.
amel. in general - agn., calc., ***calc-p.,*** elaps, ***lach.,*** naja, phos., sil., zinc.
bed, in - kali-br.
boys, premature - bar-c.
brain fag, mental torpidity, with - ph-ac.
burning - clem., sulph.
caresses, during - ***arn.,*** **CON.,** ery-a., ***gels., nat-c., nux-v.,*** petr., ***phos., sars., sel.,*** sulph., ust.
colic, during - plb.
constitution, in a, robust - **NUX-V.**
night, 3 a.m. - pip-m.
in a, weak - ***gels.***
convulsions, in - art-v., pip-m.
copious - bell., carl., ***kali-c.,*** merc-i-f., nat-m., par., petr., **PH-AC.,** ***pic-ac., staph.,*** thymol.
3 a.m. - pip-m.
night - carb-an., ***dig.,*** hipp., ign., kali-chl., ol-an., sars.
sex, after - bar-c.
daytime - arn., canth., cyna., ery-a., gels., graph., lach., **NUX-V.,** ust.
daytime, sleep, during - par., staph., thuj.
debility, backache, weak legs, with - aur., calc., calc-p., ***chin., cob.,*** con., cupr., dam., dig., ***dios.,*** ery-a., form., gels., kali-c., lyc., med., nat-p., ***nux-v., ph-ac., pic-ac.,*** sars., sel., ***staph., sulph.,*** zinc.
depression, with - agar., ***agn., calad., con.,*** nat-m., **PH-AC.,** sars., sulph.
desire for sex, during - ham.

SEMINAL, emissions

diarrhea, during - ***ars.***

dinner, after - agar., nat-c.

disturbing sleep - arn., camph., cann-s., carb-an., chel., coloc., con., crot-t., cycl., dig., ferr., kali-chl., lach., lact., nat-c., nat-m., ***nux-v.,*** par., petr., ***ph-ac.,*** phos., plat., plb., ***puls.,*** ran-b., samb., sars., ***sep., sil.,*** spig.

dreams, with - ***alum.,*** ambr., ang., ***ant-c.,*** aphis., arist-m., arn., ars., ars-s-f., aur., bar-c., bell., bism., bor., bov., ***calad., calc.,*** calc-ac., calc-p., ***camph.,*** cann-i., cann-s., canth., carb-ac., carb-an., caust., chin., ***cic., cob.,*** coloc., con., ***dig.,*** dios., euph., ferr., ***gels., graph.,*** ham., hura, hydr., ind., iod., iris, ***kali-br., kali-c.,*** kali-chl., ***kali-m.,*** kali-s., lach., lact., ***lil-t.,*** lipp., lyc., lyss., merc-i-f., merc-sul., myric., ***nat-c.,*** nat-m., nat-p., **NUX-V.,** ***olnd.,*** op., paeon., par., ***ph-ac., phos., pic-ac.,*** plb., ***puls.,*** ran-b., rhod., sabad., samb., sars., sel., senec., ***sep.,*** sin-n., spira., staph., stram., sulph., thuj., thymol., ust., **VIOL-T.**

amorous - ambr., ***calad.,*** cann-i., cob., con., dios., lyc., ***nux-v., phos.,*** sars., sel., senec., staph., thymol., ust., viol-t.

lascivious, of a perverted character - thymol.

lying on back, while - coloc.

morning - plb., spig.

sex, of - bor.

slept, feels he had not - ham.

unpleasant dreams - lach., sil.

urinate, after a dream that he must - merc-i-f.

vivid, with - viol-t.

wakening up - sel.

dreams, without - agar., aloe, ***anac.,*** anan., ant-c., arg-m., ***arg-n.,*** ars., aur., bar-c., bell., bism., calc., ***camph.,*** carb-v., cic., ***con., cor-r.,*** dig., **DIOS.,** ***gels., graph.,*** guai., ham., hep., ind., kali-c., merc., merc-i-f., nat-c., nat-p., ped., phos., ***pic-ac.,*** pip-m., puls., ran-s., ruta, sep., sin-a., ***stann.,*** staph., verb., vib., ***zinc., zinc-p.***

easy, too - arn., calad., ***chin.,*** con., ery-a., ol-an., ***sars.,*** sel.

excitement, from the least - ***con., ery-a., ph-ac.,*** plb., ***sars.***

emaciation, with - chin., ***ph-ac., phos., samb.***

enjoyment, with - calad., calc., nat-c., nat-p., plan., sel., sul-ac., tab.

erections, with - agar., anac., aur., ***calc.,*** cann-i., cann-s., ***canth.,*** carb-ac., carb-an., caust., chin., dig., dios., ery-a., form., ***gins., iod., kali-br.,*** kali-chl., kali-p., led., lyc., ***merc.,*** nat-m., ***nux-v.,*** par., phos., pic-ac., pip-m., puls., sil., staph., sulph., ther., viol-t.

feeble, with - sel.

painful, with - cann-i., ***canth.,*** grat., ign., kali-c., merc., mosch., ***nit-ac.,*** nux-v., pic-ac., puls., sabal., thuj.

violent, with - ***kali-m.***

SEMINAL, emissions

erections, without - abrot., absin., agar., ***agn.,*** arg-m., ***arg-n.,*** aven., ***bar-c.,*** bell., bism., bov., calad., ***calc.,*** canth., carb-an., caust., ***chin.,*** **COB.,** coff., coloc., ***con.,*** cor-r., dig., **DIOS.,** ***ery-a.,*** ferr., fl-ac., ***gels.,*** gins., goss., **GRAPH.,** ham., hep., ign., kali-br., kali-c., kali-p., lup., ***lyc.,*** mag-arct., mag-c., mosch., ***nat-c.,*** nat-m., ***nat-p.,*** nit-ac., ***nuph.,*** nux-v., op., ***ph-ac.,*** phos., plat., plb., puls., sabad., sal-n., sars., ***sel.,*** sep., sil., spig., stann., sul-ac., sulph., trio., visc., zinc., zinc-pic.

morning - coc-c.

sleep, during - **DIOS.,** ***nuph.***

wine, after - ***plb.***

erotic - squil.

evening - carb-an., nat-c.

evening, dream, in a - cob.

excitability of parts, from - ***cast.***

excitement, from sexual - **CALC.,** cod., con., gels., ***nat-m.,*** petr., **PIC-AC.,** stann.

exertion, over, from - ferr.

falls asleep, as soon as he - ***pic-ac.***

fancy, with excitement of - ***kali-br.***

without - dios., phos., sars.

forenoon - caust.

sitting, while - sulph.

frequent - acon., ***alum.,*** alum-sil., ***am-c.,*** ang., arg-m., arg-n., arn., aur., bar-m., ***bor.,*** bov., ***calc.,*** calc-ac., canth., carb-an., carb-v., caust., **CHIN.,** cic., cob., ***con.,*** cor-r., dig., ferr., ***graph., kali-c.,*** kali-p., lach., lact., lyc., lyss., mag-arct., mag-aust., mag-c., mag-m., ***nat-c.,*** nat-m., ***nat-p.,*** nit-ac., **NUX-V.,** op., petr., **PH-AC.,** phos., ***plb., puls.,*** sac-alb., ***sac-l.,*** sars., sel., ***sep.,*** sil., stann., **STAPH.,** sulph., tarax., zinc.

elderly man, in - bar-c., caust., nat-c., sulph.

following quickly each other - bar-c.

leaning the back against anything - ant-c.

one night - ind., ***ph-ac., puls.***

several in, a week - ***dig., sars.,*** tarent., ***ust.***

sex, after - ph-ac.

sleep, during - ***nuph.***

fright at slight noise, from - aloe.

high living, after - **NUX-V.**

impotence, with - ***uran-n.***

indigestion, from - sang.

involuntary - dios., ham., nat-p., sel., sep.

irritability, despondency, with - ***aur.,*** calad., ***calc., chin., cimic., con.,*** dios., kali-br., ***nux-v.,*** ph-ac., phos., ***sel., staph.***

leaning the back against anything, as if pollution would come, when - ant-c.

looking at passing girls, when - calad., sel.

lying on back, while - cob., coloc., hyper.

masturbation, after - agn., ***alum.,*** arg-m., bar-c., **CHIN.,** ***dig., ery-a., gels., graph.,*** lup., **NUX-V.,** ***ph-ac.,*** phos., ***puls.,*** sal-n., ***sars.,*** **SEP.,** ***sil.,*** **STAPH.,** ***tarent.,*** ust.

tendency to, with - ust.

SEMINAL, emissions
midnight, after - ran-s., samb., sil.
at - goss.
before - coloc.
morning - acon., aloe, cahin., carb-v., cham., chin-s., coc-c., eug., grat., lact., lil-t., merc-i-f., merc-i-r., nat-c., nat-m., nux-v., petr., petros., phys., pip-m., plb., psor., puls., ran-b., rhus-t., sabad., spig., thuj.
5 a.m. - coc-c.
bed in, penis relaxed - canth.
falling in sleep again, on - ol-an.
sleep, during - lact.
stool, during - amyg., helio., nat-m., ph-ac.
pressing, at - ***alum.,*** canth., ***chin.,*** cimic., digin., gels., kali-br., ***nuph., ph-ac.,*** phos., pic-ac., sel., trib.
waking, on - petr.
night, 1 a.m. - calc-p., dig., sulfonam.
3 a.m. - aloe, coff-t.
3 a.m. to 5 am., after masturbation - ***sil.***
4 a.m. - anth., cob., pip-m.
every - mag-c., ***nat-m., nat-p., pic-ac.,*** tarax., ***ust.***
almost every night - am-c., ***phos.***
other night - nat-p., ***pic-ac.,*** tarax.
third night, or - **NUX-V.**
several nights - ***agar.,*** alum., am-c., ang., aur., bov., ***calc.,*** calc-p., carb-an., caust., con., ***dig., graph.,*** ind., kali-c., lac-ac., mag-aust., plb., sars., ***staph., sulph.,*** zinc., ziz.
lying on back, on - stann.
towards morning - erech., petros.
noon - cact.
odorless - sulph.
offensive - thuj.
pungent - lach.
urine, stale like - nat-p.
pain, during - plb.
painful - ***con., kali-c.,*** mosch., nat-c., sabal., ***sars.***
paralytic symptoms set in, before - ***kali-br.***
perspiration, with - ***lach.***
premature - ***agn.,*** bar-c., ***calad., calc.,*** carb-v., ***chin., cob.,*** con., graph., hep., kali-c., ***lyc.,*** ol-an., onos., ***ph-ac.,*** phos., ***sel.,*** sep., sulph., titan., zinc.
prostatic disease, in - aesc.
rheumatic pains, with - gins.
sadness, with - agar., ***agn., calad., con.,*** nat-m., **PH-AC.,** sars., sulph.
seldom - ***kali-c.***
sensation of pollution - cer-s., ***mez.***
as before a pollution - dig., mur-ac.
suppressed, as if one had been - clem.
waking, on - am-c.
sex, after - acon., ***agn.,*** am-c., bar-c., bry., calc., ***dig.,*** gels., ***graph.,*** kali-c., lyss., **NAT-M.,** nat-p., ph-ac., ***phos., rhod.,*** sep.
desire for sex, during - ham., nat-m., ph-ac.

SEMINAL, emissions
sexual excess, after - ***agn.,*** alum., ***dig., nat-m.,*** **NUX-V.**
sitting, while - sel., sulph.
dinner, after - agar.
erection, without - nat-m., trio.
sex, after - nat-m.
sleep, during - agar., aloe, anac., ang., ***arg-m.,*** arn., aur., ***camph.,*** cann-s., clem., ***cor-r.,*** crot-t., **CYCL.,** dig., **DIOS.,** ***ferr., guai., ham.,*** ind., ***lach.,*** lact., lil-t., lyss., med., ***meph.,*** nat-a., nat-c., **NUX-V.,** ol-an., par., ***pic-ac.,*** ran-b., rhod., sel., stann., ***stram.,*** ther., ***thuj.,*** thymol., verb., vib., ***zinc.***
waking, during - ***thuj.***
waking, without - tab.
spasms, with - art-v., grat., ***nat-p.***
stiffness of linen, causing no - med.
stool, during - acet-ac., ***alum.,*** anan., ars., canth., carb-v., caust., ***chin.,*** cimic., con., ***gels.,*** kali-br., nat-m., ***nuph.,*** ol-an., ***petr., ph-ac.,*** phos., pic-ac., plb., **SEL.,** sep., sil., sulph., thymol., trib., viol-t.
difficult - agn., alum., am-c., anac., con., hep., nat-c., nit-ac., ***petr.,*** sep., staph.
straining, at - ***alum.,*** canth., ***chin.,*** cimic., digin., gels., kali-br., ***nuph.,*** ol-an., ***ph-ac.,*** phos., pic-ac., ***sel.,*** trib.
sudden, during dream of sex - sumb.
talking about women, from - ***ust.***
thick - sabal.
thrill prolonged - cann-i.
tuberculosis, in - **CALC.**
unconscious - caust., ***dios., ham.,*** ind., lach., lact., lyss., merc-i-f., nat-c., ***nat-p.,*** plan., plb., ***sel.,*** sep.
urination, during - ***alum.,*** canth., ***chin.,*** cimic., digin., ***ery-a.,*** gels., kali-br., ***nuph., ph-ac.,*** phos., pic-ac., ***sel.,*** trib., ***viol-t.***
after - daph., kali-c.
vertigo, with - ***sars.***
vision weak, with - kali-c.
voluptuous - viol-t.
sensation, without - sul-ac.
thrill long after - sel.
waking, on - acon., acon-c., aloe, arn., ars., cahin., crot-t., cycl., dig., gast., naja, petr., phos., pic-ac., ***sel.,*** sil., ***thuj.***
wasting of testes, with - ***iod.,*** sabal.
watery - led., nat-p., sel., sulph.
weakness, from - ***agn.,*** sul-ac.
wine, after - plb.
women, looking at passing girl, when - calad., pic-ac., sel.
caressing a woman, while - **CON.,** ***phos.,*** sars.
presence of a women, when in - ***con., nux-v.,*** sal-n., ust.
talking about women, from - ***ust.***
touch of a women, on - ***nux-v.***

SENSITIVENESS, genitalia - ***cocc.,*** coff., ***ph-ac.,*** **PLAT.,** ***staph.,*** tarent., verat., zinc.
unbearable, a little suffering - coff.
sensitiveness, penis - cocc., corn., crot-t., tab., thuj., verat., zinc.
glans - ***cor-r.,*** **MERC-C.,** thuj.
sex, after - eug.
prepuce - cann-s., ***cor-r., merc.***
sensitiveness, scrotum - kali-c., nat-m., ph-ac., plat., **STAPH.,** zinc.
sensitiveness, testes - clem.

SEX, general
aversion, sex, to - aeth., agar., agn., alco., am-c., arg-m., arn., astac., bar-c., bor., bufo, cann-s., carb-an., caust., chlor., clem., coff., cub., ether, ferr., ferr-ma., franz., **GRAPH.,** hell., ***ign.,*** kali-br., kali-c., kali-n., kreos., lach., **LYC.,** moly-met., morph., nat-m., nuph., nux-m., op., petr., phos., ***psor., rhod.,*** sabad., sabin., sep., spirae., stann., staph., stram., sul-ac., tarent., teucr., ther., thuj., upa., ust.
erotic dreams, ending in a pollution, with - ***plat.***
evening - dios.
forenoon - phys.
impotence, with - ***graph.***
masturbation, with - kali-br.
night - bufo.
pains, from - ***sep.***
desire, (see, Sexual desire)
enjoyment, sexual
absent - ***agar., anac.,*** anan., arg-n., bart., berb., bufo, ***calad.,*** calc., cann-i., cann-s., canna, carb-v., ***dios.,*** eug., ferr., ***graph.,*** ind., lyc., lyss., nat-c., ***nat-m.,*** nat-p., nit-ac., nux-m., onos., phos., ***plat.,*** psor., rhodi., sal-ac., sanic., ***sep.,*** sul-ac., tab., tarent.
emission, during - psor.
diminished - bart., plat., sep., tarent.
burning, with - cann-i.
extreme - agn., ambr., ***fl-ac.,*** lach., nat-m., nit-ac., ***plat.,*** stann., sulph.
feeble and too short, too - berb.
increased - agn., ambr., calc-p., lach., nat-c., ***nat-m., plat.,*** stann., sulph.
insupportable - stann.
prolonged - cann-i., ***sel.***
short - plat.
enjoyment, sexual, sensation as from sex - am-m., lach.
bathing, on - nat-c.
inner parts, in - ambr.
midnight, after - lyc.
morning on waking, before urination - ***kali-c.***
pollutions, in - lach.
sleeping and waking, between - kreos.
excesses of, agg. - acon., **AGAR., AGN.,** alum., anac., ant-c., arn., ***ars.,*** asaf., aur., bar-c., bell., bor., ***bov.,*** bry., ***calad.,*** **CALC.,** ***calc-s.,*** cann-s., canth., caps., carb-an., ***carb-v.,*** caust., cham., **CHIN.,** ***chin-a.,*** cina, cocc., coff., **CON.,** ***dig.,*** dulc., ***ery-a.,*** ferr., ***gels.,*** graph., ign., ***iod., ip., kali-br., kali-c.,*** kali-n.,

SEX, general
excesses of, agg. - **KALI-P.,** led., ***lil-t.,*** **LYC.,** mag-m., ***merc.,*** mez., ***mosch., nat-c.,*** **NAT-M., NAT-P.,** ***nit-ac.,*** **NUX-V.,** op., petr., **PH-AC., PHOS.,** plat., plb., ***puls.,*** ran-b., rhod., rhus-t., ruta., sabad., samb., sec., **SEL., SEP., SIL.,** ***spig.,*** squil., stann., **STAPH., SULPH., THUJ.,** valer., zinc.
headache, after - **AGAR.,** arn., ***bov.,*** **CALC.,** carb-v., ***chin.,*** con., kali-c., lach., merc., ***nat-c.,*** nat-m., nat-p., ***nux-v.,*** ph-ac., phos., pip-m., ***puls.,*** **SEP., SIL.,** spig., ***staph., sulph., thuj.***
mental, symptoms, from - agar., ***agn.,*** alum., ars., asaf., aur., ***bov.,*** calad., **CALC.,** ***carb-v., chin.,*** chin-a., cocc., ***con., iod., kali-c.,*** kali-p., kali-s., lil-t., **LYC.,** mag-m., ***merc., nat-c.,*** nat-m., nit-ac., **NUX-V.,** petr., **PH-AC., PHOS.,** ***puls.,*** sel., **SEP.,** ***sil.,*** spig., **STAPH.,** sulph., thuj., zinc.
excitement, agg. - ***bufo,*** **LIL-T.,** sars.
fright during, agg. - lyc.
headache, from - agar., arg-n., arn., ***bov.,*** calad., **CALC.,** ***calc-p.,*** chin., dig., graph., **KALI-C.,** ***lyc., nat-c.,*** nat-m., ***petr., phos.,*** puls., **SEP., SIL.,** staph.
impotency, (see Male, Impotency)
involuntary, almost - kali-fer.
lasciviousness - agar., aloe, ***ambr., apis,*** arund., aur., bor., ***calad., calc.,*** calc-s., ***canth., carb-v., chin.,*** coc-c., ***con.,*** cop., ***dig., fl-ac., graph.,*** **HYOS.,** hyper., ign., **LACH.,** lyc., **LIL-T.,** lyss., merc., mosch., nat-m., nit-ac., op., **ORIG., PHOS., PIC-AC., PLAT.,** ***puls.,*** raph., ***sel., sep., sil.,*** spig., **STAPH.,** ***stram., tarent., tub., verat.,*** zinc.
long, too - carb-s.
masturbation, disposition to - agn., ***alum.,*** alumn., ambr., ***anac.,*** **ANAN.,** ***apis, aur., bar-c.,*** bell., ***bell-p.,*** **BUFO,** calad., calc., ***calc-p.,*** cann-i., cann-s., **CARB-V., CARC., CAUST.,** ***chin., cina,*** cocc., ***coff., con., dig.,*** dios., dros., ***ferr., gels., grat.,*** hyos., ***kali-br.,*** kali-p., **LACH.,** ***lyc., med., meph.,*** merc., nat-m., ***nux-v., op.,*** **ORIG.,** ***ph-ac., phos., pic-ac.,*** **PLAT.,** ***plb., puls.,*** sal-n., sec., sel., **SEP.,** sil., ***stann.,*** **STAPH.,** stict., ***stram., sulph.,*** tarent., **THUJ.,** ***tub., ust.,*** zinc.
ailments from - agar., alum., ***ambr.,*** anac., ant-c., ***arg-m.,*** ars., bov., ***bufo,*** calad., **CALC.,** calc-s., ***carb-v., carc.,*** **CHIN., COCC., CON.,** ***dig.,*** ferr., **GELS.,** ***hyos., iod.,*** kali-c., ***kali-p., lyc.,*** mag-p., ***merc.,*** merc-c., mosch., nat-c., ***nat-m.,*** **NAT-P.,** nux-m., ***nux-v.,*** **ORIG.,** petr., **PH-AC.,** ***phos.,*** plb., ***puls.,*** **SEL., SEP.,** sil., ***spig.,*** squil., **STAPH., SULPH.**
childhood, since - ***hyos.***
children, in - bell-p., ***carc.,*** dys-co., hyos., ***med.,*** orig., plat., ***scirr.,*** stann., staph., thuj.
depressed, when - carc., staph., ***ust.***

SEX, general
masturbation, disposition to
epilepsy, in - ***bufo,*** **CALC.,** ***lach., plat., stram.***
excessive - ***alum.,*** bell., **CALC., CARB-V.,** ***chin., stram.***
every opportunity, at - ***hyos.***
headache, after - ***calc.,*** carb-v., ***chin., con.,*** lyc., merc., nat-m., nux-v., phos., puls., ***sep.,*** spig., ***staph.,*** sulph.
involuntary - camph.
irresistible tendency - thuj., ***ust.***
itching, from - ***staph.***
mania, in - bell.
puberty, before - plat.
sexual excesses, after - carb-v., phos., ***staph.***
sleep, during - camph., carb-v., ***plat.,*** thuj.
solitude, seeks to - ***bufo,*** ust., thuj.
worms, from - calad., cina.
onanism, ailments from - agar., alum., ***ambr.,*** anac., ant-c., ***arg-m.,*** ars., bov., ***bufo,*** calad., **CALC.,** calc-s., ***carb-v.,*** **CHIN., COCC., CON.,** ***dig.,*** ferr., **GELS.,** ***hyos., iod.,*** kali-c., ***kali-p., lyc.,*** mag-p., ***merc.,*** merc-c., mosch., nat-c., ***nat-m.,*** **NAT-P.,** nux-m., ***nux-v.,*** **ORIG.,** petr., **PH-AC.,** ***phos.,*** plb., ***puls.,*** **SEL., SEP.,** sil., ***spig.,*** squil., **STAPH., SULPH.**
prostate complaints after - sel., tarent., thuj.
motions as of - caust., phos.
painful - arg-n., bor., calc., ferr., kali-c., kreos., merc-c., nat-m., plat., sabal., sep., sulph.
weakness, after - ***agar.,*** berb., **CALC.,** chin., clem., ***con., dig., graph., kali-c., kali-p.,*** lil-t., lyc., mosch., ***nat-m.,*** nit-ac., petr., ***ph-ac., phos.,*** **SEL.,** ***sep., sil.,*** staph., tarent.

SEXUAL, desire, general
convulsions, during - canth., sabin., zinc.
decreased - acon., adlu., aeth., agar., agav-t., **AGN.,** ***alum.,*** am-c., ambr., anac., ange-s., ***anh.,*** ant-c., ant-ox., apis, aran-ix., arg-m., ***arg-n.,*** arn., arund-d., aur., bar-ac., **BAR-C.,** bell., berb., bor., ***brom., calad., calc.,*** calc-p., ***camph.,*** cann-s., canth., caps., carb-ac., carb-an., carb-s., carb-v., carl., **CAUST.,** chen-v., chin., chin-s., chlor., ***clem., coff.,*** coloc., ***con.,*** cortico., cortiso., cund., cycl., des-ac., ***dios.,*** euph., ***ferr.,*** ferr-m., fl-ac., franz., gink-b., **GRAPH.,** halo., hell., ***hep.,*** hyos., ***ign.,*** ind., indg., iod., kali-bi., kali-br., ***kali-c.,*** kali-chl., ***kali-i., kali-p.,*** kali-s., kali-sil., ***kreos., lach.,*** lact., laur., lec., levo., lil-s., lup., **LYC.,** ***mag-c.,*** mag-m., mag-p-a., man., meny., merc-c., moly-met., morph., ***mur-ac., nat-m.,*** nat-p., ***nit-ac., nuph.,*** nux-m., oci-s., **ONOS.,** op., oxyt., petr., ***ph-ac.,*** phos., pic-ac., plan., plat., ***plb., psor.,*** rauw., ***rhod.,*** rhodi., rumx., sabad., ***sabal.,*** sabin., ***sel.,*** seneg., **SEP.,** sieg., **SIL.,** spig., spong., stann., **STAPH.,** sul-ac., ***sulph.,*** teucr., thala., ther., thiop., thuj., upa., ust., vichy-h., visc., x-ray.
abnormal, from - lyss.
chilliness, with - kali-chl.

SEXUAL, desire
decreased,
diabetes, in - ***cupr.***
erections, with - lyss.
without - caust., ***coff., dios., kali-br.***
evening - dios.
excesses, after - aven., **STAPH.,** ***sulph.,*** upa.
morning - petr.
night - cocc.
relaxed parts, with - acon., coff.
spinal affections, in - ***chin.***
delirium, during - **STANN.**
eating, after - aloe, colch., lyss.
erections, with - aloe, arn., aur., calc., coloc., ***dig.,*** ferr-ma., hyos., par., puls., rhod., ***sil.***
without - acon., ***agar., agn., alum., am-c., anac., arg-m., arg-n., aur.,*** aur-s., bar-c., **CALAD.,** ***calc., camph., chin.,*** cob., **CON.,** corn., crot-h., ***dig.,*** ferr-ma., **GRAPH.,** hep., ign., kali-c., lach., **LYC.,** lyss., mag-m., meny., naja, ***nat-m.,*** nat-p., nuph., ***nux-m., nux-v.,*** op., ***ph-ac., phos., psor.,*** puls., sabad., sal-n., ***sel., sep., sil.,*** stann., ***staph.,*** sulph.
excessive - ***agar.,*** agn., ***alum., calc., calc-p.,*** camph., **CANN-I., CANTH.,** caust., colch., coloc., con., ferr., ***fl-ac., graph.,*** grat., ham., ***hyos., kali-br., kali-c., lach., lyc.,*** lyss., **MED., MERC.,** mosch., ***nat-c., nat-m.,*** nit-ac., **NUX-V.,** op., ***orig.,*** **PHOS.,** ***phys., pic-ac.,*** **PLAT.,** ***plb.,*** psor., puls., rhus-t., sabin., sal-n., seneg., sep., ***sil.,*** **STAPH., STRAM.,** sulph., ***tarent.,*** ther., ***thuj., tub., ust., verat.,*** **ZINC.,** zinc-pic.
children, in - aloe.
puberty, at - manc.
complaints, from - **LYSS.**
poor results, with - agar., am-c., graph., meny., sel.
uncontrollable - agar., canth., ***caust., chin.,*** con., ***graph.,*** kali-c., ***lyc.,*** mag-c., med., ***nat-m.,*** **PHOS., PLAT.,** sabin., **SIL.,** ***staph., verat.,*** zinc.
excitement of, easy - cinnb., con., ***graph.,*** kali-c., ***lyc.,*** mag-arct., ***nux-v.,*** **PHOS.,** ***picro.,*** plat., ***plb.,*** sumb., **ZINC.**
discharge of prostatic fluid, with - nit-ac.
falling asleep, on - merc-i-r.
increased - acon., agn., ***agar.,*** alco., ***all-c.,*** aloe, alum., ***am-c.,*** ambr., ***anac.,*** anag., **ANAN.,** ***ant-c., ant-s.,*** ant-t., apis, aran-ix., arn., ars., arund., asaf., aspar., aster., ***aur.,*** aur-i., aur-m., aur-s., bar-c., **BAR-M.,** bell., berb., bor., bov., brom., bry., ***bufo,*** cact., cahin., caj., ***calad.,*** **CALC., CALC-P.,** ***camph.,*** **CANN-I.,** ***cann-s.,*** **CANTH.,** caps., carb-ac., carb-v., **CARC.,** carl., ***cast.,*** caust., cedr., cent., cham., chen-v., chim-m., ***chin.,*** cina, ***cinnb.,*** clem., coca, ***cocc., coc-c.,*** cod., ***coff.,*** colch., coloc., colocin., **CON.,** cop., ***croc.,*** crot-h., ***cub.,*** del., dema., der., des-ac., dig., ***dios., dulc.,*** erig., ery-a., eucal., ***ferr.,*** ferr-i., ferr-m., ferr-ma., ferr-p., ***fl-ac.,*** form., ***gels.,***

SEXUAL, desire

increased - ***gins.***, gnaph., goss., gran., ***graph.***, grat., gymn., ***ham.***, helon., ***hep.***, hipp., hydr., hydr-ac., ***hyos.***, hyper., ***ign.***, ***ind.***, indg., ***iod.***, ***iris***, ***kali-bi.***, ***kali-br.***, ***kali-c.***, ***kali-i.***, ***kali-n.***, kali-p., kali-sil., ***lac-c.***, ***lach.***, lact., ***laur.***, led., lil-t., lim., **LYC.**, **LYSS.**, mag-arct., mag-aust., mag-p-a., man., manc., mang., meny., ***merc.***, merc-c., merc-i-r., merl., ***mez.***, mim-p., morph., ***mosch.***, mur-ac., murx., naja, ***nat-c.***, ***nat-h.***, ***nat-m.***, ***nat-p.***, ***nat-s.***, ***nit-ac.***, nitro-o., nuph., nux-m., **NUX-V.**, nym., oci-s., ol-an., onos., ***op.***, ***orig.***, ox-ac., par., pen., pers., petr., ***ph-ac.***, **PHOS.**, **PIC-AC.**, pip-m., **PLAT.**, ***plb.***, psor., ptel., **PULS.**, raph., rhod., rhus-t., rib-ac., rob., ruta, sabad., ***sabin.***, sac-alb., ***sal-n.***, sang., sars., **SEL.**, seneg., ***sep.***, **SIL.**, sin-n., spig., spira., spong., ***stann.***, **STAPH.**, stict., ***stram.***, sul-ac., sulph., sumb., ***tarent.***, tell., tep., teucr., thlaspi, ***thuj.***, thymol., **TUB.**, upa., ***ust.***, verat., verb., **ZINC.**, ***zinc-p.***, ***zinc-pic.***, zing., ziz.

abdomen, during distention of - ign.
ability decreased - sel.
afternoon - agar., hyper., lyss., rhodi.
2. p.m. - cinnb.
siesta, after - eug., lach., mag-aust.
sleepiness - agar.
appetite, with increased - cinnb.
attacks of increased desire - acon., ***ant-c.***, apis, cann-i., canth., caps., fl-ac., ***hyos.***, ***ign.***, lach., ***op.***, phos., ***plat.***, sel., sil., staph., stram., ***verat.***
moonlight, in the - ***ant-c.***
attempt to satisfy it, by every, until it drives him to onanism and madness - anan.
bath and on leaving it, in warm - nat-c.
bed, in - kali-br.
going to bed, on - naja.
warm, when getting - ant-c.
children, in - ***bar-c.***
chorea, in - ***verat-v.***
continued - ***nit-ac.***
days, several - sars.
daytime - crot-h., hyos., lach., sil.
delirium, during - **STRAM.**
desire for sex, without - bor.
driving, when - apis.
eating, after - lyss.
elderly man, in an - arn., calad., ***fl-ac.***, mosch., sel., staph., sulph., thuj.
but impotent - lyc., sel.
emission, after an - aloe, ars., grat., kali-c., mez., nat-m., nit-ac., ***ph-ac.***, rhod., sep.
erections, with - ferr-ma., hyos., lyss., op., par., rhod., sin-n.
with, incomplete - aran-ix., con.
erections, without - acon., ***agar.***, ***agn.***, ***alum.***, ***am-c.***, ***anan.***, aq-mar., aran-ix., ***arg-m.***, ***arg-n.***, ***aur.***, aur-s., bar-c., **CALAD.**, ***calc.***, calc-i., calc-sil., ***camph.***, carb-s., ***chin.***, cob., **CON.**, corn., crot-h., ***dig.***, ferr-ma., **GRAPH.**, hep., ign., kali-c., lach., **LYC.**, lyss., mag-m., meny., naja, ***nat-m.***, ***nat-p.***, nuph., ***nux-m.***, ***nux-v.***, op., pers., ***ph-ac.***, ***phos.***, pic-ac., ***psor.***, puls., sabad., sal-n., ***sel.***, ***sep.***, ***sil.***, stann., ***staph.***, sulph., upa.

evening - acon., ***aloe***, alum-sil., calc., hipp., nat-s., thuj.
bed, in - cic., nat-m.
lying, while - nat-c.
falling asleep, on - kali-br., merc., merc-i-r.
fancies, with - ***ign.***, sil.
without - hep., hyos., meny.
forenoon - calc., hipp., phos., plumbg.
walking, on - calc.
headache, with throbbing - ***pic-ac.***
indifference, followed by sexual - tell.
legs were crossed, while - nat-c.
midnight, after waking - ant-s.
waking, 3 a.m. - calc.
morning - agar., anac., aur., bar-c., calc., calc-p., carb-v., cob., coc-c., coca, form., kreos., lach., nat-s., ox-ac., petr., plat., puls., sil.
bed, in - aster., kali-cy., lach., sil., spirae.
beer, after - nat-c.
elderly, man, in an - arn., ***fl-ac.***, mosch., staph., sulph.
elderly, man, in an, impotent, but - lyc., sel.
erections, with - nat-s.
falling asleep, on - kali-br., merc., merc-i-r.
fancies, with - ***ign.***, sil.
fancies, without - hep., hyos., meny.
headache, with throbbing - ***pic-ac.***
indifference, followed by sexual - tell.
legs were crossed, while - nat-c.
paralytic disease, in - ***sil.***
parts relaxed, with - acon., aur-s., crot-h.
pollution, after a - aloe, ars., con., grat., kali-c., mez., nat-m., nit-ac., ***ph-ac.***, rhod., sep.
pollution, without - coff.
priapism, like - **CANN-S.**, **CANTH.**, coloc., ***graph.***, ign., kali-c., ***nat-c.***, **NAT-M.**, nit-ac., **NUX-V.**, op., ph-ac., ***phos.***, plat., ***puls.***, ***rhus-t.***, ***sil.***, staph., thuj.
restlessness, with - ant-c.
rising, after - aur., calc.
sleep, during - cann-s.
waking, after - aloe, anac., aur.
waking, on - aeth., carb-ac., coc-c., gnaph., nat-c., ptel., ***puls.***, thuj.
night - alum-sil., aur., camph., ***canth.***, cer-b., cinnb., gnaph., guare., lach., ***lyc.***, mez., nat-c., nym., ox-ac., sil., ***sulph.***, thuj., zinc.
painful erections, with - merc.
violent erections, with - ***fl-ac.***
paralytic diseases - ***sil.***
parts relaxed, with - acon., aur-s., crot-h.
perverted - agn., med., nux-v., plat., staph., ***thuj.***

SEXUAL, desire
increased,
pollution, after an - aloe, ars., con., grat., kali-c., mez., nat-m., nit-ac., ***ph-ac.,*** rhod., sep.
without pollutions - coff.
priapism like - **CANN-S., CANTH.,** coloc., ***graph.,*** ign., kali-c., ***nat-c.,*** **NAT-M.,** nit-ac., **NUX-V.,** op., ph-ac., ***phos.,*** plat., ***puls., rhus-t., sil.,*** staph., thuj.
restlessness, with - ant-c.
rising, after - aur.
sex, after - mez., nat-m., ***ph-ac.***
excess of sex, after - ***ph-ac.***
sight of erotic things, at - tarent.
strong, but futile - calc., con., lyc., phos.
tabes dorsalis, in - ***fl-ac.***
talking with women, when - am-c., clem.
touching a women, when - bor., con., graph., grat., nat-c., plat.
waking, on - aeth., carb-ac., coc-c., ptel.
weakness, with physical - aq-mar., aran-ix., calad., calc., calc-i., calc-sil., con., ferr-ma., graph., ***kali-c.,*** lyc., nat-m., ***phos.,*** pic-ac., sel.
women, in company of - zinc.
lacking (see Sex, general, aversion) - achy., **AGN.,** alco., aloe, alum., am-c., amyg., anac., anan., ***anh.,*** ant-ox., arg-m., ***arg-n.,*** asar., bar-c., bar-s., bart., bell., ***berb.,*** bor., brom., ***bufo,*** caj., calc., ***camph.,*** canth., ***caps.,*** carb-ac., ***carb-an.,*** **CARB-S.,** ***carb-v.,*** carl., cench., chen-v., chlf., cinnb., cob-n., con., ***cop.,*** cortico., cub., equis., ery-a., ery-m., ferr., ferr-ma., ferr-p., fl-ac., franz., get., ***graph., hell.,*** hep., ***ign., iod.,*** jac-c., **KALI-BI., KALI-BR.,** ***kali-c.,*** kali-p., kali-s., kali-sil., lach., lec., ***lyc.,*** lyss., ***mag-c.,*** meph., ***merc.,*** mur-ac., myric., ***nat-m.,*** nat-p., ***nit-ac., nuph.,*** nux-m., ***onos.,*** op., osm., oxyt., ***ph-ac.,*** phos., ***plb., psor.,*** ptel., rumx., ***sabal.,*** sel., sil., spira., spong., ***stann.,*** staph., sul-i., ***sulph., sumb.,*** tab., thuj., x-ray.
cold agg. - achy.
coldness of scrotum, with - aloe, berb., brom., ***caps., merc.***
continued - lach.
erections, with - ***alum.,*** bry., ***calad.,*** eug., ferr-ma., fl-ac., mag-c., nit-ac., nux-v., spig., sulph., tarent.
without - ***camph.,*** graph.
fleshy people, in - **KALI-BI.**
morning - carb-v.
waking, after - aloe, anac., ***puls.***
work, with aversion to - caust.
perverted - agn., nux-v., plat., staph.
pollutions, after - aloe, con., mez., ***nat-m., ph-ac.***
with - sars.
without - ***coff.***
sexual minded - sep., staph.
sleep, during - ***nat-c., stram.***
after - ***agar.***
disturbing - astac., **CANTH.,** ***sars.***

SEXUAL, desire
sleeplessness, during - ant-c.
stool, during - nat-c., ***nat-s.***
suppressed, then excited - **ERY-A.**
suppressing the, complaints from - **APIS,** berb., calc., **CAMPH.,** ***carb-o., carb-v.,*** **CON.,** ***hell., kali-br.,*** kali-n., ***lil-t.,*** **LYSS.,** ***mosch., ph-ac., phos.,*** pic-ac., plat., **PULS.,** sabal., **STAPH.,** ***thuj.***
amel. - calad.
headache, after - ***con., puls.***
violent - acon., am-c., ***anac.,*** **ANAN.,** ant-c., arn., bar-m., ***bufo,*** calad., camph., **CANN-I., CANTH.,** cench., ***coloc.,*** cop., crot-h., ***fl-ac., graph.,*** grat., ***kali-br., lach., lyss.,*** merc., mosch., mygal., ***nat-h.,*** **PHOS., PIC-AC., PLAT., SIL.,** stann., ***stram.,*** sulph., ***tarent.,*** **TUB., ZINC.,** zinc-p.
sexual mania - apis, canth., **PHOS.,** ***tarent.***
trembling, with - am-c., graph., **PLAT.**

SHARP, pain, genitalia - berb., bor., clem., croc., euphr., inul., rhus-t., sil.
sharp, penis - acon., anan., arn., asaf., asar., asc-t., aspar., aur., berb., bor., brach., brom., calad., calc., cann-s., caps., caul., chel., cinnb., coc-c., coloc., con., crot-t., ***dros.,*** elaps, guai., ham., ign., kali-n., ***lith.,*** lyc., mag-s., merc., merc-i-f., ***mez.,*** mur-ac., naja, nat-m., osm., petr., ph-ac., phos., plat., puls., ran-s., sabad., sep., sil., spig., stann., staph., ***sulph.,*** sumb., ***thuj., viol-t.,*** zinc.
burning - mur-ac., spig.
coughing - ign.
crawling - mez.
erection, during - alum.
extending, anus - merc.
backward - aur.
forward - asar., spig.
to, glans - asar., brom., spong.
to, testes - carb-s., thuj.
itching, stitches - kali-n., ph-ac., spig.
morning - sulph.
root - calc-p., zinc.
sitting, while - thuj.
and walking - mag-s.
tip - euph., euphr., ferr-m., mez., ph-ac., thuj.
urination, after, spasms of urethra and tenesmus of rectum - ***prun.***
urination, during - aur., ***merc.,*** nat-m., petr., prun.
sharp, penis, glans - acon., arn., ars., berb., brom., carb-ac., ***caul.,*** cinnb., clem., coc-c., dros., ***euph.,*** euphr., ferr-ma., hep., ***kali-bi.,*** lyc., ***merc.,*** mez., nat-m., ph-ac., phos., ***prun.,*** ran-s., rhod., sabin., spong., stann., ***sulph.,*** samb., ***thuj.,*** zinc.
pressing, on it, when - thuj.
urination, during - acon., sulph., thuj.
after - ***prun.***
before - aur.
sharp, penis, prepuce - ars., cham., cocc., ***hep., mang., nit-ac.,*** sep., sumb., thuj.
urination, after - berb., con., kali-bi., merc.

sharp, prostate - bov., calc-p., ***con., cycl.,*** kali-bi., kali-c., kali-n., lyc., ***puls., sabal.***
afternoon - aur., kali-bi.
bladder, and, deep in pelvis, morning, and forenoon, after sex - all-c.
extending to forward - sil.
forward - sil.
to genitals - bov.
sitting and walking, while - cycl.
urging to stool or urination, with - cycl.
urination, during - cact., caust., cop., cycl., kali-n., merc-d., pareir., sel.
walking, agg. - ***kali-bi.***

sharp, scrotum - anan., arn., berb., carb-an., chin., clem., lyc., meny., mez., ph-ac., rhus-v., spig., sulph., **THUJ.,** viol-t., zinc.
burning and stitching - spig.
itching and stitching - spig.

sharp, spermatic cord - all-c., ammc., am-m., ***arn.,*** arum-d., ***bell., berb., bry.,*** calc., carb-s., clem., goss., grat., ***merc.,*** nat-m., ***nux-v.,*** ox-ac., podo., polyg., ***puls.,*** rhod., spong., ***staph.,*** sulph., sumb., ***thuj.***
evening - ammc.
in bed - bell.
extending to, abdomen - ***grat., staph.***
to, chest - grat.
to, downward - ***berb.,*** calc., staph.
to, penis - puls.
to, upward - bell., thuj.
left, then right - calc., staph.
walking, while - ammc., ox-ac.

sharp, testes - aesc., arn., ***bar-m., bell.,*** berb., brom., bry., calc., carb-s., **CAUST.,** cocc., graph., ***ham.,*** ip., lyc., ***lycps.,*** merc., merc-c., nat-m., ***nux-v.,*** op., ox-ac., polyg., ***puls., rhod.,*** sel., ***spong., staph.,*** sulph., sumb., tarax., ***thuj.,*** zinc.
evening - ox-ac., rhod., ***sel.***
extending, spermatic cord, to - coc-c., fl-ac., ox-ac., ***spong.***
stomach, to - ***ham.***
left - carb-s., ***fl-ac.,*** merc-c., puls., staph., ***thuj.,*** zinc.
legs, crossing - ip.
night - ham.
rest, during - rhod., zinc.
right - bry., ***caust.,*** coc-c., graph., rhod., sel., spig.
sitting, while - rhod.
urination, during - thuj.
walking, while - ox-ac.
amel. - ***rhod.***

SHINING, scrotum - ***graph., merc.,*** thuj.

SHIVERING, genitalia - ang., coloc., zinc.

SHRIVELLED, genitalia genitals - **AGN.,** ***arg-n.,*** carb-s., **IGN., LYC.,** merc.

shrivelled, scrotum - berb., caps., carb-s., ***crot-t.,*** rhod., ther., zinc.

shrivelled, spermatic cord - ***caps.***

SMARTING, pain, penis - asar., aur-s., berb., crot-h., sulph.
end of - arum-t.

SMARTING, pain
glans - ***asar.,*** berb., nux-v.
prepuce - benz-ac., nux-v., puls.
underside - carb-v.

smarting, scrotum - berb., carb-s., ran-s.
between and thighs - hep., nat-c.

SMEGMA, increased - alum., ***canth.,*** **CAUST.,** nat-c., ***nux-v.,*** sang., sulph., sumb.
increased, foul - sulph.

SOFTENING, of testes - caps.

SORE, pain, genitalia, bruised - ant-s., arn., ars., arum-t., cocc., lil-t., phos., **PLAT.,** ***sulph.,*** syph., verat.
smarting, and, as from salt after urinating - caust.
urination, during - kreos.

sore, penis - asar., bor., calad., ***cann-s.,*** canth., cop., hep., ***ign.,*** lach., nat-c., rhus-t., rhus-v., sabad., sulph., tep., ***thuj.***
lower, side - cic.

sore, penis, glans - asar., caps., chel., cic., cycl., merc., nat-c., rhus-t., thuj.
urination, during - ***lyc.,*** nit-ac.

sore, penis, prepuce - ail., calad., carb-v., sep., verat.
evening - cycl., mez.
margin - chin., **IGN.,** ***mur-ac., nit-ac.***
walking, while - **MERC.**

sore, prostate - alum., **CHIM.,** ***cycl., rhus-t.,*** sul-ac.

sore, scrotum - am-c., anac., berb., ***calc-p.,*** chin., coff., cupr-ar., kali-c., ph-ac., zinc.
between scrotum and thigh - ***bar-c.,*** **GRAPH., LYC.,** ***merc., nat-c., nat-m.,*** **PETR.,** rhod., ***rhus-t., sulph.,*** zinc.
from rubbing - nat-m.
oozing fluid - calc-p., cop.
perspiring, after - plb.
sides of - petr., thuj., zinc.
spots, in - nit-ac.
thighs, between - ***caust.,*** rhod.

sore, spermatic cord - brach., **CLEM.,** equis., **PHYT.,** ***sars.***
right - ***clem.***
touch, on - chin., clem., meny., merc-i-r., sars.

sore, testes - ***acon.,*** aesc., alum., am-c., apis, **ARG-M.,** ***arg-n.,*** arn., ars., ***aur., calc., caust.,*** chel., cimic., **CLEM.,** ***cocc.,*** coloc., con., cop., ***dig.,*** echi., equis., ***ham.,*** hep., indg., kali-bi., kali-br., kali-c., kali-n., lith., med., ***merc.,*** mez., nat-a., nat-c., ***nat-m.,*** **NIT-AC.,** oci., ol-an., ox-ac., ***pall.,*** ph-ac., ***phos.,*** polyg., psor., **PULS., RHOD.,** sabad., **SPONG.,** staph., tarent., ***thuj.,*** zinc.
afternoon - calc-s.
evening - **PULS.,** sabad.
6 to 11 p.m. - **AUR.**
in bed - ***arg-m.***
extending, left - ***polyg.***
up spermatic cord - ***equis.,*** polyg., puls., **RHOD.**

sore, testes
left - ***arg-m.,*** calc., nat-a., ***nit-ac.,*** sabad., ***thuj.***
morning - sars.
right - acon., **ARG-M.,** arg-n., **AUR.,** ***caust.,*** dig., ***rhod.,*** sabin.
sitting, while - **PULS.**
walking, while - **ARG-M.,** ***clem.,*** staph., thuj.
wine - thuj.

SPERMATIC cord, general - berb., ham., ***puls.,*** rhod., spong.

SPERM, low count of, infertility - sulfa., x-ray.

SPOTS, genitalia, yellow, brown, on - cob.
spots, penis - calc.
blue - sulph.
glans - arn., ***carb-v.,*** cinnb., lach., nat-m., ***nit-ac.,*** petr., sep., ***sil.,*** ther., thuj.
granular - cinnb., thuj.
red - arn., ***carb-v.,*** caust., cinnb., con., lach., nat-m., ***nit-ac.,*** petr., sep., ***sil.,*** ther., thuj.
spots, penis, prepuce - lach., nit-ac., rhus-t., thuj.
red - nit-ac.
spots, scrotum - calc., ***sil.***
white - ***merc.,*** thuj.

SQUEEZING, pain, testes - ***sil.,*** **SPONG.,** staph., ***thuj.***

STICKING, pain, genitalia - lyc., merc., mur-ac., petr., phos., ***rhod., sulph., thuj.,*** zinc.
sticking, prostate - nit-ac.

SUPPURATION, penis, prepuce, under the - caps., **CINNB.,** ***cor-r., hep.,*** jac., jug-r., lyc., ***merc.,*** **MERC-C.,** ***nit-ac.,*** sep., sulph.
suppuration, prostate - hep., **SIL.**
suppuration, testes - phyt.

SWELLING, genitalia - aloe, ang., **ARN.,** ***ars., canth.,*** carb-o., coc-c., kali-bi., ***lach., lyc., merc.,*** plb., **RHUS-T.,** sac-alb., tarent., wies.
dropsical - ***apis, dig.,*** **GRAPH.,** ***rhus-t.***
painful - ***ars., canth.,*** plb., rhus-t.
sensation as if - zinc.
swelling, penis - anac., apoc., **ARN.,** ***ars.,*** aspar., bufo, calc-p., ***cann-s., canth., cinnb.,*** cop., cor-r., cupr., fl-ac., graph., iris, ***kali-i., kreos., lac-c., led., merc., merc-c., mez., mill.,*** nat-a., nat-c., nat-p., ***nat-s.,*** ph-ac., plb., ***rhus-t.,*** rhus-v., sabin., ***sil.,*** sol-n., sumb., tarent., ***vesp.***
bluish-red - arn., ars.
edematous - ***apis, apoc.,*** arn., ***cann-s., canth., dig., fl-ac., graph., lyc., merc., nat-s., nit-ac., nux-v.,*** puls., ***rhod.,*** **RHUS-T.,** sil., sulph., ***vesp.***
hard - arn., merc., nux-v., ph-ac., sabin., spong.
dorsum - sabin.
hot - arn., form., kali-c., puls.
lymphatics - lact., ***merc.***
vessels, along - merc.

swelling, penis
painful - arn., ars., calad., cann-s., canth., caps., graph., lact., ***merc.,*** nit-ac., nux-v., plb., puls., rhus-t., sabin., sulph., thuj.
painless - mez.
swelling, penis, glans - ***ars.,*** cann-s., ***canth., cinnb., cor-r., dor.,*** iris, ***kali-i.,*** med., ***merc., nat-c.,*** plb., **RHUS-T.,** sac-alb., sulph., sumb., thuj.
one side of - spig.
painful and inflamed - ***acon.,*** antipyrin., ***apis, arg-n.,*** arn., ars., calad., ***cann-s., canth., cop.,*** cor-r., ***cub.,*** dig., ***gels.,*** ham., merc., ***merc-c., nit-ac.,*** ph-ac., ***rhus-t.,*** sars., ***thuj.***
swelling, penis, prepuce - ***apis,*** **CALAD.,** cann-s., canth., ***caps.,*** carb-s., cham., **CINNB.,** ***cor-r., dig., fl-ac.,*** form., ***graph., jac.,*** lac-c., **MERC.,** ***merc-i-f.,*** mez., mill., ***nat-c., nat-s.,*** **NIT-AC.,** sabin., **RHUS-T.,** ***rhus-v.,*** sep., sil., ***sulph., sumb., thuj.,*** **VESP.,** ***viol-t.***
fraenum, on - sabin.
swelling, prostate - ***bar-c.,*** cann-s., chel., **CHIM.,** ***con.,*** cop., cub., ***dig.,*** dulc., hipp., ***iod.,*** med., merc-d., ***puls., sabal.,*** sel., senec., sep., staph., sul-ac., ***thuj.***
sensation, as if - senec.
swelling, scrotum - anac., anan., ***apis,*** apoc., ***arn., ars.,*** asaf., ***bell.,*** brom., calc., ***canth., carb-v.,*** carl., caust., ***chel.,*** chin., ***clem.,*** colch., con., cupr-ar., ***graph.,*** ign., jac., mez., ***nat-m.,*** nit-ac., ph-ac., plb., ***puls.,*** rhus-d., **RHUS-T.,** ***rhus-v.,*** sac-alb., ***sep.,*** sol-n., stram., syph., urt-u., ***vesp.***
edematous - anan., **APIS,** ***apoc., arg-m.,*** **ARS.,** calad., ***canth., colch., dig.,*** ferr-s., fl-ac., **GRAPH.,** ***kali-c., lach., lyc., nat-m., nat-s., phos.,*** **RHUS-T.,** zinc.
elephantiasis - sil.
gonorrhea, with chronic - brom.
inflammatory - ***apis,*** ars., crot-t., euph., ***ham.,*** ph-ac., plb., ***rhus-t.,*** verat-v.
painless - mez.
sides of - agar., **CLEM.,** mez., puls.
swelling, spermatic cords - anth., arn., ***berb., calc., cann-s., chin.,*** coloc., ***ham., kali-c., kali-i.,*** ph-ac., ***phos.,*** **PULS.,** ***sars.,*** **SPONG.,** tarent., yohim.
inguinal glands, with - clem.
left - berb.
right - **CLEM.,** puls.
sexual excitement, after - ***sars.***
walking, agg. - ***berb.***
swelling, testes - ***acon., agn.,*** alum., anan., ant-t., ***apis,*** arg-m., ***arg-n., arn., ars., ars-i., aur.,*** aur-m., aur-m-n., aur-s., ***bapt.,*** bar-c., ***bar-m., bell., brom.,*** bry., calc., ***calc-p.,*** canth., carb-an., carb-s., carb-v., ***carl.,*** chel., ***chin.,*** **CLEM.,** coloc., ***con., cop.,*** cub., ***dig.,*** elaps, ***graph., ham.,*** hippoz., ind., ***iod.,*** kali-ar., kali-br., ***kali-c., kali-i.,*** kali-s., ***lach.,*** lyc., mag-aust., ***med., merc., merc-c., merc-i-r.,*** merc-sul., ***mez.,*** mill., nat-a., nat-c.,

swelling, testes - ***nat-m.,*** nat-p., ***nit-ac.,*** ***nux-v.,*** oci., ***ol-an., ph-ac.,*** phyt., ***plb., psor.,*** **PULS., RHOD.,** rhus-t., ***sil.,*** **SPONG.,** staph., stry., sulph., tarax., tarent., tep., thuj., tus-f., vario., ***verat-v.,*** vib., yohim, ***zinc.***
alternately - ol-an.
contusion, after - vario.
left - alum., brom., cop., mez., oci., ph-ac., podo., **PULS.,** ***rhod., spong.,*** vib.
hard, painless - brom.
mumps, from - abrot., ars., ***carb-ac., piloc., merc.,*** nat-m., nux-v., phos., **PULS.,** rhus-t., staph.
painful when driving - ***brom.***
right - apis, arg-n., **AUR.,** chel., **CLEM.,** graph., iod., ***puls.,*** **RHOD.,** sul-ac., tarent.
thickening of epididymis, with - carb-s., spong., sulph.
unrequited sexual passion, from - ***iod.***

SYPHILIS, penis, ulcers on, chancres - anan., apis, arg-n., ars., ars-m., asaf., ***aur.,*** **AUR-M., AUR-M-N.,** bor., caust., **CINNB.,** ***con., cor-r., hep.,*** iod., ***jac., kali-bi., kali-chl., kali-i., lac-c., lach.,*** lyc., **MERC., MERC-C.,** ***merc-i-f., merc-i-r.,*** merc-p-r., mygal., **NIT-AC.,** ***ph-ac.,*** phos., ***phyt.,*** plat., plat-m., sil., ***staph.,*** still., ***sulph., thuj.,*** viol-t.

TEARING, pain, penis - ambr., aur., colch., coloc., con., iod., kali-c., kali-i., merc., mez., petr., ph-ac., tab., thuj.
root, walking agg, leaning against small of back while standing amel. - ign.
walking agg, to glans, after urination - sars.
walking agg. - ign., zinc.
tip - zinc.

tearing, penis, glans - ambr., cinnb., ***colch.,*** coloc., euph., kali-c., lyc., merc., ***mez., pareir.,*** petr., thuj., zinc.
urination, during - ***pareir.,*** petr., ***sars.***
to root of penis -sars.
urination, before - aur.

tearing, penis, prepuce - chin., jac.

tearing, spermatic cord - anag., ***arg-m.,*** arum-t., bell., ***berb., calc., colch., iod.,*** nit-ac., nux-v., ol-an., ***ox-ac., puls., staph.,*** sumb.
coughing - nat-m.
downward - calc., staph.
evening - bell.
in bed - bell.
left - sumb.
rest, during - arg-m.
right, 4 p.m. - arg-m.
upward in left - bell.
walking, while - ***berb.***

tearing, testes - ant-t., arum-t., caust., ***chin., con.,*** euph., hyos., nat-c., ph-ac., **PULS.,** ***rhod.,*** sep., staph., ust.
right - arum-t.
extending to abdomen - arum-t.

TENSION, genitalia - graph., nat-m., rhus-t.
touched by clothing, when - graph.

tension, penis - ant-s., calc-p., graph., kali-c., kali-i., mosch., mur-ac., nat-c., psor.

tension, prostate - clem., lyc., thuj.

tension, scrotum - arn., ***clem.,*** com.

tension, spermatic cords - cann-s., chel., ***clem.,*** kali-n., med., ol-an., ph-ac., phos., ***puls., sulph.***

tension, testes - aur., kali-c., kali-n., sulph.

THICKENING, penis, prepuce - elaps, lach., thiosin., sulph.

thickening, scrotum - ***rhus-t., sulph.***

thickening, spermatic cord - calad., carb-v., **CLEM.,** rhus-r., ***rhus-t., sulph.***
extending into abdomen - kali-n.

thickening, testes, epididymis, with swelling - carb-s., spong., sulph.

THIN, scrotum - pyrog.

THRILL, penis, prolonged - cann-i.

TICKLING, sex, during, obliging withdrawal, genitalia - calc.

tickling, penis, glans - bell., benz-ac., iod.

tickling, scrotum - sel.

TIED, penis, with a cord, sensation as if penis - plb.

TINGLING, genitalia - ***alum.,*** ang., mosch., sel., sulph.

tingling, penis - ant-t., bell., berb., cop., ferr., ham., iod., laur., puls., seneg., sumb., thuj.
root - rhus-t.

tingling, penis, glans - acon., ant-t., bell., calc., caps., carb-ac., carb-v., iod., kali-bi., lyc., lyss., merc., mez., ph-ac., puls., seneg., spig., sumb., thuj.

tingling, penis, prepuce - jac., merc., ph-ac., seneg., tarax.

tingling, scrotum - acon., arn., com., kali-n., lachn., plat., sel.

tingling, testes - agn., carb-v., euphr., merc., rhod., sulph., thuj., zinc.

TUBERCLES, genitalia - ***hydrc., thuj.***

tubercles, penis, - bov., thuj.
glans - hippoz.

tubercles, scrotum - bufo.

tubercles, spermatic cord - ambr., ***graph., iod., kali-c.,*** mang., ***merc., nit-ac.,*** ph-ac., ***phos.,*** plb., **PULS.,** sars., **SIL., SPONG.,** staph., sulph., thuj., zinc.

tubercles, testes - ambr., ***arg-m.,*** calc., carb-s., carb-v., caust., graph., hep., **IOD.,** kali-c., lyc., ***merc.,*** nat-m., ***nit-ac., petr., ph-ac.,*** phos., plb., psor., **PULS.,** sep., **SIL., SPONG.,** ***staph.,*** sulph., **TUB.,** ***zinc.***

TUMOR, penis, glans, soft - bell.
yellow, behind - lyc.

tumor, testes, indolent - tarent.

TWINGING, sensation, testes - coloc.

TWISTING, pain, testes, left - nit-ac.

TWITCHING, penis - aur., bar-c., ***calc.,*** carl., caust., ***cinnb.,*** graph., lach., lyc., mez., nat-m., nit-ac., rhod., stann., **THUJ.,** viol-t., zinc.
burning seminal vesicles to glans - ***mang.***
glans - mez.
root - zinc.
twitching, prostate - form.
twitching, scrotum - graph.
twitching, spermatic cords - ang., graph., ***mang.***
twitching, testes - lyc., meny., sil.

ULCERS, genitalia - ***ars.,*** cupr-ar., hep., ***lach., merc., phyt., thuj.***
burning - **ARS.,** hep.
chancre hard - carb-an., cinnb., kali-i., merc., merc-c., ***merc-i-f.,*** merc-i-r.
soft - cor-r., merc., nit-ac., thuj.
deep - ***merc.***
gangrenous - ***merc-c.***
groin, from incised bubos - ***carb-an.,*** chel.
painful - ***ars.,*** cann-s., ***caust.,*** cop., ***cor-r.,*** crot-t., ***hep., merc., merc-c.,*** mez., ***nit-ac.,*** osm., sep., thuj.
spreading - **ARS., MERC-C.**
ulcers, penis - ail., anan., apis, arg-n., ars., ars-h., ***ars-i.,*** ars-m., aur., aur-m., aur-m-n., calc., caust., ***cinnb., cor-r., hep., kali-bi.,*** kali-chl., lac-c., lyc., **MERC., MERC-C.,** ***merc-i-f.,*** nat-c., ***nit-ac., nux-v., ph-ac.,*** phyt., psor., **THUJ.**
bleeding - cor-r., hep., **MERC.,** ***nit-ac.,*** staph.
chancres - anan., apis, arg-n., ars., ars-m., asaf., ***aur.,*** **AUR-M., AUR-M-N.,** bor., caust., **CINNB.,** ***con., cor-r., hep.,*** iod., ***jac., kali-bi., kali-chl., kali-i., lac-c., lach.,*** lyc., **MERC., MERC-C.,** ***merc-i-f., merc-i-r.,*** merc-p-r., mygal., **NIT-AC.,** ***ph-ac.,*** phos., ***phyt.,*** plat., plat-m., sil., ***staph.,*** still., ***sulph., thuj.,*** viol-t.
burning - ***ars-m.***
cheesy base - hep., kali-bi.
complications, with - ***ars.,*** hecla., ***hep.,*** lach., merc., ***sil.,*** sulph., thuj.
deep - aur-m-n., ***kali-bi., kali-i.,*** merc., nit-ac., ***sulph.***
elevated - ***cinnb., hep.,*** merc.
lead-colored, sensitive edges - nit-ac., ***sil.***
elevated margins - ***ars.,*** kali-bi., hep., **LYC.,** ***merc., nit-ac., ph-ac.***
flat - aur-m., ***cor-r., nit-ac.,*** thuj.
painful - cor-r.
gangrenous - ars., lach.
hard - aur., carb-an., **CINNB.,** ***con.,*** jug-r., kali-chl., kali-i., **MERC., MERC-C., MERC-I-F., MERC-I-R.**
edges - ***kali-i.***
indolent - sep., sil.
indurated - cinnb.
lardaceous base, deep, round, penetrating, painful, bleeding, raw, everted edges - merc.
inflamed - cinnb.

ulcers, penis
itching - benz-ac., lyc., merc., merc-i-f., sep., ***sulph., thuj.***
lardaceous base - arg-n., cor-r., ***hep.,*** **MERC.,** ***staph.***
mercurio-syphilitic - aur., **HEP.,** kali-chl., ***lach.,*** **NIT-AC.,** ***sil., staph.,*** still., ***sulph.***
offensive - hep., merc., **NIT-AC.**
painful - ***cor-r., sil.***
painless - bapt., merc-i-r., nit-ac., op.
phagedenic - **ARS.,** ***aur-m-n.,*** caust., ***cinnb.,*** hydr., kali-p., ***lach., merc-c., nit-ac.,*** sil., sulph.
ragged edges - nit-ac.
recurrent - ***sep.***
red -cor-r., thuj.
serpiginous - **ARS.**
soft - cor-r., merc., nit-ac., thuj.
sore - ***merc.***
splinters, sticking pains, as from - arg-n., hep., **NIT-AC.,** ***thuj.***
swollen - cinnb.
ulcers, penis, fraenum, destroying - ***nit-ac.***
ulcers, penis, glans - apis, ars., ***ars-h.,*** ars-i., ***aur-m-n.,*** benz-ac., ***cinnb.,*** cor-r., kali-i., ***lac-c.,*** lyc., **MERC., MERC-C., NIT-AC.,** ***psor.,*** sep., ***sulph.,*** syph., ***thuj.***
ulcers, penis, prepuce - ail., arg-m., ***arg-n., ars., ars-h.,*** **AUR-M.,** aur-m-n., bor., cann-s., ***caust., cinnb.,*** cop., ***cor-r., hep.,*** ign., kali-bi., **MERC., MERC-C.,** merc-i-r., ***nit-ac.,*** nux-v., ph-ac., ***phos.,*** phyt., ***sep., sil.,*** staph., ***sulph., thuj.,*** viol-t.
tip - ***merc., merc-c., nit-ac.***
under surface of - lyc.
ulcers, scrotum - am-c., aur., ***aur-m.,*** cupr-ar., ***kali-i.,*** nit-ac., sep.
ulcers, sides of - crot-t.

UNEASY, feeling - kali-c.
uneasiness, prostate - ptel.

URTICARIA, genitalia - clem., cop., merc., nat-c.

VARICES, penis, prepuce - ham., lach.
varices, spermatic cords - ham.

VARIOCELE, spermatic cord - aesc., arn., ***aur.,*** bell., ***calc.,*** carb-v., colch., ***coll.,*** crot-h., fl-ac., ***ham., lach., lyc., merc-i-r., nux-v.,*** osm., ***ph-ac., podo., puls.,*** ruta., sep., ***sil., sulph.,*** tab.
strain, following a - ruta.

VESICLES, genitalia - ant-t., carb-v., chin-s., **CROT-T.,** cupr-ar., ***merc., nat-c.,*** nat-p., **NIT-AC.,** petr., ph-ac., **RHUS-T.,** ***rhus-v.,*** sep.
vesicles, penis - aloe, ars-h., ***calc.,*** carb-v., ***caust.,*** **CROT-T.,** ***graph., hep., merc.,*** **NIT-AC.,** ***ph-ac., rhus-t., rhus-v., sep.,*** tep., thuj.
burning - caust., ***merc.***
itching - calc., ***hep.,*** **NIT-AC.,** ph-ac.
ulcers, becoming - caust., **MERC., NIT-AC.,** thuj.
at meatus - merc-c., ***nit-ac.***
white - merc.

vesicles, penis, glans - ***ars-h.,*** caust., ***merc., ph-ac.,*** rhus-t., stann., thuj.

vesicles, penis, prepuce, vesicles - ars-h., carb-v., caust., graph., merc., nit-ac., thuj.

vesicles, scrotum - ars., bell., ***chel.,*** **CROT-T.,** cupr-ar., ***petr.,*** psor., ***rhus-t., rhus-v.***
painful - chel., psor.
raphe, along - ***nit-ac.***
yellowish - chel., ***rhus-t.***

VOLUPTUOUS, sensation genitalia - bor.
scratching, caused by - ***crot-t.***

WARTS, genitalia - ***calc.,*** euphr., ***lyc., merc.,*** **NAT-S., NIT-AC.,** ***sabin., sars., staph.,*** **THUJ.**

WEAKNESS, genitalia, sex, after - ***berb.***
urination, after, as if he would have an emission - berb.

weakness, genitalia, sensation of - agn., carb-an., lyc., mang., mur-ac., ***nat-m.***
stool, after - ***calc., calc-p.***

weakness, prostate - ***bar-c.,*** berb., chim., ***con., dig.,*** lyc., med., **SABAL., SEL.,** ***thuj.***

WRINKLED, scrotum - rhod.

Mind

ABANDONED, forsaken feelings, (see Isolation, feelngs) - allox., alum., anac., ***arg-n.,*** ars., asar., **AUR.,** bar-c., calc., calc-s., camph., cann-i., carb-an., carb-v., carc., chin., chin-b., coff., cortico., ***cycl.,*** dros., hell., hura, ip., kali-br., kali-c., keroso., lac-d., ***lach.,*** lact., lam., laur., lil-t., lith., lyss., ***mag-c., mag-m.,*** mag-aust., ***meny., merc., nat-c.,*** nat-m., pall., ***plat.,*** **PSOR., PULS.,** rhus-t., sabin., sars., sec., sep., spig., ***stram., thuj.,*** valer., verat.
anxiety, as if a friend had abandoned her - ars., puls., ***rhus-t.***
air, open amel. - ***puls.,*** rhus-t.
elderly people, in - aur., puls., psor.
evening - bar-c., ***puls.***
friendless, feels lonely - alum., puls., thuj.
headache, with - ***meny.***
morning - carb-an., carb-v., ***lach.***
waking, on - ***arg-n., lach.***

ABANDONS, forsakes his own children - lyc., sec.
relations - lyc., sec.

ABRUPT - **CALC.,** cham., **HEP.,** ***lyc.,*** med., nat-m., ***nit-ac., nux-v., plat.,*** **PULS.,** rauw., sil., **SULPH.,** ***tarent.***
harsh - ars., caust., **GRAPH.,** hep., ***kali-i.,*** lach., lyss., med., nat-m., nux-v., ***sep., staph.***
rough, yet affectionate - lyc., nux-v., **PULS.**

ABSENT-minded, preoccupied - abel., ***acon.,*** act-sp., adlu., aesc., agar., ***agn.,*** all-c., ***alum.,*** alum-p., alum-sil., ***am-c.,*** am-m., ambr., ***anac.,*** ang., **APIS,** aq-mar., arag., arg-m., ***arn.,*** ars., ars-s-f., art-v., arum-i., arum-t., asaf., ***asar.,*** atro., ***aur.,*** aur-a., aur-s., ***bapt., bar-c., bell.,*** berb., bol., ***bov.,*** bufo, ***calad.,*** calc., calc-p., calc-s., calc-sil., **CANN-I.,** cann-s., ***canth.,*** caps., carc., ***carl.,*** carb-ac., carb-s., **CAUST.,** ***cench.,*** cent., **CHAM.,** chel., chin., ***cic.,*** clem., ***cocc.,*** coff., ***colch.,*** coloc., con., cot., croc., crot-h., ***cupr.,*** cycl., daph., dirc., dub., dulc., elaps, ferr-ar., ***graph.,*** grat., guai., ham., **HELL.,** hep., hura, hydr., ***hyos., ign.,*** ind., jug-c., kali-bi., ***kali-br., kali-c., kali-p.,*** kali-s., kali-sil., ***kreos.,*** kres., ***lac-c.,*** **LACH.,** laur., led., ***lyc.,*** lyss., ***mag-c.,*** mag-p-a., manc., mang., med., menis., ***merc.,*** merc-cy., **MEZ.,** mosch., naja, nat-a., nat-c., ***nat-m.,*** nat-p., nit-ac., **NUX-M.,** ***nux-v., ol-an., olnd., onos., op., petr., ph-ac., phos.,*** **PLAT.,** ***plb.,*** ictod., psor., **PULS.,** quas., ran-b., ran-s., rheum, rhod., ***rhus-t.,*** rhus-v., ruta, sal-ac., sanic., sant., saroth., sars., ***sel.,*** **SEP.,** ***sil.,*** spig., spong., stann., staph., stict., stram., ***sulph.,*** sul-ac., ***syph.,*** tarent., tell., thiop., thuj., tub., valer., **VERAT.,** verb., viol-o., viol-t., zinc., zinc-c.
afternoon - ang.
coffee or wine, after, from much business - ***all-c.***
nausea, after - calc.
air, in open - plat.
albuminuria, in - ***cocc.***
alternating with animation - alum.

ABSENT-minded
become, as to what will become of him - nat-m.
cerebral irritation, in - ***all-c., cupr-ac.***
conversing, when - bol., chin., chin-b., psil.
daytime, 11 a.m. to 4 p.m. - kali-n.
dreamy - ang., arn., cann-i., cench., olnd., ***phos.,*** sep., staph.
epileptic attack, before - ***lach.***
inadvertence - ***alum.,*** am-c., cham., nux-v., staph.
lack of awareness, attacks of - **ARS.,** art-v., ***bapt., hyos.,*** ign., merc-cy., ***nat-m., phos.,*** zinc-c.
mail a letter, goes to, brings it home in her hands - ***lac-c.***
menses, during - calc., mur-ac.
morning - guai., nat-c., ph-ac., phos.
11 a.m. to 4 p.m. - kali-n.
noon - mosch.
old age, in - am-c., ***con., lyc.***
ozaena, in - ***aur.***
periodical attacks of, short lasting - chlorpr., fl-ac., ***nux-m.***
purchases, makes, and goes out without them - ***lac-c.***
reading, while - agn., lach., ***nux-m.,*** ph-ac.
sleep, on going to - ang.
senselessness, with, and intoxicated condition - ***nux-m.***
spoken to, when - am-c., am-m., ambr., bar-c., nux-v.
standing in one place, never accomplishes what he undertakes - ***nux-m.***
starts, when spoken to - aur-m., carb-ac., ptel., sulph.
stroke, in - **BAR-C.**
supposes to be in two places at a time - lyc.
thoughts, vanishing of - ***cann-i.,*** zinc.
urticaria, in - ***bov.***
vertigo, during - hep.
waking, on, does not know where he is or what to answer - ***nux-m.***
work, when at - hura
writing, while - mag-c.
yellow fever, in - ***sulph.***

ABSORBED, mentally - acon., aloe, alum., am-c., am-m., ambr., anh., ant-c., ***arn.,*** asar., bar-c., bell., bov., brucin., bufo, calc., cann-i., cann-s., canth., ***caps., carl.,*** caust., cham., chel., chin., cic., clem., ***cocc.,*** con., cupr., cycl., dig., elaps, euphr., grat., ham., **HELL.,** hyos., ign., indg., iod., ip., kali-c., kiss., lach., ***laur.,*** lil-t., mag-c., mag-m., mang., merc., **MEZ.,** mosch., mur-ac., nat-c., ***nat-m.,*** nat-p., nit-ac., **NUX-M.,** nux-v., ol-an., ***onos., op., petr.,*** phel., phos., plat., plb., ***puls.,*** ran-b., rheum, ***rhus-t.,*** sabad., sars., sel., sep., spig., stann., staph., stram., stront-c., **SULPH.,** thuj., verat., viol-o., vip.
afternoon - mang.
alternating with frivolity - arg-n.
as to what would become of him - nat-m.
daytime - elaps.
eating, after - aloe.
evening - am-m., ***sulph.***

ABSORBED, mentally
future, about - spig.
hours, for, generally in morning, in insanity - nux-v.
menses, during - mur-ac.
misfortune, imagines - calc-s.
morning - ***nat-c.,*** nux-v.

ABSTRACTION, mental - acon-l., agn., ***alum.,*** am-c., aml-n., ang., ***arn.,*** bell., berb., bov., bufo, camph., ***cann-i.,*** caps., carb-ac., caust., ***cham.,*** cic., colch., con., cortico., ***croc.,*** cycl., elaps, ***graph.,*** guai., ***hell., hyos.,*** ictod., kali-c., ***kreos.,*** laur., lyc., ***lyss.,*** mag-c., mang., ***merc., mez.,*** nat-c., ***nat-m.,*** **NUX-M.,** nux-v., ***oena., ol-an.,*** olnd., ***onos.,*** op., ph-ac., ***phos.,*** plat., plb., ran-b., sabad., sars., sec., sil., spong., stann., stram., sul-ac., ***sulph.,*** thuj., ***tub.,*** verb., vesp., ***visc.***
morning - guai.

ABUSED, ailments from being, (see Humiliation) - ***acon.,*** alum., am-m., **ANAC.,** ***arg-n.,*** ars., ***aur., aur-m.,*** bell., ***bry.,*** calc., calc-s., **CARC.,** caust., ***cham.,*** **COLOC.,** con., form., gels., grat., **IGN.,** ***lach.,*** **LYC.,** ***lyss.,*** med., merc., **NAT-M.,** ***nux-v., op.,*** **PALL.,** petr., **PH-AC.,** plat., ***puls.,*** rhus-t., ***seneg.,*** sep., sil., **STAPH.,** stram., ***sulph.,*** thuj., verat., zinc.
anger, with - anac., ***carc.,*** **COLOC.,** ***staph.***
indignation, with - anac., carc., **IGN., STAPH.**
punishment, from - ***anac.,*** **CARC.,** cham., ign., lyc., nat-m., **STAPH.,** tarent.
sexual abuse, from - **ACON.,** anac., **ARN., CARC., IGN.,** lyc., ***med.,*** **NAT-M.,** nux-v., **OP.,** ***plat., sep.,*** **STAPH.,** thuj.
shame, from - ign., ***nat-m.,*** **STAPH.,** thuj.
violence, from - acon., ***anac.,*** **ARN.,** ***aur., bry.,*** **CARC.,** coff., lyc., nat-m., ***op.,*** **STAPH.**

ABUSIVE, insulting - ***abies-n., acon.,*** alco., am-c., am-m., **ANAC.,** ***arn.,*** ars., atro., ***aur., bell.,*** bor., bufo, camph., canth., caust., **CHAM.,** chel., cic., ***con.,*** cor-r., croc., cupr-ar., dulc., elae., ***ferr.,*** gall-ac., **HEP.,** hist., ***hyos., ign.,*** ip., kali-i., **LACH., LYC.,** ***lyss.,*** mag-aust., mag-c., merc., mosch., nat-c., ***nit-ac.,*** **NUX-V.,** pall., ***petr.,*** plat., plb., raja-s., ran-b., ***seneg., sep.,*** sil., spong., staph., ***stram.,*** sulph., syph., ***tarent., tub., verat.,*** viol-t.
angry, without being - dulc.
children and family, to - kali-i., nux-v., ***sep.***
insult parents - am-m., calc-p., ***cham.,*** **CINA,** hyos., **LYC.,** nat-m., **PLAT., TUB.**
crying mood, with - ***stram.***
drunkenness, during - hep., nux-v., petr.
evening - am-c.
fever, during typhoid - lyc.
forenoon - ran-b.
husband insults wife, in front of children - ***anac.,*** ars., **LACH.,** lyc., nux-v., **VERAT.**
wife and children - lyc., lyss., ***nux-v.***
inclined to be - atro., caust., ***con.,*** elae., lyc., nux-v., ***sep.***

ABUSIVE, insulting
jealousy, from, with unchaste expressions - nux-v.
menses, before - cham.
mother - ***sep.,*** thuj.
pains, with the - ars., **CHAM.,** cor-r., nux-v.
scolds until the lips are blue and eyes stare and she falls down fainting - ***mosch.***
somebody on the road, to - con.

ACT, no longer wishes to, for herself, in nervous debility - ***cur.***

ACTIONS, behaviour
foolish - bell., **HYOS.,** ***merc.,*** sec.
hysteria, in - ***apis.***
insane, with convulsions - ***phos.***
ludicrous - bell., ***hyos.***
monkeys, like - **HYOS.**

ACTIVITY, mental
alternating with
apathy - sarr.
dullness - acon., med.
exhaustion - ***aloe.***
indifference - sarr.
laziness - ***aloe.***
amel. (see Work, general) - con., cycl., helon., iod., kali-bi., lil-t., mur-ac., sep.
business, in - brom., manc.
creative - coff.
desire for - hyper., led., nat-s.
disturbed - stram.
dream, like a - op.
emotional - viol-o.
evening - graph., lycps., rhus-t.
9 p.m. after walking in open air - chin-s.
fruitless - apis, arg-n., bor., calc., kali-br., lil-t., stann., tarent., ther.
midnight, until - **COFF.,** graph.
morning - acon.
5 a.m. - fago., lycps.
night - chin., dig., ***lach.,*** nitro-o., sin-n., ***sulph.***
4 a.m., from - cortico.
perspiration, during - op.
prostration, with physical - mosch.
restless - dig., ign., lycps., nux-v., verat., viol-o.
evening - lycps.
night - dig.
sleeplessness, with - dig., rhus-t., thea., zinc.
night, during - thea.
thinks of everything - arag.
work, at - benz-ac.

ADDICTIVE, personality - ***carc.,*** lach., ***med., nux-v.,*** op., thuj.

ADMIRATION, excessive - cic., sulph.
for things that are not admirable - sulph.

ADMONITION, agg. - ***bell.,*** calc., carc., kali-c., nit-ac., ***nux-v.,*** pall., ***plat.***
children, in - carc., med.
kindly agg. - bell., chin., ign., nux-v., ***plat.,*** stann.

ADULTEROUS - ***calc.,*** calth., caust., lach., med., phos., **PLAT., PULS., STAPH.,** ***thuj.,*** verat.

AFFECTATION, (see Haughty) - alum., carb-v., caust., con., graph., ***hyos.,*** **LYC.,** mez., nat-m., petr., **PLAT.,** ***stram., verat.***
gestures and acts, in - hyos., mez., stram., verat.
mania, in - ***stram.***
words, in - lyc., plat., verat-v.

AFFECTIONATE - acon., alum., anac., ant-c., ***ars.,*** bar-c., bor., bry., carb-an., carb-v., ***carc.,*** caust., coff., ***croc.,*** graph., hura, hyos., ***ign.,*** lach., lyc., med., ***nat-m.,*** nit-ac., ***nux-v.,*** ox-ac., par., ph-ac., ***phos.,*** plat., **PULS.,** seneg., sil., staph., thea., verat.
active - hura.
children, kiss and caress - ***puls.***
distasteful - carb-ac.
returns affection - ***phos., puls.***

AGONY, anguish - acet-ac., **ACON.,** aeth., aloe, alum., am-caust., ambr., ***anac.,*** anh., am-caust., ant-a., ant-t., ***apis,*** aran., arg-m., ***arg-n., arn.,*** **ARS.,** ars-s-f., asaf., asar., ***aur.,*** aur-a., ***bism.,*** **BELL.,** bov., bufo, buni-o., buth-a., calad., **CALC., CALC-AR.,** calc-f., camph., **CANN-I.,** carb-o., ***carb-v.,*** **CARC., CAUST.,** cedr., cham., chin., chlorpr., cob-n., coca, ***coff.,*** coloc., ***crot-c.,*** crot-h., ***cupr.,*** cyt-l., der., des-ac., **DIG.,** foll., ***gels.,*** **GRAPH.,** halo., hed., **HEP.,** hoit., ***hyos., jatr., kali-ar.,*** kali-c., kali-i., lach., lact., ***lat-m.,*** levo., ***lob.,*** **LYC.,** ***mag-c.,*** mag-m., mag-s., mosch., mur-ac., murx., naja, nat-a., nat-c., nep., nit-ac., ***nux-v.,*** oena., onop., ***op.,*** perh., ***phos.,*** plan., **PLAT.,** ***plb.,*** pneu., ***psor., puls.,*** rauw., rhus-t., saroth., ***sars.,*** sec., sep., stann., ***stram.,*** sulfonam., sulph., tarent., thala., thea., thuj-l., thyr., tril., verat., vip., vip-a., ***zinc-valer.***
afternoon - am-c., ***cupr.,*** eupi., nux-v., ph-ac., rhus-t., staph.
air, in open, amel. - **CANN-I.,** ***puls.***
alone, when - ***phos.***
amenorrhea, in - ***graph., plat.***
anger, from - ***plat.***
bed, amel. after going to - mag-c.
blood, as if in - sep.
breathing, preventing - ars.
cardiac - **ACON., ARN.,** ***ars., bell., carb-v., dig.,*** kali-ar., **SPONG.**
chill, during - ***arn.***
clothes, too tight when walking in open air, as if - arg-m.
constricted, as if everything became - ***ars.***
convulsive - nux-v.
crying, with - bell.
daytime - graph., mag-c., merc., murx., nat-c., psor., puls., stann.
5 a.m. to 5 p.m. - psor.
death, agony before - acon., alum., **ARS.,** ***carc.,*** cocc., cupr., **LAT-M.,** puls., ***rhus-t.,*** **TARENT.,** ***tarent-c., verat.***
driving from place to place - arn., **ARS.,** ***rhus-t.***
restlessness, with - **ACON., ARS., BISM.**
eating, while - hyos., sep.
after - ***asaf., sep.***

AGONY, anguish
evening - ambr., ars., bell., calc., carb-v., foll., hep., kres., ***mur-ac., phos.,*** thiop.
7 p.m. - buth-a., chlorpr.
pressing in head, during - ars.
fever, during - ***arn.,*** ars., ***calc., kali-c.***
night - arn.
forenoon - nicc., ran-b., rhus-t.
horrible things, after hearing - calc.
lamenting, moaning - tarent.
lie down, must - mez., ph-ac., phel.
loss of his friend, from - **NIT-AC.**
mania, during - ars.
menses, during - ***bell.,*** calc., coff., ign., merc., nit-ac., phos., ***plat.,*** stann., xan.
before - ***graph., murx.***
morning - ***alum.,*** calc., meph., nux-v., puls., verat.
motion, amel. from - des-ac.
nap, after - **STAPH.**
nausea, with - ail., ***ars.,*** **DIG.**
night - ambr., arn., cob-n., hep., nat-s., nux-v., plan., puls.
4 a.m. - alum., ***nux-v.***
paralysing, impossible to call and move, with heat in head - cob-n.
perspiration, during - arn.
noon - bell.
oppression, with - ***cann-i., op.,*** phos., verat.
desire to sit up or jump out of bed, and - ***verat.***
pain, during - **ACON.,** ***arn.,*** **ARS., AUR.,** ***cham., ign.,*** tarent.
palpitation, with - **ARS.,** aur., ***calc.,*** kali-ar., ***mosch., puls., verat.***
perspiration, during - ambr., ***arn.,*** chin-s.
rest, cannot in any place - ***ars.***
room, with light and people, agg. in a - levo.
shock, from injury, in - ***op.***
stool, during - merc., ***verat.***
before - acon., ***ictod.,*** merc., verat.
stormy, weather, in - ***phos.***
stretching, with, in impending menses - carl.
suicide, attempt to commit - aur., carc., ***hep., nat-s.***
tossing about, with - **ACON.,** ***ars.,*** **CHAM.,** coff.
tremulous, rest agg., motion amel. - ***puls.***
uremia, in - ***hydr-ac.***
vomiting, with - ***aeth.,*** ars., asar.
waking, on - des-ac., ***dig.,*** nat-s., nux-v.
walking, in open air - arg-m., arg-n., bell., canth., cina, plat., tab.

ALCOHOLISM, dipsomania - ***absin.,*** acon., adon., **AGAR.,** agav-t., alum., am-m., anac., ange., anis., ***ant-c., ant-t., apoc.,*** apom., arg-m., arg-n., arn., ars., ars-s-f., ***asaf., asar.,*** **AUR.,** ***aven.,*** bar-c., ***bell.,*** bism., bor., bov., bry., bufo, cadm-s., ***calc.,*** calc-ar., camph., cann-i., ***caps.,*** carb-ac., carb-an., ***carb-s., carb-v., carc.,*** card-m., caust., cham., ***chel.,*** chim., **CHIN.,** chin-m., cic., ***cimic.,*** coc-c., ***cocc., coff.,*** con., croc., **CROT-H.,** ***cupr-ar.,*** dig., ***eup-per., ferr.,*** fl-ac., ***gels.,*** glon., ***graph., hell.,*** hep., hydr., ***hyos.,*** ichth., ***ign.,*** ip., ***kali-bi.,***

ALCOHOLISM, dipsomania - kali-br., kali-c., kali-i., kola., ***lac-c.,*** **LACH.,** ***laur., led.,*** lob., lup., ***lyc.,*** mag-c., meph., merc., mez., mosch., ***nat-c.,*** nat-n., nat-s., ***nux-m.,*** **NUX-V.,** op., passi., petr., ph-ac., ***phos.,*** plat., plb., psor., puls., ***quas., querc.,*** **RAN-B.,** raph., ***rhod., rhus-t.,*** rumx., ruta, sang., sars., sec., **SEL.,** ***sep., sil.,*** staph., ***stram.,*** stront-c., ***stroph.,*** **SUL-AC., SULPH.,** syph., tarax., tub., valer., **VERAT.,** ***zinc.***

acute - acon., bell., ***op., lach.***

drinking, on the sly - ***lach., sulph.***

excitement from - stram., zinc.

habit, to overcome - ange., aven., bufo, ***cinch., querc.,*** ster., ***sul-ac.,*** sulph.

hereditary craving - asar., ***carc.,*** lach., psor., sul-ac., sulph., **SYPH.,** tub.

hypochondriasis, with - **NUX-V.**

idleness, from - lach., nux-v., sulph.

irritability, with - ***nux-v.***

menses, before - **SEL.**

pregnancy, during or after - nux-v.

recurrent - anac., aur., bell., ***chin.,*** hyos., nux-v., op., stram., thuj.

weakness of character, from - ars., petr., puls.

alcoholism, delirium tremens, mania-a-potu - acon., **AGAR.,** agar-pr., alco., anac., ant-c., ***ant-t., apoc.,*** apom., ***arn.,*** **ARS.,** ars-s-f., asar., atro., aur., **AVEN.,** ***bell.,*** bism., bry., bufo, ***calc.,*** calc-ar., calc-s., camph-br., ***cann-i.,*** cann-s., ***caps.,*** carb-v., ***carc.,*** chin., chin-m., chin-s., chim., chlf., chlol., ***chlor., cimic.,*** cocc., ***coff.,*** cori-r., ***crot-h., cupr-ar.,*** cypr., dig., dor., ether, ferr-p., fl-ac., gels., ***glon.,*** grat., hell., hydr., **HYOS.,** ***hyosin.,*** ichth., ign., ***kali-br.,*** kali-i., kali-p., **LACH.,** led., lob., lol., lup., lyc., ***merc.,*** nat-c., **NAT-M., NUX-M., NUX-V.,** oena., **OP.,** passi., ***past., phos.,*** plb., psor., puls., querc., **RAN-B.,** raph., rhod., rhus-t., scut., sel., sep., sil., spig., ster., **STRAM.,** stroph., **STRY.,** stry-n., ***sulph., sul-ac.,*** sumb., ***syph.,*** teucr., thea., thuj., tub., tus-p., verat., ***zinc.,*** zinc-ac.

chronic - sul-ac.

delusions, with - ***bell.,*** calc., cann-i., ***kali-bi., lach., op., stram.***

elderly, emaciated persons, in - **OP.**

escape, attempts to - ***bell.,*** stram.

excitement, with - chlf., ***zinc.***

face, with red, bloated - ***bell., crot-h.,*** stram.

fear, calms the - scut.

talking, excessive, with loquacity - ***lach., ran-b.***

mild attacks - ***cypr.***

oversensitiveness, with - coff., **NUX-V.**

praying, with - **STRAM.**

sleeplessness, with - aven., ***cimic., coff., gels.,*** hyos., kali-br., kali-p., ***nux-v.***

small quantity of alcoholic stimulants, from - **OP.**

sopor with snoring - **OP.**

trembling - **ARS.,** ***aven., bar-c., cedr., hyos.,*** kali-br., kali-p., lach., ***nux-v., stram.***

alcoholism, delirium tremens

trembling, of hands - ***aven., coff., kali-br., lach.,*** **NUX-V.,** ***stram.***

ALERT, mentally - ***coff.,*** op.

ALTERNATING, mental and physical symptoms, (see Generals) - ***abrot.,*** alum., ***arn.,*** astra-e., aur., bell., **CARC.,** ***cimic.,*** con., ***croc.,*** ferr., **IGN.,** lach., ***lil-t., murx., nux-m.,*** **PLAT.,** sabad., stram., ***sul-ac.,*** tub.

other mental symptoms, with - alum., ***anac.,*** aur., ***bell.,*** **CARC.,** con., croc., ferr., **IGN., NUX-M.,** ***plat.,*** stram., sul-ac., valer., ***verat.,*** zinc.

physical, symptoms, with - alum., arn., astra-e., aur., ***bell.,*** **CARC.,** ***cimic., croc.,*** ferr., **IGN.,** lach., ***lil-t., nux-m.,*** **PLAT.,** sabad., stram., sul-ac., tub.

vaginal discharge, with - murx.

ALZHEIMER'S disease - ***alum., agn., anac.,*** ant-c., arg-m., ***arg-n., ars.,*** aur., ***aur-i.,*** aza., bapt., bar-ac., ***bar-c.,*** bar-m., bell., bry., calc-p., cann-i., ***con., crot-h.,*** fl-ac., **HYOS.,** ign., iod., lach., lil-t., ***lyc., kali-br.,*** kali-p., nat-i., nat-m., nux-m., nux-v., ***ov., phos.,*** pic-ac., sec., sep., staph., sulph., thiosin., zinc.

foolish talking, with - ars., bar-c., con., ***hyos.,*** op., plb., puls.

AMATIVENESS - agn., ant-c., calc., **CANTH.,** ***caust., con.,*** **HYOS.,** ign., kali-br., ***lach.,*** lil-t., **LYC.,** ***merc.,*** murx., nat-m., orig., ph-ac., ***phos.,*** pic-ac., ***plat., sel.,*** senec., squil., stann., staph., stram., sulph., ***ust.,*** verat.

want of, in men - con., **LYC.**

women, in - caust., lyc., sulph.

AMBITION, general

ailments from deceived - anac., bell., ***ign.,*** merc., ***nux-v.,*** plat., puls., verat.

loss of ambition, (see Indifferance, Work, aversion) - acon., alum., am-m., apoc., ars., asar., calc-sil., ***calc.,*** caust., cocaine, ***con.,*** dios., erig., **GELS.,** graph., ***lach.,*** lyc., nat-p., ***nux-v.,*** pall., petr., **PH-AC.,** plat., puls., rob., ***sep.,*** staph., verat.

AMBITIOUS - acon., alum., anac., ***ars.,*** asar., aur., calc., carb-an., ***carc.,*** caust., cocaine, cocc., con., graph., ***ign., lach., lyc.,*** nat-m., **NUX-V.,** pall., plat., puls., sil., staph., ***sulph., verat.***

employed every means possible - ars., lyc., ***nux-v.,*** plat., ***verat.***

AMOROUS, (see Sexual, behaviour) - acon., agar., agn., ***ant-c.,*** apis, **BELL.,** ***bufo,*** calad., **CALC.,** camph., cann-i., **CANN-S., CANTH., CARB-V.,** caust., **CHIN.,** coff., ***coloc., con.,*** croc., dulc., fl-ac., ***graph.,*** **HYOS.,** ***ign., iod.,*** kali-c., ***lach.,*** lil-t., **LYC.,** meny., ***merc., mosch., murx.,*** nat-c., **NAT-M.,** ***nit-ac.,*** nux-m., ***nux-v., op.,*** ph-ac., **PHOS.,** pic-ac., **PLAT.,** plb., **PULS.,** rhus-t., ruta, sabin., sanic., sars., sel., ***sep., sil., stann., staph.,*** **STRAM.,** sulph., thuj., **VERAT.,** zinc.

erections, without - ambr., calad., caps., **IGN.,** meny., **SEL.**

AMOROUS, behaviour
thoughts - ant-c., canth., ***carb-an., chin., dig.,*** graph., lach., plat., sel., **STAPH., THUJ.,** verb.

AMUSEMENT, aversion to - aur., ***bar-c.,*** hep., ***ign.,*** lil-t., meny., nat-c., ***nat-m.,*** olnd., ***sulph.***
desire for - hyos., med., ***lach.,*** pip-m.

ANARCHIST - ***caust.,*** kali-c., merc., sep.

ANGER, general - abrot., acet-ac., **ACON.,** aesc., act-sp., ***aeth.,*** agar., agn., all-c., allox., aloe, alum., am-c., ***am-m.,*** ambr., am-c., **ANAC.,** ang., ***ant-c., ant-t., apis,*** arg-m., arn., ars., ars-h., ***ars-i.,*** arum-t., ***asaf.,*** asar., aster., atro., **AUR.,** aur-a., aur-s., bar-c., bar-i., bar-m., ***bell.,*** berb., ***bond., bor., bov.,*** **BRY.,** bufo, buth-a., cact., calad., ***calc.,*** calc-ar., ***calc-p., calc-s.,*** calc-sil., camph., cann-s., canth., ***caps., carb-an., carb-s., carb-v., card-m.,*** carl., cast., ***caust.,*** cench., cer-s., **CHAM.,** chel., ***chin.,*** chin-a., chlor., cic., cimic., **CINA,** cinnb., clem., coca, ***cocc., coff.,*** colch., ***coloc., con.,*** cop., cor-r., ***croc.,*** crot-h., crot-t., ***cupr-ar.,*** cur., cypr., cycl., cyna., cyt-l., daph., des-ac., dig., dirc., dros., ***dulc.,*** elae., elaps, eupi., ferr., ferr-ar., ferr-i., ferr-m., ferr-ma., ferr-p., ferul., fl-ac., form., gamb., ***gels.,*** gink-b., gran., ***graph.,*** grat., haem., ham., hell., **HEP.,** hura, ***hydr.,*** hydr-ac., ***hyos.,*** hydr., **IGN.,** indg., ***iod., ip., jatr.,*** kali-ar., kali-br., **KALI-C.,** kali-chl., kali-cy., ***kali-i.,*** kali-m., kali-n., ***kali-p.,*** **KALI-S.,** ***kreos.,*** kres., ***lach.,*** lact., laur., ***led., lob.,*** **LYC.,** lycpr., lyss., macro., mag-arct., ***mag-aust., mag-c., mag-m.,*** mag-p-a., mag-s., manc., mang., med., meli., meph., **MERC.,** merc-cy., merl., ***mez.,*** mosch., ***mur-ac.,*** myric., nat-a., ***nat-c.,*** **NAT-M.,** nat-p., ***nat-s.,*** nicc., **NIT-AC.,** nit-s-d., nuph., nux-m., **NUX-V.,** ol-an., olnd., op., osm., ***pall.,*** par., ped., **PETR.,** ***ph-ac.,*** phel., ***phos.,*** plan., plat., plb., ***psor.,*** ptel., puls., puls-n, ran-b., rat., rheum, ***rhus-t.,*** ruta, sabad., sabin., samb., sang., saroth., sars., scroph-n., sec., seneg., **SEP.,** sil., sol-m., ***spig.,*** squil., ***stann.,*** **STAPH.,** stram., ***stront-c.,*** sul-ac., **SULPH.,** sumb., syph., ***tarent.,*** tell., teucr., thea., ***thuj.,*** thyr., tril., tub., upa., valer., verat., verb., vinc., ***zinc.,*** zinc-cy.

absent persons while thinking of them, at - ***aur.,*** kali-c., lyc., ***staph.***

activity, with great physical - ***plat.***

afternoon - bov., canth., cench., kali-c.
air, in open - mur-ac.

agg. from anger - alum-sil., calc-sil., ***cham., coloc.,*** nat-a., ***staph.,*** zinc-p.

ailments, after anger - **ACON.,** agar., alum., alum-sil., am-c., anac., ***ant-t., apis,*** arg-m., arg-n., arn., ***ars.,*** ars-s-f., ***aur.,*** aur-a., ***aur-m.,*** aur-m-n., bar-c., ***bell., bry.,*** cadm-s., calc., calc-ar., ***calc-p.,*** calc-s., calc-sil., camph., carc., caust., **CHAM.,** chin., cina, cist., cimic., **COCC.,** ***coch., coff.,*** colch., **COLOC.,** croc., cupr., ferr., ferr-p., ***gels.,*** graph., grat., hyos., **IGN.,** iod., **IP.,** kali-br., ***kali-p., lach., lyc.,*** mag-c., mag-m., manc., merc., mez., nat-a., nat-c., ***nat-m.,*** nat-p., nat-s., nux-m., **NUX-V.,**

ANGER, general

anger, ailments from - ol-an., olnd., **OP.,** petr., ***ph-ac., phos.,*** **PLAT.,** ***puls., ran-b.,*** rhus-t., sac-alb., samb., scroph-n., sec., sel., ***sep.,*** sil., stann., **STAPH.,** stram., stront-c., sulph., ***tarent.,*** verat., vinc., zinc., zinc-p.

alternating with
antics playing - op.
cares - ran-b.
cheerfulness - ant-t., aur., cann-s., caps., caust., cocc., croc., ign., nat-m., op., seneg., spong., stram., zinc.
contentment - caps.
crying - bell., cann-s., lac-c.
discontentment - aur., ran-b.
discouragement - lyc., ran-b., staph., zinc.
exhilaration - bov., caps., ***op.,*** seneg.
exuberance - ant-t.
hysteria - ign.
indifference - carb-s., chin.
jesting - caps., cocc., ign.
kindness - cench.
laughing - croc., stram.
quick repentance - anac., croc., lyss., mez., olnd., **SULPH.,** tub., vinc.
sadness - ambr., coff., erig., sumb., zinc.
singing - croc.
tenderness - croc.
timidity - ran-b., zinc.
tranquillity - ***croc.,*** kali-c.
vivacity - cocc., nat-m.

answer, when obliged to - ***arn.,*** ars., ***bry.,*** cham., coloc., nat-m., **NUX-V.,** ***ph-ac.,*** puls.

anxiety, with - **ACON.,** alum., **ARS.,** aur., ***bell.,*** bry., calc., carc., ***cham.,*** cocc., coff., ***cupr., gels.,*** hyos., **IGN.,** lyc., nat-c., nat-m., **NUX-V.,** ***op.,*** petr., phos., ***plat., puls.,*** rhus-t., samb., sep., stann., stram., sulph., verat.

argued with, if - op.

aroused, when - nux-v., sil., zinc.

blame, on - ign.

business, about - bry., ip., nux-v.

business, failure, from - ambr., aur., calc., coloc., bry., ip., kali-br., nat-m., nux-v., sulph.

caressing, from - chin., ***cina,*** ign., nit-ac.

causeless - chel., cyn-d., ***mez.,*** ped.

children, in - anac., ***calc-p.,*** **CHAM., CINA,** hep., nux-v., ***phos., tub.***

chill, during - caps.

coffee agg. - calc., calc-p., ***cham.,*** nux-v., phos.
drinking coffee and wine, while - chlor.

cold, after taking - calc.

consoled, when - ars., cham., ***hell.,*** **IGN.,** ***nat-m.,*** sabal., ***sep.,*** sil.

contradiction, from - aesc., aloe, am-c., ***anac.,*** ars., **AUR.,** ***bry.,*** cact., calc-p., cocc., ***ferr., ferr-ar.,*** grat., helon., hura, **IGN., LYC.,** merc., nat-a., nat-c., nat-sil., ***nicc.,*** nit-ac., ***nux-v.,*** olnd., op., petr., **SEP.,** ***sil.,*** stram., tarent., ***thuj.,*** til., ***verat.***
blame, or - ***ign.***

conversation, from - puls., tarent-c.

convulsion, before - ***bufo.***

ANGER, general
cough, from - acon., ***ant-t.,*** arg-m., arg-n., ***arn., bell.,*** bry., ***caps., cham.,*** **STAPH.,** verat.
before - asar., bell., cina.
crying from pain, with - ***cham.,*** merc., op., staph.
delirium, in - ***cocc.***
delusions during menopause, with - **COLOC.,** ***nux-v., zinc.***
diarrhea, during - gnaph.
dinner, during - kali-c.
dreams, after - mur-ac.
easily - aesc., arg-n., ars., bell., calad., calc., ***caps.,*** **CHAM.,** ***cocc.,*** con., ***crot-h., dulc., ferr., gels., graph., hell.,*** iris, **LYC.,** meph., **NUX-V.,** ***phos., plat., psor.,*** ran-b., squil., teucr., ***thuj.,*** valer., ***zinc.***
eat, when obliged to - ars.
eating, amel. after - am-m.
epileptic attack, before - indg.
evening - ***am-c.,*** ant-t., bov., ***bry., cahin., calc.,*** canth., ***croc., kali-c.,*** kali-m., **LYC.,** nat-c., nat-m., ***nicc., op., petr.,*** sil., zinc.
6 p.m. - cench.
8:30 p.m. - cench.
amel. - nat-s., verb.
face, pale, livid - ars., ***carb-v., con.,*** **NAT-M.,** ***petr., plat.,*** **STAPH.**
red - **BELL., BRY.,** calc., **CHAM.,** hyos., **NUX-V.,** puls., spig., staph., stram.
spots in, with - am-c.
tip of nose, with - vinc.
white - ars., carb-v., nat-m., petr., plat., staph.
fear, of their own anger - anac., staph.
fever, during - hipp.
fits of - cer-s., ***staph.***
forenoon - carb-v., nat-c., phos.
11 a.m. - ***arg-n.,*** **SULPH.**
forgetfulness, during - hydr.
former vexations, thinking about - ***calc., carb-an.,*** lyc., ***nat-m.,*** sars., sep., sulph.
fright, with - **ACON.,** ***aur., bell.,*** calc., **CARC.,** cocc., coff., cupr., ***gels.,*** glon., **IGN.,** nat-c., ***nux-v., op., petr., phos., plat., puls.,*** samb., sep., **STRAM.,** sulph., zinc.
grief, with silent - ***acon.,*** alum., am-m., ars., aur., aur-a., bell., ***bry., carc.,*** cham., ***chin., cocc., coloc.,*** gels., hyos., **IGN., LYC.,** nat-c., ***nat-m.,*** nux-v., ***ph-ac.,*** phos., plat., puls., **STAPH.,** verat., zinc.
happen, at what he thinks may - sol-m.
headache, from - acon., arg-n., **BRY.,** cast., cham., coff., coloc., dulc., ign., kali-c., lyc., mag-c., mez., nat-m., ***nux-v.,*** petr., phos., plat., ran-b., rhus-t., sep., **STAPH.**
vexation, after - acon., bry., cast., cham., cocc., coff., ign., ip., lyc., mag-c., **MEZ.,** nat-m., nux-v., petr., phos., ran-b., rhus-t., **STAPH.,** verat.

himself, with - anac., ars., aur., bell., ***ign.,*** lyc., nux-v., ***staph., sulph.***
constipated, when - aloe.
indignation, with - ars., ***aur.,*** carc., **COLOC.,** ip., lyc., merc., mur-ac., nat-m., ***nux-v.,*** plat., **STAPH.**
interruption, from - bry., cench., ***cham., cocc.,*** graph., ***hell., nux-v.***
involuntary - carb-v.
jealousy and incoherent talk, with - hyos., lach.
laughing, with bursts of - ***croc.***
bursts of anger, and crying alternate - ***plat.***
light, bright, agg. - colch.
lunch, during - kali-c.
menses, during - am-c., cast., caul., cimic., hyos., kreos.
before - cham., kali-fer., ***sep.***
mental exertion, after - calc-sil.
mistakes, over his - ars., aur., bell., carc., **IGN.,** ***nit-ac.,*** nux-v., ***staph., sulph.***
misunderstood, when - ***bufo., ign.***
morning - am-m., bov., ***calc.,*** carb-an., ***kali-c.,*** mang., nat-s., ***nux-v., petr., sep.,*** staph., ***sulph.***
waking, on - ars., canth., carb-an., cast., ***kali-c.,*** **LYC.,** petr., phos., sul-ac., sulph.
news, bad, about - calc-p., caust., ign.
at unpleasant - calc-p.
night - graph., lyc., mag-s., rhus-t.
noise, at - coff., hep., ip.
sleep, during - calad.
noon - am-m., zinc.
to 2 p.m. - aster., opun-f.
odors, agg. - colch., sep.
pains, about - ars., aur., bry., canth., ***cham., coloc., hep.,*** op.
agg. - ant-t., cham.
from the - ars., ***aur.,*** **BRY., CHAM.,** ***hep.***
paralysed, felt as - calc-p., ***cist.***
past events, about - calc., carb-an., ***nat-m.,*** nit-ac., sars., sep., staph., sulph.
pinched, on being - stram.
pregnancy, during - ***nux-m.,*** nux-v., ***sep.***
recovery, if one spoke of her complete - ***ars.***
remorse, followed by - anac., croc.
reproaches, from - cadm-met., cham., coloc., croc., ***ign., staph.***
seizes, the hands of those about him - op.
sensation, as if he should be angry - mosch.
sex, after - ***calc., calc-ar.***
sleep, after - chin-s.
spoken to, when - bry., ***cham., elaps, hell.***
stabbed anyone, so that he could have - anac., chin., **HEP.,** merc., mosch., nux-v., stront-c., zinc., zinc-ac.
stitches in head, from - dulc.
stool, before - calc.
sudden - bar-ac., merc.
suffocative attack, with - ***cham.***

ANGER, general

suppressed, ailments from - anac., ***aur.,*** **CARC.,** caust., cham., ***coloc.,*** hep., ***ign.,*** **IP., LYC.,** ***nat-m.,*** sep., **STAPH.**

sympathy, agg. - ferr., ***ign., nat-m.,*** sabad.

talk, indisposed to - am-m., ***bry., ign.,*** nat-m., petr., puls., staph., sul-ac.

others, from talking of - mang., rhus-t.

tear himself to pieces, could - sulph.

temper tantrums - calc-p., ***cham., cina,*** thyr., ***tub.***

things, do not go his way - calc-p., ign., thuj,

thinking of his ailments - ***aur-m.***

throws things away - coff., ***coloc.,*** **STAPH.,** tub.

tickled, on being - ign., stram.

touched, when - ***ant-c.,*** iod., sanic., **TARENT.**

tranquility, followed by - ip.

trembling, with - alum., ambr., arg-n., ***aur.,*** cham., chel., cop., daph., ferr-p., gels., lyc., mag-aust., merc., ***nit-ac.,*** nux-v., pall., phos., ***plat.,*** ran-b., sep., **STAPH.,** yohim, ***zinc.***

trifles, at - ***acon.,*** anac., ***ars.,*** atro., aur., bell., bry., cael., calc., calc-i., cann-s., caust., cer-s., ***cham., chel.,*** chin., cina, clem., ***cocc., con.,*** croc., digin., dros., hell., ***hep., ign.,*** ip., kali-bi., kali-m., kali-sil., kreos., lach., lyc., lyss., mang., meph., ***mez.,*** nat-a., nat-c., ***nat-m.,*** nat-p., ***nit-ac.,*** **NUX-V.,** petr., phos., ***plat.,*** rhus-t., sabad., sanic., sarcol-ac., sel., seneg., sep., ***staph.,*** stram., sul-ac., thuj., tub., zinc-p.

agg. - cer-s., ***phos.,*** sep.

understood, when not - ***ign.,*** laur.

vaginal discharge ceases, as soon as - ***hydr.***

vex others, inclined to - **CHIN.**

vexation, from - **ACON.,** agar., alum., am-c., anac., ***ant-t., apis,*** arg-n., arn., ***ars., aur., aur-m., bell., bry.,*** calc., calc-ar., ***calc-p.,*** calc-s., cadm-s., carc., caust., **CHAM.,** chin., cist., cimic., **COCC.,** ***coff.,*** **COLOC.,** croc., cupr., ferr., ferr-p., ***gels.,*** hyos., **IGN., IP.,** ***kali-p., lach., lyc.,*** mag-c., mag-m., manc., mez., nat-c., ***nat-m.,*** nat-p., nat-s., nux-m., **NUX-V., OP.,** petr., ***ph-ac., phos.,*** **PLAT.,** ***puls.,*** ran-b., rhus-t., samb., sec., sel., sep., sil., stann., **STAPH.,** stram., sulph., ***tarent.,*** verat., zinc.

violent - **ACON.,** ambr., **ANAC.,** ***apis, ars.,*** **AUR.,** aur-s., bar-c., ***bell.,*** bor., ***bry.,*** bufo, cahin., ***calc.,*** camph., cann-s., canth., carb-s., ***carb-v., caust.,*** cer-s., **CHAM.,** ***chel.,*** chin-b., cimx., cocc., coff., ***croc.,*** cupr., cypr., dros., ferr., ferr-p., ***graph.,*** grat., **HEP.,** ***hyos.,*** ictod., ign., iod., ***kali-c.,*** kali-chl., kali-i., **LACH.,** led., ***lyc.,*** lyss., ***mag-aust.,*** mag-c., mag-s., ***meli.,*** mez., mosch., ***nat-m.,*** nat-s., **NIT-AC., NUX-V.,** oena., olnd., pall., ***petr.,*** ph-ac., phos., ***plat.,*** puls., seneg., ***sep.,*** sil., **STAPH.,** stram., stront-nit., sulph., **TARENT.,** tell., thyr., tub., verat., zinc., zinc-p.

ANGER, general

violent, fits of - lach., med., nux-v., staph., stram., stront-c., tub.

when things don't go after his will - thuj., tub.

voices of people - con., teucr., zinc.

waking, on - bell., carb-an., cast., caust., cham., chin-s., kali-c., **LYC.,** lyss., mag-s., **NUX-V.,** petr., phos., rhus-t., sanic., sul-ac., tub.

weakness, anger followed by - mur-ac., staph.

will, if things do not go after his - lach., thuj.

work, about - bry., ***ign.,*** nat-m., **NUX-V.**

aversion to - bov., mag-aust.

cannot work - calc-p.

worm, affections, with - ***carb-v.,*** **CINA.**

ANIMATION, agg. - ***coff.,*** **HYOS., LACH.,** ***sabad.,*** **VALER.**

ANOREXIA nervosa - **ARS.,** calc., ***carc.,*** caust., **CHIN.,** hyos., ***ign.,*** lach., levo., merc., ***nat-m.,*** perh., puls., rhus-t., ***staph.,*** **SULPH.,** tarent., verat.

refuses, to eat - ars., bell., caust., cocc., croc., grat., **HYOS.,** ***ign.,*** **KALI-CHL.,** kali-p., op., **PH-AC.,** ***phyt.,*** plat., puls., sep., **TARENT., VERAT., VIOL-O.**

ANSWERS, general

abruptly - ars., ars-h., ***cic.,*** coff., gels., ***hyos.,*** jatr., mur-ac., ***ph-ac.,*** phos., plb., rhus-t., sec., sin-a., sin-n., ***stann., sulph., tarent.***

aversion to - ***agar.,*** alum., alum-p., ambr., am-c., am-m., anac., ***ant-c.,*** ant-t., apom., ***arn.,*** ars., ars-i., ars-s-f., atro., ***aur.,*** bell., ***bry.,*** bufo, cact., calc-s., calc-sil., carb-an., carb-h., carc., caust., ***cham.,*** chin., chin-s., chlol., cimic., cocc., coff., ***coloc.,*** con., cupr., euphr., ***gels.,*** **GLON.,** hell., **HYOS.,** ign., iod., juni., kali-ar., ***kali-p.,*** lil-t., lyss., mag-m., **MANC.,** merc., mosch., mur-ac., naja, ***nat-m.,*** nat-s., **NUX-V.,** op., oxyt., petr., **PH-AC.,** ***phos., puls.,*** rhus-t., sabad., sars., ***sec.,*** sil., spong., ***stann.,*** stram., ***stry., sulph., sul-ac.,*** tab., tarent., verat., vib.

talkative at other times - cimic.

morning - mag-m.

sings, talks, but will not answer questions - agar.

civil, cannot be - **CHAM.**

confusedly as though thinking of something else - bar-m., ***hell.,*** mosch.

correctly when spoken to, during unconsciousness - ***arn., bapt., hyos.***

dictatorial - ***lyc.***

difficult - carb-o., chlol., cocc., hell., iod., ph-ac., ***phos.,*** sulph., ***sul-ac.,*** verat.

disconnected - coff., ***crot-h.,*** kali-br., phos., stram., stry.

distracted - ***lyc.,*** plect.

evasively - cimic.

foolish - ars., bell.

hastily - ars., bell., bry., bufo, carc., cimic., cocc., hep., lach., **LYC.,** rhus-t., stry.

hesitating - graph., sec.

ANSWERS, general
imaginary questions - atro., ***hyos.,*** phos., plb., stram., tarent.
imperfect - ***anac.,*** atro.
impolite - **CHAM.**
inappropriate - ***ph-ac.,*** sul-ac.
incoherently - bell., cann-i., chlol., coff-t., crot-t., cupr., cycl., hyos., ***ph-ac.,*** phos., raja-s., valer.
incorrectly - ail., ***bell.,*** carb-v., ***cham., hyos.,*** merc., nux-m., ***nux-v., op.,*** ph-ac., ***phos.,*** raja-s., stram., ***verat-v.***
indifferent - atro.
irrelevantly - bell., carb-v., cimic., ***hyos., nux-m.,*** ph-ac., ***phos.,*** stram., sul-ac., ***sulph.,*** valer.
childbirth, after - ***thuj.***
monosyllable (see Speech) - achy., agar-pa., acon., bell., carb-h., carb-s., carc., gels., kali-br., **MERC.,** mur-ac., **PH-AC.,** plb., puls., sep., ***thuj.,*** tub., **VERAT.**
"no" to all questions - crot-c., hyos., kali-br., tub.
nods, by - puls.
offensive - lyss.
"perhaps" to all questions - carc.
question, repeats first - ambr., ***caust.,*** hell., kali-br., ***med.,*** sulph., ***zinc.***
questioned, when, does not know what to answer - kali-c.
says nothing, indifferent, does not answer - ***colch.,*** tarent.
questions, in - ***aur.***
rapidly - carc., lyss., ***sep.,*** stry.
reflects long - alum., ***anac., cocc., cupr.,*** grat., **HELL.,** merc., ***nux-m., ph-ac.,*** **PHOS.**
refuses to - ***agar.,*** ambr., ***arn.,*** ars., ***atro.,*** bell., bufo, calc-sil., ***camph.,*** caust., ***chin.,*** chin-a., ***cimic., hell., hyos.,*** kali-a., led., lyss., med., nux-m., ***nux-v.,*** petr., ph-ac., **PHOS.,** sabad., sec., ***stram.,*** **SULPH.,** ***sul-ac.,*** tab., tarent., ***verat., verat-v.***
signs with hands, by - carb-s.
sleep, during - med.
sleeps at once, anguish then - bapt., hep.
slowly - acon., agar-ph., ***anac.,*** arn., ars., ars-h., ars-s-f., bapt., carb-h., ***carb-v., cocc.,*** cupr., ***con., gels.,*** **HELL.,** hyos., ***kali-br.,*** lyc., med., **MERC.,** ***nux-m.,*** op., ox-ac., **PH-AC., PHOS.,** plb., rhod., ***rhus-t.,*** sep., ***sulph.,*** sul-ac., ***thuj.,*** zinc.
snappishly - calc-p., **CHAM.,** sin-n.
spoken to, when, yet knows no one - ***cic.***
stupor returns quickly after - ***arn., bapt.,*** brom., **HYOS.,** olnd., op., ***ph-ac.,*** phos., plb.
unable to answer - ars., lon-x.
unconscious, as if - plat.
unintelligibly - ***chin.,*** coff-t., ***hyos.,*** **PH-AC.,** ***phos.***
unsatisfactory - phos.
vaguely - dig.

ANTAGONISM, with self, (see Will) - **ANAC.,** aur., bar-c., cann-i., cann-s., ***ign., kali-c.,*** lac-c., ***sep.***

ANTICIPATION, ailments from, (see Anxiety, Worry) - acon., aesc., aeth., agn., alum., am-c., ***anac.,*** apis, **ARG-N., ARS.,** ***bar-c., bry.,*** **CALC.,** calc-s., ***camph.,*** canth., ***carb-v.,*** **CARC.,** ***caust.,*** cench., ***chin.,*** chin-s., chlorpr., ***cic., cocc., coff.,*** crot-h., dig., dys-co., ***elaps, fl-ac.,*** **GELS., GRAPH., HYOS., IGN.,** kali-br., kali-c., ***kali-p., lac-c.,*** lach., levo., **LYC.,** ***lyss.,*** **MED.,** ***merc.,*** mosch., naja, ***nat-c.,*** **NAT-M.,** nux-v., ox-ac., ***petr., ph-ac.,*** **PHOS., PLB., PSOR., PULS.,** rhus-t., sep., **SIL.,** spig., staph., ***still.,*** stram., ***stront-c.,*** syc-co., ***thuj., verat.***
anxiety from an upcoming engagement - **ACON.,** anac., **ARG-N.,** ***ars., carb-v.,*** **GELS., LYC.,** med., **NAT-M.,** ph-ac., ***sil., thuj.***
anticipating for his relatives - ars., calc., carc., phos.
chill, from - ant-t., **ARS.,** bell., **BRY.,** cham., chin., chin-a., **CHIN-S.,** eup-per., gamb., **GELS.,** ign., **NAT-M., NUX-V.,** sep.
dentist or physician, before going to - ***acon.,*** calc., ***gels.,*** mag-c., ***phos., tub.***
examination, before - ***aeth.,*** anac., carb-v., ***gels.,*** lyc., sil., thuj.
excitement, with - **ARG-N., CARC.,** ***coff., gels.***
fear of failure, with - lyc.
impending evil, sense of - merc.
matters, for, before they occur, and generally correctly - ***med.***
morning - nabal.
singers and speakers, in - arg-n., **GELS.,** lyc.
stage-fright - **ACON.,** anac., **ARG-N.,** ***ars., carb-v.,*** **GELS., LYC.,** med., **NAT-M.,** ph-ac., ***sil., thuj.***
unusual ordeal, of any - **GELS.**

ANTICS, plays - apis, ***bell.,*** cic., croc., cupr., dat-m., **HYOS.,** ign., kali-bi., lact., op., merc., phos., plb., stram., verat.
delirium, during - bell., cupr., **HYOS.,** lact., op., phos., plb., stront-c.
drunkenness, during - bell., stram.

ANTISOCIAL, behaviour - ***anac.,*** caust., lach., med., stram., syph.

ANXIETY, general - ***abrot.,*** **ACON.,** acon-c., ***acon-f., acet-ac.,*** act-sp., ***aeth.,*** ether, agar., agar-ph., agn., agre., ail., alco., ***all-c.,*** all-s., allox., aloe, ***alum., alum-sil.,*** alumn., ***ambr., am-c.,*** am-m., ***aml-n.,*** amyg., ***anac.,*** ang., anh., ant-a., ***ant-c., ant-t.,*** apis, aran., aran-s., ***arg-m.,*** **ARG-N.,** ***arn.,*** **ARS.,** ***ars-h.,*** **ARS-I., ARS-S-F.,** arum-m., arund., asaf., ***asar., aspar.,*** aster., atro., **AUR.,** aur-m-n., **AUR-S.,** bar-ac., ***bar-c.,*** bar-i., ***bar-m.,*** **BELL.,** benz-ac., berb., **BISM.,** bond., ***bor., bov.,*** brom., **BRY.,** bufo, buni-o., but-ac., buth-a., **CACT.,** cadm-s., cahin., calad., **CALC.,** calc-ac., **CALC-AR.,** calc-br., ***calc-f.,*** **CALC-P., CALC-S.,** calen., calth., **CAMPH., CANN-I.,** cann-s., ***canth.,*** caps., ***carb-an.,***

ANXIETY, general - ***carb-o.,*** **CARB-S., CARB-V., CARC.,** ***carl., casc., cast.,*** **CAUST.,** cedr., ***cench.,*** cent., ***cham., chel.,*** **CHIN.,** ***chin-a., chin-s., chlol., chlor., cic.,*** cic-m., ***cimx.,*** cimic., cina, cinnam., clem., cob-n., coc-c., coca, ***cocc.,*** coch., cod., ***coff.,*** coff-t., colch., ***coloc.,*** **CON.,** ***convo-s.,*** corn., cortico., cot., croc., ***crot-c., crot-h.,*** crot-t., cub., culx., ***cupr., cupr-ar.,*** cupr-s., cur., cycl., cypr., cyt-l., der., **DIG.,** ***dros.,*** dulc., elaps, ergot., ***euph.,*** euph-c., eup-per., euon., ***ferr., ferr-ar., ferr-m.,*** ferr-p., ***ferr-i.,*** fil., ***fl-ac.,*** gamb., ***gels.,*** gins., glon., goss., gran., ***graph.,*** grat., grin., guare., haem., hed., ***hell.,*** hell-f., ***hep.,*** hip-ac., hist., hura, ***hydr-ac.,*** hydroph., ***hyos., hyper.,*** hypoth., ***ictod., ign.,*** indg., inul., **IOD.,** ip., piloc., ***jal., jatr.,*** kali-a., **KALI-AR.,** kali-bi., kali-br., **KALI-C.,** kali-chl., ***kali-i., kali-n.,*** **KALI-P., KALI-S.,** ***kalm.,*** kiss., kreos., kres., lac-c., ***lach.,*** lact., lat-m., ***laur., led.,*** lip., lipp., ***lil-t., lith.,*** lob., **LYC., LYSS.,** ***mag-arct., mag-c.,*** mag-f., ***mag-m., mag-s.,*** man., manc., mang., med., medus., meny., ***merc.,*** **MERC-C.,** merc-n., merc-s-cy., **MEZ.,** mill., morph., mosch., ***mur-ac.,*** murx., mygal., naja, **NAT-A., NAT-C.,** ***nat-p., nat-m., nat-s.,*** nicc., **NIT-AC.,** nit-s-d., nitro-o., ***nux-m., nux-v.,*** oci-s., oena., ol-an., ol-j., olnd., ***op., orig.,*** osm., ***ox-ac.,*** paeon., pall., par., ***petr.,*** phel., ***ph-ac.,*** **PHOS.,** pin-s., pituin., plan., ***plat., plb.,*** podo., **PSOR.,** ptel., **PULS.,** puls-n, ***pyrog.,*** ran-a., ran-b., ran-s., raph., rat., ***rauw.,*** reser., rheum, rhod., rosm., **RHUS-T.,** ***ruta, sabad., sabin.,*** sac-alb., sal-ac., ***samb.,*** sang., sars., **SEC.,** sel., ***seneg., sep., sil.,*** sin-n., ***spig., spong.,*** squil., ***stann.,*** staph., still., ***stram.,*** stront-c., stroph-s., stry., sul-i., sulo-ac., **SULPH.,** sul-ac., ***sumb., tab.,*** tanac., tarax., ***tarent.,*** tax., tep., ter., thea., ***ther.,*** thiop., ***thuj.,*** thyreotr., tong., trach., tub., valer., **VERAT.,** ***verat-v.,*** verb., verin., vesp., viol-o., viol-t., vip., visc., wies., wild., xan., ***zinc.***

abandoned her, as if a friend had - ars., puls., ***rhus-t.***

abdomen, with distention in - arg-n., lyc., mag-m.

accident, as if some, would happen - mag-s., phos.

afternoon - aeth., am-c., arg-n., ***ars.,*** bell., bov., cact., ***calc.,*** carb-an., carb-v., ***chel.,*** crot-t., cupr., franz., gamb., kali-n., mag-c., mag-m., nat-c., nit-ac., nux-v., phel., ph-ac., phos., puls., rhus-t., ruta, stront-c., tab., zinc., zinc-p.

2 p.m. to 4 p.m. - aq-mar.

3 p.m. to 6 p.m. - con.

4 p.m. - ***lyc.,*** tab.

4 p.m. to 5 p.m. - thuj.

4 p.m. to 6 p.m. - ***carb-v.,*** lyc.

5 p.m. to 6 p.m. - am-c.

amel. - tab.

and evening - erig.

sleep, after - **STAPH.**

until 3 p.m. - ***aster.***

until evening - con., kali-n., mag-m., nat-c.

ANXIETY, general

ailments, from anxiety - acon., ***arg-n., ars.,*** aur., calc., calc-p., ***carc,*** cimic., ***gels.,*** hyos., kali-p., lyc., nit-ac., ph-ac., ***phos.,*** samb., staph.

air, in open - acon., anac., ant-c., arg-m., bar-c., bell., cina, hep., ign., lach., plat., spig., tab.

amel. - alum., aml-n., arund., ***bry.,*** calc., calc-s., **CANN-I.,** carl., ***crot-t.,*** graph., grat., **KALI-S.,** laur., ***lyc., mag-m., puls., rhus-t.,*** spong., ***sulph., til.,*** valer., verat.

alone, when - alco., arg-n., **ARS.,** cadm-s., caust., cortico., ***dros.,*** hep., ***kali-br.,*** kali-c., ***mez.,*** nit-ac., **PHOS.,** rat., ***rhus-t.,*** sep., tab., zinc.

as if, and all about were dead and still - ***rhus-t.***

alternating with,

contentment - zinc.

exhilaration - spig., spong.

indifference - nat-m.

rage - bell.

anger, during - caps., sep., verat.

anticipating (see Anticipation)

apparition, from horrible, while awake - ***camph.,*** zinc.

ascending, steps, on - ***nit-ac.,*** ox-ac.

attacks, of anxiety - **ACON.,** aloe, alum., ang., **ARG-N.,** ars., bar-c., bell., calc-i., ***cann-i., carb-v.,*** **CARC.,** caust., ***cham.,*** chel., ***cocc., cupr., cupr-ar.,*** ferr., ***hyos.,*** ictod., ign., **KALI-AR.,** med., nat-c., nat-m., nat-s., nit-ac., **PHOS.,** plat., ruta, sep., spong., ***sulph., tab.,*** thuj.

cannot control herself - ***arg-n., cupr-ac.***

heart disease, in - ***kali-ar., spong.***

night agg. - ***ars.***

throat in, with - **SPONG.**

bathing, the feet, after - nat-c.

bed, in - alco., ***ambr.,*** am-c., anac., ant-c., **ARS.,** berb., ***bar-c., bry.,*** calad., ***calc., camph.,*** carb-an., ***carb-v., caust., cench., cham.,*** chin-s., ***cocc.,*** cupr-ac., ***ferr., graph., hep., ign.,*** kali-c., kali-n., laur., ***lyc.,*** lyss., ***mag-c.,*** mag-m., nat-a., nat-c., nat-m., nat-p., nat-sil., nit-ac., nux-v., ***phos., puls.,*** **RHUS-T.,** sabin., sep., sil., stront-c., ***sulph.,*** ter., verat.

as if she would never get awake again - ang.

driving out of - **ARS.,** bry., carb-s., caust., ***cham.,*** chin., chin-s., ***graph., hep.,*** lyss., nat-m., nit-ac., ***puls., rhus-t.***

heat of - ***ars-i.***

on going to - ter.

could with difficulty be induced to go to - caust.

passing off on sitting up in - spong.

rising, on - rhus-t.

sit up, must - carb-v.

spasms, in, after fright - ***cupr.***

tossing about, with - ***ars.,*** camph., canth., ***cupr-ac., ferr.***

turning in, when - lyc.

beer, after - ferr.

ANXIETY, general
belching, amel. - kali-c., mag-m., mez.
ending with - verat.
bleeding, with, intestinal - **ACON.,** ***crot-h., phos.***
lungs, of - ***ip., phos.***
breakfast, after - con., kali-c.
breathing, on deep breathing - acon., ***spig.***
deeply amel. - agar., caps., rhus-t.
must breath deep - caps.
breathing, difficult, from - ***acet-ac.,*** acon., **ARS.,** astac., bism., ***carb-an., carb-v.,*** coca, ***kalm.,*** lach., ***lyc., phos.,*** puls., **SPONG.,** viol-o.
clothing, must loosen - stann.
liver complaints, in - ***acet-ac.***
spasms of chest, with - ***hyos.***
stool, amel. after - ***ictod.***
tuberculosis, in - ***chin-a.***
burning of stomach, with coldness of body - **JATR.**
business, about - anac., ***ars.,*** bar-c., bry., calc., ***carc.,*** **NUX-V.,** ***psor.,*** puls., **RHUS-T.,** sulph.
dispepsia, from - **NUX-V.**
catalepsy, in - art-v.
causeless - ***carc.,*** **BRY.,** calc-f., kali-ar., ***phos.,*** plb., sabad., tab., tarent., thala., zinc-valer.
chagrin, after - lyc.
chest, rising from - kali-bi.
sharp, stitching in, from - ruta.
childbirth, during - cupr.
children, in - acon., ***ars., bor.,*** calc., calc-p., ***carc., cina, gels., kali-c., phos.***
about his - acet-ac., acon., ***ars.,*** calc., ph-ac., phos., rhus-t., sulph.
chest complaints, with - ***calc-p., phos.***
infants, in - ***acon.,*** ars., ***cham.,*** phos.
lifted from the cradle, when - calc., ***calc-p.,*** bor.
rocking, during - **BOR.**
waking, evening, in - **CINA**
morning, in - ***chin.***
night, at - ***dros.***
chill, during - **ACON.,** anh., arn., **ARS.,** ars-h., **CALC., CALC-AR.,** calen., **CAMPH.,** caps., carb-v., chin., chin-a., cimx., ***cocc.,*** cycl., gels., hura, ign., lam., laur., ***mez.,*** nat-m., nux-v., phos., plat., **PULS.,** ***rhus-t.,*** sec., sep., tub., ***verat.***
after - ***ars., chel.,*** kali-c.
before - ars., ars-h., **CHIN.**
neuralgia, with - ***mez.***
rigor, after, in valvular disease - **CHEL.**
cholera asiatica, in - **CAMPH.,** ***chin-s., cupr.***
as if cramps in calves would set in - ***jatr.***
cholerine - ***ant-t., asar.***
church bells, from hearing - ***lyss.***
closing eyes, on - calc., carb-an., **CARB-V.,** ***mag-m., psor.***
clothing, must loosen, and open window - ***nux-v.,*** **PULS.,** sulph.
tight, as if too, walking out of doors - arg-m.
cloudy, damp weather, in - sang.

ANXIETY, general
coffee, after - bart., cham., ign., nux-v., stram.
amel. - morph.
cold drinks amel. - acon., ***agar-em.,*** sulph.
becoming, from - carb-ac., manc., nux-v.
coldness of feet at night, during - thuj.
company, in - ***acon., ambr.,*** bar-c., bell., cadm-s., ***lyc., petr.,*** plat., stram.
agg. - aq-mar.
shuns, even his doctor - iod.
condition, about her - spong.
confinement, during - cupr.
after, with rash - ***cupr.***
rash, followed by, on seventh day - ***calc.***
confusedness before eyes, after - ***psor.***
confusion and cloudiness, with, typhoid - **PH-AC.**
congestion to, chest - ant-t., kali-n., ***nit-ac.,*** sep.
to, heart - nit-ac.
conscience, of (See Guilt)
constriction of, chest - ***spig.,*** stann.
caused by drawing across lower - ***chin.***
stomach, in - guai.
continence prolonged, from - ***con.***
contraction in heart region, from - ***cact.,*** nit-ac.
control over senses is lost, with feeling that - arg-n., cann-s., carc., med., ***merc-sul.***
conversation, from - alum., ***ambr.,*** plat., stram.
convulsions, before - **CIC.**
convulsive trembling or shaking, with, does not extend below waist - ***cupr.***
cough, during - ***mosch., stram.***
after - ***cina***
before - ars., ***cupr.,*** iod., lact.
loose, suddenly changes to dry, hoarseness, dyspnoea, typhoid, during - ***spong.***
rough, dry in diphtheria, during - ***merc-cy.***
tickling and expectoration of bright red frothy blood, often preceded by hawking, during - ph-ac.
whooping cough, during - ***stram.***
attack of, before - ***cupr.***
coughing, from - arund., merc-c., nit-ac., stram.
cramp, as from - calc.
as if, in calves would set in - ***jatr.***
in rectum, during - calc.
in stomach, during - kali-c.
crime, as if committed - **CHEL.,** ***ferr.***
crowd, in a - ***acon., ambr.,*** bell., ***lyc., petr.,*** plat., stram.
cruelties, after hearing of - ***calc., carc., cic.***
crying, amel. - aster., dig., graph., ***tab.***
followed by - acon., am-m., carb-v., kali-c.
daily - nat-c., verb.
dancing, when - ***bor.***
dark, in - aeth., calc., carb-an., carb-v., hypoth., nat-m., **PHOS.,** ***puls.,*** rhus-t., **STRAM.,** zinc.

ANXIETY, general

daytime - ambr., ant-c., aur-a., aur-i., ***bell.,*** caust., chin-a., laur., mag-c., mang., merc., nat-c., nit-ac., phyt., plat., psor., puls., ruta, sul-ac., zinc.
 5 a.m. to 5 p.m. - psor.
 all day - verb.
debility, with, faintness and aching in left iliac region - ***crot-h.***
dentition, during - kali-br.
diabetes, in - ***nat-s., phos.***
 makes it worse - cod.
dinner, during - mag-m.
 after - ambr., canth., gins., hyos., mag-m., nat-m., ***phos.,*** sil., verat.
 amel. - sulph.
 opression of chest, with - ***phos.***
 pregnancy, in fifth month of - psor.
diphtheria, in - ***chin-a.***
diseases, about - acet-ac., agar., am-c., **ARS.,** ***calc.,*** **CARC.,** ***chin-a., kali-ar.,*** **NIT-AC., PHOS.,** syph.
 awake at night, when - ars., ars-h.
 menopausal period, in - ***kali-br.***
 concerning recovery - ***ars.,*** aur., ***ph-ac.***
 despair of getting well, with - ***ars., aur.***
disguises, which he vainly - alco.
do something, compelled to - ars., ***bry.***
domestic affairs, during pregnancy, about - bar-c., calc., puls., ***stann.***
dread, with feeling of - phos., sang.
dreams, on waking from frightful - **ACON.,** alum., ***ars.,*** bov., calc., ***chin.,*** cina, graph., hep., lyc., mag-c., mur-ac., ***nat-m.,*** nicc., op., petr., ph-ac., phos., puls., sil., **SPONG.,** zinc.
drinking, after - ***cimx., puls.***
 cold water amel. - acon., sulph.
driving from place to place - **ARS.,** aur., bry., ***iod.,*** merc., sul-i.
duty, as if he had not done his - ars.
 religious, produced by lascivious impulses - ***orig.***
dyspepsia, causes - cypr.
eating, while - ***carb-v.,*** mag-c., mez., ran-b., sabad., ***sep.***
 after - aloe, ***ambr., arg-n.,*** asaf., bell., canth., carb-an., ***carb-v., caust.,*** cham., chin., ***coc-c.,*** con., ferr., ferr-m., ferr-p., hyos., kali-c., kali-p., kali-sil., lach., mag-m., merc., ***nat-c., nat-m.,*** nat-p., nat-sil., ***nit-ac.,*** **NUX-V.,** phel., ph-ac., ***phos.,*** psor., ran-b., sep., sil., thuj., verat., viol-t.
 irregular action of heart, from - ***cocc.***
 amel. - aur., **IOD.,** mez., sulph.
 before - mez., ran-b.
 warm food, while - mag-c.
emissions, after - carb-an., petr., ***phos.***
epilepsy, between intervals of - cupr., ***lyc.***
 threatened with a fit - alum.
evening - acon., agar., ***alum.,*** alum-p., alum-sil., ***ambr.,*** am-c., anac., ant-t., **ARS., ARS-S-F.,** bar-c., ***bar-m.,*** bell., berb., ***bor.,*** bov., bry., cact., calad., **CALC., CALC-AR.,**

ANXIETY, general

evening - **CALC-S.,** carb-an., ***carb-s.,*** **CARB-V.,** ***caust.,*** chel., chin., ***chin-a., cina,*** coca, cocc., coff., colch., **DIG.,** digin., ***dros., fl-ac.,*** graph., ***hep.,*** hipp., hura, kali-ar., kali-c., kali-i., kali-m., kali-n., kali-p., kali-s., kali-sil., lact., ***laur., lyc.,*** mag-arct., mag-c., mag-m., ***merc.,*** mez., mur-ac., nat-a., nat-c., ***nat-m.,*** nat-p., **NIT-AC.,** nux-m., ***nux-v.,*** paeon., petr., ***phos.,*** plat., podo., ***puls.,*** ran-b., ***rhus-t.,*** ruta, sabin., **SEP.,** sil., spig., ***stann.,*** stront-c., **SULPH.,** tab., tub., verat.
 6 p.m. - chel., ***dig.***
 7 p.m. - am-c., buth-a., dros., petr.
  7 p.m. to 8 p.m. - am-c., dros.
 8 p.m. - chin., dros., mur-ac.
 alone, when - ***dros.***
 amel. - am-c., chel., mag-c., sul-ac., verb., zinc.
 as evening comes on - **CALC., SEP.**
 bed, in - **AMBR.,** am-c., anac., ant-c., **ARS., ARS-S-F.,** ***bar-c.,*** bar-s., berb., ***bry.,*** calad., ***calc.,*** calc-ac., ***calc-ar., calc-s.,*** calc-sil., carb-an., ***carb-s.,*** **CARB-V.,** ***caust., cench.,*** cham., ***cocc., graph.,*** hep., kali-ar., kali-c., kali-m., kali-n., kali-p., kali-s., kali-sil., laur., lil-t., ***lyc., mag-c., mag-m.,*** mez., mur-ac., nat-a., nat-c., nat-m., nat-s., nit-ac., ***nux-v.,*** phos., ***puls.,*** sabin., sep., sil., stront-c., ***sulph.,*** ter., verat.
  amel. - ***mag-c.***
  closing the eyes, on - ***mag-m.***
  uneasiness and must uncover - ***bar-c.,*** mag-c., nat-m., ***puls.***
  violent exercise, from - ox-ac.
 breathing, with oppression of - **CARB-V.,** coca
 fever, with hectic - ***phos.***
 night, and - ***merc.***
 returns in - colch.
 twilight, in the - ambr., ***ars., calc., carb-v., caust.,*** dig., laur., nux-v., ***phos.,*** podo., ***rhus-t.,*** sep.
  nervous exhaustion, from - ***phos.***
everything, about - ars., carc., phos., sarr.
exaggerated - **ARS.,** calc., carc., chel., **LYC.,** merc., **NUX-V.,** ***phos.,*** **PULS.,** sil., **STAPH.,** ***sulph.,*** tub.
excitement, from - asaf., carc., ***phos.***
 irritable heart, with - ***asaf.***
exercise, from - ***sarcol-ac.***
 amel. - **IOD.,** tarent.
 work, manual agg. - **IOD.**
exertion of eyes, from - ruta, ***sep.***
expected of him, when anything is - arg-n., ***ars.,*** ign., ***lyc.***
faintness, with - ***arg-n.,*** ars., cic., ***crot-h., dig.,*** ign., nux-v., ***plb.,*** **SPONG.**
 after - ars-s-f.
 as if, would come on - arg-n., gels., **SPONG.**
 when walking, makes her walk faster - ***arg-n.***

ANXIETY, general

family, about his - acet-ac., ars., ***calc.,*** calc-sil., ***carc.,*** hep., petr., phos., puls.

which he left behind on a short journey, increases until he becomes inconsolable, towards evening - ***petr.***

fasting, when - ars., iod.

fear, with - **ACON.,** ***alum.,*** alum-p., am-c., ***am-m.,*** amor-r., **ANAC.,** ant-c., ant-t., **ARG-N., ARS.,** ars-s-f., ***aur., bar-c.,*** bar-s., bell., berb., bry., calad., ***calc.,*** calc-ar., calc-s., ***canth.,*** carb-s., **CARB-V., CARC., CAUST.,** chel., ***chin.,*** chin-a., ***chin-s.,*** cic., cina, clem., ***cocc., coff.,*** con., ***cupr., dig.,*** dros., dulc., ferr., ferr-ar., ferr-p., ***graph.,*** hell., ***hep.,*** hyos., ***ign., kali-ar., kali-c.,*** kali-i., kali-n., ***kali-p.,*** kali-s., kali-sil., ***kreos.,*** lach., ***lyc.,*** mag-arct., ***mag-c.,*** manc., mang., meny., ***merc.,*** mez., mosch., murx., nat-a., nat-c., ***nat-m.,*** nat-p., nicc., ***nit-ac.,*** nux-m., nux-v., onos., phel., **PHOS.,** ***plat.,*** **PSOR.,** ***puls.,*** rat., ***rhus-t.,*** ruta, sabin., samb., sang., **SEC.,** ***sep.,*** sil., ***spig.,*** spong., staph., ***stront-c.,*** sulph., tab., thuj., til., vario., ***verat.,*** vesp.

agg. till 5 a.m., with sleeplessness - ign.

stands, when he, forehead becomes covered with cold sweat, sick to vomiting - verat.

fever, during - **ACON.,** ***alum.,*** **AMBR.,** am-c., anac., arg-m., arn., **ARS.,** ars-s-f., ***asaf.,*** **BAR-C., BAR-S.,** bell., berb., bov., ***bry., calc., calc-ar.,*** calc-s., canth., carb-an., carb-v., casc., cham., chin., chin-a., ***chin-s.,*** cocc., coff., con., crot-h., cycl., dros., ***ferr.,*** ferr-ar., ferr-p., fl-ac., graph., grat., ***guare.,*** hep., hyper., ign., **IP.,** kali-c., lach., laur., ***mag-arct., mag-c.,*** mag-m., merc., ***mur-ac.,*** nat-a., nat-c., nat-m., nat-p., nat-s., nicc., nit-ac., nux-v., ol-an., op., par., ***petr.,*** ph-ac., ***phos.,*** plan., plat., plb., ***puls.,*** pyrog., rheum, rhod., ***rhus-t., ruta,*** sabad., sabin., ***sec.,*** **SEP.,** spig., ***spong., squil.,*** stann., stram., sulph., ***tub.,*** valer., verat., ***viol-t., zinc.,*** zinc-p.

2 a.m. to 5 a.m., with sleeplessness - ign.

as from - carb-v.

intermittent, during - ***ant-c., ant-t., cocc., lyc.***

prodrome, during - ars., chin.

puerperal, during - ***plat.***

yellow, during, - ***merc.***

fingers or hands, caused by tingling in, in myelitis - agar., phos., ***verat.***

fits, with - alum., arg-n., ars., bell., calc., ***carc.,*** caust., cocc., cupr., ferr., ***hyos.,*** ign., med.

before - **CIC.**

flatus, from - coff., ***lyc.,*** **NUX-V.**

emission of, amel. - calc., calc-ac., mur-ac.

obstructed flatus, with - sulph.

flushes of heat, during - aloe, ambr., arn., calc., dros., graph., ign., nat-c., op., phos., plat., puls., ***sep.,*** spong.

emphysema, in - ***carb-v.***

fly away, as if she must, no peace anywhere - ***bell.***

ANXIETY, general

foot bath, after a - nat-c.

foreboding, with gloomy - ***ferr.***

forenoon - acon., alum., alumn., am-c., bar-c., calc., canth., clem., ***lyc., nat-m.,*** paeon., plat., ran-b., sars., sulph.

11 a.m. - arg-n.

amel. by a little whiskey - ***arg-n.***

friends at home, about - bar-c., ***phos.,*** phys., ***sulph.***

fright, after - **ACON., CARC.,** ***cupr.,*** gels., ***ign., kali-br.,*** lyc., merc., nat-m., **OP.,** phos., rob., ***sil., verat.***

fear of fright still remaining - **OP.**

seventh month of pregnancy, during -***ign.***

future, about - acon., aeth., agar., allox., alum., alum-p., ***anac.,*** ant-c., ant-t., **ARG-N.,** arist-cl., arn., **ARS.,** aur., ***bar-c., bar-m.,*** bar-s., **BRY.,** buth-a., calad., **CALC.,** calc-ac., ***calc-ar.,*** calc-f., calc-s., carb-s., **CARC.,** ***caust.,*** cham., chel., ***chin.,*** **CHIN-S., CIC.,** cocc., ***con.,*** cupr., cycl., ***dig.,*** dirc., ***dros., dulc.,*** euph., euphr., ferr-ac., ***ferr-p.,*** fl-ac., ***gels.,*** gins., ***graph.,*** grat., hep., hipp., ***iod.,*** kali-c., kali-p., kalm., ***lach.,*** lil-t., mag-arct., mang., merc., ***mur-ac.,*** nat-ac., nat-a., ***nat-c., nat-m.,*** nat-p., nat-s., ***nit-ac., nux-v.,*** petr., ***ph-ac.,*** **PHOS.,** psor., ***puls.,*** ran-b., ***rhus-t., sabin.,*** scroph-n., ***sep., sil.,*** sol-t-ae., ***spig.,*** **SPONG.,** ***stann., staph.,*** stram., sul-ac., ***sulph.,*** tarent., thuj., tub., verat., vichy-h., viol-t., wies., xan.

albuminuria, in - ars., ***calc.***

beating in stomach, with - ant-t.

childbed, in, or after - **BRY.**

disgust of life, with - ***lach.***

evening, 7 p.m. - buth-a.

melancholia, with - ***sulph.***

orchitis, in chronic - ***spong.***

spermatorrhea, in - ***dig.***

ghost, as of a, from which he could not free himself after waking - ***sulph.***

green stripes, on seeing - thuj.

head, with congestion to - acon., carb-v., ***cupr.,*** cycl., ***ign.,*** puls.

headache, with - ***acon.,*** aeth., ***ars.,*** bell., bov., calc., carb-v., caust., fl-ac., glon., kali-n., lyss., nit-ac., plat., ruta, sep., tub.

agg. lying down - ***sep.***

gastric - ***caust.***

health, about - acet-ac., acon., **AGAR.,** agn., alum., alum-p., alum-sil., am-c., ***arg-m.,*** **ARG-N.,** arn., **ARS.,** aeth., ars-h., blatta, brom., bry., bufo, ***calad., calc.,*** calc-ar., ***calc-p.,*** calc-s., calc-sil., cann-i., **CARC.,** ***chin-a.,*** cocc., cop., glon., grat., ign., **KALI-AR.,** kali-c., kali-p., kali-sil., lac-c., lach., lob., **LYC.,** mag-m., med., nat-c., nat-p., **NIT-AC.,** nux-m., nux-v., ***ph-ac.,*** plat., **PHEL., PHOS.,** podo., psor., ***puls.,*** sel., ***sep.,*** sil., staph., sulph.

especially during menopausal period - ***kali-br.,*** sil.

gone when symptoms gone - cocc.

ANXIETY, general

health, of relatives - ars., calc., ***carc.,*** cocc., **HEP.,** merc., phos.

little concerned about his own - carc., cocc.

heat, with (see fever) - berb., bov., ***cham.,*** nicc., **NUX-V.,** ***sec.***

face, of - **CARB-V.,** graph.

flushes of - ***calc., dros.,*** **SEP.**

head of, with - ***cupr.***

and cold feet - ***sulph.***

sudden - **SPONG.**

hematemesis, in - ip., ***nat-m., phos.***

hemoptysis, in - **ACON.,** phos.

himself, about - lyc., ***sil.***

home, about - bry., nat-p.

hot air, as if in - **PULS.**

house, in - alum., ars., aster., ***bry.,*** carl., chel., kali-c., **LYC.,** ***mag-m.,*** plat., **PULS., RHUS-T.,** spong., ***til.,*** valer.

amel., in - ign.

on entering - alum., rhod.

household matters, about - calc., puls.

hungry, when - ars., cina, ***iod., kali-c.,*** phos.

hurried, feeling - **ARG-N., CARC.,** med., **NAT-M.**

hydrothorax, in - ***coch.***

hypochondriacal - ***acon.,*** agar., agn., alum., am-c., anac., arg-n., ***arn., ars.,*** asaf., asar., bar-c., ***bell.,*** bry., calad., ***calc.,*** cann-i., canth., **CARC.,** caust., cham., ***con.,*** cupr., dros., ferr-p., graph., ***grat.,*** hyos., ign., ***iod.,*** kali-ar., ***kali-c.,*** kali-chl., kali-p., lach., lob., **LYC.,** mag-arct., med., mosch., nat-c., **NAT-M.,** ***nit-ac., nux-v.,*** ol-an., ox-ac., ph-ac., **PHOS.,** plat., psor., ***puls., raph., rhus-t., sep.,*** squil., staph., sulph., valer.

mania to read medical books - **CALC.,** ***carc., nux-v., puls.,*** staph., sumb.

hysterical - ars., ***asaf.,*** carc., con., **THER.**

ice-cold, drinks agg. - aq-mar.

imaginary evils, about - anac., laur., **SEP.**

inactivity, with - bov., coff., laur., merc.

inconsolable - ***acon.,*** ars., nit-ac.

ineffectual desire for stool, from - **AMBR.**

inexpressible, with fainting - ***dig.***

intense - ars-s-f., carc.

joyful things, by most - ***plat.***

kidney pain, in - ars., ***berb., op.***

laryngitis, in - ***arg-m.***

laughing and crying, ending in profuse perspiration, from a - ***cupr.***

law suit or dispute, as if he was engaged in - ign., ***nit-ac.***

liver disease, in, with dropsy - ***fl-ac.***

looking, steadily - ***sep.***

lunch, after - mag-c., mag-m.

lying, while - ars., calc-s., carb-v., ***cench.,*** hep., nux-v., puls., ***sil.,*** spong., stann.

amel. - mang.

must lie down with anguish - mez., phel., ph-ac.

ANXIETY, general

lying, side, on - bar-c., kali-c., phos., puls.

left - bar-c., **PHOS.,** puls.

right, from flatulence - kali-c.

masturbation, from - cann-i.

menopausal period, during - acon., ***aml-n.,*** ars., cimic., glon., puls., sep., ***tril.***

menorrhagia, in - ***cann-i.***

menses, during - acon., ***bell., calc.,*** calc-sil., canth., caul., cimic., cina, cocc., coff., con., hyos., ign., inul., ***kali-c.,*** kali-i., kali-sil., kreos., mag-m., ***merc.,*** nat-c., ***nat-m., nit-ac.,*** nux-v., phos., ***plat.,*** sec., **SIL.,** stann., ***sulph.,*** verat., zinc., zinc-p.

amel., during - stann., zinc.

anger and anxiety, during - acon., bell., lach., nux-v., op., ph-ac., staph., verat-v.

after - ***agar., pall.,*** phos., sec.

which prevents sleep - agar.

amenorrhea, in - ***cycl., ign.***

before - acon., am-c., calc., carb-an., carb-s., carb-v., ***cocc.,*** con., ***graph., ign.,*** kali-bi., mag-arct., mag-m., mang., merc., ***nat-m., nit-ac., nux-v.,*** puls., ***stann., sulph.,*** zinc.

mental exertion, from - acon., ars., aur-m., benz-ac., calc., camph., cham., cupr., ***cupr-ac.,*** iod., mang., nat-c., ***nit-ac.,*** nux-v., phos., ***plan.,*** puls., rhus-t., sec., verat.

mind ceased to be active, after - benz-ac.

metrorrhagia, in - ***sabin.***

midnight, until 2 a.m. - carb-an.

after - acon., alum., ant-c., **ARS.,** calc., ***cench.,*** chin., cast., chin-s., colch., dulc., graph., hep., lyc., mag-arct., mang., **NUX-V.,** quas., rat., ***rhus-t.,*** **SPONG.,** squil.

waking, on - calc., ign., lyc., ph-ac.

waking, on half - con.

agg. - acon., **ARS.**

before - ambr., am-c., ars., bar-c., bar-s., ***bry., carb-s., carb-v.,*** caust., ***cocc.,*** ferr., ***graph.,*** gels., ***hep.,*** kali-c., laur., ***lyc., mag-c.,*** mag-m., merc., ***mur-ac.,*** nat-c., ***nat-m.,*** nat-p., nat-s., nat-sil., nux-v., phos., ***puls.,*** sabin., sil., stront-c., ***sulph.,*** tub., verat.

11 p.m. - ruta.

waking, on, amel. on rising - caust., sil.

moaning, with - sep.

money matters, about - ***ars.,*** calc-f., calc-sil.

morning - ***ail., alum.,*** am-c., anac., **ARS.,** ***ars-s-f.,*** bar-c., calc-s., canth., carb-an., ***carb-s., carb-v., caust., chin.,*** cocc., con., **GRAPH.,** ign., ip., kali-ar., **LACH.,** led., ***lyc.,*** mag-c., mag-m., mag-s., mez., nat-m., nat-s., nit-ac., ***nux-v.,*** **PHOS.,** plat., puls., rhus-t., sep., ***staph., sulph.,*** sul-ac., verat., zinc., zinc-p.

perspiration, during - ***sep.,*** sulph.

rising, amel. - carb-an., cast., fl-ac., nux-v., rhus-t., sep.

on and after - arg-n., carb-an., mag-c., rhus-t.

ANXIETY, general
morning, waking, on - ***alum.,*** alum-p., anac., calc-sil., carb-an., ***carb-v., caust.,*** chel., ***chin.,*** cocc., **GRAPH.,** ign., ip., kali-ar., **LACH.,** ***lyc.,*** mag-c., mag-m., mag-s., nat-m., nit-ac., ***nux-v., phos.,*** plat., puls., rhus-t., sep., squil.
motion, from - acon., aloe, berb., bor., cocc., **DIG.,** ***hyos.,*** kali-i., ***lach.,*** mag-c., nat-c., nicc., rheum, stann., stram.
airplane, of - **BOR.**
amel. - acon., act-sp., ***ars.,*** naja, ph-ac., ***puls.,*** seneg., sil., tarax.
cable-railway, of - **BOR.**
downward - **BOR.,** coff-t., ***gels.,*** sanic.
elevator, of - **BOR.**
finish hurried, forceful motions at once, if he does not - ***stram.***
heart disease, in - **DIG.**
slightest, in child in cyanosis - ***lach.***
mucus, from accumulation of, in bronchi - arund.
murder, as if he had committed, in mania - ***ars.***
music, from - bufo, dig., ***nat-c.***
nausea, from - ant-t.
diarrhea, in - **ARG-N., ANT-C.,** ***calc.,*** gels., **NUX-V.**
nervous attack, with - asaf.
neuralgia, in - ***cham.***
night - ***acon.,*** agar., ***alum.,*** alum-p., ***alum-sil., alumn.,*** ambr., am-c., am-m., ang., ant-c., arg-m., arg-n., arn., **ARS.,** ***ars-s-f., aster.,*** aur-a., aur-i., ***bar-c.,*** bar-s., ***bell.,*** bor., bov., bry., cact., ***calc., calc-ar., calc-s.,*** calc-sil., camph., cann-s., canth., ***carb-an., carb-s., carb-v., carc.,*** cast., ***caust., cham., chin.,*** chin-a., chin-s., cina, clem., cob-n., cocc., coff., con., cupr-ac., cupr-ar., cycl., dig., ***dros.,*** dulc., ***ferr.,*** ferr-ar., ferr-p., ***graph., haem., hep., hyos., ign.,*** jatr., kali-ar., kali-bi., kali-c., kali-m., kali-n., kali-p., kali-s., kali-sil., kreos., ***lach.,*** lac-ac., lact., lil-t., lith., lyc., mag-arct., ***mag-c.,*** mag-m., mang., ***merc.,*** merc-c., nat-a., nat-c., ***nat-m.,*** nat-p., nat-sil., ***nit-ac.,*** nux-v., petr., phel., ***phos.,*** pituin., plan., plat., plb., **PULS.,** ran-b., ran-s., rat., ***rhus-t.,*** sabad., sabin., ***samb.,*** sep., sil., spong., squil., stront-c., ***sulph.,*** tab., thuj., ***verat.,*** zinc., zinc-p.
11 p.m. - ***bor.***
12 p.m. - tub.
1 a.m. to 3 a.m. - ***ars.,*** kali-ar., hep.
2 a.m. - chin., graph., nat-m.
2 a.m. to 4 a.m. - coc-c.
3 a.m. - **ARS.,** sil.
after - ***ars.,*** rhus-t., verat.
3 a.m. to 5 a.m. - ant-c.
4 a.m. - alum.
5 a.m. - nat-m.
amel. - quas.
children, in - abel., ***acon.,*** agre., arg-m., **ARS., BOR.,** ***calc., carc.,*** caste., ***chlol., chlor., cina,*** convo-s., **KALI-BR.,** ***kali-p., stram.,*** **TUB.**

ANXIETY, general
night, at
children, in, wakes at 2 a.m. to 3 a.m. - calc.
emansio mensium - ***dig.***
escape, with desire to - ***merc.***
fright, in bad effects of - ***merc.***
heart disease, in - ***dig.***
heat, with - ***sulph.***
as from - ***puls.***
helplessness, with feeling - ***lith.***
metrorrhagia, after - ***sep.***
palpitation, with, caused by pressure in stomach - ***sulph.***
rheumatism, with - ***ars.***
typhoid, in - ***canth.***
visions, with frightful - ***camph.***
waking and on - ***alum.,*** arg-n., ***ars.,*** carb-o., carb-v., caust., chel., ***cina,*** con., ***dros.,*** graph., lac-ac., lyc., nat-c., ***nat-m.,*** nit-ac., ***phos.,*** plat., ***puls.,*** rat., sep., sil., **SULPH.,** zinc.
night-watching, from - caust., **CARC.,** ***cocc.,*** cupr., **NIT-AC.**
noise, from - agar., alum., ***aur.,*** bar-c., caps., ***caust.,*** chel., nat-c., petr., ***phos.,*** puls., **SIL.**
ear, in - sil.
water, of rushing - **LYSS., STRAM.**
noon - bar-c., chin-s., cic., mag-c., mez.
to 3 p.m. - aster.
nosebleed, amel. - kali-chl.
nursing, after - ***cham.,*** cocc.
oppression, with - sulph.
chest, of - ***acon., dig.,*** ph-ac., **PHOS.,** ***psor.***
oppressive - **CARB-V.**
scarlatina, in - ***calc.***
others, for - acon., ***ambr., arg-n., ars.,*** bar-c., ***calc-p.,*** **CARC.,** caust., chel., cocc., ***dulc.,*** fl-ac., hep., manc., merc., naja, ***nux-v.,*** perh., ph-ac., **PHOS.,** ***staph., sulph.***
pains, from the - ***acon.,*** **ARS.,** carb-v., ***carc.,*** caust., ***coloc., nat-c.,*** sars.
abdomen, in - ***coloc.,*** cupr., mez., spig.
anus, in - phos.
cancer, of - ars., **CARC.**
eyes, in - acon., spig.
heart, in - acon., ***kali-ar.,*** mill., ***op., phos., spig.***
sharp, stitches - **SPIG.**
stomach, in - ars., graph., sulph.
pancreatic disease, in - ***atro.***
paralysed, as if - am-m., cob-n.
periodical - arn., ***ars., calc-i., cham.,*** cocc., nat-c., nat-m., ***phos.,*** plat., sep., spong., ***sulph.***
peritonitis, in - ars., ***lyc.***
perspiration, agg. - aq-mar., merc.
amel. - agar., calc.
cold - acon., ars., ***crot-h.,*** euph-c., ***ferr.,*** ferr-m., ***nux-v., plb.,*** sep., ***tab.,*** verat.
faintness, with - ***plb., tab.***
forehead, on - ***nux-v., sep., verat.***
prolapsus uteri, during - acon.
headache, from violent, with - ***ant-c.***

ANXIETY, general
perspiration,
forehead, on, with - ars., carb-v., ***nux-v., phos.,*** sep.
profuse, during night and in morning, with - ***ph-ac.***
physical - acon., agar., alum., am-m., ambr., ***aml-n., ant-t.,*** **ARG-N.,** arn., **ARS.,** ars-i., **ARS-S-F.,** bar-c., bar-m., bar-s., bell., bor., ***brom., bry., calc.,*** calc-ar., calc-i., **CAMPH.,** cann-s., ***canth.,*** carb-v., caust., cench., **CHAM.,** ***chel., chin.,*** chlor., cic., cocc., ***coff., colch.,*** con., ***cupr.,*** **DIG.,** euph., ***ferr., ferr-ar., ferr-i., ferr-p.,*** guai., ign., inul., ***iod.,*** **IP.,** ***kali-ar.,*** kali-c., kreos., laur., lob., ***lyc.,*** mag-c., meph., merc., mez., mosch., mur-ac., nat-c., nat-m., nat-s., nux-m., **NUX-V.,** op., petr., **PH-AC., PHOS.,** plat., plb., prun., **PULS.,** ran-b., rhod., rhus-t., ruta, sabad., sabin., sars., ***sec.,*** seneg., ***sep.,*** sil., spig., squil., ***stann., staph.,*** stram., ***sul-i.,*** **SULPH.,** sul-ac., tarent., ***teucr.,*** ther., thuj., ***verat., zinc.,*** zinc-p.
pining away, from bodily and mental - ars., **AUR.**
playing piano, while - ***nat-c.***
pneumonia, in - ***ant-t.,*** **ARS.,** ***chel.,*** **PHOS.,** ***squil.***
pollutions, after - carb-an., petr., ***phos.***
pregnancy, in - acon., ***ant-t.,*** bar-c., ign., psor., stann.
continued - stann.
paroxysms, during, lasting two or three hours - ***ant-t.***
precordia, about - **ACON.**
present, about - calc-ac., ***con.***
pressure, chest, on - ***acon.,*** aur., **CARB-V.,** coca, ***dig.,*** ph-ac., **PHOS.,** ***plat., psor.,*** sabad., **SULPH.,** ***tab.***
chest, in - bell.
epigastrium, in - guai.
pulsation in the abdomen, with - lyc.
pursued, as if - ***anac.,*** hyos., kali-br.
walking, when - ***anac.***
qualmishness, with, causes, from slight, with throbbing - ferr.
evening - ***puls.***
wabbling, with - anac.
railroad, when about to journey by, amel.
while in train - arg-n., ars.
rain, during - calc., ***elaps.***
reading, while - ***mag-m., sep.***
preventing - quas.
rest, during - act-sp., hist., iod., seneg.
retching, when - ***chel.***
rheumatism, in - ***ant-t.***
riding, while - ***arg-n., aur., bor., lach.,*** psor., sep.
down hill - **BOR.,** ***psor.***
rising, after - arg-n., carb-an., chel., mag-c., rhus-t.
lying, from - verat.
seat, from a, on - berb., verat.

ANXIETY, general
rising, amel. - carb-an., mill.
risings, in esophagus, from hot - ***hyper.***
rocking, during - **BOR.**
room, air, amel. in open - ***bry.***
entering a - alum.
salvation, about - aq-mar., **ARS.,** ars-s-f., **AUR.,** aur-a., aur-s., ***calc., calc-ar.,*** calc-s., ***camph.,*** carb-s., chel., cann-i., ***graph.,*** hura, ign., kali-p., **LACH., LIL-T.,** ***lyc., med., mez.,*** nat-m., nux-v., ph-ac., plat., plb., podo., ***psor., puls.,*** **STAPH.,** ***stram.,*** **SULPH.,** ***thuj.,*** **VERAT.**
exacting, too, as to their religious practices - ign., ***lyc.,*** ph-ac., **STAPH.,** sulph.
faith, about loss of his - coloc., merc-ac., nux-v., staph., sulph.
hell, of - ***plat.***
morning - psor.
night - calc-ar.
scruples, excessive religious - ars., ign., lyc., nux-v., puls., staph., **SULPH.**
soul's welfare, about - ***lil-t.***
scarlatina, in, appearance of eruption, before - ***merc.***
delayed appearance of eruption, with - ***ip.***
sedentary employment, from - ***ars.,*** graph.
sewing - sep.
sex, during - kreos., ***lyc.***
after - sep.
thought of - ***kreos.,*** lyc., puls.
sexual desire in excess, from suppressed - **CON.**
shaving, while - calad.
shuddering, with - bell., calc., carb-an., **CARB-V.,** nat-c., plat., puls., tab., verat.
sitting, while - ant-t., benz-ac., carb-an., ***caust.,*** dig., ***graph.,*** nit-ac., ph-ac., phos., puls., sil., staph., tarax.
amel. - iod.
bent - rhus-t.
must sit, forward, if possible at open window - chin-a.
sleep, during - acon., agar., ang., arn., **ARS.,** aster., ***bell.,*** camph., cast., cham., ***cocc.,*** con., ***cocc.,*** cycl., dig., dor., dulc., ferr., ***graph.,*** hep., ip., ***kali-c., kali-i., lyc.,*** merc., ***merc-c., nat-c., nat-m., nit-ac.,*** nux-v., op., petr., ***phos.,*** phys., puls., rhus-t., samb., sil., ***spong., squil.,*** stann., stram., stront-c., verat.
after, in afternoon - **STAPH.**
before - alum., ambr., berb., carb-v., ***caust., mag-c.,*** nat-c., sil.
evening - berb.
fainting would return, as though, and he would die - ***caust.***
going to, on - acon., ***calc.,*** carb-v., ***caust.,*** cench., hep., ***lach., lyc.,*** merc., nat-m., ***puls.,*** quas., rhus-t.
rush of ideas, with, and blood to head, forcing him to rise - ***puls.***
loss of sleep, from - **CARC.,** ***cocc.,*** **NIT-AC.**

ANXIETY, general

sleep,

menses, after - agar., aster., **COCC.,** ***kali-i.,*** ***merc-c.,*** zinc.

on starting from - am-m., clem., samb.

partial slumbering in the morning, during - juni.

soul's welfare - ***lil-t.***

soup, after - ***mag-c.,*** ol-an.

speak, cannot - ***ign.***

speaking, when - alum., ***ambr.,*** nat-c., plat., stram.

agg. - aq-mar.

company, in - plat.

public, in - acon., arg-n., gels., lyc.

spermatorrhea, in - ***phos.***

standing, while - aloe, anac., berb., cina, ph-ac., sil., ***verat.***

amel. - calc., phos., tarax.

stitching in, spine, from - ruta.

stomach, from - abrot.

stool, during - acon., ars., ars-s-f., calen., camph., canth., caust., cham., jal., mag-c., merc., plat., raph., sec., sep., stram., sulph., tab., ***verat.***

after - acon., ***bor., calc.,*** carb-v., ***caust.,*** coloc., crot-t., jatr., ***kali-c.,*** kali-i., laur., merc., nat-c., **NAT-S.,** ***nit-ac.,*** nux-v., rhus-t.

bloody, after - kali-c.

as for stool - cham., sep.

before - acon., ambr., ant-c., ***ars.,*** bar-c., berb., ***bor.,*** cadm-s., calc., calen., canth., caps., caust., cham., crot-t., kali-ar., ***kali-c.,*** mag-m., ***merc.,*** mez., rhus-t., sabin., ***verat.***

ineffectual desire for, from - **AMBR., CAUST.**

while straining at, with red face - ***caust.***

stooping, when - bell., rheum

amel. - bar-m.

stormy weather, during, (see thunderstorm) - ***lyc.***

strangers, presence of - ant-c., bar-c., ***carb-v., stram.***

stretch arms, had to - ***nat-c.***

study - sel.

study, effects of too much, cannot be resisted - ***cupr-acet.***

stupidity, with - anac.

success, from doubt about - ***lac-c.***

sudden - acon., ang., bar-c., chel., ***cocc.,*** ictod., nat-m., plat., ruta, ***tab.,*** thuj.

angina pectoris, with - acon., cact., spig., ***tab.***

night, at - ang.

perspiration, with, amel. after stool - ***ictod.***

suffering, with - ars., ***dig.***

suicidal - ***aur., carc.,*** caust., ***dros.,*** hep., ***merc.,*** nux-v., plat., ***puls., rhus-t.,*** staph.

supper, after - caust., mag-c., nux-v.

swallowing, on, due to pain - ***merc-cy.***

terrible - ars., carc., vesp.

ANXIETY, general

things that happened long ago, about, with palpitation - ***sep.***

thinking about it, from - alum., ambr., bry., ***calc.,*** caust., con., ***nit-ac.,*** staph., tab.

thoughts, from - ***arg-n.,*** ars., calc., phos., rhus-t.

disagreeable - **ARG-N.,** phos., sep.

thoughts, sad - rhus-t.

thunderstorm, during - carc., caust., gels., ***lyc., nat-c.,*** nat-m., ***nit-ac.,*** **PHOS.,** sep.

before - ***nat-c., phos.***

time is set, if a - ***arg-n.,*** gels., med., nat-m.

timorous, in whooping cough - ***caust.***

tobacco, from smoking - calad., petr., sep.

touched, aversion to being - ant-c., arn., cina, hep.

trifles, about - anac., ***ars.,*** bar-ac., bar-c., bor., calc., calc-i., caust., ***chin.,*** cocc., ***con., ferr.,*** graph., kali-m., kali-sil., laur., phos., sep., ***sil.,*** thuj.

chlorosis, in - ***nux-v.***

tuberculosis, in - agar., ***chin-a.***

tunnel, when on a, going through - **STRAM.**

typhus, in - **ARS., CALC.,** ***chin-s.,*** **SPONG.**

unconquerable - **CUPR.**

urination, during - acon., cham.

after - dig.

before - alum., dig., ph-ac., ***sars.,*** sep.

desire is resisted, when the - sep.

urging to, with - cham.

vaccination, after - ***thuj.***

vexation, after - ***acon.,*** lyc., phos., sep., staph., verat.

voice, on raising the - cann-s.

vomiting, on - ant-c., dulc.

amel. - hell-f.

attacks of bloody, between - ***ip.***

wakens from - samb.

waking, on - acon., agar., ***alum.,*** alum-sil., am-c., am-m., anac., ant-t., arg-m., arg-n., ***arn.,*** **ARS.,** ars-h., ars-s-f., aster., bapt., bell., bism., bor., bry., bufo, ***cact.,*** calc., calc-ar., calc-s., carb-an., ***carb-s.,*** **CARB-V.,** cast., caust., chel., ***chin.,*** chin-a., cina, cocc., con., cub., dig., ***dios., dros., glon., graph.,*** hep., ign., ip., iris, kali-ar., kali-bi., ***kali-c.,*** kali-p., kali-s., **LACH.,** lepi., lyc., lyss., mag-c., nat-a., nat-c., nat-m., nat-p., ***nat-s.,*** nicc., nit-ac., ***nux-v.,*** ph-ac., ***phel., phos.,*** plat., psor., puls., ran-s., rat., rhus-t., ***samb.,*** sep., sil., sol-t-ae., ***spong.,*** squil., ***stram., stront-c., sulph.,*** tab., thuj., tub., verat., zinc., zinc-p.

agg. - aq-mar.

walking, while - acon., aloe, ***anac.,*** ant-c., arg-m., ***arg-n.,*** bar-c., bell., cina, clem., hep., ign., manc., mang., nux-v., plat., spong., staph., tab.

after - asc-t., dig.

air, cool, in - nux-m.

air, open, in - ***anac.,*** arg-m., ***arg-n.,*** bell., cina, hep., ign., **LYC.,** nux-v., plat., spong., tab.

ANXIETY, general
walking, while
air, open, amel. - ***iod., kali-i., kali-s., puls., rhus-t.***
amel. - colch., hist., sil., staph.
faster, which makes him walk - **ARG-N.,** fl-ac., sep.
rapidly, when - nit-ac., ***staph.***
slowly, must, otherwise something will happen - cupr.
warm bed, yet limbs cold if uncovered - **MAG-C.**
warmth, from - gamb., **KALI-S.,** lach., ***puls.***
amel. - ars., ***graph., phos.***
weariness, of life, with - ant-c., ***aur.,*** bell., carc., caust., chin., dros., hep., ***lach.,*** merc., ***nux-v.,*** plat., ***puls.,*** rhus-t., sil., spong., stel.
wild - ars., sec., tarent.
work, inclination to work, with - calc.
manual labor, during - aloe, anac., ***graph.,*** iod.
agg. - **IOD.**
preventing work - mosch.
unfit for work, to become - cean.
wounded esophagus, from - **CIC.**

APATHETIC, (See Indifferance)

APHASIA, (See Speech) - agar., alum., ***anac.,*** ant-chl., ant-t., arag., ***arg-n.,*** arn., ***ars.,*** arum-m., aur-m., bar-ac., ***bar-c., both., calc.,*** calc-p., cann-i., ***caust.,*** cham., ***chen-a.,*** chin., chin-a., ***colch.,*** con., crot-h., cupr., dios., dulc., elaps, ***glon.,*** hyos., ***kali-br.,*** kali-cy., ***kali-m.,*** kali-p., lac-c., ***lach., laur.,*** lil-t., ***lyc., mag-c., merc.,*** mez., naja, **NIT-AC.,** ***nux-m., nux-v.,*** oci., oena., olnd., ph-ac., phos., ***plb.,*** puls., stram., sulfon., sumb., syph., tab., xero, ***zinc.***
amnesia, from - kali-br., plb.
forgetful, of words while speaking, of, words hunting for - agar., alum., am-br., anh., ***arg-n.,*** **ARN.,** ***bar-c.,*** bar-s., benz-ac., **BOTH.,** cact., calc., camph., **CANN-I.,** cann-s., carb-an., carb-s., carb-v., chen-a., coca, cocc., colch., con., crot-h., dulc., glon., ham., helo., hydr., ***kali-br.,*** kali-c., kali-p., ***lach.,*** lil-t., ***lyc., med., nat-m., nux-v., onos., plb.,*** podo., **PH-AC.,** puls., rhod., sil., staph., sulph., syph., ***thuj.,*** verat.
hemiphlegia of right side, with - chen-a.
inability to articulate without any affection of the tongue - both.

APPROACH of persons, agg. - ***arn.,*** con., ign., lyc., stry.
aversion, to being approached - ***arn.,*** aur., caj., canth., cina, hell., helon., hipp., ign., ***iod.,*** lil-t., ***lyc.,*** sanic., sulph.

ARDENT - alum., caust., nux-v., sulph.

ASKS, for nothing, (see Wants) - ant-c., ***arn.,*** ars., ***bry.,*** cocc., hell., hep., hyos., linu-c., mez., mill., nicc., **OP.,** puls., rheum

ASTONISHED - coff., cori-r., ign., stram.

ATTACK others, desire to - lyss., stram.

ATTENTION, agg. (see Concentration) - ign., sil.
amel. - camph., gels., hell.

ATTITUDES, assumes strange - cic., ***cina,*** cocc., ***coloc.,*** gamb., **HYOS.,** merc., nux-v., ***plb.,*** rheum, zinc.
amel. - rheum
as if in - nat-s.
strange, does things - arg-n., cact., sep.

AUDACITY - acon., agar., alum., ant-t., ***arn.,*** bell., bov., calad., cocaine, guai., hep., **IGN.,** lach., mag-arct., merc., mez., nat-c., ***nux-v.,*** op., plat., ***puls.,*** sil., squil., staph., **SULPH.,** tarax., tub., verat.

AUTISTIC, children - ***carc.,*** cann-i., ***nat-m.,*** op., thuj.
vaccinations, after - carc., thuj.

AUTOMATIC, behaviour - anac., anh., bell., calc., hell., hyos., lyc., mag-c., ***nux-m.,*** phos., sil., ***stram.,*** zinc.
hand, right, mouth towards - nux-v.
one arm and leg, head etc. - apoc., bry., hell., iodof., mygal., pyrog., zinc.

AVARICE, (see Greedy)

AVERSION, general
approached, to being - ***arn.,*** aur., caj., canth., cina, hell., helon., hipp., ign., ***iod.,*** lil-t., ***lyc.,*** sanic., sulph.
bathing, to - am-c., ant-c., clem., rhus-t., **SULPH.**
black and sombre, everything that is - rob., stram., ***tarent.***
children, to - lyc., plat., **SEP.,** raph.
dislikes her own - glon., ***lyc.,*** phos., plat., ***sep.,*** verat.
little girls (in a woman) - raph.
darkness, to - sanic., stram.
everything, to - alumn., am-m., ant-c., ars., ***asar.,*** bism., ***bov.,*** calc., camph., canth., caps., cent., ***cocc.,*** coloc., cupr., grat., hyos., ip., lach., lyc., mag-c., merc., mez., phos., plat., plb., plumbg., ***puls.,*** rheum, rhod., ruta, sars., ***sep.,*** spong., sulph., thea., thuj.
forenoon - sars.
family members, to - am-c., am-m., aur., ***calc.,*** calc-s., con., ***crot-h., fl-ac.,*** hep., iod., ***kali-c., kali-p.,*** lyc., **MERC.,** ***nat-c.,*** nat-m., phos., plat., plb., senec., **SEP.**
female - am-c.
talks pleasantly to others - fl-ac.
friends, to - cedr., coloc., ferr., fl-ac., ***led.***
pregnancy, during - ***con., sep.***
fuss - nat-m.
going out - cycl.
herself, to - lac-c., staph., thuj.
husband, to - ***glon.,*** kali-c., kali-p., ***nat-c.,*** nat-m., **SEP.,** thuj., verat.
children, and - ***glon.,*** **SEP.,** ***verat.***
laughing faces, to - mag-aust.
light, to - tarent.
literary, persons - sulph.

AVERSION, general
men, to - bell., ***caust.,*** con., graph., ***lyc.,*** nat-m., ***plat.,*** raph., ***sep.,*** stann.
contempt for - cic., ***plat.***
loss of confidence in - cic.
shuns the foolishness of - cic.
mother, to - thuj.
night - bufo.
parents, to - fl-ac.
persons, to all - absin., calc., chin., ***merc-ac., nat-c., nux-v.,*** phos., ***staph., sulph.***
persons, to certain - ***am-m., aur.,*** **CALC.,** caust., crot-h., hep., **NAT-C.,** nat-m., nit-ac., sel., stann.
sight of - cic.
who don't agree with him - calc-s.
places - hep.
pregnancy, no affection for anybody during - acon., ***sep.***
red, to - ***alum.***
red, yellow, green and black - tarent.
religious, to the opposite sex - lyc., ***puls.,*** sulph.
school, to - calc-p., lyc., med., nat-m.
sex - ***raph.,*** **SEP.**
society - anac., ***nat-c.,*** stann., syph.
sex, to her own - raph.
opposite - am-c., ign., nat-m., puls., ***sep.,*** staph., thuj.
those, around - ars.
water - **AM-C.,** ***lyss.***
cold - phys.
running agg., from hearing or seeing - ang., apis, arg-m., bell., brom., canth., **LYSS.,** nit-ac., ***stram.,*** sulph., ter.
wife, to his - ars., ***fl-ac., med.,*** nat-s., staph., ***thuj.***
women, to - am-c., bapt., con., ***dios.,*** ign., ***lach., lyc.,*** mag-c., nat-m., ***puls.,*** raph., sulph., **THUJ.**
homosexuality, with - ***plat., thuj.***
her own sex - raph.

AWKWARD, mentally (see Generals) - aeth., agar., ambr., ***anac.,*** apis, asaf., ***bar-c.,*** bov., calc., ***camph.,*** cann-i., ***caps.,*** carb-s., cocc., con., gels., hell., ***ign.,*** ip., kali-c., kali-chl., lach., ***lol.,*** lyc., mosch., ***nat-c.,*** nat-m., nat-s., **NUX-V.,** ph-ac., phos., plb., rheum, sars., sil., stann., sulph., tarent., thuj.
drops things - aeth., **AGAR., APIS,** ars-s-r., ***bov.,*** bry., colch., hell., ign., lach., mosch., ***nat-m.,*** nux-v., plat., ***plb.,*** stann., staph., tarent.
menses, during - alum.

AWARENESS, heightened - anh., cann-i., ***coff.,*** op.

BAD, feelings, good and bad by turns - alum., carc., med., psor.
morning, in - ***lyc.,*** mag-c., ***nux-v.,*** sars.
takes everything into bad part - anac., ***ars.,*** bov., caps., cocc., nat-m., ***nit-ac.,*** nux-v., puls., staph., verat.

BAD, news (see News)

BARGAINING - ars., ***bry.,*** lyc., **PULS., SIL.,** ***sulph.,*** thuj.

BARKING, noises, makes - ***bell.,*** brom., calc., ***canth.,*** dros., nit-ac., ***nux-m.,*** spong., stann., ***stram.***
bellowing - bell., ***canth., cupr., nux-m.***
delirium, during - ***bell., canth.***
growling like a dog - alum., ***bell.,*** lyss., mag-m., phos.
sleep, during - lyc.

BASHFUL, (see Timid, Yielding) - aloe, ***ambr.,*** anac., arg-n., ars-s-f., aur., ***bar-c.,*** bar-s., bell., ***calc.,*** calc-s., calc-sil., ***carb-an.,*** carb-v., carc., caust., ***chin.,*** **COCA,** con., coff., ***cupr.,*** graph., hyos., ***ign.,*** iod., kali-bi., ***kali-p.,*** lil-t., manc., mang., meli., merc., mez., ***nat-c.,*** nat-p., nit-ac., nux-v., ***petr.,*** phos., **PULS.,** sil., ***staph., stram., sulph.,*** tab., tarent., ***zinc.***
covering their face with their hands, but look through their fingers - bar-c.
hiding - **ARS.,** ***bar-c.,*** **CUPR.,** ***hyos.,*** puls.

BATTLES, talks about - bell., hyos.
war, talks of - agar., bell., hyos.

BED, aversion to, shuns - ***acon.,*** arn., ars., bapt., calc., camph., cann-s., canth., caust., ***cedr.,*** cench., cupr., graph., kali-ar., ***lach.,*** lyc., merc., nat-c., pyrog., squil.
desires to remain in - alum., alumn., ant-c., ***arg-n.,*** con., ***hyos.,*** merc., psor., puls., rob., sil., verat-v.
morning - ferr-m., ***sep.***
sexual excitement, from - verat.
get out of, wants to - acon., ***agar., bapt., bell., bry., camph.,*** cupr., hell., **HYOS.,** op., oper., rhus-t., ***stram., verat.***
wants to, chill, during - ***hyos.***
jumps out of, and runs recklessly about - sabad., stram.
wants to destroy himself but lacks courage - chin., sabad.
slide down in, inclination to - mur-ac.
tossing about in, with anxiety - ***ars., cupr-acet.***

BEGGING, entreating - ***ars.,*** aur., bell., kali-c., plat., puls., stram.
sleep, in - stann.

BELLOWING - bell., ***canth., cupr., nux-m.***

BENEVOLENCE - bell., ***carc.,*** coff., coff-t., ign., nux-v., op., ***phos.***

BESIDE oneself, being - **ACON.,** anac., anh., ant-t., apis, arn., ***ars.,*** aur., bar-c., bell., calc., carb-an., carb-v., carc., caust., **CHAM.,** chin., **COFF.,** colch., coloc., con., cupr., cupr-ar., dros., graph., hep., hyos., **IGN.,** kali-ar., kali-c., kali-n., lyc., mag-s., merc., nat-c., nat-m., nit-ac., **NUX-V.,** ph-ac., phos., plb., ***puls.,*** sec., sep., sil., sol-n., spig., stann., stram., sulph., tarax., thuj., ***vario., verat.,*** verb.
anxiety, from - ***acon.,*** ars., ***graph.,*** mag-c.
bad weather, from - am-c.
trifles, from - kres., thuj.

BILIOUS, disposition - ars., bol., bufo, chel., ***chin.,*** coca, hell., lyc., ***nux-v.,*** sul-ac., tarent.
difficulty with someone, after - tarent.
grief, after - tarent.

BITES - acon., **AM-BR.,** ***ant-t., anthr.,*** **ARS.,** ***arum-t., aster.,*** **BAR-C., BELL.,** bufo, ***calc., camph.,*** cann-i., ***canth., carb-s.,*** carb-v., cic., ***cina,*** croc., cub., ***cupr.,*** cupr-ac., cupr-c., cur., hydr-ac., ***hyos.,*** hura, ign., ***lach.,*** lil-t., ***lyc., lyss.,*** mag-c., **MED., NAT-M.,** nit-ac., op., phos., ***phyt.,*** plb., podo., sanic., sec., senec., **STRAM., SULPH.,** tarent., ***verat.***
arms, bites own - op.
around him - phos.
children, in - **BELL.**
clothes, bites - plb.
convulsions, with - croc., ***cupr.,*** lyss., ***tarent.***
delirium, during - **BELL.,** ***canth.,*** cupr., hydr-ac., hyos., lyss., sec., **STRAM.,** verat-v., ***vero-o.***
evening - croc.
everyone who disturbs him - hyos.
everything, at - ***bell.***
father, his - carb-s.
fingernails, habit of - ***acon.,*** **AM-BR.,** ***ant-t.,*** arn., **ARS., ARUM-T., BAR-C.,** ***brom.,*** calc., calc-f., calc-p., carc., caust., **CINA,** cupr., hura, **HYOS.,** ***lyc.,*** lyss., ***mag-c.,*** **MED., NAT-M.,** nit-ac., phos., plb., puls., sanic., senec., seneg., ***sil.,*** staph., ***stram.,*** **SULPH.,** syc-co., upa., **VERAT.**
fingers - acon., ***arum-t.,*** carc, cina, med., plb., op.
sleep, in - elaps
tips, of - carc.
fists - acon.
garments - plb.
glass when fed - ars., bell., cham., ***cina, cupr., puls., verat.***
hands - hura, op.
himself - acon., arum-t., elaps, hura, lyss., op., plb., tarent.
impulse to - bell., bufo, cupr., phyt., podo., sec., stram.
night - bell.
in sleep - ***mygal.***
objects - **BELL.,** bufo, **HYOS.,** sil., **STRAM.**
paroxysmally - phos.
people - **BELL., STRAM.**
pillow - lyc., lyss., phos.
shoe and swallowing the pieces - verat.
snapping - lyss.
spits, barks and bites - ***calc.***
spoons, other things - ars., **BELL.,** cham., cina, cupr., hell., lyss., puls., verat.
tumblers, edge of, when trying to drink - ars.
worm affections, in - ***cina,*** croc.

BLACK and sombre, everything that is, aversion to - rob., stram., ***tarent.***

BLASPHEMY - **ANAC.,** calc., canth., nat-c., nat-m., nit-ac., plat., spig., staph.
and cursing - am-m., **ANAC.,** canth., chin-b., lyc., nat-c., ***nat-m.,*** nit-ac., nux-v., op., spig., staph.

BLINDNESS, pretended - verat.

BLISSFUL, feeling of, (see Peace, Tranquility) - ***cann-i.,*** coff., ***op.***

BLOOD, or a knife, cannot look at - **ALUM.**
wounds, cannot look at - acon., ign., **NUX-V.,** staph.

BOREDOM, feelings, ennui - ***alum.,*** alumn., amph., aur., bar-c., bor., cahin., calc., camph., carc., cer-s., chin., ***con.,*** cupr., cur., elaps, ferr., hura, hydrc., hydr., ign., kali-bi., kali-n., kiss., lach., laur., led., **LYC.,** mag-m., manc., **MED., MERC.,** mez., ***nat-c., nux-v.,*** paull., petr., pip-m., plat., ***plb.,*** rhus-t., ***spig.,*** spira., spirae., **SULPH.,** tarent., **TUB.,** ven-m., zinc.
afternoon - plb.
entertainment amel. - aur., lil-t., ***pip-m.***
evening - mag-m.
forenoon - alum.
homesickness, with - alum., ***caps., clem.***
menses, during - berb.
silent - **PLB.**

BORROWING, from everyone - ars., calc., lyc., phos., plat.

BORROWS, trouble - acet-ac., apis, bar-c., calc., phos., sang.

BRAGGART, boaster - alco., arn., ars., ***bell.,*** lach., **LYC.,** merc., nat-m., ***nux-v.,*** plat., ***stram.,*** **SULPH.**
rich, wishes to be considered as - lach., ***lyc.,*** verat.
squanders through ostentation - calc., nux-v., plat., puls.

BREAK things, desire to - ***apis,*** bell., carb-s., hura, hyos., ***nux-v.,*** sol-t-ae., ***staph., stram.,*** sulph., ***tarent., tub.,*** verat.
bright objects - lyss.

BROODING, (see Sulks) - alum., anh., arn., ***ars., aur.,*** aur-s., bar-i., bell., calc., calc-s., canth., caps., carb-an., caust., cham., chel., clem., cocc., cycl., euphr., ***gels.,*** goss., hell., **IGN.,** ip., kali-p., lach., lil-t., lyc., mez., mur-ac., ***naja,*** **NAT-M.,** nux-v., olnd., op., ***ph-ac.,*** plat., ***rheum,*** staph., ***stram.,*** sulph., **VERAT.**
condition, over one's sickness - ars., ***ph-ac.***
corner, brooding or moping in a - aur., aur-s., ***bar-c.,*** bar-i., bell., camph., cocc., con., cupr., hyos., nat-m., ph-ac., puls., **VERAT.**
disappointment, over - **BELL.,** ***nat-m., ph-ac.***
disease, over his - ars., ph-ac.
evening - **VERAT.**
forbidden things, over - ***plb.***
imaginary troubles, over - **IGN.**
melancholia, with - naja.
sickness, about his - ars., ph-ac.
unpleasant things - kiss.

BRUTALITY - absin., alco., **ANAC.,** ***lach.,*** nux-v., sulph.
drunkenness, during - anac., ***lach.,*** nux-v., sulph.

BUOYANCY - carc., eucal., ***fl-ac., sarr.***
alternating with despondency - ***carc., nux-v.***

BULIMIA - arg-n., ***carc.,*** ign., iod., med., nat-m., puls., staph.

BUSINESS, (see Work)
ailments from failure of - ***ambr.,*** **AUR.,** calc., cimic., coloc., ign., kali-br., **LYC.,** nat-m., ***nux-v.,*** ph-ac., puls., rhus-t., sep., sulph., verat.
averse to - acon-l., agar., am-c., anac., arn., ars., ars-h., asar., aur-m., ***brom.,*** **CALC.,** chin-s., cimic., ***con.,*** cop., fl-ac., **GELS.,** graph., hipp., kali-ar., kali-bi., kali-br., kali-c., kali-i., kali-s., lac-ac., ***lach.,*** laur., lil-t., **LYC.,** mag-s., nat-a., nat-c., nux-v., opun-v., ***ph-ac., phyt., puls.,*** rhod., rhus-t., **SEP., SIL.,** stann., ***sulph.,*** syph., ther.
desire for - ars., calc., ***carb-v.,*** carc., cer-b., con., fel., lach., ***nux-v.,*** tarent.
incapacity for - agn., caust., chin-s., kali-bi., lyc., mit., sel., sil., sul-i., tab.
neglects his - ***lyc.,*** op., ***sulph.***
talks of - ars., bell., **BRY.,** canth., cimic., dor., ***hyos.,*** Mygal., op., phos., plb., stram., sulph.
worn out, from - ***calc., coca,*** kali-p., **NUX-V., SIL.**

BUSY - acon., anac., ***apis,*** arn., ars., ***bar-c., bry.,*** calad., calc., caps., carc., cer-b., cimic., cocc., con., fel., ferr-p., ***hyos.,*** ign., ***iod., kali-br.,*** kali-i., kalm., ***lach.,*** lil-t., mag-m., merc., mosch., ***nux-m., op.,*** phos., rhus-t., ***sep.,*** stram., stront-c., ***sulph., tarent.,*** ther., ***vario., verat.,*** zinc.
fruitlessly - absin., ***apis, arg-n.,*** ars., bor., calc., canth., ***lil-t.,*** stann., sulph., tarent., ther., verat.
himself, with - mag-m., staph.
weak, and - mosch.

CALCULATING, (see Mathematics, Mistakes)

CAPRICIOUSNESS - acon., act-sp., agar., ***alum.,*** alum-sil., am-c., ant-c., ant-t., arn., ***ars.,*** asaf., aur-m., bar-c., ***bell.,*** bov., **BRY.,** brom., calc., ***calc-p.,*** calc-s., calc-sil., cann-s., caps., cann-i., canth., carb-an., carb-s., **CARC.,** caste., **CAUST., CHAM.,** ***chin.,*** chin-a., cimic., **CINA,** ***cocc., coff.,*** coloc., croc., ***cypr.,*** dig., dros., ***dulc.,*** ferr., fl-ac., goss., grat., ***hep.,*** hera., ***ign., iod.,*** **IP.,** kali-ar., **KALI-C.,** kreos., lach., led., lyc., mag-arct., mag-aust., mag-arct., mag-c., mag-m., ***mag-p., merc., merc-i-f.,*** nat-c., nat-n., nit-ac., nux-m., ***nux-v.,*** op., par., ***ph-ac., phos.,*** **PLAT.,** plb., ***puls.,*** raph., ***rheum,*** rhod., sac-alb., sarr., sars., sec., **SEP.,** sil., spig., spong., **STAPH.,** stram., ***sul-ac., sulph.,*** thuj., thyr., **TUB.,** valer., verat., **VERAT-V.,** viol-t., zinc.
afternoon - cann-s., sars.
children, in - calc-p., carc., ***cham., cina,*** ign., puls., sac-alb.
daytime - cast., ran-b.
evening - aur., bov., calc-s., cast., croc., fl-ac., ign., ran-b., zinc.
forenoon - cann-s.

CAPRICIOUSNESS,
morning - bov., ***nit-ac.,*** staph.
noon - zinc.

CAREFULNESS - **ARS.,** ***aur., bar-c.,*** bry., calc., **CHIN., GRAPH.,** ***ign., iod., lach., lyc., nux-v., puls.,*** ran-b., ***sep.,*** **SIL., STRAM., SULPH.,** ***verat.***

CARESSED, agg. - bell., calc., chin., ign., plat.
aversion to being - chin., **CINA,** ***ign.,*** **NAT-M.,** nit-ac.
caresses husband and child, then pushes away - anac., ign.
proof, against - cina
propensity for caresses - cann-i., carc

CARRIED, desires to be - acon., acet-ac., ant-c., ant-t., ***ars.,*** aspar., bell., benz-ac., bor., brom., **BRY.,** calc., carb-v., **CHAM.,** ***chel., cina,*** coff., coloc., ign., ip., kali-c., ***kreos., lyc., kali-c.,*** merc., podo., phos., **PULS.,** ***rhus-t.,*** sanic., stann., staph., sulph., vac., ***verat.***
aversion to be - ***coff.***
caressed and carried, desires to be - acon., kreos., puls.
croup, in - brom.
fast - acon., **ARS.,** bell., brom., **CHAM.,** ***cina.,*** rhus-t., verat.
fondled, and - kreos., phos., ***puls.***
rocked, and - ***cina.***
shoulder, over - ***cina,*** podo., stann.
sitting up - ant-t., ***puls.***
slowly - **PULS.**
will not be laid down - benz-ac.

CARRIES, things from one place to another and back again - mag-p.

CATATONIA - cic., cortico., rauw.

CAUTIOUS - acon., **ARS.,** bar-c., bry., cact., calc., caust., ***cupr.,*** graph., hyos., ***ign.,*** ip., mag-arct., nux-v., op., ***puls.,*** stram., verat.
anxiously - **ARS.,** am-c., bar-c., caust., ***lyc., puls.,*** sil., sulph.

CELIBACY, ailments from - ***con.,*** nat-m., phos., staph.

CENSORIOUS, (See Critical)

CHANGE, desire for (See Restlessness) - ***bry., calc-p., carc.,*** cham., hep., plat., sep., ***tub.***
dislike of - bol.
of impressions agg. - ***ign.***

CHARACTER, lack of - bar-c., ***caust.,*** **LYC.,** ***sil.***

CHARLATAN - calc., lyc., plat., thuj., sulph.

CHASES, imaginary objects - stram.
persons - cur.

CHEERFUL, feelings, happy - abrot., ***acon.,*** aesc., aeth., agar., alco., aloe, anac., anag., ang., ant-c., anth., apis, apoc., ***arg-m.,*** ars., asaf., asar., ***atro., aur.,*** aur-i., aur-m., aur-s., ***bell.,*** bor., bov., brom., bry., cact., calc-i., calc-p., **CANN-I., CANN-S.,** canth., caps., carb-ac., ***carb-an.,*** carb-o., carb-s., carb-v., ***carc.,*** carl., cast., caust., cent., chin., chin-s., chlor., **CIC.,** cinch., ***cinnb.,*** cob., coca, cocc., **COFF.,** colch., coloc., con., cot., **CROC.,**

CHEERFUL, feelings - crot-h., cupr., cycl., cypr., dros., ether, elae., ery-m., eucal., eug., eupi., fago., ferr., ferr-ma., ferr-p., ***fl-ac., form.,*** gamb., gels., glon., graph., ***grat.,*** guare., hura, hydr., hydrc., **HYOS.,** ***ign.,*** ilx-p., inul., iod., iodof., kali-bi., kali-br., kali-chl., kali-cy., keroso., kiss., kres., **LACH.,** laur., lepi., ***lyc.,*** mag-m., mag-s., manc., merc., mit., mosch., nabal., **NAT-C.,** nat-m., nat-p., nat-s., nicc., ***nit-ac.,*** nitro-o., ***nux-m., nux-v.,*** ol-an., ***op.,*** orig., ox-ac., ped., peti., petr., ph-ac., ***phos.,*** phys., pip-m., ***plat.,*** plb., prun., psor., rhod., rhodi., rhus-v., ruta, sabad., sarr., ***sars.,*** scut., sec., seneg., sep., spig., spong., squil., stann., staph., ***stram.,*** sul-i., ***sulph., sul-ac.,*** tab., ***tarax., tarent.,*** teucr., thea., ther., thuj., tong., trio., ***tub.,*** valer., ***verat.,*** verb., viol-o., visc., wies., ***zinc.,*** zing.

- **afternoon** - aster., aur-m., anac., ang., arg-m., calc., calc-s., mag-c., nat-s., ox-ac., phos., plb., sars., thuj.
  - 3 p.m. - ped.
  - 4 p.m. to 6 p.m. - merc-i-r.
  - 5 p.m. - ol-an.
- **air,** in open - ang., merc-i-f., nux-m lyss., ***mag-c.,*** mag-m., mag-aus., ***meny., merc., nat-c.,*** pall., ***plat.,*** **PSOR., PULS.,** rhus-t., sabin., sars., sec., sep., spig., ***stram.,*** valer., verat.
- **alternating** with
  - aversion to work - spong.
  - bursts of, indignation - aur., caps., croc., ign.
    - of, passion - acon., ***aur.,*** cann-s., caps., croc., hyos., ign., seneg., stram.
  - crying - acon., alum., arg-m., bell., carb-ac., graph., iod., phos., plat., spong.
  - dancing - bell.
  - destructiveness - spong.
  - distraction - spong.
  - dullness - piloc.
  - grief - calc-s., graph., ***op.***
  - impatience - tell.
  - irritability - ant-t., aur-a., ***stram.,*** zinc.
  - lachrymose mood - plb., psor., sep., spong., sumb.
  - looking down on the street - ***dios.***
  - loquacity, with - aeth.
  - mania - bell., ***cann-i.,*** cann-s., croc.
  - melancholy - zinc., ziz.
  - moaning - bell., coff., stram.
  - moroseness - acon., ant-t., ars., ***aur.,*** carb-v., cycl., form., merc., nat-c., nat-m., plat.
  - pain - plat.
  - palpitation - spig.
  - passion, burst of - ***aur.,*** caps., croc., ign., stram.
  - physical sufferings - plat.
  - quarrel - croc., spong., staph.
  - sadness - abrot., acon., agar., aran., arg-m., asar., ***aur.,*** **BELL.,** calc-s., cann-s., canth., carb-an., ***carc., caust.,*** cench., ***chin.,*** cimic., clem., coc-c., **COFF.,** croc., cupr., ferr., fl-ac., gels., graph., hell., **HYOS.,** ign., iod., ***kali-chl., kali-m., lach.,*** lyc., mag-arct., med., nat-c., ***nat-m.,*** nid., nit-ac., ***nux-m., nux-v.,*** op., ***petr.,*** plat., ***phos.,*** psor., senec., sep., spig., **STAPH., STRAM.,** sulfa., tarent., thyr., tub., zinc., ziz.
    - evening - ***graph.***
    - every other day - ferr.
    - morning - nux-v.
  - seriousness - cann-s., plat., spong.
  - shouting - chin.
  - sympathy, want of - merc.
  - timidity - mag-arct.
  - vexation - ant-t., ***bor.,*** caust., cortiso., nat-m., spong.
  - violence - aur., croc., stram.
- **bed,** in - ***hep.***
  - jumps out of - **CIC.**
- **causeless** - aur-i.
- **chill,** during - ***cann-s.,*** nux-m., phos., ***puls.,*** rhus-t., verat.
- **clapping** one's hands - cic., verat.
- **company,** in - bov.
- **constipated,** when - ***calc., psor.***
- **convulsions,** after - sulph.
- **dancing,** laughing, singing, with - bell., **HYOS.,** ***nat-m.,*** plat., ***stram.,*** tab.
- **daytime** - anac., arg-m., aur., caust., mag-m., mur-ac., sars.
- **death,** while thinking of - ***aur.***
- **desires** to be - chin.
  - ineffectually - ***manc.***
- **destruction,** with - spong.
- **dreams,** after - mur-ac.
- **drunkenness,** during - coff., op., staph.
- **eating,** while - anac., bell., carb-ac., cist.
  - after - carb-v., mez.
- **evening** - agar., ***aloe,*** alum., aster., bell., bism., bufo, calc., carb-ac., cast., chin., chin-b., chin-s., cist., clem., cupr., cycl., ferr., graph., ***lach.,*** lachn., lyss., mag-c., med., merc-i-f., merc-i-r., nat-c., ***nat-m.,*** nux-m., nux-v., ol-an., phel., plat., sulph., sumb., teucr., ***valer.,*** verb., viol-t., zinc., zinc-p.
  - 6 p.m. - calc-s.
  - 9 p.m. - asc-t.
  - bed, in - alum., ***ang.,*** ant-c., arn., aur., bor., carb-an., carb-v., ***lach.,*** laur., lyc., mag-aust., ***merc.,*** mez., ***nat-m., nit-ac., nux-v.,*** phos., ***prun., puls.,*** ran-b., ran-s., rhus-t., ***sep.,*** sil., ***spig.,*** staph., sul-ac., ***sulph., zinc.***
  - ill-humor during the day - sulph., viol-t.
  - sad in morning, and - nux-v.
- **followed** by, anxiety - ***gels.***
  - irritability - clem., hyos., nat-s., ol-an., op., seneg., tarax.
  - melancholy - gels., graph., meph., petr., plat., ziz.
  - prostration - clem., spong.
  - sleepiness - bell., calc.
- **foolish,** and - acon., agar., anac., arund., bell., calc., carb-an., carb-v., ***hyos.,*** merc., par., seneg., **SULPH.**

CHEERFUL, feelings
forenoon - aeth., bor., caust., clem., com., graph., nat-m., nat-s., phos., pip-m., plb., zinc.
headache, with - ***ther.***
heart, disease, with - cact.
heat, during - acon., mosch., ***op.,*** sabad., thuj.
hysterical - ther.
loquacious, and - aeth., lach.
manual labor, during - ang.
melancholy, with - zinc.
menses, during - ***fl-ac.,*** stram.
before - acon., coca, fl-ac., hyos.
misfortune of others, from - ars.
morbidly - aur-s.
morning - bor., bov., calc-s., carb-s., caust., cinnb., con., fl-ac., graph., hep., hura, lach., nat-s., ***plat.,*** psor., spig., sulph., zinc.
8 a.m. - hura.
air, in open - plat.
flatus, after emission of - carb-s.
rising, on - hydr.
sad in evening, and - calc-s., graph.
waking on - aloe, clem., hydr., nux-m., tarent.
music, from - ***croc.***
never - **HEP.,** ***nit-ac.***
night - alum., bell., caust., croc., cupr., cypr., hyos., kreos., lyc., nitro-o., op., ph-ac., sep., sil., stram., sulph., verat.
2 a.m. - ***chin.***
pain, with all - spig.
after - form.
paroxysms, in - aur-i.
perspiration, during - apis, ars., bell., clem.
pollutions, after - pip-m.
quarrelsome, and - ***bell., staph.***
room, in the, amel. - tarent.
sadness, after (see alternating with sadness) - cench., orig.
seriousness, with - ***chin.,*** spong.
sex, after - nat-m.
shouting - ***chin.***
simulates hilarity, while he feels wretched - apis.
sleep, during - alum., bell., caust., croc., hyos., kreos., lyc., ph-ac., sil., sulph.
stools, after - ***bor.,*** calc., nat-c., **NAT-S.,** ox-ac.
supper, after - cist.
thoughtless - arn.
thunders and lightens, when it - bell-p., ***carc.,*** lyc., **SEP.**
urination, after - erig., eug., hyos., ***bor.***
waking, on - ***sulph.,*** tarent.
walking, in open air, on and after - alum., ang., cinnb., fl-ac., plb., tarent., teucr.

CHILDBED, mental symptoms during - ***bell.,*** **PLAT.,** ***puls.,*** **SEP.,** sulph., verat., zinc.
agg. - acon., sec., ***sep.,*** stram.

CHILDISH, behavior - acon., aeth., ***agar.,*** alco., aloe, alum., ambr., **ANAC.,** ***apis, arg-n.,*** arn., ars., **BAR-C.,** ***bar-m.,*** **BELL.,** bov., ***bufo,*** calad., calc., carb-an., ***carb-s.,*** carb-v., chlol., **CIC.,** con., ***croc.,*** crot-c., ***hell.,*** **HYOS.,** ign., kali-br., kres., lach., lyc., ***nat-c., nux-m.,*** nux-v., ***op.,*** par., ***ph-ac.,*** phos., pic-ac., plb., puls., rhus-t., seneg., sep., sil., ***stram.,*** sulph., thyr., tub., verat., viol-o.
body grows, but - bufo.
childbirth, after - apis.
epilepsy, after - tab.
before - caust.
naive - bar-c., bell., bov., stram.
old age, in - **BAR-C.**

CHILDREN, (see Children, chapter)
aversion to (see Aversion) - plat., ***sep.***
abandons, his own, flies from - lyc.
covering their face with their hands, but look through their fingers - bar-c.
desires to, beat - chel.
to, have, to beget - nat-m., ox-ac.
dislikes her own - glon., ***lyc.,*** plat., **SEP.,** verat.
especially little girls - raph.
impatient with - anac., ***nux-v.***
watchful, who are on the look out for every gesture - phos.

CLAIRVOYANCE - ***acon., anac.,*** anh., arn., benz., calc., ***cann-i.,*** carc., ***crot-c.,*** dat-a., hydroph., hyos., lach., ***lyss.,*** mag-arct., ***med.,*** nabal., ***nux-m.,*** op., ***phos.,*** pyrus, sil., stann., stram., tarent., valer., ***verat-v.***
midnight - cann-i.
sleep, during - com.

CLIMB, desire to - hyos., stram.
convulsions, before - **CIC.**
walls, climbs during delirum - ***bell.***

CLINGING, child awakens terrified, knows no one, screams, clings to those near - ***acon., ars.,*** **BOR.,** cham., cina, stram.
convulsions, before - **CIC.**
grasps at others - ***ant-t.,*** ars., ***camph.,*** op., phos.
bystanders - **ANT-T.**
the nurse when carried - ***ars.,*** bor., ***gels.,*** puls.
held, wants to be - acon., ***ars., cham.,*** gels., kali-p., lach., nux-m., nux-v., **PULS.,** sang., sep., stram.
amel. being - diph., **PULS.**
restlessness, with - ***ars., carb-v.***
take the hand of mother, will always - ars., bar-c., ***bism., phos.,*** puls.
to persons or furnitiure - ***bar-c.,*** bism., bor., coff., gels., phos., stram.

CLOSING, eyes amel. mental symptoms - kali- c., zinc.

CLOTHED, improperly - hell., ***hyos.,*** sec., stram., ***sulph.***

COLORS, reaction to
aversion to, black - tarent.
blue, aversion to - tarent.
blue, green, red, charmed by - tarent.

COLORS, reaction to
bright - ***sil.***
red - ***alum.***
red, yellow, green and black - ***tarent.***

COMA, (see Brain, Coma)

COMMUNICATIVE, expansive - acon., alum., bar-c., carc., hydrc., ***lach.,*** lyc.

COMPANY, general
aversion to - achy., acon., agar., allox., ***aloe,*** **ALUM.,** alum-p., alum-sil., alumn., ***ambr.,*** **ANAC.,** anan., ant-c., ant-t., arag., ***arg-n.,*** arist-cl., arn., ***ars., ars-m.,*** atro., ***aur.,*** aur-i., ***aur-s.,*** **BAR-C.,** bar-i., bar-m., bar-s., ***bell.,*** bov., ***bry.,*** buf-s., ***bufo, cact.,*** cadm-met., calc., calc-i., ***calc-p.,*** calc-s., camph., cann-i., caps., **CARB-AN.,** carb-s., ***carb-v.,*** carc., cedr., cench., **CHAM.,** ***chin.,*** **CIC.,** cimic., cinnb., clem., coca, ***coloc., con.,*** convo-s., cop., cortico., ***cupr.,*** cur., ***cycl., dig.,*** dios., elaps, eug., euph., ***ferr.,*** ferr-i., ferr-p., fl-ac., **GELS.,** graph., grat., ham., ***hell.,*** helon., ***hep., hipp.,*** hydr., ***hyos.,*** **IGN.,** ***iod.,*** jug-c., kali-bi., kali-br., kali-c., kali-i., kali-p., kali-s., ***lac-d., lach., led.,*** lil-t., ***lyc.,*** mag-aust., mag-c., mag-m., mang., meny., meph., moly-met., murx., ***nat-c.,*** **NAT-M.,** nat-p., nat-s., nicc., **NUX-V.,** op., ***oxyt., pall.,*** pana., petr., ph-ac., phos., pic-ac., ***plat., plb.,*** prot., ptel., psor., ***puls., rhus-t.,*** sapin., sec., ***sel., sep.,*** sieg., ***stann.,*** **STAPH.,** stram., sul-i., sulfonam., ***sulph.,*** sul-ac., ***syph., tarent.,*** tep., thala., thiop., ***thuj.,*** til., trinit., tub., ust., verat., x-ray.
alone agg., when, and amel. in company - alum-sil.
amel., when - allox., ambr., ***bar-c.,*** bov., carb-an., con., convo-s., cortico., cycl., ferr., ferr-p., halo., hell., iris, ***lyc.,*** mag-c., mag-s., ***nat-c., nat-m.,*** petr., ph-ac., phos., ***plb.,*** rauw., **SEP.,** stann., staph., stram., sulph., trio., visc.
yet dreads being - ars., bufo, ***clem., con.,*** elaps, kali-br., ***lyc.,*** **NAT-C.,** ***sep.,*** stram., tarent.
alternating with, bursts of pleasantry and sarcasm - rad-br., rhus-r.
desire for company - acon.
avoids the sight of people - acon., ars., calc., **CIC.,** ***cupr.,*** cur., ferr., ***gels., iod., lac-d., led., nat-c., nat-m.,*** puls., ***sep., thuj.***
and lies with closed eyes - sep.
shuts herself up - cur.
wants to get into the country away from people, - calc., elaps.
bear anybody, cannot - merc., nux-v., staph., ***sulph.***
childbirth, after - ***sep., thuj.***
crying, with - ***rhus-t.***
agg. - ***cycl.***
desire for - acon., act-sp., aeth., agar., all-s., ant-t., ***apis,*** **ARG-N., ARS.,** ars-h., asaf., aur-m., bell., **BISM.,** bov., brom., bry., bufo, cadm-s., ***calc.,*** calc-ar., calc-p., ***camph.,***

COMPANY, general
desire for - carb-v., caust., cench., ***clem.,*** coloc., ***con.,*** cot., crot-c., crot-h., cyna., der., dros., ***elaps,*** fl-ac., ***gels.,*** hep., **HYOS.,** ***ign., kali-ar.,*** kali-br., **KALI-C.,** ***kali-p.,*** **LAC-C.,** lach., ***lil-t.,*** **LYC.,** manc., merc., ***mez.,*** naja, ***nat-c.,*** nit-ac., ***nux-v., pall.,*** ph-ac., **PHOS.,** plb., **PULS.,** rad., ran-b., rat., ***sep.,*** sil., stann., ***stram., stry.,*** sulph., syph., tab., tarent., thymol., verat., verb., zinc., zinc-p.
alone, while agg. - aeth., agar., ambr., ant-t., ***apis,*** **ARS.,** asaf., bell., bism., bov., brom., bufo, calc., cadm-s., calc-s., ***camph.,*** cedr., clem., con., ***dros.,*** elaps, ***fl-ac.,*** gels., **HEP.,** ***hyos., kali-c.,*** lach., lil-t., ***lyc., merc., mez.,*** nat-c., nat-m., ***pall.,*** ph-ac., **PHOS.,** plb., ran-b., rat., sep., sil., stann., ***stram.,*** tab., trif-r., zinc.
yet fear of people - ars., bufo, clem., con., tarent.
evening - brom., dros., kali-c., plb., puls., ran-b., tab., thiop.
friend, of a - plb.
happen, as if something horrible might - ***elaps***
headache, during - meny.
menses, during - stram.
night - ***camph.,*** **STRAM.,** tab.
spoken to, but averse to being - achy.
wants to be watched constantly - gall-ac.
yet treats them outrageously - ***kali-c.***
desires solitude to, indulge her fancy - ***lach.***
lie with closed eyes - sep.
practice masturbation - ***bufo,*** thuj., ust.
forenoon - alum.
friends, of intimate - bell., cham., coloc., ***ferr.,*** hep., ***iod., nat-c., sel.***
heat, during - con., hyos., ***puls.***
ill, at ease - coca
loathing, at company - bell., ign., lyc., nux-v., sep., staph.
meeting, of friends, amel. - alum., puls.
whom he imagines he has offended - ars.
menses, during - ***con.,*** plat., sapin., sep.
desires to be let alone - cic., nux-v.
morning - alum.
perspiration, during - ars., ***bell.,*** lach., lyc., puls., sep.
pregnant, when - lach., ***nat-m.,*** nux-m.
presence of, people intolerable to her, stool, during - **AMBR.,** ***nat-m.***
urination, during - ambr., hep., mur-ac., **NAT-M.,** tarent.
strangers, to - **AMBR.,** ***bar-c., bry.,*** bufo, ***carb-v.,*** caust., **CIC.,** cina, ***con.,*** cupr., ***iod.,*** lach., lyc., nat-m., petr., phos., ***sep., stram.,*** tarent., ***thuj.***
sits, in her room, does nothing - brom., puls.
smiling, faces - ***ambr.***
solitude, fond of - nat-c., **NAT-M.**
walk, alone, want to - caj.

COMPLAINING - acet-ac., acon., alco., aloe, ***alum.***, ambr., anac., ***ant-c.***, arn., **ARS.**, asaf., ***aur.***, bell., ***bism.***, bor., ***bry.***, ***bufo***, ***calc.***, ***calc-p.***, ***canth.***, caps., carc., caust., ***cham.***, chin., chin-a., **CINA,** cocc., ***coff.***, colch., ***coloc.***, ***cor-r.***, cori-r., crot-h., dig., dulc., goss., hell., hep., hyos., ign., indol., kali-c., kali-i., kiss., ***lach.***, ***lyc.***, mag-p., ***merc.***, merc-c., ***mosch.***, **NIT-AC.**, ***nux-v.***, op., ph-ac., petr., ***phos.***, plat., psor., puls., rheum, rhus-a., rhus-t., sep., sil., spira., staph., ***sulph.***, tab., tarent., tub., tus-f., ***verat.***, verat-v., zinc.
- alternating with screaming - bufo
- children, in - anac., ***ant-c.***, **ARS.**, bell., ***bism.***, bor., ***bry.***, ***bufo***, **CALC-P.**, caps., caust., **CHAM.**, **CINA,** ***coloc.***, hep., hyos., ***ign.***, ***lach.***, ***lyc.***, mag-p., ***merc.***, **NIT-AC.**, ***nux-v.***, psor., puls., rheum, rhus-t., sil., staph., ***sulph.***, tab., tarent., **TUB.**, ***verat.***, zinc.
- complaining and threathening - tarent.
- day and night - ***coloc.***
- disease, of - ***ant-t.***, **LACH.**, ***nux-v.***, ph-ac.
- menopausal period, during - ***kali-br.***
- morning in bed - prun.
- night in sleep - nux-v.
- offences long past - calc.
- others, of - sep.
- pain, of - ars-h., ***mosch.***, ***nux-v.***
  - on waking - prun., verat.
- pitiful - ars.
- plaintive, in sleep - stann.
- pregnancy, during - ***mosch.***
- relations and surroundings, of - ***merc.***
- sleep, in - bell., con., ign., nux-v., sulph.
  - comatose - anac., op.
- supposed injury, of - ***hyos.***
- threatening, and - tarent.
- trifles, of - ***lach.***
- waking, on - cina.

COMPLAINTS, broods over imaginary - naja.
- describe, cannot properly - puls.

COMPREHENSION, (see Understanding)

CONCENTRATION, general

active - alum., anac., ***anh.***, calc., calc-f., caust., coca, cod., ***coff.***, coff-t., hell., hyos., nat-m., nux-v., olnd., op., ox-ac., ***phos.***, rhus-t., staph., sulph., ***syph.***, thea.
- menses, after - ***calc.***
  - before - calc.

aversion, to - calc., ***gels.***, lyc., med., nux-v., phos., ***ph-ac.***, plb., ***sil.***, staph.

difficult - ***acon.***, acon-c., acon-l., ***aesc.***, ***aeth.***, agar., ***agn.***, ail., alco., alet., all-c., allox., aloe, ***alum.***, alum-p., alum-sil., am-m., ***ambr.***, **ANAC.**, ang., ant-c., ***apis***, ange-s., aq-mar., arag., ***arg-m.***, arg-n., arn., ars., ars-i., asaf., asar., atro., aur., aven., bapt., **BAR-C.**, bar-i., ***bar-m.***, bar-s., bell., berb., ***bov.***, brom., bry., bufo, buth-a., cact., cadm-met., calad., ***calc.***, ***calc-f.***, calc-sil., camph., ***cann-i.***, cann-s., ***canth.***, caps., carb-ac., ***carb-an.***, carb-o., **CARB-S.**, **CARB-V.**, **CARC.**, **CAUST.**, cench., cent., cham., chel., chin., chin-s., chlol., chlorpr., cic., ***cimic.***, cinnb., clem., cob-n.,

CONCENTRATION, general

difficult - coca, ***cocc.***, cod., coff., colch., coloc., ***con.***, coni., ***corn.***, cortico., cortiso., croc., ***cupr.***, cycl., ***dros.***, des-ac., ***dulc.***, elaps, erig., ery-a., esp-g., euph-hy., euphr., eys., fago., ferr., ferr-ar., ferr-i., ferr-p., fl-ac., ***gels.***, **GLON.**, glyc., goss., **GRAPH.**, grat., halo., ham., ***hell.***, helo., hipp., hir., hist., hura, hydr., ***hydr-ac.***, hydroph., ***hyos.***, iber., ichth., ictod., ign., indol., iod., irid., iris, jug-c., jug-r., kali-ar., kali-br., ***kali-c.***, kali-i., kali-p., kali-s., kali-sil., kalm., ***lac-c.***, **LACH.**, lact., lam., laur., **LEC.**, led., levo., lil-s., ***lil-t.***, lol., **LYC.**, lycps., lyss., macro., mag-c., mag-m., man., mang., ***med.***, meph., ***merc.***, merc-c., merl., ***mez.***, morph., mosch., myric., myris., narcot., **NAT-A.**, ***nat-c.***, ***nat-m.***, nat-p., nicot., ***nit-ac.***, **NUX-M.**, **NUX-V.**, oci-s., olnd., ol-an., onop., onos., op., orig., ox-ac., petr., **PH-AC.**, **PHOS.**, phys., ***pic-ac.***, pituin., ***plat.***, plect., psor., ptel., ***puls.***, ran-b., ran-s., raph., rhod., rauw., rhus-r., rhus-t., ***rhus-v.***, rib-ac., sabad., sang., sanic., sant., saroth., sarr., sars., scut., sec., ***sel.***, senec., seneg., **SEP.**, **SIL.**, sin-a., spig., ***spong.***, squil., stann., staph., stict., ***stram.***, sul-ac., ***sulph.***, sumb., ***syph.***, ***tab.***, tanac., tarax., ***ter.***, ***thuj.***, til., trio., tub., upa., ven-m., verat., verb., viol-o., xero, ***zinc.***, zinc-p.
- abstract things - med.
- afternoon - ang., cham., ery-a., myris., sang.
- air, amel. in open - nat-a.
- alternating with uterine pains - gels.
- attempting to concentrate it becomes dark before the eyes, on - arg-n.
- aversion to - calc., lyc., nux-v., ph-ac., plb., staph.
- calculating, while - **NUX-V.**, **SIL.**
- can't fix attention - ***aesc.***, ***aeth.***, bov., hipp., hyos., ign., med., ***phos.***, **SIL.**, **SIN-N.**, verat.
- children, in - ***aeth.***, am-c., **BAR-C.**, ***carc.***, graph., lach., med., ph-ac., ***phos.***, sil., zinc.
- conversation, during - lyc., sulph.
- crazy feeling on top of head, wild feeling in head, with confusion of ideas - lil-t.
- dark before the eyes, on attempting to it becomes - arg-n.
- drawing, when - iod.
- eating, amel., from - ***calc-f.***, cina, phos.
- evening - am-m., nat-c.
- forenoon - ptel., sil., til.
- headache, with - cob-n., ***dulc.***, ***kali-c.***
- interrupted, if - berb., mez.
- masturbation, from - aven.
- menses, after - ***calc.***
- morning - ***anac.***, canth., phos.
- studying, reading, while - acon., **AETH.**, agar., ***agn.***, alum., ambr., ang., asar., ***bar-c.***, bar-m., bell., calc-f., calc-sil., carb-ac., carb-s., caust., cham., coff., corn., ***dros.***, fago., ferr-i., **HELL.**, iod., kali-bi., kali-c., ***kali-p.***, kali-sil., lach., lyc., merc., mur-ac., nat-a., ***nat-c.***, nat-p., **NUX-V.**, olnd., ox-ac., ***phos.***, pic-ac., scut., **SIL.**,

CONCENTRATION, general
studying, reading, while - sin-a., spig., ***staph.,*** sul-i., sulph., ***syph.,*** tab., zinc-p.
learns with difficulty - **AGAR.,** agn., ***anac., ars., bar-c.,*** calc., calc-p., caste., caust., con., kali-sil., ***lyc.,*** mag-p., nat-m., olnd., okou., ph-ac., ***phos.,*** rib-ac., sil.
talking, while - merc-c., ***nat-m.***
vacant feeling, has a - ***asar., gels.,*** mez., nat-m., ***nit-ac.,*** olnd., phos., ***ran-b., staph.***
working, while - plect.
writing, while - acon., mag-c.

CONFIDENCE, lacking of self esteem - agn., alum., am-c., am-m., ambr., **ANAC.,** anan., ang., anh., arg-n., ars., **AUR.,** aur-i., aur-s., bar-ac., **BAR-C.,** bell., ***bry.,*** buth-a., calc., **CALC-F.,** calc-sil., canth., carb-an., carb-v., **CARC.,** caust., ***chin.,*** chlor., cob., cocc., dros., ferr., gels., hyos., ign., iod., ***kali-c.,*** kali-n., **KALI-P.,** kali-s., kali-sil., ***lac-c.,*** lach., **LYC.,** manc., ***med.,*** merc., mur-ac., naja, nat-c., ***nat-m.,*** nat-s., nit-ac., nitro-o., ***nux-v.,*** olnd., op., pall., **PETR.,** phos., pic-ac., plb., **PSOR.,** ***puls.,*** ran-b., ***rhus-t.,*** ruta, sant., **SIL., STAPH.,** stram., sul-i., sulph., sul-ac., sumb., syph., tab., ther., ***thuj.,*** verat., verb., viol-t., zinc.
beer amel. - thea.
children, in - ***anac.,*** arg-n., ars., aur., **BAR-C.,** ***calc.,*** **CALC-F.,** calc-p., calc-sil., carb-v., **CARC.,** caust., gels., hyos., ign., ***kali-p.,*** kali-s., ***lac-c.,*** lach., **LYC.,** ***med.,*** merc., nat-c., **NAT-M.,** nat-s., nit-ac., phos., ***psor., puls.,*** sant., **SIL., STAPH.,** stram., syph., ***thuj.,*** verat.
failure, feels himself a - **AUR.,** ***lyc.,*** naja, ***staph.,*** sulph.
performance anxiety, with - arg-n., gels., ***lyc.***
want of self, and thinks others have none which makes her unhappy - ***aur.***

CONFIDING - hydrc., kres., mur-ac., op., spig.

CONFOUNDING, objects and ideas, (see Mistakes) - calc., cann-s., hyos., nux-v., plat., ***sulph.***
present and past - anac., cann-i., cic.

CONFUSION, mental - absin., acet-ac., ***acon.,*** acon-f., act-sp., ***aesc.,*** aesc-g., ***aeth., agar.,*** agn., ail., alco., all-c., aloe, ***alum.,*** alum-sil., ***am-br.,*** ambr., am-c., am-m., aml-n., amyg., ***anac.,*** anac-oc., ang., ant-c., ***ant-t.,*** anthr., apis, ***apoc., arag.,*** aran., arg-m., **ARG-N.,** ***arn., ars.,*** ars-i., asaf., ***asar.,*** aspar., aster., astra-e., ***atro., aur.,*** aur-m., ***bapt., bar-c.,*** bar-i., ***bar-m.,*** **BELL.,** bell-p., benz-ac., berb., ***bism., bor.,*** both., ***bov.,*** brom., **BRY.,** ***bufo,*** cadm-s., calad., **CALC.,** calc-i., ***calc-p.,*** calc-s., ***calc-sil.,*** camph., **CANN-I.,** ***cann-s., canth., caps.,*** carb-ac., ***carb-an.,*** carb-h., carb-o., ***carb-s.,*** **CARB-V.,** carc., carl., caust., cham., ***chel., chin.,*** chin-a., chin-s., chlf., chlol., chlor., chloram., chlorpr., chr-ac., cic., cina, cinnb., cimx., clem., coca, **COCC.,** ***coc-c.,*** cod., ***coff.,*** coff-t., coffin., ***colch., coloc.,*** com., ***con.,*** convo-s., cop., corn., cortico., cortiso., cot., ***croc., crot-c., crot-h.,*** crot-t., cund., ***cupr.,*** cupr-ar., cur., cycl., dat-a., dig., dios., dirc., ***dros., dulc.,*** echi., ery-a., ether, eug., eup-pur., euphr., eupi., ***fago., ferr.,*** ferr-ar., ferr-p., fl-ac., form., galin., ***gels.,*** gent-l., gins., **GLON.,** gran., ***graph.,*** grat., halo., **HELL.,** hep., hipp., hura, hydr., hydr-ac., **HYOS.,** ***hyper.,*** iber., ign., indg., iod., ip., ir-foe., piloc., jatr., jug-c., kali-ar., kali-bi., kali-br., ***kali-c., kali-i.,*** kali-n., kali-p., kali-s., kalm., ***kreos., lac-c.,*** **LACH.,** lac-ac., lact., ***laur., lec.,*** led., lil-t., lob., lol., ***lyc.,*** lyss., ***mag-c.,*** mag-m., mag-s., man., **MED.,** meli., menthol, ***meny.,*** meph., **MERC.,** merc-c., ***mez.,*** moly-met., morph., ***mosch.,*** mur-ac., murx., myric., naja, narcot., nat-a., ***nat-c.,*** **NAT-M.,** nat-p., nat-s., nicc., nit-ac., nitro-o., **NUX-M., NUX-V.,** oci-s., oena., ***olnd.,*** **ONOS., OP.,** osm., par., parathyr., ped., peti., **PETR., PH-AC.,** phel., ***ph-ac.,*** **PHOS.,** phys., plan., **PLAT.,** ***plb.,*** plb-chr., ***psor.,*** ptel., ***puls., pyrog.,*** querc., ran-b., ran-s., raph., rauw., rheum, **RHUS-T.,** rhod., ruta, ***sabad.,*** sabin., sal-ac., samb., sang., sars., ***sec.,*** sel., senec., ***seneg.,*** **SEP., SIL.,** ***spig.,*** spira., spong., squil., stann., ***staph.,*** stict., **STRAM.,** stront-c., **STRY.,** sul-ac., sulfa., ***sulph.,*** syph., ***tab.,*** tanac., tarax., ter., teucr., ther., thiop., ***thuj.,*** thymol., trom., tub., vac., valer., ***verat.,*** verb., viol-o., viol-t., vip., xan., xero, ***zinc.,*** **ZINC-P.**
afternoon - agar., alumn., asaf., bry., calc., cann-s., carb-v., cham., chel., chin., clem., coloc., crot-t., ery-a., ferr., graph., hell., hyos., kali-bi., kali-c., kali-cy., lac-ac., laur., nat-m., nux-v., op., petr., phel., sabin., sep., sulph., verat-v., zinc.
air, in open - agar., caust., colch., con., crot-t., hyos., mag-c., nit-ac., nux-v., rhod., spig., sulph.
amel. - acon., am-m., ant-t., ars., aur-m., bar-c., bar-s., bell., bry., calc-s., clem., coc-c., croc., dulc., glon., grat., hydr-ac., kali-s., mag-m., mag-s., mang., meny., merc., nat-c., par., phos., ***psor.,*** phyt., rat., sulph.
arouse himself, compelled to - **CARB-V.,** ***sulph.***
ascending agg. - ptel., ***sulph.***
bed, while in - ambr., calc., phos., rhod.
amel. - nat-c.
jump out of, makes him - ars., cic., merc.
beer, from - bell., calc., chin., ***coloc.,*** con., cor-r., crot-t., ign., phos., ***zinc.***
belching, amel. - bry., gent-c., sang.
bread agg. - crot-t.
breakfast, after - calad., coc-c.
amel. - bov., mag-c.
before - calc., fl-ac.
calculating, when - nat-m., ***nux-v., psor., syph.***
carousal, after a - gran., **NUX-V.**
as after a - ph-ac.
carrying heavy loads, when - agar.

CONFUSION, mental
chill, during - acon., aloe, ***caps., cham.,*** cic., coff., con., dros., hell., hyos., kali-c., nat-c., nux-m., phos., plb., rhus-t., ruta, stram., verat., viol-t.
closing eyes, on - atro.
coffee, after - all-c., arg-n., calc-p., mill.
amel. - coca, hipp.
cold, bath, amel. - calc-p., euphr., ***phos.***
cold, taking a, after - phos.
concentrate the mind, on attempting to - asar., gels., mez., nat-c., nat-m., nit-ac., olnd., ran-b., staph.
conversation, agg. - ***sil.***
convulsions, before - ***lach.***
cough, before paroxysm of - cina
crying, amel. - ***sep.***
daily, affairs, about - lyc.
dimness, of eyes, with - til.
dinner, after - arg-n., carb-v., euphr., mag-m., nux-v., petr., phos., plan., tab., thuj., zinc.
dinner, during - mag-m.
dream, as if in - ail., arn., calc., carb-an., cupr., meli., ***cann-i.,*** cann-s., ***carb-v.,*** cham., chin., grat., guai., ign., ***lec.,*** mez., ***phos.,*** rhus-t., sep., spig., squil., sulph., thuj., zinc.
drinking, after - bell., bry., **COCC.,** con., croc.
drowsiness, while resisting - coca
duality, sense of - ***alum.,*** **ANAC.,** anh., arg-n., **BAPT.,** calc-p., cann-s., cycl., des-ac., ***gels.,*** lach., lyc., naja, nat-m., nux-m., op., paro-i., **PETR.,** phos., plat., plb., psor., puls., ***pyrog.,*** sec., sil., ***stram.,*** ther., thuj., tril., xan.
eating, after - agar., ambr., apis, aran., arg-n., bell., bufo, ***calc.,*** calc-sil., ***carb-v.,*** caust., **COCC.,** coc-c., coloc., croc., cycl., euphr., ferr., ferr-p., grat., hyos., lach., led., lob., ***lyc.,*** mag-m., meny., ***merc., mez.,*** mill., nat-c., ***nat-m.,*** nat-p., nat-sil., nit-ac., ***nux-v.,*** olnd., op., petr., ***ph-ac., phos.,*** plan., **PULS.,** sabad., sabin., ***sep., sil., sulph.,*** tab., thuj., zinc., zinc-p.
amel. - agar., apis, caust., fago., jug-r., lach., mez., phos.
emissions - ***sel.,*** sumb.
epileptic attack, after - plb., sil.
before - lach., plb., sil.
evening - aloe, am-c., aran., ars., ars-i., bar-c., bar-s., bell., bor., bov., calc., calc-ar., calc-s., calc-sil., cann-s., carb-an., ***carb-v.,*** cedr., cham., chin-s., coc-c., coloc., corn., cycl., dig., dios., dros., dulc., euphr., ferr., ferr-ar., ferr-i., ferr-p., graph., hipp., iod., ip., kali-ar., kali-c., kali-n., kali-p., kali-s., kali-sil., kalm., ***lyc.,*** mag-s., mez., mill., murx., nat-a., nat-c., nat-m., nat-p., nat-sil., ***nux-m.,*** nux-v., ph-ac., phos., psor., ptel., puls., rhus-t., ruta, sars., sep., sil., spig., stann., sul-i., sulph., sul-ac., thuj., valer., zinc., zinc-p.
amel. - sars.
excitement, amel. - chin., cycl.
forenoon - phys., sep., sulph.

CONFUSION, mental
hat, putting on, agg. - calc-p., ferr-i.
head separated from body, as if - allox., cocc., ***daph.,*** **PSOR.**
headache, with - agar., con., nat-m., petr., phos., sil., tarax., xan., zinc.
heat, during - alum., arg-m., ***bapt.,*** bry., bufo, camph., cham., chin., coc-c., coloc., dros., ***hyos.,*** ign., ip., laur., nat-c., op., phos., puls., raja-s., sep., tab., thuj., valer., verat.
identity, as to his - **ALUM.,** ***anh.,*** ant-c., aur., bapt., camph., cann-s., kali-br., lach., med., nat-m., petr., phos., plb., pyrus, stram., sulph., thuj., valer.
injury to head, after - arn., ***hell.,*** **NAT-S.**
interruption, from - berb., ***mez.***
intoxicated, as after being - acon., agar., am-m., anac., ang., arg-m., bell., ***bry.,*** camph., ***carb-v., chin.,*** clem., cocc., coloc., cor-r., croc., **DIG.,** dulc., ***glon.,*** grin., kali-c., kali-n., lam., laur., mosch., nat-m., ***nux-v.,*** op., ***ph-ac.,*** psor., puls., rheum, sabin., squil., valer.
as if intoxicated - ***acon.,*** agar., amyg., anan., ant-c., arg-m., asar., **BAPT.,** bell., bism., bufo, ***carb-o.,*** **CARB-S.,** ***carb-v.,*** chin-s., cupr., ***dig., glon.,*** graph., grat., grin., hyos., ign., kali-c., kali-n., lach., laur., led., lyc., mag-c., mag-m., mez., ***nux-m.,*** nux-v., phel., ph-ac., ran-b., rhus-t., sabad., ***sil.,*** spong., thuj., tong., visc.
spirituous liquors, from - ***alum.,*** bell., bov., ***con.,*** cor-r., **NUX-V.,** petr., stront-c.
knows not where she is nor whenever came to objects around her - ***aesc.,*** coff-t., ***mez.***
laughing, agg. - ther.
location, about - cic., ***glon., nux-m., petr.***
loses, his way in well-known streets - **GLON.,** ***merc., nux-m.,*** nux-v., ***petr.,*** plb., puls., ran-b., thuj.
lying, amel. - nat-m.
lying, when - brom., bry., ***carb-v.,*** cham., ***grat.,*** lil-t., mag-m., merc., rhus-r., sep.
masturbation, from - ***gels.***
menses, during - am-c., cimic., cocc., graph., lyc., phos.
after - graph., nat-m.
before - cimic., ***sep.***
mental exertion, from - ang., ant-t., apis, aran., ***aur.,*** aur-s., bor., ***calc., calc-p., calc-s.,*** canth., carb-s., ***carb-v., caust.,*** cham., ***cocc.,*** euon., ***gels.,*** hep., iod., ***kali-sil.,*** laur., ***lyc.,*** mag-c., mag-m., mez., **NAT-C.,** ***nat-m., nat-p.,*** **NAT-SIL.,** ***nit-ac., nux-m., nux-v.,*** olnd., ox-ac., petr., ***ph-ac., phos., pic-ac., puls.,*** ran-b., scut., ***sep., sil., staph.,*** sul-i., ***sulph.,*** thuj.
amel. - carb-v.
miscarriage, after - helon., ruta.
mixes subjective and objective - calc., cann-s., hyos., nux-v., plat., sulph.

CONFUSION, mental

morning - acon., agar., aloe, alum., alum-p., alum-sil., ambr., am-m., ***anac.,*** ant-t., arg-n., arn., ars., ars-i., arum-t., asaf., asar., aur., aur-a., aur-i., aur-s., ***bar-c.,*** bar-s., bell., bism., bov., ***bry.,*** bufo, ***calc.,*** calc-ar., ***calc-s.,*** canth., caps., ***carb-an.,*** carb-s., ***carb-v.,*** caust., cham., chel., ***chin.,*** chin-a., chin-s., ***chlol.,*** cic., clem., cob., cocc., ***colch.,*** coloc., con., corn., crot-h., euphr., ferr-ar., ferr-p., ***graph.,*** hyos., hyper., ign., iod., jug-r., kali-ar., kali-c., kali-n., kali-p., kali-s., **LACH.,** lact., lyc., mag-c., mag-m., mag-s., merc., mill., mosch., murx., ***nat-c.,*** nat-m., nat-p., nat-s., nicc., nux-v., op., ox-ac., petr., ph-ac., phos., podo., ran-b., ran-s., ***rhod., rhus-t.,*** ruta, samb., sars., seneg., sep., sil., squil., stann., staph., stry., sul-i., **SULPH.,** sul-ac., sumb., ***thuj.,*** til., trif-p., ust., verat., zinc., zinc-p.

rising, after amel. - alum., ant-t., mag-s., phos., rhus-t.

on and after - anac., arg-n., asar., aur., bell., bry., calc., ***carb-v.,*** cham., chel., cic., cina, clem., coc-c., corn., graph., ign., kali-c., kali-sil., lact., mag-c., mag-m., mag-s., merc., merl., nat-m., ped., ph-ac., ***phos.,*** plb., raph., rhod., rhus-t., sabad., samb., sep., sil., sulph.

waking, on - acon., ***aesc.,*** agar., alum., alum-p., alum-sil., ***anac.,*** ant-t., arg-n., ars., ars-s-f., ***bar-c., bry.,*** calc., calc-p., calc-s., calc-sil., cann-s., carb-an., carb-s., ***carb-v.,*** chin-a., cimic., clem., coc-c., euphr., ferr., ferr-ar., graph., hyper., ign., **LACH.,** ***lyc.,*** mag-m., mag-s., merc., merc-i-f., ***naja,*** nat-m., ***phos.,*** puls., rheum, rhod., ruta, ***sil.,*** sulph., ***thuj.,*** til., trif-p., zinc., zinc-p.

motion, from - acon., ambr., bell., bry., calc-p., cob., ign., indg., lob., mosch., nat-c., nux-v., phos., ***puls.,*** tab.

amel. - arg-n., ferr., ferr-p.

head, of - carb-an., sulph.

night - anac., arg-n., calc., cedr., ***chel.,*** corn., crot-t., fl-ac., lyc., mur-ac., phos., psor., ptel., raph., ruta, sec., sep., ***sulph.,*** til.

lying down, on - brom., lil-t., rhus-r.

waking, on - ***chel.,*** chin., ***glon.,*** kali-bi., merc-i-f., mez., phos., plat., psor., puls., sil., sulph.

walking about after midnight, on - ***stram.***

noises, in ear, from - mag-c.

nosebleed, amel. - carb-an., cham.

old age, in - ***bar-c., con.***

paroxysms of pain, during - ***acon.,*** apoc., ***cham., coff.,*** dulc., verat.

periodic - staph.

perspiration, during - ***chin.,*** samb., ***stram.***

pregnancy, during - ***nux-m.***

present for the past - cic.

CONFUSION, mental

reading, while - agar., agn., ***alum.,*** ambr., ang., ***apis, calc.,*** canth., cocc., ferr-i., lil-t., ***lyc.,*** nat-m., nux-m., ***ph-ac.***

if he attempts to understand it - ***olnd.***

riding, while - bry., sil.

rising, after - ***alum.,*** aur., bell., bov., bry., kali-c., laur., merc., nat-m., nat-s., phos., rhod.

room, in - ars., mag-c.

scratching, ear, behind - calc.

head, right side of - sul-ac.

sex, after - bov., calc., caust., mez., ***ph-ac.,*** phos., rhod., sel., sep.

sitting, while - am-c., asaf., asar., bar-c., bell., calc., calc-sil., carb-an., caust., cic., colch., kali-c., kali-sil., mang., merc., nat-c., nat-m., nit-ac., op., phos., phyt., puls., ***rhus-t.,*** sabad., sars., sep., sil., spig., sul-ac., thuj., valer., verat.

situations, of - anh.

sleepiness, with - echi., gels., nux-m., pip-m.

sleeping, after - ambr., anac., ars., bry., calc., carb-v., ***con.,*** graph., hep., lach., op., squil., ***sulph.,*** uran-n.

siesta - calc., carb-v., chel., **CON.,** graph., mill., phos.

a long - kali-c.

smoking, after - alum., bell., ferr-i., gels., petr., thuj.

spirituous liquors, from - ***alum.,*** bell., bov., ***con.,*** cor-r., **NUX-V.,** petr., stront-c.

spoken to, when - ***sep.***

standing, while - bov., bry., cic., grat., lith., plb., staph., thuj., valer., verat.

standing, while, amel. - ir-foe.

stitches in chest, from - sep.

stool amel. - ***bor.,*** mag-s., ***nat-s.***

stooping, when - bov., calc., caust., coloc., corn., ***glon.,*** hell., nat-m., nit-ac., phos., spig., valer., vinc.

stooping, when, amel. - verat.

stretching on the couch, on - hep.

sun, in the - ***nat-c.,*** nux-v.

surroundings, of - bell-p.

talking, while - glon., ***nat-m.,*** sep., ***sil.,*** staph., ***thuj.***

thinking of it agg. - hell., olnd.

time, to - halo., **LACH.**

trifles, about - carc.

urination, amel. - ter.

vertigo, with - **COCC.,** ***cupr-ar.,*** sil., stann., ***stram.***

vexation, after - nux-v.

vomiting, amel. - tab.

waking, on - acon., ***aesc.,*** agar., ambr., anac., ant-t., arg-n., ars., bar-c., berb., bov., bry., calad., ***calc.,*** calc-ar., calc-p., caps., ***carb-v.,*** cham., chel., chin., clem., cocc., coc-c., con., euphr., gels., glon., graph., grat., hell., hep., hyper., ign., kali-br., kali-c., kali-n., ***lach., lyc.,*** mag-s., merc., merc-i-f., mez., nat-c., nat-p., nat-sil., nux-m., op., ***petr., ph-ac.,***

CONFUSION, mental

waking, on - **PHOS.,** ***plat.,*** naja, psor., ***puls.,*** rheum, rhod., rhus-t., ruta, ***sep., sil.,*** squil., stann., staph., ***stram., sulph.,*** til., ***zinc.***

children - aesc.

walking, while - agar., ang., arg-n., asar., bell., bor., ***bry.,*** calc., camph., carb-an., carb-v., cic., coc-c., coff., coloc., con., dros., ferr., ***glon.,*** grat., kali-c., ***lach., mez.,*** nat-c., nat-m., nit-ac., ***nux-m., petr.,*** rhus-t., ***sabad.,*** sep., spong., sulph., tarax., thea., thuj., viol-t.

air, in open - acon., agar., ars., carb-v., caust., coff., **GLON.,** kali-chl., lyc., **NUX-M., PETR.,** sep., spig., sulph., tub.

after - nat-m.

after, amel. - caust.

amel. - bry., ***carl.,*** graph., **LYC.,** merc-i-f., merc-i-r., nat-c., par., **PULS.,** rhod., sulph.

amel. - agar., ferr-p., sulph.

midnight, about or after, on walking - ***stram.***

warm room, in - acon., bell., ***iod.,*** kali-s., **LYC.,** merc-i-f., nat-m., phos., ph-ac., **PULS.,** ***sulph.***

washing, the face amel. - ***ars.,*** calc-p., coca, cycl., euphr., ferr-p., ***phos.***

will, strong effort of, amel. - glon.

wine, after - all-c., ***alum.,*** amyg., bov., coloc., con., kali-chl., mill., ox-ac., petr., ***zinc.***

working, while - merc.

wrapping, up head amel. - mag-m.

writing, while - arg-n., brom., croc., ferr-i., gent-l., laur., lil-t., nat-c., vinc.

yawning, amel. - bry.

CONSCIENTIOUS, about trifles - anh., ***apis,*** **ARS.,** ars-s-f., aur., aur-a., aur-i., ***bar-c.,*** bry., calc., calc-p., calc-s., carb-s., **CARC.,** cham., chin., chin-a., cocc., con., cycl., ferr., ferr-ar., ferr-i., graph., hep., hyos., **IGN.,** iod., lac-d., lac-f., ***lyc.,*** med., mez., ***mur-ac.,*** nat-a., **NAT-C.,** nat-sil., ***nux-v.,*** ph-ac., ***puls.,*** sarr., sec., sep., **SIL.,** spig., **STAPH.,** ***stram.,*** sul-i., **SULPH., THUJ.,** verat.

afternoon, 4 to 8 p.m - ***lyc.***

children, in - **ARS.,** ***bar-c.,*** calc., ***calc-p.,*** calc-s., ***carc.,*** cham., hyos., **IGN.,** ***lyc.,*** nat-c., ***nux-v.,*** puls., **SIL.,** ***staph.,*** sul-i., ***sulph., thuj.,*** verat.

eating, after - ign.

morbid - spirae.

pedant - plat., puls., sil.

religious, very - carc., ***ign.,*** **LYC.,** nat-m., nux-v., **PULS.,** ***staph.,*** **SULPH.**

trifles, occupied with - ars., cocc., ***graph.,*** lil-t., nit-ac., nux-v., petr., thuj.

CONSOLATION, general

agg., from kind words - arg-n., arn., ***ars.,*** aur., ***bell.,*** cact., calc., ***calc-p.,*** calc-sil., **CARC.,** ***cham.,*** chin., coff., graph., ***hell.,*** **IGN.,** kali-c., kali-p., ***kali-s.,*** kali-sil., kalm., ***lil-t.,*** lyc., merc., **NAT-M.,** ***nit-ac.,*** nux-v., pall., ***plat.,*** sabad., sabal., sabin., **SEP., SIL.,** staph., sulph., **SYPH.,** tarent., thuj., tub., visc.

amel. - asaf., carc., ***phos.,*** **PULS.**

anger, wakes with - ***sabal.,*** senn.

CONSOLATION, general

inconsolable - **ACON.,** ambr., ***ars.,*** asar., brom., calc-p., ***caust., cham., chin.,*** cina, coff., dig., **IGN.,** kali-br., ***lyc.,*** nat-c., ***nat-m.,*** nit-ac., **NUX-V.,** ***petr.,*** phos., ***plat., puls.,*** rhus-t., sep., sil., ***spong., stann.,*** stram., sulph., ***verat.***

air, amel. in open - coff.

alone and darkness agg - stram.

anxiety about his family during a short journey, from - ***petr.***

crying from consolation, continuous - nat-c.

dreams, in his - tab.

over fancied misfortune - **VERAT.**

suicide, even to - **CHIN.**

refuses, for own misfortune - nat-m., nit-ac.

CONTEMPTUOUS, (see Scorn) - agn., anac., ***aloe,*** alum., ***arg-n.,*** arn., ***ars.,*** bry., canth., caps., cham., ***chin.,*** **CIC.,** cina, com., cycl., guai., hell., hura, hyos., ign., ***ip.,*** lac-ac., lac-c., ***lach., lyc.,*** merc., nat-m., nit-ac., ***nux-v., pall.,*** par., **PLAT.,** puls., sec., sil., spong., stram., **SULPH.,** ***verat.***

air, in open or when sun shines into room, paroxysms against her will - ***plat.***

everything, of - ***chin.,*** cina, ip., **PLAT.**

hard for subordinates and agreable-pleasant to superiors or people he has to fear - lach., lyc., plat., verat.

opponents, for - com.

paroxysms against her will - ***plat.***

ravenous hunger and greedy, hasty eating, with sudden contemptuous - ***plat.***

relations, for - sec.

self, of - ***agn.,*** anac., ***aur.,*** cop., lac-c., ***staph.,*** thuj.

alternating with eccentricity - agn.

CONTENTED, feeling, (see Cheerful) - aloe, alum., arn., aur., ***bor., caps.,*** carb-h., carl., ***cic.,*** coca, cocc., com., cycl., fl-ac., gins., laur., mag-s., meny., mez., nat-c., nat-m., **OP.,** phos., spig., staph., tarax., ***zinc.***

afternoon, after stool - ***bor.***

1 a.m. to 11 p.m. - tus-f.

forgets all his ailments and pains - op.

himself, with - caust., cic., led., mag-s., meny.

night - op.

quietly, and - op.

CONTENTIONS, (see Quarrelsome)

CONTRADICT, disposition to - alum., **ANAC.,** ***apis,*** arn., ***ars., aur.,*** aur-m., bar-c., cael., camph., ***canth.,*** **CAUST.,** ***cupr.,*** ferr., grat., **HEP.,** hyos., ictod., **IGN., LACH.,** ***lyc.,*** mag-c., ***merc.,*** nat-c., nicc., nit-ac., nux-v., ***olnd.,*** ruta, ***sep.,*** staph., sulfonam., sulph., trom., vip-a.

afternoon - ***canth.***

evening, amel. - nicc.

CONTRADICTION, is intolerant of - acon., aloe, alum., alum-sil., am-c., ***anac., ant-c.,*** arn., ars., asaf., asar., aster., **AUR.,** bell., ***bry.,*** cact., calc-p., cann-i., canth., ***caps.,*** carb-s., carc., ***cham.,*** chin., ***cina, colch.,*** coloc., con., ***cocc.,*** echi., ***ferr.,*** glon., grat., hell., ***helon.,*** **HEP.,** hura, hyos., ictod., **IGN.,** lach., ***lyc.,*** med., merc., mez., morph.,

CONTRADICTION, is intolerant of - mur-ac., ***nat-c., nat-m.,*** nicc., nit-ac., nuph., ***nux-v.,*** olnd., op., pall., petr., phos., plan., ***plat.,*** puls., sars., ***sep., sil., staph.,*** stram., ***syph.,*** tarent., thuj., ***thyr.,*** til., ***verat.***
ailments from - anac., ***aur.,*** aur-a., cael., cham., **IGN.,** sil.
agg. - aur., bry., ferr., helon., ***ign.,*** lyc., nux-v., olnd., petros.
evening amel. - nicc.
forenoon - nat-c.
restrain himself to keep from violence, has to - aloe, ***hep.,*** sil.

CONTRADICTORY, intentions are, to actions - ***ign.,*** phos., puls., ruta, sep., thuj.
to speech - acon., alum., am-c., caps., chin., ign., lyc., nux-m., rhus-t., sep.

CONTRARY, (see Irritable, Quarrelsome, Obstinate) - abrot., acon., **ALUM.,** alum-p., alum-sil., ambr., **ANAC.,** anan., ant-c., ***ant-t.,*** **ARG-N.,** ***arn., ars.,*** arum-t., aur., aur-a., ***bar-c.,*** bell., bry., calad., calc., calc-s., calc-sil., camph., canth., caps., carb-an., ***caust.,*** **CHAM.,** chin., cina, ***cocc.,*** con., croc., guai., **HEP.,** ign., ip., ***kali-c.,*** kali-p., kali-sil., kreos., **LACH.,** lact., laur., led., lyc., mag-c., mag-m., **MERC.,** ***nit-ac., nux-v.,*** petr., phos., plb., ***puls.,*** ruta, samb., sars., sep., sil., spong., ***sulph.,*** **TARENT.,** ***thuj.,*** trom.
afternoon - ***canth.***
evening - nicc.

CONTROL, lack of emotional - anac., arg-m., ***arg-n.,*** caust., cham., ign., ***med.,*** olnd., staph., stram., tarent., ***tub.,*** verat.

CONVERSATION, agg. (see Talking) - acon., alum., **AMBR.,** am-c., aur., calc., cann-s., canth., carc, chin., cocc., coff., ferr., dios., ***fl-ac.,*** graph., helon., **IGN.,** iod., kali-c., mag-m., mang., mez., **NAT-M.,** nat-p., ***nux-m., nux-v.,*** ph-ac., plat., puls., ***rhus-t.,*** sars., sep., **SIL.,** spig., staph., sulph., thuj.
amel. - aeth., eup-per., lac-c.
aversion to - ***ambr., ars.,*** ars-s-f., asim., atro., bell., calc., ***carb-an.,*** carc, chel., ferr., gels., murx., ox-ac., plb., ***ptel.,*** thea., ziz.
desire for - ars., chen-a., narcot.
imaginary beings, with - chlol.

COPROPHAGIE, (see Feces)

COSMOPOLITAN, (see Travel)

COUNTING, continually - ***hyos.,*** mosch., phys., sil.

COUNTRY, desire for the - elaps.

COURAGEOUS - acon., agar., alco., alum., ant-t., berb., ***bov., calad.,*** calc-s., caust., dros., ferr-p., gins., ***ign.,*** merc., mez., nat-c., **OP.,** phos., ***puls.,*** squil., sulph., tab., tarax., ter., valer., verat.
alternating with, discouragement - merc., op., staph.
with, fear - ***alum.***
foolish - calad.

COWARDICE, (see Confidence, lacking) - ***acon.,*** agar., agn., alco., alum., alum-sil., **AM-C.,** anac., ang., ant-t., arg-n., ars., aur., aur-s., **BAR-C.,** bar-i., bar-m., bar-s., bell., ***bry.,*** calc., calc-s., ***calc-sil.,*** camph., canth., carb-an., carb-v., caust., cham., ***chin.,*** chin-b., cocc., coloc., con., cupr., dig., dros., **GELS.,** graph., hep., hydr-ac., ign., iod., ip., kali-c., kali-n., kali-p., kali-sil., laur., led., **LYC.,** merc., mur-ac., nat-m., nit-ac., ***nux-m.,*** nux-v., olnd., **OP.,** ph-ac., phos., plat., plb., ***puls., ran-b.,*** rhus-t., ruta, sabin., sec., sep., ***sil.,*** spig., stann., staph., ***stram.,*** sul-i., sulph., sul-ac., tab., ther., thuj., ***verat.,*** verb., viol-t., visc.
anger, with sudden ebullition of - bar-c.
children, in - ***acon.,*** agar., anac., arg-n., ars., **BAR-C.,** bar-i., bar-m., calc., calc-s., ***calc-sil.,*** carb-v., caust., cham., **GELS.,** graph., ign., iod., kali-p., **LYC.,** merc., nat-m., **OP.,** ph-ac., ***phos., puls., sil.,*** staph., ***stram.,*** thuj., ***verat.***
opinion, without courage of own - graph., ign., petr., puls., staph.
sadness, with - ***sulph.***

CRAWLING, on floor - ***acet-ac.,*** bell., cann-i., ***lach.***
bed, around in - ***stram.***
child crawls into corners, howls, cries - camph.
rolling on the floor - acet-ac., ars., ***calc.,*** **OP.,** prot., ***sulph.***

CREDULOUS - bar-c., ***bell., phos., puls.,*** staph.

CRITICAL, censorious - acon., alum-sil., am-c., alum., apis, ***arn.,*** **ARS.,** ars-s-f., aur., aur-a., aur-s., ***bar-c.,*** bar-s., bell., benz., bor., ***brom.,*** calc., calc-ar., calc-p., calc-sil., caps., carl., ***caust.,*** cench., ***cham.,*** chin., chin-a., cic., cocc., cycl., der., dulc., gran., **GRAPH.,** guai., ***helon.,*** hyos., ign., ***ip.,*** iris, kali-ar., kali-c., kali-cy., lac-ac., ***lach., lyc.,*** mag-arct., mag-c., ***merc., mez.,*** morph., mosch., myric., naja, nat-m., ***nux-v.,*** par., petr., ***phos., plat.,*** plb., puls., ran-b., rhus-t., ***sep.,*** sil., sol-t-ae., staph., **SULPH.,** tarent., til., tus-f., **VERAT.**
afternoon - dulc.
close friends, with - ars-s-f., aur-s., chin-a., der.
disposed to find fault or is silent - ***verat.***
evening - rhus-t.
scolds herself - merc.
unoccupied, when, close application amel. - sapin.

CROAKING, behaviour - cina, cupr.
sleep, in - bell.
frogs, as of - cupr., cupr-ac.

CROSS, disposition - cham., ***cina,*** lyc., ***nux-v.,*** upa., tub.
waking, on - **LYC., NUX-V.**

CRUELTY, inhumanity (see Brutality, Malicious, Moral feeling) - abrot., ***absin.,*** **ANAC.,** ***ars.,*** bell., bry., canth., chin., croc., cur., **HEP.,** ***hyos., kali-i.,*** kali-p., ***lach.,*** lyss., med., nicc., ***nit-ac., nux-v.,*** op., ***plat.,*** sel., staph., ***stram.,*** syph., tarent., verat.

animals, to - anac., **ARS.,** bell., calc., med., tub.

children cannot bear to see cruelty at the movies - ***calc.,*** caust., phos.

family, to her - kali-p., sep.

suffer, loves to make people and animals - **ANAC., ARS.,** ***bell.,*** tub.

CRYING, weeping - acet-ac., ***acon.,*** aeth., ether, ail., allox., ***alum.,*** ambr., am-c., ***am-m.,*** amyg., anan., ang., anh., ***ant-c., ant-t.,*** **APIS,** apoc., arg-m., ***arg-n., arist-cl.,*** arn., ***ars.,*** ars-i., arum-m., asar., aster., ***aur.,*** aur-a., aur-i., aur-m., aur-s., bapt., bar-c., bar-i., bar-s., ***bell.,*** benz., berb., bor., brom., ***bry.,*** bufo, buth-a., ***cact.,*** **CALC.,** ***calc-ar., calc-i., calc-p.,*** **CALC-S.,** camph., cann-i., cann-s., canth., caps., carb-an., **CARB-S.,** ***carb-v.,*** **CARC.,** card-m., carl., cass., cast., **CAUST.,** cedr., cench., ***cham., chel.,*** chen-a., chin., chin-a., ***chin-s.,*** chlf., **CIC.,** ***cimic., cina,*** cinnam., cit-v., clem., ***cocc., coff.,*** colch., coloc., ***con.,*** convo-s., cop., cortiso., croc., crot-c., ***crot-h., cupr.,*** cupr-ac., cur., ***cycl.,*** der., ***dig.,*** dros., dulc., eup-per., eup-pur., ***ferr.,*** ferr-ar., ferr-i., ferr-p., ferul., gels., gent-c., gins., glon., goss., **GRAPH.,** haem., ***hell., hep.,*** hir., hist., hura, ***hydr.,*** hydroph., hyos., iber., **IGN.,** ind., iod., ***ip.,*** jug-r., kali-ar., ***kali-bi.,*** **KALI-BR.,** ***kali-c.,*** kali-chl., kali-fer., kali-i., kali-n., kali-ox., ***kali-p.,*** kali-s., kiss., kreos., **LAC-C.,** lac-d., lach., lachn., lact., lam., lat-m., laur., led., levo., ***lil-t.,*** lith., lob., lob-s., **LYC.,** lyss., ***mag-arct.,*** mag-aust., ***mag-m., mag-p.,*** mag-s., ***mang., med., meli.,*** meny., **MERC.,** ***merc-i-r.,*** merl., methys., mez., morph., mosch., naja, nat-a., nat-c., **NAT-M.,** ***nat-p., nat-s.,*** nat-sil., nicc., nid., ***nit-ac.,*** nitro-o., ***nux-m., nux-v., op.,*** **PALL.,** peti., ***petr., phel., ph-ac., phos.,*** **PLAT.,** plb., psil., psor., **PULS.,** pyrus, raja-s., ran-b., rheum, **RHUS-T.,** rib-ac., ruta, sabin., samb., sars., sec., senec., **SEP.,** sil., sol-n., spig., ***spong.,*** squil., ***stann., staph.,*** stram., ***stry.,*** **SULPH.,** ***sul-ac.,*** syph., tab., ***tarent.,*** tep., thea., thuj., thuj-l., til., tub., ust., vac., **VERAT.,** vinc., **VIOL-O.,** viol-t., wies., zinc., zinc-p., ziz.

admonition, from - bell., ***calc.,*** carc., chin., ign., ***kali-c., lyc.,*** nat-m., nit-ac., plat., ***staph.***

afternoon - bell., carb-v., cast., cop., dig., phos., ***sil.,*** tab., tarent.

4 p.m. - puls.

4 p.m. to 8 p.m. - **LYC.**

aggravates, symptoms - ant-t., ***arn., bell.,*** bor., canth., ***cham., croc., cupr., cycl.,*** hep., lach., ***nat-m.,*** nit-ac., puls., ***sep., stann., teucr., verat.***

air, in open - carb-v., hura

amel. in - coff., ***nat-s., plat.,*** **PULS.**

alone, when - ***con.,*** ign., **NAT-M.**

amel. - allox.

CRYING, weeping

aloud - acon., alum., carb-an., ***cham.,*** cic., ***cocc.,*** coff., con., crot-c., cupr., ***hep.,*** hyos., ***ign.,*** kali-c., lob., **LYC.,** lyss., ***mag-p.,*** merc., nat-c., nat-m., nux-v., ***op.,*** phos., plat., plb., plect., puls., sabin., ***sep.,*** staph., ***stram.,*** sulph.

sleep, in - mag-c.

alternating with

cheerfulness - acon., alum., arg-m., bell., bor., cann-s., carb-an., graph., ign., iod., nux-v., plat., spong., ***stram.***

dancing - bell.

hopefulness - raph.

ill humor - bell., kali-i.

irritability and laughter at trifles - graph.

jesting - ***ign.***

laughter - ***acon.,*** agar., alum., alum-p., alumn., ***asaf.,*** asar., ***aur.,*** aur-s., bell., bov., bufo, ***calc.,*** camph-br., cann-s., caps., ***coff.,*** con., ***croc.,*** graph., ***hyos.,*** hypoth., ***ign.,*** kali-p., ***lyc.,*** **MERC., MOSCH.,** nat-m., **NUX-M.,** nux-v., ***phos., plat.,*** puls., samb., sep., spig-m., ***stram.,*** sulph., sumb., tarent., ***valer.,*** verat., ziz.

and singing - stram.

queer antics - carb-an., cupr.

rage - acon., cann-s.

singing - acon., bell., stram.

vexation - bell.

ameliorates, symptoms - ***anac.,*** astac., colch., cycl., ***dig., graph.,*** **HELL.,** ign., **LACH.,** ***lyc., med.,*** merc., nit-ac., phos., ***plat.,*** **PULS.,** sep., tab.

anecdotes, from - ***lach.***

anger, with - ant-t., ars., ***ign.,*** sulph., zinc.

after - ambr., arn., bell., caust., cham., ***cocc., coff.,*** ign., lac-c., lil-t., mag-aust., ***mosch.,*** nat-m., ***nux-v., plat.,*** puls., sabin., spong., ***staph.,*** syph.

answering a question, at - **PULS.**

anxiety, after - acon., am-c., am-m., asar., bell., calc., camph., canth., carb-v., cast., dig., **GRAPH.,** ign., ***kali-c.,*** **KALI-I.,** lyc., nat-m., ***phos.,*** puls., ***spong.,*** sul-ac., sulph., zinc.

anxious - am-c., ars., caust., **GRAPH., KALI-I.,** nat-m.

attacks, before - ant-t.

bells, sound of - ant-c., cop.

bitter - hep., nat-m.

caressing, from - chin., cina, ign.

carried, when - chel., cina., sil.

causeless - acon., **APIS,** ars., bell., cact., camph., ***carc., cina, graph.,*** hura, kali-ar., kali-br., kali-c., kreos., ***lyc.,*** **NAT-M.,** nit-ac., nux-v., phos., **PULS.,** pyrog., rhus-t., **SEP.,** staph., **SULPH.,** syph., tarent., tub., viol-o., ***zinc.***

children, in - ars., ***bell., bor.,*** camph., caste., carc., caust., **CHAM.,** chin., cina, ***coff., graph., hyos., ign., jal., kali-c., lyc.,*** nit-ac., **PULS., RHEUM,** ***seneg.,*** sil.

CRYING, weeping
children, in, babies - ***acon.,*** ars., bell., bor., calc., ***carc., cham.,*** coff., ign., ip., jal., ***puls., rhod.,*** senn., syph., thuj.
birth, since - acon., carc., cham.
cries piteously if taken hold of or carried - ***cina,*** sil.
difficult dentition, from - cham., ***phyt.***
his will is not done, when - calc-p., cham., **CINA.,** tub.
night - arund., ***bor., lac-c., psor., rheum***
quiet only when carried - **CHAM.,** cina.
toss all night - ars., ***psor., rheum.***
child, like a - ars., ***bar-c., cupr-ac.,*** ign., ***puls.***
about ilness with senseless prattling - ars., calad.
childbirth, during - ars., cham., ***coff., puls.***
chill, during - acon., ars., ***aur.,*** aur-a., **BELL., CALC.,** cann-s., ***carb-v.,*** **CHAM.,** con., hep., ign., kali-c., **LYC.,** merc., nat-m., ***petr.,*** plat., **PULS.,** sel., sil., stram., sulph., verat., **VIOL-O.**
chorea, in - caust.
consolation, agg. - bell., cact., calc., ***calc-p.,*** cham., chin., hell., **IGN.,** kali-c., lil-t., lyc., merc., nat-c., **NAT-M.,** nit-ac., nux-v., ***plat.,*** **SEP., SIL.,** staph., sulph., ***tarent.,*** thuj.
amel. - ***puls.***
contradiction, from - ign., ***nux-v.,*** stram., tarent.
controlled - ign., nat-m.
convulsions, during - absin., acon., ***alum.,*** ant-t., ***bell.,*** **CAMPH.,** ***canth., caust.,*** cham., cic., cina, cocc., **CUPR.,** hyos., ***ign.,*** lach., ***lyc., merc.,*** mosch., ***nux-v.,*** op., plb., sil., sulph., vip.
after - caust., cina
epileptic - absin., **CUPR.,** ***indg., lach.***
from - bell.
convulsive - ign., mag-p.
asthma, with - bov.
coryza, during - **PULS.,** ***spig.***
coughing, during - ant-t., arn., ars., ***bad., bell., cahin.,*** cham., chin., ***cina,*** **HEP.,** ip., lyc., osm., ph-ac., samb., sep., sil., spong., sulph., verat.
after - arn., bell., caps., cina, hep., op.
before - ant-t., ***arn.,*** **BELL.,** bor., **BRY., HEP.,** phos.
whooping cough, in - ***ant-t., arn., caust.***
dark, in - stram.
day and night - apis
daytime - alum., bry., lyc., mez., stram.
delirium, after - nat-s.
delusions, after - dulc.
desire to cry - am-m., aster., ***cact.,*** chin-b., ***nat-m., puls.***
all the time - ail., ***ambr., camph., ferr., ip.,*** kali-c., ***lyc.,*** merc., merc-c., ***murx.,*** nat-m., op., **PULS.,** samb., ***stram., thuj.***
but eyes are dry - ***camph., nat-m.***
despair, from - ***ars., aur.,*** chel., ***cupr-ac.,*** hell., sil.

CRYING, weeping
difficult - carc., ign., ***nat-m.***
dinner, after - mag-m.
disappointments, about - dig., ***ign.***
discontent, with self - aur., carc., nit-ac., staph.
disease, with progressive - aeth., ars., calad.
disturbed at work, when - ***puls.***
drinking, after - ***caust.,*** nux-v., petr.
drunkenness, being sentimental during - ***caust., lach.***
easily - alum., arg-m., aster., ***bell., calc.,*** carc., **CAUST.,** chin., coff., ***kali-br.,*** lyc., ***nat-m., op.,*** **PULS.,** rhus-t., sep., staph., trinit.
eating, while - carb-an.
children, in - bell., staph.
after - arg-n., arn., iod., mag-m., puls.
elderly people for nothing - caust.
emission, after an - hipp.
emotion, after slight - aster., **CUPR.,** ign., kreos., ***lach.,*** lyc., naja. ***puls.***
evening - acon., alum., am-c., am-m., ***calc.,*** carb-an., clem., coca, ***graph.,*** hyper., kali-c., kali-chl., kali-i., kali-sil., lact., lyc., lyss., mag-arct., mez., nat-m., ***plat.,*** **PULS.,** ***ran-b., rhus-t.,*** sil., ***stram.,*** sul-i., sulph., ***verat.***
amel. - am-c., cast., zinc.
everything, about - apis., carc., puls.
evil, impended, as if - kali-i.
fever, during - **ACON.,** ***anac., ant-c.,*** apis, **BELL.,** bry., calc., ***caps.,*** cham., coff., cupr., graph., ign., ip., ***lyc., petr.,*** plat., **PULS.,** ***spig.,*** **SPONG.,** ***stram.,*** sulph., til., vac., verat.
forenoon - hura, sars.
future, about the - ars., lyc.
goes off alone and weeps as if she had no friends - bar-c.
hallucination, after - dulc.
headache, with - ***coff.,*** coloc., ***kali-c.,*** kreos., lyss., phos., plat., ran-b., sep.
hopelessness, from - arg-n., ***ars.,*** **AUR.**
humiliation, after - carc., coloc., ign., pall., puls., staph.
hysterical - ars., aur-a., cact., ***carc., coff.,*** ign., ***kali-p., nat-m.,*** sep., sumb., ***tarent., verat-v.***
illness, during - calad.
impatience, from - dulc.
interrupted, when - ***puls.***
involuntary - ***alum.,*** alum-p., ***aur., bell.,*** camph., ***cann-i., carc., caust.,*** cina, coff., croc., **CUPR., IGN.,** kali-br., lach., mang., ***merc.,*** morph., mosch., **NAT-M.,** peti., phos., **PLAT.,** plb., **PULS., RHUS-T., SEP.,** stann., stram., verat., viol-o.
amel. by vinegar - stram.
weakness, from - ars., olnd., ***vinc.***
irritable - calc., carb-s., ign., sep.
joy, from - ***coff.,*** lach., lyc., ***plat.***
joyful or sad things, at - **PULS.**
lamenting, and - ars., coff.

CRYING, weeping
laughing at the same time, and - aur., cann-i., ign., lyc., sumb.
menopausal period, at - ferr.
lonely, feeling - lith., nat-m., ***puls.***
looked at, when - ant-c., kiss., ***nat-m.***
looking at anyone - kiss.
lying, while - euphr.
meeting people, when - ***aur.***
men, in - med., staph.
menopausal period, at - ferr., puls., sep., **SULPH.**
menopause, during - **SULPH.**
menses, during - ***ars.,*** cact., calc., caust., ***cocc., coff.,*** con., cycl., graph., hyos., ***ign.,*** ind., lach., lyc., ***nat-m., petr., phyt.,*** phos., ***plat., puls.,*** sec., sep., ***stram.,*** thuj., tub., verat., zinc., zinc-p.
which does her no good - cycl.
after - alum., con., lyc., phos., ***stram.***
before - ***cact.,*** con., ***lyc., nat-m., phos.,*** **PULS.,** sep., ***zinc.***
suppression of, in - ***chen-a., cycl.***
midnight, at - mag-arct., mag-c.
after - ars., bry.
before - ars., merc., nux-v.
morning - alumn., am-c., bell., bor., canth., carb-an., dulc., kreos., peti., phos., plat., prun., puls., rhus-t., sars., sil., spong., stram., sulph., tarent.
inclined to, at 11 a.m. - **SULPH.**
waking, on - alum., alum-p.
music, from - acon., ***ambr., carc.,*** dig., **GRAPH.,** ign., kali-p., ***kreos.,*** kali-n., ***nat-c.,*** **NAT-M.,** nat-s., ***nux-v., sabin.,*** tarent., ***thuj.***
bells, of - ant-c., cop.
organ, on hearing - **GRAPH.**
piano, of - all-c., cop., ***nat-c.,*** nat-s.
need, about a fancied - ars., chin.
nervous, all day - ars., bry., caust., lac-c., lyc., stram.
feels so, feels like crying all the time, but it makes her worse - stann.
feels so, she would scream unless she held on to something - ***sep.***
news, at bad - carb-an., ph-ac.
night - alum., alum-p., am-c., anac., ant-t., arn., ars., ars-s-f., aur., aur-s., bar-c., bar-s., bell., ***bor.,*** bry., calad., calc., calc-ar., calc-sil., camph., caps., carb-an., ***cast.,*** caust., cham., chel., ***chin.,*** chin-s., ***cina, cocc.,*** con., croc., euph., graph., guai., hep., hipp., hyos., ign., indg., ip., kali-ar., kali-c., kali-i., kali-sil., lac-c., ***lach.,*** lup., lyc., mag-arct., ***mag-c.,*** mag-m., merc., merc-ac., ***nat-c., nat-m.,*** nicc., nit-ac., ***nux-v.,*** op., ph-ac., phos., ***phyt.,*** plat., ***psor., puls.,*** rheum, rhus-t., ruta, ***sep.,*** sil., spong., stann., ***stram.,*** sul-ac., sulph., tab., tarent., thuj., verat., ***zinc.***
all night, laughs all day - stram.
quiet during day - jal.

CRYING, weeping
night, at
sleep, in - alum., carb-an., caust., cham., con., ign., lach., lyc., nat-m., nit-ac., ***nux-v.,*** thuj.
waking, on - chin-s., sil.
nightmare, after - guai.
noise, at - aeth., ign., kreos., ***lach.***
nursing, while - ***lac-c.,*** **PULS.**
obstinate - cham.
offence, from - ***stram.***
former, about - caust., ign., lach., staph.
imaginary, at least - cham.
opposition, at least - nux-v.
pains, with - ***ars.,*** asaf., bell., canth., ***carc.,*** cham., cina, ***coff., glon.,*** kali-c., ***lach.,*** lyc., ***merc.,*** merc-c., mez., mosch., ***nux-v.,*** op., ***plat.,*** puls., stram., verat.
after - glon.
during intermission of - glon.
palpitation, during - phos., ***plat.***
paralysis, in - caust.
paroxysmal - **KALI-BR.,** ***lac-c.,*** phos., stry.
past events, thinking of - lyc., ***nat-m.***
periodically, every four weeks - ***con.***
perspiration, during - acon., arn., aur., **BELL.,** bry., ***calc.,*** calc-s., ***camph., cham.,*** chin., **CUPR.,** graph., **LYC.,** nux-v., **OP.,** ***petr.,*** phos., ***puls.,*** rheum, rhus-t., sep., ***spong., stram.,*** sulph., verat.
piteous - cham., ***puls.,*** stram.
pitied, if he believes he is - ***nat-m.***
poetry, at soothing - lach.
pollutions, after - hipp., ***ust.***
pregnancy, during - apis, lach., ***mag-c.,*** ign., nat-m., ***puls.,*** stann.
questioned, when - cimic.
reading, while - ***crot-h.,*** lach.
refused anything, when - bell., cham., ign., tarent., viol-o.
remonstrated with, when - bell., ***calc.,*** calc-p., carc., ign., ***kali-c.,*** nit-ac., plat., puls., staph.
reproaches, from - calc., carc., ign., nat-m., ***plat., staph.***
rising, after - am-c.
room, in - ***plat.***
sad, thoughts, at - alum., carb-v., cina, kali-c., ***nat-m.,*** phel., plat., stram.
but is impossible to cry - ***nat-m., nux-v.***
sexual excitement, with - aster., stram.
silently - cycl.
singing, when - hura
sits and, for days - ***ambr.***
sleep, in - all-s., ***alum.,*** alum-p., alum-sil., anac., ang., ant-t., ***arn.,*** ars., ars-s-f., ***aur.,*** aur-a., bar-c., bell., ***bor.,*** bry., bufo, calad., calc., calc-ac., calc-sil., camph., caps., carb-an., carb-s., ***carb-v., cast., caust.,*** **CHAM.,** chin., chin-s., cina, ***cocc., con.,*** croc., cur., euph., fl-ac., glon., graph., hep., ***hyos.,*** ign., ip., kali-ar., ***kali-c.,*** kali-i., kali-sil., kreos., ***lach.,***

CRYING, weeping

sleep, in - lyc., mag-arct., mag-c., mag-m., ***merc., mur-ac., nat-c., nat-m.,*** nicc., ***nit-ac., nux-v., op., ph-ac.,*** phos., plan., ***plat.,*** podo., ***puls.,*** rheum, rhus-t., rob., sabin., ***samb.,*** sarr., ***sep., sil., spong.,*** stann., stram., sul-ac., sulph., tab., tarent., thuj., verat., wild., ***zinc.***

aroused from - lyc.

child good during the day, screaming and restless all night - ***jal.***

loudly - kali-i.

waking, without - hyos.

sleepiness, with - cham.

spasmodic - alum., aur., bell., carb-o., **CAUST.,** cina, cupr., **IGN.,** lach., mosch., nat-m., ***phos.,*** plb., stram., thala.

spasms, after - alum., ***caust.***

speaking, when - kali-c., **MED.,** puls., sep.

speeches, when making - cupr.

spells of - sep.

spoken to, when - cimic., ign., ***med., nat-m.,*** plat., sil., **STAPH.,** thuj., ***tub.***

kindly - ***iod., sil.***

stool, before - phos., puls., rhus-t.

stool, during - ***aeth., bor., cham.,*** cina, phos., rhus-t., sil., sulph.

supper, after - arn.

sympathy with others - carl., caust., ***phos.,*** puls.

taking cold, after - ***op.***

telling of her sickness, when - bry., ***carc.,*** ign., ***kali-c.,*** kali-p., ***med.,*** **PULS., SEP.,** sil.

over again, and - med.

thanked, when - **LYC.**

toothache, with - sep., ther.

touched, when - ant-c., ant-t., cina, sil., stram.

trifles, at - ant-c., arg-m., bell., benz., bufo calc., **CAUST.,** cina, cocc., coff., con., hypoth., ***ign.,*** nat-m., petr., plat., ***puls.,*** puls-n, sil., stram., sulph., ven-m., visc.

laughing or crying on every occasion - ***caust.,*** **PULS.,** sep., ***staph.***

worry, children at the least - ***caust.,*** lyc., nit-ac., tub.

undress, and - thyr.

ungratefulness, at - ***lyc.***

urination, before - ***bor., lyc., sars.***

urination, during - erig., ***sars.***

vexation, from - calad., cham., ign., nux-v., petr., sulph., tarent., ***zinc.***

old - caust., ign., lach., staph.

violent - hydr-ac., stram.

waking, on - alum., am-c., am-m., ant-t., arn., bell., bor., bufo, carb-an., chin-s., ***cic.,*** cina, guai., hyos., kali-i., lach., lyc., ***mag-c.,*** merc., nicc., nux-v., op., paull., phos., plan., puls., raph., ruta, sabad., sep., sil., ***stram.,*** sulph.

walking, in open air, when - bell., calc., coff., ***sep.***

amel. - ***puls., rhus-t.***

washed, in cold water, when - ant-c.

CRYING, weeping

whimpering - ***ars., aur.,*** bell., calc., canth., caust., ***cham., chin.,*** cic., cocc., colch., cupr., hyos., ign., ***ip., kreos., merc.,*** nit-ac., nux-v., phos., **PULS.,** rheum, rhus-t., squil., stram., sulph., verat., zinc.

anger, with - zinc.

night - ars., phos.

sleep, during - alum., anac., ***arn., ars., aur., bar-c., bry.,*** calc., ***caust., cham.,*** chin., ***hyos., ign.,*** ip., lach., lyc., merc., nat-m., ***nit-ac., nux-v.,*** op., ph-ac., phos., puls., rheum, sil., stann., sulph., verat.

comatose - anac.

toothache, with - mag-c.

CUNNING - ***tarent.***

CURSING, swearing - alco., aloe, am-c., **ANAC.,** arn., ***ars., bell.,*** bor., bov., bufo, ***calc.,*** cann-i., canth., ***caust.,*** cer-s., chin-b., ***con.,*** cor-r., cupr., dulc., gall-ac., ***hydr., hyos.,*** ip., ***lac-c., lil-t., lyc.,*** lyss., ***mosch.,*** nat-c., ***nat-m.,*** **NIT-AC., NUX-V.,** oena., op., opun-v., pall., ***petr., phos.,*** plat., plb., puls., spig., staph., ***stram., tarent., tub., verat.***

afternoon - op.

amel. - cor-r.

children, in - **ANAC.,** ***bell.,*** hyos., ***lyc.,*** lyss., nit-ac., nux-v., plat., ***stram.,*** tarent., ***tub., verat.***

convulsions, during - ars.

curses his mother, throws food or medicine across room - ***hydr.***

evening - lil-t.

when home - nit-ac., op.

headache, during - bry., nat-m.

night - ***verat.***

all night, and complains of stupid feeling - verat.

pains, at - cor-r.

rage, in - **ANAC.,** ***nit-ac.,*** verat.

after - ***arn.***

CUT, mutilate others, desires to - lyss.

DANCING - acon., ether, ***agar.,*** apis, ***bell.,*** cann-i., **CARC.,** chlol., ***cic., cocc.,*** con., ***croc.,*** crot-t., grat., **HYOS.,** ign., merc., nat-m., nitro-o., ***ph-ac.,*** pip-m., plat., rob., sant., ***sep.,*** sil., stict., ***stram.,*** tab., **TARENT.**

agg. - bor., spong.

alternating with moaning - bell.

with sighing - bell.

amel. - cann-s., caust., ***ign.,*** nat-m., **SEP.,** sil., stann.

desire to - ***carc, sep.***

evening - nat-m.

loves to - ***carc, sep.***

grotesque - agar., ***cic., hyos., tarent.***

unconscious - ph-ac.

wild - ***bell.,*** carc., camph., tarent.

DARKNESS, agg. mental state - acon., ***aeth.,*** am-m., ars., bapt., berb., ***calc.,*** camph., cann-s., ***carb-an., carb-v., caust.,*** cupr., graph., ***lyc.,*** nat-m., ***phos.,*** plat., ***puls.,*** rhus-t., sanic., sil., **STRAM.,** stront-c., ***valer.,*** zinc.

DARKNESS, general
aversion to - phos., sanic., stram.
desire for - achy.
to lie down in the dark and not be talked to - tarent.

DAY-dreaming - ***acon.,*** arn., bry., **CANN-I.,** cham., chin., graph., hep., ***ign.,*** merc., ***nux-v., op.,*** petr., **PHOS.,** rheum, sep., ***sil.,*** stram., ***sulph.***

DEAFNESS, pretended - verat.

DEATH, general
agony before - acon., alum., **ARS.,** ***carc,*** cocc., cupr., **LAT-M.,** puls., ***rhus-t.,*** **TARENT.,** ***tarent-c.,verat.***
contempt, of - ***op.***
conviction, of - alum-p., ars-h., bapt., bell., ***canth., coff., cupr-ac.,*** kali-ar., ***phyt., psor., thuj.***
fever after, nosebleed amel. - ***psor.***
desires, death (see Loathing, Suicidal) - acon., agn., alum., alum-sil., ambr., anh., ant-c., apis, aran., ars., ars-m., ars-s-f., **AUR.,** aur-a., aur-m., ***aur-s., bell.,*** berb., calc., caps., carb-v., ***carc, caust.,*** chel., ***chin.,*** clem., cortico., der., euph-c., ***gad., glon.,*** hep., hura, hydr., kali-bi., kali-br., ***kreos.,*** **LAC-C.,** ***lac-d., lach.,*** led., lil-t., lyc., ***merc.,*** merc-aur., mez., nat-c., ***nat-m.,*** nat-s., ***nit-ac.,*** nux-v., op., phos., phyt., plat., plb., psor., puls., ran-b., rat., ***rhus-t., rob.,*** sec., ***sep., sil.,*** spong., ***staph.,*** stram., sul-ac., **SULPH.,** thuj., verat., verat-v., vip., zinc.
afternoon - ruta.
agony, from - bell., caust.
alternating with, laughing - aur.
with, rage - bell.
anxiety, from - bell., caust.
chill, during - kali-chl., spig.
convalescence, during - absin., ***aur.,*** lac-c., sep.
despair, from - aur., ***kreos.***
evening - **AUR.,** ruta.
forenoon - apis.
meditates on easiest way of self destruction - ***aur.,*** lac-d., nat-s.
menses, during - berb.
morning, on waking - nat-c., phyt.
pains, during - rat.
rage, during intervals from - bell.
walking in open air, while - bell.
dying, sensation of - acon., aesc., ether, ***agn.,*** apis, ***ars.,*** camph., cann-i., cench., cic., ***graph.,*** kali-bi., kali-n., **LAT-M.,** morph., nux-v., op., ***phos., plat.,*** sil., verat., ***zinc.***
chill, during - cann-i.
evening - ether
spasm, during - nux-v.
presentiment, of death - **ACON.,** ***agn., aloe,*** alum., anac., ***anthr.,*** **APIS,** ***arg-n.,*** arn., ***ars.,*** bapt., bar-m., **BELL.,** ***bry., cact., calc.,*** cann-i., canth., ***chel., cench.,*** cimic., ***cupr.,*** dig., ferr-br., gels., ***graph.,*** hell., ***hep.,*** kali-ar., kali-c., kali-n., lac-d., ***lach.,*** lob., ***lyc.,*** lyss., ***med.,*** **MERC.,** mosch., nat-m., ***nit-ac.,***

DEATH, general
presentiment, of death - ***nux-v.,*** petr., ***phos., plat.,*** podo., puls., ***raph.,*** rhus-t., sep., staph., stram., sul-ac., sulph., tab., thea., verat., vip., zinc., zinc-p.
alternating with, anguish - raph.
with, rage - stram.
believes that she will die soon, and that she cannot be helped - ***agn.***
predicts the time - **ACON.,** ***aloe,*** alum., ***arg-n.,*** hell., ***lac-d.,*** thea.
sudden death, of a - ***cench.***
thinks of death calmly - aur., zinc.
vomiting, with - med.
thoughts, of - **ACON.,** agn., aloe, am-c., ***apis,*** arn., ***ars.,*** ars-h., aur., camph., cann-i., carb-an., caust., ***cham.,*** chel., ***con.,*** cortico., cortiso., ***crot-c., crot-h.,*** cupr., ***dig.,*** ferr., ferr-ar., **GRAPH.,** hist., hura, kali-ar., kali-c., ***lach.,*** lat-m., ***lob.,*** merc., op., plat., ***psor., puls.,*** rauw., rhus-t., rob., spong., stram., tarent., verat., verat-v., vinc., ***zinc.***
afternoon - tarent., zinc.
alone, when - ***crot-c.***
evening - ***zinc.***
fears, without - apis, ***coff.,*** merc., verat-v.
joy, give him - aur.
morning - con., lyc.
those belonging to him, for, with anxiety - ***ferr.***
waking, on - lyc.

DEBAUCH - fl-ac., med., ***nux-v.,*** pic-ac., sep.

DECEITFUL - agar., anac., arg-n., ***ars., bell.,*** bufo, ***calc.,*** chlol., chlor., coca, cupr., dros., fl-ac., hyos., **LACH.,** ***lyc.,*** merc., ***morph., nat-m., nux-v.,*** **OP.,** plat., plb., puls., sep., sil., sulph., ***tarent.,*** **THUJ.,** ***verat.***
fraudulent - bell., calc., merc.
perjured - hep., nat-m., nit-ac.
untruthful - alco., ***arg-n.,*** lyc., ***morph.,*** **OP., THUJ.,** ***verat.***

DECEPTION, causes grief and humiliation - **AUR.,** carc., **IGN., LYC.,** ***merc.,*** **NAT-M.,** ***nux-v.,*** op., **PH-AC., PULS.,** sep., verat.
ailments from friendship, deceived - ***ign.,*** mag-c., mag-m., ***nat-m.,*** nux-v., ph-ac., sil., sulph.

DEEDS, feels as if he could do great - hell., op.
useful, desire to be - ***cer-b.***
misdeeds of other's agg. - caust., colch., ign., ***staph.***

DEFIANT - acon., alum., am-c., anac., ***arn.,*** bell., bufo, canth., **CAUST.,** ***cham., cina,*** guai., ***ign.,*** kreos., ***lyc.,*** med., nux-v., ph-ac., ruta, sec., sep., sil., spong., sulph., **TUB.**

DELICACY, feeling of - gels., ign., nat-m., nux-v., sil., ***thuj.***
emotional - nat-m.
physical - gel., sil., thuj.

DELIRIUM tremens, (See Alcoholism)

DELIRIUM, general - absin., acet-ac., ***acon.***, ***act-sp.***, aesc., ***aeth.***, ether, **AGAR.**, agar-cps., agar-pa., agar-ph., agn., ail., alco., alum., am-c., amyg., anac., anag., anh., anthr., ant-c., ant-t., anan., apis, arg-m., arg-n., arn., **ARS.**, **ARUM-T.**, astac., atro., ***aur.***, aur-m., ***bapt.***, bar-c., **BELL.**, bism., bol-lu., bomb-pr., brom., **BRY.**, bufo, calad., cact., ***calc.***, calen., ***camph.***, **CANN-I.**, cann-s., ***canth.***, caps., carb-ac., ***carb-s.***, carb-v., ***carl.***, caul., ***cham.***, **CHEL.**, chin., chin-a., chin-s., chlf., chol., chloram., chr-ac., ***cic.***, cic-m., cimic., ***cina***, clem., coff., ***colch.***, coloc., ***con.***, convo-s., cop., cor-r., croc., **CROT-C.**, ***crot-h.***, ***cupr.***, ***cupr-ac.***, cupr-ar., cyt-l., dat-f., dat-m., ***dig.***, diph., dor., dub., dub., ***dulc.***, euph., fagu., ferr-p., gall-ac., ***gels.***, glon., graph., guare., ham., hell., hep., hipp., hippoz., hydr., **HYOS.**, hyosin., hyper., ign., iod., iodof., ***ip.***, iris, ir-fl., ir-foe., jatr., juni., kali-ar., kali-bi., kali-br., kali-c., ***kali-i.***, ***kali-m.***, kali-n., kali-p., kalm., lac-c., **LACH.**, lachn., lact., lat-k., lept., lil-t., lob., lol., lup., **LYC.**, lyss., manc., ***meli.***, meny., ***merc.***, ***merc-c.***, merc-cy., merc-i-r., merc-n., merc-sul., merl., mez., ***mill.***, morph., mosch., mur-ac., mygal., naja, nat-m., nat-s., **NIT-AC.**, nit-s-d., nitro-o., ***nux-m.***, ***nux-v.***, ***oena.***, op., oper., ox-ac., paeon., par., ***petr.***, ph-ac., ***phos.***, plat., ***plb.***, podo., psor., ***puls.***, phyt., pyrog., ran-b., ran-s., rheum, rhod., **RHUS-T.**, sabad., sabin., sal-ac., samb., sang., sant., sapin., sarr., **SEC.**, sel., sil., sin-n., sol-n., spig., stigm., **STRAM.**, stry., ***sulph.***, sul-ac., sul-h., sulfa., syph., tab., tang., tarax., tarent., tarent-c., tax., ***ter.***, thea., trinit., tub., valer., vario., **VERAT.**, **VERAT-V.**, verin., vesp., vip., vip-a., xan., zinc., zinc-ac., zinc-s.

- **abandons** her relatives - sec.
- **absurd** things, does - sec.
- **addresses** objects - stram.
- **afternoon,** 4 p.m. to 12 p.m. - ***stram.***
- **alternating** with, colic - plb.
  - coma, also with somnolency - plb., stram.
  - consciousness - acon., ***phos.***
  - sadness - tub.
  - sopor - acet-ac., cocc., ***coloc.***, plb., vip.
  - tetanic convulsions, lies on his back, knees and thighs flexed, hands joined - stram.
- **angry** - ***cocc.***
- **answers,** abruptly - cimic., ***lach.***, stram., verat.
  - correctly when spoken to, but delusions and unconsciousness return at once - ***ant-t.***, diph., ***hell.***, ***op.***, ***ph-ac.***, phos., sulph., ***ter.***
  - slowly, relapses - arn., bapt., diph., ***hell.***, hyos., ***ph-ac.***, phos., sulph.
- **antics,** plays - bell., cupr., **HYOS.**, lact., op., phos., plb., stram.
- **anxious** - ***acon.***, anac., apis, ***ars.***, ***bell.***, calc., camph., cupr., hep., ***hyos.***, ign., lac-c., nux-v., ***op.***, phos., plb., puls., sil., ***stram.***, sulph., ***verat.***
- **apathetic** - ph-ac., verat.
- **arms,** extends - sep., stram.
  - throws about - bell.

DELIRIUM, general

- **aroused,** on being - dat-f., hep., phos., sep.
  - to answer questions, could be aroused - ***hyper.***
- **bed,** and escapes, springs up suddenly from - **ACON.**, ***agar.***, alco., ***ars.***, atro., ***bell.***, ***bry.***, ***chin-s.***, cic., ***coloc.***, ***crot-h.***, ***cupr.***, dig., gall-ac., hell., ***hyos.***, iod., merc-c., merc-meth., morph., **NIT-AC.**, nux-v., op., oper., past., phos., plb., puls., rhus-t., sec., sol-m., ***stram.***, sul-ac., ***verat.***, verat-v., ***zinc.***
  - creeps about in - stram.
- **bellows,** like a calf - cupr.
- **blames,** himself for his folly - op.
- **bleeding,** after - arn., ars., bell., chin., chin-a., ign., lach., lyc., phos., ph-ac., sep., squil., sulph., verat.
- **books,** endeavored to grasp - atro.
- **business,** talks of - ars., bell., **BRY.**, ***canth.***, dor., **HYOS.**, op., ***phos.***, **RHUS-T.**, stram.
- **busy** - arum-t., bapt., bell., ***bry.***, camph., ***hyos.***, kali-cy., rhus-t., ***stram.***, sulph.
- **carotids,** pulsating, with - ***bell.***
- **changing,** subjects rapidly - **LACH.**
- **cheerful** - acon., ***bell.***, cact., con., op., sulph., verat.
- **chill,** during - aeth., ***arn.***, ars., astac., ***bell.***, ***caps.***, cham., **NAT-M.**, nux-v., puls., ***sep.***, stram., sulph., ***verat.***
- **climbs** walls during - ***bell.***
- **closing** the eyes, on - bapt., ***bell.***, ***bry.***, calc., graph., ***lach.***, led., pyrog., sulph.
- **cold,** after catching - ***op.***
- **coldness,** with - ***verat.***
- **collapse,** with - colch., cupr.
- **coma** vigil - cur., ***hyos.***, mur-ac., ***op.***, phos.
- **comical** - ant-c., **HYOS.**, ***stram.***, verat.
- **congestion,** with - ***apis***, aur-m., ***bell.***, brom., iod.
- **constant** - bapt., bell., con., ***lach.***
- **convulsions,** during - acon., ***aeth.***, amyg., ars., ***bell.***, ***camph.***, crot-h., cupr., ***dig.***, ***kali-m.***, mosch., plb.
  - after - absin., bell., kali-c., kali-chl., sec.
  - before - ***kali-m.***, op., sul-h.
- **crying** - ***acon.***, agar., agar-pr., atro., bell., ***canth.***, ***caust.***, ***chin-s.***, ***cina***, crot-h., cupr., ***cupr-ac.***, dat-m., ferr-p., merc.
  - crying, for help - ***canth.***, stram.
- **dark,** in - ***calc-ar.***, ***carb-v.***, ***cupr.***, ***stram.***
- **day** and night - ***op.***, ***stram.***
- **death,** talks about - ***acon.***
- **delusions,** with - aeth., ***ars.***, ***bell.***, ***cann-i.***, ***cann-s.***, cham., dig., graph., ***hyos.***, ***kali-bi.***, op., petr., plb., sep., sil., spong., ***stram.***, ***sulph.***
- **depletion,** after - ***chin.***
- **devils,** sees - op.
- **distension** of abdomen and constipation, with - ***acet-ac.***
- **dogs,** talk about - bell.
- **eating,** amel. - anac., bell.

DELIRIUM, general
embraces the stove - hyos.
encephalitis, in - ***acon., cocc., puls.***
envy, with - lyc.
epilepsy, during - op.
after - ***arg-m.,*** plb.
erotic - camph., cann-i., ***canth., hyos.,*** kali-br., ***lach., phos., plat., sec., stram.,*** verat.
escapes in abortion - ***coloc.***
evening - ***bell.,*** bry., canth., croc., cupr., lach., lyc., phos., plb., sulph.
6 p.m. - phos.
8 p.m. - mygal.
dark, in the - ***calc-ar.,*** cupr.
nap, during - nux-v.
exaltation of strength, with - ***agar., aur.,*** hyos., sec., stram.
exhaustion, with - agar., ail., am-c., bapt., dor., hyos., lyc.
extravagant language, with - bell.
face, distorted - ***plb.***
livid - ***bell.***
muscles constantly in play - ***stram.***
pale - ***hyos.***
red - ***ail., bapt.,*** **BELL.,** dor., ***gels.,*** **HYOS.,** op.
fantastic - ***bell.,*** carb-s., cham., con., dulc., graph., hyos., op., sep., sil., spong., ***stram., sulph.***
fatigue, study, overexertion, from - lach.
fear of men, with - bell., ***plat.***
fever, during - acon., act-sp., aeth., agar., ail., anag., ant-t., ***anthr., apis, ars., arum-t.,*** bar-c., **BELL.,** ***bry.,*** bufo, **CALC.,** ***camph., canth., cham.,*** chel., ***chin., chin-s.,*** cimic., coff., colch., ***crot-h.,*** dor., ***dulc., hell., hep., hyos.,*** ign., iod., juni., ***lach.,*** merc-i-r., morph., mur-ac., ***nat-m.,*** op., ***ox-ac.,*** psor., **PYROG.,** ***sabad.,*** sal-ac., ***sec., sin-n., spong.,*** stram., sul-ac., sulph., vario., verat., verat-v.
fierce - agar., ***bapt.,*** bell., hyos., ***stram.***
fire, talks of - ***calc.***
foolish, silly - acon., aeth., agar., bell., calc-sil., cic., hyos., merc., ***op., stram.,*** sulph.
foreign, countries, talks of - cann-i.
talks in a - lach., nit-ac., ***stram.***
frightful - ***acon.,*** anac., ***atro.,*** bar-c., **BELL.,** calc., canth., cic., colch., coloc., dig., ***hep., hyos.,*** nat-m., nux-v., ***op., phos., plb., puls.,*** rhod., sec., sil., **STRAM.,** ***verat.,*** zinc., zinc-p.
furious - bell., ***bry.,*** verat.
gather objects off the wall, tries to - bell., hyos.
gay - agar., ant-t., aur., ***bell.,*** cann-s., con., hyos., lact., ***stram.,*** verat.
alternating, with laughing, singing, whistling, crying, etc. - stram.
alternating, with melancholy - agar.
giggling - hyosin.
grimaces, with - ***bell.***
groping as if in dark - plb.
head, with hot - ***bell.,*** bufo

DELIRIUM, general
headache, during - acon., agar., ail., ars., cimic., ***colch.,*** crot-h., glon., mag-c., ***meli.,*** mosch., ***nux-v.,*** sec., stram., tarent., verat.
from - atro., ***aur.,*** aur-m.
heat agg. - bry., stram.
home, wants to go - bell., bry., ***cupr-ac.***
horses, talks about - ***stram.***
hysterical, almost - bell., ***hyos.,*** ign., tarent., verat.
imperious - lyc.
injuries to head, after - bell., hyos., op., ***nat-s., stram.,*** verat.
intermittent - con., **STRAM.**
intoxicated, as if - ***agar.,*** am-c., carb-an., chin-s., cori-r., vip.
jealousy, from - **HYOS.**
jerking, with - acon.
jumping, with - acon., bell., lact., merc.
know his relatives, does not, throws wine and medicine at nurse - agar.
laughing - acon., apis, ***bell.,*** colch., con., cupr., ***hyos.,*** hyosin., ***ign.,*** lach., lact., op., plb., sec., sep., ***stram.,*** sulph., thea., verat., zinc.
lochia, during - verat.
look fixed on one point - ***acon.,*** art-v., bov., camph., canth., cupr., dor., ***ign.,*** stram., ran-b.
staring, with wrinkled face - stram.
loss of fluids, from - ***chin., lach.***
maniacal - acon., ***aeth.,*** agar., ail., ant-c., ***apis,*** ars., **BELL.,** bry., ***camph.,*** cann-i., ***canth.,*** carb-s., chin-s., ***cic., coff.,*** colch., con., cori-r., crot-h., ***cupr.,*** dig., glon., ***hell.,*** **HYOS.,** indg., ***kali-bi., lach.,*** led., lob., lyc., merc., merc-c., nat-m., nux-m., ***oena., op.,*** plb., rhod., ***sec.,*** **STRAM.,** tarent., ter., ***verat.,*** zinc.
love, from disappointed - ***phos.***
meningitis cerebro-spinal - ***apis,*** **BELL.,** ***chr-ac., hell.,*** naja, ***nat-s., sulph., verat.,*** verat-v.
menses, during - acon., apis, bell., cocc., hyos., lyc., nux-m., puls., stram., verat.
sees something alive - cocc.
before - acon., ars., bell., hyos., lyc., verat.
menstrual difficulties, with - apis.
suppressed, with - stram.
mental, exertion - ***lach.***
mild - ***apis,*** **BAPT.,** bell., ***ph-ac., puls.,*** rhus-t., sec., **STRAM.,** ***valer., vario.,*** verat.
miscarriage, after - ruta
moaning, with - bell., ***crot-h.***
morning - ambr., bry., con., dulc., hell., hep., merc., nat-c.
at daybreak - **BRY.,** con.
waking, on - ambr., dulc., hell., hep., nat-m.
mouth, moves lips as if talking - bell.
puts stones in - merc.
moves, constantly from place to place - ***oena.***
queer - **STRAM.**

DELIRIUM, general

murmuring - arn., calad., ***hyos.,*** ***lyc.,*** ph-ac., ***phos.,*** rhus-t., ***stram.,*** tab., ***zinc.***
slowly - ph-ac.
to himself - hyos., merc., tab.

muttering - agar., ***ail.,*** ***amyg.,*** ***ant-t.,*** ***apis,*** ***arn.,*** ars., arum-t., ***bapt.,*** ***bell.,*** **BRY.,** calad., calc-sil., chel., ***cic.,*** ***colch.,*** convo-s., ***crot-h.,*** dor., gels., hell., ***hep.,*** **HYOS.,** ***iris,*** kali-br., kali-cy., ***lach.,*** ***lyc.,*** ***merc.,*** ***mur-ac.,*** nat-m., nux-v., ***op.,*** ***ph-ac.,*** **PHOS.,** raja-s., ***rhus-t.,*** ***sec.,*** **STRAM.,** ***sulph.,*** ***tab.,*** ***tarax.,*** ***ter.,*** ***verat.***
himself, to - bell., hyos., rhus-t., tab.
sleep, in - ant-t., ars., bry., ***gels.,*** sulph.
slowly - ph-ac.

naked in delusions, wants to be - ***hyos.,*** stram.

night - **ACON.,** ***aeth.,*** ***apis,*** arn., **ARS.,** ars-i., ars-s-f., atro., aur., aur-a., **BAPT.,** ***bell.,*** ***bry.,*** ***cact.,*** calc., camph., cann-i., ***canth.,*** ***carb-s.,*** carb-v., ***cham.,*** ***chel.,*** chin-a., chin-s., cod., coff., colch., coloc., con., cor-r., ***crot-h.,*** dig., dulc., ether, graph., hep., hippoz., hydr., piloc., ***kali-ar.,*** ***kali-c.,*** kali-m., kali-p., **LACH.,** lyc., ***lyss.,*** ***merc.,*** merc-c., merc-cy., merc-sul., nit-ac., nux-v., op., ***plb.,*** ***puls.,*** rheum, rhus-t., sec., sep., sil., ***stram.,*** sul-i., sulph., sul-ac., syph., tub., verat.
1 a.m. to 2 a.m. - ***lachn.***
midnight, after - apis.
waking, on - ***cact.***

noisy - agar., ***bell.,*** ***camph.,*** ***hyos.,*** **STRAM.,** verat.

nonsense, with eyes open - ars., anac., bapt., ***canth.,*** cham., coll., coloc., crot-h., ***hyos.,*** op., ***stram.,*** tarent., **VERAT.**

noon - bell., bry.
until midnight - ***lach.***

pains, from - **HYOS.,** **VERAT.**
with the - acon., arg-m., arg-n., bov., cham., dulc., tarent-c., ***verat.***

paroxysmal - ***bell.,*** con., ***gels.,*** naja, phos., plb.

periodic - ***bell.,*** samb.

persecution, of - ars., calc., cupr., hyos., kali-br., ***lach.,*** merc., nat-m., rhus-t., stram., verat.

perspiration, amel. - aeth.
cold, with - ***verat.***

picking at nose or lips, with - ***arum-t.***

pupils, with dilated - acon., **BELL.,** ***cimic.,*** ***stram.***

quiet - **BRY.,** calc-sil., camph., ***carb-v.,*** ***chel.,*** chin., chlf., ***chlor.,*** croc., cupr., cupr-ac., **HYOS.,** hyosin., kali-p., op., past., ***ph-ac.,*** phos., plb., rhus-t., sec., tab., valer., verat.
alternating with restlessness - ***chlor.***

rabid - bell., canth., lyss., ***stram.***

raging - ***acon.,*** ***act-sp.,*** ***aeth.,*** **AGAR.,** agar-pa., ail., alco., anac., ant-s., ***ant-t.,*** apis, arg-m., arg-n., ars., ars-s-f., atro., **BELL.,** bry., calc., ***camph.,*** cann-i., cann-s., **CANTH.,** ***carb-s.,*** cham., chin-s., cic., chel., chin., ***cimic.,*** cina, clem., colch., coloc., ***cupr.,*** cupr-ac., dat-f., dig., dulc., ether, glon., graph., ***hell.,*** hep., **HYOS.,** hyper., jatr., juni., ***kali-i.,*** lach., lob., lol., **LYC.,** ***merc.,*** merc-cy., morph., mosch., nat-m., **NIT-AC.,** nux-m., ***oena.,*** **OP.,** par., phos., ***plb.,*** ***puls.,*** rheum, **SEC.,** ***sol-n.,*** **STRAM.,** sulph., sul-ac., ***tab.,*** tarent., trach., **VERAT.,** verat-v., vip., zinc., zinc-p.

rambling - atro., ***bell.,*** chlol., ***chlor.,*** hyos., ***nat-m.,*** plb., sec., ***sulph.***

recognizes no one - agar., **AIL.,** bell., calad., hyos., merc., nux-v., op., stram., tab., verat.

refuses to take the medicine - agar-pr., lach.

religious - agar., alco., aur., lach., **VERAT.**

repeats the same sentence - camph.

reproachful - hyos., lyc.

restless - acon., ail., atro., bry., **HYOS.,** iod., merc-sul., phos., plb., ***stram.,*** sulph., ***verat.***

rocking to and fro - bell., hyos.

rolls, on floor - ***op.***

romping, with children - agar.

running, with - bell., con.

sad - acon., bell., puls.

same subject all the time - petr.

scolding - chr-ac., hyos., merc., stram., verat-v.

screaming, with - crot-h., cupr., ***merc.***

sepsis, from - ***bapt.,*** crot-h., dor., ***lach.,*** mur-ac., **PYROG.,** ***rhus-t.,*** sec., tarent-c., ter., ***verat.,*** ***verat-v.,*** ***vip.***

shy, hides himself - **STRAM.**

silent - agar., sec.

singing - agar., cic., lact., stram.

sleep, during - acon., ant-c., **APIS,** ars., ***bar-c.,*** **BELL.,** bry., ***cact.,*** ***calc.,*** cham., cina, cupr., cupr-ac., ***gels.,*** hyper., lach., ***lyc.,*** merc., mur-ac., ***nit-s-d.,*** ***op.,*** rheum, sant., spong., stram., verat.
comatose - acon., ant-c., arn., bry., camph., coloc., puls., sec.
after - ***lach.,*** petr.
amel. - bell., ***cact.***
aroused, on being - phos., hep., sec.
falling, on - ***bell.,*** ***bry.,*** cact., calc., camph., caust., ***chin.,*** ***gels.,*** gins., guai., ign., merc., ph-ac., ***phos.,*** rhus-t., ***spong.,*** ***sulph.***

sleepiness, with - acon., ant-c., arn., ***bell.,*** ***bry.,*** calc-p., camph., coloc., ***crot-h.,*** hyos., lach., ***op.,*** **PULS.,** sec.

sleeplessness, with - cimic.

sopor, with - aeth., agar., ***ail.,*** am-c., ***ant-t.,*** ***apis,*** arn., ***bapt.,*** bell., benz-n., ***camph.,*** ***carb-ac.,*** diph., gels., ***hell.,*** ***hyos.,*** kali-c., lach., laur., lob-p., mur-ac., nit-s-d., nux-m., ***op.,*** ***ph-ac.,*** ***phos.,*** piloc., ***rhus-t.,*** stram., ter., thyr., ***verat.,*** ***zinc.***

sorrowful - acon., bell., dulc., lyc., puls.

spectres - op.

stupid - ***stram.***

DELIRIUM, general

talkative, loquacious - ***agar.,*** aur., bapt., bar-c., ***bell.,*** bry., camph., cann-i., **CIMIC.,** ***crot-h., cupr.,*** dat-m., dor., gels., ***hyos.,*** **LACH., LACHN.,** lyss., merc-cy., naja, oena., ***op.,*** oper., par., petr., ***phos., plat.,*** plb., podo., ***rhus-t.,*** **STRAM.,** ***sulph., verat.***

fever, in - lachn.

indistinct - apis, bell., ***hyos., op.***

rhyme, in - thea.

talks of business - ***bry.***

teeth, grinding - **BELL.**

terror, expression of - bell.

thirst, with - camph., ***verat.***

throwing from windows - calc., sil.

trembling, with - acon., apis, ars., bell., bry., calc., chin., hyos., ign., nat-m., op., phys., plat., ***puls.,*** rhus-t., sabad., samb., stram., sulph., valer., verat., verat-v.

urinates on the floor, tries to - plb.

outside the pot - bell.

violent - ***acon.,*** agar., alum., ***apis,*** **ARS.,** atro., ***aur.,*** **BELL.,** camph., canth., chlf., con., ***cupr.,*** **HYOS.,** ***lach., op.,*** phos., plb., puls., ***sec.,*** **STRAM.,** verat., verat-v., zinc., zinc-p.

is restrained and calmed with great difficulty - zinc.

vivid - bell., ***stram.***

waking, on - aur., bell., bry., cact., carb-v., chel., cina, coff., colch., cur., dulc., ***hyos.,*** lob., ***lach.,*** merc., nat-c., par., sep., stram., zinc.

watching, vigil, from - cur., ***hyos., lach.,*** mur-ac., op., phos.

water, jumping into - bell., sec.

wedding, prepares for - ***hyos.***

well, declares she is - apis, ***arn., ars.***

wild - atro., **BELL.,** ***bry.,*** calen., camph., canth., chlol., colch., cupr., gels., hydr-ac., ***hyos., kali-br.,*** lach., nat-sal., ***op.,*** **PLB., STRAM.,** ***valer., vario., verat.***

at night - gall-ac., plb.

wraps up in fur during summer - hyos.

wrongs, of fancied - hyos.

DELUSIONS, (see Delusions, chapter)

DEMENTIA, madness (see Insanity, Mania, Schizophrenia) - ***agar.,*** alco., alum., **ANAC.,** ant-c., ars., ***bell.,*** calc., calc-p., cann-i., carb-s., ***carc.,*** coca, con., croc., crot-h., hell., **HYOS.,** ign., kali-i., lach., ***lil-t., merc., nat-sal., nux-v.,*** op., ***ph-ac., phos., pic-ac.,*** sulph., tarent., ***verat.***

epileptics, of - acon., ***bell.,*** cimic., cupr., ***cupr-ac., ferr-i.,*** laur., ***oena., sil.,*** sol-c., stram., verat-v.

masturbation, from - ***agn.,*** calc-p., canth., caust., dam., nux-v., op., ***ph-ac.,*** phos., pic-ac., ***staph.***

paretic - ***acon., aesc-g., agar.,*** bell., cann-i., cimic., cupr., hyos., ign., iodof., merc., ***phos., plb.,*** stram., verat-v., zinc.

sadness, with - tarent.

DEMENTIA, madness

senile, (see Alzheimer's disease) - ***agn., anac.,*** ant-c., arg-m., ***arg-n.,*** ars., aur., ***aur-i.,*** aza., bapt., bar-ac., ***bar-c.,*** bell., bry., calc-p., cann-i., carc., ***con., crot-h.,*** fl-ac., ***hyos.,*** ign., iod., lach., lil-t., ***lyc.,*** nat-i., nat-m., nux-v., ***ov., phos.,*** sec., sep., sulph., thiosin.

senile, foolish talking, with - bar-c., con., ***hyos.,*** op., plb.

at night - puls.

syphilitics, of - aur-i., ***kali-i.,*** merc., nit-ac., sulph.

DEPRAVITY, dishonest - ***anac.,*** lyc., thuj.

DEPRESSION, sadness (see Despair) - ***abies-n.,*** abrot., acal., acet-ac., achy., **ACON.,** acon-f., act-sp., adlu., adon., ***aesc.,*** aeth., ether, agar., agav-t., ***agn.,*** ail., alco., alf., all-c., all-s., allox., aloe, ***alum.,*** alumn., am-br., ***ambr., am-c., am-m., aml-n.,*** ammc., ***anac.,*** anan., ang., anh., ***ant-c.,*** anthr., apis, apoc., arag., aran., ***arg-m., arg-n., arist-cl., arn.,*** **ARS., ARS-I.,** ars-m., ars-s-r., arum-d., arum-m., arum-t., ***asaf.,*** asar., asc-t., astac., aster., astra-e., atro., **AUR.,** aur-i., **AUR-M.,** ***aur-s.,*** aza., bapt., bar-ac., ***bar-c.,*** bar-i., ***bar-m., bell.,*** benz-ac., berb., bol., bor., bov., ***brom., bry., bufo,*** buf-s., buni-o., but-ac., ***cact.,*** cadm-met., caj., calad., **CALC.,** calc-ac., **CALC-AR.,** ***calc-f., calc-p.,*** **CALC-S.,** ***camph.,*** camph-br., cann-i., ***cann-s., canth., caps.,*** carb-ac., **CARB-AN.,** carb-o., **CARB-S.,** ***carb-v.,*** **CARC.,** card-m., carl., cass., cast., **CAUST.,** cecr., cedr., cench., **CHAM.,** ***chel.,*** chim., **CHIN.,** ***chin-a.,*** chin-b., ***chin-s., chlol.,*** chlor., chlorpr., chr-ac., ***cic.,*** **CIMIC.,** ***cina,*** cinnb., ***clem.,*** cob., cob-n., coc-c., coca, ***cocc.,*** coch., ***coff., colch., coloc., con.,*** convo-d., convo-s., cop., ***corn.,*** cortico., cortiso., cot., ***croc.,*** **CROT-C.,** ***crot-h.,*** crot-t., cund., ***cupr., cupr-ac.,*** cupr-ar., ***cur., cycl.,*** cypr., cyt-l., der., ***dig.,*** dirc., ***dros., dulc.,*** echi., elae., elaps, elat., ergot., erig., esp-g., eug., euon., eup-per., eup-pur., euph., euphr., fago., fagu., **FERR.,** ***ferr-ar.,*** **FERR-I.,** ferr-m., ***ferr-p.,*** ferul., fic., fl-ac., flav., flor-p., form., frax., gad., gamb., **GELS.,** glon., goss., gran., **GRAPH.,** ***grat.,*** guai., guat., haem., halo., ham., **HELL.,** ***helon., hep.,*** hera., **HIPP.,** hir., hist., ***hura, hydr.,*** hydr-ac., hydrc., hydroph., **HYOS.,** hyper., hypoth., iber., **IGN.,** ind., ***indg.,*** indol., **IOD.,** ***ip.,*** iris, jac-c., jug-c., kali-a., ***kali-ar.,*** kali-bi., **KALI-BR.,** ***kali-c.,*** kali-fer., kali-i., kali-n., **KALI-P.,** kali-s., kalm., kreos., kres., **LAC-C.,** ***lac-d.,*** **LACH.,** lachn., lact., lam., lapa., lat-m., lath., ***laur., lec.,*** led., lepi., **LEPT.,** lil-s., **LIL-T.,** lipp., lith., lob., ***lob-s.,*** luf-op., lup., **LYC.,** lycps., lyss., mag-arct., mag-aust., macro., mag-c., mag-f., mag-m., mag-p., mag-s., ***manc., man., mang.,*** med., meli., menis., meny., meph., **MERC.,** ***merc-aur., merc-c., merc-i-f., merc-i-r.,*** merl., methys., **MEZ.,** ***mill.,*** mit., moly-met., morph., mosch., ***mur-ac.,*** **MURX.,** ***mygal.,*** myric., nabal., ***naja,*** **NAT-A.,** nat-br., **NAT-C.,** nat-f., nat-hchls., **NAT-M.,** nat-n., ***nat-p.,*** **NAT-S.,** nat-sal., nep., nicc., **NIT-AC.,** nux-m., ***nux-v.,*** oena., ***ol-an.,***

DEPRESSION, sadness - olnd., onop., **OP.,** orig., oxyt., palo., parat., paull., ped., pen., penic., perh., peti., ***petr.,*** phel., phenob., ***ph-ac., phos., phyt.,*** pic-ac., picro., pin-s., plan., **PLAT.,** plect., ***plb.,*** plb-a., plumbg., pneu., podo., polyg., polyp-p., prot., prun., psil., **PSOR.,** ptel., **PULS.,** pyrog., pyrus., rad., ran-b., ran-s., raph., rauw., reser., rham-f., rheum., rhod., **RHUS-T.,** ***rhus-v.,*** rib-ac., rob., rumx., ***ruta,*** sabad., ***sabin.,*** sac-alb., sal-ac., sang., sanic., sant., sapin., sarcol-ac., saroth., sarr., sars., scut., sec., ***sel.,*** senec., seneg., **SEP.,** sieg., ***sil.,*** sol-c., sol-o., ***spig.,*** spira., ***spong.,*** squil., **STANN.,** stann-i., ***staph., still., stram.,*** stront-c., **STRY.,** ***sul-ac., sul-i.,*** sulfa., sulfonam., **SULPH.,** sumb., ***syph., tab.,*** tarax., tarent., tell., ***ter.,*** thal., thea, thiop., **THUJ.,** thymol., til., tong., tril., trinit., trio., tub., upa., ***uran-n.,*** ust., valer., **VERAT.,** ***verat-v.,*** verb., vesp., ***vib.,*** vip-a., ***vinc.,*** viol-o., viol-t., ***visc.,*** wild., wye., xan., x-ray., yuc., **ZINC., ZINC-P.,** zing., ziz.

- **acute** - aur., carc., nat-m.
- **afternoon** - aeth., alum., alum-p., ant-t., calc-s., carb-an., carl., cast., ***chin-s.,*** cimic., ***cocc.,*** coc-c., con., cop., dig., echi., ***graph.,*** grat., hydr-ac., ign., iod., mang., mur-ac., myric., nicc., ol-an., op., ***phos.,*** plat., puls-n, rhus-r., ruta, sulph., tarent., thuj., ***zinc.,*** zinc-p.
  - 6 p.m. - coca, dig.
  - amel. - agar., ***cann-s.***
- **air,** in open - aeth., con., cupr., hep., ***kali-c.,*** mur-ac., petr., ***ph-ac.,*** sabin., sep., sul-ac., sulph.
  - amel. - arg-n., arist-cl., carl., coff., **PLAT., PULS.,** rhus-t., tarent.
- **alcoholics,** in - alco., ***aur.,*** carc., cimic., lach., nat-m., nux-v., puls., staph.
- **alone,** when - aeth., all-s., allox., **ARS.,** aur., bov., ***calc.,*** con., ***dros.,*** ferr., ***ferr-ar.,*** kali-ar., kali-c., kali-n., lyc., mag-aust., mag-m., ***mez.,*** **NAT-M.,** phos., **PULS.,** sil., ***stram.,*** valer., zinc.
  - amel. - allox., nat-m.
- **alternating** with, (see Manic depression)
  - anger - aur., kali-fer., staph., zinc.
  - antics playing - ***op.***
  - contentment - zinc.
  - eccentricity - petr.
  - euphoria - aster., coff., lach., meph., nid., onop., senec.
  - exuberance - ferr., petr., plat.
  - fear - zinc.
  - fright - op., zinc.
  - indifference - sep.
  - irritability - ambr., zinc.
  - physical energy - ***aur.,carc.,*** hir., med.
  - quarrelsomeness - ***con.,*** sulfonam.
  - sexual excitement - lil-t.
  - stupor - thyr.
  - tenderness - plat.
  - tranquility - chin-b.
  - vehemence - ambr.
  - vivacity - carc., caust., psor., tarent.
- **amenorrhea,** in - anac., aur., caust., cycl., cypr., ign., kali-p., nat-m.

DEPRESSION, sadness

- **anger,** from - aur., calc-p., carc., ign., lyc., nit-ac., ***puls.,*** spig., ***staph.***
  - after - apis, ars., bell., nux-v., petr., phos., plat., puls., sep., **STAPH.**
- **annoyance,** after - kali-bi.
- **anxious** - ***acon.,*** asaf., asar., calc., carb-an., carb-v., carc., caust., cic., ***croc., crot-h.,*** crot-t., cupr., dig., dros., graph., hep., iod., ***kali-br.,*** laur., lyc., lyss., ***mag-arct.,*** merc., nit-ac., **PLAT.,** rhus-t., ruta, sep., spig., spong., stann., tab., thuj-l.
  - menopause, during - ***kali-br.***
- **aversion,** to see her children from sadness - ***con., sep.***
  - devotedly attached children become burdensome - **KALI-I.**
- **bed,** will not leave - aran.
- **bitter** - calc-s.
- **breakfast,** after - con.
- **burning,** in right lumbar region, from - nit-ac.
- **business,** when thinking of - ***aur., puls.,*** syph.
- **cancer,** with - carc., con.
- **causeless** - ***calc-sil.,*** carc., cench., nat-m., ped., phos., rhus-t., ***sep.,*** staph., sulph., tarent.
- **cheerfulness,** after - carb-s.
- **childbirth,** after - ***agn., anac.,*** arg-n., ***aur., aur-m.,*** bell., ***cimic., con.,*** ign., ***kali-br., lach., lil-t.,*** manc., nat-m., plat., ***psor., puls.,*** **SEP., SULPH.,** thuj., ***tub., verat., verat-v.,*** zinc.
- **children** - abrot., ***ars.,*** aur., ***calc., carc.,*** caust., ***lach.,*** lyc., **NAT-M.,** rhus-t., sulph.
- **chill,** during - **ACON.,** am-c., anthro., ***apis,*** **ARS.,** calc., cann-s., carb-s., cham., **CHIN.,** chin-a., cocc., **CON.,** cupr., ***cycl., graph.,*** hep., **IGN.,** kali-chl., kali-m., lach., ***lyc.,*** merc., merc-sul., **NAT-M.,** nit-ac., nux-v., ol-an., phos., plat., ***puls.,*** rhus-t., sac-alb., sel., sep., spig., staph., verat.
  - before - ***ant-c.***
- **clear,** weather - ***stram.***
- **cloudy,** weather - am-c., ***aur.,*** plat., sep.
- **cold,** from becoming - cimic., ***phos.,*** teucr.
- **company,** agg. in - euph., ***lyc., nat-m.***
  - amel. - bov.
  - aversion to, desire for solitude - alum., aur., ***con.,*** cupr., ***helon., led.,*** murx., ***nat-c., nat-m.,*** rhus-t., sep.
  - desire for - stram.
- **complaining,** amel. - tab.
- **consoled,** cannot be - ars., ***aur., nat-m.***
- **continence,** from - bell., **CON.,** hyos., stram.
- **conversation,** amel. - ***lac-d.***
- **coughing,** after - iod., sep.
- **criminal,** as if being the greatest - sabad.
- **cry,** cannot - am-m., apis, ***carc.,*** crot-c., ***gels.,*** **IGN., NAT-M.,** nux-v., staph.
- **crying,** agg. - sep., ***stann.***
  - amel. - dig., med., phos., puls.
  - palpitations, and - lac-d.

DEPRESSION, sadness
darkness - am-m., ars., calc., camph., ***phos.,*** plat., rhus-t., stram.
day and night - kali-p., sulph.
crying, with - ***caust.***
diarrhea in morning, with - lil-t.
daytime - agn., calc-sil., cench., cerv., dros., lyss., nat-m., paull., phel., stann., staph., sulph., sul-ac., zinc.
death, fear of, with - cupr.
diarrhea, during - ***apis, cocc.,*** crot-h., ferr., ***gamb., lyc., merc.***
diet, errors of - **NAT-C.**
digestion, during - iod.
dinner, after - ***ars.,*** canth., ***nat-c., nux-v.,*** til., zinc.
disappointment, from - dig., ign.
disease, about - alum., carc., cecr., sin-n., ***sulph.,*** syph.
diverted from thoughts of himself, desires to be - ***aur.,*** camph.
domestic affairs, over - sep.
dream, from - phos., plat.
drowsiness, with - coca.
drunkenness, during - nux-v., puls., staph.
dwelling, constantly on her condition - carc., nat-m., ***sulph.***
eating, after - alum., ***anac.,*** ant-c., arg-n., ***ars.,*** asaf., bar-c., canth., caust., cham., ***chin., cinnb.,*** con., graph., hyos., iod., mosch., ***nat-c.,*** **NUX-V.,** ol-an., podo., ptel., ***puls.,*** til., zinc.
amel. - am-c., am-m., clem., kali-bi., mag-m., tarent.
before - mag-m.
desire for, with - ign.
hasty eating, from - sulph.
while - sep.
emission, from - aur., dig., dios., ham., nat-c., nat-p., **NUX-V.,** ph-ac., ***puls.,*** sang., ust.
enjoys - ign., nat-m.
epilepsy, before attack of - zinc., zinc-valer.
day and night - art-v.
eruption suppressed, with - ***psor.,*** **SULPH.**
evening - aeth., agar., alum., am-c., ***ant-c.,*** ant-t., arag., ***ars.,*** ars-s-f., **AUR.,** aur-a., **AUR-S.,** bar-c., bov., ***calc.,*** carb-an., ***carb-s., carb-v., calc-s.,*** cast., caust., con., cop., cycl., dig., ferr., ferr-ar., ferr-p., fl-ac., ***graph., hep.,*** hyper., ign., kali-ar., kali-bi., kali-c., kali-chl., kali-p., kali-s., kreos., lact., ***lyc.,*** lyss., mag-arct., mag-c., mag-s., murx., nabal., naja, nat-a., nat-c., nat-m., nat-p., **NIT-AC.,** ***phos., plat.,*** **PULS.,** ran-b., ran-s., rhus-t., ***ruta,*** sel., senec., seneg., ***sep.,*** spig., stram., ***sulph.,*** ther., ***verat.,*** zinc., zinc-p.
9 a.m. - phos., sac-alb.
amel. - aloe, am-c., bism., calc., cann-s., carb-v., coca, halo., ham., kali-c., mag-c., nicc., sulph., viol-t., ***zinc.***
bed, in - ***ars., calc., graph.,*** kali-c., ***stram.,*** stront-c., ***sulph.,*** thuj.
cheerful in morning, but - graph.

DEPRESSION, sadness
evening, at
eating, when - tarent.
twilight, in - am-m., ***ars.,*** ign., ***phos., puls.,*** rhus-t.
excitement, after - ambr.
exertion, after - agar., ***ars.,*** calc., ***coca,*** hypoth.
air, in open - kali-c.
amel. - ferr.
exhilaration, after - myric., plat., ziz.
extreme - sel.
eyes closed, with - arg-n.
fault, as if in - tarent.
fear, from - sec.
fever, during the - **ACON.,** aesc., ***ant-c.,*** apis, aran., arg-n., **ARS.,** ars-s-f., aur., ***bell., bol.,*** bry., ***calc.,*** calc-ar., calc-sil., carb-s., chin., chin-a., coca, cocc., ***con., dig., elat., eup-per., gels.,*** graph., hipp., ign., ***ip.,*** kali-ar., lyc., nat-a., ***nat-c.,*** **NAT-M.,** nat-p., nat-s., ***nux-m.,*** op., ***petr.,*** ph-ac., ***phos.,*** plan., puls., ***rhus-t., samb.,*** sep., ***sil., spong.,*** stann., staph., stram., sulph., tarent., vip.
financial loss, after - ars., **AUR.,** mez., psor.
flowers, smell of - hyos.
forenoon - alum., am-c., ant-c., arg-m., apis, ***cann-s.,*** graph., nux-m., phel., sars., sel., thuj.
forenoon, amel. - graph., sars.
friends, as if having lost affection of - ***aur., puls.***
girls, before puberty - ***ars.,*** calc-p., ***hell.,*** ign., ***lach., nat-m., puls., sep.***
gloomy - aur., bov., cupr., graph., sep.
grief, after - am-m., **AUR.,** ***carc., ign.,*** **NAT-M.,** ***ph-ac.,*** staph.
hemorrhoids suppressed, after - caps.
happy, on seeing others - cic., hell., helon.
harsh word, from a - med., nat-m.
headache, during - agar., agn., aloe, ***arg-n.,*** ars., aur., caust., cimic., cod., con., ***crot-h., dulc.,*** **GUARE.,** ***ign.,*** indol., iris, kali-c., lac-d., ***lachn.,*** lil-t., merl., ***naja,*** nat-c., nat-m., ol-an., phos., pic-ac., ***plb.,*** ptel., ***puls.,*** sarr., ***sars.,*** sel., sep., stann., ***ter.,*** ther., thymol., zinc.
health, about the - acon., ars., carc., ***sep.,*** staph.
heart, sensations, from - aur., lyc.
heat flushes of, during - nat-c.
heaviness of, body - ***cedr.,*** graph.
feet - graph.
legs - calc., con.
horrid - syph.
house, in - ***plat.,*** **RHUS-T.**
driving out of - laur.
entering, on - plat., tarent.
humiliation, after - **CARC.,** ***ign., puls., staph.***
hunger, with canine - ***nat-m.***
hysterical, with occipital headache - graph.
idleness, with - calc.

DEPRESSION, sadness

impotence, with - ***agn., aur., calad., gels.,*** **KALI-BR.,** ***spong.***

infertility, from - aur., nat-m.

injuries, from - arn., ***hyper.***

head, of the - arn., ***carc., cic.,*** con., hell., hyper., **NAT-S.,** puls., rhus-t., sulph.

insult, as if from - ***cocc.***

itching, from - **PSOR.**

jealousy, with - ***kali-ar., lach.***

labor, during - cimic., ***ign.,*** lach., nat-m., puls., rhus-t., sulph., ***verat.,*** zinc.

laughing, after - plat.

involuntary, with - ***phos.***

light, subdued agg. - nat-s.

loquacity, after - aran-ix.

love, from disappointed - ***aur.,*** bell., carc., dig., ***hyos.,*** **IGN.,** ***nat-m.***

back, lumbar region, from burning in - nit-ac.

masturbation, from - agar., ***aur.,*** calad., cocc., ***con.,*** gels., ham., ***nat-m.,*** nat-p., nux-v., **PH-AC.,** ***plat.,*** sars., sil., staph., sulph.

menopause, during - anac., ***arg-m.,*** arg-n., arist-cl., ***aur., aur-m.,*** buth-a., ***cimic., con.,*** hydroph., ign., ***kali-br., lach.,*** lil-t., magn-gr., manc., nat-m., penic., ***psor.,*** puls., **SEP., SULPH.,** ***tab.,*** valer., ***verat.,*** zinc., zinc-valer.

menses, during - am-c., aur., berb., brom., cact., calc., ***caust.,*** cimic., cop., cur., ferr., graph., ign., ***lac-c.,*** lac-d., lyc., mag-m., merc., mur-ac., murx., nat-c., ***nat-m.,*** nat-sil., nit-ac., ***petr.,*** plat., plb., ***puls.,*** senec., ***sep.,*** sil., stann., ***tab.,*** thuj., tub., zinc.

after - alum., chin., ***ferr.,*** hell., sapin., sil., ust.

agg. during - ***cycl.,*** macro.

amel. - arist-cl., ***cycl., lach.,*** macro., ***stann.,*** zinc.

before - acon., am-c., ***aur.,*** bell., berb., brom., ***calc.,*** carl., ***caust., cimic., con.,*** cycl., ferr., ferr-p., hell., helon., ***ign.,*** iris, lac-c., lac-d., ***lyc.,*** manc., ***murx.,*** nat-c., **NAT-M.,** ***nit-ac.,*** phos., plat., psor., **PULS.,** sabal., **SEP., STANN.,** stram., ***verat.,*** vesp., vip-a., xan.

delayed, from - **KALI-P.,** ***lyc.***

suppressed - ars., aur., aur-a., calc., chen-a., cimic., ***con.,*** croc., cycl., nat-m., nux-m., nux-v., ph-ac., phos., puls., ***rhus-t.,*** sep., sil., staph., sulph.

the first menses - hell.

mental exertion, after - ***ars.,*** asar., ***kali-p.***

mercury, after abuse of - **AUR., AUR-M.,** ***hep., nit-ac.,*** staph.

midnight, after - manc., ph-ac., phos., rhus-t.

milk, disappearing after - agn.

misfortune, as if from - **AUR.,** ***calc.,*** chin-s., cycl., phel., ph-ac., phos., puls., rhus-t., staph., sulph.

DEPRESSION, sadness

morning - agar., aloe, ***alum.,*** alumn., am-c., amph., anac., ant-c., apis, arag., arg-m., arg-n., ***aur.,*** aur-s., bar-c., bar-m., brucin., calad., calc., calc-sil., cann-i., canth., ***carb-an.,*** cast., caust., con., cop., dulc., hep., hura, hyper., graph., kali-c., kali-p., kali-s., kali-sil., kreos., **LACH.,** lil-s., ***lyc.,*** mag-m., mag-p., mag-s., manc., mur-ac., myric., naja, ***nat-s.,*** nicc., ***nit-ac., nux-v.,*** ol-an., op., ***petr., phos., plat., plb., puls.,*** rhus-t., sarr., sars., sep., sil., sul-ac., sulph., tarax., vichy-h., zinc., zinc-p.

9 a.m. - noon - alumn.

amel. - carb-an., graph.

bed, in - dulc.

mirthful in evening - calc-s., nux-v.

rising after, amel. - sep.

waking, after - anac., ant-c., cop., hipp., nit-ac., nux-m., phel., ptel., thuj.

waking, on - **ALUM.,** alum-p., ars., bar-c., carb-an., cop., ign., kali-c., kali-p., **LACH.,** ***lyc.,*** nit-ac., ph-ac., phos., plat., ***sep.,*** tarax., tarent., verat., xan.

music, from - ***acon., ambr.,*** cham., ***dig., graph., kreos.,*** lyc., ***nat-c., nat-m.,*** nat-p., ***nat-s.,*** nux-v., phos., ***sabin.,*** sep., tarent., ***thuj.***

distant - lyc.

menses, during - nat-c., sabin.

sad music, amel. - mang.

news, bad after - calc-p., puls.

disagreeable after - calc-p., puls.

night - alum., am-c., ammc., arn., ***ars.,*** **AUR.,** bell., calc., camph., carb-an., ***caust.,*** dulc., ***graph.,*** kali-p., lach., lil-t., nat-c., ***nat-m., phos.,*** plat., ***rhus-t.***

amel. - am-c., tarent.

and day, crying, with - ***caust.***

diarrhea in the morning, with - lil-t.

bed, in - ***ars.,*** graph., kali-c., lil-t., ***nat-m.,*** rhus-t., stram., sulph.

noise, from - ant-c., nat-c., phos.

noon - canth., caust., phys., sarr., ***zinc.***

lively, in evening sad, or vice versa - ***zinc.***

nosebleed, after - puls.

old age, in - ***aur.,*** esp-g.

pain, from - ***sars.***

slightest, from - carb-v.

palpitations, with - coca.

periodical - ***ars.,*** asar., ***aur., con.,*** cop., kali-ar., plat., puls., sel., sulph.

every fourteen days - ***con.***

every third day - kali-ar.

perspiration, during - ***acon., apis,*** ars., ars-s-f., ***aur.,*** aur-a., aur-s., bell., bry., ***calc.,*** calc-ar., calc-s., carb-s., ***chin.,*** chin-a., **CON.,** graph., ign., piloc., lyc., ***nat-m.,*** nit-ac., nux-v., puls., ***rhus-t.,*** sel., ***sep.,*** spig., ***sulph.,*** thuj.

pollutions, from sexual - agar., ***agn.,*** aur., ***calad., con.,*** cypr., dig., ***dios., dys-co., ery-a.,*** ferr-br., ham., **KALI-BR.,** med., ***nat-m.,*** nat-p., **NUX-V.,** ph-ac., ***puls.,*** sang., sars., ***sep.,*** sulph., ust.

DEPRESSION, sadness
pregnancy, in - aur., chin., cimic., helon., lach., ***nat-m.***, nux-m., ***plat., puls.***, **SEP.**
pressure about chest, from - asaf., graph.
puberty, in - ant-c., ***ars.***, aur., ***calc.***, caust., ***graph., hell.***, helon., ign., ***lach.***, manc., ***nat-m.***, puls., rhus-t., **SEP.**, sulph.
quarrel, with husband, after - ***anac.***
quiet - ars., ***hell.***, ign., nux-v., ph-ac., puls., ziz.
religious - ars., ***aur.***, carc., mez., psor., ***sulph.***
respiration, with impeded - ant-c., lach., laur., ***lyc.***, sep., tab.
sex, after - ***agar.***, calc., cedr., con., ***nat-m.***, sel., ***sep.***, staph., sulph.
sexual, excesses, from - agar., ***agn.***, aur., ***cimic.***, con., ind., ***lil-t.***, nux-v., pic-ac., plat., sep., spong.
excitement, with - bell., manc.
after - tarent.
suppressed - **CON.**
psychopathy, with - ind.
shock, from - nitro-o.
sighing, with - ***agn.***, am-c., am-m., ***ant-c., aur.***, cact., calc-p., carb-an., cimic., cocc., con., ***cycl.***, dig., ***graph.***, iber., ***ign., indg.***, kali-p., lach., lil-t., mur-ac., naja, nat-c., ***nat-m.***, nat-s., nit-ac., nux-v., ph-ac., phos., plat., psor., ***puls.***, rhus-t., sec., ***sel., sep., stann.***, staph., sulph., thuj., zinc.
amel. - ***dig.***, lach.
sits in corner and does not want to have anything to do with the world - hipp.
sleep and never to wake, would like to - ars-m.
sleepiness, with - calc., calc-p., ***corn.***, eup-per., mag-p., murx., rhus-t., ***sil.***
sleeplessness, with - ars., **AUR.**, carb-an., **CARC.**, ***cimic.***, gels., ign., ***thuj.***
sadness, from - acet-ac., **AUR., CARC.**, ***ign., kali-br.***, kali-c., rhus-t., sulph., ***thuj.***
slight, an undeserved, from - arg-n.
society, agg. in - euph.
amel. - bov.
stool, amel. after - nat-m., nux-v.
stories, from sad - calc., **CIC.**
suicidal disposition, with (see Suicidal disposition) - alum., **AUR.**, calc., ***carc.***, cas-s., chin., cimic., con., graph., ***hep.***, ign., med., ***merc-aur.***, naja, ***nat-m.***, nat-s., ***psor.***, ran-b., rumx., sep., ***spig.***, **STAPH.**, sulph.
sultry, weather, in - sep.
sunshine, in - ***merc., stram.***
amel. - aur., plat.
superfluous, feeling - ***naja.***
supper, after - nux-v.
amel. - am-c., clem., tarent.
sympathy agg. - carc., con., ign., ***nat-m., sep.***
talk, indisposed to - **ARG-N.**, ***ars.***, bar-c., ***cact.***, ign., mag-c., **NAT-M.**, nit-ac., ph-ac., ***puls.***, stann., verat.
telling, it to somebody, amel. after - alum-sil.
thinking, of his position, on - hell.
thunderstorm, amel. - sep.

DEPRESSION, sadness
trifles, about - agar., bar-ac., bar-c., cocc., ***dig., graph.***, mez., saroth.
typhus, after - ***anac., hell.***
unoccupied, when - tarax.
urination, amel. - eug., hyos.
urination, s. followed by frequent - man.
vaginal discharge amel. - ***murx.***
vexation, after - calc-p., kali-bi., ***plat., puls.***
waking, on - ***alum.***, bell., bufo, calc-p., carb-an., coc-c., ign., kali-c., ***kali-p., lach.***, lepi., lyc., nit-ac., op., ***ph-ac.***, plat., plb., raph., ***sep.***, stront-c., tarent., thyr., x-ray.
walking, while and after - acon., con., tab., ther., thuj.
air, in open - ant-c., calc., coff., ***con., cupr.***, hep., kali-c., nux-v., petr., ***ph-ac.***, rhus-t., ***sep.***, sulph., tab.
air, in open, amel. - plat., ***puls., rhus-t.***
amel. - cop., hist.
only while, the longer he walks the worse he gets - ***ph-ac.***
stand still or sit down, must - cupr.
warm, room - calc., ***plat.***, **PULS.**, rhus-t., tarent.
wet, weather, during - ***elaps,*** rhus-t.
wine, amel. - thuj.
work, shyness, in - berb., bov., crot-t., dor., laur., mez., prun., zinc.
wounds, after - hyper.
wringing the hands - ars., sulph., syph.
wrong way, as if having done everything in - ***naja.***

DESIRES, general
anxious, full of - ***cast.***
cavern, to be in - elaps.
children, to beat - chel., nux-v.
to have, beget - ***nat-m.***, ox-ac.
everything, for - sant.
exercises, for - **BELL.**, cann-i., coca, crot-c., erech., eucal., orig., phos., rhus-t., ziz.
air, in open - teucr.
physical - coca.
full of - agav-t., ***ars.***, bry., carc., cina, dulc., ign., ip., ***puls.***, rheum, rhus-t., ***spig.***
grandeur, for - cur.
has no more - ***hell., op.***
impatiently many things, dislikes its favorite playthings, child - arn., calc-p., **CHAM.**, dulc., kreos., puls., **RHEUM**
indefinite - chin., ip., lach., ***puls.***, sang., sil., ***ther.***
inexpressible, full of - ***ip.***
more than she needs - ***ars.***, ars-s-f., bar-s., bry., zinc-p.
numerous, various things - ***cina,*** phos.
present, things not - bry., calc-sil., puls., rheum
this and that - coff., ***puls.***
unattainable things - bry., ign., op.
uncontrollable - alco.
vexatious things, to say - mez.
watched, to be - gall-ac.

DESIRES, general
woman, ideal - ant-c., nat-m.

DESOLATE, room appears - valer.

DESPAIR, feelings (see Depression) - ***acon.,*** aesc., agar., ***agn.,*** all-c., aloe, ***alum.,*** alum-sil., am-c., am-m., ***ambr., anac.,*** ant-c., ***ant-t., arg-n.,*** arn., **ARS.,** ars-h., ***ars-i.,*** ars-s-f., aster., **AUR.,** bad., bar-c., bell., benz., benz., bov., brom., bry., bufo, **CALC.,** calc-i., calc-s., ***calc-sil.,*** camph., ***cann-i.,*** canth., carb-an., carb-s., ***carb-v.,*** **CARC.,** ***caust.,*** cham., chel., ***chin.,*** chin-a., chin-s., clem., **COFF.,** ***cocc.,*** colch., ***con.,*** crat., ***crot-t.,*** cupr., ***cupr-ac.,*** cur., der., dig., eup-per., ***gad.,*** gamb., gels., ***graph.,*** **HELL.,** helon., hep., hura, hydr-ac., hyos., **IGN.,** iod., kali-ar., kali-br., kali-i., kali-n., ***kali-p.,*** kreos., ***lach.,*** laur., ***lept., lil-t.,*** lith., **LYC.,** med., ***merc., mez.,*** morph., naja, ***nat-a., nat-c., nat-m.,*** nat-s., nat-sil., ***nit-ac.,*** nitro-o., ***nux-v., op.,*** orig., petr., ***ph-ac.,*** phos., pic-ac., plat., plb., podo., **PSOR.,** ***puls., rhus-t.,*** ruta, sec., sel., ***sep.,*** sil., spig., stann., ***staph., stram.,*** sul-ac., sul-i., **SULPH.,** sumb., ***syph.,*** tab., ther., thuj., thymol., tub., valer., **VERAT.,** verb., vip.
alternating with hope - acon., bov., carc.
childbirth, during - ars., ***coff.***
chill, during - ***acon.,*** ant-t., **ARS.,** ***aur.,*** aur-a., bell., bry., ***calc., cham.,*** chin-a., cupr., graph., hep., **IGN.,** merc., nux-v., rhus-t., ***sep., tarent., verat.***
criticism, from the smallest - ***med.***
death, with fear of - ars., **CALC.**
existence, about miserable - ars., ***aur.,*** carc., ***sep.***
fever, during - ***acon.,*** ant-t., ***ars.,*** bell., calc-s., ***carb-v.,*** cham., chel., chin-a., con., graph., ign., petr., puls., rhus-t., sep., ***spong.,*** stann., stram., sulph., verat.
future, about - ars., ***nat-m.***
health, about their - ***ars.,*** aur., calc., ***carc.,*** staph.
hypochondriasis, in - ***arg-n.***
itching of the skin, from - **PSOR.**
life, of - ***ars., aur.,*** calc., cimic.
lost, thinks everything is - aur., ign.
love, from disappointed - ***aur.,*** caust., ***hyos.,*** ign., nat-m.
masturbation, in - ***op.***
menorrhagia, in - ***cocc.***
menses, before - verat.
night, all during the - ***aur.,*** lith.
others, about - ***aur.***
oneself, and - ***arg-n.,*** aur.
pains, with the - acon., **ARS., AUR.,** aur-a., calc., carb-v., **CARC.,** ***cham., chin.,*** chin-a., ***coff.,*** colch., hyper., lach., lil-t., mag-c., nux-v., stram., ***verat.,*** vip.
stomach, in the - ant-c., ***coch., coff.***
periodical - ***ars., aur.,*** aur-a.
perspiration, during - **ARS.,** calc., ***carb-v., cham., graph.,*** lyc., ***sep.,*** stann., verat.
pregnancy, during - nat-m.

DESPAIR, feelings
rage, bordering on - ***agar.,*** anac., nit-ac.
cursing and imprecations, with - anac., **NIT-AC.**
recovery, of - ***acon.,*** all-s., **ALUM., ARS.,** ***aur.,*** aur-a., aur-i., ***aur-s.,*** bapt., bar-c., ***bry.,*** **CALC.,** calc-ar., calc-s., cann-i., **CARC.,** ***caust.,*** cham., chlol., cimic., **COLOC.,** ***hell.,*** hura, ***ign.,*** kali-ar., kali-br., kali-c., kreos., lac-c., lach., ***lyc.,*** mag-c., ***med.,*** **MERC.,** nat-s., ***nit-ac.,*** nux-v., ***psor., sep.,*** sil., **SYPH.,** ther., ***thyr.,*** verat., zinc.
convalescence during - carc., psor.
convulsions, after - calc.
religious - ***arg-n.,*** **ARS., AUR.,** aur-a., aur-i., aur-s., ***calc.,*** calc-i., carc., ***camph., chel.,*** cycl., hell., hura, ign., ***kali-p.,*** **LACH., LIL-T.,** ***lyc.,*** med., meli., ***mez.,*** nat-m., plat., plb., podo., ***psor.,*** **PULS.,** ***stram., sulph., thuj.,*** **VERAT.**
alternating with sexual excitement - **LIL-T.**
suppressed menses, during - **VERAT.**
rising, amel. on - chloram.
screams of despair, paroxysmal - lyss.
sexual craving, from - aster.
social position of - ***aur.,*** calc., ign., ***lyc.,*** puls., rhus-t., sep., staph., sulph., **VERAT.**
trifles, over - ***graph.***
typhus, after, nosebleed amel. - **PSOR.**
vomiting, during - ars-h.
waking, in intermittent - ***ant-t.***
work, over his - anac., calc., sulph.

DESTRUCTIVE, behaviour - ***anac.,*** agar., anan., apis, ***bell.,*** bufo, calc., ***camph., canth.,*** carb-s., carc., ***cimx., con., cupr.,*** cur., hep., hura, ***hyos.,*** iod., kali-p., lach., laur., lil-t., merc-i-f., mosch., ***nux-v.,*** oena., op., phos., plat., plb., sec., sol-t-ae., ***staph.,*** **STRAM.,** stront-c., sulph., ***tarent.,*** tub., ***verat.,*** verat-v.
children, in - anac., ***bell.,*** carc., cham., ***cina,*** hep., ***hyos.,*** lach., med., ***nux-v., staph.,*** **STRAM.,** tarent., **TUB.,** ***verat.***
clothes, of - ***bell., camph.,*** hyos., ***ign.,*** nux-v., plb., ***stram., sulph.,*** **TARENT.,** ***verat.***
cuts them up - ***verat.***
cunning - ***tarent.***
drunkenness, during - bell., verat.

DETERMINATION, gloomy - pyrus.

DEVELOPMENT of children arrested - aeth., ***agar.,*** **BAR-C.,** ***calc., calc-p.,*** carc., cupr., des-ac., ***phos.,*** sil., vip.

DIRTINESS - **AM-C.,** bor., calc-s., ***caps., crot-h.,*** med., merc., ***nux-v.,*** petr., ***plat., psor.,*** sil., **STAPH., SULPH.,** verat.
dirting everything - am-c., bry., ***nat-m.***
dirty skin, with - am-c., ars., lyc., nux-v., ***psor., sulph.***
urinating and defecating everywhere, children - ***sep.,*** sil., sulph.

DISAPPOINTMENT, ailments from - acon., alum., apis, ars., **AUR.,** ***bry.,*** caust., ***cham.,*** cocc., colch., ***coloc., gels.,*** grat., hyos., **IGN.,** ***lach.,*** **LYC.,** ***merc.,*** **NAT-M.,** ***nux-v., op.,*** **PH-AC.,** plat., **PULS.,** sep., **STAPH.,** verat.
acute, or recent - **IGN.**
ailments from literary, scientific failure - calc., ***ign.,*** lyc., nux-v., puls., ***sulph.***
chronic - **NAT-M.**

DISCOMFORT - agar., ammc., ars., aur., bol-s., bry., calad., calc-p., ***camph.,*** cina, clem., colch., digin., ferr., form., glon., gran., ***grat.,*** hell., hipp., hydr-ac., kali-bi., kali-c., kali-chl., lach., lyc., mag-c., morph.
afternoon - mag-arct., sil.
bathing, after - phys.
chill, during - ars.
eating, after - bar-ac., bry., clem., olnd., ph-ac., zinc.
dinner, after - crot-t., iod., ol-an., zinc.
supper, after - petr., seneg.
evening - calc., coloc., sabad., sulph.
forenoon - agar., lyc., mag-c.
heat, during - ran-b.
morning - ang., hipp., mag-c.
walking, on - ant-c., plect.
night - nicc., petr., puls-n.
noon - mez.
pickled fish, after - calad.
walking, after - arg-m., caust.

DISCONCERTED, feelings - brom., ign.

DISCONTENTED, dissatisfied (see Depression) - acon., aeth., agar., agn., alet., all-c., aloe, alum., alum-p., alum-sil., am-c., ***am-m.,*** ammc., **ANAC.,** ang., ***ant-c.,*** ant-t., apis, arn., ***ars.,*** ars-i., ars-s-f., asaf., asar., ***aur.,*** aur-a., aur-m., aur-s., bar-c., bell., berb., ***bism., bor.,*** bov., brom., ***bry.,*** calc., calc-i., **CALC-P.,** calc-s., calc-sil., cann-s., canth., caps., carb-ac., carb-an., carb-s., **CARC.,** caust., ***cham., chel., chin.,*** chin-a., cic., ***cina,*** cinnam., cinnb., clem., cob., cocc., coff., ***colch.,*** coloc., ***con.,*** crot-t., ***cupr.,*** dulc., eug., ferr., ferr-ar., ferr-p., fl-ac., goss., graph., grat., ham., hell., ***hep.,*** hipp., hura, ign., indg., indol., iod., ip., jug-r., kali-ar., ***kali-c.,*** kali-m., kali-n., kali-p., kali-s., kali-sil., kreos., lach., laur., led., lepi., lil-t., ***lyc.,*** lyss., mag-aust., mag-c., mag-m., mag-p., mag-s., man., manc., mang., meny., **MERC.,** merc-c., mez., mur-ac., nat-a., ***nat-c.,*** **NAT-M.,** nat-p., ***nit-ac., nux-v.,*** ol-an., op., orig., ***pall.,*** pana., par., petr., ph-ac., phos., ***plat.,*** plb., prun., psor., ***puls.,*** ran-b., rheum, rhod., ***rhus-t.,*** rob., ruta, samb., sars., sel., ***sep., sil.,*** sin-n., spong., ***stann., staph.,*** stram., stront-c., sul-i., **SULPH.,** ***syph.,*** tab., tarent., teucr., ther., ***thuj.,*** til., **TUB.,** viol-t., zinc.
afternoon - grat., mur-ac., nat-m., op., zinc.
stool, before - ***bor.***
air, in open - mur-ac.
always - carc., **HEP.,** lach., **MERC.,** nit-ac.
children - calc-p., carc., ***cham., cina, tub.***
crying amel. - ***nit-ac.,*** ziz.
daytime - ars., led.
eating, after - bov., fl-ac.

DISCONTENTED, dissatisfied
evening - calc., fl-ac., hipp., ign., jug-r., ran-b., ***puls., rhus-t.***
amel. - aloe, puls.
everything, with - alum., alum-sil., am-c., ammc., anac., apis, arn., ars., bell., bism., calc-sil., cann-s., canth., carb-an., carc., cham., chin-a., cina, cocc., coff., colch., ***coloc.,*** cupr., eug., graph., grat., ham., **HEP.,** hipp., hura, ign., iod., ip., kali-c., kali-s., kreos., lach., lil-t., mag-c., meny., **MERC.,** merc-c., mez., mur-ac., nat-c., **NAT-M.,** nit-ac., nux-v., ***pall.,*** petr., ***plat., puls.,*** rheum, samb., sars., ***sep.,*** sieg., spong., stann., staph., sul-ac., ***sulph.,*** thea., ***tub.***
headache, during - ign.
health, about - phos.
himself, with - ***agn.,*** aloe, ***ars., aur.,*** bell., bry., calc-p., carc., caust., cham., cinnam., cinnb., cob., cocc., ***hep., ign.,*** kali-c., ***lyc.,*** mag-aust., mang., meny., merc., mez., mur-ac., ***nit-ac.,*** nux-v., ***ph-ac., puls.,*** ruta, **STAPH.,** ***sulph.,*** tarent., ther., viol-t., ziz.
inanimate objects - caps.
menses, during - cast., tarent.
morning - hipp., ***lyc., nux-v.,*** plb., puls.
rainy weather, during - aloe.
revolutionary - caust., **MERC.**
sex, after - ***calc.***
stool, before - ***bor.***
surroundings, with - ang., carc., ***cham.,*** chel., meny., merc., mez., par., plat., ***tub.***
wrong, everything another does is - ***cham.***

DISCORDS, ailments from, between friends - ars., **GRAPH.,** hep., ***ign.,*** lach., merc., **NAT-M.,** nit-ac., nux-v., sulph.
chief and subordinates - graph., lach., ***lyc.,*** merc., nat-m., nit-ac., nux-v., staph., sulph.
workers, between - **ARS.,** hep., **LACH.,** merc., nat-m., ***nit-ac.***

DISCOURAGED, feelings - ***acon.,*** agar., agn., aloe, alum., alum-p., alum-sil., am-br., ambr., ***anac.,*** ang., ange-s., ant-c., ant-t., ***apis,*** arg-m., arn., ***ars.,*** ars-h., ars-i., aur., bar-c., bell., brom., bry., buf-s., calad., ***calc.,*** calc-i., camph., canth., carb-an., carb-s., **CARB-V.,** carc., ***carl.,*** caust., cench., cham., ***chin.,*** chin-a., ***chin-s., cocc.,*** coff., colch., coloc., con., convo-d., cupr., der., des-ac., dig., ***dros.,*** gran., graph., hell., hep., hipp., hydr., hydr-ac., hypoth., hyos., iber., ***ign.,*** **INSULIN,** iod., ***ip.,*** iris, kali-bi., kali-c., kali-i., kali-m., kali-n., kali-p., kali-s., kali-sil., lac-ac., **LACH.,** laur., lith., **LYC.,** ***mag-arct.,*** mag-m., mang., merc., merc-c., moly-met., mur-ac., myrt-c., nat-a., nat-c., nat-m., nat-p., nat-s., nat-sil., ***nit-ac., nux-v.,*** olnd., op., pen., ***petr.,*** ph-ac., phos., plat., plb., podo., ***psor., puls.,*** pyrus, ran-b., ***rhus-t.,*** sabin., sarcol-ac., sec., ***sep., sil.,*** spig., ***stann.,*** staph., stram., sul-i., ***sulph.,*** sul-ac., tab., ***tarent.,*** ther., thuj., tub., tub-r., valer., **VERAT.,** verb., viol-t., vip., visc., zinc.

DISCOURAGED, feelings
afternoon - con.
air, in open - ***ph-ac.***
air, in open, amel. - coff.
allernating with, confidence - alum.
anger - ran-b., zinc.
courage - merc., op., staph.
exaltation - petr., sul-ac.
exuberance - petr.
haughtiness - agn.
hope - alum., kali-c., ***merc., op., staph.***
irritability - zinc.
quarrelsomeness - ran-b.
anxiety, with - ***acon.***, bar-c., canth., ***cham., graph., mag-arct.***, puls.
business, aversion to - puls.
children, in - calc-p., lyc., sil.
crying, with - bar-c., ***carb-v.***, chin-s., laur., ***lyc.***, nux-v.
amel. - nit-ac.
cursing, with - nit-ac.
daytime and night - carb-an.
disgust, with - caust.
evening - ant-t., calc., ferr-p., ran-s., ***puls., rhus-t.***
eating amel. - tarent.
future, about - ***dros.***, merc.
impatience, with - ***calc.***
irresolution, with - puls.
irritability, with - carb-v., dig.
menses, before - carl.
moaning, with - cham., nux-v., verat.
morning - hipp., plat., sep., sulph.
bed, in - puls.
morose, and - op.
night - graph.
pain, from - colch., hep., lach., nux-v.
praying, with - puls.
quiet, and - lyc.
rage, with - colch., nit-ac.
reproaches himself - ***mag-arct.***
sex, after - sep.
waking, on - ***graph., puls.***
walking, while - am-c., ph-ac.

DISCRIMINATION, lack of - **ALUM.**, con., hep.

DISCUSS, desire to - trio.

DISCUSSES her symptoms with everyone - arg-n., ars., ***pop-c.***

DISGUST, (see Aversion) - aloe, arn., ars., asar., aur., camph., caps., ***carc.***, caust., cimx., coloc., con., ***croc., hep.***, ip., ***kali-c.***, lac-c., ***laur.***, led., mag-c., mag-m., ***merc.***, mez., nux-v., petr., phos., plb., **PULS.**, samb., sars., sil., spong., ***stram.***, **SULPH.**, syph., tarent., thea., **THUJ.**
consciousness of his unnatural state of mind - tarent.
dirt, with - ars., carc., thuj.

DISGUST,
everything, with - arn., aur., carc., caust., con., ip., kali-i., ***laur., led.***, mag-c., mag-m., ***merc.***, nux-v., petr., phos., ***puls.***, samb., sars., spong., thea., thuj.
exhilaration, of others, at - mag-aust.
himself, with, has no courage to live - ***merc.***
laughing of others, at - ambr.
medicine bottle, on sight of the - visc.
nausea from her own effluvia, to - **SULPH.**

DISHONEST - ars., ***bry., calc., lach.***, lyc., op., **PULS.**, ***sil., sulph.***, **THUJ.**

DISOBEDIENCE - acon., agn., ***am-c.***, am-m., arn., bufo, calc., calc-p., canth., caps., caust., cham., ***chin.***, cina, ***dig.***, elae., guai., ***lyc.***, med., **MERC.**, nit-ac., nux-v., petr., phos., spig., ***staph.***, sulfon., sulph., ***syph.***, **TARENT.**, **TUB.**, ***viol-o., viol-t.***
children, in - cham., ***chin., cina***, med., thuj., ***tub.***, verat.

DISLIKES, her own sex - glon., ***lyc.***, plat., raph., ***sep.***, verat.

DISTANCE, inaccurate judge of, (see Mistakes) - agar., anac., arg-n., ***cann-i.***, cann-s., carb-an., dat-m., glon., hyos., ***nux-m.***, onos., op., stann., ***stram.***
distance, exaggerated, is - anac., ***cann-i.***, glon., nux-m., ox-ac., ***stram.***, sulph., ther.
runs against things which appear to him distant - stram.
time during sleepiness, and - nux-v.

DISTURBED, averse to being - agar., ***ant-c.***, ant-t., arn., bell., berb., **BRY.**, cact., carb-an., ***cham.***, chin-a., ***cocc., coloc., gels.***, graph., hell., ign., iod., mur-ac., naja, ***nat-m.***, nat-s., **NUX-V.**, op., oxyt., ***ph-ac.***, phos., puls., sars., sil., staph., ***sulph.***, tub.

DIVERSION, amel. - ign., lach., phos., pip-m.

DOMINATION, by others, a long history of, ailments from (see Abused, Humiliation) - ***anac.***, **CARC.**, **LYC.**, nat-m., sep., **STAPH.**
children, in - ***anac.***, **CARC.**, **LYC.**, med., nat-m., sil., **STAPH.**, thuj.

DOMINEERING, dictatorial - allox., **ANAC.**, apis, arn., ars., aur., ***camph.***, caust., cham., chel., ***chin.***, con., ***cupr.***, dulc., ferr., ***lach.***, lil-t., **LYC.**, ***merc.***, nux-v., phos., ***plat.***, sep., ***sulph., verat.***
command, talking with air of - arn., cupr., ***lyc., phos., plat.***
power, love of, with - ars., lach., lyc., nux-v.

DOUBTFUL, feelings - anh., bar-c., **CARB-V.**, cic., ***graph.***, ing., ***lach.***, **LYC.**, ***petr.***, sep., sil., staph.
recovery, of - ***acon.***, agn., ***alum.***, arn., **ARS.**, ars-h., ***aur.***, bry., calc., calc-sil., carc., ***ign.***, kali-c., kreos., lac-c., lach., ***lept.***, lil-t., ***lyc.***, mag-c., ***merc.***, nat-s., ***nit-ac.***, nux-v., ***ph-ac.***, phos., psor., puls., sep., ***stann.***, sulph., syph.
medicine is useless - alumn., ars., aur.
menopausal period, during - sars.

DOUBTFUL, feelings
soul's welfare, of - **ARS., AUR.,** bell., calc., chel., croc., cycl., dig., hyos., **LACH.,** ***lil-t.,*** lyc., nux-v., **PULS.,** sel., stram., ***sulph., verat.***

DREAM, as if in a - absin., acon., agar., ail., alum., ***ambr.,*** aml-n., ***anac.,*** ang., ***ant-c., apis,*** arg-n., arn., ars., atro., ***bell.,*** bry., buth-a., ***calc.,*** **CANN-I.,** ***cann-s.,*** carb-ac., carb-an., ***carb-v., cench.,*** cham., chin., coca, ***coff., con.,*** cupr., ***glon., hell.,*** hep., ***hyos., lach.,*** lil-t., ***med.,*** merc., ***nat-m.,*** **NUX-M.,** nux-v., oena., ol-an., olnd., **OP.,** ***ph-ac., phos.,*** phys., puls., rheum, sabad., sep., sil., squil., **STRAM.,** ***sulph.,*** thuj., valer., ***verat., visc.,*** zinc., ziz.
beautiful - absin.
daytime - ars., elaps
escape in a world of dreams - anh.
future, about the - ***staph.***
poetical - olnd.
night - nat-c.

DRESSES, averse to - ***con.***
indecently - ***hell., hyos.,*** stram.
unable to - bar-c., merc.

DRINKING, mental symptoms after - ***bell., cocc.,*** con., ***lyss., stram.***

DUALITY, sense of - alum., **ANAC., BAPT.,** cann-s., cycl., **GELS.,** ***lach.,*** lil-t., lyc., ***naja,*** nat-m., ***nux-m.,*** op., petr., ***phos.,*** plb., psor., puls., sec., sil., ***stram.,*** ther.
own, as if it were not his - alum., lach., nat-m., thuj.
sick, as if someone else were - gels.

DULLNESS, mental - ***abies-n.,*** abrot., acet-ac., ***acon.,*** aconin., aesc., aesc-g., aeth., ether, ***agar.,*** agn., ***ail.,*** alco., alf., ***aloe, alum.,*** am-m., ***ambr.,*** am-c., ***ammc.,*** amor-r., amyg., ***anac.,*** ang., anh., ant-c., ***apis,*** apom., arag., ***arg-m.,*** **ARG-N.,** arn., ars., ars-i., asaf., asar., asc-t., aster., atro., aur., **BAPT., BAR-C., BAR-M., BELL.,** bell-p., berb., bism., bol., ***bor., bov.,*** **BRY.,** bufo, cact., caj., ***calad.,*** **CALC.,** calc-ar., calc-caust., **CALC-P., CALC-S.,** camph., cann-i., ***cann-s.,*** canth., caps., carb-ac., carb-an., carb-o., ***carb-s.,*** **CARB-V.,** ***carc.,*** carl., ***caust.,*** cedr., cent., ***cham., chel.,*** chim., ***chin.,*** chin-a., ***chin-s., cic.,*** cimic., cimx., ***clem.,*** coca, ***cocc.,*** coc-c., cod., coff., ***colch., coloc., con.,*** coni., ***cop.,*** corn., cortico., cot., croc., ***crot-h.,*** crot-t., cupr., cupr-ar., cycl., des-ac., ***dig.,*** dros., dulc., echi., epil., euon., eup-pur., euphr., fago., ***ferr.,*** ferr-ma., ferr-p., form., gad., **GELS.,** gent-l., get., gins., ***glon.,*** glyc., gran., **GRAPH., GUAI.,** gymn., haem., halo., ham., **HELL.,** helon., ***hep.,*** hipp., hir., hist., ***hydr., hydr-ac.,*** hydroph., **HYOS.,** hyper., ign., ind., indg., indol., iod., ip., irid., iris, jug-c., juni., kali-bi., **KALI-BR., KALI-C.,** kali-i., kali-n., kali-p., ***kali-s., kreos.,*** lac-c., **LACH.,** lact., **LAUR.,** lec., led., lepi., lil-t., lim., **LYC.,** ***lyss.,*** macro., ***mag-arct.,*** mag-aust., ***mag-m.,*** mag-p., maland., manc., mang., med., ***meli.,*** meny., meph., ***merc., merc-c.,*** merl., ***mez.,*** mosch., mur-ac., myric., naja, **NAT-A., NAT-C., NAT-M.,** ***nat-p., nat-s.,*** nicc., ***nit-ac.,*** **NUX-M.,** ***nux-v.,*** ol-an., ***olnd.,*** **OP.,** par., ped., pen., penic., ***petr.,*** **PH-AC., PHOS.,** phys., **PIC-AC.,** pip-m., pisc., plat., **PLB.,** podo., psil., ***psor.,*** ptel., **PULS.,** raja-s., ran-b., ran-s., rheum, ***rhod.,*** rhus-g., ***rhus-t.,*** rhus-v., ruta, sabad., sabin., sac-l., sal-ac., sal-n., sal-p., samb., sang., sanic., saroth., ***sars., sec., sel.,*** **SENEG., SEP.,** sapin., **SIL.,** sol-m., ***spig., spong.,*** squil., ***stann.,*** **STAPH.,** still., ***stram.,*** stront-c., sulfa., **SULPH.,** sul-ac., sumb., syph., ***tab.,*** tarax., ***tarent.,*** teucr., thala., ther., ***thuj.,*** **THYR.,** til., trif-p., **TUB.,** upa., uran-n., urea, ust., valer., verb., ***verat.,*** viol-o., viol-t., vip., xero, **ZINC., ZINC-P.,** zinc-valer., ***zing.***
afternoon - all-c., anac., ang., arg-n., ars., atro., cadm-s., caj., cann-s., cimic., cod., con., dios., ferr., graph., ham., ***hell.,*** hyos., laur., lil-t., nat-m., pip-m., plan., puls., rhus-r., ***sep., sil.,*** sulph., zinc.
amel. - anac.
air, in open - hyos., nat-a., plat.
after being in - lyc.
amel. - cinnb., graph., **LYC.,** mag-m., meny.
alone, when - ph-ac.
alternating with, clearness of mind - colch.
dim vision - bell.
hilarity and mirth - piloc., spong.
singing - spong.
vivacity - crot-h.
work, desire for - cycl.
beer, after - coloc.
breakfast, after - bapt.
cares for his business, from - ph-ac.
chagrin, from - ign., lach.
children - aeth., abrot., ***agar.,*** **ARG-N., BAR-C.,** ***bar-m.,*** bufo, ***calc.,*** **CALC-P.,** ***carb-s., carc.,*** iod., lach., ***lyc., med., merc., sil.,*** **SULPH.,** ***syph., tub., zinc.***
chill, during - agar., bell., bry., ***caps., cham.,*** cic., cimx., dros., ***gels., hell., lach.,*** led., nux-m., phos., plb., rhus-t., stann.
closing eyes, on - zinc.
amel. - kali-c.
company, in - ***plat.***
condition, could not think of her - chel.
conversation, from - sil., staph.
coryza, during - ars.
cough, during - hep.
damp air, during - sulph.
from - ***calc., carb-v.,*** merc., puls., ***rhus-t.,*** sil., verat.
daytime - abies-n., cinnb., merc., nat-a.
diabetes, in - ***helon., op.,*** ph-ac., phos., sul-ac.
dinner, during - sulph.
after - carb-an., mag-c., zinc.
does what's told, waits comment - phos.
dreams, after - arn., bell., caps., chin., cocc., sil.
drunken, as if - ***bell., op.***
drunkenness, during - op., stram.
eating, after - calc-s., chel., graph., led., meny., ***rhus-t.,*** tab.

DULLNESS, mental

eating, amel. - fago., ***iod., mez., nat-c., phos.,*** sep., sil.

elderly people - **AMBR., BAR-C., *con., lyc.***

emissions, after - caust.

emotions, from - acon., op., ph-ac., ***staph.***

epilepsy, before - ***caust.***

evening - ***anac.,*** calc-s., cann-s., carb-v., coca, cod., dig., dios., dulc., hipp., ign., kali-c., lach., lyc., mag-m., mez., mill., mur-ac., myric., naja, nat-m., pip-m., puls., rhus-t., ruta, sep., stann., ***sulph.***

amel. - agar., bufo, cic., puls., sil., sulph.

going to bed, after - caj.

fever, during - ***arg-n., bapt.,*** bell., bry., caps., carb-v., ***cham.,*** chin-s., ***hyos., ign.,*** merc., nat-c., ***puls.,*** sil., sulph.

after - sep.

fog, as enveloped in a - petr.

forenoon - ***anac.,*** ars., bar-c., bism., carb-an., lach., mag-c., mur-ac., myric., nat-a., nat-m., phys., psor., sars., sep., sil., sulph.

gas light, after injurious effects of - ***caust.,*** **GLON.**

grief, from - ign., lach., ***ph-ac.***

head as if enlarged, with ill humor and nausea - meph.

headache, with - zinc.

humiliation, after - ***staph.***

hurried, cannot think at all if - med.

impotency, with - ph-ac.

injuries of head, after - arn., cic., ***hell.,*** hyper., merc., ***nat-s.,*** rhus-t.

interrupted, when - colch.

looking out the window lasting for hours - mez.

loss of fluids, after - ***chin., nux-v.,*** sulph.

lying, while - bry.

amel. - zinc.

masturbation, after - ***gels.,*** ph-ac., **STAPH.**

menses, during - calc., lyc., lycps.

mental exertion, from - agar., ***anac.,*** aur., calc., ***calc-p.,*** cocc., ***glon.,*** graph., hep., hura, ign., lach., lyc., mag-c., **NAT-C.,** nat-m., ***nux-v., olnd.,*** ph-ac., pic-ac., puls., ran-b., sel., ***sil., sulph.***

morning - aesc., agar., am-c., ***ambr.,*** **ANAC.,** arn., bar-c., berb., bor., canth., caps., carb-an., carb-s., cer-b., **CHIN.,** cycl., form., ***graph.,*** guai., hyper., ign., kali-c., kali-n., kali-p., lact., laur., manc., merc., mez., nat-a., nat-c., nat-s., nux-v., ox-ac., ***ph-ac.,*** phos., plat., phys., puls., puls-n, rhod., sarr., sep., sil., squil., staph., sulph., sul-ac., ***sumb.,*** tell., ***thuj.***

bed, in - chel., cocc.

rising on - ham., mag-m., phos., scut., stram.

waking, on - ***aesc.,*** anac., arn., bar-c., berb., caps., carb-an., carb-v., **CHIN.,** ham., ign., kali-c., kali-n., kali-sil., merc., plat., puls., ruta, sil., stann., staph., thuj.

motion, agg. - bry.

motion, amel. - rhus-t.

DULLNESS, mental

news, from bad - calc-p., gels.

disagreeable, from - calc-p.

night, amel. - ***agar.***

waking, on - aesc., bapt., com., ery-a., lyc., lyss., phos., plat., verat.

noon - ars., con., esp-g., zinc.

painful - dig., meny., nat-c., phos.

palpitation, with - kali-c.

paroxysmal - sep., zinc.

periodical - chin.

perspiration, during - ars., caps., chin., graph., hyos., sabad., sulph., thuj.

pollutions, with - **KALI-BR.**

after - caust., ind., nat-c., ph-ac., ran-b., sabad., sep.

pressing in hypogastrium, from - kali-a.

reading, while - acon., agn., alum., ambr., bism., ***carb-v.,*** cocc., coff., **CON.,** dros., ferr-i., ***glon.,*** hipp., ind., iod., kali-sil., lac-c., ***lach.,*** **LYC.,** mez., ***nat-c.,*** nat-p., nat-sil., nux-m., ***nux-v.,*** olnd., **OP.,** ***ph-ac.,*** sil., ***sulph.***

rising from bed - ox-ac.

room, in a - meny.

says nothing - arn., ***hell., lach., rheum,*** spong.

sex, after - ***sep.***

sexual excesses, after - ***agn., anac.,*** arg-n., aur., chin., nat-m., nux-v., ***ph-ac., sel., staph.***

siesta, after - bar-c., ***graph.,*** lyc.

sleep, after sound - berb., mez.

sleepiness, with - arn., cact., calad., cann-s., carb-an., carb-v., caust., chin., clem., coff., colch., croc., crot-h., ***cupr.,*** dig., ferr., ***gels., hyos.,*** kreos., lact., lyc., mag-s., ***merc.,*** nat-m., nux-m., ***phos.,*** plb., sep., staph., zinc.

sleeplessness, with - carc., dulc., lact., ran-s.

smoking, from - acon.

speaking, while - am-c., kali-c., ***lyc.,*** mez.

spoken to, when - bry., lob.

standing, agg. - bov., bry., guai.

stool, after - cycl.

stooping, on - sulph.

think long, unable to - aeth., anac., cham., cinnb., con., ery-a., ***gels.,*** med., ***ph-ac.,*** **PHOS.,** ***pic-ac.,*** stram.

think or concentrate, unable to - ***aeth.***

subject, on one - cann-i.

toothache, from - clem.

understands, questions only after repetition - ambr., ***caust.,*** cocc., hell., kali-br., med., ***phos., sulph., zinc.***

urine, copious flow of amel. - ***gels., ter.***

vomiting, amel. - asar.

waking, on - alum., alum-sil., am-m., anac., arn., bar-c., bell., berb., bov., calc., ***cann-s.,*** caps., chin., chel., clem., cocc., con., cur., dig., grat., ham., **LACH.,** ***med.,*** nat-c., nat-sil., nux-m., op., **PHOS.,** pic-ac., plat., psor., ***puls.,*** rheum, sil., sol-m., stann., staph., stram., thuj., verat.

DULLNESS, mental
walking, while - ham., ph-ac., phys., rhus-t.
amel. in open air - bor., graph., **LYC.,** nat-a., plan.
rapidly, after - nat-m., sulph.
warm room, on entering - acon., ***puls.***
washing, amel. from cold - ***calc-p.,*** cann-i.
weight, on vertex, from - med.
wine, after - acon., all-c., mill., petr., zinc.
words, with unability to find right - lil-t.
working, amel. - cycl.
writing, while - acon., arg-n., cann-s., chin-s., glon., kali-sil., mag-c., nux-m., rhus-t., ***sil.***

DUTY, lack of sense of - alum., ambr., anac., ars., **CALC.,** carc., cench., coloc., hep., lach., **LYC.,** ***merc.,*** nat-m., sil., sulph.
aversion to domestic - cench., cit-l., ***lyc.,*** sul-i.
wanting in the sense of an indelicacy of conscience - anac., ars., coloc., lach., lyc., merc., nat-m., sulph.

DWELLS, on past disagreeable occurrences - ***ambr.,*** am-c., arg-n., asar., ***benz-ac.,*** calc., ***cham., chin.,*** cob-n., ***cocc., con.,*** cop., form., glon., goss., hep., hyos., ign., kali-c., kali-p., kiss., kreos., ***lyc.,*** meny., mez., **NAT-M.,** ***nit-ac.,*** op., phos., ***plat.,*** psor., rhus-t., ***sep.,*** spong., ***staph., sulph.,*** syph., thuj., verat., visc.
disappointments, on - ***ph-ac.***
grief from past offences - calc., **NAT-M.,** staph.
grieve therefore, to - ***nat-m.***
lying awake thinking of everything that others have done to displease her, in the morning she has forgotten about it - am-c.
midnight, after - **RHUS-T.**
night - ambr., benz-n., caust., chin., graph., kali-c., ***kali-p.,*** lyc., nat-m., ***plat., rhus-t., sulph.***
offences come back to him, long forgotten - glon., nat-m.
recalls, disagreeable memories - am-c., calc., hep., hyos., ***lyc.,*** **NAT-M.,** nit-ac., phos., sep., sulph.
old grievances - glon., **NAT-M.,** phos., sars., sulph.
sexual matters, on - nat-m., staph.
thinking of everything that others have done to displease her, lying awake thinking of it, in the morning she has forgotten about it - am-c.

DYSLEXIA, (see Learning disabilities)

EAT, refuses to (see Anorexia) - ars., bell., ***bor.,*** carc., caul., caust., ***chin.,*** cocc., croc., grat., **HYOS.,** ***ign.,*** **KALI-CHL.,** kali-p., lach., op., **PH-AC.,** ***phyt.,*** plat., puls., rhus-t., sep., sulph., **TARENT., VERAT., VIOL-O.**
spoon, cannot eat with a - bar-c., bell.

EATING, amel., mental symptoms - aur., cina, **GOSS.,** iod., kali-bi., phos.
a little, amel. - bell., tarent.

EATING, amel.,
after - calc-f., caust., dicha., goss., ***iod.,*** mez., petr., ***phos.,*** tarent.
evening - tarent.

EATS, more than she should - ars., cina., iod.

ECCENTRIC, behaviour - aesc., agn., alco., am-c., ambr., ang., arg-n., ***ars.,*** ars-h., ***asar.,*** asc-t., ***bell.,*** bufo, calc., ***cann-i.,*** coff., coff-t., cub., cupr., cupr-ac., cupr-ar., cycl., form., glon., hoit., hyos., iodof., kali-c., lac-ac., **LACH.,** lact., lyss., muru., nat-m., nitro-o., nux-v., ***op.,*** pall., petr., plat., raja-s., sang., sep., spig., stram., sul-ac., **SULPH.,** sumb., ***tarent.,*** teucr., thea., valer., verat., verat-v., verb.
alternating with, sadness - petr., ***stram.***
with, timidity - sul-ac.
chorea, with - ***cupr., cupr-ac.,*** sumb.
epilepsy, before fit of - ***cann-i.***
evening - asc-t., teucr.
fancies, in - agar., apoc., arg-n., glon., lact., pall., plat., ***verat-v.***
metrorrhagia, after - ***sep.***
night, all of - op.
political - ars., caust., lach.
religious - puls., stram., verat.

ECSTASY, (see Blissful, Tranquility) - **ACON.,** ether, ***agar.,*** agn., am-c., ang., ***anh., ant-c.,*** apis, arn., astra-e., bell., berb., bry., camph., **CANN-I.,** ***cann-s.,*** canth., carb-h., cast., cham., ***cic.,*** coca, ***cocc., coff.,*** croc., crot-h., cupr., cupr-am-s., cur., cypr., ery-a., fl-ac., hyos., ign., iod., jatr., keroso., kres., ***lach.,*** lyss., nitro-o., nux-m., olnd., ***op.,*** ph-ac., **PHOS.,** plat., plb., sel., sil., stann., staph., stram., sulph., sumb., thea., valer., verat.
alternating with sadness - senec.
amorous - op., pic-ac., thea.
sleep, during - phos.
brain disorder, preliminary to incipient - cypr.
heat, during - chin., coff., laur., puls., sabad.
joy, as after excessive - lach.
morning on waking - crot-h.
night - cur.
waking, on - ***cypr.***
night, walking in moonlight - **ANT-C.**
periodical - ***cic.***
twice a day, seems to be dying - ***cic.***
perspiration, during - carb-v., iod., nit-ac., sulph.
sublime - crot-h.
waling in open air, on - cinnb.

EFFEMINATE, men - ***calc.,*** **LYC.,** med., ***plat.,*** **PULS.,** ***sil.,*** staph., ***thuj.***

EGOTISM, ailments, from - ***calc.,*** lach., ***lyc.,*** med., merc., ***pall.,*** **PLAT.,** sil., **SULPH.**

EGOTISTICAL, haughty - acon., agar., alum., anac., arn., asar., aur., bell., calc., cann-i., cann-s., ***caust.,*** chin., cic., cina, con., cupr., dulc., ferr., ferr-ma., gran., grat., guai., ham., hell., ***hyos.,*** ign., ***ip.,*** kali-i., ***lach.,*** lil-t., **LYC.,** merc., nat-m., nitro-o., nux-v., ***pall.,*** par., phos., **PLAT.,** ***puls.,*** rob., sabad., sec., ***sil.,*** squil., ***staph., stram.,***

EGOTISTICAL, haughty - stront-c., **SULPH.,** thuj., **VERAT.**
- ailments, from - ***calc., lyc.,*** merc., ***pall.,*** plat., sil., ***sulph.***
- clothes, likes to wear his best - ***con.***
- exessive, self-esteem - act-sp., anac., anan., arn., aur., ***calc., lach., lyc.,*** med., merc., nux-v., ***pall.,*** par., phos., **PLAT.,** ***sil.,*** staph., stram., **SULPH.,** ***verat.***
- looks, self-contented - ferr., ferr-ma.
- pregnancy, during - ***verat.***
- reciting their exploits - agar.
- religious, haughtiness - ***plat.***
- speaking always about themselves in company - lach., par., staph.
- stiff and pretentious - ***lyc.***
- stupid and haughty - bell., calc., lyc., plat., stram., verat.
- weening, over - grat.
- wounded, wishes to be flattered - **PALL.**

ELATED, state of mind - cann-i., coca, ***coff.,*** iod., lach.
- alternating with sadness - senec.

ELEVATION - cinnb., coca, coff., op.
- morning on waking, in the open air - cinnb.

EMBARRASSMENT, feelings of - ***ambr., bar-c.,*** carb-v., ferr., ign., **LYC., NAT-M.,** phos., staph., sulph.
- ailments, after - anac., arg-n., coloc., gels., **IGN.,** kali-br., **LYC., NAT-M.,** ***op.,*** ph-ac., plat., sep., ***staph.,*** **SULPH.**
- company, in - ***ambr., lyc.***

EMBITTERED, exasperated - ambr., anac., ang., ign., mang., nit-ac., phenob., puls., ***sulph.,*** valer.
- offences, from slight - ang.

EMBRACES, behaviour
- anything in morning, worse in open air - plat.
- companions - agar., phos., plat., puls.
- everyone - caps., ***croc., hyos.,*** man., phos., plat., stram., ***verat.***
- inanimate objects, even - ***verat.***
- menses, before - ***verat.,*** zinc.

EMOTIONS, ailments after strong (see Excitement) - acetan., acon., arg-n., ***arn.,*** aster., ***aur., calc.,*** **CAPS., CARC.,** caust., **COFF.,** ***gels.,*** hyos., **IGN.,** kali-c., kreos., lyc., lyss., med., nat-c., **NAT-M., PH-AC.,** ***phos.,*** plat., psor., ***sep.,*** **STAPH.,** zinc.
- ailments after supressed emotions - **CARC.,** ***nat-m.,*** sep., **STAPH.**
- easily exited - carc., med., morph., phos., sumb.
- predominated by the intellect - ***nat-m.,*** valer., ***viol-o.***
- slightest emotion causes palpitation - calc-ar., lith., phos.
- trembling after - carc., psor., staph.

ENEMY, thinks everyone is the (See Schizophrenia) - ***lach.,*** meli., ***merc.***

ENNUI, (See Boredom)

ENVY - ***am-c.,*** **ARS.,** bry., calc., cench., cub., cur., hell., **LACH.,** lil-t., ***lyc.,*** nat-c., nux-v., ***plat.,*** **PULS.,** sarr., sep., spig., ***staph.,*** sulph., zinc.
- avidity, and - ***ars., chin.,*** lyc., nit-ac., nux-v., ph-ac., ***puls.,*** rhus-t., sep., stann., staph., sulph.
- hate, and - am-c., am-m., **CALC.,** nat-c., nat-m., nit-ac., **PULS.**
- qualities of others, at - ars., calc., lach., ***lyc.,*** puls., sulph.

ERRATIC, chaotic, behaviour - acon., agar., am-c., ambr., anac., ant-t., ***ars.,*** asaf., asar., ***bell., bov.,*** bry., canth., **CARC.,** ***chin.,*** ferr., hell., hyos., ign., kali-c., led., mag-m., **MED.,** meny., ***merc.,*** mez., mosch., nat-c., ***nux-v., phos., ph-ac.,*** puls., ***rhod.,*** rhus-t., sabad., sec., ***seneg., spig.,*** squil., staph., thuj., verb., viol-o., viol-t., zinc.

ERRONEOUS, notions - cann-i., sulph., verat.

ESCAPE, attempts to - acon., ***aesc., agar.,*** agar-st., alco., all-s., ***ars.,*** ars-m., arum-t., bapt., bar-c., **BELL.,** ***bry.,*** camph., caust., cham., chel., chin., chlor., cic., ***cocc.,*** coloc., ***crot-h., cupr., dig., glon.,*** hell., **HYOS.,** ign., iod., kali-br., lach., lil-t., lyc., meli., merc., merc-c., mez., ***nux-v., oena., op.,*** oper., phos., plb., puls., ran-b., rib-ac., rhus-t., samb., sol-n., **STRAM.,** sulph., sul-ac., tub., valer., ***verat.,*** zinc., zinc-p.
- anxiety at night, with - ***merc.***
- crime, for a fear of having committed a - ***merc.***
- delirium, during - sol-m.
- family and children, from her - am-c., lyc., nux-v., phos., ***sep.,*** staph.
- fever, during - ***chlol., coloc., hell., op.***
- mania puerperalis, in - ***stram.***
- meningitis, in - ***verat.***
- night - merc.
- pregnancy, during - ***bar-c.***
- restrained with difficulty, is - ***stram.,*** zinc.
- run away, to - bar-c., ***bell.,*** bry., chel., ***cupr.,*** dig., glon., hyos., ***merc.,*** mez., nux-v., op., rhus-t., ***verat.***
  - run away, to, wants, and hide as she insists that everyone is looking at her - meli.
- screaming, with - stram.
- springs up suddenly from bed - ***ars.,*** bell., chin., ***crot-h.,*** glon., nux-v., oper., rhus-t., ***verat.***
  - springs up suddenly from bed, to change beds - **ARS.,** hyos.
- street, into - ***hyos.***
  - gesticulating and dancing in their shirts - ***bell.,*** hyos.
- surrounded and captured by men, as if - ***hyos.***
- waking, on - ***cupr-ar.***
  - children - ***staph.***
- wants to visit his daughter - ars.
- window, from - ***aesc., bell.,*** bry., calc-sil., glon., valer.

ESTRANGED, feels, from her family - am-c., anac., arg-n., arn., ars., con., hep., lyc., ***nat-c., nat-m.,*** nat-s., ***nit-ac.,*** nux-v., phos., plat., psor., ***sep.,*** staph., ***thuj.***
- flies from her own children - lyc.
- forgetful of relatives and friends - lyss.
- friends, from - nat-c.
- ignores his relatives - bell., hyos., merc., verat.
- society, from - anac., ***nat-c.,*** plat., **THUJ.**.
- strangers, being kind with, but not with his family and entourage - lyc., nux-v., puls.
- wife, from his - arg-n., ars., lyc., nat-s., plat., staph., **THUJ.**

EUPHORIA, (see Blissful, Tranquility) - asar., ***cann-i.,*** chloram., cob-n., cortiso., kres., ***op.,*** palo., thyr.
- alternating with, quarrel - thyr.
  - with, quiet, desire for - asar.
  - with, sadness - asar., cortiso., man.
- feeling of lightness as after an anesthesia by chlorethylene, with - asar.

EXACTING, too (see Conscientious, Fastidious) - **ARS., CARC.,** ***puls.***
- disease, in - **ARS.,** ***carc.,*** pip-m.

EXALTATION, politics - ***caust.,*** lach.
- religious - ***puls., stram., verat.***

EXCITEMENT, excitable - abrot., absin., acet-ac., **ACON.,** aeth., ether, agar., agar-st., agav-t., agn., alum., alum-p., alum-sil., alumn., ambr., am-c., aml-n., **ANAC.,** anag., anan., ang., ***anh.,*** ant-c., ant-t., anthr., ***apis,*** arg-m., **ARG-N.,** ***arn., ars., ars-h., ars-i.,*** ars-s-f., art-v., arum-t., ***asaf., asar.,*** aster., atro., **AUR.,** aur-a., ***aur-i., aur-m.,*** **AUR-S.,** bad., bapt., **BELL.,** bell-p., benz-n., benz-ac., bor., brom., ***brucin., bry.,*** bufo, calad., ***calc.,*** calc-ar., ***calc-p., calc-s.,*** calc-sil., ***camph.,*** camph-br., ***cann-i., cann-s., canth.,*** carb-ac., ***carb-s.,*** carb-v., **CARC.,** ***carl.,*** cast., caul., **CAUST.,** cedr., ceph., **CHAM.,** ***chel., chin.,*** chin-a., chin-s., chlor., ***cic., cimic.,*** cina, cist., cit-v., clem., ***cob.,*** cob-n., coca, cocaine, cocc., ***coch.,*** **COFF.,** coff-t., colch., **COLL.,** coloc., con., convo-s., cori-r., croc., crot-h., cryp., cub., ***cupr.,*** cupr-ar., cycl., cypr., cyt-l., ***daph., dig.,*** digin., dub., elaps, eucal., eup-per., ***ferr.,*** ferr-ar., ferr-i., ***ferr-p.,*** fl-ac., form., ***gels., glon.,*** gran., **GRAPH.,** guare., guare., ham., hell., **HEP.,** hipp., hoit., hura, hydr-ac., **HYOS.,** hyosin., hyper., iber., ***ign.,*** ilx-p., ***iod.,*** jug-r., ***kali-ar.,*** kali-bi., **KALI-BR.,** kali-c., **KALI-I.,** kali-m., ***kali-p., kali-s.,*** kali-sil., kreos., **LAC-C.,** kres., **LACH.,** lachn., lappa-a., laur., lec., lil-t., ***lith.,*** lob., ***lol., lyc., lycps.,*** lyss., ***mag-m.,*** mag-s., mang., meph., ***merc.,*** merc-c., merc-d., merl., meth-ae-ae., ***mez.,*** mill., **MOSCH.,** mur-ac., mygal., myric., ***naja,*** nat-a., ***nat-c.,*** **NAT-M.,** nat-p., nat-s., nat-sil., **NIT-AC., NUX-V.,** oena., ol-j., **OP.,** ox-ac., paeon., pall., palo., par., paull., ***petr.,*** **PH-AC., PHOS.,** phys., pin-s., pip-m., pisc., plan., ***plat.,*** plect., ***podo.,*** prun., ***psor.,*** **PULS.,** pyrog., rad., raph., rauw., reser., rheum, rhus-t., rumx., sabad., sal-ac., samb., sang., sant., saroth., scut., sec., sel., senec., seneg., ***sep., sil., spig., spong., stann.,*** **STAPH.,** ***stram., stry.,*** sul-i., ***sulph., sul-ac.,*** sumb., tab., tell., ***tarent., ter.,*** tere-ch., ***teucr., thal., thea.,*** ther., ***thuj.,*** thyreotr., tril., tub., ***valer., verat.,*** verat-v., verb., ***viol-o.,*** vip., voes., ***zinc.,*** **ZINC-P.,** zinc-valer., ziz.
- **absent** persons, about - aur.
- **afternoon** - aloe, ang., aspar., cann-i., iod., lyc., phos., thiop.
- **ailments** from, emotional - acet-ac., ***acon.,*** agar., anac., ***arg-n., arn.,*** asaf., aster., ***aur., bell.,*** bry., ***calc.,*** calc-ar., calc-p., **CAPS., CARC.,** ***caust.,*** cimic., ***cist., cob., cocc.,*** coch., cod., **COFF.,** coff-t., **COLL.,** ***con.,*** convo-s., cupr., cypr., epip., ferr., **GELS.,** ***glon.,*** goss., hyos., ign., ***kali-br.,*** kali-c., ***kali-p.,*** kreos., lach., lyc., ***lyss.,*** nat-c., ***nat-m.,*** nit-ac., nux-m., ***nux-v., pall.,*** **PH-AC.,** ***phos.,*** phys., plat., ***psor.,*** **PULS.,** sac-alb., samb., scut., ***sep.,*** stann., **STAPH.,** ***tarent.,*** **TUB.,** ***verat., zinc.***
  - sexual - kali-br., kali-p., ***plat.,*** staph.
- **agg.** - ***acon.,*** ambr., arg-n., aur., bor., calc., carc., ***caust.,*** **CHAM.,** chin., cist., cob., ***cocc.,*** coff., ***colch.,*** coll., coloc., con., cupr-ac., ferr., ***gels., hyos.,*** **IGN.,** kali-p., lyss., nit-s-d., ***nux-v.,*** petr., ph-ac., **PHOS.,** sel., sep., sil., spong., stann., ***staph.***
- **agreeable** - carc., pip-m., phos.
- **alternates** with,
  - convulsions - **STRAM.**
  - delirium - agar.
  - dullness - alum-p., anac.
  - indecision - cortiso.
  - prostration - ***kali-c.***
  - sadness - aster., colch., ***con.,*** cortiso., ferr-p., foll., ox-ac., phenob., ***plb.,*** rad., rauw., sul-ac., thyr., thyreotr.
  - sleepiness - ***kali-br.***
  - taciturn, afternoon - thiop.
- **amel.** - aur., lil-t., merc-i-f., ***pip-m.***
- **amnesia,** followed by transient - agav-t.
- **anticipating** events, when - **ARG-N., CARC.,** ***gels.,*** **KALI-BR.,** med.
- **bath,** during - gast.
- **beer,** after - coc-c.
- **champagne,** after - chlor.
  - as after, followed by sudden unconsciousness - amyg.
- **children,** in - aloe, ambr., ***carc.,*** hyosin., lyc., ***med., phos.***
- **chill,** during - **ACON.,** ars., aur., aur-a., calc., canth., caps., carb-v., caust., ***cean.,*** **CHAM., COFF.,** ***hep.,*** lach., lyc., ***nat-m., nux-v.,*** phos., puls., spig., sulph., verat.
  - before - ***cedr.***
- **coffee,** as after - chin., ***chin-s.,*** sulph., valer.
- **company,** in - ***lec., pall., sep.***
- **confusion,** as from - nux-m.
- **contradiction,** from the slightest - ***ferr.***
- **convulsions,** with - ***cic.***
  - after - agar-st.
- **convulsive** - canth., ***lyss.***
- **cough,** during - cadm-s.

EXCITEMENT, excitable
crying, till - ***carc.,*** **CON., LACH.**
dancing, singing and crying, with - hyos., tarent.
debate, during - ***caust., nit-ac.***
desire for - calc-p., cot., tub.
easily - carc., coff., morph., phos., sumb.
eating, amel. - bell.
epilepsy, before - ***art-v., indg.***
evening - agar., am-c., anac., atha., ***brucin.,*** calc., carb-v., chel., chin., daph., elaps, ferr., ferr-p., fl-ac., graph., hyper., kali-s., ***lach.,*** lyc., lycps., mez., ***nux-v.,*** ox-ac., phel., phos., ***puls.,*** sumb., teucr., ther., valer., zinc.
bed in - ***ang.,*** ant-c., arn., ***aur.,*** bor., ***calc., carb-an.,*** carb-v., jug-r., lach., laur., lyc., mag-aust., ***merc.,*** mez., ***nat-m., nit-ac.,*** **NUX-V.,** ***phos., prun., puls.,*** ran-b., ran-s., rhus-t., ***sep.,*** sil., spig., staph., ***sulph.,*** sul-ac., zinc.
thinking of the things others have done to displease her - am-c.
exertion, after - sulph.
face, cold perspiration of, with - iber.
heat of, with - aloe
fever, during - alum., anthro., ***apis,*** ars-h., cham., chin-s., coff., coff-t., ***ferr.,*** kali-c., lach., mag-c., mosch., op., ***petr., rhus-t., sars.,*** stram., sulph., tarent., valer., verat.
from excitement - **CAPS.**
of head, with - meph.
puerperal, during - ***cham.,*** coff., ***lach.***
feverish - ant-t., aspar., chlor., colch., cub., merc., merc-c., phos., sec., seneg., sul-i.
dinner, after - sep.
evening - merc-c.
menses, during - rhod.
night - sulph.
forenoon - aeth., chin-s., elaps.
hemorrhagia, after - ***chin.***
headache, before - cann-i.
hope, as in joyous - ***aur.***
horrible things, after hearing - ***calc., carc.,*** **CHIN., CIC.,** cocc., gels., ign., ***lach.,*** nat-c., nux-v., ***teucr., zinc.***
hungry, when - cina, kali-c., iod.
hurried, as if - arg-n., carb-v., carc., coff., med.
hydrocephalus, in - ***apis, carb-ac.***
joy, from - caust., **COFF.,** puls.
lascivious, with painful nocturnal erections - ***merc.***
melancholy, followed by - nat-m.
menopausal period, during - arg-n., cimic., coff., glon., ign., lach., phys., ther., valer., zinc.
menses, during - caul., cimic., cop., ferr., hyos., kreos., ***mag-m., nat-c.,*** nat-m., puls., rhod., senec., ***tarent.,*** verat.
after - ferr.
before - alum-sil., croc., ***kreos., lach., lyc.,*** mag-c., mag-m., nat-m., ***nux-v.,*** rob., sep., thuj.

EXCITEMENT, excitable
menses, return of, excitement brings - **CALC.**
mental work, from - ambr., kali-p., ind., med., nat-p.
moral ailments, from - ***acon.,*** **BELL., IGN., PH-AC.,** ***phos., staph.***
morning - ars., aeth., calc., canth., chin., chin-s., con., cop., kalm., lach., ***lyc.,*** mang., nat-c., nat-m., nat-s., ***nux-v.,*** sep., spong.
motions, quick, brusque, performed with uncontrollable zeal - cit-v.
music, from - ***kreos.,*** pall., sumb., ***tarent.***
nervous - absin., **ACON.,** ***ambr., anac.,*** ap-g., apis, ***arg-n., ars.,*** asaf., ***asar.,*** aur., ***bell.,*** bond., ***bor.,*** bov., but-ac., calc-br., ***camph-br.,*** caust., cedr., ***cham., cimic.,*** cina, cinnb., ***coff.,*** coffin., con., ferr., ***gels.,*** goss., helon., hyos., ***hyosin.,*** iber., ***ign.,*** iod., kali-bit., ***kali-p.,*** lac-c., lach., lil-t., mag-c., med., morph., nat-c., nitro-o., nux-m., ***nux-v., phos.,*** psor., puls., sec., ***sep., sil.,*** staph., ***stram.,*** stry., sul-ac., ***sumb.,*** tarent., teucr., thea., torula., ***valer.,*** zinc., zinc-valer.
news, after bad or disagreeable - ***apis, calc.,*** calc-p., carc., chin., cinnb., cupr., form., **GELS.,** ***ign.,*** kali-c., kali-p., lach., nat-c., nat-m., phos., puls., stram., ***sulph.***
night - ambr., am-c., ammc., ant-s., ***apis,*** arg-n., ars-s-f., ***aster.,*** berb., carb-an., carb-h., carb-s., calc., chel., chlol., ***coff.,*** cop., dig., ***ferr., graph.,*** hura, kali-br., ***lach.,*** laur., lyc., mez., mosch., nat-m., nit-ac., ***nux-v.,*** plect., ***puls.,*** saroth., sep., ***sulph., tarent.,*** ther., thuj., zinc.
sleep, during - lyc.
waking, on - berb., coc-c., thea., thuj.
noon - bry., hura, sulph.
pain, during - ars., ***aur., carc.***
palpitation, violent, with - alum., ambr., ars., asaf., ***cact.,*** calc., calc-ar., ***cocc.,*** coff., ***glon., lil-t.,*** lith., ***nit-ac.,*** ox-ac., ***plat.,*** stann., staph., stront-c.
perspiration, during - ***acon., bell.,*** **CHAM.,** ***cocc.,*** **COFF.,** ***con., lyc.,*** nux-v., ph-ac., ***sep.,*** **TEUCR.**
pregnancy, during - ***acon.,*** ambr., asar., cimic., croc., ***gels., nux-m.***
reading, while - ***coff.,*** med., ph-ac.
foreign language, in - v-a-b.
religious - ***aur.,*** lach., ***verat.***
rushing in ears, with - ther.
sadness, after - ***cann-i.,*** spig.
sex, after - ***calc.***
sexual ailments, from - med., ***nat-m.,*** plat., psor.
sleep, before - nat-m., psor.
stammers when talking to strangers - dig.
suppression of excretions, from - acon., asaf., carc., med., merc.
swallows, continually while talking - ***staph.***
talking, while - ***am-m.,*** ambr., am-c., ammc., caust., graph., merc.

EXCITEMENT, excitable
- **tea,** after - sulph.
- **trembling,** with - arg-n., aur., brucin., **COCC.,** gels., nitro-o., **NUX-V.,** petr., ***psor.,*** spig., ***teucr., valer.***
  - after - psor.
  - inward, with - gels., petr.
- **trifles,** over - chin-a., cinnb., ferr., lachn., med., morph., nit-ac., phos., sul-ac., sumb., zinc.
- **urination,** during - aloe.
- **vaginal** discharge, after suppressed - asaf.
- **waking,** on - coc-c., nat-m., sep., thuj.
  - frightened, as if - acon., ***merc.***
- **walking,** after - caust., fl-ac., nat-m.
  - after, air, in open - caust.
  - air, in open - alum., ant-c., sulph.
- **water** poured out, from hearing - **LYSS., STRAM.**
- **weakness,** with - caust., coff., ***con., phos.,*** puls.
- **wine,** after - ambr., iod., zinc.
  - as from - camph., chin-s., jug-r., kali-i., lyc., mosch., naja, valer.
- **women,** in - cedr., con., ign.
- **working,** when - mur-ac., olnd.
- **writing,** while - med.

EXCLUSIVE, too - **CALC.,** ***nat-m., plat.***

EXERCISE, mental symptoms amel., by physical - calc., ***carc.,*** ign., ***rhus-t., sep.***

EXERTION, mental agg., (see Generals) - abrot., achy., ***agar.,*** agn., ***aloe,*** ambr., am-c., aml-n., ***anac.,*** ang., **ARG-M., ARG-N.,** arn., ars., ars-i., asaf., asar., **AUR.,** aur-a., ***aur-i.,*** aur-m., aur-s., aven., bar-ac., bell., berb., bor., cadm-met., calad., **CALC.,** ***calc-ar.,*** calc-i., **CALC-P.,** calc-sil., ***carb-ac., carb-v., caust.,*** cham., ***chin.,*** cimic., cina, cist., ***cocc.,*** coff., ***colch., con.,*** cortiso., crot-h., ***cupr., cupr-ac.,*** dig., echi., ***epig.,*** ferr-pic., fl-ac., ***gels., glon., graph.,*** hell., ***hep.,*** **HYOS., IGN.,** iod., iris, kali-ar., ***kali-br.,*** kali-c., **KALI-P.,** kali-s., kali-sil., **LACH.,** laur., **LEC.,** led., lil-t., **LYC.,** mag-c., mag-m., mang., med., meny., meph., ***naja, nat-a.,*** **NAT-C., NAT-M.,** ***nat-s., nat-sil., nit-ac., nux-m.,*** **NUX-V.,** ***olnd., op.,*** par., ***petr., ph-ac., phos.,*** **PIC-AC.,** pip-m., plan., plat., plb., ***psor., puls.,*** rad., ran-b., rhus-t., ***sabad., sars.,*** **SEL., SEP., SIL.,** spig., spong., stann., **STAPH.,** ***stram.,*** sul-i., sulfon., ***sulph.,*** tarax., thymol., **TUB.,** verat., verb., vinc., vip., zinc., zinc-p.
  - amel. - calc., calc-p., ***camph.,*** cic., croc., ***ferr.,*** hell., ***helon.,*** kali-br., ***nat-c.,*** nat-m., rauw., sep., ***verat.,*** zinc.
  - puberty, agg. from mental excitement during - calc-p., kali-p.
  - weakness, from - ***aloe,*** apis, arn., ars., aur., ***bell.,*** **CALC.,** cham., cocc., **CUPR., FERR-PIC.,** ign., ***kali-c.,*** kali-n., ***kali-p.,*** **LACH., LEC.,** ***lyc.,*** **NAT-C.,** nat-m., ***ph-ac.,*** **PSOR., PULS.,** sabad., **SEL.,** sep., **SIL.,** spong., ***sulph.,*** thuj.

EXHAUSTION, mental - abrot., acet-ac., ***acon., aeth.,*** agar., agn., ail., alco., alf., ***alum.,*** alum-p., alum-sil., am-c., ambr., ***anac.,*** ang., anh., ant-c., apis, aran-s., **ARG-M.,** ***arg-n.,*** arn., ars., ars-i., ars-s-f., asaf., asar., asc-t., aster., **AUR.,** aur-a., aur-i., **AUR-S.,** aven., **BAPT.,** ***bar-c.,*** bar-i., bar-m., **BELL.,** berb., bov., ***bry.,*** bufo, buni-o., buth-a., calad., ***calc.,*** calc-ar., calc-f., calc-i., calc-p., calc-s., calc-sil., camph., cann-i., ***cann-s.,*** canth., ***caps.,*** **CARB-AC.,** carb-an., ***carb-s., carb-v.,*** carl., cast., ***caust.,*** cham., chin., chin-a., cic., cinnb., clem., cob-n., coca, ***cocc., coff.,*** coff-t., colch., coloc., **CON.,** convo-d., convo-s., corn., cortico., croc., cub., **CUPR.,** ***cupr-ac.,*** cypr., dig., digin., dulc., elaps, equis., eucal., ferr., **FERR-PIC.,** fl-ac., ***gels.,*** glon., gran., ***graph.,*** grat., ham., ***hell., hep., hipp.,*** **HYOS.,** hyper., ***ign.,*** ind., iod., ip., kali-br., kali-c., kali-i., **KALI-P.,** ***kali-sil.,*** lac-d., **LACH.,** lat-m., laur., **LEC.,** ***led., lob.,*** lol., **LYC.,** lyss., mag-c., man., mang., meli., menis., meny., merc., ***merc-c.,*** mez., morph., mosch., mur-ac., naja, nat-a., **NAT-C.,** ***nat-m.,*** **NAT-P.,** nat-s., nat-sil., nid., **NIT-AC.,** ***nux-m.,*** **NUX-V.,** ol-an., olnd., onos., op., pall., par., petr., **PH-AC., PHOS.,** phys., **PIC-AC.,** pip-m., ***plan.,*** plat., ***plb.,*** podo., ***psor.,*** ptel., ***puls.,*** pyrog., rad., ran-b., raph., rhus-t., ruta, sabad., ***sars., sel.,*** seneg., **SEP., SIL.,** sium, ***spig.,*** spong., stann., ***staph., stry-p., sul-ac.,*** sul-i., **SULPH.,** syph., tab., tanac., teucr., thuj., trio., tub., valer., **VERAT.,** verat-v., viol-o., xan., ***zinc.,*** **ZINC-P.,** ***zinc-pic.,*** zinc-valer.
  - abortion, after - ***caul.***
  - afternoon - anac., nat-m., sep., sil.
  - business, from - podo.
  - cares, from - ph-ac., pic-ac.
  - convulsions, from - aeth., ***chin-s., cic.,*** hydr-ac., sec., sil., ***staph., stry.,*** sulph.
  - eating, after - anac., lach., nat-m.
  - emissions, after - carb-an., ***sel.***
  - epilepsy, in - ***art-v.***
  - evening - am-m., astra-e., bufo, cham., ign., merc-c., nat-m., osm.
  - fever, in - ***anac., bapt., nit-s-d.,*** rhod.
  - grief, from - **IGN.,** kali-br., ***ph-ac.,*** phys.
  - headache, with - arg-n., nux-v., sil.
  - influenza, after - cypr., gels., ph-ac.
  - injuries, from - ***acet-ac.,*** camph., hell., ***hyper., sul-ac.,*** verat.
  - menses, after - **ALUM.**
    - before - ***cinnb.***
  - morning - berb., canth., carb-v., **LACH., PH-AC.,** ***phos.,*** ran-s.
  - night - ign., kali-c., nux-v., ran-s.
  - noon - carb-v., phos.
  - nursing, after - ***nit-ac., zinc.***
  - old age, in - **BAR-C.**
  - overstudy or night-watching, from - zinc.
  - pain, from - cham.
  - pollutions, after - bell-p., carb-an., ***cypr., gels.,*** ph-ac., ***phos., sel., viol-t.***
  - reading, from - aur., ***sil.***
  - scientific labour, from - graph., sulph.
  - sex, after - ***calc.,*** sep.
  - sleep, from loss of - pic-ac.

EXHAUSTION, mental
- sleepiness, with - corn-f.
- sleeplessness, with - ***aven.,*** **CARC.,** cast., caust., coff., **CUPR.,** gels.,***kali-p.,*** lach., ph-ac.
- talking, from - calc., ***calc-p.,*** **NAT-M.**
- trembling, with - arg-n., cann-i., con., ***gels.,*** ***kali-p.,*** stann.
- trifles, from - ***phos.***
- vertigo, during - ambr., ***arg-n.,*** bapt., chin., cocc., con., echi., gels., ***tab.,*** verat.
- vexation, from - ***staph.***
- waking, on - op., ***syph.***
- writing, after - pic-ac., ***sil.***

EXHILARATION - absin., acon., ether, ***agar.,*** agn., alco., allox., alum., am-c., anag., ang., ant-c., arg-m., ars-h., asar., ***bell.,*** calc-f., camph., **CANN-I.,** canth., carb-ac., ***carb-s.,*** carc., chel., chin-a., chin-s., ***cinnb.,*** clem., cob., ***coca,*** cocc., cod., **COFF.,** colch., coll., cortico., cortiso., ***croc.,*** cub., cupr., erio., eucal., eug., ***fl-ac., form.,*** ***graph.,*** gels., hydr., ign., iod., ***kali-br.,*** kali-n., **LACH.,** laur., lyss., man., med., mez., **OP.,** ***ox-ac.,*** phel., phos., ***pip-m.,*** myric., sabad., sec., senec., ***stram.,*** sul-ac., sulfa., sumb., tanac., **TARENT.,** thea., teucr., thuj., valer., visc., zinc., ziz.
- afternoon - arg-n.
- air, in open - phel.
- alternating with, grief - op.
  - with, sadness - agn., carc., croc., med., ox-ac.
- blissful - cann-i.,***op.***
- can recall things long forgotten - ***gels.***
- daytime - lyss.
- delirium, followed by horrible - absin.
- diarrhea, during - ox-ac.
- evening - anac., chin., cycl., graph., med., phos., teucr.
- morning - bov., cinnb., phys.
- night - ***med.***
- perspiration, during - op.
- sadness, after - ziz.
- sex, after - bor.
- strength, with increased - ziz.
- walking in open air, while - cinnb.

EXPANSIVE, too demonstrative - ***acon.,*** alum., bar-c.

EXTRAVAGANCE - am-c., ***bell., carb-v., caust.,*** chin., ***con.,*** croc., guare., iod., ***nat-m.,*** petr., phel., ph-ac., plat., stram., verat.

EXTROVERTED - carc., lach., lyc., med., nux-v., ***phos., puls.,*** sulph., tarent.
- too demonstrative - acon., bell., carc., ign., ph-ac., staph.

EXUBERANCE - alum-p., am-c., ***bell.,*** carb-s., cast., caust., chin-s., croc., iod., petr., ph-ac., phel., plat., **STANN.,** stram., sumb., verat.
- alternating with, moroseness - ant-t.
  - with, sadness - petr.

FACES, makes, ill mannered - ***hyos.***
- makes, strange - ars., hyos., merc., pall.

FANATICISM - ***caust.,*** puls., rob., sel., ***sulph.,*** ***thuj.***

FANTASIES, imaginations
- **absorbed,** in - arn., cann-i., cupr., sil., stram.
- **absurd** - alco., carb-s.
- **agreeable** - cann-i., op., stram.
- **anxious** - fl-ac.
  - night, during fever - sep.
- **confused** - ***ail.,*** **BAPT.,** camph., con., ***glon.,*** ham., **HYOS.,** ***lil-t.,*** phos., **STRAM.**
- **exaltation,** of - ***absin., acon., agar.,*** agn., alum., alum-sil., ***ambr., am-c., anac., ang.,*** ant-c., apoc., arg-n., arn., ***ars., asaf.,*** aur., aur-a., aur-s., bar-c., **BELL.,** ***bry.,*** bufo, buf-s., calc., calc-sil., camph., **CANN-I.,** cann-s., ***canth.,*** carb-an., ***carb-s.,*** carb-v., **CARC.,** caust., ***cham.,*** chel., **CHIN.,** chin-a., ***cic.,*** coca, cocc., ***coff.,*** coff-t., con., convo-d., croc., ***crot-c.,*** cupr., cycl., dig., elaps, euphr., fl-ac., ***graph.,*** hell., hep., **HYOS.,** ign., iod., kali-ar., kali-c., kali-p., ***lac-c.,*** **LACH.,** lact., led., lil-t., ***lyc.,*** mag-m., meph., ***merc.,*** merc-c., mosch., mur-ac., naja, nit-ac., ***nux-m.,*** nux-v., **OP.,** olnd., ox-ac., ***petr.,*** ph-ac., ***phos.,*** pic-ac., pip-m., plan., ***plat., plb.,*** psor., puls., rhus-t., sabad., samb., ***sec.,*** seneg., sep., ***sil.,*** spong., stann., staph., **STRAM., SULPH.,** thuj., valer., verat., verb., viol-o., ***zinc.,*** zinc-p., ziz.
  - afternoon - anac., ang., lyc.
  - alone, when - ars.
  - business, of - bell.
  - capricious - acon., viol-o.
  - closing the eyes in bed - bell., ***calc.,*** camph., ***graph.,*** led., lyc., sep., ***sulph.***
  - day and night - ambr., caust.
  - daytime - elaps.
  - evening - am-c., anac., ***caust.,*** chel., chin., cycl., naja, ***phos.,*** sulph.
    - bed, in - agar., alum., ambr., ***bry., calc.,*** camph., carb-an., ***carb-v.,*** carc., caust., ***chin.,*** cocc., graph., hell., ign., ***kali-c.,*** lyc., merc., nat-c., ***nux-v.,*** ph-ac., phos., ***puls.,*** rhus-t., sabad., ***sil.,*** staph., ***sulph.,*** viol-t.
    - twilight, in - ***caust.***
  - fitful - acon., viol-o.
  - frightful - **CALC.,** ***caust.,*** hydr., hydr-ac., ***lac-c.,*** merc., **MERC-AUR.,** ***op., sil.,*** **STRAM.**
  - going to bed, after - chin., hell., ign., ***phos.***
  - happened, thinks they had - ***staph.***
  - heat, during - chin., coff., laur., puls., sabad.
  - morning - canth., con., ***nux-v.***
    - bed, in - chin.
  - night - agar., ars., aur., ***bar-c.,*** bor., ***bry.,*** **CALC.,** canth., carb-an., carb-v., ***carc.,***caust., ***cham., chin.,*** coff., con., ***graph.,*** hep., hipp., hydr., ***hyos.,*** ign., ***kali-c.,*** kali-n., ***lach., mag-arct.,*** ***nit-ac., nux-v., op.,*** petr., ph-ac., phos., plat., plb., puls., sep., sil., spong., ***sulph.,*** ***zinc.***

FANTASIES, imaginations
night, at
sleeplessness, with - agar., alum., ambr., anh., ant-t., arg-n., ***bell.,*** bor., bry., calc., ***carc.,*** cas-s., ***cham., chin.,*** cocc., coff., coloc., ***graph.,*** hep., ign., kali-c., kali-n., led., ***lyc.,*** merc., nat-c., ***nux-v.,*** petr., ph-ac., phos., rhus-t., sabad., ***sep., sil.,*** spong., staph., sulph., thuj., viol-t.
walking in open air - ant-c., sulph.
working, while - ang., mur-ac., olnd.
laughable, before falling asleep - sulph.
lively - acon., coff., dig., kali-br., **LACH.,** op.
periodically returning - ars.
perspiration, during - carb-v., iod., nit-ac., sulph.
pleasant - **CANN-I.,** coca, cod., cycl., lach., ***op.,*** stram.
power, increased, of - ang., cann-i., ***carc.,*** chin., hyos., **LACH.,** op., sulph., viol-o.
wanting of, decreased - cann-s., sel.
reading, on - coff., ***mag-m.,*** ph-ac.
repulsive, when alone - fl-ac., sel., tarent.
sexual, fantasies - alum., am-c., ***ambr.,*** anac., arund., aur., bell., ***calad., calc.,*** camph., ***canth.,*** carb-v., **CARC.,** caust., ***chin.,*** cod., ***con.,*** cop., dig., ***graph.,*** hipp., ***hyos.,*** ign., ***kali-br., lach.,*** lil-t., ***lyc.,*** lyss., med., nat-c., ***nat-m., nuph.,*** nux-v., ***op., orig.,*** petr., **PLAT.,** psor., sang., ***sel.,*** sep., ***sil.,*** sin-n., **STAPH.,** stram., **THUJ.,** ***ust., verat.,*** verb., yuc., ***zinc.***
dreaming, even when - ambr.
forenoon - hipp.
impotency, with - calad., ***chin., op., sel.***
lying down, while - thuj.
night - aur.
sleeplessness, during - lyc.
sleep, falling asleep on - arg-n., bell., ***calc.,*** camph., carc., chin., ign., ***spong.,*** sulph.
preventing - ***arg-n., op.,*** phos., ***staph.,*** viol-t.
strange - **STRAM.**
pregnancy, during - lyss.
unpleasant - op., rumx.
bed, after going to - phos.
vivid, lively - acon., alco., bell., ***cann-i.,*** cann-s., carb-an., carc., cham., ***coff.,*** croc., cycl., hell., hyos., ign., ***lach.,*** lact., ***lyc.,*** meph., morph., naja, nat-m., nux-v., op., ***phos.,*** pic-ac., puls., **STRAM.,** valer., zinc.
evening - cycl., hell.
falling asleep, when - nat-m.
followed by heat - phos.
midnight, after - puls.
waking, on - calc., ign., kali-n., ***lach.,*** plat., puls., sep., sil., sulph.
wild - con.

FASTIDIOUS - alum., ***anac.,*** arg-n., **ARS.,** asar., aur., ***calc.,*** **CARC.,** con., ***graph.,*** ign., iod., lac-ac., med., ***nat-m., nat-s., nux-v.,*** phos., plat., psor., **PULS.,** sep., sil., sulph., thuj.
details, for - carc., sil.
cleanliness, for - ars., carc.

FASTIDIOUS,
menses, before - sep.
order, for - ars., calc., carc.
time, being on - carc., nat-m.

FEAR, phobias, general - abrot., absin., acet-ac., **ACON.,** act-sp., aeth., ether, agar., agn., ***all-c.,*** aloe, ***alum.,*** alum-sil., am-br., am-c., am-m., ambr., aml-n., anac., ang., ant-c., ant-s., ant-t., apis, aral., arg-m., **ARG-N.,** arist-cl., ***arn.,*** **ARS.,** ars-h., ars-i., ars-s-f., art-v., arum-m., asaf., aspar., astac., aster., atro., **AUR.,** aur-a., bapt., ***bar-c.,*** bar-m., **BELL.,** berb., bism., **BOR.,** brom., ***bry.,*** bufo, but-ac., ***cact.,*** calad., **CALC.,** calc-f., **CALC-P.,** ***calc-s.,*** calc-sil., camph., cann-i., cann-s., canth., ***caps.,*** carb-an., **CARB-S.,** ***carb-v.,*** **CARC.,** cast., caul., ***caust.,*** cham., chel., chin., chin-a., chlol., chlor., **CIC.,** cimic., cina, cist., clem., cob-n., ***coca, cocc.,*** coc-c., coff., ***coff-t.,*** colch., coloc., ***con.,*** cortico., croc., ***crot-h., cupr.,*** cupr-ac., cupr-ar., cycl., cyt-l., daph., **DIG.,** dros., dulc., echi., elaps, euph., euphr., ferr., ferr-ar., ferr-p., fl-ac., ***form., gels.,*** gent-c., gins., glon., **GRAPH.,** grat., hed., hell., ***hep.,*** hoit., hydr-ac., ***hyos.,*** hyper., iber., **IGN.,** ***iod.,*** ip., iris, jatr., **KALI-AR.,** ***kali-br., kali-c.,*** kali-i., kali-n., kali-p., kali-s., kreos., kres., lach., lact., lat-m., laur., led., ***lil-t.,*** lipp., lob., lol., **LYC., LYSS.,** macro., mag-arct., mag-c., ***mag-m.,*** mag-s., manc., mang., med., ***meli.,*** meny., ***merc.,*** merc-c., merc-i-r., mez., ***mosch.,*** murx., mur-ac., ***nat-a.,*** **NAT-C.,** ***nat-m., nat-p.,*** nat-s., nicc., nit-ac., ***nux-v., onos.,*** **OP.,** orig., ox-ac., ***petr.,*** ph-ac., **PHOS.,** ***phyt.,*** pip-m., **PLAT.,** plb., podo., **PSOR.,** ***puls.,*** pyrog., rad., ran-b., ran-s., raph., rheum, rhod., ***rhus-t.,*** rhus-v., ruta, sabad., sabin., samb., sang., sars., sec., sel., seneg., **SEP.,** sil., ***spig., spong.,*** squil., ***stann.,*** staph., **STRAM.,** ***stront-c.,*** stroph-s., stry., succ., ***sulph., sul-ac., syph., tab.,*** tarax., tarent., tell., ***ther.,*** tere-ch., thuj., til., ***tub.,*** valer., ***verat.,*** visc., wye., xan., ***zinc.,*** zinc-m., **ZINC-P.**
abandoned, of being - carc., ***puls., staph.***
abdomen, arising from - asaf., kali-ar.
accidents, of - acon., **ARG-N.,** calc., ***carb-v.,*** cupr., ***gins.,*** iod., mag-c., mag-s.
afternoon - aeth., am-c., ant-t., berb., carb-an., carb-v., cast., dig., mag-c., nat-c., nicc., ***nux-v.,*** stront-c., ***sulph., tab.***
4 p.m. - tab.
5 p.m. - nux-v.
agoraphobia, (see crowds) - ***acon., arg-n.,*** arn., calc., hydr-ac., ***kali-ar.,*** lyc., **LYSS.,** ***phos.,*** nux-v., ***sep.***
public places, of - acon., ***arg-n., arn.,*** bar-c., ***calc.,*** crot-h., ferr., **GELS.,** glon., hydr., hydr-ac., ***kali-p.,*** levo., nux-v., puls., visc.
aids, disease, of catching (acquired immune deficiency) - ars., carc., thuj.
ailments from fear, (see Fright) - **ACON.,** arg-m., ***arg-n., bell.,*** calc., calc-sil., **CARC.,** ***caust.,*** cocc., coff., cupr., ***gels.,*** glon., graph., ***ign.,*** kali-p., lyc., **OP.,** phos., puls., sil., verat.

FEAR, phobias

air, fresh, of - caps., ***coff.***

open, in - anac., cycl., ***hep.,*** nux-v.

open, in, amel. - bry., plat., ***valer.***

airplanes - ***acon.,*** **ARG-N.,** ars., **CALC.,** gels., lup., nat-m.

alcoholics, in - ***kali-p.***

alone, of being - act-sp., all-s., ant-t., ***apis,*** **ARG-N.,** ***arist-cl.,*** **ARS.,** ***ars-s-f.,*** asaf., aur-a., bell., bism., brom., bry., bufo, cadm-s., calc., calc-ar., ***camph.,*** carc., ***clem., con.,*** **CROT-C.,** cupr-s., dros., ***elaps,*** gall-ac., ***gels.,*** hep., **HYOS.,** kali-ar., kali-br., **KALI-C.,** ***kali-p., lac-c.,*** **LYC.,** ***lyss.,*** merc., mez., morg., naja, nat-c., nit-ac., nux-v., **PHOS.,** plb., ***puls.,*** ran-b., rat., ***sep., stram.,*** syc-co., tab., tarent., verat., zinc.

darkness, in - kali-br., **PHOS.,** rad-br., valer.

desire of being alone, but - con.

die, lest he - ***arg-n.,*** **ARS.,** ***ars-h.,*** bell., ***kali-c., phos.***

evening - brom., dros., kali-c., puls., ran-b., tab.

headache, with - meny.

injure himself, and - ars., merc., ***nat-s.***

left alone, to be - ars., camph., puls.

night - arg-n., ***camph., caust., hell., med.,*** **STRAM.**

alternating with, exhilaration - coff.

mania - ***bell.***

rage - bell.

sadness - zinc.

amenorrhea, from fear - ign., ***op.***

animals, of - abel., **BELL.,** bufo, **CALC.,** carc., caust., **CHIN.,** hyos., ***stram.,*** syc-co., **TUB.**

venomous, of, at night - abel.

anorexia, from fear - ars., carc., ***ign.***

approaching, others approaching him - acet-ac., ***ambr.,*** anac., **ARN.,** bar-c., ***bell.,*** cadm-s., cann-i., caust., con., ***cupr., cupr-ac., ign.,*** iod., ***lyc.,*** nux-v., op., petr., phos., plb., sep., ***stram.,*** stry., tarent., ***thuj.***

children cannot bear to have anyone come near them - ***cina, cupr.***

delirium, in - cupr., stram., ***thuj.***

lest he be touched - **ARN.,** colch., rhod.

vehicles, of - anth., hydr-ac., lyss., phos.

arrested, of being - ars., cupr., kali-br., lach., meli., plb., tab., zinc.

ascending, of - ***nit-ac.***

attacked, of being - anac., lach., op., stram.

away, from home - ign., lyc.

bed, of the - ***acon.,*** alumn., ***ars.,*** bapt., calc., ***camph.,*** cann-s., canth., ***caust.,*** cedr., cench., cupr., kali-ar., kali-c., ***lach.,*** lyc., merc., nat-c., nat-m., squil.

raised himself in, when he - ox-ac.

wetting - alum.

behind him, that someone is - anac., brom., crot-c., lach., ***med.,*** merc., ***phel.***

betrayed, being - hyos., ign., lach., ***nat-m.***

birds, of - calc-ar., calc-s., ign.

bitten, of being - ***hyos., lyss.***

FEAR, phobias

black, everything - rob., **STRAM.**

blind, of becoming - agre., nux-v., sulph.

blood, of - ***alum.,*** nux-m., plat.

brain, inflammation of - psor.

softening of - abrot., ***asaf.,*** calc-sil.

breath away, takes - acon., ***rhus-t., verat.***

bridge, crossing, a - **ARG-N.,** bar-c., ***bor., ferr.,*** lyc., puls., ter.

brilliant objects, looking-glass, etc., of, or cannot endure - cann-i., canth., lach., lyss., stram.

bugs - ***calc.,*** ign., lyc., ***nat-m.,*** phos.

burden, of becoming a - raph.

business - ***graph., lil-t.***

busy streets - **ACON.,** carc., **PSOR.**

cancer, of - agar., **ARS.,** bar-c., **CALC.,** calc-f., calc-p., **CARC.,** chin-a., ign., ***kali-ar.,*** med., ***nit-ac.,*** **PHOS., PSOR.,** ruta.

carried, being, or raised - ***bor.,*** bry., sanic.

cats, of - calc., med., syph., ***tub.***

causeless - calc-f., ***phos.,*** sabad., tarent.

cemetery - stram.

censured, of being - caps.

children, in - **ACON., ARS., BAR-C.,** ***calc.,*** **CARC.,** ***caust.,*** **LYC., PHOS.**

night, at - **ACON.,** arg-m., **ARS.,** ***aur-br.,*** **BOR., CALC.,** cham., ***chlol.,*** cic., ***cina,*** cypr., ***kali-br.,*** kali-p., **PHOS.,** scut., sol-n., ***stram.,*** tub., zinc.

dentition, during - kali-br.

worry, from - ars., calc., kali-br.

chill, during - calc., carb-an., tub.

choking, of - ars., lach., lyss.

cholera, of the - ars., jatr., **LACH., NIT-AC.,** ph-ac., verat.

church or opera, when ready to go - **ARG-N.,** ***gels.***

claustrophobia, closed places - **ACON.,** ambr., aran., **ARG-N.,** ***calc.,*** chin-a., cocc., ***ign.,*** kali-ar., ***lac-d.,*** **LYC.,** med., **NAT-M.,** nit-ac., nux-v., plb., psor., **PULS.,** ruta, staph., **STRAM.,** succ., sulph., tab., valer.

narrow places, fear in - acon., ambr., aran., aran-s., ***arg-n.,*** ars., bry., ***calc.,*** carb-an., carc., caust., cimic., cocc., dys-co., ***ign.,*** kali-c., ***lac-d.,*** lach., **LYC.,** lyss., manc., med., merc-i-f., morg., ***nat-m.,*** nat-s., nux-v., plb., **PULS.,** sep., staph., ***stram.,*** succ., sulph., tab., valer.

trains of - ***arg-n.,*** succ.

vaults, churches and cellars, of - ***ars., calc.,*** carb-an., carc., caust., ***puls.,*** sep., stram.

closet, when in - **LAC-D.**

closing eyes, on - aeth., ***caust., carb-an.***

coal-scuttle, of the - cann-i.

cockroaches, of - alum., manc., ***phos.***

cold - phys.

taking, of - nat-c., sulph., syph.

taking, of, during heat - sulph.

company, of - cic.

confusion, that people would observe her - ***calc.,*** cann-i., med.

FEAR, phobias

contamination, germs, of - ***ars.,*** bor., bov., **CALC.,** ***carc.,*** cur., ***lach.,*** sil., **SULPH.,** syph., ***thuj.***

control, losing - ***arg-n.,*** cann-i., carc., ign., med., nat-m., ***staph.,*** thea.

conversation, of - bar-s.

convulsions, before - **CUPR.,** nat-m.

corners, to walk past certain - ***arg-n., kali-br.***

cough, during - dros.

cough, of - ant-t., bry., phos.

creeping out of every corner, of something - med., ***phos.***

crossing, bridge, a - **ARG-N.,** bar-c., ***bor., ferr.,*** lyc., puls., ter.

streets - acon., hydr-ac., plat.

crowd, in a (see agoraphobia, public places) - **ACON.,** aloe, am-m., ***arg-n.,*** arn., ars., ars-s-f., asaf., ***aur.,*** aur-a., aur-i., aur-s., bar-c., bar-s., bell., bufo, calc., carb-an., carc., caust., cic., con., dios., ferr., ferr-ar., ferr-p., gels., graph., hep., hydr-ac., ***kali-ar.,*** kali-bi., kali-c., kali-p., led., levo., ***lyc.,*** nat-a., nat-c., ***nat-m.,*** nat-s., ***nux-v.,*** petr., phos., plat., plb., ***puls.,*** rhus-t., sel., stann., sulph., tab., til.

crying, with - ***ars.,*** kali-c., phos., spong.

amel. - ***aster.,*** dig., **GRAPH.,** phos., tab.

cruelties, report of, excite - calc., cic.

cutting, himself when shaving - **CALAD.**

danger, of impending - camph., caust., ***cic.,*** cimic., ***cocc.,*** ether, macro., meli.

going to sleep, on - coff.

night - ether.

dark - ***acon.,*** aeth., am-m., arg-n., ***ars.,*** bapt., bell., brom., calad., ***calc.,*** calc-ac., calc-ar., calc-p., calc-s., ***camph.,*** **CANN-I.,** ***cann-s., carb-an., carb-v.,*** carc., ***caust.,*** cham., chin-s., ***cupr.,*** gels., ***grin.,*** hyos., kali-bi., kali-br., ***lyc., manc., med.,*** morg., ***nat-m.,*** nux-m., op., **PHOS.,** ***puls.,*** rad., rhus-t., sanic., sil., **STRAM.,** ***stront-c.,*** valer., zinc.

dawn, of the return of - kali-i.

day and night - ars.

daytime, only - lac-c., ***lyc.,*** mur-ac., pip-m., sul-ac.

death, of - **ACON.,** act-sp., ***agn.,*** all-s., aloe, alum., alum-p., am-c., anac., anan., anh., ant-c., ant-t., ***apis,*** aran., ***arg-n., arn.,*** **ARS.,** ***ars-s-f.,*** asaf., ***aur.,*** aur-a., aur-s., bapt., bar-c., bar-s., ***bell., bry.,*** bufo, ***cact.,*** **CALC.,** ***calc-ar.,*** calc-s., calad., camph., ***cann-i.,*** cann-s., canth., caps., carb-an., carb-s., carb-v., **CARC.,** ***caust.,*** chel., chin., **CIMIC.,** ***cocc., coff.,*** con., cop., croc., ***crot-c.,*** culx., ***cupr.,*** cur., ***cycl., dig.,*** dros., ***elaps,*** fago., ferr., ferr-ar., ***ferr-p., fl-ac.,*** **GELS.,** glon., **GRAPH.,** ***hell., hep.,*** hydr., hydr-ac., hyos., ign., iod., ip., iris, **KALI-AR.,** ***kali-c.,*** kali-fer., ***kali-i., kali-n.,*** kali-p., kali-s., **LAC-C.,** ***lach.,*** lat-m., led., ***lil-t.,*** lob., ***lyc.,*** mag-s., med., ***merc., mosch.,*** mygal., naja, nat-c., ***nat-m.,*** **NIT-AC.,** nux-m., **NUX-V.,** ***op.,*** ox-ac., petr.,

FEAR, phobias

death, of - ***ph-ac.,*** phase., **PHOS.,** phyt., **PLAT.,** pneu., podo., ***psor., puls.,*** raph., rheum, ***rhus-t.,*** rob., sabad., ***sec.,*** sep., sium, ***spong.,*** stann., staph., still., stram., squil., sulph., syph., tab., tarax., tarent., trach., tril., vario., ***verat.,*** verat-v., vinc., visc., zinc., zinc-p.

afternoon, 5 p.m. - nux-m.

alone, when - ***arg-n., arn.,*** **ARS.,** ars-h., bell., ***kali-c.,*** med., ***phos.,*** tub.

evening in bed - ***ars., caust.,*** kali-c., ***phos.***

alternate laughing and crying, with - ***plat.***

amenorrhea, in - plat.

anger, from - ***plat.***

angina, in - ***dig.,*** squil.

cancer, from - ars., carc.

desire for death, with fear - ***aur., aur-m.***

die, fear he will, if he go to sleep, after nightmare - ***lach.,*** led.

dream, from - alum., cench.

dyspnea, with, and restlessness - psor.

evening - ***calc., phos.***

bed, in - nat-m.

heart symptoms, during - **ACON.,** ***ang., arn.,*** asaf., ***cact.,*** cench., **DIG.,** glon., kali-ar., ***naja,*** phos., ***plat., psor.***

heat, during - acon., calc., cocc., ip., mosch., ***nit-ac.,*** **RUTA**

hunger, from - ars., calc.

impending death., of - acon., ***ars.,*** asaf., **BELL.,** bry., caps., ***carc., caust., croc.,*** cupr., lach., **MERC.,** nux-v., op., **PHOS.,** sep., staph., v-a-b.

labor, during - **ACON.,** ***ars., coff., plat.***

lying down, on - mosch.

menses, during - acon., plat., verat.

before - acon., kali-bi., plat., sec., sulph., xan.

morning - alum., con., lyc.

night - act-sp., am-c., ***arn.,*** calc-ar., chel., kali-s., ***phos.***

1 a.m. to 3 a.m. - ars.

pain, from - acon., ars., **COFF.**

perspiration, during - kali-n.

predicts the time - **ACON.,** ***arg-n.***

pregnancy, during - **ACON.**

prepares farewell messages - ***lyc.***

pressure in hypochondrium, with - ph-ac.

sadness, with - ***plat.,*** vinc.

sleep, during - aeth., ign.

followed by deep - vario.

soon, that she will die - ***agn., sep.***

starvation, from - ars., calc.

strenght, with loss of - ***rhus-t.***

sudden, of - acon., ***arn., ars., cench.,*** thea.

vexation, after - ars.

vomiting - ***ars.,*** mag-c.

waking, on - alum., ***ars.,*** con.

from an afternoon sleep - ***ign.***

walking, while - ***dig.***

delusions, from - bell., **STRAM.**

dentist, of going to - acon., ***arg-n.,*** calc., ***gels.***

FEAR, phobias

destination, of being unable to reach his - **LYC.**
destruction, to all near her, of impending - ***kali-br.***
devil, being taken by the, of - anac., manc.
devoured by animals, of being - stram.
diarrhea, from - ***arg-n.,*** ars., **GELS.,** ign., ***kali-p.,*** **OP.,** ***verat.***
diarrhea, with - acon., aeth., ars., ***crot-t.,*** gels., ***puls.***
dinner, after - mag-m., phel.
dirt, of - ars., carc., thuj.
disabled, being - **ARS.,** mag-m., psor.
disaster, of - ***calc.,*** elat., lil-t., psor., puls., tab., ***tub.***
disease, of impending - acon., ether, agar., ***alum.,*** am-c., ant-t., ***arg-n., arn.,*** **ARS.,** ***bor.,*** bov., bry., bufo, calad., ***calc., calc-ar.,*** calc-s., carb-ac., carb-an., **CARC.,** chlor., cic., cimic., elaps, elat., eup-pur., hep., hydr., ign., iris, **KALI-C.,** kali-p., kali-tel., kreos., ***lac-c.,*** lach., ***lec., lil-t.,*** lyc., mag-arct., med., merc., nat-a., nat-c., nat-m., nat-p., ***nit-ac., nux-v.,*** paull., ***ph-ac.,*** **PHOS.,** ***plat.,*** pneu., podo., psor., puls., sabad., sel., staph., sulph., tab., tarent., thuj., tril.
contagious, epidemic diseases, of - ars., **CALC.,** lach., thuj.
night, in bed - carb-ac.
worse walking in open air - hep.
disfigured, of being - hep.
disturbed, of being - agar.
doctors, of going to - **ACON.,** ***arg-n., arn.,*** calc., **GELS.,** ***ign.,*** **IOD.,** nat-m., nux-v., ***phos., sep., stram.***
physician, will not see the, he seems to terrify her - iod., nat-m., ***nux-v., phos., stram.,*** thuj., verat-v.
dogs, of - **BELL.,** bufo, ***calc.,*** carc., ***caust.,*** **CHIN.,** ***hyos.,*** lach., lyss., merc., nat-m., nat-p., phos., plat., ***puls.,*** sep., sil., ***stram.,*** sulph., syc-co., ***tub.***
door, bell ringing, on hearing - lyc.
closed, lest the door should be - lac-d.
opening, in - cic., con., lyc.
downward motion, of - **BOR.,** calc., coca, cupr., gels., hyper., lac-c., lil-t., ***sanic.,*** sil., zinc.
hammock, of, while asleep - coff-t.
drawn upward, of being - camph.
dreams, terrible, of - **NUX-V.,** spong., ***sulph.***
driving, him from place to place - meny.
drowned, of being - cann-i.
duty, neglect his, to - aur.
unable to perform her, she will become - ***lac-c.***
dying, of - xan.
eating - caust., grat., hera., op., puls., tarent.
after - asaf., canth., carb-v., caust., hyos., kali-c., lach., mag-m., nit-ac., nux-v., phel., tab., thuj., viol-t.
amel. - anac., graph.

FEAR, phobias

emission, after an - aloe, carb-an., petr.
endure, cannot - lyss.
enemies, of - anac., hyos.
epilepsy - alum., arg-n., merc.
morning, in the - alum.
escape, with desire to - ***bell., bry.,*** coloc., cupr., dig., merc., puls., stram., verat.
evening - alum., alum-p., ***am-c.,*** anac., ant-t., ***ars.,*** aur-a., bar-c., bar-s., berb., brom., calad., **CALC.,** calc-ar., carb-an., ***carb-v.,*** **CAUST.,** coc-c., ***cupr.,*** dig., ***dros.,*** form., hep., hipp., ***kali-ar., kali-c.,*** kali-i., kali-p., lach., ***lyc., mag-c.,*** mag-m., merc., nat-a., nat-c., nat-m., nit-ac., nux-v., paeon., petr., ***phos.,*** plat., **PULS.,** ran-b., ***rhus-t.,*** stront-c., tab., valer., verat., ***zinc.,*** zinc-p.
amel. - mag-c., zinc.
bed, in - agar., ***ars.,*** calc., ***graph., kali-c.,*** mag-c., merc., nat-a.
twilight - am-m., berb., ***calc., caust.,*** kali-i., ***phos.,*** **PULS.,** rhus-t.
walking, while - ***nux-v.***
events, of sudden - cocc.
everything, constant - acet-ac., ars., bell., ***calc.,*** carc., hydr-ac., ***hyos., lyc.,*** nat-c., phos., ***puls.***
ringing doorbell, even at - ***lyc.***
evil, of - acon., agar., alum., am-c., ambr., **ANAC.,** ant-c., ***arg-n.,*** arn., ***ars.,*** ars-i., ars-s-f., asaf., aster., aur., aur-a., aur-i., ***aur-m.,*** aur-s., bar-c., bar-i., bar-m., bar-s., bell., bry., calad., **CALC.,** calc-p., calc-s., camph., caps., carb-an., ***carb-v.,*** cast., ***caust.,*** cham., ***chin.,*** chin-a., **CHIN-S.,** cina, ***cocc., coff.,*** colch., croc., crot-h., cupr., cycl., dig., dros., dulc., euph., ferr., ferr-ar., ferr-p., graph., hell., hep., hyos., ***iod., kali-ar.,*** kali-c., **KALI-I.,** kali-m., kali-p., kalm., ***lach., laur., lil-t.,*** lyc., ***lyss.,*** mag-arct., mag-c., ***mag-s.,*** meny., merc., mosch., mur-ac., nat-a., ***nat-c., nat-m.,*** nat-s., nicc., nit-ac., nux-v., ***onos., pall.,*** petr., ***phos.,*** puls., **PSOR.,** rad., rhus-t., ruta, sabad., sabin., sec., ***sep.,*** sil., spig., spong., squil., ***stann., staph.,*** stram., stront-c., sulph., sul-ac., tarent., ***thuj.,*** verat.
afternoon - chin-s.
evening - **ALUM.,** graph., sulph.
walking in open air, while - cina.
morning, on waking - mag-s.
night - chin-a.
examination, before - ***aeth.,*** anac., ***arg-n.,*** carc., ***gels., lyc.,*** pic-ac., sil.
exertion, of - calad., calc-sil., ***gels.,*** guai., mez., ph-ac., phos., phyt., **SIL.,** sul-i., tab., thea.
amel. - tarent.
exposure, of, at night in bed - mag-c.
extravagance, of - op.
extreme - hed.
failure, of - arg-n., arn., ***carc.,*** cob-n., gels., ign., iod., ***lac-c.,*** **LYC.,** naja, nat-m., phos., sil., sulph.

FEAR, phobias

failure, of

business, in - arg-n., arn., carb-an., gels., iod., lac-c., ***lyc.,*** nat-m., ***nux-v.,*** phos., ***psor.,*** sil., sulph.

examinations, in - aeth., arg-n., **GELS., LYC.,** sil.

fainting, of - ***acon., arg-n.,*** ars-s-f., aster., carb-an., **LAC-C.,** ***plat.***

faith, to lose his religious - coloc., merc., nux-v., staph., ***sulph.***

falling, of - acon., alum., alumn., **ARG-N.,** ars., ***bor.,*** calc., chin., coff., ***cupr.,*** cur., ***gels.,*** hyper., kali-c., kali-s., ***lac-c., lil-t.,*** lysi., nux-v., onos., sanic., sil., ***stram.,*** tab., tub., zinc.

afternoon - nux-v.

child holds on to mother - ***cupr-ac.,*** **GELS.**

downstairs - lac-c.

down- and upstairs - onos.

evening - lyss.

everything is falling on her - stram.

forwards - alum.

height, from - hyos.

high walls and building upon him - arg-n., arn.

houses, of - hydr-ac.

letting things fall, of - coca.

room, in, agg. - lil-t.

sleep, on going to - coff.

turning head, on - der.

walking, when - coca, hura, lyss., nat-m.

family, to bring up his - calc., puls., ***staph.***

fasting, of - kreos.

fever, during - acon., ***ars.,*** bell., cham., nux-m., phos., spong.

chilly, while - calc., sulph.

cold, during a - sulph.

going to bed, on - hura.

typhus, of - tarent.

fire, things will catch - cupr., ***cupr-ac.,*** stram.

fit, of having a - agar., alum., ***arg-n.,*** cann-i., carb-an., grat., lach., lyc., lyss., merc., nux-m., phos., puls.

flies, of - abel.

food, after - ars., canth., caust., mag-m., phel., tab.

forenoon - am-c., nicc., paeon.

friend, has met with an accident - ars.

friends, of - cedr.

meeting - sep.

gallows, of the - ***bell.***

germs, contamination, from - ***ars.,*** bor., bov., **CALC.,** ***carc.,*** cur., ***lach.,*** sil., **SULPH.,** syph., ***thuj.***

get talked about, to - nux-v., pall., puls.

ghosts, of - ***acon.,*** agar., ***ars.,*** ars-s-f., bell., brom., calc., cann-i., ***carb-v., caust.,*** chin., chin-a., clem., cocc., dros., ***hyos., kali-br.,*** kali-c., ***lyc., manc.,*** med., op., ***phos., plat., puls.,*** rad., ran-b., rhus-t., sep., spong., ***stram., sulph.,*** zinc., zinc-p.

FEAR, phobias

ghosts, of

conversing, thinks he is, with - ***nat-m.,*** **PLAT.**

dark, in the - brom.

evening - brom., lyc., ***puls.,*** ran-b.

night - ***acon.,*** ars., ***carb-v.,*** chin., chin-a., ***lyc., puls.,*** ran-b., ***sulph.***

waking, on - cocc., sulph.

going out, of - pneu., sep.

grieving, as if - am-m., phos.

hanged, of being - **PLAT.**

happen, something bad will - acet-ac., alum., alum-p., aml-n., anth., arn., ***ars.,*** bar-c., bufo, cact., ***calc.,*** calc-s., calen., ***carb-v.,*** carc., **CAUST.,** chel., cocc., ***coloc.,*** crot-t., elaps, fl-ac., gels., graph., ***iod., kali-ar., kali-br.,*** kali-p., ***lac-c., lil-t.,*** lyc., ***lyss.,*** mag-c., mang., med., merc., mosch., nat-a., ***nat-m., nat-p.,*** nicc., **NUX-V.,** ***onos., pall., ph-ac.,*** **PHOS.,** pic-ac., ***plat.,*** plb., pyrus, psor., scut., spong., stry., sul-i., tab., tarent., thea., **TUB.,** xan.

air, fresh, amel. - aml-n., ***crot-t.,*** rhus-t., spong., ***sulph.,*** zinc.

evening, in bed amel. - mag-c.

twilight aggr - caust.

night - ***arn.,*** nat-p.

still, cannot sit - aml-n.

terrible - ***calen., ign.,*** **LYSS.**

warmth of bed amel. - ***caust.,*** mag-c.

when alone relieved by conversation - rat.

health, of loved persons - ars., carc., hep., **MERC.,** phos.

ruined, that she has - chel.

heat from - chen-a.

heart, arising from - aur., kali-ar., lyc., meny., merc-c., mez.

pain about heart, from - ***acon.,*** cact., daph., ***kali-ar., phos.,*** spig.

will cease beating, lying down, on - lach.

unless constantly on the move - ***gels.***

unless not moving - dig.

heart, disease of - acon., arg-n., ***arn., aur.,*** bapt., cact., ***calc.,*** calc-p., daph., hed., **KALI-AR.,** lac-c., lach., ***lil-t.,*** lob., ***med.,*** nat-m., nux-m., **PHOS.,** sars., sin-n., ***spong.***

organic disease, of - ***apis, aur., kali-ar.***

heights, high places - **ARG-N.,** ***aur.,*** calc., cob-n., coca, gels., nat-m., phos., puls., staph., ***sulph.,*** zinc.

hell - manc.

home, away from - ign., lyc.

homosexuality, of - ars., manc., med., ***puls., staph.,*** **THUJ.**

humiliated, of being - ***carc.,*** lyc., puls., ***sep., staph.***

hungry, when - grat.

hurry, following - benz-ac.

hurt, of being, emotionally - ***arn.,*** carc., chin., hep., ign., kali-c., **NAT-M.,** ruta, spig.

feelings, of others - chin., ***nat-m.,*** phos.

husband, that he would never return, that something would happen to him - ***plat.***

FEAR, phobias

hydrocephalus, in - ***zinc.***

imaginary things, from - acon., ars., **BELL.,** brom., calc-sil., ***hell.,*** hydr-ac., iod., laur., lyc., merc., ***phos.,*** **STRAM.,** verat., zinc.

animals - **BELL.**

imbecile, that he would become - stram.

impotency, of - lyc., pituin.

impulses, his own - **ALUM.,** ***anac.,*** arg-n., staph.

incurable, of being - acon., alum., arg-n., arn., ***ars., aur.,*** cact., calc., calc-sil., **CARC.,** cecr., cimic., ign., lac-c., lach., lil-t., stann.

infection, of - ars., ***carc., bor.,*** bufo, calad., **CALC.,** lach., syph., thuj.

injured, of being - **ARN.,** ***calc.,*** **CALAD.,** cann-i., cupr-ac., hyos., ***rhus-t.,*** **STRAM.,** stry.

insanity, of - ***acon.,*** agar., **ALUM.,** alum-p., alum-sil., ***alumn.,*** ambr., ***anac.,*** antipyrin., aq-mar., ***arg-n.,*** ars., ars-i., bov., bry., **CALC.,** ***calc-ar.,*** calc-i., calc-s., **CANN-I.,** carb-an., carb-s., **CARC.,** ***chel.,*** chlor., **CIMIC.,** colch., cupr., ***dig., eup-per.,*** gels., glon., ***graph.,*** ham., ign., iod., kali-bi., ***kali-br.,*** kali-s., ***lac-c.,*** lach., lat-m., laur., levo., lil-s., ***lil-t., lyss.,*** mag-c., **MANC.,** ***med., merc.,*** merl., mosch., ***nat-m., nux-v.,*** ol-j., ***phos.,*** phys., pic-ac., plat., psor., **PULS.,** rhod., ***sep.,*** spong., ***staph., stram.,*** sul-i., sulph., sumb., syph., tarent., thuj., verat.

evening in bed - nat-m.

if he wants to repose, must always move - ars., iod.

menopause, during - ***cimic.***

night - calc., ***merc.,*** phys.

insects, of - abel., **CALC.,** cimic., lyc., ***nat-m.,*** phos.

job, that he will lose his lucrative - calc., ign., ***lyc.,*** puls., rhus-t., staph., sulph.

joints are weak, that - sep., thuj.

jumps, on touch - bell.

out of bed, from - ***ars.,*** **BELL.,** stann.

out of the window - ars.

killing, of - absin., alumn., am-m., ***ars., chin.,*** der., kali-br., merc., ***nux-v., rhus-t.,*** sulph., thea.

child, her - manc., nux-v., sulph., **THEA.**

knife, with a - ars., der., ***nux-v.***

mother, her - der.

someone, he might - rhus-t.

knives, of - alum., ars., chin., hyos., lyss., merc., plat.

labor, during - acon., arn., ***ars.,*** cham., coff., ign., ***op.,*** plat.

after - iod.

fear of - ars., cham., cimic., ign.

late, of being - **ARG-N.,** carc., ***nat-m.***

lifelong - am-c., am-m., ***ars.,*** calc., **CARC.,** lyc., ***op.,*** petr., puls., sil., stann., sulph., zinc.

lightning, of - bell., cycl., dig., lach., ***phos.,*** phys., sil.

liver, in affections of - ***mag-m.***

FEAR, phobias

long, lasting - ***acon.,*** hyos., ***op.,*** petr.

looked at - ***ant-c.,*** ars., bar-c., meli., nat-m., rhus-t.

looking before her, when - sulph.

losing his reason (see insanity, fear of) - alum., ***calc., cann-i.,*** carb-an., carc., chlor., lyss., ***med.,*** stram.

lung disease, in - aral., ars., phos.

lying, down, of, lest one die - mosch.

in bed, while - kali-c., sil.

maniacal - sec.

manual labor, after - iod.

medicine, of not being able to bear any kind of - all-s., ars., carc., crot-h., lach., med.

selecting remedies, when - ars., crot-h.

taking too much, of - all-s., ars., iber., lach.

men of - acon., aloe, ambr., anac., ***aur.,*** bar-c., bar-m., bell., **CIC.,** con., ***hyos.,*** ign., kali-bi., lach., **LYC.,** merc., **NAT-C.,** nat-m., phos., ***plat., puls.,*** rhus-t., sel., sep., stann., sulph.

confidence, loss of - cic.

contempt for - cic., plat.

shuns the foolishness of - cic., nat-c.

menopause, during - ***cimic., glon.***

menses, during - acon., ***bell., coff.,*** con., **IGN.,** ***lach.,*** mag-c., manc., ***nat-m.,*** nux-m., oena., op., ***ph-ac.,*** phos., plat., sec., staph., verat.

after - pall., ***phos.***

before - ***acon.,*** bor., calc., con., hep., kali-bi., kali-br., mang., plat., sec., sulph., xan.

menstrual pain, during - ant-t.

suppressed from - acon., act-sp., ***calc., lyc., nux-m.***

mental exertion, after - calc-sil.

mice, of - ***calc.,*** colch.

waking, on - colch.

midnight - acon., ars., con., manc.

3 a.m. - **ARS.,** kali-c.

after - ign., mang., rat.

before - cina.

mirrors in room, of - bufo, camph., cann-i., ***canth., lyss.,*** puls., ***stram.***

miscarriage, from threatening - ***cimic., op., sabin.***

mischief, he might do, night on waking - ***phys.***

misfortune, of - **ACON.,** agar., alco., alum., alum-p., alumn., am-c., aml-n., ***anac.,*** ant-c., arn., **ARS.,** ars-i., aster., atro., bar-c., ***bry.,*** bufo, calad., cact., **CALC.,** calc-f., calc-i., calc-s., carb-s., carc., cast., ***caust.,*** cham., **CHIN-S.,** cic., cimic., ***clem.,*** colch., crot-t., cupr., cycl., dig., digin., dros., ferr., ferr-ar., ferr-p., fl-ac., gins., glon., ***graph., hell.,*** hura, hydr-ac., ***iod.,*** ip., kali-c., kali-i., kali-m., lach., laur., lil-t., lipp., lyss., mag-c., mag-s., mang., **MED.,** meny., ***merc.,*** merc-c., mez., mur-ac., naja, ***nat-c.,*** nat-m., nat-p., nat-s., nicc., **NUX-V.,** phel., phos., plat., **PSOR., PULS.,** rhus-t., rumx., sabin., spong., stram., sul-i., sulph., tab., tarent., thuj., valer., verat., vichy-g., vichy-g., vinc., zinc.

FEAR, phobias
misfortune, of
afternoon - cast., hura, tab.
2 p.m. - hura.
chilliness, during - cycl.
daytime - phel.
evening - ferr., nat-m.
bed, in, amel. - mag-c.
forenoon - am-c.
heat, during - atro., cycl.
morning - am-c., mag-s.
night - syph.
monsters - calc.
moral obliquity alternating, with sexual excitement - lil-t.
morning - alum., anac., arg-n., ars., carb-an., carb-s., carb-v., caust., chin., ***graph.,*** ign., ip., ***lyc.,*** mag-c., mag-m., mag-s., mur-ac., nicc., nit-ac., ***nux-v.,*** phos., puls., rhus-t., sep., sul-ac., ***verat.***
bed, in - lyc., nux-v.
rising, on - arg-n.
until evening - sul-ac.
waking, on - puls.
motion, of - ***bry.,*** calad., gels., mag-p.
motoring - gins.
murdered, of being - absin., anac., ars., ***cimic.,*** lach., op., phos., ***plat.,*** plb., nat-m., rhus-t., staph., stram., tab.
music, from - ***acon., ambr.,*** bufo, dig., ***nat-c.,*** nux-v., ***sabin.,*** tarent., thuj.
narrow place, in (see claustrophobia) - acon., ambr., aran., aran-s., ***arg-n.,*** ars., bry., ***calc.,*** carb-an., carc., caust., cimic., cocc., dys-co., ***ign.,*** kali-c., ***lac-d.,*** lach., **LYC.,** lyss., manc., med., merc-i-f., morg., ***nat-m.,*** nat-s., nux-v., plb., **PULS.,** sep., staph., ***stram.,*** succ., sulph., tab., valer.
trains and closed places, of - ***arg-n.,*** succ.
vaults, churches and cellars, of - ***ars., calc.,*** carb-an., caust., ***puls.,*** sep., stram.
nausea, after - tab.
near, of those standing - bell.
neglected, of being - ars., nat-m., ***puls.,*** thuj.
new, persons, of - bar-c., lyc.
news, of hearing bad - aster., ***calc., calc-p.,*** dirc., dros., gels., ***lyss.,*** nat-p.
night - **ACON.,** am-c., arn., **ARS.,** ***ars-s-f.,*** aur-a., ***aur-br., bell., calc.,*** calc-ar., ***calc-s.,*** calc-sil., **CAMPH.,** carb-an., ***carb-s., carb-v.,*** **CARC.,** ***caust.,*** cham., ***chin.,*** chin-a., chlol., cic., ***cina,*** cocc., colch., con., ***crot-c.,*** cypr., dros., dulc., eup-per., graph., hep., ign., ip., ***kali-ar., kali-br.,*** kali-c., kali-p., kali-s., ***lach.,*** lyc., mag-c., manc., ***merc.,*** nat-c., ***nat-m., nat-p.,*** nit-ac., op., ph-ac., **PHOS.,** ***puls.,*** rat., rob., **RHUS-T.,** scut., sil., sol-n., spong., stann., ***stram., sulph.,*** syph., tab., thea., ***tub.,*** verat., zinc., zinc-p.
children, in - **ACON.,** arg-m., **ARS.,** ***aur-br.,*** **BOR.,** ***calc.,*** **CARC.,** cham., ***chlol.,*** cic., ***cina,*** cypr., ***kali-br.,*** kali-p., **PHOS.,** scut., sol-n., ***stram.,*** tub., zinc.

FEAR, phobias
night, at
children, in, dentition, during - kali-br.
worry, from - ars., calc., kali-br.
lie in bed, cannot - rhus-t.
waking, after - aesc., carb-v., con., lach., lyc., phos., samb., spong.
noise, from - acon., aloe, alum., ***ant-c., asar., aur.,*** bar-c., ***bell., bor.,*** calad., cann-s., ***caust., cham.,*** chel., chin., cic., ***cocc.,*** coff., ferr., hipp., hura, ign., kali-c., ***lyc.,*** mag-m., med., mosch., nat-c., ***nat-m., nat-s.,*** nit-ac., nux-v., **PHOS.,** sabad., sil., sulph., tab., tanac., tarent., ***ther.,*** zinc.
at door - ***aur.,*** cic., ***lyc.***
least - aur.
night - bar-c., ***caust.,*** nat-m., ***nat-s., phos.***
rattling - aloe.
rushing water - hyos., **LYSS., STRAM.**
street, in - bar-c., ***caust.***
sudden, of - ***bor., cocc.***
noon - zinc.
to 3 p.m. - aster.
observed, of her condition being - atro., **CALC.,** chel.
occupation, of - lyc., sel., sil.
occurrence, will end seriously, every little - iod.
operation, of each - calc.
opinion of others, of - ign., ***lyc.,*** **NUX-V., PULS.,** staph.
ordeal, of an - ***arg-n.,*** arn., ***gels.,*** kali-br., lyc., ***lyss., stroph.***
orgasm, sexual, of - plat., staph.
outdoors, to go (see agoraphobia) - anth.
overpowering - ***acon.,*** arg-n., ars., aur., bell., carb-v., carc., caust., cham., chin., cocc., coff., dig., nux-v., ***op., phos.,*** plat., puls., rhus-t., sulph., verat.
pain, during - acon., ***ars., carc.,*** merc-br.
of the pain - ***ars.,*** clem., cori-r., der., pip-m.
will become unbearable - all-c., ars., carc.
palpitation, with - ***acon.,*** alum., aur-m., cact., ***ferr.,*** glon., ***merc.,*** nat-m., nit-ac., ***op., phos., puls.,*** spong.
paralysis, of - ***anac.,*** arn., asaf., bapt., bell., syph.
people, of - acet-ac., ***acon.,*** aloe, alum., alum-p., ambr., am-m., ***anac., anh., arist-cl.,*** ars., ars-i., ars-s-f., ***aur.,*** aur-a., aur-i., aur-s., bar-ac., ***bar-c.,*** bar-i., bar-s., bell., buf-s., calc., calc-i., camph., carb-an., carb-s., ***carb-v., caust.,*** chin., ***cic.,*** cocc., ***con.,*** crot-h., crot-t., cupr., cupr-acet., dios., ferr., ferr-ar., ferr-p., fl-ac., gels., graph., hep., hydrc., **HYOS.,** ign., ***iod., kali-ar.,*** kali-bi., kali-br., ***kali-c.,*** kali-p., kali-s., lach., ***led.,*** **LYC.,** meli., merc., ***nat-a.,*** **NAT-C.,** ***nat-m.,*** nat-s., phos., ***plat., puls.,*** rhus-g., **RHUS-T.,** sel., ***sep.,*** sil., stann., ***staph.,*** sul-i., sulph., tab., til.
alone agg., yet if - ars., clem., con., kali-br., lyc., sep., stram., tarent.
menses, during - con.

FEAR, phobias
people, of children, in - **BAR-C., LYC.**
fever, during - cupr.
perspiration, with - ***spong.***
physician, (see doctors)
piano, when at - ***kali-br., phos.***
pins, pointed, sharp things, of - alum., ***apis,*** ars., bov., lac-f., merc., nat-m., plat., ***sil., spig.***
hunts for pointed things, although affraid of them - sil.
pitied, of being - chin.
places, buildings - ***arg-n.,*** calc., kali-p., visc.
pneumonia, of - chel., phos.
poisoned, of being - agre., all-s., anac., apis, **ARS.,** ars-m., bapt., ***bell.,*** bry., cimic., glon., ***hyos.,*** ign., ***kali-bi., kali-br.,*** **LACH.,** nat-m., ph-ac., phos., plb., **RHUS-T.,** ***verat.,*** verat-v.
night - ars., ars-m.
has been - ars., euph., glon., lach.
police, of - anac., cann-i., cupr., lach., meli.
pollutions, after - aloe, carb-an.
position, to lose his lucrative - calc., ign., ***lyc.,*** puls., rhus-t., sep., staph., sulph., verat.
poverty - ambr., **ARS., BRY.,** ***calc., calc-f.,*** calc-s., calc-sil., chlor., kali-c., meli., nux-v., **PSOR.,** puls., ***sep.,*** sulph.
spending in order to not being short of money in future, fear of - ars., ***nux-v.,*** stann.
pregnancy, during - ***acon., ars., caul., cimic.,*** con., lyc., lyss., ***nux-m.,*** stann.
prolonged, fear, ailments after - ***carc.,*** lyc., op.
public, appearing in, of - anac., arg-n., ***carb-v.,*** **GELS.,** ***lyc.,*** plb., **SIL.**
places, of (see agoraphobia, crowd) - acon., ***arg-n., arn.,*** bar-c., ***calc.,*** crot-h., ferr., **GELS.,** glon., hydr., hydr-ac., ***kali-p.,*** levo., nux-v., puls., visc.
punished, of being - anac., ***carc.,*** lyc., ***staph.***
pursuit, of - hyos., lach.
putrefy, body will - bell., thuj.
rage, to fly into a - calc., chin., ***nux-v., staph.***
rags - calc., chin., **NUX-V.,** ***staph.***
railroad travel, of - ***arg-n.,*** bar-c., ferr., puls.
rain, of - elaps, naja.
rats - ***calc.,*** cimic.
recover, he will not - all-s., ant-t., ars., aur., carc., hep.
menopausal period, during - sars.
recurrent - arn., ars., carc., cham., cocc., nat-c., nat-m., **OP.,** phos., plat., sep., spong., sulph.
red, anything - ***alum.***
reproach, of - caps., carc., dig., ***staph.***
respiration, of - osm.
responsibility, of too much - calc., carc., lyc., sil.
restlessness, from fear - ***acon.,*** am-br., aml-n., **ARS.,** aur., ***ign., iod., merc.***

FEAR, phobias
riding in a carriage - acon., ***aur., bor.,*** bry., gins., ***lach., psor.,*** sanic., ***sep.***
closed carriage, in a - cimic., succ.
robbers, of - alum., anac., ***arg-n.,*** **ARS.,** aur., aur-s., bell., ***con.,*** elaps, ***ign.,*** kali-p., ***lach.,*** mag-c., mag-m., ***merc.,*** nat-c., **NAT-M.,** ***phos.,*** sanic., sil., sol-t-ae., sulph., verat., ***zinc.,*** zinc-p.
midnight, on waking - ***ign.,*** nat-m., sulph.
night - lach.
waking, on - merc., nat-m., sil.
room, on entering - alum., lyc., plat., til., ***valer.***
run over, of being, on going out - acon., arn., anth., hydr-ac., lyss., phos.
sadness, with - ***crot-h., kali-br.,*** **KALI-I.,** ***nat-m.,*** plat., ***plb.,*** rhus-t., vinc.
say, something wrong, lest he should - ***lil-t.,*** lyc.
headache, during - med.
scorpions, of - abel.
sea, of the - ***morbill.***
self-control, losing - **ARG-N.,** ***gels., ign.,*** med., ***nat-m., staph.***
sensation, of making - med.
senses, with exalted state of, smell, taste, touch - lyss.
serious, thoughts - crot-h., plat.
sex, impotence from fear during sex - ***lyc., sin-n.***
thought of, in a woman - ***kreos., staph.***
shadows, of - acon., calad., ***calc.,*** phos., staph.
his own - calad., ***calc.,*** lyc., staph.
shivering, from fear - **GELS.**
sighing, with - ip., ***rhus-t.***
sitting, amel. - iod.
sleep, before - acon., arg-n., calad., calc., carb-v., cob-n., gels., nat-c., ***rhus-t.,*** sars.
he will never again - ***ign.***
to close the eyes lest he should never wake - aeth., ang., hypoth.
sleep, to go to - bapt., calad., calc., calc-sil., camph., coff., ***hydr-ac., lach., led.,*** merc., nat-m., ***nux-m.,*** nux-v., ***rhus-t.,*** sabal., thea.
lest he die - nux-m.
something should happen - sabal.
smallpox, of - ***vac., vario.***
snakes, of - abel., bell., calc., cench., elaps, hep., **LAC-C.,** ***lach.,*** ruta, spig.
society, of losing his position in - ***lyc.,*** nux-v., sep., staph., verat.
softening, of the brain - abrot., ***asaf.***
sold, of being - ***hyos.***
solitude, of - ***ars.,*** ars-s-f., asaf., bell., bism., cadm-s., clem., elaps, gala., kali-c., lyc., plb., puls., ran-b., sep., tab.
speak, to - arg-m., sep.
speaking, in public - acon., arg-n., gels., ***lyc.,*** op.
speechless, with - acon., op.
spiders, of - abel., calc., nat-m.
spoken, to when - kali-br., sep.

FEAR, phobias
starting, with - bar-c., bell., calc-p., ***carc., hyos.,*** kali-br., nit-ac., ***op., phos., verat.***
starving, of - ars., ***bry.,*** calc., ***sep.,*** sulph.
stomach, arising from - adon., asaf., ***aur.,*** bry., ***calc.,*** calc-s., ***cann-s.,*** canth., ***dig.,*** euph., kali-ar., ***kali-c., lyc., mez., phos.,*** thuj.
ulcer, in - ign., sabad.
stool, of involuntary - sep.
stoppage of circulation, with sensation of - ***lyc.***
strangers, of - ambr., **BAR-C.,** bufo, ***carb-v., caust., cupr.,*** lach., ***lyc.,*** stram., ***thuj.***
strangled, to be - ars., **PLAT.**
streets, of busy - **ACON.,** carc., **PSOR.**
stroke, of having a - abel., ***alum.,*** apis, ***arg-m.,*** arg-n., arn., ***aster.,*** bell., brom., carb-v., cench., ***coff.,*** elaps, ***ferr.,*** ferr-p., ferr-t., fl-ac., glon., kali-ar., kali-br., lach., nat-c., phos., plat., ***puls.,*** sel., ***sep.,*** staph., ter., thuj., verat., ***zinc.***
evening in bed - ***puls.***
night, at, with feeling as if head would burst - ***aster.***
palpitation, with - arg-m., kali-ar.
stool, during - verat.
waking, on - arn., carb-v., glon.
struck, by those coming towards him, of being - **ARN.,** bell., ign., kali-c., lach., stram.
walking behind him, by those - alum.
subways, of - **ACON.**
suffering, of - achy., ***ars.,*** bry., calc., ***carc.,*** cor-r., cori-r., der., eup-per., hep., lil-t., merc-br., pip-m., spig.
suffocation, of - **ACON.,** acon-f., am-br., amyg., apis, arg-n., ***ars., bry.,*** carb-an., carb-v., ***dig., grin., kali-i.,*** **LACH.,** ***lob.,*** merc., naja, ***phos.,*** **PULS.,** rob., samb., ***spig., spong., staph., stram., sulph.***
closing eyes - carb-an.
eating amel. - ***graph.***
evening - ether.
goitre, in - ***merc-i-f.***
heart disease, in - ***dig., spong.***
lying, while - carb-an., mosch.
mucus in throat, from - carb-an.
night - agar., ***ant-t.,*** arn., ars., aur-m., cact., ***chin., dig., lyc.,*** med., ***puls.,*** sil., ***spong., sulph.***
paralysis of respiratory muscles, from - acon-f.
sleeps, if he - bapt.
walk about, must - am-br.
suicide, (see Suicidal) - ***alum.,*** arg-n., ***ars.,*** aur., aur-m., carc., ***merc.,*** **NAT-S.,** ***nux-v.,*** plat., ***rhus-t.,*** sep.
gun, with a - ***nat-s.***
knife, with a - merc.
superstitious - ***arg-n.,*** con., med., rhus-t., stram., zinc.
supper, after - caust.
surprises, from pleasant - ***coff.***
syphilis, of - ars., ***hyos., merc.***
talking loud, as if would kill her - meli.

FEAR, phobias
telephone, of - visc.
things, of real and unreal - cann-i.
thinking of disagreeable things, when - arg-n., phos.
sad things, when - rhus-t.
thoughts, of his own - anac., ***arg-n.,*** camph., thuj.
throat, from sensation of swelling of - ***glon.,*** lach., nat-m.
thunderstorm, of - bell., bor., ***bry., calc.,*** **CALC-P.,** carc., caust., ***coloc.,*** con., cycl., dig., dys-co., electr., ***gels., graph.,*** hep., lach., lyc., ***merc., nat-c., nat-m., nit-ac.,*** **PHOS.,** psor., ***rhod., sep.,*** sil., **STAPH.,** sulph.
torturing, of - ars-s-f.
touch, of - ***acon.,*** ang., **ANT-C.,** ant-t., apis, ***arn.,*** asar., ***bell.,*** calc-sil., **CHAM.,** ***chin.,*** cina, coff., ***colch.,*** con., cupr., ***hep.,*** ign., iod., kali-c., lach., lyc., mag-p., nit-ac., nux-m., ***nux-v.,*** ph-ac., phos., ***plb.,*** sanic., sep., sieg., ***spig.,*** stram., sulph., ***tarent., tell.,*** thuj.
chest wall, on - stroph-s.
others passing, by - acon.
sore parts - tell.
train, travel, of - bar-c., ferr., puls.
trains and closed places - succ.
tread lightly, must, or will injure himself - cupr.
trembling and chattering of teeth, with - elaps
tremulous - abrot., acon., ambr., ant-c., ars., ***aur.,*** bell., calc., carb-v., caust., ***cham.,*** cina, coff., cupr., **GELS.,** graph., iber., lach., ***mag-c.,*** mosch., ***nat-c.,*** nicc., **OP.,** phos., ***plat.,*** puls., ran-b., rat., rhus-t., sars., sep., ther.
trifles - ***ars.,*** bor., calc., ign., ***kali-c., lyc., nat-c., nat-m.***
troubles, of imaginary - ars., hydr-ac., kali-c., laur.
tuberculosis, of - ***calc.,*** kali-c., lac-c., paull., sep., tarent.
tunnels, of (see claustrophobia) - arg-n., bell., nat-m., **STRAM.**
no light in carriage, with, may cause fainting - stram.
unaccountable, vague - alco., ***ars.,*** phos., samb.
unconsciousness, of - alumn.
undertaking, anything - ***arg-n., ars., lyc.,*** sil.
new enterprise, a - ***lyc., sil.***
unlovable, of being - puls., staph.
upward, of being drawn - camph.
urinating, after - sulph.
urinating, in public - ambr., nat-m.
urine, from retention of - apis, ***op.***
involuntary loss of urine, fear of - pituin.
vehicles, approaching of - hydr-ac.
vertigo, of - arg-n., sumb.
vexation, after - ***ars.,*** cham., lyc., verat.
voice, of using - cann-i.

FEAR, phobias

waking, on - acon., ***agn.,*** alum., alum-p., alum-sil., am-c., ant-t., aster., ***bell.,*** bism., ***bor., bry.,*** bufo, ***cact., calc., caps.,*** carb-an., ***cham.,*** cina, cocc., con., cupr., hep., hyos., ign., iris, kali-br., kali-c., ***lac-c.,*** lach., lepi., ***lyc.,*** lyss., mag-s., ***med.,*** nat-c., ***nat-m.,*** nat-p., nat-sil., nit-ac., ***nux-v.,*** ph-ac., psor., ***puls.,*** rat., ***sil., spong., stram., sulph.,*** ter., **TUB.,** xan., zinc., zinc-p.

agg. - syph.

dream, from a - abrot., ***acon.,*** alum., bov., ***chin.,*** cina, frax., graph., ***lyc.,*** mag-m., **NUX-V.,** phos., ph-ac., sil., spong., sulph., tarent.

fear of something under the bed - bell.

walking, of - nat-m.

across busy street - ***acon.,*** crot-h., hydr-ac., plat.

dark, in the - ***carb-s.***

people behind him may hit him - alum.

walks till perspiration amel., from fear - camph.

walking, while - alum., anac., bar-c., cina, hep., ***lyc.,*** nux-v., staph.

air, in open - anac., cina, lyc.

rapidly - staph., tarent.

warm room, in - iod.

warm room, of - valer.

water, hydrophobia - acet-ac., **BELL.,** calc., cann-i., ***canth.,*** cupr., fagu., gels., **HYOS.,** iod., jatr., ***lach.,*** **LYSS.,** nux-v., perh., phel., ***phos.,*** plb., ruta, sabad., **STRAM.,** sulph., tarent.

running - ***lyss.,*** stram.

weary of life, and fear - aur-m., carc., kali-p., ***lyc., nit-ac., plat.,*** rhus-t.

wet his bed, fears he will - alum., lyc.

wind, of - ***cham.,*** thuj.

women, of - puls., raph., thuj.

work, dread of - ***arg-n.,*** aur-i., cadm-s., ***calc.,*** calc-sil., cham., chin., coloc., ***con.,*** graph., hyos., ind., iod., ***kali-c.,*** kali-p., kali-s., kali-sil., nat-m., nat-p., ***nux-v.,*** petr., phos., plb., ***puls.,*** ran-b., sanic., sel., ***sil., sulph.,*** tab., tarax., tong., zinc.

afternoon - ***arg-n.***

daily, of - calc-f., nux-v.

headache, during - gran.

literary, of - ***nux-v., sil.,*** sulph.

mental, of - calc-p., graph., nat-p., ***sil.***

persuaded to, cannot be - ***con.***

wrong, of something - ***kali-br.***

wounds, to see - alum., calc., ign.

FEARLESSNESS (see Courageous) - ***agar.,*** bell., cocaine, **OP.,** sil.

FECES, passed on the floor - cupr., sep., sil., sulph.

licks up cow-dung, mud, saliva - merc.

swallows his own - ***camph.,*** merc., verat., visc.

urinating and going to stool everywhere, children - ***sep.,*** sil., sulph.

FEIGNING, (see Pretending)

FIGHT, wants to - bell., bov., hipp., hyos., lach., merc., nux-v., sec.

FINANCIAL, loss of wealth or property, ailments from - ambr., **ARS., AUR.,** calc., ***calc-p.,*** carc., caust., ***con.,*** dig., ***ign.,*** kali-br., lach., lyc., ***psor.,*** staph.

FIRE, desire to be near to - naja.

flame of, seemed passing through him - phos.

thinks and talks of - ***calc.***

throws things into - staph.

wants to set things on fire - alco., ant-t., **BELL., HEP.,** hyos., phos., staph., stram.

FLATTERER - arn., carb-v., **LYC.,** nux-v., petr., plat., puls., sil., staph., sulph.

FLATTERY, desires - carb-v., lyc., ***pall.***

gives everything, when flattered - lyc., puls., sulph.

FLOATING, sensation of (see Vertigo) - ***asar.,*** calc., euon-a., jug-r., ***lac-c.,*** lact., mag-aust., passi., ph-ac., phos., phys., stict., stroph., ***tarent.,*** tell., thuj., valer., visc., xan.

FOOLISH, behavior - absin., acon., ether, agar., all-c., alum., ***anac.,*** anan., ant-c., ***apis,*** arg-n., arn., ***ars., bar-c., bar-m., bell.,*** bufo, calc., ***camph.,*** cann-i., cann-s., canth., carb-an., carb-v., ***carl., chin.,*** cic., cocc., cod., con., cot., croc., cupr., der., dulc., ferr., hell., **HYOS.,** ign., kali-c., lach., lact., ***lyc., merc.,*** mosch., ***nat-c.,*** nat-h., nux-m., nux-v., op., par., ph-ac., ***phos.,*** phys., ***plb.,*** pyrus, ***sec.,*** seneg., sep., **STRAM.,** tanac., ***tarent., verat.,*** verb.

air, in open - nux-m.

epilepsy, before - caust.

fever, during - acon.

grotesque behavior - cact., cori-r.

happiness and pride - **SULPH.**

morning, on waking - aur.

night - cic.

spasms, during - sec.

talking, boys, in - tab.

drunkenness, during - petr.

FORGETFUL, (see Memory)

FORGOTTEN, something, feels constantly as if he had - arg-n., calc., caust., cham., ***iod.,*** mill., phos., sil., ***tub.***

things, come to mind during sleep - calad., sel.

FORSAKEN, feelings (see Abandoned)

FRAGILE, sensation of being - ***thuj.***

frail, as if body were - gels., sil., ***thuj.***

FRIGHT, ailments from - **ACON.,** act-sp., agar., anac., ***apis,*** arg-m., **ARG-N.,** arn., ars., ***art-v., aur.,*** aur-m., ***bell.,*** bry., ***bufo, calc.,*** calc-sil., camph., carb-s., **CARC.,** ***caust.,*** cham., cimic., cina, cocc., ***coff.,*** crot-h., ***cupr.,*** **GELS.,** ***glon., graph., hyos.,*** hyosin., ***hyper.,*** **IGN.,** iod., ***kali-br.,*** kali-c., ***lach.,*** laur., **LYC.,** lyss., mag-c., merc., morph., nat-c., **NAT-M.,** nit-ac., nux-m., ***nux-v.,*** **OP.,** ***petr.,*** **PH-AC., PHOS.,** ***plat.,***

FRIGHT, ailments from - **PULS.,** ***rhus-t.,*** sabad., samb., sec., ***sep.,*** **SIL.,** stann., stram., sulph., verat., vib., visc., zinc., zinc-p.
accident, from sight of an - **ACON.,** gels., ign., **OP.**
anxiety, after fright - **ACON.,** ***carc., cupr.,*** gels., ***ign., kali-br.,*** lyc., merc., nat-m., ***op.,*** phos., rob., ***sil., verat.***
image of fright still remaining - **OP.**
seventh month of pregnancy, during - ***ign.***
children, in highly exitable, nervous - acon., ***arg-n.,*** **CARC.,** coff., gels., hyosin., **IGN.,** ***op.,*** phos.
fear of the fright still remains - **OP.**
headache, causes - **ACON.,** ***arg-n.,*** calc., ***chin-a., coff., cupr.,*** gels., hipp., hyos., **IGN.,** ***nux-v., op.,*** ph-ac., ***plat.,*** **PULS.,** samb.
image of the fright still remains - **OP.**
menses, during - ***acon.,*** bell., **IGN.,** ***lach.,*** nux-v., ***op.,*** ph-ac., phos., staph., verat.
severe - acon., ***carc., op.***
shock, in - hyper.
weakness, causes - coff., **GELS.,** merc., op.

FRIGHTENED, easily - abrot., ***acon.,*** ether, ail., alum., alum-sil., alumn., am-c., am-caust., am-m., ambr., ang., ant-c., ant-t., **ARG-N.,** ***arn.,*** **ARS.,** ars-h., ars-i., ***ars-s-f.,*** aur., aur-a., aur-s., **BAR-C.,** bar-m., bar-s., **BELL.,** benz-ac., berb., bism., **BOR.,** brom., ***bry.,*** bufo, cact., calad., ***calc.,*** calc-p., calc-s., ***calc-sil.,*** calen., cann-i., cann-s., canth., ***caps.,*** carb-ac., ***carb-an.,*** carb-s., ***carb-v., carc., caust.,*** cham., chel., chlor., cic., ***cit-ac.,*** clem., cob., cocc., coff., con., cupr., cupr-ac., cur., daph., ***dig.,*** ferr-i., glon., **GRAPH.,** guai., hep., hura, ***hyos.,*** hyper., iber., ***ign.,*** iod., iris, juni., kali-ar., kali-br., ***kali-c.,*** kali-i., ***kali-p.,*** kali-s., kali-sil., lac-c., ***lach.,*** led., lil-t., **LYC.,** mag-aust., ***mag-c.,*** mag-m., ***merc.,*** mez., morph., mosch., mur-ac., **NAT-A., NAT-C.,** ***nat-m.,*** nat-p., nat-s., ***nat-sil., nit-ac.,*** **NUX-V.,** ***op.,*** orig., ***petr.,*** ph-ac., **PHOS.,** plat., plb., psor., ptel., ***puls.,*** rhus-t., ***sabad., samb.,*** sarr., **SEP.,** ***sil.,*** spong., ***staph.,*** **STRAM.,** stront-c., stront-c., stry., ***sulph.,*** sul-ac., sumb., thea., ***ther.,*** verat., xan., zinc.
blood, at sight of - ***alum.***
chill, during - verat.
crying amel. - phos.
delusions, from - bell., **STRAM.**
evening - carb-an., iber., merc., ol-an., sulph.
eyes, on closing - op.
falling asleep, on - ***aur., nit-ac.,*** nux-v., phos.
fever, during - sabad., verat.
menses, during - acon., bell., **IGN.,** lach., nux-v., op., ph-ac., phos., staph., verat.
menses, before - ***calc.***
night - cast., cimic., crot-c., ***ign., lyc., nat-m., phos.,*** samb., sang., sep., ***spong.,*** thea.
on waking - ***euphr., sep.***
on waking, 3 a.m. - **ARS.,** cham., con.
nocturnal emissions, after - aloe.
noon - zinc.

FRIGHTENED, easily
noon, nap, after - bar-s., ***calc-sil.,*** nat-c., nit-ac.
pains, from - ars., sulph.
pollutions, after - aloe..
roused, when - ***calc.,*** nat-a.
shadow, his own - calad.
sneezing, at - ***bor.***
touch, from - ***kali-c.,*** ruta.
trifles, at - am-c., am-m., ang., ant-t., arn., bar-c., bor., bufo, calc., calen., caust., hyper., kali-ar., **KALI-C.,** kali-i., kali-s., kiss., ***lach., lyc.,*** merc., mez., ***nit-ac.,*** nux-v., ***phos.,*** rhus-t., sep., sumb.
trifles, at, day before menses - calc.
urinating, before - alum.
waking, on - ***am-m., ambr.,*** ant-c., ***ars., bell.,*** bism., bor., ***cact., calc., caps., cham., chlol., cina, cocc.,*** dig., ***euphr.,*** eupi., ***graph.,*** hep., ***hyos.,*** ign., ***kali-c., lach.,*** led., lyc., ***med.,*** mit., ***nat-m.,*** nit-ac., nux-v., op., sil., sol-n., spong., stram., sul-i., sulph., tub., verat., zinc.
dream, from a - abrot.,acon., casc., chin., con., dicha., ***erig.,*** graph., ***ign.,*** **LYC.,** mag-m., ***meph., sulph.,*** tarent.
in a fright from least noise - nux-v.
terrified, knows no one, screams, clings to those near - ***stram.***

FRIVOLOUS, behaviour - agar., apis, ***arn.,*** bar-c., bell., calad., con., lach., **MERC.,** par., ***puls.,*** sil., spong., sulph.

FROWN, disposed to - cham., equis., hell., hyos., lyc., mang., **NUX-V.,** plb., rheum, rumx., sep., stram., sulph., verat.

FUR, behaviour, wraps up in, summer - hep., hyos., merc., ***psor.***

GAMBLING, passion for - ars., bell., calc., caust., chin., ***lyc.,*** merc., ***nux-v.,*** sulph., verat.

GESTURES, makes - anac., ars., asc-c., ***bell.,*** bufo, camph., calc., cann-i., carc., chin-s., cic., ***cocc.,*** **HYOS.,** kres., mosch., nux-m., nux-v., plat., plb., puls., sep., sil., ***stram., tarent.,*** verat., zinc.
actions, repeated - chen-a.
actor, like an - hyos.
angry, in night walking - meph.
automatic - anac., calc., cann-i., hell., hyos., nux-m., phos., tab., zinc.
sleep, during - phos.
awkward, in - caps., nat-c., nat-m., nux-v., sil., sulph.
breaks things, pins - **BELL.,** calc.
sticks - ***bell.,*** calc.
brushing the face or something away, as if - hyos.
cautious - pip-m.
childish - anac.
clapping the hands - ***bell.,*** cic., ***stram.,*** verat.
overhead - sec.
collar, pulls at - ant-c., **LACH.**

GESTURES, makes
confused - ***acon.,*** sil.
convulsive - acon., ether, alco., ant-t., apis, ars., bell., camph., cann-s., canth., cori-m., hydr-ac., ign., iod., kali-bi., merc., morph., nux-v., op., petr., plb., pyrus, sec., sol-n.
drink, at sight of - bell.
sleep, during - aeth.
thinking of motion, when - aur.
covers mouth with hands - ip., kali-bi., lach., ***rumx.***
crossing the hands - mosch.
decided - fl-ac.
drinking, as if - bell.
enthusiastic - nitro-o.
evening on falling asleep - sil.
extravagant - stram.
frightful - ***hep.,*** hyos.
furious - cann-i., ***hep.,*** sep.
grasping or reaching at something - agar., arn., ars., arum-t., atro., ***bell., bor.,*** bufo, calc-p., ***cham.,*** chin., cina, cocc., colch., con., dub., dulc., hell., **HYOS.,** hyosin., ***iod., lyc.,*** mosch., mur-ac., oena., op., paeon., phos., ***ph-ac.,*** plat., ***psor.,*** rhus-t., ***sol-n.,*** **STRAM.,** sulph., tarent., verat., ***zinc.,*** zinc-m., zinc-p.
bystanders, at - **ANT-T.,** ars., bell., phos.
noses - merc.
chewing and swallowing - ***sol-n.***
children put, everything in the mouth - ***calc.,*** merc., ***sulph.***
fingers in the mouth - ***calc., cham.,*** **IP.,** kali-p., lyc., nat-m., sil., tarent.
evening on falling asleep - sil.
genitals - ***acon.,*** bell., bufo, canth., ***hyos., merc., stram.,*** ust., zinc.
cough, during - zinc.
fever, during - hyos.
spasms, during - sec., stram.
mother, in sleep, at - **BOR.**
night - atro., sol-n.
nose, lips, at - ***arum-t., cina***
objects, at real or imaginary - dat-m.
picks at bedclothes - acon., agar., ant-c., ***arn., ars.,*** ars-s-f., art-v., atro., arum-t., ***bell.,*** cham., chin., cina, cocc., ***colch.,*** con., dulc., ***hell.,*** hep., **HYOS.,** ***iod., kali-br., lyc., mur-ac., nat-m., op., ph-ac., phos., psor., rhus-t.,*** sol-n., **STRAM.,** sulph., tarent., verat-v., ***zinc.,*** zinc-m., zinc-p.
dreams, during - op.
lips, and - hell.
quickly - ***stram.***
rest, during - alco.
sides of the bed, at - nux-v.
sleep, during - ***op.,*** phos.
spot, one - ars., ***arum-t.,*** cham., con., kali-br., lach., tarent., thuj.
bleeds, until - arg-m., arum-m., cina, con., phos.
sore, until - arum-t., ph-ac., zinc.
wrong things, at - lyss.

GESTURES, makes
involuntary, motions of the hands - alumn., ars., bell., cann-i., caust., cic., coca, fl-ac., ***hyos.,*** kali-br., merc., mosch., nat-m., ***phos.,*** puls., sang., sil., stram., sulph., tab., verat.
face, to the - stry.
folding - puls.
folding, unfolding coverings, and - plb.
hands, rubbing together - cann-i.
hasty - bell.
head, to the - phos., plb., ***stram.,*** verat.
sleep, during - ***ars.***
knitting, as if - tarent.
lifting up - ars.
sleep, during - op., phos.
spinning and weaving - hyos., sars., ***stram.***
throwing about - atro., bell., bry., canth., carb-an., mosch., nat-c., phos., sil., stram.
throwing about, over head - ars., bell., hydr-ac., mosch., stram.
waving in the air - bry., op., stram.
wild - acon., camph.
winding a ball, as if - agar., stram.
impatient - coca.
indicates his desires by - ***stram.***
intoxicated, as if - **HYOS.**
labored - coni.
light - chin., clem., coff., phel., wies.
lively - alco., ped.
nervous - phys., tarent.
nuts, as if opening - hyos.
perseverance, with great - anac.
plays with, buttons of his clothes, with the - mosch.
counting money, as if - calc., nux-v., staph.
fingers - asar., bell., calc., con., crot-c., ***hyos.,*** kali-br., lach., rhus-t., tarent., ther.
pouring from hand to hand, as if - bell.
pulls, hair of bystanders - bell.
nose of strangers - merc.
ridiculous or foolish - arg-n., ***bell.,*** cic., croc., ***cupr.,*** **HYOS.,** ign., kali-p., ***lach.,*** merc., ***mosch., nux-m.,*** nux-v., op., ***sep., stram., tarent.,*** verat.
open air, in - nux-m.
standing on the street, while - ***nux-m.***
scratching, thighs - sars.
walls - arn., canth.
shy - arg-n.
slow - chin-s., coni., **PHOS.,** plb., verat.
spinning, around on the foot - cann-s.
imitates - hyos., ***stram.***
stamps the feet - ant-c., ant-t., dulc., hyos., ***stram.,*** **VERAT.**
children during sleep - ***ign.***
strange attitude and position - agar., agar-ph., camph., caust., ***cina,*** cocc., ***coloc.,*** gamb., hyos., lyc., merc., ***nux-m.,*** nux-v., op., ***plb.,*** rheum, sep., stram., sulph., zinc.
arms, of - hyos., sep., stram.
gait, in - nux-v., sep.
head, of - agar., sulph.

GESTURES, makes

sublime - hyos., nitro-o.

talking, gesticulates while - nux-v., sep.

head, with - lyc., puls., sulph.

tapping, on head with one's finger - carc.

uncertain - acon., ***phos.,*** sil., verat.

violent - agar., ***bell., camph.,*** cic-m., ***hep., hyos.,*** kali-br., plb., ***stram.***

vocation, of his usual - ars., bell., plb., stram.

wild - camph.

wringing the hands - ars., asar., aur., kali-br., ***kali-p., phos.,*** plat., ***psor.,*** puls., ***stram., sulph.,*** **SYPH.,** ***tarent.***

GIGGLING - bufo, ***cann-i.,*** hyos., nat-m.

GLOOMY, morose - abies-c., abrot., acet-ac., ***acon.,*** adon., ***aesc.,*** aeth., ***agar.,*** agn., alco., alf., aloe, alum., alum-sil., ***am-c.,*** am-m., ambr., **ANAC.,** ang., **ANT-C.,** ***ant-t.,*** anthro., apis, ***aran.,*** arg-m., arg-n., ***arn., ars.,*** ars-s-r., ***art-v., asaf., asar.,*** asc-t., aspar., aster., **AUR.,** aur-s., bar-ac., bar-c., bell., berb., ***bism.,*** bond., ***bor., bov.,*** brom., **BRY.,** bufo, cact., **CALC.,** calc-ac., calc-br., ***calc-p.,*** calc-s., calc-sil., calen., cann-s., canth., ***caps.,*** carb-ac., carb-an., ***carb-s.,*** carb-v., card-b., carl., cast., ***caul.,*** caust., **CHAM.,** chel., chin., chin-s., chlol., chlor., cic., cimic., cina, cinnb., clem., coc-c., cocc., ***coff., colch., coloc., con.,*** cop., cor-r., ***corn., croc., crot-h., crot-t.,*** cupr., ***cycl.,*** dam., daph., des-ac., dicha., ***dig.,*** digin., dios., dirc., dros., dulc., elae., elaps, euon., euph-a., euphr., fel., ferr., ferr-ma., ferr-p., fl-ac., form., franz., gamb., gent-l., ***gran., graph., grat.,*** guai., ham., hell., helon., ***hep.,*** hera., hipp., hydr., ***hyos.,*** iber., ign., indol., ***ip.,*** iris, jatr., jug-r., kali-ar., ***kali-c.,*** kali-chl., kali-i., kali-n., ***kali-p.,*** kalm., kiss., kreos., lac-c., lachn., ***laur., led.,*** lipp., ***lyc.,*** lycpr., lyss., mag-arct., ***mag-aust., mag-c., mag-m.,*** manc., mang., med., meph., ***merc., merl., mez.,*** mosch., ***mur-ac.,*** myric., naja, ***nat-c., nat-m., nat-s.,*** nicc., ***nit-ac.,*** nit-s-d., nux-m., **NUX-V.,** ol-an., ***olnd., op.,*** opun-v., orig., osm., paeon., ***pall.,*** palo., par., ***petr., ph-ac., phel., phos.,*** pic-ac., ***plan., plat., plb.,*** plect., ***prun., psor.,*** **PULS.,** rad., ran-b., ran-s., rat., rheum, rhod., **RHUS-T.,** rhus-v., ruta, sabad., sabin., sac-alb., ***samb., sang.,*** sanic., sapin., sars., sel., ***sep.,*** serp., **SIL.,** sin-n., sol-t-ae., spig., spira., ***spong.,*** squil., stann., ***staph., stram., stront-c., stry.,*** sul-ac., sulfon., ***sulph.,*** sumb., ***syph.,*** tab., tarax., tep., teucr., thea., thuj., thymol., til., tub., upa., uran-n., ust., uva., vac., valer., ***verat.,*** verat-v., verb., vinc., viol-o., viol-t., vinc., vip., visc., wies., ***zinc., zinc-oc.,*** zinc-p.

afternoon - alum., aeth., anac., ant-c., bor., bov., cann-s., canth., chel., cinnb., colch., con., elaps, hydr-ac., kali-c., laur., mag-s., mang., merc-c., mur-ac., nat-c., nat-m., nit-ac., op., ox-ac., puls., ruta, sang., sars., zinc.

5 p.m. to 7 p.m. - ***con.***

amel. - mag-c.

siesta, after - brom., cycl.

twilight, in - am-m., ***phos.***

GLOOMY, morose

air, in open - ***aeth.,*** bor., ***con.,*** mur-ac., plat., rhus-t.

amel. - asar., calc., coff., stann.

alternating with

cheerfulness - ant-t., ars., aur., bor., bov., calc-p., ***chin.,*** chin-b., cortiso., cycl., eug., kali-c., kali-chl., mag-m., merc-c., nat-m., oena., ol-an.

crying - bell.

exuberance - ant-t.

laughing - bor., croc.

singing - croc.

tenderness - plat.

business does not proceed fast, when - ip.

caressing agg. - chin.

causeless - aloe, chel., cycl., ***nat-m.***

children, in - ***ant-c., ant-t.,*** ars., bor., calc., **CARC., CHAM.,** ***cina,*** graph., hep., psor., ***puls.,*** rheum, sac-alb., sil.

carried, desire to be - benz-ac., cham.

cry, when touched - **ANT-C.**

daytime - ***cina***

morning early - **STAPH.**

spoken to, when - ***nat-m.***

chill, during - anac., ars., calen., caps., caust., hep., ign., kreos., mag-aust., mez., nat-m., plat., puls.

cloudy weather, from - aloe, am-c.

coffee, after - calc-p.

contradiction, by - ign., tarent., ***verat.***

conversation amel. - lyss.

convulsions, before - zinc., zinc-valer.

cough, before fits of - ant-t., asaf., bell.

whooping cough, in - ***bry.,*** cupr-ac.

daytime - ***cham., cina,*** ip., iris, kreos., lyc., ***med.,*** merc., ***merc-c.,*** nat-m., phel., phos., plat., staph., sul-ac., sulph., viol-t.

dentition, in - **CHAM.**

dreams, by - op.

drunkenness, during - caust., hydr., lach., nux-v.

ear lobes, with hot - ***alum.***

eating, after - am-c., arn., ***bor.,*** bov., bry., calad., carb-v., cham., ferr-ac., ***graph.,*** iod., kali-c., merc., ***merc-cy.,*** merc-sul., nat-c., nux-v., ol-an., phos., puls., thuj.

evening - aloe, am-c., bar-c., bov., calc., cast., con., cycl., dios., fago., form., hep., ign., indg., kali-c., lyc., lyss., mag-aust., mag-c., mag-m., mur-ac., nat-c., nat-m., ox-ac., pall., phos., puls., spig., **SULPH.,** zinc.

amel. - euph-a., puls.

and next forenoon - kalm.

bed, in - chin., rhus-t., upa.

fever, during - ***acon., aran.,*** asar., bor., cic., ***ferr.,*** ip., lyc., mag-aust., mosch., petr., ***sulph.***

after - am-c., card-b., hipp.

fly in wall, by - sars.

GLOOMY, morose
forenoon - am-c., am-m., ant-t., caust., colch., con., des-ac., hipp., ***mag-c., mang., nat-m.,*** nat-p., nicc., phos., sars., seneg., sil., verat.
1 a.m. to 1 p.m. - kreos.
forgetfulness, from - ***anac.***
heat, in head, with - aeth.
house, agg in, amel. on walking in open air - calc., mag-c., **RHUS-T.**
hurry, with - carc., thuj.
hypochondriasis, in - carc., grat., ***mosch.,*** **PULS.**
interruption, from - cham.
laughing, followed by loud - stram.
menopausal period, at - ***psor.***
menses, during - am-c., cas-s., cast., ***cham.,*** ferr., ind., lyc., mag-c., plat., tarent.
after - bufo, ferr.
before - ***cham., lyc., nux-v.***
suppressed, in - cycl.
morning - am-c., am-m., ant-t., ***ars.,*** bov., brucin., bry., calc., calc-ac., canth., cast., chin., chlor., coff., con., hep., hipp., kalm., kreos., ***lach., lyc.,*** lyss., mag-c., mag-m., mang., merc-i-r., ***nat-m.,*** nat-s., nit-ac., ***nux-v.,*** ph-ac., phos., plat., sars., sep., **STAPH.,** sul-ac., sulph., tarax., zinc.
bed, in - ***ars.,*** bell., bry., cast., kali-c., ***lyc.,*** mez., nit-ac., nux-v., petr., ph-ac., plat., puls., rhus-t., thuj.
waking, on - agar., bell., carb-an., coca, kali-ar., **LYC.,** merc-i-r., nat-m., nit-ac., sul-ac., thuj.
music, during sad - ***mang.***
amel. - mang.
night - anac., ant-t., bor., camph., cham., chin., ***jal.,*** lyc., lyss., mag-arct., nux-v., phos., ***psor.,*** rheum, **RHUS-T.,** sabad.
noon - zinc.
nosebleed, amel. - kali-chl.
oneself, with - ars., aur.
pain, after - **CHAM.,** crot-t., hep., ign.
perspiration, during - mag-c.
pollutions, after - ***dig.,*** nat-c., ***thuj.***
puberty, in - ***cina,*** ph-ac.
questioned, when - nat-m.
rainy weather, from - am-c.
repentance, followed by - vinc.
sex, after - ang., calc., nat-c., ***nat-m.,*** petr., ***sel.,*** sil.
sleep, in - anac., nux-v., rhus-t.
amel. - caps.
sleepiness, with - calc., calen., carb-an., hyos., kali-c., ol-an., ph-ac., sabad., sep.
stool, before - ***bor.,*** calc.
storm, during - am-c.
talk, indisposed to - ***chin., stann.,*** viol-t.
talking of others, on - zinc.
thinking of his ailments, when alone, on - **AUR-M.**
thunderstorm, from - am-c.

GLOOMY, morose
trifles, about - aspar., ***bell.,*** carb-v., **CHAM.,** chel., con., ***cycl.,*** hep., lyc., meph., merc-i-r., ***ptel.,*** sil.
twilight, in - ***phos.***
waking, on - anac., ant-t., ***ars.,*** bell., bor., bry., calc., cass., caust., cham., chel., ***cina,*** cycl., ign., kali-c., **LYC.,** lyss., mag-aust., mez., nit-ac., nux-v., petr., ph-ac., phos., plat., plb., rhus-t., sabad., sep., tarent., thuj.
walking in open air, after - puls.
weather, from bad - am-c.
women, in - calc., nat-m., nux-v., plat., sil.
work, with inclination to - sars.
worm affection, in - ***carb-v.,*** **CINA,** ***fil.***

GLUTTONY - all-s., ant-c., ***calc.,*** caust., ***chin.,*** cina, ***merc.,*** op.

GODLESS, want of religious feeling - ***anac.,*** calc., coloc., croc., **LACH.,** ***lyc.,*** merc., plat., sil., ***sulph.***

GOING out, aversion to - acon., am-c., anth., clem., ***cycl.,*** hydr., lyc.

GOSSIPING - ars., calc., caust., hyos., lach., par., stram., verat.v

GOURMAND - calc., chin., ip., mag-c., merc., nat-c., **VERAT.**

GREEDY, avarice - alum., **ARS.,** bry., calc., calc-f., carb-an., carb-v., caust., ***chin.,*** cina, coloc., con., graph., hep., ***hyos.,*** lach., ***lyc.,*** med., meli., nat-c., nat-m., nit-ac., ***nux-v.,*** petr., ***ph-ac.,*** plat., **PULS.,** rheum, ***sep.,*** **SIL.,** staph., sulph.
alternating with squandering - calc., lach., merc., sulph.
anxiety about future, from - ***nux-v., ph-ac.,*** staph.
cupidity, grasping greedily with both hands anything offered to him - ***hyos.***
generosity towards strangers, as regards his family - carb-v., hyos., nat-m., nux-v.
squandering on oneself, but - calc., hyos., nux-v., sep.

GRIEF, ailments from - alum-p., am-m., ***ambr.,*** anac., ***ant-c., apis, arn., ars.,*** art-v., **AUR.,** aur-a., aur-m., aur-s., ***bell., bry.,*** cael., ***calc., calc-p.,*** caps., **CARC., CAUST.,** clem., **COCC.,** colch., ***coloc.,*** con., ***crat.,*** cycl., cypr., dig., ***dros., gels., graph., hura, hyos.,*** **IGN.,** ip., kali-br., kali-c., kali-p., **LACH.,** lob-c., lob-s., lyc., mag-c., nat-c., **NAT-M.,** nat-s., naja, nit-ac., **NUX-V.,** ***op.,*** **PH-AC., PHOS.,** phys., pic-ac., ***plat., puls., samb., sol-o.,*** spig., **STAPH.,** tarent., tub., ***uran-n.,*** verat., ***zinc.***
death of, loved ones or friends - calc., **CARC., CAUST.,** gels., **IGN.,** ***kali-br.,*** lach., **NAT-M.,** nux-v., ph-ac., plat., staph., sulph.
nursing loved ones with prolonged illness, after - ***carc.,*** cocc.
recent - **IGN.,** ***nat-m.***
afternoon - ***tarent.***
business, morning, when thinking of - ***puls.***
complaining, with - caust., ign.

GRIEF, general
condition, about his - ***aur.,*** staph.
constant and chronic - ***graph., nat-m.***
cry, cannot after grief - aeth., am-m., apis, ***carc.,*** crot-c., ***gels.,*** ign., kali-fer., **NAT-M.,** nux-v., op., puls.
day and night - caust.
daytime - staph.
delusions, from - ***zinc.***
devasting, grief - aur., carc.
evening - ***graph.***
amel. - nux-v., staph.
fear, at night, with - ***merc.***
feelings of grief - acet-ac., acon., agar., ail., alum., am-c., am-m., ***ambr.,*** anac., ant-c., arn., ***ars.,*** **AUR.,** aur-a., bar-c., benz-ac., bov., cael., calc., calc-p., caps., carb-an., card-m., ***carc.,*** **CAUST.,** chin., ***cic., cimic.,*** cocc., coff., ***coloc.,*** con., croc., cycl., dig., dros., ***graph., hell.,*** hyos., ***iber.,*** **IGN.,** kali-bi., kali-br., ***lach.,*** lact., laur., ***lyc.,*** mag-m., meny., ***merc.,*** mez., ***mur-ac.,*** nat-c., **NAT-M.,** nit-ac., ***nux-v., op., ph-ac.,*** phos., plat., **PULS.,** ran-s., rhus-t., ***sep.,*** sil., **STAPH.,** stram., stront-c., sul-ac., ***sulph.,*** tarent., tub., verat.
fits, of grief - asaf., ign.
future, for the - aur., mang., nat-c., ***nat-m.,*** stann.
headache, from - ***aur., calc.,*** **IGN., NAT-M.,** op., ***ph-ac., phos., puls.,*** **STAPH.**
heart, problems, with - aur., dig., lach., ***nat-m.***
hunting, for something to grieve one - lil-t.
losing, objects, after - **IGN.**
morning - alum., nux-v., phos., puls.
night, in bed - graph., ph-ac.
offenses, from long past - calc., caust., ***cham., ign.,*** lach., **NAT-M.,** ***op., staph.***
past events, about - caust., **NAT-M.,** ***plat.***
silent - am-m., ***carc., coff.,*** cycl., ***gels.,*** **IGN.,** ip., kali-fer., lyc., **NAT-M.,** ***ph-ac., puls.,*** sal-ac., staph.
indignation, with - ***carc., coloc., staph.***
submissiveness, with - **PULS.,** ***staph.***
stomach trouble, causing - **ANT-C.,** ign., ***nat-c.,*** nux-v.
trifles, over - ars., bar-c.
undemonstrative - ***carc.,*** cycl., ***ign.,*** **NAT-M.**
undermining, the constitution - ph-ac., ***phos.***
waking, on - alum., ***lac-c., lach.,*** ph-ac.
weakness, causes - **CARC.,** ***caust., ign.,*** nat-m., **PH-AC.,** ***pic-ac.***

GRIMACES, makes - agar., bell., carc., cina, ***cupr.,*** gels., hell., hyos., ign., olnd., nux-m., pall., plat., ***stram.,*** verat-v.
convulsions, before - absin.
strange faces, makes - ars., merc., pall.

GROPING, as if in the dark - croc., hyos., op., plb.

GROWLING, like a dog - alum., ***bell.,*** hell., lyc., lyss., mag-m., phos., ***stram.***
sleep, in - lyc.

GRUNTING - bell., cina, hell., ign., puls.
sleep, during - ign.

GUILT, feelings - achy., **ALUM.,** alum-p., alum-sil., ***am-c.,*** anac., arn., **ARS.,** ***ars-s-f.,*** atro., **AUR.,** aur-a., aur-s., bry., cact., calc., canth., carb-an., carb-s., ***carb-v.,*** **CARC.,** ***caust.,*** cham., **CHEL.,** chin., cina, ***cocc., coff., con.,*** cupr., cycl., **DIG.,** ***ferr.,*** ferr-ar., ferr-p., ***graph.,*** hell., hip-ac., ***hyos., ign., kali-bi., lach., mag-arct.,*** mag-aust., mag-c., mag-s., ***med., merc.,*** **NAT-M.,** nit-ac., ***nux-v., ph-ac.,*** phos., ***plat.,*** **PSOR.,** ***puls.,*** rheum, ***rhus-t.,*** ruta, sabad., sarr., ***sil., spig.,*** spira., **STAPH.,** ***stram.,*** stront-c., **SULPH.,** ***thuj., verat., zinc.,*** zinc-oc.
afternoon - ***am-c.***
dreams, in - lach., lem-m., nat-m.
evening - caust.
dinner, and after - ***verat.***
grief, with - carc., ign., ***nat-m.***
no rest night or day, prevents lying down - ***phos.***

HATRED, feelings (see Malicious)- acon., ***agar.,*** aloe, am-c., am-m., **ANAC.,** ***aur., calc., cham.,*** **CIC.,** cupr., kali-c., kali-i., ***lac-c.,*** **LACH.,** ***led.,*** lyc., mang., **NAT-M.,** ***nit-ac.,*** **NUX-V.,** ph-ac., phos., puls., rhus-t., stann., stram., sulph., tarent.
absent persons, of, better on seeing them - fl-ac.
bitter feelings for slight offences, has - ang.
children, of - anac., ***lyc., nux-v.,*** **PLAT.,** ***sep.***
men, of - bar-c., ign., led., lyc., phos., stann.
persons, of, who had offended him - ***aur.,*** calc., mang., ***merc., nat-m.,*** nit-ac., nux-v., sep., staph., sulph.
unmoved by apologies - **NIT-AC.**
persons, of, who do not agree with him - anac., calc-s.
revenge, hatred and - agar., aloe, am-c., am-m., **ANAC.,** aur., calc., cic., fl-ac., hep., hydr., **LACH.,** led., mang., mygal., **NAT-M.,** ***nit-ac., ph-ac.***
women, of - ***puls., raph.***

HEEDLESS - abies-c., agar., ail., agn., alco., ***alum.,*** alum-p., ambr., am-c., am-m., ***anac.,*** apis, arn., asaf., aur., aur-m., ***bar-c., bell.,*** bov., buf-s., calad., camph., cann-s., canth., carl., ***caust., cham.,*** cic., clem., coff., ***con.,*** cortico., croc., cupr., daph., euon., ***gels.,*** guai., ham., ***hell.,*** hep., ***hyos.,*** ign., ind., kali-c., kali-sil., kreos., ***lach.,*** laur., ***lyc.,*** mag-arct., ***merc.,*** mez., nat-c., ***nat-m.,*** nat-p., nit-ac., ***nux-m.,*** nux-v., ***op., olnd.,*** ped., ph-ac., ***phos.,*** plat., puls., rhod., rhus-t., rib-ac., ruta, sep., sil., spig., staph., stram., sulph., tarax., thuj., tub., valer., verat., zinc., zinc-p.
business, about - myris.
morning, on waking - cot.
talking and writing, in - carl.

HEIGHTS, high, places, agg. - ***arg-n., aur.,*** gels., puls., staph., ***sulph.***

HELD on to, desires to be - **ARS.,** ***gels.,*** kali-p., lach., ***nux-m., nux-v., phos.,*** **PULS.,** ***sang., sep., stram.***

HELPLESSNESS, feeling of - anac., arg-n., **ARS.,** ***calad.,*** ether, hell., jasm., kali-br., **LYC.,** petr., phos., **PULS.,** stram., tax.
afternoon - kali-br.
night - ***lith.***

HIDE, desire to - ars., ***bar-c.,*** **BELL.,** camph., chlol., ***chlor.,*** cupr., eug., ***hell.,*** hyos., ***ign.,*** lach., ***puls.,*** **STAPH.,** ***stram.,*** tarent.
child thinks all visitors laugh at it and hides behind furniture - ***bar-c.***
children, desire to - aur.
run away, and - meli.
strangers, from - bar-c.
fear, on account of - ***ars., bell.,*** cupr.
fear, on account of, assaulted, of being - tarent.
things - bell.

HIDES, true feelings - aur., carc., nat-m., staph.

HIGH-spirited - ***carc.,*** hydr., hyos., ***med.,*** op., spig., spong., ***tub.,*** verat., verb.

HOLDING or being held, amel. - ***ars., bry.,*** carb-an., diph., dros., eup-per., ***gels.,*** glon., ***lach.,*** lil-t., murx., nat-s., ***nux-m., nux-v.,*** phos., **PULS.,** rhus-t., sang., ***sep.,*** sil., ***stram.,*** sul-ac., sulph.
anything, agg. - caust.
attendant, to - ant-t.
constantly mother's hand - bar-c., ***bism., phos.,*** puls.

HOME, desires to, go - acon., ars., bell., **BRY.,** ***calc.,*** calc-p., cic., chlol., cimic., coff., cupr., ***cupr-ac.,*** hyos., ***lach.,*** meli., ***op.,*** plan., rhus-t., valer., verat., vip.
elderly, people - cic.
go out, and when there to - **CALC-P.,** ***cupr-ac.***
leave - arag., ***bry.,*** elat., lach., merc.
talks of - bell., ***bry.***

HOMESICKNESS, nostalgia - acon., ***aur., bell.,*** **BRY.,** calc-p., **CAPS., CARB-AN.,** carl., ***caust.,*** cent., chlor., cimic., ***clem., cocc., coff., crat.,*** dros., elaps, elat., eup-per., eup-pur., ***hell.,*** hipp., hyos., **IGN.,** iris-t., ***kali-p.,*** lach., lipp., mag-c., **MAG-M.,** manc., meli., **MERC.,** ***nat-m., nit-ac.,*** op., petr., **PH-AC.,** ***phos.,*** plan., plb., puls., puls-n, sac-l., sac-alb., senec., sep., ***sil., staph.,*** valer., verat.
ailments, from - ***caps., clem.,*** eup-pur., hell., ***ign.,*** mag-m., **PH-AC.,** senec.
evening - hep.
heat in throat, with - **CAPS.**
house, even when in her own - eup-pur.
morning - carb-an.
red cheeks, with - ***caps.***
silent ill humor, with - nit-ac., ***ph-ac.***

HOMOSEXUALITY, (See Sexual, behaviour)

HONOR, effects of wounded, (See Humiliation) - carc., cham., ign., ***lyc.,*** nat-m., nux-v., **STAPH.,** verat.
no sense of honor - anac., ars., hyos., lach., verat.

HOPEFUL, feelings - acon., aur., calc., ferr-ma., hydr., ***ign.,*** nat-m., op., sang., seneg., sulph., ***tub.,*** verat.
alternating with, despair - acon., kali-c.
sadness - acon., kali-c., raph.
lung, disease in - aur.
recovery, of - sang.

HORRIBLE things, sad stories, affect her profoundly - ars., ***aur., aur-m.,*** **CALC.,** calc-s., carb-v., **CARC.,** ***caust.,*** chin., **CIC.,** cocc., con., ferr., gels., ***hep.,*** ign., **IOD.,** ***lach., lyc.,*** manc., nat-c., nat-m., ***nit-ac., nux-v.,*** **PHOS.,** prot., ***puls., sep., sil.,*** **STAPH.,** ***sulph., teucr., zinc.***

HOUSE, aversion to being kept in - lyc.
agg. - bry., lyc., mag-m., ***puls.,*** rhus-t., til.
amel. - agar., cycl., ign.

HOWLING, behaviour - **ACON.,** ***alum.,*** arn., ars., ***aur., bell.,*** brom., calad., camph., caps., ***cham., cic.,*** cina, coff., cupr., ign., ip., lyc., merc., nat-m., nux-v., op., ***phos.,*** stann., **STRAM.,** verat., ***verat-v.,*** verb., viol-t.
all night - ***verat.***
anger, with - arn.

HUMILIATION, ailments from (see Abused) - ***acon.,*** alum., am-m., **ANAC.,** ***arg-n.,*** ars., ***aur., aur-m.,*** bell., ***bry.,*** calc., calc-s., **CARC.,** cas-s., caust., ***cham.,*** **COLOC.,** con., form., gels., grat., **IGN.,** ***lach.,*** **LYC.,** ***lyss.,*** merc., **NAT-M.,** ***nux-v., op.,*** **PALL.,** petr., **PH-AC.,** plat., ***puls.,*** rhus-t., ***seneg.,*** sep., sil., **STAPH.,** stram., ***sulph.,*** verat., zinc.
anger, with - ***carc.,*** **COLOC.,** ***staph.***
indignation, with - **IGN., STAPH.**
punishment, from - anac., ***carc.,*** cham., ign., lyc., **STAPH.,** tarent.
rape, after - ***anac.,*** **CARC.,** coloc., ign., ***lyc., med., nat-m.,*** op., plat., puls., sep., **STAPH.,** thuj.
sexual abuse, after - ***anac.,*** **CARC.,** coloc., ign., ***lyc., med., nat-m.,*** plat., puls., sep., **STAPH.,** thuj.
shame, from - ***carc., ign.,*** nat-m., **OP., STAPH.**

HURRIED, feelings - ***acon.,*** aloe, alum., alum-p., am-c., ambr., anac., anan., apis, **ARG-N., ARS.,** ***ars-i.,*** ars-s-f., ***aur.,*** aur-a., aur-i., aur-s., ***bar-c.,*** bar-i., bar-s., **BELL.,** benz-ac., bov., ***bry.,*** cact., calad., calc., ***calc-f.,*** calc-s., calc-sil., ***camph.,*** cann-i., cann-s., canth., caps., carb-an., ***carb-s.,*** carb-v., **CARC.,** caust., cham., chlol., cimic., coca, cocc., ***coff.,*** con., croc., ***crot-c.,*** cur., dig., **DULC.,** elaps, esp-g., graph., grat., **HEP.,** hyos., **IGN.,** ***iod.,*** ip., kali-ar., ***kali-c.,*** kali-i., kali-p., kali-s., ***lach.,*** laur., led., **LIL-T.,** lob-p., lyc., lycps., lyss., ***mag-arct.,*** mag-aust., mang., **MED.,** merl., meny., **MERC.,** mez., morph., mosch., nat-a., nat-c., **NAT-M.,** nat-p., nit-ac., **NUX-V.,** olnd., op., ox-ac., ***ph-ac.,*** phos., pip-m., plat., plb., ptel., ***puls.,*** rheum, rhus-t., sep., **SIL.,** staph., ***stram.,*** stront-c., stroph., sul-i., **SULPH., SUL-AC.,** sumb., syph., **TARENT.,** ***thuj., tub.,*** verat., viol-t., zinc., zinc-valer.

HURRIED, feelings
afternoon - ferr-p.
agg. - benz-ac., coff.
ailments from hurry - ***acon.,*** am-c., arg-n., ***arn.,*** calc., carc., ***bry., nit-ac.,*** nux-v., ***puls.,*** rhus-t., sulph.
aimless - lil-t., **SUL-AC.**
always in - ars-s-f., dulc., nux-v., sil., staph.
awkwardness from - alum., ambr., apis, ***mosch.,*** nat-m., sulph.
breath, with short - caust.
chill, during - cann-s.
complaints, from - arn.
drinking, while - anac., ***ars., bell.,*** bry., cina, ***coff.,*** hell., ***hep.,*** lyc., ***stram., zinc.***
unconsciousness, during - hell.
duties, as by imperative - **LIL-T.**
eating, while - anac., arg-n., aur., bell., berb., calad., **CAUST.,** clem., ***coff.,*** cupr., **HEP.,** kali-c., ***lach.,*** lyc., olnd., pip-m., ***plat.,*** plect., ***rhus-t.,*** **SUL-AC.,** sulph., zinc.
cannot eat fast enough - zinc.
everybody, moves too slowly - arg-n., med., nux-v., tarent.
must hurry - arg-n., cann-i., ***lach.,*** nat-p., ***nux-v.,*** **TARENT.**
execution, with slow - alum.
fast enough, cannot do things - ***sul-ac.***
menses, during - ign.
mental work, in - ambr., aur., ign., ***kali-c.,*** laur., op., ***sul-ac., thuj.***
movements, in - acon., arg-n., ars., atro., ***bell.,*** camph., cann-i., coca, con., coff., gins., ***hyos.,*** kali-c., meny., merc., merl., **STRAM.,** ***sulph.,*** **SUL-AC., TARENT.,** ***thuj.,*** viol-t.
involuntary, hurried - **SULPH.**
cannot do things fast enough - aur., **SUL-AC.**
cannot do things fast enough, angry, making him - ***nux-v.,*** sul-ac.
night - lach.
occupation, in - acon., aur., camph., carb-v., cimic., hep., ***kali-c.,*** kali-p., **LIL-T., NUX-V.,** op., puls., sep., **SUL-AC.,** ***thuj.,*** viol-t.
desires to do several things at once - aur., **LIL-T.,** petr., plan.
things do not move fast enough - alum., tarent.
time, for the appointed, to arrive - **ARG-N.**
to do, several things at once - calc., ***lil-t.***
trifle things, in - med., sul-ac., sulph.
walking, while - acon., **ARG-N.,** canth., carb-an., fl-ac., iod., med., mosch., prun., sep., stram., ***sulph.,*** **SUL-AC., TARENT.,** ***thuj.***
walks to and fro, cannot be amused by thinking or reading - lil-t.
work, in - calc-f., cimic., op., sep., sul-ac., sul-i.
afternoon - aloe.
writing, in - alum., anac., lyc., ped., ptel., sul-ac.

HYPERACTIVE, children (see Restlessness) - anac., ***ars.,*** ars-i., calc-p., **CARC.,** ***cina,*** coff., **HYOS.,** ***iod.,*** **MED.,** nux-v., **STRAM.,** ***tarent.,*** thuj., **TUB.,** ***verat.***

HYPOCHONDRIASIS - abies-n., acon., agn., alf., aloe, alum., ***ambr., anac.,*** anag., anan., ***ant-t.,*** arg-m., ***arg-n., arn., ars.,*** arum-m., ***asaf.,*** **AUR.,** aur-m., aven., aza., bell., **BENZ-AC.,** bism., brom., bry., **CACT.,** ***calc.,*** canth., ***caps.,*** caust., ***cham.,*** chin., ***cimic., cocc.,*** coff., **CON.,** croc., cupr., ***cycl.,*** dig., esp-g., euphr., ferr., ferr-p., gels., ***graph., grat.,*** hell., helon., ***hep.,*** hydr-ac., ***hyos.,*** **IGN.,** ***iod., ip.,*** kali-br., kali-c., ***kali-p., lach., lyc.,*** lycps., mag-c., merc., **MEZ.,** ***mill.,*** **NAT-C., NAT-M.,** nep., **NUX-V.,** ***ph-ac., phos.,*** plat., plb., podo., **PULS.,** ***sep.,*** sin-n., stann., ***staph., sulph.,*** sumb., tarent., ***ter.,*** thuj., ***valer., verat.,*** vib-t., viol-o., zinc., zinc-oc., zinc-valer., ***zing.,*** ziz.
afternoon - cocc., graph., zinc.
air, in open - ***con.,*** petr.
alcoholics, in - ***nux-v.***
alone, when - ars.
crying, with - am-c., calc., kali-c., mez., plat., ***puls.,*** stram., viol-o.
daytime and merry in evening - ***sulph.***
eating, after - anac., chin., ***nat-c., nux-v.,*** zinc.
evening - kreos., lyss., nux-v., phos., puls.
fever, during - nux-m.
forenoon - nux-m.
imaginary illness - calc., kali-c., sabad., sep.
interest in his surroundings, takes no - euphr.
masturbation, after - ***tarent.***
menses, during - cur.
suppression of - ***con.***
morning - alum., anac., lyc.
morose - con., graph., grat., mag-arct., petr., phos., **PULS.,** sabin., sulph.
night - alum., calc., lach., mag-arct., nat-m.
nosebleed amel. - kali-chl.
pollutions, after - anac., ***ph-ac.,*** sil., staph.
sexual - mosch.
abstinence, from - **CON.,** mosch.
excesses, from - **CON.,** ***ph-ac.,*** **STAPH.**
suicide, driving to - alum., aur., calc., caust., chin., con., graph., hep., ***nat-m.,*** sep., **STAPH.,** sulph.
suppression of eruptions, after - **SULPH.**
walking, on - ***alum.,*** lyc.

HYPOCRISY - bar-c., caust., **LYC.,** merc., nux-v., phos., **PULS.,** sep., **SIL., SULPH.,** ***thuj.***

HYSTERICAL, behaviour - abrot., absin., ***acet-ac., acon.,*** ether, agn., ***agar., aloe, alum.,*** alum-sil., am-val., ***ambr.,*** am-c., aml-n., ***anac.,*** anag., apis, aquileg., ***arg-n.,*** arn., ***ars.,*** ars-s-f., ***art-v.,*** arund., **ASAF.,** asar., asc-t., aster., **AUR.,** aur-a., aur-i., aur-s., bapt., ***bar-c.,*** bar-i., bell., benz-ac., bor., brom., bry., bufo, ***cact., caj.,*** calad., ***calc., calc-s.,*** calc-sil., ***camph.,*** camph-br., cann-i., ***canth.,*** cann-s., ***carb-s.,*** **CARC.,** ***cast., caul.,*** **CAUST.,** cedr., ***cham., chen-a.,*** chim., chin., chin-s., ***chlf.,*** chlor., cic., ***cimic., chlol., cinnam.,*** cob., ***coca,*** **COCC.,** ***coff., coff-t.,*** **CON.,** convo-s., cop., cor-r.,

HYSTERICAL, behaviour - cot., crot-h., crot-t., ***croc.,*** cupr., cypr., ***elaps,*** electr., ***eup-a.,*** eup-pur., ***ferr.,*** ferr-ar., ferr-i., ferr-p., **GELS.,** ***graph.,*** ***grat.,*** hell., hura, ***hydr-ac.,*** ***hyos.,*** ***ictod.,*** **IGN.,** ***indg.,*** iod., ip., kali-ar., ***kali-c.,*** **KALI-P.,** kali-s., kali-sil., ***lac-ac.,*** **LACH.,** lact., ***lil-t.,*** lob., ***lyc.,*** ***mag-c.,*** **MAG-M.,** man., mang., ***merc.,*** mez., ***mill.,*** morph., **MOSCH.,** mygal., nat-a., ***nat-c.,*** nat-hchls., **NAT-M.,** nat-p., nat-s., nat-sil., **NIT-AC.,** nitro-o., **NUX-M., NUX-V.,** ol-an., op., orig., ***pall.,*** par., ***ph-ac.,*** ***phos.,*** phys., **PLAT.,** ***plb.,*** polyg., ictod., **PULS.,** pyrus, ***raph.,*** ***rhus-t.,*** sabin., sac-alb., sang., scut., ***sec.,*** **SEP.,** senec., **SIL.,** spira., stann., staph., ***stict.,*** stram., stry-p., succ., sul-ac., sul-i., ***sulph.,*** ***sumb.,*** **TARENT.,** thal., ***ther.,*** thuj., thyr., ust., **VALER., VERAT.,** vib., ***viol-o.,*** visc., xan., zinc., zinc-c., ***zinc-valer.,*** ***ziz.***

- **amenorrhea,** in - ign., ***xan.***
- **attacks,** in - absin., carb-s.
- **belching,** amel. - cinnam.
- **changing,** symptoms - carc., ign., **PULS.**
- **evening** - ether, kali-s.
- **fainting** - ***acon.,*** am-c., arn., **ARS.,** asaf., ***cham.,*** cimic., **COCC.,** cupr., ***dig.,*** **IGN.,** lac-d., lach., ***mosch.,*** ***nat-m.,*** ***nux-m.,*** ***nux-v.,*** puls., samb., stict., ***sumb.,*** ter.
- **fright,** after - ign., sabad.
- **grief,** from - bar-s., ***gels.,*** ***hyos.,*** **IGN.**
- **hemorrhage,** after - stict.
- **hysterical** complaints in deep scrofulous constitution, psora, syphilis - asaf.
- **injure** herself, desire to - ***hydr-ac.***
- **lascivious** - agn., hyos., mosch., ***plat.,*** ***tarent.***
- **lie** down, must - ***stict.,*** ther.
- **light** and noise agg. - ***stict.***
- **looked,** at, when - plb.
- **loss** of fluids, after - ***chin.,*** ***cinnam.***
  - blood - chin., ***stict.***
- **ludicrous** - ***tarent.***
- **man,** in a - carc., croc., med., mosch.
- **menopause,** at - aquileg., cimic., ***ign.,*** ***lach.,*** ***ph-ac.,*** ther., valer., zinc-valer.
- **menses,** during - acon., bry., calc., caul., caust., cham., chin., ***cimic.,*** cocc., coff., cupr., form., hyos., ign., mag-m., merc., nat-m., **NUX-M.,** nux-v., puls., stram., sulph., verat.
  - after - chin., cupr., ferr., puls.
  - amel. - ***zinc.***
  - before - caul., ***cimic.,*** cocc., con., cupr., elaps, gels., ***hyos.,*** ***ign.,*** kali-c., ***mag-m.,*** ***mosch.,*** nat-m., nux-m., nux-v., ph-ac., phos., ***plat.,*** puls., senec., sep., sulph., vib.
  - copious - caul., cimic., ***mag-m.***
  - first day of - raph.
  - scanty - ign., **NUX-M.**
- **metrorrhagia,** during - caul., cimic., mag-m.
- **moaning,** agg., sighing amel. - tarent.
- **moon,** agg., increasing - ***sulph.***
- **morning,** agg., sighing amel. - tarent.
- **move,** any part of body, cannot - ter.

HYSTERICAL, behaviour

- **music,** amel. - **TARENT.**
- **night** - ***senec.***
- **pain** joints, hysterical - ***arg-n.,*** cham., cot., hyper., ***ign.,*** zinc.
- **pletoric,** subjects, in - ***acon.,*** ***gels.***
- **pollutions,** after - anac., sil., staph.
- **pregnancy,** childbirth, during - ***chel.,*** ***chlol.,*** **GELS.,** ign.
- **puberty,** at - ant-c., ign., ***lach.,*** ***ther.***
- **sex,** agg. - lac-c., staph.
  - amel. - con.
- **sexual** excesses, after - agar., anac., con., lach., ***ph-ac.,*** sep.
  - orgasm, at the height, of - lac-c.
- **sleep,** with disturbed, and anxiety - ***carc.,*** ***sep.***
- **sleeplessness,** with - ***carc.,*** croc., ***kali-br.,*** mosch., ***senec.,*** ***stict.***
- **suppression** of, discharges, after - **ASAF.,** ***lach.***
  - sexual urges, from - ***brom.,*** **CON.**
- **touch** and pressure, intolerance of - ***tarent.***
- **twitchings,** menses, during - acon., bry., calc., caust., cham., chin., cocc., coff., cupr., form., hyos., ign., ip., lyc., mag-m., merc., nat-m., nux-v., puls., sulph.
  - after - chin., cupr., puls.
  - before - cupr., kali-c., nat-m., ph-ac., phos., plat., puls., sep., sulph.
- **watched,** only when - plb.

IDEALISTIC - ***caust.,*** **IGN., NAT-M.,** ***plat.***

IDEAS, general

- **abundant** - acon., aesc., agar., alum., alum-p., ambr., am-c., aml-n., anac., anag., ang., anh., ant-c., arg-m., ***arg-n.,*** ***ars.,*** ars-s-f., ars-s-r., asaf., asar., aur., aur-a., aur-s., ***bell.,*** bor., ***bry.,*** bufo, caj., ***calc.,*** calc-f., calc-p., calc-sil., camph., **CANN-I.,** cann-s., canth., carb-ac., carb-s., carb-v., caust., cham., **CHIN.,** chin-a., ***chin-s.,*** chlor., cimic., ***cinnb.,*** cob., coca, coc-c., **COFF.,** ***coff-t.,*** colch., coloc., der., eupi., ferr-p., flor-p., gels., glon., graph., hell., hep., hyos., hyper., ign., kali-br., kali-c., kali-n., kali-p., kali-s., kreos., lac-ac., **LACH.,** laur., ***lyc.,*** lyss., med., menthol, meph., merc., mez., morph., mur-ac., nat-a., nat-c., nat-p., ***nat-s.,*** nit-ac., ***nux-m.,*** ***nux-v.,*** olnd., **OP.,** opun-v., pall., ph-ac., **PHOS.,** phys., pic-ac., ***pip-m.,*** plat., ***puls.,*** rhus-t., sabad., sep., sil., spig., spong., staph., stram., ***stry.,*** **SULPH.,** sumb., tab., ter., thea., thuj., ***tub.,*** valer., verat., verb., viol-o., viol-t., zinc., zing.
  - alternating with, deficiency of - alum-p.
  - chill, during - phys., spig.
  - closing the eyes - led., spong.
  - evening - anac., arg-n., **CHIN.,** ***coff.,*** **LACH.,** lyc., lycps., nat-p., ***nux-v.,*** phos., ***puls.,*** sabad., sil., ***staph.,*** ***sumb.,*** ***valer.,*** viol-t.
    - bed, in - agar., bry., ***calc.,*** caust., chin., cocc., graph., kali-c., **NUX-V.,** ***lyc.,*** ***puls.,*** rhus-t., sil., sulph.
  - forenoon - ox-ac.

IDEAS, general
  abundant,
    headache, after - aster.
    heat, during - op., stram., thuj.
    night - aloe, bor., ***calc.***, calc-sil., ***cham.***, ***chin.***, chin-a., ***chin-s.***, coca, ***coff.***, colch., graph., hep., kali-c., ***lyc.***, ***nux-v.***, ***op.***, pic-ac., puls., sabad., sep., sil., ***staph.***, sulph., tab., viol-t.
    perspiration, during - valer., viol-o.
    rush of - ang., **ARS.**, **BELL.**, bor., **BRY.**, calad., **CHIN.**, cocc., **COFF.**, croc., fl-ac., **IGN.**, ***lac-c.***, **LACH.**, marr., nux-m., **NUX-V.**, olnd., ***op.***, **PHOS.**, ***puls.***, **RHUS-T.**, **SABAD.**, spig., ***staph.***, **VALER.**, verat., verb., viol-o., viol-t.
    same idea repeated - ***arg-n.***, mag-m., sulph.
    uncertain in execution, but - med.
    urination, after - cann-i.
  compelling - ***lach.***, nit-ac.
  deficiency, of - acet-ac., ***acon.***, agn., all-s., alum., alum-p., alum-sil., ***am-c.***, ambr., ***anac.***, ang., anh., arg-m., arg-n., arn., arund., asaf., asar., aster., atro., aur., **BAR-C.**, bell., berb., bov., bry., caj., calc., ***calc-p.***, camph., cann-s., canth., ***carb-v.***, ***caust.***, cham., ***chin.***, cic., clem., cocc., coff., coloc., ***con.***, corn., croc., cupr., cycl., dig., glon., graph., guai., **HELL.**, hep., ***hyos.***, ign., iod., ip., ***kali-br.***, kali-p., kreos., ***lach.***, laur., lepi., lil-t., **LYC.**, mag-arct., meny., ***merc.***, merc-c., ***mez.***, nat-c., ***nat-m.***, nat-p., ***nit-ac.***, ***nux-m.***, nux-v., olnd., **OP.**, petr., **PH-AC.**, **PHOS.**, plat., ***plb.***, ***puls.***, ran-b., ran-s., rheum, rhod., ***rhus-t.***, ruta, ***sel.***, sep., sil., spig., stann., **STAPH.**, stram., sulph., ***tarent.***, thuj., trom., valer., verat., **VIOL-O.**, xan., ***zinc.***
    brain fag, in - kali-p., ***ph-ac.***
    daytime - calc-sil.
    interruption, from any - colch.
    menses, during - ***lycps.***
    overexertion, on - ***mez.***, olnd., sil.
    vomiting, amel. - asar.
  disconnected - alum., am-c., ***cann-i.***, nat-c., ph-ac., sulph., zinc.
  erroneous - sabad., valer.
  exaggerated - glon., pall., plat.
  fixed - acon., alum., anac., arg-n., **ARS.**, aur., bry., **CANN-S.**, canth., cham., chin., cic., coca, ***cocc.***, cupr., **EUPHR.**, glon., graph., **HELL.**, **HYOS.**, **IGN.**, ***iod.***, lach., lyss., **MERC.**, **NAT-M.**, ***nit-ac.***, **OP.**, ph-ac., plat., ***psor.***, ***puls.***, ***rhus-t.***, ***thuj.***, **VERAT.**
  insane - ***lyss.***
  persistent - med.
  persecution of - ***anac.***, ***chin.***, con., cycl., ***dros.***, hyos., ***lach.***, thyr.
  repeated, same ideas - arg-n., mag-m.
  ridiculous - ***arg-n.***, cann-i., kali-p., **LACH.**, ***stram.***
  strange - ***arg-n.***, ***sulph.***
  vanish - anac., ***nux-m.***, olnd., verat.
  wander - dulc., phos., thuj.

IDIOCY - absin., ***aeth.***, agar., alum., anac., anan., ant-c., apis, ars., bac., **BAR-C.**, ***bar-m.***, bell., bell-p., ***bufo***, calc., ***calc-p.***, caps., carb-o., ***carb-s.***, ***carc.***, cent., cham., chlol., cic., ***hell.***, **HYOS.**, lach., lyc., med., merc., morg., mosch., nat-m., nux-m., olnd., op., ph-ac., ***phos.***, plb., sarr., sec., stram., sulph., tab., thuj., thyr., ***tub.***, verat.
    alternating with furor - aeth.
    bite, desire to - **BELL.**, **STRAM.**
    cretinism - absin., ***aeth.***, ***anac.***, arn., bac., ***bar-c.***, bar-m., ***bufo***, calc-p., carc., hell., ign., iod., ***lap-a.***, lol., nat-c., oxyt., ph-ac., plb., sep., sulph., ***thyr.***
    down's, syndrome - **BAR-C.**, calc., carc., pituit., thyr.
    giggling - stry.
    idiotic actions - ant-c.
      epilepsy, before - caust.
    masturbation, with - bufo, med., orig.
    pulling feathers out of bed - ant-c.
    shrill shrieking, with - ***bor.***, ***lac-c.***, **TUB.**
    stroke, after - hell.

IDLENESS - calc., glon., lach., lyc., nat-m., nux-v., stann., sulph.
    afternoon - bor.
    agg. - con.

IMAGINARY disease - arg-n., ars., mosch., sabad., ***verat.***
    broods over - ars., cycl., lil-t., naja.

IMAGINATION, (see Fantasies)

IMBECILITY - absin., acon., aeth., agar., agn., alco., **ALOE**, **ALUM.**, alum-p., alum-sil., **AMBR.**, ***am-c.***, **ANAC.**, anac-oc., anil., ant-c., ant-t., apis, arg-m., ***arg-n.***, ***ars.***, art-v., asar., ***aur.***, aur-a., aur-s., bac., ***bapt.***, **BAR-C.**, **BAR-M.**, bar-s., **BELL.**, bov., brom., **BUFO**, **BUF-S.**, ***calc.***, calc-p., calc-s., calc-sil., camph., ***cann-s.***, ***caps.***, carb-an., carb-o., **CARB-S.**, carb-v., ***caust.***, cham., ***chel.***, chin., chlol., chlor., cic., ***cocc.***, **CON.**, croc., ***crot-h.***, cupr., cycl., dig., ***dios.***, dulc., ***fl-ac.***, ***hell.***, **HYOS.**, ***ign.***, iod., kali-bi., ***kali-br.***, kali-c., kali-m., ***kali-p.***, kali-sil., **LACH.**, ***laur.***, lol., **LYC.**, mang., ***med.***, meli., ***merc.***, ***merc-c.***, mez., mosch., mur-ac., nat-a., ***nat-c.***, nat-i., ***nat-m.***, ***nat-p.***, nat-sil., nit-ac., **NUX-M.**, **NUX-V.**, olnd., **OP.**, ***oxyt.***, ***par.***, ***petr.***, **PH-AC.**, ***phos.***, **PIC-AC.**, ***plat.***, ***plb.***, ***puls.***, ran-b., rheum, ***rhus-t.***, ruta, ***sabad.***, ***sabin.***, sars., sec., sel., seneg., ***sep.***, **SIL.**, sol-n., ***spig.***, spong., stann., ***staph.***, **STRAM.**, stry., sul-ac., **SULPH.**, ***syph.***, tab., tax., ***ther.***, thuj., ***thyr.***, tub., **VERAT.**, ***verb.***, viol-o., zinc., zinc-p.
    aphasia, with - ***anac-oc.***
    epilepsy, before - ***caust.***
    laughing for nothing - hyos., stram.
    negativism - hell., ign.
    old rags are as fine as silk - **SULPH.**
    rage, stamps the feet - anac., lyc., nux-v., op., verat.
    senile - ***anac.***, ant-c., ***aur.***, **BAR-C.**, **CON.**, ***lach.***, phos., sec.
    sexual excitement, with - ***bell.***, ***hep.***, ***hyos.***, ***phos.***, ***staph.***, ***stram.***

IMBECILITY,
screams when occupying with him - ***hell., ign.***

IMITATION, mimicry - bell., cupr., hyos., lach., nux-m., sars., stram., verat.
voices and motions of animals, of - ***stram.***

IMPATIENCE, (see Hurried, Restlessness) - ***acon.***, act-sp., aeth., agar-ph., alco., all-s., allox., ambr., ***anac.***, ant-c., ***apis,*** aral., **ARG-N.,** ***ars., ars-h., ars-i.,*** ars-s-f., aster., aur., aur-a., aur-i., aur-m-n., bar-c., bar-i., bar-s., bell., ***bry.,*** bufo, ***calc.,*** calc-f., calc-i., calc-s., calc-sil., ***carb-ac.,*** carb-v., **CARC., CHAM.,** chin., chin-a., cimic., ***cina,*** colch., ***coloc.,*** cub., culx., digin., dros., ***dulc.,*** ferul., gels., gins., goss., graph., hell., ***hep.,*** hura, ***hyos.,*** **IGN.,** ***iod.,*** **IP.,** kali-ar., ***kali-bi., kali-c.,*** kali-p., kali-s., kali-sil., ***kreos., lach.,*** lil-t., ***lyc.,*** lyss., manc., **MED.,** merc., mosch., murx., nat-a., nat-c., ***nat-m.,*** nat-p., nep., nicc., nid., ***nit-ac.,*** nuph., nux-m., **NUX-V.,** onos., op., osm., pall., ph-ac., ***plan., plat., psor., puls.,*** rheum, ***rhus-t.,*** sang., sars., **SEP., SIL.,** spig., spong., stann., ***staph., sul-ac.,*** sul-i., **SULPH.,** tarax., ***tarent.,*** tax., thal., thiop., thuj., vac., vip-a., viol-t., wies., zinc., zinc-p.
afternoon - nit-ac., sang.
always - merc., sil.
children, about his - kali-c., nux-v.
contradiction, at slightest - alco., nuph.
coryza, with - **NUX-V.**
cures him at once, the patient insists that the doctor - ars., cham., nit-ac.
daytime - lyss.
dinner, during - sulph.
eating, while - merc.
forenoon, 11 a.m. - sulph.
headache, during - manc., nux-v., pall., lyss., ***sulph.,*** zinc.
heat, with - ars., bell., ***cham., ip.,*** lyc., ***nat-m., nux-v., puls., viol-t.***
house, in - asar.
intermittent fever - chin-a.
itching, from - osm., sars.
morning - dulc., sulph.
noon - hura.
pain, from - ***cham.,*** hura, murx.
perspiration, during - aur., mez., sul-ac., zinc.
playing of children - anac., nux-v.
reading, while - nat-c.
room, in a warm crowded - ***plat.***
runs about, never sits or sleeps at night - ***iod.***
sitting, while - ***sep.***
slowly, everything goes too - ***cham.***
spoken to, when - ***nux-v.***
supper after - nit-ac.
talk of others, during - sulph., zinc.
tossing about - ***acon.***
trifles, about - kali-p., ***med.,*** merc., nat-m., sol-a., ***sulph., sul-ac.***
urinating, before - sulph.
waking, on - ***lyc.***
walking, while - lyc.

IMPATIENCE,
working, in - ***nux-v.,*** sep.

IMPERTINENCE - acon., bufo, canth., graph., hyos., lach., ***nat-m.,*** nit-ac., nux-v., pall., phos., spong., staph., ***stram.,*** verat.
acts, in his - stram., verat.

IMPETUOUS - acon., ***anac., bry.,*** calc-s., ***carb-v.,*** caust., ***cham.,*** croc., ferr-p., **HEP.,** ictod., ***kali-c.,*** kali-i., kali-p., kali-s., lach., laur., led., med., nat-c., ***nat-m.,*** **NIT-AC., NUX-V.,** olnd., phos., rheum, **SEP.,** ***staph.,*** stront-c., ***sulph., zinc.,*** zinc-p.
afternoon - caust.
daytime - nit-ac.
evening - ferr-p.
heat, with - sep.
morning - staph.
perspiration - ***acon., ars., bry.,*** carb-v., ferr., ***hep.,*** hyos., nat-m., phos., stram., sulph., thuj.
urination, before - sulph.

IMPOLITE - HEP., lyc., **MERC.,** ***plat.***

IMPORTANCE, feels his - glon., ***plat.,*** stram., **SULPH.,** verat.

IMPRESSIONABLE, (See Sensitive) - ant-c., ***arg-n.,*** calc., ***carc.,*** con., croc., med., **PHOS.,** tarent., viol-o.
unpleasantly by everything - ***con.***

IMPROVIDENT - alum., caust., nat-m.

IMPUDENCE - hyos., ***phos., plat.,*** verat.

IMPULSE, morbid (see Kill) - alum., anac., ***arg-n.,*** ars., caust., hep., iod., lach., lyc., merc.
contradictory - ***anac.,*** carc.
horrid - alum., ars., caust., hep., iod., lach., merc.
busy, when, amel. - iod.
pinch, to - coff.
rash - bell., ***hyos.,*** nux-v., staph., ***stram.,*** verat.
run, to - acon., all-s., arg-n., bell., cann-i., glon., **HYOS.,** ***iod.,*** mez., ***nux-v., orig.,*** phys., **STRAM.,** ***tarent.,*** **TUB., VERAT.**
away - puls.
menses, before - lach.
night, at - iod.
scream, to - sep.
set on fire, to - alco., ant-t., **BELL., HEP.,** hyos., phos., staph., stram.
stab his flesh with the knife he holds, to - ***lyss.***
to do strange things - cact.
unfit, for - sep.
unworthy - ***nat-s.,*** plat.
violence, to do - merc.

IMPULSIVE - ARG-N., ***ars., aur.,*** camph., carc., cer-b., ***cic.,*** croc., cupr., gins., hep., **IGN.,** ***med.,*** merc., nux-v., phos., **PULS.,** rhus-t., staph., stram., tarent., thea., tub.

INATTENTION, agg. - gels., ***hell.***

INCITING, others - hyos.

INCONSOLABLE, (see Consolation)

INCONSTANCY - acon., acon-l., act-sp., agar., alum., am-c., ***ambr.,*** anh., apis, arn., ars., asaf., bism., bor., cann-s., canth., ***carc.,*** cimic., coff., dros., ***graph.,*** **IGN.,** **KALI-BR.,** lac-c., lach., led., lil-t., lyc., mag-arct., mag-aust., nat-c., nux-m., nux-v., op., petr., plan., plat., sil., spig., stann., stram., sulph., syph., thuj., valer., verat., voes., zinc.

thoughts, of - alum., am-c., hell., merc., mez., thuj.

INDECISION, irresolution - act-sp., ***agar., alum.,*** alum-p., alum-sil., alumn., am-c., ***anac.,*** ang., anh., apis, ***arg-n.,*** arn., ***ars.,*** ars-i., asaf., aur., aur-a., aur-i., aur-s., bar-ac., **BAR-C.,** bar-i., ***bar-m.,*** bism., bry., buf-s., bufo, buth-a., cact., ***calc.,*** calc-ar., calc-f., calc-i., calc-p., calc-s., ***calc-sil.,*** camph., **CANN-I.,** cann-s., canth., ***carb-s.,*** **CARC.,** caust., cench., cham., chel., chin., chin-s., ***chlol.,*** cimic., cina, clem., coca, ***cocc.,*** coch., coff., coll., ***con.,*** cortico., croc., crot-h., cupr., ***cur.,*** daph., dig., dros., dulc., ferr., ferr-ar., ferr-i., ferr-m., ferr-ma., **GRAPH.,** grat., guare., guat., **HELL.,** hyos., **IGN.,** iod., ***ip.,*** kali-ar., kali-br., kali-c., kali-m., kali-p., kali-s., kali-sil., lac-c., lac-d., **LACH.,** laur., led., **LYC.,** lyss., ***mag-arct.,*** mag-aust., mag-m., mag-p-a., man., mang., ***merc., mez.,*** mur-ac., ***naja,*** nat-c., ***nat-m.,*** nat-sil., nit-ac., ***nux-m., nux-v.,*** **ONOS., OP.,** pall., **PETR.,** ***phos.,*** pic-ac., plat., plb., ***psor.,*** **PULS.,** rad., rheum, rhus-r., ruta, sanic., sant., seneg., ***sep., sil.,*** spig., ***stann.,*** staph., sul-ac., ***sulph.,*** tab., tarax., tarent., thuj., zinc., zinc-p.

acts, in - **BAR-C.,** chin., ***lyc.,*** nat-c., nat-sil., nux-m., **ONOS.,** tarent.

afternoon - hyos.

air, amel. in open - asaf.

anxious - ***graph.***

changeable - asaf., bism., cann-s., carc., ign., led., mag-aust., nux-v., op., plat., puls., sil., thuj.

debility, in nervous - ***cur.***

evening - calc., ferr-p., mag-arct., ***puls.***

ideas, in - cann-i., mag-aust., nat-m., sulph., tarent.

impulsive though, when decision is made - mag-arct.

indolence, with - puls., tarax.

marry, to - carb-v., ign., lach., **LYC.,** nat-m., ***nux-v.,*** phos., plat., puls., sil., ***staph.,*** verat.

morning - des-ac., nat-c., pall.

projects, in - ars., asaf., **BAR-C.,** buf-s., cact., cham., ign., **LYC.,** ***nux-m.,*** rhus-r.

sleepiness, with - hyos.

trifles, about - ars., **BAR-C.,** graph., ***lyc.,*** lyss.

waking, on - lyc.

INDEPENDENT - ***calc.,*** calc-p., ***bell.,*** kali-c., nat-m., ***nux-v., sulph.***

INDIFFERENCE, apathetic - absin., acet-ac., ***acon., agar., agn.,*** ail., allox., **ALUM.,** alum-p., alum-sil., alumn., am-c., ambr., am-m., amor-r., **ANAC.,** ***anac-oc., anh.,*** ant-t., **APIS,** aq-mar., arag., ***arg-n., arn., ars.,*** ars-h., ars-i., ars-s-f., arum-t., asaf., asar., aster., atro., ***bapt., bar-c.,*** bar-i., bar-m., bar-s., ***bell.,*** berb., bism., bor., ***bov.,*** brom., bry., bufo, but-ac., buth-a., cadm-met., calad., **CALC.,** calc-ar., calc-f., calc-i., ***calc-p.,*** calc-s., camph., cann-i., cann-s., caps., ***carb-an.,*** carb-o., ***carb-s.,*** **CARB-V.,** carc., caust., ***cham., chel.,*** **CHIN.,** ***chin-a., chin-s.,*** chlf., chloram., chlorpr., cic., ***cimic.,*** cina, clem., ***cocc.,*** cod., coloc., **CON.,** coni-br., corn., croc., **CROT-C.,** ***crot-h.,*** cupr., cupr-s., ***cycl.,*** cypr., cyt-l., dig., dros., ***dulc.,*** elaps, euphr., ferr., ferr-ar., ferr-i., ferr-p., fl-ac., **GELS.,** glon., glyc., ***graph.,*** guai., guare., gymn., ham., harp., **HELL.,** helo., hep., hura, hydr-ac., hydrc., ***hyos., ign.,*** ind., indol., iod., ip., jatr., jug-r., ***kali-ar.,*** kali-bi., kali-br., ***kali-c.,*** kali-chl., kali-n., ***kali-p.,*** kali-s., kali-sil., kres., lac-c., lac-d., ***lach.,*** laur., lepi., levo., lil-s., **LIL-T.,** linu-u, luf-op., ***lyc.,*** lyss., mag-c., mag-m., man., manc., ***meli.,*** meny., ***merc.,*** merc-i-f., **MEZ.,** moly-met., morph., ***mur-ac.,*** naja, nat-a., **NAT-C., NAT-M., NAT-P.,** nep., nid., ***nit-ac., nit-s-d., nux-m.,*** **NUX-V.,** olnd., **ONOS., OP.,** ped., petr., **PH-AC., PHOS.,** ***phyt., pic-ac.,*** **PLAT.,** plb., prun., psil., ***psor.,*** ptel., **PULS.,** rad-br., ran-b., raph., rheum, rhod., rhus-g., rhus-t., ruta, rumx., sabad., sabin., sac-alb., sang., saroth., sarr., sars., ***sec.,*** sel., seneg., **SEP.,** sieg., ***sil.,*** spong., squil., stann., **STAPH.,** ***stram.,*** sul-ac., sulfa., sul-i., ***sulph., syph., tab.,*** tarax., tarent., ***tell.,*** thal., ther., thiop., ***thuj.,*** **THYR.,** trinit., ***tub.,*** ven-m., ***verat.,*** verb., ***viol-t.,*** vip., visc., xan., ***zinc.,*** zinc-p., ziz.

afternoon - con., ham., mag-c.

agreeable things to - ambr., anac., cina, corn., merc., op., rhod., staph., stram.

air, in open - con., mur-ac., plat.

amel. - nat-a.

alternating with

activity - aloe, aur., sarr.

anger - carb-s., nid.

anxiety and restlessness - ant-t., nat-m.

cheerfulness - agn., meny., tarent.

excitement - alum-p., phenob., sabad.

jesting - meny.

sensitiveness - bell.

timidity - stram.

vexation - cham., chin.

weeping - phos.

anosognosia - thala.

anxiety, after - ***acon.***

boredom, with - alum., con., ***kali-n.,*** lach., lyc., med., ***nat-c., nux-v.,*** petr., ***plb.,*** sulph., zinc.

business affairs, to - agar., ***arg-n.,*** arn., calc., ***fl-ac.,*** ham., ***kali-bi.,*** kali-p., myric., nat-a., ***ph-ac.,*** phys., phyt., ***puls.,*** rhus-t., ***sep., stram., sulph.***

caresses, to - **CINA.,** nat-m.

INDIFFERENCE, apathetic

children, to her - aur-a., kali-i., ***lyc.,*** nat-c., **PHOS., SEP.**

chill, during - arn., con., ign., kali-m., **OP., PHOS., PH-AC.,** puls., sil., verat.

cold, and indifferent - anac., plat., sabad., ***sep.,*** sulph.

company, while in - **ARG-N.,** bov., kali-c., lyc., nat-c., nat-m., ***plat.,*** rhus-t.

amel. - bov.

company, to - rhod.

complain, does not - ***hyos.,*** **OP., STRAM.**

unless questioned, then say nothing of his condition - colch.

concussion of brain, after - **ARN.,** ***cic., hell.,*** nat-s., ***op.***

conscience, to the dictates of - anac., cann-i., caust., con., graph., petr.

conversation, from - sil.

crying, with - caust., ign., ***plat.***

daytime - anac., dig., merc., verat., xan.

dead, everything seems to him - **MEZ.**

desires, has none, no action of the will - hell., op., ***verat.***

disagreeable things, to - ambr., anac., bor., cina, cocc., coff., op., rhod.

done for her, about anything being - **LIL-T.**

duties, to - ars., **CALC.,** carb-v., cench., lach., merc., nat-m., ***ptel.,*** sil., sul-i., sulph.

domestic - aur-a., brom., calc., ***cimic.,*** cit-l., sep., sul-i.

eating, after - aloe, lach., lyc., ***ph-ac.,*** sel.

eating, to - merc., nat-c., nat-m., ***staph.***

epilepsy, in - ***crot-h.,*** kali-br., ***op.***

evening - aloe, dig., kali-chl., phos., tarent.

everything, to - ***acon.,*** acet-ac., agar., agn., ail., ambr., anac., ***apis,*** arg-n., arn., ***ars.,*** asaf., ***bapt.,*** bell., bism., bov., bry., buth-a., **CADM-MET.,** cann-s., canth., caps., **CARB-V.,** cham., ***chin.,*** cic., ***cimic., cina,*** con., croc., cypr., dig., fl-ac., ***gels.,*** glyc., ***hell.,*** hydr., hydr-ac., hyos., ***ign.,*** indol., kali-ar., lach., lepi., lil-t., ***lyc., merc.,*** merl., mez., nat-c., ***nat-m.,*** nat-p., nit-ac., ***nit-s-d.,*** nux-m., ***nux-v., op.,*** **PH-AC.,** ***phos., pic-ac., pituin., plat., puls., rheum,*** sec., ***sep.,*** sima., stann., **STAPH.,** sulph., syph., **THYR.,** verat., ziz.

done for her - lil-t.

excitement, after - ambr.

exciting events, to - ferr-p.

exertion, after - nat-m.

exposure of her person - **HYOS.,** ***phos., phyt., sec.,*** stram., verat.

external things, to - agn., am-c., am-m., berb., bov., cann-i., cham., cic., coca, euphr., ***hell.,*** kali-bi., lyc., merl., op., plat., rumx., sil., stann., staph., **SULPH.,** tarent., thuj., verat., vip.

impressions - con., ***hell.,*** lyc.

family, to his - carb-v., hell., nat-p., nit-ac., ***sep.***

INDIFFERENCE, apathetic

fever, during - ail., ***apis,*** aran., ***arn.,*** bapt., chin., ***chin-s.,*** **CON.,** ferr-p., **GELS.,** ***nit-s-d.,*** **OP.,** phos., **PH-AC.,** ***puls., sep.,*** stram., verat., viol-t.

fine, feeling, to - op.

forenoon - alum., sars., sep.

friends, to - kali-sil., nat-sil.

dearest, even towards - ***phos.***

future, to - syph.

happiness, to - ars-i.

himself, to - thuj-l.

household, matters, to - calc., cimic.

important things, to - calc., fl-ac.

news - ars-h.

influenza, after - ***cadm-met., gels., ph-ac.***

interrogations, to - tanac.

irritability, with - ziz.

irritating, disagreeable things, to - ambr., anac., bor., cina, coc-c., coff., op., rhod.

joking, to - sabad.

joy, to - ambr., kali-p., nat-a., ***op.***

joy and suffering - ambr., anac., carb-v., cina, hell., ***op.,*** puls.

joyless - apis, **AUR.,** bell., cann-s., ip., meny., ***nat-m.,*** nit-ac., ***op., puls.,*** sabin., **SEP.**

lies with eyes closed - arg-n., cocc., ph-ac., ***sep.***

life, to - absin., ***ars., aur.,*** bov., cham., lyc., ***merc.,*** phos., ***phyt., sep.,*** sulph., ***tab., xan.***

loved ones, to - ***acon.,*** allox., ars., ars-i., bell., carc., ***fl-ac.,*** **HELL.,** kali-sil., merc., nat-p., nat-sil., ***ph-ac.,*** **PHOS.,** plat., **SEP.,** ***syph.***

and animated to strangers - ***fl-ac.***

masturbation, after - agn., ph-ac., **STAPH.**

menopausal period, in - ***cycl., sep.***

mental exertion, after - nat-m.

money-making, to - chin., kali-c., merc., nat-c., sep.

morning - all-c., corn., mag-c., manc., **PH-AC.**

to 3 p.m. - tarent.

on waking - all-c., hep., mag-m., manc., petr., ***ph-ac.,*** phyt., staph.

morose - am-c., bov., ***con.,*** lach.

music - ign.

loves, which she - ***carb-v.,*** caust.

naked, to remain - **HYOS.**

notices, nothing - ***verat.***

onanism, after - **STAPH.**

opposite sex, to - ***puls.,*** **SEP.,** thuj.

ordinary, matters, to - com.

others, toward - plat., sabad., sulph.

pain, to - arn., arund., iod., jatr., op.

periodical - ars., chin.

personal, appearance - hyos., **SULPH.**

persons, to all - mez.

perspiration, during - ***ars.,*** bell., ***calc., lach.***

pleasure, to - alum., anac., ***arg-n., ars.,*** calc-ar., ***cham.,*** chin-a., ***chin-s.,*** cocc., croc., ferr-p., graph., **HELL.,** hep., hura, ip., kali-ar., kali-c., kali-m., kali-sil., mag-c., mag-m., meph., mez., mur-ac., nat-a., nat-c., **NAT-M.,** ***nit-ac.,*** **OP.,**

INDIFFERENCE, apathetic

pleasure, to - petr., prun., ***puls.***, sars., ***sep.***, spig., stann., staph., stram., **SULPH.**, tab., ther.

puberty, in - bar-c., lach., ph-ac.

reading, while - mez.

recovery, about his - ***ars.***, aur-m-n., ***calc.***

relations, to - acon., ***fl-ac.***, **HELL.**, hep., kali-p., nat-c., nat-p., **PHOS.**, plat., **SEP.**, ***syph.***

her children - aur-i., kali-i., ***lyc.***, nat-c., **PHOS., SEP.**

religion, to his - anac., coloc.

reprimands, to all - ***merc.***

sex, during - lyss.

after - ***calc.***

sleepiness, with - acon., am-m., ammc., ant-t., ars., carb-an., carb-v., chel., cinnb., com., croc., culx., dig., grat., ip., laur., lyc., mag-c., mag-m., nat-c., ***ph-ac.***, rat., sars., tong., verb., ***zinc.***

sleeplessness, with - ***nit-s-d.***

society, when in agg. - **ARG-N.**, bov., ***kali-c.***, lyc., nat-c., nat-m., **PLAT.**, rhus-t.

when in, amel. - bov.

stoical to what happens - ail., op.

stool, after - ***cycl., gels., ph-ac.***

every - arn.

stormy weather, in - sang., tub.

struggling, unequal, adverse circumstances, with - ph-ac.

suffering, to - ***hell.***, **OP., STRAM.**

surroundings, to - abel., allox., ars-i., bufo, levo., merc., nat-sil., ph-ac., phos., phyt., raja-s., rumx., sel., sul-i., thuj-l.

taciturn - calc., ***hell., nit-s-d.***, plat., staph.

typhoid, in - ail., ***apis, arn.***, chin., ***chin-s., colch., nit-s-d., ph-ac., verat.***

vexation with distress in stomach, after least - ***kali-bi.***

walking, in open air, while - ***con.***

welfare, of others, to - anac., ars., caust., lach., nat-m., ***nux-v.***, plat., **SULPH.**

window, looks hours at - mez.

women, to - nat-m.

work, with aversion to - agar., allox., calc., camph., ign., lach., ph-ac., rhod., sil., squil., staph.

INDIGNATION, feelings - acon., ambr., ***ars.***, aur., bry., ***calc-p.***, caps., carc., caust., cham., chin., cocc., ***coloc.***, croc., dros., ign., ip., lyc., mag-c., merc., nat-c., **NUX-V.**, phos., plat., ***spig.***, **STAPH.**, verat.

ailments from - acon., anac., carc., ***coloc.***, ign., ip., ***lyc.***, nat-m., nux-v., plat., **STAPH.**

discomfort, from general - op.

dreams, at unpleasant - calc-p.

morning - ars.

pregnant, while - nat-m.

INDISCRETION - acon., alum., arn., ***bar-c.***, bor., bov., bry., bufo, calad., calc., camph., caps., caust., con., croc., graph., hyos., ign., kali-c., laur., meny., ***merc.***, nat-m., ***nux-v.***, op., plat., puls., spong., staph., stram., ***verat.***

INDOLENCE, (see Laziness)

INDUSTRIOUS, mania for work (see Work, general)

INHIBITED - lyc., ***med., merc.***, nat-m., puls., sil., ***staph.***

INJURE, fears to be left alone, lest he should injure himself - alum., arg-n., ars., ***cimic., merc.***, **NAT-S.**, sep.

feels as if she could easily injure herself - sep.

frenzy, causing him to, himself - agar., lyss.

satiety of life, must use self-control to prevent shooting himself - ***nat-s.***

INJURIES, mental symptoms from - acon., arn., bell., ***carc.***, cic., ***glon., hell.***, hyos., hyper., mag-c., **NAT-S.**, ***op.***, stram., verat.

INJUSTICE, cannot tolerate - **CAUST.**, ign., nux-v., ***staph.***

INQUISITIVE - agar., aur., hyos., lach., laur., lyc., puls., sep., sulph., verat.

INSANITY, general - absin., acon., aeth., ether, ***agar.***, ail., alco., all-c., ***alum.***, alum-p., alum-sil., ***am-c.***, ambr., ***anac.***, anag., anan., ant-c., ant-t., ***apis, arg-m.***, arg-n., ***arn.***, **ARS.**, ars-i., ars-s-f., arum-t., atro., ***aur.***, aur-a., aur-i., aur-s., bac., bar-c., ***bar-m.***, **BELL.**, berb., bor., bov., brom., bufo, cact., calad., ***calc.***, calc-ar., calc-i., calc-s., calc-sil., ***camph.***, cann-i., cann-s., ***canth.***, carb-an., carb-s., **CARC.**, ***caust.***, cench., cer-b., ***chel.***, chin-s., chlol., ***cic., cimic., cocc.***, coff., colch., coloc., ***con.***, cortiso., ***croc., crot-c.***, crot-h., **CUPR.**, cur., ***cycl.***, dig., ***dulc.***, euph., fl-ac., gels., ***glon., hell., hep.***, **HYOS.**, ***ign.***, indg., iod., kali-ar., kali-bi., ***kali-br.***, kali-c., ***kali-chl.***, kali-i., ***kali-m.***, kali-ox., ***kali-p., lach.***, led., ***lil-t., lol.***, **LYC.**, man., ***manc.***, med., meli., **MERC.**, merc-c., mez., mosch., murx., naja, nat-c., ***nat-m.***, nat-s., ***nux-m.***, **NUX-V.**, oena., olnd., ***op.***, opun-v., ***ox-ac.***, par., passi., penic., ph-ac., ***phos.***, phys., ***plat.***, plb., ***psor., puls.***, raph., rhod., ***rhus-t.***, sabad., sec., seneg., sep., sil., sol-n., squil., stann., **STRAM.**, ***sulph.***, syph., **TARENT.**, ter., thuj., thyr., ***tub.***, **VERAT.**, verat-v., vip., zinc., zinc-p.

alcoholics, in - **ARS.**, ars-s-f., ***aur.***, aur-a., ***bell.***, calc., cann-i., carb-v., carc., chin., ***coff.***, crot-h., dig., hell., hep., ***hyos.***, **LACH.**, merc., nat-c., **NUX-V.**, ***op.***, puls., ***stram.***, sulph.

alternating, with

depressive narcosis - apis, ***hyos., op.***

fever, inflammatory - tub.

mental symptoms, with other - ***con.***, sabad.

with physical symptoms - cer-b., ***croc.***, hyos., ***lil-t.***, **PLAT.**, ***sabad.***, tub.

metrorrhagia, with - crot-c.

sadness, with - tub.

stupor, with - op.

INSANITY, general

amenorrhea, from - ***cocc.***

anger, from - anac., bell., ***ign., lach.,*** lyc., op., ***plat., staph.***

anxiety, with - ***ars.,*** bell., cupr., kali-c., nat-c., ***stram.,*** verat.

bleeding, after - carb-v., ***chin., cupr.,*** kreos., ph-ac., ***sep.,*** staph., verat.

break pins, she will sit and - bell., calc., hyos.

brutal - absin.

burrows, in ground with his mouth, like a pig - stram.

business, from failure in - aur., ***cimic., lil-t.***

busy - **APIS,** bell., ***iod.,*** kali-br.

capricious - raph.

cheerful, gay - bell., cann-s., croc., cupr., ign., mez., ***stram.,*** verat.

childbirth, after - agn., ***aur.,*** bar-c., ***bell., camph., cann-i.,*** cann-s., canth., ***chlol.,*** cic., ***cimic.,*** crot-h., ***cupr., cupr-ac.,*** ferr-p., ***hyos., kali-bi.,*** kali-br., kali-c., kali-p., ***lyc.,*** nat-m., ***nux-v., petr.,*** phos., ***plat., puls., sec.,*** senec., sep., ***stram., sulph.,*** thyr., ***verat.,*** verat-v., zinc.

chilliness, with - calc., phyt.

coldness of skin - crot-h.

company, with desire for light and - **STRAM.**

convulsions, with - cupr., ***hyos., stram., verat-v., zinc.***

crawls, on the floor - ***lach.***

crazy person, behaves like a - ***cann-s.,*** cortiso., ***croc.,*** **HYOS.,** kali-ar., ***lach., nux-m., sec., stram., tarent., verat.***

does all sorts of crazy things - ***hyos.,*** stram.

crying, with - cann-s., merc., stram.

dancing, with - bell., cic., ***hyos.,*** ph-ac.

stripping himself and dancing - ***bell., hyos.***

despair, with insanity and weariness of life from fear of mortification or of loss of position - ***aur.,*** calc., ign., puls., rhus-t., staph., sulph., verat.

dictatorial - **LYC.**

domestic calamity, after - aur., ***lach.***

dresses in his best clothes - con.

drunk, as if - agar., oena.

eat, refuses to (see Anorexia) - aur., ars., bell., ***bor.,*** carc., caul., caust., ***chin.,*** cocc., croc., grat., **HYOS.,** ***ign.,*** **KALI-CHL.,** kali-p., lach., op., **PH-AC.,** ***phyt.,*** plat., puls., rhus-t., sep., sulph., **TARENT., VERAT., VIOL-O.**

eats, dung - merc.

filth - sulph.

refuse - meli.

elderly people, in - anac., ars., ***aur-i.,*** bar-ac., ***bar-c.,*** calc-p., con., ***hyos., phos.,*** sec.

ensue, feels as if it would - ***acon.,*** ars., ***calc.,*** cimic., colch., ham., ***lac-c.,*** lil-t., med., ***merc.,*** phys., tarent.

envy, with - **LYC.**

INSANITY, general

erotic - ambr., **APIS, BAR-M.,** bell., bufo, ***calc-p.,*** camph., ***cann-i., canth.,*** ferul., gins., grat., **HYOS.,** kali-br., lil-t., lyss., manc., ***murx., nux-v., orig., phos., pic-ac.,*** **PLAT.,** ***puls.,*** rob., sal-n., ***stram., sulph., tarent.,*** **VERAT.,** zinc.

menses, after - ***kali-br.***

before - dulc., stann.

eruptions, after suppressed - bell., ***caust., hep.,*** stram., ***sulph., zinc.***

escape, desire to - ars., ***bell.,*** cupr., dig., hyos., nux-v., ***op., stram.,*** verat.

face, pale, with - camph., cortiso., merc., **STRAM.,** verat.

red, with - aur-i., calc., op., verat.

fanatics, of - aur-a., verat.

feces, passes her, on the floor - cupr.

feet, with a stamping of - ant-c., verat.

females, of - ***acon.,*** apis, ***bell.,*** cimic., ***orig.,*** plat., puls., stram., verat.

self accusation, from - hell.

stupor, alternating, with - apis

foolish, ridiculous - ***bell.,*** cic., **HYOS.,** merc., nux-m., nux-v.

fortune, gaining a, after - bell., ***caust.,*** puls., stram., verat.

losing a, after - ***aur.,*** calc., ign., rhus-t., verat.

fright or anger, caused by - **ARS., BELL.,** ***ign.,*** op., plat., staph.

gluttony, with - chin., **VERAT.**

alternating with refusal to eat - hyos., ip., stram., verat.

grief, from - **ARS., BELL.,** ***cocc.,*** **HYOS.,** ign., ***plat.***

haughty - ***hyos.,*** lach., **LYC., PLAT.,** ***stram.,*** **VERAT.**

head, washing in cold water, amel. - sabad.

heat, with - ***ars.,*** bell., cact., ***chin.,*** hyos., ***kali-p.,*** stram., verat.

humiliation, from - ***anac.,*** bell., **CARC.,** ***lach.,*** **NUX-V.,** plat., ***puls.,*** **STAPH.**

immobile as a statue - cham., fl-ac., hyos.

injuries, to the head, from - alco., carc., hell., ***nat-s.,*** stram.

insensibility, painlessness, with - **HYDR-AC.,** hyos., ***op.,*** stram.

lamenting, moaning, only - bell., hyos., stram.

lascivious - hyos., ***par., plat.,*** stram.

laughing, with - **HYOS.,** op., sec., ***stram., tarent., verat., verat-v.***

love, from disappointed - ***hyos.,*** ign., tarent.

malignant - agar., cann-s., ***cupr.,*** lyc.

masturbation, from - anan., bufo, ***cocc., hyos.,*** op., ***plb.***

megalomania - cupr., glon., ***graph., hyos., lach.,*** lyc., ***phos., plat., stram.,*** **SULPH.,** ***syph.,*** **VERAT.,** ***verat-v.***

melancholy - ars., ***aur.,*** bell., calc., caust., cic., hyos., ***ign.,*** nux-v., ***petr.,*** ph-ac., ***puls.,*** rhus-t., staph., sulph., verat.

INSANITY, general
menses, during - acon., ***bell.,*** lach., plat., puls., stram., verat.
before - cimic.
profuse, with - **IGN.,** sep.
suppressed, with - apis, ign., ***puls.***
menopausal period, during - aster., cimic., cycl., hipp., ***lach., lil-t., puls., sep., sulph.,*** ther., ***verat.***
mental labor, from - hyos., ***kali-p., lach.,*** **NUX-V.,** ***phos.,*** **TUB.**
mild - ***croc., verat.***
neuralgia, with disappearance of - cimic., ***nat-m.***
noisy - ***chlor.,*** verat.
obsession, with - anac., sulph.
obstinate in - ***dig., nux-v.***
onanism - bufo, ***cocc., hyos.***
pain, from intolerable - **ACON.,** ars., aur., ***colch., hyper.,*** **VERAT.**
paralysis, with - ars., kali-br., ***lach., phos.***
paroxysmal - ***bell.,*** cic., ***dig.,*** gels., kali-i., ***nat-m.,*** nat-s., phos., stram., ***tarent.***
periodical - ***con.,*** nat-s., ***plat., tarent.***
persecution, mania - ***anac.,*** **ARS.,** calc., caust., **LACH.,** meli., sulfon., verat.
perspiration, cold, with - stram.
following - cupr.
position, from fear to lose the - calc., ign., puls., rhus-t., staph., sulph., verat.
prayers, insists upon saying his, at the tail of his horse - euph.
raising hands and kneeling as in prayer - ***ars.,*** aur.
pregnancy, in - ***bell.,*** cimic., hyos., ***stram.***
pride, with - **HYOS.,** plat., **STRAM., VERAT.**
pulse, with frequent - ars., crot-h., cupr., ***cupr-ac.***
purchases, makes useless - con., **LACH.,** ***nux-v.***
quarrelsome - hyos.
rage - anac., ars-s-f., lach., stram.
religious - anac., ***ars.,*** aur., aur-a., bell., croc., ***hyos., kali-br., lach.,*** lil-t., lyc., merc., nat-c., nux-v., ***plat., puls.,*** **STRAM.,** ***sulph.,*** **VERAT.**
reproaches, others - **LYC.**
restlessness, with - ***ars.,*** bell., bry., canth., chin., ***hyos.,*** merc., nux-v., puls., stram., ***tarent.,*** verat., zinc.
with, legs, of - **TARENT.,** ***zinc.***
secretive - dig., tarent.
sexual excesses, from - anan., ***apis, lach.,*** lil-t., ***phos.,*** staph.
shy - agar.
signs, writes unintelligible - ars.
silent - verat., ***verat-v.***
sleeplessness, with - aur., ***bell.,*** carc., ***cocc., hyos., kali-br.,*** nux-m., op., ***stram., tarent.***
split his head in two, will - ***naja.***
stamps, the feet - ant-c., stram., verat.

INSANITY, general
staring of eyes - ***bell., camph.,*** crot-t., stram.
strength increased - agar., ***bell.,*** canth., cori-r., hyos., ***op., plb., stram.,*** **TARENT.**
stroke, after - hell.
suicidal disposition, with - ars., ***aur.,*** hyos., naja, verat.
syphilis, in - anag., merc., syph.
talkative, excessive - bell., bry., buth-a., hyos., **LACH.,** par., ***stram.***
threatens, destruction and death - **TARENT.**
tongue out, putting his, clicking, distortion of face, with - bell., lach.
touched, will not be - ***thuj.***
travel, with desire to - bell., bry., chin., hyos., nux-v., puls., stram., ***tub.,*** verat.
urine, passes on the floor - plb.
varicose veins, with - arn., ars., fl-ac., lach., lyc., sulph., ***zinc.***
after - anac., ant-c., arn., bell., caust., hyos., ign., lach., lyc., nux-v., phos., sep., sulph., verat.
wantonness, with - bell., cupr., ***hyos.,*** merc., mez., stram., verat.
wedding preparations, of - hyos.

INSECURITY - ***aml-n.,*** anh., **ARS.,** ***bry.,*** cann-s., cham., ***lyc.,*** sumb.
sense of - ail., aloe, ars.

INSOLENT - anac., bell., bufo, calc., ***canth., graph., hyos., lac-c.,*** lach., lil-t., **LYC.,** lyss., med., ***nat-m.,*** nit-ac., ***nux-v.,*** pall., par., ***petr.,*** phos., ***psor.,*** **PLAT.,** spong., staph., stram., sulph., **VERAT.**
afternoon - ***canth.***
children, in - sac-alb.
servants to chiefs, of - lyc., nat-m.

INTELLECTUAL - **ACON.,** anac., aur., bapt., **BAR-C., BELL.,** cann-i., cann-s., cocc., **HELL., HYOS.,** ign., **LACH.,** laur., **LYC.,** merc., nat-c., nat-m., nux-v., **OP., PH-AC., PHOS.,** ***plat., puls., rhus-t.,*** **SEP.,** sil., **STRAM., SULPH., VERAT.**

INTEMPERANCE, agg. - stram.

INTERRUPTION, agg. mental symptoms - colch., culx., ***nux-v.,*** staph., sulph., verat.

IRRESOLUTION, (see Indecision)

INTOLERANCE - ars., bar-c., caust., cham., cocc., con., ferr-p., merc., nux-v., psor., sulph.
afternoon - ferr-p.
ailments, of - nux-v.
hindrance, of - ferr-p.
interruption, of - cham., cocc.
spoken to, of being - cham.
vexation of - ferr-p.

INTOXICATED, as if - ***agar.,*** ail., am-c., arg-m., bapt., ***cann-s.,*** cocc., con., conch., kali-i., lil-t., meph., mosch., nux-m., rhus-t., ter.

INTROSPECTION - **ACON.**, alum., am-m., ***anh.***, arn., ***aur.***, bell., bism., bov., cann-i., canth., caps., carb-an., carl., caust., cham., ***chin.***, clem., **COCC.**, cycl., dig., dros., euph., euphr., hell., hyos., **IGN.**, ***indg.***, ***ip.***, lil-t., lyc., mag-m., meny., mez., mur-ac., nux-v., ol-an., olnd., op., phel., plb., **PULS.**, rheum, sabad., sars., ***sep.***, stann., staph., stram., **SULPH.**, verat., viol-o., viol-t.

afternoon - hell.

eating, after - aloe, ferr-ma.

forenoon - phos.

morning - nat-c.

night - ***camph.***

IRRITABILITY - abies-c., abrot., absin., ***acet-ac.***, **ACON.**, act-sp., adlu., ***aesc.***, ***aeth.***, ***agar.***, ***ail.***, alco., alf., allox., ***aloe***, **ALUM.**, alum-p., am-caust., am-m., ambr., am-c., amn-l., ***anac.***, anan., ang., anh., **ANT-C.**, ant-ox., ***ant-t.***, ap-g., **APIS**, arag., aran., ***arg-m.***, ***arg-n.***, ***arn.***, **ARS.**, ***ars-i.***, ars-s-f., ***art-v.***, arum-t., ***asaf.***, ***asar.***, asc-t., aspar., aster., atro., **AUR.**, aur-a., aur-i., aur-m., ***aur-s.***, bar-ac., ***bar-c.***, bar-i., bar-m., bar-s., **BELL.**, bell-p., benz-n., berb., ***bism.***, bol., bond., ***bor.***, **BOV.**, brach., brom., **BRY.**, bufo, but-ac., buth-a., cact., cadm-met., ***cadm-s.***, calad., **CALC.**, calc-ar., calc-br., calc-f., calc-i., ***calc-p.***, **CALC-S.**, calc-sil., calen., camph., ***camph-br.***, cann-i., cann-s., ***canth.***, ***caps.***, ***carb-ac.***, carb-an., **CARB-S.**, **CARB-V.**, ***carc.***, card-m., ***carl.***, cast., caste., ***caul.***, **CAUST.**, cedr., cench., cer-b., cer-s., **CHAM.**, chel., ***chin.***, ***chin-a.***, chin-s., chion., chlol., chlor., chlorpr., cic., cimic., cimx., ***cina***, cinnb., ***clem.***, cob-n., coca, ***cocc.***, coc-c., ***coff.***, ***colch.***, ***coloc.***, ***con.***, cop., cor-r., cori-r., corn., cortico., cortiso., crat., ***croc.***, ***crot-h.***, crot-t., cub., ***cupr.***, cupr-ac., cupr-ar., cupr-s., ***cycl.***, cyn-d., cyna., cyt-l., daph., des-ac., ***dig.***, digin., der., dios., dor., dros., ***dulc.***, elaps, equis., eup-per., euphr., eupi., euon., fago., fel., ***ferr.***, ferr-ar., ferr-i., ferr-p., fl-ac., form., gall-ac., ***gamb.***, ***gels.***, ***gran.***, **GRAPH.**, grat., guai., guat., ham., hell., ***helon.***, **HEP.**, hip-ac., hipp., hir., hist., hura, ***hydr.***, hydr-ac., hydroph., ***hyos.***, ***hyosin.***, hyper., iber., ***ign.***, ***ind.***, indol., ***iod.***, ***ip.***, iris, jatr., kali-ar., ***kali-bi.***, ***kali-br.***, **KALI-C.**, kali-chl., kali-f., **KALI-I.**, kali-n., ***kali-p.***, **KALI-S.**, kali-sil., kalm., kiss., ***kreos.***, kres., ***lac-c.***, lac-d., ***lach.***, lachn., lact., laur., ***lec.***, ***led.***, lept., **LIL-T.**, linu-c., lipp., lon-p., luf-op., **LYC.**, lycpr., ***lycps.***, lyss., macro., mag-arct., mag-aust., **MAG-C.**, mag-f., mag-m., ***mag-s.***, man., manc., ***mang.***, ***med.***, meli., menis., meph., ***merc.***, ***merc-c.***, ***merc-i-r.***, merl., ***mez.***, mill., mim-p., morph., mosch., ***mur-ac.***, ***murx.***, myric., nabal., naja, nat-a., **NAT-C.**, **NAT-M.**, nat-p., ***nat-s.***, nicc., nid., **NIT-AC.**, nit-s-d., nitro-o., nux-m., **NUX-V.**, oci., oena., ol-an., ***olnd.***, onop., ***op.***, orig., osm., ox-ac., paeon., ***pall.***, palo., par., ped., pers., **PETR.**, phel., **PH-AC.**, **PHOS.**, ***phyt.***, pic-ac., plan., **PLAT.**, plect., podo., prot., prun., ***psor.***, ptel., **PULS.**, pyrog., rad., **RAN-B.**, ran-s., rat., rheum, rhod., **RHUS-T.**, rhus-v., rumx., ***ruta***, ***sabad.***, sabin., sac-alb., sal-p., ***samb.***, sang., sanic., sant., sapin., sarcol-ac., saroth., ***sars.***, sec., sel., senec., seneg., **SEP.**, **SIL.**, sin-n., sol-m., sol-t-ae., ***spig.***, ***spong.***, squil., ***stann.***, **STAPH.**, ***stram.***, stront-c., **STRY.**, sul-i., sulfa., sulfonam., sulfon., **SULPH.**, **SUL-AC.**, ***sumb.***, syph., tab., ***tarent.***, tarax., tell., tep., teucr., thal., thea., thymol., thyr., til.

absent persons, with - aur., fl-ac., kali-cy., lyc.

after-pains, in - ***nux-v.***

afternoon - aeth., aloe, alum., anac., ant-t., ***bor.***, bov., calc-s., cann-i., cann-s., cast., chel., colch., ***con.***, cycl., elaps, graph., hydr-ac., ign., iod., lil-t., mag-c., mang., merc-c., mur-ac., nat-m., nit-ac., op., ox-ac., plb., ruta, sang., sars., sumb., thuj., zinc.

2 p.m. - mez.

4 p.m. - bor.

5 p.m. - paeon.

5 p.m. to 6 p.m. - ***con.***

air, in open - aeth., am-c., arn., bor., calc., ***con.***, kali-c., mur-ac., nux-v., plat., puls., rhus-t.

amel. - anac., calc., coff., ign., mag-c., ***rhus-t.***, stann.

alone, when - cortico., phos.

alone, wishes to be - bry.

alternating with

care - ran-b.

cheerfulness - ant-t., ars., ***aur.***, aur-a., bor., ***carc.***, caust., chin., cocc., croc., cycl., lyc., merc., merc-c., nat-c., nat-m., plat., ***ran-b.***, sanic., spig., spong., ***stram.***, sul-i., tell., zinc.

cowardice - ran-b.

crying - aur., bell.

hypochondriacal mood during day, merry in evening - sulph., viol-t.

indifference - asaf., bell., carb-an., colch., sep., ziz.

indignation - zinc.

jesting - cocc.

remorse - mez.

sadness - ambr., asar., ptel., puls., zinc.

tenderness - plat.

timidity - ran-b., zinc.

tolerance - nid.

anxiety, with - ars., **NUX-V.**, sabin.

suicide, with inclination to commit, afraid to die - **NUX-V.**

aroused, when - bufo, nux-m., op., sil.

back, lumbar region right, burning - nit-ac.

breakfast, after - con.

before - nat-p.

business, about - bor., ip., nat-m.

important, in an - ***bor.***

childbirth, during - caul., **CHAM.**, ***hyos.***, ***sep.***

children, in - abrot., ant-c., ant-t., ars., benz-ac., bor., bry., ***calc-p.***, caust., **CHAM.**, ***chin.***, **CINA**, cupr., dulc., gels., graph., ***iod.***, ip., kali-br., kali-p., kreos., lac-c., lyc., **MAG-C.**, phos., puls., rheum, rumx., sanic., sep., ***sil.***, ***staph.***, ***tub.***, zinc.

day and night, sleepless - ***psor.***

cross, good all night - **LYC.**

good, cross at night - ***jal.***

pushes nurse away - lyc.

scream by touch - **ANT-T.**

IRRITABILITY, general
children, in
sick, when - ***cham., lyc.***
sleepless day and night -carc., psor., syph.
children, towards - kali-i., ***nux-v., sep.***
chill, during - acon., alum., anac., arn., ***ars.,*** ars-s-f., aur., aur-a., bell., bor., bry., **CALC.,** calen., camph., **CAPS.,** carb-v., cast., ***caust.,*** cham., chin., chin-a., cimx., cocc., coff., **CON.,** cycl., gels., hep., hyos., ***ign.,*** kali-ar., kreos., **LYC.,** mag-aust., mag-c., merc., mez., nat-c., ***nat-m., nit-ac., nux-v., petr.,*** plan., phos., **PLAT.,** ***puls.,*** **RHEUM,** ***rhus-t., sabad.,*** sep., sil., ***spig.,*** staph., ***sulph.,*** teucr., thuj., verat.
coffee, after - calc-p., ***cham.,*** nux-v.
cold, after taking - calc.
consolation, agg. - ***bell.,*** bry., ***cact.,*** calc., ***calc-p.,*** calc-sil., chin., hell., **IGN.,** kali-c., kali-sil., lil-t., lyc., merc., **NAT-M.,** ***nit-ac.,*** nux-v., ***plat.,*** sabal., **SEP., SIL.,** staph.
contradiction, at slightest - **IGN.**
conversation, from - ***ambr.,*** plect.
convulsion, before - art-v., ***aster.,*** bufo, ***lach.***
cough, from - ***cina.***
whooping cough, in - ***bry., cupr-ac.***
day and night - ***cham.,*** ign., ip., lac-c., op., ***psor., stram.***
daytime - am-c., anac., ant-c., bism., calc., carb-v., caust., cycl., dulc., ip., iris, kreos., lyc., mag-c., med., merc., ***merc-c.,*** nat-c., nat-m., petr., phel., phos., plat., puls., sars., sep., stann., staph., sul-ac., sulph., verb., viol-t., zinc.
daytime, only - lyc., med.
dentition, during - calc., ***calc-p.,*** **CHAM.,** cina, kreos., **RHEUM,**
diabetes, in - ***helon., lycps.***
dinner, during - teucr.
after - am-c., cham., coc-c., ***hydr.,*** mill., ***nat-c.,*** teucr., til.
before - phos.
disease, before - caps.
disturbed, when - graph., op.
drinking, wine and coffe, while - chlor.
easily - ***phos., nux-v.***
eating, during - chlor., teucr.
after - aeth., am-m., ambr., am-c., arn., ars., ***bor., bry.,*** carb-v., cham., chlor., con., graph., ***hydr.,*** iod., ***kali-c.,*** kali-i., lyc., merc., merc-sul., ***nat-c., nat-m.,*** **NUX-V.,** plat., ***puls.,*** teucr., thuj.
amel. - am-c., am-m., kali-bi., nat-s., phos.
satiety, to - merc.
emission, after - coff., dig., ***lil-t.,*** nat-c., ***nux-v.,*** sang., sel., **STAPH.,** ust.
epilepsy, before - ***art-v., lach.***
evening - aesc., aloe, am-c., am-m., ant-c., ant-t., bar-c., bar-m., bar-s., bov., cahin., ***calc., calc-s.,*** calc-sil., canth., carb-s., ***cast., con.,*** cycl., dios., fago., ign., indg., jug-r., ***kali-c.,*** kali-m., kali-p., ***kali-s.,*** kali-sil., kalm., lach.,

IRRITABILITY, general
evening - lil-t., lyc., lyss., mag-c., mag-m., mur-ac., nabal., ***nat-c.,*** nat-m., nat-sil., nicc., ox-ac., pall., phos., plan., ***puls.,*** ran-b., sil., spig., **SULPH.,** sumb., trio., **ZINC., ZINC-P.,** ***zing.***
amel. in - aloe, am-c., bism., calc., mag-c., nat-m., nicc., verb., viol-t., zinc.
bed, in - upa.
children in brain affections - zinc.
excited, when - arg-n., chin.
exertion, from - ***sep.,*** sulph.
mental - pic-ac., sapin.
expression, from unintelligible - sol-t-ae.
family, to her - kali-fer., ***sep.,*** thuj.
fancied, occurences, about - meph.
fever, during - acon., anac., aran., ***ars.,*** atha., ***bry., cham.,*** carb-v., caust., chim-m., chin-m., cina, ***ferr.,*** hep., ip., lach., mag-arct., mosch., **NAT-C.,** ***nat-m., nux-v.,*** petr., ph-ac., phos., plan., ***psor.,*** puls., ***rheum,*** staph., ***sulph.,*** ust.
after - am-c., ***cina,*** hipp.
forenoon - aeth., am-c., am-m., ant-c., ant-t., arg-m., carb-an., carb-v., caust., cinnb., grat., hipp., lil-t., mag-c., mag-m., ***mang.,*** nat-m., nat-p., nicc., phos., plect., ran-b., seneg., sil., verat.
forgetfulness, because of his - carc.
grief, from - caust., ***ign., kali-br.,*** mag-c., nat-m.
hemorrhoids, with - ***apis,*** **NUX-V.**
headache, during - ***acet-ac.,*** acon., aeth., ***am-c.,*** am-m., ant-c., ***anac., ars.,*** bell., bov., **BRY.,** calc., calc-i., calc-p., calc-sil., ***cham., chin., chin-a.,*** chin-s., coca, con., cycl., dulc., graph., helon., hipp., ign., ind., iod., kali-ar., kali-c., kali-p., ***kreos., lac-c.,*** lach., lachn., laur., lyss., mag-m., ***mag-p.,*** mang., meph., merc., ***mez.,*** nat-m., ***nux-v., nicc.,*** op., pall., plat., ***phos., sang.,*** sil., spong., stann., **SYPH.,** teucr., thuj., vip., zinc., zinc-p.
before - chin-a., nat-s.
hurried, when - alum., merc., nux-v.
idle, while - calc., glon., lach., nat-m., nux-v., stann., sulph.
impotency, with - ***pic-ac.***
insults, from - canth.
itching, from - anac.
liver trouble, in (see Bilious) - ***bry., cham.,*** chel., **NUX-V.,** ***podo.***
lying, amel. on - sulfonam.
masturbation, after - ***hyos.***
medicine, at thought to take the - mim-p.
menopausal period, during - ***cimic.,*** ign., kali-br., ***lach.,*** manc., ***psor.,*** sel., **SEP.,** valer., zinc-valer.
menses, during - aeth., am-c., aran., asaf., bell., berb., bry., calc., cast., caust., ***cham.,*** cimic., cina, con., eupi., ferr., ind., kali-c., kali-p., kali-s., kreos., lyc., mag-c., mag-m., mag-s., nat-c., nat-m., nat-p., ***nux-v.,*** petr.,

IRRITABILITY, general

menses, during - ph-ac., plat., puls., sars., sep., stram., ***sulph.,*** tarent., zinc., zinc-p., zing.
an intermission of, during - eupi.
after - berb., bufo, carb-ac., cimic., ferr., nat-m.
before - berb., calc., ***caust., cham.,*** cocc., eupi., ign., kali-c., kali-fer., kreos.,***lach.,*** lil-t., ***lyc.,*** mag-m., morg-g., ***nat-m., nux-v., puls.,*** **SEP.,** thyr.

miscarriage, in - ***caul.***
threatened, in - ***cham.***

morning - am-c., am-m., ant-c., ant-t., bov., calad.,***calc.,*** canth., carb-an.,***carb-s.,*** carb-v., cast., cham., chin., cob-n., cocc., con., chlol., cycl., erig., graph., grat., hipp., ***iber.,*** kali-ar., kali-c., kali-p., kali-s., kali-sil., kalm., kreos., ***lach.,*** mag-c., mag-m., ***mang., merc-i-r.,*** myric., nat-c., ***nat-m.,*** nat-p., ***nat-s.,*** nicc., ***nit-ac.,*** nux-v., ***petr.,*** phos., plat., psor., ran-b., sabad., sang., sars., seneg., sep., sil., spong., **STAPH.,** stram., sul-ac., sulph., tarax., thuj., ***til.,*** verat., zinc., zinc-p.
7 a.m. - calad., sep.
children, in - ***chin.***
loss of blood, after - ***stict.***
rising, after - arg-n., calc., canth., carc., ***carl.,*** cham., coff., hep., mag-m., nat-s., phos., sulph.
stool, before - calc.
waking, on - agar., ant-t., arg-n., ars., ars-s-f., ***bell.,*** bov., bry., bufo, camph., carb-an., cham., coca, con., cupr., cycl., gamb., iris, jatr., kali-ar., ***kali-c.,*** kali-p., kali-s., lil-t., **LYC.,** ***mag-m., merc-i-r.,*** mez., nat-m., nat-s., ***nit-ac.,*** **NUX-V.,** petr., ph-ac., phos., plat., plb., ***puls.,*** rhus-t., sul-ac., ***sulph.,*** thuj., **TUB.**

music, during - anac., ***calc.,*** caust., ***mang., nat-c.,*** nat-m., nux-v., sep., viol-o., zinc.
harsh, from - sumb.
piano, of - anac., nat-c., ***sep.,*** zinc.
violin, of - viol-o.

night - anac., ant-t., anthr., bor., camph., cham., chin., coloc., ***jal.,*** lyc., nux-v., phos., pic-ac., rheum, **RHUS-T.,** sabad.
night, 1 p.m. to 2 a.m. - thea.
babies, in sick - ***psor.***
day and - cham., lac-c., op., psor., stram.
only - ant-t., ***jal.,*** lac-c., nux-v., psor., rheum
retiring after - bufo, cinnb.
visions, with frightful - camph.
waking, on - lyc., ***psor.***

noise, from - allox., ant-t., ars., bell., caust., cinnb., cocc., ***ferr.,*** iod., ip., kali-c., nat-m., phos., pip-m., plect., ptel., puls-n, trio., ven-m.
crackling of newspapers, even from - ***asar., ferr.,*** ign., lyc., nat-c.

noon - am-m., aster., cinnb., kali-c., nat-c., nat-m., rumx., teucr., zinc.
amel. - aeth.

pain, during - aloe, ars., **BRY.,** canth., **CHAM.,** colch., ***coloc.,*** hep., ign., ***op.***

IRRITABILITY, general

perspiration, during - ang., bry., ***calc.,*** calc-p., ***cham.,*** clem., hep., mag-c., ***merc.,*** nat-m., **RHEUM,** sep., ***sulph.,*** thuj.

pollutions, after - coff., dig., ***lil-t.,*** nat-c., ***nux-v.,*** sang., sel., **STAPH.,** ust.

pregnancy, during - ***cham., sep.***

prolapsus, uterus, in - ***lil-t., sep.***

puberty, in - ign., ***phos., sep.***

questioned, when - apis, ***arn.,*** **BRY.,** bufo, ***cham.,*** coloc., nat-m., **NUX-V.,*****ph-ac.,*** puls., ust.

reading, while - med., nat-c.

remorse, with easy and quick - ***sulph., tub.***

rocking, fast amel. - cham., ***cina.***

sadness, with - asar., **AUR.,** bov., dig., kali-br., ***kali-c.,*** **KALI-I.,** lyc., ***nat-m.,*** nit-ac., polyg., plat., ptel., puls., sal-ac., sep., sul-ac., ***sulph.,*** ziz.

sends the, doctor home, says he is not sick - ***apis,*** **ARN., CHAM.**
nurse home - cham., ***fl-ac.***
out of the room - **CHAM.**

sex, after - agar., bov., calad., **CALC.,** calc-s., calc-sil., ***chin.,*** dig., graph., ***kali-c.,*** kali-p., ***kali-sil.,*** mag-m., ***nat-c.,*** nat-m., nat-sil., nit-ac., nux-v., ***petr., phos.,*** ph-ac., ***sel.,*** **SEP., SIL.,** staph., thuj.
amel. - ***tarent.***

sexual, appetite, loss of, from - sabal.
excesses, from - ol-an.
excitement, from - ***nux-v.***
weakness, with - ***pic-ac.***

sitting, while - aeth., calc., mang., nat-m.

sleep, during, by noise - calad., ***thuj.***
after, in children - lyc., nux-v.

sleepiness, with - ind.

sleeplessness, with - bell., calc., ***coff.,*** **HYOS.,** ***kali-br.,*** mosch., ***nat-m.,*** plat., psor.
children, in - cham., psor.

spoken to, when - ars., aur., aur-a., bufo, carb-s., **CHAM.,** elaps, gels., ***graph.,*** hyos., ***kali-p., lil-t.,*** nat-m., nat-s., ***nit-ac.,*** nux-v., rhus-t., ***sep.,*** sil., staph., stram., ***sulph.,*** ter., ust., verat.

stool, after - graph., nat-c., ***nit-ac.,*** rheum.
before - aloe, ***bor., calc.,*** merc., ***nux-v.***

supper, after - arn., nat-c.

suspicious - cham., lyc., merc.

taciturn - am-c., ars., coloc., puls., sulph.

takes, everything in bad part - alum., bov., caust., ***croc.,*** nat-m., ***pall.,*** puls.

talking, while - alum., ambr., cham., mang., nicc., psor., staph., sul-ac., teucr., zinc.

thunderstorm, before - nat-c.

touch, by - ***ant-c.,*** lach., tarent.

travel, is too slow, when the - cortiso.

trifles, from - ang., ant-c., arg-m., ***ars.,*** aspar., ***bell.,*** bry., ***calc.,*** calc-sil., cann-s., carb-v., ***caust.,*** **CHAM.,** ***cimic., cina, clem.,*** cocc., croc., graph., hell., ***hep.,*** hist., ign., ip., kali-bi., kreos., lach., lyc., ***med.,*** meph., ***mez.,*** nat-c.,

IRRITABILITY, general

trifles, from - ***nat-m.,*** nat-p., **NIT-AC., NUX-V.,** petr., ***phos., plat., ptel.,*** saroth., sep., sil., stram., sulph., verat.

vaginal discharge ceases, as soon as - ***hydr.***

waking, on - agar., anac., ant-t., arg-n., ***ars., bell.,*** berb., bov., brom., bry., bufo, calad., camph., carb-an., cast., caust., cham., chel., chin., chin-a., chin-s., ***cina,*** clem., coca, cupr., ***cycl.,*** gamb., iris, jatr., ***kali-c.,*** kali-p., ***lach.,*** lil-t., **LYC.,** mag-aust., mag-m., ***merc-i-r.,*** mez., nat-m., nat-s., nat-sil., ***nit-ac.,*** **NUX-V.,** pall., petr., ***ph-ac.,*** plat., plb., ***psor.,*** puls., rhus-t., sep., sulph., sul-ac., thuj., **TUB.**

amel. - caps.

whooping cough, in - ***bry.***

walking, when - am-c., berb., ***bor.,*** clem., con., sumb., thuj.

air, amel. in open - mag-c., **RHUS-T.**

warm, room - anac., calc., ign., ***puls.***

water, hearing or seeing, on - **LYSS.**

weakness, from - mur-ac.

weakness, with - **CHIN.,** gall-ac., ***kali-p.***

weather, in rainy or cloudy - aloe, am-c.

whooping cough, in - ***bry., cupr-ac.***

working, when - plan.

worm, affections, in - **CINA,** fil.

ISOLATION, feelings of, (see Abandoned) - ***anac., anh., arg-n.,*** arist-cl., camph., cann-i., cann-s., coca, cortico., hura, ***nat-m.,*** plat., ***puls.,*** stram., ***thuj.***

JEALOUSY, feelings - anac., anan., ***apis,*** ars., bufo, calc., calc-p., ***calc-s.,*** camph., ***caust., cench.,*** cocc., coff., coloc., gall-ac., **HYOS.,** ign., ip., kali-ar., ***kali-c.,*** **LACH.,** lil-t., ***lyc., med.,*** nat-m., **NUX-V.,** op., ph-ac., ***plat., puls.,*** raph., ***staph., stram.,*** thuj., verat.

accuses wife of being faithless - ***lach., stram.***

ailments from - ***apis,*** **HYOS.,** ***ign., lach.,*** **NUX-V.,** ***phos.,*** **PULS.,** staph.

animals and objects, of - **CAUST.,** hyos., lach., nux-v.

appreciate anything, desires that others shall not - ***ip.***

brutal from, gentle husband becoming - calc., ***lach.,*** nux-v., sulph.

children, between - ars., lyc., ***nat-m., nux-v., puls.,*** sep.

crying, with - ***caust.,*** nux-v., ***petr.***

drunkenness, during - ***hyos.,*** **LACH.,** nux-v., puls.

foolish as it is irresistible - ***hyos., lach.***

happy, seeing others - hell.

images, with frightful - ***lach.***

impotency, with - calad., lyc., nux-v.

insane - ***hyos., lach.***

insult, driving to - ***nux-v.***

irrational - coca.

kill, driving to - **HYOS.,** lach.

men, between - ***ars.,*** lach., lyc., nux-v., puls., verat.

neglect, accuses husband of - ***stram.***

people around, of - op.

JEALOUSY, feelings

quarrels, reproaches, scolds, with - ***lach., nux-v.***

rage, with - **HYOS.**

sadness, with - ***kali-ar.***

sexual excitement, with - calc., caust., chin., con., nux-v., phos.

strikes his wife - ***calc., lach., nux-v.,*** sulph.

talkative, excessive, with - lach., mag-c., petr.

tearing the hair - lach.

vengeful - hyos., ***lach.***

women, between - ars., ***nat-m., nux-v.,*** sep.

JOKING, jesting - aeth., ether, agav-t., aloe, arg-m., ars., bar-c., bell., bry., calc., cann-i., ***caps.,*** carb-v., ***cic., cocc.,*** coff., **CROC.,** cupr., glon., **HYOS., IGN.,** ip., kali-cy., ***kali-i., lach.,*** lyc., meny., merc., merl., nat-m., ***nux-m.,*** op., peti., plat., psor., rhus-r., **RHUS-T.,** sars., sec., spong., ***stann.,*** staph., ***stram.,*** sul-ac., tab., ***tarent.***

alternating with, anger - caps., ign.

crying - ***ign.***

indifference - meny.

seriousness - plat.

vexation - cocc.

averse to - ***acon.,*** am-c., ang., apis, ars., bor., bov., caps., carb-an., ***cina,*** cocc., cycl., ***merc.,*** nat-m., nux-v., puls., sabin., sil., spig., staph., sulph., thuj.

erotic - bell., ***calc.,*** hyos., nux-v.

facetious, desire to do something - cact.

fun of somebody, making - ***lach.***

gravity, after - plat.

indifference, after - meny.

joke, cannot take a - ***acon.,*** ang., caps., **IOD.,** lyc., merc., nat-m., nux-v., puls., sulph.

licentious - alco.

malicious - ars.

puns, makes - cann-i.

ridiculous or foolish - bell., ***cic.,*** croc., **HYOS.,** ***stram.,*** tanac., ***verat.***

trifles with everything - agar., alum., con.

waking, on - tarent.

JOY, ailments from excessive - ***acon.,*** caust., **COFF.,** croc., cycl., helon., ***manc.,*** nat-c., ***op., ped., puls.,*** verat.

alternating with irritability - cycl.

fits of joy with bursts of laughter - ***asaf.,*** verb.

headache from excessive joy - ***coff.,*** cycl., op., puls., scut.

misfortune of others, at the - ars., anac.

sleeplessness from excessive - **COFF.**

JUMPING, behaviour

bed, out of - absin., ***acon.,*** aeth., alco., ambr., ant-t., ***arg-n., ars.,*** atro., **BELL.,** bry., calc., camph., **CHIN.,** chin-a., ***chin-s.,*** chlol., cic., ***cupr.,*** cupr-ac., dub., gall-ac., ***glon.,*** **HYOS.,** lach., lyss., ***merc.,*** merc-c., merc-meth., **OP.,** phos., plb., puls., rumx., sabad., sol-m., **STRAM.,** sul-ac., ***syph.,*** **VERAT-V.**

crawls on floor, and - acet-ac.

fever, during - chin-a., ***hyos.,*** morph.

JUMPING, behaviour
bed, out of
frightful dream, from a - dulc.
mania, in - ***cupr-ac., puls.***
returning to bed continually, and - bell.
children, in evening - **CINA.**
chairs, on , tables and stove - ***bell.***
start, scream fearfully - nat-c., sulph.
impulse, to - agar., ***aur.,*** croc., stram., tarent.
bridge, when crossing a - arg-n., merc.
dreams, in - calc-f.
epilepsy, after - arg-m.
height, from a - anac., ***arg-n.,*** **AUR.,** gels., staph.
river, into - ***arg-n.,*** sec., sil.
run recklessly, and - sabad.
suddenly, as from pain - cina.
window, from - aeth., arg-m., arg-n., ars., **AUR.,** bell., camph., ***carb-s.,*** chin., crot-c., gels., ***glon.,*** thea., thuj., verat.
pain makes her so desparate that she would like to - aur.
wall, boys will jump a straight, and try to scramble up it - petr.
wild leaps in mania puerperal - ***nux-v.***

KICKING, behaviour - ***bell.,*** carb-v., ***cham.,*** cina, ***lyc.,*** nux-v., prot., ***stram.,*** stry., tarent., verat-v.
child is cross, kicks and scolds on waking - lyc.
legs, with - ign.
sleep, in - **BELL.,** cina, nat-c., phos., ***sulph.***
stiff and kicks when carried, becomes - ***cham.,*** cina,
worm affections, in - ***carb-v.,*** cina.

KILL, impulse or desire to - agar., alco., alum., anac., ***ars., ars-i., bell.,*** calc., camph., chin., cupr., cur., **HEP., HYOS.,** ***iod.,*** kali-ar., ***lach., lyc.,*** lyss., ***merc., nux-v.,*** op., ***petr., phos., plat.,*** sec., sil., ***staph., stram.,*** syph., thea., thyr., x-ray.
alcoholics, in - ***ars.***
barber wants to kill his customer - ***ars., hep.***
child, his own - merc., ***plat.***
delirium, in - chlf.
desire to kill the person that contradicts her - ***merc.***
drunkenness, during - bell., hep., ***hyos.***
everyone he sees - ***hyos.***
herself, sudden impulse to - iod., meli., merc., ***nat-s., nux-v.,*** rumx., thea., thuj.
husband, impulse to kill her beloved - anac., ***merc., nux-v., plat.,*** thea.
menses, agg. during - ***merc.***
razor, therefore implores him to hide his - ***merc.***
knife, with a - ***alum.,*** ars., chin., ***hep., hyos.,*** **LYC.,** lyss., ***merc., nux-v.,*** plat., ***stram.***
at sight of a - ***alum., merc.,*** nux-v., plat.
at sight of a, knife or a gun - ***alum.,*** merc., plat.
loved ones - ars., chin., merc., ***nux-v., plat.***

KILL, impulse or desire to
menses, during - ***merc.,*** x-ray.
before - lach., sep., x-ray.
offense, sudden impulse to kill for a slight - ***hep., merc., nux-v.***
parents, in a child - ***der.***
poison, impulse to - ars., lach., nux-v.
rest, during - iod.
somebody, thought he ought to kill - anac., camph., ***hyos.***
something urges her to kill her husband, of whom she is very fond - anac., ***merc., nux-v., plat.,*** thea.
sudden impulse to - **ALUM.,** arg-n., ***ars., ars-i., hep.,*** iod., kali-ar., merc., ***nux-v., plat.,*** staph., sulfon., sulph., thea.
herself - merc.
threatens to - ***hep.,*** lach., meli., ***tarent.***
those who approach - meli.
wife and children - ***hep., lach.***
throw child, sudden impulse to, fire, into - hep., lyss., ***nux-v.,*** thea.
window, out of - lyss., thea.
walking in open air, while - camph., hyos.
woman, irresistible, impulse to kill a - ***iod.***

KILLED, desires to be (see Loathing, Suicidal)- ***ars.,*** **AUR.,** bell., carc., coff-t., ***phyt.,*** stram.
labor, during - ***coff-t.***
stabbing heart, by - ***ars.***

KISSES, carress children, and - ***puls.***
everyone - agar., caps., ***croc., hyos.,*** kres., man., phos., plat., stram., ***verat.***
his companions' hands - agar., anac.
menses, before - ***verat.,*** zinc.

KLEPTOMANIA - ***absin.,*** ars., ***art-v.,*** **BELL.,** bry., calc., carb-v., caust., cic., ***cur.,*** hyos., kali-br., kali-c., lyc., med., nat-m., ***nux-v.,*** **OP.,** oxyt., plat., ***puls.,*** sep., sil., staph., stram., ***sulph.,*** syph., tarent., ***thuj.***
dainties - mag-m., nat-c.
money - calc., op., puls.
steals, dainties - mag-m., nat-c.

KNEELING and praying - ***ars., aur.,*** euph., nat-s., ***stram.,*** verat.
agg. - cocc., mag-c., ***sep.***
amel. - aesc., euph.
difficult - tarent.

LAMENTING, wailing - ***acet-ac., acon.,*** act-sp., ***alum.,*** ambr., am-c., ***anac.,*** arg-n., arn., ***ars.,*** asaf., **AUR.,** aur-a., aur-s., bar-s., ***bell., bism.,*** brom., ***bry.,*** bufo, calad., ***calc.,*** calc-ar., calc-sil., camph., ***canth.,*** caps., caust., ***cham., chin., cic., cina,*** cocc., ***coff., coloc., cor-r.,*** cupr., cupr-ac., cycl., dig., dulc., hell., hyos., ign., ip., kali-ar., kali-br., kali-i., kali-p., ***lach.,*** **LYC.,** lyss., mag-p., merc., morph., ***mosch.,*** nat-a., ***nat-c.,*** nat-m., nit-ac., nux-m., **NUX-V.,** ***op.,*** petr., ph-ac., phos., plat., plb., **PULS.,** ran-b., rheum, rhus-t., rob., sec., sep., sil., stann., staph., stram., stry., ***sulph.,*** syph., tarent., thal., til., tub., **VERAT., VERAT-V.,** viol-t., zinc.
alternating with, anger - arn.
crying - bufo.

LAMENTING, wailing
alternating, with, delirium - bell.
laughing - ars-s-f.
anxiety in epigastrium, about - ars.
anxious - plb., puls.
appreciated, because he is not - calc-s.
asleep, while - alum., arn., bry., ***cham.***, ***cina,*** mag-arct., op., ph-ac., phos., stann., stram., sulph.
convulsions, during - ars.
evening - **VERAT.**
fever, during - puls., til.
future, about - lyc.
heat of whole body except hands, with - **PULS.**
hoarse - brom.
imaginary misfortune, over his - alum-p.
involuntary - ***alum.***
loud, piercing - ***ars.***
menses, during - ars., ***cocc.***
morning on waking - ***cina.***
night - stram., verat.
waking, on - sil.
others, about - merc.
pain, during - nux-v.
about the pain - ars., cham., **COLOC.,** **LACH.,** ***mag-p.,*** ***nux-v.***
perspiration, during - ign.
sadness, in - ***puls.***
sickness, about his - arg-n., ars., **LACH.,** nux-v., ph-ac.
stool, if children have urging before - **RHEUM.**
trifles, over - ***coff.***
waking, on - ant-t., cina, merc., sil., ***stram.***

LASCIVIOUSNESS, (see Sexual, behaviour)

LATE, always - ***calc.,*** plat., puls., sil.

LAUGHING, behaviour - acon., acon-l., ether, agar., alco., aloe, alum., ambr., am-c., anac., anan., apis, ***arg-m.,*** arn., ***ars.,*** arund., asaf., ***aur.,*** aur-a., bar-c., ***bell.,*** **BOR.,** ***bufo,*** ***calc.,*** **CANN-I.,** cann-s., caps., carb-v., cast-eq., caust., cic., ***coff.,*** con., cor-r., cori-r., ***croc.,*** crot-h., ***cupr.,*** cypr., elae., ***ferr.,*** ferr-ar., graph., hell., hura, **HYOS., IGN.,** kali-bi., kali-p., keroso., kreos., ***lach.,*** lepi., lil-t., ***lyc.,*** merl., nat-a., nat-c., ***nat-m.,*** ***nux-m.,*** nux-v., op., peti., **PHOS.,** ***plat.,*** plb., puls., ran-s., rob., sabad., sant., sarr., sec., ***sep.,*** sil., spong., ***stann.,*** **STRAM.,** stry., sulph., sumb., tab., tarax., ***tarent.,*** valer., verat., verb., zinc., zinc-s.
actions, at his own - iris, stram.
agg. - acon., ang., ***arg-m.,*** arg-n., ***ars.,*** aur., ***bell.,*** **BOR.,** cann-i., cann-s., ***carb-v.,*** ***chin.,*** ***coff.,*** con., cupr., ***dros.,*** hyos., kali-c., laur., ***mang.,*** mez., mur-ac., nat-m., nux-v., **PHOS.,** ***plb.,*** **STANN.,** sulph., syph., tell., ther.
aloud - calc-f.
excessive - coff.
ailments from laughing, excessive - ***coff.***
air, in open - ***nux-m.,*** ***plat.***
alternating with
agony, fear of death - ***plat.***

LAUGHING, behaviour
alternating with, anxiety - stram.
frenzy - stram.
gaiety - stram.
groaning - ars-s-f., bell., crot-c., stram., verat.
loathing of life - ***aur.***
metrorrhagia - crot-c.
quarrelsomeness - croc.
quietness - hyos.
rage, frenzy - acon., stram.
sadness - canth., caust., nat-c., nid., ***phos.,*** stram., zinc.
seriousness - nux-m., plat.
screaming - asaf., croc., ign., kali-p., mosch., ***nux-m.***
spasms - alum.
taciturnity - plat.
tenderness - croc.
vexation, ill-humor - croc., sanic., stram.
violence - croc., stram.
whining, moaning - hyos., verat.
annoying - bell.
anxiety, during - lyc., nat-m.
after - ***cupr.,*** lyc.
asthma, with - bov.
averse, to - ambr., bar-c.
barking, dog, as a - ***ether.***
bed, in - agar.
beside herself, claps hands over head - ***sec.***
causeless - arn., bar-c., bufo, cann-i., syph., tab.
childish - bar-c., bufo, croc.
children, in - aloe, cypr.
insane - camph.
chill, during - agar., calc.
followed by - hura.
chorea, in - caust.
company, in - tarent.
constant - **CANN-I.,** cann-s., ***hyos.,*** verat., ***verat-v.,*** ***zinc.***
contemptuous - alum.
convulsions, before, during or after - ***alum.,*** aur-m-n., ***bell.,*** calc., ***camph.,*** ***caust.,*** con., cypr., ***ign.,*** mosch., ***plat.,*** stram., zinc.
between paroxysms - alumn., plat.
cries, and, by turns - asaf., bov., coff., croc., ign., mosch., ***nux-m.,*** samb.
crying, and, at same time - cann-i., lyc.
or, on all occasions - calc-sil., ***caust.,*** **PULS.,** sep., ***staph.***
quickly followed by - croc.
cyanosis, with - cann-i., cann-s.
daytime - peti.
delirious - apis, bell., cupr., hyos., op., stram., verat.
desire, to - nitro-o., ***tarent.***
dream, during - alum., caust., hyos., lyc.
laughing during comic dream, continues after waking - ***sulph.***
easily - ars., arund., ***puls.***
eating, after - puls.
epilepsy, after - cupr.

LAUGHING, behaviour

evening - cupr., ether, nat-m., sulph., valer., zinc.

everything, seems ludicrous - hyos., lyc., ***nux-m.,*** sabad.

exhausted, condition, during - con.

foolish - ***hyos.***

forced - hyos.

forenoon - graph., nux-m.

gaiety, with - hyos., stram.

grinning - bell.

hysterical - acon., ***alum.,*** alum-sil., am-c., anac., ant-t., apis, arn., ***ars.,*** asaf., **AUR.,** ***bell., calc.,*** cann-s., carb-an., caust., cic., cocc., ***con., croc.,*** cupr., hyos., **IGN.,** lyc., nat-c., nat-m., nux-m., ***phos.,*** plat., sant., ***sec.,*** sel., sil., **STRAM.,** sulph., sumb., **VALER.,** verat., ***zinc.***

idiotic - ***atro.,*** merc-meth.

ill humor, with - stram.

imbecility, in - hyos., stram.

immoderately - ***am-c.,*** anac., bar-c., bell., **CANN-I.,** carb-v., coff., ***croc.,*** cupr., ferr., graph., ***hyos.,*** ign., ***mosch., nat-m.,*** nitro-o., ***nux-m., nux-v., plat.,*** ran-s., stram., ***stry., stry-p.,*** tarent., verb., zinc., zinc-oc.

involuntarily - agar., aur., bell., ***bor., cann-i.,*** carb-s., con., croc., hyos., **IGN.,** lyc., mang., ***nat-m., nit-ac.,*** op., phos., plb., puls., sep., ***tarent.,*** zinc-oc., zinc-s.
- eating, after - puls.
- joyless, yet - lyc.
- speaking, when - aur.
- spine, from pressure on - agar.
- tears, with - phos.
- yawning, after - agar.

irritation, in stomach and hypochondria, from - con.

joy, with excessive - asaf., verb.

joyless - lyc.

looked at, when - lyc.

loudly - agar., **BELL.,** cann-s., croc., hydr-ac., ***hyos.,*** op., ***stram.***

love, from disappointed - ***hyos.***

ludicrous, everything seems - coca, ***hyos.,*** lyc., ***nux-m.,*** sabad.

menopause, during - ferr.

menses, before - coca, ***hyos., nux-m.***

midnight - kreos., sil.

misfortune, at - apis

mocking - tarent.

morning - graph., hura, lach., phos., plat., psor.
- 7 a.m. to 8 a.m. - hura.

nervous - mosch., nat-m., tarent.

never - am-c., am-m., **ARS.,** aur., hep., ***nit-ac.***

night - alum., ambr., caust., cic., kreos., lyc., op., sep., sil., stram., sulph., verat.

overwork, after - ***cupr.***

pain, every paroxysm of, excites a nervous laugh - hura, nux-v.

LAUGHING, behaviour

paroxysmal - **BELL.,** stram.

peculiar, to herself - thyr.

perspiration, ending in profuse - ***cupr.***

rage, with - ***stram.***

reprimands, at - graph.

reproach, at - ***graph.***

sad, when - phos.

sadness, followed by - plat.
- ends in - ign.

sardonic - **BELL.,** camph., cann-i., ***caust., colch.,*** con., croc., hydr-ac., ***hyos.,*** ign., nux-m., ***oena.,*** phyt., plb., ran-b., ran-s., ***sec.,*** sol-n., ***stram.,*** stry., tarent., verat., zinc., zinc-p.

scornful - alum.

screaming, shrieking - croc., cypr.

screams, then - tarent.

serious matters, over - ***anac.,*** apis, arg-n., bufo, cann-i., cast-eq., ign., lil-t., lyc., ***nat-m.,*** nux-m., phos., ***plat.,*** sulph.
- air, in open - ***plat.***

sexual excitement, with - hyos., stram.

silly - apis, bell., bufo, cic., croc., crot-c., ether, **HYOS.,** ***lach.,*** lyc., merc., nux-m., ***par.,*** stram., stry., zinc-p.
- children at every occasion, in - croc.

sleep, during - alum., bell., caust., croc., cypr., ***hyos.,*** junc., kreos., **LYC.,** nat-hchls., ph-ac., sep., ***sil., stram.,*** **SULPH.**
- going to, on - sulph.

spasmodic - acon., ***alum.,*** alum-p., alumn., am-c., anac., ant-t., apis, arn., ars., asaf., **AUR.,** ***bell., calc.,*** cann-i., cann-s., carb-an., ***caust.,*** cic., cocc., colch., ***con.,*** croc., cupr., ether, hyos., **IGN.,** lyc., mosch., nat-c., nat-m., nux-m., oena., op., ***phos.,*** plat., sec., sel., sil., ***stram.,*** stry., sulph., sumb., thala., thuj., valer., verat., zinc., zinc-oc., zinc-p.
- asthma, with - bov.
- before, during or after epilepsy - ***bufo,*** caust.
- crys, and, by turns - ign., sumb.
- epilepsy, after - cupr.
- tittring - bufo.
- uncontrollable - mosch.
- wrong places, at - plat.

speaking, when - aur., bell.

speechlessness, with - stram.

stomach and hypochondria, from irritation in - con.

stupid expression, with - apis, atro., ***nux-m., tarent.***

trifles, at - am-c., anac., ars., bufo, ***cann-i., croc.,*** graph., ***hyos.,*** ign., ***lyc., mosch.,*** nux-m., ped., ***plat., stram., stry-p.,*** tarent., zinc., zinc-oc.

tritillation, all over with an irresistible desire to - zinc-s.

unbecoming - croc.

uncontrollable - mosch.

vexation, at - lyc.

violent - ran-s., stram.

LAUGHING, behaviour

waking, on - sep.

weakness, during - con.

wildly - atro., calc.

word said, at every - **CANN-I.**

wrong, places, at - plat.

LAZINESS, indolence - abrot., acon., acon-l., aesc., ***agar.,*** agar-cit., ail., alco., alet., aloe, ***alum.,*** alum-p., alum-sil., am-c., am-m., ambr., ammc., ***anac.,*** ant-c., ant-t., anth., ***apis,*** apoc., arag., arg-m., ***arg-n., arn.,*** ars., ars-h., ars-i., ars-m., ars-s-f., asaf., asar., asc-t., ***aster.,*** atro., ***aur.,*** aur-a., aur-i., ***aur-m.,*** aur-s., bapt., bar-ac., bar-c., bar-i., bell., berb., berb-a., blatta-a., bor., bov., brom., ***bry.,*** bufo, buf-s., cadm-s., cadm-met., caj., ***calc., calc-ar., calc-f.,*** calc-i., ***calc-p.,*** calc-sil., camph., ***cann-s.,*** canth., ***caps.,*** carb-ac., carb-an., **CARB-S.,** ***carb-v.,*** carl., ***caust.,*** cer-b., cham., **CHEL., CHIN.,** chin-a., chin-s., cic., cinnb., clem., cob., ***cob-n., coca,*** cocaine, cocc., coc-c., coff., colch., con., ***corn.,*** croc., crot-h., crot-t., culx., cupr., ***cycl.,*** cyn-d., dicha., dig., dios., dirc., dros., dulc., elaps, erig., eug., euon., euphr., ferr., ferr-p., ferul., ***form.,*** gamb., ***gels.,*** gins., glon., gran., **GRAPH.,** grat., guai., ***ham.,*** hell., helo., helon., ***hep.,*** hera., hura, hydr., hydr-ac., hyos., hyper., ign., ilx-p., ind., indg., indol., ***iod.,*** ip., jug-r., kali-ar., ***kali-bi.,*** kali-br., ***kali-c.,*** kali-cy., kali-n., kali-p., kali-s., kiss., ***lac-c.,*** lac-ac., lac-d., **LACH.,** lact., laur., lec., lil-t., linu-c., **LYC.,** mag-arct., mag-aust., mag-c., mag-f., ***mag-m.,*** mag-s., manc., meny., ***meph., merc.,*** merl., ***mez.,*** meli., mill., mur-ac., nat-a., nat-c., nat-h., **NAT-M.,** nat-n., nat-p., nat-s., nat-sil., nid., **NIT-AC.,** nitro-o., **NUX-V.,** ol-an., olnd., op., osm., ox-ac., pall., par., paull., petr., ***ph-ac.,*** **PHOS., PIC-AC.,** pip-m., plan., ***plat.,*** plb., plect., ***psor.,*** **PULS.,** ran-b., ran-s., rheum, rhod., rhus-g., rhus-t., rob., rumx., ruta, sabad., ***sabin.,*** sang., sarcol-ac., saroth., sarr., sars., sec., seneg., **SEP.,** sieg., ***sil.,*** spig., spira., spong., squil., stann., ***staph.,*** stram., stront-c., sul-i., **SULPH.,** sumb., syph., tab., tarax., tarent., ***teucr.,*** thea., ***ther., thuj.,*** thymol., tong., **TUB.,** uran-n., valer., verat., verb., viol-t., visc., wild., ***zinc.,*** **ZINC-P.,** zing., ziz.

afternoon - aloe, anac., ***bor.,*** bufo, buf-s., chel., erig., gels., hyos., lyc., mag-c., mag-s., nat-m., op., petr., sep., sil., viol-t.

2 p.m. - chel.

air, in open - arn.

amel. - calc., graph.

amenorrhea, in - cycl.

amused, when not - carb-s.

anger, after - ***nux-v.***

breakfast, after - nat-s.

burning in the right lumbar region, with - nit-ac.

business, when transacting - nux-v., opun-v.

changing to mania for work - aur-s.

children - bar-c., lach.

chill, during - camph.

content, with - ziz.

damp weather - sang.

LAZINESS, indolence

daytime - digin., phos., plan., ran-b.

difficulties, in face of - cocc.

dinner, after - agar., ant-c., bar-c., ***chel., chin.,*** mag-c., tong., zinc.

disappointment, from - nux-v.

eating, after - agar., anac., asar., ant-c., bar-c., bov., cann-i., chel., ***chin.,*** dig., ign., ***kali-c.,*** lach., ***lyc.,*** mag-c., ***nat-m.,*** nux-m., nux-v., ol-an., ***ph-ac., phos.,*** plat., plb., thuj., zinc.

emission, after an - nat-c., sep.

evening - agar., calc-p., cann-s., carb-v., coca, dios., erig., ferr-i., form., mag-c., mag-m., nat-m., pall., plb., puls., ran-s., spig., sulfon., **SULPH.,** viol-t.

amel. - aloe, bism., clem., sulph.

forenoon - ***alum.,*** alumn., anac., hipp., indg., lach., mag-c., nat-m.

housework, aversion to her usual - ***cit-ac.***

intelligent, although very - alum., am-c., con., ***graph., petr.***

lumbar region right, with burning - nit-ac.

masturbation, after - ***dig., gels.***

morning - all-c., aloe, alum., am-c., am-m., ambr., ammc., anac., ang., ant-t., canth., carb-an., carb-s., ***carb-v.,*** chel., clem., ***cocc.,*** ham., helo., hep., hipp., indg., kali-n., lach., lact., mag-c., merc., ***nat-m.,*** nat-s., nux-v., ox-ac., pall., phyt., plat., ran-b., ran-s., rheum, ***rhod.,*** rhus-t., rumx., sabin., ***seneg.,*** squil., sulph., syph., tarax., ther., verat., verb.

rising, on - dig., nat-c., op., verb.

waking - chin-s.

nervous exhaustion, in - ***coca***

noon - aloe, chin-s.

physical - alco., bar-c., calc., carb-ac., cham., chel., chin., cob., cycl., franz., iod., ***kali-bi., lil-t.,*** lyc., menis., nat-c., nat-m., nux-v., puls., sec., sep., ***sulph.***

pollutions, after - ***dios.,*** nat-c., sep.

postpones the work - ***nat-m.***

sadness, from - berb., bov., crot-t., dor., laur., mez., prun., zinc.

sex, after - nat-c.

siesta, after - anac., bor.

sitting, while - nat-c., nit-ac., ruta

sleep, after - bor., chin-s., mez., pip-m.

sleepiness, with - acon., am-m., ammc., ant-t., ars., carb-an., carb-v., chel., chin., cinnb., clem., colch., coloc., dig., dulc., grat., ip., laur., lyc., mag-c., mag-m., nat-c., rat., sars., ther., tong., verb., ***zinc.***

stool, after - colch.

before - ***bor.***

suddenly - calc.

waking, on - ***aloe,*** pip-m.

walking, after - caust.

walking, while - arn., caust., chin-s., coff., nit-ac., sabin.

work - helo.

harm, he thinks it would do him - ***arg-n.***

works well after beginning, but - tarax.

LEARNS, easily - camph., ***coff.,*** lach., nux-v., phos., plat., sulph.
poorly - agar., agn., ***anac., ars.,*** **BAR-C.,** ***calc.,*** calc-p., carb-v., caust., con., med., nat-m., olnd., ph-ac., ***phos.,*** tub., verat.

LEARNING, disabilities, studying, reading, learns with difficulty (see Mistakes) - **AGAR.,** agn., ***anac., ars., bar-c.,*** **CALC.,** calc-p., ***carc.,*** caste., caust., con., kali-sil., **LYC.,** mag-p., nat-m., olnd., okou., ph-ac., ***phos.,*** rib-ac., sil., ***thuj.,*** tub., verat.

LEWDNESS, (See Sexual, behaviour)

LIBERTINISM - act-sp., alum., bell., calc., ***canth.,*** carb-v., ***caust.,*** chin., con., fl-ac., hyos., lyc., merc., nat-m., ***nux-v.,*** orig., ph-ac., ***phos.,*** pic-ac., ***plat.,*** puls., sep., ***staph.,*** stram., sulph., verat.

LIES, inclination to tell - alco., arg-n., calc., carb-v., caust., coca, con., lyc., merc., **MORPH.,** nat-m., nux-v., **OP.,** puls., sil., staph., sulph., ***syph.,*** thuj., ***verat.***
charlatan and liar - calc., lyc., nat-m., puls., thuj.
believes all she says is a - lac-c.
never speaks the truth, does not know what she is saying - alco., arg-n., calc., ***morph.,*** **OP.,** ***syph., verat.***

LIGHT, aversion to - achy., stram., tarent.
desire for - ***acon., am-m.,*** asar., **BELL.,** ***calc.,*** cann-s., carb-an., **GELS.,** grin., lac-c., nat-m., phos., plb., ruta, sanic., **STRAM.,** ***stront-c.,*** valer.
full of, sees - anh.
shuns light - ambr., **CON.,** hyos., plat., tarent., zinc.

LIVELY - ***arg-n.,*** bell., cimic., coff., ***lach., phos., rhus-t., sulph., verat.***

LOATHING, feelings - acon., alum., ang., ant-t., arg-m., ***arg-n.,*** arn., asar., ***aur.,*** bell., benz-ac., bufo, ***calc.,*** canth., carb-o., carc., cham., chel., hep., hyos., ip., jatr., kali-bi., kali-c., laur., mag-m., merc., mez., myric., paull., phel., phyt., plat., ***plb., puls.,*** raph., rat., sapin., sec., seneg., ***sep.,*** staph., stram., sumb., tarent., thea., ***thuj.***
business, his - ars-h.
eruption, before - cop.
evening - alum., alumn., ***hep.,*** raph., sulph.
fear of death, during - cop.
forenoon - tong.
morning - mag-m., phyt.
waking, on - phyt.
noon - pic-ac.
pain, during - aloe.
pain, from - ars., phyt.
puberty, in - ant-c.
rising, when - plect.
smoking, when - sep.
life, of - agn., act-sp., alum., alum-p., alum-sil., ***ambr.,*** am-c., **ANT-C.,** ant-t., **ARS.,** ars-s-f., **AUR.,** aur-a., ***aur-m., aur-s., bell.,*** berb., bov., ***calc.,*** calc-ar., calc-s., calc-sil., carb-an., ***carb-v.,*** carc., caust., **CHIN.,** ***chin-a.,*** cic., cop., dros., grat., hep., hydr., hydroph., hyos.,

LOATHING, feelings
life, of - kali-bi., kali-br., kali-m., ***kali-p.,*** kreos., lac-c., lac-d., ***lach.,*** laur., led., ***lyc.,*** **MERC.,** mez., naja, nat-a., nat-c., **NAT-M.,** ***nat-s.,*** nat-sil., ***nit-ac.,*** **NUX-V.,** op., ***ph-ac.,*** **PHOS.,** ***plat., plb.,*** podo., ***puls., rhus-t., rhus-v.,*** ruta, sec., ***sep.,*** **SIL.,** spig., ***spong.,*** **STAPH.,** stram., sul-ac., ***sulph.,*** tab., ***ter.,*** **THUJ.,** ***tub., valer.,*** verat., zinc., ***zinc-p.,*** ziz.
anxiety, with - ***lach.***
eating, amel. on - cic.
evening - **AUR.,** dros., hep., kali-chl., rhus-t., spig.
menses, before - cer-b.
morning - ***lach.,*** **LYC.,** nat-c.
must restrain herself to prevent doing herself injury - **NAT-S.**
speaking - anac., dios.
oneself, at - aur., lac-c., spirae., staph.
waking, on - ***lach., lyc.,*** nat-c.
work - anac., arg-n., arn., calc., chin., con., croc., hyos., kali-c., lach., merc., nat-m., petr., ***puls.,*** ran-b., ***sil.,*** sulph., ***tab.,*** tarax., ther., tub.
evening - reser.

LONGING, knows not for what - croc., kali-c., tub.
good opinion of others, for - lyc., ***pall.***
pining for someone - plb.
repose for tranquility - nux-v., sulph.
sunshine, light and society, for - grin., stram.

LOQUACITY, (See Talkative, excessive)

LOOKED at, cannot bear to be - ambr., **ANT-C.,** ***ant-t.,*** **ARS.,** calc., ***cham., chin., cina,*** hell., ***iod.,*** kali-br., mag-c., **NAT-M.,** nux-v., rhus-t., sil., stram., sulph., tarent., **TUB.**
agg. mental symptoms - **ANT-C.,** ant-t., ***ars.,*** cham., ***cina,*** lyc., merc., ***nat-m.,*** puls.

LOOKING, backwards, as if followed - lach., staph.
bed, about, to find something - ign.
behind her - med., sanic.
others, at, in distress - tarent.
sides, on all - kali-br.
window, out of, for hours, without being conscious of objects around - mez.

LOVE, ailments, from disappointed, (see Grief) - am-c., ant-c., **AUR.,** ***bell., bufo,*** cact., ***calc-p.,*** carc., ***caust., cimic., coff.,*** com., ***con.,*** dig., ***hell.,*** **HYOS., IGN.,** iod., kali-c., ***lach.,*** lyc., **NAT-M.,** nux-m., nux-v., **PH-AC.,** phos., ***puls.,*** sep., **STAPH.,** sulph., tarent., verat.
exalted - ant-c.
jealousy, anger and incoherent talk, after - ***hyos.,*** nat-m.
rage, after - ***hyos.,*** lach.
sadness - **AUR.,** bell., ***hyos.,*** **IGN., NAT-M.**
silent grief, with - carc., **IGN., NAT-M., PH-AC.,** phos.
suicidal disposition from - **AUR.,** ***hyos.***
unhappy love - bell., calc-p., carc., caust., hyos., ***ign., nat-m.,*** ph-ac., staph., tarent.
unrequited love - ign., **NAT-M.,** tarent.

love, animals, for - aeth., carc., med., phos., sulph.
cats, for - ***sulph.***
perversity - hura, ind., kali-n., nux-v., plat.
love-sick - ***ant-c.,*** til.
jealousy, anger, and incoherent talk, with - ***hyos.,*** lach.
married person, with - ign., **NAT-M.,** staph.
one of her own sex, with - calc., calc-p., fl-ac., ***lach.,*** **MED.,** nat-m., phos., **PLAT.,** puls., ***sulph.,*** **THUJ.**
one of his own sex, with - ***med.,*** nat-m., orig., phos., plat., puls., sep., staph., ***thuj.***
of same sex, with - anh., calc., calc-p., hypoth., ***lach.,*** nat-m., phos., **PLAT.,** puls., ***sulph.,*** thiop.
with someone, unobtainable - ign., ***nat-m.***

LUDICROUS, things seem - **CANN-I.,** cann-s., ***hyos.,*** nat-m., ***nux-m.,*** plat., stram., tarent.
things, does - ***hyos.,*** sec.

MADNESS (see Dementia, Insanity, Mania, Schizophrenia)

MAGNETIC, state of mind - crot-c.

MALICIOUS - abrot., ***acon.,*** agar., alco., aloe, ambr., am-c., am-m., **ANAC.,** arn., ***ars.,*** ars-s-f., ***aur.,*** aur-a., bar-c., ***bell.,*** berb., ***bor.,*** bry., bufo, ***calc.,*** calc-s., cann-s., canth., caps., carb-an., caust., ***cham.,*** chin., cic., cina, clem., coca, cocc., coloc., com., con., croc., ***cupr.,*** cycl., cyna., fl-ac., glon., guai., haem., ***hep.,*** hydr., ***hyos.,*** ign., ip., kali-c., kali-i., ***lac-c.,*** **LACH.,** ***led.,*** levo., ***lyc.,*** mang., med., merc., mosch., ***nat-c.,*** **NAT-M.,** nicc., ***nit-ac.,*** **NUX-V.,** op., par., ped., petr., ***ph-ac.,*** phos., plat., puls., ran-b., sec., sep., sol-m., squil., stann., staph., **STRAM.,** stront-c., sulph., syph., tarent., **TUB.,** tus-f., verat., zinc., zinc-p.
anger, with - ***anac.,*** bar-c., canth., ***caps.,*** carb-an., ***chin.,*** hep., ***lyc., nat-m.,*** nicc., petr., zinc.
dogs, for - tub.
dreams, in - lach.
injure someone, desire to - anac., lach., levo., osm., stram.
insulting - hyos., merc.
laughing - cupr.
loved ones, to - sep.
night - ***calc., sulph.***
sadness, in - **KALI-I.**

MANIA - absin., ***acon.,*** acon-l., aeth., agar., ail., alco., ***alum.,*** **ANAC.,** anag., anan., anh., ant-c., ant-t., ***apis, arn., arg-m.,*** **ARS.,** ars-s-f., ***arum-t.,*** atro., ***aur.,*** aur-a., aur-i., aur-s., bapt., bar-c., ***bar-m.,*** **BELL.,** ***brom.,*** bry., bufo, cact., ***calad., calc.,*** calc-i., ***camph., cann-i., cann-s., canth.,*** carb-s., **CARC.,** caust., cham., chel., ***chin.,*** chin-s., ***chlol.,*** cic., ***cimic.,*** coca, **COCC.,** coff., colch., ***con.,*** cori-r., cortico., croc., ***crot-c.,*** crot-h., ***cupr.,*** cupr-ac., ***cycl.,*** dat-f., dat-m., der., dig., dros., dulc., ferr-p., gels., glon., grat., ***hell., hep.,*** **HYOS.,** hyosin., ***ign.,*** indg., ***iod.,*** iodof., iris-t., kali-bi., **KALI-BR.,** kali-c., **KALI-CHL.,** kali-i., ***kali-m., kali-p.,*** kres., ***lach.,*** laur., led., lil-t., **LYC.,** lyss., man., ***manc.,*** med., **MERC.,** merc-c., murx., nat-m., nit-ac., ***nux-m.,*** **NUX-V.,** oena., ***op.,*** orig., ***ox-ac.,*** par., passi., petr., ph-ac., ***phos.,*** pic-ac., pisc., ***plat.,*** plb., ***psor.,*** puls., raph., rhod., rhus-t., ruta, sabad., sec., senec., seneg., ***sep.,*** sil., ***sol-n.,*** spig-m., spong., staph., **STRAM.,** sul-h., ***sulph., tarent.,*** ter., thea., thyr., tub-k., ust., **VERAT.,** verat-v., vip., zinc.
abuses everyone - anac., ***camph.,*** lach., ***tarent.***
alternating with
depression - arg-m., ***anac.,*** bell., **CARC.,** coff., ***con.,*** cyt-l., ***hyos.,*** kres., **LACH.,** ***med., nat-s.,*** psor., **STAPH.,** stram., sulfa.
metrorrhagia, menses - ***crot-c.***
sadness - tub.
anguish, during - ars., carc.
anxiety, with - ***stram.***
cold perspiration, with - camph., stram.
demoniac - agre., **ANAC.,** bell., ***hell.,*** hyos., lach., op., plat., sil., **STRAM.,** sulph., verat.
destruction, followed by laughter and apologies, of - tarent.
erotic - calc-p., **HYOS.,** phos., ***plat.,*** stann., stram., ***tarent.,*** verat.
evening - crot-c.
excitement in gesture or speech - ***hydr-ac.***
fever, during - cact.
hands, claps - ***stram.***
wringing, runs about day and night - ***hell.,*** syph.
heat, during - cact.
held, wants to be - **ARS.**
jumps over chairs and tables - bell.
light, for, photomania - ***acon.,*** am-m., **BELL.,** calc., **GELS.,** ***lac-c.,*** ruta, **STRAM.,** valer.
delirium, with - calc., ***stram.***
lochia, from suppressed - cimic., plat., verat.
menses, alternating with - crot-c.
before - sep.
suppressed, after - ***puls.,*** stram.
mental exertion, after - lach.
monomania - ign., sil.
neuralgia, following disappearence of - cimic.
night - cic., kali-i.
dancing, laughing, striking, with - cic.
midnight, agg. about - ***staph.***
noisy - verat.
pain, from - ***ars.***
paroxysmal - ***tarent.,*** tub.
periodical - arg-n., ***nat-s., tarent.,*** tub.
puerperal - agn., bell., ***cann-i., cimic., hyos.,*** plat., sec., senec., ***stram.,*** verat., verat-v., zinc.
anxiety, with, and almost loss of consciousness - ***camph.***
rage, with - agar., ant-t., apis, ***ars.,*** **BELL.,** camph., cann-i., cann-s., croc., cupr., **HYOS.,** ***lach.,*** lol., **LYC.,** ***merc.,*** nux-v., ***op.,*** ph-ac., phos., plb., ***sec.,*** sol-n., staph., **STRAM.,** ***verat.,*** verat-v., zinc.

MANIA, behaviour
religious - anac., aur., lach., plat., plb., sulph., ***verat.***
scratching themselves - bell.
screaming, in - ***bell.,*** cic., lach., stram.
sexual, men, in - apis, hyos., **PHOS.,** ***tarent.***
sexual, women, in - **APIS, PHOS., PLAT.,** ***tarent.***
women, in, menses, before - cann-i., ***dulc.,*** lach., plat., sep., verat.
singing, with - bell., cic., ***cocc.,*** hyos., ***nux-m., tarent., verat.***
puerperal in - ***plat.***
spasms, after - arg-m.
spit and bite at those around him, would - ***bell.***
suppressed, eruptions, after - ***caust., hep., zinc.***
tears, clothes - nux-v., staph., ***tarent., verat.***
hair, own - bell., canth., stram., tarent., verat.
himself to pieces with nails - canth., stram., verat.
violence, with deeds of - **ANAC.,** ars., ***bell.,*** hyos., **LACH.,** ***plat.,*** sec., **STRAM.**
wild - anac., ***bell.,*** kali-br., lach., ph-ac., **STRAM.**
wild, look in eyes - ***cupr-s.,*** **STRAM.**

MANIC depression - agar., arg-m., ***anac.,*** aur., bell., **CARC.,** coff., ***con.,*** cyt-l., ***hyos.,*** kres., **LACH., MED.,** ***nat-s.,*** psor., **STAPH.,** stram., sulfa.

MARRIAGE, idea of, seemed unendurable - fl-ac., ***lach.,*** **LYC.,** ***med.,*** pic-ac., ***puls.,*** staph.
obsessed by idea of, girls are excited sexually - bell., ***caust.,*** plat., verat.
thought of, amel. - orig.

MASCULINE, girls, habits of - carb-v., ***nat-m., sep.,*** petr., plat.
women - fl-ac., ***nat-m., sep.***

MATHEMATICS, general, (see Mistakes)
apt for - cocc., lach., nux-v.
calculating, inability to - alum., bell., calc., calc-p., cann-i., caust., crot-h., graph., kali-c., kali-p., ***lyc.,*** merc., nat-c., nat-m., ph-ac., psor., rhus-t., ***sil.,*** staph., syph.
geometry, to do - ail., ***alum., ambr., calc.,*** caust., con., lyc., sil.
horror of - calc., ***lyc.,*** nat-m., ***sil.,*** staph., sulph.
inapt for - bell., calc., kali-c., lyc., sil., syph.
algebra - alum., caust., lyc., sil., staph.
geometry - ***alum., ambr.,*** calc., caust., con., lyc., sil.

MEDDLESOME - atro., hyos.

MEDITATION - acon., am-m., ant-c., aur., bar-c., berb., calc-s., ***cann-i.,*** cann-s., canth., **CARB-AN.,** chin., cic., clem., cocc., coff., con., cycl., eug., euph., ham., hell., ***hyos.,*** ign., ip., kali-n., ***lach.,*** led., lyss., manc., mang., meny., mez., mur-ac., naja, nat-c., ol-an., phel., phos., plb., ran-b., rhus-t., sabad., sep., spig., staph., ***sulph.,*** thuj.

MEDITATION,
deep, profound - acon., **SEP.,** staph.
night - op.

MEGALOMANIA - **CANN-I.,** cupr., glon., ***graph., hyos., lach.,*** lyc., ***lycpr.,*** **PLAT.,** ***stram.,*** **SULPH.,** ***syph.,*** **VERAT.,** verat-v.

MEMORIES, recalls disagreeable, (see Dwells) - am-c., ambr., benz-ac., ***calc.,*** carc., cham., ***hep.,*** hyos., ***lyc.,*** **NAT-M.,** nit-ac., op., phos., psor., sep., ***staph.,*** sulph., thuj.
old grievances, of - glon., ***nat-m.,*** nit-ac., staph.

MEMORY, general
active - acon., acon-f., ***agar., aloe,*** alum., anac., ang., anh., ant-c., arn., ars., ars-s-f., asaf., ***aur.,*** aur-a., bad., bapt., **BELL.,** bov., brom., bufo, calc-p., camph., cann-i., cann-s., caps., carb-v., chin., cimic., cob., coc-c., coca, cocc., coc-c., **COFF.,** coff-t., croc., cub., cupr., cycl., dig., fl-ac., ***gels.,*** glon., grat., hipp., **HYOS.,** iber., ***ign.,*** kali-p., lac-ac., **LACH.,** lyss., manc., meph., nat-m., nat-p., ***nux-m., nux-v.,*** **OP.,** ox-ac., ***phos.,*** phys., pip-m., plat., plb., puls., raph., rhus-t., senec., seneg., sil., spig., stry., sulph., ***sul-ac.,*** ter., thuj., valer., verat., verb., viol-o., zinc., zing., ziz.
afternoon - anac., ang.
alternating with, dullness - rhus-t.
lassitude - ***aloe.***
weak memory - acon., ars-s-f., cycl., rhus-t.
evening - agar., **LACH.**
midnight, until - **COFF.**
fever, during - op.
morning - fl-ac.
music, for - croc.
names, for proper - ***asar.***
past events, for - anh., bell., ***hyos.,*** nat-m., seneg.
haunted by and longing for - caps., ***kali-p.***
recollection, unvoluntary - fl-ac., ***hyos.,*** nat-m.
short, but - calc., sil., staph., sulph.
suppressing sexual desire, from - lach.
confused, seemed - anac., chin-s., cupr., naja, op., petr., sel., ***stram.***
forgetful - abrot., acet-ac., ***acon.,*** aeth., agar., ***agn.,*** ail., alum., alum-p., alum-sil., **AMBR.,** am-c., ***anac.,*** apis, arg-m., ***arg-n., arn.,*** ars., ars-s-f., arum-t., ***aur.,*** aur-a., aur-s., aza., **BAR-C.,** bar-i., ***bell.,*** bor., bov., brom., bry., cahin., calad., ***calc., calc-p.,*** calc-s., camph., cann-i., cann-s., ***canth.,*** caps., carb-ac., ***carb-an.,*** **CARB-S.,** ***carb-v.,*** carc., card-m., ***caust.,*** cench., cham., ***chel.,*** chin., chin-a., ***cic.,*** cimic., ***cinnam.,*** cinnb., clem., **COCC.,** coff., **COLCH.,** coloc., ***con., corn.,*** cortico., cortiso., ***croc.,*** crot-h., cupr., cycl., ***dig.,*** elaps, ferr., ferr-ar., ***ferr-p., fl-ac.,*** form., ***gels., glon., graph., guai.,*** gymn., ham., hell., hep., hipp., hydr., hydr-ac., hydroph., hyos., ign., iod., ip., kali-bi., ***kali-br.,*** kali-c., kali-i., kali-n., ***kali-p.,*** kali-s., kali-sil., kalm., kreos.,

MEMORY, general
forgetful - ***lac-c., lach.,*** laur., lec., led., lil-t., **LYC.,** lyss., mag-c., manc., med., meli., **MERC.,** mez., ***mill.,*** morph., mosch., naja, nat-a., nat-c., ***nat-m., nat-p.,*** nat-s., nat-sil., nit-ac., nux-m., nux-v., olnd., op., **PETR., PH-AC., PHOS.,** pic-ac., plan., **PLAT.,** plb., psor., ptel., puls., ran-b., raph., rheum, rhod., ***rhus-t.,*** rhus-v., ruta, sabin., sal-ac., sanic., sarr., sec., sel., sep., sil., spig., stann., staph., stram., stront-c., ***sulph.,*** syph., tab., tarax., tell., ***thuj.,*** trom., ***tub.,*** verat., verat-v., verb., viol-o., visc., ***zinc.,*** **ZINC-P.,** zing.
afternoon - anac., graph., laur., sep.
amel. - ***anac.***
alcoholics, forgetfulness in - ***calc.,*** lach., merc., **NUX-V.,** ***op.,*** puls., rhus-t.
business, of - sel.
busy, when - ant-c.
chill, during - bell., con., hyos., podo., rhus-t.
connection of consecutive thoughts, of - ***op.***
eating, after - calc-s., ferr., mag-c., nat-m., rhus-t.
amel. - sil.
elderly people, of - am-c., ***ambr.,*** anac., ***bar-c.,*** coff., ***con., crot-h.,*** lach., ***lyc., ph-ac.,*** rhus-t., sulph.
emotions, from - ***acon.,*** op., ph-ac., ***staph.***
epilepsy, before - ***caust.***
happened before, of what - absin.
errand - bar-c., manc., med.
evening, in - fl-ac., ***form.,*** laur., lyc., naja, nat-m., rhus-t., sep.
events, recent - absin., ail., graph., rhus-t.
everything, busy, when - ant-c.
except dreams, of - ***ign.***
that had occurred for six years - ***lach.***
friends and relatives, of - lyss.
fright, after - ***cupr.***
going, of where he is - ***cench., merc.***
headache, during - apis, bell., calc., caps., glon., zinc.
heat, during - ***alum., arn.,*** cocc., ***guare.,*** rhus-t.
after - ***mag-p.,*** podo.
house was, on which side of the street his - **GLON.,** ***nux-m.,*** nux-v., ***petr.***
immediately, of everything - ***dig.***
loss of fluids, from - ***chin.,*** **NUX-V.,** ***sulph.***
masturbation, after - ***dig.,*** kali-br., staph.
menopausal period, during - ***lach., phys.***
menses, during - raph.
mental exertion, from - anac., ***aur.,*** calc., lach., nat-c., nat-m., ***nux-v.,*** puls., sil., sulph.
morning, in - **ANAC.,** berb., buf-s., ph-ac., phos., sil., stann., stram., ***thuj.***
amel. - fl-ac.
waking, on - ***kali-br.,*** stann., ***thuj.***
motion, on - laur.
names - ***anac.,*** bar-ac., ***chlor., euon.,*** guai., hep., lyc., med., ***sulph.,*** syph., xero.
own - alum., kali-br., ***med.,*** sulph., valer.
night - chin., sil., sulph.
nosebleed, after - ***kreos.***

MEMORY, general
forgetful,
periodical - carb-v., chin., nat-m.
pollutions, after - staph.
profession, forgets her - tarent.
purchases, of, goes off and leaves them - absin., agn., anac., bell., caust., iod., ***lac-c.,*** nat-m.
seminal emissions, from - staph.
sentence, finish, cannot - ***cann-i.,*** med.
sex, after - ***sec.***
sexual excesses, after - calad., kali-br., ***nat-p., ph-ac., sec., staph.***
shaving or dressing, of - chel.
sleep, during, he remembers all he had forgotten - calad., sel.
street, which side of the, his house was on - **GLON.,** ***nux-m., petr.***
streets, of well-known - cann-i., ***crot-h.,*** **GLON.,** lach., ***petr., nux-m.***
thinking of something agg. forgetfulness, diversion amel. - lil-t.
tobacco poisoning, from - ***calad.***
waking, on - chin., cob-n., kali-br., kali-n., ptel., sil., stann., thuj.
walking, while, after eating - rhus-t.
watch, to wind - fl-ac.
words while speaking, of, word hunting - agar., alum., am-br., anh., ***arg-n.,*** **ARN.,** ***bar-c.,*** bar-s., benz-ac., **BOTH.,** cact., calc., camph., **CANN-I.,** cann-s., carb-an., carb-s., carb-v., chen-a., coca, cocc., colch., con., crot-h., dulc., glon., ham., helo., hydr., ***kali-br.,*** kali-c., kali-p., ***lach.,*** lil-t., ***lyc., med., nat-m., nux-v., onos., plb.,*** podo., **PH-AC.,** puls., rhod., sil., staph., sulph., syph., ***thuj.,*** verat.
increase, of - bell., ***coff.,*** hyos., seneg.
loss, of - **ANAC.,** bar-ac., **BELL.,** ***camph.,*** carb-s., cic., cori-r., ***dig.,*** **HYOS.,** pic-ac., **VERAT.**
aphasia, in - cann-i., hyper., kali-br.
catalepsy, after - camph.
coma, after - cori-r.
epileptic fits, after - absin., calc., cic., ***zinc.***
fear, from - anac.
imbecility, in - ***anac.***
injuries, after - am-c., **ARN.,** chin-a., cic., hyper., merc., rhus-t.
concussion of the brain, after - hell., ***hyper., nat-s.***
head, of - am-c., **ARN.,** cic., ***hell.,*** hyper., merc., ***nat-s.,*** rhus-t.
insanity, in - aur., ***merc., stram.***
mental exertion, from - ***nat-c.***
objects, naming, for - chin-s.
past life - nux-m.
stroke, after - **ANAC.,** op., ***plb.***
sunstroke, after - ***anac.,*** glon., ***lach.***
vital fluids, from loss of - **CHIN., NUX-V., SULPH.**

MEMORY, general

weakness of - abrot., absin., acet-ac., ***acon.,*** acon-c., act-sp., aesc., aeth., agar., ***agn.,*** ail., alco., all-s., allox., ***alum.,*** alum-sil., alumn., **AMBR.,** am-c., am-m., **ANAC.,** ***anac-oc.,*** anan., anh., ***apis, arg-m.,*** **ARG-N.,** ***arn.,*** **ARS.,** ars-h., art-v., arum-t., asaf., asc-t., ***atro., aur.,*** aur-a., aur-m., aur-s., aza., bapt., bar-ac., **BAR-C.,** bar-i., bar-s., **BELL.,** berb., ***bol.,*** bor., ***bov.,*** brom., ***bry.,*** **BUFO, BUF-S.,** cadm-met., calad., **CALC.,** calc-ar., ***calc-p.,*** calc-s., calc-sil., camph., **CANN-I.,** cann-s., caps., carb-ac., ***carb-an.,*** carb-o., **CARB-S.,** ***carb-v.,*** carc., card-m., carl., **CAUST.,** cench., cham., chel., ***chin., chin-a.,*** chlf., ***chlol.,*** chlor., chlorpr., ***cic.,*** cimic., ***clem.,*** cob-n., coca, **COCC.,** coff., **COLCH.,** coloc., **CON.,** convo-s., cop., cori-r., ***corn.,*** cortico., cortiso., cot., croc., crot-c., ***crot-h.,*** crot-t., cub., culx., ***cupr.,*** cupr-ac., ***cycl.,*** der., ***dig.,*** dulc., elaps, erio., ***euphr.,*** eupi., ferr., ***ferr-p., fl-ac., form., gels.,*** gins., **GLON.,** glyc., ***graph., guai.,*** guare., guat., gymn., haem., ham., **HELL.,** ***helo., helon.,*** **HEP.,** hipp., hist., ***hydr.,*** **HYOS.,** hyper., ***iber.,*** ichth., ***ign.,*** iod., ip., iris, jug-c., juni., kali-ar., kali-bi., ***kali-br.,*** kali-c., kali-cy., ***kali-i.,*** kali-n., **KALI-P.,** kali-s., kali-sil., kalm., kreos., ***lac-ac., lac-c.,*** lac-d., **LACH.,** ***laur.,*** lec., led., lil-t., linu-c., lipp., **LYC.,** lyss., mag-arct., mag-c., man., manc., mang., **MED.,** meli., **MERC.,** ***merc-c., mez.,*** mill., mit., morph., mosch., murx., naja, ***nat-a., nat-c., nat-m., nat-p.,*** nat-sal., nat-sil., nid., **NIT-AC.,** nitro-o., **NUX-M.,** ***nux-v., oena.,*** okou., ***olnd.,*** onos., ***op.,*** pall., peti., ***petr.,*** **PH-AC.,** phenob., **PHOS.,** phys., ***pic-ac.,*** pip-m., plan., **PLAT.,** **PLB.,** pneu., psil., psor., ptel., ***puls.,*** rad., ran-s., raph., rhod., rhus-g., ***rhus-t.,*** ruta, sabad., sabin., sanic., sapin., sarr., sec., ***sel.,*** seneg., **SEP.,** serp., ***sil., spig.,*** spong., ***stann., staph., stram.,*** stront-c., stry., ***sulph.,*** sul-ac., ***syph.,*** tab., tarax., ***tarent.,*** tell., ***thuj.,*** thyr., trif-p., ***tub.,*** valer., **VERAT.,** verat-v., verb., ***viol-o.,*** viol-t., visc., yuc., ***zinc., zinc-m., zinc-p.,*** zinc-pic., zing.

acute - gels.

alcoholics, in - **CALC.,** ***lach.,*** merc., **NUX-V., OP.,** puls., **SULPH.**

business, for - agn., chel., fl-ac., hyos., kali-c., kreos., phos., sabin., sel., sulph., tell., tep.

colors, for - lyc., sil., staph.

dates, for - acon., ***con.,*** crot-h., fl-ac., kali-bi., kali-br., med., merc., nux-v., staph., syph.

details, for - cadm-met.

do, for what he was about to - agn., allox., ***bar-c.,*** bell., calc-p., calc-s., ***carb-ac.,*** carb-an., carb-s., ***card-m.,*** **CANN-I.,** cann-s., ***chel.,*** cinnb., cortico., fl-ac., gran., hydr., iod., jug-c., kali-s., kreos., ***lac-c.,*** manc., nat-m., ***nux-m., onos.,*** phos., psil., ***sulph.***

MEMORY, general

weakness of

done, for what he has just - absin., ***acon.,*** agar., allox., aster., ***bar-c.,*** bor., bufo, bov., calad., ***calc-p.,*** camph., **CANN-I.,** chel., cic., fl-ac., graph., ***hyos.,*** lac-c., lach., laur., lyc., nat-m., ***nux-m., onos.,*** rad., rhus-t., sabin., thuj., zinc.

elderly, in - anac., bar-c.

everyday things, for - carc., halo.

expressing one's self, for - acet-ac., agar., am-c., arg-n., bell., cann-i., cann-s., carb-an., carb-s., cimic., ***coca,*** cocc., colch., cot., crot-h., dulc., gad., haem., ign., ***kali-br., kali-c.,*** kali-p., kiss., lac-c., lach., ***lact.,*** lil-t., ***lyc.,*** med., morph., murx., ***nat-m., nux-v., ph-ac.,*** phys., **PLB.,** puls., sep., ***stram.,*** tab., thuj.

facts, for - bell., **CALC.,** med., verat.

past - ail., bell., calc., camph., hyos., lach., lyc., nux-m., sulph.

past, elderly people, in - coff.

recent - allox., aza., bell., cael., calc., carb-ac., carb-s., carb-v., graph., hydr., hyos., nat-m., nux-v., sulph., verat.

recent, elderly people, in - lach., sulph.

forms, for - ambr., lyc., staph., sulfa., sulph.

happened, for what has - absin., buf-s., carb-ac., cocc., graph., hydr., ***lach., nat-m., nux-m.,*** rhus-t., sulph., syph.

just - allox.

remembers past events, but - syph.

headache, during - bell.

heard, for what has - agar., calc., cann-i., carb-v., **HELL., HYOS.,** ***lach., med.,*** mez., nat-m., ***nux-m.,*** plat., psor., sulph.

just - allox., iber.

labor for mental - acon., aloe, asar., bar-c., ***con.,*** cycl., ***gels.,*** graph., ign., laur., lyc., naja, **NAT-C., NAT-M.,** ***ph-ac., pic-ac.,*** sel., sep., ***sil.,*** sol-n., spig., spong., staph., ther., thuj.

child cannot be taught - ***bar-c.***

fatigue, from - calc., colch., gels., nat-c., nat-m., nux-v., ph-ac., plat., puls., sep., sil.

learned by heart, cannot repeat what he - mez.

letters, for the names of the - ***lyc.***

makes several letters, how to - chr-ac.

music, for - ign., lyc., staph., sulfa.

names, for proper - allox., alum., ***anac.,*** aza., bar-ac., bell., cann-i., carl., caust., chin-s., chlor., cortico., croc., ***crot-h., euon-a.,*** fl-ac., glon., ***guai.,*** hep., hist., kali-br., kali-p., lach., lith., ***lyc., med.,*** merc., nat-a., nat-m., nux-v., olnd., perh., ph-ac., ptel., puls., ***rhus-t.,*** sec., spig., staph., stram., ***sulph.,*** syph., tab., xero.

objects, of - chin-s., lith.

persons, of - chlor., guai.

naming, objects, for - chin-s.

occurrences of the day - acet-ac., calad., nat-m., perh., ***ph-ac.,*** plb., ***rhus-t.***

MEMORY, general
weakness of
orthography, for - con., crot-c., hydr., ***lach., lyc.,*** sil., sulph., tab.
periodical - carb-v., chin., nat-m.
persons, for - acet-ac., agar., ail., ambr., anac., bell., cedr., cham., chlor., croc., ***crot-h.,*** hyos., lyc., merc., nux-v., op., staph., stram., sulph., syph., thuj., verat.
places, for - allox., calc., ***crot-h., hep.,*** merc., nux-m., psor., sil., **STAPH.,** sulph., syph.
read, for what he has - allox., ambr., anac., arn., ars-m., bell., calc-sil., ***cann-i.,*** carb-ac., cocc., coff., colch., chlor., corn., guai., ham., halo., **HELL.,** hipp., hydr., ***hyos.,*** jug-c., lac-c., lac-d., **LACH.,** ***lyc., med., merc.,*** nat-c., ***nat-m., nux-m.,*** olnd., ***onos., op.,*** perh., ***ph-ac.,*** phos., psor., **STAPH.,** syph., tep., viol-o.
just read - **ANAC.,** ph-ac., viol-o.
said, for what has - ail., arg-m., ***arn., bar-c.,*** calc., calc-sil., ***cann-i.,*** carb-an., ***carb-v.,*** colch., croc., **HELL.,** hep., **HYOS.,** kali-n., lach., ***med.,*** merc., ***mez., mur-ac.,*** nux-m., ***psor.,*** rhod., stram., sulph., tep., verat.
just said, for what has - calc-sil.
say, for what he is about to - allox., am-c., arg-m., ***arg-n., arn.,*** atro., **BAR-C., CANN-I.,** cann-s., carb-an., card-m., carl., colch., cot., **HELL.,** hydr., hyper., iod., kali-s., lach., lil-t., ***med.,*** merc., ***mez., nat-m.,*** nux-m., ***onos.,*** ph-ac., plb., podo., rhod., rhus-t., ***staph.,*** stram., ***sulph.,*** thuj., verat.
seen, for everything what has - ***anac.***
studies, of young people in their - ***nat-c.***
sudden and periodical - calc., calc-s., ***carb-v.,*** chin., laur., ***kali-br.,*** nux-m., nux-v., syph.
pain, fright, from - am-c., anac., arg-n., bell., hep., laur., nux-m., pall., prun., puls.
thought, for what has just - acon., agar., alum., anac., bell., ***cann-i., cocc.,*** colch., fl-ac., ***hyos., med.,*** nat-m., ran-s., rob., staph., stram., sulph., verb.
time - ***lach.,*** merc.
verses, to learn - nux-v., puls., sulph.
vexation, agg. - am-c.
words, for - agar., allox., alum., ***anac.,*** anh., arag., ***arg-n., arn.,*** **BAR-C.,** cact., calc., calc-p., **CANN-I.,** ***cann-s.,*** caps., ***carb-s.,*** cham., chin., cimic., coca, ***cocc.,*** con., crot-h., cupr., dios., ***dulc.,*** ham., ***hell., hep.,*** hist., ***kali-br., kali-c., kali-p.,*** lac-c., ***lach.,*** lil-t., ***lyc.,*** lyss., med., murx., ***nat-m., nux-m., nux-v., op., ph-ac.,*** **PLB.,** podo., **PULS.,** rhus-t., sil., staph., sulfa., ***sulph.,*** sumb., thiop., thuj., xero.
write, for what is about to - **CANN-I.,** chr-ac., colch., ***croc.,*** dirc., med., ***nat-m., nux-m.,*** rhod., rhus-t.
written, for what he has - calad., cann-i., nux-m.

MEN, dread of - aloe, ***aur., bar-c.,*** bar-m., bell., ***caust.,*** **CIC.,** con., dios., graph., ign., lach., ***led., lyc., nat-c., nat-m.,*** phos., plat., **PULS.,** raph., **SEP.,** stann., staph., sulph.
shuns the foolishness of - cic., ***nat-c., sulph.***

MENTAL, general affections of - ***acon.,*** **ANAC., ARS., AUR., BELL.,** bry., ***calc.,*** **CANN-I.,** cham., chin., ***coff.,*** **HYOS.,** ***ign.,*** **LACH.,** lil-t., ***lyc.,*** nat-c., ***nat-m.,*** **NUX-V.,** ***op.,*** ph-ac., ***phos.,*** plat., **PULS.,** sep., **STRAM.,** ***sulph.,*** valer., ***verat.***
acute - acon., ***coff.,*** ign., ***op.***
weakness, with physical - gels., op., ph-ac., sil.
ailments from mental shock - acon., apis, ***arn.,*** coca, gels., ign., iod., kali-p., ***op., pic-ac.,*** plat.
blank - cor-r., hell., stann.
childish, body grows - bufo.
digestive affections, with - arg-n.
evening, amel. - tarent.
filthy - merc.
heart complaints, alternating with - lil-t.
nose blowing, amel. - kali-chl.
pain agg. - cham., sars., verat.
rheumatism agg. - cimic.
shaving agg. - calad.
soles, rubbing, amel. - chel.
stool amel. - bov., cimic., nat-s.
syphilis agg. - asaf., ***aur.,*** hep., lach., merc., nit-ac., phyt.
uterine complaints, alternating with - arn., lil-t.
vaginal discharge, appearing amel. - murx.
waking, on, agg. - calc., **LACH.,** ***lyc.,*** **STRAM.,** zinc.
weakness, spasms, after - sec.
yawning, amel. - bry.

MESMERIZED, seem as if (see Magnetized) - oena.

MILDNESS, (see Yielding) - ***acon.,*** alum., alumn., ambr., amph., anac., **ARN., ARS.,** ***ars-i.,*** asar., aur., bell., **BOR.,** bov., ***cact., calad., calc.,*** calc-sil., ***cann-i.,*** caps., carb-an., cast., caust., cedr., chel., chim-m., cic., ***cina,*** clem., **COCC.,** ***croc., cupr.,*** cycl., euph., euphr., gels., hell., hydr., hyos., hypoth., ***ign., indg.,*** iod., kali-c., kali-cy., kali-p., laur., ***lil-t., lyc., mag-arct.,*** mag-m., manc., mang., mosch., mur-ac., murx., nat-a., nat-c., **NAT-M.,** ***nit-ac., nux-v.,*** op., petr., ph-ac., **PHOS.,** plat., plb., **PULS., RHUS-T.,** sars., ***sep.,*** **SIL.,** ***spong.,*** stann., **STAPH.,** ***stram., sulph.,*** sumb., ***thuj., verat.,*** viol-o., viol-t., zinc.
alternating with, anger - kali-c.
hardness - croc.
obstinacy - ***cupr.,*** tub.
complaining, bears suffering, even outrage without - ***ign.***
epileptic attack, after - ***indg.***
evening - croc.

MIRTH - acon., aeth., ***agar.,*** aloe, alum., am-c., ***anac.,*** anag., anan., ang., ant-t., apis, arg-m., arn., ars., ars-i., arund., asaf., asar., asc-t., ***aur.,*** bar-c., ***bell.,*** brom., ***calc.,*** calc-s., camph., **CANN-I.,** cann-s., caps., carb-an., ***carb-s.,*** carb-v., caust., cham., chin., chin-s., chlor., cic., cimic., clem., cob., cocc., coc-c., **COFF.,** con., ***croc.,*** cypr., cycl., dros., eupi., ***ferr.,*** ferr-ar., ferr-i., ferr-p., ***fl-ac.,*** form., gamb., gels., graph., **HYOS.,** ign., iod., ip., kali-c., kali-p., kreos., **LACH.,** lachn., laur., led., ***lyc.,*** mag-c., mag-s., meny., merc., merc-c., merc-i-f., merc-i-r., merl., mez., naja, nat-a., **NAT-C.,** nat-m., nat-p., nit-ac., ***nux-m.,*** **OP.,** ox-ac., par., ped., petr., phel., ***ph-ac., phos., plat.,*** plb., psor., puls., rhus-t., sabad., sars., seneg., sep., spig., spong., squil., stann., staph., ***stram.,*** sulph., sul-ac., sumb., tab., ***tarax., tarent.,*** ther., thuj., valer., ***verat.,*** verb., ***zinc.***

- afternoon - ang., ***ant-t.,*** arg-m., cann-s., lyc., merc-i-f., phos., ***staph.,*** verb.
- air, in open - phel., plb., teucr.
- alternating with, bursts of indignation - aur., caps., croc., ign.
  - crying - arg-m., carb-an., iod., spong.
  - irritability - caust., cocc., croc., nat-m., spong.
  - lachrymose mood - plb., psor., sep., spong., sumb.
  - mania - bell., ***cann-i.,*** croc.
  - palpitation - spig.
  - sadness - cann-i., caust., croc., ferr., hell., nat-c., nit-ac., petr., ***phos.,*** plat., sep., tarent., zinc.
  - seriousness - plat.
- chill, during - nux-m.
- daytime - ant-t.
- emission, after an - pip-m.
- evening - aloe, alum., am-c., anac., aster., bell., buf-s., calc., calc-s., carb-v., cast., chel., ***chin.,*** coc-c., cupr., cycl., ferr., **LACH.,** lachn., laur., mag-c., ***nat-m.,*** phel., pip-m., sars., ***sulph., valer.,*** viol-t., ***zinc.***
  - bed in - alum.
  - ill-humor during the day - sulph., viol-t.
- foolish - acon., agar., bell., calc., carb-v., merc., par., seneg.
- forenoon - graph., nat-m., zinc.
- heat, during - acon.
- morning - con., ***fl-ac.,*** graph., mag-m., sulph.
  - waking, on - chin.
- night - alum., bell., caust., ***chin.,*** croc., cypr., kreos., lyc., naja, ph-ac., sep., sil., stram., sulph., verat.
  - 2 a.m. - ***chin.***
- sleep, during - alum., bell., caust., croc., hyos., kreos., lyc., ph-ac., sil., sulph.
- stool, after - ***bor., nat-s.***

MISANTHROPY - acon., all-c., ***ambr., am-m.,*** **ANAC.,** ant-c., ars., ***aur.,*** bar-c., bell., ***calc.,*** cic., clem., con., cop., crot-h., cupr., grat., guai., hydrc., ***hyos.,*** iod., kali-bi., kali-c., lach., ***led., lyc.,*** mag-m., merc., **NAT-C.,** nat-m., nit-ac., pall., ***phos.,*** plat., ***puls.,*** rhus-t., sep., ***stann.,*** staph., stram., sulph., tab.

MISCHIEVOUS - ***agar.,*** aloe, **ANAC.,** arn., ***ars.,*** bar-c., bufo, ***calc.,*** calc-ar., **CANN-I.,** cann-s., ***cupr., hyos., lach., merc.,*** **NUX-V.,** puls., spong., **STANN.,** ***stram.,*** **TARENT.,** ***verat.***

- imbecility, in - ***merc.***

MISERABLE, feelings - ***ars.,*** **AUR.,** fl-ac., graph., iod., kreos., naja, ***nit-ac.,*** sabad., sep., stann., tab., zinc.

- makes himself, by brooding over imaginary wrongs and misfortunes - ars., aur., naja., nit-ac.

MISTAKES, general

- **calculating,** in (see Mathematics) - ail., ***am-c.,*** chin-s., con., ***crot-h.,*** gali., lach., ***lyc.,*** merc., ***nux-v.,*** rhus-t., ***sumb.,*** syph.
  - adding, in - chin-s.
  - cannot calculate after childbirth - ***thuj.***
- **differentiating** of objects, in - calc., cann-s., hyos., nux-v., plat., sulph.
- **localities** - aesc., anh., arg-n., atro., bell., bov., bry., camph-br., cann-i., cham., cic., fl-ac., **GLON.,** hura, ***kali-br., kali-p.,*** lach., merc., nat-m., **NUX-M.,** nux-v., par., **PETR.,** phos., plat., psor., puls., sil., stram., sulph., valer., verat.
- **measure** and weight and gives wrong answers - nux-v.
- **names,** calls things by wrong - am-c., calc., ***dios.,*** lac-c., sep., ***stram.,*** sulph.
- **persons,** in - alco., cham.
- **reading** - carc., cham., ***hyos.,*** lach., lact., lyc., merc., plb., sil., stann.
- **space** and time, in - anh., bor., bov., ***cann-i.,*** caust., cic., ***glon.,*** lach., nux-m.
- **speaking,** in - acet-ac., ***agar., alum.,*** alum-sil., am-br., ***am-c.,*** am-m., arg-n., ***arn., bell.,*** bov., bufo, ***calc.,*** calc-p., calc-s., calc-sil., cann-s., canth., carb-s., caust., cer-s., ***cham., chin.,*** chin-s., coca, ***cocc.,*** con., cortico., croc., crot-h., cupr., cycl., dios., dirc., ***dulc.,*** esp-g., graph., haem., ham., hep., hyos., hyper., ign., ir-foe., kali-br., ***kali-c.,*** kali-p., kali-sil., kiss., ***lac-c.,*** lach., lil-t., **LYC.,** mang., ***merc.,*** murx., **NAT-M.,** nat-c., nux-m., nux-v., onos., osm., ph-ac., plb., ***puls.,*** rhod., rhus-r., sec., sel., sep., sil., staph., stram., sul-ac., sulph., ***thuj.,*** visc., zinc.
  - agg., after exertion - agar.
  - hurry, from - ***ign.***
  - intend, what he does not - alum., cham., ***nat-m.***
  - misplacing words - all-c., alum., am-c., ***arn.,*** bov., bufo, ***calc.,*** calc-p., calc-s., calc-sil., cann-s., carb-s., caust., cham., **CHIN.,** cocc., con., crot-h., cycl., fl-ac., graph., hep., hyos., hyper., kali-br., kali-c., kali-p., kali-s., kali-sil., ***lac-c., lach., lyc.,*** merc., nat-c., ***nat-m., nux-m., nux-v.,*** osm.
  - mispronounces words - ***caust.***
  - old age, in - am-c.
  - omitting words - cham., helo., nux-v., ***verat-v.***

MISTAKES, general
speaking, in
reverses words - calc., caust., ***chin.,*** cycl., kali-br., onop., osm., stram., sulph.
sleeplessness, after - agar.
spelling, in - agar., all-c., allox., am-c., aza., ***cortico.,*** crot-h., fl-ac., helo., hyper., lac-ac., ***lach.,*** lob-s., ***lyc., med.,*** nux-m., nux-v., rauw., stram., sulph.
transposes sounds - caust.
writing - lach., lyc., thuj.
wrong answers, gives - cann-s., nat-m., nux-v., phos.
answers, gives, syllables - caust., **LYC.,** onop., sel.
words, (see words, wrong)
time, in - acon., alum., anac., ***anh.,*** atro., bad., bor., bov., camph., ***cann-i.,*** cer-b., cic., cocc., con., croc., dirc., elaps, fl-ac., glon., halo., hura, ***lach.,*** med., nux-m., nux-v., op., pall., petr., plb., psor., sulph., ther.
afternoon, always imagines it is - ***lach.,*** stann.
confounds future with past - anac., cic., croc., staph.
present, with future - anac.
present, with past - anac., ***cic.,*** croc., med., nux-m., staph.
far off feeling - cann-i., med., syph.
present merged with eternity - anh.
space and time, in - anh., bor., bov., ***cann-i.,*** caust., cic., ***glon.,*** lach., nux-m.
words, using wrong - agar., ***alum.,*** alum-sil., am-br., ***am-c., arg-n., arn., both.,*** bov., bufo, ***calc., calc-p.,*** cann-s., canth., caust., cham., ***chen-a.,*** **CHIN.,** ***cocc.,*** con., cortico., crot-h., cupr., ***dios.,*** dirc., ***dulc.,*** esp-g., graph., hep., ***hyos., kali-br.,*** kali-c., lac-c., **LYC.,** lyss., mang., med., merc., nat-m., **NUX-M.,** ***nux-v.,*** osm., ph-ac., sep., sil., staph., ***stram., thuj.,*** yuc., zinc.
form, right words can not - aesc.
name of objects seen instead of one desired - am-c., calc., ***lac-c.,*** sep., sulph., tub.
names, calls things by wrong - am-c., calc., ***dios.,*** lac-c., sep., ***stram.,*** sulph.
opposite, hot for cold - ***kali-br.,*** nux-m.
putting right for left or vice versa - ***chin-s., dios., fl-ac.,*** hyper., ir-foe.
says plums, when he means pears - dios., lyc., ***stram.***
spoonerism - caust., chin.
work, in - acet-ac., all-c., bell., chin-s., meli., nat-c., phos., sep.
writing, in - adlu., agar., allox., alum., alum-sil., am-br., ***am-c.,*** arag., aza., benz-ac., bov., calc., ***calc-p.,*** cann-i., ***cann-s.,*** carb-an., carb-o., carb-s., cench., cer-s., ***cham., chin.,*** chin-s., chr-ac., colch., con., croc., crot-h., dios., dirc., ***dulc.,*** fl-ac., gali., graph., hep., hydr., hyper., ign., ir-foe., ***kali-br.,*** kali-c., ***kali-p.,*** kali-s., kali-sil., lac-ac., ***lac-c.,*** **LACH.,** lil-t., lob-s., **LYC.,** mag-arct., mag-c., med., morph., nat-c., ***nat-m., nux-m.,*** nux-v., onos., opun-v., phos.,

MISTAKES, general
writing, in - ptel., puls., rauw., rhod., rhus-t., sac-alb., sep., sil., staph., sulph., stram., ***sumb.,*** tab., **THUJ.,** visc., yuc.
adds letters - ***lyc.***
confounding letters - lyc.
hurry, from - ***ign.***
old age, in - am-c., ***crot-h.***
omitting, letters - colch., erig., ***hyper.,*** kali-br., ***lac-c., lyc.,*** meli., ***nux-m.,*** nux-v., onos., op., puls., stram., ***thuj.,*** zinc.
syllables - bov., ***cham.,*** colch., kali-br., ***lyc.,*** nux-v., ***thuj.***
words - benz-ac., ***cann-s.,*** cer-s., ***cham.,*** erig., hyper., ***kali-br.,*** lac-ac., lac-c., lach., lachn., ***lyc.,*** meli., ***nux-m.,*** nux-v., ***rhod.,*** sac-alb., ***thuj.***
repeating words - ***calc-p., cann-s.,*** kali-br., lac-c., sulph.
spelling, in - agar., all-c., allox., am-c., aza., ***cortico.,*** crot-h., fl-ac., helo., hyper., lac-ac., ***lach.,*** lob-s., ***lyc., med.,*** nux-m., nux-v., rauw., stram., sulph.
transposing letters - caust., ***chin., lyc.,*** opun-v., stram.
wrong, letters, figures - am-c., galin.
wrong, words - bov., ***calc.,*** calc-p., cann-i., cench., chin-s., dirc., fl-ac., hyper., lac-c., ***lyc.,*** sars., sep., thuj., yuc.
headache, during - nux-m.

MOANING, groaning - **ACON.,** ether, alum., am-c., ambr., ang., ant-t., ***apis, arn., ars.,*** aur., aur-s., ***bar-c.,*** bar-s., **BELL.,** ***bor., bry., calad.,*** calc., **CALC-P.,** ***camph.,*** **CANN-I.,** cann-s., canth., caps., ***carb-ac.,*** carb-an., carb-o., carb-s., carb-v., caust., ***cham.,*** chin., chin-a., chlf., cimic., ***cic., cina,*** coca, ***cocc.,*** coff., ***colch., coloc., crot-c.,*** crot-h., ***cupr.,*** cupr-ac., dig., dulc., eup-per., ***eup-pur.,*** ferr-s., gels., graph., hell., hoit., hydr., hydr-ac., hydrc., ***hyos., ign., ip.,*** juni., ***kali-br.,*** **KALI-C.,** kali-cy., ***kali-i.,*** kali-m., kali-p., kreos., lac-d., lach., lachn., lat-m., laur., lyc., lyss., mag-c., mang., merc., merc-c., mez., mill., ***mur-ac.,*** naja, nat-c., nit-ac., ***nux-v.,*** oena., op., ox-ac., petr., ***phos.,*** phys., phyt., podo., plb., psor., ***puls.,*** pyrus, rheum, rhus-t., rumx-a., sars., ***sec.,*** sel., senec., sep., squil., ***stram.,*** stry., sul-ac., sulph., tab., tanac., tarent., **TUB.,** verat., **ZINC.**
abdomen, from cramping pain in - **COLOC.**
afternoon - cina.
ailments, with little - tub.
alternating with, dancing - bell.
laughing - bell., stram., verat.
songs, gambols - bell.
anxious - **ACON.,** alum., calad., plb.
stupor, with broken, in child with gastritis mucosa - ***ars.***
breath, every, with - bell.
children, in - bor., ***cham., cina,*** lach., mill., phyt., ***podo.,*** sac-alb.
carried, if desires to be - puls.
piteous, of child, because he cannot have what he wanted - **CHAM.**
wanted, piteous because they cannot have what they - **CHAM.**

MOANING, groaning
chill, during - arn., chin-a., cupr., ***eup-per., nat-m.,*** samb.
colic, during - sep.
constant and gasping for air - kreos., mang., merc., phyt.
contradicted, when - tarent.
convulsions, in - ***ign., sil., tub.***
cough, during - bell., cina, podo.
whooping-cough - ***cupr-ac.***
crying, with - ***hell.***
daytime - zinc.
dentition, in - **CHAM.,** phyt., ***podo.***
diarrhea, in - ***apis***
dreaming, while - ant-t., arn., ars., aur., ***bapt., bell.,*** carb-v., ***cham.,*** cic., cupr-ac., ***gels.,*** graph., ***hell.,*** hyos., kali-br., lach., lyc., ***mur-ac.,*** nat-m., nit-ac., ***op.,*** puls., rhus-t., verat.
frightful dreams, with - puls.
ear lobes, with hot - ***alum.***
epilepsy, in, after fall on head - cupr.
evening - ars., coca.
evening, sleep, during - ars.
fate, about the - ***kali-br.***
fever, during - acon., ***arn.,*** bell., cham., chin-a., coff., eup-per., ign., ip., lach., ***mur-ac.,*** nux-v., podo., **PULS.,** thuj., verat.
head, holds, and, vomiting, when - cimic.
hemicrania, with - cop.
honor, from wounded - ***nux-v.***
ill humor, from - cham.
illness, before - ant-t.
impulse, to - graph.
involuntary - ***alum., cham.,*** hell.
lifted, when - sul-ac.
loud - mur-ac., stram., stry.
sleep, in - calad.
measles, in, plantive moaning - ***lach.***
menses, after - ***stram.***
menses, during - ***ars., cocc.,*** lyc., plat.
morning - ***bor.***
night - ***ars.,*** cupr., hep., phyt., plat., podo., sec., sol-n., tarent., zinc.
3 a.m. - **KALI-C.**
dentition, in difficult - ***phyt.***
melancholy, with - plat.
tossing about, with - ***dulc.***
objects, about - caps.
offence happened long ago, for trifling - ***cham.***
old age, in - ***bar-c.***
pain, from - cham., ***coff., coloc., eup-per., hydr., nux-v.,*** phos., sil.
perspiration, during - acon., bar-c., bry., camph., chin., cupr., ***merc.,*** phos., stram., verat.
pollutions, after - hipp.
restlessness, with - **CHAM.,** ***stram.***
sleep, during - ***ail.,*** aloe, ***alum.,*** am-c., anac., ant-t., apis, arn., ***ars.,*** ars-h., **AUR.,** ***bapt., bell.,*** bry., bufo, cadm-s., calad., calc., calc-p., ***carb-an.,*** carb-v., caust., ***cham.,*** chin., cic., clem., coc-c., cocc., coff.,

MOANING, groaning
sleep, during - con., ***crot-c.,*** cupr., erio., eup-per., ***gels.,*** graph., ***hell.,*** hyos., ***ign., ip., kali-br.,*** kali-p., kreos., lach., led., ***lyc.,*** merc., ***mur-ac.,*** nat-m., ***nit-ac., nux-v., op.,*** ph-ac., phos., plect., ***podo., puls.,*** rheum, rhus-t., ***samb.,*** sep., sil., stann., ***sulph., thuj.***
children - **CALC-P.**
eyelids half closed, rolling of head, with - ***podo., samb.***
grinding of teeth, with - ***kali-br.***
sleepiness, with - ***cham.***
sleeplessness, with - crot-c.
stool, before - puls.
touch, on - ant-t.
trifle, about every - caust.
waking, on - am-c., cina.
weakness - graph.
whooping-cough - ***cupr-ac.***
why, does not know - ***hyos.***

MOCKING - acon., alum., anh., ars., chin., guai., hyos., ign., ip., ***lach.,*** nux-m., nux-v., par., ped., plat., stann., tarent., verat.
friends, at his - alco.
jealousy, with - ***lach.***
others are mocking him, thinks - ign., nux-v., ph-ac., sep.
relatives, his - sec.
ridicule, passion to - acon., hyos., lach., nux-v., verat.
sarcasm - ***ars.,*** bry., cann-i., carb-o., caust., cinnb., ign., lac-ac., ***lach.,*** nux-v., pall., sec., sep.
satire, desire for - ars., ***lach.***

MONOMANIA - acon., anac., anan., aur., carb-v., camph., cic., hell., ***ign.,*** nux-m., puls., ***sil.,*** stram., sulph., thuj., ***verat.***
appear in a public place in a grotesque manner, to - anan., hyos.
property, of - ***ars.,*** sep., sil., sulph.
religious - plb., stram., ***verat.***

MONEY, passion for making - calc., carc., ign., ***lyc.,*** med., **NUX-V.,** sulph.

MOODS, general
agreeable - abrot., ant-t., croc., ign., lach., meny., plat., sul-ac., zing.
alternating - ***acon.,*** agn., **ALUM.,** alum-p., anac., ***anh.,*** ant-t., arn., ars., ars-i., asaf., asar., aur., aur-i., ***bar-c.,*** bar-i., **BELL.,** bism., bor., **BOV.,** calc., cann-s., caps., ***carb-an.,*** **CARC.,** caust., ***cench., chin.,*** cob-n., con., cortico., cortiso., ***croc.,*** cupr., cycl., ***dros.,*** **FERR.,** ferr-ar., ferr-i., ***ferr-p., graph.,*** hist., hyos., **IGN., IOD.,** ***kali-c.,*** kali-s., lac-c., **LYC.,** man., med., merc., ***naja,*** nat-c., ***nat-m.,*** nid., ***nux-v.,*** op., ***phos.,*** **PLAT.,** ***puls.,*** **SARS.,** seneg., sep., stann., staph., stram., **SUL-AC.,** ***sulph.,*** tarent., ***tub.,*** valer., verb., **ZINC.**
bad, in cloudy weather - aloe., aur.

MOODS, general

changeable, variable - ***acon.,*** acon-l., agar., agn., alco., aloe, ***alum.,*** alum-p., alum-sil., am-c., ambr., anac., ang., ant-c., ant-t., ***apis,*** arg-m., ***arg-n.,*** arn., ***ars.,*** ars-h., ars-i., asaf., asar., astra-e., ***aur.,*** aur-i., aur-m., aur-s., ***bar-ac., bar-c., bell.,*** bism., ***bor.,*** bov., bry., bufo, buth-a., ***calc., calc-p.,*** calc-s., calc-sil., cann-i., cann-s., caps., carb-an., carb-o., carb-s., carb-v., **CARC.,** carl., caust., cham., ***chin.,*** cimic., cina, coc-c., coca, ***cocc., coff.,*** con., cortico., ***croc., cupr.,*** cycl., ***dig.,*** dros., eup-per., ***ferr.,*** ferr-ar., form., gels., graph., hell., hyos., **IGN.,** iod., ***kali-c.,*** kali-p., kali-s., kali-sil., lac-c., lac-d., lach., lachn., **LYC.,** ***mag-c.,*** mag-m., med., meny., ***merc.,*** merc-c., mez., morph., mosch., nat-c., nat-m., nid., nit-ac., **NUX-M.,** nux-v., onop., op., ***petr.,*** phel., ***phos.,*** pic-ac., plan., ***plat.,*** plb., ***psor.,*** **PULS.,** ran-b., rat., rheum, rhod., ruta, sabad., sabin., sang., sanic., sapin., **SARS.,** seneg., ***sep.,*** sil., spig., spong., ***stann., staph., stram., sul-ac.,*** sul-i., sulph., tab., tarax., tarent., thuj., ***tub., valer.,*** verat., verb., viol-o., yuc., **ZINC.,** zinc-p.
- dinner, after - aloe.
- evening - aur., croc., puls.
  - alternating evenings, on - ferr.
- fever, during - ***nux-m.***
- menses, before - cham.
- night - carb-v.
  - agg. - cic.
- nosebleed, amel. - bor.
- opinions, in - bell., graph., kali-c., lyc., petr., plat.
- perspiration, during - ***aur.,*** croc., ***stram.,*** **SUL-AC.,** zinc.
- rapidly - asaf., croc., ign., puls., rhod., sep., tab., tarent., tub., ***valer.***
- supper, after - am-c., carb-v.
- touch, on - asaf.

insupportable - calc.

repulsive - acon., alum., ambr., ant-c., arn., ars., aur., bell., camph., caps., carb-ac., carc., caust., con., croc., ***hep.,*** ign., ip., kali-c., lact., laur., led., lyc., mag-c., mag-m., ***merc.,*** nit-ac., nux-v., petr., phos., plb., ***psor., puls.,*** samb., sars., sep., sil., spong., sulph., ***thuj.***
- everyone, to - aloe

wills, between opposite - ***anac., ign.,*** irid., op.

MOON, general (see Environment, moon)

MORAL feelings, want of - abrot., acetan., achy., am-c., **ANAC.,** ars., aster., **BELL.,** bism., ***bufo,*** cass., cer-s., cham., chin., clem., ***coca, cocaine,*** cocc., con., coloc., convo-d., croc., cur., hep., **HYOS.,** ***kali-br.,*** lac-c., **LACH.,** ***laur., morph.,*** nat-m., nit-ac., nux-v., op., ped., ph-ac., pic-ac., ***plat.,*** psil., sabad., ***sep.,*** **STRAM.,** stry-p., ***tarent.,*** **VERAT.**
- criminal, disposition to become a, without remorse - **ANAC.,** ars., bell., hep., ***lach.,*** med., merc., stram., thuj.

MOROSE, feelings (see Gloomy)

MORTIFICATION, (See Abused, Humiliation)

MURMURING, in sleep - raph., puls., sulph.

MUSIC, general

agg. - **ACON.,** ***aloe, ambr., anac.,*** bry., bufo, cact., ***calc.,*** carb-an., ***carc.,*** caust., ***cham., coff., croc., dig.,*** **GRAPH.,** ***ign.,*** kali-c., kreos., ***lyc.,*** med., merc., **NAT-C.,** nat-m., nat-p., ***nat-s.,*** **NUX-V.,** pall., ***ph-ac., phos.,*** phys., puls., ***sabin.,*** **SEP.,** stann., staph., sumb., tarent., tub., viol-o.
- menses, during - nat-c.
- organ, of - lyc., thuj.
- piano playing - cham., ***nat-c.,*** phos., sep.
- sad - nat-m.
- violin playing - calc., ***kali-c., viol-o.***

agreeable, is - cann-i., ign., tarent.

amel. - am-m., anh., **AUR.,** ***aur-m.,*** cann-s., carc., croc., cupr., mang., merc., nat-m., sul-ac., sumb., **TARENT.,** ***thuj.,*** tub.
- restlessness of extremities - **TARENT.**
- sad - mang.

aversion to - **ACON.,** alum., bufo, carc., caust., cham., hep., merc., nit-ac., ***nux-v.,*** sabin., sep., viol-o.
- joyous, but immediately affected by saddest - mang.
- violin - viol-o.

carried by, sensation of being - anh.

cough, music agg. - **AMBR.,** ***calc.,*** cham., kali-c., kreos., ph-ac.
- piano, when playing - ambr., **CALC.,** cham., kali-c., kreos., ph-ac.
- violin, when playing on - kali-c.

desire, to playing piano - chlor., ***plat.***

drums, produce euphoria - anh.

ear-ache, from - ambr., cham., kreos., ***ph-ac.,*** tab.

faintness, on hearing - cann-i., sumb.

headache, from - acon., ambr., cact., **COFF.,** nux-v., ***ph-ac., phos.,*** podo., viol-o.

loves, to hear or play - ***carc., tarent.***

palpitation, when listening to - ***ambr.,*** carb-v., ***staph.,*** sulph.

sleepiness, from - stann.

trembling, from - aloe, **AMBR.,** nat-c., thuj.
- feet, of - thuj.

weariness, from - lyc.
- playing piano - anac.

MUTILATE, body, inclination to - agar., ***ars.,*** bell., hyos., staph., stram.

MULTIPLE, personalites disorders (see Insanity, Schizophrenia) - ***anac.,*** carc., ***plat.,*** stram., verat.
- control, under, is superhuman - agar., ***anac., lach., naja,*** op., plat., ***thuj.***
- double, delusion of being - alum., arg-n., **ANAC.,** anh., arg-n., ***bapt.,*** cann-i., ***cann-i.,*** cann-s., cycl., ***gels.,*** glon., lach., lil-t., lyc., mosch., nat-m., ***nux-m.,*** op., ***petr.,*** phos., **PLAT.,** plb., psor., puls., pyrog., sec., sil., ***stram.,*** ther., thuj., ***trill.,*** valer., xan.

MULTIPLE, personalites disorders
identity, errors of personal - ***alum.,*** anac., ant-c., bapt., cann-i., cann-s., cic., hyos., lac-c., lach., mosch., nat-m., petr., phos., plat., plb., pyrog., pyrus, stram., thuj., valer., ***verat.***
belong, to her own family, does not - ***plat.***
christ, thinks himself to be - cann-i., verat.
divine, thinks he is - cann-i., glon., stram., verat.
emperor, thought himself an - cann-i.
general, that he is a - cupr.
great, person, is - ***agar.,*** aeth., alum., bell., ***cann-i.,*** cupr., glon., ***hyos., lach.,*** lyc., lyss., phos., ***plat.,*** stram., sulph., ***verat.***
noble, thinks he is a - phos., plat.
officer, that he is an - agar., bell., cann-i., ***cupr.,*** cupr-ac.
queen, thinks she is - cann-i., plat.
some one, else, thinks she is - anac., ***cann-i.,*** cann-s., gels., ***lach.,*** mosch., phos., plat., plb., pyrog., stram., ***valer., verat.***
virgin, mary, thinks she is - cann-i., verat.
possessed, as if, by spirits - ***anac.,*** bell., canth., ***hyos.,*** man., op., ***plat.,*** sil., ***stram., sulph.,*** verat.
demoniacal, thinks he is - **ANAC., HYOS.**
devil, by a - **ANAC.,** ***hyos., plat.,*** **STRAM.**
three, persons, delusion that he is - anac., bapt., cann-i., nux-m., ***petr.***

MUTTERING - ether, ail., alum., anac., ***apis, arn.,*** ars., ars-s-f., arum-t., atro., bapt., ***bell.,*** bry., calad., calc., calc-sil., cann-s., caust., cham., chel., chlor., cic., ***cocc.,*** colch., coni., ***crot-h.,*** dulc., hell., ***hep.,*** **HYOS.,** iris, **LACH.,** ***lyc., merc.,*** morph., ***mur-ac.,*** nat-m., nux-v., ***op.,*** ph-ac., ***phos.,*** plb., ***rhus-t.,*** sang., sec., sil., stann., **STRAM.,** sul-ac., tab., tarax., ***verat.,*** vesp., vip.
evening - bell., con., ***phos.,*** plb.
bed, in - sil.
falling asleep, on - calc-sil.
himself, to - hyos., tarax.
night - ***arg-n.,*** atro.
waking, on - atro., sil.
old age, in - ***bar-c.***
sleep, in - alum., ***apis,*** ars., bar-ac., bar-c., camph., con., ***hyos.,*** indg., kali-br., merc., ***nit-s-d.,*** raph., ***rhus-t.,*** sul-ac., **SULPH.**
sleeplessness, with - **HYOS.**
stroke, in - ***arn., cocc., crot-h.***
unintelligible - ***anac-oc., ars.,*** cann-s., ***hell.,*** hyos., ***nux-v.***

NAKED, wants to be - ***bell.,*** bufo, camph., cham., **HYOS.,** merc., merc-c., ***phos.,*** phyt., puls., ***sec., stram.,*** tarent., ***verat.***
bares her breast in puerperal mania - ***camph.***

NAKED, wants to be
constantly, wants to be - ***stram.***
delirium, in - ***bell.,*** **HYOS.,** merc., ***phos.,*** phyt., ***sec., stram.***
drunkenness, during - hyos.
hyperaesthesia of skin, in - ***hyos.***
morning in bed - hyos., mag-c., phos.
sleep, in - hyos., merc., puls., sulph.

NARRATING, her symptoms agg. - **CALC.,** cic., ign., ***puls.,*** teucr.

NARROW-minded - alum., am-c., ars., bar-c., con., ***kali-c.,*** sulph.

NEGLECTS, his own appearance - coca, ph-ac., ***sulph.***
business - op., ***sulph.***
children, her - aur-a., sep.
everything - am-c., bar-c., caust., ph-ac., tell.
household, the - aur-a., sul-i.
important things - alum., con.

NEW, all objects seem - ***hell.,*** stram.

NEWS, bad, ailments from - acon., alumn., ***apis, arn.,*** ars., art-v., aur., ***bry.,*** **CALC.,** ***calc-p., caust., cham.,*** chin., cic., cinnb., cocc., colch., ***coloc.,*** cupr., dig., dros., form., **GELS.,** grat., hyos., **IGN.,** kali-c., kali-p., lach., lyss., ***med.,*** mez., ***nat-m.,*** nat-p., ***nux-v.,*** paeon., ***pall.,*** ph-ac., phos., puls., sabin., sep., ***staph.,*** stram., ***sulph.,*** tarent., teucr.
joyful, feels as if he had received - ***lyss.***
sad or depressing news, headache after - calc-p., cocc., ***gels.,*** ign., nat-m., nux-v., op., staph.

NYMPHOMANIA, (See Sexual, behaviour)

OBSESSIVE-compulsive disorder - ***anac., arg-n.,*** **ARS.,** aur., ***calc., carc.,*** **HYOS.,** ***ign.,*** iod., **MED.,** ***nat-m., nat-s.,*** **NUX-V.,** ***plat.,*** psor., **PULS.,** ***sil., staph.,*** sulph., syph., thuj., ***verat.***

OBSTINATE, stubborn - abrot., ***acon.,*** act-sp., ***agar.,*** alco., aloe, **ALUM.,** alum-p., alum-sil., alumn., am-c., **ANAC.,** ***ant-c.,*** ant-t., apis, **ARG-N.,** arn., ***ars.,*** ars-s-f., arum-t., aur., aur-a., aur-s., bar-ac., **BAR-C., BELL., BRY.,** bufo, **CALC.,** calc-f., **CALC-P.,** ***calc-s.,*** camph., canth., ***caps.,*** carb-an., carb-s., carb-v., carc., ***caust.,*** **CHAM.,** chel., ***chin.,*** chin-s., **CINA,** coca, coloc., croc., ***crot-h.,*** cycl., dig., dros., ferr., ferr-ar., ferr-p., guai., hell., ***hep.,*** hura, ***hyos., ign.,*** ip., ***kali-c.,*** kali-i., kali-m., ***kali-p.,*** kali-s., kali-sil., kalm., kreos., lach., ***lyc., mag-m.,*** menis., merc., mosch., mur-ac., ***nit-ac.,*** **NUX-V.,** ***pall.,*** petr., ***ph-ac.,*** phel., phos., plat., plb., ***psor.,*** puls., ***sanic.,*** sec., sep., ***sil., spong., staph.,*** stram., ***sulph.,*** syph., **TARENT.,** ***thuj.,*** **TUB.,** verat., viol-o., viol-t., zinc., zinc-p.
against whatever was proposed, he had the queerest objection - **ARG-N.**
appearance of menses, upon - ***cham.***
children - abrot., am-c., ***ant-c.,*** arg-n., ars., arum-t., aur., bell., **CALC.,** ***calc-p., caps.,*** carc., ***cham., chin., cina,*** hyos., kreos., lyc., nux-v., psor., ***sanic.,*** sec., ***sil.,*** syph., tarent., thuj., **TUB.**

OBSTINATE, stubborn
children,
annoy those around them - ***psor.***
chilly, refractory and clumsy - ***caps.***
inclined to grow fat - **CALC.**
masturbation, boys after - aur.
yet cry when kindly spoken to - sil.
declares there is nothing the matter with him - apis, **ARN.**
eruption, during - psor.
evening - ign., mur-ac.
execution of plans, in - dros.
fever, during - acon.
forenoon - chin-s.
friendly, tries to appear - ***pall.***
menorrhagia, in - ***nux-v.***
menses, upon appearence of - ***cham.***
night - dig.
queerest objection, against whatever was proposed, he had the - **ARG-N.**
resists wishes of others - alum., **NUX-V.**
simpleton, as a - lyc., plat., verat.
stool, during - sulph.
tossing about impatiently - ***acon.***

OCCUPATION, (see Work)

OFFENDED, easily, takes everything in bad part - ***acon.***, agar., ***alum.***, anac., ang., ***apis***, arn., **ARS.**, ars-s-f., ***aur.***, aur-a., aur-s., ***bell.***, bor., ***bov.***, ***bufo***, **CALC.**, calc-ar., calc-s., camph., cann-s., ***caps.***, carb-an., carb-s., ***carb-v.***, **CARC.**, **CAUST.**, cench., cham., ***chel.***, chin., chin-a., cic., ***cina***, cinnb., ***cocc.***, ***coloc.***, ***croc.***, ***cycl.***, dros., ***graph.***, hyos., **IGN.**, **IOD.**, kali-n., ***lach.***, lil-t., **LYC.**, lyss., mag-s., merc., nat-c., **NAT-M.**, nit-ac., **NUX-V.**, ***pall.***, ***petr.***, phos., ***plat.***, prot., ***puls.***, ran-b., ***sars.***, ***sep.***, ***sil.***, ***spig.***, stann., **STAPH.**, stram., sul-ac., ***sulph.***, syph., thuj., **TUB.**, ***verat.***, viol-o., ***zinc.***, zinc-p.
takes everything in bad part, offenses, from past - calc., ***cham.***, ***ign.***, ***op.***, ***staph.***

OPTIMISTIC - anh., ***calc.***, coff., ferr-m., fl-ac., hydrc., ign., lyc., nep., nux-v., ***op.***, puls., rib-ac., sil., ***sulph.***, visc.
weakness, in spite of the - gali., kali-c.

PAINLESSNESS, of complaints, usually painful - **ARN.**, ***hell.***, **OP.**, **STRAM.**

PANIC, attacks of anxiety - **ACON.**, aloe, alum., ang., **ARG-N.**, ars., bar-c., bell., calc-i., ***cann-i.***, ***carb-v.***, caust., ***cham.***, chel., ***cocc.***, ***cupr.***, ***cupr-ar.***, ferr., ***hyos.***, ictod., ign., **KALI-AR.**, ***lyc.***, med., nat-c., nat-m., nat-s., nit-ac., **PHOS.**, plat., ruta, sep., spong., ***sulph.***, ***tab.***, thuj.
cannot control herself - ***arg-n.***, ***cupr-ac.***
heart disease, in - acon., ***kali-ar.***, phos., ***spong.***
night agg. - ***ars.***
throat in, with - **SPONG.**

PASSIONATE - ***alco.***, ***anac.***, ars., aur., ***bar-c.***, ***bell.***, ***bry.***, calc., cann-i., canth., carb-s., ***carb-v.***, **CARC.**, ***caust.***, coff., con., croc., hep., hura, hyos., ign., ***ip.***, ***kali-c.***, **KALI-I.**, lach., laur., led., **MED.**, **NAT-C.**, nat-m., nat-s., **NUX-V.**, olnd., petr., ph-ac., phos., plat., ***psor.***, sabad., seneg., ***sep.***,

PASSIONATE - stann., stram., ***sulph.***, sumb., tarent., ***thuj.***, **TUB.**
morning - nat-s.
trifle, at every - nat-m., nux-v., ph-ac., phos., sumb.

PASSIVE (see Bashful, Mild, Timid, Yielding)

PEACE, sense of heavenly, (see Tranquility) - arg-m., ***cann-i.***, **OP.**

PERSEVERANCE - acon., bry., caps., calc., dig., dros., guare., lac-c., lyc., nat-c., nit-ac., nux-v., phos., plan., sil., sulph.
duties, in performing irksome - linu-c.
has none - alum., asaf., grat., lac-c., lach., ***lyc.***, nux-v., phos., plan., ***sil.***, sulph.

PERTINACITY, (see Obstinate, Perseverance) - caps., dros., stram.

PESSIMISTIC - agar-t., **ARS.**, **AUR.**, bar-c., calc., caust., cecr., halo., hyos., lach., **NIT-AC.**, ***nux-v.***, pers., ***psor.***, sep., stann., vip-a.
good and bad by turns - alum., med., psor.
takes everything into bad part - anac., ***ars.***, bov., caps., cocc., nat-m., ***nit-ac.***, nux-v., puls., staph., verat.
temper, in morning - lyc., mag-c., ***nux-v.***, sars.

PITIES, feelings of, self - agar., ***aur.***, **CALC.**, carc., nit-ac., **PULS.**, ***staph.***
desire to show being - tarent.

PLANS, making many - anac., agn., ang., arg-n., **CHIN.**, ***chin-s.***, ***coff.***, ***lyc.***, ***nat-s.***, ***nux-v.***, olnd., op., sep., **SULPH.**, tab., visc.
bold - agar.
carrying out, insists on - dros.
evening - ***chin.***, ***chin-s.***, ***sulph.***
gigantic - op., sulph.
night - **CHIN.**, sulph.
revengeful - agar., ***anac.***, ***lach.***

PLAY, general
alternating with, sadness - psor.
aversion to, in children - ***bar-c.***, bar-m., ***cina***, ***hep.***, ***lyc.***, merc., nat-m., **RHEUM**, ***sulph.***
sit in corner and play - bar-c., bar-m.
desire to - ***con.***, tarent.
buttons of his clothes, with the - mosch.
dirty trick on others or their teachers, schoolboys p. a - lach., zinc.
grass, in the - elaps
hide and seek, at - bell.
night - cypr., ***med.***
night, children, in - cypr.
toys, with childish - **CIC.**
inability to - merc., sulph.

PLAYFUL - aloe, bufo, cimic., cocc., croc., elaps, ign., lach., meny., naja, ox-ac., seneg., tarent.

PLAYS, with his fingers - calc., crot-c., rhus-t.
with buttons of his clothes - mosch.

PLEASURE, feeling - ang., cann-i., carb-ac., cod., ether, mate, op., til.
morning - til.
sleeplessness, during - sec.

PLEASURE, feeling
voluptuous ideas, only in - bell.
wakefulness, during - sec.
waking, on from a dream of murder - thea.

POSITIVENESS - ars., camph., ***caust.,*** ferr., ***lach., merc.,*** nux-v., sep.

POWER, love of - ***lyc., nux-v.,*** sulph.

PRAYING - ***alum.,*** arn., ***ars.,*** **AUR.,** ***bell.,*** cer-b., euph., hyos., lach., lyss., manc., med., nat-s., op., opun-v., plat., **PULS.,** rhus-t., **SEP., STRAM.,** sul-ac., sulph., **VERAT.**
fervent - alum., **SEP.**
kneeling and - ***ars.,*** aur., nat-s., ***stram.,*** verat.
loud in sadness - ***plat.***
menses, during - ***stram.***
morning - op.
nights - cer-s., stram.
others to pray for him, begged - lyss.
piety, nocturnal - stram.
quietly - arn., ars.
timidly - stann.
vomiting, constantly during paroxysm of - med.

PRECISION, of mind increased - coff., ferr-p.

PRECOCITY, mental - **ASAR.,** calc., carc., lyc., merc., phos., tub., verat.

PRESUMPTUOUS - arn., calc., ***lyc.,*** plat., staph.

PRETENDS, to be sick - arg-n., bell., ign., mosch., plb., sabad., sil., ***tarent., verat.***
deafness, to be - verat.
faintness - ***tarent.***
pregnancy, to be - verat.

PROCRASTINATES (see Laziness) - ***lyc.,*** med., sulph.

PROPHESYING - ***acon.,*** agar., anh., ant-c., camph., con., **LACH.,** med., nux-m., stram.
disagreeable events, of - med.
predicts the time of death - **ACON.,** ***arg-n.,*** thea.

PUBERTY, mental problems during - ant-c., hell., ***ign.,*** manc., ***nat-m., puls., sep.***

PULL, desires to, one's hair - ars., **BELL.,** ***cina,*** cupr., lach., ***lil-t.,*** med., mez., tarent., tub.
one's nose in the street - merc.
one's teeth - bell.
presses her head and pulls her hair - tarent.

PUNISHMENT, ailments after - agar., ***anac.,*** **CARC.,** cham., coloc., ign., lyc., nat-m., **STAPH.**

PUNS, makes - cann-i.

QUARRELSOME - acon., agar., alco., aloe, alum., ambr., am-c., ***anac.,*** anan., ang., anh., ant-t., ***arn., ars.,*** ars-s-f., ***asaf.,*** asar., aster., atro., **AUR.,** aur-a., aur-s., bar-c., ***bell.,*** bor., ***bov., brom., bry.,*** bufo, cael., calc., calc-s., ***camph.,*** canth., caps., caste., ***caust.,*** cench., **CHAM.,** chel., chin., **CINA,** coff., colch., ***con.,*** cor-r., ***croc.,*** crot-h., culx., ***cupr.,*** cyn-d., dig., ***dulc.,*** elaps, ferr., ferr-ar., fl-ac., gran., ***hep.,*** hipp., hir., ***hist.,*** **HYOS.,** ictod., **IGN.,** ip., kali-ar., ***kali-c.,***

QUARRELSOME - ***kali-chl.,*** kali-i., kali-p., ***lach.,*** lepi., lil-t., ***lyc.,*** lyss., mag-aust., mag-c., mag-s., meph., ***merc.,*** merl., mez., ***mosch.,*** nat-a., ***nat-c., nat-m.,*** nat-s., nicc., ***nit-ac., nit-s-d.,*** **NUX-V.,** olnd., op., pall., **PETR.,** ***ph-ac., phos., plat.,*** plb., ***psor.,*** puls., ***ran-b.,*** rat., reser., rheum, ***rhus-t.,*** rib-ac., ruta, sac-alb., seneg., **SEP.,** ***sil.,*** spong., stann., ***staph., stram.,*** stront-c., sulfonam., **SULPH.,** sul-ac., **TARENT.,** thea., ***thuj.,*** til., tub., upa., ***verat., verat-v.,*** viol-o., viol-t., zinc.
afternoon - alum., dulc.
4 p.m. - lyc., lyss.
ailments from quarrels - berb., caust., chion., cic., glon., ***ign.,*** kali-chl., nat-m., spig., ***staph.,*** thuj.
alternating with
care and discontent - ran-b.
gaiety and laughter - croc., ***lach.,*** spong., ***staph.***
silent depression - aur., ***con.***
singing - croc.
anger, without - bell., caust., ***dulc.,*** staph.
causeless - stram.
childbirth, during - **CHAM.**
disputes with absent persons - lyc.
disturbed, if - **NUX-V.**
evening - am-c., ant-c., nat-m., nicc., op., psor., sil., til.
face, heat of, with - mosch.
pale, with - mosch.
family, with her - kali-p., thyr.
forenoon - ran-b.
herself, with - merc.
himself and his family, with - kali-c.
intoxicated, when - ***petr.***
jealousy, from - ***cench., hyos., lach.,*** nux-v.
menses, during - am-c.
menses, at beginning of - ***cham.***
morning - ***lyc.,*** petr., psor., ran-b.
night - verat.
noon - 2 p.m. - aster.
pains, during - nux-v.
before - cor-r.
pugnatious - bell., nat-c., nicc.
recriminations about trifles - cop.
sleep, in - alum., ars., ***bell.,*** caust., cupr., hep., merc., raph., rheum
staring of eyes, heat of face, bluish lips, dry mouth, with - mosch.
waiting for answers, without - ***ambr., graph.***
waking, on - lyc.

QUESTIONS, speaks continually in - ambr., ***aur.***

QUICK, to act - ***coff.,*** ign., ***lach.***

QUIET, disposition - abies-c., aloe, ***alum.,*** am-c., ars., asar., ***aur., bell.,*** bism., brucin., caps., ***caust.,*** cham., ***cic.,*** clem., cocc., dros., euph., euphr., ***gels., hell., hyos., ign.,*** ip., ***lach.,*** lyc., mang., mur-ac., **NAT-M.,** nux-v., op., petr., **PH-AC.,** plat., ***plb.,*** puls., rheum, sabad., sars., sep., sil., stann., thuj., tub., valer., viol-t., zinc.

QUARRELSOME,
alternating with, gaiety, trilling, singing - aur., bell.
laughing - nux-m.
rage - hyos.
childbirth, after - ***thuj.***
clasped, with hands - puls.
heat, during - ***bry., gels.***
hypochondriasis, in - puls., valer.
light and noise are intolerable - con.
menses, during - am-c., mur-ac.
noise, intolerable to - con.
sleep, after - anac.
wants to be - ars., bell., **BRY.**, cadm-s., cann-i., coca, cupr-s., dios., eryt-j., euph., **GELS.**, sal-ac.
afternoon - sapin.
chill, during - ars., **BRY.**, ***kali-c.***
desires repose and tranquility - bell., con., nux-v., sulph.
walking in open air - arn., bor., calc-p., sabin.

QUIETED, cannot be - calc-p., **CHAM., CINA.**
carried, only when - **CHAM.**
rapidly - ars., ***cham.***

RAGE, feelings, fury (see Violent) - ***acon.***, acon-c., ***aeth.***, **AGAR.**, agn., alco., alumn., **ANAC.**, ant-t., arg-m., arg-n., ***arn., ars.***, ars-s-f., ***atro.***, aur., bar-c., **BELL.**, bry., bufo, calc., ***camph.***, cann-i., cann-s., **CANTH.**, ***carb-s.***, cham., chel., chin., chin-s., cic., cimic., cina, cocc., ***colch.***, coloc., cori-r., croc., crot-h., ***cupr.***, cyn-d., dig., dros., dulc., eupi., fl-ac., glon., graph., ***hell.***, hep., **HYOS.**, hyper., ign., jatr., kali-c., **LAC-C.**, **LACH.**, lob., ***lol.***, **LYC.**, mag-p-a., med., meli., ***merc.***, **MOSCH.**, ***nat-m., nit-ac.***, nux-m., **NUX-V.**, oena., **OP.**, par., petr., ph-ac., ***phos.***, plb., ***puls.***, raja-s., raph., ruta, sabad., ***sec.***, seneg., sep., ***sol-n., staph.***, **STRAM.**, stry., sulo-ac., ***sulph.***, sul-ac., ***tab.***, tarent., thyr., tub., **VERAT.**, vip., zinc.
ailments from rage, fury - ***apis, arn.***, carc., **STAPH.**
alone, while - bufo.
alternating, with,
affectionate disposition - croc.
anxiety - bell.
cheerfulness - acon., bell., cann-s., croc., hyos., seneg.
consciousness - acon., stram.
convulsions - **STRAM.**
desire for death - bell.
fear - bell.
laughing - acon.
presentiment of death - stram.
religious excitement - agar.
repose - hyos.
sleep - ars.
amourous, morning when rising - agn.
aroused, when - phos.
biting, with - bell., ***camph.***, canth., croc., cupr., sec., ***stram., verat.***
chained, had to be - ars., sec., stram.
childbirth, during - ***bell.***

RAGE, feelings
chill, during - cann-s., ***cimx.***
cold, applications to head amel. - sabad.
consolation, from - ***nat-m.***
constant - ***agar., verat.***
contradiction, from - aur., ***lac-c.***, olnd.
convulsions, after - op.
convulsive - ars., ***bell., canth., hyos., stram.***
crying, with - cann-i., cann-s.
cursing, with - anac., ***nit-ac.***, verat.
day and night - hyos.
delusion, puts him into rage - ***stram.***
drink or touching larynx, when trying to - canth.
drinking, while - bell., ***stram.***
drunkenness, during - agar.
eating, during and after - chlor.
epilepsy, with - bell., cupr., hyos., nux-v., op., plb.
after - ***arg-m.***, op.
evening - acon., anac., ars., ***bell.***, croc., ***hyos., lach.***, merc., nit-ac., op., phos., plat., puls., thyr., trio., zinc.
foaming mouth, with - ***camph.***
hair, pulls, of bystanders - ***bell.***
hallucinations, from - ***stram.***
headache, with - ***ars.***, **BELL.**, cimic., croc., ***lyc.***, nat-m., puls., **STRAM.**, ***verat.***
heat on body, with - ***verat.***
insults, after - sang., stram.
kill people, tries to - hep., **HYOS.**, lach., sec., ***stram.***
laughing, with - ***stram.***
love, after disappointed - ***hyos., lach.***
malicious - ***anac., bell.***, cann-s., cocc., cupr., ***lach.***, lyc., mosch., petr., sec.
medicine, from forcible administration of - ***bell.***
menses, during - acon., bell., hyos.
at beginning of - acon.
mischievous - agar.
morning, in bed - kali-c.
night - acon., ***apis***, ars., ***bar-c., bell.***, con., ***hyos.***, lyc., merc., nat-c., nat-m., nit-ac., plb., puls., ***verat.***
pain, from - acon., arg-m., cham., hep.
paroxysms, in - acon., camph., canth., chin-b., croc., ***cupr.***, mosch., oena., ***puls., stram., verat.***
reading and writing, by - med.
relatives, does not know his - ***bell.***
repentance, followed by - anac., croc., lyss., tub.
screaming, with - ***anac., bell.***, canth., cupr., hyos., lach., plb., sec., sol-n., ***verat.***
shining objects, from - bell., canth., hyos., lyss., ***stram.***
sleep, in - phos.
rage followed by continuous deep - sec.
spitting, with - bell., ***camph.***, cann-s.
stand, unable to - ***stram.***
staring looks, with - bell.
strength, increased - ***agar.***, **BELL.**, hyos., op.
striking, with - cupr., lyc., stram.

RAGE, feelings
suffering, from - aloe.
suicidal disposition, with - ant-t., sec., stram.
taken up, child on being - ***stram.***
tears, clothes - ***camph.***
tossing about in bed, making unitelligible signs - stram.
touch, renewed by - ***bell.,*** lach., ***op., stram.***
touching, larynx or when trying to drink - canth.
trifles, at - bar-c., cann-s., thyr.
violent - agar., **ANAC.,** bar-c., **BELL.,** canth., cocc., croc., cupr., **HYOS., LACH.,** lyc., nux-v., staph., **STRAM.,** ***verat.***
water, sight of - ***bell., canth.,*** cupr., hyos., lach., merc., ***stram.***
worm, affections, in - ***carb-v.,*** **CINA.**

RASHNESS, (see Impulsive) - ***aur.,*** caps., meny., puls.

READING, agg., symptoms from - ang., asaf., ***calc.,*** carb-ac., cina, cocc., colch., fl-ac., mag-m., med., mur-ac., nat-sil., olnd., ph-ac., stann., tarax.
averse to - ***acon.,*** alum., bar-c., brom., carb-ac., ***carl.,*** clem., coca, con., corn., cycl., hydr., kali-bi., lac-ac., ***lach.,*** lil-t., med., nat-a., ***nux-v.,*** ox-ac., phys., puls., pyrus, ***sil.***
walking in the open air, amel. - ox-ac.
desires to be read to - anth., chin., clem.
difficult, is - ***agn., coca,*** hura.
mental symptoms agg. from, amel. - agn., petr.
passion to read - alum., ***carc.,*** cocc., nat-m., ***sulph.***
medical books - ***calc., carc., nux-v., puls.,*** staph., ***sulph.***
subject, must change the - dros.
unable, to read (see Learning) - aeth., cann-i., cycl., ham., lyc., merc., narcot., nat-m., sep.
children, in - alum., lyc., mag-c.
written, what he has - lyc.
understand, does not - ***ambr., colch.,*** corn-f.

RECOGNIZE, does not, his relatives - acet-ac., agar., ***alum., anac.,*** **BELL.,** calad., cic., cupr., ***glon.,*** **HYOS.,** kali-bi., kali-br., ***lach.,*** lyc., meli., ***merc.,*** nux-m., oena., ***op.,*** phos., plb., sil., ***stram.,*** sul-ac., tab., valer., ***verat.,*** zinc.
anyone - aesc., ***glon., hyos., verat.***
friends - kali-br.
house, his own - meli., merc., psor.
speaking, the one to whom he is - stram.
surroundings - ***kali-p.***
well known streets - arg-n., cann-i., **GLON.,** lach., **NUX-M., PETR.,** plat.

RECOGNIZES, everything, but cannot move - cocc., ***cur.,*** sang.

REFLECT, mentally unable to - acon., alum., ambr., aur., bar-c., lyc., nat-c., nux-m.
old age, in - ***ambr., bar-c.***
studying, from - ***nat-c.***

REFLECTING - berb., ***carb-an.,*** eug., euph., lyss., meny., ***nat-m.,*** ol-an., ***phos.,*** plat.
sadness, in - ***cocc.,*** **NAT-M.,** ***plat.***

REFUSES, (see Eat, refuses)
help - aur., cina., ***nat-m.***
medicine, to take the remedy - ***arn.,*** ars., calad., cimic., hyos., ***kali-p.,*** **LACH.,** ***stram., verat-v.,*** visc.
treatment, every - bell., caust., lach., plat.
in spite of being very sick - arn., ars., caust., nux-v.

REJECTED, feelings - ign., **NAT-M.,** puls., staph., thuj.

REJECTION, ailments from - acon., alum., ***aur.,*** bell., **BRY., CHAM.,** coff., ***coloc.,*** ferr., hyos., ***ign.,*** ip., lyc., **NAT-M., NUX-V.,** olnd., ***par., phos., plat.,*** sep., ***staph.,*** stront-c., sulph., verat.

REJECTS, what he asks for (see Capricious) - arn., ***cham.,*** cina, puls.

RELIGIOUS, affections - ***alum.,*** alum-sil., am-c., ***arg-n., ars.,*** ars-s-f., ***aur.,*** bar-c., ***bell., calc.,*** camph., carb-s., ***carb-v.,*** carc., caust., ***cham., chel.,*** cina, coff., con., croc., cycl., dig., ferr., ferr-ar., ***graph.,*** hura, **HYOS.,** hyper., ***ign.,*** kali-br., ***kali-p.,*** **LACH., LIL-T.,** ***lyc., med., meli.,*** merc., ***mez.,*** nat-m., nux-v., ph-ac., ***plat., psor., puls., rhus-t.,*** rob., ruta, sabad., sel., **SEP.,** sil., stann., staph., **STRAM., SULPH.,** tarax., thuj., **VERAT., ZINC.**
alternating with sexual excitement - lil-t., ***plat.***
bible, want to read all day the - ***calc.,*** stram.
children, in - ***ars., calc.,*** carc., ***lach., stram., sulph.***
fanaticism - aur., med., puls., rob., sel., sulph., thuj., ***verat.***
feeling, want of religous - ***anac.,*** coloc., croc., kali-br., laur.
horror of the opposite sex - lyc., nat-m., ***puls.,*** sulph.
insane - nat-c., stram., verat.
mania - anac., aur., lach., plat., plb., sulph., ***verat.***
melancholia - ars., ***aur., aur-m.,*** con., croc., ***kali-br., kali-p., lach., lyc.,*** lil-t., ***meli.,*** mez., ***plat.,*** plb., psor., puls., sel., ***stram., sulph., verat.***
remorse, from - aur., con.
narrow-minded in religious questions - hyos., kali-c., puls., ***stram.***
night, tortured by religious ideas - aur., camph., lil-t.
penance, desires to do - aur., ***plat., verat.***
preoccupations - achy.
puberty, in - ***ars., calc., lach.,*** puls., ***sulph.***
songs - raja-s.
speculations, dwells on - **SULPH.**
taciturnity, haughtiness, voluptuousness, cruelty, religious affections with - ***plat.***
talking on religious subjects - ***hyos.,*** lach., sulph., ***verat.***

REMORSE, feelings, regret (see Guilt) - alum., alum-sil., am-c., anac., ***ars.***, ars-s-f., ***aur.***, aur-a., ***bell.***, cact., ***calc.***, calc-p., carb-an., carb-v., carc., caust., cham., chel., chin-b., cina, clem., ***cocc.***, **COFF.**, con., croc., ***cupr.***, cycl., ***dig.***, ferr., ferr-ar., graph., ***hyos.***, ***ign.***, kali-br., kalm., lach., ***med.***, merc., nat-c., **NAT-M.**, nit-ac., nux-v., olnd., ***ph-ac.***, phos., plat., psor., ***puls.***, rheum, ruta, sabad., sec., sel., ***sil.***, stram., stront-c., sulph., ***verat.***, ***zinc.***
- afternoon - am-c., carb-v.
- evening - ***puls.***
- indiscretion, over past - spirae.
- menses, after - ***ign.***

REMORSE, feelings
- night - puls.
- repents quickly - ***anac.***, croc., olnd., sulph., tub.
- trifles, about - ***sil.***
- waking, on - puls.

REPROACHES, ailments from, (see Abused, Humiliation) - agar., anac., bell., calc-sil., ***carc.***, cham., ***coloc.***, dys-co., gels., ***ign.***, **LYC.**, med., ***nat-m.***, nux-v., **OP.**, ph-ac., plat., **STAPH.**, ***stram.***, tarent.
- himself - ***acon.***, anac., ***ars.***, **AUR.**, aur-a., calc-p., cob., con., cycl., ***dig.***, gink-b., hell., hura, ***hyos.***, ***ign.***, kali-br., lach., lyc., ***mag-arct.***, med., merc., nat-a., ***nat-m.***, ***op.***, ph-ac., ***puls.***, ***sarr.***, sil., ***staph.***, stram., sulph., ***thuj.***, verat.
  - laughing at reproaches - ***graph.***
- others - ***acon.***, alum., **ARS.**, aur., bor., ***calc.***, calc-p., caps., ***carc.***, cham., **CHIN.**, cic., gels., gran., ***hyos.***, ign., **LACH.**, ***lyc.***, med., **MERC.**, mez., nat-a., ***nat-m.***, ***nux-v.***, par., rhus-t., sep., ***staph.***, sulph., **VERAT.**
  - afternoon, 4 p.m. - bor.
  - imaginary insult, for - aur-a.
  - morning - ***ph-ac.***
  - pains, during - ***cham.***, nux-v.

REPULSIVE, mood - acon., alum., ambr., ant-c., arn., ars., aur., bell., camph., caps., carb-ac., ***carc.***, caust., con., croc., ***hep.***, ign., ip., kali-c., lact., laur., led., lyc., mag-c., mag-m., ***merc.***, nit-ac., nux-v., petr., phos., plb., ***psor.***, **PULS.**, samb., sars., ***sep.***, sil., spong., sulph., ***thuj.***, upa.
- everyone, repulses - aloe.
- help, repulses - ***cina.***

RESERVED - aeth., alco., alum., alum-p., arg-n., arn., ars., asar., ***aur.***, aur-a., bell., bism., cact., ***calc.***, caps., carb-an., caust., cham., chin., clem., coloc., cycl., dros., euph., euphr., fl-ac., grat., ***hell.***, ***hyos.***, ***ign.***, indg., ip., lach., lyc., mag-c., ***mang.***, meny., ***mur-ac.***, **NAT-M.**, nit-ac., nux-v., olnd., op., petr., ph-ac., **PHOS.**, ***plat.***, plb., ***puls.***, rheum, sabad., sabin., sil., spong., ***stann.***, ***staph.***, verat.
- afternoon - anac., mang.
- air, in open - plat., stram.
- displeasure - aur., ign., ip., nat-m., ***staph.***
- eating, after - plb.
- evening - am-m.

RESERVED,
- menses, during - am-c., mur-ac.
- morning - cocc., hep., petr.
  - bed, in - cocc.
- sleep, after - anac.
- walking, in open air, while - bor., ph-ac., sabin.
  - after - arn., calc.

RESIGNATION - agar., agn., ***alum.***, anh., **AUR.**, bry., chin-b., lyc., nat-m., nit-ac., ***ph-ac.***, pic-ac., staph., sulph., ***tab.***, ***tub.***

RESPONSIBILITY, aversion to - **LYC.**, ***med.***, phos.
- burdened, with, at too young of age - ***calc.***, ***carc.***
- inability to realize - fl-ac., lyc.
- over responsible - aur., ***calc.***, calc-p., ***carc.***, ign., nat-m., nat-s.
- unusual agg. - aur., ***calc.***, ***carc.***, lyc.

REST, desire for - ***aesc.***, alum., ***anac.***, arn., bell., brom., ***bry.***, calc., clem., coca, ***colch.***, haem., kali-bi., lach., lyc., morph., nux-v., op., ***ph-ac.***, sabad., sil., ***stann.***, vesp.
- afternoon - mez., phos.
- cannot, when things are not in proper place - anac., **ARS.**, calc., sep., sulph.

RESTLESSNESS, (see Hurried) - abies-c., abies-n., abrot., absin., **ACON.**, acon-c., act-sp., adon., aeth., ***agar.***, agar-ph., agar-st., ail., alco., all-c., all-s., aloe, alum., alumn., ambr., am-c., ammc., aml-n., amn-l., **ANAC.**, anan., ang., ***anh.***, ant-a., anthr., ant-c., ant-s., ***ant-t.***, ***apis***, apoc., apom., aq-mar., arag., aran., ***arg-m.***, **ARG-N.**, arist-cl., arn., **ARS.**, ***ars-h.***, **ARS-I.**, ***art-v.***, arum-i., arum-t., ***asaf.***, asar., asc-t., aster., atro., ***aur.***, aur-a., aur-i., ***aur-m.***, aur-s., bad., **BAPT.**, bar-c., bar-i., **BELL.**, bell-p., ***bism.***, ***bol.***, bol-s., bor., both., ***bov.***, bry., bufo, buth-a., cact., cadm-s., cadm-met., calad., **CALC.**, ***calc-ar.***, ***calc-f.***, calc-i., **CALC-P.**, ***calc-s.***, ***calen.***, calo., calth., **CAMPH.**, cann-i., ***cann-s.***, canth., caps., carb-an., carb-o., ***carb-s.***, ***carb-v.***, **CARC.**, carl., casc., cast., caul., ***caust.***, cedr., ***cench.***, ceph., cer-b., cerv., ***cham.***, ***chel.***, chim., ***chin.***, chin-a., chin-s., chlol., chlor., chr-ac., cic., **CIMIC.**, ***cina***, cinnb., cist., **CIT-V.**, clem., cob., coca, cob-n., cocaine, ***cocc.***, coc-c., cod., ***coff.***, coff-t., coffin., ***colch.***, **COLOC.**, coll., colocin., com., con., convo-s., ***cop.***, cor-r., corn., croc., ***crot-c.***, crot-h., crot-t., cub., culx., **CUPR.**, cupr-ac., **CUPR-AR.**, cupr-s., cur., cycl., cyt-l., cypr., des-ac., ***dig.***, dios., dirc., dor., dros., dub., ***dulc.***, eaux, elaps, erig., eug., eup-per., euph-l., euphr., eupi., ery-a., **FERR.**, **FERR-AR.**, ***ferr-i.***, ferr-m., ferr-p., fic., fl-ac., form., frax., gast., gels., gent-c., gins., glon., goss., ***graph.***, guai., guare., haem., ham., **HELL.**, helon., hep., hipp., hist., hydr-ac., **HYOS.**, hyosin., hyper., iber., ***ign.***, ind., ***iod.***, ***ip.***, iris, piloc., jal., jatr., kali-a., kali-bi., ***kali-br.***, ***kali-c.***, kali-chl., kali-cy., kali-i., kali-m., ***kali-n.***, kali-per., ***kali-p.***, ***kali-s.***, kali-sulo., kalm., kreos., kres., lac-ac., ***lac-c.***, ***lac-d.***, ***lach.***, lachn., lact., lam., lat-m., laur., ***lec.***, ***led.***, lepi., levo., ***lil-t.***, lip., lipp., lob., lob-p., ***lol.***, **LYC.**, lyss., mag-aust., macro., mag-c.,

RESTLESSNESS, general - mag-m., mag-p., mag-s., manc., man., ***mang.,*** **MED.,** menis., menth-pu., menthol, meny., meph., **MERC.,** ***merc-c.,*** merc-cy., merc-d., merc-i-r., merc-meth., merc-sul., merl., meth-ae-ae., ***mez.,*** mill., ***morph., mosch.,*** mur-ac., mygal., myric., naja, ***nat-a., nat-c.,*** nat-f., ***nat-m.,*** nat-p., nat-s., nep., nicc., nicot., ***nit-ac.,*** nit-m-ac., nitro-o., nuph., nux-m., ***nux-v.,*** oena., olnd., ol-an., onop., onos., ***op.,*** orig., osm., ox-ac., passi., past., perh., petr., ***ph-ac., phos.,*** phys., phyt., plan., ***plat.,*** **PLB.,** plb-chr., podo., prun., ***psor.,*** ptel., **PULS.,** puls-n, **PYROG.,** pyrus, rad., rad-br., ran-a., ran-b., rat., rauw., rheum, rhod., rhus-g., **RHUS-T.,** ***rhus-v., rumx., ruta,*** sabad., sabin., ***samb.,*** samb-c., sanic., sant., sarcol-ac., saroth., sarr., scut., **SEC.,** seneg., senn., **SEP., SIL.,** sol-m., sol-n., sol-t., spig., spong., ***stann.,*** **STAPH.,** ***stict.,*** **STRAM.,** stront-c., ***sul-ac.,*** sulfa., sul-i., **SULPH.,** sumb., syph., ***tab.,*** tarax., **TARENT.,** tax., ***tell.,*** teucr., thal., ther., thiop., ***thuj.,*** thymol., thyr., tong., trom., ***tub.,*** upa., uran-n., urt-u., ust., vac., ***valer.,*** verat., verat-v., vib., vinc., viol-o., viol-t., vip., vip-a., visc., voes., wies., wye., yuc., zinc., zinc-a., zinc-o., zinc-val., zing.

afternoon - anac., ang., apis, aur., bor., calc-s., ***carb-v.,*** caul., ***chin-a.,*** cimic., coloc., dios., fago., hyos., jug-c., merc., merc-sul., naja, nicc., ruta, sapin., staph., tab., thuj., upa.
- 3 p.m. - caul., nicc.
- 4 p.m. - dios.
  - 4 p.m. to 6 p.m. - carb-v., lyc.
- 5 p.m. - chin-s., thuj.
- lying, when - aur.

air, in open amel. - ***aur-m.,*** graph., lach., laur., lyc., ***staph.,*** valer.

alone, when - all-s., ***ars.,*** mez., ***phos.***

alternating with, indifference - nat-m.
- sadness - apis
- sleepiness and stupor, during fever - ***ars.***
- stupor - thyr.

anger, from - ***cham.,*** **COLOC.,** staph.

angina pectoris, in - acon., ***aur-m., kali-ar.***

anxious - **ACON.,** adon., ***aeth.,*** alum., alum-sil., ***am-c.,*** ambr., anac., ant-a., ant-t., aq-mar., **ARG-N.,** arn., **ARS.,** ***ars-i.,*** asaf., aspar., atro., ***aur.,*** aur-a., ***bell.,*** bism., bov., ***bry.,*** **CALC.,** calc-i., calc-p., camph., canth., caps., carb-an., ***carb-v.,*** **CARC.,** ***cast., caust., cham.,*** chel., chin., chin-a., chin-s., cimic., clem., coff., coloc., con., croc., crot-h., ***cupr.,*** dros., ***ferr.,*** frax., ***graph.,*** halo., ***hell., hep.,*** hist., ***iod., jal.,*** **KALI-AR., KALI-C.,** kali-i., kali-n., lach., lact., lol., **LYC.,** ***mag-arct.,*** mag-aust., mag-m., mang., med., meny., ***merc.,*** **NAT-A., NAT-C.,** ***nat-m.,*** nat-p., nat-sil., ***nit-ac.,*** nux-v., op., ph-ac., ***phos.,*** plat., psor., ***puls.,*** plb., pyrog., ***rhus-t.,*** ruta, ***sabad.,*** sanic., sep., ***sil.,*** **SPONG.,** staph., ***sulph.,*** spig., staph., ***tab.,*** tarax., **TARENT.,** ***thuj.,*** valer., ***verat.,*** vip., wies., zinc.
- compelling, do something, to - ***bry.***
  - rapid walking - **ARG-N., ARS.,** lil-t., sul-ac., **TARENT.**

RESTLESSNESS, general

anxious,
- driving from place to place - **ARS.,** ***tab.***
- epilepsy, during intervals of - ***arg-n.***
- lying amel. - mang.
- megrim, in - ***aeth.***
- morning - ***zinc.***
- music agg. - ***nat-c.***
- no rest at any employment - ***chel.***
- perspiration on forehead and heat of head - **PHOS.**
- thunderstorm, during - ***nat-c.***
- walks about room, during headache - ***coloc.***
- yawning, and - ***plb.***

back, during tired aching in - calc-f.

bed, in - amn-l., apoc., arist-cl., **ARS.,** dios., fago., hura, iod., nit-ac., phos., **PULS.,** rad., tax., tell.
- amel. - cham., cocc.
- driving out of - arg-m., **ARS.,** ***ars-i., bell.,*** **BISM.,** bry., carb-an., ***carb-v.,*** caust., cench., ***cham.,*** chin., chin-a., chin-s., con., **FERR.,** ferr-ar., ferr-p., ***graph., hep.,*** hyos., ***lyc., mag-c.,*** mag-m., merc., nat-c., nat-m., nat-sil., nicc., nit-ac., nux-v., phos., puls., **RHUS-T.,** sep., sil., ther., tub.
- heat of, from - op.
- tossing about in - **ACON.,** agar-ph., alco., alumn., alum., ant-t., apis, ***arg-n.,*** arn., **ARS.,** ars-s-f., asaf., ***arum-t.,*** atro., bapt., ***bell.,*** benz-n., bor., ***bry., calc.,*** calc-ar., ***camph.,*** canth., carb-an., carb-o., carbn., carl., ***cast., caust., cham.,*** chen-a., ceph., ***chin.,*** chin-s., chlf., cic., ***cina,*** cinnb., cist., ***cit-v.,*** clem., coca, cocc., ***coff.,*** coloc., con., cor-r., crot-t., **CUPR.,** cur., dig., dulc., **FERR.,** ferr-ar., ferr-m., ferr-p., ***gels.,*** goss., graph., guai., hell., hydr-ac., hyos., ign., **IP.,** ***kali-ar.,*** kali-n., kreos., ***lach.,*** lachn., led., ***lyc.,*** mag-c., mag-m., manc., mang., meny., ***merc.,*** merc-c., mosch., ***mur-ac.,*** nat-a., nat-c., nat-m., nit-ac., ***nux-v.,*** op., par., petr., phos., plan., plat., podo., ***puls.,*** pyrog., ***ran-s.,*** rheum, **RHUS-T.,** senn., ***sep.,*** serp., sil., sol-t., squil., ***staph., stram., stry.,*** sul-ac., ***sulph.,*** tab., tarax., **TARENT.,** tep., ter., thea., thuj., tril., tub., ust., valer., ***vario.,*** verat., zinc.
  - convulsions, during - bar-m.
  - suddenly - chin.
- wants to go from one bed to another - **ARS.,** ***bell., calc.,*** cham., cina, ***ferr., hyos.,*** merc., mez., ***plb., rhus-t.,*** sep., stram., ***tarent.,*** verat.

belching, from insufficient - calc., kali-c.

busy - acon., ***aur.,*** bell., bry., caps., carc., dig., hyos., ***ign.,*** ip., ***lach.,*** mag-arct., ***mosch.,*** nat-c., nux-v., stann., sul-ac., ther., verat.

cares, from - kali-br.

chest, from congestion in - sep.
- heat rising up into the mouth from - nux-v.

childbirth, during - ***acon.,*** ars., ***camph.,*** chlf.

RESTLESSNESS, general
children, in (see Hyperactive) - absin., ambr., ***anac.,*** ant-t., ***arg-n.,*** **ARS.,** bor., bufo, calc-br., ***carc., cham.,*** cina, cypr., hyos., ign., ip., ***jal.,*** kali-c., mag-c., ***med.,*** **MERC.,** rheum, **RHUS-T.,** sulph., ***tarent., tub., verat.,*** zinc.
babies, in - acon., ars., kali-p., sil.
dentition, during - **RHEUM.**
eruption, with skin - ***psor.***
night - acon., ars., kali-c.
but morning fresh and lively - ***psor.***
relieved by being carried about - ant-t., ars., ***cham.,*** cina, kali-c.
roving, wandering - bell., bry., nux-v.
chill, during the - acon., aeth., anac., **ARS.,** asaf., bell., bor., cann-s., caps., carb-v., cham., eup-per., kali-ar., kreos., lam., mez., nat-c., nat-m., petr., plan., plat., rhus-t., spig.
at beginning of - ***lach.,*** phos.
clasping, amel. - med.
company, in - ***carb-v.,*** mez., staph.
conscience, of - ***chel.,*** merc., ***puls.,*** zinc-oc.
conversation, from - ***ambr.***
convulsions, after - oena.
epileptic - cupr.
before - **ARG-N.,** bufo, caust., nat-m.
between - arg-n., cham.
convulsive - guare.
coughing, with - sulph.
day and night - ars., canth., chel., iod., tarent., sulph.
daytime - ambr., kali-br., nat-c., nat-m., pip-m., plan., ***rhus-t.,*** staph., sulph.
dinner, after - am-m., nat-c., ruta, thuj.
amel. - thuj.
disguise, vainly seeks to - alco.
drink, at the sight of - bell.
drinking agg. - ***crot-c.***
drives him from place to place - acon., ***am-c.,*** **ARS.,** aur., ***bell.,*** bism., ***calc-p.,*** canth., carb-v., ***cedr.,*** cench., cimic., crot-h., ***cupr.,*** dros., graph., ***hist.,*** hyos., iod., kali-i., kres., ***lach., lyss.,*** meny., merc., nat-c., nux-v., plat., prun., puls., sep., sol-m., spig., stann., staph., ***tab.,*** tarax., tarent., verat.
air, in open - lach., nux-v., valer.
dry skin, with - thea.
eating, when - bor., petr.
after - am-m., bar-c., chin., cinnb., lach., nux-m., nux-v., petr., ph-ac., phos., rhod., rhus-t., sulph., verat.
eruption, with, in children - **PSOR.**
evening - acon., ether, agar., ***alum., am-c., ars.,*** ars-s-f., bov., ***calc.,*** calc-s., ***carb-v.,*** caul., **CAUST.,** chin-s., clem., dios., equis., fago., ferr., guare., hep., piloc., kali-ar., lach., laur., lyc., lycps., mag-c., mag-m., meph., ***merc.,*** mur-ac., ***nat-c.,*** nat-p., nicc., nit-ac., nux-v., ph-ac., phos., phys., ***rumx.,*** ruta, sabin., scut., sep., sulph., thuj., verat., zinc., zinc-p., zing.
6 p.m. to 6 a.m. - **KREOS.**
7 p.m. - am-c.

RESTLESSNESS, general
evening,
8 p.m. - calc., **MERC.**
bed, in - am-c., cham., hep., lyc., **MAG-M.,** nux-v., phos., sabin., sep., thuj.
twilight, at - caust.
exertion, after - cimic.
least - ***merc.***
exhaustion, with - chin-a.
eyes, on closing at night, agg. - **MAG-M.,** sep.
fainting, followed by - calc.
fever, during - ***acon.,*** acon-l., am-c., anac., ant-t., ***apis, arn.,*** **ARS.,** ars-s-r., atro., bapt., ***bar-c., bell.,*** calc., calc-ar., caps., ***carb-v., cham.,*** chin., chin-a., ***chin-s.,*** cina, clem., cob-n., colocin., con., cub., ***eup-per., ferr., ferr-ar.,*** ferr-p., ***gels.,*** hyper., ***ip.,*** kali-ar., lachn., ***lyc., mag-arct.,*** mag-c., mag-m., merc-c., mosch., ***mur-ac., op.,*** phos., plan., **PULS.,** pyrog., rheum, **RHUS-T.,** rhus-v., ruta, sabin., sec., sep., spong., staph., stram., ***sulph.,*** syph., thuj., valer.
after - ph-ac., puls., sep.
feverish - anac., ***ars.,*** cimic., phos., pyrog., ran-b., ruta.
forenoon - acon., am-m., anac., calad., cimic., fago., lyss., nat-c., phos., sil., thuj.
gout, with - ign.
hands, clutching tightly amel. - med.
headache, during - anac., arg-n., ***ars., bell.,*** bry., cadm-s., calad., canth., cham., chin., ***coloc.,*** daph., dulc., gent-c., hell., ign., kali-i., ***lach., lyc.,*** lyss., morph., lil-s., naja, nux-m., pyrog., ran-b., ruta, sil., spig., sulph., syph., ***tab.,*** vip.
pain in forehead, at night, from - cycl.
hunger, with - ***cina, iod.,*** kali-c., phos.
hypochondriacal - ars., ***asaf.,*** graph., valer.
hysterical - ***asaf., tarent.***
internal - ***acon.,*** agar., ang., atro., **ARS.,** carb-an., carl., chel., dros., eupi., gins., lact., lob., lyc., mag-c., mag-m., mag-s., mang., meph., nat-c., nat-m., nit-ac., op., par., plb., ph-ac., phos., ran-b., rheum, **RHUS-T.,** sep., **SIL.,** stram., sulph., viol-t.
evening, in bed - eupi.
forenoon, on walking - acon.
morning, on waking - sep.
night, on waking, with headache - par.
as if would beat about herself with hands and feet - lyc.
in dream - agar.
itching, with - ***psor.***
after - coloc.
knows not what to do with himself - stann.
lascivious thoughts, during - graph.
lying, lying, while - alum., aur., aur-a., cit-v., mag-m., merc., nux-v.
lying, on back agg., on side amel. - calc-p.
menopausal period, at - ***kali-br.***
menses, during - ***acon.,*** am-c., ant-t., apis, ***ars.,*** ars-s-f., bell., bor., ***calc.,*** calc-ar., ***cham.,*** cocc., ***coff.,*** croc., ***cycl.,*** gels., hyos., ign., ip.,

RESTLESSNESS, general

menses, during - kali-ar., kali-c., kali-p., kali-s., mag-m., merc., nat-c., nit-ac., ***nux-v.,*** op., phos., plat., ***puls., rhus-t.,*** sec., ***sep., stram.,*** sulph., tarent., thuj., vib., xan.

after - mag-c.

before - ***acon.,*** ang., arist-cl., caul., caust., ***cham., cimic.,*** coloc., con., ign., kali-c., ***kreos., lach.,*** lyc., mag-c., mag-aust., mag-m., ***mag-p.,*** mang., nit-ac., ***nux-v.,*** puls., ***sal-n.,*** senec., ***sep.,*** **SULPH.,** tril.,vib., xan.

suppressed, during - ars., cimic., kali-c., nicc., nux-v., rhus-t., sep., zinc.

mental work, during and after - bor., fago., graph., ind., ***kali-p.,*** nat-c.

amel. - ***nat-c.***

metrorrhagia, during - ***acon., apis,*** cham., hyos., stram.

midnight, at - nat-m.

waking, on - graph., phyt., plat.

after - **ARS.,** bapt., bry., ***dios.,*** lyc., merc., merc-i-r., ***nit-ac.,*** **RHUS-T.,** rhus-v., sil., sulph., zinc.

before - alum., carb-s., cot., euph., ***ferr.,*** mag-m., mur-ac., nat-m., pic-ac., plat., sars., senec.

closing eyes agg., on - **MAG-M.,** sep.

heart, from uneasiness about - phys.

morning - ail., bell., dulc., fago., gamb., ***gels.,*** hyos., hyper., iod., ir-foe., kali-br., ***lyc.,*** meph., nat-m., myric., ph-ac., phys., sulph., thuj., upa., zinc., zinc-p.

bed, in - guai., ph-ac.

rising, after - puls.

waking, on - cina, dulc., hyper., lyc., mygal., nit-ac.

motion, amel. - lyc., macro., puls., rhus-t.

move, must constantly - ***apis, ars., bell.,*** canth., caust., cench., cimic., ***hippoz.,*** ign., ***iod., kali-br., kreos., led.,*** **RHUS-T.,** sul-i., trom.

but too weak to - ***bapt.***

music, from - nat-c., tarent.

nausea, from - ars., cina, phos.

with - ars., lac-d.

night - abies-c., abies-n., abrot., acon., acon-c., adel., alum., alum-sil., am-caust., am-m., ambr., ammc., anac., ang., ***anh.,*** anil., ant-ox., anth., anthr., ant-t., ***apis,*** apoc., ***arg-m., arg-n.,*** ARS., ***ars-i., ars-s-f.,*** asaf., asc-t., aster., atro., aur., aur-a., aur-s., bad., ***bapt., bell.,*** bism., ***bor.,*** bov., brach., bry., cact., cahin., ***calc.,*** calc-ar., calc-caust., calc-sil., calen., calo., camph., canth., carb-ac., carb-an., carb-s., ***carb-v.,*** carbn., card-m., ***cast-v.,*** cast., ***caul.,*** **CAUST.,** cedr., ***cham.,*** chin., chin-a., chr-ac., cic., cimic., cina, cinnb., ***cist., cit-v.,*** clem., coca, coc-c., coff., colch., coloc., colocin., com., cop., cor-r., corn., crot-t., ***cupr.,*** cupr-s., ***cycl.,*** cypr., dig., digin., digox., dios., dirc., dor., dulc., erig., euph-a., euphr., eupi., fago., ***ferr.,*** ferr-ar., ferr-i., ferr-p., fl-ac., form., gall-ac., gels., gent-l., get., glon., gnaph., ***graph., guai.,*** hall, hell., hell-v., hep., hura, -hydr., **HYOS.,** hyper., iber., ***ign.,*** indg., ind., iod., ***iris,*** jac., jatr., jug-c., **KALI-AR.,** kali-bi., ***kali-br.,*** kali-c., kali-i., kali-n., kali-sil., kiss., **KREOS.,** ***lac-c.,*** lach., led., lil-s., **LYC.,** lycps., lyss., mag-c., ***mag-m.,*** mang., ***med., menis.,*** menth-pu., **MERC.,** ***merc-c.,*** merc-cy., merc-meth., merc-sul., morph., mosch., ***mur-ac.,*** mygal., myric., ***nat-a.,*** nat-c., nat-m., nat-p., nat-s., nat-sil., nicc., nicot., nit-ac., nux-m., nux-v., nym., op., osm., ost., ox-ac., par., ped., petr., ph-ac., ***phos.,*** phys., phyt., pip-m., plan., plb., ***podo.,*** polyp-p, psor., ptel., **PULS.,** puls-n, rad., ***ran-b., ran-s.,*** **RHUS-T.,** rhus-v., rumx., ruta, sabad., sang., sapin., sars., senec., senn., ***sep.,*** sil., sol-t-ae., spig., spira., spirae., spong., stram., stry., sul-ac., **SULPH.,** sul-i., syph., tab., tarax., thea., ***teucr.,*** thuj., tub., uran-n., ust., ***valer.,*** verat., verat-v., verb., vesp., vip., visc., yuc., zinc., zinc-p.

1 a.m. - ars., get., mang., nat-a., phos., phys., stann.

2 a.m. - ambr., com., ferr., graph., kali-ar., iod., mag-m., myric., zing.

3 a.m. - agar., calc-ar., ***chin-a.,*** cimic., coc-c., ***kreos.,*** lil-s., nat-a., nat-m., polyp-p.

everything feels sore, must move about - nicc.

3 a.m. to 4 a.m. - fago.

4 a.m. - wild.

until - nit-ac.

5 a.m. - tarent.

waking, on - caust.

noon - bell., lyss., sulph.

pacing back and forwards - ars., plan.

pain, during - **ACON., ARS.,** chr-ac., ***cham., coloc.,*** dios., kali-c., lyc., plb., syph.

pain, from - ***acon., ars.,*** bell., caust., cham., coloc., lyc., sil.

toothache - ***cham.,*** mag-c., mag-p., mang., mez.

painful - acon-f.

palpitations, with - acon., aeth., ars., calc., coff., ign., ***kali-ar.,*** lach., nat-m., phase., ***phos.,*** puls., sapo., spig., spong., verat., zinc.

paroxysms, during - plb.

after - oena.

periodical - ***ars.***

every third day - anac.

perspiration, during - bry., graph., lachn., samb.

amel. - ***sulph.***

pregnancy, during - acon., ambr., ***colch., nux-m.,*** verat.

feverish, and, during last month - colch.

pressing in liver, from - ruta..

pulse, from intermittent - digox.

rage, ending in a - canth.

reading, while - dros., ***nat-c.,*** ph-ac., sumb.

rising, on - atro., fago., ptel.

seat, from a - caust.

room, in - ***iod., kali-s.,*** **LYC.**

RESTLESSNESS, general
sadness, with - ***plat.***
sex, during - upa.
after - **CALC.,** cop., dig., mez., petr., ***sep.,*** staph.
sexual excitement, in - ant-c., cann-i., ***canth., kali-br.,*** kali-p., ***raph.,*** staph.
sitting, while - alum., ***ars.,*** cact., ***caust.,*** dirc., ***ferr., iod.,*** lipp., **LYC.,** mag-c., med., merc., nat-m., plan., **RHUS-T.,** ***sep., sil.,*** staph., sulph.
at work - ars., **GRAPH.**
sleep, before - ***acon.,*** phos., thuj.
sleepiness, with - ars., bufo, coloc., ***con.,*** crot-h., ***hep.,*** lact., ***merc., petr.,*** rhus-t., ***sep., stram.***
sleeplessness, from - ***carc., lac-d.,*** stict.
smoking, after - calad.
spine, affections, in - ip.
stool, during - bell.
after - cench.
storm, during - gels., nat-c., ***nat-m., phos.,*** psor.
before - ***gels., psor., rhod.***
strangers agg., presence of - sep.
stretching, backward amel. - bor.
study, when attempting to - fago., ind., med.
stupefaction, with - ***bapt.,*** kali-i., rhus-t.
sunlight agg. - cadm-s.
talking, after - ambr., bor.
thunderstorm, during - gels., nat-c., phos.
before - ***gels., psor., rhod.***
toothache, with - cham., mag-c., mang., mez.
tremulous - arn., aur., euph., ***plat.,*** valer.
urination, before - cahin., ph-ac.
urinary troubles, with - ***canth.,*** meny.
waiting, during - hist.
waking, on - am-m., ambr., am-c., ***ars.,*** bell., canth., carb-an., cedr., chin., chr-ac., cina, dulc., graph., guai., hyper., mag-m., merc., mur-ac., ***nat-m.,*** ph-ac., phos., rhus-t., sep., ***sil.,*** squil., stann., tarax., thea., zinc.
walking, while - acon., ambr., caust., merc., paeon., ran-b., thuj.
amel. - cench., culx., dios., nat-m., nicc.
air, in open amel. - aur-m., graph., **LYC.,** ph-ac., **PULS.**
compelling rapid - **ARG-N.,** ***ars., tarent.***
warm bed agg. - ***ars-i.,*** ferr., ***iod., kali-s., lach.,*** nat-m., ***puls.***
women, in - cast., cedr., helon., kali-br., sec., senec., xan.
urinary troubles, with - ***canth.,*** meny.
working, while - cit-v., cortico., **GRAPH.,** voes.
tedious work - passi.
worries, from - ars., calc., carc., kali-br.

REVEALS, secrets - agar., alco., hyos.
sleep, in - am-c., ***ars.***

REVELRY, feasting - agar., ambr., ang., ant-c., ip., kali-c., lach., med., ***nat-c., nux-v.,*** sel., sulph.

REVENGEFUL, (see Malicious)

REVERENCE, for those around him - cocc., ham., ***hyos.,*** lyc., nat-m., nux-v., plat., puls., sil., sulph.
lack of - anac., coloc., verat.

RIDICULE, mania to - acon., ***hyos.,*** lach., nux-v., verat.

ROMANTIC, feelings, (see Sentimental) - ambr., **ANT-C.,** ***calc-p.,*** carc., caust., ***cocc., coff.,*** con., **IGN.,** lach., med., nat-c., **NAT-M.,** ***phos.,*** plat., ***puls., staph.,*** tub.

ROOM, full of people agg. - ***ambr., ant-c., arg-n.,*** ars., bar-c., carb-an., con., ***hell., lyc., mag-c.,*** nat-c., nat-m., petr., ***phos., plb., puls.,*** sabin., ***sep.,*** stann., stram., ***sulph.***

ROVING about, aimless - arag., hyos., meli.
naked - ***hyos.***
senseless, insane - bell., bry., canth., chin., coff., ***hyos., nux-v.,*** puls., sabad., stram., verat.
wrapped in fur in the summer - hyos.

RUDENESS, (see Insolent) - ambr., ***anac.,*** arn., aur., aur-s., bar-c., bell., bufo, ***canth.,*** carc., ***cham.,*** eug., ferr., gall-ac., ***graph.,*** hell., ***hyos.,*** ign., ***lac-c.,*** lach., **LYC.,** lyss., nat-m., nit-ac., nux-m., ***nux-v.,*** op., pall., par., ***petr., phos.,*** **PLAT.,** ***psor.,*** rad., sieg., spong., **SULPH.,** ***stram.,*** tub., **VERAT.**
ailments from, rudeness of others - bar-m., ***calc.,*** carc., cocc., ***colch.,*** ign., ***lyc.,*** mag-m., mur-ac., ***nat-m.,*** nux-v., ph-ac., **STAPH.**
children, of naughty - ***ant-c.,*** cham., ***chin.,*** cina, dulc., ***merc.,*** nat-m., rheum, staph., sulph.
employees to the chiefs, of - lyc., nat-m.
fever, during - lyc.
sensitive, to (see Offended) - ***calc.,*** cocc., ***colch.,*** mag-m., ***nat-m.,*** nux-v., ph-ac., **STAPH.**
women, in - ***cham.***

RUNS, about - agar., ars., ***bell.,*** bufo, ***calc.,*** canth., con., ***chin., cupr.,*** cupr-ar., glon., hell., **HYOS.,** iod., plb., **STRAM.,** ***sulph.,*** tarent., **VERAT.**
against, people, in walking - cann-i.
against, things - bell.
dangerous places, in most - agar.
forward, when trying to walk - mang.
fright, as if in - op., ***zinc.***
lightness and rapidity, with great - clem.
menses, before - lach.
paroxysms, in, agg. evening - **VERAT.**
room, in - ***coff.,*** hyos., morph., ***plat.***
recklessly - sabad.
shirt, in - bell.
streets at night, in - ***puls.***
unsteady - ***coff.***

SADNESS, (see Depression)

SARCASM - ***ars., sulph.***

SATYRIASIS, (see Sexual, behaviour)

SCHIZOPHRENIA, (see Dementia, Insanity, Mania, Multiple personalites) - **ANAC.,** anh., **AUR.,** bell., ***carc.,*** hyos., ***kali-br.,*** **LACH.,** med., ***meli.,*** **STRAM.,** verat.

SCHIZOPHRENIA,
catatonic - chlorpr., cic., convo-s., cortico., halo., rauw., reser., thala., thiop.
hebephrenia - anh., cann-i., chlorpr., halo., ***hyos.,*** kres., rauw., reser., thala., thiop.
paranoid - ***anac.,*** anh., ars., bell., carc., cupr., ***hyos.,*** **LACH.,** kali-br., med., ***meli.,*** merc., plat., plb., rauw., ***stram.,*** verat.
conspiracies, against him, there were - ***anac., ars., lach.,*** plb., puls.
enemy, everyone is an - lach., meli., ***merc.,*** plat.
surrounded by - ***anac.,*** carb-s., ***crot-h.,*** lach., ***merc.***
under the bed, is - am-m.
wait for an, lying in - alco.
persecuted, that he is - abrot., absin., ***anac.,*** ars., aur., ***bell.,*** calc., **CHIN.,** cic., ***cocaine,*** con., crot-h., cupr., cycl., **DROS.,** hell., ***hyos.,*** **IGN.,** kali-br., **LACH.,** lyc., med., meli., merc., nat-c., nat-m., ***nux-v.,*** op., plb., puls., ***rhus-t.,*** sil., spong., staph., stram., stry., ***sulph.*** syph., thyr., verat., ***zinc.***
pursued, by enemies - absin., ***anac.,*** ars., aur., ***bell., chin.,*** cic., ***cocaine,*** con., crot-h., cupr., cycl., dros., hell., ***hyos.,*** kali-br., ***lach.,*** lepi., lyc., med., meli., merc., nat-c., nux-v., plb., ***puls.,*** rhus-t., sil., stram., stry., zinc.
watched, that she is being - anac., aq-mar., **ARS.,** ***bar-c., calc., hyos.,*** lach., med., meli., rhus-t.

SCORN, feelings (see Contempt) - acon., alum., ***aur.,*** bell., **BRY., CHAM.,** coff., ***coloc.,*** ferr., hyos., ip., lyc., ***nat-m.,*** **NUX-V.,** olnd., ***par., phos., plat.,*** sep., ***staph.,*** stront-c., sulph., verat.

SCORNED, ailments from being - acon., alum., ***aur.,*** bell., **BRY., CHAM.,** coff., ***coloc.,*** ferr., hyos., ***ign.,*** ip., lyc., **NAT-M., NUX-V.,** olnd., ***par., phos., plat.,*** sep., ***staph.,*** stront-c., sulph., verat.

SCRATCHING, with hands - bell., stram., tarent.
child, on waking - calc.
desire to - arn.
himself, raw - arum-t., psor.
lime off the walls - arn., canth.

SCREAMING, shrieking, shouting - absin., acon., aeth., agar., agav-t., alco., alum., ***anac.,*** ant-c., ***ant-t.,*** **APIS,** arg-m., arn., ars., arum-i., atro., ***aur.,*** aur-a., ***aur-m.,*** bad., ***bell., bor.,*** bry., bufo, calad., ***calc.,*** calc-hp., ***calc-p.,*** **CAMPH.,** cann-i., ***canth.,*** carb-ac., carb-an., carb-o., carb-s., carb-v., carc., cast., ***caust., cedr.,*** cench., ***cham., chin.,*** chlor., **CIC.,** ***cina,*** cocc., coff., croc., crot-c., crot-h., **CUPR.,** ***cupr-ac.,*** cupr-ar., dulc., elaps, equis-a., eup-per., ferr-p., ***gels., glon., hell.,*** hydr-ac., ***hyos.,*** hyper., ***ign., iodof., ip., jal.,*** kali-ar., ***kali-br.,*** **KALI-C.,** kali-p., kali-s., kreos., lac-c., lach., lat-m., laur., lepi., lil-t., **LYC.,** mag-c., mag-p., merc., merc-meth., meth-ae-ae., mosch., nit-ac., nux-v., olnd., op., ***phos.,*** **PLAT.,** plb., plb-chr., podo., puls., ran-s., ***rheum,*** samb., sars.,

SCREAMING - sec., seneg., sep., sil., sol-n., **STRAM.,** stry., sul-ac., ***sulph.,*** syph., tanac., tarent., thal., ***thuj.,*** **TUB.,** vac., valer., **VERAT.,** verat-v., viol-t., vip., ***zinc.***
agony, from - ars., lat-m.
anger, in - cast., ***cham.,*** ign., ***nux-v.,*** puls., sep.
anxiety, from - calc., chin-s., cocc., ***hyos., lyc.,*** ran-s.
approaches the bed, when anyone - ***ign.***
barking, like - canth., stram.
brain cry - ***aml-n.,*** **APIS,** arn., ars., ***art-v.,*** bell., calc-hp., ***carb-ac., cham.,*** cic., cupr., ***cupr-ac.,*** dig., dulc., ***glon., hell., hyos.,*** ign., ***kali-br., kali-i., lyc., merc.,*** merc-c., phos., ***rhus-t.,*** sol-n., stram., sulph., ***zinc.***
cannot, but wants to scream - ***stram.***
cheerful mood, causeless during - ***chin.***
children, in - aeth., ail., anac., ***apis,*** bell., benz-ac., **BOR.,** calc., ***calc-p.,*** camph., ***carc.,*** caste., **CHAM.,** ***cina,*** coff., cupr., dor., dulc., ***glon., hell., ign.,*** ip., ***jal.,*** kali-br., ***kali-p., kreos.,*** **LAC-C.,** lyc., mag-c., ***nux-v.,*** puls., ***rheum, senn.,*** sil., stram., syph., **TUB.**
colic with - **CHAM.,** mag-p., ***nux-v.***
consolation, agg. - bell., cham., ign.
crying and - ***cham.,*** ign., nux-v.
day and night - calc., rheum
evening - ***cham.,*** **CINA,** cinnam., zinc.
night - carc., ***cham., chlol.,*** jal., ***kali-p., lac-c.,*** nux-v., psor., rheum.
nursed, when being - bor.
playing at daytime, but - psor.
sleep, during - **APIS,** ***arn.,*** bell., bor., ***calc-p.,*** caste., ***ign.,*** inul., ***lyc., psor.,*** **PULS., SULPH.,** ***tub.***
dreams, from - acon., carc., tub.
spoken to, when - sil.
stool, during - ***kreos.,*** **RHEUM**
urging for, on - **RHEUM.**
touched, when - ant-t.
urination, before - sars.
waking, on - bor.
chorea, in - chlol., ***cupr-ac., ign., stram., zinc.***
convulsions, during - acon., ***aml-n.,*** ant-t., ***apis, art-v.,*** bell., calc., ***camph.,*** canth., ***caust.,*** cedr., ***cic., cina, crot-h., cupr.,*** **HYOS.,** ***ign., ip.,*** kali-bi., ***lach., lyc., merc.,*** nit-ac., nux-v., **OP.,** stram., sulph., vip.
after - cupr., plb., sil.
at the end - hell.
before - ***aml-n., apis,*** art-v., ***bell., bufo,*** calc., camph., canth., cedr., **CIC.,** ***cina,*** crot-c., **CUPR.,** hydr-ac., **HYOS.,** ***ip., kali-br., lach.,*** laur., ***lyc.,*** nit-ac., nux-v., ***oena., op.,*** phos., plb., sil., ***stram.,*** stry., ***sulph.,*** verat-v., ***zinc.***
between - bell., kali-bi.
epileptic - ***bufo,*** cedr., **CIC.,** crot-h., ***cupr.,*** hydr-ac., **HYOS.,** ign., ***ip., kali-bi., lach., lyc.,*** nit-ac., ***nux-v., oena.,*** op., ***sil.,*** stann., stram., sulph., verat-v.
puerperal - ***hyos., iod., lach.***
cough, with - ***arn.,*** bell., cina.

SCREAMING, shrieking
cramps, during - coloc., ***cupr.***
abdomen, in - **COLOC.,** cupr., ***jatr., lyc., mag-p.,*** plb.
day and night - stram.
delusions, from - ars., kali-c., plat., puls., stram.
with - bell., canth., hyos., ***stram.,*** verat.
dentition, during - ***apis,*** calc-p., **CHAM.,** ***kreos., rheum,*** ter.
drinking, while - nux-v.
drunkenness, during - caust., hyos., ign., stram.
evening, agg. - verat.
feels as though she must - ***anac.,*** apis, aur., ***calc.,*** calc-p., cic., cina, ***elaps,*** hell., ***lil-t.,*** nux-v., **SEP.,** sil., stann.
fever, during - bell., lyc., stram.
fraise, cry - ***apis, glon., hell., hyos., kali-br.,*** lyc., merc., zinc.
frenzy, in a - cham., lach.
help, for - ***camph., ign.,*** kali-c., ***laur.,*** plat.
sleep, in - hep., kali-c., rhus-t.
springing up from bed - hep., rhus-t.
hoarse - bell., stram.
holds, on to something, unless she - **SEP.**
hydrocephalus, in - **APIS,** ***cina, dig.,*** kali-i., ***lyc.,*** merc., ***zinc.***
imaginary, appearances, about - ***kali-c.***
impulse, to - ***calc., sep.***
laughter, after - tarent.
locomotive, like a - nux-m.
mania, in - stram.
menses, during - ***cocc., coloc.,*** cupr.
after - aur.
before - ***sep.,*** **TUB.**
suppressed, from - cupr.
midnight - lac-ac.
mirth, during - chin.
night - ant-t., calc., carc., cypr., jal., kreos., mag-c.
obstinate - ***cham.***
pain, with the - **ACON.,** ***ars.,*** **BELL.,** ***bry.,*** **CACT., CHAM.,** cic., **COFF., COLOC.,** gels., kali-n., mag-c., mag-m., mag-p., op., **PLAT.,** plb., podo., puls., sep.
feet, in - spig.
back, lumbar region, in - alum., bry., chin.
paroxysmal - ***ign., lyc.***
runs, shrieking through house - bufo.
sleep, during - ***agar.,*** alum., am-c., anac., ant-c., ***ant-t., apis, arg-m.,*** arn., ***aur., bell.,*** **BOR.,** ***bry.,*** bufo, calc., ***calc-hp., calc-p.,*** calc-sil., ***caps.,*** carb-ac., carb-an., carc., ***cast.,*** caust., ***cham.,*** chel., chin., chlol., ***cic., cina,*** cocc., croc., ***cupr-ac.,*** cypr., dig., dor., dulc., euph., ***fl-ac.,*** gran., graph., ***guai., hell., hep., hyos., ign.,*** inul., iodof., ip., ***kali-br.,*** kali-c., kreos., ***lac-c.,*** **LYC.,** ***mag-c., mag-m.,*** morg-g., ***nat-c.,*** nat-m., nit-ac., nux-m., op., phos., plat., psor., **PULS.,** ***rheum,*** sep., ***sil.,*** spong., stram., stront-c., stry., sul-ac., ***sulph.,*** thuj., **TUB.,** ***verat.,*** **ZINC.,** zinc-p.

SCREAMING, shrieking
sleep, during
jumping out of sleep and shrieks for aid - hep., rhus-t.
menses, before - carb-v., sep., sul-ac., **TUB.,** ***zinc.***
spasms, in - ***cupr.,*** hydr-ac.
stool, during - carb-v., **KREOS., RHEUM.**
before - bor.
children, in, during - ***kreos.,*** **RHEUM.**
urging for, on - **RHEUM.**
sudden - ***apis, bell.,*** bor., bry., calc., cham., ***chin., cic., cina,*** cypr., gels., ***hell.,*** iodof., kali-br., ***kali-c., stram.,*** tub., verat., ***zinc.***
thunderstorm, during - gels.
touched, when - ***acon.,*** ant-c., kali-c., ***merc.,*** ruta.
trifles, at - **KALI-C.,** rib-ac.
unconsciousness, until - bufo.
urinating, before - **BOR.,** lach., **LYC.,** nux-v., **SARS.,** thuj.
waking, on - alum., apis, arn., ars., ***bry.,*** caps., ***cham., cina,*** con., gels., guai., ***hydr-ac., hyos., ign., kali-br., kali-p.,*** kali-s., ***lyc., mag-c.,*** meny., phos., ruta, sep., sil., stram., sulph., **ZINC.**

SEARCHING - ***bar-c.,*** caust., dig., ***ign.,*** lyc., ***nat-m., sep.,*** **THUJ.,** zinc.
floor, on the - ign., plb., stram.
night, at, for thieves - ars., ***nat-m.***
after having dreamt of them - ***nat-m.***

SECRETIVE - aur., ***bar-c.,*** bov., caust., dig., ***ign.,*** lyc., ***naja,*** nat-m., nit-ac., phos., plb., ***sep.,*** syph., **THUJ.,** zinc.

SECRETS, divulges, (see Reveals)

SELFISHINESS - agar., asaf., **ARS.,** crot-t., ign., med., mosch., ***puls.,*** pyrus, sil., ***sulph.,*** valer.

SELF-torture - acon., **ANAC.,** ***ars.,*** bell., ***lil-t.,*** plb., **STAPH.,** tarent., ***tub.***

SENSES, general, (see Brain)

SENSITIVE, general - ***acon., aesc.,*** aeth., alco., all-s., aloe, alum., am-c., ***ambr.,*** **ANAC.,** ang., anh., ***ant-c.,*** ant-t., apis, aq-mar., arg-m., **ARG-N.,** arn., ***ars., ars-i.,*** ars-s-f., ***asaf.,*** **ASAR.,** atro., **AUR.,** aur-a., aur-s., bar-c., **BELL., BOR.,** ***bov.,*** bry., bufo, buth-a., cadm-met., calc., calc-ar., ***calc-p., calc-s.,*** calen., camph., cann-s., ***canth.,*** carb-an., carb-o., ***carb-s., carb-v.,*** **CARC.,** cast., **CAUST.,** cer-s., **CHAM., CHIN., CHIN-A., CHIN-S.,** cic., cimic., ***cina,*** clem., coc-c., cocc., **COFF.,** colch., **COLOC.,** con., convo-s., cop., croc., ***crot-h.,*** cupr., daph., dig., digin., dros., ***ferr.,*** ferr-ar., ferr-p., fl-ac., **GELS.,** gran., graph., haem., ham., hell., ***hep.,*** hist., hyos., hyper., hypoth., **IGN.,** ***iod.,*** ip., ***kali-ar.,*** kali-bi., ***kali-c., kali-i.,*** kali-n., **KALI-P.,** ***kali-s.,*** kreos., ***lac-c.,*** **LACH.,** ***lat-m.,*** laur., **LIL-T., LYC., LYSS.,** ***mag-arct.,*** **MAG-C., MAG-M.,** ***mag-p.,*** mag-s., man., mang., mate, ***med.,*** meph., ***merc.,*** merc-c., mez., morph., mosch., mur-ac., murx., mygal., ***nat-a., nat-c.,*** **NAT-M.,** ***nat-p., nat-s., nit-ac.,***

SENSITIVE, general - **NUX-V.,** olnd., onop., ***op.,*** paeon., **PH-AC., PHOS.,** phos-h., ***plat.,*** **PLB.,** ***psor.,*** **PULS.,** pyrog., **RAN-B.,** rhus-t., sabad., ***sabin.,*** samb., sang., sanic., sars., ***seneg., sep.,*** **SIL.,** spig., stann., **STAPH., STRAM.,** stry., ***sul-ac.,*** sul-i., **SULPH.,** tab., tarent., tell., ter., ***teucr.,*** thea., **THER.,** thuj., tub., upa., **VALER., VERAT.,** viol-t., vip., zinc.

afternoon - ph-ac., plat., sulph.

ailments, to the most trifling - nux-v.

broth, to the smell of - **COLCH.**

certain persons - am-m., aur., calc., crot-h., **NAT-C.,** sel., stann.

children - ***acon.,*** agar., ***ant-c.,*** ant-s., ant-t., ***bell.,*** bor., calc., ***calc-p.,*** calc-sil., **CARC.,** caust., **CHAM.,** chin., ***cina,*** coloc., croc., gels., **IGN.,** kali-c., ***kali-p.,*** lyc., med., **NAT-M.,** ***nux-v.,*** op., ph-ac., **PHOS.,** plat., ***puls.,*** stann., ***staph.,*** stram., tarent., ***teucr., tub.***

chill, during - bry., ***caps.,*** chin., colch., hep., nat-c., petr., phos., verat.

coffee, after - **CHAM.,** coff., nux-v.

smell of, to the - arg-n., lach., sul-ac.

colors, to - kali-c.

cooked food, smell of - ars., chin., **COLCH.,** ***dig., eup-per., sep.,*** stann.

cruelties, when hearing of - **CALC., CARC.,** cic., hep., ***phos.***

crying, of children - caust., ign., phos., puls., ***sep.***

daytime - carb-v.

drugs, from - acon., ars., ***aven.,*** cham., coff., lyc., **NUX-V.,** puls., sep., sil., sulph.

eating, during - teucr.

after - cann-s., **NUX-V.,** teucr.

evening - ***calc.,*** merc., nat-m., ph-ac., plat., ran-b.

external impressions, to all - arn., caps., ***carc.,*** cham., clem., ***cocc.,*** coff., ***colch.,*** hep., ***iod.,*** lac-c., lach., ***nit-ac., nux-v.,*** ph-ac., **PHOS.,** ***staph.,*** sul-i., tub.

fever, during - bell., carb-v., lyc., nat-m., nit-ac., **PULS.,** teucr., valer.

fish, smell of, to - ***colch.***

food, smell of - arg-n., **ARS.,** ***cocc.,*** **COLCH.,** eup-per., ***ip.,*** lach., **SEP.,** stann.

forenoon - nat-c.

headache, during - ars., ***bell., cham.,*** chin., coff., ***ign., nux-v., sil.,*** spig., tela.

light, to - ***acon., ars.,*** aur., **BELL.,** buth-a., ***colch.,*** con., ***kali-p.,*** lac-c., ***nat-m.,*** **NUX-V., PHOS.,** sang., stram.

menopausal period, during - absin., arg-n., cimic., coff., dig., ***ign.,*** kali-br., ***lach.,*** ov., ***sep., ther.,*** valer., ***zinc-valer.***

menses, during - am-c., lyc., ***nux-v.,*** phos., plat.

before - chin., ign., nat-m., nit-ac., ***nux-v.,*** puls., ***sep.***

mental exertion, after - ***lach.***

SENSITIVE, general

mental impressions, to - am-c., ***arg-n.,*** ars., aur., bar-c., calc., clem., croc., dig., graph., hep., iod., lyc., mag-c., nat-c., nit-ac., ***phos.,*** sep., sil., tarent., zinc.

moral impressions, to - all-s., chin., dig., ign., nux-v., ***phos.,*** psor., ***puls.,*** staph.

morbidly - staph.

morning - calc., graph., hyos., nat-s., ***thuj.***

music, to - ***acon.,*** aloe, ***ambr.,*** anac., bry., bufo, cact., ***calc.,*** carb-an., **CARC.,** caust., ***cham.,*** coff., cop., ***croc.,*** cupr., dig., **GRAPH.,** ***ign., kreos., lyc.,*** merc., **NAT-C., NAT-M.,** nat-p., ***nat-s.,*** **NUX-V.,** pall., ***phos., ph-ac.,*** puls., ***sabin.,*** **SEP.,** stann., sulph., ***tab.,*** **TARENT.,** thuj., tub., tub-k., viol-o., zinc., zinc-p.

church - ***thuj.***

continues to hear the music he heard during day in the evening - lyc.

every not causes stitches in ear, violent pains in head - ph-ac.

piano - anac., ***nat-c.,*** sep., zinc.

sacred - lyss., thuj.

violin - viol-o.

night - kali-c.

noise, to - achy., **ACON.,** allox., aloe, alum., alum-p., alum-sil., ambr., am-c., anac., ***ang.,*** anh., ant-c., ant-t., apis, ***arg-n., arn., ars., ars-i.,*** **ASAR.,** ***aur.,*** aur-a., aur-i., aur-m., ***bar-c.,*** bapt., bar-i., **BELL., BOR.,** ***bry.,*** bufo, buth-a., cact., ***calad., calc.,*** calc-f., calc-sil., camph., cann-i., cann-s., caps., carb-an., ***carb-s., carb-v., carc.,*** card-m., ***caust., cham.,*** chel., **CHIN., CHIN-A.,** chin-b., chlol., chol., cic., cimic., cinnb., ***cocc.,*** **COFF.,** colch., **CON.,** convo-s., cop., crot-h., cyn-d., ***ferr., ferr-ar., ferr-p., fl-ac.,*** foll., gels., glon., ***hell.,*** hep., hura, hyos., **IGN.,** ***iod., ip.,*** kali-ar., **KALI-C.,** kali-i., ***kali-p.,*** kali-s., kali-sil., lac-ac., ***lac-c., lach., lachn., lat-m.,*** lept., ***lyc.,*** lycpr., ***lyss., mag-c., mag-m., man.,*** manc., mang., ***med., merc.,*** mosch., ***mur-ac.,*** nat-a., ***nat-c., nat-m.,*** nat-p., ***nat-s.,*** nat-sil., **NIT-AC.,** ***nux-m.,*** **NUX-V.,** onos., **OP.,** ox-ac., palo., ph-ac., phel., **PHOS.,** plan., ***plat.,*** ptel., ***puls.,*** rhus-t., sabad., sang., sec., seneg., **SEP., SIL.,** ***spig.,*** stann., staph., stram., stry., sulfon., sulfonam., sulph., syph., tanac., tarent., **THER., TUB.,** visc., yuc., **ZINC., ZINC-P.**

agg. the pains - coff.

aversion to - asar., bor., bry., coff., con., ferr., kali-c., op., raph., zinc.

breath of air, to the least - lyss.

chill, during - bell., **CAPS.,** gels., ***hyos.***

crackling of paper, to - ***asar.,*** bor., ferr., ign., lyc., nat-c., tarax.

evening - ***calc.***

labor, during - bell., bor., ***chin.,*** cimic., ***coff.***

menses, during - kali-p.

morning - ***fl-ac.***

music, amel. - **AUR.,** bufo, nat-m., sul-ac., sumb., **TARENT.,** thuj., tub.

SENSITIVE, general

noise, to

others eat apples, hawk or blow their noses, cannot bear to hear - lyss.

painful sensitiveness to - am-c., arn., ***coff., con., nux-v., sang.,*** seneg., ***sil., spig.***

penetrating - ***asar.,*** bar-c., chin., cocc., ***coff.,*** con., ferr., iod., lept., lil-t., lyc., manc., mur-ac., sabin., ***ther.***

scratching linen, silk or strings, to - **ASAR.**

shrill sounds - ***calc., nit-ac., ther.***

sleep, on going to - ***calad., calc.***

slightest - acon., aloe, ant-c., arg-n., **ASAR.,** bar-c., ***bell., bor.,*** bufo, chin., cinnb., ***cocc.,*** **COFF.,** ***ferr., lyc.,*** nat-c., nat-s., **NUX-V., OP.,** petr., ***phos., sabin., sep.,*** **SIL., THER.,** uva., xan.

greatly accentuated - bad.

loud, but not - bor.

penetrates the body, especially teeth - ther.

stepping, of - **COFF.,** ***nit-ac.,*** **NUX-V.,** sang.

striking of clocks, ringing of bells, to - ant-c., **ASAR., COFF.,** dros., **THER.**

sudden reports - bor., calad., cocc., nat-c., nat-m.

talking, of - agar., am-c., cact., ***cocc., coff., con., ign.,*** **ZINC.**

voices - ***ars.,*** aur., aur-a., bar-c., ***cocc., con.,*** ferr-ar., kali-ar., ***kali-c.,*** lyss., ***mag-m.,*** mur-ac., ***nit-ac.,*** **NUX-V.,** ***sil., teucr.,*** **ZINC.**

male - bar-c., ***nit-ac.***

several - petr.

water splashing - brom., **LYSS., NIT-AC.,** stram.

thought of it, even - lyss.

noon - zinc.

odors, to - ars., aur., bell., calc-f., carb-ac., ***caust.,*** cham., coff., **COLCH.,** dros., eup-per., graph., ign., lach., lyc., lyss., man., merc., ***merc-i-f., nux-v.,*** op., ***phos.,*** sang., **SEP.,** stann., staph., sulph., ther., vario.

camphor - kali-n.

dirty clothes - carb-an.

flowers - all-c., graph., lac-c., nux-v., sabad., sang.

foul things - par.

remains for a long time - dios.

mice - sabad.

musk amel. - mosch.

sour - alum., dros.

stool - dios., ***sulph.***

strong - anac., coff., sel.

sweet, agreeable - arg-n., aur., nit-ac., sil.

wood - graph.

others, what, say about her - ign., lyc., nat-m., stann., staph.

pain, to - **ACON.,** ***arn.,*** **ARS.,** asaf., ***aur., bart.,*** cact., ***carc.,*** **CHAM.,** ***chin.,*** **COFF.,** colch., cupr., daph., ferr-p., graph., **HEP.,** ***hyper., ign.,*** lat-m., lyc., mag-p., mag-s., mang., med., meli., mez., ***morph.,*** mosch., nat-s., nit-ac., nux-m., ***nux-v.,*** op., phos.,

SENSITIVE, general

pain, to - ***phyt., pip-m.,*** ran-s., stann., stram., ther., valer., zinc-valer.

peaches, smell of - all-c.

perspiration, during - bar-c., bell., chin.

pregnancy, during, exteme - acon., asar., cimic., ***ther.***

puberty, in - ***acon.,*** ant-s., ant-t., ***bell.,*** calc., ***cham.,*** ign., ***kali-p.,*** nat-m., ***phos., puls.,*** sep., ***staph., teucr.***

reading, to - crot-h., lach., mag-m., merc.

reprimands, to - calc-sil., ***carc.,*** coloc., ***ign.,*** lyc., ***med.,*** **NAT-M., STAPH.**

rudeness, to - ***calc.,*** cocc., ***colch.,*** mag-m., **NAT-M.,** nux-v., ph-ac., **STAPH.**

sad, stories - ***calc.,*** carc., cic., phos.

sensual impressions, to - ***am-c.,*** ars., ars-i., ***aur.,*** bar-c., calc., carc., cast., ***chin.,*** dig., ***graph.,*** hep., iod., ***lyc.,*** mag-c., ***nat-c., nit-ac.,*** nux-v., **PHOS.,** ***sep.,*** sil., thuj., ***zinc.***

singing, to - lyss., nux-v.

involuntary joins in on hearing anyone sing - croc.

sneezing, to - bor.

sour, smell of - dros.

steel points, directed toward her - apis, nat-m., **SIL., SPIG.**

sweets, smell of - aur., nit-ac., sil.

touch, to - ***acon.,*** caust., chin., cina, coff., foll., ***lach.,*** meny., op., phos., staph., tell.

vinegar, smell of - agar.

want of sensitiveness - bell., cann-i., chin., con., cupr., cupr-ac., cycl., daph., euphr., ***hydr-ac.,*** hyos., ***lyc.,*** **OP.,** ***ph-ac.,*** phos., ran-b., rheum, rhod., sabin., staph., stram.

wine, smell of, to - tab., zinc.

SENSES, (see Brain, chapter)

SENTIMENTAL, (see Romantic) - acon., alco., ambr., **ANT-C.,** ars., calc., ***calc-p.,*** canth., carc., cast., caust., chin., chin-a., ***cocc., coff.,*** con., crot-h., ***cupr.,*** hydr-ac., **IGN.,** kreos., lach., laur., ***lyc.,*** manc., nat-c., **NAT-M.,** nit-ac., **NUX-V.,** ***phos.,*** plat., plb., ***psor., puls.,*** sabad., sabin., ***staph., sulph.***

diarrhea, during - ***ant-c.***

drunkenness, crying or being sentimental during - ***caust., lach.***

menses, before - ***ant-c.***

moonlight, in - **ANT-C.**

twilight, in - ant-c.

SEPARATED, feels as if - agar., anac., arg-n., calc-p., cocc., daph., dulc., hyper., ***psor.,*** sabin., sep., ***thuj.,*** tril., verat.

SERENE, (See Tranquility)

SERIOUS - aeth., ***alum.,*** alum-p., am-m., ambr., am-c., anac., ang., ant-c., arg-m., **ARS.,** ars-s-f., asar., aur., bar-c., bart., bell., bor., bov., calc., cann-s., caust., cham., ***chin., cina, cocc.,*** coff., con., cycl., ***euph.,*** euphr., ferr., ferr-ar., grat., hyos., ign., iod., lach., ***led.,*** lyc., ***merc.,*** mur-ac., naja, nat-c., nat-p., nux-m., olnd., op., orig., ph-ac.,

SERIOUS, behaviour - plat., plb., puls., rhus-t., seneg., sep., spig., ***staph., sul-ac.,*** sulph., thuj., til., valer., verat.
absurdities, over - anac.
alternating with, cheerfulness - cann-s., cycl.
foolish behaviour - sul-ac.
jesting - plat.
laughing - nux-m.
day, during, exaltation at night - med.
evening - seneg., thuj.
ludricous things, when seeing - anac.
noon amel. - aeth.

SEXUAL, behaviour, (see Female and Male)
celibacy, ailments from - ***con.,*** nat-m., phos., staph.
excesses, mental symptoms from - agar., **AGN.,** alum., ***alum-p.,*** **APIS,** arg-n., arn., ars., asaf., aur., aur-a., ***bov.,*** calad., **CALC.,** calc-p., calc-sil., carb-an., ***carb-v.,*** **CHIN.,** chin-a., cocc., ***con.,*** dig., ***iod.,*** kali-br., ***kali-c.,*** kali-p., kali-s., kali-sil., lil-t., **LYC.,** mag-m., ***merc., nat-c.,*** nat-m., nat-p., nit-ac., **NUX-V.,** ol-an., onos., petr., **PH-AC., PHOS.,** plat., plb., ***puls.,*** sec., sel., **SEP.,** ***sil.,*** spig., **STAPH.,** sulph., symph., ***thuj.,*** upa., zinc., zinc-p.
homosexuality, men - ***calc.,*** **LYC., MED.,** nat-m., orig., ***phos., plat.,*** **PULS.,** sep., ***sil.,*** staph., **THUJ.**
women - calc-p., ***fl-ac., lach.,*** **MED., NAT-M.,** phos., **PLAT.,** puls., ***sep.,*** **STAPH.,** ***sulph.,. thuj.***
lasciviousness, lustful - ***acon.,*** agar., agn., aloe, ***ambr.,*** anac., ant-c., ***apis,*** arund., aster., aur., bell., bor., bov., ***bufo, calad., calc.,*** calc-p., calc-s., calc-sil., ***cann-i.,*** cann-s., ***canth., carb-v.,*** carl., ***caust.,*** cer-s., ***chin.,*** coc-c., cod., ***con.,*** cop., croc., ***dig., fl-ac., graph.,*** **HYOS.,** hyper., ign., kali-br., **LACH.,** lyc., **LIL-T.,** lyss., **MED.,** merc., mosch., ***murx.,*** nat-m., nit-ac., nuph., nux-v., op., **ORIG.,** ph-ac., **PHOS., PIC-AC., PLAT.,** plb., ***puls.,*** raja-s., raph., ***sabin., sel., sep., sil.,*** spig., **STAPH.,** ***stram.,*** sulph., ***tarent.,*** **THUJ.,** tere-ch., ***tub.,*** ust., ***verat.,*** zinc.
afternoon - lyss.
cachexia, in - psor.
convulsions, before - ***lach.***
daytime - lach.
dreaming, after - sil.
eating with feeling of weakness in parts, after - lyss.
elderly men - dig.
emotions, with violent - cop.
epilepsy, followed by - ***lach.***
erections, with - lyss., op., sin-n.
painful - lyss.
evening - calc.
bed, in - nat-m.
impotence, with - calad., ***chin., op., sel.***
insanity, in - hyos.
menses, before - stram.
morning - coc-c.
bed, in - sil.
prostate, with enlarged - dig.

SEXUAL, behaviour
lasciviousness, lustful
uncovers sexual parts - **HYOS.**
watching, women on the street - calad., fl-ac.
women at every touch - ***murx.***
lewdness - agn., apis, bell., bufo, ***camph., canth., cub., hyos., lach.,*** lyss., nux-v., op., plat., ***phos., pic-ac.,*** rob., stram., tarent., verat.
fancies, even when dreaming - ambr.
songs - ***hyos.,*** op., ***stram.***
talk - aur., ***bell.,*** bufo, calc., camph., chlf., cub., ***hyos., lil-t., nux-v.,*** phos., plat., ***stram.,*** tub., verat.
nymphomania, women - ambr., agar., anh., ***ant-c., apis,*** asaf., aster., ***bar-m., bell.,*** calad., calc., ***calc-p.,*** camph., ***cann-i., cann-s., canth.,*** carb-v., ***cedr., chin., chlor.,*** coca, ***coff., croc.,*** cyna., ***dig.,*** dulc., ***ferul., fl-ac.,*** gins., graph., **GRAT., HYOS.,** ign., ***kali-br.,*** kali-p., **LACH.,** ***lil-t., lyc.,*** manc., ***med., merc.,*** mosch., ***murx.,*** nat-c., nat-m., ***nux-v.,*** op., **ORIG.,** ph-ac., ***phos.,*** pic-ac., **PLAT.,** plb., psil., ***puls., raph., rob., sabad.,*** sabin., ***sal-n.,*** sil., stann., ***staph.,*** **STRAM.,** stry., sulph., sumb., ***tarent.,*** thuj., valer., ***verat., zinc.,*** zinc-pic.
chorea, with - tarent.
girls - ***orig., plat.,*** raph.
young - ***orig.***
loquacity, with - ***verat.***
menopausal period, at - lach., manc., ***murx.***
menses, during - calc., coca, ***hyos.,*** kali-br., kali-c., ***plat., sec., verat.***
after - sul-ac.
before - calc., calc-p., kali-c., ***phos.,*** stram., ***verat.***
suppressed - ant-c., canth., chin., cocc., hyos., ***murx.,*** phos., ***plat.,*** stram., sil., sulph., verat., zinc.
metrorrhagia, during - mosch., murx., plat., sabin., sec.
mucus, with bluish-white - ambr.
pregnancy, during - phos., zinc.
puerperal - bell., ***chin.,*** coca, kali-br., ***plat.,*** verat., zinc.
sex agg. - ***tarent.***
obscene - agn., alum., anac., apis, bell., bufo, calc., ***camph., canth.,*** carb-v., ***caust.,*** chin., con., ***cub.,*** **HYOS.,** ***lach.,*** lil-t., lyc., lyss., ***med.,*** merc., murx., nat-m., nux-v., op., orig., ***phos., pic-ac.,*** **PLAT.,** puls., rob., staph., stram., sulph., tarent., ***thuj., verat.***
man searching for little girls - caust., phos., plat., thuj., verat.
songs - alco., canth., **HYOS.,** op., raja-s., stram., verat.
talk - aur., ***bell.,*** bufo, ***calc.,*** camph., chlf., cub., ***hyos., lil-t., nux-v.,*** phos., ***stram.,*** verat.
rape, ailments from - **ACON.,** anac., **ARN., CARC., IGN.,** lyc., ***med.,*** **NAT-M.,** nux-v., **OP.,** ***plat., sep.,*** **STAPH.,** thuj.

SEXUAL, behaviour
- **satyriasis,** men - anac., camph., cann-i., **CANTH.,** con., cyna., ***fl-ac.,*** grat., hyos., ***kali-br., lyss.,*** **MED.,** merc., nat-m., nux-v., ***phos., pic-ac., plat.,*** sal-n., saroth., ***stram.,*** sulph., **THUJ.,** thymol., ust., ***verat.,*** zinc-pic.
- **sexual** abuse, ailments from - acon., anac., arn., **CARC., IGN.,** lyc., ***med.,*** **NAT-M.,** nux-v., **OP.,** ***plat., sep.,*** **STAPH.,** thuj.

SHAMELESS - alco., ***anac.,*** bell., ***bufo,*** calc., camph., cann-s., canth., cub., cupr., hell., **HYOS.,** lyc., ***med.,*** merc-c., mosch., murx., nat-m., nux-m., ***nux-v., op.,*** **PHOS.,** ***phyt.,*** **PLAT.,** sabin., **SEC.,** ***staph., stram., tarent., verat.***
- bed, in - nat-m.
- children, in - hyos., med., plat., ***tub.***
- exposes the person - **HYOS.,** ***phos.,*** phyt., ***sec., tarent.,*** verat.
- lying-in, during - verat.

SHINING objects, agg. - **BELL.,** bufo, camph., cann-i., ***canth.,*** cocc-s., glon., ***hyos.,*** lach., **LYSS.,** mur-ac., phos., **STRAM.,** tub.
- amel. - ***stram.,*** tarent.
- averse to - bufo.
- surface of water - **LYSS.**

SHRIEKING, (see Screaming)

SIGHING, emotional (see Breathing, chapter) - acon., act-sp., ether, agar., ***agn.,*** ail., alum., am-c., am-m., aml-n., anac., ang., ant-c., apoc., arg-n., ars., atro., ***aur.,*** bell., benz-n., **BRY.,** cact., **CALC-P.,** camph., carb-ac., carb-an., ***carc.,*** cedr., ***cench.,*** cer-b., ***cham.,*** chin., chin-s., **CIMIC.,** cob., ***cocc.,*** colch., con., ***corn.,*** croc., cupr., cur., ***cycl.,*** der., dig., elae., eup-per., ***eup-pur.,*** gels., ***glon.,*** gran., ***graph., hell.,*** hura, hyos., iber., **IGN.,** ***indg., ip.,*** kali-cy., kali-p., lach., lact., lil-t., lyc., lyss., merc-c., mill., mit., morph., mur-ac., naja, nat-c., ***nat-m., nat-p.,*** nat-s., nit-ac., nux-m., ***nux-v.,*** op., ***ph-ac.,*** phos., phys., plat., plb., podo., psor., ***puls.,*** raja-s., ran-s., ***rhus-t.,*** sac-l., ***sec., sel., sep.,*** sil., spong., ***stann.,*** staph., ***stram.,*** sulph., tab., tax., ther., thuj., til., trad., verat-v., vip., zinc.
- afternoon - ant-c.
- alternating with dancing and jumping - bell.
- causeless - nux-v.
- convulsions, before - bufo, plb.
- crying, continues long after - ***ign.***
- dinner, after - arg-n.
- emptiness in stomach, during - **IGN.**
- epileptic attacks, before - ***bufo,*** cic., lyss., ***plb.***
- evening - chin.
  - 7 p.m. - lycps.
- grief, after - calc-p., **IGN.,** nat-m.
- heat, during - acon., ***arn.,*** ars., bell., bry., carb-v., ***cham.,*** cocc., ***coff., ign.,*** ip., nux-v., puls., rhus-t., sep., thuj.
  - head, of - clem.
- honor, from wounded - ***nux-v.***
- hysteria, in - ***hydr-ac.,*** **IGN.,** ***plat.***
- involuntary - ***ferr-m.,*** hell.
- menopause, during - xan.

SIGHING, emotional
- menses, during - ars., cimic., cocc., graph., ign., plat.
  - amel., during - nat-p.
  - after - stram.
  - before - ***ign.,*** lyc., nat-p.
- morning, 9 a.m. - ign.
- night - bry.
  - 2 a.m. - ign.
- perspiration, during - acon., ars., **BRY.,** ***cham.,*** chin., ***cocc.,*** cupr., ***ign., ip.,*** nux-v., phos., ***rhus-t., sep.,*** stram., thuj., verat.
- shocks from injuries, in - ***lach.***
- sleep, during - anac., ars., aur., bell., camph., ***kali-p.,*** mag-c., op., puls., ***sulph.***
  - comatose - ars.
- throat, with grasping at - ign., **STRAM.**
- vaginal discharge, during - phys.
- waking, on - puls.

SILENT, (see Talk)

SILLY, (see Foolish)

SINGING - acon., ***agar.,*** anan., apis, ***bell.,*** cann-i., cann-s., caps., ***carb-s.,*** chin., chlor., ***cic., cocc.,*** cot., ***croc.,*** cupr., der., ferr-p., gels., hipp., hydr., **HYOS.,** kali-c., ***lach.,*** lachn., lact., lob-s., lyc., lyss., ***mag-arct.,*** mag-c., manc., merc-i-f., merl., mez., nat-c., nat-m., nux-m., op., ph-ac., phos., ***plat.,*** sang., sars., sep., ***spong., stram.,*** sul-ac., sulo-ac., sulph., tab., tarent., ***teucr.,*** ther., ***verat.***
- alternating with,
  - anger - croc.
  - crying - ***acon.,*** bell., der., stram.
    - and laughing - stram.
  - distraction - spong.
  - groaning - ***bell.***
  - hatred of work - spong.
  - quarrelsomeness - croc.
  - talking - ***gels.***
  - vexation - agar., croc.
- boisterous - alco.
- dancing and crying - tarent.
- evening - nat-m.
- fever, during - bell., ***op.,*** stram., verat.
- headache, with - ther.
- hilarious, joyously - agar., ***hyos., nat-m.,*** op.
  - night - verat.
- hoarse, exhausted, and - tarent.
  - until hoarse very - ***tarent.***
- involuntarily - ***croc.,*** lyc., lyss., spong., tarent., teucr.
  - on hearing a single note sung - ***croc.***
- joyously, at night - verat.
- latin, paternoster - ***stram.***
- maniacal - cocc.
- menses, during - stram.
- monotonous - ***op.***
- morning on waking - ery-m.
- night - bell., croc., ***mag-arct.,*** ph-ac., verat.
- obscene, songs - alco., canth., **HYOS.,** op., raja-s., stram., verat.
- sadness, after - merc-i-f.
- screaming and crying, followed by - ***hyper.***

SINGING,
sleep, in - ***bell.,*** **CROC.,** hyper., lach., ***mag-arct.,*** ph-ac., stram., sulph.
trilling - acon., ***bell.,*** cocc., lyc., mag-c., nat-c., nux-v., phos., staph., ther., verat.
waking, on - ***sulph.***

SIT, inclination to - acon., ***agar.,*** alum., am-c., ***am-m., anac.,*** ant-c., ant-t., arg-m., arg-n., ***arn., ars., ars-i.,*** asar., ***aur.,*** bar-ac., bar-c., bar-m., ***bell.,*** bor., brom., bry., calc., camph., ***cann-s.,*** canth., caps., ***carb-s., carb-v.,*** caust., ***cham., chel.,*** **CHIN.,** chin-a., ***cocc.,*** cod., colch., **CON.,** croc., cupr., cycl., dulc., ***euphr., ferr.,*** **GRAPH., GUAI.,** hell., ***hep.,*** **HIPP.,** ***hyos.,*** ign., ***iod.,*** ip., jac-c., kali-ar., kali-c., kali-p., lac-c., lach., laur., lil-t., lyc., mag-c., mag-m., merc., mez., mur-ac., nat-a., nat-c., ***nat-m.,*** nat-p., ***nit-ac.,*** **NUX-V.,** ol-an., olnd., op., petr., **PHOS.,** ***ph-ac., pic-ac.,*** plat., plb., **PULS.,** ran-b., ***ran-s.,*** rheum, rhod., rhus-t., ruta, ***sec., sep.,*** sil., ***spong.,*** **SQUIL.,** stann., stront-c., ***sulph., tarax., teucr., verat.,*** verb., viol-t., ***zinc.***
muse, and sit - ham.
physical desire to sit - puls.

SITS, general
breaks pins, and - **BELL.,** calc.
crying - ***ambr.,*** calc-sil.
erect - cham., hyos., lyc., puls., stram.
head on hands and elbow on knees, with - glon., iod.
knees drawn up, resting her head and arms on knees, with - **ARS.**
looking at the ground - stram.
meditates - calc-s.
misfortune, imaginary, over - calc-s., lil-t.
moody silence, in - mag-p.
mops, sadness, with - cimic., psor., puls.
pins, and breaks - **BELL.**
place, in one, for 3 or 4 days during headache - con.
stiff, quite - ***cham., hyos.,*** kali-m., puls., ***sep., stram.***
delirium, in - sep.
long time, for a - nat-p.
still - alum-p., alum-sil., arn., aur., aur-s., bar-c., bar-i., bar-m., brom., calc., calc-sil., carb-s., cham., chin-a., cimic., ***cocc.,*** elaps, fl-ac., ***gels.,*** hell., ***hep.,*** **HIPP.,** hyos., kali-a., kali-m., kali-sil., lyc., nat-p., ***nux-v., pic-ac., plat.,*** **PULS.,** ***sep.,*** stram., thala., **VERAT.,** zinc-p.
wrapped in deep, sad thoughts, as if, and notices nothing - ***ambr.,*** aur., cench., ***cocc.,*** elaps, ***hipp.,*** plat., ***puls., stram., verat.***

SIZE, incorrect judge of (see Mistakes) - agar., carb-v., phys., ***plat.,*** staph., stram.
frame, size of, seems lessened - phys.
smaller, things appear - carb-v., phys., **PLAT.,** staph., stram.

SLANDER, disposition to - am-c., ***anac.,*** **ARS.,** bell., bor., ***caust.,*** cor-r., helon., hyos., ip., ***lach.,*** lyc., merc., nit-ac., ***nux-v.,*** par., petr., plat., sep., spig., stram., **VERAT.**
denouncer - ars., lach., nat-c., nat-m.
sneak - ars., lach., nat-c.

SLOWNESS, mental - **ALUM.,** am-m., ambr., ammc., ***anac.,*** aq-mar., **ARS., ASAR., BAR-C.,** bell., bell-p., **BRY.,** cact., **CALC.,** ***carb-v.,*** **CARC.,** chel., ***chin.,*** caust., clem., cocc., **CON.,** cortiso., cupr., dulc., echi., ferr-ma., flor-p., gels., ***graph.,*** halo., **HELL.,** hep., hist., hyos., ign., ip., kali-bi., kali-br., kali-m., kreos., lach., lyc., lycps., mag-arct., meph., merc., nat-m., nux-m., nux-v., olnd., onop., onos., ox-ac., ***op.,*** **PH-AC., PHOS.,** plb., **PULS.,** rhus-t., ruta, ***sep.,*** sil., ***sulph.,*** thuj., ***verat.,*** zinc.
always behind hand - ***cact.***
bus, sensation of sl. of - cortiso.
calculation, in - calc.
children, in - alum., ***anac.,*** **BAR-C., CALC., CARC.,** caust., con., cortiso., gels., ***graph.,*** **HELL.,** hyos., kali-bi., kali-br., lyc., merc., nat-m., ***op.,*** **PH-AC., PHOS.,** puls., ***sil.,*** thuj., ***verat.,*** zinc.
eating, while - acon.
elderly people, of - **BAR-C.,** cact., **CALC., CON.,** ***hell.,*** kali-p., ***phos.,*** zinc.
motion, in - ***anac., calc.,*** cocc., ***con.,*** crot-h., **PHOS.,** sep.
pain, to respond to - ***alum., cocc.,*** plb.
purpose, of - graph.
work, in - cact., ***calc.,*** mag-arct.

SLUGGISHNESS, (see Dullness)

SMALLER, (see Size)

SMILING - alco., ars., atro., bell., **HYOS.,** nux-v., sumb., ***verat.***
convulsions, before - bell.
foolish - bell., hyos., ***merc.,*** verat.
involuntarily - aur., bell., lyc.
speaking, when - aur.
never smiles - alum., ambr., **AUR.,** verat.
sardonic - bell.
sleep, in - cadm-s., croc., hyos., ph-ac.

SNAPPISH - ***calc-p.,*** **CHAM., CINA,** lil-t., ***nux-v., sep.***

SNEERS, at everyone, (see Contempt, Scorn)

SOBBING, (see Crying, Sighing)

SOCIETY, (see Company)

SOLEMN, (see Serious)

SOLITUDE, fond of, (see Company, aversion) - **NAT-C., NAT-M.,** sulph.

SOMNAMBULISM, (see Sleep, Sleepwalking)

SORROWFUL, (see Depression, Morose)

SPEECH, general, (see Mind, Talking or Mouth, speech) - bell., caust., crot-h., gels., glon., hyos., kali-br., **LACH.,** lyc., merc., nat-c., nat-m., nux-m., nux-v., phos., stann., stram.
abrupt - ars., cham., mur-ac., plb., sul-ac., sulph., **TARENT.**

SPEECH, general

angry - anac., zinc.

sleep, in - cast.

anxious, in sleep - alum., graph., nux-v., ***sulph.***

aphasia, (see Mind, Aphasia)

awkward - ***nat-c.***

babbling - con., cortico., dulc., gels., ***hyos.,*** lach., lyc., plb., sel., ***stram.***

benevolent - tus-f.

blundering - lach.

bombast, worthless - crot-h., ***lach.,*** nux-v., staph.

broken - camph.

childish - acon., ***arg-n.,*** bar-c., lyc.

confused - alco., bell., benz-n., bry., calc., ***cann-s.,*** carl., ***caust., crot-c.,*** crot-h., ***gels., hyos., lach.,*** lyc., med., mosch., ***nat-m.,*** nux-m., ***nux-v., op.,*** sec., sep., stram., thuj.

morning on waking - atro.

night, at - cham.

sleep, in - calc.

convincing - op.

crying, hoarse like a child - cupr.

delirious - ***bell.,*** camph., canth., ***cic., cupr-ac., hyos.,*** op., passi., plb., ***rheum,*** stram., tab., vip.

business, of - **BRY.**

chill, during - cham.

aroused during, on being - hep.

fever, during - coff., til.

menses, before - lyc.

night - dig., rheum, sil.

sleep, in - **BELL.**

asleep, on falling - phos.

midnight, before - rheum, ***sulph.***

waking, on - bry.

difficult, anger, from - kali-p.

tries, though she - cimic.

utter, every word loudly - hyos.

distorted - cupr-ac.

embarrassed - aeth., atro., carb-s., merc., morph., nat-m., pall., tab.

enthousiastic - cann-i.

excited - morph., nat-c.

extravagant - ***cann-i.,*** ether, lach., ***nux-m.,*** plb., stram., verat.

facile - hyos., lach., sil.

faster than ever before, especially during fever - pyrog.

fine - hyos.

finish sentence, cannot - ars., **CANN-I.,** lach., med., thuj.

does not - cimic.

firmer, surer in afternoon than in forenoon - anac.

fluent - cupr-ac., ped., sil., thea.

foolish - aur., ***bell.,*** bry., bufo, calc., calc-sil., caust., ***chin.,*** **HYOS.,** ***lach.,*** merl., ***nux-m.,*** par., phos., ***stram.,*** tab.

forcible - pall.

SPEECH, general

forgetful, of words while speaking, of, words hunting for (see Aphasia) - agar., alum., am-br., anh., ***arg-n.,*** **ARN.,** ***bar-c.,*** bar-s., benz-ac., **BOTH.,** cact., calc., camph., **CANN-I.,** cann-s., carb-an., carb-s., carb-v., chen-a., coca, cocc., colch., con., crot-h., dulc., glon., ham., helo., hydr., ***kali-br.,*** kali-c., kali-p., ***lach.,*** lil-t., ***lyc., med., nat-m., nux-v., onos., plb.,*** podo., **PH-AC.,** puls., rhod., sil., staph., sulph., syph., ***thuj.,*** verat.

foreign tongue, in a - camph., lach., nit-ac., ***stram.***

future, about - hyos.

hasty - acon., alco., ambr., anac., arn., ars., atro., aur., ***bell.,*** bry., bufo, ***camph.,*** cann-i., cann-s., caust., chlol., cimic., cina, cocc., fl-ac., **HEP., HYOS.,** ***ign.,*** kali-c., kali-p., **LACH.,** lil-t., lyc., lyss., **MERC.,** morph., ***mosch.,*** nux-v., op., ***ph-ac.,*** plb., ***sep.,*** stann., ***stram.,*** stry., ***thuj., verat.***

answers slowly, but - merc.

heavy - aran-s.

hesitating - absin., agar., agn., amyg., ***arg-n.,*** canth., carb-s., cortico., euphr., graph., kali-br., lat-m., laur., lyc., merc., morph., ***nux-m.,*** ph-ac., ***puls.,*** sec., staph., thuj., vip.

incoherent - absin., ***agar.,*** alco., amyg., ***anac.,*** anh., ***apis, arg-n.,*** ars., ars-s-f., ***atro., bapt., bell.,*** **BRY.,** buth-a., calad., cact., ***camph.,*** **CANN-I.,** ***cann-s.,*** carb-s., cham., chel., chlol., cimic., coca, coff., ***crot-h.,*** cub., cupr., cycl., dulc., ether, ***gels.,*** hep., hydr-ac., **HYOS.,** kali-bi., kali-br., kali-c., kali-p., **LACH.,** merc., merc-c., merc-meth., ***morph., nux-m.,*** op., par., past., ***ph-ac.,*** **PHOS.,** plb., raja-s., **RHUS-T.,** spig., spig-m., **STRAM.,** stry., ***sulph.,*** tanac., vip., visc., zinc., zinc-p.

anxiety, during, in erysipelas - ***chel.***

dozing, after - op.

epileptic attack, after - ars., plb.

evening - bell.

night - bell., gels., kali-bi., plb.

perspiration, ending with - ***cupr-ac.***

sleep, during - cub., ***gels.,*** kali-bi., phos., ***stram.***

asleep, on falling - kali-bi.

waking, on - cact., ign., op.

inconsiderate - alco., calad., mez.

indistinct - cocc., glon., lyc.

excitement, from - laur.

interesting - thea.

intoxicated, as if - amyg., carb-an., ***gels.,*** **HYOS.,** lyc., meph., nat-m., ***nux-v.,*** vip.

irrelevant - atro.

jerks, by - ***agar.,*** bov., caust., mygal.

loud - arn., ars., atro., aur., ***bell.,*** cham., ***hyos.,*** **LACH.,** nux-m., stram.

sleep, in - ***arn., bell., sil.,*** spong., ***sulph.***

low - bell., ***carb-an.,*** nux-v., ***sec.,*** staph.

merry - agar., ether, mur-ac.

sleep, in - mur-ac.

SPEECH, general

monosyllabic - ars., merc., meli., ***nux-v., ph-ac., sul-ac., thuj.***

nonsense - acon., ***anac.,*** arg-m., atro., aur., ***bell.,*** bufo, calc-sil., ***camph., cann-i.,*** canth., chlf., chlol., cupr., ether, **HYOS.,** kali-br., ***lach.,*** merc., nux-m., op., plb., ***stann., stram.,***

nonsense - ***sulph.,*** tub., ***verat.***

springing up while asleep, on - kali-c.

offensive - ***anac.,*** lyss.

pathetic - lyss.

phrases, in high-sounding - ***nux-v.***

plaintive - crot-h.

prattling - acon., aloe, ***anac.,*** atro., bell., **BRY.,** calad., cyna., **HYOS.,** ign., lach., nux-v., op., plb., ***stram.,*** tarax.

lies naked in bed - **HYOS.**

morning - **BRY.**

sleep, in - ***nux-v.***

random, at night - lach., plb., verat.

rapturous - ether.

repeats same thing - coff-t., kres., lach., plat.

respectful - agar.

sharp - cham., hyper.

short, abrupt - cham.

slow - ***aesc-g., aeth.,*** agar., agar-ph., anac., anh., ant-c., ***arg-n.,*** ars., atro., bar-c., bell., ***both., bov.,*** bufo, caj., cann-i., ***cann-s.,*** carb-an., ***caust.,*** cer-s., chin-s., chlf., cic., cocc., ***cupr.,*** gels., **HELL.,** hyos., ***ign., kali-br.,*** kali-cy., kali-p., **LACH.,** laur., lyc., mang., mang-o., merc., mez., morph., mygal., naja, nat-c., ***nat-m.,*** nux-m., olnd., ***op.,*** petr., ***ph-ac., phos.,*** phys., ***plb.,*** rhus-t., ***sec., sep., stram.,*** sulfon., syph., ***thuj.,*** vip., zinc.

hunts for words - thuj.

stammering, stuttering (see Mouth, Speech)

strange - cham., ether, gall-ac., stram.

terse - op.

threatening - stram., tarent.

unintelligible - acon., amyg., ars., **BELL.,** bufo, calen., euph., **HYOS.,** lyc., ***merc.,*** naja, nux-v., ***ph-ac.,*** plb., ***sec.,*** sil., **STRAM.,** sul-ac., tab., ***verat-v.***

convulsions, before epileptic - bufo.

midnight, before - nux-v.

sleep, in - arn., atro., cast., cham., mur-ac.

unsuitable - nux-v.

vexations, about old - cham.

desire to say - mez.

violent - cann-i., ***nat-c.,*** stram.

vivacious - cann-i., **HYOS.,** ***sulph.***

voice, in a shrill (see Larynx, voice) - cann-i., cupr., stram.

low, soft, in a - ***viol-o.***

wandering - acon., aeth., agar., ***ambr., anac.,*** arg-n., arn., ***ars.,*** ars-s-f., ***atro.,*** aur., aur-a., **BELL.,** ***bry.,*** calc., ***camph.,*** canth., cham., chin., chin-a., cic., ***cimic.,*** cina, coloc., cupr., dulc., **HYOS.,** ign., kali-c., ***kali-p.,*** **LACH., LYC.,** merc., **NUX-M.,** nux-v., ***op., par., phos., plat.,*** plb., ***puls.,*** rheum, ***rhus-t.,***

SPEECH, general

wandering - sabin., sec., spong., **STRAM.,** ***sulph.,*** tub., ***verat.***

afternoon and especially evening - ***nux-v.***

night, at - aur., bell., bry., coloc., dig., op., rheum, sep., sulph.

subject to subject, from - agar., ***lach.***

whispering - cupr., meli., stann.

says she dares not to talk loud as it would kill her - meli.

wild - anac., ars., atro., camph., lyc., plb., spig-m., stram., ***verat-v.***

sleep, in - hyper.

SPITEFUL, (see Malicious)

SPIT, desire to - aeth., bar-ac., bell., calc., ***cann-s.,*** carb-s., ***coc-c.,*** cupr., glon., lyc., merc., ***nux-v.,*** rhus-t., sec., ***sulph., tab., verat., verat-v.***

afternoon - gels.

anger, from - ***calc.***

directions, in all - lyss.

eating, after - der.

faces of people, in - ars., **BELL.,** bufo, ***calc.,*** cann-i., cann-s., ***cupr.,*** cupr-ac., hyos., merc., phos., plb., ***stram., verat.***

floor, on the, and licks it up - merc.

morning - der.

SPOKEN to, averse to being - agar., am-c., anh., ant-c., ant-t., arn., ***ars., ars-i.,*** ars-s-f., aur., aur-a., aur-s., **BRY.,** caj., calc-sil., camph., ***carb-s.,*** **CHAM.,** con., cur., cyn-d., elaps, fago., ***gels., graph.,*** ham., hell., helon., ***hipp., hyos.,*** ign., **IOD.,** kali-p., kalm., kreos., lil-t., lyc., mag-m., myric., nat-m., ***nat-s.,*** nit-ac., nux-v., op., ***ph-ac.,*** plan., plat., plb., puls-n, rhus-t., sep., ***sil.,*** sin-n., staph., stram., ***sulph., tarent.,*** tep., teucr., tub., verat., zinc.

agg. when spoken to - cham., plat.

alone, wants to be let - ant-t., aur., caj., helon., hipp., ign., ***iod.,*** lil-t., ***sulph.***

being called, agg. - sulph.

chill, during - ***hyos.***

kindly, even - ign., nat-m., sil.

morning - ars., nat-s.

SQUANDERS, money - agar., alum., ***bell.,*** calc., caust., con., hep., **LACH.,** lyc., **MERC.,** ***nux-v.,*** stram., sulph., syph., verat.

boasting, from - calc., lyc., nux-v., plat., puls.

order, from want of - lyc., plat., sil.

STAGE-fright, (see Anticipation, Anxiety) - **ACON.,** anac., **ARG-N.,** ***ars., carb-v.,*** **GELS., LYC.,** med., **NAT-M.,** ph-ac., ***sil., thuj.***

STAMPING, feet - ant-c., stram., verat.

STARING, thoughtless - brom., **CANN-I.,** carb-s., cench., cic., **HELL.,** ***hydr-ac.,*** hyos., ***merc-c.,*** op., ***phos., puls.,*** ran-b., stram.

thoughtless, morning - ***guai.***

STARTLED, starting - ***acon., agar.,*** alum., ambr., ang., ant-c., ant-t., apis, arg-m., ***arn.,*** **ARS.,** ***ars-h., ars-i., ars-s-f., asar., atro.,*** aur-m., ***bar-c.,*** bar-m., **BELL.,** benz-ac., berb., bism., ***bor.,*** brom., **BRY.,** ***bufo,*** calad., ***calc.,*** calc-ar., calc-s., calc-sil., camph., cann-s., **CAPS.,** carb-ac.,

STARTLED, starting - ***carb-an., carb-s., carb-v.,*** card-m., carc., ***caust.,*** cham., chel., chin., chin-a., ***cic.,*** cimic., ***cina, cocc.,*** colch., ***con.,*** cupr., ***cur.,*** cypr., ferr-i., graph., hep., hura, hydr-ac., **HYOS.,** hyper., ***ign.,*** inul., ***kali-ar.,*** **KALI-C.,** ***kali-i.,*** **KALI-P.,** ***kali-s.,*** kali-sil., **LAC-C.,** lach., led., lil-t., ***lyc.,*** lyss., ***med.,*** merc., mosch., mur-ac., **NAT-A.,** ***nat-c.,*** **NAT-M.,** ***nat-p., nit-ac., nux-m., nux-v., op., petr., phos., phys.,*** plat., psor., ptel., puls., rhus-t., sabad., samb., ***scut., sep., sil.,*** sol-n., spong., **STRAM., STRONT-C.,** stry., ***sulph.,*** sul-ac., sumb., tab., ***tarent., ther.,*** tub., verat., vinc., zinc.

- **afternoon** - lyss., nicc., pall., sulph.
- **anxious** - aloe, apis, cupr., hep., lyc., ***phos.,*** samb., stront-c., ***sulph.***
  - downward motion, from - ***bor.***
- **bed** in - cic., hura, merc-meth., tab.
  - awake, while lying - anac., bry., euph.
- **called** by name, when - sulph.
- **convulsive** - ars., calc-p., hyos., stry.
- **crackling** of paper, from - calad.
- **daytime** - nux-v.
- **dentition,** during - calc-p., cham.
- **door** is opened, when a - hura, mosch., phos.
  - slams - calad., ox-ac.
- **dream,** from a - acon., am-m., aur., bar-c., bov., calc., caps., carb-v., colch., cor-r., croc., dig., ***ferr-ma.,*** indg., kali-i., ***kali-n.,*** led., mag-arct., mag-aust., ***mag-c., mag-s.,*** mez., murx., nat-c., nat-s., nicc., nit-ac., peti., petr., puls., sars., ***sil.,*** staph., sulph., teucr.
  - dreams, in - ant-c., petr., ***puls.,*** sulph.
- **easily** - ***acon.,*** agar., am-c., am-m., ant-c., ant-t., apis, ars-s-f., ***asar.,*** bar-c., bar-m., ***bell.,*** **BOR.,** ***bufo,*** calad., calc., calc-s., ***camph.,*** carb-v., ***cham.,*** cic., cimic., ***cocc.,*** cypr., helon., hura, hyper., ***ign., kali-br.,*** **KALI-C.,** kali-i., **KALI-P.,** kali-s., kali-sil., med., merc., mez., **NAT-C., NAT-M., NAT-P.,** ***nit-ac.,*** nux-m., ***nux-v.,*** op., **PHOS.,** phys., ***psor.,*** sabad., samb., ***scut., sep., sil.,*** spong., ***stram., sulph.,*** sumb., tab., ***tarent., ther.,*** tub., verat., xan., zinc.
- **eating,** after - hep.
- **electric,** as if - agar., cann-s., euph., kiss., phos.
  - sleep, during - ***arg-m., ars., nat-m., nux-m.***
  - shocks through the body while wide awake - euph., mag-m., nat-p.
  - wakening her - ***arg-m., ars., nat-m.,*** nux-m.
- **evening** - ped., plat., ***puls.***
  - falling asleep, on - ambr., am-m., anac., arn., **ARS.,** ars-s-f., bar-c., ***bell.,*** bry., dulc., kali-bi., lach., merc-c., nat-c., plat., sars., ***sel.,*** stront-c., ***sulph.***
  - jerking or twitching, ceasing on falling asleep - ***agar.,*** hell.
  - sleep in - calc., kali-i., petr.
- **fall,** on hearing anything - alum.
- **falling,** as if - bell., bism., dig., mez., ph-ac.
- **feet,** as if coming from the - lyc.
  - wakening her - ***arg-m., ars., nat-m.,*** nux-m.
- **frequently** - **IGN.**

STARTLED, starting

- **fright,** from and as from - ***acon.,*** alum., ***am-c.,*** ambr., anac., apis, arn., atro., ***bar-c.,*** **BELL., BOR.,** bry., bufo, ***cact.,*** calc-p., calen., carb-s., ***carb-v., caust.,*** chin., ***cic.,*** coff., coff-t., ***con.,*** dig., euphr., **HYOS.,** hyper., jac-c., kali-ar., ***kali-br.,*** **KALI-C., KALI-P.,** kali-s., kali-sil., ***kreos., lyc.,*** macro., mag-c., mag-s., ***merc.,*** merc-c., mosch., mur-ac., naphtin., nat-a., **NAT-C., NAT-M.,** nat-p., **NAT-S.,** nat-sil., **NIT-AC.,** ***op.,*** **PHOS.,** plb., psor., ruta, sabad., sars., ***sep., sil., spong.,*** stann., staph., **STRAM.,** stront-c., ***sulph.,*** **VERAT.**
- **hawking,** at - **BOR.**
- **heat,** during - caps., cham., ferr-p., ign., nat-m., op.
- **involuntarily,** violent - stront-c.
- **itching** and biting, from - mag-c.
- **lying,** while - lyc.
  - back, on - calc-p., mag-c., nit-ac.
  - right side - mag-c.
- **menses,** during - ***bor.,*** ign., ***zinc.***
  - before - calc., sep.
- **mental** exertion, from - vinc.
- **midnight** in sleep, about - mag-c.
  - after - cast., ***teucr.***
  - before - alum., ant-t., bism., kali-i., mag-m., stront-c.
- **morning,** from sleep - chin-s., clem., hura, phos., sabad., spong.
- **night** - alum., am-c., carb-v., euph., indg., lyc., mag-c., mag-m., merc-c., morph., nat-s., nit-ac., pall., sil., spong., staph., stram., sulph.
  - menses, during - zinc.
- **noise,** from - acon., aloe, alum., ang., ant-c., apis, ars., asar., aur., bar-ac., ***bar-c.,*** **BOR.,** bufo, calad., ***calc.,*** camph., cann-s., carb-v., card-b., ***caust.,*** chel., ***cic., cocc., con.,*** cub., hipp., hura, kali-ar., **KALI-C.,** ***kali-i., kali-p.,*** kali-sil., ***lach., lyc.,*** lyss., mag-c., ***merc., med.,*** mosch., ***nat-a.,*** **NAT-C., NAT-M., NAT-P., NAT-S.,** ***nat-sil.,*** nit-ac., **NUX-V.,** ***op.,*** ox-ac., **PHOS.,** ptel., rhus-t., sabad., sabin., **SIL.,** spong., sulph., tab., ther.
- **noon** - chel., hep., mag-c., nat-c., nit-ac., nux-v., sep., ***sil., sulph.,*** zinc.
  - sleep, in - mag-c., nat-c., nit-ac., sep., sil., ***sulph.***
- **pain,** agg. - arg-n., lyc.
  - from - sulph.
- **palpitation,** from - dig.
- **paroxysmal** - ars., rhus-t.
- **perspiration,** during - caust., cham., sabad., samb., spong.
- **prick** of a needle, at the - calc.
- **recovering** consciousness - ***nux-m.,*** phys.
- **sex,** after - sep.
- **siesta,** from - mag-c., nat-c., nit-ac., sep., sil., sulph.
- **sleep,** during - acon., aeth., agn., ***alum.,*** am-m., ambr., anac., ang., ant-c., ant-ox., ***apis, arg-m.,*** arn., ***ars., ars-h.,*** ars-i., ars-s-f.,

STARTLED, starting

sleep, during - arum-i., atro., ***aur.,*** aur-m., auran., bar-c., **BELL.,** bism., bov., brom., bry., calad., ***calc.,*** calc-ar., calc-i., calc-p., calc-sil., camph., canth., caps., carb-an., carb-s., ***carl.,*** cast., ***caust., cham.,*** chel., ***chin., cocc.,*** coff., ***colch.,*** croc., ***crot-c.,*** crot-h., ***cupr.,*** cur., cycl., dig., dulc., euphr., ferr-ma., graph., ***grin.,*** guai., hep., hura, **HYOS.,** hyper., indg., iod., ***ip.,*** iris, kali-ar., kali-bi., ***kali-br.,*** **KALI-C.,** kali-i., ***kali-n.,*** kali-p., ***kali-s., kreos., lach.,*** laur., led., lob-c., lyc., ***mag-arct.,*** mag-aust., mag-c., mag-m., med., ***merc.,*** merc-c., mez., ***morph.,*** mosch., myris., nat-c., ***nat-m.,*** nat-p., ***nat-s.,*** nicc., nit-ac., ***nux-m., nux-v., op.,*** ox-ac., petr., ph-ac., ***phos.,*** plat., plb., **PULS.,** ***rat.,*** rheum, rhod., rhus-t., ruta, sac-alb., ***samb.,*** sars., ***sec.,*** seneg., sep., sil., sol-t-ae., spig., spong., stann., staph., stram., stront-c., sul-ac., sul-i., **SULPH.,** ***tab.,*** teucr., thuj., verat., ***zinc.,*** zinc-p.

before - alum.

falling asleep, on - aeth., agar., ***alum.,*** alum-p., alum-sil., am-c., ambr., am-m., arn., **ARS.,** ars-h., ars-s-f., arum-t., bapt., bar-c., **BELL.,** bism., bry., ***calc., carb-an.,*** carb-v., ***caust.,*** chin., chin-a., ***cina, coff.,*** cor-r., daph., ***dros., dulc.,*** ferr-ma., **HEP.,** ign., ip., kali-ar., kali-bi., ***kali-c.,*** kali-s., kali-sil., kreos., ***lach.,*** led., **LYC.,** mag-c., mag-m., merc., ***merc-c., nat-a., nat-c., nat-m.,*** nat-p., ***nat-s., nit-ac., nux-v.,*** op., ox-ac., paeon., petr., ***phos., phys.,*** plb., rat., rhus-t., sars., ***sel.,*** sep., ***sil.,*** stront-c., stry., **SULPH.,** ***tab.,*** tub., verat.

evening - ambr., am-m., anac., arn., **ARS.,** ars-s-f., bar-c., ***bell.,*** bry., dulc., kali-bi., lach., merc-c., nat-c., plat., sars., ***sel.,*** stront-c., ***sulph.***

feet, as if coming from - lyc.

from sleep - abrot., ***acon.,*** aesc., ***agn., alum., am-c.,*** am-m., anac., ***ant-c.,*** ant-t., ***apis,*** arn., ***ars.,*** aur., aur-m., ***bar-c.,*** **BELL.,** benz-ac., ***bism.,*** **BOR.,** bov., bry., bufo, ***cact., calad., calc.,*** cann-s., canth., caps., carb-ac., carb-s., carb-v., carc., cast., **CAUST.,** ***cham.,*** chel., ***chin.,*** chin-s., cimic., ***cina, cinnb.,*** cit-v., clem., ***cocc., coff.,*** colch., con., convo-d., cor-r., cycl., ***dig.,*** dros., dulc., ***euphr.,*** ferr-i., ferr-p., ferul., gins., graph., guai., ***hep.,*** hydroph., **HYOS.,** hyosin., ign., kali-bi., kali-br., ***kali-c.,*** kali-i., ***lach.,*** led., lup., lyc., mag-c., mag-m., ***med., menis., merc., merc-c.,*** mez., murx., mur-ac., nat-a., ***nat-c., nat-m.,*** nat-p., nat-sil., ***nit-ac., nux-v.,*** ol-an., op., ***ph-ac., phos.,*** plat., plb., psor., ***puls., rat., ruta,*** sabad., sabin., ***samb.,*** sang., ***sars., sep.,*** scut., ***sil.,*** sol-a., **SPONG.,** ***stram.,*** sul-ac., ***sulph.,*** tarent., ***ter.,*** thea., thuj., verat., zinc.

comatose sleep, from - ***ant-t.,*** hell., sec.

STARTLED, starting

menses, before - sep.

menses, during - ***zinc.***

pain in heart, with - xan.

touch, from slightest - ***ruta***

touched, when - coff., stry.

sleepiness with - ang., ant-t., ***cham.,*** chel., kali-i., mag-c., merc., plat., ***puls.,*** sars., seneg., ***tarent.,*** verat.

afternoon - sil.

sneezing of others, at - **BOR.**

spoken to, when - aur-m., carb-ac., ptel., sulph.

tossing of arms, from - merc.

touched, when - ***bell., cocc.,*** coff., **KALI-C.,** ***kali-p.,*** kali-sil., mag-c., phos., ***ruta, sil.,*** stry.

tremulous - bar-c., cham., ***sil.***

trifles at - ***arn., bor.,*** calc., cham., ***cocc.,*** hura, ***lyc., nat-c., nat-m.,*** nux-m., ***nux-v., petr.,*** phos., ***psor.,*** sabad., ***sil., spong.,*** sul-ac., ***sulph.,*** ther., zinc., zinc-m.

unexpected - arn.

twitching - con.

uneasiness, from - mur-ac.

urinate, on beginning to - alum.

waking, on - anac., ***bell., bry.,*** chin-a., ***kali-c., lach.,*** led., lyc., nit-ac., pall., sul-i.

as if suffocated - aur-m., ***lach., op.***

STRANGE, everything seems (see Delusions, chapter) - anac., ***bar-m., cann-i., cann-s., cic.,*** glon., ***graph.,*** kali-p., ***med.,*** plat., plb., sep., tub., valer.

outside of body, as if - sabad.

voices seem - alum., **CANN-S.**

things, impulse to do - ***arg-n.,*** bell., cact., calc., chin., ***hyos., lach.,*** nat-m., puls., stram., verat.

dressing, in - hell., ***hyos.,*** sil., sulph.

opinions and acts, in - arg-n., calc., ***hyos.,*** sulph., verat.

STRANGERS, presence of, agg. - ***ambr.,*** ant-t., **BAR-C.,** ***bry.,*** bufo, carb-v., caust., cina, con., lyc., nat-m., petr., phos., ***sep., stram.,*** tarent., ***thuj.***

agg., menses, during - con.

amel. - thuj.

among, as if - aster.

child coughs at sight of - ambr., ***ars.,*** bar-c., phos.

sensation as if one were a - arg-n., nat-m., plat., thuj., valer.

STRIKING - alum., ***arg-m.,*** atro., **BELL.,** bov., camph., ***canth.,*** carb-v., ***cham.,*** **CINA,** con., cub., ***cupr.,*** der., elaps, ***glon.,*** hell., hydr., **HYOS.,** ***ign., kali-c.,*** kreos., lil-t., ***lyc.,*** lyss., mosch., ***nat-c.,*** **NUX-V.,** phos., plat., ***plb.,*** scut., sieg., staph., ***stram.,*** stront-c., stry., syph., ***tarent.,*** tub., ***verat.***

abdomen, his - bell.

about him at imaginary objects - **BELL.,** canth., cupr., **HYOS.,** ***kali-c.,*** kreos., lil-t., lyc., mosch., ***nat-c.,*** nux-v., op., phos., plat., ***stram.,*** stront-c.

while dreaming - phos.

STRIKING,
anger, from - ***nat-c.***
his friends - plat., tarent.
animals, at - med.
boy clawing his father's face - **STRAM.**
bystanders, at - **BELL.,** carb-s., chen-a., ***hyos.,*** lyc.
chest, his - camph., verat-v.
children, in - **CHAM.,** chel., **CINA,** cur., lyc., ***tub.***
convulsions, after - cupr.
puerperal - ***glon.***
desires to - alum., bell., bufo, carb-s., der., elaps, hydr., **HYOS.,** lil-t., nat-c., **NUX-V.,** ***staph.***
evening amel. - hydr.
to push things - coff-t.
drunkenness, during - hep., hyos., nux-v., verat.
epilepsy, in - arg-m.
face, his - bell.
fists, with - syph.
head, his - ars., stram., tarent.
himself - ars., bell., camph., cur., plat., ***tarent., verat-v.***
knocking his head against wall - apis, ars., **BELL.,** con., hyos., mag-c., **MILL.,** rhus-t., scut., syph., **TUB.**
reprimanded, when - tub.
strikes her head with her hands, her body and others - ***tarent.***
wall, the - canth., con.

STUPEFACTION, as if intoxicated (see Dullness) - absin., acet-ac., acon., act-sp., adon., aesc., aesc-g., aeth., **AGAR.,** ***ail.,*** aloe, ***alum.,*** alum-p., am-m., ambr., aml-n., amyg., anac., anan., ang., ant-c., ant-t., arg-m., arg-n., **APIS,** ***arn., ars.,*** ars-i., ars-s-f., arum-t., asaf., asar., asc-c., aur., **BAPT.,** bar-c., **BELL.,** bism., ***bov.,*** brucin., **BRY.,** bufo, cact., calad., ***calc.,*** calc-ar., calc-p., calc-s., calc-sil., ***camph., cann-i.,*** cann-s., caps., carb-an., carb-h., carb-o., carb-s., ***carb-v.,*** caust., cench., cham., chel., chin., chin-a., chin-s., chlol., chlor., chr-ac., ***cic.,*** cina, cit-v., clem., cob., **COCC.,** ***coc-c.,*** coch., coff., colch., coloc., ***con.,*** cor-r., corn., croc., ***crot-h.,*** crot-t., ***cupr.,*** cupr-ac., cupr-ar., cur., cycl., cyt-l., dig., digin., ***dulc.,*** echi., ether, euph., euphr., ferr., ferr-ar., ferr-i., ferr-p., **GELS.,** gent-l., gins., graph., gran., haem., ***ham.,*** **HELL.,** helon., ***hep., hydr.,*** hydr-ac., **HYOS.,** ign., ind., jatr., iod., ip., just., kali-bi., kali-br., kali-chl., kali-cy., kali-i., kali-n., kali-p., kreos., lach., lact., laur., led., lil-t., lob., lol., lon-c., lup., ***lyc.,*** mag-aust., ***mag-m.,*** med., meph., ***merc., merc-c.,*** mez., morph., mur-ac., narcin., nat-c., ***nat-h.,*** nat-m., nat-p., nat-s., nicc., nicot., ***nux-m.,*** **NUX-V.,** ol-an., olnd., **OP.,** par., ***petr.,*** **PH-AC.,** phel., **PHOS.,** phys., pic-ac., plan., plat., ***plb.,*** podo., psor., ***ptel., puls.,*** raph., rat., ***rheum,*** rhod., **RHUS-T.,** rhus-v., ruta, ***sabad.,*** sal-ac., samb., sars., ***sec.,*** sel., seneg., sep., sil., sol-n., spig., squil., ***stann.,*** staph., **STRAM.,** stry., sul-ac., sul-i., ***sulph.,*** tab., tarent., ***ter., thuj.,*** uran-n., valer., **VERAT.,** verat-v., verb., vip., ***visc., zinc.,*** zinc-p.

STUPEFACTION, mental
afternoon - caj., calc., lyc., mang., phys., ***puls., zinc.***
air, in open - cina, ***nux-v.***
amel. - agar., bell., merc., mosch.
alternating with, convulsions - ***aur.***
delirium - acet-ac.
violence - absin.
anxiety, with - anac.
chill, during - bor., con., hell., ***nux-m.,*** stram.
conversation, after animated - bor.
convulsions, between - ***aur., bufo, cic., hell., hyos.,*** lach., ***oena.,*** **OP.,** ***plb., sec.,*** tarent.
daytime - nit-ac.
debauchery, as after - psor.
dinner, after - bufo, coloc., nat-m., nux-v., plan.
eating, agg. after - ***cocc.,*** hyos., morph.
emissions, after - caust.
evening - bov., dulc., lyc., merl., ***sulph.,*** zinc.
exertion, mental, agg. - mag-c., petr., raph.
head, from congestion of the - bell.
with congestion of the - ***kali-c.***
headache, during - sabin.
before - plat.
heat, during - ***apis, camph.,*** chin-a., lachn., ***sep.,*** stram.
injury, to head, after - arn., cic., con., ***hell.,*** nat-s., puls., rhus-t.
knows, not where he is - merc., ran-b., thuj.
loquacious - kali-i., meph.
menses, during - ***lycps., nux-m.***
morning - acet-ac., agar., bar-c., chin., cob., graph., lyc., nat-c., phos., rhus-t., sars., squil., ***thuj.***
11 a.m. to 6 p.m. - ars.
amel. - ***agar.***
rising, after - ***bov.,*** rhod., sabad., ***thuj.***
waking, on - am-c., cham., chel., nat-c., phos.
motion, from - ***staph.,*** thuj.
night - arg-n., bar-c., calc., chel., fagu., lyss.
11 p.m. - sulph.
waking, must rise on - psor.
noon - zinc.
nosebleed, after - zinc.
paroxysms, in - zinc.
perspiration, during - stram.
pollutions, after - caust.
reading, on - lyc.
remains, fixed in one spot - hyos., nux-m., stram.
restlessness, with - ***bapt.,*** kali-i., rhus-t.
rising, after, amel. - phos.
rising, on - sil.
rouses, difficulty, with - hell., lyc., **OP.,** sel., sul-ac.
easily and then fully conscious - ph-ac.
sits, motionless like a statue - hyos., nux-m., stram.
sitting at table, while - carb-an.
sleepiness, with - bell., cocc., con., euph., lach., mag-arct., nux-m., nux-v., ***plb.,*** ter.

STUPEFACTION, mental
 smoking, from - acon.
 stooping, on - calc., nicc., valer.
 sun, agg. in - ***nux-v.***
 suppressed, exanthemata, from - **CUPR.**
 vertigo, during - acon., aeth., agar., arn., ***aur.,*** bar-c., bell., bov., ***calc.,*** clem., croc., dulc., gels., gran., graph., hell., hydr., hydr-ac., kreos., laur., mill., mosch., mur-ac., op., phos., phyt., psor., ran-b., sabin., sec., ***sep.,*** sil., stann., staph., sulph., zinc.
 vomiting, after - aeth.
 waking, on - agar., am-c., chel., hyos., nat-c., phos., tarent.
 walking, when - alumn., **ARS.,** calc., carb-an., ip.
  air, in open - ars., aur., cina, sulph.
 warm room, in - merl., phos.
  when feet became warm, amel. - ***lach.***
 wine, after - cor-r.
 writing, while - arg-n.

STUPIDITY, (see Dullness)

STUPOR, (see Unconsciousness)

SUCCEEDS, never - am-c., asar., aur., canth., ***lyc.,*** mur-ac., nat-c., nat-s., nux-v., sulph.

SUICIDAL, depression - alco., ***alum.,*** ambr., am-c., ***anac.,*** anan., anh., ***ant-c., ant-t.,*** arg-n., ***ars.,*** asaf., **AUR.,** aur-a., **AUR-M.,** ***bell., calc.,*** calc-sil., ***caps.,*** carb-v., carc., caust., chel., ***chin.,*** chin-a., cic., ***cimic.,*** clem., crot-h., cur., der., dros., fuli., gels., graph., grat., hell., ***hep.,*** hipp., hydr-ac., ***hyos., ign.,*** iod., ***iodof.,*** kali-ar., ***kali-br.,*** kreos., ***lac-d., lach.,*** lil-t., lyc., med., meli., ***merc., merc-aur.,*** mez., morph., ***naja, nat-m.,*** **NAT-S.,** nit-ac., ***nux-m., nux-v.,*** op., orig., phos., plat., ***plb.,*** **PSOR.,** ***puls.,*** rauw., reser., rhus-t., rumx., sarr., sec., ***sep.,*** sil., ***spig.,*** staph., ***stram.,*** sulph., tab., tarent., ter., thea., thuj., thuj-l., tub., ust., verat., ***zinc.,*** ziz.
 anger, driving to suicide - carb-v.
 anxiety, from - aur., nux-v., puls.
 axe, with an - naja.
 cancer history in family, with - ***carc.***
 car, under - ars., kali-br., lach.
 courage, but lacks - alum., ***aur-m.,*** **CHIN.,** nit-ac., **NUX-V.,** phos., plat., rhus-t., ***sulph.,*** tab.
 crying, amel. - merc., phos.
 delusions, from - ars., hyos., verat.
 despair, from - ambr., ant-c., **AUR.,** carb-v., hyos.
  about his miserable existence - **AUR.,** ***sep.***
  religious - ***aur.,*** verat.
 dread, of an open window or a knife, with - arg-n., camph., chin., ***merc.***
 drowning, by - ant-c., ***arg-n., aur., bell., dros., hell.,*** hep., ***hyos.,*** ign., ***lach.,*** nux-v., ped., ***puls., rhus-t.,*** sec., ***sil.,*** staph., sulph., verat.
  love, from disappointed - ***hyos.***
 drunkenness, during - ars., bell., nux-v.

SUICIDAL, depression
 easiest way, meditates on - aur., **LAC-D.**
 erotomania, in - orig.
 evening - aur., chin., dros., hep., kali-chl., rhus-t., spig.
  twilight, in - rhus-t.
 fear of, with, death - alum., ***aur-m., chin.,*** **NIT-AC.,** ***plat.,*** rhus-t., ***staph.,*** tab.
  open window or a knife - arg-n., camph., chin., ***merc.***
 fire, to set oneself on - ***ars.***
 fright, after - ***ars.***
 gassing, by - ars., nux-v.
 hanging, by - **ARS.,** aur., ***bell.,*** carb-v., hell., nat-s., ter.
 heat, during - ***ars.,*** bell., nux-v., puls., rhus-t., stram.
 homesickness, from - caps.
 hypochondriasis, in - alum., aur., calc., caust., chin., con., graph., hep., ***nat-m.,*** sep., **STAPH.,** sulph.
 head, injury, after - **NAT-S.**
 intermittent, during - ***ars.,*** chin., lach., ***spong.,*** stram., valer.
 knife, with - alum., ***ars.,*** bell., ***calc.,*** hyos., ***merc.,*** nux-v., stram.
  razor - acon., alum., ***stram.***
 love, disappointed, from - aur., bell., caust., ***hyos.,*** staph.
 meditates, on easiest way - ***aur.,*** **LAC-D.**
 menses, before - iris.
  menses, during - ***merc.,*** sil.
 midnight, after - ***ars.,*** nux-v.
 morning - lyc., nat-c.
 music, from - nat-c.
 night, at - ant-c., ***ars., aur.,*** chin., nux-v., phos.
  bed, in - ant-c.
 pains, from - ars., **AUR.,** carc., bell., lach., ***nux-v.,*** sep.
 perspiration, during - alum., ***ars., aur.,*** aur-a., **CALC.,** hep., ***merc.,*** sil., ***spong.***
 poison, by - ***ars., bell.,*** ign., lil-t., op., puls.
 pregnancy, during - aur.
 run over, to be - alum., ars., aur., kali-br., lach.
 sadness, from - alum., **AUR.,** calc., caust., chin., cimic., con., graph., ***hep.,*** ign., med., ***merc-aur.,*** naja, ***nat-m., nat-s., psor.,*** ran-b., rumx., sep., ***spig.,*** **STAPH.,** sulph.
 seeing, blood or a knife, she has horrid thoughts of killing herself, though she abhors the idea - ***alum.***
  cutting instruments, on - ***merc.***
 shooting, by - alum., anac., ***ant-c.,*** aur., calc., carb-v., chin., hep., med., meli., nat-m., ***nat-s.,*** nit-ac., nux-v., op., puls., sep., **STAPH.,** sulph.
 stabbing, by - ars., bell., nux-v.
 starving, by - merc.
 talks, always of suicide, but does not commit - **NUX-V.**

SUICIDAL, depression
thoughts, of - agn., alum., alum-p., alum-sil., ***ant-c.,*** arg-n., **AUR., AUR-S.,** ***caps.,*** **CARC.,** dros., ***hep., ign.,*** iris, kali-ar., kali-br., lil-t., ***merc.,*** naja, **NAT-S.,** prot., **PSOR.,** ***puls., rhus-t.,*** thuj., ***thuj-l.,*** zinc-p.
drive him out of bed - ***ant-c.***
throwing, himself from, a height - anac., ***arg-n.,*** ars., **AUR., BELL.,** camph., crot-h., gels., glon., hyos., ign., iod., iodof., ***lach., lyss., nux-v.,*** orig., sec., ***sel., sil.,*** staph., ***stram.,*** sulph., x-ray.
windows - ***aeth.,*** arg-n., ***ars.,*** **AUR.,** aur-a., bell., camph., ***carb-s.,*** chin., crot-c., gels., ***glon., iod., iodof.,*** nux-v., ***sulph.,*** thea., thuj., verat.
windows, pain, from - ***aur.***
waking, on - lyc., nat-c.
walking, in open air, while - bell.

SUGGESTIONS, will not receive - helon., sulph.

SULKY - ***agar.,*** anac., **ANT-C.,** arn., ars., aur., bov., calc., canth., carb-an., carb-s., carl., ***caust.,*** chel., cina, ***con.,*** dulc., hura, **IGN.,** kali-bi., kali-br., ***kali-c.,*** kali-n., lyc., mag-c., mag-m., mang., menis., **MERC.,** mur-ac., **NAT-M.,** ***nux-v.,*** op., petr., ph-ac., ***plat.,*** sars., spig., spong., stann., staph., stront-c., sulph., sul-ac., zinc.
afternoon - cinnb.

SULLEN, (see Morose)

SUPERSTITIOUS - agar., **ARG-N.,** ars., bell., ***con., med.,*** op., rhus-t., stram., syph., zinc.

SURPRISES, ailments from pleasant - chin., **COFF.,** merc., ***op.,*** phos., verat.

SUSPICIOUS, mistrustful - **ACON.,** ambr., **ANAC.,** anan., ang., anh., ant-c., apis, ***arn.,*** **ARS.,** ars-s-f., ***aur.,*** aur-s., ***bapt.,*** bar-ac., **BAR-C.,** ***bar-m., bar-s., bell., bor.,*** **BRY.,** bufo, ***cact.,*** cadm-met., calc., ***calc-p.,*** calc-s., **CANN-I.,** cann-s., caps., carb-s., carc., canth., carb-v., carc., **CAUST., CENCH.,** cham., chin., chin-a., **CIC.,** ***cimic.,*** coca, ***cocc.,*** con., ***crot-h., cupr.,*** **DIG.,** ***dros.,*** graph., ***hell., hyos.,*** ign., ip., **KALI-AR.,** kali-bi., kali-br., ***kali-p.,*** **LACH., LYC.,** ***lycps.,*** macro., ***med.,*** meli., meny., ***merc.,*** mez., ***morph.,*** mur-ac., ***nat-a., nat-c.,*** nat-p., nat-s., ***nit-ac., nux-v., op.,*** ph-ac., ***phos.,*** plat., ***plb.,*** **PULS., RHUS-T.,** ruta, sanic., sarr., **SEC.,** sel., ***sep.,*** sil., ***spig., stann., staph.,*** still., **STRAM.,** ***sul-ac.,*** sul-i., **SULPH.,** syph., thuj., thyr., verat., ***verat-v.,*** viol-t.
afternoon - ***lach.,*** nux-v.
3 p.m. to 8 p.m. - cench.
daytime - ***merc.***
enemy, considering everybody his - ***puls.***
evening - cench., ***lach.***
fear of company - ambr., bar-c., ***nat-c.***
foolishly - apis
insulting - merc.
looks on all sides - kali-br.
medicine, will not take - ars., ***cimic., lach.***
menopausal period, during - ***cimic., lach.***

SUSPICIOUS, mistrustful
plotting against his life, people are around the house - anac., ars., ***lach.***
poisoned, of being (see Fear) - ars., hyos.
solitude, desire for - cic., crot-t.
talking about her, that people are - ***bar-c.,*** hyos., ign., pall., staph.
walking, while - ***anac.***

SYMPATHY, agg. (see Consolation) - cact., coff., hell., ign., ***nat-m.,*** sabal., sulph., syph.
aversion to - ***arn., ign., nat-m.***
desire for - **PHOS.,** ***puls.***

SYMPATHETIC, compassionate - alco., am-c., bell., calc., ***calc-p.,*** **CARC.,** carl., ***caust., cic., cocc.,*** croc., graph., ***ign.,*** iod., lach., lyc., manc., med., ***nat-c., nat-m., nit-ac.,*** nuph., ***nux-v.,*** **PHOS., PULS.,** tarent., tarent-c.
animals, only for - aeth., carc.
felt same pain his brother complained of - ***lyss., phos.***
unsympathetic - am-c., **ANAC.,** ars., ***cham.,*** chin., **DIG.,** mag-m., nat-m., nit-ac., op., ***plat.,*** puls., ***sep.***

TALK, general
anxiety, in giving a public (see Anticipation, Anxiety) - acon., ***arg-n.,*** gels., lach., ***lyc.,*** sil., sulph.
desires to, talk to some one - ***arg-m., arg-n.,*** ars., caust., lil-t., nux-m., petr., phos., puls., stict., tarax.
forenoon - caust.
inapt to, in public - ***carb-v., lyc.,*** petr.
indisposed, to - abrot., ***acon.,*** aeth., ether, ***agar.,*** alco., aloe, alum., alum-p., alum-sil., ambr., am-c., am-m., anac., anh., ***ant-c.,*** ant-t., apoc., ***arg-m., arg-n., arn., ars.,*** ars-s-f., ars-s-r., arum-m., ***arund.,*** aster., atro., **AUR.,** aur-a., aur-s., bapt., ***bar-c.,*** bar-m., ***bell.,*** berb., bism., bor., bov., brom., bry., bufo, buf-s., buth-a., cact., ***calc.,*** calc-p., calc-s., calc-sil., camph., cann-i., cann-s., canth., ***caps.,*** carb-ac., **CARB-AN.,** carb-s., ***carb-v.,*** carc., carl., cast., ***caust.,*** cham., chel., ***chin.,*** chin-a., chlol., cic., ***cimic.,*** cina, clem., **COCC.,** coff., colch., ***coloc.,*** con., cortico., cortiso., crot-c., crot-t., cupr., cycl., dig., dirc., dros., ***euph.,*** euphr., fago., ***ferr.,*** ferr-ar., ferr-p., fl-ac., ***gels.,*** gent-c., **GLON.,** graph., grat., guai., ham., ***hell.,*** helon., ***hep.,*** hera., ***hipp.,*** hist., hydr., hydr-ac., ***hyos., ign.,*** iod., ip., piloc., jatr., jug-r., kali-ar., kali-bi., kali-c., kali-m., kali-p., kali-s., kali-sil., kreos., lac-ac., lac-d., lach., led., lil-t., ***lyc., lycps.,*** mag-arct., mag-aust., mag-c., ***mag-m.,*** mag-s., manc., ***mang.,*** meny., ***merc.,*** mez., moly-met., mosch., ***mur-ac.,*** murx., myric., naja, nat-a., nat-c., ***nat-m.,*** nat-p., ***nat-s.,*** nat-sil., nicc., ***nit-ac.,*** jug-r., nux-m., ***nux-v.,*** ol-an., onos., op., orig., ox-ac., oxyt., petr., **PH-AC., PHOS.,** phys., ***pic-ac.,*** pip-m., **PLAT.,** ***plb.,*** plumbg., ptel., **PULS.,** rheum, ***rhus-t.,*** sabad., sabin., sac-alb., sars., sec., sep., sil., spig., spong., squil., ***stann., staph., stram.,*** stront-c.,

TALK, general

indisposed, to - sul-ac., **SULPH.,** tab., tarax., ***tarent.,*** thea., ***thuj.,*** tong., tub., ust., **VERAT.,** viol-o., viol-t., **ZINC.,** zinc-p.
afternoon - fago., grat., hell., mag-s., nat-a., nat-m., sep.
1 p.m. - grat.
air, in open - ph-ac., plat.
alternating with, jesting - plat.
laughing - plat.
loquacity - bell., buth-a., cimic., ign.
quarrelsomeness - ***con.***
violence - aur-a.
company, in - arg-m.
die, as if he would - ***mur-ac.***
eating, after - aloe, arg-n., ferr-m., mez., plb.
evening - am-m., kali-c., ***ph-ac., plat.,*** **ZINC.**
amel. - bism., clem.
fever, during - ars., bor., cham., ***gels.,*** lach., lyc., ***nux-m.,*** nux-v., ***ph-ac., puls., tarent.***
forenoon - aeth., hep., nat-m.
fright, after - ***ign.***
headache, during - ***anac., coff-t.,*** con., nat-a., ox-ac.
humiliation, after - ***carc., ign., staph.***
loquacity, after - bell.
loud - nux-m., sil.
menses, during - ***am-c.,*** cast., elaps, mur-ac., ***senec.***
morning - cocc., hep., mag-m., nat-s., sabin., tarax.
waking, on - cocc., thuj.
walking while - sabin., thuj.
obstinacy, from - cham.
perspiration, during - ars., bry., calc., chin., merc., mur-ac., ***op.***
pregnancy, during - ***verat.***
sadness, in - **ARG-N.,** ***ars.,*** bar-c., ***cact.,*** ign., mag-c., nit-ac., ph-ac., ***puls.,*** stann., verat.
sexual excesses, after - **STAPH.**
sickness or injuries, about - **BAPT.**
silent, desire to be, taciturn - tub.
sits, does not move - ***hep.,*** stram.
sufferings, over his - ign.
waking, on - anac., cocc.
walking in open air, after - arn.

others, of, agg. - acon., agar., alum., am-c., ambr., **ARS.,** aur., **BRY.,** ***cact.,*** carb-an., chin., ***cocc.,*** colch., ***con.,*** elaps, ferr., ferr-ar., ***hell., helon.,*** **HYOS.,** kali-c., kalm., lyss., mag-m., mang., mez., nat-a., ***nat-c.,*** nat-m., ***nat-s., nit-ac.,*** **NUX-V.,** petr., ***ph-ac.,*** rhus-t., ***sep.,*** sil., ***stram.,*** teucr., verat., ***zinc.***

questions, in - aur.

slow learning to - **AGAR.,** ***bar-c.,*** bell., bor., ***calc.,*** calc-p., caust., med., **NAT-M.,** nux-m., ph-ac., phos., sanic., sil., sulph.

TALKATIVE, (see Talking, excessive)

TALKING, general

agg. all complaints - alum., am-c., ***ambr.,*** anac., arg-m., arg-n., arn., bor., calc., cocc., ferr., mag-c., mag-p., stann., ***sulph.***

TALKING, general

excessive, loquacity - abrot., acon., aeth., ether, ***agar.,*** agn., alco., aloe, ambr., anac., anh., ant-t., apis, ***arg-m.,*** arn., ars., ars-h., ars-i., ars-s-f., ***aur.,*** aur-a., aur-s., bapt., bar-c., bar-i., bar-s., ***bell.,*** benz-n., bor., bov., bufo, buth-a., calad., calc., calc-ac., ***camph., cann-i.,*** cann-s., canth., ***carl.,*** carb-s., caust., chel., ***cimic.,*** cocaine, ***cocc.,*** coc-c., coff., con., ***croc., crot-c.,*** crot-h., ***cupr.,*** dulc., eug., eup-pur., ferr-m., ferr-p., gamb., gast., ***gels.,*** gink-b., glon., grat., guare., hep., hydrc., **HYOS.,** ***iod.,*** iodof., ip., ***kali-i.,*** kres., **LACH.,** ***lachn.,*** lil-t., lyc., lyss., mag-c., meph., merc-cy., merc-i-f., ***mosch., mur-ac.,*** nat-a., ***nat-c.,*** nat-m., nicc., nux-m., nux-v., oena., onos., ***op., par.,*** parth., past., petr., ***phos.,*** physal., ***plb., podo.,*** psor., ***pyrog.,*** rhus-t., sal-ac., sec., ***sel.,*** stann., staph., stict., **STRAM.,** sulph., tab., tarax., tarent., teucr., thea., ther., thuj., thymol., trom., valer., ***verat.,*** verat-v., viol-o., viol-t., zinc., zinc-p.
afternoon - ***nux-v.***
alternating with, laughing - bell., carb-s.
maliciousness - ars-s-f.
rage - stram.
silence - bell., buth-a., cimic., ign.
answers no questions, during which - ***agar.***
babbling - lyc.
business, of - ***bry.,*** hyos.
busy - lach., ther.
changing quickly from one subject to another - agar., ambr., arg-m., arg-n., ***cimic.,*** **LACH.,** lyc., par., stram., tub., valer.
cheerful, exuberant - croc., grat., iod., kali-i., lach., nat-c., ***par.,*** tab., verat.
chill, during - ***podo.,*** teucr., zinc.
convulsions, during - hyos.
cough, after - dros.
daytime - arg-m.
drunk, as if - meph., ***mosch.***
drunkenness, during - caust., hep., **LACH.,** mag-c., petr., sulph.
evening - calc., calc-ac., **LACH.,** nux-v., sel., sol-t-ae., sulph., teucr., verat-v., viol-t.
excited - ***cupr., lach.,*** sel., ***ther.***
exhausted, until - nat-c.
ecstasy, with - lach.
fever, during - coff., ***gels., lach.,*** lachn., mag-arct., ph-ac., ***podo.,*** stram., **TEUCR.,** ***tub.***
foolish - par.
forenoon - caust.
half smiling - zinc.
hasty - acon., hyos.
headache, during - bar-c., lach., stram.
before - cann-i.
health, about his - ars., **NUX-V.**
heedless - ***iod.***
hilarity, with - ther.
hoarseness, only kept in check by - ***lach.***
incoherent - ambr., arg-n., bry., cimic., hyos., ***lach.,*** onos., phos., podo., rhus-t., sel., stram., teucr., tub.

TALKING, general

excessive, loquacity

insane - ***apis,*** bell., ***hyos.,*** lach., ***par., staph., stram., verat-v.***

jesting, with - croc., kali-i., lach.

listen, would not - ***hep.***

makes speeches - arn., cham., ***lach.***

menopause, at and during - ***phys.***

menses, during - ***bar-c., lach., stram.***

mental exertion, after - lach.

night - ***aur.,*** lyss., plb., puls.

1 a.m. to 2 a.m. - ***lachn.***

openhearted - anh., bov.

perspiration, during - ars., bell., ***calad.,*** cocc., hyos., ***sel.,*** tarax.

precocious - stroph.

pregnancy, during - ***bar-c.***

questioning, rapid - aur.

religious objects, about - ***verat.***

selected expressions, in - lach.

self-satisfied - par.

sleep, during - ambr., cupr., ign., op.

sleeplessness with l. especially before midnight - ***lach.***

speeches, makes - arn., cham., ign., ***lach.***

stupid and irritable, then - lachn.

sweat, with - calad., cupr., sel.

unimportant matters, about - agar., cimic., lach., meph., par., stram.

vivacious - cortiso.

witty - cortiso.

hysterical - cinnam.

pleasure in his own talking - par., nat-m., stram., sulph.

prolonged talking amel. - nat-m.

sleep, in - acon., ***ail.,*** alum., alum-p., alum-sil., ambr., am-c., ant-t., apis, ***arn.,*** arg-n., ars., aur., ***bar-ac.,*** bar-c., bar-m., bar-s., **BELL.,** brach., bry., bufo, ***cact., calc.,*** camph., ***cann-i., carb-an.,*** carb-s., carb-v., cast., caste., caust., ***cham., cina,*** cinnb., dig., ***gels.,*** graph., ***hell.,*** hyos., hyper., coff., com., con., cortico., cupr., graph., ***hyos.,*** ign., indg., kali-c., kali-m., kali-sil., kalm., kali-ar., kali-bi., **KALI-C.,** kali-p., kali-s., ***lac-c.,*** **LACH.,** ***led.,*** lyc., mag-aust., mag-c., mag-m., merc., ***mur-ac.,*** nat-c., ***nat-m.,*** nit-ac., ***nux-v., op.,*** ph-ac., phos., plb., podo., psor., ***puls.,*** raph., rheum, ***rhus-t.,*** sabin., sel., ***sep., sil.,*** spig., spong., ***stann., stram., sulph.,*** thuj., tub., zinc., zinc-p.

angry exclamations, with - cast.

anxious - alum., graph., ***mag-m.***

business of - con., rhus-t., sulph.

children, in - ***ambr.,*** psor.

comatose sleep, in - nux-v., op., raph.

confess themselves loud, they - bell., **HYOS.,** stram.

excited - alum., cast., graph., nux-v., sulph.

gentle voice, all night in a - ***camph.***

loud - ***arn., bell., sep., sil.,*** spong., ***sulph.***

obstacles being removed - cham.

reveals secrets in sleep - am-c., ***ars.***

supplicates timidly - stann.

TALKING, general

sleep, in

thought when awake, what he - am-c.

war, of - hyos.

unpleasant things, of, agg - ***calc., cic.,*** ign., ***teucr.***

TALKS, general

absent persons, with - ***stram.***

night - dig.

alone, when - lach., nux-v., stram.

anxious about his condition - **NUX-V.**

wakes wife and child - ***arg-n.***

dead people, with - bell., **CALC-SIL.,** canth., hell., ***hyos.,*** nat-m., stram.

humming - lyc., nux-v., staph.

imaginary beings, with - chlol.

listens, does not care whether anyone - ***stict.***

of nothing but, murder, fire and rats - ***calc.***

of nothing but, one subject - ***arg-n.,*** cann-s., lyc., petr., stram.

rhymes, in, repeats verses - agar., ant-c., lach., stram.

sufferings, troubles constantly of his - arg-n., ***mag-p., nux-v.***

war, of - agar., bell., hyos.

talks, to himself - aeth., ***ant-t.,*** apis, ***aur.,*** bell., calc., chlol., crot-h., ***hyos.,*** ign., ***kali-bi.,*** lach., mag-arct., mag-c., mag-p., merc., mosch., mur-ac., nux-m., nux-v., oena., op., ph-ac., plb., pyrog., ran-b., rhus-t., **STAPH.,** stram., sul-ac., tab., tarax., vip.

dead people, with - bell., **CALC-SIL.,** canth., hell., ***hyos.,*** nat-m., stram.

nothing but, murder, fire and rats - ***calc.***

one subject - ***arg-n.,*** cann-i., lyc., petr., stram.

only when alone - ***lach., nux-v.,*** **STRAM.**

pains, of her - ars., mag-p.

troubles, of her - arg-n.

war, of - agar., bell., hyos.

TEARS, things - agar., **BELL.,** bufo, ***camph., canth., cimx.,*** cupr., gink-b., hyos., ign., iod., ***kali-p., lil-t.,*** merc., ***nux-v., oena.,*** op., phos., **STAPH., STRAM.,** sulph., tarent., ***tub., verat.***

away, morning - dulc., **STAPH.**

genitals, her - sec.

hair, her - ***bell., lil-t.,*** tarent.

and presses her head with hands - tarent.

himself, at - ars., bell., cur., plb., sec., **STRAM.**

his nails, at skin around - carc.

night-dress and bedclothes - ***bell., kali-p.***

pillow, with teeth - phos., **STRAM.**

THEORIZING, (see Plans) - ang., apis, arg-n., ars., ***aur.,*** **CANN-I.,** ***chin.,*** cocc., ***coff., lach.,*** lyc., op., puls., ***sel., sep.,*** sil., **SULPH.,** ***verat.***

evening - ***chin.,*** **SULPH.**

night - chin., coff., ***sulph.***

THINKING, general

aversion to - act-sp., agar., ***ail.***, ***aster.***, ***bapt.***, berb., bry., caps., ***carb-v.***, casc., ***chin.***, coca, corn., ***echi.***, ferr., ferr-p., ***gels.***, gins., kali-n., lac-ac., **LEC.**, ***lyc.***, nat-a., nat-m., ***petr.***, **PH-AC.**, **PHOS.**, ptel., plan., rumx., ***sil.***, squil., stram., thea., verat., wies.
afternoon - lyc.
after walking in open air - arn.
evening - lyc.
morning - ambr., kali-n.

complaints agg., of - agar., ***alum.***, alum-p., alumn., am-c., ambr., arg-m., ***arg-n.***, arn., ars., aur., aur-a., aur-m., bad., ***bapt.***, ***bar-c.***, bry., calc., ***calc-p.***, ***caust.***, cham., chin-a., ***colch.***, con., dros., ***gels.***, graph., ***hell.***, ***helon.***, hura, hydr., iod., lac-c., ***lach.***, laur., lycps., mag-s., **MED.**, menth-pu., merc., mosch., nat-m., ***nit-ac.***, ***nux-m.***, ***nux-v.***, pip-n., plan., sin-n., stann., sumb., thyr., zinc.
agg. - agar., ***alum.***, ambr., am-c., arg-m., arn., ars., aur., aur-m., ***bapt.***, ***bar-c.***, bry., calc., ***calc-p.***, ***caust.***, chin-a., con., dros., ***gels.***, graph., ***hell.***, ***helon.***, hura, lac-c., ***lach.***, mag-s., ***med.***, mosch., nat-m., ***nit-ac.***, ***nux-v.***, olnd., **OX-AC.**, ***oxyt.***, phos., ***pip-m.***, plb., ***ran-b.***, ***sabad.***, sars., sep., spig., ***spong.***, staph., thuj.
amel. - **CAMPH.**, cic., cocc., ***hell.***, mag-c., pall., prun.

constantly of his ailments - ***ars.***, ***ham.***

disagreeable things agg., of - calc., cic., phos.

faster than ever before, especially during fever - lach., pyrog.

little affairs, about - calc.

sad things agg., of - calc., rhus-t.

unable to talk - abies-n., ***aeth.***, alum., ***anac.***, arg-n., aur., bapt., calc., calc-ac., cann-i., caps., carb-v., ***con.***, dig., ***gels.***, glyc., kali-br., ***kali-p.***, lob., lyc., ***nat-c.***, nat-m., ***nux-m.***, ***nux-v.***, olnd., petr., ***ph-ac.***, ***phos.***, ***pic-ac.***, rhus-t., sep., sil., staph., tab., zinc.

THOUGHTS, general

abdomen, as if from - thuj.

automatic - chlorpr.

business at evening in bed, of - bell., cocc., nux-v., sulph.

circles, move in - cann-i.

control of thoughts lost - lycps., oena., puls., sulph.
afternoon, 2 p.m. - nux-m.
chilliness, during - ars.
evening - nat-m.
sitting and reflecting, while - arg-m.
undressing, while - morph.

crude - camph.

disagreeable - alum., ***ambr.***, bar-c., benz-ac., calc., carc., ***chin.***, ***cocc.***, ***hep.***, kiss., lyc., meny., mez., ***nat-m.***, nit-ac., psor., rhus-t., sec., sep., sulph., thuj., verat.
midnight, after - **RHUS-T.**
night - benz-n.
waking, on - lyc.

THOUGHTS, general

disconnected - alum., am-c., arg-n., bapt., berb., cann-i., caps., carb-o., ***chin.***, colch., ***cupr-ac.***, dig., gels., lam., laur., lyc., ***nat-c.***, ***nux-v.***, ph-ac., ***rhus-v.***, sieg., sulfa., sulph., ***syph.***, trom., ven-m., verat., viol-o., ***zinc.***
read, cannot - ***nat-c.***, **NUX-V.**
talking, when - merc-c.

disease, of - alum., ***ars.***, carc., chel., lepi., murx., nat-m., nat-p., nit-ac., phos., ph-ac., sep., sulph.
incurable, of some - ***ars.***, merc.

disgusting thoughts with nausea - carc., sang.

erroneous - sabad., verat.

foolish thoughts in the night - chin.

frightful - arg-n., calc., ***caust.***, ***iod.***, lac-c., lyss., phos., phys., ***plat.***, ***rhus-t.***, thea., ***visc.***
blood or a knife, on seeing - ***alum.***
evening - ***caust.***
bed, in - lac-c.
night - phos.
on waking - kiss., phys., ***visc.***

future, of the - arg-n., chin-b., cycl., iod., senec., sep., spig.

himself, cannot think of anyone besides - crot-t.
desires to be diverted from thoughts of himself - camph.

insane - ***lyss.***

intrude and crowd around each other - acon., arg-n., ars., camph., ***cann-i.***, canth., cinnb., ***fl-ac.***, lach., ***merc.***, mur-ac., ph-ac., phos., ***sulph.***, verb.
closing eyes, on - spong.
night - tub.
reading, on - ph-ac.
sexual - aloe, arund., con., ***graph.***, med., orig., ***phos.***, pic-ac., ***plat.***, sel., ***staph.***
too weak to keep them off or to hold on to one thought - ***ars.***
while at work - mur-ac., ***sulph.***
writing, while - ***lach.***

monotony, of - anh., chlol.

outside, of body, as if - sabad.

past, of the - cann-i., meny., ***nat-m.***
evening - senec.
journeys, of former - sol-t-ae.

persistent - acon., aeth., alum., am-c., ***ambr.***, ***anac.***, ang., ap-g., apis, ***arg-n.***, ***ars.***, ars-i., aur., ***bell.***, benz-ac., bry., ***calc.***, calc-s., **CANN-I.**, ***cann-s.***, canth., carb-s., ***carb-v.***, caust., cham., chel., ***chin.***, chin-a., coca, cocc., cupr., ***euphr.***, glon., ***graph.***, hell., hyos., ***ign.***, ***iod.***, kali-ar., kali-c., kali-i., lach., lam., laur., lyss., meli., merc., mez., mur-ac., **NAT-M.**, nit-ac., nux-m., ***nux-v.***, olnd., op., osm., petr., ***ph-ac.***, phos., phys., plat., ***psor.***, ***puls.***, ***rhus-t.***, ***sabad.***, sec., sep., ***sil.***, stann., ***staph.***, ***stram.***, sul-i., ***sulph.***, tab., tarent., thea., ***thuj.***, tub., ***verat.***, verb., viol-o., visc.
alone, when - ars., kali-c., zinc.
desires, of - bry., ign., puls.
evening - caust., graph., ign., kali-c., ***nat-m.***
evil, of - anac., ***lach.***

THOUGHTS, general
persistent,
expression and words heard recur to his mind - lam., ***sulph.***
garment made the previous day, about a - aeth.
homicide - anac., calc., iod., op., phos., stram.
humorous - nux-m.
ideas of, which first appeared in his dreams - carc., ***psor.***
injury to others, of doing - osm.
lying, while - caust., graph., kali-c., lac-c.
midnight, at - plat.
before - graph.
murder, fire and rats, of nothing but - ***calc.***
music, about, in evening - ign.
night - **PULS.**
song since 4 p.m. - nyct.
night - ant-c., calc., graph., kali-ar., kali-c., petr., **PULS.,** tub.
occurrences of the day at night, of the - asim.
offended him, of persons who had - glon.
thinks mind and body are separated - anac., sabad., thuj.
of nothing but murder, fire and rats - ***calc.***
thoughts separated from will - anac., anh.
unpleasant subjects, haunted by - ***ambr.,*** arg-n., asar., caust., ***cocc.,*** graph., kali-c., **NAT-M.,** petr., rhus-t.
waking, on - acon., bry., ign., plat., ***psor.,*** sil.
walking in open air amel. - graph.
profound - bell., calc-ar., ***cann-i.,*** cocc., cycl., grat., kres., mur-ac., ***sulph.***
future, about his - cycl., spig.
rapid, quick - acon., aesc., alco., anac., ang., anh., bell., caj., ***cann-i.,*** carb-ac., caust., chin., cimic., cob., **COFF.,** colch., ***hyos., ign.,*** kalm., lac-c., ***lach.,*** morph., nux-v., onos., ***op., ox-ac.,*** ped., ***phos., phys., pic-ac.,*** rhus-t., sabad., sulph., valer., verat., **VIOL-O.**
fever, during - cham.
repetition, of - mag-m., stram.
rush, flow of - acon., agar., alco., ***alum.,*** ambr., ***anac., ang., ars.,*** **BELL.,** bor., ***bry.,*** caj., calad., ***calc.,*** camph., ***cann-i.,*** canth., caust., ***chin.,*** cimic., coca, cocc., **COFF.,** coff-t., coloc., con., cori-r., cycl., der., eupi., fl-ac., ***glon., graph.,*** hep., ***ign., kali-c., lac-c.,*** **LACH.,** ***mag-arct.,*** meph., merc., morph., nat-m., nitro-o., nux-m., ***nux-v.,*** olnd., op., orig., ***ph-ac.,*** **PHOS.,** ptel., ***puls., rhus-t., sabad., sil.,*** spig., staph., ***sulph.,*** tab., ter., teucr., thea., **VALER.,** verat., verb., viol-o., viol-t., zinc.
afternoon - anac., ang.
5 p.m. - sol-t-ae.
air, amel. in open - coff.
alone, when - ars.
business accomplished, in evening of - sulph.
day and night - ambr., caust.
drunkenness, as in - valer.

THOUGHTS, general
rush, flow of
evening - anac., chin., nux-v., phos., ***puls.***
bed, in - agar., ***bry., calc.,*** caust., ***chin.,*** cocc., ***graph., kali-c.,*** lyc., ***nux-v., puls.,*** rhus-t., sabad., ***sil.,*** staph., ***sulph.,*** viol-t.
morning - canth., con., nux-v.
bed, in - chin.
rising, after - nux-v.
night - agar., aloe, bor., ***bry., calc., chin.,*** chin-a., coca, coff., colch., con., ***graph.,*** hep., hyos., ***kali-c.,*** kali-n., ***lach., mag-arct.,*** nat-m., ***nux-v., op.,*** ph-ac., plat., ***puls.,*** sep., ***sil.,*** spong., ***sulph.,*** tab., zinc.
partial sleep, in - hyos.
reading, while - coff., olnd., ph-ac.
sleeplessness from - agar., bor., bry., calc., carc., caust., ***chin.,*** cocc., coloc., ***graph.,*** hep., kali-c., kali-n., ***lyc., nux-v., op.,*** plat., ***puls.,*** sabad., ***sep., sil.,*** staph., sulph., viol-t.
waking, on - bor., chin., ***mag-arct.,*** ph-ac., plat., sil.
walking in open air, on - ant-c., sulph.
work, during - ang., mur-ac., olnd.
sexual, (see Sexual, behaviour) - aloe, ambr., aster., bell., calc., canth., con., ***graph., hyper., kali-br.,*** lyc., **MED.,** nat-c., orig., ***phos.,*** pic-ac., ***plat., sel.,*** sep., sil., **STAPH.,** ***stram.,*** sulph., ***thuj., ust.***
day and night - chin., dig., staph.
impotency, with - lyc., ***sel.***
masturbation, with (see Sexual, masturbation) - ust.
stagnation of (see Dullness) - ***cann-s.,*** chin., hyos., iod., lyc., mag-arct., ph-ac., seneg., sulph., thuj.
evening - rumx.
stomach, as if from - acon.
strange - **ARG-N.,** calc., cann-i., canth., ***lyss., stram.,*** sulph., thuj., verat.
pregnancy, in - ***lyss., stram.***
stroke, of - aster.
thoughtful - acon., alco., aloe, alum., am-m., arn., bar-c., bart., bell., bor., brom., calc., cann-s., canth., ***carb-an.,*** cham., chin., cic., clem., ***cocc.,*** cycl., euph., euphr., grat., ***hep.,*** hyos., ***ign.,*** ip., kali-n., ***lach.,*** lyc., mag-m., manc., mang., mez., nat-c., nit-ac., nux-v., ***phos.,*** plan., plb., ***puls.,*** ran-b., rhus-t., sabad., ***sep.,*** spig., ***staph.,*** stront-c., ***sulph.,*** thea., thuj., til., viol-o.
afternoon - hell., mang.
all night - op.
cold wet weather, in - aloe.
eating, after - aloe.
errors of others, about the - cic.
evening - senec.

THOUGHTS, general

tormenting - acon., alum., am-c., ant-c., **ARG-N.,** ***ars.,*** astra-e., calc-s., carb-s., ***caust.,*** con., graph., guat., ***lach.,*** lac-ac., lac-c., ***lyc.,*** mez., **NAT-M.,** ***nit-ac.,*** nitro-o., phos., ***rhus-t.,*** sep., sul-i., ***sulph.,*** thea.

evening - ***caust.,*** graph., kali-c.

night - ant-c., arg-n., kali-ar., kali-c., tub.

past disagreeable events, about - am-c., spong.

sexual - aq-mar., aster., con., graph., ***staph.***

two, trains of thoughts - ***anac.,*** lyss., paro-i., ***sil.***

vacancy, of - chlol., ***gels.,*** lyc., oena., phos.

vagueness, of - iod., nitro-o., sulph.

vanishing, of - am-c., ***ambr.,*** ***anac.,*** anh., ant-t., apis, apoc., ars-s-f., ***asar.,*** bapt., bell., berb., bor., ***bry.,*** ***calc.,*** calc-s., ***camph.,*** **CANN-I.,** ***cann-s.,*** canth., carb-an., cham., ***chel.,*** chin., cic., coff., croc., cupr., euon., ***gels.,*** guai., hell., hep., iod., ip., kali-bi., kali-c., kali-p., kreos., lac-c., ***lach.,*** laur., ***lyc.,*** lycps., ***manc.,*** med., ***merc.,*** ***mez.,*** ***nat-m.,*** ***nit-ac.,*** **NUX-M.,** nux-v., ol-an., op., ph-ac., pic-ac., plan., ***psor.,*** ***puls.,*** ran-b., ran-s., rhod., rhus-t., rob., saroth., staph., sulph., ***tab.,*** verat., viol-o., viol-t., zinc., zinc-p.

chill, during - bell., bry., lach., rhus-t.

closing eyes, on - ther.

company, in - ambr.

exertion, on - nit-ac.

headache, during - bell.

interrupted, when - berb., mez., ***staph.***

menses, before - ***nux-m.***

mental exertion, on - ***asar.,*** canth., caust., cham., euon., ***gels.,*** hep., mez., nat-m., ***nit-ac.,*** olnd., ran-b., staph.

morning - ***ph-ac.***

overlifting, after - ***psor.***

periodically - chin.

reading, on - ***anac.,*** asar., bry., camph., ***cann-i.,*** ***lach.,*** lyc., **NUX-M.,** ***ph-ac.,*** pic-ac., staph.

rising from stooping, on - ars.

speaking, while - ***anac.,*** asar., camph., ***cann-i.,*** ***lach.,*** lyc., med., ***mez.,*** **NUX-M.,** pic-ac., staph., ***thuj.,*** viol-o.

standing, while - rhus-t.

turning head, on - rhus-t.

when spoken to - sep.

work, at - ***asar.,*** hep.

writing while - ***anac.,*** asar., camph., ***cann-i.,*** ***lach.,*** lyc., **NUX-M.,** pic-ac., rhus-t., staph.

wandering - ***acon.,*** alco., all-s., ***aloe,*** am-c., ambr., anac., ang., anth., apoc., ***arn.,*** ars-i., atro., ***bapt.,*** bell., ***cann-i.,*** cann-s., carb-s., caust., chin-s., chlol., cic., ***colch.,*** coloc., corn., crot-h., cupr., dig., dulc., ery-a., ferr., glon., ***graph.,*** hyos., ign., iod., kali-br., lach., lyc., lycps., manc., merc., merc-c., naja, nat-c., nat-m., nat-p., nit-ac., olnd., op., peti., ph-ac., ***phos.,*** phys., pic-ac., plb., plect., ***puls.,*** sanic., sol-m., staph., sulph., tab., thuj., valer., viol-o.,

THOUGHTS, general

wandering - yuc., ***zinc.,*** zinc-p.

afternoon - ang., atro.

evening - caust.

listening, while - sol-t-ae.

menses, during - calc.

morning - mit.

night - bell.

studying, while - ham., phys.

talking, while - merc-c.

work, at - sol-t-ae.

writing, while - iris, **NUX-M.**

THREATENING - agar., ***hep.,*** **LACH.,** ***stram.,*** **TARENT.,** ***tub.,*** valer.

destroy, threatens to - lach., tarent.

kill, threatens to - ***hep.,*** lach., stram., ***tarent.***

THROWS things away - acon., ars., bry., camph., cham., ***cina,*** coloc., coff., dulc., ***kreos.,*** lyss., prot., **STAPH.,** stram., tarent., thea., ***tub.***

morning - dulc., **STAPH.**

persons, at - agar., bell., lil-t., lyss., ***staph.,*** tub.

who offend - **STAPH.**

THUNDERSTORM, loves to watch - bell-p., ***carc.,*** lyc., ***sep.***

TIDY - ars., carc., ign., nat-m.

TIME, general

desire to arrive on time - carc., ***nat-m.***

passes too quickly - ***anh.,*** atro., coca, **COCC.,** elaps, op., psil., sieg., sulph., ***ther.,*** thuj., visc.

slowly, too - aloe, ***alum.,*** ***ambr.,*** ***anh.,*** ***arg-n.,*** bar-c., camph., **CANN-I., CANN-S.,** ***cench.,*** con., dirc., **GLON.,** hep., lach., **LYC.,** mag-m., ***med.,*** ***merc.,*** nat-c., ***nux-m.,*** ***nux-v.,*** onos., pall., petr., plb.

a few seconds seem ages - cann-i.

night, at - nux-v.

waste away his - bor., cocc., crot-t., lach., ***nat-c.,*** nat-m., nux-v., stann., staph., ***sulph.,*** tub.

loss of conception of - anh.

TIMID, (see Bashful, Mild, Yielding) - ***acon.,*** aloe, ***alum.,*** alum-p., alum-sil., ***alumn.,*** am-caust., ***ambr.,*** ***am-c.,*** ***am-m.,*** anac., ang., ant-t., ***arg-n.,*** arn., ***ars.,*** ars-i., ars-s-f., ***aur.,*** aur-a., aur-i., aur-s., **BAR-C.,** bar-i., bar-m., bell., ***bor.,*** **BRY., CALC.,** calc-ar., **CALC-S.,** calc-sil., canth., carb-an., ***carb-s.,*** ***carb-v.,*** carc., carl., ***caust.,*** cham., ***chin.,*** chin-a., ***coca,*** cocc., coff., ***con.,*** cortico., croc., ***crot-h.,*** ***cupr.,*** daph., dat-m., **GELS.,** ***graph.,*** **HYOS.,** ***ign.,*** iod., ip., ***kali-ar.,*** kali-bi., kali-br., **KALI-C.,** kali-i., kali-n., ***kali-p.,*** ***kali-s.,*** ***kali-sil.,*** lach., laur., lil-t., **LYC.,** ***mag-arct.,*** mag-aust., mag-c., manc., meli., ***merc.,*** mur-ac., naja, ***nat-a.,*** **NAT-C.,** ***nat-m.,*** nat-p., ***nit-ac.,*** ***nux-v.,*** op., **PETR., PHOS.,** plat., **PLB., PULS.,** ran-b., ***rhus-t.,*** ruta, sabad., sec., **SEP., SIL.,** spig., ***spong.,*** **STAPH.,** ***stram.,*** sul-ac., sul-i., **SULPH.,** tab., thuj., ***tub.,*** verat., verb., zinc., zinc-p.

TIMID,
afternoon - carb-an., con., ferr-p., ran-b.
alone, when - sil.
alternating with,
anger - zinc.
assurance - ***alum.***
exaltation - petr., sul-ac.
hope - kali-c.
irritability - zinc.
quarrelsomeness - ran-b.
sadness - zinc.
vexation - ran-b., zinc.
awkward, and - calc., carb-v., nat-c., nat-m., nux-v., plan., sil., sulph.
bed, about going to - acon., ars., bapt., camph., cann-i., ***caust.,*** cench., lach., lyc., nat-c., squil.
business, in transacting - op.
company, in - ***ambr.,*** carb-v., chin., cortico., ph-ac., staph.
daytime - carb-an., nat-m., pip-m., verb.
delirium, during - dat-m., **STRAM.**
evening, in bed - kali-c., nat-c.
twilight, in the - phos.
fright, after - ***acon.***
morning, 9 a.m. - carl.
night - caust., kali-c., **RHUS-T.**
public, about appearing in - aeth., **AMBR.,** arg-n., ***ars., carb-v.,*** dys-co., **GELS.,** ***lyc.,*** med., ***ph-ac.,*** **PLB., SIL.,** staph., thuj.
talk, to - cupr., lach., ***lyc.,*** sil.
capable of talking, but - gels., ***lyc.,*** sil.
school, children, in - carc., lyc., puls., sil.

TORMENTS, everyone with his complaints - agar., ***ars., nit-ac., psor.,*** **ZINC.**
those around him - alumn., ars., **CALC.,** lach., nit-ac.
himself - acon., ars., bell., ***lil-t.,*** nat-m., plb., ***staph.,*** tarent., tub.

TORPOR - apis, berb., ***cic., crot-h., gels.,*** kali-br., ***lyc.,*** **NAT-M., NUX-M., OP.,** ***plb.,*** sang., ***stram.***

TORTURE, of animals, (see Self-torture) - **ANAC.**

TOUCH things, impelled to - bell., carc., hyos., lycps., ***merc.,*** sulph., ***thuj.***
children, in - carc., ***cina.***
does not know if objects are real until she has touched them - sulph.
inability to do so - sulph.

TOUCHED, emotional aversion to being - ***acon., agar.,*** **ANT-C.,** ***ant-t.,*** **ARN.,** ars., asar., ***bell., bry.,*** bufo, calc., camph., canth., **CHAM.,** ***chin.,*** cimic., ***cina,*** cocc., ***coff.,*** colch., con., cupr., gels., hell., hep., ***ign.,*** iod., **KALI-C.,** kali-fer., ***kali-i., lach.,*** lachn., lyc., mag-c., mag-m., ***med.,*** merc., mez., **NAT-M.,** nux-m., nux-v., plb., sanic., **SEP.,** ***sil.,*** stram., **TARENT.,** ***thuj., tub.,*** verat.
ticklishness - ign., **KALI-C.,** med., zinc.
caressed - chin., ***cina,*** nit-ac.

TRANCE, state - ***acon.,*** art-v., camph., camph-br., ***cann-i.,*** cham., keroso., **LACH.,** laur., ***morph., mosch.,*** nux-m., **OP.,** sabad., stram., tab., ter.
alternating with spasms every summer - ***stram.***
playing on piano with closed eyes, writes letters in an acquired language - ***camph.***

TRANQUILITY, serenity - aesc., ether, alco., aloe, apis, arg-m., arn., ***ars.,*** asar., aur., bell., caps., caust., cer-b., ***cham., chel., chin.,*** chin-s., chlor., ***cic.,*** clem., coca, cocc., ***coff.,*** croc., cycl., dros., euph., ferr., ferr-ar., fl-ac., gins., gran., ham., ***hell.,*** hydr-ac., ***hyos.,*** ign., ip., kali-br., lach., laur., led., lil-t., lyc., lyss., mag-s., manc., meny., mez., merl., mosch., mur-ac., naja, nat-c., nat-m., nat-p., **OP.,** paro-i., petr., **PH-AC.,** phos., ***plat.,*** plb., psil., seneg., **SEP.,** sil., spig., stann., staph., sul-ac., sulph., tarax., tell., thyr., tus-f., verat., viol-t., zinc.
anger, after - ip.
forenoon - aeth.
hemoptysis, hemorrhages, in - ***ham.***
incomprehensible - cann-i., morph., op.
morning, on waking - chel., manc.
reconciled to fate - aloe, cham.
stool, after - bor.

TRAVEL, desire to - am-c., am-m., anan., arag., aur., bar-c., bell., bry., calc., **CALC-P., CARC.,** caust., cimic., cur., elaps, elat., goss., ***hipp.,*** ign., ***iod.,*** lach., lyss., mag-c., ***merc.,*** sanic., thea., **TUB.,** verat.
amel. - ign., tub.

TRIFLES, seem important, (see Conscientious) - ferr., ign., ip., sil.
everything, with - agar.

TWILIGHT agg. mental symptoms - berb., ***calc.,*** caust., ***phos.,*** plat., ***puls.,*** rhus-t., valer.
terrifying apparations in the twilight - berb.

UNATTRACTIVE, things seem - chin.

UNCONSCIOUSNESS, (see Brain, Coma)

UNDERSTAND, does not, questions addressed to her - tarent.
can not, but can speak - elaps.

UNDERSTANDING, difficult - agn., ***ail.,*** alum., ***anac.,*** **BAR-C.,** ***bapt.,*** cocc., ***gels., hell.,*** kali-p., lyc., nat-c., ***nux-m.,*** olnd., ***op., ph-ac.,*** phos., plb., xero, ***zinc.***
reads or hears about, what he - sel.
easy - aesc., ambr., anac., ang., aur., bar-c., bell., bor., brom., buth-a., calc-f., camph., cann-i., cann-s., caust., **COFF.,** hyos., ign., **LACH.,** lyc., lyss., meph., **OP.,** ox-ac., ***phos.,*** pic-ac., ***pip-m., plat.,*** puls., rhus-t., sabad., sel., sulph., tab., thiop., valer., ***verat.,*** viol-o.
drunkenness, during - calc., sulph.

UNDERTAKES, lacks will power to undertake anything, (see Succeeds) - ***lyc.,*** phos., ***pic-ac., sil.***

UNDERTAKES, lacks will power to
many things, perseveres in nothing - ***acon.,*** alum., ant-c., apis, bism., bor., canth., cortico., graph., ign., ***lach., lac-c.,*** **LIL-T., LYC.,** ***nux-m.,*** petr., phos., pin-s., plan., sanic., stann., sulph., verat.
nothing, lest he fail - ***arg-n., lyc.,*** sil.
things opposed to his intentions - phos., sep.

UNFEELING, hardhearted, (see Cruelty, Moral feeling) - alco., **ANAC.,** ars., bism., cench., con., croc., hep., hyos., ***lach., laur.,*** op., plat., sabad., **SEP.,** squil., ***sulph.,*** sumb.
family, with his or her - kali-i., **SEP.**

UNFORTUNATE, feels - ***ars.,*** **AUR.,** bry., carb-v., **CARC.,** ***chel., chin.,*** cub., ***graph.,*** hell., hura, ip., kali-c., ***lyc., puls.,*** rhus-t., sars., sep., ***staph.,*** sulph., ***tab.,*** verat.

UNFRIENDLY, humor - am-c., mag-m., plat.

UNHAPPINESS, prolonged - aur., ***carc.***

UNOBSERVING - alum., asar., bar-c., ***caust., hell.,*** kali-c., merc., nat-c., op., petr., ph-ac., phos., plat., sep., sulph., thuj.

UNREAL, everything seems - ail., ***alum.,*** **CANN-I.,** cann-s., lac-c., lil-t., ***med.,*** op., staph.

UNSYMPATHETIC, (see Indifferant, Unfeeling, Sympathetic)

UNTRUTHFUL, (see Deceitful)

UNWORTHY, objects seem - ***chin.***

USEFUL, desire to be - calc., ***cer-b.***

VACILLATION, (see Mood, changeable)

VANITY, (see Egotism) - ***bell.,*** **LYC.,** ***merc.,*** nux-v., **PLAT.,** ***puls.,*** **SULPH.**

VENERATION - coff.

VERSES, makes poetry - agar., am-c., ***ant-c.,*** cann-i., carb-v., chin., coff., ***hyos., lach.,*** lyc., nat-m., staph., stram., thea.
asleep, on falling - nat-m.

VINDICTIVE, vengeful, (see Malicious) - ***anac.,*** **LACH.,** ***nit- ac.,*** ph-ac.

VIOLENCE, ailments from, (see Abused, Fright, Humiliation) - acon., ***anac.,*** **ARN.,** ***aur., bry.,*** **CARC.,** coff., lyc., nat-m., ***op.,*** **STAPH.**

VIOLENT, behaviour - abrot., absin., acon., aesc., agar., agav-t., alco., alum., ambr., am-c., **ANAC.,** ang., ***ant-t.,*** apis, arn., ars., **AUR.,** bar-c., **BELL.,** bor., ***bry.,*** calc., calc-p., camph., canth., ***carb-s., carb-v.,*** caste., caust., ***cham.,*** chin., **CIC.,** cocc., coff., coloc., con., corn., croc., cupr., cyna., dros., dulc., ferr., graph., grat., **HEP., HYOS.,** ictod., ign., ***iod.,*** kali-bi., kali-c., ***kali-i., kali-p., lach., led.,*** lil-t., ***lyc., mag-arct.,*** mag-s., mang., merc., merc-c., merl., mez., mosch., nat-c., ***nat-m.,*** nat-s., nit-ac., **NUX-V.,** olnd., ox-ac., ***petr.,*** ph-ac., ***phos.,*** plat., plb., ran-b., sabad., sac-alb., seneg., ***sep.,*** sil., spig., stann., staph., **STRAM.,** stront-c., ***sulph., tarent.,*** teucr., **TUB.,** ***verat.,*** verat-v., ***visc.,*** zinc.
activity, with bodily - ***plat.***

VIOLENT, behaviour
alternating with,
laughing - stram.
mildness - croc.
stupor - absin.
tranquillity - aur-a.
chases family out of house - ***verat.***
crossed, when - ***sil.***
menses agg. - ***oena.***
deeds of, rage leading to - agar., **ANAC.,** ars., bar-c., ***bell.,*** bry., calc., chin., cic., cocc., con., **HEP.,** hyos., ***ign., iod.,*** iodof., kali-ar., **LACH.,** lil-t., lyc., mosch., nat-c., nicc., nit-ac., nux-v., phos., plat., **STRAM.,** stront-c., tarent., ***verat.,*** zinc.
evening - mill.
dinner, after - mill.
siesta, after - caust.
trifles, at - ***hep., nat-m.***
exhaustion, to - **NAT-C.**
forenoon - carb-v.
friends, to his - kali-ar.
morning, in - calc., carb-an., carb-v., gamb., graph., nat-s., petr., psor.
pain, from - aloe, ant-t., **AUR., CHAM., HEP.,** lyc.
reproached, when hearing another - calc-p.
sick, when - bell.
sleep, before - op.
stool, before - calc.
talk of others, from - con., hep., mang.
touch, from - lach.
trifles, at - cas-s., ***hep., nat-c.***

VISIONS, (see Delusions)

VIVACIOUS - aloe, alum., ang., anh., arg-m., ars., ars-s-f., buf-s., cact., cann-s., carb-s., **CARC.,** chin., cob., cocc., cod., ***coff.,*** crot-h., cupr., cycl., dig., gels., glon., guare., hep., hipp., hydrc., ***hyos.,*** iod., keroso., **LACH., MED.,** nat-c., nit-ac., nux-v., par., peti., petr., ph-ac., sabad., seneg., sep., spig., sul-ac., sumb., tarent., thea., ***tub.,*** valer., verat., zinc.
afternoon - calc-s., ox-ac.
alternating with, absent-mindedness - alum.
muttering - ars-s-f.
sorrow - tarent.
evening - buf-s., ferr.
intoxication, as from - cann-s.
morning - fl-ac.
rising, after - gels.

WAILING, (see Lamenting)

WALKING, behaviour
aversion to - ***zinc.***
circle, walks in a - bell., ***stram., thuj.***
desire to - acon., arg-n., ***ars.,*** ferr., fl-ac., kali-i., lil-t., lyc., mag-c., merc., naja, phos., sep., tarent., ***thlaspi,*** thuj., valer.
as soon as she sets out desire gone - calc-s.
hard walking amel., mental symptoms - hist.

WALKING, behaviour
  hither and thither, walks - asaf.
  late learning to - calc-f., lyc., merc., ph-ac., phos., pin-s.
  must - cham.
  rapidly from anxiety - ***arg-n.,*** fl-ac., ***sep.***
  self-sufficient impression of importance, walks along with a - ferr-ma.
  slowly and dignified - caj.

WANDER, desires to (see Restlessness, Travel) - arag., ***bry.,*** calc., ***calc-p.,*** carc., cench., cimic., elat., hyos., ***kali-br.,*** lach., lyss., med., merc., sanic., stram., **TUB.,** verat., verat-v.
  amel. mental symptoms - hist.
  house, desires to walk about in - ***valer.***
  night - ***calc., elat.***
  pregnancy, during - ***verat.***
  restlessly, wanders about - ars., bell., canth., hyos., lyss., nux-v., ***stram., tub.,*** verat.

WANTS, nothing - arn., ***op.***

WASHED, aversion to being, in children - ***sulph.***

WASHING, always, her hands - ars., ***carc.,*** coca, ***lac-c., med., nat-m., psor.,*** sep., ***sulph.,*** **SYPH.,** thuj.
  cleanness, mania for - ars., carc., sil., sulph.
  face, amel. - ars., phos.
  feet, agg. - nat-c.

WEARISOME, burdened feeling - acon., aeth., alum., am-m., anac., ant-c., arg-n., arn., ars., asar., bell., bism., bov., bry., **CALC.,** ***calc-s.,*** cann-s., canth., caps., carb-an., ***carc.,*** caust., cham., chin., clem., cocc., colch., coloc., con., cupr., cycl., dig., ***euon.,*** graph., ***grat.,*** guai., hep., ign., indg., ip., kali-c., kali-n., kreos., lach., led., lyc., ***mang.,*** merc., mez., mur-ac., nat-c., nat-m., ***nat-s.,*** nit-ac., nux-v., olnd., petr., ***ph-ac.,*** phos., plat., puls., ran-b., rat., rheum, rhus-t., sabin., samb., sars., ***sep.,*** spong., squil., ***staph., stront-c.,*** sulph., ***sul-ac.,*** teucr., thuj., verb., viol-t., ***zinc.***
  air, in open - aeth., sabin.
  evening - mag-c., puls., ***zinc.***
  morning - am-c.

WEARY, of life - agn., aloe, alum., ambr., am-c., ant-c., ant-t., apis, **ARS., AUR.,** aur-a., ***bell.,*** berb., bov., buth-a., ***calc.,*** calc-ar., calc-sil., carb-v., **CARC.,** caust., **CHIN.,** chin-a., con., dros., euph-c., grat., hep., hipp., hyos., kali-bi., ***kali-br.,*** kali-chl., ***kali-p.,*** kreos., ***lac-d.,*** lach., laur., led., lyc., manc., ***merc.,*** mez., mur-ac., naja, nat-c., ***nat-m., nat-s.,*** nep., ***nit-ac., nux-v.,*** op., ***ph-ac.,*** **PHOS.,** phyt., pic-ac., **PITUIN.,** plat., plb., psor., ***puls., rhus-t.,*** rhus-v., rib-ac., ruta, sec., sep., ***sil.,*** spig., spong., staph., stram., sulph., sul-ac., ***ter.,*** thuj., tub., tub-r., valer., verat., zinc., ziz.
  afternoon - mur-ac., ruta
  air, in open - bell., mur-ac.
  alcoholics, in - ***ars.***
  alternating with cheerfulness - bor.
  company, in - ***lyc.***
  despair about trifles - act-sp.

WEARY, of life,
  evening - **AUR.,** dros., hep., kali-chl., rhus-t., ruta, spig.
  fear of death, but - ars., ***kali-p., nit-ac., plat., rhus-t.***
  forenoon - apis
  future, from solicitude about - ***lach.***
  heat, during - bell., chin., lach., stram., valer.
  humiliation, after - ***carc., puls., staph.***
  menses, during - berb.
    before - berb.
  morning - ***lach.,*** nat-c.
    bed, in - lyc.
    waking, on - lyc., nat-c., phyt.
  night - ant-c., nux-v.
  old age, in - aur., calc.
  pains, from the - phyt.
  perspiration, during - alum., ***aur.,*** **CALC.,** hep., ***merc.,*** sil.
  sight of blood or a knife, at - alum.
  syphilis, in - ***lyc.***
  unfit for life - aur., carc., sep., staph.
  unworthy - aur.,carc., ***nat-s.,*** plat., staph.
  waking, on - lyc., nat-c.
  walking in open air, while - bell.

WEEPING, (see Crying)

WELL, says he is when very sick - ***apis,*** **ARN.,** ars., atro., bell., cann-s., cinnb., coff., hyos., iod., kreos., merc., **OP.,** puls.
  feels not well, but knows not why - brom.
    very well, before becoming sick - bry., nux-v., phos., **PSOR.,** sep.

WHIMSICAL, (see Mood)

WHINING, (see Complaing, Moaning)

WHISTLING - agar., bell., calc., cann-i., cann-s., caps., carb-an., carb-s., ***croc., lach.,*** lachn., lyc., merc-i-f., ***plat., stram.,*** sulph.
  fever, during - caps.
  involuntary - carb-an., lyc.
  jolly - carb-an.
  low, soft voice - viol-o.

WICKED - ***anac.,*** ars., cocc., cur., lach., stram.

WILD, feeling in head - ambr., bapt., ***cimic.,*** lil-t., ***med.***

WILDNESS, (see Hyperactive) - acon., acon-l., **ANAC.,** ant-t., aur., bapt., bell., calc-p., camph., canth., carc., chlor., ***cina,*** croc., cupr., fagu., hyos., **LACH.,** lil-t., ***lob-s.,*** lyss., mag-aust., **MED.,** mosch., nat-s., op., petr., ph-ac., phos., **STRAM.,** tab., tarent., tub., ***verat.***
  bright light, odors - ***colch.***
  children, in - carc., ***cina, med.,*** petr., stram.
  convulsions, before - agar-st.
  evening - croc.
  headache, during - bapt.
  misdeeds of others, from - ***colch.***
  night on waking - cot.
  trifles, at - ign.
  vexation, from - ph-ac.

WILL, general
contradiction of - acon., **ANAC.,** ant-t., caps., ***ign.,*** naja, sep.
two, feels as if he had two wills - **ANAC.,** anh., ***lach.,*** naja.
loss of - alum., am-c., am-m., ***anh.,*** bar-c., ***bar-s., calc.,*** calc-ac., calc-sil., camph., chin-s., clem., coca, ***con.,*** cortico., croc., des-ac., grat., ***hell.,*** hypoth., lyc., ***merc.,*** nat-br., nat-c., ***nat-m.,*** nid., op., ***ph-ac.,*** phos., ***pic-ac., ptel.,*** sil., sulph., thuj-l.
control, has none, does not know what to do, feels dull in the head - alum., apis.
melancholia, from - ***arg-n.***
muscles refuse to obey the will when attention is turned away - alum., gels., ***hell.,*** lil-t.
stroke, after - ***anac.***
walking, while - chin-s.
weakness, of - abrot., acetan., ***alum.,*** alum-sil., am-c., am-m., ambr., ***anac.,*** ant-c., ars., asaf., ***bar-ac., bar-c.,*** bism., bry., **CALC.,** calc-ac., cann-s., caust., cer-s., chin., cimic., ***coca, cocaine,*** coff., coloc., ***con., cori-r.,*** dulc., graph., grat., ***haem.,*** ign., ip., kali-br., kali-c., kali-sil., ***lach.,*** laur., ***lyc.,*** merc., ***mez., morph.,*** nat-c., nat-m., nux-v., op., ***petr., pic-ac.,*** puls., rheum, ***sil.,*** staph., stry-p., sulph., ***tarent.***
exertion, from mental - ***pic-ac.***

WITTY - aeth., alco., cann-i., caps., chlol., cocc., ***coff.,*** croc., ***lach.,*** lyc., ***op.,*** spong., **SULPH.,** sumb., thea.

WOMEN, aversion to - am-c., bapt., ***dios., lach.,*** nat-m., ***puls.,*** sulph., ***thuj.***
to her own sex - raph.
to masculine - fl-ac., ***nat-m., sep.***

WORK, general
ailments, from mental work - agar., ***alum-p.,*** alum-sil., ambr., ***anac., arg-n.,*** arn., ars., ***ars-i.,*** ars-m., aven., bar-ac., bell., ***calc., calc-p.,*** calc-sil., chin., coca, cocc., con., **CUPR.,** cupr-acet., ***epig.,*** epip., fl-ac., ***gels.,*** graph., ign., iod., iris, kali-br., ***kali-c.,*** **KALI-I.,** ***kali-p., lach.,*** lyc., mag-p., med., **NAT-C.,** nat-m., nat-p., nux-m., ***ph-ac.,*** phos., ***pic-ac.,*** pip-m., psor., pyrog., rhus-t., sabad., scut., sel., sep., **SIL., STAPH., TUB.,** vinc.
laundry work, agg. - sep.
seems to drive him crazy, owing to the impotency of his mind - ind., ***kali-p.,*** med.
amel., from work or diversion - agar., alum., apis, ars., aur., bar-c., calc., calc-p., calc-sil., ***camph.,*** chin., cic., ***con., croc., cupr., cycl., ferr., hell., helon., ign., iod.,*** kali-bi., ***kali-br., lil-t.,*** lyc., ***merc-i-f.,*** merc-i-r., mez., mur-ac., ***nat-c., nux-v.,*** orig., ox-ac., pall., ***pip-m.,*** pip-n., **SEP.,** sil., spig., stram., tarent., thuj., verat.
changing constantly - ***sanic.***
desire to - naja, rhus-t., sumb., ther.

WORK, general
aversion, to - aloe, arg-n., asc-t., bapt., **CALC.,** carb-v., chel., ***chin.,*** **CON.,** cycl., gels., **GRAPH.,** ham., lach., **LYC., NAT-M.,** ***nux-v., phos.,*** ph-ac., psor., puls., rhus-t., sil., sulph., ther., zinc-chr.
business - agar., am-c., anac., ars., ars-h., aur-m., ***brom.,*** **CALC.,** chin-s., cimic., ***con.,*** cop., fl-ac., graph., hipp., kali-ar., kali-bi., kali-br., kali-c., kali-i., kali-s., lac-ac., ***lach.,*** laur., lil-t., **LYC.,** mag-s., ph-ac., ***phyt., puls.,*** **SEP., SIL., SULPH.,** syph.
customary - calc., sep.
mental work, to - acet-ac., **ACON.,** aesc., agar., agn., alf., **ALOE,** alum., alum-p., alumn., ***anac.,*** arag., arn., asar., atro., ***aur.,*** aur-m., **BAPT.,** bar-c., bar-s., bell., berb., ***bor.,*** brom., buf-s., buth-a., cadm-s., cahin., ***calc.,*** calc-p., calc-s., calc-sil., cann-i., ***caps., carb-ac.,*** carb-an., carb-v., ***carl.,*** caust., cham., **CHEL., CHIN.,** ***chin-a.,*** chin-s., cinnb., clem., cob., coca, ***colch.,*** coloc., con., cortiso., corn., cycl., dros., dulc., echi., fago., ***ferr.,*** ferr-p., ***form., gels.,*** glon., graph., grat., ***ham.,*** hell., hep., hipp., hydr., hyos., hyper., ind., indol., ip., ***kali-bi.,*** kali-c., ***kali-i.,*** kali-n., ***kali-p.,*** kali-s., kalm., lac-d., ***lach.,*** laur., **LEC.,** ***lil-t., lyc.,*** mag-m., mag-p., med., meph., merl., mez., mur-ac., nat-a., nat-c., ***nat-m., nat-n.,*** nicc-s., ***nit-ac.,*** **NUX-V.,** olnd., op., ox-ac., oxyt., pall., par., petr., ***ph-ac.,*** **PHOS.,** ***phyt., pic-ac.,*** plan., plat., plb., ptel., ***puls.,*** ran-s., raph., rham-cal., rhod., ***rhus-t.,*** rumx., sabad., sanic., scut., sel., ***sep., sil.,*** sol-n., spig., spong., squil., ***staph.,*** stry-p., sulfonam., ***sulph.,*** tanac., teucr., thea., ***thuj.,*** thymol., **THYR.,** ***tub.,*** upa., valer., viol-o., viol-t., upa., yuc., ***zinc.,*** zinc-p.
afternoon - hyos., nat-a.
forenoon - get.
forenoon, 11 a.m. - fago.
morning - kali-n.
overstudy, due to - calc., con., kali-p., sil.
desire, for mental - anth., aloe, arn., aur., bad., ***brom.,*** carb-ac., carc., chin., clem., cob., coca, gels., ham., lach., laur., naja, nat-m., nat-p., ped., pip-m., rhus-t., seneg., ***sulph.,*** sumb., **TARENT.,** ther.
evening - cic., ***lach.,*** lycps., nat-p., puls.
night, 1 a.m. - gels.
2 a.m., until - thiop.
easy, at night - ***med., lach.***
fatigue, chronic, from overwork - abrot., ***acon.,*** **AUR.,** ***calc., carc.,*** cocc., coff., **CON.,** fago., ***graph.,*** hyos., ***ign.,*** kali-p., lach., lyc., **NAT-C.,** ***nux-v., pic-ac., sel.,*** **SIL.,** staph., sulph.

WORK, general

impossible - abies-n., abrot., acon., ***aeth.,*** agar., agn., **ALUM.,** am-c., ***ambr., anac.,*** anh., apoc., arag., ***arg-m.,*** arg-n., arn., ars., asar., astra-e., aur., ***bapt.,*** bar-c., berb., bor., brom., buth-a., cadm-met., calad., **CALC.,** calc-ac., calc-ar., camph., cann-i., ***canth.,*** caps., carb-ac., ***carb-v.,*** carc., caust., cer-b., chel., chin., chin-s., cocc., coff., ***con.,*** cop., crot-h., cycl., dig., dirc., dulc., equis., ***ferr., gels.,*** gins., glon., glyc., graph., grat., gymn., haem., ham., ***hell.,*** hep., hipp., hydr., ***hydr-ac.,*** hyos., ign., ***kali-br., kali-p.,*** kalm., kiss., kreos., ***lach.,*** lact., laur., lil-t., lyc., lyss., mag-arct., mag-c., mag-m., mag-p., mang., ***med.,*** meli., merc., mez., morph., naja, nat-a., **NAT-C.,** ***nat-m.,*** nat-p., nat-s., nit-ac., ***nux-m., nux-v.,*** olnd., op., ***petr., ph-ac., phos.,*** pic-ac., ptel., ***rhus-t.,*** sabad., sars., sel., sep., sieg., **SIL.,** sol-m., ***spig.,*** spong., stann., ***staph., sumb.,*** tab., tell., ***ter.,*** thal., ***thuj.,*** tub., verat., vib., visc., ***zinc.***

afternoon - fago., hyos., sil.
air, in open - nat-a.
burning in right lumbar region, from - nit-ac.
eating, after - ars-s-f.
evening - ***ign.***
exertion, after - nat-m.
headache, during - sep.
interruption, by least - berb.
morning - agar., ***ph-ac.***
night - form.
old age, in - ***ambr.***
sexual excesses, after - ph-ac., pic-ac., ***sel.***
siesta, after - graph.

workaholic, mania for, or tendency to overwork - acon., aeth., agar., allox., aloe, amn-l., ang., apis, arist-cl., arn., ars., **AUR.,** aur-a., ***bar-c.,*** bell., brom., bry., bufo, **CALC.,** calc-ac., calc-ar., calc-f., calc-p., cann-s., caps., **CARC.,** caust., cer-b., chin., cimic., cit-v., clem., cob-n., coca, ***cocaine,*** cocc., **COFF.,** cycl., dicha., dig., ***eucal.,*** euph., euphr., fl-ac., fuc., gamb., guare., helo., helon., hura, ***hyos.,*** hyper., ***ign.,*** indg., ***iod.,*** ip., iris, kali-br., kreos., ***lacer., lach.,*** laur., led., lil-t., ***lyc.,*** mag-arct., mag-c., man., manc., menth., mez., mosch., mur-ac., murx., nat-c., nat-m., nat-s., nep., **NUX-V.,** ***op.,*** ped., phos., pic-ac., pip-m., pisc., plan., plb., rhus-t., sars., seneg., ***sep., spig.,*** stann., staph., stram., sul-ac., ***sulph.,*** **TARENT.,** ther., **TUB.,** ***valer.,*** verat., viol-o., visc., wies., zinc.

afternoon - sars.
evening - ***lach.***
heat, during - op., sars., ***thuj.,*** verb.
menses, before - ***bar-c.,*** bell., bry., ***calc., calc-p.,*** caust., chin., cocc., coloc., com., ***hyos., ign.,*** ip., kreos., **LACH.,** lyc., ***mag-c.,*** mang., mez., mosch., mur-ac., nat-c., nux-v., ***phos.,*** puls., rhus-t., **SEP.,** stann., sul-ac., sulph., **VERAT.**
morning, 7 a.m. to 9 a.m. - coca.
night - coca.
sex, after - calc-p.

WORRIES, full of - acet-ac., ambr., anac., arg-n., arn., **ARS.,** aur., ***bar-c.,*** bry., **CALC.,** calc-p., calc-sil., cann-i., carc., ***caust.,*** chel., ***chin.,*** cimic., coff., con., dig., dros., graph., hed., **IGN.,** iod., ***kali-br.,*** kali-n., kali-p., ***lyc.,*** mag-c., mang., med., mur-ac., ***nat-c., nat-m.,*** nux-v., op., petr., phos., ***ph-ac.,*** pic-ac., ***psor., puls.,*** sal-ac., sep., sil., ***spig.,*** stann., **STAPH.,** ***sulph.,*** thuj., vac.

ailments, from - ambr., ***ars.,*** **CALC.,** carc., ***caust.,*** con., **IGN.,** kali-br., kali-p., lyc., nat-m., **NUX-V.,** ***ph-ac.,*** **PHOS.,** pic-ac., ***staph.***
alone, when - hep.
alternating with, exhilaration - op.
quarrelsomeness - ran-b.
business, or work - acet-ac., ars., ***bry.,*** **CALC.,** carc., caust., kali-p., lil-t., lyc., **NUX-V.,** podo., psor., ***puls.,*** rhus-t.
business, or work, even when prosperous - ars., bry., lyc., psor.
causeless - petr.
company, with aversion to - con., nat-m.
daily cares, affected by - ambr., calc., nat-m., nux-v.
domestic affairs, about - ars., bar-c., ***calc., puls.,*** sep.
evening - dig., kali-c., puls.
bed, in - ars., graph.
midnight - dulc.
morning - ***puls.,*** staph.
bed, in - alum.
night - ***psor.***
others, about - ars., ***calc., caust.,*** cocc., lach., phos., ***puls.,*** sulph., zinc.
over-careful - ***ars., iod.***
relatives, about - ars., ***caust.,*** hep., lach., rhus-t., ***spig.,*** zinc.
sleeplessness - ars., **CALC.,** ign., kali-p.
symptoms disappear while worrying - merc-i-f.
trifles, about - ***ars.,*** aur., ***chin.***
waking, on - hep.
walking in open air - hep.

WRITING, agg. mental symptoms, (see Mistakes) - asaf., laur., med., nux-m., rhus-t., ***sil.,*** stann.

aversion to - hydr., squil., thea.
desire for - chin., lipp., spig.
difficulty in expressing ideas when - cact., calc., cann-s., carb-an., cimic., kali-c., lyc., sep., sil., zinc.
disconnectedly, writing - colch.
fatigue, from - ***sil.***
inability for - ars., caust., ign., lyc., **NUX-V.,** sil.
connectedly - colch.
learning to write in children - caust., sil.
to write as rapidly as she wishes, anxious behavior, makes mistakes - ign.
indistinctly, writes - kali-br., merc., stram.
meannesses to her friends - ***lac-c.***
talent for easier - op.

WRONG, cannot tell what is - thuj.
as if had done something - ign., ***nux-m.,*** ruta.
doing things - hell.
everything seems - calc., carc., coloc., eug., hep., ***naja,*** nux-v.

YIELDING, passive (see Mild, Timid) - alum., ***ars.,*** **BAR-C.,** calc-sil., cann-s., cocc., croc., ***ign.,*** kiss., ***lyc., nat-m.,*** murx., ***nux-v.,*** petr., ph-ac., ***phos.,*** **PULS.,** sep., **SIL., STAPH.**

Mouth

ABSCESS, gums - alum., am-c., aur., ***bufo***, euph., ***hecla.,*** **HEP.,** jug-r., lach., **MERC.,** petr., phos., plb., **SIL.**
recurring, frequently - ***bar-c.,*** calc., **CAUST., HEP.,** ***lyc.,*** **MERC.,** ***nux-v., sil., sulph..*** sul-ac.
sensation, of - am-c.
abscess, lips - ***anthr.***
upper - ***bell.***
abscess, palate - phos.

ACHING, pain, gums - crot-c., nit-ac.
morning - brom.
teething children - bry.
aching, palate - alum., bufo, chel., chin-s., eupi., hydr., ***kali-bi.,*** merc., morph., ***nit-ac., phos.,*** sars., ther.
chewing, food - aloe.
swallowing, amel. - ruta.
yawning - zinc.

ACRIDITY, upper, lips - mang.

AIR, as if filled with - acon.

APHTHOUS, ulcers - acet-ac., ***aeth.,*** agar., all-s., alum., anan., ant-c., apis, arg-m., **ARS.,** ***ars-i., arum-t.,*** asim., aur., aur-m., aur-s., **BAPT.,** ***berb.,*** **BOR.,** brom., bry., ***calc.,*** canth., caps., ***carb-ac., carb-an.,*** carb-s., ***carb-v.,*** caul., cean., cham., chin., chin-a., chlor., cic., clem., cocc., com., cub., ***dig.,*** dulc., ***ferr.,*** gamb., ***hell., hep.,*** hippoz., hydr., ill., ***iod., ip., jug-c., kali-ar., kali-bi., kali-br., kali-c.,*** **KALI-CHL.,** kali-i., kali-m., kali-s., ***kreos.,*** lac-c., lac-d., ***lach., lac-ac., lyc., mag-c.,*** **MERC., MERC-C.,** ***merc-d.,*** **MUR-AC.,** ***myric., nat-a.,*** nat-c., nat-h., **NAT-M.,** nat-p., ***nit-ac.,*** nux-m., **NUX-V.,** ox-ac., petr., phos., phyt., plan., ***plb.,*** ran-s., rhus-t., sal-ac., sanic., sars., sec., semp., sil., ***staph.,*** **SUL-AC., SULPH.,** ter., thuj., tub., vinc.
bleeding easily - **BOR.,** ***lac-c., sul-ac.***
bloody, offensive ichor - ***sul-ac.***
bluish - **ARS.**
burning - chin-a., ***nat-m.,*** sulph.
children, in - asim., bapt., **BOR.,** bry., casc., kali-br., ***kali-chl., lac-ac.,*** med., **MERC., NAT-M.,** ***mur-ac., nux-m., nux-v.,*** plan., sac-alb., **SUL-AC.,** sulph., viol-t.
babies, in - ***bor., bry.,*** calc., merc.
diarrhea, lienteric, with - hell.
extending through intestinal tract - ***ter.***
eye affections, with - brom.
food, sour and salty, after - bor.
gangrenous - ***ars.,*** carb-ac., cocc., lach., merc-d., plb.
influenza, in - ant-t., nat-m.
mothers, while nursing - bapt., hydr.
pregnancy, during - kreos.
salvation, with - hell.
small and sore - med.
white - ***ars., bor., sul-ac.***
yellowish base - ***staph.***
aphthae, gums - colch., cub., ***hep.,*** **NAT-M.,** ***sul-ac.***
aphthae, lips, on - ***ant-t.,*** cadm-s., cub., ***hydr.,*** ip.
aphthae, palate - agar., agav-a., bor., ***calc., hep.,*** kali-bi., ***nux-m.,*** **PHOS.,** sars., semp., sul-ac.
mercurial - agar., aur., sulph.

ATROPHY, gums - kali-c., ***merc.,*** plb.

BITING, general
cheek, when talking or chewing - bufo, carb-an., ***caust.,*** cic., hyos., **IGN., NIT-AC.,** ol-an.
when not - dios.
fingernails - ***acon., am-br., ant-t.,*** arn., ***ars.,*** **ARUM-T.,** ***bar-c.,*** brom., calc., calc-f., calc-p., **CARC.,** caust., **CINA.,** cupr., hura1, ***hyos., lyc.,*** lyss., med., ***nat-m.,*** nit-ac., phos., plb., puls., sanic., ***senec., sil.,*** staph., stram., ***sulph.,*** upa., verat.
glass, as if when fed, child - ars., bell., cham., ***cina, cupr., puls., verat.***
lip, lower, eating, while - benz-ac.
night, in sleep - cic., ***mygal.,*** phos.
tongue, talking, while - hyos.
tip of - ther.

BITING, pain
cheek, inside - coloc., dros.
gums, in - ars., carb-v., ***zinc.***
lips - ip.
lower - benz-ac.
palate, in - carb-v., canth., ***kali-c.,*** mez., ran-s., ***zinc.***

BITING, sensation, in - acon., ambr., am-m., asar., aur-m., cham., cupr-s.

BLEEDING - ***acon.,*** am-c., ***arn., ars.,*** ars-i., ***arum-t.,*** bar-m., ***bell.,*** canth., ***carb-s., carb-v., chel.,*** **CHIN.,** chin-a., cina, ***cor-r.,*** **CROT-H.,** cupr., dros., ***ferr.,*** ferr-ar., ferr-p., ham., **HEP.,** ***ip., kreos., lach.,*** led., lyc., manc., ***merc., merc-c.,*** nux-m., ***nux-v.,*** **PHOS.,** ***rhus-t., sec., sul-ac.,*** ter., tril., vario.
black blood - ***carb-v., crot-h., lach.***
cheek, inside, spot - mag-c.
clotted - canth., ***caust.,*** coch.
continuous, does not coagulate - anthr., crot-h.
easily - **HEP.,** lach., ***merc.,*** **PHOS.,** tub.
extraction of teeth, profuse after - calen., ***phos.***
forenoon - chel.
oozing of blood - ail., anthr., ***chel.,*** crot-h., lach., merc-c., ***phos.,*** rhus-t., ***sul-ac.,*** ter.
scarlet fever, in - **ARUM-T.**
whooping cough, in - ***cor-r.,*** dros., ip., nux-v.
bleeding, gums - ***agar.,*** ail., ***alum.,*** ambr., ***am-c.,*** anac., ***ant-c.,*** ant-t., apis, arg-m., ***arg-n.,*** ars., arum-m., arum-t., arund., aur., bapt., **BAR-C.,** ***bell.,*** berb., bor., **BOV.,** bufo, **CALC.,** carb-an., carb-s., **CARB-V.,** ***caust.,*** cedr., ***chel.,*** chin-s., cist., colch., con., crot-c., **CROT-H.,** crot-t., erig., euphr., ferr., ferr-ar., ferr-i., ferr-ma., ferr-p., ***graph., ham., hep.,*** hippoz., ***iod.,*** kali-ar., kali-bi., kali-c., kali-chl.,

bleeding, gums - kali-n., ***kali-p.,*** kali-s., kreos., lac-c., **LACH.,** lyc., mag-c., ***mag-m.,*** **MERC., MERC-C.,** mez., mur-ac., ***myric.,*** nat-a., nat-c., **NAT-M.,** nat-p., **NIT-AC.,** ***nux-m., nux-v.,*** ox-ac., petr., ***ph-ac.,*** **PHOS.,** plan., plb., ***psor.,*** ran-s., rat., rob., ruta., ***sang., sec.,*** **SEP.,** ***sil.,*** sin-n., spig., ***staph., sulph., sul-ac.,*** tarax., tell., ***ter.,*** thuj., tril., ***zinc.***
afternoon, 3 p.m. - ferr-i.
black blood - graph.
oozes out - bov., kreos.
teeth are extracted, when - ***ars.***
blood, coagulates quickly - kreos.
cleaning them, when - am-c., ***anac.,*** calc-s., calen., ***carb-v., graph.,*** kali-chl., ***lyc.,*** ox-ac., ph-ac., ***phos.,*** ruta., sep., ***staph., ter.***
copious - ambr.
easily - alum., ***am-c., anac., ant-c.,*** apis, ***arg-n.,*** ars., arum-m., asc-t., aur., berb., ***bov., carb-an.,*** **CARB-V.,** ***cist.,*** con., **CROT-H.,** gran., ***ham.,*** **HEP.,** ***iod., kali-chl., kali-p.,*** **KREOS., LACH.,** lyc., ***mag-m., merc.,*** **MERC-C., NAT-M.,** ***ph-ac.,*** **PHOS.,** rob., ruta., ***sep., sul-ac.,*** tell., ***zinc.***
extraction of teeth, profuse, after - alumn., **ARN.,** ***calen., kreos., ham.,*** **LACH., PHOS.,** tril.
menses, during - ***cedr.***
around decayed tooth - bell.
suppressed - ***calc.***
morning - sep.
night - calc., graph.
pain, with - agar.
pressing with finger, large quantity oozes - bapt., graph.
scurvy - ant-t., **ARS.,** ***carb-an., mur-ac., nat-m., nux-v., sulph.***
sucking them - ***am-c., bov.,*** **CARB-V.,** kali-bi., ***nit-ac., rat.,*** zinc.
touch, on - ***hep.,*** lyc., **MERC.,** ***nat-c.,*** ph-ac., **PHOS.,** plb., ***sep.,*** sul-ac., tub., zinc.

bleeding, lips - aloe, am-c., ***ars.,*** **ARUM-T.,** ***brom., bry.,*** carb-an., ***cham.,*** chlor., cob., ***ign.,*** kali-c., ***lach.,*** nat-m., ph-ac., plat., stram.

bleeding, palate, oozing, purpura - ***crot-h., lach., phos.,*** ter.

BLOATED, lower, lips - mur-ac.

BOILS, corners of - am-c., **ANT-C.**

boils, gums - agn., anan., arn., aur., ***bell.,*** carb-an., ***carb-v.,*** caust., chel., euph., ***hep.,*** jug-r., ***kali-chl., kali-i.,*** lac-c., ***lyc., merc.,*** mill., ***nat-m.,*** nat-p., nat-s., ***nux-v., petr.,*** ph-ac., ***phos.,*** plan., plb., ruta, **SIL.,** staph., **SULPH.**
small, near left upper canine, painful to touch - agn.

boils, lips - ***hep., lach.,*** nat-c., petr.

BORING, pain, gums - ***calc.***

boring, palate - ***aur.***

BREATH, cold - acon., ant-t., ars., **CAMPH.,** carb-o., **CARB-V.,** ***cedr., chin.,*** chin-s., cist., colch., ***cop.,*** cor-r., ***helo.,*** jatr., merc., ***phos.,*** rhus-t., ***tab.,*** ter., **VERAT.**
chill, during - **CARB-V.,** verat.

breath, hot - **ACON.,** aeth., agar., anac., ***ant-c.,*** apis, ***ars.,*** asaf., asar., ***bell.,*** calc., calc-p., cann-s., **CARB-S.,** ***cham.,*** chel., coc-c., coff., ***ferr.,*** kali-br., mag-m., ***mang.,*** med., merl., mez., naja, ***nat-m., phos.,*** ptel., raph., ***rhus-t., rhus-v., sabad.,*** squil., ***stront-c., sulph.,*** sumb., trif-p., zinc.
afternoon - ***bad., rhus-t.***
as if - rad-br.
chill, during - anac., camph., cham., **RHUS-T.**
cold limbs, with - cham.
coryza, during - mag-m.
evening - mang., sumb.
fever, during - zinc.
morning, on waking - sulph.

BREATH, mouth, odor
acrid - agar.
alkaline - ***kali-c.***
burnt, on coughing - dros.
cadaverous - ars., caps., ***hyos.,*** **NIT-AC.,** phos.
worse morning and evening - ***hyos.***
cheesy - ***aur., hep., kali-c.,*** kali-p., mez.
constipation, with - carb-ac.
cresses, like - par.
earthy, morning - mang.
eating, after - arn., aur., carb-v., cham., merc., nux-v., sil., ***sulph.,*** zinc.
ether, or chloroform, like - verat-v.
fish brine, before asthma attack - **SANIC.**
garlicky - petr., ***tell.,*** sin-n.
horse-radish - agar.
menses, during - ovi-g-p.
mercury - ant-c., bar-m., sil.
metallic - berb., ***merc-i-f.,*** mez.
musty - ***alum., crot-h.,*** eup-per., nat-c., rhus-t.
offensive odor - abies-n., acet-ac., acon., ***agar.,*** ail., ***all-c.,*** aloe, alum., ***ambr.,*** am-c., ***anac.,*** anan., ***ant-c., anthr.,*** apis, arg-m., arg-n., **ARN., ARS., ARS-I.,** asaf., ***aur., bapt., bar-c.,*** bar-m., ***bell.,*** berb., bor., bov., ***bry.,*** bufo, cact., ***calc.,*** calc-s., ***caps.,*** **CARB-AC.,** carb-an., ***carb-s.,*** **CARB-V.,** ***carl.,*** cast., ***caust.,*** **CHAM., CHEL.,** ***chin.,*** chin-a., ***cimic.,*** cina, cist., ***clem.,*** coc-c., coch., con., cop., ***croc.,*** crot-h., cupr-ar., daph., dig., ***diph.,*** dros., ***dulc., fl-ac., gels., graph.,*** hell., ***hep., hyos.,*** indol., ***iod.,*** ip., kali-ar., ***kali-bi., kali-c.,*** kali-chl., ***kali-i.,*** kali-n., **KALI-P.,** kali-per., kali-s., **KREOS.,** ***lac-c., lac-d.,*** **LACH.,** led., ***lyc., manc.,*** mang., med., meph., **MERC., MERC-C.,** merc-cy., merc-d., ***merc-i-f.,*** merc-sul., mez., ***mur-ac.,*** **NAT-M.,** ***nat-s.,*** nicc., **NIT-AC.,** ***nux-m.,*** **NUX-V.,** osm., ***petr., ph-ac.,*** phos., ***phyt.,*** plan., **PLB.,** podo., **PSOR.,** ***puls.,*** pyrog., querc., rheum,

BREATH, mouth, odor
offensive odor - rhus-t., sabin., sal-ac., sanic., sars., sec., seneg., ***sep.,*** sil., sin-a., spig., ***stann.,*** staph., stront-c., **SULPH.,** ***sul-ac.,*** tell., ter., teucr., thea., thuj., tril., **TUB.,** ust., verat-v., verb., zinc.
cough, during - all-s., ambr., arn., **CAPS.,** dros., graph., lach., mag-c., merc., mez., sang., sep., stann., sulph.
eating, after - sulph.
evening - aur., sulph.
evening or night - puls., sulph.
girls at puberty - aur., aur-m.
meals, only after - cham., ***nux-v.,*** sulph.
menses, during - bar-m., ***cedr., merc.***
menses, before - caul., ***sep.***
morning - acet-ac., agar., ambr., am-c., apis, ***arg-n.,*** arn., ***aur.,*** bapt., bell., cact., ***camph.,*** cast., chin., cimic., cop., fago., grat., hyos., lyc., mang., ***nux-v.,*** phys., **PULS.,** sang., sars., ***sil.,*** sulph., thea., verb.
morning, only - ***arn.,*** bell., ***nux-v.,*** sil., ***sulph.***
night - aur., ***podo.***
onions, like - kali-i., lyc., petr., sin-n., tell.
pepper-like - asc-t.
pitch - canth.
putrid odor - act-sp., alum., ambr., ***anac., apis, arg-m., arg-n.,*** **ARN., ARS., ARS-I.,** ***arum-t., aur., aur-m-n., bapt.,*** bar-c., ***bar-m.,*** bov., brom., bry., bufo, calc., camph., ***caps.,*** **CARB-AC.,** carb-an., carb-s., ***carb-v.,*** cedr., **CHAM.,** chin-a., chlol., ***chlor., cina,*** cist., coca, ***crot-h.,*** dig., ***dulc.,*** gels., ***graph., hell., ign.,*** iod., ***kali-bi.,*** kali-br., ***kali-chl.,*** **KALI-P., KREOS.,** ***lac-c., lach., lyc., mang.,*** **MERC.,** ***merc-c., mur-ac.,*** **NAT-M., NIT-AC.,** ***nux-v.,*** ol-j., petr., ***ph-ac.,*** **PHYT.,** plan., **PLB., PSOR.,** ***puls.,*** pyrog., ***rhus-t.,*** ruta., sabin., sang., sec., seneg., **SPIG.,** stann., stram., staph., sulph., **TUB.**
anger, after - arn.
eating, after - cham., nux-v.
eating, while - chr-ac.
menses, during - ***cedr.***
morning - ambr., arg-n., cast., camph., crot-h., grat., kali-p., lyc., med., puls.
morning, and night - aur., puls.
sickening - agar., aloe, ***arn.,*** ars-h., berb., canth., carb-h., chlol., ***croc.,*** gins., kali-br., merc., nat-c., ***nit-ac.***
sour - agar., cham., coc-c., crot-h., ***eup-per., graph.,*** mag-c., nicc., ***nux-v.,*** sep., ***sulph.,*** verat.
stool-like - bell.
sweetish - carb-an., ***merc.,*** nit-ac., uran.
unnoticed, by himself - bar-c.
urine, like - ***graph.***

BURNING, pain - acet-ac., ***acon., aesc.,*** aeth., agar., ail., alum., am-c., ant-t., ***apis,*** arn., **ARS., ARUM-T.,** arund., asaf., asar., aur., aur-m., bad., ***bar-m.,*** **BELL.,** berb., bov., ***brom.,*** bufo, calad., calc., camph., canth., ***caps.,*** carb-ac., carb-an., ***carb-s., carb-v., caust.,*** cedr., ***cham.,*** chel., chlol., clem., cob., cocc., coc-c., colch., coloc., crot-t., cupr., cupr-s., ***dig.,*** dios., ferr-i., fl-ac., gels., glon., gymn., hell., ***hydr.,*** hyper., ***ign., ip.,*** **IRIS,** ir-fl., jatr., kali-ar., kali-bi., kali-c., kali-chl., kali-i., kali-p., kreos., lach., lyc., ***mag-m.,*** manc., mang., ***merc., merc-c.,*** merc-i-r., merc-sul., merl., **MEZ.,** mur-ac., ***nat-a.,*** nat-c., ***nat-m., nat-s., nit-ac.,*** nux-m., nux-v., oena., op., ox-ac., petr., ph-ac., ***phos.,*** plat., plb., ***psor., ran-b.,*** rhus-t., rhus-v., sabad., sal-ac., **SANG.,** sec., seneg., ***sep.,*** spig., ***spong.,*** squil., stict., stram., ***sulph., sul-ac.,*** tab., tarax., ter., ***verat.,*** vesp., xan., zing.
afternoon - ***mez.***
chewing, when - ph-ac.
cold water, agg. - ***ars., bufo.***
amel. - berb., dros., dulc., merc-c.
eating, after - mez.
extending to, anus - ***iris.***
to, bronchi - ip.
to, stomach - aesc., am-c., brom., chel., gels., iris, ir-fl., ***merc-c., mez.,*** nit-ac., sin-n., sul-ac.
inside of - calc-s.
inspiration, on - mez., ***phos.***
morning - **ARUM-T.,** cupr-s., kali-c., sulph.
night - merc., nit-ac., sulph.
pepper, as from - caps., coca, dros., mez., ***nat-s.,*** sulph., verat.
spots - act-sp., ***ars.,*** kali-i., ph-ac., ran-s.
swallowing, when not - ph-ac.
touched, when - nat-c.

burning, gums - ***alum., ars.,*** asar., bell., bufo, ***caps.,*** cast., ***cham.,*** con., ***graph.,*** mag-c., **MERC.,** ***merc-c.,*** mez., mur-ac., ***nat-s.,*** nux-v., petr., ph-ac., phos., ***puls.,*** rhus-t., ***sep.,*** sil., stront-c., ***ter.,*** ther., **THUJ.**
eating, while - mag-c., **NAT-M.**

burning, lips - ***acon.,*** agar., ***all-c., am-c., am-m.,*** anac., ant-t., apis, arg-n., arn., ars., **ARUM-T.,** aur., aur-m-n., asaf., bar-c., bell., berb., bor., bry., caps., carb-ac., ***carb-an.,*** carb-s., chel., chin., chlf., ***cic.,*** con., ***crot-t., glon., ham.,*** hyos., kali-c., lac-c., lach., lyss., mag-s., ***merc., mez., mur-ac.,*** nat-s., ***nux-m., ph-ac., phos.,*** plat., ***psor.,*** rhod., ***sabad.,*** spig., ***staph., sulph.,*** tab., thuj., zinc.
air, in open - plat.
lower - am-c., anac., bar-c., bor., clem., coloc., graph., kali-c., ***mez., mur-ac., nat-m., ph-ac.,*** sang., sep.
between chin and - mag-c.
smoker's, in - bry.
touch, on - merc., ***mez.***
upper - ars., bar-c., bor., brom., ***calc-p.,*** caust., mag-c., ***mez.,*** mur-ac., nat-c., nat-m., phos., sep., spig., sulph., verat.
air, open in - plat.

burning, palate - ***aesc., all-c.,*** ambr., ant-c., arn., ***arum-t.,*** arund., ***bell.,*** benz-ac., ***bor.,*** calc., ***camph., canth.,*** carb-v., ***caust., cimx.,*** cina, cinnb., ***cocc.,*** coc-c., coloc., crot-t., dulc., ***euph.,*** glon., ***grat.,*** gymn., ign., iris, lach., laur., ***mag-c.,*** manc., merc., merc-c., ***mez.,*** mur-ac., naja, ***nat-s., nit-ac.,*** nux-m., ***nux-v., par.,*** ph-ac., ***phos.,*** podo., ***ran-b.,*** rheum, sabad., ***sang.,*** sanic., seneg., sep., spig., ***squil.,*** staph., ther., thuj., zinc.
coughing - dig.
evening and night - mur-ac.
menses, during -***nat-s.***
morning - **ARUM-T.,** coca, lyc.
pepper, as from -coca, crot-t., ***mez.***
spots - mur-ac.
velum - ***ambr.,*** arg-n., ***calc., crot-c., lach.,*** nux-m., ph-ac., ran-b.
warm drinks agg. - sanic.

BURNT, pain, as if - all-c., alum., ***am-br., apis,*** arg-n., ars., bad., bapt., **BELL.,** berb., bov., calad., camph., caps., caust., chin., chin-a., ***cimx.,*** coc-c., dios., glon., ***hydr.,*** hyos., **IRIS,** jac-c., jatr., lath., ***laur.,*** lyc., ***mag-m.,*** med., ***merc-c.,*** plat., psor., ***puls.,*** rhus-v., rumx., sabad., sal-ac., sang., seneg., sep., stict., syph., ***tarent., thuj., verat-v.,*** zinc.
dinner, after - alum.
morning - ***am-br.,*** dios., mag-m., mez.
menses, during - mag-m.
waking, on - bov., nat-c.
burnt, as if, gums - ars-m., ***cimx.,*** ign., ***sep.***
burnt, as if, palate - bar-c., ***calc.,*** cimx., lac-ac., sang., sep., tarent.

CANCER, lips - acet-ac., ***ars.,*** ars-i., aur., ***aur-m.,*** camph., ***carb-an.,*** caust., ***cic., cist.,*** clem., com., **CON., CUND.,** hydr., kali-chl., kali-s., ***kreos., lach., lyc.,*** phos., phyt., ***sep., sil.,*** sulph., tab., thuj.
epithelioma - ***cic., con., hydr.,*** lap-a., sep.
lower - ***ars.,*** clem., ***merc-i-f., phos., sep., sil.***
lower - ant-chl., ***ars., cist., clem., con.,*** dulc., ***lyc., phos.,*** **SEP.,** ***sil.***
pressure of pipe - ***con.,*** sep.
ulcers - ***ars., aur-m.,*** carb-an., ***clem.,*** **CON.,** ***kali-bi.,*** lyc., ***phos.,*** phyt.
cancer, palate - aur., hydr.
hardness, with - hydr.

CARIES, (see Decay)

CHAPPED, lips - agar., **ALUM.,** am-m., ***ant-t.,*** apis, arn., ars., **ARUM-T.,** bov., **CALC., CARB-V.,** cham., chel., chin., ***colch., cor-r.,*** fl-ac., ***graph.,*** guare., hep., ***kali-bi., kali-c.,*** kali-i., kreos., ***mag-m.,*** **NAT-M.,** ol-an., ph-ac., ***phos.,*** sel., staph., **SULPH.,** tab., tarax., zinc.

CLAMMY - bell., bufo, ***dios.,*** gamb., gels., glon., jac-c., lac-d., ***lach.,*** merc-sul., naja, nat-s., ***onos.,*** plb., sang.
waking, on - cycl., ***puls.***

CLOSE, cannot at night - chim.
desire, to keep - cob.

CLOSED - amyg., ant-t., ***cic., stram.,*** sulph.

COATED, creamy - nat-p.
white - bor., ***lac-c., sul-ac.,*** upa.

COLDNESS, sensation of - acon., ***ars.,*** bol., ***camph.,*** carb-an., ***carb-v.,*** chlf., clem., eupi., kali-n., ***lac-c., lach.,*** lyss., plat., rhus-t., tell., ***verat.***
convulsions, after - eupi.
extending to stomach - kali-n.
hot tea seems cold - camph.
icy - cocc.
peppermint, as from - ***camph., lyss.,*** rhus-t., tell., verat.
coldness, gums - phos.
upper - sil.
coldness, lips - apis, ars., ***cedr.,*** cupr., plat., verat.
menses, during - cedr.
coldness, palate - caust.

CONDYLOMATA, palate on - arg-n.

CONSTRICTION - lach., lob-s., nit-ac., phos., plb., sulph.

CONTRACTING, pain - aesc., asar., nit-ac.
spasmodic - calc.
contracting, palate - arn., cinnb., glon.

CONTRACTION, spasmodic - acon., ***ars.,*** asar., ***bell.,*** bufo, calc., cupr., hyos., mosch., sep.
sensation - aesc., asar., alum., fl-ac., seneg.

CONVULSIONS, lips - ***ambr.,*** caust., crot-c., kali-c., ran-b.

COVERS mouth with hand - am-c., arg-n., cor-r., cupr., ip., kali-bi., ***lach.,*** **RUMX.,** thuj.

CRACKED - ambr., bism., bufo, ***cocc.,*** lach., ***ph-ac., phos.***
skin, corners - ambr., am-c., ***ant-c.,*** apis, **ARUM-T.,** calc., caust., cinnb., **CUND.,** eup-per., **GRAPH.,** ***hell., hydr.,*** ind., ***iod., merc., mez., nat-a., nat-m.,*** **NIT-AC.,** ***sep.,*** **SIL.,** ***thlaspi, zinc.***
cracked, gums - plat.
cracked, lips - ***agar., ail.,*** aloe, alum., ambr., ***am-c., am-m.,*** ant-c., ant-t., ***arn.,*** **ARS., ARUM-T.,** aur., ***bapt.,*** bar-c., bell., bism., ***bov.,*** **BRY., CALC.,** calc-p., ***calc-s., caps.,*** carb-ac., ***carb-an.,*** **CARB-S., CARB-V.,** caust., ***cham.,*** chel., **CHIN.,** chin-a., cimic., clem., colch., con., cop., cor-r., ***croc., cund.,*** cupr., dros., dys-co., echi., glyc., **GRAPH.,** guare., ham., hep., ***hell., ign.,*** iris, jatr., kali-ar., kali-bi., kali-c., kali-i., kali-p., kali-s., kalm., ***kreos.,*** **LACH.,** mag-m., mag-p., mang., meny., ***merc., merc-c.,*** merc-p-r., ***mez.,*** mur-ac., nat-a., nat-c., **NAT-M.,** nicc., nit-ac., nux-v., par., ped., petr., ph-ac., ***phos., plat.,*** plb., puls., ***rhus-t.,*** sabad., sel., sep., ***sil.,*** spig., squil., ***stram.,*** **SULPH.,** syph., tab., tarax., ter., tub., ***verat., zinc.***
coryza, during - staph.
lower - apis, arag., bry., cham., cimic., ***nat-c.,*** **NAT-M.,** ***nit-ac., phos.,*** **SEP.,** sulph., zinc.

cracked, lips
middle of - calc., ***cham.,*** hep., ***nat-m.,*** phos., ***puls.,*** sep.
lower - agar., ***am-c.,*** aur-m., ***cham.,*** chin., dros., ***hep.,*** **NAT-M.,** nux-v., ph-ac., phos., ***puls.***
upper - hell., ***hep., nat-m., sel.,*** tarax.
right side - merc.
upper - bar-c., calc., hell., ***kali-c.,*** nat-c., ***nat-m.,*** tarax.

CRACKLING, of, on pressure, gums - daph.

CRAMP, lips - ambr., caust., kali-c., ran-b.
cramp-like, pain, lips - bell., caust., kali-c., ***merc.,*** plat.

CRAWLING - acon., alum., merl., nux-m., ***zinc.***
cheek inside - zinc.
crawling, gums - arn., graph., kali-c., **SEC.**
crawling, palate - acon., ars., carb-v., graph., grat., phos., polyg., ran-b., sabad., sil.

CRUSTS - ***myric.***
ulcerated - arg-n.

CUTTING, pain, gums, in - iod., mag-c., nit-ac.
cutting, lips, lower - clem., phos.
upper - lyc., nit-ac., ***sep.***
cutting, palate, in, when swallowing - hell.

DECAY, gums - calc., merc.
decay, palate - **AUR.,** guare., hippoz., ***merc.,*** merc-cy., ***nit-ac.,*** syph.

DESQUAMATION, cheek, inside - sulph.
desquamation, palate, sensation of - phos.

DETACHED, gums from teeth - ***am-c., ant-c.,*** arg-m., ***arg-n., aur-m-n., bapt.,*** bar-c., bov., brom., bufo, caps., ***calc., camph., carb-s.,*** **CARB-V.,** caust., ***cist.,*** colch., cupr., ***dulc.,*** gran., ***graph.,*** hep., ***iod., kali-c., kali-i.,*** **KALI-P.,** ***kreos.,*** lac-c., lach., **MERC.,** ***merc-c.,*** mez., nat-c., ***nat-s.,*** nit-ac., ***par., ph-ac., phos.,*** psor., rhus-t., plb., sep., **SIL.,** ***staph., sulph.,*** ter., ***zinc.***
and bleed easily - ant-c., **CARB-V.,** ***phos.***

DISCHARGE, of stinking brown ichor on making incision near second molar - anthr.
putrid - **CARB-AC.**

DISCOLORATION, of
blueness - ambr., ***gymn.,*** merc., plb.
brown-red - lyc.
paleness - acet-ac., ***chin-s.,*** eup-per., ferr., mang., merc., ***nat-m.***
purple - merc.
blotches - plb.
reddish, blue - ars.
margins - merc.
reddish, spots - berb., sars.
cheeks - mag-c.
redness - am-c., ***apis,*** ars., bell., ***bor.,*** calad., ***canth.,*** chlol., ***cupr-ac., cycl.,*** ferr-i., ***hydr., hyos.,*** ign., ***kali-bi., kali-chl.,*** kreos., ***merc.,*** merc-c., merc-cy., merc-i-r., merc-sul., nat-a., ***nat-c., nit-ac.,*** rhus-v., sal-ac.
spots - plb.

DISCOLORATION, of
white - mur-ac.
patches - sal-ac.
yellow - plb.
creamy - ***nat-p.***
patches - ***nit-ac.***
spots - lac-c., lach., lyc.

discoloration, of gums
black - ***merc.,*** plb.
blue line on margin - **PLB.**
bluish - aur-m., ***lach.,*** lyc., merc., olnd., ***plb.,*** psor., sabad.
bluish-red - con., **KREOS.,** lach.
bluish-white - olnd.
brown - chel., ***colch., plb., phos.***
dirty - ***alum.,*** merc.
gray, dirty gray - ***alum.***
greenish tint along free border - cupr-s.
pale - asc-t., carb-an., ***chel., cycl.,*** **FERR.,** med., **MERC-C.,** nit-ac., nux-v., phos., **PLB.,** senec., ***staph.***
purple - ***bapt.,*** **PLB., MERC-C.,** ***lach.***
thin border nearest teeth - **PLB.**
redness - am-c., ant-t., ***apis,*** arund., ***aur., bell.,*** berb., calc., calad., canth., ***carb-an., cham.,*** crot-h., ***dol., dulc.,*** eup-per., ferr-p., hydr., ***iod., lach.,*** kali-ar., kali-c., kali-chl., kali-n., kali-p., **KREOS.,** mag-c., **MERC.,** ***merc-c.,*** merc-i-r., mur-ac., ***nat-s., nit-ac.,*** nux-v., phel., ran-s., ***sep.***
dark - ***aur.,*** **BAPT.,** ***bor.,*** hydr., sep.
dirty - berb.
margins bright red - ***crot-h., merc.***
pale - bar-c., kali-chl.
sooty - hippoz.
violet border - merc-cy.
white - acet-ac., ars., aur-m., ***crot-h., ferr., kali-bi.,*** **MERC.,** ***nit-ac.,*** nux-v., ***ph-ac.,*** spong., ***staph.,*** zinc.
yellow - asc-t., ***carb-v., merc.***

discoloration, lips
black - acon., ant-t., **ARS.,** bry., bufo, carb-ac., ***carb-v., chin., chlor.,*** colch., con., ***hyos.,*** kali-ar., ***kali-c., lach., merc., merc-c.,*** merc-sul., ***phos.,*** ph-ac., ***psor.,*** rhus-t., squil., ***verat.***
bluish - **ACET-AC.,** ***acon.,*** agar., alum., alumn., am-c., amyg., **ANT-T.,** ***apis, apoc.,*** **ARG-N.,** ***ars.,*** ars-i., ***aur., bar-c.,*** berb., ***cact.,*** calc., **CAMPH.,** caust., ***cedr., chin., chin-s.,*** chlor., ***colch.,*** con., ***crot-h.,*** **CUPR.,** cur., ***dig., dros.,*** eup-pur., ***hep.,*** **HYDR-AC.,** ***iod., ip.,*** kali-ar., ***kali-i.,*** kreos., **LACH.,** lachn., **LYC.,** merc., merc-cy., mosch., ***nat-m.,*** **NUX-V.,** ***op., phos.,*** plan., ***prun.,*** psor., samb., sec., stram., ***stry.,*** verat., vip.
chill, during - ***ars., chin-s.,*** eup-pur., ***ip.,*** **NAT-M.,** ***nux-v., sec.***
convulsions, during - **NUX-V.**
menses, during - ***arg-n., cedr.***
scolding, from - ***mosch.***
whooping cough - carb-v., ***cupr.,*** dros., ip., ***nux-v.***

discoloration, lips
brown - ant-t., ***ars.***, ars-h., bry., ***carb-v.***, chlor., ***hyos.***, olnd., op., ***phos.***, ***psor.***, rhus-t., squil., staph., sul-ac., ***verat.***
spots upper - nat-c., sulph.
streak along lower - ***ars.***
brownish yellow forehead at edges of hair - caul., kali-p., med., nat-m.
changing color, lips - sulph.
pale - ant-t., ***apis***, ***aran.***, **ARS.**, ***calc.***, carb-ac., caust., coca, ***colch.***, cupr., ***cycl.***, dig., **FERR.**, ***ferr-ar.***, ***ferr-p.***, **HYDR-AC.**, ip., **KALI-AR.**, kali-c., ***lac-d.***, ***lyc.***, manc., ***mang.***, **MED.**, ***merc-c.***, nat-p., ***op.***, ph-ac., phos., pic-ac., ***puls.***, sec., ***senec.***, spig., sulph., thuj., valer., verat., verat-v., xan.
menses, during - cycl., ***ferr.***
menses, suppressed - ars., chin., cycl., ***ferr.***, ph-ac., rhus-t., ***senec.***, ***sep.***, sulph.
red - all-c., aloe, ***apis***, ***ars.***, arum-t., ***aur-m.***, bar-c., ***bell.***, bry., carb-v., chlol., lac-c., ***lach.***, lachn., merc., merc-c., ped., puls., rhus-t., ***sang.***, spig., stram., **SULPH.**, thyr., ***tub.***, verat.
bleeding - ***arum-t.***, kreos.
dark - bar-c., bell., gins., mez.
lower lip - sep., ***sulph.***
spot - caust., nat-m., sulph.
upper lip - ars-i., calc., nat-m.
scarlet - stroph.

discoloration, of palate
blotches - ***elaps***, ***fl-ac.***, ***syph.***, zinc.
bluish - merc-sul., ***phyt.***
red - acon., apis, cham., phos., sulph.
coppery - ***kali-bi.***, ***merc.***
grayish - lac-c., rhus-t.
purple - phyt.
red - **ACON.**, aeth., ant-t., **APIS**, arg-n., ***bapt.***, bell., berb., ***caps.***, ***caust.***, **CHAM.**, cimic., coc-c., ***colch.***, cop., ***daph.***, ***fl-ac.***, ***graph.***, ***kali-bi.***, ***kali-i.***, ***lach.***, ***merc.***, merl., morph., ***mur-ac.***, ***nit-ac.***, op., ***phyt.***, puls., sul-ac., ziz.
velum - aeth., agn., ***alum.***, ***apis***, ***arg-n.***, ***bell.***, ***calc.***, ***cedr.***, ***cham.***, chen-a., cop., cupr-ac., kali-bi., ***merc.***, ***mur-ac.***, nux-m., ***petr.***, ***puls.***
spots, in forepart as if ulcers would form - kali-bi.
white - am-caust., ***ferr.***, lac-c., ***merc.***, **NAT-P.**, rhus-t., sil.
yellow, creamy - **NAT-P.**

DISTORTED - agar., ***bell.***, bry., camph., ***cocc.***, ***con.***, ***cupr.***, cur., ***dulc.***, ***graph.***, ign., kali-n., lach., ***laur.***, ***lyc.***, merc., **NUX-V.**, op., ph-ac., plat., **PLB.**, puls., sec., stram., stry., sulph., tarent.
alternating sides - cham., lyc., nit-ac.
one-sided - dulc., graph.
right corner outward - bell.
sleep, during - bry., cupr.
talking, when - caust.

DRAWING, pain - gymn., nux-v.
drawing, gums - anac., alum., ang., caps., carb-an., caust., con., iod., lyss., nat-m., ruta, sep., staph.
drawing, lips - bell., calc., ***sep.***, spig.
drawing, palate - hydr., sars., ther.
arches on swallowing - coc-c.
convulsive, extending to fauces - cham., merc.

DRAWN, to left - phos., verat-v.
drawn, lips - ant-t., ***apis***, ***camph.***, nux-v., phyt., tab.
swollen, and - ***merc-c.***
upper, lips drawn up, exposing teeth - acon., ant-t., **CAMPH.**, ***phyt.***

DROPPING, lips - bar-c., merc., nux-v., verat.

DRYNESS, of - **ACON.**, aesc., aeth., agar., agn., all-c., aloe, ***alum.***, alumn., ambr., ***am-c.***, anac., ang., ***ant-c.***, ***ant-t.***, anthro., aphis., ***apis***, ***arg-m.***, arg-n., ***arn.***, **ARS.**, ***ars-h.***, ***ars-i.***, ***ars-m.***, **ARS-S-F.**, ***arum-t.***, asaf., asar., ***atro.***, aur-m., bapt., **BAR-C.**, **BAR-M.**, **BELL.**, berb., **BOR.**, bov., brom., **BRY.**, ***calc.***, calc-p., calc-s., ***camph.***, **CANN-I.**, ***cann-s.***, ***canth.***, **CAPS.**, carb-an., ***carb-s.***, **CARB-V.**, caul., ***caust.***, cedr., ***cench.***, **CHAM.**, ***chel.***, **CHIN.**, chin-a., chlor., cic., cimic., cina, ***cinnb.***, cist., ***cocc.***, coc-c., coff., colch., ***coloc.***, com., con., cop., cor-r., **CROT-C.**, ***crot-h.***, ***cupr.***, cur., dios., ***dulc.***, echi., euph., euphr., ***ferr.***, ***ferr-ar.***, ferr-i., ferr-p., ***gamb.***, ***gels.***, glon., ***graph.***, ham., hell., helon., hipp., hippoz., **HYOS.**, ***hyper.***, **IGN.**, ind., iod., ip., jac-c., jatr., ***kali-ar.***, **KALI-BI.**, ***kali-c.***, ***kali-chl.***, ***kali-i.***, ***kali-n.***, ***kali-p.***, kali-s., lac-c., lac-d., **LACH.**, lac-ac., lact., **LAUR.**, lec., led., ***lil-t.***, lob., **LYC.**, lyss., ***mag-c.***, ***mag-m.***, mag-s., manc., mang., med., **MERC.**, merc-c., merc-i-f., merl., ***mez.***, mill., mosch., **MUR-AC.**, ***myric.***, **NAJA**, **NAT-A.**, **NAT-AC.**, **NAT-M.**, nat-p., **NAT-S.**, nicc., ***nit-ac.***, **NUX-M.**, **NUX-V.**, oena., olnd., ol-an., onos., ***op.***, ox-ac., par., ***petr.***, phel., **PH-AC.**, **PHOS.**, pic-ac., ***phyt.***, plat., ***plb.***, ***psor.***, ptel., ***puls.***, ran-s., rat., ***rhod.***, **RHUS-T.**, rumx., ruta., sabad., sabin., sal-ac., samb., sanic., sang., sarr., ***sars.***, sec., senec., ***seneg.***, **SEP.**, **SIL.**, sin-n., sol-n., ***squil.***, staph., ***stram.***, ***stront-c.***, sul-ac., **SULPH.**, tab., ***tarent.***, tell., thea., ther., thuj., **VERAT.**, **VERAT-V.**, zinc.
afternoon - mag-c., ph-ac.
anterior part - ars., bry., nux-v.
breath offensive, evening, in - puls.
morning, in - nux-v.
chewing food agg. - ferr., thuj.
chill, during - mur-ac., petr.
coryza, during - alum.
dinner, after - kali-n.
before - kali-n.
dreams, during - apis, calc., caust., lach., ***nux-m.***, ***par.***, puls., tarent.
eating, after - sulph.
evening - aloe, am-c., bov., bry., cann-s., cycl., lyc., merc-c., mez., naja, nux-m., phos., plat., ***senec.***, verat.
fever, during - zinc.
forenoon - caust., sars., seneg.

DRYNESS, of
menses, during - ***cedr.,*** **NUX-M.,** tarent.
moisten, food, could not - ars., merl.
morning - ambr., am-c., arg-n., arn., **BAR-C.,** bar-m., berb., bry., cann-s., caps., carb-an., ***carb-s.,*** carb-v., ***cham.,*** chin., cimic., coff., cop., ***dios., ferr., graph.,*** jac-c., kali-c., kali-n., ***lyc., mag-c.,*** mag-m., manc., mang., mur-ac., nat-c., nat-s., ***nit-ac., nux-v.,*** ol-an., op., par., petr., ph-ac., plb., podo., **PULS.,** ***rhus-t., sabad.,*** sang., sars., seneg., ***sep.,*** spig., **SULPH.,** thuj., verat., zing.
waking, on - alum., ambr., ammc., am-c., apoc., calc., carb-v., clem., cob., coca, graph., kali-c., **LAC-C.,** ***lyc.,*** mag-c., mang., naja, ol-an., ***par., phos., podo., rhus-t.,*** sep., spig., stram., stront-c., tarax.
morning, waking, on, thirstless - ambr.
night - acon., am-c., ***ant-c., arum-t.,*** bell., bry., calc., ***carb-s., caust., cench., cinnb., cocc.,*** coff., eupi., glon., graph., jatr., kali-c., ***lyc., mag-c.,*** mag-m., ***nux-m., nux-v.,*** phel., ***pic-ac.,*** phos., rumx., ***rhus-t.,*** senec., sel., ***sep.,*** sil., ***sulph.,*** tarent.
waking, on - ars-i., ***carb-s., rat., rhus-t.***
posterior part only - mez., thuj.
sand in it, as if - bov.
sensation of - acon., arg-m., ars., asaf., aur., bell., caul., chin., cic., cina, ***colch.,*** dios., dros., kali-c., lyc., **NUX-M.,** rhus-t., stram., stront-c., sul-ac., viol-o., viol-t.
morning - asaf., stront.
sensation of, with moist - acon., sulph., viol-t.
coated with mucus - acon., bell., dios., kali-c.
sensation of, cough, with - phyt.
sleep, preventing - kali-c.
swallowing, on - bell., lyc.
thirst, with - acon., aloe, alum., am-c., arg-n., arn., ars., ***bar-c.,*** berb., **BRY.,** ***camph.,*** canth., ***carb-s.,*** caust., cham., chel., ***chin.,*** cinnb., cocc., coc-c., cycl., dig., kali-i., kreos., ***lach.,*** laur., ***lec.,*** lyc., lyss., mag-m., ***merc-c.,*** mez., mill., ***nat-c.,*** **NAT-M.,** nat-s., nit-ac., ***nux-m.,*** op., petr., ***phos.,*** plat., ***rhus-t.,*** sars., sec., ***stram.,*** sulph., tab., thuj., verat.
thirstlessness, with - acon., all-c., aloe, alumn., ***ambr.,*** ang., ***apis,*** arn., ars., asaf., ***bell.,*** **BRY.,** calad., ***camph.,*** cann-i., cann-s., carb-an., carb-v., caust., ***cocc.,*** dios., dulc., euph., euphr., guare., ign., jatr., kali-bi., kali-c., kali-n., lac-c., ***lach., lyc.,*** mag-c., mag-m., mez., nat-m., nit-ac., **NUX-M.,** ***nux-v.,*** onos., op., ***par.,*** ph-ac., phos., **PULS.,** rheum, sep., spig., sabad., samb., sabin., sanic., sars., ***sil., stram.,*** thuj., **TUB.,** verat.
walking, in open air, while - sil.

dryness, lips - ***acon.,*** aesc., agar., all-s., aloe, alum., ***am-c., am-m., aml-n.,*** anac., anan., ang., **ANT-C.,** ***ant-t., apis,*** apoc., ***arg-n., ars.,*** ars-m., asar., ***bar-c.,*** bar-m., ***bell.,*** berb., **BRY.,** brach., calad., ***calc., calc-ar.,*** cann-i., cann-s., ***canth.,*** carb-an., ***carb-s.,*** carb-v., card-m., caust., chel., ***chin.,*** chr-ac., cimic., cocc., con., cop., ***crot-t.,*** cub., cycl., ***dig.,*** dios., dros., ***ferr.,*** ferr-ar., ferr-p., ***gels., graph.,*** ham., ***hell., helon., hydr.,*** **HYOS.,** hyper., ***ign.,*** iodof., iris, jal., kali-ar., ***kali-bi., kali-c.,*** kali-i., kali-p., ***kalm., kreos., lach., lac-c., lyc.,*** mag-s., mang., meny., ***merc., merc-c., merc-cy.,*** merc-i-f., mez., ***mur-ac.,*** nat-c., **NAT-M.,** nat-s., ***nit-ac.,*** **NUX-M.,** ***nux-v.,*** olnd., ph-ac., ***phos.,*** phyt., plat., ***psor.,*** ptel., **PULS.,** ***rhod.,*** **RHUS-T.,** ruta., sabad., sang., senec., ***sep., sil.,*** spig., ***stram.,*** **SULPH.,** tab., thuj., ***verat.,*** **VERAT-V.,** vib., vinc., zinc.
air, open - mang.
evening - mag-s.
lower, inner side - asar.
morning - carb-an., mag-c., mang.
night - ant-c., calad., cham.
waking, on - ambr., calad., coca.

dryness, palate - acon., aesc., agar., ***all-c.,*** ang., arg-m., arg-n., arn., asar., ***apis,*** atro., ***bell., bry.,*** bufo, ***calc., camph.,*** cann-s., ***carb-an.,*** card-m., cina, ***cist.,*** chel., chin., chlor., cocc., coc-c., coloc., cop., cycl., ***dros., fl-ac.,*** glon., grat., hell., ***hyos.,*** lac-ac., lach., led., mag-c., mang., meny., merl., ***merc.,*** merc-sul., mez., myric., ***nat-m.,*** nit-ac., **NUX-M.,** olnd., op., par., ph-ac., **PHOS.,** phyt., puls., samb., ***seneg.,*** sep., staph., ***stict., stram.,*** **SULPH.,** thuj., **VERAT.,** viol-o., zing.
air, open, agg. - mang.
eating, after - bry.
evening - chlor., ***cycl.,*** fl-ac., staph.
forenoon - phos.
leather, like, soft palate - ***stict.***
morning - phyt., cann-s., tub.
on waking - mez., ***puls., sulph.,*** tub.
nausea, with - dig.
night - ***calc., nux-m.,*** tub.
one-sided - ***fl-ac.***
soft palate - ***dros.***
talking, from - graph.

ECCHYMOSES, dark red, bloody - anthr., ***ter.***

ECZEMA, around - ***mez.,*** mur-ac., ***nat-m.***
corners - ***arund., graph., hep.,*** lyc., ***rhus-t.,*** sil.

eczema, lips - ***ant-c.,*** aur-m., bov., calc., graph., lyc., ***mez., rhus-v.***

EDEMA, palate - apis, kali-i.

EGG-white, dried on lips - ol-an., ph-ac.

ELONGATION, sensation of, gums - ***nit-ac.***

elongation, palate, sensation of - stry.

ENLARGED, sensation as if - ***absin., alum.,*** bell., ***caj., card-m., phys., polyg., rat., spig., xan.***

EPITHELIOMA, (see Lips, cancer)

EPULIS - calc., ***nat-m., thuj.***
soft and painless - calc.

ERUPTIONS, around - ***agar.***, am-c., anac., **ANT-T., ARS.,** bell., ***bor., bov., cadm-s., calc.,*** calc-f., carb-s., caust., cic., cocc., crot-h., dulc., **GRAPH.,** ***hell., hep.,*** hydr., ***hyper.,*** ign., kali-ar., ***kali-bi., kali-c.,*** **KALI-CHL.,** kali-i., **KREOS.,** lach., laur., ***led., lyc., mag-c., mag-m.,*** mang., ***merc., merc-c., mez., mur-ac.,*** **NAT-A., NAT-C., NAT-M.,** nat-p., nat-s., **NIT-AC.,** ***nux-v., par., petr., phos.,*** **RHUS-T.,** rhus-v., **SEP.,** ***sil.,*** **STAPH., SULPH.,** tarax., zinc.
below - caust., graph., hep.
corners - ***ant-c., bell.,*** bov., **CALC.,** calc-f., cann-s., carb-v., caust., ***cic., cund.,*** **GRAPH.,** ***hep., ign.,*** iris, ***kreos., lyc., mang.,*** **MERC.,** mez., nat-c., ***nat-m.,*** **NIT-AC.,** nux-v., ***petr., phos.,*** ph-ac., psor., rhus-t., seneg., ***sep., sil.,*** tab., verat.
right - bell., hep., merc., sep., til.
crusty, around - **GRAPH.,** hyper., ***led., merc., mez., nat-m.,*** **NIT-AC.,** rhus-v.
corners of - ant-c., **GRAPH.,** guare., kali-p., nat-m., nit-ac., ***rhus-t.,*** rhus-v., ***sars.***
inner cheeks and lips - berb.
red and painful - berb.
pimples - dulc.
around - agar., ***bar-c.,*** bov., calc., ***dulc.,*** kali-c., ***mag-c., mur-ac.,*** phos., ***rhus-t.,*** sep., ***sil.,*** zinc.
corners, of - bar-c., bell., lyc., mag-m., mang., nat-m., petr., phos., tarax.
pustules - ant-t., ars-s-f., berb., caps., crot-t., hep., hydr.
scurfy, around - am-c., anac., calc., ***cic., graph.,*** mur-ac., ***petr.,*** sep.
corners of - ign., lyc., petr., sil.

eruptions, lips - agar., ail., alum., ***am-c.,*** am-m., ant-c., ant-t., apis, arg-n., arn., **ARS.,** asc-t., aur-m., bell., berb., ***bor.,*** bov., brom., bry., cadm-s., ***calc.,*** calc-f., calc-s., cann-s., canth., caps., carb-an., carb-s., carb-v., caust., cham., chel., chin-s., cic., cinnb., ***clem., com., con., crot-t.,*** dig., ferr-m., ***graph.,*** guai., hell., ***hep.,*** hydr., ign., ip., kali-c., kali-chl., kali-s., lac-c., lach., lyc., ***mag-c., mag-m.,*** mang., med., merc., merc-c., ***mur-ac.,*** nat-a., ***nat-c.,*** **NAT-M.,** nat-p., nat-s., nicc., ***nit-ac.,*** nux-v., pall., par., petr., ph-ac., phos., plat., rhod., **RHUS-T.,** ruta., sang., sars., seneg., ***squil.,*** **SEP.,** ***sil.,*** spong., staph., sulph., tarent., ter., thuj., valer., viol-t., urt-u.
blotches - arg-m., ars., bar-c., caust., con., hep., kali-i., mag-m., nat-c., sep., sil., sulph.
burning - am-c., aur., bov., caust., graph., mag-m., mur-ac., nat-m., nicc., plat., rat., seneg., ***staph.,*** sulph.
crusty - alum., ***apis, ars.,*** berb., bry., ***cinnb., con.,*** graph., kali-p., ***merc.,*** merc-c., ***mur-ac.,*** nat-m., nit-ac., ***nux-v.,*** **PH-AC.,** ***rhus-t.,*** sep., **SIL.,** squil., staph., ***ter.,***

eruptions, lips
crusty - thuj., valer.
itching - am-c., calc., graph., mag-m., nit-ac., sil.
lower - bor., **BRY.,** ***calc.,*** caust., ***nat-c., nat-m., ph-ac.,*** phos., **SEP.,** ***sulph.***
papular, upper - zinc.
pimples - ***agar.,*** am-m., arn., aur., bell., berb., bor., ***bov.,*** bufo, calc., ***carb-v.,*** ferr-m., ***graph.,*** guai., ***hep., kali-c.,*** kali-chl., kali-p., ***merc., mur-ac., nat-c.,*** nit-ac., nux-v., pall., par., petr., ph-ac., ruta., ***sep.,*** spig., staph., thuj.
burning - aur., hep., ph-ac., staph.
burning, itching - aur., kali-c.
itching - am-m., aur., kali-c., nit-ac., thuj.
inside - mag-m.
pimples, lower - mang., nicc., nit-ac., pall., zinc.
pimples, upper - am-m., ant-c., arn., bufo, calc., ***carb-v.,*** clem., mang., spig., ***thuj., zinc.***
burning - aphis., graph.
itching - graph., lyc.
red - zinc.
sore to touch - zinc.
pustules - ***anthr.,*** ant-c., aur., bell., berb., ***calc., cinnb.,*** clem., ***hep.,*** iris, mag-c., mur-ac., samb., sep., ***viol-t.,*** zinc.
black - **ANTHR.,** ***lach.***
upper - ***anthr.,*** ant-c., calc., carb-v., ***viol-t.,*** zinc.
rough, corners, raw - ant-c., arum-t., graph.
scurfy - ant-t., **ARS.,** bar-c., bell., berb., bor., calc., cham., ***cic., hep.,*** ign., ***kali-c.,*** merc., mur-ac., ***nat-a.,*** nux-v., petr., ph-ac., phos., plan., rhus-t., ***sep., sil.,*** squil., staph., sulph.
upper - **ARS.,** ***bar-c.,*** bell., bor., ***carb-v., cic.,*** cinnb., dig., graph., **KALI-C., KREOS.,** ***lyc.,*** mag-c., mag-m., mang., ***nat-c., nat-m.,*** nit-ac., ***par.,*** phyt., ***rhus-t., sep., sil.,*** squil., **STAPH., SULPH.,** ***thuj.,*** viol-t., zinc.

eruptions, palate, crusts, dry, scaly - myric., plb., sec., sul-ac.
crusts, dry, scaly, behind the base of the uvula - ***bar-c.***
white - ox-ac.
pimples - bapt., dulc., nux-v., rumx.
pustules - ambr., ant-t., coc-c., phos.

ERYSIPELAS, lower, lip extending from - ***anthr.,*** apis

EVERTED, lips - **APIS,** bar-c., calc., camph., graph., merc., nat-m., phyt., psor., syph.
belly, big, with - syph.
swollen - **MERC-C.**

EXCORIATION, of mucous membranes - ail., ambr., am-caust., ant-c., ars., **ARUM-T.,** arund., bell., berb., bufo, ***canth., carb-an.,*** carb-v., chlor., cina, coc-c., dig., fl-ac., hell., ip., kali-ar., kali-c., ***lach.,*** lac-ac., med., merc., merc-sul., mez., mur-ac., nat-m., nit-ac., nux-v., ph-ac., ***phos.,***

EXCORIATION, of mucous membranes - sang., sep., spong., stram., sulph., ***sul-ac., tub.***
places, in - am-caust., bell., ***lach.,*** phos.
menses, agg. - ***kreos.***
scaling, off - spig.
excoriated, as if - aesc., ambr., asim., bism., oena.
excoriated, corners of - ant-c., ***ars.,*** **ARUM-T.,** bell., bov., brach., ***caust., cocc., cund., dios.,*** eup-per., form., ***hell.,*** ind., ip., ***lyc.,*** **MERC.,** mez., nat-c., nat-m., pall., phos., ***psor., sulph.,*** zinc.
excoriated, lips - am-m., ant-t., **ARS., ARUM-T.,** calc., canth., ***caust.,*** cham., cop., cupr., ***graph.,*** ham., ***hell., iod.,*** kali-c., ***kali-p.,*** **LACH.,** lac-c., lyc., mang., merc., mez., ***mur-ac.,*** nat-m., ***nit-ac.,*** phos., ***sep.,*** stram.
inside - cupr., sep.
menses agg. - ***kreos.***
saliva, from acrid - **NIT-AC.**
upper - mag-c.
excoriation, of palate - am-c., ***canth.,*** euph., graph., par., phyt.
sensation, as if - lach., par.
shrivelled, as if burnt - bor.
spot - mur-ac.

EXCRESCENCES, painful - staph.
excrescenes, gums - ***staph.***

EXOSTOSES, roof of - asaf.

FEVER, blisters, lips (see Vesicles, lips)- **APIS.,** ars., brom., ***calc-f.,*** canth., ***crot-t.,*** graph., hyos., ***lac-c.,*** med., **NAT-M.,** phos., **RHUS-T.,** sep., urt-u.

FINGERS, in the mouth, children put - ***calc.,*** calc-ox., calc-p., ***cham.,*** **IP.,** lyc., med., nat-m., ***sil.,*** tarent., verat.

FISTULA, gums - ***aur., aur-m., bar-c., calc.,*** canth., **CAUST.,** coch., **FL-AC.,** ***kali-chl., lyc.,*** mag-c., ***nat-m.,*** nit-ac., petr., phos., **SIL.,** ***staph., sulph.***
near upper right canine - fl-ac.
upper incisors - canth.
fistula, palate to antrum of highmore - fl-ac., merc., sil.

FOAM, froth, from - absin., acet-ac., acon., aeth., agar., alet., am-m., aphis., ***ars.,*** art-v., asaf., ***bell.,*** brom., ***camph.,*** cann-i., canth., ***carb-ac.,*** carb-v., ***caust., cedr., cham., cic., cina,*** cocc., ***colch.,*** con., ***crot-c., crot-h.,*** **CUPR.,** ***glon.,*** hydr-ac., **HYOS.,** ***ign.,*** kreos., ***lac-c., lac-d., lach.,*** lact., ***laur., lyc.,*** lyss., ***mag-m.,*** mosch., naja, nux-m., ***oena.,*** olnd., ***op.,*** par., ph-ac., phos., plb., rhus-t., ***sec., sil.,*** stann., ***stram.,*** stry., sul-ac., ***tab.,*** tart-ac., teucr., ther., ***verat.***
bloody - absin., bell., canth., ***crot-c., ign.,*** merc-c., oena., sec., ***stram.***
morning - crot-c.

FOAM, froth, from
convulsions, during - agar., ars., ***art-v.,*** bell., ***bufo,*** camph., canth., ***caust., cham., cina,*** cocc., colch., ***cupr.,*** gels., ***glon., hyos.,*** lyss., lyc., ***oena., op.,*** staph., ***stry.,*** sulph., tax.
after - sil.
odor of rotten eggs - bell.
reddish - bell., canth., hyos., ***lach.,*** sec., stram.
shaking chill, during - ther.
sleep, during - sil., stram.
talking, while - ***lac-d.,*** plb.
white-milky - aeth.
yellow-green - ***sec.***

FOOD, escapes from mouth while chewing - ***arg-n.***

FORMICATION, lips - ant-c., berb., bor., calc., caust., graph., nat-c., nat-m., ph-ac., stront.
lower, bug, as if a - bor.
menses, during - graph.

FROTH, cotton-like - alet., aq-mar., bry., canth., ***lyss., nux-m.,*** nux-v., ph-ac., sulph.
white-milky - aeth.

FURRY, gums - sul-ac.

GANGRENE - ***crot-h.,*** ferr-ar., hydr., **LACH.,** merc-c., merc-d., sil., sulph., sul-ac.
children, in - **ARS.,** casc.
gangrene, gums - ***lach.,*** **MERC-C.,** ***sec.***

GINGIVITIS, inflammation of gums - acon., ***alumn.,*** am-c., arg-n., ars., ars-i., aur-m., bell., bor., bufo, ***calc-f.,*** calc-s., ***caps., cham.,*** chin-s., ***hecla.,*** hep., kali-n., **KREOS.,** lach., lyss., mag-c., ***merc., merc-c., mur-ac.,*** **NAT-M.,** naja, ***nux-v.,*** **PHOS.,** ***phyt.,*** plb., rhus-t., **SIL.,** sulph., thuj., tub.
left upper side - ***kreos.***
lower incisors, at - petr.

GLANDULAR, swelling - iod.

GLAZED, palate - atro., ***hyos.,*** lac-c.
velum -***carb-ac.***

GLUED, up sensation - mur-ac.
glued together, as if, lips - cann-i., helon., stram.

GNAWING, pain, in gums - bar-c., ***euph., puls.***

GRASPING, at mouth - sil.

GREASY, sensation of - ol-an.
greasy, gums - iris.
greasy, lips - am-m.
greasy, palate - palate - asaf., card-m., kali-p., ol-an.

HAIR, palate on, sensation of - ***kali-bi.***

HAIRY, sensation in - ther.

HARD, palate - bell., calc., hyos., ***nit-ac.,*** nux-v., ***phos.***
cancer, in - hydr.
sensation of a hard object - mang.
spot - caust.

HEAT, in - ***acon.,*** aeth., alum., anan., ***ars.,*** ars-h., aur., ***bad.,*** **BELL., BOR.,** bov., brach., brom., ***calc., calc-s., camph., carb-v.,*** **CHAM.,** chel., chin., chin-a., ***cimic.,*** cinnb., clem., ***colch.,*** croc., crot-t., cupr-s., dor., fl-ac., ***hyper., jatr., kali-chl., kali-i.,*** kali-s., lyc., mag-c., mag-m., manc., merc., merl., mez., naja, nat-m., nat-s., psor., rhus-t., ***sal-ac., senec.,*** sep., sil., ***stront-c., sulph.,*** verat.
afternoon, 5 p.m. - hyper.
coryza, during - mag-m.
morning - abrot., nat-c.
night - am-c., cinnb., phos., ***sulph.***
heat, gums - ***acon., bell., caps.,*** carb-v., ***cham., dulc.,*** eup-pur., ***kreos.,*** lyc.
cold sensation in teeth, with - anan.
heat, lips - ***acon.,*** aesc., aloe, ambr., ang., arn., ars-m., bell., gels., ***hyper., kali-chl., merc., nit-ac.,*** sabad., sep., sulph.
burning heat - arn.
upper - ***apis,*** bor., ***carb-v., kali-bi.,*** mez.
heat, palate - bol., ***camph.,*** canth., dulc., led., ***mez.***

HEAVY, feeling, lower, lips - ***graph., mur-ac.***
upper - caust.

HERPES, around (see Fever blisters, Vesicles) - am-c., anac., ***apis,*** ars., ***bor.,*** cic., con., ***hep.,*** kreos., mag-c., med., nat-c., **NAT-M.,** ***par.,*** phos., **RHUS-T.,** ***sep.,*** sulph.
corners of - carb-v., ***lyc.,*** med., **NAT-M.,** ph-ac., phos., sep., ***sulph.***
below - ***calc-f., nat-m.***
cutting - phos.
stitching - phos.
herpes, lips about - agar., anac., apis, ***ars.,*** asc-t., bor., brom., ***calc-f.,*** canth., carb-v., caust., chel., crot-t., ***dulc.,*** dys-co., ***graph., hep.,*** hyos., ip., kali-p., lac-c., lach., manc., ***med.,*** nat-a., nat-c., **NAT-M.,** ***nicc., par.,*** ph-ac., phos., **RHUS-T.,** sars., **SEP.,** sil., sang., sul-i., sulph., syc-co., ***tub.,*** upa., urt-u.
above - phos.
black - tub.
blisters - apis., nat-m.
hard, small - calc-f.
inner side - med.
menses, during - nat-m., sars.
upper - agar., med., sars.

IMPETIGO, lips - ***ant-c., ars., echi.,*** tarent.
around - ***ant-c., ars.,*** tarent.

INDENTED, gums - ***carb-v.***
indented, lips, corners - sil.

INDURATION, inside of cheek - ***caust.***
induration, gums - brom.
indurations, lips - aur-m., bell., calc-p., chin., ***con.,*** sil.
sense of - cycl.
upper - calc-p.
induration, palate - calc., ***mez., phyt.***

INFLAMMATION, of mouth - ***acon.,*** aloe, ***alum.,*** am-c., apis, arg-n., arn., ars., arum-t., aur-m., ***bapt., bell.,*** bism., ***bor.,*** brom., bufo, ***calc.,*** calc-s., ***canth., caps., carb-ac., cinnb., colch.,*** corn., crot-t., dig., guai., hippoz., ***hydr., ign.,*** ip., ***iris, kali-chl.,*** kali-m., ***kali-p.,*** lach., manc., **MERC.,** ***merc-c., merc-cy.,*** merc-sul., mez., ***mur-ac.,*** nat-a., ***nat-c.,*** nat-m., ***nit-ac., nux-v.,*** oena., ox-ac., **PETR.,** psor., ran-s., rhus-t., sac-alb., sal-ac., sep., sin-n., ***staph.,*** sulph., sul-ac., ***ter.,*** verat., ***vesp.***
burns, from - apis, ***canth.***
follicular, ulcerative - **KALI-CHL.,** myric.
vesicular - anac., anan., canth., caps., kali-chl., mag-c., ***mur-ac.,*** nat-m., rhus-t., sulph.
gangrenous - ***ars.,*** bapt., hydr., kali-chl., kreos., ***lach., merc-c.,*** merc-sul., sec., sul-ac.
mercurial - bapt., carb-v., hep., hydr., mur-ac., ***nit-ac.***
nursing women, in - ***bapt.,*** bor., caul., ***helon., hydr.***
nurslings - bapt.
sore spots inside cheek - aloe.
suppressed hemorrhoids - puls.
ulcerative - agav-a., aln., ***arg-n., ars.,*** arum-t., bapt., bor., chlor., ***cinnb.,*** cory., ***hep.,*** kali-bi., ***kali-chl.,*** kali-cy., mag-c., menthol, ***merc., merc-c., merc-sul., mur-ac.,*** nit-ac., nit-m-ac., phos., rhus-g., sul-ac., sulo-ac., tarax.
inflammation, gums (see Gingivitis)
inflammation, lips - ***acon.,*** anan., **BELL., MERC.,** mez., ph-ac., staph.
corners - sil.
left upper - mang.
inflammation, palate - ***acon., apis, bell., calc.,*** canth., cham., cimic., ***coc-c., colch., gels., lach.,*** merc., ***nux-v., ran-b.,*** seneg., zinc.
arch - bell., berb., kali-n.
suppurating spots - sars.
velum - ***acon.,*** apis, ***bell., calc., coff.,*** kali-c., kali-n., lac-c., ***lach., lyss.***

ITCHING - am-c., anac., apis, aur-m., hep., ***merc.,*** merc-i-f., psor.
cheek, inside - mag-c.
scarlatina, in - **ARUM-T.**
itching, gums - am-c., bell., calc., camph., caust., cimx., graph., kali-c., ***merc., nit-ac.,*** phos., rhod., zinc.
between the teeth - caust.
bleeding when scratched - am-c.
pain after scratching, with - cimx.
itching, lips - am-c., ***apis,*** ars., arum-t., asc-t., aur-m., berb., ***nit-ac.,*** ol-an., sabad., tub.
lower - sil.
spot - sulph.
upper - ars., bar-c., calc-ac., calc-ar., con., hell., mag-c., nat-c., nit-ac., phos., vinc., zinc.

itching, palate - apis, arum-t., arund., canth., crot-h., ferr-ma., gels., ***glon., kali-c.,*** kali-p., ***lac-c.,*** lyss., ***merc.,*** nux-v., ***phos., polyg.,*** puls., ***ran-b.,*** sabad., sil., stry., teucr., upa., ***wye.***
burning - arund.
lying, after - carb-s.
palate, and ear - teucr.

JERKING, pain, in gums - ars., hep., lyc., thuj.

LEATHER, soft, palate, feels like - stict.

LICKS, lips - agar., aloe, ars., bufo, kreos., lyc., nat-m., phys., ***puls.,*** stram., zinc.
agg. - valer.
heat, during agg. - ***puls.***
amel. - mang.

LUMPS, sensation of, on palate - carc.

MEMBRANE, false - **ARUM-T.,** bry., hippoz., ***iod., lac-c., merc-cy., mur-ac.,*** **NIT-AC.,** ***sul-ac.***
silvery, white all over mouth - ***kali-chl., lac-c.,*** sul-ac.
white, coating, like - sul-ac.
whitish, yellow - **NIT-AC.,** ***sul-ac.***

membrane, on lips - arum-t., ars-i., bry.

membrane, palate covered with a false - iod., ip., ***lac-c., lach., merc.,*** merc-cy., merc-i-f., ***mur-ac., nit-ac., sang.,*** sulph.
evening - **NAT-P.**
velum -apis, ***iod., lach., lyc.,*** merc-cy., merc-i-f., ***mur-ac., sang.,*** seneg.
white -zinc-m.
yellowish gray - nit-ac.

MERCURIAL, affections of gums - ***carb-v.,*** chin., ***hep.,*** hydr., **MERC.,** ***nit-ac.,*** phyt., staph.

MOTION, lips, speaking, as if - hell.

MUCUS, slime, in - aloe, alum., am-c., ang., aphis., apoc., arg-n., arn., ars., ars-i., asar., aur., ***bar-c., bar-m., bell.,*** bor., brom., bry., ***calc.,*** calc-s., caps., ***caust.,*** cedr., **CHEL.,** ***chin.,*** chlor., ***crot-h.,*** cupr., cycl., echi., euph., ***fl-ac.,*** graph., hep., hydr., ***ign.,*** iod., ***ip., kali-ar., kali-c.,*** kali-chl., kali-p., kali-s., kreos., ***lac-c., lach.,*** laur., lyc., mag-c., mag-m., manc., ***merc., merc-c.,*** nat-c., **NAT-M., NUX-M.,** ***nux-v.,*** oena., op., ox-ac., ***petr., ph-ac.,*** phos., plat., plb., ***psor., puls., rhus-t.,*** sel., sep., ***sil.,*** spig., squil., staph., stram., ***sulph.,*** sul-ac., ther., teucr., verat.
acid - benz-ac.
balls of - mag-p.
bloody - bism.
burning - graph.
cotton, like - **PULS.**
eating, after - hyper., ***lac-c.,*** plat., verat.
evening - alum., am-c., ang., calc.
exertion, on - chin.
flies from mouth when coughing - bad., ***chel.***
greenish expelled while sneezing - colch.
morning - agar., alum., ars-i., **BELL.,** calc., calc-s., carb-an., chin., cupr., dios., ***fl-ac., graph.,*** ign., ***iod.,*** kali-n., lyc., mag-c., mag-m., manc., merc., mur-ac., nicc., ***nux-v.,*** ph-ac., plat., plb., **PULS.,** ***podo.,*** rheum, sars., ***sep.,*** sil., spig., ***stront-c., sulph.,*** thuj., til., zinc., zing.
night - sulph.
offensive - bry., zinc.
palate, through - puls.
ropy - aesc., ail., am-m., ant-c., arg-n., chel., dulc., ***epip.,*** ferr-m., hydr., iod., iris, **KALI-BI.,** kali-br., kali-chl., ***lyc.,*** lyss., med., merc-sul., nat-m., ***phyt.,*** piloc., ***puls.,*** sul-ac., tarax.
epileptic convulsions, during - kali-bi.
salty - graph.
thick - ***aesc.,*** aloe, apis, atro., bar-c., bell., bufo, ery-a., ip., myric., ***nux-m.,*** verat., verat-v.
viscid - aesc., agn., ail., ang., apis, arg-n., ***arum-t., bar-c., bar-m.,*** bell., ***bry.,*** **CAPS.,** carb-ac., ***carb-v.,*** chel., cinnb., cop., ***crot-h.,*** cycl., ery-a., ferr-m., hell., ***hydr.,*** **KALI-BI.,** kali-br., ***lach.,*** lyc., lyss., mag-c., manc., med., ***mur-ac.,*** myric., ***nat-s.,*** nit-ac., pall., ph-ac., ***phyt.,*** plat., psor., puls., **RHUS-T.,** rhus-v., ruta., sel., squil., stann., stram., sul-ac., sumb., tab., verat.
yellowish - ***aesc.,*** hyos., plb., spig., tab.

MUCOUS, membrane, ailments of - acon., all-c., ant-t., apis, ***arg-n., ars., bell.,*** bor., ***bry.,*** caps., ***cham., dulc.,*** eucal., euph., hep., hydr., ip., kali-bi., ***merc., nux-v.,*** phos., ***puls.,*** rumx., sabad., sang., senec., seneg., squil., ***stann., sulph.,*** syph., ter., thuj.
blood oozes from - ars-h.
corrugated - carb-ac.
dark - aesc., bapt., carb-v., ham., lach., merc-i-r., mez., phos.
discolored, some places blue, others pale, covered with tough mucus which lies in brown crusts on lips - ars.
dryness - alum., ***bell.,*** bry., caust., kali-c., nux-m., sang., stict.
excoriation, menses agg. - ***kreos.***
palate - caust.
glossy, as if varnished - ***apis,*** nit-ac., ter.
inflamed - canth., colch., dulc., ign., merc-i-r.
milky - kali-i.
pale - acet-ac., ars., chin., chin-s., ***eup-per., ferr.,*** ferr-m., kali-c., mang., ***merc.,*** morph., ***nat-m.,*** phos.
patches - arg-n., lach., merc-i-f., nit-ac., puls.
purple - ***lach.***
raw - arum-t., nux-v.
red, bright - acon., bell., canth.
dusky - ***bapt.,*** lach., morph., ***phyt.***
tumid, with gray based ulcers - kali-chl.
scalded - ham.
shrivelled - bor.
spongy - camph., caps., phyt.
thickened - sul-ac.
ulcerated - arg-n., ars., hydr., kali-i., kreos., merc-c., nit-ac., phyt., sil., sul-ac.
vesicles - apis, bor., canth., carb-v.
white, in children - arg-n., bor., caust., kali-c., merc., nat-c., psor., sul-ac.

MUCOUS, membrane
wrinkled - ars., elaps, merc.
yellowish gray - **NIT-AC.**

NOSODITIES - iod., lyss., mag-c., merc-i-r., phos., stront.
bleeding and burning when touched - mag-c.
nodosities, gums - berb., caust., nat-s., ph-ac., plb., ***staph.***
nodosities, lips - bell., caust., ***con., sep.,*** sil., sulph.
upper - ars.
nodosities, palate - ***asaf.,*** mang.

NUMBNESS - ***acon.,*** ambr., bar-c., ***bov.,*** carb-s., colch., indg., jatr., ***kali-br.,*** kali-c., kali-i., lyc., mag-c., mag-m., mag-s., nat-p., nat-s., nit-ac., stram., ther.
headache, with - nit-ac.
menses, during - mag-m.
morning - bar-c., bov., kali-i., stront.
on waking - ambr., kali-i., mag-c.
one-sided - nat-m.
numbness, gums - ***acon., apis,*** ign.
numbness, lips - ***acon.,*** ambr., calc., caust., cic., crot-c., ***crot-h.,*** echi., glon., lath., ***nat-m.,*** olnd., phos., plat.
lower - calc., ***glon.***
morning on waking - ambr.
upper - cycl., olnd., phos.
numbness, palate - bapt., bar-c., verat.
morning on waking - mag-c.

ODOR, (see Breath, odor)

OPEN - ail., am-c., ant-t., apis, arum-t., **BAR-C.,** bar-m., bell., brom., ***calad.,*** camph., carb-an., caust., colch., cupr., gels., ***hell., hyos.,*** hydr-ac., kali-s., **LACH.,** ***laur.,*** **LYC.,** med., merc., mez., ***morph., mur-ac.,*** naja, nat-c., ***nux-v.,*** **OP.,** ox-ac., ph-ac., ***phos.,*** puls., samb., sil., squil., ***stram.,*** stry., **SULPH.,** ther., tub.
coryza, in - mag-c., mag-m., nat-c., zinc.,
difficult to - anthr., ant-t., ars., ***caust.,*** chin-s., cocc., colch., dig., kali-c., **LACH.,** ***merc-c.,*** mosch., nit-ac., nux-v., ***phos.,*** psor., stry., sul-ac., upa.
dreams, during - merc., rhus-t., samb.
flies open suddenly - carb-an., ign., mag-arct., ***rhus-t.***
involuntarily - ther.
sleep, during - brom., **CALC.,** caust., cham., chim., dulc., elaps, hep., ign., ***lyc.,*** merc., ***nux-v.,*** **OP.,** plan., ***rhus-t.,*** samb., sul-i., vario., zinc.
tension, in anterior throat, from - sil.
wide, after yawning remains - ***ant-t.***
before an attack of epilepsy - ***bufo.***

PAIN, mouth - acon., ail., alum., alumn., apis, ***arum-t.,*** bell., bor., caust., coloc., cop., ferr-i., fl-ac., hep., ip., kali-p., merc., mez., mur-ac., myric., ***nat-m., nit-ac.,*** par., sul-ac., upa., verat.
extending through head and down into neck - lyss.
rinsing agg. - coc-c.
salt water, in - carb-an., verb.
sleep, after - rheum.
pain, gums - act-sp., ***agar.,*** alum., ambr., apis, arg-m., arg-n., ***arn.,*** **ARS.,** ***ars-i.,*** aur., ***bell.,*** bism., ***bov.,*** bry., ***calc.,*** canth., ***carb-an., carb-v., caust., cham.,*** chel., crot-c., ***crot-h., dol.,*** graph., ***ham., hep.,*** hyos., iod., kali-br., kali-i., kali-n., ***lach.,*** lyc., ***lyss.,*** **MERC.,** merc-c., phos., plb., ruta., sep., ***sil.,*** spong., **STAPH.,** zinc.
chewing, while - arn., lach., spong., zinc.
chewing, impossible - zinc.
cold, air agg. - hyos., ***mez.,*** phos., ***sil.***
cold, drink, agg. - sars., staph., sulph.
amel. - bov., laur.
extraction of teeth, after - canth., fl-ac., ***hecla.,*** hyos., ***hyper.,*** **NUX-V.**
morning - brom.
night, preventing sleep - dol.
pulsating - arn., bell., calc., daph., sep.
salty food, from - carb-v.
scratched, when - cimx.
spots, in - aur-m., ox-ac.
tobacco, smoking, from - sars.
tooth extraction, after - arn., calen., sep.
touched, when - arg-m., ars., ars-m., ***bar-c.,*** bell., cast., **HEP.,** iod., **MERC.,** nat-m., ph-ac., ruta, sil., ***staph., ter.***
pain, lips - am-c., anan., ars., ars-m., arum-t., ***bell.,*** bry., cic., cor-r., ***hep., kali-c.,*** mag-s., merc., mez., ***mur-ac., nat-m.,*** plb., psor., ***rhus-t.,*** sep., sil., ***sulph.***
crack, as if - am-c.
excoriated, as if - caust.
lower lip - bry., ign., puls., sep.
neuralgia - apis.
rubbing, after - phos.
splinter, as from a - bov., ign., ***nit-ac.,*** par., ***sep.***
touch agg. - bry., ***hep.,*** merc., mez.
least - cadm-s.
upper lip - ars., bar-c., carb-v., kali-c., sulph., zinc.
pain, palate, in - act-sp., alum., arum-t., aur., bufo, canth., **CARB-V.,** carc., cham., chel., chin-s., coc-c., coff., eupi., hydr., ***kali-bi.,*** kali-c., merc., mez., morph., ***nit-ac., phos.,*** ran-s., ruta, sars., ther., thuj., zinc.
chewing, while - bor., zinc.
eyes and root of nose, to -phos.
plate of teeth, from, worse on touch, eating - alum., bor.
sneezing, on - ictod.
swallowing - caps., coc-c.
talking - coc-c.
velum - zinc.
yawning - zinc.

PASTY - nuph.

PARALYSIS, lips, upper - cadm-s., graph.
paralysis, palate - ***gels., lach., plb., sil.***
sensation, of, left - meny.

PATCHES, syphilitic - arg-n., hydrc., ***kali-i.,*** lach., ***merc., merc-c.,*** merc-i-f., merc-i-r., ***nit-ac.,*** phyt., puls., sang.

PEELING, lips, (see Dryness) - acon., aloe, alum., am-m., arum-t., bell., berb., camph., canth., caps., cham., cob., con., iod., ***kali-c.,*** kali-chl., kreos., ***lac-c.,*** mez., mosch., nat-c., **NAT-M.,** nat-s., nit-ac., ***nux-v.,*** plat., plb., puls., sep., stram., sul-ac., sulph., thuj., thyr.

PERSPIRATION, lips, lower - rheum
upper - acon., coff., kali-bi., kali-c., med., nux-v., rheum, sin-n.

PICKING, of lips - apis, ***arn.,*** ars., **ARUM-T., BRY., CINA,** cob., con., hell., kali-br., ***lach.,*** **NAT-M.,** ***nit-ac., nux-v.,*** ph-ac., rheum, sanic., ***stram.,*** tarent., zinc., zinc-m.
upper - acon., kali-bi.

PINCHING, pain, palate - ant-c., caps.
swallowing, agg. - ant-c., caps.

PRESSING, gums together - phyt., podo.

PRESSING, pain, in gums - arn., aur., hep., nit-ac., rhus-t., ***sil.***
leaden bullet, like a, in lower - arn.
pressing, palate, in - arum-t., aur., caps., **CARB-V.,** cham., iod., meny., ruta., sars., staph., thuj.
swallowing, when -caps.
velum - thuj.

PRICKING, pain, palate - arg-n., calc., caust., cob.

PRICKLING - anac., cedr., colch., fl-ac., manc., nat-p., nit-ac., psor., spig., seneg., ***zinc.***
prickling, gums - arn., lyc.
prickling, palate - arg-n., caust., sang.

PROTRUDING, gums - kreos., lach.

PROUD, flesh - alum.

PUCKERED, sensation, in palate - arn.

PULSATING, gums - ambr., ***arn.,*** bell., ***calc.,*** daph., kali-n., mag-m., merc., phos., puls., ***sep.,*** staph., ***sulph.,*** thuj.
menses, during - **SEP.**
pulsating, palate - glon., rhus-t.

PULSATION, lips - berb.

PURPURA - ***crot-h., lach., phos., psor.,*** ter.

PUSTULES, gums - aur., calc., ***carb-an., carb-v.,*** nat-s., petr., puls.
near diseased molar - aloe.

PUTRID, gums - am-c., cist., ***nat-m.,*** nux-v.

PUTS, children put everything in mouth - ***sulph.***

QUIVERING, lips - ars., berb., ***carb-v.,*** cast., crot-h., lact.
upper - ***carb-v.,*** nat-c.

RANULA - **AMBR., CALC.,** ***canth.,*** cham., fl-ac., hippoz., lac-c., ***lach., merc., mez., nat-m., nit-ac., plb.,*** psor., sac-alb., ***staph.,*** syph., ***thuj.,*** verat.
gelatinous - mez., nit-ac., staph.
bluish-red - ***thuj.***
periodic - chr-ac., lyss.

RASPING - ambr., asar.
eating solids, while - ph-ac.
rasping, palate - aphis., carb-v., mez., mur-ac., ran-s.

RATTLING, in - lac-c.

RECEDING, gums, from teeth - ***am-c., ant-c.,*** arg-m., ***arg-n., aur-m-n., bapt.,*** bar-c., bov., brom., bufo, caps., ***calc., camph., carb-s.,*** **CARB-V.,** caust., ***cist.,*** colch., cupr., ***dulc.,*** gran., ***graph.,*** hep., ***iod., kali-c., kali-i.,*** **KALI-P.,** ***kreos.,*** lac-c., lach., **MERC.,** ***merc-c.,*** mez., nat-c., ***nat-s.,*** nit-ac., ***par., ph-ac., phos.,*** psor., rhus-t., plb., sep., **SIL.,** ***staph., sulph.,*** ter., ***zinc.***
bleed easily - ant-c., **CARB-V.,** ***phos.***

RINGWORM - nat-m., ran-s., sanic., tarax., tub.

ROUGHNESS - am-c., berb., bov., calc., carb-an., carb-v., caust., cina, cycl., dig., ip., lyc., ***nat-s.,*** phos., sep., sulph.
roughness, palate - ang., ant-c., apis, ars., ***calc.,*** **CARD-M.,** cina, dig., ***dros.,*** guare., hyos., iris, mag-c., mez., naja, phos., sep., squil., staph., stram., thuj.
forenoon - phos.

SALIVA, (see Salivation)
acrid - agar., am-c., ars., arum-t., asaf., asar., bor., daph., hydr., ign., ***kali-chl.,*** kalm., kreos., lac-c., lact., lob., manc., ***merc.,*** merc-c., ***merc-i-f.,*** mosch., ***nit-ac.,*** ph-ac., plb., sabad., sec., stann., staph., sulph., tarax., tax., zinc., zing.
albuminous - am-caust., calad., ***stram.***
alkaline - jab., plb., sin-n.
aromatic - coca.
astringent - caps., merc-c., par., sabad.
bitter - ***ars.,*** bapt., bry., ***chel.,*** coca, kali-bi., kali-s., kalm., lyc., mang., phos., ptel., ***puls.,*** sulph., thuj., ust.
bloody - acon., am-c., arg-m., arn., ars., aspar., bad., ***bell.,*** bry., **BUFO,** calad., camph., canth., carb-s., ***carb-v.,*** cic., clem., **CROT-C.,** ***crot-h., dros.,*** eug., gels., ***hyos.,*** indg., jatr., ***kali-i.,*** **MAG-C.,** ***merc., merc-c., nat-m.,*** **NIT-AC.,** ***nux-v.,*** op., **PHOS.,** ***rhus-t., sec.,*** staph., stram., ***sulph.,*** thuj., vip., zinc.
menses, before - ***nat-m.***
morning - nit-ac.
sleep, during - rhus-t.
sweet, with - kali-i.
taste, disgusting, with - kali-i.
bluish - plb.
bluish, white - carb-ac.
brassy - kali-chl.
brownish - bell., bism., crot-c., plan.
burning - manc.
clammy - arg-m., bell., berb., camph., cann-s., eug., lob.
cool - asar., bor., chen-v., cist., merc-c., phyt.
coppery - merc., ran-b.
cotton, like - ***berb., nux-m.,*** **PULS.**
dark - merc-d.
dries on palate and lips, becomes tough - lyc.

SALIVA, general

fetid - ars., caps., ***dig.***, ***iod.***, lach., ***manc.***, **MERC.**, merc-d., ***merc-i-f.***, **NIT-AC.**, ***petr.***, phos., zinc.

hot, and - daph., sabad.

foul, water like - phos.

frothy - acon., ***apis***, bell., ***berb.***, brom., ***bry.***, ***bufo***, cann-i., canth., carb-an., caul., cham., cina, cinnb., cocc., ***crot-h.***, cub., ***cupr.***, ***dig.***, dulc., eug., gaul., ***hyos.***, ***ign.***, iod., ***ip.***, kali-bi., kali-m., ***kreos.***, lac-c., lach., lyc., lyss., morph., ***nux-m.***, ol-an., ph-ac., phel., ph-ac., phos., phys., pic-ac., plb., ***puls.***, ran-s., sabin., spig., stram., sulph.

talking, while - nat-c., sabin.

gluey - bad., bell., cimic., cinnb., lach., nux-m.

green - gins., graph., sec.

hot - asar., daph., manc., mosch., sabad., tax.

hot, nausea, during - sabad., tax.

jelly-like - sabad.

metallic, tasting - bism., cedr., ***cham.***, cimx., cimic., ***coc-c.***, jatr., kali-bi., kali-chl., lyc., merc., ***phyt.***, ran-b., thuj., zinc.

musty - kali-bi., led.

offensive - alumn., ars., atro., bry., ***caps.***, ***dig.***, ***dulc.***, ***iod.***, kali-c., ***lach.***, lob., ***manc.***, **MERC.**, ***merc-c.***, ***merc-i-r.***, **NAT-AC.**, ***petr.***, plb., valer.

morning - glon., petr.

night - merc.

oily - aesc., cub.

onions, odor of - kali-i.

reddish - sabin., sul-ac.

ropy - coc-c., ferr., ***iris***, **KALI-BI.**, lach., lyss., phyt., sabad., sanic., sulph.

saltish - am-c., ang., ***ant-c.***, ***carb-an.***, colch., **CYCL.**, dig., elaps, ***euph.***, ***hyos.***, kali-bi., ***kali-i.***, kali-p., lac-ac., ***lyc.***, mag-m., ***merc.***, ***merc-c.***, mez., nat-c., ***nat-m.***, ***phos.***, rhus-t., ***sep.***, sin-a., stram., ***sulph.***, tax., verat., verb.

collects in mouth - verb.

left - euph.

morning - rhus-t., sulph., sul-ac.

watery - verb.

scanty - arn., ars., asaf., aspar., ***bell.***, berb., calad., coca, cycl., hyos., piloc., kali-bi., ***merc-c.***, ***nux-m.***, nux-v., op., petr., phos., plb., spong., stram., sulph., tax., thea., ***verat.***

sharp, taste - ph-ac.

slimy - bell., ***camph.***, glon., lach., ***merc.***, petr., plb., rhus-t., sars.

snow-white - ol-an.

snowy - ol-an.

soapy - berb., bry., dulc., ***merc.***, ph-ac., phos.

soapy, morning - apis.

sour - agar., alum., ang., atro., ***calc.***, ***calc-p.***, carb-s., con., crot-t., hydr., **IGN.**, kali-bi., ***kali-chl.***, kreos., lact., laur., lob., lyc., manc., merc., nat-c., nat-m., nat-s., par., petr., ph-ac., phos., plb., podo., sec., stann., staph., ***sulph.***, tarax., tax., upa., uran-n., zing.

spoiled taste - bell.

SALIVA, general

suppressed - bell., cahin., cann-s., merc-c., op., phyt., stram.

teething children, in - kali-br.

swallowing, impossible - spig.

sweet - ***all-s.***, alum., alumn., aspar., aur., ***canth.***, ***carb-an.***, **CHAM.**, chin., cop., ***cupr.***, ***dig.***, hyos., iris76, ***kali-i.***, lob., nicc., nit-ac., pic-ac., ***phos.***, ***plb.***, **PULS.**, ***sabad.***, sep., sul-ac., syph., thuj.

disgustingly - canth.

meals, after - all-s.

night - ***sulph.***

thick - anan., ***ars.***, bell., bism., cahin., calad., cann-i., carb-ac., cedr., cimic., cocc., crot-c., kali-p., ***nux-m.***, op., phyt., rhus-t., rhus-v., tax.

thick, morning - glon.

thin - jatr., lyss., manc.

viscid - acon., acet-ac., agn., am-br., anag., anan., apis, arg-m., ***ars.***, asar., bapt., bell., ***berb.***, calc., camph., cann-s., caps., carb-s., carb-v., **CHEL.**, cimic., cinnb., con., ***crot-c.***, ***cupr.***, cycl., dulc., elaps, eug., fl-ac., ign., iris, jatr., **KALI-BI.**, kali-c., kali-i., lac-c., **LACH.**, lachn., lob., **LYSS.**, med., **MERC.**, **MERC-C.**, merl., nat-a., nat-c., nit-ac., ***nux-m.***, ph-ac., phos., ***phyt.***, pic-ac., ***puls.***, seneg., sep., spig., ***stram.***, sul-ac., tarax., verat.

drawing out in strings - agn.

dribbling - stram.

drinking, after beer, lemonade, orangeade - **SIL.**

morning - glon.

nap, after - euph.

night - merc.

watery - am-c., asar., aur-m., calc., calc-ar., camph., carb-an., cob., ***colch.***, coloc., ***cycl.***, dig., dros., hell., iod., ip., jatr., kreos., led., lob., lyss., mag-m., manc., ***merc.***, nat-m., ox-ac., phos., puls., ***sul-ac.***, thea.

white - ars., bell., calad., cann-i., ip., ol-an., ran-b., sabin., spig.

white, bluish - carb-ac.

yellow - cycl., ***gels.***, lyc., lyss., ***manc.***, merc., ***merc-c.***, ***phyt.***, rhus-t., sec., ***spig.***

blood, as from - ***gels.***

SALIVATION, (see Saliva) - acet-ac., acon., act-sp., aesc., aeth., agar., alet., all-s., aloe, ***alum.***, alumn., ambr., **AM-C.**, am-m., ***anac.***, anag., anan., ang., ant-c., ant-t., anthr., aphis., apis, apoc., arg-m., arg-n., arn., ars., ars-h., ***ars-i.***, ars-m., arum-m., **ARUM-T.**, arund., asaf., ***asar.***, aspar., aster., ***aur.***, ***aur-m.***, bapt., **BAR-C.**, ***bar-m.***, ***bell.***, bism., **BOR.**, bov., ***brom.***, bry., bufo, cadm-s., cahin., calad., ***calc.***, ***calc-ac.***, ***calc-p.***, calc-s., ***camph.***, ***canth.***, ***caps.***, carb-ac., carb-an., carb-s., ***carb-v.***, card-m., ***caust.***, ***cham.***, ***chel.***, ***chin.***, chin-a., chlor., ***cic.***, cimic., cina, ***cinnb.***, cinnam., ***clem.***, cob., ***coc-c.***, ***colch.***, coloc., con., cop., croc., ***crot-c.***, crot-t., ***cupr.***, cupr-ar., cycl., daph., dig., ***dros.***, ***dulc.***, eug., euph., eup-pur., ferr., ferr-ar., ferr-i., ***ferr-ma.***, ***ferr-p.***, **FL-AC.**, ***gamb.***, ***glon.***, ***gran.***, ***graph.***, grat., ***hell.***, helon., ***hep.***, hippoz.,

SALIVATION, general - hydr-ac., hyos., ***ign.***, **IOD.**, **IP.**, ***iris***, jab., jatr., kali-ar., kali-bi., kali-br., **KALI-C.**, ***kali-chl.***, ***kali-i.***, kali-n., kali-p., kali-s., kalm., ***kreos.***, lac-ac., ***lac-c.***, ***lach.***, lachn., ***lact.***, laur., led., lil-t., lob., ***lyc.***, **LYSS.**, mag-m., ***manc.***, mang., med., meny., **MERC.**, **MERC-C.**, ***merc-cy.***, ***merc-d.***, **MERC-I-R.**, mez., ***mur-ac.***, ***naja***, ***nat-c.***, **NAT-M.**, nat-p., ***nat-s.***, nicc., **NIT-AC.**, ***nux-m.***, **NUX-V.**, oena., ***ol-an.***, op., ***ox-ac.***, par., ***petr.***, phel., ***phos.***, phys., ***phyt.***, plan., plat., ***plb.***, ***podo.***, polyg., ptel., ***puls.***, ran-b., ran-s., rat., rhod., rhus-t., ruta., sabad., sang., sars., sec., ***seneg.***, ***sep.***, ***sil.***, sin-n., spig., spong., squil., stann., staph., ***stram.***, ***sulph.***, ***sul-ac.***, **SYPH.**, ***tab.***, tarax., tell., teucr., thea., thuj., uran., ust., **VERAT.**, verb., viol-t., ***zinc.***

afternoon - alum., grat., mag-c., mag-m., phos.

alternating, with dry mouth - calc., carb-v., con., ign., phos., verat.

angina, in - bar-m.

anterior part - mez.

aphthae, in - ***hell.***, **MERC.**, **MERC-C.**, nat-m.

asthma, in - ***carb-v.***

cardialgia, in - puls.

children, in - camph.

chill, before - ip., rhus-t.

chill, during - asaf., ***caps.***, cham.

concomitant symptom, as a - lob., ***merc.***

convulsions, with - bar-m., caust., ***oena.***

copious, abscess in throat, with - pyrog.

coryza, during - **ARUND.**, calc-p., cupr-ac., kali-i.

cough, with - ambr., ***am-m.***, ars., bell., carb-v., cycl., lach., merc., mez., nat-m., spig., staph., thuj., verat.

crawling, in throat, from - am-m., carb-v.

dentition, in - hell., ***merc.***, ***nat-m.***, **SIL.**

diarrhea, with - rheum

diphtheria, with - lac-c.

dribbling - stram.

dryness, of mouth, with salivation - acon.

sensation of dryness, with salivation - alum., aral., asaf., calad., calc., chin., colch., kali-c., laur., lyc., mag-m., ***merc.***, nat-m., nux-v., plb., rhod., sep., spig.

dyspnea, with - lob.

eat, on begining to - sulph.

eating, after - ***all-s.***, cast-eq., ***caust.***, cham., lyc., kali-p., mag-c., ***nat-s.***, ***nux-v.***, petr., ***rhus-t.***, staph., sulph.

evening - bry., lyc., ox-ac., sep., sulph.

evening, in bed - alum., nat-m.

expectoration, frequent - am-c., cadm-s., dig., graph., ***lyss.***, ***puls.***, rhus-t., sabad., spig.

fetid breath, with - ***kali-br.***

fever, during - arund., ***dros.***, hell., hep., ***nit-ac.***, ***stram.***, ***sulph.***

forenoon - calc.

forepart - lyc., plb.

side, right of - hep.

gushes, in, colic, with - led.

suddenly - ign., nat-m.

SALIVATION, general

headache, during - am-c., epip., hipp., ign., irid., iris, kali-bi., mang., **MERC.**, ***nat-s.***, op., phos., sep., verat.

before - ***fl-ac.***

heat, during, all over - ***cic.***

hiccough, with - lob.

hunger, with - lob.

lying, while - ip., ptel., rhus-t., trif-r.

measles, during - nat-m.

menopause, during - piloc.

menses, during - agar., eupi., kali-n., mag-c., ***merc.***, ***nux-m.***, phyt., ***puls.***

after - ***cedr.***

before - ***puls.***, pulx.

mental, work, during - merc., ***merc-c.***, nit-ac.

mercury, from - alumn., anan., asaf., bell., **CHIN.**, ***cupr.***, dig., dulc., ***hep.***, ***iris***, kali-chl., **IOD.**, lach., ***nat-m.***, ***nit-ac.***, ***phyt.***, ***sulph.***

morning - alum., aur., **GRAPH.**, iod., lac-ac., ***lyc.***, mag-c., mag-m., merc-i-f., plat., rhus-t., sars., stann., ***sulph.***, verat.

bed, in - rhus-t.

sleep, during - bar-c.

waking, on - stann.

nausea, with - **CAMPH.**, carb-s., ***chin.***, ***ip.***, ***lach.***, ***lob.***, ***sulph.***, verat.

causes nausea - colch.

taste, with - sulph.

night - ***arg-n.***, bar-c., canth., cench., crot-h., culx., dig., gran., ign., mag-arct., med., **MERC.**, merc-c., ***nat-m.***, nux-v., phos., ptel., puls., ***rhus-t.***, ruta, sulph., syph., verat.

1 a.m. - ***merc.***

lying down agg. - bell.

pains, during - cocc., epip., gran., helon., kali-c., led., mang., merc., ***phos.***, plan., rheum, sulph.

paralysis, after - agar., op., zinc.

paralysis, in - mang.

periodical - ***culx.***

pregnancy, during - acet-ac., ant-t., ars., ***coff.***, **GOSS.**, ***gran.***, ***helon.***, ***iod.***, ip., iris, ***piloc.***, ***kali-i.***, **KREOS.**, lac-ac., ***lac-c.***, lob., ***merc.***, ***nat-m.***, nit-ac., piloc., sep., sulph., zinc-s.

pressure on larynx, as if with - tarax.

profuse, with constant desire to spit - bry., cadm-s., coc-c., graph., grat., lac-c., ***lyss.***, ***puls.***

headache, during - cinnb., epip.

rage, during - canth.

retching, with - lob.

scarlatina, during - **ARUM-T.**, caps., **LACH.**, ***merc.***, ***sulph.***

shuddering, with - arg-m., arg-n., euph.

siesta, after - zinc.

sleep, during - ***arn.***, ***aur.***, ***bar-c.***, carb-an., cham., chin-b., cocc-s., ***culx.***, cupr., dios., ign., ***ip.***, ***kali-c.***, lac-ac., ***lac-c.***, lach., ***lyc.***, med., **MERC.**, nit-ac., ***phos.***, ***puls.***, rheum, ***rhus-t.***, sul-ac., ***sulph.***, ***syph.***

preventing - ign.

smoking, while - bry., kali-bi., merc., rhus-t., sep.

SALIVATION, general
sneezing, with - fl-ac.
speaking, while, constantly - graph., lach.
stomach, disorders, with - ars.
pains, during - gran.
stool, during - colch., ***rheum.***
after - crot-t., mag-m.
before - ***fl-ac.***
stooping - **GRAPH.,** nux-v.
stroke, in - ***anac.,*** ant-c., **NUX-V.**
sudden attacks - carb-v., dig., ign., nat-m.
swallow, must - ip., merc.
swelling of salivary glands, with - trif-p.
talking, while - graph., ***iris, lach.,*** mang., nat-c., sabin.
toothache, during - bar-c., bell., calc., caust., **CHAM.,** daph., ***dulc.,*** graph., kali-m., mag-c., **MERC.,** nat-m., rheum, sep.
walking, while - caust., petr.

SALTY, lips - merc., ***nat-m.,*** sulph.

SCABS, gangrenous, gums - chin., sulph.

SCORBUTIC, gums - all-s., alum., ***alumn., am-c., anan., ant-c.,*** ant-t., arn., **ARS.,** ***ars-i.,*** **ASTAC.,** ***aur-m-n.,*** bapt., ***bov., brom., calc., camph.,*** canth., ***carb-an., carb-s.,*** **CARB-V.,** chin-s., chr-ac., ***cist.,*** coch., ***dulc.,*** echi., ***hep., iod., kali-c.,*** **KALI-CHL.,** ***kali-i., kali-n.,*** **KALI-P., KREOS.,** lac-ac., lach., ***lyc.,*** **MERC., MUR-AC.,** ***nat-m., nit-ac., nux-m., nux-v., ph-ac., phos.,*** phyt., ***psor.,*** sac-alb., sep., ***staph., sulph.,*** sul-ac., ***ter.,*** thuj., ***zinc.***
salt eaters, in - coch., phos.

SCRAPING - arn., dig., gymn., lyc.
scraping, palate - cact., ***camph.,*** chin., coc-c., coloc., dig., ***dros.,*** fago., hyos., lyss., meph., ***mez.,*** phos., staph., ran-b.
scraping, pain, palate - camph., hell., meph.

SCRATCHING - alum., caust., nit-ac., phos.
scratching, palate - ambr., ant-c., aphis., ars., bell., camph., coloc., hell., mez., squil., staph.

SENSITIVE - ***apis, coc-c.,*** ip., lyc., naja, **PHYT.,** sin-n., sul-ac.
air, to - agar.
food and drink unbearable - sin-n.
touch, to - **HEP.,** ***nat-s.***
sensitive, lips - hep., kali-c., mag-c., merc., nat-m.

SHARP, pain - merc.
sharp, gums - aeth., ang., ars., asar., ***calc.,*** camph., con., graph., kali-c., lyc., nit-ac., petr., ***puls.,*** sars., sep., stront-c.
extending to left temple - am-m.
left, lower - am-m.
morning - ars.
right, upper - am-c.
touch, on - petr.
sharp, lips - ant-c., asaf., bell., bov., caust., clem., kali-c., nat-c., con., nit-ac., ph-ac., phos., sabad., sep., spong., stann., staph., sulph., thuj., zinc.
sharp, lips
extending to face, on touch - staph.
upper - phos.
extending to ear - nat-m.
sharp, palate - ***aesc.,*** bar-c., ***calc., camph.,*** caust., cob., coc-c., ign., kali-c., lach., mag-m., nit-ac., ph-ac., ran-s., sabad., ***staph.,*** stram., zinc.
dinner, after - phos.
extending to, brain - staph.
to, chin - bov.
to, ear - cob., ***ign.***
to, right parotid gland -agar.
posterior - dig.
swallowing, when -meny.
velum, in - coloc., sil.

SHINY, lips - cub.

SHRIVELLED, gums - carb-v., merc., par.
shrivelled, lips - am-m., ant-t., chim., mang.
shrivelled, palate - arn., bor., cycl.

SKIN, loose on palate - phys.

SLIMY, lips - kali-i., stram., zinc.

SMACKING, of lips - aml-n.

SOFT, palate - merc.
rim - merc-i-f.
ulcer, eating uvula - hep.

SOFTENING, gums - arg-m., cupr., iod., **KREOS., MERC.,** ph-ac., phos., plb., ***ter.***

SORDES, under left cheek - carb-ac.
sordes, on the lips - **ARS.,** ***colch., hyos., phos.,*** **STRAM.**

SORE, pain - abrot., agar., ail., aloe, alum., am-c., apis, ***ars.,*** ars-m., **ARUM-T.,** asaf., bell., bism., ***calc.,*** carb-ac., caust., chin., chlor., cinnb., coc-c., con., ***crot-h.,*** cupr., dig., dios., glon., ***helon., hep.,*** hyos., ***ign.,*** ip., kali-ar., kali-c., kali-p., ***lac-ac., lach.,*** lachn., lyc., lyss., mag-c., mag-s., ***manc.,*** mang., med., **MERC., MERC-C.,** merc-i-r., ***merc-sul.,*** naja, nat-a., nat-c., **NAT-M.,** ***nit-ac.,*** nux-v., ox-ac., petr., ph-ac., **PHOS.,** plb., podo., rhus-v., ***sabad.,*** samb., sec., sin-n., stram., verat.
cheek, inside of - bell., carb-ac.
chewing - nat-c.
right side, spot - calc-p.
eating, while - alum.
menses, before - phos.
morning - arum-t., dios., mang.
nursing, during - hydr., mur-ac., sin-a.
pregnancy, during - hydr., sin-a.
spot inside right cheek - calc-p.
spots - phos.
sore, gums - agar., alum., ambr., am-c., arg-m., ***arg-n., arn.,*** **ARS.,** ars-m., arund., asaf., ***aur.,*** aur-m., bapt., bar-c., bar-m., bell., berb., bism., brom., bry., calc., calc-s., ***caps.,*** carb-an., **CARB-V.,** ***caust., cham., chin-a.,*** clem., cob., cupr-ar., dig., dios., ***dol.,*** gamb., gels., ***glon., graph., ham., hep., iod., kali-bi.,*** kali-chl., kali-i., lach., mag-c., **MERC.,** ***merc-c.,*** mur-ac., ***myric.,*** naja,

sore, gums - ***nat-a., nat-m., nit-ac.,*** nux-v., petr., ph-ac., ***phos.,*** plb., polyg., ptel., ***puls.,*** rhod., rhus-t., ruta., sars., ***sep.,*** **SIL.,** sin-n., ***staph.,*** ter., thuj., ***zinc.***
between gums and cheek - rhod.
chewing, while - **CARB-V.,** hyos., ***nit-ac.,*** petr., sil.
cold, air, agg. - cob.
water agg. - sil.
water agg., and warmth agg. - **NAT-M.**
dentition, during - berb., dol.
eating, while - aur., ***clem.,*** mag-c., ***phos.,*** spong., zinc.
inner side of gums - graph.
morning - caust.
touch, on - aur., graph., ph-ac.

sore, lips - ***arum-t.,*** bor., calc., ill., lyc., mur-ac., ***nat-m., rhus-t., rhus-v.,*** sep.
lower lip - ***arum-t.,*** bor., calc., euph., ill., mez., nat-m., ***rhus-t., rhus-v.,*** sep.

sore, palate - agar., all-c., alum., apis, ***arum-t.,*** benz-ac., brom., calc-s., caps., carc., ***caust.,*** cinnb., eupi., ferr-s., gamb., glon., graph., ign., iris, kali-bi., ***lac-c.,*** lach., laur., ***mang., mez.,*** mur-ac., nat-m., nat-s., **NIT-AC.,** ***nux-v.,*** par., phos., ***phyt.,*** plb., sang., sil., thuj.
bread, eating amel. - mang.
extending to ear - thuj.
menses, during - nat-s.
morning - mang.
spots -***caust.,*** mur-ac.
swallowing, saliva - thuj.
touched, when - iris, merc., nat-s.
velum -ph-ac., rhus-t., ruta.
walking, on - kali-bi.

SPEECH, (see Mind, Speech)
blundering - lach.
broken - camph.
crying, hoarse like a child - cupr.
difficult - acon., aesc., ***agar.,*** am-c., ***anac.,*** anan., ant-t., arg-n., ars., ars-i., aster., aur., ***bapt.,*** bar-c., bar-m., **BELL.,** bufo, cact., cadm-s., ***calc.,*** calc-s., ***camph.,*** cann-s., carb-an., ***carb-s., carb-v., caust.,*** cedr., ***cench.,*** chel., chin., chlor., ***cic.,*** cimic., ***cocc.,*** colch., ***con.,*** cop., **CROT-C.,** ***crot-h.,*** crot-t., ***cupr.,*** cycl., ***dig., dulc., euphr.,*** **GELS.,** ***glon., graph.,*** hep., hippoz., ***hyos., kali-br.,*** lac-c., **LACH.,** ***laur., lyc.,*** lyss., ***mag-p., merc., mez.,*** morph., mosch., ***mur-ac., nat-c.,*** **NAT-M.,** nat-p., nicc., ***nux-m.,*** nux-v., **OP.,** ph-ac., ***phos., plb.,*** ruta., sec., sel., seneg., sep., sil., ***spong.,*** **STANN., STRAM.,** stry., sulph., sul-ac., tab.
breath, from want of - mez.
chorea, from - ***agar.,*** art-v., asaf., ***bufo,*** **CAUST.,** cic., ***cupr., cupr-ac., mag-p., morph.,*** mygal., sep., ***stram.,*** tarent.
eating, after - am-c.
enlarged tonsils, from (see Throat)
heaviness, of tongue - ***anac., ars., carb-v.,*** **CROT-C., GELS.,** ***glon., lach., mag-p., nat-c.,*** nicc.

SPEECH, general
difficult,
inarticulate sounds - anac., bell., ***dulc.,*** hyos.
menses, during - ***cedr.***
names, cannot pronounce - chin-s.
nasal - bar-m., bell., lach., ph-ac.
painful - am-c.
saliva, from viscid - arg-m.
spasm in throat, from - cupr., lyss., stry.
tongue, from - ***agar.,*** arg-n., cypr., lyc., ***ruta.,*** sec., ***stram.***
swelling, of tongue, from - anan., ant-t., bapt., **DULC.,** gels., morph.
typhoid, in - agar., ***ars., lach.***
weakness, from - am-c., manc.
chest, of - ***stann.***
organs of speech - ***glon., nat-m.***
throat, of - **STANN.**
words, can utter single, with great exertion - art-v., cocc., ***lach., stram.***
drawing - carb-an., tab.
faltering, tongue - nit-ac., sulph.
high - lach.
indistinct - apis, barc., bry., calc., caust., ***cocc., glon., lyc.,*** nit-ac., sec., verat.
dryness of mouth, from - lyc.
of throat, from - bry., seneg.
morning - lyc.
lisping - ***acon., ars.,*** con., ***lach.,*** nat-c., nux-v., ***verat.***
stammering, stuttering - ***acon., aesc-g.,*** agar., agar-ph., anac., anan., anh., arg-n., ars., ars-i., atro., bar-c., **BELL.,** benz-n., ***both., bov., bufo, cann-i., cann-s., carb-s.,*** carc., **CAUST.,** cer-s., cham., cic., cocc., con., ***cupr.,*** dig., dulc., dys-co., ***euphr.,*** gels., ***glon.,*** hell., hyos., ***ign.,*** iod., ***kali-br.,*** kali-cy., lac-c., ***lach.,*** laur., lyc., ***mag-c., mag-p.,*** **MERC.,** mygal., naja, nat-a., ***nat-c.,*** nat-m., nux-m., **NUX-V.,** olnd., ***op., phos., plat.,*** plb., ruta, ***sec., sel.,*** sep., ***spig.,*** **STRAM.,** sulfon., ***sulph.,*** thuj., verat., vip.
certain letters, for - lach.
children, in - bov., caust., merc., nat-m.
dentition, during - stram.
excitement - ***agar., caust.,*** dig., dys-co.
exerts himself a long time before he can utter a word - **STRAM.**
fast, talking, when - lac-c.
last, words of the sentence - lyc.
letters, for certain - lach.
loud, every word - hyos.
quick and stammering - merc.
roll out tumbling over each other - hep.
sex, after - ***cedr.***
suddenly - mag-c.
strangers, with - dig., staph.
typhoid, in - agar., ***ars., lach.***
vexation, from - ***caust.***
subdued and quick - tab.
swallows, his words - ***cic.,*** staph.
thick - aesc-g., agar., bapt., caust., **CROT-C.,** dulc., **GELS.,** ***glon.,*** **LACH.,** ***mag-p., nat-c., nat-m.,*** **NUX-V.,** ***plat.,*** syph., tub., ***verat-v.***

SPEECH, general
  uncertain - camph.
  unintelligible - ars., art-v., asaf., ***bell.,*** bufo, chel., ***fl-ac., hyos.,*** lyc., merc., naja, ***ph-ac.,*** rhus-t., sil., **STRAM.,** thuj., verat., zinc.
  wanting, (see Mind, Aphasia) - alum., ant-t., ***apis, arg-n., ars., bar-c.,*** **BELL.,** both., ***calc., caust.,*** chen-a., chin., cimic., ***cic.,*** colch., ***con., crot-c., crot-h.,*** cupr., ***glon.,*** hep., hydr-ac., ***hyos., kali-br., kali-chl.,*** kali-cy., kali-n., kali-p., ***lach., laur.,*** lyc., ***mag-c.merc.,*** mosch., **NIT-AC.,** ***nux-m., nux-v.,*** oena., olnd., onos., op., ***plb., stram.,*** stry., thuj., ***verat.,*** zinc.
    amnesia, from - kali-br., plb.
    cannot speak a syllable though she makes the effort - calc., cimic.
    fevers, like in typhus - apis, ars., op., ***stram.***
    fright, after - hyos.
    pain, stomach - laur.
    paralysis of organs, from - ***anac., cadm-s.,*** canth., **CAUST.,** ***crot-c.,*** crot-h., ***gels., glon., mur-ac.,*** staph.
    soreness of lacerated tongue, from - hyper.
    spasms in throat, from - cupr.
    stroke, after - ***bar-c.,*** caust., crot-c., ***crot-h., ip., laur.,*** **NUX-V.**
    typhus, in - agar., ***apis, ars., op.,*** **STRONT-C.**
    uterine displacement - ***nit-ac.***

SPITTING, constantly - cadm-s., cadm-met., calc., graph., grat., hydr-ac., laur., lyss., mag-m., ***mer-c.,*** mez., ***nat-m., nit-ac.,*** petr., rhus-t., sabad., sang., stram.
    foamy - phel.
    nausea, with - bar-ac.
    night - **NAT-M.**
    spasmodic - **LYSS.**

SPLINTER, like a - ***nit-ac.,*** upa.
  splinter, lips, as from a - bov., ign., **NIT-AC.,** phos., sep.

SPONGY, gums - ***alumn.,*** ant-t., ars., bry., ***canth., caps., carb-v.,*** chlol., cupr., ***dulc.,*** graph., ***ham.,*** kali-br., ***kali-chl.,*** **KALI-P., KREOS., LACH., MERC., MERC-C.,** myric., plb., ***rob., sang., staph., ter.,*** zinc.
  sticky, viscid - bell., ***berb.,*** calad., kali-c., mur-ac., ***nat-m.,*** phos., plat., ruta., squil., ***verat.***
    eating, amel. - berb.
    feverish, feeling - ***gels.***
    morning - ***berb., crot-h.,*** graph., phos., plat., ***sabad.,*** sulph.

STICKY, lips - merc-i-r., nux-m., zinc.

STIFF, lips, muscles - ***aml-n.,*** **APIS,** crot-h., ***euphr.,*** kalm., ***lach.***
    upper - ***euphr.***
  stiff, palate - crot-h., grat., nat-m.

STINGING, pain, lips - agar., am-m., ant-c., ***apis,*** ars., asaf., caust., ***graph.,*** kali-c., merc., nit-ac., petr., ph-ac., phos., sil., stann., staph., sulph., thuj.
    upper - am-m.

STOMATITIS, ulcerative - ***alum., ars., arund., asar.,*** **ASTAC.,** ***bapt.,*** bor., ***calc., canth., caps.,*** carb-ac., ***carb-v.,*** chin., ***chlol., crot-h.,*** dig., ***dulc., ferr.,*** hell., hep., hyos., iod., ***kali-bi., kali-chl.,*** **KALI-I.,** lac-ac., ***lach.,*** **MERC.,** ***merc-c.,*** mill., mur-ac., myric., ***nat-m.,*** nit-ac., **NUX-V.,** ph-ac., ***podo., sep., sil., staph.,*** **SULPH.,** ***sul-ac.,*** tril.
    cold, after a - dulc.

SUBLINGUAL, gland - ***canth.,*** kalm., **MERC.,** psor.
    inflammation - kalm., **MERC.,** psor.
    swelling - ***canth.,*** kalm., **MERC.,** psor.

SUPPURATION, gums - am-c., canth., carb-an., carb-v., caust., **HEP.,** lach., **MERC.,** mez., nat-s., petr., ***phos.,*** puls., **SIL.**

SWELLING - ***acon., am-c., anthr.,*** ant-t., ***bell.,*** bism., calad., calc., calc-s., camph., canth., carb-ac., carb-an., carb-v., ***caust.,*** cop., dulc., glon., ***hydr.,*** ign., **KALI-CHL.,** kali-p., lach., lyc., **MERC.,** ***merc-c.,*** **NIT-AC.,** nux-v., op., par., sep., sil., sul-ac., verat., vesp., vip.
    alternately, and contracting - xan.
    cheeks, inside of - am-c., calc., caust.
      sensation - chin.
    erysipelatous, after extraction of teeth - sil.
    morning, on waking - nit-ac.
    sensation of - am-c., ***camph.,*** samb.
    spasms, before - plb.
  swelling, gums - ***agar.,*** all-s., ***alum.,*** ambr., am-c., am-m., anac., anan., ***apis, arg-n.,*** arn., **ARS., ARS-I.,** arund., aur., ***bar-c.,*** bar-m., bell., bism., **BOR.,** brom., bry., **CALC.,** ***calc-s., camph., caps.,*** canth., ***carb-an.,*** **CARB-S.,** ***carb-v.,*** cast., **CAUST.,** cham., **CHIN.,** ***chin-a., cist.,*** cob., con., ***crot-h.,*** crot-t., daph., ***dol.,*** ferr., ferr-ar., ferr-p., ***gels., glon.,*** **GRAPH.,** ***ham., hep.,*** hydr., ***iod.,*** jug-r., kali-ar., ***kali-bi.,*** kali-br., ***kali-c., kali-i.,*** kali-n., kali-p., kalm., lac-c., **LACH.,** ***lyc.,*** lyss., ***mag-c., mag-m.,*** **MERC., MERC-C.,** ***merc-cy., merc-i-f., merc-i-r., mur-ac.,*** naja, nat-c., **NAT-M.,** nicc., **NIT-AC.,** nux-v., osm., ***petr.,*** phel., ***ph-ac., phos.,*** **PLB.,** puls., rhod., sabad., sabin., sal-ac., sars., **SEP.,** ***sil.,*** sin-n., spig., spong., ***staph., stront-c.,*** **SULPH.,** ***sul-ac.,*** thuj., verat., zinc.
    between gums and, cheeks - rhod.
      and, teeth - nit-ac.
    bluish-red, ecchymosis - con.
      spongy, between lower incisors, begins on left and extends to right, bleeds often - nat-m.
    convulsions, with - kreos., stann.
    decayed tooth, around - anag., bar-c., calc., calc-s., carb-v., cocc., nat-m., phos., sabin.
    extraction of teeth, after - ***arn.,*** sil.

swelling, gums
hard, painful, in socket of a tooth that has been out for years - med.
incisors, above - lyc., nit-ac.
menses, during - ***nit-ac.***
after - phos.
before - bar-c., phos.
instead, of - kali-c.
morning - nat-m.
painful - agar., ambr., aur., bar-c., bell., bor., ***bry.,*** calc., carb-an., crot-t., dol., graph., kali-c., kali-chl., kali-i., lyss., ***mag-m.,*** nux-v., par., petr., phel., ran-s., rhod., sabin., sars., sil., staph., ***sulph.,*** thuj., zinc.
chewing, while - phos., spong.
pale, red - ***bar-c.***
right - cast., ***merc.***
sensation of - am-c., ***cham.,*** chin., puls., spong.
side, inner - ambr., hep., sep.
inner, incisors - nat-m.
inner, upper - dios.
left, lower left, with stitches up to left temple - am-m.
right - aur., bell.
warmth, amel. - ***kali-i.***
white - crot-h., nit-ac., nux-v., sabin.
dirty - kali-n.

swelling, lips - acon., ail., alum., anan., ant-t., **APIS,** arg-m., arg-n., arn., ***ars.,*** **ARUM-T.,** asaf., ***aur., aur-m.,*** bar-c., **BELL.,** ***bov.,*** brach., **BRY.,** cadm-s., calad., ***calc.,*** canth., ***caps., carb-an., carb-v.,*** chin., ***clem., cor-r., crot-h.,*** dig., gels., glon., hell., hep., kali-ar., ***kali-c.,*** kali-chl., kali-p., kali-s., ***kalm., lach.,*** lachn., lyc., ***merc., merc-c.,*** mez., ***nat-c.,*** **NAT-M., NIT-AC.,** ***nux-m.,*** op., ***par.,*** ph-ac., ***phos.,*** phel., plb., ***psor.,*** puls., rhus-t., sang., **SEP.,** ***sil.,*** staph., stram., ***sulph.,*** thuj., tub., urt-u., zinc.
edematous - apis.
inside - dig.
lower - alum., arn., **ASAF.,** bor., calc., ***caust., clem.,*** com., ***kali-bi., kali-c.,*** kali-s., lach., ***lyc., merc-c.,*** mez., ***mur-ac.,*** nat-c., **NAT-M.,** nit-ac., puls., ***sep.,*** sil., stram., ***sulph.***
lower, as if - glon.
morning - lyc.
sense of - lact., olnd.
upper - **APIS,** arg-m., ars., **BAR-C., BELL.,** ***bov., bry.,*** **CALC.,** ***calc-p.,*** canth., ***carb-v.,*** graph., grat., guare., **HEP.,** ***kali-c.,*** kali-p., ***lach., lyc.,*** mang., ***merc.,*** merc-c., merc-i-f., ***mez., nat-c.,*** **NAT-M., NIT-AC.,** phel., ***phos., psor.,*** rhus-t., **STAPH., SULPH.,** ***tub.,*** vinc., zinc.
evening - sulph.
morning - ***calc.,*** grat.
turned up - merc-c.

swelling, palate - aloe, ***apis,*** arg-m., ***arg-n.,*** ars., arum-t., ***bar-c.,*** bar-m., bell., ***calc., carb-an.,*** chin., cimic., coff., crot-t., **LACH.,** ***merc.,*** nat-s., ***nux-v.,*** par., ***phyt.,*** psor., rumx., seneg., ***sil.,*** staph., **SULPH.,** ***sul-ac., zinc.***
arch - bell., berb., ***caust.,*** chin., merc., ***nit-ac.,*** seneg.
suppuration, with - ***bar-c.,*** merc., nux-v., sil., sulph.
sensation of - arg-n., ***arum-t., camph.,*** cycl., glon., ign., nux-v., puls., sulph.
tight, almost painless, size of pigeon's egg - par.
velum - acon., ***aeth.,*** bell., ***calc.,*** carb-v., cimic., coff., ***merc.,*** **MERC-C.,** ***spong., verat.***

TEARING, pain - ***bell.,*** calc., carb-v., lyc.
tearing, gums - aeth., alum., ***ars.,*** berb., calc., canth., ***colch.,*** gamb., ***hyos.,*** kali-c., laur., lyc., ***merc.,*** sabin., **SARS.,** staph., sulph., ***teucr.***
tearing, lips - agar., caust., stann.
lower - mag-c., zinc.
upper - caust., kali-c.
tearing, palate - ambr., lach.
extending, to left ear - ambr.

TENSION, of lips - apis, lachn., spig., sulph.
lower - ph-ac., plan., puls., sep.
upper - apis, **BELL.,** ***hep.,*** mag-c., mur-ac., rhus-t., sabad., spig., thuj.
tension of, lips - apis, hep., lachn., spig., sulph.
tension, palate, in arches of - coc-c.

THICK, lips - bufo, med., mez.

THRUSH (see Aphthous, ulcers) - arum-t., **BOR.,** iod., lac-c., ***kali-chl.,*** **MERC.,** merc-cy., mur-ac., **NAT-M.,** nit-ac., sang., sulph., **SUL-AC.,** syph., thuj.
bleeding easily - **BOR.,** ***lac-c., sul-ac.***
burning - chin-a., ***nat-m.,*** sulph.
children, in - asim., bapt., **BOR.,** casc., kali-br., ***kali-chl.,*** med., **MERC.,** nat-m., ***mur-ac., nux-m., nux-v.,*** plan., sac-alb., sulph., **SUL-AC.,** viol-t.
in, babies - bor., ***bry.,*** calc.
mothers, while nursing - bapt., hydr.
pregnancy, during - kreos.
small and sore - med.

TINGLING, lips - ***acon.,*** apis, arn., echi., ferr-ma., ***nat-m., pic-ac.,*** sabad.
upper - paeon.

TREMBLING, lips - ***agar.,*** aloe, ***arg-n.,*** arn., ***bell.,*** benz-ac., cann-i., crot-h., ***gels.,*** iod., lach., lact., ***nux-v.,*** op., ran-s., ***stram., sulph., ter., zinc.***
lower - ant-c., ant-t., arn., bry., con., gels., plb., ran-s., sulph.
eating, while - arn.
speaking, while - arg-n.
upper - ars., bell., hep., ox-ac.

TUBERCLES, painful, gums - ph-ac., **PLB.**

TUMORS - benz-ac., calc., ***lyc.***, ***nit-ac.***
left side behind last molar - benz-ac.
malignant - calc.
painless - calc., ***nit-ac.***
right lip, inner side - calc.
small - lyc.
spongy - calc.
ulcerated - benz-ac.
tumors, gums, inflamed - canth.
painless, movable, lower gums - nat-s.
size of walnut - ***nit-ac.***, staph.
in place of two bicuspids - **SIL.**
tumor, lips, cystic on - ***con.***, kreos., sep.
cystic on, lower - phos.
tumors, palate, hard - canth., hydr.

TWITCHING, lips - ***agar.***, art-v., bell., ***carb-v.***, ***cham.***, cimic., dulc., ***gels.***, ***ign.***, ip., lact., mygal., nicc., ol-an., op., ran-b., senec., sil., squil., stry., ***sulph.***, tell., **THUJ.**, vip.
convulsions, during - sil.
cold, air, in - dulc.
lower - cann-i., hipp., ind., ***puls.***, ***thuj.***
morning, in bed - plat.
in sleep - ol-an.
sleep, during - anac.
on falling to - **ARS.**
speaking, while - arg-n.
spasmodic - ***agar.***, art-v., cimic., ***gels.***, ***ign.***, mygal., nicc., op., stry.
twitching, up - tell.
upper - ***agar.***, ***ars.***, **CARB-V.**, ***graph.***, hep., nat-c., nicc., plat., ***thuj.***, ***zinc.***

ULCERATIVE, pain, gums - acon., bell., carb-an., graph., ***hep.***, nat-c., ***sil.***
pressing them, on - phel.
ulcerative, palate - am-c., caust., ***rhus-t.***

ULCERS, (see Aphthous) - ***agn.***, ***alum.***, ***anac.***, anan., arum-t., **ARS.**, ***bapt.***, ***bor.***, calc., calc-s., ***canth.***, ***caps.***, carb-an., carb-s., caust., chlor., ***cic.***, cop., corn., ***crot-c.***, crot-h., cupr-s., ***dulc.***, ***fl-ac.***, gamb., gran., ***graph.***, hell., hep., hippoz., ***hydr.***, **IOD.**, ***iris***, jatr., kali-ar., ***kali-bi.***, ***kali-chl.***, **KALI-I.**, **LACH.**, **MERC.**, ***merc-c.***, ***merc-cy.***, ***merc-d.***, mez., **MUR-AC.**, nat-a., ***nat-c.***, ***nat-m.***, ***nat-p.***, **NIT-AC.**, ***nux-m.***, nux-v., op., ox-ac., petr., ***phos.***, ***phyt.***, pic-ac., plb., ***psor.***, rumx., sanic., sin-n., ***staph.***, ***sul-ac.***, tab., ter., thuj., uran., zinc.
base, black - mur-ac.
lardaceous - ant-t., caps., ***hep.***, **MERC.**, **NIT-AC.**, phos., syph.
milky - **KALI-I.**
spongy - ars.
swollen - hell.
biting - nat-m.
bleeding - kreos., merc., sul-ac.
bluish - ars., aur., ***mur-ac.***
burning - alum., ***ars.***, ***caps.***, ***carb-v.***, caust., chin., cic., ***hydr.***, kali-ar., kali-i., ***kreos.***, ***merc.***, ***nat-c.***, nat-m., ph-ac., sep., sin-n.
cold water amel. - dulc.
deep - ***carb-v.***, gamb., merc-d., ***mur-ac.***, sul-ac.
dirty looking - **NIT-AC.**, ***plb.***

ULCERS, general
edges, elevated - hell.
gray - hell.
hard - ***kali-bi.***, phos.
irregular - ars., **KALI-I.**, merc.
irregular, jagged - ars., merc.
extending from throat to roof of - ars.
fetid - ***bapt.***, nux-v., nit-ac., plb., ***merc.***
flat - ***caps.***, ***nat-c.***, nat-m., merc., mez., sul-ac.
forming rapidly - ***bor.***
gangrenous - ***ars.***, ***bapt.***, ***bor.***, **LACH.**, ***sul-ac.***, syph.
grayish - carb-v., hell., merc-c.
herpetic - ars-s-f., nat-m.
itching - chin.
malignant - **ARS.**, ***lach.***, ***phos.***
mercurial - bor., hep., ***iod.***, kali-i., ***nit-ac.***
painful - ***ars.***, ***fl-ac.***, kali-bi., ***merc.***, mur-ac., nat-m., **NIT-AC.**, petr.
biting teeth together, when - petr.
morning - zinc.
sore, smarting - ars-m., bov., nat-a.
splinter, like - ***nit-ac.***
stinging stitches - ***nit-ac.***
touch, to - cic., nat-c., ***nat-m.***
painless - bapt., hell., phos.
after suppressed brown herpetic eruption on face - phos.
lower lip, inner surface - phos.
perforating - ***kali-chl.***
phagedenic - ars., ars-s-f., ***caps.***, ***merc-c.***, **NIT-AC.**, ***sul-ac.***
purple - carb-v., ***plb.***
small - ***alum.***, ***caps.***, chlor., ***merc.***, zinc.
spreading - ***alum.***, ***lach.***, merc., merc-p-r.
syphilitic - ***aur.***, ***aur-m.***, ***fl-ac.***, **HEP.**, hydr., **KALI-BI.**, **KALI-I.**, ***lach.***, **MERC.**, ***merc-i-r.***, ***phyt.***, **SYPH.**
white - cic., ***sul-ac.***
as if coated with milk - ***kali-i.***
left lower lip, inside - ars-m.
yellow - aloe, calc., hell., ***plb.***, ***sul-ac.***, zinc.
orifice of salivary glands, at - acon., bell., **MERC.**
ulcers, gums - ang., alum., aloe, anan., ars., aur., aur-m., berb., bufo, ***calc.***, caps., ***carb-v.***, caust., corn., ***crot-c.***, ***cupr.***, ***hep.***, hippoz., ***iod.***, ***kali-bi.***, kali-c., kali-chl., ***kali-i.***, **KREOS.**, lac-c., ***lach.***, ***lyc.***, **MERC.**, ***merc-c.***, mill., mur-ac., **NAT-M.**, nat-p., nicc., ***nux-v.***, ox-ac., ***ph-ac.***, **PHOS.**, phyt., **PSOR.**, sang., ***sep.***, ***sil.***, stann., ***sul-ac.***, ***staph.***, zinc.
base lardaceous - ***hep.***
blood, discharging, which tastes salty - alum.
exuding, on pressure - bov.
scorbutic - acet-ac., mur-ac.
sensation of, at root of tooth - am-c.
sloughing - ***merc.***, merc-i-r., op., staph.
yellowish - hell., sulph.

ulcers, lips - am-m., anan., **ARS.,** ***aur-m.,*** bell., bov., ***bry., caps.,*** carb-s., ***caust., cham.,*** chin., chin-a., ***cic., clem., con., graph.,*** hep., ***kali-ar., kali-bi., kali-c.,*** kali-chl., kali-p., lyc., ***mag-c., merc., mez.,*** nat-a., nat-c., ***nat-m.,*** **NIT-AC.,** nux-v., ***ph-ac., phos., phyt., psor.,*** sep., **SIL.,** staph., **STRAM.,** sulph., ***zinc.***
acrid, saliva from - ***nit-ac.***
air, open agg. - ars.
burning - ***caust.,*** chin., ***cic.,*** nux-v., staph., sulph.
cancerous - ***ars., aur-m.,*** carb-an., ***clem.,*** **CON.,** ***kali-bi.,*** lyc., ***phos.,*** phyt.
crusty - staph.
itching - chin., staph.
lower - ***caust., clem.,*** ign., ***lyc.,*** ph-ac., ***phos.,*** sep., sil., sulph., zinc.
painful on motion - ars., caps.
phagedenic - ***ars., con.***
serpiginous - bor.
splinter, with sensation of - bov., **NIT-AC.**
touch agg. - ars.
upper - caust., kali-c., merc., ***mez.,*** staph., ***zinc.***

ulcers, palate - am-c., ***apis,*** **AUR.,** ***aur-m., cinnb.,*** dulc., ***kali-bi., lach., lyc.,*** **MERC.,** ***merc-c., nat-m., nit-ac.,*** nux-v., ***ph-ac., phos., phyt., sang.,*** sanic., sil.
edges hard - kali-bi.
perforating - ***kali-bi.,*** mez., ***sil.***
punched out, looking - ***kali-bi.***
sloughing - ***kali-bi., lach., merc-c., nit-ac., phos., syph.***
syphilitic - **AUR., AUR-M.,** ***hep., kali-i., syph.***
velum, on - dros., hippoz., ***kali-i., merc., merc-cy., nit-ac., ph-ac., phyt.,*** syph.

VEINS, distended, lips - ***crot-h., dig.***

VELVET, sensation as if covered with - coc-c., dig., nux-m.

VESICLES - agar., ambr., am-c., am-m., ***anac.,*** ant-t., apis., **ARS.,** aur., ***bar-c.,*** bor., ***calc.,*** calc-s., ***canth.,*** caps., ***carb-an.,*** cham., ***chel.,*** chim., cinnb., crot-t., cupr., gamb., hell., iod., ***kali-ar.,*** kali-c., lac-c., ***mag-c.,*** manc., ***merc.,*** mez., nat-a., ***nat-c.,*** **NAT-M.,** nat-p., nat-s., nit-ac., nux-v., oena., ox-ac., phos., rhod., rhus-t., spig., spong., ***staph.,*** sulph., ***sul-ac.,*** ter., ***thuj.***
biting - nat-m., rhod.
blood - agar., led., nat-m., sec.
burning - ambr., am-c., ***am-m.,*** apis, arg-m., ars., bar-c., bry., ***caps., carb-an.,*** cycl., gamb., ***kali-c.,*** kali-chl., **KALI-I.,** kali-n., ***mag-c.,*** mang., merl., mez., mur-ac., nat-a., nat-c., ***nat-m.,*** nat-s., phel., psor., seneg., spong., sulph., thuj.
cheek, inside - calc., mag-c.
cold things amel. - ***nat-s.***
cutting - mag-s.
gangrenous - sec.
menses, before - mag-c.
painful - ***anac.,*** apis, berb., caust., kali-c., nux-v.

VESICLES, mouth
sore, smarting - apis, arg-m., lyc., sulph.
stinging, stitches - **APIS,** cham., hell., kali-chl., nat-m., spong.
suppurating - mag-c., phos.
ulcers, becoming - calc., ***carb-an.,*** clem., ***merc.***
whitish - berb., canth., mez., phos., ***thuj.***
yellow - agar., cycl., zinc.

vesicles, gums - bell., canth., daph., ***iod.,*** kali-c., ***mag-c., merc.,*** mez., nat-s., petr., rhus-v., sep., **SIL.,** staph., zing.
black - petr.
burning - bell., mag-c., mez., sep.

vesicles, lips (see Fever-blisters) - agar., ail., ***alum.,*** am-c., am-m., ant-t., asc-t., aur., berb., bor., bov., calc-s., ***carb-an.,*** chel., chin-s., cic., ***clem.,*** com., ***con.,*** hell., hep., kali-p., kali-s., lac-ac., lac-c., ***mag-c., mag-m.,*** mang., merc., nat-c., **NAT-M.,** nat-s., ***nit-ac.,*** par., plat., rhod., ***sanic.,*** sang., seneg., sil., valer.
lower - agar., ail., aur., com., mag-m., nat-s., par.
upper - ***agar.,*** alum., am-m., cic., kali-p., mag-p., mang., rat., rhus-v., seneg., valer., zinc.
blood blisters - ***nat-m.***

vesicles, palate - carb-v., iod., ***mag-c.,*** manc., nat-c., nit-ac., phos., rhus-t., spig., sulph.

WARTS - caust., ph-ac., thuj.
warts, lips - ***caust.,*** kali-s., **NIT-AC.,** thuj.
warts, palate - arg-n.

WATERY, gums, look - **APIS.**

WETTING, lips constantly - ***culx.***

WRINKLED, lips - am-c.
wrinkled, palate - **BOR.,** phos.

Muscles

ABSCESS - arn., asaf., calc., chin., ***cupr.***, ***ph-ac.***, ***sil.***, staph., ***sulph.***, symph., ***syph.***
deep, muscles, of - calc.
psoas - arn., asaf., chin., ***cupr.***, ***ph-ac.***, ***sil.***, staph., ***sulph.***, symph., ***syph.***
abscess, tendons - ***mez.***

ACHING, pain - achy., ***acon.***, agav-t., alet., am-caust., ***ant-t.***, **ARN.**, ars., aster., bell., bell-p., brach., ***bry.***, calc., calc-p., carb-s., ***caust.***, ***cimic.***, ***colch.***, ***dulc.***, eryt-j., eup-per., ferr-p., **GELS.**, harp., hist., ign., lat-m., **LAC-AC.**, led., lyc., ***macro.***, mag-s., man., ***marco.***, merc., merc-c., morph., nat-f., nat-m., op., ***phyt.***, plb., ptel., puls., ***pyrog.***, ***ran-b.***, rauw., ***rham-cath.***, ***rhus-t.***, ***ruta***, sal-ac., sil., staph., stram., stroph-s., ***stry.***, sulfa., tab., tarax., thal., thuj., valer., ***verat.***, ***verat-v.***, zinc.
attachment, of - phyt., rhod., ruta.
chill, during - aran., arn., ars., eup-per., ***ip.***, nat-m., ***nux-v.***, **PYROG.**, ***rhus-t.***, sabad., tub.
exertion, from - ***arn.***, calc., calc-p., gels., ***lac-ac.***, ***rhus-t.***, ***ruta.***
extensors - calc-p.
fever, during - arn., eup-per., **GELS.**, puls., ***pyrog.***, ***rhus-t.***, ***tub.***
flexors - anac., arn., carb-s., caust., cic., dros., gels., kalm., merc., mez., op., ***phos.***, plan., plb., ptel., rhus-t., sep.
forenoon - caust.
influenza, during - ***acon.***, arn., **BRY.**, ***caust.***, ***chel.***, ***euph.***, **EUP-PER.**, **GELS.**, rhus-t., naja.
morning - caust.
motion agg. - bry., nux-v.
amel. - am-c., ***mur-ac.***, ***puls.***, **RHUS-T.**, ***tub.***
rheumatic - merc-i-r., rhus-t.
waking, on - arn., sep.

ATONY, of muscles - calc., con., gels., **HYDR.**, op.

ATROPHY - ***ars.***, **CALC.**, ***phos.***, **PLB.**, sars.
affected parts - ***plb.***
local paralysis - plb.
progressive - **PHOS.**
alternating with colic and constipation - ***plb.***

BANDAGED, sensation as if - arund., ***chin.***, nit-ac., **PLAT.**

BANDAGING, amel. - ***arg-n.***, bry., lac-d., ***mag-m.***, pic-ac., tril.

BINDING up, amel. - apis, arg-n., bry., chin., gels., mag-m., mang., mim-p., puls., rhod., sil., tril.

BORING, pain, flexor - plan.

BURNING, pain - ***acon.***, ***alum.***, am-m., anac., ***arg-m.***, arn., **ASAF.**, aur., bar-c., bry., calc., caust., cic., cina, **COCC.**, colch., ***dig.***, euph., ign., laur., lyc., mag-c., mang., merc., **MEZ.**, mur-ac., **NUX-V.**, ***olnd.***, par., phyt., plat., plb., rhod., **RHUS-T.**, ***sabad.***, sabin., samb., sep., spig., stann., **STAPH.**, **SUL-AC.**, tarax., **THUJ.**, viol-t., zinc.
hot needles, like - alum., apis, ars., bar-c., ***kali-c.***, mag-c., naja, nit-ac., ol-an., rhus-t., spig., vesp.
tearing, in - bell., ***carb-v.***, caust., kali-c., led., lyc., ***nit-ac.***, ruta., sabin., tarax., zinc.

CONTRACTION, muscles and tendons - acon., acon-c., ***ars.***, ***bar-c.***, ***bell.***, bry., **CALC.**, canth., carb-s., carb-v., **CAUST.**, cedr., **COLOC.**, con., ***crot-c.***, ***crot-h.***, ***cupr.***, ferr., ferr-m., **GRAPH.**, ***guai.***, hydr-ac., hydrc., jatr., kali-ar., ***kali-i.***, **LYC.**, ***merc.***, mill., mur-ac., ***nat-c.***, ***nat-m.***, ***nux-v.***, oena., op., ***phos.***, ***plb.***, ***ruta.***, **SEC.**, ***sep.***, ***sil.***, still., stram., sulph., syph., vib.
chill, during - **CIMX.**
involuntary - ***op.***
night - plb.
paralysis, of extensors, from - ***ars.***, **PLB.**
parts, of, supplied with involuntary muscles, as intestines, ureters, etc., with intense pain - ***tab.***
periodic - ***sec.***
skin - cupr.
slow - stram.
stiff during exacerbation of pains - ***phos.***
sudden - sec.
contraction, muscles and tendons, of joints - ***anac.***, ***aur.***, ***caust.***, cimx., ***colch.***, ***form.***, ***graph.***, ***merc.***, ***nat-m.***, ***nit-ac.***, petr., sec., stront.

CONTROL voluntary, cannot - alum., ***anac-oc.***
loss of, so weak as to fall - amyg.

CONVULSIONS, extensor - **CINA.**
flexor muscles - ***bell.***

CRAMPS, of - acon., agar., alum., am-c., am-m., ***ambr.***, **ANAC.**, anan., **ANG.**, arg-m., ***arn.***, ***ars.***, ***asaf.***, asar., atro., aur., bar-c., **BELL.**, bism., bor., bov., bry., bufo, cact., **CALC.**, calc-s., **CAMPH.**, ***cann-s.***, caps., carb-an., carb-o., carb-s., carb-v., ***cast.***, ***caust.***, cedr., ***cham.***, chin., cic., ***cimic.***, **CINA**, clem., ***cocc.***, colch., **COLOC.**, ***con.***, coni., croc., ***crot-c.***, crot-h., **CUPR.**, ***cupr-ac.***, cyt-l., dig., ***dios.***, ***dulc.***, euph., euphr., eup-per., ferr., ***gels.***, ***graph.***, ***hell.***, hist., ***hyos.***, ***ign.***, iod., ip., ***iris***, jatr., kali-bi., ***kali-br.***, ***kali-c.***, kali-n., kali-p., kali-s., kreos., lach., lat-m., **LYC.**, mag-m., **MAG-P.**, mang., meny., **MERC.**, merc-c., merc-sul., mez., mosch., ***mur-ac.***, nat-f., nat-m., ***nit-ac.***, **NUX-V.**, olnd., ***op.***, ox-ac., ***petr.***, ph-ac., phos., ***phyt.***, **PLAT.**, ***plb.***, plb-a., puls., ran-b., rheum, rhod., ***rhus-t.***, ***rob.***, ruta, sabad., samb., sang., sarcol-ac., scop., ***sec.***, sel., **SEP.**, ***spig.***, ***spong.***, squil., ***stann.***, staph., stront-c., **SULPH.**, syph., ***tab.***, tarent., ***thuj.***, tub., ***valer.***, **VERAT.**, verb., vib., viol-o., viol-t., ***zinc.***, zinc-s.
afternoon - sulph.
air, cold agg. - bufo.
body, all over - hydr-ac., ***hyos.***, olnd.
and lower limbs, in - ***iris.***
chill, during - cupr., ***sil.***
coldness, with, of arms and legs - ***merc.***

CRAMPS, of
exertion, after - ***mag-p.***
hydrocephalus, acute, in - ***cupr-ac.***
intermittent - phyt.
left side, often only in - ***chin-s.***
limbs, upper, particularly in - ant-t.
menses, with - mag-m.
after - chin., cupr., puls.
morning - sulph.
motion, on - nux-v.
night - ***calc.,*** cupr., merc.
waking , on - calc., sulph.
paralysis, followed by - tab.
paraplegia, precede - sec.
periodic - euph.
pregnancy, during - calc., ***cupr., hyos.,*** mag-p., mill., ***phos., verat.,*** vib.
pressure, agg. - zinc.
radiating over whole body - dios., lyc., nux-v.
right - elaps.
semen discharge of - bufo.
sex agg. - coloc., cupr., graph.
stiffness, with - verat.
followed by - sec., sel.
stool, during - bell.
tension - ***cham.***
tonic, commence in hands and feet, spread all over, with rice water discharges - **VERAT.**
touched, when - ***guare.***
toxemia, sequel of, or in broken-down constitutions - ***crot-h.***
transfixion - cupr.
vomiting of dark coagulated blood - nat-m.
wandering - **CAUST.**
women and children, in - ***hyos.***

CRAMP-like, pain - **ANAC.,** ant-c., arg-m., asaf., aur., bism., ***calc.,*** caust., chel., ***chin.,*** dulc., euph., graph., iod., kali-c., mang., ***meny.,*** mosch., ***mur-ac.,*** **NAT-C.,** nat-m., nux-v., ***petr.,*** ph-ac., phos., **PLAT.,** ran-b., ruta., samb., sil., stann., stront-c., thuj., valer.

DRAWING, pain - ***acon.,*** agn., alum., ambr., anac., ang., **ANT-C., ANT-T.,** apis, arg-m., arn., asaf., asar., aur., bar-c., **BELL.,** berb., bism., bov., bry., calc., ***camph.,*** cann-s., canth., ***caps.,*** carb-ac., ***carb-v., caust.,*** **CHAM.,** ***chel., chin.,*** cic., ***cina, clem.,*** **COCC.,** coff., ***colch.,*** croc., cupr., **CYCL.,** dig., dros., dulc., euph., ferr., **GRAPH.,** hell., hep., hydr., hyos., ***ign.,*** ip., kali-bi., kali-c., kali-n., led., ***lyc., meny.,*** merc., mez., morph., ***mosch.,*** nat-m., nit-ac., ***nux-m.,*** nux-v., olnd., par., petr., ph-ac., phos., **PLAT.,** ***plb.,*** **PULS.,** ran-b., ran-s., **RHOD.,** ***rhus-t.,*** ruta, sabad., sabin., samb., sec., sep., sil., spig., spong., ***squil.,*** staph., stram., sul-ac., ***sulph.,*** tarax., ***teucr., thuj.,*** **VALER.,** ***verat.,*** verb., viol-o., viol-t., ***zinc.***
chill, during - ***ars.,*** ferr., hell., lyc., ***merc., nux-v.,*** ph-ac., ***puls.,*** **RHUS-T.**
after - puls.

DRAWING, pain
cramp-like - asaf., ***graph.,*** kali-n., petr., ***plat.,*** sil.
paralytic - ***aur., cocc., hep., mag-m.,*** mez., ***nux-v.,*** **RHUS-T.,** sabad.
drawing, tendons, in - am-m., caust., kali-bi., nat-m., rhus-t., ruta, thuj.

DUPUYTREN'S contracture - caust., cimex.

EMACIATION - ars., ***calc.,*** carb-s., clem., nit-ac., phyt., **PLB.,** ***sec.,*** stront-c., **SULPH.**
diseased part, of - ***ars.,*** bry., ***carb-v.,*** dulc., ***graph.,*** **LED.,** ***mez.,*** nat-m., nit-ac., ph-ac., phos., **PLB., PULS.,** ***sec.,*** sel., ***sep.,*** sil.
paralyzed part, of - ***kali-p.,*** nux-v., **PLB.,** ***sec., sep.***

EXCITABILITY, increased, and action in voluntary, with diminution of it in involuntary - op.

EXHAUSTED, easily, from slight exertion - ***ferr., lac-ac.***

FLABBY - am-c., **CALC.,** ***cham.,*** **PHOS.,** sars.
chlorosis, in - ***cycl.***
coldness, with - calc., verat-v.
diarrhea, with - ***bor.***
diphtheria, in - ***merc-cy.***
liver disorder, in - sil.
ophthalmia, in strumous - ***merc-d.***
parkinson's disease, in - rhus-t.
pott's curvature, in - calc., ***sulph.***
flabby, sensation, (see Generals) - ***aeth.,*** ant-t., **CALC.,** caps., carb-ac., ***chin.,*** cocc., ***gels., lyc.,*** mur-ac., ph-ac., stram., sulph.

FULLNESS - cinnb., ham.

GNAWING, pain - ***ars.,*** cocc., dros., eup-per., lach., merc., nit-ac.
flexor muscles - merc.
night - nit-ac.

HEAT - agar., bapt., brom., bufo, carb-ac., cupr., ***guai.,*** lil-t., nat-m., stann., ***sulph.,*** verat., ***zinc.***
alternating with cold - bell., ***lyc.,*** stram.
chilliness, over back, during - gins.
creeping - op.
eruption, before - nat-m.
night - arn.
in bed - fago., ***led.***
paralyzed limb - ***alum.,*** phos.
uncover, must - agar.
warmth of bed intolerable - ***led.***

HEAVINESS, tired - acon., aesc., ***agar.,*** ail., ***aloe, alum.,*** ambr., ammc., am-c., amyg., anac., ant-c., ant-t., ***apis,*** **ARG-M.,** ***arg-n., arn.,*** **ARS.,** ***ars-i.,*** asaf., atro., bar-c., bar-m., **BRY.,** bufo, calad., ***calc.,*** calc-p., camph., cann-i., cann-s., caps., carb-an., ***carb-s., carb-v., caust., cham.,*** **CHEL.,** ***chin.,*** chin-a., cimic., ***clem.,*** coff., ***coloc.,*** **CON.,** cor-r., ***crot-h.,*** crot-t., ***cupr.,*** cycl., dig., dulc., eupi., ferr., ferr-ar., ferr-i., ferr-p., **GELS.,** gins., glon., gran., ***graph.,*** **HELL.,** hep., hipp., hyos., hyper., iod., ip., ***kali-ar.,*** kali-bi., ***kali-c.,*** **KALI-P.,** kalm., kreos., lach., lact., led., ***lyc., lyss.,*** mag-c., manc., **MERC.,** ***merc-c.,*** merc-i-f., ***mez.,*** morph., nat-c., ***nat-m.,*** nit-ac., **NUX-V.,**

HEAVINESS, tired - ***onos.,*** op., osm., paeon., par., petr., **PH-AC., PHOS.,** phys., ***pic-ac.,*** pin-s., plb., ***puls.,*** ruta., ***sabad.,*** sabin., ***sec., sel., sep., sil.,*** spig., stann., stram., ***sulph.,*** tep., ter., ther., thuj., trom., verat., zinc., zing.
ascending stairs - calc., clem., lyc.
chill, during - coc-c., sep.
before - ther.
emissions, after - ph-ac., puls.
exertion, on - ***lach.***
fever, during - **CALC., GELS., NUX-V.,** pyrog., **RHUS-T.,** sulph.
mental exertion, from - ***ph-ac.***
motion, on - ***lach.,*** mez.
amel. - caps., cham.
painful - agar.
paralytic - plb.
pregnancy, during - ***calc-p.***
rest, during - caps.
rising after sitting - carb-v.
amel. - merc., nat-m.
sex, after - bufo, ph-ac., puls.
sexual excesses, from - ph-ac., ***puls.***
sitting, while - caps., ruta.
storm, during - ***phos.***
waking, on - cham., sep., tep.
walking, while - acon., ***calc.,*** paeon., **PIC-AC.**
amel. - carb-v.
walking, in open air - lyc., sil., zinc.
amel. - carb-v.

INDURATIONS, of - alum., ***anthr., bad.,*** bar-c., ***bry.,*** **CALC-F.,** carb-an., carb-v., ***caust., con.,*** dulc., hep., hyos., iod., kali-c., kali-chl., lach., ***lyc.,*** nat-c., nux-v., ph-ac., puls., ran-b., rhod., rhus-t., sars., sep., sil., spong., sulph., thuj.

INFLAMMATION, muscles, (see Myositis)
inflammation, tendons (see Tendonitis)

INJURIES, soft parts - **ARN.,** bell-p., calc., ***calen.,*** cham., **CON.,** dulc., euphr., ham., lach., nat-c., nat-m., phos., ***puls., rhus-t.,*** samb., sulph., ***sul-ac., symph.***
injuries, tendons - arn., ***anac., arg-m.,*** calen., **RHUS-T., RUTA.**

JERKING, of - acon., aesc., ***agar.,*** alum., am-c., ***anac.,*** ant-c., ***ant-t., apis, arg-m., arg-n.,*** arn., ars., asar., ***bar-c., bell., bry.,*** cadm-s., calc., **CALC-P.,** ***cann-i.,*** caps., carb-s., cham., chin., ***chion.,*** **CIC.,** ***cimic.,*** cocc., ***colch., con., croc., cupr.,*** dulc., euph., euphr., ***ferr.,*** ferr-ar., ***gels., glon., graph.,*** **HYOS.,** ip., kali-i., kali-s., ***lach., lil-t.,*** mag-c., ***meny., merc.,*** merc-c., **MEZ.,** mosch., ***nat-c.,*** nat-m., nit-ac., ***nux-m., nux-v.,*** olnd., ***op.,*** petr., ph-ac., ***phos., plat., plb., puls., rhus-t.,*** ruta, sabad., sabin., **SEP.,** sil., ***spig., stann.,*** staph., **STRAM.,** ***stront-c.,*** **SULPH., SUL-AC.,** ***tarent.,*** ter., ***valer.,*** viol-t., ***visc.,*** **ZINC.**
alternation of flexors and extensors - ***plb.***
left side paralyzed, right side convulsed - art-v.
motion, on - sep.
amel. - ***merc., thuj.,*** valer., zinc.

JERKING, of
paralyzed parts - ***arg-n.,*** merc., ***nux-v., phos., sec., stry.***
one leg, and one arm - apis, apoc., hell., stram.
side, other side paralyzed - apis, art-v., bell., ***stram.***
side lain on, in - ***cimic.***
sleep, during - agar., aloe, ***alum.,*** ambr., anac., ant-t., arg-m., ***ars., bell.,*** bry., cast., cham., cimic., cob., ***cocc., colch., con.,*** cor-r., ***cupr.,*** daph., dulc., hep., ign., ip., ***kali-c., lyc.,*** merc., nat-c., ***nat-m.,*** nat-s., nit-ac., op., phos., puls., ran-s., rheum, rhus-t., sel., sep., sil., stann., staph., stront-c., ***sulph.,*** sul-ac., thuj., viol-t., zinc.
falling asleep, on - acon., ***agar., alum.,*** arg-m., **ARS.,** cob., hyper., ***ign.,*** **KALI-C.,** phys., puls., ran-b., ***sel.,*** sil., ***stront-c., stry., sulph., sul-ac., zinc.***

JERKING, pain - arn., ***bry., calc.,*** carb-s., caust., **CINA,** cocc., coff., ***coloc.,*** euph., guai., ***lyc.,*** mang., ***meny.,*** mez., mur-ac., **NUX-V.,** ph-ac., plb., sep., sil., spong., **SQUIL.,** stann., zinc.

LAMENESS, flexor - calc-p., ruta.

LAX, muscles - agar., ars., **CAPS.,** ***chin., clem., cupr-ac.,*** dig., ***hyos.,*** **FERR.,** ***ip.,*** **PHOS.,** verat., viol-o.
affecting voluntary motion - ferr-p.
chronic headache, in leucophlegmatic people, with - ***sul-ac.***
emaciation, with - ***ferr.***
intermittent fever, in - ***ars.***
pneumonia senilis, in - ***ferr.***
sensation, of - aml-n.
sphincters - ***aloe, bell., hyper., phos.,*** podo., ***sec.***
suddenly, become - ***hell.***
syphilis, in - iod.

LIFTING, straining of muscles and tendons, ailments from - acet-ac., ***acon., agn.,*** alum., alum-sil., alumn., ***ambr.,*** arist-cl., **ARN.,** bar-c., bell., ***bell-p., bor., bov.,*** **BRY., CALC.,** calc-f., calc-p., ***calc-s.,*** calc-sil., calen., **CARB-AN.,** ***carb-s., carb-v., caust.,*** chin., ***cocc.,*** coloc., **CON.,** croc., cur., ***dulc., ferr.,*** ferr-p., ***form.,*** **GRAPH.,** ***hyper.,*** iod., ***kali-c.,*** kali-m., kali-sil., ***kalm.,*** lach., led., ***lyc.,*** merc., ***mill.,*** mur-ac., ***nat-c.,*** nat-m., nit-ac., nux-v., olnd., onos., petr., ***ph-ac.,*** phos., plat., podo., prun., psor., ***puls.,*** rhod., **RHUS-T., RUTA,** ***sec.,*** sep., **SIL.,** spig., stann., staph., stront-c., stroph., ***sulph.,*** sul-ac., thuj., ***valer.***
amel. - spig.
arms, of - rhus-t., sul-ac.
children - bor., calc-p.
headache from - ambr., ***arn.,*** bar-c., ***bry., calc.,*** cocc., ***graph., lyc., nat-c.,*** nux-v., ***ph-ac.,*** **RHUS-T.,** ***sil.,*** sulph., valer.
overlifting, agg. - agn., ambr., carb-v., graph., sep.
reaching high - sulph.

LIFTING, straining
tendency to strain in lifting - arn., bry., ***calc.***, carb-v., con., graph., lyc., ***nat-c.***, nat-m., psor., ***rhus-t., ruta,*** **SIL.,** ***symph.***

LOOSE, sensations, as if - ***am-c.***, bar-c., bov., carb-an., caust., chin., croc., hyos., ***kali-c.***, kali-m., laur., med., nat-s., **NUX-M.,** nux-v., psor., **RHUS-T.,** sec., sul-ac., thuj.
as if flesh were - staph., ***thuj.***
open, and - sec.

MOVEMENT, automatic - **COCC.**

MUSCULAR, dystrophy - caust., lath., plb.

MYOSITIS - ***arn.***, bell., bry., calc., ham., hep., kali-i., merc., mez., ***rhus-t., ruta.***

MYASTHENIA gravis - alum., con., gels.

NEEDLES, sensation, like hot - **ARS.,** ol-an.

PAIN, muscles, (see Aching, pain) - achy., ***acon.***, agav-t., alet., am-caust., ***ant-t.***, **ARN.,** ars., aster., bell., bell-p., brach., **BRY.,** carb-s., ***caust.***, **CIMIC.,** ***colch.***, dios., ***dulc.***, eryt-j., ferr-p., **GELS.,** harp., hist., ign., lat-m., **LAC-AC.,** led., lyc., ***macro., mag-p.***, mag-s., man., ***marco.***, merc., merc-c., morph., nat-f., nat-m., op., ***phyt.***, plb., puls., ***ran-b.***, rauw., ***rham-cath., rhus-t., ruta,*** sal-ac., sil., staph., stram., stroph-s., ***stry.***, sulfa., tab., tarax., thal., thuj., valer., **VERAT.,** ***verat-v.***, zinc.
attachments, at - ***phyt., rhod., rhus-t.***
chill, after - ***elat.***
exertion, from - gels.
flexor muscles - anac., arn., carb-s., caust., cic., dros., gels., kalm., merc., mez., op., ***phos.***, plan., plb., rhus-t., sep.
forenoon - caust.
hot bathing amel. - lat-m., ***mag-p.***, rhus-t.
hysterical - ign., nux-v., plb., puls.
morning - caust.
motion, on - ***bry.***, sil.
agg. - bell-p., bry., nux-v.
amel. - ***phos., rhus-t.***
numbness, with - ***lyc.***
overexertion, after - **ARN.,** gels., ***rhus-t.***
rheumatic - merc-i-r.
rheumatism, in acute - verat-v.
stitching, cramping - ***cimic.***
stretching, on - mag-s.
touched, when - cocc.
waking, on - sep.

pain, tendons - am-m., anac., arn., benz-ac., berb., ***bry.***, calc-p., caust., colch., coloc., harp., iod., kali-bi., kalm., prun., ***rhod.***, **RHUS-T.,** ***ruta,*** sabin., thuj., zinc.
attachments, at - ***phyt., rhod., rhus-t.***
expansion, from - agar., thuj.

PARALYSIS, (see Nerves, Paralysis)
coldness, of parts with - caust., ***cocc.***, dulc., graph., ***nux-v., rhus-t.***
elderly, people - ***bar-c., con., kali-c.***
emotions, after strong - ***apis,*** **IGN.,** nat-m., nux-v., stann.
exertion, after - ars., ***caust., gels.***, nux-v., ***rhus-t.***

PARALYSIS,
extensors, of - alum., ars., calc., ***cocc., crot-h.***, cur., **PLB.**
flexors - caust., mez., ***nat-m.***
hysterical - cur., **IGN.,** plb., tarent.
isolated - caust., cupr., plb.
painless - abies-c., acon., aeth., alum., ambr., ***anac., arg-n.***, arn., ***ars., aur., bapt.***, bar-c., bry., cadm-s., **CANN-I., COCC.,** colch., **CON.,** crot-h., ***cupr.***, cur., **GELS.,** graph., **HYOS.,** kalm., ***laur.***, **LYC.,** ***merc.***, nat-m., ***nux-v.***, **OLND.,** ***op., ph-ac., phos.***, **PLB.,** ***puls.***, rhod., **RHUS-T.,** ***sec.***, sil., stram., sulph., ***verat., zinc.***
partial - ***ars., nux-v.***
rheumatic - bar-c., ***caust., cocc.***, lyc., ***rhus-t.***, sulph.
single, parts - anac., ***ars.***, caust., cupr., plb.
spastic - ***benz-d-n.***, gels., ***hyper., lach., nux-v.***, plect., plb., sec., ***stry., zinc.***
stiffness, with - caust., con., lach., lyc., nat-m., rhus-t., sil.
toxic - ***apis, ars.***, bapt., gels., lac-c., ***lach.***, mur-ac., rhus-t.
weakness - ***gels.***

PARALYTIC pain, in - agn., ant-c., asaf., carb-v., cham., ***chin.***, cic., cina, cocc., con., dig., graph., ***hell.***, **KALI-C.,** mez., mosch., nat-m., nit-ac., phos., ***sabin., sars.***, seneg., sil., stann., verb.
tearing, in - agn., ant-c., asaf., carb-v., cham., ***chin.***, cic., cina, cocc., con., dig., graph., ***hell.***, **KALI-C.,** mez., mosch., nat-m., nit-ac., phos., ***sabin., sars.***, seneg., sil., stann., verb.

PINCHING, pain - brucin., cann-s., lyc., mag-aust., sulph.

PRESSING, pain - agar., agn., am-m., ***anac.***, ang., arg-m., arn., ***asaf., asar.***, aur., bell., bism., bry., calc., camph., cann-s., ***caps., carb-an.***, caust., chel., chin., cina, clem., cocc., con., ***cupr.***, **CYCL.,** dig., dros., euph., euphr., graph., hell., hep., ***ign.***, kali- n., ***led.***, lyc., mag- c., mag-m., mang., meny., merc., mez., ***mosch.***, mur-ac., nat-c., nat-m., **NUX-M.,** nux-v., ***olnd.***, petr., ***ph-ac., phos., plat.***, plb., puls., ran-b., nitro-o., ran-s., rheum, rhod., rhus-t., **RUTA.,** ***sabad.***, sabin., samb., sars., sil., spig., spong., ***stann., staph.***, stront-c., sulph., ***sul-ac., tarax., teucr.***, thuj., ***valer., verat.***, **VERB.,** viol-t., zinc.
flexor muscles - arn., cic., ***dros.***
sticking - am-m., anac., arg-m., arn., asaf., bar-c., bell., calc., chin., colch., coloc., cycl., dios., dros., euph., ***ign.***, kali-c., mez., ***mur-ac.***, olnd., phos., plat., rhus-t., ruta, sabad., sars., sep., spong., stann., staph., sul-ac., tarax., thuj., verb., viol-t., ***zinc.***
tearing - agar., anac., ***ang.***, arg-m., arn., asaf., asar., aur., ***bell.***, bism., calc., ***camph.***, cann-s., carb-v., chin., colch., cupr., cycl., hyos., led., meny., petr., ph-ac., ruta, sars., sep., spig., spong., stann., sulph., zinc.

PRESSING, pain
parts lain on, in - kali-c.
twitching - petr.

QUIVERING - ***am-c.,*** **BELL.,** berb., bism., ***calc.,*** caps., caust., ***clem.,*** com., **CON.,** dig., hep., hyos., ign., iod., kali-c., kali-n., lyc., mag-c., mosch., ***nit-ac.,*** nux-v., petr., sars., ***sep.,*** sil., stann., stront-c., **SULPH.,** verb.
all over, followed by vertigo - ***calc.***
lying, while - ***clem.***

RELAXATION, of (see Lax) - acet-ac., aeth., ***agar.,*** alum., ambr., amyg., ang., anh., ant-t., arg-m., arn., ***ars.,*** asaf., atro., bar-m., bar-s., bell., cortiso., bry., **CALC.,** calc-sil., camph., canth., **CAPS.,** carb-ac., carb-an., carb-o., carb-s., caust., ***cham.,*** chin., chin-a., chlor., cic., ***clem.,*** coca, **COCC.,** colch., ***con., croc., crot-c.,*** cupr., cur., cycl., dig., ***dios.,*** dros., euph., ***ferr.,*** ferr-ar., ferr-i., fl-ac., **GELS.,** ***graph.,*** guare., ***hell.,*** helo., hep., hydr., hydr-ac., ***hyos., iod., ip.,*** jug-r., kali-ar., **KALI-C.,** kali-m., kali-n., kali-p., kali-s., lach., laur., ***lyc., mag-c.,*** mang., merc., morph., mur-ac., murx., nat-c., nat-p., nit-ac., nux-m., nux-v., olnd., op., oxyt., ph-ac., **PHOS.,** phys., plat., plb., puls., rheum, sabad., ***sec., seneg., sep.,*** sil., sol-n., spig., ***spong.,*** stram., sul-ac., sul-h., ***sulph.,*** tab., ter., thuj., tub., ***verat.,*** verat-v., viol-o., zinc.
connective tissue - arg-m., calc., calc-br., caps., ferr-i., hep., kali-c., mag-c., merc-i-r., nit-ac., sec., spong.
sex, after - ***agar.,*** sep.

RHEUMATISM - ***bry., cimic.,*** viol-t., ***kalm.***

SARCOMA, cutis - ars., bar-c., calc-f., calc-p., carb-ac., carb-an., ***crot-h., cund.,*** cupr-s., graph., hecla., ***kali-m.,*** lach., ***lap-a.,*** nit-ac., phos., sil., symph., thuj.
lymphoid - ars., ars-i.

RIGID - ***acon.,*** apis, arg-n., arn., ars., ***cocc.,*** coff., ***hell.,*** kali-c., kali-p., ***lyc.***
chronic gout or rheumatism in elderly persons, with - ol-j.
meningeal irritation, from - ***phys.***
menses, at time for return of - phys.

SHARP, pain - ***acon.,*** agar., agn., ***alum.,*** ambr., am-c., ***am-m.,*** anac., ang., ant-c., ant-t., ***apis,*** arg-m., ***arn.,*** ars., ***ars-i.,*** **ASAF.,** asar., aur., bar-c., bar-m., **BELL.,** bism., bor., bov., **BRY.,** calad., **CALC.,** camph., cann-s., canth., caps., carb-an., carb-v., ***caust.,*** cham., chel., ***chin.,*** cic., cina, clem., ***cocc.,*** colch., coloc., ***con.,*** croc., cupr., cycl., dig., dros., dulc., euph., euphr., ferr., glon., ***graph., guai., hell.,*** hep., hyos., ***ign.,*** iod., **KALI-C.,** ***kali-m.,*** kali-n., kreos., lach., ***laur.,*** led., lyc., ***mag-c.,*** mag-m., mang., ***meny.,*** **MERC.,** merc-c., merc-i-r., mez., mosch., ***mur-ac., nat-c., nat-m., nit-ac.,*** nux-m., nux-v., olnd., ***par.,*** petr., ph-ac., ***phos.,*** plan., plat., plb., prun., **PULS.,** ran-b., ***ran-s.,*** rheum, rhod., **RHUS-T.,** ruta., ***sabad., sabin.,*** samb., sang., ***sars., sep., sil.,*** **SPIG.,** ***spong.,*** squil., ***stann.,*** **STAPH.,** stront-c., stry., **SULPH.,** sul-ac., **TARAX.,** teucr., **THUJ.,** valer., verat., verb., ***viol-t., zinc.***

SHARP, pain
burning in - ***acon., alum.,*** am-m., anac., ***arg-m.,*** arn., **ASAF.,** aur., bar-c., bry., calc., caust., cic., cina, **COCC.,** colch., ***dig.,*** euph., ign., laur., lyc., mag-c., mang., merc., **MEZ.,** mur-ac., **NUX-V.,** ***olnd.,*** par., phyt., plat., plb., rhod., **RHUS-T.,** ***sabad.,*** sabin., samb., sep., spig., stann., **STAPH., SUL-AC.,** tarax., **THUJ.,** viol-t., zinc.
hot needles, like - alum., apis, ars., bar-c., ***kali-c.,*** mag-c., naja, nit-ac., ol-an., rhus-t., spig., vesp.
jerking - arn., ***bry., calc.,*** carb-s., caust., **CINA,** cocc., coff., ***coloc.,*** euph., guai., ***lyc.,*** mang., ***meny.,*** mez., mur-ac., **NUX-V.,** ph-ac., plb., sep., sil., spong., **SQUIL.,** stann., zinc.
tearing in - acon., agn., alum., ambr., am-c., am-m., **ANAC.,** ang., arg-m., ***ars.,*** asaf., asar., aur., bell., bism., bor., **CALC.,** ***camph., cann-s.,*** canth., caps., caust., chel., ***chin.,*** cina, clem., coloc., con., cycl., dig., dros., **GUAI.,** hell., kali-c., kreos., led., **MANG.,** merc., mez., mur-ac., nat-m., nux-v., olnd., ph-ac., phos., **PULS.,** rheum, ***rhus-t.,*** ruta., sabin., samb., ***sars.,*** sep., sil., spig., spong., squil., staph., sul-ac., tarax., **THUJ.,** verb., zinc.
warm in bed, while - carb-v.
sharp, tendons - **KALI-C.**

SHORTENED, muscles and tendons (see Contractions) - ambr., am-c., **AM-M.,** anac., ars., aur., ***bar-c.,*** calc., carb-an., carb-v., **CAUST.,** cic., cimic., **CIMX., COLOC.,** con., cupr., dig., dros., **GRAPH.,** ***guai.,*** hell., hep., hyos., kali-c., kreos., lach., led., ***lyc.,*** mag-c., ***merc.,*** mez., mosch., ***nat-c.,*** **NAT-M.,** nit-ac., ***nux-v.,*** ox-ac., petr., ph-ac., phos., plb., puls., ran-b., rheum., ***rhus-t.,*** ruta., samb., ***sep.,*** sil., stann., sul-ac., sulph.
as if too short, in legs - bov.

SHRIVELLING, of body (see Immunity, Emaciation) - ***abrot.,*** alum., am-c., am-m., ambr., ***ant-c., arg-n.,*** arn., ***bar-c.,*** bism., ***bor.,*** bry., ***calc.,*** camph., cham., chin., cupr., fl-ac., hell., graph., kali-br., ***lyc.,*** merc., mur-ac., nux-v., op., ph-ac., plb., psor., rheum, rhod., rhus-t., sabad., ***sars., sec., sep.,*** sil., spig., stram., ***sulph.,*** verat., viol-o., vip., zinc.

SOFT, (see Flabby) - **CALC.**
and flabby - calc., ***fl-ac.***
pott's curvature, in - ***sulph.***

SORE, pain (see Aching, pain) - abrot., ***agar., alum.,*** alumn., ang., anac., ***apis,*** apoc., **ARG-M., ARN., AUR.,** bad., ***bapt., bell., bell-p., bov.,*** bufo, calad., ***calc.,*** carb-an., ***carb-s., carb-v., caust., cham.,*** chel., **CHIN.,** chlf., cic., ***cimic., cist.,*** clem., cob., coff., coloc., ***con., crot-h.,*** cupr., cupr-ac., ***dig., dros., ferr., gels.,*** guai., ham., ***helon.,*** hyos., ***hyper.,*** jac., kali-c., kali-i., **LAC-AC.,** ***lac-c., led., lith., magn-gr.,*** merc., ***mez., mur-ac.,*** myric., ***nat-m.,*** nat-n., nat-p., ***nit-ac.,*** **NUX-V.,** par., **PH-AC.,** phos., phys.,

SORE, pain - ***phyt.,*** pic-ac., plb., **PULS.,** ***pyrog.,*** **RHUS-T.,** ***ruta.,*** sang., ***sep., spig.,*** squil., ***sulph.,*** tub., ***verat.,*** viol-o., zinc.
bending, after - coff.
cold, from becoming - ***ph-ac.***
descending, on - ***arg-m.***
evening - cham.
7 p.m. - cham.
forenoon - aur.
lying, agg. - aur., ***nux-v.***
on painful side amel. - ***nux-v., rhus-t.***
morning - aur., caps., cob., nit-ac., **PH-AC.,** pyrus, verat.
bed, in - anac., aur., carb-v., chin., coff., **NUX-V.,** ***rhus-t.***
waking, on - abrot.
motion, on - agar., ***arg-m., arn., calc.,*** chin., nux-v.
amel. - caps., ***chin.,*** coloc., **COM., RHUS-T., TUB.**
night - ***con.,*** spig.
nosebleed, after - agar.
paralytic - ***arn., calc.***
rising, on, amel. - aur., coff., ***nux-v.***
sitting, when - coloc.
sleep, nap, after - dig.
touch, on - dulc.
sore, tendons - arn., bry., ***calc-p.***

SPASMS of sphincters (see Cramps) - **BELL.**

STICKING, pain, in - acon., agn., ambr., anac., ant-t., arg-m., arn., asaf., bar-c., bell., bry., calc., camph., cann-s., canth., caps., chin., cic., ***colch.,*** coloc., con., cycl., dros., dulc., ***euph.,*** guai., hyos., ***ign.,*** iod., kali-c., ***lyc.,*** mag-c., mang., merc., ***mur-ac.,*** nat-m., olnd., ph-ac., phos., plat., rheum, sars., sep., spong., staph., sul-ac., sulph., teucr., thuj., **ZINC.**

STIFFNESS, of - abrot., absin., acon., aeth., ***agar.,*** am-c., am-m., ***aran.,*** arg-m., **ARS.,** ars-i., ars-s-f., **ASAF.,** ***bell.,*** bov., brom., **BRY.,** ***calc.,*** calc-p., calc-s., camph., cann-i., cann-s., canth., ***caps., carb-ac., carb-an.,*** carb-o., ***carb-s.,*** carb-v., carl., **CAUST.,** ***cham.,*** **CHEL.,** ***chin.,*** chin-a., ***cic., cimic.,*** **COCC.,** ***colch.,*** **CUPR.,** cycl., dig., ***dulc.,*** eup-per., ferr-ar., graph., ***guai., hell.,*** hydr-ac., ***hyos.,*** iod., kali-ar., kali-bi., ***kali-c.,*** kali-p., **KALM.,** ***lach.,*** lath., ***laur.,*** **LED.,** lith., **LYC.,** ***med.,*** meny., ***merc., merc-c.,*** merc-i-r., merc-sul., mosch., naja, nat-a., nat-c.1, ***nat-m., nat-s.,*** nit-ac., nux-m., ***nux-v.,*** olnd., op., ox-ac., **PETR.,** ph-ac., ***phos., phyt., plat.,*** plan., plb., psor., ***puls.,*** **RHUS-T.,** ***sang.,*** sars., ***sec.,*** sel., **SEP., SIL.,** ***spong., stram., stry.,*** **SULPH.,** tab., ***thuj.,*** verat., verat-v., ***zinc.***
cerebrospinal meningitis, in - ***rhus-t.***
exercise, amel. - **RHUS-T.**
exertion, after - arn., calc., **RHUS-T.,** ***tub.***
morning in bed - calc-p., ***chin., lach., led.,*** **RHUS-T.,** staph.
move, on beginning to - ***agar., caps.,*** kali-p., ***lyc., psor.,*** **RHUS-T.**
painful - ***lyc.***
paralytic - ***cocc.,*** lith., merc-c., nat-m., plb.

STIFFNESS, of
rising, on - agar., op., plan., psor., **RHUS-T.**
sleep, after - ***lach.,*** morph., ox-ac., **RHUS-T.,** ***sep.***

STRETCHING, (see Generals, Stretching) - ***calc.,*** ind., ***ip.,*** lyss., **RHUS-T.,** ***rhus-v.,*** zinc.
afternoon, in - arum-t.
chill, before - ***ign.***
convulsions, in puerperal, on remission of symptoms - ***atro.***
gaping feeling, with tiredness all over - vac.

SUBSULTUS, tendinum - ***agar.,*** ambr., am-c., ***ars., asaf.,*** bell., ***calc., camph., canth., chel., chlor.,*** **HYOS., IOD.,** ***kali-i., lyc., mez., mur-ac., ph-ac., phos.,*** rhus-t., ***sec., stry.,*** sul-ac., **ZINC.**

TEARING, pain - acon., agar., agn., alum., ***ambr.,*** am-c., ***am-m.,*** anac., ant-c., ant-t., ***arg-m.,*** arn., ***ars.,*** ars-i., ***asaf.,*** asar., ***aur.,*** bar-c., bar-m., ***bell., bism., bor.,*** bov., ***bry.,*** **CALC.,** camph., ***canth.,*** caps., ***carb-an.,*** **CARB-S., CARB-V., CAUST.,** cham., ***chel., chin.,*** cic., ***cina,*** clem., cocc., ***colch.,*** coloc., con., croc., cupr., cycl., dig., dros., euph., ferr., ***graph.,*** guai., hell., ***hep.,*** hyos., ign., iod., ip., **KALI-C.,** kali-n., kali-s., kreos., lach., laur., led., **LYC.,** ***mag-c., mag-m., mang.,*** meny., **MERC.,** mez., mosch., ***mur-ac., nat-c., nat-m.,*** **NIT-AC.,** nux-v., olnd., par., petr., ph-ac., ***phos.,*** plat., plb., ***puls.,*** ran-b., rheum, **RHOD.,** rhus-t., ***ruta.,*** sabad., ***sabin.,*** samb., sars., sec., sel., seneg., **SEP., SIL.,** spig., spong., squil., ***stann.,*** **STAPH., STRONT-C., SULPH.,** sul-ac., tarax., ***teucr.,*** thuj., valer., verat., verb., viol-o., viol-t., **ZINC.**
and burning - bell., ***carb-v.,*** caust., kali-c., led., lyc., ***nit-ac.,*** ruta., sabin., tarax., zinc.
tearing, joints and muscles - agar., anac., arg-m., arn., asaf., asar., aur., ***bell.,*** bism., calc., ***camph.,*** cann-s., carb- v., chin., colch., cupr., cycl., hyos., led., meny., petr., ph-ac., ruta., sars., sep., spig., spong., stann., sulph., zinc.

TENDONITIS - arg-m., ***rhod., rhus-t.***

TENSION - **ACON.,** am-m., anac., ang., ant-c., arn., ars., bar-c., bell., berb., cann-i., cann-s., canth., carb-v., caust., chin., dulc., graph., ***guai.,*** kali-c., lach., led., ***mosch., nat-c., nat-m.,*** **NIT-AC., NUX-V.,** olnd., ph-ac., **PHYS.,** phyt., ***plat.,*** plb., ***puls.,*** **RHUS-T., SEP.,** ***sil.,*** stann., staph., sulph., verb., zinc.
cholera asiatica, in - ***cupr-m.***
headache in right side, to neck and shoulders - ***lach.***

TWITCHING - **AGAR.,** ***alum.,*** alumn., ambr., ***apis,*** arn., ***ars.,*** ars-i., asaf., **BELL.,** calad., calc., cann-i., carb-ac., carb-v., carl., caust., ***cham.,*** **CHEL.,** ***chin., chin-s., cic.,*** cimic., **CINA,** ***cocc., coff.,*** colch., coloc., ***crot-c., cupr.,*** cypr., dros., dulc., graph., ***hell.,*** **HYOS., IGN.,** kali-ar., kali-c., kali-i., kali-n., kali-p., kali-s., kreos., lach., lyc., ***merc., merc-c.,*** morph., mur-ac., ***mygal.,*** nat-a., ***nat-c., nat-m.,*** nat-p.,

TWITCHING - nat-s., nit-ac., ***nux-m., nux-v.,*** **OP.,** paeon., petr., ph-ac., phos., plb., puls., ran-s., **RHUS-T.,** ***rhus-v.,*** sec., ***sep., sil.,*** **STRAM., STRY.,** sulph., **VALER.,** ***visc., zinc.***
afternoon, when trying to sleep - alum.
backward and inward - cupr.
bed, in - merc-n., nux-v., stry.
chill, during - acon., dig., jatr., lyc., nux-m., ***nux-v.,*** op., ox-ac., stram., tab.
after - puls.
convulsions, during - ***op.***
after - nux-v.
cough, during - cupr.
cramp-like - plat.
daytime - carb-v., petr., ***sep.,*** sil.
electric shocks, as from - agar., ***ars.,*** colch., nat-m., plat., ***ter., verat.***
evening - caust., graph.
bed, in - ***carb-v.,*** kali-n., nux-v.
sitting, while - am-m.
fever, during - all-s.
flexor muscles - op.
forenoon - alumn.
lightning-like - stry.
manual labor amel. - agar.
menses, during - ***coff.,*** oena.
morning - phos., sulph.
after rising - alumn.
sleeping - cham.
motion amel. - ***ars.,*** cop., phos., valer.
moving them, when - ***lyc.,*** sep.
night - ambr., calc., mag-c., nat-c., phos., sep., sil., staph., stront.
in bed - **ARS.,** merc-n., stry.
followed by - **RHUS-T.**
one arm and one leg - apis, apoc., hell., stram., tub.
one side, paralysis, of the other - ***apis,*** art-v., ***bell., stram.***
paralytic - cina.
paralyzed parts - apis, ***arg-n.,*** merc., nux-v., phos., ***sec.,*** stram., ***stry.***
paroxysmal - stram.
respiration simultaneous, with - hyos.
sitting, while - **VALER.**
sleep, during - acon., alum., ambr., ***ars.,*** bell., cham., cob., ***colch.,*** cupr., ***hell.,*** hep., ***kali-c., lyc.,*** mag-c., morph., nat-c., nat-m., petr., puls., ***sep.,*** sil., ***stront-c.,*** sulph., thuj., ***zinc.***
before - alum.
on falling asleep - alum., **ARS.,** ***cham.,*** mag-c., ***nat-m.,*** puls.
waking - nit-ac.
sudden - arn.
thunderstorm, during - phos.
touched, when - puls.
vexation, after - ign., petr.
vomiting, during - stram.
waking, on - op.
wandering - am-m., cast., cocc., coloc., graph., ***merc.,*** nat-s., plat.
write, on attempting to - nat-m.

WEAKNESS, of - acon., agar., alum., ***alumn.,*** am-c., am-m., anac., ant-c., ***arn.,*** ars., asaf., aur., **BAR-C.,** bar-m., bell., berb., bry., ***calc.,*** cann-s., canth., ***carb-ac., carb-v.,*** caust., cham., ***chin., chlol.,*** cimic., cocc., colch., ***con.,*** cortico., ***croc., dig.,*** dros., ***dulc.,*** euphr., ***ferr.,*** ferr-m., ferr-p., **GELS.,** graph., hyos., iod., kali-bi., kali-c., kali-n., ***kali-p.,*** laur., ***lyc.,*** macro., mag-c., mag-m., mag-p., mang., meny., merc., mez., mur-ac., ***nat-c.,*** **NAT-M., NIT-AC.,** nux-v., olnd., ***op.,*** petr., ph-ac., phos., phys., **PIC-AC.,** ***plat., plb.,*** puls., rad-br., rheum, ***rhod.,*** sabad., sarcol-ac., sec., ***sep., sil.,*** sin-n., spig., stann., stram., stront-c., sul-ac., ***sulph.,*** ter., thuj., ***verat.,*** verat-v., zinc.
could hardly move about - ***ferr-p.***
emissions, after - ***ph-ac.***
exertion, least, after - ***anac.,*** **ARS.,** bry., ***calc.,*** **CARB-V.,** cic., gels., ***kali-c., phos.***
liver disorder, in - sil.
paralytic - alum., ***alumn.,*** am-m., ***anac.,*** ars., bell., carb-v., **CAUST.,** ***cham., con.,*** ferr-ar., gels., ***kali-bi., kali-br., kali-c.,*** merc-c., nux-v., phos., sabad., **VERAT.**
progressive - acon., ars., caust., cupr-ar., ***dig.,*** kreos., ***ol-j., phos., plb.,*** verat.
raising arm to mouth is painful - eucal.
sexual debility, in - ***dig., ph-ac.***
walking, worse, feel as if giving way after rising - arg-m., ***cupr-m., ferr., guare.,*** **HYDR.,** kali-br., ***mag-c.***

Neck

ABSCESS - ***lach., lyc., petr.,*** ph-ac., psor., sec., sil., sul-ac., ***tarent-c.***
neck and nape - sul-ac.
scars, cicatrices, old - **SIL.**
abscess, throat, external - ***cham.,*** **HEP.,** kali-c., ***kali-i., lach., lyc.,*** **MERC.,** ***nit-ac.,*** phos., psor., sep., **SIL.,** sulph., sul-ac.

ACHING, pain - acon., ***aesc.,*** ambr., bar-c., bell., ***bry., calc., calc-caust.,*** cann-i., carb-v., chin., ***cimic.,*** con., dig., dios., **GELS.,** ***guai.,*** hell., hydr., ign., iod., kali-p., kalm., ***lach.,*** lachn., lil-t., lyc., lyss., ***merl.,*** myric., naja, nat-m., onos., par., petr., ***phyt.,*** ran-b., rhus-v., sep., sil., ***syph., verat-v.,*** vesp., ***zinc.***
air, slightest draft of - calc-p.
bending head back amel. - cycl., lac-c.
coughing, on - ***bell.***
evening - alum., olnd., **ZINC.**
extending to,
arms - plect.
back, small of on going to stool - verat.
head and shoulders - dios.
occipital region - aml-n.
shoulders - ***verat-v.***
spine - hell.
forenoon - agar.
morning - aml-n., thuj.
rising - calc-caust.
waking, on - ars.
motion, on - ***aesc.,*** glon., mez., sars., verat-v.
nape - cocc., gels., ph-ac., pic-ac., stroph.
room, on entering from open air - ran-b.
supper, after, amel. - sep.
writing, while - carb-an., **ZINC.**

AIR, cannot bear a draft of, on nape - ***hep., merc., sil.***
air, throat, external, sensitive to - ail., ***caust.,*** crot-t., ***fl-ac., hep., merc., sil.,*** tub.
air, sensation of, blowing through glands and thyroid on breathing - spong.

BLOW, throat, external, as from a, upper side - ruta.

BLUISH, nape of - ars., ***lach., rhus-t.***

BOILS - aster., bell., ***calc.,*** carb-an., coloc., crot-h., cypr., dig., ***graph., hep.,*** indg., **KALI-I.,** ***lach.,*** nat-m., ***nit-ac., petr., phos., psor.,*** rhus-v., sec., **SIL.,** sul-i., **SULPH.,** thuj., ust.
nape - pic-ac., sulph.
boils, side of - caust., coloc., graph., kali-i., mag-c., nat-m., nit-ac., phyt., rhus-v., sep.
sharp pain, with - hep., sep.

BORING, pain - bar-c., ***mag-p.,*** psor., sulph.
eating, after - sulph.

BRACHIAL, neuralgia - acon., all-c., bell-p., **BRY.,** calc-f., cham., **HYPER.,** ***kalm.,*** merc., nux-v., ***rhus-t.,*** ruta.., sulph., verat.

BREAK, as though neck would - **BELL.,** ***chel.,*** form.

BROKEN, as if - acon., agar., caust., chel., gels., nux-v., sabin., thuj.
as if it would break in two, worse left side when riding in a carriage - form.
moving or raising head, on - chel.

BROWN, neck and nape - caul., sanic.
skin of brown and greasy - apis, ***lyc., petr.,*** sep., thuj.

BURNING, pain - am-c., ***apis, ars.,*** aur-m-n., ***bar-c.,*** bell., ***calc.,*** carb-v., ***caust.,*** grat., kali-bi., kali-n., lach., lil-t., lyc., lyss., ***med.,*** **MERC.,** naja, nat-c., ***nat-s.,*** nicc., pall., phel., **PH-AC.,** ***phos., rhus-t.,*** stront-c., tab., vesp.
afternoon - fago.
evening - mag-c.
extending to,
down back - ***med.***
clavicle - nat-s.
occiput - ***calc.***
external - arn., aur-m-n., ***calc.,*** colch., ign., mez.
itching, sticking - ***calc.***
morning - am-c.
moving head agg. - nat-s., plb.
paroxysms - plb.
piercing - apis
scratching, after - mag-c.
sleep, amel. - ***calc.***
spots, in - kali-br.
stinging - glon.
swallowing - ***petr.***
touched, when - nat-m.
turning as if burnt, and twisting head, on - calc.
vertebra, first - nat-m.
burning, glands - bell., **MERC.,** nit-ac.
burning, sides - alumn., berb., calc., caust., coloc., form., grat., ign., merc-i-f., nat-s., stram., sulph., stront-c., tab., vesp.
dinner, after - grat.
left - berb., coloc., form., nat-s.
motion - stront-c.
right - alum., caust., merc-i-f., vesp.
burning, throat pit - calc-p., chel., elaps, lach.
morning - elaps

CARBUNCLES - ***anthr., caust.,*** crot-h., ***hep.,*** **LACH.,** rhus-t., **SIL.,** sulph.

CLOTHING, agg., throat, external - ***agar.,*** ambr., aml-n., ant-c., ***apis,*** arg-n., ***bell., calc., cact.,*** carb-an., carc., caust., cench., chel., **CENCH.,** cocc., con., **CROT-C., CROT-H.,** ***elaps,*** glon., kali-bi., ***kali-c.,*** lac-c., **LACH.,** merc., merc-c., naja, nicc., sars., ***sep.,*** sulph., ***tarent.,*** tub.

CLUCKING, throat, external, muscles, in - rheum.

COLDNESS - ***calc.,*** cann-i., carb-s., chel., chr-ac., ***dulc.,*** fl-ac., ir-foe., kali-chl., laur., lyc., nat-s., op., ran-s., **SIL.,** ***spong.,*** zinc.
creeping - sil.
evening - dulc., ***spong.***
extending, to occiput - chel.
to sacrum on lying down - thuj.
icy, nape - chel.
morning - ran-s.

COLDNESS,
sensitive to a draft - ***hep., merc.,*** sil.
coldness, throat, external - alum., berb., nat-s., phos., ***spong.***
evening - ***spong.***
night - lyc.

COLLAR, as if too tight, throat, external - aml-n., sep.

COMPRESSING, pain - crot-h., pip-m.

CONGESTION - bell., carb-h., **GELS.,** glon., ***kali-c.,*** tell.
congestion, throat, external - kali-c.
holding hands on heart - am-c.

CONSTRICTING - ***ferr., glon.***

CONSTRICTION, or band - agar., apis, asar., ***bell.,*** cact., calc-p., chel., dulc., ***glon., lach., nux-m.,*** sep., spong.
cord, as of a - chel., spong.
constriction, throat, external - acon., arg-n., ars., asar., cact., fl-ac., ***glon.,*** iod., **LACH.,** naja, puls., rat., ***sep.,*** **STRAM.,** ***stry.,*** tab., xan.
lying - glon.
sleep, during - lach.
throat pit - apis, ign., rhus-t., valer., zinc.
eating amel. - rhus-t.
sleep, on going to - valer.
constriction, throat pit - apis, ign., rhus-t., valer., zinc.
eating amel. - rhus-t.
sleep, on going to - valer.

CONTRACTING, pain, nape of - nux-m.

CRACKING - ***agar.,*** agn., aloe, alst., anac., aur-m-n., ***chel.,*** chin., ***cocc.,*** mag-arct., ***nat-c., nicc.,*** nit-ac., nux-v., ol-an., ***petr.,*** puls., raph., sep., spong., stann., ***sulph.,*** ther., thuj., x-ray, zing.
bending head backward - sulph.
moving, when - petr.
rising from stooping, on - nicc.
stooping, on - spong.
vertebra - chel., cocc., ol-an.

CRACKLING, throat, external, in muscles - rheum.

CRAMP, throat, external, in side - bar-c., cic., graph., mang., plat., sep., spong.

CRAMPING, sternocleido., muscle - trif-p.

CRAMP-like, pain - ant-c., arn., ***asar.,*** calc., ***calc-p.,*** **CIC.,** cimic., glon., mang., meny., naja, phyt., plat., sel., ***spong.,*** verat-v.
eating, after - sep.
evening - mang.
moving head - cimic., mang.
nape - hydr-ac., nux-v.
sneezing - arn.
swallowing, when - ***zinc.***
touch amel. - meny.
yawning - arn.

CRAWLING, throat, external, glands, in - con.

CRUSHED, throat, external, as if - sep.

CURVATURE of spine - ***calc.,*** phos., ***syph.***

CUTTING, pain - canth., dig., eup-per., glon., graph., grat., ***kali-bi.,*** naja, samb., stry.
right shoulder, and - gamb.
cutting, throat, external - ruta.
left - thuj.
cutting, sides - thuj.

DIGGING, pain - mang., ***thuj.***
moving head, on - thuj.
night - mang.

DISCOLORATION, throat, external - kali-bi., kali-s., podo., rhus-v.
blue - ***lach.***
brown - kali-s.
spots, in - kali-bi., ***sep.***
itching - kali-n.
lividity - ***ars.***
purple - tarent.
redness - am-caust., apis, graph., rhus-v.
spots, in - am-c., **BELL.,** carb-v., iod., kali-n., ***sep.,*** stann., tarent.
stripe, in - mang.
white spots - nat-c.
yellow - ars., chel., hydr.
spots - ***iod.***

DISLOCATED, as if - ang., asar., calc., cinnb., lachn.
arm, when lifting the - ***ang.***
extending over head and shoulders - asar.
turning head, on - calc., lachn.

DISTENTION, throat, external, left - caust.

DRAGGING, pain - ***gels.,*** pic-ac.

DRAWING, pain - acon., ***aesc., agar.,*** ail., all-s., ***alum.,*** ambr., ***am-c.,*** anac., ***ang.,*** ant-c., apis, asaf., asar., aur., bad., bapt., ***bell.,*** berb., bor., ***bry., calc-p.,*** camph., cann-i., cann-s., canth., carb-ac., carb-an., carb-s., ***carb-v.,*** carl., caul., **CHEL.,** ***chin.,*** cic., **CIMIC.,** clem., cocc., coc-c., ***coloc.,*** con., crot-t., cur., dig., dios., ***ferr.,*** fl-ac., kali-bi., kali-c., ***kali-n.,*** lact., ***lil-t., lyc.,*** lyss., mang., med., meny., ***merc.,*** mosch., ***nat-c., nat-m., nat-s.,*** nicc., nit-ac., ***nux-m., nux-v.,*** pall., ***petr.,*** ph-ac., phys., plb., psor., ***puls.,*** raph., rat., ***rhod.,*** ruta, sep., sil., stann., ***staph., sulph.,*** tep., ter., **THUJ.,** viol-o., zinc.
afternoon - calc-p., mag-c., nux-v., thuj.
bending head backwards - cycl., dig., valer.
cold, damp air - ***nux-m.***
evening - ant-c., nat-m., thuj.
exertion, arms of, agg. - ant-c.
manual agg. - ant-c.
extending to,
downward - am-c., asaf., ***chel.,*** coloc., nat-c., nux-v., psor., rat., spong.
ear - cann-s., colch.
elbow - lyc.
epigastrium - crot-c.
head - apis, calc., ***carb-v., ferr.***
occiput - lyc., nat-m., ***petr.,*** ph-ac., pin-s., spig., valer.
scapula - ant-c.
shoulders - bor., camph., ***chel.,*** con., crot-h., kali-n., lyc., mosch., phyt.

DRAWING, pain,
extending, to
shoulders, left shoulder and scapulae while walking in open air - bor.
tendons - am-m.
upward - ambr., calc., cann-s., ***petr.,*** ter.
intermittent - spig.
menses, before - ***nat-c.,*** nux-v.
morning - ant-c., cimic., nux-v., staph.
on bending head forward - ***cimic.***
on waking - aloe, alum.
moving, when - acon., asaf., ***bell.,*** caps., ***coloc.,*** hyos., ***rhus-t.,*** vario.
amel. - alum.
head, agg. - nat-c.
paralytic - cocc., staph.
paroxysmal - sil.
reading, while - nat-c.
rheumatic - anac., bor., sep., ***staph.***
right - sulph., zinc.
sitting, while - ant-c., aur-m., nux-v.
stooping, on - ant-c., berb., canth., rhus-t.
sudden - nat-c.
turning head - ant-c., chel., hyos.
to left - ***ant-c.***
walking - calc-p., con.
in open air - camph., con.
windy weather - calc-p.

drawing, glands - alum.

drawing, sides - alumn., ant-c., asaf., bell., ***bry.,*** caul., chel., chin., cic., clem., cocc., coloc., ***crot-c.,*** cycl., dulc., grat., hell., indg., kali-c., lyc., med., nat-s., nit-ac., ***nux-v.,*** petr., ph-ac., sars., ***seneg.,*** sep., spong., squil., staph., sulph., teucr., zinc.
afternoon - ***chel.,*** fl-ac., kalm.
bending head, backward - cycl.
forward - staph.
chewing - zinc.
downward - sil., zinc.
evening - ant-c., cycl., mag-c.
extending to,
ear, behind - rhod.
elbow - lyc.
eye - ph-ac.
limbs, into - stram.
lower jaw - indg.
shoulder - ***chel.,*** con., led., lyc., rhod.
upward - lyc., thuj.
holding head erect - zinc.
jerking side - spong.
left - indg.
lancinating - ***indg.***
left - caul., chel., cic., coloc., cycl., lyc., nat-s., sulph., verat.
morning - thuj.
waking, on - thuj.
motion, on - asaf., ***chel.,*** coloc., cycl., nux-v., sulph.
right - ***caust., chel.,*** con., dulc., grat., indg., kali-c., mag-c., mag-m., nux-v., plat., sars., sil., spong., staph., sul-ac., thuj., zinc.
to lower jaw - indg.
sitting, while - ant-c., ***chel.***

drawing, sides
turning head - clem., ***crot-c.,*** ph-ac.
twitching - plat.
upward - thuj.
walking in open air - camph.

drawing, throat, external - nat-m.

ECZEMA - anac., ***lyc.,*** psor., ***sil.***

ELECTRIC shocks from - calc-p.

EMACIATION - ***calc.,*** iod., ***lyc.,*** mag-c., **NAT-M.,** ***sanic., sars.,*** senec., verat.

ERUPTIONS - ***agar.,*** ant-c., ant-t., arn., ars., bar-m., bell., berb., bry., caust., cham., chel., ***clem., graph., hep., kali-bi.,*** lyc., mang., nat-a., nat-m., ***petr.,*** psor., rhus-t., sec., sep., **SIL.,** staph., stram., sul-ac., sul-i., sulph., thuj.
acne - amph., jug-r.
dry on, peeling off in fine mealy scales - graph.
erythema - chlol., gels., hyos.
itching, menses, before - carb-v.
margins of hair - nat-m., petr.
measly spots - ars., cop., morph.
moist - caust., ***clem.***
nodules, painless - ***graph.,*** psor.
itching - sil.
red - petr.
pimples - agar., alum., berb., bor., cann-s., carb-an., carb-v., cinnb., ***clem.,*** crot-t., ***gels.,*** hep., hyos., jug-r., kali-bi., kali-c., kali-n., lyc., meph., nat-a., nat-m., nicc., pall., petr., ph-ac., psor., ***puls.,*** rhus-t., ***sil., staph., sulph.,*** sul-ac., thuj., trom., verb., zing.
burning - am-c., kali-n.
confluent - tarent.
deep-seated - til.
extending to scalp - clem.
flattened - rhus-t.
hard - crot-t.
inflamed - sulph.
itching - bar-c., kali-c., puls., ***sil., staph.***
moist - ***clem.***
painful to touch - hep., sulph.
scratching, on - carb-an., nicc., ***puls.***
scratching, from - nat-c.
suppurating - nat-c., calc-p.
purpura - ars.
pustules - ant-c., aur., bell., kali-n., nat-a., nat-c., psor., sars., tab., thuj., zinc-ac.
like cow-pox - ant-t.
scabs, bloody - ant-t.
scales, white - graph., ***sil.***

eruption, throat, external - ***anac., ars.,*** berb., bry., bov., bry., calc., canth., caust., clem., dig., ***hep.,*** kali-n., lyc., merc., ph-ac., raph., sars., sep., squil., thuj.
blotches - graph., nat-m., sars., sep., spong.
burning - kali-n.
crusts - anac.
itching - lyc., mag-c.
moist - ***caust.***
painful - lyc.

eruption, throat, external
pimples - agar., alum., ant-c., berb., bor., bov., canth., ***cinnb.,*** clem., ***hep., jug-r.,*** kali-n., lyc., mag-c., mez., mur-ac., nat-m., ph-ac., raph., ***puls.,*** spig., spong., stann., staph., sulph., ***thuj.,*** zinc.
pustules - ant-c., aur., chel., ***psor.***
row, in a - thuj.
rash - am-c., chin.
red - chin., lyc., mez., ph-ac., sep., spig., thuj.
scratching, after - mag-c.
stitching - phos.
tubercles - am-c., lach., lyc., mur-ac., nicc., ph-ac., phos., sec.
urticaria - bry., kali-i.
vesicles - clem., mag-c., ph-ac., sep., vip.
side of - alum.
side of, ear, discharge from - **TELL.**

ERYSIPELAS - graph., kali-i., ph-ac.
extending to face - rhus-t.

EXCORIATION, throat, external, from rubbing of clothes - olnd., squil.

FISTULA, throat, external - ***phos., sil.***

FORMICATION - arund., ***carl.,*** dulc., lac-c., nux-v., phos., sabin., ***sec.,*** spong.
house, on entering a - phos.
formication, throat, external - rhus-v., spong.
throat pit, causing cough - ***sang.***

FULLNESS, throat, external, in jugular - ***crot-c.***
fullness, throat pit, in - cham., con., ***lach.***

FUNGUS, growth on - thuj.

GNAWING, pain - ***nat-s., thuj.***

GRASPS, throat, external during cough - acon., ***all-c., cupr., iod.,*** lob., ***samb.***

HEAT - aesc., agar., aml-n., ***calc.,*** coloc., com., cycl., fago., ***fl-ac., glon.,*** hydr., kalm., ***lach.,*** merc-i-f., ***nux-v.,*** ol-an., ***par.,*** phel., ***phos.,*** rhus-t., sars., ***sumb.,*** tarent.
afternoon - com.
with cold hands - sumb.
evening, 7 to 8 p.m. - fl-ac.
extending, all directions - rhus-t.
down back - glon., ***par.***
up back - calc., ***fl-ac., glon.***
flushes, in spine - aesc., fl-ac., hydr., ***lach., med.,*** **PHOS.,** podo., sarr.
sitting, while - dig.
heat, throat, external - cycl., lach., sars., sulph.

HEAVINESS - ***agar.,*** asar., ***calc-p.,*** cann-i., caps., carb-ac., ***chel.,*** kali-c., meny., nux-v., **PAR.,** ***petr., phos.,*** plb., **RHUS-T.,** samb., sep., tab., verat.
morning - nux-v.
nape - meny., ***nux-v.,*** par., ***rhus-t.***
walking, after - ***rhus-t.***
weight upon - kali-c., **PAR.,** ***phos.,*** rhus-t.

HERPES - ars., carb-an., caust., clem., ***con., graph.,*** hyos., kali-n., lac-d., ***lyc.,*** nat-m., ***petr.,*** psor., ***sep.,*** sulph.
itching - caust.
moist - carb-an., caust., nat-m., sep.
herpes, throat, external - lac-d., lyc., **PSOR.,** sars., sep.

INFLAMMATION, of neck region - par., ***rhus-t.***
spondylitis - ph-ac., ***rhus-t.***
inflammation, glands - acon-l., ***am-c.,*** astac., bac., **BAR-C.,** bar-i., ***bell., brom., calc.,*** calc-chln., calc-f., calc-i., ***carb-an.,*** caust., ***cist.,*** dulc., graph., hecla., ***hep.,*** iod., kali-i., kali-m., ***lap-a.,*** mag-p., **MERC.,** ***merc-i-f., merc-i-r.,*** nit-ac., ***phyt.,*** rhus-r., ***rhus-t.,*** rhus-v., sil., spong., ***still.,*** sulph.

INJURIES - ***arn.,*** bell-p., **BRY.,** ***calc.,*** calc-f., caust., cic., **HYPER.,** mez., ***nat-s.,*** **RHUS-T.,** ***ruta, symph.***
concussion, of, spine - arn., mez., nat-s.
whiplash - arn., **BRY.,** ***calc.,*** caust., cic., **HYPER., RHUS-T.,** ***ruta.***

INDURATION of glands, throat, external - ***alum., alumn.,*** am-c., ant-c., bac., bar-c., ***bar-i.,*** **BAR-M., BELL., CALC.,** calc-f., **CALC-I.,** ***calc-p.,*** **CARB-AN.,** carb-s., ***carb-v.,*** carc., ***cist.,*** **CON.,** ***cupr., dulc., graph., hecla., hep.,*** **IOD.,** ***kali-i., lyc., merc., nat-c.,*** nat-m., ***nit-ac.,*** puls., ***rhus-t., sars.,*** sep., **SIL.,** ***spong.,*** staph., **SULPH.,** syc-co., **TAB.**
knotted cords, like - aeth., **BAR-I., BAR-M.,** berb., ***calc.,*** **CALC-I.,** ***cist., dulc.,*** hecla., hep., ***iod.,*** lyc., ***merc.,*** nit-ac., ***psor.,*** rhus-t., ***sil., sulph.,*** **TUB.**

ITCHING - agar., agn., **ALUM.,** ammc., anac., ***ant-c.,*** arg-n., ars., benz-ac., ***berb.,*** calc., carb-ac., carb-v., caust., con., cycl., ***gels.,*** grat., hydr., hydr-ac., ign., jug-c., kali-bi., kali-n., laur., lyc., mag-c., mag-m., mang., merc-i-r., mez., morph., myric., nat-a., nat-c., **NAT-M.,** nat-p., nicc., nit-ac., ox-ac., pall., ***puls.,*** rat., ***rhus-t.,*** rumx., sars., sep., sil., squil., staph., **SULPH.,** tarent., ther., thuj., trom.
burning - ***kali-bi.***
scratching, after - mag-c.
evening - calc., carb-v., fl-ac., mag-c., stront-c., ther., trom.
bed, in - calc., sulph.
before going to bed - mag-m.
undressing, while - am-m., hyper., nat-s.
extending in all directions, worse from heat, better from cold - rhus-t.
menses, during - mag-c.
morning - fl-ac., nat-m., sulph., ther.
rising, after - sulph.
night - ail., hydr.
in heat of bed - ***sulph.***
scratching, after, agg. - nat-m.
changes place - sars.
not relieved by - nicc.
stinging - carb-v., rhus-t.
touched, when - psor.
walking in open air - nit-ac.
air, in open, burning - berb., ***calc.***

itching, throat, external - **ALUM.,** ambr., am-m., anac., ant-c., apis, ars., aur., bov., ***calc.,*** canth., carb-v., caust., chel., ***cist.,*** con., fl-ac., form., ***glon.,*** kali-i., kali-n., lyc., mag-c., mez., ***nat-c.,*** nit-ac., plan., rhus-v., samb., sep., stront-c., sulph., tarent., thuj.
evening - mez.
before going to sleep - mag-c.
extending to,
chest - fl-ac.
eustachian tubes - caust.
larynx - sil., zinc.
menses, during - mag-c.
morning - mag-c.
dressing, while - mag-c.
night - kalm.
scratching amel. - mag-c., squil.
stitching - carb-v., sars.
swallowing agg. - aur., con.
walking in open air - nit-ac.

JERKING, muscles, in - aeth., coloc., sep.
muscles, in, convulsions, before - bufo.

JERKING, pain - aeth., aur., caps., ***chin.,*** tarax.
jerking, throat, external - arg-m., caps.

JERKS, throat, external, left - mez.

LAMENESS - cycl., nat-c., par., spig.
nape - zinc.

LANCINATING, pain - bell., canth., elaps

LUMP, throat pit, in - ***lob.***

NUMBNESS - berb., cast-eq., ***chel.,*** dig., hura, merc-i-f., par., ***plat.,*** rhus-t., tell.
numbness, throat, external - ***carb-an.,*** chel., olnd., sep., ***spong.***

ORGASM, in nape of, extending over top of head of forehead, afternoon, during motion - mang.

PAIN, neck - abrot., ***acon., aesc., aeth., agar.,*** ail., all-c., all-s., ***alum.,*** alumn., ambr., ***am-c.,*** am-m., ***anac.,*** ang., ant-c., ***apis,*** arg-m., arn., **ARS.,** ***ars-i.,*** arum-t., ***asar., atro.,*** aur-m-n., bar-c., **BELL.,** berb., bor., ***bry.,*** cact., ***calc., calc-p.,*** calc-s., ***camph.,*** cann-i., cann-s., canth., carb-ac., carb-an., carb-s., ***carb-v.,*** card-m., **CAUST.,** ***chel., chin.,*** chin-a., ***chin-s.,*** **CIC.,** cimic., ***cinnb.,*** clem., coc-c., ***cocc.,*** cod., colch., ***coloc., con.,*** crot-c., crot-h., cund., cupr., cupr-ar., cur., cycl., ***daph.,*** dig., dios., dol., ***dros., dulc.,*** echi., eup-per., ferr., ferr-ar., ***ferr-p., fl-ac., form.,*** gamb., **GELS.,** ***glon.,*** **GRAPH.,** grat., ***guai., hell., hep., ign., ip.,*** jac-c., ***kali-ar., kali-bi.,*** kali-c., kali-cy., kali-n., ***kali-p.,*** kali-s., ***kalm.,*** **LAC-C.,** ***lach.,*** lachn., lact., laur., led., lil-t., ***lyc., lyss.,*** mag-c., ***mag-p., med.,*** meph., ***merc., mez.,*** mosch., myric., naja, nat-m., ***nat-s.,*** nit-ac., ***nux-m.,*** nux-v., olnd., ol-an., onos., ox-ac., pall., **PAR.,** petr., **PH-AC.,** ***phos.,*** phys., ***phyt.,*** pic-ac., pip-m., plb., podo., psor., ***puls., ran-b.,*** raph., rat., **RHOD.,** rhus-t., rumx., ruta., sabin., samb., ***sang.,*** sarr., sars., sel., sep., ***sil.,*** spig., stann., stram., staph., stry., sulph., ***tab.,*** tarax., tarent., ter., thuj., vario., verat., vesp., ***zinc.***

PAIN, neck
afternoon - calc-p., chel., chin-s., mag-p., nux-v., thuj.
4 p.m. - ***chin-s.***
air, a draught of - **CALC-P.,** cimic., hep., lach., merc., psor., **RHUS-T.,** sanic., sil., stront-c.
cold damp - nux-m., ***ran-b.***
fresh, amel. - psor.
open - laur.
amel. - psor.
alternating, with headache - hyos.
amel. - spong.
ascending, steps - ph-ac.
bending, head, backward - bell., chel., cic., cinnb., cycl., kali-c., laur., lyc., valer.
backward, amel. - cycl., lac-c., ***lyss.,*** manc., syph.
forward, on - cimic., graph., lyss., rad-br., stann.
amel. - gels., laur., sanic.
left, to - par.
right, to - sulph.
blow, as of - naja.
blowing, nose - ***kali-bi.***
breathing, deeply - ***chel.***
chewing agg. - form., zinc.
chill, during - ail., ars-h.
clothing agg. - caust., lach.
cold, taken in open air - phos.
coughing - ***alum., bell., caps.,*** lact., **SULPH.**
dinner, after - con.
eating, after - ***nux-v.***
evening - alum., brach., dios., fl-ac., form., ***kali-s.,*** nat-m., ***nux-v.,*** olnd., thuj.
going to bed - alum.
looking up - form.
exertion, agg. - arg-n., ***calc.,*** lil-t., ***sep.***
mental - par., zinc.
physical - ant-c.
extending to,
arm, to - all-c., ***bry.,*** cham., cocc., corn-f., ***hyper., kalm., lach.,*** nat-m., ***nux-v., rhus-t., sulph.,*** ter., ***verat.***
and fingers, to - ***kalm.,*** nux-v., par.
left - kalm., ***lach.,*** par.
right - ferr-pic.
back, down the - aeth., am-c., chel., cimic., ***cocc.,*** graph., glon., gua., lil-t., ***kalm.,*** mag-c., nat-m., phyt., podo., psor., rat., sang., sep., stry., thuj., verat.
on going to stool - verat.
brain - ferr., kalm., ***par.***
clavicles, to - ***gels.,*** nat-s.
ear, to - bov., cann-s., calc-p., colch., elaps, lyss., thuj.
behind left - apis.
behind right - elaps.
epigastrium, to - crot-c.
eye, to - gels., sel., **SIL.,** sulph., thea.
face, to - kalm.
fingers, to - ***kalm.,*** nux-v., par.
forehead - daph., lyss., mez., rat., sars., tub.
walking, while - rat.

PAIN, neck

extending to,

head, to - apis, ***carb-v., ferr.,*** meny., ***par., puls.,*** **SIL.,** stront.

all over - carb-v., **GELS.,** grat., kalm., nat-s.

through - fl-ac.

larynx, to - **CALC-P.**

occiput, to - bell., bry., calc-p., chel., chin., chin-s., ***cinnb.,*** dulc., eup-per., ***ferr.,*** **GELS.,** glon., hell., kali-c., kalm., lat-m., nat-c., nat-m., ***nat-s.,*** nux-v., ***phyt.,*** puls., **SIL.,** spig., tub., valer., verat., zinc-p.

when head is bent back - cinnb.

sacrum, to - chel., guai., lyc.

shoulders, to - alum., bor., calc-p., camph., caust., crot-h., daph., dios., gels., graph., kalm., kali-n., ip., lach., laur., mez., mosch., nat-m., phyt., sang., stry., thuj., ***verat-v.***

between - am-m., ***apis.***

evening, after lying down - lyc.

left - bor., ran-b.

left, walking, while - bor.

motion, on - equis.

right - ***acon.,*** alum., hydr.

throat, to - chin.

upward - aml-n., berb., calc., cann-s., canth., dios., form., **GELS.,** lach., ***nat-s., petr.,*** sep., **SIL.,** stram., stront-c., ter., ***verat-v.***

vertex, to - ***bell.,*** berb., calc., carb-v., caust., ***chel., cimic.,*** ferr., fl-ac., **GELS.,** ***glon., hell., kalm.,*** puls., rhus-t., ***sang.,*** sep., **SIL.,** ***stram.,*** verat-v.

to nape, back and forth - ***chel.***

wrists, to - chel.

forenoon - agar., stry.

gargling agg. - form.

glands, from swollen - graph.

hawking agg. - form.

left - ***con.,*** thuj.

lifting, exertion agg. - arg-n., calc., lil-t., sep.

looking up, on - **GRAPH.**

lying, while - ***glon.,*** kali-i., ***lyc.***

back, on - graph., spig.

right side - ferr.

menses, during - ***calc.,*** mag-c.

before - nat-c., nux-v., sulph.

mental, exertion - par.

morning - ant-c., arg-m., asaf., bar-c., chel., eupi., ferr-ma., ferr-p., kali-c., nat-c., ***nux-v., rhod.,*** sars., sil., spig., staph., ***stram.,*** sulph., thuj., ***zinc.***

rising, amel. - alum.

waking, on - aloe, alum., ars., asaf., kali-bi., psor., thuj., verat.

motion, amel. - aur-m-n., spig.

hand, of, agg. - cimic.

moving head - ***aesc., agar., alum.,*** asaf., am-m., bad., bapt., ***bell.,*** brach., ***bry.,*** cann-s., canth., ***chel.,*** chin., cimic., ***cocc.,*** colch., ***coloc., dros.,*** form., glon., ***hyper.,*** ip., kali-bi., merc., mez., nat-s., nux-v., podo., ***ran-b.,***

PAIN, neck

moving head - ***rhus-t.,*** sabad., sars., stann., stram., ***sulph., tarent.,*** verat-v.

to either side - ***agar.***

nape of neck - nat-ch., xan.

neuralgic - chel., hydr., nux-v.

night - alum., carb-an., caust., glon., guai., ***kalm.,*** lach., merc-c., nat-s., ***olnd., puls.,*** sang., sil., stann., sulph., ***zinc.***

6 p.m. to 4 a.m. - guai.

before - sulph.

midnight - lach., mag-s.

noon - ptel.

overlifting, after - ***calc.***

paralytic - nat-c., nat-m.

paroxysmal - anac., ***kalm.,*** nux-v., sil., ***stry.***

periodic - ***chin-s.,*** colch., ***kali-s.***

perspiration, amel. - thuj.

position, as from wrong - dulc., lyc., nux-v., psor., puls., **RHUS-T.,** thuj., zinc.

pulsating - ***eup-per.,*** lyss.

raising the, arms - ***ang.,*** ant-c., ***graph.***

the, head - ars., chel., senn.

reading, while - nat-c.

rheumatic - acon., ambr., anac., ***ant-c.,*** bapt., berb., bism., bor., ***bry.,*** calc., ***calc-p.,*** carb-s., caust., **CIMIC.,** ***colch., con.,*** cycl., ***dulc.,*** gels., graph., ***guai.,*** iod., ***merc.,*** mez., ***nux-v., puls.,*** **RAN-B.,** ***rhod.,*** **RHUS-T.,** ***sang., sil., spig.,*** squil., ***staph.,*** stict., ***sulph.,*** tarent., verat.

riding, in a carriage - form.

right, side - sulph.

on turning head - carc., cinnb., ***mez.***

rising from stooping - nicc., spig.

room, agg. - psor.

seized by hand, as if - grat.

shoulder, and neck - crot-t., guai., lachn., sang., stict., sulph., verat-v.

right - nux-v., sang., zinc.

sides, alternating - calc-p., lac-c., ***puls.***

sitting, while - aur-m., lyss., nux-v.

erect amel. - rad-br.

sleep, preventing - sil.

sneezing, when - am-m., arn., mag-c.

amel. - calc.

standing, amel. - rad-br.

in one position, agg. - cham.

sternomastoid muscle, left - elat.

stool, after, amel. - asaf.

stooping - agar., ant-c., berb., canth., gran., graph., kali-bi., lac-ac., manc., par., ***rhus-t.,*** spig., sulph.

sublingual glands - arund., iod.

swallowing, when - calc-p., colch., nat-c., petr., zinc.

talking - ***calc.,*** sulph.

touch, from - chin., lach., ***nux-v.,*** tell.

PAIN, neck
turning, head - acon., agar., alumn., am-c., am-m., ant-c., aur-s., bell., ***bry., calc.,*** canth., carb-s., chel., chin., coloc., dulc., eup-per., graph., hyos., nat-m., nat-s., plat., ***ran-b.,*** sanic., sep., spong., stram., tarent., verat.
to left - ***alum., ant-c.***
uncovering amel. - sars.
waking, on - psor., thuj.
walking, while - calc-p., con., ph-ac., tab.
after - cur.
wandering - **LAC-C.**
warm, room - ***kali-s.,*** psor.
warmth, external, amel. - ***rhus-t.***
windy, weather - ***calc-p.***
writing, while - carb-an., lyc., **ZINC.**
yawning, on - arn., cocc., nat-s.

PAIN, glands - arn., **BELL.,** bor., ***calc., caps., carb-v.,*** caust., hell., hura, kali-c., ***merc., nat-m.,*** psor., puls., **SIL.,** thuj.
coughing, when - nat-m.
night - merc., thuj.
turning head, when - ign., kali-c.

PAIN, sides - abrot., alum., arg-m., ***bell.,*** calc-p., chin-s., ***chel.,*** cinnb., coloc., crot-c., jac-c., kali-c., kali-i., kali-n., kalm., lyss., merc-i-f., nat-s., ***par.,*** phys., psor., sars., sel., tarent., verat-v., vesp.
afternoon - chel., iris
bending head to right - sulph.
blowing nose - merc.
extending to,
behind ear - rhod.
eye - sel.
pectoral muscles - ars.
shoulder - ***chel.,*** par., zinc.
wrist - chel.
forenoon - fl-ac.
heat amel. - trif-p.
left - sel.
morning - sars., tarent., zinc.
motion, on - ***chel., colch.,*** ham., kali-c., phys., tarax.
cramping - cimic.
head, of - com.
jaw, of - tarax.
night - vesp.
paroxysmal - ***sel.***
pulsating - manc.
rheumatic - calc-s., ***chel.,*** cycl., iod., phys., rhus-t., staph.
right - ph-ac., sars.
turning head to, on - arg-m., cinnb., nat-m., ***tarent.***
painful side - vesp.
right - arg-m., chin-s., psor., ***tarent.***
waking, on - phys.
yawning - plat.

PAIN, throat, external - ***bar-c.,*** caps., fago., kreos., ***merc., nat-m.,*** op., phos., ***puls.,*** sul-ac.
extending to sternocleidomastoideus, upper part - gels.
morning - phos.
motion, on - phos.

PAIN, throat, external
touch, on - phos.

PAIN, throat, pit - ***caust.,*** iod., ***lach.,*** spong.
anger, after - staph.
drinking, when - nit-ac.
hawking of mucus - **CAUST.**

PARALYSIS, throat, external - gels., spig.
diphtheria, after - ***lac-c.***
sterno-mastoid - plb.

PARALYTIC, morning - sel.

PERSPIRATION - ***anac.,*** ars., **CALC.,** cann-s., chel., **CHIN.,** elaps, ferr., fl-ac., lach., mag-c., mang., med., mosch., ***nit-ac.,*** nux-v., phel., **PH-AC.,** sanic., ***sep., sil.,*** spig., **STANN., SULPH.,** tub.
cold, nape of neck - con.
daytime - ph-ac.
evening - fl-ac.
menses, before - ***nit-ac.***
morning - nux-v., stann., sulph.
motion, least - **CHIN.**
night - ***calc., sulph.,*** tub.
sleep, in - **CALC.,** ***lach.,*** med., ph-ac., ***phos., sanic.***
amel. - samb.
walking - camph.
perspiration, throat, external - alum., bell., cann-s., cham., clem., coff., euph., ip., kali-c., lach., **MANG.,** nux-v., par., petr., **RHUS-T.,** samb., spig., **STANN.,** sulph.
evening - chel.
6 p.m. to 9 p.m. - chel.
midnight - rhus-t.
night - nit-ac.
one-sided - nit-ac.
waking, on - mang., nit-ac.

PINCHING, pain, throat, external - ph-ac., phos.
side - hep., iod., lyc., zinc.

PRESSES, throat, external, with both hands - bell.

PRESSING, pain - agar., agn., ambr., ***anac.,*** ant-s., ***ars., bar-c.,*** **BELL.,** benz-ac., bism., bry., canth., ***carb-v.,*** card-m., ***chel., cocc., coloc.,*** crot-t., cupr., dig., ***elaps*** euph., ***glon.,*** graph., grat., guai., ip., ***lach., laur.,*** lyc., lyss., meny., merc., mez., mosch., ***nat-m., nat-s.,*** nit-ac., ol-an., **PAR.,** petr., ph-ac., **PHOS.,** ***puls.,*** rhus-t., samb., sars., sil., spong., ***sulph.,*** tarax., thuj.
air, open, in - ***laur.***
bandaged, as if - asar.
bending head, backward - bell., cupr., dig.
backward amel. - cycl.
forward - rhus-t.
forward, compelling - ***laur.***
collar, as from a tight - asar.
coughing - ***bell., caps.***
evening - fl-ac., sep.
extending to,
clavicle - nat-s.
head - ambr., grat.
occiput - guai., nat-c., nat-s., ph-ac.
shoulders - ip.

PRESSING, pain
finger, as by a - rheum.
intermittent - ***anac.,*** dulc.
lying, while - ***glon., lyc.***
on back- dulc.
morning - dulc., sil.
waking, on - anac., asaf.
motion, agg. - petr.
of head, on - mez.
night - sulph.
rising from bed - cinnb.
small spots - lyc.
stooping, on - canth.
swallowing - colch.
talking, on - sulph.
turning head - canth., ***coloc., nat-s.***
vertebra, seventh - sep.
walking, air, in open - meny., sep.
weight, as from - anac., caps., coloc., **PAR.**
after walking - **RHUS-T.**

pressing, glands - alum.

pressing, sides - anac., ant-c., arg-n., asaf., aur., bell., bism., cocc., ***coloc.,*** crot-t., dig., form., kalm., lach., led., lyc., mag-c., ***merc.,*** nat-s., nit-ac., phos., ***ph-ac.,*** sabin., ***sars.,*** spong., squil., staph., tarax., zinc.
extending, ear, behind - nat-s.
shoulder, to - sul-ac.
impending swallowing - anac.
intermittent - spong.
left - sil., sul-ac., verat.
motion, agg. - sars.
amel. - led.
right - anac., carb-v., cocc., kali-c., thuj., zinc.
talking, while - zinc.
touch agg. - sars.
turning head - ***coloc.***
upward - thuj.
walking in open air - arg-m.
rapidly amel. - caust.

pressing, sublingual glands - iod.

pressing, throat pit - aesc., anac., **BROM.,** ***caust.,*** cic., graph., **LACH.,** lob., phos., sars.
anger, after - ***staph.***
foreign body, as of - ***caust.***
inspiration, on - caust.
swallowing agg. - staph.

PRICKLING - ***carb-an.***

PROLAPSE, of cervical disc - bry., prot.

PULSATING - **APIS,** ***calc-p.,*** chel., con., cur., daph., ***eup-per.,*** ferr., glon., lyss., manc., nat-m., ***nat-s., nit-ac.,*** op., ***phos.,*** raph., staph., sulph., sumb., **VERAT-V.**
extending to,
forehead and occiput - chel.
forehead on moving or stooping - ter.
lumbar region - cur.
shoulder - **APIS,** con.
holding head backward amel. - lyss., manc.
lying down, on - plb.
menses, during - ***nit-ac.,*** **VERAT-V.**
before - ***nit-ac.***
motion agg. - ***ferr.***

PULSATING,
raising head from stooping - kali-n.
sitting, while - ***calc-p.***
vertebra - kali-n.
writing agg. - manc.

pulsation, carotids, throat, external - ***acon.,*** aml-n., arg-n., ***aur., bad.,*** **BELL.,** ***bry., cact., calc.,*** calc-p., chin., cocc., colch., cupr., dirc., elaps, fago., ***gels., glon., hep.,*** hyos., hyper., lac-ac., lil-t., meli., olnd., ***op.,*** phos., phys., rumx., sabad., sep., sol-n., spig., spong., stram., ***stront-c., tarent.,*** tub., usn., ***verat-v.,*** thuj.
excitement, from - ***bad.***
left - sulph.
walking rapidly after dinner - carb-ac.

pulsation, glands - ***am-m.,*** bell., lach.

pulsation, sides - cycl., ***gent-c.,*** hura, lac-ac., nat-m., sars., sulph., sumb., ***tarent.***
evening - cycl.

QUIVERING, in - ***ang.***

RASH - ant-c., bry., caust., **CHEL.,** mez., nat-c., sec.
erysipelatous - hydr.
heat - **SULPH.**
itching - calc., ***mez.***
miliary - nat-a.
purple - hyos.
red - nat-a.

rash, front - am-c., chin.

REDNESS - aml-n., ***bell., crot-h., graph.,*** iod., lac-d., merc., phos., ***rhus-t.,*** verat., vesp.

SENSITIVE, throat, external, angles of jaw, at - thyr.
slightest touch, to - ***lac-c.,*** **LACH.,** ***nicc.***

SHARP, pain - acon., aeth., agar., alum., ang., arn., aur., bad., bar-c., bell., ***bov.,*** bry., calc., ***carb-an.,*** carb-s., carb-v., caust., chel., ***chin.,*** cocc., coc-c., con., dig., dros., elaps, ferr-p., graph., guai., ign., kali-c., lach., lyc., lyss., mag-s., merc., nat-c., ***nat-m., nat-p.,*** nat-s., nicc., ph-ac., psor., puls., ***rhus-v.,*** samb., ***sars.,*** senec., sep., sil., spong., ***stann.,*** staph., ***stry.,*** sul-ac., ***sulph.,*** tarax., thuj., verat., zinc.
afternoon - stry.
ascending steps, on - ph-ac.
bent over - sulph.
coughing - alum.
evening - bov., coc-c., nat-c., thuj.
in bed - lyc.
extending to,
ear - bov., thuj., stry.
eye - sel.
head - kalm.
lumbar region - tep., stry.
occiput - kali-c., ph-ac.
sacrum - lyc., stry.
shoulder - am-m., laur., stry., thuj.
shoulder, right - alum.
upward - berb., lyc.
vertex - rhus-r., ***sil.***
itching - stann.
lying, while - caust., kali-i.

SHARP, pain
moving, on - alum., camph., dig., guai., merc., sars.
head - acon., am-m., bad., dig., samb., sars., thuj.
head, forward and backward - cocc.
morning in bed - stann.
night - caust., kalm., nat-m., nat-s.
pulsating - cocc.
sitting, while - lyc.
amel. - tarax.
sneezing, on - am-m., lyc., mag-c.
stinging - ***apis,*** bar-c., calc., lyss., phyt.
stooping, on - agar., sulph.
stretching out amel. - sulph.
swallowing amel. - ***spong.***
talking while - ***calc.***
turning head, on - alum., verat.
vertebra, between last cervical and first thoracic - staph.
walking, on - ph-ac.
sharp, glands - alum., bell., bor., carb-an., kali-c., lyc., sil.
sharp, sides - alum., aur., berb., bor., chin., clem., form., ***graph.,*** guai., kali-bi., kalm., meny., nat-c., phos., rat., ***sars.,*** spig., spong., staph., stront-c., stry., sul-ac., tarax., ***thuj.,*** zinc.
afternoon - canth.
boring - tarax.
evening - clem.
extending to arms - ***berb.***
left - kali-c., phos.
morning - thuj.
motion of, head - am-m., graph., sars.
of, throat - dig.
night - kalm.
right - ang., carb-ac., nat-c., sars., spig.
swallowing amel. - spong.
touch agg. - sars.
turning head - coc-c., dig.
sharp, submaxillary glands - iod.
sharp, throat, external - alum., am-m., ***anac.,*** ant-c., chin., colch., hep., kalm., nat-m., rhus-v., sars., tep., ***thuj.***
extending to ear - alum., phos., tep.
intermittent - cupr.
turning head, when - hep.
sharp, throat, pit - bell., ran-s., ***spong.,*** thuj.
inspiration, on - thuj.

SHOCKS - corn., ***manc.***
waking, on - ***manc.***

SHORTNESS, region, of - alum., bell., cic., cimic., syph.
fat neck, in children - kali-bi.
nape - ign., nat-m., tub.

SORE, pain - acon., ***aesc., agar.,*** ambr., arg-m., arn., ***ars.,*** ars-i., ***bad.,*** bapt., ***bell.,*** bov., brach., calc-p., ***carb-ac.,*** caust., chin., cic., coloc., cycl., dig., dros., dulc., ***ferr.,*** fl-ac., ***gels.,*** graph., ham., iod., kali-bi., ***kalm., lach.,*** lec., lyc., merc-i-f., naja, nat-c., ***nat-m.,*** **NAT-S.,** ***nit-ac.,*** nux-m., nux-v., **PH-AC.,** ***phos.,*** phys., podo., psor., puls., ruta., sabin., sang., sep., **SIL.,** sol-n., stram., sulph., tarent., tep., ***thuj., zinc.***
bending head backwards - ***bad.,*** cic., hep.
burning - ph-ac.
evening - sep.
lying down - lyc.
morning after rising - am-m.
after waking agg. - arg-m., ph-ac.
motion, on - am-m., asar., nux-v.
amel. - ***sulph.***
moving head - kali-c., ***kalm.,*** merc-i-f., podo.
spine - ***aesc., ang., arn.,*** carb-ac., ***card-m.,*** **CHIN-S.,** ***cimic.,*** cinnb., ***cocc., coloc.,*** con., dios., ***gels., ham., hyper., lach.,*** nat-a., ***nat-s.,*** ox-ac., **PAR.,** plan., stram., **SULPH.,** ***tell.***
stooping, on - nux-v.
stretching, on - nat-s.
vertebra - ham.
seventh - carb-ac., con., ***gels.,*** sep.
seventh at joint with first thoracic - dig.
walking amel. - mag-s.
air, in open - sep.
yawning - nat-s.
soreness, glands - aesc., ail., **BELL.,** canth., clem., ***hep.,*** kali-bi., merc., mur-ac., nat-m., ***phyt., psor.,*** rhus-t., vesp.
left - ang.
soreness, throat, external - ***bar-c., bell., calc.,*** chel., ***chin-s.,*** clem., cob., cycl., ***hep.,*** kali-bi., **LACH.,** med., merc-i-f., ***nicc.,*** sul-ac., tarent., verat.
deep in throat - cycl.
forenoon - iod.
motion, on - bry., cic.
touch - cic.
turning head - calc.

SPASMODIC, drawing (see Torticollis) - ***acon.,*** alum., ant-c., ***apis,*** **BELL.,** calc., camph., cann-i., **CAUST.,** cedr., ***cham.,*** chin., **CIC., CIMIC.,** ***cina, cupr.,*** eup-per., ***gels., glon., hell., hep.,*** hyos., hyper., ***ign., ip.,*** kreos., ***lyc., mez.,*** mur-ac., ***nat-m., nat-s., nux-v.,*** **OP.,** ***phel.,*** samb., stram., ***tab.,*** verat-v., ***zinc.***
afternoon - mag-c.
chin to sternum - ***cann-s.,*** med.
evening - ant-c.
left, to - asar., ***bell.,*** caul., **LYC.,** ***nux-v.,*** **PHOS.**
lying - ant-c.
right, to - caust., ***cupr., lachn., lyc.***
rigidly - ran-b.
sleep, during - alum.

SPASMS, head bend forward - med.
sides of neck - ***carb-ac., med.***

SPONDYLITIS - ph-ac.

SPOTS - ***carb-v.,*** hyos., petr.
red - ***carb-v., lyc.,*** sep., stann.
yellow - iod.
spots, throat, external - ars., bell., bry., carb-v., cinnb., cocc., iod., lach., lyc., ***sep.,*** stann., vip.

SPRAINED, as if - ***agar., ars., calc.,*** cinnb., ***con.,*** kali-n., lyc., nat-m., nicc., ***ruta.***, sep., ***sulph.***
left - asar., ***con.***
rising from stooping - nicc.
sprained, as from a, in sides - petr.
left - ***con.,*** sars.
sprained sensation, throat, external - carb-an.

STIFFNESS - acon., ***aesc.,*** **AGAR.,** ***alum.,*** am-c., ***am-m.,*** **ANAC.,** anan., ***ang., ant-t., apis,*** **ARG-M.,** ***ars.,*** arum-t., asar., aur., bad., ***bapt.,*** **BAR-C., BELL.,** berb., brach., ***brom., bry.,*** calad., **CALC.,** ***calc-p.,*** calc-s., camph., cann-i., ***canth.,*** caps., carb-ac., carb-an., carb-s., ***carb-v.,*** caul., **CAUST.,** ***cedr.,*** **CHEL.,** ***chin.,*** chin-a., **CIC., CIMIC.,** ***cocc.,*** colch., ***coloc.,*** com., ***con.,*** cor-r., cupr-ac., cupr-ar., cycl., ***dig., dros., dulc.,*** elaps, **EUPH.,** eup-pur., fago., ***ferr.,*** ferr-ar., ferr-i., ferr-p., ***fl-ac.,*** form., ***gels.,*** get., ***glon., graph., guai.,*** **HELL.,** ***hep.,*** hura, hyos., **IGN., IND.,** kalm., ***kali-bi.,*** **KALI-C.,** ***kali-chl., kali-i., kali-n.,*** kali-p., ***kali-s., lac-c.,*** **LACH., LACHN.,** laur., ***led.,*** **LYC.,** ***lyss.,*** **MAG-C.,** ***manc., mang.,*** meny., ***merc.,*** merc-i-f., merc-i-r., ***mez.,*** morph., mur-ac., myric., nat-a., ***nat-c., nat-m.,*** nat-p., ***nat-s.,*** **NIT-AC., NUX-V.,** ol-an., pall., ***par., petr.,*** ph-ac., ***phos., phys., phyt., plat.,*** plb., ***podo., psor., puls., rat., rhod.,*** **RHUS-T.,** ***rhus-v., sang.,*** sec., sel., ***sep.,*** squil., **SIL.,** ***spig., spong.,*** stann., ***staph.,*** stict., stram., ***stry., sulph., syph., tab., tarent.,*** tep., ***thuj.,*** tub., vario., verat., vib., x-ray, ***zinc.,*** zing.
afternoon - brom., ptel., thuj.
waking, on - bar-c.
air, draft of - **CALC-P.,** ***cimic.,*** **RHUS-T.**
alternating, with toothache - mang.
bending head forward agg. - kali-bi.
cold, after taking - ***dulc., guai., nit-ac.,*** **RHUS-T.**
coryza, during - ars., ***bell.,*** dulc., **LACH.,** lachn., ***lyc., nux-v., rhus-t.,*** sulph.
cracks when moving - petr.
eating, after - ***nux-v.***
evening - acon., am-m., cast., cimic., meny., sel.
extending, down - anac.
headache, during - am-c., ant-c., arg-m., bar-c., ***bell., calc.,*** caps., carb-s., crot-h., cur., cycl., ***glon., graph., ign.,*** kali-c., kali-n., ***lach.,*** mag-c., merc-i-f., mur-ac., myric., nat-c., ph-ac., sang., sep., sil., spig., tarent., verat.
in occiput - graph.
intermittent, during - ***cocc.***
left - bell., carb-an., chel., coloc., glon., guai., kreos., lyc., nat-m., squil., zinc.
extending to temples - spig.
spine, and - adon.
yawning, on - nat-m.
lifting, from - **CALC.,** lyc., **RHUS-T.,** sep.
lying on back - spig.
menses, during - ***calc.***

STIFFNESS,
morning - alum., ang., ars., asar., bell., bor., ***brom.,*** bufo, ***calc., chel.,*** dig., ferr., hell., ***kali-c.,*** lyss., manc., ***rhod.,*** ruta, spig., ***sulph., zinc.***
rising, on - bov., rhod.
rising, on amel. - spig.
waking, on - anac., arg-m., ***calc.,*** eupi., graph., ***kali-c.,*** manc., ***phyt., rhod.***
motion amel. - alum., caps., ph-ac.
night - ars., ***dulc.,*** gels., kali-c., **PHYT.**
3 to 4 a.m. - spig.
one-side - coloc., guai., stict.
painful - hell., phos.
rest, during - ph-ac., rat., ***rhod., rhus-t.***
right - agar., caust., lachn., nat-m.
extending to temples - chel., spig.
sleep, during - ***alum.***
stool, after - ***puls.***
stooping - calc.
turning head, on - alum., am-c., ***am-m.,*** aur., bell., ***bry.,*** calad., ***calc., chel., coloc., dulc.,*** kali-n., par., rat., spong., tarent.
to left - alum.
to painful side - anac.
violent motion amel. - rat.
waking, on - anac., graph., kali-c., ***lach., manc.,*** phys.
walking in open air - ***camph., lyc.***
washing from - ***dulc.,*** **RHUS-T.**
yawning, on - cocc., nat-m.
stiffness, sides - aesc., alum., anac., asc-t., ***bell.,*** benz-ac., **BRY.,** calc., camph., ***caust.,*** cham., ***chel.,*** coloc., ***dig., guai.,*** hura, kreos., ***lachn.,*** laur., led., ***lyc., mang.,*** merc-i-f., ***mez.,*** nat-a., nat-m., nat-s., ***nux-v.,*** petr., ph-ac., phys., phyt., ***puls.,*** sec., ***sil., spong.,*** squil., staph., ***stront-c., stry.,*** thuj., zinc., zing.
left - asc-t., ***bell.,*** carb-an., chel., coloc., hura, laur., lyc., ph-ac., kreos., ***puls.,*** spong., ***stry.,*** thuj.
morning - ***chel.,*** zinc.
right - **CAUST.,** ***chel.,*** lyss., mez., nat-m., nit-ac., petr.
waking, on - asc-t.

STRAINING, throat, external, muscles - sep.

STRETCHING, throat, external - sep.

SUBMAXILLARY, glands
abscess - calc., hippoz., kali-i., lach., phos., sil.
boring - led., lyc., nat-m., puls., sabad.
boring, night - nat-m.
cancer - ***anthr.,*** calc-s., carb-an., ferr-i.
contraction - sil.
digging - ***rhus-t.***
drawing - am-m., ***arg-m.,*** cob., ign., lyc., ***sil.***
eating, after - lyc.
enlarged - asim., ***bar-m., kali-c.,*** **KALI-I.,** ***merc-c., merc-i-f.,*** **RHUS-T.,** sil.
indurations - **BAR-C., BAR-M.,** ***carb-v., cocc., con., cupr.,*** graph., kali-n., ***merc-i-f.,*** nat-m., ***psor., rhus-t.***

SUBMAXILLARY, glands
inflammation - ars., **BAR-M.,** ***bell.,*** chin., crot-t., ***dulc.,*** graph., kali-ar., kali-c., ***kali-i.,*** kali-s., kalm., ***lach.,*** lyc., mag-c., **MERC.,** nit-ac., ***phyt., psor., puls.,*** **RHUS-T.,** sep., ***sil.,*** spong., stram., ***sulph., sul-ac.,*** tarent., ***verat-v.***
lancinating - am-m.
pain - ambr., ***ars., aur., aur-m.,*** **BAR-C., BAR-M.,** brom., bry., carb-s., **CHIN.,** cina, clem., coc-c., ***cor-r., crot-t., dulc.,*** graph., ign., kali-n., led., lyc., mag-c., mez., nat-m., ***nit-ac., phos.,*** plb., puls., ***rhus-t.,*** sabad., sep., ***sil., staph., stram., sulph., sul-ac.,*** verat.
chewing, when - ***calc.***
night - nat-m.
swallowing, when - cor-r., stram.
swelling, with - staph.
pulsation - am-m., cham., lyc., stram., tarent.
sensitive - ars., lyc., merc-cy., psor.
sharp - am-m., arg-m., bell., ***calc.,*** merc., ***mez.,*** nux-v., ph-ac., sil., ***sulph., sul-ac.***
swallowing, when - nux-v., ***rhus-t.***
sore - cop., crot-t., graph., kali-c., lyc., mag-c., merc-c., nat-m., ***nit-ac.,*** psor., puls., sep., ***sil., spong., staph., sulph.,*** vesp.
stinging - am-m., kali-i.
stinging, swallowing, on - nux-v.
swelling - ambr., am-c., ***am-m., anan., anthr., arg-m., ars.,*** **ARS-I., ARUM-T.,** aur., ***aur-m.,*** **BAR-C., BAR-M.,** bell., bov., **BROM.,** bufo, calad., **CALC.,** ***calc-p., calc-s., carb-an.,*** carb-s., **CHAM.,** chlol., **CHIN.,** chin-a., chin-s., clem., ***cocc., con., cor-r., crot-h., crot-t., ferr-i., graph., hep.,*** hippoz., ign., ***iod., jug-c., kali-ar., kali-c., kali-i.,*** kali-n., kali-p., kali-s., ***lach., lac-c.,*** led., **LYC.,** mag-m., med., ***merc., merc-c.,*** merc-cy., merc-i-f., ***merc-i-r., mur-ac.,*** **NAT-C.,** ***nat-m.,*** nat-p., ***nat-s.,*** **NIT-AC.,** ***nux-v., petr., phyt., plb., psor.,*** **RHUS-T.,** ***sep.,*** **SIL.,** spong., stann., ***staph.,*** stram., ***sulph., sul-ac.,*** syph., tab., tarent., verat., zinc.
hard - **BROM., CALC.,** ***graph., kali-c., merc.,*** **RHUS-T.,** syph.
left - arum-t., **BROM.,** ***cor-r.,*** vesp.
painful - am-m., arum-t., aur., aur-m., **BAR-C.,** ***bar-m.,*** bufo, **CALC.,** ***graph.,*** merc-i-r., ***nit-ac.,*** **SIL.,** ***sulph.***
right - bufo, kali-br., sep., spong., stram., ***sulph.***
ulcers - ***kali-i.***

SWELLING of neck - ***iod.,*** nux-v., ***phos.***
nape of neck - apis, ars., ***bar-c.,*** berb., carb-v., der., lach., puls., sep., sumb., tub.
cords, with pain at base of brain - med.
fatty - am-m.
vertebra seventh cervical - calc.
talking, while - iod.
swelling, glands - aesc., aeth., ***agar., alum., alumn., am-c., am-m.,*** ant-c., ant-t., ***apis,*** arn., **ARUM-T.,** astac., bac., **BAR-C., BAR-M., BELL.,** bov., **CALC.,** calc-s., camph., canth., ***carb-an.,*** carb-s., ***carb-v., cham.,*** cinnb., **CIST.,** ***con.,*** cupr., dros., ***dulc.,*** ferr., ferr-i., **GRAPH.,** ***hell., hep.,*** ign., ***iod.,*** kali-bi., **KALI-C.,** ***kali-i.,*** kali-m., kali-p., kreos., ***lac-ac., lach.,*** lap-a., led., ***lith.,*** **LYC.,** ***mag-m.,*** **MERC.,** ***merc-c.,*** merc-i-f., mur-ac., ***nat-c., nat-m.,*** nat-p., ***nat-s., nit-ac., petr., phos., phyt., psor., puls.,*** **RHUS-T.,** ***sep.,*** **SIL.,** ***spig., spong.,*** **STAPH.,** stict., **SULPH.,** sul-ac., syph., tarent., tep., ***thuj., tub.,*** vesp., viol-t., zinc.
evening agg. - ***kali-c.***
extending to shoulder - ***graph.***
hard - ***bar-m., calc.,*** **CON.,** ***iod.,*** lyc., merc., ***sars.,*** **SIL.**
knocking - cist.
left - stict.
malignant - cist.
milk crusts, with - viol-t.
painful to touch - cupr.
string of heads, like a, around neck - aeth.
suppurative - **CALC.,** ***cist., hep., lith.,*** **MERC.,** ***nit-ac.,*** **SIL.,** ***sulph., tub.***
swelling, sides - ***ail.,*** alum., ***am-c., apis,*** **BELL.,** calc., chel., ***glon.,*** hyos., kali-ma., ***lach., lyc.,*** merc., merc-c., nat-c., nit-ac., **RHUS-T.,** ***sars.,*** sil., spig., stry., thuj., vesp.
right - sars., sil.
sensation of - alum., mang., sep., xan.
stripe - mang.
suppurative - hyos.
swelling, throat, external - aesc., ***ail., am-c.,*** am-m., anan., ***apis,*** ars., ***bell.,*** cann-s., caust., chel., cic., ***crot-c.,*** ferr., hyper., ***iod.,*** kali-i., kali-n., **LYC.,** ***merc.,*** op., **RHUS-T.,** rhus-v., sars., ***spong.,*** sulph., **TARENT.,** zinc.
coughing, when - ars.
cramp, after - graph.
menses, before - iod.
sensation - mang.
speaking loud, when - iod.
swelling, veins - hyos., nat-m., op., sil., stry., thuj.

TEARING, pain - **ACON.,** asaf., aeth., **AM-M.,** arn., aur., berb., ***calc.,*** calc-caust., camph., ***canth., caps.,*** carb-s., **CARB-V.,** ***caust.,*** chel., ***chin.,*** cic., clem., coc-c., coloc., con., cupr., dig., gels., ***glon.,*** graph., ***kali-c.,*** kalm., ***lach.,*** laur., led., ***lyc.,*** lyss., mag-c., mag-m., meny., ***merc.,*** nat-c., ***nat-s., nux-v.,*** olnd., phos., plb., psor., rat., ***rhod.,*** rhus-v., sars., sel., sil., ***spig.,*** stront-c., sulph., verat., ***thuj., zinc.***
afternoon - mag-c.
bending head forward - camph.
chill, during - ars-h.
coughing - alum.
evening - ***nux-v.***
extending to,
down back - mag-c., rhod.
ear - thuj.

TEARING, pain
extending to,
forehead - rat., sars.
shoulder - alum., am-m., thuj., til.
shoulder, right, in evening after lying down - lyc.
vertex - rat.
up either side to top of head - ***lach.***
upward - berb., canth., ***lach.***
jerking - aur., ***caps.,*** rat.
left - rat., sulph.
lying, while - ***lyc.***
menses, during - am-m., mag-c.
midnight, before, on waking - sulph.
morning - kali-c., ***stram.***
motion, on - carb-v., dig., ign., kali-bi., verat.
of head - ***am-m.,*** canth., nat-c., ***sulph.***
nape of neck - xan.
night - rhod.
paroxysmal - nux-v.
pressure amel. - zinc.
sneezing - am-m.
spine - ***lach.***
spine, at night - caust.
stool, after, amel. - asaf.
sudden - nat-c.
walking, while - rat.
warm room, in - caust.

tearing, sides - aeth., am-m., anac., ***aur.,*** berb., **BRY.,** calc., ***caps., carb-v.,*** grat., indg., iod., kali-bi., nat-c., petr., phos., rat., sabin., ***sel.,*** staph., tarax., teucr., zinc.
evening - mag-c., olnd.
extending to,
axilla - phos.
ear - mez., zinc.
occiput - berb.
left - lyc., mez., phos., ***sel.,*** sulph.
morning - zinc.
motion, on - ***carb-v.,*** sulph., verat.
of head - am-m.
night - olnd.
paroxysmal - ***sel.***
pressure amel. - zinc.
rheumatic - berb.
right - aeth., kali-c., mag-c., nat-c.

tearing, throat, external - aeth., am-m., bov., ***carb-v.,*** par., tep., thuj.
blood vessels - phos.
intermittent - cupr.

TENSION - agar., aloe, **ALUM.,** am-m., ant-c., ***apis,*** aur., ***bar-c.,*** **BELL.,** berb., bism., bov., ***bry.,*** calc., camph., carb-an., ***carb-s., carb-v., caust., chel.,*** **CIC., CIMIC.,** cinnb., colch., con., cupr., dig., dulc., elaps, euph., ***gels.,*** glon., graph., ***hell.,*** hyos., hyper., iod., ip., kali-c., kali-s., ***lac-c., lyc., mag-s.,*** mang., med., mez., mosch., ***nat-c., nat-m., nat-s.,*** nicc., nit-ac., ***nux-m., ol-an.,*** par., ***plat.,*** plb., psor., ***puls., rat., rhod.,*** **RHUS-T.,** sars., sep., sil., ***spong., staph., stram.,*** stront-c., ***sulph., thuj.,*** verat., verat-v., ***zinc.***
afternoon - alum.
cold, damp air - ***nux-m.***
evening - am-m., nat-m., rat.

TENSION,
extending to eye - sulph.
to shoulder - sulph.
left - rat.
lifting, from - sep.
menses, before - iod., ***nat-c.,*** nux-v.
midnight, before - ***sulph.***
morning - mag-s., sulph.
on rising - mag-s.
on waking - anac.
motion, on - bry., camph., graph., kali-c., nat-c., nicc., ***rhus-t.,*** sars.
amel. - con., ***rhod., rhus-t.***
of head - nat-c., sulph., thuj.
night, lying on side - staph.
numbness, with - plat.
raising up quickly - caust.
right - caust., zinc.
sitting, while - nat-c., sulph.
while, bent - sulph.
sleep, during - alum.
standing, when - rat.
stooping - am-c., ant-c., aur., ***canth.,*** lyc.
stretching out amel. - sulph.
turning head - caust., mur-ac., spong., ***verat.***
waking, on - anac., psor.
walking while - nat-c.
amel. - mag-s., ***rhod., rhus-t.,*** sulph.
in open air - ***lyc.,*** meny.
warm, becoming, amel. - mosch.
writing, while - lyc.

tension, glands - ambr.

tension, sides - agar., arg-m., bar-c., bell., berb., bov., ***calc., caust., chel., dig.,*** iod., kali-bi., kreos., laur., mag-m., ***med.,*** meph., nat-m., ph-ac., plb., ***rhod.,*** sars., sep., ***spong., sulph., zinc.***
bending head backward - cic.
convulsive - agar., raph.
evening - rat.
standing - rat.
left - cic., sulph., zinc.
lying on side - thuj.
morning - coc-c.
moving head, on - bov., graph., sars., verat.
night - staph.
painful - sulph.
rheumatic - iod.
right - ang., **CAUST.,** mag-m., sars., spong.
swallowing, on - colch.
waking, on - coc-c.
walking, after - nat-m.

tension, throat, external - caust., cic., mag-c., ***nux-m.,*** sep., verb.

TICKLING, throat, external, in gland - kali-c.

TIGHT, throat, external, cannot bear anything around collar and waist - **LACH.,** ***sep.***

TINGLING, throat, external- calc.

TORTICOLLIS, (see Spasmodic) - ***acon.,*** alum., ant-c., ***apis,*** ars., asar., **BELL.,** ***calc.,*** camph., cann-i., caul., **CAUST.,** cedr., ***cham.,*** chel., chin., **CIC., CIMIC.,** ***cina, colch., cupr.,*** con., dulc., eup-per., eup-pur., ***gels., glon., graph.,*** guai., ***hell., hep.,*** hura, ***hyos.,*** hyper., ***ign., ip.,*** kreos., lac-ac., lac-c., lach., **LACHN., LYC.,** mag-c., merc., ***mez.,*** mur-ac., ***nat-m., nat-s., nux-v.,*** **OP.,** ***phel.,*** **PHOS.,** ***ran-b.,*** **RHUS-T.,** samb., stram., sulph., syc-co., ***tab.,*** verat-v., ***zinc.***
afternoon - mag-c.
cattle, in - aesc-g.
chronic - bar-c.
contraction of muscles on one side, twisting neck to one side - ***hyos.***
diphtheria and scarlet fever, in - **LACHN.**
chin to sternum - ***cann-s.,*** med.
evening - ant-c.
fright, after, due to spinal disease - ***nux-v.***
left, to - asar., ***bell.,*** caul., **LYC.,** ***nux-v.,*** **PHOS.**
lying - ant-c.
obliquely, turned - ***hyos.***
right, to - **CAUST.,** ***cupr., lachn., lyc.***
right shoulder, drawn to - ***cupr-m.***
to, by hard swelling - ***aur-m.***
rigidly - ran-b.
shock, from - nux-v.
sleep, during - alum.
spondylitis suboccipital is, from - asaf., mez., nat-m., phos., sil., sulph.
swelling, head drawn to one side by - ***cist.***
twisted by hard, to right shoulder - con.
throat, with sore - lachn.
waking, on - asc-t.

TOUCHING agg., throat, external - apis, brom., bry., lac-c., **LACH., PHYT.,** spong.

TREMBLING, throat, external - graph.

TUBERCLES - ant-c., carb-an., caust., nicc., zinc.
tubercles, front - am-c., lach., lyc., mur-ac., nicc., ph-ac., phos., sec.

TUMORS, lipomas, fatty, on - **BAR-C.,** calc., ***thuj.***
malignant on - calc-p.
cystic, on both sides - brom.
tumors, throat, external, cystic - bar-c., ***brom.,*** sil., thuj.
fatty - ***bar-c.***
recurrent fibroid - ***sil.***
side - ***brom.***

TWITCHING - aeth., arn., bufo, caust., coloc., mag-c., mag-m., nat-m., ph-ac., ran-b., sep., sulph., tarax.
extending down the back - mag-c.
raising, head - ph-ac.
rest, during - ph-ac.
tearing, extending into vertex, while walking - rat.
twitching, throat, external - ***agar.,*** arg-m., asaf., bism., carb-ac., crot-c., graph., mez., phos., spong.
left - mez., sars.
from left side of the neck to the left side of the throat - agar.
twitching, throat, external right - lyc.
twitching, side - ang., kali-c., tarax.

ULCERS - sil.
ulcers, throat, external - ars., lyc., ***sil.***

UNCOVERING, throat, external agg. - alum., berb., **HEP.,** ***kali-ar.,*** **KALI-C.,** ***merc., nat-m., nat-s.,*** **NUX-V.,** ***phos.,*** **RHUS-T.,** ***rumx.,*** **SIL.,** ***spong.,*** **SQUIL.,** ***thuj.,*** **ZINC.**

URTICARIA, front - bry., kali-i.

VESICLES - calc-caust., camph., clem., mag-c., naja, nat-h., nat-p., petr., zinc-s.
vesicles, front - clem., mag-c., ph-ac., sep., vip.
side of - alum.
from ear, discharge - **TELL.**
red - chin., lyc., mez., ph-ac., sep., spig., thuj.
scratching, after - mag-c.
stitching - phos.

VICE, throat, external, sensation as in a - xan.

WARTS - nit-ac., thuj.
warts, throat, external - nit-ac., sil., thuj.

WEAKNESS - abrot., acon., ***aesc., aeth., agar.,*** aloe, ant-t., arg-n., ars-m., ***cact.,*** calc-p., caps., caul., cimic., **COCC.,** ***gels., glon., kali-c., lach.,*** nat-m., nit-ac., ***par.,*** petr., phos., pic-ac., **PLAT.,** sanic., sep., ***sil., stann.,*** staph., sulph., ***verat.,*** verat-v., viol-o., ***zinc.***
falling forward - nux-m.
headache, with - fago.
manual labor, from - ***agar., kali-c., lach.,*** nit-ac., ***sil.,*** verat.
stupor, with - hyos., zinc.
writing, while - **ZINC.**

WIND, as if blowing, on, as if - olnd.

WRINKLED skin, region - sars.
wrinkled, throat, external - sanic.

Nerves

AMYOTROPHIC, lateral sclerosis - ***arg-n., ars.***, cupr., hyper., kali-p., ***lach., lath.***, merc., ***phos.***, **PLB.**, sec., sep., sulph.
softening of spinal cord, with - ***arg-n.***, cupr., hyper., ***lath.***, plb.

ANALGESIA, sensation - bell., chel., ***cic.***, **COCC.**, con., hell., ***hyos.***, ign., kali-br., laur., **LYC.**, merc., mosch., **OLND., OP., PH-AC.**, phos., pic-ac., ***plb.***, puls., ***rhus-t., sec.***, **STRAM.**, ***sulph.***
inner parts - ars., bell., bov., hyos., **OP., PLAT.**, spig.
parts affected - anac., asaf., ***cocc.***, con., ***lyc., olnd.***, **PLAT.**, puls., rhus-t.

ANESTHESIA, sensation - abrot., absin., ***acon.***, alco., ambr., ant-t., arg-n., ***ars.***, ars-i., atro., bar-m., bell., berb., cadm-s., ***camph.***, cann-i., ***caps.***, carb-ac., carbn-chl., carb-h., carb-o., carb-s., caul., ***caust.***, cham., chlf., chlol., ***cic.***, cocc., crot-chlol., cupr-ac., cycl., ***eucal.***, **HYDR-AC.**, hyos., ***hyper.***, ign., kali-br., ***kali-i.***, keroso., laur., lyc., mag-arct., man., merc., meth-ae-ae., methyl-b., nitro-o., ***nux-m.***, nux-v., ***olnd., op.***, ox-ac., ph-ac., **PLB.**, puls., ran-a., rhod., ***sec.***, spig., stram., stront-c., tab., ter., verat., ***verat-v.***, vip., zinc.
affected parts, of - plb.
right side, of - plb.

APOPLEXY, (see Stroke)

ASLEEP feeling (see Numbness)

ATAXIA, general - ***agar.***, **ALUM.**, arag., ***arg-n.***, ars., ***calc., caust., cocc.***, crot-c., ***fl-ac., gels., graph., hell., helo., kali-br., lach., lil-t.***, naja, nux-m., ***nux-v., onos., phos., plb., sil., stram., sulph., zinc.***

BRACHIAL, neuralgia - acon., all-c., bell-p., **BRY.**, calc-f., cham., **HYPER.**, ***kalm.***, merc., nux-v., ***rhus-t.***, ruta.., sulph., verat.

CATALEPSY - acon., ***agar.***, aran., ***art-v.***, bell., cann-i., cham., chlol., ***cic., cocc., coff., con., cur., ferr., gels.***, **GRAPH.**, hyos., ign., ***ip.***, lach., ***nat-m., nux-m.***, **OP.**, ***petr., ph-ac., plat.***, staph., stram., sulph., thuj., verat.
fright, after - ***acon.***, bell., ign., ***gels.***, **OP.**
grief, after - ***ign., ph-ac.***, staph.
jealousy, from - ***hyos.***, **LACH.**
joy, from - **COFF.**
love, unrequited from - hyos., ***ign.***, lach., nat-m., ***ph-ac.***
religious excitement, from - stram., sulph., verat.
sexual excitement, from - ***con., plat.***, stram.

CEREBRAL palsy - arn., hell., ign., op.

CEREBRO-spinal axis, ailments of - agar., arg-n., chin., cocc., ***gels.***, ign., ***nux-v.***, phos.

CHOREA, general - ***abrot.***, absin., acon., **AGAR.**, agar-ph., agarin., ***ambr., aml-n., ant-t.***, apis, ***arg-n., ars.***, ars-i., ars-s-f., **ART-V.**, ***asaf.***, aster., ***atro.***, aven., ***bell., bufo, cact.***, **CALC.**, calc-i., ***calc-p., colch., cast.***, caul., **CAUST.**, ***cham.***, cedr., ***chel.***, **CHIN.**, chlol., **CIC., CIMIC., CINA**, cocaine, ***cocc.***, coch., ***cod.***, coff., con., ***croc., crot-c.***, crot-h., **CUPR.**, ***cupr-ac., cupr-ar.***, cypr., ***dios.***, dulc., eup-a., ***ferr.***, ferr-ar., ferr-cit., ferr-cy., ***ferr-i., ferr-r., ferr-s.***, form., ***gels., guare., hipp., hyos.***, **IGN.**, ***iod.***, ip., kali-ar., ***kali-br.***, kali-c., kali-i., kali-p., ***kali-s.***, **LACH.**, lat-k., lat-m., laur., levo., ***lil-t.***, lyss., ***mag-p., mang.***, merc., mez., ***mill., morph.***, mur-ac., **MYGAL.**, ***nat-m., nit-ac., nux-m., nux-v.***, ol-an., ***op.***, passi., ph-ac., ***phos.***, phys., phyt., picro., plat., plb., psor., ***puls.***, rhod., ***rhus-t.***, russ., sabin., ***sant., scut., sec., sep., sil., sin-n.***, sol-n., ***spig.***, stann., ***staph.***, stict., **STRAM.**, ***stry.***, stry-p., sul-ter., sulfon., ***sulph., samb., sumb.***, tanac., **TARENT.**, ***ter.***, thal., thiop., thuj., ***tub.***, valer., verat-v., visc., ***zinc.***, zinc-ar., ***zinc-br.***, zinc-cy., zinc-p., zinc-valer., ziz.
afternoon - ***nat-s.***
anemia, from - ars., chin., ***ferr-r.***, hyos.
anxiety, from - stram.
backward, motions, with - ***bell.***
begins, in face and spreads to body - ***sec.***
bleeding, after - chin., stict.
children, who have grown too fast - calc-p., ign., phos.
cold, agg. - ign.
bath, after agg. - ***rhus-t.***
colors, bright, from - tarent.
amel. - tarent.
cordis - tarent.
dancing, excessive - bell., hyos., stram., ***tarent.***
daytime - art-v., tarent.
dentition, in second - bell., ***calc.***, calc-p.
dinner, after - zinc., ziz.
dry, weather - ***caust.***
ear, piercing from - lach.
eating, after - ign.
emotional - agar., arg-n., ***caust.***, cimic., **IGN.**, ***laur.***, mag-p., ***op., phos.***, **STAPH.**, ***tarent.***
evening, agg. - ***zinc.***
exercise, amel. - ***zinc.***
face, in - ***caust.***, cic., cina, ***cupr.***, hyos., ***mygal.***, nat-m., zinc.
begins in, and spreads to body - ***sec.***
cold and clammy, up to knee - laur.
falling, with - ***calc.***
fear, from - calc., op.
fluids, loss, of animal - ***chin.***
foot, from suppression of sweat of - form., sil.
fright, from - acon., agar., arg-n., ***calc.***, **CAUST.**, cimic., cupr., ***cupr-ac.***, cupr-ar., ***gels.***, **IGN.**, ***kali-br., laur., nat-m.***, **OP.**, phos., ***stram.***, visc., ***zinc.***
grief, after - cimic., ***cupr-ac.***, **IGN.**, tarent.
gyratory, motions, with - stram.
hands, of - cina.
holding, amel. - asaf.
hyperaesthesia, with excessive - ***tarent.***
imitation, from - ***caust., cupr.***, mygal., ***tarent.***
jerks, constant, cannot keep still - laur.

CHOREA, general
left, side - ***cimic., cupr.,*** rhod.
light, agg. - ign., tarent., ziz.
loss, of animal fluids, from - ***chin.***
lying, on back amel. - ***cupr.,*** cupr-ac., ***ign.***
masturbation, from - agar., ***calc.,*** chin., cina
menopausal period, during - cimic.
menses, during - caul., caust., **ZINC.**
absent or difficult - puls.
after amel. - sep.
before - caul.
misses, laying hold on anything - asaf.
moon, new, at - cupr.
full agg. - nat-m.
morning - arg-n., mygal.
motion, agg. - ***cupr-ac.,*** ziz.
muscles, local - hyos.
music, amel. - ***tarent.***
nervous, disturbances, from - ***asaf.,*** bell., ***cimic., cocc.,*** croc., gels., hyos., ***ign.,*** kali-br., op., stict., stram.
night - ***arg-n.,*** **CAUST.,** cupr.
amel. - ***art-v., tarent.***
noise, agg. - ign., ziz.
noon - arg-n.
numbness, of affected parts, with - nux-v.
nymphomania, with - ***tarent.***
onanism, from - agar., ***calc.,*** chin.
one sided - ***calc., cocc., cupr.,*** nat-s., phys.
side lain on - cimic.
periodic - ***cupr., cupr-ac.,*** nat-s.
every seven days - croc.
same hour returning - ign.
pocket, keeping hand in, amel. - aster.
pollutions, with - ***dios.***
pregnancy, during - bell., ***caust., chlol., cupr.,*** gels.
puberty, in - agar., ***asaf.,*** caul., ***cimic.,*** ign., ***puls.***
punishment, from - ***ign., staph.***
rest, during - ***zinc.***
rheumatic - **CAUST.,** ***cimic.,*** kali-i., ***rhus-t.,*** spig., stict.
rhythmical, motions, with - agar., caust., cham., cimic., lyc., ***tarent.***
right, side - ***ars., caust., nat-s.,*** phys., ***tarent.,*** zinc.
run or jump, must, cannot walk - bufo, kali-br., ***nat-m., stram.***
running, better than walking - tarent.
sex, after - ***agar., cedr.***
side, crosswise left arm and right leg - agar., cimic., ***stram.***
crosswise left arm and right leg, right arm and left leg - tarent.
left - ***cimic., cupr.,*** rhod.
one-sided - ***calc., cocc., cupr.,*** nat-s., phys., tarent.
right - ***ars., caust., nat-s.,*** phys., ***tarent.,*** zinc.
tongue affected, staccato speech - caust.

CHOREA, general
side lain on - cimic.
sight of bright colors amel. - tarent.
sleep, during - cupr., tarent., verat-v., ***ziz.***
amel. - **AGAR.,** cupr., hell., mag-p., mygal., ziz.
spasms, in, partial, changing constantly - stram.
spinal - asaf., cic., cocc., cupr., mygal., nux-v.
stool, during - mag-p.
strabismus, with - ***stram.***
suppressed, eruptions - ***caust.,*** cupr., **SULPH.,** ***zinc.***
swallowing, impossible - art-v.
sympathetic - caust.
thinking of it, when - ***caust.***
thunderstorm, during - ***phos.***
before - ***agar., rhod.,*** sep.
tongue, with protrusion of - sumb.
touch, agg. - ziz.
tubercular - calc., ***calc-p.,*** caust., ***iod.,*** phos., psor.
uterine ailments, with - ***caul.,*** **CIMIC.,** croc., ***ign., lil-t., nat-m., puls.,*** sec., ***sep.***
waking, on - ***chlol.***
wet, after getting - ***rhus-t.***
wine, agg. - ***zinc.***
worms, after - asaf., ***calc., cina,*** sant., ***spig.***

COLLAPSE, (see Emergency)

COMA, (see Mind, Unconsciousness)

CONDUCTION of nerves delayed - alum., cocc.

CONVULSIONS, general (see Epilepsy) - absin., acet-ac., ***acon.,*** aconin., aesc., aesc-g., aeth., aether, ***agar.,*** agre., alco., ***alet.,*** alum., alum-p., alum-sil., am-caust., am-m., ambr., am-c., ***aml-n.,*** amyg., ang., anis., ***ant-c., ant-t., anthr.,*** antipyrin., ***apis, aran.,*** arg-m., ***arg-n.,*** arist-cl., ***arn., ars., ars-s-f.,*** arum-m., ***asaf.,*** **ART-V.,** aster., **ATRO.,** aur., aur-a., bar-c., ***bar-m.,*** bar-s., bart., **BELL.,** benz-n., bism., bor., both., bov., brom., brucin., ***bry.,*** **BUFO,** buth-a., cact., **CALC.,** calc-i., carb-an., carb-h., ***carb-s., camph.,*** cann-i., cann-s., ***canth., carb-ac.,*** carbn., cast., caul., **CAUST., CHAM.,** chen-a., chin., ***chlf.,*** chlor., **CIC.,** cic-m., ***cimic.,*** **CINA,** cit-ac., clem., coca, ***cocc.,*** coc-c., cod., coff., colch., colchin., coloc., ***con.,*** convo-s., cop., cortico., cortiso., croc., ***crot-c., crot-h.,*** cryp., cub., **CUPR.,** ***cupr-ac.,*** cupr-s., cur., ***cypr.,*** cyt-l., dat-m., dat-s., ***dig.,*** dor., dulc., euon., ***eupi.,*** fagu., ferr., ferr-ar., ferr-m., ferr-s., form., frag., ***gels., glon.,*** gran., ***graph.,*** grat., guare., ***hell., hydr-ac.,*** **HYOS.,** hyper., ***ign.,*** indg., iod., ***ip.,*** ir-fl., jasm., jatr., juni., ***kali-br., kali-c., kali-chl.,*** kali-cy., kali-i., kali-m., kali-ox., kali-p., kalm., keroso., lach., **LACT.,** lat-m., laur., linu-c., linu-u, **LOB.,** lol., lon-x., ***lyc., lyss., mag-c.,*** mag-m., ***mag-p.,*** man., manc., med., meli., meny., meph., ***merc., merc-c.,*** merc-d., merc-n., merc-p-r., methyl-b., mez., mill., morph., ***mosch., mur-ac.,*** nat-f., ***nat-m.,*** nat-s., nit-ac., nitro-o., **NUX-M., NUX-V.,** ***oena.,*** oest., ol-an., ol-j., olnd., **OP.,** ox-ac., passi., petr., ***phos.,***

CONVULSIONS, general - ***phyt.,*** picro., pituin., plat., **PLB.,** ***podo., psor., puls.,*** ran-b., ran-s., ***rat.,*** rauw., rhus-t., ric., rob., rumx-a., russ., ruta, sabad., sal-ac., ***salam.,*** samb., ***sant., sec.,*** sep., ***sil.,*** sin-n., sium, ***sol-c., sol-n.,*** spig., spirae., squil., **STANN.,** staph., **STRAM.,** stront-c., stroph., **STRY.,** ***stry-s.,*** sul-ac., sul-i., ***sulph.,*** tab., tanac., tarent., tax., ***ter.,*** thal., thea., thuj., thymol., ***tub., upa.,*** upa-a., urea, ust., ***valer., vario., verat.,*** verat-v., vesp., vib., vip., **ZINC.,** zinc-cy., zinc-i., zinc-m., zinc-p., zinc-valer., zing., ziz.

addison's, disease, in - ***calc., iod.***

afternoon - arg-m., stann.

air, draft of - ars., cic., ***lyss.,*** **NUX-V., STRY.**

alcohol drinks, after - ran-b.

alcoholics, in - ***anthr.,*** glon., ***hyos., nux-v., ran-b.***

alternating, with
- cerebral congestion - bell., hyos.
- excitement of mind - **STRAM.**
- rage - **STRAM.**
- relaxation of muscular system - acet-ac.
- rigidity - stry.
- trembling - arn., merc., nux-v.
- unconsciousness - agar., aur.

amenorrhea, in - art-v., ign.

anger, after - bufo, **CHAM.,** cina, ***kali-br.,*** lyss., **NUX-V.,** ***op.,*** plat., **STAPH.,** sulph.
- epilepsy, from - art-v., **CALC.**
- mothers milk, affects - cham., nux-v.

anxiety, from - stram.

apoplectic, see strokes

bathing, amel. - gels., jasm.

begin, in the
- abdomen - aran., ***bufo.***
- arm - arum-t., ***bell.***
  - left - sil.
- back - ars., sulph.
- calf muscles - lyc.
- face - absin., cina, ***bufo,*** dulc., ***hyos., ign., lach.,*** sant., ***sec.***
  - left side - ***lach.***
- fingers - ***cupr-ac.***
  - and toes - ***cupr., cupr-ac.***
- head - cic.
- legs - ***cupr-ac.***
- toes - ***cupr-ac., hydr-ac.***

belching, amel. - ***kali-c.***

bending, elbow amel. - nux-v.
- head backwards, from - **NUX-V.**

biting, with - croc., ***cupr.,*** lyss., ***tarent.***

bleeding, with - ***chin.,*** hyos., ip., ***plat., sec.***
- after - ars., bell., bry., calc., cina, con., ign., lyc., nux-v., puls., sulph., verat.
- during - chin., plat., plb., sec.

brain, tumors, in - plb.

bone, in the throat, from - ***cic.***

bright, light, from - bell., ***canth.,*** lyss., nux-v., op., **STRAM.**

cerebral, softening - ***bufo, caust.***

changing, in character - ***bell.,*** ign., ***puls.,*** **STRAM.**

CONVULSIONS, general

childbirth, during - ***acon.,*** aeth., aml-n., arn., ***bell., canth.,*** cham., ***chin.,*** chin-s., chlf., ***chlol.,*** **CIC.,** cimic., cinnam., cocc., coff., ***cupr., cupr-ar.,*** gels., glon., ***hydr-ac.,*** **HYOS., IGN.,** ip., **KALI-BR.,** merc., merc-d., mosch., ***oena.,*** op., piloc., ***plat., sec.,*** sol-n., spirae., stram., **VERAT-V.,** ***zinc.,*** ziz.
- after - ***acon.,*** ambr., ***ant-c.,*** ant-t., apis, ***arg-n.,*** arn., ars., art-v., ***atro.,*** **BELL.,** benz-ac., **CALC.,** canth., ***carb-v.,*** caul., caust., ***cham., chin., chin-s.,*** chlf., chlol., **CIC.,** cimic., cinnam., ***cocc., coff.,*** crot-c., ***crot-h., cupr., gels., glon., hell., helon.,*** hydr-ac., **HYOS.,** ***ign., ip., piloc.,*** **KALI-BR., KALI-C.,** kali-p., ***lach., laur., lyc.,*** lyss., mag-p., ***merc., merc-c., mill.,*** mosch., ***nat-m., nux-m., nux-v.,*** oena., ***op.,*** ph-ac., ***phos., piloc., plat.,*** puls., ***sec.,*** sol-n., **STRAM.,** ***sulph., ter.,*** thyr., ***verat.,*** verat-v., zinc.
- bleeding, with - ***chin.,*** hyos., ***plat.,*** phos., ***sec.***
- blindness, with - aur-m., cocc., cupr.
- perspiration and fear, with - stram.
- screaming, shrieking, with - ***hyos., iod., lach.***

children, in - absin., acon., ***aeth.,*** agar., ***ambr., aml-n.,*** ant-t., ***apis,*** arn., ars., **ART-V.,** asaf., **BELL.,** bry., bufo, **CALC.,** ***calc-p., camph.,*** canth., caust., ***cham., chlol., cic.,*** cimic., **CINA,** cocc., ***coff.,*** colch., ***crot-c., cupr., cupr-ac., cypr.,*** dol., ***gels.,*** glon., ***guare.,*** **HELL.,** ***hep., hydr-ac., hyos., ign., ip., kali-br.,*** kali-c., kali-p., kreos., ***lach.,*** laur., ***lyc., mag-p.,*** meli., merc., mosch., nux-m., ***nux-v.,*** oena., **OP.,** passi., ph-ac., phos., plat., scut., sec., ***sil., stann.,*** **STRAM.,** ***sulph.,*** ter., upa., **VERAT.,** ***verat-v.,*** **ZINC.,** ***zinc-cy.,*** zinc-s., ***zinc-valer.***
- approach of strangers, from - lyss., op., tarent.
- dentition, during - ***acon., aeth.,*** art-v., arum-t., ***bell.,*** **CALC.,** ***calc-p., caust.,*** **CHAM.,** ***cic., cina,*** coff., ***colch., cupr., cupr-ac., cypr.,*** gels., hyos., ***ign., ip.,*** **KALI-BR.,** ***kreos., lach.,*** mag-p., ***meli.,*** merc., mill., nux-m., passi., ***podo.,*** rheum, sin-n., ***stann., stram.,*** sulph., thyr., ***verat-v., zinc.***
- diarrhea, with - nux-m.
- holding, when, amel. - nicc.
- infants, in - ***art-v.,*** **BELL.,** bufo, ***cham., cupr.,*** **HELL.,** ***hydr-ac., mag-p., meli.***
- newborns, in - ***art-v., bell., cupr.,*** nux-v.
- nursing, angry or frightened mother - bufo.
- playing or laughing excessively from - coff.
- strangers, approach of - op.

chill, during - ***ars., camph., lach.,*** merc., nux-v.

choreic - stict.

CONVULSIONS, general

clonic - acon., **AGAR.,** alum., alum-p., ambr., am-c., am-m., anac., ang., ant-c., ant-t., ***anthr.,*** antipyrin., apis, ***arg-m.,*** arn., ***ars.,*** ***art-v.,*** asar., aster., aur., ***bar-c.,*** bar-m., bar-s., **BELL.,** bor., bov., brom., ***bry.,*** **BUFO,** ***calc.,*** calc-i., ***calc-p.,*** camph., cann-s., canth., carb-ac., carb-o., ***carb-s.,*** carb-v., caul., ***caust.,*** **CHAM.,** chin., ***chin-s.,*** ***chlf.,*** **CIC.,** cimic., ***cina,*** clem., cocc., coff., coloc., ***con.,*** croc., **CUPR.,** dig., dol., dulc., gels., graph., guai., hell., hep., **HYOS.,** ign., iod., ***ip.,*** kali-ar., kali-bi., ***kali-c.,*** kali-m., ***kalm.,*** kreos., lach., lat-m., laur., ***lyc.,*** **LYSS.,** mag-c., mag-m., ***mag-p.,*** mang., meny., ***merc.,*** ***mez.,*** mosch., mur-ac., mygal., nat-c., nat-f., ***nat-m.,*** ***nicot.,*** nit-ac., ***nux-m.,*** nux-v., ***oena.,*** ol-an., ***olnd.,*** **OP.,** petr., ph-ac., phos., phys., ***plat.,*** **PLB.,** podo., puls., ran-b., ran-s., rheum, rhod., rhus-t., russ., ruta, sabad., samb., sars., ***sec.,*** sel., seneg., **SEP.,** ***sil.,*** spig., spong., squil., ***stann.,*** staph., **STRAM.,** ***stront-c.,*** stry., ***stry-s.,*** ***sulph.,*** sul-ac., tab., tarent., tarax., teucr., thuj., thymol., upa-a., ust., valer., verat., verat-v., visc., ***zinc.,*** zinc-p., zinc-valer.
- alternating with tonic - bell., ***cimic.,*** con., ***ign.,*** ***mosch.,*** nux-v., plat., sep., stram., ***tab.,*** verat-v.

closing, a door, on - stry.

cold, air, from - ***ars.,*** bell., ***cic.,*** ***indg.,*** merc., nux-v.
- becoming - bell., ***caust.,*** cic., mosch., ***nux-v.***
- drinks, from - caust., cupr., lyc.
- water amel. - ***caust.,*** lyc.

cold, during a - cupr.
- taking a cold - bell., ***caust.,*** cic., ***mosch.,*** ***nux-v.,*** thyr.
  - at night, worse right side - caust.

coldness, of the body - aeth., anan., **BELL.,** ***camph.,*** caust., cic., ***hell.,*** hydr-ac., hyos., mosch., ***nicot.,*** **OENA.,** op., stram., ***verat.***
- feet, of - bell., ***cupr.***
- hands, of - ***cupr.***
- head hot, feet cold - bell.
- one side, of body - ***sil.***

colic, during - bell., **CIC.,** ***cupr.,*** plb., sec.

compression, on spinal column - tarent.

concussion of the brain, from - **ARN., CIC.,** ***hyper.,*** **NAT-S.**

congenital - hell., ***kali-br.,*** verat.

consciousness, with - ang., ars., aur-a., bar-m., bell., calc., camph., ***canth.,*** caust., **CINA,** cupr., grat., ***hell.,*** hyos., ***ign.,*** ***ip.,*** kali-ar., ***kali-c.,*** lyc., ***mag-c.,*** merc., mur-ac., ***nat-m.,*** nit-ac., ***nux-m.,*** ***nux-v.,*** ***phos.,*** ***plat.,*** plb., sec., ***sep.,*** sil., **STRAM.,** stry., sulph.

consciousness, without - absin., acet-ac., acon., ***aeth.,*** agar., agre., aml-n., ant-t., **ARG-N.,** ***ars.,*** ***aster.,*** aur., ***bell.,*** **BUFO, CALC.,** ***calc-ar.,*** ***calc-p.,*** ***calc-s.,*** ***camph.,*** **CANTH.,** carb-ac., cham., ***caust.,*** chin., **CIC.,** cina, ***cocc.,*** crot-h., ***cupr.,*** cupr-ac., cupr-ar., cur., dig., ferr., glon., ***hydr-ac.,*** **HYOS.,** ign., ***ip.,*** ***kali-c.,*** lach., laur., led., lyc., merc., ***mosch.,*** nat-m., nit-ac., nux-v., **OENA.,** op., phos., ***plat.,*** **PLB.,** sec., ***sep.,*** ***sil.,*** ***stann.,*** staph., ***stram.,*** ***sulph.,*** tanac., ***tarent.,*** verat., vesp., **VISC.**

contradiction, from - ***aster.***

cough, during - bell., ***calc.,*** ign., meph., stram., ***sulph.***
- after - cina, ***cupr.,*** hyos., ***ip.,*** just., ***verat.***
- whooping cough, in - ***brom.,*** ***calc.,*** ***cupr.,*** ***hydr-ac.,*** ***ip.,*** **KALI-BR.**

croup, in - ***lach.***

cyanosis, with - ***cupr.,*** cupr-ac., ***hydr-ac.,*** ***verat.***
- daytime - ***art-v.,*** ***kali-br.***
- degenerative - aur-m., ***phos.,*** zinc-p.
- delirium tremens, in - ***hyos.***

dentition, (see children)

diarrhea, after - mag-p., zinc.
- amel. - lob.
- with - nux-m.

diet, errors, in - ***cic.***

downwards, spread - ***cic.,*** sec.

draft, agg. - ars., cic., ***lyss.,*** **NUX-V., STRY.**

drawing up of legs, alternately - cyt-l.

drinking, after - ars., art-v., bell., ***hyos.,*** ***stram.***
- water - calc., canth.
- water, cold amel. - bry., caust., lyc.

drugs, after - acon., **ARN.,** ***nux-v.***

dyspnea, alternating with convulsions - plat.

eating, while - plb.
- after - aster., ***calc-p.,*** cina, grat., hyos., nux-v.

emission, of semen during - urt-u., grat., ***nat-p.***
- of semen, from - ***lach.***

epilepsy, (see Epilepsy, general)

epileptic, like, convulsions - ***absin.,*** acon., aeth., **AGAR.,** alum., alum-sil., am-c., aml-n., ***anac.,*** ant-c., ant-t., ***arg-m.,*** **ARG-N.,** arn., ***ars.,*** art-v., asaf., aur., aur-a., **BELL.,** bism., bry., ***bufo,*** **CALC.,** calc-i., calc-p., calc-s., ***camph.,*** canth., carb-s., caul., **CAUST.,** ***cedr.,*** ***cham.,*** chin., ***chin-a.,*** chlorpr., **CIC., CINA,** ***cocc.,*** coloc., con., ***convo-s.,*** cortico., cub., **CUPR.,** ***cur.,*** dig., dros., dulc., ferr., ferr-ar., gall-ac., ***gels.,*** **GLON.,** graph., hell., ***hydr-ac.,*** **HYOS.,** ***hyper.,*** hypoth., ign., indg., iod., ***ip.,*** kali-br., ***kali-c.,*** kali-i., kali-m., kali-s., ***lach.,*** laur., led., lob., lol., ***lyc.,*** mag-c., mag-p., ***med.,*** merc., mosch., mur-ac., ***nat-m.,*** ***nit-ac.,*** ***nux-m.,*** ***nux-v.,*** oena., op., passi., petr., ph-ac., phos., ***phys.,*** ***picro.,*** ***plat.,*** **PLB.,** prot., ***psor.,*** ***puls.,*** ***ran-b.,*** ran-s., rauw., rhus-t., ruta, salam., ***sec.,*** ***sep.,*** ***sil.,*** stann., staph., **STRAM.,** ***stry.,*** sul-i., **SULPH.,** tarax., ***tarent.,*** teucr., thuj., valer., verat., verat-v., verb., verbe-h., vip., **VISC.,** zinc., zinc-cy., zinc-p., ***zinc-valer.***

eruptions, fail to break out, when - ***ant-t.,*** **CUPR., ZINC.**
- from suppressed eruptions - agar., bry., ***calc.,*** ***caust.,*** ***cupr.,*** ***stram.,*** ***sulph.,*** ***zinc.***

CONVULSIONS, general

evening - alum., ***alumn.***, **CALC.**, ***caust.***, ***croc.***, gels., graph., kali-c., laur., merc-n., nit-ac., ***op.***, plb-chr., stann., stram., sulph.

8 p.m. - ars.

9 p.m. - ***lyss.***

open air - caust.

exanthemata, suppressed or does not appear, convulsions when - ant-t., apis, ars., ***bry.***, ***camph.***, ***cupr.***, ***cupr-ac.***, ***gels.***, ***hep.***, ***ip.***, op., ***stram.***, ***sulph.***, **ZINC.**, zinc-s.

excitement, from - acon., ***agar.***, art-v., ***aster.***, ***bell.***, cann-i., ***cham.***, cic., cimic., ***coff.***, ***cupr.***, ***gels.***, **HYOS.**, ***ign.***, ***kali-br.***, ***nux-v.***, **OP.**, phos., plat., ***puls.***, sec., tarent., ***zinc.***

from religious - ***verat.***

exertion, after - alum., alumn., ***calc.***, ***glon.***, kalm., ***lach.***, ***lyss.***, nat-m., petr., sulph.

exhaustion, great, after convulsion - ars., art-v.

extension, of body, forcible, amel. - nux-v., stry.

extensor, muscles - **CINA.**

eyelids, while touching - coc-c.

falling, with - ***agar.***, alum., alum-p., am-c., ***ars.***, ***aster.***, **BELL.**, bufo, ***calc.***, calc-i., ***calc-p.***, camph., canth., ***caust.***, ***cedr.***, **CHAM.**, ***chin-a.***, cic., cina, cocc., ***con.***, **CUPR.**, dig., dol., dulc., **HYOS.**, ign., ***iod.***, ip., lach., laur., lyc., lyss., merc., nit-ac., **OENA.**, op., petr., ph-ac., phos., plb., sec., sep., sil., ***stann.***, staph., ***stram.***, sulph., verat., zinc.

backwards - ang., ***bell.***, camph., canth., chin., cic., cic-m., ***ign.***, ***ip.***, kalm., nux-v., ***oena.***, **OP.**, rhus-t., spig., ***stram.***

forward - arn., ***aster.***, calc-p., canth., cic., cupr., ferr., rhus-t., sil., sulph., sumb.

left side - bell., caust., lach., sabad., sulph.

right side - bell.

runs in a circle to - ***caust.***

sideways - bell., ***calc.***, con., nux-v., sulph.

fear, from - acon., arg-n., art-v., **CALC.**, ***caust.***, cupr., glon., hyos., kali-p., oena., ***op.***, phos., sil.

fever, during the - ars., **BELL.**, camph., carb-v., ***caust.***, ***cic.***, ***cina,*** cur., ***ferr-p.***, ***hyos.***, ign., ***nat-m.***, **NUX-V.**, op., sep., **STRAM.**, verat.

fingers, spread - sec.

fluids, from - ***bell.***, canth., hyos., **LYSS.**, **STRAM.**

forcibly, aroused from a trance, when - ***nux-m.***

fright, from - ***acon.***, ***agar.***, apis, ***arg-n.***, ***art-v.***, bell., ***bufo,*** **CALC.**, ***caust.***, cham., cic., ***cupr.***, ***gels.***, glon., **HYOS.**, **IGN.**, **INDG.**, ***kali-br.***, ***kali-p.***, laur., lyss., nat-m., **OP.**, ***plat.***, ***sec.***, sil., ***stram.***, sulph., tarent., verat., ***zinc.***

of the mother during pregnancy - bufo, **OP.**

goitre, suppression of - iod.

grasping tight amel. - mez., nux-v.

grief, after - ***ars.***, art-v., ***hyos.***, **IGN.**, indg., nat-m., nux-v., ***op.***

heart disease, from - calc-ac.

CONVULSIONS, general

heat, during the - ars., **BELL.**, camph., carb-v., ***caust.***, ***cic.***, ***cina,*** cur., ***ferr-p.***, ***hyos.***, ign., ***nat-m.***, **NUX-V.**, op., sep., **STRAM.**, verat.

hiccough, followed by - cic.

humiliation, from - ***calc.***, cham., ***staph.***

hydrocephalus, with - ***arg-n.***, ***art-v.***, ***calc.***, ***kali-i.***, ***merc.***, ***nat-m.***, ***stram.***, ***sulph.***, ***zinc.***

hydrophobia, with - ***bell.***, ***canth.***, ***cur.***, gels., ***stram.***

hypochondriasis, with - mosch., stann.

hysterical - absin., acet-ac., acon., ***alum.***, alum-p., ambr., ***apis,*** ars., **ASAF.**, asar., ***aur.***, aur-a., aur-s., ***bell.***, ***bry.***, ***calc.***, calc-s., cann-i., cann-s., cast., caul., ***caust.***, ***cedr.***, cham., chlf., ***cic.***, ***cimic.***, ***cocc.***, coff., ***coll.***, **CON.**, croc., cupr., dig., ***gels.***, graph., hydr-ac., hyos., **IGN.**, ***iod.***, ***ip.***, kali-ar., kali-p., lach., lact., ***lil-t.***, lyc., ***mag-c.***, ***mag-m.***, meph., merc., ***mill.***, **MOSCH.**, ***nat-m.***, nit-ac., ***nux-m.***, nux-v., oena., op., petr., phos., ***plat.***, plb., puls., ruta, sec., ***sep.***, ***sol-c.***, stann., staph., ***stram.***, sul-i., sulph., sumb., tarent., thyr., valer., ***verat.***, ***verat-v.***, visc., zinc., zinc-p., ***zinc-valer.***

menses, before - hyos., ign., lach.

indigestion, from - **IP.**

indignation - ***staph.***

injuries, from - ***ang.***, **ARN.**, art-v., **CIC.**, con., cupr., cupr-ac., hep., **HYPER.**, meli., **NAT-S.**, ***op.***, oena., puls., ***rhus-t.***, sil., sulph., ***valer.***

head, of the - **ARN.**, art-v., **CIC.**, ***cupr.***, ***hyper.***, ***led.***, meli., **NAT-S.**

slight - valer.

spinal - hyper., tarent., zinc.

intermittent - absin.

internal - acon., agar., alum., ambr., am-c., anac., ang., ant-c., ant-t., arg-m., arn., ars., ***asaf.***, asar., bar-c., ***bell.***, bism., bor., bov., ***bry.***, calad., ***calc.***, camph., canth., caps., carb-an., ***carb-v.***, **CAUST.**, ***cham.***, cina, **COCC.**, coff., colch., coloc., con., ***cupr.***, dig., dulc., euph., ***ferr.***, graph., hep., **HYOS.**, **IGN.**, iod., ***ip.***, ***kali-c.***, kali-m., kali-n., kreos., lach., laur., led., ***lyc.***, mag-c., ***mag-m.***, merc., ***mosch.***, mur-ac., nat-c., nat-m., nit-ac., nux-m., **NUX-V.**, op., petr., ph-ac., ***phos.***, ***plat.***, plb., **PULS.**, rhod., rhus-t., sabad., sars., ***sec.***, seneg., ***sep.***, sil., spong., **STANN.**, ***staph.***, stram., stront-c., sulph., sul-ac., teucr., thuj., valer., verat., ***zinc.***, zinc-p.

interrupted, by painful shocks - stry.

isolated groups of muscles, of - acon., ***cic.***, cina, cupr., ign., nux-v., ***stram.***, ***stry.***

jealousy, from - ***lach.***

knocking body, from - hyper.

labor, during - ***acon.***, aeth., aml-n., arn., ***bell.***, canth., cham., chin., chin-s., ***chlol.***, ***cic.***, cimic., cocc., coff., cupr., ***cupr-ar.***, gels., glon., ***hydr-ac.***, ***hyos.***, ign., ip., kali-br., merc-c., merc-d., mosch., ***oena.***, op., piloc., plat., ***sec.***, sol-n., spirae., stram., ***verat-v.***, ***zinc.***

CONVULSIONS, general

laughing - ***coff., cupr.,*** graph.
laughing, with - coff., graph.
left, side of body - ***calc-p.,*** cupr., elaps, graph., ***ip.,*** nat-m., plb., ***sulph.***
light, agg. - ***bell.,*** **LYSS.,** ***op.,*** nux-v., **STRAM.**
lightning, like, head to foot - hydr-ac.
love, disappointed, from (see grief) - hyos., **IGN.**
lying, on abdomen, with spasmodic jerking of pelvis upward - cupr.
back, on, agg. - calc-p., nux-v., phos.
convulsively turned on the back - ***cic.***
side, on - puls.
convulsively turned on the back - ***cic.***
masturbation, from - ***bufo,*** calad., ***calc.,*** dig., elaps, kali-br., ***lach.,*** naja, nux-v., **PLAT.,** plb., sep., sil., stram., ***sulph.***
meningitis, in cerebrospinal - ***ant-t., apis, arg-n., crot-h., glon., hell., tarent., verat.***
menopausal period, during - glon., ***lach.***
menses, during - apis, ***arg-n., art-v., bell.,*** bufo, ***caul.,*** caust., ***cedr., cimic., cocc., coll., cupr.,*** gels., glon., ***hyos., ign., kali-br.,*** kali-m., ***lach., mill.,*** mosch., ***nat-m.,*** nux-m., ***nux-v.,*** **OENA.,** phys., ***plat.,*** plb., puls., ***sec.,*** sol-c., stram., ***sulph.,*** tarent., ***zinc.***
after - kali-br., syph., verat-v.
before - ***bufo,*** canth., carb-v., ***caust., cupr.,*** cupr-ac., ***hyos., kali-br.,*** nux-v., oena., ***puls.,*** thyr., verat-v.
painful, with - caul., nat-m.
instead of - cic., oena., puls.
suppressed, from - ***bufo, calc-p., cocc.,*** cupr., ***gels.,*** glon., ***mill., puls.***
mental exertion, after - bell., cann-i., ***glon.***
mercurial vapors, from - stram.
metastasis - ***cupr.***
midnight - bufo, cina, ***cocc.,*** sant., zinc.
after - nit-ac.
milk, suppressed, from - agar.
mirror, from a - lyss.
miscarriage, after - ruta.
moon, full, at - arg-n., **CALC.,** caust., luna, ***nat-m.***
new, at - ***bufo, caust., cupr., kali-br., sil.***
morning - arg-n., art-v., ***calc., caust.,*** cocc., crot-h., kalm., ***lyc., mag-p.,*** nux-v., plat., sec., sep., sulph., tab.
4 a.m. to 4 p.m. - ***calc.***
5 a.m. - plb.
9 to 10 a.m. - ***nat-m.,*** plb.
motion, agg. - ars., bell., ***cocc.,*** graph., ***nux-v., stry.***
limbs, on - cocc., **PIC-AC.**
amel. - merc., ther.
music amel. - calc., tarent.
nausea, vomiting, followed by - bell.
nervousness, from - ***arg-n.***

CONVULSIONS, general

night - ***arg-n.,*** ars., ***art-v.,*** aur., bufo, ***calc.,*** calc-ar., ***caust., cic., cina, cupr.,*** dig., ***hyos.,*** kali-c., kalm., lach., lyc., ***merc., nit-ac.,*** nux-v., oena., **OP.,** ***plb., sec.,*** **SIL.,** ***stram.,*** sulph., zinc.
3 a.m. - ***stram.***
vertigo during daytime - nit-ac.
noise, from - ang., ant-c., arn., ***cic.,*** ign., ***lyss., mag-p.,*** nux-v., stry.
arrests the paroxysm - ***hell.***
amel. - hell.
odors, from strong - brucin., ***lyss.,*** sil., stram., ***sulph.,*** stry.
old age, in - plb.
onanism, after - ***bufo,*** calad., ***calc.,*** dig., elaps, kali-br., ***lach.,*** naja, nux-v., **PLAT.,** plb., sep., sil., stram., ***sulph.***
one-sided - apoc., ***art-v.,*** bell., ***calc-p.,*** caust., dulc., elaps, gels., graph., hell., ***ip., plb.***
paralyzed side - ***phos.,*** sec.
paralysis of the other - apis, ***art-v.,*** bell., lach., phos., ***stram.***
opisthotonos (see back) - verat-v.
painful - rhod.
urination agg. - elat.
pains, during - ars., ***bell.,*** coloc., ign., kali-c., lyc., meny., nux-v.
after - chin., plat.
renewed at every - bell.
palpitation, after - glon.
paralysis, with - arg-n., bell., **CAUST.,** cic., cocc., cupr., ***hyos.,*** lach., laur., ***nux-m., nux-v., phos.,*** plat., ***plb., rhus-t.,*** sec., ***stann., tab.,*** vib., zinc.
followed by paralysis - acon., **CAUST.,** cupr., ***elaps,*** plb., sec.
paralysed, part in - sec.
paresis, followed by - acon., ***elaps,*** plb.
periodic - ***agar.,*** ars., bar-m., calc., ***cedr.,*** chin., chin-s., cupr., ***ferr.,*** ign., indg., ***kali-br.,*** lach., lyc., nat-m., nux-v., ***op.,*** plb., sec., stram., vip.
periodic every, day - camph., ***cupr., ferr., op.,*** stram.
5 or 6 days - ***lyc.***
7 days - ***agar.,*** chin-s., ***indg., kali-br.,*** nat-m.
10 days - ***kali-br.***
14 days - cupr., ***kali-br.,*** oena.
18 or 20 days - ***tarent.***
perspiration, during - ars., ***bell.,*** **BUFO,** camph., nux-v., op., sep.
after - ***bry.***
cold, with - camph., ***cupr., ferr.,*** stram., ***verat.***
pregnancy, during - ***acon.,*** aeth., aml-n., arn., ***bell.,*** canth., cast., ***cedr., cham., chlol., cic.,*** cimic., ***cina,*** croc., ***cupr., cupr-ar., gels., glon.,*** hell., ***hydr-ac., hyos.,*** ign., ***ip.,*** kali-br., lyc., lyss., mag-c., mag-m., merc-c., merc-d., mill., mosch., nux-m., ***oena.,*** op., piloc., pituin., plat., ***rhus-t.,*** sec., sol-n., spirae., stram.,

CONVULSIONS, general

pregnancy, during - stry., tarent., thyr., ***verat-v., zinc.***
pressure, on a part, from - cic.
on spine - ***tarent.***
on stomach, from - canth., cupr., cupr-ac., nux-v.
prodrome, as a - verat-v.
prostration, followed by - aeth., ***chin-a., cic.,*** hydr-ac., sec., sil., ***stry.,*** sulph.
puberty, at - art-v., caul., caust., cupr., hypoth., lach., puls., zinc., zinc-valer.
girls, in - art-v., caul., caust.
punishment, after - agar., ***cham.,*** cina, ***cupr.,*** **IGN., STAPH.**
rage, automatic impulse, followed by - op.
recent cases - ***bell.,*** caust., cupr., ***hydr-ac., ign.,*** op., plb., stram.
recurrent, several times daily - art-v., cic.
religious excitement, from - verat.
reproaches, from - agar., cham., ign., staph.
restlessness, followed by - cupr.
riding, carriage, in a amel. - ***nit-ac.***
right, side of body - ***bell.,*** caust., **LYC.,** ***nux-v.***
left paralyzed - ***art-v.***
to left - visc.
rubbing, amel. - ***phos., sec.,*** stry.
running, after - sulph.
in circle, before - caust.
scleroses, brain tumor, from - plb.
screaming, shrieking, with - acon., ***aml-n.,*** ant-t., ***apis, art-v.,*** bell., calc., ***camph.,*** canth., ***caust.,*** cedr., ***cic., cina, crot-h., cupr.,*** **HYOS.,** ***ign., lach.,*** lyc., ***merc.,*** nit-ac., ***nux-v.,*** oena., **OP.,** stann., ***stram.,*** sulph., verat-v., vip., ***zinc.***
sex, during - ***bufo.***
after - ***agar.***
sexual, excesses, from - bufo, ***kali-br., phos.***
excitement, from - art-v., bar-c., ***bufo,*** calc., **KALI-BR.,** ***lach., plat.,*** stann., sulph., visc.
shining, objects, from - bell., **LYSS., STRAM.**
shock, after - aesc., ***op.***
shrieking, (see Screaming)
side, lain, on - cimic.
left side of body - bell., ***calc-p.,*** chin-s., colch., cupr., elaps, graph., ***ip.,*** nat-m., nit-ac., plb., sabad., stram., ***sulph.***
to right - ***sulph.***
not, lain on - onos.
one-sided - art-v., brom., calc-p., chin-s., cina, ip., plb.
paralysis of the other - apis, ***art-v.,*** bell., hell., lach., phos., ***stram.***
side - ***phos.,*** sec.
right side of body - ***bell.,*** caust., chen-a., **LYC.,** ***nux-v.,*** sep., tarent.
left paralyzed - ***art-v.***
to left - visc.
speechlessness, with - dulc.

CONVULSIONS, general

sleep, during - ***arg-n.,*** **BELL.,** bufo, calc., ***caust.,*** cham., ***cic.,*** cina, cocc., ***cupr.,*** cupr-ar., ***gels., hyos., ign., kali-c., lach.,*** mag-c., merc., oena., ***op.,*** puls., ***rheum, rhus-t.,*** sec., sep., ***sil., stram., sulph.,*** tarent.
after loss of - **COCC.**
amel. - agar.
ending in deep - aeth., hyos., kali-br., lach., ***op.***
on falling, to - ***ars.,*** cupr., ign., ***kali-c.***
on going to - aeth., arg-m., sulph.
sleeplessness, with or after - alum., art-v., bell., bry., calc., carb-an., carb-v., ***cic.,*** cupr., cypr., hep., hyos., ign., ip., **KALI-BR.,** kali-c., merc., mosch., nux-v., passi., ph-ac., phos., puls., rheum, rhus-t., sel., sep., sil., stront-c., thal., verbe-h., zinc., zinc-valer.
smallpox, fails to break out, when - **ANT-T.**
speak, on attempting to - ***lyss.***
spinal, origin - thuj.
stool, during - nux-v.
stooping, amel. - hyos.
strange person, sight of - lyss., op., tarent.
stretching, out, parts, of amel. - sec.
limbs, of, during - bell.
before convulsions - ***calc.***
strokes, apoplectic - aster., ***bell., crot-h., cupr., lach.,*** nux-v., stram., ***verat-v.***
sudden - ars., ***bell.,*** hydr-ac., mez., oena., stry., ***verat-v.***
suppressed, discharges - ***asaf.,*** cupr., stram.
agg. - absin., caust., mill.
discharges - ***asaf.,*** cupr., mill., stram.
eruption - ***agar., ant-c., bry., calc., camph., caust., cupr., cupr-ac., hyos., ip., kali-m.,*** psor., ***stram., sulph., urt-u., zinc.***
footsweat, after - **SIL.**
mother's milk - ***agar.***
perspiration - ***sil.***
secretions and excretions - ***stram.***
suppuration, during - ***ars., bufo,*** canth., lach., ***tarent.***
swallow, during attempt to - **LYSS.,** ***mur-ac.,*** nux-m., nux-v., ***stram.***
swing, letting legs, excites convulsion - calc.
syphilitic - aur., iod., ***kali-br.,*** **KALI-I.,** merc-c., mez., ***nat-ac., nit-ac.***
tubercular - kali-br.
tetanic rigidity - abel., absin., acet-ac., ***acon.,*** aconin., aesc., agar-ph., agre., alum., ***am-c.,*** am-m., ***aml-n.,*** amyg., ***anac., ang., ant-t., arn., ars.,*** asaf., ***atro., bell.,*** benz-n., both., brucin., bry., ***calc.,*** calc-p., ***calen., camph.,*** cann-i., cann-s., ***canth.,*** carb-h., carb-o., carb-s., carbn., ***cast.,*** caust., ***cham., chin-s.,*** chlf., ***chlol.,*** **CIC.,** cina, ***cocc., con.,*** cori-m., cortico., crot-h., ***cupr.,*** cupr-ac., cupr-ar., ***cur.,*** dig., dros., dulc., ***gels.,*** grat., ***hell.,*** hep., ***hydr-ac., hyos.,*** **HYPER.,** ***ign., ip.,*** jasm., juni., kali-bi., ***kali-br.,*** kali-c., kali-cy., kali-n., Kreos., ***lach., laur., led.,*** linu-c., ***lob., lyc.,***

CONVULSIONS, general

tetanic rigidity - ***lyss.***, mag-c., ***mag-p.***, meph., ***merc.***, methys., ***mill.***, morph., ***mosch.***, mur-ac., nat-f., nicot., nux-m., **NUX-V.**, ***oena.***, ol-an., ***op.***, **PETR.**, phos., ***phys.***, ***phyt.***, **PLAT.**, ***plb.***, ***puls.***, rhod., ***rhus-t.***, sant., buth-a., ***sec.***, seneg., **SEP.**, ***sol-n.***, stann., ***stram.***, ***stry.***, stry-p., sul-ac., sulph., tab., tanac., ***ter.***, teucr., ***ther.***, thyr., ***upa.***, valer., verat., verat-v., verin., vib-p., zinc.

dashing cold water on face amel. - benz-n.

injured parts become cold as ice and spasms begin on the wound - **LED.**

traumatic - acon., **ARN.**, ***chlol.***, ***cic.***, ***cur.***, ***hell.***, ***hydr-ac.***, **HYPER.**, ***led.***, nat-s., ***nux-v.***, stram., tetox., teucr.

trismus, with - ***ant-t.***, ***bell.***, ***cupr-ac.***, ***oena.***, ***stram.***, ***verat-v.***

wiping perspiration from face agg. - nux-v.

wounds in the soles, finger on palm - ***bell.***, **HYPER.**, ***led.***

thunderstorm - agar., ***gels.***

tight, grasp amel. - nux-v.

tightly, binding the body amel. - mez.

tobacco, swallowing, from - ip.

together - ther.

tonic - acon., agar., alum., alum-p., alum-sil., am-c., am-m., ambr., anac., **ANG.**, ant-t., apis, arg-m., arn., ars., asaf., asar., **BELL.**, bor., bry., **BUFO**, ***calc.***, camph., cann-s., canth., caps., carb-o., ***caust.***, ***cham.***, chin., chlf., **CIC.**, cina, clem., cocc., coloc., con., cupr., ***cur.***, cycl., dig., ***dros.***, dulc., euph., ***ferr.***, ferr-ar., graph., guai., hell., hep., hydr-ac., hyos., ***ign.***, ***ip.***, kali-c., lath., laur., led., ***lyc.***, mag-p., mang., med., meny., ***merc.***, mez., ***mosch.***, nat-c., nat-m., nit-ac., nux-v., olnd., ***op.***, **PETR.**, ph-ac., ***phos.***, ***phys.***, phyt., **PLAT.**, ***plb.***, puls., rhod., rhus-t., sabad., sars., ***sec.***, seneg., **SEP.**, sil., spig., spong., stann., ***stram.***, stry., ***stry-s.***, sumb., ***sulph.***, tab., thuj., upa., ***verat.***, verat-v., visc., zinc.

single parts - ign.

tooth, extraction, after - bufo.

touched, when - acon., ***bell.***, ***carb-o.***, **CIC.**, cocc., ***lyss.***, ***mag-p.***, ***nux-v.***, ***stram.***, ***stry.***

tumor, followed by - arg-n., cic.

touched, when - acon., bell., carb-o., **CIC.**, cocc., lyss., nux-v., stram., stry.

turning, the head - cic.

bed, in - chen-a.

twitching, with - verat.

unjustly, accused, after being - caust., ***staph.***

uremic - apis, apoc., ars., ***carb-ac.***, chlf., cic., crot-h., ***cupr.***, cupr-ar., ***dig.***, glon., hell., hydr-ac., **KALI-BR.**, ***kali-s.***, merc-c., ***mosch.***, oena., ***op.***, piloc., ***plb.***, stram., ***ter.***, urea, urt-u., ***verat-v.***

vaccination, after - apis., ant-t., bell., ***cic.***, **SIL.**, ***thuj.***

vaginal discharge, with - ***caust.***, ***lach.***

valvular disease, from - calc-ar.

vertigo, after - hyos., tarent.

CONVULSIONS, general

vexation, from - agar., ars., bell., ***calc.***, camph., cham., **CUPR.**, ***ign.***, ***ip.***, nux-v., ***staph.***, sulph., verat., zinc.

vital fluids, from loss of - lach.

vomiting, during - aeth., ***ant-c.***, **CUPR.**, guar., ***ip.***, oena., op., upa.

amel. - agar., dig., sec.

waking, on - bell., ***ign.***, lyss.

warm, bath agg. - ***apis,*** glon., lach., nat-m., op.

room, in - op.

water, at sight of - ***bell.***, **LYSS.**, **STRAM.**

waving of arms, with - cyt-l.

weakness, during - hura, kali-c.

during nervous - sep.

wet, from becoming - calc., ***cupr.***, rhus-t.

whooping cough, with - hydr-ac.

worms, from - art-v., asaf., bar-m., ***bell.***, ***cham.***, ***cic.***, **CINA**, cupr., cupr-o., ***hyos.***, ***ign.***, ***indg.***, kali-br., sabad., ***sant.***, sil., spig., ***stann.***, stram., sulph., tanac., ***ter.***, teucr.

yawning - graph.

CONVULSIVE movements - acon., ***agar.***, ***alum.***, alum-p., ang., ant-t., apis, ***arg-n.***, arn., ars., ars-i., ***asaf.***, bar-c., bar-i., **BELL.**, brom., bry., ***bufo***, cact., ***calc.***, calc-i., ***camph.***, cann-s., ***canth.***, ***caust.***, **CHAM.**, **CIC.**, ***chin-s.***, ***cina***, **COCC.**, coff., ***con.***, croc., **CUPR.**, cupr-ar., dig., dulc., ***hell.***, **HYOS.**, **IGN.**, ***iod.***, **IP.**, kali-ar., lach., laur., lyc., mag-arct., ***mag-p.***, meny., merc., mosch., ***mygal.***, nat-c., nux-m., ***nux-v.***, olnd., **OP.**, phyt., ***plb.***, petr., ph-ac., phos., plat., ran-b., ran-s., ***rheum***, rhus-t., ***ruta***, sabad., samb., **SEC.**, spig., spong., ***squil.***, ***stann.***, staph., **STRAM.**, sulph., tab., ***tarent.***, ***verat.***, ***zinc.***

beginning in extremities - verat.

in face - dulc.

COORDINATION, disturbed (see Incoordination)

DIZZINESS, (see Vertigo, chapter)

EPILEPSY, general (see Convulsions) - ***absin.***, acet-ac., acon., ***aeth.***, ***agar.***, alco., all-c., ***alum.***, alum-p., alum-sil., alumn., ***am-br.***, am-c., ***ambr.***, ambro., ***aml-n.***, amyg., ***anac.***, ***anag.***, ang., anil., anis., ant-c., ant-t., antipyrin., apis, **ARG-M.**, **ARG-N.**, arn., ***ars.***, ***art-v.***, asaf., ***aster.***, ***atro.***, aur., aven., ***bar-c.***, **BAR-M.**, bar-s., **BELL.**, benz-n., bism., bor., bry., **BUFO**, caj., **CALC.**, **CALC-AR.**, ***calc-p.***, ***calc-s.***, camph., cann-i., ***canth.***, ***carb-an.***, carb-s., carb-v., ***cast.***, ***cast-eq.***, caste., caul., **CAUST.**, ***cedr.***, ***cham.***, chen-a., ***chin.***, chin-a., chin-s., ***chlol.***, chlorpr., ***cic.***, cic-m., ***cimic.***, ***cina***, cinnam., ***cocc.***, coloc., ***con.***, convo-s., cori-r., ***crot-c.***, ***crot-h.***, **CUPR.**, ***cupr-ac.***, ***cupr-ar.***, ***cur.***, ***cypr.***, dat-m., des-ac., dig., dros., dulc., fago., ferr., ***ferr-cy.***, ferr-p., ***form.***, ***gels.***, ***glon.***, graph., ***hell.***, hep., hydr-ac., **HYOS.**, ***hyper.***, ***ictod.***, ***ign.***, ***indg.***, iod., ***ip.***, irid., kali-ar., kali-bi., **KALI-BR.**, kali-c., ***kali-chl.***, ***kali-cy.***, kali-m., ***kali-p.***, kali-s., kres., ***lach.***, ***laur.***, led., levo., lith-br., lol., ***lyc.***, ***lyss.***, ***mag-c.***, ***mag-p.***, man., ***med.***, meli., merc., methyl-b., mill., mosch., mur-ac., naja, ***nat-m.***

EPILEPSY, general - ***nat-s.,*** nicot., nit-ac., nitro-o., nux-m., ***nux-v.,*** **OENA.,** oest., onis., onon., ***op.,*** passi., perh., petr., ***ph-ac., phos.,*** phys., ***picro., plat.,*** **PLB.,** polyg-p., ***psor., puls.,*** ran-b., ran-s., rauw., rhus-t., rib-ac., ruta, ***salam.,*** sant., ***sec.,*** sep., **SIL.,** sin-n., ***sol-c.,*** sol-n., spirae., ***stann.,*** staph., ***stram., stry.,*** sulfon., **SULPH.,** sumb., ***syph.,*** tab., tanac., tarax., ***tarent., ter.,*** thea., thiop., thuj., tub., valer., verat-v., verb., verbe-h., **VISC.,** verat., vip., ***zinc.,*** zinc-oc., zinc-p., ***zinc-valer., ziz.***

abdomen, epilepsy begins in - bufo.
night - ***bufo, cupr., sil.***
status epilepticus - ***acon.,*** aeth., ***bell.,*** cocc., oena., plb., zinc.

epilepsy, attack of, after
automatic impulse - op.
blind - sec.
ear noises - ***caust.***
headache - ***calc., caust.,*** cina, cupr., kali-br.
hiccough - cic.
nausea - bell.
prostration - aeth., ***chin-a., cic.,*** hydr-ac., sec., sil., ***stry.,*** sulph.
rage - op.
ravenous appetite - calc.
restlessness - cupr.
sleep, deep - aeth., hyos., kali-br., lach., ***op.***
tumor - arg-n., cic.
urine, copious - caust., ***cupr.,*** lach.
vomiting - acon., ***ars.,*** bell., ***calc.,*** colch., ***cupr.,*** glon.

epilepsy, attack of, during
biting tongue - ***art-v., bufo,*** camph., ***caust.,*** cocc., ***cupr., oena., op.,*** sec., stram., tarent., valer.
eyes turned upwards to right - ***hydr-ac.***
downwards - aeth.
face, bluish - absin., agar., atro., ***bell.,*** cina, **CUPR.,** ***hyos.,*** ign., ***ip.,*** nux-v., ***oena.,*** **OP.,** phys., plb., stry., ***verat.***
pale - am-c., ars., bell., calc., caust., chin., cic., cina, ***cupr., ip.,*** lach., mosch., nat-m., plb., puls., sil., stann., sulph., ***verat.***
red - aeth., ***bell.,*** bufo, camph., caust., **CIC.,** cina, cit-ac., cocc., ***cupr.,*** ign., ip., lyc., nux-v., ***oena.,*** **OP.,** stram.
yellow - cic., plb.
froth, foam from mouth - aeth., agar., ***art-v., aster.,*** bell., ***bufo,*** camph., canth., ***caust., cham., cic., cina,*** cocc., colch., ***cupr.,*** gels., ***glon.,*** hydr-ac., ***hyos.,*** ign., ***ind., lach.,*** laur., lyc., lyss., med., ***oena., op.,*** plb., ***sil.,*** staph., ***stry.,*** sulph., tax., vip.
involuntary discharges - cocc.
urination - art-v., **BUFO,** ***caust.,*** cocc., cupr., **HYOS.,** lach., nat-m., nux-v., ***oena., plb.,*** stry., ***zinc.***
jaws locked - aeth.
pupils, contracted - cic., ***op.,*** phyt.
dilated - aeth.
fixed - aeth.

EPILEPSY, general
epilepsy, attack of, during
screaming, shrieking - ***bufo,*** cedr., **CIC.,** crot-h., ***cupr.,*** hydr-ac., **HYOS.,** ign., ***ip., kali-bi.,*** lach., ***lyc.,*** nit-ac., ***nux-v., oena.,*** op., ***sil.,*** stann., stram., sulph., verat-v.
swelling of stomach, screaming, unconsciousness, trismus, distorted limbs, frequent during night, recurrent tendency - cic.
teeth, grinding of - ***bufo,*** **HYOS.,** sulph., tarent.
throwing body backwards - ***camph.***
forwards - ***cupr.***
thumbs clenched - aeth.
vertigo, with - arg-n., bell., calc., caust., cocc., cupr., hydr-ac., nit-ac., op., sil., stram.
winking of eyes - kali-bi.

epilepsy, aura of
abdomen to head, with - ***indg.***
absent - ars., art-v., atro., bell., camph., canth., cham., cic., cupr., cupr-ar., dios., hydr-ac., lach., nat-s., oena., plb., podo., tarent., valer., zinc., zinc-valer.
several fits, close together - art-v.
arms, in - bell., calc., ***calc-ar., lach.,*** sil., ***sulph.***
forearms, in - bell., calc., sulph.
left arm, in - ***calc-ar.,*** cupr., ***sil.,*** sulph.
auditory disturbances - ***bell.,*** calc., cic., hyos., sulph.
back, in - ars., sulph.
and left arm - ***calc-ar.,*** sulph.
creeping down spine - ***lach.***
belching - ***lach.***
blind - ***cupr.***
brain, wavy sensation, in - cimic.
cold air over spine and body - agar.
coldness - cina, sep., sil.
feet, of - cina, ***lach.***
feet, of, on left side before epilepsy - ***sil.***
on left side before epilepsy - ***sil.***
running down spine - ars.
scapula, between - sep.
confusion - ***lach.***
congestion of blood to head - calc-ar., op., sulph.
creeping down spine - ***lach.***
descending - bry., calc., carb-v., kali-c., lyc., phos., sulph., tub.
drawing in left chest - nit-ac..
in limbs - ars.
in limbs, chest, in left - nit-ac.
ear, noises in - hyos.
epigastrium to uterus and legs, from - **CALC.**
expansion of body, sensation of, before - ***arg-n.***
of feet and toes, sensation of - gels.
eyes, sparks before - ***hyos.***
turned upwards to left - bufo
face, chewing motion - ***calc.***
formication in - nux-v.
twitching - laur.
fear - aml-n., arg-n., cupr., nat-m.

EPILEPSY, general

epilepsy, aura of

female, extending from uterus to, stomach - bufo

to, throat - lach.

fingers and toes, in - cupr.

formication - bell., calc., nit-ac., nux-v.

genitalia, from - bufo.

glow, from foot to head - visc.

hand, in right - cupr.

to head, from - ***sulph.***

head, from - caust., lach., stram., sulph.

trembling sensation - ***caust.***

headache - ***bell.,*** calc., ***calc-ar.,*** cann-i., caust., cina, ***lach.,*** staph., zinc.

heart, from - **CALC-AR.,** lach., naja

heat, flushes of - calc-ar., indg.

heel to occiput - ***stram.***

right - ***stram.***

jerk in nape - ***bry.,*** bufo.

knees - cupr., cupr-ac.

ascending - cupr.

legs, in - lyc., plb.

right leg to abdomen, from - lyc.

limbs, in - bell., calc., cina, cupr., lyc., plb., sil., sulph.

left - cupr., sil., sulph.

morose - zinc., zinc-valer.

mouse, running like a, up limb, heat from stomach, visual or aural disturbance - ars., aur., **BELL., CALC.,** ign., nit-ac., sep., ***sil.,*** stram., ***sulph.***

mouth wide open - ***bufo.***

nausea, with - cupr., ***sulph.***

nervous feeling, a general - arg-n., ***nat-m.***

numbness of brain - bufo, indg.

palpitation - absin., ars., ***calc., calc-ar.,*** cupr., ferr., ***lach.,*** nat-m.

perspiration scalp - ***caust.,*** hell-v.

pupils dilated - **ARG-N.,** bell., ***bufo.***

ravenous appetite - ***calc.,*** **HYOS.**

restlessness - arg-n., bufo, caust.

sadness - art-v., zinc., zinc-valer.

screaming, shrieking - **CIC.,** ***cupr.,*** hydr-ac., stram.

shocks - ars., ***laur.***

shoulders, pain between, begins as, or dizziness, flashes of heat, from abdomen to head - indg.

solar plexus, from - am-br., art-v., bell., ***bufo, calc., caust.,*** **CIC.,** cupr., ***indg.,*** **NUX-V.,** ***sil.,*** **SULPH.**

extending to both sides, chest, and throat - am-br.

solar plexus, from, head, to - calc., ***sil.***

speech, unintelligible - bufo.

stomach, in - art-v., bell., bism., bufo, ***calc.,*** calc-ar., ***caust.,*** **CIC.,** cupr., **HYOS.,** ***indg.,*** **NUX-V.,** ***sil.,*** **SULPH.**

rising from stomach to head - **CALC.**

teeth, grinding of - ***sulph.***

throat, narrow sensation in - lach.

tongue swelling - plb.

trembling - absin., arg-n., aster.

urging for stool - calc-ar.

EPILEPSY, general

uterus - bufo.

to throat - ***lach.***

to stomach - bufo.

various symptoms - bufo.

vertigo - ars., ***calc-ar., caust.,*** **HYOS.,** indg., ***lach., plb.,*** sil., ***sulph., tarent.,*** visc.

visual disturbance - ***bell.,*** calc., hyos., lach., sulph.

voice, loss of - calc-ar.

vomiting - ***cupr.,*** op.

warm air streaming up spine - ***ars.***

waving sensation in brain, begins as - cimic.

FAINTING, faintness (see Vertigo, chapter) - abies-c., acet-ac., acetan., **ACON.,** ***aesc.,*** aeth., aether, agar., agar-em., alco., alet., all-c., aloe, ***alum.,*** alum-p., alum-sil., alumn., am-br., ambr., am-c., am-m., ***aml-n.,*** amyg., anac., ant-c., ant-m., ***ant-t.,*** apis, ***apoc.,*** apom., ***arg-n., arn., ars.,*** ars-h., ***ars-i.,*** ars-s-f., ars-s-r., asar., atro., bapt., bar-c., bar-i., ***bar-m., bar-s.,*** bell., benz-n., benz-ac., berb., beryl., bism., bol., bol-s., bor., bov., brom., **BRY.,** bufo, cact., **CADM-S.,** calad., calc., calc-ar., calc-i., calc-mur., calc-p., calc-sil., calo., ***camph.,*** cann-i., ***cann-s., canth.,*** carb-ac., ***carb-o., carb-s., carb-v.,*** carl., cass., cast., cast-eq., **CAUST.,** cedr., cench., cer-s., **CHAM.,** ***chel.,*** chim., **CHIN.,** ***chin-a.,*** chin-s., chlol., ***chlor.,*** cic., ***cimic.,*** cina, cinnam., cit-v., **COCC.,** ***coch.,*** coff., colch., ***coll., coloc., con.,*** coni., conv., convo-d., cot., croc., ***crot-c.,*** **CROT-H.,** crot-t., culx., cupr., cupr-ac., ***cupr-ar.,*** cupr-s., cur., cycl., **DIG.,** digin., digox., dios., dros., dubo-h., dub., dulc., elaps, ery-a., eucal., eup-pur., ***euph.,*** euph-c., ***ferr., ferr-ar., ferr-i.,*** ferr-p., ***form.,*** gamb., gels., gent-c., **GLON.,** gran., ***graph.,*** grin., hedeo, hell., hell-f., **HEP.,** hippoz., hura, ***hydr.,*** hydr-ac., ***hyos.,*** **IGN., IOD.,** iodof., **IP.,** iris, piloc., jal., jasm., jug-c., kali-ar., kali-bi., kali-br., kali-c., kali-cy., kali-n., kali-ox., kali-p., kali-sil., kalm., ***kreos.,*** **LAC-C.,** ***lac-d.,*** **LACH.,** lac-ac., lat-k., ***laur., led.,*** lept., ***lil-t., lina.,*** lob., luf-act., lup., ***lyc.,*** lycps., lyss., mag-arct., mag-c., ***mag-m.,*** magn-gr., manc., mang., merc., ***merc-c.,*** merc-cy., merc-d., merc-n., merc-p-r., mez., **MOSCH.,** mur-ac., ***naja,*** narc-po., narc-ps., ***nat-h., nat-m.,*** nat-ns., nat-p., nit-ac., nitro-o., **NUX-M., NUX-V.,** oena., ol-an., olnd., ***op.,*** ox-ac., paeon., pana., parth., ped., ***petr., ph-ac.,*** phase., ***phos.,*** phys., ***phyt.,*** picro., pip-m., plan., plat., **PLB., PODO.,** ***psor.,*** ptel., **PULS.,** puls-n, ran-b., ran-s., rhus-t., rob., ruta, sabad., sal-ac., ***sang.,*** sapin., ***sars.,*** sec., senec., ***seneg.,*** **SEP.,** sieg., ***sil.,*** sin-n., sol-t., sol-t-ae., ***spig.,*** spong., stann., staph., **STRAM.,** stroph., stry., sul-i., **SULPH.,** sul-ac., **SUMB.,** ***tab.,*** tarent., tax., ***ter.,*** ther., thuj., ***thyr.,*** til., ***tril.,*** tub., uran-n., ust., valer., **VERAT.,** ***verat-v.,*** verin., vesp., ***vib.,*** viol-o., vip., zinc., zinc-m., zinc-p., zing.

addison's disease, in - ***calc., sep.***

after-pain, after every - hep., ***nux-v.***

FAINTING, faintness

afternoon - anac., ***asar.,*** bor., dios., phys., seneg., sulph.
1 p.m. - lycps.
2 p.m. after chill - gels.
4 p.m. after mental exertion - rhodi.
5 p.m. - nux-m.
aggravated, after fainting - acon., ars., chin., ***mosch.,*** nux-v., ***op.,*** sep., stram.
air, in open - ***mosch.,*** nit-ac., ***nux-v.***
amel. - bor., crot-c., dios., trif-p.
amenorrhea, in - glon.
anemia, in - acet-ac., ferr-i., ***mosch., spig.,*** trinit.
anger, after - ***cham., gels., nux-v.,*** phos., staph., vesp.
angina pectoris, in - ***arn., hep., spong.***
precordial, anguish with - ***aml-n., merc-i-f.,*** plb., tab.
anguish, after - nux-v., verat.
anxiety, with, when walking, makes her walk faster - ***arg-n.***
ascending, hill, on - agar.
mountains, on - ***coca.***
stairs - aether, ***anac.,*** calc., iod., lycps., plb.
asthma, from - ***ars., atro.,*** berb., kreos., lach., morph.
bed, in - caust., dios.
belching, from - ***arg-n.,*** **CARB-V.,** nux-v.
after - ***arg-n., nux-v.***
amel. - mag-m.
bending, head backwards amel. - ol-an.
bleeding, from - ***acon.,*** cann-s., carb-v., **CHIN.,** crot-h., ***ip., lach.,*** verat.
childbirth, after - calc., chin., sep.
rectum - chin., ***ign., nux-v.***
uterine - ***apis,*** **CHIN.,** ***coc-c., kreos.,*** merc., ***phys.,*** tril.
blindness, after - nux-m.
blood, at sight of - **ALUM.,** nux-m., nux-v., ***verat.***
blood loss, from - **CHIN.,** ***ferr.,*** ferr-p., ***ip.,*** op., tril.
blowing, an instrument - kali-n.
breakfast, after - bufo, naja.
before - ***calc.***
breath, deep, amel. - asaf.
cause, without - asaf.
childbirth, with - cimic., ***coloc.***
chill, during - alum., dios., hedeo, ***merc-i-f., nux-v., sep.***
chilliness, with - zing.
church, in - ***ign.,*** merc-i-f.
closed, room, in - ***acon., asaf.,*** ip., ***lach.,*** **PULS.,** ***tab.,*** vesp.
clothes, from tight - kali-n.
cold, from taking - petr., ***sil.***
water amel. - glon., vip.
weather - sep.
coldness of skin, with - ***camph.,*** carb-v., ***chin., laur.,*** mosch., ***tab., verat.***

FAINTING, faintness

colic, during intestinal - asaf., ***cast., coll., coloc.,*** hydr., ***manc., nux-m.,*** stram.
constriction of chest - acon., ars.
convulsions, after - ars-s-f., ***verat.***
cough, during - ***ars.,*** coff., ip., kali-c., ***phos.***
between spells of - ***ant-t.***
crowded, in a, room - ambr., ***am-c.,*** ars., bar-c., con., ***ign., lyc.,*** nat-c., ***nat-m., nux-m., nux-v., phos., plb.,*** **PULS.,** sulph.
street, in a crowded - asaf.
dark, places, in - ***stram.***
dehydration, from - ars., bar-c., ***carb-v.,*** **CHIN., IP.,** kreos., merc., nux-m., nux-v., **PH-AC., TRIL.,** ***verat.***
diarrhea, during - ars., crot-t., ***cupr-ac., nux-m.,*** paeon., podo., ***puls.,*** verat.
after - aloe, ars., colch., **NUX-V.**
before - ars., sulph., sumb.
die, as if would - vinc.
dinner, during - asaf., lyc., ***mag-m., nux-v.***
after, when taking exercise in open air - am-m., ***kali-c., nux-v.***
diphteria, in - ***brom., canth.,*** kali-m., ***lach., sulph.***
discouraged, when - ars.
disturbed, when - asaf.
drowsy - ars.
drug, on thinking of - asaf.
eating, after - bar-c., bufo, ***caust., mag-m., nux-v., ph-ac.,*** plan., sang., sil., sul-ac.
before - asaf., bufo, ***culx.,*** ind., phos., ***ran-b.,*** sulph.
egg, on smelling freshly beaten - ***colch.***
emission, after - **ASAF.,** ***ph-ac.***
emotional, upset after - **IGN.,** puls., ***staph.***
evening - ***aesc-g.,*** alet., am-c., asaf., ***calc.,*** coff., glon., ***hep.,*** kali-n., ***lac-d.,*** lach., lyc., lycps., mosch., ***nat-m.,*** nux-v., phos., rhus-t., ***sep.***
5 p.m. - nux-m.
5:30 p.m. - nux-m.
6 p.m. - glon.
7 p.m. - lycps., seneg.
8 to 9 p.m. - ***nux-v.***
9 p.m. - mag-m., meli., rhus-t.
cardiac depression, from - lycps.
exertion, on - nat-m.
stiffness of fingers and arms, with - petr.
stool, during - sars.
undressing, on - chel.
excitement, on - ***acon.,*** am-c., ***asaf.,*** aster., camph., ***caust., cham.,*** cocc., **COFF., IGN.,** kali-c., **LACH.,** mosch., ***nat-c., nux-m.,*** **OP.,** ***ph-ac.,*** **SUMB.,** ***verat.,*** vesp.
exertion, on - ***arn., ars.,*** calc., ***calc-ar., carb-v., caust., cocc.,*** ferr., hyper., ***iod., lach., lob.,*** mosch., nat-m., nux-v., plan., plb., ***rhus-t., senec.,*** **SEP.,** sulph., ***ther., verat.***
on, slight - verat.
eyes, closing agg. - ant-t.

FAINTING, faintness
face, blue, with - morph.
pale - chin., ferr., ***ip.,*** op., tril.
red - acon., ***ptel.***
falling, with - ***ars., camph., stach.***
backward - ***lac-d.***
left side, to - mez.
fasting, amel. - alum-sil.
fever, during - ***acon., arn.,*** ars., bell., ***eup-per., ign., nat-m.,*** nux-v., op., ***phos., puls.,*** **SEP.**
after - sal-ac.
before - ars.
childbirth, during - cimic., ***coloc.***
intermittent, during - ***phos.***
food, if delayed in the least - **CULX.**
forenoon - kali-n., phos., sep., staph., stram.
9 a.m. - ped.
10 a.m. - ven-m.
tuberculosis, in - ***kali-c.***
11 a.m. - ind., ***lach.,*** **SULPH.**
11 to 12 a.m. - zinc.
standing erect, on - dios.
walking in open air - lycps.
frequent - **ARS.,** ***bapt., camph.,*** carb-s., ***hyos., merc., merc-cy., murx., op., phos.,*** **SULPH.**
fright, after - **ACON.,** ***gels.,*** **IGN.,** ***lach., nux-v.,*** **OP.,** ***phos., staph., verat.***
fruit, acid, amel. - naja
gastric affections, in - ***alumn.,*** **ARG-N.,** bufo, dios., ***dor.,*** elaps, ***kali-bi., mag-m., mez., nat-s.,*** ol-an., sang., **SULPH.**
grief, from - ***ign., staph.***
headache, during - ars., ***calc.,*** carb-v., cast., ***gels.,*** glon., graph., hippoz., lyc., mez., mosch., nat-m., ***sil.,*** stram., ***sulph., ter.,*** verat., zing.
heart disease, in - ***arn., ars., cact., chel.,*** crat., ***dig., kali-p.,*** lycps., ***spig.***
heart weakness, from - am-c., ars., carb-v., cratag., dig., hydr-ac., lach., laur., verat.
pressure about, with - cimic., ***manc.,*** petr., plb.
heat, with flushes of - ***crot-t., sep.,*** **SULPH.**
hematemesis, from - **ARS.**
hemoptysis, after - sil.
heat then coldness, from - **CARB-V.,** ***iod.***
with fainting - **SEP.**
heated, when - ip., ***puls.,*** tab.
summer, from - ***ant-c., ip.***
hour, at a certain - lyc.
hunger, from - cocc., croc., crot-c., **CULX.,** iod., ***phos., sulph.,*** tub.
hysterical - am-c., arn., ars., asaf., cench., ***cham.,*** cimic., **COCC.,** cupr., ***dig.,*** **IGN.,** kali-ar., lac-d., lach., **MOSCH.,** ***nat-m., nux-m., nux-v.,*** puls., ***sep.,*** stict., sumb., ter.
injury, from shock in - ***arn.,*** atro., ***camph., cham.,*** dig., ***hyper., nat-s.***
concussion of brain, from - ***hyos.,*** **NAT-S.**
injuries, with slight - verat.
kneeling in church, while - **SEP.**
labor, during - cham., ***cimic.,*** cinnam., ***coff.,*** ign., **NUX-V., PULS., SEC.,** ***verat.***

FAINTING, faintness
lights, from being in a room with many - nux-v.
listening, to reading, from - agar-em.
looking, steadily at any object directly before eye - sumb.
looking, upwards - tab.
loss of fluids, from - ars., bar-c., ***carb-v.,*** **CHIN., IP.,** kreos., merc., nux-m., nux-v., **PH-AC., TRIL.,** ***verat.***
blood loss - **CHIN.,** ***ferr.,*** ferr-p., ***ip.,*** op., tril.
lungs, weakness from - am-c., carb-v.
lying, while - berb., calad., **CARB-V.,** caust., iod., lyc., sulph.
after - calad., mag-c.
amel. - alum., dios., ***merc-i-f., nux-v.***
on the side, while - lyc., sil.
medicine, taking, on - asaf.
meditating, while - calad., ***calc.,*** coff., ***nux-v., par.***
meningitis, in - ***ant-t., dig., glon.***
menopausal period, during - **ACON.,** chin., cimic., cocc., ***coff.,*** crot-h., ferr., ***glon., kali-c.,*** **LACH.,** ***mosch., nit-ac.,*** nux-m., nux-v., ***phys.,*** sep., ***sulph.,*** tab., tril., valer., ***verat.,*** viol-t.
menses, during - ***acon.,*** apis, berb., ***calc.,*** cham., chin., cimic., ***cocc.,*** glon., ***ign.,*** **LACH.,** laur., lyc., mag-c., mag-m., ***mosch.,*** murx., nat-m., ***nux-m.,*** **NUX-V.,** plb., ***puls.,*** raph., ***sars.,*** **SEP.,** sulph., tril., tub., uran-n., verat., ***vib.,*** wies.
coldness, with - laur.
after - ***chin., lach., lyc.***
before - am-c., ars., chin., cimic., cocc., ign., lach., ***lyc., mosch., mur-ac., nat-m., nux-m., nux-v., sep., thuj.,*** verat.
from pain - ***cocc.,*** ign., kali-s., ***lap-a., nux-v., sars., sep.***
from suppressed - cocc., kali-c., ***nux-m.,*** op.
metrorrhagia with - apis, ***chin.,*** ferr-m., ***tril.***
morning - alumn., **ARS.,** bor., ***carb-v., cocc., con.,*** culx., dios., kali-c., kali-n., ***kreos.,*** lach., med., nat-m., nit-ac., **NUX-V.,** petr., plb., puls., ***sang.,*** sep., staph., stram., stry., **SULPH.**
7 a.m. - dios.
8 a.m. - dios., ped.
8 to 9 a.m. - phos.
air, in open - mosch., nux-v.
bed, in - carb-v., ***con.***
eating, during - lach.
amel. - nux-v.
before - ***calc.***
house, on entering - petr.
rising, on - **BRY.,** calc., **CARB-V., COCC.,** ***iod., kreos., lac-d., lach.,*** nat-m., petr., sep.
quickly from stooping or turning head quickly - ***sang.***
stool, during - phys.
waking, on - graph.

FAINTING, faintness

moving, on - **ARS., BRY., COCC.,** ***croc.,*** cupr., cupr-ac., ***hyos.,*** kali-c., ***lob.,*** nat-hchls., ***nit-ac.,*** nux-v., phys., spig., **SPONG.,** ***verat.***
amel. - jug-c.
quickly - samb., sumb.
music, on hearing - cann-i., sumb.
mydriasis, with - morph.
nausea, during - ail., alum., alumn., ang., ***arg-n., ars.,*** calad., calc., carb-an., carb-s., caust., cham., chel., **COCC.,** coff-t., fago., ***glon.,*** graph., **IP.,** ***kali-c.,*** **LACH.,** lob., nat-m., **NUX-V.,** op., petr., picro., plan., sep., sul-ac., sulph., ***tab.,*** valer., verat., vesp.
after - ***kali-bi.***
before - ***verat.***
nervous - cench., ign.
night - am-c., ars., bar-c., calc., carb-v., dios., graph., ***mosch.,*** nit-ac., nux-m., ***nux-v.,*** sep., ***sil.,*** ther., vip.
3 a.m. - dios.
midnight - sep.
noise - ant-c., asaf., bor., lyc., merc., nat-m.
noon - bov., cic., ign.
nosebleed, with - ***calc.,*** cann-i., cann-s., carb-v., chin., croc., ferr., lach., ***phos.***
before - ***carb-v.***
from - ***acon., cann-s.,*** croc., crot-h., ***ip., lach., phos.***
numbness, tingling, with - **ACON.,** bor., nat-m., nux-v.
nursing child, when - vip.
odors, from - ***colch.,*** ign., **NUX-V., PHOS.,** sang.
cooking food, from - **COLCH.,** ip.
eau de cologne amel. - sang.
eggs, of - ***colch.***
fish - colch.
flowers - **PHOS.,** sang.
tobacco - ***ign.***
perfume or vinegar - agar.
stool, of - dios.
operations, on talking of - alum., calen.
pain, from - ***acon.,*** apis, ars., asaf., bism., bol., ***cham., cocc.,*** coff., coloc., ***gels.,*** **HEP.,** ***ign.,*** iod., morph., mosch., ***nux-m., nux-v.,*** phos., phyt., ran-s., sil., ***stront-c.,*** stroph., ***valer., verat.,*** vib., vip.
abdomen in - ***cocc., coll.,*** plb., stram.
after every - hep., ***nux-v.***
anus, in - sulph.
ear, in - ***cur., hep., merc.***
head, in - mez.
heart, in - arn., ***cact.,*** **LACH.,** ***manc.***
prick of a needle, from - calc.
sacrum, in - dios., hura.
spermatic cords, in - calc-ar.
stomach, in - ***ars., coll.,*** cupr-s., ***dios.,*** puls., ran-b., ran-s., sin-n., ***sulph.***
stool, during - ***cocc.***
teeth, in - chin., ***puls.,*** verat.
testicles, in - ***laur.***

FAINTING, faintness

palpitation, during - **ACON.,** ***am-c.,*** arg-n., beryl., cact., cham., cimic., ***coc-c., hydr., iod., kalm.,*** **LACH.,** ***manc.,*** nat-m., **NUX-M.,** petr., sul-i., tab., ***verat.***
after - am-c.
periodical - cact., ***coll.,*** fl-ac., lyc., nit-ac., staph.
every day - ***hydr.***
perspiration, during - agar., ant-t., apis, ***ars., calc.,*** carb-v., ***ign.,*** hyos., ***lob., sep.***
after - arn., sal-ac.
amel. - ***olnd.***
cold, with - ***bry., camph.,*** caps., carb-v., ***chin.,*** **DIG.,** ***hydr.,*** lach., ***tab.,*** ther., ***verat.***
suppressed foot sweat, from - ***sil.***
pregnancy, during - ***bell., kali-c., nux-m., nux-v., puls.,*** sec., ***sep., verat.***
slightest motion of child, from - ***lach.***
pressure, around the waist, from - ***lac-d., merc.***
prolonged - ***hydr-ac., laur.***
pulse, with imperceptible - ***chin., crot-h.,*** morph.
irregular - **DIG.,** morph.
slow - **DIG.**
raising, arms above head - ***lac-d.,*** lach., spong.
the head - apoc., ***bry.,*** ip.
read, when attempting to, while standing - glon.
reading, after - asaf., cycl., tarax.
riding, while - ***berb.,*** grat., ***sep.,*** sil.
after - berb.
rising, on - acon., ambr., ***bry.,*** cadm-s., calad., ***calc.,*** cer-b., chel., crot-h., cupr., ind., ***iod., lach.,*** merc-i-f., phyt., plb., ran-a., vac., vario., ***verat-v.,*** vib.
after - **CARB-V.,** ***iod.***
from bed, on - acon., apoc., berb., **BRY.,** calad., ***calc., carb-v., cina,*** colch., ***iod.,*** nat-m., op., **PHYT.,** rhus-t., rob., sep., trom.
seat, from - carb-v., staph., sumb., trom.
room, entering - plb.
running up stairs - sumb.
sex, during - murx., orig., ***plat.***
after - **AGAR., ASAF.,** ***dig., nat-p., sep.***
sexual excesses, after - ***dig.,*** ol-an.
scolding, from - ***mosch.***
shaking, after - asaf., arn., colch., kali-br., kreos., lyc., merc-c., sec., stry.
shock, from - ***atro.***
sitting, while - iod., kali-n., nat-s., nux-v.
down, on - bov., kali-n.
up, from - **ACON.,** arn., **BRY.,** carb-v., chin., ***dig.,*** dios., ***ip., nux-v.,*** **PHYT.,** ***ran-b., sep.,*** sulph., verat-v., ***vib.,*** vip.
suddenly - ery-a., ***verat-v.***
upright, while - acon., calad.
sleep, after - **CARB-V.**
followed by - syph.
loss of, by - carc., cocc., syph.

FAINTING, faintness
- **sleeping,** on left side - asaf.
- **smoking,** on - ***ign., ip.,*** sil.
  - after - ***caust., lob.***
- **snoring,** with - stram.
- **speaking,** from - ***ars.***
- **standing,** while - **ALUM., ALUMN.,** ant-t., apis, aur., berb., bov., ***bry.,*** chin., ***dig.,*** dios., glon., kali-n., lil-t., lyc., ***nux-m.,*** nux-v., phyt., rhus-t., sars., sil., sep., ***sulph., zinc.***
  - menses, during, in church - ***lyc., nux-m., puls., sep.***
  - prolapse of uterus, from - ***lil-t.***
  - urinating, while - acon.
- **starting** at something falling to the floor, from - merc.
- **stomach,** sensation of something rising from - am-br., **CALC.**
- **stool,** during - aloe, ***ars.,*** bor., colch., coll., crot-h., crot-t., ***dulc.,*** dios., ***merc., nux-m.,*** ox-ac., petr., plan., ***puls., sars.,*** spig., stann., ***sulph.,*** tub., ***verat.,*** verat-v.
  - after - ***aloe,*** apis, ***ars., ars-s-f., bol., calc., cocc.,*** colch., **CON.,** crot-t., cur., dig., dios., gall-ac., hydr., kiss., ***lyc., merc.,*** morph., nat-s., ***nux-m.,*** nux-v., paeon., ***phos.,*** plan., phyt., **PODO.,** sarr., sars., sulph., ***ter., verat.***
  - amel. by - rhodi.
  - before - ***ars.,*** dig., glon., puls., sars., samb., ***sulph.***
  - odor of, from - dios.
  - urging, from - ***cocc.***
- **stooping,** on - elaps, sumb.
- **storm,** before a - petr.
- **sudden** - ant-c., camph., cham., hydr-ac., ip., kali-cy., ***phos.,*** podo., ran-b., rhus-t., ***sep.,*** valer.
- **summer** heat, from - ***ant-c., ip.***
- **temples,** on rubbing with both hands - merc.
- **tendency** to - aether, carb-o., carb-s., colch., cupr-s., dig., elaps, euph., iod., kali-ox., ***magn-gl.,*** nux-m., ol-an., sol-t-ae., sulph., ***sumb.,*** tab., thea., verat.
- **tetanic** spasm, after - nux-v.
  - before - sul-h.
- **thinking,** after - calad.
- **thunderstorm,** before - petr., sil.
- **transient** - ***mur-ac.,*** nux-m.
- **trembling,** with - asaf., caust., ***lach.,*** nux-v., petr.
- **trifles,** from - ***sep.,*** sumb.
- **turning** the head, on - ery-a., ptel.
- **urinating,** during - ***med.,*** stann.
  - after - **ACON.,** all-c., med.
- **uterine** affection, in - ***cimic., cocc.,*** murx.
- **vaginal** discharge, with - bar-c., cycl., ***lach., nux-m.,*** sulph.
- **vertigo,** with - acon., alet., berb., bry., camph., ***carb-v.,*** gels., glon., ***hep.,*** mag-c., ***nux-v.,*** phos., sabad., tab.

FAINTING, faintness
- **vomiting,** with - agar., apom., crot-t., **IP.,** ***kali-c.,*** nit-ac., ***phyt.,*** **TAB., VERAT.**
  - after - **ARS.,** bism., ***cocc.,*** dig., elaps, ***gamb.,*** kali-c., nux-a., **NUX-V.,** ***stict.,*** verat.
  - before - **ARS.,** crot-h., **IP.**
- **waking,** on - **CARB-V.,** dios., graph., lach., ptel., ther.
  - waking, on, if sleeping on left side - asaf.
- **walking,** while - aether, arn., ***ars.,*** berb., bov., ***con.,*** cur., dor., ferr., get., merc., nat-s., ***verat-v.***
  - after - berb., ***con.,*** nux-v., paeon.
  - continuing amel. - ***anac.***
  - downstairs, from going - ery-a., stann.
  - upstairs, from going - ***anac.***
- **walking,** open air, agg., in - berb., bor., caust., lycps., mosch., sep., seneg.
  - after - ***nux-v.***
  - amel. - am-c.
    - rapidly - petr.
- **warm,** bath - ***lach.***
  - room - ***acon.,*** ant-c., calc-i., ***ip.,*** kreos., ***lach.,*** **LIL-T.,** lyc., ***nat-m.,*** nux-v., **PULS., SEP.,** spig., tab., trif-p., ust., vesp.
- **washing,** clothes, on - ther.
- **water** on, amel. by dashing cold - glon.
- **weakness,** from - ant-t., ***ars., carb-v.,*** caust., ***coca, ferr., hydr., lach.,*** nux-m., nux-v., ran-b., ***sang., verat., zing.***
- **well,** feels especially before the attack - psor.
- **wet,** after getting - ***sep.***
- **wine,** agg. - sumb.
- **wounds,** from slight - ign., ***verat.***
- **writing,** after - calad., ***calc.,*** mosch., op.

GUILLAIN-barre syndrome - carc., con., thuj.

INCOORDINATION, general - ***agar.,*** **ALUM.,** arag., arg-n., bell., ***calc.,*** carb-s., caust., chlol., coca, cocc., **CON.,** ***cupr., gels.,*** merc., ***onos., ph-ac., phos., plb.,*** sec., ***stram., sulph.,*** tab., ***zinc.***
- coordination disturbed - ***agar., alum.,*** arg-n., bar-c., bell., caust., ***cimic., cocc.,*** con., echi., ferr., gels., glon., graph., hyos., ign., kali-p., lach., merc., nux-v., onos., phos., plat., ***rhus-t.,*** sulph.
- legs - ***alum.,*** bell., chlol., crot-c., ***nux-m., onos., phos., plb., sil., sulph.***
- limbs - ***agar.,*** **ALUM.,** ***arag.,*** arg-n., bell., ***calc.,*** carb-s., caust., chlol., coca, cocc., **CON.,** ***cupr., gels.,*** merc., ***onos., ph-ac., phos., plb.,*** sec., ***stram., sulph.,*** tab., ***zinc.***

INFLAMMATION, of nerves, (see Neuritis)

LOCKJAW, (see Emergency, Tetanus)

MULTIPLE, sclerosis - ***alum.,*** arg-m., ***arg-n., atro., aur.,*** aur-m., bar-c., bar-m., bell., calc., cann-i., carb-s., **CAUST.,** ***con., crot-h.,*** des-ac., **GELS.,** halo., irid., ***lath., lyc.,*** man., merc., **NAT-M.,** nux-v., ox-ac., **PHOS.,** ***phys., pic-ac., plb.,*** psil., sil., ***stry.,*** sulph., tarent., thal., thuj., syph., wild., xan., zinc.

MULTIPLE, sclerosis
begins, in lower limbs - con.
double vision, with - gels.
grief, from - caust., con., phos., nat-m.
shots, influenza, after - gels.
softening of spinal cord, with - ***arg-n., atro., aur.,*** bar-c., bell., calc., caust., chel., ***crot-h.,*** gels., ***lath.,*** lyc., nux-v., ox-ac., ***phos., phys., plb.,*** sil., ***stry.,*** sulph., tarent., thuj.
vertigo, with - con.

MYATROPHY, progressive spinal - ars., carb-s., hyper., kali-hp., **PHOS.,** phys., ***plb.,*** sec.

NEURITIS - **ACON.,** ***alum-sil., ant-c., ars.,*** **BELL.,** ***cact.,*** caust., ***cic., coca,*** **COFF.,** ***gels., hep.,*** **HYPER.,** iod., ***ip.,*** kali-i., ***kalm.,*** lac-c., ***lec., led., merc., nat-m., nux-v.,*** **PHOS.,** ***puls., rhus-t., sil.,*** stram., sulph., zinc.

NUMBNESS, sensation
coldness, with - plat., sumb.
diagonal - thyr.
epilepsy, before - bufo.
external - abrot., absin., ***acon.,*** ail., agar., alum., ***ambr.,*** am-c., am-m., **ANAC.,** ant-c., ***ant-t., apis, arg-n.,*** arn., ars., ars-i., asaf., asar., aur., ***bapt., bar-c.,*** bar-m., ***bell.,*** **BERB.,** bism., bov., brom., bry., bufo, cact., caj., calc., camph., cann-i., cann-s., canth., carb-ac., ***carb-an.,*** **CARB-S.,** ***carb-v., caust.,*** cedr., ***cham., chel.,*** chin., chlor., ***cic.,*** cimic., cinnb., coca, **COCC.,** colch., coloc., **CON.,** croc., ***crot-c., crot-h.,*** cupr., cur., dig., dios., dulc., elaps, euphr., ferr., fl-ac., ***gels., glon., gnaph.,*** **GRAPH.,** ***hell.,*** hydr-ac., **HYOS.,** ***hyper., ign.,*** iod., ip., iris, kali-br., **KALI-C.,** ***kali-fer., kali-n.,*** kali-p., kalm., lach., laur., ***led.,*** **LYC.,** mag-m., ***merc., mosch., nux-m., nux-v.,*** **OLND.,** onos., **OP.,** ***ox-ac.,*** oxyt., par., petr., **PH-AC., PHOS.,** phys., ***pic-ac., plat.,*** **PLB.,** ***puls.,*** rhod., ***rhus-t.,*** **SEC.,** ***sep., sil.,*** spig., spong., staph., **STRAM.,** sulph., tab., thea., ***urt-u.,*** valer., verat., verat-v., verb., ***zinc.***
alternating with, hypersensitiveness - plat.
bruised part, in the - arn.
epilepsy before - bufo.
evening - ped.
feels neither heat nor cold - berb.
inspiration, on - ped.
left half of body - ***caust., lach.,*** mez., xan.
menopause, during - ***cimic.***
morning - ambr.
music, from - sabin.
night - sil.
waking, on - mez.
right half of body - ars., lyc.
whole body - acon., ambr., apis, arg-n., asc-t., ***bar-m.,*** bell., caj., caps., cedr., chel., crot-c., gels., gymn., kali-bi., **KALI-BR.,** kreos., lyss., merc., nitro-o., nux-v., **OLND.,** ***ox-ac.,*** pic-ac., tab., tarent.
feels neither heat nor cold - berb.
grasping objects agg. - cocc.

NUMBNESS, sensation
headache, during - cedr.
heat or cold, to extreme - berb.
internally - acon., ambr., am-c., ***ars.,*** asaf., bar-c., ***bell., bov.,*** calc., carb-an., carb-s., caust., cham., chin., cina, coff., colch., con., crot-t., cupr., dig., ferr., **GELS.,** graph., ***hyos.,*** ign., ***kali-br.,*** kali-c., laur., lyc., mag-c., mag-m., merc., mur-ac., nat-m., nit-ac., nux-m., olnd., ***op.,*** petr., phos., **PLAT.,** plb., puls., ran-b., rheum, sars., seneg., sil., ***spig.,*** stann., stram., stront-c., thuj., valer., verat.
lower half of body, of - spong.
lying down agg. - zinc.
news, after bad - calc-p.
pains, from - asaf., cham., ***coloc.,*** gnaph., hyper., kalm., mez., nat-m., plat., puls., rhus-t.
after - acon., agar., graph., mez., plat.
part, lain on - ***ambr.,*** am-c., arg-m., ***arn.,*** ars., ***bar-c.,*** bry., bufo, ***calc.,*** calc-sil., carb-an., ***carb-s.,*** **CARB-V.,** ***chin.,*** cop., croc., glon., ***graph.,*** hep., ign., kali-c., ***lach.,*** lyc., mag-c., mez., ***nat-m.,*** pall., phel., ***phos.,*** **PULS.,** ***rheum,*** **RHUS-T.,** samb., sep., ***sil., sumb.,*** zinc.
not lain on - fl-ac., mag-m.
places, changing - raph.
prick, heat sensation, painful - kreos., ***plb.,*** thuj.
pricking, with - tarent.
single, parts, in - ***acon.,*** agar., alum., ***ambr.,*** am-c., am-m., ***anac.,*** ant-c., ***ant-t., arg-m., arg-n.,*** arn., ars., ars-i., asaf., asar., aur., ***bar-c.,*** bell., bor., bov., bry., ***calc., calc-p.,*** camph., cann-s., canth., caps., **CARB-AN., CARB-S.,** ***carb-v.,*** caust., ***cham.,*** chel., ***chin.,*** cic., cina, **COCC.,** colch., ***coloc.,*** con., **CROC.,** dig., dros., dulc., euph., euphr., ***ferr.,*** ferr-p., **GRAPH.,** ***guai.,*** hep., hyos., ***ign.,*** iod., ip., kali-ar., **KALI-C.,** ***kali-fer.,*** **KALI-N.,** kali-p., kreos., laur., led., **LYC.,** mag-c., ***mag-m.,*** mang., **MERC.,** mez., mosch., ***mur-ac.,*** nat-c., ***nat-m.,*** nat-p., nit-ac., ***nux-v.,*** olnd., op., ***par., petr., phos.,*** ph-ac., plat., plb., **PULS.,** ***rheum, rhod.,*** **RHUS-T.,** sabad., sabin., samb., ***sars., sec., sep.,*** **SIL.,** spig., spong., squil., stann., staph., ***stram., sulph.,*** sul-ac., teucr., thuj., valer., ***verat., zinc.,*** **ZINC-P.**
spinal affections, in - fl-ac.
spots, in - ambr., bufo8, cadm-s., caust., ***lyc., plat.,*** sul-i.
stretching part agg. - rad-br.
spots, in - ***lyc., plat.***
suffering, parts, of - ***acon.,*** alum., ambr., ***anac.,*** ant-t., arn., ***ars.,*** ars-i., ***asaf.,*** aur., bell., bor., bov., bry., calc., cann-s., carb-an., carb-v., caust., **CHAM.,** chel., chin., cic., cina, ***cocc.,*** coff., colch., coloc., **CON.,** croc., cupr., cycl., dig., dulc., elaps, euphr., ferr., ferr-ar., ferr-p., ***gnaph., graph.,*** hell., hep., hyos., ign., iod., kali-c., **KALI-N.,** kreos., ***lyc.,*** mag-m., merc., mez., mur-ac., nat-m., nux-m.,

NUMBNESS, sensation

suffering, parts, of - nux-v., ***olnd.,*** petr., ph-ac., phos., **PLAT., PLB., PULS.,** rheum, rhod., ***rhus-t.,*** ruta, samb., sec., sep., sil., spong., stann., staph., stram., stront-c., sulph., sul-ac., thuj., verat., verb., viol-o., zinc.

bruised parts - ***arn.***

unilateral - ars., caust., chel., **COCC.,** nat-m., phos., ***puls.***

left - ars., sumb., xan.

right - caust., elaps, naja

upper half of body - ***bar-c.***

waking, on - aran., cham.

wooden feeling - kali-n., petr., ***thuj.***

PAINLESSNESS, of complaints, usually painful - **ARN.,** ***hell.,*** **OP., STRAM.**

PAINS, (see Generals)

PARALYTIC, pain, (see Generals)

PARALYSIS, agitans (see Parkinson's disease)

PARALYSIS, general - absin., ***acon.,*** agar., ang., arag., arg-i., ***arg-n., arn.,*** ars-i., asaf., astra-e., aur., ***aur-m., bar-ac., bar-c., bar-m., bell.,*** calc-caust., ***calen.,*** carb-o., carb-s., **CAUST.,** chen-a., chin-s., cic., **COCC.,** colch., **CON.,** ***cupr., dulc.,*** elaps, **GELS.,** graph., grin., ***gua.,*** helo., hydr-ac., hyos., ***hyper.,*** ign., ir-fl., kali-br., ***kali-c.,*** kali-i., kali-p., **LACH.,** ***lath.,*** lol., merc-c., nat-m., ***nux-v., olnd., op., ox-ac.,*** oxyt., **PHOS.,** ***phys., phys.,*** pic-ac., plat., **PLB.,** ***plb-a., plb-i.,*** plect., ***rhus-t.,*** sec., stann., staph., stry-f-c., sulph., tab., ***thal.,*** verat., xan., zinc., zinc-p.

alcohol, after abuse of - ant-t., ***ars.,*** calc., ***lach.,*** nat-s., ***nux-v.,*** **OP.,** ran-b., sep., ***sulph.***

agitans, (see Parkinson's Disease)

anger, after - nat-m., ***nux-v.,*** staph.

one-sided - staph.

arsenic, from - ***chin.,*** ferr., graph., ***hep., nux-v.***

ascending, spinal - alum., ars., bar-ac., ***con.,*** gels., lath., led., mang., ***ox-ac., phos.,*** pic-ac., sec., vip.

atrophy, with - cupr., **GRAPH.,** ***kali-p., plb., sec., sep.***

change of weather from warm to cold-wet - ***caust., dulc.,*** rhus-t.

childbirth, after - **PHOS., RHUS-T.**

cold, bathing amel. - caust., con.

taking, after - dulc., rhod.

wind or draft, after - caust.

contractions of limbs, with - chen-a.

convulsions, followed by - tarent-c.

convulsions, side, of other - hell., stram.

cramps, after - tab.

descending - ***bar-c.,*** merc., zinc.

diptheria, after - ant-t., apis, arg-m., ***arg-n.,*** arn., ***ars.,*** aur-m., aven., ***bar-c.,*** camph., carb-ac., ***caust.,*** **COCC.,** ***con., crot-h., diph., gels.,*** helon., ***hyos.,*** kali-br., kali-i., kali-p., ***lac-c., lach., nat-m.,*** nux-v., ***phos., phys.,*** phyt., ***plb.,*** plb-a., rhod., ***rhus-t.,*** sec., sil., sulph., thuj., zinc.

PARALYSIS, general

diphtheritic - arg-n., caust., ***cocc.,*** diph., gels., lac-c., ***lach., rhus-t.***

elderly people, of - ***bar-c., con., kali-c.,*** **OP.**

emission agg. - mag-aust.

emotions, after strong - ***apis,*** gels., **IGN.,** lach., nat-m., nux-v., stann., stram.

epilepsy, after - cur., ***hyos.***

extends, from above downwards - ***bar-c.,*** merc.

upwards - alum., ***ars.,*** bar-ac., bar-c., ***con.,*** gels., hydr-ac., lath., led., lyss., mang., ***ox-ac.,*** pic-ac., sec.

flaccid - plb.

formication, with - cadm-s., phos., sec.

fright, as if, from - nat-m.

gradually, appearing - **CAUST., CON.,** syph.

hemiplegia - acon., ***alum., anac., apis,*** arg-n., ***ars.,*** bapt., bar-m., ***both., cadm-s.,*** **CAUST.,** ***cocc.,*** coc-c., cop., elaps, ***graph.,*** hyos., ***kali-c., kali-i.,*** kali-p., ***lach., mur-ac.,*** nat-c., ***ph-ac., phos.,*** plb., **RHUS-T.,** ***sars., stann.,*** staph., stront-c., ***sul-ac.,*** tab., thuj.

anger, after - staph.

left - acon., anac., **APIS,** arg-n., arn., ***bapt.,*** bar-m., bell., brom., caust., ***elaps,*** **LACH.,** lyc., nit-ac., **NUX-V.,** ox-ac., petr., podo., **RHUS-T.,** ***stann.,*** stram., sulph.

mental excitement - stann.

shock, after - apis.

onanism - stann.

one side, numbness, the other - cocc.

pain, caused by - nat-m.

right - ***apis,*** arn., bell., calc., **CAUST.,** colch., **CROT-C.,** ***crot-h.,*** elaps, ***graph.,*** nat-c., op., phos., ***plb., rhus-t.,*** sang., sil., stront-c., sulph.

spasms, after - stann.

twitching of one side, the other is paralyzed - ***apis,*** art-v., ***bell., stram.***

hemorrhage, with - plb.

hyperesthesia of other side - plb.

hysterical - acon., arg-n., asaf., cocc., ***ign.,*** phos., ***tarent.***

infantile paralysis - ***acon., aeth.,*** bung., ***caust.,*** chr-s., ***gels.,*** kali-p., lath., nux-v., phos., ***plb.,*** rhus-t., sec., sulph., vip.

dentition, during - kali-p.

paresis, after - olnd.

infectious diseases, after - caust., gels.

insane, in - ant-c., ars., aur., ***bell.,*** caust., crot-h., hyos., kali-br., kali-i., merc-c., nat-i., nux-v., op., ***phos.,*** phys., plb., stram., sulph., verat.

intermittent fever, after - arn., ***ars., lach.,*** **NAT-M.,** ***nux-v.***

internally - ***acon.,*** ant-c., arg-n., ***ars.,*** bar-c., **BELL.,** calc., cann-s., canth., caps., caust., chin., cic., ***cocc.,*** coloc., ***con.,*** cycl., dig., **DULC.,** euphr., ***gels.,*** graph., helo., **HYOS.,** ip., kali-c., lach., ***laur.,*** lyc., meny., merc., mur-ac., nat-m., ***nux-m., nux-v., op.,*** petr., phos., plb., ***puls.,*** ran-b., rheum, ***rhus-t.,*** sec., sel., seneg., sep., sil., spig., **STRAM.,**

PARALYSIS, general

internally - sulph., tab., tarent., zinc.

laundry's ascending paralysis - aconin., con., lyss.

lead-poisoning, from - alum., ***alumn., ars.,*** cupr., kali-i., nux-v., ***op.,*** pipe., ***plat., plb., sul-ac.***

legs, (see Legs, chapter)

lower half of body, of - alum-p., alum-sil., ars., graph.

lying on a moist ground - rhus-t.

masturbation, agg. from - ***chin.,*** stann.

mental shock, from - apis, caust.

mercury, from - **HEP.,** ***nit-ac.,*** staph., stram., ***sulph.***

moistness, with - stann.

motion, with disorderly - merc.

motor nerves, in - cur., ***gels., ox-ac., phos., phys.,*** xan.

muscles, of, extensor - alum., ars., calc., ***cocc., crot-h.,*** cur., **PLB.**

flexor - caust., mez., ***nat-m.***

isolated - cupr.

nettle rash, after disappearence of - cop.

neuragials, with - abrot.

nicotine, from abuse of - calad., nux-v.

numbness, with - sec.

of other side - cocc.

one-sided - acon., acon-c., adren., agar., ***alum., alum-p.,*** alumn., am-m., ambr., ***anac., apis,*** arg-m., arg-n., arn., ars., ars-s-f., asar., ***aur.,*** bapt., bar-c., bar-m., ***bar-s., bell., both.,*** bov., bufo, cadm-s., caj., calc., carb-o., carb-s., carb-v., **CAUST.,** chel., chen-a., chin., chin-s., cob-n., ***cocc., coc-c.,*** colch., coni., cop., cur., cycl., dig., dulc., ***elaps, graph.,*** guai., hell., hep., ***hydr-ac.,*** hyos., ign., irid., ***kali-c., kali-i.,*** kali-m., kali-p., ***lach.,*** laur., led., lyc., mag-aust., merc., mez., ***mur-ac.,*** nat-c., nat-m., nit-ac., nux-v., olnd., ***op.,*** ox-ac., perh., petr., ***ph-ac., phos.,*** phys., pic-ac., plb., podo., rhod., ***rhus-t.,*** sabin., ***sars., sec.,*** sep., spig., stann., staph., ***stram.,*** stront-c., stry., ***sul-ac.,*** syph., tarax., thuj., verat-v., vip., xan., zinc., zinc-p.

anger, after - staph.

aphasia, with - cench.

coldness of the paralyzed part with - ars., ***caust.,*** cocc., ***dulc.,*** graph., nux-v., plb., rhus-t., zinc.

convulsions, after - ***hyos.***

convulsions, paralyzed side, of - ***phos.,*** sec.

convulsions, well side, of the - apis, ***art-v.,*** bell., hell., ***stram.***

headache, after - ars.

heat in the paralyzed part - alum., phos.

here and there, now - bell.

hyperesthesia of the well side - plb.

involuntary motion of the paralyzed limb - arg-n., merc., phos.

PARALYSIS, general

one-sided,

left - acon., ***all-c.,*** ambr., ***anac., apis,*** arg-n., ***arn.,*** ars., art-v., bapt., ***bar-m.,*** bell., brom., cocc., cupr-ac., cupr-ar., elaps, gels., hydr-ac., lacer., **LACH.,** lyc., ***nit-ac.,*** **NUX-V.,** op., ox-ac., petr., phys., ***plb.,*** podo., **RHUS-T.,** sant., stann., ***stram.,*** stront-c., stroph., sulph., verat-v., vip., xan.

mental excitement - stann.

numbness of the paralyzed side, with - ***apis,*** cann-i., ***caust., coc-c., rhus-t.,*** staph.

numbness of the paralyzed side, with, well side, of - cocc.

onanism - stann.

one side, numbness, the other - cocc.

pain, caused by - nat-m.

right - acon., apis, ***arn., bell.,*** both., bufo, ***calc., canth.,*** carb-s., **CAUST.,** ***chel.,*** chen-a., colch., crot-h., cur., ***elaps, graph.,*** irid., ir-fl., ir-foe., kali-i., merc-i-r., ***nat-c.,*** nat-m., ***op.,*** plb., ***rhus-t.,*** sil., stront-c., sulph., thuj., vip.

right, aphasia, with - canth., chen-a.

shock, after - apis

spasms, after - stann.

of the other side, with - bell., lach., phos.

stroke, after - acon., ***alum.,*** anac., apis, arn., ars., ***bar-c.,*** bell., both., bufo, cadm-s., caj., calc-f., calen., ***caust., cocc.,*** con., ***crot-c., crot-h.,*** crot-t., ***cupr.,*** form., ***gels.,*** glon., ***hyos.,*** kali-br., lach., laur., merc., nux-v., **OP., PHOS.,** ***plb.,*** sec., sep., stann., stram., ***stront-c.,*** sulph., verat-v., ***vip.,*** zinc.

suppression of eruption - ***caust.,*** hep.

twitching of one side, the other is paralyzed - ***apis,*** art-v., ***bell., stram.***

organs, of - absin., ***acon.,*** agar., agn., alum., ambr., am-c., am-m., ***anac.,*** ant-c., ant-t., arn., ars., asaf., asar., aur., ***bar-c.,*** **BELL.,** bism., bor., bov., ***bry., calc.,*** camph., cann-s., canth., ***caps.,*** carb-ac., carb-an., carb-s., carb-v., **CAUST.,** cham., chel., chin., cic., ***cocc.,*** colch., coloc., con., croc., cupr., cycl., dig., dros., **DULC.,** euphr., gels., graph., hell., hep., hydr-ac., **HYOS.,** ign., iod., ip., kali-br., kali-c., kreos., lach., laur., led., ***lyc.,*** mag-c., mag-m., mang., meny., merc., mez., mur-ac., nat-c., nat-m., ***nit-ac.,*** nux-m., nux-v., ***olnd., op.,*** par., ***petr.,*** ph-ac., ***phos., plb.,*** **PULS.,** rheum, rhod., ***rhus-t., ruta,*** sabad., sabin., sars., **SEC.,** seneg., ***sep.,*** **SIL.,** spig., spong., squil., stann., staph., ***stram.,*** stront-c., ***sulph., sul-ac.,*** thuj., ***verat.,*** verb., zinc.

pain, from - nat-m.

painful - ***agar.,*** alum-sil., ***ant-t.,*** arn., ***ars.,*** bell., cact., cadm-s., calc., carb-v., **CAUST.,** chin., cina, ***cocc.,*** colch., con., crot-t., dulc., ***gels.,*** hell., helo., hyos., ***kali-n.,*** kali-p., ***lach., lat-m.,*** lath., lyc., mang., **NUX-V.,** ***op., phos.,*** phys., **PLB., RHUS-T.,** sang., sec., sil., staph., sulph., thal., verb., **ZINC.,** zinc-p.

PARALYSIS, general

painless - absin., acon., aeth., alum., alum-p., ambr., ***anac.,*** ang., ***arg-n.,*** arn., ***ars.,*** ars-s-f., ***aur.,*** aur-a., aur-s., ***bapt., bar-c.,*** bell., bov., ***bufo,*** bry., cadm-s., calc., camph., **CANN-I.,** cann-s., ***carb-s.,*** carb-v., ***caust.,*** cham., chel., chin., chin-s., chlor., cic., **COCC.,** colch., coloc., **CON.,** crot-h., ***cupr., cur.,*** ferr., **GELS.,** graph., hell., hydr-ac., ***hyos.,*** ign., ip., kali-c., kalm., laur., led., **LYC.,** mag-arct., ***merc.,*** nat-m., nux-m., nux-v., **OLND.,** ***op.,*** ph-ac., phos., **PLB.,** ***puls.,*** rhod., **RHUS-T.,** ***sec.,*** sil., staph., stram., stront-c., sulph., ***verat.,*** zinc., zinc-p.

paraplegia - agar., anh., ***arg-n., ars.,*** bapt., caul., gels., kali-t., kalm., lath., mang., nat-m., **NUX-V.,** phys., pic-ac., pip-m., plb., rhus-t., rhus-v., ruta, sec., stry., sulph., thal., thyr., vip., wild.

atrophy, with - ars.

childbirth, after - caul., caust., plb., rhus-t.

diphtheria, after - ars.

exertion, after - nux-v., rhus-t.

fever, after - rhus-t.

hunger, with - cina

hysterical - cocc., ign., tarent.

progressive - mang.

rigidity of muscles, with - chel.

sensation of - aesc., aur.

sexual excess, after - rhus-t.

spastic - gels., hyper., ***lath.,*** nux-v., sec.

perspiration, from suppressed - ***colch., gels., lach., rhus-t.***

poliomyelitis, (see Nerves, Poliomyelitis)

post-diphteritic, (see diphteria)

pseudo-hypertrophic - cur., ***phos.,*** thyr., verat-v.

rheumatism, after - bar-c., chin., ***ferr., ruta.***

river bath in summer, from - bell-p., ***caust.,*** rhus-t.

sensation of - phos.

senses, of - ***cocaine,*** cyt-l., hell., kali-n., plat.

sex, after - phos.

sexual excesses, from - ***nat-m., nux-v.,*** **PHOS.,** ***rhus-t.,*** sil.

single parts, organs, localized - ***am-t.,*** anac., ***ars.,*** bar-c., bell., **CAUST.,** ***dulc.,*** gels., hyos., nux-v., ***op.,*** phos., plb., puls., sec., sil., sulph.

slowly advancing - caust., ***con.,*** syph.

spasms, after - cocc., cupr., cur., elaps, hyos., ***sec.,*** stann., vib.

spasms, then paralysis - tarent.

spasms, with paralysis - nux-m., plb., zinc.

spastic spinal paralysis - benz-d-n., gels., hyper., kres., lachn., lath., ***nux-v.,*** phos., plect., sec.

sphincters, of - ars., ***caust.,*** gels., naja, nux-v., phos., phys.

spine, from diseased - med.

stroke, after - ***arn., bar-c., bell., caust., cocc., lach.,*** nux-v., op., **PHOS.,** stann., zinc.

PARALYSIS, general

suppressed eruptions - caust., ***dulc.,*** hep., lach., ***psor., sulph.***

suppressed footsweat - colch.

sweat, with - stann.

touch, sensitive to - plb.

toxic - ***apis, ars.,*** bapt., crot-h., gels., lac-c., ***lach.,*** mur-ac., rhus-t.

arsenic - ***chin.,*** ferr., graph., ***hep., nux-v.***

lead - alum., ***alumn., ars.,*** caust., cupr., kali-i., nux-v., ***op.,*** pipe., ***plat.,*** plb., ***sul-ac.***

mercurial - **HEP.,** ***nit-ac.,*** staph., stram., ***sulph.***

tremors, after - plb.

twitching, with - stram.

typhoid-like disease, in - ***agar.,*** caust., ***lach., rhus-t.***

wet, after getting - **CAUST.,** ***rhus-t.***

PARKINSON'S disease - ***agar.,*** ant-t., aran., aran-ix., arg-m., ***arg-n.,*** ars., aur., ***aur-s.,*** aven., bar-c., bufo, ***camph-br.,*** cann-i., chlorpr., cimic., cocaine, cocc., ***con.,*** dub., ***dubo-m., gels.,*** halo., ***helo., hyos., hyosin., kali-br.,*** kres., lath., levo., lil-t., ***lol.,*** lyc., ***mag-p.,*** mang., **MERC.,** merc-sul., nicot., nux-v., perh., ***phos., phys., plb.,*** prun., psil., ***puls.,*** rauw., reser., **RHUS-T.,** scut., stram., syph., tab., ***tarent.,*** thiop., ***thuj.,*** **ZINC.,** ***zinc-pic.***

right side - ***phos., thuj.***

POLIOMYELITIS, infection - ***acon.,*** aeth., alum., arg-n., arn., ars., bell., ***bung., calc.,*** carb-ac., ***caust.,*** chin-a., chr-s., cur., dulc., ferr-i., ferr-p., **GELS.,** hydr-ac., hydroph., hyos., kali-i., kali-p., karw-h., kres., lach., **LATH.,** merc., nux-v., phos., phys., ***plb.,*** plb-i., ***rhus-t.,*** sec., stry-p., sulph., verat., verat-v.

neuralgic pains, after - rhus-t.

paralysis of diaphragm, with - cupr., op., sil.

REFLEXES, general

diminished - ***alum.,*** arg-n., cur., kali-br., oena., op., oxyt., phys., plb., ***sec.***

increased - anh., bar-c., cann-i., cic., cocc., lath., mang., morph., nux-v., stry.

lost - alum., morph., nat-br., sulfon.

SENSES, (see Brain, chapter)

SHOCKS, electric-like - ***acon., agar.,*** ail., alum., ***ambr.,*** anac., ang., apis, **ARG-M.,** ***arg-n.,*** arn., **ARS.,** ***art-v.,*** bar-c., ***bar-m.,*** bell., bufo, calad., calc., ***calc-p., camph.,*** cann-s., carb-ac., carb-v., caust., ***cic.,*** cimic., ***cina, clem., cocc.,*** colch., con., croc., cupr., ***dig.,*** dulc., ***fl-ac.,*** graph., hell., hep., kali-c., kreos., ***laur., lyc.,*** mag-m., manc., mang., mez., mur-ac., nat-a., nat-c., ***nat-m.,*** nat-p., ***nit-ac., nux-m., nux-v.,*** ol-an., olnd., ***phos.,*** plat., puls., ***ran-b., ruta.,*** sep., spig., squil., stram., ***stry.,*** sulph., sul-ac., sumb., ***tab., thal.,*** **VERAT.,** xan., zinc.

concussion of brain, from - **CIC.**

convulsions, before - ***bar-m., laur.***

interrupted by painful shocks - stry.

epilepsy, before - ars.

SHOCKS, electric-like
evening in bed - sulph.
lying, while - ***clem.***
morning - mang.
motion or rest, during - graph.
move, on beginning to - ***arg-n.***
return of the senses, on - cic.
right side of body - agar.
sleep, during - **ARG-M.,** ***ars.,*** kreos., lyc., mez., ***nat-m., nux-m.***
on going to - agar., alum., **ARG-M., ARS.,** ***bell.,*** calc., ***ip.,*** kali-c., nat-a., ***nat-m., nit-ac., phos., stry.,*** thuj.
slow pulse, with - ***dig.***
touching anything - alum.
waking, while - lyc., ***mag-m.,*** manc.
wide awake, while - mag-m., nat-p.

SHUDDERING, nervous - acon., anac., ***am-m.,*** **ARN.,** asar., aur., ***bell.,*** benz-ac., calc., camph., cann-s., caust., chin., cic., cimic., cina, ***cocc.,*** cupr., ***gels.,*** hyos., kreos., laur., ***led.,*** lyc., mag-m., mang., ***merc., mez., nat-m.,*** nux-m., **NUX-V.,** ph-ac., phos., ***puls., rhus-t.,*** seneg., sep., ***sil., spig.,*** staph., valer., verat., viol-t.
air, cold, in - cham.
belching, with - ip.
bruised, if - spig.
eating, while - lyc.
after - lyc., rhus-t., sulph.
emptiness in stomach, after - phos.
epileptic convulsions, before - cupr.
headache, from - bor., sars.
imaginations, at - phos.
menses, before - sep.
nausea, with - mag-c., stann.
pains, with - sep., sil.
with, umbilical - chin., ip.
part touched - ***spig.***
starting, with - sulph.
stool, during - alum., ***bell.,*** calad., cast., con., ind., kalic., mag-m., nat-c., nit-ac., plat., stann., spig., verat.
after - mez.
thinking of disagreeable things - ben-ac., phos.
twitching of legs, after - con.
vomiting, with - sulph.
waterbrash, with - sil.
wine, drinking - cina.
yawning, when - arn., ***cina,*** hydr., ip., laur., mag-m., nux-v., olnd., sars.

SUPPRESSED, discharge, nervous illness after - **ASAR.,** ***zinc.***

TETANUS, lockjaw, (see Emergency)

TREMBLING, general - abrot., absin., acet-ac., ***acon.,*** acon-f., ***agar.,*** agn., alum., alumn., **AMBR.,** am-c., am-m., aml-n., ***anac.,*** ant-c., **ANT-T.,** ***apis,*** aran., ***arg-m.,*** **ARG-N.,** ***arn.,*** **ARS.,** ars-i., asaf., ***aur.,*** bar-c., bar-m., ***bell.,*** bism., ***bor.,*** bov., brom., ***bry.,*** bufo, cadm-s., ***calad., calc., calc-p., camph.,*** cann-s., canth., caps., ***carb-ac., carb-s.,*** carb-v., ***caust., cedr.,*** cham., ***chel.,*** chin., ***chin-a., chin-s.,*** **CIC., CIMIC.,** ***cina,*** clem., **COCC.,** cod., ***coff., colch.,***

TREMBLING, general - coloc., **CON.,** croc., **CROT-C.,** ***crot-h.,*** crot-t., ***cupr.,*** cur., dig., dios., dros., ***dulc.,*** euphr., ***ferr.,*** ferr-ar., ferr-p., **GELS.,** glon., ***graph.,*** helo., hep., ***hyos., ign., iod., kali-br., kali-c., kali-fer.,*** kali-n., kali-s., ***kalm.,*** kreos., lac-ac., **LACH.,** laur., ***lec., led.,*** lyc., ***lyss.,*** mag-c., mag-m., mag-p., mag-s., mang., ***med.,*** meny., meph., **MERC.,** ***merc-c., mez., mosch.,*** mygal., **NAT-A.,** nat-c., ***nat-m., nat-s., nit-ac.,*** nux-m., ***nux-v., olnd.,*** onos., **OP.,** ox-ac., pall., par., petr., ***ph-ac., phos., phyt., pic-ac.,*** plan., **PLAT.,** ***plb.,*** polyg., ***psor.,*** **PULS.,** ran-b., ran-s., rheum, rhod., **RHUS-T.,** ruta., ***sabad.,*** sabin., samb., sars., ***sec., seneg., sep., sil.,*** spig., spong., ***stann.,*** staph., **STRAM.,** stront-c., ***stry.,*** **SULPH.,** sul-ac., sumb., ***tab., tarent.,*** teucr., thea., **THER.,** ***thuj.,*** valer., ***verat.,*** verb., viol-o., ***visc.,*** **ZINC.**
afternoon - carb-v., ***gels.,*** lyc., lyss., pic- ac.
air, open - calc., kali-c., laur., ***plat.***
amel - clem.
anger, from - acon., ambr., arg-n., ***aur.,*** chel., cop., daph., lyc., merc., ***nit-ac.,*** pall., phos., ran-b., sep., **STAPH.,** ***zinc.***
with anger - petr.
anxiety, from - **ARG-N.,** ars., ambr., aur., bell., bor., ***calc.,*** canth., carb-v., caust., ***cham.,*** chel., ***coff., con.,*** croc., cupr., euph., **GELS.,** graph., ***lach.,*** lyc., mag-c., mez., mosch., ***nat-c.,*** nit-ac., nux-m., phos., ***plat.,*** psor., ***puls., rhus-t.,*** samb., sars., sep., sulph., valer.
anxiety, with - agar., petr.
ascending, on - merc.
breakfast, after - arg- n.
amel - ***calc., con.,*** nat-m., nux-v., staph.
caressing, while - caps.
chill, during - ang., anac., ars., bry., chin., chin-s., cina, **COCC.,** con., eup-per., ferr., **GELS.,** merc., ***par.,*** petr., plat., sabad., sul-ac., zinc.
cold drinks, amel - phos.
coldness, during - bor.
company, agg - ***ambr.,*** lyc.
conversation, from - ***ambr.,*** bor.
convulsive - acon., asaf., carb-h., crot-h., op.
coughing, from - am-c., bell., ***cupr., phos.,*** seneg.
dinner, during - mag- m.
drinking, excessive, after - plb.
eating, after - alum., ant-c., lyc.
emotions, after - arg-n., **COCC.,** ferr., hep., merc., nat-c., nat-m., ***plb., psor.,*** **STAPH.,** stram., ***zinc.***
evening - chel., lyc., mez., mygal., nat-m., nit-ac., pic-ac., plb., stront-c., sulph.
bed, in - eupi., lyc., nux-v., samb.
sleep, after - carb-v.
walking, after - ***sil.***
exertion, after - ***merc.,*** nat-m., ***phos.,*** **RHUS-T.,** sec.

TREMBLING, general
exertion, on slight - bor., ***cocc.,*** ferr., ***merc.,*** phos., ***plat., plb.,*** polyg., ***rhus-t.,*** sec., ***stann., zinc.***
fatigue, after - gels., plb.
fever, during - ars., calc., camph., cist., eup-per., kali-c., lach., mag-c., mygal., sep.
forenoon - ars., carb-o., lyc., nat-m., ***plat.,*** sars.
exertion, on - gels.
fright, from - arg-n., ***aur., coff.,*** glon., hura, ign., mag-c., merc., nicc., ***op.,*** puls., rat., rhus-t., sep.
frightened, as if - gels., **OP.,** paeon., tarent.
headache with chill, during - carb-v.
hungry, when - ***alum., crot-h.,*** iod., olnd., phos., stann., ***sulph., zinc.***
internally - ambr., ***ant-t., arg-n.,*** asaf., bell., ***brach.,*** bry., calad., **CALC.,** ***camph.,*** caps., carb-s., carb-v., ***caul., caust.,*** cina, ***clem.,*** cocc., colch., ***con., crot-h.,*** cycl., ***eup-per.,*** **GRAPH.,** hep., **IOD.,** ***kali-c., kali-n.,*** kreos., ***lec.,*** lil-t., ***lyc.,*** meph., merc., mosch., nat-a., ***nat-c., nat-m.,*** nit-ac., nux-m., ***nux-v.,*** par., petr., ***phos., plat., puls.,*** **RHUS-T.,** ruta., ***sabad.,*** sabin., samb., ***seneg., sep.,*** sil., ***spig.,*** **STANN., STAPH.,** ***stront-c., sulph.,*** **SUL-AC.,** ***teucr.,*** valer., zinc.
night - nat-m., plat.
standing, while - merc.
joy, from - acon., aur., coff., merc., valer.
looking down, on - kali- c.
lying, while - clem.
meeting friends - tarent.
menses, during - arg-n., calc-p., ***graph., hyos., lec.,*** merl., ***nit-ac.***
after - ***chin.***
before - alum.
mental exertion, from - aur., ***bor.,*** plb., vinc.
morning - alumn., ***arg-m., arg-n.,*** ars., bar-c., calc., cimic., ***con., dulc.,*** graph., lyc., mag-c., nat-m., ***nux-v.,*** petr., phos., sil., sulph.
breakfast, before - ***calc., con.,*** nat-m., nux-v., staph.
rising from bed - petr.
amel. - mag-c.
waking, on - ***arg-m.,*** calc., caust., ***dulc.,*** hyper., mag-c., nit-ac., phos., tarent.
motion, on - anac., arg-n., iod., phyt., sulph., zinc.
amel - merc., plat.
music - **AMBR.**
night - ***bell.,*** hyos., lyc., phos.
3 a.m - ***rhus-t.***
dreaming, after - phos., sil.
half awake while - sulph.
sleep, after - ***sil.***
noise, from - bar-c., caust., ***cocc.,*** hura, ***kali-ar.,*** mosch., tab.
noon, after sleep - nat- m.
nursing infant, after - ***olnd.***
pains, with the - ***cocc.,*** **NAT-C.,** ***plat.,*** puls.

TREMBLING, general
paroxysmal - lyc., ***merc.***
periodical - **ARG-N.**
perspiration, with - ars.
playing the piano, while - nat- c.
rising from sitting, affected parts - **CAUST.**
side lain on - clem.
sleep, during - con., kali-c.
before - nat-m., sep.
startled from - petr.
smoking, from -aven., ***hep.,*** nat-m., sil., sulph.
something is to be done, when - **KALI-BR.**
stitching in ear, from - thuj.
stool, during - carb- s.
after - ars., carb-v., caust., **CON.,** lil- t.
before - hydr., merc., sumb.
supper, after - alum., caust.
thunderstorm - agar., ***morph.,*** nat-p., ***phos.***
touch, unexpected - ***cocc.***
urination, after - ars.
vexation, from - acon., ***aur.,*** lyc., nit-ac., petr., ran-b.
voluptuous - calc.
waking, on - abrot., calc., ***cina,*** lach., ***merc.,*** nit-ac., rat., samb., tarent.
walking, while - am-c., lact., merc., nux-v.
after - cupr., ust.
wine - ***con.***
writing, while - ***phos., sil.***

VERTIGO, (see Vertigo, chapter)

WEAKNESS, nervous - acon., aesc., ***agar., agn., alet., alum.,*** alum-p., alumn., am-c., am-m., ambr., ***anac.,*** ang., ***aran., arg-n.,*** arn., ars., asaf., ***asar.,*** aur., ***aven., bar-c.,*** bar-i., ***bell.,*** bry., ***calc.,*** calc-p., calc-sil., calen., camph., carb-an., carb-v., carb-s., cast., caust., cham., **CHIN.,** chin-a., chin-s., cic., ***cimic.,*** **COCA, COCC.,** ***coff.,*** colch., ***con.,*** croc., ***cupr.,*** cur., cycl., cypr., dig., dios., ***fl-ac., form.,*** **GELS.,** graph., ***guai.,*** hedeo, ***helon.,*** hell., hep., hydr-ac., hydrc., hyos., ***ign., iod.,*** kali-br., kali-n., **KALI-P.,** lac-c., lach., lact., laur., **LEC.,** led., ***lil-t.,*** lyc., mag-m., meph., ***merc.,*** mosch., mur-ac., **NAT-C.,** nat-m., **NAT-P.,** nat-s., **NAT-SIL., NIT-AC.,** nux-m., **NUX-V.,** op., petr., **PH-AC., PHOS.,** phys., **PIC-AC.,** pip-m., ***plat., plb.,*** **PULS.,** rhus-t., sabin., sars., scroph-n., sec., **SEL., SEP., SEP., SIL.,** spig., spong., squil., **STANN., STAPH.,** stram., stry-n., stry-p., sul-ac., ***sulph.,*** sumb., tab., ***tarent., teucr., ther.,*** tub., ***valer.,*** verat., vib., ***viol-o.,*** xan., zinc., zinc-m., **ZINC-P.,** ***zinc-pic.***
afternoon - cimic.
walk, after a - petr.

Nose

ABSCESS - ***calc.,*** **HEP.,** ***lac-c.,*** lach., ***merc.,*** **SIL.,** still.
root, at - ***puls.***
septum, at - acon, ***bell.,*** calc., ***hep.,*** sil.
tip, at - acon., am-c., anan.

ACHING, pain - asar., cimic., ***elaps,*** merc-i-f.
above root of nose - ***acon.,*** agar., am-m., ant-t., arn., ***ars., ars-i.,*** aster., ***bapt.,*** bar-c., ***bell., bism.,*** bor., brom., ***calc.,*** calc-p., camph., canth., ***caps.,*** chel., coc-c., coloc., **CUPR.,** dig., dulc., ferr., ***glon.,*** guai., ham., ***hep., ign.,*** kali-bi., ***kali-c.,*** kali-chl., **KALI-I.,** kreos., ***lach.,*** merc., ***merc-i-f.,*** mosch., nux-v., plat., ***prun.,*** puls., raph., ***rhus-v.,*** **STAPH.,** stict., ***ther.,*** viol-t., xan.
evening - ferr.
left half - mur-ac.
menses, during - arn., hep., ***ign.,*** kali-bi., ***lach.***
night - rhus-v.
pulsating - **ARS.**
bones - bell., cast-eq., cycl., mosch., sulph.
dorsum - agn., canth.
morning - canth.
root - agn., asar., bapt., chin., hell., ***hep., kali-bi.,*** nat-a., puls., sang., sulph.
at root begins and extends gradually over the head, with delirium and vomiting - cimic.

ACNE - am-c., ars., ***ars-br.,*** aster., bor., calc-p., caps., cann-s., **CAUST.,** clem., elaps, graph., kali-br., nat-c., sel., ***sep.,*** sil., ***sulph., thuj.,*** zing.

ADENOID, growth, (see Throat, Adenoids) - ***agra.,*** bar-c., ***calc-f., calc-i., calc-p.,*** chr-ac., iod., kali-s., lob-s., mez., psor., sang-n., sulph., thuj., tub.

AGGLUTINATION, of nostrils - **AUR.,** bar-c., carb-an., lyc., phos.
morning - lyc.
sensation of - phos.

AIR, as if, a light current passing over the dorsum - spig.
too much, passed into nose and mouth, as if - ther.
air, sensitive to cold - ant-c., camph., cimic., cor-r., dulc., fago., hep., ***ign.,*** kali-bi., kali-i., ox-ac., phos., rumx., stict.
inhaled, to - acon., ***aesc.,*** am-c., ***ant-c.,*** ars., aur., brach., brom., bufo, camph., ***cimic.,*** cist., cor-r., echi., fago., gins., ***hep.,*** hydr., ***ign.,*** kali-bi., kali-i., kreos., lith., mag-s., med., nat-a., nux-v., osm., ox-ac., phos., psor., ***ran-b.,*** rumx., sep., syph., thuj.
frontal sinus - zinc.
post nasal - kreos.

ALLERGIC rhinitis, (see Hay fever) - **ALL-C., ARS.,** ars-i., carb-v., **EUPHR.,** iod., kali-i., ***nat-m.,*** **NUX-V.,** puls., ***sabad.,*** sang., sil., wye.

BITING, pain - ambr., ang., arn., ***aur.,*** bar-m., berb., bry., calc-p., ***carb-v.,*** chin., euph., grat., hell., hep., kali-c., kali-n., lach., lyc., mez., plat., ran-s., ***sabad.,*** spig., teucr., thuj.
left nostril, in evening - chin.
septum - asar.
skin, on - ***mez.***
suffocative - euph.
wings, on - aphis.

BLOOD, congestion of, to the - alum., am-c., calc., **CUPR.,** hep., osm., samb., sulph.
on stooping - am-c.

BLOW, the, compelled to, in the evening - lith.
compelled to, in the evening, sensation of a large body in nose - am-m., **TEUCR.**
constant inclination to - agar., am-c., ***am-m.,*** bar-c., ***bor.,*** bov., calc., carb-an., echi., hep., ***hydr., kali-bi.,*** lac-c., lyc., mag-c., mag-m., mang., nat-m., phos., psor., **STICT.,** ***sulph.,*** **TEUCR.,** ther., tritic.
relief, but no - ***kali-bi.,*** lach., psor., ***stict., teucr.***
inability in children - am-c., aur., bar-c.

BOILS - acon., alum., am-c., anan., cadm-s., carb-an., con., ***hep.,*** mag-m., phos., sars., sil.
as from a - hep.
inside - alum., am-c., carb-an., sep., sil., ***tub.***
tip - acon., am-c., anan., apis, bor., carb-an.

BORING, pain - asaf., **AUR.,** bism., brom., ***kali-i.,*** merc-i-r., nat-m., ruta, spig., sulph.
bones - **AUR.,** aur-m-n., led., mez., nat-m., phos.
extending, to forehead - ***kali-i.***
extending, to root of nose - ***coloc.***
night - phos.
night - **AUR.,** phos.
right side - camph., psor., spig.
root - agar., bism., ***hep.,*** nat-m., phos., sulph.
morning - ***hep.***
7 to 12 a.m. - hep.

BORING, in nose, with fingers - anac., **ARUM-T.,** aur., bufo, carb-v., caust., **CINA,** con., hep., lyc., merc., nat-c., ***nat-m.,*** nat-p., ***ph-ac.,*** phos., psor., sabad., sel., **SIL.,** spig., stict., sulph., teucr., thuj., verat., ***zinc.***
brain symptoms, with - cina, sulph.

BUBBLING, sensation - sars., sulph.

BURNING, pain - ***aesc.,*** aeth., ***agar., all-c.,*** aloe, alum., ambr., ***am-c.,*** anan., ang., ant-c., apis, aphis., ***arg-m., arg-n.,*** **ARS.,** ***arund.,*** aur., aur-m., bar-c., ***bell.,*** berb., bor., bov., brach., bufo, calad., ***canth.,*** caps., ***carb-an., carb-v.,*** card-m., ***caust.,*** chel., chlor., cimic., cina, ***cist.,*** clem., coc-c., ***coloc., con.,*** cop., crot-c., ***crot-t.,*** gamb., ***gels.,*** gran., grat., ***hep., hydr.,*** kali-ar., ***kali-bi., kali-c.,*** **KALI-I.,** ***kali-n.,*** kali-p., kali-s., led., lyc., ***mag-m., med., merc-c.,*** merl., ***mez.,*** nat-a., ***nat-m., nat-s.,*** nicc., ***nit-ac.,*** ol-an., pall., petr., phel., ph-ac., ***phos.,*** phys., plat., psor., rat., sabad., sars., senec., ***seneg.,*** stann., **SIL.,** sin-n., stry., ***sulph.,*** syph., tab.
air, open - kali-c.
around, nose - phos.

BURNING, pain
blowing, on - carb-v., graph., kali-n., sars.
after blowing out thick mucus - aesc., ant-c., cist., nat-a., ***nit-ac.***
bones - **KALI-I.,** kali-n., ***mez.,*** nat-m., phos.
cold air - bufo, cist.
coryza, during - ***aesc., all-c.,*** aloe, ***am-c.,*** **ARS.,** calad., ***caust., gels.,*** mez., ***senec., seneg., sulph.***
dorsum - bar-c., coloc.
drop of hot grease, like a - bar-c.
edge of wings - sulph.
evening - pall.
inhaling on - mag-m., med.
cool air - aesc.
left - caps., cina, cist., coff., ***gels.,*** grat., kali-c., ***sep.***
margins - arn., chel., sulph., thuj.
menses, during, agg - carb-an.
morning - mag-m.
narina - caps., caust., con., kali-c., mag-m., med.
nosebleeds, with - hydr., led.
pepper, as from - calad., ***seneg.***
post nasal - ***aesc.,*** arg-n., ***cist.,*** crot-t., ***kali-bi., merc-i-r.,*** phos.
left, like scalding water - ***gels.***
right - card-m., crot-t., hydr., kali-bi., kali-n.
root, inside - carb-s., ***kali-bi.,*** nat-m.
extending to ear - elaps.
left side - kali-c.
right side - lachn.
septum - aphis., cina, ***kali-bi.,*** mez., sil., ***sulph.***
left - cina.
morning - ***sulph.***
touch, on - sil., staph.
side of nose - aeth., alum., graph., petr., sil.
sinuses - kali-i.
spots - bar-c., graph., iod.
throbbing - kali-i.
tip - bell., bor., caps., ***carb-an.,*** carb-s., nicc., ol-an., ox-ac., rhus-t., sil.
menses, during, agg - ***carb-an.***
touch - kali-n., mag-m., phos.
wings - all-c., aphis., ars., caps., chel., clem., coc-c., kali-c., kali-n., ***nit-ac.,*** sang-n., seneg., sin-a., sulph., syph.
edge of - sulph.
left - hell., sulph.
right - sulph.
right, evening - alum.

BURROWING, pain - coloc., kali-n.
tip - sil.

BURSTING, pain - asaf., bar-c., kali-bi.
right wing, in - asaf.

CANCER - alumn., ***ars.,*** **AUR.,** ***aur-m., calc.,*** carb-ac., ***carb-an.,*** cund., ***kreos.,*** merc., ***phyt., sep.,*** sulph.
epithelioma - ***ars.,*** ars-i., ***carb-ac.,*** cund., ***hydr.,*** **KALI-S.,** ***kreos.***
nose wing - med.
flat, on right side - euphr.
noli me tangere on - cist., jug-c., phyt., thuj.

CATARRH - acet-ac., ***acon.,*** aesc., ***agar.,*** ail., aloe, ***alum., alumn.,*** ambr., am-c., ***am-m., ant-c., ant-s.,*** ant-t., ***apis, arg-m., arg-n.,*** **ARS.,** ***ars-i., asaf.,*** asar., aspar., ***arum-t.,*** **AUR.,** ***aur-m.,*** bapt., ***bar-c., bar-m.,*** **BELL.,** berb., ***bor., bov.,*** **BROM.,** bry., calad., **CALC.,** calc-ar., ***calc-p., calc-s.,*** camph., canth., caps., ***carb-ac., carb-an.,*** **CARB-S., CARB-V.,** ***cast.,*** caust., cham., chel., chin., chin-a., cic., cimic., cina, cinnb., ***cist.,*** clem., cocc., coc-c., coff., colch., coloc., ***con.,*** cop., cor-r., crot-h., crot-t., cupr., cycl., dros., elaps, **EUP-PER.,** euph., ***euphr., ferr., ferr-ar., ferr-i.,*** ferr-p., ***fl-ac., form.,*** gels., **GRAPH.,** guai., hell., **HEP.,** ***hippoz., hydr.,*** ign., ***iod.,*** jal., ***kali-ar.,*** **KALI-BI.,** ***kali-c., kali-chl., kali-i., kali-p.,*** kali-s., kreos., lac-ac., ***lac-c.,*** lac-d., ***lach.,*** laur., lem-m., led., **LYC.,** mag-c., ***mag-m., mang., med.,*** meny., **MERC., MERC-C.,** ***merc-i-f., merc-i-r., mez.,*** mosch., mur-ac., naja, **NAT-A.,** ***nat-c.,*** **NAT-M.,** nat-p., ***nat-s., nicc.,*** **NIT-AC., NUX-V.,** ***nux-m., ol-j., osm.,*** par., **PETR.,** ph-ac., ***phos.,*** plat., plb., **PSOR., PULS.,** ran-b., ran-s., rhod., **RHUS-T.,** ***rumx., sabad., samb., sang., sars.,*** **SEL.,** seneg., **SEP., SIL.,** ***spig.,*** spong., ***squil.,*** stann., staph., ***stict.,*** still., stront-c., **SULPH.,** sul-ac., tab., ***teucr., ther., thuj., tub.,*** uran., ust., verat., zinc.
air, open, amel. - ***aur.,*** bry., carb-v., ***mag-m.,*** **PULS.**
cold, weather - ***ars.***
constant - med.
damp, weather - ***nux-m.***
dry, chronic - ***carb-v., dulc., nat-m.,*** **SIL.,** ***spong.,*** **STICT.,** ***sulph.***
elderly, of old age - ***alum.,*** am-c., bar-c., eup-per., ictod., kali-s., ***kreos.,*** merc-i-f.
evening - mang., ***puls.***
extending to, antrum - berb., kali-c., kali-i., merc., phos., spig.
antrum, left - mez.
chest, to - bry.
frontal sinuses, to - ***ars.,*** berb., bry., ***calc., cupr.,*** ferr., hep., ***hydr.,*** **KALI-BI.,** ***kali-chl., kali-i.,*** kali-m., **LYC.,** med., **MERC.,** merc-i-f., ***nat-m.,*** nat-s., ***nux-v., puls., sang.,*** **SIL.,** stict., **THUJ.,** verb.
left - kali-s., lach., sep., teucr.
measles, scarlatina and variola, after - ***thuj.***
mercury, after - asaf., kali-chl.
morning - ***ferr-i.***
nosebleeds, with - ip., kali-bi.
one-sided - hippoz., kali-c., nat-c., phos., phyt.
retrocession, of eruptions, from - ***sep.***
right - ***lyc.***
seaside, agg - nat-m.
silver, nitrate, abuse of - ***nat-m.***

catarrh, sinuses, of - ***ars.,*** berb., bry., ***calc., cupr.,*** ferr., hep., ***hydr.,*** **KALI-BI.,** ***kali-chl., kali-i.,*** kali-m., **LYC.,** med., **MERC.,** merc-i-f., ***nat-m.,*** nat-s., ***nux-v., puls., sang.,*** **SIL.,** stict., **THUJ.,** verb.
left - kali-s., lach., sep., teucr.

catarrh, post-nasal - acon., aesc., ***alum.,*** alumn., ant-s., ***arg-n., aur.,*** aur-m., bar-c., bry., ***calc., calc-s., canth.,*** caust., cinnb., ***cor-r.,*** euphr., ***ferr.,*** **FERR-P., HEP., HYDR.,** ***iod.,*** **KALI-BI.,** ***kali-c., kali-chl., kali-i.,*** kreos., lith., ***lyc.,*** mag-s., ***manc., mang.,*** med., ***merc-i-f., merc-i-r., merl., mez.,*** nat-a., **NAT-C., NAT-M.,** nat-s., ***nit-ac.,*** petr., ***phyt.,*** phos., ***plb.,*** **PSOR.,** ***rhus-t.,*** sang., ***sel.,*** **SEP.,** ***sil.,*** spig., staph., ***ther., thuj.,*** zinc.

CHAPPED - arum-t., carb-an.
nostril - aur., graph.

CLAWING, pain - arg-n., kali-n.

COLDNESS - aloe, anan., apis, arn., ***ars.,*** ars-h., bell., brom., calc-p., **CAMPH.,** cann-i., ***carb-s.,*** **CARB-V.,** ***chin.,*** cist., cocc., colch., ***crot-h.,*** cycl., dros., ictod., ***ign.,*** iod., **LAC-C.,** laur., mang., murx., ***nux-v.,*** op., ph-ac., ***plb.,*** polyg-p., ***puls.,*** sep., ***sil., spong.,*** stram., sulph., tab., tarax., **VERAT.,** verat-v., zinc.
chill, during - apis, ant-c., bol., cedr., chel., colch., iod., meny., sil., sulph., ***tarax.***
icy - ***cedr., verat.***
inside, blowing, after - ***cist.***
inhaling, when - ***aesc.,*** anan., ***ant-c., ars.,*** brom., camph., cimic., ***cist.,*** **COR-R.,** hipp., ***hydr., kali-bi.,*** lith.
knees, with hot - ign.
root - cinnb.
sores - ars.
tip of - aloe, anac., ant-c., **APIS,** ***arn., ars., calc-p., camph.,*** carb-v., ***cedr., chin.,*** crot-h., hell., kali-c., ***lach.,*** lob., med., meny., polyg-p., ***tab., verat.***
walking in room, while - ***camph.***
wings, both - laur.

COLDS, tendency to take (see Coryza) - **ACON.,** aesc., agar., all-c., **ALUM.,** alum-p., alum-sil., alumn., am-c., am-m., anac., ***ant-c.,*** ant-t., aral., aran., ***arg-n.,*** arn., ***ars., ars-i.,*** ars-s-f., **BAC., BAR-C.,** bar-i., bar-m., bar-s., ***bell.,*** benz-ac., bor., **BRY.,** calad., **CALC.,** calc-i., **CALC-P.,** ***calc-s.,*** calc-sil., ***calen.,*** camph., caps., carb-an., ***carb-s., carb-v.,*** carc., caust., **CHAM.,** chin., chin-a., cimic., cinnb., cist., clem., cocc., coc-c., coff., colch., coloc., ***con.,*** croc., cupr., cycl., dig., dros., **DULC.,** dys-co., elaps, eup-per., euphr., ***ferr.,*** ferr-ar., ferr-i., ferr-p., ***form.,*** gast., ***gels.,*** goss., ***graph.,*** ham., hed., **HEP.,** hyos., hyper., ign., iod., ip., kali-ar., ***kali-bi.,*** **KALI-C., KALI-I., KALI-P.,** kali-s., kali-sil., ***lac-d.,*** lach., led., **LYC.,** mag-arct., mag-aust., mag-c., mag-m., **MED., MERC.,** mez., naja, **NAT-A.,** ***nat-c.,*** **NAT-M.,** nat-p., nat-sil., **NIT-AC.,** ***nux-m.,*** **NUX-V.,** ol-j., op., osm., ***petr., ph-ac.,*** **PHOS.,** plat., **PSOR.,** ***puls.,*** rhod., ***rhus-t.,*** **RUMX.,** ruta, sabad., sabin., samb., sang., sars., sel., senec., **SEP., SIL.,** solid., spig., stann., staph., sul-i., ***sulph., sul-ac.,*** syph., **THUJ., TUB.,** valer., verat., verb., zinc.
chilled, easy - acon., ars., bry., hep., ***merc.,*** nat-m., nux-v., phos., puls.

COLDS, tendency to take
cold, air agg. - ***acon.,*** all-c., ars., dulc., hep., merc., ***nux-v.,*** phos.
dry weather agg. - acon., bry., caust., hep., nux-v.
feet, from - con., ***sil.***
wet weather agg. - calc., ***dulc.,*** rhus-t., nat-s.
colds, go to the chest - ant-t., ars., ***bac.,*** carb-v., ip., ***phos., tub.***
drafts, from - kali-c., nux-v., ph-ac.
chest on, from - ph-ac.
menses, during - bar-c., graph., mag-c., senec.
first, agg. - calc-p.
overheated, from - kali-c.
sneezing, with alot of - ***all-c.,*** dulc., hep., ip., kali-i., merc., ***nat-m.,*** phos., rhus-t., sulph.
sweating, after - nit-ac.

CONGESTION, to nose - am-c., sulph.
root of nose, to - nit-ac.

CONSTRICTION - graph., hell., kali-n., nat-m.

CONTRACTING, pain - anac., caps., fago., graph., hell., hep., ***kali-n.,*** sabad.
blowing, on - kali-c.
extending to eye - zinc.
from left to above left eye - caps.
o occiput - kali-c.
left - caps.

CONTRACTION - hep., lyc., nit-ac.,

CORROSIVE, nostril - lyc.

CORYZA, general - ***acon., aesc.,*** aeth., agar., ail., **ALL-C.,** all-s., aloe, alum., **AMBR.,** ammc., ***am-c., am-m., anac.,*** anan., ant-c., ant-t., aphis., apis, ***apoc.,*** aran., arg-m., arg-n., arn., **ARS.,** ***ars-i., arum-t.,*** **ARUND.,** asaf., ***asar., aspar.,*** asc-t., astac., ***aur., aur-m.,*** aur-s., ***bad.,*** bapt., bar-c., bar-m., **BELL.,** ***benz-ac., berb., bor.,*** bov., ***brom., bry.,*** bufo, ***cact.,*** cahin., calad., ***calc.,*** calc-ar., calc-f., calc-p., calc-s., camph., canth., ***caps., carb-an., carb-ac.,*** **CARB-S., CARB-V.,** cast-eq., ***caust., cean., cham.,*** **CHEL.,** ***chin.,*** chin-a., ***chlor., cic.,*** cimic., cimx., ***cina, cinnb.,*** clem., cocc., coc-c., coff., ***colch.,*** coloc., con., corn., ***cor-r.,*** croc., crot-h., crot-t., cupr., ***cycl.,*** daph., dig., dros., dulc., eucal., **EUP-PER.,** eup-pur., euph., **EUPHR.,** ***ferr., ferr-ar., ferr-i.,*** **FERR-P.,** fl-ac., ***gels.,*** glon., ***graph.,*** guai., **HEP.,** ***hydr.,*** ign., ill., ***iod.,*** ip., ***jab.,*** jac-c., ***kali-ar., kali-bi., kali-c., kali-chl.,*** **KALI-I.,** kali-n., kali-p., ***kali-s., kalm.,*** kreos., lac-ac., ***lac-c., lach.,*** laur., ***lyc.,*** lyss., ***mag-c., mag-m.,*** mag-s., mang., med., meph., **MERC.,** ***merc-c., merc-i-r.,*** merc-sul., ***mez.,*** mur-ac., myric., ***naja,*** **NAT-A.,** ***nat-c., nat-m.,*** nat-p., nat-s., nicc., ***nit-ac.,*** **NUX-V.,** ***osm.,*** par., ***petr.,*** phel., ***ph-ac.,*** **PHOS.,** ***phyt.,*** plat., plb., psor., **PULS.,** rhod., **RHUS-T.,** rhus-r., ***rumx., sabad., sang.,*** sars., sel., ***senec.,*** seneg., ***sep.,*** **SIL.,** sin-n., spig., ***spong., squil.,*** stann., **STAPH.,** ***stict.,*** still., **SULPH.,** sul-ac., tarent., tell., ter., ***teucr.,*** thuj., til., vac., verat., verb., zinc.

CORYZA, general

acrid, dry in warm room, fluent in open air - hydr.

afternoon - agar., alum., lach., lyc., sin-n., staph., stict.

4 p.m. - apis.

air, agg. in cold - ***calc-p.,*** coff., ***dulc.,*** graph., hyos., ***kali-ar.,*** mang., **MERC., PH-AC.**

draft of, from a - acon., ***dulc., elaps,*** kali-ar., kali-c., med., ***merc., nat-c.,*** nit-ac., nux-v.

post nasal, sensitive to - kreos.

snow - ***puls., rhus-t.***

warm - ant-c., ***apis,*** **MERC.**

agg., yet, dreads cold - apis, ***merc.***

air, open - ***aeth.,*** alumn., ars-i., ***calc-p.,*** carb-ac., carb-s., coloc., ***dulc.,*** euphr., ***graph.,*** hydr., iod., ***kali-bi.,*** lith., merc., nat-a., nat-c., **NIT-AC.,** plat., ***phos.,*** **PULS.,** sabad., sulph., tarax., teucr., thuj.

amel. - ***acon., all-c.,*** bry., ***calc-s.,*** chin-a., ***cycl.,*** euphr., mag-m., merc., merc-i-r., **NUX-V.,** phos., ***puls.,*** stict., tell., thuj.

after a while - tell.

dry, cold - acon., hyos.

alternating, days - nat-c.

with cutting pain in abdomen - calc.

amel., the general symptoms - thuj.

annual, (see Hay fever, Allergic rhinitis)

ascending - arum-t., brom., lac-c., merc., sep.

asthmatic, breathing, with - **ALL-C., ARS.,** ***ars-i., bad., carb-v., dulc., euphr.,*** **IOD.,** kali-i., lach., ***naja, nat-s., nux-v., sabad.,*** sang., ***sin-n.,*** sil., stict.

autumn, in - merc.

bathing, in cold water amel. - calc-s.

sea, in, amel. - med.

bloody, in infants - calc-s.

change of season or of temperature - all-c., gels.

changeable - ***puls.,*** staph.

children, in - merc-i-r.

chill, during - calad., elat., merc., nux-v.

chilled, from becoming, while overheated, snow or ice, from - ant-c., dros., iod., laur., puls., seneg., verat., verb.

chilliness, with - ***acon.,*** aphis., arg-n., ***ars., bry.,*** calc-p., carb-s., caust., graph., **MERC.,** nat-c., nit-ac., **NUX-V.,** ***puls., sarr., sil., spig., spong., sulph.***

back, in - aphis.

chronic, long-continued - ail., alum., am-br., am-c., am-m., anac., ***apis,*** ars-i., aur-m., bals-p., berb., **BROM.,** bry., ***calc.,*** calc-i., calc-p., ***canth.,*** coch., ***colch.,*** cist., coloc., ***con.,*** cub., ***cycl.,*** elaps, eucal., fl-ac., graph., hep., ***hippoz.,*** hydr., ***kali-bi.,*** kali-c., kali-i., kreos., lem-m., ***lyc.,*** mang., med., merc-i-r., merc-sul., nat-a., nat-c., nat-m., nat-s., nit-ac., ol-j., phos., psor., puls., sabad., ***sang.,*** sang-n., sars., sep., ***sil.,*** spig., spong., stict., ***sulph.,*** ther., thuj., ***tub., teucr.***

asthma, causing - ars., sil.

left side - ***berb.***

CORYZA, general

cold, on becoming - benz-ac., graph., ***kali-ar.,*** kali-i., ***merc.,*** nat-c., nux-v., petr.

constant - bar-c., calc., carb-s., graph., kali-n., nat-c., sil.

cough, with - acon., ***all-c.,*** alum., ambr., am-c., ***ars.,*** ars-i., bad., bar-c., **BELL.,** ***calc.,*** canth., carb-an., carb-s., carb-v., ***caust., cham.,*** cimx., ***colch.,*** con., dig., **EUPHR.,** ***ferr-p., gels., graph.,*** hep., ign., iod., **IP.,** ***kali-bi.,*** kali-c., kali-chl., ***kali-i.,*** kali-n., kali-p., lach., ***lyc.,*** mag-c., mag-s., meph., merc., nat-a., nat-c., ***nat-m., nit-ac.,*** ph-ac., ***phos.,*** rumx., ***rhus-t., sang.,*** sarr., sars., ***seneg.,*** sep., sil., spig., ***spong., squil.,*** staph., ***sulph.,*** sul-ac., ***tell., thuj.***

agg. - agar., bell., euphr., ip., ***lach.,*** nit-ac., nitro-o., ***squil.,*** sulph., thuj.

after - kali-n.

croup, with - ***acon., ars.,*** cub., ***hep., nit-ac., spong.***

cutting, the hair, from - ***bell.,*** **NUX-V.,** puls., ***sep.,*** sil.

daytime - carb-v., caust., cimic., euphr., merc., ***nux-v.,*** stann.

damp agg. - kali-i.

descending - ars., bry., carb-v., iod., kali-c., phos., stict., sulph., tub.

diarrhea, followed by - alum., calc., carb-v., chin., psor., rumx., ***sang.,*** sel., sulph., tub.

dinner, after - nat-c.

diphtheria, during - am-c., ***ars.,*** **ARUM-T.,** ***carb-ac.,*** chlor., crot-h., ***ign.,*** **KALI-BI.,** kali-ma., ***lac-c., lach., lyc., merc-c., merc-cy., merc-i-f., mur-ac.,*** **NIT-AC.**

discharge, with, nosebleeds - ant-t., ars., graph., kali-bi., puls.

discharge, without, dry - ***acon.,*** agar., all-c., all-s., alum., ambr., ***am-c.,*** am-m., anac., ***ant-c.,*** apis, ***ars.,*** asar., asc-t., aur., aur-s., ***bell.,*** bov., ***bry., cact.,*** **CALC.,** calc-s., ***camph., caps., carb-an., carb-s., carb-v.,*** **CAUST.,** cham., chel., **CHIN.,** ***chin-a.,*** coff., cor-r., croc., cupr., cycl., dig., dros., ***dulc., graph.,*** hep., ***ign., iod., ip.,*** kali-ar., ***kali-c.,*** kali-chl., kali-n., kali-p., kreos., lach., ***lyc., mag-c.,*** mag-m., ***mang.,*** merc., mez., mosch., ***nat-a., nat-c., nat-m.,*** nat-s., ***nit-ac.,*** **NUX-V.,** ol-an., ol-j., op., ***par.,*** petr., **PHOS.,** ***plat.,*** psor., ***puls.,*** rat., sabin., sac-alb., **SAMB.,** sars., ***sep., sil., spig., spong.,*** squil., stann., **STICT.,** ***sulph., sul-ac.,*** teucr., ***thuj.,*** uran., verb., ***zinc.***

afternoon - mag-c.

air, open, in - calc-p., naja, **NUX-V.**

alternating with watery - alum., am-c., ant-c., ant-t., ***apis, ars.,*** bell., cund., euphr., kali-n., ***lac-c.,*** lach., mag-c., ***mag-m., mang., nat-a., nat-c., nat-m.,*** nit-ac., **NUX-V.,** par., ***phos.,*** **PULS.,** quillaya, sang., ***sil.,*** sin-a., spong., ***sulph.,*** sul-ac., zinc.

annual, (see hay fever)

day - carb-an.

CORYZA, general

discharge, without

eating - spig.

evening - calc., carb-s., carb-v., cimic., euphr., iod., lach., mang., nicc., nux-v., puls., ***sulph.***

with discharge during the day - cimic., dig., euphr., ***nux-v.***

bed, in - kali-c.

followed by watery - asc-t., cor-r., plat.

indoors - thyr.

left - calc-caust., ***sep.***

morning - ***apis,*** calc., ***carb-an.,*** carb-v., con., dig., iod., kali-c., lach., laur., mag-s., nat-m., nux-v., ***sil.***

rising, after - bov.

rising, after, amel. - carb-an.

watery daytime - ***sil.***

watery in evening - apis

night - alum., am-c., calc., ***caust.,*** dig., euphr., lach., ***mag-c.,*** mag-m., nat-c., nicc., nit-ac., **NUX-V.** sep.

watery during the day - caust., dig., euphr., merc., nat-c., nicc., **NUX-V.**

nose, obstruction, with - mang.

warm room - ***ars., coloc.,*** hydr., ***iod.,*** plat., ***puls., sulph., thuj.,*** zing.

dyspnea, with - ars-i., kali-i., nit-ac.

eating, after - cann-i., clem., fl-ac., **NUX-V.,** ***plb.,*** sanic., spig., sulph., ***zinc.***

agg - carb-an., nux-v., sanic., trom.

elderly, people - am-c., anac., ant-c., ars., camph., sul-i.

palpitations, with - anac.

evening - ***all-c.,*** anac., aphis., ***apis,*** arn., ***carb-an., carb-v.,*** chlor., dulc., euphr., iod., kali-bi., lach., lith., mang., mag-c., phos., ***puls., rumx.,*** sel., sin-n., ther., trom., ***zinc.***

fluent, dry in morning - apis

lying down, after - zinc.

excitement, amel. - fl-ac.

exhausting - arg-m., arg-n.

extending to, chest - all-c., am-c., ant-c., ars., carb-v., euphr., iod., ip., mang., merc., lap-a., nux-v., phos., sang.

frontal sinuses - ***ars.,*** calc-p., cimx., ***kali-i., sil., stict.***

fever, with - ***acon.,*** all-c., anac., ***ars.,*** bar-m., ***bell.,*** **BRY.,** chlor., gels., graph., ***hep.,*** iod., jab., lach., **MERC.,** nat-c., nit-ac., ***seneg.,*** sep., spig., ***tarent.***

flowers - **ALL-C.,** phos., sabad., sang.

chamomille - ***wye.***

odors of, agg. - phos., sabad., sang.

fluent, dry and, alternately - nat-m.

indoors - all-c., calc-p., nux-v.

thick and, alternately - staph.

hot - cham., iod.

hunger, with - all-c., ars-i., hep., ***sul-ac.***

intermittent - nat-c.

CORYZA, general

laryngitis, with - acon., alum., am-m., ***ars.,*** ars-m., bar-c., ***benz-ac.,*** **BRY.,** calc., ***calc-p.,*** calc-s., carb-s., **CARB-V., CAUST.,** cham., ***dig.,*** dulc., eup-per., ferr-p., graph., ***hep., kali-bi.,*** kali-c., ***kalm., mag-m.,*** mag-s., **MANG., MERC.,** ***merc-i-r.,*** nat-a., ***nat-c.,*** nat-m., ***nit-ac., petr.,*** phel., **PHOS.,** puls., ***ran-b., rumx., seneg., sep., spig., spong.,*** sulph., sul-ac., ***tell.,*** thuj., zinc.

left - agar., ***all-c.,*** alum., **ARUM-T.,** bad., berb., cist., cop., jug-c., mang., thlaspi, thuj., zinc.

to right - agar., all-c.

light, strong - ***puls.***

lying - chin-a., euphr., mag-m., sin-n., spig.

amel. - merc.

flows into fauces and rattle while breathing - phos.

watery, while - ***spig.***

menses, during - alum., ***am-c.,*** am-m., bar-c., ***graph., kali-c.,*** kali-n., ***lach.,*** mag-c., phos., senec., sep., zinc.

before - graph., ***mag-c.,*** tarent.

with cough and hoarseness - ***graph.***

suppressed - seneg.

milk agg. - lac-d.

morning - aeth., alum., all-c., ant-c., ars-m., ***arum-t.,*** asc-t., ***bar-c.,*** bufo, ***calc.,*** calc-ar., calc-p., ***carb-v.,*** con., corn., cycl., dig., euphr., ferr-i., iod., kali-bi., lach., ***mag-c.,*** myric., nat-m., **NUX-V.,** onos., puls., sars., sep., ***squil.,*** sumb.

amel. - stict.

and evening - mag-c.

waking - ars., ***aster.,*** carb-v., dulc.

motion, amel. - ***dulc.,*** phos., ***rhus-t.,*** thuj.

newborns, in - ars., cham., dulc., nux-v., samb.

night - alum., bry., ***calc., carb-an.,*** carb-v., caust., cham., euphr., ferr., mag-m., **MERC.,** naja, ***nat-c.,*** nat-s., nicc., ***nit-ac., nux-v.,*** phos., rumx., sang., thuj.

3 a.m. agg - am-c.

air, in open - ***aeth.,*** calc-p., calc-s., nat-c.

noon - cina.

nosebleeds, with - ant-t., ars., graph., kali-bi., puls.

nose, obstruction, with - ars.

obstinate, with soreness beneath nose and on margin of nose - **BROM.,** iod.

one-sided - alum., am-m., aur-m., bell., hep., kali-c., nux-v., **PHOS.,** ***phyt.,*** plat., rhod., staph., stann.

overheated, from becoming - acon., ars., bry., ***carb-v., puls., sep.,*** sil.

peaches, from the odor of - **ALL-C.**

periodical attacks - ars., brom., chin., ***graph.,*** nat-m., sang., sil.

alternate days - aran., nat-c.

every fourth day - iod.

twenty-one days - ars-m.

perspiration, with - eup-per., jab., ***merc.***

amel. after - nat-c., nat-m.

polyuria, with - calc.

CORYZA, general
recurrent - bac., carc.
right - **ARS.**, brom., ***calc-s.,*** euphr., kali-bi., ***kali-i.,*** merc-i-r., ***sang.,*** sars., tarent.
bath, after a - calc-s.
to left - brom., ***carb-v.,*** chel., dros., euphr., lyc.
rose, cold - ***all-c.,*** phos., ***sabad., sang., tub.,*** wye.
salivation, with - calc-p., kali-i.
scarlatina, during - **AIL.,** ***all-c., am-c.,*** **ARUM-T.,** ***caps., mur-ac., nit-ac.,*** phos., phyt., rhus-t.
short - graph., nit-ac., sep., sulph.
side, one - nux-v., phos., phyt.
singer's - all-c.
sitting, on cold stone - nux-v.
up amel. - mag-m., sin-n.
sleep, fluent in - ***fl-ac.,*** lac-c.
smell, acute, with - kalm.
sneezing, then, with - ***all-c.,*** carb-an., naja., ***nat-m.***
sleeplessness, with - ars., ***calc-ar.***
sore, throat, with - ***carb-an., calc-p.,*** cimic., ***lach.,*** **MERC., NIT-AC., NUX-V., PHOS.,** ***phyt.***
spring - gels., lach., naja
stool, during - thuj.
stooping, agg - laur.
sudden, attacks - agar., alum., apis, bar-c., cycl., fl-ac., ***plan., iod.,*** spig., staph., sulph., ***thuj., zinc.***
evening after lying down - ***zinc.***
summer - ***gels.***
diarrhea, with - dulc.
suppressed - ***acon.,*** ambr., am-c., ***ars., arum-t.,*** **BELL.,** brom., ***bry., calc.,*** carb-v., cham., ***chin., cina,*** graph., kali-bi., kali-c., **LACH.,** ***lyc.,*** nat-m., nit-ac., ***nux-v.,*** par., puls., sep., ***sil.,*** teucr.
as if - osm.
air, from least contact of cold - dulc.
swallowing, agg - carb-an.
talking, agg - acon.
uncovering, the head, from - ***hep., nat-m.***
urination, burning, with - ran-s.
violent, attacks - ***all-c.,*** alum., **ARS., ARUM-T.,** ***bry., calc., carb-v.,*** chlor., cocc., cycl., **LYC.,** mag-c., mez., nat-c., nit-ac., ph-ac., sil., ***staph.,*** thuj.
walking, amel. - ***dulc.,*** merc-i-r., phos., ***puls., rhus-t.***
warm, room - **ALL-C.,** ***ant-c.,*** carb-v., cycl., ***merc., merc-i-r., nux-v.,*** phos., puls., sep.
amel. - ***ars.,*** calc-p., coloc., ***dulc., sabad.***
becoming, when walking, amel. - merc-i-r.
washing, after - fl-ac.
amel. - calc-s., phos.
watery, discharge - ***acon., aesc.,*** aeth., ***agar.,*** ail., **ALL-C.,** alum., **AM-C.,** ***am-m.,*** anac., anan., ant-c., ***ant-t.,*** aphis., apis, **ARG-M., ARS.,** ***ars-i., arum-t.,*** asaf., ***asc-t., aspar.,***

CORYZA, general
watery, discharge - aur., aur-m., bad., ***bar-c.,*** bar-m., **BELL.,** berb., ***bor., bov., brom., bry.,*** bufo, cact., cahin., calad., **CALC.,** ***calc-ar.,*** calc-f., ***calc-p., calc-s., camph.,*** carb-ac., ***carb-an.,*** carb-s., ***carb-v.,*** cast., cast-eq., ***caust., cham., chel., chin.,*** chin-a., chlor., cimic., cimx., cina, cinnb., clem., coc-c., coff., colch., ***coloc., con.,*** cop., ***cor-r.,*** crot-t., ***cupr., cycl.,*** dig., ***dros., dulc., elaps, eup-per.,*** eup-pur., euph., **EUPHR.,** ferr-i., ***fl-ac.,*** form., ***gels., glon.,*** graph., guai., ***hep., hydr.,*** **IGN.,** ***iod.,*** jac., **KALI-AR.,** ***kali-bi., kali-c., kali-chl.,*** **KALI-I.,** kali-n., ***kali-p.,*** kali-s., kalm., kreos., **LAC-C.,** ***lach.,*** lil-t., ***lyc.,*** mag-c., ***mag-m., mag-s., mang.,*** meph., med., meny., **MERC., MERC-C.,** merc-i-r., merc-sul., ***mez.,*** mur-ac., naja, ***nat-a.,*** **NAT-C., NAT-M.,** nat-p., ***nat-s.,*** **NIT-AC., NUX-V.,** ol-j., ***osm.,*** ox-ac., par., ***petr.,*** ph-ac., phos., ***phyt.,*** plat., plb., **PULS.,** ***ran-b.,*** ran-s., rhus-t., rhus-r., rumx., **SABAD.,** ***sang.,*** sarr., sars., sel., ***sep., sil.,*** sin-n., ***spig., spong.,*** squil., staph., **SULPH.,** sul-ac., ***syph.,*** **TELL., THUJ.,** xan., ***zinc.***
afternoon - alum., **ARUM-T.,** calc-p., kali-c., mag-s., plb., sulph., trom., wye.
amel. - nat-c.
air, in open - ***ars., carb-ac.,*** calc-s., ***coloc.,*** dulc., euphr., hydr., ***iod.,*** **NIT-AC.,** plat., **PULS.,** sabad., ***sulph.,*** tell., ***thuj.,*** trom., zinc., zing.
amel. - ars-i., ***calc-s.,*** carb-v., cycl.
alternating sides - **LAC-C.**
cold, room - ***carb-ac., calc-p., merc.***
water - fl-ac.
daytime - carb-v., caust., cimic., dig., euphr., merc., nat-c., **NUX-V.,** stann.
evening - agar., **ALL-C.,** aphis., ***apis,*** bufo, ***carb-an., carb-v.,*** coff., fl-ac., kali-c., mez., nat-a., ***puls., rumx.,*** sel., sulph., ther., thuj., trom., ***zinc.***
followed by coryza without discharge - zinc.
forenoon - calc-p., cimic., merc-i-r., nat-c.
10 a.m. - med.
11 a.m. - ***tell.***
morning - ***acon.,*** alum., ant-c., calc-p., carb-v., caust., coloc., ***cycl.,*** dros., ***euphr.,*** mag-c., **NUX-V.,** puls., sars., ***sep., squil., sulph.,*** thuj.
bed, in - carb-v.
dry in afternoon - mag-c.
rising, after - caust., **NUX-V.**
with cough and expectoration - **EUPHR.**
night - aur-m., fl-ac., iod., ***kali-bi.,*** merc., ***nat-c., rumx.***
noon - ***cina.***
nosebleeds, with - ant-t., ars., graph., kali-bi., puls.
stooping, on - agar., ***merc.***
warm room - **ALL-C.,** cycl., ***merc., nux-v.,*** **PULS.**
windy weather - euphr.

CORYZA, general
  weather, dry cold - acon., nux-v.
    changeable, in - dulc., gels., hep.
    wet, during - all-c., dulc., hep., mang., ***merc., puls.,*** sin-n.
    windy, in - acon., euphr.
  wet, after getting - sep.
  whooping, cough, in - all-c., dros.
  wind, caused by, cold west - ***kali-bi.***
    cold, dry - **ACON.,** ***spong.***
    north east, after - **ALL-C.**
  yawning, with - carb-an., cupr., lyc.

CRACKLING, in - acon., sulph.

CRACKS, in, corners - fago., ***graph.,*** mag-p., merc.
    nostrils - **ANT-C.,** anthro., arum-t., ***aur., aur-m.,*** fago., ***graph.,*** merc., nit-ac., ***petr.,*** thuj.
    septum - merc.
    tip - **ALUM.,** carb-an.
      menses, during - carb-an.
    wings - aur-m., caust., hep., lac-c., ***merc.,*** sil., ***thuj.***

CRAMPING, pain - nux-m., plat., sulph.
    bone, right side - laur., plat.
    root - ***acon.,*** arn., bapt., bell., colch., kali-c., hyos., ***mang., plat.,*** zinc.
      right side - kali-c.
    tip - stront.
    wings - kali-n., plat., zinc.
      left - plat.
      right - ambr.

CRAMPS, nose - sulph.
    muscles - lyc.
    wing - ambr.

CRUSHING, pain in root - anan.

CRUSTS, bloody - hydr., thuj.
    cold, parts becoming, agg. - chin., sulph.
    foamy - sil.
    glue-like - hep.
    hard, plugging nose - mur-ac.
    hot - kali-i.
    post nasal - bufo, caust.
    sudden - ***fl-ac., hydr., kali-bi., lach., nat-c.,*** nat-m., phos., ***sil., staph.,*** thuj.
    watery, watery, eating on nose - plb., ***trom.***
    yellow-orange - kali-bi.

CUTTING, pain - arn., bry., caust., ***kali-bi.,*** kali-i., nit-ac., zinc.
    bones - indg., ***kali-bi., kali-i.,*** merc-i-f., teucr.
    evening - lyc.
      bed, in - lyc.
    left nostril - agar., sep.
    right nostril - lyc.
    root - ***kali-c., teucr.***
      to occiput - ferr-i.
    septum - lyc., merc-i-f.
      left, on inspiration - agar.
      upper part of - lyc.

CUTTING, pain
    wing - caust., stram., zinc.
      left - zinc.
      right - caust.

DECAY, bones, of (see Ozaena) - **ASAF., AUR.,** ***aur-m.,*** aur-m-n., cadm-s., calc-s., fl-ac., ***hecla., hep., hippoz.,*** kali-i., merc-i-r., nit-ac., ***phos., phyt.,*** **SIL.,** ***still.***
    septum - hecla., ***hippoz., kali-bi.***
    syphilitic - ***kali-bi., sil.***

DESQUAMATION - ars., aur., aur-m., canth., carb-an., crot-t., ***nat-c., nat-m.,*** nit-ac., phos.
    septum - crot-t., kali-bi.
    tip - carb-an., nat-c.

DIGGING, pain - ***coloc.,*** kali-n.
    from left side to root - ***coloc.***
    tensive in right nostril - lach.

DILATED, nostrils (see Motion) - ***ant-t., ars.,*** cupr., hell., iod., ***lyc.,*** op., ox-ac., phos., phys., ***spong.***
    expiration, during - ***ferr.***
    inspiration, each - ***merc-i-f.***
    sensation of - iod.

DIPHTHERIA, in - ***am-c., hydr., kali-bi., lyc.,*** merc-c., merc-cy., nit-ac., ***petr.***
    begin in nose - lyc., merc-c., merc-cy.
    extends to lips - am-c.
    post nasal - lac-c., lach.

DIRTY, (see Sooty)

DISCHARGE, general
  afternoon - lyc.
  air, open, amel. - hydr., puls.
  albuminous - ***aur.,*** hippoz., ***iod.,*** **NAT-M.,** ***nat-s.***
  bitter - ars., ph-ac.
  bland - ***calc.,*** **EUPHR.,** jug-c., kali-i., plan., **PULS.,** ***sep., sil.,*** staph.
  blood-streaked - phos.
  bloody - acon., act-sp., ***agar.,*** **AIL., ALL-C., ALUM.,** ambr., **AM-C.,** ***am-m.,*** ant-t., ***apis,*** arg-m., arg-n., **ARS.,** ars-h., ***ars-i., arum-t.,*** asar., ***aur., aur-m., aur-m-n.,*** bar-c., **BELL.,** bor., bry., bufo, calad., ***calc.,*** **CALC-S.,** canth., caps., carb-ac., carb-s., ***carb-v., caust.,*** chel., **CHIN., CHIN-A.,** cimic., cinnb., clem., ***cocc., con.,*** cop., ***croc., crot-c.,*** crot-h., cupr., dros., euphr., ***ferr., ferr-ar.,*** ferr-i., ferr-p., gels., ***graph.,*** **HEP.,** hippoz., ***hydr.,*** ind., iod., ip., ***kali-ar., kali-bi., kali-c.,*** **KALI-I.,** kali-n., kali-p., kali-s., kaol., kreos., ***lac-c., lach.,*** laur., led., ***lyc.,*** mag-c., mag-m., ***mang.,*** **MERC.,** ***merc-i-r., mez.,*** myric., ***nat-m.,*** **NIT-AC.,** nux-m., ***nux-v.,*** op., par., petr., ph-ac., **PHOS.,** phyt., **PSOR.,** puls., ran-b., rhus-t., sabad., sabin., sanic., sarr., sel., ***sep., sil., sin-n.,*** spig., spong., ***squil., stict., sulph.,*** sul-ac., ***thuj., tub.,*** zinc.
    coryza, during - sulph.
    coughing, when - caps.

DISCHARGE, general

bloody,

morning - ***am-c.,*** arum-t., calc., kali-c., ***lach.,*** lyc., petr., spig., sulph.

on blowing nose - calad., caust., chel., graph., lach., meny., nit-ac., phos., puls., sep., sulph., thuj., zinc.

night - sulph.

one side, from - asc-t.

post nasal - cor-r., ***hep.,*** nux-v., puls., sabad., spig., tell.

blue - am-m., arund., ***kali-bi., nat-a.***

brownish - ***kali-s.,*** sin-n., thuj.

burning - agar., **ALL-C.,** alum., ***am-c.,*** am-m., **ARS.,** ***ars-i., ars-m.,*** arum-t., brom., calad., calc., canth., carb-an., ***caust.,*** chen-a., cina, ***cinnb.,*** con., euph., ham., iod., ***kali-ar.,*** kali-bi., kali-c., kali-i., kali-s., kreos., merc., mez., mosch., **PULS.,** ***sulph.,*** sul-ac.

changeable - calc., ***puls.,*** staph.

clear - ***acon.,*** agar., all-c., am-m., asar., ars., aur., calc., carb-s., cast., cedr., con., graph., hydr., ***iod.,*** kali-m., lac-ac., mag-c., mang., ***nat-m.,*** phos., sulph.

hot water - acon.

constant - agar., hydr., iod., kali-bi., lac-c., phos., teucr.

cold - ambro., ichth., kali-i., lach.

copious - acon., aeth., agar., ail., **ALL-C.,** alum., ***alumn.,*** anac., anan., **ARS.,** ***ars-i.,*** arum-t., aspar., bar-c., bar-m., berb., bor., ***bry.,*** calc., calc-f., canth., carb-s., caust., cedr., chlor., cic., coc-c., coff., cop., cor-r., crot-c., cupr., cycl., dros., ery-a., euph., euphr., eup-pur., ferr-i., ***graph.,*** guai., hydr., ***iod., kali-bi.,*** kali-c., kali-chl., **KALI-I.,** lac-ac., lac-c., lyc., mag-m., mur-ac., ***nat-a., nat-c.,*** **NAT-M.,** nat-s., ***nit-ac.,*** nux-v., **PHOS.,** plan., plat., ***puls.,*** rhod., ***rumx., sabad., senec., sep.,*** sil., ***spig., stict., sulph.,*** staph., teucr., ***tub.,*** verat-v., ***zinc.***

air, in open - hydr.

coryza, without - mag-m., phos.

morning, after rising - rhus-t.

post nasal, from - carb-v., **COR-R.,** euph., ***spig.***

stuffing of head, with - ***acon.,*** agar., ***arum-t., calc.,*** hep., **KALI-I.,** ***nit-ac., nux-v.,*** phos., sapo., spig.

morning, in - ***arum-t.***

coughing, agg. - agar., caps., lach., nat-m., nit-ac., ***squil.,*** sul-ac., sulph., thuj.

creamy - ***hippoz.***

crusts, scabs, inside - ***agar.,*** ail., ***alum., alumn.,*** ant-c., apis, arg-n., ***ars.,*** arund., ***aur., aur-m.,*** aur-s., bar-c., ***bor.,*** **BOV.,** ***brom.,*** bry., ***calc., calc-s., carb-an.,*** carb-s., caust., cic., coc-c., con., cop., crot-t., culx., daph., ***elaps, ferr.,*** ferr-ar., ***ferr-i.,*** ferr-p., **GRAPH.,** hep., ***hippoz.,*** **HYDR.,** hyper., ***iod.,*** **KALI-BI.,** ***kali-c.,*** kali-p., ***kaol.,*** lac-c., ***lach.,*** lith., ***lyc.,*** mag-c., ***mag-m.,*** **MERC.,** ***merc-i-f.,*** merc-i-r., ***mez., nat-a., nat-c., nat-m.,*** nat-p., nat-s., ***nit-ac.,*** nux-v., petr., ***phos., phyt.,***

DISCHARGE, general

crusts, scabs, inside - psor., ***puls.,*** ran-b., rhod., rat., rhus-r., ***sanic.,*** sars., **SEP.,** ***sil.,*** staph., **STICT.,** stront-c., ***sulph.,*** syph., teucr., **THUJ.,** trom., **TUB.,** vinc., xan.

adhere, tightly - phos.

black - calc., rhod.

bloody - ambr., am-c., am-m., calc., ***kali-bi.,*** nat-a., ***phos.,*** puls., sep., stront.

bran-like - sulph.

brown crusts - ***kali-c., thuj.,*** vinc.

cold agg., parts becoming - chin., sulph.

detach, hard to, and leave raw and sore - ***ars., bov.,*** **KALI-BI.,** nit-ac., ***phos.,*** phyt., psor., stict., ***thuj.***

detached, bleeding, cause - ***arg-n., kali-bi.,*** lac-c., ***nat-a., nit-ac.***

easily, but if pulled away too soon cause soreness at root and intolerance of light - **KALI-BI.**

leaving nostrils raw and bleeding until others form, when - ***ars.,*** brom., ***nit-ac.***

re-form if - ***ars.,*** bor., **KALI-BI.,** lac-c., ***psor.***

detaching, causes pain and soreness - ***kali-bi.,*** nit-ac., teucr., ***thuj.***

elastic plugs - **KALI-BI.,** ***lyc.***

foamy - sil.

gluey - hep., kali-bi.

gray - ail., hippoz., kali-c.

green, every morning - ***nit-ac., thuj.***

masses - ***elaps,*** **KALI-BI.,** ***phos.,*** **SEP.,** ***teucr., thuj.***

greenish, seem to come from an ulcer - ***nat-s.***

hard - mur-ac.

high up - arum-t., crot-t., ***sil.,*** staph.

discharge of a large scab from gathering high up beyond the nasal bones - arum-t.

large, must discharge through post-nasal - alum., ***sep.***

hot - kali-i.

left - cob., nat-p.

painful - graph., ***sil., thuj.***

post nasal - alum., ***bar-c.,*** bufo, calc-ar., caust., culx., elaps, hydr., ***sep.***

right - ***alum., aur.,*** hep., ***iod.,*** lith., nit-ac., sars., ***sil.,*** uran., xan.

septum, on - anac., ***kali-bi., lac-c., psor.,*** sel., ***sil.,*** **THUJ.**

right - ***lac-c.,*** uran.

shining - lith.

sudden - ***fl-ac., hydr., kali-bi., lach., nat-c.,*** nat-m., phos., ***sil., staph.,*** thuj.

watery eating on nose - plb., ***trom.***

whitish - kali-bi.

yellow - aur., aur-m., ***calc., cic., hydr., kali-bi., iod.,*** kali-c., mag-m., rhod.

coryza, in - ***bar-c.,*** brom., ***kali-c.***

dry - aur-m.

orange - kali-bi.

thick, heavy, high up - crot-t.

dark, nostrils - ant-t., colch., crot-h., hell., hyos.

DISCHARGE, general

daytime - arum-t., caust., nat-c.

dinner, after - trom.

dries, quickly, forming scabs - psor., ***stict.***

dripping - acon., agar., ***all-c.***, am-c., ***ars.***, arum-t., cham., calc., chin., con., eup-per., euphr., graph., ***hep.***, kali-i., lach., mag-c., nat-m., nit-ac., nux-v., phos., rhus-t., sep., squil., ***sulph.***, tab.

post nasal - all-c., **HYDR., KALI-BI.,** merc-c., spig., ***thuj.***

eating, while - carb-an., clem., nux-v., plb., sanic., sulph., ***trom.***

agg. - plb.

evening - ***puls.***

excoriating - agar., ***ail.***, **ALL-C.,** ***alum.***, ***am-c.***, **AM-M.,** anac., ant-c., ant-t., apis, **ARS.,** ***ars-h.***, **ARS-I.,** ars-m., **ARUM-T.,** ***aur-m.***, bor., ***brom.***, cact., cahin., calad., ***calc.***, ***calc-s.***, cann-s., canth., carb-an., ***carb-s.***, ***carb-v.***, cast., ***caust.***, cedr., ***cham.***, chin., chlor., cinnb., ***con.***, euphr., eup-pur., ***ferr.***, ferr-ar., **FERR-I.,** ferr-p., fl-ac., ***gels.***, **GRAPH.,** ham., ***hep.***, ***hippoz.***, ***hydr.***, ign., **IOD.,** kali-ar., ***kali-bi.***, ***kali-c.***, ***kali-i.***, kali-n., kali-p., kali-s., **KREOS.,** ***lac-c.***, ***lach.***, ***lyc.***, mag-c., ***mag-m.***, mag-s., mang., **MERC.,** ***merc-c.***, ***merc-i-f.***, ***mez.***, ***mur-ac.***, ***naja***, nat-m., **NIT-AC., NUX-V.,** ph-ac., ***phos.***, ***phyt.***, puls., ***ran-b.***, ***rhus-t.***, ***sang.***, sep., ***sil.***, ***sin-n.***, spig., ***squil.***, stann., staph., stict., ***sulph.***, sul-ac., ***sul-i.***, thuj., uran., ***zinc.***

air, in open - kali-s.

bland, discharge from eyes, with - **ALL-C.**

corners, of nose - chin-a.

daytime - cahin.

left, nostril, from - **ALL-C.**

menses, during - am-c.

morning - ars-m., ***squil.***

11 a.m. - ars-m.

night - **NIT-AC.**

right - kali-bi., sang.

upper, lip and around nose - **ALL-C.**

washing, in cold water amel. - calc-s.

expectoration, with - sabal.

fish-brine, smelling like - elaps.

flocculent - am-c., ***ars.***, carb-v., ferr., puls., sep., sil., sulph.

forenoon - erig.

frothy - merc., sil.

gelatinous - hep., sel.

glairy - alum., ***aur.***, kali-m., **NAT-M.,** ***petr.***

glassy - cedr., iod.

glue-like - hep., ***kali-bi.***, hydr., ***merc-c.***, ***psor.***, sel., stict., ***sulph.***

post nasal, from - caps., ***kali-bi.***, ***merc-c.***, sumb.

gray - **AMBR.,** anac., ars., asim., carb-an., chin., hippoz., kali-c., kreos., **LYC.,** mang., med., nux-v., rhus-t., sang., seneg., sep., thuj.

grayish-white - sang.

DISCHARGE, general

greenish - ***alum.***, anan., arn., ars., ***ars-i.***, arund., asaf., aur., aur-m., ***berb.***, ***bor.***, bov., ***bry.***, bufo, calc., ***calc-f.***, cann-s., carb-an., carb-s., ***carb-v.***, cimic., colch., cop., culx., dros., ferr., ferr-ar., ***ferr-i.***, graph., hep., hippoz., hydr-ac., hyos., ind., iod., kali-ar., **KALI-BI.,** ***kali-c.***, **KALI-I.,** kali-p., kali-s., kreos., **LAC-C.,** led., lyc., lyss., mang., **MERC.,** ***nat-c.***, ***nit-ac.***, nux-v., par., ***phos.***, plb., **PULS.,** ***rhus-t.***, sanic., **SEP.,** ***sil.***, spig., stann., ***stict.***, sulph., ***sul-i.***, syph., ***teucr.***, ***ther.***, **THUJ.**

blood-streaked - **PHOS.**

light, on exposure to - ***nat-s.***

stains pillow in sleep - lac-c.

greenish-black - **KALI-I.**

brown - ***hydr-ac.***

greenish-yellow - ***alum.***, arund., ***aur-m.***, bufo, ***calc-f.***, ***calc-s.***, caust., cop., ***hep.***, **HYDR., KALI-BI.,** ***kali-c.***, ***kali-i.***, lac-c., ***mang.***, ***med.***, **MERC.,** ***nat-c.***, ***nat-s.***, par., ***phos.***, plan., psor., **PULS.,** rhus-t., sabad., sars., **SEP.,** ***sil.***, syph., ***ther.***, **THUJ., TUB.**

night, at, staining pillow - lac-c.

gummy - sumb.

gushing, fluid - agar., bac., dulc., euphr., fl-ac., hydr., kali-bi., lach., ***nat-c.***, **NAT-M.,** phos., sel., squil., ***thuj.***

morning - squil.

hard, dry - agar., ***alum.***, **ALUMN.,** ant-c., ars., arund., **AUR.,** ***aur-m.***, bar-c., ***bor.***, brom., ***bry.***, calc., carb-s., ***con.***, elaps, ***graph.***, guare., hydr-ac., ***iod.***, **KALI-BI.,** ***lach.***, lyc., ***merc.***, merc-i-f., mez., ***nat-a.***, ***nat-c.***, nat-s., petr., phos., sec., **SEP., SIL.,** staph., **STICT.,** stront-c., ***sulph.***, tell., thuj., xan.

menses, during - sep.

morning - asim., **SIL.**

plugs - mur-ac.

post nasal - ***merc.***

hot - acon., ars-i., ars-m., iod., kali-i., lyc., rhus-t.

ichorous - **AIL.,** all-c., ars., ars-i., arum-t., aur-m-n., ***lyc.***, merc., ***nit-ac.***, ***rhus-t.***

singing, while - all-c.

left, nostril, from - all-c., kali-s., lach., sep., teucr.

lumpy - alum., cinnb., ***hydr.***, **KALI-BI.,** merc-d., osm., petr., phos., puls., sel., sep., sil., solid., teucr., zinc-i.

blowing nose - merc-d.

post nasal, from - calc., cimic., ***hydr.***, **KALI-BI.,** merc-i-f., osm., sep., syph., teucr., zinc.

yellow - hydr., puls.

morning - berb., kali-p., mang., phos., puls., squil.

5 a.m. - ***ars.***

musty - nat-c.

night - crot-c., kali-bi., **LAC-C.,** nat-s., **NIT-AC.**

DISCHARGE, general

offensive - agar., alum., anan., ars., **ASAF.,** asim., **AUR.,** ***aur-m., bar-c.,*** bell., berb., bufo, **CALC.,** ***calc-f., calc-s., carb-ac.,*** carb-s., caust., chim., con., cop., cub., cur., ***elaps,*** fl-ac., ***graph.,*** guai., ham., **HEP.,** ***hippoz., iod.,*** **KALI-BI.,** ***kali-c., kali-i., kali-p., kali-s.,*** kreos., ***lach.,*** led., ***lyc., mag-m.,*** **MERC.,** merc-i-f., nat-a., **NAT-C.,** nat-s., ***nit-ac.,*** nux-v., petr., ph-ac., ***phos.,*** phyt., **PSOR., PULS.,** rhus-t., sarr., sabin., sang., ***sep.,*** **SIL.,** spig., stann., stram., **SULPH.,** syph., tell., teucr., ***ther., thuj.,*** ust.

fetid - ***agar.,*** anthr., apis, ***asaf.,*** **AUR.,** ***aur-m-n.,*** berb., ***calc., carb-ac.,*** caust., cop., cur., eucal., ***graph., hep., iod., kali-c., kali-n., kreos.,*** led., lyc., mag-m., ***merc., myric.,*** nat-c., ***nit-ac.,*** petr., ***puls.,*** rhus-t., sil., tell., ***ther.,*** thuj.

burnt - berb.

cheese, like - hep., merc., **TUB.**

herring pickle - ***elaps.***

pungent - berb.

putrid - agar., arund., asaf., bufo, **CARB-AC.,** ***elaps,*** graph., **PSOR.**

sour - alum., hep.

menses, during - ***graph.,*** sep.

sickly, sweetish - nit-ac., thuj.

urine, like - graph.

one-sided - calc-s., hippoz., phyt., puls.

orange - puls.

post nasal, (see Catarrh, post nasal) - ***all-c., alumn.,*** anac., ***ant-c., arg-n.,*** arn., ars., arum-t., bar-c., bry., bufo., ***calc., calc-s., canth.,*** **CAPS.,** carb-ac., ***carb-an.,*** carb-v., chin., cinnb., cop., **COR-R.,** elaps, euph., euphr., ***ferr.,*** gran., hep., **HYDR.,** iod., **KALI-BI.,** ***kali-chl.,*** lach., lac-ac., ***mang.,*** med., ***merc.,*** merc-c., merc-i-f., ***merc-i-r.,*** mez., ***nat-a.,*** **NAT-C., NAT-M.,** ***nat-p., nat-s., nit-ac.,*** osm., paeon., ***petr.,*** ph-ac., ***phos., plb., psor., phyt.,*** rhus-t., rumx., ***sel.,*** sep., sin-n., ***spig.,*** staph., ***stict.,*** sulph., tell., thuj., ***tub., zinc.,*** zing.

forenoon - ***arg-n.***

morning - aur., ***mang., nat-m.,*** petr., tell.

night - nat-p., nat-s.

profuse, (see copious)

purulent - ail., ***alum.,*** am-c., anac., anan., arg-m., ***arg-n.,*** ars., ***ars-i., asaf.,*** asar., **AUR.,** ***aur-m.,*** aur-m-n., ***bar-m.,*** bell., ***berb.,*** **CALC., CALC-S.,** ***carb-s.,*** cham., chin., chin-a., cic., cina, ***cocc., coloc.,*** **CON.,** cop., cur., dros., eucal., euph., euphr., ***ferr., ferr-ar., ferr-i., ferr-p., graph.,*** guai., **HEP.,** ***hippoz., hydr.,*** ign., ***iod.,*** ip., ipom., kali-ar., **KALI-BI.,** ***kali-c., kali-i.,*** kali-n., ***kali-p.,*** **KALI-S.,** kreos., lac-c., **LACH.,** led., **LYC.,** mag-c., ***mag-m.,*** **MERC.,** merc-i-f., mur-ac., ***nat-a., nat-c., nat-m., nat-p., nat-s., nit-ac.,*** nux-v., ***petr., ph-ac., phos.,*** **PSOR.,** ***puls., rhus-t.,*** sabin., samb., ***sang., sep.,*** **SIL.,** stann., staph., ***stict.,*** still., ***sulph., thuj.,*** **TUB.,** ***uran.,*** zinc.

DISCHARGE, general

purulent,

children - alum., arg-n., ***calc.,*** cycl., hep., iod., ***kali-bi., lyc.,*** nat-c., nit-ac.

forenoon - ail.

left - uran.

morning, early, on blowing the nose - am-c.

right - ***kali-c., puls.***

sudden - aur-m.

weekly - kali-s.

reading aloud, when - verb.

reddening upper lip - ***all-c.,*** ars-i.

reddish - par.

reddish-yellow - calc.

right, nostril, from - crot-c., kali-bi., kali-c., kali-p., lyc., puls., sang.

salty - aral., cimic., ***nat-m.***

taste - aral., tell.

scanty - kali-bi., kaol., mag-c., sin-n.

room, in a - hydr.

singing, when - all-c.

starch, like boiled - ***arg-n., nat-m.,*** nat-s.

stool, during - thuj.

stooping, agg - am-c.

sudden - fl-ac., hydr., kali-bi., lach., nat-c., nat-m., phos., sel., staph., thuj.

suppressed - ail., all-c., alum., ambr., am-c., am-m., ***arg-n., ars., aur.,*** **BRY., CALC.,** ***carb-s., carb-v.,*** caust., cham., ***chin.,*** cina, con., ***dulc., graph., hep., hydr., ip.,*** **KALI-BI.,** ***kali-c., kali-i., lach., lyc.,*** mag-c., mang., **MERC.,** ***nat-a., nat-c., nat-m., nit-ac., nux-v., petr., phos.,*** **PULS.,** samb., sars., ***sep., sil.,*** stann., sulph., thuj.

talking, while - kali-bi., nat-c.

tallow, like, leaving grease spots on linen - ***cor-r.,*** lyc.

thick - acon., aeth., agar., all-c., ***alum.,*** ambr., ***am-m.,*** ant-c., apis, apoc., arg-n., **ARS.,** ***ars-i.,*** ars-m., ***arum-t.,*** arund., asim., ***aur., bad., bar-c., bar-m.,*** bapt., bor., bov., ***calc., calc-f.,*** **CALC-S.,** caps., ***carb-s., carb-v.,*** caust., cinnb., cist., ***coc-c.,*** colch., cop., cor-r., croc., dig., dulc., ery-a., euphr., ferr-i., graph., ***hep., hippoz.,*** **HYDR.,** iod., ip., ***kali-ar.,*** **KALI-BI.,** kali-br., ***kali-c., kali-i.,*** **KALI-P.,** ***kali-s.,*** kreos., **LAC-C.,** lach., lac-ac., lyc., lyss., mag-c., mag-m., mang., med., ***merc.,*** merc-i-f., ***mur-ac., nat-a., nat-c., nat-m., nat-p.,*** **NAT-S.,** nit-ac., nux-v., op., par., petr., ph-ac., ***phos.,*** plb., **PULS.,** ***rhus-t., ran-b., sabad.,*** samb., sanic., ***sang.,*** sars., sel., ***sep.,*** **SIL.,** sin-n., ***spong., stann., staph., sulph., sul-ac., sul-i.,*** syph., ***ther.,*** teucr., **THUJ., TUB.,** zinc.

clear, headache if it ceases - ***kali-bi.***

daytime - ***arum-t.***

post nasal, from - alum., ant-c., ***carb-an.,*** **HYDR., KALI-BI.,** ***nat-p., nat-s.,*** petr., ***phyt.***

then thin - staph.

DISCHARGE, general

thin - aesc., aphis., ars., arum-t., bov., camph., caps., coc-c., colch., crot-c., ***graph.,*** hep., hippoz., hydr., ind., **IOD.,** kali-s., lac-c., lach., lil-t., mez., mur-ac., naja, nat-c., nat-m., ***phyt.,*** rhod., ***sabad.,*** sin-n., ***sulph.***
evening on going to bed -camph.
morning, on rising - camph.
relieving the burning - psor.

viscid, tough - agar., alum., arg-n., ars., **BOV.,** brom., ***cann-s., canth.,*** carb-an., ***caust.,*** **CHAM.,** cinnam., coc-c., ***colch.,*** croc., dros., gran., ***graph.,*** hep., ***hippoz.,*** **HYDR., KALI-BI., KALI-I., KALI-S.,** lac-ac., ***mez.,*** mur-ac., ***nat-a.,*** nat-c., ***par., phos., plb., psor., ran-b., sabad., samb.,*** sanic., sel., ***sep., sil.,*** spig., ***spong.,*** **STRAM.,** ***sulph.,*** sul-ac., ***thuj.***
post nasal, from - alum., calc., canth., **CAPS.,** ***carb-an.,*** **HYDR., KALI-BI.,** ***nat-a., nat-p., phyt.,*** plb., psor., staph., sumb.

watery, (see Coryza, watery) - abrot., ***acon.,*** aesc., ***agar.,*** ail., **ALL-C.,** aloe, alum., ambr., am-c., am-caust., am-m., anag., ant-c., ant-t., aphis., apis, arg-m., **ARS.,** ***ars-i.,*** **ARUM-T.,** arund., asar., ***aur-m.,*** bad., bell., berb., bov., ***brom., bry.,*** bufo, cahin., ***calc.,*** calc-p., calc-s., carb-an., ***carb-v.,*** cast., **CHAM.,** chel., ***chin.,*** chin-a., chlor., cinnb., clem., cob., coca, coc-c., coff., colch., coloc., con., cub., cupr., cupr-ar., ***cycl.,*** dios., dros., dulc., elaps, euph., **EUPHR.,** eup-pur., ferr., ferr-ar., ***ferr-i., fl-ac.,*** gels., **GRAPH.,** guai., ham., ***hydr.,*** ind., ign., **IOD.,** ***kali-bi., kali-i.,*** kali-m., kali-n., ***kali-p.,*** kreos., lac-c., lach., lil-t., lyss., mag-c., mag-m., mag-s., meny., **MERC.,** mez., mur-ac., ***naja,*** **NAT-A., NAT-M.,** nat-s., **NIT-AC., NUX-V.,** osm., ox-ac., pall., par., petr., phos., ***phyt.,*** **PLAN.,** plb., puls., ran-s., rumx., ***sabad., sang., seneg.,*** sep., ***sil.,*** sin-n., spig., squil., staph., ***sulph.,*** sul-ac., **TELL.,** ter., teucr., thuj., zinc.
air, in open - ***ars.,*** calc-s., carb-ac., dulc., euphr., hydr., ***iod.,*** nat-m., **NIT-AC.,** ***phos.,*** **PULS.,** sabad., ***sulph.,*** tell., thuj., zinc.
chorea, with - ***agar.***
cold room, in - carb-ac.
coryza, watery, without - ***agar.,*** alum., am-c., kali-n., ter.
drinking, after - caust.
eye pain, during - euphr., mag-c.
left - am-br., chlor.
night, at - calc-s.
menses, during - am-c.
morning, 5 a.m. - ***ars.***
night - nat-s.
5 a.m. - ***ars***
nosebleeds, after - agar.
right - alum., calc-s., ***kali-bi.,*** nit-ac.
day, during - calc-s.
sudden copious from eyes, nose and mouth - **FL-AC.**
warm room, amel. - calc-s., carb-ac.
washing in cold water amel. - calc-s.

DISCHARGE, general

whey-like - ferr.

white - agar., apis, ***arg-n.,*** ars-s-r., arund., ***aspar.,*** berb., elaps, graph., hippoz., ***hydr., kali-chl., kali-m.,*** kali-p., **LAC-C.,** lyc., merc., **NAT-M.,** nux-v., ***sabad.,*** sanic., sin-n., spig.
daytime - cimic.
left - graph.
lumpy, post nasal, from - zinc.
milky - ***kali-chl.,*** **SEP.**
white of eggs, like - alum., ***aur.,*** kali-m., **NAT-M.,** ***petr.***

yellow - acon., ***alum.,*** am-m., anag., ant-c., ***arg-n., ars., ars-i., ars-m.,*** **ARUM-T., AUR.,** ***aur-m., bad., bar-c., bar-m.,*** bell., ***berb.,*** bov., brom., bufo, **CALC., CALC-S.,** chin-a., chlor., ***cic.,*** cinnb., ***cist.,*** coc-c., ***con., cop.,*** cupr., ery-a., ***ferr-i., graph.,*** **HEP.,** ***hyper.,*** **HYDR.,** ind., ***iod.,*** kali-ar., **KALI-BI.,** ***kali-c.,*** kali-chl., **KALI-I., KALI-P., KALI-S.,** ***lach.,*** lac-ac., lil-t., **LYC.,** ***mag-m.,*** mag-s., mang., med., ***mez.,*** mur-ac., ***nat-a., nat-c., nat-m., nat-p., nat-s.,*** **NIT-AC.,** ***phos.,*** plan., **PULS.,** rhus-t., sabin., sanic., sang., sel., seneg., **SEP.,** ***sil.,*** sin-n., spig., stann., ***stram.,*** **SULPH.,** teucr., ***ther., thuj.,*** **TUB., URAN.**
afternoon - bad.
alternately, watery - kali-s.
daytime - ***arum-t.***
dirty - teucr.
post nasal, from - cinnb.
evening - calc-s., **PULS.,** sulph.
honey, like - **ARS-I.**
left - calc-s., kali-bi., sumb.
morning - berb., **KALI-BI.,** kali-p., ***lach., mang.,*** phos., **PULS.,** sulph.
post nasal, from - ant-c., ***calc-s.,*** cinnb., **HYDR., KALI-BI.,** meny., merc-i-f., ***nat-s., nat-p.,*** puls., ***rumx.,*** sep., spig., sumb.
right - plan.

yellowish-green - ***alum.,*** arund., ***aur-m.,*** bufo, ***calc-f., calc-s.,*** caust., cop., ***hep.,*** **HYDR., KALI-BI.,** ***kali-c., kali-i.,*** lac-c., ***mang., med.,*** **MERC.,** ***nat-c., nat-s.,*** par., ***phos.,*** plan., psor., **PULS.,** rhus-t., sabad., sars., **SEP.,** ***sil.,*** syph., ***ther.,*** **THUJ., TUB.**
stains pillow at night - lac-c.
yellowish-white - calc., merc-i-r.

DISCOLORATION, general

black (see Sooty) - merc.

bluish - agar., aur., crot-h., ***lach.,*** verat-v.
root - calc.
tip - agar., carb-an., ***crot-h., dig.***
wings - hydr-ac.

brown - ***aur.***
across, nose - ***carb-an., lyc.,*** op., sabad., **SEP.,** sulph., ***syph.***
red, in spots - ***aur.***

copper colored spots - ars., cann-s.

DISCOLORATION, general

redness - ***agar.,*** aloe, **ALUM.,** anan., anthr., ***ars.,*** ars-i., ***apis,*** arund., ***aur.,*** aur-m., bar-c., ***bell., bor., calc.,*** cann-s., canth., carb-an., carb-s., carb-v., caust., chel., **CHIN.,** cycl., ferr-m., ***ferr-p.,*** fl-ac., graph., ***hep.,*** hippoz., iod., ***kali-bi., kali-c.,*** kali-i., kali-n., ***lach.,*** led., lith., mag-c., ***mag-m.,*** mag-p., mang., ***merc., merc-c., nat-a., nat-c.,*** nat-m., **NIT-AC., PHOS.,** ***plb.,*** psor., ran-b., rhus-t., sarr., ***stann.,*** **SULPH.,** thuj., ***zinc.***

across - lappa-a.
afternoon - kali-c.
air, in cold open - aloe, ***sulph.***
alcoholics, in - agar., crot-h., ***lach.,*** led.
anger, after - vinc.
children, raw and dirty - merc.
eating on - ***sil.***
erysipelatous - **APIS,** ***rhus-v.***
left side - lac-ac.
evening - mag-c.
excitement, after - vinc.
exertion, after - sil.
freezing, after - ***zinc.***
inside - acon., act-sp., ail., apis, ***ars.,*** bar-c., bell., bry., carb-an., cocc., gels., hep., kali-bi., kali-c., ***kali-i.,*** lach., **MERC.,** nux-v., petros., phel., phos., polyg., stann., **SULPH.**
bloody - ***kali-c.***
left - ***nat-m.,*** stann.
post nasal - ***arg-n.,*** phyt.
right - aur.
septum - alum., bov., bor., ***lil-t.***
left side - aur-m., nat-m.
mercury, abuse of - lach.
painful to touch - bell., ***carb-an.***
right side - aur., lith., ox-ac.
extending to cheek - anthr.
saddle - ictod.
septum - alum., berb., lil-t., sars.
shining - bor., canth., merc., ***ox-ac., phos.***
tip - bell., bor., ***phos.,*** sulph.
wing, right - canth.
spots, in - aur., calc., ***iod.,*** ph-ac., rhod., ***sars.,*** sil., verat.
right side - euphr.
sudden - bell., bor.
swollen - lith., mag-m.
across - ictod.
tender to touch - aur., calc., rhod.
women, in young - bor.

redness, tip - agar., alum., ***aur., bell.,*** bor., ***calc.,*** caps., **CARB-AN.,** ***carb-s., carb-v.,*** chel., clem., con., ***crot-h., kali-c.,*** **LACH.,** led., mag-p-a., merc., nat-m., nicc., ***nit-ac.,*** phos., ***rhus-t.,*** sep., sil., **SULPH.**
alcoholics - agar., carb-an., lach., ***led.***
anger, from - vinc.
begins at tip and spreads - ***ox-ac.***
evening - caps.
menses, during - carb-an.
purple, in cold air - aur., phos.
stooping, when - ***am-c.***

DISCOLORATION, general

redness, wings - all-c., aur., ***caj.,*** calc., chin-a., ***kali-bi., kali-c., mag-m.,*** ph-ac., ***phos.,*** sabin., **SIN-N.**
corners - benz-ac., plb.
edges - coc-c., ***gels.,*** ph-ac.
left - nat-m., stann., zinc.
right - canth., gins., mag-m.

yellow saddle - carb-an., lyc., op., sanic., **SEP.,** sulph.
spots - cadm-s., ***sep.***

DISTENDING, pain - bar-c.

DISTENSION - lyc.

DOUBLE, feels as if she had two noses - merl.

DRAGGING, pain in bones - merl.

DRAWING, pain - agar., anac., ant-c., bapt., bell., camph., canth., caul., caust., clem., colch., crot-h., crot-t., ***hep., kali-n.,*** lach., laur., mez., nat-s., sil.
bones - clem., ***colch.,*** lach., mez.
like a saddle - cinnb., thuj.
extending to eyes - hep.
left - bell., camph.
night - ***crot-h.,*** hep.
right - aesc., lyc., nat-c., zinc.
root - ***calc., carb-v.,*** kali-chl., nat-m., petr., ***phyt.,*** rheum, ***sil.***
extending to tip - rheum
extending upward - nat-m.
rubbing, amel. - nat-c.
wings - caust.

DRAWN up as if by string, tip of nose - crot-c.

DRIPPING, nose - ***all-c., ars.,*** ars-i., arum-t., calc., euphr., graph., nit-ac., nux-v., rhus-t., sabad., sulph.

DRYNESS, inside - abrot., ***acon.,*** aesc., ***agar.,*** ail., ***all-c.,*** aloe, alum., alumn., ***ambr.,*** am-c., am-m., anac., ant-t., ***apis,*** **ARS., ARS-I.,** arum-t., ***arund.,*** atro-s., aur., **BAR-C.,** bar-m., **BELL.,** ***berb.,*** bism., bor., brom., ***bry.,*** bufo, ***cact.,*** **CALC.,** ***calc-s., cann-s.,*** **CARB-S., CARB-V.,** ***caust., cham., chel.,*** chin., chin-a., chlor., cic., cimic., ***cimx.,*** clem., cob., ***coc-c., colch.,*** con., cop., cor-r., crot-t., cund., ***cycl., dig.,*** dios., dros., dulc., ***euphr.,*** eup-per., ferr-i., gamb., gran., **GRAPH.,** hipp., hydr-ac., hydr., ***hyos.,*** hyper., ign., ***iod.,*** ip., kali-ar., **KALI-BI.,** ***kali-c.,*** kali-n., kali-p., ***kali-s.,*** lac-c., lach., lact., laur., lil-t., lith., **LYC.,** ***mag-m.,*** manc., ***mang.,*** meli., meph., merl., ***merc., merc-i-r., merc-i-f., mez.,*** mur-ac., nat-a., nat-c., **NAT-M.,** ***nat-s.,*** nicc., ***nit-ac.,*** **NUX-M.,** ***nux-v.,*** ol-an., op., ***petr.,*** ph-ac., **PHOS.,** ***psor.,*** puls., ***quillaya,*** rat., rhod., ***rhus-t.,*** rhus-v., ***rumx.,*** sabad., **SAMB.,** senec., ***seneg., sep.,*** **SIL.,** sin-n., spig., **SPONG., STICT.,** stram., **SULPH.,** tab., tell., ***ther.,*** **THUJ.,** til., trom., ust., ***verat.,*** vinc., ***wye.,*** xan., ***zinc.,*** zing.
afternoon, 3 p.m. - ***sulph.***
air, in warm - calc-p., kali-bi.
air, open, on walking in the - ant-c., lyc., sulph.
amel. - ***thuj.***

DRYNESS, inside
alternating with discharge, sides - sin-n.
anterior part - spig.
blowing compelled, but no discharge - agar., cimic., **KALI-BI.,** lac-c., ***lach.,*** mag-c., naja, ***psor.,*** **STICT., TEUCR.**
dry sensation, when - bar-c.
breath through mouth, must - meli.
chronic - ambr., am-c., caust., ***sil.***
cool air, amel. - kali-bi.
coryza, with - nit-ac.
discharge, after - bar-c.
evening - apis, cur., dulc., graph., kali-bi., paeon., tell., thuj., trom.
footsweat, after suppressed - **SIL.**
forenoon, in open air - ***sulph.***
headache, during - dulc.
heat, with - cann-s., clem.
indoors - nux-v., thyr.
left - calc-s., cob., chel., cist., merl., ***sep.,*** sin-n.
morning - apis, ***calc.,*** ferr-i., ***lyc.,*** mag-c.
bed, in - aloe, paeon.
waking, on - am-c., ***calc.,*** carb-an., kali-bi., lyc., mag-c., sulph., thuj.
walking, while - hydr.
night - am-m., ***bor.,*** cact., ***calc.,*** calc-s., lyc., mag-c., nux-v., phos., ***sil.,*** spig., thuj.
moist, during day - calc.
prevents sleep - ***bor.***
wakes her - ammc., mag-c., stict.
outside - carb-an., caust.
painful - calc., **GRAPH.,** kali-bi., ***phos.,*** sep., ***sil., stict.,*** sulph
coryza, during - sulph.
post nasal - ***acon., aesc.,*** alumn., calc-p., carb-ac., carb-v., ***cinnb., coc-c.,*** fago., graph., lyc., merc-c., nat-c., ***nat-m.,*** nux-m., onos., rumx., ***sep., sil.,*** sin-n., stram., ***wye.,*** zinc., zing.
air, in open - nat-c.
morning - carb-ac., nat-m.
night - cinnb.
right - gamb., kali-bi., petr.
sensation of - mez., nat-m., ***petr.,*** phos., seneg., **SIL.**
blowing nose - bar-c.
stuffed sensation, with - trinit.
swallowing, amel. - sin-n.
tip - carb-an.
warm, room - ***kali-bi., kali-s., thuj.***

DYSPNEA, in nose - ***ars.,*** kreos., lach., puls., sabad., sulph.

ECZEMA - ***ant-c.,*** caust., ***cist.,*** rhus-t., ***sep.,*** sulph.
fissure of right wing - ***thuj.***

EDEMA - **APIS,** bapt.

ELECTRIC, sparks, sensation of, at left wing with desire to rub - carb-ac.

ENLARGING, sensation - cann-s.

EPISTAXIS, (see Nosebleeds)

ERUPTIONS - agar., agn., ***alum.,*** am-c., am-m., anac., ant-c., arn., ars., ars-i., arum-t., ***aur.,*** aur-m-n., bar-c., bar-m., bell., bor., bov., brom., bry., cadm-s., calc., canth., caps., ***carb-an.,*** carb-s., ***carb-v.,*** **CAUST.,** cham., chel., chin., cina, ***cist., clem.,*** con., crot-t., dulc., ***elaps,*** euphr., graph., guai., hep., ign., iod., iris, kali-ar., ***kali-c.,*** kali-n., kali-s., lach., laur., ***led.,*** lyc., mag-c., mag-m., meny., ***merc.,*** mez., mur-ac., ***nat-a.,*** **NAT-C.,** nat-m., **NAT-P.,** nicc., ***nit-ac.,*** nux-v., olnd., par., petr., **PH-AC.,** phos., plat., plb., ***puls.,*** ran-b., ***rhus-t.,*** sars., sel., **SEP., SIL.,** ***spig.,*** staph., stront-c., **SULPH.,** sul-ac., syph., tarax., thuj., verat., viol-t., zinc.
acne - am-c., ars., ***ars-br.,*** aster., bor., calc-p., caps., cann-s., **CAUST.,** clem., elaps, graph., kali-br., nat-c., sel., ***sep.,*** sil., ***sulph., thuj.,*** zing.
around, nose - alum., am-c., ***ant-c.,*** bar-c., bov., calc., ***caust.,*** dulc., elaps, mag-m., ***nat-c.,*** par., **RHUS-T.,** ***sep.,*** sil., sulph., sul-ac., tarax., zinc.
blotches - bell., iod.
burning - alum., apis, caust., graph., nat-c., nat-m., ol-an., phos.
comedones - dros., ***graph., nit-ac.,*** sabin., sel., ***sulph.,*** sumb., ***thuj., tub.***
coppery - ***carb-an.***
corners, of - anac., carb-v., dulc., euphr., led., mang., mill., plb., ***rhus-t.,*** thuj.
crusty, nose - ail., ***alum., aur.,*** aur-m-n., ***calc.,*** carb-an., carb-s., carb-v., ***caust.,*** chin., ***cic.,*** graph., hyper., ***iod., led., lyc., mag-m.,*** mang., **MERC.,** ***merc-i-r., nat-m., nit-ac.,*** ph-ac., ran-b., rat., sars., ***sep., sil.,*** spong., ***staph., sulph.,*** syph.
around - led.
below - sulph.
extend down lip with deep fissure, very sore and sensitive to touch - ***hep.***
inside and on - ***ant-c.,*** aur., bor., **BOV.,** carb-an., chel., cic., crot-t., **GRAPH.,** ***hep., kali-c.,*** **LACH.,** ***lyc.,*** mag-m., ***merc., merc-c., nat-s.,*** phos., **PULS.,** rat., sars., **SEP.**
margins - ***calc-s.,*** kali-bi., nit-ac., phos., sulph.
of nostrils, bloody on - ***phos.***
tip - ***carb-an.,*** carb-v., **CAUST.,** ***nit-ac.,*** sep., ***sil.***
under nose - bar-c., ***kali-c., rhus-t.,*** sars., ***sil.***
wing, near the - aur., ***merc-i-r., nit-ac.,*** petr., rhus-t.
excoriating, nose - agar., bov., caust., graph., phos., sil.
inside - am-m., mag-c., phel., podo., sars., sel., sil.
left - bell., bor., calc., cob., sars.
right - calc., carb-an., dulc., gamb., kali-n., lach.
itching - apis, carb-v., iod., lyc., nat-c., nit-ac., pall., phel., sil., squil., ***sulph.***
below - sars.

ERUPTIONS,
moist, alae - thuj.
nose - aur-m-n., carb-v., **GRAPH.,** nat-c., thuj.
septum - vinc.
nodular, nose - bar-m., nat-m.
painful, nose - calad., caps., cor-r., mag-c., phos., sel., sep.
stinging - apis, squil.
touched, when - chin., clem., kali-c., petr., ph-ac.
pimples, nose - agar., alum., **AM-C.,** ***anac.,*** arum-d., aur., bar-c., ***bell.,*** bor., brom., **CALC.,** caps., cann-s., carb-an., carb-v., **CAUST.,** clem., cub., dulc., euphr., ***fl-ac., graph.,*** guai., ***kali-c.,*** kali-i., kali-n., lach., ***lyc.,*** mag-arct., mang., ***merc., nat-c., nat-m.,*** ol-an., ox-ac., pall., petr., ***ph-ac., phos.,*** podo., plan., plb., ***psor.,*** rhus-t., sars., sel., ***sep., sil., sulph.,*** **SYPH.,** ***teucr.,*** thuj.
about - carb-v., nat-m., par.
below - caps., dig.
burning - alum., aphis., canth., kali-n.
when touched - canth.
corners, in - dulc., tarax.
dorsum, on, with inflamed base - fl-ac.
inside - arn., calad., calc., carb-an., graph., guai., kali-c., petr., ox-ac., sil., tub.
nostrils - chin., sep.
left - calc., dulc., graph., kali-c.
left, below - dig.
painful only when muscles of face and are moved - calc.
right - aphis., ox-ac., phos., rat.
oozing - ol-an.
red - ant-c., aur., calc-p., ph-ac., plan.
root - bell., caust., ***led.***
septum - arg-n., asc-t., calad., chin., nat-m., ol-an., ***teucr.***
below - nat-m.
oozing - ol-an.
side - aster., sil.
left - caps., nat-c.
right - alum., euphr., lach., ox-ac., sars.
small and hard - agar.
tip - am-c., asaf., **CAUST.,** coc-c., cund., ***lyc.,*** nit-ac., pall., ph-ac., spong.
tip, bleeding when pressed - pall.
sore - ***lyc.***
white - carb-v., kali-c., ***nat-c.***
wings - bar-c., chin., nat-m., phos., tarax., zing.
left - fl-ac.
perforation, size of a pea - fl-ac.
pustules, nose - ***am-c.,*** ant-c., asc-t., bell., bov., bufo, clem., cocc., euphr., hippoz., ***iris,*** mag-c., merc., nat-c., nit-ac., petr., ph-ac., ***phos.,*** plb., podo., sars., tarax., ***tub.***
corner - mang.
inside - arn., hippoz., ***tub.***
left - kali-n., nat-c.
right - con., cund., fl-ac., mag-c., mang., sars.
root - clem.

ERUPTIONS,
pustules,
septum - am-c., ***anac.,*** hippoz., lycps., petr., psor.
perforation, with - hippoz.
right - anac., sars., tarax.
tip - am-c., clem., kali-br., lyc., mag-c.
under the nose - arn., bor., bov., mag-c., squil.
wings - anac., euphr., mang., tarax.
left - nat-c.
right - petr.
red, on - aur., bell., carb-s., crot-t., lach., ph-ac., samb., syph., thuj.
root, of - caust.
scurfy, nose - aur-m-n., iod., nat-m., sil.
tip - caust., nit-ac., sep.
under - bar-c.
septum - bar-c., bov., calad., caps., crot-t., ol-an., psor., teucr., thuj., vinc.
tip - acon., ***aeth.,*** am-c., anan., asaf., carb-an., carb-v., ***caust.,*** clem., kali-n., lyc., nit-ac., pall., ph-ac., ***sep.,*** sil., spong.
tubercles, nose, side of - nat-c.
root, of - sep.
wings, of - hippoz.
under, nose - arn., bor., bov., sars., squil.
wings, on - ars., aur-m., carb-v., chin., cor-r., dulc., euphr., fl-ac., hipp., ***merc-i-r.,*** nat-m., ***nit-ac.,*** petr., rhus-t., sep., ***sil.,*** spig., thuj.

ERYSIPELAS - am-m., ***apis, aur.,*** cadm-s., ***calc., canth.,*** hippoz., graph., plb., rhus-t., stram.
redness, of - **APIS,** ***rhus-v.***

EXCORIATED, (see Discharges)
corners of - chin-a.
inside, of - nat-m

EXOSTOSES - merc., phos.

EXPANSION, sensation of, in nasal passage while walking in open air - carb-ac., carb-an.
post nasal - ***fl-ac.***

FAN-like, (see Motion)

FOOD, sensation of, post nasal, in - ***nit-ac.,*** petr., ***sil.***
swallowing, on - ***nit-ac., sil.***

FOREIGN, body, sensation - am-m., calc., con., hep., kali-bi., nat-c., psor., ruta, sep.
as from a - calc-p., con.
root - spig.
upper part - am-m.

FORMICATION, (see Itching) - aesc., arg-m., arn., merc., nat-m., ran-b., rhus-t., ***sulph.,*** teucr., thuj.
dorsum - con.
inside - am-c., aur., carb-v., con., hep., med., mez.
root - ***teucr.***
tears flow, until - cham.
tip - con., kali-n., mosch.

FRECKLES - phos., **SULPH.**

FROST-bitten - ***agar., zinc.***
easily - agar., ***zinc.***

FULLNESS, sense of - aesc., agar., all-c., asaf., **BAPT.,** ***cham.,*** echi., **KALI-I.,** lac-ac., ***lac-c.,*** laur., par., ***phos.,*** puls., ***senec.***
around nose - calc.
frontal sinuses, from inflammation - ***kali-bi.***
left nostril, high up - phos.
root - aesc., cann-i., cund., ***gels., kali-bi.,*** lac-c., nat-p., ***par.,*** phos., sang., **STICT.**
extending to neck and clavicle - gels.

GANGRENE - ***ars.,*** hippoz.

GNAWING, pain - fago., merc., **SIL.**
above, nose - calc-ac., merc., ph-ac., phos., raph.
nasal bones, in - bufo, **KALI-I.**
outer part, as of something acrid - plat.
root - calc., merc., raph.
tip - berb.

GRIPING, pain - kali-n.
tip - kali-n.
wings - kali-n.

GUMMY nostrils - bor.

HAIR, of nostrils falls out - calc., ***caust., graph.,*** iod.

HARDNESS, of - aur-m-n., calc., calc-f., canth., carb-an., con., **KALI-C.,** thuj.
mucous, surface, of - iod.
wings, of - aur-m., ***thuj.***
left, of - alum., ***thuj.***

HAY fever, (see Allergic rhinitis, Coryza) - agar., ail., **ALL-C.,** ***ambro., aral.,*** **ARS.,** ***ars-i., arum-t.,*** **ARUND.,** aspar., bad., benz-ac., ***brom.,*** calc., camph., ***carb-v.,*** chin-a., chrom-k-s., ***cocain., con., cupr-a.,*** cycl., ***dulc.,*** euph-pi., ***euphr., gels.,*** graph., grind., hep., iod., ***just.,*** kali-bi., kali-c., ***kali-i., kali-p.,*** kali-s., lach., linn-u., lyc., mag-m., **MED.,** meph., merc., merc-i-f., ***naja,*** naph., **NAT-M., NAT-S.,** nux-v., phel., phos., **PSOR.,** ***puls., ran-b.,*** ros-d., rhus-t., **SABAD.,** ***sang.,*** sang-n., senec., sep., sin-a., **SIN-N.,** ***sil.,*** skook., ***stict.,*** sul-ac., sul-i., sulph., syc-co., teucr., tong., trif-p., **TUB.,** ***wye.***
annual, prophylactic - ars., kali-p., ***psor.***
asthmatic breathing, with - ambro., ambro., **ALL-C., ARS.,** ***ars-i., bad., carb-v.,*** chin-a., ***dulc., euphr.,*** **IOD.,** kali-i., lach., linn-u., ***naja,*** nat-c., ***nat-s., nux-v.,*** op., ***sabad.,*** sang., ***sin-n.,*** sil., stict., sulph.
august, in - **ALL-C.,** dulc., gels., naja
until the fall - sin-n.
autumn, in - wye.
chronic, coryza - ail., alum., am-c., anac., ***apis, ars.,*** ars-i., berb., **BROM.,** bry., ***calc.,*** calc-p., ***canth.,*** coch., ***colch.,*** cist., coloc., ***cycl.,*** eucal., fl-ac., graph., hydr., kreos., ***lyc.,*** mang., nat-a., nat-c., nat-m., ol-j., phos., ***psor.,*** puls., ***sang.,*** sars., sep., ***sil.,*** spig., spong., ***sulph., tub., teucr.***
dryness of mucus membranes of nose, mouth and throat, with - wye.
grass, newly mown - dulc.

HAY fever
spring, in - ***all-c., ars., gels.,*** lach., naja, ***sabad.,*** sang., tub.

HEAT, in - ***apis,*** arn., bar-m., ***bell.,*** calad., cann-i., cann-s., canth., ***cham.,*** **CHIN.,** clem., colch., cor-r., crot-h., daph., euphr., eup-pur., ***graph.,*** guare., hell., ***hep.,*** hyos., ***kali-bi.,*** kali-c., lyc., mag-m., merc-i-r., naja, ***nux-v.,*** psor., rhus-r., ruta., sang., stront-c., thuj., vinc., verat.
air expired feels hot - **KALI-BI.,** rhus-t.
bleed, as if would - cann-s.
breath seems hot - **KALI-BI.,** ptel., rhus-t.
burning - ars., carb-an., chin., kali-fer., kali-i., merc., sang., sil.
cold to touch - arn.
fever, in - arn.
left - cina, coff., nat-m.
below - rhus-t.
nostrils - cina.
hot - ***acon.,*** aesc., lyc., sep., zinc-i.
right - ***merc-i-r.***
root - **KALI-BI.**
sneezing, when - com.
tip - bell., caps., con., mag-arct., ***nat-m.***
evenings - ***caps.,*** sin-n.
warm weather, in - bell.

HEAVINESS - am-c., carb-v., ***caust., cham.,*** colch., ***crot-h.,*** euphr., ***ind.,*** kali-bi., merc., ***phyt.,*** samb., ***sang.,*** sil., ***stann.***
as of a weight hanging down - ***kali-bi.,*** merc.
bones, in - colch.
root - bism., cinnb., ***sang.,*** stann., ther.
sinuses - stann.
stooping, when - am-m., sil.

HERPES, nose - acon., **AETH.,** aloe, alum., aur., bell., ***calc.,*** chel., clem., conv., dulc., graph., gins., iod., lyc., mur-ac., ***nat-c., nat-m., nit-ac.,*** ph-ac., ***rhus-t., sep.,*** sil., spig., sulph.
around, nose - sep., sulph.
itching - nit-ac.
wings, of - dulc., nat-m., nit-ac., phys., sil.

INFLAMMATION, nose - acon., agar., alum., apis, ***arn., ars., asaf.,*** asar., ***aur.,*** aur-m., ***bell.,*** bor., ***bry.,*** cadm-s., ***calc.,*** cann-s., ***canth.,*** carb-an., ***caust.,*** coch., cist., ***con., crot-h.,*** ferr-i., ferr-pic., ***fl-ac.,*** graph., ***hep., hippoz.,*** ip., kali-i., kali-n., **LACH.,** mang., med., medus., ***merc.,*** merc-c., ***merc-i-r.,*** naphtin., ***nat-c., nat-m., nit-ac.,*** nux-v., ped., phel., **PHOS.,** plb., ***puls.,*** ran-b., rat., ***rhus-t., sep.,*** sil., **SULPH.,** verat.
alcoholics, in - ***ars.,*** bell., ***calc.,*** hep., ***lach.,*** merc., ***puls., sulph.***
bones - anan., asaf., **AUR.,** ***aur-m.,*** **HEP.,** merc., ***phos.,*** still.
inside - ***agar.,*** am-m., ***bell.,*** bor., ***bry.,*** canth., ***calc.,*** chel., cham., cist., cocc., con., goss., ***hep., kali-bi., kali-i.,*** mang., merc., ***nat-m., nux-v.,*** **PHOS.,** polyg., ran-b., rhus-t., sil., stann., ***sulph.,*** verat.
left - cist., goss., ***nat-m.***
margins - bar-c., mez.

INFLAMMATION, nose
post nasal, acute - ***acon.,*** camph., cist., gels., kali-bi., menthol, ***merc-c.,*** nat-a., wye.
chronic - aur., calc-f., elaps, fago., ***hydr., kali-bi.,*** kali-c., merc-c., pen., sep., ***spig., stict.,*** sulph., thuj.
mucus, with dropping of - ***alum.,*** am-br., ant-c., ars-i., aur., calc-sil., ***cor-r.,*** echi., glyc., ***hydr.,*** irid., ***kali-bi.,*** kali-m., lem-m., merc-i-r., nat-c., ***pen., phyt., sang-n.,*** sin-n., ***spig.,*** stict., teucr., ther., wye.
right - **AUR.,** merc-i-r.
septum - alum., psor., sars.
tip - ***aur.,*** bell., bor., bry., ***carb-an.,*** **CAUST.,** crot-h., kali-c., ***kali-n., lach.,*** lyc., merc., nicc., ***nit-ac.,*** phos., ***sep.,*** sulph., ***rhus-t.***
wings - nit-ac., sulph.
inflammation, sinus, (see Sinusitis)

ITCHING - ***agar.,*** ail., alum., am-c., am-m., apis, ***arg-n.,*** arn., ars-m., **ARUM-T.,** arund., asc-t., ***aur.,*** aur-m., aur-s., bar-c., bell., berb., bor., ***bov.,*** brach., brom., ***calc., calc-p., calc-s.,*** camph., caps., carb-ac., carb-s., ***carb-v.,*** card-m., **CAUST.,** ***cham., chel.,*** chin., cinnb., **CINA,** cob., coc-c., colch., com., con., ***crot-c.,*** ferr-m., fl-ac., grat., hell., hydr., ign., ip., jatr., kali-ar., ***kali-c., kali-n.,*** kali-p., kali-s., lac-c., ***lyc.,*** lyss., ***mag-m.,*** med., ***merc.,*** merc-sul., merl., ***mez., nit-ac., nux-m., nux-v.,*** olnd., ***ph-ac.,*** phos., puls., rat., samb., sanic., sep., ***sil., spig.,*** squil., staph., stry., **SULPH.,** ***teucr.,*** ther., thuj., tub., uran., urt-u., vinc., zinc.
bones - spong.
burning - ***agar., aur.***
dorsum - alum., chin., con., samb., spig.
eating, while - jatr., lach.
evening - carb-v., coloc., kali-n., lach., puls., sil.
extending to pharynx - rumx.
inside - ***agar.,*** ambr., am-c., am-m., anac., ***arg-m., arg-n.,*** arn., ***ars.,*** ars-h., asar., **ARUND.,** ***aur.,*** aur-m., bar-m., bell., benz-ac., berb., bor., brach., brom., bufo, ***calc.,*** calc-p., camph., ***caps., carb-v.,*** card-m., **CAUST.,** ***cham.,*** chel., **CINA,** ***colch.,*** con., corn., cupr., eug., euphr., gamb., gran., graph., ***hep.,*** hyper., ign., kali-ar., ***kali-bi.,*** kali-c., kali-n., ***kali-s.,*** kalm., lac-c., laur., ***lyc.,*** lyss., mag-c., mag-m., med., merl., ***merc.,*** mosch., mur-ac., nat-c., ***nat-m.,*** nit-ac., **NUX-V.,** ol-an., petr., ph-ac., phos., plat., ***puls., ran-b.,*** ran-s., rat., rhod., ***sabad.,*** sang., ***sel.,*** seneg., sep., ***sil.,*** sin-n., ***spig., stict.,*** stram., ***stront-c.,*** **SULPH.,** syph., tab., ***teucr.,*** ther., ***thuj.,*** uran., urt-u., ust., ***zinc.,*** zing.
left - arg-m., asc-t., bell., benz-ac., brom., calc., camph., carb-v., card-m., caust., cob., coloc., grat., kali-bi., mag-c., mang., med., ol-an., rhus-r., spong., sars., syph., zinc.
left, then right - brom.

ITCHING,
inside, right - ***all-c.,*** am-c., card-m., con., dros., hydr., kali-c., kali-n., nat-m., ***teucr.,*** zinc.
right, then left - aur-m., card-m., verat-v.
left - bad., carb-v., chel., cob., grat., hell., laur., nat-m., pall., rhus-r., sars., staph.
menses, after - ***sulph.***
night - am-m., arg-n., ***gamb.***
nosebleed, before - am-m., arg-m.
nostrils - carb-v., caust., con., ph-ac., plat.
painful - mag-c.
post nasal - arg-m., kali-p., lyc., ***ran-b., wye.***
right - fl-ac., gins., hydr., merl., sars., spig., ***teucr.***
root - con., inul., merc., olnd.
rubs - agar., bell., bor., caust., sabad.
before attacks - bufo.
child starts out of sleep and - lyc.
constantly - arg-n., bor., **CINA,** med., sil.
septum - benz-ac., bry., ***iod., kali-bi.***
tip - agn., ars-m., calc-p., carb-an., carb-s., **CAUST.,** ***chel.,*** colch., ***con.,*** laur., kali-n., merc., mosch., mur-ac., ol-an., paeon., ***petr.,*** ph-ac., rat., rheum, rhus-v., ***sep., sil.,*** sulph.
wings - agar., alum., aur., **CAUST.,** calc., cann-s., carb-v., ***cina,*** merc., nat-m., nat-p., ***nat-s.,*** sars., sel., sil., sulph.
left - ars-m., bad., bell., hell., laur., mag-c., nat-m., staph.
right - fl-ac., laur., spig., staph., thuj.
worms, from - **CINA,** spig.

JERKING, pain - con.
from above down - hyos.
left - caps.
right - zinc.
sudden in root - hyos.

KNOBBY, tip - ***aur.***

LACERATING, pain - cadm.

LACERATION, of - ***calen.,*** hyper.

LIPOMA - ***sulph.***

LIQUIDS, come out through the nose on attempting to swallow - anan., **ARUM-T.,** aur., ***bar-c.,*** bell., bism., canth., ***carb-ac.,*** caust., cupr., cur., gels., hyos., ign., kali-bi., ***kali-ma.,*** **LAC-C., LACH., LYC.,** ***merc., merc-c., merc-cy., nat-m.,*** op., petr., ***phyt., plb.,*** puls., sil., ***sul-ac.***

LUMP, post nasal - cist., hydr., kali-bi., ***lach.,*** nat-m., phos., sep., spig., stict., sulph., teucr., zinc.
post nasal, as if - aesc., cist., hydr., kali-bi., ***lach.,*** nat-m., phos., sep., spig., stict., sulph., teucr., zinc.

LUPUS - alumn., ars., ***aur-m.,*** calc., ***caust.,*** cic., hydr., ***hydrc., kali-bi.,*** kali-chl., **KREOS.,** merc., ***phyt.,*** rhus-t., sulph., thuj., tub., x-ray.
exedens - cist., ***hydrc.,*** jug-c., phyt., thuj.
left side - caust., ***kreos.***
wing, on - ***aur-m., hydrc.***

LYING, agg. - puls.

MEMBRANE, mucous, destroyed - am-m.
detached - ***elaps***
gangrenous - ***ars.***

MOIST, after eating - caust.

MOTION, wings, fan-like - ammc., **ANT-T.,** ars., bapt., bell., ***brom.,*** bry., ***chel.,*** chlor., cupr., diph., ferr., gad., hell., ***iod.,*** kali-bi., kali-br., **LYC.,** merc-i-f., ol-j., **PHOS.,** phys., pyrog., rhus-t., ***spong.,*** sul-ac., thuj., zinc.
palpitation, with - lyc.
snoring, with - diph.
constant, of - ***ammc.,*** bapt., chlor., ***kali-bi., ol-j.***
pneumonia, in - ***ammc.,*** **ANT-T.,** ***kreos.,*** **LYC.,** ***phos., sulph.***

NECROSIS - ***phos.***

NODOSITIES - **ARS., AUR.,** bar-m., merc-i-r., ***sulph.***
root, painless - sep.
surrounded by red swelling, like acne., rosacea - cann-s.

NOSEBLEEDS, epistaxis - abrot., acet-ac., **ACON.,** ***agar.,*** ail., ***all-c.,*** aloe, alum., ***alumn.,*** **AMBR., AM-C.,** am-m., anac., anag., anan., **ANT-C.,** ant-s., ant-t., apis, aran., ***arg-m.,*** arg-n., **ARN.,** ***ars., ars-i.,*** asaf., asar., astac., aster., aur., ***bapt., bar-c., bar-m.,*** **BELL.,** benz-ac., ***berb.,*** bism., bor., **BOTH., BOV.,** ***brom., bry., bufo,*** cadm-s., **CACT., CALC., CALC-P., CALC-S.,** camph., ***cann-s.,*** canth., ***caps., carb-an.,*** **CARB-S., CARB-V.,** card-m., **CAUST.,** ***cham.,*** **CHIN.,** chin-a., ***chin-s.,*** cic., ***cina, cinnb.,*** cinnam., clem., cocc., coff., colch., coloc., ***con., cop.,*** cor-r., **CROC.,** crot-c., **CROT-H.,** ***cupr., dig., dros., dulc.,*** echi., ***elaps, erig.,*** eupi., euphr., ferr., ferr-ar., ferr-m., **FERR-PIC.,** gamb., gels., ***glon., graph.,*** **HAM.,** ***hecla., hep., hydr.,*** **HYOS.,** ign., indg., ***iod.,*** **IP.,** kali-ar., ***kali-bi., kali-c.,*** kali-chl., **KALI-I.,** ***kali-n.,*** kali-p., kali-s., ***kreos., lac-ac.,*** **LACH.,** lachn., ***led.,*** lil-t., lob., ***lyc., lyss., mag-c.,*** mag-m., mag-s., **MED., MELI.,** ***meny.,*** meph., **MERC.,** ***merc-c., mez.,*** **MILL.,** ***mosch.,*** mur-ac., nat-a., ***nat-c.,*** nat-h., ***nat-m., nat-p.,*** nat-s., **NIT-AC.,** ***nux-m., nux-v.,*** oena., op., ox-ac., par., ***petr., ph-ac.,*** **PHOS.,** pic-ac., plat., plb., ***prun.,*** **PULS.,** ran-b., ***rat., rhod., rumx.,*** ruta., sabad., **SABIN.,** samb., ***sang.,*** sarr., ***sars.,*** **SEC.,** senec., seneg., ***sep., sil.,*** sin-n., spig., ***spong.,*** squil., ***stann.,*** staph., stict., stram., stront-c., **SULPH.,** ***sul-ac.,*** tarax., ***tarent., ter.,*** teucr., ***thuj.,*** til., ***tril.,*** **TUB.,** ***ust.,*** vac., valer., ***verat.,*** vinc., viol-o., vip., zinc.
afternoon - ***ant-t., calc-p.,*** carb-an., cham., indg., kali-n., ***lyc.,*** mag-arct., ***nat-s., sulph.,*** tab., thuj., trom.
3 p.m. - ***sulph.***
4 p.m. - ***lac-c., lyc.***
alcoholics, in - ***carb-v.,*** hyos., ***lach.,*** nux-v., **SEC.**
alternating, with spitting of blood - **FERR.**
amel. mental symptoms - bor., lach.

NOSEBLEEDS, general
amenorrhea, with - ***bry., cact.,*** con., ham., lach., ol-j., ***phos., puls.,*** sep.
anemia, with - bry., chin., ferr., hydr., kali-c., nat-n., ***puls.***
anger, from - ***ars.***
bleeders - bov., crot-h., lach., ***phos.***
blood, type of
acrid - kali-n., nit-ac., sil.
bright - ***acon.,*** am-c., ant-t., arn., ars., bapt., bar-c., **BELL.,** bor., bry., calc., canth., ***carb-ac.,*** carb-an., carb-v., ***chin.,*** cic., ***crot-c.,*** dig., dios., dros., ***dulc., elaps, erig.,*** ferr., ***ferr-p.,*** graph., **HYOS., IP.,** kali-n., kreos., ***lach.,*** laur., ***led.,*** mag-m., merc., mez., ***mill.,*** nat-a., nat-c., nat-s., nux-m., ***ph-ac.,*** **PHOS.,** puls., ***rhus-t.,*** sabad., ***sabin.,*** sec., sep., sil., stram., stront-c., sulph., ***tub.,*** zinc.
clotted, coagulated - acon., ***arg-n.,*** arn., bapt., **BELL.,** bry., cann-i., canth., carb-an., ***carb-s.,*** caust., **CHAM., CHIN.,** con., ***croc.,*** dig., dios., dulc., ***ferr., ferr-m.,*** hep., hyos., ign., **IP.,** kali-n., kreos., ***lach.,*** lyc., lyss., mag-c., ***merc.,*** nat-h., ***nat-m., nit-ac.,*** nux-v., ph-ac., ***phos.,*** **PLAT.,** ***puls.,*** **RHUS-T.,** sabin., **SEC.,** sep., stram., stront-c., ***sulph., tarent., tub.***
livery - sabin.
nose, continually full of - ferr.
quickly - croc., merc., nit-ac., puls., rhus-t.
slowly - ham., lach.
dark - acon., am-c., ant-c., ***arn.,*** asar., bapt., ***bell.,*** bism., bry., calc., canth., ***carb-s.,*** **CARB-V.,** ***cham.,*** chin., ***cina,*** cinnb., cocc., con., **CROC.,** ***crot-h.,*** cupr., dig., dros., ***elaps,*** ferr., graph., ***ham.,*** ign., ***kali-bi., kali-n., kreos.,*** **LACH.,** led., lyc., mag-c., mag-m., ***merc.,*** mill., mur-ac., nat-h., ***nit-ac., nux-m.,*** **NUX-V.,** ***ph-ac.,*** phos., plat., ***puls.,*** **SEC.,** sel., ***sep., stram.,*** sulph., sul-ac., ***tarent.***
dark, and thin - carb-an., ***carb-v.,*** **CROT-H., HAM.,** ***lach., nit-ac.,*** **SEC.,** ***sul-ac.***
fluid - arn., ***carb-v.,*** **CROT-H.,** ***erig., ham.,*** **SEC.,** ***sul-ac.,*** ter.
hot - acon., ***bell.***
offensive - ***sec.***
pale - arn., bar-c., bell., ***carb-ac.,*** carb-an., ***carb-v.,*** crot-h., dig., dulc., ***ferr., graph.,*** hyos., ***kreos.,*** lach., lachn., led., phos., puls., rhus-t., ***sabad.,*** sabin., sec., ***sulph.,*** ter.
stringy - bapt., **CROC.,** ***cupr.,*** kali-bi., ***kreos., lach.,*** mag-c., ***merc.,*** naja, ***sec.,*** sep., verat.
warm - dulc.
blow, from a - acet-ac., **ARN.,** ***elaps,*** ferr-p., ***ham.,*** **MILL.,** phos., ***sep.***
blowing, the nose, from - ***agar.,*** alum., ***alumn.,*** ambr., am-c., am-m., anac., ant-c., arg-m., arg-n., **ARN.,** asar., asc-t., aur., ***aur-m.,*** bapt., ***bar-c.,*** bor., ***bov.,*** brom., ***bry.,*** bufo, ***calad.,***

NOSEBLEEDS, general
blowing, the nose, from - calc., calc-p., canth., caps., carb-ac., ***carb-an.,*** **CARB-S.,** ***carb-v.,*** caust., chin., cinnb., ***croc., crot-h.,*** cupr., dros., elaps, ferr., ferr-i., ferr-p., ***graph.,*** hep., indg., iod., kali-c., kali-p., kali-s., **LACH.,** led., lyc., mag-c., mag-m., meny., merc., mez., nat-a., nat-c., ***nat-m.,*** nat-p., nat-s., nit-ac., ***nux-v.,*** par., **PH-AC., PHOS.,** ***puls.,*** ran-b., rhus-t., ruta., sabad., sars., ***sep.,*** sil., spig., spong., stront-c., **SULPH.,** teucr., ***thuj.,*** zinc.
evening - bor., graph., sep.
left - am-c., bapt., kali-n., sars.
morning - ***agar.,*** arn., ***bov.,*** bor., ***caust.,*** **LACH.,** nat-c., nit-ac., ***puls.,*** sulph., thuj.
night - arg-n., graph., nit-ac.
playing of wind instruments, due to - rhus-t.
right - arg-n.
wind instruments, from blowing, - ***rhus-t.***
boring, with finger - ***ferr-m., lach., sil.***
children, in - abrot., bell., calc., chin-s., ***croc.,*** **FERR., FERR-P.,** ferr-pic., ***ham.,*** merc., ***mill.,*** nat-n., **PHOS.,** ***sil., ter.,*** tub.
chill, during - bell., bry., calc., kreos., puls., rhus-t.
after - ***eup-per., hep.***
in place of - nat-m.
clotted - ham.
coffee, agg. - nux-v.
convulsions, during - caust.
coryza, during - graph., nit-ac., sulph.
cough, with - acon., arn., bell., bry., carb-an., carb-v., cina, cupr., **DROS.,** dulc., ferr., ferr-i., ferr-p., hyos., kali-bi., ***indg.,*** iod., ip., kreos., lach., ***led.,*** merc., mosch., mur-ac., nat-m., nit-ac., nux-v., phos., ***puls.,*** rhus-t., sabad., sep., sil., spong., ***sulph.,*** sul-ac.
night - nat-m.
whooping cough - **ARN.,** ***bry., cina, cor-r., crot-h.,*** **DROS., IP.,** ***led., merc., mur-ac., nux-v.,*** **PHOS.,** spong., stram.
after the paroxysm - cina, indg.
crying, while - ***nit-ac.***
after - nit-ac.
diphtheria, in ars., ***carb-v., chin., crot-h., hydr., ign., kali-chl., lach., merc-cy., nit-ac.,*** phos.
dinner, during - kali-bi., spong.
after - am-c., arg-m., zinc.
ear, noises, with - bell., chin., graph., nux-v.
easily - ferr-p., **PHOS.**
amel., which - tub.
eating, after - am-c., arg-n., kali-c., ***zinc.***
amel. - tarax.
elderly, people - ***agar., carb-v.,*** chin., ferr., ham., ***phos.,*** **SEC.,** sul-ac., verat.
emotions, from - carb-v., **PHOS.**
evening - ***ant-c.,*** bor., bufo, ***carb-s., coff., colch.,*** dros., ***ferr.,*** gamb., ***graph.,*** kali-bi., ***lach., lyc.,*** mez., ***ph-ac., phos., puls.,*** sars., ***sep., sulph., sul-ac.,*** thuj., til.
6 p.m. - coff.
exertion, from - **ARN.,** carb-v., ***croc., rhus-t.***

NOSEBLEEDS, general
fever, during - bry., carb-v., ***ferr-p.,*** ham., meli., phos.
flushes, after - ferr.
habitual - ***mill.,*** ferr., ferr-p., nat-n., **PHOS.,** sil.
hawking - rhus-t.
headache, during - **ACON., AGAR.,** alum., ambr., am-c., aml-n., ant-c., asaf., bell., ***bry.,*** cadm-s., carb-an., cham., chin., ***cinnb.,*** crot-h., dig., dulc., ferr-p., ham., kreos., lach., mag-c., ***meli.,*** mill., nux-v., rhus-t., tub.
after - am-c., ant-c., bell., carb-an., croc., lach., mag-arct., meli., nux-v., rhus-t., sabin., **SEP.**
heated, when he becomes - thuj., thyr.
hemoptysis, with - ***ham.***
hemorrhoids, with - **SEP.**
flow of, suppressed - ***nux-v.,*** sulph.
hot, weather - **CROC.**
itching, with - ***arg-n., arn.,*** bell., ***carb-v.,*** kali-bi., lach., ***rhus-t.***
after - ***am-m.***
followed by - ***hydr.***
jarring, from - ***carb-v.***
left - am-c., am-m., aml-n., bapt., berb., caust., dios., dulc., ***ferr.,*** hydr., ***kali-n.,*** merc., rhod., sars., tarent.
left, after a bath - calc-s.
left, to right - ham.
lifting, agg. - ***rhus-t.***
lying, when - hura, puls.
measles, agg. - bry., puls., sabad.
menopause - arg-n., bell., bry., ***ham.,*** **LACH.,** nux-v., ***puls., sep., sulph., sul-ac.***
menses, during - acon., **AMBR.,** ***bry.,*** dig., gels., ham., nat-c., ***nat-s.,*** puls., ***sep., sulph.,*** verat.
after - sulph.
before - ***bar-c., ip.,*** **LACH.,** ***nat-s.,*** nux-v., ***puls., sulph.,*** thea., ***verat.,*** vib.
instead of - ***bry.,*** dulc., graph., ***ham., lach.***
intermittent - nat-c.
intermits, when flow - ***eupi.***
profuse - acon., ambr., calc., croc., sabin.
scanty - bry., corn., graph., ***phos.,*** puls., sep.
suppressed - acon., bell., **BRY.,** ***cact.,*** calc., ***con., croc., gels.,*** ham., hyos., kali-i., **LACH.,** nit-ac., ol-j., ***phos.,*** **PULS.,** ***rhus-t., sabin.,*** senec., ***sep.***
morning - acon., agar., ***agn.,*** aloe, **AMBR.,** am-c., ant-c., apis, arn., ***arum-t.,*** bell., berb., bor., **BOV.,** ***bry.,*** bufo, ***calc., calc-s.,*** canth., caps., **CARB-AN.,** ***carb-s., carb-v., caust., chin.,*** coff., colch., croc., dros., ***ferr.,*** ferr-p., ***graph.,*** **HAM.,** hep., hipp., hyos., kali-bi., ***kali-c.,*** kali-p., kali-s., kreos., ***lac-ac., lach., mag-c., meny.,*** merc., ***nat-c., nat-m.,*** **NIT-AC.,** ***nux-v., petr., phos.,*** puls., rhus-r., ***rhus-t.,*** sabin., sec., ***sep., stann.,*** **SULPH.,** thuj.
6 to 7 am - ***chin.***

NOSEBLEEDS, general
morning,
8 am - ***bry.***
9 a.m. - kali-c.
10 to 12 a.m. - carb-v.
bed, in - ambr., bar-c., bov., ***caps., carb-v.***
amel. - mag-m.
rising, after - agar., berb., **BRY., CHIN.,** coff., ferr., sep., stann., thuj.
stooping, on - ***ferr.***
waking, on - aster., bell., ***bry.,*** mag-c., stann.
motion, agg. - carb-v., ***rhus-t.***
night - aloe, ant-c., arg-m., arn., ***bell.,*** bry., calc., caps., carb-an., **CARB-V.,** con., cor-r., croc., graph., hyos., kali-chl., mag-m., mag-s., ***merc.,*** mill., nat-m., nat-s., **NIT-AC.,** ***puls., rhus-t.,*** sars., ***verat.***
3 a.m. to 4 a.m. - bry.
10 p.m. - graph.
toward morning - apis
noon - kali-bi., tarax.
numbness, with - acon., bell., med.
oozing - crot-h., ham., phos.
overheating, from - sep., thuj.
ozaena, in - sang.
periodic - carb-v., chin., croc., kali-c., puls.
persistent - camph., ***carb-v., croc., crot-h., ferr.,*** led., mill., mur-ac., **PHOS.,** ***sulph.,*** tril.
perspiration, with - **PHOS.**
forehead, on - crot-h.
plethoric, patients - abrot., ***acon.,*** nux-v.
pregnancy - cocc., phos., ***sep.***
purpura, hemorrhagica, with - ***crot-h., ham., lach.,*** **PHOS.,** rhus-t.
right - am-c., arg-n., bry., calc., cic., con., cupr., gamb., ind., kali-bi., kali-c., kali-chl., mag-c., sars., ***verat.***
to left - coca, cor-r.
rubbing, after - phos.
salivation, with - hyos.
sight, with loss of - indg., ox-ac.
singing, after - hep.
sitting, while - carb-an., sul-ac.
sleep, during - bell., bov., ***bry., crot-c.,*** graph., **MERC.,** ***merc-c.,*** nat-s., ***nit-ac., nux-v.,*** puls., sulph., ***verat.***
smell, lost - ***ip.***
sneezing, when - am-c., bapt., ***bov., con., indg., mag-c.,*** rumx., ***sabad.***
after - zinc.
spasms, with - mosch.
spring, in the - con.
standing, agg. - sul-ac.
stool, during - carb-v., coff., phos., rhus-t.
straining at, while - ***coff., rhus-t., phos.***
straining, after - ***carb-v.***
stooping, when - dros., ***ferr., nat-m., nux-v.,*** ol-j., ***rhus-t.,*** sil.
after - carb-v.
swallowing - lac-c.
sweat, on forehead, with - crot-h.

NOSEBLEEDS, general
talking, while - lac-c.
touch, from slight - cic., hydr., ind., ***sec.***
typhoid fever, during - **ARN., BAPT.,** ***bry., chin-s.,*** **CROT-H.,** gels., kali-p., **LACH.,** ***ph-ac., rhus-t., ter.***
vertigo, with - bell., bry., carb-an., lach.
after - carb-an.
before - carb-v.
vicarious - ***bry.,*** **HAM.,** ***lach.,*** mill., **PHOS.,** puls.
vomiting, with - sars.
after - ars.
walking, while - elaps, lyc., nat-c.
air, in open - lyc., nat-c.
warm, becoming - carb-v.
room - ***puls.,*** sep.
washing face, from - am-c., ant-s., **ARN.,** ***calc-s., dros.,*** kali-bi., ***kali-c.,*** phos., tarent.
feet - carb-v.
watery, discharge, after - agar.
weakened, by - ***chin.,*** corn., ferr., ferr-p., sec., verat.
wet, after being - ***dulc., puls., rhus-t.***
wine, from - ars.
women, young - **PHOS., SEC.**

NUMBNESS - acon., ars-h., ars-m., asaf., bell., cadm-s., ferr., jug-c., kali-bi., lyc., med., nat-c., nat-m., nux-m., olnd., phys., plat., ran-b., sabad., samb., sang., sil., spig., stict., viol-o.
bones, of - aml-n., arn., ***asaf.***
right - plat.
inside - nat-m.
nosebleeds, with - acon., bell., med.
one-sided - ***nat-m.***
tip, of - gels., viol-o.

OBSTRUCTION - acon., aeth., ***agar.,*** ail., ***all-c., alum., ambr.,*** am-br., ***am-c.,*** am-caust., ***am-m.,*** anac., ant-c., apis, apoc., arg-m., ***arg-n.,*** **ARS., ARS-I.,** ars-m., **ARUM-T.,** asaf., **AUR.,** ***aur-m.,*** bad., bapt., bar-c., ***bar-m., bor., bov.,*** brom., bry., bufo, cact., cadm-s., calad., **CALC.,** ***calc-s.,*** cann-s., **CAPS.,** ***carb-ac., carb-an.,*** **CARB-S., CARB-V.,** cast., **CAUST.,** ***cham.,*** chel., ***chin.,*** chin-a., chlor., cic., cimic., cina, cob., coc-c., coff., ***coloc.,*** **CON.,** cop., cor-r., crot-t., ***cupr., dig.,*** dios., dros., ***dulc.,*** echi., ***elaps,*** eup-per., ferr-i., fl-ac., gels., **GRAPH.,** grat., ***ham., hell., hep., hydr.,*** ign., ***iod., ip., kali-ar.,*** **KALI-BI.,** ***kali-c., kali-chl., kali-i.,*** kali-n., ***kali-p.,*** kali-s., kalm., kreos., lac-c., lac-ac., ***lach.,*** laur., **LYC.,** mag-c., ***mag-m., mang.,*** med., ***merc., merc-c., mez.,*** mosch., mill., ***mur-ac., nat-a.,*** **NAT-C., NAT-M.,** nat-p., ***nat-s.,*** nicc., **NIT-AC.,** ***nux-m.,*** **NUX-V.,** ol-an., op., par., ***petr.,*** phel., ph-ac., **PHOS.,** ***phyt.,*** pic-ac., plat., plb., ***psor.,*** **PULS.,** ran-b., raph., rat., ***rhod., rhus-t., rumx., sabad.,*** **SAMB.,** ***sang.,*** sars., sec., sel., ***seneg., sep.,*** **SIL.,** spig., ***spong., stann.,*** staph., ***stict.,*** stram., ***sulph., sul-ac., sumb.,*** syph., tab., tell., **TEUCR.,** thuj., verb., vinc., ***zinc.,*** zing.
afternoon - mag-c.

OBSTRUCTION,
air, in the open agg. - arg-n., ***nat-m., rhod., rhus-t., sulph.***
agg. cold, from - dulc.
amel. - arg-n., kali-c., ***phos.***, phyt., pic-ac., rhod., rhus-t., ***sulph.***
alternates, with discharge - ***ars.***, bell., mag-c., mang., nat-m., sang., ***sil.***
alternating sides - acon., am-c., bor., **LAC-C.**, mag-m., mez., nux-v., ***phos.***, phyt., plat., pyrog., rhod., rhus-t., sabad., sin-n., sulph., upa.
anterior, part - arg-m.
blowing, after - carb-v.
blood pressure, from high - iod.
breathes through mouth - am-c., kali-c., lyc., mag-c., mag-m., nux-v., samb.
adenoids removal, after - kali-s.
dreams, during - am-c., lyc., nux-v., samb.
children - am-c., ambr., apoc., ***ars.***, asc-t., aur., kali-bi., ***lyc.***, med., ***nux-v.***, osm., phos., sabad., ***samb., syph.***
obstinate - med.
nursing infants - ***aur., kali-bi.***, **LYC.**, **NUX-V.**, ***samb.***, teucr.
chronic - bry., **CALC.**, ***con.***, fl-ac., lem-m., sars., sel., ***sil., sulph.***, teucr., ***thuj.***
obstinate - med., sars., thuj.
cold, after every - ***sil.***
coryza, amel. - sil.
day - mag-c., ***naja.***
diphtheria, in - am-c., hydr., ***kali-m., lyc., merc-cy.***
discharge, with - ars., bry., calc., chin., cic., graph., ***kali-bi., lach.***, mag-m., merc., nit-ac., nux-v., osm., puls., sil., ***thuj.***
fluent, with - arum-t.
fetid, with - arum-t.
drink, inability to - lach.
eating, after - nat-c., spig.
evening - ant-c., ***carb-v.***, cimic., ***cina***, euphr., ***iod., kali-bi., kali-c.***, kalm., ***lyc., mag-m.***, **PULS.**, ***ran-b.***, sep., staph., ***teucr., thuj.***
footsweat, suppressed, from - **SIL.**
forenoon - carb-an., sars.
headache, with - calc., lach., phos., sang., thuj.
high places, in - nat-m.
hot, wet applications amel. - dulc.
lachrymation, with - bor.
leaflet, as from a - ign., kali-i., mur-ac.
left - alum., am-c., anac., ***arum-t.***, asar., chin-a., cimic., carb-an., carb-v., chlor., mag-c., ***mag-m.***, mag-s., nit-ac., nux-m., rhod., sec., sep., ***sin-n.***, stann., stram., ***thuj.***, uran.
with water dropping out - bov.
lying, while - bov., caust., chin-a., mag-m., ***nux-m.***, puls., rhus-t.
menses, before - ***mag-c.***

OBSTRUCTION,
morning - aeth., apoc., arn., arum-t., bell., bov., ***calc., carb-an.***, con., dig., ferr-i., ***hep., kali-bi.***, kali-i., lach., lith., ***lyc.***, mag-c., ***mag-m., nat-a.***, nit-ac., par., ***phos.***, rhod., sep., ***sil.***, trom.
fluent during day - ***sil.***
waking, on - aeth., apoc., ***calc.***, carb-an., kali-bi., ***kali-i.***, nit-ac., phyt., sil.
night - ***agar.***, **AM-C.**, am-m., arg-n., ***ars., bov., calc., caust., ferr-i.***, glon., ip., ***kali-p.***, **LYC.**, ***mag-c., mag-m., nat-a., nat-c.***, nicc., nit-ac., **NUX-V.**, phel., phos., ***samb.***, sec., sep., sil., stict., tell., zinc-i.
head, from uncovering, during day - ***nat-m.***
wakes him - ***mag-c.***, nit-ac., ***phyt.***, stict.
wakes him, 3 a.m. - ***phyt.***
nosebleed, with - acon., calc., puls.
one-sided - alum., bell., chel., coc-c., ferr-m., ***hep.***, ign., lac-c., ***lach.***, mez., ***nux-v.***, phos., phyt., plat., ***pyrog., rhod.***, sabad., ***sin-n., staph., sulph.***, sul-ac., teucr., vinc.
alternately - ***gels., kali-bi.***, lac-c., manc., mez., nux-m., phyt., plat., rhod., sabad., sin-n.
side he is lying, on - ***rhus-t.***
post nasal - anac., ***calc-s.***, hydr., iris, kali-bi., kali-i., med., nat-a., petr., puls., sin-n., staph., ***thuj.***, zing.
pus, with - ***calc.***, chin-a., lach., led., ***lyc.***, nat-c., puls., sep., **SIL.**
night - **LYC.**
reading aloud, while - kali-bi., sil., teucr., verb.
riding, in a carriage - asaf., ***phyt.***
right - alum., bapt., ***bor.***, brom., camph., carb-v., chel., croc., ***gels.***, kali-bi., kali-c., kali-n., lac-c., lil-t., mag-c., ***merc.***, nat-a., nicc., phyt., ***sars.***, sep., stict., ***sulph.***, **TEUCR.**, thuj., xan.
fluent, left - alum.
then left - ***bor.***, brom., chel.
rising, from bed amel. - nux-m.
room, amel. in - dulc.
root, at - arg-n., **ARS.**, ***kali-i.***, lith., ***lyc.***, med., mur-ac., par., sin-n., stict., sulph.
painful - arg-n., ***kali-bi.***
speaking, reading aloud, while - kali-bi., sil., teucr., verb.
sleep, during - ***am-c.***, ars., **LYC.**, ***stict.***
nose, obstruction, wet weather agg. - calc., ***dulc.***, elaps, lem-m., ***mang.***
sneezing, when, nostrils stick together - carb-an.
after - brom., carb-v., phos., sul-ac.
stool, after - hep.
stooping, when - agar.
sudden - sep.
swelling, from - cadm.
syphilitic - phyt.
talking, while - nat-c., sil.
walking, in open air amel. - ***kali-c., puls.***

OBSTRUCTION,
warm, damp weather - ***kali-bi.***
room - **ANT-C.**, arg-n., ***ars-i.***, calc-p., carb-v., cycl., ***hydr.***, **IOD.**, kali-c., **KALI-I.**, op., phos., pic-ac., plat., **PULS.**, ran-b., sabad., ***sulph.***, ***thuj.***
watery, discharge, with - am-m., calc., mag-m., nit-ac.
wet, weather agg - calc., ***dulc.***, elaps, lem-m., ***mang.***

obstruction, sensation of - agar., arum-t., **AUR.**, ***aur-m.***, bar-c., cann-s., ***cham.***, cob., cupr., eucal., ferr-i., ***ham.***, ***hydr.***, kali-bi., laur., mag-m., meny., merc-c., nat-a., nat-c., nat-s., **NUX-V.**, stann., stram., thuj., zinc., zing.
post nasal - hydr., lac-ac.
right nostril - aur., teucr.
sinuses - stann.
watery discharge, with - am-m., **ARS.**, arum-t., bov., brom., calc., cham., chin., ***cupr.***, graph., kali-i., mag-m., ***merc-c.***, nit-ac., nux-v., sec., sin-n.

ODORS, imaginary and real - ***agn.***, ***anac.***, apoc-a., ars., aur., ***bell.***, calc., colch., cor-r., dios., euph-a., graph., ign., ***kali-bi.***, mag-m., manc., ***merc.***, nit-ac., ***nux-v.***, op., par., ***phos.***, ***puls.***, sang., ***sep.***, sulph., valer., zinc-chr., zinc-m.
acid - alum., bell.
agreeable - ***agn.***, puls.
almonds, bitter - laur.
animals, in back part of nose - con.
bad in the morning - kreos., puls.
beer, sour - ***bell.***, thuj.
blood, of - nux-v., psor., sil.
brandy - aur.
burning, something - anac., aur., graph., nux-v., sulph.
tinder in the morning - anac.
burnt, hair - graph., sulph.
feathers - bapt.
horn - sulph.
sponge - anac.
cabbage, of - benz-ac.
cancerous - cadm-s., sulph.
catarrh, as of - graph., puls., sulph.
chalk, food smells like - sulph.
cheese, of - ***nux-v.***
chicken, dung - anac.
coffee, of - puls.
corpse, like - vichy-g.
coryza, in post nasal - con.
cucumbers, like a - chin., vichy-g.
drinks, smell putrid - ***nux-v.***
dust, of - benz-ac., mag-arct.
earth, as of - calc., verat.
eggs, like rotten - mag-arct.
feces, of - ***chel.***
fermented, beer, of - agn., bell., thuj.
fetid - arg-n., asaf., ***aur.***, **BELL.**, ***calc.***, ***carb-s.***, ***chel.***, chlor., chr-ac., crot-t., elaps, ***graph.***, iod., **KALI-BI.**, kreos., lac-c., meny., merc., nit-ac., nux-v., **PAR.**, ph-ac., **PHOS.**, ***plb.***, ***puls.***, sarr., ***sep.***, sil., **SULPH.**, verat.

ODORS, imaginary and real
fetid, blowing nose - aur.
breathing through when - nit-ac.
fish-brine, of - agn., ***bell.***, colch., elaps, thuj.
blowing nose - bell.
food, of - nat-m.
garlic, sensitive to - sabad., ***thuj.***
gunpowder - ***calc.***, manc.
honey, everything smells like - ***apoc-a.***
horse-radish - raph.
lime, and whitewash - mag-arct.
lobster, when expectorating - lyc.
manure, of - anac., bry., ***calc.***, mag-c., verat.
milk, of, nauseating - bell.
musk - agn.
musty, discharge - nat-c.
nauseating - canth., meny.
offensive - agar., anac., ars., asaf., benz-ac., ***calc.***, ***calc-s.***, ***chel.***, ***cina***, dros., elaps, ham., mag-c., mez., nat-p., ***nit-ac.***, par., ***phos.***, sep., **SULPH.**, verat.
blowing on - ***aur.***, kali-bi., **SULPH.**
evening - nit-ac.
hollow teeth, from - mez.
lying down - nit-ac.
morning - kreos., nat-p., puls.
oil, burning - raph.
old, catarrh - ars., ***graph.***, merc., ***puls.***, **SULPH.**
onions - cor-r., ***manc.***, plat.
roasted - sang.
peas, soaked - sulph.
pigeon, dung - anac.
pine-smoke - ***bar-c.***
pitch - ars., con.
pus, of - arg-n., gamb., seneg., sulph.
night - arg-n.
putrid - anthr., asaf., aur., ***bell.***, benz-ac., calc., cob., graph., ***kali-bi.***, kreos., mag-arct., meny., merc., ***nit-ac.***, par., phos., **PULS.**, seneg., sep., ***sulph.***, verat.
blowing on - ***aur.***, kali-bi.
bread and milk smell - par.
eggs, of - aur., bell., ***calc.***, kali-bi., mag-arct., meny., merc., nux-v., phos., sep., ***sulph.***
food, and milk, smell - ***nux-v.***, par.
food, smells - sulph.
morning on waking - kreos.
remain for a long time - dios.
sickly - aur., cob., nit-ac., ***nux-v.***, sil.
smoke of - bar-c., cor-r., mag-p-a., ***sulph.***, verat.
smoked, ham - colch.
snuff - graph., **SULPH.**
soot, of - graph.
sour - alum., bell.
bread smells - bell.
morning, early - alum.
sulphurous - anac., ***ars.***, calc., graph., ***nux-v.***, plb., sulph.
sweetish - aur., nit-ac., nux-v.
syrup, dislikes - sang.
tallow - valer.
tar - ars., con.

ODORS, imaginary and real
tinder - anac., nux-v.
tobacco - puls.
ulcerous - cadm-s., seneg.
whiskey - aur.

OILY - calc., ***hydr., iris,*** puls.

OPEN, sensation, post nasal, on walking in open air - fl-ac.

OZAENA - all-s., ***alum., am-c., arg-n., ars.,*** **ASAF., AUR., AUR-M.,** ***aur-m-n.,*** **CALC.,** ***calc-f., calc-p., carb-ac., carb-an., carb-s.,*** chr-ac., ***con.,*** crot-h., ***cur., elaps,*** fl-ac., ***graph.,*** **HEP.,** ***hippoz., hydr.,*** **KALI-BI., KALI-I.,** ***kali-p., kali-s., lach.,*** mag-m., **MERC.,** ***merc-c., merc-i-f.,*** mez., ***myric., nat-a., nat-c., nat-m.,*** nat-p., ***nat-s., nit-ac.,*** ol-j., ***petr., ph-ac.,*** phos., ***phyt.,*** **PULS.,** ***sang.,*** **SEP., SIL.,** ***stict., sulph., syph., teucr., ther.***
acrid - lyc., mag-m.
crusty - mag-m.
menses, during - graph.
suppressed itch, after - calc.
syphilitic - **AUR.,** ***aur-m., asaf.,*** crot-h., ***fl-ac.,*** **HEP.,** kali-bi., ***kali-i., merc.,*** **NIT-AC.,** ***phyt.,*** **SIL.,** ***syph.***

PAIN, nose - acon., aesc., agar., agn., alum., anac., ant-t., ***arg-m., arg-n., ars.,*** ars-i., ars-m., ***arum-t.,*** arund., asaf., asar., aspar., **AUR.,** ***aur-m.,*** bar-c., bell., benz-ac., ***bor.,*** brom., bufo, ***calc.,*** cann-i., carb-an., ***carb-s.,*** carb-v., chin., cimic., ***cinnb.,*** coff., ***colch.,*** coloc., cor-r., ***crot-h.,*** cycl., ***elaps, euphr.,*** fl-ac., glon., **GRAPH.,** grat., guai., hell., **HEP.,** ign., ***iod.,*** kali-ar., **KALI-BI., KALI-I.,** kali-n., kali-s., kalm., lach., laur., lyc., lyss., mag-c., mag-m., ***merc., merc-i-f.,*** nat-a., nat-m., nat-s., ***nit-ac.,*** olnd., petr., phos., phyt., prun., **PULS.,** ran-b., rheum, ruta., sang., sars., ***sep.,*** **SIL.,** spig., ***sulph.,*** teucr., ***thuj.,*** verat.
air, on inhaling - ***aesc.,*** am-c., ***ant-c.,*** brach., bufo, gins., ***hep.,*** hydr., mag-s., osm., ox-ac., phos., ***psor.,*** sep., thuj.
open amel. - acon., ***all-c.,*** hydr., iod., nux-v., ***puls.,*** tell.
alternating sides - kali-i., ***lac-c.,*** lach., mez., nux-v., ***phos.,*** phyt., rhod., ***sin-a., sin-n.,*** sulph.
blowing the nose - aur., euphr., **GRAPH.,** ***hep.,*** iod., kali-bi., kali-c., kali-i., ***led.,*** mang., ***nat-m.,*** nit-ac., ***sil.,*** teucr.
bones - ***aesc.,*** arg-n., ***ars.,*** **AUR.,** aur-m-n., benz-ac., ***carb-an.,*** cast-eq., colch., cor-r., cycl., guai., **HEP.,** indg., **KALI-BI.,** ***kali-i.,*** kali-n., lach., led., merc., mez., mosch., nat-m., onos., phos., ***puls.,*** **SIL.,** ***sulph.,*** thuj., verat.
daytime - ***sulph.***
pulsating - anan., **KALI-I.**
right side - aesc., aur.
breathing, strongly, while - am-c., bor., op.
cartilage, junction of - **KALI-BI.**
pressure, from - calc.
coughing, when - nit-ac.

PAIN, nose
dorsum - agn., canth., chin., ***hep.,*** kali-bi., kalm., ***phos.***
right nostril - lyc.
dryness, from - calc., **GRAPH.,** ***kali-bi., phos., sep., sil., stict.,*** sulph.
evening - alum., ars-m., cycl.
extending, to
brain, to, like rays - ***sil.***
chin, to - chin.
downward from above - arn.
ear, to - berb., elaps, fago., psor.
swallowing, on - berb., elaps, fago., psor.
eyebrows, to - inul.
eyes, to - **HEP.,** lyc.
forehead, to - bufo, calc., kali-i., nat-s., sil.
head, to - kali-bi., kali-i.
malar bone, to - kali-bi., thuj.
neck, to - gels.
occiput, to - acon., agar., kali-c.
post nasal, to - bapt.
root, of nose, to - ***coloc.,*** ferr-p., ***kali-i.,*** lach., sang.
from, along orbital arch to external angle of left eye - kali-bi.
temples, to - kali-bi., mag-c.
face-ache, with - spig.
flea-bites, like - asc-t.
forenoon - phos.
headache, with - **AGAR.,** ferr., glon., hep., merc., mez.
inside - **GRAPH.,** ill., led.
left - alum., arg-m., ars-m., arum-m., bell., carb-v., nat-m., rhod., sep., stann.
lying down, agg. - ***bor.,*** puls.
amel. - cupr.
menses, before - con.
motion, agg - cupr., lyc.
night - am-m., **AUR.,** bell., cor-r., lach., phos.
sleeplessness, with - cor-r.
nosebleed, with - mill., rumx.
nostril, anterior angle, of - cocc.
left - bell.
interior angle of - coff.
one-sided - am-m., hep., ign., nux-v., phos., phyt., ***sabad.,*** sil., sin-a., sin-n.
operations, after - calen., ferr-p.
paroxysmal - plat., zinc.
post nasal - ***elaps,*** kali-ma.
as if air streamed in on coughing or talking - mag-s.
belching, after - sulph.
blowing, nose - ***carb-v.***
coughing - ***carb-v.***
swallowing - ***carb-v.***
pressure, agg. - chin., con., cupr-ar., led.
amel. - agn., kali-bi.
glasses, of, agg. - arg-n., chin., cinnb., con., cupr-ar., fl-ac., kali-bi., ***merc.,*** phos.
pulsating - ars., bor., ***coloc.,*** kali-bi., ***kali-i.,*** ph-ac., plat.

PAIN, nose
right - am-m., brom., camph., con., mez., psor., spig., teucr.
right, to left - euphr.
root, in - ***acon.,*** agn., ***alum., ant-t.,*** arg-n., ***ars., arum-t.,*** arund., aspar., ***bapt.,*** calc., cann-i., ***carb-v., chin.,*** chion., cimic., cinnb., ***con.,*** crot-t., ***cupr., dig.,*** dys-co., ***elaps,*** euphr., ***ferr.,*** ferr-p., ***gels., glon.,*** hell., **HEP.,** hyos., ***ign.,*** iod., **KALI-BI.,** kali-i., lach., ***merc., merc-i-f., mez., nat-a., nat-m., nat-s.,*** nicc., par., ***petr., phos., phyt.,*** plat., ***puls., sang.,*** sarr., sars., ***sep., sil.,*** stict., sulph., ther., thuj., verat-v., zinc.
extending to
ears on swallowing - elaps
forehead - ***mez.,*** sabal.
occiput - acon., agar.
headache, with - **AGAR.,** ***cupr.,*** ferr., glon., hep., **KALI-BI.,** ***merc., merc-i-f., mez.***
menses, before - ***con.***
paroxysmal - arn., hyos., zinc.
pulsating - kali-bi., sarr.
vomiting, after - dig.
rubbing, amel. - bell., nat-c.
septum - alum., caust., plb., kali-bi., sel., ***sil.***
sinus, pulsating - sil.
right, night - am-m.
ulcerative - sil.
sneezing, on - ***nit-ac.***
spectacles, agg. - cinnb., lyc.
pressure of glasses, agg. - arg-n., chin., cinnb., con., cupr-ar., fl-ac., kali-bi., ***merc.,*** phos.
talking, agg. - canth.
tip - bar-c., bell., carb-an., ***cist.,*** kali-n., lyc., plb.
menses, during - carb-an.
touch, on - sulph.
touch, on - alum., ***aur.,*** bar-m., bell., bry., canth., carb-an., caust., colch., ***hep.,*** kali-bi., kali-n., led., lyc., ***mag-m.,*** mag-s., **MERC.,** nat-c., ***nat-m.,*** **NIT-AC.,** petr., ph-ac., ***phos.,*** rhus-t., sabin., ***sil.,*** sulph., stann.
weather, changing of - ars.
wings - bar-c., calc., gels., hep., stram.
left - alum., zinc.
touch, on - alum., stann.
just above - lach.
right - arg-n.
from motion - calc.
touch - mag-m.
touch - mag-m., stann.
winter agg. - am-c., ars., sulph.

PARCHMENT, sensation as if nose were - ***kali-bi.,*** sulph.

PERFORATION, septum, of - alum., kali-bi., kali-i., merc., merc-c., sil., syph.

PERSPIRATION, on - bell., cimx., cina, laur., ***nat-m.,*** rheum, ruta., ***tub.***
cold, around nose - **CHIN.,** rheum.
morning - cimx.

PICKING, the nose with fingers (see Boring) - **ARUM-T., CINA,** ***con., cop.,*** hell., hyper., lac-c., **LYC.,** nat-p., nit-ac., nux-v., ph-ac., **PHOS., SIL., TEUCR.,** thuj., zinc.
affected parts, the - mag-m.
bleeds, until it - **ARUM-T., CINA,** ***con., lach., phos., sil.***
constant desire - **CINA,** ***con.,*** lil-t., rumx., stict., symph., ter.
brain affections, in - **CINA,** ***con., hell.,*** **SULPH.**

PINCHED - ***camph., kali-bi., lyc., spig.,*** spong., verat., verat-v.

POINTED - anan., ***ant-t., ars.,*** **CAMPH.,** ***carb-v.,*** cocc., ***cupr., hell., lach.,*** myos., nux-v., ***ph-ac.,*** plb., rhus-t., spong., staph., **VERAT.**

POLYPS - agra., ***all-c.,*** alumn., ***apis,*** arum-m., aur., bell., cadm-s., **CALC.,** calc-i., ***calc-p., carb-s.,*** caust., ***con.,*** form., ***graph.,*** hecla., hep., hydr., ***kali-bi.,*** kali-i., ***kali-n., kali-s., lem-m.,*** lyc., med., merc., merc-c., ***merc-i-r.,*** nit-ac., ***phos.,*** puls., ***psor.,*** **SANG.,** ***sang-n., sep., sil.,*** staph., ***sulph.,*** syc-co., **TEUCR., THUJ.,** wye., zinc-chr.
bleeds easily - calc., calc-p., ***phos.,*** thuj.
left - alumn., apis, calc., merc-i-r.
post nasal - ***teucr.***
right - ***caust., kali-n., sang.***

POST nasal, ailments of - cinnb., elaps, ***hydr., kali-bi., lyc., merc., merc-c.,*** merc-i-r., ***nat-c., nat-m.,*** phos., rumx., sep., ***spig., staph.,*** sulph., ther., thuj., zinc-i.

PRESSING, pain - acon., agn., agar., alum., asaf., ***aur-m., bor.,*** calc., ***cinnb., colch.,*** coloc., con., ***cor-r.,*** cycl., grat., ***kali-bi.,*** kali-c., kalm., laur., mag-c., mag-m., merc., olnd., phos., prun., puls., ran-b., ***sil., sulph.,*** teucr., verat.
above nose, changing to tearing, followed by dulness in back of head - ambr., cupr.
alternately sticking - laur.
as if, brain were forcing its way out - am-c., ***bor.***
nostril were pinched - ***kali-bi.,*** lachn., spong.
bones - agar., arn., bell., carb-v., cinnb., cycl., **KALI-BI.,** lyc., ***sulph.,*** verat.
bones, evening - sulph.
bones, pressed asunder - colch., cor-r., laur., ***puls.,*** prun.
dorsum like a stone - agn., coloc., kalm.
as from spectacle - ***cinnb.***
pressure amel. - agn.
downward - mag-s., merc.
through right side - bor.
extending to side - chin.
lying agg - ***bor.***
post nasal - lyc.
right - lyc., plat.
root, in - acon., aesc., agar., agn., all-c., all-s., alum., am-c., anan., ***ant-t.,*** arum-t., aspar., aster., ***bapt.,*** bar-c., benz-ac., bism., ***brom.,*** calc., cann-s., caps., carb-v., cimic., chel., ***chin.,*** cimx., ***cinnb.,*** coloc., cund., ***cycl., dulc., gels.,*** grat., hell., hep.,

PRESSING, pain
root, in - hipp., ***hyos., iod.,*** **KALI-BI.,** ***kali-c.,*** kali-i., ***kali-p.,*** kalm., ***lac-d.,*** lyc., mag-s., manc., mang., meny., ***merc.,*** mez., ***nat-a., nat-m.,*** nux-v., olnd., onis., par., phos., plat., prun., ptel., ***puls., ran-b.,*** raph., rhus-v., ruta, sang-n., sarr., ***sep.,*** spong., stict., ther., ***thuj., zinc.***
extending to side of forehead - chin.
followed by nosebleed - bry., ***dulc.,*** kali-bi., ***ruta.***
followed by vertigo - ***zinc.***
nosebleeds, with - ruta.
pressure, amel. - ***kali-bi.***
stupefying - acon., cann-s., olnd., zinc.
tip - lact.

PRESSURE of glasses agg. - arg-n., chin., cinnb., con., cupr-ar., kali-bi., ***merc.,*** phos.

PROTUBERANCES - ***iod., nit-ac.,*** syph.

PUFFINESS - bell., caust., kali-c., merc., nat-c., ph-ac., plb., puls., rhus-t., sep.

PULLED, as if - ***nat-c.***

PULLING, sensation in left side as if a hair were pulling - plat.

PULSATION - acon., ***agar.,*** all-c., arg-m., **ARS.,** bor., brom., ***coloc.,*** cor-r., **KALI-I.,** mag-m., sil.
left - arg-m.
root - bor., **KALI-BI.,** phos., sarr.
tip - ph-ac.

QUIVERING - agar., chel., mosch., stront.
left side - am-c.
root, extending to cheek - calc-s.
visible - mez.

RATTLING - alum.

RAWNESS, pain - ***aesc.,*** ail., all-c., ars., ars-h., **ARUM-T.,** bar-m., calc., cop., echi., ***hydr.,*** kali-ar., ***lach.,*** lec., mag-m., ***merc-c., mez.,*** nat-m., ***sep., sil., sul-i.***
blowing, when - hep.
after - aesc., ant-c., cist., ***hep.,*** nat-a., ***nit-ac.***
coryza, during - aesc., **ALL-C., ARS.,** ail., ant-c., sep., uva., ***sil.***
inspiration, during - ***aesc.,*** agar., ***ant-c., sep.***
left - ***sep.***
margin - sulph.
morning - mag-m.
nostrils - ***ail., arum-t.,*** bar-c., **BOV., BROM.,** cast., calc., ***calc-p.,*** iod., **LACH.,** ***mag-m.,*** merc., merc-c., phos., rhus-t., ***sep.***
post nasal - ***acon., arum-t.,*** **CARB-V.,** chlor., ***cist.,*** dig., hydr., iris, ***kali-bi.,*** kali-n., lac-ac., ***merc-i-r.,*** pen., ***quillaya,*** sep.
afternoon - nat-a.
evening - dig.
inspiration agg - ***ferr-p.,*** kreos.
morning - chlor.
saddle, like a - cinnb., thuj.
septum - lac-c., ***mag-m.***

RAWNESS, pain
tip - calc., carb-s.
wings, inner surface - ***mag-m.,*** med., nat-m.

RESPIRATION, noisy - chin.

RHINOSCLEROMA, stony hard growths - aur-m-n., ***calc-p.,*** con., guare., rhus-r.

ROSACEA - calc-p., cann-s., carb-an., **CAUST.,** kali-i., ***psor.,*** rhus-t.

ROUGHNESS, inside - mez.
inside, night - carb-v.
post nasal - am-m., gall-ac., hyper., staph.

SCRAPING, pain - nux-v.
sensation, post nasal - ***kali-bi., kali-chl., kali-p.,*** **MED.,** nat-c., **NAT-M.,** nat-s.

SCRATCHING - ruta.
post nasal, in - staph.

SCURFY, nostrils - ***alum.,*** am-m., ***ant-c.,*** **AUR.,** bor., **BOV., CALC.,** carb-an., chel., cic., crot-t., ferr., **GRAPH.,** ***hep., hippoz., iod., kali-bi., kali-c.,*** **LACH.,** ***lyc.,*** mag-m., ***merc., merc-c., nat-m., nat-s., nit-ac., petr., phos.,*** **PULS.,** rat., sars., **SEP., SIL.,** ***sulph., thuj.***
nostrils, side of - petr.

SHARP, pain - ***aesc.,*** anan., **APIS,** asc-t., ***aur.,*** bar-m., bell., berb., calc., calc-p., camph., caps., con., euph., euphr., ill., ipom., kali-bi., ***kali-c.,*** mur-ac., **NIT-AC.,** nux-m., olnd., puls., ***sang.,*** spig., tarent., teucr., thuj.
alternating with pressure - laur.
blowing nose - ***kali-bi.,*** kali-c., ***nit-ac.,*** sulph.
bones - ars., calc., cham., ***cina,*** kali-bi., kali-i., lach., led., spong., teucr.
left - spong.
corners - camph.
coughing - ***nit-ac.***
dorsum, right side - con., inul.
extending, radiating to top of head - tarent.
to ears - merc-c.
to occiput - cic.
to occiput on blowing nose - kali-c.
inside - bufo, calc., ***con.,*** hydr-ac., merc-c., mur-ac., sang.
extending to ear on blowing nose - calc.
extending to ear on blowing extending to forehead - ***staph.***
extending to forehead - bufo, ***kali-bi., kali-i.***
left - arg-m., calc., carb-ac., chin., grat., ***spong.***
inspiration, during - chin.
post nasal - ***aesc.***
right - psor., sulph.
extending to forehead on blowing nose - sulph.
blowing the nose as if bones rubbed together, on - kali-bi.
breathing, on - op., ox-ac.
root, in - acon., inul., ***kali-bi.,*** merc-i-f., mill., nicc., nat-m., ***nit-ac., phos., rhus-t.,*** sil., teucr.

SHARP, pain
root, in, alternating with stitching in occiput - acon.
before he falls with vertigo - ***kali-c.***
extending, to external angle of eye - ***kali-bi.***
extending, to tip - camph.
left - agar.
sneezing, on - nit-ac.
septum - aur., chin., ***cinnam.***, con., ***iod.***, ***sil.***
septum, on touch - con., sil., zinc.
side - aeth., alum., sil., sul-ac.
sneezing - ***nit-ac.***
tip - bell., ***con.***, ill., kali-c., kali-n., sars., sep., sil.
extending to forehead - sil.
touch, on - sep.
touching - calc., **NIT-AC.**, ***sil.***, zinc.
upper part - teucr.
wings - kali-c., stram.
junction of, with face - all-s.
junction of, with face, left side - all-s.

SHINY, (see Swelling) - aur-m-n., ***calc.***, canth., ***hydr.***, ***iris***, merc., ***mez.***, ox-ac., **PHOS.**
tip - ***bell.***, bor., ***phos.***, ***sulph.***
wing, right - canth.

SIDES, alternating - phyt., sin-n., sulph.

SINUSITIS, infection - ***ars.***, berb., bry., ***calc.***, cinnb., ***cupr.***, ferr., **HYDR.**, **KALI-BI.**, ***kali-chl.***, ***kali-i.***, kali-s., lach., **LYC.**, ***med.***, **MERC.**, merc-i-f., nat-s., ***nux-v.***, phos., **PULS.**, ***sang.***, **SIL.**, stict., syph., **THUJ.**, verb.
catarrh, of - ***ars.***, ***asaf.***, aur-m., bell., berb., bry., cact., ***calc.***, calc-p., camph., cimx., cinnb., cist., coch., cori-r., eucal., ferr., ***hep.***, **HYDR.**, ***iod.***, ***kali-bi.***, kali-c., ***kali-chl.***, ***kali-i.***, kali-m., **LYC.**, med., **MERC.**, ***merc-i-f.***, mez., ***nux-v.***, ph-ac., ***phos.***, ***puls.***, pyrog., ***sang.***, **SIL.**, spig., ***stict.***, teucr., ***thuj.***, verb.
constant - med.
extending to, antrum - berb., kali-c., kali-i., merc., phos., spig.
left - mez.
headache, from sinus catarrh - acon., aesc., ***all-c.***, ***alum.***, ambr., am-m., ***ars.***, ***ars-i.***, ***aur.***, bell., ***bry.***, ***calc.***, **CALC-S.**, camph., carb-s., ***carb-v.***, caul., cham., chin., chin-a., ***chlor.***, cic., cimic., cina, **DULC.**, **EUPHR.**, ***ferr.***, ***ferr-ar.***, ferr-p., ***gels.***, **GRAPH.**, gymn., hell., **HEP.**, **HYDR.**, ign., ***iod.***, ***kali-ar.***, **KALI-BI.**, ***kali-c.***, **KALI-I.**, ***kali-s.***, kalm., ***lach.***, laur., ***lyc.***, ***mang.***, **MERC.**, merc-i-f., mez., nat-a., ***nat-m.***, **NUX-V.**, ***phos.***, ***puls.***, ran-b., rumx., sabad., samb., sang., sil., staph., ***stict.***, still., ***sulph.***, teucr.
nosebleed, with - ip., kali-bi.
sinusitis, frontal sinuses - ***ars.***, berb., bry., ***calc.***, ***cupr.***, ferr., **HYDR.**, **KALI-BI.**, ***kali-chl.***, ***kali-i.***, **LYC.**, **MERC.**, merc-i-f., ***nux-v.***, **PULS.**, ***sang.***, **SIL.**, stict., **THUJ.**, verb.
sinusitis, frontal sinuses
coryza, in - ***ars.***, calc-p., cimx., ***kali-i.***, ***sil.***, ***stict.***
sinusitis, post-nasal catarrh - acon., aesc., ***alum.***, alumn., ant-s., ***arg-n.***, ***aur.***, aur-m., bar-c., bry., ***calc.***, ***calc-s.***, ***canth.***, caust., cinnb., ***cor-r.***, euphr., ***ferr.***, **FERR-P.**, **HEP.**, **HYDR.**, ***iod.***, **KALI-BI.**, ***kali-c.***, ***kali-chl.***, ***kali-i.***, kreos., lith., ***lyc.***, mag-s., ***manc.***, ***mang.***, **MED.**, ***merc-i-f.***, ***merc-i-r.***, ***merl.***, ***mez.***, nat-a., **NAT-C.**, **NAT-M.**, ***nat-s.***, ***nit-ac.***, petr., ***phyt.***, phos., ***plb.***, **PSOR.**, ***rhus-t.***, sang., ***sel.***, **SEP.**, ***sil.***, spig., staph., ***ther.***, **THUJ.**, zinc.
acute - ***acon.***, camph., cist., gels., kali-bi., menthol, ***merc-c.***, nat-a., wye.
chronic - aur., calc-f., elaps, fago., ***hydr.***, ***kali-bi.***, kali-c., merc-c., pen., sep., ***spig.***, ***stict.***, sulph., thuj.
mucus, with dropping of - ***alum.***, am-br., ant-c., ars-i., aur., calc-sil., ***cor-r.***, echi., glyc., ***hydr.***, irid., ***kali-bi.***, kali-m., lem-m., merc-i-r., nat-c., ***pen.***, ***phyt.***, ***sang-n.***, sin-n., ***spig.***, stict., teucr., ther., wye.

SMELL, general (see Odors) - aur., **BELL.**, calc., ***colch.***, graph., hep., lyc., nat-m., **NUX-V.**, **PHOS.**, **PULS.**, ***sep.***, sil., **SULPH.**
acute - **ACON.**, ***agar.***, alum., ***anac.***, ant-c., arn., ***ars.***, **AUR.**, asar., ***bar-c.***, **BELL.**, bry., ***calc.***, canth., caps., carb-ac., ***carb-s.***, ***cham.***, **CHIN.**, cina, ***cocc.***, **COFF.**, **COLCH.**, ***con.***, cycl., cupr., **GRAPH.**, ham., ***hep.***, hyos., ***hyper.***, **IGN.**, kali-ar., kali-c., kali-p., kali-s., ***kalm.***, lac-ac., lach., **LYC.**, ***lyss.***, mag-c., mez., nat-a., nat-c., nat-p., ***nux-m.***, **NUX-V.**, **OP.**, petr., ph-ac., **PHOS.**, ***plat.***, ***plb.***, puls., sabad., sel., **SEP.**, sil., stann., ***sulph.***, tab., thuj., valer., viol-o., zinc.
everything smells too strong, - aur.
headache, during, smell acute - **PHOS.**
pregnancy, during - colch., ***sep.***, stann.
diminished - ***alum.***, **ANAC.**, ***arg-n.***, asaf., **BELL.**, benz-ac., **CALC.**, calc-s., ***caps.***, ***cocc.***, ***coloc.***, con., ***cycl.***, ***hell.***, ***hep.***, **HYOS.**, kali-ar., kali-c., laur., ***lyc.***, menthol, ***merc.***, ***mez.***, mur-ac., nat-a., **NAT-M.**, nit-ac., ***nux-v.***, olnd., op., phos., ***plb.***, **PULS.**, rhod., rhus-t., ruta., sang., sec., **SEP.**, **SIL.**, sulph., tab., teucr., zinc.
epilepsy, with - plb.
leaflet at root, with sensation of - kali-i.
taste, and - anac., crot-t., just., mag-m., ***nat-m.***, ***puls.***, sil.
coryza, after - mag-m.
coryza, with - med.
lost, wanting - ail., ***alum.***, ***am-m.***, ***anac.***, ***ant-c.***, ***ant-t.***, ***ars.***, ***ars-i.***, arund., aspar., ***aur.***, **BELL.**, ***bry.***, bufo, **CALC.**, **CALC-S.**, camph., ***caps.***, carb-an., ***carb-s.***, card-m., ***caust.***, ***cham.***, chlor., cod., ***cupr.***, cycl., ***elaps***, ***graph.***, **HEP.**, ***hyos.***, ***ign.***, ***iod.***, ***ip.***, ***kali-bi.***, ***kali-i.***, kali-n., kali-p., ***kali-s.***, lach., ***lyc.***,

SMELL, general
lost, wanting - ***mag-m.,*** mag-p., mang., med., ***mez.,*** **MERC.,** ***nat-a.,*** ***nat-c.,*** **NAT-M.,** ***nux-m.,*** ***op.,*** phel., **PHOS.,** **PLB.,** ***psor.,*** **PULS.,** rhod., ***rhus-t.,*** ***sang.,*** ***sarr.,*** sec., **SEP.,** **SIL.,** spig., ***sulph.,*** ***sul-ac.,*** stram., ***teucr.,*** verat., ***zinc.***
perverted - anac., colch., mag-m., mag-p., sang., sep.
sensitive, to odors (see Odors)
broth - **COLCH.**
coffee - arg-n., lach., sul-ac.
cooking, food - chin., **COLCH.,** ***dig.,*** ***eup-per.,*** ***sep.,*** stann.
eggs - **COLCH.**
fish - ***colch.***
flowers - all-c., chin., **GRAPH.,** hyos., ***lac-c.,*** lyc., **NUX-V.,** **PHOS.,** sang.
food - arg-n., **ARS.,** ***cocc.,*** **COLCH.,** eup-per., ***ip.,*** lach., **SEP.,** stann.
gas, causes vertigo - **NUX-V.,** **PHOS.**
mice - sabad.
peaches - all-c.
soot - bell.
sour, odors - dros.
stool - **SULPH.**
strong, odors - ***acon.,*** ***agar.,*** anac., asar., **AUR.,** bar-c., **BELL.,** bry., calc., canth., carb-s., ***cham.,*** ***chin.,*** ***cocc.,*** **COFF.,** **COLCH.,** ***con.,*** cupr., **GRAPH.,** ***hep.,*** **IGN.,** kali-c., **LYC.,** ***lyss.,*** mag-c., nat-c., nat-m., **NUX-V.,** petr., **PHOS.,** plb., puls., sabin., sel., ***sep.,*** spig., ***sulph.,*** valer.
syrup - sang.
tobacco - ***bell.,*** chin., **IGN.,** lyss., ***nux-v.,*** phos., ***puls.,*** ***sep.***
unpleasant, odors - ***acon.,*** all-c., pall., **SULPH.**
vinegar - agar.
wine - tab.

SMOKE, as if in - bar-c.

SNEEZING, general - ***acon.,*** ***aesc.,*** aeth., ***agar.,*** ail., ***all-c.,*** aloe, alum., alumn., ambr., ***am-m.,*** ammc., ***anac.,*** anag., ***ant-t.,*** aphis., apis, ***arg-m.,*** ***arg-n.,*** arn., **ARS.,** ***ars-i.,*** ars-s-r., arum-d., arum-t., ***arund.,*** asar., aspar., ***aur.,*** ***bad.,*** bapt., ***bar-c.,*** bar-m., ***bell.,*** benz-ac., berb., bor., brach., ***brom.,*** **BRY.,** bufo, ***calc.,*** ***calc-ar.,*** ***calc-p.,*** ***calc-s.,*** ***camph.,*** ***caps.,*** ***carb-an.,*** carb-ac., **CARB-V.,** **CARB-S.,** cast., ***caust.,*** chel., ***chin.,*** ***chin-a.,*** ***chin-s.,*** chlor., ***cic.,*** cimic., **CINA,** ***cist.,*** clem., cob., cocc., **COC-C.,** coch., colch., ***con.,*** cop., crot-t., crot-h., cupr., ***cycl.,*** dig., ***dros.,*** ***dulc.,*** euph., ***euphr.,*** **EUP-PER.,** eup-pur., ferr., ***ferr-ar.,*** ferr-i., ***ferr-p.,*** form., ***gamb.,*** gels., glon., ***graph.,*** grat., ham., hell., hep., hydr., hyper., ill., ***indg.,*** ***ind.,*** ***iod.,*** ***ip.,*** ipom., iris, jac-c., ***kali-ar.,*** ***kali-bi.,*** kali-c., kali-chl., ***kali-i.,*** kali-n., kali-p., kali-s., ***kalm.,*** ***kreos.,*** ***lac-c.,*** ***lach.,*** lac-ac., lil-t., ***lyc.,*** lyss., mag-m., meph., **MERC.,** merc-i-f., merc-sul., mez., mur-ac., ***nat-a.,*** ***nat-c.,*** **NAT-M.,** ***nat-p.,*** ***nat-s.,*** nicc., ***nit-ac.,*** ***nux-m.,*** **NUX-V.,** olnd., ol-j., ox-ac., ***osm.,*** ***petr.,*** ***ph-ac.,*** ***phos.,*** phys., ***plan.,*** prun., psor., ptel., **PULS.,** ran-s., rat., ***rhus-r.,*** **RHUS-T.,** ***rumx.,*** **SABAD.,** ***sal-ac.,*** sac-alb., **SANG.,** sanic., sars., sec., ***senec.,*** ***seneg.,*** ***sep.,*** ***sil.,*** ***spong.,*** ***squil.,*** ***staph.,*** stict., **SULPH.,** ***tarax.,*** tarent., ***teucr.,*** ther., thuj., verat., zinc., zing.
abortive - ars., calc-f., carb-v., nux-v., ***sabad.,*** sil.
afternoon - bad., fl-ac., laur., mur-ac., zinc.
air, amel. in the - ***all-c.,*** calc-i., calc-s., phos., puls.
cold, in - anan., ars., hep., sabad.
open, in - alumn., ***kali-bi.,*** sabad., tarax.
ascending, agg. - sol-v., tub.
asthma, alleric, hay, with - ***ars.,*** ***carb-v.,*** ***dulc.,*** ***euphr.,*** lach., ***naja,*** ***nat-s.,*** ***nux-v.,*** sin-n., stict.
belching, with - ham., lob., ***phos.***
blowing, nose agg. - carb-v.
burning in with - senec.
chalk, from - ***nat-p.***
chronic tendency - nat-m., sil.
combing, or brushing the hair, from - sil.
concussive - cast., sulph.
constant - all-c., anac., ars., ***dulc.,*** gamb., ***indg.,*** iris, merc., nat-c., squil.
forenoon - cimx.
night, during - carb-v., rhus-t.
coryza, without - acon., aesc., ***agar.,*** alum., ***am-m.,*** ars., **CALC.,** ***carb-v.,*** caust., cic., cist., con., dig., dros., euph., ***euphr.,*** hell., hyos., iod., kali-c., lyc., meny., ***merc.,*** mur-ac., nat-c., nicc., ***nit-ac.,*** petr., phos., ***sep.,*** sil., stann., staph., sulph., ***teucr.,*** zinc.
coughing, with - agar., bad., bell., just., psor., squil.
after - **AGAR.,** ***arg-n.,*** bad., ***bell.,*** bry., caps., ***carb-v.,*** hep., lyc., psor., seneg., ***squil.,*** sulph.
before - ***ip.***
between the coughs - bry.
whooping, cough, with - cina.
daytime - gamb., ther.
dinner, during - grat.
after - agar., phos., zinc.
dizzy, until - seneg.
dry, nose, with - ambr., chin., graph.
dust, causes - benz-ac., brom., lyss.
ear, itching, with - cycl.
eating, agg. - kali-p., zinc.
evening - all-c., bar-c., ***cist.,*** glyc., ***iod.,*** lyss., mag-c., mur-ac., nit-ac., petr., phos., ***puls.,*** rumx., **SULPH.,** ther.
bed, on going to - bufo
eyes, opening - am-c., ***sang.***
closed - gamb.
forenoon - cimx.
frequent - acon., agar., ***all-c.,*** alum., ambr., am-c., **AM-M.,** anac., arg-m., arn., **ARS.,** asaf., aspar., ***aur.,*** bar-c., bar-m., ***bell.,*** ***brom.,*** ***bry.,*** calc., carb-an., **CARB-S.,** **CARB-V.,** cast., ***caust.,*** chin-s., cic., cist., **COC-C.,** con., cor-r., crot-h., cupr., ***cycl.,*** dig., ***dros.,*** ***dulc.,***

SNEEZING, general

frequent - euph., gins., graph., gymn., ***hep.,*** hyos., kali-ar., ***kali-c.,*** kali-i., kali-n., kali-p., kalm., ***kreos.,*** lact., laur., lil-t., ***lyc.,*** mag-c., mag-m., mag-s., mang., **MERC.,** mez., mosch., mur-ac., nat-a., nat-c., nat-m., ***nit-ac.,*** nux-m., **NUX-V.,** petr., ***phos., plan.,*** prun., **PULS.,** ran-s., rhus-t., ruta., ***sang.,*** sep., ***sil.,*** spig., stann., ***squil.,*** staph., ***stict.,*** stront-c., **SULPH.,** ther., verat., ***zinc.***
morning - alum., calc., sulph.
evening - petr.
heat, before - chin.

ineffectual, efforts - acon., aeth., alum., asar., benz-ac., calc., **CALC-F.,** canth., **CARB-V.,** caust., cocc., colch., euph., guare., hell., indg., ***kali-i.,*** laur., lyc., ***mez.,*** mur-ac., ***nat-m., nit-ac.,*** osm., phos., ***plat.,*** plb., sars., **SIL.,** sulph., sul-ac., zinc.
air in open - cocc.

inhaling, from - brom.

irritation, in larynx, from - ***agar., arg-n., carb-v.***

itching, with - ***stry.***
ear, in - cycl.

looking, at shining objects - lyss.

lying, agg. - kali-bi.
amel. - merc.

menses, during - mag-c.

morning - agar., ***all-c.,*** **AM-C.,** aspar., benz-ac., bov., bry., calc., calc-ar., **CAUST.,** chlor., ***cimx., cist.,*** clem., fl-ac., ***gels.,*** hell., ***kali-bi.,*** kali-n., ***kreos.,*** laur., lyc., lyss., ***mag-c.,*** merc., mez., ***nat-m.,*** nit-ac., ***nux-v.,*** onos., phos., ***puls.,*** sars., ***sep.,*** sin-n., stict., **SULPH.,** zinc.
2 a.m. - kali-p.
5 a.m. - nicc.
6 a.m. - ***sep.***
bed, in - agar., **AM-C.,** aspar., **NUX-V.,** ***puls., sep.***
evening, and - nit-ac., sulph.
fasting - hell.
prevents talking - rhus-t.
rising, after - all-c., bov., caust., hell., nux-v., rhod., sars.
waking, on - **AM-C.,** ars., aster., bov., calc., chin., graph., hydr., kali-c., spig.

night - ***arum-t.,*** carb-v., ***elaps,*** ferr-i., petr., rhus-t., ***rumx.,*** sin-n.
2 a.m. - kali-p.
lying down, while - sin-n.

odors, from - phos.
strong, from - gamb., phos.

opening, eyes - am-c., ***graph.,*** sang.

painful - carb-an., cina, dros., kali-i.

paroxysmal - ***agar.,*** arn., bell., calc., con., ***gels.,*** glon., ham., hell., ***ip., kali-i.,*** lach., lyss., ***nat-m.,*** nux-v., phos., ***rhus-t., sabad.,*** sil., staph., ***stram., sulph.,*** sul-ac., tab., ther.
morning - gels.
prolonged attacks - nux-v.
lasting 4 to 6 hours with sinking of strength - petr.

persistent - cycl., sabad., sang.
rapid, and - verat.
weakness, for hours with - petr.

rising, from bed agg. - staph.

salivation, with - fl-ac.

sleep, during - bar-m., ***nit-ac.,*** puls.
wakes him from - **AM-M.**

sleepiness, with - ***petr.***

sneezing, agg. - carb-v.

stomach, as from - ***dig.***

sudden - glon., rumx.

sunshine, in - agar., hydr., ***merc.,*** merc-sul., **NAT-M.,** ***sang.***

talking, prevented - rhus-t.

throat, vapor in, as from - sal-ac., thuj.

tickling, in the trachea, from - caps.

tingling, in nose - bor., carb-v., ferr., kali-bi., paeon., plat., rumx., stict., teucr.

uncovering, from - **HEP.,** ***merc.,*** nat-m., nux-v., pyrog., ***rhus-t.,*** sil.
hands - **HEP.,** pyrog., rhus-t., ***rumx.***

unsatisfactory - ars-i.

violent - acon., ***all-c.,*** am-c., anag., aphis., arg-m., ***ars.,*** ars-h., asaf., asar., aspar., ***bar-c.,*** brom., ***bry.,*** calad., canth., caps., carb-v., chin., chlor., ***cina,*** cist., coc-c., con., croc., crot-h., dig., fl-ac., ***gamb.,*** gels., gymn., ictod., ***ind.,*** indg., ***ip.,*** kali-ar., ***kali-c., kali-i.,*** kali-p., laur., lyc., mag-c., merc., mosch., ***nat-a., nat-c., nat-m.,*** nicc., nit-ac., ***nux-v.,*** olnd., puls., rhus-t., rumx., sabad., seneg., sil., ***squil.,*** sulph., ther., ***thuj.,*** verat.
lasting 5 minutes - seneg.

walking, in open air - cocc., plat., tarax.

warm, room, in - ***all-c.,*** **PULS.**

water, putting hands in, on - phos.

yawning, with - astac., bry., cycl., lob., mag-c.

SNUFFLES - alum., am-c., apoc., ***ars., asc-t., aur.,*** aur-m., cupr., elaps, kali-bi., kali-i., **LYC.,** ***med.,*** merc., nat-m., **NUX-V.,** osm., phos., puls., sabad., **SAMB.,** sep., syph., ***thuj.,*** vib.
averse to - spig.
infants, in new-born - acon., ***dulc.,*** **LYC.,** ***merc.,*** **NUX-V.,** ***puls.,*** **SAMB.,** ***thuj.***
coryza, with - acon., ***am-c.,*** bell., ***cham.,*** dulc., elaps, hep., merc-i-f., ***nux-v., samb.,*** stict., sulph.

SNUFFLING, constantly, but no discharge - iodof.
speaking, while - kali-bi.
warm, damp weather, in - ***kali-bi.***

SOOTY, nostrils - ***ant-t., chlor., colch.,*** crot-h., ***hell., hyos., lyc.,*** med., merc., ***zinc.***

SORE, pain
bones, in - arg-n., **AUR.,** ***aur-m., aur-s.,*** chel., cupr-ar., guai., ***hep.,*** jab., ***lac-c.,*** merc., ***nat-m., sil.***
in, left - aesc., anac., arg-n., nat-m.
in, right - **AUR.**
dorsum - **HEP.,** ***kali-bi., nat-c., petr.,*** **PHOS.,** ***sil.***

SORE, pain
externally - act-sp., agar., am-m., arg-n., ***arn., ars.,*** **AUR.,** bell., benz-ac., brach., ***brom., calc.,*** cic., ***cina,*** coloc., con., crot-t., cupr-ar., ***hep.,*** iod., ***kali-bi.,*** kali-n., lac-c., led., lyss., ***nat-m., petr., phos., puls.,*** **SIL.,** viol-o., zinc.
blowing, on - ***aur.,*** **GRAPH.,** led., mag-s., ***nat-m., sil.***
compressing wings, when - arg-n., colch., nat-m.
evening - alum.
spots, in - merc-i-f.
touch - ***alum.,*** am-m., anac., **AUR.,** ***aur-s.,*** bell., bry., ***calc.,*** caust., cic., colch., euphr., graph., ***hep.,*** ictod., ***kali-bi.,*** kali-i., lyss., ***mag-m.,*** mang., ***merc., nat-m., nit-ac.,*** **PHOS.,** ***sil.,*** sulph., thuj., zinc.
inside - ***aesc.,*** agar., ***alum.,*** ambr., ***am-m.,*** anac., ang., ant-c., aphis., arn., ***ars.,*** **ARUM-T., AUR.,** bapt., bar-c., bar-m., bor., ***bov., brom., calc., calc-p.,*** camph., carb-an., carb-s., caust., cham., chel., cic., cocc., colch., ***con.,*** cop., crot-t., dios., ***euphr.,*** gels., **GRAPH.,** hep., ***hyper., ign.,*** jab., **KALI-BI.,** ***kali-c.,*** **KALI-I.,** ***kali-n.,*** kali-p., kali-s., kaol., lac-c., ***lach.,*** lact., lith., ***mag-m.,*** mag-s., **MANG.,** med., ***merc.,*** merc-c., ***mez.,*** mur-ac., nat-a., ***nat-m.,*** nat-p., nat-s., nicc., **NIT-AC.,** ***nux-v.,*** ol-an., ***petr.,*** phos., podo., psor., ptel., puls., ran-b., rhod., ***rhus-t.,*** sars., sec., sep., **SIL.,** sulph., stann., staph., syph., teucr., ***thuj., tub.,*** uran., zinc.
left - agn., **ARUM-T.,** coff., fl-ac., ictod., med., nat-p., staph.
left, inspiration, at - ant-c.
right - ***alum.,*** am-c., ant-c., ***aur.,*** calc., colch., kali-bi., ***kali-n.,*** kali-p., lac-c., mag-c., ***sil., thuj.***
margin - am-m., calc., ***calc-p.,*** kali-bi., nux-v., squil., sumb., thuj.
nostrils - nux-v.
post nasal - am-m., bapt., cop., kreos., lec., mag-c., ox-ac., par., ph-ac.
coughing, on - carb-v.
morning - dig.
root - ***ant-t.,*** carb-an., kali-bi., nicc., ***nit-ac.,*** raph.
operation, after - arn., ferr-p.
septum - ***alum.,*** bor., ***bov.,*** calc., caust., ***colch.,*** con., hep., ***hydr.,*** **KALI-BI.,** kali-s., ***lac-c., mag-m., merc-i-f., mur-ac.,*** nat-m., sep., ***sil., staph., sulph.,*** thuj.
right side - lac-c., lyc., ***merc-i-f.***
right side, from a pimple - calad.
tip - bell., ***bor.,*** calc., carb-an., cist., ***con.,*** hep., kali-bi., ***lith.,*** lyc., merc-sul., op., rhus-t., sil., tax.

SORE, pain
wings - am-m., aur., brom., calc., calc-p., calc-s., gels., iod., kali-bi., ***nat-m.,*** nit-ac., rhus-t.
left - calc., med., nat-m.
right - cic., daph., hydr., mez.
touch agg. - ***ant-c.,*** ars., ***arum-t.,*** aur-m., calc., cop., cori-r., fago., ***graph., hep., kali-bi.,*** merc., merc-c., ***nit-ac.,*** petr., squil., uran-n.

SPARKS, sensation of electric, left wing - carb-ac.

SPASM, in wings - ambr.
muscles - lyc.

SPLINTER-like, pain - ***aur.,*** hep., kali-bi., ***nit-ac.***
touch, on - ***nit-ac., sil.***

SQUEAKING, sensation - nat-c., teucr.

STICKING, pain, septum when touched - zinc.

STIFF, cold, from, as if - phos.

STINGING, pain - sep.

STRING-like, pain, to ear - lem-m.

SUNKEN - ***aur.,*** hep., merc., ***psor.,*** sil., syph.
infants, in - ***aur-m.***

SWELLING, of - ***alum.,*** am-c., am-m., anan., anthr., **APIS, ARN., ARS., ARS-I., ARS-M.,** asaf., **AUR., AUR-M.,** aur-s., ***bapt.,*** **BAR-C.,** ***bell.,*** bor., bov., brom., bry., cadm-s., **CALC.,** ***calc-p., calc-s.,*** cann-s., ***canth., carb-an., carb-s.,*** caust., cham., cist., cocc., **COC-C.,** cor-r., crot-h., ***ferr-i.,*** fl-ac., ***graph., guai.,*** **HEP.,** hippoz., ictod., ign., ***iod., kali-ar., kali-bi.,*** **KALI-C.,** kali-chl., ***kali-i.,*** kali-n., ***kali-p.,*** kali-s., ***lach.,*** lith., **LYC.,** mag-c., ***mag-m.,*** meph., **MERC.,** ***merc-c.,*** merc-i-r., ***naja, nat-m.,*** nicc., nit-ac., petr., ***ph-ac.,*** **PHOS.,** ***puls.,*** ran-b., rat., ***rhus-t., rhus-v.,*** sarr., **SEP.,** ***sil.,*** sol-n., **SULPH.,** thuj., ***tub.,*** urt-u., ***zinc.***
air, after walking in - aur.
below, senation, of - rhus-t.
bones - anan., asaf., **HEP.,** ***hydr.,*** ictod., **KALI-I.,** ***merc., merc-i-r.,*** **PHOS.,** sulph.
cold - ph-ac.
coryza, with - phos.
hot - merc-i-r.
dorsum - calc., kali-bi., ***ph-ac.,*** rat.
evening - alum., mag-c., ***puls.***
amel. - caust.
hard - alum., aur-m-n., calc., thuj.
inside - ***acon.,*** am-c., aspar., bell., cadm-s., ***calc.,*** canth., carb-ac., cist., cocc., ***euphr., ign., kali-bi., kali-c.,*** kali-n., ***lach., merc., nat-m.,*** rhus-t., sang., **SEP.,** ***sil.,*** stann., ***teucr.,*** zinc.
inside, sensation, of - kali-n., mag-c.
knotty - **ARS., AUR.**
ridge, on - calc.
left - ***alum.,*** am-m., ***aur-m.,*** brom., ***calc.,*** cist., ***hydr.,*** lach., merc., ***nat-m.,*** sep., stann., thuj.
when pressed - brom.
morning - aur., caust.
one-sided - cocc., croc., hippoz., ***phos., zinc.***
post nasal - bry., hydr., ph-ac.

SWELLING, of
red, like a saddle - ictod.
right - ***aur.,*** aur-m., cocc., cor-r., ***kali-bi., lith., mez., merc-i-f., merc-i-r.,*** ox-ac., zinc.
sensation of - kali-n., rat.
room in, after walking in air - aur.
root - ***calc.,*** hippoz., ***kali-bi.,*** merc., ***nit-ac., petr.,*** sars.
coming and going - ***calc.***
septum - ***alum.,*** caust., elaps, ham., merc., ***merc-i-f.***
shining - ***aur-m-n.,*** bor., lith., ox-ac., sulph.
red - bor., merc., ox-ac., phos., sulph.
red, left - aur-m.
red, right side to tip - ox-ac.
spongy, vascular, distending it - kali-bi.
spot, on right lachrymal bone which throbs - kali-bi.
throbbing - cor-r., kali-bi.
tip - ***bell., bor., bry.,*** calc., **CAUST.,** ***chel.,*** clem., ***crot-h., kali-c.,*** lyc., merc., merc-sul., nicc., ox-ac., ***sep., sulph.***
warm weather, in - bell.
touch painful to - alum., ***calc.,*** hippoz., ***nat-m., phos.***
wings - aur., brom., cann-s., carb-an., hydr-ac., kali-bi., ***kali-c.,*** lach., mag-m., ***nat-m., nit-ac.,*** ox-ac., phos., phel., stann., ***sulph.,*** thuj.
left - ***alum.,*** merc., nat-m., stann., thuj., zinc.
left, spot - calc., zinc.
right - arg-n., calc., hydr., ***mag-m.,*** merc-i-f., mez.

SYPHILITIC affections - asaf., aur., aur-m., cinnb., fl-ac., kali-bi., kali-i., ***merc.,*** merc-c., sil.

TEARING, pain - alum., arn., cadm-s., ***calc.,*** chel., ***chin.,*** colch., euphr., ind., kali-bi., kali-i., lach., lyc., mag-c., mag-m., mang., nat-s., nicc., ***sep.,*** sil., spong., ***sulph.,*** zinc.
above, nose - aeth., agar., ambr., chel., lyc., nat-c., nat-m.
pressing upon eyelids - chel.
bones - ***aur-m., con.,*** gamb., indg., ***kalm.,*** mez.
nausea, with - ***kalm.***
dorsum - ***chin.***
left - am-c., aur-m., mang., ol-an.
post nasal - zinc.
pressure amel. - alum., sulph.
right - alum., zinc.
root - cast., chin., coloc., ***kalm., mang., merc-c.,*** nicc., ***phos.***
to forehead - ***nat-m.***
septum - plb.
side - carb-an., carb-v.
extending to eye - lyc.
extending to temple - mag-c.
left - mag-c.
right - lyc.
wings - caust., sil., stram.
left - sil., thuj.
right - caust.

TENSION - ***acon.,*** asaf., bor., cadm-s., caps., carb-an., kali-bi., merc., ***petr.,*** ph-ac., ran-b., sulph., ***thuj.***
above nose - ***glon.,*** hep.
across - merc.
below - rhus-t.
bones - thuj.
dorsum - ph-ac.
inside - cadm-s., canth., graph., ***lac-d.***
nostrils - caps.
painless over nasal bones - asaf.
root - ***all-c., ant-t.,*** cadm-s., carb-ac., cupr., ***graph.,*** ham., ***kali-bi., kali-i.,*** lac-d., meny., merc., nat-p., petr., spong.
above, as from a band - ant-t.
above, as from a saddle - thuj.
skin - acon., arg-m., ***petr., phos.***
tip - ***carb-an.***
wings - thuj.

THICK - ***ferr-i.,*** kali-c.

TINGLING - aesc., agar., all-c., ambr., am-c., arg-m., arn., berb., calc., canth., caps., colch., corn., dros., gran., lach., mag-c., nat-p., ol-an., rhus-r., sul-ac.
bones - cinnb., corn., spong.
inside - agar., ***all-c.,*** ambr., am-c., arg-m., **ARN.,** berb., bor., ***caps.,*** carb-ac., carb-v., cham., ***colch., con.,*** daph., ***gels.,*** hep., hydr-ac., laur., mag-c., nat-p., nit-ac., ol-an., ph-ac., plat., ***ran-b.,*** ran-s., rat., ***rumx., sabad.,*** sep., spig., stry., sul-ac., sulph., tab., ***teucr.***
blowing the on - hep.
cobweb, as from - brom.
evening - carb-v.
left - arg-m., carb-v., dros., hep., nat-p.
nosebleed, before - arg-m.
right - agar., ***all-c.,*** ars-s-r., mag-c., ***stict.,*** sul-ac.
spreading through whole body - sabad.
sudden, sharp, followed by sneezing - ***rumx.***
tears, with - nat-p.
post nasal - arg-n., mag-c., ran-b.
root - ambr.
septum when blowing the nose - bry.
tip - aesc., bell., berb., carb-an., carb-v., caust., con., kali-n., lach., mosch., paeon., ran-s., rheum, sars., ***sep.***
amel. by rubbing - bell.
wings - carb-ac.

TORPOR, sense of - asaf., plat., samb., viol-o.

TREMULOUS, sensation at tip - ***bry.,*** chel.

TUMORS, hard - ars.
inside - ars., kali-bi.
left side - merc-i-r.
post nasal - chr-ac., osm.
root - bell.
tip - anan., carb-an., sulph.

TWITCHING - am-a., ***ambr.,*** aur., bry., ***calc., chel., con., glon., hyos., kali-bi., lyc.,*** mosch., nat-m., phys., ***plat.,*** puls., zinc.
creeping under skin, left side - arg-n.

TWITCHING, of
left, side - am-c., nat-m.
seems to draw up the wing - am-c.
right, side - brom., zinc.
root - phos.
left side - nat-m.
visible - con., glon., ***hyos., mez.,*** nat-m.
septum - aur.
tip - ***bry.,*** chel.
wing, right - lyc.
left - plat., kali-bi.

ULCERATIVE, pain - aeth., arn., ***hep.,*** ign., ***kali-c.,*** mag-s., ***puls., staph.***
corners - camph., nux-v.
inside - ***am-m.,*** ars., **AUR.,** bell., bor., bry., ***hep.,*** ign., ***kali-bi., nit-ac., nux-v.,*** puls., ***sil.,*** verat.
left - am-m., cocc., puls., staph.
right - **AUR.,** ***graph., kali-c.,*** thuj.
root on, stooping - puls.
touch - petr.
septum, on touch - staph.
touch, on - am-m., **AUR.,** bry., petr., ***sil.***
wings - nux-v.
evening - nux-v.
left - laur.
motion, on - nux-v.

ULCERS - anan., ***anthro.,*** ars., asaf., aur-m-n., bry., caust., cocc., cor-r., ***fl-ac., hecla.,*** hep., ***kali-bi., kali-c.,*** merc., nat-c., nat-m., ***puls.***
inside - ***alum.,*** anan., ang., **ANT-C.,** arg-n., ***arn., ars., ars-i.,*** **AUR., AUR-M., AUR-M-N.,** ***bor.,*** brom., bry., bufo, cadm-s., ***calc.,*** calc-p., carb-an., ***carb-s., cham., crot-c.,*** ferr-i., ***fl-ac., graph., hippoz.,*** hyos., ign., ***iod.,*** jatr., **KALI-BI.,** kali-c., ***kali-i.,*** kali-n., kali-p., lyc., ***mag-m., merc., merc-c., nat-c.,*** **NIT-AC.,** ***petr., phos.,*** puls., sang., **SEP., SIL.,** ***squil.,*** staph., ***sulph.,*** syph., tab., **THUJ.**
burning - ***ars., sil.***
malignant - carb-an., kali-bi.
painful - **SIL.**
perforating - fl-ac., ***kali-bi.,*** merc., ***merc-c.***
right - aur., bry., gamb., kali-n., ***sil.,*** thuj.
right, high up - ***nat-c., sil., thuj.***
yellow, crusted - arg-n.
left - ***aur-m.,*** bell., bor., bry., calc., lyc.
nostrils - alum., bell., bufo, cadm-s., ***cocc., cor-r.,*** kali-c., mag-m., merc., nit-ac., petr., phos., **SEP.**
outer angle - bell.
under nose - arund.
post nasal - arg-n., arum-t.
right - cor-r., gamb.
septum, around - alum., ***nit-ac.***
round ulcers - alum., ***aur.,*** brom., calc., calc-p., cop., carb-ac., ***fl-ac., hippoz., hydr.,*** **KALI-BI.,** ***kali-i.,*** merc., ***merc-c., nat-c.,*** nit-ac., sars., ***sep.,*** **SIL.,** syph., **THUJ.,** vinc.

ULCERS,
syphilitic - ***aur.,*** aur-m., cor-r., kali-bi., ***kali-i.,*** lach., ***merc., nit-ac.***
tip - ***bor., bry.,*** **CAUST.**
wings - kali-c., psor., **PULS.,** ***sanic.,*** thuj.
wings, borders - ***kali-bi.,*** mag-m.
left - dulc., fl-ac., kali-bi., kali-c.
right - ***ars.,*** cor-r.

UNEASY feeling around - ail.

UPWARD, tip feels drawn - crot-c.

VEINS, varicose - aur., ***carb-v., crot-h.,*** mez.

VESICLES - am-c., ant-c., clem., crot-t., ***lach.,*** lac-ac., ***mag-c.,*** mag-m., ***mez.,*** nat-c., ***nat-m.,*** nit-ac., petr., phel., phos., ***plb.,*** **RHUS-T.,** sil., verat.
around - phos.
centre, on - ***carb-ac.***
inside, right - **CARB-AN.,** lach., phos.
menses, before - mag-c.
nostril, under - sil.
root - nat-m.
septum - am-c., crot-h., thuj.
side, bloody - sep.
tip - nit-ac.
wings - chel., **NAT-M.,** sil., thuj.
right - nat-c.

WARTS, on - **CAUST.,** ***nit-ac.,*** **THUJ.**
inside, nose - nit-ac.
tip of, nose - ***caust.***

WATER flowing from, as if hot - acon., gels.
nostrils - gels.

WHISTLING - alum.

WRINKLED, skin - cham.

Pelvis

ABSCESS, buttocks - carb-o., ***sulph.,*** thuj.
abscess, coccyx, just below - paeon.
abscess, perineum - ***hep., merc., sil.***

ACHING, pain, buttocks - bry., ***calc.,*** calc-p., cupr., staph.
aching, coccyx - calc-p., carb-v., caust., ***fl-ac., kali-bi.,*** sulph., xan., ***zinc.***
menses, during - zinc.
sitting, while - petr., plat.
stool, after - sulph.
aching, iliac - agar., alum., berb., calc., ***carb-ac., carb-v.,*** cimic., crot-t., cupr., dios., dulc., elaps, eupi., gels., grat., iris, kreos., lil-t., lith., nat-a., ox-ac., phos., plan., plat., plb., ptel., spig., stann., ***ter.,*** zinc., zing.
bending, on - puls-n
breakfast, after - zinc.
coughing on - ***caust.,*** eupi.
dinner, after - phos.
eating, amel. - phys.
evening - bor., dios., naja, rhus-t., zinc.
supper after - zinc.
extending, ilium to ilium - asar., cimic., lil-t.
thighs, down - ***thuj.***
to knee - ***kali-c.***
left - ***caust.,*** cimic., ***coloc.,*** crot-h., cupr., dios., eupi., gels., naja, nat-a., ox-ac., puls-n, **THUJ.**
lying on left side - ***com.,*** phys.
morning - sumb.
stool, before - sumb.
motion, on - ptel., puls-n.
night - dios., pic-ac.
11 p.m. - pic-ac.
noon - thuj.
paroxysmal - ***cocc.***
pressure amel. - phys.
raising arm - eupi.
right - ***cocc., kali-c.,*** phos., phys., ***pic-ac.,*** ptel., sumb.
sitting, while - agar.
stool, before - sumb.
supper, after - zinc.
walking, while - eupi.
in open air amel. - phys.
in room - thuj.
aching, ilium, crest of - bell., berb., brom., calc., camph., carb-an., cham., eupi., form., ip., ***iris, kali-c.,*** led., plan., rhus-t., sabad., sang., staph., tell., ***ter.,*** zinc.
coughing - eupi.
extending to knee - **KALI-C.**
to thigh - staph.
left - eupi.
morning - staph.
motion - ***ter.***
night - sang.
pressure amel. - sabad.
raising arm - eupi.
rising from seat - bell.
sitting, while - sabad., zinc.
aching, ilium, crest of
walking, while - eupi., led.
amel. - sabad., staph.
warmth amel. - staph.
aching, sacro-iliac, junction - **AESC.,** ant-t., apis, arg-n., bry., calc-p., cimic., coloc., dios., ferr., gels., hep., jug-c., nat-p., ol-j., plb., rhus-t., rumx., sabad., spong., sulph., thuj.
symphyses - aesc., coloc., jug-c., sulph.
aching, sacrum - acon., **AESC., AGAR.,** alum., arg-n., aur., ***bapt.,*** calad., ***calc., calc-p., calc-s.,*** canth., carb-an., carb-s., ***carb-v.,*** cham., chin., ***cimic., coff.,*** colch., con., eug., eup-pur., fl-ac., **GELS.,** graph., ***helon.,*** hep., ***ign., kali-bi.,*** kali-c., ***lach.,*** lil-t., lyc., ***merc.,*** **MUR-AC.,** nat-m., ***nux-v.,*** ol-j., op., ***phyt.,*** ptel., **PULS.,** ***rhus-t., sep., sil.,*** staph., stram., ***sulph.,*** vario., verat.
as if flesh were detached from bones - acon., kali-bi.
evening - led., ter., ***sep.***
extending into lower extremities - calc-ar., ***cimic., lil-t., sep.***
menses, before - ***vib.***
morning - ang., calad., kali-n., nat-m., sel., ***staph.,*** thuj.
motion, on - ***aesc., colch.***
night - arg-n.
pressure amel. - colch., ***sep.***
sitting - **AGAR.**
stooping - **AESC.**
walking - **AESC.,** ***colch.***

ALIVE, iliac, sensation of something, right region - **THUJ.**

BENT, back as if, in coccyx - mag-p.

BOILS, buttocks - agar., alum., am-c., aur-m., bart., bar-c., bor., cadm-s., calad., graph., indg., ***hep., lyc.,*** nit-ac., ***ph-ac.,*** phos., plb., psor., ***rat.,*** sabin., sars., sec., sep., ***sil., sulph.,*** thuj.
blood - aur-m., hep., lyc.
boils, perineum - alum., ant-c.
boils, sacrum - aeth., thuj.

BORING, pain, buttocks - cina, coloc., merc.
sitting, while - cina.
boring, sacrum - aloe, ***berb.,*** cimic., kali-c.
break, as though the back would - ***aesc., alumn.,*** **BELL.,** chel., cocc., ***kali-c.,*** kalm., kreos., ***nat-m., nux-v.,*** vario.
lying, while - berb.
menses, during - **BELL.,** ***nux-v., vib.***
suppressed - **BELL.,** ***nux-v.***
sacral region - acon., calad., led.
sitting, while - berb.

BROKEN, as if, coccyx - cist.
broken, as if, sacrum - acon., ***aesc.,*** agar., alum., am-m., ang., arn., ***ars.,*** bry., ***calc-p., eupi.,*** graph., hep., nux-m., nux-v., meli., ***phos.,*** plat., rhus-t., ruta., ***staph.,*** verat.
cough, with - ***phos.***
morning, in bed - staph.
night, in bed, amel. by rising and walking - ang.
walking, while - ***calc-p.***

BUBBLING, sensation, buttocks - ant-c., zinc.
standing, while - ant-c.

BURNING, pain, buttocks - bar-c., bry., calc-p., coloc., lyc., mag-m., mang., **MERC.,** mez., sep., staph., sulph., stront.
between - arg-m., sep., thuj.
while walking - thuj.
buttocks and thighs - nat-c.
evening, after lying down - sulph.
scratching, after - mag-m.
sitting, while - mang.

burning, coccyx - apis, canth., cist., colch., mur-ac., laur., ***phos.,*** staph., sulph.
evening - apis
extending up the spine - mur-ac.
menses, during - carb-v., mur-ac.
sitting, while - ***apis,*** cist.
touched, when - ***carb-an.,*** cist.

burning, perineum - ant-c., mur-ac., nit-ac., plb., ***rhod.,*** sil., thuj.
sex, after - sil.

burning, sacro-iliac, symphyses - rumx.

burning, sacrum - bor., ***carb-v.,*** colch., coloc., ***ferr., helon.,*** kreos., lachn., mur-ac., murx., ph-ac., phos., ***podo.,*** rhus-t., sabin., sep., sil., staph., sulph., tarent., ter., thuj.
afternoon, 4 p.m. - lachn.
menses, during - carb-v., ferr.
sitting, while - bor.
sticking - mur-ac.
stool, after - coloc.
warmth of bed agg. - ***coloc.***

BURROWING, pain, iliac - dulc.

burrowing, sacrum - calad.

BURSTING, pain, perineum - sanic.
stool, after - sanic.

CARBUNCLES, buttocks - agar., thuj.

COLDNESS, buttocks - agar., daph., hydr.
gluteal region - agar., calc.
menses, before - mang.
night, 1 a.m - hydr.
in bed - ***cench.***

coldness, sacrum - arg-m., benz-ac., ***dulc.,*** hyos., laur., ***lyc.,*** ox-ac., ***puls., sanic.,*** stront-c., sulph.
chill, during - aesc., asaf., eup-pur., ***puls.,*** sulph.
chilliness - lyc., **PULS.,** sulph.
extending upwards - **SULPH.**
menses, during - ***puls.***
stool, during - ptel.
wet cloth, as if - sanic.

CONSTRICTION, buttocks - plat., thuj.

constriction, perineum, closure - lyc., sil., sulph.

CONTRACTION, of muscles and tendons, buttocks - rhus-t.

CONVULSION, buttocks - bar-c., calc., nux-v., sep.

CRAMP-like, coccyx - ***bell.,*** grat.
menses, during - ***bell.***

cramp-like, sacrum - ***bell.,*** thuj.

CRAMPS, buttocks - bell., bry., cann-s., caust., graph., rhus-t., ***sep.***
night, in bed - ***sep.***
standing, while - rhus-t.
stooping, while - bell., cann-s.
stretching, out limbs - sep.

cramps, perineum - sulph., thuj.

CRUSHED, sacrum, as though - sil.

CUTTING, pain, buttocks, forenoon - alum.

cutting, coccyx - canth.

cutting, iliac - ***agn.,*** nat-p., thuj.
extending into testicle - hydr.
fossa, right to left - sang.
extending to rectum - sang.

cutting, ilium, morning - cina.
morning, anterior superior spinous process - sulph.
extending to scapula - nat-m.
extending to thigh - ruta., thuj.

cutting, perineum - am-m., aur., bov., lyc., nux-v., thuj.
evening - am-m.
morning - lyc.

cutting, sacro-iliac, symphysis - nat-p.

cutting, sacrum - ail., all-s., alum., ***bell., calc-p.,*** dig., gamb., ***gels.,*** guare., helon., kali-bi., lob., mag-m., nat-m., nat-p., nat-s., rhus-t., samb., senec., ***sulph.***
bending, backward, when - rhus-t.
forward - samb.
hips and - ail.
menses, during - ***senec.***
morning - all-s.
standing, while - rhus-t.
stooping agg. - samb.
warmth amel. - sulph.

DIAPER, rash, buttocks - ***bapt., bor.,*** bry., ***kali-chl., merc., merc-c., mur-ac., nit-ac., sulph.,*** **SUL-AC.**
excoriation, between buttocks - arg-m., arum-t., ***berb.,*** bufo, calc., calen., ***carb-s.,*** carb-v., **GRAPH.,** ***kreos.,*** nat-m., ***nit-ac.,*** puls., ***sep., sulph.***

DISCOLORATION, buttocks, redness - cann-s., hyos.
spots, in - cann-s., mag-c.

DISLOCATED, as if, sacrum - agar., nux-v.

dislocated, sacro-iliac, symphyses as if separated - calc-p.
walking, while - calc-p.

DRAGGING, pain, coccyx - ***ant-t., caust.,*** graph., kreos.

dragging, perineum - cann-s., graph., nat-a., puls., ther.

dragging, sacrum - ***carb-v.,*** helon., ***sep.,*** ust.

DRAWING, pain, buttocks - agar., aloe, bar-c., berb., bry., calc., ***camph., chin.,*** crot-t., cupr., dig., mang., mez., nat-m., nit-ac., ph-ac., ***rhus-t.,*** sep., sil., zinc.
cramp-like - calc., mang., ph-ac.

DRAWING, pain, buttocks
extending to feet - nit-ac.
gluteal muscles - camph., cycl., gels., mosch., ***sulph.,*** verat.
left - agar., ph-ac.
pressure amel - ***rhus-t.***
right - ***rhus-t.,*** sep.
rising from seat - mang.
sitting, while - ***chin.,*** cycl.
amel - mang.
standing, while - chin., mang.
amel - cycl.
waking - agar.
walking, while - ph-ac.
wine, after - zinc.

drawing, coccyx - ***calc.,*** carb-v., **CAUST.,** graph., kreos., lil-t., mur-ac., ***rhus-t., thuj.***
evening - ***caust.,*** graph.
extending, to rectum and vagina - ***kreos.***
to thighs - ***thuj.***
upwards - mur-ac.
menses, during - caust., ***cic.,*** graph., kreos., thuj.
paroxysmal - thuj.
rising from a seat, amel. - kreos.
sensation of pulling upwards from tip of - lil-t.
sitting, while - ***kreos., thuj.***
standing erect impossible - thuj.
sticking while walking - bry.
urination, preventing - thuj.

drawing, ilium, crest - lyc., ruta., thuj.
extending to thigh -ruta., thuj.

drawing, perineum - berb., ***cycl., kali-bi.,*** mez., sulph.
sitting, while - ***cycl.***
walking, while - cycl.

drawing, sacrum - acon., ***am-c.,*** ang., ***ant-c.,*** arg-n., aster., **BAR-C.,** bell., ***chel., chin.,*** cocc., colch., croc., dig., ***dios.,*** dulc., ***helon.,*** hep., ign., kali-bi., **KALI-C.,** led., lyc., mur-ac., nat-c., nat-m., **NUX-V.,** sabin., samb., sil., spong., stram., ***sulph.,*** sul-ac., ter., ***thuj.,*** valer., verat., zing.
bending backward - bar-c.
evening - bar-c.
extending into thighs - nux-v.
to lumbar region - mur-ac.
flatuence, as from obstructed - nat-c.
lying on back - bell.
menses, during - cham., con., zing.
morning - kali-bi., lil-t.
pressure amel. - led.
rising from a seat, agg. - ***bar-c., thuj.***
sitting, while - ***bell.,*** staph., ***thuj.***
standing, while - led.
amel. - bell.
erect, impossible - thuj.
stool, before - zing.
walking, rapidly agg. - bell., ***bry.***
slowly amel. - bell., kali-bi.

EMACIATION, buttocks - bar-m., ***lath.,*** nat-m., sac-alb.
gluteal muscles - lath., plb.

ERUPTIONS, buttocks - ant-c., bor., canth., caust., ***graph.,*** mez., ***nat-c.,*** nat-m., nux-v., sel., thuj., ***til.***
between - olnd.
moisture - arum-t., thuj.
pimples - sulph.
pustules - phos.
upper part of - hep.
blotches - ant-c., bry., sars.
dry - nat-c.
elevations - mez.
excoriation - ***rhus-t.,*** thuj.
itching - calc-p., caust., graph., mag-m., nat-c., thuj., til.
knots - ther.
leprous spots, annular - ***graph.***
painful - graph.
pimples - ant-s., ars-h., bar-c., berb., calc., canth., chel., cob., graph., ham., hura, kali-n., lyc., mag-c., mang., meph., merc., nat-p., nux-v., ***petr.,*** plan., rhus-t., sel., sulph., thuj., ***til.***
itching - kali-n., lyc., mag-m., thuj., ***til.***
painful - ham., sulph.
pustules - ant-c., calc., grat., hyos., jug-c., ph-ac.
red - mag-m.,
scabs - chel., ***graph.,*** psor.
scratching, after - kali-n.
scurfy - calc-p.

eruptions, coccyx - bor., graph., merc.
itching - ***graph.,*** led., nat-c.
moist, on - ***arum-t.,*** graph., led., nit-ac.
scabs, bloody - bor., ***graph., sil.***

eruptions, sacrum, moist, on - graph., led.
scabs, bloody - ***sil.***

eruptions, perineum - brom., graph., ***petr.,*** sars., ***sulph.,*** tell., tep.
dry - ***petr.***
itching - alum.
newborn, in - med.
pimples - nit-ac., sep., sulph., sul-ac.
squeaking - kali-i.
walking, when - myric.

EXCORIATION, buttocks, between - arum-t., arg-m., ***berb.,*** bufo, ***carb-s.,*** **GRAPH.,** ***kreos.,*** nat-m., ***nit-ac.,*** puls., ***sep., sulph.***
walking, from - arg-m., **CAUST.,** nat-m., ***nit-ac.***

excoriation, of perineum - alum., arum-t., aur-m., ***calc.,*** carb-an., ***carb-v., caust., cham., graph., hep.,*** ign., **LYC.,** ***merc.,*** petr., puls., rhod., sep., ***sulph.,*** thuj.
female - ***calc., carb-v., caust.,*** **GRAPH.,** hep., **LYC.,** ***merc., petr., sep., sulph.,*** thuj.

EXOSTOSES, on sacrum - rhus-t.

FLUTTERING, commencing in sacrum and gradually rising to occiput - ol-j.

FORMICATION, buttocks - ang., ars.

formication, perineum - acon., chel., petros., rhod.

formication, sacrum - bor., chin., crot-t., graph., ph-ac., sars.

FULLNESS, perineum - alum., ***chin.,*** berb., bry., cycl., nux-v.

GNAWING, pain, buttocks, as if gnawed by dogs - hura.

gnawing, coccyx - agar., alum., ***gamb., kali-c.,*** ph-ac.

menses, during - kali-c.

gnawing, sacrum in - alum., phos.

evening - canth.

after going to bed - naja.

stretching amel. - alum.

HEAT, coccyx - agar., alum., arn., ars., bor., ***calc.,*** carb-an., carb-v., caust., chin., colch., graph., hep., ign., laur., led., merc., mur-ac., ph-ac., phos., plat., rhus-t., spig., staph., sulph., zinc.

heat, perineum, in - alum., aur.

heat, sacrum - sars., sep., sulph.

HEAVINESS, coccyx - ant-c., ***ant-t., arg-n.***

sensation as if a heavy weight were tugging at - ***ant-t.***

standing amel. - arg-n.

stool, during - arg-n.

heaviness, sacrum - ***arg-n.,*** berb., **CHIN.,** cimic., con., dios., ***ferr.,*** hura, mag-s., ***phyt., rhus-t., sec., sep.,*** zing.

genitals, and - lob.

sitting, while - aloe, ***arg-n.,*** hura, **RHUS-T.**

standing amel. - ***arg-n.***

stool, during - ***arg-n.***

walking - arg-n.

weight - **ARG-N., CHIN.,** ***cimic., con., ferr.***

HERPES, buttocks - bor., caust., kreos., ***nat-c.,*** nat-m., nicc.

herpes, iliac -***tell.***

herpes, perineum - kali-c., **PETR.,** tell.

INDURATION, buttocks, muscles - ph-ac., thuj.

INFILTRATION, buttocks, with bloody serum - vip.

INJURIES, coccyx - aesc., arn., bell-p., ***carb-an.,*** **HYPER.,** led., ***mez.,*** **SIL.,** tell.

injuries, perineum, lacerated - ***calen.,*** hyper., staph.

penetrating - calen., hyper., symph.

injuries, sacrum - aesc., arn., ruta, symph.

ITCHING, buttocks - ***am-c.,*** ant-t., asc-t., bar-c., calc., ***calc-p.,*** carb-ac., ***caust.,*** cham., con., dulc., gran., kali-c., lyc., ***mag-c.,*** mag-m., mez., olnd., ***petr.,*** prun., sel., ***sil.,*** staph., stront-c., **SULPH.,** ther., thuj., zinc.

air, open - rumx.

bed, in - rumx.

between - alum., ***bar-c.,*** con., kali-c.

burning - am-c.

cold water amel - petr.

corrosive - sulph.

dinner, after - laur.

evening - sars.

bed, in - lyc., staph.

undressing - mag-c.

ITCHING, buttocks

gluteal region - coloc., fl-ac., mur-ac., ph-ac., tarax.

morning, rising, on - nat-c.

night - con., petr.

bed, in - merc-i-f.

scratching, agg - petr.

amel - kali-i., olnd., thuj.

itching, coccyx - agar., alum., am-c., bar-c., bor., ***bov.,*** chin., con., fl-ac., ***graph.,*** lyc., spig.

burning - fl-ac.

corrosive - ph-ac.

evening in bed - carb-an.

menses, during - dros., graph., ph-ac.

warmth of bed agg. - ***petr.***

itching, iliac - osm., sulph., ***tell.***

right - stront.

itching, perineum - agn., ***alum.,*** ars., bell., canth., cann-s., carb-v., ***chel.,*** cina, con., ***fl-ac.,*** gran., ign., kali-c., mur-ac., nat-c., ***nat-s.,*** nux-v., **PETR.,** plb., ***sars.,*** seneg., **SULPH.,** tarax., tep., thuj.

forenoon - thuj.

night - ***carb-v.,*** con., kali-c., petr.

scratching, after, pain - alum., tarax.

agg. - alum.

stool, during - ***sulph.***

touched, when - ***carb-v.***

walking, while - ign.

itching, sacrum - agar., alum., bor., bov., fl-ac., graph., laur., led., med., merc., par., plb.

burning - kali-c.

walking, while - merc.

JERKING, pain coccyx - alum., calc., carb-an., caust., chin., ***cic.,*** rhus-t., sulph.

menses, during - ***cic.***

jerking, sacrum - chin., petr.

sacral region - chin., fl-ac.

LABOR-like, pain, sacrum - ***cham., cimic.,*** croc., ***kali-c.,*** kali-i., kreos., **PULS.,** ***sars.,*** sec., sep., ***sulph.***

extending to thighs - cham.

morning - ***puls.***

LAMENESS, sacrum - **AESC.,** ***calc-p.,*** com., phos., ***rhus-t.,*** **SIL.**

rising from a seat, when - **AESC.,** phos., **SIL.,** ***sulph.***

straining or lifting, as from - **RHUS-T.,** staph.

walking, while - **AESC.,** com.

LANCINATING, coccyx - ***canth., tarent.***

lancinating, sacrum - cupr., ***plb., zinc.***

LUMP, sensation of, perineum - arg-n., cann-i., cann-s., **CHIM.,** kali-m., ***ther., sep.***

sitting on it, as if - chim.

MOISTURE, perineum - carb-an., ***carb-v.,*** thuj.

night - ***carb-v.***

NUMBNESS, buttocks - ***calc-p.,*** dig., plb., raph., spong., sulph.

lying, while - sulph.

rising, on, after sitting - calc-p.

NUMBNESS, buttocks
sitting, while - ***alum., calc-p.,*** dig., guai., ***sulph.***
numbness, coccyx - berb., **PLAT.**
menses, during - plat.
sitting, while - **PLAT.**
numbness, iliac, fossa, right, amel. lying on it - ***apis.***
numbness, sacrum - berb., ***calc-p., graph.,*** ox-ac., plat., spong.
lower limbs, and - ***calc-p.***
sitting, while - plat.

PAIN, buttocks - agar., **BAR-C.,** bry., ***calc.,*** calc-p., **CAMPH.,** caust., cina, cist., coca, coloc., cupr., euph., eup-per., guai., hep., iod., kali-bi., kali-c., kalm., merc., mez., mill., nit-ac., ***phos.,*** plb., ***puls.,*** sep., staph., **SULPH.,** tarent.
afternoon, 5 p.m. on open air - coca
evening - mill.
gluteal region - am-m., eup-per., euphr., hura, kalm., laur., lepi., med., nit-ac., puls., rhus-t., sol-t-ae., spig., tab.
sitting, after - laur., puls.
sitting, while - am-m., sulph.
sleep, during - am-m.
walking - spig., tab.
hindering labor - ***kali-c.***
lying, while - sulph.
morning - mill.
6 a.m. until midnight - tarent.
night, while riding in a carriage - nit-ac.
sitting, after - staph.
pressure agg - mill.
right - nit-ac.
sitting, while - cann-s., chin., cina, cycl., **HEP.,** ***phos.,*** sep., ***staph.,*** sulph.
from - kali-c.
stepping - mez.
ulcerative - calc., kali-c., phos., ***puls.***
walking - ***mez.***

PAIN, coccyx - aesc., agar., agn., alum., am-c., ***am-m.,*** ant-t., **APIS,** arg-n., arn., ars-i., asaf., bell., bell-p., bor., bov., ***bry., calc., calc-caust., calc-p.,*** calc-s., cann-i., ***cann-s., canth.,*** cast., cast-eq., ***carb-an., carb-s., carb-v.,*** **CAUST.,** cic., cimic., ***cist.,*** colch., ***con.,*** dios., ***euph., ferr-p., fl-ac., gamb.,*** graph., grat., hep., ***hyper.,*** ign., iod., ***kali-bi., kali-c.,*** kali-i., ***kali-p.,*** **KREOS.,** lac-c., ***lach.,*** lact., led., lil-t., lob., ***mag-c., med., merc.,*** mur-ac., nat-m., ***nit-ac.,*** nux-m., ***par., petr.,*** ph-ac., ***phos.,*** pic-ac., plat., plb., ***rhus-t., ruta., sep., sil.,*** staph., sulph., syph., tarent., ***thuj.,*** verat., xan., **ZINC.**
childbirth, confinement, after - tarent.
dislocated, as if - agar., sulph.
evening - alum., ***apis, cast-eq., caust.,*** graph., ***kali-bi.***
extending, spine up, after stool - euph.
through spine to vertex during stool, drawing, head backward - euph., ***phos.***
to rectum and vagina - ***kreos.***
to thighs - rhus-t.
to urethra before urination - ***kali-bi.***

PAIN, coccyx
fall, after a - **HYPER.,** ***mez.,*** **SIL.**
as from a - kali-i., ruta.
lying, while - ***carb-an.***
on back - bell.
menses, during - bell., canth., carb-an., ***caust., cic., cist.,*** graph., kali-c., kreos., merc., ph-ac., thuj., zinc.
instead of - ars.
suppressed - bell., caust., kali-c., mag-c., merc., petr., phos., plat., ruta., thuj., zinc.
morning on waking - ***kali-bi.***
motion, on - ***caust.,*** euph., fl-ac., kali-bi., ***phos.,*** tarent.
impeding - lach., ***phos.***
pressure - ***arum-t., calc-p., carb-an., carb-v., euph.,*** fl-ac., ***kali-bi., petr.,*** **SIL.,** tarent., xan.
on abdomen, amel. - merc.
pulling, from up - lil-t.
riding, as after a long carriage ride - **SIL.**
in a carriage - nux-m., ***sil.***
rising from a seat - ***caust., euph., kali-bi.,*** **LACH., SIL.,** ***sulph.***
amel. - kreos.
sex, during - kali-bi.
sitting, while - ***am-m., apis,*** arg-n., bell., ***carb-an., cast-eq.,*** cist., **KALI-BI.,** ***lach.,*** led., ***par., petr.,*** plat., syph., rhus-t., tarent., thuj., xan., zinc.
after, unable to rise - bell.
on something sharp, as if - ***lach.***
sleep, during - ***am-m.***
standing - verat.
amel. - arg-n., bell., tarent.
erect - thuj.
stool, during - phos., sulph.
after - grat., sulph.
stooping, when - sulph.
stretching amel. - alum.
touched, when - alum., bell., ***carb-an., calc-p.,*** cist., ***euph.,*** fl-ac., ***kali-bi.,*** lach., petr., phos., **SIL.,** xan.
ulcerative - ***carb-an., phos.***
urinating, while - ***graph.***
before - kali-bi.
walking, while - bry., ***kali-bi.***
slowly amel. - bell.

PAIN, ilium - agar., eupi., form., hell., iris
crest of right, worse in morning on sitting down, better standing and walking, extending to thigh - staph.
muscles, attachment - camph., ***form., tarent.***

PAIN, loins - canth., plb., rheum, thuj., zinc.
hollow of - pall.
sticking - berb., plb.

PAIN, perineum - agn., alum., ant-c., aur., ***berb.,*** bov., calc-p., ***canth.,*** carb-an., carb-v., **CAUST.,** chel., chim., cupr-ar., ***cycl.,*** kali-bi., ***lyc.,*** nux-v., ol-an., paeon., phos., plb., ***puls.,*** sanic., sel., sulph., thuj.

PAIN, perineum
erection, during - alum.
extending to, genitals - bov.
penis - phyt.
rectum - bov.
rising from a seat - alum.
sex, after - alum.
sitting - alum., lyc., puls.
standing - alum.
stool, agg. - sanic.
urging to urinate - ant-t., aran., cop.
urinating while - phos.
walking agg. - chel.

PAIN, sacro-iliac, junction - **AESC.,** ***ant-t.,*** apis, ***arg-n., bry., calc-p., cimic., coloc.,*** dios., ferr., gels., hep., hyper., jug-c., mag-p-a., nat-p., ol-j., plb., rhus-t., rumx., sabad., spong., sulph., tell., thuj.
extending, down region of sciatics during labor. - ***cimic.***
to groin - ***thuj.***
right - nat-p.
separated, as if - calc-p.
standing - spong.

PAIN, sacrum - abrot., absin., acon., act-sp., **AESC., AGAR.,** ail., aloe, all-s., ***alum.,*** am-c., am-m., ang., ant-c., **ANT-T.,** ***apis, arg-m.,*** arg-n., arn., ***ars.,*** ars-i., asaf., aur., bad., ***bapt., bar-c., bell.,*** **BERB.,** bor., ***bry.,*** calad., **CALC.,** ***calc-p.,*** calc-s., canth., ***caps.,*** carb-ac., ***carb-an.,*** carb-s., ***carb-v.,*** caul., ***caust.,*** cham., chel., ***chin.,*** chin-a., cic., ***cimx., cimic.,*** cina, cinnb., cob., cocc., coc-c., colch., ***coloc.,*** coff., con., cor-r., croc., cupr., cupr-ar., dig., ***dios., dulc.,*** eup-per., eup-pur., ferr., ferr-i., fl-ac., form., gamb., **GELS.,** glon., ***graph.,*** ham., ***helon., hep., hyper., ign.,*** iod., kali-ar., ***kali-bi., kali-c.,*** kali-i., kali-n., ***kali-p.,*** kali-s., ***kreos., lac-c., lach.,*** lact., lam., ***laur.,*** lec., led., ***lept.,*** lith., ***lil-t., lob.,*** **LYC.,** ***lyss.,*** mag-c., mag-m., mag-s., ***med.,*** meli., meny., ***merc.,*** mez., mosch., murx., **MUR-AC.,** naja, nat-a., nat-c., ***nat-m.,*** nat-p., ***nat-s.,*** **NIT-AC., NUX-M.,** ***nux-v.,*** ol-an., ol-j., **ONOS.,** op., ox-ac., petr., phel., ***phos.,*** phys., ***phyt.,*** pic-ac., plat., plan., ***podo., psor.,*** ptel., **PULS.,** ran-b., ran-s., rhod., ***rhus-r., rhus-t., ruta.,*** sabin., samb., sang., sarr., sars., ***sec.,*** seneg., **SEP.,** ***sil.,*** spong., staph., stram., stront-c., ***sulph.,*** sul-ac., tarax., **TELL.,** ter., ***thuj.,*** ust., valer., **VARIO.,** verat., vib., xan., zinc., zing.
after-pains - hyper., sulph.
afternoon - colch.
alternating with aching in occiput - alum., carb-v.
bed, in - visc.
bending backward - bar-c., con., plat., puls., rhus-t.
backward, amel. - lac-c., puls.
forward, amel. - sang.
blowing nose - arg-n.
breathing, when - berb., carb-an., carb-v., **MERC.,** ruta, sel., spig., sulph., tarax.
childbirth, after - ***hyper.,*** nux-v., phos.

PAIN, sacrum
chill, during - ars., gamb., hyos., **NUX-V.,** psor., verat.
cold, from taking - dulc., nit-ac.
coughing, when - am-c., bry., ***chel.,*** merc., nit-ac., sulph., ***tell.***
daytime - lil-t.
dysentery, with - ***caps., nux-v.***
emissions, after - ***graph.***
evening - agar., bar-c., lac-c., led., naja, nit-ac., puls., sep., ter.
amel. in - lil-t.
exertion, during - agar.
extending to,
coccyx while sitting - kreos.
down legs - ***agar.,*** arn., cimx., ***coloc., graph., lac-c.,*** lyc., ***med., pic-ac.,*** plat., plb., ***sep.***
stool, after - rhus-t.
to great toe - arn.
feet - cob., kali-m., lyc.
front - ***arg-n.***
groin - plat., ***sabin.,*** **SULPH.**
menses, during - arn., ***sabin.,*** **SULPH.**
pelvis, around, before menses - plat., puls., sep., vib.
hips - **AESC.,** berb., cimx., coloc., ***lac-c.,*** pall., phyt., puls., **SEP.,** ust.
and pelvis - arg-n.
and thighs - ***cimic., lac-c., sep.***
labor, during - ***cimic.***
right - ***sulph.***
sitting, while - thuj.
lower extremities - ***cimic.,*** cimx., ***lac-c., lil-t., sep.***
ovarian region - ust.
pelvis - visc.
pubis - arg-m., helon., ***laur.,*** **SABIN.,** ***sulph.***
one bone to another, and from - sabin.
right hip - ***sulph.***
thighs - arn., berb., ***cimic., coloc.,*** kali-c., kreos., nux-v., ***sec., sep., sulph., tell.***
left - kali-c.
right - colch., tell.
right agg. by pressing at stool or cough - **TELL.**
sitting, while - thuj.
uterus - ***cham.,*** helon., nat-m.
fall, as from a - ruta.
falling, from - kali-c.
forceps, delivery, after - **HYPER.**
heat, during - chin.
instrumental delivery, after - **HYPER.**
laughing when - ***tell.***
leaning against a chair - agar.
lifting, from - ***calc., puls., rhus-t., sang.,*** staph.
lifting, when - anag., bry.
lying, while - agar., **BERB.,** chin., naja, nux-v., puls., tarax., thuj., zing.
amel. - **AGAR.,** kali-c.
with body bent forward - bry.

PAIN, sacrum
lying, while
back, on the - bapt., bell., ***ign.,*** lyc., puls., ***tell.***
amel. - ***agar.,*** calc-p., puls.
compelled - agar., calc-p., cimx.
not able to rise - **AGAR.,** sil.
side - act-sp., ***nat-s.,*** puls.
amel. - puls.
right, agg. - agar.
menses, during - ***am-c., am-m., berb.,*** bor., calc., calc-s., carb-s., carb-v., ***caust.,*** cham., cimic., con., ferr., ***kali-c.,*** kali-n., ***kali-p.,*** kreos., ***lob.,*** lyc., mag-c., mag-m., ***nat-c.,*** nat-p., phos., prun., ***puls.,*** rat., ***sabin.,*** sang., ***sars., senec., sulph.,*** zinc., zing.
before - am-c., bar-c., carb-an., caust., kali-n., lach., mag-c., nux-v., puls., spong., ***vib.***
beginning of - asar.
instead of - spong.
morning - ang., calad., ign., kali-n., lac-c., lil-t., nat-m., petr., phos., ***puls.,*** sel., ***staph.,*** sulph., thuj., verat.
sex, during - kali-bi.
waking, on - carb-s., carb-v., ***kali-bi.***
motion, during - ***aesc., agar.,*** caust., chel., ***chin.,*** coloc., form., hura, kali-bi., lil-t., lyc., phos., phys., psor., phyt., plan., **PULS.,** sars., sec., tell.
amel. during - ang., aloe, coloc., fl-ac., ***lac-c., lyc.,*** **NUX-M.,** psor., **PULS., RHUS-T.**
gentle, amel. - **PULS.**
moving arm, on - chel.
night - am-c., ang., arg-n., cham., chin., colch., lach., lyc., mag-c., mag-s., nat-s., nux-v., ***puls.,*** staph.
1 am - staph.
bed, driving out of - mag-c.
waking him frequently - colch.
paralytic - arg-n., ***graph.***
periodic, into pelvis, with pains in thighs and upper limbs - visc.
pressure amel. - kali-c., led., mag-m., ***sep.***
raising leg, on - bry.
rheumatic - kali-bi., sulph., zinc.
riding in a carriage - lac-c., **NUX-M.**
rising from, sitting - **AESC.,** ant-c., bar-c., **CALC.,** ***caust.,*** con., ferr., ***kali-bi., lac-c.,*** **LYC.,** petr., phos., psor., ***puls.,*** rhod., **SIL.,** ***staph.,*** **SULPH.,** tell., thuj., verat.
stooping - ***lyc., phos.,*** sars., verat.
sex, from - ***agar.,*** calc., ***calc-p., kali-c.,*** nat-c., ***petr., phos.,*** **SEP., SIL.,** staph.
sitting, while - **AGAR.,** aloe, ang., ant-t., ***apis, arg-m., arg-n.,*** asaf., asar., bar-c., ***bell.,*** **BERB.,** bor., bufo, carb-an., caust., cist., cob., kali-bi., ***kreos., lac-c., lyc.,*** meny., merc., nat-a., nat-c., nat-s., ol-an., phel., prun., ***puls.,*** **RHUS-T.,** ruta, sabad., spig., ter., ***thuj.***
a while, after - aloe, asaf., berb., phos., puls.
erect - lyc.
must sit bent forward - lyc.
sneezing - arg-n.

PAIN, sacrum
standing, while - ***agar.,*** **CON.,** led., ***lil-t., lith.,*** merc., ***phos.,*** plan., puls., rhus-t., spong., verat.
amel. - arg-n., bell.
erect - petr.
stool, during - ***agar., arg-n.,*** **CARB-AN.,** ***merc-c.,*** **NUX-V.,** ***podo.,*** sars., ***tell.***
after - aesc., ***podo.,*** tab.
amel. - berb., indg.
before - berb., carb-v., ***dios.,*** kali-n., nat-c., sars., zing.
inability to - aesc., bor., puls.
pressing at - ***agar., carb-an., tell.***
with urging to - am-be., lil-t., ***merc-c.,*** **NUX-V.**
stooping, when - **AESC.,** bor., buf-s., kali-bi., lac-c., lyc., meny., ol-an., plb., ruta, sars., sulph., ***tell.,*** thuj., verat.
stretching amel. - alum.
out leg, on - bry.
touch agg. - colch.
slight agg. - lob.
turning, in bed - ***bry., nux-v., staph.***
to left amel. - agar.
ulcerative - ***puls.***
urinating, while - ***graph.,*** sulph.
urine, on retaining - ***nat-s.***
vaginal discharge, agg. - aesc., psor.
amel. - murx.
walking, while - acon., **AESC.,** ***agar.,*** bor., bry., form., ham., kali-bi., ***kali-c., phos.,*** sabad., sars., spong., sulph., verat., zinc.
amel. - ang., arg-m., arg-n., ***lyc.,*** merc., nat-a., psor., staph., ***tell.,*** thuj.
air, in open amel. - ruta, ***tell.***
slow amel. - bell., **PULS.**
stepping with left foot, when - spong.

PARALYSIS, sensation of, muscles, sacrum - ***phos.***

PERITONITIS, pelvic, (see Female)

PERSPIRATION, buttocks, nates - thuj.
perspiration, perineum, about the anus and - agar., ***alum.,*** bell., carb-an., con., ***hep.,*** kali-c., psor., rhus-t., ***thuj.***
morning - ***thuj.***
night - kali-c.
stool before and during - sep.
perspiration, sacrum - plan.
cold - plan.

PINCHING, pain, perineum, in - carb-an., lyc., ***puls.***

PRESSING, pain, buttocks - cupr., iod., lyc., mill., sars., sep., zinc.
forenoon - mill.
gluteal region - cact., cimic., iod., mez.
plug, as from - ***anac.***
pulsating - chin.
walking, while - mill.
pressing, coccyx - aloe, apis, calc., calc-p., cann-i., ***cann-s., carb-an., carb-v.,*** chin., hep., iod., merc., ph-ac., phos., ***sep.,*** valer., zinc.

pressing, coccyx
evening - ***apis,*** kali-bi.
sitting, while - ***apis.***
pressing, ilium - chel.
pressing, perineum - ***alum., asaf.,*** berb., cycl., ***lyc.,*** mez., olnd., sulph., ***thuj.***
pressing, sacrum - acon., agar., ***all-c.,*** aloe, ang., arg-m., ***berb.,*** bor., cann-s., **CARB-AN.,** ***carb-v.,*** caust., chel., ***ferr., ign.,*** iod., ***lyss.,*** meny., mosch., **NUX-V.,** ***puls.,*** ruta., sabin., samb., ***sec.,*** sep., spong., tarax., thuj., verat., zinc.
dull instrument, as from a - mosch.
evening - ***puls.***
extending to ilium - thuj.
leaning back against chair - agar.
lying - ***berb.***
menses, during - ferr.
motion amel. - aloe
night - ang.
pressing down - bell., berb., merl., **NUX-V.,** sec., ***sep.***
sitting, while - agar., aloe, ***berb.***
stepping, on - acon., spong.
urging to stool, with - ***merc-c.,*** **NUX-V.**
walking, while - acon., spong.

PRICKLING, sacrum - mez.

PULSATION, buttocks - phos., prun., rumx., sol-t-ae., zinc.
afternoon, 2 p.m - sol-t-ae.
pulsating, coccyx - agar., par.
pulsation, perineum - bov., ***caust.,*** polyg.

PULSATING, sacrum - ***bar-c.,*** berb., caust., graph., ign., kali-c., lach., **NAT-M.,** nit-ac., nux-v., ol-an., sabin., sars., sep., ***sil.,*** tab.

SACRO-iliac, syndrome - **AESC.,** ***ant-t.,*** apis, ***arg-n., bry., calc-p., cimic., coloc.,*** dios., ferr., gels., hep., hyper., jug-c., mag-p-a., nat-p., ol-j., plb., rhus-t., rumx., sabad., spong., sulph., tell., thuj.
extending, down region of sciatics during labor. - ***cimic.***
to groin - ***thuj.***
right - nat-p.
separated, as if - calc-p.
standing - spong.
sacro-iliac, junction, separated, as if - calc-p.

SENSITIVE, buttocks - ***ars.***
sensitive, sacrum, extremely, to touch of clothing - lob.

SHARP, pain, buttocks - ***alum.,*** ang., ant-c., bar-c., berb., ***calc.,*** **CALC-P.,** carb-o., caust., cham., dulc., euphr., ***guai.,*** laur., lyc., merc., ol-an., par., plb., prun., staph., sulph., zinc.
afternoon, 3:30 p.m - ol-an.
dinner, during - laur.
evening in bed - staph.
extending to hips and groin - nat-m.
gluteal muscles - asaf., aur., cham., chin-s., con., hyos., meny., mur-ac., staph., tab., viol-t.
jerking - meny.

SHARP, pain, buttocks
itching - stann.
scratching, from - prun.
amel - staph.
sitting, while - alum., calc-p., guai., mang.
small spots - **CALC-P.**
standing, while - berb.
sharp, coccyx - agn., am-c., arg-m., calc., calc-p., ***canth., caust.,*** colch., dios., lact., ***mag-c.,*** mur-ac., nat-m., nicc., ***par.,*** ph-ac., phos., ***pic-ac., rhus-t.,*** **SIL.,** ***tarent., thuj.,*** verat., zinc.
extending, to anus - carb-v., thuj.
up back - mur-ac., ***phos.***
itching - dros., ph-ac., verat.
jerking - carb-v., rhus-t.
menses, during - caust., ph-ac.
pressure on - ***sil.***
pulsating - ign., par.
rising from seat - **SIL.**
sitting, while - dros., lach., par.
itching, while - ***par.***
standing, while - verat.
startling - calc-p., mur-ac.
stinging - sil.
stool, during - ***phos.***
before - sep.
sharp, iliac - agar., alum., anac., ***berb.,*** brom., cham., kali-chl., kali-n., laur., led., lyc., merc., mez., sil., spig., thuj.
extending, down leg - kreos.
ilium to ilium - lil-t.
left - ***con.***
menses, during - ***con.***
morning -berb.
sitting, while - kali-n.
sharp, ilium, crest of - berb., brom., eupi., kali-n., kreos., manc., merc., naja, nat-m., olnd., plan., spig., stront-c., thuj.
extending, downward - zinc.
to chest - lach.
to gluteal muscles - ***berb.***
to small of back - mag-m.
inspiration, on - mill.
walking while - eupi.
sharp, perineum - alum., am-m., aur., berb., bov., ***calc-p.,*** carb-v., chel., chin., mag-m., merc., nat-c., nit-ac., sep., spig., sulph., thuj.
evening - am-m., sep.
extending to, anus - nit-ac.
to, penis - ***calc-p.***
to, uterus - berb.
sharp, sacro-iliac, symphyses - phos.
sharp, sacrum - acon., **AGAR.,** agn., aloe, ambr., ang., arn., ars., asaf., bar-c., bell., berb., ***bry.,*** calc., ***calc-p.,*** calc-s., ***carb-an.,*** carb-v., chin., cocc., coloc., **CON.,** dulc., hyper., ign., jug-r., kali-bi., kali-c., kali-i., kali-n., ***lith.,*** lyc., mag-c., merc., mur-ac., nat-c., nat-m., nat-s., nicc., nit-ac., ox-ac., ***phos., phyt.,*** plb., puls., ruta., sil., squil., spong., staph., ***sulph.,*** tarax., tell., thuj., verat., ***zinc.***
breathing, when - **MERC.,** spig.
burning - mur-ac., thuj.

sharp, sacrum
coughing - bry.
extending, down outside of hips to feet - coloc., ***phyt.***
from left side to left testes - thuj.
to anus - asaf.
to ilium - thuj.
to gluteal and hips - **KALI-C.**
jerking - thuj.
lie on the back, compelled to - ***agar.,*** calc-p.
motion - coloc.
pregnancy - **KALI-C.**
rubbing amel. - thuj.
sitting, while - bar-c., nat-s., spig., staph.
standing, while - **CON.,** ***lith.***
stool, after, amel. - indg.
walking, while - ***agar.,*** calad.
amel. - staph.
in the open air - ***agar.***

SHOCKS, buttocks, nates - cocc.
shocks, sacrum, in - cupr.

SHOOTING, buttocks - carb-o.

SHUDDERING, buttocks - croc.
sitting, while - croc.

SORE, pain, buttocks - agar., arg-m., ***ars.,*** calc-p., card-m., caust., cist., ***hep.,*** lyc., mag-m., mag-s., merc., nat-m., nit-ac., nux-v., ***puls.,*** sanic., sel., sulph., zinc.
between - sulph.
sitting, while - agar., caust., ***hep.,*** phos., sel., sep.
after - agar., puls.
touch on - sulph.
walking, while - mag-s.
sore, coccyx - alum., ***am-m., arn.,*** calc-p., ***carb-an., carb-v.,*** **CAUST.,** ***cist., euph.,*** fl-ac., **HYPER.,** ***kali-bi., kali-i.,*** lach., ***mez.,*** nat-m., ***petr.,*** phos., ***ruta.,*** **SIL., SULPH.,** xan.
extending to sacrum - ruta.
injury, from - ***carb-an.,*** **HYPER.,** ***mez.,*** **SIL.**
lying agg. - am-m., carb-an.
menses, during - bell., carb-an., caust., kreos.
rising from a seat - **SULPH.**
sitting, when - ***am-m.,*** carb-an., ***cist., kali-bi.,*** **SIL.**
preventing - cist.
sleep, during - ***am-m.***
stooping agg. - sulph.
touch, on - alum.
sore, iliac, bruised, tenderness - aur., carb-an., cic., kreos.
drawing up thigh amel. - aur.
sitting, while - aur.
standing amel. - aur.
sore, ilium, bruised, tenderness - nat-c., sulph.
sore, perineum - alum., echi.
sore, sacro-iliac, junction - ***calc-p.,*** rumx.
menses, during - thuj.
symphyses - ***calc-p.,*** coc-c., hep., rumx., verat.
menses, during - thuj.
sore, sacrum - ***acon., agar.,*** **ALUM.,** am-c., ***am-m.,*** ang., arg-m., ***arn.,*** ars., bapt., berb., ***bry., calad.,*** carb-s., ***caust.,*** chin., cina, cinnb., ***colch.,*** coloc., cor-r., dig., eup-per., ferr., ***fl-ac.,*** gamb., ***graph., hep.,*** hyper., ign., kali-bi., kali-i., kreos., lact., ***lob.,*** mag-c., mag-m., meny., ***merc.,*** nat-a., nat-c., ***nat-m., nat-s., nux-m., nux-v.,*** ox-ac., phel., ***phos.,*** phyt., ***plat.,*** ran-b., ran-s., rhod., **RHUS-T.,** ***ruta., sabad.,*** sars., ***sep.,*** sil., spong., staph., stront-c., ***sulph., tell.,*** thuj., ***verat.***
lying, on side, when - act-sp., ***nat-s.***
quietly on the back - **RHUS-T.**
menses, before - ***spong.***
moving amel. - **RHUS-T.**
paralytic pain in knees on rising from seat - ***verat.***
sitting, while - ***merc.,*** **RHUS-T.**
spine - am-c., ang., ***berb., colch.,*** kali-bi., ***lob.,*** nat-a., rhus-t., sarr., ***sep., sil.***
menses, before - ***spong.***
stooping or walking agg. - nat-a.
stooping - nat-a.
touch of clothing, sensitive to - ***lob.***
walking - nat-a.

SPRAINED, coccyx, as if, after stool - grat.
sprained, sacrum, as if - agar., ***calc.,*** lach., ol-an., rhod., sulph.

STICKING, pain, perineum - alum., bell., bov., carb-v., mag-m., merc., sep., thuj.

STIFFNESS, sacrum - acon., ***aesc.,*** am-m., apis, ***bar-c.,*** berb., ***bry., caust., lach.,*** laur., ***led., lyc.,*** manc., meph., prun., puls., rheum, ***rhus-t.,*** sil., ***sulph.,*** thuj.
evening - bar-ac., petr.
morning - thuj.
move, beginning to - ***lach.***
sitting, after - ambr.
standing erect impossible - rheum.

SWELLING, buttocks - ***coloc.,*** crot-t., dulc., ph-ac., sulph.
swelling, coccyx, sensation of - syph.
swelling, perineum, raphe of - thuj.

TEARING, pain, buttocks - agar., ambr., ***bar-c.,*** berb., chin., cina, colch., dros., kali-c., kali-n., lyc., mag-m., merl., mez., mill., nat-c., thuj., zinc.
between - ambr.
crawling - kali-c.
evening - nat-c.
extending, downwards - aur-m., ***bar-c.,*** thuj.
to anus - colch.
to hips and groin - nat-m.
forenoon - mill.
gluteal muscles - agar., coc-c.
motion, amel - kali-n.
periodically - ***bar-c.***
rising, when - dros.
amel - agar.
sitting, amel - mag-m., nat-c.
standing, while - nat-c.
waking - agar.
walking, while - berb., mag-m.

tearing, coccyx - ant-c., ***bell., calc-caust., calc-p., canth., cic.,*** kali-bi., ***mag-c., mag-p., merc.,*** nat-s., ***sil.***
menses, during - canth., ***cic.,*** merc.
pressing, on abdomen amel. - ***merc.***
sitting, while - par., rhus-t., zinc.
tearing, iliac - crot-t.
tearing, ilium, crest of - ***berb.,*** zinc.
extending, into gluteal muscles - ***berb.***
upward - berb.
sitting, while -zinc.
tearing, perineum - am-m., mez.
tearing, sacro-iliac, symphyses - ***bry.***
tearing, sacrum - ***aesc.,*** asar., ***bry., coloc.,*** helon., ***lyc.,*** mag-m., ***mez.,*** mur-ac., spong., zinc.
extending, down the sciatic nerve - ***coloc.***
down to coccyx and thighs - thuj.
to occiput - led.
toward lumbar - mur-ac.
pressure amel. - mag-m.
sacrum and hips while walking - **AESC.**
sitting, while - spong.
erect, while - lyc.
walking - asar.

TENSION, buttocks - ant-c., arg-m., arn., bell., berb., ***merc.,*** sil.
gluteal region - spig.
lying on back amel - merc.
night - merc.
during sleep - merc.
stooping - bell.
tension, iliac - arg-m., chel., grat.
left - arg-m., grat.
tension, perineum - echi.
tension, sacrum - ***bar-c.,*** berb., caps., caust., puls., samb., sars., ***sulph.,*** tarax., ***zinc.***
ascending agg. - carb-s.
evening - bar-c.
lying - ***berb.***
sitting - ***berb.***

THRUSTS, sacrum - samb.
thrusts, spine - dig.

TINGLING, buttocks, prickling, asleep - ***alum.,*** calc-p., dig., sulph.
gluteal muscles - calc-p.
sitting, while - ***alum.,*** calc., dig., sulph.

TUBERCLES, buttocks - hep., mag-m., mang., phos.
tubercle, perineum on - ***thuj.***

TWITCHING, buttocks - **AGAR.,** ant-c., calc., kali-c., mag-c., mag-m., nat-c., ph-ac., phos., prun., sep., spong., stann., tarax.
evening - ant-c.
sitting, while - ant-c., calc., nat-c.
twitching, coccyx - alum., ***cic.***
menses, during - ***cic.***
painful - alum.
twitching, ilium, crest, and jerking -***cina.***
twitching, sacrum, sitting - staph.

ULCERS, buttocks - bor., sabin., sulph., vinc.
burning - vinc.
upper part of - sabin.
ulcers, coccyx - paeon.
ulcers, sacrum - arg-n., ars., crot-h., paeon., zinc.
burn like fire - ***ars.***

URTICARIA, buttocks - hydr., lyc.

VESICLES, buttocks - bor., cann-s., carb-an., crot-t., iris, olnd., ph-ac., rhus-t.
corroding - bor.

WARTS, buttocks - con., thuj.

WEAKNESS, sacro-iliac, synchondroses - ***aesc.,*** arg-n., ***sep.***
weakness, sacrum - ***aesc.,*** ars., calc-p., coloc., helo., kalm., lith., merc., nat-a., nat-m., nux-m., petr., ***phos.,*** pic-ac., ***sep.,*** sil., sulph., ***zinc.***
evening - petr.
night - ***lith.***

WEIGHT, perineum - cact., **CON.,** cop., graph., hydrc., puls.

WOUNDS, perineum - ***calen.,*** hyper., staph., symph.

Perspiration

PERSPIRATION, general - ***acet-ac., acon.,*** aesc., aeth., ail., ***agar.,*** all-c., alst., alum., ambr., am-c., am-m., aml-n., anac., ang., anthr., anthro., ***ant-c.,*** **ANT-T.,** apis, apoc., arn., arg-m., arg-n., ***ars.,*** ars-i., arund., asc-c., asaf., aur., bapt., ***bar-c., bell.,*** benz-ac., berb., bol., bov., brom., ***bry.,*** bufo, cact., cahin., calad., **CALC.,** camph., cann-i., canch., ***caps.,*** carb-ac., ***carb-an., carb-v.,*** caust., ***cedr.,*** cham., chel., **CHIN.,** ***chin-s.,*** cimx., cic., cina, cinnb., clem., coff., ***cocc.,*** colch., coloc., con., corn., crot-c., crot-h., crot-t., cupr., cur., cycl., daph., ***dig.,*** dios., dros., ***dulc., elaps, elat.,*** eupi., eup-per., eup-pur., **FERR.,** fl-ac., gamb., ***gels.,*** glon., ***graph.,*** grat., ***guai.,*** hell., **HEP.,** hydr-ac., ***hyos.,*** ign., ***iod.,*** **IP.,** iris, jab., jatr., kalm., kali-bi., kali-c., kali-i., kali-n., kali-s., kreos., lac-ac., lach., lachn., laur., led., lil-t., lob., **LYC.,** ***mag-c.,*** mag-s., mang., meny., ***merc.,*** merc-c., merc-cy., merl., ***mez.,*** morph., mosch., mur-ac., myric., naja, ***nat-a.,*** nat-c., **NAT-M.,** nicc., nit-ac., nux-m., **NUX-V., OP.,** ***ox-ac.,*** par., ***petr., ph-ac.,*** **PHOS.,** phys., plan., plat., plb., ***podo.,*** **PSOR.,** puls., ***ran-s.,*** rheum, rhod., rob., ***rhus-t.,*** sabad., sabin., sal-ac., **SAMB.,** sang., sarr., sel., ***sec.,*** senec., **SEP., SIL.,** spig., spong., stann., staph., stram., stry., ***sulph.,*** sul-ac., sumb., tab., tarent., tarax., tax., teucr., ther., thuj., trio., ***valer.,*** **VERAT.,** ***verat-v.,*** vip., zinc., ziz., ***zing.***

ACRID - all-s., ***caps.,*** **CHAM.,** coff., ***con.,*** fl-ac., graph., ***hell.,*** iod., ip., ***lac-ac.,*** lyc., merc., nat-m., ***nit-ac.,*** par., ran-b., rhus-t., sil., tarax., tarent., zinc.

AFFECTED, parts, on - acon., **AMBR., ANT-T.,** anthro., ars., asar., bry., calc., ***caust.,*** chin., ***cocc., coff.,*** fl-ac., guai., hell., kali-c., lyc., **MERC.,** nat-c., nit-ac., nux-v., petr., puls., **RHUS-T.,** ***sep.,*** sil., ***stann.,*** stram., stront-c., thuj.
- morning - ***ambr.***

AFTERNOON - all-s., am-m., ars., ***berb.,*** calc-s., canth., cina, ferr-i., fl-ac., ***hep.,*** kali-n., mag-m., mag-s., nat-a., ***nat-m.,*** nat-p., nicc., nit-ac., ***nux-v.,*** op., ptel., sil., staph., sulph.
- 1 to 3 p.m. - kali-c.
  - 1 to 4 p.m. - phos.
- 3 p.m. - ferr., mag-s.
  - 3 to 5 p.m. - sil.
- 4 p.m. to midnight - bell.
- 5 p.m. - puls., sarr.
- coldness, during - gels.
- fever, during - ferr., gamb., nit-ac.
- sleep, during - ant-t., calad., carb-an., nat-m., nit-ac.

AGGRAVATES, after, in general - ars., bell., bry., ***calc.,*** carb-v., **CHIN.,** con., ign., iod., kali-c., lyc., **MERC.,** nat-c., nat-m., nux-v., petr., **PH-AC.,** ***phos., puls.,*** sel., **SEP.,** sil., spig., squil., ***staph., sulph.***

AIR, cold - ars., **BRY., CALC.,** carb-an., ***lyc.,*** sep., verat.

AIR, cold
- exercise in - ***bry.,*** calc., carb-an., caust., ***chin.***
- open, in the - ***bry.,*** **CALC.,** caps., ***carb-an.,*** carb-v., ***caust., chin.,*** guai., hep., ip., kali-c., lach., **PSOR.,** rhod., ruta., ***sil.,*** thuj., valer.
  - amel. - alum., graph.

ALTERNATING, with heat - apis.

AMELIORATES, in general - ***ars., bov.,*** **BRY.,** ***calad.,*** calc., **CUPR.,** ***iod.,*** lyc., nat-c., rhus-t.
- after, amel. - ***acon.,*** aesc., ambr., am- m., ant-t., ***ars.,*** bar-c., bell., bov., ***bry., calad., canth.,*** **CHAM.,** chel., clem., cocc., coloc., **GELS.,** ***graph.,*** hell., ***hep.,*** hyos., ip., kali-n., led., lyc., mag-m., **NAT-M.,** nit-ac., nux-v., ***olnd.,*** op., **PSOR.,** puls., rhod., **RHUS-T.,** sabad., sabin., samb., sel., spong., stram., ***stront-c., sulph.,*** sul-ac., tarax., ***thuj.,*** valer., ***verat.***

ANGER, from - acon., bry., ***cham.,*** cupr., lyc., ***petr.,*** **SEP.,** staph.

ANXIETY, during - alum., ***ambr.,*** am-c., ant-c., arn., **ARS.,** bar-c., bell., benz-ac., berb., bry., **CALC.,** calc-p., cann-s., carb-s., ***carb-v., caust.,*** **CHAM., CHIN.,** chin-a., clem., cic., cimx., cocc., **FERR.,** ***ferr-ar.,*** **FL-AC.,** graph., kali-bi., kali-n., kreos., ***lyc., mag-c.,*** **MANG.,** ***merc., merc-c.,*** mez., mur-ac., ***nat-a., nat-c.,*** nat-m., ***nat-p.,*** nit-ac., ***nux-v.,*** **PH-AC.,** ***phos.,*** plb., ***puls., rhus-t.,*** samb., sel., **SEP.,** ***sil.,*** spong., stann., staph., stram., ***sulph.,*** sul-ac., tab., tarent., ***thuj.,*** verat.
- dinner, after - calc.
- evening - ambr., sulph.
- night - **ARS.,** carb-an., ***carb-v.,*** nat-m.

ASCENDS - arn., ***bell.***

AWAKE, only, while - **SAMB.,** sep.

BED, in - ***alum.,*** am-m., ang., ars., ars-i., asar., bry., bufo, **CALC.,** ***camph.,*** caps., ***cham.,*** dirc., dulc., eug., **FERR.,** ferr-ar., ferr-i., ***hell.,*** iod., kali-ar., kali-c., kali-n., lyc., ***merc., mur-ac.,*** nat-a., nat-c., ***nit-ac.,*** nux-v., phos., plb., ***rhus-t., samb., sel.,*** sep., sol-n., ***sulph.,*** verat.
- getting out of, amel. - ars., bell., ***calc., camph.,*** hep., ***hell.,*** lach., lyc., ***merc., puls.,*** **RHUS-T.,** ***sep.,*** sulph., **VERAT.**
- sweat and chilliness as soon as he gets warm in - arg-n.

BLOODY - ***anag.,*** arn., ars., calc., cann-s., cham., chin., clem., cocc., **CROT-H.,** ***cur.,*** hell., **LACH.,** ***lyc., nux-m., nux-v.,*** petr., phos.
- night - ***cur.***

BODY, except the head - bell., merc., nux-v., **RHUS-T., SAMB.,** ***sep.,*** thuj.

BURNING - merc., ***mez.,*** **NAT-C.,** verat.

CLAMMY, sticky, viscid - abies-c., absin., acet-ac., acon., act-sp., ***aeth.,*** aloe, aml-n., anac., ant-a., ant-c., ***ant-t.,*** apis, arn., **ARS.,** ars-s-f., benz-ac., benz-n., brom., ***bry.,*** cact., **CALC.,** calc-p., **CAMPH.,** canth., carb-ac., carb-an., carb-h.,

CLAMMY, sticky, viscid - carb-v., ***cench.,*** **CHAM.,** chin., cimic., cocc., coff., coff-t., colch., coloc., ***corn., crot-c.,*** crot-h., cub., cupr., ***cupr-ar.,*** daph., dig., dulc., elaps, elat., fago., **FERR., FERR-AR.,** ***ferr-i.,*** **FERR-P.,** ***fl-ac.,*** formal., gast., glon., guat., ***hell., hep.,*** hydr., hydr-ac., hyos., ign., iod., ip., jatr., kali-cy., kali-n., kali-ox., lach., lachn., laur., lil-t., lob., lup., **LYC.,** lyss., med., **MERC.,** ***merc-c.,*** merc-cy., merc-p-r., ***merc-sul.,*** mez., morph., ***mosch.,*** mur-ac., ***naja,*** naphtin., nat-c., nat-m., ***nux-v.,*** op., ox-ac., **PH-AC., PHOS.,** phys., ***plb., psor.,*** pyrus, sanic., ***sec.,*** sol-t., ***spig., spong.,*** stann., ***sul-ac.,*** sul-i., sulph., sumb., tab., tanac., tela, ter., trach., ***tub.,*** **VERAT.,** verat-v., vip., zinc., zinc-m., zinc-s.
- evening - clem., sumb.
- menopause, at - ***crot-h., lach., lyc., sul-ac., ter.***
- morning - mosch.
- night - cupr., fago., hep., ***lyc., merc.***
- starting from sleep, with - daph.

CLOSING, the eyes, on - ***bry.,*** calc., carb-an., **CON.,** ***lach.,*** thuj.

COLD, sweat - abies-c., acet-ac., ***acon.,*** act-sp., aeth., ***agar.,*** agar-ph., ail., alco., aloe, **AM-C.,** ambr., ***anac.,*** anh., ***anthr., ant-c.,*** **ANT-T.,** apis, ***arn.,*** **ARS.,** ars-i., ars-s-f., asaf., aur., ***aur-m.,*** bar-c., bar-m., bar-s., bell., benz-ac., bol-lu., both., ***bry., bufo,*** buth-a., cact., cadm-s., calad., **CALC.,** calc-p., calc-s., calc-sil., **CAMPH.,** ***cann-i.,*** cann-s., ***carb-ac., carb-s.,*** **CARB-V.,** canth., caps., cast., ***cench.,*** cent., cham., **CHIN., CHIN-A.,** chlol., ***chlor.,*** cimic., ***cina, cist.,*** **COCC.,** coff., coff-t., colch., coloc., con., corn., croc., ***crot-c.,*** crot-h., cupr., ***cupr-ac., cur.,*** dig., digin., dulc., ***dros., elaps,*** esp-g., ***euph.,*** euphr., **FERR.,** ***ferr-ar., ferr-i.,*** ferr-p., formal., frag., gels., ***graph., hell.,*** **HEP.,** ***hydr-ac., hyos.,*** hura, ***ign.,*** iod., **IP.,** jatr., kali-ar., kali-bi., ***kali-c.,*** kali-cy., kali-n., kali-p., kalm., lac-c., ***lach.,*** lachn., laur., lil-t., ***lob.,*** lol., lup., **LYC.,** mag-arct., manc., mang., med., ***merc.,*** **MERC-C.,** merc-cy., merc-p-r., merc-sul., ***mez.,*** morph., mur-ac., ***naja,*** narcot., ***nat-a., nat-c.,*** nat-m., nat-p., nit-ac., ***nux-v.,*** op., ox-ac., paeon., ***petr., ph-ac., phos.,*** plan., plb., podo., ***psor., puls.,*** pyrog., ran-s., ***rheum,*** rhus-t., ***ruta,*** sabad., sang., **SEC.,** seneg., **SEP.,** sil., ***spig., spong.,*** stann., ***staph., stront-c.,*** sul-i., ***sulph.,*** sul-ac., sulo-ac., sumb., ***tab.,*** tela, ***ter.,*** tere-ch., thea., ***ther., thuj., tub., vip.,*** **VERAT., VERAT-V.,** wye., zinc.
- afternoon - **GELS.,** phos., verat-v.
- cigar, after - op.
- clammy sweats, with, chill - corn., cupr., lyss., **VERAT.**
  - with, bleeding - **CHIN.**
- convulsions, during - camph., ***cupr., ferr.,*** stram., ***verat.***
- diarrhea, in - aeth., ant-t., ***ars.,*** calc., ***camph.,*** cupr., hell., jatr., pic-ac., ***sec., sil.,*** sulph., ***tab.,*** ter., ***verat.***
- dysmenorrhea, in - ***sars., verat.***
- eating, while - **MERC.**
  - after - digin., sul-ac.

COLD, sweat
- evening - anac., hura, phos.
  - 6 p.m. - psor.
- exertion of body, or mind, after the slightest - act-sp., ***calc.,*** **HEP., SEP.**
- headache, with - **GELS.,** graph., ***verat.***
- heat, with sensation of internal - anac.
- increases the coldness of the body - cinnb., cist.
- lying, while - thea.
- menses, during - ars., coff., phos., ***sars., sec.,*** **VERAT.**
- morning - ***ant-c.,*** canth., chin., esp-g., euph., ruta.
- motion, on - ant-c., sep.
- nausea, with - ***calc., ip., lach.,*** **PETR.,** ***tab., verat.,*** verat-v.
  - and vertigo, with - ail.
- night - aeth., am-c., buth-a., chin., coloc., croc., cupr., cur., ***dig.,*** fago., iod., lob., mang., op., rhus-t., **SEP.,** thuj.
- over the body, warm sweat on the palms - ***dig.***
- rising from bed, on - bry.
- stool, during - merc., sulph., thuj., verat.
- sudden attacks of - ***crot-h.***
- urination, after - bell.
- vertigo, with - ail., ***merc-c.,*** ther.
- vomiting, with - **CAMPH.,** ***ip.,*** thea., **VERAT.,** ***verat-v.***
- walking, on - rhus-t.
  - in cold open air - rhus-t.

COLDNESS, during - ***arg-n.,*** gels., lachn., psor., raph., ***puls.,*** **VERAT.**
- after - aml-n., carb-s., corn., kali-cy., mur-ac., petr., senec., sil., sulph., thuj.
- legs, of, with coldness - calc.
- hands, of - nit-ac.

COLIC, during - mez., nux-v., plan., plb., sulph.

COLLIQUATIVE, wasting of body - acet-ac., **ANT-T.,** ***ars., ars-h.,*** camph., carb-an., ***carb-v.,*** cast., **CHIN.,** eup-per., **EUPI.,** ferr., ferr-m., gels., ***iod.,*** **JAB.,** ***lach., lyc.,*** mill., ***nit-ac.,*** op., ph-ac., phel., ***psor.,*** pyrog., rhus-g., salv., ***samb., sec.,*** stann., sulph.

CONVERSATION, from - ***ambr.***

CONVULSIONS, during - ars., art-v., ***bell.,*** **BUFO,** camph., nux-v., op., sep.
- after - acon., ars., art-v., cedr., cupr., sec., stry.

COUGHING, from - acon., ant-c., ant-t., apis, **ARS.,** arg-n., bell., brom., bry., ***calc.,*** caps., carb-an., carb-s., ***carb-v., caust., cham.,*** chin., chin-a., cimx., dig., ***dros.,*** eug., eupi., ***ferr.,*** ferr-ar., guare., **HEP.,** ***ip.,*** kali-c., ***kali-n.,*** lach., lyc., ***merc.,*** nat-a., nat-c., nat-m., nat-p., ***nux-v.,*** ph-ac., **PHOS.,** psor., puls., ***rhus-t., sabad.,*** **SAMB.,** sel., seneg., **SEP.,** sil., ***spong.,*** squil., sulph., tab., ***thuj.,*** tub., ***verat.***
- night - chin., dig., eug., kali-bi., lyc., ***merc.,*** nat-c., nit-ac., psor., sulph.
- paroxysms of, end with - ars., brom., ***ign.***

COVERED, parts - **ACON., BELL.,** ***cham.,*** **CHIN.,** ***ferr.,*** led., lyc., ***nit-ac.,*** nux-v., ***puls.,*** sec., spig., ***thuj.***
perspiring, yet wants to be - aeth.

CRITICAL - ***acon.,*** bapt., bell., bry., ***canth.,*** chlor., pneu., ***pyrog.,*** rhus-t.

DAYTIME - agar., ambr., am-c., am-m., anac., ***ant-t.,*** bell., bry., **CALC.,** ***carb-an.,*** carb-s., ***chin., con., dulc.,*** **FERR.,** ferr-ar., ***ferr-p., graph.,*** guai., ***hep.,*** kali-bi., **KALI-C.,** lach., laur., led., **LYC.,** ***merc.,*** **NAT-C., NAT-M.,** ***nat-p., nit-ac.,*** **PH-AC.,** puls., ***rheum, sel.,*** **SEP.,** sil., ***staph., stram.,*** **SULPH.,** sul-ac., verat., zinc.
awake, while - **SAMB.**
closing the eyes, when - **CON.**
day and night without relief - apis, ars-s-f., chin-a., ***colch.,*** **HEP.,** lach., ***pyrog., sal-ac.,*** samb., sep., syph., tub.
nausea and languor, with - **MERC.**
sleep, during - bell., caust., con., lyc.

DEBILITATING - acon., ambr., ***ant-t.,*** **ARN., ARS.,** ***bar-c.,*** **BRY.,** ***calad., calc.,*** **CAMPH.,** canth., ***carb-an.,*** **CAUST., CHIN.,** ***cocc.,*** **CROC.,** dig., **FERR.,** graph., ***hyos.,*** **IOD., KALI-N.,** lyc., **MERC.,** ***nat-m.,*** **NUX-V., PH-AC., PHOS.,** psor., ***rhod.,*** **SAMB., SEP.,** ***sil., stann., sulph., tarax.,*** **TUB.,** verat.

DESCENDING - sep.

DIARRHEA, with - ***acon.,*** con., sulph., **VERAT.**

DISEASE, acute, after - piloc., psor.

DRINKING, after - aloe, ars., carb-v., cast., cham., chin., ***cocc.,*** con., kali-c., kali-p., ***merc., puls.,*** rhus-t., ***sel.,*** sulph., sumb.
amel. - ***caust., chin-s.,*** cupr., nux-v., ***phos.,*** sil., thuj.
warm drinks - bry., kali-c., ***merc.,*** phos., sul-ac.
wine amel. - acon., apis, con., lach., ***op.,*** sul-ac., thuj.

DYSPNEA, with - anac., ***ant-t.,*** apis, **ARS.,** arund., **CARB-V.,** ***lach.,*** lyc., mang., meny., nux-v., psor., sep., sil., sulph., thuj., verat.
chronic - tub.

EATING, while - ant-t., arg-m., ars., ***bar-c., benz-ac.,*** bor., bry., ***calc.,*** **CARB-AN., CARB-S., CARB-V.,** cocc., ***con.,*** graph., guare., ign., kali-ar., **KALI-C.,** ***kali-p.,*** **MERC.,** nat-c., ***nat-m.,*** **NIT-AC.,** nux-v., ol-an., phos., ***puls.,*** sars., **SEP.,** sil., sul-ac., valer., viol-t.
amel. - anac., ***ign.,*** lach., mez., **PHOS.,** zinc.
anxiety and cold sweat - **MERC.**
eating, after - arg-m., ars., **BRY., CALC., CARB-AN., CARB-S., CARB-V.,** ***caust., cham.,*** con., ***crot-c.,*** crot-h., ferr., ferr-ar., graph., ***kali-c., laur., lyc.,*** nat-m., **NIT-AC.,** ***nux-v.,*** petr., ph-ac., **PHOS.,** psor., sel., **SEP.,** ***sil.,*** **SULPH.,** thuj., ***viol-t.***
amel. - ***anac.,*** alum., ***chin.,*** cur., ***ferr.,*** **LACH.,** ***nat-c., phos., rhus-t.,*** sep., verat.
breakfast - ***carb-v.,*** grat.
eating, after
dinner - ***carb-an.,*** dig., mag-m., phos., ptel., sep., thuj.
warm food - ***bry.,*** carb-an., ***carb-v.,*** cham., ***ferr., kali-c.,*** lach., ph-ac., **PHOS.,** puls., sep., **SUL-AC.,** ***thuj.***

EMISSIONS, after - ***calc.,*** puls., ***sep.,*** sulph.

EVENING - ***agar.,*** anac., anthro., ars., bar-c., bell., berb., bov., cahin., calad., calc-s., canth., carb-s., carb-v., chel., chin-s., cocc., coloc., con., lach., kali-n., mag-c., mag-m., ***meny.,*** merc., merc-c., ***mur-ac.,*** nat-m., nat-p., ***phos.,*** psor., rat., rhus-t., ***sarr.,*** sep., spig., ***sulph.,*** sumb., thuj., verat.
6 p.m. - dig., plb., ***psor.***
to 8 p.m. - ***sulph.***
7 p.m. - elaps, mag-s.
to 1 a.m. - **SAMB.**
8 p.m. - ferr., mag-s., sumb.
with nausea and heat - ferr.
bed, in - ***agar.,*** ars., asar., calc., eug., ferr., ***meny.,*** **MERC.,** rat., **SULPH.,** verat.
every alternate - ***bar-c.***
evening, lasting all night - anthro., meny.
heat, with the - carb-v.
lasting all night - bol., chel., cocc., led., ***meny.,*** **HEP.,** ***kali-c.,*** **PULS.**
rest, even when at - cahin., ***sarr.***

EXCITEMENT, after - bar-c., graph.

EXERTION, during slight - acon., aeth., **AGAR.,** ambr., aml-n., ***ars.,*** **ARS-I.,** asar., bapt., bell., benz-ac., berb., ***brom., bry.,*** but-ac., **CALC., CALC-S.,** camph., canth., caps., carb-an., ***carb-s.,*** carb-v., caust., ***chel.,*** **CHIN.,** ***chin-a.,*** chin-s., cinnb., ***cist., cocc.,*** corn., ***cupr.,*** eup-pur., ***eupi.,*** **FERR.,** ferr-ar., **FERR-I.,** ***ferr-m.,*** ferr-p., ***gels.,*** **GRAPH.,** ***hep.,*** **IOD.,** kali-ar., **KALI-C.,** kali-n., **KALI-P.,** ***kali-s.,*** kreos., lach., led., **LYC.,** mag-c., med., ***merc., merc-sul., nat-a.,*** **NAT-C.,** ***nat-m., nat-p.,*** **NAT-S., NIT-AC.,** op., petr., ph-ac., **PHOS.,** phyt., **PSOR.,** rheum, **RHUS-T.,** sabad., sel., **SEP.,** ***sil.,*** spig., stann., **SULPH.,** sul-ac., tab., thuj., **TUB.,** valer., verat.
after, amel. - agar., bry., polyg., ***sep.***
front part of body, often only in, after exertion - agar.
mental - act-sp., aur., bell., bor., **CALC.,** graph., **HEP.,** hyos., ***kali-c.,*** **LACH.,** ***lyc.,*** nat-m., nux-v., phos., ***psor.,*** **SEP.,** sil., **STAPH.,** ***sulph.,*** tub.
amel. - ferr., nat-c.

FACE, of the whole body except the - ***rhus-t., sec.***

FEET, except - chin., phos.

FEVER, after the - ant-t., **ARS.,** ***bell.,*** bov., bry., ***calad.,*** calc., carb-v., coloc., ***chin., chin-a., chin-s., cupr., ferr., gels.,*** glon., graph., hell., ***hep.,*** kali-n., ***lach., lyc.,*** merc., nat-a., nat-c., nat-m., ***nat-s., nux-v.,*** op., ph-ac., ***phos., puls.,*** pyrog., ***rhus-t.,*** spig., spong., stram., sulph., tab., thuj., tub., verat-v., ***zinc.***

FLATUS, when passing - kali-bi.

FLIES, attracting the - bry., ***calad.,*** puls., sumb., thuj.

FORENOON - **AGAR.,** ars., **FERR.,** ign., sep., sulph., sul-ac.
- 7 a.m. to 12 a.m. - phos.
- 9 a.m. after stool - sumb.
- exertion, on - gels., sulph., valer.
- menses, during - agar., ars., sep., sulph.
- sleep, during - nux-m.

FRIGHT, from - ***anac., bell.,*** **GELS.,** lyc., **OP.,** sep., sil.

HEAD, except the - ***bell.,*** merc., mur-ac., nux-v., **RHUS-T., SAMB.,** ***sec., sep.,*** **THUJ.**

HEADACHE, during - ant-c., apis, arg-m., arn., ***ars., bry.,*** canth., carb-v., caust., chin-s., eup-per., glon., graph., hyos., kali-n., lachn., lyc., mag-s., ***merc.,*** nat-m., nat-s., op., ox-ac., phel., plat., puls., rhus-t., ***sulph.,*** tarent., thuj.
- after - calc., ***chim.,*** merc., puls., ***sep.,*** staph., sulph.
- amel. - bov., carb-s., chin-a., clem., graph., mag-m., ***nat-m.,*** nat-s., nux-v., psor., spong., ***sulph.,*** tarent., thuj.
- preceded by headache - ferr., lyc.
- suppressed, from - ***ars., bell.,*** bry., ***calc.,*** **CARB-V.,** ***cham., chin.,*** lyc., merc., ***nux-v.,*** phos., ***puls.,*** rhus-t., sep., **SIL.,** ***sulph.***

HOT, sweat - **ACON.,** ***aesc.,*** aml-n., anac., ant-c., aphis., asar., asc-t., aur., ***bell.,*** bism., bry., calc., calc-sil., camph., canth., ***caps., carb-v.,*** **CHAM.,** chel., chen-a., chin., cocc., ***coff.,*** **CON.,** corn., dig., dros., ***hell.,*** **IGN., IP.,** kreos., lach., led., lyc., merc-i-r., nat-c., **NUX-V., OP.,** par., penic., ***ph-ac.,*** phos., pip-n., **PSOR.,** puls., ***pyrog.,*** rauw., ***rhus-t.,*** sabad., sang., **SEP.,** sil., ***stann.,*** staph., ***stram., sulph.,*** thuj., til., verat., verat-v., viol-t.
- gives no relief - til.

INTERMITTENT - ant-c., bell., coloc., cupr-ar., ferr., kali-n., nux-v., ***sep.,*** sil.

LONG-LASTING - am-c., am-m., anthro., ***ars.,*** **CAUST.,** cimx., con., cupr., dulc., **FERR.,** ***ferr-ar., gels.,*** **HEP.,** ***led.,*** **SAMB.,** ***verat.***
- continuing through apyrexia - ***verat.***

LOWER, limbs, except - lyc.

LUMINOUS - phos.

LYING, while - ars., ***caps.,*** chel., **FERR.,** ferr-ar., ham., hep., lyc., ***mag-s.,*** **MENY.,** merc., op., podo., puls., **RHUS-T., SAMB.,** ***sep.,*** tarent., tarax.

MENSES, during - agar., ars., asar., bell., ***bor.,*** coff., ***caust., graph., hyos.,*** kali-c., kreos., mag-c., ***mag-m.,*** murx., phos., sars., sec., ***sep.,*** stram., sulph., tell., **VERAT.**
- after - ph-ac.
- before - bell., calc., ***graph., hyos.,*** nat-s., phos., sil., ***sulph., thuj.,*** **VERAT.**

MIDNIGHT - acon., alum., am-m., arg-m., arn., ***ars.,*** bar-c., bar-m., berb., canth., clem., con., dig., dros., ***ferr., fl-ac.,*** hep., ip., kali-ar., kali-c., lach., lyc., mag-m., mag-s., merl., ***mur-ac.,*** nat-m., nux-v., op., par., ph-ac., ***phos.,*** plat., rhus-t., sabad., ***samb.,*** sil., staph.
- after - acon., ***agar.,*** alum., ***ambr.,*** am-m., arg-m., ars., ***bar-c.,*** bell., bol., carb-an., ***chel.,*** clem., coloc., con., ***dros.,*** **FERR.,** graph., hell., hep., kali-c., kali-s., lachn., lyc., mag-c., ***mag-m.,*** merc., merl., nicc., nux-v., phos., puls., sabad., samb., ***sil.,*** staph., sulph., **TUB.**
  - on waking - bell.
- before - ***calc.,*** carb-v., hep., ***mur-ac.,*** nat-m., ph-ac., phos., staph.
- lasting until morning - mag-c., mag-m., ***phos.***
- lying on the back, while - cham.
- waking, on - bell., bol., colch., con., phos., sulph.

MORNING - acon., ***alum.,*** ambr., **AM-C.,** am-m., ang., ***ant-c., arg-n., ars.,*** ars-i., aur., bell., bor., bov., ***bry.,*** bufo, **CALC.,** canth., caps., carb-an., ***carb-s.,*** **CARB-V.,** cham., ***caust., chin., chin-a.,*** chin-s., ***chel.,*** cic., cimx., clem., cocc., ***coff.,*** coloc., con., dros., dulc., elaps, eug., ***euph.,*** eupi., **FERR.,** ***ferr-ar.,*** ferr-i., ferr-p., gamb., graph., grat., guai., ***hell.,*** **HEP.,** hyper., iod., kali-ar., kali-c., kali-n., kali-p., kali-s., kreos., lachn., ***lyc., mag-c.,*** mag-m., mag-s., **MERC.,** merl., mez., ***mosch.,*** mur-ac., nat-a., nat-c., nat-m., nat-p., nicc., **NIT-AC.,** nux-v., op., ox-ac., par., ***ph-ac.,*** **PHOS.,** ***puls.,*** ran-b., ***rhus-t., sabad.,*** **SAMB.,** sang., senec., ***sep.,*** **SIL.,** spig., spong., ***stann., sulph.,*** sul-ac., thuj., **VERAT.,** zinc.
- 5 to 6 a.m. - bov.
- 6 a.m. - alum., sil.
  - 6 to 7 a.m. - sulph.
- bed, in - alum., am-m., ant-c., benz-ac., bufo, **CALC.,** caps., chin., con., **FERR.,** graph., kali-c., kali-i., kali-n., lyc., nat-c., nicc., phos.
- breakfast, after - carb-v., grat.
- coffee after - cham.
- early in - stann.
- every alternate - ***ant-c., ferr.***
- heat, after - ars., graph., nit-ac., **PULS.**
- lasting until noon - ***ferr.***
- menses, before - nat-s.
- restless night, after a - arg-n., lyc.
- side, sweat every morning agg., on the affected - ambr.
- sleep, during - **ANT-C.,** bell., bor., ***bov.,*** bufo, ***chel., chin., chin-s.,*** con., **FERR.,** ign., lachn., nat-m., ph-ac., **PULS.,** zinc.
- waking, on - am-m., ant-c., carb-v., con., dig., euphr., iod., sep., spong.
  - after - acon-c., ***ant-c.,*** ant-t., bry., carb-an., carb-v., chel., chin., con., dig., ferr., gamb., hyper., mag-s., ***nux-v.,*** ph-ac., phos., phys., **SAMB., SEP., SULPH.**

MOTION, on - agar., alum., ***ambr.,*** am-m., anac., ant-c., ant-t., ***ars.,*** ars-i., arund., bell., **BRY., CALC.,** camph., canth., ***carb-an.,*** **CARB-S.,** carb-v., ***caust.,*** cham., **CHIN.,** chin-a., ***chin-s., cocc.,*** cur., **FERR.,** ferr-ar., ferr-i., gels., **GRAPH., HEP.,** iod., ip., kali-ar., ***kali-bi.,*** **KALI-C.,** mag-c., mag-m., **MERC.,** nat-a., ***nat-c., nat-m., nit-ac.,*** **NUX-V.,** phos., **PSOR.,** puls., ***sel.,*** **SEP.,** sil., **STANN.,** ***stram.,*** **SULPH.,** sul-ac., thuj., **VERAT.,** ***zinc.***

amel. - ***ars.,*** **CAPS.,** con., ferr., **MERC.,** ***puls.,*** **RHUS-T.,** sabad., **SAMB.,** sep., ***sul-ac.,*** sulph., thuj., ***valer.,*** verat.

brings on chilliness - eup-per., eup-pur., hep., **NUX-V.,** psor., ***tub.***

making any, sweat disappears and heat, comes on - ***lyc.***

NEWS, bad, from - calc-p.

NIGHT, sweats - acon., ***acet-ac., agar.,*** agn., aloe, ***alum., ambr.,*** am-c., ***am-m., anac.,*** ang., ant-t., anthr., anthro., arg-m., ***arg-n., arn.,*** **ARS.,** ars-h., ***ars-i.,*** asar., asc-t., aur., bar-c., bar-m., bell., berb., bol., bor., bry., ***calc., calc-p.,*** calc-s., ***canth.,*** carb-ac., **CARB-AN.,** ***carb-s.,*** **CARB-V., CAUST.,** casc., cham., ***chin., chin-a., cic.,*** cina, cimx., cist., ***clem.,*** coca, ***cocc.,*** colch., coloc., **CON.,** cupr., cur., cycl., dig., dios., dros., ***dulc., eup-per.,*** euphr., eupi., fago., ***ferr., ferr-ar., ferr-i., ferr-p.,*** gamb., ***graph.,*** guai., hell., **HEP.,** hura, ign., ***iod., ip.,*** **KALI-AR.,** kali-bi., **KALI-C.,** kali-n., ***kali-p.,*** **KALI-S., LACH.,** laur., lec., ***led.,*** lob., ***lyc.,*** mag-c., mag-s., manc., mang., med., **MERC.,** merc-c., ***mur-ac., nat-a., nat-c., nat-m.,*** nat-p., nat-s., ***nit-ac.,*** nux-v., ox-ac., op., petr., ph-ac., phos., phyt., plb., psor., ptel., **PULS.,** raph., rat., rheum, ***rhus-t.,*** sabin., **SAMB., SEP., SIL.,** spig., spong., stann., ***staph.,*** stram., ***stront-c.,*** **SULPH.,** sumb., tab., **TARAX.,** tarent., ther., **THUJ.,** til., ***valer., verat.,*** viol-t., zinc.

10 p.m. - bor.

during chilliness - ***bry.***

lasting until morning - laur.

to 10 a.m. - ***bry.***

11 p.m. - sil.

until 2 a.m. - carb-an.

1 a.m. - mag-c.

2 a.m. to 3 a.m. - merc.

to 5 a.m. - puls.

3 a.m. - bry., ***calc.,*** calc-ar., carb-an., clem., ferr-m., merl., nat-c., nux-v., par., **PSOR.,** stann., sulph.

during sleep - ***merl.,*** nat-c.

to 4 p.m. - eupi., rhus-t.

4 a.m. - ***caust., chel., ferr.,*** gamb., sep., ***stann.,*** tell.

during sleep - ***carb-an.,*** **CHEL.**

alternating with dryness of skin - ***apis,*** **NAT-C.**

apyrexia, during - cimx.

covering, when - nit-ac.

ever so little, when - ***chin.***

every other night - bar-c., kali-n., **NIT-AC.**

fever, during - carb-v., stront-c., sulph.

NIGHT, sweats

lasting all night, without relief - **HEP.,** kali-c., **MERC.**

with loquacity - **PULS.**

long lasting musty night, sweats - ***cimx.***

lying down, after - ang., ***hep.,*** meny., rhus-t., sabad., sil.

menses, during - asar., bell., bor., kali-c., sulph.

before - bell., graph., sulph., **VERAT.**

miliary itching, eruptions, with - ***rhus-t.***

sleep, during - agar., anac., ant-t., ***bell.,*** **CALC.,** carb-an., chel., ***chin.,*** chin-s., con., cycl., dig., eup-per., euphr., hyos., kali-n., mur-ac., merc., nat-c., nit-ac., phos., **PULS.,** thuj., ***tub.***

stupid slumber, during - **PULS.**

stupor, with - puls.

tuberculosis, in - ***acet-ac., agarin., ars.,*** ars-i., atro., bac., ***chin.,*** erio., gall-ac., hep., ***jab.,*** kali-i., lyc., myos., ***ph-ac., phos.,*** piloc., salv., samb., sec., ***sil.,*** stann., tub.

wakefulness, with - calc., cham., hep.

waking, on - alum., anac., bell., canth., ***chin., cycl.,*** dros., led., ***mang.,*** merc-c., nat-m., nit-ac., nux-v., sep., sil., staph., sulph., thuj.

NOON - acon., cham., cinnb., clem., valer.

ODOR, general

aromatic - all-c., benz-ac., guare., petr., rhod., sep.

bitter - dig., ***verat.***

morning, in the - verat.

blood, like - ***lyc.***

burnt - **BELL.,** ***bry.,*** mag-c., sulph., thuj.

cadaverous - ***ars.,*** art-v., lach., ***psor.,*** pyrog., thuj.

camphor, like - camph.

carrion, like - lach.

cheesy - con., ***hep.,*** phos., plb., sanic., sep., sulph.

old - bry., hep., sanic.

drugs, like corresponding - asaf., benz., carb-h., camph., chen-a., iod., ol-an., phos., sulph., tab., ter., valer.

eggs, like spoiled - plb., staph., sulph.

elder-blossoms - ***sep.***

eruptions, with - med.

fetid - aesc., all-s., aloe, am-c., am-m., ambr., anac., arn., ***ars.,*** aur-m., ***bapt.,*** **BAR-C.,** bell., bov., ***canth., carb-ac.,*** carb-an., ***carb-v.,*** cimic., coloc., con., crot-h., ***cycl.,*** dios., ***dulc.,*** eucal., ***euphr.,*** ferr., fl-ac., **GRAPH.,** ***guai.,*** **HEP.,** ***kali-c., kali-p.,*** lac-c., lach., led., lyc., ***mag-c.,*** mag-m., med., ***merc.,*** merc-c., **NIT-AC., NUX-V.,** ***petr.,*** **PHOS.,** plb., ***psor.,*** **PULS., PYROG.,** ***rhod., rhus-t.,*** rob., **SEL.,** ***sep.,*** **SIL.,** spig., **STAPH.,** stram., sulph., tell., ***tub.,*** thuj., vario., ***verat.,*** zinc.

coughing, after - ***hep.***

eruptions, with - ***dulc.***

ODOR, general
honey, like - thuj.
garlic, like - ***art-v., bov.,*** kali-p., ***lach.,*** osm., **SULPH.,** tell., thuj.
leek, like - thuj.
lilac, like - sep.
mice, like - tub.
musk, like - ***apis,*** bism., mosch., puls., ***sulph.,*** sumb.
musty - arn., bor., ***cimx.,*** crot-h., merc., merc-c., nux-v., ***psor., puls., rhus-t.,*** sanic., ***stann.,*** staph., syph., teucr., thuj., thyr.
old rain water - sanic.
offensive - acon., aloe, all-s., am-c., ambr., apis, **ARN.,** ***ars.,*** ars-s-f., art-v., asar., aur-m., ***bapt.,*** bar-c., **BAR-M.,** bar-s., bell., bov., bry., but-ac., calc., calc-sil., camph., ***canth.,*** carb-ac., **CARB-AN., CARB-S.,** ***carb-v.,*** caust., cham., chin., cimx., cimic., cocc., coloc., con., cycl., daph., ***dulc.,*** euphr., ***ferr.,*** ferr-ar., ***fl-ac.,*** **GRAPH.,** guai., **HEP.,** hyos., ign., iod., ip., kali-a., kali-ar., kali-c., kali-i., kali-p., ***lach.,*** led., **LYC.,** ***mag-c.,*** man., med., ***merl.,*** **MERC.,** mosch., murx., nat-m., **NIT-AC., NUX-V.,** oci-s., oena., ol-an., osm., **PETR.,** ***phos.,*** plb., podo., ***psor.,*** **PULS.,** pulx., ***pyrog.,*** rheum, ***rhus-t.,*** rob., rhod., sac-l., ***sel.,*** **SEP., SIL.,** sol-t-ae., spig., stann., ***staph.,*** stram., **SULPH.,** ***syph.,*** tarax., tax., ***tell.,*** **THUJ.,** vario., ***verat.,*** zinc.
afternoon - ***fl-ac.***
cheese, like old - sanic.
cough, after - hep., merl.
exertion, on - nit-ac.
menses, during - psor., stann., stram.
morning - carb-v., dulc., merc-c., nux-v.
motion, on - eupi., mag-c.
night - ars., **CARB-AN.,** carb-v., con., cycl., dulc., euphr., ***ferr.,*** graph., ***guai., lyc.,*** mag-c., **MERC.,** nit-ac., nux-v., puls., rhus-t., ***sep.,*** spig., staph., ***tell.,*** thuj.
night, morning - mag-c., merl.
night, sleep, during - cycl.
on one side - **BAR-C.**
wash it off, cannot - lac-c., med.
onions, like - art-v., bov., ***calc.,*** kali-i., kali-p., lach., ***lyc.,*** osm., petr., phos., sin-n., tell., ***thuj.***
pickled herring, like - vario.
pungent - ***cop.,*** gast., ***ip.,*** rhus-t., ***sep.,*** sulph., thuj.
putrid - ***bapt.,*** **CARB-V.,** con., led., ***mag-c.,*** med., nux-v., **PSOR.,** rhus-t., sil., ***spig.,*** **STAPH.,** stram., verat.
rancid, smelling at night - thuj.
rank - art-v., ***bov.,*** cop., ferr., goss., ***lach., lyc., sep., tell.***
during menses - ***stram., tell.***
sickly - ***chin.,*** thuj.
smoky - bell.

ODOR, general
sour - ***acon.,*** alco., all-s., ***arn.,*** **ARS.,** ars-s-f., ***asar., bell.,*** **BRY.,** bufo, **CALC.,** calc-s., calc-sil., ***carb-s., carb-v., caust., cham.,*** chel., chin., ***cimx.,*** clem., **COLCH.,** colos., ***cupr.,*** ferr., ferr-ar., ferr-m., ***fl-ac.,*** gast., ***graph.,*** **HEP.,** hyos., ign., **IOD.,** ***ip., iris,*** kali-c., kalm., kreos., lac-ac., lac-d., ***lach.,*** led., **LYC., MAG-C., MERC.,** nat-m., ***nat-p.,*** **NIT-AC.,** ***nux-v.,*** piloc., **PSOR.,** puls., pyrog., **RHEUM,** ***rhus-t.,*** rob., ***ruta, samb.,*** sanic., **SEP., SIL.,** spig., staph., ***sul-ac.,*** sul-i., **SULPH.,** sumb., tarent., tep., ***thuj.,*** **VERAT.,** zinc.
afternoon - ***fl-ac.***
forenoon - sulph.
morning - ***bry., carb-v., iod.,*** lyc., nat-m., rhus-t., sep., **SULPH.,** sul-ac.
night - ***arn.,*** ars., asar., bry., carb-s., ***caust.,*** cop., ***graph.,*** **HEP.,** iod., ***kali-c.,*** lyc., mag-c., **MERC.,** nat-m., nit-ac., ***phyt.,*** plect., ***sep.,*** sil., ***sulph., thuj., zinc.***
night, sleep, during - bry.
sour-sweet - bry., **PULS.**
spicy - rhod.
sulfuric acid, like - plb., ***staph.,*** sulph.
sulphur, like - phos., ***sulph.***
sweetish - apis, ***ars., calad.,*** merc., puls., ***sep.,*** thuj., ***uran-n.***
urine, like - berb., bov., **CANTH.,** card-m., caust., coloc., ery-a., graph., lyc., nat-m., **NIT-AC.,** plb., rhus-t., sec., thyr., urt-u., ust.
wine, like - sec.
yeasty - torula.

OILY - agar., arg-m., arn., ***ars.,*** aur., **BRY.,** bufo, calc., carb-v., **CHIN.,** fl-ac., lup., lyc., **MAG-C.,** med., **MERC.,** merc-c., ***nat-m.,*** nux-v., ol-j., petr., plb., ***psor.,*** raph., rhus-t., ***rob.,*** sanic., ***sel.,*** **STRAM.,** sumb., **THUJ.,** thyr.
daytime - bry.
morning - bry., chin.
night - ***agar.,*** bry., croc., mag-c., **MERC.**

PAINFUL, parts - kali-c.

PAINS, from - acon., ***ant-t.,*** bell., ***bry.,*** calc., caust., ***cham., chel.,*** chin., cocc., ***coloc.,*** dios., dulc., form., ***hep.,*** hyos., iris, **LACH.,** lyc., mag-p., **MERC., NAT-C.,** phos., ***podo., rhus-t.,*** sel., **SEP.,** spig., still., stram., ***sulph.,*** sul-ac., sumb., ***tab.,*** thuj., til., verat.
after disappearance of - chel.

PALPITATION - agar., ars., caust., ***lach.***

PERIODICAL - ***ars.,*** sil.
hour, at the same - ant-c.

PROFUSE - abrot., ***acet-ac., acon.,*** aesc., aeth., agar., ***agarin.,*** alum., ambr., am-c., am-m., aml-n., ant-c., **ANT-T.,** anthro., apis, arg-n., **ARS.,** ars-i., asar., asc-c., aur., ***aur-m.,*** **AUR-M-N.,** bapt., ***bar-c.,*** **BELL.,** benz., bol., **BRY.,** bufo, cact., **CALC.,** calc-s., ***camph.,*** canth., ***caps.,*** carb-ac., **CARB-AN., CARB-S., CARB-V.,** casc., cast., ***caust.,*** **CEDR.,** cham., chel., **CHIN.,**

PROFUSE, sweats - **CHIN-A., CHIN-S.,** ***cist.,*** chlor., clem., cocc., coc-c., ***colch., coloc.,*** con., cop., corn., croc., ***crot-c., cupr., dig.,*** dulc., elaps, elat., eup-per., eup-pur., **FERR., FERR-AR.,** ***ferr-i.,*** ferr-m., ***ferr-p., fl-ac., gels.,*** graph., guai., **HEP.,** hyos., hyper., iod., ***ip., jab,*** **KALI-AR., KALI-BI., KALI-C.,** kali-n., **KALI-P.,** kali-s., ***lac-ac.,*** lac-c., ***lach.,*** lact., lith., lob., **LYC.,** ***mag-c.,*** mang., **MERC.,** merc-c., ***mez.,*** morph., ***nat-a., nat-c.,*** **NAT-M.,** ***nat-p., nit-ac., nux-v., op.,*** par., petr., **PH-AC.,** ***phos.,*** piloc., podo., polyp-p, pyrog., **PSOR.,** ***puls.,*** rob., ***rhus-t., sabad.,*** sal-ac., **SAMB.,** sang., sanic., sars., ***sec., sel.,*** **SEP., SIL.,** ***spong.,*** stann., staph., stram., sul-ac., ***sulph., tarax., thuj., thyr.,*** til., **TUB.,** ust., valer., **VERAT.,** verat-v., zinc., zinc-m.

affected parts, on - **ANT-T.**
afternoon - ***fl-ac.***
with heat - staph.
awake, only while - ***samb.,*** sep.
diarrhea, increased and frequent, profuse urination - acon.
chill, congestive, after - nux-v.
covered parts, on - bell., **CHAM., CHIN.,** ***ferr., nit-ac.,*** nux-v., sec., ***thuj.***
day and night, without relief - **HEP.,** ***merc., samb.***
daytime, during sleep - ***caust.***
debilitating - bry., ***chin.,*** chin-s., gels., ***merc., ph-ac., phos.,*** rhod.
and fetid - carb-an., merc.
not - casc., rhus-t., **SAMB.**
delirium, during - carb-ac., stram.
diarrhea, with and copious flow of urine - ***acon.***
dyspnea, with - mang.
evening - bar-c., chel., con., fl-ac., samb., sarr., sulph.
7 p.m. lasting until 1 p.m. dry heat, returns on going to sleep - **SAMB.**
every alternate - bar-c.
high fever, with - con.
lasting all night - bol.
heart symptoms, with relief of - dig.
menopause, during - aml-n., bell., crot-h., hep., ***jab.,*** lach., nux-v., ***sep.,*** til., valer.
menses, during - ***hyos., graph., murx., verat.***
before - hyos., thuj.
midnight, after - acon., alum., ambr., am-m., ars., bol., clem., coloc., graph., **KALI-C.,** mag-c., mag-m., phos., sil., sulph.
before - ***carb-v.***
lasting until morning - graph., mag-c., ***phos.***
morning - acon., am-c., am-m., ars., bry., carb-v., caust., chin., **CHIN-S.,** dulc., **FERR.,** ***ferr-ar.,*** **MAG-C.,** ***merc.,*** nat-c., nat-m., nat-p., ***nit-ac.,*** **OP.,** ***ph-ac.,*** **PHOS.,** ***puls., rhus-t.,*** sep., **SIL.**
bed, in - am-m., **FERR.**
hot, dry - ***cham.,*** chin., **OP.,** phos.
lasting all day - ferr.
sleep, during - ***chin-s., puls.***
waking, after - ***ferr., sep.,*** **SULPH.**

PROFUSE, sweats
music, from - ***tarent.***
night - acet-ac., am-m., anthro., ant-c., ***ant-t.,*** arg-n., ***ars.,*** ars-i., asar., bar-c., benz., berb., bol., ***bry.,*** cact., ***calc-p.,*** canth., caps., carb-ac., ***carb-an., carb-s., carb-v.,*** casc., caust., cham., chel., ***chin.,*** chin-s., ***cic., clem.,*** coloc., cupr., fago., ***ferr-p.,*** gall-ac., graph., **HEP.,** iod., **KALI-AR., KALI-C.,** ***kali-p., lob., lyc.,*** mag-c., med., **MERC.,** merc-i-r., merc-sul., nat-a., ***nat-c., nat-m.,*** nat-p., **NIT-AC.,** petr., ***ph-ac.,*** **PHOS.,** ***psor.,*** sabad., ***samb.,*** sarr., sars., **SIL.,** ***spong.,*** stram., stront-c., **SULPH.,** syph., ***tarax.,*** **THUJ.,** valer., ***verat.,*** xan.
after 3 a.m. - bry., clem., nat-c., par.
after 4 a.m. - ***stann.***
every alternate night - bar-c., kali-n., ***nit-ac.***
on waking the sweat ceases, and returns again on falling asleep - cham.
sleep, during - carb-an., ***chin.,*** chin-s., nat-c., ***phos., thuj.,*** til.
sleeplessness, with - bar-c., ***cham.,*** cic., corn., iod., **SULPH.**
rage, during - acon., ant-t., ars., ***bell.,*** hyos., lyc., merc., nat-c., nat-m., nit-ac., nux-v., ***op.,*** ph-ac., phos., puls., ***stram.,*** verat.
sex, after - ***agar.***
siesta, during - ***caust.,*** sel.
sitting quietly, while - **KALI-BI.**
sleep, during - aral., camph., carb-an., ***chin.,*** chin-s., hyos., merc., nat-c., ***op., phos.,*** podo., ***thuj.***
uncovered parts, on, except the head - ***thuj.***
urine, copious flow and diarrhea - ***acon.***
vomiting, with - acon.
waking, on - am-m., canth., chin., ***ferr.,*** **SAMB.,** ***sep.,*** **SULPH.**
walking, while - bry., canth., chin-s., kali-c., ***merc.,*** **PSOR.,** sel., ***sep., sulph.***
in the open air - **CAUST.,** ***chin.,*** lyc., ph-ac., rhod., sel., ***zinc.***

RAGE, during - acon., ant-t., ars., ***bell.,*** hyos., lyc., merc., nat-c., nat-m., nit-ac., nux-v., ***op.,*** ph-ac., phos., puls., ***stram.,*** verat.

RELIEF, gives no - ***acon.,*** anac., ***ant-c., ant-t.,*** arn., **ARS.,** bar-c., bell., benz-ac., ***calc.,*** camph., cann-s., carb-v., **CAUST., CHAM.,** chel., ***chin.,*** cimx., cina, cinnb., ***cocc.,*** coff., colch., coloc., con., croc., ***dig.,*** dros., dulc., eup-per., ***ferr.,*** ferr-ar., **FORM.,** graph., ***hep.,*** hyos., ***ign., ip., kali-c.,*** kali-n., kreos., led., lyc., ***mang.,*** **MERC.,** mez., mosch., mur-ac., nat-a., ***nat-c.,*** nat-m., ***nit-ac.,*** **NUX-V., OP.,** par., ph-ac., ***phos.,*** plb., psor., ***puls.,*** ran-b., rhod., **RHUS-T.,** ***sabad.,*** sabin., samb., sel., **SEP.,** spong., stann., staph., **STRAM.,** stront-c., **SULPH.,** tarax., thuj., ***til.,*** valer., **VERAT.,** ***verat-v.***

ROOM, in the - acon., ***apis,*** bry., caust., cist., ***fl-ac.,*** **IP.,** ***nux-v., phos.,*** **PULS.,** rhod., rhus-t., sep., sulph., valer.
warm - carb-v.

SADNESS, from - calc-p.

SALTY, deposits after perspiration - sel.

SCANTY, sweat - alum., ant-c., apis, calad., chin-s., cimx., ***cina,*** casc., conv., croc., cycl., dulc., elaps, ***eup-per.,*** eup-pur., gamb., ign., ***ip.,*** kali-c., kali-i., lach., led., nat-m., nux-m., nux-v., phel., ran-b., sep., sil.

chill, after a severe - eup-per.

viscid - abies-c., fl-ac., hep., ***lyc., merc.,*** phal., phos.

SCRATCH, must - mang.

SENSATION, as if about to perspire, but no moisture appears - alum., ***am-c.,*** bapt., bor., bov., camph., calc., cimx., croc., ***ferr.,*** glon., **IGN.,** iod., nicc., phos., puls., ***raph.,*** sars., senec., **STANN.,** sul-ac., sulph., thuj.

SEX, after - ***agar., calc.,*** chin., ***eug.,*** **GRAPH.,** nat-c., sel., **SEP.**

SHIVERING, with - ant-t., aml-n., arg-n., cedr., coff., eup-per., hell., led., lyc., ***merc.,*** **NUX-V.,** puls., pyrog., raph., ***rhus-t.,*** sep., sulph., tab., verat.

SHUDDERING, after - rhus-v., stry., thuj.

SIDES, one sided - acon., alum., ***ambr.,*** anac., ant-t., arn., aur-m-n., ***bar-c.,*** bell., ***bry.,*** carb-v., ***caust.,*** cham., ***chin., cocc.,*** fl-ac., ign., lyc., merc., merl., nux-m., **NUX-V.,** ***phos.,*** **PETR.,** piloc., **PULS.,** ran-b., rheum, rhus-t., sabin., ***spig.,*** stann., stram., ***sulph.,*** **THUJ.**

left - ambr., anac., **BAR-C.,** ***chin.,*** fl-ac., kali-c., phos., piloc., **PULS.,** rhus-t., spig., stann., sulph.

right - aur-m-n., bell., bry., fl-ac., merl., nux-v., ***phos.,*** piloc., ***puls.,*** ran-b., sabin.

SINGLE, parts - ***acon., ambr.,*** ars., bar-c., bell., ***bry.,*** **CALC.,** ***calc-p.,*** cann-s., caps., **CAUST.,** ***cham.,*** chin., con., fl-ac., hell., hep., **IGN.,** ip., ***led., lyc.,*** merc., **MEZ.,** nux-v., par., ***petr.,*** phos., phos., plect., ***psor.,*** **PULS.,** ***pyrog.,*** rhus-t., ***sel.,*** **SEP.,** ***sil., spig.,*** spong., ***stann., sulph., thuj., tub.,*** verat., zinc.

back of body - sep.

contact, in, with another - nicc-s.

front of body - agar., **ARG-M.,** arn., ***calc.,*** canth., **COCC.,** ***graph.,*** kali-n., merc., nux-v., **PHOS., SEL.**

lain on - ***acon.,*** bry., ***bell.,*** **CHIN., NIT-AC.,** nux-v., puls., ***sanic.***

lower part of body - am-c., am-m., apis, ars., asaf., aur., bry., calc., cinnb., coloc., con., **CROC.,** cycl., dros., euph., ferr., ***hyos., iod.,*** kali-n., mang., merc., nit-ac., nux-v., ***phos.,*** ran-a., sanic., sep., sil., thuj., ***zinc.***

not lain on - ***benz.,*** thuj.

posterior parts - sep.

side not reclined upon - benz., thuj.

uncovered parts - thuj.

unilaterally - nux-v., piloc., puls.

upper part of body - acon., agar., ***anac., ant-t.,*** arg-m., arn., **ASAR.,** aza., bar-c., bell., berb., ***bov.,*** calc., camph., canth., ***caps., carb-v.,*** caust., ***cham.,*** chin., cina

SINGLE, parts

upper part of body - coc-c., dulc., dig., eup-per., euphr., fl-ac., graph., ***ign.,*** ip., **KALI-C.,** lat-m., laur., mag-c., mag-m., mag-s., merc-c., mosch., mur-ac., nat-c., ***nit-ac.,*** nux-v., **OP., PAR.,** petr., ph-ac., phos., ***piloc.,*** plb., puls., ***rheum,*** rhus-t., ***ruta,*** sabad., ***samb., sars., sec.,*** sel., sep., sil., spig., sul-ac., thuj., tub., valer., verat.

sleep, before - berb.

spots, in - merc., ptel., tell.

SITTING, while - am-c., ***anac.,*** **ARS.,** ***asar., calc.,*** caps., caust., chin., ***con., ferr., kali-bi.,*** lyc., mang., nat-c., ph-ac., phos., rhod., ***rhus-t.,*** sep., spong., ***staph.,*** sul-ac., sulph., tarax., valer.

SLEEP, during - ***acet-ac.,*** aeth., agar., am-c., anac., ***ant-c., ant-t.,*** aral., ***ars., ars-i.,*** bar-c., **BELL.,** bol., bor., bry., bufo, **CALC.,** camph., ***carb-an.,*** carb-s., carb-v., ***caust.,*** **CHAM., CHEL., CHIN.,** ***chin-a., chin-s.,*** cic., cina, clem., **CON.,** corn-f., cycl., dig., dros., dulc., euphr., eup-per., ***ferr., ferr-ar., ferr-p.,*** hep., **HYOS.,** ign., ***iod.,*** ip., kali-ar., kali-c., kali-i., ***kali-p., lac-c.,*** lachn., lyc., ***merc.,*** **MEZ.,** mur-ac., ***myos.,*** nat-c., ***nat-m.,*** nit-ac., nux-v., ***op.,*** petr., ***ph-ac., phos.,*** phyt., picro., ***piloc.,*** **PLAT., PODO.,** psor., **PULS., RHUS-T.,** ***sabad., salv.,*** sang., sanic., **SEL.,** ***sep.,*** **SIL.,** stann., staph., stram., stront-c., ***sulph.,*** syc-co., ***tarax.,*** thal., **THUJ.,** til., **TUB.,** verat., zinc., zinc-m.

amel. - ars., bell., bry., carb-an., chin., hep., ***merc., nux-v.,*** ph-ac., ***phos.,*** puls., **SAMB.**

dry heat, on waking - **SAMB.**

even when closing the eyes - carb-an., **CON.**

on beginning to - aeth., am-c., ant-c., **ARS.,** ***calc.,*** carb-an., ***con.,*** hep., lyc., ***mag-c.,*** **MERC.,** mez., **MUR-AC.,** op., ***phos.,*** rhus-t., puls., ***sanic.,*** sars., ***sep.,*** sil., **SULPH.,** tab., **TARAX., THUJ.,** til., verat.

on going to amel. - bry., ***merc.,*** nux-m., ph-ac., phos., **SAMB.,** ***sep.***

waking, during - con., hep., merc., ph-ac., phos., ***samb.***

after, and on - alum., anac., ***ant-c.,*** ant-ox., arn., ***ars.,*** bar-c., bell., bov., bry., ***calc., calad.,*** canth., carb-an., carb-s., carb-v., caust., cedr., ***chel., chin., chin-a.,*** cic., ***clem.,*** colch., con., corn., cycl., dig., ***dros.,*** eupi., euphr., ***ferr.,*** ferr-ar., glon., graph., hep., hyper., jug-c., ign., lac-c., lach., led., lyc., mag-c., mag-m., mang., ***merc.,*** merc-c., nat-m., nicc., ***nux-v.,*** ph-ac., ***phos.,*** pip-m., ptel., ran-b., rat., rumx., **SAMB., SEP.,** sil., stann., staph., **SULPH.,** ***tarax.,*** til.

amel. - ant-c., ***ars.,*** bell., ***cham.,*** **CALC.,** chin., cycl., ***euphr., hell.,*** **NUX-V.,** op., **PHOS.,** ***plat.,*** **PULS.,** sel., ***sep.,*** sil., stram., ***sulph.,*** **THUJ.**

SMOKING - nat-m., thuj.

SPOTS, in - merc., ptel., tell.

STAINING the linen - ***arn.,*** ars., bar-c., bar-m., **BELL.,** benz-ac., ***calc.,*** carb-an., carl., cham., chin., clem., dulc., ***graph., lac-c.,*** **LACH.,** ***lyc.,*** mag-c., med., ***merc.,*** nux-m., ***nux-v.,*** rheum, ***sel.***
bloody - anag., ***arn.,*** ars., calc., cann-i., ***cham.,*** chin., ***clem.,*** cocc., crot-h., ***cur.,*** dulc., hell., **LACH.,** ***lyc.,*** merc., **NUX-M.,** ***nux-v.,*** phos., ***sel.***
night - cur.
blue - ***indg.,*** iod., kali-i.
brown - iod., nit-ac., sep., wies.
brownish-yellow - ars., ***bell.,*** carb-an., graph., lac-c., ***lach.,*** mag-c., sel., thuj.
dark - bell.
difficult to wash out - ***lac-d., mag-c., merc.***
green - agar., cupr.
red - ***arn., calc., carb-v.,*** cham., chin., clem., ***crot-h., dulc.,*** ferr., gast., **LACH.,** ***lyc.,*** **NUX-M.,** ***nux-v.,*** thuj.
yellow - ars., ***bell.,*** benz-n., bry., cadm-s., **CARB-AN.,** carl., ***chin.,*** chin-a., ***crot-c.,*** elat., ***ferr.,*** ferr-ar., **GRAPH.,** guat., hep., ***ip.,*** lac-c., lac-d., **LACH.,** lyc., ***mag-c.,*** **MERC.,** ***rheum,*** **SEL.,** ***thuj.,*** tub., ***verat.***

STICKY - agar., anthr., anthro., ant-t., ars., both., brom., cann-i., canth., caust., chlor., crot-h., ferr., fl-ac., hep., iod., kali-bi., kali-br., lachn., op., plb., phos., tab., tax.
evening - anthro., fl-ac.

STEAMING - bell., psor.

STIFFENING the linen - **MERC.,** nat-m., sel.

STOOL, during - acon., agar., ars., bell., calc., carb-v., cham., chin., crot-t., ***dulc.,*** ferr., ferr-ar., hep., ip., **MERC.,** nat-m., rhus-t., sep., ***stram., sulph.,*** trom., **VERAT.**
cold - merc., sulph., verat.
after - acet-ac., **ACON.,** aloe, ant-t., ars., calc., camph., carb-v., **CAUST.,** chin., crot-t., kali-c., lach., ***merc.,*** ph-ac., phos., rhus-t., ***samb., sel.,*** sep., sulph., sumb., tab., tub., **VERAT.**
amel. - thuj,
increased sweat - acon.
warm sticky, becomes cold and - **MERC.**
before - ***acon.,*** ant-t., ***bell.,*** bry., calc., caps., caust., dulc., kali-c., **MERC.,** op., phos., rhus-t., **TROM.,** ***verat.***

STRANGERS, in the presence of - ambr., **BAR-C.,** lyc., ***sep.,*** stram.

SUDDEN - aml-n., apis, ars., bell., ***carb-s.,*** clem., ***crot-h.,*** hyos., ***ip.,*** merc-cy., valer.
afternoon - clem.
and disappearing suddenly - **BELL.**
while walking in the open air, with chilliness - led.

SUPPRESSED, sweat, ailments from - ***acon.,*** am-c., anthr., apis, arn., ***ars., aspar.,*** atro., ***aur-m-n.,*** **BELL.,** bell-p., **BRY.,** cadm-s., ***caj.,*** **CALC., CALC-S.,** calc-sil., cann-s., ***carb-s., carb-v.,*** cary., caust., **CHAM., CHIN.,** ***clem.,*** coff., **COLCH.,** coloc., cupr., **DULC.,** ***eup-per., ferr.,*** ferr-p., ***graph.,*** hep., hyos., iod., ip., kali-ar., ***kali-c.,*** kali-sil., lach., led., ***lyc.,*** mag-c., ***merc.,*** mill., nat-c., ***nat-m., nat-s.,*** nit-ac., ***nux-m., nux-v.,*** olnd., op., ph-ac., ***phos.,*** plat., ***plb.,*** **PSOR.,** puls., **RHUS-T.,** sabad., sec., sel., senec., seneg., **SEP., SIL.,** spong., squil., staph., **STRAM., SULPH.,** teucr., thuj., verb., verat., viol-o.

SYMPTOMS, agg. while sweating - ***acon.,*** ant-t., arn., **ARS.,** calc., **CAUST., CHAM.,** ***chin.,*** chin-a., cimx., croc., eup-per., ***ferr.,*** ferr-ar., **FORM.,** ign., ***ip.,*** lyc., **MERC.,** nat-a., nat-c., ***nux-v.,*** **OP.,** phos., puls., ***psor.,*** **RHUS-T., SEP.,** spong., **STRAM., SULPH., VERAT.**
after - ***acon.,*** ant-t., calc., cham., **CHIN.,** ***con.,*** ip., ***merc.,*** **PH-AC.,** phos., ***puls.,*** **SEP.,** sil., ***staph., sulph.***
amel. while sweating - ***acon.,*** aesc., aeth., ***ars.,*** apis, bapt., bell., ***bov.,*** **BRY.,** ***calad.,*** camph., canth., ***cham., chin-s.,*** cimx., **CUPR.,** elat., eup-per., **GELS.,** ***graph., hep., lach.,*** lyc., **NAT-M.,** psor., **RHUS-T.,** samb., sec., ***stront-c., thuj., verat.***
except the headache - ***nat-m.***
except the headache, which is made worse - ars., chin-s., **EUP-PER.**

TALKING, while. - ambr., graph., ***iod.,*** sil., ***sulph.***

THIGHS, except - lyc.

TUBERCULOSIS, in - acet-ac., ars., ars-i., bac., bry., calc., carb-v., ***chin.,*** erio., ferr., gall-ac., hep., jab., ***ph-ac., phos.,*** samb., sep., ***sil.,*** stann., sulph., tub.
night, at - ***acet-ac., agarin., ars.,*** ars-i., atro., bac., ***chin.,*** erio., gall-ac., hep., ***jab.,*** kali-i., lyc., myos., ***ph-ac., phos.,*** piloc., salv., samb., sec., ***sil.,*** stann., tub.

UNCOVERED, desire to be - ***acon.,*** calc., ***camph.,*** ferr., iod., **LED.,** mur-ac., ***nat-m., op.,*** **SEC.,** spig., staph., verat., ***zinc.***
uncovered, parts, on - bell., ***puls., thuj.***

UNCOVERING, agg. - staph.
amel. - acon., ***bell.,*** calc., ***camph.,*** **CHAM.,** ***chin., led.,*** **LYC.,** ***nit-ac., puls., staph.,*** spig., sulph., ***thuj.,*** verat.
aversion to - acon., aeth., ars., arn., aur., bar-c., ***calc.,*** carb-an., chin., ***clem.,*** colch., con., ***eup-per.,*** gels., ***hell.,*** hep., mag-m., nat-a., ***nat-c.,*** nux-m., **NUX-V., RHUS-T., SAMB.,** sil., squil., ***stram., stront-c.,*** tub.

VEXATION, after - acon., bry., ***cham.,*** lyc., ***petr.,*** **SEP.,** staph., verat.

VOMITING, with - aeth., sulph.

WALKING, while - ***agar.,*** ambr., benz-ac., ***bry.,*** **CALC.,** canth., carb-an., caust., chin-s., ***coc-c.,*** coloc., eug., ferr., ferr-m., hydr-ac., ip., ***kali-c.,*** led., ***merc.,*** nat-m., **NUX-V.,** op., **PSOR.,** sel., **SEP.,** sil., **SULPH.,** sumb., ther., til., valer.
after - rhus-t.

WALKING, while
air, in open - ant-c., bell., **BRY.,** ***calc.,*** ***carb-an.,*** carb-v., **CAUST.,** coloc., **CHIN.,** ***guai.,*** hep., led., lyc., nat-c., nit-ac., ***phos.,*** ph-ac., rhod., ruta., ***sulph.,*** sumb., zinc.
amel - alum., **ARS.,** bry., graph., puls., thuj.
amel. - cham., chel., ***puls.,*** sulph., ***thuj.***

WARM, sweats - acon., ant-c., asar., benz., calc., camph., carb-v., cham., cocc., dig., dros., ign., kali-c., kreos., lach., led., nat-m., nux-v., op., phos., puls., sep., sil., staph., stram., sulph., thuj., til., verat.
causing uneasiness - **CALC.,** cham., nux-v., ***puls.,*** **SEP.,** ***sulph.***
convulsions with - sil.
epilepsy, after - sil.
evening - anac., puls.
every other morning - ant-c.
morning - carb-v.
night - staph., thuj.
sitting, in - asar.
somnolence with - op.
waking, amel. on - thuj.

WARMTH, of room unbearable - plan.

WASH off, difficult to - ***lac-d., mag-c., merc.,*** sep.

WEAKNESS, causes - acon., agar., ambr., am-c., aml-n., ant-c., anthr., apis, ***ars.,*** bar-c., benz., **BRY.,** bov., ***calad., calc.,*** **CAMPH., CARB-AN.,** carb-v., **CHIN.,** ***chin-a.,*** **CHIN-S.,** cocc., croc., dig., **FERR.,** ***ferr-ac., ferr-i.,*** ferr-p., graph., hyos., ign., **IOD.,** kali-bi., kali-n., lac-c., lyc., **MERC.,** nat-m., ***nit-ac.,*** op., **PH-AC., PHOS., PSOR.,** puls., ***pyrog.,*** rhod., **SAMB.,** ***sec.,*** **SEP.,** ***sil., stann., sulph., tarax.,*** **TUB.,** ***verat., verat-v.***

WIND, cold, agg. - cur.

WORK, during - berb.

WRITING, while - bor., ***hep., kali-c., psor.,*** **SEP.,** ***sulph., tub.***

Pregnancy

PREGNANCY, general (see Childbirth) - **ACON.,** aesc., ***agar.,*** **ALET.,** alum., am-c., ***am-m.,*** ambr., ***ant-c.,*** **ANT-T.,** ***apis, arg-m.,*** arg-n., ***arn.,*** ars., asaf., ***asar., bar-c.,*** **BELL.,** bell-p., ***benz-ac., bism., bor., bry.,*** **CALC.,** calc-p., **CAMPH.,** ***canth., caps.,*** carb-ac., ***carb-v., caul.,*** **CAUST., CHAM.,** ***chel., chin.,*** cic., **CIMIC., COCC.,** coff., coll., coloc., con., **CROC.,** cupr., cycl., ***dros.,*** dulc., equis., ***ferr., ferr-p., gels.,*** glon., ***goss.,*** graph., ***ham.,*** **HELL.,** helon., hydr., ***hyos.,*** ign., **IP.,** piloc., kali-bi., kali-br., kali-c., ***kali-fer.,*** kali-i., kalm., kreos., ***lac-ac., lach., lam., laur., lyss.,*** mag-m., ***merc., mosch., murx.,*** nat-c., ***nat-m.,*** nit-ac., ***nux-m.,*** **NUX-V.,** op., ph-ac., plat., plb., podo., pop., ***psor.,*** **PULS.,** pyrog., rat., ***rhus-t., sabad.,*** sabin., sec., **SEP.,** ***stann.,*** stram., sulph., tab., ***tarent.,*** verat., vib., viol-o.
- affections, in second and fifth months - psor.

ABDOMEN, during
- aching - ***con.***
  - every night after going to bed, better by getting up and moving about - con.
- bruised pain, in - arn., ***nux-m., sep.***
  - great, in bowels - lyss.
  - in walls of - ***puls.***
- colic - ***ars.,*** mill., **NUX-V., SEP.**
  - frequent, which draws the patient nearly double - ***coloc.***
- colicky paroxysmal pains after blow received in abdomen and getting feet wet - nux-m.
- congested condition of viscera - ***podo.***
- cramps - ***gels., vib.***
  - cannot remain covered - ***camph.***
  - distressing - ***cupr-m.***
- cutting pain, dysuria - ph-ac.
- dragging, in - ***kali-c.***
- flattened in front and bulging out in each lumbar region - puls.
- lying on abdomen amel. - podo.
- pain, during - arn., ***ars., bell., bry., cham., coloc., con.,*** hyos., ***ip., kali-c.,*** lach., **NUX-V.,** plb., puls., sep., ***verat.***
- room enough, feeling as if there were not, at night in bed, must stretch violently - plb.
- sharp pains across - ***cimic.***
- shooting - **KALI-C.**
  - across, either right to left, or left to right - ***cinnb.***
- soreness, in - arn., ***nux-m., sep.***
  - great, in bowels - lyss.
  - in walls of - ***puls.***
- spasmodic pains with chill, particularly after anger - ***bry.***
- spasms - puls.
- stitching - **KALI-C.**
- tearing tensive pain in spot, in lower, corresponding to seat of placenta, worse at night when lying on affected side, and sore to touch, as if ulcerated - puls.
- tender - ***nux-m.***
- throbbing - sel.

ABDOMEN, during
- tight, sensation as if something, would break if too much exertion were made at stool - ***apis.***
- tympanitic - ***psor.***

ABORTION, spontaneous, (see Miscarriage)

AFFECTION, has no, for anybody - **ACON., SEP.**

ALBUMINURIA, (see Urine, chapter) - am-c., ***apis,*** apoc., ***ars., ars-i.,*** bell., benz-ac., berb., bry., cact., calc-ar., ***canth.,*** cinch., colch., dig., dulc., ferr., ***gels.,*** hell., ***helon.,*** kali-br., ***kali-c., kali-m.,*** kalm., lach., led., ***lyc., merc-c., nat-m.,*** phos., phyt., rhus-t., senec., sep., sulph., ***ter.,*** uran-n.
- retinitis, with - ***apis, ars.,*** colch., gels., kalm., ***merc-c.,*** phos., zinc.

APPETITE, ravenous, during, at night - ***par.***

APPREHENSION - ***lyss.***

ANGER, worse from - ***nux-m.***

ANUS, burning - ***caps.***
- stool, after, contracts around prolapsed rectum, which becomes constricted and sensitive to touch, painful, like a sore - ***mez.***
- painfully sore, and hot feeling - ***zing.***

AWKWARD, falls easily - **CALC.**

BACK, pain, during - ***aesc.,*** kali-c.
- aching - lyss.
- burning, lumbar, during - rhus-t.
- drawing in sacral region - ***sars.***
- pains - arg-n.
- pains, severe, in small of, particularly forcing and pressing, as if a heavy weight came into pelvis, low down - ***kali-c.***
- shooting, after diarrhea, with colic - calc-ar.
- sore, lumbar, during - lyss.
- soreness, great, in lower part - lyss.

BEARING, down, pain, pregnancy, during - calc-ar., ***kali-c.,*** lyss.
- come out, as if everything would, during - ***kali-c.***
- frequent and prolonged forcing pain, particularly in thin, ill-conditioned women - **SEC.**
- labor-like pains - ***puls.***
  - discharge of serous fluid, with - sep.
  - night watching and mental disturbance, after - puls.
  - seventh month, at - ***sep.***
- painful, prolonged - **UST.**
- spasmodic, distressing, preventing sleep - ***cham.***

BELCHING - acet-ac., ***nat-m.***
- eggs, spoiled, like, during - mag-c.
- relieve - **ANT-T.**
- sour, during - nux-v.
- sweetish, during - nat-m., ***zinc.***
- tasting like rotten eggs - ***mag-c.***
- water-brash, during - acet-ac., dios., ***lac-ac.,*** lob., ***nat-m., nux-m., tab.***

BLADDER, cramp-like pains - ***lyc.***
- symptoms - puls.

BLEEDING, uterine, during, (see Labor, Miscarriage) - ***apis***, bell., ***cann-i.***, caul., ***cham.***, chin., cimic., ***cinnam.***, ***cocc.***, croc., ***erig.***, ham., **IP.**, kali-c., **KREOS.**, ***nit-ac.***, ***phos.***, ***plat.***, ***puls.***, ***rhus-t.***, ***sabin.***, sec., ***sep.***, ***tril.***
cervical os dilated to size of half a dollar - tril.
fifth and seventh month - **SEP.**
first part, in - nit-ac.
fright, after - ***ign.***
lying amel. - ***ign.***
overexertion, from - ***cinnam.***, ***erig.***, ***nit-ac.***
sixth month - ***cann-i.***, erig.
third month - **KREOS.**, ***sabin.***
miscarriage, threatening - ***cinnam.***
in third month - **KREOS.**
first half, in, after overexertion and mental depression - ***nit-ac.***
fright, after, better lying on back without pillow, lower end of mattress elevated - ***ign.***
labor-like pains, bloody discharge, with - ***cham.***
lifting, from, straining, overstretch ing arms, or taking false step - ***cinnam.***
months, especially fifth and seventh - **SEP.**
painless flow, steady, at sixth month, from overexertion - ***erig.***

BREASTS, hard knots - ***calc-f.***
painful - ***sep.***
nodules, during - ***fl-ac.***
breasts, pain, during - calc-p., cimic., ***sep.***
burning, during - ***calc-p.***
inflammatory pain - ***bell.***, ***bry.***
neuralgic pain - ***con.***, puls.
nipples, under, during - ***cimic.***
sore, during - ***calc-p.***

BREATHING, difficult, from upward pressure - **NUX-V.**
dyspnea - viol-o.
with upward pressure - ***nux-m.***

CHEST, congestion, during - ***glon.***, ***nat-m.***, ***sep.***
rush of blood upward - lyss.
pains in lower ribs - arg-n.

CHILDBIRTH, general (see Labor, Lochia) - ***acon.***, ***arn.***, ***aur.***, ***bell.***, bor., calc., calc-f., ***calen.***, carb-v., **CAUL.**, **CAUST.**, **CHAM.**, ***chin.***, ***cic.***, ***cimic.***, cocc., ***coff.***, ***coff-t.***, ***coll.***, cupr., ferr., ***gels.***, goss., graph., hyos., hyper., ign., ip., ***kali-c.***, ***lyc.***, mag-m., mill., mosch., nat-c., nat-m., ***nux-m.***, ***nux-v.***, ***op.***, plat., **PULS.**, ***pyrog.***, ***rhod.***, rhus-t., ruta, sabin., **SEC.**, **SEP.**, stann., stram., sulph., verat., vib.
abdomen, tenderness - chlf.
after, to speed recovery - ***arn.***, **BELL-P.**, ***calen.***, ***caul.***, chin., kali-c., puls., ***sep.***
after-pains of - ***acon.***, aml-n., **ARN.**, asaf., ***atro.***, aur., **BELL.**, bor., ***bry.***, ***calc.***, carb-an., carb-v., ***caul.***, **CHAM.**, chin., cic., ***cimic.***, cina, cinnam., cinnb., cocc., ***coff.***, coloc., ***con.***, croc., **CUPR.**, cupr-ar., cycl., **DIOS.**, ***ferr.***, ***gels.***, ***graph.***, hyos., **HYPER.**, ***ign.***, iod., ip., **KALI-C.**, kreos., ***lac-c.***, lach., lil-t., lyc., ***mill.***

CHILDBIRTH, general
after-pains - nat-c., nat-m., nux-m., nux-v., ***op.***, **PAR.**, ***phos.***, plat., ***podo.***, **PULS.**, pyrog., **RHUS-T.**, ***ruta***, **SABIN.**, **SEC.**, ***sep.***, sul-ac., ***sulph.***, ter., ust., ***vib.***, ***vib-p.***, vinc., ***xan.***, zinc.
child nurses, pain when - ***arn.***, ***cham.***, con., puls., **SEC.**, **SIL.**
distant parts, in - carb-v.
distressing, severe - **CUPR.**
extending, to
abdomen, across, into groins - caul., cimic.
calves and soles, in - cupr.
groins, into - caul., ***cimic.***
shins, into - carb-v., cocc.
thights, into - ***lac-c.***
fear of death, with - ars., **COFF.**
frequent - rhus-t.
headache, with - hyper.
intolerable - cimic.
hip, in - cimic., sil.
instrumental delivery, after - ***arn.***, calen., ***hyper.***, ***rhus-t.***
insupportable - ***coff.***
menses, with offensive - ***crot-h.***
motion agg., least - ***bry.***
multipara, in - cupr., sep.
prolonged - arn., calc.
evening agg. - ***puls.***
sensitive women, in - ign., ***gels.***, ***nux-v.***, ***op.***
violent, persistent - vib.
weak - arn., caul., **PAR.**, puls.
anus, tenesmus, child's head presses against symphysis pubis - ***cinnb.***
sense of weight - ***sep.***
atony of uterus, after - am-m., ***caul.***, op., plb., puls., sec., ***sep.***
breathing, air, desires fresh - ***cham.***
difficult - ***sep.***, ***stann.***
fanned, wishes to be, wants air - ***carb-v.***, ***sulph.***
oppressed - ***chin-s.***
suffocating spells - **HYOS.**, puls.
cervix, os
contracted, spasmodically - ***bell.***, ***sep.***
amniotic fluid gone - ***bell.***
dilated, widely, complete atony, face flushed, patient drowsy dull - ***gels.***
flabby, os open, no pains, bag of waters bulging, patient more and more drowsy, speech thickens, convulsions seem threatening - ***gels.***
half open - ***sep.***
hard - ***sep.***
rigid - ***cimic.***, ***caul.***, chlf., ***con.***, **GELS.**, ***lob.***, ***verat-v.***
scarcely able to endure pains - **CHAM.**
rounded and hard, feels as if it would not dilate - **GELS.**
soft - ***ust.***
tenderness - ***plat.***, sep.
anterior lip, of - ***sep.***
widened, not, correspondingly - ***bell.***

CHILDBIRTH, general
confinement, problems during - acon., agn., ant-c., ant-t., **ARN.,** asaf., asar., aur., **BELL., BELL-P.,** bor., bov., ***bry., calc.,*** **CALEN.,** camph., canth., ***carb-an.,*** carb-v., **CAUL.,** caust., **CHAM.,** chin., cina, cocc., ***coff.,*** colch., coloc., con., ***croc.,*** cupr., cycl., dros., dulc., equis., ***ferr., gels.,*** glon., graph., helon., rhod., **SEP.**
lesions of parts - arn., ***calen.***
chilliness - coff.
nervous, chatters in first stage - **GELS.**
shivers, in first stage - **CIMIC.**
shuddering, with pains, better when warmly covered - ***sep.***
coldness, of skin - ***camph.***
covered, cannot bear to be - ***camph.***
cramps, legs, in - ***bell.***
fingers and toes - cupr-m.
crying - ***coff.***
despair - ***coff.***
difficult - abrot., acon., ***cimic.,*** arn., ***aur., bell.,*** bor., calc., **CAUL., CAUST.,** ***cham., coff-t., gels.,*** goss., ***hyos., kali-c., lyc.,*** nux-v., puls., rhod., ***sec.,*** sep., sulph., verat., vib.
enraged - ***bell.***
eyes, glittering - ***coff.***
extreme sensibility to light - ***con.***
face, pinkish, as if uniformly flushed - ***gels.***
puffed - ***coff.***
fainting - cinnam., **SEC.**
fear of death - ***coff.***
fear, from - ign., ***op.***
feet, cold - ***sep.***
fever, after - ***apis, arg-n.,*** arn., ars., ***bapt.,*** bell., ***bry.,*** **CARB-S.,** cham., cimic., coff., coloc., **ECHI.,** ***ferr.,*** gels., ***hyos.,*** ign., ip., kali-c., **LACH., LYC.,** mill., ***mur-ac.,*** nux-v., op., phos., plat., **PULS., PYROG., RHUS-R., RHUS-T.,** sec., sil., **SULPH.,** verat., verat-v.
lochia, from suppressed - ***lyc.,*** mill., puls., **SULPH.**
fright, from - ign., ***op.***
grief, symptoms from - ***caust.,*** ign.
hands, cannot bear to have them touched - ***cinch.***
head, hot - ***coff.***
heart, neuralgia - ***cimic.***
heat - ***coff-t.***
feverish - ***caul.***
flushes - ***sep.***
hysteria, since - ***chel.,*** **GELS.**
hysterical, during - ***chlol.***
rigid, with, unyielding os, nervous excitement - **GELS.**
irritable, snappish - **CHAM.**
irritability, nervous - ***hyos.***
lamenting - ***coff.***
limbs, violent moving - ***coff.***
muscles, rigidity - coff.
in first delivery, in women who have married late - ***bell.***

CHILDBIRTH, general
nervous - ***chlol.,*** chlf.
perineum, rigid - ***lob.***
position, abnormal - ***puls.***
child lying transversely, during first stage in thirty minutes, vertex presented - puls.
labor pains, ineffectual, from defective position of child - ***acon.***
pulse, intermittent - ***chin-s.***
rapid - ***chin-s.***
slow and full - ***gels.***
weak - ***chin-s.***
rapid, too - ***lyc.***
recovery, slow - arn., ***bell-p.,*** caul., ***graph., sep.***
restlessness - ***acon., camph.,*** chlf.
shooting, upward, in vagina - ***sep.***
skin, dry - ***acon., coff-t.***
sleepless - ***con.***
spains very distressing - ***coff.***
slow - ***bell., caul.,*** chlol., chlf., ***ign.,*** **PULS.,** ***sec.***
long and painful - ***arn.***
almost painless, uterine contraction, feeble, insufficient - goss.
sad feelings and forebodings - **NAT-M.**
speech, thick tongue, like one intoxicated - ***gels.***
suppressed - cact.
stillborn babies, women who deliver - cimic.
subinvolution, of genitalia, after - ***bell.,*** bry., ***calc., carb-v., caul.,*** chin., **CIMIC.,** cycl., ***hydr., kali-bi.,*** **KALI-BR.,** kali-c., ***kali-i., lil-t.,*** mill., ***nat-h.,*** nat-s., ***op.,*** plat., podo., psor., **PULS.,** ***sabin., sec.,*** **SEP.,** staph., **SULPH.,** ter., ***ust.***
twitching - cinnam.
convulsive - ***chin-s.***
unconscious - ***chin-s.***
sank into semi-stupid state, could be roused by shaking, soon relapsed - ***gels.***
uterus, atony - caul., ***gels.***
constriction of lower part - **BELL.**
contractility hindered by sycotic complications - ***thuj.***
contraction, causing pain in small of back - ***coff.***
prolonged, tonic - ***sec.***
with every, violent dyspnea, seeming to neutralize labor pains - ***lob.***
contractions feeble - caul.
feeble and weak - ruta
insufficient - ***acon.***
interrupted by sensitiveness of vagina and external parts - ***plat.***
want of, with persistent bleeding of brownish blood - ***ust.***
darting, fine needle-like, upward from cervix - ***sep.***
expulsive power, want of - ***puls.***
flabby - ***sec.***
hour-glass contractions - ***cham., sec., sep.***

CHILDBIRTH, general
  uterus,
    inactive - ***puls.***
      insufficient pains - ***gels.***
    inertia - ***puls.***
      child's head is in the opening of pelvisand the action of womb is insufficient for expulsion - **PULS.**
    loose, everything seems, and open, no action - **SEC.**
    shooting in cervix - ***sep.***
    spasmodically, head, held inside, after body is born - ***bell.***
    split open, appears as if, from top to bottom, longitudinal fibres alone contracting, leaving a sulcus in middle - 2sec.
    strength weakened by too early or perverted efforts - ***sec.***
    throat, to, like a wave, ending with choking feeling, impeded labor, impending spasm - ***gels.***
  vagina, hot, dry, tender, undilateable - ***acon.***
    vagina, great sensitiveness on examination - ***plat.***
    vulva, tenderness - ***plat.***
  weakness, after - ***arn.,*** ars., asaf., **BELL.,** bor., bry., calc., camph., carb-an., carb-v., **CAUL.,** caust., ***cham.,*** chin., cimic., cocc., coff., ***con.,*** gels., **KALI-C., KALI-P.,** kreos., lyc., mag-c., mag-m., merc., mosch., nat-c., ***nat-m.,*** nux-m., ***nux-v.,*** **OP.,** phos., plat., **PULS.,** rhus-t., ruta, sabad., **SEC., SEP.,** stann., sul-ac., sulph., thuj., zinc.
    night watching, from - caust.
    pain in back, with - kali-c.
    shiver, finished with - caul.

CHILLINESS, constant, after night watching and mental disturbance - puls.

CHLOASMA - cadm-s., card-m., caul., ***lyc.,*** nux-v., rob., ***sep., sol.***
    sun, agg. - cadm-s., sep., sol.

CHOREA, during - ***caust.,*** chlol., ***cupr.***

CONCEPTION, easy - ***bor.,*** canth., merc., nat-c., nat-m.

CONFUSION, during - ***nux-m.***

CONGESTION, in general - ***psor.***

CONSTIPATION, during - ***agar.,*** **ALUM.,** ***ambr., ant-c., ant-t., apis, bry., calc.,*** carb-v., cocc., **COLL.,** coloc., ***con.,*** **DOL.,** ***graph., hydr., kali-c., lyc.,*** meny., merc., nat-m., **NAT-S.,** ***nit-ac.,*** **NUX-V.,** ***op., phyt.,*** **PLAT., PLB.,** ***podo., puls.,*** sabad., **SEP.,** stann., ***sulph., verb.***
    bowels, alternating with loose - ***dios.***
    crumbling stool - ***am-m.***
    difficult stool - ***nux-m.***
    feces hard - ***verat.***
    hemorrhoids from inertia of lower bowel - coll.
    manual assistance must be rendered - **SEP.**
    nausea, with - ***coll.***
    night, after, watching and mental disturbance - puls.

CONVULSIONS - ***bell., cic.***
    seventh month, in a woman with albuminuria, dropsy, headache, etc., in quick succession, with unconsciousness - oena.
    unconsciousness, with - ***gels.***

COUGHS, during - calc., ***caust., con.,*** ip., kali-br., ***nat-m., nux-m.,*** phos., puls., sabin., sep., vib.
    deep and loose - apoc.
    hacking - ***nux-m.***
      constant - ***kali-br.***
    loose, in morning - ***sep.***
    month, during second, worse at night, and morning, and on lying down - vib.
    nervous, threatening miscarriage - ***kali-br.***
    night, worse at - ***con.***
    short and dry - apoc.
    spasmodic, constant, dry, worse from speaking, walking or mental exertions - ***con.***
      hacking - ***bell.***
    urine, with ejection of - ***ferr-p.***

CRAMPS, metrorrhagia, with - ***hyos.***
    abnormal craving - ***lyss.***

CRYING, during - apis, ***mag-c.,*** ign., nat-m., **PULS.,** ***sep.,*** stann.
    tendency to - ***mag-c., puls.***

DEPRESSION, during - chin., cimic., lach., **NAT-M.,** nux-m., plat., ***puls.,*** **SEP.**

DERANGEMENT, emotional - ***bell.***

DIARRHEA, during - alum., am-m., ***ant-c., apis, cham., chel., chin.,*** dulc., ferr., gels., hell., hyos., ***iris, lac-ac., lyc., nux-m.,*** nux-v., petr., **PHOS.,** ***puls., sep., sulph.***
    chronic, with fainting and sluggish flow of ideas - ***nux-m.***
    colic - calc-ar.
    face, with earthy color of - lyc.
    hard, then, difficult stools - olnd.
    mucous - ***caps.***
    rectum, with prolapsus - ***mez.***
    riding, worse from - petr.

EARS, affections - ***caps.***

ECLAMPSIA, toxemia - **APIS,** apoc., ***ars.,*** ars-i., ***aur-m.,*** benz-ac., berb., bry., cact., ***calc-ac., canth., chin.,*** cinnb., ***colch., crot-h., cupr-ar.,*** dig., dulc., ferr., ***gels.,*** glon., hell., ***helon.,*** ind., ***kali-ar.,*** kali-br., ***kali-c., kali-chl.,*** kalm., ***lach.,*** led., ***lyc., merc.,*** **MERC-C.,** ***nat-m., ph-ac., phos.,*** rhus-t., sabin., senec., ***sep.,*** sulph., ***ter.,*** thlaspi, thyr., uran., ***verat-v.***
      and after delivery - ***merc-c.,*** ph-ac., ***pyrog.***
    kidneys inflammation, with - ***crot-h.***

EDEMA, during pregnancy - **APIS,** ***apoc., ars.,*** aur-m., colch., ***dig.,*** dulc., hell., helon., ***jab.,*** lyc., merc., merc-c., nat-m., sanic., uran-n.
    hydrops amnia - apis.
    labia swollen - jab.

EPIGASTRIUM, gone feeling - ***nat-m.***
every morning at two or three o'clock, tensive, stitching pain, must rise and walk about - puls.
tightness across - **KREOS.**

ERUPTION, skin disease - ant-c.
eruption - ***sep.***

ESOPHAGUS, burning - ars.

EXPECTORATION, putrid taste and smell - con.

EYES, dim, after night watching, mental disturbance - puls.
diplopia and dim vision - ***gels.***
hemeralopia - ran-b.
mist before - ***calc.***
nephritic retinitis - ***merc-c.***
retinitis albuminurica - ***kalm.***
sunken, after night watching and mental disturbance - puls.
spots, yellow - am-c.

FACE, aching - ***ign., sep., stram.***
discoloration, bluish, during - ***phos.***
earthy - ***mag-c.***
erysipelas, during - ***bor.***
pain, during - ***ign., sep.,*** stram.
alternately, and red, after night watching and mental disturbance - puls.
pale, bluish, puffed - ***phos.***
turned, on slightest excitement - nux-m.
spots, yellow brown - ***sep.***
syncope - ***nux-v.***
twitching, during - ***hyos.***

FAINTNESS, with - ***bell.,*** ign., ***nux-m., nux-v., puls.,*** sec., ***sep., verat.***
excitement, on slightest - nux-m.
faintness - ***ars.***

FALSE conception - ***caul.,*** puls.
all symptoms of former pregnancies, except she had a regular monthly flow, lasting three or four days, somewhat scanty, painless and too pale - puls.
imaginary - croc., verat.

FEAR, during - **ACON.,** ***ars., caul., cimic.,*** con., lyc., lyss., ***nux-m.,*** stann.
death of, during - **ACON.,** ***ars.***

FEELING as in beginning of pregnancy - apis.

FEET, cramp in soles and toes - **CALC.**
coldness, during - ***lyc.,*** **VERAT.**
lame, with soreness from instep to sole - sil.
lameness, during - sil.
swollen, with heartburn and varicose veins - ***zinc.***
tearing, during - phos.

FETUS, general
arrested, development of the - ***sec.***
crosswise, as if lying - ***arn.***
dead, expelled - ***canth.,*** cimx., ***puls.,*** ruta.
retained - arist-cl., man., pyrog., sec.
eighth month in, child moves so violently it awakens her, causing cutting in bladder, with urging to urinate - thuj.

FETUS, general
position, abnormal - ***acon.,*** **PULS.**
breech - **PULS.**
crosswise, as if lying - ***arn.***
room, as if fetus had lack of - ***plb.***

fetus, motions, of
ceased, have - ***caul.***
desire to urinate, pain in bladder and cutting pain, with - thuj.
disturbing sleep - con., ***thuj.***
feels, too sensitively - ***sep.***
fist of a fetus, like the - ***nat-c., sulph.,*** **THUJ.**
movements hurt or make her sore - ***arn., op., sep.***
nausea and vomiting, cause - arn.
painful - ***arn.,*** con., op., puls., ***sep.,*** **SIL.**
produce rawness - sep.
says child turns over and does not lie right, it pains her - ***puls.***
sleep, motion disturbs - ***con., thuj.***
somersaults, seems to be turning - ***lyc.***
tympanic abdomen, with - psor.
urinate, with desire to, pain, in bladder and cutting pain - thuj.
violent - arn., ***ars.,*** croc., ***lyc., op., psor.,*** **SIL.,** ***thuj.***
felt too violently and are painful - croc.
somersaults, as - ***lyc.***

FEVER, pains threatening miscarriage during febrile stage of intermittent - ***puls.***
yellow - ***cadm-s.,*** plat.

FOOD, general
aversion, bread, to - ***sep.***
food, to - ant-t., ***laur.***
thought of food sickens her - ***sep.***
desire, acids, for - ***verat.***
cold, wants everything - ***verat.***
food, for certain kinds of - ***mag-c.***
food, for salt - ***verat.***
food, for salt and salted - ***nat-m.***
strange - lyss.
unusual articles, for, of food - ***chel.***
loathing, of during (see Nausea) - colch., ip., ***laur., sep.***

FRIGHT, worse from - ***nux-m.***

GENITALIA, general
edema of vulva - ***merc.***
inflamed - ***coll.***
itching - acon., ambr., ars., bell., bor., bov., calc., ***calad.,*** carb-ac., ***chlol.,*** con., ***dol.,*** graph., helon., hydr., kreos., lyc., ***merc., nat-m., plat.,*** sabin., sep., sil., sulph., thuj.
almost delirious - ***coll.***
at eighth month - ***coll.***
onanism, inducing - **CALAD.**
parts smell bad, are swollen dark red and protruding, she cannot lie down - ***coll.***
sore, she could neither walk, lie down nor sit, except on edge of chair - ***coll.***
swelling - ***coll.***

GENITALIA, general
swelling of labia - podo., ***sep.***

HAIR, falling, during - **LACH.,** ***sep.***

HANDS, nails blue - ***phos.***

HAUGHTY - ***verat.***

HAUNTED by seeing a man who had a disfiguring nasal cancer, she was sure her child would be marked - ***nat-m.***

HEAD, burst, as if it would - ***lyc.***
congestion - fl-ac., ***glon., lyss.***
enlarged, sensation, during - **ARG-N.**
expanded, feels - **ARG-N.**

HEADACHE, during - acon., ***cimic.,*** alumin., ***bell., bry.,*** calc., caps., caust., ***cham.,*** cocc., ***coff., gels., glon.,*** hyos., ***ign.,*** kalm., nux-m., ***nux-v., op., phos.,*** plat., ***puls.,*** rhus-t., ***sep., spig.,*** sulph., verb.
dandruff, with - ***calc.***
during third month - ***ferr-p.***
frequently recurring tearing stitching in right side - ***sep.***

HEARING, impaired, periodic, during - caps.

HEART, anxiety about precordia - **ACON.**
cease, sensation as if, had ceased, during - arg-m.
palpitations, during - ***arg-m., con., laur.,*** **LIL-T.,** ***nat-m., sep.***

HEARTBURN - ***apis, caps.,*** ox-ac.
night, at, while going to bed - con.
palpitation, with - nat-m.
with swollen feet - ***zinc.***

HEAT, thighs, during - podo.

HEMOPTYSIS - **ACON.**

HEMORRHOIDS - ***aesc., am-m., ant-c., caps., coll.,*** crot-h., ***hydr.,*** lach., ***lyc., nat-m.,*** **NUX-V., SEP.,** ***sulph., zinc.***
childbirth, since agg. - ***ign.,*** **KALI-C.,** ***lil-t., mur-ac., podo., puls.,*** **SEP.,** ***sulph.***
first month - ***lach.***

HICCOUGHS, during - ***cycl., op.***
continued - ***op.***
eating, while - ***cycl.***

HUNGER, appetite, without - ***nat-m.***
painful - ***sep.***
canine - ***verat.***

HYPOCHONDRIA, stitches in left - ***mag-c.***
soreness and pain in right - phyt.

IDEAS, full of strange - ***stram.***

IMAGINARY - apis, ***caul., croc.,*** cycl., ign., nux-v., ***op., puls., sabad.,*** sulph., thuj., ***verat.***

IMAGINING, frightful, usually caused by engorged condition of brain - ***kali-br.***

IRRITABILITY - ***cham.***

INFERTILITY, (see Female, chapter)

INGUINAL region, latter months sharp pain in right, preventing motion - ***podo.***

ITCHING, general, during - chlol., cocc., dol., sep., tab.
all over, worse at night, preventing sleep, worse scratching, no perceptible eruption on skin - ***dol.***
insupportable pruritus over whole body - ***tab.***
itching, genitalia, during - ambr., chlol., ***calad., fl-ac., helon., merc.,*** **SEP.,** urt-u.
swollen, during - ***merc., podo.***

JAUNDICE - **ACON.,** aur., **NUX-V.,** ***phos.***

JOINTS, swollen - ***nit-ac.***

LABOR, pains, (see Childbirth, general) - acon., ambr., arn., ***ars.,*** aur., bell., **CAUL.,** caust., **CHAM.,** cimic., ***coff.,*** con., ferr., **GELS., IGN., KALI-C.,** kali-p., lyc., ***nux-v.,*** op., phos., plat., **PULS.,** rhus-t., ***sec.,*** **SEP.**
absent, cervical os dilated, membranes protruding - ***gels.***
agony and sweat, with desire to be rubbed - ***nat-c.***
alternate, with bleeding - puls.
atony of uterus, during - am-m., ***caul.,*** op., plb., ***puls.,*** sec., sep.
back, extending down the, into gluteal muscles - cimic., ***kali-c.***
paroxysmal in - cimic., gels., ***kali-c., nux-v., sep.***
through to, and up the - ***gels.***
worse in - cimic., ***kali-c., nux-v.***
belchings, with - bor.
between pains, no freedom from suffering - chlf.
bleeding, uterine, during and after labor - ***acet-ac.,*** acon., adren., alet., alum., am-m., aml-n., apis, ***arn.,*** ars., ***bell.,*** bry., ***cann-i.,*** cann-s., carb-v., caul., ***cham., chin., cinnam.,*** cocc., coff., ***croc.,*** crot-h., cycl., **ERIG.,** ***ferr., gels.,*** ger., **HAM.,** ***hydr., hyos., ign.,*** **IP.,** kali-c., kalm., kreos., lach., lyc., merc., ***mill.,*** nit-ac., nux-m., nux-v., op., ph-ac., **PHOS.,** ***plat.,*** plb., puls., ***rhus-t.,*** **SABIN., SEC.,** senec., sep., ***thlaspi,*** tril., ***ust.***
alternating with, and restlessness - ***puls.***
bright red - bell., ***hyos., ip.,*** mill., ***ust.***
fluid and painless - mill.
clotted - phos., sabin., tril.
constant - ***ip.,*** **NUX-M.,** ***sabal., ust.***
dark - bell., caul., chin., ***gels., ip., sabin.,*** sec., tril., ***ust.***
fluid - sec.
eight days after - ***sabin.***
hot - bell., ip.
profuse, collapsic symptoms, with - ip.
profuse, gushes - bell.
inertia uteri, with - am-m., caul., puls., sec., ***ust.***
motion agg., slightest - **CROC.,** sec.
offensive - ***nit-ac.***
putrid - ***ust.***
one week after - ***kali-c.***
paroxysmal flow - chin.

LABOR, pains
bleeding, uterine
prevents hemorrhagia - ***arn.***
profuse - **APIS,** bell., ***ip., plat., sabin.,*** tril.
some days after - **CINNAM.**
thick - chin.
two weeks after - ***ust.***
blood, with more or less discharge of dark - ***cham.***
breath, loss of, fifth month - puls.
cease nearly or entirely - ***nux-v.***
and fly all over body - ***gels.***
bleeding, from - ***cinch.***
convulsions begin - ***sec.***
with complaining loquacity - ***coff.***
ceased for thirty-six hours - ***cimic.***
ceasing - acon., arn., asaf., **BELL.,** ***bor.,*** bry., cact., calc., ***camph.,*** carb-an., ***carb-v., caul., caust., cham.,*** chin., **CIMIC.,** cinnam., cocc., ***coff., gels., graph., guare.,*** hyos., ign., **KALI-C.,** kreos., lach., lyc., mag-c., mag-m., merc., mosch., nat-c., ***nat-m.,*** nux-m., ***nux-v.,*** **OP.,** phos., plat., **PULS.,** rhus-t., ruta., **SEC.,** ***sep.,*** stann., sulph., sul-ac., ***thuj.,*** zinc.
bleeding, with - ***chin.,*** cimic., puls., sec.
convulsions come on - bell., cham., cic., cupr., hyos., ign., ***sec.***
cramps in hip, from - cimic.
excitement, from emotional - cimic.
exhaustion, from - caul.
loquacity, with - ***coff.***
nervous shivering, with - cimic.
wave from uterus to throat stops the pains - gels.
weak - ***bell.,*** caul., cimic., gels., ***kali-c.,*** kali-p., nat-m., ***op.,*** **PULS., SEC.**
shivering, nervous, with - caul., cimic.
cervix, during labor
contracted, spasmodically - acon., aml-n., **BELL.,** cact., **CAUL., CIMIC.,** con., **GELS.,** hyos., lach., lyc., sec., ***sep.,*** vib., xan.
dilated - ***gels.***
half open - ***sep.***
rigidity of - acon., ant-t., ***bell.,*** **CAUL., CHAM.,** chlf., cimic., ***con.,*** **GELS.,** ign., jab., lob., lyc., nux-v., sec., ***verat-v.***
soft - ***ust.***
stenosis - con.
child, seems to ascend with every pain - ***gels.***
complains - cham., ***coff-t.***
cramp in flexor tendons of fingers and toes - **DIOS.**
cramps in abdomen, shooting down legs - vib.
cutting - asaf.
across, left to right - ***ip.***
umbilical region in, interfere with true pains - **IP.**
darting, fine needle-like, shooting upward from cervix - ***sep.***
deficient - ***bell., caul.,*** **PULS.,** sep., ***ust.***

LABOR, pains
desperate, make her - **ARS.,** ***aur., cham.***
desire to jump from window or dash herself down - ***aur.***
distracted, feels as if she would go - coff.
distressing - acon., ambr., arn., **ARS.,** aur., bell., ***caul.,*** caust., **CHAM.,** chin., cimic., ***coff.,*** con., **GELS.,** hyos., **IGN., KALI-C.,** lyc., nux-v., phos., plat., puls., sec., **SEP.**
but of little use - ***phos.***
can hardly bear them, wishes to get away from herself - ***cham.***
escape, wants to - bell.
easing - caul., cimic., vib.
escape, tries to - ***bell.***
evening agg. - ***puls.***
worse towards - ***puls.***
everything, as if, would come out - ***sep.***
excessive - acon., ambr., arn., art-v., ***bell.,*** **CHAM.,** chlol., ***cimic., coff., coff-t.,*** con., cupr., ***nux-v.,*** puls., rhus-t., sec., **SEP.,** ust.
discharge of dark coagulated blood - ***cham.***
in rapid succession - ***acon.***
exhausting - arn., ***caul.,*** gels., puls., sep., ***stann., verat.***
extending, groin, into - cimic., thuj.
heart, to - cimic.
knees and up to sacrum - phyt.
thighs, into - ***kali-c.,*** vib.
upward - **CALC.,** gels., puls.
run upwards - ***bor.,*** **CALC., CHAM.,** gels., lyc.
fainting, causing - ***cimic.,*** ign., **NUX-V.,** ***puls.***
fainting with, or cramps - ***cimic.***
faint, tendency to - **NUX-V.**
false, labor - arn., **BELL.,** bor., **CALC., CAUL.,** ***cham., cimic., cinnb.,*** cinnam., coff., ***con.,*** **DIOS.,** ***gels., kali-c.,*** kali-p., mit., ***nux-m., nux-v., op.,*** **PULS.,** sec., sep., vib.
fourth month, in - mit.
interrupt true pains, which seem insufficient - **GELS.**
prophylactic - caul.
seventh month, in - nux-v.
spasmodic - **BELL.**
fear of death, with - ars., ***coff.***
flagging, from protracted labor - ***caul.***
foot against a support, better by placing, and pressing and relaxing alternately, so as to agitate whole body - ***lyc.***
get up, says she must and will - ***cham.***
groin, felt in - cimic.
hip, leaving the uterus, going to the - cimic.
hour-glass contraction - bell., cham., sec.
incessant - sec.
ineffectual - acon., arn., bell., **CAUL.,** ***caust.,*** cimic., cinnam., ***coff.,*** eup-pur., gels., goss., **KALI-C.,** kali-p., ***op.,*** mit., nux-v., phos., plat., **PULS.,** sec., sep., ***ust.***
in small of back - ***coff.***
violent - arn.

LABOR, pains
- **inefficient** - caul., coff., ***kali-c.***, nux-v., ***puls.***
- **insupportable** - ***coff., thuj.***
  - walking agg. - ***thuj.***
- **interrupted** - ***caul., mag-m., plat.***
  - hysterical spasms, by - ***mag-m.***
- **irregular** - aeth., arn., ***caul.***, caust., cham., cimic., cocc., ***coff.***, cupr., ***nux-m.***, nux-v., **PULS.**, ***sec.***
- **irritability,** with - ***caul.***
- **left**-sided - plat.
- **long** and painful - ***arn., sep.***
- **motion,** must keep in constant, walks the room crying - ***lyc.***
- **nausea,** during - ant-t., caul., cham., ***cocc.***, **IP.**, mag-m., ***puls.***, **SEP.**
- **noise,** agg. - cimic.
- **painful**, too - acon., ant-c., arn., ***aur.***, **BELL., CHAM.**, ***chin.***, cimic., ***cocc.***, **COFF.**, ***con.***, cupr., hyos., ***lyc.***, mag-c., nat-c., **NUX-V.**, ***phos.***, puls., sec., **SEP.**, sulph.
- **painless,** almost - goss.
- **palpitation,** cause, fainting and suffocation - ***puls.***
- **places,** felt in wrong - cham., cimic.
- **point,** reach a certain, then cease - ***plat.***
- **position,** wants to change, often - arn.
- **premature** - ***caul.***, nux-v., puls.
- **pressing** urging, as during menses - ***graph.***
- **prolonged** - ***cinnb.***, kali-c., puls., **SEC.**
  - unsuccessful, caused by a particular condition of placenta - spong.
- **pubes,** above - ***sep.***
- **rapid,** too - ***lyc.***
- **restlessness,** with - ***acon., arn., ars., camph.***, chlf., coff., ***lyc.***
  - between pains - cupr.
- **rigidity** of muscles, with (see cervix) - ***bell.***, caul., cod., ***gels.***
- **running** upward - ***bor.***, **CALC., CHAM.**, gels., lyc.
  - sluggish - ***puls.***
- **sacro**-illiac, left, articulation running into groin - ***thuj.***
- **sacrum,** in, to knees and ankles, then up to sacrum - ***phyt.***
  - slight pressure on, only periodic, - ***bell.***
  - from, into region of stomach, causing pain and vomiting - ***puls.***
- **scold,** inclined to - **CHAM.**
- **screaming,** overwhelming, with - ***acon.***
- **shooting** - ***kali-c.***
- **short** - ***caul., puls.***
- **shiver,** passing off with a, causing much distress - ***caul.***
- **slow** - arn., ***bell.***, **CAUL.**, chlf., chlol., gels., ***ign.***, mit., **NAT-M., PULS.**, ***sec., sep.***, visc.
- **sluggish** - mit., ***puls.***
  - or irregular - ***puls.***
- **soreness,** with - ***arn.***, ars., ***caust.***

LABOR, pains
- **spasmodic** - acon., ambr., arn., asaf., ***bell.***, bor., ***bov., bry.***, carb-an., calc., carb-v., **CAUL., CAUST., CHAM., CIMIC.**, ***cocc.***, coff., con., cupr., ferr., **GELS., HYOS.**, ign., ***ip.***, kali-c., lob., lyc., ***mag-p.***, mag-m., mosch., ***nux-m., nux-v., op.***, phos., plat., **PULS.**, ***sec., sep.***, stann., stram., vib., zinc.
  - causing urging to stool or to urination - ***nux-v.***
  - exhausting, out of breath - ***stann.***
  - ineffectual - ***plat., puls.***
  - stomach, felt more in, than in uterus - bor.
  - stool, causing urging to - **NUX-V.**, plat.
  - suppressed and wanting - cact., carb-v., caul., cimic., ***op., puls.***, sec.
- **spasms,** appear like tonic - ***chin-s.***
- **stand,** must, or walk about, wants back rubbed, likes to have room warm - ***nux-v.***
- **stomach,** worse in, than uterus - ***bor.***
- **stool,** causing urging to - **NUX-V.**, plat.
- **suppressed** and wanting - cact., carb-v., caul., cimic., ***op., puls.***, sec.
- **tardy** - hyper.
- **thirst,** with - ***caul.***
- **tormenting,** useless, at beginning - caul.
- **twitches,** accompanied by convulsive - ***chin-s.***
- **twitching,** with - ***chin-s.***
- **upward,** run - **CALC., CHAM.**, ***lyc.***
  - dart, head of child goes back - ***bor.***
- **urination,** with frequent - ***cham.***
- **vomiting,** during - ant-t., caul., cham., ***cocc.***, **IP.**, mag-m., ***puls.***, **SEP.**
- **walking,** agg. - thuj.
  - from, insupportable, must lie down - ***thuj.***
- **wandering** about - caul., cimic.
- **weak,** too - aeth., arn., bell., ***camph.***, cann-i., ***carb-s., carb-v.***, **CAUL.**, ***cimic.***, cinnam., ***gels., graph., guare., kali-c.***, kali-p., mit., ***nat-c.***, **NAT-M.**, ***nux-m.***, op., **PULS., SEC.**, ***thuj.***
  - especially after disease, or great loss of fluids - ***carb-v.***
  - or ceasing, with somnolence - ***puls.***
- **weakness,** after - aeth., **ARN.**, asaf., ***bell.***, bor., bry., calc., ***camph.***, cann-i., cann-s., carb-an., ***carb-s., carb-v.***, **CAUL.**, ***caust., cham.***, chin., **CIMIC.**, cinnam., cocc., coff., **GELS.**, ***graph.***, goss., ***hyos., ign.***, **KALI-C.**, kali-p., kreos., lyc., mag-c., mag-m., merc., mit., mosch., ***nat-c.***, **NAT-M.**, ***nux-m., nux-v.***, **OP., PHOS.**, plat., **PULS.**, rhus-t., ***ruta.***, sabad., **SEC.**, sep., sulph., sul-ac., stann., ***thuj.***, ust., zinc.
  - pain in back, with - kali-c.
  - shiver, finished with - caul.
- **wriggling** about, at seven and a half months - sec.

LAMENESS, all over - ruta.

LEGS, cramps, during - ***gels.***, ham., ***vib.***
with cold sweat - ***verat.***
cramps in calves - **SEC.**, ***sep.***
latter months - ***sep.***
drawing down thighs, third month - ***podo.***
stiffness, sensation of swelling and weakness of left - ***ham.***
tearing pains in ankles, on motion - ***lyc.***
varicose veins - acon., apis, ***arn.***, ars., ***carb-v.***, ***caust.***, **FERR.**, ***fl-ac.***, ***graph.***, ***ham.***, ***lyc.***, ***lycps.***, ***mill.***, ***nux-v.***, ***phos.***, **PULS.**, sep., sulph., ***zinc.***
cramping pains at night, preventing sleep - ***ham.***
attributable to high living - **NUX-V.**
veins, swelling of, of ankles - ***lyc.***
walk, cannot, muscles will not obey will - ***gels.***
weariness - calc-p.

LIMBS, heaviness, during - ***calc-p.***
pulling, upper, during - plb.
varicose, lower, during - acon., apis, ***arn.***, ***ars.***, **CARB-V.**, ***caust.***, ***ferr.***, **FL-AC.**, ***graph.***, ***ham.***, ***lyc.***, ***mill.***, ***nux-v.***, phos., **PULS.**, sep., ***zinc.***
weakness, during - calc-p.
lower - plb.

LIPS, blue - ***phos.***

LOCHIA, discharge
abdomen, prolonged bearing down - **SEC.**
acrid - bapt., ***carb-an.***, con., **KREOS.**, ***lil-t.***, ***merc.***, ***nit-ac.***, plat., ***pyrog.***, rhus-t., ***sep.***, ***sil.***
black and clotted - ***plat.***
blackish - **KREOS.**
bloody - acon., arn., bell., bry., calc., ***caul.***, ***cham.***, chin., chr-ac., crot-h., ***erig.***, ham., ip., kreos., nit-ac., pyrog., rhus-t., ***sec.***, sil., ***tril.***, ust.
after growing light, it again becomes bloody - ***calc.***, **ERIG.**, ***kreos.***, ***rhus-t.***, sil.
child nurses, when - ***sil.***
motion, after least - erig.
return after least motion, better by rest - ***erig.***
brown - ***carb-v.***, ***kreos.***, ***sec.***
cheese, like - bell.
clotted - ***chin.***, cimic., **KREOS.**, ***ust.***
partly - **UST.**
copious - abrot., acon., benz-ac., bry., calc., carb-an., ***cham.***, chin., ***coff.***, ***con.***, ***croc.***, erig., hep., lil-t., mill., ***nat-c.***, nat-m., oci-s., ***plat.***, puls., ***rhus-t.***, ***sec.***, senec., **SIL.**, sulph., tril., ***ust.***, xan.
dark - caul., caust., ***cham.***, ***chin.***, ***croc.***, **KREOS.**, nit-ac., ***plat.***, pyrog., **SEC.**, ust.
almost black - ust.
fever, in puerperal - ***kreos.***
stingy, and - ***croc.***
genitals, swelling, lochia worse at night - ***merc.***
green - lac-c., sec.
gushing - erig., ***plat.***
motion agg. - erig.

LOCHIA, discharge
fetid - ***bapt.***, ***bell.***, ***bry.***, **CARB-AN.**, ***carb-v.***, **CHR-AC.**, ***cinch.***, **KREOS.**, ***rhus-t.***, **SEC.**, sep., sil.
bloody, slimy - acon.
cadaverous - ***stram.***
character, suddenly changes, becomes dirty brown or chocolate colored - **SEC.**
excoriating - ***sep.***
fever, in septic - sal-ac.
vitiated - ***rhus-t.***
peritonitis, in puerperal - ***lach.***
hot - ***bell.***
ichorous - ***carb-an.***, rhus-t., ***sec.***
intermittent - ***calc.***, con., ***kreos.***, ***plat.***, pyrog., rhus-t., sulph.
limbs, numb - **CARB-AN.**
loose, as if - hedeo
lumpy - cimic., **KREOS.**
cheesy - ***cinch.***
partly fluid, partly clotted - **UST.**
milky - ***calc.***, ***puls.***, ***sep.***
miscarriage, after - ruta.
motion, agg. - erig.
night, agg. - ***merc.***
with swelling and inflammation of genitals - ***merc.***
nursing, while - **SIL.**
pure blood flows every time the baby nurses - **SIL.**
offensive, fetid - acon., ars., ***bapt.***, bell., ***bry.***, carb-ac., ***carb-an.***, ***carb-v.***, ***chin.***, **CHR-AC.**, ***crot-h.***, crot-t., ***echi.***, erig., kali-chl., **KALI-P.**, **KREOS.**, lach., nit-ac., nux-v., oci-s., ***pyrog.***, ***rhus-t.***, **SEC.**, ***sep.***, sil., stram., sulph.
fetid, cadaveric - stram.
putrid - ***ars.***, bapt., ***bell.***, carb-ac., **CARB-AN.**, echi., kali-chl., kali-p., ***kreos.***, lach., pyrog., rhus-t., ***sec.***
profuse - art-v., bry., coff., erig., ***mill.***, **SEC.**, tril., **UST.**, ***xan.***
bloody - ***cham.***
excoriating - ***lil-t.***
fever, in puerperal - ***cham.***
nursing, while - **SIL.**
womb, burning in region of - ***bry.***
protracted - bapt., bell., bell-p., ***benz-ac.***, ***calc.***, carb-ac., **CARB-AN.**, ***caul.***, ***chin.***, croc., helon., hep., **KREOS.**, lil-t., merc., mill., **NAT-M.**, ***plat.***, ***rhus-t.***, **SEC.**, **SENEC.**, sabin., **SEC.**, ***sep.***, sulph., tril., ***ust.***
limbs, numb, with - carb-an.
with pain in back and hips - ***lil-t.***
purulent - ***chin.***, ***lach.***
ichorous - ***lach.***
red - acon., bry., calc., chin., psor., ***sil.***, sulph.
returning - acon., ***calc.***, erig., helon., ***kreos.***, ***psor.***, ***puls.***, ***rhus-t.***, senec., sulph.
almost ceasing, freshening up again - **KREOS.**
motion, after least - ***erig.***
when going about after confinement - ***acon.***

LOCHIA, discharge
scanty - ***acon., bell.,*** bry., cham., coloc., dulc., guare., mill., ***nux-v., pyrog.,*** **PULS., SEC.,** stram., ***sulph.***
suppressed - ***acon.,*** alet., aral., art-v., ***bell.,*** **BRY.,** ***camph., carb-ac.,*** caul., ***cham., chin., cimic.,*** coloc., ***dulc.,*** echi., ***hep., hyos.,*** kali-c., leon., mill., mur-ac., ***nux-v.,*** op., plat., psor., **PULS., PYROG.,** ***sec.,*** sil., ***stram.,*** **SULPH., TER.,** verat., zinc.
anger, from - cham., coloc.
cancer - **SEC.**
cold, from - ***acon., bry.,*** cham., ***cimic., dulc.,*** **PYROG.,** ***sulph.***
cold or damp, by - ***dulc.***
colic, with - ***coloc.,*** nux-v.
dampness from - ***dulc.***
day, third - ***mill.***
draft, by - ***verat-v.***
emotions, by - ***cimic., ign.***
excitement, by - cimic.
fever, with - ***acon.,*** mill., sec.
fright, from - ***acon.,*** ign., op.
grief, from - ign.
head as if it would burst - **BRY.**
irritability, diarrhea, colic or toothache, causing - ***cham.***
metritis and peritonitis puerperalis, in - **TER.**
nymphomania, with - ***verat.***
puerperal mania - ***camph.***
sexual desire, with increased - ***verat.***
suddenly on fourth day, from exposure to a draft - verat-v.
suddenly, in puerperal fever - ***cimic., verat-v.***
temple, followed by boring in left, left supraorbital nerve and orbit of eye, worse talking or mental exertion - sil.
vexation, after - acon., cham., coloc.
thin - bell., **CARB-AN.,** cimic., lach., ***pyrog., rhus-t., sec., ust.***
partly clotted - **UST.**
puerperal peritonitis, in - ***lach.***
watery, with small clots - ***cimic.***
white - ***nat-m., puls., sep.,*** sulph.

MANIA - ***stram.***

MASTITIS, painful, during - ***bell., bry.***

MELANCHOLY, with occasional uterine bleedings and cramps - ***plat.***
suicidal - aur.

MENSES, during - cocc., ***croc.,*** kali-c., kreos., ***nux-m.,*** phos., plat., rhus-t., sec.
first month, flows with much pain - ***calc.***

MENTAL problems, during - ***bell.,*** chin., con., ign., lyss., nat-m., nux-m., ***puls., sep.***

MISCARRIAGE, spontaneous, abortion - abrot., absin., acon., ***alet.,*** aloe, ambr., ant-c., **APIS,** arg-n., arist-cl., ***arn.,*** ars., art-v., asaf., ***asar.,*** asc-c., aur-m., **BELL.,** bor., ***bry., calc.,*** calc-f., calc-s., camph., cann-s., ***canth.,*** caps., carb-an., carb-s., carb-v., **CAUL.,** caust., cedr., **CHAM.,** ***chin.,*** chin-s., ***cimic.,*** cina, cinnam., ***cocc.,*** coff., coloc., con., **CROC.,** crot-h., cupr., cycl., dig., dulc., **ERIG.,** ***eup-per., eup-pur., ferr., ferr-i.,*** ferr-p., fil., **GELS., GOSS.,** ham., ***helon., hep.,*** hippoz., ***hyos., ign.,*** iod., **IP.,** ***iris, kali-c.,*** kali-m., kali-p., kali-s., kou., kreos., lach., lip., ***lyc., merc., mill.,*** morph., murx., nat-c., nit-ac., **NUX-M.,** ***nux-v., op.,*** parth., ***phos., pin-l., plat., plb.,*** podo., **PULS.,** pyrog., ***rat., rhus-t.,*** rosm., ***ruta,*** **SABIN., SEC., SEP.,** ***sil., stram.,*** sul-ac., ***sulph., syph.,*** tanac., tarent., ***ter.,*** thlaspi, thuj., ***tril., ust.,*** verat., **VIB.,** wies., zinc.
agg. - helon., kali-c., ***lil-t.,*** murx., pyrog., rheum, ruta, sabin., sec., sep.
ailments, from miscarriage or abortion - aur., calen., ***caul.,*** chin., **CIMIC.,** ***helon.,*** **IGN.,** ***kali-c., kali-s., lac-c., merc., nat-m., plat., podo.,*** rheum, ***sabin.,*** sec., **SEP., STAPH.,** stram., ***sulph., thlaspi.***
back, weakness of - ***kali-c.***
breasts, knots and cakes in - lac-c.
chilliness, resembling ague - ***kali-c.***
cough, dry - ***kali-c.***
exhausted, system - ***merc.***
eyes weak - **KALI-C.**
bleeding, much, stool only after an injection - plat.
legs, weakness of - ***kali-c.***
kidneys secrete less urine - ***stram.***
metrorrhagia - **ERIG.,** ***plat., thlaspi.***
paralysis, partial of right leg - lac-c.
spasms with full consciousness, followed by exhaustion - sec.
stool, involuntary, with retention of urine and partial paraplegia - sulph.
stool, muco-gelatinous, preceded by undefined pain all over abdomen, worse after stool - podo.
sweats - ***kali-c.***
tongue red and pointed - podo.
urinary complaints - rheum
weak, debilitated constitutions, especially in - ***kali-c.***
anemia, with - alet., carb-v., chin., ***ferr.,*** ferr-ac., kali-c., kali-n., kali-per., sec., ***sep.,*** sulph.
anger, from - cham.
bleeding, uterine, threatening miscarriage (see Bleeding, pregnancy) - anac., apis, ***bell., calc., chin.,*** cimic., ***croc.,*** erig., goss., ***ham.,*** **IP., KREOS.,** ***lyc., nit-ac., phos., puls.,*** ruta, ***sabin., thlaspi, tril., ust.***
bright red, flowing steadily - ***hyos.***
coagula - **KALI-C.**
long continued - ***lyc.***
mental or sexual excitement agg. - ***sil.***
motion, worse from slightest - **CROC.**
passive - caul.
in lumps for days and weeks - ***ust.***

MISCARRIAGE, general

bleeding, profuse - erig.

after or when threatening, painless draining from uterus, nose or lungs, bright red, no pains in joints - ***mill.***

exhausting, black, clotted - ***plat.***

flow worse at three a.m. - ***nux-v.***

for four months after, when an alarming bleeding took place - ***ip.***

cold, from - acon.

exposure to cold damp weather and places - ***dulc.***

constitution, in flabby persons - ***ust.***

cough, by - ip., ***kali-br., rumx.***

dry shaking, spasmodic cough, in paroxysms, helps to produce - rumx.

death, querulous, fear of - ars., coff.

emotions, from - bapt., cham., **GELS.,** ***helon., op.***

excitement - **GELS.,** helon.

exertion, from - ***arn.,*** bry., **ERIG.,** helon., mill., nit-ac., ***rhus-t.***

false, labor, from - arn., **BELL.,** bor., **CALC., CAUL.,** ***cham., cimic., cinnb.,*** coff., ***con., dios., gels., kali-c.,*** kali-p., ***nux-m., nux-v., op.,*** **PULS.,** sec., sep., vib.

fear, from - acon.

fear of death, with - ars., coff.

fever, from low - bapt.

fright, from - **ACON.,** cham., cimic., ***gels., ign., op.***

last months, in - op.

grief, from - ign.

suppressed, from - ign., nat-m.

hemorrhoids, painful, not bleeding - ***ham.***

influenza, during - camph., ***gels.***

epidemic, during - camph.

injuries, after - ***arn.,*** bell-p., cinnam., ham., puls., ***rhus-t.,*** ruta.

iron, poisoning, from - ferr.

labor pains, from false - ***caul.,*** nux-m.

lead, poisoning, from - plb.

if born the child lives but a year or two - plb.

menorrhagia, characterized by abundant - plb.

mental shock, depression and low fever, from - bapt.

news, bad - ***bapt., gels.***

from sudden bad - ***gels.***

night-watching, from - bapt.

ovarian disease, from - apis.

ovaries, inflammation supervening - ***coloc.,*** **SABIN.**

overheated, from becoming - bry.

pains, with, flying across abdomen, doubling her up, chills, pricking in breasts, pains in loins - cimic.

frequent, labor-like, no discharge - sec.

irregular, feeble, tormenting, scanty flow, or long continued, passive oozing, backache, weakness, internal trembling - caul.

MISCARRIAGE, general

pains, with, small of back, from, extending, abdomen, around to, ending in crampy, squeezing, bearing down, tearing down thighs - vib.

extending, pubes, to, agg. from motion, blood partly clotted - sabin.

extending, thighs, to, weak back, agg. from motion, subsequent debility and sweat - kali-c.

placenta, fatty degeneration of, from - phos.

placenta praevia, from (see Placenta) - ***nux-v., sabin., sep., verat-v.***

placenta retained - sabin., sep., verat-v.

with constant feeling in rectum as if bowels ought to be moved - ***nux-v.***

reaching up, from - aur.

septicemia, with - pyrog.

sexual frequency - cann-i., cann-s.

shock, from - bapt.

sixth, week - ***ip., spong.***

syphilis, from - ***aur.,*** kali-i., ***merc., merc-c., nit-ac.,*** phyt., staph., syph., thuj.

tendency, to - ***alet.,*** aloe, ***apis,*** arg-n., asar., aur., ***aur-m.,*** bac., ***bapt.,*** bufo, ***calc.,*** cann-s., carb-v., ***caul., cimic.,*** cocc., erig., ***eup-pur.,*** ferr., ferr-ac., ferr-m., ***helon.,*** hyos., ign., **KALI-C.,** kali-chl., kali-i., kali-n., kali-per., kreos., ***lyc.,*** merc., merc-c., ***mill.,*** nux-m., nux-v., phyt., **PLB.,** puls., rhus-t., ruta, ***sabin., sars., sec.,*** **SEP.,** sil., sul-i., ***sulph.,*** syph., thuj., **VIB.,** ***vib-p., zinc.,*** zinc-m.

atonic condition, from - caul., ***helon.***

back and loins painful - caul.

back into buttocks and thighs, with pains from - **KALI-C.**

backache, severe - ***kali-c.,*** vib.

bearing-down pains, spasmodic - caul.

bleeding - ***cinnam.***

continues after pains have stopped - ***ham.***

dark, now fluid, now coagulated - puls.

of dark stringy blood - ***croc.***

with uterine - ip., phos., sulph.

blood, alternately bright thin, and dark, or in clots on motion - sabin.

copious, flow of thin black - ***sec.***

dark - ***cham.***

from vagina, in eighth month - ***cann-i.***

cervical os considerably dilated - puls.

children, especially in women who have had - ***plat.***

convulsions, with - ***ip.***

convulsive movements - ***sec.***

cough, by - rumx.

cough, by nervous - ***kali-br.***

debility, from uterine - ***caul.***

depressing emotions, sudden - **GELS.**

emotion, slightest overexertion or irritating - ***helon.***

epoch, repeating at same - cedr.

exposure in a damp cold place - ***dulc.***

falls, shocks, etc., from - **ARN.**

MISCARRIAGE, general
tendency, to
feeble, cachectic women, having a wan, anxious countenance - ***sec.***
venous women, in - asaf., sep.
flabby women, in - asaf., calc., ***caul., sec., ust.***
flow ceases and returns with double force - **PULS.**
flow slight - caul.
fourth month - caul.
frequent and early, ovum expelled at every menstrual period causing infertility - ***vib.***
fright, from - ***acon., gels., op.***
especially in latter part of pregnancy - ***op.***
gonorrhea patients, in - ***cann-s.***
hysterical women, disposed to faint, feel chilly and catch cold easily - **NUX-M.**
labor pains, during, had to hold on to objects - ***caul.***
false labor pains, with bloody discharge - ***sec.***
menorrhagia, with - sulph.
month, at third or fourth - eup-pur.
mercury, after abuse of - ***hep.***
month, fifth to seventh - ***sep.***
second - apis, ***kali-c.***
third - ***cimic.,*** croc., ***sabin., sec.,*** thuj., ust.
nausea and vomiting - ***verat.***
pains in loins extending through epigastrium and iliac region down thighs - sang.
navel to uterus, sharp pain around - ***ip.***
nerves, from sensibility of - ***asar.,*** ferr.
neuralgia, with - ***sulph.***
ovarian irritation and inflammation, after a fall - ham.
pains, excessively severe - ***coff.***
excited by walking - ***helon.***
with cold sweat - ***verat.***
prevented, if given before membranes are injured and when the pains are spasmodic and threatening - ***vib.***
rectum as though bowels ought to be moved, constant uneasiness in - ***nux-v.***
straining or overexerting, from - ***rhus-t.***
tired and nervous women, in - kali-p.
typhus, in - ***bapt.***
uterine debility, from - ***caul.,*** sep.
vagina discharge, with - ***plb.***
dry and constricted - puls.
varicosed condition of uterus from frequently recurring congestion - ***nux-v.***
vascular excitement - caul.
vexation, from - ***acon.***
weakness, tremulous - caul.
women who have had children, in - ***plat.***
tenesmus, rectal agg. - bell., calc., cocc., con., ip., lyc., merc., nux-v., rhus-t., sep., sulph.
thunderstorm, from - cinnam., nat-c., rhod.

MISCARRIAGE, general
threatened - ambr., ***apis, arn., bell., bry., calc.,*** **CAUL.,** caust., ***cham., cimic., chin., cinnam., eup-pur., ferr., helon., ip., kali-c.,*** kali-m., ***merc., nux-m.,*** nux-v., ***op., plb.,*** **PULS.,** rat., ***rhus-t., sabin., sec.,*** **SEP.,** ***sil., stram., tril., vib.***
time, month, or week
early months - alco., **APIS,** ***caul., sep., vib.***
eighth month - cann-i., ***puls.***
week - ***spong.***
fifth month - plb.
to seventh - kali-c., plb., ***sep.***
to sixth month - ars.
first month - alco., **APIS,** vib.
fourth month - **APIS,** ***eup-pur.,*** sep.
last months - op.
repeating same time as before - cedr.
second month - agar-se., apis, ***cimic.,*** **KALI-C.,** kali-n., plb., sep., vib.
second or third month - apis, ***cimic.,*** **KALI-C.,** ***sabin., sec.,*** sep., thuj., tril., vib.
seventh month - ***ruta,*** sep.
(expulses dead fetus) - ***ruta.***
six or eight weeks, at, flowing like menses - spong.
sixth month - lac-c., ***ruta,*** sep.
week - ***ip., ang.,*** spong.
sixth week of pregnancy, with acute pains - ***ip.***
seventh month, dead foetus - ***ruta.***
third - apis, bell., cimic., ***croc., eup-per., eup-pur.,*** **KALI-C.,** ***kreos., merc., nux-v.,*** plb., ***sabin., sec., sep.,*** thuj., tril., ***ust.***
at end of - ***merc.***
bleeding, with - tril.
bleeding, worse at three a.m. - ***nux-v.***
discharge of bright red partly clotted blood, from motion - sabin.
end of, on the - merc.
trauma, from - ***arn.,*** cinnam.
unconsciousness, with - sec.
urination, with constant desire for - canth.
uterus, atony, from - ***cimic., alet.,*** **CAUL.,** cinch., ferr., **HELON.,** ***puls.,*** sabin., sec., ***sep., ust.***
bearing-down pains as if everything would come from her - sep., ***ust.***
chronic inflammatory condition, with nausea and vomiting - ***kali-c.***
difficult contraction, after - ***sec.***
discharge, thin, black, foul-smelling - ***sec.***
indurations, causes - aur-m-n.
metritis - **SABIN.,** verat.
prolapsus after - **NUX-V.,** sep.
vagina discharge, with - ***acon.***
vexation, from - ***acon.,*** cham.
vomiting, from - ***ip.***
vulva, itching causes - ***sep.***

MISCARRIAGE, general
weakness, of uterus, from - alet., ***carb-v.,*** **CAUL.,** chin., chin-s., cimic., ferr., ***helon.,*** merc., puls., sabin., ***sec.,*** senec., **SEP.,** sil., ***ust.***

MOLES, hydatids, to promote expulsion - ***ars., bell.,*** cinch., ***ferr., lyc.,*** merc., ***nat-c., puls., sabin.,*** sec., ***sil.,*** sulph.
darting, shooting pain - ***calc.***
to remove disposition - ***calc., sil.***

MORNING sickness, (see Nausea, Vomiting) - acon., alet., anac., ars., bar-c., carb-ac., cast., ***con.,*** ferr., ***goss., graph., ign., ip., iris, jatr., kali-br., kreos.,*** lac-c., ***lac-d.,*** lach., **LAC-AC.,** ***lil-t., lob.,*** mag-m., **MERC.,** ***merc-i-f., nat-m., nux-m.,*** **NUX-V.,** petr., phos., plat., plb., ***podo.,*** psor., ***puls.,*** sabin., senec., **SEP.,** sil., tarent., verat.
appetite, with loss of, and diarrhea - ***sabin.***
faintness, could not rise from bed - ***goss.***
months, during early - ***goss.***
during first - asar.
vomiting watery fluid - bov.
frothy watery mucus - ***nat-m.***
white mucus - ***kali-m.***
sour masses or fluids - nat-p.
not amounting to, with faint, sickish spells during forenoon - ***sulph.***
protracted - ***iris.***
walk, sick during a, feels as if she must lie down and die - ***kali-c.***

MUSCLES, myalgic pains, like false pains - ***alet.***

NAUSEA, during - acet-ac., acon., ail., alet., ***amyg.,*** anac., ***ant-c., ant-t., apom.,*** arg-n., ***ars.,*** **ASAR.,** ***bry.,*** cadm-s., carb-ac., ***carb-an.,*** cast., ***cer-ox.,*** **CIMIC.,** ***cocc.,*** cod., ***colch., con., cuc-p.,*** cupr-ac., ***cupr-ar.,*** cycl., ferr., ferr-ar., ferr-p., gnaph., ***goss., hell.,*** ingluv., **IP.,** ***iris, jatr.,*** kali-ar., kali-br., ***kali-c.,*** kali-m., kali-p., **KREOS., LAC-AC.,** ***lac-c., lac-d.,*** lac-v-c., ***lach.,*** laur., ***lil-t., lob., lyc., mag-c., mag-m.,*** med., merc., ***merc-i-f., nat-m.,*** nat-p., ***nux-m.,*** **NUX-V.,** ***ox-ac., petr.,*** ph-ac., ***phos.,*** piloc., plat., plb., ***podo., psor., puls.,*** **SEP.,** ***sil.,*** staph., stry., sulph., ***sul-ac., sym-r.,*** **TAB.,** tarent., ther., ***thyr.,*** verat.
constant - ip., ***mag-c.***
eating, worse before and after, better while eating - ***anac.***
frequent, with vomiting after eating - ***op.***
night, after, watching and mental disturbance, after eating - puls.
women, in, suffering from scirrhosities - con.

NECK, pulsating carotids - ***gels.***
undulation of jugular veins - ***phos.***

NERVOUSNESS - ***acon.,*** ambr., ***gels.,*** nux-m.

NEURALGIA - ter.

NOSE, bleeding - ***sep.***

NOTIONS, strange - ***lyss.***

OVARIES, pain, during - kali-p., podo., ***xan.***
numb aching, in left, third month - ***podo.***

PALPITATION - ***arg-m., lil-t., nat-m., sep.***
violent, with morning sickness - ***con.***

PELVIS, bones, as if, were getting loose - ***murx.***
feeling of lameness - **CALC.**
pain between crest of right ilium and sacrum - ***arn.***
sacro-illiac symphysis gives out walking, must sit down, feels best lying - ***aesc.***
stiff, articulations, when beginning to move - ***rhus-t.***

PERIODICITY, all symptoms worse every third day - ***mag-c.***

PLACENTA, (see Childbirth)
bleeding, arterial, from partial separation - ***ip.***
labor pains, during - ***ip.***
removal, after - ***ip.***
pains, as from an ulcer over seat of, when lying on right side and on pressure - puls.
placenta praevia - ***erig., ip., nux-v., sabin., sep., verat.***
bleeding, from - ip., nux-v., sabin., sep., verat-v.
retained - ***agn.,*** all-s., ***arn., ars.,*** art-v., ***bell.,*** **CANTH.,** carb-v., ***caul.,*** chin., cimic., croc., ergot., gels., ***goss., hydr., ign., ip., kali-c., nux-v.,*** phos., plat., ***puls., sabin., sec.,*** **SEP.,** visc.
action, want of, or spasmodic contraction - ***puls.***
atony, from - ***sabin.***
bearing down, with constant strong - ***sec.,*** sep.
bleeding from - **BELL.,** ***canth., carb-v.,*** caul., ***ip.,*** mit., phos., ***puls.,*** **SABIN.,** sec., sep., stram.
bleeding, postpartum - ***croc.***
blood, with profuse flow of hot, speedily coagulates - ***bell.***
especially during early months of pregnancy - sec.
high up in fundus, could not be removed by gentle traction - puls.
miscarriage, after - ***sabin.,*** sec., ***sep., verat-v.***
miscarriage, after - sabin., sep., verat-v.
rectum, with constant feeling in, as though bowels ought to be moved - ***nux-v.***
relaxed feeling, with, of parts - ***sec.***
removed eighteen hours after delivery - ***kali-c.***
secondary - ***puls.***
spasmodically - ***bell.***
urination, with painful - **CANTH.**

POSTPARTUM, general
abdomen, contracted into little knots or bunches about size of walnut - ***cham.***
pain, in a primipara - nux-v.
pressing pain in left lower, towards back, worse from motion - ***agar.***
sensitiveness - ***bell.***

POSTPARTUM, general

after pains - ***acon.***, ***cimic.***, **ARN.**, **BELL.**, ***bry.***, caul., **CHAM.**, cinnam., cycl., **DIOS.**, ferr., ***gels.***, hyos., hyper., ***ign.***, kali-c., lac-c., lil-t., mill., nux-v., par., podo., puls., rhus-t., sep., ust., vib., ***xan.***

abdomen, with sensitiveness of - ***sabin.***

bearing down, strong - ***podo.***

blood, discharge of fluid, and clots in equal proportions with every pain - ***sabin.***

cramps in limbs - ***cupr-m.***

day, on second, after delivery of fourth child, unbearable when child nurses - cham.

distant, in parts, from pelvis - carb-v.

distressing, particularly in women who have borne many children - **CUPR-M.**

exhausting, after, lengthy labor - ***caul.***

fear, with, of death - **COFF.**

groins, into - ***caul.***

groins, worse in - ***cimic.***

bleeding, with, from irregular contractions - sec.

heat, with, and flatulency - ***podo.***

intense, but very imperfect contractions - **PAR.**

instrumental, after, delivery - ***arn.***, ***hyper.***, ***rhus-t.***

insupportably intense - ***coff.***

irritable, in, women - ***nux-v.***

long, last too - ***acon.***, ***cham.***, ***coff.***, ***gels.***, **SEC.**

long, too, and too violent, worse towards evening - ***puls.***

long, too, after severe labor with much and excessive straining - ***rhus-t.***

menses, with offensive - ***crot-h.***

motion, worse from least, or deep inspiration - ***bry.***

nausea, with, and vomiting - ***cimic.***

nursing, excited by, pains left to right - con.

nursing, return while - ***arn.***

nursing, worse when - **SEC.**

oversensitiveness - ***cimic.***

primipara, in a - ***atro.***

sacrum, in - ***phos.***

sacrum, in and hips, violent, with headache, after instrumental delivery - hyper.

sensitive, in, women - ***op.***

sensitive, in, women who cannot compose themselves to sleep - ***gels.***

spasmodic - ***caul.***

shoot into thighs - lac-c.

anus, prolapsus - ***podo.***

atony of bladder - **ARS.**

back, aching - ***hyper.***

nettle-like pains over back where it touched bed, sixty hours after labor - ***kali-c.***

pain in sacral region - ***phos.***

bleeding - acet-ac., alet., ***alum.***, ***arn.***, **BELL.**, bry., ***cann-i.***, ***cann-s.***, caul., **CHAM.**, ***cinch.***, cinnam., cocc., ***croc.***, erig., **FERR.**, ***ham.***, ***hydr.***, ***hyos.***, **IP.**, kalm., lyc., merc., **NIT-AC.**, nux-m., nux-v., op., ph-ac., **PLAT.**, plb., puls., rhus-t., **SABIN.**, sec., sep., ***thlaspi***, tril., ***ust.***

POSTPARTUM, general

bleeding,

atony, from, of blood vessels - ***kali-c.***

one week after labor - ***kali-c.***

bright red, more blood comes with every start - ***hyos.***

flowing steadily - ***hyos.***

clots, in large - ***croc.***

coffee-ground, offensive discharge - ***nit-ac.***

constant, every few minutes, a large clot of bright red blood, with bearing-down pains - ***ust.***

continued and obstinate - **NUX-M.**

contractions, from irregular, with violent after-pains - sec.

days, some, after delivery - **CINNAM.**

eighth, day, reappearance of blood - sabin.

fluid and gushing, severe, - ***ip.***

hard delivery, following a - ***mill.***

hasty labor, after - caul.

malaise - ***mez.***

motion, worse from slightest - **CROC.**

painless, dark red - ***sabin.***

passive - caul., ***gels.***

or lumpy for days and weeks, after miscarriage - ***ust.***

placenta adhering - ***ip.***, ***kali-c.***

prevents - **ARN.**

primipara, in a, after first few pains, when the os has dilated about an inch - cinnam.

profuse - **APIS,** ***plat.***

containing large number of clots, worse on rising, causing loss of consciousness - sabin.

puerperal peritonitis, with, constant, putrid - ***ust.***

relaxation of uterus temporarily better by compression - sec.

repeated, small - **CINNAM.**

septicaemia, in - sal-ac.

secondary, from retained placenta in coagula - ***puls.***

steady flow, bright red - ***ip.***

tampon, relieved by a, constant, but when removed bleeding returned, occasional labor-like pains, cause some strings and shreds to pass - sabin.

uterus, flabby from, atonic condition of - ***ust.***

week, one, after confinement, with adherent placenta - ***kali-c.***

two, after labor, large bright red clots, no pain - ust.

breasts, left inflamed and hard, with fever and prostration - ***crot-h.***

stitching in a hard lump which formed in lower outer part of breast - ***crot-h.***

bruised, parts feel - **ARN.**

chill, chilliness - ***mez.***

followed by heat intermingled with chilliness, particularly when turning in bed - puls.

within sixty hours - ***kali-c.***

POSTPARTUM, general
cough, as if something would be torn out of chest - rhus-t.
diarrhea, stools offensive - sulph.
dysentery, with faintness after effort at stool - aloe
epilepsy, brought on by a fall immediately before delivery - rhus-t.
face, pale - ***mez.,*** sec.
yellow spots - ***crot-h.***
flatulence, with labor-like pains - ***nux-m.***
hands, fingers spasmodically flexed - rhod.
hemorrhoids - phys., ***ham., ign., kali-c., lil-t.,*** **NUX-V.,** ***podo.,*** puls., sep., ***sulph.***
hiccough, for fourteen days constant, preventing eating, drinking and sleeping, in primipara - nux-v.
hips, coxalgia - hyper.
coxarthrocace - ***calc.***
legs, pain in right, with numbness from hips to feet - rhus-t.
paralysis, with atrophy - plb.
paralysis - PHOS., RHUS-T.
membranes, retained - ***canth.,*** caul.
paralysis, of right side, apparent total abolition of functions of voluntary motion and special sensation - rhus-t.
paraplegia - caul.
perineum, ruptured - ***arn.,*** **CALEN.**
phlegmasia alba dolens - acon., apis, arn., ars., ***bell., bry., calc., cham., ham., kali-c., led.,*** lyc., nux-v., ***puls.,*** sep., ***stram.,*** sulph.
after forceps delivery, swelling of whole lower limb, painful, worse in thigh - ***all-c.***
left leg - crot-h.
typhoid symptoms, with - **RHUS-T.**
pulse, small - lyc.
and rapid - ***crot-h.***
recovery, slow - ***graph.***
rectum, during stool, painful, burning, passing over into a kind of sore - ***mez.***
protrusion - ***ruta.***
soreness - ARN.
sweat, debilitating, retarding convalescence - ***samb.***
excessive - ***cham.***
tongue, trembling - ***crot-h.***
unconsciousness - ***chin-s.***
urine, constant dribbling - ***arn.***
retention - **ARS.,** ***op.,*** puls.
kidneys secrete less or none at all - ***stram.***
no will to urinate - **HYOS.**
uterus, anteversion - ***nux-m.***
burning, alternates with pain in limbs - rhod.
dilated - ***croc.***
metritis - ***nux-v., sabin.***
metritis, threatened, in consequence of catching cold - puls.
metritis with typhoid symptoms - **RHUS-T.**
prolapsus - ***podo., rhus-t.***

POSTPARTUM, general
relaxed, difficult contraction, after miscarriage - ***sec.***
relaxed, with bleeding - sec.
rupture of cervix - ***calen.***
soft, bleeding - ***croc.***
uncontracted - ***nux-m.***
vaginal discharge - sars.
lesions, with septic fever - calen., sul-ac.
lesions - ***calen.***
vulva, sensitive, cannot bear touch of napkin - ***plat.***

PUERPERAL, general
abdomen, colic - ***nux-m.***
flatulency - ***lyc.,*** **NAT-S.**
pendulous - bell., ***calc.,*** croc., podo., sec., **SEP.**
puffed, causing anxiety - ***ambr.***
rhagades on surface - hep., sep., sil., sulph.
constipation - ***ambr., ant-c.,*** **PLAT.**
four weeks after - ***lil-t.***
six weeks after, hydrogenoid constitution - ***nat-s.***
convulsions - acon., cimic., ***ant-c.,*** ant-t., apis, ***arg-n.,*** arn., ars., art-v., ***atro.,*** **BELL.,** benz-ac., canth., carb-v., caul., caust., cham., chin-s., chlol., chlf., **CIC.,** cinnam., ***cocc., coff.,*** crot-h., ***cupr-m., gels., glon., hell., hydr-ac.,*** **HYOS.,** ***ign.,*** **KALI-BR.,** ***kali-c.,*** kali-p., ***lach.,*** laur., mag-p., ***merc-c.,*** mill., mosch., nat-m., nux-m., nux-v., ***oena., op., phos.,*** ph-ac., ***plat.,*** puls., sec., stram., ***verat., verat-v.,*** zinc.
albuminuria, with - ***atro., gels.***
torpidity, coma, blue, bloated face, septic or zymotic influence, or in hemorrhagic or broken-down constitutions - crot-h.
alternate convulsive action and opisthotonos - ***plat.***
anger, after - **CHAM.**
apoplectic form - ***gels.***
begin when labor ceases - ***sec.***
blood-letting, after - verat-v.
bright object, from presence of - ***canth.***
brilliant object, renewed by sight of some, or contact - ***stram.***
cerebral congestion, hot, dry skin, thirst, restlessness, fear of death - ***acon.***
caused by sudden - verat-v.
violent, with - **BELL.,** ***verat.***
conscious during paroxysm - ***cocc.***
consciousness, loss of - ***stram.***
and drowsiness, mouth open - ***op.***
continue after birth of foetus - ***ant-t.***
convulsive motion of limbs, third day - ***mill.***
drinking, from, water - ***canth.***
epileptic, after fright - ***art-v.***
head attacked after - ***atro.***
epileptiform - stram.
in a primipara, seventh month - ***cedr.***
eruption, if an, especially a chronic one, has recently disappeared - zinc.
escape, attempts to - ***stram.***

PUERPERAL, general

convulsions,

excited whenever she attempted to drink water, or if she hears it poured from one vessel to another - ***lyss.***
eyes immovable, open - ***cocc.***
face, after delivery convulsions with red - ***glon.***
fear, with great - ***stram.***
frequent, paroxysms more and more, and last longer - ***cocc.***
fright, from - art-v.
frightened appearance before and during - ***stram.***
grin, sardonic - ***stram.***
groaning, commence and end with, and stretching of limbs - ***ign.***
head, particularly where there is convulsive motion of, from behind forward - ***nux-m.***
hysterical, especially in, women who easily faint and suffer from languor in back and knees, drowsy before and after spasms - ***nux-m.***
immediately after delivery - ***aml-n.***
knew every one but her child, during intervals - ***gels.***
labor protracted - ***gels.***
larynx, touch of, reproduces spasms - ***canth.***
lassitude, after, dull feeling in forehead and vertex, fullness in region of medulla - ***gels.***
latter stage, during, of pregnancy - ***apis***
laughter - ***stram.***
limbs, violent movements of - caust.
minutes, last four or five, during intervals turns restlessly in bed - ***glon.***
mouth, with frothing at, followed by variable spasms during eighth month - sec.
muscles, action of, of face, eyes, etc. - ***chin-s.***
rigid, and distorted features - ***op.***
nervous excitement, from - ***cimic.***
opisthotonos, with - ***sec.***
os uteri rigid - ***gels.***
pain, worse at every - sec.
phosphorus, after, apparently indicated, had failed, symptoms felt mostly during rest, worse after dinner and towards evening - zinc.
position, brought on by changing - ***cocc.***
screams - caust.
sensibility, loss of - ***stram.***
shoots passing through whole body - ***laur.***
sigh, passing off with a, after several minutes - ***cocc.***
singing - ***stram.***
sleep, during - ***cocc.***
sound, from, or sight of water - ***canth.***
speech, loss of, or stammering - ***stram.***
suppuration suspected - bufo
sweat, with copious - ***stram.***
teeth, gnashing of - caust.
terror, spells cause - ***cocc.***
thirteen, times in twenty-four hours, senseless to sopor - ***plat.***
threatened - ***gels.***

PUERPERAL, general

convulsions,

uremia, from, or reflex irritation - ***chlf.***
visions, frightful - ***stram.***
vomiting, with - ***cupr-m.***
water, from sight of - ***canth.***

diarrhea - ***coll., hyos., rheum, stram.***

edema- am-m., apis.

eruption, vesicles, of, as large as peas on neck, shoulders, chest and abdomen, down as far as navel, after fourteen days - ***merc.***

rash - ***bry.***, cham., ***ip.***
red, seventh day - ***calc.***
third day, with convulsions - ***cupr-m.***
violent headache after - ***hyper.***

eyes, iritis from loss of blood - ***cinch.***
sensitive to light, six weeks after, hydrogenoid constitutions - ***nat-s.***
sudden blindness - aur-m.

fever, during - cimic., ***acon.***, apis, ***arn.***, **ARS.**, ***bapt.***, **BELL.**, **BRY.**, ***calc., canth., carb-ac.***, cham., cocc., coff., ***colch.***, coloc., ***hyos., kali-c.***, kreos., ***lach., mur-ac.***, nux-v., op., plat., ***puls., rhus-t., sec.***, sulph., ter., verat., **VERAT-V.**, zinc.
abdomen distended - **BRY.**
abdomen, stitches in - **BRY.**
albuminuria, torpidity, coma, blue, bloated face, septic or zymotic influence, or in hemorrhagic or broken-down constitutions - crot-h.
breasts, distended - **BRY.**
sore - ***cham.***
cerebral congestion - ***verat-v.***
day, fourth, severe chill, followed by fever - ***phyt.***
delirium - ***verat-v.***
emotion, particularly after violent, or suppression of milk - ***bell.***
excitement - ***cham.***
fetid discharge - ***op.***
fright, especially when caused by - ***op.***
high, fever - ***verat-v.***
indignation, brought on by, or grief because of unkind treatment - ***coloc.***
inhalations, deep, painful - **BRY.**
intermittent, on fifth day, - ***lach.***
lie, cannot, on either side - **BRY.**
lochia, sudden suppression of - ***verat-v.***
malignant - ail.
milk, absence of - ***cham.***
sudden cessation of - ***verat-v.***
notions, with absurd, or mania - kali-p.
ovaritis, with - crot-h.
overexcitement of senses - ***op.***
pain, excessive - ***verat-v.***
peritonitis - ***bell., bry., kali-c.***, spig.
ascites, with - ***ars.***
at onset, heat seems to issue from body of patient - bell.
constant flooding, secretion putrid, with - ***ust.***

PUERPERAL, general
fever, during
pulse bounding hard - ***verat-v.***
quick - ***verat-v.***
weak - ***verat-v.***
putridity, with - ***kreos.***
pyaemia - ***arn.***
restlessness, with great - ***cham., verat-v.***
septicemia, ovaritis - crot-h.
signs of dissolution of blood - **ARS., LACH.**
skin cold and clammy - ***verat-v.***
stage, first - ***kali-m.***
second - kali-p.
tenesmus, with - ***verat-v.***
thirst, with, for large quantities of water - **BRY.**
tympanitis, with - ***verat-v.***
typhoid symptoms - ***bapt.***
vagina moist - ***kreos.***
weeks, after six, followed by vulvitis with herpes, vesicles size of lentils, filled with purulent matter, hydrogenoid constitution - ***nat-s.***
hair, losing - ***nat-m., sep.***
mania - **CIMIC.,** ***aur., bell., camph.,*** chlol., ***cupr-ac., hyos., kali-br.,*** kali-c., ***stram., sulph., verat.***
bed, when in, in dark room, delusion that there is another baby in bed which requires attention, also that she had a third leg which would not remain quiet - petr.
head feels strange, tries to injure herself - ***cimic.***
impudent, behavior - ***verat.***
melancholia - ***anac.***
timid - stram.
nymphomania - ***cinch., kali-br., verat., zinc.***
spasms, with, during seventh month - phos.
voluptuous tingling from genitals into abdomen - ***plat.***
ovaries, painful - **LACH.**
stool, nervous, cannot attempt in presence of nurse - ***ambr.***
urine, bloody - **BUFO.**

PULSATION, externally, body, during - ***kali-c.***

PULSE, small, after night watching and mental disturbance - puls.
small, slow - ***gels.***

RECTUM, burning pain, during - ***caps.***
sharp pain, during - ***kali-c.***

RECTUM, pressing stitching proctalgia - ***kali-c.***
inactive - ***verat.***

RESTLESSNESS, during - acon., ambr., nux-m., verat.
in last months - ***colch.***

SACRUM, pains, in - led., ***sars., xan.***
indescribable, like a gnawing stiffness in sacrum and hip bone, down over whole thigh, worse standing, in last months - ***led.***

SACRUM, pains
radiating until fingers, hands, feet and toes are involved and cramped from darting, drawing pains, with anxiety, palpitation and faintness - ***sars.***
severe, in sacral region before and during stool - ***sars.***
writhing in sacral region - ***sars.***

SALIVATION, during, ptyalism - acet-ac., ant-t., ***coff., helon., iris,*** jab., kali-bi., ***kali-i.,*** **KREOS.,** ***lac-ac., merc., nat-m.,*** puls., sin-n., sulph., ***sul-ac.***
salty, viscid - ***kali-i.***

SEPSIS puerperalis - ***arn.,*** ars., echi., lach., lyc., ***op.,*** phos., ***puls., pyrog.,*** **RHUS-T.,** ***sec.,*** **SULPH.**
suppressed lochia, from - lyc., sulph.

SEXUALITY, desire, increased, during - bell., lach., merc., plat., puls., stram., verat.
nymphomania, during - zinc.

SKIN, coldness, during - ***nux-m.***
discoloration, yellow, jaundice, during - aur.
dry - ***nux-m.***
itching - ***dol.***
symptoms worse - ***cham.***

SLEEP, groaning, crying out - alum.

SLEEPINESS, during - ***gels., helon., nux-m.***
drowsy, yet unable to sleep - nux-m.

SLEEPLESSNESS, insomnia - acon., ***cimic.,*** ambr., ***bell.,*** cact., cham., cinch., ***coff.,*** cypr., gels., hyos., ign., ***kali-br.,*** lyc., mag-p., mosch., nux-v., ***op.,*** puls., rhus-t., staph., stram., tarent.
from cramps in calves - calc., cham., ***cupr-ac.,*** coff., ferr., nux-v., ***verat.***

SORENESS, all over - arn., ruta

STOMACH, symptoms - cadm-s., ***sabad., tab.***
and abdominal symptoms - ***alum.***
and bilious complaints - ***nux-v.***
troubles, especially when head symptoms are prominent - ***petr.***
burning in - ars., ***dios.***
pylorus in, with vomiting - ***canth.***
burst, as if it would, with wind - **ARG-N.**
can lie comfortably only on, in early months - ***podo.***
constriction or sensation of heavy weight pressing upon, pain constant but remittent in character, worse by cough - ***con.***
cramps - ***con.***
dyspepsia, flatulent - ***nux-m.***
emptiness, sensation of - ***sep.***
fullness, sensation of, during - **NUX-M.**
full and distended, as after over eating - ant-c.
gastro-intestinal affections - ant-c.
heartburn, during - apis, ***caps.,*** con., ***merc.,*** nat-m., ox-ac., zinc.
night, at - ***merc.***
pain, during - con., dios., ip.
sweetish belchings - ***zinc.***
water, accumulation of acrid, with cramps - ***lyc.***

SWELLING, face, during - ***merc-c., phos.***

TACITURN - ***verat.***

TASTE, bloody, during - ***zinc.***
metallic, during - zinc.
sour, during - ***lac-ac., mag-c.,*** ox-ac.

THIRST, during - phos., ***verat.***

THROAT, burning, roughness, stinging, with desire to vomit - ***mag-c.***

TONGUE, tingles - alum.
white, after night watching and mental disturbance - puls.

TOES, cramps, during - ***calc.***

TOOTHACHE, during - ***acon.,*** alum., apis, ***bell.,*** bry., ***calc., cham., hyos.,*** **LYSS.,** ***mag-c., merc., nux-m.,*** nux-v., ***puls., rat.,*** rhus-t., **SEP.,** ***staph., tab.***
breath, with short - **SEP.**
ebullition, with internal, of blood from chest to head - ***lyss.***
stinging, tearing in front teeth, worse during cold, damp weather, from washing, from touch or sucking teeth, better from warmth - ***nux-m.***
tearing, during - nux-m.
terrible, during early months, must get up at night and walk - ***rat.***
worse - ***puls.***

TOXEMIA, (see Eclampsia)

UMBILICUS, aching, during - plb.

UNCONSCIOUSNESS, during - ***nux-m., nux-v., sec.***

URINATION, difficult - ***acon.,*** bell., cann-s., ***canth.,*** equis., helon., hell., ***lyc.,*** merc-c., ***nat-m., nux-v., puls.,*** ter., uva.
escape, too quick, of urine - ***sep.***
frequent desire - ***cocc.***
copious - ***lil-t.***
night, during - podo.
urging - **NUX-V.**
involuntary, during - **ARS.,** bell., canth., caust., clem., kreos., ***nat-m.,*** podo., **PULS.,** ***sep., syph.***
rise, must, between twelve and three a.m. - ***acon.***
strangury - eup-pur., ***lyc.***
urging, during - acon., ***puls.,*** sulph.
constant, and pressure, with tension in abdomen - ***puls.***

UTERUS, during
bearing, down, come out, as if everything would, during - ***kali-c.,*** sep.
burning - ***bry.***
cervical os patulous - ***sabin.***
cramping, during - ***cupr-ar.***
pain, during - bry., kali-p., lyss., plat.
from inflammation of os and cervix - lyss.
prolapsus, with much aching pain in region of left ovary, heat running down to left thigh, must lie on stomach - ***podo.***

UTERUS, during
rheumatic pains, worse evening and night, disturbing sleep - ***puls.***
soreness - ***puls.***

VAGINA, burning, during - bor.
itching, during - bor., **CALAD.**
prolapus, during - calc-ar., ***ferr.***
swelling - bor.

VAGINAL discharge - ***cocc.,*** **KREOS.,** ***murx., puls.,*** **SEP.**
bloody mucus, profuse discharge of, third month - ***cocc.***
gonorrhea, discharge like - bor.
mucous, runs down limbs - **ALUM.**
painless, from uterus - ***cocc.***
serous, from uterus - ***cocc.***

VERTIGO, during - ars., ***gels.,*** ip., **NAT-M.,** phos.

VISION, double, during - bell., cic., ***gels.***

VOMITING, during - acet-ac., acon., alet., ***amyg.,*** anac., ***ant-c.,*** ant-t., ***apis, apom., ars.,*** **ASAR.,** bism., ***bry., calc., cadm-s., canth., caps., carb-ac.,*** card-m., cast., **CHEL.,** ***cic.,*** cinnam., cocaine, cocc., cod., ***colch., con.,*** cupr-ar., ***cycl.,*** dios., ***ferr.,*** ferr-ar., ***ferr-p.,*** goss., graph., ***helon.,*** ign., ***ip., iris,*** **JATR.,** ***kali-bi., kali-br.,*** kali-c., kali-p., **KREOS., LAC-AC.,** lac-d., ***lac-c., lach., lil-t.,*** lob., ***lyc., mag-c., mag-m.,*** **MED.,** ***merc-i-f., nat-m.,*** nat-p., **NAT-S., NUX-M., NUX-V.,** ***op., ox-ac., petr., ph-ac., phos.,*** piloc., plat., plb., ***podo., psor., puls.,*** **SEP.,** ***sil., sulph., sul-ac.,*** stry., ***sym-r.,*** **TAB.,** tarent., **THYR.,** tub., ***verat., verat-v.,*** zinc.
blood - ip., phos., ***sep.***
congestion, with, of pelvic viscera - ***podo.***
fetus, from movements of - arn.
frequent and severe attacks, first of food, then mucus, and finally blood, worse in morning, during latter half of - ***nat-m.***
latter, in, half, violent and frequent, first food, then mucus, and finally blood, worse in morning - ***nat-m.***
long and continued, cannot retain food on stomach - ***kali-bi.***
mucus, in - sul-ac.
nausea, in some cases more, than vomiting - **IP.**
nausea, with deathly - **TAB.**
persistent - med., piloc., psor.
persistent, late in afternoon and evening - ***lach.***
pylorus, with burning at - ***canth.***
retching - ars., ***canth.***
riding, worse - 2petr.
sour - ***mag-c.***
stomach rejects everything - asar.
suffering, in women, from scirrhus - ***con.***
supper, after - **KREOS.**
taste, with bitter - ***nat-s.***
water - sep.
water, of sweetish, before breakfast - **KREOS.**

WANDER, wants to, about house - ***verat.***

WATER-brash - ***dios.***, lob., ***nat-m.***, ***nux-m.***, ***tab.***

WEAKNESS, general, during - alet., alum., alumn., arn., calc-p., ***caul.***, ***helon.***, murx., ***puls.***, ***sep.***, ***sulph.***, ***verat.***

- faintish - alum.
- languor - calc-p.
- walk, tired from a short - **CALC.**
- uncertainty in walking, joints weak - murx.

Pulse

ABNORMAL - **ACON.,** agar., agn., ambr., am-c., am-m., ant-c., ***ant-t.,*** arg-m., ***arg-n., arn.,*** **ARS., ARS-I.,** asaf., asar., aur., bar-c., **BELL.,** bism., bor., bov., ***bry.,*** calad., calc., ***camph.,*** cann-s., canth., caps., carb-an., ***carb-s., carb-v.,*** caust., cham., chel., ***chin.,*** cic., cina, cocc., colch., coloc., ***con.,*** croc., **CUPR., DIG.,** dulc., ferr., ***gels., glon.,*** graph., guai., hell., ***hep.,*** **HYOS.,** ign., **IOD.,** ip., ***kali-c.,*** kali-n., **KREOS., LACH.,** ***laur.,*** led., lyc., mang., meny., ***merc.,*** mez., mosch., mur-ac., nat-m., nit-ac., nux-m., nux-v., olnd., **OP.,** par., petr., **PH-AC., PHOS.,** plat., plb., puls., ran-b., ran-s., rheum, rhod., **RHUS-T.,** sabad., sabin., samb., ***sec.,*** seneg., ***sep.,*** **SIL.,** spig., spong., squil., stann., staph., **STRAM.,** stront-c., ***sulph.,*** sul-ac., thuj., valer., **VERAT.,** viol-o., viol-t., zinc.

ABSENT - amyg., ant-t., ***arg-n., ars.,*** ars-h., ars-s-f., cit-l., colch., con., hell., **HYDR-AC.,** ***mosch., phyt., podo.,*** stram.
- cholera, in - ***bry., camph., cupr-ac., cupr-m., hydr-ac., laur., op., verat.***
- gastritis, in - nux-v.
- labor, in - ***lach.***
- metrorrhagia, in - croc., ***kreos.***
- rheumatism, in cardiac - ***cact.***
- spotted fever, in beginning of - ***am-c.***
- suffocation, with - **CACT.**
- sunstroke, in - ***glon.***
- suppressed, with strong palpitation - ***puls.***
- sweat, with cold - ***camph., carb-v.,*** med., ***verat.***

AUDIBLE - ant-t., ***camph.,*** con., ***dig.,*** hell., iod., kali-c., kreos., merc., op., phos., plb., sep., **SPIG.,** sulph., ***thuj.***

BOUNDING - ***acon.,*** aether, alco., ars., atro., ***bell.,*** benz-ac., camph., cann-i., canth., chin-s., chlor., colch., corn-f., dulc., eup-per., ***eup-pur.,*** fago., glon., iod., jatr., kali-chl., lil-t., naja, paro-i., plan., raph., trif-p., visc.
- ascending stairs, on - petr.
- awaking at two a.m. - benz-ac.
- dysmenorrhea, in - verat-v.
- intermittent, in - calad.
- walking, on - petr.

CHEST, feels beating in left, while sitting - ***calc-p.***
- with each beat a broad stitch upward in muscles - ***calc.***

COMPRESSIBLE, easily, (see Soft) - iber., kali-m., ***lycps., phos., plb.,*** stram., sumb., zinc.
- apoplexy, in - ***aster.***
- diphtheria, in epidemic - ***lach.***
- endocarditis, in - ***aur.***
- scarlatina, in malignant - ***lach.***
- shock, in - ***hyper.***

CONTRACTED - acon., acet-ac., agar., ant-t., arn., ars., ***asaf., aster.,*** bell., bism., bor., calc., calth., cann-i., canth., chin., cina, colch., crot-t., cupr., cupr-ac., hyos., iod., ***kali-bi., kali-br.,*** kali-s., kiss., lach., laur., merc-cy., morph., nit-ac., op., ox-ac., paeon., petr., plb., russ., phos., ***sec.,*** spira., squil., stann., stram., stry., sul-ac., ***tarent.,*** vip., zinc., zinc-m.
- chill, with shaking, in evening - ox-ac.
- chorea, in - ***asaf.***
- full and powerful, over 100 - ***acon.***
- liver, in inflammation of - ***merc.***
- melancholy and jealousy, with - ***kali-a.***
- nosebleed, with - ***kali-bi.***
- palpitation, with - ***sec.***
- peritonitis, in - ***atro.***
- smallpox, in - mill.
- toothache, in - ***cocc-s.***

DISCORDANT, with fever - lil-t., **PYROG.,** thyr.

DOUBLE - acon., agar., aml-n., amyg., anan., apis, apoc., bell., cycl., ferr., gels., glon., iber., ***kali-c., phos.,*** piloc., plb., rhod., ***stram.,*** zinc., zinc-s.
- angina pectoris, in - ***aml-n.***
- beats seem to run into each other - iber.
- sometimes intermitting when heart's action is accelerated - ***ferr-m.***
- typhus, in - ***apis, arg-n.***

DRINKING, affected by alcohol - ***rhus-t.,*** sul-ac.
- affected by beer or coffee - ***rhus-t.***
- increased by wine - zinc.

EATING, quieter after meals - cinch.

EMPTY - alco., camph., chin., ferr., ***lach.,*** petr., ***sec., verat.***

EPIGASTRIUM, beat felt - ***nat-m., puls.***

EVENING, violent, cannot lie on left side - brom.

EXCITED - ant-t., anth., cyt-l., dig., iod., ***nux-v.,*** petr., plumbg., sol-t-ae.

FAST, pulse, accelerated, elevated, exalted - **ACON.,** aesc., ***aeth., agar., ail.,*** aloe, all-c., alum., ambr., am-c., am-m., anac., ant-c., ***ant-t.,*** **APIS,** arg-m., ***arg-n.,*** **ARN., ARS., ARS-I.,** ***asaf.,*** asar., aster., **AUR.,** ***aur-m., bapt.,*** bar-c., bar-m., **BELL.,** ***benz-ac.,*** **BERB.,** bism., bor., bov., brom., **BRY.,** calad., calc., ***camph.,*** cann-i., ***canth.,*** carb-v., caust., cedr., ***cham.,*** chel., chin., chin-a., ***chin-s., cina,*** clem., cocc., coc-c., coff., ***colch.,*** **COLL.,** coloc., **CON., CROT-C.,** crot-t., **CUPR.,** cycl., **DIG.,** ***echi.,*** euph., ***ferr.,*** ferr-i., **FERR-P.,** fl-ac., **GELS., GLON.,** grat., guai., ham., ***hell.,*** hep., hipp., ***hyos., hyper., ign.,*** **IOD.,** ip., kali-bi., kali-c., kali-i., kali-n., kreos., ***lach., laur.,*** lob., lyc., ***lycps., manc.,*** mang., **MERC.,** merc-c., merc-cy., ***mez.,*** mill., ***mosch., mur-ac., naja,*** nat-a., ***nat-c.,*** **NAT-M.,** ***nat-s.,*** nicc., ***nit-ac., nux-m.,*** **NUX-V.,** olnd., onos., **OP.,** osm., ox-ac., par., petr., phel., **PH-AC., PHOS.,** ***phys., phyt.,*** pic-ac., ***plat., plb.,*** podo., ***puls.,*** **PYROG.,** ran-b., ***ran-s.,*** rheum, rhod., **RHUS-T.,** ***rhus-v.,*** sabad., samb., ***sang.,*** sars., **SEC.,** seneg., ***sep.,*** **SIL., SPIG.,** ***spong.,*** **STANN.,** staph., **STRAM., SULPH.,** sul-ac., ***tab., tell.,*** ter., thuj., ***valer., verat.,*** **VERAT-V.,** vesp., **ZINC.**
- **beats** per minute,
  - 80 - aphis., ars-i., arum-d., ***phos.,*** ran-s.
    - 84 - thlaspi
    - 85 - **LACH.**
    - 86 - ***kali-c.***

FAST, pulse
beats per minute
87 - ***agar.***
88 - chlol.
89 - ***merc-c.***
90 - ant-a., arund., colch., merc-sul., still.
92 - ars-h.
96 - **TARENT.**
96 to 104 - chin-b.
98 - chin-a.
100 - agar., amyg., daph., ***ign.,*** kali-br., ***kreos.,*** lac-c., med., sarac.
107 - ars-h.
108 - ***cycl., kali-i.***
110 - hippoz., ***phyt.,*** puls., rumx.
120 - ant-chl., ***bapt., cina, cupr-m.,*** hippoz., ***ign.,*** lac-c., ***lach., lyc., merc-cy.,*** rumx., sars., sulph., vario., verat-v.
125 - sulph.
126 - vesp.
128 - ars-h.
130 - amyg., asim., merc-sul., mygal., sil.
140 - amyg., ***cina,*** coll., dor., lac-c., sulph., tarent.
143 - coca
144 - psor.
150 - merc., verat-v.
160 - lyss., verat-v., vesp.
170 - colch.
200 - chin-a.
afternoon - agar., bapt., chel., chin-s., chr-ac., ferr-i., gels., gins., kali-chl., kali-n., lyc., merc-sul., nat-m., oena., phos., phys., podo., ptel., sumb.
2 p.m., at, 100 - bapt.
3 p.m., at, 90 - agar.
4 p.m., at, 84 - chr-ac.
slow in the morning, but - **KALI-N.,** thuj., zinc.
albuminuria, in, 112 - ***apis***
120, easily compressed - ***calc-ar.***
amenorrhea, in, 120 - verat-v.
anemia, in - trinit.
anger, by - sep.
angina, in - ox-ac.
120 - ***bar-m.***
arteries, visible throbbing of - bell., jab.
ascites, in - ***apis***
asthma, in - bapt.
100 - tab.
congestion to heart, with - ***asaf.***
millari - ***cupr-m.***
awaking, on - sil.
bladder, in catarrh of, 110 - uva.
bleeding of lungs, in - ***ip.***
chronic passive, 120 - **SEC.**
postpartum, in - ***croc.***
bowels, in inflammation of, 110 - ***verat-v.***
brain, affection of, small and empty, 106 - ***glon.***
cerebrospinal disease, in - verat-v.
inflammation of brain - **BELL.,** ***merc.,*** puls.
irritation of, 90 - ***lach.***

FAST, pulse
brain, traumatic meningitis, in, 140 - ***hyper.***
breast tumor, in - ***ars-i.***
bronchial catarrh, in, 150 - ***lach.***
and vesical, 100 - ***cop.***
bronchitis, in - ***phos.***
burns, in, 160 - calen.
cancer labii, in - ***camph.***
catarrh, in acute, 120 - ***ant-t.***
chest affection, in, after miscarriage - ***nux-m.***
troubles, in, after repelled itch - ***hep.***
childbirth, after - ***crot-h.***
chill, during - chin-s., coloc., crot-t., gels., zinc.
cholera, in - zinc.
130 - verat.
cholera infantum, in - coff-t.
cholerine, in - ***phos.***
coffee, after - agar.
colic, in - ***iris,*** nux-v.
lead colic, in, 120 - op.
convulsions, during - aeth., oena., op., stry.
epileptiform, in, 190 - verat-v.
puerperal, in - op., stram.
counted, could not be - ***ant-t., arg-n., ars.,*** camph., ***cedr., dig., lach., lyc., merc-c., merc.,*** plat., zinc.
scarcely to be, in scarlatina, in diphtheria, after failure of lachesis - ***lac-c.***
croup, in - ***acon., ant-t., bell., brom., hep.,*** sang., spong.
diphtheritic, 100 - ***kali-bi.***
daytime - nat-a., nat-m.
debility, with general - ter.
delirium tremens, in, 120 - chlol.
diabetes, in, 90, relieved - uran-n.
diarrhea, in chronic, 100 - sulph.
130 - ***coloc.***
diphtheria, in - ***bapt., chin-a., kali-br.,*** kali-i., kali-m., ***kali-per., lac-c., lach., lyc., merc-cy., mur-ac., phyt.,*** spong., ***sul-ac.***
drinking, after - nat-m.
dropsy, in - ***aur-m.***
dysentery, in - ***colch.***
eating, after - ***arg-n., iod.,*** **LYC.,** mez., nat-m., ***nux-v., phos., puls.,*** rhus-t., ***sulph.***
ebullitions, with - ambr.
sitting, while - ***mag-m.***
enterocolitis, in - ***nuph.***
erysipelas, in - rhus-t.
100 - ***hydr.***
of face and scalp, 120 - ***cinch.***
evening - acon., alum-sil., am-caust., anth., anthro., aphis., ***arg-m., arg-n.,*** ars., arum-i., aster., atha., bry., ***carb-an.,*** **CAUST.,** chin-s., ***cinnb., crot-h., dulc.,*** euph., euphr., ***ferr.,*** gent-l., ham., hell., hyper., jug-r., ***lach., lyc.,*** mez., mill., ***mur-ac.,*** murx., ***nat-c.,*** nat-sil., ***nux-v.,*** oena., olnd., ox-ac., ***ph-ac., phos.,*** plan., ***puls.,*** ran-b., rheum, sars., sep., ***sil., sulph.,*** sumb., teucr., ***thuj., tub.,*** upa., ***zinc.***

FAST, pulse
evening, in
bed, in - arg-m., sul-ac.
blood vessels, with distended, pulse slower mornings - ***puls.***
dysentery, in - ***caps.***
especially in - ***carb-an.***
tuberculosis, in - ***iod.***
slow in the morning, but fast in evening - arg-m., arn., asar., carb-an., caust., chin., ***kali-c.,*** **KALI-N.,** ***lyc.,*** mez., **OLND.,** petr., phos., puls., **RAN-B.,** ***sars.,*** sep., **SPIG.,** teucr., **THUJ., ZINC.**
towards - teucr.
aphonia, in - ***ferr.***
excited - anthro., bar-m., cahin.
at night, with ebullitions - ***nat-c.***
dentition, in - ***verat-v.***
pneumonia, in - ***lach.***
towards evening, with orgasm of blood - caust.
excitement, from - anthro., bar-m., cahin., con., digox., merc.
great, of heart and circulation, in pneumonia - ***ran-b.***
exercise, only during - fl-ac.
exertion, by every slight - iod.
face and feet, with coldness of - ***lyc.***
facial neuralgia, in - spig.
falls down suddenly as if dead, 100, after singing - lyss.
faster than the heart - beat - acon., arn., ***rhus-t., spig.***
fever, during - chin-s., meny., ruta, ***sec.***
without - camph.
fit, before the - oena.
forenoon - aphis., calc., chin., com., lyc., merc-sul., mez., nat-p., oena., op., plan., ptel., trom.
gonorrhea, after - ***camph.***
hay catarrh, in - stict.
head, with pains in - ***crot-h.***
headache, in - ***glon.***
full and tense, 86 - ***glon.***
heart affection, in, 160 - ***lach.***
88 - ***cact., lycps.,*** mosch.
cardiac distress, in, in night - ***arn.***
hyperesthesia, in, 100 to 110 - ***ign.***
nerves, in irritation of, 140 - ***coll.***
carditis, in - ***carb-v.***
disease, in, 90 - ***lycps.***
pericarditis, in, 120 - spig.
rheumatism of, in, 105 - ***cact.***
heartbeat, quicker than - acon.
heartbeat, reminds one of, in beginning of phthisis - sal-ac.
heat in face, with flushes of, and congestion to chest - seneg.
heat of skin, with, in jaundice - ***acon.***
heat, with dry - sec.
tuberculosis florida, in - merc-c.
hematemesis, in - ***sec.***
120 to 130 - ***ars.***

FAST, pulse
hemoptysis, in, 100 to 120 - acal.
hepatic disorder, in - sil.
hip disease, in, 120 - staph.
hysteria, in - ***cinnam.***
influenza, in, 130 - chel.
insanity, in - nux-v., verat-v.
intermittent fever, in - ***ars., dig.,*** nat-m.
intermittent, and fast pulse - acon., agar., aloe, alum., am-m., ars., ***aur.,*** bell., benz-ac., bism., cann-i., canth., chin., chin-s., colch., cupr., ***dig.,*** gels., glon., grat., hyos., ign., kali-chl., lob., merc-c., merc-cy., mez., mur-ac., nat-a., nit-ac., nux-m., ***nux-v.,*** olnd., op., ox-ac., plb., phos., phys., sep., stram., ***sulph.,*** tab., verat-v., zinc.
irregular, and - visc.
kidneys, in haematuria from, 100 - ter.
labor, during - ***chin-s.,*** coff-t.
liver, in functional derangement of, 96 - sep.
lying, when, 80, when sitting 93 - spig.
lyssophobia, in - ***lyss.***
mania, during second of stage of attack of - tarent.
mania, in - ***anac., bell., cupr-ar.***
meals, after - ars-h., ***lyc.***
melancholia, in - ***anac., arg-n.***
meningitis, in - ***bell., phys., cic., hell.***
basilar, in incipient, 90 to 100 - ***kali-br.***
menses, during - ***croc.***
after - ***nat-m.***
metrorrhagia, after, 110 - ars-h.
midnight, after - ***benz-ac.,*** hyper.
miscarriage, in - ***coloc.***
120 - ust.
morning - agar., ail., ***ars., ars-m.,*** asaf., atro., ***canth.,*** cedr., chin., chin-s., fago., ***graph.,*** ign., ***kali-c.,*** merc-c., ***mez.,*** mit., myric., oena., onop., ox-ac., phos., phys., podo., sang., sulph., sumb., ther., thuj., upa.
100, at 9 a.m. - trom.
slow during the day and in the evening, but - **AGAR.,** alum., **ARS.,** calc., canth., chin., graph., ***ign.,*** **KALI-C.,** lyc., mez., nux-v., phos.
slower at night - ***ars.***
during day and evening - ***ign.***
waking, on - alumn.
motion, by - **ANT-T.**
motion agg. - alum-sil., ant-t., ***arn., bry., dig.,*** digin., fl-ac., ***gels.,*** glon., ***graph., iod., lycps.,*** **NAT-M.,** ***nux-v.,*** petr., ***phos.,*** sep., staph., stram.
by every - petr., sep.
moving, while, sinks to its accustomed slowness during rest - dig.
myelitis, in, 100, hard - ***dulc.***
perimyelitis, in, 120 - sep.
neuralgia, in - ***cham.***
of intestines, with - ***gels.***
neuropathies, in - kali-a.

FAST, pulse

night - alum-sil., anthro., arum-i., aster., cinnb., con., dulc., nat-sil., nux-v., plect., ptel.

slow by day, but - am-c., bor., ***bry.,*** calc., carb-an., dulc., hep., kali-n., mag-c., ***merc.,*** mur-ac., nat-c., nat-m., phos., ran-s., sabin., **SEP.,** ***sil.,*** sulph.

slower during day - bry.

noon - mit., oena., ox-ac.

112 - ars-h.

noticing it, when - ***arg-n.***

ovarian cyst, in - ***iod.***

ozaena, in, 120 - ***elaps***

pain, from - tarent.

phlebitis, in, small, wiry, 120 - ***ham.***

pleurodynia, in, 120 - ran-b.

pleurisy, in, 110 - seneg.

pleuritic with plastic exudation, 136 - ***hep.***

pneumonia, in - ***ant-t., iod., merc.,*** nux-v.

100 - sulph.

102 - stram.

106 - ***kali-c.***

110 - ***iod.***

110, small, thin, hard - lachn.

112 - ***ant-t.,*** sulph.

115, small - ***chel.***

120 - ***ant-t., iod.***

120 to 130 - ***lyc.***

130 - sulph.

132 - ***ant-t.,*** stram.

150, in evening - phos.

184 - sulph.

bronchial, in 145 - ***lyc.***

catarrhal, over 100 - ***bapt.***

hepatization, stage of - phos.

typhoid, 110, small, wiry - ***lachn.***

pyaemia, in - ***ars.***

quicker, harder - calc-ar.

than beat of heart - ***spig.***

rest, during - ***mag-m.***

rheumatism, acute, 100 - chel.

rising up, on - ***bry., dig.***

scarlatina, in, 136 - ***cina***

140 - arum-t.

after, 140 - ***lach.***

dropsy, in, 120, small - ***dig.***

malignant, 150 - stram.

septicemia, in, 130 - sal-ac.

siesta, especially after, all day - cahin.

sitting while - aspar., gins., indg., ***mag-m.,*** nat-m., oena.

skin dry, not hot, 90 - elaps

silver nitrate for gonorrhea, after injecting, 100 - tarent.

slow and faint, afterwards - bapt.

and back again, suddenly to, often changing - ***glon.***

small, and fast - **ACON.,** **aeth.,** alum., apis, arn., **ARS.,** ***ars-i.,*** asaf., ***aur., aur-m.,*** bell., benz-ac., bism., bry., cahin., ***camph.,*** canth., chin., cocc., colch., coloc., ***con.,*** crot-t., ***dig.,*** ferr-m., fl-ac., gels., glon., grat., ***hell.,*** hyos.,

FAST, pulse

small, and fast - ign., ***iod.,*** kali-bi., kali-chl., kali-n., ***lach.,*** lach., led., **LAUR.,** lob., lyc., ***lycps.,*** merc-c., merc-cy., ***mur-ac.,*** nat-m., nit-ac., ***nux-m.,*** **NUX-V.,** olnd., op., ox-ac., petr., phos., phyt., pic-ac., puls., ran-s., raph., rhod., rhus-t., samb., **SIL.,** sol-t-ae., staph., **STRAM.,** sul-ac., tab., **VERAT.,** zinc.

125-130 - bar-c.

and often irregular - ***fl-ac.***

and strong - acon., apis, arn., ars., bell., chin., crot- t., gels., hyos., merc-c., merc-cy., op., raph., stram.

and tremulous - ***hell.***

contracted - acet-ac.

scarcely to be counted, surface cold and dry - ***ail.***

weak, in evening - ***lob.***

smallpox, in - mill.

120 - chin-s.

soft, intermittent - ***hell.***

soft, weak, sometimes filiform - ***gels.***

speech, with confusion of, and disconnected answers - crot-h.

spinal irritation, in, 100 - ***chin-s.***

stairs, mostly when going up - rumx.

standing, on - nat-m.

stomach, affection of, 100 - ***lac-c.***

gastric disorder, in, 80 to 88 - ***atro.***

gastro-enteritis and albuminuria, in - ***apis***

stomach pain, with 100 - ***kali-c.***

ulcer of stomach, in - mez.

stroke, in - ***aster., crot-h., laur.,*** phos.

100 - ***cocc.***

precursor of - aster.

stool, after - ***agar.,*** **CON.,** glon.

strong and small - acon., apis, arn., ars., bell., chin., crot-t., gels., hyos., merc-c., merc-cy., op., raph., stram.

angina, in - ***merc.***

study, effects of over - ***cupr-ac.***

suddenly, gradually decreases - ***verat-v.***

summer complaint, in, 120 to 160 - ***ferr-p.***

sunstroke, with - ***verat-v.***

supper, after - cupr.

synanche cellularis, in - anthr.

temperature, out of proportion to - lil-t., ***pyrog.,*** thyr.

tetanus, in traumatic, 80 - ***hydr-ac.***

after a burn, 133 - ***aml-n.***

thinking of past troubles - nat-m., sep.

thread like, in epilepsy - ***bufo***

becomes constantly more rapid and smaller until at length it is, and finally no longer can be felt - lyss.

throat, in sore, 130 - ***lac-c.***

quinsy, in, 100 - ***hep.***

ulcerated, in 120 - ***lyc.***

tonsillitis, 130 - ***lac-c.***

tonsils, in chronic hypertrophy of, 120 - ***bar-m.***

thrombosis, in, 130 - ***apis***

FAST, pulse

tuberculosis, in - ***ars-i., brom., lach., nat-a.,*** samb., sep., stann.

tumultuously - acon., aml-n., lycps.

perspiration, with - coca

unconsciousness, with sudden - ***cocc.***

uremia, asphyctic form - ***hydr-ac.***

urine, with copious - dig.

urticaria, in, 104 - rhus-t.

uterus, in induration of - ***carb-an.***

uterine neuralgia, in, 100 - nux-v.

vertigo, with - tell.

vexation, after - acon., arg-n., **CHAM.,** coloc., ign., ***nat-m., nux-v., petr.,*** **SEP.,** ***staph.***

warm applications, from - sulph.

weak - nat-m.

intermittent, in - rhus-t.

quinsy and old age, in - ***bar-c.***

typhus, in - ***camph.***

FEELS, pulse

beating, feels, not frequent, but quick - ***calc-p.***

fingers, in - ***aml-n., glon.***

lying down, when - calad.

meningitis, in, every beat is felt - ***glon.***

nape, in, while sitting - ***calc-p.***

feels, pulse, in body

all over - glon., lil-t., ***puls.,*** sep.

and from time to time like a slow rising wave through throat into head, followed by a sensation of momentary rush of blood - lyss.

especially in hysterical women - ***kali-c.***

feels beating through whole, particularly left chest - sep.

different parts of, in - nat-p.

like tick of a watch, in - ambr.

over body, in sick headache - sang.

parts, in all, most in epigastrium - agar.

through whole, strong - alum.

fever, during - ***cocc.***

heat stage of intermittent, in - ***ars.***

whole, especially about heart - clem.

even during rest -

FEVERISH - ***acon.,*** alum., alumn., anthro., ***ars., bell.,*** bov., croc., gins., lac-ac., merc-c., mez., morph., plb., ***pyrog.,*** sars., sec., ***stram., sulph.,*** thuj., vip.

aphthae, in - ***hell.***

caries, in, of tarsal and metatarsal bones - ***merc.***

coxarius, in morbus - ***kali-c.***

synanche cellularis, in - ***anthr.***

gonorrhea, in - ***merc.***

FLICKERING - carb-ac.

FLUTTERING - arn., ***crot-h., kali-bi.,*** verat.

pericarditis, in - colch.

seventh to ninth day of pneumonia, on - ***phos.***

120 - gels.

FLOWING - ferr-p., gels., syph., verat-v.

FLUTTERING - apis, ***arn., ars.,*** cann-i., carb-ac., cimic., coff., colch., ***crot-h.,*** dig., gels., gins., juni., ***kali-bi.,*** kali-n., morph., **NUX-V.,** op., ph-ac., ***phos.,*** ptel., pyrog., ***sec.,*** stann., stram., sul-h., thea., ***verat.,*** zinc., zinc-m.

FREQUENT, (see Fast)

FULL - acet-ac., **ACON.,** aesc., aeth., aether, agar., agar-pa., alco., aloe, ***all-c.,*** **ALUM.,** alumn., am-m., ***aml-n., amyg.,*** anan., **ANT-T.,** anth., antipyrin., antipyrin., apis, apoc., ***arn.,*** ars., ars-h., ars-i., ars-m., arum-d., arum-t., asaf., asar., asc-c., asim., atro., ***aur.,*** bapt., bar-c., bar-i., bar-m., **BELL.,** benz-ac., **BERB.,** bism., brom., **BRY.,** ***cact.,*** cahin., caj., **CALC.,** camph., ***canth.,*** carb-ac., carb-o., cedr., celt., cent., cham., **CHEL.,** ***chin.,*** chin-a., chin-s., chlf., chr-ac., cimic., cocc., coff., colch., coloc., con., cor-r., cori-r., crot-c., crot-h., crot-t., cub., ***cupr.,*** cupr-ac., cupr-s., cycl., cyt-l., daph., dat-f., **DIG.,** digin., dirc., dor., ***dulc., eup-per., eup-pur.,*** fago., ferr., ferr-m., ferr-p., gast., **GELS.,** gins., ***glon.,*** **GRAPH.,** ham., hell., ***hep.,*** hydr-ac., **HYOS.,** iber., ictod., ***ign.,*** iod., piloc., jug-r., juni., kali-bi., ***kali-c.,*** kali-chl., kali-i., kali-m., **KALI-N.,** kali-ox., kreos., lac-ac., ***lach.,*** laur., ***led., lil-t.,*** linu-c., lipp., lyc., lycps., menth., ***merc.,*** merc-c., merc-cy., merc-pr-a., merl., ***mez.,*** mill., morph., ***mosch.,*** mur-ac., myric., ***naja,*** nat-m., ***nat-n.,*** nit-ac., nitro-o., ***nux-v.,*** olnd., ol-an., onos., ***op.,*** ox-ac., par., ***petr.,*** phel., ***ph-ac., phos., phys.,*** phyt., piloc., plan., plb., plect., puls., ran-b., ran-s., raph., rat., rhus-t., sabad., ***sabin.,*** samb., sang., sarr., sars., scroph-n., sec., seneg., ***sep., sil.,*** sin-n., sium, sol-n., ***spig.,*** spira., spong., **STRAM.,** stront-c., ***sulph.,*** sumb., sul-ac., ***tab.,*** tanac., tarax., tarent., ter., tep., thea., thuj., til., toxi., trif-p., trom., valer., ***verat., verat-v.,*** vinc., viol-o., vip., visc., yuc., zinc., zing.

accelerated with erethism, and, frequent at night, slower by day - ***merc.***

afternoon - iod., nat-a., phyt., zinc., zing.

3 p.m., at - agar.

ague, in - eup-pur.

bleeding, in - ***ferr.***

bounding than acon., less, not so flowing as gels - ***ferr-p.***

cancer labii, in - ***camph.***

chill, during, and heat - chin-s.

cold, after catching, after labor - puls.

compressed, easily, in concussion of brain - ***hell.***

croup, in - ***hep.***

delirium, in - ***bell.,*** stram.

diphtheria, in - ***merc-cy.***

dysentery, in - ***caps.***

ebullitions, and accelerated, with - ***mosch.***

evening - acon., anth., anthro., hell., myric., olnd., ran-b., scut., seneg., sulph., thuj., zinc., zing.

excited - ***ferr.***

fast, with violent beating in arteries - ***merc.***

FULL, pulse
fever, during - chin-s., ***coloc.,*** vinc.
and violent thirst, with, followed by general sweat, mostly on forehead - ran-b.
bilious remittent - ***crot-h.***
childbed - ***coloc.***
intermittent fever - bar-m., ***cedr.,*** chin-a., ***cinch.***
forenoon - nat-a., trom., zing.
frequent - colch.
frequent and tense - ***gels.***
hallucinations, in - ***hyos.***
hard - ***graph.***
after-pain, with - ferr.
eclampsia, in - ***glon.***
mumps, in - dor.
somewhat accelerated - ***dulc.***
uterine bleeding - ***ferr.***
head, with congestion to, in ague - podo.
towards evening - ***croc.***
headache, in - ***gels.***
heart disease, in - **AUR.**
heat, with, at night - ran-s.
hydrocephalus and bronchitis, in incipient - ***apis***
intermitting every six beats, with cardiac heaviness - ***acon.***
irritable in evening and in hysteria - ***camph.***
labored - ***op.***
laryngitis, in acute pharyngolaryngitis - ***naja***
lung affections, in - ***kali-n.***
mania, hystero-mania, during second stage of attack of - tarent.
mania, in - ***cupr-ac.***
meals, after - ars-h.
metrorrhagia, in - sabin.
morning - ***canth.,*** jac-c., phos., phyt., sep., zinc.
9 a.m. - trom.
night - com., ***merc.,*** sep.
nosebleeds, in - croc.
palpitation, with - tell.
paralysis, with imbecility - ***anac-oc.***
pneumonia, in - ***merc.,*** zinc.
in typhoid - ***sang.***
quick - ***glon.***
quinsy, in - ***bar-c.***
rapid - ***aeth.,*** camph., ***led.***
rheumatism, acute - ***chel.***
right - kali-chl.
round, in phthisis pulmonalis - ***ferr-p.***
soft-flowing, with slight fever - ***gels.***
scarlatina, in - arum-t.
scarlet fever, after - ***hep.***
sitting, when - ***arg-n.***
slow - nat-m., par.
slow and intermittent, sunstroke - ***glon.***
snoring, with - ***op.***
soft - ***phyt.***
fever, at night, with - raph.

FULL, pulse
spasm, after - ***bry.***
stroke, in - ***arn., chin-s.,*** **NUX-V.,** ***verat-v.***
strong, and - acon., bell., ***bry.***
but only 28 - ***dig.***
throat and chest, with pains in - ***lac-c.***
typhus, in - ***arn., calc.***
and albuminuria, in - ***apis***
weak, and full - ***ferr-p.,*** gels., verat.
thin, contracted - ***cham.***
vacillating, about 100 - ***gels.***

HARD - **ACON.,** aesc., aeth., aether, agar-cps., agar-pa., agro., alco., ***all-c.,*** all-s., am-c., am-caust., am-m., ***aml-n.,*** ammc., ***amyg.,*** anan., ant-c., ant-m., ***ant-t.,*** apis, ***arn.,*** ars., ars-h., ars-i., ars-s-f., arum-d., asaf., asar., aster., atro., ***bar-c.,*** bar-i., bar-m., **BELL.,** ***benz-ac.,*** **BERB.,** bism., brom., **BRY.,** ***cact.,*** calad., calth., camph., ***canth.,*** carb-ac., carb-s., cent., cham., **CHEL.,** ***chin.,*** chlor., cimic., ***cina,*** clem., cocc., coff., colch., coloc., con., cor-r., corn., crot-h., ***cupr.,*** ***cupr-ac.,*** cupr-s., cycl., cyna., daph., ***dig.,*** digin., ***dulc., ferr.,*** gast., gels., glon., gran., **GRAPH.,** ham., hell., ***hep.,*** **HYOS.,** hyper., iber., ***ign.,*** indg., iod., jatr., kali-bi., ***kali-c.,*** kali-i., kali-m., ***kali-n., kreos., lach.,*** laur., ***led.,*** lyc., ***lycps.,*** ***merc.,*** merc-c., merc-cy., merc-d., ***merc-p-r.,*** mez., morph., ***mosch.,*** mur-ac., nat-c., nat-m., ***nit-ac.,*** nit-s-d., nitro-o., ***nux-v.,*** olnd., op., ox-ac., par., petr., phel., ph-ac., ***phos.,*** phyt., plect., plumbg., puls., plb., ran-b., ran-s., rauw., sabin., samb., sang., sec., seneg., ***sep.,*** serp., ***sil.,*** sin-a., sol-m., sol-t-ae., spig., spira., spong., squil., **STRAM., STRONT-C.,** stroph., ***stry.,*** sul-h., ***sulph.,*** tab., tanac., tarent., tep., ***ter.,*** thuj., til., uva., valer., verat., verat-v., vinc., viol-o., vip., wies., zinc., zinc-m.
accelerated, somewhat - ***dulc.***
afternoon, 3 p.m., at - agar.
awaking at 2 a.m. - benz-ac.
breathing, with anxious - ***op.***
climbing, after - rauw.
colic, in - op.
compressible, not easily - ***lycps.***
conjunctivitis, in - sep., ***sulph.***
consciousness, on recovering, in evening - aster.
convulsions, epileptic, in - aeth.
puerperal, in - ***lach.***
cord-like - tab.
croup, in - ***hep.,*** spong.
delirium tremens, in - ***kali-bi.,*** stram.
delirium, in - ***bell.***
elderly people, in - **ANT-T.**
evening - all-c., ***bapt.,*** dulc., plb., plumbg., ran-b., zing.
typhus, in - ***bapt.***
excited - ***ferr.***
excitement, with - stroph-s.
exertion, after sudden - rauw.

HARD, pulse
fever, in childbed - ***coloc.***
gastric, in - puls.
puerperal, in - puls.
full - calad.
at beginning of paroxysm - ferr.
gastritis, in acute, after taking cold - ***coloc.***
heat, with - ***coloc.,*** vinc.
hepatitis - cocc., ***merc.***
incompressible - colch.
scarlet fever, in - sulph.
insanity, in - nux-v.
lung affections, in - ***kali-n.***
mania, in - ***cupr-ac.***
meningitis infantum, in - **APIS**
morning - petr., phyt., zinc.
11 a.m. - zing.
noon - ox-ac.
pneumonia, in - **ANT-T.,** ***cact., kali-c., phos.,*** rhus-t., sulph., **VERAT-V.**
quick, with every fever - ***calc.***
without being frequent - cact.
rapid, in scarlatina - arum-t.
shot, like, gliding along under fingers - ***apis***
single beats - aur., cact., lach., lil-t., zinc.
slow, and - stroph-s.
stroke, in - ***aster.,*** **NUX-V.,** ***plb.***
stroke, in congestive, as iron - ***verat-v.***
tense - ***dulc.***
thrombosis and typhus, in - ***apis***
tuberculosis, in - ***ars-i.***
typhoid, in - ***lach.***
typhus, in - ***arn.,*** **NIT-AC.**
abdominalis, in - nux-v.
unconsciousness, with sudden - ***cocc.***
unrhythmical - ***aeth.***
90 to 100 - ***alum.***

HEAVY - crot-c., phos., stram., ***verat-v.,*** yuc.
night - com.
reverberates, with dilatation of heart - ***ant-t.***

HEAVY - verat-v.

IMPERCEPTIBLE, (see Low) - **ACON.,** aeth., agar., agn., amyg., anil., ant-t., ***apis, arg-n.,*** arn., ***ars.,*** ars-h., ars-s-f., bell., benz-ac., ***cact.,*** cadm-br., **CAMPH.,** cann-i., cann-s., ***canth., carb-ac.,*** carb-h., **CARB-V.,** chel., chin., chlor., cic., cic-m., cit-l., ***cocc.,*** **COLCH.,** coloc., con., crot-h., **CUPR.,** cupr-ar., cyt-l., digin., dulc., ferr., gins., gels., guai., hell., **HYDR-AC.,** hyos., kali-cy., lach., ***ip.,*** kalm., kreos., laur., ***led.,*** man., ***merc.,*** merc-c., morph., ***mosch., naja,*** nux-v., oena., ***op.,*** ox-ac., petr., ph-ac., phos., ***phyt.,*** plb., plat., ***podo.,*** puls., rhus-t., ***sec.,*** **SIL.,** stann., stram., stry., sulph., sul-ac., tab., tax., verat., zinc.
almost - **ACON.,** aeth., agar., agn., am-c., aml-n., ant-t., ***apis, ars.,*** bell., **CAMPH.,** carb-o., chin., chlor., cic-m., coff-t., crot-h., cub., cyt-l., dig., digin., ferr., **GELS.,** glon., ham., hell., ***hydr-ac.,*** hydrc., ***ip.,*** kali-bi., ***lach., laur.,*** man., mang., ***merc.,*** merc-c., morph., ***naja,*** olnd., op., ox-ac., ph-ac.,

IMPERCEPTIBLE, pulse
almost - phos., plb., ***podo., puls., rhus-t., ric.,*** seneg., sol-n., sol-t., ***spong., stram., tab.,*** tere-ch., thea., ther., ***verat.,*** vip., zinc.
convulsions, during - olnd., nux-v.
stupor, during - hep.

INTERMITTENT - acet-ac., ***acon., aeth., agar.,*** agar-pa., aloe, alum., am-c., am-m., amyg., ang., ant-t., apis, ***apoc., arg-n.,*** arn., ***ars.,*** ars-h., ars-i., ars-s-f., asaf., ***atro., aur.,*** bapt., bell., benz-n., benz-ac., bism., brom., ***bry., cact.,*** calth., ***camph.,*** cann-i., ***canth., caps.,*** carb-ac., carb-an., ***carb-v., cedr.,*** **CHIN.,** chin-s., ***chlol.,*** chlor., cic-m., ***cimx.,*** cinnb., coff., ***colch., con.,*** conv., ***crat., crot-h.,*** cupr., cupr-ac., daph., **DIG.,** digin., digox., fago., ferr., ferr-m., frag., gast., ***gels.,*** glon., grat., ***hep.,*** hyos., hura, iber., ign., ***iber., iod.,*** jatr., juni., kali-bi., ***kali-c.,*** kali-chl., ***kali-i.,*** kali-m., kali-p., ***kalm.,*** keroso., ***kreos., lach.,*** lapa., ***laur., lil-t.,*** lipp., lob., ***lycps.,*** lyss., mag-p., meny., **MERC.,** ***merc-c.,*** merc-cy., merc-sul., meth-ae-ae., mez., morph., mur-ac., murx., naja, nat-a., **NAT-M.,** ***nit-ac.,*** nit-s-d., nitro-o., nux-m., nux-v., olnd., ***op., ox-ac.,*** **PH-AC.,** phos., phys., phyt., pip-n., plan., ***plb.,*** prun-v., ***ptel., ran-s., rhus-t.,*** sabin., ***samb.,*** scut., **SEC.,** ***sep., spig.,*** staph., ***stram., stroph.,*** stry., ***sulph.,*** sul-ac., ***tab., tarent.,*** ter., thea., thuj., trif-p., trinit., trom., verat., **VERAT-V.,** xan., ***zinc.,*** zinc-m., ***zinc-p.***
angina pectoris, in - phyt.
asthma thymicum, in - ***samb.***
bed, on going to, with weakness - ter.
carditis, in - ***carb-v.***
chronic - ***cact.***
chest trouble, in, after suppressed itch - ***hep.***
with tensive pains across - ***kali-i.***
collapse, with threatened - ***nat-m.***
delirium, in - amyg.
diarrhea, in - thuj.
dinner, after - nat-m.
diphtheria, in - ***kali-per., mur-ac., naja, nat-a.***
dysentery, in - colch.
dyspnea, from - ***phos.***
eight or ten minutes, every, after attack for weeks - ***dios.***
elderly people, in - tab.
endocarditis, in - ***aur.***
face ache, after - ***cocc-s.***
fear of death, they excite, so long - ***nux-m.***
frequently, with palpitation - ***sec.***
heart disease, in - ***ars.***
with acute darting pain in - lycps.
with sensation of constriction in - ***nat-m.***
hemiplegia, in - hydr-ac.
hemorrhoids, after operation for - ***croc.***
hydrocephalus acutus, in - ***dig.***
intervals, at - ***cact.***
stooping at - vario.
labor, during - ***chin-s.***
long interval, exciting fear of death - nux-m.
meningitis, in, and typhus - ***apis, verat.***

INTERMITTENT, pulse
menses, before - ***kali-c.***
metritis, in - sec.
metrorrhagia, in - croc.
morbus brightii, in - ***lycps.***
nosebleed, with - ***carb-v.***
omitted before single strong beat - aur.
palpitation, during - ***arg-m.***
pneumonia, in - ***ant-t., verat.,*** verat-v.
typhoid - ***ter.***
protracted, growing more - ***lach.***
rheumatism, in cardiac - ***cact.***
scarlatina, in malignant, or diphtheria - ***mur-ac.***
stroke, in - ***sep.***
typhoid, in - ***lyc., ter., zinc.***
typhus, in - ***apis, verat.***
uneven - ***merc-c.***
volume and rhythm, in - rhus-t.
waking at night, when - ars-h.
yellow fever, in - ***merc.***
intermittent, beats
every other beat - nat-m., ph-ac., ***spig.***
fifth beat - ars-h., ***chel., coca,*** crot-h., dig., nit-ac., ***nux-v.***
every, in heart disease - ***coca***
fifth or sixth stroke, missed every - chel.
fifty or sixty beats one omits, every, gradually oftener, evening fifth or sixth or third - ars-h.
fortieth to sixtieth beat - agar., ars-h.
fourth beat - ***apis, calc-ar.,*** cimic., dig., iber., **NIT-AC.,** ***nux-v., sulph.,*** tab.
or fifth beat, every - ***nux-v.***
one or two - ph-ac.
seventh beat - dig., ***mur-ac.***
seventeenth beat, every - ***cina***
single beats omit - ***stram.***
sixth beat - acon., ars-h., ***chel.,*** dig., ***mur-ac.***
suspending two or three beats each minute - cub.
tenth beat after exertion or vexation - gels.
to thirtieth beat - agar., ***cina,*** kali-m., lach.
third beat - ***apis,*** arum-t., ars-h., cimic., dig., iber., kali-c., ***mur-ac., nat-m.,*** nit-ac., phase., ***sulph.,*** vib.
every, in typhoid fever - **MUR-AC.**
third or fifth beat - crot-h., ***nit-ac.***
third or fourth beat - apis, ***cimic.,*** sulph.
third or fourth beat, every, in organic disease of heart - ***apis.***
third or seventh beat - dig., ***mur-ac.***
thirty or forty beats, after - agar.
twenty-fifth or thirtieth beat, every - kali-m.

IRREGULAR - acetan., ***acon.,*** acon-c., ***adon., adren.,*** aeth., ***agar.,*** agar-pa., agarin., aloe, alum., alum-p., am-caust., aml-n., anac., ang., anh., anil., **ANT-C.,** ant-t., antipyrin., antipyrin., apis, apoc., arg-m., ***arg-n.,*** arn., **ARS.,** ars-h., ***ars-i.,*** ars-s-f., arum-d., ***asaf., aspar., atro., aur.,*** aur-a., ***aur-s.,*** bapt., bar-ac., bar-c., bar-m., bell., bell-p., benz-n., benz-ac., bism., bol-lu., ***bry.,*** bufo, ***cact.,*** cael., calc., calen., camph., cann-i., cann-s., canth., ***caps.,*** carb-ac., carb-an., carb-v., carb-o., caust., cham., chel., **CHIN.,** chin-s., ***chlol.,*** chlor., chlorpr., chr-ac., ***cimic.,*** cimx., cina, clem., coff., coffin., ***colch., con., conv.,*** convo-s., cor-r., cortico., ***crat., crot-h.,*** cub., cupr., cupr-ac., cyt-l., **DIG.,** ***digin.,*** digox., dirc., dulc., euph., fago., ferr., ferr-m., ferr-p., form., ***gels.,*** gins., glon., guare., ham., hed., hell., ***hep.,*** hir., hist., home., ***hydr-ac., hyos., iber.,*** ign., iod., piloc., jatr., juni., ***kali-bi., kali-c.,*** kali-chl., kali-cy., ***kali-i.,*** kali-m., kali-n., kali-p., kali-s., ***kalm.,*** **LACH.,** lachn., laur., ***lil-t.,*** lob., lol., ***lycps.,*** mag-p., mag-s., manc., mang., meny., meph., ***merc., merc-c.,*** merc-cy., merc-i-f., merc-sul., mez., morph., ***mur-ac.,*** myric., ***naja,*** nat-a., nat-f., **NAT-M.,** nat-n., nat-s., nicc., nit-ac., nit-s-d., nux-m., nux-v., oena., ***olnd.,*** onop., ***op.,*** ox-ac., penic., **PH-AC.,** ***phase., phos.,*** phys., ***phyt.,*** pic-ac., piloc., pip-n., ***plan., plb.,*** prun-v., ptel., puls., **PYROG.,** rauw., ***rhus-t.,*** sabad., sabin., sac-alb., ***samb., sang.,*** sant., ***saroth.,*** **SEC.,** seneg., ***sep.,*** ser-ang., ***sil.,*** sol-n., sol-t-ae., ***spig., squil.,*** stann., ***still.,*** **STRAM.,** stroph., stroph-s., stry., stry-ar., stry-p., sul-ac., sul-h., sulfa., sulo-ac., ***sulph., sumb., tab.,*** tanac., tarent., tax., thea., thiop., thuj., trach., trif-p., ***tub.,*** uva., valer., ***verat.,*** **VERAT-V.,** vib., vip., vip-a., visc., wies., xan., yuc., zinc., zinc-m., ***zinc-p.***
accelerated, now, then slow, changing every few beats - ant-c.
angina pectoris, in - ***dig., tab.***
asthma thymicum, in - ***samb.***
bed, in going to, with weakness - ter.
beats, in strength of - zinc.
boring, with, in region of heart - still.
carditis, in - ***carb-v.***
cerebrospinal meningitis, in - ***glon.***
chest, with tensive pains across - ***kali-i.***
cholera, in - ***tab.***
coldness and insensibility, with - ***sang.***
delirium, with - ***verat.***
diarrhea, with - ***cupr-ac.***
epileptiform eclampsia, in - ***cedr.***
excitement in chest, with great, especially in cardiac region - ***phyt.***
exertion, on slight - ***arg-n.,*** meny., ***nat-m.***
fatty heart, with - kali-f.
fluttering, with - ***lil-t.***
forceps delivery, after - cact.
hemoptysis, in - ***dig.***
hard rapid and small beats, alternate - **NIT-AC.**
heart disease, in - ***ars.,*** op.
in organic disease of - ***apis***
in functional disturbance of - ***lach.***
with violent action of - glon.
hepatic disorder, in - sil.
hydrocephalus acute, in - ***cupr-ac.***
hydrocephaloid, in - ***carb-ac.***
hysteria, in - ***cedr.***
imperceptible - ***laur.***
influenza, in - chel.
intermittent - nat-m.
intermitting, yet full - gels.
left side, worse lying on - ***nat-m.***

IRREGULAR, pulse
lying down, on - lycps., still.
on back, while - arg-n.
on back, while, left side, on - ***nat-m.***
meningitis, in cerebrospinal - ***verat.***
morbus brightii, in - ***lycps.***
morning - caust.
normal, one, followed by two small rapid beats - ***nit-ac.***
nosebleed, with - ***kali-bi.***
palpitation, during - ***arg-m., cact.***
with, on going to bed - ter.
pendulum, like, of a clock placed obliquely, every other beat stronger - ars-h.
pleurodynia, in gouty - colch.
pneumonia, in typhoid - ***ter.***
quick, now, now slow - ***kali-c.***
rapid, sometimes, sometimes slow - mang.
retarded, some beats, felt for more than a second, followed by a few quicker beats - ars-h.
retinitis albuminurica, in - ***ars.***
rhythm, in, in angina pectoris - ox-ac.
in hypertrophy of heart - ***cact.***
scarlet fever, after, and in ascites - ***apoc.***
slow, and - acon., arn., ars., asaf., bell., camph., cann-i., chel., chin., cimic., colch., **DIG.,** dulc., ham., hell., hyos., iod., **KALM.,** laur., lob., merc-c., merc-cy., mez., ***naja,*** nit-ac., nux-v., olnd., op., ox-ac., plb., ph-ac., phys., phyt., rhus-t., seneg., sul-ac., tab., verat., **VERAT-V.,** zinc.
slow, then - ***sil.***
small - **DIG.**
soft, and, 60 to 68 - cact.
sputa, with brownish bloody - ***nit-ac.***
stool, after - ***agar.***
stroke, in - ***laur.***
study, effects of over - ***cupr-ac.***
sweat, with general - still.
thorax is violently contracted and expanded, while - ***mosch.***
typhoid, in - ***nit-ac., zinc.***
typhus, in abdominal - **STRAM.**
variable, with great rapidity - lyss.
weakness, with - sang.
yellow fever, in - **LACH.,** ***merc.***

IRRITABLE - agar., ant-t., arg-m., ars., bar-m., camph., chlol., colch., cupr-ar., dig., iod., kali-bi., meny., ox-ac., puls., stram., tab.
abscesses on neck, indicating return of - psor.
brain affection, in - ***cupr-m.***
bronchial and vesical catarrh, in - ***cop.***
conjunctivitis, in - sulph.
dysmenorrhea, in - tarent.
face pale now red, with, with sharp pointed nose - nux-v.
ovarian cyst, in - ***iod.***
smallpox, in - vario.

JERKING - acon., agar., aml-n., ***arn.,*** ars., arum-d., aur., bar-c., calad., canth., con., dig., digin., dulc., fago., gins., glon., **IBER.,** jatr., nat-m., nat-p., nux-v., plb., thuj.
hydrocephalus acute, in - ***dig.***
periodic - arg-m.
smaller, weaker, on rising from reclining position to sitting position - dig.

LABORED - crot-h., cupr., cupr-ac., hydr., iris, kreos., merc., merc-c., merc-i-f., mit., morph., op., stram.

LARGE - **ACON.,** ant-t., **APIS,** ***arn.,*** asaf., asar., atro., bar-c., **BELL.,** bism., ***bry.,*** camph., canth., cench., ***chel.,*** chin., chin-s., colch., coloc., **CON.,** ***cupr.,*** cupr-ac., dig., dulc., ferr., ferr-p., gels., glon., hell., hep., **HYOS.,** ign., **IOD.,** ip., jatr., kali-cy., **KALI-N.,** lach., led., lycps., manc., merc., mez., mosch., mur-ac., nat-m., nat-p., nux-v., olnd., op., par., petr., ph-ac., phos., plb., ran-b., ran-s., ***sabin.,*** samb., ***sep.,*** sil., ***spig.,*** spira., spong., **STRAM.,** stry., sul-ac., sulph., syph., ***tab.,*** verat., ***verat-v.,*** viol-o.
angina pectoris, in - ***aur-m.***
full, quick, not hard - ***gels.***
soft - ***gels.***

LIMPING - ars-h.

LOW, pulse (see Imperceptible) - colch., petr.
ailments, after disappointment - ph-ac.
almost ceases - ***ant-t.***
angina pectoris, in - ***tab.***
asiatic cholera, in, gradual extinction - ***hydr-ac.***
brain, in anaemia of - kali-br.
cardiac dropsy, in - ***dig.***
cholera, collapse in - ***ars-h.,*** **CAMPH.,** ***cupr-m.,*** sec., ***verat.***
cholera infantum, in - ***laur.,*** verat.
cholera morbus, in - ***jatr.***
coldness and collapse, with - kali-br.
colic, in, lumbago - ***coloc.***
collapsed - dulc., kali-p.
in stroke - puls.
complexion, with earthy - ***sil.***
diarrhea, with muco-purulent - kali-br.
diphtheria, in - ***merc-cy.***
in larynx - ***brom.***
enteritis, in - ter.
fainting, with - ***crot-h.***
feeble, in sunstroke - glon.
fever, after - **ANT-T.**
gastro malacia, in - ***kreos.***
gastritis mucosa, colic in - ***ars.***
bleeding, with - ***cinch.***
hemorrhoids, in - ***graph.***
limbs cold - ***kalm.***
liver, in cirrhosis of - ***sulph.***
meningitis, in - rhus-t.
menorrhagia, in - ***apoc.***
menses irregular - ***dig.***
menorrhagia, intermittent after, quick - ***gels.***
neuropathies, in - kali-a.
pneumonia, of, on seventh to ninth day - ***phos.***

LOW, pulse
prostration, with - ***ter.***
puerperal convulsions, in - nux-v.
respiration, with simperceptible - chlol.
scarlet fever, in - sulph.
spasm, in, following pneumonia and typhoid fever - nux-v.
stroke, in - ***laur.***
syncope, in - amyg.
tetanus, in - ***cic.***
typhoid, in - ***phos., zinc.***
typhus, in - ***camph.***
warmth of body, with - ***merc.***

QUICK - ammc., amyg., aml-n., anthro., ***ant-t.,*** ars-s-f., asaf., asar., asc-c., atro., bry., ***chel.,*** cocc., colch., ***coloc.,*** con., cop., corn., ***crot-h.,*** cupr-s., daph., ferr-p., ***gels.,*** glon., ***ham.,*** hyper., iod., ***lach.,*** lyss., ***mez.,*** olnd., ***op.,*** plb., rumx., ***sang., stram., tab.,*** vesp.
angina pectoris, in - ***aml-n., lyc.***
beat of heart, than - arn.
breathing, with anxious - ***op.***
carditis and cardiac rheumatism, in - ***cact.***
catarrh, in acute bronchial - ***kali-bi.***
cerebrospinal disease, in - verat-v.
cholera, in - ***ph-ac.***
consciousness, on recovering, afternoon - aster.
cough, in whooping - ***cor-r., verat.***
croup, in - ***phos.***
delirium tremens, in, first stage - ***kali-bi.***
diaphragmitis, in - ***dig.***
diphtheria, in - ***kali-br., nat-a., sulph.***
140 - ***apis.***
dysentery, in - ***merc-c.***
dysmenorrhea, in - tarent.
dyspepsia, in - ***dig.***
facial erysipelas, in - rhus-t.
feeble, and, during fever, at night - chin-b.
vomiting during pregnancy - ***cupr-ar.***
fever, in childbed - ***coloc.***
force lessened, but - coff-t.
gastritis, in acute, after taking cold - ***coloc.***
full - ***cimic.***
gastro malacia, in - ***kreos.***
head, with congestion of blood to, towards evening - ***croc.***
hard, small - ***acon.***
headache, with - corn.
in chlorotic - zinc.
in nervous - ***naja***
heart's beat, than - ***rhus-t.***
heart disease, in - **AUR.,** op.
heat at night, with - ran-s., raph.
and violent thirst, with, followed by general sweat mostly on forehead - ran-b.
hepatitis, in - ***ars., chion.***
hydrocephalus acutus, in - ***dig.***
intermittent fever, in - ***cedr.***
irritable - lyss.
irritation of cardiac nerves - ***coll.***
laryngitis, pharyngolaryngitis, in acute - ***naja***
lung affections, in - ***kali-n.***

QUICK, pulse
melaena, in - ***ham.***
meningitis, in incipient basilar - ***kali-br.***
menses irregular - ***dig.***
metrorrhagia, in - sabin.
moment, but varying every - ***kali-i.***
moved, when - apoc.
morning, in, 9 a.m. - trom.
night, during - sep.
nosebleeds, in - croc.
palpitation, with - ***cact.***
peritonitis, in - ***atro.***
pneumonia, in - ***cact., merc., phos.,*** puls., ***verat-v.***
scarlatina, in - ***apis, cupr-m.***
small, irregular - ***cupr-ac., glon.***
soft, irregular - ***gels.***
spasmodic - ***nux-v.***
stroke, in - **NUX-V.**
strong, and - asar.
supraorbital nerve, beginning of pain at exit of, diffused over forehead - ***lac-d.***
sweats, then - ***gels.***
throat and chest, with pains in - ***lac-c.***
tuberculosis, in incipient - ***lycps.***
typhoid, in - nux-v.
typhus, in - ***nit-ac.***
and ascites, in - ***apis***
unequal - cupr-m.
weak, but, with shooting stabbing in region of heart through to left scapula - ***kalm.***
whitlow, in - ***nit-ac.***
yellow fever, in - ***merc.***

ROLLING, under finger, requiring pressure in order to count - arum-d.

ROUND - bapt.

SENSIBLE, (see Feels)

SHARP - colch., rhus-t.
puerperal convulsions, in - stram.

SHORT - nit-s-d.

SLOW - ***abies-n.,*** acet-ac., achy., ***acon.,*** acon-c., acon-f., acon-l., adon., adren., aesc., aeth., aether, ***agar.,*** agar-cps., agar-pa., agn., ***all-c.,*** am-caust., aml-n., ***amyg.,*** anan., anh., anil., ant-c., ***ant-t.,*** apis, apoc., arn., ars., ars-m., ars-s-f., asaf., asc-t., ***aspar.,*** atro., bapt., bar-ac., bar-i., ***bell.,*** benz-n., benz-ac., **BERB.,** both., brom., cact., cahin., ***camph.,*** **CANN-I.,** ***cann-s., canth., caps.,*** carb-ac., carb-o., carb-s., catal., caust., cench., ***chel.,*** chin., ***chin-s.,*** chlor., chr-ac., cic., cimic., coca, coff-t., colch., coloc., ***con.,*** croc., ***crot-h.,*** cryp., cub., cund., ***cupr.,*** cupr-am-s., cur., cyt-l., daph., dat-f., delphin., **DIG.,** digin., digox., dirc., dub., dulc., eryt-j., esin., euph-c., eupi., fago., ferr., ferr-ma., gast., **GELS.,** gins., glon., grat., ham., ***hell.,*** helo., hep., hippoz., home., hydr., hydr-ac., hyos., ign., iod., iris, piloc., jac-c., jatr., juni., kali-bi., ***kali-br.,*** kali-c., kali-chl., kali-cy., kali-n., kali-s., **KALM.,** kreos., kres., lach., lachn., lact., lat-k., lat-m., ***laur., lob.,*** lon-x., ***lup.,*** lycpr., ***lycps.,*** mag-c., mag-s., ***manc., mang.,*** mec., meny., meph., merc., merc-c., merc-cy., merc-sul., meth-ae-ae., mez., ***morph.,*** mosch., mur-ac.,

SLOW - myric., ***myrt-c., naja,*** narcot., nat-a., nat-c., ***nat-m.,*** nat-n., nit-ac., nit-s-d., nitro-o., ***nux-m.,*** nux-v., oena., ol-an., olnd., **OP.,** ox-ac., par., pen., petr., ph-ac., phel., phos., phys., phyt., pic-ac., pip-n., pituin., plb., ***podo.,*** prop., prun., prun-p., puls., ran-b., raph., rauw., rhod., rhus-t., ruta, samb., ***sang.,*** sars., ***sec.,*** **SEP.,** sil., sol-n., **STRAM.,** stroph-s., stry., sulo-ac., sumb., ***tab.,*** tanac., ***tarent.,*** tax., thea., thiop., thuj., thymol., trif-p., trinit., trio., uva., upa., valer., **VERAT., VERAT-V.,** verb., vip., visc., wies., wye., zinc., zing.

30 - amyg., ***dios.***
40 - kali-br., ***kalm.,*** zinc.
40, about - plb.
45 - colch.
48 - lycps.
48, seven a.m. - chr-ac.
48, varied between, and 84, normal 52 - chr-ac.
50 - kali-br.
50, below - chr-ac.
50 to 60 - chin-s.
50 in morning, later 80 - astac.
52 - chr-ac.
52, in morning - ars-h.
55, afterwards 70, on eighth day, 92 - asc-t.
56 - bar-c.
56, in evening - ars-h.
58 - lycps.
58, in afternoon - chr-ac.
58 to 68 - lachn.
60 - agar., ars-m., asc-c., ***atro., crot-h.***
60 to 94 - iber.
60, in morning - ars-h.
60, in paralysis, with imbecility - ***anac-oc.***
60, below, in rest, above 120 after motion - **ARN.**
60, from 80 to, even to 47 - kreos.
60, after operation for hemorrhoids - ***croc.***
61 - sarac.
62 - ant-t.
62 to 64, in afternoon and evening - chr-ac.
64 - ars-h., med., vesp.
64 to 88 - asc-t.
64, in morning - ars-m.
65 - ***mosch.***
66 - sumb.
66, in purpura - led.
66, regular, feeble, sitting - aml-n.
67 to 70, in purpura hemorrhagica - ter.
68 - aphis., aster., sarac.
68, sitting - ***aml-n.***
80 to 64, fro - ***ars-i.***

afternoon - aloe, chin-s., gins., myric., ox-ac.
albuminuria intermitting, in - ***dig.***
alternating with, frequent pulse - bell., chin., cic., cimic., dig., ***gels.,*** iod., ***morph.,*** rhus-t., stroph.
anemia, in, 52 - carb-s.

SLOW, pulse
angina, in - ***dig.***
beat of heart, slower than - dulc., ***hell., verat.***
bounding, full and - visc.
cardialgia, in - phos.
cerebral disturbance, in, scarcely 60 - croc.
chill, during - ***hydr.,*** meny., mur-ac.
50 - brach.
cholera, in - ***jatr., hell., ip.***
colic, in - alum., op.
lead colic, in - ***alum.***
contracted, small - lact.
croup, in bronchial - ***ant-t.***
daytime, during - dulc., graph., mur-ac., sep.
and evening - ***graph.***
in forepart of - cinnb.
more frequent at night - ***mur-ac.***
in morning - agar.
diabetes, in - ***op.***
diarrhea, in, in typhus - ter.
intermittent fever, in - ***dig.***
diminishing rapidly - calen.
diphtheria, in - **BAPT.**
epidemic, in - ***lach.***
dropsy, general anasarca, in, 60 - ***naja***
intermittent fever, in - ***dig.***
dyspepsia, in - ***dig.***
eating, particularly after - chin-s.
evening - ars., cund., ***graph.,*** mez., myric., phyt., nat-a.
feeble - ***op.***
small - ***acon.***
fever, during - alum., lil-t., karw-h., pyrog.
after - **ANT-T.**
apyrexia, in - cinch.
bilious fever, in, 50 - ***crot-h.***
typhus, in - ***arn., stram.***
forenoon - cinnb., myric.
full - euph., lept.
hard, and - squil.
often, corresponding powerful beat of heart, sometimes intermittent and small - ***dig.***
headache, in - zinc.
heart beat, with violent - verat-v.
hurried, then - cub.
hydrocele, in - ***dig.***
hydrocephalus, in - ***apis, grat.***
hypertrophy with dilatation and aortic obstruction, with severe pain in cardiac region - ***kalm.***
insanity, in - ***hyos.***
intermittent fever, in - ***acon., gels.***
less than 50 - ***nat-m.***
or stroke - ***chin-s.***
irregular, with fainting - **DIG.**
jaundice, in - ***phos.***
liver problems or hepatitis, in - dig., ***mag-m.***
lying, in - dig.
mania, during first part of attack of - tarent.
meningitis, in - verat.
at first, later frequent and soft - ***gels.***

SLOW, pulse
menses, during - ars-m.
metrorrhagia, in - ***hyos.***
after confinement - ***ip.***
morning - arg-m., chin-s., grat., jac-c., lycps., myric., olnd., petr., ran-b., sars., thuj., zinc.
nephralgia, in - op.
nephritis, in desquamative - plb.
neuralgia, with - kalm.
48 - ***kalm.***
night - phys.
nymphomania, in - ***dig.***
paralysis, in, with imbecility - ***anac-oc.***
pneumonia, in - ***verat-v.***
poisoning by foul breath, in - ***anthr.***
pregnancy, during, small - ***gels.***
puberty, at - dig.
quick, changing from - ars-h.
or too, not in relation to temperature - alum., graph., lil-t., pyrog., vario.
rest, during - petr.
scarlatina, in, 50 - rhus-t.
shock, in - dig., hyper., op.
54 - ***hyper.***
sinks to forty beats - cann-i., cann-s., naja, plb.
slower than the beat of heart - agar., cann-s., ***dig.,*** dulc., hell., **KALI-I.,** ***kali-n.,*** kres., laur., lyc., nat-m., sec., verat.
sluggish - ***gels.***
68 - kali-m.
small, feeble, 62 - lac-ac.
in stroke - ***laur.***
snoring, with - ***op.***
soft, regular, 66 - aesc.
spasm, in, from fright - ***cupr-m.***
stroke, in - ***arn., op.***
after, weak, small - ***cupr-m.***
congestive - ***verat-v.***
50 to 60 - ***plb.***
sluggish - **NUX-V.**
taste, with flat - merc-sul.
tetanus, in - ***cic.***
vertigo, with - ther.
worse standing than sitting, going off when lying - ***petr.***
vomiting, between attacks of - ***apoc.***
vomiting, on - squil.
vomiting, with - squil., ***verat-v.***
waking, on - ther.
weak - agn., **DIG.**
after typhoid - ***hell.***
hydrocephalus, in - ***dig.***
trembling - ***merc.***

SMALL - **ACON.,** acon-s., aeth., aether, ***agar.,*** agar-pa., agro., ail., ald., alco., alum., am-c., am-caust., ammc., amyg., ant-c., ant-m., ***ant-t.,*** apis, apoc., arn., **ARS.,** ars-h., ***ars-i.,*** ars-s-f., arum-d., asaf., asc-t., aspar., aster., atro., ***aur.,*** aur-a., ***aur-m., aur-s.,*** bar-c., bar-i., bar-m., ***bell.,*** benz-n., benz-ac., bism., bol-lu., bry., caj., calad., calc., calth., **CAMPH.,** cann-i., cann-s., canth., carb-ac., carb-an., **CARB-V.,** carb-h., catal., ***cham.,*** **CHEL.,** ***chin., chin-a.,*** chin-s., ***chlor.,*** cic., ***cina,*** clem., coca, ***cocc.,*** cod., coff., ***colch., coloc., con.,*** coni., cop., croc., ***crot-h.,*** crot-t., cub., cund., **CUPR.,** cupr-ar., cupr-s., cyt-l., delphin., **DIG.,** digin., ***dulc.,*** euph-l., ferr., ferr-m., fl-ac., frag., gels., glon., graph., grat., **GUAI.,** gymn., haem., ***hell.,*** helo., hippoz., hydr-ac., ***hyos.,*** iber., ign., ***iod.,*** ip., juni., kali-a., kali-bi., ***kali-br., kali-c.,*** kali-chl., kali-cy., kali-fer., kali-i., kali-m., kali-n., ***kali-p.,*** kali-s., keroso., ***kreos.,*** lac-ac., ***lach.,*** led., **LAUR.,** lil-t., ***lob.,*** lyc., ***lycps.,*** mang., meny., ***merc.,*** merc-br., merc-c., merc-cy., merc-d., ***merc-p-r.,*** merc-n., merc-sul., meth-ae-ae., ***mez.,*** morph., mosch., ***mur-ac.,*** naja, narcot., nat-br., nat-m., nat-n., nat-s., nit-ac., nit-s-d., ***nux-m.,*** nux-v., oena., ***ol-j.,*** olnd., ***op.,*** ox-ac., past., peti., petr., ***ph-ac., phos.,*** phys., phyt., pic-ac., ***plat.,*** plb., plumbg., podo., prun., prun-p., ptel., puls., ran-a., ran-b., ran-s., ***raph.,*** rhod., rhus-t., ric., rumx-a., russ., ruta, sabad., sal-ac., ***samb., sang.,*** sarr., **SEC.,** seneg., serp., **SIL.,** sol-n., sol-t., sol-t-ae., solin., spig., spirae., spong., squil., ***stann.,*** staph., **STRAM.,** stroph., stry., ***sul-ac., sulph.,*** tab., tanac., ***tarent.,*** tax., ***ter.,*** thea., thuj., til., tub., upa., uva., valer., **VERAT.,** vesp., viol-o., vip., visc., wies., zinc., ***zinc-m., zinc-p.,*** zinc-s.
accelerated - **AUR.,** cahin., ferr-m., glon.
ascites, in - **APIS**
and hydrothorax, in - apoc.
asthma millari, in - ***cupr-m., samb.***
bleeding of lungs, in - ***ip.***
blennorrhea, cysto-blenorrhea, in - uva.
brain, in inflammation of - puls.
bronchial catarrh, in acute - ***kali-bi.***
chest affection, in after miscarriage - ***nux-m.***
with great excitement in, especially in heart region - ***phyt.***
childbirth, after - ***crot-h.***
chill in evening, with shaking - ox-ac.
cholera, in - verat.
cholera infantum, in - coff-t.
sporadic, in - ***tab.***
colic and lumbago, in - ***coloc.***
confinement, after - ***lyc.***
convulsions, epileptic, in - aeth.
cough and typhus, in - ***bapt.***
counted, could not be - **CUPR-M.**
croup, in - ***brom., phos.***
debility, with general, in metritis and peritonitis puerperalis - **TER.**
delirium, in - ***phos.***
delirium tremens, in - ***coff.,*** **STRAM.**
depressed - acal.
diabetes, in - uran-n.
diphtheria, in - ***chin-a., crot-h.,*** lac-c., ***lach., merc-cy., mur-ac., sul-ac.***
after failure of phyt. and lyc. - ***lac-c.***
of lips - rhus-t.
dropsy, in - ***aur-m.***

SMALL, pulse
dysentery, in - ***merc-c.***
chronic - nux-v.
erysipelas, in - sulph.
evening, particularly in - ***iod.***
feeble, with cold face - ***merc-c.***
fever, in intermittent - ***ars., cocc.***
in puerperal - puls.
frequent, in affection of liver, with dropsy - fl-ac.
hard - camph.
headache, in chlorotic - zinc.
nervous, in - ***naja***
heart disease, in - ***cact., lach.,*** op.
and circulation, with great excitement of - ***ran-b.***
pain, in - stram.
region, with severe pain in - ***kalm.***
hyperaesthesia, in cardiac - ***ign.***
hepatized left lung, in - ***camph.***
imperceptible, almost - cupr-m.
influenza, in, diarrhea of children and pneumonia - ***ant-t.***
insanity, in - nux-v., verat-v.
intermittent, in - grat.
in croup - ***carb-v.***
with cold skin - ***merc-c.***
intermitting, irregular - ***acon.***
irregular, rapid - lyss.
labor, in - ***coff-t.***
left - kali-chl.
liver, in affection of - ***mag-m.***
inflammation of - cocc.
meningitis, in - ***ant-t., sulph.***
menses, during - ***croc.***
menopause, during - murx.
nephritis, in desquamative - plb.
neuralgia, in - ***cham.***
in uterine - chin-s., nux-v.
neuropathies, in - kali-a.
night-watching, after, and mental disturbance during pregnancy - puls.
nosebleeds, in - ***carb-v., kali-bi.,*** **SEC.**
orgasm of blood, with - kreos.
pain, though, suddenly abates - ***nit-ac.***
palpitation, with - ***cact.***
hysterical - ***nux-m.***
parkinson's disease, in - rhus-t.
peritonitis, in - ***atro., verat.***
pleuritis, in, with plastic exudation - ***hep.***
pleurodynia, in - ran-b.
pneumonia, in - ***ant-t., kali-c., phos.,*** puls.
quick, after working in sun - ***glon.***
and, in cystitis - ***hell.***
scarlatina, in - ***cupr-m.***
sitting, when - ***aml-n.***
slow, 60 - camph.
anasarca, in - ***hell.***
soft - ***cupr-ac.***
spinal irritation, in - ***chin-s.***

SMALL, pulse
stomach, in ulcer of - mez.
with cramp in - ***coch.***
sweat, with cold - calad.
synanche cellularis, in - anthr.
thread like, in heart disease - ***ferr-m.***
pneumonia, in - ***dig.***
tuberculosis, in - ***guai.***
typhoid fever, in - ***lach., ter., zinc.***
typhus, in - ***agar., arg-n., camph.,*** zinc.
unconsciousness, sudden - ***cocc.***
uneven - ***cham.***
vomiting of bile, with - bism.
weak - ***glon.,*** gymn., merc-sul., plat.
and frequent - camph.
and slow - ***lob.***
in peritonitis - ***lyc.***
intermittent, uneven - ***ferr.***
with sudden rise of temperature during desquamative stage of scarlet fever - ***lyc.***
whooping cough, in - ***verat.***
wiry, in hydrothorax - ***hell.***

SOFT - acal., acet-ac., ***acon.,*** aesc., aeth., aether, agar., agn., ant-c., ant-s., **ANT-T.,** anth., apis, apoc., arn., ***ars.,*** ars-h., arum-d., aspar., aster., atro., ***aur.,*** bapt., bar-c., bar-m., bell., bism., bry., calc-ar., calc-i., camph., cann-i., cann-s., canth., ***carb-ac.,*** **CARB-V.,** carb-o., carb-s., cham., chin., ***chlor.,*** cic., cit-l., cocc., ***coffin., colch.,*** con., conv., crot-h., cub., **CUPR.,** cupr-s., cyt-l., **DIG.,** digin., digox., dulc., ery-a., euph., ferr., ferr-m., ***ferr-p., gels.,*** glon., ***guai.,*** ham., hell., hep., hydr-ac., hyos., iber., iod., ip., piloc., jal., jatr., juni., kali-bi., kali-c., kali-chl., kali-cy., ***kali-m.,*** kali-n., ***kalm.,*** kreos., lac-ac., **LACH.,** lat-m., laur., ***lob.,*** lyc., ***lycps., manc.,*** mang., ***merc.,*** merc-cy., mez., morph., **MUR-AC.,** ***naja,*** narcot., nat-a., nat-m., nat-n., nitro-o., nux-v., oena., ***ol-j.,*** olnd., **OP.,** ***ox-ac.,*** ph-ac., ***phos.,*** phys., phyt., ***plat.,*** plb., polyp-p, puls., ran-s., rhod., rhus-t., ***sang.,*** sant., sec., seneg., sil., sin-n., sol-n., ***spig.,*** spirae., **STRAM.,** stry., sul-ac., ***sulph., sumb.,*** syph., ***tab.,*** tarax., **TER.,** thuj., toxi., trio., uva., valer., **VERAT.,** ***verat-v.,*** vip., zinc., zinc-m.
angina pectoris, in - phyt.
blennorrhoea, cysto-blenorrhoea, in - uva.
breath, in poisoning by foul - ***anthr.***
chest affection, in, after miscarriage - ***nux-m.***
chlorosis, in - sep.
cholera, in - ***jatr.***
compressible, in typhoid pneumonia - ***sang.***
consumption, in - ***guai.***
diphtheria, in - ***brom.***
scarcely perceptible - ***crot-h.***
dyspepsia, in - ruta
fever, in intermittent - ***ars.***
full - ***gels.***
headache, in - zinc.
heart, hyperesthesia, in - ***ign.***
heat at night, with - ran-s.
and violent thirst, followed by general sweat, mostly on forehead - ran-b.

SOFT, pulse
insanity, in - ***hyos.***
irregular, with palpitation - ***puls.***
lumbago, in - kali-c.
measles, before, in repercussion - ***lach.***
metrorrhagia, in - sabin.
paralysis agitans, in - rhus-t.
pneumonia senilis, in, quick, occasionally slow - ***ferr.***
typhoid, in - ***sang.***
quick - ***laur.***
sitting, when, in hypochondriasis - ***arg-n.***
slow, intermittent - ***hell.***
trembling, in yellow fever - ***merc.***
typhus, in - crot-h.
and albuminuria, in - ***apis***
uremia, in, asphyctic form - ***hydr-ac.***
vertigo, with cardiac - crot-h.
weak - aesc.
weakness, with general, worse in back part of neck - cact.
yellow fever, in - ***merc.***

SOUND, audible - ***glon.***
whistling, in heart disease - ***ars.***
whizzing - kali-p.

SPASMODIC - ***ang.,*** arn., ars., bism., carb-s., chin., **COCC.,** cupr., cupr-ac., ***dig.,*** indg., iod., kali-bi., merc., ***merc-c.,*** nux-m., nux-v., plb., sabad., ***sec.,*** sep., ***stram.,*** zinc., zinc-s.
asthma millari, in - ***cupr-m.***
headache, in - ***carb-s.***
measles, in - ***verat.***

STRONG - achy., acon., aether, agar., agar-pa., alco., aloe, am-c., aml-n., amyg., ant-t., apis, arn., ars., ars-h., ars-i., asar., aster., aza., ***bell.,*** bism., ***bry.,*** caj., cann-i., canth., catal., chel., chin., chin-a., cinnb., coca, con., crot-t., ***cupr.,*** dig., fago., ferr-p., gast., gels., gins., hell., hoit., hydrc., hyos., iber., iod., jatr., ***kali-m.,*** kreos., lach., lappa-a., laur., lycps., ***merc.,*** merc-c., merc-cy., merc-i-r., mill., morph., nat-s., op., par., paro-i., petr., **PH-AC.,** phys., ***puls.,*** ran-b., raph., sabad., **SABIN.,** sang., sarr., seneg., serp., sium, sol-t-ae., **SPIG.,** stram., stront-c., stry., tanac., ter., uva., valer., ***verat.,*** **VIOL-O.**
stroke, in - ***arn.***
chest and throat, with pain in - ***lac-c.***
with pulsation in upper part of, at night in bed - cact.
dysentery, in - ***caps.***
erysipelas, in phlegmonous - verat-v.
fever, typhus, in - ***apis***
full, hard - **ACON.**
hard - ***led.***
heart disease, in - op.
intermittent, in yellow fever - ***merc.***
pneumonia, in - ***lach., verat-v.***
slow - ***spig.***

SYNCHRONOUS, not synchronous between larger arteries - ***dig.***
disagrees with heart sounds - ars.
femoral beats faster than radial - ***ham.***

SYNCHRONOUS, pulse
head, crackling in one side, synchronous with pulse, particularly in morning and in open air, better indoors - ***coff.***
heart stroke, not synchronous with - ***apis,*** aur., ***dig.,*** kali-m., pyrog., spig.

TENSE - acon., adren., agro., all-c., all-s., am-c., ***am-m.,*** ammc., ***ant-t.,*** aphis., ars., atro., bell., benz-n., bism., **BRY.,** cann-i., camph., canth., cham., chel., chin., clem., coca, coff-t., colch., con., corn-f., ***cupr.,*** dig., **DULC.,** ferr., hyos., kali-i., merc-c., ***mez.,*** morph., nat-c., nit-ac., ox-ac., petr., plb., sabad., **SABIN.,** sang., sec., sol-t-ae., spira., squil., stram., til., ***valer.,*** verat., verat-v., zinc.
colic, in - op.
hard, in carditis and cardiac rheumatism - ***cact.***
intermittent, in - ***cocc.***
measles, in, with pneumonic symptoms - ***cupr-m.***
neuralgia, in - ***cham.***
night, especially at - dulc.
perimyelitis, in - sep.
pleuro-pneumonia biliosa, in - rhus-t.
turned and twisted evenings, as if - ars-h.
whitlow, in - ***nit-ac.***

THIN, dysmenorrhea, in - ***graph.***
erysipelas, in - sulph.
tobacco poisoning, in - nux-v.

THREADY - acon., agar-pa., ***ail.,*** alum., aml-n., amyg., ***apis,*** arn., ***ars.,*** ars-s-f., ars-s-r., bell., camph., canth., carb-v., carb-h., chlf., colch., cop., crat., **COLCH.,** ***crot-h.,*** cupr., **DIG.,** digin., hell., ***hydr-ac.,*** hyos., iod., jatr., kali-bi., kali-n., lach., **LAT-M.,** merc-c., merc-n., morph., naja, nat-f., olnd., op., ox-ac., petr., ***phos.,*** phys., phyt., ***plat.,*** plb., ptel., ***pyrog.,*** raja-s., rhus-t., sal-ac., sant., sec., sol-t-ae., solin., ***spig.,*** stram., sul-ac., sulph., tab., tax., ***ter.,*** **VERAT.,** verat-v., ***verb.,*** vip., ***zinc.,*** zinc-m.
anxiety, with - ***acon.***
asphyxia, in - ***ant-t.***
bleedings, in - ***sec.***
catarrh, in acute - ***ant-t.***
cholera, in - ant-t.
colic, in - alum., ***hell.***
diarrhea, during, 65 - asc-t.
diphtheria, in - ***merc-cy., naja***
of lips, in - rhus-t.
intermittent fever, in - ***cinch.***
tertian, in - ***lach.***
typhus, in - ***bapt.,*** zinc.
hematemesis, in - **ARS.**
heart disease, in - op.
carditis, in, and cardiac rheumatism - ***cact.***
beating, not, but like a thread quickly pulled through artery, in cardiac rheumatism - spig.
liver complaint, in - ***phos.***
measles, in, with pneumonia symptoms, 100 - ***cupr-m.***
meningitis, after - ***cupr-m.***
nosebleed, in - **SEC.**

THREADY, pulse
pneumonia, in typhoid - ***phos.***
prostration, with - ***ter.***
scarlet fever, in - ***zinc.***
after - **ACON.**
shock, in - ***hydr-ac.***
injuries, from - ***lach.***

THRILL, peculiar, under finger - **IBER.**

THUMPING - ***nux-v.***

TREMULOUS - acon., ambr., **ANT-T.,** apis, ***ars., bell.,*** **CALC.,** camph., cann-i., canth., carb-ac., ***cic.,*** cina, cinnb., cocc., colch., ***crot-h.,*** dig., fago., gels., gins., ***hell., iber.,*** iod., kali-c., ***kreos.,*** lach., merc., ***merc-c.,*** merc-sul., nat-m., nux-m., op., ox-ac., phos., plat., plb., ***rhus-t.,*** ruta, ***sabin., sep.,*** **SPIG.,** ***staph., stram.,*** sul-ac., valer.
cholera, in - ant-t.
and bronchial catarrh, in - **ANT-T.**
cough, in - ant-t.
dropsy, in - ***ars.***
dyspepsia, in - ***dig.***
eating, after - ***calc.***
hematemesis gastritis, in - ***ars.***
meningitis, in - rhus-t.
night - ***calc.***
overworking, from - agar.
paroxysm, at close of - chin-s.
tetanus, in - ***cic.***
typhoid fever, in - **CALC.,** crot-h.
yellow fever, in- ***merc.***

TUMULTUOUS, with tensive pains across chest - ***kali-i.***

UNCHANGED - asim., clem.
delirium, in - amyg.
irritation of cardiac nerves, in - ***coll.***
mucous irritation, in, et morbus medicinalis - ***hydr.***

UNDULATING - agar., amyg., ***ars.,*** camph., carb-ac., carb-o., chlf., crot-h., dig., digin., gins., iber., op., plb.
anasarca, in - ***ars.***
measles, in repercussion of - ***lach.***
wavy - ***crot-h.***
waves, in long, in convulsions - ***zinc.***
weak - camph.

UNEQUAL - agar., ars-m., ***calc.,*** cinch., con., cupr-m., ***kali-c., lach.,*** lyss., mang., ***op.,*** sabin., thlaspi
angina pectoris, in - ***lyc.***
catarrh of a child, in - ***ant-t.***
cyanosis, in - ***dig.***
hysteria, in - ***hyos.***
weak - ***cham.***

VARIABLE - ant-t., ***canth.,*** colch., ***cupr-m., glon., ign.,*** nat-a., ***nit-ac.,*** olnd., ***op.,*** plb., ***spig., stram.,*** zinc.
heart distress in night, with - arn.
inflammation of diaphragm, in - morph.
meningitis, in - ***apis***
shifts according to phantoms which offer themselves to her imagination - ***hyos.***
tuberculosis, in - ***kali-c.***

VARIABLE, pulse
typhoid fever, great and sudden changes in - ***verat-v.***
typhus, in - ***bapt.***
and scarlatina, in - ***apis***

VIBRATING - amyg.
pneumonia, in - ***cact.***
typhoid, in - ***sang.***

WEAK, pulse - acet-ac., ***acon.,*** acon-f., ***adon.,*** adren., aesc., aeth., aether, agar., agar-cps., agar-em., ***agarin.,*** **AGN.,** ail., ald., aloe, alum-p., am-caust., am-m., amyg., ampe-qu, ***ant-a.,*** ant-c., ant-m., **ANT-T.,** anth., apis, apoc., apom., ***arn.,*** **ARS.,** ars-h., ***ars-i.,*** ars-s-f., arum-d., asaf., asc-c., ***aspar.,*** aster., ***atro.,*** **AUR.,** aur-a., aur-m., ***aur-s.,*** aza., bapt., **BAR-C.,** bar-m., bar-s., bell., benz-ac., **BERB.,** bism., bry., buth-a., ***cact.,*** caj., calad., **CAMPH.,** cann-i., **CANN-S.,** ***canth.,*** carb-ac., carb-an., **CARB-V.,** carbn-chl., carb-o., cass., catal., cedr., cench., ***cham.,*** chen-a., ***chin.,*** chin-s., ***chin-a.,*** chlol., chlor., **CIC.,** cimic., ***cimx.,*** coca, ***cocc.,*** cod., coff., coff-t., colch., coll., ***coloc.,*** con., coni., ***conv., crat.,*** **CROT-H.,** crot-t., cub., ***cupr., cupr-ac.,*** cupr-ar., cycl., cyt-l., ***dig.,*** digin., digox., dios., diph., dirc., dor., erio., ery-a., eryt-j., fago., fagu., ferr., ***ferr-m.,*** gast., **GELS.,** ***glon.,*** guai., ham., hell., ***hydr-ac.,*** hydrc., hyos., hyosin., iber., ***ign., iod., ip.,*** iris, jasm., jatr., juni., kali-ar., ***kali-bi., kali-br., kali-c.,*** kali-chl., ***kali-n.,*** kali-x., kali-t., ***kalm.,*** keroso., kreos., lac-ac., ***lac-c.,*** **LACH.,** lact., lat-k., ***lat-m.,*** **LAUR.,** lil-t., lob., lyc., ***lycps., lyss., manc.,*** mang., ***merc., merc-c., merc-cy.,*** merc-i-f., merc-n., merc-p-r., merc-sul., mez., mom-b., morph., ***mosch., mur-ac.,*** **NAJA,** narcot., nat-f., nat-m., nit-ac., nit-s-d., ***nux-m.,*** nux-v., oena., olnd., op., ox-ac., past., peti., **PH-AC.,** ***phase., phos.,*** phys., phyt., **PLAT.,** plb., plumbg., podo., polyp-p, prop., psor., ***puls.,*** pyrog., raja-s., rhod., ***rhus-t.,*** rhus-v., ric., rumx-a., sabin., sac-alb., sal-ac., sal-p., ***sang.,*** sant., sapin., ***sapo., sec.,*** seneg., sep., sil., sol-t-ae., solin., ***spig.,*** spira., spong., ***staph., still., stram.,*** stront-c., stry., sul-ac., sul-h., sulo-ac., ***sulph.,*** sumb., ***tab.,*** tanac., ***tarent.,*** tart-ac., tax., ter., tere-ch., thea., ***thuj.,*** thymol., ***thyr.,*** trif-p., upa., ***ust.,*** uva., ***valer., vario., verat., verat-v.,*** verb., vesp., vip., vip-a., visc., xan., zinc., ***zinc-m.,*** zinc-p., zinc-s., zing.
accelerated, in stroke and old age - ***bar-c.***
anasarca, in - chlol.
angina pectoris, in - ***dig.,*** phyt.
apyrexia, in - cinch.
blood, with great want of - ***mosch.***
breathing, with quick labored - crot-h.
bronchial catarrh, in - **ANT-T.**
cardialgia, in - stram.
children, in - ***ant-t.***
chlorosis, in - ***ferr., ip.***
cholera, in - ***jatr., tab.,*** verat.
sporadic - tab.
second stage - ***cupr-m.***
cholerine, in - ***aeth.***
beginning to fall - ***ferr.***

WEAK, pulse

coldness, with, and collapse - dor.
colic, in - ***iris***
cough, in - ant-t.
cough and typhus, in - ***bapt.***
croup, in - ***brom.***
delirium tremens, in - stram.
depressed - ars-s-r.
diabetes mellitus, in - kali-br.
diarrhea, chronic - ***coloc.***
diphtheria, in - ***crot-h., kali-per., lach., merc-cy., nat-a.,*** **PHYT.,** ***sul-ac.***
dropsy, in - ***aur-m.***
dysentery, in - ***ars., merc-c.***
chronic, in - nux-v.
flatulent indigestion, in - ***lyc.***
dyspepsia, in - ***dig.***
dyspnea, in - ***cact.***
eating, after - dios.
erysipelas, in - rhus-t.
faint - ***carb-v., rhus-t.***
fainting, in - ***camph., laur.***
fever, during, afternoon - chin-b.
bilious - ***crot-h.***
intermittent - polyp-p, puls.
nervous, sinking - ***camph.***
intermittent, in, small, scarcely perceptible during apyrexia - ***ferr.***
typho-malaria, in, 140, from twentieth day - ***ham.***
typhoid, in - nux-v., ***zinc.***
rapidly sinking - anthr.
typhus, in - ***apis, bapt.,*** crot-h.
frequent, irregular - ***ail.***
gonorrhoea, after - ***camph.***
heart disease, in - ***cact., lach.,*** op.
cardiac distress, in, in night - arn.
cardiac rheumatism, in - ***cact.,*** spig.
dilated heart, in - ***tab.***
pericarditis, in - spig.
fatty, with - kali-f., phos.
hepatic disorder, in - ***chion., mag-m., phos.,*** sil.
hydrothorax, in - ***apoc.***
indistinct, in dropsy, after scarlatina - ***apis***
influenza, in - eup-per., gels.
labor, during - ***chin-s.***
lungs, in paralysis of - ***mosch.***
melancholy, with, and jealousy - ***kali-a.***
meningitis, in - verat.
cerebrospinal, hardly perceptible, in - ***gels.***
sinking - ***stram.***
menorrhagia, in - ***apoc.,*** croc., ***verat.***
when moved - apoc.
morning, in - cimic., olnd., sep., thuj.
motion, on - bar-s.
old age, in - ***aur.***
orgasm of blood, with - kreos.
overworking, from - agar.
palpitation, with - cinch.
hysterical, in - ***nux-m.***

WEAK, pulse

paroxysm, at close of - chin-s.
perceptible, scarcely - puls.
peritonitis, in - ***coloc.***
phlegmasia alba dolens, in - ***nat-s.***
pleurodynia, in - ran-b.
pneumonia, in - ***sulph.***
hepatization stage - phos.
typhoid - ***phos.***
quick - ***crot-h.***
after pain in abdomen - ***ham.***
and intermittent - lyss.
quicker, gradually weaker and, 120 to 180, especially after paroxysms - lyss.
quickly, in renal colic - ***dios.***
regular - plan.
dropsy and hectic fever, in - ***eup-pur.***
rheumatism, in acute - colch.
scarlatina, in - zinc.
scarlet fever, after - apoc.
sexual debility, in - ***dig.***
shock from injuries, in, dying away - chlf., ***lach.***
of injury, as if dying - chlf.
sighing, with occasional deep - hell.
silver nitrate of, after injecting, for gonorrhea - tarent.
sinking - bism., chlol., euph.
sitting - ***aml-n.***
slow - cupr-m., glon.
in tertian intermittent - ***dig.***
small - acet-ac.
chlorosis, in - ***abrot.***
emansio mensium, in - ***dig.***
spine, in concussion of - ***hyper.***
stool, after, subdued - caust.
with watery - jal.
stroke, in, and typhus - ***arn.***
study, effect of over - ***cupr-ac.***
sunstroke, in - ***glon.***
tetanus, in - ***cic.***
thread like, almost imperceptible, in bleeding - ***ham.***
tobacco poisoning, in - nux-v.
tuberculosis, in - ***ars-i.,*** samb., stann.
incipient, in - ***lycps.***
vertigo, with cardiac - crot-h.
vomiting, after - aloe, asc-c.
with bilious - ***crot-h.***

WIRY - amyg., ars., benz-n., bol., cupr., cupr-ac., dig., gels., ***glon.,*** ham., iber., kreos., ***lac-c., lycps.,*** oena., ox-ac., phos., phys., sec., tax., ter., zinc.
ascites, in, and gastro-enteritis - ***apis***
cerebrospinal disease, in - verat-v.
corded - ammc.
meningitis, in incipient basilar - ***kali-br.***
pleuro-pneumonia, in - seneg.
pneumonia, in - ***lach.***
stroke, in - ***plb.***

Rectum

ABSCESS - ***calc., calc-s., hep., merc.,*** paeon., rhus-t., ***sil.,*** syph., thuj.
just below the coccyx - ***paeon.***

APHTHOUS, anus, condition of - ***bapt., bor.,*** bry., ***kali-chl., merc., merc-c., merc-d, mur-ac., nit-ac., sulph.,*** **SUL-AC.**

BALL, sensation of, (see Lump) - ***sep.***

BITING, pain - agar., alum., ambr., bar-c., canth., caps., carb-v., caust., chin., dulc., hell., kali-c., lach., led., lyc., merl., mez., nat-c., nux-v., ph-ac., phos., rhod., sabin., sep., ***sulph.***
worms, as from - cinch-b.

BLACK- merc-c.

BLEEDING, from anus and rectum - acal., acet-ac., **ACON.,** ***aesc.,*** agar., ***aloe,*** alum., ***alumn.,*** ambr., ***am-c.,*** am-m., anac., ***ant-c., apis,*** arn., **ARS.,** asar., aur., aur-m., bapt., **BAR-C.,** bar-m., ***bell.,*** berb., ***bism., bor.,*** bufo, **CACT., CALC.,** calc-f., ***calc-p., calc-s.,*** camph., ***canth., caps.,*** carb-an., ***carb-s., carb-v.,*** card-m., carl., **CASC.,** caust., ***cham., chin.,*** chin-a., chin-s., chlor., chr-ac., ***cinnam.,*** cob., cocaine, ***cocc.,*** **COLL.,** coloc., **CROT-H.,** cupr., ***cycl.,*** dios., elaps, elat., ***erig., eug., ferr.,*** ferr-ar., ferr-m., ferr-p., ***fic., fl-ac., graph.,*** **HAM.,** ***hep.,*** hydr., hyper., ***hyos., ign., ip., kali-ar., kali-bi., kali-c., kali-chl.,*** kali-i., kali-m., kali-n., kali-p., ***kali-s.,*** **LACH.,** led., ***lept.,*** lob., **LYC.,** lyss., manc., med., ***merc., merc-c., mill.,*** morg., morg-g., ***mur-ac.,*** **NAT-M.,** ***nat-s.,*** **NIT-AC.,** ***nux-m.,*** **NUX-V.,** op., paeon., ph-ac., **PHOS.,** ***phyt.,*** plat., ***podo.,*** **PSOR.,** ***puls.,*** pyrog., ***rat.,*** rhus-t., rhus-v., ***ruta.,*** sabin., scroph-n., ***sep.,*** sil., stram., sul-ac., **SULPH.,** ter., thlaspi, thuj., valer., verat., yohim, zinc.
afternoon - sulph.
amel. - aesc.
black - aloe, alumn., ant-c., colch., crot-h., ***ham.,*** hydr., kali-m., merc-c., ***sec., sulph.***
liquid - elaps.
strings - croc.
bright - caust.
clotted - am-m., nat-m., stram.
large - alum., alumn.
congestion to head, with - calc.
constant in drops, no blood with stool - cob., puls.
coryza, during - ***calc.***
dark - alum.
evening alum., calc., sulph.
stool, during - calc.
exertion, after - berb.
exhausting, slight - hydr.
flatus, during emission of - ***phos.***
meat scraping, as if - am-m.
menses, during - am-c., ***am-m.,*** ars-m., ***graph.,*** **LACH.,** lyss.
after - graph.
before - am-c.
scanty, during - lach.
suppressed - graph., ham., zinc.

BLEEDING, from anus and rectum
morning - con., mur-ac., plan.
stool, after - puls.
night - **NIT-AC.**
periodic - ***mur-ac., nit-ac.***
rubbing, on - aesc.
removal of hemorrhoids, after - nit-ac.
standing agg. - crot-h.
stool, during - ***alum.,*** alumn., ***ambr.,*** **AM-C.,** am-m., asar., aur., aur-m., bufo, ***calc-p., carb-an., carb-v.,*** caust., con., **HAM.,** ***hep.,*** ign., iod., ***ip., kali-c.,*** lyc., mur-ac., **NAT-M.,** ***nit-ac.,*** nux-v., plan., **PHOS.,** psor., ***puls.,*** rheum, ruta, sep., ***tub.***
after - ***agar., aloe, alum.,*** **AM-C.,** bor., ***calc-p.,*** carb-s., ***carb-v.,*** chel., cycl., fl-ac., grat., ***ign., kali-c.,*** kali-n., ***lach.,*** merc., mez., nat-m., ***phos.,*** rhus-v., sel., sep., spong., sulph.
difficult, from - petr.
hard, from - ***fl-ac., kali-c.,*** kali-n., morg., morg-g., **NAT-M.,** prun., sabin., ***tub.***
urination, during - kali-c., merc.
walking, while - alum., crot-h., sep.

BOILS, anus, in - calc-p., carb-an., caust., petr.
near - caust.

BORING, pain - bry., cina, zinc.

BUBBLES, sensation - coloc., nat-m.

BURNING, pain - abies-c., **AESC.,** aeth., **AGAR., ALOE,** ***alum.,*** ambr., am-c., ***am-m.,*** ant-c., ***apis,*** apoc., arg-n., arn., ***ars., ars-i.,*** arum-t., aspar., aur., aur-m., bapt., ***bar-c.,*** bar-m., bell., **BERB.,** bor., ***bov., bry.,*** cahin., **CALC.,** calc-p., calc-s., canth., **CAPS., CARB-AN., CARB-S., CARB-V.,** ***card-m.,*** carl., ***cast.,*** caust., cham., ***chel.,*** chin., chin-a., clem., cocc., coc-c., ***coch.,*** coff., colch., coll., ***coloc.,*** con., ***cop., crot-t.,*** cub., cupr., cycl., der., dig., dor., ***dulc.,*** erig., ***euph., eup-per.,*** ferr., ferr-ar., ferr-i., ferr-p., ***gamb.,*** gels., **GRAPH.,** grat., ham., hell., ***hep.,*** hydrc., hyos., ign., ***iod.,*** ip., **IRIS,** jug-r., **KALI-AR.,** ***kali-bi.,*** **KALI-C.,** kali-n., kali-p., **KALI-S.,** ***lach.,*** lact., laur., ***lil-t., lyc.,*** lyss., ***mag-m.,*** mag-s., ***manc.,*** med., **MERC.,** ***merc-c.,*** merc-i-f., merc-sul., merl., ***mez., mur-ac.,*** naja, **NAT-A.,** ***nat-c.,*** **NAT-M.,** nat-p., nat-s., nicc., **NIT-AC.,** nuph., **NUX-V.,** ol-an., ***olnd., op., paeon., petr.,*** petros., ph-ac., ***phos.,*** plat., plb., ***prun., psor.,*** ptel., **PULS.,** ***rat.,*** rheum, rhus-t., rhus-v., sabad., sabin., sars., **SEP., SIL.,** sin-a., ***spong.,*** stann., staph., ***stront-c.,*** **SULPH.,** ***sul-ac.,*** sumb., tarent., tep., ***ter.,*** **THUJ.,** urt-u., verat., verat-v., ***zinc.***
afternoon - coloc., euphr., ***sulph.***
2 p.m., - dios.
sleeping, after - chin.
cold application amel., - ***aloe,*** apis, euphr., ***kali-c., ter.***
constant - ars., ***kali-c.,*** lyc., nat-m.
daytime, walking, while - nat-m.
diarrhea, during - **ALOE,** alum., ***ars., aur.,*** aur-m., bov., bry., canth., **CAPS.,** carb-an., caust., chin., chin-a., ***dulc., gamb.,*** glon., graph., grat., **IRIS,** jug-c.,

BURNING, pain
diarrhea, during - ***kali-ar., kali-c.,*** kali-s., ***lach., manc.,*** **MERC.,** ***mur-ac., nuph.,*** op., ***rat.,*** **SULPH.**
after - ***canth., dulc.,*** grat., laur., nicc., op., ***rat.***
dysentery, in - aloe, ***ars.,*** **CAPS.,** ***carb-v., coloc., lach., urt-u.***
evening - bar-c., ***carb-an., iod.,*** kali-c., ***mur-ac.,*** nit-ac., ***sulph.,*** thuj., zinc.
exercise, after - sulph.
fissure, in - **GRAPH.**
flatus, after - ***agar.,*** **ALOE,** ant-t., bapt., ***carb-v.,*** cham., cocc., dios., phos., plb., psor., ***puls., staph., sulph.,*** sumb., ***teucr., zinc.***
agg., - ***iod.***
amel., - ***ars.***
lying, while - ***puls.***
menses, during - berb., carb-v., zinc.
after - graph.
midnight, before - thuj.
stool, after - op.
morning - carb-ac., colch., hyper., mag-m., **MUR-AC.,** nicc., **NIT-AC.,** ***sulph.,*** thuj.
bed, in - colch.
moving, after - crot-t., kali-n.
night - am-c., ant-c., ***ars., iod.,*** nat-m., ***nit-ac.,*** ox-ac., puls., **SULPH.**
noon - dios.
paroxysmal - colch., ***puls.***
pregnancy, during - ***caps.***
pressure amel., - kali-c.
prolapsed, in the - ***apis.***
rhagades - **GRAPH.**
rubbing, after - carb-v., phel., ***sabad.***
sitting, while - ip., **SULPH.,** thuj.
standing, while - crot-h., ***lach.,*** ter.
stool, during - agar., ***aloe,*** **ALUM.,** am-c., am-m., **ARS.,** ***bar-c.,*** bar-m., ***berb., bor., bry., calc.,*** calc-s., cann-s., ***canth.,*** caps., carb-an., ***carb-s.,*** carb-v., cast., caust., cham., chin., chin-a., chion., clem., cob., cocc., coloc., **CON.,** corn., crot-t., cycl., dios., ferr., ferr-ar., ferr-p., ***fl-ac.,*** gamb., ***graph.,*** grat., hep., ***hydr.,*** **IRIS,** kali-ar., kali-bi., kali-c., kali-p., kali-s., ***lach.,*** lil-t., ***lyc.,*** mag-m., ***merc., merc-c., merc-sul., mur-ac.,*** nat-a., nat-c., ***nat-m.,*** nat-p., ***nat-s.,*** nicc., **OP.,** osm., ***phos.,*** phys., pic-ac., ***plat.,*** plb., ***puls., rat.,*** rheum, rhus-t., sabad., sep., ***sil.,*** sin-a., ***staph.,*** stram., ***stront-c.,*** **SULPH.,** ***sul-ac.,*** tab., tep., ter., ***verat.,*** vinc., ***zinc.***
tickling - ***ran-s.***
urination, after - ***nit-ac.***
vexation agg., - ***cham.,*** nat-m.
walking while - ***carb-an., mez.,*** nat-m., sulph., ***thuj.***
stool, after - **AESC.,** agar., **ALOE,** alumn., am-c., ***am-m.,*** ant-t., ***apis,*** **ARS.,** ***ars-i.,*** arund., asc-t., aster., bar-c., bar-m., ***berb.,*** bov., **BRY.,** ***calc.,*** cann-s., ***canth.,*** caps., ***carb-s., carb-v., carl., cast.,*** **CAUST.,** cic., clem., cob., coc-c., ***coloc.,*** cop., ***corn.,***

BURNING, pain
stool, after - crot-t., dirc., dulc., euphr., ferr., ferr-ar., ferr-i., ferr-p., **GAMB.,** ***graph.,*** grat., hell., hep., ***hydr.,*** ign., ind., iod., ***iris,*** jug-c., jug-r., ***kali-ar., kali-bi., kali-c.,*** kali-n., kali-p., kali-s., kalm., ***lach.,*** laur., ***lil-t., lyc., mag-c., mag-m., merc., merc-c., mur-ac., nat-a., nat-c., nat-m.,*** nat-p., ***nat-s.,*** nicc., **NIT-AC.,** nuph., nux-m., ***nux-v., olnd.,*** osm., paeon., ***petr.,*** phel., ***phos., pic-ac.,*** ptel., ***puls.,*** **RAT.,** rheum, rhod., rhus-t., sars., sec., sep., **SIL.,** sin-a., sol-t-ae., stann., ***staph., stront-c.,*** **SULPH.,** tarent., ter., ***thuj., trom.,*** urt-u., ***zinc.***
amel. - clem., verat-v.
hard, after a - aesc., agar., ***aloe,*** alumn., am-m., ***ars.,*** coc-c., ***kali-bi.,*** kali-c., lil-t., lyc., mag-m., nat-c., ***nat-m.,*** phos., **RAT.,** sabad., sec., **SIL.,** ***sulph.,*** til., ter., ***thuj.***
stool, before - ***berb.,*** dios., iod., jug-c., ***nat-m., olnd., rat.,*** sabad., ***sulph.,*** verat.
urination, after - ***nit-ac.,*** rhus-t.
burning, anus, in, with nausea - kali-bi.

CANCER - ***alum., ars.,*** carb-v., graph., **HYDR.,** ***kali-c.,*** laur., lyc., mur-ac., nat-s., ***nit-ac.,*** paeon., phyt., ***ruta,*** sang., ***sep.,*** spig., tub.

CATARRH, of the (see Mucus, Moisture) - ***arg-n.,*** aur., ***nit-ac.***

CAULIFLOWER, excrescence - ***thuj.***

CHILLINESS, before stool - ars., camph., elat., ***lyc.,*** merc., ***phos.***
constipation, during - lac-d.
chilliness, anus, in, after stool - kali-c.

CHOLERA, (see Intestines)

CLAWING, pain, anus, in - ***ferr.,*** lach., nat-c., phel.
dinner, after - phos.
stool, during - aeth., ***thuj.,*** zinc.

COLDNESS, anus, in - all-c., kali-bi., nat-m., sil., sulph.
afternoon - kali-bi.
drops, cold - cann-s.
flatus and stool, during - ***con.***
waking, after - nat-m., sulph.
walking in open air, after - sil.

CONDYLOMATA - ***arg-m., arg-n.,*** aur., benz-ac., ***caust.,*** **CINNB.,** ***euphr.,*** jac-c., kali-br., ***lyc.,*** merc., ***merc-d., mill., nat-s.,*** **NIT-AC.,** petr., phos., pic-ac., sabin., sep., staph., sulph., syc-co., **THUJ.**
bleeding, copious - ***mill.***
dry - thuj.
extremely sensitive - **STAPH.**
flat - ***euphr.,*** sulph., **THUJ.**
sore - benz-ac., ***thuj.***
on touch - euphr.
sharp, stitching - euphr., thuj.

CONGESTION, (see Redness) - sep., sul-ac.

CONSTIPATION, general, (see Inactivity) - abies-c., abies-n., ***abrot.,*** **AESC.,** ***aeth., agar., agn.,*** alet., ***aloe,*** **ALUM., ALUMN.,** ***ambr., am-c., am-m.,*** ammc., ***anac.,*** anan., ***ang.,*** ant-c., **APIS,** ***arg-m., arg-n.,*** arn., **ARS.,** ***ars-i.,*** arund., asaf., asc-c., asc-t., aster., ***aur.,*** aur-m., bad., ***bar-c., bar-m.,*** bell., ***berb.,*** bol., bor., bov., brach., **BRY.,** ***cact.,*** calad., **CALC.,** ***calc-p., calc-s.,*** camph., cann-s., caps., ***carb-ac., carb-an.,*** **CARB-S.,** ***carb-v., card-m.,*** casc., caul., **CAUST.,** ***chel., chim., chin.,*** chin-a., chin-s., chr-ac., cimx., cina, **CLEM.,** ***coca,*** **COCC., COFF.,** colch., **COLL.,** ***coloc.,*** **CON.,** ***cop.,*** cor-r., ***croc., crot-c., crot-h.,*** crot-t., cub., cupr., cycl., ***daph., dig., dios., dulc., elaps,*** ery-a., euon., euph., ***ferr., ferr-ar., ferr-i.,*** ferr-p., ***fl-ac., form., gamb.,*** **GRAPH.,** ***guai., hell.,*** hep., hippoz., ***hydr., hydrc.,*** hyos., ***hyper., ign., iod., iris,*** jab., jac-c., ***jatr., kali-ar., kali-bi., kali-br., kali-c., kali-chl., kali-i.,*** kali-n., kali-p., ***kali-s., kreos.,*** **LACH., LAC-D.,** ***lac-ac., laur.,*** led., ***lept., lil-t.,*** **LYC.,** lycps., ***mag-c.,*** **MAG-M.,** mag-s., ***manc.,*** mang., med., meli., ***meny., merc.,*** merc-c., ***merc-d., merc-i-f.,*** **MEZ.,** ***mosch.,*** murx., ***mur-ac.,*** myric., naja, ***nat-a., nat-c.,*** **NAT-M.,** nat-p., nat-s., nicc., **NIT-AC.,** ***nux-m.,*** **NUX-V., OENA.,** olnd., **OP.,** osm., ***ox-ac.,*** paeon., pall., petr., ph-ac., **PHOS.,** ***phyt.,*** **PLAT., PLB.,** ***podo., psor., ptel., puls., pyrog., raph., rat.,*** rhus-t., rob., **RUTA.,** ***sabad., sabin.,*** sang., **SANIC.,** ***sars., sec., sel., seneg.,*** **SEP., SIL.,** spig., ***spong.,*** squil., ***stann.,*** **STAPH., STRAM., STRY., SULPH.,** ***sul-ac.,*** sumb., ***tab., tarent.,*** tell., ***ter., ther.,*** **THUJ.,** tril., ***tub.,*** urt-u., ust., vario., ***verb.,*** **VERAT.,** ***vib.,*** viol-o., vesp., **ZINC.**

absolute - ***op.***

alternate, days, agg. - alum., calc., cocc., con., kali-c., lyc., ***nat-m.***

alternating, with diarrhea - ***abrot.,*** acet-ac., agar., ail., aloe, am-m., **ANT-C.,** ant-t., ***arg-n., ars.,*** ars-i., ***aur.,*** aur-m-n., berb., ***bry.,*** calc., ***carb-ac.,*** carb-s., ***card-m., casc.,*** **CHEL.,** ***cimic.,*** cina, ***cob.,*** coff., ***coll., con.,*** cop., cor-r., crot-h., ***cupr., dig.,*** dios., ferr., ***ferr-i.,*** gamb., gnaph., grat., ***hep.,*** ho., ***hydr., ign., iod.,*** kali-ar., kali-bi., ***kali-c.,*** kali-s., ***lach., lac-d., lact., lec.,*** lil-t., ***lyc.,*** mag-s., ***manc., mang.,*** merc., mez., nat-a., nat-c., ***nat-m.,*** nat-p., ***nat-s.,*** **NIT-AC.,** ***nux-m.,*** **NUX-V., OP.,** ***phos., plb.,*** **PODO.,** polyg., ***ptel., puls.,*** rad., rhus-t., ***ruta.,*** sang., sars., sep., stram., ***sulph.,*** sumb., ***tab., tub.,*** verat., zinc.

children, in - lyc., nux., verat.

elderly people, in - **ANT-C.,** bry., nux-v., op., ***phos.***

amel. physical symptoms - ***calc.,*** merc., ***psor.***

anus very sore, with - graph., nat-m., nit-ac., sil.

backache, with - ***aesc.,*** euon., ***ferr.,*** kali-bi., sulph.

bedwetting, with - caust.

bleeding, with - alum., am-m., anac., calc-p., ***coll.,*** lac-d., lam., morph., nat-m., ***nit-ac., nux-v.,*** phos., psor., sep., vib.

CONSTIPATION, general

bowels, action lost, as if with - aeth.

breath, with offensive - carb-ac.

cheese, from - coloc.

children, in - acon., ***aesc.,*** **ALUM.,** ***ant-c.,*** apis, bell., **BRY., CALC.,** caust., ***cham., coll.,*** croc., ***graph., hep., hydr.,*** hydr-ac., kreos., **LYC.,** ***mag-m.,*** meph., ***nat-m., nit-ac.,*** **NUX-V.,** nyct., **OP.,** ***paraf., plat., plb., podo., psor.,*** sanic., ***sep., sil.,*** sulph., verat.

infants, in - aesc., ***alum.,*** bry., ***calc.,*** caust., coll., lyc., mag-m., ***nux-v., op.,*** plb., psor., sel., sep., verat.

bottle fed, from artificial food - alum., calc., nux-v., op.

newborn, in - alum., ***calc.,*** caust., med., **NUX-V., OP.,** ***sulph.,*** verat., ***zinc.***

chronic - **ALUM.,** bry., calc., graph., lac-d., ***nat-m., nux-v.,*** **OP.,** plb., ***sep.,*** sul-i., sulph., verat.

cloudy weather agg. - aloe.

coffee, after - ***mosch.***

colds agg. - ign.

confinement, after - mez., sep.

constant, desire, with - aloe, anac., coloc., ***con., mag-c., mag-m.,*** nat-p., **NUX-V.,** ***plb., puls.,*** ruta., ***sil., sulph.***

contraction, spasmodic of anus, with - caust., ***lach., lyc., nat-m.,*** nit-ac., plb., sil.

cramps, colic, with - ***coll., cypr.,*** glon., op.

stool, during - ***aloe,*** alst., bry., camph., ***canth.,*** caps., cean., ***cham., chin., coloc., cupr., cupr-ar.,*** dulc., ***elat.,*** gamb., ***ip., jatr.,*** lept., ***merc., merc-c.,*** merc-d., podo., rheum, ric., sec., sulph., trio., ***trom., verat.,*** zinc.

dentition, during - dol.

diarrhea, after - asc-t.

followed by, with cramps - trinit.

difficult, stool, (see Inactivity) - ***aesc.,*** agar., ***all-c.,*** aloe, **ALUM., ALUMN.,** ***am-c.,*** **AM-M.,** ***anac.,*** ang., **ANT-C,** ***apis, aur., aur-m.,*** bapt., ***bar-c.,*** **BAR-M.,** ***berb.,*** bov., **BRY.,** ***cact., calc.,*** calc-p., ***calc-s., camph.,*** canth., carb-an., **CARB-S.,** ***carb-v.,*** **CAUST.,** cham., chel., chin., cimx., ***clem., cocc.,*** colch., coll., coloc., **CON.,** cop., crot-t., dulc., ***ferr.,*** ferr-i., ferr-p., gels., **GRAPH.,** grat., ***hell.,*** **HEP.,** ***ign., ind.,*** iod., ***kali-bi., kali-c.,*** kali-n., ***kali-p.,*** **KALI-S.,** kalm., kreos., **LACH.,** ***lac-c.,*** **LAC-D.,** lact., laur., ***lyc.,*** lyss., mag-c., **MAG-M.,** mag-s., mang., meli., ***merc.,*** merc-c., ***mez., mur-ac.,*** naja, ***nat-c.,*** **NAT-M.,** nat-p., nat-s., **NIT-AC., NUX-M., NUX-V.,** ***oena.,*** ol-an., olnd., **OP.,** ph-ac., ***phos.,*** **PLAT., PLB.,** ***podo., psor., puls., rat., rhod.,*** **RUTA.,** ***sabin.,*** **SANIC.,** ***sars.,*** **SEL.,** senec., **SEP., SIL.,** ***stann.,*** staph., ***stram.,*** stront-c., **SULPH.,** sul-ac., sumb., ***tarent.,*** **THUJ.,** valer., ***verb., vib.,*** **ZINC.**

natural appearing stool - graph., **PSOR., SIL.**

CONSTIPATION, general

difficult, stool, with

soft stool - agn., **ALUM.,** ***anac.,*** calad., ***calc-p., carb-v., chin.,*** colch., dulc., gels., graph., ***hell.,*** **HEP.,** ***ign., kali-c., kali-s.,*** lach., ***lac-c.,*** lob., lyc., mag-c., mag-m., ***nat-c., nat-m., nat-s.,*** nicc., nit-ac., **NUX-M.,** petr., ph-ac., phos., plat., ***psor., puls., rhod., ruta.,*** sars., **SEP.,** ***sil.,*** spig., ***stann.,*** staph., sulph., tarax., verb., zinc.

stool, recedes - agn., eug., kali-s., ***lac-d., mag-m., mur-ac., nat-m.,*** **OP.,** ***sanic.,*** **SIL.,** sulph., ***thuj.***

urinating, can pass stool only when - aloe, alum.

drinking amel. - caps., mosch.

drugs, after abuse of - agar., ant-c., ***bry.,*** chin., **COLOC.,** ***hydr.,*** lach., **NUX-V.,** ***op.,*** ruta., sulph.

dryness, of rectum, from - **ALUM.,** ***bry.***

elderly, people - aloe, ***alum.,*** alumn., ***ant-c., bar-c., bry.,*** calc., ***calc-p., con.,*** cycl., hydr., ***lach.,*** lyc., nat-m., ***nux-v., op., phos., phyt.,*** rhus-t., ruta., ***sel.,*** sep., ***sulph.***

emaciation, with - kreos.

enemas, abuse of, from - ***op.***

fainting, with - verat.

fetor oris, with - ***carb-ac.,*** op., psor.

gall-stones, jaundice, with - chion.

gastric derangements, from - ***bry.,*** hydr., ***nux-v.,*** puls.

hard, stool from (see Stool)

heart, weakness - phyt.

hemorrhoids, from - ***aesc., aesc-g., aloe,*** alumn., ***calc-f.,*** caust., ***coll.,*** euon., glon., graph., hydr., kali-s., lyc., nat-m., nit-ac., ***nux-v.,*** paraf., podo., ***rat.,*** sil., ***sulph.,*** wye.

headache, during - aloe, alum., **BRY.,** euon., gels., hydr., iris, lac-d., ***nat-m.,*** nicc., nux-v., op., plb., sep.

heart weakness - phyt., spig.

heat of body, with - cupr.

hernia, umbilical, with - cocc., nux-v.

home, when away from - alum., nat-m., ***lyc.***

impaction, from - **OP.,** plb., pyrog., sel.

incomplete, (see insufficient)

ineffectual, urging and straining - acon., ***aesc.,*** agar., ***all-c.,*** aloe, ***alum.,*** **AMBR., ANAC.,** ant-c., ant-t., arg-m., ***arn., ars.,*** ars-i., asaf., aster., ***bar-c., bell.,*** benz-ac., berb., bism., bov., brach., ***bry., cact.,*** cahin., ***calc., calc-s.,*** cann-i., ***cann-s.,*** canth., ***caps.,*** carb-ac., ***carb-an.,*** carb-s., ***carb-v.,*** carl., **CAUST.,** cedr., chel., ***chim.,*** chin., chin-a., chin-s., cimx., clem., ***cocc.,*** coc-c., colch., **COLL.,** ***coloc.,*** **CON.,** corn., crot-t., cupr., cycl., dios., dirc., dros., dulc., elat., eupi., eup-pur., fago., ***ferr.,*** ferr-ar., ferr-i., ferr-p., fl-ac., form., glon., gran., ***graph.,*** grat., ham., hell., hep., hura, **HYDR.,** hyper., ***ign., iod.,*** kali-ar., ***kali-bi., kali-c.,*** kali-n., kali-p., ***kali-s., kalm.,*** kreos.,

CONSTIPATION, general

ineffectual, urging and straining - **LACH.,** ***lac-c., lac-d.,*** laur., **LIL-T.,** lob-s., **LYC.,** ***mag-c.,*** **MAG-M.,** mag-s., **MERC.,** merc-c., mosch., myric., nat-a., ***nat-c.,*** **NAT-M.,** ***nat-p.,*** nicc., **NIT-AC., NUX-V.,** ***oena.,*** ol-an., olnd., ***op.,*** ox-ac., par., petr., phel., ph-ac., ***phos.,*** phys., phyt., **PLAT.,** plb., podo., psor., ptel., **PULS.,** ***rat.,*** rheum, rhod., rhus-t., rob., ***ruta.,*** sabad., ***sang., sanic.,*** **SARS.,** sec., **SEL., SEP., SIL.,** sol-n., spig., ***stann., staph.,*** stram., **SULPH.,** sul-ac., sumb., tab., **TARENT.,** ter., **THUJ.,** til., ***verat.,*** viol-o., ***zinc.***

evening - ***sil.***

menses, during - calc., puls.

plugged up, as if - anac.

infants, in (see children)

injuries, from mechanical - arn., ruta

insufficient, incomplete, unsatisfactory stools - **ALOE,** ***alum., alumn., anac.,*** ang., apis, ***arn.,*** ars., ***bar-c.,*** bell., ***benz-ac., bry.,*** calc., calc-s., caps., carb-ac., carb-an., carb-s., carb-v., **CARD-M.,** ***caust., cham., cheir.,*** colch., coloc., euphr., ***gamb.,*** gels., glon., graph., hep., hyos., ***ign., iod.,*** **KALI-C.,** ***kali-s.,*** lact., **LYC.,** mang., ***mag-m.,*** **MERC-C.,** mez., naja, **NAT-C., NAT-M., NIT-AC.,** ***nux-m.,*** **NUX-V.,** ***oena.,*** **OP.,** par., petr., plat., ***plb., pyrog.,*** rhod., sabad., ***sars.,*** **SEL.,** seneg., ***sep.,*** **SIL.,** spong., squil., stann., ***staph.,*** **SULPH.,** ***thuj., zinc.***

itching, with intense - dol.

lead poisoning, from - ***alum.,*** op., plat., plb.

lean, far back to pass a stool, must - ***med.***

lightheadedness, sensation of, with - indol.

menses, during - alum., ***am-c.,*** am-m., ant-c., **APIS,** ***aur.,*** bov., bry., chel., coll., cycl., **GRAPH., KALI-C.,** kali-s., kreos., **NAT-M.,** ***nat-s., nux-v.,*** phos., **PLAT.,** ***plb.,*** **SEP., SIL.,** sulph., thuj.

after - dirc., graph., lac-c.

amel. - aur.

before - am-c., bry., ***graph.,*** **KALI-C.,** lac-c., ***lach.,*** mag-c., nat-m., nat-s., nux-v., sep., **SIL.,** sulph., vesp.

instead of - ***graph.***

suppressed, during - ***graph., ham.***

mental shock, from nervous strain - mag-c.

milk amel. - iod.

monday, every - stann.

neurastenia, with - alum., ign.

newborn, (see children)

obstinate - aeth., ***alum.,*** hydr., ***op.,*** sul-i., syph.

with flatulence and hemorrhoids - **COLL.**

years, for - alum., op., syph.

operation, after, (see surgery)

painful, (see cramps) - nat-m., **NIT-AC.,** ***tub.***

compels child to desist from effort - ign., lyc., ***sulph.***

CONSTIPATION, general

painful, persistent rectal pain, with - ***aesc.,*** aloe, alumn., caust., hydr., ***ign.,*** lyc., mur-ac., ***nat-m., nit-ac.,*** rat., sep., sulph., thuj.

passes better, standing - caust.

periodic - ***kali-bi.***

every three weeks - ***kali-bi.***

portal, stasis, from - **AESC.,** ***aloe,*** **NUX-V., SULPH.**

pregnancy, during - ***agar., alum., ambr., ant-c., apis, bry., coll.,*** coloc., ***con.,*** **DOL.,** ***hydr., lyc.,*** nat-m., **NAT-S., NUX-V.,** ***op.,*** **PLB., PLAT.,** ***podo., puls.,*** **SEP.,** ***sulph.***

after - lil-t., ***lyc.,*** mez., **SEP.,** verat.

preoccupation, with bowels - ***mag-m.***

prolapse, with rectal - ***aesc.,*** alum., ferr., ***ign.,*** lyc., med., podo., ruta, sep., sulph.

uterus, from - stann.

prostate enlarged, with - arn., sil.

prostatic fluid, with - alum., hep.

puerperal - ***bry., coll.,*** nux-v., **SEP.,** verat., zinc.

purgatives or enema, from - aloe, ***hydr., nux-v.,*** op., sulph.

amel. - lac-d.

does not amel. - tarent.

retention - alum., cocc., sil., ***stram.***

pain, from - sil.

riding agg. - ign.

seashore, at - aq-mar., bry., lyc., mag-m.

sedentary, habits, from - aloe, ***ambr., bry., lyc.,*** **NUX-V.,** ***op.,*** **PLAT.,** ***podo., sep., sulph.***

seminal, emission, after - sep., thuj.

something remaining behind, sensation of, with constipation - aloe, alum., lyc., nat-m., ***nux-v.,*** sep., sil., sulph.

standing, passes stool easier when - alum., **CAUST.**

stool, after, agg., which is induced only with cathartics - **COLL.**

must be removed, mechanically - aloe., ***alum.,*** bry., calc., con., lyc., med., nat-m., ***op.,*** plat., sanic., sel., ***sep.,*** sil., sulph.

recedes - agn., aloe, alum., eug., kali-s., ***lac-d.,*** lyc., ***mag-m.,*** med., ***mur-ac., nat-m.,*** nux-v., **OP.,** ***sanic.,*** sep., **SIL.,** sulph., ***thuj.***

menses, during - sil.

remains long in the rectum with no urging - ***alum.,*** am-c., bry., carb-an., cocc., **GRAPH.,** ***lach.,*** **OP.,** sep.

awful anxiety, with - **TARENT.**

general amel., with - calc., merc., psor.

scanty, with profuse urination - alum., bry., caust., graph., hep., kali-c., kreos., lyc., nat-c., nux-v., rhus-t., sabin., samb., sep., spig., sulph.

soft, with - **ALUM.,** anac., chin., ***hep.,*** ign., **NUX-M.,** plat., psor., puls., ***sep.,*** sil., staph.

strain, must (see ineffectual) - ***alum.,*** chin., coll., ***nat-m., nux-v.,*** rat., ***sep.,*** sil.

surgery, after - ***op.***

CONSTIPATION, general

torpor of from - aloe, **ALUM.,** ***anac.,*** caust., chin., lach., lyc., nat-m., **OP.,** psor., sel., ***sep., sil., verat.***

travelling, while - ***alum.,*** lyc., nat-m., ***nux-v., op., plat.***

unable, to pass the stool in presence of nurse or others - **AMBR.,** ***nat-m.***

unsatisfactory, (see insufficient)

urging, to stool, with

absent, no desire, with - **ALUM.,** ***bry.,*** graph., hydr., indol., **OP.,** sanic., sulph., verat.

abortive - anac., con., lyc., mag-m., nat-m., ***nux-v.,*** puls., sep., sil., sulph.

constant, not for stools - lach.

urination amel. - lil-t.

crampy - plb.

eating, on - sanic.

erection, with - ign., thuj.

felt in, lower abdomen - aloe

felt in, upper abdomen - anac., ***ign.,*** verat.

ineffectual - caps., merc., ***merc-c.,*** rheum, rhus-t., ***sulph.***

irresistible - ***aloe,*** nat-c.

neuralgia, with - iris

passes flatus only - **ALOE,** carb-v., mag-m., myric., nat-c., nat-s., phos., ruta, sep.

prolapsus, with - ruta, sep.

sex, after - nat-p.

sleep, in - phyt.

stool, after - merc.

urination amel. - lil-t.

urinating, can pass stool only when - aloe, alum.

with frequent - sars.

urine, retention, with - canth.

vexation, after - bry., mag-c., nux-v., staph.

wine, after - ***zinc.***

women, in - aesc., alet., ***alum.,*** ambr., anac., arn., ***asaf.,*** bry., calc., ***coll.,*** con., ***graph., hydr.,*** ign., lach., lyc., mez., ***nat-m.,*** nux-v., op., ***plat., plb., podo.,*** puls., **SEP.,** sil., sulph.

worse after stool, which is induced only with cathartics - **COLL.,** ***nux-v.***

CONSTRICTION, cramp, contraction, closure, etc. - acon., ***aesc.,*** aeth., ***agar.,*** alum., am-c., ang., arg-n., ars., ***bell.,*** benz-ac., berb., bor., ***cact., calc.,*** calc-s., ***camph., cann-s.,*** carb-an., carb-v., carc., **CAUST.,** ***chel.,*** chin., cic., cimx., ***cocc.,*** coff., ***colch.,*** coloc., cop., crot-t., der., ferr., ferr-ar., ferr-i., ferr-p., ***fl-ac., form.,*** gall-ac., graph., grat., guare., hipp., hura, ***hyos.,*** **IGN.,** kali-ar., ***kali-bi., kali-br.,*** kali-c., **LACH.,** laur., **LYC.,** mag-arct., mag-aust., mag-p-a., mang., med., meli., ***merc-c.,*** mez., nat-c., ***nat-m.,*** nat-p., **NIT-AC., NUX-V.,** ***op., phos.,*** **PLB.,** rat., ***rhus-t.,*** sars., sec., ***sep.,*** sil., sol-t-ae., staph., stront-c., ***sulph.,*** sumb., syph., ***tab.,*** ther., thuj., tub., verb.

afternoon - ***cocc.,*** coloc.

alternating with itching - ***chel.***

with pressure - bell.

CONSTRICTION, cramp, contraction, closure
breakfast, after - calc-s.
evening - chin., ign.
walking, while - ign.
extending, glans, to - chin.
perineum, to - sep.
rectum, into - sil.
testes, to - chin., sil.
upward - laur., sep., sil.
vagina, to - sep.
flatus, passing - fl-ac.
forenoon - ***calc.***
lying amel., - ***mang.***
menses, during - ***cocc.,*** thuj.
mental exertion, after - nux-v.
morning - nux-v.
in bed - phos.
rising, after - nux-v.
motion, agg. - caust.
amel., - coloc.
night - sec.
painful - bell., brach., ***calc., caust., cocc.,*** coloc., **IGN., LACH.,** ***lyc.,*** mag-aust., ***mang., mez.,*** **NUX-V., PLB.,** sars., ***sep., sil., thuj.,*** tub.
prolapsed rectum, anus - ***lach., mez.***
sex, during - merc-c.
after - caust.
sitting, while - chin., ***cocc., mang.***
amel. - ***ign.***
rising from - thuj.
spasmodic - anac., chel., coff., grat., ***ham., hipp., lach., lyc.,*** merc-c., nat-m., **NIT-AC., NUX-V., OP.,** ***phos.,*** **PLB.,** sil., ther., verb.
standing, agg. - arn., ***ign.***
amel., - sanic.
stool, during - ***alum., ars., chel.,*** chin-s., coloc., ferr., glon., hell., ***kreos.,*** mang., **NAT-M., NIT-AC.,** nux-m., mur-ac., ***nux-v.,*** phos., **PLB.,** rat., sep., **SIL.,** ***thuj.***
after - aesc., chel., colch., elaps, ***ferr.,*** form., grat., **IGN.,** kali-bi., **LACH.,** ***mez.,*** **NIT-AC.,** nux-m., ***phos.,*** plat., ***sep.,*** stront-c., ***sulph.,*** thuj.
after, hard, from - ferr.
before - aeth., ***aloe,*** alst., ***bell.,*** bor., casc., ***cham., chin.,*** cina, ***coloc.,*** crot-t., ***cupr-ar., dios.,*** dulc., elat., gamb., ***ham., ip.,*** iris, lach., lept., ***mag-c.,*** merc., ***merc-c.,*** merc-d., ***nat-m., nux-v.,*** phos., plb., rheum, senn., sep., sulph., trom., ***verat.***
preventing - all-c., ***berb., chel., lach.,*** **LYC.,** ***nat-m., nit-ac., nux-v.***
urging to, during - caust.
stooping, on - caust.
amel. - carc.
urinating, on - carb-s., nat-m.
at close of - ***cann-s.***
uterine cancer, from - kreos.
walking, on - ***caust.,*** crot-t.
preventing - caust.
weather, due to cold - verat.

CORD, extending from anus to navel - ferr-i.

CRAMP, sitting, when, (see Constriction) - mang.

CUTTING, pain - aesc., aloe, **ALUM.,** ***ars.,*** calad., calc., calc-p., canth., carb-v., ***caust., chel.,*** con., ***graph., ign.,*** indg., ip., ***kali-ar., kali-c.,*** kali-s., laur., ***lyc.,*** mag-c., mang., meli., ***merc.,*** mur-ac., nat-a., nat-c., nat-h., ***nit-ac.,*** **NUX-V.,** ***phos.,*** plan., plat., ***rat.,*** sars., sec., sep., **SIL.,** stann., staph., ***sulph.,*** sumb., thuj., zinc.
afternoon - sep., sulph.
diarrhea, during - **ARS.**
dysentery, in - ***merc-c.***
evening - nat-h., phos.
extending through coccyx - carb-an.
up rectum - hell., mur-ac., ***sep., sulph.***
flatus or passing stool amel. - canth.
forenoon, walking, while - ***sulph.***
jerking - zinc.
morning - graph., lyc., mang.
bed, in - ***graph.***
rising, after - mang.
night - sep.
10 a.m., - aloe.
sitting - **RAT.**
standing agg., - ***lach.***
stool, during - agar., asar., all-c., alum., am-c., ant-t., ars., canth., carb-an., carb-v., caust., dios., hell., mag-c., mang., ***mur-ac.,*** nat-a., nat-c., ***nat-m.,*** nat-p., **NIT-AC.,** ***phos., pic-ac., plat.,*** plb., ***puls., sars.,*** sep., stann., staph., **SULPH.,** sumb., vib.
after - ***aesc.,*** agar., ***aloe,*** alumn., am-m., calc., chel., ***graph.,*** hell., ***hydr., ign.,*** merc-cy., mur-ac., nat-m., **NIT-AC., NUX-V.,** paeon., pic-ac., ***puls.,*** **RAT.,** sep., ***sil.,*** sin-a., staph., sulph., sumb., thuj., vib.
before - ***asar.,*** mag-c., mur-ac., sep., sulph., verat-v.
walking, while - mag-c., meli., ***sulph.***

DIAPER, rash, of anus - ***bapt., bor.,*** bry., ***kali-chl., merc., merc-c., mur-ac., nit-ac., sulph.,*** **SUL-AC.**

DIARRHEA, general - ***acet-ac., acon., aesc.,*** aeth., **AGAR.,** alet., all-s., **ALOE,** ***alum.,*** am-m., ammc., anan., ang., anthr., ant-a., **ANT-C., ANT-T., APIS,** apoc., ***aran.,*** arg-m., **ARG-N.,** ***arn.,*** **ARS.,** ars-i., arum-m., asaf., ***asar.,*** asc-t., astac., aster., aur., aur-m., **BAPT., BAR-C.,** bar-m., ***bell., benz-ac.,*** berb., bism., ***bor., bov.,*** brach., ***brom.,*** **BRY.,** bufo, cact., **CALC.,** ***calc-ar., calc-p.,*** calc-s., **CANTH.,** ***caps.,*** carb-ac., ***carb-s.,*** **CARB-V.,** ***casc.,*** cast., ***caust.,*** cean., **CHAM.,** chel., chim., **CHIN.,** ***chin-a.,*** chin-s., cic., ***cina,*** cinnam., ***cist.,*** clem., cob., ***cocc., coff., colch., coll., coloc., con., cop.,*** **CORN.,** ***crot-h.,*** **CROT-T.,** cub., ***cupr.,*** cupr-ar., cycl., ***dig.,*** dios., dros., **DULC.,** ***echi.,*** euph., **FERR., FERR-AR., FERR-I.,** ***ferr-p., ferr-s.,*** **FL-AC., GAMB.,** gels., ***gran., graph., grat.,*** guai., ham., **HELL., HEP.,** ***hydr., hyos., ign., ill.,*** ind., **IOD., IP., IRIS,** jab., ***jatr.,*** jug-c., ***kali-ar.,*** **KALI-BI.,** ***kali-c.,*** kali-chl., ***kali-i.,*** kali-n., kali-p., ***kali-s.,*** kreos., ***lach.,*** lac-ac.,

DIARRHEA, general - ***lac-c., lac-d.,*** laur., lec., led., ***lept., lil-t.,*** lith., **LYC.,** lyss., ***mag-c., mag-m., mag-p.,*** maland., manc., med., meli., **MERC., MERC-C.,** merc-sul., mez., morph., mur-ac., naja, ***nat-a., nat-c.,*** **NAT-M.,** ***nat-p.,*** **NAT-S.,** nicc., **NIT-AC.,** ***nuph., nux-m., nux-v.,*** ol-an., ***olnd., ol-j.,*** op., ox-ac., par., ***petr.,*** phel., **PH-AC., PHOS.,** phyt., pic-ac., plan., ***plb.,*** **PODO.,** prun., ***psor., ptel., puls.,*** raph., rat., **RHEUM,** rhod., rhus-t., rumx., sabad., samb., ***sang., sanic.,*** sars., **SEC.,** sel., seneg., ***sep.,*** **SIL.,** spong., squil., ***stann.,*** staph., stram., stry., **SULPH.,** ***sul-ac.,*** sumb., tab., tarax., ***tarent., ter.,*** **THUJ.,** trom., ***valer.,*** **VERAT.,** xan., ***zinc., zing.***

acids, after - ***aloe, ant-c.,*** apis, ars., ***brom.,*** bry., cist., coloc., lach., **NAT-P.,** nux-v., ***ph-ac., sulph.***
- acid foods, amel. - arg-n.

acute, diseases, after - ars., ***carb-v., chin.,*** gels, ***ph-ac., psor., sulph.***

afternoon - aloe, alum., am-c., ***ars., bell., bor.,*** calc., carb-an., **CHIN.,** ***chin-a.,*** corn-s., dulc., ***ferr.,*** ferr-ar., ferr-p., gent-l., hell., kali-ar., kali-c., laur., lec., lept., lyc., mag-c., mag-s., ***manc.,*** merc-c., mur-ac., petr., phos., phyt., ***psor.,*** stann., sulph., sul-ac., ter., zinc.
- 4 p.m. - ***benz-ac.***
  - to 6 p.m. - carb-v., rhus-t.
  - to 8 p.m. - hell., ***lyc.***
- 5 p.m. to 6 p.m. - dig.
  - to 7 p.m. - ***benz-ac.***
- regularly - ***ferr.***

air, cold, in - nat-s., ***sil.***
- evening - **MERC.**
- on abdomen - ***caust.***
- on abdomen, currents of - ***acon.,*** **CAPS., NUX-V.,** ***sil.***

air, open, in - agar., am-m., coff., cycl., grat.
- amel. - dios., iod., lyc., nat-s., **PULS.**

alcoholic, drinks, after - ant-t., ars., lach., **NUX-V.,** sulph.
- abuse, of - ars., lach., nux-v.

alcoholics, in - ant-t., ***apis, ars.,*** chin., **LACH.,** nux-v., ***phos.***

aloe, after abuse of - aloe., mur-ac., ***sulph.***

alone, when - stram.

alternating, catarrh of chest, with - seneg.
- eruptions, with - calc-p., crot-t.
- headache, with - ***podo.***
- rheumatism, with - cimic., dulc., kali-bi.

alternating with, catarrh of chest, with - seneg.
- with, eruptions - calc-p., crot-t.
- with, headache - aloe, ***podo.***
- with, rheumatism - cimic., dulc., ***kali-bi.***

alternating with constipation - ***abrot.,*** acet-ac., agar., ail., aloe, am-m., **ANT-C.,** ant-t., ***arg-n., ars.,*** ars-i., ***aur.,*** aur-m-n., berb., ***bry., carb-ac.,*** carb-s., ***card-m., casc.,*** **CHEL.,** ***cimic.,*** cina, ***cob.,*** coff., ***coll., con.,*** cop., crot-h., ***cupr., dig.,*** dios., ***ferr-i.,*** gamb., gnaph., grat., ***hep.,*** ho., ***hydr., ign., iod.,*** kali-ar., kali-bi., ***kali-c.,*** kali-s., ***lach., lac-d., lact., lec.,*** lil-t., ***lyc.,*** mag-s., ***manc., mang.,***

DIARRHEA, general

alternating with constipation - merc., mez., nat-a., nat-c., ***nat-m.,*** nat-p., ***nat-s.,*** **NIT-AC.,** ***nux-m.,*** **NUX-V., OP.,** ***phos., plb.,*** **PODO.,** polyg., ***ptel., puls.,*** rhus-t., ***ruta.,*** sang., sars., sep., stram., ***sulph.,*** sumb., ***tab., tub.,*** zinc.
- children, in - lyc., nux., verat.
- elderly, people, in - **ANT-C.,** bry., nux-v., op., ***phos.***

ameliorates, all symptoms - abrot., nat-s., ph-ac., ***zinc.***

anger, after - acon., ***aloe,*** ars., bar-c., bry., ***calc-p., cham.,*** **COLOC.,** ip., ***nux-v., staph.***

anticipation, after - ars., **ARG-N., GELS.,** ***ph-ac.***

anxiety, with - ***arg-n.,*** ars., gels., thuj.
- after - ***ars.,*** camph., ***gels.,*** sil., tab.

apyrexia, during - ***iod.***

autumn, in - ***ars.,*** asc-t., bapt., chin., **COLCH.,** ip., **IRIS,** merc., ***merc-c., nux-m., verat.***

bathing, after - ***ant-c.,*** calc., rhus-t., ***podo.,*** sars.
- cold, after - ***ant-c.***

battle, on going into - **GELS.**

beer, after - aloe, chin., gamb., ind., ip., kali-bi., lyc., mur-ac., **SULPH.**
- amel. - phos.

belching, amel. - ***arg-n.,*** carb-v., grat., hep., lyc.

bilious - agar., apis, ***asc-t., bry.,*** cact., cham., colch., ***con.,*** eup-pur., ***fl-ac., ip., iris,*** med., ***merc., merc-c., mur-ac.,*** **NAT-S.,** ***nit-ac., ph-ac.,*** **PODO.,** ***psor., ptel.,*** ter.

boils, begin to heal, as soon as - rhus-v.

breakfast, after - aeth., agar., aloe, alum., ***arg-n.,*** bor., calc., carb-s., cycl., iris, kali-p., kalm., led., lyc., mag-p., mez., nat-m., **NAT-S.,** nuph., nux-v., ox-ac., phos., psor., ***rhod.,*** **THUJ.**
- amel. - bov., nat-s., trom.

burns, after - ars., calc.

cabbage, after - bry., petr., podo.

camping, from - ***alst.,*** jug-c., podo.

cancer of rectum, with - card-m.

castor oil, after - bry.

catarrh, or coryza, after - ***sang.***

cathartics, after - carb-v., ***chin., hep.,*** nit-ac., **NUX-V.**

chagrin, after - aloe, bry., cham., coloc., ***staph.***

chamomile, abuse of - cham., ***coff.,*** valer.

chest, after pains in the - sang.

children, in - ***acon.,*** **AETH.,** ***agar.,*** agn., apis, ***arg-n.,*** **ARS.,** arund., bapt., bar-c., bell., ***benz-ac.,*** bism., ***bor.,*** **CALC.,** calc-ac., ***calc-p.,*** **CALC-S.,** camph., **CHAM.,** ***cina,*** chin., ***coloc.,*** colos., ***crot-t., dulc.,*** elat., ***ferr., form.,*** gamb., grat., hell., hep., **IP.,** ***iris,*** jal., kali-br., kreos., laur., lyc., lyss., ***mag-c.,*** **MAG-M.,** med., **MERC.,** ***merc-c., merc-d., mez., nat-m.,*** nit-ac., nux-m., ***nux-v.,*** olnd., paull., ***ph-ac.,*** **PHOS., PODO., PSOR.,** ***puls.,*** **RHEUM,** sabad., samb., senn., sep.,

DIARRHEA, general

children, in - **SIL.,** stann., ***staph.,*** **STRAM.,** **SULPH.,** sul-ac., ***valer.,*** verat., zinc.

nursing - arund., calc-p., cham.

chill, during - ars., chin., cina, elat., nux-v., **PHOS.,** puls., rhus-t., **VERAT.**

after - sec.

before - verat.

chocolate, after - **ARG-N.,** bor., ***lith.***

cholera, epidemic, during - camph., chin., cupr., **IP.,** ***phos.,*** puls., sec., verat.

after an attack of - sec.

chronic - acet-ac., all-s., aloe, ang., ant-c., ***arg-n.,*** arn., ***ars.,*** ars-i., bapt., ***calc.,*** calc-p., cet., ***chap., chin., coto,*** crot-t., ***cupr-ar.,*** elaps, ferr., ***ferr-m.,*** gamb., ***graph.,*** hep., ***merc.,*** merc-d., ***nat-s.,*** nit-ac., olnd., ***ph-ac., phos., podo.,*** psor., puls., ***rhus-a.,*** rhus-t., rumx., sulph., ***thuj., tub.,*** urt-u.

chronic, mucus, with large amounts of - urt-u.

cider, after - ant-c., calc-p., podo.

coffee, after - canth., caust., ***cist.,*** coloc., corn., ***cycl.,*** fl-ac., hyper., ign., nat-m., osm., ox-ac., phos., ***thuj.***

amel. - brom., ***coloc.,*** corn., phos.

smell of, after - sul-ac.

cold, general

applications amel. - cycl., lyc., ***puls.***

after, taking - acon., ***aloe,*** ant-t., ars., bar-c., ***bell., bry., calc.,*** camph., ***caust., cham.,*** chin., chin-a., coff., con., cop., **DULC.,** elat., gamb., graph., ***ip., jatr.,*** kali-c., merc., ***nat-a., nat-c.,*** nat-s., nit-ac., **NUX-M.,** ***nux-v.,*** op., ***ph-ac.,*** puls., ***rhus-t.,*** sang., sel., sep., ***sulph.,*** verat., zing.

as after taking cold - coloc.

summer, in - aloe, ant-t., bry., ***dulc.,*** **PH-AC.**

becoming, after - arg-n., ***cocc., dulc.,*** nat-a., ***ph-ac.***

drinks, after - ***acon.,*** agra., aloe, ant-c., arg-n., **ARS.,** asaf., bell., ***bry.,*** calc-ar., camph., ***caps., carb-v.,*** caust., cham., chin., chin-a., cinnam., cocc., crot-t., ***dulc., ferr., ferr-ar.,*** fl-ac., grat., ***hep.,*** kali-ar., lept., ***lyc.,*** manc., nat-a., nat-c., ***nat-s.,*** nit-ac., ***nux-m.,*** nux-v., ***ph-ac., puls., rhus-t.,*** sec., sep., ***sil., staph., sul-ac.,*** trom., verat.

amel. - ***phos.***

summer, in - ***carb-v., nat-s.,*** **NUX-M.,** verat.

coryza, ceasing - sang.

nights - acon., ***dulc.***

place amel. - ***puls.***

weather, from - asc-t., ***calc.,*** **DULC.,** ip., merc., nat-s., ***nit-ac., nux-v., polyg.,*** rhod., ***rhus-t.***

confinement, after - hyos.

coryza, during - chlor., sep.

following - ***sang., sel.***

cucumbers, after - verat.

DIARRHEA, general

damp, weather - agar., aloe, ars., ***calc.,*** cist., ***dulc.,*** lach., ***lept.,*** **NAT-S.,** puls., ***rhod.,*** rhus-t., sulph.

amel. - alum., asar.

cold weather - asc-t., ***calc.,*** **DULC.,** ***merc.,*** nux-m., rhod., rhus-t., zing.

darkness, agg. - ***stram.***

daytime, only - am-m., ang., arg-n., bapt., ***bry.,*** canth., cina, ***cocc., con.,*** crot-t., ***elaps,*** fl-ac., ***form., gamb.,*** glon., ***hep.,*** jab., ***kali-c.,*** kali-n., mag-c., nat-a., **NAT-M.,** nat-s., ***nux-v.,*** **PETR.,** squil., sul-ac., ***thuj., trom.***

and night - calc-p., coloc., hyos., kali-c., merc-c., sil.

debauch, after a - ant-c., **NUX-V.**

dentition, during - acet-ac., ***acon., aeth., apis,*** apoc., ***arg-n., ars.,*** arund., ***bell.,*** benz-ac., ***bor.,*** **CALC.,** calc-ac., ***calc-p.,*** canth., carb-v., **CHAM.,** chin., chlol., ***cina, coff.,*** colch., ***coloc.,*** corn., cupr., **DULC., FERR.,** ferr-ar., ***gels.,*** graph., hell., ***hep.,*** ign., ***ip.,*** jal., ***kreos., mag-c., merc.,*** nux-m., olnd., ph-ac., phyt., ***podo., psor.,*** **RHEUM,** ***sep.,*** **SIL.,** ***sulph.,*** sul-ac., zinc.

diet, indiscretion, in eating, after the slightest - aesc., all-s., ***aloe, ant-c.,*** arg-m., **ARS.,** ***asaf.,*** brach., ***bry., carb-v.,*** **CHIN.,** cimic., ***colch.,*** fl-ac., ***gamb.,*** graph., ***iod., ip.,*** kali-chl., naja, nat-m., ***nux-v., petr., ph-ac.,*** **PHOS.,** ***podo., psor.,*** ptel., **PULS.,** ***sulph.,*** zing.

least change of, from - ars., all-s., nux-v.

dinner, after - alum., am-m., caps., carb-s., chin., coloc., **GRAT.,** ***lil-t.,*** **MAG-C.,** nat-m., nit-ac., nux-v., ped., trom., verat.

domestic, cares, from - ars., ***coff.***

drainage, bad - ***carb-ac., pyrog.***

drinking, water, from - ***aloe,*** ant-c., ant-t., ***apis,*** **ARG-N., ARS.,** ***asaf.,*** bry., calc-ar., caps., ***cina,*** coloc., ***crot-t.,*** cub., ***elat.,*** **FERR., FERR-AR.,** fl-ac., gamb., ***grat.,*** kali-ar., kali-n., lach., laur., manc., nux-m., **NUX-V.,** ***podo.,*** rhod., sec., sep., staph., sulph., ***sul-ac., trom.,*** verat., ***zing.***

bad, water, after - ars., ***zing.***

immediately after - ***arg-n.,*** cina, ***crot-t., podo.***

drugging, after - ars., ***nux-v.***

dry, weather - alum., asar.

eating, while - ars., chin., ***crot-t.,*** **FERR.,** ***kali-p.,*** podo., puls., rad-br., trom.

after - aesc., aeth., ***agar.,*** **ALOE,** alum., ***alst.,*** am-m., ant-c., ***apis,*** apoc., ***arg-n.,*** **ARS.,** ars-i., ***asaf.,*** asar., aur-m., aur-m-n., bor., ***brom., bry., calc.,*** calc-s., canth., caps., carb-s., ***carb-v.,*** caust., cedr., ***cham.,*** **CHIN., CHIN-A.,** ***cina,*** cist., **COLOC.,** con., ***corn.,*** **CROT-T.,** cub., ***dulc., ferr., ferr-ar., ferr-i.,*** ferr-ma., ***ferr-m.,*** ferr-p., ***fl-ac., form., gamb.,*** hep., hyper., ign., ***iod., kali-ar.,*** kali-n., ***kali-p., lach.,*** laur., **LYC.,** mur-ac., **NAT-A.,** ***nat-c.,*** nat-p., ***nat-s.,***

DIARRHEA, general

eating,

after - nit-ac., nux-m., ***nux-v., petr., ph-ac., phos.,*** **PODO., PULS.,** raph., ***rheum,*** rhod., rhus-t., sanic., sars., sec., ***staph.,*** sulph., ***sul-ac.,*** tab., tanac., ***thuj.,*** **TROM.,** verat., zinc.

amel. - arg-n., ***brom., chel.,*** dios., grat., ***hep.,*** iod., jab., ***lith., lyc.,*** nat-c., nicc., nit-ac., ***petr.,*** plan., sang.

effluvia, noxious, from - ***crot-h., pyrog.***

eggs, after - chin-a.

elderly, people - **ANT-C., ARS.,** ars-i., bov., ***carb-v., chin.,*** coff., con., ***fl-ac.,*** **GAMB.,** iod., kreos., nat-s., **NIT-AC.,** nux-v., op., ***ph-ac.,*** phos., sec., sulph.

prematurely, with syphilitic mercurial dyscrasia - ***fl-ac.***

women - kreos., nat-s.

emaciated, people, in - ***ars., calc., calc-p.,*** iod., nat-m., phos., ***rheum,*** **SIL.,** sulph., ***sul-ac.***

emotional - ***acon., aloe,*** **ARG-N.,** ***arn., ars., bry., calc-p., cham., coloc.,*** **GELS.,** hyos., ***ign., kali-p.,*** **OP.,** ***ph-ac.,*** puls., ***staph.,*** verat., zinc.

eruptions, suppressed, after - ant-t., apis, bry., dulc., ***hep., lyc.,*** mez., petr., ***psor.,*** **SULPH.,** ***urt-u.***

evening - ***aloe,*** alum., bor., ***bov.,*** bry., ***calc.,*** calc-p., calc-s., canth., carb-an., caust., colch., cycl., dig., dulc., gels., ign., iod., ip., ***kali-c.,*** kali-n., kali-p., kali-s., ***lach.,*** lept., lil-t., mag-m., mang., merc., mez., mur-ac., nat-a., nat-m., nat-s., nuph., ped., phel., ***ph-ac., phos.,*** pic-ac., puls., rhus-t., ***sang.,*** senec., stann., sulph., ter., thuj., valer., verat., zinc.

cold air, in - colch., **MERC.,** nat-s.

exanthemata, during - ant-t., ars., chin., squil.

after suppression of - ant-t., ***bry.,*** graph., hep., merc., psor., sulph.

excitement, from - **ACON.,** aloe, ant-c., ***arg-m.,*** **ARG-N., ARS.,** camph., ***carb-v.,*** caust., ***cham.,*** chin., cina, coch., coloc., ***crot-h.,*** **GELS.,** hyos., ign., ip., ***kali-p., lach., lyc.,*** op., petr., ***ph-ac.,*** phos., puls., sep., sil., tab., ***thuj.,*** verat.

fear, with - **ACON.,** ***arg-n., gels.***

theatre, before going to - **ARG-N.,** gels.

exertion, bodily, during - ***rheum.***

after - ars., ***calc.,*** ferr., nat-s., ***puls., rhus-t.***

fat, flabby people - caps.

fever, with (see typhoid) - aesc., ars., chin., nux-m., phos., puls.

after - phos.

hectic, during - aesc.

after - phos.

intermittent, during - ant-c., ars., chin-a., **CINA,** cocc., con., gels., puls., ***rhus-t.,*** thuj.

puerperal - carb-ac., ***pyrog.,*** sulph.

pernicious - camph., cupr., pyrog.

fish, after - ars., chin-a.

DIARRHEA, general

flatus, after - nat-m.

fluids, loss of after - ***carb-v., chin.,*** ph-ac.

food, acids, agg. - lach., ***nat-p.***

amel. - arg-n.

artificial, after - alum., calc., mag-c., sulph.

aversion to, with - ars., chin., nux-m., phos., puls.

change of, after - all-s., nux-v.

cold, agg. - ant-c., **ARS.,** bry., ***carb-v.,*** cocc., coloc., **DULC.,** hep., ***lyc., nat-s., nit-ac.,*** nux-m., ***nux-v., ph-ac., puls., rhus-t.,*** sep., sul-ac.

amel. - **PHOS.**

crude - cham.

farinaceous, after - lyc., nat-c., **NAT-M., NAT-S.**

fat, after - ant-c., carb-v., cycl., ***kali-chl.,*** kali-m., mag-s., ***puls.,*** thuj.

rancid, after - ***ars.,*** carb-v.

rich, after - arg-n., ***ip.,*** kali-chl., ***nat-s.,*** phos., **PULS.**

solid, after - bapt., ***olnd.,*** **PH-AC.,** ***podo.***

warm agg. - ***phos.***

forenoon - ***aloe,*** apis, ***cact.,*** carb-an., ***gamb.,*** kali-c., lil-t., mag-c., mur-ac., ***nat-m., nat-s.,*** plan., **PODO.,** sabad., stann., ***sulph., thuj., tub.***

8 a.m. - ***ferr.. nat-m***

8 to 10 a.m. - plan.

9 a.m. - ***nat-s.***

10 a.m. - ***nat-m.***

to 10 p.m. - aloe.

fright, after - acon., ***arg-n.,*** **GELS.,** ign., ***kali-p., op., ph-ac.,*** phos., ***puls.,*** verat.

fruit, after - acon., ***aloe,*** ant-t., **ARS.,** ***bor.,*** **BRY.,** calc., ***calc-p., carb-v.,*** **CHIN.,** ***chin-a., cist.,*** **COLOC.,** ***crot-t., ferr., ip., iris,*** lach., lith., ***lyc.,*** mag-c., ***mur-ac.,*** nat-p., **NAT-S.,** ***olnd., ph-ac., podo.,*** **PULS.,** rheum, ***rhod.,*** sul-ac., trom., **VERAT.,** zing.

sour, after - ***ant-c., cist., ip., lach.,*** nat-p., ***ph-ac.***

with milk, after - ***podo.***

stewed, after - bry.

unripe fruit, after - aloe, chin., ***ip.,*** rheum, ***sul-ac.***

game, high, after - **ARS.,** ***carb-v., crot-h., lach.,*** pyrog.

gastric derangements, from - ***ant-c.,*** bry., chin., coloc., ip., lyc., ***nux-v., puls.***

ginger, after - ***nux-v.***

glistening, objects, looking at - *stram.*

gouty, subjects - benz-ac., iod.

grief, after - calc-p., ***coloc., gels., ign.,*** op., merc., **PH-AC.**

ground, standing on damp, after - **DULC.,** elat., ***rhus-t.***

hair, cutting, after - ***bell.***

heat, dry, amel. - sulph.

amel. - ***ars., hep.***

moist external, amel. - ***nux-m.***

sun, of - agar., camph., carb-v.

DIARRHEA, general
hot, weather - ***acon., aeth., aloe,*** ambro., ***ant-c., ars.,*** bapt., ***bell.,*** **BRY.,** calc., **CAMPH.,** caps., ***carb-v., cham.,*** **CHIN.,** chin-a., coff., colch., ***crot-h.,*** **CROT-T.,** ***cuph., cupr., cupr-ar., ferr.,*** ferr-p., **GAMB.,** ***hyper., iod., ip.,*** iris, ***jatr., kali-bi.,*** lach., mag-c., mag-s., merc., ***mez.,*** mur-ac., ***nat-m.,*** nat-p., **NUX-M., OLND.,** ***ph-ac., phos.,*** **PODO.,** ***psor.,*** rheum, ***sec.,*** sil., ***sul-ac.,*** verat.
hot days and cold nights - acon., dulc., merc-c.
hydrocephalus, acute, during - ***apis,*** bell., ***calc., carb-ac., hell., zinc.***
hyperacidity, from - cham., ***nat-p.,*** rheum, rob.
ice cream, after - arg-n., **ARS.,** bry., calc-p., ***carb-v.,*** dulc., **PULS.**
amel. - ***phos.***
imagination, from exalted - ***arg-n.***
indignation, from - ***coloc., gels., ip., staph.***
injuries, after - ***arn.***
intestinal atony, debility, from - ***arg-n.,*** ars., caps., ***chin., ferr.,*** oena., oreo., ***sec.***
jaundice, during - ***chion., dig., lycps., merc., nat-s., nux-v.,*** sep., ***sulph.***
joy, sudden, from - ***coff.,*** **OP.**
lemonade, after - ***cit-ac., phyt.***
light, bright, from - ***bell.,*** colch., ***stram.***
loss of fluids, after - ***carb-v., chin.,*** ph-ac.
lying, agg. - ***dios.,*** ox-ac., raph.
amel. - ***bry.,*** merc., podo., sabad.
abdomen, on the, amel. - aloe, alum., calc., coloc., phos., rhus-t.
back, on the, agg. - phos., podo.
amel. - ***bry.***
lying, side, on the, agg. - ***bry.,*** nit-ac.
left, agg. - ***arg-n.,*** arn., ***phos.***
amel. - phos.
right, agg. - ph-ac.
amel. - podo.
magnesia, after - bry., ***nux-v.,*** puls., rheum
measles, during - squil.
after - ***carb-v.,*** chin., merc., ***puls.,*** squil.
meat, from - ***caust.,*** ferr., lept., sep.
calf - kali-n.
putrescent, from - ars., crot-h.
smoked, from - calc.
melons, from - ***zing.***
menopause, during - apis, ***lach.,*** sulph., tab.
morning - rumx.
menses, during - alum., am-c., ***am-m.,*** ant-c., ars., **BOV.,** bry., calc-p., ***caust.,*** cham., chel., cinnb., clem., glon., graph., kali-c., kali-i., kali-p., kali-s., ***kreos.,*** lach., lac-c., mag-c., nat-a., nat-c., ***nat-p.,*** nat-s., nicc., nux-v., ***phos.,*** plat., podo., ***puls., sars.,*** sil., stront-c., sul-ac., ***tab.,*** tub., **VERAT.,** ***vib.,*** zinc.
after - ars., bov., graph., ***lach.,*** mag-m., nat-m., puls., ***tub.***
before - aloe, alum., ***am-c.,*** apis, **BOV.,** ***cinnb.,*** cocc., hyper., **LACH.,** ***nat-s., sil.,*** tub., ***verat.***

DIARRHEA, general
menses,
before and during - am-c., ***am-m., bov.,*** verat.
beginning, at - **AM-C.**
mental, exertion, after - ***arg-n., nux-v., pic-ac.,*** sabad.
amel. - kali-p.
mercury, after abuse of - asaf., ***hep., kali-i.,*** lach., merc., ***nit-ac.,*** sars., staph., ***sulph.***
milk, after - aeth., ars., bry., **CALC.,** con., iod., ***kali-ar., kali-c.,*** lac-d., ***lyc., mag-c.,*** **MAG-M., NAT-A., NAT-C.,** ***nicc.,*** nit-ac., ***nux-m.,*** podo., **SEP.,** ***sil., sulph.,*** valer.
boiled, after - ***nux-m., sep.***
hot, amel. - chel., crot-t.
sour, after - ***podo.***
morning - acet-ac., aeth., ***agar.,*** all-c., ***aloe,*** alum., am-c., am-m., ang., ant-c., ant-t., ***apis, arg-n., ars., ars-i.,*** aur., ***bor.,*** **BOV.,** brom., **BRY.,** ***cact.,*** calc-s., carb-an., carb-s., caust., chin., chin-a., chlor., cimic., cist., ***coloc., cop.,*** **CORN.,** crot-t., ***dig., dios., dulc.,*** eup-per., ***ferr., ferr-ar.,*** ferr-i., ferr-m., ferr-p., fl-ac., ***gamb.,*** gnaph., graph., ***grat., guai.,*** hep., hura, ***hydr.,*** ichth., ***iod.,*** iris, kali-ar., **KALI-BI.,** ***kali-c.,*** kali-i., kali-n., kali-p., kali-s., kalm., lach., ***lil-t., lith., lyc.,*** lyss., **MAG-C.,** mag-m., mag-s., manc., med., ***merc., mur-ac.,*** nat-a., nat-c., nat-m., nat-p., **NAT-S.,** nicc., nit-ac., ***nuph.,*** nux-m., ***nux-v.,*** ol-j., olnd., osm., ox-ac., ***petr., ph-ac.,*** **PHOS.,** phyt., plan., **PODO.,** psor., ***puls.,*** rhod., rhus-t., rhus-v., **RUMX.,** sang., sarr., senec., sil., squil., staph., stict., **SULPH.,** sumb., ***tab., thuj.,*** trom., ***tub.,*** valer., ***verat., zinc.,*** zing.
4 a.m. - mang., petr.
5 a.m. - aloe, ***phos.,*** **SULPH.,** syph., tub.
6 a.m. - aloe, arg-n., kali-p., lach., ox-ac., petr., ***sulph.***
to 10 a.m. - chin-a.
to noon - ***rumx.***
7 a.m. - xan.
10 a.m. to noon - ***rumx.***
afternoon, until - bor., ***nat-m.***
bed, driving out of - **ALOE,** bell., bov., bry., chin., cic., dios., hep., hydr., hyper., ***kali-bi., lil-t.,*** med., nat-a., nat-s., nuph., petr., ***phos.,*** phyt., ***podo., psor., rumx., sil.,*** **SULPH.,** syph., ***tub., zinc.***
rising, after - aeth., agar., aloe, ars., ***bry.,*** cahin., calc., ***cocc.,*** fl-ac., lept., lyc., mag-s., nat-c., ***nat-m.,*** **NAT-S.,** ***nux-v.,*** ox-ac., ***phos.,*** plan., ***psor., sulph.,*** verat.
and moving about - ars-i., **BRY.,** lept., ***nat-m.,*** **NAT-S.**
waking with urging - ***cench.,*** form., graph., kali-bi., kali-i., lyc., petr., phos., **SULPH.,** zinc.

DIARRHEA, general

motion, agg. - aloe, **APIS,** arn., ars., ***bell.,*** **BRY.,** cadm-s., calc., chin., ***colch.,*** coloc., ***crot-t.,*** **FERR.,** ***ferr-ar.,*** hura, ip., merc-c., mur-ac., ***nat-m.,*** nat-s., ***nux-v.,*** ox-ac., phos., ***podo.,*** puls., rheum, rumx., tab., ***tub.,*** **VERAT.**

amel. - coloc., cub., cycl., ***dios.,*** nit-ac., plan., rhod., ***rhus-t.,*** zinc.

downwards - ***bor.,*** cham., sanic.

nephritis, from - ter.

news, bad, from - **GELS.**

exciting from - **GELS.**

nervousness, agg. - acon., **ARG-N.,** ***ars.,*** ***cham., coff.,*** **GELS.,** hyos., ign., ***op.,*** phos., podo., ***puls., verat.***

night - abrot., acon., aeth., aloe, anac., ang., ant-c., ant-t., **ARG-N.,** ***arn.,*** **ARS.,** arum-t., asaf., asc-t., ***aur.,*** aur-m., bar-c., bell-p., bor., bov., brom., ***bry.,*** canth., ***caps., carb-s.,*** carb-v., ***caust., cham., chel.,*** **CHIN., CHIN-A.,** ***chin-s., cinnb.,*** cist., colch., ***con., crot-t.,*** cub., **DULC.,** ***ferr.,*** **FERR-AR.,** ***ferr-m.,*** ferr-p., fl-ac., ***gamb., graph., grat.,*** hep., ***hyos.,*** ign., ip., **IRIS,** jal., **KALI-AR.,** kali-bi., ***kali-c.,*** kali-p., kali-s., kreos., **LACH.,** lith., lyss., ***mag-c.,*** mag-m., manc., **MERC.,** merc-c., ***mosch.,*** **NAT-A.,** ***nat-c.,*** nat-m., nat-n., ***nat-p.,*** **NUX-M.,** petr., ph-ac., ***phos.,*** **PODO., PSOR., PULS.,** ***rhus-t.,*** sel., senec., ***sil., stront-c., stry.,*** **SULPH.,** ***tab.,*** ther., ***tub.,*** verat., wye., zinc.

1 a.m. to 3 a.m. - asc-t.

to 4 p.m. - ***psor.***

2 a.m. - aran., ***ars.,*** cic., phos., rhus-v., tab.

to 3 a.m. - ***iris,*** phos.

3 a.m. - cimic., mag-c., nat-c., petr., phos.

amel. - stront-c.

to 4 a.m. - aeth., ***kali-c.,*** lyc.

to 11 a.m. - nat-m.

4 a.m. - fl-ac., form., mang., ***petr.,*** phos., **PODO.,** ***rhus-t.,*** sec.

to 6 a.m. - ***all-c.,*** phos.

to 7 a.m. - nuph.

5 to 6 a.m. - ***nuph.***

lying agg. - ***lach.***

midnight, after - aloe, ***arg-n.,*** **ARS.,** arum-t., asc-t., bry., ***chin., chin-a.,*** cic., cist., dros., **FERR-AR.,** ferr-p., fl-ac., gamb., iris, **KALI-AR.,** kali-c., kali-s., lyc., manc., merc-c., nat-a., nat-m., ***nux-v.,*** sec., squil., staph., stront-c., **SULPH.**

before - mag-c., nux-m., puls., rhus-t.

noon, to - ars., cist.

night, only - chin.

noise, from - colch., ***nit-ac., nux-v.***

sudden, from - bell., bor.

noisy - lem-m.

noon - alum., ant-c., bor., carb-s., crot-t., jab., mag-m., sulph.

noxious effluvia, from - bapt., carb-ac., ***crot-h.***

nursing, after, infants - ant-c., ***crot-t.,*** nat-c., ***nux-v.***

women, in - ***chin., rheum.***

DIARRHEA, general

onions, after - lyc., nux-v., ***puls., thuj.***

opium, after - ***mur-ac., nat-m.,*** nux-v., **PULS.**

oranges, after - ***ph-ac.***

overheated, after being - acon., aloe, **ANT-C.,** elat., **PULS.**

oysters, after - ***aloe, brom., lyc., podo., sul-ac.***

painless - ***aloe,*** anthr., ***apis,*** arg-n., arn., ***ars.,*** ars-i., arum-t., **BAPT.,** bar-m., bell., **BISM., BOR.,** bry., ***calc.,*** calc-s., ***camph.,*** cann-i., carb-an., carb-s., ***cham., chel., chin.,*** cinnb., clem., ***cocc.,*** coch., ***coff.,*** colch., coloc., con., ***crot-t., dulc.,*** **FERR.,** ***ferr-ar., ferr-p.,*** gamb., ***gels.,*** graph., ***grat.,*** hell., **HEP., HYOS.,** ***ign.,*** ip., iris, jab., ***jatr., kali-ar.,*** kali-bi., ***kali-c.,*** kali-n., kali-p., kali-s., ***lach.,*** laur., ***lyc., mag-c.,*** merc., **NAT-M.,** ***nat-p., nat-s.,*** nit-ac., ***nuph.,*** nux-m., nux-v., ***olnd.,*** op., petr., **PH-AC., PHOS.,** plat., **PODO.,** ***psor.,*** puls., ***pyrog.,*** ran-b., rhod., ***rhus-t.,*** rumx., sec., sep., ***sil.,*** **SQUIL.,** stann., stram., **SULPH.,** ***sul-ac.,*** tab., **TUB.,** thuj., ***verat.,*** zinc.

night - ars., bor., bry., canth., cham., ***chin.,*** dulc., merc., puls., rhus-t., sulph., verat.

only after eating in daytime - **CHIN.**

palpitation, with - jatr.

pastry, after - arg-n., ***ip., kali-chl., lyc., nat-s., ph-ac.,*** phos., **PULS.**

pears, after - bor., bry., ***verat.***

periodical - apis, ars., ***chin.,*** euph-c., iris, ***kali-bi.,*** mag-c., thuj.

alternate days, on - ***alum., carb-ac.,*** **CHIN.,** dig., fl-ac., ***iris,*** nit-ac.

every fourth day - sabad.

three weeks - mag-c.

hour later each day - fl-ac.

nightly - iris.

same hour, at - apis, sabad., sel., thuj.

summer - ***kali-bi.***

perspiration, amel. - stram.

suppressed, from - acon., cham., ferr-p.

pneumonia, in - ant-t.

pork, after - acon., acon-l., ant-c., cycl., lyc., nux-m., ***puls.***

potatoes, after - ***alum.,*** coloc., sep., verat.

sweet, after - ***calc-ar.***

pregnancy, during - alum., am-m., ***ant-c.,*** apis, ars., cham., ***cham., chel., chin.,*** dulc., ferr., ferr-m., hell., ***hyos., lyc., nux-m.,*** nux-v., petr., ph-ac., **PHOS.,** psor., ***puls., sec., sep.,*** stram., ***sulph.***

puerperal - ***cham.,*** hyos., puls.

quinine, after abuse of - ferr., hep., lach., nat-m., pall., **PULS.**

rhubarb, after - ***cham., coloc.,*** merc., nux-v., puls.

riding, from - **COCC.,** mag-s., nux-m., ***petr.,*** psor.

amel. - ***nit-ac.***

train, in a - med.

DIARRHEA, general
rising up, agg. - acon., ***bry.,*** cocc., op., trom.
bed, from, amel., - cub., dios., mez.
rubbing, amel. - dios., lyc.
salmon, after eating - ***fl-ac.***
sauerkraut, after - ***bry., petr.***
school, girls, in - ***calc-p., ph-ac.***
sea, bathing, from - mag-m., sep.
seashore, while at - ***ars.,*** bry.
sensation, as before a - agar., **ALOE,** apoc., carl., colch., crot-t., dig., dros., **DULC.,** eupi., form., gels., glon., grat., ind., iris, kali-n., lyc., merc-i-f., mez., nat-m., ***nit-ac.,*** phos., pip-m., plan., plb., sulph.
smoking, while - bor.
walking, while - nat-m.
septic, conditions, from - **ARS.,** ***carb-ac., carb-v., crot-h., lach.,*** **PYROG.,** ***sulph.***
shell-fish, from - carb-v.
shining, objects agg. - ***stram.***
sitting, agg. - crot-t., dios.
amel. - cocc.
erect agg. - ***bry.***
sleep, during - bry., ***sulph., tub.***
after - bell., **LACH.,** pic-ac., sulph., zing.
amel. - alum., crot-t., ***phos.***
small-pox, during - ant-t., ***ars.,*** **CHIN.,** thuj.
smoking, agg. - bor., brom., cham.
soup, from - mag-c.
spices, from - phos.
spring, in - ***bry.,*** iris, ***lach.,*** sars.
standing, agg. - ***aloe,*** ars., bry., ***cocc.,*** ign., lil-t., rheum, **SULPH.**
amel. - merc.
stormy, weather - petr.
strain, after a - ***rhus-t.***
sugar, after - **ARG-N.,** calc., calc-s., crot-t., gamb., ***merc.,*** ox-ac., ***sulph.,*** trom.
maple sugar - calc-s.
sundown to sunrise agg., from - colch.
supper, after - hyper., iris, kali-p., trom.
suppressed, gonorrhea, after - **MED.**
sweets, from, (see sugar) - ***arg-n.,*** calc-s., crot-t., ***gamb.***
thinking, of it - ox-ac.
thunderstorm, during - nat-c., phos., rhod.
before - rhod.
tobacco, from - brom., cham., ign., puls., tab.
tuberculosis, during - acet-ac., arg-n., ***arn., ars., ars-i., bapt.,*** bism., calc., ***chin.,*** coto, ***cupr-ar.,*** elaps, ferr., ferr-p., iod., iodof., **PH-AC.,** ***phos.,*** rumx., sil.
typhoid fever, from - ***ars., bapt.,*** echi., eucal., ***hyos.,*** lach., ***mur-ac.,*** nuph., op., ph-ac., ***rhus-t.,*** stram.
ulceration of intestines, from - kali-bi., merc-c.
urinating, agg. - ***aloe,*** **ALUM.,** apis, canth., ***hyos.,*** squil.
uterine, bleeding with - tanac.
vaccination, after - ant-t., sil., ***thuj.***
vaginal discharge, with - puls.

DIARRHEA, general
veal, after - ***kali-n.***
vegetables, after - ars., bry., cist., cupr., hell., lept., ***lyc.,*** nat-a., nat-c., ***nat-m., nat-s.,*** petr., podo., verat., zing.
vexation, from - aloe, ***calc-p.,*** cham., ***coloc., petr., staph.,*** sulph.
vinegar, after - ***ant-c.***
walking, agg. - ***aloe,*** alum., ***calc., gels.,*** merc.
warm, application amel. - alum., ***nux-m.,*** podo., rhus-t.
drinks, agg. - ***fl-ac.***
food, agg. - ***phos.***
room, agg. - apis, ***iod.,*** nat-s., **PULS.**
warmth, agg. - ***puls.,*** sec.
bed, of amel. - coloc., ***nux-v.,*** **SIL.**
washing, the head, after - podo., tarent.
water, hearing running, agg. - **LYSS.**
polluted, from - ***alst.,*** ars., camph., ***zing.***
weakness, without - **PH-AC.,** puls., ***sulph., tub.***
weaning, after - arg-n., **CHIN.**
weather, change of, from - ***acon., bry.,*** calc., calc-s., caps., colch., ***dulc.,*** ip., ***merc., nat-s., ph-ac., psor.,*** rhus-t., sil.
wet, after getting - ***acon., calc.,*** **RHUS-T.**
feet, after getting - acon., nux-m., **RHUS-T.**
whooping cough, during - cast-v.
wind, after exposure to, cold - ***acon., dulc.***
east wind - psor.
wine, from - lach., lyc., ***zinc.***
amel. - chel., dios.
sour - **ANT-C.**
winter - asc-t., nat-s., ***nit-ac.***
wrapping, up warmly amel. - **SIL.**

DIPHTHERIA, ailments since - lac-c., phyt., pyrog.
prophylactic - apis, diph., merc-cy.

DISCOLORATION, anus, green, mucous stains skin around and scrotum - cinnb.

DISTENSION - agar., merc., op., staph., sulph.

DRAGGING, sensation, heaviness, weight - acon., **AESC.,** agar., **ALOE,** ang., ant-c., arn., bar-c., bell., berb., bry., ***cact.,*** calc., cann-s., ***carb-v.,*** caust., chel., coll., con., ***crot-t.,*** cycl., euphr., graph., hep., hyos., inul., kali-bi., kali-c., kali-n., kali-p., kreos., lach., lact., laur., led., lil-t., lob., lyc., mag-m., manc., merc., ***nit-ac.,*** nux-m., ***nux-v.,*** phos., plan., plb., puls., rhus-t., sac-alb., sep., staph., sulph., sumb., ther., thuj., verat., ***zinc.***
afternoon - cycl.
dinner, after - cycl.
sleep, after - cycl.
evening, during loose stool - op.
flatus, amel. - zinc.
menses, during - ***aloe.***
before - phos.
morning - lyc.
stool after - lyc.
standing, while - ***zinc.***

DRAGGING, sensation
stool, during - mez., ***nit-ac.,*** op.
after - hell., kali-bi., nat-m., rhus-t., ruta., zinc.
amel., after - kreos.
before - hell., merc.

DRAW, in anus, desire to - agar.

DRAWING, pain - ant-c., aur-s., calc., cann-s., carb-v., chel., chin., ***cycl.,*** eupi., kreos., lach., lact., mang., mez., phos., rhod., zinc.
downwards - phos.
extending, abdomen, into - aloe, zinc.
coccyx, through - carb-an.
genitals through - carb-an., rhod.
genitals, through, before stool - carb-an.
umbilicus, to - ***lach.***
upwards - mez., plb., thuj.
urethra, through - hipp., mez.
sex, after - caust.
sitting, while - chin., ***cycl.***
walking, while - ***cycl.***

DRIPPING from, sensation of - aloe, ferr-i., sulph.

DROPPING, of something cold out of anus - cann-s.

DRYNESS - **AESC.,** aeth., agar., alum., ***alumn.,*** calc., carb-v., ***graph.,*** hyper., ***kali-chl., nat-m.,*** rat., sulph., sumb.
sensation of - agar., calc., carb-v.

DYSENTERY, (see Intestines)

EMPTINESS, sensation of - podo.

ERUPTIONS, anus, about - ***agar.,*** am-c., am-m., ant-c., ars., berb., ***calc.,*** carb-an., carb-s., carb-v., ***caust., graph., hep.,*** ign., kali-c., lyc., med., merc., **NAT-M.,** ***nat-s.,*** **NIT-AC., PETR.,** sep., ***staph., sulph.,*** thuj.
blotches - carb-v., stann., ***staph., thuj.***
burning - ars., calc., petr.
crust - berb., paeon., ***petr.***
eczema - berb.
itching - ars., cinnb., lyc., **PETR.,** staph., sulph.
newborn, in - med.
pimples - ***agar.,*** brom., carb-v., ***cinnb.,*** kali-c., kali-i., nit-ac., polyg., staph.
pustules - am-m., calc., caust.
hard, small - caust.
scurfy - ***petr.***
stinging - kali-c., nit-ac.
ulcerous - kali-c.
vesicular - brom., carb-an., carb-v.
warmth of bed agg. - ***petr.***

EXCORIATION, anus - ***aesc., agar.,*** agn., all-c., alum., am-c., ***apis,*** arg-m., ***ars.,*** asc-c., aur-m., ***bar-c., berb., calc.,*** calc-s., carb-an., **CARB-S., CARB-V., CAUST.,** ***cham.,*** coloc., dirc., ferr., ***gamb.,*** **GRAPH.,** grat., hep., ***hydr., ign.,*** kali-ar., kali-c., lach., **LYC.,** med., ***merc., merc-c.,*** mur-ac., nat-a., ***nat-m., nat-p., nit-ac.,*** nux-v., ***petr.,*** phos., ***plan., podo., puls., sanic., sep.,*** **SULPH.,** sumb., ***syph., thuj., tub.,*** urt-u., zinc.
acrid, moisture, from - carb-v., ***merc-c., thuj.,*** zinc.

EXCORIATION, anus
must rub, until raw - ***agar.,*** alum., am-c., ***arg-n., bar-c., calc., carb-s.,*** **CARB-V., CAUST., GRAPH.,** kali-c., **LYC.,** ***merc.,*** **PETR.,** phos., ***puls., sep.,*** **SULPH.**
riding, in a wagon - psor.
on horseback - carb-an.
stools, from the - **ALOE, APIS,** ***ars., bapt.,*** coloc., dirc., ***kreos., merc.,*** mur-ac., **NIT-AC.,** nux-m., ***nux-v.,*** rheum, sang., ***sulph., tub.***

excoriation, buttocks, between - arum-t., arg-m., ***berb.,*** bufo, ***carb-s.,*** **GRAPH.,** ***kreos.,*** nat-m., ***nit-ac.,*** puls., ***sep., sulph.***
walking, from - arg-m., **CAUST.,** nat-m., ***nit-ac.***

excoriation, of perineum - alum., arum-t., aur-m., ***calc.,*** carb-an., ***carb-v., caust., cham., graph., hep.,*** ign., **LYC.,** ***merc.,*** petr., puls., rhod., sep., ***sulph.,*** thuj.
female - ***calc., carb-v., caust.,*** **GRAPH.,** hep., **LYC.,** ***merc., petr., sep., sulph.,*** thuj.

FECES, remained in, as if - carb-an., ***graph., lyc.,*** nat-c., **NAT-M.,** ***nit-ac.,*** **SEP.,** stann., ***verat.***
something remaining behind, with constipation, as if - aloe, alum., lyc., nat-m., ***nux-v.,*** sep., sil., sulph.

FISSURE - aesc., ***agn., all-c., aloe,*** alum., anac., ant-c., apis, arg-m., ***ars.,*** arum-t., berb., calc., calc-f., ***calc-p.,*** carb-an., ***carb-v., caust.,*** **CHAM.,** cimx., ***cund.,*** cur., ***fl-ac.,*** **GRAPH.,** grat., ham., ***hydr., ign.,*** iris, kali-c., kali-i., ***lach.,*** led., med., ***merc., merc-d.,*** merc-i-r., mez., morph., mur-ac., ***nat-m.,*** **NIT-AC.,** nit-m-ac., ***nux-v., paeon., petr., phos., phyt.,*** plat., ***plb.,*** **RAT.,** rhus-t., sang-n., sanic., **SEP., SIL.,** ***sulph.,*** syph., **THUJ.,** vib.
bleeding after stool - lac-d., ***nat-m., nit-ac.***
children, tall - calc-p.
infants - kali-i.
sensation of hammers in - ***lach.***
ulcerate - graph.

FISTULA - ***aloe, alum.,*** ant-c., aur., **AUR-M.,** bar-m., bell., **BERB.,** bry., cact., **CALC., CALC-P.,** calc-s., carb-s., **CARB-V., CAUST.,** ***fl-ac., graph., hep., hydr.,*** ign., **KALI-C.,** ***kreos., lach., lyc., merc.,*** myris., **NIT-AC.,** nux-v., paeon., ***petr., phos.,*** puls., querc., ***rat., sep.,*** **SIL.,** ***staph., sulph., syph., thuj.***
alternates with chest disorders - berb., calc-p., ***sil.***
itching, with - berb.
palpitation, with - cact.
recto-vaginal - thuj.
perineum - thuj.
vagina, and - thuj.
pulsating - ***caust.***

FLATUS, rectal (see Intestines) - ***aesc.,*** **AGAR., ALL-C., ALOE,** ***alum.,*** am-c., ***am-m.,*** ambr., ant-c., ***ant-t., apoc.,*** **ARG-N., ARN.,** ***ars., ars-i., asaf.,*** asar., ***aur.,*** aur-m., ***bar-c.,*** bar-m., ***bell., bism.,*** bor., brom., ***bry.,*** calad., calc., camph., carb-ac., carb-an., **CARB-S., CARB-V.,** card-m., casc., ***caust.,*** **CHAM.,** ***chel.,*** **CHIN.,** ***chin-a.,*** cic., chlor., **COCC.,** ***coc-c., colch.,*** **COLOC.,** ***con.,*** cop., **CORN.,** ***crot-h., crot-t.,*** cycl., dig., **DIOS.,** ***dulc.,*** elat., euph., fago., ***ferr., ferr-ar.,*** ferr-i., ***ferr-p.,*** fl-ac., ***gels.,*** gnaph., **GRAPH.,** ham., ***hep.,*** hydr., hyos., **IGN.,** ***indg.,*** iod., ***kali-ar.,*** kali-bi., ***kali-c.,*** kali-i., kali-n., ***kali-p., kali-s., lach.,*** led., ***lil-t.,*** **LYC.,** mag-c., ***mag-m.,*** mang., **MERC.,** meny., mez., mur-ac., ***nat-a., nat-c., nat-m., nat-p.,*** **NAT-S.,** ***nit-ac.,*** nux-m., **NUX-V., OLND., OP.,** ox-ac., pall., **PH-AC., PHOS.,** phys., **PIC-AC.,** plat., **PLB.,** ***podo., psor.,*** **PULS., RAPH.,** rhus-t., ***rhod.,*** ruta., sabad., samb., ***sang.,*** sars., ***sec., sel., sep.,*** **SIL.,** spig., **STAPH.,** stram., **SULPH.,** sul-ac., tarent., tell., tep., ter., **TEUCR.,** ***thuj.,*** thyr., torula., valer., **VERAT.,** vib., ***zinc.***

acids, after - ***ph-ac.***

afternoon - am-c., aur-m., benz-ac., cast., cham., carb-v., dig., fl-ac., iod., mag-c., myric., nat-c., nat-s., nicc., osm., phos., plb., stront-c., zinc.

amelioration, from - acon., all-c., aloe, ambr., anac., ant-t., ***arg-n.,*** arn., asaf., asar., aur., bism., bor., bry., calc-p., canth., caps., ***carb-s.,*** **CARB-V.,** ***cham.,*** chel., ***chin.,*** cic., ***cocc.,*** coff., ***colch., coloc.,*** con., crot-t., eup-per., ***graph.,*** guai., hep., hyos., ***ign.,*** kali-c., kali-s., lach., laur., **LYC.,** meny., mez., nat-m., **NAT-S.,** nit-ac., nux-m., **NUX-V.,** ***ph-ac., phos.,*** plat., ***plb.,*** **PULS.,** rheum, ***rhod.,*** rhus-t., ruta., sabin., **SANG.,** sel., sep., sil., spig., spong., squil., **STAPH.,** stram., **SULPH.,** teucr., thuj., ***verat.,*** verb., zinc.

amel., without - camph., **CHAM., CHIN.,** graph., mang.

burning - mag-m.

cold - ***con.***

coughing, on - graph., ***nux-v.,*** sang., ***sulph.***

daytime - aloe, nat-m., ox-ac., plat., **SULPH.**

delusion of, everybody notices his - zinc-p.

diarrhea, during - ***agar.,*** **ALOE,** am-m., ***arg-n.,*** asaf., bor., bov., ***bry., calc-p.,*** **CARB-V.,** ***chin., colch., coloc.,*** cub., cupr., ***dios., kali-c.,*** kali-n., ***lach., lyc.,*** mag-m., ***manc., mur-ac.,*** nat-p., **NAT-S.,** ***nicc.,*** nit-ac., nux-v., **OLND.,** ***phos.,*** plan., plat., rhus-t., sabin., sang., sars., sep., sil., squil., tab., zing.

difficult - all-c., anac., calc-p., camph., cocc., coff., hep., hyos., kali-c., lyss., mez., nat-s., op., ox-ac., phos., plat., sil., sul-ac.

dinner after - alum., ant-c., ***arg-n., cycl.,*** grat., hell., nat-m., nit-ac., sulph., verat.

dysmenorrhea, with - vib.

eating, after - ***aloe,*** ant-c., con., ign., op., plat., sep., tab.

FLATUS, rectal

evening - aesc., aloe, alum., am-c., carb-an., cast., chel., chin-s., ***colch.,*** crot-t., fago., ***gamb.,*** kali-n., lyc., nat-m., nat-s., nicc., phos., ***ph-ac.,*** sarr., sol-t-ae., stront-c., **SULPH.,** thuj., zinc.

stool, during - gels.

forenoon - calc-p., carb-an., nat-m.

10 a.m., - fl-ac.

stool, before - fl-ac.

hot - acon., ***agar.,*** **ALOE,** ant-t., bapt., ***carb-v.,*** cham., cocc., dios., phos., plb., ***psor., puls., staph., sulph.,*** sumb., ***teucr., zinc.***

hysterical - valer.

inspiration, during - caust.

involuntary - phos.

nearly - graph.

loud - **ALOE,** alum., am-m., **ARG-N.,** berb., calad., carb-v., **CAUST.,** coloc., con., fl-ac., hydr., kali-n., ***lach.,*** mag-c., merc., ***mez.,*** **NAT-S.,** ox-ac., phos., plan., squil., ***teucr.,*** verat., ***zinc.***

night, at - **ARG-N.**

stool, after - aloe, ox-ac.

stool, during - ***aloe, hydr., indg., ip.,*** **NAT-S.,** ***ph-ac.,*** thuj.

stool, sputtering - **ALOE,** eug., **NAT-S.,** ***thuj.***

sugar, after - **ARG-N.**

menses, during - clem., kali-c., mag-c., nicc.

moist - ***all-c., ant-c., carb-v.,*** zinc.

morning - **ALL-C.,** aloe, bov., bufo, caust., cedr., fl-ac., hell., hep., lyc., mag-m., mag-s., **NAT-S.,** nit-ac., plb., ***puls.***

stool, during - chel.

waking, on - ***carb-v.,*** rheum.

night - all-c., alum., am-c., arg-m., bry., cast., coloc., hep., hom., ign., kali-c., lyc., mag-c., ox-ac., sol-t-ae., **SULPH.,** verat.

menses, before - mang.

stool, during - psor.

noon - ox-ac., sulph.

odorless - **AGAR.,** ambr., arg-n., ***bell.,*** carb-v., lyc., mang., nicc., ***phos., plat.,*** **SULPH.,** ***thuj.,*** zinc.

offensive - ***aesc.,*** agar., ***all-c.,*** **ALOE,** alum., am-m., ammc., ant-c., **ARN., ARS.,** ars-i., **ASAF.,** ***aur.,*** bar-c., bar-m., ***bor., bov.,*** **BRY.,** ***calc., calc-p.,*** camph., carb-ac., ***carb-an.,*** **CARB-S., CARB-V., CAUST.,** cedr., ***chin.,*** chin-a., ***cocc., coff., colch., coloc.,*** con., cop., ***corn.,*** crot-t., ***dios.,*** dirc., ***dulc.,*** ferr-ma., form., glon., ***graph.,*** hell., hipp., ***hydr., ign.,*** kali-c., kali-n., ***kali-p.,*** kali-s., **LACH.,** lact., lec., lith., lyc., mag-c., merc., ***mez.,*** mur-ac., ***nat-c.,*** **NAT-M., NAT-S.,** nicc., **NIT-AC.,** nux-m., ***nux-v., olnd.,*** op., petr., ***ph-ac., phos., plb., podo., psor.,*** **PULS.,** rhod., ruta., ***sanic.,*** sang., sep., sarr., sars., **SIL.,** squil., stann., ***staph., stram.,*** **SULPH.,** sumb., tell., ***teucr., valer., zinc.***

FLATUS, rectal
offensive, ammoniacal odor - agn.
cheese-like - ***sanic.***
eating, after - puls.
garlic odor - agar., ph-ac.
night - sep.
sour odor - calc., mag-c., nat-c., nat-m., rheum.
spoiled eggs - ant-t., **ARN.,** ***cham.,*** coff., fl-ac., ***hep.,*** nat-c., nat-m., olnd., ***psor.,*** spig., ***staph.,*** **SULPH.,** ***tell.***
writing, after - ant-c.
pneumonia, in, noisy - sulph.
pressing, against coccyx - zinc.
retained in rectum - hep., nux-v., sep.
sensation, as if flatus would pass - mag-c.
but stool comes - mag-m.
short - mez., plat., squil., sul-ac.
stool, during - ***agar.,*** **ALOE,** am-m., am-m., apoc., ***arg-n.,*** asaf., ***bry., calc-p., carb-v.,*** caust., ***chin.,*** cocc., **COLL.,** ***coloc., con., corn.,*** **CROT-T.,** cub., eug., **FERR.,** fl-ac., gamb., gels., hydr., indg., ip., hipp., ***hydr., ign., indg., ip., iris,*** jatr., mang., mur-ac., **NAT-S.,** ***nit-ac.,*** nux-m., **OLND.,** osm., ***ph-ac.,*** plat., **PODO.,** ***psor.,*** ruta., sabin., sang., **SEC.,** squil., ***staph.,*** stroph., sul-ac., **THUJ.,** thyr., tub., zing.
after - aloe, am-m., colch., con., hep., ox-ac.
before - aesc., aloe, am-m., ***apis,*** arg-n., asaf., calad., carb-v., cocc., ***colch.,*** coloc., ***crot-t.,*** dig., ferr., fl-ac., ***gamb.,*** gels., kali-c., mag-c., mez., nat-m., ***nat-s.,*** olnd., petr., phos., plat., ***podo.,*** puls., sabad., sang.
urging for stool, but only flatus is passed - ***aloe,*** ant-c., cahin., ***carb-an., carb-v.,*** caust., chin., ***colch.,*** kali-n., ***lac-c.,*** laur., mag-c., mag-m., mez., myric., osm., **NAT-S.,** ruta., ***sang.,*** sep.
sugar, after - **ARG-N.**
touching, abdomen - squil.
violent - graph.
walking - mag-c., sep.

FOREIGN, body, sensation of - lil-t., nat-m., rumx., sep., sulph.
something hard - caust.

FORMICATION, anus - ***aesc.,*** agar., ail., aloe, all-c., alum., ambr., ant-c., ant-t., arg-m., arg-n., ***bar-c.,*** benz-ac., ***berb.,*** bov., **CALC., CALC-S.,** canth., carb-s., ***carb-v.,*** caust., chel., chin., ***cinnb.,*** coc-c., colch., ***croc.,*** elaps, fago., ferr-i., ferr-ma., gran., grat., hep., ***ign.,*** **KALI-C.,** kali-p., kreos., mez., mosch., ***mur-ac., nat-c., nux-v.,*** ol-an., petros., phos., ***plat.,*** plb., rhod., rhus-t., ***sabad., sep.,*** sil., spig., spong., **SULPH.,** ter., ***teucr.,*** verat-v., ***zinc.***
bug, crawling from - aesc., ferr-i., sulph.
stools, after - kali-m.
evening - euphr., kali-c., plat., spong., ***sulph.,*** teucr.
in bed - plat., ***teucr.***

FORMICATION, anus
night - ***nux-v.***
sitting, while - **SULPH.**
stool, after - aloe, berb., chin., mez., teucr.
before - kali-c., phos.
walking - phos.
after - phos.
worm in, as from - cina, cinnb.

FULLNESS - acon., **AESC.,** agar., **ALOE,** alum., apis, ars., bell., berb., bry., carb-v., caust., cycl., ferr., **HAM.,** kali-bi., ***lach.,*** lil-t., manc., med., meli., **NIT-AC.,** phos., plan., sabin., stram., **SULPH.,** thuj.
alternating with sensation of emptiness - thuj.
stool, after - **AESC.,** alumn., ***lyc., sep.***
walking, after - aesc.

GNAWING, pain - ***carb-v.,*** elaps, ferr., merc., phos., stann.

GRIPING, pain - ***calc.,*** carb-v., ***cocc.,*** **IGN.,** kali-c., mur-ac., nat-m., nit-ac., ox-ac., thuj.
afternoon - ***cocc.***
driving, while - glon.
evening - mez.
extending to abdomen - mez.
forenoon - ***calc.***
sitting - ***calc., cocc.***
stool, when not at - carb-v.
amel. - ***nat-a.***

GRUMBLING - mang.

GURGLING, in - calc., carb-an., hep., laur., stry., ***sulph.***

HEAT - **AESC.,** agar., **ALOE,** apis, ars., berb., bry., calc-p., clem., colch., ***con.,*** cycl., ***eup-per.,*** glon., iod., ***lach.,*** lil-t., ***merc.,*** naja, nat-m., nit-ac., phyt., ***rat., rumx.,*** sep., sulph.
afternoon - cycl.
morning - glon.
rising, on - glon.
noon - agar.
stool, during - ***aloe,*** ant-t., form., ***glon.,*** **PODO.**
after - calc., calc-s., caps., euphr., sol-t-ae., zinc.
urination, after - rhus-t.

HEMORRHOIDS - abrot., acet-ac., acon., **AESC.,** ***aesc-g.,*** aeth., **AGAR.,** agn., **ALOE,** alum., alumn., am-br., ***am-c.,*** am-m., anac., anan., ang., ***ant-c.,*** ant-t., ***apis,*** apoc., arg-n., arn., **ARS.,** ***ars-i.,*** arum-t., arund., aster., aur., aur-m., bapt., ***bar-c., bell.,*** berb., bor., bov., ***brom.,*** bry., ***bufo, cact., calc., calc-f., calc-p., calc-s.,*** cann-s., canth., ***caps.,*** carb-ac., **CARB-AN., CARB-V.,** carb-s., ***card-m.,*** carl., casc., **CAUST.,** cham., ***chel.,*** chim., chin., chin-a., chr-ac., cic., cimic., ***cimx.,*** clem., ***coca,*** cocc., ***coff.,*** colch., **COLL.,** ***coloc.,*** con., cop., croc., crot-h., cycl., ***dios.,*** dol., elaps, ***erig., eug.,*** euphr., ***ferr., ferr-ar.,*** ferr-m., ferr-p., ***fl-ac.,*** gels., **GRAPH.,** grat., **HAM.,** ***hell., hep., hydr., hyos., hyper., ign., iod., ip.,*** **KALI-AR.,** ***kali-bi.,*** **KALI-C.,** ***kali-m.,*** kali-n., kali-p., **KALI-S.,** kreos., **LACH.,** lact., ***lept.,*** lil-t., lob., **LYC.,** mag-c., ***mag-m.,*** manc., med.,

HEMORRHOIDS - ***merc.,*** **MERC-I-R.,** mez., mill., mosch., **MUR-AC.,** ***nat-m., nat-s.,*** **NIT-AC., NUX-V., PAEON.,** ***petr.,*** ph-ac., **PHOS.,** phys., ***phyt.,*** pin-s., plan., plat., plb., ***podo., polyg., psor.,*** **PULS.,** rad., **RAT.,** ***rhus-t.,*** rhus-v., rumx., ***ruta., sabin., sang.,*** scroph-n., sec., ***semp.,*** **SEP.,** ***sil.,*** stann., ***staph.,*** stront-c., **SULPH.,** ***sul-ac.,*** sumb., syph., ***ter.,*** ther., ***thuj., tub.,*** verat., verat-v., verb., ***wye.,*** yohim, zinc., ***zing.***

alcoholics, in - ***ars., carb-v., lach.,*** **NUX-V.,** ***sul-ac.,*** **SULPH.**

alcohol abuse, in sedentary persons agg. - aesc-g., nux-v., sulph.

alternating with, lumbago - aesc., ***aloe.***

palpitation - **COLL.**

abdominal plethora, with - aesc., ***aloe,*** coll., ham., nux-v., sep., ***sulph.***

bathing, agg. - sulph.

backache, with - ***aesc.,*** aesc-g., ***bell.,*** calc-f., chr-ac., euon., ham., ign., ***nux-v.,*** sulph.

beer agg. - ***aloe,*** bry., ferr., nux-v., rhus-t., **SULPH.**

bleeding, as soon as the rheumatism is better - ***abrot., ham.***

amel. - aesc.

vicarious bleeding - ham., mill.

blind - aesc., anac., ant-c., ars., asc-t., brom., calc-f., caps., ***calc-p.,*** cham., ***coll.,*** coloc., dulc., ferr., grat., ***ign.,*** mag-p-a., nit-ac., ***nux-v.,*** podo., ***puls., rhus-t., sulph.,*** verat., wye.

bluish - aesc., aesc-g., aeth., ***aloe,*** ars., caps., **CARB-V.,** dios., ***ham.,*** **LACH.,** ***lyc.,*** manc., **MUR-AC.,** phys., ***sulph.,*** verat-v.

burning - ham., rat., sulph.

bursting - ham.

cherries, like a bunch - aesc., aloe, calc., dios., mur-ac.

childbirth, agg. or since - acon., ***aloe,*** bell-p., ***ign.,*** **KALI-C.,** ***lil-t., mur-ac., podo., puls.,*** **SEP.,** ***sulph.***

children, in - ***mur-ac.***

chills up and down back, with - aesc.

chronic - **AESC.,** ***aloe,*** am-c., apis., calc., carb-v., ***carb-s.,*** caust., **COLL.,** dios., graph., **HAM.,** ***lach., lyc.,*** **MERC-I-R.,** ***nit-ac.,*** **NUX-V.,** petr., ***phos.,*** phyt., ***podo.,*** **SULPH.,** ***tub.***

cold, amel. - aesc., aloe, apis, brom., kali-c., nux-v.

water - ***aloe,*** nux-v., rat.

confinement, after - aloe, apis., sep.

congested - ***acon.,*** aesc., agar., ***aloe,*** alum., apoc., arg-n., ars., ***bell., carb-s.,*** carb-v., ***caust., cham.,*** cop., ferr-p., graph., ham., ***hep.,*** **KALI-C.,** kali-n., ***merc., mur-ac.,*** **NUX-V., PAEON.,** podo., ***puls., rhus-t.,*** sil., ***sulph.,*** verat-v., verb., zing.

constipation, with - ***aesc.,*** aesc-g., am-m., anac., ***coll.,*** euon., kali-s., ***nux-v.,*** paraf., sil., sulph., verb.

HEMORRHOIDS, general

coughing, sneezing agg. - caust., ign., ***kali-c.,*** lach.

debility, with - ars., chin., ham., hydr., mur-ac.

diarrhea, with - lach., merc.

excitement - arg-n., gels., hyos., nat-c., nux-v., sumb.

external - abrot., **AESC.,** all-c., **ALOE,** alum., ***am-c.,*** anac., ***ang.,*** ant-c., apis, apoc., arn., ars., ars-i., aur., ***bar-c., bar-m.,*** berb., ***brom.,*** bry., cact., ***calc., calc-p.,*** calc-s., caps., carb-ac., carb-an., ***carb-s.,*** carb-v., ***caust., coll.,*** coloc., dios., ***ferr., ferr-ar.,*** ferr-i., ferr-p., fl-ac., ***gran., graph.,*** grat., **HAM.,** ***hep., iod.,*** kali-ar., kali-c., kali-n., kali-p., kali-s., **LACH.,** ***lyc.,*** med., ***merc.,*** **MUR-AC.,** nat-m., ***nit-ac.,*** nux-v., ***paeon.,*** ph-ac., ***phos.,*** phys., ***plat., podo., puls.,*** **RAT.,** rumx., ***rhus-t., sep., sil.,*** **SULPH.,** sul-ac., ***ter.,*** thuj., ***tub.,*** verat., zinc.

fissures, soreness of anus, with - caps., cham., ***nit-ac.,*** rat.

fullness of right hypochondrium, with - aesc.

flatuence, from - caust., zinc.

protrude, when passing flatus - ***bar-c., phos.***

glass, like broken in - rat.

grapes, like - aesc., ***aloe,*** dios.

hard - ail., alum., ambr., **CAUST.,** ***lach., lyc.,*** phys., ***sep.***

heat, agg, - aesc., sulph.

heart disease, with - cact., coll., dig.

hypochondriasis, with - aesc., grat., ***nux-v.***

internal - **AESC., ALOE,** ***alum.,*** ant-c., arn., **ARS.,** bor., **BROM.,** ***calc., caps.,*** caust., **CHAM.,** cimic., **COLOC., HAM.,** hep., **IGN.,** kali-ar., kali-c., kali-p., kali-s., ***lach.,*** lyc., **NUX-V.,** ***petr., ph-ac., phos., plan.,*** **PODO., PULS.,** ***rhus-t.,*** sep., stront-c., **SULPH.,** ***ter.,*** verat.

irritability, with - ***apis,*** **NUX-V.,** sulph.

large - **AESC.,** agar., **ALOE,** alum., ang., arn., ars., bry., ***cact., calc.,*** caps., **CARB-AN.,** ***carb-s., carb-v.,*** **CAUST.,** clem., ***coloc.,*** cycl., ***dios.,*** euphr., ***ferr.,*** ferr-ar., gall-ac., ***graph.,*** **HAM.,** kali-ar., **KALI-C.,** kali-n., kali-s., ***lach.,*** lyc., manc., ***merc., mur-ac.,*** nat-m., **NIT-AC., NUX-V.,** ***podo., puls.,*** sep., **SULPH.,** sul-ac., thuj., ***tub.***

impeding stool - caust., sul-ac.

lifting agg. - rhus-t.

lying, agg. - puls.

down amel. - am-c.

menopause, agg. - aesc., **LACH.,** sep.

menses, during agg. - ***aloe,*** am-c., calc., ***carb-s., carb-v.,*** cocc., ***coll., graph., ign., lach.,*** lyss., phos., ***puls., sulph.***

after, agg. - cocc.

before - cocc., phos., puls.

suppressed, during - phos., ***sulph.***

mental, exertion - ***caust.,*** nat-c.

mercury, after abuse of - ***hep., sul-ac.***

milk, agg. - ***sep.***

HEMORRHOIDS, general
morning, agg. - aloe, **DIOS.,** mur-ac., sabin., sulph., sumb., thuj.
amel. - alum., coll.
bed, in, agg. - graph., rumx.
waking him - aloe, kali-bi., petr., sulph.
motion, agg. - apis, carb-an., euphr., merc., ***mur-ac.,*** nat-m., puls.
mucous piles, continually oozing - am-m., ant-c., calc-p., caps., carb-v., caust., puls., sep., sul-ac., sulph.
night, agg. - aesc., aloe, alum., am-c., ant-c., ars., carb-an., carb-v., coll., euphr., ferr., graph., ***merc.,*** phys., ***puls.,*** rhus-t., **SULPH.**
nosebleed, with - carb-v.
offensive - carb-v., manc., med., podo.
operations, agg. after - coll., croc.
pain, burning, smarting - ***aesc.,*** aloe, am-m., ***ars.,*** calc., ***caps.,*** carb-an., carb-v., caust., ***fl-ac.,*** graph., ***ign.,*** mag-m., ***nux-v.,*** psor., ***rat.,*** sul-ac., sulph.
stitches in rectum, when coughing - ign., ***kali-c.,*** lach., nit-ac.
painful, very - ***aesc.,*** aesc-g., ***aloe,*** ars., ***bell.,*** cact., ***caps.,*** carb-v., ***cham., coll., cub.,*** ferr-p., graph., ***ham., hyper.,*** kali-c., ***lach., lyc.,*** mag-m., ***mur-ac.,*** nat-m., nit-ac., ***nux-v.,*** paeon., plan., puls., ***rat., scroph-n., sed-ac.,*** sep., ***sil.,*** staph., sulph., thuj., verb., zing.
stand, cannot - plan.
pelvic congestion, with - ***aloe, coll.,*** ham., hep., nux-v., ***podo.,*** sep., sulph.
pendulous - nit-ac.
pregnancy, during - ***aesc., am-m.,*** ant-c., ars., ***caps.,*** carb-v., ***coll., lach., lyc.,*** mur-ac., ***nat-m., nux-v.,*** podo., puls., **SEP.,** ***sulph.***
after - ham., sep.
pressure of buttocks agg. - mur-ac.
prolapsus, anus and uterus, with - podo.
protruding, grape-like, swollen - abrot., **AESC.,** ***aloe,*** am-c., calc., caps., ***carb-v., caust., coll., dios.,*** graph., ham., kali-c., lach., ***mur-ac.,*** nux-m., ***nux-v.,*** rat., scroph-n., sep., sulph., symph., thuj., zinc.
bleeding, with - lach., lept.
flatus passing, while - bar-c., ***mur-ac.,*** phos.
lying, when - puls.
menses, during - puls.
stool, during - calc-p., rat., sil.
stool, preventing - sul-ac., verb.
urinating, when - ***bar-c.,*** kali-c., ***mur-ac.***
walking agg. - sep.
pulsating - ham.
purgations, after - aloe, ***nux-v.***
purple - aesc., aloe.
reflex, from - coll.
rheumatism, abates, after - abrot.
riding, amel. - ***kali-c.***
sitting, agg. - caust., graph., ign., ***thuj.***
amel. - ars., calc., ign., lach.
spasm of sphincter, with - lach., sil.
splinter, like - aesc., ***nit-ac.,*** rat.

HEMORRHOIDS, general
standing, agg. - ***aesc., am-c., caust., sulph.***
stepping, wide, agg. - graph.
sticking, cough, during - ign., ***kali-c.,*** lach., nit-ac.
sticks, as if in - aesc.
stool, after - ***aloe,*** ham., mur-ac., sulph.
after, for hours agg. - aesc., am-m., ign., rat., sulph.
preventing - ***aesc., caust., lach., paeon.,*** sul-ac., ***thuj.***
protrude during - aesc., alumn., ***am-c.,*** ang., ***bar-c., calc.,*** **CALC-P.,** fl-ac., ***kali-bi., kali-c., lach., lyc., mur-ac., nit-ac.,*** phos., ph-ac., plat., **RAT.,** ***rhus-t.,*** sep., ***sil.***
strangulated - acon., ***aesc.,*** **ALOE,** ars., ***bell., ign.,*** **LACH.,** ***nux-v.,*** **PAEON.,** ***sil., sulph.***
stricture, from - bapt.
suppressed, ailments from - aloe, am-m., apis, ars., ***calc., caps.,*** carb-v., ***coll.,*** cupr., ***ign.,*** lycps., ***mill.,*** **NAT-M., NUX-V., OP.,** phos., puls., ran-b., **SULPH.**
suppurating - anan., ***carb-v., hep., ign., merc.,*** **SIL.**
tenesmus, with, anal and visceral, diarrhea - caps.
dysenteric stools - aloe, sulph.
pregnancy, during - coll.
thinking, of them agg. - ***caust.***
touch, agg. - abrot., **BELL.,** berb., calc., carb-an., ***carb-s.,*** **CAUST.,** graph., ***hep., kali-c.,*** lil-t., lyc., merc., **MUR-AC.,** nit-ac., nux-v., phos., **RAT.,** sep., sil., stann., **SULPH.,** sul-ac., syph., **THUJ.**
ulcerating - aesc., ***cham., hep.,*** **IGN.,** kali-c., ***lach.,*** nit-ac., ***paeon.,*** phos., **SIL.,** staph., syph.
urination, agg. - kali-c.
after, agg. - merc.
protrude during - aloe, **BAR-C.,** ***bar-m.,*** canth., ***kali-c.,*** merc., ***mur-ac.,*** nit-ac.
vaginal discharge, suppressed, from - am-m.
vicarious bleeding, with - ham., mill.
walking, agg. - **AESC.,** agn., alum., ars., **BROM.,** calc., **CARB-AN., CAUST.,** cycl., kali-ar., kali-c., **MUR-AC.,** nit-ac., phos., phys., rumx., sep., sil., **SULPH.,** sumb., ther., thuj., zinc.
amel. - **IGN.**
warm, amel. - ***aesc.***
hot water, amel. - ***ars.,*** mur-ac.
weather agg. - nit-ac.
warmth, external, amel. - ***ars.,*** lyc., ***mur-ac.,*** petr., phos., ***sep.,*** zinc.
white piles - carb-v.
wiping, after stool agg. - **AESC., GRAPH., MUR-AC., PAEON.,** puls., ***sulph.***

HERPES, anus, about - ***berb., graph.,*** lyc., med., ***nat-m.,*** **PETR.,** ***thuj.***

INACTIVITY, of rectum - ***aesc.***, aeth., agn., alet., **ALUM., ALUMN.,** am-c., am-m., **ANAC.,** ant-c., ant-t., arg-n., ***arn.,*** asaf., aur., ***bar-c.,*** bar-m., bell., bov., **BRY.,** ***calc., calc-s., camph.,*** canth., ***carb-an.,*** **CARB-S.,** ***carb-v.,*** carc., caust., **CHAM.,** ***chin., coca, cocc.,*** coff., ***coll.,*** colch., crot-t., dulc., euphr., ferr., fl-ac., ***gels.,*** **GRAPH.,** hell., **HEP., HYDR.,** hyos., ***ign.,*** iod., ***kali-br.,*** **KALI-C.,** kali-n., ***kali-p.,*** kali-s., kreos., lac-d., ***lach., lap-a., lyc.,*** mag-c., ***mag-m.,*** mang., med., meli., merc., mez., mosch., mur-ac., ***nat-c.,*** **NAT-M.,** ***nat-p.,*** nit-ac., **NUX-M., NUX-V., OENA.,** olnd., **OP.,** par., ***petr., ph-ac.,*** **PHOS.,** ***phyt., plat.,*** **PLB.,** podo., ***psor.,*** ptel., ***puls., pyrog., rat.,*** rheum, rhus-t., **RUTA.,** sabad., **SANIC.,** sars., **SEL.,** seneg., ***sep.,*** **SIL.,** spig., squil., stann., ***staph.,*** stram., stront-c., sul-ac., ***sulph.,*** sumb., ***tab.,*** tarax., **TARENT.,** ***thuj.,*** til., valer., ***verat.,*** verb., vib., zinc.
- morning - staph.

INEFFECTUAL urging, (see Constipation)

INFLAMMATION, (see Proctitis)

INSENSIBILITY - ***aloe,*** alum., phos.

INVOLUNTARY, stool - **ALOE,** alum., am-c., ant-t., ***apis,*** apoc., arg-n., **ARN.,** ***ars., bapt.,*** bar-c., bar-m., **BELL.,** bor., ***bry.,*** bufo, ***calc.,*** calc-s., ***camph., carb-ac., carb-v., caust., cedr., chel., chin.,*** chin-a., chin-s., ***cina, colch., coloc.,*** con., ***cop., crot-h.,*** crot-t., ***cub., cupr.,*** cycl., ***dig.,*** dulc., ferr., ferr-ar., ferr-p., gamb., gels., glon., grat., ***hell.,*** hippoz., hydr-ac., **HYOS.,** ign., iris, kali-ar., kali-bi., ***kali-c.,*** kali-p., kali-s., ***lach., laur.,*** lyss., manc., med., merc., merc-c., mosch., ***mur-ac.,*** **NAT-M., NAT-P.,** ***nux-v.,*** oena., **OLND., OP.,** ***ox-ac.,*** petr., **PH-AC., PHOS.,** ***plb.,*** podo., ***psor., puls., pyrog.,*** **RHUS-T.,** rob., ruta., ***sanic.,*** **SEC.,** sep., staph., stram., stry., **SULPH.,** sul-ac., tab., tarent., thuj., trom., **VERAT.,** zinc.
- bending over, on - ***ruta.***
- convulsion, during - cupr., ***oena.***, stry.
- coughing or sneezing, on - bell., merc., ph-ac., ***phos.,*** rumx., spong., ***squil., sulph.,*** verat.
- eating, while - ferr.
  - after - ***aloe,*** chin.
- excitement, from - ***hyos.***
- fetus movement, from - ph-ac.
- flatus, as if - ars., sulph.
- flatus, on passing - acon., **ALOE,** ***apoc.,*** bell., calc., ***carb-v., caust.,*** cench., ferr-ma., ign., iod., jatr., kali-c., mur-ac., ***nat-c., nat-m.,*** **NAT-P.,** ***nat-s.,*** nux-v., **OLND., PH-AC., PODO.,** pyrog., ***rhus-t.,*** sanic., staph., sulph., ***tub.,*** **VERAT.**
- formed stool - ***aloe, bell., coloc.,*** hyos.
- fright, after - **OP.,** ***phos., verat.***
- grief, from - op.
- hard stools - bell., caust., coloc.
- headache, with - mosch.
- labor, after - hyos.
- laughing, on - ***sulph.***
- lumps of - ***aloe, coloc.***

INVOLUNTARY, stool
- lying, when - ox-ac.
- morning - ***zinc.***
- motion on - apis, bry., ***ph-ac., phos.***
  - beginning of - ***rhus-t.***
- move, on beginning to - ***rhus-t.***
- mucus, on passing flatus - spig.
- night - arn., bry., carb-ac., ***chin.,*** con., hyos., mosch., psor., puls., ***rhus-t.***
  - and after eating in daytime - chin.
  - bed, in - carb-ac., ***plb., sulph.***
  - bed, in, stool hard - **ALOE, BELL.**
- open, as if anus were wide - ***apis,*** apoc., ***phos.,*** sec., trom.
- paralysis from - ***alum.,*** bell., hyos., laur., ***nux-v.,*** op.
- sex, after - cedr.
- sleep during - ***arn., ars.,*** arum-t., bell., ***bry.,*** cench., chin., colch., ***con., hyos.,*** lach., laur., merc., mosch., ***mur-ac.,*** nat-m., nat-s., ***phos., ph-ac.,*** **PODO., PSOR.,** ***puls., rhus-t., sulph.,*** thuj., ***tub.,*** verat., zinc.
- sneezing, on - ***sulph.***
- solid. although - , ars., caust., coloc., ***hyos.***
- standing, on - aloe, ars., ***coloc.***
- stooping, on - ***ruta.***
- urination, during - ail., ***aloe,*** bell., ***carb-ac.,*** carb-s., ***hyos.,*** ind., ***mur-ac.,*** nat-s., phos., squil., ***sulph.,*** verat.
  - and stool - acon., apis, ***arg-n., arn., ars.,*** atro., aur., bar-c., bell., bry., calc., camph., carb-v., ***chin.,*** chin-a., cina, colch., con., dig., ***hyos., laur.,*** mosch., **MUR-AC.,** nat-m., ***olnd., ph-ac., phos.,*** puls., pyrog., rhus-t., sec., stram., sulph., verat., zinc.
  - and stool when not straining, voluntary defecation impossible - agar., arg-n.
- urine, and - ail., ***mur-ac.***
- vomiting, during - arg-n., ars.
- walking, on - aloe
- yellow, watery - hyos.

ITCHING, anus and rectum - acon., **AESC., AGAR.,** agn., ***all-c.,*** **ALOE,** ***alum.,*** alumn., ***ambr.,*** **AM-C.,** ***am-m.,*** anac., anan., ang., ***ant-c.,*** apis, apoc., arg-m., ***arg-n., ars., ars-i.,*** aur-s., bar-c., bar-m., ***bell., berb.,*** bor., bov., brom., bry., bufo, cact., cahin., **CALC.,** ***calc-ar.,*** calc-f., ***calc-p.,*** **CALC-S.,** ***caps.,*** carb-ac., **CARB-S., CARB-V.,** card-m., ***carl.,*** casc., **CAUST.,** cham., ***chel.,*** chin., chin-a., chin-s., ***cic.,*** **CINA,** cinnb., cist., ***clem.,*** cocc., coc-c., coff., ***colch., coll.,*** coloc., con., cop., ***croc.,*** crot-t., cub., cupr., dios., ***dulc.,*** elaps, elat., ***euph.,*** ferr., ferr-ar., ferr-i., ferr-ma., ferr-m., ferr-p., **FL-AC.,** glon., **GRAPH.,** ***gran.,*** grat., ***ham.,*** hep., hom., hydrc., ***ign., indg., iod., ip.,*** jac-c., jug-r., ***kali-ar.,*** kali-bi., **KALI-C.,** kali-n., kali-p., **KALI-S.,** ***lach.,*** led., lil-t., lith., **LYC.,** mag-c., ***mag-m.,*** med., meny., ***merc., mez., mill.,*** morg-g., morph., ***mur-ac.,*** naja, ***nat-a.,*** **NAT-C.,** ***nat-m., nat-p.,*** nat-s., **NIT-AC., NUX-V.,** op., ox-ac., ***paeon., petr.,*** phel., ph-ac., **PHOS.,** ***plat.,*** plb., polyg., prot., prun., psor., **PULS.,** rad., ran-s., ***rat.,*** rhus-t., ***rhus-v., rumx.,***

ITCHING, anus and rectum - ***ruta.***, ***sabad.***, sabin., sang-n., ***sars.***, sec., ***sep.***, serp., ***sil.***, sin-a., ***spig.***, ***spong.***, squil., ***stann.***, ***staph.***, **SULPH.**, ***sul-ac.***, ***sul-i.***, syph., tab., tell., ***teucr.***, ther., ***thuj.***, ***tub.***, uran-n., urt-u., ***verb.***, viol-o., wye., ***zinc.***, zing.
alternating, with ear - sabad.
ascarides, from - ***calc.***, calc-f., chin., ***cina.***, dol., ferr., graph., ign., ***nat-p.***, nit-ac., ***sabad.***, sin-a., sulph., ***teucr.***, ***urt-u.***
burning - ***agar.***, ***alum.***, ant-c., ***berb.***, bufo, calc., carb-s., chin., cocc., euph., ***iod.***, jug-r., kali-c., lyc., mur-ac., nat-c., paeon., rhus-v., sars., **SULPH.**, ***thuj.***
cold, bathing amel., - aloe, caust., fl-ac.
daytime - **SULPH.**
dinner, after - caust.
discharge, of moisture, after - ***sulph.***
eczematous - nit-ac.
evening - alum., bor., ***calc-p.***, cham., croc., ***iod.***, kali-bi., kali-c., lyc., nux-v., phos., ***plat.***, ***puls.***, ran-s., sil., ***sulph.***, thuj., zinc.
bed, in - ant-c., cahin., calc-p., cinnb., ***ign.***, ***lyc.***, ***nat-m.***, petr., plat., ***sulph.***, ***teucr.***
extending, into urethra during stool - thuj.
forenoon - dios., paeon.
menses, during - carb-v., phos.
before - graph.
morning - agar., carb-v., carb-s., cench., jac-c., lach., nat-m., ***sulph.***
bed, in - carb-v.
night - agar., aloe, alum., alumn., ant-c., calc-f., carb-s., con., ***ferr.***, fl-ac., ***ign.***, ***nat-p.***, petr., phos., rhus-v., ***sulph.***
midnight, before - thuj.
pain, ending in - ***zinc.***
painful - bell.
perineum, stool, after - tell.
riding, while - bov.
rubbing agg., - ***alum.***, petr.
scratching, agg. - ***agar.***, ***alum.***, arg-m., ars., bar-c., calc., ***caps.***, carb-v., ***caust.***, chel., con., merc., ***mez.***, mur-ac., nat-c., petr., ph-ac., phos., **PULS.**, rhus-t., rhus-v., sep., ***sil.***, stann., ***staph.***, **SULPH.**
sex, after - anac.
sitting, while - jac-c., ***staph.***, sulph.
sleep, after - carb-v., ***lach.***
on going to - petr.
sleeplessness, causing - ***aloe,*** alum., coff., ign., ***indg.***, teucr.
stick, as of, with - rumx.
stool, during - kali-c., merc., mur-ac., nat-m., phos., pic-ac., sil., ***sulph.***, teucr.
after - agar., aloe, alum., berb., bov., cahin., calc., carb-s., carb-v., clem., ***euph.***, eupi., ***kali-c.***, kali-m., lyc., mag-m., ***merc.***, ***mur-ac.***, ***nat-m.***, nicc., nit-ac., pic-ac., plat., ptel., sec., ***sil.***, ***staph.***, sulph., tell., ter., ***teucr.***, thuj., zinc.
amel. - clem.
before - euph., ***spong.***
urging to - euph.

ITCHING, anus and rectum,
stooping, on - arg-m.
voluptuous - ***agar.***, ***alum.***, ambr., arg-m., ***carb-v.***, cina, merc., mur-ac., petr., plat., ***puls.***, sep., ***sil.***, spig., **SULPH.**
walking, while - aesc., kali-bi., nat-m., nit-ac., nux-v., phos.
air, in open - arg-m., bell., nit-ac.
warm bed, in - ***alum.***, cahin., calc-p., carb-v., ***ign.***, ***lyc.***, ***nat-p.***, ***petr.***, ***sulph.***, ***teucr.***
itching, anus, around - agn., ***berb.***, bry., buf-s., **CINA,** euph., ***fl-ac.***, lyc., ***mez.***, nat-s., ***nux-v.***, op., **PETR.**, serp., **SULPH.**, tarax.
warmth of bed - ***petr.***

JERKS - chin.

LUMP, sensation of (see Weight) - aloe, anac., apoc., bry., cann-i., ***caust.***, chin., crot-h., ***crot-t.***, gamb., hell., ***kali-bi.***, ***lach.***, lil-t., med., nat-c., ***nat-m.***, phos., plat., rumx., sac-alb., sang., sarr., **SEP.**, ***sil.***, sul-ac., sulph., ther., thuj.
menses, during - ***sil.***
sitting agg., - cann-i., kali-bi., lach., nat-m.
sphincter, posterior side - med.
standing agg., - ***lil-t.***
stool, before - ***lach.***
not amel., by - **SEP.**

MOISTURE, from - acon., ***aesc.***, agar., ***aloe***, ***alum.***, am-c., anac., **ANT-C.**, apis, ars., aur., bapt., ***bar-c.***, ***bar-m.***, bell., ***bor.***, bry., ***calc.***, calc-p., ***calc-s.***, ***canth.***, ***caps.***, ***carb-an.***, **CARB-S.**, **CARB-V.**, carl., **CAUST.**, chel., chin., chin-a., clem., coc-c., coff., ***colch.***, coloc., cor-r., ***dios.***, dulc., ferr., ferr-ar., ferr-p., **GRAPH.**, ***hell.***, **HEP.**, ign., ***lach.***, led., lyc., med., meli., ***merc.***, ***merc-c.***, mill., ***mur-ac.***, ***nat-m.***, **NIT-AC.**, ***nux-v.***, ***paeon.***, ***petr.***, ***phos.***, ***phyt.***, podo., ***puls.***, ran-s., ***rat.***, rhus-t., **SEP.**, **SIL.**, spig., stann., **SULPH.**, sul-ac., syph., **THUJ.**, zinc.
acrid - carb-v., merc-c., nit-ac., thuj., zinc.
black - merc-i-f.
bloody - alum., apis, carl., op., sabad., sil., thuj.
constant - sep.
staining yellow - ant-c.
dark - med., merc-i-f.
evening - carb-an., dios.
fetid - ***ant-c.***, ***calc.***, hep., med., paeon., sep., sul-i.
flatus, from - all-c., ant-c., carb-v., zinc.
glutinous - carb-v., **GRAPH.**
herring brine, smelling like - calc., med.
ichorous - ferr.
menses, during - **LACH.**
mucus, urinating, when - carb-ac.
musty odor - carb-v.
night - carb-v., nat-m., sulph.
orange colored - kali-p.
perineum - carb-an., ***carb-v.***, paeon., thuj.
scratching - alum., **CARB-V.**, ***caust.***, dulc., **GRAPH.**, lyc., merc., nat-m., nit-ac., petr., rhus-t., sep., sil., **SULPH.**, sul-ac., thuj.
staining yellow - ant-c.

MOISTURE, from
stool, after - bar-c., bor., ***graph.,*** hep., paeon., ***sep.,*** stann., sumb., zinc.
before - kali-c.
warm, escaping - acon.

NAUSEA, felt in - ruta.

NUMBNESS, anus, of - acon., carb-ac., phos.

OPEN, anus - aesc., aloe, ***phos., sec.,*** sol-t-ae.
open, anus, sensation of - ail., **ALOE,** alum., ***apis,*** apoc., ign., kali-c., op., ***phos.,*** puls., sec., sumb., trom.
stool, after - apoc., sumb.
passes right through - aloe, apoc.

PAIN, rectum - acon., **AESC.,** agar., all-c., ***aloe, alum., alumn.,*** **AM-C.,** am-m., anac., ant-c., arn., ***ars.,*** ars-i., bar-c., bar-m., bell., berb., **BROM.,** bry., ***bufo,*** cact., calad., calc., calc-p., calc-s., camph., canth., ***caps., carb-an., carb-s., carb-v.,*** carl., **CAUST.,** cham., chel., chin., chin-a., chr-ac., cimic., cocc., colch., **COLL.,** ***coloc.,*** con., ***croc.,*** cupr., cycl., dios., dulc., euphr., ferr., ferr-ar., ferr-p., **GRAPH.,** grat., ham., hell., **IGN.,** iod., iris, ***kali-ar.,*** kali-bi., **KALI-C.,** kali-chl., ***kali-n.,*** kali-p., kali-s., lac-ac., lach., ***lil-t.,*** **LYC.,** mag-c., med., ***merc.,*** mez., mill., ***mur-ac.,*** nat-c., nat-m., nat-p., ***nit-ac., nux-v.,*** **PAEON.,** phel., ph-ac., ***phos.,*** phys., phyt., plb., ***podo., psor.,*** **PULS.,** ***rat.,*** rhus-t., rhus-v., rumx., ***ruta.,*** sabad., sars., sec., seneg., ***sep.,*** sil., stann., stront-c., **SULPH.,** sul-ac., sumb., syph., tarent., ther., **THUJ.,** valer., zinc., zing.
afternoon - chel., ***cocc.,*** cycl.
alternating with pain in wrists - sulph.
bladder, and, at the same time - ambr.
childbirth, after - gels., podo., ruta.
continuous - am-c., am-m., calc., graph., ign., kali-c., kali-chl., lyc., ***nit-ac.,*** nux-v., phyt., sep., stront-c.
diarrhea, in - kali-chl.
stool, long after - aesc., agar., aloe, alum., am-c., am-m., calc., ***colch.,*** graph., ***ign.,*** mur-ac., nit-ac., ***paeon.,*** rat., sil., stront-c., sulph.
walk about, must - paeon.
convulsive - ***lach.,*** lyc., psor., sang.
cough, from - ign., ***kali-c., lach.,*** nit-ac., puls., tub.
diarrhea, with - ars., mag-m., sul-ac.
as after long - rheum.
drawing, anus in, when - sulph.
eating, after - lyc., nux-v.
evening - carb-v., dios., ***lach.,*** mez., nux-v., ***sulph.***
lying, while - ***ign.***
extending to,
abdomen - aloe, ***mez.,*** phos., zinc.
ankles, to - alum.
genitals, to - carb-an., chin., lil-t., phyt., rhod., ***sep.,*** sil., zinc.
genitals, to, before stool - carb-an.
heels, to - fago.
liver, to - ***dios.,*** lach.
penis, to - zinc.
testes, to - sil.

PAIN, rectum
extending to,
thighs, down - alum., alumn., cann-i., gran., plb., rhus-t., sabin.
thighs, down - alumn.
umbilicus, to - coloc., ***lach.***
upward - graph., ***ign.,*** lach., phos., ***sep.,*** sulph.
urethra, through - hipp.
urethra, to - bry., thuj.
vulva - ars.
flatus, on passing - camph., ***carb-v.,*** nat-c.
forenoon - kali-bi., nat-m., thuj.
10 a.m., sitting, while - **SEP.**
hot applications amel. - rat.
kneeling amel. - ***aesc.***
laughing agg. - lach.
lying, agg. - aesc., crot-t., phos., ***puls.,*** zinc.
abdomen, on amel. - nux-v.
back, on - chel.
back, on amel. - alumn., ***am-c.,*** mang.
side, on agg. - puls.
menses, during - ***aloe,*** ars., berb., phos.
before - ign., petr.
mental exertion, after - ***caust.,*** nux-v.
morning - calc-p., dios., ***kali-bi.,*** podo.
7 a.m. - nat-m.
stool, after - ***kali-bi.***
stool, during - ***podo.***
motion, agg. - ***nux-v., thuj.***
amel. - ***puls.***
neuralgic - plb.
night - mosch., nat-m., ox-ac., ***puls.***
4 a.m. - ***mag-c.***
morning - nux-v.
periodical, every day - ***ign.***
pregnancy, during - caps., kali-c.
pressing, asunder, as if - op.
down, on - crot-t., podo., ***sulph.***
umbilicus, on, agg. - **CROT-T.**
umbilicus, on, amel. - kali-c.
pressure amel. - carc.
pulsating - aloe, ***bell.,*** caps., ham., lach., ***meli.,*** merc., sil., ***sulph.,*** thuj.
sex, after - caust., merc-c., sil.
sitting, while - ***aesc., aloe,*** ammc., am-m., ars., bar-c., berb., calc., cann-s., caust., chel., cocc., coloc., cycl., euphr., **LYC.,** ***mang., mur-ac., ph-ac.,*** phos., **RAT.,** ***ruta.,*** sars., **SEP.,** staph., sulph., ther., thuj.
amel. - ars., ***ign.,*** lach.
sleep, during - kali-c.
sneezing agg. - lach.
standing agg. - ***aesc.,*** arn., ferr., ***ign.***
erect - ***petr.***
stool, during - aeth., aloe, ***alum.,*** alumn., ambr., am-c., am-m., anac., ***ant-c.,*** asaf., **ARS.,** aur., bar-c., bar-m., bell., ***berb.,*** brom., ***bry.,*** **CALC.,** calc-p., calc-s., canth., caps., carb-an., ***carb-s., carb-v.,*** casc., cham., ***chel.,*** chin., chin-a., cimx., **COLCH., COLL.,** coloc., con., crot-t., ***cupr.,*** dros., ferr., ferr-ar., ferr-p., ***fl-ac.,*** **GRAPH.,** grat., hep., hyos., ***ign.,***

PAIN, rectum
stool, during - ***kali-ar., kali-bi.,*** kali-c., kali-p., kali-s., kreos., ***lac-c., lach., lil-t.,*** **LYC.,** lyss., mag-m., manc., med., ***merc.,*** merc-i-r., mez., mur-ac., nat-c., nat-m., **NIT-AC.,** nux-v., ***ox-ac., paeon.,*** ph-ac., phos., plan., plat., ***plb.,*** **PODO.,** puls., **RAT.,** rhus-t., sabin., ***sanic., sep.,*** **SIL.,** stann., **SULPH.,** sul-ac., sumb., ***syph.,*** tarent., ***thuj., tub., zinc.***
after - **AESC., ALOE,** ***alumn., am-c., am-m.,*** apoc., ***ars.,*** asaf., bar-c., bell., ***berb.,*** bov., ***brom.,*** cact., calc., calc-p., calc-s., canth., carb-s., ***carb-v.,*** carl., casc., caust., cic., cocc., ***colch.,*** crot-t., dios., elaps, ***graph.,*** grat., hydr., **IGN.,** ***kali-ar.,*** kali-bi., kali-c., kali-p., kali-s., ***kalm., lach.,*** lil-t., lob., ***lyc.,*** manc., **MERC.,** merc-c., merc-i-r., mez., **MUR-AC.,** ***nat-c.,*** nat-m., nat-p., **NIT-AC.,** ***podo., psor.,*** puls., **RAT.,** rhus-t., rhus-v., ***ruta.,*** sabad., ***sep.,*** seneg., sil., staph., stront-c., **SULPH.,** ***sul-ac.,*** sumb., tarent., thuj., verat-v.
after, long, agg. - nit-ac., paeon.
amel. - acon., aesc., aloe, alum., ant-t., arn., ars., asaf., bapt., bry., cahin., calc-p., canth., cham., colch., ***coloc.,*** corn., dulc., ***gamb.,*** hell., lept., nat-s., nuph., **NUX-V., RHUS-T.,** sanic.
before - am-c., ***berb., carb-an.,*** iod., ***kali-c.,*** lec., lach., lil-t., ***lyc.,*** merc., nat-m., nat-s., nit-ac., ***nux-v.,*** podo., ruta., sulph.
straining at, after - ***aesc.,*** lach., med., nux-v., phos., plb., ruta., ***sil., thuj.***
urination, during - rhus-t.
stooping, agg. - caust., ruta.
amel. - chel.
urinating agg. - ***mur-ac.,*** valer.
vomiting, after - kali-c.
vomiting, agg. - mur-ac., podo.
walking, while - **CAUST.,** coloc., cycl., ***ign.,*** kali-c., ***mez.,*** ran-s., sep., sulph., sumb.
warm, bathing, agg. - brom.
amel. - ***ars., lach., mur-ac.,*** phos., ***rat.***
drinks amel. - carc.
wiping - aloe, ***graph.,*** lach., mur-ac.

PARALYSIS - acon., aeth., agar., aloe, **ALUM.,** arn., ars., ars-i., atro., ***bar-m., bell.,*** bry., ***calc., caust.,*** chin., chin-a., coll., coloc., cupr., ***erig.,*** ferr., ***gels., graph., hyos.,*** kali-ar., kali-c., kali-p., ***laur.,*** manc., **MUR-AC.,** op., oxyt., nat-m., ph-ac., **PHOS., PLB.,** puls., rhus-t., **SEC.,** sel., **SIL.,** sulph., syph., ***tab.,*** tarent., thuj., verat.
hemorrhoids, after removal of - kali-p.
paralysis, sensation of - **ALOE,** alum., ***anac.,*** apoc., cann-i., cocaine, erig., ferr-m., graph., kali-bi., kali-c., med., ***nux-v.,*** petr., ph-ac., plat., plb., rhod., sabad., sanic., sec., ***sep.,*** sul-ac.

PERSPIRATION, about the anus and perineum - agar., ***alum.,*** bell., carb-an., con., ***hep.,*** kali-c., psor., rhus-t., sep., thuj.

PINCHING, pain - eug., merc., nat-m., ***nit-ac.***

PLUG, sensation of, wedged between pubis and coccyx - aloe.
plug were pressing out, as if - bry., ***crot-t.,*** kali-bi., ***lach.,*** lil-t., ***sep., sil.***

POLYPS - am-m., ***calc., calc-p.,*** kali-br., ***nit-ac.,*** nux-v., **PHOS.,** ruta., sang., teucr., **THUJ.**
bleeding - phos., nit-ac., sabin.

PRESSING, pain - acon., **AESC.,** ***aloe,*** alum., ang., ant-c., apoc., arg-m., ***arn., ars.,*** asaf., ***bar-c.,*** bar-m., ***bell., berb.,*** bry., cact., cahin., calc., ***calc-s.,*** carb-an., carl., carb-s., carb-v., **CAUST.,** chel., ***chin.,*** chin-a., cob., coll., coloc., con., cop., ***crot-t., cycl.,*** dulc., eug., eup-pur., ferr-i., form., gran., ***graph.,*** hell., hydr., **IGN.,** iod., ***iris,*** kali-ar., ***kali-bi.,*** kali-c., ***kali-n.,*** kali-p., kali-s., kreos., ***lach.,*** lact., laur., **LIL-T.,** ***lyc.,*** mag-c., ***mag-m., merc.,*** merc-i-f., merl., mez., ***murx.,*** mur-ac., nat-c., nat-m., **NIT-AC., NUX-V.,** op., ox-ac., **PETR.,** phel., ***phos.,*** plat., ptel., ***puls.,*** rhus-t., ***sars.,*** seneg., ***sep.,*** sil., spig., ***stann.,*** staph., stry., **SULPH.,** ***valer.,*** verat., verb., zinc.
afternoon - chel., cycl., sep., sulph.
sleep, during - cycl.
alternating with contraction - bell.
diarrhea, as in a - calc., nat-m.
would come on, as if - calc., ***crot-t.,*** mag-c.
dinner, after - sep.
downward - agar., ***aloe,*** alum., ars., bell., berb., bry., ***cact.,*** calc-p., cann-s., ***carb-v.,*** cean., cimic., cob., ***corn.,*** **CROT-T.,** dios., dros., euph., hyper., ***ip.,*** kali-c., kali-n., ***lach.,*** lil-t., lyc., mag-c., med., ***nit-ac., nux-m.,*** nux-v., op., ox-ac., pic-ac., **PODO.,** prun., ***puls., sep.,*** sul-ac., **SULPH.,** verat., xero.
evening - calc., chin-s., ran-s.
bed, in - iod.
extending to abdomen - zinc.
feces were lodged in, as if - ***caust.***
flatus, during - ***carb-v.***
amel. - ant-c.
before - kali-c.
from - zinc.
forenoon - kali-bi.
lying, while - crot-t., nux-v., ptel.
menses, during - ***aloe.***
before - ign., petr.
mental exertion - caust.
morning - ***kali-bi.***
motion, agg. - ***nux-v.***
night - ***lyc.***
noon - agar., kali-bi.
rising from seat - phos.
sitting, while - ammc., calc., ***cann-s., cycl.,*** euphr., staph., sulph., thuj.
standing, while - arn., ***ferr.***

PRESSING, pain
stool, during - alum., ant-c., asaf., corn., ***kali-bi.,*** ***lil-t.,*** **LYC.,** nat-m., ox-ac., phos., ***podo.,*** sin-a., staph., sul-ac., **SULPH.,** ***zinc.***
after - apoc., bar-c., ***calc.,*** caust., ***ign.,*** ***kali-bi.,*** ***kalm.,*** ***merc.,*** nit-ac., ph-ac., phos., plat., ***podo.,*** ***puls.,*** seneg., sil., stann., sul-ac., ***sulph.***
before - ant-c., cob., ***nat-m.,*** ***nit-ac.,*** ***nux-v.,*** phos., **PLAT.,** sul-ac., til.
not for - ***dros.,*** **LACH.,** mez.
walking - ***cycl.,*** ***ran-s.,*** sulph.

PRICKLING - agar., bry., cact., colch., grat., lact., **NIT-AC.,** ***ter.***
stool during - cact.
after - grat.

PROCTITIS, inflammation of rectum and anus - ***aesc.,*** aloe, alum., ambr., ***ant-c.,*** colch., coll., ferr-p., ***hep.,*** hydr., ip., kali-bi., kali-i., ***merc.,*** merc-c., ***nit-ac.,*** ***op.,*** paeon., ***phos.,*** podo., ric., sabal., ***sulph.,*** zing.
syphilitic - bell., merc., ***nit-ac.,*** sulph.

PROLAPSUS, of rectum - ***aesc.,*** all-c., ***aloe,*** alumn., ant-c., **APIS,** apoc., aral., arg-n., arn., ***ars.,*** arund., ***asar.,*** aur., ***bell.,*** **BELL-P.,** bufo, **CALC.,** ***calc-s.,*** canth., ***carb-s.,*** carb-v., ***carc.,*** caust., cic., cocc., ***colch.,*** ***coll.,*** ***crot-c.,*** crot-t., ***dig.,*** dios., ***dulc.,*** elaps, ***ferr.,*** ***ferr-ar.,*** ***ferr-i.,*** ***ferr-m.,*** ferr-p., fl-ac., ***gamb.,*** ***gels.,*** gran., ***graph.,*** ham., ***hep.,*** ***hydr.,*** **IGN.,** ***iris,*** ***kali-bi.,*** kali-c., kali-n., kali-p., ***lach.,*** lept., ***lyc.,*** ***mag-m.,*** mag-p., mag-p-a., ***mang.,*** med., **MERC.,** ***merc-c.,*** mez., morg-g., **MUR-AC.,** ***nat-m.,*** ***nat-s.,*** ***nit-ac.,*** nux-m., **NUX-V.,** ***phos.,*** phyt., ***plb.,*** **PODO.,** psor., rad-br., rhus-t., ***ruta.,*** **SEP.,** ***sil.,*** sol-t-ae., ***sulph.,*** sumb., syc-co., syph., tab., ther., thuj., trom., valer., zinc.
burning, with - ***alum.***
childbirth, after - **BELL-P.,** ***podo.,*** ***ruta.,*** **SEP.**
children - bell., carc., chin-s., ***ferr.,*** ***ferr-p.,*** ***hydr.,*** ign., mur-ac., ***nux-v.,*** **PODO.,** syph., tub.
contracted - mez.
convulsive - ***ars.***
coughing - caust.
diarrhea, during - ***calc.,*** **DULC.,** gamb., mag-m., **MERC.,** ***mur-ac.,*** **PODO.**
evening - **IGN.**
excitement, from mental - podo.
flatus, when passing - ***mur-ac.,*** valer.
forenoon - rhus-t.
hemorrhage of after - ***ars.***
kneeling - ail., podo., ruta.
menses, during - aur., podo.
mental excitement, from - podo.
morning - podo.
night - ***aesc.***
overlifting, from - ign., nit-ac., podo., ruta.
painful - ***ars.,*** ther.
paralysis, with - plb.
pregnancy, during - podo.
replacing difficult - mez.

PROLAPSUS, of rectum
sensation of - ***aesc.,*** chel., dios., iris
sitting agg. - ther.
smoking agg. - ***sep.***
sneezing, after - podo.
squatting - ruta.
standing - ***ferr-i.***
stool, during - aesc., ***aloe,*** ***ant-c.,*** ail., asar., bell., bry., ***cinnb.,*** ***calc.,*** carb-v., colch., crot-t., dulc., ferr., ferr-ar., ferr-p., ***fl-ac.,*** ***gamb.,*** ham., **IGN.,** kali-c., kali-n., **LYC.,** mag-m., mez., mur-ac., ***nux-v.,*** phos., plan., **PODO.,** ***rhus-t.,*** ***ruta.,*** **SEP.,** ***sulph.,*** ***trom.***
after - ***aesc.,*** ***aloe,*** alum., ant-c., apoc., ars., asar., calc-ac., canth., carb-v., ***cocc.,*** crot-t., euph., ham., ***hep.,*** ***ign.,*** ***indg.,*** iris, kali-bi., ***lach.,*** ***merc.,*** mez., mur-ac., ***nat-m.,*** ***nit-ac.,*** ***phos.,*** plat., **PODO.,** ***sep.,*** sol-t-ae., ***sulph.,*** ***trom.***
before - ***podo.,*** ***ruta.***
urging, with - ruta.
stooping, on - podo., ruta
straining, from - ign., nit-ac., ***podo.,*** ruta
without - ***graph.,*** kali-c., ***ruta.***
urination, during - **MUR-AC.,** ***podo.,*** ***valer.***
difficult - ***sep.***
vomiting, when - ***mur-ac.,*** ***podo.***
walking, after - arn.
washing body amel. - arn.

PULSATION - aloe, alum., alumn., am-m., apis, benz., berb., calc-p., caps., caust., crot-t., cycl., grat., ***ham.,*** **LACH.,** lyss., manc., meli., ***nat-m.,*** rhod., seneg., ***sulph.***
eating, after - aloe.
evening - am-m.
sitting, amel. in bed - am-m.
menses, during - lach., ***lyss.***
sitting, while - ***aloe,*** am-m.
small hammers, like - **LACH.**
stool, during - nat-m.
after - aloe, alumn., apis, berb., caps., ***lach.,*** manc., sang., seneg., ***sulph.***
pulsation, anus, walking, on - cench.

RASPING, pain - ant-c., grat., nat-m., verat.

REDNESS of anus, congestion - ***aesc.,*** aloe, alumn., ars., cham., ***coll.,*** hyper., med., merc-cy., nat-m., nit-ac., paeon., ***petr.,*** sabad., ***sep.,*** **SULPH.,** valer., ***zinc.,*** zing.
around anus - ***cham.,*** merc-cy., paeon., sulph., zing.
rash, fiery red in babies - med.
fiery - med.

RELAXED, anus - **ALOE,** apis, apoc., ***carb-v.,*** chin., kali-c., kali-p., mur-ac., ***petr.,*** **PHOS.,** puls., rhod., ***sec.,*** sumb., zing.
relaxed, sensation of, anus, after stool - lept., podo.

RETRACTION - agar., bapt., bry., ***kali-bi.,*** ***op.,*** plb., tell.
draw in, desire to - agar.
drawn up - plb.

RETRACTION,
painful - ***kali-bi.***
stool, after - ***kali-bi.***
retraction, anus - agar., bapt., bry., ***kali-bi., op.,*** plb., tell.
painful - ***kali-bi.***
stool, after - ***kali-bi.***

SCRAPING, pain - am-c., ant-c., calc-p., carb-an., crot-t., grat., nat-m., puls., verat.
stool, after - nit-ac., phos.

SCRATCHING, pain - ars., kali-n., sep.

SENSITIVE - ***aloe, bell.,*** berb., calc., ***caust.,*** cina, ***graph., hep., lach.,*** lil-t., ***lyc.,*** **MAG-M., MUR-AC., NIT-AC.,** nux-v., ***podo.,*** rat., ***sep.,*** sil., sul-ac., sulph., syph., thuj.
stool, after - mag-m., phos.

SHARP, pain - ***acon.,*** **AESC.,** agar., ***all-c., aloe,*** alum., alumn., ambr., am-m., ang., ant-t., ***apis,*** arg-n., arn., **ARS.,** arund., aur., aur-s., ***bar-c., bar-m.,*** bell., ***benz-ac., berb.,*** bor., bov., brom., bry., cact., calad., ***calc., calc-p.,*** calc-s., cann-i., cann-s., canth., ***caps.,*** **CARB-AN.,** ***carb-s., carb-v.,*** carl., **CAUST.,** cham., chel., chin., chin-a., coc-c., colch., coloc., **CON.,** ***cop., croc.,*** crot-t., cupr., cycl., euphr., ferr-ar., ferr-i., ferr-ma., gins., ***graph.,*** grat., **IGN.,** indg., ip., jac-c., jatr., ***kali-ar.,*** kali-bi., **KALI-C.,** kali-n., kali-p., **KALI-S.,** kreos., **LACH.,** led., **LYC.,** lyss., mag-c., ***mag-m., mag-p., med.,*** meli., **MERC.,** merc-c., merc-i-f., ***mez.,*** mosch., ***mur-ac., nat-c., nat-m.,*** nicc., **NIT-AC.,** nuph., nux-m., nux-v., ol-an., petr., phel., ***ph-ac., phos., phyt.,*** plat., plb., ***puls.,*** ran-b., ran-s., ***rat., rhus-t., ruta., sabad.,*** **SEP., SIL.,** spong., stann., stram., stry., **SULPH.,** ***sul-ac.,*** tarent., teucr., ***thuj.,*** til., zinc.
afternoon - agar., chin-s., lyc., nat-m., sulph.
alternating, with burning, in prepuce - thuj.
with itching, in glans, penis - thuj.
coughing, on - ***ign.,*** **LACH.,** nit-ac.
dinner, after - kali-n., phos.
drawing in anus - sep., sulph.
eating, after - **NUX-V.**
before - ***caust.***
erect, when body is - **PETR.**
evening - benz-ac., bor., calc-p., carb-s., carb-v., gran., iris, kali-c., merc-c., nat-m., ***nit-ac.,*** **SULPH.,** thuj., zinc.
bed, in - ***nat-m.***
extending to,
abdomen - aloe, mag-m., ***sep.***
back - carl.
bladder - mosch., thuj.
downwards and outwards - asar., ***carb-v.,*** lith.
genitals, while walking - sil.
ilium and glans, penis - petr., ***thuj.***
inguinal region, left - croc., kreos.
inwards - zinc.
inner side of thigh - alumn.
liver - ***dios.***
loins - aloe
outward - ***carb-v.,*** lith.
penis - carl.
pudendum, after stool - cast.

SHARP, pain
extending, to
pudendum, during menses - aloe, ars.
root of penis - zinc.
upward - aesc., ***graph.,*** hell., **IGN.,** ***lach.,*** mag-c., ***mez., rhus-t., sep.,*** thuj.
upward, stool, after - alumn., ***mez.,*** sulph.
urethra - carb-s., cocc., thuj.
flatus, on passing - bry., phos.
amel. - coloc., ***mag-c.***
forenoon - calc., lach., sep.
itching - alum., bry., coloc., nat-m., ph-ac., puls., stann., sulph.
lying, while - nat-c., **SULPH.**
menses, during - aloe, ***ars.,*** phos.
mental exertion, after - **NUX-V.**
motion, on - bell., kali-n.
morning - lyc., mag-c., zinc.
waking, after - mag-c.
night - sep., thuj., stry.
midnight - thuj.
periodical - agar., ***ign.***
pregnancy, during - ***kali-c.***
pressure, on - sep.
rising, from seat - phos.
sex, during - calc.
sitting, while - ***ars., calc.,*** gran., iod., kali-c., nat-c., ***ruta.,*** **SULPH.,** ***thuj.***
sneezing, when - ***lach.***
standing, while - ***sulph.,*** valer.
stool, during - am-c., am-m., ***berb.,*** calc-s., carb-an., carb-s., ***carb-v.,*** caust., chin., coc-c., ferr-i., **GRAPH.,** ***ign.,*** ip., laur., mag-m., mur-ac., ***nat-c.,*** nat-m., **NIT-AC.,** nux-m., ***nux-v.,*** pic-ac., ***sep.,*** sil., ***staph.,*** sul-ac., sulph.
after - ***aloe,*** am-m., ***berb.,*** calad., ***calc.,*** canth., cham., chin., hell., kali-n., laur., ***lyc.,*** mag-m., ***mez.,*** nat-m., nicc., **NIT-AC.,** pic-ac., ***plat., rat.,*** sep., stann., ***thuj.***
before - asar., ***berb., con.,*** gamb., ***kali-c.,*** kali-n., phos., ***plat.,*** spong., sul-ac.
difficult stool, after - alum., ***plat., rat.***
hard, during - bar-c., bell., hell., prun., sul-ac., sulph.
urging, during - mag-c.,
tearing - graph., nat-m.
twitching - zinc.
urination, during - carb-s., sulph.
walking, while - ***ars.,*** coc-c., crot-t., kali-c., meli., nat-p., petr., phos., ***sil.,*** squil., sulph., zinc.
after - mag-c., thuj.
air, in open amel. - thuj.

SHOCK, electric-like - apis, stry.
stool, before - apis.

SORE, pain - **AESC.,** ***agar.,*** agn., alet., **ALOE,** alum., alumn., ambr., am-br., am-c., am-m., ant-c., ant-s., **APIS,** arn., ***ars.,*** aspar., ***atro.,*** aur., ***bar-c.,*** **BAR-M., BELL., BERB.,** ***bry., calc., calc-p.,*** calc-s., ***caps., carb-an., carb-s., carb-v.,*** **CAUST.,** colch., coll., coloc., crot-t., ***cycl.,*** dios., elaps, gall-ac., **GAMB., GRAPH., HAM.,** hep., **IGN., IRIS, KALI-AR.,** kali-bi., **KALI-C.,** kali-m., ***kali-p.,*** **KALI-S., LACH.,** lact., lil-t., **LYC., MERC.,** ***merc-c.,*** merc-i-f., merc-sul., **MUR-AC.,** nat-a., nat-c., ***nat-m.,*** nat-s., nat-p., **NIT-AC.,** nux-m., ***nux-v.,*** onos., ox-ac., **PAEON.,** petr., ph-ac., phos., phys., plb., ***podo.,*** prun., psor., **PULS.,** rad-br., **RAT.,** ***rhus-t.,*** sars., ***sep.,*** **SIL.,** sol-t-ae., spong., stann., staph., ***stry.,*** **SULPH.,** sul-ac., syph., tab., thuj., verat., vib., ***zinc.,*** zing.

- evening - bar-c., ***carb-an.,*** kali-bi., ***sulph.,*** zinc.
- jerking - sep.
- lying, while - sulph.
  - on back - chel.
- menses, during - ars., ***berb.,*** carb-v., mur-ac.
- morning - ***calc-p.,*** thuj.
- moving, after - crot-t., ***puls.***
- night - ant-c., phel., sars.
- ovaries, with pain in - onos.
- sitting, while - ***am-m., berb.,*** **CAUST.,** chel., ***cycl.,*** mag-c., ***mur-ac.,*** **RAT.,** ***sulph.***
- stool, during - ***aesc., agar.,*** **ALOE, ALUM.,** ***ant-c.,*** brach., caust., coloc., ***graph., grat.,*** nat-c., ***nat-m.,*** phos., spong., ***sulph.***
  - after - ***aesc.,*** **ALOE,** ***alum.,*** ant-c., **APIS,** apoc., calc-s., ***carb-s., cham.,*** chel., colch., crot-t., gamb., **GRAPH.,** hep., **IGN.,** iod., kali-bi., kali-c., mag-m., ***merc.,*** mez., ***mur-ac., nat-m.,*** **NIT-AC.,** nux-m., nux-v., phos., ***podo.,*** puls., **RAT.,** stann., staph., ***sulph.***
  - diarrheic after - nat-m., phel., **SULPH.,** tab.
  - hard stool, during - ***nat-m., sulph.***
- thinking of agg. - caust.
- touch, on - ars.
- walking, while - arg-m., **CAUST.,** cycl., ***kali-bi.,*** kali-m., mag-c., ***mez., nit-ac.***

SPASMS, in - ***caust., colch., ferr., tab.***

- sex, during - merc-c.
- urinate, with urging to - ***caust.***
- walking - caust.

SPLINTER, pain, like a - acon., **AESC.,** agar., ***alum.,*** am-m., ***arg-n., bar-c.,*** bell., ***carb-v.,*** caust., coll., graph., hell., ***ign.,*** iris, ***kali-c., lach.,*** lyc., merc., mez., ***nat-m.,*** **NIT-AC.,** nux-v., plat., **RAT.,** ruta, sanic., ***sep., sil.,*** sulph., thuj.

- flatus passing amel. - coloc., ***mag-c.***
- menses, during - ars.
- vomiting, on - agar.

STANDING, stool passes better, on - **CAUST.**

STICKING, pain - acon., **AESC.,** aloe, ant-c., ***ars.,*** cact., calc., ***carb-v.,*** **CAUST.,** chel., ***coll., coloc.,*** ferr-i., **GRAPH.,** grat., **IRIS,** jac-c., kali-c., kali-n., lact., lyc., nat-a., ***nit-ac.,*** **NUX-V.,** phos., puls., ***rat.,*** rumx., ***sil.,*** **SULPH.,** sumb., ***teucr., thuj.***

- stool, during - ferr-i., **NIT-AC.**
  - after - **NUX-V., RAT.**

STINGING, pain, in - **AESC.,** acon., ***am-m., apis, ars., caps.,*** carb-an., ***caust.,*** coch., lyc., mag-m., ***nat-m.,*** nit-ac., **NUX-V.,** ***phos., puls.,*** sil., ***staph.,*** sulph.

- menses, during - phos.
- night, lying - **ARS.,** ***puls.***
- stool, during - berb., caps., caust., coc-c., ip., ***lyc.,*** mag-m., nat-c., nat-m., nicc., **NIT-AC.,** ***sil.,*** sulph.
  - after - aloe, berb., ***canth.,*** kali-n., **NIT-AC.,** ***puls., sulph.***
- walking, while - carb-an.

STRICTURE - ***aesc.,*** agar., ***aloe,*** alum., ang., ***bar-m.,*** bell., ***bor.,*** calc., ***calc-sil., camph.,*** coff., colch., con., crot-t., elaps, fl-ac., hep., hydr., ign., kreos., ***lach., lyc.,*** med., mez., ***nat-m.,*** nit-ac., phos., plb., ***ruta,*** sec., ***sil.,*** syph., tab., thiosin., thuj., tub.

- hemorrhoids, from - bapt.

SWELLING, anus, of - ***aesc., apis,*** aur., bell., bor., bufo, ***coll.,*** crot-t., cur., ***graph., hep.,*** ign., kali-i., lach., med., mur-ac., nux-v., ***paeon., podo.,*** phys., sarr., sep., ***sulph.,*** teucr.

- black - ***carb-v., mur-ac.***
- menses, during - sep.

swelling, sensation of - ***aesc.,*** cact., graph., hep., nat-m., nux-m., sulph.

TEARING, pain - ***all-c.,*** alumn., aur., ***berb.,*** calc., carb-s., carb-v., chin., ***colch.,*** erig., eupi., ferr., grat., ign., ***kali-c.,*** kreos., lach., laur., led., ***lyc., mez.,*** nat-m., **NIT-AC., NUX-V.,** ph-ac., phos., ***ruta.,*** sars., sep., sulph., sul-ac., thuj., tub., zinc.

- after hard stool - lyc.
- bed, in - chin.
- bending forward amel. - alumn.
- coughing, on - lach.
- dinner, after - mang.
- evening - ph-ac.
- extending, into abdomen - mag-c.
  - into abdomen, during stool - mag-c.
  - through urethra - mez.
  - upward - ***lach.,*** sep.
- jerking - thuj.
- lying on back amel. - alumn.
- morning - ph-ac.
- moving, on - valer.
- sitting, while - ***ruta.***
- stool during - agar., ***calc.,*** colch., ferr., ***lach.,*** mez., nat-a., **NAT-M.,** ***nit-ac., sars., sel., sep., sul-ac.***
  - after - aesc., alumn., ***kali-c.,*** lyc., ***nat-m.,*** **NIT-AC.**
  - though soft - nit-ac.
- twitching - thuj.
- urinating, while - ***ruta.***
- warm clothes, amel. - phos.

TENESMUS, [illegible]
agar., **ALOE,** [illegible]
ant-c., **APIS,** apoc., [illegible]
arum-t., asaf., atro., aur-m., [illegible]
benz., berb., ***bov.,*** brom., bry., cact., [illegible]
cann-i., cann-s., ***canth.,*** **CAPS.,** [illegible]
carb-an., carb-s., ***carb-v., caust.,*** cham., chin-s., cinnb., cob., cocc., **COLCH.,** ***coll., coloc.,*** con., ***corn., crot-t.,*** cuph., cupr., cupr-ac., cupr-ar., ***cycl.,*** der., dig., dios., dirc., erig., ***euph.,*** eup-per., eupi., gamb., fago., ferr., ferr-ar., ferr-i., ferr-m., ferr-p., gels., graph., grat., ***ham.,*** hep., hyos., ign., iod., ***ip., iris,*** kali-ar., ***kali-bi.,*** kali-c., ***kali-i., kali-n.,*** kreos., ***lach.,*** lac-c., lact., laur., liatr., **LIL-T.,** ***lyc.,*** lycps., ***lyss.,*** mag-c., mag-s., manc., **MERC., MERC-C.,** merc-cy., merc-d., merc-sul., ***mez.,*** mill., morph., mur-ac., ***nat-a., nat-c., nat-m.,*** nat-p., nat-s., nicc., **NIT-AC.,** nux-m., **NUX-V.,** oena., ol-an., op., ox-ac., petr., phel., ph-ac., phos., phys., ***phyt.,*** pic-ac., ***plat.,*** plb., podo., psor., ptel., puls., rat., rheum, rhod., ***rhus-t.,*** rumx., ruta., sang., sel., senec., ***sep., sil.,*** sol-n., sol-t-ae., spig., spong., squil., stann., **STAPH.,** ***stront-c.,*** **SULPH.,** sumb., tab., ***tarent.,*** ter., thuj., trom., tub., verat., verat-v., vip., xan., zinc.
- bladder, and - alum., **CAPS.,** lil-t., ***merc-c.,*** **NUX-V.**
- coffee, after - ***nat-m.***
- constipation, during - asaf., ***con.,*** plb., ***nux-v.,*** vib.
- diarrhea, during - ***alum.,*** **ARS.,** carb-s., carb-v., cimic., ***coloc.,*** cop., com., crot-t., form., ***gamb.,*** hydr., mag-m., mag-s., ***merc.,*** **MERC-C.,** mur-ac., ***nit-ac.,*** op., phys., phyt., plb., ptel., sarr., sel., ***sulph.,*** tab., verat.
  - after - bell., caps., carb-an., ***dulc.,*** hydr., kali-c., kali-n., laur., ***lil-t.,*** mag-c., phel., phos., rhus-t., stront-c., sulph., tab., zinc.
  - before - hydr.
  - hemorrhoids, with - caps.
- dinner, after - alum., nat-m.
- dysentery, during - acon., **APIS,** arn., ars-i., **CAPS., COLCH.,** con., cop., dios., ip., ***merc.,*** **MERC-C.,** ***nit-ac.,*** rheum, sulph., ter., xan.
  - after - calc.
- eating - ***coloc.,*** crot-t.
- evening - ferr., plat.
- extending to, bladder - canth., ***caps., med.,*** merc-c., ***nux-v.***
  - to, perineum - mez.
  - to, urethra - mez.
- flatus, on attempting to suppress - acon.
- hard stool, with - ***con.***
- jerking - sep.
- menses, during - ***am-c.,*** nat-s.
  - before - thuj.
- milk, after - nicc.
- morning - aeth., nicc.
  - rising, after - aeth.
- night - bov., ***merc.,*** zinc.
- sitting, while - crot-t., staph., ***sulph.***

[illegible]SMUS, ineffectual straining
- stool, during - ***acon.,*** aesc., ***aeth.,*** **ALOE, AGAR.,** alum., am-c., am-m., ang., ant-t., apis, apoc., arg-n., ***arn., ars.,*** arum-t., asc-t., aster., bapt., ***bell., calc.,*** calc-s., canth., ***caps.,*** carb-ac., carb-s., ***caust., cedr.,*** cob., coff-t., ***colch., coll., coloc.,*** con., cop., ***corn.,*** crot-t., ***cupr.,*** dios., fago., ferr., ferr-ar., ferr-m., fl-ac., form., gamb., gran., graph., grat., hell., hep., hipp., hydr., hyper., **IP.,** iris, kali-ar., ***kali-bi.,*** kali-chl., kali-i., kali-n., kalm., lach., ***lac-c.,*** laur., ***lil-t.,*** lob-s., lyc., lyss., ***mag-c.,*** mag-m., mang., **MERC., MERC-C.,** ***morph.,*** myric., ***nat-a., nat-c., nat-m., nat-s.,*** nicc., ***nit-ac.,*** **NUX-V., OP.,** ox-ac., petr., phys., phyt., pic-ac., plan., plat., plb., ***podo.,*** ptel., rob., ***rhus-t.,*** senec., sep., ***spong.,*** staph., ***sulph.,*** tab., ther., thuj., ***trom.,*** verat., zinc.
  - after - ***aeth.,*** **AGAR.,** aloe, ambr., am-m., ant-t., ***apis,*** apoc., ars., aster., bapt., ***bell.,*** bov., calc-p., calc-s., ***canth., caps.,*** cob., ***cocc., colch.,*** corn., cupr-ac., dios., dros., dulc., erig., fago., fl-ac., gamb., gins., grat., hell., ***ign.,*** ind., indg., ip., jug-c., kali-ar., ***kali-bi.,*** kali-c., kali-n., kali-p., ***kali-s.,*** lach., laur., lil-t., lyc., lyss., ***mag-c., mag-m.,*** mag-s., manc., **MERC., MERC-C.,** ***merc-d.,*** merc-i-r., ***merc-sul., mez., nat-m.,*** nicc., nit-ac., nux-v., phel., phos., ph-ac., phys., plat., plb., ***podo.,*** ptel., **PULS.,** ***rheum, rhus-t.,*** sars., senn., sil., **SULPH.,** tab., ***trom.,*** zinc.
  - amel. - acon., aesc., aloe, alum., ant-t., arn., ars., asaf., bapt., bov., bry., cahin., calc-p., canth., cham., colch., ***coloc.,*** corn., dulc., **GAMB.,** hell., lept., nat-s., nuph., **NUX-V., RHUS-T.,** sanic., tarent.
  - amel., during - verat-v.
  - before - acon., aeth., **AGAR.,** alum., arn., berb., cham., ***coloc.,*** crot-c., dirc., fago., grat., mag-m., ***merc.,*** **MERC-C.,** ***nux-v.,*** phys., plat., plb., sep., **SULPH.,** tarent., verat.
  - relieved by stool - nux-v.
- urination, during - carb-v., ferr., med., ***prun.***
  - after - coloc., mur-ac.
- walking, while - ***sulph.***
- warmth, amel. - coloc., sulph.
- water, on hearing running - **LYSS.**

TENSION - ***calc.,*** chin., euphr., graph., ***ign., lyc., nux-v.,*** rhus-t., ***sep.,*** **SIL.**
- convulsive - ign.
- stool, after - berb., sep.

TINGLING - ***carb-v., colch.,*** ferr-ma., plat., ter.
- evening - plat.
- stool, during - ***carb-v.***

TREMBLING, anus, in - con.

TWINGING, pain - caust., kali-c., lact., lyc., mag-c., nat-c., zinc.
exercise, after - coc-c.
flatus amel. - kali-bi.
stool, during - spong.
after - canth., grat.
twinging, anus, writhing in - ***croc.***

TWITCHING - agn., ars., bry., calc., carb-ac., colch., ***coloc.,*** iod., ***merc.,*** nat-m., ***sil., staph.***
afternoon - coloc.
bed, in - chin.

ULCERATION - ALUMN., ***calc., carb-v.,*** caust., **CHAM.,** cub., ***hep., hydr., kali-bi.,*** kali-c., ***kali-i., nat-s., nit-ac., paeon., petr.,*** phos., ***phyt.,*** puls., sars., **SIL.,** staph., ***sulph.,*** syph.

ULCERATIVE - mag-c., mez., sulph.

URGING, desire to stool - abrot., acon., **AESC.,** aeth., **AGAR.,** all-c., **ALOE,** ***alum.,*** alumn., ambr., ***anac.,*** ang., ***apis,*** arg-m., ***arg-n., arn., ars.,*** ars-h., ars-i., arum-t., asc-t., ***asar.,*** atro., aur., aur-m., bar-c., ***bell.,*** benz-ac., ***berb., bism.,*** bor., bov., ***bry.,*** bufo, cadm-s., cahin., calad., calc., calc-p., camph., cann-s., canth., caps., carb-an., carb-s., carb-v., cast-eq., cast-v., cast., caust., cham., ***chel.,*** chin., chin-s., cic., ***cimx.,*** cimic., cist., clem., cob., cocc., coc-c., coff., ***colch., coloc.,*** com., ***con., corn.,*** croc., crot-c., crot-t., cupr., cycl., dig., dios., ***dulc.,*** elaps, eug., fago., ferr., ferr-ar., ferr-i., ferr-ma., gamb., gent-l., glon., ***graph.,*** gran., grat., ham., ***hep.,*** hydr., hyos., hyper., **IGN.,** indg., iod., iris, kali-bi., ***kali-c.,*** kali-chl., ***kali-n.,*** kalm., kreos., lach., lact., **LIL-T.,** lyc., mag-c., ***mag-m.,*** mag-s., manc., meny., **MERC.,** ***merc-c.,*** merc-i-f., merc-i-r., mez., naja, ***nat-a., nat-c.,*** nat-m., nat-p., nat-s., nit-ac., nux-m., **NUX-V.,** oena., ***op.,*** osm., ox-ac., pall., petr., phel., ***phos.,*** phys., **PIP-M.,** plan., ***plat.,*** **PLB.,** ***podo.,*** prun., ptel., ***puls., ran-s.,*** rat., ***rheum, rhod.,*** rhus-t., ***ruta.,*** sabad., sabin., sars., sec., senec., ***sep.,*** serp., **SIL.,** sol-t-ae., spig., spong., squil., stann., ***staph.,*** stram., stront-c., **SULPH.,** sul-ac., sumb., ***tab.,*** tarent., tell., ther., ***thuj.,*** trom., verat., verb., vib., vinc., ust., zinc.
absent in company - **AMBR.**
anxious - acon., arg-n., ars., gels., ***merc., nux-v.,*** ol-an., sulph.
belching, on each - aesc.
breakfast, during - dios.
after - carb-s., grat., mag-c., mag-m., spong.
chilliness, in hand and thighs, in - **BAR-C.**
clothing, on tightening - bry.
coffee, after - nat-m.
colic, during - coloc., ind., **NUX-V.**
constant - aesc., anac., ant-s., arn., ars., asaf., bar-c., bell., ***berb.,*** bry., calc., cob., con., cop., **CROT-T.,** ger., ham., hyos., ***ign.,*** kali-a., ***lil-t.,*** mag-c., ***mag-m.,*** **MERC., MERC-C.,** ***merc-d.,*** nat-a., nat-m., ***nat-s., nux-v.,*** phyt., ***pip-m.,*** plat., ptel., ruta., sep., sin-a., ***sulph.,*** sumb., zinc-s.

URGING, desire to stool
diarrhea, with - ars., canth., mag-c., ***merc-c.,*** nit-ac.
dinner, during - dios.
after - ant-c., cann-s., caps., caust., colch., coloc., ***ferr-ma.,*** kali-bi., mag-m., nat-m., par., phel., ran-s., sulph.
drinking, after - caps.
eating, after - **ALOE,** alum., ***anac.,*** ant-c., apoc., aur., bar-c., cham., clem., **COLOC.,** crot-t., ferr-ma., fl-ac., phos., ***rheum,*** rhus-t., sulph., zinc.
effort, great desire passes away with - **ANAC.**
evening - bism., carb-v., lyc., sep., stann., sulph.
in sleep - phyt.
flatus, for - alum., carb-an., caust., kali-c., lyc., mag-c., mag-m., meny., mez., osm., phos., sep.
flatus, when passing - **ALOE,** spig., ruta.
passing amel. - caps., carb-v., ***colch.,*** kali-c., kali-n., mag-c., mez., nat-a., ruta.
frequent - abrot., **ALOE,** ***ambr., apis, arg-m.,*** arn., asaf., **BAR-C.,** bell., berb., bor., brom., cahin., calc-p., carb-an., ***caust., coloc.,*** **CON., CORN.,** dios., ham., ***hep.,*** hura, ***hyos., ign.,*** kreos., lac-c., lac-d., **LIL-T., MERC., MERC-C.,** ***nat-m.,*** nat-s., nit-ac., **NUX-V.,** ox-ac., petr., ***ph-ac.,*** phos., **PLAT.,** ***puls., rheum,*** ruta., sars., stann., staph., stram., sulph., tab., verb.
fright, from - ***caust.***
hang down, letting feet - rhus-t.
ineffectual, then involuntary stool - agar., arg-n.
labor pain, with every - nux-v., plat.
lying bent up amel. - staph.
menses, during - calc., mang., puls., sep.
before - eupi.
miscarriage, during - calc.
morning - aloe, nat-s.,sulph.
motion, on - ars-i., ***bry., crot-t., mur-ac., rheum.***
news, exciting, after - gels.
night - ***aloe,*** am-c., carl., coloc., graph., kali-c., lyc., mag-c., merc-i-r., nat-m., phys., sil., **SULPH.,** sul-ac., thuj., zinc.
11 p.m. - gels., mag-c., merc-i-r., pip-m.
2 a.m. - uran-n.
menses, before - mang.
midnight - dios., lach.
waking - ***aloe,*** ferr-i.
rising from - rheum, rumx.
on rising - ***aloe.***
sex, after - nat-p.
sitting on - crot-t.
smoking, while - calad., thuj.
standing, while - aloe, bry., lil-t.
startled, when - ***gels.***

URGING, desire to stool

stool, during - abrot., ***aesc.,*** aeth., agar., am-m., anac., ***ant-c.,*** arg-m., ars-i., bar-c., bell., bov., bry., calad., calc., carb-s., carl., coca, ***coll.,*** con., cycl., dios., dirc., dros., dulc., eupi., ferr., form., gamb., graph., grat., hep., inul., iris, lycps., mag-m., merl., mez., nat-c., nat-p., nicc., nit-ac., ox-ac., phys., phyt., pic-ac., pip-m., plan., plat., ptel., ran-s., rat., rhus-t., sars., sep., sil., spong., stann., stram., **SULPH.,** sul-ac., tab., tarent., verb.

after - aesc., ***aeth.,*** agar., **ALOE,** ambr., ars., ars-i., bar-c., bell., berb., bry., calc-p., camph., chin., cic., cocc., colch., crot-t., cycl., dig., dios., dros., ferr., ferr-ar., ferr-i., form., grat., ign., iod., iris, kali-c., kali-p., ***lach.,*** lyc., mag-c., ***mag-m.,*** **MERC., MERC-C.,** merc-i-r., mez., naja, nat-a., nat-c., nat-m., ***nat-p.,*** nicc., ***nit-ac.,*** nux-v., petr., **RHEUM,** ruta., samb., sol-t-ae., spig., stann., **SULPH.,** tab., tarax., til., verat.

amel. - acon., aesc., aloe, alum., ant-t., arn., ars., asaf., bapt., bry., cahin., calc-p., canth., cham., colch., ***coloc.,*** corn., dulc., **GAMB.,** gels., hell., lept., nat-s., nuph., **NUX-V., RHUS-T.,** sanic., tarent.

before - all-s., ***aloe,*** alum., ***ars., bell.,*** berb., calc-f., camph., cist., coloc., con., ***crot-t.,*** euphr., ferr-i., fl-ac., form., gamb., grat., hell., hep., ***ign.,*** kali-bi., kali-n., lact., lept., ***merc-c., merc-d.,*** mez., nat-c., nat-m., nat-s., ***nux-v.,*** olnd., osm., phos., ***podo., rheum, rhus-t.,*** sil., stront-c., **SULPH.,** verat.

hard, during - mag-c.

yellow, during - mag-c.

sudden - aesc., agar., ***aloe,*** ant-s., bar-c., bry., carb-v., cic., cocc., **CROT-T.,** cycl., dig., dirc., ***ferr.,*** gent-c., gent-l., graph., ign., kali-bi., kali-c., kali-n., lac-ac., ***lach.,*** lil-t., mag-m., manc., naja, ***nat-c., nat-p., nat-s.,*** plat., ***podo., psor.,*** ptel., rhus-t., rob., sep., **SULPH.,** sumb., tab., verat., zinc.

after - ***cann-s.***

evening - gent-c., gent-l.

morning - manc., **SULPH.**

night - nux-v.

supper, after - calc-p., ox-ac., podo.

thinking about it, on - iris, ***ox-ac.,*** oxyt.

tormenting, but not for stool - ***lach.***

urination, during - **ALOE,** alum., aphis., cann-s., ***canth.,*** carb-v., caust., crot-h., cycl., dig., merc., ***mur-ac.,*** **NUX-V.,** prun., ***puls.,*** squil., staph., sumb., thuj.

after - alum., ***cann-s.***

amel. - nat-m.

urine is discharged, but only - lil-t.

vertigo, during - spig., zinc.

waking, on - alum.

URGING, desire to stool

walking, while - cob., coloc., laur., pall., rheum

water, on hearing running - **LYSS.**

WEAKNESS, weak feeling - ***agar.,*** **ALOE,** alum., apoc., bry., ***calc.,*** coloc., kali-c., lept., ***petr., phos.,*** tab., ***sep.***

stool, after - lept., ***podo.***

before - nat-p.

urination, during - inul.

WEIGHT, in, and a feeling as if a plug were wedged between the pubis and coccyx (see Lump) - ***aloe, cact.,*** caust., hep., **SEP.,** sil., thuj.

WORMS, (see Intestines)

Shoulders

ABSCESS, axilla - am-c., ***apis***, ars., bell., bufo, cadm-s., ***calc***., calc-s., cedr., coloc., ***crot-h***., **HEP.,** kali-bi., kali-c., lac-c., **MERC.,** ***merc-i-r.***, nat-m., ***nat-s***., **NIT-AC.,** petr., ph-ac., prun., **RHUS-T.,** ***sep.,*** **SIL.,** ***sulph.,*** thuj.

ACHING, pain - abrot., acon., aesc., agar., ail., arg-m., ***arn.,*** asaf., bor., ***calc.,*** calc-p., cann-i., carb-an., ***caust.,*** chel., coca, coloc., crot-t., cur., dios., ferr-i., hura, hydr., jatr., jug-c., kali-bi., kali-p., lac-c., lach., laur., led., lil-t., lob-s., lyss., merc-i-f., mez., mosch., myric., naja, ***nat-m.,*** ***nit-ac.,*** pip-m., plan., prun., sep., sil., sin-n., ***staph.,*** sumb., teucr., trom., ust., verat., verat-v., zinc.

afternoon - coloc., dios.
1 p.m. - dios.
1:30 p.m. - chel.
bed, in - fago., sumb.
bending arm - laur.
cold, on becoming - sil.
evening - mez., still.
when bending forward - carb-ac.
extending, to arm - brom.
to elbow - abrot., plb.
to fingers - elat.
lying on painful side agg. - nat-m.
morning, 4 a.m. - fago.
bed, in - sumb.
waking, on - coca
motion amel. - calc., kali-p., verb.
move on beginning to - ind.
moving arm, on - calc., croc., nat-a.
night - sil.
noon - phyt.
raising arm - coloc.
respiration, deep - ***chel.***
rheumatic - ***caust.,*** nat-a., plan.
walking, while - arg-m., brom.

aching, axilla - asaf., bry., chel., dios., ind., lat-m., phys., staph., thuj.

AIR, passing down from shoulder to finger, sensation as if - ***fl-ac.***

ALIVE, something in - berb.

ARTHRITIC, nodosities - ***calc., kali-i.***

BOILS - am-c., am-m., bell., hydr., ***kali-n.,*** nit-ac., ph-ac., sulph.

blood, large - ***calc.,*** jug-r., lyc., zinc.

boils, axilla - bor., **HEP.,** ***lyc., merc., nat-s.,*** petr., ***phos.,*** ph-ac., sep., ***sil., sulph.,*** thuj.
left - bor., lyc., ***phos., sep.***
painful, small - sep.
recurrent - lyc.
right - thuj.
tearing, pain - petr.

BORING, pain - arg-m., arg-n., aur., aur-m-n., coloc., ***ferr.,*** hell., ***mez.,*** nat-s., ph-ac., phos., ***rhod.***

afternoon, 4 p.m. - arg-n.
dinner, after - mez., phos.
evening - mez.

BORING, pain
extending to,
elbows - ferr.
finger ends - ferr.
heat amel. - ferr.
left - aur., bar-c., ph-ac.
lying on painful side - ph-ac.
morning - arg-m., arg-n.
bed, in - mez.
waking, on - nat-m.
motion, agg. - ***ferr.,*** mez., phos.
amel. - mez.
paralytic - nat-m.
right - arg-m., arg-n.
sitting, while - aur.
walking, while - mez.
weight of bed clothes - ***ferr.***

boring, axilla - arg-m., plb.

BROKEN, sensation, as if - ***chel., cocc.,*** nat-m.
left - mag-m.

BUBBLING, sensation - berb., mang., puls., tarax.
afternoon - puls.

BURNING, pain - alumn., am-m., ant-t., ***ars.,*** aur-m-n., berb., carb-s., ***carb-v.,*** clem., cocc., dios., graph., grat., ***iris,*** kali-bi., kali-c., mag-m., mang., meny., merc., mez., mur-ac., par., ph-ac., ***phos.,*** puls., ***rhus-t.,*** sep., spong., stront-c., sulph., tab., tep.

acromion - mez.
beneath - **AIL.,** lyc., sulph.
evening - alumn., dios., sep., sulph.
lying down, after - sulph.
walking, while - rhus-t.
extending, over the arm - mag-m., puls., sulph.
to hip - mag-m.
to scapula - mag-m.
night - puls.
right - am-m., ***carb-v.***
scratching, after - kali-c.
sitting, while - merc.
spots, in - kali-bi., mang.
top, on - ***carb-v.***

burning, axilla - am-c., berb., calc-p., ***carb-v.,*** caust., coloc., jug-r., kali-c., nat-m., sep., spig., thuj., zinc.
right - cocc., ruta.

BURSITIS - ant-c., ***apis.,*** ars., bell., ***bell-p., bry.,*** graph., hep., iod., ***lycpr.,*** puls., rhus-t., **RUTA..,** **SIL.,** ***stict., sulph.***

CANCER, axilla - ***aster.,*** con., ***phyt.***

CHILLINESS - lept.

COLDNESS - arg-n., aur., bry., ***caust.,*** cocc., hell., hydr., hyper., ***kali-bi., kreos.,*** lyc., phos., sep., sil., spig., stry., tep., verat.

eating, after - arg-n.
epilepsy, in - ***caust.***
evening, 9 p.m. - hydr.
10 p.m. - sep.
supper, after - ran-b.
extending to small of back - kreos.
morning - aur., sil.

coldness, axilla - agar., lact.

CONSTRICTION - agar., bov., ***cact.,*** nit-ac., plat., sep.
left - agar.

CONTRACTION, muscles and tendons - brom., elaps, kali-c., ***mag-c.,*** plb., rhod.
convulsive - cit-v.
extending to,
back - mag-c.
hand - elaps
morning - mag-c.
extending to back - mag-c.
sudden - alum.

CRACKED, skin - petr.

CRACKING, joints, in - aloe, anac., ant-t., bar-c., brach., ***calc.,*** carb-s., ***cic.,*** cinnb., ***croc.,*** ferr., gins., ***kali-c.,*** merc., mez., nat-a., nat-m., phos., sabad., sars., thuj.
elevation of arm - ***kali-c.,*** nat-a.
as if would crack - mur-ac.
morning - aloe.
night in bed - mez.
right - carb-s., sars.
stretching - sabad.

CRAMPS - cimic., elaps, lil-t., naja, ***plat.***
evening, 6 p.m. - elaps
extending to hand - elaps.
cramp, axilla - com., hura, iod.

CUTTING, pain - anac., ***bell.,*** colch., ***coloc., dig.,*** eup-pur., manc., merc-i-f., sil., sulph., sul-ac., thuj., verat.
bending arm forward - ign.
forenoon - sulph.
while walking - sulph.
right - sulph.
stabbing from within out - bell.
cutting, axilla - ang., dios., kali-c., ruta., sul-ac., thuj.
across from right to left - ***elaps.***
right - ***crot-c.,*** kali-c.
scar, in, of an old abscess - thuj.

DECAY, of bone, joint - sil.

DISCOLORATION, of
blackness in spots - vip.
brown, liver spots - ant-c.
mottled - berb.
redness - berb., chin., chin-s., lac-c., lach., ph-ac., puls-n, tab.
spots - berb., ph-ac., ***sul-ac.,*** tab.
yellow spots - ant-c.

DISLOCATION, as if, feeling - agar., anac., ant-t., caps., caust., ***ign., mag-c.,*** mag-m., merc., olnd., puls., ***sep.,*** sulph.
menses, during - mag-c.

DRAWING, pain - ***acon.,*** aeth., agar., ambr., am-c., am-m., anac., anag., ang., apis, ***arg-m., arg-n.,*** arn., ars., aur-m., aur-m-n., bapt., berb., bor., brom., ***bry.,*** camph., canth., carb-s., ***carb-v.,*** caust., cham., chel., cimx., clem., coc-c., colch., coloc., crot-h., cupr., dios., dros., dulc., elaps, euph., ferr-m., ferr-p., gent-c., gins., glon., hell.,

DRAWING, pain - hep., ign., iod., ***iris,*** jatr., kali-bi., ***kali-c.,*** kreos., lact., led., lil-t., ***lyc., mag-m.,*** mang., mez., naja, nat-c., ***nat-m.,*** nat-p., nat-s., nux-v., ol-an., pall., petr., ph-ac., ***phos.,*** phys., ***plat., puls.,*** ran-s., ***rhod.,*** rhus-t., sabad., sang., sanic., ***sep.,*** sil., stann., staph., ***sulph.,*** tab., teucr., thuj., verat., zinc.
air, open - nat-c.
alternating side - mag-m.
drawing, pain in hips - bry.
scraping in fauces - sulph.
bed, in, agg. - aur-m., coloc., lyc., nat-m., staph.
cramp-like - ***plat.***
dinner, after - sep.
evening - ambr., chel., lach., lyc., nat-m., nat-s.
extending to,
arm - anag.
arm - bry., chel., cimx., mang.
back of chest - dios.
deltoid region - zinc.
elbow - carb-ac., petr.
finger ends - apis, chel., elaps, ***nux-v., rhus-t.***
hand - ***lyc.,*** plat.
head - nat-m.
neck - anag.
neck, nape of - anag., apis
thighs - nux-v.
wrist - chel., ***puls.***
forenoon - cham., lyc.
left - nat-p.
then right - aeth.
lying, agg. - stann.
arm under head - staph.
on painful side - thuj.
morning - carb-v., dios., hyper., kali-c., naja, rhod., ***sep.,*** staph.
bed, in - ***nat-m.,*** staph.
waking, on - coloc., kali-c., ***nat-m.***
motion, agg. - caust., ferr-p., ***iris,*** mag-m., staph.
agg. of arm - staph.
amel. - am-m., ***arg-m.,*** carb-v., cocc., ign., ***rhus-t.,*** sep., thuj.
night - acon., coloc., thuj., zing.
bed, in - coloc.
paralytic - chel., kali-bi., ***phos.,*** staph., thuj.
paroxysmal - lyc.
pressure agg. - crot-h.
raising arms, on - anag., bry., calc., cocc., coc-c., ***iris,*** mag-m., sanic., zinc.
after eating - cocc.
rheumatic - agar., caust., carb-v., lyc., naja, phys.
right - am-c., am-m., carb-v., coc-c., euph., ferr-p., ***lyc.,*** nat-c., sep., thuj.
rising, after - cocc., coloc., thuj.
sitting, while - coloc., led.
standing erect - arn.
stooping, when - bor.
thread, as by a - plat.
uncovering the part - nat-m.

DRAWING, pain
walking, after - pall.
amel. - euph.
in open air - brom.
wind, in - carb-v.
drawing, axilla - ***bell.,*** cact., chin., coloc., com., lil-t., mang., nat-s., seneg., sil.
extending to,
down spine to lowest ribs - guai.
elbow - thuj.
upper arm - led.
upper arms, on raising - arn., rhus-t.
wrist - elaps
glands - sil.
paralytic - am-c.
right - carb-v.

DRYNESS, axilla - hep.

ECZEMA - petr.
eczema, axilla - ***hep.,*** jug-r., merc., ***nat-m.,*** petr., **PSOR.,** sep., sil.

EMACIATION, of - ***plb.,*** sumb.

ERUPTIONS - alumn., ars., nux-v., sep.
black pores - ***dros.***
desquamation - ***ferr.,*** merc.
elevations - alumn.
pimples - ***ant-c.,*** berb., chel., ***cist.,*** cob., cocc., com., fl-ac., hura, jug-r., kali-c., kali-chl., kali-n., mag-c., mag-m., puls., sulph., tab., zinc.
bleeding when scratched - cob., mosch.
boils, like - zinc.
burning - mag-m.
burning, scratching, after - kali-c.
indolent - chel.
itching - hura, mag-m.
itching, scratching, after - kali-c., mag-c.
painful - kali-chl., thea.
red - ant-c., chel., com., hura, jug-r., kali-chl.
stitching - kali-n.
pustules - ant-c., ***calc.,*** kali-br., rhod.
scabs - ars.
eruptions, axilla - brom., calc., elaps, ***hep.,*** jug-r., lyc., ***merc.,*** nat-m., nicc., petr., psor., ***rhus-t., sep., sulph.,*** thuj.
burning - ***merc.***
burning, scratching, after - phos.
cracks - ***hep.***
crusts - anac., jug-r., **NAT-M.**
dry - ***hep.***
itching - elaps, ***hep.,*** phos., ***psor.***
moist - brom., carb-v., jug-r., nat-m., ***sep.,*** sulph.
painful - ***merc.***
pimples - cocc., phos.
pustules - crot-c., viol-t.
scaly - jug-r.

EXCORIATION, axilla - ars., aur., carb-v., con., ***graph.,*** mez., sanic., ***sep., sulph.,*** zinc.

FISTULOUS, axilla, openings in - ***calc., sulph.***

FORMICATION - ars-h., arund., berb., caust., chin-s., cocc., fl-ac., lac-c., lyc., mag-c., osm., sarr., thuj., urt-u.
evening, in bed - osm., thuj.
morning - mag-c.
urination, during - hep.
formication, axilla, in - berb., cocc., con.

FROZEN, shoulder - ferr., rhus-t., ruta, sang., ***thiosin.***

FULLNESS- bry.

GANGRENE - ***crot-h.***

GNAWING, pain - am-c., nicc., sulph.
night - sulph.

HEAT - aesc., brom., nux-v., spong., urt-u.
acromion - phos.
heat, axilla - aur.

HEAVINESS - carb-an., ***ferr.,*** hep., kali-n., mag-m., ***nat-m.,*** nat-s., ***nux-m.,*** par., phos., ***puls.,*** sulph., thuj., zinc.
motion, on - mur-ac.
waking, on - zinc.

HERPES- kali-ar.
herpes, axilla - carb-an., elaps, lac-c., lyc., mez., nat-m., rhus-t., sep.
herpes zoster - dol.

INDURATION, axillary, glands - am-c., bufo, calc., **CARB-AN.,** clem., ***con.,*** **IOD.,** ***kali-c.,*** lac-c., ***phyt.,*** **SIL.**

INFLAMMATION, axillary, glands - acon-l., ***aster., bar-c.,*** bell., calc., carb-an., ***con.,*** elaps, graph., hep., jug-r., ***lac-ac.,*** nat-s., **NIT-AC.,** petr., phos., ***phyt.,*** raph., rhus-t., sil., sulph.

INJURIES - ***arn., bry.,*** calc., ***calen., ferr-m., rhus-t.,*** **RUTA,** zinc.
straining, after - arn., ***rhus-t.,*** ruta..
rheumatic, lameness, with - ***ferr-m., rhus-t., ruta.,*** thiosin.

ITCHING - alumn., am-c., ars., bar-c., berb., bov., brom., carb-ac., caust., cob., coloc., cund., cycl., dios., fl-ac., ***gels.,*** hep., jug-c., kali-bi., kali-br., kali-c., mag-c., mag-m., mang., mez., ***mill.,*** myric., nat-c., nicc., op., osm., pall., puls., sars., stront-c., sulph., ther., thuj., ***urt-u.***
afternoon - fl-ac., mag-c.
2 p.m. - ol-an.
menses, during - mag-c.
burning - mez.
evening - fl-ac., hura, osm.
lying down, on - mur-ac., osm.
sleep, before going to - mag-c.
forenoon - mag-c.
menses, during - mag-c.
morning - fl-ac.
dressing, while - mag-c., mag-m.
scratching, agg. - stront.
amel. - bov., ol-an.
itching, axilla - agn., ***anac.,*** arg-n., asar., aster., berb., calc-p., carb-an., ***carb-s., carb-v.,*** caust., cocc., con., cop., cycl., dig., elaps, form., grat., ham., ***hep.,*** hura, jug-r., kali-c., kali-n., mag-c., nat-m., ***nit-ac., phos.,***

itching, axilla - sang., sep., spig., spong., squil., stann., **SULPH.**, viol-t.
below - asar.
heated, when body becomes - arg-n., ***hep.***
menses, before - sang.
morning - form.
perspiration agg. - jug-r.
sitting - spong.

JERKING - ars., alum., ***lyc.,*** puls., sil., spig., zinc.
sudden - alum.

LAMENESS - abrot., aesc., ***all-c.,*** ambr., bism., bry., carb-ac., cimic., coc-c., dios., ***fl-ac.,*** kali-i., ***lach.,*** laur., ***merc-i-f., nat-m.,*** phyt., psor., ***rhus-t.,*** **RUTA.**, sep., zing.
evening, when heated - coc-c.
morning, on waking - abrot., calc-ar.
night, on waking - coc-c.
raising arm, on - bry.
right - merc-i-f.
smoking, while - carb-ac.
walking, while - carb-ac.
writing - merc-i-f.

MOISTURE, axilla, humor in, from - ***carb-v., sulph.***

NODULES, axilla, in - lyc., mag-c., phyt.

NUMBNESS - alumn., merc., ox-ac., plb., ***puls.,*** sep., ***urt-u.,*** zinc.
morning - zinc.
night - sep.

PAIN, shoulders - abrot., acon., aesc., ***agar.,*** all-c., ***alum.,*** alumn., ammc., am-c., am-m., anag., apis, ***arg-m.,*** arn., ***ars.,*** asc-t., aspar., aster., aur., aur-m., bad., bapt., bar-c., ***berb.,*** brom., ***bry., cact., calad., calc., calc-p., calc-s.,*** carb-ac., ***carb-s.,*** carb-v., card-m., ***caust.,*** cham., **CHEL.**, chin., chin-a., chin-s., ***cimic.,*** cimx., ***cist.,*** coc-c., ***colch.,*** coloc., com., cop., ***crot-c., crot-h.,*** cupr., daph., dig., dios., dirc., dros., ***dulc., echi.,*** eup-per., fago., **FERR.**, ***ferr-ar.,*** **FERR-M.**, ***ferr-p.,*** fl-ac., gels., gins., glon., ***graph.,*** guai., ***ham.,*** hell., ***hep.,*** hura, hyper., ***ign.,*** ind., ***iod., iris,*** jatr., jug-c., kali-ar., ***kali-bi.,*** kali-c., ***kali-i., kali-n.,*** kali-p., ***kalm.,*** kreos., lac-c., lac-ac., ***lach.,*** lachn., laur., lec., ***led.,*** lil-t., lob., ***lyc.,*** lyss., ***mag-c., mag-m.,*** mang., ***med., merc.,*** merc-c., merc-i-f., merc-sul., ***mez.,*** mosch., mur-ac., myrt-c., naja, ***nat-a., nat-c.,*** nat-m., nat-s., nit-ac., nux-m., ***nux-v.,*** ol-an., olnd., pall., ph-ac., ***phos.,*** phys., ***phyt.,*** plan., ***plb.,*** prun., psor., ptel., ***puls., ran-b.,*** raph., ***rhod.,*** **RHUS-T.**, rumx., **SANG.**, sars., sep., sil., ***staph.,*** stram., stront-c., stry., **SULPH.**, tab., tarent., ***thuj.,*** tril., trom., verat., vesp., vip., zinc.
abducting, arm agg. - ***chel.***
acromion - cham.
afternoon - cham., chel., cupr., dios., mag-c.
alternating - **LAC-C.**
with hip - kalm.
asleep, as if - caust.
bending, forward - graph.
head, on - puls.
cold, air, amel. - thuj.

PAIN, shoulders
cold, becoming, on - ***calc., calc-p., chel., dulc.,*** **HEP.**, ***kali-c., merc.,*** **NUX-V.**, ***phos., psor., rhod.,*** **RHUS-T.**, **SIL.**, ***sulph.***
cough, during - am-c., ars., ***bry.,*** chin., dig., ***ferr., lach., phos., puls.,*** rhus-t., sang., thuj., xan.
damp, weather - **DULC.**, ***phyt., ran-b.,*** **RHUS-T.**, thuj.
dinner, after - asc-t., mez., phos., phys.
dislocation, as of - ant-t., caps., cor-r., ***croc.,*** fl-ac., ign., mag-c., mag-m., mez., myrt-c., nicc., olnd., **RHUS-T.**
evening - calc., chel., cist., fl-ac., led., lyc., mag-c., ***mez.,*** nat-s., pall., puls., sang., stry.
6 p.m., while walking - rhus-t.
7 p.m. - dios., stry.
bed, in - nux-v.
extending to,
arm - ars., bapt., brom., bry., cimx., glon., ind.
back - ars., dios.
chest - sars.
deltoid muscle - bol., chel.
elbow - abrot., cupr-ar., dros., ferr., fl-ac., ind., petr., phos., plb.
fingers - apis, ***calc-p., cocc.,*** elat., ferr., fl-ac., naja, nux-v., rhus-t., thuj.
hand - ***arn.,*** chin-s., glon., jatr., lat-m., mag-m.
head - ind.
neck - anag., apis, lac-ac.
ribs, upper - phos.
side, down - fago.
wrist - chel., ***cimic., guai.,*** lyc., ***puls.***
fallen out, as if - sulph.
fatigue, as from - kali-n., mez., petr.
forenoon - cham., dios., hyper., ***lyc.***
9 a.m. until evening - lyc.
10 a.m. - kalm.
11 a.m. - lac-ac.
glands, from - graph.
hanging down the arm - mez., nux-v., ruta., thuj.
amel. - ***phos.***
holding anything firmly with hand - bry.
humerus, head of, too large, as if - mez.
jerking - arn., ars., fl-ac., mez., mosch., puls., sil., tarax.
lain, on - graph., sil.
left - ***agar.,*** alumn., ammc., arg-m., cinnb., guai., ind., ***iod.,*** kali-c., ***kalm.,*** **LED.**, mag-m., mang-m., merc-c., nat-m., ***ph-ac., rhus-t.,*** **SULPH.**
and right hip - **LED.**, nux-m.
cough, during - ***ferr.,*** rhus-t.
lying on painless side agg. - nat-m.
to right - asc-t., ***calc-p.,*** lach., ***med.,*** naja
lifting - coloc., ***ferr.,*** ind., ***sang.,*** sep., stann., staph.
as after - mez.
on painful side, agg. - ***lach.,*** nat-m., nux-v., ***ph-ac., rhod., thuj.,*** zinc.

PAIN, shoulders

lifting,

on painful side, amel. - coc-c., kali-bi., ***lyc.,*** nux-v., puls.

quiet amel. - sang.

menses, during - mag-c.

instead, of - ars.

morning - arg-m., arg-n., ars., ***caust.,*** dios., kalm., ol-an., ***phos.,*** ran-b., sumb.

5 to 6 a.m. - fago.

bed, in - mez., ol-an., staph.

rising, on - kalm., phos., ran-b.

rising, on amel. - sil.

waking, after - phos.

waking, on - caust., fl-ac., kali-bi., kali-c., kalm., sil.

motion, on - am-m., asc-t., ***bry.,*** carb-v., caust., chel., echi., fago., ***ferr.,*** ferr-p., ***guai.,*** iris, kali-bi., kali-i., kali-n., kalm., lac-ac., ***led.,*** mag-m., mez., nat-m., ***phos., ran-b., staph.***

amel. - alumn., arg-m., bapt., calc., cham., colch., dios., dros., euph., **FERR.,** ***ferr-p.,*** kali-p., ***lyc.,*** mag-m., mez., mur-ac., ***ph-ac.,*** **RHUS-T.,** ***sep.,*** stann., verb.

arm, of - asar., bell., calc., cann-s., caust., chel., croc., ***ferr., iris, kali-bi.,*** kali-c., kali-n., kreos., ***lach.,*** lac-ac., ***led.,*** mag-c., med., merc., mur-ac., nat-a., nat-m., olnd., petr., phyt., puls., ***rhod.,*** ruta., ***sang.,*** sars., sep.

arm, of backwards - berb., dros., ***ign., kali-bi.,*** laur., mag-c., puls., sep., zinc.

shoulders, of, amel. - ph-ac.

night - abrot., bell., calc., cast., ***caust.,*** dig., ***kali-bi.,*** kali-c., ***kali-n.,*** mag-c., ***merc., phos.,*** **SANG.,** sep., sil., stict., sulph.

2 to 8 a.m. - ***ph-ac.***

bed, in - naja, ***sang.***

lying on it, while - sulph.

turning in bed - **SANG.**

waking - caust.

warm wrapping amel. - sil.

paroxysmal - ind., lyc., ***puls.,*** sarr.

pectoralis, tendon - sep.

perspiration amel. - thuj.

pressing, on something - kali-c.

pressure, amel. - coc-c., nat-c.

pulsating - ***led.,*** mag-m., mez., mur-ac., ph-ac., thuj.

putting the arm behind him agg. - **FERR.,** ***rhus-t.,*** **SANIC.,** sep.

raising the arm, agg. - ***alum., bar-c., bry.,*** calc., card-m., chel., cocc., dros., ***ferr.,*** hep., ***ign., iris, kali-bi.,*** kali-n., kreos., lac-c., ***led.,*** lyc., mag-c., mag-m., nat-c., nat-m., ***nit-ac.,*** petr., ***phos.,*** phyt., prun., puls., ***rhus-t.,*** **SANG.,** ***sanic.,*** sep., ***sulph.,*** sul-ac., syph., thuj., zinc.

amel. - ph-ac.

respiration, during - bry., sulph.

riding, while - cund., ***rhus-t.***

PAIN, shoulders

right - ammc., am-m., apis, berb., ***calc.,*** carb-v., **CHEL.,** ***cimic.,*** cimx., ***coloc., crot-c.,*** **FERR-M.,** fl-ac., iris, ***kalm.,*** lact., ***led., lept.,*** lob., ***lyc.,*** lyss., mag-c., med., ***nit-ac.,*** pall., phos., ***phyt.,*** **SANG., SARS.,** thuj., urt-u., wild.

then left - am-m., ***apis,*** bad., jatr., lac-c., lob., ***lyc.,*** lyss.

side, lain on - graph., rhod., sil.

not lain on - kali-bi.

sitting, after long - all-c., aur., coloc., led., rhod.

swallowing, food - ***rhus-t.***

thinking, of it - bapt.

thunderstorm, before - ***rhod.***

touching, when - acon., bry., mang., mur-ac., phos., sep.

turning in bed - ***sang.***

over, after amel. - nux-v.

ulcerative - berb., thuj.

vexation, after - ***coloc.***

waking, on - abrot., rumx., zinc.

walking, while - arg-m., aur-m-n., brom., hydr., kali-n., nat-s., pall., phos., sulph.

after - phos.

amel. - calc-s., euph., ***rhod.,*** **RHUS-T.**

slow amel. - ***ferr.***

wandering - cact., hyper., ***kali-s., phyt.,*** senec.

warmth, external agg. - ***guai.***

amel. - echi., ***ferr.,*** **HEP.,** ***lyc.,*** **RHUS-T.,** ***sil., thuj.***

warmth, of bed - thuj.

wine, agg. - ***ph-ac.***

writing, while - fl-ac., ***merc-i-f., valer.***

PAIN, axilla - ***agn.,*** arg-n., asaf., asar., ***aster.,*** bell., bry., cact., carb-an., carb-v., chel., cic., clem., ***crot-c.,*** con., dios., graph., ***hep.,*** ind., iod., nat-s., nit-ac., phos., phys., plb., seneg., sep., ***sil.,*** staph., sul-ac., sulph., thuj., verat., vip.

alternating sides - colch.

glands - am-c., asar., ***aster.,*** **BAR-C.,** kali-c., prun., rhus-t., ***sulph.,*** sul-ac.

menses, before - ***calc.,*** sang.

motion, amel. - dulc.

muscles of, right side - prim-v.

pulsating - dulc.

right to left - elaps.

swelling, with or without - jug-c.

pain, axilla, region of - kali-bi., meny., zinc.

extending, down arms - jug-c., ***nat-a.***

to little finger - nat-a.

to pectoral muscles - ***brach.***

intermittent - dulc.

morning - ran-b.

motion agg. - ran-b.

pulsating - squil., zinc.

raising, arm - caps.

touch, on - caps., squil.

PARALYSIS, of - ***caust., cur.***

paralysis, sensation of - aeth., ambr., aur-m., bry., elaps, euph., ***ferr-i.,*** kreos., lact., mang., mez., mur-ac., nat-m., nux-v., puls., ***rhus-t.,*** sep., sars., stann., staph., sulph., tep., valer., verat.
evening - ***ambr.***
left - aur-m., brom., ***ign., rhus-t.***
morning, rising, on - lach.
right - laur., merc-c., pall., psor.
rising, after - aur-m.
walking, while - arn.

PARALYTIC, pain - asar., ***berb.,*** brom., ***caust., chel., ferr.,*** ind., kali-bi., kali-i., kali-n., laur., lyc., lyss., mang., mez., mur-ac., ***nat-m.,*** nux-v., ph-ac., phos., prun., ***rhod.,*** sars., stann., staph., stront-c., valer.

PERSPIRATION - chin.
sex, after - agar.
under, dinner amel. - phos.

perspiration, axilla - ***all-c.,*** aloe, asar., ***bov.,*** **BRY.,** ***calc.,*** cadm-s., caps., carb-ac., carb-an., carb-s., ***carb-v.,*** **CEDR.,** chel., ***cur.,*** **DULC.,** gymn., ***hep., hydr.,*** hyos., **KALI-C.,** kali-p., ***kali-s., lac-c.,*** lach., laur., lil-t., merc-c., ***nat-m., nit-ac.,*** ox-ac., ***petr.,*** phos., **RHOD.,** sabad., sanic., **SEL., SEP., SIL.,** squil., **SULPH.,** sul-ac., tab., ***tell., thuj.,*** tub., verat., viol-t., zinc.
acrid - sanic.
air, cool, in - bov.
brown - ***lac-c.,*** thuj.
coldness, during - tab.
copious - ***sanic.,*** sel.
daytime - dulc.
eats holes in the clothing - iod., sep., sil., psor.
evening - sabad.
frosty deposit in hair, with - sel., thuj.
offensive - apis, bov., ***calc.,*** carb-ac., con., dulc., **HEP.,** ***hydr.,*** kali-c., ***lac-c., lach.,*** lappa-a., ***lyc.,*** merc-c., nat-s., **NIT-AC.,** ***nux-m.,*** osm., **PETR.,** phos., ***rhod., sel., sep.,*** **SIL.,** ***stry-p.,*** **SULPH.,** ***tell.,*** thuj., tub.
garlic, like - ***bov., kali-p., lach.,*** osm., **SULPH.,** ***tell.,*** thuj.
menses, between - sep.
menses, during - stram., tell.
red - arn., ***carb-v.,*** dulc., **LACH., NUX-M.,** nux-v., thuj.
sour smelling - asar.
yellow - lac-c.

PINCHING, pain - cina., colch., kali-c., mez., ph-ac., sep., sulph.
right deltoid - ***ferr.***

PRESSING, pain - acon., aloe, am-c., am-m., ammc., ***anac.,*** ang., ***arg-m.,*** arg-n., arum-t., aur-m-n., ***bell.,*** bism., bor., bov., brom., ***bry.,*** calc., camph., carb-an., card-m., **CAUST.,** chel., clem., coloc., cop., cor-r., crot-t., dig., fl-ac., ***hell.,*** hydr., hyper., ind., kali-bi., kali-c., kali-n., kali-p., kalm., lach., ***laur.,*** **LED.,** ***lyc.,*** mag-c., mag-m., merc., mez., mur-ac., ***nat-c.,*** nat-m., nat-p., ***nat-s., nit-ac.,*** nux-m., olnd., petr., ph-ac., phos., plat., prun., puls., ***ran-b., rhus-t.,*** sabad., **SEP.,** sil., stann., ***staph.,*** stront-c., **SULPH.,** thuj., verb., verat., zinc.
cold, from becoming, on uncovering - sil.
cough, during - dig.
evening - chel., fl-ac., nat-s.
sitting, while - mez., ***rhus-t.***
extending to elbow - sil.
to hand - sil.
forenoon, 10 a.m. - kalm.
inspiration, on - kali-c.
intermittent - sul-ac.
left - anac., bell., staph., sul-ac.
lifting - coloc., ind., sep., staph.
morning - ***phos.,*** staph.
motion, agg. - staph.
amel. - verb.
moving, arm - chel., dig., kali-bi., led.
amel. - calc.
night - cop., sep.
pressing, amel. - nat-c., sep.
raising, arm - kali-bi.
right - apis, laur., ph-ac., prun., sil.
tearing - ***led.,*** zinc.
tremulous - sul-ac.
waking, on - zinc.
walking, while - aur-m-n., hydr., ***led.,*** nat-s., staph., sulph.
after sitting - ran-b.

pressing, axilla - ***agn.,*** ang., asar., astac., camph., carb-v., chin., dros., led., lyc., mang., spong.
below - kali-c., lyc., mang.
left, in - chel., led.
region, of - sep., squil., thuj.
of paroxsmal - rhus-t.
right, in - ***agn.,*** carb-v., sil., staph.

PULSATION - am-m., arg-m., bar-c., bar-m., berb., brach., cocc., ***coloc.,*** dig., hura, ***kali-c., led.,*** mez., mur-ac., ph-ac., ***rhod.,*** rhus-t., sol-t-ae., stann., sulph., tab., tarax., thuj.
acromion - merc.
alternating with tearing - bar-c.
cold air, amel. - rhus-t.
evening - dig., mez.
motion, agg. - mez.
amel. - am-m., arg-m.
right - am-m., ***led.***
walking, while - dig.
amel. - rhus-t.
warmth agg. - rhus-t.

pulsation, axilla - am-m., cocc., dulc., spong.

RAISED - ferr., nat-m.
dyspnea, with - ant-c., eup-per.

RASH - berb., ***calc.,*** puls., tep.

rash, axilla - ***hep., sulph.***

RHEUMATIC, pain - acon., agar., alumn., ammc., am-m., ant-t., apis, ars., aur., bapt., ***berb.,*** brom., ***bry., cact., calc., calc-p.,*** carb-ac., carb-s., carb-v., card-m., ***caust., chel., chim., chin.,*** chin-s., ***cimic.,*** **COLCH.,** coloc., crot-c., dig., ***dulc.,*** ery-a., fago., **FERR.,** ***ferr-i., ferr-m., ferr-p., fl-ac.,*** form., graph., grat., ***guai., ham.,***

RHEUMATIC, pain - ign., ind., ***iod., iris,*** jatr., jug-c., ***kali-bi., kali-c., kali-i., kali-n., kalm., lac-ac., lac-c.,*** lach., ***led., lyc.,*** lyss., mag-c., mag-m., mang., **MED.,** ***merc.,*** merc-i-f., naja, ***nat-a., nat-c., nat-m.,*** nat-p., nit-ac., nux-m., nux-v., ol-an., olnd., pall., ph-ac., ***phos., phyt.,*** plan., ***puls.,*** ran-b., **RHOD., RHUS-T.,** ruta, sabin., ***sang., sanic., staph.,*** stict., stram., stront-c., stry., **SULPH.,** ***thuj.,*** trom., ust., zinc.
up the neck - lac-ac.

SENSITIVE - ***apis,*** aspar., cina, con., ferr., lach., pall.
sensitive, axilla - kali-c., nit-ac., sul-ac.

SHAKING - agar.

SHARP, pain - acon., aesc., ***agar.,*** ail., **ALUM.,** alumn., ambr., am-c., ammc., ang., ars., ars-i., asaf., asar., asc-t., aur., **BELL.,** berb., bor., brom., ***bry.,*** **CALC.,** calc-p., calc-s., camph., canth., carb-an., **CARB-S.,** ***carb-v.,*** caust., cham., ***chel., chin.,*** chin-a., ***cic.,*** cina, clem., ***cocc.,*** colch., crot-h., crot-t., cupr., dig., dulc., elat., euphr., **FERR.,** ferr-ar., ***ferr-i.,*** ferr-p., form., glon., ***graph.,*** grat., ***guai.,*** hell., hura, hydr., hyper., indg., inul., iod., ***iris, kali-c.,*** kali-n., kali-p., kreos., lach., ***laur., led.,*** lith., lob., ***lyc.,*** mag-c., mag-m., med., ***merc.,*** mez., mill., mur-ac., nat-c., nat-m., nat-p., nat-s., nicc., nit-ac., nux-m., ***nux-v.,*** ox-ac., pall., petr., ***phos.,*** phys., phyt., plat., plb., ptel., puls., **RAN-B.,** ran-s., raph., ***rhus-t.,*** ruta., sabad., sars., senec., ***sil.,*** squil., stann., ***staph.,*** stront-c., stry., sulph., sul-ac., tab., tep., ***thuj.,*** trom., ***valer.,*** verat., verb., viol-t., zinc.
afternoon - canth., chel., euphr., indg., kreos., mag-c., nicc., stront.
2 p.m. - hyper., laur.
4 p.m. - indg., ptel.
alternating, shoulders - mag-m.
burning - graph., mez., mur-ac., plb., stann.
in acromion - berb.
chill, during - ***hell.***
chilly, when - nit-ac.
cold damp weather - carb-s.
coughing, from - bor., carb-an., hyper., merc., puls., ***sep.,*** sulph., verat.
dinner, after - calc., phos., zinc.
evening - calc-s., fl-ac., lyc., merc., mur-ac., puls., sulph.
expiration, on - caust., sulph.
downward - carb-s., caust., ***ferr., kreos., rhus-t.,*** squil., sabad., sil., sulph.
to cervical muscles - cham., chel.
to chest - ***camph., sulph.***
to fingers - ***kreos., rhus-t.***
to hand - caust.
to hip - mag-m.
inspiration, on - berb., hyper., nit-ac., sulph.
left - ***bell., graph.,*** med.
on coughing - sulph.
lying, while - **RHUS-T.**
on it - sulph.
menses, instead of - ars.

SHARP, pain
morning - carb-an., carb-v., colch., gels., hura, lyc., nat-m., phys., sil., trom.
10 a.m. - sil.
bed, in - sulph.
cough, during - carb-an.
eating, after - gels.
moving arm - puls.
motion, during - carb-v., ign., ***iris,*** staph., sulph.
amel. - ***cocc.,*** iod., ***kali-c.,*** med., phos., **RHUS-T.,** sulph.
moving, arm - ***puls.,*** **RHUS-T.,** staph.
head from side to side - cupr.
night - alum., graph., phyt., ***sulph.***
noon, before eating - senec.
raising arm - agar., cic., ***iris, led.,*** mag-m., sars., sul-ac.
respiration, on - berb., nit-ac., stann.
right - ***apis,*** brom., carb-s., carb-v., caust., ***chel.,*** colch., iris, merc-i-f., pall., **RAN-B.**
on coughing - bor.
sitting, while - ox-ac.
sleep, before - sulph.
tearing - asar., caust., mosch., petr., sil., sul-ac.
touch, agg. - nit-ac., staph.
walking, while - dig., lac-ac.
amel. - **RHUS-T.,** thuj.
warm bed - ***sulph.***
sharp, axilla - agar., alum., ant-c., arg-m., arg-n., ars., asaf., aur., aur-m-n., berb., brom., bry., calc., canth., ***caust.,*** con., elaps, graph., kali-bi., kali-c., kalm., lact., laur., ***lyc.,*** mag-c., mang., mez., nat-m., nat-s., olnd., petr., phos., puls., sil., spong., staph., ***sulph.,*** thuj., verat., zinc.
evening - hura, rat., stront-c., zinc.
extending to, breast - caust.
chest, to - canth., cop., laur., mag-s., meny.
shoulder, to - phos.
upper arm, to - squil.
glands - lyc.
itching - staph., stann.
lifting - sul-ac.
motion, agg. - stann.
of arm - meny.
night - petr.
noon - bry.
raising the arm - kali-c., mag-c.
rest, during - aur-m-n.
right - arg-m., ***crot-c.,*** laur., stann.
sitting - aur-m-n., chel., nat-s., spong.
sharp, axilla, region, of - anac., bor., brom., dros., gamb., olnd., spig., tab., thuj.
afternoon, 3 p.m. - bell.
coughing, on - dros.
inspiration agg. - ruta.
intermitting - thuj.
inward - thuj.
left - calc., dig., ruta, sang., zinc.
lying on painful side - nat-c.
motion, on - mang.
pressure, amel. - dros.

sharp, axilla, region, of
right - bor., brom., carb-v., colch., nat-c.
rubbing, amel. - anac.
sitting - spong.
walking - nat-c.

SHOCKS - arg-m., manc.
evening, while writing - manc.
left - agar.
right - ***alum.,*** stann., sul-ac.
writing, while - sul-ac.

SHOOTING, pain - ail., alum., alumn., asc-t., bell., ***calc.,*** calc-p., crot-t., elat., ***ferr.,*** form., iris, lith., phys., ptel., ***rhus-t.,*** sulph., trom.
alternating with shooting in elbow - tep.
downward - ***ferr.***
evening - sulph.
heat, agg. - rhus-t.
joint - am-c., ferr., ox-ac., tep.
extending to arm - calc-p., ferr.
lying, on side - rhus-t.
morning - phys., trom.
bed, in - sulph.
breakfast, after - gels.
night, before falling asleep - sulph.
right - iris.
walking, on - lac-ac.

SHUDDERING - mag-m., verat.

SORE, pain - abrot., acon., aesc., alum., am-c., aml-n., arg-m., arn., aur., bapt., berb., brach., brom., calc-p., calc-s., camph., cann-s., chel., ***chin., cic.,*** cocc., coloc., ***con.,*** cop., crot-c., crot-h., cupr., ***dros.,*** elaps, fago., ***ferr.,*** fl-ac., gels., ***gran.,*** ham., hep., ***ign.,*** ind., iod., ***kali-c.,*** kali-i., kali-n., laur., ***led., lyc.,*** lyss., mag-c., merc-i-f., mez., mur-ac., nat-c., nat-m., nit-ac., **NUX-V.,** phos., pic-ac., plat., ***podo.,*** psor., ruta., sanic., sarr., sep., spig., staph., stram., stry., sulph., thuj., verat.
air, open, amel. - calc-s.
belching, amel. - mag-c.
bending, arm - crot-h.
evening - am-c., calc-s., mag-c.
exercise - pic-ac.
extending, to hand - sarr.
to wrist - brach., verat.
joint - cic., cupr., ign., ***nux-v.***
lain on - dros., ***ign., lach.***
left - ind., kali-c., ***kali-i.,*** mag-c., sulph.
lifting - nat-m.
lying, while - ***lyc.***
morning - kali-n.
rising, on - cupr.
waking, on - abrot., calc-s., chel., fl-ac.
motion, amel. - kali-c.
moving, arm - ***arg-m.,*** cann-s., dros., fago., ***ham.,*** ign., kali-c., mag-c., nat-m., sanic., sars., stram., sulph.
amel. - ***lyc.,*** sulph.
night - ***sulph.***
lying on side - acon., merc-i-f.
paralytic - ***led.,*** mag-c.
paroxysmal - crot-h.
placing arm behind back impossible - ***ferr.***

SORE, pain
raising the arm - dros., gran., nat-m.
right - coloc., ***merc-i-f.,*** psor.
sitting, while - coloc.
sleeping, after - acon.
touch, on - kali-c.
under, left - kali-i.
right - kali-c.
waiting - merc-i-f.
waking, on - acon., chel., fl-ac., nux-v.
walking, while - arg-m., carb-ac.
yawning, when - mag-c.

sore, axilla - ars., brach., ***carb-v.,*** dios., form., kali-c., lac-ac., ***mez.,*** nux-v., ran-s., sul-ac., zinc.
evening - sep.
raising arm - caps.

SPRAINED, as if - agar., **ALUM.,** ***ambr.,*** arn., asar., arg-m., berb., bry., caust., coc-c., croc., cycl., hep., ***ign.,*** lyc., mag-c., mang., merc., mur-ac., ***nat-m.,*** nicc., pall., petr., phos., puls., rhod., **RHUS-T.,** ***ruta., sabin.,*** sep., spig., stann., ***staph., sulph.,*** ter., thuj.
dinner, after - sep.
evening - ***ambr.***
extending to wrist - puls.
lying, while - coc-c.
motion, on - mag-c.
amel. - arg-m., mur-ac., nicc., stann.
moving arm - asar., mag-c., petr., ruta., sep., ***staph.,*** vesp.
night - sep.
paralytic - stann.
raising the arm - **ALUM.,** alumn., mag-c., petr., phos., ***sulph.***
amel. - ruta.
walking, amel. - arg-m.

STIFFNESS - bapt., **CALC-S.,** caust., com., ***cupr.,*** elaps, euph., ***fl-ac.,*** graph., guai., ***ham., ind.,*** jatr., kali-bi., kali-c., ***lyc., merc-i-f., nat-c.,*** nat-s., ***petr., phos.,*** **RHUS-T.,** sep., sil., staph., stry., verat.
evening - calc-s., com.
left - sep.
morning - calc-s., phos., ***rhus-t.,*** staph.
night - calc., kali-c.
putting arm over head, must - calc.
right - ***merc-i-f.***
walking, amel. - calc-s.
in open air - lyc.

SWELLING - acon., apis, bry., calc., calc-p., carb-o., ***coloc.,*** crot-h., crot-t., kali-c., kali-chl., kali-i., lac-c., lach., merc., thuj., vip.
pustules, after - kali-c.
vaccination, after - apis, bell., led., thuj.

swelling, axilla, scratching, after - nat-m.

swelling, axillary, glands - aesc., aeth., am-c., **AM-M.,** anan., anthr., ***ars., aster., aur.,*** **BAR-C.,** ***bell.,*** brom., cadm-s., calc., ***carb-an., clem., coloc., con.,*** **HEP.,** iod., ***kali-bi.,*** **KALI-C.,** kali-p., **LACH.,** ***lyc.,*** **MERC.,** ***merc-i-r., nat-c., nat-m., nat-s.,*** **NIT-AC.,** petr., ***ph-ac.,*** **PHOS.,** ***phyt., puls., rhus-t., sep.,*** **SIL.,** ***staph.,*** sul-ac., ***sulph.***

swelling, axillary, glands
breasts, with pain in - lac-ac.
damp weather, in - aster.
hard - aster., carb-an., iod., sil.
menses, before - aur.
night - aster.
painless - ***lach.***
right - nat-m.
sensation, of - benz-ac.
suppurative - coloc., sep., sulph.

TEARING, pain - acon., aesc., agar., agn., ***alum.,*** alumn., ***ambr.,*** am-c., ***am-m.,*** arg-m., ***ars.,*** aur-m., bar-c., ***bell., berb.,*** bism., bor., ***bov., bry.,*** cact., calc., calc-p., cann-s., carb-an., carb-s., ***carb-v.,*** caust., cham., chel., ***chin.,*** chin-a., cic., cist., cocc., coc-c., colch., coloc., crot-t., dulc., ***euon.,*** **FERR.,** ferr-ar., ***ferr-m., ferr-p., gamb., graph.,*** grat., hell., hep., ***hyper.,*** inul., kali-ar., kali-bi., **KALI-C.,** kali-i., ***kali-n.,*** kali-p., kalm., lach., lachn., ***laur., led.,*** **LYC.,** ***lyss., mag-c., mag-m.,*** mag-s., ***mang., merc.,*** merc-c., ***mez.,*** mosch., mur-ac., nat-c., ***nat-m.,*** nat-p., ***nat-s.,*** nicc., nux-m., nux-v., par., phel., ph-ac., ***phos.,*** plb., psor., ***puls., rat., rhod., rhus-t.,*** sang., sars., sec., sep., sil., stann., ***staph., stront-c.,*** **SULPH.,** sul-ac., tep., ***thuj.,*** verat., verb., **ZINC.**
afternoon - chel., kali-n., mag-s., psor.
4 p.m. - indg., ***lyc.***
5 p.m. - arg-m., mag-c., sulph.
raising arm - nicc.
air, cold amel. - thuj.
open, in - lact.
alternating with pulsation - bar-c.
belching, amel. - sep.
cold, becoming - **HEP.,** ***lyc.,*** **NUX-V.,** ***phos.,*** **RHUS-T.,** ***sil., sulph.***
dinner, after - phos., sep.
drawing - alum., coc-c., dulc.
evening - kali-n., lyc., mez., psor., rhod., zinc.
bed in - nat-m., rhod., sil., zinc.
extending to,
arms - ars., calc-p., coc-c., ferr., lach., ***lyss.,*** mag-m., mang., nat-c., ol-an., rat., stront-c., sulph.
arms, upper, bone - sulph.
arms, upper, bone, middle - mag-c.
back of hand - ***crot-t.***
chest - am-c., mag-c.
clavicle - arg-m., mag-c., par., sars.
elbow - ars., ***crot-c., ferr-m.,*** mag-c., nat-c., sars.
fingers - chin., ***lachn.,*** lyss., mag-m., par., thuj., zinc.
fingers, little - nat-c.
fingers, joints, of - mag-c.
head - kali-n.
neck - arg-m., berb.
palm - mag-m.
occiput - berb.
scapula - mag-c., mag-m.
wrist - kali-n., mag-c., rat.
forenoon - mag-c.
hanging down arm - thuj.
amel. - mag-m.

TEARING, pain
house, on going into - bry.
inspiration, on - agn.
jerking - am-c., ***chin.,*** sulph.
knitting, while - kali-c.
left - alumn., cic., ferr., graph., nat-c., ***phos.***
lying, on left side amel. - nux-v.
on painful side, agg. - thuj., zinc.
on painful side, amel. - lyc., puls.
morning - bry., coloc., lyc., mag-c.
2 to 5 a.m. - kali-n.
6 a.m. - bry.
bed, in - am-m., rhod., sulph.
waking, on - ***carb-v.,*** puls., sulph., verat.
motion, on - agn., am-m., berb., ***camph.,*** carb-v., chel., ***ferr-m.,*** ferr-p., ***graph., led.,*** mag-m., ***merc.,*** mez., nat-c., sil., ***stann.,*** sulph., verat.
amel. - arg-m., carb-an., cocc., ***ferr.,*** ferr-p., kali-c., lyc., mag-s., nat-c., psor., **RHUS-T.,** sulph., thuj., verb.
paralytic - agar., carb-v., ***ferr., ferr-m.,*** kali-n., rhod.
slow amel. - ***ferr., ferr-m., ferr-p., puls.***
night - bell., coloc., ***crot-t.,*** graph., kali-bi., kali-n., lyc., ***merc., sulph.,*** tep.
bed, in - bar-c., coloc., ***phos.***
before going to bed - am-m.
midnight - ammc., cast.
warm in bed, when - caust., ***merc.,*** thuj.
paralytic - agar., carb-v., chin., ***ferr., ferr-m.,*** kali-n., rhod., stann.
placing, arm over head - thuj.
posterior, part - nat-m.
pressing, arm down - mag-m.
pulsating - sil.
raise arm, cannot - **FERR.,** ***ferr-m.,*** mag-m.
rheumatic - ***bry., ferr., ferr-m.,*** ferr-p., grat., kali-bi., nat-m., nux-m., puls., **RHUS-T.**
right - agar., am-c., arg-m., cact., carb-v., ***coc-c., ferr-p.,*** mag-c., mag-m., ***rat.***
rising, from bed, amel. - kali-n.
rubbing, amel. - carb-an., laur.
side, lain on - zinc.
not lain on - kali-bi.
stooping, on - bor.
touch - ***chin.,*** mur-ac.
walking slowly amel. - ***ferr., ferr-m.***
warmth, amel.- graph.
of bed - caust., ***ferr., thuj.***
wet, cold weather - **RHUS-T.**

tearing, axilla - alum., arg-n., **ARS.,** aur., bell., calc., canth., chel., chin., kali-bi., kali-c., nat-m., petr., psor., sabin., thuj., zinc.
boils - petr.
night- petr.
pulsating - lyc.
raising the arm - kali-c.

TENSION, in - aeth., anac., ***apis,*** asar., berb., ***bov., bry.,*** carb-v., casc., coc-c., coloc., crot-h., dig., ***euph.,*** eupi., hyos., iris, kali-bi., ***kali-c.,*** kali-i., kali-n., lach., lact., laur., ***lyc.,*** mag-m., mang., mez., nat-c., nat-m., nat-p., nit-ac., petr., phos., ***sep.,*** staph., sulph., verat., ***zinc.***
brushing the teeth, while - phos.

TENSION, in
burning - mag-m.
menses, during - berb.
morning - calc., kali-c., sulph.
in open air - nat-c.
in bed - nat-m.
rising, after - euph.
motion, amel. - sep.
motion, of arm, on - dig.
mouth, closing, agg. - mag-c.
moving on, of arm - coloc., crot-h., euph., phos.
paralytic - euph.
raising the arm, on - bry., euph., hyos., ***iris.***
rest, during - euph.
rheumatic - ***lyc.,*** puls., zinc.
right - sulph.
stooping agg. - mag-c.
uncovering - nat-m.
waking, on - coloc.
walking, air, in open, while - lyc.
amel. - euph.
writing, while - bov.
tension, axilla - aur., spig.

THROWN, back, shoulders - acon.

TINGLING, prickling, asleep - cham., mez., verat., zinc.

TREMBLING - aesc., asaf., com., dros., sulph.

TUBERCLES - crot-h., kali-chl., phos., rhus-t.
tubercles, axilla - nit-ac., phos.

TUMORS, fatty - am-m.
tumors, axilla - ars-i., aster., ***bar-c.,*** con., petr., phyt.
encysted - bar-c.
hard bluish lump - calc-p.
tumors, axillary glands - aster., ***carb-an.,*** **CON.,** ***cund.,*** kali-i., ***lach., phos., phyt.,*** sang., sec., ***sil.***

TWISTING, sensation - hura.

TWITCHING - agar., alum., arg-m., arn., ars-h., asaf., bell., calc., chel., cic., dios., ***dros.,*** fl-ac., graph., hyos., ign., ***lyc.,*** mag-c., merc., mez., ox-ac., petr., puls., sep., sil., spig., ***spong.,*** stry., sulph., sul-ac., tarax., zinc.
posterior margin of axilla - arg-m.
rest, during - **DROS.**
sleep, during - hyos.
writing, while - sul-ac.
twitching, axilla, posterior margin of - arg-m.

ULCERS, axilla - bor.

URTICARIA - lach.

VESICLES - am-m., ant-c., chlor., crot-h., lach., mag-c., mang., ***merc.,*** rhus-t., vip.
after scratching - mag-c., mang.
burning - am-m.

WEAKNESS - acon., aloe, alumn., arg-m., bapt., bor., bov., brom., carb-an., carb-v., cedr., chin-a., cic., clem., ***com.,*** cupr-ar., gins., kali-n., laur., mag-c., nat-m., nux-v., phos., pic-ac., plat., ran-s., ***rhus-t., ruta,*** sep., sil., stry., thiosin., thuj., zing.

WEAKNESS, of
bending, forward - alumn.
left - alumn.
morning, on waking - arg-m.
paralytic - arg-m., carb-v.
right - carb-v.
walking, after - bapt.

WIND, sensation of, blowing on - lyc.
passing over and extending to fingers - fl-ac.

Skin

ABSCESSES, suppurations, (see Generals)

ACNE, general (see Face)

chin - ***hydr.,*** prot., verat., ***viol-t.***

pregnancy, after - sep.

forehead - ant-c., ***ars.,*** aur., bar-c., bell., ***calc.,*** calc-pic., ***caps.,*** **CARB-AN., CARB-S., CARB-V., CAUST.,** ***cic.,*** clem., **HEP.,** ***kreos.,*** led., ***nat-m., nit-ac.,*** **NUX-V.,** ***ph-ac.,*** **PSOR., RHUS-T., SEP., SIL., SULPH.,** viol-t.

lips - bor., psor., sars., ***sul-i.***

nose - am-c., ars., ***ars-br.,*** aster., bor., calc-p., caps., cann-s., **CAUST.,** clem., elaps, graph., kali-br., nat-c., sel., sep., sil., ***sulph.,*** zing.

rosacea - agar., ***ars., ars-br.,*** ars-i., aur., ***aur-m.,*** bell., ***calc-p.,*** **CALC-SIL.,** canth., ***caps.,*** carb-ac., ***carb-an.,*** carb-s., **CARB-V., CAUST.,** chel., chrysar., ***cic.,*** clem., eug., ***hydr-ac., hydrc.,*** iris, kali-br., kali-i., ***kreos.,*** **LACH.,** led., mag-p., ***mez.,*** nux-v., ov., ***petr., plb.,*** **PSOR.,** ***rad.,*** rhus-r., **RHUS-T.,** ***ruta, sep., sil., sul-i., sulo-ac., sulph.,*** sul-ac., syc-co., ***tub., verat.,*** viol-o., ***viol-t.***

bluish - ***lach., sulph.***

groups, in - **CAUST.**

nose, on - calc-p., cann-s., **CAUST.,** ***psor.***

vulgaris - ***ant-c., ars., ars-i.,*** **AUR.,** bar-c., bell., ***calc.,*** **CALC-SIL.,** ***calc-s.,*** **CARB-AN., CARB-S., CARB-V., CAUST.,** chel., ***con., cop., crot-h., eug.,*** graph., **HEP.,** iod., **KALI-BR.,** ***kreos., lach.,*** led., med., ***nat-m., nit-ac.,*** **NUX-V.,** ***ph-ac., psor., puls.,*** sabin., sanic., sel., **SEP., SIL.,** ***sulph.,*** sul-i., ***thuj., tub.,*** uran.

chin - ***hydr.,*** verat., ***viol-t.***

fire, near a - ***ant-c.***

heated agg. becoming - ***caust.***

ACTINOMYCOSIS - hecla., hippoz., kali-i., ***nit-ac.***

ADHERENT - arn., par.

bone to - arn., ***asaf.,*** aur., chin., hell., Merc., ***ph-ac.,*** puls., ruta., sabin., ***sil.,*** staph.

ALLERGY, to milk - **TUB.**

ANESTHESIA - acon., ***all-s., alum.,*** ambr., ***anac., arg-n.,*** arn., ***ars.,*** ars-i., bell., bry., calc., ***camph.,*** cann-i., ***caps., carb-ac., carb-s.,*** carl., caul., caust., cham., **CHIN.,** chin-a., chin-s., chlol., ***cic., cocc.,*** con., cupr-ar., cycl., hell., hyos., iod., ***kali-br., kali-i.,*** laur., lyc., meph., ***merc.,*** mosch., nat-m., **NUX-V.,** oena., **OLND.,** ***op., petr.,*** ph-ac., ***phos.,*** plat., ***plb.,*** **PULS., RHUS-T.,** ***sec.,*** sep., stram., sulph., tarent., ter., verat-v., vinc., ***zinc.***

morning, on waking - ***ambr.***

spots, in small - bufo.

suppressed eruptions, after - ***zinc.***

ANGIOMA - lyc., sulph.

ATROPHY of skin - ars., cocc., graph., sabad., sulph.

of dermal - thal.

BEDSORES, decubitus - ***agar.,*** ambr., am-c., am-m., ant-c., ***arg-n.,*** **ARN.,** ars., bapt., bar-c., bell., bov., ***calc.,*** calc-p., canth., carb-an., ***carb-v.,*** caust., cham., **CHIN.,** coff., colch., crot-h., dros., ***echi.,*** euph., fl-ac., **GRAPH.,** ***hep.,*** hydr., **HYPER.,** ***ign.,*** kali-ar., kali-c., kreos., **LACH., LED.,** ***lyc.,*** mag-m., mang., ***merc.,*** mez., ***nat-c.,*** nat-m., nit-ac., nux-v., olnd., op., **PETR.,** ph-ac., phos., plb., ***puls.,*** rhus-t., ruta., sel., **SEP., SIL.,** spig., squil., ***sulph., sul-ac.,*** ter., zinc.

BIRTHMARKS, nevi - **ACET-AC.,** arn., ars., ***calc.,*** calc-f., carb-an., ***carb-v.,*** **CARC.,** cund., **FL-AC.,** lach., ***lyc.,*** med., nux-v., **PHOS.,** plat., rad., ***sep.,*** sol, ***sulph.,*** **THUJ.,** ust., vac.

smooth - con., phos., sep., sulph.

spidery - carb-v., lach., ***plat.,*** sep., thuj.

red - med.

BITING, sensation - ***agar.,*** agn., alum., am-c., ***am-m.,*** ant-c., arn., bar-m., berb., bell., bor., bov., ***bry., calad., calc.,*** camph., canth., caps., carb-an., ***carb-v., caust.,*** cham., chel., chin., cocc., coc-c., ***colch.,*** coloc., ***con.,*** dros., **EUPH.,** ***gamb.,*** hell., ***ip.,*** kreos., ***lach.,*** **LED.,** ***lyc.,*** lyss., mag-c., mang., merc., ***mez.,*** mur-ac., nat-c., nat-m., nat-p., nicc., ***nux-v., olnd.,*** op., pall., petr., phel., ph-ac., phos., plat., **PULS.,** ran-b., ran-s., rhod., rhus-t., ruta., sel., sep., sil., spig., ***spong.,*** stront-c., ***sulph.,*** thuj., verat., viol-t., zinc.

chill, during - gamb.

night, in bed - coc-c., mag-c., sulph.

before sleep - coc-c.

perspiration, from - cham., tarax., thuj.

scratching, after - am-c., ***am-m.,*** bry., calc., canth., carb-an., carb-s., carb-v., ***caust.,*** chin., con., dros., ***euph.,*** hell., ip., kreos., **LACH.,** ***led., lyc.,*** mang., merc., ***mez.,*** nat-c., nat-m., nux-v., **OLND.,** petr., ph-ac., ***puls.,*** ran-b., ruta., sel., sep., sil., ***spong., sulph.,*** zinc.

changing place on scratching - sulph.

spots, in - nat-m.

BLISTERS - alum., am-c., ***anac.,*** **ANT-C.,** ***ars.,*** aur., bor., bry., ***bufo,*** **CANTH.,** carb-an., carb-s., **CAUST.,** ***cham., clem.,*** crot-h., ***dulc., graph.,*** hep., ***kali-ar., kali-c.,*** kali-s., lach., ***mag-c.,*** manc., ***merc.,*** nat-a., ***nat-c.,*** nat-m., nat-p., nit-ac., ***petr.,*** phos., ***ran-b., ran-s.,*** **RHUS-T.,** rhus-v., ***sep., sil., sulph.,*** syph., verat., vip., zinc.

blood - sec.

burn, as from a - ambr., aur., bell., **CANTH.,** carb-an., clem., lyc., nat-c., phos., sep., sulph.

small - apis, ***canth.,*** nat-m., ***rhus-t.,*** sec.

BLOTCHES, (see Eruptions)

BOILS - abrot., aeth., agar., alum., alumn., am-c., am-m., ***anac.,*** anan., anth., ***ant-c.,*** ant-t., **ANTHR.,** ***apis,*** **ARN.,** ***ars., ars-i.,*** aur., ***bar-c.,*** **BELL.,** ***bell-p.,*** brom., bry., bufo, ***calc.,*** calc-hp., calc-p., ***calc-pic.,*** **CALC-S.,** carb-an., carb-s., carb-v., chin., chin-a., cist., cocc., coc-c., ***con., crot-h.,*** dulc., ***echi.,*** elaps, ***euph., ferr-i.,*** gels.,

BOILS - ***graph.***, **HEP.**, hippoz., ***hyos.***, ***ichth.***, ign., ***iod.***, jug-r., ***kali-i.***, kali-n., kreos., **LACH.**, laur., ***led.***, luf-op., **LYC.**, mag-c., mag-m., ***med.***, **MERC.**, ***mez.***, mur-ac., nat-a., nat-c., ***nat-m.***, nat-p., ***nit-ac.***, nux-m., ***nux-v.***, ol-myr., oper., **PETR.**, ***ph-ac.***, ***phos.***, ***phyt.***, pic-ac., **PSOR.**, puls., pyrog., rhus-r., **RHUS-T.**, sars., ***sec.***, ***sep.***, **SIL.**, spong., stann., staph., stram., sul-i., **SULPH.**, ***sul-ac.***, syph., **TARENT.**, ***tarent-c.***, ***thuj.***, tub., zinc., zinc-oc.

blood - alum., ***anthr.***, arn., ars., ***bell.***, bry., ***calc.***, **CROT-H.**, euph., hyos., ***iod.***, iris, kali-bi., ***lach.***, ***led.***, lyc., mag-c., mag-m., ***mur-ac.***, ***nat-m.***, nit-ac., **PHOS.**, ph-ac., pyrog., sec., sep., ***sil.***, sulph., sul-ac., thuj., zinc.

small - alum., iris, ***sil.***

blue - ***anthr.***, bufo, crot-h., lach., tarent.

body, all over - viol-t.

crops of - ***calc-s.***, echi., sil., sulph., syph.

children, disposition to - ***calc-s.***, mag-c., sil.

greenish, pus - ***sec.***

impotency, with - pic-ac.

injured, places - ***dulc.***, ***sil.***

large - ant-t., ***apis***, bufo, ***hep.***, hyos., ***lach.***, ***lyc.***, merc., nat-c., ***nit-ac.***, nux-v., phos., sil., viol-t.

maturing, not - sanic.

slowly - hep., sil., sulph.

menses, at - merc.

periodical - **ARS.**, hyos., ***iod.***, ***lyc.***, ***merc.***, nit-ac., phos., phyt., sil., staph., ***sulph.***

receding - lyc.

recurrent tendency - ***arn.***, ars., berb., calc., calc-mur., calc-p., ***calc-s.***, echi., hep., sil., ***sulph.***, torula., tub.

scarring - kali-i.

small - **ARN.**, bar-c., dulc., ***fl-ac.***, **KALI-I.**, lappa-a., ***lyc.***, mag-c., mag-m., nat-m., nux-v., pic-ac., sec., sulph., tarent., tub., viol-t., zinc.

menses, during - med.

spring, in the - bell., ***crot-h.***, ***lach.***

stinging, when touched - mur-ac., sars., sil.

successions, of - anthr., arn., sulph.

BRUISED, pain - arg-m., **ARN.**, ***ars.***, cic., dros., dulc., olnd., plat., rhus-t., sul-ac.

BRUISES, ecchymosis - aeth., anthr., arg-n., **ARN.**, ars., bad., bar-c., bar-m., ***bell-p.***, both., ***bry.***, calc., ***carb-v.***, cham., chin., chlol., coca, ***con.***, ***crot-h.***, dulc., euphr., ***ferr.***, **HAM.**, ***hep.***, kreos., ***lach.***, laur., **LED.**, ***nux-v.***, par., **PH-AC.**, **PHOS.**, plb., ***puls.***, rhus-t., ruta., **SEC.**, sep., ***sulph.***, **SUL-AC.**, ***tarent.***, ***ter.***, trinit., uran-n.

contused - **ARN.**, ham., **LED.**, sul-ac., symph.

persistence of ecchymosis, with - arn., ham., led., ***sul-ac.***

returning yearly - crot-h.

tendency to bruise easily - arn., ham., lach., sep., ***phos.***

venous stasis, from - ham., sep.

BUBBLING, sensation - calc.

BURNING, sensation - acet-ac., **ACON.**, agar., all-c., alum., ***ambr.***, am-c., am-m., anac., anan., ***anthr.***, ant-c., **APIS,** ***arg-m.***, ***arn.***, **ARS.**, ars-i., asaf., asar., aur., bapt., bar-c., bar-m., **BELL.**, berb., bism., bov., **BRY.**, ***bufo,*** calad., ***calc.***, ***calc-s.***, camph., cann-s., canth., ***caps.***, ***carb-an.***, ***carb-v.***, ***caust.***, cham., chel., chin., chin-a., ***cic.***, clem., ***cocc.***, coff., colch., coloc., con., cop., ***crot-t.***, cupr., cycl., dig., dros., ***dulc.***, elat., ***euph.***, ***ferr.***, ferr-ar., ferr-i., ferr-p., fl-ac., ***form.***, graph., grin., guai., hell., ***hep.***, ***hyos.***, ***ign.***, iod., kali-ar., **KALI-BI.**, ***kali-c.***, ***kali-n.***, kali-p., ***kali-s.***, kreos., **LACH.**, laur., led., **LYC.**, mag-arct., mag-c., mag-m., mang., medus., meny., ***merc.***, ***mez.***, mosch., mur-ac., nat-a., nat-c., ***nat-m.***, nat-p., nit-ac., ***nux-v.***, ol-an., olnd., ***op.***, par., petr., ph-ac., **PHOS.**, plat., plb., ***puls.***, rad., ***ran-b.***, rhod., **RHUS-T.**, ruta., sabad., sabin., samb., sang., sars., sec., sel., seneg., ***sep.***, **SIL.**, ***spig.***, spong., ***squil.***, stann., ***staph.***, stram., stront-c., **SULPH.**, sul-ac., tarent., ***ter.***, teucr., thuj., urea, ***urt-u.***, ***ust.***, valer., verat., vesp., viol-o., viol-t., zinc.

cold water, after working in - thuj.

coldness, with - verat-v.

evening, rising - mang.

fever, without - graph., lach.

flames, as from - viol-o.

hand, has laid on, where - hyos.

heated, getting - bry.

lying, amel. - mang.

mental excitement, from - ***bry.***

morning, in bed - carb-v.

mustard plaster, like - kali-c.

nettles, as from - calc-p., cocc., **URT-U.**

night - ***ars.***, ***carb-v.***, cinnb., clem., ***con.***, ***dol.***, ***merc.***, nux-v., ***olnd.***, rhus-t.

parts lain on - lyss., manc., ***sulph.***

perspiration, from - merc., **MEZ.**, **NAT-C.**, verat.

scratching, after - agar., ambr., ***am-c.***, am-m., anac., ant-c., arn., ***ars.***, bar-c., ***bell.***, bov., ***bry.***, calad., calc., cann-s., canth., caps., carb-an., carb-s., carb-v., **CAUST.**, chel., cic., cocc., coff., con., crot-t., cycl., dros., ***dulc.***, euph., graph., ***hep.***, kali-ar., kali-c., kali-p., ***kali-s.***, ***kreos.***, ***lac-c.***, **LACH.**, laur., ***led.***, ***lyc.***, mag-c., mag-m., mang., **MERC.**, mez., mosch., nat-c., nat-m., nat-s., nit-ac., nux-v., **OLND.**, par., ***petr.***, ph-ac., ***phos.***, puls., ran-b., rhod., **RHUS-T.**, sabad., sabin., samb., sars., sel., seneg., **SEP.**, **SIL.**, spig., spong., ***squil.***, ***staph.***, stront-c., **SULPH.**, thuj., ***til.***, verat., viol-t., zinc.

sex, after - agar.

sleep, after - ***urt-u.***

sparks, as from - agar., arg-m., calc., ***calc-p.***, nat-m., **SEC.**, sel.

spots - agar., am-c., ***am-m.***, apis, ***ars.***, bell., canth., ***carb-v.***, caust., chel., croc., cupr., ferr., ***fl-ac.***, iod., kali-ar., ***kali-c.***, lach., lyc., mag-c., mag-m., ***merc.***, ***mez.***, nat-s., **PH-AC.**, plat., ***rhus-t.***, sel., **SULPH.**, ***sul-ac.***, tab., thuj., viol-o., zinc.

sedentary habits, from - ran-b.

BURNING, sensation
- sun, from - bufo, canth., kali-c., rob., sol, verat.
- touch, on - ***canth.,*** caust., ***ferr.,*** sabin.

BURNS, (see Emergency, Burns)

BURNT, scorched, as if - ***ars., canth.,*** ran-b., verat-n., verat-v.

CALLOUSES, skin (see Hardness) - am-c., **ANT-C.,** bor., ***dulc.,*** elae., ***ferr-pic.,*** **GRAPH.,** hydr., lach., led., lyc., ***nit-ac.,*** petr., ***ran-b., rhus-t.,*** sal-ac., sars., **SEP.,** ***sil.,*** sulph., ***thuj.***
- hands, on - ***am-c., ant-c.,*** **GRAPH.,** kali-ar., rhus-v., sil., **SULPH.**
  - cracks, deep, with - cist., graph.
- soles, on - **ANT-C.,** ***ars., calc.,*** plb., sil., sulph.
  - tenderness - ***alum.,*** lyc., med., ***nat-s.***
- toes, on - **ANT-C.,** ***graph.***

CANCER, epithelioma - acet-ac., alum., alumn., arb., arg-m., arg-n., ***ars.,*** **ARS-I.,** ars-s-f., aur., aur-a., ***bell.,*** brom., calc., calc-p., calc-sil., carb-ac., carb-an., ***carc.,*** chr-ac., cic., clem., **CON.,** ***cund.,*** euph., fuli., ho., ***hydr., hydrc.,*** kali-ar., kali-chl., kali-m., ***kali-s., kreos., lap-a.,*** **LYC.,** mag-m., mag-s., merc., merc-c., methyl-b., nat-m., nectrin., nit-ac., phos., ***phyt.,*** puls., rad., rad-br., raja-s., ***ran-b.,*** ran-s., scroph-n., sep., ***sil., sol.,*** sulph., ***thuj.,*** uran-n.
- flat - cund.
- melanoma - ***arg-n.,*** ars., ***carc.,*** card-m., ***lach., sol,*** ph-ac.
- sunlight, from - carc., sol.

CARBUNCLES - acon., agar., ***apis, anthr.,*** ant-t., ***arn.,*** **ARS., BELL.,** both., bry., ***bufo,*** calc-chln., **CALC-S.,** caps., ***carb-ac.,*** carb-an., carb-v., ***chin.,*** coloc., ***crot-c., crot-h.,*** cupr-ar., ***echi.,*** euph., ***hep.,*** hippoz., ***hyos.,*** jug-r., ***lach.,*** lappa-a., lappa-m., ***led.,*** mur-ac., nit-ac., phyt., pic-ac., ***pyrog., rhus-t., scol., sec.,*** **SIL.,** sul-ac., ***sulph., tarent-c.***
- bluish, red - ***anthr.,*** lach., tarent.
- burning - ***anthr., apis, ars., crot-c.,*** crot-h., coloc., hep., **TARENT-C.**
- impotency, with - pic-ac.
- purple, with small vesicles around - ***crot-c.,*** **LACH.**
- scarlet - apis, ***bell.***
- stinging - **APIS,** carb-an., ***nit-ac.***

CHAPPING - ***aesc.,*** alum., alumn., ant-c., arn., aur., bry., **CALC.,** cham., ***cycl.,*** **GRAPH., HEP.,** ***kali-c.,*** kreos., ***lach.,*** lyc., mag-c., mang., merc., nat-c., nat-m., nit-ac., olnd., petr., **PULS., RHUS-T.,** ruta., **SARS., SEP.,** sil., **SULPH.,** viol-t., zinc.

CHICKENPOX, eruptions - acon., **ANT-C.,** ***ant-t.,*** ars., asaf., ***bell.,*** canth., ***carb-v.,*** caust., coff., con., cycl., hyos., ip., ***led., merc.,*** nat-c., nat-m., **PULS., RHUS-T.,** ***sep.,*** sil., **SULPH.,** ***thuj.***

CHILBLAINS, (see part affected)

CHLOASMA - card., caul., ***lyc.,*** nux-v., rob., ***sep.***
- sun, agg. - cadm-s., sep., sol.

CICATRICES, (see Scars)

CLAMMY - calc., carb-v., cub.

COLDNESS - abies-c., acet-ac., acon., aeth., agar., agn., ail., alum., ambr., am-c., am-m., anac., ***anan.,*** ant-c., ant-chl., ***ant-t.,*** apis, arn., **ARS.,** ***ars-i.,*** asaf., asar., aur., bar-c., bar-m., ***bell.,*** bism., both., bov., bry., ***cact.,*** calad., **CALC., CALC-P., CAMPH.,** cann-s., canth., ***caps.,*** carb-ac., carb-an., **CARB-S.,** ***carb-v., caust., cham., chel., chin., chin-a., cic.,*** cina, cocc., ***coff., colch.,*** coloc., con., crat., croc., ***crot-h., cupr.,*** cycl., **DIG.,** ***dios.,*** dros., dulc., euph., euphr., eup-pur., ***ferr.,*** ferr-ar., ***ferr-i.,*** ferr-p., ***graph., hell.,*** **HELO.,** hep., **HYDR-AC.,** hyos., ***ign., iod.,*** **IP.,** jatr., ***kali-ar.,*** kali-br., ***kali-c.,*** kali-chl., kali-m., kali-n., kali-p., ***kali-s.,*** kreos., ***lach.,*** lachn., lat-m., lath., **LAUR.,** ***led., lyc.,*** mag-c., mag-m., mang., med., meny., ***merc., merc-c., merc-cy., mez.,*** mosch., mur-ac., nat-a., nat-c., nat-m., nat-p., ***nit-ac.,*** **NUX-M.,** ***nux-v.,*** olnd., ***op.,*** **OX-AC.,** par., petr., ph-ac., ***phos., phyt., plat., plb., podo.,*** puls., pyrog., ran-b., rhod., **RHUS-T.,** ruta., sabad., sabin., ***samb.,*** sang., sars., **SEC.,** sel., seneg., **SEP.,** ***sil.,*** spig., spong., squil., stann., staph., stram., stront-c., **SULPH.,** sul-ac., ***sumb., tab.,*** tarax., teucr., ***ther.,*** thuj., valer., **VERAT.,** verat-v., verb., zinc.
- alternates with heat - stram.
- convulsions, during - anan., ***camph.,*** caust., cic., ***hell.,*** hyos., mosch., **OENA.,** op., stram., ***verat.***
- diarrhea during - aeth., ***camph., jatr., laur.,*** tab., ***verat.***
- dry, and - camph., nux-m.
- eating, after - camph., ran-b.
- exercise, during - plb., ***sil.***
- fever, during - ***camph., iod.***
- heat, with internal - bar-c., euph., ***ferr., ign., iod.,*** mosch., ***verat., zinc.***
- icy - ant-t., ***ars.,*** cadm-s., ***calc.,*** **CAMPH., CARB-V.,** chlol., cupr., hell., lachn., ***nat-m., sec.,*** tarent., ***verat.***
  - in spots - ***agar.,*** arg-m., berb., caust., mosch., ***par.,*** petr., tarent., **VERAT.**
- injured parts - **LED.**
- labor, during - coff.
- left - caust., dros., ***lach., sil.***
  - before epilepsy - ***sil.***
- menses, during - coff., dig., ***led., tab.,*** thuj., ***verat.***
  - after - graph.
  - before - ***sil.***
- night - ***ars., camph., carb-v., hyos., mosch.***
- one side of body during convulsions - ***sil.***
- pain, during - ars.
- painful, nerves, along - ***led.,*** merc., sil.
- pregnancy, during - ***nux-m.***
- scratching, after - agar., mez., petr.
- sensation of - arn., ***calc.,*** caust., chel., led., ***merc., mosch., plat.,*** puls., ***rhus-t.,*** sec., ***verat-v.***
- spots - ***agar.,*** arg-m., berb., caust., mosch., ***par.,*** petr., tarent., **VERAT.**
- stool, after - crot-t.
- suffering parts - caps., caust., ***led.,*** merc., mez., ***sil.***

COLDNESS,
trembling, with - mosch., op.
uncover, must - ***camph., sec.***
upper part of body - ip.

COMEDONES, (see Face)

CONDYLOMATA, (see Excrescences) - acet-ac., alumn., anac., ant-t., ***apis, arg-n., aur., aur-m.,*** aur-m-n., benz-ac., ***calc.,*** caust., cham., ***cinnb.,*** euph., ***euphr., fl-ac.,*** **HEP.,** ***kali-chl., kali-i.,*** lac-c., ***lyc.,*** **MED.,** ***merc.,*** **MERC-C.,** ***merc-d.,*** merc-sul., ***mill.,*** **NAT-S., NIT-AC., PH-AC.,** ***phos.,*** phyt., psor., ***sabin., sars., sep.,*** sil., ***staph., sulph.,*** syph., ***teucr.,*** **THUJ.**
bleeding - ***cinnb., med.,*** **NIT-AC.,** sulph., **THUJ.**
broad - nit-ac., ***thuj.***
burning - apis, ***cinnb., nit-ac.,*** ph-ac., sabin., ***thuj.***
dry - lyc., merc., merc-c., nit-ac., sars., staph., sulph., thuj.
fan-shaped - ***cinnb.,*** sulph., ***thuj.***
flat - acet-ac.
fleshy - ars., ***staph., thuj.***
horny - thuj.
itching - lyc., psor., ***sabin.,*** staph., thuj.
moist - ***apis,*** caust., euphr., med., merc., merc-c., **NIT-AC.,** psor., sabin., staph., sulph., **THUJ.**
offensive - calc., hep., med., ***nit-ac.,*** thuj.
pediculated - caust., lyc., nit-ac., ph-ac., staph., thuj.
rapid growing - ***thuj.***
sticking pain - **NIT-AC.**
suppurating - ***thuj.***
syphilitic - aur., aur-m., aur-m-n., ***cinnb.,*** kali-i., ***merc.,*** **NIT-AC.,** staph., syph., ***thuj.***

CONTRACTIONS - alum., am-m., anac., asar., bell., bism., bry., carb-v., ***chin.,*** cocc., cupr., ferr., ***graph.,*** kali-c., kreos., lyc., merc., nat-m., nit-ac., ***nux-v.,*** olnd., par., petr., phos., ***plat.,*** plb., puls., ran-s., rhod., **RHUS-T.,** ruta., sabad., sec., ***sel.,*** sep., sil., spig., stann., stront-c., sulph., sul-ac., zinc.

COPPERY spots, remaining after eruptions - med.

CORD, thin, as if under skin - euph.

COWPOX, vaccinia - ***acon.,*** ant-t., apis, ***bell.,*** merc., phos., ***sil.,*** sulph., ***thuj.,*** vac.

CRACKS - ***aesc.,*** aloe, alum., am-c., ***ant-c.,*** anthro., ***arn.,*** ars-s-f., ***aur., bad.,*** bar-c., bry., cact., **CALC.,** calc-s., ***carb-an.,*** **CARB-S.,** carb-v., ***cham., cist.,*** com., cund., ***cycl.,*** eug., **GRAPH.,** ***hep.,*** hydr., iris, kali-ar., kali-c., ***kali-s., kreos., lach.,*** led., ***lyc.,*** mag-c., ***maland., mang., merc.,*** merc-i-r., merc-p-r., ***nat-c., nat-m., nit-ac.,*** olnd., osm., ***paeon.,*** **PETR.,** phos., pix., ***psor.,*** **PULS.,** ran-b., rat., ***rhus-t.,*** ruta., **SARS., SEP.,** ***sil.,*** **SULPH.,** teucr., viol-t., x-ray, xero, ***zinc.***
bloody, deep - ***merc.,*** **NIT-AC., PETR.,** puls., ***sars., sulph.***
burning - petr., sars., zinc.
fetid - ***merc.***
humid - aloe.

CRACKS, in
itching - merc., ***petr.***
mercurial - ***hep., nit-ac., sulph.***
new skin cracks and burns - ***sars.***
painful - ***graph.,*** mang., nit-ac., petr., sars., x-ray, zinc.
summer agg. - coc-c.
ulcerated - bry., merc.
washing, after - alum., ***ant-c.,*** bry., **CALC.,** ***calc-s.,*** cham., kali-c., lyc., nit-ac., ***puls.,*** rhus-t., sars., **SEP., SULPH.,** zinc.
winter, in - alum., **CALC.,** ***calc-s.,*** **CARB-S.,** ***graph.,*** **PETR.,** ***psor.,*** **SEP., SULPH.**
yellow - merc.

CUTTING, sensation - **BELL.,** calc., calen., dros., graph., ign., lyc., mur-ac., ***nat-c.,*** ph-ac., rhus-t., sep., sil., sul-ac., ***viol-t.***

DECUBITUS, (see Bedsores)

DERMATITIS - ***acon.,*** agn., alum., ***anac.,*** ant-c., ***apis, arn., ars., asaf., aur.,*** bad., bar-c., ***bar-m.,*** bell., bor., bry., ***calc.,*** camph., cann-s., canth., caust., **CHAM.,** chlol., cina, cocc., colch., com., con., croc., crot-h., ***dulc.,*** euph., ***gels.,*** graph., **HEP.,** hyos., ***kali-s.,*** kreos., lach., lyc., mang., **MERC.,** mez., nat-c., nat-m., ***nit-ac.,*** petr., phos., ***plb.,*** **PULS.,** ran-b., **RHUS-T.,** ruta., sep., **SIL.,** ***staph., sulph.,*** tarent-c., verat., zinc.
edema, malignant, with - com.
sebaceous glands - lyc., psor., raph., sil., sulph.
tendency to - alum., ars., ***asaf., bar-c.,*** bell., ***bor.,*** calc., camph., canth., **CHAM.,** chel., con., croc., euph., graph., ***hep.,*** hyos., lach., mang., ***merc.,*** nat-c., nat-m., ***nit-ac., petr.,*** plb., ***puls.,*** ran-b., **SIL.,** staph., ***sulph.***

DISCOLORATION, skin

blackish - acon., ant-c., ***apis, arg-n.,*** **ARS.,** asaf., aur., ***carb-v.,*** chel., ***crot-h., lach.,*** nit-ac., ph-ac., phyt., **PLB., SEC.,** spig., trinit.
bleeding, from - trinit.
pares - sabin.
spots - aeth., ***ars., crot-h.,*** ferr., ***lach.,*** rhus-t., sec., ***vip.***

bluish - acon., ***aeth.,*** agar., ail., am-c., ***ant-t., apis, arg-m.,*** arn., ***ars.,*** aur., ***bapt., bell.,*** bism., ***brom.,*** bry., bufo, cadm-s., calc., ***camph., carb-an., carb-s.,*** **CARB-V.,** chin., chin-a., coca, cocc., con., cop., crat., **CROT-C.,** ***crot-h., cupr.,*** cur., **DIG.,** elaps, ***ferr-p.,*** gels., hell., ***hydr-ac.,*** ip., ***kali-br.,*** kali-i., kreos., **LACH.,** ***laur.,*** led., mang., merc., merc-cy., morph., ***mur-ac.,*** naja, nat-m., ***nux-m.,*** **NUX-V., OP.,** ***ox-ac.,*** ph-ac., phos., ***phyt.,*** plb., puls., rhus-t., samb., ***sec.,*** sil., spong., ***stram.,*** sul-ac., sulph., syph., ***tarent.,*** thuj., **VERAT., VERAT-V.,** vip.
affected parts - carb-an., lach., led., sec.
burning, with - anthr., ars., lach.
injuries, from - ***arn.,*** bell., con., lach., ***led.,*** puls., sul-ac.
washing, after - phos.

DISCOLORATION, skin

bluish, spots - aeth., anan., anthr., ant-c., apis, arg-n., **ARN.,** ***ars.,*** bad., bar-c., bar-m., berb., bor., ***bry.,*** calc., ***carb-an., carb-v.,*** chlol., ***con.,*** **CROT-H.,** dulc., euphr., ***ferr.,*** hell., ***hep., lac-c.,*** **LACH.,** laur., ***led., lyc.,*** merc., mosch., nit-ac., ***nux-m., nux-v., op.,*** **PH-AC., PHOS.,** ***plat.,*** plb., ***puls.,*** rhus-t., ruta., ***sars.,*** **SEC.,** sil., ***sulph.,*** **SUL-AC.,** tarent., ter.
- indurated - ***sars.***
- recurring annually - ***crot-h.***
- red - phyt., plb.

bluish-black - aeth.

brown, liver spots - am-c., ***ant-c.,*** ant-t., ***arg-n.,*** arn., ***ars.,*** ars-i., ***aur.,*** bac., bad., bapt., berb., bor., ***bry.,*** cadm-s., calc., calc-p., calc-s., canth., ***carb-s., carb-v.,*** carc., card-m., ***caul.,*** caust., chel., cob., ***con.,*** cop., cor-r., crot-h., **CUR.,** dros., ***dulc.,*** ferr., ferr-i., graph., guare., ***hyos., iod.,*** kali-ar., kali-bi., kali-c., kali-p., kreos., **LACH.,** ***laur.,*** **LYC.,** lycps., man., **MERC.,** merc-i-r., ***mez.,*** nat-a., ***nat-c., nat-h.,*** nat-p., **NIT-AC.,** ***nux-v.,*** op., paull., petr., ***phos., plb.,*** puls., ***rhus-t.,*** rob., ruta, sabad., sanic., **SEP.,** sil., stann., staph., **SULPH.,** sul-ac., tarent., ***thuj., thyr., tub.,*** verat.
- elevated - caust.
- inflamed - ferr.
- itching - caust., lyc., sulph.
- suppurating - ferr.

chloasma - card-m., caul., ***lyc.,*** nux-v., rob., ***sep.***
- sun, agg. - cadm-s., sep., sol.

copper-colored - carb-an., carb-v., cortiso., syph.

dark spots, in elderly people - ars., aur., bar-c., ***carb-an., con., lach., lyc.,*** op., ***sec.***

dirty - ***ars.,*** bor., bry., bufo, ***ferr., ferr-i.,*** ferr-pic., ***iod.,*** merc., ***nat-m., nit-ac.,*** petr., phos., ***plb.,*** **PSOR.,** sec., stram., **SULPH.,** tarent., ***thuj.,*** tub.
- elevated - caust.
- gray - ***iod.***
- inflamed - ferr.
- itching - caust., lyc., sulph.
- spots - berb., sabin., ***sec.***

dusky - ars-i., calc-p., merc.

gray, spots - iod., nit-ac.

green, spots - ***arn.,*** ars., ***bufo,*** carb-v., **CON.,** crot-h., ***lach.,*** med., nit-ac., sep., sul-ac., verat., vip.

liver, spots (see Discoloration, brown spots)

mottled - **AIL.,** ars., ***carb-v.,*** con., cop., chlol., **CROT-H.,** glon., kali-bi., kali-m., **LACH.,** led., lil-t., manc., ***nat-m.,*** nux-m., ***nux-v.,*** ox-ac., phos., rhus-t., sars., syph., ***thuj., verat-v.***
- chill, during - arn., crot-h., ***nux-v.,*** rhus-t.
- spots, in - tarent-c.
- washing, after - kali-c.

DISCOLORATION, skin

pale - ***acet-ac., anan., apis, ars.,*** bar-c., **BELL.,** benz-ac., **CALC.,** ***calc-s., carb-ac.,*** carb-an., ***carb-v.,*** caust., ***chin., chin-a.,*** **COCC.,** ***con., cupr., dig.,*** **FERR.,** ***ferr-ar., ferr-p., fl-ac.,*** graph., ***hell., helon.,*** ign., kali-ar., ***kali-c., kreos.,*** **LYC.,** mang., ***merc., merc-c., nat-m., nat-s.,*** **NIT-AC.,** ***nux-v.,*** olnd., op., ph-ac., ***phos.,*** **PLAT.,** ***plb., podo.,*** **PULS.,** sabin., sang., **SEC.,** ***sep., sil., spig.,*** staph., **SULPH.,** ***sul-ac.,*** sumb., tab., valer., **VERAT.,** zinc.
- spots - agav-a., ***ail.,*** bapt., both., lach., ***morph.,*** ox-ac., sec., ***sul-ac.***

purple - ail., ham., lach.

red - ***acon.,*** **AGAR.,** agn., ***ail., am-c.,*** ant-c., **APIS,** ***arn.,*** **BELL.,** bov., ***bry.,*** calc., camph., canth., carb-v., chin., cinnb., cocc., coc-c., coll., ***com.,*** con., cop., ***crot-c., crot-h., crot-t.,*** cur., cycl., ***dulc.,*** euph., ferr-p., **GRAPH.,** hyos., ign., kreos., lach., led., ***lyc., manc.,*** **MERC.,** ***nat-m.,*** nit-ac., ***nux-v.,*** olnd., ***op.,*** paeon., petr., ***ph-ac., phos.,*** phyt., plb., ***puls.,*** **RHUS-T.,** ruta., ***sabad.,*** sec., sep., sil., spong., squil., stann., **STRAM.,** ***sulph.,*** sul-ac., ***tarax.,*** tell., teucr., til., zinc.
- bee sting, from - apis, bell.
- flush over whole body, a - cub.
- heat, with - ars., bell.
- scratching, after - agar., am-c., ant-c., arn., ***bell.,*** bov., canth., chin., dulc., ***graph.,*** kreos., lyc., ***merc., nat-m.,*** nux-v., ***olnd.,*** op., petr., ph-ac., puls., **RHUS-T.,** ruta., spong., tarax., teucr.
  - streaks, after - calc., carb-v., euph., par., ph-ac., ***phos.,*** sabad.

red, spots - acon., aeth., agn., ***alum., ambr.,*** **AM-C.,** am-m., ***ant-c.,*** ant-t., ***apis, arn.,*** **ARS.,** ars-i., aur., bar-c., **BELL.,** benz-ac., brom., ***berb., bry.,*** calad., **CALC.,** canth., caps., ***carb-an., carb-v.,*** caust., cham., chel., chin., ***chlol.,*** cinnb., cist., clem., **COCC.,** ***coc-c.,*** coff., ***con.,*** cor-r., croc., ***crot-h., crot-t.,*** cupr., ***cycl., dros., dulc.,*** elaps, ferr., ferr-ar., ferr-i., ***graph.,*** hep., hyos., iod., ***ip., jug-c.,*** kali-ar., kali-c., kali-i., kali-n., kali-s., **LACH.,** led., ***lyc., mag-c.,*** mag-m., mang., **MERC.,** mez., nat-a., nat-c., nat-m., nat-p., **NIT-AC.,** nux-v., oena., ol-j., op., par., ***petr., ph-ac.,*** **PHOS.,** phyt., ***plb.,*** puls., rhod., ***rhus-t.,*** **SABAD.,** ***samb.,*** sars., sec., **SEP.,** ***sil.,*** spong., squil., ***stann., stram.,*** **SULPH., SUL-AC.,** sumb., ***tab., teucr.,*** thuj., verat., vip., zinc.
- air, cold - sabad.
- bathing, after - ***am-c.,*** phos.
  - with soap - sulph.
- bluish-red - ***anthr.,*** apis, ***ars., bell.,*** crot-h., elaps, ***lach.,*** **PHOS.**
- bluish-red, nodules - acon.
- brownish-red - calc., cann-s., ***carb-v.,*** **NIT-AC.,** ***phos.,*** **SEP.,** thuj.
- burning - lyc., sulph.

DISCOLORATION, skin

red, spots

coppery - alum., ***ars.,*** calc., cann-s., **CARB-AN.,** carb-v., ***cor-r.,*** crot-t., ***kreos.,*** **LACH.,** led., ***mez.,*** ***nit-ac.,*** phos., phyt., ***rhus-t.,*** ruta., syph., ust., ***verat.***

coppery, after desquamation - ***carb-an.,*** chol.

desquamation, after - ***carb-an.,*** ***fl-ac.***

fiery red - acon., bell., ferr-ma., stram.

itching - con., dulc., graph., lyc.

moist - crot-t.

pale red - nat-c., phos., ***sil.,*** teucr.

red wine, like - ***cocc.,*** **SEP.**

rose-colored - cann-s., carb-an., carb-v., cocc., cop., rhod., sars., sep., teucr., tep.

scarlet - acon., **AM-C.,** am-m., arn., ***ars.,*** bar-c., **BELL.,** ***bry.,*** ***carb-an.,*** carb-v., caust., cham., coff., ***croc.,*** dulc., euph., hep., ***hyos.,*** iod., ip., lach., **MERC.,** ph-ac., phos., rhus-t., ***stram.,*** ***sulph.***

smooth, indurated - ***carb-an.***

violet - ***ferr.,*** nit-ac., phos., verat.

warmth agg. - fl-ac.

red, streaks - apis, bell., bufo, calc., carb-v., euph., lach., merc., par., ph-ac., ***phos.,*** pyrog., rhus-t., sabad.

spots, general

burnt, as if - ant-c., ***ars.,*** carb-v., caust., ***cycl.,*** euph., hyos., kreos., rhus-t., sec., stram.

circumscribed pigmentation following eczematous inflammation - berb., lach., ***lyc.,*** med., merc., merc-d., ***nit-ac.,*** sil., sulph., ust.

death spots, in old people - ars., aur., bar-c., ***con.,*** ***lach.,*** ***lyc.,*** op., ***sec.***

flea-bites, like - ***acon.,*** led., pall.

glistening - ***calc.,*** phos.

lenticular - calc., rhus-t., vip.

moist - ant-c., ars., carb-v., ***crot-t.,*** ***hell.,*** kali-c., lach., sel., **SIL.,** ***sulph.,*** tarax.

scratching, after - ***am-c.,*** ant-c., bell., calc., cocc., cycl., graph., mag-c., mang., merc., nit-ac., ph-ac., ***phos.,*** ***rhus-t.,*** ***sabad.,*** sep., sil., ***sulph.,*** sul-ac., verat.

small - ant-t., bry., lach., led., lyc., merc., op., rat., squil., ***sul-ac.,*** vip.

smarting - bry., ***ferr.,*** hep., ***led.,*** nat-m., ph-ac., ***puls.,*** sil., verat.

smooth - carb-an., carb-v., cor-r., lach., mag-c., petr., sumb.

star shaped - stram.

stinging - canth., chel., lach., lyc., merc., ***nit-ac.,*** ***puls.,*** **SIL.**

tint, of, every - crot-c.

yearly, returning - ***crot-h.***

streaks - ph-ac.

violet - bell.

white - **APIS,** **ARS.,** calc., carb-v., ***fl-ac.,*** **KALI-C.,** lac-c., sumb.

DISCOLORATION, skin

white, spots - ***alum.,*** am-c., **ARS.,** ars-s-f., ***aur.,*** ***berb.,*** ***calc.,*** calc-f., carb-ac., carb-an., coca, graph., ***merc.,*** ***nat-c.,*** nat-m., nit-ac., ***phos.,*** sel., ***sep.,*** **SIL.,** ***sulph.,*** sumb., syph., zinc-p.

becoming bluish - ***calc.***

with dark borders - ***calc.***

yellow, (see Yellow, skin)

DISEASES, concomitant with kidney affections - cub.

DRY, (see Inactivity) - acet-ac., ***acon.,*** acon-f., ***aeth.,*** agar., **ALUM.,** ambr., ***am-c.,*** ***anthr.,*** ant-c., ***ant-t.,*** ***apis,*** apoc., arg-m., arg-n., ***arn.,*** **ARS.,** ***ars-i.,*** asaf., bar-c., bar-m., **BELL.,** ***berb-a.,*** ***bism.,*** bor., **BRY.,** bufo, cahin., **CALC.,** calc-s., ***camph.,*** ***cann-s.,*** canth., carb-an., ***carb-s.,*** ***carb-v.,*** caust., **CHAM.,** ***chel.,*** **CHIN.,** ***chin-a.,*** clem., cocc., ***coff.,*** **COLCH.,** coloc., con., ***crot-h.,*** crot-t., diph., **DULC.,** **EUP-PER.,** ***ferr.,*** ferr-ar., ferr-p., fl-ac., **GRAPH.,** hell., hep., hydrc., ***hyos.,*** ***hydr-ac.,*** ign., ***iod.,*** ***ip.,*** **KALI-AR.,** kali-bi., **KALI-C.,** kali-i., kali-n., kali-p., kali-s., kreos., ***lach.,*** laur., **LED.,** ***lith.,*** **LYC.,** ***mag-c.,*** ***maland.,*** mang., merc., mez., mosch., mur-ac., ***nat-a.,*** ***nat-c.,*** **NAT-M.,** nat-p., ***nit-ac.,*** **NUX-M.,** nux-v., **OLND.,** **OP.,** par., **PETR.,** ***ph-ac.,*** **PHOS.,** ***phyt.,*** piloc., ***plat.,*** **PLB.,** ***psor.,*** ***puls.,*** ran-b., ran-s., rhod., ***rhus-t.,*** rumx., ruta., ***sabad.,*** samb., sang., sanic., sars., **SEC.,** **SENEG.,** ***sep.,*** **SIL.,** skook., spig., ***spong.,*** ***squil.,*** ***staph.,*** **STRAM.,** stront-c., **SULPH.,** sul-ac., ***sumb.,*** **TEUCR.,** thuj., ***thyr.,*** ***tub.,*** ust., vac., valer., vario., ***verat.,*** **VERB.,** ***viol-o.,*** viol-t., x-ray, zinc.

alternating, with, sweat gushing - apis.

burning - **ACON.,** alum., ambr., am-m., anac., ant-c., ant-t., ***apis,*** arg-m., ***arn.,*** **ARS.,** bar-c., bar-m., **BELL.,** bism., **BRY.,** ***calc.,*** camph., cann-s., canth., caps., carb-s., carb-v., caust., cham., ***chel.,*** chin., clem., ***cocc.,*** ***coff.,*** colch., coloc., con., croc., cupr., cycl., ***dulc.,*** ferr., graph., ***hell.,*** hep., hyos., ign., ip., ***kali-ar.,*** ***kali-c.,*** kali-n., kali-s., kreos., **LACH.,** laur., ***led.,*** **LYC.,** mang., ***merc.,*** mosch., mur-ac., nat-c., nat-m., nat-p., ***nit-ac.,*** nux-m., **NUX-V.,** **OP.,** par., ***ph-ac.,*** **PHOS.,** **PULS.,** ran-b., rheum, rhod., ***rhus-t.,*** ruta., sabad., sabin., ***samb.,*** ***sec.,*** sel., ***sep.,*** ***sil.,*** spig., spong., ***squil.,*** stann., ***staph.,*** **STRAM.,** stront-c., ***sulph.,*** sul-ac., tarax., thuj., **VALER.,** verat., viol-t., zinc.

cracking, as if - murx.

hot - tell., ust.

jaundice, in - sang.

morning, in bed - mag-c.

night - nat-c.

perspire, inability to (see Inactivity) - acet-ac., acon., ***aeth.,*** **ALUM.,** ambr., am-c., ***anac.,*** apis, apoc., arg-m., arg-n., arn., **ARS.,** ***ars-i.,*** **BELL.,** ***berb-a.,*** bism., bry., calc., cann-s., ***cham.,*** ***chin.,*** coff., **COLCH.,** ***con.,*** crot-t., cupr., ***dulc.,***

DRY, skin

perspire, inability to (see Inactivity) - eup-per., **GRAPH.,** hyos., iod., ip., kali-ar., **KALI-C.,** kali-i., kali-s., lach., laur., ***led., lyc.,*** mag-c., ***maland.,*** merc., merc-c., nat-c., **NAT-M.,** nit-ac., **NUX-M.,** nux-v., olnd., op., ***petr., ph-ac.,*** phos., plat., **PLB.,** ***psor.,*** puls., ***rhus-t.,*** sabad., ***samb.,*** sanic., sars., sec., seneg., sep., **SIL.,** spong., **SQUIL.,** ***staph.,*** sulph., teucr., thuj., thyr., verb., viol-o.

exercising, when - arg-m., ***calc., nat-m.,*** **PLB.**

pollution, after - bar-c.

rough - iod., ***lith.,*** merc., nat-c.

ECCHYMOSIS, (see Bruises)

ECZEMA - ***aethi-m.,*** aln., alum., am-c., am-m., anac., ***ant-c.,*** arb., arg-n., **ARS., ARS-I.,** astac., aur., ***aur-m.,*** **BAR-M.,** bell., berb., berb-a., bor., ***bov.,*** brom., bry., ***calad.,*** **CALC., CALC-S.,** canth., caps., carb-ac., carb-s., ***carb-v., carc.,*** cast-eq., ***caust.,*** chrysar., **CIC.,** clem., com., con., cop., **CROT-T.,** cycl., **DULC.,** fl-ac., frag., fuli., **GRAPH., HEP.,** hippoz., hydr., hydrc., ***iris,*** **JUG-C., JUG-R.,** ***kali-ar.,*** kali-bi., ***kali-c., kali-chl.,*** kali-m., ***kali-s.,*** kreos., lach., **LAPPA-M.,** led., ***lith., lyc., mang., merc.,*** merc-d., merc-p-r., merc-sul., **MEZ.,** mur-ac., nat-m., nat-p., ***nat-s.,*** nit-ac., nux-v., **OLND., PETR.,** ***phos., phyt.,*** piloc., ***plb.,*** podo., prim-v., **PSOR.,** ***ran-b.,*** **RHUS-T.,** rhus-v., ***sars., sep., sil.,*** skook., ***staph.,*** **SULPH., SUL-I.,** tarent-c., tell., ***thuj., thyr.,*** tub., ust., ***vinc., viol-t.,*** x-ray, xero.

acute form - acon., anac., bell., canth., ***chin-s., crot-t.,*** mez., ***rhus-t.,*** sep.

alternating, with internal affections - ***graph.***

children, in - carc., graph., nat-m., sulph.

gastric symptoms, with - ant-c., iris.

madidans - cic., con., dulc., graph., hep., kali-m., merc-c., merc-p-r., mez., sep., staph., tub., viol-t.

menopause agg. - mang.

menses, agg. - mang.

neurasthenic persons, in - ***anac.,*** ars., phos., stry., stry-p., viol-t., zinc-p.

pigmentation in circumscribed areas, following with - berb.

rheumatic-gouty persons, in - alum., arb., lac-ac., ***rhus-t.,*** urea

seaside, at the, ocean voyage, excess of salt - ***nat-m.***

sore, as if excoriated - ***skook.***

strumous persons, in - ***aethi-m., ars-i.,*** calc., ***calc-i.,*** calc-p., caust., cist., crot-t., ***hep.,*** merc., merc-c., rumx., sep., sil., tub.

suppressed menses, from - kali-m.

urinary, gastric, hepatic disorders, with - lyc.

vaccination, after - skook.

agg. - mez.

whole body, over - crot-t., rhus-t.

EDGES - graph., hep., nat-p., nit-ac., petr., psor., ***sulph.***

itching - ambr., caust., petr.

ELASTICITY, lack of (see Inelasticity)

ELECTRIC, sparks, as from, sensation - agar., ***arg-m.,*** calc., ***calc-p.,*** nat-m., **SEC.,** ***sel.***

ERUPTIONS - acet-ac., ***acon.,*** agar., agn., alum., alumn., ambr., ***am-c.,*** am-m., anac., ***ant-c.,*** ant-t., ***apis,*** arg-m., arn., **ARS., ARS-I.,** arund., asaf., asar., aster., aur., **BAR-C.,** bar-m., bell., bism., bor., bov., ***bry.,*** calad., **CALC., CALC-S.,** camph., cann-s., canth., caps., ***carb-an., carb-s., carb-v.,*** **CAUST.,** cham., chel., chin., chin-a., chin-s., chlor., ***cic.,*** cimic., cina, ***cist.,*** clem., cob., cocc., coff., colch., coloc., ***con.,*** cop., croc., ***crot-t.,*** cupr., ***cycl.,*** dig., dros., ***dulc.,*** elaps, euph., euphr., fl-ac., ***graph.,*** guai., ***hell.,*** hep., hyos., ign., iod., ***ip.,*** **JUG-C., JUG-R.,** ***kali-ar.,*** kali-bi., ***kali-br.,*** **KALI-C.,** kali-n., kali-p., **KALI-S.,** ***kreos.,*** lach., laur., led., **LYC.,** mag-c., **MERC., MEZ.,** mosch., mur-ac., ***nat-a.,*** nat-c., **NAT-M.,** nat-p., ***nit-ac., olnd.,*** op., par., **PETR.,** ph-ac., phos., plat., plb., **PSOR.,** ***puls.,*** ran-b., ran-s., rheum, rhod., **RHUS-T.,** ***rhus-v., rumx.,*** ruta., sabad., samb., sars., sec., sel., seneg., **SEP., SIL.,** spig., spong., squil., stann., ***staph.,*** stram., stront-c., **SULPH.,** sul-ac., ***sul-i.,*** tarax., teucr., ***thuj.,*** tub., valer., verat., verb., ***viol-t.,*** zinc.

allergic - apis, dulc., med., puls., urt-u.

alternating with - ant-c., ars., calad., graph., hep., staph., sulph.

asthma - ***ars.,*** calad., mez., rhus-t., ***sulph.***

diarrhea - calc-p.

digestive symptoms with - graph.

dysentery - rhus-t.

internal affections - ars., crot-t., graph., rhus-t.

pain in limbs - crot-t., staph.

respiratory symptoms - ***ars., calad.,*** crot-t., kali-ar., kalm., lach., mez., psor., rhus-t., sulph.

tightness of chest - calad., kalm., rhus-t.

bathing, cold amel. - ant-c.

biting - agn., alum., am-c., ***am-m.,*** ant-c., arn., ars., bell., bor., bov., ***bry., calc.,*** camph., canth., caps., carb-an., carb-s., carb-v., ***caust.,*** cham., chel., chin., cocc., ***colch.,*** coloc., con., dros., **EUPH.,** hell., ***ip., lach.,*** **LED.,** ***lyc.,*** mag-c., mang., merc., ***mez.,*** mur-ac., nat-c., nat-m., nux-v., ***olnd.,*** op., petr., ph-ac., phos., plat., **PULS.,** ran-b., ran-s., rhod., ***rhus-t.,*** sel., sil., spig., ***spong.,*** still., stront-c., ***sulph.,*** thuj., verat., viol-t.

night - ars.

blackish - ant-c., **ARS.,** asaf., ***bell., bry.,*** chin., con., crot-h., hyos., ***lach.,*** mur-ac., nit-ac., ran-b., ***rhus-t., sec.,*** sep., ***sil.,*** spig., ***still.,*** vip.

bleeding - aeth., alum., ant-t., apis, ars., calc., dulc., euph., hep., kali-ar., kali-c., kali-n., ***lach.,*** lyc., med., **MERC.,** merc-c., ***nit-ac.,*** olnd., ***par., petr., psor., sep.,*** **SULPH.**

ERUPTIONS, general

bleeding,

scratching, after - alum., ***ars., bov., calc.,*** chin., cocc., cupr-ar., ***dulc., lach., lyc.,*** mez., nux-v., petr., ***psor.,*** **SULPH.,** ***til.***

blotches - anac., ***ant-c.,*** arn., ***ars., asaf.,*** bar-c., ***bell.,*** berb., ***bry.,*** calc., caps., chel., chlol., cocc., coff., con., croc., ***crot-h.,*** crot-t., dulc., fl-ac., hell., ***hep., hyos.,*** ign., kali-c., kreos., ***lach., led.,*** lyc., ***mag-c., mang., merc.,*** nat-c., nat-m., ***nit-ac., nux-v.,*** op., ***petr.,*** ph-ac., ***phos., puls., rhus-t., rhus-v.,*** ruta., sabin., ***sars., sec.,*** sel., sep., ***sil.,*** spig., ***squil.,*** staph., stram., sulph., sul-ac., valer., verat., vip.

indurated - am-m., phos., sars.

inflamed - hep., mang., ***merc., phos., sil.***

itching, oozing - **GRAPH.,** sul-ac., thuj.

livid - sul-ac.

red - arg-n., carb-v., crot-t., fl-ac., merc., mur-ac., op., phos., sul-ac., urt-u.

desquamating - fl-ac., thuj.

elevated - fl-ac., ***rhus-t.***

scratching, after - kali-c., lach., lyc., merc., nat-c., nit-ac., op., rhus-t., spig., verat., zinc.

stinging - ***petr.,*** sars., stram., zinc.

watery - graph., mag-c.

yellow - ant-c., sulph.

blue, dark - ***ail.,*** arg-n., ***crot-h., lach., ran-b.,*** sars., ***sulph.***

body, all over - ars., **DULC.,** ***psor.,*** sulph., tub.

breast-feeding, during - ***sep.***

brownish - anag., dulc., nit-ac., ph-ac., phos.

burning - agar., alum., ***ambr., am-c.,*** am-m., anac., ant-c., ant-t., **APIS,** arg-m., **ARS.,** aur., bar-c., ***bell.,*** berb., bov., ***bry.,*** bufo, calad., ***calc., calc-s.,*** cann-s., canth., caps., **CARB-AC.,** ***carb-an., carb-s., carb-v.,*** **CAUST.,** chin., chin-a., **CIC.,** ***clem.,*** cocc., coff., colch., com., ***con.,*** crot-t., cub., dig., dulc., euph., **GRAPH.,** guai., hell., ***hep.,*** ign., kali-ar., ***kali-bi., kali-c.,*** kali-i., kali-n., kali-s., kreos., ***lach.,*** laur., led., ***lyc.,*** mang., **MERC.,** ***mez.,*** nat-a., nat-c., nat-m., nat-p., nit-ac., ***nux-v.,*** olnd., par., petr., ph-ac., ***phos.,*** plat., plb., ***psor., puls., ran-b.,*** **RHUS-T.,** sabad., sars., seneg., sep., ***sil.,*** spig., spong., squil., stann., ***staph.,*** stram., stront-c., ***sulph.,*** teucr., thuj., urt-u., verat., viol-o., ***viol-t.,*** zinc.

air, open in - led.

night - ars., caust., ***merc.,*** **RHUS-T.,** staph., til.

rubbing, after - sars.

scratching, amel. - ***kali-n.***

touch agg. - cann-s., canth., ***merc.***

washing, when - ***merc.***

in cold water, after - clem., thuj.

clustered - ***agar., calc.,*** ph-ac., ran-b., rhus-t., staph., verat.

cold, agg. - agar., lac-d., petr., ***psor., rhus-t.***

air, from - ***apis,*** ars., caust., dulc., kali-ar., kali-c., mang., ***nit-ac.,*** psor., **RHUS-T.,** rhus-v., ***rumx.,*** sep.

ERUPTIONS, general

cold, agg.

bathing agg. - ***ant-c.,*** thuj.

becoming cold, from - **ARS.,** dulc., sars.

disappearing, from - calc.

confluent - agar., ***ant-t., caps., chlol., cic.,*** hyos., ***ph-ac.,*** phos., rhus-v., valer.

coppery - alum., ***ars., ars-i.,*** aur., ***calc.,*** cann-s., **CARB-AN.,** carb-v., cor-r., ***kali-i., kreos.,*** led., ***lyc., merc., mez., nit-ac.,*** phos., ***psor., rhus-t.,*** ruta., syph., ***verat.***

covered parts - ***led., thuj.***

dense - agar., calc.

spots - benz-ac., lach., med., ***merc., mez., nit-ac.,*** ust.

covered, parts - ***led.,*** thuj.

crusty - ***agar., alum.,*** ambr., am-c., am-m., ***anac.,*** anag., ***anan., anthr.,*** **ANT-C.,** ant-t., apis, **ARS., ARS-I.,** ***aur., aur-m., bar-c.,*** bar-m., ***bell.,*** bov., ***bry.,*** **CALC., CALC-S.,** caps., ***carb-an.,*** **CARB-S.,** carb-v., ***caust.,*** cham., ***chel., cic., cist., clem.,*** com., **CON., DULC.,** elaps, ***fl-ac.,*** **GRAPH.,** hell., ***hep., jug-c., kali-ar., kali-bi., kali-c.,*** kali-chl., ***kali-i.,*** kali-p., ***kali-s.,*** kreos., ***lach., lappa-a., led., lith.,*** **LYC.,** mag-c., **MERC.,** ***merc-i-r.,*** **MEZ.,** mur-ac., **NAT-M.,** nat-p., **NIT-AC.,** nux-v., **OLND.,** paeon., par., **PETR.,** ph-ac., ***phos., phyt.,*** plb., ***psor., puls.,*** **RAN-B., RHUS-T.,** ***rhus-v., sabad.,*** sabin., sang., ***sars., sep.,*** **sil.,** ***spong.,*** squil., ***staph.,*** **SULPH.,** sul-ac., tell., thuj., vac., verat., vinc., ***viol-t.,*** zinc.

allergic, hay - **GRAPH.**

black - ***ars.,*** bell., chin., vip.

bleeding - merc., ***mez.***

body, over whole - ars., **DULC.,** ***psor.***

brown - am-c., ant-c., berb.

burning - am-c., ***ant-c.,*** calc., cic., puls., sars.

dry - ***ars., ars-i.,*** **AUR., AUR-M.,** ***bar-c., calc.,*** chin-s., graph., lach., led., merc., ***ran-b.,*** sulph., thuj., ***viol-t.***

fetid - graph., lyc., med., ***merc.,*** plb., ***psor.,*** staph., **SULPH.**

gray - ars., merc., ***sulph.***

greenish - ant-c., calc., petr., sulph.

hard - **RAN-B.**

hay, allergic - **GRAPH.**

honey colored - carb-v., graph.

horny - ***ant-c.,*** graph., **RAN-B.**

inflamed - **CALC.,** ***lyc.***

mercury, after abuse of - **KALI-I.**

moist - alum., anac., ***anthr.,*** **ARS.,** ***bar-c.,*** **CALC., CARB-S.,** ***cic.,*** clem., **GRAPH.,** ***hell., hep., kali-s.,*** **LYC., MERC., MEZ.,** ***olnd.,*** phos., plb., ran-b., **RHUS-T.,** ruta., sep., ***sil.,*** **STAPH., SULPH.**

oozing, greenish, bloody - ant-c.

patches - hydr., kali-c., ***merc.,*** **NIT-AC.,** sabin., sil., thuj., zinc.

renewed daily - crot-t.

ERUPTIONS, general

scratching, after - alum., am-c., am-m., ant-c., ars., ***bar-c.,*** bell., bov., bry., ***calc.,*** caps., carb-an., carb-s., carb-v., cic., ***con., dulc., graph., hep.,*** kali-ar., kali-c., kali-s., kreos., led., **LYC.,** ***merc.,*** mez., nat-m., petr., phos., puls., ran-b., **RHUS-T.,** sabad., sabin., sars., sep., sil., ***staph.,*** **SULPH.,** thuj., verat., viol-t., zinc.

serpiginous - ***clem., psor.,*** sulph.

smarting - puls.

suppurating - ***ars.,*** plb., sil., ***sulph.***

thick - bov., calc., merc-aur.

warm weather - bov.

white - ***alum., calc., mez.,*** **NAT-M.,** tell., thuj.

yellow - ***ant-c.,*** aur., aur-m., ***bar-m., calc., calc-s.,*** carb-v., ***cic.,*** cupr., dulc., hyper., iod., ***kali-bi., kali-s.,*** kreos., med., ***merc., mez.,*** nat-p., ***petr.,*** ph-ac., ***spong., staph.,*** sulph., ***viol-t.***

yellow-white - ***mez.***

dentition, during, itching eruption - calc.

desquamating - acet-ac., agar., **AM-C.,** ***am-m.,*** ant-t., apis, ***ars., ars-i., arum-t., aur.,*** bar-c., **BELL.,** bor., ***bov.,*** calc., calc-s., canth., caps., carb-an., caust., cham., ***clem., coloc.,*** con., crot-h., crot-t., cupr., dig., ***dulc.,*** elaps, euph., ferr., ferr-p., ***graph., hell.,*** iod., ***kali-ar., kali-c.,*** **KALI-S.,** kreos., lach., ***laur., led., mag-c.,*** manc., ***merc.,*** **MEZ.,** mosch., ***nat-a.,*** nat-c., nat-m., nat-p., **OLND.,** op., par., ***ph-ac., phos.,*** plat., plb., **PSOR.,** ***puls.,*** ran-b., ran-s., ***rhus-t., rhus-v.,*** sabad., ***sec.,*** sel., **SEP.,** ***sil.,*** spig., ***staph., sulph.,*** sul-ac., tarax., teucr., thuj., urt-u., verat.

peeling off, as if - agar., bar-c., **KALI-S.,** lach., ph-ac., phos., phyt., rhus-t., ***sulph.***

dirty - merc., ***psor., sulph.,*** syph.

discharging - ***aethi-a.,*** alum., ***anac.,*** anag., ***ant-c.,*** ant-t., ***ars., ars-i., bar-c.,*** bell., ***bov.,*** bry., bufo, cact., cadm-s., ***calc., calc-s.,*** canth., caps., carb-an., **CARB-S., CARB-V.,** ***caust.,*** cham., chrysar., ***cic.,*** cist., ***clem., con.,*** crot-h., ***crot-t.,*** cupr., **DULC., GRAPH.,** ***hell., hep.,*** hydr., iod., ***jug-c., kali-ar., kali-br., kali-c.,*** kali-p., ***kali-s., kreos., lach.,*** led., **LYC.,** ***manc., merc.,*** **MEZ.,** mur-ac., nat-a., nat-c., **NAT-M.,** nat-p., ***nat-s.,*** nit-ac., olnd., ***petr., ph-ac., phos.,*** phyt., ***psor.,*** ran-b., **RHUS-T.,** rhus-v., ruta., sabin., ***sars., sel.,*** **SEP., SIL., SOL-N.,** squil., ***staph.,*** still., stront-c., ***sulph.,*** sul-ac., ***sul-i.,*** tarax., ***tell., thuj.,*** vario., vinc., viol-t., zinc.

bloody - ant-c., calc., crot-h., lach., merc., nux-v.

corrosive - ***ars., calc.,*** caps., carb-s., ***clem.,*** con., ***graph.,*** merc., ***nat-m.,*** ran-s., ***rhus-t.,*** **SULPH.,** ***thuj.***

destroying hair - ars., graph., lyc., merc., mez., ***nat-m.,*** petr., ***rhus-t.,*** sil.

glutinous - ***calc., carb-s.,*** **GRAPH.,** ***nat-m.,*** sulph.

greenish - ant-c., ***kali-chl.,*** rhus-t.

honey, like - graph.

ERUPTIONS, general

discharging,

ichorous - ant-t., clem., ran-s., ***rhus-t.***

pus - ***calc-s.,*** clem., dulc., graph., ***hep.,*** lyc., nat-c., nat-m., ***nit-ac., sil., sulph.***

scratching, after - alum., ars., bar-c., bell., bov., bry., calc., carb-an., ***carb-v.,*** caust., cic., con., dulc., **GRAPH.,** hell., hep., ***kali-c., kreos.,*** **LACH.,** led., **LYC.,** merc., mez., nat-c., nat-m., nit-ac., ***olnd., petr.,*** **RHUS-T.,** ruta., sabin., sars., sel., ***sep.,*** sil., squil., ***staph.,*** sulph., sul-ac., tarax., thuj., viol-t.

thick - bov., calc.

thin - cupr., ***dulc.,*** hell., **NAT-M.,** ***rhus-t.,*** rhus-v., sol-n.

white - bor., **CALC.,** ***carb-v.,*** caust., ***dulc.,*** graph., lyc., merc., ***nat-m., phos.,*** **PULS.,** sep., **SIL.**

yellow - ***alum., anac.,*** **ANT-C.,** ars., bar-c., ***calc.,*** canth., carb-an., **CARB-S., CARB-V.,** caust., ***clem.,*** cupr., ***dulc., graph., hep.,*** iod., ***kali-c., kali-s.,*** lach., ***lyc.,*** merc., ***nat-m.,*** nat-p., **NAT-S., NIT-AC., PHOS., PULS.,** ***rhus-t.,*** **SEP., SIL.,** sol-n., **SULPH.,** ***thuj., viol-t.***

dry - ***alum.,*** alumn., anac., anag., ant-c., **ARS., ARS-I., AUR., AUR-M., BAR-C.,** ***berb-a., bov., bry.,*** bufo, cact., cadm-br., calad., **CALC., CALC-S.,** canth., ***carb-s., carb-v.,*** caust., clem., cocc., com., cory., ***cupr., dulc., fl-ac., graph., hep.,*** hydr-ac., hydrc., hyos., ***iod., kali-ar., kali-c., kali-chl.,*** kali-i., kali-m., kali-s., ***kreos.,*** **LED.,** lith., ***lyc., mag-c., maland., merc.,*** **MEZ.,** morg., nat-c., nat-m., nat-p., nit-ac., par., ***petr., ph-ac.,*** **PHOS.,** phyt., pip-m., pix., ***psor.,*** rhus-t., ***sars.,*** sel., **SEP., SIL.,** stann., ***staph., sulph.,*** teucr., thuj., tub., valer., **VERAT.,** ***viol-t.,*** x-ray, xero, ***zinc.***

bleeding after scratching - alum., ***ars., calc., lyc., petr., sulph.***

eating, away, (see phagedenic)

ecthyma - ant-c., ant-t., arg-n., ars., bell., bor., cham., cic., cist., ***crot-t.,*** hydr., ***jug-c., jug-r., kali-bi.,*** kali-br., kali-i., kreos., ***lach.,*** lyc., ***merc.,*** nit-ac., petr., rhus-t., sec., ***sil.,*** staph., sulph., thuj.

elevated - anac., ars., asaf., ***bry.,*** calc., carb-v., caust., cop., crot-h., cupr-ar., dulc., graph., lach., merc., mez., op., phos., sulph., tab., tarax., valer.

emotions, after - elaps.

excoriated - alum., ***arg-m.,*** aur., bry., calc., colch., dros., ***graph., hep.,*** **MERC., NAT-M.,** ***nit-ac.,*** par., **PETR.,** ph-ac., puls., ***rhus-t.,*** sabin., ***sep.,*** sil., **SULPH.,** viol-t.

fetid - ***ars., graph., hep.,*** kali-p., ***lach., lyc., merc.,*** mez., ***nit-ac.,*** **PSOR.,** rhus-t., ***sep., sil.,*** staph., **SULPH.,** zinc.

fish, after - ars., sep.

ERUPTIONS, general
flat - ***am-c.,*** ant-c., ant-t., ***ars., asaf.,*** **BELL.,** carb-an., euph., **LACH.,** ***lyc.,*** merc., ***nat-c.,*** nit-ac., petr., ***ph-ac.,*** phos., puls., ***ran-b., sel., sep., sil.,*** staph., sulph., thuj.
flea, bites, like - calc., graph., led.
friction, slight agg. - sulph., vinc.
clothes, of agg. - bad., olnd.
constant agg. - sep.
gastric symptoms, with - ant-c.
granular - ***agar.,*** am-c., ars., ***carb-v.,*** cocc., graph., hep., kreos., led., nat-m., nux-v., par., phos., valer., zinc.
grape, shaped - agar., **CALC.,** rhus-t., staph., verat.
gritty - am-c., graph., ***hep.,*** nat-m., phos., zinc.
hairy, parts, on - agar., calc., kali-i., lach., ***lith.,*** lyc., ***merc., nat-m.,*** nit-ac., ph-ac., **RHUS-T.,** sil.
hard - agar., ***ant-c.,*** aur., caust., mez., ***ran-b.,*** rhus-t., spig., valer.
humid, see discharging
horny - ***ant-c., ran-b.***
hydroa - kali-i., kreos., mag-c., ***nat-m.,*** rhus-v.
inflamed - am-c., ars., calc., ***lyc.***
injured, parts - calc-p.
injury, slight agg. - alum., psor., sil.
itching, eruptions - acon., ***agar.,*** agn., ***alum.,*** ambr., ***am-c.,*** am-m., ***anac.,*** anag., ***ant-c., ant-t.,*** arg-m., ***arn.,*** **ARS.,** ***ars-i.,*** asaf., bar-c., bell., bov., ***bry.,*** bufo, ***calad., calc., calc-p., calc-s., canth.,*** caps., carb-an., carb-s., carb-v., **CAUST.,** ***cham.,*** chel., chin-s., cic., cimic., cina, **CLEM.,** cocc., con., ***crot-t.,*** cupr., dig., dulc., **GRAPH.,** guare., ***hep., ign.,*** ip., iris, ***jug-c., jug-r., kali-ar.,*** kali-bi., kali-br., ***kali-c., kali-i.,*** kali-n., kali-p., ***kali-s., kreos., lach.,*** laur., ***led., lyc.,*** mag-c., mag-m., mang., ***merc.,*** **MEZ.,** nat-a., nat-c., **NAT-M., NIT-AC., NUX-V.,** ***olnd., par., petr.,*** ph-ac., ***phos., phyt.,*** plb., ***psor., puls., ran-b.,*** ran-s., **RHUS-T.,** sabad., sabin., ***sars., sel.,*** **SEP.,** ***sil.,*** spig., spong., ***squil.,*** stann., **STAPH.,** stram., stront-c., **SULPH.,** sul-ac., tarax., teucr., thuj., valer., verat., ***viol-t.,*** x-ray, zinc.
air, cold, in - ***kali-ar., psor., rumx.***
amel. - kali-bi., kali-i.
evening - ***alum.,*** bor., graph., kreos., mag-m., mez., staph.
heat, agg. - **KALI-I.**
of stove amel. - ***rumx., tub.***
menses, during - carb-v., ***kali-c.,*** med.
before - apis, aur., carb-v., con., dulc., kali-c., mag-m., mez., nat-m., sang., sars., sep.3, verat.
night - ant-c., ant-t., ***ars.,*** ars-i., ***clem.,*** crot-t., graph., ***iris,*** kali-bi., kreos., **MERC.,** ***mez.,*** olnd., ***rhus-t.,*** staph., ust., verat., viol-t.
open air, in - led., ***nit-ac.***
overheated - ***kali-i.***
patches, bleeding after scratches - **SULPH.**
storm, before - graph.

ERUPTIONS, general
itching, eruptions
touch, agg. - mez.
undressing, when - ***ars-i., kali-ar.,*** nat-s., **RUMX.**
warm, room agg. - ***sep.***
warmth, agg. - ***alum.,*** bov., ***caust., clem., kali-i., led., lyc.,*** **MERC.,** ***mez.,*** nat-a., ***psor., puls.,*** **SULPH.,** verat.
of bed agg. - aeth., ***alum.,*** anac., ant-c., caust., ***clem.,*** cocc., ***kali-a.,*** kreos., mag-m., merc., mur-ac., **PSOR.,** ***puls., rhus-t.,*** sars., staph., **SULPH.,** ***til.,*** verat.
of fire - ***mez.***
washing, agg. - mez., sulph.
in cold water agg. - ***clem.***
jerking pain, with - asar., calc., ***caust.,*** cham., chin., cupr., lyc., ***puls.,*** **RHUS-T.,** sep., sil., ***staph.***
mealy - am-c., **ARS.,** aur., bov., bry., bufo, **CALC.,** cic., ***dulc.,*** graph., kreos., led., ***lyc.,*** merc., mur-ac., nit-ac., **PHOS.,** ***sep.,*** **SIL.,** sulph., thuj., verat.
white - ***ars., calc.,*** dulc., **KALI-CHL.,** lyc., sep., sil., thuj.
menses, during - all-s., apis, ***bell.,*** bell-p., calc., ***cimic.,*** con., ***dulc.,*** eug., ***graph.,*** hyos., ***kali-ar.,*** kali-c., kali-n., mag-m., mang., ***med.,*** nux-m., petr., psor., sang., ***sars.,*** sep., sil., ***thuj.,*** verat.
after - kreos.
before - apis, carb-v., con., dulc., dulc., graph., sars.
menstrual eruption - apis, dulc., kreos., sep., thuj.
metastasis, lungs, to - acon., apis, ars., carb-v., dulc., hep., ip., psor., puls., sec., sulph.
miliary - ***acon.,*** am-m., ars., ***bry.,*** cact., cent., hura, led., ***piloc.,*** raph., syzyg., urt-u.
milium - ***calc-i.,*** staph., tab.
milk, from - calc., sep.
morphea - ars., ***phos.,*** sil.
nettlerash, (see Urticaria, hives)
overheated, from being - ***bov., carb-v., con.,*** **NAT-M.,** ***psor., puls.***
painful - agar., alum., ambr., ant-c., apis, arg-m., **ARN.,** ***ars., asaf.,*** aur., bar-c., **BELL.,** berb., bov., calc., cann-s., canth., caps., chel., ***chin.,*** cic., ***clem., con., cupr., dulc.,*** guai., ***hep.,*** kali-ar., ***kali-c.,*** kali-s., ***lach.,*** led., ***lyc., mag-c., mag-m.,*** merc., nat-a., nat-c., nat-p., **NUX-V.,** par., petr., **PH-AC.,** phos., ***puls.,*** ran-b., ran-s., rhus-t., ruta., sel., seneg., ***sep.,*** **SIL.,** ***spig., spong.,*** squil., **SULPH.,** thuj., valer., ***verat.,*** verb.
splinters, as from, when touched - ***hep., nit-ac.***
painless - ***ambr.,*** anac., ant-c., ant-t., bell., cham., ***cocc., con.,*** cycl., dros., ***hell., hyos.,*** lach., laur., **LYC.,** ***olnd.,*** ph-ac., phos., puls., rhus-t., samb., ***sec.,*** spig., staph., ***stram., sulph.***

ERUPTIONS, general

papular - aur., ***calc., caust.,*** cham., cycl., gels., ***grin.,*** hippoz., ***hydrc., iod., kali-bi., kali-c.,*** **KALI-I.,** kali-s., lyc., ***merc., petr.,*** phos., pic-ac., ***sep.,*** sil., ***sulph., syph.,*** zinc.

patches - agar., ail., ars., berb., ***calc., carb-v., graph., iris,*** jug-c., ***kali-bi., kali-c., lith.,*** mang., phos., ***puls., sars., sep.,*** thuj., ***viol-t.***

petechiae - apoc., ***arn.,*** **ARS.,** aur-m., ***bapt.,*** bell., berb., **BRY.,** calc., ***camph.,*** canth., ***con., crot-h.,*** cupr., cur., dulc., eup-per., ***hyos., lach.,*** led., mur-ac., nat-m., nux-v., phel., ***ph-ac.,*** **PHOS., RHUS-T.,** ruta, ***sec.,*** sil., squil., stram., sul-ac., ter., vario.

elderly people, in - ***con.***

moist, after scratching - ars.

painful, in evening - ars.

phagedenic - alum., am-c., ***bar-c., bor., calc.,*** carb-s., carb-v., caust., **CHAM.,** chel., ***clem., con.,*** croc., **GRAPH.,** hell., ***hep.,*** kali-ar., kali-c., lach., lyc., mag-c., mang., merc., mur-ac., ***nat-c.,*** nat-m., nat-p., ***nit-ac.,*** nux-v., olnd., par., **PETR.,** ph-ac., phos., plb., ***rhus-t.,*** sars., ***sep.,*** **SIL.,** ***squil., staph.,*** sulph., tarax., ***viol-t.***

pimples - ***acon., agar.,*** aloe, alum., ambr., am-c., am-m., anac., **ANT-C.,** ***ant-t.,*** aran., arg-m., arn., **ARS.,** ars-i., aster., ***aur.,*** bar-c., ***bar-m., bell.,*** berb., bov., brom., ***bry.,*** bufo, ***calad.,*** calc., ***calc-p., calc-s., canth.,*** caps., ***carb-an., carb-s.,*** carb-v., **CAUST.,** ***cham.,*** chel., chin., chin-a., cimic., cina, ***cist.,*** clem., ***cocc.,*** coc-c., ***con.,*** crot-h., crot-t., cub., cupr., cycl., dros., ***dulc.,*** euphr., ***fl-ac.,*** gels., ***gamb., graph.,*** hell., ***hep.,*** iod., ***kali-ar.,*** kali-br., ***kali-c.,*** kali-chl., kali-n., kali-p., kali-s., ***kreos., lach., led., lyc.,*** mag-c., mag-m., mang., meph., **MERC.,** ***merc-c., mez.,*** mosch., ***mur-ac.,*** nat-a., ***nat-c.,*** **NAT-M.,** ***nat-p., nat-s.,*** **NIT-AC.,** ***nux-v.,*** pall., par., petr., **PH-AC., PHOS.,** plb., **PULS., RHUS-T.,** ruta, sabad., ***sars.,*** sel., ***seneg.,*** **SEP.,** ***sil.,*** spig., ***spong., squil.,*** stann., ***staph.,*** stront-c., **SULPH.,** sul-ac., tab., tarax., tarent., tell., ***thuj., til.,*** valer., verat., viol-t., **ZINC.**

alcoholics, in - kreos., lach., led.

black - carb-v., ped., spig.

bleeding - ***cist.,*** par., rhus-t., stront-c., thuj.

burning - agar., **ARS.,** bov., canth., caust., graph., kali-c., mag-m., merc., nat-s., ph-ac., ***rhus-t.,*** squil., staph., stront-c., sulph., til.

after scratching - caust., graph., mag-m., sulph.

close together - cham., staph., thuj., verat.

confluent - cic., mur-ac., ph-ac., tarent., valer.

copper-colored - kali-i.

crusts, with - calc., merc., squil.

green - ***calc.***

gnawing, itching - ant-c., ant-t., ***caust.,*** mang., nit-ac.

hard - agar., ***bov.,*** nit-ac., rhus-t., sabin., valer., verat.

ERUPTIONS, general

pimples,

inflamed - agar., berb., bry., ***chel.,*** nit-ac., petr., stann., sulph.

itching - acon., ambr., ammc., ***ant-c., apis, ars.,*** bar-c., bov., ***bry.,*** calc., carb-an., carb-s., ***caust.,*** cham., cocc., ***con.,*** dulc., **GRAPH.,** ***hep.,*** kali-c., laur., led., lyc., mag-c., mag-m., merc., mur-ac., nat-c., nat-m., nat-s., ***nit-ac.,*** ph-ac., ***psor.,*** puls., ***sep., sil.,*** squil., staph., stront-c., ***sulph.,*** **TELL.,** til., zinc.

when warm - caust., **KALI-I.,** sars., ***tell.,*** til.

menses, during - lac-c.

moist - ***calc.,*** graph., kali-c., nat-s., ol-an., puls., sil., sulph., thuj., zinc.

painful - ant-c., apis, arg-m., arn., ***cist.,*** cocc., con., dulc., graph., kali-c., kali-chl., kali-i., lach., mur-ac., nat-c., nit-ac., nux-v., phos., plb., puls., seneg., spong., squil., staph., sulph., verat.

perspiring parts, on - con.

scratching, after - agar., am-c., am-m., ***ant-c.,*** bar-c., bry., ***caust.,*** chin., cocc., con., cycl., dros., dulc., graph., hep., kali-c., laur., merc., nat-c., nat-m., ***nit-ac.,*** petr., ph-ac., phos., ***puls., rhus-t.,*** sabad., sabin., sars., sel., **SEP.,** sil., spong., squil., staph., stront-c., ***sulph.,*** verat., ***zinc.***

white, after - agar., ***ars.,*** bov., bry., ip., sulph.

smarting - agar., bell., calc., cham., coloc., dig., kali-c., kali-n., lyc., merc., teucr., verat.

sore, as if excoriated - alum., arg-m., bell., bov., calc., clem., guai., ***hep.,*** hyos., mez., ph-ac., ***rhus-t.,*** sabin., sel., spig., stann., teucr., verat., zinc.

splinter, pain like a - arn., hep., ***nit-ac.***

stinging - alum., ant-c., arn., ***bell.,*** calc-p., ***canth.,*** caps., caust., cocc., hell., kali-c., kali-n., kreos., mez., nat-c., squil., staph.

tearing - dulc.

tensive - arn., bov., con., mang., nat-s.

tingling - canth.

titillating - bell., caust., mag-m., verat.

touch, sensitive to - berb., calad., **HEP.**

ulcerated - ***merc.,*** nit-ac., ph-ac., sabin., sep.

pocks - ***ant-c., ant-t., arn., ars.,*** bell., bry., caust., clem., cocc., euon., hyos., ***kali-bi., kreos., merc.,*** mill., psor., puls., ***rhus-t.,*** sil., sulph., ***thuj.***

black - ***ars.,*** bell., hyos., lach., mur-ac., ***rhus-t.,*** sec.

burning - **ARS.,** lach., merc.

suppurating - bell., ***merc.,*** sulph.

whitish - iod., lyc.

pustules - agar., aln., am-c., am-m., anac., ***ant-c.,*** **ANT-T.,** ***ant-s.,*** arn., **ARS.,** ars-i., ***aur., bell., berb.,*** bry., bufo, calad., ***calc.,*** calc-p., ***calc-s., carb-ac., carb-s., carb-v., caust.,*** cham., ***chel., cic.,*** cina, cinnb., ***clem.,*** cocc., ***con.,*** cop., ***crot-h., crot-t.,*** cupr-ar.,

ERUPTIONS, general

pustules - cycl., ***dulc.,*** echi., euph., fl-ac., gnaph., ***hep.,*** hippoz., ***hydrc., hyos.,*** iod., ***iris,*** jug-c., jug-r., kali-ar., ***kali-bi., kali-br.,*** kali-c., ***kali-i.,*** kali-s., ***kreos.,*** lach., ***merc.,*** merc-c., ***mez., nat-m., nit-ac.,*** nux-v., ***petr.,*** ph-ac., phos., phyt., podo., ***psor., puls.,*** ran-b., **RHUS-T.,** rhus-v., ***sars.,*** sec., ***sep., sil.,*** squil., **STAPH.,** sul-i., **SULPH.,** tab., tax., tell., thuj., vac., vario., viol-t., zinc.

bathing agg. - ***dulc.***

black - **ANTHR.,** ant-t., bry., kali-bi., **LACH.,** ***mur-ac.,*** nat-c., rhus-t., thuj.

bleeding - ant-t.

blue, spots, leaving - rheum.

bluish - rheum.

brown - ant-t.

burning - am-c., jug-r., petr.

when touched - canth.

when uncovering - mez.

confluent - ant-t., **CIC.,** ***merc.***

cracked - rhus-t.

dry - ***merc.***

fetid - anthr., ars., bufo, viol-t.

greasy - kreos.

green - jug-r., ***sec.,*** viol-t.

hard - anac., ant-c., crot-h., nit-ac.

humid - bell.

indolent - ***kali-br., psor.***

inflamed - anac., crot-t., ***kali-bi.,*** rhus-t., sep., stram.

itch-like - clem., grat.

itching - anthro., ant-t., berb., ***crot-t., dulc.,*** graph., hydr-ac., ***kali-bi.,*** merc., nux-v., petr., ***rhus-t.,*** sars., ***sulph.***

night - ***kali-bi.***

lumpy - anthro., cham.

malignant - **ANTHR.,** apis, **ARS.,** ***bell., bufo,*** canth., ***carb-v.,*** cench., ***crot-h.,*** **LACH.,** ***ran-b., rhus-t., sec., sil., tarent-c.***

mixed with vesicles - ant-t.

painful - ant-t., ars., berb., ***kali-br.,*** stram., viol-t.

pityriasis versicolor - ***sulo-ac.***

red - anac., ant-t., ars., berb., caust., **CIC.,** cimic., crot-h., crot-t., graph., hydrc., hydr-ac., kali-c., mez., ***nit-ac.***

areola - anac., ant-t., bor., calad., lach., nit-ac., par., thuj.

rose-colored - ars., dulc.

scaly - merc.

scratching, after - am-m., ant-c., ars., bell., bry., cycl., hyos., merc., puls., **RHUS-T.,** sil., staph., ***sulph.***

scurfy - anac., ant-c., ant-t., bov., crot-t., dulc., ***kali-chl.,*** merc.

small - ant-t., hydrc., kali-i., kali-n., puls.

sore - calad., merc.

spots, covered with - jug-r., lyc.

stinging - am-c., berb., dros., rhus-t., ***sep.***

syphilitic - ***kali-bi.***

tensive - ant-t., crot-h., mag-s., kali-n.

tetters, on the - kreos.

ERUPTIONS, general

pustules,

thin, which break and send out ichorous pus, which corrodes the skin and spreads - ant-t.

titillating - mez.

ulcerated - ant-t., ***ars.,*** crot-t., cupr-ar., ***dulc.,*** mag-m., ***merc.,*** nat-c., ***sars.,*** sil.

water, containing - kali-i., rhus-t., stram.

white - calad., cimic., cop., cycl.

tips - ***ant-c.,*** ant-t., puls.

yellow - anac., carb-v., hyos., ***merc.,*** staph., viol-t.

red - acon., ***agar.,*** **AM-C.,** anac., ***anan.,*** ant-c., apis, ***arn., ars.,*** aur., berb., ***calc.,*** cham., chel., chin-s., ***chlol.,*** cic., ***clem.,*** cocc., ***com.,*** con., cop., crot-t., cycl., ***dulc.,*** fl-ac., ***graph., kali-bi.,*** **KALI-C.,** kali-s., lach., lyc., ***mag-c.,*** **MERC.,** ***mez., nit-ac.,*** ox-ac., petr., ph-ac., **PHOS.,** ***rhus-t.,*** sabad., sars., sep., sil., spig., staph., ***stram.,*** **SULPH., SUL-AC.,** thuj., til., valer., vip.

areola - anac., ant-t., bor., cocc., tab.

insect, stings, like - apis, bell., sep.

scarlet - ***anan.,*** cop.

spotted - merc., verat.

rupia - aethi-m., alum., ant-t., **ARS.,** berb-a., bor., calc., caust., cham., clem., ***fl-ac., graph., hep.,*** hydr., kali-c., ***kali-i.,*** lach., lyc., ***maland.,*** merc., merc-i-r., ***mez.,*** nat-c., ***nat-m., nat-s.,*** nit-ac., petr., ***phyt.,*** rhus-t., sec., sep., sil., staph., sulph., ***syph.,*** thuj., thyr.

scabby - ant-c., ars., calc., chrysar., ***cic.,*** dulc., graph., ***hep., lyc.,*** merc., ***mez.,*** mur-ac., nat-m., petr., staph., ***sulph.,*** vinc., viol-t.

scaly, (see Ichthyosis) - agar., ***am-m.,*** anac., ant-c., **ARS.,** ***ars-i., aur., bar-m., bell.,*** bor., bufo, cact., cadm-s., ***calad., calc.,*** calc-s., canth., cic., **CLEM.,** com., cupr., cycl., dulc., ***fl-ac.,*** graph., hep., ***hydrc.,*** hyos., iod., kali-ar., ***kali-bi.,*** kali-c., kali-i., kali-m., ***kali-s.,*** kreos., ***led.,*** lyc., ***mag-c.,*** manc., med., ***merc.,*** mez., ***nat-a.,*** nat-c., ***nat-m., nit-ac.,*** oena., ***olnd.,*** petr., **PHOS., PHYT.,** platan., ***plb., psor., rhus-t.,*** sang., ***sars.,*** **SEP.,** ***sil.,*** staph., ***sulph., syph.,*** teucr., thuj., thyr.

bran-like - agar., alum., am-c., anac., arg-m., **ARS.,** ars-i., aur., bac., berb-a., bor., bry., **CALC.,** calc-p., canth., carb-ac., carb-an., carb-v., chlor., ***cic.,*** clem., ***colch., dulc., fl-ac., graph.,*** iod., graph., ***kali-ar.,*** **KALI-CHL.,** kali-i., **KREOS.,** lach., led., ***lyc.,*** mag-c., mang., merc., merc-p-r., ***mez., nat-a.,*** nat-m., ***nit-ac.,*** olnd., petr., phos., **PHYT.,** pip-m., ran-b., rhus-t., sanic., ***sep.,*** **SIL.,** staph., sul-ac., sul-i., sulph., tell., ter., ***thuj.,*** thyr.

spots - hydrc., kali-c., ***merc.,*** **NIT-AC.,** ***puls.,*** sabin., sil., thuj., zinc.

white - anac., ***ars.,*** graph., **KALI-CHL.,** lyc., thuj., zinc.

yellow - **KALI-S.**

ERUPTIONS, general

scarlatina - acon., **AIL., AM-C., APIS,** arn., ***ars., arum-t.,*** bar-c., **BELL., *bry., calc., carb-ac., carb-v., cham., crot-h., cupr., gels.,*** hep., ***hyos.,*** **LACH., LYC., MERC.,** mur-ac., **NIT-AC., *ph-ac., phos.,*** phyt., **RHUS-T., *stram., sulph., zinc.***

gangrenous - ***ail.,*** **AM-C., *ars.,* CARB-AC., *lach., phos.***

patches, in - ***ail.***

receding - ***am-c., phos., sulph.,*** **ZINC.**

smooth - ***am-c.,*** **BELL.,** euphr., hyos., merc.

scorbutic, spots - anan., merc., merc-c.

scratching, after - agar., alum., **AM-C.,** am-m., ant-c., arn., ***ars., bar-c.,*** bell., bov., bry., ***calc.,*** canth., carb-an., carb-s., carb-v., **CAUST.,** chin., cic., con., ***cycl., dulc.,*** euph., graph., hell., ***hep.,*** ip., ***kali-c.,*** kali-s., ***kreos.,*** lach., laur., **LYC.,** mag-c., ***merc.,*** mez., nat-c., nat-m., nit-ac., nux-v., ***olnd., petr.,*** ph-ac., phos., plb., ***puls.,*** rhod., **RHUS-T.,** sabin., ***sars., sep., sil.,*** spong., squil., ***staph.,*** stront-c., **SULPH.,** sul-ac., thuj., verat., viol-t., zinc.

scurfy - merc.

sensitive - ant-c., arg-m., bell., **HEP.,** lach., led., nit-ac., par., sabad., spig., stann., valer.

serpiginous - ***clem., hep., psor., sars., sulph.***

shining through - merc.

smarting - acon., agar., ***alum.,*** ambr., ant-c., apis, **ARG-M.,** ars., ***aur.,*** bar-c., ***bry., calc.,*** cann-s., canth., caps., carb-an., carb-s., chel., chin., ***cic.,*** coff., ***colch.,*** dol., ***dros.,*** ferr., **GRAPH.,** hell., **HEP.,** ign., kali-c., ***kali-s.,*** lach., led., lyc., mag-c., ***mang.,*** merc., mez., nat-c., ***nat-m., nit-ac.,*** nux-v., olnd., ***par., petr., ph-ac.,*** phos., plat., ***puls.,*** ran-b., ***rhus-t.,*** ruta., sabin., sars., sel., **SEP.,** sil., ***spig.,*** spong., ***squil.,*** staph., ***sulph.,*** teucr., valer., ***verat., zinc.***

spring - graph., ***nat-s.,*** **PSOR.,** rhus-t., ***sars., sep.***

agg. - nat-s., psor., sang., ***sars.***

stinging - acon., alum., am-m., ***anac.,*** ant-c., **APIS,** arn., ***ars.,*** asaf., ***bar-c.,*** bar-m., ***bell.,*** bov., ***bry.,*** calc., camph., canth., caps., carb-v., caust., cham., chin., **CLEM.,** cocc., ***con., cycl.,*** dig., ***dros.,*** graph., guai., hell., ***hep.,*** ign., kali-ar., kali-c., kreos., ***led.,*** lyc., mag-c., ***merc.,*** mez., mur-ac., nat-a., nat-c., ***nat-m.,*** **NIT-AC.,** nux-v., petr., phos., ***plat.,*** **PULS., *ran-b.,*** ran-s., ***rhus-t.,*** sabad., ***sabin.,*** sars., sel., **SEP., SIL.,** spong., squil., ***staph.,*** stram., stront-c., **SULPH.,** thuj., ***urt-u.,*** verb., ***viol-t.,*** zinc.

sting, of insects, like, red - apis, bell., sep.

strophulus - apis, ***bor.,*** calc., ***cham.,*** cic., led., merc., rhus-t., ***spira.,*** sulph., sumb.

sudamina, (see vesicular)

summer, in - bov., graph., ***kali-bi.,*** led., mur-ac., sars., sel.

sun, from - ***nat-m., sol.***

ERUPTIONS, general

suppressed, eruptions, ailments from - acon., ail., alum., am-c., ambr., anac., ant-c., ant-t., ***apis,*** **ARS., *ars-i.,*** ars-s-f., asaf., bad., bar-c., ***bell.,*** **BRY.,** calad., calc., ***camph.,*** caps., carb-an., ***carb-v., caust., cham.,*** chin., ***cic.,*** clem., con., ***cupr.,*** cupr-ac., cupr-ar., **DULC., *gels., graph., hell., hep.,*** hyos., iod., **IP., KALI-BI.,** kali-c., ***kali-s., kreos.,*** lach., laur., ***lyc.,*** mag-c., mag-s., merc., ***mez., nat-c.,*** nit-ac., ***nux-m.,*** **NUX-V.,** op., **PETR., PH-AC.,** phos., plb., **PSOR.,** ptel., ***puls., rhus-t.,*** sars., sel., senec., ***sep.,*** sil., ***staph.,*** **STRAM.,** sul-ac., **SULPH.,** thuj., ***tub., tub-k.,*** verat., verat-v., ***viol-t.,*** x-ray, **ZINC.**

fail to break out - ***ail.,*** am-c., ant-t., ***apis., stram., sulph., zinc.***

exanthemata - ***ail., apis,*** hell., verat.

suppurating - alum., am-c., **ANT-C.,** ant-t., apis, ***ars., bar-c.,*** bell., ***bor.,*** cadm-s., ***calc.,*** calc-s., ***carb-s.,*** carb-v., caust., **CHAM.,** chel., ***cic., clem.,*** cocc., ***con.,*** croc., cycl., ***dulc.,*** euphr., **GRAPH.,** hell., ***hep.,*** jug-c., kali-c., ***kali-s.,*** lach., led., **LYC.,** mag-c., mang., **MERC.,** mur-ac., ***nat-a., nat-c.,*** nat-m., nat-p., **NIT-AC.,** nux-v., olnd., par., **PETR.,** ph-ac., phos., plb., ***psor.,*** puls., **RHUS-T., *samb., sars.,*** sec., **SEP., SIL., *squil.,*** spig., ***staph., sulph.,*** tarax., thuj., verat., viol-o., ***viol-t., zinc.***

swelling, with - acon., am-c., arn., ars., ***bell.,*** bry., calc., canth., carb-v., caust., chin., cic., con., euph., hep., ***kali-c.,*** lyc., mag-c., **MERC.,** nat-c., nat-m., nit-ac., petr., ph-ac., phos., ***puls.,*** **RHUS-T.,** ruta., ***samb.,*** sars., ***sep.,*** sil., ***sulph., thuj.***

syphilitic - arg-n., ars., **ARS-I., *aur.,*** bad., dulc., ***fl-ac., guai., hep., kali-bi.,*** kali-chl., **KALI-I.,** kreos., ***lach., lyc.,*** **MERC., MERC-C., MERC-I-F., MERC-I-R., NIT-AC.,** petr., ***phyt.,*** plat., rhus-t., rumx., sang., sars., sep., ***sil.,*** staph., still., **SYPH., *thuj.***

tearing pain, with - acon., arn., ars., ***bry., calc.,*** canth., carb-v., caust., clem., cocc., dulc., graph., kali-c., **LYC.,** merc., ***mez.,*** nat-c., nit-ac., phos., puls., ***rhus-t., sep., sil., staph., sulph.,*** zinc.

tense - alum., ant-t., ***arn.,*** bar-c., bell., bry., canth., carb-an., **CAUST.,** cocc., con., hep., kali-c., mez., olnd., ***phos.,*** puls., **RHUS-T.,** sabin., sep., spong., staph., ***stront-c.,*** sulph., thuj.

transparent - cina, ***merc.,*** **RAN-B.**

ulcerative, pain, with - am-c., ***am-m.,*** ant-c., ars., bar-c., caps., caust., con., graph., kali-c., laur., ***mang.,*** merc., ***phos., puls., rhus-t., sep.,*** **SIL., *staph.,*** sulph., tarax., zinc.

vaccination, after - mez., sars., sil., skook., thuj.

washing agg. - canth., **CLEM., *dulc.,*** hydr., mez., phos., ***psor.,*** sars., **SULPH.,** urt-u.

cold water, in - **CLEM., *dulc.,*** lac-c., sulph.

ERUPTIONS, general

whitish - agar., anan., ant-c., **ARS.,** ***ars-i.,*** bor., bov., bry., com., con., hep., ip., merc., ***mez.,*** phos., ***puls.,*** sulph., thuj., ***valer.,*** zinc.

winter, agg. - ***aloe,*** alum., ars., ***calc., dulc., hep.,*** kali-c., ***mang., merc., mez.,*** **PETR.,** ***psor.,*** **RHUS-T.,** sabad., ***sep., stront-c.,*** sulph.

amel. - kali-bi., sars.

yellow - ***agar.,*** anac., ***ant-c.,*** ars., aur., ***bar-c.,*** bar-m., bufo, cadm-s., ***calc-s.,*** chel., ***cic.,*** cocc., cupr., ***dulc., euph.,*** hell., kali-c., ***kali-chl.,*** kreos., lach., led., lyc., **MERC.,** ***nat-c.,*** nat-s., ***nit-ac.,*** par., ph-ac., ran-s., raph., ***rhus-t.,*** sep., ***spong.,*** tab., valer.

ERYSIPELAS - **ACON.,** ***am-c.,*** am-m., ***anac.,*** anac-oc., anan., ant-c., ***anthr.,*** **APIS,** ***arn., ars., ars-i.,*** arund., atro., ***aur.,*** bar-c., bar-m., **BELL.,** ***bor., bry.,*** bufo, ***calc.,*** cadm-s., ***camph., canth.,*** carb-ac., ***carb-an., carb-s.,*** carb-v., caust., ***cham.,*** chel., ***chin., clem.,*** colch., com., cop., ***crot-c., crot-h.,*** crot-t., cupr., dulc., ***echi.,*** elat., **EUPH.,** ***gels.,*** **GRAPH.,** ***hep.,*** hyos., ***iod., ip., jug-c.,*** jug-r., kali-ar., ***kali-c., kali-chl.,*** kali-i., ***kali-p.,*** kali-s., **LACH.,** led., ***lyc.,*** mag-c., mang., **MERC.,** mur-ac., nat-a., nat-c., nat-m., nat-p., nat-s., ***nit-ac.,*** petr., ***ph-ac., phos.,*** plb., podo., prim-o., ***puls.,*** ran-b., rhod., **RHUS-T.,** ***rhus-v., ruta.,*** sabad., samb., sars., sep., ***sil., sulph.,*** syph., ***tarent-c.,*** tax., ***ter., thuj.,*** verat., verat-v., vesp., ***xero,*** zinc.

afebrile - ***graph.,*** hep., lyc.

biliary, catarrhal duodenal symptoms, with - hydr.

brain symptoms, with - am-c.

chronic - ***graph., ter.***

constitutional tendency, with - calen., ***graph.,*** lach., psor., sul-ac.

edema, persisting, with - ***apis,*** ars., aur., graph., hep., lyc., sulph.

elderly people - ***am-c.,*** carb-an.

erratic - apis, arn., ***ars.,*** bell., chin., ***graph.,*** hep., hydr., mang., ***mur-ac., puls.,*** rhus-t., sabin., sulph.

gangrenous - acon., ***anthr., apis,*** **ARS.,** ***bell., camph.,*** **CARB-V.,** chin., com., **CROT-C.,** ***hippoz.,*** hyos., **LACH.,** mur-ac., ***rhus-t., sabin.,*** **SEC.,** ***sil.,*** ter.

left to right - lach., ***rhus-t.***

menses, during - ***graph.***

neonatorum - apis, bell., camph.

traumatic, umbilical, newborn - apis.

phlegmonous - acon., anthr., arn., ***ars.,*** bell., both., crot-h., ferr-p., graph., ***hep.,*** hippoz., ***lach.,*** merc., ***rhus-t.,*** sil., ***tarent-c.,*** verat-v.

prophylactic - graph.

recurrent, chronic, and - ***apis, crot-h.,*** ferr-p., ***graph.,*** nat-m., ***rhus-t., sulph.***

repercussion, with - cupr-ac.

right to left - ***apis,*** arund., ***graph., lyc.,*** sulph.

ERYSIPELAS,

scratching, after agg. - ***am-c.,*** ant-c., arn., ars., ***bell.,*** bor., bry., calc., canth., carb-an., carb-v., ***graph., hep.,*** hyos., ***lach., lyc.,*** mag-c., **MERC.,** nat-a., nat-c., nit-ac., petr., phos., puls., ran-b., **RHUS-T.,** samb., sil., spong., ***sulph.,*** thuj.

smooth - ***apis,*** **BELL.**

streaks, running in - ***graph.***

swelling, with - ***acon.,*** am-c., **APIS,** ***arn., ars.,*** **BELL.,** bry., ***calc.,*** canth., carb-s., carb-v., caust., chin., **CROT-C.,** euph., ***graph., hep.,*** kali-c., ***lach.,*** lyc., mag-c., **MERC.,** nat-a., nat-c., nat-m., nit-ac., petr., ph-ac., phos., puls., **RHUS-T.,** rhus-v., ruta., samb., sars., sep., sil., ***sulph., thuj., verat-v.,*** zinc.

swelling, with, marked, with burning, itching and stinging - rhus-t.

traumatic - calen., psor.

umbilical, newborn - apis.

vesicular - astac., am-c., ***anac., ars.,*** bar-c., ***bell.,*** bry., ***canth.,*** carb-an., ***carb-s.,*** com., crot-t., **EUPHR.,** ***graph., hep., kali-chl.,*** kali-s., ***lach.,*** mez., petr., phos., puls., ran-b., **RHUS-T.,** ***rhus-v.,*** sabad., ***sep.,*** staph., stram., ***sulph.,*** urt-u.

ERYTHEMA, general

exsudativum multiforme - antipyrin., bor-ac., vesp.

nodosum - acon., ant-c., ***apis, arn.,*** ars., chin., chin-a., ***chin-s.,*** ferr., led., nat-c., ptel., ***rhus-t., rhus-v.***

simplex - ***acon.,*** antipyrin., apis, ***arn.,*** ars-i., ***bell.,*** bufo, ***canth.,*** chlor., echi., gaul., grin., kali-c., lac-ac., ***merc.,*** mez., narc-ps., nux-v., rhus-t., rob., ter., urt-u., ust., verat-v., xero

EXCORIATION, (see Intertrigo) - ***arn., ars., ars-i.,*** **ARUM-T.,** ***aur.,*** **BAR-C.,** bell., **CALC., CALC-S.,** canth., **CARB-S.,** ***carb-v., caust.,*** **CHAM.,** ***chin.,*** clem., **GRAPH.,** ***hep.,*** hydr., **IGN.,** iod., kali-ar., kali-c., ***kali-chl.,*** kali-s., laur., **LYC.,** ***merc., merc-c., nat-m.,*** nat-p., **NIT-AC.,** ***olnd., petr.,*** ph-ac., phos., ***psor.,*** **PULS., RHUS-T.,** ruta., sars., **SEP., SULPH.**

scratching, after (must scratch it raw) - agar., ***alum.,*** am-c., ant-c., arn., ***bar-c.,*** bov., calc., ***carb-s.,*** caust., chin., dros., **GRAPH.,** hep., kali-c., kreos., ***lach., lyc.,*** mang., merc., ***olnd.,*** **PETR.,** phos., plb., puls., rhus-t., ruta., sabin., ***sep.,*** sil., squil., sul-ac., ***sulph.,*** tarax., ***til.***

EXCRESCENCES, growths, (see Condylomata, Warts) - ***ant-c.,*** ant-t., ars., aur., bell., **CALC.,** ***carb-an., carb-s., carb-v.,*** carc., **CAUST.,** clem., cocc., ***fl-ac.,*** **GRAPH.,** ***hep.,*** iod., lach., **LYC.,** med., nat-m., **NIT-AC.,** nux-v., ph-ac., phos., plb., puls., ran-b., rhus-t., sabin., ***sil.,*** **STAPH.,** ***sulph.,*** syph., **THUJ.**

fibroma - calc-ar., ***con., iod.,*** kali-br., lyc., sec., thuj.

fleshy - ars., calc., ***staph., thuj.***

EXCRESCENCES, growths
fungus, cauliflower - **ANT-C.,** ***ars.,*** clem., ***con.,*** iod., ***kreos.,*** lac-c., **LACH.,** ***nit-ac.,*** petr., phos., rhus-t., sabin., sang., **SIL.,** ***staph.,*** sulph., **THUJ.**
haematodes - ant-t., **ARS.,** bell., calc., **CARB-AN.,** ***carb-v.,*** clem., ***kreos., lach., lyc., merc., nat-m., nit-ac.,*** nux-v., **PHOS.,** ***rhus-t.,*** sep., **SIL.,** staph., ***sulph.,*** **THUJ.**
medullary - bell., ***carb-an., phos.,*** sil., sulph., ***thuj.***
syphilitic - ***ars.,*** **ARS-I.,** aur., aur-m., aur-m-n., ***iod.,*** **LACH.,** ***manc.,*** **MERC., MERC-C., NIT-AC.,** staph., **SIL.,** thuj.
granular - calc., nit-ac., staph., thuj.
hard - ran-b.
horny - **ANT-C.,** mez., ***ran-b.,*** sep., sulph., thuj.
humid - merc-c., ***nit-ac.,*** psor., ***sabin.,*** staph., sulph., **THUJ.**
ragged - nat-c., ph-ac., rhus-t., thuj.
red - **NAT-S.,** thuj.
smooth - ***thuj.***
spongy - calc., lyc., nit-ac., staph., thuj.
swelling, inflamed, puffy bunches - ars., carb-an., hep., ***nat-c., phos., sil.,*** sulph.

FILTHY - ***apis, ars.,*** bry., ***caps.,*** ferr., ferr-pic., iod., merc., nat-m., petr., phos., petr., **PSOR.,** ***sanic.,*** sec., **SULPH.,** thuj.

FLABBINESS - abrot., agar., ant-t., ***apis,*** ars., aster., bar-c., bor., **CALC.,** ***camph., caps.,*** cham., chel., ***chin., clem., cocc.,*** con., croc., ***cupr.,*** dig., euph., ***ferr.,*** graph., hell., ***hep., hyos.,*** iod., ip., ***lach., lyc.,*** mag-c., merc., morph., nat-c., nat-m., op., puls., rheum, sabad., salv., sanic., sars., sec., seneg., sil., ***spong.,*** sul-ac., sulph., thyr., ***verat.***

FORMICATION, sensation - ***acon.,*** acon-f., aesc., ***agar.,*** agn., all-s., ***alum.,*** ambr., am-c., anac., ap-g., apis, ***aran.,*** arg-m., ***ars., ars-i.,*** arund., aur., ***bar-c.,*** bar-m., bell., bor., bov., bufo, calad., calc., calc-p., calc-s., calen., cann-i., cann-s., canth., caps., ***carb-s.,*** carb-v., caust., cham., chel., chin., ***chin-a.,*** cist., ***coca, cocaine, cocc.,*** cod., con., croc., ***crot-c.,*** dulc., ***ferr.,*** ferr-p., ***hyper., iod.,*** kali-c., kali-s., lach., ***laur.,*** led., **LYC.,** mag-c., ***mag-m.,*** mang., ***med.,*** medus., merc., merc-c., ***mez., morph.,*** mur-ac., nat-a., ***nat-c., nat-m.,*** nat-p., nit-ac., ***nux-v., olnd.,*** onos., **PH-AC.,** ***phos., pic-ac., plat.,*** plb., ***puls., ran-b.,*** ran-s., **RHOD., RHUS-T.,** rumx., ***sabad.,*** **SEC.,** ***sel., sil.,*** spig., spong., ***staph.,*** sul-ac., **SULPH.,** tab., **TARENT.,** thuj., tub., ***urt-u.,*** valer., ***viol-t., zinc.,*** zinc-m.
beginning at feet and extending upwards - nat-m.
chill, during - gamb.
crawling like a bug or worm - calc., ***coca,*** oena., stram., vario.
clothes, touch agg. - oena.
emission, after - ph-ac.
erection, during - tarent.

FORMICATION, sensation
evening - gent-c., mag-c., **SULPH.**
lying - ***cist.,*** ph-ac.,
undressing - sil.
flesh, between and - cadm-s., phos., sec., zinc.
forenoon - mag-c., sars.
hairs, at root of - ph-ac.
house, on entering - phos.
itching, with - colch.
morning - ferr., mag-c., staph.
night - bar-c., ***cist.,*** mag-m., sulph.
chill, during - gamb.
lying down, after - ***cist.,*** ph-ac.
waking - bar-c.
waking, on - carb-v.
numbness, with - euphr.
paralyzed parts, in - cadm-s., ***phos.,*** plb.
perspiration, during - rhod.
rubbing amel. - sec., zinc.
scratching, agg. - dulc.
amel. - croc., zinc.
sexual excitement, during - mez., tarent.
under skin - cadm-s., ***coca, sec.,*** zinc.
warmth amel. - acon.

FRECKLES - ***am-c., ant-c.,*** ant-t., bad., bry., bufo, ***calc.,*** canth., carb-v., carc., con., dros., ***dulc., ferr., graph.,*** hyos., iod., kali-c., lach., laur., **LYC.,** merc., mez., ***mur-ac., nat-c.,*** nat-p., ***nit-ac.,*** nux-m., petr., **PHOS.,** plb., ***puls.,*** rob., sec., ***sep.,*** sil., **SOL,** stann., ***sulph.,*** tab., thuj., verat.
dark - nit-ac.

FUNGUS, (see Tinea)

GANGLION - am-c., arn., aur-m., ***carb-v.,*** ph-ac., ***phos.,*** plb., rhus-t., ***ruta.,*** sil., sulph., zinc.

GANGRENE, (see Generals)

GNAWING, sensaation - agar., **AGN.,** alum., ambr., anac., ant-c., arg-m., ars., ***bar-c.,*** bell., bism., bry., canth., caps., cham., clem., cocc., con., ***cycl., dig., dros.,*** euph., graph., guai., hell., hyos., kali-c., led., **LYC.,** ***meny.,*** merc., mez., nat-c., nat-p., nux-v., **OLND.,** par., ph-ac., phos., **PLAT.,** puls., ***ran-s.,*** rhod., rhus-t., ***ruta.,*** sep., spig., ***spong.,*** squil., stann., **STAPH.,** sulph., tarax., thuj., ***verat.***
scratching, after - agar., alum., ant-c., bar-c., canth., caps., cycl., dros., kali-c., led., ***lyc.,*** **OLND.,** par., ph-ac., phos., puls., rhus-t., ruta., spong., ***staph.,*** tarax., verat.

GOOSEBUMPS, goose-flesh - ***acon.,*** aesc., aeth., agar., ***ang.,*** ant-t., arg-n., ***ars.,*** asar., aur., bar-c., bar-m., ***bell.,*** berb., bor., bov., ***bry., calc., camph., cann-s.,*** canth., carb-an., ***caust.,*** chel., chlor., ***chin.,*** chin-a., ***croc.,*** crot-t., **HELL.,** ign., kali-i., ***lach.,*** lachn., laur., ***led., lyc.,*** mag-m., mang., **MERC.,** merl., mez., mur-ac., ***nat-m., nat-s.,*** nit-ac., **NUX-V.,** ***par.,*** ped., ***phos.,*** plat., ruta., ***sabad.,*** sabin., sars., ***sil.,*** spig., stann., staph., sul-ac., tab., tarent., ***thuj.,*** tub., **VERAT.**
air, in open - agar., caust., chin., sars.
drinking, after - cadm-s., ***chin.,*** verat.

GOOSEBUMPS,
eating, while - mag-m.
evening - mang.
house, in - calc., tub.
morning - chin-s., mang., sep.
stool, after - grat.
sudden chill with hair standing on end - bar-c., dulc., merc.
walking, while - lyc.
warm room, in - mez.

GRANULATIONS, exuberant - calen., nit-ac., sabin., ***sil.,*** thuj.

GRASPED together, as if - acon., ther.

HAIR, falls out, (see Generals, Hair) - ***alum.,*** ars., ***calc.,*** carb-an., ***carb-v., graph.,*** hell., kali-c., lach., ***nat-m.,*** op., phos., sabin., ***sec., sel.,*** sulph., thal.
hair, unusual parts, on - carc., lyc., med., thuj., thyr., tub.

HAIRY, skin - med., thuj., tub.

HARDNESS, of skin, (see Indurations, Scleroderma) - ***ant-t.,*** calc-f., cist., clem., dulc., graph., petr., phos., ***rhus-t.,*** sars., ***sep.,*** sil.
callosities like, (see Callouses) - am-c., **ANT-C.,** bor., ***dulc.,*** elae., ***ferr-pic.,*** **GRAPH.,** hydr., lach., led., lyc., ***nit-ac.,*** petr., ***ran-b., rhus-t.,*** sal-ac., sars., **SEP.,** ***sil.,*** sulph., ***thuj.***
parchment, like - acon., aeth., **ARS.,** calc-f., camph., ***chin.,*** crot-h., dig., dulc., kali-c., led., ***lith., lyc.,*** op., petr., phos., rhus-t., ***sars., sil.,*** squil.
thickening, with - am-c., anac., **ANT-C.,** ***ars.,*** bor., ***calc.,*** cast-eq., cic., cist., clem., ***dulc.,*** **GRAPH.,** hydr-ac., hydrc., kali-c., ***lach., lyc.,*** par., petr., phos., rad., ***ran-b.,*** **RHUS-T., SEP.,** ***sil.,*** sulph., thuj., verat.
purple, peeling off - am-c., ant-c., bor., dulc., ***graph., lach.,*** ran-b., ***rhus-t., sep., sil.,*** sulph.

HEAT, sensation, without fever - aloe, arn., ars., bell., bor., bry., chin., cocc., coloc., dulc., ***graph.,*** hep., hyos., iod., kali-bi., ***lach.,*** lyc., mag-c., mur-ac., nit-ac., nux-v., phos., puls., rhus-t., sang., sep., sil., sulph.
convulsions, before - bell.
exercising, while - calc., nat-m.
feverish tingling over whole body - cub.
night - fl-ac., **GRAPH.,** nat-m.
scratching, after - spong., sulph.
sex, after - ***graph.***
under skin - ter.
waking, on - fl-ac., nat-m., puls., sil.

HERPES, simplex, (see Generals)
herpes, zoster, shingles (see Generals)

HIDEBOUND, sensation as if - ***crot-t.***

ICE, or ice-cold needles, sensation of - ***agar., ars.***
water on the skin - acon., gels.

ICHTHYOSIS, (see Eruptions, scaly) - agar., ***am-m.,*** anac., ant-c., **ARS.,** ***ars-i., aur., bar-m., bell.,*** bor., bufo, cact., cadm-s., ***calad., calc.,*** calc-s., canth., cic., **CLEM.,** com., cupr., cycl., dulc., ***fl-ac., graph.,*** hep., ***hydrc.,*** hyos., iod., kali-ar., ***kali-bi.,*** kali-c., ***kali-s., led., mag-c., merc.,*** mez., ***nat-a., nat-m., nit-ac., olnd.,*** petr., **PHOS., PHYT.,** ***plb., psor., rhus-t.,*** sang., ***sars.,*** **SEP.,** ***sil.,*** staph., ***sulph.,*** teucr., thuj.

IMPETIGO - aln., alum., am-c., **ANT-C.,** ant-s., ant-t., ***ars.,*** ars-i., arum-t., bar-c., calc., calc-mur., calen., carb-ac., carb-v., caust., cic., clem., con., crot-t., ***dulc.,*** **ECHI.,** euph., graph., ***hep., iris, jug-c., kali-bi.,*** kali-n., kreos., lact., lyc., maland., merc., ***mez.,*** nat-c., nat-m., ***nit-ac.,*** olnd., ***ph-ac.,*** phos., ***rhus-t.,*** rhus-v., sars., sep., ***sil.,*** staph., sulph., thuj., tub., viol-t.
face - **ANT-C.,** ars., calc., ***cic., con., crot-t., dulc., graph., hep., kali-bi.,*** kreos., ***lyc., merc., mez., nit-ac., rhus-t.,*** sep., ***viol-t.***
head - ***ant-c.,*** bar-c., calc-p., ***caust.,*** con., ***iris,*** **MERC.,** ***petr.,*** rhus-t., rhus-v., sil., sulph., ***viol-t.***
margin of the hair - ***nat-m.***
forehead - ant-c., kreos., led., ***merc., rhus-t.,*** sep., sulph., ***viol-t.***
lips - ***ant-c., ars., echi.,*** tarent.
around - ***ant-c., ars.,*** tarent.

INACTIVITY, of skin (see Dryness) - **ALUM.,** ambr., **ANAC.,** ant-c., ant-t., ***ars.,*** ars-i., bell., ***bry., calc.,*** camph., carb-an., carb-v., caust., cham., chin., cocc., **CON.,** cycl., dig., ***dulc.,*** graph., hell., hep., iod., ***ip.,*** **KALI-C., KALI-P.,** kali-s., lach., ***laur.,*** led., **LYC.,** merc., mur-ac., ***nat-c., nat-m., nat-p., nit-ac.,*** nux-v., ***olnd.,*** op., petr., **PH-AC.,** phos., plat., plb., ***psor.,*** puls., rhod., rhus-t., ruta., sabin., sars., ***sec.,*** sep., ***sil.,*** spong., squil., staph., stram., ***sulph.,*** thuj., verat., zinc.

INDENTED, easily from pressure - **APIS,** ars., **BOV.,** caps., phos., verat.

INDURATIONS, of (see Hardness) - ***agar.,*** am-c., ant-c., arg-n., ars., ***ars-i.,*** aur., ***bar-c.,*** bor., bufo, calc., ***carb-an.,*** caul., caust., ***chel.,*** chin., cic., cinnb., ***clem.,*** con., ***dulc., graph.,*** guai., ***iod., kali-c.,*** kali-s., lach., ***led.,*** lyc., mag-c., mag-m., ***mang., merc.,*** mez., ***mur-ac.,*** par., phos., ***puls., ran-b.,*** rhod., **RHUS-T.,** ruta, sars., **SEP., SIL.,** squil., ***staph.,*** **SULPH.,** ther., ***thuj.,*** tub., verat.
bluish - ***mang.,*** mur-ac.
spots - ***phos., sars.***
burning - ***hep.***
after scratching - staph.
chagrin, after - ***coloc.***
hard - kali-i., mag-c., nat-s., sil.
burning - hep.
joints, around - form.
painful - phyt.
red and sore - petr.
horny - ***ant-c.,*** graph.
itching - staph.
moist, after scratching - staph.
red - med., sabad., trinit.
hard and tender - petr.

INDURATIONS, of
scratching, after - kali-c
site of an old boil - lyc.
stitching - caust..
under - alum., kali-a., mag-c.

INELASTICTY, (see Scleroderma) - ant-c., ars., ***bov.,*** calc., ***cupr.,*** dulc., graph., lach., ran-b., ***rhus-t.,*** sep., verat.
morphea - ars., ***phos.,*** sil.

INFLAMMATION, (see Dermatitis)

INTERTRIGO, (see Dermatitis) - acon., ***aeth.,*** agn., ***ambr., am-c.,*** arn., ars., ***bar-c.,*** bell., ***bor.,*** calc., ***calc-s., carb-v.,*** **CAUST.,** ***cham., chin.,*** fago., **GRAPH.,** ***hep., hydr., ign.,*** jug-r., kali-ar., kali-br., ***kali-c.,*** kali-chl., **KREOS.,** ***lyc., mang., merc.,*** mez., morg., ***nat-m., nit-ac.,*** nux-v., ol-an., olnd., ox-ac., ***petr.,*** ph-ac., phos., ***phyt.,*** plb., psor., puls., rhus-t., ruta, sabin., ***sep., sil.,*** squil., **SULPH.,** ***sul-ac.,*** syc-co., syph., tub.
dentition, during - caust.

IRRITABLE - rad-br.

ITCHING - acon., **AGAR.,** ***agn.,*** ail., aloe, ***alum., ambr., am-c.,*** am-m., anac., anac-oc., anag., ***anan., anthr., ant-c.,*** ant-t., ***antipyrin.,*** **APIS,** ***arg-m.,*** arn., **ARS.,** ***ars-i.,*** asaf., asar., ***astac.,*** aur., aur-m., aur-m-n., ***bar-c.,*** bar-m., bell., bism., bor., **BOV.,** ***bry., calad., calc., calc-p.,*** calc-s., camph., cann-s., canth., caps., ***carb-ac., carb-an.,*** **CARB-V., CARB-S., CAUST.,** cham., **CHEL.,** chin., ***chin-a.,*** **CHLOL.,** chlor., chrysar., ***cic.,*** cina, cinnb., ***cist., clem., cocc.,*** coc-c., coff., colch., coll., coloc., ***con.,*** croc., ***crot-h., crot-t., cupr.,*** cupr-ar., ***cycl., dig.,*** dios., **DOL.,** dros., ***dulc.,*** elae., elat., euph., euphr., ***fago., fl-ac.,*** form., ***gall-ac., gamb., gels.,*** glon., gran., **GRAPH.,** grin., guai., guano, hell., hep., hyos., ***hydrc.,*** hyper., ichth., ign., indg., iod., ***ip.,*** jug-c., ***jug-r., kali-ar., kali-bi.,*** kali-br., ***kali-c.,*** kali-n., kali-p., ***kali-s., kreos., lach.,*** laur., ***led.,*** **LYC., MAG-C.,** mag-m., maland., mang., ***med.,*** meny., **MERC.,** merc-i-f., **MEZ.,** mosch., mur-ac., ***nat-a., nat-c.,*** **NAT-M.,** nat-p., ***nat-s.,*** nicc., ***nit-ac., nux-v., olnd.,*** **OL-AN.,** ***op.,*** ped., ***petr.,*** ph-ac., ***phos., pix., plat.,*** prim-o., plb., **PSOR.,** ptel., **PULS.,** pulx., rad-br., ran-b., ran-s., rheum, rhod., **RHUS-T.,** ***rhus-v., rumx., ruta., sabad.,*** sabin., sal-ac., samb., ***sars.,*** sec., sel., seneg., **SEP., SIL.,** spig., **SPONG.,** ***squil.,*** stann., **STAPH.,** stram., stront-c., **SULPH.,** sul-ac., sul-i., syzyg., ***tab.,*** tarax., **TARENT.,** tarent-c., tell., teucr., ***thuj., til.,*** **TUB., URT-U.,** valer., verat., ***vesp.,*** viol-o., ***viol-t.,*** visc., xero, zinc.

air, cold, agg. - apis, cadm-s., dulc., ***hep.,*** kali-ar., lac-ac., nat-s., nit-ac., ***olnd.,*** petr., rhus-t., ***rumx.,*** sep., spong., ***staph.,*** tell., ***tub.***
amel. - berb., fago., graph., ***kali-bi.,*** mez., stroph.

air, open, agg. - ars., hep., olnd., petr., ***rumx.***
amel. - stront-c.

alcoholics - carb-v., lach., nux-v., sulph.

bathing, after - bov., calc., clem., ***mag-c.***
agg. - ***mag-c.***

ITCHING, general

bathing, after
amel. - clem.
cold agg.- ***fago.***
hot amel. - rhus-t., syph.

bed, in - kali-ar., led., pic-ac., ***psor.,*** sil., ***sulph.***

biting - **AGAR.,** ***agn.,*** alum., am-c., ***am-m.,*** ant-c., arn., bar-m., berb., bell., bor., ***bov., bry., calc.,*** calc-p., camph., canth., caps., carb-an., ***carb-v., caust.,*** cham., chel., chin., cimic., cocc., coc-c., colch., coloc., ***con.,*** dros., ***dulc., euph.,*** hell., ip., kali-n., ***lach.,*** **LED.,** ***lyc.,*** mag-c., mang., ***merc., mez.,*** mur-ac., ***nat-c.,*** nat-m., nat-p., nicc., ***nux-v.,*** **OLND., OL-AN.,** op., ***paeon., petr., ph-ac.,*** phos., plat., ***psor.,*** ptel., **PULS.,** ran-b., ran-s., rhod., rhus-t., ***rumx.,*** ruta., sel., sep., ***sil.,*** spig., ***spong.,*** stront-c., ***sulph., tarent., tell., thuj.,*** **URT-U.,** verat., viol-t., zinc.
perspiration, after - cocc., mang.

bleeding, after scratching - sulph.
ceases when itching - alum., ***ars., crot-t.,*** murx., pix., psor., sep., ***sulph.,*** til.

burning - ***acon., agar., agn.,*** alum., ambr., am-c., anac., ant-c., ***apis,*** arg-m., arn., **ARS.,** ars-i., asaf., aur., ***bar-c., bell.,*** berb., bism., ***bov.,*** **BRY.,** ***calad., calc., calc-p.,*** calc-s., camph., cann-s., ***canth.,*** caps., carb-an., carb-v., ***caust.,*** cham., chin., chin-a., ***cic.,*** cinnb., **CHLOL.,** clem., cocc., coff., colch., coloc., ***com., con.,*** cupr., dig., dros., dulc., euph., **GRAPH.,** guai., hell., ***hep.,*** hyos., ign., iod., ***jug-c., kali-ar., kali-bi., kali-c.,*** kali-n., ***kali-s.,*** kreos., **LACH.,** lachn., laur., led., **LYC.,** mag-c., mang., meny., ***merc., mez.,*** mur-ac., nat-a., nat-c., nat-m., nat-p., nit-ac., nux-v., olnd., op., pall., petr., phel., ph-ac., ***phos.,*** plat., plb., **PULS.,** ran-b., rhod., **RHUS-T.,** ruta., sabad., samb., sars., sec., sel., seneg., ***sep.,*** **SIL.,** ***spig.,*** spong., ***squil.,*** stann., staph., stram., stront-c., **SULPH.,** sul-ac., teucr., thuj., ***urt-u.,*** valer., verat., viol-o., viol-t., zinc.
as from nettles - bry., calc-p., **CHLOL.,** cocc., **URT-U.**
ceases when itching - alum., ***ars., crot-t.,*** murx., pix., psor., sep., ***sulph.,*** til.
night - ***bov.,*** lachn., ***mez., til.***

changing site of itching, followed by - mez., ***staph.***

chill, during - ***hep., petr.***
after - graph.

cold, agg. - clem., thuj., tub.
amel. - berb., calad., fago., graph., mez.

cold, air, in - apis, cadm-s., kali-ar., lac-ac., nit-ac., ***rumx.,*** sep., spong., ***staph.,*** tell., ***tub.***
amel. - ***kali-bi.***

contact, from, agg. - ran-b.

crawling - ***acon.,*** **AGAR.,** agn., ***alum.,*** ambr., am-c., ant-c., ***arg-m., arn.,*** ars., asaf., aur., ***bar-c.,*** bell., bor., bov., bry., calad., calc., calc-s., camph., cann-s., canth., caps., ***carb-s.,*** carb-v., ***caust.,*** chel., chin., cina, cocc., **COLCH.,** ***con.,*** croc., ***dig.,*** euphr., graph.,

ITCHING, general

crawling - guai., hep., ign., kali-ar., ***kali-c.,*** kali-p., kali-s., lach., laur., led., **LYC.,** mag-c., mag-m., mang., ***merc.,*** mur-ac., nat-a., ***nat-c.,*** nat-m., nat-p., nit-ac., ***nux-v., olnd.,*** pall., par., ***ph-ac.,*** phos., **PLAT., PLB., PULS.,** ***ran-b.,*** ran-s., ***rhod.,*** **RHUS-T.,** ***sabad.,*** sabin., ***sec.,*** sel., **SEP.,** ***sil.,*** **SPIG.,** spong., squil., **STAPH., SULPH.,** sul-ac., **TARENT.,** teucr., thuj., verat., viol-t., zinc.

despair, from - **PSOR.**

desquamation, with - clem.

diabetes, in - mang.

eating, while - crot-t.

after - calc-p.

amel. - chel.

elderly, people - alum., ars., bar-ac., dol., dulc., fago., merc., ***mez., olnd., psor., sulph.,*** urt-u.

senile - dol., fago.

erosive - ruta.

eruptions, had been, where - calc-ac.

without - **ALUM., ARS.,** cist., cupr., **DOL.,** ***gels.,*** lach., med., ***merc.,*** **MEZ.,** ***petr., psor., sulph.,*** thyr.

night, agg. - thyr.

evening - alum., am-m., anac., ant-c., apis, calad., ***carb-an.,*** carb-v., chin., cocc., coloc., ***con.,*** cycl., fl-ac., kali-c., kali-n., **KREOS.,** lyc., mag-m., med., ***merc.,*** mez., mur-ac., ***nux-v.,*** olnd., ***puls.,*** sars., sel., sil., thuj., zinc.

amel. - cact.

bed, in - ***alum.,*** ang., bar-c., bell., calad., calc., camph., ***carb-an.,*** carb-v., coloc., con., cycl., kali-n., lyc., merc., mez., mur-ac., nat-c., nux-v., ph-ac., plat., ***puls.,*** sars., tell., thuj., til., zinc.

amel. - kali-c., sars.

excitement, on - bry.

exertion, after - ***nat-m.***

fever, during - kali-br.

folds of skin - sel.

hairy parts - dol., fago., rhus-t.

heat, after flushes of - sep.

of stove amel. - clem., ***rumx.,*** **TUB.**

here and there - am-c.

intolerable - podo.

intense - cub.

jaundice, during - dol., ***hep.,*** myric., pic-ac., ran-b., thyr., trinit.

jerking - calc., ***carb-s.,*** caust., ***lyc.,*** nat-m., puls., rhus-t.

lying, amel. - urt-u.

meat, after eating - rumx., ruta

menopause, during - calad.

menses, during - ***graph., kali-c.,*** phos.

after - con., lyc., ***tarent.***

amel., during - cycl.

before - calc., ***graph.,*** hep., inul., kali-c., ***sil.,*** sulph.

mental exertion - ***agar.***

ITCHING, general

morning - am-c., kali-c., ***rhus-t.,*** sars., staph., stram., sulph.

bed, in - ***calc.,*** coloc., petr., ***rhus-t.,*** spong., sulph.

rising, on - coloc., hep., ***rumx.,*** ruta, ***sars.***

waking, on - coloc., led., spong., stram.

mosquito bite, after - calad., led.

nausea, with - calad., ip., lob.

before - sang.

must scratch until he vomits - ***ip.***

nervous - arg-m.

night - ail., am-c., am-m., arg-n., bar-c., berb., bov., **CARB-S.,** cadm-s., card-m., ***caust.,*** **CHLOL.,** ***cist., clem.,*** cocc., croc., ***dol.,*** dulc., euphr., gamb., gels., ***graph.,*** iris, kali-ar., ***kali-bi.,*** kreos., ***lach.,*** lachn., ***led.,*** lyss., mag-c., manc., merc., merc-i-f., ***mez.,*** nux-v., olnd., petr., phos., plan., plat., puls., sars., ***sil.,*** stram., **SULPH.,** thuj., **URT-U.,** zinc.

12 pm to 3 am - dulc.

noon - ***alum.,*** ant-c., ***ars.,*** asim., bell-p., bov., carb-v., card-m., cist., dulc., jug-c., ***kali-ar.,*** kreos., led., lyc., ***menis.,*** merc., merc-i-f., ***mez., nat-s., olnd.,*** psor., puls., rhus-t., rumx., sang., sep., sulph., tub.

orifices, of - fl-ac.

overheated, when - ign., ***lyc.***

pain ceases, when - alum., ***ars., crot-t.,*** ign., lyc., murx., pix., psor., sep., stront-c., sulph., til.

alternating, with - stroph.

scratching, after - ars., bar-c., sulph.

painful - bar-c., sil., sulph.

parts - carb-s., ign., thuj.

paralyzed, parts, in - phos.

paroxysmal - cortiso.

parts, affected, over - agar.

lain on - carb-v., chin., con.

not lain on - chin.

suffering - dig.

perspiration, agg. - **MANG-M., MANG-M., MERC.,** mur-ac., nat-m., rhod.

perspiring, parts - all-s., am-c., benz-ac., calc., cann-s., cedr., ***cham.,*** coloc., fl-ac., ip., led., ***lyc.,*** **MANG.,** op., par., rhod., rhus-t., sabad., spong., sulph.

pleasurable - sulph.

prairie itch - led., rhus-t., rumx., sulph.

pregnancy, in - chlol., cocc., dol., sabin., sep., tab.

prickling, with - lob.

prurigo - acon., aln., ***ambr.,*** anthr., ***ars., ars-i.,*** carb-ac., chlor., dios., dol., kali-bi., ***lyc., merc., mez., nit-ac., olnd.,*** ped., ***rhus-t., rhus-v., rumx.,*** sil., sulph., ter.

respiration, with short - lob.

right, side - con.

rubbing, changes place on - tub.

gently, from, amel. - crot-t., dios., med.

ITCHING, general

scratch, must - agar., arg-m., coff., psor., staph.

until it bleeds, must - ***agar., alum., arg-m.,*** **ARS.,** ***bar-c., bov., chlol.,*** carb-v., kali-n., led., ***med.,*** mez., nit-ac., phos., ***psor., puls.***

until it is raw - ***agar., alum.,*** am-c., ant-c., arn., bar-c., bov., calc., ***carb-s.,*** caust., chin., dros., **GRAPH.,** hep., kali-c., kreos., ***lach., lyc.,*** mang., merc., ***olnd.,*** **PETR.,** phos., plb., ***psor.,*** puls., ***rhus-t.,*** ruta., sabin., ***sep.,*** sil., squil., ***sulph.,*** sul-ac., ***til.***

scratching, agg. - ***agar., alum.,*** am-m., **ANAC.,** anag., ***arg-m.,*** arn., **ARS.,** asar., bar-c., berb., ***bism., bov., calad.,*** calc., cann-s., canth., **CAPS.,** carb-an., carb-v., ***caust.,*** cham., chel., cinnb., coff., ***con.,*** crot-t., cupr., ***dol.,*** dros., graph., guai., ip., kali-c., kreos., lach., lachn., ***led.,*** lyss., mag-c., mang., merc., ***mez.,*** mur-ac., nat-a., olnd., nat-c., par., ph-ac., phos., phyt., **PULS., RHUS-T.,** rhus-v., sars., seneg., sep., ***sil.,*** spig., spong., squil., stann., ***staph.,*** stram., ***stront-c.,*** **SULPH.,** ***til.,*** tub.

bumps form, after - ***dulc.,*** lach., ***mez., rhus-t.,*** verat.

changes, places - mez., staph.

eruptions, follows - am-c., olnd.

moisture, follows - graph., olnd., rad-br., rhus-t., sel.

amel. - agar., ***ang.,*** alum., ambr., am-c., am-m., anac., ant-c., ant-t., apis, arn., ars., **ASAF.,** bell., bor., bov., ***brom., bry.,*** cadm-s., **CALC.,** calc-s., camph., ***cann-s., canth.,*** caps., carb-an., caust., chel., chin., cic., ***cina,*** clem., coloc., com., con., ***crot-t.,*** **CYCL.,** dig., ***dros.,*** form., ***guai.,*** hep., hydr., ***ign., jug-c.,*** kali-ar., ***kali-c.,*** kali-n., kali-s., ***kreos.,*** laur., led., ***mag-c.,*** mag-m., ***mang.,*** meny., merc., mez., mosch., **MUR-AC., NAT-C.,** nat-p., nit-ac., nux-v., ***olnd.,*** ph-ac., **PHOS.,** plat., ***plb.,*** prun., ran-b., ***rhus-t., ruta.,*** sabad., sabin., sal-ac., samb., ***sars.,*** sec., sel., seneg., ***sep.,*** spig., spong., stann., staph., squil., ***sulph.,*** sul-ac., tarax., ***thuj.,*** valer., viol-t., ***zinc.***

changing place, on - ***agar.,*** alum., anac., arn., asaf., calc., ***canth.,*** carb-an., chel., con., cycl., ***ign.,*** mag-c., mag-m., ***mez.,*** pall., sars., ***spong., staph., sul-ac.,*** tub., zinc.

unchanged by - acon., agar., agn., ***alum.,*** ambr., am-c., am-m., ant-c., ant-t., ***arg-m.,*** arn., asaf., aur., ***bar-c.,*** bell., bism., bor., ***bov., calad.,*** camph., carb-an., carb-v., caust., cham., chel., cina, clem., cocc., coff., colch., coloc., croc., cupr., dig., euph., euphr., ***hell.,*** hyos., iod., ***ip.,*** laur., ***mag-m., med.,*** mur-ac., nat-c., nux-v., op., ***plat.,*** prun., **PULS.,** ***ran-s.,*** rheum, rhus-t., ruta., samb., sars., sec., seneg., sil., ***spig.,*** **SPONG.,** stann., stram., sul-ac., tarax., teucr., valer.

ITCHING, general

sex, after - ***agar.***

sleep, during - am-c., ars., ***bar-c.,*** carb-v., caust., con., dulc., mag-m., ***phos.,*** sars., ***sulph.,*** zinc.

on going to sleep - ***osm.***

smarting - alum., ambr., am-m., ***arg-m.,*** arg-n., aur., berb., bry., calc., cann-s., colch., dros., ***graph.,*** hep., kali-c., led., lyc., mag-c., mang., merc., mez., mur-ac., nat-c., nux-v., olnd., par., petr., **PLAT.,** puls., ***rhus-t.,*** ruta., sabin., sars., ***sep.,*** sil., squil., staph., ***sulph.,*** valer., verat., ***zinc.***

spots - agn., alum., am-m., arn., aster., ***berb.,*** caps., ***con.,*** dros., euph., ***fl-ac., graph., iod.,*** jug-c., ***kali-c., lach., led., lyc.,*** merc., mez., ***nat-m., nit-ac.,*** op., par., sep., ***sil.,*** spong., **SULPH.,** ***sul-ac., zinc.***

liver spots - ***caust.***

perspire, which - ***tell.***

spring, in the - fl-ac., lach.

month of march - fl-ac.

stinging - acon., ***agar.,*** agn., alum., am-c., anac., ant-c., **APIS,** arg-m., ***arn.,*** ars., ars-i., asaf., asar., aur., ***bar-c.,*** bell., bov., **BRY.,** calad., calc., camph., cann-s., canth., caps., carb-an., carb-s., carb-v., ***caust.,*** cham., chel., chin., **CHLOL.,** clem., ***cocc.,*** coc-c., coff., colch., ***con., cop.,*** crot-h., ***cycl.,*** dig., ***dros.,*** dulc., euph., euphr., **GRAPH.,** guai., hell., hep., hyos., ign., iod., kali-ar., ***kali-c.,*** kali-n., kali-p., kali-s., kreos., lach., laur., led., lyc., mag-c., mag-m., mang., meny., ***merc.,*** mez., mosch., ***mur-ac.,*** nat-c., ***nat-m.,*** nat-p., nit-ac., nux-v., olnd., op., par., petr., ph-ac., phos., plat., plb., **PULS.,** ran-b., ran-s., rheum, rhod., **RHUS-T.,** ruta., ***sabad.,*** sabin., samb., sars., sel., ***sep., sil., spig.,*** **SPONG.,** squil., ***stann., staph.,*** stram., stront-c., ***sulph.,*** sul-ac., tarax., tell., teucr., ***thuj., til.,*** **URT-U.,** verat., **VIOL-T.,** zinc.

evening - petr., sars.

in bed - nat-m.

morning, on rising - sars.

scratching, after - sulph.

suppressed eruptions, after - ***ars.***

tearing - ***bell.,*** bry., ***lyc.,*** sil., ***staph.,*** sulph., zinc.

scratching, after - bell.

thinking of it agg. - med.

tickling - acon., agar., alum., ***ambr.,*** am-m., apis, ***arg-m.,*** bry., bufo, calc., canth., caps., caust., ***cham.,*** chel., chin., cist., cocc., ***colch.,*** con., dig., dros., euph., euphr., ferr., hyos., ign., **IOD.,** ip., kali-bi., kali-c., ***lach.,*** mang., ***merc.,*** mur-ac., nat-m., **NUX-V., PHOS.,** ***plat.,*** prun., ***puls.,*** ran-b., ***rhus-t., rumx.,*** ruta, ***sabad.,*** sang., sec., sel., ***sep.,*** **SIL.,** ***spig.,*** spong., squil., stann., staph., ***sulph.,*** sumb., tarax., teucr.

intolerable - coc-c.

scratching, after - agar., ambr., caps., chin., cocc., merc., **SABAD.,** ***sil.,*** spig., teucr.

ITCHING, general

touched, when - cadm-met., cocc., mez., nat-m., rhus-t.

undressing, agg. - ***alum.,*** am-m., anac., ant-c., ***ars.,*** asim., bell-p., bov., cact., carb-v., carc., card-m., cist., ***cocc., dros.,*** dulc., gamb., hep., hyper., jug-c., kali-ar., kali-br., kreos., led., lyc., mag-c., med., menis., ***merc.,*** merc-i-f., mez., mur-ac., nat-m., ***nat-s.,*** nit-ac., nux-v., ***olnd.,*** pall., ph-ac., ***psor.,*** puls., rhod., rhus-t., **RUMX.,** sang., sep., sil., stann., ***staph.,*** sulph., tell., ***tub.***

violent - agar., dros., dulc., graph., ip., lach., merc., mez., op., ***psor., sulph.,*** ther.

voluptuous - ambr., anac., arg-m., meny., ***merc.,*** mur-ac., plat., puls., rhus-t., sabad., sep., ***sil.,*** spig., spong., **SULPH.**

vomits, not relieved until he - ***ip.***

walking, in open air - cinnb., ***sulph.***

wandering - ***agar., bar-c.,*** berb., camph., ***canth.,*** caust., cham., ***con.,*** dulc., graph., jug-c., kali-c., mag-m., mang., ***merc.,*** mez., olnd., ***puls.,*** rat., rhus-v., sil., spong., staph., ***sulph.,*** tub., zinc.

warm, on becoming agg. - ***aeth., alum.,*** arg-n., bov., clem., cob., cocc., com., ***dol.,*** gels., ign., ***kali-ar., led., lyc.,*** mang., **MERC.,** mez., mur-ac., ***nat-a.,*** **PSOR.,** ***puls.,*** sars., **SULPH., URT-U.**

becoming, in bed - ***aeth., alum., anac., ant-c., apis,*** arg-n., ***ars.,*** asim., bar-c., bell-p., ***bov.,*** cadm-s., calad., ***calc.,*** calc-s., carb-an., ***carb-s., carb-v.,*** card-m., caust., cinnb., cist., ***clem.,*** cob., ***cocc.,*** coloc., cupr-ar., ***cycl.,*** dulc., ***gels., graph.,*** jug-c., ***kali-ar., kali-bi.,*** kali-br., kali-c., kali-chl., ***kali-s.,*** kreos., ***led., lyc.,*** lyss., mag-c., menis., ***merc.,*** merc-i-f., ***mez.,*** mur-ac., ***nat-m., nat-p., nat-s.,*** nux-v., ***olnd.,*** ph-ac., ***phos.,*** **PSOR.,** ***puls., rhus-t., rumx.,*** sang., sars., ***sep.,*** spong., **SULPH.,** thuj., ***til.,*** tub., ***urt-u.,*** zinc.

warmth amel. - apis, ars., caust., dulc., hep., kali-ar., kali-c., kreos., mang., nat-s., nit-ac., petr., psor., rhus-t., ***rumx.,*** sars., sep., sil., spong., staph., still., tell., **TUB.**

fire, of - tub.

washing, cold water agg., with - clem., tub.

hot water amel., with - rhus-t., rhus-v.

wiping with hand amel. - dros.

wool agg. - com., ***hep.,*** morg., phos., **PSOR.,** puls., **SULPH.,** tub.

JAUNDICE, (see Yellow skin)

KELOIDS, (see Scars) - alumn., ars., ***bad.,*** bell-p., calc., ***calen.,*** carb-v., **CARC.,** ***caust.,*** crot-h., ***fl-ac.,*** **GRAPH.,** hyper., ***iod.,*** junc., lach., merc., nit-ac., nux-v., phos., phyt., psor., rhus-t., sabin., **SIL.,** sul-ac., sulph., ***thiosin.,*** tub., vip-t.

LEPROSY, skin - alum., anac., ant-t., ***ars., bad.,*** bar-c., ***calc.,*** calo., ***carb-ac., carb-an., carb-s., carb-v., caust., chaul.,*** com., con., crot-h., cupr-ac., cur., ***dip.,*** elae., form., ***graph.,*** guano, haem., hell., ***ho.,*** hura, ***hydrc.,*** iod., ***iris,*** jatr.,

LEPROSY, skin - kali-c., ***kali-i., lach.,*** mag-c., mang., ***meph.,*** merc., ***nat-c.,*** nat-m., nit-ac., ***nuph.,*** oena., petr., ***phos., pip-m., psor.,*** **SEC.,** ***sep., sil.,*** **SULPH.,** thyr., ***tub.,*** zinc.

spots, on

buttocks, annular - ***graph.***

chin - calc.

face - ***ant-t., graph.,*** phos., **SEC.**

leg - ***graph., nat-c.***

LICE - am-c., ars., lach., ***lyc., merc.,*** nit-ac., olnd., ***psor., sabad.,*** staph., ***sulph.,*** vinc.

head, of - am-c., apis, ars., bell-p., ***carb-ac.,*** lach., led., lyc., ***merc.,*** nit-ac., olnd., ***psor.,*** **STAPH.,** sulph., tub., vinc.

LICHEN, planus - agar., anac., ***ant-c.,*** apis, ***ars., ars-i.,*** chin-a., iod., ***jug-c., kali-bi.,*** kali-i., led., merc., sars., staph., ***sul-i.***

lichen, simplex - alum., am-m., ***anan.,*** ant-c., apis, ***ars., bell.,*** bov., bry., ***calad.,*** cast-v., dulc., ***jug-c.,*** kali-ar., ***kreos.,*** lach., ***led., lyc.,*** merc., nabal., nat-c., ***phyt., plan., rumx.,*** sep., sul-i., ***sulph.,*** thuj., til.

LIVER spots, brown - am-c., ***ant-c.,*** ant-t., ***arg-n.,*** arn., ***ars.,*** ars-i., ***aur.,*** bad., bor., bry., cadm-s., calc., calc-p., calc-s., canth., ***carb-s., carb-v.,*** caust., ***con.,*** cop., cor-r., crot-h., **CUR.,** dros., ***dulc.,*** ferr., ferr-i., graph., ***hyos., iod.,*** kali-ar., kali-bi., kali-c., kali-p., **LACH.,** ***laur.,*** **LYC., MERC.,** merc-i-r., ***mez.,*** nat-a., ***nat-c.,*** nat-p., **NIT-AC.,** ***nux-v.,*** petr., ***phos., plb.,*** puls., ruta., sabad., **SEP.,** sil., stann., **SULPH.,** sul-ac., tarent., ***thuj., tub.***

elevated - caust.

gray - ***iod.***

inflamed - ferr.

itching - caust., lyc., sulph.

spots - berb., sabin., ***sec.***

LOOSE, sensation as if the skin were hanging - ant-c., bell., kreos., **PHOS.,** sabad.

LUPUS - agar., alum., alumn., ant-c., arg-n., **ARS.,** ars-i., aur-m., ***bar-c.,*** bell., calc., ***carb-ac., carb-v., caust.,*** cic., ***cist.,*** graph., guare., hep., ***hydrc.,*** kali-ar., ***kali-bi.,*** kali-c., ***kali-chl., kali-s., kreos.,*** lach., **LYC.,** mag-arct., merc-i-r., ***nat-m.,*** **NIT-AC.,** ol-j., ***phyt., psor.,*** rhus-t., sabin., sep., ***sil.,*** spong., staph., sulph., **THUJ.**

lupus, erythematosum - apis, cist., guare., ***hydrc., kali-bi.,*** paull., ***phos.,*** sep., ***thyr.***

lupus, face - alumn., ***arg-n.,*** **ARS.,** aur-m., carb-ac., ***carb-v.,*** cist., **HYDRC.,** kali-ar., ***kali-bi.,*** kali-chl., kreos., lach., psor., ***sep., sil.***

lupus, vulgaris - abr., apis, ***ars., ars-i.,*** aur-i., ***aur-m.,*** calc., calc-i., calc-s., ***cist.,*** cund., ferr-pic., form., graph., guare., ***hep., hydr., hydrc.,*** irid., kali-bi., kali-i., lyc., nit-ac., paull., phyt., staph., ***sulph.,*** thiosin., thuj., ***tub.,*** urea, x-ray.

MEASLES, (see Fevers)

MENSES, before, agg. the skin - bor., carb-v., ***dulc., graph.,*** kali-c., mag-m., ***nat-m.,*** sang., sars., ***sep.,*** stram., verat.

MOISTURE - alum., ars., bar-c., bell., ***bov.***, bry., calc., carb-an., **CARB-V.**, caust., cic., ***clem.***, con., cub., dulc., **GRAPH.**, hell., hep., kali-ar., ***kali-c.***, ***kreos.***, ***lach.***, ***led.***, **LYC.**, merc., mez., nat-c., nat-m., nit-ac., olnd., ***petr.***, ph-ac., phos., **RHUS-T.**, ruta, sabin., ***sel.***, ***sep.***, sil., squil., ***staph.***, sulph., sul-ac., tarax., thuj., viol-t.
scratching, after - ***alum.***, ars., bar-c., bell., bov., bry., calc., carb-an., ***carb-v.***, caust., cic., cocc., con., dulc., **GRAPH.**, hell., hep., kali-ar., ***kali-c.***, kali-s., ***kreos.***, **LACH.**, led., **LYC.**, merc., ***mez.***, nat-c., nat-m., nit-ac., ***olnd.***, ***petr.***, **RHUS-T.**, ruta., sabin., sars., sel., ***sep.***, sil., squil., ***staph.***, sulph., sul-ac., tarax., thuj., viol-t.
spots - ant-c., carb-v., ***hell.***, kali-c., lach., led., petr., sabin., sel., **SIL.**, ***sulph.***, tarax., vinc.

MOLES, (see Discoloration, Excrescences) - ***calc.***, carb-v., ***carc.***, graph., nit-ac., petr., ph-ac., **PULS.**, **SEP.**, sil., sol., ***sulph.***, sul-ac., tarent., **THUJ.**
itching and stinging - thuj.

MOULD forming over body, as if - sil.

MOLLUSCUM contagiosum, (see Generals)

MOTTLED, skin - **AIL.**, ars., bapt., bell., ***carb-v.***, con., ***crot-h.***, glon., kali-bi., kali-m., **LACH.**, led., lil-t., manc., ***nat-m.***, ***nux-v.***, ox-ac., phos., puls., rhus-t., sars., sulph., syph., ***thuj.***, verat-v.

NETWORK, of blood vessels - berb., ***calc.***, ***carb-v.***, ***caust.***, ***crot-h.***, clem., lach., lyc., nat-m., ox-ac., plat., sabad., stram., thuj.

NEVI, (see Birthmarks)

NODULES, (see Tubercles) - ***agar.***, am-c., ant-c., arg-n., ars., ***ars-i.***, aur., ***bar-c.***, bor., bufo, calc., ***carb-an.***, caul., caust., ***chel.***, chin., cic., cinnb., ***clem.***, con., ***dulc.***, ***graph.***, guai., ***iod.***, ***kali-c.***, kali-s., lach., ***led.***, lyc., mag-c., mag-m., ***mang.***, ***merc.***, mez., ***mur-ac.***, par., phos., ***puls.***, ***ran-b.***, rhod., **RHUS-T.**, ruta, sars., **SEP.**, **SIL.**, squil., ***staph.***, **SULPH.**, ther., ***thuj.***, tub., verat.
bluish - ***mang.***, mur-ac.
spots - ***phos.***, ***sars.***
burning - ***hep.***
after scratching - staph.
chagrin, after - ***coloc.***
hard - kali-i., mag-c., nat-s., sil.
burning - hep.
joints, around - form.
painful - phyt.
red and sore - petr.
horny - ***ant-c.***, graph.
itching - staph.
moist, after scratching - staph.
red - med., sabad., trinit.
hard and tender - petr.
scratching, after - kali-c
site of an old boil - lyc.
stitching - caust..
under - alum., kali-a., mag-c.

NUMBNESS - acon., ***ambr.***, **ANAC.**, ant-t., arg-n., cann-i., cham., con., ***crot-c.***, cycl., euphr., ***hyos.***, lach., ***lyc.***, ***nux-v.***, ***olnd.***, ***ph-ac.***, phos., plat., plb., ***puls.***, **SEC.**, sep., stram., sulph.
itching, after - cycl.
morning, on waking - ***ambr.***
scratching, after - ambr., ***anac.***, cham., con., cycl., ***lach.***, lyc., **OLND.**, ph-ac., phos., plb., sep., ***sulph.***
spots, in - bufo.

ODOR, offensive, (see Perspiration)

OOZING - ***calc.***, ***gran.***, ***lyc.***, ***merc.***, ***petr.***, ***sul-ac.***

PAIN, general
bones, near - cycl., merc., sang.
cold, to - agar., aur., plb., rhus-t.
in cold open air - rhus-t.
pressure, amel. - ign.
scratching, after - agar., ***alum.***, ***ars.***, **BAR-C.**, bell., calc., caps., chin., cocc., con., euphr., kreos., led., nat-m., nux-v., par., ***petr.***, ph-ac., plb., puls., rhus-t., sel., sep., **SIL.**, squil., staph., **SULPH.**, thuj., verat.
spots - aloe, **SULPH.**

PARCHMENT, like, (see Hard)

PELLAGRA - ***ars.***, ars-s-r., bov., chin., gels., hep., ped., psor., ***sec.***, ***sedi.***, sulph.
cachexia, with - ars., sec.
fissures, desquamation, skin eruptions - graph., ***hep.***, ign., phos., puls., sep.

PEMPHIGUS, (see Generals)

PETECHIAE, (see Eruptions)

PINCH, remains raised - caps.

PITYRIASIS, (see Eruptions, scaly) - ***ars.***, ars-i., bac., berb-a., calc., carb-ac., clem., cocc., ***colch.***, ***fl-ac.***, ***graph.***, ***kali-ar.***, mang., merc., merc-p-r., ***mez.***, nat-a., ***nat-m.***, olnd., phos., pip-m., psor., ***sabad.***, ***sep.***, staph., sul-ac., sul-i., ***sulph.***, tell., ter., thyr.
versicolor - caul.

POISON, oak or ivy (see Rhus poisoning)

POLYPS - ambr., ant-c., ***aur.***, bell., **CALC.**, **CALC-P.**, ***calc-s.***, ***carb-an.***, ***caust.***, **CON.**, graph., ***hep.***, ***lyc.***, ***med.***, ***merc.***, ***mez.***, nat-m., nit-ac., petr., ph-ac., **PHOS.**, puls., sang., sep., ***sil.***, **STAPH.**, sulph., sul-ac., **TEUCR.**, **THUJ.**
bleed profusely on slight provocation - ***phos.***, ***sabin.***
cartilage like, undergo retrograde metamorphosis - ***carb-an.***
fibroid, particularly nasal, of all kinds - **TEUCR.**
fibrous - calc-s.
fleshy, retrograde slowly - ***carb-an.***
soft - kali-s.
women, especially among old and middle-aged, in ear and nose - ***teucr.***

PRICKLING - ***acon.***, ***agar.***, ant-t., **APIS**, bar-c., bell., berb., cann-i., carb-ac., cimic., ***colch.***, croc., dros., **HAM.**, kali-ar., kali-c., **LOB.**, **LYC.**, mag-arct., mag-m., med., mez., mosch., nat-m.,

PRICKLING - nit-ac., nux-v., phos., **PLAT.**, ***ran-s.***, **RHUS-T.**, sabad., sel., sep., **SULPH.**, sul-ac., sumb., ***urt-u.***, zinc.
- single parts - sel.
- walking in open air - ***sulph.***
- warm, when - kali-ar., sumb.
  - in bed - **SULPH.**

PRURIGO - acon., aln., ***ambr.***, anthro., ***ars.***, ***ars-i.***, ars-s-f., carb-ac., ***chlol.***, ***dol.***, kali-bi., ***lyc.***, ***merc.***, ***mez.***, ***nit-ac.***, ***olnd.***, ov., ped., ***rhus-t.***, ***rhus-v.***, ***rumx.***, sil., ***sulph.***, ter.

PSORIASIS - alum., ambr., am-c., ant-t., ***ars.***, **ARS-I.**, aster., aur., aur-m-n., berb-a., ***bor.***, bry., bufo, ***calc.***, ***calc-s.***, ***canth.***, ***carb-ac.***, ***chin.***, ***chrysar.***, cic., ***clem.***, cortiso., cor-r., cupr., cupr-ac., dulc., dys-co., fl-ac., **GRAPH.**, hep., hydrc., iod., ***iris***, ***kali-ar.***, kali-br., ***kali-c.***, kali-p., ***kali-s.***, led., ***lob.***, **LYC.**, mag-c., ***mang.***, ***merc.***, merc-c., merc-i-r., ***mez.***, **MORG-G.**, mur-ac., naphtin., nat-a., **NAT-M.**, ***nit-ac.***, nit-m-ac., nuph., olnd., ***petr.***, ph-ac., ***phos.***, **PHYT.**, plat., ***psor.***, ***puls.***, ran-b., ***rhus-t.***, ***sarr.***, ***sars.***, **SEP.**, ***sil.***, **STAPH.**, stel., stry-p., ***sulph.***, tell., ter., teucr., thuj., ***thyr.***, tub., ust., x-ray
- diffusa - ars., ars-i., calc., cic., clem., dulc., ***graph.***, lyc., merc-i-r., ***mez.***, mur-ac., rhus-t., sulph., thuj., thyr.
- inveterata - calc., carb-ac., clem., ***kali-ar.***, ***mang.***, merc., petr., puls., rhus-t., ***sep.***, ***sil.***, sulph.
- syphilitic - ***ars.***, **ARS-I.**, aur., ***cor-r.***, kali-br., **MERC.**, ***nit-ac.***, **PHYT.**, ***sars.***, thuj.

PURPURA hemorrhagica - aln., ***arn.***, ars., ars-i., bell., berb., both., bov., bry., ***carb-v.***, chin-s., chlol., cor-r., ***crot-h.***, ***cupr.***, ferr-pic., ***ham.***, hyos., iod., ip., ***kali-i.***, **LACH.**, **LED.**, merc., merc-c., mill., naja, nat-n., nux-v., ***ph-ac.***, **PHOS.**, ***rhus-t.***, rhus-v., ruta, **SEC.**, sil., stram., sulph., **SUL-AC.**, **TER.**, thlaspi.
- discoloration, legs - kali-i., ***lach.***, **PHOS.**, ***sec.***
  - limbs, upper and lower - ***lach.***, ***phos.***, ***sec.***, ***sul-ac.***, ter.
- formication, with - phos.
- idiopathica - acon., ***arn.***, ***ars.***, bapt., bell., bry., carb-v., chin-s., chlor., ***crot-h.***, ***ham.***, jug-r., kali-i., ***lach.***, merc., ph-ac., ***phos.***, rhus-t., sal-ac., sec., ***sul-ac.***, sulfon., ter., verat-v.
  - colic, with - bov., coloc., cupr., merc-c., thuj.
  - debility, with - arn., ***ars.***, carb-v., lach., merc., sul-ac.
- itching, with - phos.
- miliaris - acon., am-c., am-m., arn., bell., coff., dulc., sulph., sul-ac.
- rheumatica - acon., ars., ***bry.***, merc., ***rhus-t.***, rhus-v.
- senilis - ars., bar-c., bry., con., ***lach.***, op., rhus-t., **SEC.**, sul-ac.

RASH, (see Granular) - **ACON.**, ***agar.***, ***ail.***, alum., **AM-C.**, am-m., anac., ***anan.***, ***ant-c.***, ***ant-t.***, ***apis***, ***arn.***, **ARS.**, ars-i., arund., asaf., bar-c., bar-m., **BELL.**, bov., **BRY.**, bufo, ***calad.***, ***calc.***, ***calc-s.***,

RASH - camph., ***canth.***, carb-s., ***carb-v.***, **CAUST.**, **CHAM.**, chel., chin-s., ***chlol.***, ***clem.***, cocc., ***coff.***, ***com.***, con., cop., corn., crot-t., cupr., dig., dros., ***dulc.***, elaps, euph., euphr., ***graph.***, hell., ***hep.***, ***hyos.***, iod., ***ip.***, ***jug-c.***, ***kali-ar.***, ***kali-bi.***, ***kali-br.***, ***kali-s.***, kreos., ***lach.***, ***led.***, lyc., **MERC.**, **MEZ.**, ***nat-m.***, nit-ac., nux-v., op., par., petr., **PH-AC.**, phos., phyt., ***psor.***, **PULS.**, rheum, **RHUS-T.**, sars., ***sec.***, ***sel.***, ***sep.***, ***sil.***, spong., ***staph.***, **STRAM.**, **SULPH.**, syph., tab., teucr., urt-u., valer., verat., viol-t., zinc.
- bee sting, after - ***apis***, sep.
- belladonna, after abuse of - hyos.
- black - ***lach.***
- blotches - ***agar.***, lyc.
- bluish - **ACON.**, ***ail.***, am-c., bell., ***coff.***, **LACH.**, ***led.***, ***phos.***, sep., stram., ***sulph.***
- brownish - mez.
- burning - ph-ac.
  - and itching, with - agar., clem., teucr.
- changing air - ***apis.***
- children, in - acon., ***bry.***, ***cham.***, ip., sulph.
- chronic - am-c., clem., mez., ***staph.***
- close, and itching - agar., bry., calad., sulph.
  - white, with burning - agar., bry., nux-v.
- cold air, in - apis, dulc., sars., sep.
- excoriated with - ***sulph.***
- fiery red - **ACON.**, **BELL.**, stram., sulph.
- itching - sep.
- lying-in, women, in - ***bry.***, cupr., ***ip.***
- menses, during - ***con.***
  - before - ***dulc.***
- moist - carb-v.
- night - chlol.
- nodules, with - tub.
- overheated, when - apis, lyc.
- patches - ***ail.***
- receding in eruptive fevers - **BRY.**
- scarlet - **ACON.**, **AM-C.**, ars., **BELL.**, **BRY.**, calc., carb-v., caust., ***chlol.***, ***coff.***, con., dulc., hyos., iod., ***ip.***, ***kali-bi.***, lach., ***merc.***, ph-ac., phos., rhus-t., sulph., zinc.
- scratching, after - am-c., am-m., ant-c., bov., bry., calc., carb-s., caust., dulc., graph., ip., ***lach.***, led., ***merc.***, mez., ph-ac., phos., puls., ***rhus-t.***, sars., sel., sil., spong., staph., ***sulph.***, verat., viol-t., zinc.
- slow evolution of rash in eruptive fevers - **BRY.**
- stinging, biting - nat-m., viol-t.
- suppressed - ip.
- tightness of chest alternating with asthma - ***calad.***
- warm room from the open air, on coming into - apis, ars.
- white - agar., ***apis***, **ARS.**, bov., ***bry.***, calad., ip., nux-v., ***phos.***, rhus-v., ***sulph.***, **VALER.**
  - air, in open - sars.
  - room, in - calc.

RAWNESS, (see Excoriation)

RHAGADES, (see Cracks)

RHUS poisoning, oak or ivy - agar., am-c., **ANAC.**, anag., arn., ***bry.***, **CLEM.**, **CROT-T.**, cupr., ***graph.***, ***grind.***, kali-s., led., lob., ***nuph.***, plan., **RHUS-T.**, rhus-v., ***sang.***, ***sep.***, sulph.

RINGWORM, general - anac., anag., ars-s-f., **BAC.**, ***bar-c.***, ***calc.***, calc-ac., chrysar., clem., dulc., dys-co., equis., ***eup-per.***, ***graph.***, hell., hep., iod., ***lith.***, mag-c., med., ***nat-c.***, **NAT-M.**, phos., **PHYT.**, ***sanic.***, **SEP.**, spong., sulph., syc-co., **TELL.**, **THUJ.**, torula., **TUB.**

rings, in intersecting - tell.
spots, in isolated - sep.
spring, every - **SEP.**

ringworm, beard - ant-t., anthr., ars., aur-m., ***bac.***, ***calc.***, calc-s., chrysar., ***cic.***, cinnb., cocc., cypr., ***graph.***, ***kali-bi.***, kali-m., lith., ***lyc.***, mag-p., med., merc-p-r., nat-s., ***nit-ac.***, petr., phyt., plan., ***plat.***, rhus-t., sabad., sep., sil., ***staph.***, stront-c., sul-i., ***sulph.***, tell., **THUJ.**

ringworm, face - anag., ***bac.***, bar-c., calc., cinnb., clem., dulc., ***graph.***, hell., kali-chl., lith., lyc., ***nat-c.***, ***nat-m.***, phos., **SEP.**, sulph., tarent., ***tell.***, ***thuj.***, **TUB.**

ringworm, head - **CALC.**, **DULC.**, ***phyt.***, ***sep.***, tell., thuj., tub.

ROSEOLA - **ACON.**, ***bell.***, **BRY.**, carb-v., ***coff.***, ***hyos.***, ip., ***merc.***, nux-v., phos., **PULS.**, rhus-t., sars., sulph.

syphilitic - **KALI-I.**, ***phos.***

ROUGH - ***alum.***, anag., ars., ***ars-i.***, bar-c., bell., bry., **CALC.**, calen., crot-t., fl-ac., ***graph.***, hep., ***iod.***, kali-i., ***lith.***, merc., mez., ***nat-c.***, ***nat-m.***, nit-ac., olnd., **PETR.**, ph-ac., phos., phyt., ***plb.***, psor., ***rhus-t.***, sabad., sars., ***sec.***, **SEP.**, stram., **SULPH.**, tub., zinc.

knots, small, as from - hyper.
winter, in - alumn.

RUPIA, (see Eruptions)

SCABIES - aloe, ambr., ***ant-c.***, ant-t., anthro., **ARS.**, ***aster.***, ***bar-m.***, bry., ***calc.***, canth., carb-ac., carb-an., **CARB-S.**, **CARB-V.**, **CAUST.**, ***clem.***, coloc., con., cop., crot-t., ***cupr.***, ***dulc.***, ***graph.***, guai., ***hep.***, **KALI-S.**, ***kreos.***, ***lach.***, led., ***lyc.***, ***mang.***, ***merc.***, merc-i-f., mez., ***nat-c.***, nux-v., olnd., petr., ***ph-ac.***, **PSOR.**, puls., rhus-v., sabad., **SEP.**, **SEL.**, ***sil.***, squil., staph., **SULPH.**, ***sul-ac.***, tarax., valer., ***verat.***, ***zinc.***

bleeding - calc., dulc., ***merc.***, sulph.
dry - ***ars.***, calc., carb-v., caust., clem., cupr., dulc., graph., ***hep.***, kreos., ***led.***, lyc., ***merc.***, merc-i-f., nat-c., petr., ph-ac., ***psor.***, **SEP.**, **SIL.**, staph., ***sulph.***, valer., ***verat.***, zinc.
fatty - ant-c., ***caust.***, clem., cupr., ***kreos.***, **MERC.**, sel., ***sep.***, squil., sulph.
moist - calc., ***carb-v.***, caust., clem., con., dulc., ***graph.***, kreos., ***lyc.***, merc., petr., sep., sil., squil., staph., sulph.
prairie - ***apis,*** rumx.
suppressed - alum., ambr., ant-c., ant-t., ***ars.***, ***carb-v.***, ***caust.***, ***dulc.***, graph., kreos., lach., nat-c., nat-m., ph-ac., ***sel.***, ***sep.***, sil., **SULPH.**, verat., zinc.

SCABIES,

suppressed, with mercury and sulphur - agn., ars., bell., calc., carb-v., **CAUST.**, ***chin.***, dulc., hep., iod., nit-ac., **PSOR.**, ***puls.***, rhus-t., sars., ***sel.***, **SEP.**, sil., ***staph.***, thuj., valer.

SCARLATINA - acon., **AIL.**, **AM-C.**, **APIS**, arn., ***ars.***, ***arum-t.***, bar-c., **BELL.**, ***bry.***, ***calc.***, ***carb-ac.***, ***carb-v.***, ***cham.***, ***crot-h.***, ***cupr.***, ***gels.***, hep., ***hyos.***, **LACH.**, **LYC.**, **MERC.**, ***mur-ac.***, **NIT-AC.**, ***ph-ac.***, ***phos.***, phyt., **RHUS-T.**, ***stram.***, ***sulph.***, ***zinc.***

gangrenous - ***ail.***, **AM-C.**, ***ars.***, **CARB-AC.**, ***lach.***, ***phos.***
patches, in - ***ail.***
receding - ***am-c.***, ***phos.***, ***sulph.***, **ZINC.**
smooth - ***am-c.***, **BELL.**, euphr., hyos., merc.

SCARS, general (see Keloids) - ars., ***bad.***, ***bell-p.***, calc., calc-f., **CALEN.**, carb-v., caust., crot-h., cupre-l., **FL-AC.**, gast., **GRAPH.**, hyper., ***iod.***, kali-bi., ***lach.***, maland., merc., naja, **NIT-AC.**, nux-v., petr., phos., psor., rhus-t., sabin., **SIL.**, sul-ac., sulph., syph., **THIOSIN.**, tub., vac., vip.

adherent - dros.
affections - ***caust.***, ***fl-ac.***, ***graph.***, ***iod.***, nit-ac., phyt., sil., sul-ac., ***thiosin.***
black - asaf.
bleed - ***lach.***, mag-p-a., phos., sep.
blisters, form on - mag-c.
blue - ant-c., ***bad.***, cench., lach., sul-ac.
break open - asaf., ***bor.***, calc-p., **CALEN.**, ***carb-an.***, carb-v., ***caust.***, con., croc., ***crot-h.***, fl-ac., glon., ***graph.***, ***iod.***, ***lach.***, mag-p-a., nat-c., ***nat-m.***, **PHOS.**, **SIL.**, sulph., thios., vib.
  cracks and burns - sars.
  suppurates - calen., croc.
burn, from - ars., ***carb-an.***, ***graph.***, lach., tell.
depressed - carb-an., ***kali-bi.***, kali-i., sil., syph.
drawing - graph., sep.
elevated - ***bad.***
green - led.
  turn - led.
hard - calc-f., fl-ac., ***graph.***
itching - alum., ***fl-ac.***, ***iod.***, led., naja.
nodules - sil.
painful, become - ***carb-an.***, con., crot-h., eug., graph., ***hyper.***, kali-c., ***lach.***, lyss., mag-n., ***nat-m.***, ***nit-ac.***, nux-v., phos., **SIL.**, sul-ac.
  air, open in agg. - graph.
  bones - mag-m.
  change of weather, on - carb-an., ***nit-ac.***
  touch, on - hep., puls.
pimply - iod.
pressing - carb-v., kali-c., petr., sulph.
purple - asaf.
raised, discolored - bad.
red, become - ant-c., bad., ***fl-ac.***, **LACH.**, ***merc.***, nat-m., sil., stram., ***sul-ac.***
  around edges - ***fl-ac.***
  blue, or - sul-ac.

SCARS, general
sharp - chin., mez., petr., ***sil.***
shining - sil.
sore, become - caust., ***fl-ac.,*** nux-v., **SIL.**
stinging - ***carb-an., sil., sul-ac.***
tearing - carb-v., graph., petr., sep.
tension, in - kali-c.
thick - graph.
ulcerate - asaf., calc-p.
veins, studded with - cench.
vesicles, around - ***fl-ac.***
white - rad-br., syph.

SCLERODERMA - alum., ***ant-c.,*** arg-n., berb-a., ***bry., calc.,*** caust., ***crot-t.,*** echi., ***graph., hydrc.,*** lyc., petr., phos., ran-b., rhus-r., sars., sil., still., sulph., thiosin., ***thyr.***

SEBACEOUS cysts, wens - ***agar.,*** am-c., anac., ant-c., **BAR-C.,** ***benz-ac.,*** brom., **CALC.,** calc-sil., caust., coloc., ***con.,*** daph., **GRAPH.,** ***hep.,*** kali-br., kali-c., ***kali-i.,*** mez., ***nit-ac.,*** ph-ac., phyt., rhus-t., ***sabin.,*** **SIL.,** spong., sulph., thuj.
scalp, of - agar., ***bar-c., calc.,*** **GRAPH.,** ***hep., kali-c., lob.,*** lyc., nat-c., **SIL.**

SENSITIVENESS - ***acon., agar.,*** alum., am-m., ant-c., ant-t., **APIS,** ***arg-n.,*** arn., ars., asaf., aur., ***bad.,*** aur., bar-c., **BELL.,** bell-p., bov., ***bry.,*** bufo, ***calc., calc-s.,*** camph., cann-s., canth., caps., carb-an., carb-v., cham., **CHIN.,** ***chin-a.,*** chin-s., cimic., ***chlor., coff.,*** colch., ***con., crot-c.,*** crot-t., cupr., cycl., ***ferr.,*** ferr-ar., ***ferr-p.,*** gels., ***dol.,*** **HEP.,** ***hyos.,*** ign., ***ip.,*** kali-ar., kali-c., ***kali-p., kali-s., kreos.,*** **LACH.,** ***led.,*** lyc., **LYSS.,** ***mag-c.,*** mang., **MERC.,** mez., ***mosch.,*** nat-c., ***nat-m.,*** nat-p., ***nit-ac., nux-m., nux-v.,*** olnd., osm., ox-ac., paeon., par., **PETR., PH-AC.,** phos., plan., **PLB.,** ***psor.,*** puls., ran-b., ran-s., ***rhus-t.,*** rumx., ruta, ***sang., sec., sel.,*** semp., ***sep.,*** **SIL.,** ***spig.,*** spong., squil., stann., staph., **SULPH.,** sul-ac., tarent-c., ***ther., thuj.,*** tub., verat., ***vinc.,*** xero, ***zinc.***
cold objects, to - **LAC-D.,** sep.
diminished or lost - acet-ac., ***acon.,*** ars., aur., bufo, ***cann-i., carb-o.,*** carb-s., elae., hyos., ***ign.,*** kali-br., merc., nux-v., plb., pop-c., sec., ***zinc-m.***
increased to atmospheric changes - dulc., hep., kali-c., psor., sulph.
left side - ***lach.***
right side - ***crot-h.***
spots in - ferr., hep.
sun, to - nat-m., sol., tub.

SHINING - acon., **APIS, BELL.,** ***chel., colch., kreos.,*** med.

SHRIVELLED, (see Wrinkled)

SMALLPOX, (see Fevers)

SMARTING, (see Burning)

SMOOTH - alum., phos., ter.

SOFT, boggy - ars., caps., kali-ar., lach., sil., thuj.

SORE, pain - ***agar.,*** all-c., ambr., am-c., am-m., ant-c., ***arg-n.,*** **ARN.,** ars., bapt., bar-c., bell., bov., ***calc.,*** calc-p., canth., carb-ac., carb-an., ***carb-v.,*** caust., cham., **CHIN.,** coff., colch., crot-h., dros., echi., euph., fl-ac., **GRAPH.,** ***hep.,*** hippoz., hydr., ***ign.,*** kali-ar., kali-c., kreos., **LACH., LED.,** ***lyc.,*** mag-m., mang., ***merc.,*** mez., mur-ac., ***nat-c.,*** nat-m., nit-ac., nux-m., nux-v., olnd., op., paeon., **PETR.,** ph-ac., phos., plb., ***puls.,*** pyrog., rhus-t., ruta., sel., **SEP., SIL.,** spig., squil., ***sulph., sul-ac.,*** ter., tub., vip., zinc.
child, in a - ant-c., bar-c., bell., ***calc.,*** **CHAM.,** ***chin.,*** ign., kreos., ***lyc.,*** merc., puls., ruta., ***sep.,*** sil., squil., **SULPH.**
feeling - acon., ***alum.,*** ambr., ***ant-c.,*** arg-m., **ARN.,** ***ars.,*** aur., bar-c., bor., ***bry., calc.,*** cann-s., canth., caps., carb-an., carb-v., caust., chel., chin., chin-a., ***cic.,*** **CIMIC.,** coff., colch., crot-h., ***dros.,*** **EUP-PER.,** ferr., ferr-ar., ferr-p., ***glon., graph.,*** ham., hell., **HEP.,** ***ign.,*** kali-c., kali-s., led., lyc., mag-c., mang., ***merc.,*** mez., mosch., nat-c., ***nat-m., nat-p., nit-ac., nux-v.,*** olnd., par., ***petr.,*** ph-ac., phos., ***plat., puls.,*** ran-b., ***rhus-t.,*** ruta., sabin., sars., sel., **SEP.,** sil., spig., spong., squil., staph., ***still., sulph.,*** sul-ac., teucr., valer., verat., **ZINC.**

SPLINTER, pain, as from - calad., **HEP., NIT-AC.**

SPOTS, (see Discoloration) - agar.

STICKING - ***acon., agar.,*** ang., alum., am-c., am-m., anac., ant-c., **APIS,** ***arn.,*** ars., ars-i., ***asaf.,*** **BAR-C.,** bell., **BRY.,** bufo, ***calc.,*** cann-s., ***canth.,*** caps., ***carb-s.,*** carb-v., ***caust.,*** chel., ***chin.,*** chin-a., clem., ***cocc.,*** coc-c., coff., ***colch.,*** con., ***crot-h., crot-t., cycl.,*** dig., dios., dros., dulc., euphr., **GRAPH.,** guai., hell., hep., hyos., ign., iod., kali-ar., kali-c., kali-n., kali-p., kali-s., kreos., lach., **LYC.,** mag-c., meny., ***merc.,*** mez., mur-ac., nat-c., nat-m., nat-p., ***nit-ac.,*** nux-v., olnd., par., ph-ac., ***phos.,*** plan., plat., plb., **PULS.,** ran-b., ran-s., rhod., **RHUS-T.,** ruta., ***sabad.,*** sabin., sars., sel., ***sep., sil.,*** spig., **SPONG.,** squil., ***stann., staph.,*** stront-c., ***sulph.,*** sul-ac., ***tarax.,*** tell., teucr., ***thuj.,*** verat., **VIOL-T.,** zinc.
electric - agar.
evening, in bed - alum., cycl., thuj., zinc.
night - am-c., anac., cann-s., merc., thuj.
scratching, after - alum., am-m., arn., ars., asaf., **BAR-C.,** bell., ***bry.,*** calc., cann-s., canth., carb-s., ***caust.,*** chel., chin., cocc., con., ***cycl.,*** dros., dulc., ***graph.,*** hell., kali-ar., kali-c., kali-s., ***lach.,*** lyc., ***merc.,*** mez., nit-ac., nux-v., par., ph-ac., ***puls.,*** ran-b., **RHUS-T.,** ruta., ***sabad.,*** sars., sel., sep., sil., ***spong., squil.,*** staph., stront-c., **SULPH.,** tarax., teucr., thuj., ***viol-t.,*** zinc.

STICKY - phos.

STIFF - kalm., ***rhus-t.,*** verat.

STINGING - ***acon.,*** alum., anac., **APIS,** arg-m., arn., ars., ars-i., **ASAF.,** bar-c., bell., ***bry.,*** calc., cann-s., canth., caps., carb-v., caust., cina, ***cocc.,*** colch., con., dig., dros., dulc., **HAM.,** hell., hep., hyos., ign., iod., ***kali-bi.,*** kali-c., lach., ***lyc.,*** mag-c., meny., ***merc., mez., nux-v.,*** olnd., ph-ac., phos., plat., ***puls.,*** ran-b., ran-s., ***rhus-t.,*** sabad., samb., sel., sep., ***sil.,*** spig., spong., squil., stann., **STAPH.,** ***sulph., sul-ac.,*** **THUJ., URT-U.,** viol-t.

evening, becoming warm in bed - sep., sulph.

excitement, from - ***bry.***

heat, during - chin.

STINGS, of insects, eruptions like (see Emergency) - graph.

STRIPES, streaks on - ***bell.,*** bufo, ***carb-v.,*** ceph., ***hep.,*** merc., mygal., ***phos., pyrog.,*** sabin., sil.

SWELLING, of - acal., ***acet-ac.,*** acon., ***agar.,*** agn., aloe, am-c., ***anac., ant-c.,*** **APIS,** ***arn.,*** **ARS.,** ***ars-i., asaf.,*** aur., ***bar-c.,*** bar-m., ***bell.,*** bell-p., bor., both., **BRY.,** calc., canth., caps., carb-an., carb-v., caust., chel., ***chin.,*** chin-a., **CIC.,** cina, clem., cocc., colch., coloc., ***con., cop.,*** crot-h., cupr., dig., ***dulc.,*** elat., **EUPH.,** ferr., ferr-ar., ferr-i., fl-ac., graph., hell., ***hell.,*** hep., hippoz., ***hydrc.,*** hyos., iod., ***kali-ar.,*** kali-bi., kali-br., kali-c., kali-n., kali-s., kreos., ***lach., led., lyc.,*** mag-c., mang., **MERC.,** mez., mur-ac., nat-a., nat-c., ***nat-m.,*** nat-p., nat-sal., nit-ac., **NUX-V.,** olnd., op., petr., ph-ac., ***phos.,*** plb., prim-o., ***prun.,*** **PULS.,** rhod., **RHUS-T.,** ruta., ***sabin., samb.,*** sars., sec., seneg., sep., sil., spig., spong., squil., stram., stront-c., **SULPH.,** sul-ac., syph., thuj., ***thyr.,*** verat.

affected part, of - acon., agn., ant-c., **APIS.,** arn., ars., asaf., aur., **BELL.,** ***bry., calc., canth.,*** carb-an., carb-v., ***caust.,*** chin., clem., cocc., con., dig., dulc., euph., ferr., graph., hell., ***hep.,*** iod., **KALI-C.,** lach., led., ***lyc.,*** mag-c., mang., **MERC.,** mur-ac., nat-c., nat-p., ***nit-ac.,*** nux-v., petr., ph-ac., ***phos.,*** plb., **PULS.,** rhod., **RHUS-T.,** ruta., sabin., ***samb.,*** sars., sec., **SEP.,** ***sil.,*** spig., ***spong.,*** stram., **SULPH.,** thuj.

angioneurotic - agar., antipyrin., hell.

bluish-black - acon., am-c., ***arn.,*** **ARS.,** aur., ***bell.,*** carb-v., con., ***dig.,*** hep., **LACH.,** mang., ***merc.,*** nux-v., ***op.,*** ph-ac., phos., plb., **PULS.,** samb., sec., seneg., sil., sul-ac., ***verat.***

brownish - ***thyr.***

burning - ***acon.,*** ant-c., ***arn.,*** **ARS.,** ***bell.,*** **BRY.,** calc., carb-an., carb-v., caust., chin., cocc., colch., coloc., crot-h., dulc., euph., hell., hep., hyos., iod., kali-ar., kali-c., ***lach.,*** led., **LYC.,** mang., ***merc.,*** mez., nat-a., nat-c., nux-v., op., ph-ac., **PHOS.,** ***puls., rhus-t.,*** samb., sec., sep., ***sil., spig.,*** spong., squil., stann., **SULPH.**

cold - ***ars.,*** asaf., bell., cocc., ***con.,*** cycl., dulc., lach., rhod., sec., spig.

SWELLING, of

crawling - acon., ***arn.,*** caust., chel., colch., con., lach., ***merc.,*** nat-c., nux-v., ph-ac., ***puls.,*** **RHUS-T.,** sec., ***sep.,*** spig., ***sulph.***

edema - acal., ***acet-ac.,*** acon., ***agar., anac.,*** **ANT-C., APIS., ARS.,** ***ars-i.,*** aur., ***bell.,*** bell-p., both., **BRY.,** cahin., canth., chel., **CHIN.,** chin-a., ***colch.,*** coloc., con., ***dig., dulc.,*** elat., euph., eup-per., ***ferr., ferr-ar.,*** ferr-m., guai., **HELL.,** hippoz., hyos., iod., kali-ar., kali-c., kali-n., kali-s., lach., ***led., lyc., merc.,*** mez., mur-ac., nat-c., ***nat-m.,*** nat-p., ***nat-s.,*** nat-sal., nit-ac., ***nux-m.,*** olnd., op., phos., plb., prim-o., prun., **PULS.,** rhod., ***rhus-t.,*** ruta., ***sabin., samb.,*** sars., sec., seneg., sep., sil., **SQUIL.,** stram., **SULPH., TELL.,** thyr., verat.

anxiety, with continued - ***ars.***

menses, suppressed with - cham.

gangrene, like - anthr.

hard - acon., agn., ant-c., ***arn.,*** ars., asaf., bell., **BRY.,** calc., ***caust.,*** chin., cina, con., dig., dulc., graph., hell., hep., lach., ***led.,*** lyc., merc., mez., nux-v., ph-ac., **PHOS.,** plb., **PULS., RHUS-T.,** sabin., ***samb.,*** sep., sil., spong., squil., ***stront-c., sulph., ther.***

inflamed - ***acon.,*** agn., am-c., ant-c., arn., ***ars.,*** asaf., bell., bor., **BRY.,** calc., canth., carb-v., caust., cocc., colch., con., crot-h., ***hep.,*** hyos., lach., lyc., mang., **MERC.,** mez., mur-ac., nat-c., nit-ac., petr., phos., **PULS.,** ***rhus-t.,*** sars., sep., ***sil., sulph.,*** thuj., verat.

tetter, of (exanthema) - graph.

pale - ***ant-c.,*** **APIS,** ***arn., ars.,*** bell., **BRY.,** calc., chin., cocc., con., dig., euph., ferr., graph., hell., hep., ***iod.,*** kali-c., kreos., lach., **LYC.,** merc., nit-ac., nux-v., phos., plb., ***puls.,*** rhod., ***rhus-t., sabin.,*** sep., sil., spig., ***sulph.***

scratching, after - ant-c., arn., ars., bell., bry., calc., canth., caust., chin., con., dulc., hep., kali-c., kreos., **LACH.,** led., ***lyc.,*** mang., ***merc.,*** mez., nat-m., nit-ac., phos., ***puls., rhus-t.,*** sabin., samb., sep., sil., ***sulph.,*** sul-ac.

shining - ***arn., ars.,*** **BELL., BRY.,** merc., ***rhus-t.,*** sabin., ***sulph.***

spongy - ***ant-c.,*** **ARS.,** ars-i., bell., calc., ***carb-an.,*** carb-v., caust., clem., con., graph., iod., kreos., **LACH.,** lyc., merc., nit-ac., nux-v., petr., ph-ac., ***phos.,*** rhus-t., sabin., sep., **SIL.,** ***sulph.,*** thuj.

stinging - acon., agn., ant-c., **APIS,** arn., ars., **BRY.,** canth., **CAUST.,** chel., chin., ***cocc.,*** con., cycl., dig., ferr., graph., kali-n., lach., led., mag-c., mang., mez., ***nit-ac.,*** nux-v., **PULS.,** ***rhus-t.,*** ruta., sabad., sep., sil., spong., ***sulph., thuj.***

SWELLINGS, on skin - ant-c., arg-m., ars., bar-c., graph., thuj.

SWOLLEN, sensation - alum., ***am-m.,*** ant-c., arn., ***ars.,*** aur., **BELL.,** ***bry.,*** canth., caps., carb-v., ***chin.,*** cocc., con., dig., dulc., guai., hep., hyos., ign., ***kali-n.,*** kreos., lach., ***laur.,*** merc., nit-ac., nux-m., nux-v., ***par.,*** plat., **PULS., RHUS-T.,** sabin., sars., seneg., sep., sil., ***spig.,*** spong., stann., ***staph.,*** sulph., sul-ac., verat., zinc.

TEARING, pain - ambr., anac., arg-n., bar-c., bell., berb., ***camph.,*** cann-s., chlor., coloc., ***graph., kreos.,*** mag-arct., ***nit-ac., phos.,*** plan.
  scratching, after - ars., bell., bry., calc., cycl., ***lyc.,*** puls., rhus-t., sep., sil., staph., **SULPH.**

TENSION - acon., agn., alum., am-c., am-m., anac., ant-c., arg-m., ***arg-n., arn.,*** ars., ars-i., asaf., asar., aur., ***bapt., bar-c.,*** bar-m., bell., berb., bor., bry., calc., canth., carb-an., carb-v., **CAUST.,** cham., chin., colch., ***coloc., con.,*** crot-h., dig., dulc., euph., guai., hell., hep., iod., kali-c., kali-s., kreos., lach., laur., led., lyc., mag-m., mang., meny., merc., mez., mosch., mur-ac., nat-c., nat-m., nat-s., **NIT-AC.,** ***nux-v.,*** olnd., par., petr., ph-ac., **PHOS.,** ***plat.,*** plb., ***puls.,*** rhod., ***rhus-t.,*** ruta., sabad., sabin., sars., ***sep.,*** sil., ***spig.,*** spong., stann., staph., **STRONT-C.,** ***sulph.,*** tarax., thuj., verat., verb., ***viol-o.,*** viol-t., zinc.
  scratching, after - caust., ***lach.,*** ph-ac., ruta., spig., ***stront.***

THICK, (see Hard), skin becomes, after scratching - ant-c., ars., cic., ***dulc.,*** **GRAPH.,** ***iod., kali-bi., lach., ran-b.,*** **RHUS-T.,** sep., thios., thuj., verat.

THIN, as if - thuj.

TINEA, capitis, tinea favus - ***ars.,*** brom., calc., dulc., graph., hep., kali-c., lyc., med., mez., ***phos.,*** sep., ***sulph.,*** sul-ac., thuj., viol-t.
  tinea, circinate - aesc., ant-c., calc., graph., hep., lyc., merc., mez., psor., rhus-t., sep., sulph., thuj.
  tinea, tonsurans - ars., chrysar., graph., hep., mez., nat-m., petr., psor., puls., rhus-t., sep., tell.
    scaley eruption of head - alum., ***ars.,*** arund., bell., ***calc.,*** carb-s., ***cic., fl-ac.,*** **GRAPH.,** ***kali-bi.,*** kali-n., ***kali-s., kreos., lyc.,*** merc., mez., naja, nat-m., **OLND.,** phos., phyt., ***sep., sil., staph.,*** sulph., ***thuj.***
  tinea, versicolor - ars., ars-i., calc., carb-an., carb-v., kali-s., mez., nit-ac., phos., phyt., sep., sil., psor., **THUJ.**

TINGLING, (see Prickling)

TRICHOPHYTOSIS, (see Ringworm) - ant-c., ant-t., ***ars., bac.,*** calc., calc-i., ***chrysar., graph.,*** hep., jug-c., jug-r., kali-s., lyc., mez., psor., rhus-t., semp., ***sep.,*** sulph., ***tell.,*** tub., viol-t.
  all over body - psor., ran-b.
  intersecting rings over great portion of body, with fever and great chronic disturbances - tell.
  isolated spots on upper part of body, in - sep.

TUBERCLES, (see Nodules) - agar., alum., am-c., ***am-m.,*** anac., ang., ***ant-c.,*** apis, aran., ***ars.,*** aur., ***bar-c.,*** bar-m., ***bry.,*** **CALC.,** calc-p., calc-s., ***carb-an.,*** carb-s., ***carb-v.,*** **CAUST.,** ***cic.,*** cocc., ***con.,*** crot-h., ***dulc., fl-ac., graph.,*** hell., ***hep.,*** hydrc., kali-ar., ***kali-bi., kali-br.,*** kali-c., ***kali-i.,*** kali-n., kali-s., **LACH., LED.,** ***lyc.,*** mag-c., mag-m., mag-s., mang., ***merc.,*** merc-c., ***mez., mur-ac.,*** nat-a., ***nat-c., nat-m., nit-ac.,*** nux-v., ***olnd., petr.,*** ph-ac., ***phos., rhus-t.,*** sec., sel., sep., ***sil.,*** stann., ***staph., sulph.,*** sul-ac., tarax., ***thuj.,*** valer., verat., zinc.
  burning - am-c., am-m., calc., ***carb-an.,*** cocc., dulc., kali-i., mag-m., mag-s., mang., ***merc.,*** mur-ac., nicc., ***nit-ac.,*** phos., ***staph.***
  drawing, painful - cham.
  erysipelatous - ***nat-c., phos.,*** sil.
  gnawing - rhus-t.
  hard - am-c., am-m., ant-c., bar-c., bov., ***bry.,*** con., ***lach., mag-c., mag-s.,*** nat-m., phos., rhus-t., valer.
  humid - kali-n., sel.
  inflamed - am-m., rhus-t.
  itching - am-m., aur., canth., carb-an., cham., cocc., dulc., graph., kali-c., kali-n., lach., lyc., mag-c., mag-s., mur-ac., nat-m., nit-ac., op., rhus-t., staph., stram., stront-c., tub., zinc.
  leprous - ***nat-c.,*** phos., ***sil.***
  malignant - ars.
  miliary - nat-m.
  mucous - ***fl-ac., nit-ac., thuj.***
  painful - am-c., ars., bell., bov., lach., lyc., ph-ac., zinc.
  painless - arn., bell., graph., ign., led., olnd., squil., verat.
  purple - tub.
  raised - olnd., rhus-v., valer.
  red - ***am-c.,*** berb., bov., carb-an., carb-v., dig., ***hep.,*** kali-chl., kali-i., ***lach., led.,*** mag-c., mag-m., ***merc.,*** mur-ac., nat-m., nit-ac., op., ph-ac., puls., sep., spig., sulph., ***thuj.,*** verat.
    areola - cocc., dulc., ph-ac.
  scratching, after - mang., zinc.
  scurfy - sulph.
  smooth - ph-ac.
  soft - **BELL.,** crot-h., lach.
  sore, painful, as if - ant-c., caust., ph-ac.
  stab wound, after - sep.
  stinging - calc., caust., dulc., kali-i., led., mag-c., phos., rhus-t., squil., stram.
  summer - ***kali-bi.***
  suppurating - am-c., bov., ***caust., fl-ac., kali-bi.,*** nat-c., nit-ac., ***sil.***
  syphilitic - ars., ***ars-i.,*** dulc., fl-ac., hep., kali-bi., ***kali-i., merc., nit-ac.,*** phyt., sil., thuj.
  tearing - cham., con.
  tensive - caust., mur-ac.
  tuberous - ***kali-bi., nat-c.,*** phos., sil., ***tub.***
  ulcerating - am-c., bov., ***caust., fl-ac., ant-c.,*** sec.
  umbilicated - ***kali-bi., kali-br.***

TUBERCLES, general
wart-shaped - lyc., ***thuj.***
watery - graph., mag-c.
white - ant-c., dulc., sep., sulph., valer.
winter - ***kali-br.***
yellow - ***ant-c.,*** rhus-t.

TWITCHING - mang., phos., sec., tab.

ULCERATIVE, pain - alum., ambr., am-c., **AM-M.,** anac., ars., bell., bov., ***bry.,*** canth., caps., carb-s., caust., cham., ***chin., cic.,*** cocc., dros., ferr., **GRAPH.,** hep., ign., kali-ar., ***kali-c., kali-i.,*** kali-n., kali-s., kreos., lach., laur., mag-c., mag-m., ***mang.,*** merc., mur-ac., nat-c., ***nat-m.,*** nat-p., nit-ac., nux-v., petr., ph-ac., ***phos.,*** **PULS., RHUS-T.,** ruta., sars., ***sep.,*** sil., spig., spong., stann., staph., sulph., ***sul-ac.,*** tarax., ***thuj.,*** verat., zinc.
scratching, after - am-c., **AM-M.,** arn., asaf., bar-c., bell., bry., calc., carb-v., caust., chin., cic., con., cycl., ***graph.,*** hep., kali-c., led., mag-m., mang., merc., nat-m., petr., ***phos., puls.,*** ran-b., **RHUS-T.,** sep., **SIL.,** spig., staph., ***sulph.,*** sul-ac., thuj., verat., zinc.
touched, when - ***canth.***

ULCERS, general - acon., agar., all-c., ***alum.,*** alumn., ambr., ***am-c.,*** anac., anac-oc., ***anan., anthr.,*** ant-c., ant-t., arg-m., ***arg-n.,*** arn., **ARS., ARS-I., ASAF.,** aster., ***aur.,*** bals-p., bar-c., ***bar-m., bell.,*** benz-ac., berb., bor., bov., ***brom., bry., calc., calc-p., calc-s.,*** calc-sil., ***calen.,*** camph., canth., ***carb-ac.,*** carb-an., carb-s., **CARB-V.,** ***caust., cham.,*** chel., chin., chin-a., chlor., cic., cina, ***cinnb.,*** cist., clem., cocc., coff., colch., com., ***con.,*** croc., crot-h., ***cupr.,*** cupr-ar., cycl., dig., dros., dulc., ***echi.,*** euph., ferr., ferr-ar., ferr-p., ***fl-ac.,*** gali., ***ger., graph.,*** guai., ham., **HEP.,** hippoz., ***hydr.,*** hyos., ign., ***iod.,*** ip., jug-r., ***kali-ar.,*** **KALI-BI.,** ***kali-c.,*** **KALI-CHL.,** kali-i., kali-p., **KALI-S.,** ***kreos.,*** **LACH.,** led., **LYC.,** mang., **MERC.,** ***mez.,*** mur-ac., ***nat-a., nat-c., nat-m.,*** nat-p., nat-s., **NIT-AC.,** nux-m., nux-v., ***paeon.,*** par., ***petr., ph-ac., phos.,*** **PHYT.,** plb., ***psor.,*** **PULS.,** ***pyrog.,*** rad., ran-a., ran-b., ran-s., ***rhus-t.,*** ruta, sabin., samb., sang., ***sars.,*** scroph-n., ***sec.,*** sel., seneg., ***sep.,*** **SIL.,** spong., squil., ***staph.,*** stram., stront-c., sul-i., **SULPH.,** sul-ac., syph., tarax., tarent-c., ***thuj.,*** verat., xan., ***zinc.***
aching - bell., camph., carb-v., chin., ***graph.,*** par., sil.
areola, edges, margins, with - ars., asaf., hep., lach., lyc., merc., ***puls., sil.***
dark - aesc., ***lach.***
hanging over - kali-bi.
hard - fl-ac., graph., puls., sil.
red - puls.
bases - ars., hep., ***merc.,*** nit-ac.
bed-sores - arn., chin., ***fl-ac.,*** graph., lach., petr., sep., sil., sul-ac.
children, in - cham., sulph.
early - valer.

ULCERS, general
biting - ars., bell., bry., calc., carb-an., caust., cham., chin., colch., dig., ***euph.,*** graph., ***lach., led., lyc.,*** mang., merc., mez., nat-c., nat-p., petr., ph-ac., **PULS.,** ran-b., rhus-t., ruta., sel., sil., staph., ***sulph.,*** thuj., zinc.
night - cham., rhus-t.
walking in open air - rhus-t.
black - **ANTHR.,** ant-t., **ARS.,** ***asaf.,*** bell., bism., ***carb-s.,*** **CARB-V.,** ***con.,*** euph., grin., ham., ip., kali-ar., **LACH., LYC.,** ***mur-ac., plb.,*** rhus-t., sars., **SEC.,** ***sil.,*** squil., ***sulph., sul-ac.***
base - **ARS.,** calc-f., carb-an., ip., lach., mur-ac., plb., sil., sulph., tarent-c., thuj.
margins - ***ars.,*** con., **LACH.,** sil., sulph.
spots, on centre - ***kali-bi.***
bleeding - ant-t., arg-m., ***arg-n.,*** arn., **ARS.,** ***ars-i., asaf.,*** bell., ***calc.,*** calc-s., carb-an., carb-s., ***carb-v.,*** caust., ***con.,*** croc., ***crot-h.,*** dros., ***graph.,*** ham., **HEP.,** hydr., hyos., ***iod.,*** kali-ar., ***kali-c.,*** kali-s., kalm., kreos., **LACH., LYC., MERC.,** ***mez.,*** nat-m., **NIT-AC., PH-AC., PHOS.,** ***puls., ran-b.,*** rhus-t., ruta., sabin., ***sec.,*** sep., ***sil., sulph., sul-ac.,*** thuj., zinc.
black clotted - ars.
edges - **ARS.,** asaf., caust., hep., lach., ***lyc., merc.,*** ph-ac., phos., puls., sep., ***sil.,*** sulph., thuj.
menses, during - **PHOS.**
night - ***kali-c.***
touched, when - ***carb-v.,*** ham., **HEP.,** ***hydr., lach.,*** merc-c., ***mez., nit-ac.***
easily - ars., ***carb-v.,*** dulc., hep., kreos., ***lach.,*** merc., mez., ***nit-ac., petr., phos.***
blue or black base, with - ***ars.,*** calc-f., carb-an., lach., mur-ac., tarent-c.
bluish - arn., **ARS.,** ***asaf., aur.,*** bell., bry., calc., carb-an., ***carb-v., con.,*** crot-h., ***hep., kali-i.,*** **LACH.,** ***lyc., mang., merc.,*** mur-ac., ph-ac., sec., seneg., **SIL.,** staph., tarent-c., thuj., verat., vip.
base - ***ars.,*** calc-f., carb-an., lach., mur-ac., tarent-c.
edges - ***asaf.,*** kali-s., ***mang.,*** nit-ac.
bluish, red - ars., lach., sil.
boils, from - ***calc-p.***
boring, with - arg-m., aur., bell., calc., caust., chin., hep., ***kali-c.,*** nat-c., nat-m., puls., ran-s., sep., ***sil., sulph.,*** thuj.
bruised, pain, with - ***arn.,*** cham., chin., cocc., ***con.,*** **HEP.,** hyos., nat-m., nux-v., rhus-t., ruta., ***sulph.***
motion, from - hyos.
burning - ambr., alumn., **ANTHR., ARS.,** asar., aur., bar-c., bar-m., bell., bov., bry., ***bufo,*** calc., calc-s., canth., ***carb-ac.,*** carb-an., **CARB-S., CARB-V., CAUST.,** ***cham.,*** chin., chin-a., cinnb., ***clem., con., dros.,*** ferr-ar., graph., ***hep., hydr.,*** ign., kali-ar., ***kali-c.,*** kali-p., kali-s., ***kreos.,*** lach., **LYC.,** mang., **MERC.,** ***mez.,*** mur-ac., ***nat-a., nat-c.,*** nat-m.,

ULCERS, general

burning - nat-p., ***nit-ac.***, nux-v., petr., ph-ac., ***plb.***, **PULS.**, ***ran-b.***, **RHUS-T.**, sars., sec., sel., sep., **SIL.**, squil., ***staph.***, stront-c., **SULPH.**, syph., tarent-c., ***thuj.***, ***zinc.***

around about - ***ars.***, ***asaf.***, bell., ***caust.***, cham., hep., ***lach.***, ***lyc.***, ***merc.***, mez., mur-ac., nat-c., nux-v., petr., phos., **PULS.**, ***rhus-t.***, sep., ***sil.***, staph.

margins, in - **ARS.**, asaf., carb-an., ***caust.***, clem., ***hep.***, ***lach.***, **LYC.**, **MERC.**, mur-ac., petr., ph-ac., phos., puls., ran-b., sep., **SIL.**, staph., sulph., thuj.

menses, during - ***carb-v.***

night - ***anthr.***, bell., ***carb-v.***, cham., ***hep.***, ***lach.***, ***merc.***, rhus-t., sep., ***staph.***

touched, when - ars., bell., canth., carb-v., ***lach.***, ***lyc.***, merc., mez., puls., rhus-t., sil., sulph.

burnt, as if - alum., ant-c., **ARS.**, bar-c., bell., bry., calc., ***carb-v.***, caust., ***cycl.***, hyos., ign., kreos., lach., ***nux-v.***, puls., sabad., ***sec.***, sep., stram.

burrowing - ***asaf.***, bell., bry., calc., carb-v., chin., lyc., nat-c., phos., ruta., sep., stront-c., sulph.

cancerous - ***ambr.***, ***anthr.***, ant-c., apis, **ARN.**, **ARS.**, ***ars-i.***, **ARS-S-F.**, ***aster.***, aur., aur-a., aur-i., **AUR-S.**, ***bell.***, **BUFO**, calc., ***calc-s.***, ***carb-ac.***, ***carb-an.***, ***carb-s.***, ***carb-v.***, caust., chel., chim., chin-s., clem., **CON.**, ***crot-c.***, cund., dor., dulc., ***ferr.***, fl-ac., fuli., ***gali.***, ***graph.***, **HEP.**, ***hippoz.***, hydr., kali-ar., kali-c., ***kali-i.***, ***kreos.***, ***lach.***, **LYC.**, ***lyss.***, mang., ***merc.***, merc-i-f., ***mill.***, mur-ac., ***nit-ac.***, ***petr.***, ***ph-ac.***, ***phos.***, ***phyt.***, ***rhus-t.***, rumx., sars., ***sep.***, **SIL.**, spong., squil., ***staph.***, **SULPH.**, sul-ac., sul-i., syph., tarent-c., ***thuj.***, ***zinc.***

cold, air, amel. - ***dros.***, **LED.**, **PULS.**

application, amel. pain - ***cham.***, ***fl-ac.***, **LED.**, ***lyc.***, **PULS.**

cold, feeling in - ***ars.***, **BRY.**, hep., merc., **NAT-M.**, petr., phos., plb., ***rhus-t.***, sep., ***sil.***, thuj.

crawling, with - acon., ant-t., **ARN.**, bell., caust., ***cham.***, ***clem.***, colch., ***con.***, croc., graph., hep., kali-c., ***lach.***, merc., nat-c., nat-m., nat-p., nux-v., ph-ac., plb., puls., ran-b., **RHUS-T.**, sabin., sec., **SEP.**, spong., staph., sulph., sul-ac., thuj.

crusty - ars., bar-c., ***bell.***, bov., bry., **CALC.**, ***calc-s.***, carb-an., cic., clem., **CON.**, ***graph.***, ***hep.***, ***kali-bi.***, ***kali-s.***, led., **LYC.**, **MERC.**, **MEZ.**, mur-ac., olnd., ***ph-ac.***, puls., ran-b., **RHUS-T.**, sars., ***sep.***, **SIL.**, staph., **SULPH.**, viol-t.

black scab - bell., **KALI-BI.**

cutting, with - ***arn.***, **BELL.**, ***calc.***, cic., ***clem.***, dros., graph., ign., kali-ar., ***lyc.***, mag-m., merc., mur-ac., ***nat-c.***, ph-ac., plat., rhus-t., ***ruta.***, sep., ***sil.***, sul-ac.

ULCERS, general

deep - ***agar.***, ***ant-c.***, ***anthr.***, **ARS.**, ***asaf.***, ***aur.***, ***bell.***, ***bov.***, **CALC.**, **CALC-S.**, carb-s., ***carb-v.***, caust., chel., clem., ***com.***, ***con.***, ***hep.***, ***hippoz.***, ***hydr.***, kali-c., **KALI-BI.**, ***kali-i.***, kreos., **LACH.**, led., ***lyc.***, **MERC.**, ***merc-c.***, mez., ***mur-ac.***, nat-a., nat-c., nat-m., nat-p., **NIT-AC.**, ***petr.***, ph-ac., phos., ***psor.***, **PULS.**, rad-br., rat., rhus-t., ruta., sabin., ***sars.***, sel., ***sep.***, **SIL.**, staph., stram., **SULPH.**, ***syph.***, tarent., tarent-c., thuj.

regular edges, punched out - kali-bi., phos.

dirty - ***arn.***, ***ars.***, calc., **LACH.**, ***lyc.***, **MERC.**, mosch., **NIT-AC.**, sabin., ***sulph.***, ***thuj.***

pus, without pain or redness, uneven, jagged base, with - ph-ac.

discharges, from ulcers

albuminous - ***calc.***, ***puls.***

blackish - ***anthr.***, bry., chin., lyc., ***sulph.***

bloody - ***anthr.***, ant-t., arg-m., arn., **ARS.**, ***ars-i.***, **ASAF.**, bell., calc-s., canth., carb-an., carb-s., ***carb-v.***, ***caust.***, com., ***con.***, croc., ***dros.***, graph., **HEP.**, hyos., iod., kali-ar., ***kali-c.***, kali-s., kreos., lach., ***lyc.***, **MERC.**, mez., nat-m., ***nit-ac.***, ***petr.***, ph-ac., phos., ***puls.***, pyrog., rhus-t., ruta., sabin., ***sars.***, sec., sep., ***sil.***, sulph., sul-ac., thuj., zinc.

brownish - anac., ***anthr.***, ars., ***bry.***, calc., carb-v., con., puls., rhus-t., ***sil.***

cheesy - merc.

copious - acon., arg-n., ***ars.***, ***asaf.***, bry., ***calc.***, canth., carb-s., ***chin.***, cic., ***fl-ac.***, graph., **IOD.**, ***kali-c.***, kreos., lyc., mang., ***merc.***, mez., nat-c., ph-ac., ***phos.***, **PULS.**, ***rhus-t.***, ruta., sabin., **SEP.**, ***sil.***, squil., ***staph.***, sulph., thuj.

corrosive - agar., am-c., anac., **ARS.**, **ARS-I.**, bell., calc., carb-an., ***carb-v.***, **CAUST.**, cham., chel., clem., con., crot-c., cupr., ***fl-ac.***, ***graph.***, ***hep.***, hippoz., ign., ***iod.***, **KALI-BI.**, ***kali-i.***, kreos., lach., ***lyc.***, **MERC.**, mez., nat-c., nat-m., ***nit-ac.***, nux-v., ***petr.***, ***phos.***, plb., puls., ***ran-b.***, ***ran-s.***, **RHUS-T.**, ruta., sep., **SIL.**, spig., ***squil.***, ***staph.***, sulph., sul-ac., zinc.

gelatinous - arg-m., arn., bar-c., cham., ferr., merc., sep., ***sil.***

gray - ambr., ars., carb-ac., **CAUST.**, chin., ***kali-chl.***, lyc., merc., sep., ***sil.***, thuj.

green - ***ars.***, ***asaf.***, aur., ***carb-v.***, ***caust.***, clem., com., kali-chl., ***kali-i.***, kreos., ***lyc.***, merc., naja, nat-c., ***nat-s.***, ***nux-v.***, par., ***phos.***, ***puls.***, rhus-t., sec., sep., ***sil.***, staph., ***sulph.***

ichorous - am-c., ***anthr.***, ant-t., **ARS.**, ***asaf.***, aur., bov., calc., ***carb-an.***, ***carb-s.***, **CARB-V.**, ***caust.***, ***chin.***, cic., clem., ***con.***, ***dros.***, graph., ***hep.***, ***kali-ar.***, ***kali-c.***, kali-i., ***kali-p.***, kreos., ***lach.***, **LYC.**, mang., **MERC.**, ***mez.***, mur-ac., **NIT-AC.**, nux-v., ph-ac., ***phos.***, plb., ***psor.***, ***ran-b.***, ***ran-s.***, **RHUS-T.**, ***sang.***, sec., sep., **SIL.**, squil., ***staph.***, sulph.

ULCERS, general
discharges, from ulcers
maggots, with - ars., calc., merc., ***sabad., sil.,*** sulph.
offensive - alum., ***am-c., anan., anthr., apis,*** **ARS.,** ***asaf.,*** aur., **BAPT.,** bell., bov., ***bry., calc.,*** calc-f., calc-p., ***calc-s., calen., carb-ac.,*** **CARB-AN., CARB-S., CARB-V.,** caust., ***chel., chin.,*** cic., clem., com., ***con.,*** crot-h., crot-t., cycl., echi., eucal., fl-ac., gels., ***ger., graph.,*** grin., ***guai.,*** **HEP.,** hydr., ***hyper., kali-p.,*** kreos., **LACH., LYC.,** mang., ***merc.,*** merc-c., merc-sul., ***mez., mur-ac.,*** nat-c., ***nat-p.,*** **NIT-AC.,** nux-m., nux-v., **PAEON.,** ***petr.,*** **PH-AC.,** ***phos.,*** plb., ***psor., puls., pyrog.,*** pyrus, rhus-t., ruta., sabin., ***sars., sec., sep.,*** **SIL., STAPH., SULPH.,** sul-ac., thuj., vinc.
rotten eggs, like - calc.
herring brine, like - ***graph., tell.***
old cheese, like - ***hep.,*** sulph.
putrid - ***am-c., anthr.,*** **ARS., ASAF.,** bapt., bell., bor., ***calc., calc-s.,*** **CHEL.,** chin., cycl., graph., **HEP.,** lach., lyc., ***merc.,*** **MUR-AC.,** ***nit-ac., ph-ac., phos.,*** **PSOR., PULS.,** rhus-t., ***sars., sep.,*** **SIL.,** sulph.
purulent, fetid, sloughing - ***anan., anthr.,*** ars., asaf., bapt., calc-f., ***calen., carb-ac., carb-v.,*** con., crot-t., ***echi.,*** eucal., fl-ac., gels., ***ger., hep.,*** lach., ***merc.,*** merc-c., ***mez.,*** mur-ac., ***nit-ac.,*** paeon., ph-ac., psor., puls., pyrog., sil., sulph., ***thuj.***
scanty - acon., ***ars.,*** bar-c., ***bell.,*** bov., bry., **CALC.,** carb-v., caust., chin., cina, clem., ***coff., cupr.,*** dros., ***dulc., graph., hep.,*** hyos., ign., ip., kreos., **LACH.,** led., lyc., ***mag-c.,*** **MERC.,** nux-v., ***petr., phos., plat.,*** plb., puls., rhus-t., sars., ***sep.,*** **SIL.,** spong., ***staph.,*** sulph., ***verat.***
sour smelling - calc., graph., **HEP.,** ***merc.,*** nat-c., sep., ***sulph.***
tallow, like - ***merc., merc-c.***
tenacious - ars., asaf., ***bov.,*** cham., ***con., graph., hydr.,*** merc., mez., ph-ac., phos., sep., sil., staph., viol-t.
thin - ant-t., ***ars.,*** **ASAF.,** ***carb-v.,*** **CAUST.,** dros., ***iod., kali-c., kali-i., lyc.,*** **MERC.,** nit-ac., ***phos.,*** plb., puls., ***pyrog.,*** ran-b., ran-s., rhus-t., ruta., ***sil.,*** staph., ***sulph.,*** thuj.
watery - ant-t., ***ars.,*** ars-i., ***asaf.,*** calc., carb-v., **CAUST.,** clem., con., ***dros., graph., iod., kali-c.,*** lyc., **MERC.,** nit-ac., nux-v., ***petr.,*** plb., puls., ***ran-b., ran-s., rhus-t.,*** ruta., ***sil.,*** squil., staph., sulph., thuj.
whitish - ***am-c.,*** ars., ***calc.,*** carb-v., hell., ***lyc.,*** **MEZ.,** ***puls.,*** sep., sil., sulph.
yellow - acon., alum., ambr., am-c., anac., arg-m., ars., aur., bov., bry., ***calc.,*** calc-s., caps., carb-s., ***carb-v., caust.,*** cic., ***clem.,*** con., croc., dulc., graph., hep., ***hydr.,*** iod., **KALI-BI.,** kali-n., ***kali-p.,*** kali-s., ***kreos.,***

ULCERS, general
discharges, from ulcers
yellow - lyc., mang., ***merc.,*** **MEZ.,** nat-a., nat-c., nat-m., nat-p., ***nit-ac.,*** nux-v., ***phos.,*** **PULS.,** ran-b., rhus-t., ruta., sec., sel., ***sep., sil.,*** spig., ***staph.,*** sulph., sul-ac., thuj., viol-t.
dotted - arg-n., ars., kali-bi., med.
drawing, pain, with - mez.
dropsical persons, in - ars., graph., hell., lyc., merc., rhus-t., squil., sulph.
dry - **KALI-BI.,** mang., phyt., sang.
edges - ***sang.***
hard - mang.
lardaceous, dry base, with - phyt.
eczematous edges, copper colored - kali-bi.
elevated, indurated margins, with - ***apis,*** **ARS.,** asaf., bry., calen., carb-an., caust., cic., cina, cinnb., clem., ***hep.,*** hydr., ***kali-ar., kali-bi.,*** lach., **LYC.,** ***merc.,*** mur-ac., ***nit-ac., petr.,*** ph-ac., ***phos., puls.,*** ran-b., sep., **SIL.,** staph., ***sulph.,*** thuj.
exuberant, granulations, with - ap-g., ars., carb-an., ***caust.,*** fl-ac., ***nit-ac.,*** petr., ph-ac., ***sil.,*** thuj.
fistulous - ***agar.,*** ant-c., ars., ***asaf.,*** aur., bar-c., ***bell.,*** **BRY., CALC.,** ***calc-f., calc-p.,*** calc-s., calen., carb-ac., carb-s., ***carb-v.,*** **CAUST.,** chel., ***cinnb.,*** clem., ***con., fl-ac., hep., hippoz.,*** kali-i., kreos., led., **LYC.,** ***merc.,*** nat-c., ***nat-m.,*** nat-p., ***nit-ac., petr.,*** **PHOS.,** phyt., **PULS.,** rhus-t., ruta., sabin., sel., sep., **SIL.,** ***staph.,*** stram., ***sulph., thuj.***
flat, (see superficial) - ***am-c., ars., asaf.,*** bell., ***chin.,*** cor-r., **LACH., LYC., MERC., NIT-AC.,** ***ph-ac., puls., ran-b.,*** sel., ***sep., sil., thuj.***
menopause, at - polyg.
flowing - kali-ar., kali-c., nat-s., ***rhus-t.,*** zinc-s.
yellow water - kali-s.
foul - ***am-c., anthr., ars., asaf.,*** aur., bell., bor., bry., ***calc., calc-s., carb-v.,*** caust., chel., ***chin.,*** cic., con., cycl., ***graph.,*** **HEP.,** kali-ar., kreos., lyc., mang., merc., mez., **MUR-AC.,** nat-c., nit-ac., nux-m., nux-v., ***ph-ac.,*** phos., plb., puls., ***rhus-t.,*** ruta., sabin., sec., sep., **SIL.,** staph., ***sulph.,*** sul-ac., thuj.
fungous - alum., alumn., ant-c., ***arg-n.,*** **ARS.,** bell., ***calc., carb-an., carb-s., carb-v.,*** caust., ***cham.,*** cinnb., clem., ***crot-c.,*** graph., ***hydr.,*** kreos., ***lach., merc., nit-ac., petr., phos.,*** sabin., **SEP., SIL.,** staph., ***sulph., thuj.***
areola - lach.
gangrenous - am-c., ***anthr.,*** **ARS.,** ***asaf., bapt.,*** bism., ***carb-v., chin., cinnb., con., crot-c., crot-h.,*** euph., ***kali-bi.,*** kali-p., ***kreos.,*** **LACH., LYC.,** mill., ***mur-ac.,*** rhus-t., sabin., ***sars.,*** **SEP.,** ***sil.,*** squil., sul-ac.
edges - anthr., ***ars., carb-v.,*** kreos., lach., nit-ac., sec., ***sul-ac.,*** tarent-c.
glistening, (see shining)

ULCERS, general

gnawing, pain, with - agar., ***agn.,*** bar-c., bell., calc., ***cham.,*** cycl., **DROS.,** ***hep.,*** hyos., ***kali-c.,*** lach., led., lyc., manc., ***merc.,*** mez., nat-c., ph-ac., ***phos., plat., puls., ran-s.,*** rhus-t., ***ruta.,*** sep., **STAPH.,** ***sulph.,*** sul-ac., thuj.

heat, agg. - cham., fl-ac., ***led.,*** lyc., ***puls.***

amel. - ars., clem., con., **HEP.,** ***lach.,*** rhus-t., ***sil.,*** syph.

herpetic - ***sars.***

honeycombed - cinnb.

indolent - ***agar.,*** agn., alum., ***alumn.,*** anac., ***anag.,*** **ARS.,** ***ars-i.,*** aster., bar-c., ***calc.,*** calc-f., ***calc-i., calc-p.,*** calc-s., camph., carb-an., carb-s., ***carb-v.,*** chel., com., **CON.,** crot-h., cupr., ***dulc.,*** eucal., ***euph.,*** fl-ac., fuli., ***ger., graph.,*** hep., ***hippoz., hydr., iod.,*** ip., kali-ar., kali-bi., kali-c., kali-i., kali-s., **LACH.,** ***laur.,*** **LYC.,** ***merc., mur-ac., nit-ac.,*** olnd., ***op.,*** paeon., petr., **PH-AC.,** phos., phyt., plb., ***psor., puls.,*** pyrog., rhus-t., ***sang., sars., sec., sep.,*** **SIL.,** ***still.,*** stram., **SULPH.,** syph., syzyg., xan., zinc.

tumors, after removal of - hydr.

indurated - agn., ***alumn., arg-m.,*** arn., ***ars.,*** ars-i., ***asaf., aur.,*** bar-c., **BELL.,** brom., ***bry.,*** **CALC.,** calc-s., ***carb-an., carb-s., carb-v.,*** caust., cham., chel., ***chin.,*** cic., cina, ***clem., con.,*** cupr., cycl., ***dulc., fl-ac.,*** graph., ***hep., hydr.,*** hyos., iod., ***kali-bi., lach.,*** led., **LYC.,** ***mang., merc., merc-i-f., merc-i-r.,*** mez., nat-c., nux-v., petr., phos., plb., **PULS.,** ran-b., ran-s., sel., sep., **SIL.,** staph., sulph., thuj., verat.

areola - arn., ***ars.,*** **ASAR.,** ***bell.,*** caust., cham., cina, hep., **LACH.,** ***lyc.,*** merc., mez., nat-c., nux-v., petr., phos., **PULS.,** sep., sil., staph., sulph.

base, with - ***alumn., calc-f.,*** com., con.

edges - calc-f., ***carb-an.,*** com., nit-ac., paeon., ph-ac.

margins - alum., **ARS.,** ***asaf.,*** bry., **CALC.,** calc-f., ***carb-an., carb-v., caust.,*** cic., cina, clem., ***com., fl-ac., hep., lach.,*** **LYC., MERC.,** ***nit-ac.,*** paeon., petr., ***phos.,*** ph-ac., ***puls.,*** ran-b., ***sang.,*** sep., **SIL.,** staph., **SULPH.,** thuj.

shining - fl-ac., phos., ***puls.,*** sil.

inflamed - **ACON.,** agn., ant-c., arn., **ARS.,** asaf., bar-c., ***bell.,*** bor., bov., ***bry., calc.,*** calen., carb-an., caust., ***cham.,*** cina, cinnb., cocc., colch., con., croc., cupr., dig., **HEP.,** hyos., ign., kreos., ***lac-c., lach.,*** led., ***lyc.,*** mang., **MERC.,** mez., nat-c., ***nat-m.,*** nat-p., ***nit-ac.,*** nux-v., petr., **PHOS.,** phyt., plb., ***puls.,*** ran-b., ***rhus-t.,*** ruta., sars., sep., **SIL.,** ***staph., sulph.,*** thuj., verat., zinc.

injury, after slight - mang.

insensibility, in - ***iod.,*** op.

irregular edges, with - ars., kali-bi., ***merc.,*** nit-ac., ***ph-ac.,*** phyt., sars., sil.

ULCERS, general

itching - alum., ambr., am-c., anac., ant-c., ant-t., arn., ***ars.,*** bar-c., bell., bov., bry., calc., canth., carb-v., ***caust.,*** cham., chel., ***chin.,*** clem., con., dros., ***graph.,*** **HEP.,** ip., kali-n., kreos., lach., led., **LYC.,** ***merc.,*** **MEZ.,** nat-c., nat-m., ***nit-ac.,*** nux-v., petr., ***ph-ac.,*** phos., ***psor., puls., ran-b., rhus-t.,*** ruta., sabad., sars., sel., ***sep.,*** **SIL.,** squil., ***staph., sulph., thuj.,*** verat., viol-t., zinc.

around about - ang., ars., bell., caust., clem., **HEP.,** ***lach., lyc.,*** merc., mez., nat-c., nux-v., petr., ph-ac., phos., **PULS.,** ***ran-b.,*** rhus-t., sabin., sep., **SIL.,** staph., sulph.

night - ***lyc., staph.***

jagged, margins, with - ***ars., carb-v.,*** hep., lach., **MERC.,** merc-sul., ***nit-ac., petr.,*** **PH-AC.,** ***sil.,*** staph., sulph., ***thuj.***

zigzag - ***nit-ac.***

jerking, pain, with - arn., ***asaf.,*** aur., bell., bry., ***calc.,*** **CAUST.,** cham., chin., clem., cupr., graph., lyc., merc., nat-c., ***nat-m.,*** nit-ac., ***nux-v.,*** petr., phyt., **PULS.,** ***rhus-t.,*** ruta., sep., **SIL.,** ***staph.,*** sulph.

around about - staph.

lardaceous - ant-c., ***ars.,*** cupr., ***hep.,*** kali-bi., kreos., **MERC.,** ***nit-ac., phyt.,*** sabin., sulph., thuj.

left side - aster.

maggots, with - sabad., sil.

malignant - arg-n., ***ars.,*** carb-an., ***carb-v.,*** caust., chel., hydr., lyc., merc., ***merc-c.,*** **NIT-AC.,** petr., ran-b., ran-s., ***sil.,*** thuj.

borders, with blue - mang.

mercurial - ***asaf., aur., carb-v., cist.,*** **HEP.,** ***kali-bi.,*** **KALI-I.,** ***lach., lyc.,*** merc., **NIT-AC., PH-AC., PHYT., SARS.,** sep., **SIL.,** ***sulph.***

mottled, areola - arn., ***ars.,*** **CARB-V., CON.,** ***crot-h.,*** ip., **LACH.,** ***led.,*** **PULS.,** ***sul-ac.***

multiple - ***bar-m.***

mustard poultice, from - calc-p.

painful - ang., arn., **ARS.,** ***asaf.,*** aur., **BELL.,** calc-s., ***carb-an.,*** carb-s., ***carb-v., caust.,*** chin., con., cor-r., cupr., dulc., ***fl-ac., graph., hep.,*** hyos., ***kali-bi., kreos., led., lyc., merc., mur-ac.,*** nat-m., ***nit-ac., nux-v., ph-ac.,*** phos., ***phyt., puls.,*** ran-b., ***sil.,*** sulph., zinc.

around about - ***ars.,*** asaf., hep., ***lach.,*** **PULS.**

on touch - mez.

cold application amel. - ***led.***

weather, in - ***kali-bi.***

coughing - con.

eating, before - puls.

lightnings-like, in small spot, worse from warmth - fl-ac.

margins - ***ars.,*** asaf., hep., lach., lyc., ***merc., sil.***

menses, during - ***cham.***

morning - ars.

night - ***asaf.,*** cham., ***cinnb., con., merc.***

splinter-like - ham., hep., ***nit-ac.***

warmth of bed, from - cinnb., dros., ***merc., puls.***

ULCERS, general

painless - ambr., anac., ant-t., arn., ***ars.,*** aur., ***bapt.,*** bar-c., ***bell.,*** bov., ***bry., calc.,*** camph., carb-an., ***carb-v.,*** cham., chel., chin., cic., ***cocc.,*** **CON.,** croc., ***dulc.,*** fl-ac., graph., ***hell., hyos.,*** ign., ip., ***lach.,*** laur., led., **LYC.,** merc., nit-ac., nux-m., nux-v., ***olnd.,*** **OP., PH-AC.,** ***phos.,*** plat., ***puls.,*** rhus-t., ***sec., sep.,*** staph., ***stram.,*** sulph., verat., zinc.

uneven, jagged base, dirty pus, no redness, with - ph-ac.

phagedenic - agar., ***anthr.,*** **ARS.,** aur-m-n., bor., ***calc.,*** **CARB-V., CAUST.,** cham., **CHEL.,** cic., cinnb., clem., con., ***crot-c., crot-h.,*** dulc., ***graph., hep.,*** hydrc., ***hyper., kali-ar., kali-c., kali-p., lach.,*** led., **LYC., MERC.,** merc-c., merc-cy., merc-d., ***merc-i-r., mez.,*** nat-a., ***nat-c., nat-m.,*** **NIT-AC., PETR.,** ***puls.,*** **RAN-B., RAN-S.,** ***rhus-t.,*** sars., ***sep.,*** **SIL.,** squil., staph., ***sulph., sul-ac.,*** zinc.

pimples, surrounded by - acon., ***ars.,*** bell., **CARB-V.,** ***caust.,*** cham., fl-ac., grin., ***hep.,*** **LACH.,** lyc., merc., merc-sul., ***mez.,*** mur-ac., nat-c., ***petr.,*** phos., ***puls.,*** ran-s., ***rhus-t., sep.,*** sil., staph., ***sulph.***

pressing - camph., carb-v., chin., ***graph.,*** mez., **PAEON.,** par., ***phyt.,*** **SIL.**

proud, flesh - ars., graph.

pulsating - acon., arn., ars., ***asaf.,*** bar-c., bell., bov., bry., ***calc.,*** calc-s., caust., cham., chin., clem., con., ***hep.,*** hyos., ign., ***kali-c.,*** kali-s., kalm., ***lyc.,*** **MERC.,** mez., mur-ac., ***nat-c.,*** nat-m., nit-ac., petr., ph-ac., phos., puls., rhus-t., ruta., sabad., sars., sep., ***sil.,*** staph., **SULPH.,** thuj.

night - ***hep.,*** **MERC.**

walking, when - mur-ac.

pustules, around - calc., caust., clem., ***hep., mez., mur-ac.,*** ph-ac., rhus-t., ***sil.,*** sulph.

raised edges, with - ars., calen., nit-ac., ph-ac., ***sil.***

raw flesh-like base, with - ars., merc-sul., ***nit-ac.***

red, areola - ***acon.,*** ant-c., arn., **ARS.,** ***asaf.,*** bar-c., bell., bor., bry., ***calc., cham.,*** cocc., cupr., fl-ac., **HEP.,** hyos., ign., ***kali-bi.,*** kreos., ***lach.,*** led., ***lyc., merc.,*** **MEZ.,** nat-c., nat-p., nit-ac., nux-v., ***petr.,*** ph-ac., phos., plb., **PULS.,** ran-b., ***rhus-t.,*** sars., sep., **SIL., STAPH., SULPH.,** thuj., verat., zinc.

regular, margins - kali-bi.

reopening, of old - ***ars.,*** calen., carb-v., crot-h., ***kreos., lach., sep.,*** sil., vib.

spring, in the - cench., ***lach.***

healed, when partly - **KREOS.**

round, punched - kali-bi., merc., phyt.

rubbing, from - ang.

salt rheum, like - **AMBR., ARS.,** ***graph.,*** lyc., merc., petr., phos., puls., sep., ***sil., staph.,*** sulph.

sarcomatous - ant-c., ***apis, ars.,*** **HEP.,** kreos., ***merc.,*** **NIT-AC.,** ***phos.,*** sabin., sulph., thuj.

scarlet fever, from - cham.

ULCERS, general

scooped out - vario.

scratching, after - ant-c., ***ars., asaf.,*** bar-c., bell., bry., calc., carb-an., carb-v., ***caust.,*** chin., con., graph., ***hep., iod.,*** kreos., **LACH.,** ***lyc.,*** mang., ***merc.,*** mez., nat-c., ***nit-ac., petr.,*** ph-ac., phos., puls., ran-b., ***rhus-t.,*** sabin., sep., ***sil.,*** staph., **SULPH.,** thuj.

scrofulous - bar-i., calc., calc-ac., calc-ar., calc-br., calc-caust., calc-f., calc-hp., calc-i., calc-lac., calc-mur., calc-ox., calc-p., calc-pic., calc-s., calc-sil., chin., ferr-i., hep., iod., kali-i., mag-i., merc-i-f., merc-i-r., nat-i., nit-ac., plb-i., sil., sul-i., sulph., zinc-i.

senile - tarent-c.

sensitive - alum., am-c., anac., ang., **ARN.,** ***ars.,*** ars-i., **ASAF.,** aur., ***bell., calen.,*** carb-an., carb-s., carb-v., ***caust.,*** cham., ***chin.,*** chin-a., cic., ***clem., cocc.,*** coff., con., croc., ***cor-r.,*** cupr., dig., ***dulc., graph.,*** **HEP.,** ***hydr.,*** hyos., ***iod.,*** kreos., **LACH.,** led., **LYC.,** ***merc., mez.,*** mur-ac., nat-c., nat-m., nat-p., nit-ac., ***nux-v., paeon., petr., ph-ac.,*** phos., **PULS.,** ran-b., ran-s., rhus-t., sabin., ***sec.,*** sel., ***sep., sil.,*** squil., ***staph.,*** sulph., tarent-c., thuj., verat.

around about - ***ars.,*** **ASAF.,** bell., caust., cocc., ***hep.,*** **LACH.,** lyc., merc., mez., mur-ac., nat-c., nux-v., petr., phos., **PULS.,** rhus-t., sep., sil.

margins - **ARS., ASAF.,** caust., clem., **HEP.,** ***lach., lyc.,*** **MERC.,** mur-ac., petr., ph-ac., phos., puls., ran-b., sep., **SIL.,** sulph., ***thuj.***

touch, to, causing convulsions - staph.

serpiginous - ***ars.,*** bor., calc., chel., ***merc.,*** merc-c., ph-ac., ***phyt.,*** sabad., ***sars., sil.,*** staph.

sex agg. - kreos.

shining - ***lac-c., phos.,*** puls., staph., syph.

margins - fl-ac., phos., puls., sil.

shooting - **ARS.,** ***asaf.,*** clem., ***hep.,*** **LYC.,** ***phyt., puls., staph.***

small ulcers surrounding it - calc., hep., mez., phos., rhus-t., sil.

smarting - alum., ambr., ant-c., arn., ars., bell., bry., calc., canth., caust., ***cham.,*** cic., ***graph.,*** **HEP.,** hyos., ign., kali-c., ***lyc., merc.,*** mez., ***nat-m.,*** nux-v., ***ph-ac., phos.,*** **PULS.,** ***rhus-t., sep.,*** sil., ***staph., sulph.,*** sul-ac., ***thuj.,*** zinc.

night - ***hep.,*** lyc., ***merc.,*** rhus-t.

spongy - alum., ***ant-c.,*** ant-t., **ARS.,** bell., calc., **CARB-AN.,** ***carb-s., carb-v.,*** caust., cham., ***clem.,*** con., graph., ***hep., iod., kreos.,*** **LACH.,** ***lyc.,*** **MERC.,** nit-ac., nux-v., ***petr., ph-ac., phos.,*** rhus-t., sabin., ***sep.,*** **SIL.,** ***staph., sulph., thuj.***

margins, at - **ARS.,** ***carb-an.,*** caust., clem., ***lach.,*** lyc., merc., petr., ph-ac., phos., sep., **SIL.,** staph., sulph., thuj.

spring, in the - ***calc., cench., lach.***

ULCERS, general
stinging, sharp - acon., alum., ant-c., ***apis,*** arn., **ARS.,** ***asaf.,*** bar-c., ***bell.,*** bov., ***bry.,*** calc., camph., canth., ***carb-an.,*** carb-s., carb-v., ***caust.,*** cham., chin., chin-a., ***cinnb.,*** clem., cocc., con., cycl., ***graph., hep., hydr.,*** kali-n., led., ***lyc.,*** mag-c., mang., **MERC.,** mez., mur-ac., nat-a., ***nat-c.,*** nat-m., nat-p., **NIT-AC.,** nux-v., ***petr.,*** ph-ac., phos., **PULS.,** ran-b., ***rhus-t.,*** sabad., sabin., sars., sel., ***sep.,*** **SIL.,** spong., squil., ***staph.,*** **SULPH.,** ***thuj.***
areola, in - acon., ***ars.,*** **ASAF.,** bell., cham., cocc., hep., lyc., ***merc.,*** mez., mur-ac., nat-c., nit-ac., nux-v., petr., phos., **PULS.,** rhus-t., sabin., sep., ***sil.,*** staph., ***sulph.***
evening - mez.
laughing - hep.
margins - **ARS.,** ***asaf.,*** bry., clem., ***hep., lyc.,*** **MERC.,** mez., mur-ac., petr., phos., ***puls.,*** ran-b., sep., **SIL.,** staph., ***sulph.,*** thuj.
when touched - clem.
night - mang., rhus-t., sep.
splinters, as from - hep., **NIT-AC.**
stupor, low delirium and prostration, with - bapt.
superficial - am-c., ant-c., ant-t., ***ars., asaf.,*** bell., carb-an., carb-v., ***chin.,*** cor-r., **LACH., LYC.,** ***merc., mez.,*** nat-c., ***nat-m., nit-ac.,*** petr., ***ph-ac.,*** phos., puls., ran-b., ***sel., sep., sil.,*** staph., sulph., thuj.
suppressed - clem., lach., sulph.
suppurating - acon., ambr., am-c., anac., ant-c., ant-t., arg-m., arn., **ARS.,** ars-i., **ASAF.,** aur., bar-c., ***bell.,*** bov., bry., calc., ***canth.,*** caps., carb-an., carb-s., ***carb-v.,*** **CAUST.,** cham., chel., chin., cic., clem., cocc., con., croc., dros., dulc., graph., hell., **HEP.,** hyos., ign., **IOD.,** ip., kali-ar., kali-c., kali-n., ***kali-s.,*** kreos., lach., led., ***lyc.,*** mang., **MERC.,** mez., mur-ac., nat-c., nat-m., nat-p., ***nit-ac.,*** nux-v., petr., ***ph-ac., phos.,*** plb., **PULS.,** ran-b., ran-s., **RHUS-T.,** ruta., sabad., sabin., sars., sec., sel., ***sep.,*** **SIL.,** spig., spong., squil., ***staph.,*** **SULPH.,** sul-ac., thuj., viol-t., zinc.
pain, with - am-c., anac., arn., ars., ***asaf.,*** aur., bar-c., ***bry., calc., carb-v.,*** chin., colch., ***con.,*** cycl., dros., euph., ***graph.,*** hep., hyos., iod., kali-c., kreos., led., nat-m., nit-ac., nux-v., par., petr., **PHOS., PULS.,** ***ran-b., rhus-t.,*** ruta., sars., sec., **SIL.,** staph., ***sulph.,*** valer., verat., zinc.
swollen - acon., agn., arn., ***ars.,*** aur., bar-c., ***bell., bry., calc.,*** carb-an., carb-v., caust., cham., cic., cocc., ***con.,*** dulc., graph., ***hep.,*** iod., ***kali-c.,*** led., **LYC.,** mang., **MERC.,** nat-c., ***nat-m.,*** nat-p., ***nit-ac.,*** nux-v., ***petr.,*** ph-ac., ***phos.,*** plb., **PULS., RHUS-T.,** sabin., samb., **SEP., SIL.,** staph., **SULPH.,** ***vip.***
areola - acon., ars., ***bell.,*** caust., cham., graph., ***hep.,*** lyc., ***merc.,*** nat-c., nux-v., petr., phos., **PULS.,** ***rhus-t., sep.,*** sil., staph.

ULCERS, general
swollen, margins - ***ars.,*** bry., ***calc.,*** carb-an., caust., cic., ***hep.,*** lyc., **MERC.,** petr., ph-ac., phos., ***puls., sep.,*** **SIL.,** ***sulph.***
syphilitic - anan., **ARS.,** asaf., ***aur., aur-m., aur-m-n., carb-v., cinnb., cist.,*** cortiso., ***crot-c., fl-ac.,*** graph., ***hep.,*** **IOD.,** ***kali-bi., kali-chl.,*** **KALI-I.,** lac-c., ***lach.,*** lyc., **MERC., MERC-C.,** ***merc-i-r.,*** merc-sul., mez., **NIT-AC.,** ***petr.,*** **PHYT.,** rumx., sang., ***sars., staph., still.,*** stram., ***syph.,*** **THUJ.**
tearing, with - ***ars.,*** bell., bry., ***calc.,*** canth., carb-v., caust., clem., cocc., ***cycl., graph.,*** kali-c., **LYC.,** ***merc.,*** mez., nat-c., nit-ac., ***nux-v.,*** phos., puls., rhus-t., ***sep.,*** sil., ***staph.,*** **SULPH.,** zinc.
around about - calc., staph.
motion, on - bell.
tense - arn., ***asaf.,*** aur., ***bar-c.,*** bell., bry., calc., carb-an., carb-v., ***caust.,*** cham., chin., clem., cocc., **CON.,** graph., hep., ***iod.,*** kali-c., kreos., ***lach.,*** lyc., ***merc.,*** mez., mur-ac., nat-c., nit-ac., nux-v., petr., ph-ac., ***phos., phyt.,*** **PULS.,** ***rhus-t.,*** sabin., sep., sil., ***spong.,*** staph., **STRONT-C., SULPH.,** thuj., zinc.
areola - ***asaf.,*** bell., caust., cham., cocc., hep., ***lach.,*** lyc., merc., mez., mur-ac., nat-c., nux-v., petr., phos., ph-ac., **PULS.,** rhus-t., sabin., sep., sil., staph., ***stront-c., sulph.***
thin skin over bones, on - merc.
tingling - acon., arn., bell., caust., cham., clem., con., hep., lach., phos., rhus-t., sec., sep., sulph.
night - rhus-t.
traumatic - arn., con.
tumors, after removal of - hydr.
unhealthy - alum., am-c., bar-c., bor., ***calc.,*** carb-v., caust., ***cham.,*** **CHEL.,** clem., ***con.,*** croc., ***graph.,*** hell., **HEP.,** ***hippoz.,*** kali-c., ***lach.,*** lyc., mag-c., mang., ***merc.,*** mur-ac., nat-c., nat-p., **NIT-AC.,** nux-v., ***petr.,*** ph-ac., phos., plb., ***rhus-t., sep.,*** **SIL.,** squil., ***staph., sulph.,*** viol-t.
varicose - ant-t., anac., ***ars., calc.,*** calc-f., calen., ***carb-v.,*** **CARD-M., CAUST.,** cinnb., clem-vit., crot-h., cund., eucal., **FL-AC.,** graph., grin., ***ham.,*** hydr., kreos., ***lach.,*** **LYC.,** merc., mez., phyt., psor., **PULS.,** pyrog., ***rhus-t.,*** sars., ***sec., sil., sulph.,*** sul-ac., thuj., ***zinc.***
vesicles, surrounded by - ***ars.,*** bell., caust., ***fl-ac., hep.,*** **LACH.,** merc., **MEZ.,** nat-c., ***nat-m.,*** petr., phos., ***rhus-t.,*** sep., ***thuj.***
surrounded by, red, shining areola, with - fl-ac., hep., ***mez.***
warmth, agg. - ***cham.,*** dros., euph., ***fl-ac.,*** hydr., led., ***lyc., merc., sabin., sec.***
amel. - ***ars.,*** **LACH., SIL.,** ***syph.***
wart, shaped - ars., calc., ***nat-c.,*** phos.
washing, agg. - ***hydr.***
white, spots, with - ***ars.,*** calc., con., **LACH., MERC.,** phos., sep., **SIL.,** sulph., thuj.

ULCERS, general

yellow - calc., cor-r., nit-ac., plb., staph., sulph., zinc.

UNHEALTHY, skin, every scratch festers or heals with difficulty - alum., am-c., ant-c., ***apis, arn., ars., bar-c., bar-m.,*** **BOR.,** ***bufo,*** **CALC.,** calc-s., calen., caps., **CARB-S.,** ***carb-v.,*** **CARC., CAUST., CHAM.,** chel., clem., con., croc., crot-h., ***fl-ac.,*** **GRAPH.,** ham., hell., **HEP.,** hydr., kali-bi., kali-c., **LACH.,** ***lyc.,*** mag-c., ***mang.,*** merc., merc-sul., mez., mur-ac., nat-c., nat-p., nit-ac., nux-v., **PETR.,** ph-ac., ***phos.,*** pip-m., plb., **PSOR.,** puls., pyrus, **RHUS-T.,** ***sars.,*** sel., ***sep.,*** **SIL.,** squil., ***staph.,*** still., **SULPH.,** tarax., ***tarent.,*** thuj., x-ray.

joints, around - mang.

URINARY affections, with skin - viol-t.

URTICARIA, hives - ***acon.,*** agar., all-c., am-c., am-m., anac., ***ant-c.,*** ant-t., anthro., antipyrin., ap-g., **APIS,** arn., **ARS.,** ***ars-i.,*** **ASTAC.,** aur., bar-c., bar-m., bell., benz-ac., berb., bomb-pr., ***bov., bry.,*** bufo, ***calad.,*** **CALC., CALC-S.,** ***camph.,*** carb-an., **CARB-AC., CARB-S.,** ***carb-v.,*** **CAUST.,** cham., chin., chin-a., ***chin-s.,*** **CHLOL.,** chlor., cic., ***cimic.,*** coca, cocc., ***con.,*** **COP.,** ***corn., crot-h.,*** crot-t., cub., cund., ***cupr.,*** **DULC.,** dys-co., ***elat.,*** fago., ferr-i., ***frag.,*** gall-ac., ***galph., graph.,*** **HEP., HIST.,** hom., hydr., ***ichth.,*** ign., iod., ip., ***kali-ar., kali-br., kali-c.,*** kali-chl., kali-i., kali-p., kali-s., ***kreos.,*** lach., **LED.,** ***lyc.,*** lycps., mag-c., medus., merc., ***mez.,*** nat-a., nat-c., **NAT-M.,** ***nat-p.,*** nit-ac., ***nux-v.,*** pall., ***petr.,*** ph-ac., ***phos.,*** polyg., ***psor., puls.,*** **RHUS-T.,** rhus-v., rob., rumx., ruta, ***sal-ac.,*** sanic., sars., sec., sel., ***sep.,*** sil., skook., stann., staph., stram., stroph., stry., **SULPH.,** ***sul-ac., sul-i.,*** ter., tet., thuj., ***til., trio.,*** tub., **URT-U.,** ust., valer., vario., ***verat.,*** vesp., zinc.

afternoon - chlol.

ailments, after suppressed - apis, ars., urt-u.

air, cold, in - ars., caust., dulc., kali-br., nat-s., ***nit-ac.,*** **RHUS-T.,** rumx., ***sep.***

amel. - ***calc.,*** dol., ***dulc.***

air, open in - nit-ac.

amel. - calc.

from - nit-ac., sep.

alcoholics, in - chlol.

alternating with

asthma - apis, ars., calad., graph.

cramps - ars.

croup - ars.

rheumatism,with - ***rhus-t., urt-u.***

antibiotics, after - apis, ars., moni., nit-ac., pen.

ascarides, with - urt-u.

asthmatic, troubles, in - ***apis.***

bathing, after - bov., lach., phos., ***urt-u.***

cold, after - calc-p.

catarrh, with - all-c., dulc.

catarrh, from - dulc.

cement, of - calc., petr., rhus-t., sil.

change of air and weather - ***apis.***

URTICARIA, hives

children, in - apis, cop., ***urt-u.***

chronic - apis, cop., puls., ***urt-u.***

chill, during - apis, ***ars.,*** ign., **NAT-M., RHUS-T.**

after - ***elat., hep.***

before - ***hep.***

intermittent, with - ign., nat-m.

chronic - ***anac., ant-c.,*** antipyrin., ***ars., astac., bov.,*** calc., chlor., ***cop.,*** cund., ***dulc.,*** hep., ichth., ***lyc.,*** nat-m., ***rhus-t.,*** sep., stroph., ***sulph.,*** urt-u.

recurring - hep.

clothes, from pressure of - med.

cold air, in - caust., kali-br., nat-s., ***nit-ac.,*** **RHUS-T.,** rumx., ***sep.***

amel. - ***calc., dulc.***

bath, after - ***calc-p.***

water amel. - apis, dulc.

cold taking, from - ars., calc., calc-p., **DULC.,** rhus-t., rumx., sep.

colds agg. - ***dulc.***

constipation, with - cop.

diarrhea, with - apis, bov., ***puls.***

drinking, cold water agg. - bell.

hot drinks, water, agg. - apis, chlol.

amel. - chlol.

edema, with - ***apis,*** urt-u., vesp.

emotion, from - anac., bov., dys-co., ign., kali-br., ***nat-m.***

erosion on toes, with - sulph.

evening - ***kreos., nux-v.***

exercise, exertion, from - apis, calc., hep., nat-m., psor., sanic., urt-u.

violent, after - apis, calc., ***con.,*** hep., ***nat-m., psor.,*** sanic., ***urt-u.***

exposure, from - chlor., ***dulc.,*** rhus-t.

fever, during - **APIS,** chlor., ***cop.,*** cub., **IGN., RHUS-T.,** ***rhus-v., sulph.***

suppressed, from - elat.

fish agg. - ars., astac., lyc.

flat, in plaques - form., lob.

flour, from - pot-a.

fruit, pork or buckwheat, from - puls.

gastric derangement, from - ***ant-c.,*** ars., carb-v., cop., dulc., kali-s., nux-v., ***puls.,*** rob., trio.

insect bites, from - ***apis.***

itching, burning after scratching, no fever, with - dulc.

without itching - uva.

liver symptoms, with - astac., myric., ptel.

livid - ***apis.***

lying, amel. - urt-u.

malaria, from suppressed - elat.

meat, after - **ANT-C.**

menopause at, agg. - morph., ust.

menses, during - bell., ***cimic., dulc., kali-c.,*** mag-c., puls., sec., ust.

after - kreos.

before - cimic., ***dulc., kali-c.,*** mag-c., nat-m.

URTICARIA, hives
menses, during
delayed - puls.
profuse, with - bov.
morning - ***bell.***
waking, on - bov.
nausea, after - sang.
before the - sang.
night - ant-c., **APIS,** ars., ***bov., chlol., cop.,*** hydr., ***nux-v., puls.***
nodular - ***agar., alum.,*** am-c., am-m., anac., ***ant-c.,*** ant-t., **APIS,** arn., ars., aur., bar-c., bar-m., bell., ***bry.,*** **CALC.,** cann-s., canth., caps., ***carb-an.,*** carb-s., ***carb-v.,*** **CAUST.,** ***chel.,*** chin., ***chlol.,*** chlor., cic., cocc., con., ***cop.,*** dig., dros., **DULC.,** graph., hell., ***hep.,*** ign., ***iod.,*** ip., ***jug-c.,*** kali-ar., ***kali-br.,*** kali-c., kali-i., kali-n., kali-s., kreos., **LACH.,** ***led., lyc., mag-c.,*** mag-m., ***mang.,*** merc., **MEZ.,** mur-ac., nat-a., nat-c., ***nat-m.,*** nat-p., nit-ac., nux-v., olnd., op., pall., ***petr.,*** ph-ac., phos., ***puls.,*** **RHUS-T.,** rhus-v., ***ruta.,*** sabin., ***sec.,*** sel., ***sep., sil.,*** spig., spong., squil., stann., ***staph.,*** stram., ***sulph.,*** sul-ac., tarax., thuj., ***urt-u.,*** valer., ***verat.,*** verb., viol-t., zinc.
rosy - ***bell., bry., chlol., chlor.,*** coca, cop., crot-t., gels., jug-c., kali-br., kali-i., merc., ***nat-c.,*** petr., phos., phyt., **RHUS-T.,** sil., **STRAM.,** ter.
oxyures, with - rhus-t., urt-u.
palpitation, with - bov.
periodical, every year - urt-u.
perspiration, during - **APIS, RHUS-T.**
pinworm, with - urt-u.
purple - chin-s.
receding - stroph.
recurring - hep.
rheumatic lameness, palpitation and diarrhea, with - ***bov.,*** dulc., rhus-t.
rheumatism, during - **RHUS-T., URT-U.**
rubbing amel. - elat.
sequelae, from suppressed hives, with - apis, urt-u.
scratching, after - agar., alum., am-c., am-m., ant-c., ars., bar-c., bry., ***calc.,*** carb-an., carb-s., carb-v., ***caust.,*** chin., chin-a., cic., cocc., con., **DULC.,** ***graph.,*** hell., ***hep.,*** ip., **LACH.,** led., ***lyc.,*** mag-c., mag-m., mang., merc., **MEZ.,** nat-c., nat-m., nit-ac., nux-v., olnd., ***petr.,*** puls., **RHUS-T.,** ruta., sel., sep., sil., spig., ***staph.,*** sulph., thuj., verat., zinc.
seashore, at - ars., mag-m.
shellfish, after - apis, astac., camph., lyc., ox-ac., ter., ***urt-u.***
shuddering, with - urt-u.
spring, every - rhus-t.
spirituous liquors, after - chol.
strawberries, from - ***apis,*** bry., frag., ***ox-ac., urt-u.***
sudden, coming and going - antipyrin., dys-co.
violent onset, syncope, with - camph.

URTICARIA, hives
suppression of, agg. - apis, ars., urt-u.
touch, very sensitive to - hep.
tuberosa - ***anac.,*** bol.
uncovered, parts - apis.
undressing, agg. - puls.
vegetables, from - cypr., urt-u.
vomiting, with - apis, cina.
walking, in cold air, while - ***sep.***
warmth, and exercise, agg. - ***apis, bov., con., dulc.,*** kali-c., ***kali-i., led., lyc.,*** **NAT-M.,** nit-ac., ***psor., puls., sulph.,*** **URT-U.**
amel. - ars., chlol., ***hep.,*** lyc., ***sep.***
wet, becoming, from - **RHUS-T.**
white - nat-m.
wine, from - ***chlol.***
yearly, same season - rhus-t., urt-u.

VACCINIA, (see Cowpox)

VALVE, leaf, as of a - alum., ant-t., ***bar-c.,*** ferr., iod., kali-c., kali-i., lach., mang., ***phos.,*** sabad., ***spong.,*** thuj.

VARICELLA, (see Chickenpox)
eruptions like, on limbs - ***ant-t.***

VARIOLA, (see Smallpox)

VESICLES, eruptions - agar., alum., am-c., ***am-m., anac.,*** anthr., ***ant-c., ant-t.,*** arg-m., arn., **ARS.,** aur., ***bar-c., bell., bov., bry., bufo,*** calad., ***calc.,*** calc-p., ***calc-s.,*** cann-s., **CANTH.,** caps., **CARB-AC.,** ***carb-an., carb-s.,*** carb-v., **CAUST.,** cham., ***chin.,*** chin-a., ***cic.,*** cist., **CLEM.,** cocc., com., con., cop., ***corn.,*** crot-h., **CROT-T.,** cupr-ar., cycl., dig., **DULC., EUPH.,** ***fl-ac., graph.,*** grin., ***hell., hep.,*** hyos., ign., ***iris, jug-r.,*** kali-ar., ***kali-bi., kali-c., kali-chl., kali-i., kali-n., kali-s., kreos.,*** lac-c., **LACH.,** ***lact.,*** laur., ***lyc., mag-c.,*** **MANC.,** mang., ***merc., merc-c., mez.,*** nat-a., **NAT-C., NAT-M.,** ***nat-p.,*** nat-s., **NIT-AC.,** olnd., op., osm., ***petr.,*** ph-ac., **PHOS.,** plat., plb., ***psor., puls.,*** **RAN-B.,** ***ran-s.,*** rheum, **RHUS-T.,** ***rhus-v., rumx.,*** ruta., sabad., ***sabin.,*** sal-ac., sars., ***sec., sel.,*** seneg., ***sep., sil.,*** spig., spong., ***squil.,*** staph., stram., **SULPH.,** sul-ac., tarax., ***tell.,*** ter., thuj., verat., vip., zinc.
black - ***anthr.,*** arg-n., **ARS., LACH.,** nat-c., petr., vip.
blood, filled with - ***ail.,*** **ARS.,** aur., bry., camph., canth., carb-ac., fl-ac., graph., kali-p., **LACH.,** nat-c., ***nat-m., sec.,*** sulph.
bluish - ***anthr.,*** **ARS.,** bell., con., **LACH., RAN-B.,** rhus-t., vip.
brown - anag., ant-c., carb-v., lyc., mez., nit-ac., phos., sep., thuj.
burning - agar., am-c., am-m., ***anac.,*** anag., ars., aur., ***bar-c.,*** bov., calc., carb-ac., caust., ***crot-t.,*** graph., guare., hep., kali-n., lach., mag-c., mag-m., mang., merc., ***mez., mur-ac.,*** nat-c., nat-m., nit-ac., phos., plat., ***ran-b.,*** rhus-t., seneg., sep., sil., ***spig.,*** spong., staph., sulph.
close to each other - ran-b., rhus-t., verat.
cold air - ***dulc.***

VESICLES, general,
confluent - alum., ***cic.***, phel., rhus-t., ***sulph.***
convulsions, before - cic.
cracked, breaking - ***bry.***, ***crot-h.***, ***lach.***, phos., ***vip.***
cutting - graph.
denuded surface, forming on - anag., rhus-t., staph.
drawing, painful - clem.
dry - rhus-t.
gangrenous - ***ars.***, bell., ***bufo***, ***camph.***, carb-v., **LACH.**, mur-ac., ***ran-b.***, ***sabin.***, ***sec.***, sil.
grape shaped - bufo, rhus-t.
grouped - rhus-v., sulph.
hard - lach., ph-ac., phos., sil.
heat of sun, as from - clem.
humid - hell., hep., lach., mang., ***merc.***, phos., ran-b., ran-s., **RHUS-T.**, sulph., vip.
inflamed - am-m., anac., bar-c., bell., ***crot-t.***, dulc., kali-n., rhus-t., rhus-v.
itching - aeth., am-c., am-m., ***anac.***, ant-c., ant-t., apis, ars-h., bry., **CALC.**, ***canth.***, ***carb-ac.***, caust., crot-t., daph., ***fl-ac.***, ***graph.***, ***jug-r.***, ***lach.***, mag-c., ***mez.***, ***nat-c.***, ***rhus-t.***, ***rumx.***, sel., ***sep.***, sil., sulph., tell.
around old scars - ***fl-ac.***
cold air, in - ***rumx.***
evening - kali-c.
night - ***graph.***
uncovered, when - ***rumx.***
warm, bed, in - aeth.
warm, room - apis.
milary - acon.
painful - bell., clem., kali-c., phos.
painful, as if ulcerated - mez., mur-ac.
shooting pains - ***nat-c.***
painless - stront-c., sulph.
peeling off - ***bry.***, puls., rhus-t.
phagedenic - am-c., ars., bor., ***calc.***, caust., cham., clem., graph., hep., kali-c., ***mag-c.***, merc., nat-c., ***nit-ac.***, ***petr.***, sep., ***sil.***, ***sulph.***
red - ***ant-c.***, calc-p., cic., crot-h., cycl., fl-ac., lach., mang., merc., nat-c., ***nat-m.***, ol-an., sil., valer.
areola - anac., ***calc.***, cann-s., crot-h., crot-t., kali-c., kali-chl., ***nat-c.***, sil., sulph., tab., vip.
scratching, after - ***am-c.***, ***am-m.***, ant-c., ars., bar-c., bell., bry., calc., caust., chin., ***cycl.***, dulc., graph., grat., ***hep.***, kali-ar., kali-c., kreos., **LACH.**, laur., mag-c., mang., merc., nat-c., nat-m., nicc., ol-an., ***phos.***, ***ran-b.***, **RHUS-T.**, sabin., sars., sel., sep., spong., ***sulph.***
scurfy - anac., hell., kali-bi., nat-c., nat-m., nit-ac., ran-b., sil., sulph.
small - am-m., cann-s., fl-ac., graph., hell., lach., mang., merc., nat-m., nit-ac., rhus-t., thuj.

VESICLES, general,
smarting - con., graph., hell., mag-c., mang., nat-c., ph-ac., phel., plat., rhod., rhus-t., rhus-v., sil., staph., thuj.
spots, covered with - dulc., iod., lach., merc., rhus-t., spong.
leaving - caust.
stinging - am-c., calc., cham., crot-t., nat-m., **NIT-AC.**, sil., spong., ***staph.***, ***tell.***
sudamina - ***acon.***, am-m., apis, am-c., ars., bell., ***bry.***, cact., canth., cent., chin-s., crot-t., graph., ***hep.***, hura, lac-c., lach., led., **NAT-M.**, ph-ac., ***piloc.***, raph., **RHUS-T.**, ***spong.***, sul-ac., syzyg., urt-u., valer.
sun, from exposure to - acon., camph., ***kali-i.***, sol., sol-t., ***staph.***
suppurating - ***am-m.***, aur., bov., calc., carb-v., graph., mag-c., ***nat-c.***, nit-ac., petr., phos., puls., ran-b., ran-s., rhus-t., sars., sulph., vip., zinc.
tensive - am-m., kali-n., mag-c., mag-m., mur-ac., nat-c.
transparent - con., kali-c., lach., ***mag-c.***, mag-m., mang., merc., ***ran-b.***
ulcerated - ***calc.***, caust., ***clem.***, cupr-ar., graph., ***merc.***, nat-c., **SULPH.**, ***zinc.***
watery - ars., ***bell.***, bov., canth., clem., cupr., graph., kali-c., kali-n., merc., nat-c., ol-an., plat., plb., ***rhus-t.***, rhus-v., sec., ***sulph.***, tab., vip., zinc.
white - am-c., berb., cann-s., caust., clem., con., graph., hell., hep., ***kali-chl.***, ***lach.***, ***merc.***, mez., ***nat-c.***, phos., rhus-t., sabad., sulph., ***thuj.***, valer.
wound, around a - ***lach.***, rhus-t.
yellow - ***agar.***, am-m., anac., anag., ant-c., anthr., ars., bufo, calc-p., carb-s., chel., cic., clem., com., crot-h., crot-t., **DULC.**, ***euphr.***, ***hydr.***, ***kali-n.***, kreos., lach., ***manc.***, ***merc.***, mur-ac., nat-c., nat-s., ph-ac., psor., ran-b., ran-s., raph., **RHUS-T.**, ***rhus-v.***, sep., sulph., tab., vip.

VESICLES, eruptions,
yellow, spots - cur., lyc., nux-v., sep., sulph.

VITILIGO - sep., thuj.

WARM - cub.

WARTS, general (see Condylomata, Excrescences) - acet-ac., alum., ambr., am-c., anac., anac-oc., anag., anan., ***ant-c.***, ant-t., arg-n., ***ars.***, ars-br., ***aur.***, aur-m., aur-m-n., **BAR-C.**, **BELL.**, ***benz-ac.***, ***bov.***, bufo, **CALC.**, **CALC-S.**, carb-an., carb-v., cast., cast-eq., **CAUST.**, chel., chr-ox., cinnb., cupr., **DULC.**, euphr., ferr., ferr-p., ***ferr-pic.***, ***fl-ac.***, graph., ***hep.***, kali-ar., kali-c., ***kali-chl.***, kali-m., kali-per., ***lac-c.***, ***lach.***, lyc., ***mag-s.***, ***med.***, **MERC-C.**, merc-i-f., mill., ***nat-c.***, nat-m., nat-p., **NAT-S.**, **NIT-AC.**, ***ox-ac.***, petr., ***ph-ac.***, phos., phyt., pic-ac., ***psor.***, ran-b., ***rhus-t.***, ruta, sabin., sars., semp., ***sep.***, ***sil.***, spig., staph., **SULPH.**, sul-ac., syph., **THUJ.**, verat., x-ray

WARTS, general
bleeding - **CAUST.,** cinnb., hep., lyc., nat-c., **NIT-AC.,** ph-ac., ***rhus-t., sabin.,*** staph., **THUJ.**
easily, jagged, large - caust., ***nit-ac.***
washing, from - ***nit-ac.***
brown - ***sep., thuj.***
burning - am-c., ars., cinnb., hep., lyc., ***petr.,*** phos., ***rhus-t.,*** sabin., sep., sulph.
cold, washing agg. - dulc.
cracked, ragged, with furfuraceous areola - lyc.
drawing - con.
dry - ***staph.***
fan-shaped - cinnb.,
filiform - med.
flat - acet-ac., berb., calc., ***caust.,*** **DULC.,** fl-ac., lach., merc-i-f., ruta., ***sep., thuj.***
smooth and sore - ruta.
fleshy - ***calc., caust., dulc.,*** sil., thuj.
genitalia, (see Female, Male) - calc., euphr., lyc., merc., nat-s., nit-ac., sabin., sars., staph., ***thuj.***
girls, in young - sep., sulph., thuj.
granular - arg-n.
growing - kali-c.
hard - **ANT-C.,** ***calc., caust.,*** dulc., fl-ac., lach., ran-b., ***sep., sil., sulph.***
hollow, become - ***calc.***
horny - **ANT-C.,** ***calc., caust.,*** dulc., graph., nat-c., ***nit-ac.,*** ran-b., rhus-t., ***sep., sulph.,*** thuj.
broad - rhus-t.
indented - calc., euphr., lyc., nit-ac., ***ph-ac.,*** rhus-t., sabin., sep., staph., ***thuj.***
inflamed - am-c., bell., bov., ***calc., caust., hep.,*** lyc., nat-c., ***nit-ac.,*** rhus-t., sars., sep., ***sil.,*** staph., sulph., thuj.
isolated - ***lyc., thuj.***
itching - euphr., graph., ***kali-c.,*** kali-n., ***nit-ac.,*** phos., psor., ***sep.,*** sulph., thuj.
jagged - **CAUST.,** ***lyc.,*** **NIT-AC.,** ph-ac., rhus-t., ***sep.,*** staph., **THUJ.**
large - ***caust.,*** **DULC.,** kali-c., nat-c., **NIT-AC.,** ph-ac., ***rhus-t., sep., sil.,*** **THUJ.**
seedy - thuj.
soft - dulc., mag-s.
lupoid - ferr-pic.
mercury, after abuse of - ***aur., nit-ac., staph.***
moist - ***caust.,*** lyc., **NIT-AC.,** ph-ac., psor., ***rhus-t.,*** staph., **THUJ.**
itching, flat and broad - thuj.
oozing - nit-ac.
old - ***calc., caust., kali-c., nit-ac.,*** rhus-t., sulph., ***thuj.***
painful - ambr., am-c., ***bov., calc., caust.,*** hep., kali-c., kali-s., lach., lyc., nat-c., nat-m., ***nit-ac.,*** petr., phos., rhus-t., ruta., sabin., sep., sil., sulph., ***thuj.***
hard, stiff and shiny - sil.
sticking - ***nit-ac.,*** staph., thuj.

WARTS, general
pedunculated - **CAUST.,** ***dulc., lyc., med.,*** **NIT-AC.,** ph-ac., ***rhus-t.,*** sabin., sil., ***staph., thuj.***
plantar - caust., ***nat-m.***
pulsating - ***calc.,*** kali-c., lyc., ***petr.,*** sep., ***sil.,*** sulph.
red - ***calc.,*** nat-s., ***thuj.***
all over body - nat-s.
round - ***calc.***
sensitive, to touch - ***caust.,*** cinnb., ***cupr.,*** hep., ***nat-c.,*** nat-m., ***nit-ac.,*** **STAPH.,** ***thuj.***
sharp, in - ***bov.,*** **HEP., NIT-AC.**
shooting - bov.
situated on, face and hands - calc., carb-an., caust., dulc., kali-c.
neck, arms and hand, soft and smooth - ant-c.
nose, fingertips and eyebrows - caust.
small - bar-c., berb., ***calc., caust.,*** dulc., ferr., ferr-p., hep., lach., ***nit-ac.,*** rhus-t., ***sars., sep., sulph., thuj.***
all over body - caust.
smelling, like old, cheese - ***calc., graph., hep.,*** **THUJ.**
smooth - **ANT-C.,** calc., caust., **DULC.,** nat-m., ruta.
soft - ***ant-c., calc.,*** **NIT-AC.,** sil., ***thuj.***
stinging - am-c., ant-c., bar-c., ***calc.,*** caust., graph., ***hep.,*** lyc., **NIT-AC.,** rhus-t., sep., sil., staph., sulph., **THUJ.**
suppressed, ailments after - meny., merc., nit-ac., staph., ***thuj.***
discharges, after - med.
suppurating - ars., ***bov., calc., caust., hep., nat-c., sil., thuj.***
sycotic - nit-ac.
syphilitic - ***aur.,*** aur-m., aur-m-n., ***hep., merc., merc-d.,*** **NIT-AC.,** staph., ***thuj.***
tearing - am-c.
thin, epidermis, with - ***nit-ac.***
ugly - ant-c., cinnb., ***thuj.***
ulcerating - caust., hell.
ulcers, become - calc.
surrounded by a circle of - ant-c., ***ars., calc., nat-c.,*** phos.

WAXY - **ACET-AC., APIS, ARS.,** chin., ***cupr.,*** **FERR.,** ***ip.,*** lyc., **LYCPS.,** ***phos., sil.***

WENS, (see Sebaceous cysts)

WITHERED, skin - alum., ***ars.,*** calc., camph., caps., cham., **CHIN.,** clem., cocc., croc., ***ferr., ferr-ar., ferr-p.,*** hyos., ***iod.,*** kali-c., lyc., merc., nat-m., ***ph-ac.,*** phos., rheum, rhod., ***sars.,*** **SEC.,** seneg., sel., sil., spong., sulph., syph., ***verat.***

WOOL, agg. - com., merc., phos., **PSOR.,** puls., rhus-t., **SULPH.**
clothing agg. - phos., ***psor.,*** puls., ***sulph.***

WORMS, skin - ars., coca, merc., nat-c., nit-ac., sel., sil., sulph.

WRINKLED, shrivelled - abrot., ***alum.,*** ambr., am-c., ***ant-c.,*** apis, ***ars., bor.,*** bry., calc., camph., cham., ***chin.,*** chlor., ***cocc., con., cupr.,*** graph., hell., hep., ***iod., kali-ar., kreos., lyc.,*** manc., merc., ***mez.,*** mur-ac., nat-m., nux-v., ph-ac., phos., phyt., plb., rheum, rhod., rhus-t., rumx., sabad., ***sars.,*** **SEC.,** sel., ***sep.,*** sil., spig., stram., sul-ac., ***sulph.,*** syph., urt-u., ***verat.,*** verat-v., viol-o., x-ray.

YELLOW skin, (see Liver, jaundice) - **ACON.,** aesc., agar., agn., ***aloe,*** alum., ***ambr., am-m.,*** ant-c., ***ant-t.,*** arg-n., arn., ***ars.,*** ars-i., asaf., astac., ***aur., aur-m-n., bell., berb., bry.,*** bufo, ***calc., calc-p.,*** calc-s., cann-s., ***canth.,*** carb-s., ***carb-v.,*** **CARD-M.,** casc., ***caust., cean.,*** cedr., ***cham.,*** **CHEL.,** chen-a., **CHIN.,** ***chin-a.,*** **CHION.,** chol., cina, coca, cocc., **CON.,** ***corn.,*** corn-f., croc., **CROT-H.,** cupr., ***dig.,*** dol., ***dol.,*** dulc., elat., euph., eup-per., ***ferr.,*** ferr-ar., ***ferr-i.,*** gels., graph., hell., ***hep., hydr., ign.,*** **IOD.,** iris, jug-c., kali-ar., kali-bi., kali-c., kali-p., **LACH.,** laur., ***lept.,*** **LYC.,** mag-m., mang., med., **MERC.,** ***merc-c., merc-d., merc-sul.,*** myric., nat-a., nat-c., ***nat-m.,*** nat-p., **NAT-S., NIT-AC., NUX-V.,** olnd., ***op.,*** ost., petr., ph-ac., **PHOS.,** pic-ac., **PLB.,** ***podo., ptel., puls.,*** ran-b., rheum, rhus-t., rumx., ruta, sabad., ***sang., sec.,*** **SEP.,** ***sil., spig.,*** still., ***sulph.,*** sul-ac., tab., ***tarax.,*** tarent., thuj., thyr., verat., ***vip., yuc.***
- abdomen, itching, with - cham.
- anemia, brain disease, pregnancy - phos.
- anger, after - ***bry.,*** cham., ***nat-s.,*** **NUX-V.**
- brain, affection, in - phos.
- chronic - aur., chel., ***con.,*** iod., ***phos.,*** sulph.
  - relapsing - sulph.
- cider, from - chion.
- concomitant as a - phos.
- convulsions, with - agar.
- diarrhea, after - chin.
- extension of catarrhal process - am-m., ***chel.,*** chion., ***chin.,*** dig., ***hydr.,*** lob., ***merc.,*** nux-v., podo.
- fever, during - card-m., ***ferr.,*** lach., ***nux-v.,*** vip.
- fright, from - acon.
- fruits, unripe, from - rheum.
- gallstones, with - podo.
- haematogenous - phos.
- headache, with - sep.
- humiliation, after - bry., ***lyc.***
- intermittent fever, after - am-c., ***ars., chin-s., con.,*** ferr., nat-c., nat-m., ***nux-v., sang.,*** **SEP.,** ***tub.***
- itching - thyr.
- loss of vital fluids, from - chin.
- lung symptoms, with - card-m., chel., hydr.
- malignant - acon., ***ars., crot-h.,*** lach., merc., ***phos.***
- masturbation, after - chin.
- menses, arrested, with - chion.
- mental emotion, from - bry., ***cham.,*** lach., nux-v., vip.
- nervous, excitement from - phos.

YELLOW skin
- newborn children - ***acon., bov.,*** cham., ***chel., chin.,*** chion., coll., elat., merc., merc-d., myric., ***nat-s.,*** nux-v., podo., sep.
  - stool, with bilious - elat.
- pregnancy, during - aur., phos.
- rings - ***nat-c.,*** nat-m.
- sexual excess, after - chin.
- spots - ambr., ant-t., **ARN.,** ars., canth., **CON.,** crot-c., cur., dol., cur., elaps, **FERR.,** hydrc., iod., kali-ar., kali-c., ***lach., lyc., nat-c.,*** nat-p., nux-v., **PETR., PHOS.,** plb., ***psor., ruta.,*** sabad., **SEP.,** stann., **SULPH.,** ***thuj.,*** vip.
  - turning green - con.
- summer, every - chin-a., ***chion.***
- urinary symptoms, with - carb-v., cham., chin., ign., lyc., nux-v., plb.
- vexation - ***cham.,*** kali-c., ***nat-s.***

Sleep

ANXIOUS, during - acon., agar., ang., arn., **ARS.**, aster., ***bell.***, bry., camph., cast., cham., ***cocc.***, con., cycl., dig., dor., dulc., ferr., ***graph.***, hep., ip., ***kali-c.***, ***kali-i.***, kali-n., lat-m., ***lyc.***, mag-c., merc., ***merc-c.***, ***nat-c.***, ***nat-m.***, ***nit-ac.***, nux-v., op., petr., ***phos.***, phys., puls., rhus-t., samb., sil., ***spong.***, stram., verat., zinc.
after, afternoon - **STAPH.**
before - alum., ambr., berb., ***mag-c.***, nat-c., sil.
before, evening - berb.
going to, on - acon., ***calc.***, ***caust.***, cench., hep., ***lach.***, ***lyc.***, merc., nat-m., ***puls.***, rhus-t.
loss of sleep - ***cocc.***, ***nit-ac.***
menses, after - agar., aster., **COCC.**, ***kali-i.***, ***merc-c.***, zinc.
morning, towards - inul.
partial slumbering in the morning, during - junc.
starting from, on - clem., samb.

BAD - acet-ac., ***agar.***, aloe, asar., bell., bell-p., caj., canth., chin., dirc., ferr-i., gran., gymn., ham., iod., inul., lach., lyc., lycps., mag-c., meli., merc-c., mill., merc., mit., morph., naja, nat-a., nit-ac., nux-v., tab., trif-p.
midnight, after - arum-t., merc., **RHUS-T.**
before - naja.
morning amel. - lyc.
sleepiness in evening, after - aloe.

CHILL, during - ambr., ant-c., ant-t., **APIS**, cimx., ***gels.***, ***kali-i.***, lyc., merc., ***mez.***, ***nat-m.***, **NUX-M.**, nux-v., **OP.**, ***phos.***, podo., psor., sil.
after - ***ars.***, ***camph.***, gels., ***lyc.***, ***mez.***, spong., ***verat.***

CLAIRVOYANT state, like a - com., stann.

COMATOSE - acon., aeth., ***agar.***, ***agn.***, **AIL.**, alco., anac., ang., ***ant-c.***, **ANT-T.**, ***anthr.***, ***apis***, **ARG-N.**, ***arn.***, ***ars.***, ars-s-f., ***art-v.***, ***asaf.***, atro., aur., aur-m., aur-s., **BAPT.**, ***bar-c.***, **BELL.**, ***bor.***, ***bry.***, ***bufo***, ***calad.***, ***calc.***, ***camph.***, canth., ***caps.***, carb-ac., carb-v., casc., ***caust.***, ***cench.***, cham., ***chin.***, chlf., chlf., ***chlol.***, ***cic.***, ***cimic.***, clem., cocc., ***colch.***, coloc., ***con.***, **CROC.**, ***crot-c.***, ***crot-h.***, cub., ***cupr.***, cupr-ac., cycl., cyt-l., ***dig.***, ***dor.***, euph., euphr., ferr., ferr-p., ***gels.***, ***graph.***, ***hell.***, ***hep.***, hydr-ac., hyos., ***ign.***, ***iris***, kali-c., kali-chl., ***kali-i.***, kali-n., ***kali-per.***, kreos., ***lach.***, ***lact.***, ***laur.***, ***led.***, lup., ***lyc.***, mag-arct., merc., merc-c., ***merc-cy.***, mosch., ***mur-ac.***, ***nat-m.***, nit-ac., **NUX-M.**, nux-v., olnd., **OP.**, petr., ***ph-ac.***, ***phos.***, ***phys.***, plat., ***plb.***, ***puls.***, ran-b., ***rhus-t.***, ruta, sabad., ***sec.***, seneg., sep., spig., spong., stann., ***stram.***, ***sulph.***, tab., ***tarent.***, ter., urt-u., valer., **VERAT.**, vip., ***zinc.***, ***zinc-p.***, zing.
afternoon - euph., kali-c., zing.
alternating with, delirium - plb.
with, sleeplessness - ***camph.***
with delirium - plb.
breathing, with ailments of - acon., cham., op., stram., vip.

COMATOSE, sleep
children, in - sep.
chill, during violent - op.
continued - anac., lach., op.
2 days - hyos.
3 days - ***hyos.***, ***verat.***
week, a whole - ***hell.***
convulsions, during - bufo, caust., cham., lach., op., ***plat.***, ***sulph.***
after - aeth., ***atro.***, ***bufo***, ***caust.***, cupr-ar., ***ign.***, ***kali-br.***, nat-s., plb., zinc.
before - ***sulph.***
between - agar., aur., ***bufo***, ***ign.***, **OENA.**, **OP.**, plb.
day, and night - anac., bar-c., lup.
and night - bar-c.
every other day - sep.
daytime - aeth., dig., hep., lup., plb., sabad.
delirium, with - acon., ant-c., **ANT-T.**, arn., **BAPT.**, ***bry.***, camph., coloc., puls., sec., ***verat.***
dinner, after - dig., ign.
evening - ant-t., ars., asaf., verat.
evening to evening, from - lup.
eyes, one eye open - verat.
open, with - caps., coloc., samb.
opening difficult - aeth., cham., cocc., mag-arct.
forenoon - ant-c., ant-t., verat.
all forenoon - sel.
heat, with - ***agar.***, anac., bell., bry., cham., coloc., gels., ***op.***, ***puls.***, spong., ***tarent.***
hunger, with - bell.
labor, during - lach.
menses, during - nux-m., phos.
morning - euphr., ***nux-v.***, phos.
sunrise, after - euphr., merc., nux-v., puls.
night - **PULS.**
noon - ther.
elderly people, in - op.
pains, after - lach.
perspiration night, with - **PULS.**
sitting - aur.
snoring, with - bell., carb-v., laur., ***op.***, rhus-t., ***stram.***
spasms during - op.
strokes, in - ***crot-h.***, ***op.***
sudden - mag-arct.
sunstroke, from - ***op.***
suppressed eruption, after - ***zinc.***
thirst, with - anac., bell., cham., op., verat.
uremia, in - agar., ***am-c.***, anac., ars., aur., bell., bry., ***carb-ac.***, cupr-ar., ***hell.***, lach., lact., merc-c., ***morph.***, ***op.***, ter., verat-v.
vomiting, after - aeth., cupr.
vomiting, with - dig.
yawning, with - cimic., laur.

COMA, vigil - **ACON.,** ***agar.,*** alum., ***anac.,*** ang., ant-c., ars., bell., ***bry., cham., cocc.,*** croc., cur., cycl., hydr-ac., hyos., ign., lach., laur., lon-x., lyc., merc-c., nat-m., nux-m., **OP.,** petr., ***phos.,*** plat., rheum, sep., sil., spig., ***spong.,*** stann., stram., ***sulph.,*** teucr., verat.

CONFUSED - dios., kali-bi., lyc., op.
morning, before 6 am., alternating with delusions - ars.

CONVULSION, sleep, during - bufo, caust., cham., lach., op., rheum.
after - aeth., ***art-v.,*** cupr., cupr-ar., ***hyos.,*** kali-br., ***lach.,*** nat-s., **NUX-V.,** ***oena.,*** **OP.,** ***tarent.,*** zinc.

DEEP, sleep - acon., aesc., aeth., aether, agar., agar-cit., agn., ail., alco., all-c., ***alum.,*** alum-p., ***alumn.,*** am-c., ambr., ampe-qu, amyg., anac., ant-c., ant-s., **ANT-T.,** ***apis,*** apoc., aran., **ARG-N.,** ***arn., ars.,*** ars-s-f., atro., aur., **BAPT.,** ***bar-c.,*** **BELL.,** benz-ac., berb., bor., bov., brom., ***bry.,*** cact., ***calad., calc., camph.,*** cann-i., canth., carb-ac., **CARB-H., CARB-O., CARB-S., CARB-V.,** ***carl., caust.,*** cedr., ***cench.,*** cham., ***chel., chin.,*** chin-a., chin-s., chlol., chlf., ***chlor., cic., cina,*** cinnam., coca, cocc., coch., coff., ***colch.,*** **CON.,** corn., **CROC.,** crot-c., ***crot-h.,*** crot-t., cund., ***cupr.,*** cupr-ac., ***cycl.,*** dig., dios., elaps, erig., eug., euph., ***fl-ac., gels.,*** gins., glon., **GRAPH.,** grat., guano, ***hell., hep.,*** hydr-ac., ***hyos., ign.,*** piloc., jal., kali-bi., kali-br., kali-i., ***kali-n.,*** kali-p., **KREOS.,** ***lach., lact., laur.,*** **LED.,** lepi., linu-u, lob., lol., lup., lupin., ***lyc., mag-arct.,*** mag-c., **MERC.,** ***merc-c.,*** mez., morph., ***mosch., naja,*** nat-a., nat-c., ***nat-m.,*** nat-p., **NUX-M., NUX-V., OP.,** ox-ac., peti., petr., ***ph-ac., phos., phys.,*** pip-m., pisc., plat., ***plb., podo.,*** psor., ptel., **PULS.,** ***rhod., rhus-t.,*** ruta, sabad., ***sec.,*** sel., ***seneg., sep.,*** sol-m., sol-n., spig., spong., stann., ***stram.,*** sul-ac., ***sulph.,*** tab., tax., ther., thuj., ***valer.,*** **VERAT.,** xan., ***zinc.***
afternoon - bor., euph., ign., merc-i-r., sel., sil.
catalepsy, after - grat.
heat, after - cina.
alternating with, delirium - cocc., plb., vip.
with, excitement - phos.
with, headache and dyspnea - plb.
with, sleeplessness, periods of - benz-ac.
amenorrhea, in - ***cina.***
beer, after - sulph.
children, in - cupr., cupr-ac.
chill, during - bell., ***hep.,*** laur., ***nat-m., nux-m.,*** **OP.**
after - ***ars.***
coma vigil, after - hell.
convulsions, after - aeth., ***bufo,*** canth., ***caust.,*** cupr-ac., ***hell., ign., hyos.,*** kali-br., ***lach.,*** **NUX-V.,** ***oena.,*** **OP.,** plb., sec., ***sulph.,*** tarent., zinc.
between - agar., ***bufo, ign.,*** **OENA., OP.,** plb.

DEEP, sleep
daytime - ant-t., bor., dig., erig., eug., ign., ***lact.,*** led., manc., ***merc., ph-ac.,*** phos., sel., tab.
delirium - cocc., plb., stram., vip.
after - bry., phos., stram.
dinner, after - agar., chel., til.
disturbed, yet - kali-br.
drunken, as if - kali-n.
evening - arg-n., ***ars.,*** astac., ***lyc.***
first sleep, in - ambr., aur., bell., cycl., mang., puls., thuj.
excitement or exertion, from - podo.
exhausting, with dreams - zinc.
fear of death, after - vario.
fever, during - ***all-c.,*** **APIS,** aran., ***arn.,*** ars., cact., ***calad.,*** chin-a., con., gels., ign., ***lach.,*** laur., ***mez., nux-m., nux-v.,*** **OP.,** ***phos.,*** **ROB.,** sec., spong.
interrupted by dreams, with chilliness - ***lyc.***
menses, during - **NUX-M.,** ***phos.,*** sulph.
midnight, after - nat-m., stram.
before - rhod.
morning - alum., bell., brom., bry., calc., calc-ar., **CALC-P.,** carb-s., con., gels., gins., ***graph.,*** hep., led., lyc., mag-arct., nat-c., ***nux-v.,*** op., ph-ac., phos., sulph., thuj.
5 a., after - phys.
6 a.m. - atro., calad., euphr.
10 a.m. - peti.
toward morning amel. - op.
night - asc-c., tab.
3 a., till - bapt.
sleeplessness, after - ***nep.***
noon - eug., eup-per.
afternoon, and - bor., eug., ign., sel., tab.
palpitation, with - ***podo.***
rage, after - sec.
sitting, while - ox-ac.
sudden - chin-b.
unrefreshing - ***zinc.***
uremic - agar., ***am-c.,*** anac., ars., aur-m., bell., bry., ***carb-ac.,*** cupr-ar., ***hell.,*** lach., lact., ***merc-c., moly-met., op.,*** ter., verat-v.
vomiting, after - crot-t.
writing, while - ph-ac.

DELIRIOUS - ail., morph.

DISTURBED, sleep - acon., acon-c., ail., alco., alum., amn-l., amph., anis., ***apis,*** arist-m., arn., ***ars.,*** asaf., aster., bar-ac., ***bell.,*** bell-p., cact., calad., ***calc-p.,*** carc., cham., cimic., cob., coca, cupr-ar., dig., dirc., dulc., equis., fago., form., gels., **GRAPH.,** ham., hyos., iber., ind., jal., kali-bi., kali-br., kali-i., ***laur.,*** lycps., mag-arct., mag-p-a., merc., morph., myris., naja, nat-a., nat-m., op., phys., pip-m., plan., plb., plect., polyg-p., puls., puls-n, ran-b., rhus-g., sant., sarcol-ac., sep., sol-t-ae., **SULPH.,** tab., tarent., thea., torula., valer., vesp.

DISTURBED, sleep

anxiety, from - **ACON.**, alum., am-c., ambr., ant-c., arg-m., arg-n., **ARS.**, bar-c., ***bell.***, bov., ***bry.***, calc., calc-f., cann-s., carb-an., ***carb-v.***, ***carc.***, ***cast.***, ***caust.***, cham., ***chin.***, ***cocc.***, coff., con., cycl., dig., dulc., ***ferr.***, ***graph.***, ***hep.***, ***hyos.***, ***ign.***, ***kali-c.***, kreos., lach., lact., lyc., ***mag-c.***, mag-m., mang., ***merc.***, merc-c., nat-c., ***nat-m.***, nicc., ***nit-ac.***, nux-v., op., petr., ph-ac., phel., **PHOS.**, plat., puls., ran-s., rat., sabin., ***sep.***, ***sil.***, spong., squil., ***sulph.***, tab., verat., zinc.

full moon, at - arg-n., sulph.

child-bed, in - lyc.

chill, by - alum., ***am-c.***, calc., caust., daph., graph., grat., hep., mag-c., nat-c., ***phos.***, rhus-t., sep., sil., ***sulph.***, verat.

ciphers before eyes - ph-ac., sulph.

coldness, by - ars., bor., cor-r., euphr., ferr-ma., kali-c., kreos., mang., nit-ac., sabad., sars., sulph., tab., tart-ac.

congestion, by - alumn., am-c., asar., bor., brucin., ***bry.***, calc., carb-an., dulc., graph., hep., ign., mag-c., ***merc.***, mosch., ***nat-m.***, phos., rhus-t., sabin., samb., senn., ***sil.***, sulph.

convulsions, by - cocc., hyos., kali-c., mag-c., ***puls.***, ***rhus-t.***, ***sil.***

cough, by - ***acon.***, agar., alum., am-m., ars., caust., con., hep., kali-c., kali-n., ***lach.***, lact., lyc., mag-s., mur-ac., nat-c., nat-m., ***nit-ac.***, phos., rhod., rumx., ***sep.***, ***sil.***, sul-ac., ***sulph.***

delirium, by - ***acon.***, arn., bapt., ***bell.***, ***bry.***, coloc., kali-c., ***nux-v.***, op., ***puls.***, pyrog., sec., sulph.

delusions, by - ***bell.***, calc., canth., carb-v., cham., coff-t., dulc., merc., par., ***plb.***, sulph.

dreams, by - ***acon.***, agar., alco., allox., ***alum.***, am-m., ambr., ammc., ang., ant-s., **ANT-T.**, ***apis***, arg-m., ***arg-n.***, arn., ***ars.***, ars-s-r., atro., ***bell.***, benz-ac., berb., bol., bov., brach., brucin., bry., cact., cahin., **CALC.**, calc-ar., calc-f., calc-p., calc-s., cann-i., ***caps.***, carb-an., ***carb-v.***, ***card-m.***, carl., carb-s., cast-eq., caust., cham., ***chel.***, ***chin.***, chin-s., cimic., cit-v., ***clem.***, coc-c., cocc., coff., coloc., com., ***con.***, ***cori-r.***, cor-r., croc., crot-t., cupr., ***cycl.***, cyt-l., daph., dig., dulc., euphr., ***ferr.***, ferr-i., gamb., glon., ***gran.***, ***graph.***, guare., ham., hell., ***hep.***, ign., ind., iod., kali-ar., kali-chl., kreos., ***laur.***, ***lob.***, lyc., lyss., mag-arct., mag-c., mag-m., mag-s., man., ***menis.***, merc., mez., mosch., mur-ac., myric., nat-c., nat-m., ***nat-s.***, nicc., nit-ac., nux-m., nux-v., op., par., paeon., peti., petr., ph-ac., ***phos.***, pip-m., plan., plat., plb., prun., psor., ptel., ***puls.***, ***raph.***, rhod., rhus-g., ***rhus-t.***, rhus-v., seneg., ***sep.***, ***sil.***, sin-n., sol-n., spig., ***spong.***, stront-c., sulph., tab., tarax., ***tarent.***, ***ter.***, teucr., ***thuj.***, valer., vario., verat., verb., wies., ***zinc.***, zinc-oc.

frightful - ***acon.***, alumn., ***calc.***, calc-f., lach., petros.

menses, during - ***kali-c.***

midnight, after - ph-ac., stront.

before - ***chel.***

DISTURBED, sleep

dreams, by

morning - aur., ***cycl.***, ***fl-ac.***, ***kali-m.***

5 a.m. - ham.

noon - ther.

siesta, during - **NAT-M.**

robbers, of - nat-m.

driven out of bed, sensation of being - rhus-t.

easily - coff., ***lach.***, ***lyc.***, merc., nicc., ***op.***, puls., saroth., sel., ***sulph.***

ebullitions - alumn.

erections, by - alum., ambr., ant-c., aur., carb-v., coloc., hep., kali-c., lach., led., lith., merc., merc-ac., ***nat-c.***, nat-m., ol-an., op., par., ph-ac., pic-ac., plat., plb., ran-b., sep., ***sil.***, ***stann.***, thuj.

painful - cact.

fainting, by - ars., bar-c., calc., carb-v., ***sep.***, sil., ***ther.***

fear, by - ***acon.***, am-c., ***ars.***, bell., ***con.***, ip., lyc., merc., nat-c., nat-m., ***op.***, ph-ac., ***phos.***, rat., ***sil.***, stann., ***sulph.***, zinc.

future, of the - dulc.

ghosts, of - cocc., sulph.

mice, of - colch.

robbers, of - merc., nat-m., sil.

stroke, of - arn., carb-v., nat-c.

heat, by - acon., alum., am-c., anac., arn., ars., ***bar-c.***, ***bell.***, bor., ***bry.***, ***calc.***, cann-s., carb-an., carb-v., caust., cham., ***chin.***, cina, clem., coff., ***con.***, cor-r., cycl., dulc., ferr-ma., ***graph.***, grat., hep., ign., kali-br., kali-c., kreos., **LACH.**, lact., laur., led., mag-arct., ***mag-c.***, ***mag-m.***, mang., meph., merc., merc-c., mosch., mur-ac., nat-c., ***nat-m.***, ***nicc.***, ***nit-ac.***, ***op.***, paeon., petr., ph-ac., phos., **PULS.**, ran-b., ran-s., rheum, ***rhus-t.***, sabad., sanic., sec., sep., ***sil.***, sol-t-ae., staph., sul-ac., **SULPH.**, teucr., ***thuj.***, ***verat.***, viol-t., wies.

hunger, from - ant-c., berb., bry., carb-v., caul., ***cina***, ***iod.***, kali-c., lyc., ***phos.***, raph., sabin., sulph.

menses, before - ***alum.***

midnight, after - stront.

before - calc-p., phyt.

moon, at full - nat-c., sulph.

morning - rhod., sabin.

3 a.m. to 5 a.m. - cimic.

5 a.m. - ham.

nausea, by - am-c., ambr., bar-c., bry., carb-v., cham., con., cycl., ***graph.***, hell., hep., ip., kali-c., ***lach.***, lyc., mang., mez., ***mur-ac.***, nicc., nit-ac., phel., phos., rat., rhus-t., ruta, seneg., ***sep.***, sil., squil., ***sulph.***, ther., thuj., vip.

newborn, in - acon., ***cham.***

nightmare, by - ***acon.***, alum., bell., **CALC.**, carc., cast., cinnb., con., cycl., daph., guai., kali-n., ***lyc.***, meph., mez., ***nat-c.***, ***nat-m.***, ***nit-ac.***, op., puls., ***sil.***, sulph., ter.

full moon, at - nat-c.

DISTURBED, sleep

noise, by slightest - acon., alum., alumn., am-c., ang., apis, ars., ***asar., bell., calad.,*** carb-v., cham., chin., cocc., **COFF.,** grat., ***ign.,*** kali-n., lach., ***merc.,*** narcot., nat-p., nux-v., ol-an., op., ***phos.,*** ruta, saroth., sel., sep., sul-ac., ***sulph.,*** tarent., valer., zinc-valer.

oppression of chest, by - alum., am-c., carb-v., kali-c., lach., lact., mag-m., nat-c., nat-m., nit-ac., **PHOS.,** seneg., sulph.

pains, by - alum., ars., ***aur.,*** bell., cann-i., ***cham.,*** coc-c., kali-n., lach., ***lyc.,*** mag-m., ***merc.,*** mosch., mur-ac., ***nit-ac.,*** passi., puls., sin-n., vip.

abdomen, in - am-m., bry., calc., caust., cina, cycl., dor., kali-c., lach., mag-m., mag-s., merc., mur-ac., nat-c., phos., ***rhus-t.,*** sep., zinc.

headache - alum., chin-s., con., eug., grat., lact., ***lyc.,*** mag-m., mur-ac., nat-m., nat-s., nicc., ***nit-ac.,*** phos., rhus-t., stram., ***sulph.***

stomach, in - ***nit-ac., sil.,*** valer.

palpitations, by - ***acon.,*** alum., am-c., ***cact.,*** calc., calc-ar., dig., ign., ***iod.,*** kali-ar., lact., lil-t., ***lyc.,*** nat-c., ***nat-m., nit-ac.,*** **PHOS.,** rhus-t., sep., ***sil., sulph.,*** zinc.

lying on side, when - ign., lyc., nat-c.

left side - lyc., nat-c., ***phos.***

perspiration, by - alum., am-c., bar-c., cann-s., carb-v., ***caust.,*** chel., ***chin., chin-s., cic.,*** con., croc., daph., ***dros., dulc.,*** ferr-ma., graph., ***hyos.,*** ign., kali-c., kali-n., kreos., lach., led., mang., **MERC.,** ***mur-ac., nat-m.,*** nat-s., nicc., ***nit-ac.,*** ph-ac., puls., ran-b., ***raph.,*** rat., rhus-t., sabal., sabin., sars., sep., ***sil., sulph.,*** thuj., verat., vip., zinc-oc.

cold - am-c., mang., sabad., ther.

cold, sweat - bell., calc., ***carb-an.,*** carb-v., merc., ***nux-v.,*** sil., sulph.

pollutions, by - arn., camph., cann-s., carb-an., chel., coloc., con., crot-t., cycl., dig., ferr., kali-chl., lach., lact., nat-c., nat-m., ***nux-v.,*** par., petr., ***ph-ac.,*** phos., plat., plb., ***puls.,*** ran-b., samb., sars., ***sep., sil.,*** spig., stann., staph., stram., ***sulph., thuj.***

pulsations, by - nat-m., nit-ac., rhus-t., sabad., sep., sil., sulph.

shuddering, by - ant-c., berb., bry., carb-v., caust., kali-c., raph., sabin., sulph.

sliding in bed, by - mur-ac.

suffocation, by - carb-v., lach., puls., samb.

thoughts, by activity of - acon., agar., ap-g., apis, ***arg-n.,*** bor., ***bry.,*** **CALC.,** caust., **CHIN.,** cocc., ***coff.,*** coloc., con., gels., ***graph.,*** hep., ***hyos.,*** ign., kali-c., kali-n., lyc., ***mag-arct.,*** meph., nat-m., ***nux-v.,*** ph-ac., plat., ***puls.,*** rhus-t., sabad., ***sep.,*** sil., spong., ***staph.,*** **SULPH.,** viol-t., yohim, zinc.

business, of - bell., calc., ham., hyos., ***nux-v.,*** sulph.

scientific thoughts - spong., ***sulph.***

DISTURBED, sleep

twitching, by - ***agar.,*** alum., ant-t., ***ars., bell.,*** calc., carb-v., cast., crot-h., ***cupr.,*** dulc., ***graph.,*** hyos., ***kali-c., lyc.,*** mag-c., nat-c., ***nat-m., nit-ac., op., puls.,*** rhus-t., sel., ***sep., sil.,*** sul-ac., ***sulph.,*** viol-t., zinc.

uneasiness - agar., ars., cina, clem., cocc., lach., merc., nat-c., nicc., petr., puls., sabad.

4 a.m. agg., after - plan.

vertigo, by - am-c., calc., caust., chin., ***con.,*** cor-r., lach., lyc., merc., nat-c., nicc., op., ***phos.,*** sep., ***sil.,*** stront-c., ***sulph., ther.***

visions, by - acon., alum., alum-sil., apis, ***arg-n., arn., bell., calc.,*** camph., ***carb-an.,*** carb-v., ***cham.,*** chin., coff., dulc., ***graph.,*** hell., ign., lach., led., lyc., merc., nat-c., nat-m., nit-ac., nux-m., ***op.,*** ph-ac., phos., plat., puls., rhus-t., ***sep.,*** sil., spong., sulph., thuj.

anxious - calc., phos., sep.

closing the eyes, on - apis, bell., ***calc.,*** camph., ***graph.,*** lach., led., lyc., spong., ***sulph., thuj.***

erotic - ambr., calc., sil.

frightful - bell., calc., ***carb-an.,*** carb-v., chin., lyc., merc., ***nux-v., op.,*** sil., spong., sulph.

vivacity, by - ang., ant-c., arn., aur., bor., ***calc.,*** caps., **CARC., COFF.,** ***lach.,*** lam., lyc., mag-aust., ***merc., nat-m., nicc-s., nux-v.,*** phos., ***prun., puls.,*** ran-b., ran-s., rhus-t., sel., sep., sil., ***spig.,*** staph., sul-ac., ***sulph.,*** zinc.

voluptuous images, by - ambr., calc., sil.

vomiting, by - hep., ***ip.,*** kali-c., ***lach.,*** mur-ac., nit-ac., rat., ***sil., ther.,*** thuj., verat., vip.

walking in bed, child is - rheum.

DOZING - acon., alum., ambr., ant-c., arn., ***ars.,*** aur., bell., bor., bry., calc., canth., **CHAM.,** chel., cic., cob., coc-c., ***cocc.,*** coloc., dig., dulc., euph., ferr., ***graph., hep.,*** hyos., ign., juni., kali-bi., kali-br., kali-c., ***kali-n., lach.,*** merc., naja, narcot., nat-c., nat-m., nit-ac., op., ***par., petr.,*** phos., plat., ***puls.,*** ran-s., raph., rhus-t., sabad., samb., sel., sil., sol-m., staph., sul-ac., sulph.

afternoon - chin-s., euph.

alternating with waking, afternoon - cann-i.

constantly - merc.

convulsions, with - aeth.

daytime - anac., coloc., euph., ***hep.,*** ign., ***nux-v.,*** raph.

eyes are closed, as soon as - adon.

menses, during - goss.

midnight, after - coff., ran-s.

morning - aloe, coff., pic-ac.

night, 3 am., after - ***coff.***

towards morning - ambr., coff., nux-v., ran-s.

noon - aloe.

sitting, while - narcot.

sitting, while, reading or studying, and - coca.

stool, after - aeth.

vomiting, after - ***aeth.***

waking, after - aeth., clem.

DREAMS, (see Dreams, chapter)

DULL - aesc., anac., ant-t., bell., bry., calad., calc., chin., ***con.,*** cupr-ac., dig., eug., ***graph.,*** grat., ***hep.,*** kali-n., led., lyc., merc., nux-v., op., petr., ***phos., puls.,*** zinc.
daytime - ***hep.***
eating, after - carb-v.
morning - alum., euphr., graph., phos.

EXHAUSTING - aeth., cann-s., ***ph-ac.,*** phos., sec., zinc.
deep, with dreams - zinc.
pollution, after - cann-s.

FAINTING, with palpitation - ***nux-m.***

FALLING, asleep
afternoon - aur., bar-c., cina, dios., fago., hyos., mag-c., nat-m., phys., pip-m., sabad., sep., sin-a.
1 p.m. to 2. p.m. - pip-m.
4 p.m. - cas-s., ferr-p.
sitting, while - aur., nat-m.
studying, while - gels.
work, during - zinc.
answering, when - **ARN., BAPT.,** ***hyos.***
beer, after - thea.
breakfast, after - sumb.
chill, during - op., ***verat.***
conversation, during - caust., tarax.
daytime - erig., meph., merc., thuj.
difficult, (see Insomnia) - ***arg-m., carl.,*** cham., cupr., dig., hep., lach., laur., lyc., mag-c., mag-m., mag-s., merc., mez., mur-ac., ***nat-c.,*** nat-m., nit-ac., ***phos.,*** plan., ptel., ruta, saroth., sel., sil., ***sulph.,*** thyr., upa., ust.
sex, after - bov.
perspiration, with - ***sulph.***
sleepiness, with - nat-c.
waking, after - mag-s., nat-c., ***nat-m.,*** ph-ac., ***phos.,*** thal.
3 a.m. - pic-ac.
dinner, after - ant-t., aur., calc., caust., coca, cur., **KALI-C.,** ***mag-c.,*** ph-ac., tab.
early - alum., am-m., ant-c., bor., graph., grat., lact., laur., mez., nat-m., ph-ac., sep., spong., stann., sulph.
supper, after - gels.
weakness, as from - ph-ac.
easy - lyc., mag-c., mit., plat.
11 a.m. to 3 p.m. - nat-c.
disturbed, after being - form.
evening - form.
knitting and talking, when - plb.
eating, after - arum-t., bor., calc-p., der., gamb., graph., lyc., mur-ac., nat-m., ruta
evening - am-c., graph., mez., plat., sol-m.
5 p.m. - nat-m.
bed, on going to - staph.
eating, after - am-c., gels.
reading, while - mez., plat.
sitting, while - apis, hep., **NUX-V.,** plat., tell.
twilight, at - bor.
falling, with sensation of - calen.

FALLING, asleep
fever, during - ***acon., ant-t., apis,*** **CALAD.,** caps., cedr., chel., chin., **EUP-PER.,** gels., ign., **LACH.,** lachn., laur., lyc., **MEZ., NAT-M.,** ***nux-m.,*** **OP., PODO., ROB.,** rhus-t., **SAMB.,** stram.
flushes of heat, with - ***carb-v.***
heat and chill, between - **NUX-V.**
forenoon - ***calc.***
9 a.m. - coca,
reading, while - agar., nat-s.
late - acon., agar., agn., alum., alum-p., ***am-c., am-m., ambr.,*** ammc., anac., anag., ***ang., anh.,*** ant-c., ant-t., apis, arn., **ARS.,** ars-s-f., asar., asc-t., aur., bapt., bar-c., bart., ***bell.,*** berb., bism., ***bor.,*** **BRY.,** ***calad.,*** **CALC.,** camph., cann-i., canth., caps., ***carb-an.,*** carb-s., **CARB-V.,** ***carl.,*** cast., caust., cench., cham., chel., ***chin.,*** chin-a., cimic., clem., cob., ***cocc., coff.,*** coloc., ***con.,*** cor-r., ***crot-t.,*** cupr., ***cur.,*** cycl., dig., dirc., dulc., euph., euphr., ***ferr., ferr-ac., ferr-p.,*** fl-ac., gels., ***gent-l., graph.,*** grat., guai., ***hep.,*** hipp., hyos., hyper., ***ign.,*** indg., ip., ***kali-ar., kali-c.,*** kali-n., kreos., ***lac-c., lach.,*** lam., ***laur., led., lyc.,*** lycpr., mag-arct., ***mag-c., mag-m., mag-s.,*** mang., meph., **MERC.,** ***mez.,*** mill., mosch., ***mur-ac., nat-c., nat-m.,*** nat-n., ***nat-s., nit-ac.,*** nux-m., **NUX-V.,** ***ol-an., op.,*** par., ***petr., petros., ph-ac.,*** phel., **PHOS.,** ***plat., plb., prun.,*** **PULS.,** ***ran-b.,*** ran-s., rat., rheum, rhod., **RHUS-T.,** sabad., sabin., samb., sarcol-ac., saroth., ***sars., sel.,*** seneg., **SEP.,** ***sil., spig.,*** spira., spong., ***stann., staph.,*** stront-c., ***sul-ac., sulph.,*** tab., tarax., ter., ***teucr.,*** thea., ther., ***thuj., valer.,*** verat., verb., viol-t., visc., ***zinc.,*** zinc-p.
excitement, after - chlor.
four hours, after - phos., ran-b.
going to bed late, after - am-c., sep.
heat, from - caust.
one hour, after - sulph.
one hour and a half, after - sil.
rising late, and - aster.
sex, after - bov.
sleepiness daytime, with - ammc., carb-v.
evening - ang., bor., clem., nat-n., ***nux-v.,*** sel.
three hours, after - ferr.
two hours, after - ferr., graph., ***merc.,*** phos., ran-b., ter., thuj.
waking early, with - bor., cycl., dios., guai., ***lyc.,*** ol-an., prun., puls., ran-b., sel., sep., staph., sul-ac., sulph., visc., zinc.
from dreams - bell., lach., sil., sulph.
laughing, after - phos.
listening to conversation - cinnb., tarax.
lying on back, with right arm clamped between legs, when - plb.
menses, during - phos.
mental exertion, from the least - **ARS.,** chlor., ferr., **HYOS.,** ign., kali-br., ***kali-c.,*** nat-s., ***nux-v.,*** tarax.

FALLING, asleep

morning - ***atro.,*** coca, hep., kali-c., lyc., spig.
reading in chair, after - coca.

noon - aloe
eating, while - puls.

pain, after - phyt.

palpitation, with - calc., nat-m., sil., **SULPH.**

perspiration, with - **ARS.,** tarax., ***thuj.,*** verat.

reading, while - ang., aur., cimic., ***colch.,*** ign., iris, lyc., mez., ***nat-m.,*** nat-s., phos., plat., prun., ruta, sep., sil.
fast - sil.

sewing, while - ferr.

sex, during - bar-c., ***lyc.***
after - bov.

shocks, with electric-like - ant-t., ***arg-m., ars., cupr.,*** ign., ***ip.,*** **NIT-AC.**

sitting - acon., ang., ant-t., apis, ars., arum-t., aur., calc-p., chin., cimx., ***cina,*** fago., ferr., ferr-ma., form., hep., ign., kali-br., kali-c., lyc., merc., mur-ac., nat-c., ***nat-h., nat-m.,*** nat-p., **NUX-V.,** petr., phos., puls., ***sep.,*** staph., sulph., tell., thuj., tarent., verat.
floor, on - tarent.
heat, during - chel.
soup, after - form.
work, at - nat-c.

society, in - caust., meph.

standing, while - acon., cor-r., mag-c., morph., nit-ac.
after dinner - ***mag-c.***

stool, after - ***aeth.,*** elaps, sabad., ***sulph.***

suffocation, with - ***am-c.,*** ars., bad., bell., carb-an., ***cur., dig.,*** graph., **GRIN.,** kali-i., lac-c., **LACH.,** ***merc-p-r.,*** morph., naja, ***op., samb., spong.,*** sulph., teucr., valer.

talking, while - caust., ***chel.,*** mag-c., morph., ph-ac., plat., puls.
animated talking, after - thea.
chattering, while - puls.
dinner, after - ***mag-c.,*** ph-ac.

thinking, after - nat-s.
thinking, after, intense - ***op.***

vertigo, with - tell.

vomiting - ***aeth.,*** ant-t., bell., cupr., nat-m., sanic.
after - aeth., ant-t., bell., cupr., nat-m., sanic.

walking, while - acon., nit-ac.

weakness, from - petr., phos., piloc.

wine, after - thea.

work, during - bism., lact., mur-ac., phel., ran-b., sulph., zinc.

writing, while - ph-ac., thuj.

FEIGNED - ***sep.,*** tarent.

FEVER, intermittent, during - anac., **ANT-T., *apis, arn., bell.,*** calad., caps., cedr., ***chin.,*** chin-a., dulc., **EUP-PER.,** gels., ***hep., ign.,*** **LACH.,** laur., lyc., med., merc., merc-c., **MEZ., NAT-C., NAT-M., *nux-m.,* OP., *petr.,* PODO., ROB.,** rhus-t., ***sabad.,*** **SAMB.,** stram., ***verat.***
between heat and chill - **NUX-V.,** rhus-t.
children and elderly people, in - ***op.***

FEVER, intermittent, during
stupefying, sleep - ***acon.,*** **ANT-T., APIS, *bell.,*** calc., ***camph.,*** cic., con., croc., hep., hyos., ign., led., ***nux-m.,*** **OP., *ph-ac., phos.,*** puls., rhus-t., sec., ***spong., stram.,*** valer., ***verat.***

HEAVY - acon., aesc., agar., ail., all-c., ant-c., **ANT-T.,** asc-c., bell., berb., bufo, carb-ac., carb-s., coloc., crot-t., ferr., gels., glon., hydr-ac., hydrc., iodof., piloc., kali-c., kali-n., ***lach.,*** lact., lepi., lob., lol., lyc., manc., morph., nat-c., nit-ac., nux-v., **OP.,** pic-ac., pip-m., ***podo.,*** ptel., plan., phys., rhus-t., spig., stann., sulph., tab., thuj., til., verat., xan.
afternoon, 2 p.m. - pip-m.
children, in - lach.
delirium, after - sec.
lying down in evening, after - seneg.
morning - ferr., gels., glon., hydr-ac., iber., kali-i., ***lach.,*** meny., nat-hchls., thuj.

INSOMNIA, sleeplessness - abrot., absin., ***acon.,*** acon-c., acon-f., adon., aeth., aether, ***agar.,*** agav-t., agn., agra., alco., alet., alf., allox., ***aloe,*** alum., alumn., am-caust., ambr., am-br., am-c., am-m., ***ammc.,*** anac., ang., anh., anil., ant-c., ant-ox., ant-t., anthr., ant-c., aphis., ***apis,*** apoc., apoc-a., apom., aquileg., aran., arg-c., arg-m., **ARG-N., *arn.,* ARS.,** ars-h., ***ars-i.,*** **ARS-S-F., *arum-t.,*** arund., asaf., asar., asc-t., asim., ***aster., atro., aur.,*** aur-m., aur-s., ***aven.,*** aza., ***bapt.,*** bar-c., bar-m., **BELL.,** bell-p., benz., ***benz-ac.,*** bism., ***bor.,*** brach., **BRY.,** buf-s., but-ac., **CACT.,** cadm-s., cahin., calad., **CALC.,** calc-ar., calc-caust., calc-i., ***calc-p.,*** calc-s., calo., ***camph., camph-br.,*** canch., cann-i., cann-s., ***canth.,*** caps., **CARC., *carl.,*** carb-an., ***carb-s., carb-v.,*** cast., caul., ***caust.,*** cean., cedr., cer-b., **CHAM.,** chel., **CHIN., *chin-a., chin-s.,*** chlf., chlol., chrysan., ***cic.,*** cimic., ***cina,*** cinnb., **CIT-V.,** clem., cob., coca, cocaine, ***cocc.,*** coc-c., ***cocc-s.,*** coch., **COFF.,** coff-t., coffin., colch., ***coloc., con.,*** cop., corn., cot., croc., crot-c., ***crot-h.,*** crot-t., ***cupr.,*** cupr-ac., **CYCL., CYPR.,** cyt-l., daph., ***dig.,*** dios., dip., dirc., ***dros., dulc.,*** elaps, ery-a., eucal., eug., eup-per., eup-pur., euph., euph-pe., euphr., fago., ***ferr., ferr-ar.,*** ferr-i., ferr-p., fil., ***fl-ac.,*** form., gad., gamb., ***gels.,*** get., ***glon.,*** gran., ***graph.,*** grin., ***guai.,*** guare., haem., ***hell.,*** helon., **HEP.,** hipp., hippoz., hura, hydr., hydr-ac., **HYOS., *hyosin.,*** iber., ***ign.,*** inul., ***iod.,*** iodof., ***ip.,*** iris, piloc., jac-c., ***jal.,*** jatr., jug-c., jug-r., **KALI-AR., *kali-bi., kali-br.,* KALI-C.,** kali-cy., ***kali-i.,*** kali-n., kali-p., ***kali-s.,*** kalm., ***kreos.,*** lac-ac., ***lac-c., lac-d.,*** **LACH., *lachn.,*** lact., lat-m., laur., lec., ***led.,*** lept., lil-t., ***lup.,*** lupin., ***lyc., lycps.,*** lyss., ***mag-c., mag-m.,*** mag-p., ***mag-s.,*** manc., mang., ***med.,*** meph., **MERC., MERC-C.,** merc-cy., merc-i-f., merc-i-r., merl., mez., morph., mosch., mur-ac., myris., naja, nat-a., ***nat-c., nat-m., nat-p., nat-s.,*** nicc., ***nit-ac., nux-m.,*** **NUX-V.,** olnd., **OP.,** ox-ac., passi., petr., ***ph-ac.,*** phel., **PHOS.,** phys., phyt., pic-ac., plan., ***plat.,*** **PLB., *podo.,*** prun., psor., ptel., **PULS.,** ran-b., ran-s., raph., rheum, rhod.,

INSOMNIA, sleeplessness - **RHUS-T.,** rhus-v., ***rumx.,*** ruta, sabad., sabin., samb., sang., sarcol-ac., saroth., sarr., sars., ***scut., sec., sel., senec.,*** **SEP., SIL.,** sin-n., sol-t-ae., spig., spong., squil., **STANN., STAPH.,** stict., stram., stront-c., stry., sul-ac., sulfon., ***sulph.,*** sul-ac., sumb., **SYPH.,** ***tab.,*** tarax., ***tarent.,*** tax., tela, tell., teucr., thal., **THUJ.,** thea., til., ***tub., ust., valer.,*** verat., verb., vesp., vinc., viol-o., ***viol-t.,*** vip., x-ray, xan., yohim, zinc., zinc-oc., zinc-p., zinc-valer., zing.

abdominal disturbances, from - ***alum.,*** ambr., ant-t., ars., bar-c., calad., calc., canth., caust., ***cham.,*** cina, coff., coll., ***coloc.,*** cupr., cycl., ***dulc.,*** ferr., gent-l., graph., kali-c., ***lach., lyc., mag-c.,*** mag-m., mag-s., mang., nat-m., nit-ac., nux-m., **NUX-V.,** ox-ac., phos., plan., ***plb., puls.,*** sars., sep., sulph., verat.

accident, after an - ***stict.***

aching, in, bones, from - daph.

in, legs, yet cannot keep them still - med.

in, muscles, too exhausted, tired out - helon.

afternoon - ***ars-s-f.,*** pip-m., sil.

1 p.m. to 2 p.m. - pip-m.

2. p.m. - pall.

4 p.m., till - nat-p.

agony, in - ***acet-ac.***

alcohol agg. - agav-t., ars., aven., cann-i., ***cimic., gels., hyos., nux-v.,*** op., stram., ***sumb.***

habitual - sec.

alcoholics, in - ars., aven., cann-i., ***cimic., gels., hyos.,*** lach., ***nux-v.,*** op., passi., ***sec.,*** stram., ***sumb.***

all day - chel.

alternate night - anac., lach.

alternating with

coma - ***camph.***

delirium - ***tub.***

dreams - coff-t.

sleep - crot-h.

sleepiness - asim., ***hyos.***

amenorrhea, in - ***senec., xan.***

anger, after - ***acon., cham.,*** coff., **COLOC.,** ign., lyc., ***nux-v.,*** op., ***staph.***

anxiety, from - abrot., ***acon.,*** agar., alum., arn., **ARS.,** atro., bar-c., bell., ***bry.,*** calc., carb-an., carb-v., ***caust.,*** cench., ***cham.,*** **COCC.,** coff., coloc., con., ***crot-h.,*** cupr., cupr-ar., ***dig., ferr.,*** graph., ***hyos.,*** ign., ***kali-br.,*** kali-c., kali-i., ***lach.,*** laur., lyss., mag-arct., mag-c., mag-m., mang., merc., ***merc-c.,*** nat-c., nat-m., nux-v., phos., puls., ran-b., ran-s., rhus-t., sabin., samb., ***sep., sil.,*** stram., sulph., thuj., verat., vip.

3 a.m. to 4 a., until - ***bry.***

driving out of bed, aggravates after midnight - ars.

menses, after - agar.

midnight agg., after - ars.

aortic disease, in - crat.

INSOMNIA, sleeplessness

bed, feels too hard - ***arn.,*** bapt., bry., mag-c., ***pyrog.***

late, when going to bed - am-c.

must sit up in bed - ars.

too hot - op.

beer, amel. - thea.

belching, from - bar-c., carb-v.

bleeding, from - ***chin.,*** phos.

loss of blood, after - chin., phos.

blood rushed through the body, from sensation as if - alumn.

breathing, with difficult - ***arg-n.,*** ars., ***bor.,*** carb-an., ***cham., chlol.,*** grin., ***kali-br., kali-c., kali-i., lach.,*** lact., ***morph., ran-b., stann., syph.***

children, in - ***ars., kali-br.***

burning, burning in the veins - ***ars.***

soles, from - ***lach.***

stomach, in - am-c.

ulcers, sores, in, from - staph.

calamity, after domestic - aur., calc., ***lach.***

cares, from daily - ***ambr.,*** **CALC.,** graph., ign., kali-p.

business, of - ***ambr., calc.,*** **HYOS.**

imaginary - **HYOS.**

caressed, unless - ***kreos.***

carriage, in - ***alum., calc.,*** sel.

carried, unless - cham.

causeless - ambr., aur., kali-c., mag-c., merc., mur-ac., spig., ***squil.,*** sulph.

child must be carried - ***cham.***

childbed, in - acon., bell., ***coff.,*** hyos., ign., mosch., nux-v., op., puls.

children, in - ***absin., acon., ars.,*** arund., ***bell.,*** calc., **CARC., CHAM.,** ***cina,*** **COFF.,** ***cypr.,*** hyos., ***kali-br., mag-m.,*** passi., phos., ***puls., stict.,*** sulph., tub.

caressed, child must be caressed - ***kreos.***

carried, child must be - cham.

evening - lyc.

fretful from bedtime to morning, next day lively - ***psor.***

laughing, with - cypr.

nervous children, during cough - stict.

rocked, child must be - ***carc.,*** cina, ***stict.***

wants to play and laughs, child - cypr.

chill, with - acon., am-c., ambr., anac., ant-c., **ARAN.,** ars., bell., bor., bry., calc., carb-v., ***cham.,*** chin., coff., euphr., graph., ***hep.,*** ip., kreos., ***lach.,*** lyc., mang., merc., ***mur-ac.,*** nat-m., nit-ac., nux-v., phos., plat., ***puls.,*** rhod., rhus-t., sabin., sep., sil., sulph., thuj.

chilliness, with - ***lac-c., lyc.***

cholera infantum, in - ***cadm-s.***

chronic - apis, ***ars-h., crot-h.,*** cupr-ar., hydr-ac., ***hyos.,*** **LACH.,** ***plat., verat.***

coffee, abuse of, after - cham., **COFF.,** nux-v.

coffee, abuse of, after, unless he drinks - merc.

INSOMNIA, sleeplessness
coldness, from - ***acon.,*** aloe, alum., ambr., am-c., arg-n., ars., bov., calc., camph., carb-v., cist., daph., euph., ferr., graph., ip., kreos., lac-c., mag-s., merc., mur-ac., nat-m., nat-s., nux-v., phos., plect., puls., staph., sulph., thuj., ***verat.***
feet, of - aloe, am-m., aran., ***carb-v.,*** chel., ***nit-ac.,*** petr., ***phos.,*** raph., rhod., sil., verat., zinc.
hands, of - aloe, verat., verat-v.
knees, of - apis, ***carb-v., cocc.***
taking cold, after - ***jatr.***
congestion, from - acon., alumn., am-c., ambr., asar., bry., ***calc., carb-v.,*** dulc., eucal., graph., hep., ign., kali-c., mag-c., ***merc.,*** mosch., mur-ac., nat-m., nit-ac., ***phos., puls.,*** ran-b., rhus-t., sabin., sars., senn., ***sep.,*** **SIL.,** spong., ***sulph.,*** wies.
head, to - ***bor., carb-v.,*** cycl., ***puls.,*** sil.
convalescence, during - alf., aven., cast., coff., cypr., ***hyos.,*** kali-br., scut., stann., ***tub.***
conversation, after - **AMBR.,** hep.
amel. - thea.
convulsions, before or with - alum., art-v., bell., bry., calc., carb-an., carb-v., ***cic.,*** cupr., cypr., hep., hyos., ign., ip., **KALI-BR.,** kali-c., merc., mosch., nux-v., ph-ac., phos., puls., rheum, rhus-t., sel., sep., sil., thuj.
coryza, from - ***ars.,*** mag-m.
cough, from - am-m., ***apis,*** ars., bism., calad., ***caps., caust., chlol., daph.,*** eup-per., ***hyos., kali-bi., kali-cy.,*** lyc., **NIT-AC.,** ***nux-v., ol-j., phel., phos.,*** puls., ***rhus-t.,*** sabad., sep., ***stict., sulph., syph.,*** teucr.
children, in - ***stict.***
lying down, on - ***ol-j.***
midnight, after - ***kali-c.***
urging to cough, from - ars.
whooping-cough, in - ***caust.***
country agg., in the - prot.
cramps, from - arg-m., **CALC.,** coloc., ***cupr., mag-p.***
calves, in - **CALC.,** cham., coff., ***cupr-ac.,*** ferr., mag-p., ***meny., mez.,*** nux-v., staph., ***verat.***
hands and feet, in - valer.
crawling in calfs and feet, from - sulph.
dark room - calc., grin., **PULS.,** staph., **STRAM.,** ***sulph.***
day and night, children - passi., psor.
delirium tremens, in - aven., ***cimic.,*** **GELS.,** hyos., kali-p., ***nux-v.***
delirium, with - acon., ail., aur., ***bapt., bell.,*** bry., cact., calc., ***cann-i.,*** chin., cimic., coloc., cyt-l., dig., dulc., ***gels., hyos.,*** ign., kali-br., lyc., nat-c., nux-v., op., passi., ph-ac., phos., plat., ***plb.,*** puls., rhus-t., sabad., sel., spong., ***stram.,*** sulph., ***tub.,*** verat.
delusions, with - arg-n., ***bell.,*** op.
dentition, during - acon., ***bell.,*** bor., **CHAM.,** coff., cypr., ferr-p., ***gels.,*** mag-c., phos., ter.
depression, with - **AUR.,** lyss., ***nat-m.,*** psor.

INSOMNIA, sleeplessness
despair, in - **AUR.,** carc., lyss., ***psor.***
diabetics, in - ***uran-n.***
diarrhea, during - **BUFO,** ***coloc., dulc., merc-c., nat-s.,*** **PHOS.**
autumn, in - ***merc.***
diphtheria, in - ***chin-a., kali-m.***
disorder, when room is in - ars.
doubt, from - psor.
drawing in legs - carb-v.
dreams, from - ambr., carb-an.
drugs, after - ars., **AVEN.,** cann-i., chlol., ***cimic., gels., hyos.,*** mosch., **NUX-V.,** op., sec., ***sumb.***
habitual - ***aven., nux-v.,*** sec.
mercury - ***kali-br.***
nicotinism, chronic - plan.
opium - ***aven., bell., nux-v.***
dysmenorrhea, in - ***cocc.***
eating, after - acon., agar., am-c., anac., arn., ars., aur., bar-c., bell., bor., bov., bry., ***calc.,*** canth., carb-an., ***carb-v.,*** cast., caust., cham., chel., **CHIN.,** cic., clem., croc., crot-h., cycl., dig., euph., fel., ferr., graph., grat.
amel. - ***phos.***
too late and much - ***puls.***
elderly people - ***acon.,*** ars., ***aur., bar-c.,*** **CALC.,** op., passi., ***phos.,*** sulph., **SYPH.**
erection, from - ant-t., ***plat.,*** sep., ***thuj.***
painful - **THUJ.**
erysipelas, during - ***apis, verat-v.***
evening - aloe, ***arn., ars-s-f.,*** bor., brom., bry., cact., calc., calc-p., calc-s., canth., carb-an., cob., coca, ***coff.,*** dios., dor., ***ferr.,*** fl-ac., grat., guai., **LACH.,** lyc., ***mag-c.,*** merc., mez., nat-c., ol-an., petr., ***phos.,*** psor., **PULS.,** ***rhus-t.,*** sang., spirae., staph., stront-c., **SULPH.,** tab., ***valer.,*** zing.
bed, after going to - aloe, **AMBR.,** bell., bor., carb-v., carc., mag-c., ***mag-m., ph-ac., phos.,*** sulph.
closing eyes, and - ***mag-m.***
congestion, from - rhus-t.
cough, from - phos.
heat - calc., **PULS.,** rhus-t.
joyful news, from - aloe.
menses, during - mag-m.
pulsation in vessels, from - rhus-t.
restlessness, with - phos.
sleepiness in morning, with - ***teucr.***
starting, from - ***puls.***
thoughts, from activity of - fl-ac.
toothache, from - rat.
walk, after a - fl-ac.
wine, after - fl-ac.
excitement from - abrot., agar., ***ambr.,*** anac., ***arg-n., aur-m., calc.,*** camph., canth., caps., carb-an., **CARC.,** chin., cimic., coca, **COFF.,** ***colch.,*** croc., cupr-ar., cypr., dys-co., ferr., gels., ***hep.,*** **HYOS.,** kali-p., ***lach.,*** laur., ***lyc.,*** lyss., mag-aust., mag-c., meph., ***merc.,*** mez., mosch., nit-ac., **NUX-V.,** ***op., phos.,*** plat., ***puls.,*** ran-b., senec., ***sep.,*** spong., staph.,

INSOMNIA, sleeplessness
- **excitement** from - sulph., sul-ac., teucr.
  - theater, at - arg-n., ***phos.***
- **exertion,** agg. - ***calc.,*** chin., cimic., ***nux-v., sil.***
  - after mental - agar., ambr., **ARS.,** ***aur-m.,*** aven., calc., cocc., ***coff.,*** ferr., **HYOS.,** ign., kali-br., ***kali-c., kali-p., lach., lyc., nux-v., ph-ac., pic-ac., sil.***
  - physical - **ARS.,** ***chlol., dig.,*** helon.
  - strain, after mental - ***chlol.,*** **NUX-V.**
- **exhaustion** agg. - aven., chlol., coca, cocc., ***coff.***
- **eyes,** closed eyes, with - staph.
  - inability to open, with - carb-v.
  - will not close eyes - phos.
- **fatigue,** from excessive, mental and physical - ***carc., chlol.,*** chol., cocc., gels.
- **fatigued,** yet - aur.
- **faintness,** with - ars., calc., graph.
- **falling,** sensation of - ***bell.***
- **fantasies,** from - alum., ambr., anh., ant-t., arg-n., ***bell., cham.,*** chin., coff., ign., led., merc., nat-c., ***op.,*** petr., ph-ac., phos., rhus-t., ***sil.,*** spong., thuj.
- **fear,** from - **ACON.,** alum., am-c., arn., ***ars.,*** bell., ***bry.,*** calc., carb-v., caust., cham., ***cocc.,*** coff., dig., graph., hyos., ***ign.,*** kali-c., laur., lyc., mag-c., mag-m., merc., merc-c., ***nat-m.,*** nit-ac., nux-v., **PHOS.,** ***puls.,*** ran-s., ***rhus-t.,*** sep., sil., sulph., thuj.
  - die, she must - cench.
  - falling, of - cimic.
- **fever,** during - acon., aloe, alum., alumn., am-c., am-m., **ANAC.,** ang., ant-t., **APIS,** ***aran.,*** arg-m., arn., ***ars., ars-h., bapt., bar-c.,*** bell., **BOR.,** ***bry., cact., calc.,*** cann-s., carb-s., ***carb-v., caust., cham.,*** chin., chin-s., ***cina,*** cit-v., clem., cocc., coc-c., ***coff.,*** colch., ***coloc.,*** con., eucal., ***ferr.,*** graph., hep., ***hyos.,*** ign., iod., kali-n., kreos., ***lachn.,*** laur., led., ***mag-c.,*** mag-m., mang., merc., merc-c., mosch., nat-m., nat-p., ***nit-ac.,*** nux-m., ***nux-v.,*** ol-an., ***ol-j., op., petr., ph-ac., phos.,*** plect., puls., ran-b., ran-s., **RHOD.,** ***rhus-t.,*** sabad., ***sabin.,*** sars., sep., ***sil., staph., stram.,*** **SULPH.,** thuj., verat.
  - after - ***hell.***
  - anxious - bry., ign., ***puls.***
  - dry - ***caust.,*** nit-ac., wies.
  - low, from - ***cact., stram.***
- **flatulence,** from - ambr., cocc., coff., ***nux-m.,*** nux-v.
- **flushes** of heat, from - puls., ran-b.
- **formication,** from - bufo, carb-v., guare., lyc., osm., zinc.
  - legs, of - sulph., zinc.
- **fracture,** after reposition of - ***stict.***
- **fright,** after - **ACON.,** ***ign., op.***
  - in pregnancy - ***ign., op.***
- **frightened** easily - am-m., arn., bism., bry., canth., ***chin.,*** guai., hep., ign., kali-c., led., merc., nat-m., nux-v., phos., plb., ***rhus-t.,*** sep.

INSOMNIA, sleeplessness
- **girls,** in - calc-p., puls.
- **going** to bed, but sleepy before, after - **AMBR.,** bell.
- **gonorrhea,** in - ***tarent.***
- **gout,** in - ***mang.***
- **grief,** from - aur., ***gels.,*** graph., **IGN.,** ***kali-br.,*** lach., **NAT-M.,** ***sulph.***
- **hemorrhoids,** from - ***ars., kali-c.***
- **headache,** from - acon., am-c., ammc., ***arg-n.,*** ars-i., **AUR.,** brach., bry., bufo, calc-caust., carb-o., caust., ***chel.,*** **CHIN.,** ***chlol., coff., croc.,*** elaps, ind., ***lach.,*** lyc., mag-s., manc., ***merc., merl.,*** mosch., mur-ac., nat-m., nicc., nit-ac., osm., pall., ***phys., puls.,*** sars., ***sil.,*** sol-n., ***spig.,*** spong., staph., stram., **SULPH.,** ***syph.,*** tarax., verat., zinc-valer.
- **heart,** with disease of - **AUR.,** ***aur-m.,*** **BOR.,** ***colch.,*** crat., ***dig.,*** merc., merc-c., naja, ***op.,*** spig., ***tab.,*** verat.
- **heat,** from - carb-an., kali-n., mag-c., mur-ac.
  - in head - am-m., **BOR.,** verat.
  - sensation of, with - ran-b.
- **heavy** blow, after - ***ambr., con.***
- **heavy** feeling, in arms, from - alum.
  - in limbs - ***caust.,*** gran., mag-c.
    - lower - caust.
- **hiccough,** with - ***nux-v.***
- **homesickness,** from - **CAPS.,** ***ign.***
- **humiliation,** after - ***calc., coloc., ign.,*** **STAPH.**
- **hunger,** from - abies-n., ap-g., ***chin., cina, ign.,*** lyc., ***phos.,*** psor., sanic., sulph., teucr.
- **hydrophobia,** in - ***lyss.***
- **hypochondriasis,** in - ***arg-n., bar-c.,*** graph., valer.
- **hypogastrium,** from oppression in - mag-c.
- **hysterical** - ***croc.,*** mosch., ***senec., stict.***
- **illusions** of fancy - alum., ***arg-n., bell.,*** calc., merc., nat-c., ph-ac., phos., thuj.
- **influenza,** after - ***aven.***
- **injuries,** from - ***arn.,*** nat-s., op., ***rhus-t., stict.***
- **insane** people, in - aur., bell., carc., cocc., ***hyos., lach., manc.,*** op., ***tarent.***
- **intermittent** - carb-s.
- **irritability,** from - ***acon., arg-n., bapt., chin-s., chlol., coff., gels.,*** **HYOS.,** ***kali-p., lach.,*** lyss., mosch., ***nat-m.,*** plat., ***stict.,*** valer.
- **itching,** from - acon., ***agar.,*** alum., am-c., anac., ant-c., ***apis, arn.,*** bar-c., bell., ***bov.,*** calad., carb-v., caust., chlol., ***cit-v.,*** cocc., con., cop., dol., dulc., euphr., ***gels.,*** kali-c., kreos., lach., lyss., ***merc., mez.,*** **PSOR.,** ***puls.,*** ran-b., raph., sars., staph., ***sulph.,*** teucr., valer., zinc.
  - anus, of - ***aloe,*** alum., coff., ign., ***indg.***
  - herpes - staph.
  - pregnancy, during - ***dol.***
  - scrotum - urt-u.
  - senilis, pruritus - ***mez., psor.***

INSOMNIA, sleeplessness
jerks, from - agar., alum., arg-m., arg-n., ***ars.,*** **BELL.,** calc., carb-v., cham., cimic., colch., dulc., hyos., ***ign., kali-c.,*** lyc., nat-m., op., ***puls., rhus-t.,*** sel., ***sep.,*** sulph.
joy, excessive - **COFF.**
kidney affections, in - ars., ***hyos., plb.***
labor, during - ***coff., con.***
after - ***nat-s.***
lasting several nights - anac.
late, if going to bed - am-c.
legs crossed, unless - ***rhod.***
liver complaints, in - acet-ac., ***dol.***
loss of sleep, after - ***cocc.***
sensation as from loss of sleep - cocc., euph., guai., op., ost., puls.
morning - graph., naja, sol-n.
rising, after - merc.
lying, while - ***cham.,*** chin., lyss., puls.
because unable to lie on left side - ***colch.***
uncomfortable - mag-c.
lying, side, on - card-m., ferr.
on, left - card-m., ter., thuj., x-ray.
because unable to lie on the left side - ***colch.***
on, right - merc.
mania, in - apis, cocc., nux-v., stram., verat-v.
maniacal - ***cocc.***
measles, in - ***ferr-p.***
menopause period, during - ***acon., arn., bell., cimic.,*** cocc., ***coff.,*** dig., ***gels., kali-br., senec., sulph.,*** valer., ***zinc.***
prolapsus uteri or uterine irritation, with - senec.
menses, during - agar., am-c., cimic., eupi., gent-c., ign., mag-m., nat-m., senec., sep.
dysmenorrhea, with - ***cocc.***
menorrhagia, in - cann-i.
after - cimic., kali-br., thuj.
before - agar., cycl., goss., kreos., senec., tub.
beginning, at - agar.
mental, exertion, after - agar., ***aur-m.,*** ambr., **ARS.,** ***coff.,*** ferr., **HYOS.,** ign., kali-br., ***kali-c., kali-p., lach., lyc., nux-v.,*** passi., ***ph-ac., pic-ac.***
mental, strain, after - nux-v., passi.
midnight, (see night)
miscarriage, during - ***helon.***
after - ***cypr.***
moon, full - nux-v., ***sil.***
at new - ***sep.***
morning - cinnb., cycl., dulc., kali-i., med., merc-i-r., ***nat-m.,*** ol-an., sol-t-ae.
5. a.m., after - chin., fago., nat-m., nat-s., sapin., ***ph-ac.,*** **SULPH.**
images, from - acon.
motion, sensation as if bed in - clem.
fetus, from painful motion of - arn.
muttering, with - **HYOS.**
narcotics, after - ***bell., nux-v.,*** stram.
in spite of - ***kali-i.***
without - ***kali-i.***

INSOMNIA, sleeplessness
nausea, from - am-c., ambr., cham., chin-s., cocc., ***ip., graph.***
nervousness, caused by - acon., ***ars.,*** calc., chin., coff., gels., hyos., lach., lyc., mosch., nux-v., plat., scut., stict., teucr.
neuritis, multiple, from - con.
newborn, in - acon., ***bell.,*** cham., coff., cypr., op., psor., puls., sulph.
news, after surprising - ***coff.***
night - am-c., ambr., ant-t., aphis., ***ars.,*** aur., bor., bry., camph., caps., carb-v., ***caust.,*** cham., ***chin., cina,*** cinnb., clem., cocc., ***coff.,*** coloc., ***con.,*** dros., dulc., ***ferr., graph.,*** hep., hydr-ac., ***hyos.,*** ign., jal., kali-m.
all night - yohim.
bed, after going to - form., gent-l., ham., lycps., ran-b., wies.
every other night - anac., chin., lach.
first part of - cinnb., dig., form., frax., ham., gent-l., lyc., lycps., pip-m., ***podo.,*** ran-b., tab.
agg. - pip-m.
thoughts, from activity of - cact.
latter part of in - calc-ar., lina., pip-m., zing.
middle part of in - sel.
except for middle part - ***crot-h.***
reading, amel. - sel.
sleepiness, with, afternoon and evening - abrot., **SULPH.**
sleepiness, with, daytime - ***agar.,*** am-c., ammc., anh., ant-c., arg-n., arn., aur-s., bar-ac., bell., bry., carb-s., carb-v., ***carc.,*** chin., cinnb., clem., ferr., fl-ac., ***graph.,*** hura, hyos., kali-c., lac-d., lach., mag-c., **MED.,** merc., mosch., mur-ac., nat-hchls., nat-m., nux-v., op., ***petr.,*** ph-ac., ***phos.,*** pic-ac., plan., psor., puls., ran-b., rhus-t., sep., ***sil.,*** spig., **STAPH.,** stram., sul-i., **SULPH.**
body aches all over - **STAPH.**
mental exertion, after - pic-ac.
night, midnight, after - ***acon.,*** adlu., alum., am-c., am-m., ambr., ang., ant-c., ant-t., apis, arn., **ARS.,** ars-i., ars-s-f., ***asar., asaf., aur.,*** aur-a., aur-s., bar-c., bell., ***benz-ac.,*** bor., bry., calad., calc., camph., ***cann-s.,*** canth., **CAPS.,** carb-v., caust., cham., chin., cocc., **COFF.,** colch., con., croc., cycl., cypr., dros., ***dulc.,*** esp-g., euphr., ferr., graph., guai., hell., **HEP.,** ign., ***iod.,*** **KALI-AR., KALI-C.,** kali-n., kali-p., kali-sil., kreos., lach., laur., lyc., ***mag-c.,*** mang., merc., merc-sul., mez., mosch., mur-ac., ***nat-a., nat-c.,*** nat-m., nat-p., nit-ac., **NUX-V.,** olnd., **PH-AC.,** phos., plat., plb., ***psor.,*** puls., ***ran-b., ran-s.,*** rat., ***rhod., rhus-t.,*** sabad., sabin., samb., sars., sel., ***sep.,*** **SIL.,** spong., squil., staph., ***sul-ac.,*** sul-i., sulph., ***syph., thuj.,*** v-a-b., verat., verb., viol-t.
1 a.m. at - spig.
after - ambr., ***cocc.,*** kali-n., mag-c., nat-c., nit-ac., ***nux-v.,*** sep.
until - ambr., ***cocc.,*** kali-n., merc-i-f., nat-c., sep.

INSOMNIA, sleeplessness
 night, midnight, after
  1 a.m. to 2 a.m. - ***sulph.***
   after - **KALI-C.**
   except for - calc.
   until - **CALC.**
  1 a.m. to 3 a.m. - am-m., chlorpr.
   except for - am-m., calc.
  1 a.m. to 4 a.m. - bor., phos.
   1 a.m. to 5 a.m. - mag-c.
   1 a.m. or 2 a.m., after - ***kali-c.***
  1:30 a.m. to 2:30 a.m. - agar., perh.
  2 a.m. - ***cham., puls.***
   after - all-c., bapt., benz-ac., caust., coff., cypr., dios., graph., kali-bi., **KALI-C.,** kali-sil., ***lec., mag-c.,*** mag-m., mez., nat-m., **NIT-AC.,** pall., ***ptel.,*** puls., sars., ***sil.,*** thuj., ***verat.***
   until - bor., carb-an., cupr., graph., mag-c., sil.
  2 a.m. to 3 a.m. - ***arn.,*** bapt., calc., calc-p., gink-b., kali-c., mag-m., merc.
   after - am-m., ap-g., **ARS.,** ars-s-f., ***bapt.,*** bell-p., bry., ***calc.,*** chin., ***coff.,*** gels., ***kali-c.,*** kalm., mag-c., mag-s., nat-c., nat-m., nit-ac., ***nux-v.,*** raph., ***sel., sep.***
   until - **CALC.**
  2 a.m. to 4 a.m. - am-c., am-m., arist-cl., merc., ph-ac.
   2 a.m. to 5 a.m. - arist-cl., ***bell.,*** bor., chloram., sulph.
  2:30 a.m., till - lyc., pip-m.
   after - arg-m., carb-an., lyc., pip-m.
  3 a.m. - am-m., ars., aur., bry., chin., chin-a., com., euphr., eupi., mag-c., ***merc.,*** mez., mill., nat-p., ran-s., rhus-t., sil.
   after - am-m., ammc., **ARS.,** ars-s-f., ***bapt., bell-p., bor., bry., calc.,*** calc-ar., ***calc-s., chin.,*** clem., coff., euphr., graph., jug-c., kreos., **MAG-C.,** mag-m., mag-s., mez., nat-m., nicc., ***nux-v.,*** ol-an., op., plat., ***psor.,*** ran-s., raph., rhus-t., ***sel.,*** **SEP.,** staph., **SULPH., THUJ., TUB.,** zinc-p.
   until - nat-p., sulph.
  3 a.m. to 4 a.m. - arist-cl., chel., nux-v., rib-ac.
  3 a.m. to 5 a.m. - arist-cl., bell-p., calc-f., cob-n., man.
   except for - chin.
   heat, from - **BOR.**
  3:30 a.m. until, after - arg-m.
  4 a.m. - acon-c., aloe, ***am-c., bor.,*** cocc., cupr-s., nit-ac., tarent., puls-n.
   after - bor., bufo, caust., cycl., hyper., lyc., ***mur-ac.,*** nit-ac., ***petr.,*** ph-ac., phos., plan., ruta, sep., staph., **SULPH.,** tab., thuj., trom., verb., zinc.
   pollution, after - pip-m.
   until - ***nicc.,*** op.
  4 a.m. to 6:30 a.m. - cycl.
  4:30 a.m., after - sep.

INSOMNIA, sleeplessness
 night, midnight, after
  5 a.m. - carb-an., tarent.
   after - chin., fago., nat-m., ***ph-ac.,*** **SULPH.**
   until - aloe, ran-b.
  morning, until - **ANT-T.,** ***cact., hyos.,*** psor., puls., valer., zing.
 night, midnight, before - acon., ***agar., aloe, alum., alum-p.,*** alum-sil., **AMBR.,** am-c., am-m., anac., ***ang.,*** ant-c., ant-t., ***arg-n.,*** arn., **ARS.,** ars-s-f., asar., aur., aur-a., aur-s., bar-c., bar-m., ***bell.,*** bism., ***bor.,*** **BRY.,** bufo, cact., ***calad.,*** **CALC., CALC-P.,** calc-s., ***calc-sil.,*** camph., cann-s., canth., caps., ***carb-an., carb-s.,*** **CARB-V.,** caust., cench., ***cham.,*** chel., ***chin.,*** chin-a., clem., coc-c., coca, cocc., **COFF.,** coloc., **CON.,** cor-r., cupr., cycl., dig., dor., dulc., euph., euphr., ***ferr.,*** ferr-ar., ferr-p., ***gels., graph., guai.,*** guare., ***hep., hydr.,*** hyos., ***ign.,*** ip., kali-ar., **KALI-C.,** kali-n., kali-s., kali-sil., kreos., ***lac-c., lach.,*** laur., ***led.,*** lil-t., **LYC.,** ***mag-aust.,*** mag-c., **MAG-M.,** mag-s., mang., ***med.,*** **MERC.,** merc-i-f., ***mez.,*** mosch., ***mur-ac.,*** **NAT-A., NAT-C.,** ***nat-m., nat-p.,*** nit-ac., nux-m., ***nux-v.,*** par., petr., ***ph-ac.,*** **PHOS.,** phys., **PIC-AC.,** plat., plb., **PULS.,** ***ran-b.,*** ran-s., rheum, rhod., **RHUS-T.,** sabad., sabin., samb., sars., ***sel.,*** seneg., **SEP., SIL.,** sin-n., ***spig.,*** spong., ***stann., staph., stront-c.,*** **SULPH.,** ***sul-ac.,*** tab., tarax., tarent., ter., ***teucr.,*** ther., ***thuj., valer.,*** verat., verb., viol-t., zinc., zinc-p.
  9 p.m. - kali-cy.
  10 p.m., after - pip-m.
  10 p.m. to 1 a.m., except for - nux-v.
   10 p.m. to 2 a.m. - thea.
   10 p.m. to 4 a.m., except for - sep.
  11 p.m., after - chel.
   11 p.m., until - chel., ***kali-c.,*** laur., mag-m., ***nux-v.,*** staph.
  11 p.m. to 1 a.m. - am-c., carb-v., kali-c., kreos., laur., merc., nit-ac.
   except - nux-v.
  11 p.m. to 2 a.m. or 3 a.m. - arn.
  until after midnight - lyc., plat.
 night, midnight, until - aloe, alum., ***am-m.,*** ambr., ***ang.,*** ant-c., ant-t., ars., ***bry.,*** caust., chin., coc-c., coca, coff., con., cor-r., dor., euph., euphr., graph., guare., kali-c., kali-n., kreos., lach., led., ***lyc., mag-aust.,*** mag-c., mag-s., merc., mur-ac., ***nux-v.,*** phos., phys., plat., puls., ***rhus-t.,*** sars., sep., sil., sin-n., spig., spong., ***staph.,*** **SULPH.,** teucr., thuj., verat.
  1 a.m., until - am-c., ang., atro., bry., calad., ***carb-v.,*** caust., cench., con., gels., kali-c., kreos., laur., mag-c., merc., merc-i-f., nat-p., nit-ac., plan., plat., phos., thuj.
   restlessness, from - phos.
   sensation of heat, from - still.
  1 a.m. or 2 a.m. until - bry., kali-c., kreos., ***sulph.***
   1 a.m. to 2. a.m. until - agar.

INSOMNIA, sleeplessness

night, midnight, until

2 a.m., until - all-c., allox., anac., arn., berb., bor., bry., calc., calc-p., carb-an., ***cham.,*** coca, com., cupr., cupr-ar., euphr., dulc., graph., hist., kali-c., kreos., lyss., macro., ***merc.,*** morph., nat-m., pall., phel., phos., ***puls.,*** raph., sil.

thoughts, from activity of - ***sil.***

2 a.m. or 3 a.m., until - ***arn.,*** calc., calc-p., hist.

2 a.m. or 4 a.m., until - ph-ac.

3 a.m., until - am-m., arn., ars., aur., ***bell-p.,*** bry., calc., calc-p., cench., chin., chin-a., com., eupi., euphr., mag-c., ***merc.,*** mez., mill., nat-p., ran-s., rhus-t., sil.

rising, after - aloe.

thoughts, from activity of - nat-p.

3 a.m or 4 a.m., until - bry., cupr-s., nit-ac.

3 a.m. to 5 a.m., except for - chin.

4 a.m., until - acon-c., aloe, ***am-c., bor.,*** bry., calc., ***chel.,*** cocc., cupr-s., kreos., nit-ac., tarent., thuj., wild.

4 a.m. or 5 a.m., until - aloe.

5 a.m., until - arn., carb-an., tarent.

5 a.m., except 2 hours in evening - arn.

daybreak, till - hyos., ***nux-v.***

fixed thoughts - puls.

heat and anxiety, from - graph.

morning, towards - ang., **ANT-T.,** ***arn., atro.,*** **AUR.,** buni-o., ***cact.,*** cahin., chin., chin-s., cimic., ***coff.,*** crot-h., cycl., ***fl-ac.,*** hyos., kali-i., ***kreos., lyss.,*** mag-aust., meph., merc., ***nat-c.,*** nat-m., nit-ac., puls., ***prun., psor., puls.,*** sil., spirae., ***staph.,*** sul-ac., sulph., thuj., ***valer.,*** zinc., zing.

sleepiness, with - bar-s.

talkativeness, with - ***lach.***

thirst, with - bry.

thoughts, from activity of - calc.

till after midnight - lyc., plat.

weakness, with - ***lach.,*** mosch.

without, morning - cinnb.

noise from slight - acon., alum., alumn., am-c., ang., apis, ars., ***asar., bell., calad., calc.,*** carb-v., cham., chin., **COFF.,** ***ign.,*** kali-n., lach., ***merc.,*** narcot., nat-p., ***nux-v.,*** ol-an., phos., ruta, saroth., ***sel.,*** sep., sul-ac., ***sulph.,*** tarent., valer., zinc-valer.

numbness, from - cimic., cina.

nursing, child, after - bell., ***cimic.***

sick, the - **COCC.,** ***coff.,*** zinc-ac.

nurslings - carc., syph.

open the eyes, with inability to - carb-v.

oppression of, chest, from - kali-c., nux-v., physal., ***phos.,*** ran-b., ran-s.

of, hypogastrium - mag-c.

orgasm of blood - alum., asar., bry., ***calc.,*** hep., ign., mag-c., ***merc.,*** mur-ac., ***phos., puls.,*** ran-b., rhus-t., ***sep.,*** **SIL.,** ***sulph.***

pain, on falling asleep, from - lil-t., **MERC.**

INSOMNIA, sleeplessness

pains, from - acon., ars., arum-t., ***aur.,*** bufo, cann-i., **CHAM.,** cimic., coloc., ***dol.,*** eup-per., eupi., ***ferr-p., iris,*** kreos., ***lach.,*** mag-c., mag-m., ***merc.,*** passi., phyt., plb., ptel., puls., ***rhus-t.,*** sin-n., stram., ***sulph.***

abdomen, in - bar-c.

arms, in - calc., caust., mag-s., mosch., thea.

back, in - am-m., bell., con., ***dulc.,*** lac-ac., ***lac-c.,*** mag-s., nat-m., ptel., sin-n., ***syph.***

body sore, whole - caust., staph.

bones, in - anac., daph., ***kalm., merc.,*** plb.

calves, in - staph.

chest, in - lyc., mag-m., nux-v.

eyes, in - carb-v., rheum.

face, in - caps., plan., verb.

feet, in - lach., phos.

gums, in - ***dol.,*** stann.

head, in - acon., am-c., ammc., ***arg-n.,*** ars-i., **AUR.,** brach., bufo, calc-caust., carb-o., caust., ***chel.,*** **CHIN.,** ***chlol., croc.,*** elaps, ***lach.,*** lyc., mag-s., manc., merc., ***merl.,*** mosch., mur-ac., nat-m., nicc., nit-ac., osm., pall., ***phys., puls.,*** sars., ***sil.,*** sol-n., ***spig.,*** spong., staph., stram., **SULPH.,** ***syph.,*** tarax., verat.

heart, in - man.

hips, in - sin-n.

joints, in - sol-t-ae.

knee, in - spig.

legs, in - agar., carb-v., daph., ***kali-bi.,*** med., ***mez., rhus-t.,*** staph., ***syph.***

limbs, in - aeth., bar-c., bell., caust., cham., chin., con., hep., kali-c., kreos., mag-c., merc., nat-c., nit-ac., phos., plb., ***puls.,*** ran-s., ***rhod.,*** rhus-t., sil., spig., sulph., syph., zinc.

lower - agar.

sore - cham.

lumbar region, in - mag-m.

mouth, in - merc-p-r.

muscles, in - helon.

parts lain on - ***thuj.***

rectum, in - am-c.

rheumatic pains - ***ant-t., ars.,*** atro., cact., ***caul., coloc., dulc., puls., stict.***

skin, in - petr.

stomach, in - carb-o., cocc., phos., rhus-t.

teeth, in - ***aur., bar-c.,*** canth., ***cham., cocc-s.,*** hell., mag-m., merc-c., rat., **SEP.,** ***sil.,*** spig., staph., trom.

palpitation, from - acon., adon., alum., am-c., ***aur-m.,*** bell., ***benz-ac., cact., calc.,*** cimic., coca, ***coff.,*** crot-t., dig., ***ign., iod.,*** jatr., kali-bi., ***kali-p.,*** lact., lil-t., lyc., lycps., ***nat-m.,*** **PHOS.,** psor., puls., rhus-t., saroth., sars., sep., sil., spig.

pecuniary loss, from - aur., stann.

periodic, every three hours - puls.

for half hours - anac.

perspiration, from - ***ars.,*** bry., cham., chel., chin-s., ***coff.,*** **CON.,** dulc., ferr., graph., ***merc.,*** mosch., ***nux-v.,*** petr., ph-ac., ran-b., ***rhus-t.,*** sabad., sabin., ***sel.,*** sulph., tarax., verat.

INSOMNIA, sleeplessness

perspiration, from

forehead - sars.

perspiration, with - alum., am-c., am-m., **ANAC.,** ***apis,*** arn., ***ars.,*** bar-c., bell., bor., ***bry., calc.,*** canth., carb-v., caust., ***cham., chel.,*** **CHIN.,** cic., ***clem.,*** cocc., **COFF.,** con., graph., hep., ign., kali-n., kreos., laur., led., mag-c., mag-m., mang., ***merc., merc-c.,*** nat-m., ***nit-ac.,*** nux-m., nux-v., petr., **PH-AC.,** ***phos., puls.,*** ran-b., ran-s., ***rhod.,*** **RHUS-T.,** ***sabad., sabin.,*** sars., sel., sep., sil., staph., stront-c., ***sulph., tarax., thuj., verat.***

playing and laughing, child is - cypr.

pneumonia, in - ***ant-t., bell.,*** bry., ***chel., elaps,*** kali-c., ***merc.,*** phos.

after - ***kali-c.***

position is right, no - ars., kali-c., lach., laur., lycpr., nat-c., plat., ran-b., staph.

pregnancy, during - ***acon.,*** ambr., ***bell.,*** cact., cham., chin., ***cimic., coff.,*** cypr., gels., hyos., ign., kali-bi., ***kali-br.,*** lyc., mag-p., mosch., nux-v., ***op., puls.,*** rhus-t., staph., stram., sulph., tarent.

cramps in calves, from - ***calc.,*** cham., coff., ***cupr-ac.,*** ferr., nux-v., ***verat.***

sleepiness, with - ***nux-m.***

prodrome, as a - chin.

pulsation, from - acon., ammc., ***bell., cact., glon.,*** rhus-t., sabad., sec., ***sel.,*** sulph., thea.

ear, in - sil.

head, in - ars.

lower limbs, in - agar.

of body and particularly in the abdomen - ***sil.***

reading, after - sel.

remaining up later than usual, on - grat.

restlessness, from - abies-n., abrot., **ACON.,** ***alum.,*** am-c., anac., anthro., **APIS,** arn., **ARS.,** arum-t., asaf., asar., aur., bell., bor., ***bry.,*** calc., canth., carb-an., ***carb-v.,*** caust., **CHAM.,** ***chin., cic., cina,*** cocc., ***coff.,*** coloc., ***con.,*** cor-r., ***cupr., cypr.,*** dulc., euph., euphr., eupi., ferr., gels., gent-l., graph., guai., hyos., ***ign.,*** iod., ***ip.,*** jal., kali-c., kali-n., ***kreos., lach.,*** lam., laur., ***led., lyc.,*** lycpr., mag-aust., mag-c., mag-m., mag-s., mang., ***meph., merc.,*** **MERC-C.,** mosch., mur-ac., nat-c., ***nat-m.,*** nat-s., ***nit-ac.,*** nux-m., nux-v., olnd., ***op.,*** par., ***petr., phos., plat., psor.,*** **PULS.,** ran-b., ***rhod., rhus-t.,*** ruta, sabin., sars., sec., senn., ***sep., sil., spig.,*** spong., stann., ***stram.,*** sulph., tarax., tarent., ter., thal., ***thuj.,*** vinc., zinc., zinc-valer.

and twitching in abdomen - caust.

legs, in - agar., graph., lyc., med., rhus-t., saroth., stann., ***zinc.***

retiring, after, but sleepy before - **AMBR.**

riding in a carriage, on - alum., calc., sel.

amel. - tarent.

rocked, child must be - ***bor., carc.,*** cham., cina, ***stict.***

INSOMNIA, sleeplessness

room, in dark - calc., **PULS.,** staph., **STRAM.,** ***sulph.***

illuminated - ***coff.,*** lach., nux-v., **STAPH.**

sad events, from - ***nat-m.***

sadness, from - **AUR.,** ***ign., kali-br.,*** kali-c., nat-m., ***thuj.***

saliva running down throat, from - kali-c., merc.

with constant flow of - ***ign.***

scarlatina, in - ail., bell., merc-i-r., phyt., verat-v.

screaming, with - ***cham.,*** cina, hyos., jal., senn.

children, in - ***cham.,*** cina, passi.

scruples, from - ferr.

sex, after - bov., calc., cop., nit-ac., sep., sil.

sexual excitement, from - ant-c., kali-br., ph-ac., raph.

thoughts, from - calad., calc., canth., dros., kali-br., raph., staph.

shivering, from - bry.

shocks, from - agar., alum., **ARG-M., ARS.,** ***bell.,*** ip., nat-a., ***nat-m., nit-ac., phos.***

sick feeling, from - phos.

sleepiness, with - ***acon., agar.,*** am-c., am-m., ambr., ***ant-t.,*** apis, apoc., arg-n., arn., ars., ars-m., bar-ac., bar-c., **BELL.,** bor., ***bry.,*** bufo, calad., ***calc.,*** calc-sil., camph., cann-i., canth., carb-an., carb-s., carb-v., ***caust.,*** **CHAM., CHEL.,** chin., chr-ac., cic., cina, clem., coca, cocc., cod., ***coff., con.,*** corn., ***crot-h.,*** crot-t., ***cupr.,*** daph., dirc., elaps, euphr., eupi., ***ferr.,*** ferr-ar., ferr-p., **GELS.,** gent-l., graph., ***hep.,*** hyos., kali-ar., ***kali-c.,*** kali-p., kali-sil., ***lach.,*** lact., laur., lyc., mag-aust., mag-m., med., ***merc.,*** morph., mosch., nat-a., ***nat-c., nat-m.,*** nat-p., nit-ac., ***nux-m., nux-v.,*** **OP.,** ***petr., ph-ac.,*** **PHOS.,** ***phys.,*** plb., **PULS.,** ran-b., rhod., ***rhus-t.,*** sabad., sabin., ***samb.,*** sel., ***senec.,*** **SEP.,** ***sil.,*** sol-m., spig., staph., ***stram., sulph.,*** sul-ac., syph., ***tarent.,*** ter., teucr., thuj., verat., viol-o., zinc.

afternoon - abrot.

heat, during - **PULS.**

measles, after - ***caust.***

morning - cycl.

5 a.m. - myric.

and after sunset - **SULPH.**

pregnancy, during - ***nux-m.***

restlessness, with - ***graph., petr.***

thougths, from activity of - agar.

without - ars-s-r., aur., chin-b., ***fl-ac.***

sleepy all day, sleepless all night, body aches all over - am-c., ant-c., ***arg-n.,*** ferr., lac-d., lach., med., mosch., op., ph-ac., rhus-t., sil., **STAPH.,** sulph.

smallpox, in - ***sarr.***

soreness, with - carb-v., mag-s.

mouth and throat, in - arum-t., merc.

sounds in the heart, from - x-ray.

spells of, few nights - anac.

INSOMNIA, sleeplessness

starting, from - am-m., ambr., arn., ***ars.,*** bell., bism., bry., calc., canth., ***chin., dig.,*** dulc., hyos., ign., kali-bi., kali-c., led., lyc., mag-c., merc., nat-c., nit-ac., nux-v., ***phos.,*** plb., psor., ***rhus-t.,*** sars., sel., sep., sulph., verat.

stroke, before - ***aster.***

stupefaction, with - calc., ***nux-v.***

sudden - scut.

supper, after late - ***puls.***

suppressed secretion, from - ***lach.***

surgery, after - arn., calen., ***op., stict.***

after setting broken leg - stict.

talk, with desire to - ***cypr., lach.***

tea, after abuse of - camph-br., chin., ***nux-v.,*** puls.

thinking amel. - thea.

thirst, from - all-s., calad., ign., mag-m., nit-ac., phos.

menses, during - ***sep.***

thoughts, from - acon., ***aesc.,*** agar., aloe, alum., ***ambr.,*** anh., ant-t., ap-g., apis, **ARG-N., ARS.,** aur., bar-c., bell., bor., ***bry.,*** cact., calad., **CALC.,** calc-f., ***calc-s.,*** calc-sil., canth., ***carb-s.,*** **CARC.,** caust., **CHIN.,** cinnb., ***cocc.,*** **COFF.,** coloc., con., cupr., cupr-ac., ***cypr.,*** dios., fago., ***ferr., fl-ac., gels., graph.,*** grat., ham., hell., **HEP.,** ***hyos.,*** hyper., ign., jatr., kali-ar., ***kali-c.,*** kali-n., kali-sil., ***lach., lyc.,*** meph., ***nat-m.,*** nat-p., nux-m., **NUX-V., OP.,** ***pic-ac.,*** plat., plb., podo., ***psor.,*** **PULS.,** ***pyrog., rhus-t.,*** sabad., saroth., ***sep., sil.,*** spig., ***staph.,*** **SULPH.,** teucr., thuj., ***tub.,*** verat., viol-o., viol-t., yohim, ***zinc.***

business, of - bell., ***cocc.,*** phos.

erotic - calad., staph.

events of whole past life - yohim.

morning, towards - ars.

same idea always repeated - ***arg-n.,*** bar-c., ***calc., coff., graph.,*** petr., plat., **PULS.,** ***sulph.,*** thuj.

melody repeated - ***puls.***

thunderstorm, before - agar., rhod., phos., sil.

tiredness of lower limbs, from - agar., con., gels.

tobacco, chronic abuse of, after - aven., calad., gels., nux-v., plan.

toothache, from - ***aur., bar-c.,*** canth., **CHAM.,** ***cocc-s.,*** hell., mag-m., ***mag-p.,*** merc-c., rat., **SEP.,** ***sil., spig.,*** staph., trom.

total - am-c., ambr., ars., ***aur., calc., canth.,*** carc., chin., cic., clem., **COFF.,** coloc., ***daph.,*** dulc., ***graph.,*** hep., iod., ip., kreos., mag-c., merc., mosch., nat-c., ***nit-ac., nux-v.,*** prun., rhus-t., sars., sep., sil., spong., staph.

trembling, from - calc., euph., lyc., sil.

tuberculosis, in - ***iod., sang.***

twitching of the limbs - ambr., ***alum.,*** arg-n., **ARS.,** bell., calc., canth., carb-v., carc., cham., ***cypr.,*** ign., ***kali-c.,*** lyc., merc-c., nat-m., op., **PULS.,** rhus-t., sel., sep., stront-c., sulph., tab., valer.

INSOMNIA, sleeplessness

uneasiness, from - agar., ***bry., carb-v., cina,*** cycl., hell., ***merc.,*** nat-c., phos., ***puls.,*** rhus-t.

and anxiety with heat, must uncover, which causes chilliness - ***mag-c.***

urging to urinate, with - dig., graph., nat-c., ran-b., ruta4

uterine colic, by - cann-i.

complaints, from - senec.

vaccination, after - ***mez.,*** sil., ***thuj.***

vaginal discharge, before - ***senec.***

vertigo, from - am-c., arg-m., arg-n., calad., calc., con., lac-ac., ***merc-c.,*** nat-c., nat-m., phos., rhus-t., spong., sulph., tell., ther.

vexation, after - acon., ars., calc., cham., ***coloc.,*** kali-p., nux-v., petr., ***staph.***

visions, from - ambr., ***arg-n.,*** bry., ***calc.,*** carb-an., ***cham., ign.,*** lyc., merc., ***op.,*** sulph.

anxious - ***carb-an.***

closing eyes, on - ***led., thuj.***

vivacity, from - ***ang.,*** ant-c., ***apis,*** arn., aur., bor., ***calc.,*** caps., ***carc.,*** caust., chin., ***coff.,*** cypr., graph., hyos., kali-c., lach., lam., lyc., mag-aust., ***med.,*** merc., mez., ***nat-m., nit-ac.,*** nux-v., phos., ***prun., puls., ran-b., ran-s.,*** rhus-t., ruta, sel., sep., sil., spig., staph., sul-ac., ***sulph.,*** teucr., verat.

vomiting, with - ***chin-s., ip., nux-v.***

waking, after - aeth., agar., am-c., am-m., **ARS.,** ars-s-f., ***aur.,*** aur-a., bar-c., ***bell.,*** bell-p., berb., bor., brach., calc., calc-f., calc-sil., caps., carb-s., carb-v., carc., caust., chr-ac., clem., cocc., con., cycl., ***dulc., ferr.,*** ferr-m., ferr-p., graph., jug-c., kali-ar., kali-c., kali-n., kali-sil., laur., **LACH.,** led., lyc., **MAG-C.,** mag-m., mang., ***merc.,*** mez., mur-ac., **NAT-M.,** ***nit-ac.,*** nux-m., ***nux-v.,*** ol-an., ox-ac., petr., ***phos.,*** ph-ac., phyt., pip-n., prun., psor., puls., ***ran-b.,*** ran-s., rat., rhod., rhus-t., ruta, sabin., ***sars.,*** sel., ***sep.,*** **SIL.,** spong., stront-c., ***sulph.,*** sul-ac., zinc., zinc-p.

midnight, before - ***mur-ac.***

noise, by a - ***coff.,*** ox-ac.

walking in open air, after - kali-c.

warm, coverings though limbs are cold - **CAMPH., LED.,** ***med.,*** **SEC.**

warmth, from - carb-an., kali-n., mag-c., mur-ac.

of bed - ***puls.,*** **SULPH.**

weakness, from - ammc., aven., coca, cocc., ***coff.,*** cypr., ***gels.,*** gran., helon., ***kali-br., kreos., mag-p.,*** meph., merc., ***ph-ac.,*** phos., ***pic-ac.,*** stann., ***tub.***

weaning child, of - bell., puls.

weariness, from - **ARS.,** cact., ***chlol.,*** helon.

in spite of weariness - ambr., apis, apoc., ***bell.,*** calc., cham., dulc., **GELS.,** helon., hep., kali-c., kreos., lach., meph., mur-ac., nat-m., nux-v., op., ph-ac., phos., pic-ac., puls., ran-s., ***senec., sep.,*** sil., stann., sulph., ***tarent.,*** ter.

wine, after abuse of - coff., fl-ac., **NUX-V.,** ***zinc.***

women, esp., excited - senec.

exhausted - cast.

INSOMNIA, sleeplessness

worms, from - ***cina***, ***ferr.***, teucr., ***valer.***

worries, due to - ambr., ars., **CALC.**, carc., kali-br., kali-p., ***nux-v.***, xan.

yawning, with spasmodic - cimic., croc., plat.

INTERRUPTED, (see Disturbed) - acet-ac., acon., agar., ***alum.***, alum-sil., ***am-m.***, ambr., am-c., ***anac.***, ang., ant-t., aran., ars., asaf., ***bar-c.***, berb., bov., cact., ***calc.***, calen., ***camph.***, cann-i., ***cann-s.***, canth., caps., carb-ac., carb-an., ***carb-v.***, carc., caust., ***chin.***, chin-a., chlol., coca, cocc., coc-c., ***coff.***, colch., con., croc., cund., cycl., dig., ***dros.***, dulc., equis., ***euph.***, euphr., ferr., form., ***graph.***, grat., hura, hydr-ac., ***hyos.***, ign., indg., ip., kali-c., kali-chl., kali-cy., kali-i., ***kali-n.***, kreos., lach., lact., led., lyc., mag-c., mag-m., mag-s., mang., merc., merc-c., mez., morph., mosch., ***mur-ac.***, myric., naja, nat-c., nat-m., nat-s., nicc., nit-ac., ***nux-v.***, ***ol-an.***, op., par., petr., ph-ac., phel., ***phos.***, ptel., ***puls.***, ***ran-b.***, ran-s., raph., ***rat.***, ***rhod.***, rhus-t., rumx., ruta, sabin., samb., sars., ***sec.***, sel., ***seneg.***, ***sep.***, sil., sol-n., ***spig.***, spong., squil., stann., ***staph.***, ***stram.***, ***stront-c.***, sul-ac., sulph., sumb., tab., tarax., ***ter.***, teucr., thuj., verat., viol-t., zinc.

- anxiety, from - ars., verat.
- breakfast, after - peti.
- burning in veins - verat.
- children, in - bor.
- cramps, jaw, by - carb-h.
  - by, toes - carb-h.
- dreams, by - ars.
- emissions - petr.
- hot weather, during - sel.
- jerking in limbs - merc., sumb.
- menses, during - am-c.
  - after - agar.
- midnight, after - ars., euph., lyc., mez., nat-m., pip-m., ran-s., teucr.
  - before - tab.
- morning - ambr., ars., coff., euph., merc-c., mez., teucr.
- oppression of chest - seneg.
- pain, from - stann.
- restlessness, by - agar.
- sensation of heat, by - ***bar-c.***
  - by, hands and head - verat-v.
- thirst, by - nat-m.
- toothache - cast.
- urination, by, desire for - ***nat-m.***, petr.
  - by, urging for - petr.

JERKING, of muscles, sleep, during - agar., aloe, ***alum.***, ambr., anac., ant-t., arg-m., ***ars.***, ***bell.***, bry., cast., cham., cimic., cob., ***cocc.***, ***colch.***, ***con.***, cor-r., ***cupr.***, daph., dulc., hep., ign., ip., ***kali-c.***, ***lyc.***, merc., nat-c., ***nat-m.***, nat-s., nit-ac., op., phos., puls., ran-s., rheum, rhus-t., sel., sep., sil., stann., staph., stront-c., ***sulph.***, sul-ac., thuj., viol-t., zinc.

- on going to - acon., ***agar.***, ***alum.***, arg-m., **ARS.**, cob., hyper., ***ign.***, **KALI-C.**, phys., puls., ran-b., ***sel.***, sil., ***stront-c.***, ***stry.***, ***sulph.***, ***sul-ac.***, ***zinc.***

LIGHT, sleeper, (see Disturbed, Semi-conscious) - ***acon.***, agar., ***alum.***, alumn., am-c., anac., ant-t., ***ars.***, bell., brom., brucin., **BRY.**, calad., ***calc.***, cann-s., canth., carb-an., carl., caust., ***cham.***, ***chin.***, **COFF.**, com., cortiso., crot-t., dig., ***ferr.***, ferr-ac., ***gels.***, ***graph.***, grat., **HELL.**, hyos., ***ign.***, kali-n., **LACH.**, ***lyc.***, ***merc.***, merc-c., mur-ac., narcot., nat-m., nicc., nux-m., ***nux-v.***, ol-an., ***op.***, ***phos.***, puls., ***ran-s.***, raph., ***rhus-t.***, ruta, sarcol-ac., saroth., sec., ***sel.***, senec., sep., ***sil.***, sol-t-ae., ***stram.***, sul-ac., ***sulph.***, sumb., tab., tarent., thal., ***zinc.***

- breakfast, after - peti.
- hears every sound - acon., alum., alumn., am-c., ang., apis, ars., ***asar.***, ***bell.***, calad., carb-v., cham., chin., cocc., ***coff.***, grat., ***ign.***, kali-n., lach., ***merc.***, narcot., nat-p., nux-v., ol-an., op., phos., ruta, saroth., sel., sep., sul-ac., ***sulph.***, tarent., valer., zinc-valer.
- midnight, 5 a.m., till - pip-m.
  - after - ant-s., carl., coc-c., grat.
  - agg. - carl.
  - before - canth.
  - towards morning - ***ars.***
- morning - kali-n., lycps., mag-s.
- noon - ang.

LONG, to - bell., hyos., phos., verat.

MURMURING, in sleep - raph., puls., sulph.

NARCOLEPSY, overpowering sleepiness - aeth., agar., alco., all-c., alum., ***ant-c.***, **ANT-T.**, ***ars.***, arum-m., ***aur.***, bar-ac., bar-c., calc., camph., cann-s., canth., carb-s., carb-v., ***caust.***, ***chin.***, ***cimx.***, cina, cocc., coff., coloc., coni., ***cor-r.***, ***crot-h.***, crot-t., cycl., euph., euphr., ferr., ***gels.***, grat., ***haem.***, ***hydr-ac.***, hyos., kali-c., ***kali-n.***, ***lach.***, lact., laur., lina., lyc., mag-s., ***merc.***, ***mez.***, naja, nat-c., nat-m., nat-n., nit-ac., **NUX-M.**, ***nux-v.***, **OP.**, petr., phos., ***phys.***, pimp., pip-m., plb., ***puls.***, rhod., ***rhus-t.***, ***sabad.***, scroph-n., sel., ***sep.***, ***sil.***, sol-t-ae., spig., stann., sulph., tab., ***tarax.***, tarent., verb., ***zinc.***

- afternoon - kali-c., nat-c., **PULS.**
  - 1 p.m. - lyc.
  - 3 p.m. - pall.
  - 5 p.m. - hyos.
- air, in open - merl.
- dinner, after - aur., carb-v., laur., mez., phos.
- eating, after - calc., carb-v., lyc., nit-ac., ***nux-v.***
- evening - carb-v., kali-c., lyc., mag-s., spig.
- forenoon - cann-s., lyc., spig.
- morning - mag-s., nux-v.
- noon - lyc.
- reading by light, on - mang.
- same hour, returns at - tarent.
- waking, on - ferr.
- working, while - bism., lact., mur-ac., phel., ran-b., sulph., tarent., zinc.

NIGHTMARE, (see Dreams, chapter)

NEED of sleep, great - carc., ***caust.***, chin., **COCC.**, nux-v., saroth., ***staph.***, ***sulph.***

OPPRESSIVE, (see Comatose, Deep, Dull, Heavy) - am-c., cham., mur-ac., op.
work, while at - mur-ac.

PAINS, sleep during - ***ars.,*** aur., bell., carb-an., cham., graph., kali-c., kali-n., lach., lyc., merc., mur-ac., ***nit-ac.,*** nux-m., petr., phos., rhus-t., sul-ac., sulph., til.
abdomen, in - ant-t.
after pains - phyt.
noon - kali-i.

PERSPIRATION, during - acon., anac., ***ant-t., apis,*** arn., ***ars.,*** bell., ***calad.,*** **CALC.,** ***camph.,*** **CAPS.,** carb-an., chel., chin., cic., cina, con., croc., cupr., cycl., dulc., euph., ferr., hep., hyos., ign., kali-c., lach., led., lob., ***merc.,*** merc-c., mez., mur-ac., nat-c., nat-m., nit-ac., nux-m., nux-v., **OP.,** petr., ph-ac., phos., plat., **PODO.,** psor., ***puls.,*** **RHUS-T.,** sabad., sec., ***spong.,*** stram., tub., valer., verat.
after sleep - ***ant-t.,*** arn., **ARS.,** ars-h., bor., ***calad., cham.,*** ign., mez., nat-m., nux-m., **OP.,** plb., ***rhus-t.,*** sabad., sep.
stupefying sleep during - acon., **ANT-T.,** ***apis,*** bell., calc., camph., ***chin.,*** cic., con., croc., hep., hyos., ip., led., nux-m., **OP.,** ph-ac., phos., **PULS., RHUS-T.,** sec., spong., stram., valer., verat.

POSITION, of body
abdomen, on - abrot., acet-ac., am-c., ars., ***bell., bell-p.,*** bry., calc., ***calc-p., carc.,*** caust., cina, cocc., ***coloc.,*** crot-t., cupr., ign., ***lac-c.,*** lach., ***lyc.,*** **MED.,** ***nat-m., phos.,*** phyt., ***plb.,*** podo., **PULS.,** ***sep.,*** stann., ***stram., sulph., tub.***
falling asleep, on - ***lac-c.***
pregnancy, only on beginning of - acet-ac., podo.
spasmodically throwing up the pelvis - ***cupr.***
with one arm under the head - cocc.
over the head - dig.
arms
abdomen, on - bell., calc., cocc., coloc., ign., **PULS.,** stram.
apart - ***cham.,*** plat., psor.
head, over - ***arg-m.,*** ars., calc., cast-eq., chin., cimic., coloc., dig., euph., ferr-ma., ***lac-c.,*** med., nit-ac., ***nux-v., plat.,*** **PULS.,** rheum, ruta, sulph., thuj., verat., viol-o.
under - acon., ambr., ant-t., ars., bell., caj., cedr., chin., cocc., coloc., ign., meny., ***nux-v.,*** ph-ac., plat., ***puls.,*** rhus-t., sabad., sanic., spig., viol-o.
back, on - acet-ac., acon., aloe, am-c., ambr., ant-c., ant-t., ***apis,*** arn., ars., aur., bism., **BRY.,** ***calc.,*** carb-h., cham., chin., chlor., ***cic.,*** cina, ***coca, colch.,*** coloc., crot-t., cupr., cupr-ac., cupr-ar., dig., dros., ***ferr.,*** guai., ***hell.,*** hep., hyper., ***ign.,*** ir-foe., kali-chl., kali-p., kreos., ***lac-c., lyc.,*** mag-arct., mag-aust., mang., med., **MERC-C.,** mez., morph., mur-ac., nat-a., nat-m., nit-ac., ***nux-v.,*** op., ox-ac., par., ***phos., plat.,*** **PULS.,** rhod., **RHUS-T.,** ruta, sabad., sars., sol-n.,

POSITION, of body
back, on - spig., stann., ***stram., sulph.,*** verat., viol-o., zinc.
arm over head, left - dig.
right arm clamped between legs, on falling asleep - plb.
evening, impossible - mag-m.
feet drawn up - ***puls.***
hand, crossed over abdomen - **PULS.**
hand, flat, under occiput - ambr., ars., coloc., ign., ***nux-v.,*** phos.
left hand - acon.
other arm over the head - coloc.
hand, over the head - ars., ***lac-c.,*** med., nux-v., plat., **PULS.,** sulph., verat., viol-o.
hand, thighs drawn up upon abdomen, hands above hand, head, lower limbs, uncovered - ***plat.***
head low - cench., ***dig.,*** nux-v.
upright - mag-aust.
impossible - acet-ac., acon., lact., mag-m., ***sulph.***
knees, bent - **MERC-C.**
drawn up - bry., hell., lach., merc-c.
drawn up, spread apart - plat.
midnight, after - mez.
only on back - dig., ***ferr.,*** rhus-t., sulph.
cannot find any position from palpitation - cact.
changed frequently - **ARS.,** aur., ***cact.,*** calen., ***eup-per.,*** form., ***hep., ign.,*** kali-c., lach., lyc., lycpr., mag-aust., mosch., ***nat-s.,*** phos., plat., ***pyrog.,*** rhus-t., sabin.
evening - kali-c., lach.
midnight and after midnight - plat.
palpitations, because of - cact.
morning - aur.
curled up like a dog - ars., bapt., bry.
diagonally - con.
face, on the - ***lac-c.***
genupectoral - ***calc-p., carc.,*** con., euph., ***lyc.,*** **MED.,** ***phos.,*** sep., ***tub.***
hands - cham.
hands, and knees - cina.
hands, head, left hand - dig., viol-o.
one hand - rheum.
over, one under the head - coloc., ign.
over head (see arms) - ars., cast-eq., nit-ac., nux-v., plat., puls., rheum, sulph., verat., viol-o.
under head - acon., ars., bell., chin., coloc., ign., ir-foe., phos., plat.
morning - cocc., ph-ac.
hands, nape of neck, on - ***nux-v.***
hands, pit of stomach, on - plat.
left hand - ant-t., mag-aust., phos., viol-o.
right hand - acon., plat.
hard, every position seems - laur., mag-c., phos.
head
bored into pillow - ***apis,*** arn., bell., ***hell., hep.,*** hyper., lach., ***spong.,*** verat., ***zinc.***
occiput - ***zinc.***
covered with sheet - ***cor-r.***

POSITION, of body
head
inclined, backward - alum., ***bell.,*** chin., cic., ***cina,*** cupr., dig., ***hep.,*** hyos., hyper., ign., ***nux-v.,*** rheum, sep., ***spong.,*** stann., viol-t.
forwards - acon., cic., crot-h., cupr., phos., puls., ***stann.,*** staph., viol-o.
low - absin., arn., cadm-s., cedr., ***dig.,*** hep., ***nux-v.,*** sil., **SPONG.,** sulph., zinc.
dislikes - mag-aust.
occiput impossible, lying on - dulc.
side, to one - cina, spong., tarax.
right - ars., ign.
table, on the - ***ars.***
upright - ant-t., led.
kneeling - carc., med., stram.
knees
bent - ambr., ***plat.,*** viol-o.
knees and elbows - ambr., lyc., stram., viol-o.
body bent backward, with - nux-v.
elbows, and knees - calc-p., carc., cina, lyc., ***med.,*** phos., sep., tub.
face forced into pillow, with - ***calc-p., carc.,*** cina, con., eup-per., euphr., ***lyc.,*** **MED.,** ***phos., sep., tub.,*** zinc.
spread apart - ***cham., plat.,*** puls., viol-o.
limbs, crossed - rhod.
crossed, cannot uncross - bell., ther.
drawn up - abies-c., anac., ***carb-v., cham.,*** chin., ***hell., lac-c.,*** mang., meny., **MERC.,** nat-m., op., ox-ac., ***plat.,*** plb., **PULS.,** rhod., ***stram.,*** viol-o.
left - stann.
spread apart - bell., ***cham.,*** hell., mag-c., nux-v., plat., psor., ***puls.,*** rhod., rhus-t., sulph., viol-o.
stretched out - agar., bell., cham., chin., dulc., plat., ***puls.,*** rhus-t., ***stann.***
the other drawn up - lac-c., stann.
the other drawn up, right - stann.
uncovered, inclined to have - con., plat.
lying impossible - ***cham.,*** glon., lyc., sulph., tarent.
motionless - lyc.
moves feet constantly - zinc.
naked - merc., plat., puls., **SULPH.**
odd - plb.
reverse - coff.
side, on - acon., alum., ***arn.,*** **BAR-C.,** bor., ***calc.,*** caust., colch., ***coloc.,*** ferr., kali-n., merc., mosch., nat-c., ***nat-s.,*** nux-v., ***phos.,*** ran-b., sabad., sabin., spig., sulph.
impossible - acon., aur., dig., ferr., ***lach.,*** med., ***merc.,*** mosch., nat-c., phos., puls., ran-b., rhus-t., sabad., sulph.
lain, as if not - fl-ac.
left - acon., am-c., atro., bar-c., bor., bry., bufo, calc., carc., cench., chin., gels., iris, ***kali-ar., mag-m.,*** nat-c., ***nat-s., phos.,*** psor., sabin., sep., ***sulph.***
feet drawn up - phos.
head on left arm - cob.

POSITION, of body
side, on
left, side, impossible - ***ars., cocc.,*** colch., coloc., ***kali-s., lach.,*** lyc., naja, nat-c., op., **PHOS.,** puls., sep., tab., thea.
painful side, on - bry., coloc., ***cupr-ar.***
right - ail., ***ars.,*** cham., chin., ign., ir-foe., kali-c., ***kali-s.,*** **LACH.,** ***lyc.,*** merc., ***nat-s., phel.,*** **PHOS.,** sulph., sumb.
back on waking, but on - ***lyc.***
impossible - ***acet-ac.,*** arg-n., aur., ***bor.,*** bry., chin., merc., prun., psor., puls., ran-b., sulph.
sitting - acon., ***ars.,*** bar-c., bell., bor., cann-s., caps., carb-v., chin., cic., ***cina,*** dig., hep., ***kali-c.,*** kali-n., ***lyc.,*** nat-m., phos., puls., ***rhus-t.,*** sabin., spig., ***stram., sulph.***
erect, head a little backward - ***cina, phos.***
head on the table - ***ars.***
head on the table, bent foreward, head - acon.
or to side - puls.
right side, to - ***cina.***
only sleep possible - acon., puls., sulph.
sitting up and retching during sleep - rhus-t.
up, and again - hyos.
stiff - ***cham.,*** mag-s., plat.
straight - abrot.
strange - berb., cina, plb.

PROLONGED, sleep - acon-l., aeth., agar., alum., anac., ***ant-c., apis,*** arn., bell., berb., ***bor.,*** calc., camph., cann-i., carb-an., carb-h., carb-o., carb-s., carb-v., carl., ***caust.,*** chin., chlol., chin-s., ***cob.,*** cocc., con., daph., dig., ferr., fl-ac., gels., gins., goss., ham., ***hep.,*** hura, ***hyos.,*** hydr-ac., ign., ***kali-c.,*** kreos., ***lach.,*** lact., laur., led., linu-c., ***mag-arct.,*** mag-aust., mag-m., mag-s., **MERC.,** mez., merl., mill., morph., nat-c., nat-hchls., nat-m., ***nux-m.,*** nux-v., ol-an., op., ox-ac., peti., petr., ph-ac., phel., phos., plat., ***puls.,*** sec., sel., senec., sep., sil., ***stann., staph.,*** stram., ***sulph.,*** sumb., tarent., ther., verat., zinc.
amenorrhea, with - ***cycl.***
children, in - ***bor.***
continuous - anac., lach., merc., petr.
day and night - mag-c.
days, during - ***verat.***
daytime - calc., eug., ***hep., hyos., lact.,*** meph., merc., saroth., scroph-n., ther., verat.
dinner, after - agar., til.
morning - apis, ***cycl.,*** plat., zinc.
noon - calc., spig.
and afternoon - calc., eug., ***hyos.,*** scroph-n., ther.
siesta, during - eug.
sensation as after a prolonged sleep - bapt.

RESTLESS, sleep - **ACON.,** aeth., agar., agn., ***all-c.,*** all-s., aloe, ***alum.,*** alumn., ***ambr., am-c.,*** am-m., aml-n., anac., anag., ang., ant-c., ***ant-t., apis,*** apoc., aran., ***arg-m., arg-n., arn.,*** **ARS.,** ***ars-i.,*** arum-t., ***asaf.,*** asar., aster., atro., ***aur.,*** **BAR-C.,** ***bar-m.,*** **BELL.,** berb., ***bism.,*** brach., brom., bor., bov., ***bry., cact.,*** cahin., calad., ***calc.,*** **CALC-AR.,** calc-p., calc-s., camph., cann-s., carb-ac., carb-an., ***carb-s., carb-v.,*** carc., ***card-m., carl.,*** cast., cast-eq., ***caust.,*** cedr., ***cham., chel.,*** **CHIN.,** ***chin-a.,*** chin-s., cic., cimx., ***cimic.,*** **CINA,** ***cinnb.,*** clem., coca, **COCC.,** coc-c., coff., colch., ***coloc.,*** con., ***cop.,*** croc., crot-t., **CUPR.,** ***cycl., dig.,*** dirc., dios., dor., ***dulc.,*** elaps, ***eup-pur.,*** euphr., ***ferr.,*** ferr-ar., ferr-i., ferr-m., ferr-p., gamb., ***gels.,*** gran., **GRAPH.,** guai., ham., hell., ***hep.,*** hura, ***hydr., hyos.,*** hyper., ***ign.,*** inul., iod., ip., iris, jac-c., jug-c., jug-r., **KALI-AR.,** ***kali-c.,*** kali-chl., kali-i., ***kali-n.,*** kali-p., ***kali-s., kreos., lach.,*** lachn., lact., led., lil-t., **LYC.,** mag-arct., ***mag-c., mag-m.,*** mag-s., manc., mang., med., meny., merc., merc-c., merl., mez., morph., mosch., ***mur-ac., nat-a., nat-c., nat-m.,*** nat-p., ***nat-s.,*** nicc., ***nit-ac.,*** nux-m., ***nux-v.,*** ol-an., **OP.,** ox-ac., paeon., par., ped., ***petr.,*** ph-ac., phos., phys., phyt., ***pic-ac.,*** plan., plat., ***plb., podo.,*** prun., psor., ptel., **PULS.,** ran-b., ***ran-s., raph.,*** rat., ***rheum,*** rhod., **RHUS-T.,** rhus-v., rob., ***rumx.,*** ruta, ***sabad., sabin.,*** samb., sang., sarcol-ac., sars., sec., ***sel.,*** senec., seneg., ***sep.,*** **SIL.,** ***spig.,*** spong., ***squil., stann.,*** staph., ***stram., stront-c., sul-ac.,*** **SULPH.,** tab., tarent., tax., ter., teucr., ***ther., thuj.,*** til., torula., trom., upa., uran-n., valer., verb., viol-t., zinc.

afternoon - colch., glon., mez., tarent.

anxiety, with - ***ars.,*** cham.

bodily restlessness, from - alum., am-c., anac., ars., asaf., ***bar-c.,*** caust., chin., cina, graph., hell., ign., kali-n., laur., mag-c., merc., mur-ac., nat-c., nat-m., petr., ph-ac., phos., ***rhus-t.,*** ruta, seneg., ***sep.,*** sulph., thuj.

children, in - acon., ***ars.,*** bell., bry., ***cham., cina,*** coff., hyos., ign., ***jal.,*** kali-c., lach., rheum, senn., sil., staph., valer.

chill, during - ***anthr.***

after - ***eup-pur.,*** spong.

before - anthr., arn., ***chin.***

chorea, in - ***chlol., mygal.***

coldness of body, from - ambr.

cool place, tries to find a - ***sulph.***

digestive problems, from - but-ac.

dreams, from - acon., agar., ambr., ang., ant-c., arn., ***asaf.,*** aster., ***aur., bry.,*** calad., caps., carb-v., chel., **CHIN.,** clem., coloc., dig., dulc., euph., ferr., ***ferr-p.,*** gran., guai., ign., ip., ***kali-c., lach.,*** led., lyc., mag-arct., meph., merc-sul., mosch., nat-c., nat-m., nit-ac., ***nux-v., olnd.,*** op., par., petr., phos., plb., ***puls.,*** pyrog., ran-s., rhod., rhus-t., ruta, ***sabad.,*** sabin., samb., sars., sec., sel., seneg., ***sep.,*** sil., ***spig.,*** spong., ***stann.,*** staph., stram., stront-c., sulph., teucr., thuj., valer., verb., zinc.

RESTLESS, sleep

eating, after - carb-v.

to satiety - phos.

emission, after - aloe

epilepsy, in - ***cic.***

erections, with - ol-an.

evening - caust., mur-ac., pin-s., thuj.

until 11 p.m. - pic-ac.

feet constantly, must move - zinc.

going to bed early, when - am-c.

heat, from - **ARS.,** ***calc., carb-v., cimx., dig.,*** mag-c., ph-ac., rhod., sabin., sep., spong.

from, body, of - bar-c.

before - ***chin.***

shivering, and - uran-n.

heaviness in abdomen, from - mag-m.

humiliation, after -carc., ***ign., staph.***

imagines to have to go through deep water - carb-v.

liver complaints, in - ***podo., sep.***

loss of sleep, from - ***lac-d.***

lying on left side - lyc.

menses, during - am-c., calc., goss., kali-c., nat-p.

agg., during - am-c., calc.

after - nat-p.

before - alum., calc., caust., con., ***kali-c.,*** sep.

mental derangement, in - ***con.***

metrorrhagia, in - ***sabin.***

after - sep.

morning - aur., calc., dulc., ham., hell., inul., kali-bi., kreos., mag-s., mygal., nit-ac., ran-b., ran-s., rhod., sulph., teucr., zinc.

night, before paroxysms - ***chin.***

every other - asar.

night, midnight, after - alum., am-m., aster., bry., caps., coc-c., coff., coloc., dor., dulc., ***gels.,*** iodof., ***kali-c., lach.,*** lyc., mag-c., mag-s., ***nit-ac.,*** nux-v., pic-ac., pip-m., ran-b., **RHUS-T.,** ran-s., sabin., sep., sil., sulph., teucr., verat., zinc.

until 2 a.m. - puls.

until 3 a.m. - verat.

1 a.m. to 4 a.m. - mag-c.

2 a.m., after - bapt., dios.

3 a.m., after - **ARS.,** ***dulc.,*** sulph.

3 a.m. to 5 a.m. - cimic.

4 a.m., after - aur., dulc.

4 a.m., agg. - plan.

towards morning - ***gels.***

night, midnight, at - zinc.

night, midnight, before - aeth., alum., ***arg-n., ars.,*** ars-h., asc-t., ***bell., calc-p., chel.,*** coloc., cor-r., euph., lach., ***lil-t.,*** mur-ac., nat-m., ph-ac., phos., pic-ac., nux-v., op., ***puls., rhus-t.,*** sel., teucr., thuj.

until 2 a.m. - puls.

overstudy, from - ***cupr-ac.***

pain, with - aur., glon.

limbs, in - sil.

RESTLESS, sleep
perspiration, during -merc., ***sulph.***
head, on - ***calc.***
pollution, after - aloe.
amel. - phos.
puts feet out of bed, towards morning - cur., sulph.
sexual causes, from - cann-i., ***canth., kali-br., raph.***
stroke, in - ***arn.***
summer complaints, in - ***ferr-p.***
tea abuse, from - camph-br., chin., ***nux-v.,*** puls.
tobacco, from - calad., gels.
tootache, from - alum., cham.
twitching of limbs - ambr.
uncovering, with - alum., calad., mosch., ***rhus-t.***
vaccination, after - sil., ***thuj.***
vexation, after - petr.
visions, with - bell., ***stram.***
worms, from - ***nat-p.***

RISE, indisposed to - aesc., ambr., ars., bry., canth., ***carb-v., card-m.,*** cob., crot-h., cycl., dros., ferr-ma., graph., lach., ***nat-m., nux-v., sep., sulph., thuj.,*** verat.
waking, after - bry., nux-v., puls.
rise, must - acon., ***ars.,*** bry., carb-an., ***carb-v.,*** cham., con., ***graph., lyc., mag-c.,*** mag-m., nat-c., nat-m., nicc., nit-ac., puls., ***rhus-t.,*** sep., sil., ther.
evening, before falling asleep - ***carb-v.,*** puls.
midnight, after - mag-m.
sleeplessness, during - con., ***nux-v.,*** phos., ***rhus-t.***
thunderstorm, during - ***nat-m.***
waking, on - anac., ***lac-c.***

SEMI-conscious - ***acon.,*** agar., alum., ambr., anac., ant-c., ars., aur., bapt., **BELL.,** berb., bry., calc., canth., carb-v., casc., **CHAM.,** chel., chin., chin-s., ***coff.,*** coloc., con., dig., ferr., ***gels., graph.,*** grat., hipp., hydr-ac., hyos., ign., kali-br., ***kali-c., kali-n.,*** lach., lact., led., ***mag-arct.,*** manc., merc., merc-i-r., morph., nat-c., nat-m., ***nit-ac.,*** olnd., ***op., par., petr.,*** phos., plat., prun., ***puls., ran-s.,*** raph., rhus-t., ruta, sabad., sec., ***sel.,*** sil., spig., spong., staph., ***sulph.***
daytime - verat.
evening and before midnight - rhus-t., sabad., verat.
first sleep, in - bell.
hears everything - acon., alum., alumn., apis, ars., ***bell.,*** carb-v., cham., cocc., ***coff.,*** grat., ***ign.,*** kali-n., lach., ***merc.,*** op., ruta, saroth., sep., sul-ac., ***sulph.,*** tarent., valer., zinc-valer.
conversation around, semiconscious of - dios.
midnight - mang.
after - coff., pip-m., ran-s.
night, sleepy by day - bry.
sitting, but sleepy while - ign.

SHORT, sleep - acon., agar., anag., ant-c., ant-t., ***anthr.,*** apis, ***arg-n.,*** arn., ars., ars-i., ***bar-c., bor.,*** bov., ***bry., calc., camph.,*** carb-ac., ***caust.,*** chin., ***croc.,*** cund., cupr., ***fl-ac.,*** kali-c., ***lach., laur.,*** lyc., ***lyss.,*** mag-c., mag-m., meph., merc., morph., myric., nat-a., nat-c., nit-ac., nux-v., ol-an., ox-ac., par., ped., ***petr., ph-ac.,*** **PHOS.,** plat., plb., ***prun., rhus-t., rumx.,*** ruta, ***sal-ac., sec.,*** sep., sin-n., spong., staph., sul-ac., ther., thuj., tus-f., verat-v., verb., ***zinc.***
afternoon - teucr.
amel. - meph., **PHOS.**
catnaps, in - ***camph.,*** carb-ac., ***rhus-t., rumx., sec., sel.,*** sulph.
dinner, after - aloe.
evening - cast.
midnight till morning - merc.
morning, 4 a.m. to 6. a.m. - ham.
5 a.m., after - phys.
night, 10 p.m. to 4 a.m. - sep.
11 p.m. to 4 a.m. - staph.
pain, from - plb.
refreshes - cob., ***fl-ac.,*** form., med., meph., mez., ***nux-v.,*** ph-ac., **PHOS.**
repeated, sitting while - narcot.
sensation of short sleep - dig., dros., glon., mosch., myric., ost.
evening - grat.
morning - ***ars.,*** carb-an., con., grat., kali-bi., kali-c., phos., til.
sitting and reading, while - euphr.
waking, on - myric., trif-p.

SITTING up and retching - rhus-t.

SLEEPINESS, general - abel., abies-c., abies-n., abrot., ***acon.,*** acon-a., acon-c., acon-f., acon-l., aconin., aesc., ***aeth., agar.,*** agar-cpn., agar-cps., agar-pa., agar-ph., agar-pr., agn., ail., alet., all-c., ***aloe,*** **ALUM.,** am-caust., ambr., am-br., ***am-c.,*** am-m., aml-n., ***ammc.,*** amyg., ***anac., anag.,*** anh., anil., ***ant-a.,*** **ANT-C., ANT-T., APIS,** ***apoc.,*** apoc-a., apom., arg-m., arg-n., ***arn.,*** **ARS.,** ***ars-h.,*** ars-i., ars-s-r., arum-m., arum-t., arund., ***asaf.,*** asar., asc-c., asc-t., aspar., atro., aur., aur-i., aur-m., **BAPT.,** bar-ac., ***bar-c., bar-m.,*** bart., **BELL.,** benz-ac., benz-n., ***berb.,*** bism., bor., both., ***bov.,*** brach., ***brom.,*** brucin., ***bry.,*** buf-s., bufo, cact., cadm-m., cahin., ***calc.,*** calc-ar., calc-f., ***calc-p.,*** calc-s., calen., ***camph.,*** **CANN-I.,** cann-s., ***canth.,*** caps., carb-ac., carb-o., **CARB-S., CARB-V.,** ***carl.,*** casc., cast., **CAUST.,** cedr., cench., cent., cer-b., ***cham.,*** **CHEL.,** chim., **CHIN.,** ***chin-a.,*** chin-s., chlol., chlor., chlf., chr-ac., cic., ***cimx.,*** cina, cinnam., cinnb., cist., ***clem.,*** coca, ***cocc.,*** coc-c., cod., coff., corn-f., ***croc., crot-h.,*** cycl., cyt-l., dub., eucal., ***ferr-p., fl-ac.,*** form., ***gamb., gels.,*** gent-l., gins., ***glon.,*** gran., **GRAPH.,** ***grat.,*** guai., guare., ***haem.,*** ham., hecla., hell., ***helon., hep.,*** hip-ac., hipp., hura, hydr., hydr-ac., hydrc., ***hyos.,*** hyper., ign., ***ind.,*** indg., ***indol.,*** iod., iodof., ip., iris, piloc., jac-c., jatr., jug-c., jug-r., **KALI-AR.,** ***kali-bi., kali-br., kali-c.,*** kali-chl., kali-cy., kali-i., ***kali-m., kali-n.,*** kali-p., kali-s., kalm., ***kreos.,*** lac-c., lac-d., **LACH.,** lachn., lact., lath., ***laur., led.,*** lept., lil-t., lina.,

SLEEPINESS, general - lob., lob-p., lup., ***lyc.,*** lyss., ***mag-arct.,*** mag-aust., ***mag-c., mag-m.,*** mag-s., man., ***manc.,*** mang., med., meph., ***merc.,*** **MERC-C.,** merc-cy., merc-i-f., merc-sul., ***merl.,*** mez., mill., morph., ***mosch., mur-ac.,*** myric., naja, nat-a., ***nat-c., nat-h., nat-m.,*** nat-p., nat-s., nicc., ***nit-ac.,*** nit-s-d., **NUX-M., NUX-V.,** oena., ***ol-an.,*** olnd., **OP.,** osm., ox-ac., ***par.,*** petr., ***phel.,*** **PH-AC., PHOS.,** phys., phyt., **PIC-AC.,** plan., plat., ***plb.,*** **PODO.,** psor., ptel., **PULS.,** pyrog., ran-b., ran-s., raph., rat., rheum, ***rhod., rhus-t.,*** rob., rosm., rumx., ***ruta,*** sabad., ***samb.,*** sang., sarcol-ac., saroth., sarr., sars., ***scroph-n., sec.,*** sel., ***senec.,*** seneg., ***sep., sil.,*** sol-m., spig., spong., ***stann., staph.,*** still., ***stram.,*** stront-c., stry., sulfon., **SULPH.,** ***sul-ac.,*** sul-i., sumb., tab., tarent., tarax., tax., tep., ter., thea., ther., **THUJ.,** thymol., til., trom., tub., upa., uran-n., valer., ***verat.,*** verat-v., verb., vesp., viol-o., vip., visc., x-ray, xan., zinc., zing., ziz.

- **abdominal** complaints, during - ant-c., cupr-s., ***nux-m.,*** podo.
- **accompanied** by - ant-t., nux-m., puls.
- **afternoon** - ***acon.,*** aeth., ***agar.,*** alum., am-c., amyg., ***anac.,*** ant-c., ant-t., apoc., ***arg-n., ars., arum-t.,*** asar., asc-t., aur., aur-a., aur-m-n., bar-ac., bar-c., bar-m., bart., bell., bor., bov., brom., ***brucin.,*** bry., cahin., calc., calc-s., cann-i., canth., caps., carb-ac., carb-an., carb-s., carb-v., caust., chel., **CHIN.,** chin-a., chin-s., cic., cimic., cina, clem., coc-c., coff., colch., con., ***croc.,*** crot-t., cycl., dios., dulc., euph., euphr., fago., ***ferr.,*** ferr-ar., fl-ac., form., gels., graph., ***grat.,*** guai., ham., hera., hyos., ign., ind., indg., kali-ar., kali-c., kali-i., kali-m., kali-n., kali-s., kali-sil., ***lach.,*** laur., lec., lyc., lyss., mag-c., meli., merc., merc-c., merc-sul., mez., mosch., mur-ac., nat-a., nat-c., nat-m., nat-p., nat-s., nicc., nit-ac., nux-m., **NUX-V.,** ol-an., paeon., pall., par., petr., ***ph-ac., phos.,*** phys., pip-m., plat., ***puls.,*** puls-n, ran-b., raph., rheum, rhod., **RHUS-T.,** ***ruta,*** sabad., sep., sil., spig., ***spong.,*** squil., ***staph.,*** stront-c., sul-ac., **SULPH.,** sumb., teucr., thuj., verat., verb., viol-o., viol-t., zinc., zinc-p., zing.
    - 1 p.m. - corn., hura, mag-c., phys.
        - to 2 p.m. - ail., clem.
    - 2 p.m. - ***chel.,*** elaps, equis., glon., hura, ign., kali-cy., lyc., zinc.
        - after - kali-i.
        - agg. - elaps.
        - air, amel. in open - cast.
        - house, in - lyc.
        - streetcar, in - chin-s.
    - 2 p.m. to 3 p.m. - sulph.
    - 2 p.m. to 4 p.m. - ign., staph.
        - agg. - ign.
    - 2 p.m. to 5 p.m. - clem., sil.
    - 2:30 p.m. - carb-v., grat.
    - 3 p.m. - kalm., murx., pall., phys., pip-m., ptel., tell.
        - after - carb-s.
        - agg. - nit-m-ac.
        - until evening - nat-p.

SLEEPINESS, general

- **afternoon,**
    - 3 p.m. to 4 p.m. - pall.
        - to 7 p.m. - carb-s., nat-m.
    - 4 p.m. - coca, ol-an.
        - to 6 p.m. - ind.
    - 4:30 p.m. - ferr-p., sep.
    - 5 p.m. - arg-n., bov., clem., dios., equis., hyper., piloc., lach., nat-m., thuj.
    - agg. - arum-t., ery-a.
    - air, amel. in open - myric., zing.
    - carriage, in a - chin-s., lyc.
    - church, in - chin-s.
    - eating, after - chin-b., rumx., sep.
    - evening, but sleepless at night, and - **SULPH.**
        - till evening - asc-t.
    - every other day - **LACH.**
    - lecture, during - myric.
    - reading, while - anac.
    - sitting, while - anac., ant-c., nicc., staph.
    - studying, while - gels.
    - sunset and wakeful at night, on - **SULPH.**
    - walking, while - ars-m.
    - work, at - nat-a.
- **air,** in open - acon., ant-t., bufo, chel., guare., kali-bi., mosch., nux-v., plat.
    - amel. - aeth., agar., alum., cast., chel., clem., ***ol-an.,*** plb., tab., zinc.
        - after being - bufo
        - disappearing - alum.
        - walking amel. - asar.
- **albuminuria,** in - helon.
- **alcoholics,** in - ***op.***
- **all day,** from debility, with vertigo - **NIT-AC.**
- **alone,** when - ***bry., hell.***
- **alternating** with, restlessness - ***ars.***
    - with, sleeplessness - asim., caust., ***hyos.,*** lach., sep.
    - with, vertigo - ant-t.
- **anemia,** in - hyper., ***sabin.***
- **anxiety,** with - ars., led., nux-v., rhus-r.
- **bed,** going to bed amel. - euphr.
    - in - eupi.
    - too hard - psor.
- **beer** after - sulph., thea.
- **breakfast,** after - calad., clem., lach., manc., nat-s., still., sumb., ther., verat.
    - before - ***calc.***
- **brooding,** with - carb-an.
- **caused** by other complaints - ant-t., nux-m., op., rhus-t., verat.
- **cheerfullness,** after - bell., calc.
- **childbirth,** after - phel.
- **children,** in - all-s., bor., podo.
- **chill,** during - acon., aeth., am-c., ambr., ant-c., ***ant-t.,*** apis, ars., aster., bell., bor., ***calad.,*** calc., camph., caps., cham., cimic., cimx., cina, croc., cycl., ***gels.,*** hell., hyos., hyper., ign., iris, kali-bi., ***kali-i.,*** kali-n., led., lept., lyc., merc., mez., ***nat-m.,*** nit-ac., ***nux-m.,*** nux-v., **OP.,** ph-ac., phos., plan., puls., ***rhus-t.,*** sabad., ***sabin.,*** sars., sep., staph., tarax., ter., verat.

SLEEPINESS, general
chill, during
after - gels., hipp., nux-v., ***sabin.***
before - ars., nicc., puls., sabad., ther.
between - ***nux-m.***
chilliness, during - ang., ars., aspar., calad., croc., cycl., hell., led., mez., nat-m., phos., plat., sabin., sumb., thuj.
after - nux-v.
cholera infantum, in - ***arn.***
after - ***chin.***
cloudy weather, in - physal.
coffee, after - bart.
coldness, with - crot-h.
confusion, with - echi.
consciousness, losing, as if - phys.
constant - ***bell., brucin.,*** caust., chin., clem., ferr., kali-c., kreos., mag-arct., spig., thuj., zinc.
conversation, during - caust., cench., chin-s., tarax.
convulsions, during - ***hydr-ac., op.,*** **TARENT.,** vib.
after - aeth., cur., hyos., ***stram.***
before - ***nux-v.***
and after - ***nux-m.***
coryza, during - ***cham.,*** **GELS.,** nux-v., petr.
cough, with - ant-c., **ANT-T.,** ***ip., kreos.,*** nux-m., op.
after - ***anac., ant-t., ign.***
whooping cough, after - ***ant-t., caust.***
dark, at - cench.
daytime - ***agar.,*** alum., ***am-c.,*** anac., ***ant-c., calc.,*** calc-p., cann-s., carb-v., ***chin.,*** cinnb., ***colch.,*** euphr., graph., indol., kali-c., lupin., ***lyc.,*** mag-m., merc., merc-c., ***nat-c.,*** nat-m., nux-m., ***op., phos., sep.,*** sil., spong., staph., ***sulph.,*** tub.
afternoon awake - ***abies-n.,*** cinnb., colch., graph., lach., ***lyc.,*** merc., ph-ac., sil., staph., thea.
evening awake, night sleepless - puls.
every other day - bry., lach.
third day - sep.
falling asleep late - ammc., carb-v.
restless sleep at night - hyos.
sleeplessness at night, and - ***agar.,*** am-c., ammc., anh., ant-c., ***arg-n.,*** arn., aur-s., bar-ac., bell., bry., carb-s., carb-v., chin., cinnb., clem., ferr., fl-ac., ***graph.,*** gua., hura, hyos., kali-c., lac-d., lach., mag-c., merc., mosch., mur-ac., nat-hchls., nat-m., nux-v., op., ***petr.,*** ph-ac., ***phos.,*** pic-ac., plan., psor., puls., ran-b., rhus-t., sep., sil., spig., **STAPH.,** stram., sul-i., **SULPH.**
body aches all over - **STAPH.**
new moon, at - sep.
delirium, during - acon., ant-c., arn., ***bell., bry.,*** camph., coloc., ***crot-h.,*** **OP.,** ***puls.,*** sec.

SLEEPINESS, general
diarrhea, during - ***ant-t.,*** asim., ***calc., corn.,*** nux-m.
children, in - ***ant-t.***
after - ars-m., ***nux-v.***
tenesmus, after - ***colch.,*** **SULPH.**
dinner, during - ang., bor., bov., ***calc-p.,*** cham., chin., hyper., ***kali-c.,*** nux-v., puls., rat., rhus-t., sarr.
4 p., till - coca.
after - acon., **AGAR.,** alum., alum-p., alum-sil., ***am-c., anac.,*** ant-c., ant-t., ***apis,*** arn., ars., arum-m., ***aur.,*** aur-s., bapt., bar-c., bar-m., bell., berb., bor., ***bov.,*** brucin., bry., cadm-m., calc., ***calc-p.,*** calc-sil., cann-s., canth., caps., carb-an., carb-s., ***carb-v.,*** caust., cham., chel., ***chin., cic.,*** cimic., cinnb., clem., coca, croc., crot-h., crot-t., cur., cycl., dios., eug., euph., euph-a., euphr., ferr., graph., grat., ham., hura, hydr-ac., ign., kali-bi., kali-c., kali-n., kali-sil., ***lach.,*** laur., linu-c., **LYC.,** mag-c., mag-m., mez., morg-g., mur-ac., nat-c., ***nat-m.,*** nat-p., nat-s., nit-ac., ***nux-m.,*** **NUX-V.,** ol-an., ox-ac., par., peti., ph-ac., ***phos.,*** phys., plat., plb., prun., ***puls.,*** ran-b., ***raph., rhus-t., ruta,*** scroph-n., seneg., sep., sil., squil., staph., stict., sulph., tab., tarax., thuj., til., **TUB.,** verb., vib., zinc.
agg. - arum-m., carb-an., phys.
air, amel. in open - kali-c., ol-an., rat.
before - calad., calc-p., lach., phos., scroph-n., thuj.
cold showers amel. - cadm-m.
reading, when - prun.
writing, while - coca.
drinking, after - nux-m., ph-ac.
alcohol - ***glon.***
wine - ail.
dropsy, in - apoc., ***hell.***
dullness, with - arn., cact., calad., calc-p., carb-an., caust., coff., ***cupr.,*** dig., ferr., ***gels., hyos.,*** kreos., lac-ac., ***merc.,*** nat-m., nux-m., ***phos.,*** plb., sep., staph., zinc.
eating, during - agar., bov., calc-p., cham., ***phos.,*** **KALI-C.,** puls., sarr.
after - acon., **AGAR.,** aloe, all-s., am-c., ***anac.,*** ant-c., ant-t., ***apis,*** arn., ars., arum-m., ***arum-t.,*** asaf., aur., bar-ac., bar-c., berb., bism., ***bov.,*** bry., bufo, **CALC.,** calc-p., ***calc-sil.,*** canth., caps., ***carb-s., carb-v., carl.,*** caust., chel., ***chin.,*** chin-s., cic., cinnb., clem., coc-c., coff., con., croc., cycl., dig., ***echi.,*** ferr., gamb., graph., grat., guare., hyos., ign., ***kali-c., kali-m.,*** kali-p., kali-s., lach., ***lyc.,*** lyss., meph., morg-g., ***mur-ac., nat-c., nat-hchls., nat-m.,*** nit-ac., ***nux-m.,*** **NUX-V.,** ***op.,*** par., paull., petr., ph-ac., ***phos.,*** plat., puls., ran-b., rheum, ***rhus-t.,*** rumx., ***ruta,*** scroph-n., sep., ***sil.,*** sin-a., ***squil., staph.,*** still., ***sulph.,*** tarax., ***tell., thuj., verb.,*** vib., zinc., zinc-p.

SLEEPINESS, general
eating,
before - calad., nat-m.
drinking, and - ph-ac.
motion amel. - ***caps.***
evening - ***agar.,*** aloe, ***alum.,*** alum-p., alum-sil., am-c., **AMBR., AM-M.,** anac., ang., **ANT-C., ANT-T.,** ***apis, arn., ars.,*** ars-i., arum-t., asaf., bapt., bar-c., bar-m., bell., benz-ac., berb., bor., ***bov.,*** brom., brucin., bry., calad., **CALC.,** calc-ac., ***calc-ar.,*** calc-caust., calc-i., ***calc-p.,*** **CALC-S.,** calc-sil., camph., cann-i., canth., carb-an., ***carb-s., carb-v.,*** cast-eq., caust., chel., chin., chin-a., chin-s., chlol., chr-ac., cimx., ***cic.,*** cimic., cina, ***clem.,*** cob., coca, cocc., coff., colch., ***con.,*** convo-d., ***croc.,*** crot-h., cycl., dig., dros., dulc., euphr., fago., ferr., ferr-ar., ferr-i., ferr-p., ***fl-ac.,*** form., glon., ***graph.,*** gran., grat., hecla., hell., ***hep.,*** hipp., hura, ictod., ign., ind., indg., iod., kali-ar., kali-bi., **KALI-C.,** kali-m., kali-p., ***kali-s., kali-sil.,*** lac-c., ***lach.,*** lact., ***laur.,*** lil-t., lith., lyc., mag-c., mag-m., mag-s., mang., merc., merc-c., merc-i-r., merl., mez., mosch., mur-ac., murx., naja, ***nat-c.,*** nat-m., nat-n., nat-s., nit-ac., nux-m., **NUX-V.,** pall., par., ***petr., ph-ac., phos.,*** pip-m., plat., pic-ac., plb., podo., polyp-p, psor., phys., **PULS.,** ran-b., ran-s., rhod., rhus-t., ruta, sars., sel., seneg., ***sep., sil.,*** sol-m., spig., squil., ***stann.,*** staph., stram., sul-i., ***sulph.,*** tab., tarent., ter., thuj., valer., wild., xan., yuc., zinc., zing.
5 p.m. - arg-n., bov., clem., dios., equis., hyper., piloc., lach., nat-m., thuj.
after - nat-m.
5 p.m. to 11 p.m. - bell.
or 6 p.m. - coca.
6 p.m. - alum., ant-c., hyper., laur., myric., ***nat-m.,*** sumb.
6:30 p.m. - pip-m.
7 p.m. - ***ant-c.,*** sil.
to 9 a.m. - chel., narcot.
7:30 p.m. - sol-t-ae.
8 p.m. - agar., kali-cy., lyc., mang., sep., sol-t-ae., trom., tarax.
9 p.m. - coca, lyss., nat-m., nat-s., pic-ac.
until - ang., sil.
11 p., until - nit-m-ac.
agg. - bell., ph-ac.
alternate days - lach.
anger, after - puls.
conversation amel. - fago.
early - am-m., ***apis, arn.,*** ars-i., berb., bov., calad., calc., ***carb-v.,*** cast-eq., glon., ictod., ***kali-c.,*** lil-t., mang., ***nux-v.,*** phos., puls., ***sep., sulph.***
eating, after - rumx.
every other day - lach.
falling asleep late and difficult - ang., bor., clem., nat-n., ***nux-v.,*** sel.
heat, after - nit-ac.
light amel. by - am-m.
reading, while - ang., nux-v.
riding in a carriage - pall.

SLEEPINESS, general
evening,
room, in a warm - ind.
agg. - merl.
sitting, while - ang., arg-n., ***nux-v.,*** petr.
and reading - nux-v.
sunset - anis., arum-t., dros., **SULPH.**
thirst, with - benz-ac.
twilight - **AM-M.,** bor.
walking, after - nat-m., sumb.
warmth agg. - ant-t.
wine, after - carb-s.
writing, when - brom.
excitement, after - ***nux-m., podo.,*** stram., ziz.
exertion, mental, from - **ARS.,** ferr., ***gels., hyos.,*** kali-c., nat-s., nux-m., nux-v., ph-ac., ***podo.,*** sabad., sel., tarax.
amel. - croc.
exertion, physical, from - ars., bar-c., nux-m., sel.
amel. - phys., sep.
as after - anac.
eyelids, contraction of - acon., agar., ***ant-t.,*** chel., chin., cic., cocc., ***con.,*** croc., euphr., ferr., ham., kali-c., merc., plat., sabad., staph., tarax., verb., viol-o., viol-t.
eyes closed - ***acon.***
half-closed - ***bry., kreos.***
heat, with the sensation of - plat.
opening difficult - am-m., ant-c., ant-t., ars-h., bar-c., canth., cast., chin., cic., cocc., coff., ***con.,*** grat., hell., ign., ***lach.,*** mag-arct., merc., mosch., mur-ac., nux-m., ph-ac., ***phel.,*** prun., ***sabad.,*** spig., stann., ***staph.,*** tarax., thuj., verb.
face, hot, with - ***glon.***
pallor - ***glon.***
redness - am-m.
faintness, with - stram.
after - merc.
air, agg. in open - ***crot-t.***
fever, during - ***acon.,*** ail., ***ambr., ant-c.,*** **ANT-T.,** ***apis,*** aran., **ARN.,** ***ars.,*** asaf., bell., bor., **CALAD.,** calc., camph., caps., cedr., ***cham.,*** chel., chin., cocc., croc., crot-h., cycl., **EUP-PER.,** ***gels., hell.,*** hep., hyos., ign., kali-c., ***kali-i.,*** **LACH.,** lachn., laur., ***lyc.,*** **MEZ.,** mosch., nat-c., **NAT-M.,** nit-ac., ***nux-m.,*** nux-v., **OP.,** petr., ***ph-ac., phos.,*** **PLB., PODO.,** ***puls.,*** rhus-t., **ROB.,** ruta, sabad., **SAMB.,** ***sep.,*** stram., sulph., ***ter.,*** thuj., verat., verat-v., viol-t.
before - ***puls.,*** rhus-t.
paroxysms, after - podo.
septic - stram.
forenoon - agar., ail., alum., alum-p., alum-sil., am-c., ang., **ANT-C.,** ant-t., arn., ars., bar-ac., bart., bell., ***bism.,*** brucin., cadm-s., ***calc., calc-p.,*** calc-sil., ***cann-s., carb-an., carb-v.,*** chel., chin-s., con., crot-h., cycl., dros., dulc., fl-ac., gels., graph., hell., hydr., kali-c., kali-n., lach., lyc., mag-c., mag-m., merc-sul., ***mosch.,*** myric., narcot., ***nat-c.,*** nat-m., ***nat-p., nat-s.,*** nicc., ***nux-v., phos.,*** phys., plat., ***podo.,*** puls.,

SLEEPINESS, general

forenoon - rhus-t., ruta, **SABAD.,** sars., buth-a., scroph-n., sel., sep., sil., sol-n., spig., spong., staph., sul-ac., tab., thuj., til., zinc.

8 a.m. - op., sulph.

9 a.m. - cench., phys., pip-m., sep.

sitting, while - indg.

10 a.m. - ant-t., chel., hydr., merc., merc-d., nat-p.

to 12 a.m. - calc-s.

10:30 a.m. - equis.

11 a.m. - arum-t., hydr., nux-v., rhus-t., thuj.

listening to a lecture, while - cinnb.

11 a.m. to 12 a.m. - kali-n.

11:30 a.m. - crot-h., phys., stry.

agg. - nat-p., pin-s., podo., sabad., ***sep.***

motion, agg. - ***carb-v.***

reading, while - agar., carb-v., nat-s.

rumbling in bowels - ***podo.***

sitting, while - carb-v., indg., nicc.

smoking, after - bufo

standing, while - chin-s.

until 11 a.m. - phos.

walking, while - rhus-t.

writing, while - nat-s.

fullness, with sensation of - scroph-n.

grief, when oppressed by - ***op.***

groaning, with - ***cham.***

hallucinations, with - lachn.

head to one side, child hangs - cina.

headache, during - acon., aesc., agar., ail., aml-n., ammc., ars., asar., ***bell.,*** bism., ***brucin.,*** calc., calc-p., camph., cham., chel., chin-s., ***coll.,*** con., ***corn., crot-h.,*** cub., equis., ***gamb.,*** gels., gins., glon., grat., hipp., hydr., ign., ind., iodof., ip., jug-r., kali-n., kreos., ***lach.,*** laur., lob., merc-i-r., mur-ac., myric., ***nat-m.,*** nat-s., ***nux-m., nux-v.,*** **OP.,** pall., ***ph-ac.,*** phos., plb., puls., ran-b., sep., ***stann.,*** still., stront-c., sul-ac., tanac., ter., vip., zinc.

before - sulph.

heaviness, with - aesc., carb-ac., caust., ***kreos., puls.,*** staph.

head of - ***bar-c.,*** corn., hydr.

hot weather, during - **ANT-C.,** ***corn., gels., nux-v.,*** sel.

house, in - plat., tab.

hypochondriasis, in - ***arg-n.***

hysteria, in - **NUX-M.**

impatience, with - nit-ac.

indifference, with - corn.

indolence, with - acon., am-m., ammc., ***ant-t.,*** ars., carb-an., carb-v., chel., cinnb., croc., dig., dulc., grat., ip., laur., lyc., mag-c., mag-m., nat-c., rat., sars., tong., verb., ***zinc.***

influenza, in - bapt., ***gels., sabad.***

injuries, after - op.

intermittent, sleepiness - ars., cann-i., guare.

afternoon - fl-ac.

intoxication, as from - agar., ***led.,*** **NUX-M.**

irresolation, with - hyos.

irritability, with - ind.

SLEEPINESS, general

labor pains, during - ***puls.***

after each contraction - gels.

late to bed, if he goes - calc.

laughing, after - phos.

inclination to, with - ***nux-m.***

lectrophobia, with - cann-s.

liver troubles, in - **CHEL.,** ***lept., myris., nat-m., sil.***

looking long at one place, on - cic.

lying, when - lyc., plat.

agg. - sel.

inclination to lying down - ***alum.,*** am-c., berb., bism., calad., **CAUST.,** cina, clem., ***cocc.,*** coff., coloc., con., crot-t., cycl., ***graph., hell.,*** hep., ***ign.,*** kali-c., lachn., led., ***mur-ac.,*** nat-c., nat-m., ol-an., olnd., petr., rhus-t., staph.

quietly amel., lying - phos.

side, on, left - thuj.

measles, in - ***apis,*** xan.

meeting, in interesting - pip-m.

menses, during - eupi., ***kali-c.,*** mag-c., **NUX-M.,** ***phos., sulph.,*** uran-n.

before - calc-p., puls.

suppressed, when - cycl., senec.

mental exertion - **ARS.,** ferr., ***gels., hyos.,*** nat-s., nux-v., tarax.

metrorrhagia, in - ***sec.***

morning - ***agar.,*** aesc., ail., ***all-c.,*** aloe, alum., alum-p., alum-sil., ***am-c.,*** ambr., ammc., anac., ang., ant-c., ***ant-t., apis,*** arn., ars., arum-i., asaf., ***asc-t.,*** aspar., aur., bart., bell., berb., bism., bor., bry., cact., cahin., calad., **CALC.,** calc-ac., calc-ar., **CALC-P.,** calc-sil., camph., canth., **CARB-S.,** carb-v., ***carl.,*** cast-eq., ***caust.,*** chin., cinnam., cinnb., ***clem.,*** coc-c., coca, cocc., ***con.,*** corn., croc., cur., crot-c., cycl., dig., dros., dulc., ***echi.,*** equis., ***euphr.,*** ferr-i., fl-ac., form., gamb., **GRAPH.,** grat., guare., hell., hep., hyos., ign., ind., indg., kali-c., kali-n., kreos., lach., laur., led., lith., lyc., lyss., ***mag-arct.,*** mag-aust., mag-c., ***mag-m.,*** menis., ***meph., merc.,*** merc-d., mur-ac., myric., ***nat-c.,*** nat-m., ***nat-n., nat-s.,*** nit-ac., nux-m., **NUX-V.,** op., ox-ac., petr., ***ph-ac., phos.,*** phys., plat., ***podo., puls.,*** ran-b., rat., rhod., rhus-t., sabad., scroph-n., sel., **SEP.,** ***sil.,*** sin-n., ***spig.,*** staph., stram., **SULPH.,** sul-ac., sumb., tarent., ***teucr.,*** ther., thuj., **TUB.,** upa., verat., verb., wies., xan., zinc., zing.

6 a.m. - hyos.

waking - sep.

7 a.m. - calad., wies.

8 a.m. - op., sulph.

agg. - cast.

air, amel. in open - asc-t.

bed, in - con., hell., hep., petr.

breakfast, before - ***calc.***

diarrhea, after - ***nux-v.***

eating, after - lach.

heat, after - nit-ac., sep.

nausea, with - calad.

SLEEPINESS, general
morning,
reading or writing, when - nat-s.
restless night - zinc.
riding, while - phys.
rising, on - aesc., ammc., cact., con., merc-sul., nit-ac., nux-v., ph-ac., rhod.
after - agar., all-c., ant-c., ars., bell., bism., calad., cocc., con., kali-n., mag-c., mur-ac., nat-m., nit-ac., plat., sil., spig., sulph., verb., zinc.
amel. - kali-c., nat-m.
sitting, while - cimx., phos.
sleepless night, from - ***teucr.***
turning over in bed amel. - ***meph.***
waking, on - bry., carb-v., clem., con., grat., hura, sep.
after - sul-ac.
moroseness, with - calc., calen., carb-an., carb-v., hyos., kali-c., ol-an., ph-ac., sabad., sep.
motion, on - ***carb-v.,*** sil.
amel. - caps., carb-v., ***mur-ac.,*** nicc., phos., tarax.
music, from - stann.
musing - am-c., nat-m.
nausea, with - ant-t., calad., ind., ip., ***nux-m.,*** ran-b.
after - ip.
nervousness and, in children, with cough - stict.
new moon, at - sep.
news, after sad - gels., ign.
noon - acon., agar., aloe, asc-t., aur., bor., bry., buf-s., bufo, calc., calc-ar., camph., ***chin.,*** clem., coloc., crot-h., crot-t., dros., eupi., ferr-i., graph., gymn., hura, kali-c., ol-an., op., pana., petr., phos., phys., sep., sulph., tab.
chilliness, during - ferr-i.
eating, after - cycl., ***euph., graph., puls.***
until 3 p.m. - hyos.
walking, after - puls.
nursing, after - cocc.
old people, in - ant-c.
overestimating time and distance, with - nux-m.
overpowering (see Narcolepsy) - aeth., agar., alco., all-c., alum., ***ant-c.,*** **ANT-T.,** ***ars.,*** arum-m., ***aur.,*** bar-ac., bar-c., calc., camph., cann-s., canth., carb-s., carb-v., ***caust., chin., cimx.,*** cina, cocc., coff., coloc., coni., ***cor-r., crot-h.,*** crot-t., cycl., euph., euphr., ferr., gels., grat., ***haem., hydr-ac.,*** hyos., kali-c., ***kali-n., lach.,*** lact., laur., lina., lyc., mag-s., ***merc., mez.,*** naja, nat-c., nat-m., nat-n., nit-ac., **NUX-M.,** ***nux-v.,*** **OP.,** petr., phos., ***phys.,*** pimp., pip-m., plb., ***puls.,*** rhod., ***rhus-t., sabad.,*** scroph-n., sel., ***sep., sil.,*** sol-t-ae., spig., stann., sulph., tab., ***tarax.,*** tarent., verb., ***zinc.***
afternoon - kali-c., nat-c., **PULS.**
1 p.m. - lyc.
3 p.m. - pall.

SLEEPINESS, general
overpowering
afternoon, 5 p.m. - hyos.
air, in open - merl.
dinner, after - aur., carb-v., laur., mez., phos.
eating, after - calc., carb-v., lyc., nit-ac., ***nux-v.***
evening - carb-v., kali-c., lyc., mag-s., spig.
forenoon - cann-s., lyc., spig.
morning - mag-s., nux-v.
noon - lyc.
reading by light, on - mang.
same hour, returns at - tarent.
waking, on - ferr.
working, while - bism., lact., mur-ac., phel., ran-b., sulph., tarent., zinc.
pain, during - carb-an., nux-m., op., phos.
after - lach., phyt.
hypochondrium - sep.
in abdomen, during - ant-t.
in limbs, from - aeth.
teeth - sulph.
palpitation of heart - aur., chin., crot-t., merc., nux-v., ***podo.,*** tab.
periodical - fl-ac.
afternoon - fl-ac.
every other day - bry., lach.
third day - sep.
perspiration, with - ***acon.,*** ant-c., **ANT-T.,** ***apis,*** arn., ars., ***asaf.,*** **BELL.,** bor., **CALAD.,** caps., **CHAM.,** ***cina, corn.,*** croc., cycl., ***hep., ign.,*** kali-c., lach., lyc., **MEZ.,** mosch., nat-c., nat-m., ***nit-ac., nux-m.,*** nux-v., **OP.,** petr., ***ph-ac., phos., plb.,*** podo., **PULS.,** rhus-t.
after work amel. - phys.
face, of - calc-p.
pneumonia, in - ***ant-t.,*** chel., ***op.,*** phos.
pollutions, after - aq-mar., ***sep.***
prattling, with - lach.
pregnancy, during - gels., ***helon., nux-m.***
prostration, with - cann-s., canth., con., croc.
puerperal - phel.
purpura, after - ***hell.***
reading, while - alum., anac., ang., aster., aur., bism., brom., ***carb-s., carb-v.,*** cimic., ***colch.,*** coloc., ***con., gels.,*** ign., iris, lyc., mang., mez., mosch., nat-c., ***nat-m.,*** nat-s., plat., prun., ruta, ***sabad.,*** sang., sel., sep., sil., ***sulph.,*** tab., tarax., urt-u., verat.
amel. - croc.
rest, during - kali-n.
restlessness, with - ars., bufo, coloc., ***con.,*** crot-h., ***hep.,*** lact., ***merc., petr.,*** rhus-t., ***sep., stram.***
rheumatism, in - ***lyc., puls.***
riding, while - bapt., brom., carb-ac., card-m., chin-s., lyc., op., pall., phys., sulph.
carriage, in a - bapt., pall., phys., ***sulph.***
horseback, on - lyc.
street car, on - chin-s.
strong air, in - ant-t.

SLEEPINESS, general

rising, on - merc.
amel. - nat-m., nicc.
room, in - asar., plb.
warm - ant-t., chin-s., cinnb., ind., merl.
sad news - ign.
sadness, with - calc., calc-p., ***corn.,*** eup-pur., murx., rhus-t.
scarlatina, in - ***nat-m.***
after - ***ter.***
sedentary habits, in persons of - ***gels.***
setting broken leg, after - stict.
sewing, while - ferr.
sex, during - bar-c., ***lyc.***
after - agar., sep.
shock, after mental - ***pic-ac.***
sitting, while - acon., aesc., agar., am-c., anac., ang., ant-c., ant-t., apis, aran-s., arg-m., arg-n., ars., ars-m., arum-t., aur., bapt., brucin., cadm-s., calc., calc-p., carb-v., caust., ***cham.,*** chin., chin-s., cimx., cina, clem., coca, coff., cycl., fago., ferr., ferr-ma., form., gels., ***hep.,*** ign., indg., kali-br., kali-c., lyc., merc., mez., mur-ac., narcot., nat-c., ***nat-h., nat-m.,*** nat-p., nicc., ***nux-m.,*** **NUX-V.,** par., petr., phel., plat., plb., psor., puls., ran-b., rat., rhus-t., ***sabad., sep.,*** spig., staph., ***sulph.,*** tarax., tarent., tell., thuj., verat., ***zinc.***
conversation, in - chin-s.
room, while sitting in a warm - ind.
sleepless, lying while - cham.
sleepless, walking, after - rhus-t.
lying, while - cham.
work, after - ***sulph., zinc.***
sleeplessness, during - ***acon., agar.,*** am-c., am-m., ambr., ***ant-t.,*** apis, apoc., arg-n., arn., ars., ars-m., bar-ac., bar-c., **BELL.,** bor., ***bry.,*** bufo, calad., ***calc., calc-sil.,*** camph., cann-i., canth., carb-an., carb-s., carb-v., ***caust.,*** **CHAM., CHEL.,** chin., chr-ac., cic., cina, clem., coca, cocc., cod., ***coff., con.,*** corn., ***crot-h.,*** crot-t., ***cupr.,*** daph., dirc., elaps, euphr., eupi., ***ferr.,*** ferr-ar., ferr-p., ***gels.,*** gent-l., graph., ***hep.,*** kali-sil., ***lach.,*** lact., laur., lyc., mag-aust., mag-m., med., ***merc.,*** morph., mosch., nat-a., ***nat-c., nat-m.,*** nat-p., nit-ac., ***nux-m., nux-v.,*** **OP.,** ***petr., ph-ac.,*** **PHOS.,** ***phys.,*** plb., **PULS.,** ran-b., rhod., ***rhus-t.,*** sabad., sabin., samb., sel., ***senec.,*** **SENN.,** ***sil.,*** sol-m., spig., staph., ***stram.,*** sul-ac., ***sulph.,*** syph., ***tarent.,*** ter., teucr., thuj., ***verat.,*** viol-o., zinc.
afternoon - abrot.
heat, during - **PULS.**
measles, after - ***caust.***
morning - cycl.
5 a.m. - myric.
and after sunset - **SULPH.**
pregnancy, during - ***nux-m.***
restlessness, with - ***graph., petr.***
thoughts, from activity of - agar.
smallpox, in - ***nat-m.***
smoking, while - bufo.

SLEEPINESS, general

society, in - caust., meph.
sopor - anh., cyt-l.
soporific, as after an - ***man.***
soreness, with - eug., mag-arct.
speaking, while - ***chel.***
difficult - arn.
standing - acon., alum., cor-r., mag-c., merc., morph., nit-ac., phel.
standing, at work - phel.
starting, with - ang., ant-t., ***cham.,*** chel., kali-i., mag-c., merc., plat., ***puls.,*** sars., seneg., ***tarent.,*** verat.
stool, during - ant-t., bry., elaps, ***manc.,*** nux-m., puls.
after - aeth., bry., colch., coloc., elaps, ferr-p., ***nux-m.,*** nux-v., ***sulph.***
amel. - grat.
as soon as tenesmus ceases - colch., ***sulph.***
storm, during - sil.
before - form., gels., sil.
stretching, with - am-c., ant-t., bar-c., bell., chin., hell., lach., mag-c., meph., nit-ac., ph-ac., phos., sabad.
stroke, in - apis, ***bar-c.,*** hell., ***hyos.,*** kali-i., ***nux-v., op.***
as before an apoplexy - coff.
students, in - ferr., ***gels.,*** mag-p.
stupefaction, with - bell., cocc., ***con.,*** euph., lach., mag-arct., nux-v., ***plb.***
stupor, with - cyt-l.
sudden - ***fl-ac.,*** grat., mag-aust., merc., rumx.
evening - fl-ac.
6 p.m. - rhus-t.
wine, after - fl-ac.
summer heat, with general debility, in - ***corn.***
colds, in - ***gels.***
supper, after - am-c., arum-t., **CALC.,** carb-v., chim-m., chin., clem., colch., hep., lach., mag-c., mez., nit-ac.
surgical operations, after - phos., stict.
syphilis, in - ***syph.***
talking, while - ars., caust., ***chel., mag-c.,*** morph., ph-ac., plat., plb.
thoughts, with activity of - teucr.
thunderstorm - sil.
uneasiness, with - am-c., nicc.
urine, retention, with - ter.
uteri, with prolapsus - ***agar.***
vertigo, with - aeth., alum., aml-n., ang., ant-t., arg-m., arg-n., bell., ***con.,*** crot-h., ***crot-t., gels., glon., kali-br., kali-n.,*** laur., myric., nit-ac., ***nux-m.,*** phos., puls., rhod., ***sil., stram.***
vision, affected - zinc.
vomiting, during - ant-t., ***apoc.,*** dig., ip., ran-b., urt-u.
after - ***aeth.,*** ant-c., ant-t., apom., ars., bell., cupr., dig., **IP.,** kali-bi., sanic.
drowsiness, with - apoc.
weakness and slow pulse, with - apoc.

SLEEPINESS, general
waking, on - bell., bry., calad., calc., calc-f., caust., chel., laur., lyc., ***nux-m.,*** stram.
after - bell., sul-ac.
walking, while - acon., arg-m., chin-s., caust., kali-n., lyc., nat-c., nit-ac., rhus-t., verat.
after - alum., arn., bar-c., carb-an., con., lach., lyc., nat-m., phos., phys., rhus-t., stann., ***sulph.,*** sumb.
air, in open - arn., carb-an., con., lach., lyc., nat-m., phos., phys., puls., rhus-t., sep., stann., ***sulph.,*** sumb.
as after a long walk - anac.
air, in open - ant-t., ars., ars-m., ***chel.,*** con., eug., kali-c., mosch., nux-v., rhus-t., sil., stann.
amel. - asar.
amel. - merc., nat-m., ph-ac.
warm room - ant-t., chin-s., cinnb., ind., merl.
weakness, with - aeth., am-c., anac., ang., arg-m., aur., bism., brucin., canth., chin., clem., ***croc.,*** cupr., ***cycl.,*** echi., eucal., grat., hell., kali-n., lach., lact., laur., merc-sul., ***mez.,*** nat-c., ***nit-ac.,*** pall., petr., ph-ac., phel., plat., puls., ran-b., scroph-n., sil., squil., ***sulph.,*** valer., verat.
literary occupation in evening amel. - ***croc.***
nursing or night watching, after - ***sulph.***
vertigo, with - **NIT-AC.**
weakness, as from - anac.
weariness, with - am-c., anac., ant-c., ars., bar-c., berb., bor., calad., calc., camph., caust., chen-v., ***cic.,*** clem., **COCA,** croc., dig., ferr., **GELS.,** graph., grat., hell., hep., ign., ip., ***kreos.,*** lact., laur., led., mag-arct., mang., murx., nat-c., nat-m., ***nux-v.,*** pall., petr., ph-ac., sang., sel., sep., sil., sin-n., sol-m., spig., still., ***sulph.,*** ziz.
weather, during hot - ***gels.,*** sel.
at first hot weather - vip.
weep, with inclination to - cham.
wine, after - ail., carb-s., phos., thea.
work, during - am-c., aur-m., bism., caust., euphr., ign., lact., lyc., mur-ac., nat-c., phel., ran-b., sulph., zinc.
amel. - am-c., bar-c., nat-c.
aversion to work, with - am-m., clem., colch., coloc., mag-m., ther.
scientific work, during - tarax.
amel. - croc.
when not at - am-c., mosch.
worms, with - ***nux-m.***
writing, while - bapt., brom., nat-s., ph-ac., thuj.
yawning, with - ***all-c.,*** alum., am-c., ars., aspar., bar-c., bell., bov., calc., carb-an., carb-v., cham., chel., ***chin.,*** cina, clem., coff., con., croc., ***cupr.,*** dulc., euphr., ***graph.,*** grat., haem., hell., indg., kali-bi., ***kali-c., kali-n., kreos.,*** lact., ***laur.,*** lyc., ***mag-arct., mag-aust., mag-c., mag-m.,*** mag-s., mang., merc., mez., mill., mosch., mur-ac., ***nat-c.,*** nat-m., nicc., ***nux-v.,*** ol-an., ***par.,*** ph-ac., phel., phos., plb., rat., ***rhus-t.,*** ruta, senec., spig., ***spong., squil.,*** stann.,

SLEEPINESS, general
yawning, with - ***sulph.,*** verb., zinc.

SLEEPING, sickness - ars., gels., nux-m., op.

SLEEPLESSNESS, (see Insomnia)

SLEEP-talking, during - acon., ***ail.,*** alum., alum-p., alum-sil., ambr., am-c., ant-t., apis, ***arn.,*** arg-n., ars., aur., ***bar-ac.,*** bar-c., bar-m., bar-s., **BELL.,** brach., bry., bufo, ***cact., calc.,*** camph., ***cann-i., carb-an.,*** carb-s., carb-v., cast., caste., caust., ***cham., cina,*** cinnb., dig., ***gels.,*** graph., ***hell.,*** hyos., hyper., coff., com., con., cortico., cupr., graph., ***hyos.,*** ign., indg., kali-c., kali-m., kali-sil., kalm., kali-ar., kali-bi., **KALI-C.,** kali-p., kali-s., ***lac-c.,*** **LACH.,** ***led.,*** lyc., mag-aust., mag-c., mag-m., merc., ***mur-ac.,*** nat-c., ***nat-m.,*** nit-ac., ***nux-v., op.,*** ph-ac., phos., plb., podo., psor., ***puls.,*** raph., rheum, ***rhus-t.,*** sabin., sel., ***sep., sil.,*** spig., spong., ***stann., stram., sulph.,*** thuj., tub., zinc., zinc-p.
angry exclamations, with - cast.
anxious - alum., graph., ***mag-m.***
business of - con., rhus-t., sulph.
children, in - ***ambr.,*** psor.
comatose sleep, in - nux-v., op., raph.
confess themselves loud, they - bell., **HYOS.,** stram.
excited - alum., cast., graph., nux-v., sulph.
gentle voice, all night in a - ***camph.***
loud - ***arn., bell., sep., sil.,*** spong., ***sulph.***
obstacles being removed - cham.
reveals secrets in sleep - am-c., ***ars.***
supplicates timidly - stann.
thought when awake, what he - am-c.
war, of - hyos.

SLEEP-walking, somnambulism - **ACON.,** agar., alum., alum-sil., ***anac.,*** ant-c., arg-m., ***art-v.,*** bell., ***bry.,*** calc., ***cann-i.,*** caste., cham., cic., croc., crot-h., cur., cycl., des-ac., dict., hyos., ign., ***kali-br.,*** kali-c., kali-p., kali-s., kalm., lach., luna, lyc., lyss., mag-arct., meph., mosch., **NAT-M., OP.,** paeon., petr., **PHOS.,** plat., rheum, rumx., sep., ***sil.,*** spig., ***spong.,*** stann., ***stram., sulph., tarent.,*** teucr., verat., ***zinc.***
disappearence of old eruptions, after - ***zinc.***
children, in - kali-br.
climbing the roofs, the railings of bridge or balcony - luna, lyc., phos., sulph.
emotions, suppressed, from - zinc.
honor, from wounded - ign.
make day-labor, to - bry., nat-m., sil., sulph.
mental work - phos., sep.
new and full moon, at - ***sil.***
strike sleepers, from vengeance, to - **NAT-M.,** nit-ac.
suppressed emotions, after - ***zinc.***

SNORING, respiration - acon., aeth., amyg., ***ant-t.,*** arn., ars., bapt., benz-ac., bell., ***brom.,*** calc., ***camph., carl., cham., chin., cic.,*** con., cund., ***cupr.,*** cycl., dros., dulc., fl-ac., glon., ***hep.,*** hydr-ac., hyos., ***ign.,*** kali-bi., kali-chl., **LAC-C.,** ***lach., laur.,*** lyc., mag-m., mez., mur-ac., nat-m., nit-ac., nux-m., ***nux-v.,*** **OP.,** petr., rat., rheum, ***rhus-t.,*** sabad., samb., sep., sil., stann., ***stram.,***

SNORING, respiration -stry., ***sulph.,*** teucr.
adenoids removal, after - carc., kali-s.
afternoon, nap, during - alum.
awake, while - chel., sumb.
children, in - chin., mez.
chill, during - ***chin.,*** laur., **OP.**
delirium, after - sec.
evening in bed - sil.
expiring, while - arn., camph., chin., ***nux-v., op.***
fever, during - apis, con., ign., laur., **OP.**
insensible, while - ***op.***
inspiration in sleep - bell., caps., cham., chin., hyos., ign., rheum.
lying on the back, while - dros., dulc., kali-c., mag-c., sulph.
midnight - mur-ac., nux-v.
morning, while sleeping - petr.
nose, through - puls.
sleep, in restless - chin., laur., ***op.,*** sil., stram., tub., ***zinc.***
swoon, during - stram.

SOMNAMBULISM, (see Sleep-walking)

STARTLED, during - acon., aeth., agn., ***alum.,*** am-m., ambr., anac., ang., ant-c., ant-ox., ***apis, arg-m.,*** arn., ***ars., ars-h.,*** ars-i., ars-s-f., arum-i., atro., ***aur.,*** aur-m., auran., bar-c., **BELL.,** bism., bov., brom., bry., calad., ***calc.,*** calc-ar., calc-i., calc-p., calc-sil., camph., canth., caps., carb-an., carb-s., ***carl.,*** cast., ***caust., cham.,*** chel., ***chin., cocc.,*** coff., ***colch.,*** croc., ***crot-c.,*** crot-h., ***cupr.,*** cur., cycl., dig., dulc., euphr., ferr-ma., graph., ***grin.,*** guai., hep., hura, **HYOS.,** hyper., indg., iod., ***ip.,*** iris, kali-ar., kali-bi., ***kali-br.,*** **KALI-C.,** kali-i., ***kali-n.,*** kali-p., ***kali-s., kreos., lach.,*** laur., led., lob-c., lyc., ***mag-arct.,*** mag-aust., mag-c., mag-m., med., ***merc.,*** merc-c., mez., ***morph.,*** mosch., myris., nat-c., ***nat-m.,*** nat-p., ***nat-s.,*** nicc., nit-ac., ***nux-m., nux-v., op.,*** ox-ac., petr., ph-ac., ***phos.,*** plat., plb., **PULS.,** ***rat.,*** rheum, rhod., rhus-t., ruta, sac-alb., ***samb.,*** sars., ***sec.,*** seneg., sep., sil., sol-t-ae., spig., spong., stann., staph., stram., stront-c., sul-ac., sul-i., **SULPH.,** ***tab.,*** teucr., thuj., verat., ***zinc.,*** zinc-p.
before - alum.
falling asleep, on - aeth., agar., ***alum.,*** alum-p., alum-sil., am-c., ambr., am-m., arn., **ARS.,** ars-h., ars-s-f., arum-t., bapt., bar-c., **BELL.,** bism., bry., ***calc., carb-an.,*** carb-v., ***caust.,*** chin., chin-a., ***cina, coff.,*** cor-r., daph., ***dros., dulc.,*** ferr-ma., **HEP.,** ign., ip., kali-ar., kali-bi., ***kali-c.,*** kali-s., kali-sil., kreos., ***lach.,*** led., **LYC.,** mag-c., mag-m., merc., ***merc-c., nat-a., nat-c., nat-m.,*** nat-p., ***nat-s., nit-ac., nux-v.,*** op., ox-ac., paeon., petr., ***phos., phys.,*** plb., rat., rhus-t., sars., ***sel.,*** sep., ***sil.,*** stront-c., stry., **SULPH.,** ***tab.,*** tub., verat.
evening - ambr., am-m., anac., arn., **ARS.,** ars-s-f., bar-c., ***bell.,*** bry., dulc., kali-bi., lach., merc-c., nat-c., plat., sars., ***sel.,*** stront-c., ***sulph.***
feet, as if coming from - lyc.

STARTLED,
from sleep - abrot., ***acon.,*** aesc., ***agn., alum., am-c.,*** am-m., anac., ***ant-c.,*** ant-t., ***apis,*** arn., ***ars.,*** aur., aur-m., ***bar-c.,*** **BELL.,** benz-ac., ***bism.,*** **BOR.,** bov., bry., bufo, ***cact., calad., calc.,*** cann-s., canth., caps., carb-ac., carb-s., carb-v., carc., cast., **CAUST.,** ***cham.,*** chel., ***chin.,*** chin-s., cimic., ***cina, cinnb.,*** cit-v., clem., ***cocc., coff.,*** colch., con., convo-d., cor-r., cycl., ***dig.,*** dros., dulc., ***euphr.,*** ferr-i., ferr-p., ferul., gins., graph., guai., ***hep.,*** hydroph., **HYOS.,** hyosin., ign., kali-bi., kali-br., ***kali-c.,*** kali-i., ***lach.,*** led., lup., lyc., mag-c., mag-m., ***med., menis., merc., merc-c.,*** mez., murx., mur-ac., nat-a., ***nat-c., nat-m.,*** nat-p., nat-sil., ***nit-ac., nux-v.,*** ol-an., op., ***ph-ac.,*** **PHOS.,** plat., plb., psor., ***puls., rat., ruta,*** sabad., sabin., ***samb.,*** sang., ***sars., sep.,*** scut., ***sil.,*** sol-a., **SPONG.,** ***stram.,*** sul-ac., ***sulph.,*** tarent., ***ter.,*** thea., thuj., verat., zinc.
comatose sleep, from - ***ant-t.,*** hell., sec.
menses, before - sep.
menses, during - ***zinc.***
pain in heart, with - xan.
touch, from slightest - ***ruta***
touched, when - coff., stry.
sleepiness, with - ang., ant-t., ***cham.,*** chel., kali-i., mag-c., merc., plat., ***puls.,*** sars., seneg., ***tarent.,*** verat.
afternoon - sil.

SUDDEN, daytime - ***chin.***
evening - fl-ac.
7 p.m. to 9 p.m. - calc.
sitting while - chin.

TALKING, during (see Sleep-talking)

UNREFRESHING - abrot., acon., aesc., agar., ail., alco., ***alum.,*** alum-p., alum-sil., am-m., ambr., ***am-c.,*** ammc., anac., anag., ant-c., ant-ox., ant-t., anthr., ap-g., apis, apoc-a., ***arg-m., arg-n.,*** arn., ***ars.,*** ars-h., ars-s-f., asaf., asim., aster., aur., aur-a., aur-m., bar-ac., ***bar-c., bell.,*** berb., bism., bor., bov., brom., bry., calad., **CALC.,** calc-f., calc-sil., camph., cann-s., ***caps.,*** carb-ac., ***carb-an.,*** carb-s., carb-v., carc., ***carl.,*** **CAUST.,** cham., ***chel., chin.,*** chin-a., chin-s., chlol., cic., cina, cinnb., ***clem., cob., cocc.,*** cod., coff., colch., coloc., con., corn., croc., culx., cupr., cupr-ac., cupr-ar., ***cycl.,*** daph., ***dig.,*** dros., dulc., ***echi.,*** equis., ***erig.,*** euph., euphr., ferr., ferr-ma., ***fl-ac.,*** form., glon., gnaph., graph., ***guai.,*** ham., **HELL.,** ***helon.,*** hep., hipp., hyos., hyper., ign., ip., jac-c., jug-c., kali-bi., **KALI-C.,** kali-i., kali-n., kiss., kreos., **LACH.,** lact., laur., ***lec.,*** led., lil-t., **LYC.,** ***mag-aust.,*** **MAG-C., MAG-M.,** man., meny., merc., merc-c., merl., mez., mit., mosch., mur-ac., myric., nat-a., nat-c., ***nat-m.,*** nat-n., nat-p., nicc., **NIT-AC.,** nux-m., **NUX-V.,** olnd., ***op.,*** paeon., ***petr.,*** **PH-AC., PHOS.,** pic-ac., plan., plat., ***podo.,*** prun., psor., ptel., ***puls.,*** puls-n, ran-b., rheum, rhod., rhus-t., rumx., ruta, sabad., ***sal-ac.,*** samb., sant., sarcol-ac., saroth., sarr., sars., sec., sel.,

UNREFRESHING - ***sep., sil., spig.***, spong., squil., stann., staph., ***stram.***, stront-c., sul-ac., ***sulph.***, sul-i., syph., tarax., teucr., ***thuj.***, thymol., **TUB.**, upa., vac., valer., verat., vib., viol-t., visc., wies., x-ray, xan., ***zinc.***, zinc-p., zing.
- afternoon - bar-c., colch., glon., ign., nat-m.
  - 3 p.m. to 4 p.m. - ruta.
  - 3 p.m. to 5 p.m. - cimic.
- daytime - caust., ign.
- deep - zinc.
- dreams, from - calc-f., ***chel., cod.***
- fever, in - ***ars., dig., ip., phos.***
- menses, during - ***nux-m.***
- morning - aml-n., ang., brom., bry., ***clem., cocc., cod.***, con., ***graph.***, hep., **LYC., MAG-M.**, mill., ***nat-m.***, **NUX-V.**, op., **PH-AC.**, ***podo., sep.***, **SULPH.**
  - more tired in morning than in evening - **MAG-C.**
- noon - ign.
  - and afternoon - ign.
- overstudy, effects of - ***cupr-ac.***
- rising, indisposed to - aesc., ambr., ars., bry., canth., ***carb-v., card-m.***, crot-h., cycl., dros., ferr-ma., graph., lach., ***nat-m., nux-v.***, **PH-AC.**, saroth., ***sep., sulph., thuj.***, verat.
- siesta, after - calc-s.
- sound, though - pic-ac.

VOMITING, sleep after - stram.

WAKING, general
- **abdominal** troubles, from - kali-c.
- **afternoon,** 4 p.m. to 5 p.m. - ***kali-i.***
- **agg.,** general, on waking - acon., agar., agn., alum., **AMBR.**, ***am-c.***, **AM-M.**, anac., ***ant-c.***, ant-t., ***arn.***, **ARS.**, aur., bar-c., bell., ***benz-ac.***, bism., bor., bov., bry., bufo, cact., cadm-s., calad., **CALC.**, calc-p., calc-s., cann-s., canth., ***caps., carb-an., carb-v.***, **CAUST.**, ***cench.***, cham., ***chel., chin.***, cic., cina, clem., ***cocc.***, coc-c., coff., colch., ***con.***, com., croc., ***crot-h.***, crot-t., cupr., cycl., ***dig.***, dros., dulc., euph., ferr., form., ***graph.***, guai., **HEP.**, ***hydr.***, **HYOS.**, ***ign., ip., kali-ar.***, **KALI-BI.**, ***kali-c.***, kali i., kali-n., ***kali-s.***, kreos., **LACH.**, laur., led., ***lyc.***, mag-c., mag-m., mang., meny., ***merc., merc-i-f.***, mez., mosch., mur-ac., naja, nat-c., ***nat-m.***, **NIT-AC.**, nux-m., **NUX-V.**, op., **ONOS.**, petr., ph-ac., **PHOS.**, ***phyt.***, plat., psor., **PULS.**, ***ran-b.***, ran-s., rheum, rhod., ***rhus-t.***, ruta., sabad., sabin., ***samb., sang.***, sars., sel., seneg., **SEP.**, ***sil.***, spig., spong., squil., ***staph.***, stram., stront-c., **SULPH.**, sul-ac., tarax., thuj., **VALER.**, verat., viol-o., viol-t., ***zinc.***
  - falling asleep, both agg. - stann.
  - night, at - ambr., bry., carb-v., chin., **COCC.**, ***colch.***, ip., lach., nat-c., nat-m., **NUX-V.**, ph-ac., ***puls.***, ruta, sabin., ***sel.***, sep.
    - siesta, from - caust.
  - roused - spong.
- **alarmed** - ***agn.***, cact.

WAKING, general
- **amel.,** general, on waking - ambr., am-m., ***ars.***, bry., ***calad.***, calc., cham., chin., cocc., ***colch.***, hell., ign., ip., kreos., lach., meph., nat-c., ***nux-v., onos.***, ph-ac., **PHOS.**, puls., rad-br., ruta, sabal., sabin., samb., sel., **SEP.**, spig., thuj., valer., vip.
- **anger,** with - cham., lyc.
- **anxiety,** as from - agar., con., dig., zinc.
- **bed** were in motion, as if - ***lac-c.***
- **brain** shock, in, with - coca.
- **breath,** wakens to get - ant-t.
- **call,** as from - dulc., kreos., rhod., ***sep.***
- **cause,** without - ang., caust., ***cina,*** ign., mag-c., merc., nat-c., sul-ac., sulph., thyr., viol-t.
- **chill,** with - sil.
- **clothes** feel damp or tight - ***guai.***
- **coldness,** from - all-s., ambr., arn., clem., con., ferr-ma., mang., sabad., sabal., sars., sulph.
  - feet, of - puls.
  - limbs, of - **CARB-V.**
    - left leg - agar.
- **confusion,** with - chin.
- **congestion,** with - am-c., calc., kali-c., mag-c., ***nat-m.***, nux-v., sep., sil., sulph.
- **cough,** from - **ACON.**, alum., alum-sil., ***anac., arg-n.***, ars., ***bell.***, bism., brom., calc., card-m., caust., ***chel.***, chin., coc-c., cocc., con., dios., graph., ***hep.***, **HYOS.**, ***kali-c., lach.***, mag-m., mang., nit-ac., ***nux-v., op., phos.***, psor., **PULS.**, rhus-t., ***rumx., ruta,*** samb., ***sang., sel.***, sep., sil., spong., stront-c., **SULPH.**, tab., tell., thuj.
  - menses, during - zinc.
- **daybreak** - lyc., lycps.
- **difficult** - agar., aloe, ***alum.***, amyg., ***ant-t.***, arge., bell., berb., bry., calc-f., ***camph., calc., calc-p.***, carb-s., ***carb-v., cench.***, cham., ***cic.***, clem., con., cupr-ac., ferr., gels., gins., ***glon.***, graph., hydr., hyos., iodof., ***kali-br.***, kreos., lact., led., lob., lyc., mag-m., mur-ac., nat-c., nat-m., nit-ac., ***nux-v.***, **OP.**, ph-ac., phos., phys., podo., ruta, ***sep.***, sulph., sumb., stram., ***tab.***, teucr., viol-t., visc.
  - afternoon - ferr.
    - siesta, after - eug.
  - morning - ***alum., calc.***, **CALC-P.**, caust., lyc., nit-ac., ***nux-v., ph-ac.***, stram., thuj.
- **disturbance,** as from some - calc-ac.
- **dreams,** from - ***acon.***, agar., am-c., ***am-m.***, ang., ant-c., ***ant-t.***, arg-m., arg-n., ***ars.***, asc-t., atro., ***arn.***, aur., bad., bar-c., ***bell., bov.***, bry., cahin., ***calc.***, calc-f., ***camph.***, cann-s., carb-v., carc., casc., ***cham.***, chel., ***chin.***, chr-ac., ***cic., cina,*** cinnb., clem., coca, coff., colch., coloc., con., corn., cupr., cycl., ***dig.***, dros., dulc., ***erig.***, euph., ***ferr-ma.***, gran., graph., grat., ***hep.***, hyper., ***ign.***, indg., ip., kali-bi., ***kali-c., kali-chl., kali-i.***, kali-n., ***kreos., lach.***, lam., laur., led., lob., lyc., lycpr., lyss., ***mag-arct.***, mag-aust., mag-c., ***mag-s., mang., meph., merc., mez.***, mur-ac., murx., ***nat-c.***, nat-m., ***nat-s., nicc.***, nit-ac., ***nux-v.***, olnd., ***op.***, par.,

WAKING, general

dreams, from - ***petr., ph-ac.,*** phos., plan., plat., puls., rat., rheum, rhus-t., ruta, sabad., ***sabin.,*** sars., ***sep.,*** sil., ***spig.,*** spong., stann., staph., ***stront-c.,*** **SULPH.,** tab., ***teucr., thuj.,*** verat., verb., ***zinc.***

early - acon., agar., aloe, alum., alum-sil., am-c., ambr., am-m., anag., ang., ant-c., ant-t., arn., ***ars.,*** ars-i., ars-s-f., asaf., astac., ***aur.,*** aur-a., aur-i., bar-c., bart., bell., bell-p., berb., ***bor.,*** brach., brom., bry., bufo, cadm-m., calad., ***calc.,*** calc-f., calc-i., calc-p., calc-sil., cann-s., canth., caps., carb-an., carb-s., carb-v., ***caust.,*** cham., chel., chin., chin-a., chin-s., chr-ac., cob., coca, ***cocc., coff.,*** con., cop., corn., croc., cycl., dios., dros., ***dulc.,*** ery-a., euphr., ferr., ferr-ar., ferr-i., fl-ac., ***form.,*** gels., glon., ***graph.,*** grat., guai., hell., hep., hura, hydr., hyos., hyper., ign., ind., iod., junc., ***kali-ar.,*** kali-bi., **KALI-C.,** kali-m., kali-n., kali-p., kali-s., kali-sil., kreos., ***lach., lyc.,*** lycps., ***mag-c.,*** mag-s., mang., ***meph., merc.,*** merc-i-f., mez., morph., ***mur-ac.,*** **NAT-A., NAT-C.,** ***nat-m., nat-p.,*** **NIT-AC., NUX-V.,** ol-an., olnd., ped., phel., ***ph-ac.,*** phos., **PIC-AC.,** plat., plb., prun., ptel., puls., **RAN-B.,** ran-s., rhod., rhus-t., sabad., sabin., samb., sang., saroth., sars., ***sel.,*** seneg., ***sep., sil.,*** spong., squil., staph., sul-i., **SULPH.,** ***sul-ac.,*** syph., ***thuj.,*** trom., verat., verb., viol-t., ***zinc.,*** zinc-p., zing.

down in evening, if she doesn't lie - sep.

falling asleep late, and - bor., cycl., dios., guai., ***lyc.,*** ol-an., prun., puls., ran-b., sel., sep., staph., sul-ac., sulph., visc., zinc.

feels worse if he sleeps again - ***nux-v.***

easy - ars-s-f., aur-s., brom., euph., fl-ac., merc., merc-cy., ***petr.,*** sul-ac.

midnight, before - puls.

erections, by - ambr., arn., bor., carb-v., ***card-m.,*** gnaph., ***hep.,*** kali-c., lach., nat-c., nat-m., ox-ac., petr., ***ph-ac.,*** sil., stann., thuj.

evening, falling asleep, soon after - ambr., bry., ferr., hydr-ac., kali-c., phos., ***prun.,*** puls., sul-ac.

falling sensation, with - bell., bism., dig., ***guai., ph-ac.,*** sang.

frequent - ***acon.,*** aeth., agar., agn., all-s., allox., **ALUM.,** ***alum-p., alum-sil., ambr.,*** am-c., am-m., aml-n., ammc., anac., ang., ***ant-c.,*** ant-t., anth., apis, aran., ***arg-n.,*** arn., ***ars.,*** ars-s-f., asaf., atro., aur., aur-a., bapt., bar-ac., **BAR-C.,** ***bar-m.,*** bart., ***bell.,*** benz-ac., berb., bism., ***bor., bov., bry.,*** bufo, cahin., calad., **CALC.,** ***calc-ar.,*** calc-p., calc-sil., calen., cann-s., canth., caps., ***carb-ac., carb-an., carb-s., carb-v.,*** carc., ***card-m., carl.,*** cast., ***caust.,*** cedr., cham., chel., ***chin.,*** chin-a., ***cic.,*** cimic., ***cimx.,*** cina, cinnb., clem., coca, cocc., cod., ***coff.,*** colch., coloc., con., cop., croc., culx., cupr., cycl., daph., ***dig., dros.,*** dulc., ***euph., euphr.,*** ferr., ferr-i., fl-ac., gins., ***graph.,*** grat., guai., guare., ham., **HEP.,** hura, hydr-ac., hyos., ign., indg., ip., kali-ar., ***kali-c.,*** kali-chl., ***kali-i.,*** kali-n., kali-s., kali-sil., kreos., ***lach.,*** lact., lam., laur., led., ***lyc.,*** lycpr., lyss., mag-arct., mag-aust., ***mag-c.,*** mag-m., mag-s., mang., meny., **MERC.,** merc-c., merl., mez., mosch., **MUR-AC.,** myric., naja, nat-a., nat-c., ***nat-m.,*** nat-p., nat-s., nicc., ***nit-ac.,*** nux-m., ***nux-v., ol-an.,*** olnd., op., orig., ox-ac., par., ped., petr., phel., ph-ac., **PHOS.,** phys., plan., ***plat.,*** plect., **PULS.,** ***ran-b.,*** ran-s., raph., rheum, rhod., rat., ***rhus-t.,*** ruta, sabad., sabin., samb., sang., sarcol-ac., sars., sel., senec., seneg., **SEP.,** ***sil., spig.,*** spong., ***stann.,*** squil., ***staph.,*** stram., ***stront-c.,*** **SULPH.,** sul-ac., ***tab.,*** tarax., ter., teucr., thal., thea., thuj., til., upa., valer., verat., viol-o., viol-t., wies., wild., ***zinc.,*** zinc-p.

afternoon - cann-i.

anxiety, with - ***dig.,*** lyc.

causeless - caust.

dreams, from - ***alum.,*** cina, euphr., lyc., nat-m., stront-c., tab.

every, half hour - agar., am-c., mosch., nat-m., ***sulph.***

hour - allox., ***arg-n.,*** arn., ars-h., carb-v., ferr., nat-m., staph., ***sulph.***

quarter of an hour - cic., lact., merc., mur-ac.

regular hour, at - ***sel.***

three hours - nat-m., puls.

two hours - nat-m.

falling, as if - guai.

fright, as from - coff., graph., guai., merc., nat-c.

heat, as from - cocc.

of bed - culx.

menses, during - mag-c.

midnight, about - bell.

after - am-m., caps., grat., lyc., mag-s., mez., sep., sil., spig., staph., **SULPH.**

before - alum., chel.

morning, toward - chin-s., coff., myric., rhod.

newborn, in - ***bor.***

night, 3 a.m., after - euphr.

4 a.m., after - aur.

oppression of chest, with - stann.

pain, before midnight agg., from - ***ars.***

restlessness, with - ***lach.***

sleep, as from sufficient - calc-ac., **MERC.,** ***ruta,*** tarax.

thinking of business, with - ham.

fright, as from - achy., **ACON.,** aesc., agn., ***am-m., ambr., am-c.,*** anac., ***ant-c.,*** ant-t., ***apis,*** arn., ***ars.,*** aur., bar-c., ***bell., bism.,*** **BOR.,** bov., ***bry.,*** bufo, cact., **CALC.,** calc-s., cann-s., canth., ***caps.,*** carb-ac., ***carb-an., carb-v.,*** cast., ***caust., cham.,*** chel., chlol., cic., cimic., ***cina, chin., cocc.,*** coff., colch., ***con., cupr-ar., cypr.,*** daph., ***dig.,*** dros., ***dulc., euphr.,*** ferr-ma., gins., graph., guai., ***hell.,*** **HYOS.,** ***ign., indg.,*** iodof., ***ip.,*** kali-bi., kali-br., ***kali-c.,*** kali-i., kali-n., kali-p., ***lach.,*** laur., led., **LYC.,** ***mag-arct., mag-aust.,***

WAKING, general

fright, as from - ***mag-c., mag-m., mag-s., med.,*** meny., merc., mez., ***murx.,*** nat-a., nat-c., ***nat-m.,*** nat-p., nat-s., nicc., ***nit-ac.,*** nux-m., ***nux-v.,*** op., paeon., ***petr., phos.,*** plat., psor., ***puls.,*** rat., ruta, ***sabad.,*** sabin., ***samb.,*** sang., sars., sec., sep., ***sil., spong., sep.,*** stann., staph., ***stram., stront-c.,*** **SULPH.,** sul-ac., tell., ter., teucr., ***thuj.,*** **TUB.,** ***verat.,*** xan., **ZINC.**

11 p.m. - cimic.

dreams, frightened from - bell., corn., ***erig.,*** **LYC.,** ***meph., sulph.***

lump which lodges in her throat, imagines she has swallowed a - ***sep.***

noise, from slightest - apis, ***nux-v.,*** sars.

trembling, with - abrot.

trifling, about something - ***lach.***

heart symptoms, with - abrot., chr-ac., ***kali-i., lach., merc., phos., phyt., stict.***

midnight, after - **SPONG.**

heat, from and with - alum., anac., ars., **BAR-C.,** ***bell., benz-ac.,*** bor., calc., carb-v., caust., chin-s., cina, con., ferr., graph., ***kali-bi.,*** kali-c., kali-n., ***mag-arct., mag-c.,*** mag-m., mosch., nat-m., nicc., **NIT-AC.,** petr., ph-ac., **PHOS.,** puls., ran-s., sabad., sep., sil., sulph., sul-ac., teucr., thuj.

2 a.m. - ***benz-ac.***

3 a.m. - ***ars.,*** bapt.

head, from heat in - arn.

morning - alum., ***arn.***

which passes off - calad.

hepatic symptoms, with - bry., ***carb-v.,*** ptel.

4 a.m. - ptel.

hunger, from - abies-n., ***aeth.,*** alum., am-c., ***ant-c., aran.,*** chin., ***ign.,*** iod., **LYC.,** ***lyss., petr., ph-ac.,*** phos., ***psor.,*** teucr.

impossible - acon., bell., chlf., coff., con., ***crot-h., op.,*** tab.

morning - bell., ***ph-ac.,*** tab.

impression of having slept for hours, although it was only thirty minutes, with - ***med.***

itching, from - agar., ant-c., dulc., gamb., ***jug-c., led., merc.,*** sabad., ***stram.***

jerks, by - **BELL.**

just awakened, sensation as if - cycl.

dream, from a - atro.

late - agar., alum., ambr., ***anac.,*** ang., ant-c., ant-t., ***apis,*** arn., asaf., aster., bell., berb., bism., bor., brom., bry., bufo, **CALC., CALC-P.,** canth., carb-s., carb-v., ***caust.,*** cham., clem., ***coca,*** cocc., coloc., ***con.,*** corn., croc., cur., ***cycl.,*** dig., dulc., ***euphr.,*** ferr., fl-ac., glon., **GRAPH.,** hep., hyos., hyper., ign., indg., kali-c., kali-n., kreos., ***lach.,*** laur., led., lyc., mag-c., ***mag-m.,*** mag-s., manc., menis., ***merc.,*** mez., morph., ***nat-c.,*** nat-m., ***nat-p.,*** nit-ac., **NUX-V.,** ol-an., peti., petr., phel., ***ph-ac., phos.,*** plat., puls., ran-b., rhod., rhus-t., sang., scut., **SEP.,** ***sil.,*** spig., stann., stram., **SULPH.,** sul-ac., sumb., verat., verb., zinc.

limbs, starting, by - cann-i.

WAKING, general

lying on painful side, while - ***bor.***

menses, during agg. - mag-c.

flowing in gushes, from - coca

pain, from - sel.

menses, before - sars., sul-ac.

morning, toward - ***am-m.,*** arg-n., arum-d., bell-p., chel., chr-ac., ***form.,*** mur-ac., phel., phos., squil., staph., stront.

5 a.m. - aloe, aml-n., aspar., chr-ac., con., fago., helon., kali-i., lycps., lyc., mez., nat-m., nat-p., ***sulph.***

5 a.m. to 6 a.m. - ***kali-c.***

5 a.m. with urging to stool - ***aloe,*** op., **SULPH.**

6 a., dream, from - rhus-t.

6 a.m. - ***arg-n.***

dreams, from - lyc.

heat of face, coldness of hands and soles, with - con.

immediately on falling asleep - nat-m.

move, unable to - erig., lyc., sil.

movements of child in **pregnancy,** from - con., ***thuj.***

nausea, from - alum., ***ambr.,*** ars., arund., aspar., bry., calad., ***con.,*** cupr-ar., euphr., ferr-p., ***goss., ham., hyper.,*** lach., lyc., mag-c., merc., mez., nicc., olnd., op., phel., phos., ***rat.,*** ruta, sep., sil., squil., ***sulph., ther.,*** thuj.

night - alum., astac., cann-i., ***kali-c.,*** merc-c., ***mur-ac., puls.***

midnight, at - agar., am-m., amph., ant-t., ***arg-n.,*** bar-c., bry., ***calc.,*** camph., chel., cimic., con., crot-t., gent-l., graph., laur., ***lyc.,*** mag-arct., ***mag-c.,*** mang., merc-c., nat-c., nat-m., nat-p., nicc., nit-ac., phos., plat., plect., rat., rhus-t., ruta, sep., sil., spong., sul-ac., sulph., thuj., vac.

dream, after - fl-ac., zinc.

midnight, after - alum., ***am-c.,*** am-m., calc., canth., caps., carb-an., chin., euphr., ***graph.,*** grat., ***ign.,*** kreos., ***lach.,*** lam., laur., ***lyc.,*** mag-arct., mag-c., ***merc., mez.,*** nat-m., nux-v., phel., phos., ran-b., ***ran-s.,*** sabin., sars., sel., ***sep., sil.,*** spig., **SPONG.,** squil., staph., sul-ac., syph.

midnight, before - bor., chel., chin., merc., mez., mur-ac., nat-m., nicc., phel., phos., plb., puls., sil., tab.

11 p.m. - ***bell.,*** chel., cimic., **COC-C.,** nat-m., sil., ther.

urging to stool, with - mag-c.

vertigo, with - ther.

1 a.m. - ant-t., bor., caul., ***cocc.,*** **KALI-C.,** kali-n., ***mag-c.,*** mang., ***merc.,*** merc-sul., nat-c., nat-m., nit-ac., nux-v., ph-ac., phos., rat., ***sep.,*** spig., squil., stann., stront-c., ter.

1 a.m. to 2 a.m. - rumx.

or 2 a.m. - lach.

to 3 a.m. to ***ph-ac.***

1:30 a.m. to 2. a.m. - sel.

WAKING, general
night,
2 a.m. - agar., ***all-c., am-m.,*** ant-c., ***bapt., benz-ac.,*** carb-an., ***caust., dios.,*** ferr., graph., ***kali-bi.,*** **KALI-C.,** kreos., lach., lachn., lyc., ***mag-arct.,*** mag-m., merc., mez., nat-c., nat-s., **NIT-AC.,** phys., **PTEL.,** ***rat.,*** sil., stront-c., rumx., sars., staph., sulph.
before - ferr.
2 a.m. to 3 a.m. - bapt., kali-ar., kali-bi., mag-c., nat-c., sep.
or 3 a.m. - ***samb.***
to 4 a.m. - berb., **KALI-C.,** kali-fer., merc.
to 6 a.m. - visc.
3 a.m. - am-c., am-m., ars., bell-p., benz-ac., ***bor.,*** bry., calc., calc-f., carb-v., carl., ***chin., coff.,*** dys-co., euphr., ferr-ma., glon., graph., ham., jug-c., kali-bi., ***kali-c.,*** lil-t., ***lyc., mag-c.,*** mag-m., mag-s., mez., nat-c., nat-m., nicc., nit-ac., **NUX-V.,** ***phyt., pic-ac.,*** plat., ran-s., ***raph., rat.,*** rhus-t., saroth., sel., seneg., sep., sil., **SULPH.,** zinc-p., zing.
cough, from - cahin., op.
or 4 a.m. - bufo, fago., form., ind.
to 4 a., constriction of heart, with - saroth.
to 4 a.m. - bad., bufo, fago., ind., nat-m., ***nux-v., sulph.***
urging to stool, with - mag-c.
3 a.m. to 5 a.m. - man., saroth., **SULPH.**
thoughts, from activity of - calc-f.
3:30 a.m. - ind., nat-m.
4 a.m. - ars., aur., bor., carb-v., carc., caust., chel., coloc., con., cycl., kali-c., ***lyc., mag-c.,*** mang., merc., mur-ac., nat-m., nit-ac., ***nux-v.,*** pen., per., peti., petr., phos., plb., ptel., ruta, sars., sep., sil., stann., staph., ***sulph.,*** tab., thuj., trom., ***verb.,*** zinc.
aggravation, with - cycl.
headache, from - stram.
toothache, with - nat-c.
urging to stool, with - rumx.
4 a.m.to 5 a.m. - ptel., sulph., verat.
menses after - kali-c.
toothache, with - nat-m.
noise, as from a - merc., nat-c., nat-m., sars.
fancied noise, by - bell.
from slight - acon., alum., alumn., am-c., ang., apis, ars., asar., ***bell., calad.,*** carb-v., cham., chin., ***coff., ign.,*** kali-n., lach., ***merc.,*** narcot., nat-p., nux-v., ol-an., phos., ruta, saroth., sel., sep., sul-ac., ***sulph.,*** tarent., valer., zinc-valer.
rattling of paper - calad.
nose, as if pulled by - nat-c.
numbness, with - ambr., bry., ***erig.,*** lyc., mez., phel., puls.

WAKING, general
pain, from - **ARS.,** ars-h., aur., bapt., cham., ***chin.,*** chr-ac., eup-per., ***kali-c.,*** kali-n., **LACH.,** lyc., merc-c., mur-ac., myric., ***nat-m.,*** ph-ac., ran-a., raph., sars., sel., staph., tell.
midnight especially - **ARS.**
palpitation, with - agar., alum., am-c., ***ars.,*** benz-ac., bufo, ***calc., camph., cann-i., carb-an.,*** chin., coc-c., hyos., iris, kali-bi., ***lyc., merc., merc-c.,*** mur-ac., ***nat-c.,*** nat-m., nit-ac., ox-ac., petr., **PHOS.,** rad-br., rhus-t., sars., ***sep., sil., spong.,*** stram., sulph., thuj., zinc.
paralysed feeling, with - ferr-i., kreos., nat-c., phos.
perspiration, from - am-m., ant-c., ant-t., ars., astac., bar-c., ***bell.,*** berb., calc., calc-p., ***caust., chel.,*** chin., ***chin-a., cic.,*** clem., **CON.,** croc., daph., **DROS.,** euphr., ***ferr.,*** ferr-ma., form., gamb., ***hep.,*** kreos., ***lac-c., lac-d., lach.,*** laur., ***led., lyc., merc., nat-m.,*** nat-s., nicc., ***ptel., puls.,*** ran-b., ***rat.,*** rumx., sabad., ***samb.,*** sep., ***sil.,*** sulph., tarax., ther., ***tub.***
pollutions, from - aloe, arn., cahin., crot-t., cycl., dig., petr., phos., ***sel.,*** sil., ***thuj.***
sensation as before a pollution, with - mur-ac.
pulled on the nose, as if - mur-ac., nat-c.
regular hour - ***sel.***
same hour, at the - rhod., ***sel.***
scratching in larynx, from - bov.
sensation as after a deep sleep, with - phys.
sexual excitement, from - carb-ac., lyc.
shocks through the body, while - ***arg-mur.,*** ars-h., carc., dig., ***mag-m.,*** manc., merc.
head and neck, in - mag-arct.
singing in sleep, by - mag-arct., sulph.
slept one's fill, as having - agar., calc-ac., caps., cycl., dig., dros., ***ferr., form.,*** ip., kreos., ***lyc.,*** **MERC.,** prun., ***puls., ran-b.,*** ran-s., ruta, samb., ***sel.,*** spig., stann., sul-ac., tarax., viol-t.
3 a.m. - form.
obliged to rise and occupy himself - ***lac-c.***
short sleep, even after - med., meph., ph-ac.
slightest touch, from - ruta.
sneezing, from - dig., hep.
soreness, with - ***arn., rhus-t.***
sudden - ars., bry., carb-ac., cinnb., crot-t., ferr-ma., kali-c., ***kali-i.,*** kreos., mag-arct., nat-c., phys., sec., spira., sulph., til.
2 a.m. - benz-ac., kreos.
3 a.m. - bry.
called, as if - kreos.
dream, as from a - cinnb.
dropping, by postnasal - hydr.
nightmare, from - thea.
pollution, after a - crot-t.
stool, from desire for - ***bry., dios., kali-bi.***
1 a.m. - caul.
5 a.m. - **SULPH.**
6 a.m. - arg-n.

WAKING, general
suffocation, from - ant-t., kali-i., lach., samb., spong., valer.
falling asleep, when - naja.
menses, during - spong.
talking, with - arn., bry., ***sulph.***
thirst, by - aloe, ant-t., berb., bor., ***calad.,*** carb-v., chin-s., **COFF.,** dros., eug., kali-n., ***lil-t.,*** mag-c., ***nat-s.,*** nit-ac., plat., ran-s., ***rat.,*** rhus-t., ***sel.,*** sep., ***stram.,*** sul-ac., sulph., thuj.
thoughts of business, with - hyos.
with, careful - ***ambr., calc.***
tight, every seems too - ***guai.***
toothache, by - am-m., ars., bell., ***calc., carb-an.,*** cast., cham., ***glon.,*** lach., mag-p., mez., nat-c., nat-m., phos., sabin., sep., spig.
touch, from slightest - ruta.
twitching, from - carc.
urinate, with desire to - ant-c., ant-t., carb-v., card-m., caust., croc., ***hep., kali-bi., kali-c.,*** kreos., mag-c., nat-m., sarr., sil.
vertigo, from - ant-t., chin., ***dulc.,*** euphr., ***hyper., kali-c.,*** kali-i., lach., lyc., ***med.,*** merc., nicc., **NUX-V.,** op., ***phos.,*** sil., stram., ***sulph.,*** ther.
warmth, from - cocc., kreos., sep.
of bed - culx.
worms, from - calc-f.

WALKING in bed, child is - rheum.

YAWNING - abies-c., abrot., ***acon.,*** acon-c., ***aesc.,*** agar., all-c., alum., alum-sil., am-c., ambr., ammc., am-m., amyg., anac., ang., ant-c., ***ant-t., apis,*** apom., ***aran.,*** arg-m., ***arg-n., arn.,*** **ARS.,** ars-h., ars-i., arum-t., arund., asaf., asar., aspar., astac., atro., aur., aur-m., bar-c., bell., bol., bor., bov., brach., ***brom., bry.,*** bufo, cahin., calad., ***calc., calc-ar.,*** calc-caust., ***calc-p.,*** calc-sil., camph., cann-s., canth., caps., carb-ac., carb-an., carb-s., carb-v., card-b., card-m., ***carl.,*** cast., **CAUST.,** cedr., cer-b., ***cham.,*** **CHEL.,** chen-v., chin., chin-a., chin-s., chlf., cic., cimic., cimx., **CINA,** ***cit-v., clem.,*** cob., coca, ***cocc.,*** coc-c., coff., colch., coloc., con., cor-r., **CROC.,** crot-c., crot-h., crot-t., ***cupr.,*** cupr-ac., cycl., daph., dig., dros., dulc., elat., eup-pur., euph., euphr., eupi., fago., ferr., ferr-ma., form., gamb., gels., gent-l., glon., gran., **GRAPH.,** grat., guai., haem., hecla., hell., hep., hipp., hura, hydr., hydrc., hydr-ac., hyos., hyosin., hyper., **IGN.,** ind., iod., ip., piloc., jatr., jug-c., jug-r., **KALI-AR.,** kali-bi., ***kali-c.,*** kali-cy., kali-i., kali-n., kali-p., kiss., **KREOS.,** lach., lachn., lact., ***laur.,*** led., lepi., ***lil-t.,*** lim., lina., lob., lol., ***lyc.,*** lycps., lyss., ***mag-c.,*** mag-m., mag-p., ***mang.,*** menis., meny., med., meph., merc., ***merc-c.,*** merc-sul., merl., mez., mill., morph., mosch., ***mur-ac.,*** naja, nat-a., nat-c., ***nat-m.,*** nat-s., nicc., nit-ac., nux-m., **NUX-V.,** ***ol-an., olnd.,*** **OP.,** ost., ox-ac., ***par.,*** ped., peti., petr., phel., ph-ac., ***phos.,*** phys., phyt., pimp., plat., plb., podo., polyp-p, psor., ptel., ***puls.,*** puls-n, quas., ran-b., raph., rat., rheum, rhod., **RHUS-T.,** rumx., ruta, ***sabad.,*** sabin., ***sal-ac.,*** sang., ***sars.,*** sec., sel., senec., seneg., ***sep., sil.,*** spig., spong., ***squil., stann., staph.,*** stram., stront-c., sulph., sul-ac., tab., tarent., tarax., tart-ac., tax., tell., ter., teucr., thea., thuj., til., tong., trom., vac., valer., ***verat.,*** verb., vinc., ***viol-o., viol-t.,*** vip., xan., zinc., zinc-valer.
abdominal symptoms, with - bov., ***cast.,*** caust., haem., hep., mag-arct., puls.
accompaniment, as an - agar., cast., cina, kreos., sars.
afternoon - ***arg-n.,*** arum-t., ***asar.,*** bell., bov., canth., caust., erig., ign., jug-r., kali-c., kali-chl., laur., mag-c., nat-a., nat-c., nicc., nux-v., par., plat., ran-s., sang., sep., spirae., ***spong.,*** stry., tong.
1 p.m. - form.
2 p.m. - chel., grat.
3 p.m. - com.
3 p.m. to 8 p.m. - ped.
4 p.m. - plan.
walking in open air am - plan.
4 p.m. to 6 p.m. - ph-ac.
5 p.m. - arg-n., euphr.
agg. - arum-t.
amel. - phel.
sitting, while - nicc.
walking, after - sep.
air, in open - eug., euphr., stann.
amel. - clem., ol-an.
walking in open air, after - sep.
all-day - aspar., kreos., mag-m., ph-ac., zinc.
alternating with cough - ***ant-t.***
with cough, belching - berb.
anemia, in - ***graph.***
anxiety, during - ***plb.***
appetite, with wanting - kreos.
belching, with - berb., lol., nat-m., phos., tell.
alternating with belching - berb.
amel. - thuj.
breakfast agg. - carl.
bulimia, with - ***lyc.***
childbirth, after - ***plat.***
children, in - ***cham.,*** ign.
chill, during - acon., agar., am-c., ant-t., apis, arn., ars., ars-h., bol., bol., **BROM.,** ***bry.,*** calad., caps., caust., chin., cimx., cina, cob., croc., cycl., dig., **ELAT., EUP-PER.,** gamb., graph., ip., kali-c., ***kreos.,*** laur., lyc., mag-aust., mag-m., ***meny.,*** merc., mez., ***mur-ac.,*** murx., **NAT-M.,** nat-s., **NUX-V.,** ***olnd.,*** par., phos., plat., puls., rhus-t., ruta, ***sep.,*** sil., teucr., thuj., zinc.
before - aesc., ant-t., ***aran.,*** arn., ars., elat., ***eup-per.,*** chin., ign., ip., nat-m., nicc., nux-v., rhus-t.
mouth remains open for a long time - ant-t.
chilliness, with - acon., am-c., ant-t., ars., bar-ac., bol., ***bry., calc.,*** caps., chin., chin-s., ***cina,*** cob., croc., daph., dig., ***gels., ip., kreos.,*** lyc., mag-m., merc-sul., ***nat-m., nat-s.,*** olnd., par., phos., puls., rhus-t., ruta, sep., sil., teucr.
menses, before - **PULS.**

YAWNING, general
church, in - pic-ac.
coldness, with - caust., nat-c.
coma, in - aml-n.
complaints, during other - agar., ant-t., cast., cina, kali-c., kreos., sars.
abdominal symptoms, with - cast.
conference, during a - caust.
constant - am-m., asar., ***bry.,*** calc., caps., chin., chin-s., ***cocc.,*** eug., hep., lath., mag-c., nat-c., nux-v., op., par., phos., plat., sars., spig., staph., sulph., trom., zinc.
lying down, after - ***cocc.***
constriction of throat, from - nat-m.
conversation, listening to a - ***caust., lyss.***
convulsions, in - agar., ***aml-n., graph., ign.,*** kali-bi., ***op.***
before - agar., ***tarent.***
convulsive - hep.
coryza, during - bry., carb-an., cupr., hell., laur.
coughing, when - anac., ***ant-t.,*** arn., ***bell.,*** brom., cham., ign., kreos., lyc., nat-m., nux-v., ***op.,*** phos., puls., rhus-t., zinc.
after - ***anac.,*** ant-c., **ANT-T.,** arn., ***ip.,*** **KREOS.,** nux-v., op., sang.
alternating with coughing - ***ant-t.***
causes cough - arn., ***nux-v.***
children especially - **ANT-T.**
cramps in stomach, with - calc.
crying, while - staph.
laughter, then - agar.
daytime - agar., aspar., brach., croc., lyc., ***nat-c.,*** **NUX-V.,** ph-ac., phys., phyt., ***sulph.***
delirium, before - agar.
diarrhea, after - nux-v.
pendant - ***caps., cupr.***
dinner, during - ***calc-p.,*** ign., lact., zinc.
after - ant-t., ars., bry., canth., cob., colch., dig., ***ign.,*** laur., ***lyc.,*** kali-bi., mag-c., mag-m., nat-c., nat-m., nit-ac., phel., phos., plat., plb., rat., ***squil.,*** sul-ac., tab., zinc.
before - alum., ***bry., calc-p.,*** lyc., merc.
drinking, agg. - carl.
cold water - thuj.
dyspnea - bapt., ***brom.,*** sulph.
after - sulph.
eating, after - ambr., ***aran.,*** ars., aur-m., caps., chin., chin-s., con., ign., ip., ***kali-c., nat-c.,*** nat-s., nit-ac., plat., squil., ***sulph.***
amel. - chen-v.
emptiness of stomach, from - ammc.
evening - aloe, am-c., am-m., ***arn.,*** bell., bov., ***calc.,*** cann-s., carl., cast., caust., ***cedr.,*** chel., chin-s., cocc., coc-c., cupr., cycl., erig., euphr., graph., hecla., ***hep.,*** hura, ign., ip., lach., lyc., mag-c., merc., mez., nat-c., nit-ac., nux-v., ox-ac., ph-ac., phos., psor., rat., rhus-t., sulph., sumb., thuj., verat., zinc.
5 p.m. - arg-n., euphr.
5 p.m. to 6 p.m. - fago.

YAWNING, general
evening,
7 p.m. - mag-c.
amel. after - nat-m.
8 p.m. - aloe
9 p.m. to 10 p.m. - ph-ac.
agg. - mill., ph-ac.
bed, in - nat-m.
reading, after - lyc.
twilight, in the - bell.
fever, during - aesc., arn., ***ars.,*** bry., calc., calc-p., chin-s., cina, croc., ***ign.,*** kali-c., kreos., **NIT-AC.,** nux-v., ***op., phos.,*** plat., ***rhus-t.,*** ruta, sabad., sep., thuj.
before - ars., ***elat., ip., nux-v., rhus-t.***
forenoon - agar., aloe, ant-t., bart., ***calc-p., carb-an.,*** caust., cham., coca, crot-t., graph., hell., hep., hyos., indg., kali-c., kali-n., lyc., mag-c., mag-m., mez., nat-c., rhus-t., sars., senec., spig., zinc.
9 a.m. - carl., lyc.
10 a.m. - arg-n.
11 a.m. - arum-t., caust., mit., rhus-t.
frequent - ***acon.,*** agar., alum., am-c., am-m., ang., alum., am-c., am-m., ant-c., ant-t., ***arn., ars.,*** asar., bar-ac., bar-c., ***bell.,*** blatta-a., ***brom.,*** bry., calc., camph., cann-s., canth., ***caps., carb-v.,*** caust., ***cham.,*** **CHEL.,** chin., chin-a., chin-s., cic., cina, ***cit-v.,*** cimx., ***cocc.,*** coff., colch., con., cor-r., croc., crot-h., ***crot-t., cupr.,*** dig., dros., dulc., elat., euph., euphr., ***gran.,*** grat., **GRAPH.,** ***guai.,*** haem., ***hep., hydr-ac., ign.,*** ip., kali-c., kali-i., kali-sil., kreos., lach., ***lact.,*** laur., ***lyc.,*** lyss., ***mag-arct.,*** mag-aust., mag-c., mag-m., ***mang.,*** meny., meph., ***merc-c.,*** merc., mosch., myric., nat-a., nat-c., nat-m., nat-s., nit-ac., nux-v., ol-an., ***olnd.,*** onis., par., phel., ph-ac., ***phos.,*** plat., ***plb., puls.,*** rheum, rhod., rhus-t., ruta, sabad., sars., ***sep., sil.,*** spig., squil., stann., staph., stront-c., sul-ac., **SULPH.,** tab., tarax., tart-ac., tax., ***verat.,*** verb., vinc., xan., zinc., zinc-ac.
afternoon - mag-c.
menses, during - nat-m.
dinner, after - lyc.
evening - bell., hep., lyc., mag-c., nat-c., ph-ac.
6 p.m., after - mag-c.
reading, after - lyc.
restlessness, with - aran.
riding in a carriage - nat-m.
sleepiness and restlessness, with - ***con., kali-i.***
forenoon - indg., lyc., nat-c., nat-m., ph-ac., sars.
listening to others, when - caust., lyss.
menses, during - mag-m.
morning - ***cocc.,*** lycps.
sleep, after - ign.
sleeping off the intoxication, after - alco.
supper, after - ***lyc.***
wine amel. - nat-m.

YAWNING, general
fruitless efforts to yawn - lach., ***lyc.***
children, in - ***lyc.***
giddiness, with - agar.
girdle sensation, with - stann.
headache, with - ***all-c.,*** am-c., chin-a., cycl., form., ***glon.,*** ign., nux-v., ***phos.,*** staph.
before - agar.
hemorrhage, with - apis.
hiccough, with - aml-n., caust., cocc., mag-c., nat-m.
honor, from wounded - ***nux-v.***
hysteria, in - ***kali-p.,*** tarent.
indoors - ruta.
ineffectual - acon., ambr., ant-t., cham., cocc., croc., ign., lach., ***lyc.,*** manc., phos., ruta, spira., stann.
oppression of chest, from - ***phos.***
injuries, from - ***lach.***
interrupted - ars., cham., cocc., ign., lyc., ruta.
intoxication, as from - bell.
lachrymation, with - ammc., ant-t., bar-c., calc-p., ferr., hell., ign., ***kali-c.,*** kreos., mag-p., meph., ***nux-v.,*** ph-ac., rhus-t., ***sabad.,*** sars., staph., viol-o.
laughter, involuntary, followed by - agar.
leaning towards left amel. - phel.
listening to, conversation - ***caust., lyss.***
others - med.
loud - ferr-ma.
siesta, after - aloe.
lying down, after - ***cocc.,*** plan.
menorrhagia, in - ***apis.***
menses, during - am-c., anac., carb-an., nux-v., op.
after - ***cit-v.***
before - am-c., carl., phel., **PULS.**
metrorrhagia, in - jatr., meph.
midnight, after - ***thuj.***
miscarriage, in threatening - ***cham.***
morning - agar., alum., am-m., ang., ant-t., apis, aspar., bar-c., brom., bry., carl., cedr., ***cocc.,*** croc., crot-t., cycl., ferr., hyper., ign., kreos., lach., mag-arct., mag-c., mag-m., mang., mur-ac., nat-c., nat-m., nicc., ***nux-v.,*** rat., rhus-t., sep., tab., tarent., verat., viol-o., zinc., zing.
7 a.m. - cedr.
8 a.m. - nicc.
9 a.m., till - mag-c.
air, in open - croc.
bed, in - mag-arct., mag-m., sep.
every morning - viol-o.
incessantly - ***cocc.***
noon, till - hep.
rising, on - acon., alum., ign., mag-arct., mag-c., mag-m., plat., rhus-t., senec.
after - apis, mag-c., ***nux-v.***
room agg., in - croc.
waking, on - agar., alum., bar-c., cocc., mag-m., nux-v., verat.
walking in open air - agar.

YAWNING, general
nausea, with - ***kali-bi., kali-c.,*** lol., nat-m.
near objects seem distant, when - all-c.
neuralgia, before the attack of - ***chel.***
night - bell., ***caust.,*** nit-ac.
9 p.m. - ***cedr.***
9 p.m. to 10 p.m. - ph-ac.
eating agg., after - ruta.
noon - bry., ign., menis., merc., psor., sep., verat.
and afternoon - ars., asar., bell., bov., bry., canth., caust., ***ign.,*** lact., laur., mag-c., mag-m., merc., nat-c., nicc., nit-ac., par., phel., phos., plat., plb., rat., sep., sul-ac., tab., tong.
after walking - sep.
riding, while - mill.
siesta, after - bar-c., ign., verat.
oppression of chest, with - croc., ign., stann.
pain, during - aran., nux-v., phos., puls.
before - agar.
paroxysms, in - agar., ph-ac.
paroxysmal - agar., ang., ferr., til.
paying attention to others - caust., lyss.
periodical - arum-t.
perspiration, during - arn., ***ars.,*** bry., caust., cina, croc., ign., ***kali-c.,*** kreos., ***nit-ac.,*** **NUX-V.,** op., phos., plat., ***rhus-t., sabad.,*** **SEP.**
pulsations in chest, with - calc.
head, in - calc.
reading, while - euphr., nat-c., tarax.
aloud - hyos., thuj.
respiration, with difficult - bapt., ***brom.,*** sulph.
after - sulph.
restlessness, with - ***lach.,*** plb.
rheumatism, in - ***bry.***
sadness, in - merc-sul.
shuddering - arn., calad., ***cina,*** hydr-ac., ip., kali-c., laur., mag-m., meny., mez., nux-v., ***olnd.,*** phos., sars., sep.
sighing - ign.
sitting, while - atro., bor., carl., clem., cocc., nat-c., nicc., tarax.
sleep, during deep - ***all-c.,*** all-s., cast.
sleepiness, during - ***all-c.,*** alum., am-c., ang., ars., aspar., bar-c., bell., bov., calc., carb-an., carb-v., cham., chel., ***chin.,*** cic., cina, clem., coff., con., croc., ***cupr.,*** dulc., euphr., grat., haem., hell., indg., kali-bi., ***kali-c., kali-n., kreos.,*** lact., ***laur.,*** lyc., ***mag-arct., mag-aust.,*** mag-c., ***mag-m.,*** mag-s., mang., merc., mez., mill., mosch., mur-ac., ***nat-c.,*** nat-m., nicc., ***nux-v., ol-an., par.,*** ph-ac., phel., phos., plb., rat., ***rhus-t.,*** ruta, senec., spig., ***spong., squil., sulph.***
cough, after - anac.
sleepiness, without - acon., alum., am-m., ang., ant-t., arn., bry., canth., caust., cham., chin., ***croc.,*** cupr., cycl., grat., hep., ***ign.,*** indg., kali-i., lach., lact., laur., lyss., mag-arct., mag-c., mang., mosch., nat-m., ol-an., phel.,

YAWNING, general

sleepiness,without - phos., **PLAT.**, rhod., **RHUS-T.**, ***sep.***, spig., squil., staph., sulph., tax., viol-o., zinc.

soreness, with - bar-c.

spasmodic - acon., agar., am-c., ang., ant-t., arn., ars., bov., bry., calc., carl., chin-a., ***cina,*** cocc., coloc., ***cor-r.,*** croc., cupr., euphr., gran., ***hep.,*** hipp., ***ign.,*** lach., laur., ***mag-arct.,*** ***mag-p.,*** med., mosch., ***nat-m.,*** nux-v., pana., **PLAT., RHUS-T.,** sep., ***staph.,*** squil., sulph., tarent.

amenorrhea, in - ***cina.***

evening - am-c., ign., sulph.

fever, during - ars., nux-v., rhus-t.

morning - ign.

sleep, after deep - nat-m.

wine amel. - nat-m.

spasms, before - agar., merc., tarent.

stool, after - anac., nux-v., op.

before - form., lyc., sulph., verat.

stretching, with - acon., aesc., ***agar.,*** all-c., ***alum., am-c.,*** ambr., aml-n., ang., ant-t., arn., **ARS.**, asar., bar-c., ***bell.,*** bor., bov., ***bry.,*** calc., calc-p., camph., cann-s., canth., caps., ***carb-v.,*** carl., cast., ***caust.,*** **CHAM.,** ***chel., chin.,*** chin-s., ***cina,*** coca, cocc., crot-h., cupr-ac., cur., dig., dros., elat., euphr., ferr., ***form., gels.,*** gran., ***graph., guai.,*** hell., hep., hydr-ac., ***ign., ip.,*** kali-c., kreos., ***lach.,*** lact., lyc., mang., meph., morph., nat-m., **NUX-V.,** onis., plb., rhod., rhus-t., sec., sil., ***staph.,*** ***sulph.,*** tab., tart-ac., tong., viol-o.

forenoon - ant-t.

hiccough, with - aml-n.

indoor - ruta.

menses, before - puls.

wretched feeling, with - form.

stupefaction, with - jatr., meph.

suffocating, as from - ***cit-v.***

summer complaints, in - ***ars.***

supper, after - coca, ***lyc.,*** ruta

before - merc.

thirst, with - bry.

trembling, with - ***cina,*** olnd.

internal - nux-v.

jaw, of lower - olnd.

uneasiness, with - am-c., ang., nicc.

uninterrupted, nearly - ars.

vehement - agar., am-c., ant-t., ars., caust., cham., cina, ***cocc.,*** coff., ***cor-r.,*** croc., euphr., ferr-ma., gran., hep., hyos., ***ign.,*** indg., lach., ***mag-arct.,*** mag-c., mag-p., mez., mosch., nat-m., nit-ac., nux-v., ***plat.,*** rat., rhus-t., staph., sulph., til., verat.

repeated, in coma - aml-n., kali-c.

siesta, after - aloe.

wine amel. - nat-m.

vomiting, between the acts of - apom.

wakefulness, with - cham., kali-bi.

waking, on - alum., bar-c., cocc., dig., mag-m., nux-v., verat.

YAWNING, general

walking, while - bart., camph., chlf.

after - alum., nat-m.

amel. - berb., ox-ac., **PLAN.**

in open air - eug., euphr., kali-c., lycps., stann.

warm, bed - chin-s.

rooms - mez.

weakness, with - alum., camph.

weariness, with - ars., bar-c., ***calc.***

wine amel. - nat-m.

work, with aversion to - ang., mag-m., tong.

not at work, when - mosch.

Stomach

ACHING, dull, pain, (see Pain, general)

ACRIDITY - calc., carb-v., hep.

AIR, as if was forcing through - bar-c., cob., coc-c., crot-c.
sternum, below - bell.

ALIVE, sensation as if something, in - anac., chel., cocc., coloc., **CROC.,** sang., tarent.

ANTIPERISTALTIC, (see Reversed)

ANXIETY, in - ***acon.,*** am-m., ant-t., arg-m., ***arg-n.,*** **ARS.,** bry., ***calc.,*** calc-ar., ***calc-p., cann-s., carb-v., caust., cham., chel.,*** cic., cocc., coff., ***colch.,*** crot-t., ***cupr., dig.,*** dros., ***ferr.,*** ferr-ar., gran., ***grat.,*** guai., haem., hydr., hydr-ac., ***jatr., kali-ar.,*** kali-bi., kali-br., ***kali-c.,*** kali-s., lact., laur., ***lyc.,*** merc., merc-c., mez., mosch., mur-ac., nat-m., ***nux-v., op., paeon.,*** phos., plb., ***puls.,*** rhus-t., sang., ***sec.,*** sep., ***sil.,*** squil., ***stann., stram.,*** sulph., sul-ac., sumb., tab., **TARENT.,** ter., teucr., thuj., ***verat.,*** vesp.
asthma, in - ***ferr.***
cramps, with - ***aran., calc.***
diarrhea, before - mez.
eating, after - chin., osm., petr.
small quantity - osm.
excitement, after - calc., dig., ***kali-c.,*** mez., phos.
extending to head - nat-m., thuj.
menses, during, agg. - sil.
morning, on waking, in alcoholics - **ASAR.**
night, rising upwards - **ARS.**
pain extending to back, with, vomiting amel. - ***sep.***
people, on approach of - lyc.
periodically, recurs with weakness - ars.
pressure - **BAR-M.**
rising up, on - ars.
sitting, when - calc.
standing, while - teucr.
amel. - calc.
stomachache, with - ***bry.***
stool, before - mez.
twisting, 8 a.m. to 9 a.m. - ***cocc.***
vexation, after - **LYC.**
waking, on - **ASAR.** ferr.
walking, amel. - calc.
anxiety, epigastrium - calc-ac., ***dig., kali-ar.,*** kali-c., phos.
children, in - ***calc-p.***
gastralgia, with - ***lyc.***
oppression of breathing, with - sabad.
pressure, with, in hysteria - nux-v.

APPETITE, (see Food chapter, Appetite)

APPREHENSION, fear, in - asaf., ***aur.,*** bry., calc., ***cann-s.,*** canth., ***dig.,*** kali-ar., ***kali-c., lyc.,*** mag-c., **MEZ.,** ***phos.,*** thuj.

ATROPHY - bism., kreos., ox-ac.

BALANCED, up and down, as if stomach were - ph-ac.

BALL, sensation of - ***bell.,*** coc-c., lach., senec.
burning - ***bell.***
rising up into throat - ***lach., senec.***
rolling in - arn., phos.

BAR, laid over stomach - ***haem., quillaya.***

BELCHING, general, (see Heartburn) - abies-c., absin., acet-ac., **ACON.,** ***aesc.,*** aeth., ***agar.,*** agn., ***all-c.,*** aloe, alum., **AMBR.,** am-c., anac., ang., ***ant-c., ant-t.,*** apis, apoc., **ARG-N., ARN.,** ***ars.,*** ars-h., ars-i., **ASAF., ASAR.,** asc-t., aur., bapt., ***bar-c.,*** bar-i., bar-m., **BELL.,** benz-ac., berb., ***bism.,*** bov., brach., brom., **BRY.,** bufo, cahin., ***calc.,*** calc-s., ***camph.,*** cann-i., cann-s., ***canth.,*** caps., ***carb-ac., carb-an.,*** **CARB-S., CARB-V.,** carl., ***caust., cham., chel.,*** **CHIN.,** chin-a., cimx., ***cinnb.,*** clem., ***cimic.,*** cina, cist., **COCC.,** coc-c., coff., ***colch.,*** coloc., com., **CON.,** cop., ***croc.,*** crot-c., crot-t., **CUPR.,** cupr-ar., ***cycl.,*** dig., ***dios., dulc., eup-per.,*** eup-pur., eupi., fago., ***ferr.,*** ferr-ar., ***ferr-i.,*** ferr-p., ***fl-ac., gels.,*** gent-c., gent-l., gins., glon., gran., ***graph.,*** grat., **GUAI.,** gymn., ham., hell., ***helon., hep., hydr.,*** hydrc., hyos., hyper., ***ign.,*** **IOD.,** indg., ***ip.,*** **IRIS,** jatr., ***jug-c.,*** kali-ar., **KALI-BI., KALI-C.,** kali-chl., kali-i., kali-n., ***kali-p., kali-s., kalm.,*** kreos., ***lac-ac., lac-d., lach.,*** lact., ***laur., lec.,*** led., lil-t., lith., lob., **LYC.,** lyss., **MAG-C.,** ***mag-m.,*** mang., **MED.,** meph., merl., **MERC.,** merc-c., merc-i-r., ***mez.,*** mosch., ***mur-ac.,*** **NAT-A., NAT-M.,** ***nat-p., nat-s.,*** nicc., ***nit-ac.,*** nux-m., **NUX-V.,** ol-an., olnd., osm., ***ox-ac.,*** pall., par., ***petr., ph-ac.,*** **PHOS.,** phys., pic-ac., plat., ***plb.,*** **PSOR., PULS.,** ***ran-b., ran-s.,*** raph., rat., rheum, rhod., **RHUS-T.,** rhus-v., rob., rumx., ***ruta., sabad.,*** sabin., sang., ***sars.,*** sec., sel., ***seneg.,*** **SEP.,** ***sil.,*** spig., sol-t-ae., spong., ***squil., stann., staph.,*** stram., ***sul-ac.,*** **SULPH.,** sumb., tab., ***tarax.,*** **TARENT.,** tep., ter., ***thuj., valer.,*** **VERAT.,** ***verb.,*** vesp., ***zinc.,*** zing.
acids, after - ph-ac., staph.
acrid - aloe, alum., ***ambr., apis,*** arg-m., ars., asaf., bell., bufo, cact., ***calc., calc-s., cann-s., carb-an.,*** carb-s., carb-v., caps., carb-v., ***caust.,*** cham., cop., crot-h., crot-t., cupr., ***dig.,*** dios., dor., echi., fago., ***fl-ac., graph., lac-ac., lach.,*** lact., lob., **LYC.,** mang., ***merc.,*** mez., ***nit-ac., nuph., nux-v.,*** ol-an., ox-ac., petr., phos., ***phyt.,*** raph., ***rhus-t., sang., sep., sul-ac.,*** ter., ther., thuj., verat., zinc.
afternoon - ***caust.,*** chin.
alcoholics, in - ***sul-ac.***
bread, after - crot-h.
dinner, after - aloe, petr.
eating, after - all-s., anac., carb-s., spig.
evening - alum., ***ambr., caust.***
fever, during - cub.
night - merc.
sweets, after - raph., zinc.
afternoon - aeth., agar., am-m., ars., ars-i., bar-c., calc., ***carb-v., caust.,*** chel., chin-s., ***cic.,*** con., crot-t., cupr., fago., fl-ac., hydr., ***lyc.,*** mag-c., mag-m., merc., ***nat-c.,*** op., ox-ac., sang., thuj.
3 p.m. - gels., sumb.

BELCHING, general
afternoon,
4 p.m. after - coff., nat-m., valer.
night, until - bar-c.
eating, after - petr.
aggravated, from - agar., cann-s., **CHAM., CHIN.,** ***cocc., kali-c., lach.,*** phos., ***rhus-t.,*** sep., stann., ***sulph.,*** zinc.
air, in open - nat-m.
alcoholics, in - ***ran-b., sul-ac.***
almonds, tasting like - ***caust., laur.***
alternating with, hiccough - agar., sep., wye.
with, yawning - berb., lyc.
ameliorated, from - acet-ac., ***acon.,*** aesc., agar., aloe, alum., all-c., ambr., am-m., **ANT-T., ARG-N.,** ars., ***aur., bar-c.,*** bar-i., berb., bry., cann-s., ***canth.,*** **CARB-S., CARB-V.,** ***chel.,*** cocc., coc-c., colch., coloc., cop., ***dig., dios., fl-ac.,*** **GRAPH.,** ***hydr.,*** **IGN.,** iod., **KALI-BI., KALI-C.,** ***kali-i.,*** kali-n., ***kali-s., lac-ac., lach.,*** **LYC.,** mag-c., mag-m., mosch., ***nat-c.,*** nat-m., ***nit-ac., nux-v.,*** op., par., petr., ph-ac., phos., ***pic-ac., plat.,*** rumx., **SANG.,** ***seneg., sep., sil., sulph.,*** sul-ac., ***tarent.,*** ter., zinc.
apples, tasting of - agar.
apyrexia, during - ant-c.
asthma, with - ambr.
astringent - merc-c.
beer, after - aur., ferr., sulph.
bitter - acet-ac., aesc., ***aloe, alum., ambr., am-c., am-m.,*** ant-c., ant-t., ***apis,*** arg-m., arg-n., **ARN.,** ars., aur., bar-c., bar-m., bell., ***berb.,*** bism., ***bry., calc.,*** calc-i., calc-p., ***calc-s., cann-s.,*** carb-ac., carb-an., carb-s., ***carb-v., carl.,*** caul., cham., ***chel.,*** **CHIN.,** ***chin-a.,*** chin-s., ***chion.,*** cob., ***cocc.,*** coloc., corn., crot-t., cupr., ***dios.,*** dros., eup-per., ferr., ferr-ar., ferr-i., ***ferr-m.,*** ferr-p., fl-ac., ***grat.,*** graph., hell., hep., ***hydr.,*** hyos., hyper., ***ign.,*** indg., ip., kali-ar., kali-c., kali-i., kali-n., kali-p., kali-s., ***lac-c.,*** laur., ***lyc.,*** mag-c., mag-m., mag-s., ***merc., merc-i-r.,*** mur-ac., nat-c., nat-m., nat-n., nat-p., **NAT-S.,** nicc., ***nit-ac.,*** nit-m-ac., **NUX-V.,** op., ox-ac., petr., ***ph-ac.,*** phos., phys., ***pic-ac.,*** plb., **PODO.,** ptel., **PULS.,** raph., rhod., ***rob.,*** sabad., sabal., sal-ac., ***sars.,*** senec., ***sep.,*** sil., sin-a., spong., squil., ***stann.,*** staph., stict., stry., sul-ac., sulph., ***sul-ac.,*** tarent., tarax., teucr., thuj., tong., upa., verat., verat-v., verb., xero, zinc.
afternoon - am-m., kali-n.
almonds, like - tong.
anger, after - arn.
bread and butter, after - chin.
cough, after - sul-ac.
dinner, during - sars.
after - bar-c., fl-ac., sars., sul-ac.
amel. - ferr.
before - sars.
drinking, after - sars.
water, after - aloe, chin.
eating after - ars., bell., ***bry., chin.,*** cina, kali-p., kreos., lach., led., **LYC.,** ***nat-m., nat-s., sars., sep., stann.,*** thuj., verat.

BELCHING, general
bitter,
eating, amel. - am-m.
evening - bell., cast., dios., kali-n., ***puls.,*** sars.
milk soup, after - alum.
potatoes, after - ***alum.***
fasting, while - ***nux-v.***
fat food, after - ***ferr., ferr-m.***
food comes up - **LYC.,** ***nat-s.***
forenoon - am-m., ign., nat-c., nicc.
menses, during - ***sep.,*** sulph.
milk, after - sulph.
morning - am-m., calc-s., hyper., lyc., sars., sil.
breakfast, after - pic-ac., ***sep.***
coughing, after - sul-ac.
rising, on - cedr., sep.
night - calc-s., cast., chel., ***merc., nux-v.,*** ox-ac., **PULS.,** tong.
potatoes, after - ***alum.***
rich food, after - ferr., ***ferr-m.***
soup, after - sars.
sour food, after - mag-m., ph-ac.
stool, during - cham.
stooping, when - cast.
supper, after - zinc.
walking in open air, while - grat.
bitter-sour - chin., kali-c., mag-m., sars., sul-ac.
bitter-sweetish - plat.
bloody - merc-c., nux-v., phos., raph., ***sep.***
bread, after - bry., chin., crot-h., merc., nat-m.
and milk, after - zinc.
breakfast, during - ox-ac., zinc.
after - ars., calc-p., carb-ac., carb-v., cham., con., cycl., grat., hell., hyper., kali-br., phos., pic-ac., ***plat.,*** sars., sep., sulph., verat.
before - ***bov., ran-s.***
burning, (see Heartburn) - ***caust.,*** coff., crot-t., ferr., ***iod., lyc.***
butter, after eating - **CARB-V., PULS.**
cabbage, after - **MAG-C.**
chill, during - nux-v.
after - zinc.
chilliness, with - ***sil.***
choking, after - op.
chronic - alum.
coffee, after - ***caust., coca,*** cycl., ***puls.***
constant - ars., ***chel., con.,*** cupr., euph., graph., mur-ac., nat-c., nit-ac., sars., sulph.
convulsions, before - ***arg-n.,*** lach., nux-v., psor., sulph.
convulsive - ars-h., coc-c., ham., kali-bi., nux-v., phos., sang., til.
cool - cist.
coughing, after - **AMBR.,** arn., carb-v., chin., lob., rumx., **SANG.,** ***sul-ac.,*** verat.
daytime - bry., **IOD.,** petr.
desire for belching - mang., vario.
difficult - **ARG-N.,** ***con., graph., nux-v.***

BELCHING, general
dinner, during - grat., mag-m., ol-an., sars.
after - agar., aloe, am-c., ang., apis, ars., bar-c., carb-v., carl., coca, cycl., dig., fl-ac., ham., kreos., lach., lyc., mag-m., merc., nat-m., nicc., nit-ac., petr., rat., sars., sul-ac., ***sulph.,*** zinc.
amel. - mang.
before - ran-b.
rising from stooping, when - cast.
walking, while - mag-m.
drinking, after - aeth., aloe, anac., apis, arg-n., ars., bism., canth., ***carb-v.,*** coloc., crot-t., hyper., ***kali-c.,*** lyc., merc., mez., ***nat-m.,*** nux-v., rhus-t., ***sep.,*** tarax., zinc.
cold water - chin., mez., phos.
amel. - carl.
eating, while - alum., dulc., grat., merc., nat-c., nit-ac., olnd., phos., ***sars.***
after - acon., aesc., agar., all-s., ambr., am-m., ***anac.,*** ang., apis, **ARG-N.,** ars., asaf., ***bar-c.,*** bar-m., bell., berb., ***bry.,*** bufo, calc., calc-s., ***camph.,*** carb-an., **CARB-S.,** **CARB-V.,** card-m., ***caust.,*** cham., ***chin.,*** chin-a., cic., cina, ***colch.,*** coloc., com., con., cop., cycl., daph., dig., dulc., echi., **FERR.,** ferr-ar., ferr-i., ferr-p., grat., gymn., ham., ***hep.,*** hydr., kali-ar., kali-bi., ***kali-c.,*** kali-p., kali-s., ***kreos., lach.,*** lec., ***lyc.,*** merc., mur-ac., nat-a., ***nat-c.,*** **NAT-M.,** nat-p., ***nat-s., nit-ac., nux-m., nux-v.,*** onos., ***ox-ac.,*** petr., ph-ac., ***phos., pic-ac.,*** plat., ***podo.,*** **PULS.,** ***ran-s.,*** rat., rhus-t., ruta., sang., ***sars., sep., sil., spig., stann.,*** staph., **SULPH.,** tarax., thuj., ***verat., zinc.***
hour after - aeth.
immediately - mag-p.
amel. - am-m., sulph.
before - carb-v., croc., nit-ac., nux-v., plat., ran-b., ran-s., sel., sulph.
eggs, spoiled, like - acon., ***agar.,*** ant-t., **ARN.,** brom., bufo, coff., dios., elaps, kali-c., ***lyc.,*** mag-m., mag-s., med., petr., phos., plan., podo., ***psor.,*** ptel., rhus-t., ***sep.,*** stann., **SULPH.,** ***valer.***
evening - carl.
morning - stann.
on rising - **ARN.,** graph., mag-c., ***mag-s.,*** petr., sulph., valer.
on waking - valer.
night - ***ant-t.,*** mag-c., phos.
pregnancy, during - mag-c.
smelling like - ***cham.,*** elaps, elat., ferr., ***podo.,*** psor., rhus-t., sulph.
night - mag-c.
tasting like yolk of - apis.
empty - abies-n., acon., ***aesc., aeth.,*** **AGAR.,** all-c., aloe, alum., ***ambr.,*** am-br., **AM-C.,** am-m., anac., anan., **ANT-C.,** ant-t., **ARG-N.,** **ARN., ARS., ARS-I.,** arund., ***asaf., asar.,*** bapt., ***bar-c., bar-i.,*** bell., ***berb.,*** **BISM.,** bov., brom., ***bry.,*** cahin., ***calad., calc.,*** calc-s., camph., cann-i., **CANN-S.,** canth.,

BELCHING, general
empty - **CARB-AC.,** ***carb-an.,*** **CARB-S.,** **CARB-V.,** card-m., carl., ***casc.,*** cast., caul., **CAUST.,** ***cham., chel., chin.,*** chin-a., chin-s., chlol., cimx., cinnb., cist., clem., cob., ***cocc.,*** coc-c., coff., ***colch., coloc.,*** **CON.,** cop., corn., ***croc.,*** crot-t., ***daph., dios.,*** dulc., elat., erig., euph., eup-per., eupi., fago., ***ferr.,*** ferr-ar., ferr-i., ferr-p., fl-ac., gamb., gent-c., gins., ***glon.,*** gran., grat., ***guai.,*** gymn., ham., hell., helon., hep., ***hydr.,*** hyos., hyper., ign., indg., **IOD., IP.,** iris, jatr., ***kali-ar.,*** **KALI-BI.,** kali-c., kali-chl., **KALI-I.,** kali-p., kali-s., ***kalm., kreos., lac-c.,*** lac-d., ***lach.,*** lact., laur., ***lec.,*** led., lob., **LYC.,** mag-c., mag-m., mag-s., manc., mang., med., ***meny.,*** merc., merc-i-f., ***mez.,*** mill., mosch., myric., ***nat-a., nat-c.,*** nat-m., nat-p., nat-s., nicc., ***nit-ac.,*** nux-m., olnd., ol-an., ox-ac., pall., petr., ph-ac., ***phos.,*** phys., phyt., **PIC-AC.,** plan., ***plb.,*** podo., ptel., **PULS.,** ran-b., ran-s., raph., rhod., rhus-t., rumx., ruta., sabad., sabin., sang., sars., sec., senec., ***seneg.,*** sep., sil., sin-a., sol-n., spig., spong., squil., stann., staph., stront-c., stry., **SULPH.,** sul-ac., sumb., tab., tarax., **TARENT.,** thuj., til., ***valer., verat.,*** verat-v., verb., vinc., viol-t., xan., zinc., zing.
afternoon - aeth., ambr., ars., bar-c., ***carb-v.,*** crot-t., dios., hydr., hyper., iris, lyc., mag-m., nat-m., op., ox-ac.
5 p.m. - dios., hyper., ox-ac.
6 p.m. - iris.
coffee, after - nat-m.
while stomach is empty - op.
air, open, in - nat-m.
alternating with hiccough - agar.
beer, after - vinc.
breakfast, after - ars., grat., hell., sulph.
before - ***bov., ran-s.***
coldness, during - gamb.
cough, after - **AMBR., SANG.,** sul-ac., verat.
dinner, after - am-c., alum., ars., cact., cycl., lyc., mag-m., ***sulph.,*** zinc.
drinking, after - bism., carb-v., coloc., nat-m., rhus-t., tarax., vinc., zinc.
cold water - phos.
eating, after - ***acon.,*** ars., bry., calc., ***camph.,*** carb-an., card-m., coloc., cycl., grat., ***hydr.,*** nat-c., ***nat-m., ox-ac.,*** ph-ac., ***phos., plat., ran-s.,*** rhus-t., ***sep.,*** spig., **SULPH., VERAT.**
evening - abrot., am-c., coc-c., dios., hyper., rumx., sars., sulph., verat., zinc.
hiccough, during - sulph.
lying, while - verat.
fasting, while - plat., valer.
forenoon - cast-eq., colch., com., ***con.,*** hydr., ign., kali-c., myric., naja, par., ***pic-ac.,*** sars., zinc.
9 a.m. - com.
10 a.m. - cast-eq., ign.
11 a.m. - hydr.
headache, during - apis, ***calc.***
hysteria, during - mang.
menses, before - mang.

BELCHING, general
menstrual colic, during - mang.
mental exertion - ***hep.***
morning - alum., anac., bar-c., bov., bry., calc., cedr., cina, cob., coloc., con., croc., dios., kali-c., mag-c., nat-m., ***pic-ac., plat.,*** stann., ***sulph.,*** sul-ac.
7 a.m. - dios.
fasting, after - bov., cina, croc., nit-ac., ***plat.***
rising, on - cedr.
rising, on, after - nat-m.
waking, on - bar-c., calc.
nausea, during - arn., coc-c.
night - dios., dirc., mang., mur-ac., phys., phos., sumb., tanac.
7 p.m. - dios., phys.
9 p.m. until midnight - phos.
9 p.m. until midnight, while walking in open air - phos.
9:30 p.m. - dirc.
11 p.m. - sumb.
menses, before - mang.
noon - olnd., ox-ac.
eating, while - olnd.
rising up - coloc.
soup, after - carb-v., mag-c.
stool, after - bar-c.
sugar, from - raph.
supper, after - alum., lyc., sep.
waking, on - bar-c., calc., rumx.
evening - abrot., ***alum., ambr.,*** am-c., bell., calc., carb-v., ***caust.,*** coc-c., con., crot-h., cupr., cycl., dros., eupi., fl-ac., gels., grat., ham., hyper., kali-bi., mag-c., mez., phos., **PULS.,** ran-s., rhus-t., rumx., sars., sep., sil., sin-n., sol-t-ae., stram., sulph., verat., zinc., zing.
evening, eating, while - cham.
excitement - arg-n.
faintness, causing - ***arg-n.,*** ars., **CARB-V.,** chin., mosch., nux-m., nux-v., ph-ac.
fever, during - ant-c., cub., lach., ran-b.
farinaceous food, after - carb-v., lyc., nat-c., sulph.
fasting, while - acon., bov., cina, croc., ***nit-ac., nux-v.,*** plat., valer.
fats, after - ***caust.,*** chin., ***ferr.,*** ferr-m., nat-m., **PULS., SEP.,** thuj.
fever, during - cub., lach., ran-b.
fishy - carb-an.
fluid, (see water) - abies-n., agar., all-c., alum., anac., ant-c., ant-t., ars., aur-s., ***calc.,*** cann-s., carb-s., carl., caul., cham., chlol., coc-c., crot-h., cycl., dig., fago., form., gent-c., graph., gran., gymn., ham., hell., ***lac-ac.,*** lyc., mez., mosch., nicc., nux-v., ***plat.,*** plb., ptel., **PULS.,** raph., rhod., rob., ***sulph.,*** ust., verat., verb.
afternoon - valer.
4 p.m. - ***valer.***
coffee, after - puls.
dinner, after - cast.
eating, after - cina, staph.
forenoon - ***carl.***

BELCHING, general
fluids,
greenish - ars., graph.
morning - all-c., verat., verb.
breakfast, after - phos.
night - nux-v.
white bread, after - ***crot-h.***
painless, in diphtheria - carb-ac.
yellow - cic.
food, of, (see Regurgitation) - ***aesc.,*** aeth., ***alum.,*** am-m., ***ant-c., arg-n.,*** ars., ***arum-t.,*** asaf., ***bell., bry.,*** bufo, ***calc., calc-s.,*** camph., ***cham.,*** canth., carb-an., carb-s., ***carb-v., caust.,*** **CHIN.,** chin-a., coff., ***con., cop.,*** cycl., ***dig.,*** echi., **FERR.,** ferr-i., **FERR-P.,** glon., graph., ***hep.,*** ign., ***ip.,*** iris, kali-ar., ***kali-bi.,*** kali-c., kali-p., kali-s., kalm., ***lach.,*** lob., ***lyc.,*** mag-m., ***mag-p.,*** mang., ***merc., mez., mur-ac., nat-m.,*** nat-p., nit-ac., ***nux-v.,*** **PHOS., PH-AC.,** pic-ac., plat., plb., ***podo.,*** **PULS.,** quas., ran-b., rob., ***rhus-t.,*** sars., senec., spig., ***sulph.,*** sul-ac., tab., tell., teucr., thuj., ust., valer., verat.
tasting, like - aesc., aeth., agar., aloe, ambr., am-c., am-m., anan., **ANT-C.,** ***apis,*** arn., ars., arg-n., aur-s., bell., **BRY.,** ***calc.,*** camph., **CARB-AN.,** carb-v., carl., cast., **CAUST.,** cham., chel., **CHIN.,** cic., cocc., colch., ***con.,*** cop., croc., crot-h., cycl., echi., euphr., **FERR.,** ***ferr-ar., graph., grat.,*** ham., hep., ign., ***ip.,*** kali-bi., kali-c., kali-i., lac-ac., lach., laur., lyc., mag-m., mang., nat-a., nat-c., **NAT-M.,** nux-v., olnd., phel., ***phos.,*** phyt., plb., **PULS.,** ***ran-s.,*** rat., rhus-t., ***rumx.,*** ruta., sars., sep., ***sil.,*** sin-a., spig., squil., staph., still., ***sulph.,*** sumb., tab., tell., ***thuj.,*** til., trom., verat., zinc.
afternoon - coff., euphr., petr.
afternoon, 1 p.m. - chel.
afternoon, after dinner - canth., cina, sars., squil.
drinking water agg. - **APIS.**
morning - agar., mag-c.
smoking, while - thuj.
forenoon - agar., am-m., calc-p., carl., colch., hep., ign., mag-c., mag-m., myric., naja, nat-c., nicc., par., sars., sulph., zinc.
foul - acet-ac., anan., ant-c., ***ant-t.,*** **ARN.,** ars., **ASAF.,** asar., aur-m., ***berb., bism.,*** bufo, calc., calc-ar., calc-s., carb-an., carb-s., ***carb-v.,*** caust., cina, ***cocc.,*** con., cop., cub., ***dig., ferr.,*** ferr-ar., ferr-p., ***fl-ac., graph., hep.,*** hydr., ***kali-bi.,*** lact., merc., mosch., mur-ac., naja, nat-m., nat-s., nit-ac., nux-v., olnd., phos., ***plb., psor., puls.,*** raph., sang., sec., ***sep., sulph., sul-ac.,*** thuj., valer.
alcoholics, in - sul-ac.
evening - nat-s., phos., stram., thuj.
fat or rich food, after - **ASAF.,** ***caust.,*** nat-m., ***puls.***
forenoon - cocc.
milk, after - nat-m.
morning - ***nux-v.***
night - merc.

BELCHING, general

foul,

pastry or pork, after - ***puls.***

peaches, after - psor.

frequent - ambr.

frothy - alet., all-c., ***canth.,*** kreos., ***lach.,*** lyc., ***mag-m.***

morning - all-c.

white - mag-m.

garlic, like - aesc., **ASAF.,** ***mag-m.,*** mosch., sulph., sul-ac.

garlic, after a spasm - mag-m.

greasy - aesc., carb-v., ***cycl.,*** ferr-i., lyc., **MAG-C.,** ***puls.,*** zinc.

headache, with - apis, arg-n., ***calc.,*** camph., iod., **MAG-M.,** phos., sil.

headache, during - psor.

hiccough, like - ant-t., calc., ***cycl.,*** mez., plat., sars., sulph.

after - ars.

dinner, after - carb-an., plat.

hot - acet-ac., apis, ars., aur., canth., carb-v., ***caust.,*** cob., cop., ***hep.,*** kali-bi., ***lac-ac.,*** naja, ***petr., phos.,*** phys., ***podo.,*** puls., sil., sin-a., zinc.

eating, after - hep., ***podo.***

morning - tab.

ineffectual, and incomplete - acon., agar., alum., ambr., am-c., anac., ang., ***arg-n.,*** arn., ***ars.,*** arund., asar., bar-c., ***bell.,*** calad., canth., carb-ac., carb-an., carb-s., ***carl., caust.,*** chel., **CHIN.,** ***cocc.,*** con., cycl., ferr., ferr-ar., ferr-m., **GRAPH.,** grat., hyos., indg., kali-c., kali-p., ***lach.,*** laur., ***lyc.,*** mag-c., ***manc.,*** **MED.,** mez., mur-ac., **NAT-M.,** nux-v., petr., phel., ph-ac., ***phos., phyt.,*** pic-ac., plat., plb., ***puls.,*** rhus-t., sabad., sars., spig., sulph., sul-ac., zinc., zing.

evening - dios.

forenoon - sil.

morning - ol-an.

after breakfast - con.

night - caust., sulph.

before menses - mang.

on going to bed - sulph.

large, quantities of wind - **ARG-N.,** asaf., bapt., ***carb-v., hep., lyc., phos.***

labor pains, during - bor.

lead, tastes like - sulph.

lime, water, tasting like - kali-c.

long, continued - glon., sul-ac.

loud - ***abies-n.,*** acet-ac., acon., agar., alum., ambr., ***anac.,*** ant-c., **ARG-N.,** arn., **ASAF.,** ***bism.,*** bor., ***bry., caj., calc.,*** calc-p., caps., carb-ac., carb-an., carb-s., ***carb-v.,*** caust., cham., ***chin., coca, coloc.,*** com., con., ***cycl., dios.,*** fago., ferr-i., ferr-m., ferr-p., glyc., gran., ***graph.,*** grat., ***hep.,*** hydr., ind., ***iod.,*** ip., iris, jug-c., jug-r., kali-bi., ***kali-c.,*** kali-n., lach., lact., ***lyc.,*** mag-c., manc., merc., ***merc-i-r.,*** mosch., ***nat-c.,*** nat-m., nat-p., nit-ac., ***nux-m., nux-v.,*** petr., ***phos.,*** **PLAT.,** plb., podo., ***puls., rob.,*** rumx., sal-ac., sang., ***sep., sil.,*** sin-n., sul-ac., sulph., sumb., tab., til., upa., uran-n.,

BELCHING, general

loud - valer., verat., verb., zinc.

afternoon - carb-s.

eating, after - calc., plat., tab.

fasting, while - **PLAT.**

involuntary - asaf.

milk, after - sulph.

stooping, when - manc.

uncontrollable - ***sil.***

lying, agg. - verat.

amel. - aeth., rhus-t.

meat, after - carb-an., ruta.

tasting of - mez., zinc.

spoiled meat - **PULS.**

menses, during - ant-t., ars., carb-an., ***graph.,*** kali-c., kali-i., **LACH.,** lyc., ***nit-ac., sep.,*** sulph., vib.

before - bry., chin., ***kali-c.,*** kreos., lach., mag-c., mang., ***nat-m., nux-m.,*** phos., ***puls.***

mental, exertion - hep.

milk, after - alum., am-c., ant-t., ***calc.,*** carb-ac., carb-s., ***carb-v., chin., cupr.,*** iris, lyc., ***mag-c., nat-m.,*** nat-s., petr., phos., ***sulph., zinc.***

milk, of - ant-t., calc., carb-ac., carb-v., lyc., sulph., zinc.

afternoon - zinc.

walking, while - mag-m.

morning - all-c., anac., arg-n., arn., aster., bar-c., bry., calc., calc-s., cob., coloc., ***con.,*** croc., dulc., hep., hyper., ***kali-c., kalm.,*** lyc., mag-c., mang., nat-m., nit-ac., nux-v., **PETR.,** plat., puls., sars., sil., stann., ***sulph.,*** sul-ac., tab., thuj., valer., verat.

breakfast, before - ***bov., ran-s.***

rising, on - cedr., nicc., ruta., sep., sin-a., verat.

after - led.

stool, after - cob.

waking, on - bar-c., calc.

motion, on - cann-i., kreos.

mouldy - ign.

mouthful, by - ferr., ***phos.***

mucus - aesc., alum., ***arn.,*** ars., bry., calc., ***canth.,*** carb-v., coca, cupr., graph., hydr., hyper., ***kali-c., lach.,*** lyc., mag-s., ***phos.,*** puls., raph., sabad., staph., sul-ac., sulph., verat.

evening - bry., hyper.

frothy - sep.

morning - all-c., bry., graph., hyper.

coughing, after - sul-ac.

mouthful - carb-v.

mucus like - sulph.

throat, from - staph.

musk, tasting of - ***caust.,*** sumb.

nauseous - am-m., ant-t., calc., carb-s., ***carb-v.,*** chin., fl-ac., ***graph.,*** grat., helon., kali-br., nat-m., ol-an., onos., par., ptel., ***PULS., sep.,*** verat., verb., zinc., zing.

nauseous, after rich food - nat-m., sep.

BELCHING, general

night - ant-t., calc., calc-s., canth., ***carb-v.,*** chel., ***crot-h.,*** ham., ***kali-c.,*** lyc., mang., ***merc.,*** mur-ac., ***nux-v.,*** ox-ac., phos., pip-m., **PULS.,** sulph., tanac., ther.
- 9 p.m. until midnight - phos.
- first, half of - nit-ac.
- lying, while - calc.
- midnight on waking - ferr.
- sleep, during - sulph.
- waking, on - calc., mur-ac., sil.

noon - indg., ox-ac., ran-b.
- eating, while - olnd.

nose, through - lyc., merc-c., phos.

olive oil, odor - phos.

oranges, like - phos.

oysters, after - bry.

painful - acon., anan., ant-c., ***bry., carb-an.,*** caust., **CHAM.,** chin., coca, cocc., con., lob., nat-c., nicc., ***nux-v.,*** ox-ac., ***par.,*** petr., phos., plb., sabad., sep.

paroxysmal - ***arg-n.,*** bell., coff., lyss., ***nat-m.,*** petr., **PHOS.,** sang., sep., sulph.

peaches, after - psor.

periodical - aesc., ip.

pork, after - psor.

potatoes, after - ***alum.,*** gran.

pressing, on, painful parts, when - ***bor.***
- stomach, from - ***sulph.***

pungent - sabad.
- pungent, coughing, on - caps.

putrid - ***acet-ac., arn.,*** asar., aur-m., bell., cocc., graph., mag-s., merc., mur-ac., nux-v., olnd., ***psor.,*** puls., sep., sulph., tab., thuj., ***valer.***

radishes, after - osm.

rancid - aeth., alum., ***arn.,*** **ASAF.,** bar-c., bism., cadm-s., ***calc.,*** calc-i., carb-s., ***carb-v., cham., croc., cycl.,*** dios., ferr-i., ***graph.,*** grat., hydr., kali-bi., ***kali-c.,*** laur., mag-m., ***mag-s.,*** merc., mez., nux-m., ornithog., phos., plumbg., ***psor.,*** **PULS.,** ran-s., raph., rhod., sabad., sang., sanic., ***sep.,*** sulph., ter., thuj., ***valer.,*** xero.
- afternoon - crot-h.
- dinner, during - alum.
- eating, after - ***graph.***
- evening - ran-s.
  - 4 p.m. - ***valer.***
  - after eating - mez.
- morning, after soup - alum.
- night - ***merc.***
- rich food, after - thuj.
- tallow, like - **PULS.**

regurgitation, (see Regurgitation)

rich, food, after - ***bry.,*** **CARB-V.,** ferr., nat-m., **PULS.,** ***sep.,*** staph., thuj.

rising, from lying, when - rhus-t.
- rising, up, on - arg-n., coloc.

salty - agar., arn., ant-t., cadm-s., ***carb-an.,*** caust., cham., ***kali-c.,*** lyc., mag-m., nux-v., sep., sil., staph., sul-ac.
- vomiting, before - sul-ac.

BELCHING, general

sardines, after - eupi.

scratchy - sulph.

shooting, pain, with - bry.

sitting, while - gels., phos.
- bent, while - rob., sabin.

sleep, after - hep.
- amel. - chel., chin.

smoking, while - agar., ***lac-ac.,*** thuj.
- after - sel.

sneezing, with - ham., lob., mag-c., phos.

sobbing - ant-t., bell., chin., coloc., cycl., meph., staph.

stomach, pain in with - ***ars.,*** **BISM.,** ***coll., nux-v.,*** puls., sang., **SULPH.**

soup, after - alum., anac., carb-v., mag-c.

sour - abrot., ***acet-ac.,*** aesc., agar., ail., ***all-c.,*** aloe, ***alum., ambr.,*** am-c., am-m., ant-t., ***bry.,*** bufo, cact., ***cadm-s.,*** **CALC.,** ***calc-p., calc-s.,*** cann-s., ***canth., carb-ac., carb-an., carb-s.,*** **CARB-V.,** caul., ***caust., cham., chel.,*** chlol., **CHIN.,** ***chin-a., chion., cimx.,*** cina, cob., ***cocc.,*** coff., coloc., com., ***con.,*** cop., crot-h., cub., cupr-ac., ***cycl., dig., dios.,*** dros., echi., elaps, ***ferr., ferr-ar., ferr-i., ferr-m., ferr-p.,*** fl-ac., form., ***gels.,*** gent-c., gins., ***graph.,*** guare., gymn., ***hep., hydr.,*** hydrc., hyos., **IGN.,** indg., ***iod.,*** **IRIS,** kali-ar., **KALI-BI.,** ***kali-c.,*** kali-chl., kali-n., kali-p., **KALI-S.,** ***kreos.,*** lac-ac., ***lac-d., lach.,*** laur., lept., **LITH.,** ***lob.,*** **LYC., MAG-C.,** mang., mez., **NAT-A., NAT-C., NAT-M., NAT-P., NAT-S.,** nicc., ***nit-ac.,*** **NUX-V.,** ***op.,*** ox-ac., pall., ***petr., ph-ac.,*** **PHOS.,** phyt., pic-ac., pip-m., plb., ***podo., psor.,*** ptel., ***puls.,*** ran-s., **ROB.,** sabad., sabin., sanic., sec., senec., ***sep., sil.,*** sol-t-ae., spig., spong., squil., stann., staph., stram., **SULPH., SUL-AC.,** tab., thuj., ust., verat, verat-v., ***zinc.,*** zing.
- afternoon - ammc., am-m., carb-s., fl-ac., kali-c., lyss., ***nat-c.,*** podo., sars.
  - after dinner - nat-m.
- alcoholics, in - ***sul-ac.***
- bread, after - crot-h., ***hydr.,*** merc., zinc.
- breakfast, during - ox-ac.
  - after - petr., sars.
- cabbage, after - **MAG-C.**
- coffee, after - ***cycl., puls.***
- cough, after - raph., sul-ac.
- daytime - ***nux-v.,*** **SULPH.**
- dinner, after - ars., fl-ac., lyc., mag-m., petr., rumx., ***sulph.,*** sumb., ***zinc.***
- drinking, after - canth., zinc.
  - water, after - psor.
- eating, after - bar-c., ***bry.,*** caps., carb-v., cham., chin., cina, ***con.,*** dig., dios., ***ferr.,*** ferr-m., ***hydr.,*** kali-c., kali-s., kreos., lyc., ***nat-a.,*** **NAT-M.,** ***nit-ac.,*** petr., ph-ac., ***phos.,*** podo., puls-n, sabin., sars., ***sil.,*** sulph., zinc.
  - 1 to 3 hours after - ***puls.***
  - 2 hours after - com.

BELCHING, general
sour,
evening - calc., chin-s., con., dios., nat-m., ox-ac., phos., ran-s., sars., sil.
air, open, in - carb-v.
bed, in - ***alum.***
eating, after - stann.
fluid - nat-m.
farinaceous food, after - ***caust., nux-v.***
fat food - ***caust., nit-ac., rob.***
forenoon - agar., alum., nicc.
fruit, after - **CHIN.**
headache, with - pall., pic-ac.
hypochlorhydria, alternating, with hyperchlorhydria - chin-a.
intermittents, in - ***lyc.***
lying on the back, while - carb-v.
menses, during - ***mag-c.***
before - ***kali-c.***
milk, after - am-c., ***calc., carb-v., chin.,*** iris, ***lyc., mag-c.,*** merc., ***nux-v.,*** phos., ***sulph.,*** zinc.
morning - calc., kali-c., ***puls.,*** sil., tab., tarent.
after rising - mag-m.
after walking - nux-v.
nausea, during - gamb.
night - calc-s., ***con.,*** kali-c., lyc., ***nux-v.,*** tanac.
pregnancy, during - nux-v.
rich food, after - chin., sulph., zinc.
sitting bent, while - ***rob.,*** sabin.
sugar, after - ***caust.,*** sulph.
supper, after - sep.
vertigo, during - sars.
waking, on - rumx.
walking, while - carb-v.
in open air - stann., sulph., sul-ac.
stool, during - cham., con., dulc., ***kali-c., merc., puls.,*** ruta.
after - aesc., anac., ***ars.,*** bar-c., ***calc-s.,*** cob., ***coloc.,*** merc., sil.
before - sumb.
stooping, on - cic., ip., phos.
sudden - ***carb-an.***
supper, after - alum., ***carb-v.,*** chin-s., ferr., ham., lyc., sars., sep., sil., zinc.
suppressed - **AM-C.,** ***calc., con.***
followed by pain in stomach - ***con.***
swallowing, air after - spig.
swallowing, when - agar.
sweetish - acon., alum., bar-c., carb-v., dulc., grat., ind., lachn., merc., plat., ***plb.,*** sulph., ***sul-ac.,*** zinc.
fluid - ***acon.,*** bar-c., ***iris,*** lachn., ***plb.***
menses, before - ***nat-m.***
morning - alum., sulph., sul-ac.
pregnancy, during - nat-m., ***zinc.***
water - ***plb.***
sweets, after - **ARG-N.,** ***caust.,*** raph., zinc.
tallow, tasting of rancid - **PULS.**
tobacco, from - ***sel.***
urination, during - rhus-t.
urinous - agn., ol-an., phos., verat.

BELCHING, general
vexation, after - ferr-p., petr.
vomiting, when - phos., phyt.
violent - **ARG-N.,** chin., graph., phos., verat.
vomiting, when - phos., phyt.
after - arg-n., ars., caust., con., sulph.
followed by - sulph.
waking, on - bar-c., calc., con., ferr., mur-ac., puls., rumx., sil.
walking, while - caps., carb-s., ***graph.,*** lyc., lycps., ***mag-m.,*** sulph.
air, in open, while - grat., phos., stann., sulph., sul-ac.
amel. - lyc.
water, of - acon., ant-c., ant-t., arn., ars., bar-c., bry., cann-i., carl., cast., caust., cob., ***colch.,*** crot-t., ***graph.,*** grat., kali-n., ***mag-m.,*** mag-s., ***merc., merc-c., mez.,*** nat-s., ol-an., phos., plat., ***plb.,*** sil., stann., ***sulph.,*** sul-ac., verat.
afternoon - am-m., kali-n.
drinking, after - graph.
eating, after - graph.
evening - kali-n., sars.
forenoon - nicc.
green - graph.
morning - graph.
nausea, during - ***mag-m.,*** mag-s.
rising, after - carb-an., mag-m.
motion, on - mez.
nausea, during - gamb., kali-n., **MERC.**
night - mang., **MERC.**
before menses - mang.
potatoes, after - mag-s.
sitting, while - phos.
urinous - agn.
water-brash - acet-ac., acon., aesc., alum., ***alumn.,*** ambr., ***am-c., am-m.,*** anac., ant-c., ***ant-t., apis,*** arn., **ARS.,** ars-i., asar., **BAR-C.,** ***bar-i.,*** bar-m., bell., ***bism.,*** bov., **BRY., CALC.,** ***calc-p., calc-s.,*** cann-s., canth., ***caps., carb-an.,*** carb-s., **CARB-V.,** ***caust.,*** chel., ***chin.,*** chin-a., ***cic., cina,*** cob., ***cocc.,*** colch., con., croc., cupr., cur., cycl., ***daph.,*** dig., ***dros.,*** dulc., euph., ferr., ferr-ar., ferr-i., ferr-p., ***graph.,*** grat., hell., ***hep., ign.,*** iod., ***ip.,*** kali-ar., ***kali-bi., kali-c.,*** kali-p., kali-s., lach., ***lac-ac.,*** laur., ***led.,*** lil-t., ***lob.,*** **LYC.,** mag-c., ***mag-m.,*** mang., meny., ***merc.,*** **MEZ.,** mosch., mur-ac., ***nat-a., nat-c., nat-m.,*** nat-p., ***nat-s., nit-ac.,*** nux-m., **NUX-V.,** olnd., **PAR., PETR.,** ph-ac., ***phos.,*** phys., pic-ac., plat., plb., podo., psor., **PULS.,** ***ran-b.,*** ran-s., rat., ***rhod., rhus-t.,*** **SABAD.,** sabin., **SANG.,** ***sars.,*** sec., seneg., ***sep.,*** **SIL.,** spig., spong., squil., stann., **STAPH., SULPH.,** ***sul-ac.,*** tab., tarax., ter., thea., thuj., valer., **VERAT.,** verb., zinc.
acids, after - phos.
afternoon - sep.
4 p.m. - ars.
while walking - nat-s.
alternating days - lyc.

BELCHING, general
water-brash
bitter - am-m., arg-m., arg-n., bar-c., calc., chel., cic., coloc., graph., grat., ign., lach., lyc., mang., merc., nat-c., ***nux-v.,*** phos., rhod., sulph., sul-ac., valer., zinc.
sour, and, with stomach pain - kreos.
breakfast, after - petr.
burning - sumb.
chilliness, with - sil.
colic, with - nux-v.
convulsions, before - hydr-ac.
cool water - caust., verat.
coryza, with - nit-ac.
cough, after - abies-n.
coughing, when - am-m., ars.
dinner after - am-m.
before - sulph.
drinking, after - nit-ac., sep.
eating, after - am-c., am-m., ***bry., calc.,*** chin., con., croc., ferr., ***kali-c.,*** lyc., merc., nat-m., ***nux-v.,*** phos., sang., ***sep., sil., sulph.***
amel. - sep., sulph.
evening - anac., caust., cycl., nat-s., podo., still., sulph., ter.
fasting agg. - grat.
hawking, when - sulph.
headache, with - mag-m.
heat of body, with - cic.
lying, while - caust., ***psor.***
meat, fresh - ***caust.***
menses, during - puls.
before - ***nux-m., puls.***
milk, after - ***calc., cupr.,*** phos.
morning - mag-m., sulph.
rinsing mouth - sulph.
night - carb-an., ***carb-v.,*** genist., graph., kali-c.
menses, during - ***puls.***
midnight after - kali-c.
noon, after eating - sulph.
periodical, every other day - hep., lyc.
same hour - hep.
pregnancy, during - acet-ac., dios., ***lac-ac.,*** lob., lyc., ***nat-m., nux-m., tab.***
riding, in a carriage - ***nux-m.***
salty - carb-an., caust.
sensation of - kali-i.
sour food, after - phos.
stool, after - caust.
strong food, after - ***mag-c.***
sudden - bar-c.
supper, after - am-m.
sweetish - ant-c.
tobacco amel. - ol-an.
tongue, with brown - sil.
wine, after - lyc.

BITTER, as if something, in stomach - cupr.

BLOWS, in pit of, sensation of - crot-c., nat-c., nux-v., plat.

BUBBLING - caust., lyc., lyss., rheum, phos.
bubbling, sensation, esophagus, in - chel.

BURNING, pain (see Heartburn) - abies-c., abrot., acet-ac., acon., ***aesc.,*** aeth., agar., ail., all-s., alum., alumn., ambr., am-c., am-m., ***anthr.,*** ant-c., ant-t., ***apis,*** apoc., arg-m., arg-n., arn., **ARS.,** ***ars-h., ars-i.,*** asaf., asc-t., aur., aur-m., bapt., ***bell., benz-ac., berb., bism.,*** bol., brom., ***bry.,*** bufo, cact., ***cadm-s., calad.,*** calc., ***calc-p.,*** calc-s., ***camph.,*** cann-i., **CANTH., CAPS.,** ***carb-ac., carb-an.,*** carb-s., **CARB-V.,** ***card-m.,*** caul., caust., cedr., ***cham.,*** chel., chin., chin-a., chin-s., chlf., chr-ac., **CIC.,** cimic., cocc., coc-c., coff., **COLCH.,** ***coloc., con.,*** cop., ***corn.,*** croc., crot-h., ***crot-t.,*** cub., cund., ***cupr., cupr-ar., dig., dios., dulc.,*** elaps, ***erig., euph.,*** ferr., ferr-ar., ferr-i., ferr-p., fl-ac., ***form.,*** gels., gent-c., gran., ***graph.,*** grat., guai., gymn., ham., hell., helon., ***hep.,*** hura, ***hydr.,*** hyos., ***ign.,*** indg., iod., ***iris,*** jab., ***jatr.,*** jug-c., jug-r., ***kali-ar.,*** kali-bi., kali-br., ***kali-c., kali-i., kali-n.,*** kali-p., kali-s., ***kreos.,*** lac-ac., ***lac-c.,*** lach., lact., ***laur.,*** lec., ***lept., lob., lyc.,*** manc., mang., med., ***merc., merc-c.,*** merc-i-f., ***mez., mill.,*** mosch., mur-ac., myric., ***nat-a.,*** nat-c., ***nat-m.,*** nat-s., nicc., ***nit-ac., nux-m., nux-v.,*** ol-an., ***ox-ac.,*** paeon., par., petr., ph-ac., **PHOS.,** phyt., plat., plb., ***ptel.,*** puls., ***ran-b., ran-s.,*** raph., rhus-t., rob., rumx., ruta., ***sabad., sabin., sang.,*** sars., **SEC.,** seneg., ***sep., sil.,*** sin-n., sol-n., ***stram., stry.,*** **SULPH.,** ***sul-ac.,*** tab., ***tarent., ter.,*** thuj., til., ***uran.,*** ust., valer., verat., verat-v., ***zinc.***
afternoon - alum., am-m., bar-c., iris, kali-bi., lyss.
after stool - fago.
alcoholics, in - ***sul-ac.***
belching, after - ***calc-p.,*** kali-c., sep., sol-n.
amel. - ***ambr.,*** ferr.
bending forward - bry.
bread, after - sars.
breakfast, during - apoc.
after - agar., caps., dig., lyc., podo., sabad., sol-n.
amel. - ***kali-bi., nat-s.,*** zinc.
chilliness, during - sang.
circumscribed - gymn.
cold drinks, after - ***ars., ars-s-r.,*** lept., ***plb., rhus-t.***
amel. - apis
cold, from a - sep.
cough, during - hep.
digestion, during - kali-i.
dinner, after - lyc., podo., zinc.
amel. - aesc.
drinking after - kali-c., ***lach., led.,*** lept., merc-c., rhus-t.
eating, after - arg-n., ars., bufo, ***caps., calc., carb-an., carb-v., daph.,*** dios., euph., graph., kali-ar., kali-bi., ***kali-c.,*** kali-i., kreos., ***lach.,*** mez., tarent.
amel. - aesc., ***graph., mez.,*** nat-s.
some hours after - agar., ***nat-m.,*** phos., ***plb.***
evening - abrot., calad., dios., ferr-i., iris, sang., sulph., verat., zinc.
8 p.m. - calc-p.
9 p.m. - lyc.

BURNING, pain
extending, to,
axilla, right - am-m.
back - ***carb-v.***
chest - arg-m., aeth., mang., mill., ol-an., ***phos.***
downward - nux-v.
larynx - kali-c.
left - ph-ac.
mouth - ***acon.,*** caps., cupr-ac., ***gels.,*** kali-bi., kali-c.
palate - mang.
throat - am-m., anac., ars., berb., ***carb-v.,*** cupr., hep., kali-bi., ***kali-c., lac-ac., lyc., nat-m.,*** phos., sang., tep.
throat, after eating - ***calc., kali-c.***
throat, pit, in - sabad.
up the esophagus - dig., hell., ox-ac., sabad., zinc.
upward - arg-n., ***calc.,*** dig., hell., mang., nux-m., nux-v., ox-ac., sabad., ***sec.,*** sep., sol-n., sulph., tril., verat., zinc.
fasting, while - graph., zinc.
fever, during - ***ars., lach.,*** nux-v., sep.
fish, on eating in evening - thuj.
forenoon - carb-s., kali-c.
fright, after - ***acon.***
headache, during - ***sang.***
inspiration - bry.
lying down, on - puls., sang.
on abdomen amel. - acet-ac.
menses, during - tarent.
morning - arg-n., ***dios.,*** hyper., ***kali-bi.,*** merc., nat-s., ***sulph.,*** zinc.
motion, on - ***bry.,*** kali-bi., thuj.
of child in utero - ars.
night - ***abrot., ars., ars-s-r.,*** kali-c., paeon., podo., sulph.
midnight, after - sil.
waking, on - hyper.
noon - nicc.
paroxysmal - ***bry.,*** mez., ***nat-m.,*** plb.
periodical - graph., sulph.
pressure agg. - kali-c., kali-n., mez., phos., zinc.
reading, while - arg-m.
rising amel. - sulph.
sitting, while - calc.
standing, while - arg-m., ***sulph.***
stool, after - ***calc-p., carb-s.,*** sol-n.
amel. - crot-h., sulph.
before - fl-ac.
sudden - nit-ac., sul-ac.
supper, after - ***carl.***
tea, after - calad.
upper arm, to right - am-m.
vomiting, when - bar-m., jatr., sul-ac.
amel. - ars., tarent.
waking, after - hyper., sabad., sulph.
walking, while - aesc., bell., sulph.
warm drinks amel. - ***ars.***
warm things, after - nat-a.

burning, esophagus - ***acon.,*** aesc., aeth., agar., ***alumn.,*** ammc., ***am-c.,*** ant-t., ***arn., ars.,*** arund., ***asaf., aster.,*** bell., bov., brom., cahin., camph., cann-i., canth., ***carb-ac.,*** carb-s., cedr., chel., chin-s., ***cocc.,*** coc-c., con., cupr-ar., ***cycl.,*** dig., ***euph.,*** gels., gymn., ***hep.,*** hydrc., iod., kali-i., kreos., lac-ac., laur., lyc., manc., merc., **MERC-C.,** ***mez.,*** mur-ac., nat-m., ***nit-ac.,*** nux-v., ***ol-an.,*** ox-ac., petr., ***phos., phyt., plb.,*** ran-s., raph., sabad., sars., **SANG.,** seneg., stry., ***sul-ac., tarent.,*** ust., verat., verat-v., zinc.
afternoon - nux-m.
belching, from - aeth., calc-ar., ol-an.
drinking, while - calc-caust., canth., mez.
eating, after - con., tarent.
some hours later - ***plb.***
evening - sin-a.
extending, to stomach - acon., ars., euph., ***gels.,*** iris, kali-bi., lyc., nit-ac., sul-ac.
upward - ***cocc.,*** crot-t., mez.
forenoon - carb-s.
morning - cupr-s.
noon - rhus-t.
pressure, on - **MERC-C.**
prickling - hydrc.
swallowing, when - **ARS.,** carb-s., ox-ac.
water - calc-caust., mez.

BURSTING, pain - kali-c.

CANCER - ***acet-ac.,*** am-m., arg-n., **ARS.,** ***ars-i.,*** bar-c., bell., **BISM., CADM-S.,** calc-f., ***caps.,*** **CARB-AC., CARB-AN.,** ***carb-v.,*** **CON.,** ***crot-h.,*** **CUND.,** form-ac., graph., **HYDR.,** ***iris,*** kali-bi., kali-c., ***kreos., lach.,*** **LYC.,** mag-p., ***merc-c., mez.,*** nux-v., ***ornithog.,*** **PHOS.,** plat., plb., sec., ***sep., sil., staph., sulph.***
pylorus - acet-ac., graph.

CHOKING, esophagus, (see Throat) - acon., ***aesc.,*** agar., ***alum., alumn.,*** anac., ***arg-m., ars., bell.,*** **CACT.,** cadm-s., ***calc.,*** canth., ***carb-ac.,*** cham., chel., chin., ***cic., cimx.,*** cocc., ***coch.,*** crot-c., ***cupr.,*** dig., dros., ***hyos.,*** **IGN.,** iod., **KALI-C.,** kali-chl., lob., lyc., lyss., **MERC-C.,** naja, ***nat-a., nat-m.,*** nit-ac., ox-ac., ***phos., plb., sabad.,*** stram., sul-ac., zinc.
below upwards - ***lob., plb.***
inspiration, on - zinc.
morning on waking - alum.
night - alum.
pressure in larynx, from - chel.
swallowing - ***alum.,*** zinc.
fluids - hyos., ***manc.***
solids - caj.

CHURNING - lyc.

CIGAR-makers, affections in - ign.

CLAWING, pain - anan., arn., calc., ***carb-an.,*** carb-v., **CAUST.,** ***cocc., graph.,*** lyc., ***nat-m.,*** nit-ac., **NUX-V.,** petr., puls., rhod., sil., ***stann.,*** sulph., ***sul-ac.,*** tab., zinc-m.
breakfast amel. - puls.
eating, after - tab.
evening - petr., sul-ac.

CLAWING, pain
morning - petr., puls.
on waking - sulph.
rising from bed - puls.

CLOTHING, disturbs - am-c., **BOV.,** ***bry., calc.,*** carb-v., caust., ***chin.,*** coff., ***crot-c., crot-h.,*** cupr., gins., ***graph., hep., kali-bi.,*** kreos., **LACH.,** lith., **LYC.,** ***nat-s.,*** **NUX-V.,** ***petr., ph-ac., puls.,*** spong., sulph.
amel. - cupr., nat-m.

CLUCKING, sound - am-c., anac., carb-an., mag-m., phos., rheum.
eating, after - zinc.

clucking, sound, esophagus - ***cina.***

COLDNESS - abrot., absin., acon., agar., alum., ***ambr.,*** am-c., arg-n., **ARS.,** arund., bar-c., ***bell.,*** berb., bol., bov., cadm-s., cahin., ***calc.,*** **CAMPH.,** cann-s., **CAPS.,** ***carb-an.,*** carb-s., ***carb-v., cast.,*** cham., chel., **CHIN.,** chin-a., chin-s., ***cist.,*** clem., coc-c., ***colch.,*** coloc., con., crot-c., crot-h., elaps, graph., grat., helon., ***hipp.,*** ign., kali-ar., ***kali-bi.,*** kali-c., kali-i., kali-n., kali-p., kali-s., ***kreos., lach., lact.,*** laur., lyss., mag-c., mag-s., ***nat-m.,*** nit-ac., ol-an., op., ***petr.,*** ph-ac., ***phos.,*** phyt., rhus-t., sabad., sec., sep., ***sil.,*** spig., spong., sulph., ***sul-ac.,*** tab., ***tarax.,*** verat., vesp.
alternating with heat - phos.
chilliness, in pit of - **ARS.,** bell., calc., cist., hipp.
cold drinks, after - ***ars.,*** **CHIN., ELAPS,** ***rhus-t., sul-ac.***
water, as from - caps., grat.
diarrhea during - nat-m., ptel.
eating, after - ***carb-an., cist., crot-c.,*** nit-ac.
before - ***cist.***
evening - alum., nat-m.
amel., in bed - kali-n
extending to body - sec.
to esophagus - meny.
forenoon - nat-m.
belching, during and after - alum.
riding, while - puls.
fruit, after - ***ars.,*** elaps
heat, after - grat.
ice cream, after - chin-s.
ice, like, after cold drinks - **ELAPS.**
pain, with - ***bov.,*** caust., ***colch.,*** ol-an.
icy - acon., **CAPS.,** caust., ***colch., hipp.,*** lachn., lact., ***phos.***
extending to esophagus - meny.
lump - bov.
pain, with - colch.
perspiration, with - zinc-i.
rubbing and pressure amel. - carb-an.
loosening clothing amel. - chin-s.
menses, after - kali-c.
morning, in bed - bov., con., mag-s.
noon - zinc.
stone, as of a cold - acon.
warm applications amel. - sul-ac.
water drinking, after - sul-ac.

coldness, esophagus - acon., agar., anan., cahin., lact., lyss., ***meny.***
hot, and or coldness, ascending - all-s.
icy - anan.

CONSTRICTION - ***aesc., agar., alum.,*** am-c., anan., ***arg-n., ars.,*** asaf., ***bell.,*** bor., cact., calc., calc-s., carb-s., carc., caul., **CHEL.,** chin-s., clem., ***cocc.,*** colch., ***coloc., con.,*** crot-h., crot-t., dig., dros., elat., ***euph., ferr., ferr-ar.,*** gent-l., **GRAPH.,** ***guai.,*** **GUARE.,** ign., hyos., ***kali-bi.,*** kali-c., kali-n., kreos., lach., lact., laur., ***lyc., mag-c.,*** mag-m., ***manc.,*** meny., merc., merc-c., merc-i-f., ***mez.,*** morph., mur-ac., nat-a., ***nat-c.,*** nat-m., nux-v., ol-an., olnd., ***op.,*** petr., phos., pip-m., plat., plb., ran-s., rat., rhod., rob., sang., sars., sec., sep., sil., spig., stront-c., sulph., ***sul-ac.,*** tell., thea., thuj., tub., zinc.
afternoon - bar-c.
afternoon, 4 p.m. - bry.
belching amel. - sep.
cardiac orifice - euph.
paroxysmal - nat-m.
on swallowing - all-c., led., ***phos.***
convulsion, before - ***aesc.***
convulsive - apoc-a., cham., kali-c., nat-m., nit-ac., sec.
dinner, after - gamb., nat-c.
eating, after - tab.
amel. - rat., ***sep., thuj.***
evening - nat-m., rat., zinc.
extending to, chest - alum., sep.
to, liver - dig.
to, pharynx - plb.
to, spine - bor.
to, throat - alum., kali-c.
fasting, when - carl.
fluid passing through intestines, as if, with - meli.
forenoon - nicc., osm.
forenoon, before belching - thuj.
inspiration, on - viol-t.
deep, agg. - bry.
menses, before - sulph.
morning - ***kali-bi.,*** kali-n., nat-m.
rising, after - mang.
night - mag-c., rat.
before midnight - nat-m.
periodic - ***arg-n.***
pressure, of finger agg. - carb-v.
pylorus, of - bry., cann-i., ***chin.,*** hep., ***nux-v.,*** ornithog., ***phos.,*** sil.

constriction of, esophagus, swallowing, impossible - ***alum., alumn., bapt.,*** **BAR-C.,** cact., ***cic., hyos., kali-c.,*** **PHOS.**

CONTRACTION - ***aeth.,*** agar., alum., am-c., anac., arg-n., ***arn.,*** **ARS.,** ***ars-i.,*** atro., bar-c., bor., calc., **CARB-V.,** caust., chel., coca, ***cocc.,*** coloc., con., **CUPR.,** cupr-ac., euphr., eup-per., gamb., gran., hydrc., iod., kali-bi., kali-c., kali-i., ***laur.,*** lyc., mag-c., merc-c., mez., nat-a., nat-c., ol-an., op., osm., ***phos., plb.,*** psor., ptel., rheum, sep., sulph., ***sul-ac.,*** tril., thuj., zinc.
bend double, must - nat-c.

CONTRACTION,
cardiac orifice - alum., ***bar-m.,*** bry., dat-a., ***phos.,*** plb.
spasmodic, painful, cardio-spasm - aeth., ***agar.,*** am-c., ***arg-n.,*** ars., ***bell.,*** calc., caul., ***con.,*** hyos., ***ign.,*** nat-m., ***nux-v.,*** phos., puls., rhus-t., sep., sil.
coughing, after - ars.
dinner, after - bar-c., mag-c., nat-c.
eating, after - bell., bry., osm.
evening - ***ars.,*** hyper., nat-c., rhus-t., zinc.
extending to back - mag-m.
to hypochondria - nat-c.
to spine - bor.
morning - alum., ferr.
until noon - bor.
wakes - con.
night - con., kali-c., mag-c., merc., nat-c.
raising arm, agg. - anac.
sitting, while - cast., nat-c.
spasmodic - ***carb-v.***
stimulants, after - osm.
stooping - nat-c.
amel. - anac.
stretching - am-c.
turning body, agg. - anac.
vomiting, while - crot-t., dig.
walking, while - cast., coloc.
amel. - nat-c.

CORROSIVE, pain - arg-n., cupr., iod., nux-v.

CRAMP, esophagus, (see Constriction) - zinc.
palpitation, with - coloc.
swallowing, on - op.

CRAMPING, pain - abrot., acon., act-sp., aesc., ***aeth.,*** agar., agn., ***alum.,*** alumn., ambr., am-c., anac., anan., ***ant-c.,*** ant-t., apis, aran., ***arg-n., arn.,*** **ARS.,** ars-i., arum-m., arum-t., asc-t., asaf., asar., ***aur-m.,*** bapt., ***bar-c.,*** bar-i., bar-m., ***bell.,*** **BISM.,** bor., brom., ***bry.,*** bufo, ***cadm-s.,*** calad., **CALC.,** ***calc-p.,*** calc-s., camph., cann-i., cann-s., canth., ***carb-an.,*** carb-h., **CARB-S., CARB-V.,** card-m., cast., ***caul.,*** **CAUST.,** ***cham.,*** **CHEL.,** ***chin.,*** chin-a., ***cina,*** **COCC.,** coc-c., coff., ***colch.,*** coll., **COLOC., CON.,** crot-t., **CUPR.,** cupr-ar., daph., dig., ***dios., dros.,*** dulc., ***euph.,*** eup-per., ***ferr.,*** ferr-ar., ferr-p., fl-ac., ***gels.,*** **GRAPH.,** grat., guai., ham., hell., ***helon.,*** hydr-ac., hydrc., ***hyos.,*** ign., iod., **IP.,** ***iris, jatr.,*** kali-ar., kali-bi., kali-br., ***kali-c., kali-n.,*** kali-p., kali-s., ***kalm., lac-d., lach.,*** lact., laur., ***lob.,*** **LYC.,** ***mag-c.,*** **MAG-P.,** mang., med., meny., merc., merc-c., merc-i-f., mez., mill., mur-ac., naja, ***nat-a., nat-c.,*** **NAT-M.,** ***nat-p.,*** nat-s., nicc., nit-ac., nux-m., **NUX-V.,** ol-an., ***op.,*** ox-ac., ***par.,*** petr., ***ph-ac., phos.,*** phys., phyt., ***pic-ac.,*** plat., ***plb.,*** **PODO.,** psor., ***ptel., puls.,*** ran-s., ***rat.,*** rhod., rhus-t., sang., sarr., sars., sec., sel., seneg., ***sep.,*** **SIL., STANN.,** staph., ***sulph., sul-ac.,*** tab., tarent., teucr., thuj., valer., **VERAT.,** verat-v., zinc.
afternoon - alum., calc., calc-s., par., puls.
1 to 2 p.m. - con.
4 p.m. - alumn.
5 p.m. - nat-m.

CRAMPING, pain
afternoon, 6 p.m. - lach.
ascending stairs - chin-s.
bed, after going to - dios., laur.
belching, with - sep.
amel. - ambr., ***bar-c., calc.,*** calc-p., coloc., kali-c., par., rat.
after - sil.
bending, backwards, amel. - dios.
double, must - **COLOC.,** kali-c.
forward, amel. - carb-v., ***chel.,*** **COLOC.,** ***lyc.,*** verat-v.
breakfast, after - bufo, verat.
after, amel. - nat-s.
breathing, deep agg. - zinc.
cheese, spoiled - ***ars.***
clothing, tight - calc., lyc.
amel. - cupr., ***nat-m.***
coffee drinkers, in - ***cham., nux-v.***
cold drinks, after - **ARS.,** ***calc.,*** ferr., ***graph., kali-c., rhus-t.***
food, from - kali-c.
cold, from a - dulc., nit-ac., sep.
as if - nit-ac., petr., sul-ac.
deathly feeling below sternum - **CUPR.**
dinner, during - bell., thuj., zinc.
before - sulph.
after - graph., ham., ***nux-m.,*** sil.
disposition to - bell., chin., **CUPR.,** stann.
drawing, up limbs amel. - chel.
drinking, after - bell., nat-c., ***nux-v.***
eating, after - bism., bry., ***calc.,*** chel., chin., cic., ***cina, cocc., coloc., crot-h.,*** daph., ***ferr.,*** ferr-i., graph., grat., ham., iod., ***kali-c., nat-m.,*** **NUX-V.,** phos., plb., puls., sil., ***sulph.,*** tab.
after, amel. - ***brom., chel., graph., ign.,*** iod.
before - lyc.
evening - agar., coloc., dulc., form., led., merc., nat-c., thuj.
bed, in - alum., phos.
extending to,
abdomen - con.
chest - kali-c., lyc., nit-ac., phos.
downward - sulph.
hypogastrium - ars.
left side - nat-c.
lumbar region - sars., nat-c.
throat - kali-c., sulph.
fasting, while - ***calc.,*** gran.
fever, during - bell., carb-v., ***cocc.,*** nux-v., puls.
forenoon - graph., podo., thuj.
fruit, after - ***lyc.***
hiccoughs, from incomplete - mag-c.
inspiration - ***caust.,*** dros.
intermittent - kali-c., phos.
loss of animal fluids, after - ***chin.***
lying - ***carb-v.,*** chel.
amel. - graph., ***lyc.,*** sil.
back amel. - laur.
side - laur.
side, left amel. - ***chel.***

CRAMPING, pain
menses, during - ars., ***cupr.,*** kali-c., phos., ***sars.***
after - ***bell.,*** bor., kali-c.
before - ***bell.,*** cupr., lach., ***puls., sep.***
morning - con., dig., gran., hyper., kali-c., nat-c., ***nux-v.,*** puls., rat., sep.
bed, in - carb-an., con., phys.
rising, after - iod., nat-s., nit-ac.
waking, on - caust., lyc., nat-m., petr.
motion, on - bufo, ***ip., nux-v.***
amel. - dios.
nausea, before - tarent.
night - abrot., calc., ***camph., carb-v., coloc., graph.,*** kali-c., nat-m., nit-ac., phos., seneg., sulph.
1 to 2 a.m., between - con.
2 a.m. - ***ars.,*** nat-c.
3 a.m. - podo.
4 a.m. till noon daily - bor.
bed, driving out of - calc.
bed, in - ptel.
midnight - lyc.
noon - agar., alumn.
nursing, mothers - carb-v.
paroxysmal - ***carb-v., coloc.,*** kali-c., nit-ac., sil.
periodic - ***arg-n.,*** ars., cupr., hyos., phos., rhod.
pork, after - ham.
pregnancy - ***con.***
pressure amel. - ***am-c.,*** dios.
riding amel. - ***gels.***
rye bread, after - merc-c.
salad, after - til.
sausage, spoiled - ***ars.***
sitting, while - ***all-c.,*** ang., hell., nat-c.
bent while - agn., bor., caps.
bent while, amel. - staph.
soup, after - zinc.
standing, erect, amel. - bry., chin-s., phys.
stool, during - bell., ***kali-c.***
after - ferr.
before - ***coloc.,*** kali-c.
causing urging to - **NUX-V.**
stooping, on - anac., jatr., nat-c.
straightening up amel. - hell.
stretching amel. - nat-c.
supper, after - phos., rhod.
before - phos.
talking - ptel.
transversely across - ***arg-m.***
touch, agg. - chel.
vomiting, during - podo.
before - apis, hyos.
walking, while - cocc., nat-c., verat.
amel. - ***all-c.,*** hell., kali-c., nat-c.
wakes - con., kali-c.
warmth, amel. - ***mag-p., nux-v.***
of bed amel. - graph.
wine, from - lyc.
worm, as from a - nat-c.

CRAWLING - agar., alum., ***ars., bry.,*** cast., caust., ***cocc.,*** colch., hyper., kali-c., lact., lyc., nat-c., nux-m., nux-v., ***puls.,*** raph., rhod., rhus-t.
crawling, esophagus, in - anan., kali-c., plb., zinc.

CROAKING, like frogs - nat-m.
turning in bed, on - nat-m.

CUTTING, pain - ***abrot.,*** aesc., aloe, alum., alumn., ambr., am-br., anac., ant-c., ***arg-n., ars.,*** ars-h., ars-i., asar., aur., aur-m., bar-c., ***bell.,*** bol., bry., ***cadm-s.,*** cahin., calad., ***calc., calc-p.,*** calc-s., cann-s., canth., caust., ***cham.,*** chel., cimic., colch., coll., ***coloc.,*** cupr., cupr-ar., dig., **DIOS.,** crot-t., gamb., glon., grat., ***hydr., ign.,*** iod., jatr., ***kali-ar.,*** kali-bi., ***kali-c.,*** kali-chl., kali-p., kali-s., laur., lepi., ***lyc.,*** mag-m., mang., ***merc., nat-a., nat-c.,*** nicc., ***nux-m.,*** nux-v., ***op.,*** paeon., petr., ***phos., phyt.,*** plb., psor., ptel., puls., raph., rat., rob., rumx., seneg., sep., ***sil.,*** sol-n., stann., stront-c., ***sulph.,*** sul-ac., sumb., ter., thuj., ust., valer., zinc.
afternoon - alum., ptel., stront-c., sulph.
1 p.m., while yawning - chel.
4 p.m. - alumn.
5 p.m. - puls.
belching, amel. - ambr., mag-m., phos.
bending, backward amel. - ***bell.***
double amel. - **COLOC.,** sol-n.
breakfast, after - kali-c., kali-n.
breathing, agg. - ***bell.,*** rat.
cold, drinks, after - ***calc-p.***
taken in open air, from - phos.
convulsive, before stool - calc-s.
coughing, on - verat.
dinner, after - ang., hydr.
amel. - caust.
eating, while - cupr-ar., zinc.
after - ang., bry., caust., chel., con., cupr-ar., hydr., ***kali-c.,*** rhod.
amel. - ang.
begining to - ang.
evening - bar-c., indg., kali-c., mang., nat-m.
extending, to
abdomen, on stretching - mag-c.
back - cupr.
chest - coloc., sep.
hypogastrium - ars.
left side - nat-c.
lumbar region - nat-c.
spine - sep.
umbilicus, navel - phos., nat-c.
flatus, emission of, amel. - asar.
forenoon - nat-c.
inspiration, on - rat.
intermittent - verb.
fever - ***aran.***
lying, agg. - cupr.
menses, during - ars., cocc.
morning - dios., kali-c., merc-i-f.
motion, agg. - ang.
night - abrot., bar-c., lyc.
1 a.m. - mag-m.
2 a.m. - kali-bi.
driving out of bed - lyc.
midnight, after - calad., ***kali-c.***
paroxysmal - ant-c., ***asaf.,*** kali-c., ***phos.,*** sul-ac.

CUTTING, pain
pressure amel. - cupr., dios., sol-n.
riding in the open air - rumx.
sitting, while - alumn., dios., sul-ac.
soup, after - indg.
stool, as from - nat-c.
before - calc-s.
urging for, with - petr.
stooping, on - dios.
sudden - chin-s.
uncover, must - mag-m.
urinating amel. - ***phos.***
vomiting, when - ars.
walking, while - sul-ac.
warm milk, after - ang.

DEATH-like, sensation - ***ars.***, **CUPR.**, ip., mez., pic-ac., ***tab.***

DIGESTION, slow - aur-m., berb., ***calc.***, **CHIN.**, ***corn.***, corn-f., cycl., eucal., ***lyc.***, nuph., ***nux-v.***, ***op.***, ***par.***, ***sabin.***, sanic., ***sep.***, **SIL.**, **TARENT.**
weak - alst., ***anac.***, ***ant-c.***, ***arg-n.***, ars., asaf., bism., ***bry.***, caps., ***carb-an.***, ***carb-v.***, ***chin.***, coch., coff., colch., ***cycl.***, ***dios.***, eucal., gran., ***graph.***, ***hydr.***, ip., kali-bi., **LYC.**, merc., **NAT-C.**, nat-m., **NUX-V.**, prun., ***puls.***, spong., zing.

DILATATION, cardiac orifice - bism., graph., ***hydrin-m.***, kali-bi., ***nux-v.***, phos., puls., xanrhi.

DISORDERED, stomach (see Indigestion) - **ANT-C.**, ant-t., **ARG-N.**, **ARS.**, **ASAF.**, **BRY.**, ***caps.***, **CARB-V.**, ***caust.***, ***cham.***, **CHIN.**, ***chin-a.***, ***coff.***, ***graph.***, ***hep.***, **IP.**, kali-ar., **KALI-BI.**, ***kali-c.***, kali-p., kali-s., lac-c., ***lob.***, **LYC.**, **MERC.**, ***mez.***, nat-a., ***nat-c.***, **NAT-M.**, ***nat-p.***, **NAT-S.**, **NUX-V.**, ***petr.***, ***phos.***, ***psor.***, ***ptel.***, **PULS.**, **ROB.**, ***sars.***, ***sep.***, ***sul-ac.***, ***tarent.***, ***thuj.***, **VERAT.**
acids, after - ***ant-c.***, caust., ferr., ***sep.***
beer, after - aloe, ferr., kali-bi., ***sulph.***
bread, after - bry., **CAUST.**, lyc., ***merc.***, nat-m., sars., ***sep.***
cheese, mouldy - ***ars.***
cold, after a - ***ant-c.***, ***bry.***
dinner, after - mag-c.
eggs - chin-a.
evening, every - ambr.
excitement, from - ***bry.***, ***cham.***, chin., coloc., ***nux-v.***, ph-ac., staph.
fat food, after - ***caust.***, chin., ***kali-m.***, ***nat-p.***, nux-v., ***ptel.***, **PULS.**, ***sep.***, ***sulph.***
fish - chin-a.
fresh meat - ***caust.***
fruit, after - act-sp., **ARS.**, ***bry.***, **CHIN.**, ***lyc.***
ice cream - **ARS.**, ***calc-p.***, ***carb-v.***, **PULS.**
menses, before and during - arg-n., ars., ***bry.***, kali-c., lach., ***lyc.***, nux-m., ***nux-v.***, ***puls.***, sep., sulph.
mental exertion - arn., calc., cocc., ***lach.***, ***nux-m.***, **NUX-V.**, ***puls.***, ***sulph.***, verat.
milk, after - aeth., alum., ars., ***bry.***, ***calc.***, ***chin.***, kali-c., ***iris***, ***lyc.***, nat-a., **NAT-C.**, nat-p., **NIT-AC.**, ***sep.***, sil., ***sulph.***, sul-ac., zinc.
night, sensation - phos.
oysters - ***bry.***, **LYC.**
peaches, after - ***psor.***
sauerkraut, after - ***bry.***, petr.
sex, after - ***dig.***
simplest food, from - alet., amyg., ***ant-c.***, carb-an., ***carb-v.***, ***chin.***, dig., ***hep.***, ***kali-c.***, lach., lyc., ***nat-c.***, ***nux-v.***, puls.
strawberries, after - ox-ac.
stromy weather, in - petr.
sweets, from - ***arg-n.***, merc.
vexation, after - **CHAM.**, ***ip.***
warm soup, amel. - nat-c.

DISAGREEABLE, sensation - nat-m., phos.
stooping, amel. - nat-m.

DISTENTION - abrot., acon., aesc., aloe, alum., alumn., ant-c., ant-t., apis, ars., ars-i., **ARG-N.**, ***asaf.***, aur., bar-m., ***bell.***, berb., ***bor.***, ***bry.***, bufo, calad., **CALC.**, ***calc-ar.***, ***calc-s.***, caps., carb-an., **CARB-V.**, carl., ***cham.***, cedr., chel., **CHIN.**, ***chin-s.***, **CIC.**, cimic., clem., ***cocc.***, coc-c., coff., **COLCH.**, ***con.***, ***croc.***, cupr., cycl., daph., ***dig.***, dios., ***dulc.***, echi., elaps, eup-pur., ferr., ferr-ar., ferr-i., ferr-m., ferr-p., ***gels.***, gent-l., gran., ***graph.***, grat., gins., ***hell.***, ***hep.***, ***hydr.***, hydrc., hydr-ac., ***ign.***, iod., kali-ar., kali-bi., **KALI-C.**, kali-p., kali-s., ***lac-d.***, ***lach.***, laur., lec., led., lil-t., **LYC.**, mag-c., ***manc.***, mang., **MED.**, ***merc.***, ***merc-c.***, merl., ***mez.***, mosch., nat-a., nat-c., ***nat-m.***, ***nat-p.***, ***nat-s.***, **NUX-M.**, ***nux-v.***, ol-an., op., petr., ***phos.***, phys., phyt., plat., plb., ***prun.***, psor., ***puls.***, raph., **RAT.**, rob., sabad., sabin., sang., sanic., sec., sep., stann., ***stram.***, **SULPH.**, sul-ac., tarent., thuj., zinc.
afternoon - nat-m., petr., sulph.
belching, amel. - ***arg-n.***, **CARB-V.**, mag-c., ***nat-s.***
does not amel. - **CHIN.**, echi., ***lyc.***, phos.
chill, during - ***cocc.***
contradiction, after - ***nux-m.***
convulsion, during - ***cic.***
dinner, after - alum., ant-c., dig., kalm., zinc.
before - rat.
drinking, after - calc., manc., nat-m., tab.
eating, while - con.
after - agar., alum., ***ambr.***, ***anac.***, ***apoc.***, ***arg-n.***, aur-m., bar-c., **BOR.**, ***bry.***, calad., ***calc.***, calc-s., cann-i., carb-an., carb-s., **CARB-V.**, ***caust.***, cham., **CHIN.**, cimic., coc-c., **COLCH.**, ***cop.***, dig., dios., dulc., ferr., ferr-p., graph., ***grat.***, ***hep.***, ***lach.***, **LYC.**, nat-m., **NAT-S.**, ***nux-m.***, **NUX-V.**, op., ***phos.***, ***puls.***, rumx., ***sanic.***, sars., sin-a., ***stann.***, sulph., sul-ac., tab.
amel. - cedr., rat.
evening - calc., dios., eupi., ***kali-bi.***, osm.
9 p.m. until midnight - phos.
bed, in - bell.
excitement, after - ***arg-n.***, nux-m.

DISTENTION,
exertion, mental, during - hep.
physical, after - ***arg-n.***
fish, after pickled - arg-n., calad.
flatus, passing, amel. - rat.
forenoon - myric.
grief, after - calc.
lying on abdomen amel. - con.
menses, before - zinc.
suppressed - cham.
midnight, after - ambr.
milk, after - ***con.***
morning - nux-v., ***phos.***
motion amel. - cedr., chin.
night, on waking - asaf.
oysters, after - ***bry., lyc.***
rising, after - coc-c.
stool, amel. - corn.
before - ars.
supper, after - zinc.
walking amel. - calad., cedr.
distension, sensation of, esophagus - aur., hyper., op., phyt., upa., verat.

DRAWING, pain - agar., all-c., ***alum.***, am-m., ***anac.***, apis, arg-m., ***arg-n.***, aur-m., bar-c., bufo, canth., cham., card-m., chel., con., cupr., dig., elaps, ferr., gins., hell., hep., ign., iod., jatr., kali-c., kali-i., lach., lyc., manc., mang., merc., nat-c., nit-ac., ***phos.***, ph-ac., plat., plb., puls., ran-s., rhod., sep., sil., ***stram.***, verat., zinc., zing.
chills, after - gins.
dinner, after - alum., mur-ac., sep.
drinking - aur-m.
eating, while - aur-m., led.
extending, to
chest - aur-m., ***phos.***
left clavicle - agar.
pharynx - alum.
small of back - ph-ac.
sternum - aur-m.
throat - con.
inwards - dros., hell., mur-ac.
lifting, as from - plat.
morning - dig., kali-c., puls.
after stool - con.
motion agg. - aloe.
night- sep.
paroxysmal - aur-m.
riding in carriage, after - phos.
stooping agg. - aur-m.
talking - kalm.
walking in open air, while - anac.

DRYNESS, in - calad., chin., ox-ac., raph.
dryness, esophagus, in - acon., ars., bell., bufo, ***cocc.***, kali-br., ***lach.***, merc-i-f., ***mez.***, nat-m., op., ptel., ***sep., sulph.***, sumb.

EMOTIONS, are felt in stomach - calc., cham., coloc., ***kali-ar.***, kali-c., mez., nux-v., phos.

EMPTINESS, weak, hungry feeling - abrot., acon., ***aesc., agar.***, ail., ***all-c.***, all-s., aloe, alum., alumn., ***ambr.***, am-c., am-m., anac., ang., **ANT-C.,** ant-t., apoc., ***aran., arg-m., arg-n.***, arn., ***ars., ars-i., asaf.***, aster., atro., aur., aur-m., ***bapt., bar-c.***,

EMPTINESS, weak, hungry feeling - bar-i., bar-m., bell., ***brom.***, bry., ***bufo,*** cact., ***calad., calc., calc-p.***, calc-s., ***camph.***, cann-s., canth., ***caps.***, carb-ac., ***carb-an.***, carb-s., carb-v., card-m., ***carl.***, cast., ***caust.***, chel., ***chin.***, chin-a., chin-s., chlol., ***cimic., cina,*** cinnb., clem., coca, coc-c., **COCC.,** coff., colch., ***coloc.***, con., cop., corn., ***croc., crot-h., crot-t.***, cupr., cupr-ar., **DIG.,** dios., ***elaps,*** ery-a., euphr., fago., ferr., ***fl-ac., gamb., gels.***, gent-c., gent-l., ***glon., graph., grat.***, **HELL.,** hep., ***hipp.***, **HYDR.,** ***hydr-ac., hyos.***, **IGN.,** ind., indg., ***iod.***, ip., jatr., ***kali-ar.***, kali-bi., ***kali-c., kali-chl., kali-fer.***, kali-i., kali-n., ***kali-p., kali-s.***, kalm., **LAC-C.,** lac-ac., ***lach., laur.***, lil-t., ***lob., lyc.***, lyss., ***mag-c.***, manc., meph., **MERC.,** merc-i-f., merc-i-r., merl., mez., ***mosch.***, **MURX.,** ***mur-ac.***, myric., naja, nat-a., ***nat-c., nat-m., nat-p., nat-s.***, nicc., nit-ac., **NUX-V.,** ***olnd., op.***, ox-ac., ***petr.***, **PHOS.,** phel., phys., phyt., plan., plat., plb., **PODO.,** ptel., **PULS.,** raph., rheum., ***rhus-t.***, rumx., ruta., sabad., ***sang.***, sarr., sars., sec., seneg., **SEP.,** sil., spig., squil., **STANN.,** staph., stram., **SULPH.,** ***sul-i.***, sumb., **TAB.,** ***tarent.***, tell., ***teucr.***, thea., thuj., til., tril., ***tub.***, ust., valer., **VERAT.,** verb., vinc., **ZINC.**
afternoon - ambr., fago., lach., puls., sulph.
1 p.m. - fago.
2 p.m. - ***grat.***
3 p.m. - phys.
air, open, amel. - bapt.
aversion to food - ***bar-c.***, bor., calc., caust., carb-s., carb-v., ***chin., cocc.***, coff., dulc., ***grat., hell., hydr., nat-m., nux-v., rhus-t., sil.***, stram., ***sulph.***, verb.
belching, after - ambr.
amel. - ***sep.***
brandy, after - olnd.
breakfast, after - am-m., coca, colch., ***dig.***, lyc., mez., puls.
breakfast, amel. - mag-m.
chill, during - ail., ***ars.***
cough, with - croc., ign., mur-ac., stann.
daytime - nat-p., stann.
diarrhea, with - ***fl-ac., lyc., petr., stram., sulph.***
dinner, after - graph., lyc., ptel., thea., zinc.
amel. - mag-c.
before - lyc., mag-c., nux-v., phos., **SULPH.**
drowsiness during - corn.
eating, while - crot-t., verat., zinc.
after - agar., alum., arn., bov., calad., carb-v., chlol., **CINA,** coloc., ***dig., grat., hydr.***, kali-p., lach., ***laur., lyc., myric.***, nat-p., olnd., op., phos., plan., ptel., puls., raph., sang., sars., sil., ***stann.***, sul-ac., thuj., **VERAT.,** zinc.
amel. - iod., mag-c., verat.
before - alumn., crot-t., ***sulph.***
eating, not relieved by - agar., ***alf.***, alum., ***ant-c., arg-m., ars.***, asc-t., aur., calc., calc-p., cann-i., ***carb-an.***, casc., cast-eq., cic., **CINA,** coc-c., coloc., dig., ***hydr.***, **IGN.,** indol., iod., kali-bi., kali-i., **LAC-C.,**

EMPTINESS, weak, hungry feeling,
eating, not relieved by - **LACH., LYC.,** mag-m., med., ***merc.,*** **MUR-AC.,** nat-m., ***nux-m.,*** olnd., par., **PHOS.,** phyt., ***psor.,*** sang., sars., **SEP.,** sil., ***staph.,*** stront-c., sulph., ***teucr.,*** **VERAT.,** zinc.
epilepsy, before - **HYOS.**
evening - ambr., calc-p., lac-c., olnd.
8 p.m. - kali-c., kalm.
eating, after amel. - **SEP.**
sleep, before - dig.
supper, before - graph.
extending to heart - **LOB.**
fever, during - zinc.
forenoon - caust., jatr., mag-c., ***nat-c.,*** nat-m., nicc., puls., sulph.
10 a.m. until evening - mur-ac., ***nat-c.***
11 a.m - alumn., ***asaf.,*** coloc., hydr., ign., ind., lach., ***nat-c.,*** nat-m., nat-p., op., petr., ***phos.,*** sep., **SULPH.,** ***zinc.***
11 a.m, with dull pain - hydr.
fruit, after - nat-c.
grief, after - ign.
headache, during - cocc., kali-p., ***nat-m.,*** nit-ac., ***phos.,*** ptel., ***sang.,*** **SEP.**
before - ign.
heart weak or dilated, with - chlol.
hunger, without - act-sp., ***agar., alum.,*** am-m., ars., ***bar-c.,*** berb., bry., carb-an., chin., chin-s., cocc., dulc., hell., kali-n., **LACH.,** ***mur-ac., nat-m.,*** nicc., ***olnd.,*** op., phos., psor., ***rhus-t., sil., sulph., sul-ac.,*** tax.
inspiration agg. - calad.
intermittent - mur-ac.
loathing of food, with - hydr.
lying down amel. - ambr., ign., murx., sep.
meeting a friend, when - cimic.
menses, before - ***ign.,*** sep., sulph.
menses, during - kali-n., kali-p., spong., tab.
menopause period - cimic., ***crot-h.,*** dig., ign., ***lach.,*** sep., ***tab.,*** tril.
midnight - mag-c., rhus-t.
after - mag-c.
milk, sips in amel. - diph.
morning - ***aesc.,*** agar., anac., apoc., arg-m., bufo, carb-v., cast., cimic., coloc., dios., hell., hydr., kali-bi., lac-c., lyc., mag-c., mag-m., mez., nat-m., nat-p., nicc., op., phos., plat., sang., sep., tarent.
2 a.m. - podo., tell.
5 a.m. - nat-c.
anxiety with - lyc., nat-m.
breakfast, before - aesc., alumn., apoc., arg-m., calc-p., carb-v., cimic., ***kali-bi.,*** lac-c., murx., sulph.
menses, during - cast.
rising, after - phos.
rising, on - nat-p., phos.
waking, on - ant-c., apoc., ***lac-c.,*** mill.
nausea, during - agar., ***arg-m.,*** arg-n., asaf., berb-a., bry., calc-p., caust., chel., cimic., cocc., ***cycl., hell.,*** hep., hydr., ***ign.,*** ip., kali-bi., kali-c., kali-p., lach., lyc., mag-m., meph., mosch., olnd., phel., **PHOS.,**

EMPTINESS, weak, hungry feeling,
nausea, during - rheum, ***rhus-t., sep., sil.,*** spig., **TAB.,** ***valer.,*** verat., zinc.
night - dios., lyc., petr., tarent.
noon - fago., nat-c.
nursing, after - ***carb-an.,*** olnd.
pains, from - ars.
paroxysmal - arg-m., glon.
pressure, from - **MERC.**
rising, after - coca
siesta, after - ang.
sighing - **IGN.**
sitting, while - acon., alumn.
sleep, during - lyc., ph-ac.
before - dig.
stool, after - ***aloe,*** ambr., dios., fl-ac., **PETR.,** ***ph-ac.,*** podo., puls., ***sep.,*** sul-ac., sulph.
talking agg. - ***rumx.***
thinking of food, when - **SEP.**
throbbing, with - ant-t., ***asaf.,*** calad., hydr., ***kali-c.,*** mag-m., nat-c., nat-m., sep., sulph.
trembling - am-c., cimic., lyc., zinc.
urination, after - apoc.
vomiting, after - ther.
walking, while - chel., chin-s., rat., sep.
about the room agg. - lyc.
after - coca, ferr.
fast amel. - myric.
wine amel. - sep.

ENLARGED - bar-c., sil.

ENLARGEMENT, upper part - elat.

EPILEPTIC aura - art-v., bell., bufo, ***calc.,*** caust., **CIC.,** cupr., ***indg.,*** **NUX-V.,** sil., **SULPH.**
extending from stomach to uterus - **CALC.**
rising from stomach to head - **CALC.,** lyc., ***sil.***

ERUCTATIONS, (see Belching)

ESOPHAGITIS, inflammation of esophagus - acon., alum., arn., **ARS.,** asaf., bell., bufo, ***carb-v.,*** cocc., euph., ***gels., iod.,*** laur., merc., merc-c., mez., naja, ***nit-ac.,*** oena., ***phos.,*** **RHUS-T.,** sabad., sec., sul-ac., verat., ***verat-v.,*** vesp.
swallowing corrosive things, from - caust., rhus-t.

EXPANDING, pain - calc.

FAINTNESS, with stomach affections - ***alumn.,*** **ARG-N.,** bufo, dios., ***dor.,*** elaps, ***kali-bi., mag-m., mez., nat-s.,*** sang., **SULPH.,** tab.
metrorrhagia, during - crat., tril.
pain in stomach, with - ***ars.,*** **BISM.,** ***coll., dios., nux-v.,*** puls., ran-s., sin-n., ***sulph.***

FALL, out, as if would - bell., hell., mag-c.

FEAR, felt in - ***kali-ar., kali-c.,*** phos.

FERMENTATION - acet-ac., apoc., ***caust.,*** **CHIN.,** croc., graph., lyc., ***plat.***
fruit, after - **CHIN.**

FLABBINESS, (see Abdomen) - **CAPS.,** euph., **IGN.,** ip., **KALI-BI.,** merc., spong., tab., thea.

FLAMES, in, sensation, as if - manc.

FLOATING, in water, as if - abrot.

FOOD, as if full of dry - calad.

food, lodges in, at cardia - phos.

food, sensation, of, lodged in esophagus - am-m., ***ars., bar-c., calc., caust.,*** cham., ***chin.,*** dig., ***gels., kali-c.,*** lac-ac., ***puls.***

going through, feels - alum.

lodged in cardia - ign.

food, is felt until it enters the stomach - alum., ambr., bry., phos.

turned, like a corkscrew on swallowing - elaps.

passed over raw places - bar-c.

FOREIGN body - cupr., grat., hep., nat-m., phos., raph.

foreign body, esophagus, sensation - anac., bell., ***gels., lyc.,*** nit-ac., phos., verat-v.

FORMICATION - aloe, ant-t., apis, colch., kali-c., laur., plat., rhus-t., sulph., verat.

dust, as from - plat.

FULLNESS, sensation of - acon., aesc., agar., aloe, alum., alumn., am-c., am-m., anan., ***ant-c.,*** ant-t., apis, ***arg-n.,*** arn., ars., ars-i., asar., asaf., bapt., ***bar-c.,*** bar-i., bar-m., ***bell., bov.,*** brach., brom., ***bry., calc., calc-p.,*** calc-s., camph., canth., carb-ac., carb-an., **CARB-S., CARB-V.,** casc., ***cast-eq.,*** **CAUST.,** cedr., cham., **CHIN.,** chin-a., ***chin-s.,*** cob., ***cocc.,*** coc-c., coff., ***colch., coloc., con.,*** corn., crot-t., ***cycl.,*** daph., dig., ***dulc.,*** euphr., eup-per., eup-pur., ***ferr.,*** ferr-ar., ferr-i., ***ferr-p., fl-ac.,*** gent-c., gent-l., ***graph., grat.,*** gymn., ***hell., hydr.,*** hyos., hyper., ***ign.,*** ind., iod., ip., iris, jac-c., kali-ar., kali-bi., **KALI-C.,** ***kali-n., kali-p.,*** kali-s., ***kreos.,*** lach., lachn., laur., lec., lith., ***lob.,*** **LYC.,** mag-c., ***manc.,*** mang., ***merc.,*** merl., mez., mill., ***mosch.,*** mur-ac., myric., ***nat-c., nat-m.,*** nat-p., ***nat-s.,*** nicc., **NUX-M.,** ***nux-v., ol-an., op.,*** par., petr., phel., **PHOS.,** plat., plb., ***prun., puls.,*** ran-s., raph., rat., ***rheum, rhus-t., rob.,*** rumx., sabad., ***sabin., sec.,*** sil., spong., squil., ***stann.,*** staph., **SULPH.,** ***sul-ac.,*** tarent., tell., tep., tril., valer., zinc.

afternoon - am-m., calc., chin-s., coca, ***sulph.***

belching amel. - ***carb-v.,*** euphr., iris, mag-c., ***nux-v.,*** phos., sil.

bread, after - **CAUST.**

breakfast, after - alum., phos., ptel., sulph.

with sensation of hunger - am-m.

chill, during - cocc.

clothing agg. - ***gels.***

coffee, after - canth.

contradiction, after - ***nux-m.***

damp weather agg. - merc.

dinner, after - agar., alum., ant-c., cast., ***clem.,*** dig., grat., kalm., nat-m., petr., zinc.

drinking, after - aloe, aspar., ***manc.,*** nat-m., sin-n., tab.

dry food, as if - cadm-s.

eating, while - cham.

FULLNESS, sensation

eating, after - aesc., agar., alum., ***ambr.,*** **AM-C.,** ***anac.,*** ant-c., ***apoc., arg-n.,*** arn., ***ars.,*** aspar., aur., aur-m., ***bar-c., bism., bor., bry., calad., calc.,*** calc-s., carb-ac., carb-an., carb-s., **CARB-V.,** cham., **CHIN.,** ***chin-s.,*** cimic., **COLCH.,** ***cop.,*** dig., **FERR.,** ***ferr-i.,*** ferr-p., ***grat., hep., hydr.,*** kali-ar., kali-bi., ***kali-c.,*** kali-s., ***lach., lac-ac.,*** lil-t., **LYC.,** mez., mosch., myric., nat-a., nat-c., ***nat-m.,*** nat-p., ***nat-s.,*** nicc., ***nit-ac., nux-m.,*** **NUX-V.,** petr., ph-ac., ***phos., pic-ac.,*** plb., ***ptel.,*** **PULS.,** rheum, ***rhus-t.,*** sep., ***sil., spong., stann., sulph.,*** sul-ac., tab., verat., zinc.

after, ever so little, after - agar., alet., alum., ***apoc.,*** bar-c., ***carb-an.,*** **CHIN.,** croc., crot-t., cycl., ***dig.,*** elaps, **FERR.,** ***ferr-i., kali-c., kali-s.,*** **LYC.,** ***manc.,*** morg-g., nat-a., ***nat-m., nux-v.,*** petr., ***ptel.,*** rhus-t., senec., sep., ***sil., sulph.,*** thuj., verat.

amel. - arg-n., ferr., mang.

evening - ars., dios., eupi., hyos., nat-c., phos.

bed, in - ***nat-s.***

eating, after - kali-bi.

eating, while - cham.

hunger, during - am-m., arg-m., asaf., asar.

menses, during - am-c., kali-c., ***kali-p.***

morning - am-m., asaf., nat-c., phos., ran-s., rhod., sulph.

fasting, when - bar-c., plat.

waking, on - sulph.

night, midnight - crot-t.

on going to bed - rumx.

noon - ox-ac., sep., sulph.

bread and milk, after - arg-n.

eating, after - ox-ac.

pregnancy, during - **NUX-M.**

oppression of breathing, with - ***nat-s.,*** nux-m., ***nux-v.,*** prun.

sleep, amel. - ***phos.***

soup, after - prun.

supper, after - carb-v., chin-s.

urination, with frequent - ferr-pic.

vomiting, amel. - kali-c.

waking, on - myric., sulph.

walking, after - colch., ferr.

water, after - aloe.

as if - kali-c., ol-an.

wine, after - rhus-t.

GANGRENE - ars., euph., sec.

GASTRITIS, inflammation, stomach - acon., ***aeth.,*** all-c., alum., alumn., ***ant-c.,*** **ANT-T.,** ***apis, arg-n.,*** **ARS.,** ars-i., asar., aur., aur-m., bar-c., bar-i., ***bar-m.,*** **BELL.,** ***bism.,*** brom., **BRY.,** ***cact., camph., canth.,*** carb-ac., carb-an., chel., cic., ***cocc.,*** colch., cund., cupr., ***dig.,*** **EUPH.,** ferr-p., ***graph.,*** hell., ***hydr.,*** hydr-ac., **HYOS.,** indg., iod., ***ip.,*** kali-ar., kali-i., kali-n., kali-s., ***lac-d.,*** lach., laur., **LYC.,** mez., **NUX-V.,** ox-ac., **PHOS.,** ***plb.,*** puls., ran-b., ran-s., sabad., ***sang., sec.,*** squil., stram., ***ter.,*** **VERAT.,** ***verat-v.***

GASTRITIS, inflammation
acute - acon., agar-em., ***ant-t.,*** **ARS.,** ***bell.,*** bism., bry., canth., ferr-p., hedeo, ***hydr.,*** hyos., ***ip.,*** iris, ***kali-bi.,*** kali-chl., merc-c., ***nux-v., ox-ac.,*** **PHOS.,** puls., sant., sin-a., verat., zinc.
alcohol abuse, from - arg-n., ***ars.,*** bism., crot-c., ***cupr., gaul.,*** lach., **NUX-V.,** phos.
chronic - alum., ***ant-c., ant-t., arg-n.,*** arn., ars., ***bism.,*** calc., calc-chln., caps., carb-ac., ***carb-v., chin., colch.,*** dig., ***graph., hydr.,*** hydr-ac., ill., iod., ip., ***kali-bi.,*** kali-c., lyc., ***merc-c., nux-v.,*** op., ox-ac., ***phos.,*** podo., ***puls.,*** rumx., sang., sep., sil., sulph., verat., zinc.
cold, after taking - ***bry., coloc.***
cold, things, after - **ACON.**
when overheated - ***acon., kali-c.***
gastroenteritis, acute - alum., ***arg-n., ars., bapt.,*** bism., bry., ***cupr.,*** merc., merc-c., ***rhus-t.,*** sant., zinc.
pylorus - iod.

GASTROENTERITIS, acute - alum., ***arg-n.,*** **ARS.,** ***bapt.,*** bism., bry., ***cupr.,*** ip., merc., merc-c., ***rhus-t.,*** sant., zinc.

GNAWING, pain - abies-c., abrot., acet-ac., aesc., agar., alum., am-c., **AM-M.,** anan., apis, apoc., **ARG-M.,** ***arg-n.,*** arn., ***ars.,*** ars-i., aur-m., bar-c., bar-i., bell., calad., ***calc.,*** calc-s., cann-i., caps., carb-an., carb-s., carb-v., ***chel.,*** chin., ***cimic.,*** **CINA,** cocc., colch., ***cupr.,*** eup-pur., ***gamb., glon.,*** graph., grat., hep., iod., ***kali-bi., kali-c.,*** kali-n., kali-p., kalm., ***kreos., lach.,*** lith., ***lyc., mag-m., merc-c.,*** mill., nat-a., nat-c., nat-p., ***nat-s.,*** nicc., ***nit-ac.,*** nux-v., op., ox-ac., ph-ac., phos., plb., ptel., ***puls., ruta.,*** sabad., seneg., **SEP.,** sil., spig., staph., **STANN.,** ***sulph.,*** verat., zinc.
afternoon - kali-c.
bending forward - plb.
chill, during - ***ars.***
dinner, after - alum., sep., ***trom.***
amel. - kali-c.
before - ***graph.***
drinking agg. - bell.
eating, after - alum., bell., cocc., ***grat., kali-bi.***
eating, amel. - ***chel., graph., hep., ign.,*** iod., ***kali-bi., lach., lith.,*** lyc., mag-m., mez., ***nat-c.,*** nat-s.
before - ***graph., mag-m.,*** rhod., seneg.
evening - nat-m., seneg.
extending to back - sep.
forenoon - nicc.
left side - arg-n.
lying amel. - sil.
morning - aesc., carb-v., nat-c., plat., ruta.
5 a.m. - kali-p., nat-c.
rising, after - nat-s.
while fasting - carb-v., nit-ac.
night - abrot., ruta.
noon, after eating - euphr.
pain in during - ***lyc.***
paroxysmal - nat-m.

GNAWING, pain
sitting bent agg. - bar-c., caps.
standing - bar-c.
sudden - chin-s.
supper amel. - **SEP.**
walking, while - bar-c.
worm, as from a - nat-c.

GOUT, metastasis to - **ANT-C.,** benz-ac., ***nux-m.,*** sang.

GURGLING - agar., am-c., anac., ***arn., ars.,*** bov., carb-an., chel., cina, ***colch.,*** croc., crot-t., **CUPR.,** fl-ac., ***hydr-ac.,*** kali-c., kali-i., lact., ***laur.,*** lob., meny., sac-alb., teucr., thuj., verb., zinc.
drinking, when - arn., ***ars.,*** cina, **CUPR.,** elaps, **HYDR-AC.,** laur., thuj.
drinking, after - **PHOS.**
eating, while - bov.
morning - bov.
nausea, with - aeth.
walking, while - carb-an.
yawning, while - zinc.

gurgling, esophagus, drinking when, in - arn., ars., ***cina, cupr.,*** cupr-ac., ***elaps, hell.,*** **HYDR-AC., LAUR.,** sil., thuj.
convulsion, during - **CINA,** ***oena.***
coughing, after - **CINA.,** mur-ac.
sleeping, while - lyc.

HACKING, sensation - sulph.

HANGING, down, sensation of, relaxed - abrot., aesc., agar., alum., arg-n., ***bar-c., bism., calc., calc-p., carb-v.,*** crot-t., echi., ***euph., hep.,*** **IGN., IP.,** lob., ***lyc.,*** mag-c., merc., mez., petr., raph., rhus-t., ***sep.,*** spong., ***staph., sul-ac., tab.***
morning - ***sulph.***
stool, after - bar-c., ***sep.***
walking, while - hep.

HARD, as if something, over the - mag-m.

HARDNESS - ars., ***bar-c., bar-m.,*** carb-v., chim., cob., lept., merc-i-f., puls., sep.
belching amel. - carb-v.
sensation of, in the pylorus - kreos.
pylorus - sep.

HEARTBURN, general (see Belching) - ***aesc.,*** agar., all-s., ***alum.,*** alumn., **AMBR., AM-C.,** ***anac.,*** ant-c., ***apis,*** arg-m., arg-n., arn., **ARS.,** ***ars-i.,*** asaf., asar., bar-c., bar-i., bar-m., bell., ***berb.,*** bor., ***bry.,*** cadm-s., **CALC.,** calc-p., ***calc-s., canth., caps., carb-an.,*** **CARB-V.,** carb-s., card-m., ***caust.,*** cham., ***chel., chin.,*** chin-a., ***chin-s.,*** **CIC.,** cocc., coc-c., coff., colch., **CON.,** corn., **CROC.,** crot-h., crot-t., dig., dulc., echi., ferr., ferr-ar., ferr-i., **FERR-P.,** ***fl-ac., graph.,*** guai., hell., ***hep.,*** hyos., ign., ***iod., iris,*** kali-ar., ***kali-c., kali-i.,*** kali-n., kali-p., kali-s., ***lach., lob.,*** **LYC., MAG-C.,** mang., ***merc.,*** mosch., mur-ac., nat-a., ***nat-c., nat-m.,*** **NAT-P.,** ***nat-s.,*** nit-ac., nux-m., **NUX-V.,** op., ox-ac., par., petr., ph-ac., ***phos.,*** plat., ***podo.,*** **PULS.,** ran-s., ***rob., sabad., sabin.,*** sec., ***sep., sil., sin-n.,*** squil., staph., ***sulph., sul-ac., syph.,*** tab., tarax., tell., ter., thuj., ***valer., verat-v., zinc.***
acids, after - **NAT-P.,** nux-v.

HEARTBURN, general
- afternoon - bry., chel., chin., crot-h., cupr., dig., hydr., nat-m., phos., sep., sol-n., sulph.
- air, open, agg. - ambr.
- alcoholics, in - ***nux-v., sul-ac.***
- beer, after - phos.
- belching, after - bar-c., ***calc.,*** con., mang., valer.
- coffee, after - calc-p., ferr-p.
- daytime - crot-h.
- dinner, after - acon., calc-p., crot-t., ham., kali-bi., lyc., mag-m., merc-i-r., nat-m., sol-n., sulph.
- drinking, after - ***alum.***
- eating, after - ***aesc.,*** agar., ***am-c.,*** anac., ***calc., calc-p.,*** carl., ***chin.,*** coc-c., con., croc., ***graph., iod.,*** lyc., merc., ***nat-m., nit-ac., nux-v.,*** sep., sil.
- eggs, boiled, after - sulph.
- evening - ambr., bell., caust., crot-h., con., dig., mang., ***nat-m., ox-ac., petr.,*** sulph., ter.
  - bed, after going to - ***con.,*** sol-n.
  - smoking, after - lach.
  - wine, after - bry.
- fat, food, after - nat-c., nit-ac., nux-v., phos.
- flatulent food, after - kali-c.
- forenoon - carb-v., coc-c., coloc., sep.
- hard dry food, after - calc.
- meat, after - agar., ***ferr-p.***
- menses, before - ***sulph.***
- milk, after - ambr., ***chin.***
- morning - arg-m., petr., phos., sulph.
  - breakfast, before - ***nux-v.***
  - rising, on - mang.
  - smoking, while - lyc.
- nausea, with - ***calc.,*** iod., ***puls., sang.***
- night - coc-c., kali-bi., ***merc.,*** ptel., ***rob.***
  - lying down, on - ***rob.***
- night, midnight - calc.
- palpitation, with - nat-m.
- pregnancy, during - acet-ac., anac., apis, calc., canth., ***caps.,*** con., dios., lac-ac., ***merc.,*** nat-m., ***nux-v.,*** ox-ac., ***puls.,*** rob., tab., zinc.
  - night, during - ***merc.***
- rancid - con., graph.
- scraping - staph.
- sitting bent, while - sabin.
- smoking, while - bell., lach., lyc., puls., staph.
- soup, after - anac.
- sour things, after - ferr-p.
- stool, after - merc.
- stooping, on - thuj.
- sugar, after - zinc.
- supper, after - ***alum.,*** caust., crot-h., kali-c., puls.
- sweets agg. - zinc.
- tobacco, from - chel., staph., tarax.
- walking in open air, while - ***ambr.***
- water, burning - ars.
- wine, after - bry., coc-c., zinc.

HEAT and flushes, in (see Burning, pain, Heartburn) - abrot., acet-ac., ***acon.,*** aesc., aeth., agar., aloe, alum., ***alumn.,*** am-c., ***anth.,*** anthr., ***apis, arg-n.,*** **ARS.,** ars-h., ars-i., aur-s., bapt., bar-c., bar-i., bell., benz-ac., brom., **BRY.,** ***calc., camph.,*** cann-i., ***canth.,*** carb-ac., carb-an., carb-s., caust., cedr., cham., chel., chin-s., chlf., ***cic.,*** cimic., cina, cinnb., coca, cocc., coc-c., cod., colch., coloc., con., corn-f., crot-t., cupr., dig., euph., eup-per., fago., ferr., ***ferr-ar.,*** ferr-i., ferr-p., fl-ac., gels., ***glon.,*** grat., gymn., hell., helon., hydr-ac., ***hydrc.,*** hyos., iod., ip., iris, jatr., kali-ar., kali-bi., kali-c., kali-chl., kali-n., kali-s., kalm., ***lac-ac., lac-c.,*** lach., laur., led., ***lob.,*** mag-m., ***manc.,*** mang., meny., merc., mez., myric., mur-ac., nat-a., nat-c., ***nat-m.,*** nat-p., nat-s., ***nit-ac., nux-m.,*** **NUX-V.,** ol-j., olnd., op., ox-ac., par., petr., ***phos.,*** phyt., plat., plb., ***podo.,*** ptel., puls., raph., rat., ***rob.,*** ruta., sabin., sang., ***sars.,*** sec., seneg., sep., squil., stry., sulph., sul-ac., sumb., tab., tarent., ***ter., thuj.,*** valer., verat., verat-v., vesp., zinc-m.
- afternoon - fago.
- belching, after - sumb.
  - amel. - fago.
- bread, after - sars.
- dinner, during - hyper.
- eating, after - con., ***ferr., sep.***
  - amel. - arg-n., ferr.
  - before - fl-ac.
- empty, when - naja
- evening - coloc., ferr-i., hyper.
- extending, to
  - abdomen - am-c., carl., chin., verat.
  - arms and fingers - con.
  - eyes - stram.
  - fauces - caps.
  - head - alum., bar-m., ***calc.,*** chin., cinnb., ***glon.,*** hell., ***lyc.,*** mag-m., mang., sumb.
  - over body - ars., ***camph.,*** op.
  - over chest - bar-m., chin., nat-m., ol-an., verat.
  - throat - cinnb., nit-ac., sumb., tarent.
  - throat pit - plat.
  - upwards - asaf., ars., ***calc.,*** carb-ac., cinnb., ***ferr., glon.,*** iris, kali-bi., laur., ***manc.,*** mang., phos., ***valer.***
  - upwards, suffocation, causing - valer.
- forenoon - alum.
- glowing - all-c.
- morning - am-m., apis, lith-m., mang.
- night in bed - cinnb.
- noon - fago.
- pit, of, during fever - cub.
- sitting - phos.
- waking, on - acon-f.
- water, cold, after - alum.
  - amel. - alumn., hyper.

heat, esophagus - aesc., aeth., aml-n., arg-n., ***ars.,*** bell., benz-ac., brom., ***camph.,*** canth., carb-ac., ***colch.,*** crot-t., guare., hydr-ac., iod., kali-chl., merc-c., nat-s., ***phos.,*** plb., ptel., rhus-t., sul-ac., wye.
- rising, after fright - hyper.

HEAVINESS, sensation - abies-n., acon., aesc., aeth., ***agar.,*** all-s., aloe, alum., am-c., am-m., ant-c., ***ant-t., apis, apoc., arg-m., arg-n., arn.,*** asc-t., ***ars.,*** bapt., ***bar-c.,*** bar-m., bell., bism., bor., ***brom., bry., cact.,*** calad., calc., calc-s., cann-i., ***carb-an., carb-s., carb-v., carl.,*** cast., cham., chel., **CHIN.,** chin-a., chin-s., cimic., cit-v., clem., coca, cocc., coc-c., ***coff.,*** colch., com., ***crot-c., crot-h., cycl.,*** dig., fago., ferr-i., ***fl-ac.,*** form., ***gels.,*** gent-c., gent-l., grat., hura, ***hydr.,*** hyos., ign., iod., ***kali-bi., kali-c.,*** kali-chl., kali-i., kali-n., kali-p., ***kali-s.,*** kreos., lac-ac., lac-c., lach., led., lil-t., ***lob.,*** **LYC.,** manc., ***mag-m.,*** merc., mur-ac., nat-a., ***nat-c., nat-m.,*** nat-p., ***nat-s.,*** nit-ac., **NUX-V.,** ***op.,*** osm., ox-ac., par., petr., phel., ***ph-ac., phos.,*** phys., **PIC-AC.,** ***plat.,*** plb., prun., psor., ***ptel.,*** puls., rat., rhus-t., ***rob.,*** rumx., sabad., ***sang.,*** sec., seneg., sep., ***sil.,*** sol-t-ae., spig., stann., stram., ***stry.,*** **SULPH.,** sul-ac., ***tab., tarent.,*** teucr., thea., upa., valer., wye., xan., zinc., zing.
- afternoon - am-m., fago., **LYC.,** ***sang.,*** stront.
  - eating, after - ***lyc.***
- ascending stairs - nux-m.
- back of - ham.
- beer, after - acon., **KALI-BI.**
- belching amel. - aloe, chel., fago., par.
- bread, after - kali-c., merc., zing.
- breakfast, after - agar., crot-h., fago., gels., lyc., petr., ph-ac., sang.
  - amel. - bar-c.
- breathing, deeply amel. - bar-c.
- carrying, agg. - bar-c.
- chill, during - sulph.
- cold drinks, after - acet-ac., ***ars.,*** podo., rhod.
- damp, weather - kali-c., nat-s., sil.
- digestion, during - hep.
- dinner, after - grat., lyc., nat-a., ptel.
- eating, while - cann-i.
  - after - ***abies-n.,*** absin., agar., alum., alumn., ***am-c., ant-c.,*** arg-n., apis, ***ars.,*** ars-i., bar-c., ***bar-i.,*** bar-m., ***bry., cact.,*** calc-ar., carb-ac., cham., **CHIN.,** chin-a., ***chin-s.,*** cimic., cycl., ***elaps,*** ferr., ferr-i., fl-ac., ***hep., hydr.,*** ign., ***iod.,*** kali-ar., **KALI-BI.,** ***kali-c., kali-p., lach.,*** lob., **LYC.,** merc., nat-a., ***nit-ac.,*** **NUX-V.,** osm., ***ph-ac., phos.,*** plan., phys., plb., ***psor., ptel., puls., rumx.,*** rhus-t., sang., ***sil.,*** **SULPH.,** ***tarent.***
- empty, while - ***fl-ac.***
- evening - alum., bell., kali-bi., rhus-t., sulph.
- forenoon - sulph.
- leaning, backwards, when - con.
- meat, after - ***kali-bi.***
- menses, during - nat-p., zinc.
  - before - tarent.
- morning - am-c., bar-c., calc-s., dios., sang., sulph.
  - waking, on - ***carb-an., puls.,*** zing.
- nausea, during - lyc.
- night - ***aesc., chin.,*** colch., crot-t., tarent.
  - walking, on - sulph.

HEAVINESS, sensation
- noon - alum., fago., ***lyc.,*** mur-ac.
  - eating, after - ***lyc.***
- palpitations, with - upa.
- potatoes, after - ***alum.***
- pressure agg. - phos., ptel.
- sleep, after - ***lach.***
- standing, long, from - hura.
- stooping, after - bar-c.
- supper, after - chin-s., plan.
- trembling, with - iod.
- waking, on - carb-an., ptel., puls., sulph.
- walking in open air amel. - bor., petr.
- water, after - chel.

HICCOUGH, general - acet-ac., acon., aeth., ***agar.,*** agn., all-c., ***alum.,*** am-c., **AM-M.,** ***ambr.,*** aml-n., anac., ang., ant-c., ant-t., ***arn.,*** **ARS.,** ars-h., **ARS-I.,** asar., arund., aur., ***bar-c., bar-i.,*** bar-m., ***bell.,*** benz-ac., berb., bism., bor., bov., brom., bufo, ***bry., caj.,*** calad., ***calc.,*** calc-f., calc-i., canth., caps., carb-an., carb-s., carb-v., carl., cast., caust., ***cham.,*** chel., ***chin.,*** chin-a., ***chin-s., chlf.,*** **CIC.,** cina, cimx., cob., ***cocc., coff.,*** colch., coloc., con., crot-t., cupr., ***cupr-s.,*** cur., **CYCL.,** ***dios.,*** dig., ***dros.,*** dulc., eup-per., ***euph.,*** euphr., ferr-p., ***gels., gins.,*** graph., grat., ham., hell., hydr., **HYOS.,** hep., hydr., hydr-ac., **IGN.,** indg., **IOD.,** ***ip.,*** jab., ***jatr.,*** jug-r., kali-ar., kali-bi., ***kali-br.,*** kali-c., kali-i., kali-n., kali-s., ***kreos., lach., laur.,*** led., lob., **LYC.,** lyss., mag-c., ***mag-m.,*** **MAG-P.,** ***med.,*** meny., **MERC.,** merc-c., mez., mill., ***morph., mosch.,*** mur-ac., **NAT-A., NAT-C., NAT-M.,** nat-s., **NICC.,** nicot., nit-ac., **NUX-M., NUX-V.,** ***op.,*** ox-ac., ***par., phos.,*** phys., phyt., plb., ***psor., puls., ran-b.,*** rat., ***ruta.,*** sabad., sabin., samb., ***sars.,*** **SEC.,** sel., ***sep.,*** sil., ***sin-n., spong., stann., staph.,*** **STRAM.,** ***stront-c.,*** sulph., ***sul-ac.,*** sumb., tab., ***tarax.,*** tarent., **TEUCR.,** ***verat., verat-v., verb.,*** zinc., zinc-valer.
- **afternoon** - agar., canth., ***ign.***
  - 1 p.m. - bov., ***verat-v.***
  - 2 p.m. - tarent., ***verat-v.***
- **agg.,** from hiccough - am-m., bry., cycl., hyos., ign., nux-v., stroph., zinc-valer.
- **alcoholic** drinks, after - **RAN-B.,** sul-ac.
- **alcoholics,** in - ***ran-b.,*** nux-v.
- **alternating,** spasms of chest, with - cic.
- **asthma,** begins with - cupr.
- **back** pain, with - teucr.
- **bed,** in - lachn., nat-m., nicc., sil., ***sulph.***
  - pain in back, with - teucr.
- **belching,** with - ant-c., ***caj.,*** cic., chin., cycl., ***dios.,*** ign., ***nux-v.,*** wye.
  - after - alum., bry., carb-an., cycl., til.
  - amel. - carb-an.
  - bitter - ign.
  - empty - ign.
- **biliary** colic, with - ***chin.***
- **brain,** affections, in - arn., cina.
  - concussion, from - hyos.
- **bread** and butter, after - nat-s.
- **breakfast,** after - tarent., zinc.
- **breath,** shortness of, with - phys.

HICCOUGH, general
cancer of stomach, in - carb-an.
chest, pain, with - stroph.
children, in - bor., ign., ip.
chill, after - am-c., ars.
cholera, in - aeth., arg-n., cic., cupr., kreos., mag-p., ph-ac., verat.
cold fruit, after - ars., dulc., graph., ***puls.***
cold taken, after - phos.
colic, with - hyos.
concussion of brain, with - hyos.
convulsions, with - bell., **CIC.,** cupr., **HYOS.,** ***ran-b.***
after - cic.
before - cupr.
convulsive - aeth., ars., bell., **GELS.,** ***mag-p.,*** nux-v., ***ran-b.,*** stram., tab.
cough, during - tab.
after - ang., tab., trif-p.
cramps, with - cupr-ar.
daytime - nit-ac., petr., phos.
dinner, during - cycl., grat., ***mag-m.,*** nat-c.
after - alum., am-m., arn., bov., carb-ac., carb-v., cob., graph., grat., hyos., indg., ***mag-m., mur-ac.,*** phos., sars., ***teucr.***
before - mag-m., mur-ac., nux-v.
drinking, after - ***ign.,*** lach., merc-c., ***nux-v.,*** puls., sul-ac.
cold drinks - ars., puls.
cold water - thuj.
hot drinks - stram.,***verat.***
earache, with - tarent.
eating, while - ***cycl.,*** eug., mag-m., merc., samb., teucr.
after - acon., ***alum.,*** ars., bar-c., bell., bor., bov., ***bry., carb-an.,*** carb-v., carl., cob., con., cop., ***cycl., graph.,*** hep., hura, **HYOS.,** ***ign.,*** lyc., mag-m., merc., nat-a., nat-c., nat-m., nat-s., ***nux-v.,*** par., phos., psor., rat., samb., ***sep.,*** sil., stann., staph., ***teucr.,*** thuj., sulph., verat., zinc.
amel. - carb-an.
before - bov., ***phos.,*** sil.
emotion, after - ***ign.***
esophagus, spasms of - verat-v.
evening - aeth., graph., kali-bi., ***kali-i., lob.,*** mag-c., nat-c., nat-s., **NICC.,** petr., rhus-t., sars., sil., sulph., ***zinc.***
5 to 8 p.m. - phys.
6 p.m. - ham., nat-c., sars.
6:30 p.m. - mag-c.
bed, in - nat-m., nicc., sil., sulph.
fasting, while - sulph.
exercise, after - carb-v.
fever, after - ars., lach.
at the hour when the fever ought to come - **ARS.**
during, fever - crot-h., ***mag-p.***
typhoid, in - phos.
yellow, during - ars-h.
forenoon, eating, after - bar-c., nat-s.
eating, after, 11 a.m. - ox-ac.

HICCOUGH, general
gastrialgia, in - sil.
gastric affections, in - kali-bi.
hawking, agg. - calc-f.
hepatitis, in - bell.
incomplete - caust., dig., mag-c.
injury to head, from - hyos.
inspiring, when - ang.
intermittent - caust.
after - ***hyos.***
intussusception, with - **HYOS.,** plb.
laughing agg. - calc.
loud - cic., graph., grat., hyos., indg., ***mag-m., mur-ac.,*** phos., sars., ***teucr.***
meningitis, in - arn.
migraine headache, in - aeth.
morning - all-c., apoc., cann-s., kali-n., verat.
fasting, while - kali-n., sulph.
rising, after - gamb., graph., mag-c.
motion, on - carb-v., merc-c.
nervous, hysterical symptoms, with - gels., ***ign., mosch.,*** nux-m., zinc-valer.
night - apoc., ars., bell., **HYOS.,** merc., merc-c., puls., sul-ac.
midnight - bell., hyos.
midnight, before - kali-c.
restlessness, with - stram.
sleep, during - puls.
noon - kali-c., sil., sulph.
nursing, babies, in - hyos., teucr.
painful - ***acon.,*** bell., carb-v., ***cimx.,*** mag-m., mag-p., nat-c., ***nicc., phos., rat., sul-ac.,*** tab., teucr., ***verat-v.***
pain in back, with, after eating, nursing - teucr.
peritonitis, in - ***hyos.,*** lyc.
persistent - kali-br., laur., merc-cy., nux-v., sul-ac., zinc-valer.
perspiration, after - ars.
pork, after - ham.
pregnancy, during - ***cycl., op.***
quinine, after - ***nat-m.***
reading, aloud, while - cycl.
salivation, with profuse - lob.
sitting up, when - kreos.
sleep, during - cina, ign., ***merc-c.***
smoking, while - ambr., ant-c., arg-m., calad., calen., ***ign.,*** lach., psor., ***puls.,*** ruta, ***sang.,*** scut., sel., sep., stann., ***staph.,*** sul-ac., verat.
after - ant-c., calc., ***ign.,*** ip.
before eating - sel.
soup, after - alum.
spasm, before - cupr.
esophagus, spasms of - verat-v.
spine affections, in - ***stram.***
strokes, in - cupr., ol-an.
supper, after - alum., cob., con., lyc., sep., staph.
at begining of - con.
surgery, after - ***hyos.,*** ign., teucr.
abdominal, after - hyos.

HICCOUGH, general
thinking, about it, on - ox-ac.
tuberculosis, in - lyc.
typhoid, in - phos.
unconscious, when - cupr.
violent - ***am-m.,*** calc-f., chin-s., ***cic., cycl.,*** hyos., lob., ***lyc., mag-p., merc-c.,*** **NAT-M., NICC., NUX-V.,** ***rat.,*** **STRAM.,** stront-c., teucr., verat., verat-v., zinc.
painful - rat., verat-v.
vomiting, while - bell., ***bry.,*** cupr., jatr., lach., mag-p., merc., merc-c., ***nux-v.,*** piloc., ruta, **VERAT.**
after - bism., bry., jatr., **VERAT.,** verat-v.
before - cupr., jatr.
fever, after - lach.
yawning, while - aml-n., carl., cocc., cycl., mag-c.
before - caust.
stretching, and, with - aml-n., mag-c.

HORRIBLE, sensation, morning, on waking, in alcoholics - **ASAR.**

HUNGER, (see Food, chapter)

HUNGRY, feeling (see Emptiness, weak)

INACTIVITY, of - ail., aloe, bell., ***carb-v., hydr.,*** manc., ***op.,*** ran-s., ***sil.***

INDIGESTION, general - ***abies-c., abies-n.,*** abrot., acet-ac., aesc., aeth., agar., alet., alf., all-c., all-s., aln., aloe, **ALUM.,** ambr., anac., ***ant-c.,*** ant-t., apoc., ***arg-n.,*** arist-cl., ***arn.,*** **ARS.,** ***ars-i.,*** atro., bapt., **BAR-C.,** ***bar-i.,*** **BAR-M.,** bell., berb., **BISM.,** bor., brom., ***bry.,*** calad., **CALC.,** calc-ar., **CALC-S.,** caps., ***carb-ac., carb-an.,*** **CARB-V.,** carc., ***card-m.,*** casc., ***cham.,*** **CHEL., CHIN.,** ***cina, coca,*** coch., ***coff., colch., coll.,*** corn-f., cupr-ac., ***dios.,*** fel., ferr-m., ***ferr-p.,*** gent-l., ***graph.,*** **HEP.,** ***hom.,*** **HYDR.,** ***ign.,*** iod., **IP.,** iris, ***kali-bi., kali-c.,*** kali-m., **LAC-D.,** ***lach.,*** lept., lob., **LYC.,** ***mag-c., mag-m., merc.,*** mez., mur-ac., nat-a., **NAT-C.,** ***nat-m.,*** nat-s., nit-ac., ***nux-m.,*** **NUX-V., OLND.,** ***op.,*** par., ped., **PETR.,** ***ph-ac., phos.,*** pic-ac., podo., pop., prun., prun-v., ***ptel.,*** **PULS.,** ***rob.,*** sal-ac., ***sang., sep.,*** sil., spong., squil., stann., sul-ac., **SULPH.,** ***tarent.,*** uran-n., valer., xero, zinc., zing.
acids - ***ant-c.,*** ars., chin., nat-m., **NAT-P.**
beer, from - ant-t., bapt., bry., ***kali-bi.,*** lyc., ***nux-v.***
bread, from - ant-c., bry., lyc., nat-m.
breast-feeding, during - ***chin.,*** sin-a.
bright's disease, in - apoc.
buckwheat cakes, from - puls.
cheese, after - ars., carb-v., coloc., nux-v., **PTEL.**
coffee, after - aeth., ***cham.,*** cycl., kali-c., lyc., **NUX-V.**
cold, after taking - ***ant-c., bry., camph.***
bathing, from - ant-c.
food, after - alum., ***ph-ac.***
weather, from - ***dulc.***

INDIGESTION, general
diet, indiscretions in - all-s., ***ant-c., bry., carb-v.,*** chin., coff., ***ip.,*** lyc., ***nat-c., nux-v., puls.,*** xan.
digestion, weak, from - alst., ***anac., ant-c., arg-n.,*** ars., asaf., bism., ***bry.,*** caps., ***carb-an., carb-v., chin.,*** coch., coff., colch., ***cycl., dios.,*** eucal., gran., ***graph., hydr.,*** ip., kali-bi., **LYC.,** merc., **NAT-C.,** nat-m., **NUX-V.,** prun., ***puls.,*** spong., zing.
drugs, abuse of, after - **NUX-V.**
eggs - chin-a., colch., ferr., ferr-m., nux-v.
elderly people - abies-n., ant-c., ars., bar-c., calc., ***carb-v.,*** chin., ***chin-s.,*** fl-ac., hep., ***hydr.,*** kali-c., ***lyc., nat-c.,*** puls., ***sep.,*** sil., sul-ac., sulph.
emotions, from unpleasant - cham., nux-m., nux-v.
evening - ambr., chin.
excesses - ant-t., carb-v., ***chin.,*** kali-c., nat-s., ***nux-v.***
farinaceous food, from - ***caust., lyc., nat-c.,*** **NAT-M.,** ***nat-s., nux-v., sulph.***
fat food, from - ant-c., ***calc.,*** carb-v., ***cycl.,*** ip., ***kali-m., puls.,*** thuj.
after - carb-v., ***puls.***
fatigue, brain fag, in children - calc-f.
fear, from - **PHOS.**
fevers, after acute - chin., quas.
fish, after - ***chin-a.***
decayed - ars., carb-v.
flatulent food - carb-v., chin., ***lyc.,*** puls.
fruit, after - act-sp., ***ant-c.,*** ars., ***chin.,*** elaps, ***ip., puls.,*** verat.
gastric juice, scanty - aln., ***alum.,*** lyc.
gout - ant-t., chin., ***colch.,*** nux-m., thuj.
grief, after - **IGN.,** tarent.
hasty eating, drinking - anac., coff., ***olnd.***
ice cream - ***ars., carb-v.,*** elaps, ip., ***kali-c.,*** nat-c., **PULS.**
ice, water, from ices - ***ars., bell-p.,*** carb-v., elaps, ip., kali-c., nat-c., ***puls.***
meat - ***caust., carb-v., ferr., ferr-p.,*** ip., ***ptel.,*** puls., sil.
decayed - ars., carb-v.
salt, after - act-sp.
melons - ars., chin., zing.
menses, during - arg-n., cop., sep.
mental, exertion, after - arn., calc., cocc., ***lach.,*** **NUX-V.,** ***puls., sulph.,*** verat.
milk, after - **AETH.,** ambr., ***ant-c., calc.,*** carb-v., **CHIN.,** ***iris, mag-c.,*** **MAG-M., NAT-C., NIT-AC.,** ***nux-v.,*** sul-ac., **SULPH.**
morning - bufo.
mussels, after - ***bell.,*** cop., ***ip.***
night-watching, from - nux-v.
onions, after - acon-l., **LYC.,** nit-ac., ***puls., thuj.***
pastries, after - ant-c., carb-v., ***ip.,*** kali-m., lyc., **PULS.**
pears, after - bor.

INDIGESTION, general
pork, after - ars., chin., **CYCL.,** ***ip.,*** **PULS.**
potatoes, after - **ALUM.**
pregnancy, during - ant-c., carb-v., chin., ***ip.,*** lyc., ***nux-v.,*** **PULS.**
salt, abuse of - carb-v., nat-m., phos.
salty, food from - carb-v.
sedentary life - nux-v.
sex, after - dig., phos.
simplest food, from - alet., amyg., ***ant-c.,*** carb-an., ***carb-v., chin.,*** dig., ***hep.,*** kali-c., lach., ***nat-c., nux-v.,*** puls.
sour food, after - aloe, **ANT-C.,** carb-v., ***nat-p., nux-v.***
sprain, from - ruta.
stooping, from - merc.
sweets - ant-c., ***arg-n.,*** ip., lyc., ***puls.,*** zinc.
tea - abies-n., ***chin., dios.,*** puls., thea., thuj.
tobacco - abies-n., calad., ***nux-v.,*** sep.
urticaria, from - cop.
vegetables, from - ars., asc-t., nat-c., nux-v., ***sep.***
vexation, after - **CHAM., IP.,** nux-m., nux-v., tarent.
warm, drinks, after - ambr.
food, after - am-c.
weather, from - ant-c., ***bry.***
water, from - ars.
bad, after - ***all-s., ars.,*** bapt., ***podo., zing.***
wines, liquors, from - ***ant-c.,*** caps., carb-v., coff., nat-s., ***nux-v.,*** sul-ac., sulph., ***zinc.***
yawning, amel. - cast.

INDURATION, of the walls - ***acet-ac.,*** **ARS.,** bar-c., con., ***kreos., mez., nux-v.,*** phos., thuj., verat.
pylorus - bism., ***cund.,*** graph., ***phos.,*** sep., ***sil., stry-p.***

INFLAMMATION, (see Gastritis)
inflammation, esophagus (see Esophagitis)

INSENSIBILITY, sensation - sars.

IRRITATION - ***acon.,*** all-c., ant-t., ***arg-n., ars.,*** aur-m., **BISM.,** carb-ac., cob., dros., ***ip.,*** kali-ar., kali-n., ***merc.,*** merc-c., ox-ac., ***phos.,*** plb., ***podo.,*** sec., stram., verat-v.
irritation, esophagus - ***cocc.,*** crot-t., phos.

ITCHING, epigastrium - con., kali-c., plat.
itching, esophagus - aeth., cahin.

JERKING - calc., mez., nat-c., ***nat-m.,*** nux-v., phos., plat., sang., ***stry.***
extending from epigastrium to rectum - ars.
to throat - phos.
mouth, on opening the - stry.

JUMPING, sensation of - croc.

LANCINATING, pain - all-s., ***ars.,*** aur-s., bad., bol., cadm-s., canth., ***carb-v., gins.,*** plb., tarent., thal.
inspiration, deep, agg. - bad.
midnight, after - ***kali-c.***
night - ars.

LIQUIDS, taken are forced into nose, (see Throat)

LUMP, sensation of - abies-n., acon., ***agar.,*** anan., ***ant-c.,*** arg-n., arn., ***ars.,*** bar-c., bell., bism., bov., ***bry.,*** calc., ***carb-v.,*** cham., ***chin.,*** colch., dig., dirc., ferr., ***graph., hep., hydr.,*** hydr-ac., ***kali-bi., kali-c., lec.,*** lil-t., ***lob., lyc.,*** manc., med., naja, nat-c., nat-m., ***nux-m., nux-v.,*** osm., passi., ***phos.,*** piloc., plb., ***puls., rhus-t.,*** rob., rumx., sang., **SANIC.,** ***sep.,*** sil., spig., sulph., xero, zing.
as if a, had fallen to back on rising from seat - laur.
belching amel. - bar-c.
cardia, in - ***abies-n., liatr.***
cold drinks, after - acet-ac., ***ars.***
eating, after - ***abies-n., ars.,*** med., nat-c., nat-m., ***nux-v., ph-ac.,*** puls., rumx.
flatuent food, after - sil.
hard - nux-m.
hot, burning - bell.
icy - bov.
lying on back, while - ***sulph.***
midnight, after - ***arg-n.***
pulsating - ***graph.***
sharp - hydr.
supper, after - calc.
lump, plug, sensation of, esophagus - ***all-c.,*** anac., ars., bar-c., bell., calc., ***caust.,*** chel., ***chin., coc-c., con., croc.,*** dig., der., ***gels.,*** lac-ac., ***lob.,*** lyc., ***merc-c.,*** nit-ac., phos., ***plb., puls.,*** rumx., sabin., tab., verat., verat-v.
cardiac opening, sensation - abies-n., tus-f.,
eating, after - elaps, ***lac-ac.***
hard - lyc.
middle, of - chin., puls.
periodical - tab.
swallowing amel. - phos.
preventing - upa.
upper part - calc-ac.

KNOT, sensation in - chin., ign., nux-v., plb.

MOVEMENT, in, sensation of - arn., chel., ***cocc.,*** colch., coloc., **CROC.,** iod., kali-n., laur., ***lyss.,*** mag-m., nat-m., nicc., ol-an., phos., sul-ac., tarent.

NARROW, pylorus feels too - calc., chin., ***lyc.,*** nux-v., phos., sulph.

NAUSEA, general - absin., acet-ac., ***acon.,*** act-sp., ***aesc., aeth., agar.,*** agn., ail., ***all-s., alum.,*** alumn., ambr., am-c., ***am-m., anac.,*** anan., ang., **ANT-C., ANT-T.,** apis, apoc., apom., ***aran., arg-m.,*** **ARG-N.,** arn., **ARS.,** ars-h., ars-i., arund., asaf., ***asar.,*** aster., aur., aur-m-n., ***bapt., bar-c.,*** bar-i., bar-m., **BELL.,** benz-ac., ***berb., bism., bol.,*** bor., both., ***bov.,*** brach., brom., ***bry.,*** bufo, cact., ***cadm-s., calc., calc-p., calc-s.,*** cahin., ***camph.,*** cann-s., ***canth., caps., carb-ac., carb-an.,*** **CARB-S.,** ***carb-v., card-m.,*** carl., cast., caul., ***caust.,*** **CHAM.,** ***chel.,*** **CHIN.,** chin-a., ***chin-s., chion., chr-ac., cimic., cina, cist.,*** clem., **COCC.,** ***cod.,*** coff., **COLCH.,** ***coll., coloc.,*** com., ***con.,*** cop., ***corn.,*** cor-r., ***crot-c., crot-h., crot-t., cub.,*** cund., **CUPR.,** ***cupr-ar., cupr-s., cycl.,*** daph., **DIG.,** dios., dros., **DULC.,** ***echi.,*** elaps, ***elat.,*** eug., euon., ***euph.,*** euphr.,

NAUSEA, general - ***eup-per.,*** eupi., ***ferr., ferr-ar.,*** ferr-i., ***ferr-p., fl-ac., form., gamb., gels.,*** gent-c., gent-l., glon., ***gran., graph.,*** grat., ***guai.,*** ham., **HELL., HEP.,** ***hydr.,*** hydrc., hyos., hyper., hura, ***ign.,*** indg., ***iod.,*** **IP., IRIS, IRIS-F.,** jatr., jug-r., **KALI-AR.,** ***kali-bi.,*** **KALI-C.,** kali-chl., kali-i., kali-n., kali-p., ***kali-s.,*** kalm., kreos., ***lac-c., lach.,*** lachn., ***lac-ac.,*** lact., ***laur.,*** lec., led., lil-t., lith., **LOB.,** ***lyc.,*** lyss., mag-c., ***mag-m., mag-p.,*** mag-s., maland., manc., mang., med., meny., meph., ***merc.,*** merc-c., ***merc-i-f.,*** merc-i-r., merl., ***mez., mosch., mur-ac.,*** mygal., ***naja, nat-a., nat-c.,*** **NAT-M.,** ***nat-p.,*** nat-s., nicc., ***nit-ac.,*** nux-m., **NUX-V.,** ***ol-an.,*** olnd., onos., op., ***ox-ac.,*** paeon., par., **PETR.,** phel., ***ph-ac., phos.,*** phys., ***phyt., pic-ac.,*** plan., ***plat., plb., podo., prun., psor.,*** ptel., **PULS.,** ***ran-b., ran-s., raph.,*** rat., ***rheum, rhod.,*** **RHUS-T.,** ***rhus-v.,*** rumx., ruta., ***sabad.,*** sabin., ***samb.,*** **SANG.,** ***sars., sec.,*** sel., senec., ***seneg.,*** **SEP., SIL.,** spig., spong., ***squil., stann.,*** staph., stram., stront-c., stry., **SULPH.,** ***sul-ac.,*** sumb., syph., **TAB.,** ***tarax.,*** tarent., tax., ***ter., ther., thuj.,*** upa., uran., ust., **VALER., VERAT.,** ***verat-v.,*** vesp., vinc., viol-t., vip., wye., xan., **ZINC.,** zing.

abdomen, in - agar., agn., ail., ant-t., asar., bell., bry., cadm-s., cic., cocc., croc., cupr., cycl., fago., gels., graph., grat., hell., hep., ip., iris, lact., mang., mur-ac., nit-ac., nux-m., par., phyt., pic-ac., plan., ***phel., puls.,*** rheum, ruta., samb., sep., sil., spong., stann., staph., sumb., teucr., thuj., valer., zing.

compressing, on - agar.

lower, abdomen - merc-i-f., puls., rhus-t.

pain, during, in abdomen - ant-t., ***arg-n., arn.,*** ars., arund., bism., chel., **COLOC.,** crot-t., ***gran.,*** grat., haem., hep., **IP.,** ***kali-c., kreos.,*** **NUX-V.,** ***ox-ac., ph-ac.,*** plb., sep., staph., sulph., ter., zing.

uncovering abdomen, in open air amel. - tab.

afternoon - aesc., arg-m., bor., calc., carb-s., caust., chin., **COCC.,** con., cycl., dros., fago., graph., grat., indg., kali-c., kali-n., lyc., mag-c., merl., mez., nat-a., ***phos.,*** podo., ***ran-b.,*** rob., sang., sars., ***sil.***

1 p.m. - corn., grat., hura, phys.

2 p.m. - grat., hura, nux-m., phys., sulph.

3 p.m. - **ARS.**

until evening - bor.

until 10 p.m. - lyc.

4 p.m. - anac., calc-p., lach., phys.

5:30 p.m. - lec.

air, amel. - am-m., anth., ant-t., bor-ac., carb-v., ***croc.,*** dig., glon., grat., hell., kali-bi., **LYC.,** naja, phos., ***puls.,*** **TAB.,** tarax.

amel., draft, in a - hipp.

open, in - acon., ang., arg-m., ars., bell., carb-s., crot-t., grat., lyc., puls., seneg., thuj.

air, travel, during - arg-n., cocc., gels., petr.

alcoholics, in - ***ars., asar.,*** carb-s., cimic., graph., nux-v., **KALI-BI.,** ***sul-ac.***

alternating, with hunger - berb., nit-ac.

amorous, caresses, from - ant-c., sabad.

NAUSEA, general

anxiety, with - ***ars.,*** bar-c., bell., calc., caust., chin., graph., ***ip.,*** kali-c., lob., nit-ac., nit-ac., puls., sep., squil., ***tab.***

after - caust., ***chel.,*** nux-v.

causing - **ANT-T.,** ***calc.,*** **NUX-V.**

deathly, with - all-c., ant-c., ant-t., arg-n., ***ars., cadm-s., camph.,*** cocc., **CROT-H.,** cupr., ***dig.,*** ferr-p., hell., **IP., LOB.,** ***med.,*** puls., **TAB.**

exerting eyes, on - **SEP.**

night, at - cycl.

weakness, and, recurs periodically - ars.

apyrexia - ant-c., chin-s., puls.

ascending, stairs rapidly - glon.

backache, during - coloc., phys., zing.

bed, in, amel. - nat-c.

beer, after - bry., cadm-s., kali-bi., lach., mur-ac., nux-v.

odor of, agg. - phos.

belching, during - cimic., cocc., coloc., crot-t., goss., grat., ***kali-c.,*** nit-ac., ol-an., ptel.

after - alum.

amel. - agar., all-c., am-m., ant-t., camph., carb-s., ***caust.,*** chel., cinnb., fago., ferr., glon., grat., kali-p., lac-c., lil-t., lyc., mag-m., nicc., ol-an., osm., phos., rhod., rumx., sabad., sul-ac., verat-v.

mucus, of amel. - kali-n.

blowing, nose - ***hell.,*** sang., sulph.

agg. - sang.

brandy, amel. - ars.

bread, after - **ANT-C.,** zinc.

black, after - ph-ac.

breakfast, during - agar., ***carb-ac.,*** ind., med., naja, plan., sang., zinc.

after - agar., ambr., bell., calc-p., ***cham.,*** coca, dig., dios., gamb., indg., kali-bi., mez., nat-m., onos., par., sabin., ***sars.,*** spig., sulph., verat., zinc.

amel. - alum., bar-c.

before - alum., alumn., anac., arg-n., aur-m., bar-c., ***berb., bov., calc.,*** eupi., fago., goss., ***lyc., nit-ac.,*** petr., phos., **SEP.,** sin-n., spig., ***tub.***

brushing, teeth, on - ars-i., coc-c.

burning in anus, with - kali-bi.

chest, in - acon., anac., arg-m., asaf., bry., cadm-s., calc., ***calen., croc.,*** glon., lach., mang., ***merc.,*** nux-v., par., ph-ac., ***rhus-t.,*** sec., staph.

pain in, from - croc.

chill, during - alum., arg-n., ***ars.,*** bell., bov., bry., calc., ***cham.,*** chel., cina, cob., ***cocc.,*** con., dros., **EUP-PER.,** hyper., ign., ***ip., kali-ar.,*** kali-c., kali-s., kreos., lach., ***lyc.,*** mag-c., ***nat-m.,*** nit-ac., petr., puls., raph., rhus-t., rumx., sabad., sang., sec., sep., sul-ac., verat., zinc.

after - elat., eup-per., ip., kali-c.

lasting until next chill - ***chin-s.***

before - ***ars., carb-v., chin., eup-per., ip.,*** lyc., nat-m., puls.

NAUSEA, general
chill, with
close of - ***eup-per.***
death-like - xan.
chilliness, with - alum., am-c., bov., cocc., con., dulc., echi., eup-per., hep., kali-m., ***kreos.,*** sul-ac., xan.
after - ***camph.,*** corn., ***eup-per., kali-bi., kreos., lach., mag-s., puls.,*** sabad., sal-ac., verat-v., xan.
closing, the eyes - ***lach.,*** sabad., ***ther.***
closing, amel. - con.
coffee, after - bry., ***calc-p., caps., caust., cham.,*** cycl., nat-m., rhus-t., vinc.
smell of - arg-n.
amel. - alet.
cold, drinks, after - agar., anac., ***ars., calc.,*** camph., carb-ac., ***cupr., kali-ar., kali-c.,*** kali-i., kali-s., lach., lac-d., ***lyc., nat-a., nat-m.,*** nux-v., puls., ***rhus-t., sul-ac.,*** teucr., ther.
amel. - ***bism., phos., puls.***
heated, when - ***kali-c.***
warm, not after - lyc., ther.
cold, when - cadm-s., **COCC.,** crot-t., ***hep.,*** kali-c., valer.
coldness, in stomach, with - kali-n.
concomitant, as a - ***ip.,*** lob., nat-s.
constant - ***ant-c., ant-t.,*** arg-n., ars., cadm-s., carb-v., coloc., ***dig.,*** graph., hep., **IP.,** iris, jatr., ***kreos.,*** lac-ac., ***lac-c.,*** lil-t., ***lob., lyc.,*** mag-m., nat-a., nat-c., nat-m., **NUX-V.,** petr., phos., plat., **SIL.,** stront-c., verat., vib.
clean tongue, with - ***ip.***
constipation, with - **COCC.,** ***hyper.***
convulsions, after - bell.
before - hydr-ac.
cough, during - ant-t., ars., aspar., bry., ***calc.,*** caps., ***coc-c.,*** coloc., cupr., dros., elaps, hep., hydr., ***ign.,*** **IP.,** kali-ar., ***kali-bi., kali-c.,*** kali-p., kali-s., lach., ***merc.,*** nat-a., nat-c., nat-m., nat-p., nit-ac., ***nux-v.,*** petr., ***ph-ac.,*** **PULS.,** ruta., sars., ***sep.,*** squil., thuj., ***verat.***
cramps, with - ***ip.,*** trio.
crowd, in a - sabin.
daytime - ars., aur., mez., mosch., ***nit-ac.,*** phos., pic-ac., sulph.
deathly - all-c., ant-c., ***ant-t.,*** arg-n., ***ars., cadm-s., camph.,*** cocc., colch., **CROT-H.,** ***dig.,*** ferr-p., hell., **IP.,** lept., **LOB.,** ***med., nux-v.,*** puls., **TAB.**
anxiety, with - all-c., ant-c., ant-t., arg-n., **ARS.,** ***cadm-s., camph.,*** cocc., **CROT-H.,** cupr., ***dig.,*** ferr-p., hell., **IP., LOB.,** ***med.,*** puls., **TAB.**
descending, agg. - bor., nat-s.
diarrhea, with - cist.
anxiety, and - ant-t.
dinner, during - am-c., bry., calc., colch., grat., hyper., lyc., mag-m., merc-i-f., ***nux-v.,*** ol-an., ox-ac., thuj.

NAUSEA, general
after - agar., am-c., am-m., ***ant-t.,*** arg-m., ***arg-n.,*** ars., berb., calc., caps., cast., colch., ***coloc., cycl.,*** con., grat., ham., kali-ar., ***kali-c.,*** kali-n., lach., nat-m., **NUX-V.,** ol-an., phos., ptel., sars., seneg., squil., spig., verat., zinc.
amel. - alet., mang., med.
before - ars., carb-v., nux-v., sabad.
draft, agg. - hippoz.
dreams, from - arg-n.
drinking, after - agar., anac., ant-t., arn., ***ars.,*** bry., camph., carb-an., chin., ***cimx.,*** **COCC.,** crot-t., cycl., dig., ***eup-per.,*** gamb., kali-bi., ***lach.,*** lyc., nat-a., ***nat-m.,*** nit-ac., ***nux-v., phos.,*** **PULS.,** rhus-t., sil., teucr.
amel. - **BRY.,** euphr., ***lob., med., paeon., phos.,*** samb.
champagne, aerated, after - digox.
drinking, while - bry.
ice water, after - lach., laur.
ice water, amel. - calc.
water, after - apoc., ars., calc., verat.
drowsiness, with - ant-t., apoc.
dryness in pharynx, from - **COCC.**
ear, felt in - dios.
eating, while - agar., am-c., ang., aur., ***bar-c.,*** bell., bov., bor., brom., calc., canth., carb-v., ***caust.,*** chin-s., ***cic., cocc.,*** coff., colch., dig., ***ferr.,*** hell., ***jac-c.,*** kali-c., mag-c., merc-i-r., morph., nux-v., olnd., phos., ptel., ***puls.,*** ruta., sabad., sil., thuj., verat.
amel., while - ***anac.***
after - acon., aesc., ***agar.,*** agn., all-c., ***alum.,*** ambr., **AM-C.,** am-m., anac., ant-t., apis, aran., ***arg-n.,*** ars., ars-i., asar., aur-m., ***bism., bor., bov., bry.,*** bufo, ***calc.,*** cann-i., carb-an., carb-s., carb-v., cast., ***caust., cham.,*** chin., chin-a., ***chin-s., cic.,*** clem., **COCC.,** ***colch.,*** coloc., ***con.,*** cur., cycl., dig., dios., dros., elaps, euphr., ***ferr., ferr-ar., ferr-i., ferr-p.,*** gent-c., gent-l., graph., grat., gymn., ham., hell., hep., hyper., ign., ind., iod., ip., jatr., ***kali-ar., kali-c.,*** kali-i., kali-p., kali-s., lac-ac., ***lach.,*** led., ***lyc.,*** mag-c., ***med.,*** merc., mosch., nat-a., ***nat-m.,*** nat-s., ***nit-ac.,*** **NUX-V.,** ol-an., ***op.,*** ox-ac., petr., ph-ac., ***phos.,*** plb., podo., ***ptel.,*** **PULS.,** rheum, ***rhus-t.,*** rumx., ***ruta.,*** sabin., sang., sars., **SEP.,** ***sil., stann., sulph.,*** sul-ac., ***tarent.,*** ter., thea., verat., ***zinc.***
amel., after - acon., alum., arg-n., aur-m., brom., bry., cham., chel., chin., fago., grat., iod., ***kali-bi., lac-ac., lob.,*** mag-c., mez., ***nat-c.,*** phos., phyt., rad., sabad., sang., **SEP.,** sil., spig., verat., verat-v.
before - anac., ars., berb., carb-v., ***caust.,*** chin., ferr., ferr-ar., graph., lyc., ***nat-s.,*** nux-v., ***ph-ac.,*** sabad., ***sulph.,*** tell.
eggs, after eating - lyss.
smell of - **COLCH.**
thought of, at the - upa.
erect, on becoming - acon., colch., eupi.

NAUSEA, general
erection, with - kali-bi.
evening - ***alum.,*** alumn., anac., arg-n., asar., bapt., bell., brach., bor., bry., ***calc.,*** calc-s., canth., carb-v., chel., coloc., con., cycl., echi., eug., fl-ac., gent-l., glon., grat., hell., ***hep.,*** ind., kali-bi., kali-n., kalm., kreos., lyc., lycps., mag-c., merc., merc-i-r., naja, nat-c., nat-m., nat-p., nit-ac., nux-m., nux-v., ***pall.,*** petr., ph-ac., phos., plan., plb., ***puls.,*** ran-b., raph., sang., senec., sep., sil., sin-n., stram., sulph., tell.
bed, in - graph., phos.
drinking, after - ***nux-v.***
eating, while - caust., cham., phos.
after amel. - tell.
supper, before - graph.
walking in the open air - lycps., phos., ***sep.***
excitement, after - **KALI-C.**
exercising, from - aloe, ars., colch., spong., tab., ther.
exertion, after - aspar., ***iris, sil.,*** spong.
expectoration, after - ars.
eyes, symptoms, with - calc., ***kalm.,*** laur., manc., nat-m., nat-s., puls., raph.
closing, from - lach., ***ther.,*** thuj.
exertion, after, vision, of - con., ***sars., sep., ther.***
using, the - con., graph., jab., piloc., puls., sep., ***ther.***
faint-like - alum., ang., ***arg-n.,*** bor., ***bry.,*** calad., calc., carb-an., carb-s., caust., cham., chel., **COCC.,** coff., colch., fago., ***glon.,*** graph., hep., hyper., ip., ***kali-c.,*** **LACH.,** mag-m., nat-m., **NUX-V.,** op., petr., phos., pic-ac., plan., plat., ***puls.,*** stict., sul-ac., sulph., **TAB.,** ***tub.,*** valer., verat., vesp.
false teeth, from - cocc.
fasting, while - alum., aur-m., bar-c., ***calc.,*** graph., **LYC.,** mag-m., meph., puls., sep., sil., valer.
fats, agg. - dros., ip., puls.
eating, after - ***ip.,*** lyss., nit-ac., ***puls.,*** sep.
fever, during - arg-n., **ARS.,** ***bry., carb-v.,*** cham., ***cimx.,*** cocc., dros., ***eup-per.,*** eup-pur., ***guare., ip.,*** kali-c., lyc., nat-c., **NAT-M.,** nit-ac., ***nux-v.,*** op., phos., ptel., ***sang.,*** sel., sep., thuj., vinc., zinc.
after - **ARS.,** dros., ***fl-ac.***
close, at - ***eup-per.***
fish, after - nat-m.
smell of - **COLCH.**
flatus, passing, agg. - ant-t.
amel. - bell.
food, on looking at - aeth., ant-t., **COLCH.,** ip., ***kali-bi., kali-c., lyc.,*** merc-i-f., mosch., ***ph-ac.,*** sabad., ***sep.,*** sil., squil., spig., ***sulph.,*** tub., xan.
relish for, with - dig.
rich, from - ant-c., carb-an., cycl., dros., ***ip., nit-ac.,*** **PULS.,** sep., ***tarax.***

NAUSEA, general
food, smell of - aeth., ***ars., cocc.,*** **COLCH.,** ***dig.,*** eup-per., ***ip.,*** merc-i-f., nux-v., ph-ac., podo., ptel., puls., **SEP.,** stann., sym-r., ***thuj.,*** tub., vario.
thought of - ***ars.,*** bor., bry., carb-v., ***chin.,*** **COCC., COLCH.,** graph., ***ip.,*** mag-c., mosch., nat-m., ***sars., sep.,*** sulph., ***thuj.,*** upa., zinc.
food eaten - arg-m., cann-s., graph., ***sars.***
forenoon - agar., arn., ars., bell., bor., bov., bry., calc., canth., carb-v., fago., ferr., hep., ign., jug-c., kali-c., lach., lyc., mag-c., mag-m., naja, nat-c., nat-m., nat-s., nicc., nux-m., op., phos., plat., puls., sars., sep., sulph.
10 a.m. - ***bor.,*** corn., sep.
11 a.m. - **ARS.,** calc., clem., hura, ign., ind., jug-c., lac-ac., puls-n
fruit, after - ***ant-t., ip.,*** nat-c.
hawking, when - ambr., anac., ***caust.,*** coc-c., ***lac-ac.,*** manc., osm., ***stann.,*** tarent.
head, in - colch.
headache, with - acon., aesc., ail., ***alum.,*** alumn., ambr., ***am-c.,*** **ANT-C.,** ant-t., apis, arg-m., arg-n., arn., ***ars.,*** asar., aur., benz-ac., ***bor., bry.,*** calc., ***calc-p.,*** calc-s., camph., cann-s., ***caps., carb-ac., carb-s., carb-v.,*** **CAUST.,** ***cedr.,*** chel., chin., chin-a., chin-s., cic., cimic., cob., **COCC.,** ***coloc.,*** **CON.,** cor-r., croc., crot-h., ***cupr.,*** cycl., dros., ***dulc.,*** epiph., ***eug.,*** eup-per., eup-pur., ferr., fl-ac., form., gels., ***glon., graph.,*** grat., hep., hipp., ign., ind., **IP., IRIS,** kali-ar., ***kali-bi., kali-c.,*** kali-p., ***kali-s.,*** kalm., kreos., ***lac-c., lac-d., lach., lept.,*** lith., ***lob.,*** lyc., mag-c., ***merc.,*** mez., mill., ***mosch.,*** nat-a., nat-c., ***nat-m.,*** nat-p., nat-s., ***nit-ac., nux-m.,*** **NUX-V.,** ***op.,*** petr., ***phos.,*** phyt., plat., ***puls.,*** ran-b., rhus-t., ruta., **SANG.,** ***sars.,*** seneg., ***sep.,*** sil., spig., ***stann.,*** stram., stront-c., ***sulph., tab.,*** tarax., tep., ter., ther., thuj., verat., zinc., zing.
trembling of body, with - bor.
heat of body, with - kali-bi.
hemorrhage, with - **IP.**
hiccough, with - ***lach.***
humiliation, after - ***puls.***
hunger, agg. - ***berb-a.,*** cocc., ign., petr., valer., verat.
hyacinths, from the odor of - lyc., phos.
ice cream, after - ***ars., ip.,*** **PULS.,** rhus-t.
amel. - cench.
ices, cold, from - ars.
inability, to vomit - ***nux-v.***
intermittent - aesc., ***ant-c.,*** **ANT-T.,** ***cina, dros.,*** elat., eup-per., hep., iod., mosch., plat., sabad., ***sep.,*** **TAB.**
night before paroxysm of - ***eup-per.***
itching, until he vomits - ip.
with, before urticaria - sang.
kidney origin, from - senec.
labor, during - ant-t., caul., cham., ***cocc.,*** **IP.,** mag-m., ***puls.,*** **SEP.**

NAUSEA, general

leaning, abdomen on something, when - samb.
head on table amel. - plat.
lemonade, amel. - cycl., puls.
light, agg. - lach.
lips, touching on - cadm-s., nux-m.
liquids, from - **MERC-C.**
looking, at moving objects - asar., cocc., ip., ***jab., piloc.***
steadily - con., ***sars., sep., ther.***
lying, while - mag-m.
down, on - ars., hep., lac-d., mill., nat-h., nat-m., phos., phys., ptel., puls., raph., rhus-t., sin-a.
amel. - ***alum.,*** alumn., arn., ***caust.,*** echi., hep., ***kali-c., nux-v.,*** phos., ph-ac., puls., sep., sil.
abdomen, on amel. - caust., mag-aust.
back, on - merc.
left side, on - ant-t., cann-s., crot-h., ferr., iris., kali-br., lach., puls., sang., sep., sul-ac., verat-v.
amel. - cann-s.
right side, on - bry., ***cann-i., cann-s.,*** crot-h., iris, sang., sul-ac.
amel. - nat-m.
side, on - bry., ip.
amel. - ant-t., nat-m.
meat, after - ***carb-an., caust.,*** cupr., lyss., merc., sulph., ter.
smell of - ***colch.,*** eup-per.
menopause, during - ***ferr.,*** glon., sars., sep.
menses, during - am-c., am-m., ant-c., arn., ars., bell., ***bor., bry., calc.,*** canth., ***caps.,*** carb-v., caul., cham., chel., cocc., ***colch.,*** con., cupr., eupi., fago., gels., ***graph., hyos.,*** hyper., **IP.,** kali-ar., ***kali-bi., kali-c.,*** kali-p., lob., ***lyc., mag-c.,*** mang., mosch., nat-a., nat-c., nat-m., **NUX-V.,** phos., pic-ac., ***puls.,*** sep., tarent., thuj., verat., ***vib.***
after - chin-s., crot-h.
before - am-c., ant-t., aur-s., berb., bufo, caul., cocc., crot-h., cupr., ***hyos., ip.,*** kreos., ***lyc.,*** mag-c., ***nat-m., nicc.,*** nux-v., phos., ***puls.,*** sep., verat., vib.
profuse, with - caps.
suppressed, with - alum., ars., caust., cocc., croc., cupr., cycl., ***ip.,*** lob., lyc., nat-m., nit-ac., ***nux-v.,*** petr., phos., **PULS.,** rhus-t., sang., sulph., verat., zinc.
mental, exertion, from - asar., ***aur., bor.,*** cupr-ar., ***lach.***
metrorrhagia, during - apoc., caps., ***ip.***
milk, after - aeth., **CALC.,** crot-t., lach., nat-c., nat-m., **NIT-AC.,** ***puls.***
amel. - chel.
morning - absin., acon., agar., ***alum.,*** alumn., am-c., ***anac.,*** ant-t., apoc., ***arn.,*** ars-m., bar-c., benz-ac., berb., bor., ***bov.,*** bry., bufo, ***cact.,*** calad., **CALC.,** camph., caps., ***carb-ac.,*** carb-s., **CARB-V.,** caust., ***cham., cic.,*** cocc., ***con.,*** crot-h., cupr-ac., ***cur.,*** cycl., ***dig.,*** dios., elaps, euph., fago., form., ***graph.,*** hep., hyos.,

NAUSEA, general

morning - hyper., inul., ***kali-bi., kalm.,*** kreos., ***lac-c., lac-d., lach., lac-ac.,*** laur., led., lob., lyc., ***mag-c.,*** mag-m., mang., ***med.,*** merc., ***mez.,*** mosch., nat-c., ***nat-m.,*** nat-p., nicc., **NUX-V.,** onos., ox-ac., ***petr.,*** phos., plat., podo., ***psor.,*** **PULS.,** ran-s., rhus-t., rumx., sabad., sars., senec., **SEP.,** ***sil.,*** spig., staph., sul-ac., ***sulph.,*** ter., ther., thuj., ***tub.,*** verat., zinc., zing.
bed, in - alum., arg-m., graph., kali-n., mag-s., **NUX-V.,** sabin., zinc.
continues whole day - cact.
early - lob.
lying down amel - rhus-t.
menses, before - ***am-m.,*** bor., ***cocc., cycl.,*** graph., ichth., ***ip.,*** kreos., meli., nat-m., ***nux-v.,*** puls., ***sep.,*** thlaspi, verat.
rising, on - asc-t., bry., calc., carb-an., dios., ferr-p., graph., hydr., iod., lac-ac., ***lac-d.,*** lyc., mag-c., mag-m., mang., nat-m., nicc., ***nux-v.,*** phos., pic-ac., podo., rhus-t., senec., ***sep.,*** sil., ther., valer., verat-v.
rising, on, amel. - sabin., zinc.
waking, on - ail., ***alum.,*** ambr., ars., ***asar., bor., con.,*** euphr., ***lac-ac.,*** nat-m., ***petr.,*** phyt., sep., sulph.
motion, on - alum anac., ***arn.,*** bov., ***bry.,*** bufo, calc., calc-p., carb-v., **COCC.,** crot-h., ***eup-per.,*** euph., dig., fago., glon., ***graph.,*** hep., ***ip., kali-bi.,*** **KALI-C.,** kali-s., kalm., ***lac-ac.,*** mag-c., med., nat-c., nat-s., ***nux-v., op.,*** phos., pic-ac., ptel., puls., sep., sil., sin-a., spong., sulph., **TAB.,** ther., ***verat., zinc.***
amel. - mez., nit-ac.
eyes, of agg. - bry., con., graph., jab., puls., ***sep.***
least, at - tab., ther.
mouth, in - aeth., agar., cadm-s., ***cocc.,*** ip., ***mag-m., puls.,*** rhod., ***stann.,*** staph., sul-ac.
mucus, in chest, from - sulph.
mucus, in throat, from - ***caust.,*** guai.
music, from - phys., sulph.
mutton, smell of - ov.
night - alum., alumn., am-c., apis, arg-m., calc., ***carb-an.,*** carb-s., carb-v., cham., chel., con., dig., ***dulc.,*** elaps, eupi., form., glon., graph., guai., hell., hep., iod., jug-c., kali-c., kali-bi., kali-n., ***lob.,*** lyc., mag-c., mag-s., ***merc., merc-c.,*** naja, nat-a., nit-ac., phos., plat., puls., rat., rhus-t., ***sep.,*** sil., sulph., tarent., ther., thuj.
2 a.m. - indg., sep.
3 a.m. - ars., mur-ac.
4 a.m. - alum., alumn.
5 a.m. - dios., nat-m.
lying down, after - chel., con., dig., ind., kali-c., naja, nat-m., nit-ac., phos., pic-ac., sang., ***tarent.***
amel. - phos.
midnight - ambr., bry., calc., crot-t., eupi., ferr., phel., ran-s., sil.
after - ambr., mang., ran-s., squil.

NAUSEA, general
night, midnight
rising, on - ambr., nat-m.
until morning - dros.
rising amel. - kali-c.
rising from sleep, on - cimic., op., puls.
waking, on - alum., alumn., ambr., hyper., ***lob.,*** lyc., mez., mur-ac., phyt., ruta, sep., spong., sulph.
noise, from - ***cocc., ther.***
noon - agar., arg-n., coloc., graph., grat., hyper., ign., mang., phos., pic-ac., sulph., stry., zinc.
nose blowing, agg. - sang.
odors, from - **COLCH.,** ***dig.,*** eup-per., ***ph-ac., sep.,*** vario.
body, of his own - thuj., **SULPH.**
opening, eyes, after - ther.
siesta, after - arn.
operation on abdomen, after - arn., calen., **BISM.,** staph.
oranges, odor of - ***cit-v.***
organ, from sound of - phys.
overheated, after being - ***ant-c.***
pain, during - acon., aloe, ant-t., ars., cadm-s., calc., carb-v., caust., ***chel.,*** coloc., crot-t., graph., hep., ***ip.,*** kali-n., lyc., nat-m., nux-v., sep., spig.
abdomen, in - lyc.
back, in - coloc., nux-v., ***sep.***
chest, in - croc.
heart, in - spig.
neck, in - carb-v.
nose, in - kalm.
sacrum, in - glon.
stomach, in - ars., kali-n.
throat, in - arag.
palate, in - ph-ac.
pale, twitching face, with, no relief from vomiting - ip.
palpitation, with - alum., arg-n., bar-c., bov., brom., bufo, kali-c., mygal., nit-ac., nux-v., ***sil.,*** thuj.
after - brom., nux-v.
causes - ***arg-n.,*** sil.
faintish nausea causing her to become sick - arg-n.
paroxysmal - dig hep., iod., mang., nat-m.
pastry, after - ant-c.
periodic - ign., ***ip.,*** nat-m., nux-v., phos., raph., ***sang.***
perspiration, during - ***corn., ferr., graph., lob.,*** merc., **NUX-V.,** ***sep.,*** sulph., tab., zinc.
amel. - glon.
pessarium, from - nux-m.
piano, playing from - sulph.
plums, after - mag-c.
pork, after - ham., ***ip.,*** **PULS.**
potatoes, after - ***alum.***

NAUSEA, general
pregnancy, during - acet-ac., acon., ail., alet., ***amyg.,*** anac., ***ant-c., ant-t., apom.,*** arg-n., ***ars.,*** **ASAR.,** ***bry.,*** cadm-s., carb-ac., ***carb-an.,*** cast., ***cer-ox., cimic., cocc.,*** cod., ***colch., con., cuc-p.,*** cupr-ac., ***cupr-ar.,*** cycl., ferr., ferr-ar., ferr-p., gnaph., ***goss., hell.,*** ingluv., ***ip., iris, jatr.,*** kali-ar., kali-br., ***kali-c.,*** kali-m., kali-p., **KREOS.,** ***lac-c., lac-d.,*** lac-v-c., ***lach.,*** **LAC-AC.,** laur., ***lil-t., lob., lyc., mag-c., mag-m.,*** med., merc., ***merc-i-f., nat-m.,*** nat-p., ***nux-m.,*** **NUX-V.,** ***ox-ac., petr.,*** ph-ac., ***phos.,*** piloc., plat., plb., ***podo., psor., puls.,*** **SEP.,** ***sil.,*** staph., stry., sulph., ***sul-ac., sym-r.,*** **TAB.,** tarent., ther., ***thyr.,*** verat.
pressure, abdomen, on - asar., lac-c., ***tub.,*** zinc.
neck, on - cimic.
painful spot, on, nausea from - nat-m.
spine, on - cimic.
stomach, on - ant-t., ars., bar-c., euph., gamb., grat., hell., hyos., kali-c., phys., ptel., sulph.
throat, on - ***lach.***
prickling, all over, with - lob.
prolonged - bar-c.
putting, hands in warm water - **PHOS.**
quiet, amel. - cadm-s.
raditiation, treatment from - ars., ***cadm-s.,*** ip.
raising, head from pillow - ***ars., bry.,*** colch., ***nux-m., stram.***
reading, while - ***arg-m.,*** arn., con., glon., jab., lyc., ph-ac., plan., sep.
rectum, felt in - ruta.
respiratory, symptoms, with - lob.
restlessness, with - lac-d.
riding, in a carriage or on the cars, while - bor., ***calc., calc-p.,*** **COCC.,** ***cycl., hep., iris, lyc., mag-c.,*** naja, ***nux-m., nux-v.,*** **PETR.,** phos., sel., **SEP.,** sulph., **TAB.,** ***ther.,*** zinc.
amel. - ***nit-ac.***
breakfast, before - hura.
rinsing, the mouth, on - bry., ***sep.,*** sul-ac.
rising, on - acon., ***arn.,*** arg-n., asar., bry., carb-an., chel., ***cocc.,*** coloc., cor-r., ferr., glon., ind., nat-s., nit-ac., olnd., phos., plat., senec., ***verat.,*** zing.
after - graph., zinc.
amel. - sabin.
up in bed - ***ars.,*** asar., **BRY., COCC.,** ***colch.,*** cor-r., ***nux-m.,*** phos., plat., sulph.
room, closed, in a - lyc., nat-c., tab.
when entering a - alum.
salivation, with - ars., calc., camph., carb-v., cocc., crot-t., cycl., euph., gran., hep., ip., **LOB.,** lyc., mag-c., mag-m., mang., meny., merc., mez., nat-c., ***nux-v., petr.,*** ph-ac., puls., ***sang.,*** sep., spong., staph., sulph., zinc,
salt, on thinking of - ***nat-m.***

NAUSEA, general
seasickness - ***carb-ac.,*** **COCC.,** colch., **CON., EUPH-C.,** ***glon.,*** hyos., ***kali-bi., kreos.,*** lac-ac., nat-m., **NUX-V., PETR.,** sanic., ***sep., staph.,*** **TAB.,** ther.
closing eyes, agg. - ther.
amel. - cocc.
nausea, without - kali-p.
sensation as if - tab.
sewing, from - lac-d., sep.
sex, during - sabad., sil.
after - kali-c., mosch.
thought of - sep.
shivering, with - kali-m., sul-ac.
shuddering, when - am-m., asar., calc., dulc., euph., hyper., ***ip.,*** mag-c., mez., nat-c., nat-m., phos., stann., ***tab.,*** zinc.
singing, agg. - ptel.
singing, when - ptel.
sinking, feeling, with - ip., ***tab.***
sitting, while - acon., alum., ars., bry., calc-ar., carb-an., cor-r., hep., mag-c., mag-m., phos., rhus-t., rob., tarax.
down, when - calc-ar., zinc.
bent over amel. - zinc.
up in bed - ***bry.,*** **COCC.,** cor-r., phos., rhust., sulph., zinc.
sleep, during - arg-m., ferr-p., nux-m., puls., seneg.
after - alum., apoc., arund., asar., bor., caust., cupr., cupr-ar., dig., ham., kali-c., ***lach., lob.,*** mur-ac., op., spong., squil., sulph., tarent., thuj., **VERAT.,** zing.
amel. - rhus-t.
before - apoc., bry., lach., nat-m., sol-n.
siesta, after - zinc.
smoking, while - bry., caj., calad., ***carb-an.,*** clem., cycl., euphr., kali-c., lac-c., ***lyc.,*** nat-m., **NUX-V.,** phos., ran-b., ruta., spong., sil., tab.
after - agar., brom., ***calc., calc-p., clem.,*** cycl., euphr., ign., **IP.,** ***kali-bi.,*** lach., ***lob.,*** **NUX-V.,** op., ***puls.,*** sars., sep., thuj., ***tab.***
amel. - ***eug.,*** sanic.
sneezing, before - sulph.
sneezing, when - hell., **LACH.,** sang., ***sulph.***
speaking, agg. - ther.
soup - acon., ***carb-v.,*** chel., stann.
amel. - cast., kali-bi., mag-c.
odor and thought of - **COLCH.**
sour, things amel. - arg-n.
spitting, from - led.
standing, while - ***agn., alum.,*** alumn., arg-m., arn., colch., crot-h., dict., hep., ***ign.,*** mag-m., merc., petr., ph-ac., puls., tarax.
amel., while - tarax.
stool, during - agar., ant-t., apis, ***ars., bell.,*** cham., chel., coloc., crot-h., crot-t., ferr., ***glon.,*** graph., grat., guai., hell., ***ip.,*** jatr., ***kali-ar., kali-c., merc.,*** merc-i-f., ***nit-ac., podo., puls., rhus-t.,*** sang., ***sil., sulph., verat.***

NAUSEA, general
stool,
after - acon., ant-t., apoc., bufo, cahin., ***caust.,*** con., crot-t., hyper., ***kali-bi.,*** kalm., ***lyss.,*** mag-c., mag-m., merc-c., mur-ac., ***nat-m.,*** nit-ac., ox-ac., petr., ***sil.,*** ter., thuj., verat., zing.
amel. - con., ferr., ip., raph., sang., thuj.
before - acon., ant-t., bry., calc., chel., cimic., cycl., dulc., grat., hell., hydr., ip., ***merc.,*** oena., ***podo., rhus-t.,*** rumx., ruta., ***sep.,*** staph., ***verat.***
desire for - ***dulc.***
stooping, on - bar-c., calc-p., carb-s., ***ip.,*** lach., mill., olnd., petr., rhod., rhus-t., ruta., sang., zinc.
amel. - hyos., petr.
stove, near - laur.
sudden - agar., chin-a., coloc., cupr., ferr-p., ind., ip., ***kali-bi., lyc.,*** mosch., petr., sulph., sul-ac., tab.
eating, while - ***bar-c., ferr., hell., ruta.***
sun, heat of - ant-c., ***carb-v.***
supper, after - alum., am-m., cast., cycl., ferr-i., graph., nat-m., psor.
swallowing, amel. - cocc.
empty, on - colch.
preventing - arn.
saliva - ant-t., ***colch.,*** dig., dios., lach., lyc., rhod., spig., sulph.
sweets - acon., **ARG-N.,** cycl., **GRAPH.,** ***ip.,*** merc., tarax.
swinging, from - coff., ***cocc., petr.***
talking, while - alum., bor., ptel., ther.
tea, after - ***aesc.***
thinking, of it agg. - arg-m., bor., calc., dros., graph., lach., mosch., sars., ***sep.***
throat, in - acon., alum., anac., ant-c., arg-m., arn., ***ars.,*** asar., aur., ***bell.,*** cann-s., carb-ac., carb-an., caust., chin., cocc., coc-c., ***coff.,*** colch., ***croc., cupr.,*** **CYCL.,** ferr., ferr-p., lyc., merc., ***mez.,*** nit-ac., olnd., **PH-AC.,** ***puls., rhus-t.,*** sars., sil., spig., ***squil.,*** **STANN.,** staph., sulph., tarax., valer.
dryness, with - cocc.
collar, by tight fitting - hyos., lach.
spasm in throat, from - ***graph.***
tobacco, odor of - ign., phos.
thought of - kali-br.
touching, lips - ***cadm-s.,*** nux-m.
trembling, with - ***ars., calc.,*** carb-v., chel., cimic., eup-per., ***plat.,*** vesp.
uncomfortable - ars-i.
uncovering, amel. - ***tab.***
amel., abdomen in open air - tab.
urinating, agg. - dig.
after - ant-c., cast., merc., pareir.
profuse - dig.
amel. - nat-p.
urine, if retains - cur.
urticaria, preceeding - sang.
vaccination, after - **SIL.**

NAUSEA, general
vertigo, during - ***cocc.,*** hyos., lach., petr., puls., ***tab., ther.***
after - calc.
vexation, after - cham., ign., ip., ***kali-c.,*** nat-m., phos.
vision, with dim - mygal.
vomiting, amel. - phyt.
does not amel. - ***dig.,*** **IP.,** sang.
inability to - **NUX-V.**
walking, while - acon., am-c., bar-c., bell., bry., calc., chin-s., con., euph., ferr., ferr-p., gamb., kali-bi., ***kali-c.,*** kali-n., led., lyc., mag-m., merc., mez., nat-s., op., ph-ac., phos., phyt., plat., ptel., rhod., ***sep.,*** sil., sulph., thuj.
after - alum., calc-s., carb-an., con., graph., plat., ***puls.,*** sep.
air, in open, while - acon., am-m., ang., bell., ***gamb.,*** graph., lach., led., lycps., nat-s., petr., phos., plat., sep., sil.
after - alum., graph., nit-ac.
amel. - ars.
amel. - acon., am-c., chr-ac., grat., puls.
warm, drinks, agg. - ***bism., lach.,*** **PHOS., PULS.**
amel. - pyrog., ther.
warm, room, in - agar., carb-v., euphr., **LYC.,** ***mez.,*** **NAT-C.,** paeon., ***phos., puls.,*** sep., **TAB.,** verat., vesp., zing.
room, in, on entering, after being in open air - ***alum., am-m.,*** calc-s., ***puls.,*** sep.
stove - ***laur.***
washing, while - bry., ther., zinc.
water, sight of water, from - phos.
thinking, of - ars-h., ip.
waves, in - ant-t., tab.
wind, walking against - plat.
wine, after - ***ant-c.,*** bry., carb-an., phos., **ZINC.**
amel. - coc-c.
sour, from - **ANT-C.**
worm, rising in throat, as if with - spig.
yawning, when - arn., nat-m.

NEURALGIC, pain - abies-n., acet-ac., aesc., alum., anac., ***arg-n., ars., atro., bell., bism., bry., carb-v., cham.,*** chel., ***chin-a.,*** cina, ***cocc.,*** cod., colch., **COLOC.,** cund., ***cupr-ar.,*** dig., ***dios.,*** ferr., gels., glon., ***graph., hydr-ac.,*** ign., ***ip.,*** kali-c., lob., **MAG-P.,** menthol, nicc., nux-m., ***nux-v., ox-ac.,*** petr., ***plb.,*** ptel., puls., quas., rham-cath., ruta, spig., stann., ***stry.,*** sul-ac., tab., ***verat.,*** zinc.

NUMBNESS - acon., bry., cast., plat., sars.

OBSTRUCTION, of pylorus, sensation of - lach., nux-v., phos.

OPEN, sensation, as if were - spong.

OPPRESSION - mur-ac., nat-c., nat-m., phos., plat., zinc.
leaning backward - con.
menses, during - plat.

PAIN, stomach - abies-n., ***abrot., acet-ac., acon., aesc., aeth.,*** agar., ail., all-c., aloe, alum., alumn., ambr., am-c., ***aml-n.,*** anac., anan., ***ant-c., ant-t., apis, arg-m.,*** **ARG-N.,** ***arn.,*** **ARS.,** ars-h., ars-i., arund., ***asaf.,*** asar., asc-t., aur., aur-m-n., bapt., ***bar-c., bar-i., bar-m.,*** **BELL.,** benz-ac., **BISM.,** bol., bor., brach., ***brom.,*** **BRY.,** ***cact.,*** cadm-s., calad., ***calc., calc-p., calc-s., camph.,*** cann-s., ***canth., caps., carb-ac., carb-an.,*** **CARB-S., CARB-V., CARD-M.,** carl., caul., **CAUST.,** ***cham.,*** **CHEL., CHIN.,** chin-a., ***chin-s.,*** cic., cimic., ***cina,*** clem., cob., **COCC.,** coc-c., coff., **COLCH., COLOC.,** ***con.,*** cop., ***corn.,*** cor-r., croc., ***crot-c., crot-h.,*** crot-t., **CUPR.,** ***cupr-ar.,*** cur., cycl., ***dig., dios.,*** dulc., echi., ***ferr., ferr-ar.,*** ferr-i., ferr-p., ***gels., gran.,*** **GRAPH.,** glon., ***grat.,*** ham., hell., hep., hura, ***hydr., hydr-ac., hyos., ign., iod., ip., iris, kali-ar., kali-bi., kali-c.,*** kali-chl., kali-i., ***kali-n.,*** kali-p., ***kali-s., kalm., kreos., lach., laur.,*** led., ***lept., lob.,*** **LYC.,** ***mag-c., mag-m., mag-p.,*** mag-s., manc., mang., ***med., merc.,*** merc-i-f., mez., mosch., mur-ac., naja, **NAT-A.,** ***nat-c., nat-m., nat-p., nat-s.,*** nicc., ***nit-ac., nux-m.,*** **NUX-V.,** ol-an., olnd., ***op.,*** ox-ac., ***petr.,*** **PHOS.,** phys., ***phyt.,*** plan., **PLB.,** podo., ***ptel.,*** prun., **PULS.,** ran-b., ran-s., rhod., rhus-t., rob., rumx., ruta., sabin., ***sang., sec.,*** senec., seneg., ***sep.,*** **SIL.,** sol-t-ae., ***spig.,*** squil., **STANN.,** ***staph., stram.,*** stront-c., ***stry.,*** **SULPH.,** ***sul-ac.,*** sumb., **TAB.,** ***tarent., ter.,*** teucr., thuj., ***uran.,*** ust., valer., **VERAT.,** ***verat-v., zinc.,*** zing.
acids, after - ***ant-c.,*** kreos., ***nat-p.,*** sulph.
afternoon - alum., alumn., am-m., arg-n., ars., bry., ***calc.,*** calc-s., canth., ferr., ***iris,*** **LYC.,** merc-c., nicc., nux-v., par., petr., ***puls.,*** sang., ***sep.,*** spong., sulph., tarent., ust.
air, cold, blowing on abdomen - caust.
open - lyc., nux-v., ol-an., phos.
amel. - adon., naja.
alcoholics, in - ***calc.,*** carb-s., ***carb-v.,*** graph., ***lach., nux-v.,*** sulph., sul-ac.
alternating with
gout - ***ant-c.,*** nux-m.
head or face, pain in - bism.
headache - nat-c.
limbs, pain in - ***kali-bi.***
skin problems - graph.
anemia, with - ferr., glon., graph.
anger, after - cham., **COLOC.,** staph.
anxiety, with - ***abrot., cham.,*** chel.
despondency and sallow face, with - nit-ac.
appears, and disappears gradually - ***stann.***
gradually and disappears suddenly - ***arg-m.***
apples, sour, after - merc-c.
apyrexia, during - ant-c.
ascending, steps, on - chin-s., ph-ac.
bandaging, abdomen amel. - cupr., nat-m.
bed, covers, from - sulph.
beer, after - carb-s., ***nux-v.***
behind, stomach - arn., cact., ham., kali-c., stram.

PAIN, stomach
belching, agg. - ant-c., ***cham.,*** cocc., phos.
amel. - aloe, ***bar-c., bry., calc., calc-p.,*** **CARB-V.,** ***chel.,*** chin., chin-s., cimic., coloc., dig., ***dios.,*** glon., ***graph.,*** hep., iod., kali-c., ***lyc.,*** nicc., nit-ac., paeon., par., plb., sep., ***tarent.***
suppressed, after - bar-c., con.
bending, backward amel. - ***bell.,*** bism., caust., ***chel., dios.,*** kali-c.
backward, must - mag-m.
bending, double, on - kalm., lyc.
amel. - alumn., carb-v., cham., ***chel.,*** colch., **COLOC.,** lach., lyc., nux-v., psor., ptel., ***sil.,*** sulph., ***verat-v.***
blowing, nose, on - **HEP.,** kali-n.
bread, after - acon., ***ant-c., bar-c.,*** **BRY., CAUST.,** coff., kali-c., merc., ***phos.,*** puls., rhus-t., ruta., sars., staph., sul-ac., zinc., zing.
amel. - nat-c.
rye, bread - merc-c.
breakfast, after - agar., aloe, all-c., anac., ars., calc-s., carb-s., caust., crot-h., cycl., kali-bi., myric., ***nat-c.,*** puls., sulph.
before - arg-n., bufo, ***iris.***
breast-feeding, from - ***carb-v.,*** chin.
breathing, on - ***anac., ars.,*** bar-c., caps., coc-c., ***lyc.,*** mang., ***puls.***
breathing, deep - arg-n., **CAUST.,** kali-n., merc., puls.
amel. - rumx.
inspiration - **ARG-N.,** asar., bry., carb-an., ***caust.,*** cor-r., dros., ign., kali-n., nat-m., op., ***phyt., puls.,*** zinc.
cardiac orifice - ***agar., arg-n.,*** asaf., bar-c., bism., cann-i., ***carb-v.,*** caul., ***cupr., ferr-cy.,*** ferr-t., form., ign., mag-m., nat-m., nit-ac., ***nux-v., onis.,*** stront-c., thea.
cheese, after - ptel.
chill, during - ***ars., bry.,*** **COCC.,** ***eup-per.,*** lob., lyc., merl., ***nux-v.,*** **PULS.,** rhus-t., sil., sulph.
clothing, from - ***am-c.,*** calc., kali-bi., lyc., nat-m., sep.
coffee, after - canth., **CHAM.,** cocc., dig., ign., ***nux-v.,*** ox-ac.
after - brom., coloc.
amel. - ol-an.
cold, after taking - lyc., sep.
food, after - carb-v., caust., kali-c., kreos., lyc., ***mang., sul-ac.***
amel. - ***phos.***
cold, drinks, after - **ACON.,** aloe, am-br., ant-c., arg-n., **ARS.,** ***bell-p.,*** bry., calad., calc., ***calc-ar., calc-p.,*** carb-s., carb-v., ***caust.,*** elaps, ferr., ***ferr-ar., graph., iris,*** kali-ar., kali-c., lyc., ***manc.,*** nat-c., nit-ac., nux-v., ol-an., ***ornithog., phos.,*** rhod., **RHUS-T.,** sil., ***sal-ac.,*** tarent., tep.
amel. - alumn., apis, arg-n., bism., ***calc-s., caust.,*** **PHOS.,** ***puls.,*** tep.
water - calc.
when overheated - acon., ***kali-c.,*** nat-c.

PAIN, stomach
constipation, with - alumn., bry., graph., nux-v., phys., ***plb., sep.***
contradiction, from - carb-v.
convulsions, with - agar., caust.
before - cupr.
cough, an attack of, before - ant-t., arn., bell., cham.
coughing, from - am-c., apoc., ***arn., ars.,*** arund., bell., **BRY.,** cadm-s., calc., ***camph., chin.,*** chin-a., chlor., cor-r., ***dros., hell.,*** hyos., ***ip.,*** kali-bi., ***lach.,*** lob., **LYC.,** mang., nit-ac., ***nux-v., phos.,*** puls., ***rhus-t.,*** rumx., ruta., ***sabad., sep.,*** sil., squil., **STANN.,** tab.
damp weather, in - ***kali-c.,*** mang., nat-s., ***sulph.***
depression, with - arg-n., gaul., nux-v.
descending stairs - bry.
diarrhea, agg. - ars.
dinner, during - corn., thuj.
after - acon., agar., alum., am-c., arg-n., ars., **CALC-P.,** cast-eq., chin., clem., cob., coc-c., coloc., crot-h., dig., elaps, graph., hyper., laur., mag-c., ***mez.,*** myric., ***nat-c., nux-m.,*** petr., phos., rhod., sep., sulph., trom., verat.
amel. - **ANAC.,** caust., **CHEL.,** graph., mang.
before - graph., lyc., nat-m., phos.
disappointment, after - carb-v., ***ign.***
drawing, up the limbs amel. - ***bry.,*** chel., coloc.
drinking, after - acon., aloe, ***apis,*** **APOC.,** arn., bell., canth., chel., ***chin., coloc.,*** daph., ferr., iris, kali-c., kali-s., lac-ac., ***lac-c., manc.,*** merc-c., nat-c., ***nat-m.,*** nit-ac., nux-v., ol-an., plb., rhus-t., rhod., sec., sil., sul-ac., sulph.
amel. - graph.
quickly agg. - sil.
eating, while - acon., ant-t., arn., ***ars.,*** bry., ***calc-p.,*** cic., coff., con., corn., crot-c., led., mang., merc., op., phos., plb., puls., sep., thuj., verat.
after - ***abies-n.,*** acon., aesc., ***agar.,*** alum., ***am-c., anac., ant-c.,*** ant-t., ***apis,*** **ARG-N.,** arn., **ARS.,** ***ars-i., asaf.,*** aur-m., **BAR-C.,** ***bar-i., bell.,*** berb., ***bism., bry.,*** cact., ***calc.,*** **CALC-P.,** calc-s., ***caps.,*** carb-ac., carb-an., carb-s., ***carb-v., caust., cham.,*** **CHIN.,** ***chin-a., chin-s., cic., cina, cist., cob., cocc.,*** coc-c., colch., ***coloc.,*** con., ***cur.,*** cycl., daph., dig., dios., ***eup-per., ferr.,*** ferr-ar., ***ferr-i.,*** ferr-ma., ferr-p., fl-ac., glon., graph., grat., gymn., ham., ***hep.,*** hura, ***hydr., iod.,*** iris, ***kali-ar., kali-bi., kali-c.,*** kali-p., kali-s., ***lac-c.,*** **LACH.,** ***led.,*** lob., ***lyc.,*** mang., ***merc.,*** merc-c., mez., mosch., **NAT-A.,** ***nat-c., nat-m.,*** nat-p., ***nat-s.,*** nit-ac., ***nux-m.,*** **NUX-V.,** osm., ox-ac., ***petr., ph-ac.,*** **PHOS.,** ***plat., plb., ptel.,*** **PULS.,** ***rob.,*** rhod., rhus-t., rumx., ***sang.,*** **SEP.,** ***sil.,*** staph., ***stront-c.,*** **SULPH.,** sul-ac., tab., ***tarent.,*** ter., thuj., verat., zinc.

PAIN, stomach

eating, 1 hour after - ***carb-v., mag-m.,*** phos., ***puls.***

2 hours to 3 hours, after - aesc., ***agar.,*** anac., bry., calc-hp., ***con.,*** mag-m., nat-p., nux-v., ox-ac., phos., ***puls.***

amel. - aesc., agar., anac., arg-n., aur., bov., ***brom., calc-p.,*** cann-i., cham., ***chel.,*** chin-a., ***cina,*** dios., fago., gamb., **GRAPH.,** ***hep., ign., iod.,*** iris, ***kali-bi., kalm., lach., lith., mag-m., mag-p.,*** mang., ***med.,*** mez., ***nat-c.,*** nat-s., nicc., ox-ac., ***petr., phos., raph.,*** rob., verat., zinc.

every bit, hurts - ars., calc-p.

immediately - ***abies-n.,*** arn., ars., calc., ***carb-v.,*** chin., cocc., ***kali-bi., kali-c., lyc., nux-m.,*** phys.

too, much - ant-c., coff., ip., ***puls.***

empty stomach, from - ***anac.,*** cina, hydr-ac., ***petr.***

evening - agar., alum., alumn., ars., calc., calc-s., carb-an., ***carb-v.,*** cast-eq., chel., coloc., dig., dios., dulc., euphr., kali-bi., kali-n., lob., lyc., mag-m., merc., nat-c., nat-m., phos., plan., **PULS.,** ***rhus-t.,*** sang., sep., sil., ***sul-ac.,*** tarent., thuj., zinc.

5 to 7 p.m. - ***staph.***

8 p.m. walking in open air - alumn.

bed, in - alum., bell., carb-an., ***carb-v., lyc.,*** phos.

amel. - kali-n.

chill, during - sulph.

menses, before - mag-c.

singing, while - sars.

excitement, after - **CHAM., COLOC.,** ***nux-v., staph.,*** zinc.

exercising while - ang., bry., calc., cann-s., caust., cupr.

extending, to

abdomen, over - **ARN.,** calc., caust., cocc., colch., cupr., nux-v., phos., puls.

to left side of - colch.

arm, to - con., indg., ***kali-c.***

axilla and upper arm - am-m.

back - absin., aloe, am-c., bell., bor., chel., ***con.,*** cupr., cycl., ***ferr.,*** hep., ign., indg., kali-c., mag-m., nat-m., ornithog., ph-ac., phos., puls., ***sulph.,*** ter.

between shoulders - **BELL.**

spine - arn., verat-v.

backward - berb., bism., con., kali-c., sulph.

backward, reverse, or - berb.

bladder and testes - ***kali-c.***

breast, nipple, to - am-c.

cardia orifice - nit-ac., sep.

chest, into - aloe, alum., arg-n., bar-c., dulc., grat., hyos., ign., ***kali-c.,*** lach., mag-c., merl., nat-m., nux-v., par., phos., plb., raph., rumx., sep.

after dinner - nat-m.

when coughing - raph., rhus-t.

clavicle, left - agar.

downward - phos., ***sep., zinc-s.***

PAIN, stomach

extending, to

esophagus, to - ***aeth.,*** brom.

groins - **PLB.**

head, to - calc., carb-v., plb.

heart, to - ***arg-n.,*** lach., ornithog., sol-n., stry.

hypochondria, to - ***aesc.,*** phos., verat.

limbs to - kali-c., **PLB.**

liver, to - arg-n., asaf., hyper., mill., nat-m., rhus-t.

lumbar region, to - am-c., carb-v.

scapula, left - arg-n.

shoulders, to - ***kali-bi., kali-c.,*** nicc., phos.

left - sol-n.

right - sang.

sides, to, than to back - coch.

sternum, to - nat-m., rheum, zing.

throat - aloe, alum., chion., con., cupr-ac., grat., mag-m., nat-m.

transversely - arn., **CHEL.,** ***cina,*** ip.

umbilicus, to - brom., lyc., nit-ac.

upward - ferr., phos.

fainting, with - **BISM.,** ***nux-v.,*** ran-s.

fasting, while - ***anac., bar-c., calc.,*** caust., cina, ***cocc.,*** fago., **GRAPH.,** hura, hydr-ac., ***ign., lach.,*** lob., nit-ac., ***petr.,*** petros., prot., psor., rhod., seneg., sep.

eating, and, after agg. - bar-c.

fat food, after - ars., caust., **PULS.**

fever, during - **ARS.,** bell., **BRY.,** carb-v., ***cham., cocc., eup-per., nat-m.,*** **NUX-V.,** ***puls., sep.***

amel. - **ARS.,** bry., carb-an., caust., ***cham., chel., lyc.,*** mag-p., ***nux-v., sil.***

flatulence, as from - ars., ***carb-v.***

flatulent, food, after - ***carb-v.***

flatus, passing, amel. - agar., carb-an., chel., dig., ***hep.,*** kali-c., lact., ***tarent.***

fluids, after - ars., merc.

loss of animal, after - ***carb-v.,*** **CHIN.**

food, from - ***arg-n.,*** bell., ***bry.,*** ign., kali-bi., ***nux-v.***

warm - bar-c.

forenoon - bapt., ***graph.,*** helon., lyc., mag-m., nat-m., nicc., podo., stann., sep., spong., thuj., ust.

8 to 9 a.m. - cocc.

stool, after - calc., sulph.

fright, from - carb-v., ***ign.***

fruit, after - ars., bor., chin., ***lyc.,*** nat-p.

gastritis, chronic with - alum., atro., bism., lyc.

gout, with - colch., urt-u.

hemorrhoids, operation, after - calen., croc.

heat, amel. - **ARS.,** bry., carb-an., caust., ***cham., chel., lyc.,*** mag-p., ***nux-v., sil.***

honey, agg. - nat-c., **SULPH.**

hot, things - chel.

drinks agg. - brom., ***graph.,*** kali-c.

humiliation, after - caust., cham., ***coloc.,*** lyc., nux-v., ***staph.***

hunger, during - hura, ***petr., psor.***

ravenous, after - mag-c.

PAIN, stomach
- **hysteria,** with - asaf., ign., plat.
- **ice** cream, after - ***arg-n.,*** **ARS.,** calc-p., ***ip.,*** **PULS.**
  - amel. - ***phos.***
- **injury,** after - nux-v.
- **jar** of walking agg. - aloe, alumn., anac., **BELL.,** bry., hell., kali-s., mang-m., ***sep.***
- **jolting,** in a carriage, from - **BELL.,** lob-s.
- **knee**-elbow position amel. - con., med.
- **laughing** - lyc.
- **lifting,** after - ***bor.,*** cadm-br., lyc., ***rhus-t.***
  - as from - plat.
- **lying,** while - bell-p., ***carb-an., carb-v.,*** chel., coc-c., lach., puls., rhus-t., stann., sulph.
  - abdomen, on agg. - ambr.
    - amel. - ***elaps,*** mag-aust.
  - amel. - am-c., bell., ***caust.,*** chin., ***graph.,*** kali-i., lach., ***lyc.,*** sil., stann.
  - back - alumn., ***lyc.***
    - amel. - ***calc.,*** laur.
  - legs, drawn up amel., with - carb-ac., sil.
- **lying,** side - bry., cupr., laur.
  - amel. - ***lyc.***
  - left - kali-br., com.
    - amel. - squil.
  - right - ***arg-n.***
    - amel. - merc.
  - with legs drawn up amel. - ***chel.***
- **meat,** after - calc., ferr., ***kali-bi.,*** ptel.
  - boiled, after - ***graph.***
- **menses,** during - am-c., ars., ***bor.,*** caps., ***carb-s.,*** caul., ***caust., cham., cocc., cupr., graph.,*** kali-c., kali-i., kali-p., lac-c., nux-m., ***nux-v.,*** phos., ***puls., sars.,*** **SULPH.,** thuj., zinc.
  - after - ***bell.,*** bor., canth., gels., kali-c., kreos., lach., nat-p., nux-v., puls., sulph.
  - before - aur-s., ***bell.,*** bor., cupr., lach., mag-c., ***nux-m., puls.,*** sep., sulph., tarent.
  - instead of - ***lach.***
- **mental** exertion, on - anac., ***arg-n.***
- **milk,** after - alum., ***ars., ferr.,*** hyper., ***mag-c.,*** **MAG-M.,** nat-c., petr., samb., ***sulph.***
  - amel. - graph., merc., merc-c., mez., ruta
  - sweet milk amel. - ars., mez.
- **misstep,** from - aloe, bar-c., ***bry.,*** puls., rhus-t.
- **morning** - aesc., anac., ant-c., asar., carb-an., carb-s., ***caust., chin., cina,*** colch., cupr., cupr-s., dig., dios., graph., hyper., iod., ***kali-bi., kali-c., lach.,*** lyc., mag-c., mag-s., nat-c., ***nat-m.,*** nat-s., **NUX-V.,** petr., ***phos.,*** plat., puls., ran-s., sep., staph., ***sulph.,*** tarent., zinc.
  - bed, in - con., phos., plb., staph.
  - eating, after - nux-v., tarent.
    - amel. - mag-c., nat-s.
  - fasting, while - caust., petr.
  - rising, on - caust., ***cina,*** nat-s., zinc.
  - stool, after - con.
  - until 1 p.m. - sep.
  - waking, on - agar., caust., con., cycl., ***lach.,*** lyc., nat-m., nicc., nit-ac., phyt., staph.

PAIN, stomach
- **morning,**
  - walking, while - agar., carb-an., cycl., nit-ac., phos., phyt.
- **motion,** on - aloe, **BELL., BRY.,** ***calc.,*** calc-p., ***caust.,*** cham., ***chel., colch., ip.,*** kali-bi., kalm., mang., nat-c., nux-v., ph-ac., rhus-t., rumx., thuj., zinc.
  - amel. - **CHIN.,** cycl., dios., kali-c., nat-c., uran-n.
  - arms, of - arg-n., nux-v.
- **nausea,** during - ***glon.***
- **nervous** depression with - ***agar.,*** arg-n., bell., gaul., ***mag-p., nux-v.,*** sang.
- **night** - ***abrot.,*** agar., alum., ***am-c., arg-n.,*** ars., bapt., ***bell., calc.,*** camph., ***carb-s., carb-v.,*** cham., cina, ***coloc.,*** con., ***graph.,*** ign., kali-ar., ***kali-c.,*** lach., merc-sul., nat-m., nit-ac., nux-v., ornithog., phos., podo., puls., rhod., rhus-t., seneg., sep., sil., ***sulph.,*** tarent., thuj.
  - 1 a.m. - mag-m.
  - 2 a.m. - ***ars., kali-c.,*** lyc., **MED.**
  - 3 a.m. - ox-ac.
  - 9 p.m., until midnight - phos.
  - bed, in - cocc., nat-s., ptel.
  - lying on the back, while - lyc.
  - midnight - ambr., ***chin.,*** lyc.
    - after - mag-c., puls., ***sulph.***
  - sleep, during - nit-ac.
  - waking, on - caust., hyper.
    - amel. - nit-ac.
- **noon** - agar., alumn., ***aur.,*** mez., seneg., zinc.
- **nursing** from - aeth.
- **nuts,** after - **SIL.**
- **over** loading agg. - nux-v., staph.
- **oysters,** after - brom.
- **pain,** with, limbs, in - ptel.
  - throat and spine alternately, in - paraf.
- **paroxysmal** - arg-n., ars., ***bell., carb-v.,*** carl., caul., ***coloc., cupr., guai., ign.,*** ip., mez., ***nit-ac., nux-v., phos., pic-ac., plb.,*** ruta.
- **passing** of sand - thuj.
- **pears,** after - bor.
- **periodical** - ***arg-n.,*** bell., calc., cupr., ***graph.,*** hyos., ign., ***iod.,*** lyc.
  - third day, every - iod.
- **potatoes,** after - ***alum., coloc.***
- **pregnancy,** during - con., dios., ip., petr.
- **pressing,** on spine, from - ***bell.***
- **pressure** - agar., alum., am-c., ant-c., arn., ars., bar-c., brom., bry., ***calc.,*** canth., caps., ***chel.,*** chin-s., dig., guai., iod., kali-bi., led., mag-m., mang., merc-c., mez., nit-ac., ***op.,*** ox-ac., phos., ran-s., tarent., vip.
  - amel. - alumn., ***coloc.,*** dios., mag-p., mang., ***plb.,*** puls., ***stann.***
- **pylorus** - all-c., canth., ***hep.,*** lyc., merc., ***ornithog.,*** tus-f., ***uran-n.***
- **radiating** - arg-n., dios., ***kali-c., plb.***
- **raising,** arm high - anac., arg-n.
- **raw** food, after - ruta.

PAIN, stomach

recurrent - graph.
rich food, after - ars., ***ip., ptel.,*** **PULS.**
riding, in a carriage - lyc., puls.
after - phos.
rising, after - caust., graph., sulph., zinc.
amel. - gels., phys., phyt.
from bed, on - ***cina, graph.***
rolling, body hard about - lil-t.
spot, painful at - kreos.
rubbing, amel. - ***lyc.***
back, amel. - bism.
sand, passing - thuj.
sex, after - ***ph-ac.***
sickening - ost.
sitting, while - acon., ambr., ***ars.,*** asaf., caust., dros., elaps, hep., nat-c., nat-s., phos., puls., sulph.
bent over - agn., bar-c., caps., ***kalm.,*** **LYC.,** sin-n.
amel. - bry., ***coloc.,*** ox-ac., staph., sulph.
erect - gels.
amel. - dios., kalm.
soup, after - ars., indg.
speaking, from - caps., hell., kalm., mag-m., nat-c., ***rumx.***
spine, pressure on - ***lach.***
spot - arg-n., bar-c., bism., kali-bi., lyc.
stepping, hard - bar-c., mag-c.
standing, while - acon., agar., carb-v., merc., rhod., **SULPH.**
amel. - kalm.
erect - bell., ***dios.***
when still amel. - alumn., kalm.
stool, during - bell., con., dios., kali-c., ***lyc.,*** mag-m., puls., ran-b., rhod., sars.
after - ambr., calc., calc-s., con., ferr., ***puls.,*** sul-ac., sulph.
amel. - carb-an., ***chel.***
before - alum., ars., ***coloc.,*** nat-c., rhus-t.
stooping - alum., aur-m., bar-c., dios., dros., glon., ***kali-c.,*** kalm., nat-c., rhod., rhus-t.
amel. - anac.
straightening, up agg. - nit-ac.
strain, from - arn., bry., rhus-t.
stretching, amel. - dios., nat-c.
sudden - cic., ***cupr.,*** elaps
sugar, after - arg-n., ign., ox-ac., sulph., zinc.
summer agg. - guai.
supper, during - am-c.
after - bry., ***calc.,*** lyc., ptel., puls., rhod., seneg., ***sep.***
amel., after - am-c., sep.
swallowing, on - bar-c., ***calc-p.,*** cor-r., nit-ac., sep.
cardiac end of stomach, at - abies-n., all-c., alum., bry., dys-co., led., ***nit-ac., phos.,*** sep.
talking, agg. - caust., hell., kali-c., rumx.
tightening, clothes amel. - fl-ac.

PAIN, stomach

touch - am-c., ant-c., bar-c., bell., calc., euph., hyos., ign., kali-bi., kali-c., kali-n., lyc., merc., **NAT-C.,** nat-m., nux-v., ***ox-ac.,*** petr., phos., sulph., thuj.
turning, bed, in - alum., bapt.
body - anac.
urination, during - ***ip.,*** laur.
amel. - carb-an.
uterine disorders, with - bor.
vaccination, after - **THUJ.**
vertigo, with - cic.
vexation, after - acon., ars., cham., ign., phos., **STAPH.**
violent - ***acon.,*** arg-n., ***arn., ars.,*** anthr., aur., ***bell.,*** **BISM.,** camph., cham., cocc., **COLOC.,** ***cupr., cupr-ar.,*** hell., hydr-ac., hyos., ***iod., ip., iris, lac-d.,*** lach., **MED.,** merc., ***nux-v.,*** phos., ***plb., podo.,*** ran-b., ran-s., sec., squil., stann., ***verat.***
going to the back - bad., cupr.
vomiting, agg. - ars., cadm-s., sep.
amel. - hyos., plb., sep.
waking, on - agar., ambr., caust., cycl., hyper., nat-m., nicc., nit-ac., phyt., rumx., sil., staph.
amel. - nit-ac.
walking, while - acon., alumn., am-c., anac., ars., **BELL., BRY.,** calc., carb-v., cocc., hell., hep., kali-n., mag-m., myric., nux-v., ***phos., phyt.,*** sep., verat.
agg., jar of - aloe, alumn., anac., **BELL.,** hell., kali-s., mag-m., ***sep.***
air, in open - anac., bell., bry., nit-ac., sil.
8 p.m. - alumn.
amel. - ambr.
amel. - all-c., bor., bov., dios., elaps, lyc., nat-c., op., ***stann.***
warm, applications, amel. - chel., **MAG-P.,** nux-m., ***nux-v., sil.***
drinks amel. - alum., ***ars.,*** bry., carc., ***graph.,*** kali-bi., kali-c., mang., nux-m., **NUX-V.,** ***ph-ac.,*** rhus-t., ***spong.,*** sulph., verat., verat-v.
food agg. - brom., chin., ***fl-ac.,*** ign., **PHOS., PULS.**
amel. - ornithog.
milk amel. - ***chel., graph.***
warmth of bed amel. - carb-v., graph., lyc., **NUX-V.**
wine, after - bry.
worms, from - ***cina,*** gran.
yawning, agg. - **ARS.,** phyt.
amel. - lyc., nat-m.

PAIN, esophagus - ***alum.,*** alumn., ant-t., caj., carb-v., caust., colch., crot-c., crot-t., hydr-ac., kali-bi., kali-chl., nit-ac., merc., mur-ac., phos., raph., sul-ac.
extending to stomach - ars., ***crot-c.,*** merc-c., mur-ac., sul-ac.
to stomach, on sneezing - ictod., poth.
pressure on larynx, agg. - iod.

PAIN, esophagus
swallowing, on - ***alum., bar-c.,*** ox-ac., ***nat-m., nit-ac.,*** verat.
solids - caj.

PARALYSIS, esophagus - ***alum., alumn.,*** **ARS.,** ***bapt.,*** bell., calc., caps., **CAUST.,** chlol., crot-c., ***gels., hydr-ac., kali-c.,*** lach., ***nux-m., op.,*** petr., ***plb., stram.,*** tab., ***verat.***
paralysis, sensation of - **ARS.,** cocc., ip., kali-c., ***lach.,*** lact., puls., ***sil.***

PERSPIRATION - bor., hyos., ***kali-m.,*** ol-an.
pit of, on - bell., bor., nux-v., sec.

PRESSING, pain - ***acon.,*** act-sp., ***aesc., agar.,*** all-c., ***all-s.,*** aloe, ***alum.,*** alumn., ***ambr., am-c.,*** am-m., ***anac.,*** anan., ant-c., ***ant-t.,*** apis, arg-m., arg-n., ***arn.,*** **ARS.,** ars-h., ars-i., ***asaf.,*** asar., ***aur.,*** aur-m., aur-m-n., bad., bapt., **BAR-C.,** bar-i., bar-m., ***bell., benz-ac.,*** berb., ***bism.,*** bor., ***bov.,*** brom., ***bry.,*** cahin., calad., **CALC.,** ***calc-p.,*** calc-s., ***camph.,*** cann-i., cann-s., canth., caps., ***carb-an.,*** **CARB-S.,** ***carb-v.,*** **CARD-M.,** carl., ***casc.,*** **CAUST., CHAM.,** ***chel.,*** **CHIN., CHIN-A.,** chin-s., chr-ac., ***cic., cina,*** clem., coc-c., coff., ***colch., coloc., con.,*** cop., cor-r., crot-h., crot-t., cub., **CUPR.,** ***cupr-s.,*** cycl., ***dig.,*** dulc., elat., euph., euphr., ***ferr.,*** ferr-ar., ferr-p., ***fl-ac.,*** gent-c., ***gent-l.,*** gins., glon., ***graph., grat.,*** guai., guare., haem., hell., helon., ***hep.,*** hyos., hydr-ac., hyper., ***ign.,*** ind., ***iod.,*** ip., jac-c., jatr., jug-r., kali-bi., ***kali-c.,*** kali-chl., kali-i., ***kali-n.,*** kali-p., kali-s., ***kalm.,*** kreos., lac-ac., ***lach., lact., laur., led.,*** lob., **LYC.,** lyss., mag-c., mag-m., mag-s., mang., ***meny., merc.,*** merc-c., merl., ***mez., mosch.,*** mur-ac., ***myric., nat-a., nat-c.,*** **NAT-M.,** ***nat-p.,*** nat-s., nicc., ***nit-ac.,*** nux-m., ***nux-v.,*** ol-an., ***op., osm.,*** ox-ac., paeon., par., ***petr.,*** phel., ***ph-ac.,*** **PHOS.,** phys., ***pic-ac., plat., plb.,*** prun., ***ptel.,*** **PULS.,** ran-b., ***ran-s., raph.,*** rheum, ***rhod., rhus-t., rob.,*** sabin., ***samb., sang., sarr.,*** sars., ***sec., seneg., sep.,*** **SIL.,** sol-n., spig., ***spong., squil., stann.,*** staph., stram., ***stront-c., sulph., sul-ac.,*** sumb., tab., tarent., ter., teucr., ***thuj., valer., verat.,*** verb., xan., zinc.
afternoon - alum., am-m., arg-n., canth., dig., kali-c., kali-c., ***lyc.,*** nicc., petr., spong.
2 p.m. - ferr.
4 to 5 p.m. - bry.
air, in open - ol-an.
alternating with headache - chel.
bandaging abdomen amel. - cupr.
beer, after - carb-v., ***nux-v.***
belching, amel. - aloe, alum., ambr., ***bar-c.,*** bry., calc-p., ***carb-v.,*** chel., chin-s., cycl., euphr., gamb., ***graph.,*** helon., hep., kali-c., kali-n., lach., mag-c., nat-c., nicc., ol-an., par., phos., sulph., zinc.
before - staph.
bending, backward amel. - kali-c.
forward agg. - bry.
bread, after - ***bar-c., bry.,*** **CAUST.,** ***phos.,*** sep., sul-ac., zing.
breakfast, after - agar., aloe, anac., ars., carb-s., caust., cycl., kali-bi., myric., ***nat-c.,*** nux-v., puls., sulph.

PRESSING, pain
breathing, deeply - carb-an.
inspiration agg. - asar., con., cor-r., ign., lyc., nat-m.
chill, during - ars., ars-h., sulph.
chillying - caust.
clothing, agg. -
clothing, from - ***am-c., ph-ac.***
coffee, after - ***cham.***
cold - caust.
food, after - ***mang.***
if, touches abdomen - caust.
coughing, on - calc., cor-r., ***phos.***
dinner after - agar., am-c., ars., carb-s., chin., ***clem.,*** coc-c., hyper., kali-n., mez., ***nat-c.,*** petr., phos., rhod., rhus-t., sulph., verat.
before - lyc., nat-m., phos.
drawing in abdomen, when - zinc.
drinking, after - ant-t., chel., ***chin-s.,*** hyos., ph-ac.
after, cold drink - acet-ac., ol-an., rhod.
rapidly - sil.
eating, while - acon., ***bry.,*** coff., con., mang., rhod., thuj., verat.
after - agar., alum., ambr., **AM-C., ANAC.,** ant-t., ars., ***asaf.,*** bar-c., bar-m., ***bell.,*** berb., ***bism.,*** bor., bov., ***bry.,*** calc., calc-s., ***canth.,*** caps., carb-ac., carb-an., carb-s., ***carb-v., cham.,*** **CHIN.,** ***chin-s.,*** cic., ***cina,*** cocc., coc-c., coloc., colch., con., dig., euph., equis., ***ferr.,*** ferr-ar., ferr-i., ferr-p., fl-ac., graph., grat., ***hep.,*** hura, hyper., iod., kali-ar., ***kali-bi., kali-c.,*** kali-p., **LACH.,** led., ***lob.,*** **LYC.,** ***lyss.,*** merc., mez., ***nat-c., nat-m., nat-p.,*** nit-ac., **NUX-V.,** op., ***ph-ac.,*** **PHOS.,** plat., plb., ***ptel., puls.,*** rhod., rhus-t., rumx., ***sang.,*** sec., ***sep., sil.,*** staph., ***stront-c., sulph., tarent.,*** ter., til., thuj., verat., zinc.
after, a little - cham., **CHIN.,** ***chin-s., ferr., hep.,*** hyper., laur., **LYC.**
amel. - anac., chin., hep., kali-c., nit-ac., petr., ptel., stront-c., verat.
evening - alum., calc., carb-an., carb-v., chel., dig., euphr., kali-bi., mez., nat-m., phos., sars., sep., sil., spong., sulph., zinc.
bed, in - carb-an., carb-v., kali-c., **LYC.,** ter.
exertion, on - carl.
expiration agg. - ***aur.***
extending, sternum - verat.
to back - mag-m., sulph., sul-ac.
to chest - alum., kali-c., mag-c., mag-m., nat-m., staph.
to downward - nat-m., plat.
to neck - arn., mag-m.
to sternum - rheum., verat.
to throat - con., mag-m.
fasting, while - carb-an., caust., nit-ac., ***petr.,*** sep.
fat food, after - **PULS.**

PRESSING, pain
fermentation amel. - sep.
flatuent food, after - lyc., sil.
flatus, as from - mag-m., plat.
forenoon - calc., ***graph.,*** lyc., mag-m., nat-m., nicc., sep., spong., stann., sulph., thuj.
hand, as by a - arn.
hawking, amel. - kali-c.
headache, before - sep.
heart, as if, were being crushed - ars., carb-v., cham., nux-v.
heat, after - grat.
jerking - dig.
lifting, after - ***calc.,*** lyc., ***rhus-t.***
lifting, as from - plat.
lying, while - carb-an., sulph., stann.
abdomen, on amel. - ambr.
back, on - caust.
back, on, amel. - ***calc.,*** chin., lyc.
side, on - chin.
side, on, left - ter.
menses, during - am-c., caps., ***caust.,*** nat-p., nux-m., puls., **SULPH.,** thuj.
after - bor., nat-p.
before - ***nux-m.***
mental exertion, after - anac.
milk, after - alum., ***ferr.,*** hyper., petr., samb.
morning - am-c., ant-c., ***carb-an.,*** caust., ***chin.,*** graph., hyper., kali-c., lach., led., nat-c., ***nat-m., nux-v.,*** petr., puls., ran-s., ruta, sep., sulph., zinc.
bed, in - kali-c., kali-n., phos., staph.
rising, after - caust., mang.
waking, on - agar., anac., ***carb-an.,*** cycl., hep., kali-c., nicc., nit-ac., phyt., staph.
motion, agg. - **BRY.,** ***calc., calc-p., chel.,*** con., ph-ac., ptel., rhus-t., zinc.
motion, amel. - nat-c.
night - ***am-c., calc.,*** caust., ***cina,*** graph., kali-c., ***lach.,*** nit-ac., ox-ac., phos., ruta, sep., sil., ***sulph.***
2 a.m. - ***kali-c.***
drives out of bed - calc., lach.
lying on back, while - lyc.
midnight - ambr.
midnight, after - sulph.
noon - alum., ***aur.,*** mez., zinc.
nursing mothers - carb-v.
paroxysmal - kali-c., mez., nat-m., ph-ac., sulph.
pears, after - bor.
potatoes, after - alum.
pressure agg. - agar., brom., ***calc.,*** caust., chel., dulc., indg., mang-m., mez., nit-ac., ***ph-ac.,*** ran-s.
amel. - carb-an., nat-m., spig., stann., sulph.
pulsating - caust.
reading aloud - caust.
riding, while - lyc., puls.
rising from bed, on - caust., graph., zinc.
rubbing amel. - lyc., phos.
sex, after - ph-ac.
singing - sars.

PRESSING, pain
sitting, while - ambr., bor., caust., chin., dig., nat-s., phos.
bent - bar-c., bor., ***kalm.***
bent, amel. - bry., sulph.
erect amel. - ***kalm.***
sleep, after - rheum.
preventing - rhus-t.
smoking amel. - kali-bi.
soup, after - alum., ars., indg., stann.
spots, in - phos.
standing, while - bar-c., merc.
amel. - dig.
step, at every - hell.
stool, during - sars.
after - ***calc.,*** carb-s., crot-t., ***pic-ac., puls.,*** sulph.
after amel. - alum.
before - alum.
stooping agg. - aur-m.
straightening out, after - dig.
supper, after - am-c., ***calc.,*** carl., lyc., nat-c., puls., seneg., zinc.
swallowing agg. - cor-r.
sweet things, after - zinc.
talking - ars., caust.
touch agg. - carb-v., chel., cupr., lyc., mang., ph-ac., plat., sars., sep.
vexation, after - cham., ign., phos.
vomiting, amel. - kali-c.
waking, on - agar., ambr., ant-s., caust., cycl., hyper., ***lach.,*** nicc., nit-ac., phyt., sil.
walking, while - bar-c., bell., ***bry.,*** mang., nat-c., ***nux-v.,*** stront.
amel. - ambr., bor., bov., bry.
in open air - anac., bry., nit-ac., sil.
in open air, amel. - ambr.
warm food amel. - ph-ac.
warmth of bed amel. - graph.
weight, as from - abies-n., ***acon.,*** arn., ars., bar-c., brom., ***bry.,*** cact., ***calc., carb-an., cham.,*** dig., elaps, fl-ac., grat., hep., kali-bi., lob., lyc., merc., ***nux-v.,*** par., phos., ***ph-ac., ptel., puls., rhus-t.,*** sec., ***sep.,*** sil., squil., ***spig.,*** spong., staph., zinc.
cardia - ars., lyc., phos.
pressing, esophagus - alum., bar-c., brom., cahin., calc., caust., cimx., ferr-ma., graph., kali-c., lach., lob., merc., nat-c., ***nux-v.,*** ol-an., phos., tab., verat.
as if, pressed on by the larynx - chel.
swallowing - ***alum.***
ball, as if - anac.
eating, while - ars.
after - alum., ars.

PRICKLY, extending down esophagus - cedr.

PULSATION - **ACON.,** agar., alumn., ***ant-c.,*** **ANT-T.,** ***arg-n.,*** ars., ars-i., ***asaf., bell.,*** bov., ***cact.,*** calad., **CALC.,** calc-s., cann-s., carb-s., carb-v., chel., **CHIN.,** chin-a., **CIC.,** coloc., cop., ***corn.,*** croc., crot-h., cupr., ***dig.,*** dros., **FERR.,** ferr-ar., ***ferr-i.,*** gamb., gins., **GLON.,** ***graph.,***

PULSATION - ***ham.,*** hura, ***hydr.,*** hydr-ac., hyos., ***iod.,*** ip., jac-c., kali-ar., **KALI-C.,** kali-i., kali-n., kali-s., ***lac-c.,*** lach., lachn., laur., lyc., ***mag-m.,*** med., ***meny.,*** meny., mosch., mur-ac., naja, nat-a., nat-c., ***nat-m.,*** nat-s., ***nit-ac.,*** **NUX-V.,** olnd., op., **PHOS.,** plat., plb., **PULS.,** rheum, ***rhus-t.,*** sel., **SEP., SIL.,** ***stann., sulph.,*** tab., thuj.
- air, open, amel. - naja
- belching amel. - ***sep.***
- cough with - acon., asaf., bell., cact., carb-v., cic., coloc., dros., ferr., graph., iod., kali-c., lyc., nat-m., puls., sulph.
  - coughing, from - ip.
- dinner, after - cact.
- eating, while - nat-m., ***sep.***
  - after - alumn., ***asaf.,*** cact., cop., kali-c., lyc., mez., ***nat-m.,*** phos., **SEL.,** ***sep.***
- evening - alumn.
  - while lying on the back - alumn.
- extending over whole abdomen - bruc.
- faintness, with - sulph.
- gastric and abdominal sufferings, during - ***asar.***
- headache, with - ***kali-c.***
- leaning against anything - gamb.
- lying on back, while - alumn., ***dios.,*** op.
- meditation, during - raph.
- menses, after - ferr.
- morning - asaf., kali-c., kali-n., ***sep.***
- nausea, with - nat-c.
- night - eup-per., ***puls.***
- noon - sulph.
- pit of stomach, in pulsation, perceptible to sight - asaf.
- rising amel. - op.
- sitting - sulph.
- straightening up - lycps.
- supper, after - nux-v.
- trembling - arg-n., calc., kali-c.
- walking, after - calad.
  - amel. - op.

PYLORIC stenosis - aeth., ornith.

RAWNESS, pain, esophagus - am-c., ars., ***calc., carb-an., caust.,*** merc., **MERC-C.**

REGURGITATION of food, (see Belching) - ***aesc.,*** aeth., ***alum.,*** am-m., ***ant-c., arg-n.,*** ars., ***arum-t.,*** asaf., ***bell., bry.,*** bufo, ***calc., calc-s.,*** camph., ***cham.,*** canth., carb-an., carb-s., **CARB-V.,** ***caust.,*** **CHIN.,** chin-a., coff., ***con., cop.,*** cycl., ***dig.,*** echi., **FERR.,** ferr-i., **FERR-P.,** glon., graph., ***hep.,*** ign., ***ip.,*** iris, kali-ar., ***kali-bi.,*** kali-c., kali-p., kali-s., kalm., ***lach.,*** lob., ***lyc.,*** mag-m., ***mag-p.,*** mang., ***merc., mez., mur-ac., nat-m.,*** nat-p., nit-ac., ***nux-v.,*** **PHOS., PH-AC.,** pic-ac., plat., plb., ***podo.,*** **PULS.,** quas., ran-b., rob., ***rhus-t.,*** sars., senec., spig., ***sulph.,*** sul-ac., tab., tell., teucr., thuj., ust., valer., verat.
- afternoon - euphr., ferr., lyc., nat-p., sulph.
- bitter tasting - chin., **LYC.,** ***nat-c.,*** ph-ac., sulph.
- child, vomits milk after nursing - acet-ac., ***aeth., ant-c.,*** calc., cham., ***nat-c., ph-ac., sanic.,*** **SIL.,** ***valer.***
- coughing, after - ***raph.,*** sul-ac.

REGURGITATION of food
- dinner, after - lyc., nat-p., sars., sulph.
  - while walking - mag-m.
- eating, while - cupr-s., grat., mag-p., merc., phos., sars.
  - nauseous taste - calc.
- eating, after - aesc., bry., **FERR.,** mag-m., mag-p., med., ***nat-m.,*** phos., podo.
  - five hours after - ***caust.***
  - immediately after - ferr., ***mag-p., phos.***
  - one hour after - aesc., aeth., sulph.
  - two hours after - ferr., lyc., sulph.
- evening - sulph.
- morning - ***sulph.***
- mouthful, by the - aesc., arg-n., ars., ***dig., ferr., hydr., hyos.,*** lach., lyc., **PHOS.,** sulph., sul-ac.
- night - ***canth., phos.,*** zinc.
  - midnight, after - sil.
  - what was eaten at noon - kali-c., ***zinc.***
  - soup eaten at noon - graph.
- noon - ***ferr.***
- rancid - puls.
- sour - graph., mag-m., zinc.
- stooping, when - cic., ip., ***phos.***
- supper, after - phos.
- vexation, after - ferr-p.
- walking, while - ***mag-m.***

regurgitation, esophagus, liquids, taken are forced into nose - anan., **ARUM-T.,** aur., ***bar-c.,*** bell., bism., canth., ***carb-ac.,*** caust., cupr., ***cur.,*** gels., hyos., ign., kali-bi., ***kali-ma., lac-ac.,*** **LAC-C., LACH., LYC.,** ***lyss., merc., merc-c., merc-cy., nat-m.,*** petr., phos., ***phyt., plb.,*** puls., sil., ***sul-ac.***

RELAXATION, of pylorus - ***ferr-p., phos.***

RESTLESSNESS - hep., kali-c., sil.

RETCHING, general (see Vomiting) - acet-ac., ***acon., aesc.,*** ail., ***agar.,*** alum., alumn., am-c., anac., ant-c., ***ant-t.,*** arg-m., ***arg-n., arn., ars.,*** ars-h., ***asar.,*** atro., aur., aur-m., bapt., bar-c., bar-i., bar-m., **BELL.,** bism., bor., brom., ***bry.,*** cact., ***cadm-s.,*** cahin., calad., camph., canth., cann-i., caps., carb-ac., carb-o., ***carb-v.,*** card-m., **CHAM.,** ***chel., chin.,*** chin-a., chin-s., chion., chlor., chr-ac., cimic., cimx., ***cocc.,*** coc-c., coch., coff., **COLCH.,** ***coloc.,*** con., crot-h., crot-t., ***cupr., dig., dros.,*** dulc., **EUP-PER.,** fl-ac., gels., glon., ***graph., hep.,*** hyos., hyper., ign., indg., iod., **IP.,** iris, jab., kali-bi., kali-c., kali-c., kali-i., kali-n., kali-p., kali-s., kalm., ***kreos.,*** lac-ac., ***lach.,*** led., lil-t., ***lob., lyc.,*** mag-c., mag-m., meny., merc., merl., mez., morph., mosch., myric., naja, ***nat-a., nat-c.,*** nat-m., nat-p., ***nat-s.,*** nit-ac., nux-m., **NUX-V.,** oena., olnd., ***op.,*** ox-ac., petr., phos., phys., ***phyt.,*** plan., ***plb., podo.,*** psor., ptel., ***puls., raph.,*** rhus-t., sabad., sabin., ***sec.,*** seneg., ***sep.,*** sil., sin-a., sol-n., squil., ***stann.,*** stram., stront-c., **STRY.,** ***sulph.,*** sul-ac., ***tab.,*** tarent., tax., tell., ter., ther., thuj., ***verat.,*** viol-t., vip., zinc.
- afternoon - raph.
- agg. from - asar.
- air, in open - graph.
- alcoholics, in - ***ars., nux-v., op.***

RETCHING, general
belching, from - coloc., sep.
chill, before - ip.
coffee, after - caps., cham.
cold drinks, after - anac., ip., ***nux-v.,*** puls., rhus-t., teucr.
constant - podo.
convulsive - dig., mag-c., merc-c., vip.
cough, with - agar., ***ambr., ant-t., apis, arg-n.,*** ars., ars-i., aspar., bell., ***bor.,*** brom., ***bry.,*** bufo, carb-s., **CARB-V.,** caust., cench., cham., ***chin.,*** chin-a., chlor., cimx., **CINA,** ***coc-c.,*** con., crot-h., crot-t., cupr., ***daph.,*** **DROS.,** dulc., ferr-m., hell., **HEP.,** ***hyos.,*** ign., ***iod.,*** **IP.,** ***kali-ar.,*** kali-bi., ***kali-c.,*** kali-i., ***kali-s., kreos., lach.,*** lob., lyc., mag-m., mag-p., ***merc., mez., nat-m.,*** **NIT-AC.,** ***nux-v., ol-j.,*** plan., **PULS.,** ruta., sabad., sang., ***seneg., sep., sil., squil.,*** stann., sulph., ***sul-ac., tab.,*** tarent., thuj., verat.
daytime - ***stann.***
diarrhea, during - **ARG-N.,** crot-t., ***cupr.***
dinner, before - carb-v.
drinking, after - anac., ars-h., gamb., hep., nat-m., plb.
dyspnea, from - am-c.
eating, when - verat.
after - agar., am-c., bism., bry., cann-i., ***cham.,*** chin., cop., cycl., graph., kali-c., lac-ac., lyc., mag-c., nat-s., plb., puls., rhus-t.
amel. - ***ign.,*** nat-c.
emotions, from - op.
empty - asar., sec.
epilepsy, before - ***cupr.***
evening - dig., hyper., kali-c., nat-m., phos., stann., stram.
walking, while - raph.
excitement, from - kali-c.
fasting. while - berb., kali-c.
food, thought of - merc-cy.
happy surprise - kali-c.
hawking mucus from fauces - ***ambr., anac.,*** **ARG-N.,** bor., ***bry., calc-p., coc-c., kali-c.,*** ip., ***merc-i-f.,*** nat-a., **NUX-V.,** osm., sulph., ***stann.***
ineffectual - ***ant-t., arn., ars., asar.,*** bar-m., ***bell.,*** brom., ***bry.,*** chin., crot-t., dig., grat., hyos., ip., kreos., nat-a., ***nux-v.,*** op., plb., ***podo.,*** puls., sabin., sil., sulph., sul-ac., ther., verat., verat-v.
and anxious, with vomiting - ars., bism., cupr., podo.
liquids, after - petr., sulph.
menses, during - ***puls.,*** thuj.
milk, after - ***calc.***
morning - alum., dig., graph., hep., kali-c., kreos., ***nat-c.,*** nat-m., ***nux-v.,*** phos., sulph.
rinsing mouth when - sulph.
rising, after - led.
rising, on - mosch.
walking, on - coc-c.
motion, during - cadm.

RETCHING, general
motion, amel. - nat-c.
night - arg-n., ***arn.,*** gamb., graph., ***merc.,*** nat-m., nux-v., ***puls.,*** ran-s., rat., rhus-t., sulph., ther.
1 a.m., on waking - rat.
midnight - bell.
noon, after soup - ant-t., mag-c.
painful - card-m., ***merc-c.,*** sec., tab.
salivation, with - ant-t., hep.
smoking, after - ***ip.,*** tab.
soup, after - ars.
spasmodic - ***merc-c.***
stool, during - ***arg-n., cupr., ip., nux-v.,*** podo.
after - phos.
swallowing, on - ***graph., kali-c., lach., merc-c.,*** tab.
on, empty, agg. - ***graph.***
touching inside of throat - ***coc-c.***
violent - ***ars.,*** asar., brom., cadm-s., dig., med., phyt., squil.
vomiting, after - ant-t., ***apis, ars.,*** **COLCH.,** ***sep.,*** stram.
waking, after - rat., sil.
walking, in open air, during and after - graph.
warm drinks - ***coc-c.,*** nat-m.
amel. - ther.
yawns, then - tell.

RETRACTION - nat-c.
sense of - calad., dig., ***dulc.,*** hell., ***kali-i.,*** lach., lact., mur-ac., ***op.***

REVERSE, esophagus, peristaltic action of - ***asaf.***

ROLLING, sensation, over in - phos.

ROUGHNESS, sensation - hell., mang.
roughness, esophagus - calc., hydrc., iod., ***nat-c.,*** sulph.

SAND, as if in - ptel.

SCRAPING, pain - **ARS.,** bry., carl., ***chel.,*** cic., crot-t., hell., nat-m., ***nux-v.,*** plat., **PULS.,** ter.
stool, after - alum.

SCREWING, together, pain - alum., kali-c., sil., sulph., zinc.

SENSITIVE - carb-v., kali-c., kali-n., sul-ac.
bad news - ***dig.***
menses, during - kali-n.
pressure, to - alum., kali-n., mag-c., mag-m., nat-c.
stepping, to hard - bar-c.
talking, to - caust., hell., kali-c.
touch, to - carb-v., nat-c.
sensitive, esophagus - kali-c.

SHAKING - anac., mag-m., mez.

SHARP, pain - abrot., ***acon.,*** aeth., agar., ail., alum., ambr., am-c., am-m., ***anac.,*** anan., ant-t., arg-n., ***arn.,*** **ARS.,** ars-i., arund., aur., aur-m., bar-c., bar-i., bar-m., ***bell., berb., bism.,*** bor., bov., ***bry.,*** buf-s., cahin., calad., calc., calc-ar., calc-s., camph., cann-i., canth., caps., ***carb-an.,*** carb-s., ***carb-v.,*** card-m., ***caust., cham., chel.,***

SHARP, pain - chin., chin-a., cic., cimic., cocc., coff., colch., coloc., com., con., croc., crot-h., crot-t., cupr., cur., cycl., dig., dros., dulc., eug., euon., euph., ***gamb.,*** gran., graph., grat., hydr-ac., hyper., ***ign.,*** iod., ip., jac-c., ***kali-ar.,*** kali-bi., ***kali-c., kali-n.,*** kali-p., kali-s., kreos., lach., laur., lept., ***lyc., mag-c.,*** mag-m., med., merc-c., mur-ac., ***nat-a., nat-c.,*** nat-m., nat-p., nicc., ***nit-ac.,*** ol-an., ***ph-ac., phos.,*** phyt., ***plat.,*** podo., ***psor., puls.,*** ran-s., raph., rheum, rhod., ***rhus-t., rumx.,*** ruta., sabin., samb., senec., ***sep.,*** sil., spig., squil., staph., stram., stry., ***stront-c., sulph.,*** sul-ac., ***tab.,*** thuj., ***zinc.***

afternoon - alum., am-m., nat-m., nicc., petr., sep.
1 p.m. - rhus-v.
3 p.m. - nicc., sulph.
on lying down - coc-c.
belching, during - bry., cocc., sep.
amel. - phos.
before - staph.
bend body backward, forcing to - ***bell.***
bending to the right - bry.
breakfast, after - kali-n.
breathing, on - **ANAC.,** calc., ***caps.,*** euphr., lyc., spig., ***sulph.***
between breaths - caps.
expiration, on - anac., spig.
inspiring, on - anac., ***bry.,*** card-m., chin., coc-c., con., mag-m., puls., sep., sulph.
clothes, from tight - aur.
cold, on taking - phos.
coughing, on - am-c., ars., ***bry.,*** phos., ***podo.,*** sep., ***tab.***
daytime - nat-m.
descending, on - carl.
dinner, after - calc., dig., ***kali-bi.,*** mez., naja
drawing - mang.
drawing in abdomen, when - zinc.
eating, after - calc., lepi., phos.
evening - cocc., con., grat., nux-v., sulph., zinc.
10 p.m. - phos.
bed, in - thuj.
sitting, while - euphr.
extending to,
abdomen - ant-t.
ankle - kreos.
arm, upper, right - am-m.
axilla, left, and back - kali-c.
axilla, right - am-m.
back - bar-c., **BOR., CHEL.,** kali-c., laur., nicc., plb., ran-b., sabin., tab.
back, around left side of - con.
breasts - lach.
chest - alum., anan., ***calc.,*** carb-an., ***lach.,*** mag-c., nat-m., ***rumx.,*** sep., staph.
downward - calc., nat-m.
ear - mang.
flank - sulph.
hip-joint - sil.
hypogastrium - ars.
inward - stram.
sacrum - anac.

SHARP, pain
extending to,
spine - tab.
sternum - chin., nat-m.
stomach, below - euphr.
upwards - phys.
false step, on a - ***bry.,*** puls.
forenoon - indg., nicc.
intermittent - verb.
jarring - zinc.
jerking - chin.
laughing, on - mang.
lifting, on - sil.
lying down, after - nux-v., sil.
amel. - spig.
on side - bry.
on side, left - com.
menses, during - ars.
morning - calad., carb-an., merc-c., nat-m.
standing, while - sulph.
waking, on - con.
motion agg. - ***bry.,*** con., ***puls.,*** sep.
moving arms - calc-ar.
night - com., mag-m.
paroxysmal - arg-m., cop., chin., manc., plb.
periodical - paeon.
pressure, on - aur., calc., merc-c.
pressure, on, amel. - podo.
rising, from stooping - carb-an., mang., plat.
sitting, while - calad., spig.
bent - aeth.
up amel. - coc-c.
soup, after - merc-c.
standing, while - dig., sulph.
stepping, on - ***bry., puls.,*** zinc.
stool, after - calc.
stooping, on - sep.
stretching - mang.
swallowing food quickly - sep.
talking, while - caps.
transversely - mag-m., zinc.
uncovering, on - coc-c.
vexation, from - lyc.
walking, while - anac., bry., grat., myric., puls., spig., til.
warm milk, after - ***ang.***
yawning - phyt.

sharp, pain, esophagus - calc., carb-s., kali-c., merc-c.
as if, a bone had lodged in it - carb-s.

SHOCK - CIC., kali-c., nat-c., nux-v., plat., tab.
convulsions, before - **CIC.**
eating - teucr.
lying on the side - camph.
sleep, during - tab.
stitching - plat.

SHOOTING, pain, in epigastrium - bell., bry., chin., puls.

SINKING, sensation, (see Emptiness, weak) - abrot., ***acon.,*** aesc., agar., ail., alum., alumn., ant-t., apoc., arum-d., ***bapt.,*** brom., bufo, cact., calad., cann-i., carb-ac., chlol., ***cina,*** colch., cop., ***cimic.,*** clem., ***cocc.,*** croc., ***crot-h., crot-t.,*** cupr., **DIG.,** dios., elaps, ***glon.,*** **HELL.,** hep., ***hydr.,***

SINKING, sensation - ***hydr-ac., ign.,*** jatr., jug-c., kali-ar., ***kali-bi.,*** kali-chl., ***kali-fer.,*** kali-i., laur., ***lept., lob., lyc.,*** mag-c., ***med., merc.,*** merc-i-r., mosch., **MURX.,** myric., naja, nat-a., ***nat-m.,*** **NUX-V.,** olnd., op., ***petr.,*** phos., phys., pic-ac., plan., ptel., puls., rhod., sabad., sec., **SEP.,** sil., ***stann., staph., sulph.,*** **TAB.,** tell., teucr., thea., til., uran., ***verat.,*** zinc.
bad news - ***dig.***
breakfast, after - colch.
before - ***kali-bi.***
waking, on - apoc.
deathly - dig., ip., lob., tab.
eating, after - ars., calc., cina, dig., ***iod.,*** lyc., ***petr.,*** plan., sil., staph., urt-u.
amel. - alumn., ***anac., bar-c., chel.,*** iod., murx., nat-c., phos., ***sep.,*** sulph.
before - alumn., ***sulph.***
evening - colch.
extending to heart - **LOB.**
forenoon - jatr., nat-m.
11 a.m. unable to wait for lunch - ***sulph.,*** zinc.
after acids - zinc.
hemorrhage, from any - ip.
inspiration, agg. - calad.
lying down, amel. - sep.
meeting a friend, when - ***cimic.***
menopause, during - cimic., crot-h., dig., hydr-ac., ***ign., sep.,*** tril.
morning - apoc., cimic., dios., hydr., ***kali-bi.***
night - dios., ***lyc.,*** tarent.
palpitations, with - cimic.
paroxysmal - glon.
pressure, from - **MERC.**
sitting, while - acon.
stool, after - ambr., dios., ***ph-ac.,*** **PODO.**
waking, on - apoc.
walking amel. - acon.
wine amel. - sep.

SLAKING, lime, sensation of - ***caust.***
spits up food - caust.
mouthful until stomach is empty - arg-n., ***ferr.,*** **PHOS.**

SLOW, (see Digestion)

SOFTENING, of - calc., kreos., merc-d.

SORE, pain - abies-n., acet-ac., ***acon.,*** aesc., ***agar.,*** all-s., aloe, alum., alumn., am-br., am-c., am-m., anac., ant-c., ant-t., ***apis,*** arg-n., **ARN., ARS.,** arund., asaf., **BAR-C., BAR-I.,** bar-m., **BELL.,** ***bov.,*** brach., brom., **BRY.,** calad., ***calc., calc-p.,*** calc-s., ***camph.,*** cann-s., canth., ***caps., carb-ac., carb-an., carb-s.,*** **CARB-V.,** card-m., carl., ***caust.,*** cham., ***chel.,*** **CHIN.,** ***chin-a., chin-s.,*** chlor., cina., cinnb., ***cocc.,*** coc-c., coff., **COLCH.,** ***coloc., con., cop., crot-c., crot-h., crot-t., cupr.,*** cupr-ar., daph., ***dig.,*** dios., elat., ***eup-per.,*** euph., eupi., fago., ***ferr., ferr-ar., ferr-i., ferr-p.,*** fl-ac., ***gamb., glon.,*** grat., ***guare., hep., hyos.,*** ign., ind., ***iod., ip.,*** **KALI-AR.,** ***kali-bi.,*** **KALI-C.,** kali-n., ***kali-p.,*** kali-s., ***kalm.,*** kreos., **LACH., LYC.,** mag-c., **MAG-M.,** ***manc.,*** mang., ***merc.,*** **MERC-C.,** merc-sul., mosch., mur-ac., myric., ***nat-a.,*** **NAT-C.,** ***nat-m., nat-p., nat-s.,*** nit-ac., **SORE,** pain - ***nux-m.,*** **NUX-V.,** ol-an., op., ox-ac., paeon., ***petr., ph-ac.,*** **PHOS.,** ***phyt.,*** plan., plb., podo., ptel., ***puls.,*** ran-b., ***raph., ruta., sabad., sang., sec., sep., sil., spig.,*** spong., ***stann.,*** stram., stry., ***sulph., sul-ac.,*** tab., tarent., ter., ther., thuj., ***verat., zinc.,*** zing.
afternoon - alum.
belching, on - cocc.
bending, from - mag-m.
breathing, deep - ***merc.***
expiration, on - kali-c.
inspiration, on - ars., kali-c.
clothing agg. - bell., ***bry., calc., coloc., crot-h., hep.,*** **LACH., LYC.,** ***nat-m.,*** **NUX-V.,** ***ph-ac.,*** spong.
coughing, on - agar., alum., ambr., am-c., ***arn., ars.,*** arum-t., arund., asc-t., bell., **BRY.,** cob., dios., **DROS.,** hell., hyos., ip., lach., mang., **NUX-V.,** ***phos.,*** sep., sil., squil., **STANN.,** thuj.
dinner, during - mag-m.
after - calc-p., mosch., phos.
drinking, after - nit-ac.
eating, after - bar-c., ***calc-p.,*** cocc., crot-h., nat-m., ***sang.***
amel. - lec., nux-v.
evening - abrot., alum., dig., dios., fago., phos., thuj.
extending to abdomen - alum.
to mouth - kali-bi.
to palate - mang.
to throat - mang.
morning - alum., chin., dios., fago., **PHOS.,** sang.
bed, in - con.
bed, in, turning in - con.
on rising - crot-h.
motion amel. - fago.
night - sep.
bed, in - mag-c.
sitting still, on - fago.
sleep, after - rheum.
stepping, on - ***aloe, bar-c., bell.,*** hell., kali-s.
stooping agg. - glon., meny.
swallowing a morsel, after - **BAR-C.**
talking, on - hell., nat-c., nat-m.
touch agg. - euph., hell., mag-c., nat-m.
turning in bed - alum.
walking, while - anac., bar-c., calc., kali-s., phos., ***sep.***
amel. - fago.

sore, pain, esophagus - alum., ars., calc., caust., caj., dig., kali-n., nit-ac., sul-ac.
feels food, whole length of esophagus - ***alum.***
swallowing, as if, over a sore, spot - ***bar-c.,*** caj., ***nat-m.***

SPASMS, esophagus - ***alum., alumn., arg-n., ars., asaf.,*** **BAPT., BAR-C., BELL.,** ***calc., carb-ac.,*** carb-s., carb-v., ***caust.,*** cham., cic., ***cimx., cocc.,*** coc-c., coloc., ***con., crot-c., crot-h.,*** **CUPR.,** ***elaps, gels.,*** graph., hydr-ac., ***hyos., ign.,*** iris, kali-ar., kali-bi., kali-c., **LACH., LAUR.,** ***lyss., manc.,*** **MERC-C.,** ***naja,*** nat-m., nicc., nit-ac., ***nux-v.,*** ox-ac., ***phos., plat., plb.,*** ran-b., rat., sars., ***stram., sulph.,*** verat., ***verat-v.,***

SPASMS, esophagus - zinc.
belching, during - coloc.
elderly, people can only swallow liquids - alum., ***bar-c.,*** caust.
evening - ***ars., asaf.,*** cham.
night - ***lach., nux-v.***
periodical - ***lyss.***
swallow, liquids, can only - **BAPT.,** ***bar-c., plb.***
swallowing, on - **BAPT., BAR-C.,** ***hyos.,*** **MERC-C.,** ***phos., sulph.,*** zinc.
liquids - ***bell.,*** coc-c., elaps, ***graph., manc., merc-c.***

SPLINTER, pain, esophagus - ars.

SPLIT, as if, esophagus, on belching - coca.

SPONGY, sensation, esophagus - elaps.

STINGING, pain, esophagus, in - ars.

STRICTURE - con.

stricture, esophagus - acon., am-m., **ARS., BAPT., BAR-C.,** ***bell., cact., calc.,*** cic., cund., gels., ***kali-c., lyss., naja,*** **NAT-M.,** ***nux-v., ox-ac., phos., stront-c., verat-v.,*** zinc.

SQUEEZING - coloc., lyc.

STENOSIS - dys-co.
pylorus - aeth., ornith.

STONE, sensation of - ***abies-n.,*** acon., ***aesc.,*** agar., all-s., alum., anac., ant-t., ***arg-n.,*** arn., **ARS., BAR-C.,** ***brom.,*** **BRY.,** cact., **CALC.,** calc-s., carb-an., carb-v., cedr., ***cham.,*** chin., coc-c., cocc., colch., coloc., dig., dios., elaps, eup-per., ferr., fl-ac., gent-c., graph., ***grat.,*** hep., ign., kali-ar., ***kali-bi.,*** kali-c., kali-p., lach., lob., lyc., manc., mang., ***merc.,*** mez., mill., naja, nat-a., ***nat-c.,*** nat-m., nux-m., **NUX-V.,** olnd., op., osm., ox-ac., par., ***ph-ac.,*** phos., ***ptel.,*** puls., ran-b., ***rhus-t.,*** rumx., sang., sec., sep., sil., spong., squil., staph., sul-ac., sulph., ter., zing.
belching amel. - alum., ***bar-c.,*** nat-c., par.
bread, after - sep.
cold - sil.
after vomiting - ***acon.,*** sil.
dinner, after - ptel.
eating, after - ***ars., bar-c.,*** **BRY.,** naja, nat-m., **NUX-V.,** ***ptel., puls.,*** rhus-t., sil.
amel. - ptel.
hawking amel. - kali-c.
morning - par.
bed, in - kali-c.
waking, on - puls.
motion agg. - ***bry., calc., nux-v.***
pressure, as from - squil.
rising sensation - sul-ac.
rubbing together - cocc., coloc.
salivation amel. - sul-ac.
sharp, as if - coloc., hydr.
supper, after - alum., ***calc.***

SUMMER, agg. - ***guai.***

SWASHING - arn., mez.
morning - mez.

SWIMMING in water, as if - abrot.

TEARING, pain - ***aeth.,*** agar., aloe, alum., alumn., am-c., ***anan., ars.,*** bar-c., chin., chin-a., ***cocc., colch., coloc., con., cupr., daph.,*** dig., dios., iod., graph., kalm., lyc., merc., merc-c., nux-v., petr., plat., plb., rhus-t., ruta., sep., ***tarent.,*** thuj., verat., ***zinc.***
anger, after - **COLOC.**
belching, during - phos., sep.
cardia - phos.
bending body to right - thuj.
amel. - merc-c.
breathing, inspiration, on - mez.
clucking-tearing - lyc.
dinner, after - ang.
drinking, after - nit-ac.
evening, in bed - thuj.
extending to,
abdomen - alum.
abdomen, side of - con.
back - sep.
chest - carb-an.
esophagus, into - ***aeth.***
intermittent - lyc.
menses, during - graph.
morning - con., sep.
motion agg. - ang., kalm.
paroxysmal - plb., ruta.
pressure agg. - iod.
rising from stooping - carb-an.
stooping, after - bar-c.
sudden - cic.
talking - kalm.
transverse - ars.
walking, while - ars.

tearing, esophagus - kali-c.

TENSION - acon., aesc., agar., ambr., anac., ***ant-t.,*** arg-n., ***ars.,*** ars-i., asaf., bar-c., bar-i., bar-m., bell., bry., cahin., calc., ***caps.,*** carl., carb-s., **CARB-V.,** cast., caust., cham., ***chel.,*** cic., clem., cocc., coff., colch., coloc., crot-t., dros., dulc., ferr., ferr-i., gent-l., grat., guare., helon., ***hep.,*** hura, iod., ***ip.,*** kali-ar., ***kali-c.,*** kreos., ***lact., lob.,*** **LYC.,** ***mag-m.,*** merc., mez., mur-ac., nat-a., nat-c., nat-m., nit-ac., **NUX-V.,** op., ph-ac., phos., plat., ***plb., puls.,*** ran-s., **RUTA.,** sabad., sel., sep., ***sil.,*** **STANN.,** ***staph., stram.,*** sul-ac., sulph., sumb., tarax., ***ter.,*** verat., zinc.
breathing, when - lyc.
deep inspiration agg. - dros., mez.
hold on - dros.
clothing agg. - ***hep., kreos.***
dinner, after - nit-ac., phos., sep.
eating, after - anac., ***iod.,*** phos., ruta, sul-ac.
before - mez.
erect position agg. - mag-m.
evening - hura, mag-m., sulph.
extending to back - sulph.
forenoon - puls.
menses, during - zinc.
milk amel. - **RUTA.**
morning - arn., kali-n.
in bed - arn., staph.
motion, agg. - caps., sep.
amel. - ***puls.***
night, 2 a.m. - ars.

TENSION,
noon - euphr.
riding in a carriage, while - phos.
sitting, agg. - hep.
stool, after - dros., sep.
before - ars., dros.
stooping, when - sep.
walking, agg. - cocc., colch.
tension, esophagus - cham., cycl.

THIRST, (see Food, Thirst)

TICKLING - anac., bry., crot-t., nat-m., sang., thea., tarent.

TIGHT, around the waist, cannot have anything - **LACH.**, lyc., ***sep.***

TINGLING - ant-t., colch., indg., ***puls., rhus-t.***
tingling, esophagus - ***acon.***

TOBACCO, sensitiveness to - asc-t., calad., ***ign., lob.***

TREMBLING - aesc., aeth., agar., am-c., arg-m., ***arg-n., ars.,*** ars-i., brach., cact., calad., **CALC.,** caps., carb-v., cimic., chin-s., ***crot-h., elaps,*** ferr., ***ham., ign.,*** **IOD.,** ***lyc.,*** mag-m., mag-s., med., nat-m., nat-s., **NUX-V.,** ***phos.,*** phys., ***rhus-t., sulph., tab.,*** verat., xan.
breakfast, after - cimic.
chilly, when - phos.
conversation, from - mag-m.
coughing, when - aesc., nux-v.
daytime - calad.
eating, on - elaps
extends all over body - iod., ***lyc.***
fever, during - caps., ign., **IOD.,** lyc.
lying down, on - agar., cocc.
menses, during - am-c., arg-n., ferr.
morning, on waking - agar.
nausea, with - aeth., calad.
noise, from - agar.
noon - ***sulph.***
urination, after - ars.

TURNING - aeth., am-m., hydr., kali-n., nat-m., ol-an., plb., sulph.
lying on it, while - hydr.
morning, after rising - kali-n.
motion, on - bell.
over, seems to, on coughing - ***puls.,*** ruta., tab.
swallowing liquids, after - plb.

TWISTING - agar., ***alum., arg-n.,*** ars., ***bar-c.,*** bry., calc., chin., cic., ***cocc.,*** crot-c., dios., gran., grat., iris, kali-bi., kali-c., kali-chl., ***lyc.,*** mez., nat-m., ***nux-m., nux-v.,*** ol-an., ox-ac., ph-ac., phos., plat., ***plb.,*** sars., sep., stry., sulph., zinc-m.
breakfast, after - agar., sol-t-ae.
dinner, after - sars., sol-t-ae.
eating agg. - grat.
extending into, abdomen - ***arg-n.***
into, chest - alum.
into, throat - sep.
forenoon - nat-c.
lying on it, while - hydr.
morning - plat., sil.
nausea, before - ph-ac.

TWISTING,
night - phos., sulph.
paroxysmal - nit-ac., plb.
sudden - chin.

TWITCHING - aesc., aloe, alumn., ars., bry., cann-s., chin-s., coloc., ***hydr., ign.,*** kali-c., lyc., mez., petros., phos., plat., puls., rat., sil., stry., tab.
convulsive - ars.
eating amel. - puls.
extending to, larynx - puls.
to, rectum - ars.
to, throat - phos.
sitting, while - phos.
walking about amel. - alumn.

ULCERATIVE, pain - ***acet-ac.,*** alum., anan., ***arg-n.,*** cann-s., cast-eq., gamb., hell., ***lach., mag-c., mag-m.,*** merc-c., ***nat-m., rat., rhus-t.,*** spong., stann.
coughing, on - ***lach.***
dinner, after - ***arg-n.***
eating amel. - gamb.
evening, lying - mag-m.
motion, on - stann.
pressing - bar-c.
touch, on - nat-m.
turning in bed, on - alum.

ULCERS - ***aloe,*** alum., anac., ***arg-n., ars., atro.,*** bell., bism., cadm-met., calc., ***calc-ar.,*** calc-p., calen., carb-v., carc., caust., chin., crot-h., ***cur., dys-co.,*** ferr-ac., ***ger.,*** graph., grin., ham., **HYDR.,** iod., ip., **KALI-BI.,** ***kali-c.,*** kali-i., ***kreos.,*** **LYC.,** med., ***merc-c., mez.,*** morg., morg-g., nat-c., nat-m., nat-p., nat-s., ***nit-ac.,*** **NUX-V.,** op., ***ornithog.,*** petr., ph-ac., **PHOS., PSOR.,** puls., ran-b., rat., ruta, **SEP.,** sil., sin-a., sul-ac., sulph., symph., syph., thuj., ***uran-n.,*** vario., verat.
anger, from - anac., nux-v., staph.
bleeding, with - caps., merc-c., ***phos.***
burning, with - ars., atrop., bism., ***phos.***
intolerable pains, with - bism., euph., kali-cy.
painless - carb-ac.
ulcers, esophagus - ***iod.***

UNEASINESS - aeth., alumn., ars., bell., ***canth.,*** carb-ac., cimic., cinnb., ***colch.,*** crot-t., cycl., dig., dios., fago., glon., grat., gymn., iris, kalm., kali-bi., kali-i., lith., lob., mur-ac., naja, osm., phos., ptel., ruta., sabad., sec., sep., sol-t-ae., tarent., verat-v., zinc.
drinkers, in hard - alumn.
stooping amel. - nat-m.

UPSIDE down, sensation - aeth.

URGING - alum.

VARICES, of esophagus - **HAM.**

VOMITING, general - absin., acet-ac., **ACON.,** ***aesc.,*** **AETH.,** ***agar.,*** alet., all-c., alumn., ambr., am-c., ***am-m.,*** anac., ***anthr.,*** **ANT-C., ANT-T., APIS,** ***apoc.,*** **APOM.,** aran., arg-c., **ARG-N.,** ***arn.,*** **ARS.,** ars-h., ars-i., arum-m., ***asar.,*** asc-t., aur., aur-m., bapt., ***bar-c.,*** bar-i., ***bar-m., bell., bism., bor., both.,*** **BRY.,** bufo, ***cact.,*** **CADM-S.,** cahin., ***calc., calc-p., calc-s., camph.,*** cann-i., cann-s., ***canth.,*** carb-ac., carb-s., **CARC.,** caust., **CHAM.,** ***chel.,*** **CHIN.,** chin-a., ***chin-s.,*** chlol., cic., ***cimic., cina, cocc., coc-c.,*** coff., **COLCH.,** coll., coloc., ***con.,*** cop., ***crot-c.,*** crot-h., crot-t., ***cub.,*** **CUPR.,** ***cupr-ar., cupr-s.,*** cycl., ***dig., dor., dros., dulc.,*** elaps, ***eup-per., euph.,*** **FERR.,** ***ferr-ar., ferr-i.,*** ferr-p., ***form.,*** **GAMB.,** gels., glon., ***gran., graph., grat., hell., hep.,*** hydr., ***hyos., ign.,*** indg., ***iod.,*** **IP., IRIS,** kali-ar., ***kali-bi., kali-br.,*** kali-c., ***kali-i.,*** kali-p., kali-s., kalm., **KREOS.,** ***lac-d., lach., laur.,*** **LOB.,** ***lyc., mang., merc., merc-c., merc-d., mez.,*** mosch., mur-ac., naja, ***nat-m.,*** nat-p., ***nit-ac., nux-m.,*** **NUX-V.,** olnd., op., ***ox-ac.,*** paeon., ***petr.,*** ph-ac., **PHOS.,** phyt., **PLB.,** podo., ***psor.,*** ptel., **PULS.,** rat., rhod., rhus-t., ruta., sabin., sal-ac., ***samb., sang., sec.,*** seneg., sel., ***sep.,*** **SIL.,** squil., sol-n., ***stry.,*** **SULPH.,** sul-ac., **TAB.,** ***tarent.,*** tep., ***ter., ther.,*** thuj., ***tub.,*** uran., ***valer.,*** **VERAT., VERAT-V.,** wye., ***zinc.***

- **abdominal,** rumbling, with - podo.
- **acids,** after - ferr., guare., nat-p.,
- **acrid** - arg-m., ***ars.,*** bufo, calad., chion., coloc., colch., con., crot-t., dor., ferr., gent-c., ***hep.,*** ip., ***iris,*** kali-c., kali-m., **KREOS.,** lyc., med., mez., phys., phyt., podo., rob., **SANG.,** sil., ther., thuj.
  - morning, while coughing - thuj.
  - night - ther.
- **afternoon** - bell., chin-s., con., graph., hep., kali-chl., mag-s., phyt., ***sulph.***
  - 2 to 3 p.m. - plb.
  - 4 p.m. - sulph.
- **aggravation,** after - cupr., dros., olnd.
- **albuminous** - ars., ip., ***jatr.,*** kali-bi., ***merc-c., plb., verat.***
- **alcoholics,** of - ***alumn.,*** ant-t., **ARS.,** ***cadm-s.,*** calc., ***caps.,*** carc., ***carb-ac., crot-h.,*** cupr., ***cupr-ar.,*** ip., **KALI-BI.,** ***kali-br., lach.,*** lob., **NUX-V.,** op., ***sang.,*** sulph., ***sul-ac.,*** zing.
- **alternating,** with convulsions - ***cic.***
  - diarrhea, with - carc.
- **amel.** - ant-t., puls.
- **anger,** after - carc., **CHAM., COLOC., NUX-V.,** staph., ***valer.***
  - indignation, with - carc., cham., coloc., staph.
  - nursing mother, in, affecting milk - calc-p., valer.
- **anticipation,** from - carc.
- **anxiety,** with - ars., ip., samb., tab.
- **appetite,** with - iod., lob., verat.
- **apyrexia,** during - ant-c., ***ip.***
- **bed,** after going to - **TARENT.**

VOMITING, general

- **beer,** after - cupr., ferr., ip., ***kali-bi., mez.,*** sulph.
  - but not after water - mez.
- **belching,** with - mur-ac.
  - as if would again, with - goss.
  - sour - nit-ac.
- **bile,** of - ***acon.,*** alum., amyg., anan., anthr., ***ant-c.,*** ant-t., ***apis, arg-n.,*** arn., apoc., **ARS.,** ars-h., ars-i., asar., asc-t., aspar., aur., bar-c., bar-i., bar-m., ***bell., bism.,*** bor., **BRY.,** bufo, ***cadm-s.,*** cahin., ***calc.,*** calc-s., camph., canth., cann-s., carb-s., carb-v., cast., **CHAM., CHEL.,** ***chin., chin-a., chion., cic.,*** cina, cocc., coch., ***coff.,*** **COLCH.,** ***coloc.,*** con., ***crot-c., crot-h.,*** crot-t., ***cupr.,*** cupr-ar., cur., cycl., ***dig.,*** dros., dulc., elaps, **EUP-PER.,** fago., ***ferr-p.,*** fl-ac., ***grat.,*** hep., hyos., ***ign., iod.,*** **IP.,** ***iris,*** jab., jatr., ***kali-ar., kali-bi.,*** kali-c., kali-i., kali-p., kali-s., ***lac-d., lach., lept., lyc.,*** lyss., mag-c., med., **MERC., MERC-C., MERC-CY.,** mez., ***morph.,*** mur-ac., ***nat-a., nat-c., nat-m.,*** nat-p., **NAT-S.,** nit-ac., **NUX-V.,** olnd., **OP.,** ox-ac., ***petr.,*** **PHOS.,** phyt., ***plb., podo.,*** **PULS.,** ***pyrog.,*** raph., rhus-t., sabad., ***sabin.,*** **SANG.,** sars., ***sec.,*** **SEP.,** sil., stann., stram., ***sulph.,*** sul-ac., sumb., tarent., tax., ***ter.,*** thuj., ***tub.,*** valer., **VERAT.,** ***verat-v.,*** zinc., zinc-m.
  - afternoon - phyt.
  - anger, after - cham., nux-v.
  - anxiety, with - ***crot-h.***
  - blood, then - agar., carb-v., verat.
  - chill, during - ***ant-c.,*** arn., ***ars., cham., cina,*** chin., ***dros.,*** **EUP-PER.,** ign., ip., lyc., ***nux-v., puls.,*** verat.
    - after - **EUP-PER.,** kali-c., **NAT-M.**
    - before - cina, ***eup-per.***
  - cold water, after - ***eup-per., rhus-t.***
  - colic, with - cham., ***chin.,*** coloc., hyos., ***iod., nux-v.***
  - cough, during - anan., cadm-s., carb-v., cham., **CHIN.,** ***puls.,*** sabad., sars., sep., stram., sulph.
  - eating, after - ant-c., bism., ***crot-h.,*** merc., stann.
  - errors in diet, from - fl-ac.
  - evening - phos., stram.
    - 9 p.m. - tax.
  - exertion, after - stram.
  - fever, during the - ***ars.,*** bry., ***cham.,*** chin., ***cina,*** crot-h., cupr., dros., **EUP-PER.,** ign., ip., iris, merc., ***nat-m., nux-v.,*** op., phos., psor., ***puls.,*** sec., sep., sulph., thuj., verat.
  - food, then - bry.
  - headache, with - arg-n., aur., ***bry.,*** cadm-s., ***calc.,*** **CHEL.,** crot-h., eup-per., **IP., IRIS,** kali-c., ***lac-d., lept., lob.,*** nat-m., ***nat-s.,*** nicc., petr., ***plb., puls.,*** rhus-t., **SANG.,** spig., sulph., verat., zinc.
    - sweets, after - arg-n., ***iris.***
  - lying on right side or back - ***crot-h.***
  - mental exertion, after - nat-m.

VOMITING, general

bile, of

morning - aspar., dros., hep., merc-c., **SEP.,** tarent., ther., zinc.

10 a.m. to 11 a.m. - cur.

on waking - stann.

motion on least - ***crot-h., stram.***

night - chin., cur., lyc., ***merc.,*** phos., ***podo.***

3 a.m. - mur-ac.

perspiration, during - ant-c., ***ars.,*** bry., **CHAM., CHIN.,** ign., ip., iris, merc., ***nux-v.,*** puls., sep., verat.

rising, on - ars.

sitting up in bed - ***stram.***

soup, after - stann.

stooping, from - ip.

tea, after - sel.

trembling and great nausea, causing prostration - ***eup-per.***

vexation, after - ***nat-s.***

bitter, of - ***acon.,*** agar., ant-c., ant-t., apis, arn., ***ars.,*** benz-ac., bol., bor., **BRY.,** bufo, cadm-s., calc., calc-s., cann-s., ***carb-s.,*** cast., ***cham.,*** chin., clem., ***cocc.,*** coc-c., colch., ***coloc.,*** con., ***crot-c., crot-h.,*** crot-t., cupr., ***eup-per.,*** form., gent-c., ***grat.,*** hydr., iris, ***kali-bi.,*** kali-c., lyc., mag-c., manc., med., ***merc.,*** merc-c., mez., ***nat-a., nat-c., nat-m.,*** nat-p., ***nat-s.,*** nit-ac., **NUX-V.,** olnd., op., ***petr.,*** **PHOS.,** phyt., ***plb.,*** ptel., ***puls.,*** raph., rhod., samb., **SANG.,** ***sars., sep.,*** sil., ***stann., sulph.,*** tab., thuj., ***verat.,*** vinc., vip., zinc.

afternoon - sulph.

breakfast, before - tab.

chill, during - ***cham.***

at close of - ***eup-per.***

coffee, after - ***cham.,*** verat.

coughing, on - ***sep.,*** verat.

drinking, after - bor., bufo, eup-per.

cold water - podo.

cold water, greenish - rhod.

eating, after - mag-c., nit-ac., stann.

evening - hell., verat.

evening, during cough in bed - ***sep.***

headache, during - form., nit-ac., ***sang.,*** sulph., thuj.

humiliation, after - puls.

fever, during - ***eup-per.,*** thuj.

menses, during - ***sars.***

before - ***caul.***

morning - bor., ***bry.,*** cham., colch., form., tab., thuj.

cough, during - thuj.

waking, on - form., sil., thuj.

night - crot-t., hell., phyt., sil.

noon, while eating soup - mag-c.

soup, from - ***mag-c.,*** stann.

standing, on - colch.

waking, on - sil.

black, of - acon., alum., ant-t., ***arg-n.,*** **ARS., CADM-S.,** ***calc.,*** camph., carb-ac., card-m., ***chin., chin-a., con., crot-h.,*** cur., dor., hell., hydr-ac., ***hyos., ip.,*** kali-i., kali-n., kali-ox., ***lach.,*** lat-m., laur., ***lyc.,*** manc., med., merc-c., ***nat-s.,*** nit-ac., **NUX-V.,** op., ox-ac., ***petr.,***

VOMITING, general

black, of - **PHOS.,** phyt., ***plb.,*** puls., raph., ***sec.,*** sil., ***sulph.,*** sul-ac., **VERAT.,** zinc.

menses, on appearance of - sulph.

blood, at sight - ph-ac.

blood, of - acet-ac., ***acon.,*** agar., aeth., aloe, alum., alumn., ***am-c.,*** anan., ant-c., ant-t., arg-n., **ARN.,** ***ars.,*** ars-h., aur-m., bar-m., bell., brom., ***bry.,*** bufo, **CACT.,** ***calc.,*** calc-s., camph., cann-s., ***canth.,*** carb-ac., carb-s., **CARB-V.,** card-m., ***caust.,*** cham., **CHIN.,** ***chin-a., cic.,*** colch., coloc., con., **CROT-H.,** ***cupr., cycl.,*** dig., dros., ***erig.,*** **FERR.,** ***ferr-ar.,*** ferr-i., ***ferr-p.,*** guai., **HAM.,** hep., ***hyos.,*** ign., iod., **IP.,** kali-bi., kali-chl., kali-i., kali-n., kali-p., ***kreos., lach.,*** led., lob., lyc., merc., ***merc-c.,*** mez., ***mill., nat-a.,*** nat-m., nat-s., ***nit-ac., nux-v.,*** olnd., op., ox-ac., ***petr.,*** **PHOS.,** ***phyt., plb., podo., puls.,*** pyrog., rat., rhus-t., ruta., **SABIN.,** samb., ***sang., sec., sep., sil., stann.,*** stram., ***sulph.,*** sul-ac., tab., ***ter.,*** uran., ust., ***verat., verat-v.,*** vip., ***zinc.***

alcoholics, in - alumn., ***ars.***

black - card-m., ***ham.***

blue - ars.

close of, at - verat.

clotted - arn., ars., caust., ham., lyc., ***merc-c.,*** nux-v., phyt., sec.

cough, with - anan.

drinking, after - merc-c.

eating, after - stram.

evening - guai., merc-c.

exertion, after - ***phos.***

infants - lyc.

lying agg. - ***stann.***

lying on the back - merc-c.

menses, during - sulph.

begining, on - sulph.

instead of, in girls - ***ham.***

suppressed, during - bell., ***bry., ham.,*** nat-m., ***phos.,*** puls., sulph.

morning - dros.

motion - ***erig.***

night - ***caust.,*** phyt., podo.

splenic affections, from - card-m.

summer evenings - guai.

suppressed hemorrhoidal flow, after - acon., ***carb-v.,*** **NUX-V.,** ***phos., sulph.***

thin - ***erig.***

bluish, of - ars., kali-c.

bowels, impacted - op., plb., pyrus.

brain, affections, in - apom., bell., glon., kali-i., plb.

bread, after - bry., nit-ac.

black, after - nit-ac., ph-ac.

breakfast, after - agar., ***bor., carb-v.,*** colch., cycl., daph., ***ferr.,*** kali-c., sars., trom.

before - eupi., ***kreos., nux-v.,*** psor., sel., **TAB.**

bright, light, from - stram.

VOMITING, general

brownish - arg-n., ***ars.,*** bar-c., bism., bry., carb-v., colch., cupr., kali-bi., mez., ***nat-s.,*** nit-ac., op., ox-ac., phos., phyt., ***plb.,*** rhus-t., sec., sulph., sul-ac., tab., zinc.
children, in nursing - aeth.
evening, after coffee - verat.
after milk - mur-ac.

brushing, teeth, on - ***coc-c.***

burning, hot - mez., podo.

cancer, from - ars., carc., cadm-s., carb-ac., kreos.

chemotherapy, from - ars., carc., cadm-s., ip., nux-v.

chill, during - ail., alum., arn., asar., bor., ***caps., cina, dros.,*** **EUP-PER.,** ferr., gamb., ***ign., ip.,*** lach., lyc., ***nat-m.,*** nux-v., ***puls.,*** rhus-t., sep., thuj., ***verat.***
after - ant-t., ***aran., bry., carb-v.,*** **EUP-PER.,** ***ip.,*** kali-c., ***lyc.,*** **NAT-M.,** rhus-t.
before - apis, arn., ars., chin., cina, eup-per., ferr., lyc., nat-m., puls., sec.

chilliness, with - ars., dulc., puls., tab.

chloroform - ***phos.***

chocolate, colored - bry., ***con.,*** mez., sec.

cholera, with - ***ars.,*** camph.

chronic, tendency - lob.

clear - colch., crot-t., elat., ferr., ***fl-ac.,*** petr., phyt., sabad., sulph., sul-ac.

clearing, throat of mucus in morning - bry., euphr.

closing, eyes, on - ***ther.***
amel. - tab.

coffee, after - camph., cann-s., ***cham.,*** glon., verat.

coffee, grounds, like - ***arg-n.,*** ars., ars-h., brom., **CADM-S.,** colch., ***con.,*** crot-h., ***cupr.,*** echi., ***iris,*** lac-d., lach., lyc., lyss., med., ***merc-c.,*** mez., mur-ac., ***nat-m.,*** nat-p., ornithog., **PHOS.,** plb., pyrog., sec., stry., sul-ac.

cold, on becoming - cocc.

collapse, weakness with - aeth., ***ant-t., ars.,*** crot-h., euph-c., ***lob.,*** **TAB.,** ***verat., verat-v.***

constant - ars., carc., hell., **IP.,** merc., plb., pyrog., syph.

constipation, with - nux-v., op., plb.

convulsions, during - ant-c., ***hyos.,*** op.
after - acon., ***ars.,*** bell., calc., colch., ***cupr.,*** glon.
before - ***cupr.,*** hydr-ac., op.

convulsive - **BISM.,** ***cupr.,*** dig., hep., lach., merc-c., sul-ac., tab., vip.

coughing, on - agar., **ALUM.,** ***anac.,*** **ANT-T.,** ***arg-n., arn., ars., ars-i.,*** bell., **BRY.,** bufo, calc., cann-s., caps., carb-s., ***carb-v., cham.,*** chin., chin-a., ***cimx., coc-c.,*** con., ***cupr.,*** cur., ***daph., dig.,*** **DROS.,** ***ferr.,*** ferr-ar., ferr-i., ferr-p., ***form.,*** gels., **HEP.,** ***hyos.,*** indg., iod., **IP.,** ***kali-ar.,*** kali-bi., **KALI-C.,** ***kali-p.,*** kali-s., ***lach.,*** laur., lob., ***meph.,*** merc., merc-c., mez., mill., myos., nat-a., nat-c.,

VOMITING, general

coughing, on - ***nat-m.,*** nat-p., ***nit-ac., nux-v., ph-ac.,*** phos., plb., ***puls.,*** rhod., rhus-t., ***sabad.,*** sang., sarr., seneg., ***sep., sil., sulph.,*** sul-ac., syph., ***tarent.,*** thuj., verat., zinc.
after - sul-ac.
whooping cough, during - ant-t., carb-v., cupr., dros., ferr-p., **IP.,** kali-br., phos.

cramps, colic with - bism., cham., coloc., ***cupr., cupr-ar.,*** op., ***nux-v.,*** pix., plb., sarr., ***verat.***

curds, in - aeth., calc., nat-p., sanic., sil., valer.

cyclic, in adults - ars., ***carc.,*** ip., ***nux-v.,*** staph.
infants, in - aeth., carc., cupr-ar., ingluv., iris, ip., kreos., merc-d.

dark - am-caust., ant-t., ***ars.,*** cadm-s., cupr., dor., merc-c., nit-ac., op., ox-ac., ***phos.,*** raph., sec., stann., sul-ac.
drinking, after - mur-ac.

death, desires, during - ip., phyt.

delayed, after a while - bism., **PHOS.**

dentition, during - calc., cham., bism., hyos., phyt.

depression, emotional, with - carc., nux-v.

diarrhea, during - ***aeth.,*** ant-c., ***apis,*** arg-m., **ARG-N., ARS.,** asar., ***ars.,*** bell., bism., ***carb-ac.,*** chin., ***colch.,*** coloc., crot-t., ***cupr.,*** cupr-ar., cycl., dios., ***dulc.,*** elaps, **GAMB.,** ***gnaph.,*** gran., ***graph., grat., hell.,*** indg., ***iod.,*** **IP.,** ***jatr.,*** kali-n., ***kreos.,*** lach., merc., merc-c., phos., ***phyt.,*** plb., ***podo., puls.,*** rob., sang., seneg., sep., stann., stram., sulph., tab., **VERAT.**
before - ars., colch., crot-t., dig., lach., phos., phyt.
with - ars., nit-ac.

difficult (see Retching) - **ANT-T.,** ***ars.,*** asar., bor., bry., cic., clem., coff., cupr., elat., grat., ***nux-v.,*** plb., raph.

dinner, during - mag-c.
after - acon., agar., anac., ant-t., graph., ***lach.,*** ol-an., ***sel.***
before - dros., sulph.

drinking, after - ***acon.,*** alum., anac., **ANT-C.,** ***ant-t.,*** apoc., ***arn.,*** **ARS.,** ars-i., bar-c., bell., ***bism., bor.,*** **BRY.,** bufo, ***cadm-s.,*** calc., camph., canth., cham., chel., chin., ***chin-a., cina,*** cocc., colch., con., crot-t., ***cupr.,*** dig., dros., ***dulc., eup-per.,*** ferr., ferr-ar., ferr-i., ferr-p., hep., ***hyos.,*** iod., ***ip.,*** kali-ar., kali-c., ***kreos., lyc.,*** merc., merc-c., merc-cy., mez., nat-m., nit-ac., ***nux-v.,*** olnd., ***op.,*** **PHOS.,** plb., puls., rhod., rhus-t., sars., ***sec.,*** sel., ***sil.,*** sulph., ***sul-ac.,*** **TAB., VERAT.,** ***verat-v.,*** zinc.
cold water, after - anac., apoc., arn., ars., ***bry.,*** bufo, chel., cina, cocc., crot-t., ***cupr., dulc., eup-per.,*** ferr., gels., ip., kali-ar., ***kali-c., lyc.,*** mez., nux-v., podo., rhod., ***sil., sul-ac., verat.,*** **VERAT-V.**
immediately, after - apoc., **ARS., BISM., BRY., CADM-S.,** crot-t., ***eup-per.,*** ip., ***nux-v.,*** sanic., sep., ***zinc.***
not after eating - sil.

VOMITING, general
drinking, after
smallest quantity - ant-t., **ARS.**, ars-h., **BISM.**, **BRY.**, **CADM-S.**, cina, **IP.**, **PHOS.**, plb., pyrog., verat., verat-v., zinc.
soon as water becomes warm in stomach - ***chlf.***, kali-bi., **PHOS.**, ***pyrog.***
warm drinks - ***bry.***, ***phos.***, ***puls.***, pyrus, sanic.
water - sars.
drinking, amel. - anac., nit-ac., tab.
cold water - ***cupr.***, phos., puls.
hot water - ars., ***chel.***, sul-ac.
drawing, catarrhal plugs from drawing, posterior nares - ***sep.***
drowsiness, with - ***aeth.***, ***ant-t.***, ip., mag-c.
easy - agar., alum., ant-t., apoc., **ARS.**, bapt., ***calc-p.***, **CHAM.**, chel., colch., dig., ***ferr.***, graph., ***ign.***, ip., jatr., ***kali-bi.***, mez., ***nux-v.***, ***phos.***, ***phyt.***, ***ran-s.***, sec., ***tab.***, zinc., zinc-m.
eating, while, sudden vomiting - am-c., ***ars.***, dig., **FERR.**, iod., puls., rhus-t., sep., sil., stann., verat.
after - acet-ac., alumn., ***am-c.***, anac., ***ant-c.***, ***ant-t.***, **ARS.**, aur-s., bell., **BRY.**, bufo, ***calc.***, calc-s., carb-an., ***carb-s.***, ***carb-v.***, cham., ***chel.***, **CHIN.**, **CHIN-A.**, chin-s., ***cina***, coloc., crot-h., crot-t., ***cupr.***, dig., ***dros.***, ***ferr.***, ***ferr-ar.***, ferr-i., ferr-m., ***ferr-p.***, ***gamb.***, ***graph.***, ***hydr.***, ***hyos.***, ***ign.***, ***iod.***, **IP.**, ***iris***, kali-ar., ***kali-bi.***, ***kali-br.***, kali-c., kali-p., kali-s., ***kreos.***, lach., lob., ***lyc.***, mag-c., **MEPH.**, merc., nat-a., ***nat-m.***, ***nat-s.***, ***nit-ac.***, ***nux-v.***, olnd., ***op.***, ***ph-ac.***, **PHOS.**, plb., psor., ***puls.***, ruta., ***sanic.***, sec., **SEP.**, **SIL.**, ***stann.***, stram., **SULPH.**, sul-ac., tab., **TARENT.**, **VERAT.**, ***verat-v.***, ***zinc.***
amel. - anac., ant-t., ferr., ign., mez., nux-v., puls., sep., tab.
only after - ***ferr.***
undigested food - aeth.
eggs, after - colch., **FERR.**, ***ferr-m.***, sulph.
smell of - ***colch.***
emotions, from - kali-br.
exhausting - aeth., ant-t., podo., verat., verat-v.
erect, on becoming - colch.
eruptions, from receding - ***cupr.***
evening - agar., anac., bell., bry., ***carb-v.***, dig., elaps, eug., kali-chl., merc., merc-c., morph., nat-s., nux-v., phos., phyt., psor., ***puls.***, sec., stram., ***sulph.***, verat.
everything - apoc., **ARS.**, ars-h., bar-m., ***crot-h.***, ***eup-per.***, ***ip.***, merc-c., op., sec., sul-ac.
excitement, after - ferr., kali-br., kali-c.
exertion, on - colch., crot-h., ferr., stram., tab., ther., verat., zinc.
expectoration, on - ***coc-c.***, dig., kali-c., lach., ***sil.***
fainting, with - cocc.
fatty, food, after - ***puls.***, sin-n.
fearful - ant-c.

VOMITING, general
fecal matter - ars., ***bell.***, bry., cahin., ***colch.***, cupr., ***nux-v.***, **OP.**, ***plb.***, pyrus, raph., rhus-t., sulph., tab., thuj.
fever, during - acon., aeth., all-s., ***ant-c.***, **ANT-T.**, ***ars.***, bapt., bell., ***bry.***, cact., ***cham.***, ***cina***, ***cocc.***, con., crot-h., dor., ***elat.***, **EUP-PER.**, eup-pur., ferr., ferr-p., hep., ign., ***ip.***, kali-c., lach., ***lyc.***, **NAT-M.**, nux-v., puls., ***stram.***, thuj., tub., ***verat.***
after - calc., ***eup-per.***
filamentous - iod., ox-ac., ***phos.***, sul-ac.
fish, after fried - kali-c.
smell of - ***colch.***
fluids, only - ars., bism.
food - acon., aeth., agar., ail., alum., ***am-c.***, anac., anan., ***ant-c.***, ***ant-t.***, apis, ***arn.***, **ARS.**, ars-i., ***bell.***, berb., bism., bor., **BRY.**, bufo, ***cact.***, ***cadm-s.***, ***calc.***, calc-p., calc-s., canth., caps., ***carb-s.***, ***carb-v.***, caust., ***cham.***, ***chel.***, **CHIN.**, chin-a., ***cina***, ***cocc.***, coff., ***colch.***, coloc., con., ***crot-h.***, crot-t., ***cund.***, ***cupr.***, ***cycl.***, dig., ***dros.***, elaps, **EUP-PER.**, **FERR.**, **FERR-AR.**, ***ferr-i.***, ***ferr-p.***, ***graph.***, grat., hydr-ac., ***hydr.***, ***hyos.***, **IGN.**, indg., iod., ***ip.***, ***iris***, jatr., kali-ar., ***kali-bi.***, ***kali-c.***, ***kali-p.***, kali-s., **KREOS.**, ***lac-d.***, ***lach.***, ***laur.***, led., lob., **LYC.**, lyss., mag-c., mag-s., manc., merc., merc-c., mill., mosch., mur-ac., ***nat-m.***, nit-ac., **NUX-V.**, olnd., ***op.***, phel., ***ph-ac.***, **PHOS.**, phyt., ***plb.***, podo., psor., **PULS.**, raph., rat., rhus-t., ruta., sabin., samb., **SANG.**, ***sec.***, ***sep.***, ***sil.***, squil., ***stann.***, ***sulph.***, sul-ac., tab., tell., ter., thuj., **VERAT.**, ***verat-v.***, zinc.
afternoon - calc., mag-s.
animal all - phos.
bile, then - ant-t., bell., ***bry.***, ***colch.***, dig., ***nat-m.***, samb.
blood, then - nux-v.
breakfast, after - ***ferr.***, sel., ***sil.***
chill, during - ail., ign., phos.
after - phos.
before - ***ars.***, ***cina***, eup-per., **FERR.**
cough, from - anac., anan., ***ant-t.***, **BRY.**, ***coc-c.***, dig., ***dros.***, ***ferr.***, **IP.**, ***kali-c.***, laur., ***mez.***, ***nat-m.***, ***nit-ac.***, ***ph-ac.***, ***puls.***, rhus-t., sep.
dark, food - mag-c.
dinner, after - anac., calc., graph., sel.
drink, not of - ***bry.***
eating, while - am-c., ars., iod., rhus-t., sep., sil., stann., verat.
eating, after - mag-c.
2 or 3 hours - aeth., ***ant-c.***, apoc., atro., bism., ***bry.***, cer-ox., ***chin.***, colch., cupr., ferr., ***ferr-m.***, ferr-p., graph., ***ip.***, iris, **KREOS.**, lac-c., nux-v., petr., phos., ***puls.***, sang., sulph., verat.
5 or 6 hours - atro., puls.
7 hours - sulph.

VOMITING, general
food, eating, after
immediately, after - ant-c., ant-t., ***apis, ars.,*** ars-h., ***bry.,*** carb-an., carb-v., cupr., dig., ***ferr., ferr-p., graph., kali-bi.,*** mosch., olnd., plb., ruta., sanic., sil., sulph., verat., zinc.
intervals of days after has filled the stomach - **BISM.**
long after - aeth., ars-i., ***ferr.,*** kreos., plat., puls., sabin., sang.
long after, whooping cough, in - meph.
one day after - cimx., sabin.
some hours after - meph., puls.
evening - carb-v., ***kreos.,*** phos., ***puls., sulph.***
sunset, after - stram.
fever, during - cina, ***eup-per.,*** ferr., ign., nux-v., thuj.
hot after - lob.
intermittents, in - ***ferr., ferr-p., nat-m.***
lying, while - olnd.
back, on the - rhus-t.
milk, except - hydr.
morning - crot-h., ***plb.,*** **SEP.,** sil., ***sulph.***
waking, on - aspar.
mucus, then - dros., mag-c., nux-v., puls., sil.
night - crot-t., kali-c., lyc., phyt., rat., sil.
1 a.m., on waking - rat.
midnight - agar., **FERR.,** nat-m.
smallest quantity - verat-v.
solid only - bry., cupr., verat.
sour - calc., hep., ***kali-bi.,*** nat-m., ***nat-s.,*** podo., sulph., thuj.
supper, after - cupr-s.
undigested - aeth., ***ant-c.,*** apoc., atro., bals-p., bell., bism., ***bry.,*** calc., cer-ox., ***chin.,*** colch., cupr., ***ferr., ferr-m.,*** ferr-p., graph., ***ip.,*** iris, ***kali-bi.,*** **KREOS.,** lac-c., ***lac-d., lyc.,*** merc., nat-m., nux-v., petr., phos., ***puls.,*** sabin., sang., stann., stry-f-c., verat.
eaten previous day - sabin.
water, then, bitter - lac-d.
vexation, after - acon., cham., ign., ip., lyc., verat.
waking, on - jug-r.
water, except - lyc.
water, then - puls.
forcible - acon., **AETH.,** ant-t., apoc., ars., ***con.,*** glon., iod., ip., jatr., manc., merc-c., mez., mosch., ***nux-v., petr., sanic.,*** stry., **VERAT.,** verat-v.
shortly after eating - ***sanic.***
sudden - ant-t., kali-bi., kali-chl., pic-ac.
fever, with - bapt.
forenoon - chin., elat., nat-s., nux-v., op., psor., sang.
7 a.m. - elat.
9 a.m., during headache - form.
10 a.m. - cur., psor.
11 a.m. - chin., cur.
frequent - **ARS.,** bar-c., canth., **CHIN.,** colch., ***con.,*** cupr., hyos., lyc., mez., ph-ac., phos.

VOMITING, general
frothy - acet-ac., acon., ***aeth.,*** all-c., ant-t., ***apis,*** **ARG-N.,** ars., arund., cadm-s., ***canth.,*** cic., coc-c., ***con.,*** crot-t., cupr-ac., ferr., glon., ***ip.,*** kali-br., kali-s., **KREOS.,** led., ***lyc.,*** mag-c., mag-m., med., ***merc-c.,*** mur-ac., nat-c., nat-p., ***nux-v.,*** phos., ***podo., puls.,*** sil., ***tub.,*** urt-u., **VERAT.,** verat-v., zinc.
hot - podo.
gastric irritation, from - ant-c., ***ars.,*** bism., ferr., ip., nux-v., phos., puls., verat.
glairy - alumn., ***arg-n., ars.,*** canth., carb-s., crot-t., cupr-ac., dig., ***iris, jatr., kali-bi.,*** kali-n., mur-ac., phos., ***sil.,*** sul-ac., ***verat-v.***
greasy - ars., ***iod.,*** manc., ***mez., nux-v.,*** sabad., thuj.
green - ***acon., aeth.,*** ant-t., aquileg., ***arg-n.,*** arn., **ARS.,** asar., bry., bufo, cadm-s., ***cann-s., canth.,*** carb-ac., carb-s., ***card-m.,*** **CHEL.,** cimic., ***cocc.,*** colch., ***coloc., crot-c., crot-h.,*** cupr., cupr-ar., cur., cycl., dig., ***dulc.,*** elaps, elat., ferr-p., guare., ***hell., hep.,*** **IP.,** jatr., kali-bi., ***lach., lyc.,*** manc., ***merc., merc-c.,*** mez., morph., ***nat-s., nux-v.,*** olnd., ***op.,*** ox-ac., ***petr., phos.,*** phyt., ***plb., puls.,*** raph., rhod., rhus-t., sabad., ***sabin.,*** sec., ***stram., teucr.,*** **VERAT.,** vip., zinc.
bitter, and, after cold drinks - rhod.
blackish - cupr., dulc., hell., osm., petr., phos., plb., sol-n., teucr.
olive - carb-ac.
dark - ***crot-h.,*** op., sec., stann., verat.
evening - stram.
fluid - ***acon.,*** asar., ***aur-m., card-m., coloc., cupr., cycl., hep., lach., nat-s.,*** olnd., ***stram.***
grass, as - ars.
mucus - kali-chl., plb.
night - ars., ***cur.***
watery - olnd.
yellowish - ***ars.,*** colch., crot-h., ***cupr., iris,*** nat-p., ***nat-s.,*** olnd., phos., plb., sabin., verat.
hawking, up mucus, when - ***ambr., anac.,*** **ARG-N.,** bor., ***bry., calc-p., coc-c.,*** euphr., ip., ***kali-c.,*** lach., merc-i-f., nat-a., **NUX-V.,** osm., ***sep., sil., stann.***
headache, during - ***aeth.,*** agn., alum., ant-t., anan., ***apis,*** arg-n., arn., ***ars.,*** asar., bar-m., ***bell., bry., cact.,*** cadm-s., ***calc.,*** calc-s., ***caps.,*** carb-s., caust., chin., chin-s., ***chlf.,*** cimic., cimx., cocc., ***coff.,*** coloc., con., corn., ***crot-h.,*** crot-t., ***cupr.,*** dulc., eug., ferr., ferr-ar., ferr-p., ***form., gels.,*** glon., ***graph., grat.,*** **IP.,** ***iris,*** jatr., kali-ar., kali-bi., kali-c., kali-chl., kali-p., kali-s., kreos., ***lac-c., lac-d., lach., lob.,*** med., **MELI.,** mez., mosch., ***naja, nat-a., nat-m.,*** nat-p., ***nat-s., nux-m., nux-v.,*** op., ***phos.,*** plat., ***plb.,*** **PULS.,** rhus-r., **SANG.,** sarr., sars., ***sep., sil.,*** spig., ***stann., stram.,*** sulph., tab., ***ther.,*** thuj., verat-v., vip., xan., zinc.
heart, with weak - ars., camph., ***dig.***
hiccough, after - cupr., jatr.

VOMITING, general

hot, drinks, can only retain - apoc., ***ars.***, ars-i., calad., casc., ***chel.***, verat.

water amel. - ***ars.***, ***chel.***, sul-ac.

hysterical - ***aquileg.***, ign., kali-br., ***kreos.***, plat., valer.

ice cream, after - **ARS.**, ***calc-p.***, ***ip.***, ***puls.***

impossible - bell., lac-d.

incessant - acon., ant-c., ant-t., ***arg-n.***, ***ars.***, ars-h., ars-i., bar-m., ***cadm-s.***, carb-v., ***carc.***, colch., crot-t., cupr., dig., grat., ***iod.***, **IP.**, kali-bi., lac-d., mag-p., ***merc-c.***, meph., mez., ***nit-ac.***, op., ***phos.***, ***plb.***, ruta., sabin., sec., squil., verat.

intermittent, in - **ANT-C.**, **ANT-T.**, **CINA**, ***elat.***, eup-per., ***ferr.***, ***lyc.***

intoxication, during - crot-h., **NUX-V.**

itching, with nausea, must scratch until he vomits - ***ip.***

kidney, origin - kreos., nux-v., senec.

labor, during - ant-t., caul., cham., ***cocc.***, **IP.**, mag-m., ***puls.***, **SEP.**

larynx, from irritation - tab.

lifting, after - sil.

light, agg. - sang., stram.

lime, water, as if - nat-c.

liquids - ***acon.***, ant-t., aran., arn., ars., ***bism.***, bry., cham., chin., dulc., ip., kreos., nux-v., phos., sil., spong., sul-ac.

as soon as liquids become warm in stomach - ***bism.***, chlf., **PHOS.**

cold water only - sil.

lying, after - olnd., puls.

amel., lying, down - bry., colch., nux-v., sym-r.

right side, on - ant-t.

back, on, while - crot-h., merc-c., nux-v., rhus-t.

amel. - bry., colch., nux-v., sym-r.

side, agg. - ferr.

left - ant-t., sep., sul-ac., verat-v.

right, back, or - crot-h.

side, agg., right in liver affections - bry., crot-h.

amel. - ant-t., colch.

measles, during - **ANT-C.**

meat, after - kreos.

meat, fresh, from - caust.

membrane - canth., merc-c., nat-s., nit-ac., ox-ac., phos., sec., sul-ac.

menopause - aquileg.

menses, during - ***am-c.***, ***am-m.***, ant-c., **APOC.**, ***calc.***, carb-s., ***carb-v.***, cham., cocc., coff., con., ***cupr.***, gels., ***graph.***, ign., ***kali-c.***, kali-i., kali-p., kali-s., ***lach.***, ***lyc.***, nux-v., ***phos.***, ***puls.***, sars., sep., ***sulph.***, tarent., ***verat.***, ***vib.***

after - bor., canth., crot-h., gels., kreos., nux-v., puls.

before - ***calc.***, caul., cham., chin., ***cupr.***, gels., ***kreos.***, ***nux-v.***, ***puls.***, sulph., verat.

suppressed - ars., bell., bry., cupr., ***ip.***, nux-v., plb., puls., verat.

VOMITING, general

mental, exertion - ferr., nat-m., tab.

milk, after - **AETH.**, ***ant-c.***, ant-t., arn., ***ars.***, ars-i., atro., bar-c., bell., bor., bov., bry., ***calc.***, ***calc-p.***, carb-v., ***cham.***, ***cina***, ferr., ***iod.***, ***iris***, kali-bi., kreos., lach., lyc., mag-c., mag-m., mag-p., merc-c., ***merc-d.***, merc-sul., morph., nux-v., ***ph-ac.***, phos., phyt., ***podo.***, rheum, samb., ***sanic.***, ***sep.***, **SIL.**, spong., sulph., **VALER.**, vario., vip.

persistently - aeth., calc-p., ph-ac.

undigested - mag-c.

child, vomits milk after nursing - acet-ac., **AETH.**, ***ant-c.***, ***calc.***, ***calc-p.***, ***nat-c.***, ***ph-ac.***, ***sanic.***, **SIL.**, ***valer.***

mother's, anger, after - calc-p., cham., valer.

curdled - **AETH.**, ***ant-c.***, ant-t., **CALC.**, ip., ***mag-c.***, mag-m., merc-d., merc-c., ***nat-m.***, nat-p., podo., sabin., **SIL.**, ***sulph.***, sul-ac., **VALER.**

sours, after anger of mother - calc-p., cham., valer.

milky - aeth., ant-c., arn., ars., ***calc.***, ip., ***mag-c.***, mag-m., merc., merc-d., ox-ac., podo., sanic., **SEP.**, valer.

pregnancy, during - sep.

month, every - crot-h.

more, than he drinks - kali-bi.

morning - absin., ambr., ant-t., ars., bar-c., bar-m., bry., calc., camph., **CAPS.**, carb-s., ***cocc.***, colch., ***con.***, ***cycl.***, ***dig.***, ***dros.***, dulc., ***ferr.***, ferr-ar., ***ferr-p.***, form., graph., ***guai.***, **HEP.**, ***ign.***, kali-ar., kali-bi., ***kali-br.***, ***kali-c.***, kali-p., kreos., ***lyc.***, merc-c., mosch., ***nat-m.***, nux-v., ***petr.***, phos., phyt., plb., psor., sec., sep., ***sil.***, ***sulph.***, ***sul-ac.***, tab., ***tarent.***, thuj., ***verat.***, zinc.

alcoholics - ant-t., ars., carb-ac., cupr., ***cupr-ar.***, ip., lob., **NUX-V.**

early - stann.

menses, before - ***am-m.***, bor., ***cocc.***, ***cycl.***, graph., ichth., ***ip.***, kreos., meli., nat-m., ***nux-v.***, puls., ***sep.***, thlaspi, verat.

rising, on - ***cocc.***, mosch., verat., verat-v.

motion, on - ***ant-t.***, **ARS.**, **BRY.**, bufo, **CADM-S.**, ***colch.***, ***cupr.***, ***ferr.***, iod., kali-bi., kalm., ***lac-d.***, ***lach.***, ***lob.***, ***nux-v.***, ***petr.***, stram., **TAB.**, ther., ***verat.***, zinc.

moving, from right side - ant-t.

least, from - tab.

mucus - ***acon.***, agar., aeth., alum., alumn., anthr., ***ant-c.***, ant-t., ***apis***, **ARG-N.**, ***ars.***, bar-c., bar-m., ***bell.***, bor., bov., brom., bry., cact., cadm-s., calad., calc., calc-s., cann-s., canth., carl., carb-s., ***carb-v.***, cast., ***cham.***, ***chel.***, ***chin.***, chin-a., ***chin-s.***, ***cina***, cinnb., ***cocc.***, coc-c., ***coff.***, colch., ***con.***, ***cop.***, crot-t., cor-r., ***cupr.***, cupr-ar., cupr-s., ***cycl.***, ***dig.***, **DROS.**, ***dulc.***, elaps, elat., form., glon., grat., ***guai.***, hell., hep., hydr-ac., ***hyos.***, ***ign.***, ***ip.***, indg., ***iris***, ***jatr.***, kali-ar., **KALI-BI.**, ***kali-c.***, kali-chl., kali-n., kali-p., kali-s., kreos., ***lach.***, lil-t., ***lyc.***, ***mag-c.***, mag-s., ***merc.***, ***merc-c.***,

VOMITING, general

mucus - ***mez.,*** mosch., mur-ac., nat-a., nat-c., ***nat-m.,*** nat-p., ***nat-s., nit-ac.,*** **NUX-V.,** olnd., ***op.,*** osm., ox-ac., **PHOS.,** ***phyt.,*** plb., ***podo.,*** psor., **PULS.,** raph., rat., rhus-t., sabad., ***sec.,*** sel., seneg., ***sil.,*** sin-a., sol-n., stann., stram., ***sulph.,*** sul-ac., tab., tax., ***ter.,*** ther., thuj., ***tub.,*** valer., **VERAT.,** verat-v., vip., zinc.

afternoon - bell., con., mag-s.

siesta, after - lyc.

blood - acon., ars., brom., dros., hep., hyos., ***kali-bi.,*** kali-n., lach., merc-c., ***nit-ac.,*** phos., zinc.

chill, before - ***puls.,*** verat.

coffee, after - ***cham.,*** cann-i., verat.

cough, from - ant-t., con., ***dros., ip., nit-ac., puls., sil.,*** thuj., ***verat.***

diarrhea, during - **ARG-N.**

drinking, after - aloe

eating, after - crot-t., ferr., sul-ac.

evening - bry., elaps, psor., nat-s., stram.

6 p.m. - nat-s.

coffee, after - verat.

forenoon - nux-v., psor.

10 a.m. - psor.

fever, during - thuj.

headache, during - con., kalic.

jelly, like - indg., ***ip.,*** jatr., ***kali-bi.***

lumps, of - canth.

morning - ars., camph., dulc., ***guai.,*** kali-bi., sec., sulph., tab., thuj.

after coffee - ***cham.***

waking, on - form., thuj.

night - phos., sil., stram., ther., verat.

rinsing, mouth, when - ***coc-c.***

sour - kali-bi., kali-c.

stool, on going to - aloe.

strings, in - arg-n.

thick - ant-t., ars.

waking, on - sil.

watery, mass of - guai.

white - ars., dig.

nausea, with - aeth., amyg., ant-t., ars., bry., **IP.,** iris, ***lob., nux-v.,*** petr., ***puls.,*** sang., sym-r., verat.

without - ant-c., apoc., apom., arn., ars., chel., kali-bi., lyc., med., sabin., ***verat-v.,*** zinc.

neuralgia, with - aran.

night - agar., ***ant-t., arg-n., ars.,*** bar-c., bell., bry., **CALC.,** calc-s., ***chin.,*** chin-a., ***cocc., con.,*** crot-t., cupr-ar., dig., dros., elat., **FERR.,** ***ferr-ar.,*** hell., hep., ***ign.,*** kali-ar., kali-c., ***lach., lyc., lyss., merc.,*** merc-c., mur-ac., nat-m., nicc., nit-ac., ***nux-v.,*** ox-ac., ph-ac., phos., ***plb., podo.,*** puls., rat., sec., seneg., sep., ***sil., stram., sulph.,*** tab., thea., ther., valer., ***verat.***

alternate nights - lach.

midnight - acet-ac., agar., ***arg-n.,*** lyc., phos.

after - **FERR.,** nat-m.

after, 1 a.m., on waking - ***rat.***

noon - ***mag-c.,*** mag-s., phos., ***verat.***

obstinate, for days - oena.

VOMITING, general

odor, of food - stann.

offensive, smelling - acon., ***ant-t.,*** arn., **ARS.,** bar-m., bell., bism., ***bry., calc., canth., cocc.,*** coff., crot-t., ***cupr.,*** guai., ***ip., led.,*** merc., nat-c., **NUX-V.,** ***op.,*** ph-ac., ***phos., plb.,*** podo., sec., **SEP.,** ***stann., sulph.,*** thuj., valer., verat.

fluid - abrot.

morning - bry.

purulent - kali-s., merc-c., ***nit-ac.***

olive oil, taste like - phos.

opium, after - aven., **CHAM.,** ***ip., nux-v.***

overheated, after - ***ant-c.***

painful - ant-t., arn., ***ars.,*** cupr-s., dig., hyos., ***ip.,*** kali-i., kali-n., ***nux-v.,*** ox-ac., phos., phyt., ruta., sul-ac., verat., verat-v.

painless - sec.

palpitation, with - ars., ***crot-h.,*** **LACH., NUX-V.**

paroxysmal - **ARS.,** bry., carc., **LOB.,** osm., ***nux-m., phos., plb., uran.***

periodic - ars., carc., ***chel., cupr., iris, lept., nat-s.,*** nux-v., plb., sang., sulph.

intervals of days between attacks - bism.

peritonitis, in - ars., op.

perspiration, during - **ARS.,** camph., chin., cina, dros., ***eup-per.,*** ip., merc., sulph.

cold, during - ars., cupr-ar., tab., ***verat.***

fails, when - ***cact.***

pessary in vagina, from - nux-m.

plums, after - ham.

pregnancy, during - acet-ac., acon., alet., ***amyg.,*** anac., ***ant-c.,*** ant-t., ***apis, apom., ars.,*** **ASAR.,** bism., ***bry., calc., cadm-s., canth., caps., carb-ac.,*** card-m., cast., **CHEL.,** ***cic.,*** cinnam., cocaine, cocc., cod., ***colch., con.,*** cupr-ar., ***cycl.,*** dios., ***ferr.,*** ferr-ar., ***ferr-p.,*** goss., graph., ign., **IP.,** ***iris,*** **JATR.,** ***kali-bi., kali-br.,*** kali-c., kali-p., **KREOS., LAC-AC.,** lac-d., lac-c., ***lach., lil-t.,*** lob., ***lyc., mag-c., mag-m.,*** **MED.,** merc-i-f., ***nat-m.,*** nat-p., **NAT-S., NUX-M., NUX-V.,** ***op., ox-ac., petr., ph-ac., phos.,*** piloc., plat., plb., ***podo., psor., puls.,*** **SEP.,** ***sil., sulph., sul-ac.,*** stry., sym-r., **TAB.,** tarent., **THYR.,** tub., ***verat., verat-v.,*** zinc.

blood - ip., phos., ***sep.***

fetus, from movements of - arn.

mucus, in - sul-ac.

persistent - ip., med., piloc., psor.

water - sep.

pressure, on abdomen, from - zinc.

spine or neck region, on - cimic.

projectile (see forcible) - ***aeth.,*** acon.

purching, with - aeth., ant-t., apis, arg-n., **ARS.,** asar., bor., camph., cham., colch., cupr., ip., ***iris,*** merc., phos., ***podo.,*** sec., seneg., sul-ac., sulph., **VERAT.,** verat-v.

bilious - eup-per.

blood - erig.

black - ars.

fright, from - op.

headache, with - graph.

VOMITING, general

purching, with
menses, during - am-m.
urination, and - crot-h.
putting, hands in warm water - ***phos.***
raising, the head - apom., ***ars., bry.,*** colch., ***stram.***
reflex - apom., cer-ox., cocc., ***ip.,*** kreos., valer.
relief, without - ant-c., ***ip.***
respiratory, symptoms, with - ip., lob.
retching, (see Stomach, Retching)
rice, vomiting after - tell.
rice, water, like - colch., ***cupr., kali-bi., verat.***
rich, food, after - aeth., ***ip., puls.,*** samb., spong., sulph.
riding, in a carriage, while - ***apom.,*** arn., ***ars.,*** bell., bor., **CARB-AC., COCC.,** coff., ***colch., ferr.,*** ferr-p., glon., ***hyos.,*** ip., kreos., mag-s., nux-m., nux-v., op., **PETR.,** phos., sanic., sec., sep., ***sil.,*** staph., sulph., **TAB.,** ther.
rinsing, mouth, when - ***coc-c.,*** sep.
rising, after - ambr., ars.
bed, from - ***lac-d.,*** sang., verat-v.
bed, up in - ***acon.,*** ail., ars., ***colch.,*** nat-m., ***stram.***
sago, like matter - phos.
salty - benz-ac., ***iod.,*** mag-c., ***nat-s.,*** puls., sil., sulph.
saliva, from - anac.
running down the throat saliva, while sitting, from - am-m.
salivation, with - graph., ign., ***ip.,*** iris, kreos., lac-ac., ***lob.,*** puls.
scarlet fever - ail., ***bell.***
scratching, when - ip.
septic - bapt., crot-h., lach., vip.
sex, after - mosch., sabad., sil.
stomach, from full, after interval of days - ***bism.,*** grat.
shivering, with - dulc.
sitting, upright - zinc.
sleep, followed by - ***aeth.,*** ant-t., cupr., nat-m.
smell, from bad - kreos.
smoking, from - agar., bufo, ***calad.,*** clem., cocc., ***ip.,*** nat-s., tab.
solids, only - arn., bry., cupr., ferr., sep., verat.
soup - mag-c.
after - ars., ***mag-c.***
sour - acet-ac., act-sp., aesc., am-c., ***ant-t.,*** arg-n., ***ars.,*** asar., bar-c., ***bell.,*** bol., ***bor.,*** brom., bry., cact., cadm-s., calad., **CALC.,** calc-s., ***camph.,*** caps., carb-s., ***carb-v., card-m.,*** **CAUST.,** ***cham., chel.,*** **CHIN.,** ***chin-a., cimic.,*** cimx., ***cocc.,*** con., crot-t., ***daph., ferr., ferr-ar., ferr-p.,*** gels., gent-c., ***graph., grat., hep.,*** hydr., ign., ***ip.,*** **IRIS,** kali-ar., ***kali-bi., kali-c.,*** kali-p., kali-s., kreos., ***lac-d.,*** lac-ac., **LYC., MAG-C.,** ***manc., merc-d., mez., nat-a.,*** nat-c., ***nat-m.,*** **NAT-P.,** ***nat-s.,*** nit-ac., **NUX-V.,** olnd., ***op.,*** osm., petr., ***ph-ac.,*** **PHOS.,** plb., podo., **PSOR., PULS., ROB.,** sabin., sang., sars.,

VOMITING, general

sour - sec., sel., sep., stann., stram., **SULPH., SUL-AC., TAB.,** thuj., ***tub.,*** **VERAT.,** zinc.
afternoon - hep., sulph.
afternoon, 4 p.m. - sulph.
bitterish - ant-t., bism., cann-i., cast., chel., cic., cina, dros., grat., ip., mag-m., nux-v., plat., puls., sars., sul-ac., sulph.
breakfast, after - bor., sel.
breakfast, before - psor.
chill, during - **LYC.,** rob.
after - lyc.
coffee, after - cann-s.
coughing, while - cimx., nat-c., phos., thuj.
curds, in - calc., nat-p.
drinking, after - bufo
eating, after - ***iris,*** nat-s., nit-ac., sel., ***sul-ac.***
epilepsy, after - ***calc.***
evening - nux-v., phos., puls.
fever, during - hep., **LYC.,** rob.
fluid - card-m., ***caust., ip., nat-m.,*** nat-p., ***nux-v.,*** phos., thuj.
forenoon - nux-v.
headache, during - apis, kali-c., ***nat-p.,*** nux-v., op., sars.
menses, during - am-c., ***calc.,*** lyc., ***nux-v., phos., puls.,*** tarent.
before - ***calc.,*** nux-v., ***puls.,*** sulph.
morning - camph., graph., kali-bi., nux-v., tab.
breakfast, before - psor.
stool, after - phos.
motion, on - kali-bi.
night - ***calc.,*** chin., crot-t., kali-c.
smoking, after - calad.
stool, after - phos.
water - con.
vomiting, spasms, with - ***cupr.,*** hyos., op.
staining black - arg-n.
speaking, loud - ***coc-c.***
spitting, after - dig.
standing, up, on - colch.
starting, from sleep, after - petr.
stool, during - apis, arg-m., ***arg-n., ars.,*** bry., ***cocc.,*** colch., crot-t., ***cupr.,*** dulc., elat., ***ip., merc.,*** ox-ac., stram., ***verat.***
after - aeth., arg-n., colch., cupr., eug., ***ip., iris, nux-v.,*** phos., verat.
before - ars., dig., glon., ip., ox-ac., podo., verat.
ineffectual, after - eug., sang.
straining, after - ther.
stool, of - nux-v., plb.
stooping, after - ***cic.,*** **IP.**
stringy - alum., ***arg-n.,*** ars., bar-m., ***chel.,*** colch., **COR-R.,** croc., cupr., ***dros.,*** dulc., ***iris, kali-bi., kreos.,*** lac-ac., med., ***merc-c., nat-m., nit-ac.,*** plb., ***sil.,*** verat.
stupor, during - hep.
sudden - acon., aeth., agar., ant-t., apoc., ***ars.,*** bell., cadm-br., crot-h., crot-t., ***cupr.,*** ferr., kali-bi., kali-chl., ***op.,*** pic-ac., sec., zinc.
sugar amel. - op.

VOMITING, general
supper, after - caul., jab., rob.
surgery, after - aeth., all-c., ***bism., nux-v., phos.,*** staph., stry.
swallow, on trying to - ***merc-c.***
empty - graph.
saliva, on - colch.
sweetish - cupr., ***iris,*** kali-bi., **KREOS.,** ***plb.,*** psor., ***tub.***
mucus - calc., ***iris,*** psor.
swoon, after - ars.
talking loudly, when - cocc.
tenacious - alumn., ant-t., arg-n., ars., bor., canth., chel., colch., cupr., dulc., hep., hyos., ***kali-bi.,*** kali-c., lach., ***merc-c.,*** nit-ac., osm., phos., rhus-t., sec., verat.
thick - acet-ac., ars., colch., merc-c., ox-ac., podo., verat-v.
morning - colch.
rinsing the mouth, on - ***coc-c.***
stool, on going to - aloe.
water, after a glass of - aloe.
thirst, with - ars., canth.
tongue clean, with - cina, dig., ***ip.***
tuberculosis, in - kali-br., kreos.
tumors, brain, from - coc-c., cocc.
unconsciousness, during - ars., benz-n.
uncovering, abdomen amel. - ***tab.***
amel., in fresh open air - tab.
uremia, in - apoc., ***ars.,*** iod., kreos., nux-v., samb., scop., senec.
urine, of - op.
urticaria, during - ***apis,*** cina.
suppression, from, of - ***urt-u.***
uterine origin, from - caul., kreos., lil-t., senec.
vertigo, during - ail., ***ars.,*** calc., ***canth., chel.,*** cimic., cocc., crot-h., crot-t., ***glon.,*** gran., ***graph., hell.,*** kali-bi., kali-c., ***lach., merc.,*** mosch., ***nat-s., nux-v.,*** oena., ***petr., puls., sang.,*** sars., sel., sep., tell., ther., **VERAT.,** ***verat-v.,*** vip.
vexation, after - acon., ***cham.,*** ign., ***ip.,*** lyc., nat-s., staph., ***verat.***
violent - aeth., ant-t., apoc., **ARS.,** ars-i., bell., bism., ***cic., cina,*** **COLCH.,** con., **CROT-T.,** ***cupr.,*** dig., ***ferr.,*** ferr-p., ***iod.,*** **IP.,** ***jatr.,*** kali-n., lach., lob., merc., mez., mosch., ***nux-v.,*** **PHOS.,** ***plb.,*** raph., **TAB., VERAT.**
sitting up, on - sil.
waking, on - acon., aeth., ant-t., apis, apoc., bry., form., graph., lach., nit-ac., rat., sil., thuj.
walking, while - am-c., crot-h.
air, in open - am-m.
warm, food - lob.
water - ***acon., aeth.,*** agar., all-c., alum., anac., ant-t., apis, arg-m., ***arn.,*** **ARS.,** ars-i., asar., aur-m., bar-c., bar-i., bar-m., ***bell., bism.,*** bor., **BRY.,** calc., ***camph., cann-s.,*** carb-ac., ***carb-s.,*** card-m., carl., **CAUST.,** ***chin.,*** chin-a., cina, clem., ***cocc., coc-c.,*** colch., ***coloc., con.,*** crot-h., crot-t., ***cupr., cupr-ar.,***

VOMITING, general
water - cupr-s., cycl., dig., dulc., elat., euph., fl-ac., graph., ***grat., guai.,*** hell., hep., hyos., hydr-ac., iod., ***ip., iris, jatr.,*** kali-ar., kali-c., ***kali-bi.,*** kali-i., kali-n., ***kreos.,*** lyc., mag-c., manc., merc., merc-c., mez., mur-ac., nat-a., ***nat-m.,*** nat-s., nit-ac., ***nux-v.,*** olnd., op., osm., ox-ac., petr., phos., phys., ***phyt.,*** plb., raph., rat., rhus-t., **ROB.,** sabad., sang., ***sec.,*** sel., seneg., ***sil.,*** sin-a., sol-n., ***stann., stram.,*** stry., ***sulph., sul-ac., tab.,*** ther., ***thuj.,*** **VERAT.,** verat-v., vinc., vip., zinc.
afternoon, 4 p.m. - sulph.
as soon as water becomes warm in stomach - kali-bi.
breakfast, before - tab.
coughing, on - dros., nat-c.
dinner, before - sulph.
drunk then, food - nux-v.
eating, on - ferr., nat-a.
after - crot-t., ferr.
evening - merc-c.
fever, during - hep.
food, then - ***iod.,*** ip., nux-v., sep., sil., sulph., sul-ac.
forenoon - nat-s.
lying on the back - merc-c.
menses during - am-c., sulph.
morning - ars., bry., elaps, ***guai.,*** sil., ***sulph.,*** thuj.
waking, on - eupi., thuj.
night - **CALC.,** crot-t., ox-ac., sul-ac., ther.
9 p.m. to 5 p.m. - phyt.
sight of, from the - ***phos.***
soup, after - ***mag-c.***
standing, on - colch.
walking, in open air - kali-bi.
water, from sight of - ***phos.***
must close eyes while bathing - lyss., phos.
white - ars., bell., carb-ac., cast., colch., crot-t., cupr-ar., dig., fl-ac., kali-bi., kali-s., ***merc-c.,*** nat-s., ox-ac., stram., sul-ac., tab., verat., verat-v.
morning - ars., colch.
night - verat.
noon - ***verat.***
wine, agg. - ***ant-c.***
amel. - kalm.
sour, after - **ANT-C.**
worms - ***acon.,*** anac., ars., bar-m., ***cina,*** coff., ***ferr.,*** hyos., merc., nat-m., ***phyt., sabad.,*** **SANG.,** sec., sil., spig., verat.
drinking milk, after - vip.
lumbrici - acon., ***cina,*** sabad., sec.
sensation of - cocc., ***lach.***
yellow - acet-ac., aeth., apis, arn., ***ars.,*** ars-i., bry., cadm-s., camph., cina, ***colch., coloc., con.,*** crot-t., ***dulc.,*** form., ***grat., iod.,*** ip., kali-bi., kali-i., lil-t., merc., merc-c., olnd., osm., ox-ac., **PHOS.,** phyt., plb., sin-a., ***ter.,*** **VERAT.,** vip., zinc.
bright - kali-bi.
daytime - merc-c.
headache, with - form., glon., verat.

VOMITING, general

yellow, vomit

morning - form.

night - ox-ac.

walking in open air, while - kali-bi.

WATER, sensation as if full of - grat., **KALI-C.,** laur., mag-c., mill., ***ol-an.,*** phel.

WEAK, feeling (see Emptiness, weak) - alumn., am-c., bar-c., caust., dig., ***ign.,*** lyc., kali-c., mag-m., petr., phos., sep., verat.

eating, after - sil.

stool, after - ambr.

urination, after - ars.

vertigo, during, compelled to lie down - ambr.

WEAKNESS, of - bell., ign., phos., stry-p., sul-ac., tell.

WINE, unable to bear any - ars., nux-v., phos., ***zinc.***

WORM, crawling up throat, as if - zinc.

Stool

ACRID, corrosive, excoriating - acon., ***aloe,*** alum., am-c., ***ant-c., arn.,*** **ARS.,** ars-i., ***bapt.,*** bar-c., bry., calc., canth., carb-an., carb-s., carb-v., ***cham., chin.,*** colch., ***coloc.,*** colos., cuph., ***dulc., ferr.,*** ferr-ar., ferr-p., ***gamb., graph., hep., hydr.,*** ign., **IRIS,** kali-ar., kali-c., kali-p., kali-s., kreos., ***lach.,*** lept., **MERC.,** ***merc-c.,*** merc-sul., ***mur-ac.,*** **NAT-M.,** ***nit-ac., nux-v., phos.,*** plan., podo., **PULS.,** rheum, sabin., sars., scop., sep., ***staph., sulph.,*** syph., ter., ***tub.,*** **VERAT.**
destroys hair - coll.

ALBUMINOUS - asc-t., **BOR.,** carb-an., ***dios.,*** merc., merc-c., ***nat-m.***
coagulated - carb-an., merc-c.

BALLS, like - aesc., **ALUM., ALUMN.,** am-c., aster., brach., calc., ***calc-p.,*** cob., cop., euphr., form., hipp., hydr., **MAG-M.,** ***med.,*** **MERC.,** ***mez.,*** **NAT-M., NIT-AC.,** ***nux-v.,*** **OP.,** phos., **PLB.,** psor., ptel., ***sil.,*** **SULPH.,** thuj., verat., vib.
black - **ALUMN., OP.,** ***plat.,*** **PLB.,** ***pyrog., verat.***
brown - ***nux-v.,*** thuj.
light colored - coll.

BILIOUS - acon., aeth., ***agar., aloe,*** ant-t., apoc., ***ars.,*** ars-h., bism., ***bry.,*** cact., calc-p., carb-ac., card-m., ***cham., chin.,*** chin-a., chel., cina, ***colch.,*** coll., ***coloc., corn.,*** **CROT-H.,** crot-t., cub., dig., dios., ***dulc.,*** elaps, elat., ***fl-ac.,*** gamb., gels., ***ip., iris,*** jug-c., kali-i., lept., ***lil-t.,*** lyc., med., **MERC.,** ***merc-c., merc-d.,*** mez., naja, **NAT-S.,** nyct., op., osm., ***phos.,*** phyt., **PODO.,** psor., **PULS.,** ***sang.,*** sec., sep., ***sulph.,*** tarax., **VERAT.,** vip., yohim., yuc., zinc.
daytime and from warm drinks agg. - fl-ac.

BLACK - acet-ac., acon., aesc., aeth., agar., aloe, alum., ***alumn.,*** ant-t., apis, ***arg-n.,*** arn., **ARS.,** ***ars-i.,*** asc-t., ***berb.,*** bol., ***brom., bry.,*** cact., ***calc.,*** calc-s., camph., canth., ***caps.,*** carb-ac., carb-s., carb-v., ***card-m.,*** caust., chin., ***chin-a.,*** chin-s., ***chion.,*** cic., ***cina, cocc.,*** colch., **COLL.,** ***crot-h.,*** cub., ***cupr.,*** dios., dulc., echi., elat., elaps, ***ferr.,*** glon., graph., ham., ***hep.,*** iod., ip., iris, jac-c., kali-ar., kali-bi., ***kali-s., lach., lac-ac.,*** lat-m., **LEPT.,** manc., med., **MERC., MERC-C.,** ***merc-d.,*** merc-i-f., morph., ***nat-m., nit-ac.,*** nux-m., ***nux-v.,*** **OP.,** ph-ac., ***phos., plat.,*** **PLB.,** ***podo.,*** psor., ***pyrog.,*** rhod., rhus-v., rob., ***rumx.,*** sec., sep., squil., stann., ***stram.,*** sulph., sul-ac., tab., tell., ***thuj.,*** ust., **VERAT.,** vip., yohim., zinc.
clots, in - cadm-s.
fecal - ant-t., **BROM.,** camph., cub., ***ferr.,*** hipp., iris, ***lept.,*** sulph., tab.
foul - chion., crot-h., lept.
tarry - chion., lept., phys., ptel.

BLOODY - ***acon.,*** aesc., aeth., agar., ail., alco., ***aloe,*** **ALUM.,** ***alumn., am-m.,*** anac., anan., ant-t., ***apis, arg-n., arn.,*** **ARS.,** ars-i., asar., arund., ***bapt., bar-m., bell.,*** benz-ac., bol., both., ***bry., bufo,*** cadm-s., calad., ***calc.,*** calc-s., **CANTH., CAPS.,** ***carb-ac.,*** carb-an., carb-s., carb-v., ***caust., cham.,*** chel., ***chin.,*** chin-a., cina, cinnb., **COLCH.,** ***coll.,*** **COLOC.,** ***con.,*** cop., ***crot-c., crot-h.,*** cub., cupr., cupr-ar., dros., ***dulc.,*** elaps, elat., ferr., ferr-ar., ferr-i., ***ferr-p., graph.,*** **HAM.,** hep., hipp., ***hydr.,*** ign., iod., ***ip.,*** iris, jal., ***kali-ar., kali-bi.,*** kali-br., ***kali-c., kali-chl.,*** kali-i., kali-n., ***kali-p.,*** kali-s., ***kreos., lac-d.,*** lach., led., ***lept., lyc.,*** lyss., mag-c., ***mag-m., manc., med.,*** **MERC-C.,** ***merc-d., merc-i-f.,*** merc-i-r., mill., ***mur-ac., nat-a., nat-c.,*** nat-m., nat-p., nat-s., ***nit-ac., nux-m.,*** **NUX-V.,** ox-ac., petr., **PHOS.,** ***phyt.,*** pic-ac., plat., ***plb., podo.,*** psor., ***puls.,*** raph., rat., ***rhus-t., ruta.,*** sabad., sabin., sarr., ***sars.,*** sec., senec., ***sep., sil.,*** staph., ***sulph., sul-ac.,*** tarent., **TER.,** ***thuj.,*** trom., urt-u., valer., ***verat.,*** vip., zinc.
charred straw, like - ***lach.***
clots - cadm-s.
bright - alum.
end, at - daph.
frothy - zinc.
menses, during - am-m., ars-m.
pure blood - acon., aloe, alum., erig., ham., merc-c., rhus-t., tril.
stool of - aloe., phos.
shivering, followed by - med.
spots, in - nat-c.
streaks, in - agar., ***aloe,*** am-c., arg-n., arn., bell., bry., calc., ***canth.,*** carb-an., cina colch., ***coloc.,*** con., ***cupr-ar.,*** euph., ***ip., kali-bi.,*** kreos., led., lil-t., mag-c., mag-m., **MERC.,** ***merc-c.,*** merc-d., ***nat-s.,*** **NIT-AC., NUX-V., PODO.,** ***psor.,*** puls., ***rhus-t.,*** squil., sul-ac., ***sulph.,*** thuj., tril., ***trom.***
tarry - ham.
frothy - elaps.
water - ferr-p., merc-c., phos., ***rhus-t.***

BLUISH - bapt., colch., phos.
clay-like - indg.
green on standing, changes to - phos.

BROWN - acon., ***aesc.,*** anac., aloe, ant-t., ***apis,*** **ARG-N.,** ***arn., ars.,*** ars-i., asaf., asc-t., bapt., bell., bor., ***bry.,*** calc., ***camph.,*** canth., carb-s., carb-v., ***chel., chin., chion.,*** coloc., cop., corn-s., cupr-ac., cupr-ar., dulc., ***ferr., ferr-ar.,*** ferr-i., ferr-m., ferr-p., fl-ac., gamb., ***graph.,*** grat., hydr., iod., ip., ***iris,*** kali-ar., kali-bi., kali-c., kali-p., kreos., ***lach., lept., lil-t.,*** **LYC.,** ***mag-c.,*** **MERC.,** merc-c., merc-sul., ***mez., mur-ac.,*** nat-m., ***nat-s.,*** nit-ac., nux-v., ***op.,*** ox-ac., petr., ***phos.,*** phyt., ***plan.,*** podo., ***psor., pyrog., raph., rheum, rhod., rumx., sabad.,*** **SEC.,** senec., sep., squil., sulph., ter., thuj., trom., tub., vario., **VERAT.,** zinc., zing.
fecal - aesc., aloe, ant-t., asaf., bapt., bor., ***bry.,*** coloc., dulc., ***ferr.,*** fl-ac., graph., kali-c., lil-t., lyc., mez., ox-ac., petr., rheum, rhod., rumx., sulph., trom.
gushes - astac., kali-bi.

CHANGEABLE - aesc., am-m., berb., cham., colch., ***dulc.,*** euon., mur-ac., ***podo.,*** **PULS.,** sanic., sil., ***sulph.***

CHOPPED - ***acon.***, arg-n., ars., bar-m., ***cham.***, nat-p., rhus-t., sul-ac., viol-t.
beets - ***apis.***
eggs - ***cham.***, **MERC.**, ***merc-d.***, ***nux-m.***, **PULS.**, ***sulph.***
spinach - **ACON.**, ***arg-n.***, ***cham.***, ***merc.***

CLAY-colored - aloe, aur-m-n., bell., benz-ac., ***berb.***, **CARD-M.**, ***chel.***, chin-a., ***chion.***, cop., ***dig.***, euph., ***gels.***, ***hep.***, ***iod.***, kali-c., ***kali-bi.***, kali-p., ***lach.***, lept., ***merc.***, ***merc-d.***, myric., **NAT-S.**, ***nit-ac.***, petros., ***ph-ac.***, phos., ***podo.***, sep., tab.

CLAY-like - **CALC.**, dig., ***lac-c.***, lycps., mag-c., med., ***podo.***, ***sil.***

COFFEE, grounds, like - ant-t., cadm-s., camph., cench., ***crot-h.***, ***dig.***, ferr-m., phos.

COLD - con., cub., lyc.

COLDS, agg. - rumx., tub.

COLORS, several - aesc., colch., euon., kali-p., menis., puls., sulph., zinc-cy.

CONSTANT, discharge - ***apis***, ip., ox-ac., ***phos.***, sep., ***trom.***

CONSTIPATION, (see Rectum, Constipation)

COPIOUS - acet-ac., aeth., ***aloe***, alumn., am-m., ang., ant-c., ***ant-t.***, ***apis***, ***apoc.***, arg-n., arn., **ARS.**, ars-h., ars-i., ***asaf.***, aur., **BAPT.**, ***benz-ac.***, berb., bry., cact., cahin., ***calc.***, ***calc-p.***, **CAMPH.**, canth., **CARB-V.**, ***cench.***, chel., **CHIN.**, chin-a., cimic., cob., coc-c., ***coff.***, ***colch.***, coll., coloc., colos., con., cop., corn., **CROT-T.**, cub., cupr., cycl., dios., ***dulc.***, **ELAT.**, euph., ***ferr.***, ***ferr-ar.***, **GAMB.**, glon., gnaph., ***gran.***, ***grat.***, guar., hep., hydr., ***ign.***, ***iod.***, ***ip.***, **IRIS**, jal., ***jatr.***, kali-ar., kali-bi., kali-c., ***kali-chl.***, ***kali-p.***, ***kreos.***, ***lach.***, ***lept.***, lil-t., ***lyc.***, ***lyss.***, mag-c., med., ***merc.***, merc-c., merc-i-f., merc-i-r., ***mez.***, mosch., ***mur-ac.***, nat-a., nat-m., **NAT-S.**, ***nux-m.***, **OLND.**, ***ox-ac.***, petr., **PH-AC.**, **PHOS.**, phyt., pic-ac., plb., **PODO.**, ***psor.***, ***ran-b.***, raph., rhus-t., ***rumx.***, sars., **SEC.**, senec., ***sep.***, ***sil.***, staph., stry., ***sulph.***, ***sul-ac.***, tab., tarax., ***tarent.***, ***ter.***, ***thuj.***, **VERAT.**, ***verat-v.***, ***vib.***, zinc.
evening - aur.
exhaust, which does not - calc., graph., **PH-AC.**, puls.
night - chel., chin., **CROT-T.**, graph., ***ign.***, ox-ac., plb., sulph., verat-v.

CREAM-colored - aloe, arg-m., arg-n., calc., ***gels.***, ***ph-ac.***

CRUMBLING - agar., aloe, alum., **AM-M.**, bapt., bry., calc., cann-s., carb-an., caust., chin-s., crot-t., cycl., ***guai.***, lach., lyc., ***mag-c.***, **MAG-M.**, **MERC.**, nat-c., **NAT-M.**, nat-p., ***nit-ac.***, olnd., ***op.***, phos., ph-ac., ***plat.***, ***podo.***, ruta., ***sulph.***, ***tell.***, ***zinc.***

CURDLED - ars., bell., bufo, ***calc.***, calen., cham., iod., mag-c., med., merc., murx., nat-p., ***nit-ac.***, nux-m., puls., ***rheum***, sanic., ***stann.***, sulph., sul-ac., tab., **VALER.**, viol-t.
milk, like, forcibly expelled - aeth., ***gamb.***

DARK - ***aesc.***, agar., aloe, **ALUM.**, arg-n., ***arn.***, ***ars.***, ***bapt.***, ***berb.***, bol., ***bry.***, carb-v., chin., chin-s., ***chion.***, cimic., colch., ***corn.***, ***ferr.***, **GRAPH.**, ham., hipp., ill., iod., kali-ar., kali-c., kali-n., kali-p., ***lach.***, lil-t., lyss., maland., mur-ac., ***nat-a.***, ***nat-s.***, ***nux-v.***, op., ***plb.***, ptel., ***rhus-t.***, ***sec.***, squil., stram., tarent., tub., verat.
fecal - ***bapt.***, carb-v., chin., ***ferr.***, hipp., mur-ac., nux-v., podo., ptel., tarent.

DIAPER, running through - benz-ac., ***podo.***

DIARRHEA, (see Rectum, Diarrhea)

DOG'S, like a - ***cimx.***, **PHOS.**, staph.

DRY - aesc., **ALUM.**, ***am-c.***, ***ant-c.***, ***arg-m.***, ***arg-n.***, ars., bapt., brach., **BRY.**, cact., ***calc.***, calc-s., ***cimx.***, cob., coc-c., ***coloc.***, ***con.***, com., ***cupr.***, dios., dulc., eupi., ***guai.***, ***ham.***, ***hep.***, iris, kali-ar., ***kali-bi.***, kali-br., ***kali-c.***, kali-chl., ***kali-s.***, kreos., **LAC-D.**, lact., **LYC.**, lycps., mag-m., mang., **NAT-M.**, **NIT-AC.**, **NUX-V.**, **OP.**, osm., **PHOS.**, ***plat.***, ***plb.***, ***podo.***, ***prun.***, puls., ***sanic.***, seneg., **SIL.**, ***stann.***, staph., ***sulph.***, ter., tril., ust., verat., vib., **ZINC.**
must be mechanically removed - aloe, ***alum.***, bry., calc., indol., ***op.***, ***plb.***, ruta, sanic., ***sel.***, sep., ***sil.***, verat.
sand, like - ***arg-m.***

EARLIER, every day - hyos.

EVENING - sep., sulph., zinc.

FALLING, out - ***aloe.***

FATTY - aloe, ars., asc-t., caps., ***caust.***, dulc., ***iod.***, iris, kalm., lil-t., lycps., ***mag-c.***, nat-s., onos., ***phos.***, pic-ac., sulph., tarent., thuj.
oily-looking fecal - bol., caust., ***iod.***, iris, ***phos.***, pic-ac., thuj.

FERMENTED - ***acal.***, agar., alf., ***aloe***, apoc., ***arg-n.***, ***arn.***, benz-ac., bor., ***calc-p.***, cham., **CHIN.**, coloc., corn-s., ***crot-t.***, ***elat.***, euph., ***gamb.***, graph., ***grat.***, iod., ***ip.***, ***jatr.***, kali-bi., ***mag-c.***, mez., ***nat-s.***, op., ***ph-ac.***, phos., plan., ***podo.***, puls., rheum, rhod., rhus-t., sabad., sanic., sec., stict., sulph., ***thuj.***, trio., verat., yuc.

FILAMENTS, like hair in feces - ***sel.***

FLAKY - ***arg-n.***, calc-p., ***chel.***, colch., cupr., ***dulc.***, ferr., guar., ***ip.***, lac-c., ***nit-ac.***, ***phos.***, sec., sulph., **VERAT.**

FLAT - aesc., arg-n., arn., chel., dig., ***merc.***, **PULS.**, sep., sulph., verat.

FLOCCULI - con., dulc., kali-m., sec.

FOOD, undigested, in stool, lienteric - abrot., acet-ac., aesc., ***aeth.***, aloe, am-m., ***ant-c.***, ***apoc.***, arg-m., ***arg-n.***, ***arn.***, **ARS.**, asar., bar-c., bor., **BRY.**, cahin., **CALC.**, ***calc-p.***, calc-s., ***carb-s.***, cham., **CHIN.**, **CHIN-A.**, chion., ***cina***, ***coloc.***, ***con.***, cop., crot-t., dulc., ***elaps***, **FERR.**, **FERR-AR.**, ***ferr-p.***, ***gamb.***, **GRAPH.**, ***hep.***, ind., iod., iodof., ip., ***iris***, jab., kali-c., kali-p., kreos., lach., laur., ***lept.***, ***lyc.***, lyss., ***mag-c.***, **MAG-M.**, ***merc.***, merc-c., mez., ***nit-ac.***, ***nux-m.***, ol-j., **OLND.**, ox-ac., ***petr.***, **PH-AC.**, **PHOS.**, phys., phyt., ***plat.***, **PODO.**, ***psor.***, ***puls.***, ***raph.***, rheum,

FOOD, undigested - ***rhod., rhus-t.,*** rhus-v., ***sang., sec., sil.,*** squil., stann., staph., stram., ***sulph.,*** sul-ac., thuj., ***tub.,*** valer., verat.
brown - kreos., psor.
food of the previous day - ***olnd.***
fruit, after - **CHIN.**
hard - ***calc.***
milk, after - ***mag-c.,*** **MAG-M.**
morning - ***chin.,*** olnd.
night - ***aeth.,*** am-m., bor., bry., **CHIN.,** coloc., **FERR.,** verat.

FORCIBLE, sudden, gushing - ail., aloe, ant-c., ***apis,*** aran., ***apoc., arg-n.,*** arn., ars., astac., bar-c., bry., calc-f., calc-p., canth., cench., cic., cist., cob., ***colch., crot-h.,*** **CROT-T.,** ***cupr.,*** cycl., dirc., ***dulc.,*** **ELAT.,** ***ferr., gamb.,*** **GRAT.,** iod., ***iris,*** jal., **JATR.,** ***kali-bi.,*** lac-c., lach., lyc., lycps., ***mag-m.,*** merc., merc-sul., naja, **NAT-C., NAT-M.,** ***nat-s.,*** nicc., ***ox-ac.,*** petr., ***phos.,*** plat., **PODO.,** psor., puls., ***ran-b., raph.,*** rhus-t., sang., **SEC.,** seneg., ***sep.,*** sil., ***sulph.,*** tab., ***thuj.,*** trom., tub., **VERAT.**
all at once in somewhat prolonged effort - ***gamb.***
impacted - calc., nat-m., sanic., sel., sep., sil.
torrent, in - nat-c.

FREQUENT - acet-ac., acon., agar., ail., aloe, alum., alumn., ***am-m., anac.,*** ant-c., ***ant-t.,*** apis, arg-n., ***arn.,*** **ARS.,** ars-i., asar., asc-t., aster., aur., bapt., bar-m., ***bell., bor.,*** bov., ***bry.,*** cact., cadm-s., ***calc.,*** calc-ac., calc-p., ***canth.,*** **CAPS.,** carb-ac., carb-an., carb-s., ***carb-v., caust.,*** **CHAM.,** chel., ***chin., chin-a.,*** cic., ***cina, cocc.,*** coc-c., coff., ***colch., coloc., con.,*** corn., ***crot-t.,*** cuph., ***cupr., cupr-ar.,*** dig., dros., ***dulc.,*** **ELAT.,** ***ferr.,*** ferr-ar., ferr-p., ***gamb.,*** glyc., ***graph.,*** grat., hell., hep., hyos., ign., iod., ***ip.,*** iris, kali-ar., ***kali-bi.,*** kali-br., ***kali-c.,*** kali-i., kreos., lac-d., ***lach.,*** lob., ***lyc.,*** mag-c., **MERC., MERC-C.,** mez., nat-a., nat-c., ***nat-m.,*** nat-p., nat-s., ***nit-ac.,*** **NUX-V.,** olnd., paraf., ***petr., ph-ac.,*** **PHOS.,** ***plat.,*** **PODO.,** ***psor.,*** puls., ***ran-b.,*** rheum, rhus-t., rob., ruta, samb., sec., ***sep., sil.,*** spig., ***sulph.,*** sul-ac., ***ter., thuj.,*** trom., **VERAT.,** yohim, zinc.
bloody water - ferr-p.
normal - psor.
scanty - ars., merc., nux-v.
work, unfitness for, causing - asc-t.

FROTHY - ***acon.,*** arn., asc-t., ***benz-ac.,*** bol., ***bor., bry., calc.,*** canth., ***caps.,*** carb-s., cedr., cench., chin., chion., cimic., colch., ***coloc.,*** crot-t., elaps, elat., ferr., fl-ac., form., ***graph., grat.,*** hell., ***iod.,*** ip., ***kali-ar.,*** **KALI-BI.,** ***lach.,*** **MAG-C.,** mag-m., **MERC.,** merc-i-f., ***nat-m.,*** nat-s., ***op., plan.,*** **PODO.,** ran-b., ***raph., rheum, rhus-t.,*** ruta., sabad., sanic., ***sil., squil.,*** stict., still., **SULPH.,** sul-ac., verat., zinc.
fluent coryza, with - calc., cham., chin., coloc., iod., lach., mag-c., merc., op., rhus-t., ruta, sul-ac., sulph.
gushing - chin., crot-t., elat.

GLISTERING - aloe, alum., calc., caust., mez.
particles - cina, mez., phos.

GRANULAR - apis, arg-m., bar-c., bell., cupr., hydr., lac-c., lyc., mang., mez., ***phos.,*** plb., podo., sars., zinc.

GRAY - aloe, **ARS.,** asar., ***aur.,*** bapt., ***calc., carb-v.,*** cench., ***chel.,*** chin., cist., crot-t., cupr., ***dig.,*** dulc., ***hydr., kali-c.,*** kreos., ***lach.,*** lycps., mag-m., **MERC.,** myric., ***nat-m.,*** nat-s., **OP., PH-AC., PHOS.,** pic-ac., plb., psor., rheum, sec., sep., sulph.
lumpy - cop.

GREEN - ***acon.,*** aesc., ***aeth., agar.,*** aloe, alum., ***am-m.,*** ant-t., ***apis,*** **ARG-N.,** ***ars., asaf.,*** asc-t., arund., aur., bar-m., ***bell., bor.,*** brom., bry., ***calc.,*** calc-ac., **CALC-P.,** ***canth., caps.,*** carb-an., carb-v., **CHAM.,** chel., ***chin., chion.,*** cinnb., colch., **COLOC.,** ***con., cop., corn.,*** **CROT-T.,** ***cupr., dulc., elat., eup-per.,*** **GAMB.,** gels., glon., **GRAT.,** guar., ***hep., hydr.,*** iodof., **IP.,** ***iris, kali-ar.,*** kreos., lac-ac., ***laur., lept., lyc.,*** **MAG-C.,** ***mag-m.,*** manc., **MERC., MERC-C.,** ***merc-d.,*** merc-i-f., ***mez., mur-ac.,*** naja, **NAT-M.,** ***nat-p.,*** **NAT-S.,** ***nit-ac., nux-v.,*** paull., petr., ***ph-ac.,*** **PHOS., PLB., PODO.,** ***psor.,*** **PULS.,** rheum, ***rhus-t.,*** rob., sal-ac., ***sanic.,*** **SEC.,** ***sep., stann.,*** **SULPH.,** ***sul-ac.,*** tab., ***ter.,*** valer., **VERAT.,** vip., zinc.
blackish - ars., op., merc., phos., sul-ac., verat.
blue, turning to - calc-p., phos.
brownish - ars., calc., crot-t., dulc., mag-c., mag-m., merc., sulph., verat.
fecal - ars., mag-m., podo., valer.
grass - acon., **ANT-T., ARG-N.,** calc-p., cham., ***ip., mag-c.,*** merc., merc-d., thuj.
hard - ***agar., chin.,*** cupr., kreos., ***stann.***
olive green - ***apis,*** ars., ***elat.,*** **SEC.**
scum on a frog-pond, like - asc-t., bry., grat., hell., ***mag-c.,*** merc., ***phos., sanic.***
spinach in flatus, like - **ARG-N.**
stains skin around anus and scrotum coppery, mucous - cinnb.
tea - gels.
turns - arg-n., bor., calc-f., nat-s., psor., rheum, sanic.
water - cupr., kali-br.
yellow, turning to - ip.

GURGLES, pops out - aloe, crot-t., gamb., grat., jatr., podo., thuj.

HARD - abies-n., ***aesc.,*** aeth., ***agar., agn.,*** aloe, **ALUM., ALUMN., AM-C., AM-M.,** anan., ang., **ANT-C.,** ***apis,*** arg-m., ***arg-n.,*** arn., ***ars.,*** ars-i., arund., asaf., asar., ***aur., aur-m-n., bar-c., bar-m., bell.,*** berb., bor., ***bov.,*** brom., **BRY.,** bufo, cact., **CALC.,** ***calc-p., calc-s.,*** camph., ***carb-an.,*** **CARB-S.,** ***carb-v.,*** **CARD-M.,** ***caust.,*** cham., ***chel.,*** chin., chin-a., chin-s., ***cimx., cina, clem., cocc.,*** coc-c., colch., **COLL.,** ***coloc., con.,*** cop., corn., crot-h., cub., ***cycl.,*** dios., dulc., eug., euphr., euph., eupi., ***ferr.,*** ferr-ar., ***ferr-i.,*** ferr-p., fl-ac., form., ***gamb.,*** glon., glyc., **GRAPH.,** ***grat., guai., ham.,*** hell., ***hep.,*** hipp., ***hydr.,*** hyos., ***ign.,*** ill., indol., ***iod., kali-ar., kali-bi.,*** **KALI-BR.,** ***kali-c., kali-i., kali-n.,*** kali-p., ***kali-s., kalm.,*** kreos., **LAC-D., LACH.,** ***lac-ac.,***

HARD - lact., ***laur.***, lil-t., **LYC.**, lycps., mag-arct., ***mag-c.***, **MAG-M.**, mag-s., med., meny., ***merc.***, merc-c., merc-i-f., merc-sul., **MEZ.**, mur-ac., nat-a., naja, nat-c., **NAT-M.**, nat-p., ***nat-s.***, nicc., **NIT-AC.**, **NUX-V.**, ***oena.***, olnd., **OP.**, ox-ac., ped., ***petr.***, ***ph-ac.***, **PHOS.**, phyt., pic-ac., ***plat.***, **PLB.**, ***podo.***, prun., ***puls.***, pyrog., ran-b., ***rat.***, rhus-t., rhus-v., rumx., ***ruta.***, ***sabin.***, sal-ac., sang., ***sanic.***, sarr., sars., **SEL.**, senec., ***seneg.***, **SEP.**, **SIL.**, sol-n., spig., spong., squil., ***stann.***, staph., ***stront-c.***, **SULPH.**, sul-ac., sumb., tab., ***tarent.***, ter., thuj., trom., ***tub.***, tril., **VERAT.**, **VERB.**, vib., **ZINC.**
- alternating hard and soft - ars., bor., iod., lach., mag-s., nit-ac., phos.
- burnt, as if - **BRY.**, ***plat.***, plb., **SULPH.**, sul-ac.
- covered with mucus - alum., am-m., casc., ***caust.***, ***coll.***, cop., ***graph.***, ***hydr.***, nux-v., sep.
- first hard, then fluid - agar., aloe, bar-c., bor., **BOV.**, **CALC.**, calc-f., calc-p., carb-s., lact., **LYC.**, mag-c., nat-c., ***nat-m.***, nat-s., rheum, spig., staph., sulph., ***sul-ac.***, tarent.
  - then paste - pall., ***ph-ac.***, stann.
  - then soft - aeth., alumn., am-m., berb., carb-an., carb-v., caust., graph., kali-c., mag-c., mag-m., mez., mur-ac., nat-c., ph-ac., sars., sep., spong., staph., sul-ac., zinc.
  - then thin - stann.
- menses, during - ***am-c.***, **APIS**, kali-c., kreos., ***nat-m.***, nat-s., sil., sulph., sul-ac.
- tough and greasy - ***caust.***
- yellow moisture, with - hep.

HEADWASHING, agg. - tarent.

HEAVY - sanic.

HOLDS back - nit-ac., sil., sulph., thuj.

HOT - ***aloe***, ***ars.***, asc-t., bell., bry., ***calc-p.***, caps., ***cham.***, cist., dios., ferr., gamb., **IRIS**, kali-p., lec., med., ***merc.***, **MERC-C.**, merc-sul., nux-v., phos., pic-ac., podo., puls., rat., sabad., scop., ***staph.***, stroph., ***sulph.***

INTESTINES, like - ant-c.

INVOLUNTARY, stool (see Rectum)

KNOTTY - ***aesc.***, aesc-g., agar., **ALUM.**, **ALUMN.**, am-c., am-m., anag., anan., ang., ***ant-c.***, apis, arn., ars., ars-i., aster., ***aur.***, bapt., ***bar-c.***, berb., brach., ***calc.***, calc-p., ***calc-s.***, carb-an., **CARB-S.**, card-m., ***caust.***, **CHEL.**, chin., chin-a., chlol., coc-c., ***coll.***, ***con.***, ***cycl.***, dios., euph., euphr., ***glon.***, glyc., **GRAPH.**, grat., ***hydr.***, indol., ***iod.***, ip., kali-ar., ***kali-bi.***, ***kali-c.***, kali-p., ***kali-s.***, kalm., ***lach.***, ***lept.***, ***lil-t.***, **LYC.**, **MAG-M.**, mang., ***merc.***, merc-c., mez., morph., nat-m., ***nat-s.***, nit-ac., ***nux-v.***, op., petr., ***ph-ac.***, phos., ***plat.***, **PLB.**, prun., ptel., pyrog., rhus-v., sang., sanic., senec., ***sep.***, **SIL.**, spig., ***stann.***, stront-c., **SULPH.**, sul-ac., sumb., ***thuj.***, ust., verat., verb., xero, ***zinc.***
- first, then soft - ***lyc.***
- green - ***chin.***, ***stann.***

KNOTTY,
- mucus, covered with - ***alum.***, caust., ***graph.***, ***mag-m.***, nux-v., ***plb.***, sep., ***spig.***
- united by threads of mucus - cham., **GRAPH.**

LARGE - ***aesc.***, alet., aloe, ***alum.***, **ALUMN.**, ***agn.***, ***ant-c.***, ***apis***, ***arg-n.***, ars., ars-i., ***asaf.***, ***aur.***, berb., **BRY.**, **CALC.**, calc-s., caust., chel., ***cob.***, cop., ***coloc.***, crot-t., cupr., ***dulc.***, **ELAT.**, euphr., fl-ac., gamb., glyc., **GRAPH.**, grat., hydr., ***ign.***, kali-ar., ***kali-bi.***, **KALI-C.**, kali-p., **KALI-S.**, ***kalm.***, **LAC-D.**, lach., **LEPT.**, mag-arct., **MAG-M.**, meli., merc., **MEZ.**, naja, ***nat-m.***, ***nux-m.***, **NUX-V.**, ***oena.***, op., ox-ac., ***petr.***, ***phos.***, ***podo.***, puls., pyrog., ***raph.***, ***rhus-t.***, ***rhus-v.***, ruta., ***sanic.***, sarr., **SEL.**, seneg., **SEP.**, **SIL.**, stann., **SULPH.**, sul-ac., sumb., tub., ***thuj.***, **VERAT.**, ***vib.***, ***zinc.***

LATER every day - carb-v., hyos., kali-c., ruta., sul-ac.,

LIENTERIC, (see food, undigested)

LIGHT-colored - acon., ***aesc.***, alum., alumn., ambr., anac., apis, **ARS.**, ars-i., ***aur-m-n.***, ***bar-c.***, ***berb.***, **BOR.**, **CALC.**, carb-an., carb-s., ***carb-v.***, **CARD-M.**, caust., cham., **CHEL.**, **CHIN.**, ***chin-a.***, ***chion.***, ***coll.***, **DIG.**, dol., eup-per., ***gels.***, gnaph., ***hep.***, ***hydr.***, iber., indol., ***iod.***, iris, kali-ar., ***kali-bi.***, ***kali-c.***, ***kali-p.***, kali-m., ***kali-s.***, **LYC.**, lycps., **MERC.**, merc-c., ***merc-d.***, ***myric.***, naja, nat-p., ***nat-s.***, ***nit-ac.***, petr., **PH-AC.**, ***phos.***, pic-ac., plb., ***podo.***, rhus-v., **SANIC.**, sep., **SIL.**, stel., sulph., **TAB.**, ***tub.***, ust., zinc.

LIME, like connected - plat.

LONG, narrow - ***alum.***, alum-p., ***bor.***, calc-sil., ***caust.***, ***graph.***, hyos., merc., ***mur-ac.***, nat-c., **PHOS.**, puls., sep., staph., sul-ac., sulph.

LUMPS, chalk, like - bell., **CALC.**, dig., hep., lach., **PODO.**, **SANIC.**, spong.

LUMPY, and liquid - aloe, **ANT-C.**, apis, ***ars.***, calc., ***con.***, graph., ip., kali-bi., **LYC.**, nat-a., nux-v., ***pic-ac.***, sec., sil., sulph., sul-ac., trom.
- and soft - euph.

MEAL-like, sediment, with - bry., chin-a., ph-ac., **PODO.**

MEMBRANOUS - aloe, ***arg-n.***, ars., asar., bol., ***brom.***, **CANTH.**, ***carb-ac.***, **COLCH.**, **COLOC.**, ***ferr.***, ferr-m., iod., kali-bi., kali-n., ***lach.***, ***lept.***, merc., merc-c., mur-ac., ***nit-ac.***, petr., phos., phyt., podo., puls., sil., sul-ac.

MISSHAPEN, angular, square, etc. - nat-m., plb., sanic., sel., sep.

MOLASSES, like - ip.

MUCUS - acon., aesc., ***aeth.***, agar., aloe, alum., am-c., ***am-m.***, ang., ant-c., ant-t., ***apis***, **ARG-N.**, ***arn.***, ***ars.***, ars-i., ***asar.***, asc-t., ***bapt.***, ***bell.***, ***berb.***, ***bor.***, ***brom.***, ***bry.***, cact., calc., calc-ac., ***calc-p.***, ***canth.***, **CAPS.**, ***carb-ac.***, carb-an., carb-s., ***carb-v.***, ***caust.***, ***cham.***, ***chel.***, cic., cimic., cina, ***cocc.***, **COLCH.**, **COLL.**, ***coloc.***, ***corn.***, ***crot-c.***, ***crot-t.***, dig., dios., dirc., dros., ***dulc.***, elat., ferr., ferr-ar., ferr-i., ferr-p., gall-ac., **GAMB.**, **GRAPH.**,

MUCUS - guai., ham., **HELL.**, ***hep.***, ***hyos.***, ign., ***iod.***, ***ip.***, ***kali-bi.***, ***kali-c.***, ***kali-chl.***, kali-i., kali-m., kali-n., **KALI-S.**, lach., laur., led., lyc., ***mag-c.***, mag-m., **MERC.**, **MERC-C.**, ***mur-ac.***, naja, nat-a., nat-c., nat-m., ***nat-s.***, nicc., ***nit-ac.***, nux-m., **NUX-V.**, ox-ac., petr., ***ph-ac.***, **PHOS.**, ***phyt.***, ***plb.***, ***podo.***, ***psor.***, **PULS.**, raph., ***rheum***, ***rhus-t.***, ric., ***ruta.***, sabad., ***sec.***, sel., sep., ***sil.***, solid., spig., ***squil.***, ***stann.***, staph., stict., **SULPH.**, ***sul-ac.***, tab., ter., trom., tub., urt-u., vario., **VERAT.**

acrid - phos.
alternates with constipation - acon.
balls of - ip.
black - ars., cocc., elat.
bloody - ***acon.***, ***aeth.***, ail., ***aloe***, alum., ***anan.***, apis, arg-n., arn., ***ars.***, ars-i., asar., bapt., bar-c., ***bar-m.***, bell., bol., ***bry.***, calc., ***canth.***, ***caps.***, ***carb-ac.***, ***carb-v.***, cham., chim., ***cinnb.***, **COLCH.**, coll., ***coloc.***, cub., dros., ***dulc.***, elaps, elat., erig., ferr-p., ***gamb.***, ham., hep., ign., ***iod.***, ***ip.***, iris, ***kali-chl.***, kali-i., ***lach.***, led., lept., lil-t., lyss., ***mag-m.***, **MERC.**, **MERC-C.**, **NAT-C.**, nit-ac., **NUX-V.**, ox-ac., petr., phyt., plb., **PODO.**, ***psor.***, ***puls.***, rhus-t., sabad., sabin., sars., sil., ***sulph.***, sul-ac., trom.
stool, after - sep.
boiled starch - arg-n., bor.
brown - **ARS.**, bapt., bor., ***carb-v.***, ***dulc.***, grat., ***nux-v.***, rheum, zing.
cheesy - phos.
chopped, eggs and spinach - cham.
colorless - **HELL.**
copious - ter.
involuntary - solid.
covered, with mucus - ***alum.***, ***am-m.***, bar-m., ***carb-v.***, caust., cham., graph., ***ham.***, hydr., ip., kali-n., ***mag-m.***, nat-m., nit-ac., nux-v., ***plb.***, phos., puls., sep., ***spig.***, tell.
cream-colored - aloe.
dark - arg-n., ***ars.***, bol., ip., lil-t., mur-ac., tarent.
dark, like frothy molasses - ip.
fetid - con., lach., merc-c., pyrog., sulph., sul-ac.
granular - bell., ***phos.***
grayish - rheum.
green - **ACON.**, aesc., ***aeth.***, agar., am-m., ***ant-t.***, apis, **ARG-N.**, **ARS.**, aur., ***bell.***, ***bor.***, ***bry.***, ***calc-p.***, ***canth.***, caps., carb-v., ***cast.***, **CHAM.**, ***chel.***, cina, ***cinnb.***, colch., ***coloc.***, corn., ***dulc.***, elat., eup-per., ferr-p., **GAMB.**, guar., hep., ***ip.***, iris, kreos., **LAUR.**, lyc., **MAG-C.**, med., **MERC.**, **MERC-C.**, mur-ac., naja, nit-ac., ***nux-v.***, petr., ph-ac., ***phos.***, podo., psor., **PULS.**, ***rheum***, rhus-t., sanic., sep., stann., ***sulph.***, sul-ac., tab., urt-u.
jelly-like - ***aloe***, ***apis***, **ASAR.**, asc-t., ***arn.***, ***bar-m.***, ***cadm-s.***, calc., caust., ***chel.***, **COLCH.**, ***coloc.***, dios., dulc., euph., ***hell.***, ***jatr.***, ***kali-bi.***, mag-c., mur-ac., nat-p., oxyt., ***phos.***, ***plat.***, podo., ***rhus-t.***, sep.

MUCUS,

jelly-like, frog-spawn, like - hell.
liquid - alum., bor., laur., ter.
lumpy mucus - aloe, carb-an., cop., graph., ip., mag-c., merc-c., phos., spig.
pea like lumps - nat-c.
offensive - sep.
only - ant-c., asaf.
red - arg-n., bor., canth., ***cina***, colch., graph., **LYC.**, merc., ***rhus-t.***, sil., sulph.
shaggy, masses - arg-n., ***asar.***, caps., lyc.
shreddy - colch.
stools, after - bry., sep., thuj.
tenacious - **ASAR.**, bor., **CANTH.**, ***caps.***, ***crot-t.***, **HELL.**, ***kali-bi.***, spig.
thick - mag-m., nat-c., spig.
transparent - aloe, am-m., asc-t., **BOR.**, carb-an., **COLCH.**, cub., dios., **HELL.**, merc., merc-c., ***nat-m.***, ***rhus-t.***
watery - arg-n., coloc., ***iod.***, lept., ter.
white - ***ars.***, asc-t., bell., **BOR.**, canth., carb-an., caust., ***cham.***, cina, cocc., colch., dios., ***dulc.***, elat., ***graph.***, ***hell.***, ***iod.***, ip., kali-c., **KALI-CHL.**, kali-m., mag-m., merc., merc-c., **NAT-M.**, ***ph-ac.***, ***phos.***, podo., puls., rheum, sulph.
like little pieces of popped corn - **CINA.**
masses - cop.
milk white - **KALI-CHL.**
worm, like a - stann.
yellow - agar., ***apis***, **ASAR.**, bell., ***bor.***, brom., ***carb-v.***, ***cham.***, chin., ***colch.***, ***cub.***, ***dulc.***, ign., **KALI-S.**, mag-c., mag-m., nicc., osm., podo., puls., ***rhus-t.***, spig., staph., sulph., ***sul-ac.***

MUSHY - aesc., agar., anac., ant-t., anth., ***bapt.***, ***berb.***, **BRY.**, cact., calc-p., carb-v., chin., erig., ***hyos.***, ***hydr.***, iris, ***kalm.***, lac-c., lept., myric., nit-ac., onos., phos., ***pic-ac.***, podo., puls., **RHUS-T.**, sars., seneg., ***sep.***, ***sil.***, ***spig.***, ***sulph.***, ter.

brown - aesc.
white - ***calc-p.***, podo., ***rhus-t.***, sep., spig.
yellow - ant-t., ***arum-t.***, ***bapt.***, ***berb.***, **BRY.**, carb-v., ***hydr.***, ***hyos.***, iris, lept., ***pic-ac.***, ***podo.***, rhus-t.

MUSTY - coloc.

NOISY - aloe, plat.

ODOR, of stool

brassy - apis.
brown, paper, burning, like - ***coloc.***
burnt, meat - carb-an.
cadaveric - ail., ant-c., ant-t., apis, arg-n., ***arn.***, **ARS.**, ***asaf.***, asc-t., ***bapt.***, ***benz-ac.***, ***bism.***, bor., ***bry.***, calc., calc-p., carb-ac., **CARB-V.**, ***cham.***, ***chin.***, coloc., corn-s., ***graph.***, ***hep.***, **KALI-P.**, kreos., **LACH.**, ***lept.***, ***merc-c.***, ***merc-d.***, mur-ac., nit-ac., nux-m., op., petr., ph-ac., ***phos.***, ***podo.***, ***psor.***, ***ptel.***, pulx., pyrog., rheum, ***rhus-t.***, rumx., sanic., ***sec.***, ***sil.***, stram., sul-ac., ***sulph.***, ***ter.***, tub.
camphor, like - petr.

ODOR, of stool
cheese, rotten, like - **BRY., HEP.,** ***sanic.***
old, like - tub.
coppery - ***iris.***
eggs, like rotten - arg-n., arn., ***ars.,*** asc-t., ***calc., carb-ac.,*** carl., **CHAM.,** hep., med., phos., podo., **PSOR.,** ***staph.,*** sulph., sul-ac.
musty - ***coloc.,*** sarr.
offensive - acet-ac., acon., ***agar.,*** ail., ***aloe,*** alumn., ant-c., ant-t., ***apis,*** apoc., arg-m., **ARG-N.,** arn., **ARS.,** ***ars-i.,*** **ASAF.,** asc-t., ***aur.,*** **BAPT.,** ***bar-m.,*** **BENZ-AC.,** ***bism.,*** **BRY.,** ***calc., calc-p., carb-ac.,*** **CARB-S., CARB-V.,** casc., cham., chin., chin-a., chlol., cic., cimic., coca, cocc., coff., ***colch.,*** coloc., con., cop., ***corn.,*** **CROT-H.,** crot-t., cupr., cupr-ar., dig., dios., dros., dulc., eug., fago., fl-ac., **GAMB.,** gnaph., **GRAPH.,** grat., ***guai.,*** hep., ***hura,*** hyos., ind., iod., ***ip.,*** iris, **KALI-AR.,** kali-c., **KALI-P.,** kali-s., kreos., **LACH.,** ***lept.,*** lil-t., lith., lob., lob-s., lyc., lycps., manc., merc., **MERC-C.,** merc-cy., merc-i-f., mez., mur-ac., nat-m., ***nat-p.,*** **NAT-S.,** ***nit-ac.,*** **NUX-M.,** ***nux-v.,*** **OP.,** par., petr., ***ph-ac., phos.,*** phys., plb., **PODO., PSOR.,** ptel., pulx., ***puls., pyrog.,*** ran-s., rheum, rhod., rhus-t., rumx., sant., sarr., sec., sep., serp., **SIL.,** sin-n., sol-t-ae., **SQUIL.,** stann., staph., **SULPH.,** ***sul-ac.,*** sumb., tab., ***tarent., ter.,*** teucr., thuj., til., tril., **TUB.,** vario., verat., vip., zinc.
night only - ***psor., sulph.***
sticking to patient - podo., psor., sulph., zinc-s.
putrid - acet-ac., agar., ***apis,*** **ARS., ASAF., BAPT., BENZ-AC.,** ***bor., bry.,*** calc., calc-f., ***carb-ac.,*** **CARB-V.,** cham., ***chin.,*** cic., cocc., ***coloc.,*** elat., graph., ip., **KALI-P.,** ***lach., mag-c., merc-c.,*** mur-ac., ***nat-s.,*** nit-ac., nux-m., nux-v., **OLND.,** par., **PODO., PSOR.,** ptel., puls., ***pyrog.,*** pulx., rhus-t., sanic., sep., **SIL.,** ***stram.,*** sul-ac., sulph., **TUB.**
sour - aeth., arg-n., ***arn.,*** bell., **CALC.,** camph., carb-s., cham., colch., ***coloc., colos.,*** con., cop., ***dulc., graph.,*** **HEP.,** iris, ***jal.,*** lyc., ***mag-c.,*** **MERC.,** mez., ***nat-c., nat-p., nit-ac.,*** olnd., ***phos.,*** podo., **RHEUM,** rob., sep., sil., **SULPH.,** verat.
milk, like - tab.
sweetish - mosch.
urine, like - benz-ac.

ODORLESS - aeth., apis, ***asar., cur.,*** cycl., ferr., ferr-s., gamb., guar., ***hell., hyos.,*** jatr., ***kali-bi.,*** merc., phos., ph-ac., ***rhus-t.,*** **VERAT.,** xan.

ORANGE, tomato sauce like - apis, nat-c.

PASTY, papescent - acon., aesc., ***agar., aloe,*** alumn., ammc., anag., anthr., ant-c., ant-t., ***apis,*** apoc., arg-m., arg-n., ***arn.,*** ars., ars-i., ***asaf., bapt.,*** bar-c., bell., ***berb.,*** bism., bor., brom., **BRY.,** cact., calad., ***calc.,*** calc-p., cann-s., canth., carb-s., ***card-m.,*** cedr., **CHEL.,** chin., chin-s., cimic., cist., clem., coc-c., colch., coll., **COLOC.,** con., cop., cor-r., crot-h., **CROT-T.,** cycl., dig., dios., dirc., dros., eug., ***euph.,*** fago., fl-ac., form., gamb., gels., gent-c., ***graph.,*** grat., hell., ***hep.,*** hydr., hyos., ign., ind., iod., ip., iris, kali-bi., ***kali-n.,*** kalm., kreos., ***lach.,*** lact., laur., led., ***lept.,*** lob., lyc., lycps., ***mag-m.,*** mang., **MERC., MERC-C.,** ***mez.,*** myric., nat-a., nat-c., ***nat-m.,*** nat-p., nit-ac., nux-m., nux-v., ***op.,*** osm., ox-ac., paeon., par., petr., ***ph-ac.,*** phos., phyt., ***plat.,*** **PODO.,** ***psor., ptel.,*** **RHEUM,** rhod., rhus-t., rhus-v., sabad., sec., sel., seneg., sep., sil., squil., stann., stram., **SULPH.,** ***sul-ac.,*** sumb., tab., tarax., ter., ther., thuj., til., trom., ust., valer., verat., verat-v., zinc.

PITCH, like - sars.

PURULENT - ***apis,*** **ARN.,** ***ars.,*** calc., ***calc-p., calc-s.,*** canth., carb-v., chin., cocc., dulc., ***hep., iod.,*** ip., kali-ar., kali-c., ***kali-p.,*** kali-s., ***lach., lyc.,*** **MERC.,** ***phos.,*** **PULS.,** pyrog., ***sec.,*** sep., ***sil., sulph.,*** trom.

REDDISH - aloe, ***canth.,*** chel., cina, colch., lyc., **MERC.,** nat-s., phos., **RHUS-T.,** ***sil.,*** sulph.

RICE, grains, like - cub.

RICE water, like - ant-t., apis, ***ars.,*** **CAMPH.,** carb-ac., cham., chel., colch., **CUPR.,** ***ferr.,*** iris, kali-br., kali-i., ***kali-p.,*** merc-sul., ***nat-m.,*** **PH-AC.,** ***phos.,*** ran-b., ***sec.,*** **VERAT.**

SAGO like - colch., phos.

SAND or gravel in - cina, hydr., lyc., rhus-t., urt-u.

SCANTY - acon., aeth., agar., aloe, ***alum.,*** alumn., ambr., ammc., **AM-M.,** apis, ***apoc.,*** arg-m., arg-n., arn., ***ars.,*** ars-i., ***asar.,*** asc-t., bar-c., ***bell.,*** benz-ac., berb., bor., ***bry.,*** cahin., ***calad.,*** calc., calc-p., calc-s., camph., cann-s., canth., carb-ac., ***carb-an., carb-s., carb-v., card-m.,*** carl., chel., chin., chin-s., cimic., coc-c., ***colch., coloc.,*** con., cop., corn., crot-t., cupr., dig., dirc., dros., ***dulc.,*** eug., euph., euphr., ferr., ferr-i., fl-ac., ***gamb.,*** gels., ***glon.,*** grat., hell., hep., hura, hydr., hyos., hyper., ***ign.,*** indg., iod., ***ip.,*** jug-r., kali-ar., ***kali-bi., kali-c.,*** kali-n., kali-s., kalm., lach., lact., led., lyc., lycps., mag-c., ***mag-m.,*** mag-s., mang., **MERC.,** ***merc-c.,*** merc-i-f., merc-sul., mez., ***nat-a., nat-c., nat-m.,*** nat-s., ***nit-ac.,*** **NUX-V.,** olnd., ***op.,*** ox-ac., par., petr., phos., pic-ac., ***plat.,*** **PLB.,** puls., ran-b., rat., rhod., rhus-t., rumx., ruta., sang., sars., seneg., sep., **SIL.,** spong., squil., ***stann.,*** staph., stront-c., **SULPH.,** sumb., tab., tarent., ter., ther., thuj., til., trom., verat., verb., ***zinc.***

SCRAPINGS, of intestines, like - asc-t., brom., ***bry.,*** **CANTH.,** ***carb-ac.,*** **COLCH., COLOC.,** ***ferr., merc.,*** nux-v., petr., phos., phyt.
meat, of, like - am-m.

SHEEP, dung, like - **ALUM., ALUMN.,** am-m., anth., bapt., ***bar-c., berb.,*** bor., brom., ***carb-an.,*** carb-s., ***caust.,*** **CHEL.,** chin-s., cob., ***coll.,*** cop., ***graph.,*** hydr., ***kali-c.,*** kali-n., ***kali-s., lach.,*** lyc., mag-c., **MAG-M., MERC.,** nat-c., **NAT-M.,** ***nat-s.,*** **NIT-AC.,** ***nux-v.,*** **OP.,** plat., **PLB.,** pyrog., ruta., sanic., ***sep., sil., spig.,*** stann., stront-c., **SULPH.,** ***sul-ac.,*** syph., tab., thuj., ***verat., verb.***
chalky - bell., calc.
green - chin., stann.
tallow, like - mag-c.

SHOOTING, out - acon., ***aloe, apis,*** arn., ars., aster., bell., calc-p., canth., cist., cob., **CROT-T.,** cycl., eug., **GAMB., GRAT.,** iod., iris, jab., **JATR.,** kali-bi., lach., lept., lyc., mag-m., merc., naja, ***nat-c.,*** nat-p., ***nat-s.,*** phys., phos., **PODO.,** psor., puls., rhod., sars., ***sec.,*** seneg., sil., sulph., thuj., verat.
all at once in a somewhat prolonged effort - **GAMB.**
torrent, in a - ***nat-c.***

SLATE-colored - ***bapt.,*** ferr-p., phos., rad-br.

SMALL - acon., aloe, **ALUM.,** am-c., ***ant-c., arg-m.,*** arg-n., ***arn.,*** **ARS.,** asaf., asar., ***bapt.,*** **BELL.,** calc-p., canth., **CAPS.,** carb-s., carb-v., ***cham.,*** cocc., ***colch., coloc., con.,*** com., ***crot-t., dig.,*** dulc., erig., eug., ferr-p., fl-ac., form., hyos., ign., ind., kali-ar., kali-c., kali-s., ***lyc.,*** **MAG-M., MERC., MERC-C.,** merc-i-f., mez., naja, nat-c., nat-m., nit-ac., **NUX-V.,** olnd., op., osm., phos., podo., puls., rhus-t., ***sars.,*** sec., sil., stann., sulph., tab., trom., urt-u., vib., zinc.

SOFT - acon., aesc., aeth., agar., ***agn.,*** ail., all-c., all-s., ***aloe,*** **ALUM.,** ambr., am-c., **AM-M.,** ammc., ***anac.,*** ang., ant-t., ***apis,*** apoc., ***arg-m.,*** arg-n., arn., ***ars.,*** ars-i., arum-t., asar., asc-c., asc-t., aster., aur., ***bapt., bar-c.,*** bar-m., bell., benz., berb., bism., bor., bov., brom., bry., bufo, cact., cahin., ***calad., calc., calc-p.,*** calc-s., canth., caps., carb-an., ***carb-v.,*** carl., ***cast-v.,*** caul., caust., chel., ***chin., chin-a.,*** chlol., cic., cimx., cinnb., cob., coca, ***cocc.,*** coc-c., coff., colch., ***coloc.,*** con., cop., crot-t., cupr., cycl., ***dig.,*** dios., dros., dulc., erig., ***euph.,*** fago., ferr-i., ferr-ma., ferr-p., fl-ac., form., gamb., gels., genist., gins., glon., gran., ***graph.,*** grat., ***guai.,*** ham., hell., **HEP.,** hipp., hydr., hyos., hyper., ictod., ***ign.,*** indg., iod., ip., iris, jatr., jug-c., kali-bi., kali-br., kali-c., kali-chl., kali-i., ***kali-n.,*** kali-s., kalm., kreos., ***lac-d.,*** lac-ac., ***lach.,*** lact., laur., lept., lith., lob., lyc., lyss., mag-c., mag-m., mag-s., mang., **MERC.,** ***merc-c.,*** merc-i-f., merc-sul., merl., ***mez.,*** mill., morph., mosch., mur-ac., nat-a., nat-c., nat-m., ***nat-s.,*** nicc., **NIT-AC.,** nuph., ***nux-m.,*** nux-v., ***olnd.,*** op., osm., paeon., pall., par., petr., phel., ***ph-ac.,*** **PHOS.,** phys., phyt., pic-ac., ***plat., psor.,*** ptel., ***puls., ran-s.,*** raph., ***rat., rheum, rhod.,*** rhus-v., ruta., sabin., sang., sars., sel., ***sep.,*** sil., spong., stann., staph., stront-c., **SULPH., SUL-AC.,** sumb., tab., tarent., ***thuj.,*** til., trom., upa., ust., verb., verat., verat-v., ***viol-t.,*** wye., zinc., zing.
dinner, after - zinc.
hard, then - anac., ant-c., nux-v., sabin.

SOFT, stool
night - zinc.

SPRAYING - thuj.

SPUTTERING - ***aloe,*** arg-n., coloc., eug., ferr., gamb., **NAT-S.,** stroph., thuj., thyr., tub.

STARCH, like - arg-n., bor.

STRINGY - ***asar., carb-v.,*** colch., **GRAT.,** lept., ox-ac., sel., **SUL-AC.,** verat-v.

SUDS, like - benz-ac., colch., elat., glon., iod., sulph.

SUPPRESSED - bell.

TALLOW, like - ars.

TARRY-looking - canth., ***chion., lept.,*** nit-ac., phys., plat.

TENESMUS, (see Tenesmus, general)

TENACIOUS - ars., ***asar.,*** bor., bry., ***caps.,*** carb-v., chel., coloc., crot-t., **HELL.,** ign., inul., kali-bi., kali-c., ***lac-c.,*** lach., mag-s., mang., med., ***merc., merc-c.,*** mez., nat-c., nat-m., op., ox-ac., **PLAT.,** plb., podo., rheum, rhus-t., sars., spig., sulph., verat., ***zinc.***

TENDINOUS, parts - ars.

THIN - acet-ac., acon., ***aeth.,*** agar., ***aloe,*** alst., **ALUM.,** ammc., anan., ang., **ANT-C.,** ant-t., **APOC.,** ***aran., arn., ars.,*** **ASAF.,** asc-t., aster., aur., bapt., bar-m., ***bell.,*** **BENZ-AC.,** bism., bor., ***bov., bry.,*** **CALC.,** cahin., calad., calc-ac., ***calc-p.,*** camph., ***carb-ac.,*** carb-an., carb-o., **CARB-S.,** ***carb-v.,*** cast-eq., ***caust., cedr.,*** clem., ***cham., chel., chin., chin-a., cic.,*** cist., ***cocc., coff.,*** **COLCH.,** ***coloc., con.,*** cop., corn., **CROT-T.,** cuph., ***cupr-ar.,*** cycl., dig., dios., dros., dulc., ***elat.,*** euph., ferr., ferr-p., **GAMB., GRAPH.,** ***grat., hep., hydr.,*** hyos., ign., ind., iod., iodof., ip., ***iris,*** jal., **JATR.,** ***kali-bi.,*** kali-c., kali-n., ***lac-ac., lach.,*** laur., lept., **LYC.,** mag-aust., ***mag-c.,*** mag-m., med., meph., ***merc.,*** merc-i-f., ***mur-ac.,*** nat-a., nat-c., ***nat-p.,*** **NAT-S.,** nicc., nit-ac., ***nuph., nux-m., nux-v.,*** **OLND.,** ***op.,*** osm., petr., **PH-AC., PHOS.,** phyt., **PIC-AC.,** plat., **PODO.,** ***psor.,*** ptel., puls., rat., ***rheum,*** rhod., ***rhus-t.,*** rhus-v., rumx., sabad., sang., sec., sel., senec., ***sep., sil., spig., spong., squil.,*** stann., staph., **SULPH.,** tab., ***tarent.,*** ter., **THUJ.,** trom., tub., vario., **VERAT.,** yohim., zinc.
fecal - aloe, alum., ant-c., ant-t., arg-n., arn., ars., bapt., bar-c., bor., bov., bry., carb-v., caust., cedr., chel., cist., colch., coloc., con., dios., dulc., **GAMB.,** hep., hydr., ign., iris, kali-n., lept., lil-t., lyc., **NAT-S.,** nicc., nux-v., **OLND.,** osm., **PIC-AC.,** phos., **PODO.,** ptel., rheum, rhod., rhus-t., rumx., samb., sang., sars., sel., **SULPH.,** trom., verat., zinc.
black - acon., apis, **ARS.,** asc-t., brom., carb-ac., carb-v., cocc., crot-h., kali-s., lept., squil., stram.
brown - apoc., arg-n., arn., ars., asaf., aster., bry., **GRAPH.,** mag-c., mag-m., nat-s., nux-v., phos., psor., raph., squil.

THIN,
copious, not - med.
dark - ars., crot-h., op., nat-s., squil.followed by hard - agar., alum., am-c., bar-c., calc., carb-an., euph., graph., lyc., mag-c., mag-m., mur-ac., nat-c., ph-ac., plat., sars., sep., sulph., sul-ac., zinc.
formed then thin - agar., aloe, **BOV., CALC.,** calc-f., lact., **LYC.,** nat-s., ph-ac., phos., stann.
green - aeth., agar., ant-c., apis, chin., crot-h., crot-t., **GRAT.,** podo., raph.
liver-colored - mag-c.
lumpy and liquid - aloe, **ANT-C.,** apis, ars., calc., con., graph., ip., kali-bi., **LYC.,** nat-s., pic-ac., sil., sulph., sul-ac., trom.
pouring, out - apis, arn., ars., benz-ac., calc-p., canth., **CROT-T., GAMB.,** grat., iod., lach., lyc., merc., **NAT-S., OLND., PH-AC., PODO.,** puls., **SEC.,** sil., sulph.
red - kali-i., rhus-t.
yellow - agar., aeth., aloe, bapt., bov., bufo, cocc., coloc., cop., crot-t., **DULC., GAMB.,** hydr., iris, lyc., merc., nat-c., **NAT-S.,** nit-ac., nux-m., **OLND., PIC-AC., PODO.,** raph., rhus-t.

TOUGH - agar., ***am-m.,*** arn., asar., bar-c., brom., ***canth., caps., caust.,*** merc-i-f., **SULPH.**

UNNOTICED, passes stool - acon., **ALOE,** ars., carl., colch., coloc., cur., ferr-ma., grat., ***hyos., mur-ac.,*** ph-ac., ***plb., staph.,*** tab., verat.
hard stool - **ALOE,** ***coloc.***
thin, watery, passes while urinating - ***mur-ac.***

WATERY - acet-ac., ***acon.,*** aesc., ***aeth.,*** **AGAR.,** ail., ***aloe,*** alum., am-m., anac., anag., **ANT-C.,** ant-t., **APIS, APOC., ARG-N.,** arn., ***ars., ars-i., arum-t.,*** **ASAF.,** asar., aur-m., bapt., bar-c., ***bar-m.,*** bell., **BENZ-AC.,** berb., ***bism., bor., bufo, cact.,*** cahin., **CALC.,** ***calc-p.,*** camph., canth., carb-ac., **CARB-S.,** ***carb-v.,*** cast., cast-eq., caul., caust., cench., **CHAM.,** ***chel., chin., chin-a.,*** chin-s., ***chr-ac., cina,*** cist., cob., ***cocc., coff.,*** **COLCH.,** ***coll., coloc.,*** **CON.,** cop., ***corn.,*** crot-h., ***crot-t.,*** cupr., cur., cycl., ***dig.,*** dios., dirc., **DULC.,** elaps, **ELAT., EUPH.,** ***ferr.,*** ferr-ar., ferr-i., ferr-p., fl-ac., **GAMB.,** gnaph., ***graph.,*** **GRAT.,** guai., ***hell., hep.,*** hipp., ***hydr., hyos., iod.,*** ip., **IRIS,** ***jal.,*** **JATR.,** ***kali-ar.,*** **KALI-BI.,** kali-br., kali-c., ***kali-i.,*** kali-n., kali-p., ***kali-s.,*** kreos., ***lac-c., lach., lec., lept., lob.,*** lyss., **MAG-C.,** mag-m., mag-s., manc., **MERC.,** ***merc-d.,*** merc-i-r., ***merc-sul., mez.,*** mosch., ***mur-ac.,*** nat-a., ***nat-c.,*** **NAT-M.,** ***nat-p.,*** **NAT-S.,** ***nit-ac.,*** nux-m., **NUX-V., OLND., OP.,** osm., ox-ac., petr., ***ph-ac.,*** **PHOS., PIC-AC.,** plan., plb., **PODO., PSOR., PULS.,** ran-b., ran-s., ***raph.,*** rat., rhus-t., ***rhus-v., rumx.,*** samb., sang., sars., **SEC.,** sel., senec., seneg., sep., ***sil.,*** spig., squil., stram., stront-c., stry., **SULPH.,** sumb., sul-ac., tab., ter., **THUJ.,** ***tub.,*** valer., **VERAT., VERAT-V.,** vib., zinc.
afternoon - ferr.

WATERY,
black - ***apis,*** arn., **ARS.,** asc-t., bapt., camph., carb-ac., ***chin.,*** chin-s., ***crot-h., cupr., iod., kali-bi., lept.,*** nat-s., ***psor.,*** rumx., sec., stann., ***stram., verat.***
bloody - aloe, am-m., apis, ars., ***canth., carb-v.,*** ferr-p., lach., petr., ***phos.,*** **RHUS-T.,** sabad.
bloody, meat washings, like - canth., ***phos.,*** **RHUS-T.**
brown - ant-t., apis, ***apoc.,*** **ARS.,** arum-t., aster., ***bapt.,*** camph., canth., carb-v., ***chel.,*** chin., dulc., ferr., ferr-ar., ***gamb.,*** gels., **GRAPH.,** ***kali-bi.,*** kreos., mag-c., petr., ***phos.,*** plan., ***rumx.,*** sulph., ***verat.***
clay-colored - ***kali-bi.,*** kali-p.
clear - apis, ***benz-ac.,*** coloc., ***merc.,*** sec., tab.
dirty - ars., brom., ***cact.,*** ferr-p., jal., lept., ox-ac., ph-ac., podo.
flakes, with - cupr., paull., ***verat.***
frothy - benz-ac., ***elat., graph., kali-ar.,*** kali-bi., ***mag-c.,*** ran-b.
gelatinous, on standing - podo.
green - acon., aeth., am-m., ars., bell., bry., **CHAM.,** ***chion.,*** colos., cupr., dulc., ***elat.,*** eup-per., ferr-p., gamb., **GRAT.,** hep., ip., iris, kali-br., kali-i., kreos., ***laur.,*** lept., ***mag-c.,*** med., ***merc-d.,*** nat-m., nat-s., ***nit-ac., phos., podo., puls.,*** rob., sanic., sec., sulph., sul-ac., ter., ***verat.***
green, scum, with - **MAG-C.,** ***merc.***
jaundice, with - berb.
lumpy, and watery - ant-c., lyc., sanic.
and, black - thuj.
muddy - lept.
meat, like washing of - ***canth.,*** phos., rhus-t.
morning - agar., ant-c., ant-t., cact., caust., cop., dios., ***fl-ac.,*** glon., hep., iod., kali-bi., kali-c., kali-n., mag-c., mur-ac., nat-m., **NAT-S.,** nux-m., nux-v., olnd., ox-ac., petr., phos., **PODO.,** ***rumx.,*** squil., **SULPH.,** tab.
night - acet-ac., agar., ant-t., **ARG-N.,** ars., cast., chel., ***chin.,*** gnaph., merc-c., mosch., nat-m., puls., senec., sulph.
perspiration, after - bell.
prune juice, like - ars., ter.
rice water, like - ant-t., apis, ***ars.,*** **CAMPH.,** carb-ac., cham., chel., colch., **CUPR.,** ***ferr.,*** iris, kali-br., kali-i., ***kali-p.,*** merc-sul., ***nat-m.,*** **PH-AC.,** ***phos.,*** ran-b., ***sec.,*** **VERAT.**
white - ang., **BENZ-AC.,** ***calc., camph., cast., caust., cina, cop.,*** dulc., kali-ar., ***kali-bi.,*** kreos., merc., nat-m., **PH-AC.,** ***phos.,*** ran-b., sec.
yellow - aesc., am-m., ***apis, apoc.,*** ars., ***bapt.,*** bor., ***calc.,*** canth., cham., ***chel., chin., cocc., colch.,*** colos., cop., crot-h., ***crot-t.,*** cycl., **DULC.,** elaps, ferr-p., **GAMB., GRAT.,** ***hydr., hyos.,*** ip., ***iris,*** jab., kali-c., kali-i., lach., ***lec.,*** merc-sul., nat-a., ***nat-c., nat-s.,*** nuph., **OLND., *ph-ac.,*** phos., pic-ac., plb., **PODO.,** puls.,

WATERY,
yellow - ***rhus-t.,*** sanic., sec., ***stront-c.,*** **THUJ.,** trom.

WAXY - kali-bi., lept.

WHEY-like - cupr., iod.

WHITE - acon., aesc., am-m., ang., anth., anthr., ***ant-c., apis,*** arg-n., ars., ***ars-i.,*** asc-t., aur-m., ***aur-m-n.,*** bar-m., ***bell.,*** **BENZ-AC.,** ***bor.,*** bufo, ***calc.,*** calc-p., calc-s., **CANTH.,** carb-s., ***cast.,*** caul., ***caust.,*** cedr., ***cham., chel.,*** chin., ***cina,*** cocc., ***colch., cop., crot-h., dig.,*** dios., dol., dros., ***dulc.,*** elat., ***form.,*** gels., ***graph., hep., hell.,*** hydr., iber., ign., ***iod., kali-ar., kali-bi., kali-c., kali-chl.,*** kreos., lac-c., lach., lyc., mag-c., manc., mang., med., merc., naja, nat-m., nat-s., **NUX-M.,** ***nux-v.,*** op., pall., petr., **PH-AC.,** ***phos.,*** plb., podo., **PULS.,** ran-b., ***rheum, rhus-t.,*** rhus-v., rob., ***sanic.,*** sec., ***sep.,*** spig., ***spong.,*** still., sulph., tarax., thuj., urt-u., verat.
chalk like - ant-c., aur-m-n., bell., **CALC.,** ***chel.,*** cimx., ***dig.,*** hep., lach., **PODO.,** rhus-t., **SANIC.,** ***sil.,*** spong.
curdy - calen.
dentition, during - ***calc.***
eggwhite, like boiled - urt-u.
fecal - aesc., aur-m-n., bar-m., **CALC.,** ***calc-p., chel.,*** cop., ***crot-h., dig., hep.,*** kali-bi., ***lyc., pall.,*** **PODO.,** rhus-t., sanic., ***sil.***
alternating with black - aur-m-n.
glassy - ars-i.
grains or particles - ***cina,*** cub., dulc., mez., ***phos.***
gray, streaked with blood - ***calc.***
grayish white - asar., aur-m-n., ***phos.,*** **PH-AC.**
greenish white - ***ph-ac.***
hard - bar-m., ***chel.,*** berb., eup-per., ***hydr.,*** iod., ***mag-c., mag-m.,*** sulph.
jelly-like - ***hell.***
masses like tallow - dulc., ***mag-c.,*** phos.
milk-like, chyle-like - ***aesc.,*** arg-n., arn., bell., berb., bufo, **CALC.,** carb-ac., carb-v., ***card-m.,*** **CHEL., CHIN.,** coloc., cop., **DIG.,** dulc., gels., hell., ***hep., kali-bi.,*** lept., ***mag-c.,*** **MERC.,** myric., nux-v., petr., plat., **PODO.,** rheum, **SANIC.,** stront-c., sulph., tab., valer.
parts in - phos.
putty, like - mag-c.
shreddy particles - **COLCH.**

YEAST, like - arn.

YELLOW - aesc., ***aeth.,*** agar., ***aloe, alumn.,*** ambr., am-m., ang., ant-c., ant-t., ***apis, apoc., arg-n.,*** arn., ***ars., ars-i.,*** arum-t., asaf., ***asar.,*** asc-t., bapt., bar-c., bar-m., bell., ***berb.,*** bol., bor., bov., brom., ***bry.,*** bufo, cahin., ***calc.,*** calc-s., canth., carb-s., carb-v., cham., **CHEL.,** ***chin.,*** cist., cocc., ***colch.,*** coll., ***coloc.,*** colos., cop., crot-c., crot-h., ***crot-t.,*** cub., cycl., dig., dios., **DULC.,** ***echi.,*** elaps, euph., fl-ac., **GAMB.,** ***gels.,*** **GRAT.,** helon., ***hep.,*** hyos., ign., iod., ip., ***iris,*** jab., ***kali-ar., kali-bi., kali-c., kali-i.,*** kali-p., kali-s., **YELLOW** - ***lach.,*** laur., lept., lil-t., **LYC.,** mag-c., mag-m., mang., **MERC., MERC-C.,** ***merc-sul., nat-a., nat-c.,*** nat-m., nat-p., ***nat-s.,*** nicc., nuph., ***nux-m.,*** nux-v., olnd., ***petr.,*** **PH-AC.,** ***phos.,*** phys., **PIC-AC.,** ***plb.,*** **PODO.,** puls., raph., rheum, **RHUS-T.,** rob., samb., ***sang.,*** sanic., **SEC.,** staph., stront-c., sulph., ***sul-ac.,*** tab., ter., **THUJ.,** urt-u.
bright - aeth., aloe, chel., colch., fl-ac., gels., ***kali-p.,*** nux-m., **PH-AC.,** ***phos.,*** podo., sul-ac., sul-i.
brownish - anan., apis, asar., coloc., fl-ac., merc-i-r., nat-p.
fecal - ***agar., aloe, alumn.,*** am-m., ant-t., ***apis,*** arum-t., asaf., bapt., bol., bor., bov., ***calc.,*** **CHEL.,** cist., cocc., colch., coloc., crot-t., cub., dig., dios., fl-ac., **GAMB.,** gels., ***hep.,*** iris, kali-c., lach., laur., lith., myric., nat-c., ***nat-p., nat-s.,*** **OLND.,** ***ph-ac.,*** **PIC-AC.,** plb., **PODO., RHUS-T.,** samb., ***sulph.***
fecal, painless immediately after eating - calc.
forenoon - mag-c.
granular - bell., mang.
green on standing, turning - arg-n., rheum
greenish - aloe, apis, cadm-s., coloc., crot-t., ***dulc.,*** **GRAT.,** jug-c., kali-bi., kali-p., lac-ac., med., merc., nat-s., puls., sec., **SULPH.,** tab., ter., verat.
hard - agar.
orange - aeth., apis, chel., cocc., ***colch.,*** coloc., dios., gels., ip., kali-bi., merc., nat-m., nuph., osm., phos., **SUL-AC.,** syph.
like pulp of - ***nat-c.***
pale - mang., zinc.
saffron, like - coloc., croc., merc., **SUL-AC.**
salmon - lac-d.
whitish - acon., aur., cocc., dig., ign., lyc., nit-ac., **PH-AC.,** phos., puls., rhus-t., ***sulph.,*** sul-ac.

Teeth

ABSCESS, teeth, of roots - am-c., ***bar-c.,*** bell-p., calc., calc-f., canth., caust., euph., ***hecla.,*** **HEP.,** lach., ***lyc.,*** **MERC.,** merc-i-f., petr., phos., plb., **PYROG., SIL.,** sulph., zinc.
abscess, jaws - ars., phos.

ACHING, pain, (see Pain, jaws)
aching, pain, (see Pain, teeth)

ADHERE, teeth, together - arg-m., ***psor.,*** **PYROG.,** zinc.

AIR, sensation, as from cold air blowing on teeth - coc-c.
if forced into them - ambr., cocc.
streaming from - nat-c., nat-s.

BITES, tumbler when drinking - **ARS.**

BITING, chewing, agg. general - aloe, ***am-c.,*** am-m., bry., chin., euphr., hep., ign., meny., ***merc., mez.,*** nat-m., nit-ac., phos., podo., puls., **RHUS-T.,** ***sep., staph., verb.,*** zinc.
amel. - bry., cocc., cupr-ac., seneg., ***staph.***
biting, teeth together, agg. - alum., **AM-C.,** anac., bell., bry., carb-an., caust., chin., coff., colch., dig., graph., ***guai.,*** hell., ***hep., hyos., ip.,*** lach., mang., merc., petr., puls., ***rhus-t.,*** sars., ***sep.,*** sil., spong., staph., ***sul-ac.,*** sulph., ***verb.***
amel. - ars., chin., cocc., coff., euph., mag-m., **PHYT.,** ***staph.***
afraid, to, for fear they would fall out - nit-ac.
cannot, at night - chim.
sends a shock through head, ears and nose - am-c.
sudden, involuntary - apis.
wants to, on something hard which relieves pains during dentition - **PHYT.**

BITING, pain, teeth - calc., cocc., phel., rhod.

BLEEDING, in hollow teeth - ph-ac., ***phos.,*** tarax.

BLOWS, teeth, sensation of - calc., nux-v., tarax.

BORING, pain, teeth - alum., ***bar-c., bell.,*** bor., ***bov.,*** bufo, calad., calc., ***calc-p.,*** camph., cann-i., cast., ***caust.,*** chel., chin., con., ***cycl.,*** daph., euph., grat., ***ign.,*** indg., kali-bi., ***kali-c.,*** kali-n., ***lach., laur.,*** lyc., mag-c., mag-m., ***mez.,*** mur-ac., ***nat-c., nat-m., nat-p.,*** nicc., ***nit-ac., nux-v.,*** petr., ph-ac., ***phos.,*** plan., rhod., sel., ***sil., sulph.,*** verat.
air, open amel. - mag-m.
cold, amel. - mag-m.
dinner, after - kali-c.
evening - nat-c.
lying, while - phos.
tearing and digging, with - alum.
molars - sel.
morning, while lying - phos.
noon - kali-n.
night - phos.
roots, in - ***cham.,*** mur-ac.
in sound teeth - alum., plan.

boring, jaws, lower - aur., aur-m-n., bov., brom., ***cocc.,*** coloc., indg., kali-bi., ***lach.,*** led., mag-c., ***mez.,*** plb., sabad.
left - mez., plb., sabad.
night - ***mez.***
ramus - agar., merc-i-f.
right - aur., brom., coloc., elaps, indg., led.
extending to ear - elaps.
boring, jaws, upper - aur., aur-m-n., led., ***mez.,*** rhus-v., thuj.

BREAK, off, pain, as if teeth would - bell., sulph.

BREAKING, off of teeth - euph., lach., nat-h., plb., sul-ac.

BRUSHING, cleaning teeth, agg. - carb-v., coc-c., lyc., merc., ruta, ***staph.***

BRUXISM, (see Grinding teeth)

BUBBLING, sensation, teeth - berb., carb-v., lyc., nit-ac., spig.

BURNING, pain, teeth - bar-c., ***caust.,*** cham., ***coloc.,*** dulc., graph., kali-c., ***mag-c.,*** merc., mez., ***nat-m.,*** nit-ac., ***nux-v.,*** phel., ***ph-ac.,*** phos., puls., rhus-t., rob., sil., spig., spong., sulph., ther., urt-u., zinc.
burning, jaws - anac., bov., caust., daph., fl-ac.
joints, of - op.
lower - ars., caust., mang.
upper - chin.

BURST, pain, teeth, as if would - bar-c., chin., ph-ac., sabin., thuj.

BUZZING, pain, teeth - hyos., sep., sulph.

CANCER, of jaws - ***ant-c.,*** arg-n., ***ars.,*** aur., calc., fl-ac., graph., ***hecla.,*** merc., phos., rhus-t., sil., symph.
bones - ***hecla.,*** symph.
left - ***ars., hecla.,*** merc., phos., sil.
right - ***ant-c.,*** arg-n., ars., aur., calc., fl-ac., graph., hecla., rhus-t.

CARIES, (see Decayed)

CHATTERING, teeth - agar., alum., bar-c., calc., carb-v., cocc., gels., ip., kali-p., phos.
chill, with - am-c., camph., caps., cupr., hep., ip., kali-n., phos., plat., sars., stann., sulph.
inward, trembling, with - ant-t.
morning, on waking - phos.
trembling, with, from fear - elaps.

CHEWING, motion of the jaws - ***acon.,*** asaf., aster., ***bell.,*** **BRY.,** ***calc.,*** caust., ***cham.,*** cic., cupr., fl-ac., gels., ***hell.,*** ign., ***lach., lyc., merc.,*** mosch., nat-m., ***phos.,*** plb., ruta, sec., sep., sol-n., ***stram.,*** verat., verat-v.
brain affections, in - bry.
chill, during - nat-m.
chorea, in - asaf.
convulsions, during - hell.
epilepsy, before an attack - ***calc.***
loud, in lower jaw - plb.
sleep, during - calc.
sleep, during - bry., **CALC.,** cina, ***ign.,*** podo., sep., zinc.

CLAWING, pain, teeth - stront.

CLINCH, teeth, together, constant inclination to - acet-ac., acon., agar., ambr., anan., bufo, camph., cann-i., caust., cina., cob., cocc., cupr., ***hyos.,*** iod., lach., laur., ***lyc.,*** mang., merc-i-f., nux-v., **PHYT.,** ***podo.,*** stry., tarent.
dentition, during - ***phyt.***
molars - sep.

CLINCHED, teeth, firmly - aeth., alum., ***bell.,*** camph., cic., ***hyos.,*** merc., **PHYT.,** podo., stram., sulph.
midnight, after - chin-s.
night - ***hydr-ac.,*** sep., ***ther.***

clinched, jaws - acet-ac., acon., act-sp., agar., ars., **BELL.,** camph., cann-i., cann-s., carb-ac., carb-h., cham., ***cic.,*** cob-n., colch., ***cupr.,*** dig., dios., ***glon.,*** hydr-ac., ***hyos., hyper., ign.,*** laur., mag-arct., mag-p., ***merc.,*** merc-i-f., **NUX-V.,** ***oena., op.,*** ox-ac., phos., phyt., ***rhus-t.,*** sec., ***sil.,*** staph., ***stram.,*** sulph., tab., tarent., ***verat.,*** vip.
emotional - ign.
grinding of the teeth, with - canth., cic.
morning - ther.
newborn, in - ambr., camph.
sunstroke, from - glon.

CLUCKING, jaws, lower - bell.

COLDNESS, teeth - acon., alum., alumn., anag., anan., aran., asar., astac., ***carb-v.,*** cocc., cocc-s., colch., cop., dros., ***gamb.,*** grat., ir-foe., kali-chl., led., ***mez., nit-ac.,*** ol-an., ox-ac., par., petr., ***ph-ac.,*** rat., rheum, sel., sep., ***spig.***
afternoon - mez.
roots - ph-ac.
chewing - ph-ac.
morning - ph-ac.
upper teeth - spig.

coldness, jaws, lower - **PLAT.**

CONTRACTING, pain, teeth - bor., cann-s., carb-an., carb-v., nit-ac., petr. stann.

CONVULSIONS, jaws - agar., ars., asaf., ***bell.,*** carb-an., coloc., crot-c., hydr-ac., ign., kali-c., mang., oena., op., ran-b., stram., sulph.
joints, of - colch., kali-c., nicc., ol-an., rhus-t., sil., spong., stann.

CORROSIVE, pain, teeth - calc., carb-v., cham., con., kali-c., merc., nicc., phos., puls., spig., staph., sul-ac., thuj.

CRACKING, when rubbing teeth - sel.

cracking, jaws, in, when chewing - ***am-c.,*** brom., chin-s., ***cor-r., gamb.,*** gran., ***lac-c., lach., meny., mez.,*** **NIT-AC.,** ol-an., **RHUS-T.,** sabad., sel., spong., ***stry.,*** sulph., ***thuj.***
as if, it would crack - petr., sep.
maxillary joints - nit-ac., rhus-t.
opening mouth wide, when - sabad., thuj.

CRAMP, jaws - tab., verat.
chewing, on - verat.
eating, while - mang., spong.
after - mang.

CRAMP, jaws
masseters - cocc., cupr., hydr-ac., stram., stry.
muscles, mouth opening agg. - cocc.
maxillary, joints - asaf., ***bell.,*** carb-h., crot-h., fl-ac., kali-c., kali-i., nit-ac., ox-ac., plat., rhus-t., sep., sil., ***spong.,*** sulph.

CRAWLING, teeth - bar-c., bor., cast., ***cham.,*** graph., kali-i., mag-m., mur-ac., ol-an., rhus-t., stront.
cold - nat-c.
root, at - sars.

CRUMBLING, of teeth - anan., ant-c., arg-n., ***bor., calc., calc-f., calc-p.,*** crot-h., epig., ***euph., fl-ac., kreos., lach.,*** med., ***plb.,*** sabad., spig., ***staph.,*** sul-ac., syph., ***thuj.***

CRUSHED, pain, teeth, as if - lyc.
molars - ***ign.***

CUPPED, teeth in children - calc-f., syph.

CUTTING, pain, teeth - alum., arn., ***aur.,*** bell., benz-ac., calc., ***camph.,*** daph., graph., ham., kali-c., ***lach., mez.,*** olnd., petr., ran-b., ***rhod.,*** rhus-t., rob., sep., sulph.
draft, as if from a cold - sulph.
evening, when lying in bed - alum.
lying, while - alum.
open air, in the - alum.
roots, in - camph., iod.
shooting through gums to roots of incisors and canines - camph.
swollen, submaxillary gland, seems to originate in - camph.
thunderstorm, before - ***rhod.***

cutting, jaws, maxillary articulation - asar.

DECAYED, teeth, rotten, hollowed - abrot., acon., alum., ***ambr., am-c.,*** anac., anan., ang., **ANT-C.,** ars., asar., aur., ***bar-c.,*** **BELL., BOR.,** ***bov.,*** bry., ***calc.,*** calc-f., **CALC-P.,** ***calc-s.,*** carb-an., carb-s., ***carb-v.,*** caust., ***cham., chin.,*** clem., cocc., coff., con., euph., **FL-AC.,** graph., ***glon., hecla., hep., hyos.,*** ip., ***kali-bi., kali-c., kali-i.,*** kali-n., kali-p., ***kreos., lach., lyc., mag-c.,*** mag-m., mang., med., meph., **MERC., MEZ., NAT-C.,** nat-m., nat-p., nat-s., ***nit-ac., nux-v.,*** ox-ac., par., petr., ***ph-ac., phos.,*** plat., **PLB.,** ***puls.,*** rheum, ***rhod., rhus-t.,*** ruta., sabin., sabad., sang., sel., **SEP.,** ***sil.,*** spig., **STAPH.,** ***sulph.,*** sul-ac., tab., ***tarax.,*** thuj., **TUB.,** verat., zinc.
appears, as soon as they - ***kreos.,*** staph.
crown, at - merc., ***staph.***
enamel, loss of - ***calc-f.***
gums, at edge of - calc., syph., ***thuj.***
internal - sel.
premature in children - ***calc., calc-f., calc-p.,*** cocc., coff., ***fl-ac.,*** hecla., **KREOS.,** merc., ***mez.,*** phos., ***plan.,*** sil., **STAPH.,** tub.
rapid - ars., bar-c., ***calc., calc-p., carb-v.,*** **FL-AC.,** med., mez., phos., plan., **SEP.**
roots, at - am-c., fl-ac., ***merc.,*** mez., sil., ***syph.,*** **THUJ.**
sensation of - asar.
sides of teeth - mez., staph., thuj.

decay, of jaws, lower - asaf., ***aur., aur-m., aur-m-n., cist., con., fl-ac., kali-i., merc.,*** mez., ***nit-ac., phos., phyt., sil.,*** staph.

DENTITION, difficult teething - **ACON.,** ***aeth.,*** am-c., ***ant-c., ant-t., apis, arn.,*** **ARS.,** arund., **BELL.,** ***bism.,*** **BOR.,** ***bry.,*** **CALC.,** calc-f., **CALC-P.,** ***canth., caust.,*** **CHAM.,** cheir., chlor., cic., cimic., ***cina, coff., colch., coloc.,*** cupr., cypr., ***dol., dulc., ferr., ferr-p., gels., graph., hecla., hell.,*** hep., hyos., ***ign., ip., kali-br., kreos., lyc., mag-c.,*** **MERC.,** ***merc-c.,*** mill., nat-m., nit-ac., op., passi., ***phyt.,*** plat., ***podo.,*** puls., ***rheum,*** scut., sec., sep., **SIL.,** sol-n., stann., **STAPH., SULPH.,** syph., ***ter.,*** tub., tub-k., zinc., zinc-br.

ailments from - ***acon., cham., coff.,*** mag-c., mag-p., ***nux-v.,*** rheum, ***rhus-t.,*** stann., staph.

brain and nervous symptoms, with - acon., agar., ***bell., cham.,*** cimic., cypr., dol., ***hell.,*** kali-br., ***podo.,*** sol-n., ter., ***zinc.***

compression of gums, with - cic., phyt., podo.

constipation, general irritation and cachexia, with - ***kreos.,*** nux-v., op.

convulsions, with - ***bell.,*** calc., ***cham., cic.,*** cupr., glon., kali-br., ***mag-p.,*** sol-n., stann.

cough, with - acon., bell., ferr-p., kreos.

deafness, otorrhea and stuffiness of nose, with - cheir.

diarrhea, with - acet-ac., aeth., apoc., arund., ***calc.,*** calc-ac., ***calc-p., cham.,*** ferr-p., ip., jal., kreos., mag-c., ***mag-p.,*** merc., olnd., phos., ***phyt.,*** podo., puls., rheum, ***sil.***

effusion of brain, with threatening - ***apis,*** hell., tub., ***zinc-m.***

eye symptoms, with - bell., calc., puls.

insomnia, with - bell., cham., ***coff., cypr.,*** kreos., passi., scut.

intertrigo, with - caust., lyc.

milk indigestion, with - aeth., calc., ***mag-m.***

salivation, with - bor.

slow - aster., **CALC.,** calc-f., **CALC-P.,** ***fl-ac.,*** mag-c., mag-m., mag-p., merc., nep., phos., **SIL.,** sulfa., ***sulph.,*** thuj., **TUB.,** zinc.

sour smell of body, pale face and irritability, with - kreos.

weakness, palor, fretfulness and must be carried rapidly, with - ars.

wisdom teeth, ailments from - ***calc.,*** ferr-pic., ***fl-ac., mag-c.,*** **SIL.**

worms, with - ***cina,*** merc., stann.

DIGGING, pain, teeth - ambr., anan., ant-c., arg-n., bell., berb., bor., ***bov.,*** bry., bufo, calc., cast., ***caust., cham.,*** chin., fl-ac., ***glon.,*** ign., kali-c., lyc., mag-m., ***nat-c.,*** nux-v., plan., plat., ***puls.,*** rat., rheum, ruta., seneg., sep., sil., spig., sul-ac., sulph.

evening - alum., nat-c.

walking, while - nat-c.

pressure, sensation as if pain were felt below left lower molars, with - ambr.

digging, lower - cocc., ***plat.***

rami of lower - ***kali-bi.***

DIRTY, look, teeth - ***all-c.,*** aur-m-n., caps.

DISCHARGE, from decayed tooth - sulph.

DISCOLORED, teeth

black - ***arg-n.,*** **CHIN.,** ***chlor., con.,*** ign., kreos., merl., **MERC.,** ***nit-ac.,*** phos., plb., puls., sep., ***squil.,*** **STAPH.,** syph., ***thuj.***

after aching - sep.

in streaks - staph.

brown, sooty - chlor.

dark - ***chin.,*** **FL-AC.,** sabin.

spots - kreos.

gray - **MERC.,** phos., plb.

yellow - ***all-c.,*** ars., asc-t., ***iod., lyc.,*** med., ***merc.,*** nit-ac., ph-ac., plb., ***sil., thuj.***

DISLOCATION, of jaws, easy - caust., mez., petr., rheum., ***rhus-t.,*** staph.

maxillary joints - ign., petr., ***rhus-t.,*** staph.

laughing agg. - tab.

sensation of - mag-arct., petr., rhus-t.

DISTORTION, lower jaw - tab.

DRAWING, pain, teeth - abrot., agar., all-c., all-s., alum., ***ambr., am-c., anac.,*** anan., ang., ant-c., arg-n., ars., asaf., astac., aur., aur-s., bad., bar-c., ***bell.,*** berb., bism., bor., ***bov., bry.,*** calad., ***calc.,*** calc-p., camph., cann-s., canth., caps., carb-an., ***carb-s.,*** **CARB-V.,** ***caust.,*** **CHAM.,** ***chel.,*** chim., chin., ***clem., coc-c., cocc.,*** colch., ***con.,*** crot-t., cycl., daph., fl-ac., ***glon.,*** **GRAPH.,** guai., hep., hyos., hyper., iod., kali-bi., kali-c., kali-n., kalm., kreos., ***lach.,*** led., lyc., lyss., ***mag-c.,*** mag-m., meph., **MERC.,** ***merc-c.,*** merc-i-f., mez., naja, nat-c., ***nat-m.,*** nat-s., nit-ac., nux-m., ***nux-v.,*** ol-an., olnd., par., petr., ph-ac., phos., ***plat., puls.,*** ran-b., ***ran-s., rhod.,*** rhus-t., sabad., sabin., sars., ***sep.,*** sil., spig., ***staph., sulph.,*** tab., tarax., ter., thuj., verat., zinc.

afternoon - canth., carb-an., cocc.

5 p.m - zing.

air, in open - chin., ***nux-v.,*** sep., ***sulph.***

amel. - chin., hep., puls.

bed, agg. in - aphis., ***kali-c.***

biting, only when - am-c.

biting, pain - carb-v.

bubbling - berb.

cold, from - ***nux-v.,*** **SEP.**

amel. from - ambr.

finger, amel. by - ang.

eating, while - am-c., bry., carb-an., con., sep., verat.

after - bry., ***cham., hep.,*** kali-c., nat-m., staph.

amel. - ambr., am-c., ***cham.***

cold food - ***con.***

evening - alum., bov., bry., hep., puls.

in bed - ***kali-c.***

preventing sleep - lyc.

right side, going off after lying down - alum.

exertion of mind - ***nux-v.***

DRAWING, pain, teeth
extending, to,
cheek - am-c., sep.
ear - alum., am-c., ***ammc.,*** anac., aphis., bar-c., cocc-s., iod., kali-c., **KREOS.,** ***nat-m.,*** sep.
eyes - chel., kali-c., nat-m.
head, side of - alum., apis
larynx - alum., nit-ac.
lower incisors to malar bone and temple, from - alum.
malar bone - alum., aphis., con.
neck - ***alum.***
other parts - alum.
other right side - aphis.
shoulders - alum.
temple - alum., con.
temple, right - bar-c., kreos.
throat - nat-m.
incisors, lower - agar., alum., asaf., kreos., sil., ***zinc.***
one of - ambr.
upper - agar., ang., camph., carb-v., grat., kreos., petr., sep., zinc.
intermittent - calc., sil.
jerking - zinc.
lancinating, as if a current of air rushed into - ambr.
lower canine - crot-t.
teeth - fl-ac.
menses, during - **AM-C.,** sep.
molars - asar., bism., bry., carb-an., carb-v., graph., olnd., petr., sep., sulph.
left - calad., carb-an., con., kreos.
lower - anac., camph., mag-c., phos., sep., zinc.
right - ambr., bell., caust., mang.
molars, upper - ambr., ang., bell., mez., **SEP.,** zinc.
extending to forhead - sep.
extending to temple - caust
morning - mang., phos., ***ran-s.,*** staph., sulph.
10 a.m. - anac.
music, from - ph-ac.
night - ambr., am-c., bell., calc., carb-an., mag-c., nat-c., nat-m., nit-ac., sep., sulph.
when lying down - canth., olnd.
noon, toward - aphis., zinc.
paroxysmal - kali-c.
pressure - ars.
pulsating - hyos., sep., zinc.
reading - all-s.
roots, in - anac., caust., iod., staph.
sound teeth, of - ther.
stretched, as if nerves were - anac., coloc., **PULS.**
sudden - carb-an., coc-c.
sweat amel. - aphis.
tearing - abrot.
thunderstorm, before - rhod.
twitching - plat.
upper amel. by cold finger - ang.
right side, all night - bell.
teeth - ang., bell.

DRAWING, pain, teeth
walking, while - camph.
in open air - ***con.***
wandering - ambr., hyos.
warm, fluids - am-c., nux-v., **SEP.**
room - hep., **PULS.**
warmth agg. - ambr.

drawing, jaws - acon., ***alumn.,*** anac., ***aur.,*** bry., calc., **CARB-V.,** caust., cham., ***con.,*** lyc., mez., mur-ac., nat-c., nit-ac., ***nux-v.,*** ph-ac., phos., puls., ***rhus-v.,*** sabad., sil., sulph., zinc.
chilliness, during - sep.
crampy, drawing - sulph.

drawing, jaws, joints - am-m., bell., daph., nat-c., ***rhus-t.,*** sars., verb.
extending to ear - agar., ol-an.

drawing, jaws, lower - agar., alum., am-m., anac., arg-n., bell., bry., calad., calc., carb-s., cham., chin., cupr., euphr., eupi., fl-ac., guai., indg., kali-bi., kali-n., lach., led., lob., lyc., nat-m., nat-s., petr., phos., stann., sulph., tab., thuj., til., viol-t., zinc.
afternoon - euphr., sulph.
drinking, after - con.
evening - anac., thuj.
extending, to
angle of lower jaw - ph-ac.
chin - phos.
ear to head - con.
side of head - viol-t.
morning - sulph.
night - sil.

drawing, jaws, upper - acon., agar., chel., dros., euphr., graph., nat-m., rhus-v., sulph., thuj., zinc.

DROPPING, of jaws - acet-ac., apis, ***arn., ars., bapt., carb-v., chel.,*** cimic., colch., cupr., gels., glon., ***hell., hyos., kali-i.,*** **LACH., LYC.,** merc-cy., **MUR-AC., OP.,** ***nux-v.,*** ph-ac., ***phos.,*** podo., sec., ***stram.,*** **SULPH.,** tab., vario., verat-v., zinc.

DRY, tooth, sockets - arn., plan., ***ruta.***

dry, teeth, sensation, as if - merc-i-f.

DULL, pain, teeth - aur., chin., clem., cocc-s., daph., dol., hyos., kali-i., kalm., lob., lyc., lyss., sep., sil., zinc.
as if soft and became bent on chewing - coch.
griping - bor.
trembling of heart, with - anag.
upper molars, with tearing, pain in cheek bone - anag.
mastication, during - aur.

DWARFED, teeth - calc-f., ***syph.***

EDGE, teeth, feel as if on - acon., agar., **AM-C.,** ars., asaf., ***aur.,*** bell., berb., brom., cahin., caps., carb-s., caust., chin., colch., cop., cor-r., daph., ***dulc.,*** ferr-ma., fl-ac., ***iod.,*** kali-c., kali-chl., **LACH.,** lith., lyss., merc., **MEZ.,** ***nat-m.,*** ox-ac., ph-ac., phos., ran-s., rob., ***sep.,*** sil., spong., staph., stront-c., ***sulph., sul-ac., tarax., zinc.***
as if covered with lime - nux-m.
chewing - spong., tarax.

EDGE, teeth, feel as if on
left side - cor-r.
menses, during - ***merc.***
night - mez.
painful - lyc.
sour belching, with - petr.
vomiting, with - sac-alb.

EDGES, teeth feel sharp and hurt gums - aloe.

ELONGATION, teeth, sensation of - agar., all-c., ***alum., am-c.,*** anac., **ANT-T.,** arg-n., arn., ***ars.,*** ars-i., ***aur.,*** bell., berb., ***bor.,*** brom., ***bry.,*** bufo, ***calc., camph.,*** calad., caps., carb-an., ***carb-v.,*** caul., **CAUST., CHAM.,** chel., chin-s., chr-ac., cinnb., clem., cob., cocc., ***colch.,*** com., crot-h., daph., form., gamb., ***glon.,*** gran., hell., ***hep.,*** hyos., iod., iris, kali-c., ***kali-i.,*** kreos., **LACH.,** lachn., laur., ***lyc.,*** **MAG-C.,** mag-m., ***merc., merc-c., merc-i-f.,*** **MEZ.,** mur-ac., ***nat-m.,*** nat-s., nicc., ***nit-ac.,*** nux-m., ***nux-v.,*** pall., petr., ***phyt., plan.,*** ptel., rat., ***rhus-t.,*** sanic., ***sep., sil.,*** spig., spong., stann., ***staph., sulph.,*** vip., ***zinc.***
air, open, agg. - alum., cob.
canines - petr.
chewing, when - alum., brom., chel., hyos.
decayed teeth - carb-an., ***hep.,*** hyos., ***plb..*** rheum, rhus-t.
incisors - agar., bell., gamb., mag-m., pall., rat., sep., sulph.
morning - ars., petr.
night in bed - anac., lachn., mag-c.

ENAMEL, teeth, deficient - **CALC-F.,** ***sil.***
yellow - sil.

ENLARGED, jaws - hecla., ***phos.***

ERUPTIONS, jaws, lower, blotches - stann., staph.

EXOSTOSIS, jaws, lower - **ANG., CALC-F., HECLA.,** ***hep.***

EXTRACTION, complaints after tooth - **ARN.,** calen., hecla, **HYPER.,** ***phos.,*** staph.

FALLING out, sensation, as if teeth - hyos.

FISTULA dentalis - calc-f., caust., ***fl-ac.,*** nat-m., ***sil.,*** staph., sulph.

FLY, teeth, to pieces, as if would, on biting together - cinnb.

FORMICATION, teeth - bar-c.
evening - bar-c.
painful - bar-c.
formication, jaws, lower - alum., alumn., buf-s., grat., ol-an., **PLAT.**

FUNGUS, jaws, lower, growth - ***hep., phos.,*** thuj.

FUZZY, teeth, as if - calc., caust., hyper.

GNAWING, pain, teeth - agar., **ANT-C.,** bar-c., berb., **CALC.,** camph., canth., carb-v., cast., ***cham., con.,*** daph., euph., indg., kali-bi., ***kali-i.,*** lac-c., mag-c., naja, nicc., ***nux-v.,*** op., phos., **PULS.,** rhus-t., sec., **STAPH.,** sul-ac., ***thuj.***
air, cold inhaling - ***rhus-t.***
amel. - ***nux-v.***
eat, on begining to - euph.
eating, after - **ANT-C.,** staph.

GNAWING, pain, teeth
evening - ***calc.,*** phos., **PULS.**
9 p.m - alum.
hollow tooth - bell.
molars - sep.
molars, lower - cast., ***nicc.***
alternating with itching in ear - agar.
left - phos.
right - cast., ***nicc.***
with violent tearing, behind ear - alum.
with violent tearing, in right ear - nicc.
molars, upper - agar., ***calc.***
morning, in bed - phos.
night - ***cham.,*** coff., mag-c.
sitting up in bed amel. - alum.
warm room - ***nux-v.***
gnawing, jaws - naja, nat-m.
lower - bar-c., fl-ac., ind., kali-i., par.
ramus - sul-ac.
upper, jaw - kali-n., samb., thuj.

GRINDING, of teeth, bruxism - ***acon.,*** ant-c., **APIS,** ***arn., ars., art-v.,*** asaf., atro., aur., bar-c., **BELL.,** ***bry., calc.,*** camph., cann-i., ***canth., carb-ac., caust., cham., cic.,*** **CINA,** coff., colch., con., ***crot-h., cupr., glon., grat., hell.,*** **HYOS.,** ign., ***laur., lyc.,*** lyss., ***merc.,*** morph., mygal., nux-v., op., phos., ***phys.,*** plan., ***plb., podo., sant.,*** sec., ***sep.,*** spig., ***stram., sulph.,*** syph., tab., thuj., **TUB.,** ***verat., zinc.***
anger, from - kali-c.
chill, during - ant-c., apis, ars., ***calc.,*** cham., lyc., phos., stram.
convulsive - ars., ***bell., caust., coff.,*** ferr., lyc., phos., ***zinc.***
epilepsy - ***bufo,*** **HYOS.,** sulph., tarent.
maniacal rage, during - acon., ars., ***bell., hyos.,*** lyc., phos., sec., ***stram.***
menses, toward close of - verat.
morning soon as awake - ant-c., conv.
sitting, while - ant-c., ars.
sleep, during - ***acon.,*** agar., ***ant-c.,*** **ARS.,** asaf., **BELL.,** ***bry.,*** calc., **CANN-I.,** carc., caust., **CINA,** ***coff.,*** colch., con., ***crot-h., hell., hyos., ign., kali-br., kali-c.,*** kali-p., lac-d., ***merc., mygal.,*** nat-p., plan., ***plb., podo.,*** psor., ***sant.,*** sep., ***stram., sulph.,*** thuj., **TUB.,** ***verat., zinc.***
worms, from - **CINA.**

GRIPING, pain, teeth - carb-an., kali-c.

GRUMBLING, pain, teeth - alum., aur., bar-c., cann-s., carb-an., cham., kali-i., kali-n., lil-t., mag-s., meny., nit-ac., ph-ac., **RHOD.,** sep.
eating, after - lyc.
left side, upper - agar.
lower left side - arg-n.
molars, night - sep.
right side, one lower molar, with sensation as if headache came from that side - aeth.

HACKING, pain, teeth - aur.

HEAVINESS, sensation, teeth - cocc., fl-ac., sabin., sep., verat.

INCRUSTATIONS, teeth - plb.

INDURATION, jaws, lower, periosteal - aur-m-n., graph., staph.

INFLAMMATION, teeth, dentine - bell., **MERC.**

inflammation, jaws, lower, periosteum - calc-f., ***merc., ph-ac., phos.,*** ruta.

IRREGULAR, teeth, formation, of - calc., **CALC-F.,** calc-p., ***syph.,*** tub.

formation of lower teeth in a scrofulous child with mesenteric disease - calc-f., phos.

order, in - tub.

ITCHING, in teeth - alum., anac., cham., clem., ***kali-c.,*** kali-n., mur-ac., puls., spong.

air, open in - mag-c.

agg. - anac.

supper, after - kali-c.

itching, jaws, lower - phos.

biting, burning - arg-m., nat-c., par.

JERK, teeth - caust., mang., petr.

eating, while - nat-c., sep.

JERKING, pain, teeth - all-c., all-s., alum., ***am-c.,*** anac., ***ant-c.,*** apis, ars., aur-m., ***bar-c.,*** bar-m., ***bell.,*** benz-ac., berb., bov., ***bry.,*** **CALC.,** ***carb-an.,*** carb-s., carb-v., ***caust.,*** **CHAM.,** ***chin.,*** chin-a., ***clem., coc-c.,*** cocc-s., ***coff., con.,*** cycl., **EUPH.,** hep., ***hyos.,*** hyper., indg., kali-c., kali-i., kali-n., kali-p., kreos., ***lach.,*** laur., ***lyc.,*** mag-c., mag-m., mag-s., mang., meph., ***merc.,*** mez., nat-c., nat-s., nit-ac., nux-m., ***nux-v.,*** ox-ac., petr., ***phos.,*** plat., plb., prun., ***puls., ran-s.,*** rat., ***rhus-t., sep.,*** sil., spig., stram., stront-c., ***sulph.,*** syph., tarax., zinc.

afternoon - sep.

canines, upper - carb-an.

drinking cold water - agar.

eating, after - kali-c., stann., sulph.

evening - mag-m., sep.

in bed - ***bry.,*** zinc.

in bed, now in upper, now in lower molars, when in upper and they are pressed by tip of finger, suddenly changes to lower - ***bry.***

extending to, ear - anac.

to, head - rhus-t.

to, temples - ars., hyos.

menses, during - graph.

molars - crot-h., sil., zinc.

molars, upper, right side - all-s., lyc.

morning - sulph.

9 a.m. - carb-s.

rising, after - mag-c.

night - cycl., mag-c., **MERC.,** rhus-t., sep.

after midnight - alum., sulph.

rising from bed, after, amel. - alum.

root, in - bell., lach., meph.

sitting up in bed amel. - ***ars.***

smoking, while - bry.

amel. - spig.

stretch and let loose, as if nerves were put on - **PULS.**

stroking head amel. - ***ars.***

torn out, as if tooth would be - berb., cocc., ind., ip.

jerking, sensation, jaws, lower - lyss.

KNOCKING, pain, teeth - ars., carb-an., kali-c.

LARGE, and swollen, teeth, sensation - bor., calc., caust., cinnb., nux-m., sil., spong., vip.

LOCKJAW (see Emergency, tetanus)

LOOSENESS, of teeth - ***alumn., am-c.,*** arn., ***ars., aur.,*** aur-m., ***aur-m-n.,*** bar-c., bar-m., ***bufo, bry.,*** calc., camph., **CARB-AN.,** ***carb-s.,*** **CARB-V., CAUST.,** cham., chel., ***chin.,*** cocc., com., ***con.,*** crot-h., dros., elaps, gels., gran., graph., ***hep.,*** **HYOS.,** ign., iod., ***kali-bi., kali-c.,*** kali-n., kali-p., lac-c., lach., ***lyc., mag-c.,*** mag-s., **MERC., MERC-C.,** ***mur-ac.,*** naja, nat-a., nat-c., nat-h., ***nat-m.,*** nat-p., nat-s., **NIT-AC.,** ***nux-m., nux-v.,*** olnd., op., ***ph-ac., phos.,*** phyt., plan., ***plb., psor.,*** puls., ***rhod., rhus-t.,*** sang., ***sec., sep.,*** **SIL.,** spong., stann., ***staph., sulph., tarent.,*** thuj., verat., **ZINC.**

falling out - ***am-c.,*** ars., bufo, cupr., ***merc.,*** nux-v., ***plb., sec.***

sensation of - acon., ***con.,*** hyos., ***nit-ac.,*** stram.

incisors - lyc., nat-m., rhus-t.

lower - graph., phos., rhus-t., sep.

molars - con., kali-n., nat-c.

morning - ars., naja, puls., thuj.

painful - ***ars.,*** aur., bar-c., camph., **CAUST.,** coloc., con., gels., mag-c., merc., plat., ***puls.***

sound teeth - ***am-c.,*** bar-c., **MERC.,** nux-v.

sudden paroxysm - aur.

looseness, sensation of - acon., ***alum., am-c.,*** arn., ***ars.,*** bism., bry., calc-f., carb-v., com., ***con.,*** graph., ***hyos.,*** ign., kali-c., lachn., lith., ***lyc., merc., merc-c.,*** nat-m., nicc., ***nit-ac., nux-m., nux-v.,*** olnd., ***rhus-t.,*** sil., spig., spong., stann., ***sulph.,*** syph., tarent., tub., ***zinc.***

biting teeth together - calc.

chewing, when - alum., ***con.,*** hyos., ***spong.***

evening - sulph.

rush of blood to head, with - hyos.

MUCUS, on teeth (see Sordes) - ail., alum., ant-t., arg-m., arn., bov., cham., cimic., hyos., iod., mag-c., mag-m., mez., plb., podo., psor., sel., senec., sulph., ***syph., ther.,*** tub.

black - apis, ***ars., chin.,*** con.

crusts - con.

brown - apis, ars., ***chel.,*** chlol., ***colch., fl-ac., hyos., kali-p.,*** sulph.

morning - iod., mag-c.

offensive - alum., mez.

sticky - ***phos.,*** verat.

thick - alum., cahin., cimic., ***dulc.,*** vario.

yellow - ***apis,*** asc-t., hyos., iod., ***plb., sul-ac.***

NECROSIS, of jaws, lower - ***hep.,*** merc., **PHOS.,** ***sil.***

upper - ***merc-c.***

NERVES, teeth, exposed, as if - ***cham.,*** coff., ***hyper., kalm.***

injuries to from dental work - calen., cham., **HYPER.**

NEURALGIC, pain, teeth - **BELL.**, bor., ***carb-s.***, **CHAM.**, ***chel.***, chlol., cimic., **COFF.**, ***coloc.***, gels., **HYPER.**, ***iris***, ***kali-p.***, **MAG-P.**, ***nux-m.***, ***plan.***, ***phyt.***, rhod., ***sil.***, ***staph.***
decayed teeth, from - ***plan.***, staph.

NOTCHED, (see Serrated)

NODOSITIES, jaws, lower - ***graph.***

NUMBNESS, of teeth - ars., asaf., aur-s., bell., ***chin.***, ***dulc.***, ign., lith., nat-m., petr., phos., plat., ***rhus-t.***, ruta., thuj.
morning, after rising - plat.
numbness, jaws - fl-ac., gran., hura, phos.

ODOR, offensive, from teeth - calc., carb-v., ***caust.***, graph., kali-c., **KREOS.**, merc., mez.

OIL, feel as if teeth covered with - aesc.

PAIN, jaws - acon., agar., alum., am-m., am-pic., ambr., am-c., ***amph.***, arum-t., aur-m., calc., carb-an., carb-v., **CAUST.**, cimic., con., crot-h., hecla, hyper., ign., lach., lyc., merc., merc-c., merc-i-r., nit-ac., phos., phyt., ***rhus-t.***, rumx., sang., seneg., spig., xan.
angles, of - ign., merc., phyt., sang.
behind - chel., sang.
right - rad.
articulation, right - xan.
bones - phos., sil.
clenching, in sleep, from - merc-i-f.
condyle - **PSOR.**
coughing - am-c.
masseters - hydr-ac., ign.
painful - caust.
rheumatic - nat-c., rhus-t.
screwed together or asunder, as if being - ambr.
pain, jaws, joints, in - agar., acet-ac., alum., alumn., ***arum-t.***, asaf., asar., brom., calc., ***caust.***, cimic., cist., cor-r., dros., fl-ac., glon., hyper., ***ign.***, laur., mang., nicc., op., ***rhus-t.***, spig., spong., ***stry.***, sul-ac., vesp.
chewing, on - acon., alum., am-c., bell., calc., coc-c., cor-r., sil.
morning - vesp.
opening mouth - alum., am-c., **CAUST.**, cor-r., dros., hep., nicc., sabad., verat.
rest, during - ***rhus-t.***
rheumatic - ***rhus-t.***
shutting mouth - ***bar-c.***
swallowing, when - ***arum-t.***
yawning - cor-r., ign., rhus-t., staph.
pain, jaws, lower - acon., agar., aloe, ambr., arg-m., ***ars.***, caps., ***carb-v.***, ***caust.***, cham., chin., cimic., cupr-ar., ***dulc.***, echi., graph., guai., ***hecla***, iod., kali-p., ***lach.***, lyss., mang., ***merc.***, merc-c., merc-i-r., ***mez.***, nit-ac., op., pall., ph-ac., ***phos.***, ***plat.***, phys., rhod., ***rhus-t.***, rumx., sep., ***sil.***, ***spig.***, stram., stry., sulph., sul-ac., tarent., zinc.
break, as if it would - ph-ac.
clenching in sleep, from - merc-i-f.
evening - nit-ac., ***plat.***
extending to ear - lyc., ol-an., sol-n.
extending to, temples - mang.
gouty - caust.

PAIN, jaws
mental, exertion - lyss.
motion, of agg. - alum., am-c., bor., bry., cham., cocc., ***coloc.***, cor-r., ign., kali-c., mag-arct., mag-p., mang., ***merc.***, nat-a., nat-m., phos., rhus-t., sabad., spig., spong., thuj., verat., ***verb.***
splinter, as of a - agar.
toothache, with - sil.
touch, on - nat-m., spong.
pain, jaws, upper - am-c., aster., brom., ***calc-p.***, ***calc-s.***, carb-v., chel., chin., cimic., cycl., euph., ***fl-ac.***, iod., kali-n., kreos., led., mang., merc-i-r., merl., olnd., op., ***phos.***, phyt., polyg., ***spig.***, stann., zinc.
extending to temple - med.
maxillary joints - bell., ign., merc., ***rhus-t.***, thuj.

PAIN, teeth, toothache - ***acet-ac.***, **ACON.**, ***agar.***, ***ail.***, all-c., alum., ***ambr.***, am-c., am-m., anac., anag., ang., ***ant-c.***, ant-t., apis, ***aran.***, arg-m., ***arg-n.***, arn., ***ars.***, ars-h., ***ars-i.***, asar., asc-t., ***aspar.***, aur., aur-m., ***bar-c.***, bar-m., **BELL.**, berb., ***benz-ac.***, bism., ***bor.***, bov., **BRY.**, ***bufo***, calad., ***calc.***, calc-f., calc-p., canth., ***carb-ac.***, carb-an., ***carb-s.***, ***carb-v.***, ***caust.***, **CHAM.**, ***chel.***, chen-a., **CHIN.**, chin-a., clem., cocc., coch., **COFF.**, colch., coloc., con., cor-r., croc., cycl., dios., dros., dulc., ***echi.***, ***euph.***, ***ferr.***, ferr-i., ferr-p., ***fl-ac.***, **GLON.**, ***graph.***, grat., guai., guare., ***hell.***, **HEP.**, ***hyos.***, hyper., ign., ***iod.***, ip., ***kali-c.***, ***kali-i.***, kali-n., ***kali-p.***, kali-s., ***kalm.***, ***kreos.***, **LACH.**, laur., led., lob., ***lyc.***, ***mag-c.***, ***mag-m.***, mag-p., ***mag-s.***, mag-arct., mag-aust., mang., **MERC.**, ***merc-c.***, merl., ***mez.***, mur-ac., ***nat-a.***, **NAT-C.**, ***nat-m.***, ***nat-p.***, ***nat-s.***, nicc., ***nit-ac.***, ***nux-m.***, ***nux-v.***, olnd., par., ***petr.***, ph-ac., ***phos.***, ***phyt.***, plat., ***plan.***, plb., prun., ***puls.***, ran-s., raph., rat., rheum, **RHOD.**, ***rhus-t.***, ruta., sabad., ***sars.***, sel., seneg., **SEP.**, sil., spig., spong., squil., **STAPH.**, stront-c., stry., ***sulph.***, sul-ac., tab., tarax., ***tarent.***, teucr., ther., thuj., ***valer.***, verat., verb., vinc., **ZINC.**
afternoon - agar., anan., calc., caust., ***form.***, ip., mag-c., merc., ***nux-v.***, phos., sulph., ther., thuj.
after dinner - berb., lach., ***nux-v.***, puls.
air, cold - all-c., ***alum.***, ***agar.***, ***anan.***, ant-c., ***bell.***, bor., bry., bufo, **CALC.**, camph., **CHAM.**, **CAUST.**, chin., cina, fl-ac., ***hep.***, hyos., ***mag-c.***, ***mag-p.***, **MERC.**, nat-m., ***nux-m.***, ***nux-v.***, ***phos.***, plat., ***puls.***, plan., ***rhus-t.***, sabad., ***sars.***, seneg., ***sep.***, ***sil.***, ***spig.***, ***staph.***, **SULPH.**, ***sul-ac.***, ***ther.***, thuj., trom.
cold, amel. - chel., ***clem.***, kali-s., mag-m., mez., ***nat-s.***, ***nux-v.***, **PULS.**, sars., ***sel.***, thuj.
draft, from a - ***bell.***, **CALC.**, calc-p., ***cham.***, ***chin.***, gymn., ***mag-c.***, sars., sep., **SULPH.**

PAIN, toothache
air, cold
drawn in mouth, from - acon., alum., ***am-c.,*** ant-c., arn., ***aur., bell.,*** berb., ***bry.,*** **CALC.,** ***calc-p.,*** **CAUST.,** chin., cina, cic., cob., fl-ac., grat., kali-n., **MERC.,** ***mez., nat-m.,*** nux-m., ***nux-v., petr., rhod.,*** rhus-t., sabin., sel., ***sil.,*** spig., ***staph., sulph.,*** thuj.
amel. - ***clem.,*** mez., nat-s., nux-v., ***puls.,*** sars., sel.
open, in the - ***acon.,*** alum., ambr., ***am-c.,*** anac., ant-c., bell., carb-an., carb-v., cast., caust., ***cham., chin.,*** con., hyos., mez., nat-c., nat-m., nux-m., ***nux-v.,*** petr., ***phos.,*** rhus-t., sep., spig., ***staph.,*** **SULPH.**
amel. - all-c., ant-c., bry., bov., hep., mag-m., ***puls.,*** sep., stann., ***sulph.,*** thuj.
air, sensation as from cold air - cedr., coc-c., par.
rushed out of - nat-c.
and in - kali-n.
were forced into - ambr., cocc-s.
alternating with, catarrh - all-c.
dizziness - merc.
headache - kali-p.
itching, in ear - agar.
sharp, pain in left breast - ***kali-c.***
sides - ambr., chel., clem., coloc., ***dulc.,*** lac-c.
tearing, in limbs - merc.
vertigo - merc.
anger, after - cham., nux-v.
anxiety, with - acon., ***coff., merc-c.***
sleep, disturbing - ***merc-c.***
autumn, in the - aur., bry., chin., colch., merc., nux-m., nux-v., rhod., rhus-t., verat.
bed, in - **ANT-C.,** ***aphis., bar-c.,*** bell., ***bov.,*** bry., ***carb-an., cham., clem.,*** com., ***graph., kali-c.,*** **MAG-C.,** ***mag-p.,*** **MERC.,** nux-v., olnd., ***petr.,*** ph-ac., ***phos., puls.,*** rhus-t., sabin., **SULPH.,** ***sul-ac.***
driving out of bed - mag-c., petr., spig.
on going to - carb-an., kali-c.
beer - nux-v., rhus-t., sulph., zinc.
amel. - camph.
belching, on - sulph.
bending, backward, from - calc.
forward with forehead on table, agg. - nit-ac.
amel. - mang.
side, to either, from - calc.
binding, tightly amel. - kali-c., sep.
biting, on elastic substance amel. - mang.
biting, teeth together, when - aesc., ***alum.,*** **AM-C.,** ars., ***aur.,*** bell., bor., ***bry.,*** calc., carb-an., caust., chin., chin-a., coc-c., colch., fl-ac., graph., ***guai.,*** hell., ***hep.,*** hyos., ***ip.,*** lach., lyc., lith., mag-m., mang., ***merc.,*** **MEZ.,** nux-v., petr., ph-ac., phos., ***puls., rhus-t.,*** **SEP.,** ***sil.,*** spong., ***staph., sulph., sul-ac.,*** tab., ***verb.,*** zinc-oc.
afraid for fear teeth would fall out - nit-ac.

PAIN, toothache
biting, teeth together, when
amel. - ars., bell., brom., bry., ***chin.,*** cocc., coff., euph., ign., mag-m., mur-ac., nat-m., ol-an., phos., **PHYT.,** puls., rhus-t., sanic.
menses, during - am-c.
desire to - merc-i-f.
bleeding, of gums amel. - bell., caust., sanic., sars., sel.
blowing, the nose, on - culx., phos., thuj.
amel. - acon.
bread, from eating - carb-an.
breakfast, after - petr.
breathing - carb-v.
deep agg. - ***nux-v.***
brushing, teeth agg. - ***bry.,*** carb-v., coc-c., **LACH.,** lyc., ***staph.***
canines - am-c., anac., calc., calc-p., ***carb-an.,*** laur., mag-m., mur-ac., nat-c., petr., ***rhus-t.,*** sep., staph., stront-c., sul-ac., zinc.
catarrh, when catarrh is better toothache is worse and vice versa - all-c.
chamomile, from - alum., cham., ***puls.***
change of weather - anan., aran., mag-c., merc., ***rhod.***
chewing, from - ***alum., am-c.,*** ant-c., anan., arg-m., arg-n., ***arn.,*** ars., aur., bell., ***bry.,*** calc., ***calc-p.,*** carb-an., ***carb-s., carb-v., caust.,*** **CHAM.,** chel., ***chin., cocc., coff.,*** con., crot-t., ***euph.,*** ferr-ma., ***graph., hyos.,*** hura, ***ign.,*** kali-ar., ***kali-c.,*** kali-p., ***lach., lyc.,*** mag-c., ***mag-m., merc.,*** **NAT-M., NIT-AC.,** ***nux-m., nux-v.,*** olnd., ***ph-ac., phos., puls.,*** rhus-t., sabin., ***sang., sil.,*** spig., spong., ***staph.,*** sulph., ***sul-ac.,*** syph., ***thuj.,*** verat., zinc.
after - nat-m., sabin., staph.
amel. by - bry., rhod., seneg.
only when - calc., lyc., olnd., sabin.
not from empty chewing - cocc.
children, in - acon., ***ant-c., bell., calc., calc-p.,*** **CHAM., COFF., HECLA,** ign., ***mag-p., merc.,*** nux-v., ***puls.,*** rheum.
chill, during - agar., ***carb-v., graph.,*** hell., kali-c., nat-m., **RHUS-T.,** sep., staph.
after - hyos.
chilliness, with - daph., euph., hell., lach., puls., rhod., rhus-t.
chronic - ***caust.***
clinch, together, desires to (see biting) - lyc., ***phyt.***
coffee, from - anan., ***bell., camph.,*** carb-v., **CHAM.,** cocc., ***ign.,*** lachn., merc., ***nux-v., puls.,*** rhus-t., sil.
cold, anything - agar., anan., ant-c., arg-n., ***ars., bar-c.,*** bov., ***calc.,*** calc-p., carb-s., ***carb-v.,*** cast., coc-c., ***colch., con.,*** grat., hell., **KALI-C.,** kali-i., kali-n., kali-p., ***lyc., mag-c.,*** mag-m., ***mag-p.,*** mang., ***merc.,*** **NAT-M.,** ***nit-ac.,*** nux-m., par., ph-ac., ***phos., plan.,*** plb., psor., puls., **RHUS-T.,** rob., **SEP.,** sil., ***spig., staph.,*** sulph., ***sul-ac.,*** syph., thuj.

PAIN, toothache

cold, anything

amel. - ***ambr.,*** bell., bism., bry., calc., caust., cham., chin., ***coff., ferr-p., glon.,*** mag-c., mag-m., merc., nat-s., nux-v., phos., ***puls.,*** sep., staph., sulph.

drinks, from - agar., anan., **ANT-C.,** arg-n., ***ars.,*** bar-c., bry., ***calc.,*** carb-an., carb-s., ***carb-v.,*** cast., caust., cench., ***cham.,*** chin-a., cina, coc-c., ***fl-ac.,*** graph., gymn., **HEP.,** kali-ar., **KALI-C.,** kali-p., **LACH.,** mag-p., ***mang., merc., mur-ac.,*** **NAT-M.,** ***nux-m., nux-v., phos., plan.,*** puls., rhod., **RHUS-T.,** rumx., sabad., ***sars.,*** sel., sil., spig., **STAPH.,** ***sulph., ther.,*** thuj., til.

amel. - ***bism., bry.,*** chim., ***coff.,*** ferr-m., nat-s., ***puls***

food, from - agar., bov., bry., ***calc.,*** carb-v., ***con., glon.,*** hell., merc., nux-v., par., plb., rhus-t., rob., sabad., sulph.

from a cold - ***acon., bar-c.,*** bell., camph., carb-v., ***caust., cham.,*** chin., colch., dulc., ***gels.,*** glon., grat., ***hyos.,*** ign., kali-c., kali-p., ***merc.,*** mez., nat-c., nit-ac., nux-m., ***nux-v.,*** phos., ***puls.,*** rhus-t., staph., sul-ac., zinc.

in the spring - puls.

hand applied amel. - ang., rhus-t.

head, on - kali-c.

overheating, after - ***cham., glon.,*** kali-c., ***rhus-t.***

water agg. - mag-c.

water amel. - ***aesc., all-c., ambr.,*** ap-g., bell., ***bism.,*** bry., camph., ***caust., cham.,*** chel., ***chin., clem.,*** **COFF.,** ***ferr., ferr-p.,*** fl-ac., ***lac-c.,*** laur., ***mag-c.,*** mag-m., merc., ***nat-s.,*** nux-v., phos., **PULS.,** rhus-t., sel., sep., sulph., thuj.

icy-cold - ferr.

weather, from - ars., nux-m., ***phos.***

coryza, with - am-m.

coughing, agg. - bry., lyc., sep.

crumbs, of bread, from - clem., nux-v., ***staph.***

damp, places, from working in - ***ars.,*** **CALC.,** ***dulc.,*** **RHUS-T.**

weather - acon., all-c., am-c., aran., ***bor., calc., dulc.,*** **MERC.,** nat-c., ***nat-s., nux-m., phos., rhod.,*** **RHUS-T.,** seneg., ***sil.***

daytime - bar-c., bell., calc., carb-an., ***cocc-s.,*** nux-v., ust.

dental, work, after - acon., **ARN.,** ***calen., hecla.,*** hep., **HYPER.,** led., merc-i-f., staph.

diverted, when, amel. - bar-c., pip-m., thuj.

drinking, from - bar-c., ***caust., cham.,*** con., ***mag-p.,*** sabin., sil.

amel., from - sel., spig.

dry, weather - ***caust.***

eating, during - ***am-c.,*** anan., ant-c., aur., bar-c., ***bry., calc.,*** canth., carb-an., carb-s., carb-v., ***cast., caust.,*** cocc., ***con.,*** crot-h., crot-t., euph., graph., hep., ign., **KALI-C.,** ***lyc., mag-c., mag-m.,*** mag-s., **MERC.,**

PAIN, toothache

eating, during - ***nat-c.,*** nux-m., phos., psor., puls., sabin., sep., ***sil., staph.,*** sulph., thuj., trom., verat.

amel. - am-c., bell., ***cham.,*** chin., coff., ip., ph-ac., sel., sil., ***spig.***

only - calc., kali-c.

after - ***alum.,*** am-c., **ANT-C.,** ars-i., bar-c., ***bell.,*** bor., ***bry.,*** carb-s., ***carb-v., cham.,*** chel., ***chim.,*** chin., coff., ferr-p., ***graph., hep., ign.,*** iod., ***kali-c., lach., lyc., mag-c.,*** mag-s., ***merc., nat-c., nat-m., nux-m., nux-v.,*** puls., rhus-t., ***sabin.,*** sil., spig., stann., **STAPH.,** ***sulph.,*** zinc.

amel. - ambr., am-c., arn., calc., carb-v., ip., ph-ac., **RHOD.,** rhus-t., sil.

dinner, before - nux-v., sulph.

evening - ail., ***alum.,*** ambr., **AM-C.,** anac., ***ant-c.,*** arum-t., apis, bar-c., ***bell.,*** bov., bry., bufo, calad., ***carb-s.,*** caust., cham., chel., ferr., graph., hep., ***hyos.,*** ign., kali-c., ***kali-i.,*** kali-n., kali-p., kali-s., ***kalm., lyc.,*** mag-c., ***mag-s.,*** mang., ***merc.,*** meph., mez., nicc., nit-ac., nux-m., ***nux-v., phos.,*** **PULS.,** ***rat., rhus-t.,*** sars., sabin., ***staph., sulph., sul-ac.,*** tab., ther., thuj.

6 p.m., lasting till 1 or 2 a.m. - sep.

in bed - alum., **AM-C., ANT-C.,** ang., aran., bar-c., bell., bov., ***bry., calc.,*** carb-ac., ***cham.,*** chr-ac., graph., ***ign., kali-c.,*** led., kali-n., **MAG-C.,** mag-m., ***merc.,*** nat-c., nit-ac., phos., ***puls.,*** sel., **SULPH.,** ***sul-ac.,*** zinc.

amel. - alum.

smoking amel. - spig.

excitement, from - ***acon.,*** bell., ***cham., coff., gels.,*** hyos.

excitement, from, amel. - thuj.

exertion, of mind and body, with - chim., nux-v.

agg. - chim.

extending to

arms - mang., sep.

left arm - coloc.

bones, to, cheek - alum., caust., chen-a., con., ham., hyos., kali-c., mag-c., mag-m., ***mang.,*** mez., nux-v., phos., rob., ***sil.***

maxillary - calc., cupr-ar., gels., sel.

maxillary, lower - hyos.

cheeks, to - bry., cham.

chest, to - kali-c.

downward - ant-c., calad., cann-i., carb-v., caust., coff., crot-h.

ear, to - alum., ***ammc.,*** am-c., anac., aphis., ***arn.,*** ars., bar-c., bell., bor., brach., bry., ***calc.,*** calc-ar., ***caust., cham.,*** chel., ***chr-ac.,*** chin., clem., cocc-s., coloc., con., hep., indg., kali-ar., kali-c., **KREOS.,** ***lach.,*** lyss., mag-c., **MANG., MERC.,** meph., mez., ***nat-m.,*** nicc., nux-m., nux-v., ol-an., petr., ***plan.,*** puls., ran-s., rat., **RHOD.,** rhus-t., sabad., sang., **SEP., STAPH., SULPH.,** thuj., viol-o.

right - glon., nicc., spig.

esophagus, to - nat-m.

PAIN, toothache
extending, to
eyes, to - bar-c., bell., calc., ***calc-p.,*** **CAUST.,** cham., chel., chim., clem., con., hyos., kali-c., kreos., lach., ***mag-c.,*** merc., nat-m., nicc., nux-v., puls., rob., sel., spig., staph., sulph., tarax.
on going into cold air - camph.
face, to - alum., am-c., ***bry.,*** caust., cham., cocc., gels., glon., ***hyos.,*** kali-c., kreos., lyss., mag-c., **MERC.,** nux-v., phos., puls., rhus-t., sabad., ***sil.,*** staph., sulph., tarax.
during menses - sep.
left side - plan.
fingers, to - coff., sep.
forehead, to - chr-ac., ***hyos.,*** kali-c., phos., rhus-t., sil., zinc.
head, to - alum., **ANT-C.,** apis, ***ars.,*** bar-c., bor., ***bry.,*** calc., caust., ***cham.,*** clem., cupr., glon., grat., ***hyos.,*** kali-ar., kali-c., ***kreos., mag-c.,*** merc., mez., nux-m., nux-v., ***ph-ac.,*** phos., psor., puls., rhus-t., ***sang.,*** staph., sulph.
larynx, to - ***alum.,*** com., ***mang.,*** nit-ac.
lower limbs, to - chen-a., kali-c., lycps., lyss.
neck, to - ***alum., bry., mang.,*** spig., thuj., zinc.
nose, to - bar-c., calc., **CAUST.,** cham., hyos., rhus-t.
occiput, to - cocc-s.
other parts, to - **MANG.**
outwardly, to - chin.
shoulder, to - ***alum.,*** rhus-t.
side, to, entire left - sep.
temples, to - act-sp., alum., ars., bar-c., calc., cham., chel., clem., con., cupr., daph., gels., glon., iod., kali-ar., kali-c., **KREOS.,** mag-c., mez., nat-m., nux-m., phos., puls., rhus-t., rob., sel., sil., spig., zinc.
throat, to - **MANG.,** ***nat-m.***
tongue, to - cic.
tooth, to another, from one - **BRY.,** ***mang.,*** nux-m., prun., ***puls.,*** rhod., til.
upward - caps., caust., clem., nat-c., nit-ac., ol-an., syph., thuj.
zygoma, to - **CAUST.,** chin-s., phos.
extraction, after - **ARN.,** calen., **HYPER.,** staph.
filled tooth, in a - cic., dios., merc-i-f., plan.
fillings, after - **ARN.,** hyper., merc., ***merc-i-f.,*** **NUX-V.,** plan., sep.
forenoon - all-s., carb-v., caust., cham., kali-c., kali-p., mang., nat-m., nux-v., puls., staph., sulph.
fruit, after eating - nat-c., nat-s.
gradually, increasing and decreasing - bell., stann.
healthy teeth, in - **ACON.,** alum., am-c., arg-n., arn., ars., bell., bry., carb-v., caust., ***cham., coff.,*** con., ham., hyos., ***mag-c.,*** nux-v., plan., rhus-t., rhod., spig., staph., sulph., zinc.
heat of bed, from - sabin.
of stove, amel. - **ARS.**
heated, when - phos., zinc.

PAIN, toothache
hot food, from - ***carb-v.,*** **COFF., KALI-C.,** lach., ph-ac., sabad., sep.
liquids amel. - ***mag-p.***
incisors - ***agar.,*** alum., ambr., am-c., am-m., ang., arg-m., asaf., asar., aur., bell., bor., bov., calc., canth., carb-v., caust., cham., chel., chin., cocc., coff., ***colch.,*** dig., dros., ign., iod., ***kali-c.,*** kreos., lyc., mag-c., ***mag-m.,*** mag-arct., ***merc.,*** mez., mur-ac., nat-c., ***nat-m.,*** nit-ac., ***nux-m., nux-v.,*** petr., ph-ac., phos., plat., ran-s., rhod., ***rhus-t.,*** sars., seneg., **SEP.,** sil., spig., spong., staph., ***stront-c., sulph.,*** sul-ac., tarax., thuj., ***zinc.***
incisors, lower - chin., nat-m.
injury, from - **ARN.,** hyper., ***nux-m.***
inspiration, on - carb-v., ***nux-v.***
intermittent - **ANT-T.,** ars-i., astac., ***bell., bor.,*** bry., calc., ***chin., cham., coff.,*** merc., nux-v., ***puls.,*** rhod., rhus-t., sabad., sil., ***staph., sulph.***
jarring, agg. - nux-m.
laying, forehead on table amel. - mang.
leaning, against pillow - nit-ac.
left - ***acon.,*** agar., ***apis,*** arg-n., ***arn.,*** arum-t., ***aur.,*** bar-c., brom., carb-v., cast., **CAUST., CHAM.,** chel., ***chin.,*** **CLEM.,** ***form., guai.,*** hyos., ***kali-c.,*** laur., merc., **MEZ.,** ***nux-m., olnd., phos.,*** rhus-t., **SEP.,** ***sil.,*** **SULPH.,** syph., **THUJ.,** ***zinc.***
to right - all-c., gamb.
loose, teeth - der., merc.
lower, teeth - aesc., ***agar.,*** alum., ambr., am-c., am-m., anac., ang., ***arn.,*** arum-t., asaf., asar., asc-t., astac., ***aur.,*** bar-c., **BELL.,** bor., bov., ***bry.,*** calc., camph., **CANTH.,** carb-an., ***carb-v.,*** **CAUST., CHAM.,** chel., ***chin.,*** cic., clem., cocc., coff., colch., coloc., con., dros., euph., graph., guai., hell., hep., hyos., ign., kali-c., kali-n., kreos., ***lach.,*** **LAUR.,** lyc., mag-arct., mag-c., mag-m., ***mang.,*** merc., mez., mur-ac., **NAT-C.,** nat-m., nit-ac., nux-m., nux-v., olnd., par., petr., ph-ac., ***phos.,*** plat., ***plb.,*** puls., ran-s., rheum, rhod., ***rhus-t.,*** ruta., sabad., ***sabin., sars.,*** sel., seneg., **SEP.,** ***sil.,*** spig., spong., squil., **STAPH.,** stront-c., sulph., sul-ac., thuj., teucr., ***verat.,*** verb., **ZINC.**
first bi-cuspid - ars.
one incisor - anac.
second molar - aesc.
lying, while - aran., ars., bell., bry., ***cham., clem., graph., hyos.,*** ign., merc., nux-v., olnd., ***phos., petr.,*** puls., ***rhus-t.,*** sep., staph., sulph., ***sul-ac.,*** trom.
amel. - alum., am-m., ***bry.,*** lyc., nat-c., ***nux-v.,*** spig.
head high, with, agg. - spig.
low, with, agg. - puls.
immediately after - ***aran.,*** bell., canth., hell., ign., puls., rat., sanic.
painful side, agg. - ars., ign., guare., nux-v., puls.

PAIN, toothache

lying, while

painful side, amel. - **BRY.,** chin-s., hyper., ign., kali-n., mag-c., puls.

painless side, agg. - **BRY.,** ***cham.,*** ign., puls.

amel. - nux-v.

right side, on - spig.

menses, during - ***am-c., ars.,*** bar-c., ***bov., calc.,*** carb-v., cast., ***cedr., cham., coff., graph.,*** kali-ar., ***kali-c., lach.,*** laur., mag-c., ***nat-m., nit-ac.,*** phos., ***puls.,*** **SEP., STAPH.,** sul-ac.

if the flow diminishes - **LACH.**

menorrhagia - ***ferr-s.***

after - am-c., ***calc.,*** cham., mag-c., mag-p., phos., thuj.

at beginning - ***nat-m., puls.***

at beginning, and end - ***puls.***

before - agar., am-c., ***ant-c.,*** ars., bar-c., calc., cham., mag-c., ***nat-m.,*** phos., ***puls.,*** sep., ***sulph.,*** thuj., zinc.

mental, exertion, from - bell., ***ign., nux-v.***

mercury, from - colch., ***hep., merc., nit-ac., staph.***

midnight, after - alum., am-c., ***ars.,*** bar-m., bell., bry., carb-v., cham., chin., ***merc.,*** nat-m., puls., rhus-t., ***staph.,*** sulph.

before - alum., am-c., bov., bry., ***cham.,*** chin., graph., ***nat-m.,*** petr., puls., rhus-t., sep., stry., sulph., sul-ac., thuj., zinc.

molars - aesc., agar., all-c., alum., ambr., ***am-c.,*** anac., ang., ant-t., arg-n., arn., asar., asc-t., aur., bar-c., bell., bism., bor., bov., **BRY.,** calad., calc., camph., canth., carb-an., ***carb-v.,*** cast., ***caust.,*** cham., **CHIN.,** clem., cocc., coff., colch., coloc., croc., cycl., dios., euph., graph., guai., hell., hyos., ign., iod., kali-c., kali-n., **KREOS.,** laur., lyc., mag-arct., mag-c., ***mag-m.,*** mang., merc., mez., mur-ac., ***nat-c., nit-ac.,*** nux-m., nux-v., olnd., par., petr., ph-ac., ***phos.,*** plat., plb., puls., ran-s., rheum, ***rhod.,*** rhus-t., sabad., sabin., sars., seneg., **SEP.,** sil., spig., spong., ***staph.,*** stront-c., sulph., sul-ac., teucr., thuj., verat., verb., **ZINC.,** zing.

left - arg-n., cast., chel.

right - cinnb.

morning - ant-t., arg-n., ars., bar-c., bry., calad., camph., carb-v., caust., chin., clem., ***ferr., hyos.,*** kreos., lach., mag-c., merc., nat-m., nux-v., ph-ac., phos., plat., ***puls.,*** rhod., ***rhus-t.,*** sulph.

3 a.m. - bry.

bed, in - kali-c., kreos., lach., mang., mez., nux-v., ran-b., ***staph.***

wakes him - calad., nat-c.

waking, on - bell., carb-v., coc-c., ***ign.,*** kali-c., ***lach.,*** mag-c., ***nux-v.,*** sil.

rising, after - bar-c., mag-c., plat., sep.

when washing - arg-n.

rising, amel. - sil.

PAIN, toothache

motion, agg. - ***bry.,*** chel., ***chin.,*** clem., daph., hyper., kali-c., merc., ***mez., nux-v.,*** sabin., spig., staph.

amel. - ***mag-c.,*** phos., ***puls., rhus-t.***

music, agg. - ph-ac.

nervous, patients - ***acon., ars., bell.,*** **CHAM., COFF.,** ***gels.,*** hyos., **HYPER.,** ***ign., mag-p., puls.,*** staph.

night - ambr., ***am-c.,*** alum., anac., ***ant-c.,*** aran., ***ars., aur.,*** bar-c., ***bell.,*** berb., bov., bry., bufo, calc., calc-p., carb-an., **CARB-S.,** ***carb-v., cedr.,*** **CHAM.,** ***chel.,*** chin., chin-a., ***clem.,*** coff., ***colch.,*** crot-c., ***cycl., glon.,*** **GRAPH.,** grat., hell., ***hep.,*** hyper., ip., kali-c., kali-i., kali-n., ***kali-p.,*** **LYC., MAG-C.,** mag-m., **MERC.,** ***merc-c., mez.,*** naja, nat-a., nat-c., nat-h., ***nat-m.,*** nat-p., ***nat-s.,*** nicc., ***nit-ac.,*** nux-m., ***nux-v., olnd.,*** par., petr., ***ph-ac., phos., psor., puls., rhod., rhus-t.,*** rob., sabad., sabin., ***sep., sil., spig., staph.,*** **SULPH.,** sul-ac.

9 p.m - **MERC.**

10 p.m - rhus-t.

10 to 12 pm - mang.

3 a.m. - bry., cham., kali-n.

chilliness as it disappears - merc.

lying, when - ***aran.,*** ars., graph., phos.

noise, agg. - calc., ***coff.,*** tarent., ***ther.***

noon - cocc., rhus-t.

nursing, mothers, in - acon., ars., bell., ***calc.,*** dulc., merc., nux-v., phos., staph., sulph.

while the infant nurses - ***chin.***

one-sided - acon.

opening, mouth from - bry., caust., hep., nux-v., petr., phos., puls., sabin.

paroxysmal - all-s., anac., bor., calc., ***cham.,*** gels., glon., hyper., ip., lac-c., lyc., merc., ***nux-m.,*** petr., ***plat.,*** rumx., sep., sulph.

pears, after eating - nat-c.

periodical - aran., ars., cham., chin-a., chin-s., coff., coloc., lach.

every other day - ***cham.,*** nat-m.

every seven days - ars., calc-ar., phos., sulph.

perspiration, during - **CHIN.,** hyos.

amel. - all-c., aphis., carb-ac., carb-an.

suppressed, from - cham.

tendency to perspire - daph.

picking, amel. by - ***all-c.,*** am-c., bell., ph-ac., sanic.

picking, excited by - kali-c., ***puls., sang.***

pregnancy, during - ***acon.,*** alum., apis, ***bell.,*** bry., ***calc., cham., hyos.,*** **LYSS.,** ***mag-c., merc., nux-m.,*** nux-v., ***puls., rat.,*** rhus-t., **SEP.,** ***staph., tab.***

pressure, agg. - carb-an., **CHAM.,** hyos., kali-bi., mag-m., nat-c., nat-m., phos., sep., spig., sulph., sul-ac., zinc.

PAIN, toothache

pressure , amel. - ail., ***alum.,*** am-c., am-m., ars., bell., ***brom.,*** bry., chin., clem., cocc., coloc., com., euph., grat., ign., indg., ***kali-c.,*** laur., kali-n., ***mag-m., mag-p.,*** merc-i-f., mur-ac., nat-c., nat-m., nat-p., ol-an., ***phos.,*** puls., rhus-t., sep., ***staph.,*** tab.
of cold hand amel. - rhus-t.

pulse, synchronous, with - clem.

quinine, from abuse of - ***hep., nit-ac.,*** **PULS.**

reading, while - calc., ign., ***nux-v.,*** thuj.

riding, in a carriage, while - calc., ***mag-c.***

right - astac., **BELL.,** brach., ***bry., calc.,*** cann-s., ***carb-ac., caust.,*** chr-ac., cinnb., coff., com., ***cycl.,*** dios., dol., **FL-AC.,** lach., lyss., ***mag-c.,*** nat-m., nit-ac., ***nux-v., petr.,*** phos., ***psor.,*** spig., **STAPH.,** verb.
to left - **ACON.,** lyc.

rising, from bed amel. - clem., mag-c., olnd., ***phos.,*** sabin.

rubbing, cheek amel. - **MERC.,** ***phos.***

saliva, with involuntary flow of - bell., ***cham.,*** daph., ***dulc.,*** **MERC.,** nat-m.

salt, amel. - mag-c.

salty, food, from agg. - carb-v.
amel. - ***carb-an.***

sex, after - daph.
relieved after - camph.

sitting, agg. - am-m., ant-c., cocc-s., graph., merc., ***puls.,*** rhus-t.
erect agg. - mang.
quiet amel. - spig.
up in bed amel. - alum., ***ars.,*** bar-m., merc., petr., rhus-t.

sleep, after - bar-m., bell., bry., calc., carb-v., ***caust.,*** con., graph., ***kali-c.,*** kali-p., ***lach.,*** nux-v., ***phos.,*** sabin., sil., spig., sulph., zinc.
amel. - merc., nux-v., puls., sanic.
on going to - ant-t., ars., ***merc.,*** sulph.
wakes from, with pain - ars., bell., calc., ***carb-an.,*** chel., lach., mag-c., mez., spig., sulph., zinc.

sneezing, agg. - thuj.

something, in, as if - nat-m.

sounds, shrill, from - ther.

sour, things, from - arg-n., cimic., cupr., dulc.
amel. - puls.

spring, in the - acon., aur., ***bell., bry., calc.,*** carb-v., ***dulc.,*** **LACH.,** lyc., ***nat-m.,*** nux-v., ***puls.,*** rhod., ***rhus-t.,*** sep., sil., sulph., verat.

standing, up, after - ign., plat., sep.
amel. - alum., nux-v., olnd., phos., sabin., spig.

stimulants, agg. - acon.

stooping, agg. - sep., spig.
amel. - arn.

sucking, agg. - bell., ***bov., carb-v.,*** cast., kali-c., mang., ***nux-m.,*** nux-v., sil., zinc.
amel. - all-c., bov., caust., ***clem.,*** mang., sep.

suddenly, begins and goes - ***bell.,*** sanic.
ceases, begins slowly - sul-ac.

PAIN, toothache

summer, in the - ant-c., bell., bry., calc., carb-v., cham., lach., lyc., nat-c., ***nat-m.,*** nux-v., puls., sel.

suppressed, footsweat, after - **SIL.**
gout, after - sabin.

swallowing, agg. - alum., chin-s., phos., staph.

sweets, after - am-c., ***nat-c.,*** phos., sep.
amel. - cham., chelo.

swelling of, cheek, with toothache - all-c., am-c., ***ant-c.,*** arn., ars., aur., **BELL.,** bor., **BRY.,** ***calc.,*** calc-f., ***calc-s.,*** caps., caust., **CHAM.,** colch., ***euph.,*** **HECLA.,** ***hep., kali-c.,*** **LACH.,** ***lyc.,*** mag-arct., ***mag-c.,*** **MERC.,** nat-c., ***nat-m.,*** nux-v., petr., ph-ac., phos., ***puls.,*** samb., **SEP., SIL.,** ***spig.,*** staph., stront-c., sulph., ***verat.***

talking, from - am-c., ars., bry., ***cham.,*** chel., nux-m., ***nux-v.,*** sep., trom.
of others agg. - ars., bry.

tea, drinking - chin., coff., ferr., ign., lach., ***sel., sep.,*** thuj.

thinking, about, it - bar-c., ***nux-v., spig.,*** thuj.

thunderstorm, before - **RHOD.**

tobacco, chewing - ***bry.***
smoking - ***bry., caust., cham.,*** chin., clem., ***ign., merc., nux-v.,*** sabin., sars., **SPIG.,** thuj.
amel. - aran., bor., camph., ***merc., nat-c., nat-s.,*** sel., spig.

touch - alum., am-c., anac., anag., ant-c., ***arn.,*** ars., aur., bar-c., ***bell.,*** bor., ***bry., calc.,*** camph., carb-an., carb-s., ***carb-v.,*** cast., caust., chel., **CHIN.,** chin-a., clem., coc-c., coff., daph., ***euph., graph., hep.,*** ign., kali-n., ***lyc.,*** mag-c., mag-m., mag-s., ***mang.,*** merc., ***merc-c., mez., nat-m., nux-m., nux-v., ph-ac., phos.,*** plan., psor., ***puls.,*** rat., rhod., rhus-t., sabin., **SEP.,** ***staph., sulph.,*** thuj.
amel. - bry., nat-m., nux-v., sep.
cheek, of - mag-m., nat-c.
food of, from - alum., bell., camph., kali-c., mag-m., mag-s., nit-ac., rob., sang.
tongue, of - am-c., anac., **ANT-C.,** bor., bry., calc., carb-v., cast., chin., ign., mag-c., ***merc., mez.,*** nat-c., nat-m., phos., rhus-t., sep., thuj.

travelling, while - ars., ***bry., cham.,*** puls., rhus-t., staph., sulph.

uncovering, body amel. - puls.

upper, teeth - ***agar., alum.,*** ambr., **AM-C.,** am-m., ang., arn., asar., ***aur., bell.,*** bor., bov., ***calc.,*** canth., carb-ac., carb-an., **CARB-V.,** ***caust., cham.,*** chel., **CHIN.,** clem., cocc., coff., colch., con., cycl., dios., euph., graph., guai., hell., hyos., kali-n., **KREOS.,** lyc., mag-arct., mag-aust., mag-c., ***mag-m.,*** mang., merc., ***mez.,*** mur-ac., ***nat-c., nat-m., nit-ac.,*** nux-m., nux-v., ***phos.,*** ph-ac., plat., puls., ran-s., rheum, rhod., rhus-t., sabad., sars., seneg., sep., sil., ***spig., spong.,*** staph., stry., sulph., ***sul-ac.,*** teucr., ***thuj.,*** verat., verb., **ZINC.**

PAIN, toothache
upper, teeth
left - arn., chel., rheum., stry.
second bi-cuspid - olnd.
right bi-cuspid - cinnb.
bi-cuspid, molar - dios.
vexation, after - ***acon., cham.,*** rhus-t., ***staph.***
vinegar amel. - puls.
walking, while - camph., guare., nux-v., ***phos.***
amel. - ***mag-c., puls.,*** rat., ***rhus-t.,*** spig.
open air in - agn., cham., con., dros., graph., kali-c., kali-n., mag-s., ***nat-c.,*** nux-v., phos., sabad., sabin., staph.
amel. - **ANT-C.,** bov., bry., clem., hep., ***kali-s.,*** lyc., mag-arct., mag-m., ***nux-v.,*** par., **PULS.,** rhus-t., sep.
in the wind - graph.
wandering - ambr., graph., hyos., mag-p., mang., nux-v., puls., thuj., til.
warm, drinks, from - aesc., agn., ***all-c.,*** am-c., am-m., bism., ***bry., carb-v.,*** **CHAM., COFF.,** ***dros., ferr-p.,*** fl-ac., **LACH.,** ***merc.,*** mill., ***nat-s., nit-ac.,*** ph-ac., **PULS.,** rhus-t., sabad., **SEP.,** sil., syph., trom.
amel. - ***ars.,*** bry., cast., ***lyc., mag-p.,*** nux-m., ***nux-v.,*** puls., ***rhus-t.,*** sang., sil., staph., sulph., sul-ac., trom.
food, from - agn., ***ambr., bar-c.,*** bell., ***bism., bry., calc., carb-s.,*** carb-v., ***caust.,*** **CHAM.,** ***clem., coff., graph.,*** guare., ***hell.,*** **KALI-C.,** mag-arct., mag-aust., mag-s., merc., ***nat-m., nux-v.,*** par., ph-ac., ***phos.,*** **PULS.,** rhod., sabad., sep., ***sil.***
things - agn., ***ambr.,*** am-c., anac., ***bar-c., bry.,*** **CALC.,** calc-p., carb-s., ***carb-v.,*** **CHAM.,** chel., clem., colch., **COFF.,** ***ferr-p.,*** glon., ***graph.,*** hell., **KALI-C.,** lach., lachn., mag-m., mag-s., ***merc.,*** nat-m., ***nit-ac.,*** par., ph-ac., ***phos., plan.,*** **PULS.,** prun., ***sep., sil.,*** spig., staph., ***sulph.***
amel. - bov., calc., ***com.,*** kali-i., ***lyc.,*** **MAG-P.,** mur-ac., nit-ac., ***nux-m., nux-v.,*** psor., ***rhod., rhus-t., sil.,*** sul-ac.
warmth, external - ***ambr.,*** arn., all-c., ***bry.,*** carb-s., carb-v., chel., **COFF.,** ***cor-r., ferr., ferr-p.,*** graph., hell., hep., lach., mag-c., mag-s., nux-m., ph-ac., ***phos.,*** **PULS.,** sabin., ***sulph.***
external, amel. - am-c., arg-n., ***ars., ars-h.,*** bov., ***calc., cast., chin., com., kali-ar., kali-c.,*** lach., ***lyc.,*** mag-m., **MAG-P., MERC.,** ***mur-ac.,*** nat-a., ***nat-c.,*** nat-p., **NUX-M., NUX-V.,** phos., ***puls., psor.,*** **RHOD., RHUS-T.,** sabad., staph., ***sil., sul-ac.***
wrapping up head amel. - **NUX-V.,** phos., **SIL.**
bed, of, agg. - ant-c., bell., bry., **CHAM.,** chel., clem., graph., jug-r., led., ***mag-c.,*** **MERC.,** ***ph-ac.,*** phos., **PULS.,** rhod., sabin., sulph.

PAIN, toothache
warmth, external
bed, of, amel. - ***lyc.,*** mag-s., ***nux-v., sil., spig.,*** vinc.
room, agg. - ***all-c.,*** nat-c., apis, bry., ***cham.,*** ham., ***hep., iris, kali-s., mag-c.,*** merc., nicc., nux-v., ph-ac., **PULS.,** rhod., sep., spig., sulph., thuj.
amel. - ***ars.,*** nux-v., phel., ***phos.,*** sulph.
washer, women, in - ***phos.***
washing, after - ant-c., bry., ***calc.,*** cham., ***merc., nux-m.,*** nux-v., phos., ***rhus-t.,*** sil., staph., **SULPH.**
with cold water, from - calc., cham., graph., kali-c., merc., nux-m., nux-v., puls., sep., ***spig.,*** staph., **SULPH.**
amel. - ***all-c.,*** asar., bell., bry., cham., clem., kali-c., laur., ***puls.***
water, from having hands in, warm or cold - ***phos.***
feet in water, from - nat-n.
held in mouth, agg. - camph., kali-c.
wet, from getting - bell., ***calc.,*** **LACH.,** rhus-t.
fingers - cham.
wind, amel. - calc.
in dry, cold - **ACON.,** ***caust.***
in raw - **ACON.,** all-c., caust., ***graph., puls., rhod.,*** rhus-t., sil.
wine, agg. - ***acon.,*** anan., ***camph.,*** ign., nux-v.
winter - ***acon.,*** **ARS.,** bell., bry., calc., carb-v., caust., cham., dulc., **HEP.,** hyos., ign., **MERC.,** ***nux-m.,*** **NUX-V.,** ***ph-ac., phos.,*** puls., **RHUS-T., SIL.,** sulph.

PARALYSIS, jaws, as if - nux-m.
paralysis, jaws, lower - arn., ars., bapt., carb-v., colch., crot-h., dulc., ***hell., hyos.,*** lach., ***lyc., mur-ac., nux-v.,*** op., ***phos.,*** ran-b., ***sec., stram., sulph., zinc.***
evening - ran-b.

PERIOSTITIS, teeth, inflammation of periosteum - agar., ant-c., ***apis, ars., asaf.,*** aur., ***aur-m.,*** bell., chin., **FL-AC.,** ***kali-i.,*** led., ***mang., merc., merc-c.,*** **MEZ.,** ***nit-ac.,*** **PH-AC.,** ***phos.,*** phyt., ***psor.,*** puls., rhus-t., **RUTA.,** ***sil., staph.***

PICKING, teeth - zinc.

PIERCING, pain, teeth - acon., ant-c., bell., ***bry.,*** calc., caust., ***cham.,*** chin., ***lach., merc.,*** nux-m., nux-v., ph-ac., ***puls.,*** rhus-t., sil., staph.

PINCHING, pain, teeth - am-c., ***aran.,*** carb-v., iod., kali-c., lyc., mag-c.
cold drinks, from - carb-an.
pinching, jaws, in, articulation of - ***bry.,*** colch., gran.

PRESSING, pain, teeth - acon., ***all-c.,*** am-c., anac., aran., ***arn.,*** ars., bism., bor., bov., bry., ***calc.,*** carb-v., caust., cham., chel., chin., ***coloc.,*** con., cor-r., euph., ***graph.,*** guare., guai., hyos., ign., iod., ***kali-c.,*** kali-p., ***kalm.,*** led., lob., **MERC.,** mez., ***nat-c., nat-m.,*** nat-p., nux-m., nux-v., olnd., petr., phos., ***rhod., rhus-t.,*** sep., ***sil.,*** spig., ***staph., sulph.,*** tarax., verat.

PRESSING, pain, teeth
asunder, expansive - anan., kalm., mur-ac., nat-m., ph-ac., ran-b., sabin., spig., spong., thuj.
dinner, after - ***kali-c.***
filling, of the - chlol.
incisor, in one - alum., sul-ac.
inward - rhus-t., staph.
molars - mez., petr., sep., zinc.
outward - arn., bell., berb., ***phos.***, ***puls.***, spig., zinc.
roots, in - alum., caust., ***kali-c.***, staph., zing.
swallowing, when - alum.
together send a shock through head, ears and nose - am-c.
transitory jerking, in upper molars and jaws, right side, in afternoon - all-s.
upper teeth - acon., aran., calc., nat-m.
warm room, on entering - all-c.

pressing, jaws, angle of - ph-ac., sil., spig.
evening - nat-c.

pressing, jaws, joints, of - asaf., dros., kali-n., nat-m., op., paeon., verb.
behind - tarax.
motion, on - kali-n.
swallowing, on - kali-n.

pressing, jaws, lower - ambr., ang., aur., berb., chin., cupr., guai., led., lyss., mag-m., petr., phos., ***sars.***, sil., spig., stront-c., ***verb.***
extending, backward - lyc.
inward - led.
nape - petr.
to chin - phos.
to ear - petr.
night - graph., sil.
right, night - chin.

pressing, jaws, upper - acon., ars., aster., calc., chel., graph., iod., kali-bi., lach., zinc.
right, night - chin

PRESSING, sensation, as if, teeth
blood were forced into them - arn., calc., chin.
held in a grip - nux-m., ***sil.***
into, sockets - alum., am-c.
pressed into, old stumps - alum.
shred of meat were between the teeth, as if a - ***caust.***, ***cor-r.***, ***lach.***, ptel.
too close - acon., arn., bell., calc., cham., chin., ***coff.***, hep., hyos., ***nux-v.***, puls.
wedged - anan., ***caust.***, ***cor-r.***, ***lach.***, ptel., ***rhus-t.***, spong.

PRICKING, pain, teeth - am-c., ant-c., bar-m., calc., caust., hell., mag-s., nux-m., phos., prun.
chewing, agg. - am-c.
molars, especially - am-c.
night, waking him - calc.
touching decayed teeth - am-c.

PROUD, flesh, teeth surrounded by - alumn.

PULLED, out, sensation, as if teeth were being - anan., ***arn.***, astac., bell., berb., bov., bufo, ***calc.***, caust., coc-c., cocc-s., com., con., ip., mag-arct., ***mag-c.***, mang., ***mez.***, mur-ac., nat-c., nux-m., nux-v., ph-ac., prun., puls., ***rhus-t.***, sabin., sel., stront-c., sulph., zinc.

PULLED, out, sensation,
and left in their sockets, as if - sanic.

PULSATING, pain - ***acon.***, agar., ***agn.***, ***all-c.***, aloe, am-c., ang., apis, arn., ***ars.***, bar-c., bar-m., **BELL.**, brom., ***calc.***, cann-i., carb-an., ***carb-s.***, ***carb-v.***, **CAUST.**, **CHAM.**, **CHIN.**, ***chin-a.***, coc-c., cocc-s., ***coff.***, ***coloc.***, daph., ***euph.***, euphr., ***glon.***, hep., ***hyos.***, kali-ar., ***kali-c.***, kali-n., kali-p., **LACH.**, ***lyc.***, ***mag-c.***, mag-s., ***merc.***, mur-ac., nat-a., nat-c., ***nat-m.***, nat-p., ***nat-s.***, ***nit-ac.***, nux-m., par., phos., plat., psor., ***puls.***, rat., ***rhus-t.***, sabad., sabin., **SEP.**, ***sil.***, ***spig.***, ***staph.***, stram., **SULPH.**, ***tarent.***, thuj., ***verat.***, zinc.
roots, in - mag-m., sep.

PULSATION, jaws, lower - bov., carb-an., cham., cupr-ar., ind., ***lach.***, nat-c., nat-m., petr., plat., stram.
biting agg. - nat-m.
evening - ind.

pulsation, jaws, upper - phos.

PULSATIONS, teeth, painless - alum., ars., sanic.

QUIVERING, jaws, lower - agar., nat-c.

RHEUMATIC pain, teeth - acon., **ANT-T.**, bell., ***bry.***, calc-p., ***cham.***, chin-s., ***cimic.***, coch., ***colch.***, guai., indg., ***mag-c.***, ***mag-p.***, ***merc.***, mill., nux-v., ***phyt.***, ***puls.***, rhod., sep., sil., staph.

RIGG'S disease, teeth - merc.

ROUGHNESS, sensation of teeth - fl-ac.
tartar, from - ***mez.***

SCRAPING, pain, teeth - berb., cham.
roots, as if scraped with a knife - arn.

SCREWING, pain, teeth - ***bry.***, **EUPH.**, mag-c.
better momentarily, from cold water - bry.

SENSITIVE, teeth, tender - agar., alum., ***am-c.***, ***ant-c.***, arg-n., aur-m., bar-c., bol., ***bry.***, carb-an., card-m., caust., **CHAM.**, coc-c., **COFF.**, ***colch.***, ferr., ***fl-ac.***, gymn., **HYPER.**, kali-bi., kali-c., ***kalm.***, **LACH.**, lyss., ***mag-c.***, **MAG-P.**, manc., mang., **MERC.**, merc-c., merc-i-r., mez., ***nat-c.***, ***nat-m.***, pall., plan., phos., sars., senec., seneg., ***sil.***, staph., ***sulph.***, zinc.
air, to - ***acon.***, aran., ***bell.***, berb., bry., **CALC.**, calc-p., calc-s., cina, mag-p., **NAT-M.**, ox-ac., sin-n., sulph.
brushing - nat-m.
chewing, when - ***agar.***, aur., ***calc-p.***, ***carb-an.***, clem., olnd., sars., sil.
cold, filled tooth - sin-n.
the least - ***carb-an.***, coc-c.
water to - acon., ***arg-n.***, ***ars.***, brom., ***bry.***, **CALC.**, calc-s., cina, gymn., hell., **LACH.**, merc., nat-m., ***nux-v.***, sep., ***sil.***, ***staph.***, sulph., ***ther.***
dental operation, cannot bear - **ANT-C.**, ***arn.***, ***fl-ac.***, **HYPER.**, ign., ***mag-c.***, phos., ***staph.***
evening - agar.
hollow tooth - aloe, caps., card-m., ***cham.***, plan., ***staph.***
incisors - agar., aur., aur-m., ***mag-m.***, pall., sars.

SENSITIVE, teeth, tender
molars, decayed - aeth., aloe.
upper - manc., zinc.
worse from eating - aloe.
morning - caust.
painful, in decayed lower molars - aeth.
points of - sulph.
pressure, to - agar., ars., ***hecla., kali-bi.,*** sulph.
sounds reverberate painfully in - ***ther.***
touch, to - agar., aloe, berb., carb-an., coc-c., **LACH.,** ***lyc.,*** mag-c., **NAT-M.,** staph.
warmth, to - **LACH.,** ***nat-m.***

SERRATED, teeth - calc-f., lach., med., plb., syph., tub.

SHARP, pain, teeth - acon., aesc., ***agar.,*** all-c., alum., ambr., ***am-c.,*** am-m., ant-c., ***apis, asaf.,*** aur., aur-s., ***bar-c.,*** bar-m., bell., benz-ac., berb., bor., ***bov.,*** **BRY.,** bufo, ***calc.,*** calc-p., ***carb-an., carb-s.,*** carb-v., **CAUST., CHAM.,** chin., cist., ***clem.,*** coff., colch., con., crot-h., cub., ***cycl.,*** daph., ***dros.,*** echi., ***euph.,*** euphr., gels., **GRAPH.,** grat., guai., haem., hell., hep., **HYPER.,** ***iris,*** kali-bi., ***kali-c.,*** kali-chl., kali-n., kali-p., kalm., **LACH.,** laur., led., **LYC.,** lyss., mag-c., **MAG-P.,** mang., ***merc., mez.,*** nat-c., ***nat-m., nit-ac.,*** nux-m., ***nux-v.,*** ol-an., ***petr.,*** phel., ***phos.,*** ph-ac., prun., psor., ***puls.,*** ran-s., raph., rat., rhod., ***rhus-t., sabad.,*** sabin., ***samb.,*** sars., **SEP.,** ***sil.,*** spig., spong., squil., ***staph., stront-c., stry., sulph.,*** tab., valer., zinc.
air, when drawing, in - am-c., ant-c.
biting, when - am-c., caust.
canines - sep., zinc.
cold, touched by anything - ***nit-ac., sulph.***
dinner, after - ambr., calc.
drinking - con., ***sulph.***
eating, while - carb-an., con., psor., sil.
after - mag-c.
amel. - calc.
edges seem, and hurt tongue - aloe.
evening - bell., bor., bufo, kali-c., zinc.
sleep preventing - lyc.
extending to,
ear - bor., bry., calc., gels., lil-t., mang., ***nat-m.,*** rhod., **SEP.,** ***sulph.,*** **THUJ.**
eyes - bov., calc., camph., nat-m., samb., sulph.
nose - calc.
right side of head - ***agar.***
side of face - clem.
zygoma - gels.
food, when touched by warm - bar-c., nit-ac.
forenoon - nat-m.
incisors - ambr., ***kali-c.,*** lach., nat-m., petr., rhod., sep., thuj.
upper - am-m.
intermittent - ***asaf.,*** bor.
left - ail., anac., bell., iod., phos., samb., ***sulph.,*** sul-ac., zinc.
upper and lower, worse lying down, compelling him to walk, better from external pressure - ail.

SHARP, pain, teeth
lower - aesc., ***carb-an.,*** euphr.
right side - ***agar.***
menses suppressed, with - **PULS.**
molars - am-c., calc., carb-an., ***kali-c.,*** zinc.
left - alum.
lower - aesc., ***caust.,*** coloc., zinc.
lower, root - sars.
lower, root, later only in right - aesc.
morning - ***camph., dros.,*** sulph.
on waking - bell., kali-c.
night - bufo, clem., ***sil.***
after midnight - alum., bar-m.
after midnight, better after rising - alum.
outward - **ASAF.**
rasping - sang.
right - aesc., bar-c., ***caust.,*** cycl., echi., gamb., teucr., zinc.
upper - arn.
roots - mag-c., sep., zinc.
tickling - carb-v., staph.
upper teeth - bell., cycl., mez., nit-ac.
right - chin., hell., lyc., phos.
vinegar amel. - puls.
warm bed amel. - ***lyc.***

sharp, jaws - acon., ambr., berb., carb-an., cimx., kalm., op., thuj., verat., zinc.

sharp, jaws, joints of - agar., bell., ***cham.,*** hep., kali-n., nat-m., nit-ac., staph., tab.
extending to,
ear - bell., ***cham.,*** **SEP.**
neck - zinc.
teeth - ***cham.***
temple - alum., mang.
motion, on - kali-n., zinc.
opening mouth - verat., zinc.
swallowing - kali-n.

sharp, jaws, lower - acon., aur., bar-c., ***bell.,*** berb., ***carb-an., caust., cham.,*** chin., cina, ***cocc.,*** colch., ***coloc.,*** cupr., dig., dros., euphr., ***gels.,*** graph., guai., kali-chl., kali-i., kalm., lact., **MANG.,** nat-p., plb., psor., rhus-v., sabin., ***sars.,*** sep., sil., staph., ***thuj.,*** zinc.
angle, of - mang.
dinner, during - euphr.
extending to
ear - sep.
ear, out of - sulph., thuj.
forehead - phos.
temples - mang.
evening - berb.
itching - mang.
laughing - mang.
morning - thuj.
night - sil., zinc.
walking, while - euphr., zinc.

sharp, jaws, upper - chel., clem., coloc., ***kali-bi.,*** kalm., meny., merc., rhus-v., ***spong.***
afternoon - indg.
evening, in bed - spong.
extending to
ear - kali-bi., phos., spong.
vertex - spig.
synchronous to pulse - clem.

SHOCKS, electric, teeth - aeth., thuj.

SHORTENED, jaws, lower, seems - alum.

SMOOTH feeling, teeth - carb-v., phos.

SNAPPING, jaws - bell., cic., ***ign.,*** lyss., merc., nux-v., plat., rhus-t.

SOFT, feel, teeth - ***caust.,*** cinnb., coch., lepi., med., merc., ***nit-ac.,*** nux-m., zinc.

SORDES, teeth - **AIL.,** alum., ***apis,*** **ARS., BAPT.,** ***bry., cact.,*** cadm-s., ***camph., carb-ac., carb-v.,*** **CHIN.,** ***dig., gels.,*** **HYOS.,** ***iris, kali-p., merc., merc-c., mur-ac.,*** ox-ac., ***petr.,*** **PH-AC., PHOS.,** ***plb., pyrog.,*** **RHUS-T.,** sec., ***stram.,*** sulph., ***sul-ac.,*** tab.
- black - **CHIN.,** ***con.***
- bloody - plan., sec.
- brown - ***apis, cact., colch., kali-p., vario.***
- dark - ***chin.,*** **FL-AC.,** tab.

SORE, pain, teeth - alum., apis, ***arn.,*** ars., aur., bapt., bar-c., bell., ***bry., calc.,*** carb-an., carb-v., caul., caust., cham., cina, cinnb., colch., crot-h., crot-t., graph., ***ign.,*** kali-ar., kali-c., kali-p., ***lyc.,*** mang., med., **MERC.,** mez., ***nat-m., nux-v., phos.,*** phyt., ***plan.,*** psor., ***puls.,*** rhod., ***rhus-t.,*** sep., ***staph.,*** tab., thuj., ***zinc.***
- air, from drawing, in - bell.
- chewing, when - ars., ***aur.***
- cold drink, from - ***ars.,*** bry.
- eating amel. - ***ign.***
- eye tooth - med.
- meals, between - ign.
- molars, right upper - alum.
- pressure amel. - alum.
- roots, in - iod.

sore, jaws - ***caust.,*** crot-h., phos., plan., sars.
- lower - agar., **AUR.,** coc-c., ***lach.,*** lyss., mang., merc-i-f., mur-ac., nat-c., ***nat-m.,*** nat-p., sabad., sars., sil., spong., verat., zinc.
  - chewing - verat.
  - morning - zinc.

SPLINTERED, pain, teeth as if - sabin.

SPONGY, teeth, feel - nit-ac.

SPRAINED, teeth, as if - ***arn.***

STICK, together, as if teeth, glued - arg-m., eupi., ***psor.,*** syph., zinc-oc.

STICKY, teeth - arg-m., iod., sang., syph.

STIFFNESS, jaws, muscles of lower - acet-ac., acon., anthr., ars-m., bad., bell., calc., cann-i., carb-s., carc., **CAUST.,** chim., cic., cocc., crot-h., daph., dios., euphr., form., ***gels.,*** glon., graph., helo., hyos., ***ign., kali-i., lach.,*** lyss., med., ***merc., merc-c., merc-i-f., mez.,*** nat-a., nat-s., nux-m., **NUX-V.,** op., petr., ***phyt.,*** **RHUS-T.,** sang., sars., sep., **STRY.,** sumb., sulph., ***ther.,*** thuj., ***verat.***
- chewing - euphr.
- morning - ***ther.***
  - after rising - nat-s.
- talking - euphr.
- tired, and - cham., merc-i-f.
- swallowing, when - ***arum-t.***

SUPPURATION, of jaws, lower - phos.

SWELLING of cheek, with toothache - all-c., am-c., ***ant-c.,*** arn., ars., aur., **BELL.,** bor., **BRY.,** ***calc.,*** calc-f., ***calc-s.,*** caps., caust., **CHAM.,** colch., ***euph.,*** **HECLA.,** ***hep., kali-c.,*** **LACH.,** ***lyc.,*** mag-arct., ***mag-c.,*** **MERC.,** nat-c., ***nat-m.,*** nux-v., petr., ph-ac., phos., ***puls.,*** samb., **SEP., SIL.,** ***spig.,*** staph., stront-c., sulph., ***verat.***

swelling, jaws - amph., ***calc-f.,*** hecla., plb., thuj.
- beneath, right - ol-an.
- hard - anthr.

swelling, jaws, lower - acon., alum., ***anthr.,*** ars., ***aur.,*** calc., ***calc-f.,*** calc-s., caust., ***crot-h., fl-ac., kali-c.,*** **LACH.,** mag-c., merc., ***nit-ac.,*** ol-an., petr., **PHOS.,** ***sil.,*** sulph., verat., zinc.
- angle, hard - lyc.
- morning - zinc.

swelling, jaws, upper - alum., ***nit-ac.,*** phos., stann.

SWOLLEN, sensation, teeth - spong.

TEARING, pain, teeth - abrot., **ACON.,** act-sp., aesc., ***agar.,*** agn., ail., alum., ambr., **AM-C.,** am-m., anac., anag., anan., ang., ant-t., aphis., apis, arg-n., arn., ***ars.,*** ars-i., arum-t., ***aur.,*** bar-c., bar-m., ***bell.,*** berb., benz-ac., bor., ***bry.,*** bufo, calc., calc-p., camph., canth., ***carb-an., carb-s.,*** **CARB-V.,** cast., **CAUST.,** ***cham.,*** chel., ***chin.,*** chin-a., clem., ***coc-c., coff., colch., coloc.,*** con., ***cupr.,*** cupr-ar., ***cycl.,*** daph., gamb., gels., ***graph.,*** grat., ***guai.,*** hell., ***hyos.,*** hyper., indg., iod., ip., kali-ar., kali-bi., ***kali-c.,*** kali-i., kali-n., ***kali-p.,*** kreos., ***lach.,*** laur., ***lyc., mag-c., mag-m.,*** mang., meph., **MERC.,** merl., ***mez.,*** nat-a., ***nat-c., nat-m.,*** nat-s., ***nicc., nit-ac., nux-m., nux-v.,*** olnd., ol-an., petr., phel., ***ph-ac., phos.,*** plb., prun., ***psor., puls.,*** ran-b., ***rat., rhod., rhus-t.,*** sabin., ***samb.,*** **SARS., SEP.,** ***sil., spig.,*** **STAPH.,** stront-c., ***sulph.,*** sul-ac., tab., tarent., teucr., ***thuj.,*** verb., viol-o., vinc., zinc.
- afternoon - agar., carb-s., sep., zinc.
- air, as from a current of - ambr.
- air, open agg. - caust., kali-n., phos.
  - amel. - mag-m.
- bed, worse after going to - **ACON.**
  - from warmth of - graph., ***ph-ac.***
- biting together, when - **AM-C.,** hell.
- cold, air - bufo, carb-s.
  - amel. - mag-m.
  - water - agar., arg-n., bor., mag-c., ***nux-m.,*** phos., ***sars.,*** staph.
- dinner, after - mag-c., nat-c.
- eating, while - aur., bry., carb-an., euph., kali-c., ***sep.,*** sil., ***staph.***
  - after - sep.
- evening - ail., alum., am-m., bell., cahin., carb-an., kali-n., mag-c., mag-s., nat-c., sep., tab., zinc.
  - bed amel. - am-m.
- extending, to,
  - ear, out through left ear - sep.
  - ears - am-c., anac., aphis., lach., nat-m.
  - malar bones - alum.

TEARING, pain, teeth
extending, to
temple - alum., calc., indg., mez.
zygoma - caust., mag-m., phos.
glowing-tearing - sulph.
forenoon - kali-n.
incisors - carb-v., stront.
lower - alum., lyc., ***teucr.,*** zinc.
morning - carb-v.
upper - kali-n., mag-m., phos., sul-ac.
jerking-tearing - nat-c., ph-ac., zinc.
left - samb., sul-ac.
lying on, painful side - **ARS.**
sound side - puls.
menses, during - ars., mag-c., nat-m., sul-ac.
before - ***ars.***
midnight, after - alum., ***bell., sulph.***
before - am-c., merc., petr., sul-ac.
molars - alum., am-c., anag., apis, bar-c., benz-ac., ***carb-v.,*** cycl., ***gamb.,*** grat., hell., kali-c., mag-c., mag-m., phos., rhod., zinc.
after getting wet - acon.
dinner, during - mag-m.
left, alternating with itching, in left ear - agar.
left, alternating with right - am-m.
lower - aesc., agar., alum., bell., mag-c., mag-m., staph., zinc.
lower, left - colch., lyc., thuj., zinc.
lower, right - canth., mag-c., verb.
right - hell.
upper - mur-ac.
upper, left - agar., am-c., arn., berb., caust., chin., cupr-ar., guai., zinc.
upper, right - aur., chin., mez., ph-ac., phos.
upper, right extending to temple - mez.
wet, after getting - acon.
morning - arg-n., caust., hyos., mang., hyper.
after walking - mag-c., ***mez.***
after washing - arg-n.
motion amel. - am-c.
night - alum., ***ars., calc.,*** calc-p., carb-an., hell., mag-c., ***merc.,*** nat-c., nat-m., nicc., nux-m., sep., sil., sulph., sul-ac.
lying on painful side agg. - ars.
opening mouth, when - caust., indg.
paroxysmal - anac., calc.
pregnancy - nux-m., sep.
pressure amel. - mag-m.
pulsating - agar., agn., bell.
rising from bed, on, amel. - alum.
roots - am-m., ant-t., camph., caust., colch., graph., lach., mag-c., meph., ***merc.,*** ol-an., sabin., staph., stront-c., ***teucr.,*** zinc.
tension in - merc-i-f.
touch, on - aur., bor.
wandering - mag-c.
warmth amel. - **ARS.**

tearing, jaws, joints, of - anac., nat-c., sep.
chewing, on - spig., zinc.

tearing, jaws, lower - aeth., ***agar., agn.,*** am-m., ***anac., anthr.,*** arg-m., ***aur.,*** bar-c., bell., berb., ***bov., bry.,*** calc., calc-ar., canth., carb-an., carb-v., ***caust., cham.,*** chin., ***colch., dros.,*** graph., indg., kali-c., kali-i., kali-n., ***kalm., lach.,*** laur., led., lyc., ***lyss.,*** mag-m., meph., ***merc.,*** mez., nat-c., nat-m., ***nux-v., phos.,*** plb., puls., ***rat.,*** rhus-v., ***sel.,*** sep., spig., stront-c., sul-ac., ***sulph.,*** viol-o., zinc.
chewing, on - ph-ac.
evening - merc., nat-c., phos., sulph., thuj.
extending, to,
chin - phos., thuj.
ear - am-c., cham., ***lyss.,*** mag-m., **SPIG.,** viol-o.
head - kali-n.
jerking, on - lyc.
left - kali-n.
lying - phos.
night, during menses - sul-ac.
right, at night - chin.

tearing, jaws, upper - agar., arg-m., berb., calc-ac., ***calc-ar.,*** carb-an., ***carb-v.,*** caust., kali-chl., ***lyc.,*** meny., merl., mur-ac., plb., rhus-v., sep., stront-c., sulph., thuj.
angle of - **BELL.,** kali-n., laur., thuj.
evening - sulph.
morning - carb-v.
night, lying - phos.
right, at night - chin., lyc.

TEMPOR-mandibular joint, jaws, (see TMJ)

TENSION, in teeth - anac., coloc., hyper., merc-i-f., nat-m., **PULS.,** sil., ther.
right side - bar-c.

tension, jaws - caust., ***ign.,*** meny., ***rhus-t.***

tension, jaws, joints, of - alum., colch., ***merc.,*** nat-m., sars., spig.
chewing - alum., am-m.
opening mouth - alum., am-m.

tension, jaws, lower - alum., aur., bar-c., ***bell.,*** carb-s., **CAUST.,** lach., lyc., merc., op., petr., ***phos.,*** sars., seneg., stram., ***stry.,*** sulph.
extending to ear - bell.
morning - lyc.

TETANUS, lockjaw (see Emergency)

THICK, jaws, lower - hecla.

TINGLING, pain, teeth - alum., bor., calc., carb-v., cast., indg., lach., mur-ac., ***rhus-t.,*** sulph.
in points of crowns in evening - bar-c.

TINGLING, jaws, lower - caust., mur-ac.

TIRED, jaws, feeling, in the - alum., cham., iod., nicc., nit-ac., tarent., vip.

TMJ, jaws, pain in joints - agar., acet-ac., alum., alumn., ***arum-t.,*** asaf., asar., brom., calc., **CAUST.,** cimic., cist., cor-r., dros., fl-ac., glon., hyper., ***ign.,*** laur., mang., mez., nicc., op., **RHUS-T.,** spig., spong., staph., ***stry.,*** sul-ac., vesp.
chewing, on - acon., alum., am-c., bell., calc., coc-c., cor-r., sil.
morning - vesp.
opening mouth - alum., am-c., **CAUST.,** cor-r., dros., hep., nicc., sabad., verat.
rest, during - ***rhus-t.***
rheumatic - ***rhus-t.***

TMJ, jaws, pain in joints,
shutting mouth - ***bar-c.***
swallowing, when - ***arum-t.***
yawning - cor-r., ign., rhus-t., staph.

TORN, out, pain, as if teeth, being - ***calc.***
dinner, during - arn.
amel. after - arn.
eating, during - sep.
after - ant-t., sep.
left side posteriorly - ant-t., cycl.
pressure of finger amel. - am-m.

TORPOR, teeth, sense of - chin., petr.

TREMBLING, jaws - agar., alum., ***ant-t.,*** cadm-s., carb-v., ***cocc., gels.,*** ign., op., phos., stry.
trembling, jaws, lower - alum., ant-t., cadm-s., carb-v., cocc., gels., ol-an., ***phos.***
speak, attempting, to, on - cocc.
yawning, while - olnd.

TUBERCLES, jaws, lower - graph., nat-c., staph., verat.

TWISTED, feeling as if teeth - lact.

TWITCHING, pain, teeth - all-c., nat-c., apis, ars., aur., aur-m., bell., bry., calc., caust., cham., cist., ***clem.,*** coff., coloc., cupr-ar., hep., hyos., ***lach., merc., mez.,*** nit-ac., ***nux-v., phos., puls.,*** sulph., thuj.
extending to ear - hep.
to ear and eye - clem.
left - calc.
right side - spig.
warmth of bed amel. - spig.
twitching, jaws, lower - alum., bell., carb-v., chin., con., kali-chl., lach., mang., merc-i-r., mill., phos., ol-an., ***sulph.***
evening - lyc.
falling, asleep, when - sulph.
left - sulph.
night - sil.
right - nit-ac.
walking, while - sabin.

ULCERATION, teeth, of roots - alum.

ULCERATIVE, pain, teeth - am-c., bell., carb-v., caust., coc-c., kali-i., kali-n., lyc., mag-c., mang., petr., phos., ***sil.***
ulcerative, at roots - am-c., alum., merc., ***sil.***
touch, from - mang., sil.
worse when chewing - alum., ***sil.***

WARM, feeling, teeth - chel.
warm, feeling, jaws - chel.
left upper jaw - ***fl-ac.***

WATER, sour, fetid, coming from teeth - nicc.

WEAKNESS, in teeth - am-c., merl.
weakness, jaws, of lower - bar-c., nit-ac.
eating, after - ***bar-c.,*** kalm.

WEDGE, shaped teeth - ***kreos.,*** syph.

WISDOM, teeth, ailments from, eruption of - ***calc.,*** calc-p., **CHAM.,** chap., ***fl-ac., mag-c., sil.***

WRENCHING, pain, teeth - nux-v., prun.

Throat

ABSCESS, predisposition to - calc., calc-i., calc-s., ferr-p., ***kali-i., sil.***

abscess, retropharyngeal - antipyrin., bell., bry., ***hep.,*** lach., ***merc.,*** nit-ac., phos., ***sil.,*** tub.

abscess, throat, external - ***cham.,*** **HEP.,** kali-c., ***kali-i., lach., lyc.,*** **MERC.,** ***nit-ac.,*** phos., psor., sep., **SIL.,** sulph., sul-ac.

abscess, tonsils - aesc., ***alumn.,*** am-m., ***anac.,*** anan., ***apis,*** aur., ***bar-c.,*** **BAR-M.,** ***bell.,*** calc., ***calc-s., canth., cham.,*** cub., cupr., cur., daph., ***guai.,*** **HEP.,** ign., ***kali-bi., lac-c., lach., lyc., manc.,*** **MERC.,** merc-c., ***merc-i-f., merc-i-r.,*** nat-m., phyt., ***plb.,*** psor., ***sabad., sang., sep.,*** **SIL.,** ***sulph., tarent.,*** tub.

left - ***lach.,*** sep.

peritonsillar - calc-s.

right - bar-c., ***lyc.***

ADENOIDS, problems with - agra., ***bar-c., bar-m., calc.,*** calc-f., calc-i., calc-p., ***carc.,*** chr-ac., iod., kali-s., lob-s., merc., mez., phyt., psor., sang-n., sulph., ***thuj., tub.***

post nasal - mez.

removal, after - carc., kali-s.

ADHESIVE, sticky, as if - caust., kali-n.

AEROPHAGIA, swallowing of air, excessive - plat.

AIR, throat, external, sensitive to - ail., ***caust.,*** crot-t., ***fl-ac., hep., merc., sil.,*** tub.

air, blowing through glands and thyroid on breathing - spong.

ANESTHESIA - ***acon., all-c.,*** arg-m., ***gels., kali-br.,*** kali-c., mag-s., olnd., verat-v.

anesthesia, fauces - kali-br.

ANTIPERISTALTIC, (see Peristalsis, reversed)

ANXIETY, and apprehension in - cann-s.

tonsils, with oppression in - am-m.

APHTHAE, (see Mouth) - ***aeth.,*** ars., arum-t., ***bell., bry., canth., gels.,*** **IGN.,** ***kali-chl.,*** med., plb., sulph.

tonsils - ***bell.,*** calc., ***gels.***

APPLE, core had lodged, sensation as if - phyt.

ASTRINGENT, sensation - ail., naja, phyt.

BITING, pain - ambr., dros., hyos., mez., nat-m., sep., verat.

sensation in back parts of fauces between swallowing - ambr.

tonsils - iod.

BLACK, (see Discoloration)

BLISTERED - canth.

BLOOD, hawks up clotted dark - zinc.

blood, oozing - **ACON.,** ***arn.,*** ars., ***bell., canth., carb-v., chin., crot-h.,*** cur., ***ferr., ferr-p., ham., ip., lach.,*** merc-c., merc-cy., ***mill., phos., sang., sec.,*** sep.

sensation of - zinc.

BLOOD, hawks up clotted dark - zinc.

blood, oozing,

tonsils - ***crot-h., lach., phos.,*** sec., ter.

uvula - lac-c.

BLOTCHES, (see Mucus patches)

BLOW, throat, external, as from a, upper side - ruta.

BONE, in, sensation of - bapt., ***calc.,*** **HEP.,** ign., lach., ***nit-ac.,*** phys.

BORING, pain - arg-m.

BREAD, crumbs, sensation of - ***coc-c.,*** dros., **LACH., NIT-AC.,** pall., ***sabad.,*** sanic.

hawking amel. - **LACH.**

BURNING, pain - absin., **ACON.,** ***aesc., aeth.,*** agar., ***alum.,*** alumn., ***am-c.,*** am-m., ammc., anan., ant-c., ant-t., ***apis,*** arg-m., ***arg-n., arn.,*** **ARS.,** ars-h., ars-i., ***arum-t., asaf.,*** astac., aur., bapt., bar-c., bar-m., ***bell.,*** berb., bism., bor., ***bov.,*** brom., cahin., ***calad., calc.,*** calc-p., calc-s., ***camph.,*** cann-i., **CANTH., CAPS.,** ***carb-ac., carb-an., carb-s., carb-v.,*** cast., **CAUST.,** cedr., cham., chel., chin., chin-a., chin-s., ***cimic.,*** cist., clem., ***coc-c.,*** cocc., colch., coloc., con., cop., ***crot-c., crot-t.,*** cupr., cupr-ar., cur., cycl., dig., dios., dros., echi., eup-per., **EUPH.,** ferr., ferr-ar., ferr-i., ferr-m., ferr-p., fl-ac., ***gels., guai.,*** hell., ***hep., hura, hyos.,*** iod., ip., iris, jatr., jug-c., kali-ar., ***kali-bi., kali-c.,*** kali-chl., kali-i., kali-ma., kali-n., kali-p., kali-s., kreos., lac-ac., **LAC-C.,** ***lach., laur.,*** lob., **LYC.,** lyss., mag-c., manc., mang., ***merc.,*** **MERC-C.,** ***merc-i-f., merc-i-r.,*** merl., **MEZ.,** ***mur-ac.,*** myric., nat-a., nat-c., **NAT-M.,** nat-p., ***nit-ac.,*** nux-v., olnd., op., ***ox-ac.,*** paeon., ***par., petr.,*** ph-ac., ***phos., phyt.,*** plb., podo., ***psor.,*** puls., ran-b., ran-s., raph., ***rhod., rhus-t.,*** rhus-v., ***sabad.,*** sal-ac., **SANG.,** ***sec., seneg., sep.,*** sil., ***spong., squil.,*** still., ***stram.,*** **SULPH.,** sul-ac., ***syph., tab.,*** tarax., tarent., tep., ter., thuj., upa., urt-u., ***verat.,*** verat-v., vesp., vip., zinc.

afternoon, 5 pm - caust.

belching, after - alum., ***sulph.***

bread, after - rhod.

cold drinks, after - ***ars.,*** calc-f., canth., hep., ***merc-c.***

amel. - ***apis.***

amel., shortly after - iris.

cough, after - cast., coc-c., hep., mag-m., ***mur-ac.,*** phos., ph-ac., sulph.

daytime - lyss.

dinner, after - dig., dros., lyc.

drinking - canth., par.

amel. - kali-n..

dryness, with - cub.

eating, after - amc., ant-t., ***calc.,*** con., ***lyc., nit-ac.,*** par., sep.

amel. - carb-an., mez.

evening - alum., carb-an., dig., ox-ac., rhus-t., sulph.

expiration - crot-t., iris, mez.

extending to,

abdomen, to - iod.

chest, to - agar., sang.

BURNING, pain
extending, to
lips, to - mez.
nostrils, left - ***gels.***
esophagus, to - ***acon.,*** agar., ***am-c.,*** anan., ant-t., carb-s., kali-ma.
mouth, to - ph-ac.
stomach, to - ***acon.,*** anan., ant-c., ***apis, arn.,*** ars., carb-ac., ***carb-s., con.,*** dor., euph., ***kali-bi.,*** mag-s., psor., sec., still., sul-ac.
forenoon - cic., rhod., spong.
hawking, when - lyc., sep.
inspiration, on - cann-i., mez., ran-b.
amel. - crot-t., iris, mez., ***sang.***
itching, menses, during - mez.
smarting - bar-c., carb-v., cist., kali-bi., merc., mez., mur-ac., phos., ph-ac., puls., teucr., zinc.
lying down, on - puls.
menses, during - calc., sulph.
before - sulph.
morning - ***arum-t., carb-an.,*** coc-c., ***kali-bi.,*** lyc., mur-ac., sulph.
night - **BAR-C.,** carb-an., mur-ac., nux-v.
cold drinks, from - calc-f.
midnight - ***arum-t.,*** kali-bi.
noon - rhus-t.
peppery - caps., coloc., crot-t., euph., ***mez.,*** ol-an., plat.
pressure, on - **MERC-C.**
seashore, at - iod.
sleep amel. - crot-t.
smoking - coc-c., tarax.
sneezing, with - verat-v.
supper, after - nit-ac.
swallowing, when - aesc., arn., ***ars.,*** aur., **BAR-C.,** canth., carb-s., caust., ***hep.,*** kali-bi., kali-c., lyc., mag-c., mez., sil., sulph.
empty, on - **BAR-C.,** merc-i-f., merc-i-r.
sweets, after - sang.
thirst, with - hyper.
vomiting, after - agar., phos., puls., sul-ac.
waking, on - puls-n
warm, drinks amel. - alum., ***ars.,*** calc-f., hep.
food, from - kali-c.
burning, fauces - ***acon.,*** aesc., ***bell.,*** canth., caps., gels., jug-c., ***nux-m., phos., phyt.,*** sin-n., still.
burning, pharynx - ars., bell., carb-v., phos.
menses, during - nat-s.
burning, throat pit - ars.
burning, tonsils - ***bell.,*** dios., iris, merc., phys., raph.
cold air amel. - iris.
burning, uvula - ***apis,*** caust., colch., lact., mez., ***sang.***

CALCAREOUS, deposit - ***calc.***

CANCER, (see Larynx) - ***carb-an.,*** led., tarent.

CASEOUS, deposits in tonsils - ***chen-a., kali-m.,*** vip.
inflamed, while - chen-a.

CATARRH, of (see Larynx) - acon., ***all-s.,*** alum., alumn., ***am-c., am-m.,*** **ANT-T.,** arn., **ARS.,** aur-m., ***bad., bar-c., bar-m.,*** bell., ***brom.,*** **CALC.,** ***calc-p.,*** **CALC-S.,** camph., cann-s., canth., carb-an., ***carb-s.,*** **CARB-V.,** ***caust., cham., chim.,*** chin-a., ***coc-c., coff., colch.,*** con., crot-t., dros., ***dulc.,*** ferr., ferr-ar., ***ferr-p., fl-ac.,*** gels., ***graph., hep., hippoz.,*** **HYDR.,** hyos., ign., ip., **KALI-AR., KALI-BI.,** ***kali-br.,*** **KALI-C.,** ***kali-chl.,*** kali-i., kali-p., ***kali-s.,*** kreos., lob., ***lyc.,*** **MANG.,** meph., **MERC.,** ***nat-a.,*** **NAT-M., NUX-M., NUX-V.,** phel., ***ph-ac., phos., phyt., puls., rhod., rumx.,*** **SANG., SENEG.,** ***sil.,*** spig., ***spong.,*** **STANN., SULPH.,** verat., verb.
alternating with, uterine complaints - ***arg-n.***
change of weather, before - ***dulc., kali-bi.***
damp weather - ***calc., dulc., kali-bi.***
elderly people, in - ***ammc., ant-t., ars.,*** **BAR-C.,** ***hydr., kali-bi.,*** **SENEG.**
evening - carb-an.
measles, after - ***carb-v.***
morning - nux-v.
night - carb-an., carb-v., spig.
sudden - **ARS.**

CHEESY, looking spots - ***bell.,*** bry., ***kali-bi., psor.***
tubercles, hawked out - mag-c., psor.

CHOKING, general - abies-n., absin., ***acon., aesc.,*** aeth., agar., aloe, ***alum.,*** ambr., am-c., am-m., anan., ***apis, arg-n., ars.,*** ars-h., ars-i., arum-t., asaf., asar., asc-t., ***bapt., bar-c.,*** **BELL.,** benz-ac., both., ***brom.,*** bry., ***bufo,*** **CACT.,** caj., ***calc., calc-s., canth., caps.,*** carb-ac., carb-an., ***carb-s., carb-v.,*** cast., **CAUST.,** cedr., **CHAM.,** chel., chin., chin-a., chin-s., chlor., cic., cimic., cinnb., ***cimx.,*** cocaine, ***cocc.,*** coc-c., coff., colch., con., cop., ***crot-c., crot-h., crot-t., cupr.,*** cur., cycl., dig., dios., dros., elaps, eup-per., ***ferr.,*** ferr-ar., ferr-p., ***fl-ac.,*** gamb., ***gels.,*** gent-c., ***glon., graph., hell., hep.,*** hura, **HYOS., IGN.,** indg., ***iod., ip.,*** iris, jac-c., kali-ar., kali-bi., ***kali-c.,*** kali-chl., kali-i., kali-n., kali-p., ***kali-s.,*** kreos., lac-ac., **LAC-C., LACH., LAUR., LYC.,** lycps., lyss., ***mag-p., manc.,*** med., ***meph.,*** merc., merc-c., merl., ***mez.,*** morph., ***mosch.,*** myric., **NAJA,** nat-a., ***nat-m.,*** nat-s., nicc., ***nux-v.,*** oena., op., ox-ac., ped., petr., ph-ac., phos., phys., ***phyt., plat.,*** **PLB.,** ptel., ***puls.,*** ran-s., raph., rat., rheum, ***rhod.,*** rhus-t., sabad., sabin., sang., sang-n., sarcol-ac., sars., seneg., ***sep., sil.,*** **SPONG.,** still., ***stram., stry.,*** **SULPH.,** sul-ac., sumb., syph., ***tab., tarent.,*** ter., ***thuj.,*** thyr., trif-p., tub., valer., vario., ***verat.,*** vip., ***zinc.***
afternoon - nat-a., nicc., sang., stry.
3 p.m. - lyss.
angina pectoris - cact., tab.
bending head, backwards, amel. - hep., lach.
the neck - ph-ac.
bowing, the head - con.
bread, eating, while - ran-s.
cardiac pain, with - arg-n., ***cact.***

CHOKING, general
clearing, the throat, when (see Retching) - ***ambr., anac.,*** **ARG-N.,** bor., ***bry., calc-p., coc-c., ip., kali-c.,*** **NUX-V.,** osm., ***stann.***
clothing, agg. - agar., ambr., ***apis, bell., cact.,*** chel., elaps, kali-bi., kali-c., **LACH.,** ***sep.***
compelling - bor., cact., ***lach., sep.***
convulsions, during - crot-h., lach.
convulsive - acon., ars., ***bell., calc., caps., carb-v., cic., con.,*** **HYOS.,** ***mag-p.,*** nat-s., puls., sars.
coughing, on - ars., coc-c., lach., tarent.
daytime - nat-s.
dinner, during - ***bar-c.***
distended, as if throat were - mag-c.
distortion of face, with - nit-ac.
drinking, when - acon., cimx., **HYOS.,** iod., kali-n., manc., meph., **NAT-M.,** phos., rhus-t.
if looked at - ***ph-ac.***
but not for solids - kali-br.
eating, while - acon., anac., kali-bi., ***kali-c.,*** kali-n., ***lach., meph., merc-c.,*** nit-ac., zinc-valer.
after - agar., sil., sulph.
bread - ran-s.
evening - alum., chin-s., **IGN.,** mag-c., ol-an., phys.
expectoration, with - ambr.
forenoon - fl-ac.
froth, from - lyss.
goitre, in - meph.
hawing up mucus, when, in morning - ambr.
headache, with - ***glon.***
heart trouble, with - cact.
injuries of pharynx, after - cic.
liquids - **HYOS.,** lyss., ***mag-p.,*** nat-s., rhus-t.
lying down, on - apis, ***kali-bi.,*** ol-j.
on back amel. - ***spong.***
menses, before - puls.
morning - agar., aster., cham., ***fl-ac.,*** naja, ol-an., stry.
4 a.m. - sumb.
5 a.m. - raph.
waking, on - agar.
mucus in mouth, from - sul-ac.
post nasal, from - spig.
night - arg-n., arum-t., cop., ***gad.,*** glon., kali-n., nit-ac., phos., ran-s., spig., sul-ac., ***tab.***
os hyoides, region of - ***all-c.***
palpitation, from - lec.
paroxysmal - verat.
raising arm - plb.
rising sensation - bell., carb-an.
sleep, on going to (see Larynx) - **BELL.,** ***cench., crot-h.,*** kali-c., ***lac-c.,*** **LACH.,** ***naja,*** **NUX-V.,** sep., teucr., valer.
smoking - sep.
solids - ***carb-v.,*** **PULS.,** lach.
speaking, when - dros., ***manc.,*** meph.
sudden - samb.

CHOKING, general
swallowing, on (see Stomach, Retching) - acon., ambr., ars., ***bar-c.,*** bell., bry., chen-a., ***cic., cupr.,*** gent-c., ***graph., hyos.,*** kali-c., ***laur.,*** **LYC.,** mag-p., manc., meph., ***merc.,*** mur-ac., ***nat-m.,*** onos., par., ***plb.,*** **PULS.,** rhus-t., stry., tarent., verat., zinc.
liquids, children, in - kali-br.
liquids, warm - lach.
solids - ***carb-v.,*** kali-bi., **PULS.,** lach.
vertigo, with - iber.
vomiting, after - thuj.
walking, while - nat-s.
amel. - dros.
wind in, as from - plat..
water, sight or thought of - anan., ***lyss.,*** stram.
writing, while - ***bar-c.***

choking, esophagus - acon., ***aesc.,*** agar., ***alum., alumn.,*** anac., ***arg-m., ars., bell.,*** **CACT.,** cadm-s., ***calc.,*** canth., ***carb-ac.,*** cham., chel., chin., ***cic., cimx.,*** cocc., ***coch.,*** crot-c., ***cupr.,*** dig., dros., ***hyos.,*** **IGN.,** iod., **KALI-C.,** kali-chl., lob., lyc., lyss., **MERC-C.,** naja, ***nat-a., nat-m.,*** nit-ac., ox-ac., ***phos., plb., sabad.,*** stram., sul-ac., zinc.
below upwards - ***lob., plb.***
inspiration, on - zinc.
morning on waking - alum.
night - alum.
pressure in larynx, from - chel.
swallowing - ***alum.,*** zinc.
fluids - hyos., ***manc.***
solids - caj.

CHOKES, easily - ***acon.,*** anac., **ARG-M., BELL.,** calc., cann-s., cocc., gels., **HYOS.,** ign., kali-c., kali-n., **LACH.,** meph., nat-m., nux-m., op., plat., ***rhus-t.,*** sil., sul-ac., verat.

CLEARING, the throat - abrot., acon., ***aesc.,*** aloe, ***alum., ambr.,*** ammc., ***am-c.,*** **ANAC., ANAG.,** ant-c., arg-m., ***arg-n., ars.,*** ars-i., asar., aur., aur-m., bapt., bell., berb., bol., bov., ***brom.,*** brach., bry., ***calc.,*** calc-p., calc-s., camph., ***carb-an., carb-v., caust.,*** chel., **CHIN.,** chin-s., cic., cimic., cocc., ***coc-c.,*** colch., ***coloc.,*** con., ***croc.,*** crot-h., cycl., dig., dros., euph., gent-c., ***graph.,*** hell., ***hep.,*** hura, hydr-ac., hyos., iod., kali-ar., kali-bi., ***kali-c.,*** kali-chl., kali-n., kali-p., ***kalm.,*** kreos., ***lach.,*** lact., laur., lyc., mag-c., mang., merc., **MEZ.,** naja, nat-a., nat-c., nat-p., nit-ac., nux-m., **NUX-V.,** ol-an., op., ox-ac., ***par.,*** petr., ph-ac., ***phos.,*** phyt., pic-ac., plat., podo., ***psor., puls.,*** ran-b., ran-s., raph., rat., ***rhod.,*** rhus-t., ***rumx., sabad.,*** sars., seneg., sep., sil., squil., stann., staph., stront-c., **SULPH.,** sumb., ***tab., teucr.,*** thuj., valer., **VERAT.,** zinc.
afternoon - bol., phos., tab.
beer, after - merc-c., staph.
bread after - ***lach.,*** ph-ac., rhus-t.
coughing, with - bell.
dryness, from - **ALUM.**

CLEARING, the throat
evening - **ALUM.,** bol., brom., ***carb-an.,*** caust., kali-n., nat-c., phos., sil., stann., sulph., zinc.
bed, in - plat., sulph.
forenoon - sep., sil.
ices, after - thuj.
morning - ***ail.,*** berb., bov., ***caust.,*** chin-s., kali-n., lyc., mur-ac., petr., sars., stann.
night - calc., ***carb-an.,*** naja, nat-m., phyt., sil.
lying on side, while - sil.
reading aloud, after - nit-ac.
sleep, after long - hep.
speak, before able to - carc.
swallowing, after - bar-c., ***carb-an.,*** caust., fago., jab., hep., hydr., lach., laur., nux-m., pic-ac., stram.
empty, after - ***ars.***
tobacco, from - osm.

CLERGYMAN, sore throat from overuse of the voice (see Larynx) - acon., alum., ***arg-m.,*** **ARG-N.,** ***arn.,*** **ARUM-T., CAPS.,** carb-v., **CAUST.,** ***coca,*** coll., ferr-p., ferr-pic., ***hep.,*** iod., ***kali-p., mang.,*** med., merc-cy., merc-sul., ***nat-m., phos.,*** **RHUS-T.,** ***sel.,*** seneg., spong., ***still.,*** sulph., tab., ter.
chronic hoarseness, with - ampe-qu, ***arg-n.,*** bar-c., calc., carb-v., ***caust.,*** graph., ***mang., phos.,*** sil., ***sulph.***
irritation, of, in public speakers and singers - wye.
lost of voice, with - arg-m., ***arg-n., arum-t.,*** caps., ***caust., ferr-p., graph., merc.,*** **RHUS-T.,** ***sel., seneg.,*** stann.
singers, in - alum., ***arg-n.,*** arn., **ARUM-T.,** caps., cupr., ferr-p., ***lach.,*** **RHUS-T.,** sil., ***stann.,*** zinc.
lost of voice, in - **ARG-N.,** arum-t., **CAUST.,** graph., mang., rhus-t., sel.
lost of voice, periodically - cupr., rhus-t.
singing, hoarseness, from - **AGAR.,** alum., ***arg-m., arg-n.,*** arn., **ARUM-T.,** ***bry.,*** caps., ***caust.,*** hep., ***mang., nat-m., nit-ac.,*** osm., **SEL.,** sep., spong., ***stann.***
amel. - rhus-t.
high notes causes cough - arg-n.
talking, from - ***alum.,*** alumn., am-c., ant-t., **ARG-M., ARG-N.,** arn., **ARUM-T.,** ***calc.,*** **CAPS.,** ***carb-v.,*** **CAUST.,** ***coc-c., ferr., kali-bi.,*** lach., ***mang.,*** morph., naja, ***nat-m., nit-ac., ph-ac., phos.,*** psor., **RHUS-T.,** sel., ***stann.,*** staph., stram.
a while, improves after - coc-c., ***rhus-t.***
amel. - ant-c., caust., graph., ***rhus-t.,*** tub.
painful - merc-cy.

CLOTHING, agg., throat, external - ***agar.,*** ambr., aml-n., ant-c., ***apis,*** arg-n., ***bell., calc., cact.,*** carb-an., carc., caust., cench., chel., **CENCH.,** cocc., con., **CROT-C., CROT-H.,** ***elaps,*** glon., kali-bi., ***kali-c.,*** lac-c., **LACH.,** merc., merc-c., naja, nicc., sars., ***sep.,*** sulph., ***tarent.,*** tub.

CLUCKING, throat, external, muscles, in - rheum.

COATED - ars., lil-t., petr., sep.
coated, tonsils - merc-c.

COLDNESS, sensation of - agar., ***all-c.,*** all-s., caj., carb-v., caust., chel., ***cist.,*** cor-r., cur., kali-bi., kali-chl., lact., lyc., lyss., mang., meny., mez., ol-an., plan., raph., ***rhus-t.,*** sanic., sep., sulph., ter., verat.
chilliness, beginning in throat - sep.
cold, air, as from - ***aesc.,*** coca, cor-r., ol-an.
water were dropping down, as if - tarent.
wind, in - lyc.
evening - sep.
expiration, on - rhus-t.
extending to sternum - vac.
icy coldness - coc-c., cur.
inspiration, on - ***cist.,*** sulph.
left, sensation of cold wind - olnd.
peppermint, as from - agar., form., mez., tell., ***verat.***
swallowing, on - nat-m.
warm drinks, seem cold - nat-m.
coldness, throat, external - alum., berb., nat-s., phos., ***spong.***
evening - ***spong.***
night - lyc.

COLLAR, as if too tight, throat, external - aml-n., sep.

CONDYLOMATA - ***arg-n., merc-c., nit-ac.,*** **THUJ.**

CONGESTION, throat, external - kali-c.
holding hands on heart - am-c.

CONSTRICTION, (see Choking, Spasms) - ***cact.,*** med., sep.
right side - nat-m.
constriction, throat, external - acon., arg-c., ars., asar., cact., fl-ac., ***glon.,*** iod., **LACH.,** naja, puls., rat., ***sep.,*** **STRAM.,** ***stry.,*** tab., xan.
lying - glon.
sleep, during - lach.
constriction, throat-pit - ***apis,*** **BROM.,** ***ign.,*** ph-ac., rhus-t., ***staph.,*** valer., zinc.
anger open - ***staph.***
bending neck agg. - ph-ac.
eating amel. - rhus-t.
sleep, on going to - valer.
swallowing, when - staph.

CONTRACTION, (see Choking)

CRACKING, in - caust.

CRACKLING, throat, external, in muscles - rheum.

CRAMP - acon., ars., chel., ***gels., graph.,*** kali-c., kali-i., nat-m., phos., ***sars.,*** sep., sul-ac.
night - sars.
swallowing, on, food compelling him to retch - graph.
cramp, throat, external, in side of - bar-c., cic., graph., mang., plat., sep., spong.

CRAWLING, sensation - acon., aesc., am-m., bry., ***carb-v.,*** cedr., colch., ***crot-c.,*** dros., glon., grat., hyper., ***ign.,*** **KALI-C.,** ***lach.,*** lob., lyc., merc., mez., pall., petr., phos., plb., prun., puls., sabad., sabin., samb., sec., sep., spong., stann., sul-i., tab., thuj.
cough, causing - am-m., bry., ***carb-v.,*** euph., ***kali-c., lach.,*** prun., stann.
evening - nux-v.
menses, during - nux-v.
morning - lach.
bed, in - iod., lach.
nausea, during - lyc.
swallowing, on - tab.
worm, as if, were squirming in - hyper., merc., ***puls.***
crawling, throat, external, glands, in - con.

CRUSHED, throat, external, as if - sep.

CRYPTS, grayish-white, tonsils - calc-i., ***ign.***

CUTICLE, (see Membrane)

CUTTING, pain - bufo, chin-s., kali-n., mang., ***merc-c.,*** merc-cy., plan., plb., puls., rob., sep., stann., staph., sulph., sul-ac., thuj., uran-n., ust.
coughing, on - calc., lyc., sulph.
extending to stomach - plb.
hawking, on - sep.
swallowing, on - stann., sul-ac.
cutting, throat, external - ruta.
left - thuj.

DENUDED, (see Erosion)

DIGGING, pain - arg-m.

DIPHTHERIA, infection, (see Membrane) - ***acet-ac.,*** ail., ***am-c.,*** ant-t., **APIS,** arg-n., **ARS.,** ars-i., ***arum-t., bapt.,*** bar-c., ***bell.,*** **BROM.,** bry., calc-p., ***canth., caps., carb-ac., con., crot-c., crot-h.,*** cupr-ac., ***diph., echi., elaps,*** guai., hep., ign., iod., **KALI-BI., KALI-CHL.,** kali-ma., ***kali-m.,*** kali-p., ***kali-per., kreos.,*** **LAC-C., LACH.,** ***lachn.,*** led., lob., **LYC.,** ***merc., merc-c., merc-cy., merc-i-f., merc-i-r., mur-ac.,*** naja, ***nat-a., nat-m., nit-ac.,*** **PHOS., PHYT., RHUS-T.,** sabad., sal-ac., ***sang., sec., sulph., sul-ac., thuj,*** vinc., zinc-m.
blood-streaked - kali-bi.
bluish - carb-ac., chin-a., lach., merc-cy., merc-i-r.
brownish - iod.
yellow, like wash leather, or firm, fibrinous and pearly - kali-bi.
curdy - lac-c.
dark - bapt., phyt.
deep-seated - ail., apis, kali-bi., nit-ac.
dirty-looking - apis, lac-c.
dry and shrivelled - ***ars.***
elastic - kali-bi.
entire throat - am-c., ars., kali-ma., merc-cy.
extending to, larynx - brom., **KALI-BI.**
to, nose - kali-bi., lyc., merc., ***merc-c.,*** merc-cy., ***nit-ac.,*** sulph.
gangrenous - bapt.

DIPHTHERIA, infection
gray - apis, carb-ac., ***con., iod.,*** kali-bi., lac-c., lach., lyc., merc., merc-cy., merc-i-f., ***mur-ac.,*** nat-a., nit-ac., **PHYT.,** sanic., sul-ac.
dirty, with fiery red margins - apis.
patch on tonsils - kali-m.
white in crypts - ign.
yellow, slight, easily detached, worse on left - merc-i-r.
greenish - elaps, ***kali-bi., merc-cy.***
irregular - lac-c., merc-i-f.
leathery - kali-n., merc-cy.
left - bell., brom., crot-h., ***lac-c.,*** **LACH.,** ***manc., merc-i-r.***
alternating sides - **LAC-C.**
extending to right - lac-c., **LACH.,** naja, petr., xan.
small patches - ***ars.,*** lach.
small patches, white - lach.
loose - lac-c., merc-i-f., merc-i-r.
migratory - ***lac-c.***
nose, in - ***am-c., hydr., kali-bi., lyc.,*** merc-c., merc-cy., nit-ac., ***petr.***
begins in - lyc., merc-c., merc-cy.
extends to lips - am-c.
post nasal - lac-c., lach.
obstruction, with - am-c., hydr., ***kali-m., lyc., merc-cy.***
nosebleeds, with - ars., ***carb-v., chin., crot-h., hydr., ign., kali-chl., lach., merc-cy., nit-ac.,*** phos.
detachment of membrane, after - ***phos.***
paralysis after - ant-t., apis, arg-m., arn., ***ars.,*** camph., carb-ac., ***caust., cocc., crot-h.,*** gels., kali-br., kali-p., lac-c., ***lach., nat-m.,*** nux-v., phos., sec., sulph.
limps, lower, of - **ARS.,** ***cocc., con.,*** gels., ***lach.,*** nat-m., nux-v., ***phos., plb., sec., sil.***
patches - canth., merc-i-r.
isolated - kali-bi.
right tonsil and inflamed fauces, easily detached - merc-i-f.
small (specks) - ail., apis, ***ars.,*** canth., iod., kali-bi., lac-c., lach., merc-i-r.
small, white - lach.
pearly - **LAC-C.,** kali-bi., ***sang.***
plugs of mucus constantly form in crypts - calc-f.
profuse - carb-ac., lach., lyc., merc-c., sul-ac.
putrid - bapt., carb-ac., merc-cy.
right - ***apis,*** ign., lac-c., **LYC.,** ***merc., merc-i-f.,*** phyt., rhus-t.
extending to left - ferr-p., lac-c., **LYC.,** ***sulph.***
scanty - merc-i-f., merc-i-r.
shining, glazed, white or yellow patch - ***lac-c.***
thick - ars., iod., sul-ac.
dark gray or brownish black - diph.
thin - lac-c., merc-cy.
false, on yellowish red tonsils and fauces - merc-sul.
then dark and gangrenous - merc-cy.

DIPHTHERIA, infection
transparent - merc-i-f., merc-i-r.
varnished, shining - ***lac-c.***
wash leather - bapt., **PHYT.,** rhus-t.
white - am-caust., ***apis, ars.,*** iod., kali-bi., **KALI-CHL.,** kreos., **LAC-C.,** ***lach.,*** lyc., ***merc., merc-c., merc-cy.,*** merc-i-f., ***mur-ac.,*** nat-a., **NIT-AC.,** nux-m., ox-ac., **PHYT.,** stram., ***sul-ac.,*** zinc.
wrinkled - **ARS.**
yellow - apis, kali-bi., lac-c., lach., merc., ***merc-cy., merc-i-f.,*** **NAT-P.,** nit-ac., rhus-t., ***sulph., sul-ac.,*** zinc.

DISCOLORATION, general
black - merc-sul.
copper-colored - ***kali-bi.,*** **MERC.**
dark - ***aesc.,*** arag., ***bapt.,*** **PHYT.**
livid - alum.
mottled - ail., bapt., kali-per., ***lach.***
pale - bar-c.
purple - **AIL.,** am-c., ***bapt.,*** fl-ac., ***kali-bi.,*** kali-chl., **LACH.,** ***merc., nat-a.,*** nit-ac., ***nux-v.,*** ox-ac., ***puls., sanic.,*** sulph., tarent.
redness, (see Redness)
white spots - ***mur-ac.,*** nit-ac.
uvula - carb-ac.
yellow spots - lac-c., lach., lyc., ***nit-ac.***

discoloration, throat, external - kali-bi., kali-s., podo., rhus-v.
blue - ***lach.***
brown - kali-s.
spots, in - kali-bi., ***sep.***
itching - kali-n.
lividity - ***ars.***
purple - tarent.
redness - am-caust., apis, graph., rhus-v.
spots, in - am-c., **BELL.,** carb-v., iod., kali-n., ***sep.,*** stann., tarent.
stripe, in - mang.
white spots - nat-c.
yellow - ars., chel., hydr.
spots - ***iod.***

discoloration, tonsils
bluish - am-c.
gray - kali-m., merc-cy.
purple - lach., phyt.

DISTENSION, sensation - mag-c., sulph.

distention, throat, external, left - caust.

DRAWING, pain - alum., apis, ***arg-n.,*** aur., calc-p., caps., croc., cupr., kali-bi., laur., merc-c., nat-m., plat., plb., sabad., stann., ***stram.,*** sulph., teucr., verat., zinc.
extending to ear - all-c., alum., bry.
moving the tongue - alum.
night - alum.
sitting up amel. - spong.
swallowing when not - ***caps.***

drawing, throat, external - nat-m.

DRAWN, out, sensation - mag-c.

DRIPPING, uvula - all-c., aral., hydr., kali-bi., merc-c., spig.

DRYNESS, of - ***acon.,*** **AESC.,** aeth., ***agar.,*** ail., ***all-c.,*** aloe, ***alum.,*** alumn., ambr., am-c., ***ammc.,*** am-m., ***anac.,*** **ANAG.,** ant-c., ***apis, arg-n., ars.,*** ars-i., ***asaf.,*** asar., ***atro.,*** aur-m-n., bapt., ***bar-c.,*** bar-m., **BELL.,** berb., both., bor., ***bov.,*** brom., **BRY.,** ***bufo,*** cadm-s., cahin., **CALAD., CALC.,** calc-p., calc-s., **CANN-I.,** cann-s., **CANTH.,** caps., carb-ac., ***carb-s., carb-v.,*** **CAUST.,** cham., ***chel.,*** chin., chin-a., chin-s., chlor., ***cic.,*** cimic., ***cimx., cinnb.,*** **CIST.,** clem., cob., ***cocc.,*** **COC-C.,** coca, ***colch., coloc., con.,*** cop., ***cor-r., crot-h.,*** crot-t., cub., cupr., cycl., dig., dios., ***dros., dub.,*** dulc., eug., eup-per., eupi., fago., ferr-p., gamb., ***gels.,*** glon., graph., ***guai.,*** ham., hell., ***hep.,*** hydr., ***hyos., ign., iod., ip., iris,*** jac-c., jatr., ***kali-ar.,*** **KALI-BI.,** kali-br., ***kali-c., kali-chl., kali-i.,*** kali-ma., kali-p., ***kali-s., kalm.,*** kreos., lac-ac., ***lach., lachn.,*** **LAC-C.,** laur., lem-m., lob., lob-c., **LYC., MAG-C.,** ***mag-m.,*** mag-s., ***manc.,*** mang., med., meny., **MERC.,** ***merc-c.,*** merc-i-f., merc-sul., **MEZ.,** morg., morph., mosch., ***mur-ac.,*** myric., ***naja, nat-a., nat-c.,*** **NAT-M.,** ***nat-p., nat-s., nit-ac.,*** **NUX-M.,** ***nux-v.,*** ol-an., olnd., onos., ***op.,*** ox-ac., par., petr., phel., ph-ac., **PHOS.,** ***phyt.,*** plan., ***plat.,*** plb., ***podo., psor.,*** ptel., **PULS.,** raph., **RHUS-T.,** rhus-v., rumx., **SABAD.,** ***sabin.,*** samb., **SANG.,** sanic., ***sars.,*** sec., sel., ***senec.,*** **SENEG., SEP., SIL.,** sin-n., sol-n., ***spong.,*** squil., ***stann.,*** staph., **STICT.,** still., **STRAM.,** stroph., stry., **SULPH.,** sul-ac., sumb., tab., tarax., tell., ***thuj.,*** thyr., tub., ust., valer., **VERAT., VERAT-V.,** verb., wye., xan., ***zinc.,*** zing.
afternoon - am-c., canth., ***cist.,*** mang., phyt., sang., sep., sulph.
5 p.m. - phyt., sulph., tell.
waking, on - sel.
air, open, in - ammc., gins., mang.
bed, in - phyt., rhus-t.
chill, during - phos., thuj.
coughing, from - rhus-t., squil.
amel. - stann.
daytime - mez.
dinner. after - zinc.
drinking does not amel. - sang., sep., verat.
dust, as if in - coc-c.
eating, after - aesc., nat-m.
amel. - anac., ***cist.,*** phos.
epiglottis - lach., lyss., wye.
evening - **ALUM.,** am-c., ***bar-c.,*** brom., cist., dulc., kali-p., lyc., ox-ac., phos., sel., senec., sep., stram., tell., ***zinc.***
6 p.m. - mang.
sleep, before - sep., staph.
excitement, with - prot.
fauces - acon., aesc., ***bell.,*** canth., caps., gels., jug-c., ***nux-m., phos., phyt., sabad.,*** senec.
fever, during - asar., nit-ac., olnd., op., sep., sulph.
forenoon - anac.
hawking agg. - ***spong.***
inspiration, on - ham., nat-a.
itching - mang.
lying, while - caust., lyc.

DRYNESS, of
midnight - ***arum-t., kali-bi.,*** puls., sul-ac.
after - puls., sul-ac.
morning - ***ail.,*** all-c., alum., ambr., am-c., ***ammc.,*** ant-c., arg-n., berb., bufo, calc., cann-s., caust., hyos., lach., lyc., mag-c., mag-m., mag-s., mang., mez., nat-a., ol-an., petr., phyt., plan., plb., **PULS.,** ran-s., sars., stann., stram., stront-c., sulph., tell., ust., zinc.
waking, while - alum., ambr., bor., carb-ac., coc-c., hep., kali-i., mag-c., ol-an., phos., **PULS.,** sars., ***seneg.,*** sep., zinc.
naso-pharynx - lem-m.
night - acon., alumn., arg-n., ars., ***calc.,*** calc-p., caust., ***cinnb., cist.,*** coc-c., glon., graph., kali-c., **LACH.,** lyc., mag-m., nat-c., nit-ac., phel., phos., plat., ***puls.,*** rhus-t., ***senec., seneg.,*** sep., sil., ***sulph., ust.***
noon - mag-m.
painful - anac., ***lach.,*** tell.
pharynx - bell., nux-m.
posterior part - caust., cimic., **DROS.,** kali-c., merc., rhus-t., mez.
rest, during - con.
right - stann.
rising, when - cob., ham.
roughness - ang., **DROS.**
soft palate - ***dros.***
speaking very difficult - bry., merc., seneg.
swallowing, on - carb-v., caust., lyc., mag-c.
amel. - stann.
saliva, amel. - ***cist.***
talking, difficult - xan.
talking, from - alum., graph., merc-ac., sil.
thirst, without - ***apis,*** asaf., calc., ***calad.,*** carb-an., caust., kali-c., ***lach.,*** lyc., mag-m., mang., meny., nat-c., **NUX-M.,** pall., par., ph-ac., psor., samb., sep.
urination, after - nit-ac.
waking, on - ***alum., ambr.,*** am-c., ***bov., cinnb., cist.,*** coc-c., ***lac-c.,*** **LACH.,** ***lachn.,*** lyc., mag-c., ***manc.,*** morph., naja, nat-a., **NUX-M.,** ol-an., par., phos., sars., sel., sep., sil., sulph., zing.
walking in open air - tell.

DUST, as if in - coc-c.

EDEMA, glottidis - **APIS,** ars., arum-t., bell., chin., chin-a., chlor., ***crot-h.,*** hippoz., ign., iod., jab., **KALI-I.,** ***lach.,*** merc., ***sang.,*** staph., ***stram., vip.***
vocal cords - **LACH.**

ELONGATED, uvula - acon., ***alumn., apis,*** aur., bapt., **BAR-M.,** brom., calc., ***caps., coff., croc.,*** **CROT-T.,** ***hep.,*** hydr., **HYOS.,** ind., ***iod., kali-c.,*** **KALI-I.,** lac-ac., ***lac-c.,*** **LACH.,** lyc., lyss., ***manc., merc.,*** merc-c., merc-i-f., merc-i-r., mill., nat-a., ***nat-m.,*** nux-v., **PHOS.,** psor., sil., **SULPH.,** thuj.
hawking, from constant - coc-c.
pressing on something hard - caps.

elongated, uvula, sensation of - coc-c., croc., dulc., plat., sulph.

EMPTINESS - calc-p., chin., elat., fl-ac., iris, lob., lyc., nat-a., ptel., sanic., xan.
swallowing, on - lyc.

ENLARGEMENT, tonsils, of - ***alumn.,*** am-c., **BAR-C.,** bar-i., **BAR-M.,** ***calc.,*** **CALC-F., CALC-I., CALC-P.,** carc., ***cedr., chen-a.,*** chin., con., ***ferr., hep.,*** ign., iod., ***kali-bi., kali-c., kali-i.,*** kali-m., **LACH., LYC.,** med., ***merc.,*** merc-i-f., merc-i-r., nat-a., ***nat-m., nit-ac.,*** petr., phos., ***phyt., sep., sil., staph., sulph.,*** syc-co., ***syph.,*** **TUB.,** vesp.
children, in pale, scrofulous - chen-a.
coryza, after - sabad.
hardness of hearing, with - ***bar-c.,*** calc-p., ***hep.,*** lyc., plb., psor.
mouth opening agg. - calc-p.
pus, plugs, with - calc-f.

EROSION - ***aesc., apis,*** ars., brom., sumb.
spots - brom.

ERUPTION, throat, external - ***anac., ars.,*** berb., bry., bov., bry., calc., canth., caust., clem., dig., ***hep.,*** kali-n., lyc., merc., ph-ac., raph., sars., sep., squil., thuj.
blotches - graph., nat-m., sars., sep., spong.
burning - kali-n.
crusts - anac.
itching - lyc., mag-c.
moist - ***caust.***
painful - lyc.
pimples - agar., alum., ant-c., berb., bor., bov., canth., ***cinnb.,*** clem., ***hep., jug-r.,*** kali-n., lyc., mag-c., mez., mur-ac., nat-m., ph-ac., raph., ***puls.,*** spig., spong., stann., staph., sulph., ***thuj.,*** zinc.
pustules - ant-c., aur., chel., ***psor.***
row, in a - thuj.
rash - am-c., chin.
red - chin., lyc., mez., ph-ac., sep., spig., thuj.
scratching, after - mag-c.
stitching - phos.
tubercles - am-c., lach., lyc., mur-ac., nicc., ph-ac., phos., sec.
urticaria - bry., kali-i.
vesicles - clem., mag-c., ph-ac., sep., vip.
side of - alum.
side of, ear, discharge from - **TELL.**

EXCORIATION - ***aesc.,*** ant-c., ars., canth., ***caust.,*** dig., fago., hell., ***merc.,*** mur-ac., ***nit-ac.,*** phyt., sul-ac.

excoriation, throat, external, from rubbing of clothes - olnd., squil.

FINGER, puts in - bell.

FISHBONE, (see Splinter, pain, as if)

FISSURED, pharynx - bar-c., elaps, kali-bi., ph-ac., phos.

FISTULA, throat, external - ***phos., sil.***

FOOD, lodges in - acet-ac., bry., ***caust.,*** chin., croc., crot-h., ign., iris, kali-c., **LACH.,** lyc., **NIT-AC.,** petr., sep., sil., sulph., ***zinc.***
bread, crumb - graph.
passes into choanae - lyc., nit-ac., petr., ***sil.***
turned, like a corkscrew on swallowing - elaps.
passed over raw places - bar-c.
sensation of - ambr., arg-n., arn., ***calc.,*** ferr-i., zinc.

FOREIGN object, in, sensation of (see Lump) - ***abies-n.,*** aesc., agar., ail., ambr., am-c., ***ant-c., apis,*** arg-n., arn., bar-c., **BELL.,** brom., bry., bufo, calc., carb-v., chel., chin-s., cic., coloc., ***con.,*** **CROT-C.,** ***crot-t.,*** graph., ign., kreos., **LACH.,** led., mag-c., ***merc.,*** mez., myric., nat-c., ***nux-m.,*** ol-an., phos., plan., plb., sabad., sabin., ***sep.,*** sol-t-ae., sulph., zinc.
afternoon - phos.
apple core - phyt.
bone, (see Bone)
evening - am-c.
morning - am-c., cob.
rhinopharynx, as if something hanging - **YUC.**
skin hanging loose in, and he must swallow over it - ***alum., sabad.***
smoking, while - plb., sep.
sneezing, while - bar-c.
stone - bufo
string, as if a - sabad., valer.
swallowing - graph., ust.
does not amel. - agar., ant-c., ***crot-c., kali-bi.,*** **LACH.,** ***sep.***
walking, rapidly - nat-c.

FORMICATION, throat, external - rhus-v., spong.
throat pit, causing cough - ***sang.***

FULLNESS, sensation - aesc., ail., aloe, am-m., anan., ***apis,*** bapt., ***bell.,*** brom., carb-an., carb-s., carb-v., caust., chin-s., cimic., ***cinnb., con., eucal.,*** eup-pur., glon., ***iber.,*** iod., kali-p., ***lach.,*** lac-c., lac-ac., phos., phys., ***phyt.,*** puls., raph., ***sang., sil.,*** sulph., syph., ***thuj.,*** zinc.
afternoon - bapt.
lying down - apis
swallowing, on - ***sang.***
turning head to left - phyt.
writing - phyt.
fullness, throat, external, in jugular - ***crot-c.***
fullness, throat pit, in - cham., con., ***lach.***

GAGGING, general - agar., benz-ac., bry., calc-p., ***carb-v., chin.,*** chin-s., cop., ***kali-c.,*** kali-chl., ***lyc.,*** par., ***podo.***
breakfast, after - calc-p.
coughing, from - ***agar., arg-n.,*** bry., calc., carb-v., caust., cench., cimx., **CINA,** coc-c., cupr., dirc., ferr., hell., **IP.,** kali-c., ***lach., lyss.,*** merc-c., sanic., sep.
drinking, when - ***cimic.***
eating, after - agar., ***ambr., kali-c., lach.***
expectoration, during - ***arg-n., coc-c.,*** par.
morning - carb-v., ***corn.,*** kali-c.

GAGGING, general
mucus in fauces, from - anac., ***ant-t., arg-n., carb-v.,*** ip., ***lyc.***
night - ***arg-n.***

GANGRENE - **AIL.,** ***am-c., anth.,*** arn., **ARS., ARUM-T.,** bapt., bell., canth., carb-ac., ***carb-s., carb-v., chin.,*** chin-a., con., **CROT-H.,** euph., ***kali-p., kreos., lach.,*** merc., ***merc-c.,*** merc-cy., ***mur-ac., nit-ac., phyt., sang., sec., sil., sulph.,*** sul-ac., tarent.
uvula - chin-a., ***lach.,*** lac-c.

GARGLING, agg. - carb-v.

GLAZED, appearance - **APIS,** arag., bell., ***carb-ac.,*** cist., ***hydr., kali-bi.,*** **LAC-C.,** ***nat-a., nat-m.,*** petr., ***phos.,*** phyt.

GLUEY - sep.

GRANULATED - bar-c., ***hydr., kali-bi., phyt.***

GRASPS, throat, external during cough - acon., ***all-c., cupr., iod.,*** lob., ***samb.***

GURGLING, drinking, after - **PHOS.**

HAIR, throat, sensation of - aesc-g., all-s., ambr., arg-n., ars., carb-s., caust., coc-c., cocaine, dros., hepat., ***kali-bi.,*** lach., nat-m., nit-ac., nux-v., pulx., ***sabad.,*** sang., buth-a., ***sil., sulph.,*** thuj., uran-n., valer., yuc.
afternoon - ***sulph.***

HANGING, sensation as if mucous - ***carb-an.,*** lach., ***merc-c.,*** phos., thuj.
thread, a - ***coc-c., valer.***
hanging, uvula, of, to one side - lach.
right side, to - apis, nat-m.

HARD, as if - ***cupr.***

HAWK, disposition to - aesc., aeth., ***ail.,*** all-c., ***alum.,*** ambr., am-m., anac., ***arg-m.,*** **ARG-N.,** ***arum-t., bar-c., bell.,*** berb., bor., ***bry.,*** bufo, cahin., calad., calc., calc-ar., calc-f., calc-p., carb-ac., ***carb-an., carb-s., carb-v., caust.,*** chel., chin-a., cimic., ***cimx., cist., coc-c.,*** colch., con., **COR-R.,** ***crot-t.,*** cycl., ***dulc.,*** eug., ferr-i., ferr-ma., ***fl-ac., gels.,*** gent-c., ***graph.,*** grat., ***guai.,*** gymn., **HEP.,** ***hydr., kali-bi.,*** **KALI-C.,** ***kali-chl.,*** kali-ma., kali-n., kali-p., kali-s., **LACH.,** lac-ac., laur., ***lil-t.,*** lob., **lyc.,** mag-c., ***mag-m., manc.,*** mang., merc., ***merc-i-f., merc-i-r., mez.,*** naja, ***nat-a.,*** **NAT-C., NAT-M.,** nat-p., ***nat-s., nit-ac.,*** **NUX-V.,** onos., paeon., pall., par., petr., ph-ac., **PHOS.,** ***phyt.,*** plat., plb., ***psor.,*** ptel., rhus-t., ***rumx., sabad.,*** sars., ***sel.,*** senec., ***seneg.,*** **SEP.,** ***sil.,*** spig., ***stann., stram., sulph.,*** teucr., ***thuj.,*** viol-t., wye., xan., ***zinc.***
air, in open - ***carb-ac.,*** nat-a.
breakfast, after - calc-p.
breathing, deep - sulph.
dryness, from - alum.
eating, after - hep., ol-an., tub.
evening - ***alum.,*** caust., hep., kali-n., stann.
forenoon - arg-n.
11 a.m. - ***viol-t.***
ineffectual - **CAUST.,** mag-c., ***mez.,*** phos., thuj.

HAWK, disposition to
morning - ***ail.,*** ambr., am-m., ***calc.,*** bor., **CAUST.,** ***cist.,*** cob., fl-ac., grat., **KALI-BI.,** kali-n., nat-c., ***nat-m., petr., phos.,*** phyt., rhus-t., sars., ***sep.***
mucus, from post-nasal - **CAPS., MED.**
night - aur., sulph.
roughness, from - ***alum.***
sleep, during - calc-p.
sleep, after - ***lach.***
talking, while - calc-p.
tickling, from - sulph.
walking, in open air - ant-c., carb-ac.

HAWKS, up, cheesy lumps, from - ***agar.,*** arg-n., bell., bry., calc-f., ***chen-a.,*** coc-c., ign., ***kali-bi.,*** **KALI-M.,** kali-p., lyc., ***mag-c.,*** merc-i-r., nit-ac., ***phos., psor.,*** sec., sil., syc-co., tub.

HEAT - ***acon.,*** aesc., aeth., alumn., ant-c., arg-n., ***ars.,*** aster., ***bell.,*** benz-ac., bol., brom., cahin., camph., canth., ***caps.,*** carb-an., carb-v., ***cham.,*** chin., chin-a., ***cist.,*** clem., cob., coca, cocc., colch., cop., crot-t., ***euph.,*** dulc., ***ferr.,*** ferr-ar., ferr-p., fl-ac., ***gels., glon.,*** hell., hep., hydr-ac., hyos., hyper., hura, ir-fl., iris, jatr., kali-ar., kali-c., kali-chl., kali-n., kali-s., laur., led., lyc., lyss., manc., ***merc.,*** merc-c., merc-sul., **MEZ.,** mosch., nat-m., nat-s., ***nit-ac.,*** **NUX-V.,** oena., ox-ac., paeon., phos., plb., pic-ac., raph., ***rhus-t.,*** samb., ***sang., senec.,*** sep., squil., stry., ***sulph.,*** sul-ac., sumb., tab., tarent., ter., teucr., ust., verat., verat-v., vesp., vip., zinc.
air, open, in - ant-c.
afternoon - sep.
2 p.m. - nat-c.
breathing, on - mang.
cold air amel. - ***sang.***
coryza, during - mag-m.
cough, after - aur-m.
evening - nux-m., ox-ac., sumb.
6 to 7 p.m. - sang.
extending to stomach - all-c., crot-t., iod., manc., merc., naja, tab.
forenoon - carb-v.
morning - fl-ac., sulph.
night - cinnb., nit-ac.
swallowing, on - ferr., tab.
walking in open air, while - led.

heat, throat, external - cycl., lach., sars., sulph.

HERPES - ***apis,*** arn., bor., hydr., jac., ***kali-bi.,*** kali-chl., ***lach.,*** merc-i-f., nat-s., ***phyt.,*** sal-ac.

herpes, throat, external - lac-d., lyc., psor., sars., sep.

HOARSENESS, (see Larynx, voice)

HOLLOW feeling, as if pharynx had disappeared - lach., phyt.

HUNGER, sensation in - mang.

INDURATION of glands, throat, external - ***alum., alumn.,*** am-c., ant-c., bac., bar-c., ***bar-i.,*** **BAR-M., BELL., CALC.,** calc-f., **CALC-I.,** ***calc-p.,*** **CARB-AN.,** carb-s., ***carb-v.,*** carc., ***cist.,*** **CON.,** ***cupr., dulc., graph., hecla., hep.,*** **IOD.,** ***kali-i., lyc., merc., nat-c.,*** nat-m., ***nit-ac.,*** puls., ***rhus-t., sars.,*** sep., **SIL.,** ***spong.,*** staph., **SULPH.,** syc-co., **TAB.**
knotted cords, like - aeth., **BAR-I., BAR-M.,** berb., ***calc.,*** **CALC-I.,** ***cist., dulc.,*** hecla., hep., ***iod.,*** lyc., ***merc.,*** nit-ac., ***psor.,*** rhus-t., ***sil., sulph.,*** **TUB.**

induration, tonsils - ***agar.,*** alum., alumn., ars-i., aur., bac., **BAR-C.,** ***bar-i.,*** **BAR-M.,** brom., calc., ***calc-i.,*** calc-p., ***cham.,*** con., cupr., ferr-p., ***graph.,*** hep., ***ign., iod., kali-bi.,*** merc-i-f., ***merc-i-r., nit-ac.,*** petr., phyt., ***plb.,*** sabad., sil., ***staph., sul-i.,*** thuj.

INFLAMMATION, sore throat (see Pain, throat or Sore, pain) - **ACON.,** aesc., ***ail.,*** all-s., aloe, ***alum., am-c., am-m.,*** anan., ant-c., ***apis, arg-m.,*** **ARG-N.,** ***ars., arum-t., aur., aur-m.,*** bad., ***bapt.,*** **BAR-C.,** ***bar-m.,*** **BELL.,** berb., bism., brom., ***bry., bufo,*** cahin., ***calc., calc-p., calc-s.,*** canth., **CAPS.,** carb-s., carb-v., caust., ***cham.,*** chin-a., cimic., ***cinnb., cist.,*** coc-c., ***coff., colch.,*** com., con., cop., ***crot-c., crot-h.,*** crot-t., ***cupr., dulc.,*** elaps, fago., **FERR-P.,** fl-ac., ***gels., graph.,*** ham., **HEP.,** hippoz., ign., ***iod.,*** ip., kali-ar., ***kali-bi., kali-c., kali-i., kali-ma.,*** kali-n., kali-p., kali-s., ***lac-c.,*** **LACH.,** lob-c., **LYC.,** ***lyss.,*** mag-c., mang., **MERC.,** ***merc-c., merc-cy., merc-i-f., merc-i-r., mez., mur-ac., naja,*** nat-a., nat-c., ***nat-m.,*** nat-p., ***nat-s.,*** nicc., **NIT-AC.,** nux-m., ***nux-v.,*** oena., ol-an., pall., **PETR.,** ph-ac., ***phos., phyt.,*** plb., psor., ptel., ***puls.,*** ran-b., ***rhus-t.,*** sabad., ***sang.,*** seneg., sep., sol-t-ae., still., stront-c., ***sulph.,*** sul-ac., tarent., tell., ***thuj.,*** vip., ***zinc.***
alternating with sore, eyes - par.
atropic - aesc., arg-n., ars-i., dub., kali-bi., ***nux-v.,*** sabal.
burning, pressing, dark - **CAPS.**
children - cham., merc., phos.
chronic - aesc., ***alum.,*** am-br., ***am-caust., arg-m., arg-n.,*** ars., arum-t., aur., ***bar-c.,*** brom., ***calc.,*** calc-p., cann-i., ***carb-s., carb-v.,*** caust., cinnb., cist., ***cob.,*** cub., elaps, ferr-p., ***fl-ac.,*** fuc., graph., ***ham., hep., hydr., iod., jug-c., kali-bi.,*** kali-c., kali-chl., ***kali-i., lach., lyc.,*** mang., med., **MERC.,** merc-c., merc-i-f., ***nat-c., nat-m., nit-ac., nux-v.,*** ol-j., ox-ac., petr., **PHOS.,** ***phyt.,*** psor., puls., ***rumx.,*** sabad., sabal., ***sang.,*** sec., seneg., ***sep., sil.,*** stann., ***sulph.,*** sumb., tab., ***thuj., wye.***
cold, after - ***bar-c., bell., cham., dulc.,*** petr.
erysipelatous - **APIS,** bapt., ***bell.,*** crot-c., ***lach.,*** lyc., ***merc.,*** phyt., ***rhus-t.***
extending, downwards - merc.
to nose - ***nit-ac.***
upwards and downwards - ***merc.***
fauces - ail., apis, ***bell., ferr-p., kali-bi.,*** menthol, merc-i-f., merc-sul.
follicular - aesc., ***ail.,*** **BELL.,** cop., guai., **HEP.,** ***hydr.,*** **IGN., IOD.,** ***kali-bi., kali-chl., kali-i., lac-c., merc., merc-cy., merc-i-r., mur-ac.,*** **NAT-M.,** ***nit-ac., phyt., sec.***

INFLAMMATION, sore throat
follicular, acute - aesc., ***alum.,*** am-br., ***arg-n.,*** arn., ars-i., ***arum-t.,*** calc-f., calc-p., caps., caust., cinnb., cist., ***hep., hydr.,*** ign., kali-bi., ***lach.,*** merc., merc-cy., ***merc-i-r.,*** nat-m., nux-v., phos., phyt., ***sang-n.,*** still., ***sulph., wye.***
forenoon - jab.
left - ***crot-h., elaps,*** form., ***lac-ac., lac-c.,*** **LACH.,** ***merc-i-r., naja,*** nicc., sec., ***sep.,*** thuj.
menses, during - ***lac-c.***
before - ***mag-c.,*** senec.
mercury, after - ***arg-m.,*** **HEP.,** ***nit-ac.***
night - ***cinnb.,*** **MERC.**
painless - **BAPT.,** carb-ac.
phlegmonous - ***acon., alumn.,*** apis, bar-c., bar-i., ***bell.,*** calc., caps., cinnb., guai., ***hep.,*** lac-c., ***lach.,*** lyc., ***merc.,*** merc-i-f., merc-i-r., merc-sul., ***nux-v., phyt.,*** sang., sang-n., sil., ***sulph.,*** thuj., vesp.
predisposition to acute catarrhal - alumn., ***bar-c.,*** lach., sulph.
rheumatic - acon., bry., colch., guai., phyt., rhus-t.
right - ars-m., **BELL.,** ham., ***lac-c.,*** lyss., **LYC.,** ***merc., merc-i-f., phyt.,*** sars., stront-c., tarent., xan.
septic - am-c., bapt., ***hep.,*** merc., mur-ac., pyrog., ***sil.***
singers, in (see Clergyman)
speakers, in (see Clergyman)
tubercular - merc-i-r.
voice, overuse of (see Clergyman)
waking, on - kali-bi., ***lach.***
warmth of bed agg. - apis, coc-c.

inflammation, epiglottis - all-c., chlor., hepat., wye.
inflammation, pharynx (see Pharyngitis)
inflammation, tonsils (see Tonsillitis)
inflammation, uvula - ***acon., alum.,*** amyg., **APIS,** ars., ***bell.,*** berb., brom., calc., caps., ***carb-v.,*** chin-s., cimic., cist., colch., cupr-ac., ***gels.,*** iod., kali-bi., kali-n., ***kali-per., lac-c., merc-c., merc-i-f., nat-s.,*** nux-v., ***phyt.,*** plb., puls., ***seneg.,*** sul-i., sulph.

IRRITATION - ***ail.,*** aster., **BELL.,** ***bov.,*** carb-ac., ***carb-v.,*** chin-s., cimic., **CON.,** ***crot-t.,*** gels., ***glon., hep.,*** hura, ip., iod., kali-br., ***kali-i., lach.,*** morph., nat-a., ***nux-v.,*** puls., rhus-t., rhus-v., sang., sars., sec., sil., sul-ac., tab., ust.
evening - chel.
extending to eustachian tube - phyt.
morning - chel., nat-c., ***sulph.***
night - tab.
public speakers and singers - wye.

irritation, fauces, deep in, causes cough - **DROS.**
irritation, pharynx - aesc., bov., olnd., verat.
irritation, throat pit - ***apis,*** bell., card-m., ***cham.,*** croc., ***hyos.,*** **IGN.,** iod., kreos., lac-c., mang., ph-ac., rhus-r., **RUMX., SANG.,** ***sil.,*** squil.

ITCHING - aeth., agar., ambr., am-m., anac., ***apis,*** arg-m., cahin., calc-s., ***cist.,*** colch., con., cop., ***glon.,*** kali-c., kali-i., ***plan.,*** samb., ***spong., wye.***
coughing, when - ambr.
periodical - ***cist.***
swallowing agg. - nux-v.

itching, fauces - phyt., rhus-t.
itching, pharynx - cahin., spig.
swallowing, when - lachn., stront.
itching, throat, external - **ALUM.,** ambr., am-m., anac., ant-c., apis, ars., aur., bov., ***calc.,*** canth., carb-v., caust., chel., ***cist.,*** con., fl-ac., form., ***glon.,*** kali-i., kali-n., lyc., mag-c., mez., ***nat-c.,*** nit-ac., plan., rhus-v., samb., sep., stront-c., sulph., tarent., thuj.
evening - mez.
before going to sleep - mag-c.
extending to, chest - fl-ac.
to, eustachian tubes - caust.
to, larynx - sil., zinc.
menses, during - mag-c.
morning - mag-c.
dressing, while - mag-c.
night - kalm.
scratching amel. - mag-c., squil.
stitching - carb-v., sars.
swallowing agg. - aur., con.
walking in open air - nit-ac.
itching, throat-pit - phos.
itching, uvula - sabad.

JERKING - nat-m., plat.
to pit of stomach - sep.
jerking, throat, external - arg-m., caps.

JERKS, throat, external, left - mez.

LANCINATING, pain - am-caust., ars., aur-s., bufo, manc., ust.
lancinating, tonsils - ust.

LEAF, sensation in pharynx, as if leaf lay before posterior nares, morning after waking - ***bar-c.***

LIQUIDS, taken are forced into nose - anan., **ARUM-T.,** aur., ***bar-c.,*** bell., bism., canth., ***carb-ac.,*** caust., cupr., ***cur.,*** diph., gels., hyos., ign., kali-bi., ***kali-ma.,*** kali-per., ***lac-ac.,*** **LAC-C., LACH., LYC.,** ***lyss., merc., merc-c., merc-cy., nat-m.,*** op., petr., phos., ***phyt., plb.,*** puls., sil., ***sul-ac.,*** verat.

LUMP, plug, sensation in - aesc., agar., ail., ***all-c., alum., ambr.,*** am-c., anan., ***ant-c.,*** apis, ***arg-n.,*** arn., ars., **ASAF.,** aur., aur-m., ***bar-c.,*** bell., benz-ac., berb., ***brom.,*** bry., bufo, ***calc.,*** calc-s., ***carb-s.,*** carb-v., ***caust.,*** cham., chel., chin-s., cic., ***cina,*** cocc., ***coc-c., con.,*** croc., ***crot-c., crot-h.,*** crot-t., cur., ***ferr., ferr-ar., ferr-p., gels., graph., hep.,*** hyos., **IGN.,** kali-ar., ***kali-bi., kali-c.,*** kali-n., kali-p., kali-s., kreos., lac-ac., ***lac-c.,*** **LACH.,** laur., ***led., lil-t., lob.,*** mag-c., med., merc., ***merc-i-f., merc-i-r.,*** mez., myric., nat-a., ***nat-c.,*** **NAT-M.,** nat-p., ***nit-ac., nux-m., nux-v.,*** ol-an., par., ph-ac., phos., ***phyt.,*** plan., ***plb.,*** **PSOR.,** ***puls.,*** rumx., ruta., ***sabad.,*** sabin., ***sep., sil.,*** sol-t-ae., still., stry., ***sulph.,*** sul-ac., tab., ***thuj.,*** ust., verat-v., zinc.

LUMP, plug, sensation in
afternoon - ***bar-c.***
belching amel. - kali-ar., ***mag-m.***
bitter, lump - sul-ac.
coughing amel. - kali-c.
eating, while - sulph.
evening - am-c., ***asaf.***, sep.
swallowing, on - sep.
forenoon - phos., phyt.
riding, while - phyt.
grief, after - ***ign.***
hard, lump - sul-ac.
hysterical - acon., con., ***ign.***, ***mag-m.***, mosch., plb., senec., valer., zinc.
belching amel. - mag-m.
unconsciousness, ending in - mosch.
left - bar-c., calc., kali-c., sil.
menopause, during - aml-n., ***lach.***, valer., zinc-valer.
middle throat - chin., puls.
morning - am-c., cob., hep.
night - graph., mag-m., nat-m.
painful - **LACH.**
right - sil., vario.
rising sensation - ***ars.***, **ASAF.**, cact., cann-i., cham., ***chel.***, ***coloc.***, ***con.***, ***gels.***, **IGN.**, kali-ar., ***kalm.***, ***lac-d.***, lach., ***lec.***, ***lob.***, **LYC.**, mag-c., ***mag-m.***, mur-ac., **MOSCH.**, **NAT-M.**, nit-ac., ***nux-m.***, **NUX-V.**, phys., ***plat.***, ***plb.***, ***puls.***, ***senec.***, ***sep.***, spong., ***stram.***, ***sulph.***, sul-ac., tarent., ***valer.***, verat-v., zinc.
sleep, during - ***crot-c.***, **LACH.**, **NUX-V.**, ***sep.***, valer.
smoking, while - plb., sep.
speech, preventing - nat-p.
stone - bufo.
swallowing, on - ***bar-c.***, calc., ***gels.***, ***graph.***, ***lach.***, ***merc.***, ***nat-m.***, nat-s., ***nux-v.***, pic-ac., puls., ***sep.***, sil., ust.
empty - caust., ***ferr.***, nit-ac., ***nux-v.***, ruta., sabad., ***sulph.***
left to right - xan.
not amel. by - agar., ant-c., crot-c., ***kali-bi.***, **LACH.**, ***nat-m.***, ***sep.***
returns after - calc., ign., ***lac-c.***, **LACH.**, ***rumx.***
when not - ferr., ***ign.***, ***nat-m.***, sulph.
upper throat - lac-ac.

lump, throat pit - benz-ac., **LACH.**, ***lob.***
eating, after - ambr.
swallowing, in - benz-ac.

MEMBRANE, fauces, exudation, (see Diphtheria) - caps., merc-cy.

membrane, pharynx, posterior wall - am-caust., canth., merc-i-f., mur-ac., ***sulph.***

membrane, tonsils - ail., am-caust., ***apis,*** carb-ac., cupr-ar., iod., ign., ***kali-bi.***, ***kali-i.***, kali-p., ***lac-c.***, **LACH.**, **LYC.**, merc., merc-i-f., **NIT-AC.**, **PHYT.**
left - lac-c., **LACH.**, merc-i-r.
right - ign., lac-c., ***lyc.***, merc-i-f., rhus-t.

membrane, uvula - ***apis,*** carb-ac., ***kali-bi.***, lac-c., merc-c., merc-i-f., ***nit-ac.***, **PHYT.**

MUCUS, in throat (see Catarrh) - acon., aesc., agar., ail., ***all-c.***, ***alum.***, ***alumn.***, ***ambr.***, am-m., ***anac.***, ant-c., ***ant-t.***, aphis., **ARG-M.**, **ARG-N.**, arn., ars., ***ars-i.***, arum-d., ***arum-t.***, asar., aur., bapt., bar-c., bar-m., bell., benz-ac., ***berb.***, bism., bor., bov., bry., bufo, cact., ***calc.***, calc-ar., calc-p., ***calc-s.***, calo., carb-ac., ***carb-an.***, carb-s., ***carb-v.***, **CAUST.**, ***cere-b.***, chel., cimic., ***cinnb.***, ***cist.***, colch., con., croc., ***crot-h.***, crot-t., cupr., cur., cycl., dros., dulc., echi., ***elaps,*** ery-a., eupi., ferr-i., ***fl-ac.***, glon., ***graph.***, grat., guai., gymn., hep., hydr., hyos., ***iod.***, ind., jug-r., kali-ar., **KALI-BI.**, **KALI-C.**, kali-i., ***kali-p.***, **KALI-S.**, kalm., kiss., kreos., **LACH.**, lac-ac., lact., laur., lob., lob-s., lyss., mag-c., mag-m., mag-s., ***merc.***, ***merc-c.***, ***merc-i-f.***, ***merc-i-r.***, ***mez.***, ***mur-ac.***, myric., **NAT-A.**, **NAT-C.**, **NAT-M.**, ***nat-p.***, ***nat-s.***, ***nit-ac.***, **NUX-V.**, ol-an., op., osm., ox-ac., par., petr., phel., ph-ac., ***phos.***, phys., ***phyt.***, plan., ***plat.***, ***plb.***, podo., ***psor.***, ptel., ***puls.***, ***ran-b.***, raph., ***rhus-t.***, ***rumx.***, sabad., samb., sars., ***sel.***, ***seneg.***, **SEP.**, ***sil.***, sol-t-ae., ***spig.***, stann., stram., ***sulph.***, sul-ac., sumb., tab., tarax., teucr., ***thuj.***, til., verat., viol-t., wild., ***zinc.***, zing.
air, open in - carb-ac.
albuminous - all-c., am-m., bor., ***caust.***, coca, merc-c., **NAT-M.**, ***nat-s.***, sel., spig., sulph.
bed, in - iod.
bitter - arn., ars., ***cist.***, cupr., ferr-ma., grat., merc., nat-m., tarax.
black - elaps, sulph.
bloody - alum., am-br., bad., bism., bor., chel., fl-ac., ***gels.***, hep., ***kali-ar.***, ***kali-ma.***, ***lyc.***, mag-c., mag-m., sars., sep., ***stann.***, thuj.
breakfast, before - sabad.
breathing, hindered - aur.
cheese, tasting like old - psor.
cool - phos.
difficult to detach - ***alum.***, ***ambr.***, am-m., ***merc-i-f.***
dinner, after - caust.
drawn from post nasal - ***alum.***, ***alumn.***, anac., ***ant-c.***, ***arg-n.***, bry., ***calc.***, calc-s., canth., carb-ac., ***carb-v.***, ***caust.***, chin., cinnb., **COR-R.**, ***elaps,*** euph., euphr., gran., ***hep.***, ***hydr.***, **KALI-BI.**, ***kali-chl.***, merc., merc-c., merc-i-f., merc-i-r., mez., ***nat-a.***, **NAT-C.**, **NAT-M.**, nat-p., ***nit-ac.***, onos., osm., paeon., ph-ac., phyt., ***plb.***, ***psor.***, rhus-t., rumx., sin-n., **SPIG.**, ***stict.***, sulph., tell., thuj., zinc., zing.
easily discharged - ***arg-m.***, bor., ***carb-v.***, nat-c.
eating, while - caust., thuj., verat.
evening - ***alum.***, ang., bry., calc-p., hep., merl., stann.
4 p.m. - nat-c.
6 p.m. - phys.
false membrane, like - bell., ***caust.***, puls.
forepart of throat - merc.
foul - ***carb-v.***, ***phyt.***
frothy - am-caust., am-m., aphis., brom., bry., caust., kali-bi., plat., ***sil.***, urt-u.

MUCUS, in throat
gelatinous - ***arg-m.,*** berb., ***caust.,*** **KALI-BI.,** ***nat-a.***
gluey - bad., ***caust.***
grayish - ***ambr.,*** **ARG-M.,** ars., ***nat-a.,*** nat-s., phos., seneg., stann., sulph.
greenish - ail., ars., bor., ***colch.,*** dros., ***lyc.,*** nat-m., ***sil., stann.,*** sumb., zinc.
hanging down - ***carb-an.,*** lach., med., ***merc-c.,*** phos., thuj.
lumps - ***agar.,*** coca, merc-i-f., seneg., ***zinc.***
sensation of - ars.
metallic taste - calc., merc., rhus-t.
morning - all-s., ***alum.,*** ambr., am-m., apis, **ARG-M., ARS.,** bad., ***bar-c.,*** bor., bov., ***calc.,*** carb-s., ***caust.,*** cimx., cina, ***cist.,*** cob., cupr., eupi., fl-ac., ***graph.,*** hep., **KALI-BI.,** ***kali-c.,*** kali-s., kreos., lact., laur., lyc., mag-c., mag-m., ***merc-i-f., nat-c., nat-m.,*** nat-s., nux-v., ***petr.,*** phos., plat., **PULS.,** rhus-t., sabad., sars., ***sel.,*** seneg., ***sep., sil.,*** spig., stram., sulph., tarax., teucr., ***thuj.***
11 a.m. - ***viol-t.***
waking, on - ***alum.,*** carb-an., nat-c.
night - alum., nat-c., nat-p., ***nat-s.,*** puls., sep.
midnight - arum-t.
waking, on - alum.
offensive - am-c., bry., ***carb-v.,*** mag-c., mur-ac., psor., ***sil.,*** thuj.
patches - ars-i., ***fl-ac.,*** kali-chl., ***merc., mur-ac., nit-ac.,*** phyt., syph.
putrid - ***carb-ac.,*** cham., lach
qualmishness, during - ***graph.***
rattling - podo.
red as blood - thuj.
ropy, (see tenacious)
saltish - alum., am-m., anac., ars., ***calc., carb-s.,*** kali-p., ***lach.,*** merc., ***nat-m., nat-s.,*** nux-v., phos., sil., sulph., tell., ther.
sensation of - grat., mez., pen., **RHOD.,** tub.
sour - crot-t., laur., mag-m., mag-s., phos., plb., tarax., teucr.
swallow, must - **CAUST.,** mag-c., mur-ac., zinc.
can neither swallow nor hawk up - am-m., kali-c., mag-s.
sweetish - aesc., all-c., cop., lach., sabad., sumb.
tenacious - aesc., agn., ***all-c., alum.,*** ambr., am-br., am-m., ***anac.,*** ant-c., ***apis,*** **ARG-M., ARG-N.,** arn., arum-t., asar., **BAR-C.,** ***bell.,*** berb., ***bor.,*** bry., bufo, ***calc.,*** calc-ar., canth., caps., carb-ac., carb-s., ***carb-v.,*** **CAUST.,** chin-s., cimic., cimx., ***cinnb., cist.,*** clem., cop., cycl., dulc., ferr-i., ferr-m., graph., grat., ***hydr.,*** ind., iod., **KALI-BI.,** ***kali-c., lach.,*** lact., laur., lith., lob., lyc., lyss., ***mag-c., mag-m., mag-s.,*** merc., merc-c., ***merc-i-f.,*** merc-i-r., mez., ***mur-ac., myric.,*** naja, nat-a., nat-c., nat-p., **NAT-S.,** ***nux-v.,*** ol-an., onos., ox-ac., paeon., pall., ***ph-ac.,*** phos., **PHYT.,** plan., ***plb., psor., puls.,*** ran-b., raph., ***rhus-t., rumx., sabad.,*** sars., ***seneg.,*** sep., **SIL.,** ***stann.,*** sul-ac., sumb., tab., ***thuj.,*** verat., zinc.
evening - alum., ran-b.
morning - ***alum., apis, arg-m.,*** bar-c., cupr., **KALI-BI.,** kali-c., lact., mag-m., **PULS.,** sars., seneg., sumb.
night - **PULS.**
thick - aesc., aloe, alum., ***anac.,*** ant-c., apis, ***arg-m.,*** **ARG-N.,** ***bell.,*** berb., bry., calc., caps., carb-ac., **CAUST.,** cimic., ***cist.,*** cur., ***glon.,*** grat., **HYDR., KALI-BI.,** kali-i., ***mag-c.,*** mag-m., merc., ***nat-a.,*** **NAT-C.,** nat-m., nat-p., nicc., nux-m., petr., ***phyt.,*** plb., psor., ran-s., ***sil.,*** stann., sumb.
morning - mag-m., petr., ***sil.***
watery - aesc., chel., laur., thuj.
morning - thuj.
white - ambr., am-m., ***bell.,*** berb., ***bor.,*** carb-ac., **CAUST.,** cob., kali-chl., kali-m., lach., mag-c., merc-c., ***merc-i-r.,*** nat-a., **NAT-M.,** nat-p., ***nat-s.,*** nux-v., raph., sel., seneg., spig., sulph.
milk white - kali-chl.
morning - spig.
yellow - aesc., ant-c., apoc., berb., ***calc., calc-s.,*** cast., ***cist.,*** cop., dros., eug., hydr., **KALI-BI.,** lach., ***nat-a.,*** nat-p., nux-v., ol-j., rumx., ***sil.,*** spig., sumb.
forenoon - lyc.
lower part - alum., graph., zinc.
morning - spig.

mucus, uvula - sep.
white tenacious mucus - am-caust.

mucus, tonsils form plugs of, constantly - calc-f.

NARROW, sensation - acon., ***alum.,*** alumn., **BELL.,** bry., ***calc., caust.,*** chin., merc., ***mez.,*** nat-m., ***nux-v.,*** phos., rhus-t., sulph.
coughing, when - coc-c.
night - phos.
swallowing, when - **BELL.,** ***calc.,*** lyc., puls.

NAUSEA, in the - acon., alum., anac., ant-c., arg-m., arn., ***ars.,*** asar., aur., ***bell.,*** cann-s., carb-ac., carb-an., caust., chin., cocc., coc-c., ***coff.,*** colch., ***croc., cupr.,*** **CYCL.,** ferr., ferr-p., lyc., merc., ***mez.,*** nit-ac., olnd., **PH-AC.,** ***puls., rhus-t.,*** sars., sil., spig., ***squil.,*** **STANN.,** staph., sulph., tarax., valer.
collar, by tight fitting - hyos., lach.
spasm in throat, from - ***graph.***

NECROSIS, fauces - merc-cy.

NUMBNESS - acon., all-c., arg-m., bor., bov., gels., ***kali-br.,*** kali-c., mag-s., nit-ac., olnd., sep., verat-v.
right, tonsil - sep.

numbness, throat, external - ***carb-an.,*** chel., olnd., sep., ***spong.***

OBSTRUCTION - anan., calc., ***con.,*** kali-bi., iod., merc-c., mur-ac., puls., pyrus, sumb.
morning - mag-c.
swallowing, when - arund., ***calc.,*** elaps, nat-s.
waking, on - led.

PAIN, throat - acon., ***aesc.,*** agar., aloe, ***alum., alumn.,*** am-c., am-m., ***anan.,*** ant-c., anthr., ***apis,*** arg-m., **ARG-N.,** ars., ars-i., **ARUM-T.,** asaf., aur-m., **BAPT.,** bar-m., **BELL.,** ***benz-ac.,*** berb., bov., brom., bry., ***calc.,*** calc-p., ***calc-s.,*** cann-s., canth., **CAPS.,** carb-ac., carb-an., carb-s., carb-v., caul., ***caust.,*** cham., chel., chin-s., cinnb., coc-c., ***coff.,*** colch., coloc., ***con.,*** cop., ***crot-c., crot-h.,*** crot-t., ***cupr.,*** cycl., ***dulc.,*** fago., ferr., ferr-i., graph., ham., ***hep., ign.,*** iod., iris, jatr., kali-ar., ***kali-bi., kali-c., kali-chl., kali-i.,*** kali-ma., kali-n., kali-p., ***kali-s.,*** kalm., kreos., ***lac-c.,*** **LACH.,** lac-ac., laur., ***lyc.,*** lyss., mag-s., ***merc., merc-c.,*** merc-i-f., merc-i-r., merl., mez., mur-ac., naja, nat-a., ***nat-m.,*** nicc., ***nit-ac.,*** nux-v., ox-ac., pall., par., ph-ac., ***phos., phyt.,*** plat., psor., **RHUS-T.,** rhus-v., rumx., ruta., ***sabad.,*** sabin., seneg., ***sep.,*** **SIL.,** stann., ***sulph.,*** sul-ac., tarent., tell., teucr., verat., vip., ***zinc.***
afternoon - chin-s., lach., naja
air, cold - bell., chin., cist., crot-h., diphtox., ***fl-ac., hep., merc.,*** mez., nux-v.
amel. - all-c., ***coff.,*** kali-bi., sang.
inspiring - sang.
inhaling - cist.
alcoholics, of - caps.
alternate days - lac-c., lach.
alternating with,
anal pain - sin-a.
headache and pain in limbs - alum., lac-d.
sore eyes - par.
apple, core, as from - ***merc.,*** phyt.
bathing agg. - lach.
bed, in - merc., merc-i-f.
belching, after - sulph.
bending, head forwards - brom., phyt.
blowing, nose - ***carb-v.,*** merc.
change, of weather - **CALC., DULC.**
chill, during - thuj.
before - eup-pur.
clearing, the throat, on - alum.
cold, drinks - arg-n., ars., calc-f., canth., ***cist.,*** fl-ac., **HEP.,** lac-c., ***lyc.,*** merc-c., ***sabad., sulph.,*** **SYPH.**
amel. - ***apis,*** carc., coc-c., diphtox., ind., lac-c., ***lach., lyc.,*** merc-i-f., onos., ***phos., phyt.***
cold, on becoming - ***ars., calc., calc-p., dulc.,*** **HEP., KALI-C.,** ***lyc., merc., nit-ac., phos., phyt.,*** **SIL.**
from a - acon., bar-c., bell., cham., ***dulc.***
things, from - ***ars.,*** **HEP., LYC.,** sabad., ***sulph.***
cough, with - kali-n.

PAIN, throat
coughing, on - acon., ambr., **ARG-M.,** ***arum-t.,*** calc., camph., **CAPS.,** carb-an., carb-s., ***carb-v.,*** chin., chin-s., cist., coc-c., cycl., fl-ac., hep., iod., kali-bi., kalm., ***lach.,*** lyc., mag-s., nat-m., ***nux-v., phos.,*** psor., ran-s., ***rumx.,*** sep., sil., spong., sulph., ***tarent.***
after - coc-c., naja
damp, weather - **CALC., DULC.,** ***hep.,*** lach., **RHUS-T.**
daytime - lyss.
alternate days - lach.
depressing, the tongue - merc-c.
dinner, after - sulph.
draft, of air - ***ambr.,*** chin., ***hep.***
drinking, agg. - canth.
amel. - bry., ign., tell.
water, on - mez.
eating, while - aloe, carb-v., ferr., phos.
amel. - acon., apis, benz-ac., carb-an., ***lach.,*** onos., pic-ac., tell.
evening - ***alum.,*** am-c., ars., caust., ***hep.,*** kali-i., lact., mag-m., nat-m., nicc., nit-ac., puls., raph., sul-ac., viol-t.
exertion, from - caust., lac-c.
expectoration, agg. - bell.
after - arund.
expiration, on - ***arg-m.***
extending to,
ear - agar., all-c., alum., ***ambr.,*** apis, ***arg-n., bell.,*** berb., bry., ***calc.,*** carb-ac., carb-an., cham., elaps, ferr-i., guai., ***hep.,*** ign., ip., iris, kali-bi., kali-ma., kali-n., kali-p., ***lac-c., lach., lith., lyc.,*** mag-c., mag-m., merc., ***merc-cy.,*** nat-m., ***nit-ac.,*** nux-v., par., petr., ***phyt., podo.,*** psor., sars., sec., sil., staph., sul-ac., sulph., tarent., tell., thuj., tub.
swallowing, on - agar., ail., alum., ***arg-n.,*** brom., ***elaps,*** ferr-i., ***gels.,*** guai., ***hep.,*** ign., kali-bi., kali-c., kali-ma., kali-n., ***lac-c.,*** lach., merc., **NIT-AC., NUX-V.,** par., petr., ph-ac., ***phyt.,*** psor., sil., staph., tarent.
eyes - merc-c., tarent.
glands of neck - sep.
submaxillary - ***merc.***
head, to - hep., merc-c., plat.
larynx - fl-ac., ***lach.***
nares, to - phos.
stomach - crot-c., lach., sul-ac.
fever, during - phos., ph-ac., sep.
foreign, object, as from a - mag-c.
hawking, on - ***bell.,*** canth., cob., **LACH.,** thuj.
inspiration, on - ail., apis, arg-n., arum-t., hep., hura, mez.
laughing - nat-m.
left - brom., ***crot-h., lac-c.,*** **LACH.,** merc-i-r., naja, nit-ac., ph-ac., phos., sabad., sep., sul-ac., teucr., tub., upa., verat.
left to right - acon., lac-c., ***lach.,*** sabad., xan.
lifting, from - calc., caust.

PAIN, throat
lying, while - bell., ***lach.***
amel. - calc., canth., lach.
menses, during - arn., bar-c., ***calc.,*** dulc., gels., ***lac-c.,*** nat-s., nux-v., ***sulph.***
before - canth., lac-c., ***mag-c.,*** nat-s.
mental, exertion, during - caust.
morning - alum., am-c., berb., calc-p., caust., chin-s., cist., graph., kali-bi., ***lach.,*** lyc., naja nat-m., nicc., ox-ac., phos., ***rhus-t.***
waking, on - caust., kali-bi., ***lach.,*** rhus-t.
motion, on - ***bell.,*** merc., merl., psor.
head, of - phos.,
throat, of - cham.
moving, the tongue - alum., ambr.
night - ***alum.,*** am-m., arg-n., camph., canth., cimic., ***cinnb.,*** cycl., graph., kali-n., mag-m., mag-s., ***merc.,*** phyt., sulph.
noon - phos.
opening, mouth - ***kali-c.***
paroxysmal - phos., sep.
peppery - coloc., ol-an., plat.
pressure, agg. - lach., merc-c.
putting, out the tongue - cocc., ***kali-bi.,*** sabad.
right - ***arg-n.,*** am-c., ***bar-m.,*** carb-v., guai., iod., kali-p., **LYC.,** ***merc-i-f.,*** meph., nicc., phyt., plat.
right to left - all-c.
rising, on - calc.
singers, in (see Clergyman)
sitting, amel. - spong.
sleep, after - kali-bi., lac-c., lach., merc-i-r.
smoking, after - coc-c.
sneezing, on - hyper., ictod., mag-c., **PHOS.**
amel. - am-br.
sore, uvula - colch., ***kali-bi.***
speakers, in (see Clergyman)
speaking, on - acon., bell., berb., calc., dros., **KALI-I.,** mag-c., merc., nicc., rhus-t., staph.
spirituous liquors, after - nux-v.
stiffness of neck, with - caust., lachn., phyt., ***rhus-t.***
stooping, on - **CAUST.,** nat-c.
suppressed foot sweat, from - ***bar-c.,*** psor., sil.
swallowing, on - acon., aesc., ***ail.,*** **ALUM.,** ambr., **AM-C.,** am-m., ***anan.,*** ant-c., ant-t., ***apis,*** **ARG-M.,** arg-n., **ARS.,** **ARUM-T.,** **AUR.,** ***bad.,*** ***bar-c.,*** bar-m., **BELL.,** bor., brom., ***bry.,*** bufo, ***calc.,*** ***calc-p.,*** calc-s., camph., ***canth.,*** caps., carb-ac., ***carb-an.,*** carb-s., ***carb-v.,*** cast., caust., ***cham.,*** chel., **CHIN.,** ***chin-a.,*** cimic., cinnb., **COFF.,** colch., con., cor-r., cupr-ac., cycl., dig., dirc., dios., dros., ***elaps,*** ferr., ferr-ar., ferr-p., ***fl-ac.,*** form., gels., gins., glon., ***graph.,*** grat., ham., hell., **HEP.,** hydr-ac., ign., ind., inul., ip., jug-c., kali-ar., ***kali-bi.,*** ***kali-c.,*** ***kali-chl.,*** **KALI-I.,** kali-n., kali-p., kali-s., kreos., **LAC-C.,** lac-d., ***lach.,*** laur., led., **LYC.,** lyss., mag-c., mag-s., mang., **MERC.,** ***merc-c.,*** merc-cy., ***merc-i-f.,*** ***merc-i-r.,*** merl., ***mez.,*** mill., mur-ac., myric., ***nat-a.,*** ***nat-c.,*** nat-m.,

PAIN, throat
swallowing, on - ***nat-p.,*** ***nat-s.,*** nicc., **NIT-AC.,** ***nux-v.,*** oena., ***onos.,*** op., ox-ac., par., ***petr.,*** ***ph-ac.,*** ***phos.,*** ***phyt.,*** pic-ac., podo., puls., ***rhus-t.,*** rumx., ruta., ***sabad.,*** ***sang.,*** ***sars.,*** sep., ***sil.,*** ***staph.,*** stict., ***stront-c.,*** ***sulph.,*** ***sul-ac.,*** tab., ***tarent.,*** ***thuj.,*** verat., zinc.
after - ambr., bry., cadm-br., ***calc.,*** ***nux-v.,*** phos., puls., rhus-t., sulph., vinc., zinc.
amel. - alum., ambr., arn., bapt., bell., **CAPS.,** cist., gels., **IGN.,** kali-bi., ***lach.,*** lac-c., led., mang., merc., mez., nux-v., puls., ***rhus-t.,*** sabad., spong., sulph., tell., ***zinc.***
behind hyoid bone, when - **CALC.**
empty - agar., ***ail.,*** alum., ambr., arg-n., ***ars.,*** **BAR-C.,** ***bell.,*** berb., bry., calc., calc-p., carb-ac., carb-s., ***cench.,*** ***cinnb.,*** cob., ***cocc.,*** ***crot-h.,*** ferr., glon., graph., ***grat.,*** ham., hep., kali-bi., **KALI-C.,** ***lac-c.,*** **LACH.,** lyc., mag-c., mang., ***merc.,*** merc-c., ***merc-i-f.,*** merc-i-r., nat-a., nux-v., phel., plat., psor., ***puls.,*** rat., ***rhus-t.,*** ruta., sep., sulph., tell., thuj., vario., vesp., zinc.
amel. - alum., gels., ***ign.,*** ip.
eating, drinking amel. - ol-an., tell.
food - bad., bapt., bar-c., bry., dirc., dros., hep., ***kali-c.,*** ***lac-c.,*** lach., merc-sul., morph., nit-ac., nux-v., petr., ph-ac., phos., rhus-t., sep., ***sulph.***
amel. - ***ign.,*** ***lach.***
liquids - **BELL.,** bry., canth., dirc., ign., **LACH.,** lyc., **MERC-C.,** nat-p., sul-ac.
amel. - cist.
solids amel. - ign., ***lach.,*** nat-p.
when not - aeth., alum., ***apis,*** arn., **CAPS.,** carc., cina, cocc., grat., **IGN.,** iod., lac-c., lach., laur., led., mag-s., mang., ***mez.,*** nux-v., phel., plat., puls., sabin., sulph., thuj., ***zinc.***
sweets, agg. - arg-n., lach., sang., **SPONG.**
amel. - ars.
swollen, glands, as from - nat-m., phyt.
talking - ambr., ***fl-ac.,*** hep., **KALI-I.,** merl., nicc., par., ph-ac., staph., tarent.
amel. - calc.
touched, when - apis, bar-c., bell., brom., bry., chin-s., cic., gamb., ign., lac-c., **LACH.,** mez., nicc., phyt., spong., teucr., zinc.
turning, the head - ***bell.,*** brom., bry., hep., ***lach.***
ulcerative - ***arg-n.,*** carb-an., ***graph.,*** ***hep.,*** ph-ac.
urine, with scanty - apis, ars., canth., lac-c., merc-cy., naja
voice, lost (see Clergyman)
waking, on - cimic., ***kali-bi.,*** ***lach.,*** myric., plan., raph.
warm, bed - ***coc-c.,*** mag-s., ***merc.***
food - gels.
warm, drinks - ***apis,*** canth., **LACH.,** ***lyc.,*** merc-i-f., **PHYT.,** spong.

PAIN, throat
warm, drinks, amel. - ***alum.,*** **ARS.,** calc-f., calc-p., ***cham.,*** guare., **HEP.,** lac-c., **LYC.,** morph., nux-v., ***rhus-t.,*** sabad., ***sulph.***
warm, room - ***apis, bry.,*** sapo.
amel. - mag-c.
warmth, in general - ***coc-c.,*** guai., **LACH.,** merc., phyt.
amel. - alum., ***ars., cham., hep., rhus-t.***
washing, bathing agg. - lach.
yawning, when - aloe, am-m., ***arg-m., arg-n.,*** calc-p., hep., mag-c., ***nat-c.,*** nat-m., nicc., phos., rhus-t., tarent., zinc.
amel. - manc.

PAIN, pharyx - alimn., ant-t., apis, ars., bell., canth., cop., cupr-a., iod., kali-chl., kali-n., kreos., merc-c., mur-ac., ox-ac., ph-ac., ran-s.
cough, during - mag-m.
sneezing - ant-t.
turning, head - ***bell.***
lower part - iod., kreos.

PAIN, throat, external - ***bar-c.,*** caps., fago., kreos., ***merc., nat-m.,*** op., phos., ***puls.,*** sul-ac.
extending to sternocleidomastoid, upper part - gels.
morning - phos.
motion, on - phos.
touch, on - phos.
pain, throat-pit - ***caust.,*** iod., ***lach.,*** spong.
anger, after - staph.
drinking, when - nit-ac.
extending to root of tongue and into hyoid bone - ***lach.***
hawking of mucus - **CAUST.**

PAIN, tonsils - aesc., alum., am-c., ***benz-ac.,*** calc-p., ***caust.,*** crot-t., graph., ***hep.,*** kali-bi., kali-p., lach., ***merc-i-f.,*** naja, raph., tarent.
drawing - con., gymn., nat-m.
left, extending to ear - ***calc.***
menses agg. - lac-c.
morning - bry.
8 a.m. - naja.
on waking - bry.
right - ***merc-i-f.***
yawning - calc-p.

PAIN, uvula - apis, colch., ***kali-bi.,*** sang., trif-p.
coughing agg. - ham.

PALENESS - ***ail., arum-t., bar-c.,*** crot-h., ox-ac., plb., ***sulph.***

PARALYSIS - ***apis,*** **ARS.,** bapt., bell., caps., ***caust., cocc.,*** cur., ***gels.,*** kali-p., ***lac-c.,*** **LACH.,** lact., ***lyc., nat-m., nux-m., op.,*** phos., ***phyt., plb., rhus-t.,*** **SEC.,** ***sil.,*** **STRAM.**
paralysis, pharynx - ***apis,*** **ARS.,** caps., ***caust., cocc.,*** **LACH.,** morph., nux-m., ***rhus-t., sil., stram.***
post diphtheritic - ***apis, arg-n.,*** **ARS.,** ***caust., cocc.,*** con., cur., diph., ***gels.,*** kali-p., **LAC-C., LACH., NAJA,** ***nat-m.,*** olnd., ***phos., plb.,*** rhus-t., **SEC.,** sil.
paralysis, throat, external - gels., spig.
diphtheria, after - ***lac-c.***
sterno-mastoid - plb.

PERISTALSIS, reversed - ambr., asaf.

PHARYNGITIS, inflammation of pharynx - bar-m., bell., ***calc., fl-ac.,*** kali-i., ***lac-c.,*** lach., merc., naja, ***nat-m., petr., phyt., sep.,*** **SIL.,** sulph.

PHTHISIS, (see Tuberculosis)

PIMPLES, on uvula - kali-bi., rumx.

POLYPS, (see Larynx)

POWDER, sensation of a - crot-c.

PRESSING, pain - acon., agar., ***alum.,*** alumn., am-c., am-m., ant-t., asaf., bar-c., ***bell.,*** berb., brom., bry., calc., calc-s., canth., **CAPS.,** ***carb-an.,*** carb-v., caust., cham., cinnb., clem., coc-c., cop., crot-t., dulc., ferr., ferr-i., ferr-ma., gent-c., ***graph.,*** grat., hell., hyos., ign., iod., kali-ar., kali-bi., kali-c., kali-chl., kali-i., kali-n., kali-p., ***kalm.,*** kreos., lac-ac., ***lach.,*** lyc., mang., ***merc., merc-c.,*** merc-i-r., merl., ***mez.,*** naja, nat-c., ***nat-m.,*** nit-ac., ***nux-v.,*** par., phel., phos., plat., rat., rhus-t., ruta., sabad., sabin., seneg., sep., sulph., tab., tarax., teucr., thuj., verat., zinc.
asunder - anac., kali-ar.
coughing, when - caps.
daytime - nit-ac.
evening - alum., ***hep.,*** nit-ac.
extending to, abdomen - zinc.
to, back - sep.
to, ear - alum., bry., carb-an., nat-m.
to, stomach - carb-an., ***nux-v.,*** phos.
morning - aloe, am-c., caust., graph., lach., naja, phos.
8 to 9 a.m. - aloe
rising, on - graph.
waking, on - caust.
night - arg-n., sars., sulph.
in bed - arg-n.
sneezing, when - led.
speaking, while - **KALI-I.**
swallowing, on - alum., am-m., ***bar-c., calc., carb-an.,*** hell., **KALI-I.,** mez., **NIT-AC.,** nux-v., par., ph-ac., puls., rhus-t., sabad., sep., sil., sulph., thuj.
vomiting, when - anac.
pressing, throat-pit - graph., mag-c., phos.
breathing, deep - caust.
pressing, tonsils - alum., bell., cann-i., cham., ***cocc.,*** nux-v., par., merl., sep., tell., zinc.
evening and night - zinc.
swallowing, when - zinc.
yawning, when - zinc.

PRESSURE, in throat-pit - aesc., anac., **BROM.,** ***caust.,*** cic., graph., **LACH.,** ***lob.,*** phos., ***rumx.,*** sarr.
anger, after - ***staph.***
inspiration, on - caust.
swallowing agg. - staph.

PRICKLY - acon., alumn., calc-f., cedr., lach., manc., sulph., tell., verat.
extending down esophagus - cedr.

PULSATING - ***am-m.***, arg-n., ***bell.***, bufo, cham., chel., coc-c., euphr., ***glon.***, **HEP.**, ind., kalm., ***lach.***, nit-ac., ph-ac., rhus-t., tarent., xan.
after cough - coc-c.
pulsating, tonsils - ***am-m.***, kalm., nit-ac.
left - nat-p.

PUSTULES - ***aeth.***, ant-t., psor., sep.
pustules, tonsils, on - ***sep.***

RAWNESS, pain - acon., ***aesc.***, all-c., aloe, ***alum.***, alumn., ***ambr.***, am-c., am-m., ***anac.***, apis, **ARG-M., ARG-N.**, ars., ***arum-t.***, bapt., **BELL.**, berb., bol., bov., ***brom., bry.***, bufo, cahin., ***calc.***, calc-s., canth., ***carb-an., carb-s., carb-v.***, **CAUST.**, chel., **CHIN.**, chin-a., cimic., cist., ***coc-c.***, cod., ***coloc.***, crot-h., dig., dor., dros., dulc., euph., ferr., ferr-ar., gamb., gent-c., ***graph.***, grat., ***hep.***, hydr., ign., ip., iris, ***kali-bi.***, kali-c., kali-chl., kali-i., kali-ma., kali-n., kali-p., kali-s., kalm., kreos., lac-ac., ***lac-c., lach.***, laur., **LYC.**, ***mag-c., mag-m.***, med., ***merc.***, **MERC-C.**, merl., ***mez., mur-ac., naja***, nat-a., nat-c., ***nat-m.***, nicc., nux-m., **NUX-V., NIT-AC.**, ol-an., onos., op., ox-ac., petr., ph-ac., ***phos.***, phel., ***phyt.***, plan., ***plat.***, plb., ***puls., sang.***, sars., ***seneg.***, sep., sil., sol-n., ***spong., stann.***, **STILL.**, stront-c., ***sulph., sul-ac.***, sumb., tab., ***thuj., zinc.***
clearing, when - seneg.
cold, air, drawing - ***bufo***, **NUX-V.**
coughing, when - ***ambr.***, anac., **ARG-M.**, carb-v., caust., chin., cob., nat-m., phos., rumx., sep., sil., **SPONG.**, stront.
damp weather - phos.
dinner, after - dros.
eating, after - ***anac.***
amel. - onos.
evening - alum., bol., bov., brach., ham., kali-bi., maag-m., mang., nat-c., ***phos.***, sulph., zinc.
expiration, on - ***arg-m.***, ph-ac.
extending to stomach - calc., ***carb-an.***, petr.
forenoon - bol., mag-c.
hawking, when - cob., mang.
morning - all-c., aloe, alum., am-m., bov., ***carb-an.***, caust., fl-ac., mez., mur-ac., puls., sars., stann., stront-c., zinc.
night - ***anac.***, **BAR-C.**, mur-ac., sumb.
sleep, after - ***lach.***
smoking, while - nat-m.
swallowing, when - **ARG-M., BAR-C.**, bry., fago., hep., nat-c., nux-v., petr., **STANN.**, sumb., zinc.
waking, on - plan.
walking, while - lyc.
air, in open - stann.
rawness, epiglottis - bell.
rawness, throat pit - arg-m.
rawness, tonsils - phyt.
rawness, uvula - ambr., calc.

REDNESS, of - absin., **ACON.**, ***aesc.***, aeth., ***ail., alum.***, am-br., ant-t., ***apis***, **ARG-N.**, ***ars.***, atro., aur-m., bapt., **BELL.**, berb., brom., bry., calc., ***calc-p., calc-s.***, canth., **CAPS., CARB-AC.**, carb-an., carb-v., caust., ***cist.***, clem., chlol., coc-c., colch., cop., crot-t., cupr., cycl., ferr-p., ***fl-ac., gels.***, gent-c., gins., ***guai.***, hippoz., ***hyos.***, ign., ind., iris, ***kali-bi., kali-chl.***, kali-i., kali-n., ***lach.***, lac-ac., **LYC.**, ***merc., merc-c., merc-i-f., mur-ac., nat-a., nat-c., nit-ac.***, nux-m., ***nux-v.***, op., ox-ac., ***petr.***, phos., **PHYT.**, pic-ac., rhus-t., rhus-v., sec., sep., sil., **STRAM.**, ***sulph.***, sul-ac., tab., tarent., verat.
dark red - acon., ***aesc., ail.***, alum., ***am-c.***, am-caust., amyg., ***apis***, arag., **ARG-N.**, **BAPT.**, bell., brom., ***canth.***, caps., **CHAM.**, ***crot-h.***, diph., ***gymn.***, ham., ***kali-bi., kali-i.***, kali-s., ***lach.***, merc., merc-c., ***merc-cy., merc-i-r., mez.***, mur-ac., ***naja***, nat-a., pen., phos., ***phyt., puls., rhus-t.***, wye., zinc-c.
glossy, as if varnished - alum., ***apis***, arag., bell., cist., hydr., kali-bi., ***lac-c.***, phos.
network - brom.
spots, in - kali-chl., merc.
redness, fauces - ***bell.***, carb-ac., ferr-p., gymn., menthol, ***merc-cy.***, merc-i-r., mez., naja, puls.
redness, pharynx - ***acon.***, alumn., ant-t., **APIS**, ars., bell., bry., calc-p., calc-s., coc-c., cop., gent-c., iod., kali-n., ***merc., merc-c., merc-i-f.***, merl., nat-a., ***nat-m.***, ox-ac., phos., stram., sul-ac., ust., verat.
back part - ***hep., kali-bi., merc-i-f.***, nit-ac.
redness, tonsils - ***acon., apis, aur., bapt.***, **BELL., CARB-AC.**, ***con.***, cop., ***ferr-p.***, fl-ac., gymn., ***kali-bi., lach., merc., merc-i-f., phyt., puls., sulph.***
bright red - acon., ***bell.***, phyt.
redness, uvula - **ACON.**, ***apis***, **ARG-N.**, ars., **BAPT., BAR-M., BELL.**, calc., ***calc-p.***, caust., cimic., colch., ***crot-t.***, cupr., ***fl-ac.***, gent-c., ***kali-bi.***, kali-br., ***lach.***, merc., ***merc-i-f.***, nat-m., petr., sulph.
dark red - ***arg-n.***, **BAPT.**, ***calc.***, caust., cupr-ac., ***lach.***

RELAXATION, sensation of - aesc., ***alum.***, alumn., am-m., bar-c., ***calc-p.***, eucal., pen., spong.
relaxation, uvula - canth., ham., ***kali***-bi.

RHEUMATIC pain - ambr., ***caust.***, gran., mez.

RIGIDITY - chel., lach.

ROUGHNESS, sensation of - ***aesc.***, agar., ail., ***aloe, alum., ambr.***, ammc., ***am-c.***, am-m., anac., ant-c., ***apis***, ang., **ARG-M.**, ***arg-n.***, ars., aspar., ***bar-c., bell.***, bor., cahin., ***calc.***, calc-ar., calc-p., cann-i., canth., caps., carb-an., carb-s., ***carb-v., caust.***, chel., **CHIN.**, cimic., ***cist.***, clem., cob., cocc., coc-c., ***coloc.***, com., ***croc.***, dig., **DROS.**, euph., eup-per., glon., ***graph.***, grat., ***hep.***, hyos., ***ip.***, iris, kali-bi., ***kali-c.***, kali-n., kreos., lac-ac., lach., laur., ***lyc.***, lyss., ***mag-c., mag-m.***, mang., meny., ***merc.***, merc-c., mez., nat-a., ***nat-c., nat-s.***, **NUX-V.**, ph-ac., ***phos., phyt., plat.***, plb., ran-b., rat., ***rhod.***, rhus-t., rob., ***sabad.***, sars., ***seneg., sep.***, sil., spong., squil., stann., staph., stront-c., ***sulph., sul-ac.***, sumb., tab., tell., ***thuj.***, ust., verat., verb., zinc.
cough, causing - **DROS.**

ROUGHNESS, sensation
coughing, from - anac., arn., carb-v., caust., cob., cop., dig., gels., hep., kali-c., kali-n., kreos., laur., merc-c., nat-s., nicc., phos., rhod., sars., seneg., sep., spong.
daytime - mez.
dinner, amel. - mag-c.
eating after - anac.
amel. - am-m., nat-c.
evening - ***alum.,*** kali-n., mang., nat-c., ***seneg.,*** stann., suph.
expiration, on - arg-m., ph-ac.
forenoon - mag-c.,
hawking, from - sep., thuj.
hiccough, from - bor.
morning - agar., ***ail.,*** alum., ant-c., ars., bor., caust., kali-n., mang., rhod., sars., seneg., sep., sulph., thuj., zinc.
rising, on - mang., sulph.
waking, on - alum., sars., seneg., sulph.
night - alum., arg-n., sil.
swallowing, on - ***arg-m., arg-n.,*** calc-p., cocc., ***hep.,*** lyc., petr., pic-ac., ***staph.,*** sulph.
talking, from - graph., sil., ***staph.***
roughness, fauces - aesc., cocc., dros., ***nux-v.,*** phos., phyt.
roughness, throat-pit - bor.
roughness, uvula - sulph.

SCAB, posterior wall of, greenish yellow - elaps

SCRAPING, (see Clearing the throat)

SCRATCHING - agar., agn., alum., ambr., ***arg-m., arg-n.,*** arn., arum-t., aur-m., ***bar-c.,*** bell., benz-ac., berb., bor., calad., calc-p., cann-s., carb-s., carb-v., chel., ***cist.,*** con., graph., ***hep.,*** hyos., ***kali-bi., kali-c., kreos., lyc., mag-c.,*** mang., ***nit-ac., nux-m.,*** **NUX-V.,** petr., ***phos., plat.,*** puls., ***rhod.,*** rob., ***seneg., sep., spong., sulph., sul-ac.,*** tab., tell., ter.
coughing - bell.
crumbs of bread, like - dros., ***lach.,*** pall.
dinner, after - dig.
evening - dig., led.
morning - cob.
night - con.
sand, as from - ***cist.***
scratching, pain - berb., kali-bi., mag-c., ph-ac., sars.
swallowing, on - mez., sep., stram.

SENSITIVE - ***acon.,*** aesc., ail., am-caust., ***apis,*** arg-m., arn., ***arum-t.,*** atro., bar-c., ***bell.,*** brom., bry., calc-p., ***canth., caps.,*** carb-ac., ***caust.,*** cocc., ***coc-c.,*** crot-h., dol., fago., ferr-p., fl-ac., graph., gymn., ***hep.,*** hom., hydr., ign., ***kali-bi.,*** kali-c., kali-i., kali-per., lac-c., ***lach.,*** lachn., led., menthol, **MERC.,** merc-c., merc-i-f., merc-i-r., mur-ac., naja, nit-ac., ***nux-v.,*** ox-ac., petr., **PHOS.,** ***phyt.,*** pop-c., quillaya, rhus-t., sabad., ***sang.,*** sang-n., spong., sul-ac., sulph., trif-p., verb., wye., zinc.
air, to - ail., crot-h.
cold, to - ***fl-ac.***
fauces - coc-c.
sensitive, uvula - clem., sulph.

SHARP, pain - **ACON.,** ***aesc., aeth., alum.,*** am-c., ***am-m.,*** anan., apis, arg-n., arn., ars., ***asar.,*** aur., ***bar-c.,*** **BELL.,** berb., ***bov.,*** brom., ***bry., calc.,*** calc-s., canth., caps., carb-ac., carb-an., carb-s., ***carb-v.,*** carl., caust., cham., chel., ***chin.,*** chin-a., ***cist.,*** coloc., cupr., ***dig.,*** ferr-ma., gamb., glon., ***graph.,*** gymn., hell., **HEP.,** ***hyos., ign.,*** iod., ***ip.,*** kali-ar., kali-bi., **KALI-C.,** kali-i., ***kali-n.,*** kali-p., kali-s., ***lach.,*** laur., ***led., lyc.,*** mag-c., mag-s., manc., mang., meny., ***merc.,*** merc-c., ***merc-i-r.,*** mez., nat-a., ***nat-c., nat-m.,*** nat-p., nicc., **NIT-AC.,** nux-m., ***nux-v.,*** par., ***petr.,*** phel., ***ph-ac.,*** phos., podo., psor., **PULS.,** ran-s., rat., ***rhus-t., sabad.,*** sabin., ***sars.,*** seneg., ***sep., sil.,*** spig., ***spong., stann.,*** staph., stram., ***sulph., sul-ac.,*** tarax., tarent., teucr., ***thuj.,*** verat.
afternoon - nat-c.
as from something sharp - glon., ***nit-ac.,*** rhus-t.
ascending steps - nux-v.
asthma, before - ***bov.***
boring-stitching - stann.
breathing - bell., chin.
cold, on becoming - **KALI-C.**
coughing, on - bor., bry., hep., kali-c., lach., lyc., nit-ac., nux-v., phos., sil.
amel. - stann.
deep breathing, on - hep.
eating, while - kali-n., sulph.
after - kali-n.
amel. - spong.
evening - alum., bar-c., ***carb-an.,*** chin., mag-c., mag-m., nat-c., sil., sulph., sul-ac.
exertion, on - manc.
extending to, ear - ambr., berb., bry., calc., **HEP.,** ign., ip., iris, ***kali-bi.,*** kali-p., mag-c., merc., ***merc-cy.,*** nux-v., sars., sol-n., thuj.
coughing, when - mag-m.
swallowing, when - calc., con., ***gels., ign.,*** lyc., mag-m., ***merc.,*** **NUX-V.,** petr., ***phyt., sulph.***
talking, when - calc.
turning head, when - hep.
yawning, when - hep., nat-m.
extending to, neck - stann.
extending to, root of tongue, when swallowing - ***phyt.***
forenoon - led.
hawking, on - plat.
inspiration, on - hep., mag-m.
left - arum-t., bell., cupr., glon., grat., kali-bi., kali-n., mag-c., mag-m., nat-c., nat-m., psor., sil., sul-ac.
mental excitement, after - ***cist.***
morning - alum., alumn., hep., kali-n., nat-c., nicc., ph-ac., ptel.
rising, on - graph., kali-n., ptel.
motion of the throat, from - graph.
tongue, from - ambr.
night - mag-m., mag-s., manc., nat-c., nat-m.
pressing, on larynx, when - kali-n.
rest, during - sabin.

SHARP, pain
right - am-c., *gamb.,* sars., stann., tarent.
sneezing on - lyc., mag-c.
stooping, on rising - graph.
swallowing, on - aeth., alum., *alumn.,* am-m., **APIS,** aur., *bar-c., bell.,* bov., **BRY., CALC.,** carb-s., caust., cham., chel., chin., chin-a., coff., gamb., graph., **HEP.,** ind., iod., kali-bi., kali-c., kali-n., kali-p., *lach.,* led., lob., lyc., mag-c., mag-m., mag-s., mang., meny., **MERC.,** mez., nat-m., **NIT-AC.,** petr., ph-ac., phos., rhus-t., *sabad.,* sars., *sep.,* **SIL.,** spig., staph., stram., **SULPH.,** sul-ac., thuj.
amel. - *kali-bi.,* rhus-t., stann.
empty, on - alum., con., mag-c., *sep., sulph.*
pressing on swollen glands amel. - spig.
when not swallowing - aeth., graph., **IGN.,** *puls., zinc.*
talking, while - am-c., graph., kali-n., mag-c., mag-m., nit-ac.
after - kali-bi.
touched externally, when - agar., bell.
turning head, on - hep.
walking rapidly - bry.
yawning, when - am-m., mag-c., nat-c., rhus-t., sil.
sharp, throat-pit - bor., phos.
sharp, tonsils - alum., *bell.,* kali-bi., *merc.,* naja, nit-ac., *ran-s.,* raph., sulph., tarent.
left - cupr., grat., kali-bi., lach.
right - lyc.
sharp, uvula - caust., nat-m., rhod., seneg., sep.

SHOCKS, in, on waking - manc.

SHRIVELLED, uvula - carb-ac.

SKIN, sensation of a, hanging in the - acon., ang., ant-c., kreos., *lach.,* ol-an., phos., plat., sabad.

SOFTNESS - cist.

SORE, pain (see Clergyman, Pain, throat) - acon., *aesc., ail., all-c., alum., ambr., am-c.,* am-m., anac., *ant-c., apis,* **ARG-M., ARG-N.,** *ars., arum-t., asaf.,* **BAPT., BELL.,** *benz-ac.,* brom., *bufo,* caj., **CALC.,** *calc-p., calc-s.,* cann-s., *caps., carb-ac.,* carb-an., carb-s., *carb-v., caust., cham.,* chlor., cimic., *cist.,* coc-c., coff., con., cop., **CROT-C.,** crot-h., crot-t., cupr., cupr-ar., cycl., dios., dor., echi., eup-per., fago., ferr., ferr-ar., **FERR-P.,** *fl-ac.,* form., **GELS.,** glon., *guai.,* ham., haem., hell., hydr., hydr-ac., **IGN.,** ind., *ip.,* jab., jac-c., jatr., jug-c., kali-ar., kali-c., kali-chl., kali-i., kali-ma., kali-p., kali-s., lac-ac., **LACH.,** lachn., *led.,* lob., **LYC.,** *lyss.,* mag-c., mag-s., **MERC.,** *merc-c., merc-cy., merc-i-f., merc-i-r., mez.,* myric., naja, *nat-a.,* nat-m., nat-p., nat-s., nicc., **NIT-AC.,** *nux-m., nux-v.,* oena., *ox-ac.,* petr., ph-ac., phos., phys., *phyt.,* pic-ac., plan., *psor.,* ptel., puls., ran-s., **RHUS-T.,** rhus-v., samb., sang., seneg., *sep., sil.,* stann., *sulph., sul-ac.,* tarent., tep., upa., verat., vesp., vinc., xan., zinc., zing.

SORE, pain
afternoon - canth., dios., op., phys., ptel.
4 p.m. - *arum-t.*
5 p.m. - caust.
air, cold, from - **BELL.,** bufo, *cist., coff., fl-ac., hep.,* mez.
air, draft of - *ambr., hep.*
every - lach.
air, open - mez.
amel. - kali-bi.
alternating sides - **LAC-C.**
change of weather - **CALC.**
clearing the, on - alum.
cold, from every - lach.
coryza, during - mag-m.
coughing, on - ambr., ant-s., ant-t., **ARG-M.,** ars., carb-v., fl-ac., *lach.,* lyc., phos., ran-s., sep., spong., tarent.
damp weather, in - *calc., dulc., hep., rhus-t.*
daytime - **LACH.,** lyss.
drinking, after - nit-ac.
eating, while - carb-v., ferr., phos.
after - sep.
amel. - apis, carb-an., pic-ac.
evening - am-c., brach., bov., calc-p., carb-an., *carb-v.,* dios., ham., ind., kali-p., lith., mez., nat-m., podo., stann., *sul-ac.,* tell., viol-t., zinc.
expiration, during - *arg-m.*
extending to,
chest - nat-c., **STANN.**
ears - bell., carb-o., form., lith., ph-ac., *podo.*
larynx - fl-ac.
neck, nape - *lach.*
stomach - lach.
forenoon - aesc., jug-c.
10 a.m. - lyss.
hawking, after - cob., thuj.
inspiration, on - mez.
left - *crot-h.,* echi., *form.,* kali-bi., **LAC-C., LACH.,** manc., *merc-i-r., naja,* ph-ac., *phos.,* rumx., sabad., *sec., sul-ac.*
extending to ear - *sec.*
extending to right - **LAC-C., LACH.,** plb., *sabad.*
lump - calc., caust., cham., ign., laur., nux-v., *sil.*
menses, during - arn., *calc.,* **LAC-C.,** sul-ac., *sulph.*
before - *lac-c., mag-c.*
morning - alum., arg-n., bov., bry., *calc-p.,* carb-v., chel., cinnb., *cist.,* cob., dios., *form.,* lyc., myric., nat-m., ph-ac., phos., phyt., puls., sil., sul-i., ust.
7 a.m. - sep.
swallowing, when not - puls.
waking, on - arg-n., aster., bov., calc-p., chel., hydr.
night - camph., canth., carb-an., crot-h., erig., *merc.,* nat-m., zinc.
opening mouth, difficult, with - kali-c.
pressure, on - *lach.*

SORE, pain
right - ***ars.,*** **BELL.,** calc-p., carb-ac., ham., ind., ***lac-c.,*** lith., **LYC.,** lyss., mag-c., ***merc., merc-i-f.,*** nat-p., nicc., **PHYT.,** plat., ptel., sars., tarent., ter., xan.
extending to left - ***arum-t.,*** bar-c., **LYC.,** ***podo., sulph.***
singers, in (see Clergyman)
sneezing - hyper.
speakers, in (see Clergyman)
speaking, from - act-sp.
stooping, after - nat-c.
straining throat after - **RHUS-T.**
swallowing (see Pain, throat)
sweets, after - sang., **SPONG.**
talking, agg. (see Clergyman) - tarent.
voice, overuse, of (see Clergyman)
waking, on - arg-n., aster., bov., calc-p., chel., ***crot-h.,*** hydr., kali-bi., ***lach.,*** merc-i-r., myric., plan., raph.
sore, pharynx - alumn., apis, ars., canth., cop., cupr-ac., kali-chl., kali-n., merc-c., mur-ac., ox-ac., ph-ac., ran-s.
cough, during - mag-m.
lower part - iod., kreos.
sneezing - ant-t.
turning head - ***bell.***
sore, uvula - caust.

SPASMS, of (see Choking, Constriction) - acon., ***ant-c., arg-n.,*** ars., ***bell.,*** brom., ***calc.,*** **CHAM.,** chel., chlol., ***cic., cocc.,*** coff., ***con.,*** **CUPR.,** ***gels., graph., hyos.,*** **IGN.,** ***iris,*** kali-ar., ***kali-i., lach.,*** **LAUR.,** ***lyss.,*** naja, nicc., ***nux-v.,*** op., sars., **STRAM., STRY.,** staph., ***sulph.,*** sul-ac., ***zinc.***
anger, after - ***cham., staph.***
headache, during - cadm-s.
swallowing, on - ***iris, mur-ac.,*** nicc., **STRAM.,** stry., ***sulph.***
compelling him to retch - **GRAPH., MERC-C.**
water, at sight or thought of - anan., ***lyss.***

SPEECH, (see Mouth)

SPLINTER, pain, as from a - ***alum., apis,*** **ARG-N.,** berb., calc., caust., ***chel.,*** **DOL., HEP.,** ign., **KALI-C.,** lac-c., ***lach.,*** mag-c., merc., ***nat-m.,*** **NIT-AC.,** phys., ***sil.,*** sol-n.
awns of barley in the pharynx - berb., mag-c.
breathing, when - arg-n.
cold, from becoming - ***kali-c.***
moving, neck when - arg-n.
extending to ear, on turning head - **HEP.**
yawning, on - **HEP.**
swallowing, on - alum., ***apis, arg-n.,*** **HEP.,** petr.

SPONGY, appearance - merc.
sensation - ***cist.***

SPOT, in, dry, sore - ***cimic.,*** cist., con., hep., lach., nat-m., phyt., sil.
spot, in pharynx - ***bufo, fl-ac., mur-ac.,*** phys.

STIFFNESS, sensation - aesc., ***bell.,*** berb., ***caust., hydr.,*** kali-m., lac-c., ***lach., lyss.,*** mag-c., mag-p., meny., mez., nit-ac., ***nux-m.,*** phyt., ***spong.,*** **RHUS-T.,** stry.

STINGING, pain - ***acon.,*** aesc., **APIS,** ***arum-t.,*** asar., ***bell.,*** led., lyss., ***mag-c., nit-ac.,*** par., spong., still., stram.
menses, before - ***mag-c.***
swallowing, on - alum., am-m., arum-t., apis, aur., dros., kali-c., **KALI-I.,** lyss., mag-c., merc., puls., thuj.
when not - aeth., **APIS,** arn., dig., ***ign., led.***
talking, while - **KALI-I.,** mag-c.
yawning, when - am-m.

SUFFOCATIVE, sensation - anan., ***apis,*** calc-f., caust., **LACH.,** lact., lyss., nux-v., phyt., sang., stry., upa., verat.
cold drinks - calc-f.
night - calc-f.
pressing left side of - upa.
pulsation in, from - upa.
warm drinks amel. - calc-f.

SULPHUR, vapor in, sensation of, on coughing - ***brom.,*** lyc., ***puls.***
inspiration - croc., lyc.

SUPPURATION, tonsils (see Abscess)

SWALLOWING, general
constant, disposition to - ***aesc.,*** aeth., apis, arum-t., ***asaf.,*** bapt., ***bell., bry., calc.,*** cact., carb-ac., carb-s., **CAUST.,** ***cedr.,*** cimic., ***cina, cinnb.,*** cist., cob., ***coc-c., con.,*** cop., crot-h., culx., cur., euph., ferr., fl-ac., ***gels.,*** glon., **GRAPH.,** grat., haem., hell., ***hep.,*** ip., ***lac-c., lach.,*** lac-ac., ***lyc., lyss., merc.,*** **MERC-C.,** merc-i-f., ***nat-m.,*** nat-s., ***nux-m.,*** phyt., plb., ***sabad.,*** seneg., **SEP., STAPH.,** stram., sulph., sul-i., sumb., thuj., til., verat., ***verat-v.,*** zinc.
bitter taste, from - chin.
choking, from - cina, **GRAPH.,** ***lyc.,*** **MERC-C.,** ***sep.***
choking, with - bell.
contraction, in larynx, from - coloc., **GRAPH.,** plat.
deep in throat - calc.
eating amel. - ***caust.,*** **MERC-C.**
evening - ***asaf.***
excitement, agg. - ***staph.***
foreign body, as from - ant-c.
fullness in throat, from - ***cinnb.,*** lac-ac., **LACH.**
lump in throat, from - aesc., agar., ***asaf.,*** calc., calc-f., ***coc-c.,*** coff., ***con.,*** ign., lac-ac., **LACH.,** ***lyss., nat-m., sabad., sep.,*** sulph.
large, as of a - ceph.
larynx, behind - ust.
mucus, from thick - ***alum.,*** **CAUST.,** sep.
night - cimic., glon., naja
pain in larynx, from - fl-ac.
sleep, in - calc., cina.
sour, bitter fluid, vertigo, with - caul.
spasm in throat, from - **GRAPH., MERC-C.**
speaking, while - ***cic., staph.,*** thuj.
walking in wind, while - ***con.***

SWALLOWING, general
difficult - acet-ac., ***acon., aesc.,*** aeth., agar., ***alum., alumn.,*** ambr., **AM-C.,** ant-c., ant-t., anthr., ***apis, arg-m., arg-n., ars.,*** ars-i., arum-t., asar., ***aur.,*** aur-s., ***bapt.,*** **BAR-C.,** bar-m., ***bell.,*** benz-ac., bism., ***brom.,*** bry., bufo, ***cact.,*** caj., ***calc.,*** calc-p., calc-s., camph., cann-s., ***canth., caps.,*** carb-s., ***carb-v.,*** card-m., ***caust.,*** cedr., cham., ***chel.,*** **CHIN.,** chin-a., chlol., chlor., ***cic.,*** cimic., cimx., cina, ***coc-c., cocc., colch.,*** coloc., con., ***cop., crot-c.,*** crot-t., ***cupr.,*** cur., dig., dios., dros., ***dulc., elaps,*** fago., ferr., ferr-ar., fl-ac., form., gent-c., ***gels.,*** glon., graph., grat., ***hell., hep.,*** **HYOS.,** ***ign.,*** ind., ***iod., ip.,*** iris, jac-c., kali-ar., kali-bi., **KALI-C.,** kali-chl., kali-ma., ***kali-n.,*** kali-s., ***kalm., lac-ac.,*** **LACH.,** lact., ***lyc.,*** **LYSS.,** manc., meny., ***merc., merc-c.,*** merc-cy., merc-i-f., ***merc-i-r.,*** meli., mez., mur-ac., myric., ***naja,*** nat-a., nat-c., nat-m., nicc., **NIT-AC.,** nux-m., **NUX-V.,** ***op.,*** ox-ac., paeon., phos., ***phyt.,*** pic-ac., ***plb., psor.,*** puls., raph., **RHUS-T.,** rhus-v., rumx., ***sabad., sep., sil.,*** **STRAM., STRY.,** sulph., ***sul-ac.,*** sumb., ***tab.,*** tarax., tarent., thuj., ust., vesp., vip., ***wye.,*** zinc.
acrid foods - **LACH.**
bending forward amel. - nit-ac.
breakfast - merc-c.
chorea, from - ***agar.***
drink, must, in order to swallow - bar-c., ***bell., cact.,*** calad., cur., elaps, guai., kali-c., ***nat-c.,*** nat-m.
evening - am-c., coc-c., fl-ac., lyc.
forenoon - fl-ac.
liquids - alumn., anan., anth., bell., bism., ***canth., cic.,*** cina, coc-c., con., ***crot-c.,*** crot-h., ***cupr., hyos., ign., iod., kali-br.,*** **LACH.,** ***lyc.,*** **LYSS.,** mag-p., ***merc.,*** merc-c., mez., nat-m., ***nit-ac.,*** nux-v., ***phos.,*** **STRAM.,** sul-ac., ***upa.,*** zinc.
amel. - kali-c.
more difficult than solids - ***alum., bell., both.,*** brom., bry., cact., canth., cocc., coc-c., gels., hyos., ign., ***lach., lyss., merc-c.,*** sil., stram.
regurgitate through the nose (see Liquids)
only, can swallow, but solid food gags - ***bapt.,*** bar-c., calad., cham., ***crot-c., crot-h.,*** nat-m., ***plb., sil.***
lying, when - sec.
amel. - canth.
menses, during - calc.
morning - am-c., arum-t., canth., cham.
nervous, when - cocc., gels., nux-v., phys.
night - ***alum.,*** naja
noon - ferr-i., phos.
press neck, must, with hands - acon.
saliva - haem., **LACH.,** meny., myric., spig.
scarlatina, smallpox, in - rhus-t.

SWALLOWING, general
difficult,
solids - ***alum., alumn., apis, arg-n.,*** atro., **BAPT., BAR-C.,** ***bell.,*** bry., ***carb-v., cham., crot-c., crot-h., dros.,*** hep., ***kali-c.,*** lac-ac., ***lac-c., lach.,*** lyc., ***nat-m.,*** nat-p., ***nux-v., plb., rhus-t., sil.,*** stram.
descends wrong way - ***anac.,*** cann-s., kali-c., ***meph.,*** nat-m.
morning - stram.
stiffness of muscles, throat - hyos.
sweets - **LACH.**
waking, on - ***alum.,*** sulph., zing.
impeded - alum., ambr., **AM-C.,** ang., ant-c., ***arn., ars., bapt.,*** bell., bufo, cact., cadm-s., caj., ***canth., carb-v., chel.,*** chlor., cic., ***cina,*** con., crot-h., cupr., elaps, hep., **HYOS.,** iod., kali-bi., kali-c., kali-n., lach., ***laur.,*** lob., lyc., meny., naja, ***nat-s., nux-v., op., plb., sabad., stram.,*** sulph., vesp.
foods only, solids can swallow, least gags, reach a certain point and are violently ejected - **NAT-M.**
liquids only, can swallow, least gags - ***bapt.,*** bar-c., ***crot-c., crot-h., plb., sil.***
lying amel. - canth.
lying while - cham., sec.
must drink at every mouthful to wash down the food - ***bell., cact.,*** cur., elaps, kali-c., ***nat-c.,*** nat-m.
night - alum.
pressure on larynx, from - ***chel.***
solids - ***alum., apis, bry.,*** cur., dros., ***graph., ign., lyc.,*** nit-ac., rhus-t., zinc.
impossible - acet-ac., acon., aeth., ***alum., alumn., ant-t., apis, arum-t., bapt.,*** bar-c., ***bell.,*** bism., ***camph.,*** cann-i., carb-ac., ***carb-v.,*** cham., chlor., ***cic., cina, crot-c., crot-h.,*** cupr., cur., dulc., ***gels., graph.,*** hydr-ac., **HYOS.,** ***ign.,*** ip., iris, kali-bi., kreos., **LAC-C.,** ***lach.,*** laur., ***lyc.,*** lyss., manc., merc-c., mur-ac., naja, **NIT-AC.,** ***nux-v.,*** oena., ***op., phos.,*** phys., ***plb.,*** psor., ***sabad.,*** spong., **STRAM.,** ***sulph., tab.,*** thuj., ***verat.***
choking, from - ***hyos., iod., kali-c.,*** manc., mur-ac.
cold things - kali-c.
constriction of, esophagus - ***alum., alumn., bapt.,*** **BAR-C.,** cact., ***cic., hyos., kali-c.,*** **PHOS.**
cardiac opening - **PHOS.**
liquids, anything but - bapt., bar-c., ***cina,*** crot-c., ***crot-h., kali-c.***
even a teaspoonful of - ***lyc.,*** **NIT-AC.**
lying, while - cham., sec.
menses, during - petr.
mucus is hawked out, until - ***thuj.***
paralysis, from - ***alum., alumn., apis,*** ars., bapt., caust., ***cocc.,*** cur., ***gels.,*** lac-ac., lach., lact., lyc., ***nat-m., nux-m., nux-v.,*** op., phyt., **STRAM.,** ***tab.***
saliva - spig.
swelling, of the tongue - apis
typhus in - bapt., ***camph.***
warm soup - lyc.

SWALLOWING, general
incomplete - benz-ac.
involuntary - ***cina,*** con., merc., mur-ac., **SEP.,** ***staph.***
walking in the wind, when - con.
sleep, in - ***calc.,*** cina.
wrong way, solids descends - ***anac.,*** cann-s., kali-c., ***meph.,*** nat-m.

SWELLING - acon., aesc., **AIL.,** am-c., am-m., anan., ant-t., **APIS,** arg-m., arn., ***ars.,*** ars-i., aur., **BELL.,** benz-ac., ***brom.,*** bufo, ***calc.,*** calc-p., ***calc-s., canth.,*** carb-s., carb-v., caust., chin-a., chlor., cic., coc-c., crot-h., crot-t., cupr-ac., dios., gamb., glon., ***graph.,*** **HEP.,** iod., jug-c., kali-ar., kali-c., kali-ma., kali-n., kali-p., kali-s., kalm., **LACH.,** led., ***lyc.,*** **MERC., MERC-C.,** ***merc-cy., mur-ac.,*** nat-a., ***nat-m., nit-ac., nux-v.,*** op., ox-ac., petr., ***phos.,*** **PHYT.,** ***plb.,*** psor., puls., ***rhus-t.,*** rhus-v., rumx., sabad., samb., sars., sec., ***seneg., sep.,*** sil., spig., **SPONG.,** ***stann.,*** stram., stry., ***sulph.,*** sul-ac., sul-i., ***thuj.,*** verat., vesp., ***wye.,*** xan., zinc.
coughing, on - ars.
edematous - ***ail.,*** anthr., **APIS,** crot-t., kali-bi., ***lac-c., nat-a., nit-ac.,*** phos., rhus-t., sul-ac.
evening - aesc., mez.
left - spig.
morning - bry.
night - merc.

swelling, tonsils - acon., alum., alumn., ***am-c.,*** ant-t., ***apis,*** arum-t., ***aur.,*** **BAPT.,** bar-ac., **BAR-C., BAR-M., BELL.,** berb., brom., bufo, **CALC.,** ***calc-p., calc-s.,*** canth., caps., ***carb-ac.,*** carb-s., carc., cedr., **CHAM.,** ***chel.,*** cinnb., cist., coc-c., ***colch.,*** cop., ***crot-t.,*** diph., ***dulc.,*** fago., ferr-p., ***fl-ac., gels., graph., guai.,*** guare., ham., **HEP.,** hippoz., ign., ***iod., kali-bi.,*** kali-c., ***kali-chl., kali-i.,*** kali-m., kali-p., kali-s., **LAC-C., LACH.,** led., **LYC.,** ***manc., merc., merc-c., merc-cy., merc-i-f., merc-i-r., mur-ac.,*** nat-a., nat-s., nicc., **NIT-AC.,** nux-v., **PHOS., PHYT.,** plat., ***plb.,*** puls., psor., ***ran-s.,*** raph., ***sabad.,*** sang-n., sep., **SIL.,** sol-n., stann., ***staph.,*** **SULPH.,** tarent., tep., thuj., **TUB.,** verat., zinc.
hardness of hearing, with - calc-p., ***hep.,*** lyc., plb., psor.
left - aesc., apis, bar-c., cist., iod., kali-c., kali-p., ***lac-c.,*** **LACH.,** ***merc-i-r.,*** nux-m., phos., sep., sulph., ust.
right - am-c., apis, bar-c., ***bell.,*** dulc., gels., ham., hep., lac-c., ***lyc.,*** merc., merc-d., ***merc-i-f.,*** naja, nat-c., nicc., phos., ***phyt.,*** plat., sabad., spong., tarent., thuj.
while writing - upa.

swelling, uvula - acon., ***alumn.,*** **APIS,** arg-n., bar-m., bell., calad., ***calc., calc-p., carb-v.,*** caps., chel., chin., ***coff.,*** crot-t., ***fl-ac., hep.,*** ind., ***iod., kali-bi.,*** **KALI-I.,** lac-c., ***lach.,*** lyc., ***merc.,*** **MERC-C.,** ***mur-ac.,*** nat-a., nat-s., ***nit-ac., nux-v.,*** par., **PHOS.,** ***phyt.,*** puls., rhus-t., rumx., sabad., **SIL.,** spong., ***sulph.,*** sul-ac., zinc.

swelling, uvula
edematous - **APIS,** crot-t., **KALI-BI.,** kali-br., ***kali-i.,*** kali-ma., lach., merc-c., ***mur-ac., nit-ac.,*** phos., phyt., rhus-t., ***sul-ac.,*** tab.
sac-like - ***apis,*** ars., caps., ***kali-bi., phyt.,*** sabad., wye.

SWOLLEN, sensation - acon., aloe, ***arg-n.,*** ars., bapt., bar-c., bell., benz-ac., ***bry.,*** calc., carb-v., casc., ***caust.,*** chin., coff., colch., dig., ***glon., hep.,*** ign., ip., kalm., lac-c., **LACH.,** led., lyc., merc., nit-ac., nux-v., ***plb.,*** puls., ***rhus-t.,*** sabad., ***sabin., sang.,*** stann., ***sulph.,*** tarax., verat., ***wye.***
swollen, throat-pit - ***lach.***
swollen, uvula - arg-n., puls.

SYPHILITIC, affections of - ***ars-i., asaf., aur.,*** **AUR-M.,** bell., cinnb., ***fl-ac.,*** **HEP.,** hydr., ***kalm., kali-bi.,*** **KALI-I.,** ***lach., lyc.,*** **MERC.,** merc-c., ***merc-i-f., merc-i-r.,*** **MEZ., NIT-AC., PHYT.,** sulph., syph.

TEARING, pain - act-sp., ***aeth.,*** agar., ambr., am-c., ars., ***bism., camph., carb-v.,*** caust., cham., cist., ***colch.,*** crot-h., hura, iod., kali-c., lyc., nat-s., sol-t-ae., staph., teucr., ***zinc.***
coughing, on - chin-s., ***cist.***
drinking, after - nit-ac.
inspiration, on - hura.
cold air - act-sp., crot-h.
jerking - zinc.
left - zinc.
lifting, on - caust.
mental exertion - caust.
morning - phos.
sneezing, when - phos.
swallowing, on, (see Pain)
saliva - agar.
upward - lyc.
tearing, tonsils - **BELL.**
swallowing, on - **BELL.**

TENSION - acon., alum., asaf., ***arg-m.,*** bov., brom., ***caust.,*** chel., chin., dig., ***glon.,*** iod., kali-n., lyc., **MERC.,** merc-c., mez., naja, nat-m., nux-m., nux-v., ph-ac., phos., puls., sabad., sec., sep., stann., tab., ***verb.***
afternoon - tab.
menses, before - ***iod.***
pit of throat - cham., puls., sulph.
right side - alum., **ARG-M.**
swallowing, when - ***asaf., lyc.,*** mez., nat-m., ***puls.***
yawning, when - ***arg-m.***

THICK, sensation - ail., sep.

THREAD, hanging in, sensation of - coc-c., ***valer.***

THROBBING, pain, tonsils - am-m., bell., phyt.

THYROID, gland, (see Glands, chapter)

TICKLING, throat to ear, swallowing - petr.
tickling, pharynx - stict.

tickling, throat-pit - **APIS,** aspar., bell., cann-s., caust., **CHAM.,** cinnb., cocc., coloc., ***con.,*** crot-h., ign., ***iod.,*** kreos., lac-c., lach., lith., mag-m., nat-c., nat-m., ph-ac., phos., ***puls.,*** rhus-r., **RUMX., SANG., *sil.,*** squil., tarax.

TINGLING, (see Formication) - acon., carb-ac., echi.

tingling, fauces, in - ***acon.,*** echi., phyt.

TONSILLECTOMY, ailments after - arn., calc., calen., strept., sulph.

TONSILLITIS, inflammation of tonsils - ***acon.,*** aesc., ***ail.,*** **ALUMN**., aml-n., anan., ant-t., anthr., ***apis, ars.,*** bad., ***bapt.,*** **BAR-C., *bar-m.,* BELL.,** benz-ac., berb., bufo, ***canth., caps.,*** cedr., ***cham.,*** chel., ***chen-a., colch., crot-h., cupr.,*** cur., ***dulc.,*** ferr-p., ***fl-ac., gels.,*** **GUAI.,** ham., **HEP., *ign., iod., kali-bi., kali-chl.,*** kali-p., **LAC-C., LACH., *lyc.,* MERC., *merc-cy.,* MERC-D., *merc-i-f., merc-i-r.,*** naja, ***nat-s.,*** **NIT-AC., *phyt., plb., psor.,*** puls., ***sabad., sang.,*** sep., **SIL., *staph.,*** still., ***sulph.,*** tarent., ust., verat., vesp., zinc.

chronic recurrent - ***alumn.,*** **BAR-C., *bar-m.,*** brom., bry., calc-f., calc-p., carc., diph., dys-co., fuc., graph., guai., ***hep.,*** kali-i., lach., lyc., mez., morg., morg-g., nat-m., phyt., **PSOR., *sang.,*** sep., ***sil.,*** sul-i., sulph., syc-co., syph., thuj., **TUB.**

cold weather, every spell of - bell., calc., ***dulc.,*** hep.

extending to, nose - **NIT-AC.**

upward and downward - merc.

painless - **BAPT.**

subacute - chen-a.

TURNING, about in - lach.

TWITCHING - ***arg-n.,*** chel., crot-t., cycl., sep.

extending to pit of stomach - sep.

ULCERATIVE, pain - ph-ac.

ULCERS - acet-ac., all-s., alum., ***alumn.,*** anan., **APIS,** arg-n., **ARS.,** ars-i., ***arum-t., aur., aur-m., bapt.,*** bell., bor., cahin., ***calc., calc-s., caps.,*** carb-s., carb-v., chel., chlor., ***cinnb.,*** clem., dros., ***elaps, fl-ac.,*** **HEP., *hippoz., hydr.,*** ign., ***iod.,*** kali-ar., ***kali-bi., kali-chl., kali-i.,*** kali-ma., kreos., ***lac-c.,*** lach., ***lyc., manc.,*** **MERC., MERC-C., *merc-cy., merc-d., merc-i-f., merc-i-r.,*** mez., mill., ***mur-ac.,*** nat-m., **NIT-AC.,** nux-v., petr., ***phyt., psor.,*** ptel., sal-ac., ***sang.,*** sanic., sars., sil., ***sulph.,*** thuj., vinc., viol-t., zinc.

aphthous - ***canth.,*** eucal., nit-ac.

burning - ***caps., manc.***

cold agg. - anan.

deep - ***apis, kali-bi., kali-i.,*** lach.

gangrenous - ail., am-c., ***ars.,*** bapt., echi., kali-chl., kali-n., kali-per., ***lach.,*** merc., ***merc-cy.,*** mur-ac., sil.

left - elaps, ***lach.***

menses, before - ***mag-c.***

mercury, after - aur., hep., hydr., ***iod., kali-i.,*** lyc., ***nit-ac.***

offensive - alum.

right - lyc., ptel.

ULCERS, in

scarlet fever does not come out, when - apis

spreading - apis, ***ars., kali-bi.,*** lach., **MERC-C.**

stinging in - kali-bi., ***lac-c., merc., nit-ac.***

syphilitic - aur-m., calc-f., ***fl-ac.,*** hippoz., ***kali-bi., lach.,*** lyc., merc., ***merc-c.,*** merc-i-f., merc-i-r., ***nit-ac.,*** phyt., still.

ulcers, fauces - ***ail.,*** arum-t., **BAPT., *bor., canth.,*** caps., ***carb-v.,*** chlor., ***fl-ac.,*** **KALI-BI., KALI-I., LACH., MERC., MERC-C., *merc-i-r., nat-s.,* NIT-AC., *phyt.,*** sars., sol-t-ae.

burning, with - ***caps.***

ulcers, pharynx - kali-bi., merc-c., mez., nit-ac., sulph., zinc.

ulcers, tonsils - **AIL., *am-c., apis, aur., aur-m.,*** bar-c., bell., ***calc., fl-ac., hep.,*** hippoz., ign., ***kali-bi., lac-c., lyc., manc., merc., merc-c., merc-i-f., merc-i-r.,*** nat-s., **NIT-AC., *phyt.,*** sep., zinc.

behind - ars., merc.

yellow - calc., zinc.

ulcers, uvula - aur., bism., fl-ac., ind., kali-bi., merc., merc-c., nit-ac., phos., phyt., sulph.

spreading - bism., ***kali-bi.,*** **MERC-C.**

syphilitic - ***aur., fl-ac., kali-bi., merc., merc-c., nit-ac.,*** phyt.

VAPOR, fumes, etc, rising in - apis, asaf., brom., bry., carb-v., chin., colch., ferr., hep., ign., ip., kali-chl., lach., lyc., merc., mosch., nux-v., ol-an., op., par., puls., rhus-t., sabad., sars., thuj., zinc.

VARICOSIS - ***alumn., bar-m.,*** brom., ***fl-ac.,*** **HAM., *puls.,*** thuj.

pharynx - **AESC., *carb-v., fl-ac.,* HAM., *kali-bi., lach., lyc., mang.,*** nat-a., phyt., ***puls.,*** vesp.

tonsils - ***bar-c., bar-m., ham., lach.***

VESICLES - ant-t., ***apis,*** ars., ***rhus-t.,*** sep.

pharynx - ant-t., canth.

tonsils - aur-m-n., iris, nit-ac.

vesicles, uvula - calc.

VOICE, (see Larynx)

WART-like, growths (see Condylomata)

WATER, as if, full of - hep.

WEAKNESS, exertion, agg. - arn., lac-c., rhus-t.

WORM, crawling up throat, as if - zinc.

Tongue

ACHING, pain - all-c., ***sang.,*** sulph., vesp.
evening - sulph.

ADHERES, to roof of mouth - alum., arg-m., bell., ***bry.,*** caust., kali-p., nit-ac., **NUX-M.,** sanic., sulph.

ANESTHESIA, sensation - carb-s.

APHTHAE - aeth., agar., ars., arum-d., aur., **BOR.,** camph., carb-v., hydr., ***ill., jug-c.,*** kali-chl., ***lach.,*** med., ***merc., merc-cy., mur-ac., nat-m.,*** nux-v., ox-ac., ***phos.,*** plb., sars., ***sulph., sul-ac.,*** tarent., thuj., tub.
edges of - arg-n.
sensitive, and bleeding - **BOR.**
spots, in - ***sul-ac.***
tip - agar., ***bry., ham., lach.,*** med.
under - med.

ATROPHY - ***mur-ac.***

BITING, pain - absin., arn., asar., bell., carb-ac., ***cham.,*** chin., coch., dios., dros., ign., jal., mez., ol-an., sulph., teucr.
anterior part - ars., sep.
border - coloc., ip.
peppery - indg., sep., teucr.
root - mez.
tip - ars., dros., ip., nat-c., puls.
tobacco - anac.
under - zinc..
biting, sensation in - absin., acet-ac., agar., alum., **BUFO,** carb-ac., ***caust., cic.,*** colch., dig., dios., glon., ***hyos.,*** **IGN.,** lach., merl., mez., ***nat-m., nit-ac.,*** petr., ***ph-ac., puls.,*** sec., sulph., thuj., verat.
morning - art-v.
night, sleep, in - alum., apis, ***cic.,*** med., mez., ***ph-ac.,*** ther., zinc.
spasms, in - ***art-v., bufo,*** camph., ***caust.,*** cocc., ***cupr., oena., op.,*** sec., tarent., valer.

BITTEN, pain as if - caust., chin-b., plb.

BLACK - aeth., ***arg-n.,*** **ARS.,** bapt., bar-c., bufo, cadm-s., camph., ***carb-ac.,*** **CARB-V., CHIN.,** ***chin-a.,*** chlol., ***chlor.,*** crot-h., cupr., dig., elaps, gymn., hippoz., hyos., ***kali-c., lach.,*** lept., ***lyc.,*** **MERC.,** ***merc-c., merc-cy.,*** merc-d., merc-sul., ***nux-v., op.,*** **PHOS.,** plb., rad-br., rhus-t., ***sec.,*** sin-n., stram., ***verat.,*** vip.
center - chlol., lept., ***merc.,*** **PHOS.,** sec.
streak like ink - arn., bapt., chlol., lept., mur-ac.
crusts - ***phos.***
edges dark streaked - petr.
gangrenous - ars., bism.
posterior part - ***verat.***
purple-black - ***op.***
red edges - **MERC.,** nux-v.

BLEEDING - anan., arg-m., ars., **ARUM-T., BOR.,** bry., cadm-s., calc., caps., cham., chlol., clem., cur., guare., kali-bi., kali-chl., lac-ac., ***lach.,*** lyc., med., ***merc.,*** nat-m., nat-p., nit-ac., nux-v., phos., ***podo.,*** sars., sec., sep., spig., ter.
tip - lach., phos.

BLOTCHES, under the, like vegetable growths - ambr.

BLUE - ***agar.,*** **ANT-T., ARS.,** benz-ac., bufo, ***carb-v.,*** colch., cupr-s., **DIG.,** gymn., ***iris, mur-ac.,*** op., ***plat., podo.,*** spig., tab., thuj.
spots, in - arg-n., sars.

BLUISH-black - bufo.
bluish-white - ars-h., gymn.

BORING, pain in - clem.
night - con.
right edge - ars.

BROAD - mag-m., merc., nat-m., puls.
seems too - ***kali-bi.,*** **NAT-M.,** par., ***podo.,*** plb., **PULS.,** vib., ziz.

BROWN - aesc., **AIL.,** am-c., ant-t., ***anthr., apis, arn.,*** **ARS.,** ars-i., atro., aur., **BAPT.,** ***bell.,*** **BRY.,** ***cadm-s., carb-ac., carb-v., chel., chin.,*** **CHIN-A.,** coc-c., ***colch., crot-h., cupr.,*** cupr-ar., ***dig.,*** dios., dor., echi., elat., gels., guai., ***hep.,*** **HYOS.,** iod., ***kali-bi.,*** kali-br., **KALI-P.,** ***lac-c.,*** **LACH.,** ***lyc.,*** med., ***merc., merc-cy., merc-i-f.,*** morph., mur-ac., nat-s., ***nux-v., op.,*** ox-ac., ph-ac., **PHOS.,** phyt., **PLB.,** ptel., ***pyrog.,*** **RHUS-T.,** rumx., sabin., sanic., **SEC.,** ***sep., sil., spong., sulph.,*** tarent., ter., verb., vip.
base, at - lyss., pyrog., torula.
center - ail., ***arn.,*** ars., ***bapt., bry.,*** canth., ***colch., crot-h., eup-pur.,*** hyos., iod., ***lac-c.,*** nat-p., ***phos., plb.,*** pyrog., vib.
morning, in rising - rhus-t.
sides moist - ***apis.***
sides moist, white - arn., nat-p.
dry - ail., ant-t., ***ars., bapt., bry.,*** kali-p., ***lach., rhus-t.,*** spong., tart-ac., vip.
morning - ***bapt.,*** **RHUS-T.,** tarax.
red tip and edges - ***lyc.,*** rhus-t.
reddish-brown - rumx., sul-ac., ***zinc.***
sides - ***kali-bi.,*** phyt.
thick - med.
yellowish-brown - ant-t., ***bapt.,*** brom., ***carb-v.,*** chel., cina, crot-h., dios., merc-i-f., ***pyrog.,*** rumx., verb.
with shining edges - bapt.

BURNING, pain - acet-ac., **ACON.,** aesc., all-c., alum., alumn., am-caust., ***am-m., apis,*** ang., arn., **ARS.,** ***ars-i., aur.,*** **ARUM-T.,** asar., bad., ***bapt., bar-c., bell.,*** benz-ac., berb., ***bov., calc., calc-s., canth.,*** carb-ac., ***carb-an., carb-s., carb-v.,*** cast., ***caust.,*** cedr., ***cham.,*** chel., chim., **CHIN.,** chin-a., chlor., ***cimx.,*** cocc., coch., coff., ***colch., coloc.,*** con., crot-t., cupr., ***dros., echi.,*** ferr., ferr-ar., ferr-i., ferr-p., gamb., gels., glon., graph., ham., ***hydr.,*** hyos., indg., iod., ***ip.,*** **IRIS,** jac-c., jatr., ***kali-ar.,*** kali-bi., kali-c., kali-chl., kali-p., kali-s., lac-ac., ***lach., laur.,*** led., ***lyc., mag-m.,*** manc., ***mang., merl., merc., merc-c.,*** merc-sul., ***mez.,*** mur-ac., naja, nat-s., ol-an., op., ***ox-ac.,*** pall., petr., phel., ph-ac., ***phos., phyt., plat.,*** plb., ***podo.,*** prun., ***psor., ran-s.,*** raph., rat., rhod., rhus-t., rumx., ***sang.,*** sanic., sars., sec., seneg., ***sep.,*** sin-n., spig., ***sulph., sul-ac.,***

BURNING, pain - tarax., thuj., verat., **VERAT-V.,** vesp., xan., zinc.
afternoon - mag-m.
anterior half - gamb.
center, of - bar-c., bry.
spot toward tip - kali-ar.
eating, after - graph.
eating, while - ***ign., nat-m.***
edges - acon., agar., apis, ***camph.,*** cycl., kali-i., mur-ac., nat-s., plat.
left - ***lach.,*** nat-s., ox-ac.
right - phos.
evening - alum., cycl., kali-n.
extending to, palate - phos.
to, stomach - apis, ars., brom., gels., ***mez.,*** puls.
fissures in - mag-m.
left side - jac-c.
morning - ***mag-m.,*** stann., sulph.
night - nat-m., ***phos.***
pepper, as from - ang., lach., merl., ***mez.,*** op., sanic., sep., teucr.
protrudes it to cool it - sanic.
root - am-caust., **ARUM-T.,** bapt., benz-ac., ***crot-c.,*** manc., med.
right - phos.
under - sel.
salt food, from - petr.
sides, one - ***calc.***
spots - act-sp., ***ars.,*** kali-i., ph-ac., ran-s.
sour food, from - petr.
tip - ***acon.,*** agar., am-c., am-m., arg-m., arg-n., aur., ***bar-c.,*** bell., bov., calc-ar., ***calc.,*** **CALC-P.,** ***camph.,*** carb-ac., ***carb-an.,*** carb-v., cast-eq., caust., ***coloc.,*** croc., crot-c., cycl., ***dros.,*** gamb., glon., hep., indg., iod., ***kali-c., kali-i.,*** kali-n., led., merc., merc-sul., mez., ***nat-c., nat-m.,*** **NAT-S.,** ox-ac., ***phos., phyt.,*** plb., psor., rat., ***sabad.,*** sang., sel., seneg., sulph., sul-ac., ter., ***thuj.***
night, at - hep.
pepper, as from - agar., ang., ***camph.,*** **CHIN.,** con., mez., ***nat-s.,*** teucr.
touch, agg. - am-c., bar-c., bell., nit-ac.
waking - nat-m.
under surface - brom.
waking, on - nat-m.

BURNS, of tongue and lips - apis., **CANTH.,** ham.

BURNT, as if - aesc., all-c., alum., apis, ***arg-n.,*** **ARS.,** bad., bapt., carb-v., ***caust.,*** chin., chlor., ***cimx., coloc.,*** cupr-s., daph., dios., ferr., glon., ***ham.,*** hydr., hyos., ign., ***iris,*** kreos., lac-ac., ***laur., lyc., mag-m., merc., mez., phos., phyt., plat.,*** podo., prun., ***puls.,*** psor., ***rhus-v., rumx.,*** sabad., ***sang.,*** sep., sin-n., sul-ac., ther., **VERAT-V.**
center - chin., hyos., plat., psor., puls., sabad., sep., ter.
eating, while - ign.
eating, or drinking, while not - ferr.
edges - apis, caust., puls.
morning - mez.
smoking, when - sep.

BURNT, as if
spots, in - aloe, ***ars.***
tip - arg-n., ars., calc-p., caps., caust., lact., lath., merc-sul., mez., ***phos., psor.,*** puls., sang., ***sep.,*** syph., vip.

CANCER - ***alumn., apis, ars., aur., aur-m.,*** benz-ac., calc., ***carb-an.,*** caust., ***con.,*** crot-h., cund., ***hydr.,*** kali-chl., **KALI-CY.,** ***kali-i., lach., mur-ac., nit-ac., phos., phyt.,*** sep., ***sil.,*** sulph., thuj.
epithelioma - ars., carb-ac., chr-ac., ***hydr., kali-cy.,*** mur-ac., ***thuj.***

CHOREA - cina.

CLEAN - ***ars., asar.,*** chin., ***cina,*** cory., dig., ***hyos., ip.,*** mag-p., nit-ac., ***pyrog., rhus-t.,*** sec., sep.
anteriorly, coated posteriorly - nux-v.
menses, at, foul after flow ceases - sep.
nausea, during - ip.
urination, when profuse - solid.
vomiting, during - ip.

COATED - ***ant-c.,*** bapt., bell., ***bry.,*** chin., merc., ***nux-v.,*** phos., puls., sulph.
diagonally - rhus-t.
edges, with clean - arg-n.
furrow, across - merc.
centre - nit-ac.
green at base - caps.
salivation, with - nit-ac.
headache, during - calc-ac., card-m., euon., gymn., ***puls.***
one-side - daph., mez., rhus-t.
white - **ANT-C.,** ant-t., ***ars., bell.,*** bism., bry., calc., ***chin.,*** hyos., kali-bi., ***kali-m.,*** merc., nit-ac., phos., ***puls., sulph.,*** tarax.
centre - petr.
yellow - bry., chel., chin., hydr., kali-p., ***mag-m.,*** merc., nux-m., rhus-t., spig.
edges indented, with - chel., hydr.
greenish - chion.
moist, filmy - merc-i-f.
mustard, as if were spread on - kali-p., podo.
patchy - lil-t.

COLD - acet-ac., acon., am-c., ***ars.,*** bar-c., bell., calc., **CAMPH.,** carb-s., ***carb-v., colch.,*** cupr-ar., ***cupr-s., iris,*** kali-br., ***laur.,*** merc., ***nat-m.,*** naja, op., ***ox-ac., ph-ac.,*** sec., **VERAT.,** zinc.
icy - ars., zinc.
morning - zinc.

COLDNESS, sensation of - acet-ac., acon., anag., ant-t., ars-h., bell., **CAMPH.,** carb-s., **CARB-V.,** cist., guare., helo., hydr-ac., iris, kali-chl., laur., naja, sec., ***verat.,*** zinc.
cold air - ***acon.***
left - aloe.
near fraenum - anag.
peppermint like, after - lyss., verat.
right half - ***gels.***
tip - bell., cupr.

CONDYLOMATA - aur., ***aur-m.,*** aur-m-n., lyc., mang., staph.

CONSTRICTING, low down in region of hyoid bone - ***all-c.***

CONTRACTED - ***carb-v., merc-c.***

CONTRACTING, pain - arum-t., bor.
anterior half, right side - ars-h.
root - acon., bell., carb-v., hydrc., lach.
tip - **ARG-N.,** hep., ***psor.,*** sil., stront-c., tub.

CONTRACTION, spasmodic cylindrical - cina.

CORRUGATED - nat-a.

CRACKED, fissured - **AIL.,** anan., ***apis,*** **ARS., ARS-I., ARUM-T.,** aur., atro., bar-c., bar-m., ***bapt., bell., benz-ac., bor., bry.,*** bufo, ***calc.,*** calc-p., calc-s., ***camph.,*** carb-ac., carb-s., ***carb-v., cham.,*** chel., ***chin.,*** chin-a., cic., clem., cob., ***crot-h.,*** cupr., cur., **FL-AC., HYOS.,** iod., ***kali-bi.,*** kali-i., ***lach., lyc., mag-m., merc.,*** mez., ***mur-ac., nat-a.,*** **NIT-AC.,** nux-v., ph-ac., **PHOS.,** plat., ***plb., podo.,*** puls., ***pyrog.,*** ran-s., raph., **RHUS-T.,** rhus-v., sac-alb., **SPIG.,** stram., ***sulph., tub., verat., zinc.***
across - lach., merc.
all directions, in - **FL-AC., NIT-AC.**
bleeding - arum-t.
centre - bapt., bry., bufo, ***cob.,*** cub., lept., ***mez., nit-ac.,*** raph., ***rhus-v.,*** sin-n., syph.
across - cob., lach., merc.
dysentery, in, and red - kali-bi.
edges - anan., clem., hydr., ***lach., nux-v.***
left - ***bar-c.***
painful with hard margins - clem.
peeling, with - ran-s.
tip - bar-c., lach.

CRAWLING - kali-n., ***plat.,*** sec.

CUT, feels on edges - anan.
off, as if - anan.

CUTTING, pain in - ***bov.,*** euon., guare., thuj.
in, edges - mag-s.

DENUDED, spots - ran-s.

DIRTY - all-c., anthro., arg-n., bapt., calc., ***camph.,*** carb-v., card-m., cean., **CHIN.,** croc., cub., ***kali-chl.,*** lac-c., **NAT-S.,** syph., zinc.
headache, during - card-m.

DISTORTED - con.

DOTTED - ant-t., bell., graph., stram.

DRAWING, pain - aster., cast.
as by a string to the hyoid bone - cast.

DRAWN, backward - tarent.
drawn, up - chion.

DRYNESS, of - acet-ac., **ACON.,** aeth., aloe, **AIL., AGAR.,** alumn., ambr., ***ant-t.,*** **APIS,** apoc., arg-m., ***arg-n., arn.,*** **ARS.,** ***ars-h., ars-i., ars-s-f.,*** art-v., ***arum-t.,*** atro., aur., aur-m., ***bapt.,*** bar-c., ***bar-m.,*** **BELL., BRY.,** bufo, cact., cahin., **CALC.,** calc-ar., ***calc-p.,*** calc-s., **CAMPH.,** ***carb-an., carb-s., carb-v.,*** **CAUST., CHAM.,** ***chel.,*** **CHIN.,** chin-a., chlor., ***cic., cist.,*** **COCC.,** coc-c., com., con., croc., ***crot-t.,*** **CUPR.,** daph., dios., ***dulc.,*** ferr-m., ***fl-ac.,*** gels., graph., guare., **HELL.,** helon., ***hydr.,*** **HYOS.,** ***iod., ip., kali-ar., kali-bi.,*** kali-br., kali-c., ***kali-i., kalm., kreos.,***

DRYNESS, of - ***lac-ac.,*** **LACH.,** laur., ***lyc., mag-m.,*** manc., **MERC.,** ***merc-c.,*** merc-i-f., ***merc-i-r.,*** merc-sul., merl., mez., **MUR-AC.,** ***nat-a., nat-c., nat-m., nit-ac.,*** **NUX-M.,** ***nux-v.,*** op., ox-ac., par., petr., ***ph-ac., phos., phyt., pic-ac., plb., podo.,*** **PSOR.,** ptel., **PULS., RHUS-T.,** rumx., sarr., ***sec., sep.,*** sin-n., ***spong.,*** staph., stram., ***stront-c.,*** **SULPH.,** ***sul-ac.,*** tab., tarent., **TER.,** ***tub.,*** vac., ***verat.,*** **VERAT-V.,** vib., zinc.
center - ***acon.,*** ant-c., ant-t., arg-m., ***arum-t., bapt., colch., crot-h.,*** hyos., ***lach.,*** **PHOS.,** phyt., seneg., ***stram.,*** sul-ac., verat.
sides moist - ***apis.***
evening - aloe, arg-n., iod., petr., **NUX-M.,** senec., tarent.
forepart - ***rumx.***
half - bell., sang.
menses, during - ***cedr.,*** sul-ac.
middle - ant-t.
morning - arg-n., ***bapt., bar-c.,*** calc., canth., ***cist.,*** clem., graph., hell., kali-c., kali-p., naja, ***nit-ac.,*** **OP.,** ***puls.,*** sep., ***sulph.***
on waking - arg-n., ***calc., clem.,*** coc-c., ***mez.,*** ol-an., **OP.,** ***par., phos., podo.,*** **PULS., RHUS-T.,** sanic., sep., **SULPH.,** tarax.
night - all-s., ang., ***calc., carb-s.,*** mez., **NUX-M.,** nux-v., ***pic-ac.,*** rumx., tarent.
root - all-c., camph.
side - cocc., sang.
thirst, without - caps., ***nat-m.,*** par., **PULS.**
tip - apis, arn., bell., ***carb-v.,*** cod., ind., mez., ***nux-v.,*** phos., ***phyt.,*** psor., puls., ***rhus-t., rumx., sec.,*** valer.
moist - bry.
sensation of - caps.
dryness, sensation of - arg-m., arn., ***ars.,*** bell., brom., ***calc.,*** cimic., ***cocc.,*** colch., mang., **NAT-M., NUX-M.,** ph-ac., puls.

ECCHYMOSES - ***phos.,*** plb.

ELONGATION, sensation of - mur-ac.

ENLARGED - acon., ars., ars-h., ars-i., colch., crot-h., cupr., dig., glon., graph., hydr., iod., kali-bi., kali-br., kali-i., lac-c., lyss., merc-c., nat-a., nat-m., ***nit-ac.,*** ox-ac., par., phos., petr., plb., sep.
base - bapt., cocc., kali-chl., spig.
enlarged, sensation as if - acon., ars., colch., crot-t., cupr., dig., glon., hydr., kali-bi., kali-i., lac-ac., merc-c., nat-a., ox-ac., par., petr., phos., plb., puls., sep.

ERUPTIONS - nat-m., sars., zinc.
papillae like strawberry - arg-n., ars., ***bell.,*** caust., kali-bi., ter.

EXCORIATION, of mucous, membrane - agar., ars., ***aur., calc., canth., carb-ac.,*** carb-v., ***cist.,*** kali-ar., ***lach.,*** lyc., ***merc., merc-c., mur-ac., nit-ac., nux-v.,*** ox-ac., ***phos., ran-s.,*** **SEP.,** ***sil.,*** sulph., sul-ac., tarax.
as if - arum-m., aur-m.
edges - ant-c.

EXCORIATION, of mucous, membrane
center - am-c.
fraenum - kali-c.
tip - kali-c.

FILMY - merc-i-f.

FISHBONE, pain, in root, on swallowing - ars.

FLABBY - ant-t., **CAMPH.,** chin-s., cimic., ***cub., hydr.,*** ign., kreos., ***lyss., lycps., mag-m.,*** **MERC.,** nat-a., ***ph-ac.,*** rhus-t., sanic., ***sep.,*** stram., ter., xan.
moist, with imprints of teeth - ars., chel., ***hydr.,*** kali-bi., ***merc., merc-c., merc-d., merc-sul.,*** nat-p., ***podo.,*** pyrog., ***rhus-t.,*** sanic., stram., yuc.

FOLDED, like little bags on edges - anis.
lead colic, in - alumn.

FROTH, edges of - am-c., apis, apisin., ***nat-m.,*** phos.

GANGRENE - ***ars.,*** kali-c., lach., merc., ***sec.***

GLOSSITIS, inflammation of tongue - ***acon.,*** am-c., anan., ang., **APIS,** ***arg-n., arn., ars.,*** arum-t., aur-m., bell., ***benz-ac.,*** brom., calc., ***calc-s., canth.,*** carb-v., caust., cocc., con., **CROT-C., CROT-H.,** ***cupr.,*** ferr-p., hep., kali-ar., kali-chl., **LACH.,** lyc., ***mag-m.,*** mang., ***merc., merc-c.,*** mez., ***nat-m., nit-ac.,*** nux-v., ox-ac., petr., ***ph-ac., phyt., plb., prun.,*** ran-s., sep., ***sil., staph., sulph., sul-ac.***
center - gels.
chronic - ***cupr.***
gouty - ***benz-ac., merc.***
induration, with - ars., ***aur-m.,*** carb-v., con., ***cupr.,*** lyc., ***merc.,*** mez., sil.
left side - ars-s-r.
mercury, after abuse of - ***calc., hep., nit-ac.,*** phyt., staph., ***sulph.***
one-sided - nux-v.
papillae - bell.

GRAY - ***ambr.,*** anan., ant-t., ars-h., bry., ***chel.,*** cupr-ac., ***kali-c.,*** lac-c., ***merc-cy.,*** ph-ac., ***phos.,*** phyt., puls.
center - phos.
grayish-yellow - ***ambr.,*** phyt.

GREASY, sensation - ***iris.,*** phys.

GREEN - ars-m., calc-caust., caps., chin., chion., cupr., led., **NAT-S.,** ***nit-ac., plb., rhod.***
base, at - caps., chion.
salivation, with - nit-ac.

GREENISH-brown - nat-s.
greenish-gray - **NAT-S.**
greenish-yellow - ***calc-caust.,*** guare., kali-p., merc-sul.

HAIR, on - all-s., ***kali-bi., nat-m.,*** nat-p., **SIL.**
anterior part - **SIL.**
posterior part - kali-bi.
reading, while - all-s.
tip - nat-p., sil.
trachea, to - sil.

HARD - alum., aur-m., ***calc-f.,*** mur-ac., semp., ***sil.***

HEAT, in - acon., am-c., ***apis,*** ars., **BELL.,** caps., caust., cimic., crot-t., manc., merc-c., ***mez., phyt.,*** plb., puls., sec., stram., stry., sulph., tax.
edges and tip - sin-n.
tip - carb-v.

HEAVINESS, of - ***anac.,*** ars., ***bell., carb-v., colch.,*** guare., hyos., ***lyc.,*** merl., ***mur-ac., nat-c.,*** **NAT-M.,** ***nux-m., nux-v., plb.,*** sec., stram., ***verat.***
difficulty in moving - aesc., ***ars.,*** calc., ***carb-v.,*** cic., con., **LACH.,** ***lyc.,*** merc., op., ***stram.***
velum palatinum - thuj.

HERPES, on - ***nat-m., rhus-t., zinc.***

INDENTED - ant-t., **ARS.,** ars-m., atro., bapt., bor., ***calc., carb-v.,*** **CHEL.,** ***crot-c.,*** crot-t., dulc., glon., ***hydr.,*** hydrc., ign., ***iod.,*** kali-bi., kali-br., kali-i., mag-m., **MERC.,** merc-i-f., nat-p., ***pip-m.,*** plb., ***podo., puls.,*** pyrog., **RHUS-T.,** sanic., ***sep.,*** stram., sumb., ***syph.,*** tell., vib., yuc.

INDURATION - ***arg-n.,*** ars., ***atro., aur., aur-m., bar-c.,*** carb-an., ***carb-v.,*** con., cupr., gamb., **HYOS.,** kali-i., lyc., ***merc.,*** mez., mur-ac., **NUX-M.,** sul-i.
center - bar-c., bry.
knotty - carb-an.
places in tongue - kali-chl., ***sulph.***

INFLAMMATION, (see Glossitis)

ITCHING - alum., apis, cedr., crot-c., dulc., ph-ac., sulph.
tip - dulc.

JERKING, in - cham.

JERKING, pain, in - aster., cast.
tip - ang.

LAME - calc., ***dulc.,*** euphr., hydr-ac.
as if - aesc-g., ***mur-ac.***
fright, after - hydr., hyos.

LACERATED - anan., art-v., ***calen.,*** hyper.

LEATHER, feels like - acon.
hard - aur.
leather, looks like burnt - hyos.

LONG, feels too - acon., aeth., ***mur-ac.,*** sumb.

MAPPED - ant-c., ***ars.,*** cham., dulc., hydr., ***kali-bi.,*** kali-m., ***lach.,*** lil-t., lyc., ***merc., merc-c.,*** **NAT-M.,** ***nit-ac.,*** ox-ac., petr., phys., phyt., ***ran-s., rhus-t.,*** sep., sul-ac., syph., **TARAX.,** ***ter.,*** thuj., ***tub.***

MEMBRANE, on, thick - thyr.
tough and yellow - ***nit-ac.***

MOTION, difficult - ***aesc.,*** anac., ***ars., bell.,*** bufo, cadm-s., calc., carb-v., ***cic., colch.,*** con., **HYOS.,** ***kali-br.,*** **LACH.,** ***lyc., merc., mur-ac., mygal., nat-c.,*** op., **PHOS.,** phys., ***puls., stram.***
constant - acon., clem., op., stram.
crusty coat, on account of - myric.
disorderly - merc.
hanging out - apis, ***lach.,*** sil., stram.
lapping - ***bufo.***
to and fro - ***cupr., hyos., lach., sulph.***

MOTION, difficult
painful from - aloe, ant-t., berb., chin., spig., ***sulph.***
side to side - ***hell.,*** lach., ***lyc.***
wanting - ars-s-f., ***aur., carb-v.,*** cic., con., op., ***phos., stram.***

MUCUS, slime, etc, collection of, on - all-c., alum., ***alumn.,*** arg-n., ars-h., ars-m., arum-d., ***bar-c.,*** bar-m., ***bell.,*** berb., calc., canth., carb-ac., carb-an., chel., chin-a., ***cocc.,*** colch., cupr., dulc., fl-ac., grat., ***hydr.,*** jug-r., kali-n., kali-p., kali-s., kreos., ***lach.,*** lact., mag-c., mag-m., ***merc.,*** merc-c., **NAT-M.,** ***nat-s.,*** nux-m., ***petr.,*** ph-ac., ***phos.,*** phyt., **PULS.,** rhus-t., sec., **SEP.,** ***sulph., verb.,*** viol-t., zinc.
eating, after - sep., verb.
morning - agar., mag-m., sang., sulph., verb.
salty - sulph.
sensation of mucus - chin.
string, can be pulled off in - bell.
tough - bell., cupr., dulc., lach., merc., nux-v., ph-ac., puls., sulph., verb.

MUCOUS membrane, excoriation - agar., ars., ***aur., calc., canth., carb-ac.,*** carb-v., ***cist.,*** kali-ar., ***lach.,*** lyc., ***merc., merc-c., mur-ac., nit-ac., nux-v.,*** ox-ac., ***phos., ran-s.,*** **SEP.,** ***sil.,*** sulph., sul-ac., tarax.

NEEDLE-like, pain - nux-v.
tip, of - merc.

NOSODITIES - ambr., aur., **CARB-AN.,** dros., eupi., iod., kali-i., lyc., mang., mur-ac., ***sil.***
hard - mur-ac.
on tip, forming vesicle, resulting in unclean ulcer with hard edges - ph-ac.
right side coming to a point - ars-h.
under - ambr.

NEURALGIC, pain - apis, crot-t., kali-ar., mang.

NUMBNESS - ***acon.,*** agar., ambr., ***apis, ars.,*** bapt., bell., bor., bov., brach., ***calc-p.,*** camph., carb-s., ***colch., crot-h.,*** eup-pur., ferr., ferr-ar., ***fl-ac.,*** **GELS.,** ***glon., hell., hyos.,*** ictod., ***ign.,*** jatr., kali-ar., ***laur.,*** lyc., mang., meph., merc., merc-c., merl., nat-a., nat-c., ***nat-m.,*** nat-p., **NUX-M.,** puls., ***rheum,*** sep., sil., sul-ac., ther., vip., zinc.
morning on waking - am-c., bov., kali-c., mag-c.
one-sided - gels., ***nat-m.,*** nux-v.
vertigo, with - agar.
posteriorly - **BOV.**

PAIN, tongue - acon., all-c., alumn., ambr., am-caust., ***apis,*** arg-m., ars., ***arum-t.,*** astac., bell., brach., ***calc.,*** carb-an., ***con.,*** crot-c., cund., eupi., ***ham.,*** hura, hyos., iod., jatr., kali-ar., kali-bi., ***kali-c.,*** kali-i., lyc., ***merc.,*** mur-ac., nit-ac., ox-ac., phos., ***phyt., plb., puls.,*** ran-s., ruta, sabad., sang., semp., sulph., ***thuj.,*** ust., ***vesp., vip.***
across - acet-ac., asar., cob., kali-p., **LACH.,** merc.
bitten, as if - caust., chin-b., plb.
chewing, when - calc., sep.

PAIN, tongue
edges, left - lach., nat-s., ox-ac.
right - phos.
extending, to
abdomen - crot-c.
fraenum - phos.
palate - all-c.
fraenum - phos.
motion agg. - aloe, ant-t., berb., chin., kalm., spig., sulph.
stiff and red - merc-i-r.
pressing with teeth - arum-m., croc.
root - anan., bapt., ***crot-c.,*** kali-bi., **KALI-I.,** lach., nat-s., ***phyt.,*** rhus-v., lyss., sel.
night before going to sleep - **KALI-I.**
putting out the tongue - cocc., ***phyt.***
swallowing, on - ars., bapt., ***calc-p.,*** cinnb., cocc., colch., gels., ***phyt.***
yawning - lach.
sides - ***calc.***
spiting - calc.
spots on - act-sp., ***ars.,*** kali-i., ph-ac.
swallowing, on - calc., ***calc-p.***
talking, when - acet-ac., ***fl-ac., kalm.,*** lyc.
tip - **ARG-N.,** hep., ***psor.,*** sil., stront-c., tub.
night, at - hep.
touch, on - thuj.
tubercles under sore - ambr.
warm or cold agg. - osm.
warmth amel. - ***sil.***

PALE - ***ail.,*** ant-t., ***ars., chel., ferr.,*** hydr., ***ip.,*** kali-br., ***kali-c., lyss.,*** **MERC.,** nat-c., ***nat-m.,*** phos., raph., ***sep., verat.,*** xan.
and flabby - acet-ac., xan.
edges - chin-s.

PAPILLAE, erect - agar., **ARG-N.,** apis, ***ars., arum-t.,*** arum-m., **BELL.,** caust., chel., croc., cupr., ham., ***hydr.,*** ictod., kali-bi., ***lach.,*** lyc., ***merc., merc-c.,*** merc-i-f., merc-sul., mez., ***nux-m.,*** olnd., podo., ***phos.,*** plb., ptel., ***rhus-t.,*** sep., stram., stry., ***tab., tarent.,*** ter., zinc.
absent at tip - carc.
back part - agar., ***kali-bi.,*** nat-a.
enlarged - ***agar., bell.,*** cupr., ***ign., kali-bi.,*** phos., tub.
root, at - ham.
tip, at - **ARS.,** sulph.
pale, effaced - all-s.
reddened - ant-t., ars., **BELL.,** ign., mez., ***nux-m.,*** ptel.
sore - ***arg-n.***

PARALYSIS - absin., ***acon.,*** anac., ***apis, arn.,*** ars., bapt., ***bar-c.,*** bar-m., ***bell.,*** brom., bufo, ***cadm-s.,*** caps., carb-s., **CAUST.,** ***cocc., con., crot-c., cupr., dulc.,*** **GELS.,** graph., guare., ***hell., hydr-ac., hyos.,*** ip., lac-c., ***lach.,*** **LYC.,** meph., merc-c., ***mur-ac., naja, nux-m.,*** nux-v., **OP., PLB.,** ***rheum, rhus-t.,*** sec., ***stram.,*** syph., verat., vesp.
creeping - kali-p.
damp, cold weather - ***dulc.***
drawn to, left - ***bell., glon., op., plb.***
to, right - ***cur., nux-m.,*** **OP.**
elderly people - ***bar-c.,*** gels., ***plb.***

paralysis, sensation of - cedr., ***cocc.,*** ip., merl., phys.
menses, during - ***cedr.***

PASTY - am-m., bufo, nux-m.

PIMPLES - bell., berb., brom., ***calc-p.,*** lyc., manc., ***nux-v.,*** plb., tarax.
edges - apis, arg-n., hura, nat-c., **NIT-AC.,** osm., sulph.
painful - bell., arg-n., graph., **NIT-AC.,** nux-v., sulph.
bleeding - graph.
tip - ***bell.,*** caps., ***hell., kali-c., nat-c.,*** sep.

PINCHING, pain - nux-v.
tip - ang.

POINTED - calc., ***chel.,*** cimic., ***lach., petr.,*** plb., podo., spig-m.

PRESSING, pain in - astac., chin., ***ham., merc.,*** ust.
root - carb-v.
under tongue - mag-m.

PRICKLING - **ACON.,** agar., ***alum.,*** apis, ars-h., arum-m., bell., bor., brach., bry., cact., carb-ac., cedr., ***chr-ac.,*** dros., dulc., echi., elaps, eup-pur., ***fl-ac., glon.,*** hell., ***kali-bi.,*** kali-n., lach., ***lyss.,*** manc., ***merc.,*** merl., nat-m., nat-p., nux-m., phos., plat., ptel., puls., rhod., rhus-t., sang., sec., spig., thuj., ***ust.,*** verat.
edges - ped.
fraenum - phos.
menses, during - ***cedr.***
tip - ars-h., cact., crot-c., crot-t., dulc., elaps, eup-pur., nat-m., phys., sang.
like a hundred needles - arum-m., carb-ac., nux-v.
under - ***lyss.***

PROTRUDED - absin., acet-ac., acon., ***apis,*** bell., cina, cocc., **CROT-H.,** ferr-m., ***hell.,*** hydr-ac., hyos., ***lach., lyc., merc-c.,*** nux-v., oena., op., **PHYT.,** plb., sec., stram., stry., sumb., syph., tab., vip.
agg. other complaints - cist., cocc., ***kali-bi., phyt.,*** syph.
amel. other complaints - med.
brain affections, in - apis, hydr-ac.
can hardly draw it in mouth - hyos., vario.
cannot be protruded - ***apis,*** brom., carb-ac., dulc., hyos., ***lyc., merc-c., nux-v., plb.,*** sabad., vesp.
catches on the teeth - ***apis, hyos.,*** **LACH.,** lyc.
convulsions, during - lach.
cool, to keep it - sanic.
difficulty, with - anac., ***apis,*** ars., calc., ***caust.,*** colch., dulc., ***gels.,*** gua., ***hyos.,*** **LACH.,** ***lyc.,*** mag-c., merc., mur-ac., ***mygal.,*** nat-m., phos., plb., pyrog., stram., sulfon., ter.
jerking, with - kali-br.
sore throat, with - sabad.
headache, in - lach.
oscillating - ***hell.,*** lach., ***lyc.***
right side - crot-h., op.
sleep, during - vario.

PROTRUDED,
snake, like a - absin., crot-h., cupr., cupr-ac., ***lach.,*** lyc., ***merc.,*** sanic., ***vip.***
rapidly, darting in and out - absin., ***cupr., lach.,*** lyc., ***merc.,*** sanic., ***vip.***
spasmodically - cina, cocc., sec.
spasms, during - sil.
suffocation, with - ars.

PSORIASIS - ***cast-eq.,*** graph., kali-bi., ***mur-ac., sep.***

PUCKERED, sensation - ars.

PULSATING - vesp.

PURPLE - ***cact.,*** hydr., ***kali-chl., lach., op., petr.,*** raph., stry.
black - op.

PUSTULES - ant-t., cund., **HEP.,** med., mur-ac., sep., vario.
burning, and stinging - am-c.
tip - cund., med., thuj.
under - am-c., med., nat-c.

RANULA - **AMBR., CALC.,** ***canth.,*** cham., fl-ac., hippoz., lac-c., ***lach., merc., mez., nat-m., nit-ac., plb.,*** psor., sac-alb., ***staph.,*** syph., ***thuj.,*** verat.
gelatinous - mez., nit-ac., staph.
bluish-red - ***thuj.***
periodic - chr-ac., lyss.

RATTLING - hyos.

RED - acet-ac., ***acon.,*** aloe, ant-c., ant-t., **APIS,** arg-n., **ARS.,** arum-t., aur., ***aur-m., bapt.,*** **BELL.,** ***bism.,*** bry., cahin., ***calc., calc-s.,*** calen., ***camph., canth.,*** carb-ac., ***carb-v., cham., colch.,*** coloc., ***crot-c., crot-h.,*** crot-t., ***cupr.,*** cur., elaps, ***ferr-p.,*** fl-ac., ***gels.,*** glon., ***hydr., hyos.,*** ictod., ***kali-bi., kali-c.,*** lac-ac., lac-c., ***lach., lyc., mag-m.,*** **MERC.,** ***merc-c.,*** mur-ac., nat-a., nat-m., ***nat-s.,*** **NIT-AC.,** ***nux-v.,*** ox-ac., pall., **PHOS.,** ***plb.,*** podo., ***pyrog.,*** ran-s., **RHUS-T.,** rhus-v., sang., sars., spong., stann., stram., ***sulph.,*** syph., tarent., ***ter., tub., verat.,*** verb.
anterior half - lach.
base, at - bry.
centre - cham., kali-bi., ***phos., rhus-t.,*** sulph., verat-v.
edges - acon., amyg., ant-c., ant-t., **ARS.,** ***bapt.,*** bar-c., bell., bry., ***canth.,*** carb-an., cadm-s., card-m., **CHEL.,** colch., conv., cop., ***crot-h.,*** cupr., echi., ***fl-ac., gels.,*** helon., ictod., ***iris, kali-bi.,*** kali-p., lac-c., ***lach.,*** lyss., **MERC.,** merc-c., merc-cy., ***merc-i-f.,*** mur-ac., ***nit-ac.,*** nux-v., op., ox-ac., ***phos., plb.,*** podo., raph., ***rhus-t.,*** rhus-v., ruta, stram., sec., sep., **SULPH.,** sul-ac., tarax., verat-v., vip.
white centre, and - bell., rhus-t.
tip, and - apis, sulph.
dots, fine - stram.
fiery-red - **APIS,** ***bell., canth.,*** calc-s., pyrog., sang.
tip - fl-ac., ***phyt., rhus-t.***

RED,
glistening - apis, ***canth.,*** com., crot-t., glon., jal., **KALI-BI.,** ***lach., nit-ac., phos.,*** pyrog., rhus-t., ***ter.***
spots - apis, manc., ***merc.,*** raph., ter., verat.
sensitive - ran-s., ***tarax.,*** ter.
streaks, middle - ant-t., cham., ph-ac.
streaks - ant-t., arg-m.
stripe down centre - ant-t., arg-m., ***arg-n.,*** arn., ***ars.,*** bapt., ***bell.,*** **CAUST.,** ***cham.,*** colch., iris, ***kali-bi.,*** lach., merc-c., mur-ac., osm., pall., ***ph-ac., phos., plb., pyrog., rhus-t., sang., tub.,*** verat., **VERAT-V.**
tip - amyg., ***apis,*** **ARS., ARG-N.,** card-m., chel., chin-a., com., conv., crot-h., cycl., eupi., ferr., ***fl-ac.,*** helon., hipp., hyos., ictod., ip., ***lach., lyc.,*** merc-i-f., merc-i-r., mez., morph., ***nit-ac.,*** oena., ox-ac., **PHYT.,** plb., **RHUS-T., RHUS-V.,** rob., sars., sec., stram., **SULPH.,** sul-ac., sul-i., verat-v., vip.
dark spot - diph.
painful - arg-n., cycl.
triangular - arg-n., **RHUS-T.,** sep.

REDDISH-blue - ars., raph.
tip - ***hyos.***

RHEUMATIC , pain- ambr.

RINGWORM - nat-m., sanic.
right side - ***nat-m.***

ROUGHNESS - alum., alumn., anac., ang., ***arg-n.,*** arum-t., bar-c., bell., ***bry.,*** calc., carb-v., casc., cocc., coc-c., coloc., cupr., dulc., graph., ***grat.,*** hyos., ***kali-bi.,*** laur., ***nux-v.,*** olnd., par., phos., ***phyt., podo.,*** ptel., sars., sep., sil., ***sulph.,*** sul-ac., thuj., x-ray.
edges - osm.
morning - bar-c., cocc., sars., sep.
streaks, in - ***calc.***
tip - carb-v., mez., phos.

SANDY, feeling tongue - apis, cist.

SENSITIVE - ***carb-v.,*** croc., ***crot-t., fl-ac.,*** gamb., graph., kali-i., ***merc.,*** merc-c., merc-i-r., ***nat-m., nit-ac.,*** osm., ***ox-ac.,*** petr., ***phyt.,*** stront-c., **TARAX.**
even to soft food - ***nit-ac.,*** osm.
tip - ***crot-t.,*** phyt.

SCRAPING, pain - bapt., camph., caust., graph.

SHARP, pain - ***acon.,*** aloe, alum., alumn., ant-c., ***apis,*** aran., ***arum-m., arum-t.,*** asar., aspar., aster., bell., berb., brach., brom., calc., carb-v., cham., ***chin.,*** clem., colch., cycl., dros., elaps, eup-pur., gamb., ***glon.,*** guare., ip., jal., ***kali-bi., kali-c.,*** kali-chl., ***kalm.,*** **LACH.,** led., mag-m., mang., meny., merc-sul., merl., mez., murx., nit-ac., ph-ac., phos., phys., prun., ran-s., sabad., sars., sep., **SPIG.,** staph., ***sulph.***
borders - ant-c., nux-v., ph-ac.
on pressure - staph.
burning - ***chin.***
fraenum - ign.
morning - cedr.

SHARP, pain
motion, during - ***sulph.***
amel. - meny.
night - ph-ac.
right side - dros., spig.
root - arn., ars., clem., ferr-i., ***nat-s., nit-ac.***
swallowing, when - ars.
turning, head - ars.
tip - acon., agar., aloe, alumn., ang., arg-n., asaf., aur., brom., canth., chin., con., ***cori-r.,*** cycl., dios., ***dros.,*** eup-pur., form., glon., ***hell.,*** ign., led., ***merc.,*** merc-sul., nat-p., ***nat-s.,*** nux-v., ph-ac., phos., ran-b., sabad., sabin., staph., verat., zinc.
under tongue - thuj.

SHRIVELLED - ars., mur-ac., sul-ac.

SMOOTH - ***apis, arg-n., ars.,*** atro., carb-ac., ***crot-h.,*** crot-t., cupr., eucal., gamb., ***glon.,*** ip., **KALI-BI.,** kali-br., **LACH.,** mur-ac., ***nat-m., nux-v., phos., plb., pyrog.,*** rob., ***sec.,*** stram., ***sul-ac.,*** sumb., ***ter.***
edges - bapt.

SOFT - merc., rhus-t., stram.
sensation as if - daph., mez.

SORE, pain - abrot., acet-ac., ***agar.,*** aloe, alum., ant-c., ***apis,*** arn., ars., ars-i., ***arum-t., bapt.,*** bar-c., bell., benz-ac., berb., brach., ***calc.,*** canth., ***carb-v.,*** caust., chel., chim., chin-a., cic., ***cist.,*** cop., ***crot-h.,*** cupr-ar., ***dig.,*** fl-ac., gamb., gels., ***glon.,*** graph., ictod., ip., kali-c., kali-p., kali-s., ***lach.,*** laur., ***lyc.,*** merc., ***merc-c., mur-ac.,*** nat-m., **NIT-AC.,** nux-v., osm., ox-ac., rhus-t., rumx., ***sabad.,*** sang., ***sep.,*** sil., sin-n., staph., ***thuj., tub.,*** zinc.
back part - benz-ac., form., lyc., ***nux-v.***
center - chin., samb.
evening - kali-n.
fraenum - all-c., kali-c.
lacerated wounds, from - hyper.
root, at, when yawning - lach.
salt, food from - petr.
sides - ant-c., calc., carb-v., dios., ictod., ***lach.,*** laur., ***puls.,*** rumx., sep.
left - graph., ***kalm., lach.,*** phys.
near tip - arum-t., ***calc-p.,*** chin., dios., ***hep., kali-c.,*** sep.
on putting out tongue - ***graph.***
right - carb-v., merc., phos., plat., sabad.
sour, food from - petr.
spots - ***agar.,*** aloe, ant-c., ap-g., bar-c., cinnb., ind., iod., nit-ac., nux-v., op., ran-s., ***sil., tarax.***
swallowing agg. - benz-ac.
tip - aesc., agar., am-c., arum-t., calc., calc-p., carb-an., dios., hep., ictod., kali-c., kali-n., merc-sul., phys., **RHUS-T.,** sabad., sang., ***sep., sil.,*** sin-n., ***ter.,*** **THUJ.,** zinc.
touch, on - nat-c.

SPASMS - acon., ***arg-n.,*** bell., bor., carb-v., ***cocc., con.,*** glon., ***lyc.,*** ruta, sec., syph.

SPLINTER, pain like a - staph.

SPONGY - benz-ac.

STICKY, viscid - ***am-m.,*** ars., bell., berb., ***bry., carb-v., con., lac-ac., merc-i-r.,*** nat-m., **NUX-M.,** ***ph-ac.,*** puls., sin-n., ***verat.***
back of - laur.

STIFF - aloe, am-c., anac., apis, ***ars.,*** ars-s-f., arum-t., aur-m., ***berb.,*** **BELL.,** bor., ***calc-p., carb-v.,*** coc-c., ***colch., con., crot-c., crot-h.,*** dulc., euphr., fl-ac., ***hell.,*** hyos., hydr-ac., kali-p., lac-c., ***lach., laur., lyc.,*** med., ***merc-c.,*** merc-i-r., merl., mur-ac., ***nat-c., nat-m.,*** nicc., nit-ac., nux-m., phys., **RHUS-T.,** sec., sep., ***stram.,*** vario.
morning, on waking - nit-ac.

SUPPURATION - canth., carb-ac., lach., ***merc.,*** merc-c.

SWELLING - acet-ac., **ACON.,** ***am-m.,*** anac., anan., ant-t., **APIS,** arg-n., ***ars., ars-i., ars-s-f.,*** arum-m., arum-t., asaf., aster., ***aur., bapt.,*** **BELL.,** berb., bism., bor., caj., calad., calc., ***calc-p., camph., canth.,*** cast., caust., ***chin., chin-a.,*** cic., ***cimic.,*** coc-c., con., **CROT-H.,** ***dig.,*** diph., dros., ***dulc.,*** elaps, ferr-m., ferr-p., ***fl-ac.,*** glon., guare., ***hell., helo.,*** hippoz., ***hydr., iod.,*** kali-ar., kali-c., kali-chl., kali-i., kali-p., ***lach., lyc., lyss.,*** mag-p., **MERC.,** ***merc-c., merc-cy.,*** merc-sul., mez., mill., ***mur-ac., naja, nat-h., nat-m.,*** oena., ***op.,*** ox-ac., ph-ac., ***phos.,*** phyt., ***plb., podo.,*** polyg., ptel., puls., ruta, sec., sil., stram., tell., ter., thuj., vesp., verat., ***vip.,*** zinc.
base, externally and internally - **ARS.**
center - ***phos.***
small, round swelling - ***dros.***
fills whole mouth - arum-m., calad., crot-h., ***kali-chl.***
mercury, after - ***kali-i.***
one-sided - apis, calc., bism., merc., ***sil.***
left - lach., laur., zinc.
right - am-be., apis, mez., thuj.
painful when, talking - ***ph-ac.***
touched - con., ph-ac., thuj.
painless - mez.
root of - bapt., caust., cimic., cocc., ferr-i., merc-c., phos.
sensation of - anac., ***bapt., camph., cimx.,*** cocc., crot-h., gels., glon., kali-ar., merl., ***mur-ac., nux-v.,*** par., petr., puls.
alternating with contraction - xan.
root at - spig.
side, of - chin.
sting of insects, after - ***acon.,*** **APIS.,** arn., bell., ***carb-ac.,*** crot-h., merc., nat-m.
tip - phos., ***nat-m.***
under - ***nat-m.***
with stinging pain - ***nat-m.***

TASTE, general
acrid - all-c., alum., anthro., apoc., asaf., berb., brom., cact., calc-s., caps., crot-t., fl-ac., hydr-ac., kali-chl., lac-ac., laur., ***lob.,*** mur-ac., nat-c., osm., plan., plb., rhus-t., seneg., verat.
teeth, from roots of - fl-ac.
tobacco, tastes - stann.
saliva, tastes - agar.
acute, sensitive - ***bell.,*** calc., ***camph.,*** **CHIN., COFF.,** glon., kali-bi., ***lyc.,*** lyss., nat-c.

TASTE, general
alkaline - am-c., calc-ar., kali-chl., ***kalm.,*** mez., zinc-m.
almonds, like sweet - coff., crot-t., dig.
after smoking - dig.
bitter - laur.
aromatic - glon.
astringent - acon., agar., ***alum., alumn.,*** am-m., arg-n., ars., aur., bar-c., brom., calc-i., caps., card-m., chin., chion., clem., coc-c., coloc., dulc., gall-ac., graph., iod., kali-bi., kali-c., kali-cy., kali-i., lach., merc., merc-c., merc-d., mur-ac., ox-ac., ***phos.,*** plb., sang.
bad - acon., agar., ***all-c.,*** all-s., alumn., ***ang.,*** anthr., anthro., ant-t., ***ars.,*** ars-i., asaf., atro., aur-m., bad., ***bapt.,*** bar-c., bar-m., bov., brom., ***bry.,*** **CALC.,** ***calc-p., calc-s.,*** camph., caust., ***cann-s.,*** carb-s., cedr., chel., chin., chin-a., cimic., cinnb., cob., ***coc-c.,*** con., ***crot-t.,*** echi., ferr-i., fl-ac., ***gels., graph.,*** ham., ***hydr.,*** hyper., ign., iod., iris, ***kali-ar., kali-bi., kali-c.,*** kali-chl., kali-n., kali-p., kreos., lac-ac., led., lyc., med., **MERC.,** ***merc-i-f., merc-i-r.,*** mez., myric., naja, nat-m., nat-p., **NAT-S.,** nux-m., **NUX-V.,** op., petr., phos., ***phyt.,*** pic-ac., podo., psor., **PULS.,** raph., sabad., sang., ***sars.,*** sel., seneg., sep., sil., sin-n., squil., stann., stry., **SULPH.,** ***sul-ac.,*** tab., tarent., thuj., vib., zinc.
bread, tastes - phos.
coughing, on - caps.
eating amel. - sil.
eating, after - agar., ars., cann-i., cann-s., con., ign., ***lyc.,*** rhus-t., sil.
apples, after - bell.
too much - sulph.
evening - bad.
meat, after - puls., zinc.
menses, during - kali-c.
milk, after - aran.
morning - am-c., arum-d., ***bar-c.,*** bry., ***calc., calc-p., camph.,*** cann-i., carb-an., echi., fago., ferr-i., graph., hydr., jac., lyc., mag-m., med., ***merc., nat-m.,*** **NAT-S., NUX-V.,** phos., **PULS.,** rhus-t., sang., ***sep.,*** sulph., tab., zing.
on waking - ***calc-p.,*** guai., ***merc., merc-i-f.,*** merc-i-r., nat-c., nat-p., nicc., sang., sul-ac., **VALER.**
night - gall-ac.
teeth, from hollow - mez.
base of - agar., nat-c.
water, tastes - ***acon., aran.,*** ars., arund., chin., chin-a., colch., coloc., ***ferr.,*** kali-bi., ***nat-m.,*** puls., ***sil.,*** sumb.
biting - nat-c.
bitter - **ACON.,** aesc., aeth., agar., agn., ail., aloe, ***alum.,*** alumn., ***am-c., am-m.,*** amyg., anac., anan., ***ang., ant-c.,*** ant-t., ***apis,*** apoc., aran., ***arg-n., arn.,*** **ARS.,** ars-h., ars-i., ars-s-f., asaf., asar., ***aur.,*** aur-m-n., bapt., ***bar-c.,*** bar-m., ***bell.,*** benz-ac., berb., ***bol., bor., bov.,*** brom., **BRY.,** bufo, cahin., ***calc.,*** calc-s., camph., ***canth., carb-an.,*** **CARB-V.,**

TASTE, general

bitter - **CARB-S.,** ***card-m.,*** casc., cast., ***caust., cham.,*** **CHEL., CHIN.,** ***chin-a.,*** chin-s., cinnb., ***cocc., coc-c., colch.,*** coll., **COLOC.,** ***con., corn.,*** croc., crot-t., ***crot-h.,*** cupr., cupr-ar., cupr-s., cycl., ***dig.,*** dios., dros., ***dulc., elaps,*** elat., ***euph., eup-per.,*** eup-pur., ferr., ferr-ar., ferr-i., gamb., gels., glon., ***graph., grat., hell., hep.,*** hipp., hydr., ***ign.,*** iod., ip., iris, ***jab., kali-ar.,*** kali-bi., ***kali-c.,*** kali-i., kali-p., kalm., kreos., ***lach.,*** lact., led., ***lept.,*** lob., ***lyc., mag-c., mag-m., mag-p., mag-s., manc.,*** mang., **MERC.,** ***merc-c., merc-i-r.,*** merl., ***mez.,*** mosch., ***mur-ac., myric.,*** naja, nat-a., ***nat-c.,*** **NAT-M.,** nat-p., **NAT-S.,** nicc., ***nit-ac., nux-m.,*** **NUX-V.,** onos., op., ***par., petr., phos.,*** phyt., pic-ac., ***plb., podo.,*** polyg., ***prun., psor., ptel.,*** **PULS.,** ran-b., ***raph., rheum, rhus-t.,*** sabad., ***sabin., sal-ac., sars., sep., sil., spong.,*** stann., staph., ***stram.,*** stry., **SULPH.,** tab., ***tarax.,*** thuj., ust., valer., ***verat.,*** viol-o., zinc.

- afternoon - nat-c., nit-ac.
- apples, tastes - bell.
  - after eating - alum.
- apyrexia, during - ***arn.,*** bol.
- beer, tastes - alum., ars., chin., stann.
  - after - coloc., euph., mez., ***puls.***
- bread tastes - anac., asar., bell., ***calc-p.,*** camph., ***chin., chin-s.,*** cina, dig., dros., ferr., merc., merl., nux-v., ph-ac., phos., ***rhus-t.,*** puls., squil., sulph., sul-ac., thuj.
- breakfast - phos.
  - after - petr.
  - amel. - ***kali-i.,*** kali-m.
- butter - chin., puls.
- chewing, when - dros., ***puls.***
- chill, during - ars., ***spong.***
  - after - ***hep.***
  - before - cina, ***hep.***
- coffee, tastes - chin., merc., puls., sabin., spong.
  - after - ***cham.,*** puls.
- drinking, after - acon., ***ars., bry., chin., gins.,*** ign., **KREOS.,** mang., ***puls.***
  - amel. - **BRY.,** ***psor.***
- eating, during - acon., ang., ars., asar., bor., ***bry., camph.,*** cham., ***chin.,*** chin-a., coloc., dig., dros., ferr., hell., hep., ***ign.,*** kreos., lyc., merc., ***nat-m.,*** nit-ac., nux-v., ph-ac., phos., **PULS.,** ran-b., rheum, ***rhus-t., sabin.,*** sars., sep., stann., staph., ***stram.,*** sulph., teucr., valer.
  - after - am-c., ang., **ARS.,** berb., ***bry., carb-v.,*** dros., hell., hep., kreos., lyc., mang., merc., ***nat-m.,*** nit-ac., ***phos.,*** **PULS.,** ran-b., stann., staph., ***sulph.,*** teucr., valer.
  - amel. - nat-c., sep., sulph.
  - before - ***carb-v., tarax.***
- evening - alum., ***am-c.,*** arn., bell., bry., kreos., lyc., petr., phos., **PULS.,** rhus-t., stann.
- everything, even saliva - bor., kreos.
  - except water - **ACON., STANN.**

TASTE, general

bitter,

- food, tastes - camph., **CHIN.,** con., graph., hep., ign., lach., lyc., ***nat-c., nat-m.,*** puls., rheum., rhus-t., sabin., sars., sep., ***sil.,*** squil., stann., staph., stram., sulph.
  - intermittents, in - ***ant-c., ars., ferr., nat-m.***
  - morning - mang.
  - swallowing, after - ars., **PULS.,** ***sil.,*** sulph.
  - swallowing, only, when - chin., kreos., rheum
- forenoon - nit-ac.
- hawking, mucus, amel. - sulph.
- hawking, when - sep.
- humiliation, after - puls.
- meat tastes - camph., puls.
- menses, at beginning of - ***calc-p., caul.***
- milk tastes - sabin.
- morning - alum., am-c., ***am-m.,*** arn., ars., ***bar-c., bry.,*** calc., ***calc-p., carb-an.,*** carb-s., ***carb-v.,*** cast., **CHAM.,** chin., cinnb., dios., dros., euphr., ***hep.,*** hyos., ip., kali-bi., kali-c., kali-i., kali-p., kreos., lach., ***lyc.,*** lyss., ***mag-c.,*** mag-m., mag-s., mang., merc., mur-ac., nat-a., nat-c., nat-m., nicc., ***nux-v.,*** petr., ph-ac., ***phos.,*** **PULS.,** rhus-t., rumx., ***sars.,*** sec., ***sep., sil.,*** stront-c., ***sulph.,*** tab., thuj., zinc.
  - better after rising - carb-an.
  - waking, on - ambr., am-c., ars-s-r., arund., dios., ***helon., kali-i.,*** lyss., mang., merc-i-r., nat-c., ***sulph.,*** zinc.
- night - ***ant-t.,*** lach., **LYC.,** rhus-t.
- noon - bell.
- periodic, every second day - ars.
- plums taste - iod.
- sleep, after - manc.
- smoking, while - asar., casc., chin., **COCC., PULS.**
  - after - anac., ang., cocc., euphr., **PULS.**
  - amel. - aran.
- soup - iod.
- sour things, taste - chin., rhus-t.
- sugar tastes - sang.
- supper, after - zinc.
- sweet things taste - aesc., chin., dulc., rheum, sang., sulph.
- throat and in mouth - con., nat-c., sep., sulph.
  - not in mouth - ars., calc., dros., phos., sep., sil., spong.
- tobacco, tastes - anac., ***camph.,*** **CHIN.,** ***cocc., euphr.,*** mag-arct., nat-m., ***spong.***
- tobacco, from - ***asar.,*** euphr., puls.
- vexation, after - petr.
- water tastes - ars., calc-p., chin-a., sil.
- wine tastes - puls., iod.

bitter-putrid - carb-an., euph.

bitter-saltish, bread - chin.

bitter-sour - aloe, bism., carb-an., caust., con., kali-c., kali-chl., lyc., petr., ran-b., rhus-t., sabad., sep., stann., sulph.

- milk - bell.

TASTE, general

bitter-sweet - arg-n., aspar., chim., crot-t., kali-i., mag-c., mag-s., meny.

bloody - acon., alum., ***am-c.,*** anan., asc-t., ***ars., bell.,*** berb., benz-ac., bism., bov., bufo, canth., carb-v., chel., dol., elaps, ***ferr.,*** ham., hyper., ***ip.,*** jatr., kali-c., kalm., ***lil-t.,*** manc., ***nat-c.,*** nit-ac., osm., phos., puls., rhus-t., sabin., sil., sulph., thuj., zinc.

coughing, when - **BELL.,** dol., elaps, ham., ***kali-bi.,*** nit-ac., **RHUS-T.**

before - elaps.

evening - zinc.

expiration - nat-c.

morning - bism., ***sil.***

pregnancy, during - ***zinc.***

sex, during - hura.

sleep, after, agg. - ***manc.***

bread, tastes like dough - phos.

burning - all-c., kali-chl., mez., osm.

meal, after every - mez.

burnt, empyreumatic - berb., bry., calad., chin-s., cycl., kali-chl., ***nux-v.,*** ph-ac., **PULS.,** ran-b., sars., sal-ac., squil., ***sulph.***

dry food, after - ran-b.

meals. during - squil.

morning - berb.

carrot tops, like - nux-v.

catarrh, like old - sep.

chalky - ign., ***nux-m.***

changeable - coff., mag-aust., ***puls.***

cheesy - aeth., chin., ***lyc.,*** phel., phos., zinc.

clammy - berb., chin-s., crot-t., gels., grat., ***nat-m.,*** nux-m., ***phos.,*** plan., prun., **PULS.,** zinc.

during sweat - gels.

morning - nicc.

clay-like - agar., aloe, caps., ***chin.,*** euphr., ***hep.,*** ign., phos., **PULS.,** stann.

food tastes like - chin., sil.

coppery, gold plate tastes - canth.

coryza, like old - upa.

diminished - cic.

disordered stomach, as from - asaf., asar., caust., ***ign.,*** nux-v., olnd., puls., rhus-t.

dry, bread tastes - ferr., ph-ac., rhus-v., thuj.

food - ars., ferr., ruta., stront.

tobacco - stann.

earthy - aloe, cann-s., chin., ***ferr.,*** hep., ***ip., nux-m.,*** phos., puls., stront-c., tell.

eggs, like rotten - acon., ant-t., **ARN.,** ***ferr.,*** goss., hep., kali-bi., **MERC., MUR-AC.,** ***sil.,*** thuj.

cough, with - ***sep.***

morning - acon., am-c., ant-t., **ARN.,** goss., **GRAPH.,** ***hep.,*** ph-ac., ***phos.,*** sil., thuj.

fatty, greasy - aesc., agar., alum., ***asaf.,*** cahin., ***caust., cham.,*** cycl., euph., glon., ip., iris, ***kali-i., lyc.,*** mang., ***mur-ac.,*** ol-an., petr., phos., ***psor., puls.,*** rhus-t., sabin., sang., ***sil.,*** sulph., thuj., valer., verat.

fishy - acon., astac., graph., lach.

TASTE, general

flour, like, in morning - nicc., lach.

especially bread - zing.

food, of - agar., am-c., **ANAC.,** benz-ac., tell.

eaten, a long time before - caust., nat-m., nit-ac., phos., ph-ac., sil., sulph.

several hours before - am-br.

game, like spoiled - aur.

garlic, like - asaf., calc-ar., merl.

herby - calad., nat-m., nux-v., ph-ac., puls., ***sars.,*** stann., verat.

beer tastes - nux-v.

herring, pickle, like - anac.

honey, everything tastes like - apoc-a.

ink, like - aloe, arg-n., ***calc.,*** fl-ac.

insipid - acon., agar., ail., ***alum.,*** ambr., ammc., **ANAC.,** ang., anan., ant-c., ***ant-t.,*** ars., arund., asaf., asar., aspar., ***aur.,*** aur-m., ***bapt.,*** bell., benz-ac., berb., bol., bor., ***bry.,*** bufo, cahin., calad., calc., calc-ar., calc-p., ***caps.,*** carb-v., caust., chel., ***chin.,*** chin-a., cob., ***cocc., colch.,*** con., corn., cor-r., crot-t., cycl., dig., dios., dulc., elaps, eup-per., euph., euphr., ***ferr.,*** ferr-ar., ferr-i., ferr-m., ferr-p., gnaph., ***guai.,*** ham., hydr., hyper., ign., ***ip.,*** iris, jac-c., kali-ar., kali-bi., ***kali-c.,*** kali-p., kali-s., kalm., kreos., laur., lyc., lyss., mag-m., mang., **MERC.,** merc-sul., mez., mur-ac., naja, ***nat-c., nat-m.,*** nit-ac., nux-m., olnd., ol-an., op., par., ***petr.,*** ph-ac., ***phos., psor.,*** **PULS.,** ran-b., rat., ***rheum,*** rhus-t., ruta., sabin., ***sanic.,*** sars., sel., seneg., sep., spig., ***stann., staph., sulph.,*** sul-ac., tab., ***thuj.,*** verb., valer., verat., vinc., zinc.

beer, after - chin., nat-c.

tastes - anac., ars., ip., nat-m., nux-v., stann.

butter tastes - caps.

drinking after - chin., coloc., mang.

eating, after - mang., petr., thuj., verb.

amel. - nat-c., phos.

evening - ***alum.,*** nat-m., olnd., thuj.

food tastes - alum., am-c., anac., arund., calc., chin., colch., cupr., ***cycl.,*** ferr., ferr-m., jac-c., olnd., ruta., stram., vinc.

menses, during - mag-c.

morning - alum., nat-c., nat-m., phos., puls., rat., ***sanic.,*** **SULPH.,** sul-ac., valer., verb.

breakfast, after - euph.

rising amel. - nat-c., sul-ac.

night - nat-c.

soup tastes, although it is salted as usual - card-m., ***cocc.,*** lyss., ***thuj.***

water, after drinking - ail., benz-ac., vario.

liver, like fried, of - podo.

loss, of - aeth., all-c., alum., am-m., ***anac., ant-c., ant-t., apis,*** ars., ***aur.,*** aur-m., bar-c., **BELL.,** ***bor., bry.,*** cact., ***calc.,*** calc-ar., cann-s., ***canth.,*** chin., cocc., coff., ***crot-h.,*** cupr., ***cycl.,*** dros., ***hep., hyos.,*** ip., ***kali-bi.,*** kali-br., kali-s., kreos., lyc., mag-c., ***mag-m.,*** merl., ***merc.,*** **NAT-M.,** nat-s., ***nux-m., nux-v.,*** op., ox-ac., ***par.,*** **PHOS.,** ph-ac., plan., podo., ***psor.,*** ptel., **PULS.,** rheum, rhod., sabad.,

TASTE, general
loss of - sang., sec., ***sep.,*** **SIL.,** stram., ***sulph., sul-ac.,*** syph., ***ther.,*** thuj., ***verat., zinc.***
morning - coca, kali-c., ***nat-s.***
manure, like - ***calc.,*** carb-an., ***merc., plb., sep.,*** verat.
mealy - nicc.
metallic - ***aesc.,*** aeth., agar., ***agn.,*** aloe, alum., ***am-c., arg-n., ars.,*** aspar., aur., aur-m., bism., bol., bufo, cadm-s., ***calc.,*** calc-s., cann-i., ***canth.,*** carb-ac., carb-s., card-m., cedr., chel., chin-a., chr-ac., cimic., cimx., ***cinnb.,*** **COCC.,** ***coc-c.,*** coch., ***coloc.,*** conv., ***cupr., cupr-ar., cupr-s.,*** echi., ferr-i., ham., hep., hyos., indg., iodof., jatr., kali-bi., kali-chl., kali-i., kali-n., lac-ac., ***lach., lyc.,*** manc., med., meph., **MERC.,** ***merc-c.,*** merc-i-r., merc-p-r., merc-sul., naja, ***nat-a.,*** **NAT-C.,** nat-h., nat-m., nat-p., ***nux-v.,*** phos., ***phyt., plb.,*** psor., puls., ran-b., **RHUS-T.,** sars., **SENEG.,** ***sep.,*** sil., ***sulph.,*** tell., ***tub., zinc.***
afternoon - nat-c.
cough agg. - cocc.
dinner, before - chr-ac.
food tastes - **AM-C.**
morning - alum., calc., sulph.
pregnancy, during - zinc.
stool, before - kali-bi.
tobacco tastes - kali-c.
milky - ***aur.***
like burnt - tab.
moldly - rhus-t.
musty - kali-bi., ***led., lyc.***
after hawking up mucus - ***teucr.***
throat, in - bor., teucr.
tobacco - thuj.
nauseous - acon., agar., ***all-c.,*** anthro., aran., bapt., bism., bol., bov., bry., canth., ***carb-an.,*** carb-s., cocc., coc-c., crot-t., gnaph., hyos., ***ip.,*** kali-n., lach., lyc., merl., ***myric.,*** **PULS.,** rheum, sabad., sec., sel., seneg., ***sulph.,*** thuj., verb., zinc.
eating, after agg. - psor.
food and meat taste - chin-s., olnd., squil.
flat, in evening - olnd.
morning - ***bry.,*** **PULS.**
smoking, from - **PULS.**
smoking, on - ip.
stool, during - ***crot-t.***
offensive - agar., am-c., **ANAC.,** asar., bar-c., bell., canth., cham., cocc., coc-c., ***coloc.,*** cycl., ferr-i., form., hydr-ac., puls., ***sep.,*** spig., **STANN.,** ***valer.***
breakfast, after - agar.
food and drink - ***coloc.***
milk, after - aran.
tobacco - camph.
onions, like - aeth., crot-c., meph.
pappy - am-m., arg-n., astac., atro., bell., bruc., calc., carb-s., chel., cocc., dios., eup-pur., graph., hep., kali-s., laur., mag-c., mag-m., ***nat-m.,*** nux-m., petr., ***puls.,*** raph., ***sanic.,*** sul-ac., ***sulph.***

TASTE, general
pasty - bry., ***cycl.,*** kali-bi., lec., merc., nux-m., ***raph., sulph.,*** verat.
tobacco tastes - staph.
peas, like raw - zinc.
peppermint, like - ferr-i., ***verat.***
peppery - acon., chin., euph., hydr., lach., lyss., manc., mez., ol-an., plat., sulph., tarax., xan.
perverted, in general - aesc., ***alum.,*** ant-t., ***arg-n.,*** arn., ars., calc., camph., carb-v., chel., ***chin.,*** cycl., fago., guai., ***gymn., hydr.,*** kali-c., lyc., mag-c., mag-m., merc., merc-c., merc-sul., ***nat-m.,*** nit-ac., ***nux-v.,*** par., podo., ***puls.,*** rheum, ***sep., sulph.,*** zinc-m.
eating, after - ars., carb-v., ***nat-m.,*** nit-ac., zinc.
morning - fago., graph., hydr., ***nux-v.,*** puls.
sleep, after - rheum
pinewood - glon.
pitch, like - ***cadm-s.,*** canth.
pungent - chim., corn., cupr-ac., hydr., puls., verat.
purulent - dros., ***puls.***
throat, in - merc., ***nat-c.***
putrid - ***acon.,*** agar., am-c., ang., **ANAC.,** ant-t., ***arn., ars., ars-i.,*** asc-t., ***aur.,*** bapt., bar-m., bell., bov., ***bry., calc.,*** calc-p., **CAPS.,** carb-s., **CARB-V.,** ***caust., cham., cinnb., cocc.,*** con., ***crot-c.,*** cupr., cycl., ***dros.,*** euph., ***ferr., ferr-ar.,*** ferr-i., ferr-p., gels., glon., graph., ***hep.,*** hydr-ac., ***hyos., ign., iod.,*** iris, kali-ar., ***kali-i., kali-c.,*** kali-p., kali-s., lac-ac., ***lac-c.,*** laur., lil-t., ***merc.,*** merc-c., mosch., ***mur-ac., nat-m.,*** **NUX-V.,** ***petr., ph-ac., phos.,*** plan., ***podo.,*** **PSOR., PULS.,** ***pyrog.,*** rhod., ***rhus-t., sep.,*** sil., spig., stict., ***sulph., sul-ac.,*** valer., ***verat.,*** zinc.
afternoon - ferr.
beer, after drinking - euph., sep.
beer, tastes - ***ign.***
eating, while - bell., con.
after - bell., rhus-t.
epileptic fit, after - caust.
before - syph.
food tastes - anac., bar-m., ign., mosch., podo., rhus-t.
hawking, when - **NUX-V.**
intermittent fever, in - **ARN.,** ***ars., puls.***
meat tastes - **PULS.**
as from spoiled - ars., petr.
menses, during - ***kali-c.***
morning - **ARS.,** ***chin.,*** iod., mag-m., ***merc-c.,*** nat-m., nux-v., ***rhus-t.,*** sil., ***sulph.***
rising - lem-m.
night - ***cham.***
pharynx, low down in when hawking up mucus - nux-v.
sex, after - ***dig.***
sleep, after - rheum.
swallowing - con.
throat, taste in - coloc.
water tastes - aur., bell., nat-m.

TASTE, general
rancid - agar., alum., ambr., asaf., bry., carb-v., caust., ***cham.,*** euph., ip., kali-bi., ***kali-i.,*** lach., ***mur-ac.,*** petr., ***puls.,*** tell., thuj., tub., ***valer.***
after food or drink - ***kali-i.***
swallowing, when - ip.
throat, in - phos., sulph.
resinous - coc-c.
rough, bread tastes - rhus-t.
salt, enough, food does not taste - ars., ***calc.,*** canth., card-m., cocc., lyss., ***thuj.***
food, only tastes natural - **LAC-C.**
salty - agar., alum., am-c., ant-c., ant-t., ***ars., ars-i.,*** bar-c., bell., benz-ac., brom., bry., bufo, cadm-s., ***calc., carb-s., carb-v., carl.,*** chin., chin-a., coff., con., croc., crot-c., cupr., ***cycl.,*** elaps, ***euph.,*** fl-ac., ***graph.,*** hydr., ***hyos.,*** iod., kali-bi., kali-br., ***kali-chl.,*** lach., lyc., mag-m., mang., **MERC., MERC-C.,** merl., nat-a., nat-c., **NAT-M.,** nat-p., nit-ac., ***nux-m., nux-v.,*** op., ***ph-ac., phos.,*** prot., ***puls., rheum,*** rhod., rhus-t., rhus-v., ***sep.,*** spig., ***sulph., tarax.,*** ther., tub., verat., ***zinc.,*** zinc-m.
eating, amel. - sulph.
evening, p.m. - bar-c., kali-bi.
food tastes - ***ars.,*** bell., benz-ac., cadm-s., ***calc., carb-v.,*** **CHIN.,** cocc., **CYCL.,** merc., puls., ***sep., sulph.,*** tarent., thuj.
morning, a.m. - brom., cupr., fl-ac., ***puls.***
noon, after - bar-c., kali-bi.
before - brom., cupr., fl-ac., ***puls.***
tip of - cupr.
water tastes - brom., merc., nit-ac.
salty-sour - alum., bell., cupr., lach., sulph.
butter tastes - tarax.
salty-sweet - croc., mez., phos.
saw-dust, food tastes like - cor-r., nux-m.
scratchy - ars., nat-c., staph.
slimy - abrot., acon., ***arn.,*** ars-h., bell., carb-an., ***cham., chel.,*** chim., ***chin.,*** dig., hell., hep., kali-c., laur., lyc., **MERC.,** ***merc-c.,*** merc-i-r., nat-c., ***nat-s., nux-m., nux-v.,*** pall., par., ***petr.,*** phel., ***phos.,*** plat., prun., **PULS.,** ***rheum,*** rhus-t., sabin., sang., sars., seneg., ***sep.,*** sil., tab., ust., **VALER.,** zing.
beer tastes - asaf.
eating, after - thuj.
drinking, after - chin.
morning - hep., lyc., merc-i-r., seneg., **VALER.,** zing.
on waking - merc-i-r., **VALER.,** zinc.
smoky - ph-ac.
bread tastes - benz-ac., nux-v.
soapy - arg-n., cact., calc-s., chlor., dulc., iod., merc., ***rhus-t.,*** sil.
drinking, after - benz-ac.
sooty - ars.

TASTE, general
sour - abrot., acet-ac., aloe, ***alum., alumn.,*** am-c., am-m., ***ant-c.,*** **ARG-N.,** ***ars., ars-i.,*** asar., aur., ***bar-c.,*** bar-m., bell., berb., bism., brom., bufo, **CALC.,** calc-ar., ***calc-s.,*** canth., ***caps., carb-s., carb-an., caust., cham., chin., chin-a., chel.,*** clem., ***cocc.,*** con., ***croc., crot-h.,*** crot-t., cupr., daph., ferr., ferr-i., fl-ac., ***graph.,*** hell., ***hep.,*** **IGN.,** iod., jac-c., kali-ar., kali-bi., kali-c., ***kali-chl.,*** kali-n., kali-p., kali-s., ***kalm.,*** kreos., lac-ac., ***lach.,*** lec., **LYC., MAG-C.,** ***mag-m., mang., merc.,*** merl., mez., ***mur-ac.,*** naja, **NAT-A., NAT-C.,** ***nat-m., nat-p., nit-ac., nux-m.,*** **NUX-V.,** ol-an., op., ***ox-ac.,*** pall., ***petr., ph-ac.,*** **PHOS.,** pic-ac., podo., ***puls.,*** rheum, rhod., rhus-t., ***sars., sep., sil., stann., sulph.,*** sul-ac., tab., ***tarax.,*** thuj., verat.
afternoon - mag-m.
beer, tastes - merc., puls., stann.
bread, tastes - ang., ***bell.,*** cham., chin., cocc., merl., nit-ac., nux-v., puls., staph.
broth, tastes - caps.
butter, tastes - puls., tarax.
coffee, tastes - chin., vac.
coughing, when - cocc.
drinking, after - berb., chin., graph., lyc., **NUX-V.,** phos., sulph.
eating, after - am-m., berb., bry., ***carb-v.,*** chlor., cocc., con., graph., lyc., mag-m., ***nat-m.,*** nit-ac., ***nux-v., phos.,*** puls., sabin., sec., ***sep., sil.***
amel. - phos.
before - bar-c., ***nat-m.***
evening - bar-c., nit-ac., sulph.
food, tastes - **AM-C.,** ars., ***calc., caps.,*** chin., iris, jac-c., lappa-a., lyc., nux-v., podo., puls., squil., tab., tarent.
meat tastes - caps., lappa-a., puls., tarax.
milk, after - am-c., ambr., carb-v., calad., lyc., ***phos.,*** rhus-t., ***sulph.***
milk, tastes - calad., calc., nux-v.
morning - am-m., bar-c., berb., carb-an., ferr., kali-n., ***lyc.,*** mang., merc., nat-c., nat-m., nit-ac., **NUX-V.,** ol-an., phos., ptel., ***puls.,*** sars., ***sep., sulph.,*** valer., zinc.
after breakfast - con., sars.
after breakfast amel. - mang.
night - kali-c., mag-m.
pregnancy, during - ***lac-ac., mag-c.,*** ox-ac.
sweet things taste - aesc., chin., dulc., sulph.
eating, after - ***lach.***
throat, in - alum.
tobacco - staph.
sour-bitter - **ASAR.,** ***kali-chl.,*** mang., samb., ***sep.***
spoiled, food - stram.
game - ***aur.***
meat - bell.
stale - bry., chin-s., petr., puls., staph., thuj.
sticky, after taste - ars-h., **PULS.,** ***psor.***

TASTE, general

straw, like - chin., cor-r., kali-i., kreos., rhod., rhus-t., ***stram., sulph.***

dishes made of flour - cor-r.

tobacco tastes - mez.

sulphur, like - ***cocc., ham.,*** nux-v.

sweet - ***acon.,*** aesc., aeth., agar., ***all-c., alum., alumn.,*** am-c., anan., arg-m., ***ars.,*** ars-i., arund., asar., aspar., astac., aur., bar-c., bar-m., ***bell.,*** bism., bol., brom., ***bry.,*** calc., calc-p., calc-s., carb-s., chel., ***chin.,*** chin-a., chlf., cob., ***coc-c., coff.,*** colch., croc., **CUPR.,** cupr-s., dig., dios., **DULC.,** ferr., ferr-ar., ferr-i., ferr-p., fl-ac., gamb., glon., gnaph., hydr-ac., iod., ip., iris, kali-ar., kali-bi., ***kali-c., kali-i.,*** kali-s., lach., laur., ***lyc.,*** mag-c., **MERC.,** mez., ***mur-ac.,*** nat-a., nat-c., nit-ac., nuph., nux-v., op., osm., phel., ***phos., plat., plb., podo.,*** **PULS.,** ***pyrog.,*** ran-b., rhus-t., ***sabad., sars., squil.,*** seneg., sep., ***spong., stann.,*** **SULPH.,** sul-ac., sumb., ***thuj.,*** verat-v., ***zinc.***

beer, tastes - cor-r., ***mur-ac., puls.***

after - nat-c.

bread, tastes - **MERC.,** squil.

broth, tastes - indg.

butter, tastes - ***puls.,*** ran-b., sang., squil.

coughing, after - aeth., astac., chin-a.

drinking, after - lyc., phel., vario.

eating, after, bitter - phos., thuj.

evening, and after meals - thuj.

food, tastes - mur-ac., puls., squil., thuj.

meat, tastes - ***puls.,*** squil.

milk, tastes - ***puls.***

morning - aeth., alum., ***ars.,*** bufo, lyc., nit-ac., ran-s., sulph.

after breakfast - agar., sulph.

on waking - aeth., cupr-s., kali-c., sulph.

mouth, posteriorly - lil-t., thuj.

night - fl-ac.

smoking, when - agar., chin., sars.

after - sel.

soup, tastes - squil.

sweets, taste too sweet - ars-h.

throat in - phos., sulph., zinc.

tobacco, tastes - sel.

tip - plat.

under - zinc.

water - lyc.

sweet-bitter and burning, then - cadm-s.

sweet-sour - bism., chin., crot-t., kali-i., mag-s., meny.

tallow, like - ***valer.***

tar, like - con.

tastelessness, of food - ***alum., amyg.,*** ant-t., apis, arg-n., ars., aster., aur., aur-m., bar-c., bell., bor., bry., ***cact., calc.,*** camph., carb-v., ***colch., cor-r.,*** cycl., dros., eup-per., ferr-m., formal., gymn., **HELL.,** ***ign.,*** just., kali-bi., kali-i., merc., morg., **NAT-M.,** nux-v., ph-ac., plan., ptel., **PULS.,** rhod., ruta., sal-ac., sars., seneg., sep., sil., squil., staph., stict., ***stram.,*** syc-co., tub., ***verat.,*** viol-t., zinc.

beer - puls.

TASTE, general

tastelessness, of food

bread - alum.

butter - puls.

coffee - nux-v.

coryza, in - alum., ***ant-t., calc.,*** cycl., ***hep.,*** mag-m., ***nat-c.,*** **NAT-M.,** nux-v., **PULS.,** ***rhod., sep., sil., sulph., sul-ac.***

cough, with - anac.

influenza, in - mag-m.

meat - alum., nux-v., puls., squil.

milk - alum., mosch., nux-v., puls.

salt - ***calc.,*** canth.

things which formerly had strong taste - acon.

tobacco - ant-t., anac., chin., puls., squil.

throat, in not in mouth - podo., ptel.

tobacco, juice as from - nat-c.

wine, like - seneg.

water tastes like wine - tab.

wood, like - ars.

foul, like - sulph.

TEARING, pain - carb-v., colch., guare., puls., ***rhus-v.,*** sep.

root - carb-v.

THICK, sensation - ars., ***bapt., bell., camph.,*** **GELS.,** ***glon., hyos., lach.,*** laur., lyc., merc-c., merl., ***mur-ac., op., phyt., plat.,*** rhus-t., ***stram.,*** syph.

TREMBLING - absin., ***agar., apis,*** arn., ars., ***aur., bell.,*** bry., **CAMPH.,** ***canth.,*** carb-ac., cimic., colch., ***crot-h.,*** cupr., cupr-ar., ***gels., hell.,*** hyos., ***ign.,*** **LACH.,** ***lyc.,*** med., **MERC.,** mur-ac., oena., ***op., ph-ac.,*** phos., ***plb.,*** rhus-t., sec., sil., stram., tab., ***tarax.,*** vip., zinc.

protruding it, when - apis, ***bell.,*** crot-h., ferr., ***gels., hell., hyos.,*** ign., **LACH.,** merc., ***nat-m., plb.,*** stram.

tip of tongue - ***thuj.***

sensation of - nat-m.

TUBERCLES - ***graph.,*** lyc., mang.

TUMORS, rounded elevation in center size of pea, sensitive, to touch, with drawing, sensation as if a string were pulling center of tongue toward hyoid bone - cast.

TWITCHING - glon., sec., sulph.

ULCERATIVE - arg-n.

tip - aesc., calc.

ULCERS - agar., aloe, ant-t., ***apis, ars.,*** ars-h., arum-t., ***aur.,*** aur-m., **BAPT.,** ***bar-c., bar-m.,*** benz-ac., bov., ***caps., calc., chin.,*** chlol., cic., cinnb., clem., corn., ***dig.,*** dros., ***fl-ac.,*** graph., hydr., ***kali-bi., kali-chl.,*** **KALI-I.,** ***kreos., lach., lyc.,*** merl., **MERC.,** ***merc-i-r., mur-ac., nat-m., nit-ac.,*** op., ***plb., phyt.,*** **PSOR.,** sil., ***sin-n., staph., sulph.,*** sul-ac., tarent., verat.

black ground, with - mur-ac.

bleeding - merc.

blue - ***ars.,*** mur-ac.

center - cupr-s., ***fl-ac.***

deep - mur-ac.

ULCERS,
edges - agar., ars., bov., ***calc.***, caust., ***cic.***, cupr., ***kali-bi.***, kali-chl., ***lach.***, ***merc.***, merc-cy., **NIT-AC.**, ***thuj.***
left, then right - ***thuj.***
right side - bov., cinnb., sil.
fraenum - agar., ***kali-c.***, naja, sep.
indurated - merc., ***merc-i-r.***, thuj.
margins undetermined, with - mur-ac.
painful - agar., bov., ***calc.***
to touch - bov., ***cic.***, thuj.
phagedenic - ***agar.***, benz-ac., ***caps.***, ***fl-ac.***, sil.
syphilitic - fl-ac., ***kali-bi.***, ***kali-i.***, **MERC.**, **NIT-AC.**, ***phyt.***
tip - am-c., cinnb., cupr., dros., lyc., merc., plb.
under - ***fl-ac.***, ***graph.***, **LYC.**, plb., **SANIC.**, thuj.
white - graph.
yellow - aloe, cupr., ***hell.***, plb.

VARICOSE, veins - calc., ***dig.***, ***fl-ac.***, ***ham.***, ***puls.***, ***thuj.***

VESICLES - acon., **AM-C.**, ***am-m.***, ant-c., **APIS**, ***arg-m.***, **ARS.**, ***bar-c.***, ***bell.***, berb., ***bor.***, brom., bry., ***calc.***, ***canth.***, ***caps.***, ***carb-an.***, carb-v., ***caust.***, cham., chim., chin., chin-a., chlol., clem., cupr., ***graph.***, ***ham.***, ***hell.***, indg., kali-ar., ***kali-c.***, kali-chl., kali-i., ***lach.***, ***lac-ac.***, **LYC.**, ***mag-c.***, mag-m., manc., mang., med., merl., ***merc.***, mez., ***mur-ac.***, ***nat-a.***, nat-c., **NAT-M.**, nat-p., nat-s., **NIT-AC.**, ***nux-v.***, phel., phos., phyt., puls., rhod., **RHUS-T.**, rhus-v., sal-ac., sars., ***sep.***, spig., spong., squil., ***staph.***, stram., ***thuj.***, verat., vip., zinc., zing.
bleeding from slightest touch - ***mag-c.***
burning - ***acon.***, am-c., **APIS**, arg-m., ars., bar-c., bry., ***calc.***, calc-p., ***caps.***, ***carb-an.***, ***graph.***, kali-chl., **LYC.**, ***mag-c.***, mang., mez., ***mur-ac.***, nat-s., ***nit-ac.***, sep., **SPIG.**, spong., ***sulph.***, ***sul-ac.***, ***thuj.***
like fire, right side - ***phel.***
eating, after - phos.
edges - am-c., ***calc.***, ***carb-an.***, caust., mag-c., mang., merc-cy., nat-c., nit-ac., ***phyt.***, sep., ***spong.***, sulph., ***thuj.***
which become ulcers - ***calc.***
fraenum - plb.
painful - ***ars.***, canth., **CAUST.**, graph., kali-c., mag-c., nux-v., sal-ac., sep., zinc.
raw - lyc.
red - bor.
scalded, as if - lyc.
stinging - ***cham.***, kali-chl.
suppurating - mag-c.
tip - am-c., ***am-m.***, aphis., ***apis***, ***bar-c.***, ***bell.***, berb., ***calc-p.***, carb-an., **CAUST.**, cycl., **GRAPH.**, ***hydr.***, indg., ***kali-i.***, kali-n., ***lach.***, **LYC.**, merc-i-r., **NAT-M.**, ***nat-p.***, nat-s., ***puls.***, sal-ac.
burning - kali-n., mur-ac., phos.
sensation as if - bell., sin-n.
ulcers, becoming - ***calc.***, clem., ***lach.***

VESICLES,
under the - am-c., bar-c., bell., ***cham.***, chin., graph., ***ham.***, ***lach.***, rhod., rhus-v.
burning - nit-ac.

WARTS - aur., ***aur-m.***, aur-m-n., kali-s., lyc., mang., staph.

WHITE - ***acon.***, ***aesc.***, agar., agn., ail., all-s., alum., ambr., am-c., am-m., anac., ang., **ANT-C.**, ***ant-t.***, ***apis***, ***arg-n.***, ***arn.***, **ARS.**, ***ars-i.***, ***ars-m.***, asaf., asar., asc-c., atro., aur-m-n., ***bapt.***, bar-c., bar-m., **BELL.**, berb., ***bism.***, bol., bor., bov., **BRY.**, cact., cahin., **CALC.**, calc-p., cann-s., ***carb-ac.***, carb-s., ***carb-v.***, caul., caust., ***cham.***, ***chel.***, ***chin.***, chin-a., chin-s., cic., ***cimx.***, ***cina***, cinnb., clem., cob., ***cocc.***, coch., ***colch.***, coll., ***coloc.***, cop., coc-c., cor-r., croc., crot-t., cupr., cupr-ar., cycl., ***dig.***, dios., echi., elaps, euph., ***eup-per.***, ***ferr.***, ferr-ar., ferr-p., ***fl-ac.***, ***gels.***, ***glon.***, gnaph., ***graph.***, guai., ham., hell., hydr-ac., hydr., **HYOS.**, ***hyper.***, ign., iod., ip., iris, jug-r., ***kali-ar.***, **KALI-BI.**, kali-br., kali-c., ***kali-chl.***, ***kali-i.***, ***kali-n.***, ***kali-p.***, ***kalm.***, ***kreos.***, lac-ac., lac-c., ***lach.***, lact., laur., lec., ***lyc.***, mag-c., mag-m., manc., mang., **MERC.**, ***merc-c.***, ***merc-i-f.***, merc-sul., ***mez.***, ***mur-ac.***, naja, ***nat-a.***, ***nat-c.***, ***nat-m.***, ***nat-s.***, **NIT-AC.**, nuph., ***nux-m.***, ***nux-v.***, olnd., ***op.***, ox-ac., par., ***petr.***, ***ph-ac.***, ***phos.***, phyt., ***plb.***, ***podo.***, ***psor.***, ptel., **PULS.**, ran-b., ran-s., raph., ***rhus-t.***, ***rumx.***, ***sabad.***, sabin., sang., sars., sel., ***seneg.***, ***sep.***, ***sil.***, **SPIG.**, ***stann.***, **SULPH.**, sul-ac., ***syph.***, **TARAX.**, tell., verat., verat-v., verb., viol-t., zinc.
border, moist and red - vip.
center - arg-n., bell., ***bry.***, canth., card-m., chin-s., gels., helon., ***kali-chl.***, nat-a., ***petr.***, phos., rhus-v., sabad., sin-n., sulph.
dark brown - ail., nat-p.
dark streaks along edges - petr.
red stripe down center - caust., cham., ***verat-v.***
cheesy - lac-c., merc-i-f., zinc.
dinner, after - nit-ac.
dirty - cahin., chin., dig., nat-p., olnd., podo., rhus-t.
with elevated papillae - olnd.
evening - bism.
milk white without coating - ***glon.***
milky - **ANT-C.**, ***bell.***, ***glon.***, kali-i., merc-cy.
moist - arg-n.
morning - agar., benz-ac., calc-p., **CHIN.**, cinnb., dig., echi., elaps, ***hell.***, kali-c., mag-m., mur-ac., nat-c., ***nit-ac.***, phos., **PULS.**, ran-s., sel., seneg., sulph.
painted, as if - **ARS.**
pale - acon., aloe, ambr., anac., ang., ars., berb., kreos., olnd., phos.
patches - cham., **TARAX.**
red insular, with - **NAT-M.**
right side - ***lob.***
root - kali-m., med., nat-m., sep., tub.
sides - **CAUST.**, ***cham.***, iod., ***kali-s.***
one side - ***daph.***, irid., lob., mez., **RHUS-T.**
patches, on - sang.

WHITE,
silvery, all over - arg-n., **ARS.,** carb-ac., glon., lac-c.
spots, clean - am-m., manc., **TARAX.**
stripes - bell., phel.
tip - canth.

WITHERED - kreos., verat.

WRINKLED - calc-p., nat-a., phos., sul-ac.
morning - calc-p.

YELLOW - ***aesc.,*** aloe, **ANT-C.,** ant-t., ***apis, arn.,*** ars., ars-h., asc-t., ***aur-m., bapt.,*** bell., ***bol.,*** bov., bry., ***camph.,*** cann-s., ***carb-v.,*** **CHEL.,** ***cham., chin.,*** chin-a., chin-s., ***cocc., colch.,*** coll., ***coloc.,*** com., corn., ***crot-h.,*** cupr., dios., ***eup-per.,*** ferr-i., ***gels., hell., hep., hyper., ip., kali-bi., kali-s.,*** lac-ac., ***lach., lept.,*** lyc., ***mag-m.,*** **MERC.,** ***merc-c., merc-i-f., merc-i-r., mez.,*** myric., ***nat-a.,*** nat-m., ***nat-p., nit-ac.,*** **NUX-M.,** ***nux-v., phos., phyt., plb., podo., psor.,*** ptel., pyrog., ***puls.,*** **RHUS-T.,** rumx., sabad., sabin., sanic., sec., ***sep.,*** **SPIG.,** ***stann., sulph.,*** thuj., ***verat., verat-v.,*** verb., vip., xan.
base - agar., ars., bol., calc-s., chin., chin-s., kali-bi., kali-s., ***merc.,*** merc-cy., **MERC-I-F.,** merc-sul., **NAT-P.,** ***nux-v., sanic., sin-n.,*** ter.
bright - merc-i-f.
shining - **APIS.**
center - bry., carb-an., chin-s., fl-ac., hell., ***lept.,*** puls., stram., verat-v.
greenish - merc-sul.
edges red - hell., merc-i-f.
dirty - ***ars., bapt.,*** com., ***kali-chl., lach., mag-c.,*** **MERC., MERC-C., MERC-I-F.,** ***myric., op., pyrog., sep.,*** verat-v.
thick coating - ***aesc., bapt.,*** bry., carb-v., cham., ***chel., chin.,*** chion., ferr., ***hydr.,*** indol., ***kali-bi.,*** kali-s., lept., lyc., ***merc., merc-d., merc-i-f.,*** nat-p., nux-v., ***ost.,*** podo., ***puls.,*** sang., sulph., yuc.
edges, center, gray - phos.
indented, with - chel., hydr.
greenish- yellow - chion.
root - nat-s.
golden yellow - ***nat-p.***
looks like half dried clay - calc-s.
gray - ambr., arg-n., phyt.
moist, filmy - merc-i-f.
mustard, as if were spread on - kali-p., podo.
patch in centre - ***bapt.,*** phyt.
patches - petr.
yellow-white - aloe, alum., ***arg-n., ars.,*** bell., ***cocc., cupr.,*** cycl., dios., ***gels., hydr., kali-bi.,*** lac-c., lyss., merc-c., mez., nit-ac., **RHUS-T.,** sec., seneg., zinc.
base - **RHUS-T.,** zinc.
thick - acon., ***ars.,*** ars-s-f., bapt., carb-s., gels.

Toxicity

ACIDS, foods, agg. - **OLND.,** ***nat-p.***
amel. - **PTEL.**
aversion, to - abies-c., arund., ***bell.,*** chin., clem., ***cocc., con.,*** dros., elaps, ***ferr.,*** ferr-m., ***fl-ac.,*** ign., kali-bi., lyc., man., nat-m., nat-p., nux-v., ph-ac., ***sabad., sulph.,*** tub.
citric acid, agg. - nat-p.
desires - puls., verat.

ADDICTIVE, personality - carc., lach., med., nux-v., op., thuj.

ACONITE, abuse of - sulph.

AIR, pollution, ailments, from - ars., sil., ***sul-ac.***

ALCOHOL, general
abuse of, ailments from - acon., ***agar.,*** alum., alumn., am-m., anac., ***ant-c.,*** apom., ***arg-n.,*** arn., **ARS., ASAR., AUR., BAR-C.,** ***bell.,*** bor., bov., cadm-s., ***calc., calc-ar.,*** carb-an., ***carb-s., carb-v.,*** card-m., caust., ***chel., chin.,*** chlol., coca, cocc., ***coff.,*** colch., ***con., crot-h.,*** dig., eup-per., ***gels.,*** hep., hydr., hyos., ***ign.,*** ip., kali-bi., **LACH.,** laur., ***led., lob., lyc.,*** naja, ***nat-c., nat-m., nux-m.,*** **NUX-V., OP.,** ***petr., puls.,*** querc., **RAN-B.,** ***rhod., rhus-t., ruta.,*** sabad., ***sang.,*** **SEL.,** sep., ***sil., spig., stram.,*** stront-c., stroph., stry., **SULPH., SUL-AC.,** tab., thuj., ***verat.,*** zinc.
paralysis, after abuse of - ant-t., ***ars.,*** calc., ***lach.,*** nat-s., ***nux-v.,*** **OP.,** ran-b., sep., ***sulph.***
agg. - acon., aeth., ***agar.,*** agav-t., aloe, alum., alumn., ***am-c.,*** am-m., anac., ang., ***ant-c.,*** apom., ***arg-n.,*** arn., **ARS., ASAR.,** aur., **BAR-C.,** ***bell.,*** berb., bor., bov., ***calc., calc-ar.,*** calc-f., calc-sil., ***cann-i.,*** caps., ***carb-ac.,*** carb-an., ***carb-s., carb-v.,*** card-m., ***caust., chel., chin.,*** chlol., cimic., ***coca,*** cocc., ***coff.,*** colch., ***con., crot-h., dig.,*** eup-per., ***ferr.,*** ferr-i., fl-ac., gels., ***glon.,*** gran., grat., guare., ***hell.,*** hep., hydr., hyos., ***ign.,*** ip., kali-bi., ***kali-br.,*** **LACH.,** laur., ***led., lob., lyc., merc.,*** naja, ***nat-c., nat-m.,*** **NAT-P.,** ***nux-m.,*** **NUX-V., OP.,** ***petr.,*** **PHOS.,** phyt., ***puls.,*** querc., **RAN-B.,** ***rhod., rhus-t., ruta,*** sabad., ***sang.,*** **SEL.,** sep., ***sil., spig., stram.,*** stront-c., stry., ***sul-ac., sulph., syph.,*** trinit., **ZINC.**
abstaining, after - calc-ar.
easily intoxicated - **CON.,** naja, phos., ***zinc.***
amel. - ***acon.,*** agar., canth., ***con., gels.,*** lach., op., sel., sul-ac.
aversion to, alcoholic stimulants - ail., alco., ang., ant-t., ars., ars-m., bell., bry., calc., calc-ar., carb-v., cham., chin., cocc., ***hyos.,*** ign., lec., man., manc., ***merc., nux-v.,*** ph-ac., phos., phyt., psor., ***rhus-t.,*** sil., spig., spong., stram., stroph., ***sul-ac.,*** sulph., zinc.

ALCOHOL, general
beer, agg. - acon., act-sp., ***aloe,*** alum., ant-t., ars., asaf., bapt., bell., ***bry.,*** cadm-s., calc-caust., carb-s., card-m., chel., chlol., chin., chlor., coc-c., cocc., coloc., crot-t., euph., ***ferr.,*** fl-ac., ign., ***kali-bi.,*** kali-m., ***led., lyc.,*** merc-c., mez., mur-ac., nux-m., **NUX-V.,** ***puls., rhus-t.,*** sec., sep., ***sil.,*** stann., staph., stram., ***sulph.,*** teucr., ***thuj., verat.***
easily intoxicated - ***chim.,*** coloc., ign., kali-m.
new - ***chin., lyc., puls.***
smell of - ***cham.***
ailments from - kali-bi., rhus-t., thuj.
bad - nux-m.
amel. - aloe, **LOB.,** mur-ac., nat-p., ***verat.***
aversion to - ***alum.,*** alum-p., asaf., atro., **BELL.,** bry., calc., carb-s., ***cham.,*** **CHIN.,** cinch., ***clem.,*** **COCC.,** crot-t., ***cycl., ferr., kali-bi.,*** med., nat-m., ***nat-s.,*** **NUX-V.,** pall., ph-ac., ***phos.,*** puls., ***rhus-t.,*** sang., sep., spig., spong., ***stann., sulph.***
evening - bry., nat-m., sulph.
morning - ***nux-v.***
desires - **ACON.,** agar., aloe, am-c., ant-c., arn., ars., asar., ***bell., bry.,*** calad., calc., camph., carb-s., carc., ***caust.,*** chel., chin., ***cocc.,*** coc-c., ***coloc.,*** cupr., dig., ***graph., kali-bi., lach.,*** mang., ***med., merc.,*** mosch., nat-a., ***nat-c.,*** nat-p., ***nat-m., nat-s.,*** **NUX-V.,** op., ***petr., phel.,*** ph-ac., phos., psor., ***puls., rhus-t., sabad.,*** sep., ***spig.,*** spong., staph., stram., ***stront-c.,*** **SULPH.,** tell., zinc.
afternoon - psor., sulph.
bitter - aloe, cocc., ***kali-bi.,*** nat-m., nux-v., puls.
chill, during - ant-c., ***nux-v.***
colic, after - ph-ac.
evening - coc-c., ***kali-bi.,*** mang., ***med.,*** nux-v., sulph., ***zinc.***
fever, after - puls.
fever, during - acon., nux-v., puls.
forenoon - agar., phos.
morning - ***nux-v.,*** phel., ***puls.***
thirst, with - ***calad.***
thirst, without - ***calad.***
brandy, agg. - agar., ***ars.,*** ars-m., bell., calc., carb-ac., chel., chin., cocc., fl-ac., hep., hyos., ign., lach., laur., ***led.,*** med., **NUX-V., OP.,** puls., ***ran-b.,*** rhod., ***rhus-t.,*** ruta, spig., ***stram.,*** sul-ac., **SULPH.,** verat., zinc.
ailments from bad - carb-v.
amel. - olnd., sel.
aversion to - ant-t., ***carb-ac.,*** ign., lob., lob-e., ***merc.,*** ph-ac., rhus-t., stram., zinc.
brandy drinkers, in - ***arn.***
desires - acon., ail., arg-n., ars., ars-m., aster., bov., bry., bufo, calc., chin., cic., coca, cub., ferr-p., ***hep.,*** lach., mosch., mur-ac., **NUX-V.,** olnd., **OP.,** ***petr., phos.,*** puls., ***sel., sep., spig., staph.,*** stram., stront-c., ***sulph., sul-ac.,*** ther.

ALCOHOL, general

desires, alcohol - acon., agav-t., ail., alco., aloe, am-c., ant-t., arg-m., ***arn.***, **ARS.**, ***ars-i.***, **ASAR.**, aster., ***aur.***, aur-a., aur-i., bov., bry., bufo, ***calc.***, ***calc-ar.***, calc-s., **CAPS.**, ***carb-ac.***, carb-an., ***carb-v.***, ***chin.***, cic., ***coca***, cocc., **CROT-H.**, cub., cupr., ferr-p., fl-ac., gins., hell., **HEP.**, iber., ign., ***iod.***, kali-bi., ***kreos.***, lac-c., **LACH.**, lec., ***led.***, ***lyc.***, ***med.***, merc., mosch., ***mur-ac.***, naja, nat-m., nat-p., nux-m., **NUX-V.**, olnd., ***op.***, ***phos.***, plb., ***psor.***, ***puls.***, rhus-t., ***sel.***, ***sep.***, sil., sol-t-ae., ***spig.***, ***staph.***, stront-c., stry-n., **SULPH.**, ***sul-ac.***, sumb., ***syph.***, tab., ter., ther., ***tub.***, ziz.
disgust for, but - thiop.
menses, before - **SEL.**

edema, from - ars., ***card-m.***, fl-ac., sulph.

liquor, agg. - ant-c., ars., bell., bov., ***cann-i.***, ***carb-v.***, cimic., led., ***ran-b.***, rhod., rhus-t., sel., sulph., verat.
desires - med.

whiskey, aversion to - ant-t., ***ign.***, merc., ph-ac., rhus-t., zinc.
desires - acon., ***arn.***, ***ars.***, calc., carb-ac., ***carb-an.***, chin., cub., fl-ac., hep., **LAC-C.**, ***lach.***, merc., nux-v., op., ***phos.***, puls., ***sel.***, ***spig.***, staph., **SULPH.**, ther.

wine, agg. - acon., acon-l., aeth., agar., alum., am-m., ***ant-c.***, ***arn.***, **ARS.**, aur., aur-m., bell., benz-ac., ***bor.***, bov., bry., cact., ***calc.***, calc-sil., carb-an., carb-s., carb-v., **CHIN.**, chlol., coc-c., **COFF.**, coloc., ***con.***, cor-r., eup-per., ign., ***fl-ac.***, ***gels.***, ***glon.***, hyos., ign., kali-chl., ***lach.***, ***led.***, **LYC.**, mag-m., ***merc.***, ***naja***, ***nat-a.***, ***nat-c.***, ***nat-m.***, ***nux-m.***, **NUX-V.**, **OP.**, ox-ac., petr., phos., puls., **RAN-B.**, ***rhod.***, rhus-t., ruta., ***sabad.***, sars., ***sel.***, **SIL.**, staph., stront-c., sul-ac., ***sulph.***, thuj., verat., **ZINC.**
champagne - calc., zinc.
red - fl-ac., zinc.
sulphureted - ***ars.***, chin., ***merc.***, **PULS.**, ***sep.***
white - **ANT-C.**, ant-t., ***ars.***, ferr., sep., sulph.
ailments from - carb-v., coff., lyc., nat-m., ***zinc.***
bad, from - carb-v.
amel. - ***acon.***, agar., ars., bell., brom., bry., ***canth.***, ***carb-ac.***, chel., chen-v., coca, cocc., ***con.***, gels., glon., graph., lach., mez., nat-m., nux-v., onos., ***op.***, osm., phos., ran-b., sel., sul-ac., sulph., thea.
sour, white - ferr.
aversion to - **ACON.**, agar., alum., ars-m., carb-s., carb-v., coff., fl-ac., glon., hyper., ***ign.***, jatr., jug-r., **LACH.**, lact., man., manc., ***merc.***, nat-m., nux-v., ph-ac., puls., ***rhus-t.***, **SABAD.**, sil., ***sulph.***, tub., ***zinc.***, zinc-p.
desires - ***acon.***, ***aeth.***, arg-m., arg-mur., ***ars.***, asaf., bov., ***bry.***, **CALC.**, calc-ar., calc-s., **CANTH.**, chel., chin., chin-a., chlor., ***cic.***, colch., cub., eup-per., fl-ac., ***hep.***, hyper., iod., kali-bi., kali-br., kali-i., ***lach.***, ***lec.***, **LYCPS.**, merc., ***mez.***, nat-m.,

ALCOHOL, general
desires - nux-v., op., **PHOS.**, puls., sec., sel., ***sep.***, ***spig.***, ***staph.***, sul-i., **SULPH.**, ***sumb.***, syph., ther., thiop., verat., vichy-g.
claret - calc-s., staph., ***sulph.***, ther.
sensitive to the smell of - tab.
sour agg. - **ANT-C.**, ant-t., ***ars.***, ferr., sep., sulph.

ALCOHOLISM, general, dipsomania - ***absin.***, acon., adon., **AGAR.**, agav-t., alum., am-m., anac., ange., anis., ***ant-c.***, ***ant-t.***, ***apoc.***, apom., arg-m., arg-n., arn., ars., ars-s-f., ***asaf.***, ***asar.***, **AUR.**, ***aven.***, bar-c., ***bell.***, bism., bor., bov., bry., bufo, cadm-s., ***calc.***, calc-ar., camph., cann-i., ***caps.***, carb-ac., carb-an., ***carb-s.***, ***carb-v.***, ***carc.***, card-m., caust., cham., ***chel.***, chim., **CHIN.**, chin-m., cic., ***cimic.***, coc-c., ***cocc.***, ***coff.***, con., croc., **CROT-H.**, ***cupr-ar.***, dig., ***eup-per.***, ***ferr.***, fl-ac., ***gels.***, glon., ***graph.***, ***hell.***, hep., hydr., ***hyos.***, ichth., ***ign.***, ip., ***kali-bi.***, kali-br., kali-c., kali-i., kola., ***lac-c.***, **LACH.**, ***laur.***, ***led.***, lob., lup., ***lyc.***, mag-c., meph., merc., mez., mosch., ***nat-c.***, nat-n., nat-s., ***nux-m.***, **NUX-V.**, op., passi., petr., ph-ac., ***phos.***, plat., plb., psor., puls., ***quas.***, ***querc.***, **RAN-B.**, raph., ***rhod.***, ***rhus-t.***, rumx., ruta, sang., sars., sec., **SEL.**, ***sep.***, ***sil.***, staph., ***stram.***, stront-c., ***stroph.***, **SUL-AC.**, **SULPH.**, syph., tarax., tub., valer., **VERAT.**, ***zinc.***
acute - acon., bell., ***op.***, ***lach.***
drinking, on the sly - ***lach.***, ***sulph.***
excitement from - stram., zinc.
habit, to overcome - ange., aven., bufo, ***cinch.***, ***querc.***, ster., ***sul-ac.***, sulph.
hereditary craving - asar., lach., psor., sul-ac., sulph., **SYPH.**, tub.
hypochondriasis, with - **NUX-V.**
idleness, from - lach., nux-v., sulph.
irritability, with - ***nux-v.***
menses, before - **SEL.**
pregnancy, during or after - nux-v.
recurrent - anac., aur., bell., ***chin.***, hyos., nux-v., op., stram., thuj.
weakness of character, from - ars., petr., puls.

delirium tremens, mania-a-potu - acon., **AGAR.**, agar-pr., alco., anac., ant-c., ***ant-t.***, ***apoc.***, apom., ***arn.***, **ARS.**, ars-s-f., asar., atro., aur., ***aven.***, ***bell.***, bism., bry., bufo, ***calc.***, calc-ar., calc-s., camph-br., ***cann-i.***, cann-s., ***caps.***, carb-v., chin., chin-m., chin-s., chim., chlf., chlol., ***chlor.***, ***cimic.***, cocc., ***coff.***, cori-r., ***crot-h.***, ***cupr-ar.***, cypr., dig., dor., ether, ferr-p., fl-ac., gels., ***glon.***, grat., hell., hydr., **HYOS.**, ***hyosin.***, ichth., ign., ***kali-br.***, kali-i., kali-p., **LACH.**, led., lob., lol., lup., lyc., ***merc.***, nat-c., **NAT-M.**, **NUX-M.**, **NUX-V.**, oena., **OP.**, passi., ***past.***, ***phos.***, plb., psor., puls., querc., **RAN-B.**, raph., rhod., rhus-t., scut., sel., sep., sil., spig., ster., **STRAM.**, stroph., **STRY.**, stry-n., ***sulph.***, ***sul-ac.***, sumb., ***syph.***, teucr., thea., thuj., tub., tus-p., verat., ***zinc.***, zinc-ac.
chronic - sul-ac.
delusions, with - ***bell.***, calc., cann-i., ***kali-bi.***, ***lach.***, ***op.***, ***stram.***

ALCOHOLISM, general
delirium tremens
elderly, emaciated persons, in - **OP.**
escape, attempts to - ***bell.,*** stram.
excitement, with - chlf., ***zinc.***
face, with red, bloated - ***bell., crot-h.,*** stram.
fear, calms the - scut.
talking, excessive, with loquacity - ***lach., ran-b.***
mild attacks - ***cypr.***
oversensitiveness, with - coff., **NUX-V.**
praying, with - **STRAM.**
sleeplessness, with - aven., ***cimic., coff., gels.,*** hyos., kali-br., kali-p., ***nux-v.***
small quantity of alcoholic stimulants, from - **OP.**
sopor with snoring - **OP.**
trembling - **ARS.,** ***bar-c., cedr., hyos.,*** kali-br., kali-p., lach., ***nux-v., stram.***
hands - ***coff., kali-br., lach.,*** **NUX-V.,** ***stram.***
weakness, in - ***ars., carb-s., kali-br., nat-s., phos., ran-b., sel., sulph.***

ALUMINIUM, poisoning - ***alum., bry.,*** cadm-m., camph., cham., ip., ***plb.,*** puls.

ANESTHESIA, ailments, from - ***acet-ac.,*** am-c., am-caust., aml-n., ***carb-v., chlf.,*** hep., ph-ac., **PHOS.**
weakness, from - acet-ac., hyper., ***phos.***

ANTIBIOTICS, worse from - apis., ars., chin., lyc., nat-p., ***nit-ac.,*** thuj.

ARSENIC, poisoning - ***ars.,*** camph., ***carb-v.,*** chin., chin-s., dig., euph., ***ferr.,*** graph., **HEP.,** iod., ***ip.,*** lach., ***merc.,*** nux-m., nux-v., ***phos.,*** plb., samb., sulph., tab., thuj., ***verat.***
chill, from - ip.
paralysis, from - ***chin.,*** ferr., graph., ***hep., nux-v.***

ARTIFICIAL, food, agg. - ***alum.,*** calc., mag-c., sulph.

BELLADONNA, abuse of - hyos., op.

BROMIDES, abuse of - am-c., camph., cham., ***kali-br.,*** lach., mag-c., op., phos., zinc-p.

CAMPHOR, abuse of - camph., canth., coff., op.

CANTHARIS, abuse of - apis, camph., canth.

CARBON, gas poisoning - acet-ac., acon., am-c., bell., bry., **CARB-V.,** lach., op., phos.,
carbon monoxide, from - acon., bell., bry., ***carb-v.,*** op.

CAUTERY, silver nitrate, to antidote - arg-n., ***nat-m.***

CHEMICALS, hypersensitive to - apis., **ARS.,** ***coff.,*** med., ***merc.*** nat-c., ***nit-ac.,*** nux-v., **PHOS.,** psor., sul-ac., sulph.
pesticides - ars.

CHEMOTHERAPY, treatment, for side effects, of - ars., **CADM-S.,** chin., ***ip.,*** nux-v.

CHINA, abuse of (see Quinine) - ant-t., aran., arn., ***ars., bell., calc., carb-v.,*** cham., coff., eup-per., ***ferr., hell.,*** **HEP.,** iod., ***ip.,*** lach., led., meny., merc., nat-c., ***nat-m.,*** nux-v., ph-ac., ***puls.,*** rhus-t., salv., ***sel.,*** sep., ***sulph.,*** thea., ***verat.***

CHLORALUM, abuse of - cann-i.

COAL gas, ailments from - acet-ac., am-c., arn., bell., bor., bov., ***carb-s.,*** carb-v., coff., ip., lach., ***op.,*** phos., sec.

COCAINE, addiction - aven., coca.

COD liver oil, abuse of - hep.

COFFEE, agg. - ***aeth.,*** agar., alet., all-c., anac., ars., arum-t., aster., aur-m., bell., bov., bry., ***cact.,*** calc., ***calc-p.,*** cann-i., **CANTH.,** ***caps.,*** carb-v., caul., **CAUST., CHAM.,** chin., cist., clem., ***cocc.,*** coff., colch., coloc., cycl., fl-ac., form., glon., grat., guare., ***hep.,*** **IGN.,** ***ip.,*** kali-bi., kali-c., kali-n., lyc., mag-c., mang., ***merc.,*** nat-m., ***nat-s.,*** nit-ac., **NUX-V.,** ox-ac., ***ph-ac.,*** plat., psor., ***puls.,*** rhus-t., sep., stram., sulph., sul-ac., ***thuj.,*** vinc., xan.
hot - caps.
menopause period, during - **LACH.**
smell of - fl-ac., lach., ***nat-m.,*** osm., sul-ac., tub.
odor of - sul-ac.
ailments from - **CHAM.,** grat., ***ign., nux-v.,*** ox-ac., thuj.
amel. - acon., agar., arg-m., ***ars.,*** brom., cann-i., canth., **CHAM.,** chel., **COLOC.,** eucal., ***euph.,*** euphr., fago., glon., hyos., ***ign.,*** lach., mag-c., mosch., ***nux-v.,*** op., phos., til.
aversion to - ***acon.,*** alum-sil., ***bell., bry.,*** **CALC.,** calc-s., carb-v., ***caust., cham.,*** chel., ***chin.,*** cinnb., coc-c., ***coff.,*** con., ***dulc.,*** fl-ac., kali-bi., kali-br., kali-i., kali-n., lec., lil-t., lol., ***lyc.,*** mag-p., man., ***merc., nat-c., nat-m.,*** **NUX-V.,** osm., ox-ac., ph-ac., ***phos.,*** phys., puls., rheum, rhus-t., sabad., ***spig., sul-ac., sulph.***
morning - lyc.
noon - ox-ac.
smell of - fl-ac., lach., ***nat-m.,*** osm., sul-ac., tub.
sweetened - aur-m.
unsweetened - ***rheum.***
desires - ***alum.,*** **ANG.,** arg-m., arg-n., ***ars.,*** aster., ***aur., bry.,*** calc-p., ***caps., carb-v., carc.,*** cham., chel., ***chin.,*** colch., ***con.,*** gran., lach., lec., lob., ***mez.,*** mosch., nat-m., ***nux-m.,*** **NUX-V.,** ph-ac., sabin., ***sel.,*** sol-t-ae., sulph.
beans of - chin., nux-v., sabin.
dysmenorrhea, in - ***lach.***
nauseates, which - caps.
strong - ***bry.,*** mosch.

COLCHICUM, abuse of - colch., led.

COPPER, fumes, agg. - camph., ***ip.,*** lyc., ***merc.,*** nux-v., op., ***puls.***
vessels agg. - hep.

DIGITALIS, abuse of - chin., crat., dig., nit-ac.

DRUG, overdose, of - ars., ***gels.***, ip., ***nux-v., op.***

DRUGS, general (see Narcotics)
abuse, of - aloe, ars., **AVEN.**, bapt., camph., carb-ac., carb-v., coff., hep., ***hydr., ip.***, kali-i., ***lob.***, mag-s., nat-m., nit-ac., **NUX-V.**, paeon., ***puls., sulph.***, teucr., thuj.
herbal - camph., ***nux-v.***
addiction to - ***aven., nux-v.***, tab.
overacts, without curing - ars., carc., cupr., med., ***ph-ac., teucr.***
oversensitive, to - acon., arn., asar., cham., ***chin.***, coff., cupr., ***ign.***, lyc., ***merc.***, nit-ac., **NUX-V., PULS.**, sep., sil., **SULPH.**, teucr., ***valer.***
high potencies - ars-i., ***ars.***, caust., hep., lyc., med., **NIT-AC.**, nux-v., **PHOS.**, sep.
quick reaction - ***bell., cupr., nux-v.***, **PHOS.**, ***zinc.***
thinking of it, agg. - asaf.
wants of susceptibility, to - carb-v., laur., ***mosch., op.***

DRUGGING, weakness, from - aven., carb-v., helon., ***nux-v.***

DUST, agg. - blatta., ***brom., lyss.***, poth., ***sil.***

ERGOTINE, abuse of - chin., lach., nux-v., sec., sol-n.

FOOD, poisoning - ant-c., **ARS.**, bapt., bry., ***carb-v.***, chin., ***coloc.***, crot-h., ***ip.***, lach., lyc., nat-p., ***nux-v.***, ph-ac., ***podo.***, psor., ***puls.***, pyrog., sul-ac., ***urt-u.***, zing.
bad, water - ***ars.***, bapt., zing.
fish, spoiled - ars., ***carb-v.***, chin., ***puls.***
fruit, acid, sour - ***ant-c., ip.***, ox-ac., **NAT-P.**, ***ph-ac., psor.***
shellfish, agg. - ***aloe***, ars., ***brom.***, bry., fl-ac., **LYC.**, ***podo., sul-ac., urt-u.***
spoiled, fatty, rich - ars., ***carb-v.***, chin., ***ip.***, nux-v., **PULS.**
meat, agg. - **ARS.**, ***carb-v.***, chin., ***crot-h., lach., puls., pyrog.***

HANGOVER, reveling, from a night of - ambr., ant-c., ***ars.***, bry., ***carb-v.***, coff., colch., **IP.**, ***laur.***, led., **NUX-V.**, ***puls., ran-b.***, rhus-t., sulph.

HEROIN, addiction - ailments from - agar., apom., ars., aur., **AVEN.**, bell., calc., cann-i., ***cham.***, cic., cimic., coff., hyos., ***ip.***, kali-per., ***lach.***, lob., ***macro.***, merc., mur-ac., nat-p., ***nux-v.***, **OP.**, ox-ac., ***passi.***, phos., plat., puls., stram., zinc.
craving for - apom., **AVEN.**, lob., ***ip.***, nat-p., ***nux-v., op.***, ox-ac., passi., upa.

HYPERSENSITIVE, (see Chemicals) - apis., ***ars., coff.***, med., ***merc.*** nat-c., ***nit-ac.***, nux-v., ***phos.***, psor., sul-ac., sulph.
drugs, to allopathic (see Drugs) - acon., arn., ***ars.***, cham., coff., lyc., **MED., NIT-AC.**, nux-v., **PULS.**, sep., sil., **SULPH.**
remedies, to homeopathic potencies, (see Toxicity, Remedies) - acon., **ARS.**, ars-i., cham., coff., **MED., NIT-AC.**, nux-v., **PHOS.**, sep., ***thuj.***

INTOXICATION, ailments, after - abies-c., absin., acet-ac., acon., aether, agar., agn., ***am-m.***, aml-n., amyg., arg-m., ars., atro., bart., bell., ***bry.***, camph., cann-s., ***caps.***, carb-an., ***carb-v.***, chel., chin., chin-s., cic., coca, ***cocc., coff.***, con., coni., cori-r., dat-m., eucal., fagu., ferr., ***gels.***, grat., hyos., ign., ip., kali-bi., kali-c., kali-i., kali-n., kiss., kreos., lach., lact., ***laur.***, led., lol., merc., mez., mill., morph., nabal., naja, nat-m., nux-m., **NUX-V., OP.**, ph-ac., phel., pip-m., ***puls.***, ran-b., rheum, rhod., sabad., samb., sec., ***spong.***, squil., ***stram.***, tab., tax., ter., teucr., thea., til., tus-f., valer., verat., vip., zinc.
cold perspiration of forehead, with - verat.
easy - bov., con., phos., ***zinc.***
headache, after - ***ant-c.***, bell., ***bry., carb-v.***, cocc., coff., glon., laur., **NUX-V.**, ***puls.***, spong., stram., sulph., tarax.
medications, drugs, intoxication from - aven., lob., nux-v.

IODINE, poisoning or abuse of - ant-c., ant-t., ***ars.***, bell., camph., chin., chin-s., coff., ***conv., hep.***, hydr., ***iod.***, lycps., merc., ***op., phos., sec.***, spong., sulph.

IRON, poisoning or abuse of - ars., calc-p., ***chin.***, chin-a., cupr., ***ferr., ferr-p., hep.***, iod., ip., merc., nat-m., ***puls., sulph.***, thea., verat., ***zinc.***

LEAD, poisoning - **ALUM.**, alum-sil., ***alumn.***, ant-c., ars., ***bell.***, carb-s., **CAUST.**, chin., cocc., ***coloc.***, crot-t., cupr., gels., hep., iod., kali-br., ***kali-i.***, kreos., lyc., mang., merc., ***nat-s.***, nux-v., op., petr., ***plat., sul-ac., sulph., ter.***, **TUB.**, uran., ***verat.***, zinc.
chronic effects of - ***alum.***, alum-sil., ***alumn.***, ant-c., ars., ***bell.***, carb-s., **CAUST.**, chin., cocc., ***coloc.***, crot-t., cupr., gels., hep., iod., kali-br., ***kali-i.***, kreos., lyc., mang., merc., ***nat-s.***, nux-v., ***op.***, petr., ***plat.***, plb., ***sul-ac., sulph.***, zinc.
paralysis, from - alum., ***alumn., ars.***, caust., cupr., kali-i., nux-v., ***op.***, pipe., ***plat.***, plb., ***sul-ac.***

MAGNESIA, abuse of - nux-v., rheum..

MERCURY, poisoning, abuse of - acon., agn., alumn., anan., ang., ***ant-c., arg-m.***, arn., ars., ***asaf.***, **AUR.**, aur-m., aur-s., ***bell., bor.***, bry., calad., ***calc.***, calo., camph., carb-an., **CARB-V.**, caust., ***chel., chin.***, cic., cina, ***clem.***, cocc., coff., ***colch.***, con., ***cupr.***, dig., dulc., ***euph.***, euphr., ferr., fl-ac., graph., ***guai.***, **HEP.**, ***hydr., iod.***, iris, kali-bi., ***kali-chl.***, **KALI-I., LACH.**, laur., ***led., lyc.***, lycps., **MERC.**, merc-i-r., ***mez., mur-ac., nat-m.***, **NAT-S., NIT-AC.**, nux-v., op., ***ph-ac.***, **PHYT.**, plat., plat-m., podo., ***puls.***, rheum, rhod., rhus-g., rhus-t., sabad., ***sars.***, sel., sep., ***sil.***, spong., **STAPH.**, still., stram., stront-c., sul-i., **SULPH.**, thuj., valer., verat., viol-t., zinc.
headache, from - arg-n., ***asaf., aur.***, carb-v., chin., clem., fl-ac., **HEP.**, ***iod., kali-i.***, led., merc., mez., **NIT-AC.**, podo., puls., ***sars.***, staph., still., sulph.
paralysis, from - **HEP.**, ***nit-ac.***, staph., stram., ***sulph.***

MINING, general, ill effects of - ant-t., carb-s., card-m., nat-a., ***sil.,*** sulph.

MORPHINE, addiction, ailments from - agar., apom., ars., aur., **AVEN.,** bell., calc., cann-i., ***cham.,*** cic., cimic., coff., hyos., ***ip.,*** kali-per., ***lach.,*** lob., ***macro.,*** merc., mur-ac., nat-p., ***nux-v.,*** **OP.,** ox-ac., ***passi.,*** phos., plat., puls., stram., zinc.

MUSHROOMS, aversion to - lyc., nat-m., nat-s.
poisoning from - ***absin.,*** agar., ***ars.,*** atro., ***bell.,*** camph., pyrog.

NARCOTICS, abuse of, (see Drugs) - acet-ac., acon., agar., am-c., apom., ars., aur., ***aven.,*** **BELL.,** bry., calc., ***camph.,*** cann-i., canth., carb-v., caust., **CHAM.,** chin., cic., cimic., **COFF.,** colch., croc., cupr., ***dig.,*** dulc., euph., ***ferr.,*** ***graph.,*** hep., ***hyos.,*** ign., ***ip.,*** kali-per., **LACH.,** lob., ***lyc.,*** macro., mag-s., merc., mosch., mur-ac., nat-c., nat-m., nat-p., nit-ac., nux-m., **NUX-V.,** ***op.,*** ox-ac., ozone, passi., ph-ac., phos., plat., plb., ***puls.,*** rhus-t., seneg., ***sep.,*** staph., sulph., thuj., ***valer.,*** verat., zinc.
addiction, to - aven., nux-v., op., tab.
ailments from - ***aven.,*** ip., ***nux-v., op.,*** ozone, verat.
headache, after drug abuse - bell., cham., coff., dig., graph., hyos., lach., lyc., nux-v., op., puls., sep., valer.

PHOSPHORUS, abuse of - lach., nux-v., phos.

POTASH, chlorate of, abuse of - hydr.

POTASSIUM, bromide, abuse of - camph., helon., kali-br., nux-v., zinc.

PTOMAINE poisoning, ailments from - absin., acet-ac., all-c., ***ars.,*** camph., carb-an., carb-v., crot-h., ***cupr-ar.,*** gunp., kreos., lach., puls., ***pyrog.,*** urt-u., ***verat.***

PURGATIVES, abuse of - aloe, hydr., ***nux-v.,*** op., sulph.

QUININE, poisoning (see China) - am-c., ***ant-t.,*** ***apis,*** **ARN.,** ***ars.,*** asaf., aza., ***bell.,*** bry., **CALC.,** calc-ar., caps., carb-an., **CARB-V.,** cham., chelo., ***chin., chin-s., cina,*** coloc., cupr., cycl., dig., eucal., **FERR.,** ferr-ar., gels., hell., ***hep.,*** **IP.,** kali-ar., ***lach.,*** mang., meny., merc., **NAT-M.,** nat-p., nat-s., nux-v., parth., ***ph-ac., phos.,*** plb., **PULS.,** ran-s., samb., sel., ***sep.,*** stann., ***sulph.,*** sul-ac., ***verat.***
weakness, from - ars-s-f., chin., chin-s.

RADIATION, sickness, for side effects, of - ars., **CADM-S.,** calc-f., chin., fl-ac., ***ip.,*** nux-v., phos., rad-br., **SOL.,** x-ray.
burns, from - calc-f., fl-ac., phos., rad-br., ***sol.,*** x-ray.

REMEDIES, reactions to, homeopathic
overacts, without curing - ars., carc., cupr., med., ***ph-ac., teucr.***
oversensitive, to - acon., arn., asar.,carc., cham., ***chin.,*** coff., cupr., ***ign.,*** lyc., ***merc.,*** nit-ac., **NUX-V., PULS.,** sep., sil., **SULPH.,** teucr., ***valer.***

REMEDIES, reactions to
oversensitive, to
high potencies - ars-i., ***ars.,*** caust., hep., lyc., med., **NIT-AC.,** nux-v., **PHOS.,** sep.
quick reaction - ***bell., cupr., nux-v.,*** **PHOS.,** ***zinc.***
wants of susceptibility, to - carb-v., laur., ***mosch., op.***

SALT, abuse of - ars., carb-v., ***nat-m., nit-s-d., phos.,*** sel.
agg. - ***alumn.,*** ars., bell., calc., ***carb-v.,*** coca, ***dros.,*** lyc., mag-m., **NAT-M.,** nit-s-d., nux-v., **PHOS.,** puls., ***sel.,*** sil.
ailments from - carb-v., nat-m., nit-s-d., phos., sel.
sight of - sil.
amel. - mag-c., nat-m.
aversion to - acet-ac., allox., arund., bufo, ***carb-v., carc.,*** card-m., chin., clem., ***con.,*** **COR-R.,** cortico., dros., elaps, ***fl-ac.,*** **GRAPH.,** lyc., lyss., ***merc., nat-m.,*** nit-ac., phos., puls., ***sel., sep.,*** sil.
desires - acet-ac., aeth., ***aloe,*** aq-mar., **ARG-N.,** atro., aur-m-n., ***bac., calc.,*** calc-f., ***calc-p.,*** calc-s., **CARB-V.,** ***carc., caust., chin.,*** cocc., ***con., cor-r.,*** dys-co., **LAC-C.,** ***lycps., lyss., manc., med., meph.,*** merc., merc-i-f., merc-i-r., morg., **NAT-M., NIT-AC.,** ***ph-ac.,*** **PHOS.,** ***plb.,*** prot., ***sanic.,*** scarl., sel., sil., staph., sulph., ***tarent.,*** teucr., ***thuj., tub.,*** uva., **VERAT.**
pregnancy, during - ***nat-m., verat.***
salt and sweets - **ARG-N.,** ***calc.,*** calc-p., calc-s., carb-v., ***med.,*** nat-m., ***phos.,*** plb., sulph., tub.

SEWER-gas, poisoning - anthr., ***bapt.,*** phyt., pyrog., ***tub.***

SILICA, poisoning, silicosis - agar-t., ars., brom., **CALC.,** camph., **FL-AC.,** hep., ictod., ip., ***lyc.,*** mag-m., merc., nat-c., nat-a., nit-ac., penic., ph-ac., ***puls.,*** **SIL.,** sulph.

SILVER nitrate, abuse of - arg-n., ***nat-m.***
cauterization, to antidote - arg-n., ***nat-m.***

SMOKE, agg. - calc., caust., carb-v., ***euphr.,*** **IGN.,** nat-m., nux-v., olnd., ***sep.,*** **SPIG.,** sulph.

STIMULANTS, agg. - agar., ant-c., chion., fl-ac., ***glon.,*** ign., lach., led., naja, ***nux-v.,*** op., thuj., ***zinc.***
amel. - gels., glon.
desires - alco., aloe, ant-t., ars-s-f., aster., aur., aur-s., calc-i., caps., caust., chin., crot-h., ***fl-ac.,*** gins., hep., iber., iod., kali-i., mur-ac., naja, nat-p., **NUX-V.,** ***puls.,*** sol-t-ae., staph., sul-i., ***sulph.,*** sumb., tab., ziz.

STONE-cutters, ailments in - **CALC.,** ip., ***lyc.,*** nat-c., nit-ac., ph-ac., ***puls.,*** **SIL.,** sulph.
stone cutter's tuberculosis - calc., lyc., sil.

STRAMONIUM, abuse of - acet-ac., ***bell., hyos.,*** stram., nux-v., tab.

STRYCHNINE, abuse of - cham., cur., ***eucal.,*** kali-br., ***nux-v.,*** phys.

SUGAR, (see Sweets) abuse of - **ARG-N.,** ***lyc.,*** merc., nat-p., phos.
agg. - **ARG-N.,** bell., ***calc.,*** **LYC.,** ***merc.,*** nat-p., ox-ac., ***phos.,*** sang., ***sel.,*** **SULPH.,** thuj., zinc.
aversion to - ars., caust., chloram., ***graph.,*** merc., phos., rauw., sin-n., ***zinc.***
desires - am-c., am-m., **ARG-N.,** ***calc.,*** cann-i., carc., dys-co., ***kali-c.,*** **LYC.,** op., ***phos.,*** prot., ***sec.,*** sulph.
can only digest if eats large amounts of sugar - nux-v., **STAPH.**
evening - ***arg-n.***
sugared water - bufo, sulph.

SULPHUR, abuse of - acon., ars., ***calc.,*** camph., cham., chin., iod., ***merc.,*** nit-ac., nux-v., **PULS.,** rhus-t., sel., sep., sulph., thuj.

TAR, abuse of, from local applications - bov., zinc.

TEA, abuse of - abies-n., ***chin., dios.,*** ferr., puls., ***sel.,*** thuj.
agg. - abies-c., ***abies-n., aesc.,*** agar., ars., aur-m., calad., cham., ***chin.,*** cocc., coff., dios., ***ferr.,*** fl-ac., hep., kali-bi., lach., lob., ***nux-v.,*** ph-ac., puls., ***rhus-t.,*** rumx., **SEL., SEP.,** ***spig.,*** stroph., ***thuj.,*** verat.
ailments from - abies-n., ***chin.,*** cocc., dios., lob., ***nux-v.,*** sel., thuj.
amel. - aloe, carb-ac., dig., ferr., glon., kali-bi., pyrus.
aversion to - carb-ac., carb-an., chin., dios., ferr-m., kali-p., ***phos., sel.,*** thea., thuj., trinit.
desires - alum., aster., calc-s., ***chin.,*** hep., hydr., lepi., nux-v., ***puls.,*** pyrus, sel., thuj., uran-n.
tea grounds - ***alum.***

TOBACCO, general
abdomen, colicky pains after smoking - bufo.
heat in abdomen rises into chest, rest of body chilly, after smoking - ***spong.***
pain in bowels, better after smoking - ***coloc.***
abuse of - ***abies-n.,*** arg-n., ***ars.,*** **CALAD.,** calc-p., camph., chin., chin-a., coca, ***gels., ign., ip.,*** kalm., lob., lyc., mur-ac., ***nicot., nux-v., phos., plan.,*** plb., scut., ***sep., spig.,*** staph., stroph., tab., thuj., verat.
boys, in - arg-n., ars., calad., verat.
addiction, nicotine - aven., calad., ign., nicot., nux-v., tab.
agg. - ***abies-n.,*** acon., act-sp., agar., ***alum., alumn.,*** ambr., anac., ang., arg-m., arg-n., **ARS.,** ars-i., asc-t., aur-m-n., bell., bor., brom., ***bry.,*** cact., ***calad.,*** calc., calc-caust., calc-p., ***camph.,*** cann-i., carb-an., carb-s., caust., cham., chel., chin., chin-a., chin-m., cic., ***clem.,*** coca, coc-c., ***cocc., coff.,*** coloc., con., conv., cupr., ***cycl.,*** dig., dor., ***euphr.,*** ferr., ***gels., hell.,*** hep., hydr., **IGN.,** iod., ***ip.,*** kali-bi., kali-br., kalm., lac-ac., ***lach.,*** lob., ***lyc., mag-c.,*** mag-m., man., ***meny.,*** merc., mur-ac., naja, nat-c., ***nat-m.,*** nicot., **NUX-V.,** okou.,

TOBACCO, general
agg. - olnd., osm., ***par.,*** petr., ***phos.,*** **PLAN.,** plb., psil., **PULS.,** rad-br., ran-b., rhus-t., ***ruta,*** sabad., sabin., sars., scut., sec., ***sel.,*** sep., sil., sol-m., **SPIG., SPONG., STAPH.,** stel., stroph., sulph., tab., ***tarax., thuj.,*** verat.
smokers, in - sec.
smoking, from - alum., ***chin.,*** dor., gels., lac-ac., sec.
when breaking off - aven., ***calad.***
ailments, from - abies-n., arg-n., ***ars.,*** **CALAD.,** chin-a., coca, con., ***ip., lach.,*** lob., ***lyc., nicot.,*** **NUX-V.,** ***phos., plan.,*** scut., sep., spig., staph., stroph., ***thuj.,*** verat.
amel. from tobacco - aran., aran-ix., arn., bor., carb-ac., ***coloc., hep.,*** levo., merc., naja, nat-c., plat., ***sep.,*** spig., stront-c., tarent., tarent-c.
angina pectoris, from - ***nux-v.***
aversion, to - acon., acon-l., alum., ***ant-t.,*** arg-n., ***arn.,*** asar., bell., bor., brom., bry., **CALC.,** ***camph., canth., carb-an.,*** chin., chlor., cimic., clem., cocc., coff., con., grat., **IGN.,** ip., jug-r., kali-bi., ***lach.,*** led., ***lob., lyc.,*** mag-aust., mag-s., man., meph., mez., nat-a., ***nat-m.,*** nux-m., **NUX-V.,** olnd., ***op.,*** par., ***phos.,*** phyt., plan., plat., psor., **PULS.,** rhus-t., sars., sep., ***spig.,*** stann., staph., stry., ***sulph.,*** tarax., thuj., til., valer., zing.
morning - meph.
sensitive to smell of - agar., ars-h., ***asc-t., bell., casc.,*** chin., **IGN.,** ***lob., lyc.,*** lyss., ***nux-v.,*** phos., puls., sol-n., tab.
cannot bear the smell - ign., ***lob.***
tobacco smoke - ant-t., arn., brom., calc., carb-an., ***casc.,*** coc-c., ign., lach., lyc., nux-v., puls., spig., tarax.
aversion, to smoking - alum., alum-p., ant-t., arg-m., ***arn.,*** asar., bell., bor., ***brom.,*** bry., ***calc.,*** calc-p., ***camph.,*** canth., carb-an., ***casc.,*** chen-a., chin., clem., coc-c., cocc., coff., con., crot-h., euphr., ferr., ferr-i., grat., **IGN.,** ip., jug-r., kali-bi., kali-n., lac-ac., lach., led., lob., ***lyc.,*** mag-s., meph., mez., nat-a., nat-m., nat-s., nicc., nux-m., ***nux-v.,*** olnd., op., ox-ac., par., phos., plat., psor., ***puls.,*** rhus-t., sars., sep., spig., stann., staph., ***sulph.,*** tarax., tell., thuj.
afternoon - ign.
bitter taste - ang.
breakfast, after - psor.
evening - ***arg-n.***
forenoon - kali-bi.
morning - ox-ac.
smoke does not taste well - ang., hyper.
smoking without relish - ars-h.
taste of his cigar, to - brom., chen-a., ferr., ***ign.***
bladder, strangury and retention of urine - ***op.***
belching, after smoking, alternating with hiccough - agar.
burning, in syphilis - ***lyc.***
breathing, agg., after smoking - ***op.***
asthma, after smoking - asc-t., calad., lob.

TOBACCO, general
- **chewing,** agg. - **ARS.,** carb-v., ign., lyc., nux-v., ***plan.,*** sel., tab., ***verat.***
  - bad effects from - ***ars.,*** carb-v., lyc., ***nux-v., plan., sep.,*** tab., ***verat.***
- **cough,** smoke agg. - brom., ***coloc., nux-v.***
  - attacks after smoking - agar., arg-n., bry.
  - causes and aggravates - ***iod.***
  - smoke excites cough - staph.
- **convulsions,** tetanic, from swallowing - ***ip.***
- **desire,** for smoking - ***ars., asar.,*** bell., **CALAD.,** ***calc-p., camph.,*** carb-ac., carb-an., carb-v., card-m., cast-eq., ***chin.,*** chlor., ***coca,*** coff., con., daph., eug., ***glon.,*** ham., kreos., led., lyc., manc., med., nat-c., ***nicot., nux-v.,*** ox-ac., ***phos.,*** plan., plat., plb., rhus-t., ***spig., staph.,*** **TAB.,** ther., ***thuj.***
  - dinner, after - nat-c.
  - evening - ox-ac.
  - smoking unpleasant first day, but after first week a crazy, insatiable desire to smoke, does not allow pipe to cool - lyss.
  - snuff - ***bell.***
  - wants to do nothing but smoke all day - eug.
- **diarrhea,** after smoking, agg. - ***cham.***
  - as if it would set in after smoking - bor.
- **disgust** for, remedies to stimulate - arg-n., ars., **CALAD.,** calc., cal-p., camph., ***caust.,*** con., ign., lach., nep., nicot., nux-v., petr., plan., **STAPH.,** stry., sulph., tab.
- **dyspepsia,** from smoking - acon., ant-c., arn., ***ars.,*** bry., cham., chin., clem., cocc., coloc., cupr., euph., ign., ***ip., lach., lyc., merc.,*** nat-c., nat-m., **NUX-V.,** phos., ***plan.,*** puls., sep., spong., staph., verat.
- **eyes,** weak sighted, after smoking - asc-t.
  - pressure in eyes, after smoking - calad.
- **feet,** smoking causes cramp in soles - calad.
- **fingers,** itching after smoking, when lying down - calad.
- **headache,** from smoking - acet-ac., acon., alum., ***ant-t., bell.,*** brom., calad., calc., caust., clem., cocc., coc-c., ferr., ferr-i., ***gels.,*** glon., **IGN.,** ***lob.,*** mag-c., **NAT-A.,** nat-m., nux-v., op., par., petr., plan., ***puls.,*** sil., spig., thuj., zinc.
  - smoking tobacco, amel. - am-c., ***aran.,*** calc-p., ***carb-ac.,*** naja
- **heart,** symptoms of circulation worse after smoking - ***spong.***
  - palpitation - ***acon.,*** **NUX-V.,** ***phos.***
  - slow soft pulse - apoc.
- **hiccough,** during smoking - puls., sang.
  - smoking, after - calen., ***ign.,*** puls.
- **impotence,** from - ***lyc.***
- **intoxicated,** feeling, after smoking - asc-t.
- **legs,** weakness, from smoking - ***clem.***
- **mouth,** smoking causes dryness - chlor.
  - peeling of inside of lips, after smoking - agar.
- **nausea,** smoking, after - agar., brom., calad., ***calc., calc-p., clem., ign.,*** **IP.,** ***kali-bi., lob.,*** **NUX-V.,** spong., ***tab.***
  - nauseous taste, from smoking - **PULS.**

TOBACCO, general
- **neurosis** cordis, from - agarin., ars., calad., ***conv.,*** dig., ***kalm.,*** lyc., nux-v., ***phos., spig.,*** staph., ***stroph.,*** tab., verat.
- **nervous** depression - ***ars., coca, gels., nux-v.,*** sep.
- **neuralgia** - ***plan.***
- **paralysis,** from abuse of nicotine - nux-v.
- **prostatorrhea,** worse after smoking - ***daph.***
- **restless,** after smoking cannot control himself - calad.
- **sensitive** to - ars-h., ***asc-t., ign., lyss.***
  - smell to, tastes snuff while box is one foot distant - lyss.
- **sleep,** insomnia - ***nux-v.***
- **snuff,** aversion to - spig.
  - desires - ***bell.***
- **stomach,** gastro-intestinal symptoms worse after chewing - ***ars.***
- **stool,** smoking causes urging to - calad.
- **sweat,** and trembling after smoking - ***nat-m.***
- **tastes** bitter - ***cocc.***
  - after smoking - asar.
  - rough, after smoking - casc.
  - when smoking - **CHIN.**
  - biting on tongue - cocc-s.
  - scratchy, bitter in mouth and fauces - ***spong.***
  - smoking, tasteless - ars-h.
  - tasteless - ant-t.
- **thirst,** violent, after smoking - 2spong.
- **throat,** burning and acidity from cardia - chel.
  - chronic inflammation in smoker - ***nat-m.***
  - smoking makes dry, and he does not enjoy it - verat.
- **toothache** - clem., ***spig.***
  - aggravates - ***ign.***
  - better painful jerks in nerve of a hollow tooth - spig.
  - jerking toothache after smoking - ***bry.***
  - smoking relieves - bor., ***nat-c.***
- **vomiting** - ***ip.***
  - smoking, after - agar., calad.
- **weakness,** from - calad., clem., hep.

TONICS, agg. - carb-ac.
- aversion to - sul-ac.
- desires - aloe, caps., carb-ac., carb-an., caust., ***cocc.,*** gels., med., ***nux-v., rhus-t., ph-ac.,*** phos., ***puls.,*** rheum, sul-ac., sulph., ***valer.***

TURPENTINE, abuse of - ter., nux-m.

VACCINATIONS, ailments, after - ***acon., ant-t., apis, ars., bell.,*** bufo., ***calc.,*** **CARC.,** crot-h., echi., graph., hep., kali-chl., ***kali-m.,*** lac-v., **MALAND.,** ***merc.,*** merc-sul., **MEZ.,** ***ped., per.,*** phos., plan., ***psor.,*** puls., rhus-t., sabin., sarr., **SARS.,** sep., **SIL.,** skook., **SULPH.,** syc-co., **THUJ., TUB., VAC.,** ***vario.***
- abscess in axilla - **SIL.**
- acute reactions - acon., apis., arn., bell., calen., cic., ***hyper., led.,*** plan., thuj.,
- allergy, shots, ailments from - ***thuj.***
- asthma, after - **ANT-T.,** carc., ***sil.,*** **THUJ.**

VACCINATIONS, ailments
atrophy of right arm, after revaccination - thuj.
backache, since - **SIL.**
condylomata, consists of a number of pointed, which could be separated by a fine probe, roundish, ulcerating edge - thuj.
conjunctivitis - thuj.
convulsions - **SIL.**
cough, after - ant-t., carc., sil., ***thuj.***
whooping cough, immediately, in two scrofulous boys - ***thuj.***
diarrhea - ***sil.,*** thuj.
eruptions, after - mez., sars., sil., skook., thuj.
itch like, depriving child of sleep - ***mez.,*** psor.
erysipelas, dark and thickened, skin - crot-h.
fever, with backache, headache - **SIL.**
headache, after - sil., thuj.
imbecility, after - thuj.
influenza shots, ailments, after - carc., gels., thuj.
keratitis - vac., vario.
nausea, from - **SIL.**
preventive, for side effects - **HYPER., LED.,** sil., sulph., ***thuj.,*** vario.
pustular eruption - ***crot-h.***
on head - sulph.
pustules, itching, burning - psor.
redness, erysipelatous - ***apis***
sleeplessness - carc., ***thuj.***
speech, loss of - thuj.
swellings over whole arm, red and inflamed - **SIL.**
tuberculosis, incipient - tub.

Urine

ACETONURIA - acetan., ars., aur-m., calc., ***calc-mur.,*** carb-ac., ***caust.,*** cic., colch., cupr-ar., euon., ***insulin,*** nat-sal., phos., ***senn.***

ACRID - acon., ail., alum., alumn., ant-t., **ARN.,** arund., asaf., astac., atro., aur-m., **BENZ-AC.,** ***bor.,*** brach., ***calc., cann-s.,*** canth., caps., carb-s., ***card-m., caust., chel.,*** chin-s., ***clem.,*** colch., ***coc-c., cupr., cycl.,*** dig., ***dulc.,*** euon., ***fl-ac., graph.,*** **HEP.,** ign., ***iod., kali-bi., kali-c., kreos.,*** **LAUR.,** ***lith.,*** lyc., med., **MERC., MERC-C.,** mur-ac., ***nat-m., nat-s., nit-ac.,*** nit-m-ac., nux-v., oci., par., petr., ***phos., plan.,*** prun., puls., rhus-t., sabin., ***sars.,*** senec., ***seneg., sep., staph.,*** stann., **SULPH.,** tell., ***thuj., uran.,*** urt-u., ***uva.,*** verat.
- menses, during - ***alum.,*** apis, nat-m.

ALBUMINOUS, proteinuria - acetan., acon., adon., all-c., all-s., alum., ***am-be.,*** am-caust., ant-c., ***ant-t.,*** **APIS,** apoc., arg-m., ***arg-n.,*** **ARS.,** ***ars-i., aur.,*** **AUR-M.,** ***aur-m-n., berb.,*** bism., ***brach.,*** bry., cahin., ***calc.,*** **CALC-AR.,** ***cann-s., canth., carb-ac., carb-s., carb-v.,*** caul., chel., ***chim., chin., chin-a.,*** chin-s., cinnb., chlol., coc-c., coch., ***colch.,*** conv., cop., ***crot-c., crot-h., cupr.,*** cupr-ac., cupr-ar., cupr-s., ***dig., dulc.,*** equis., ***euon.,*** eup-pur., ***ferr., ferr-ar., ferr-i.,*** ferr-p., ferr-pic., form., fuch., ***gels.,*** **GLON., HELL.,** ***helon., hep., hippoz., iod., kali-bi., kali-c., kali-chl., kali-i.,*** kali-n., kali-p., kali-s., ***kalm.,*** **LAC-D.,** ***lach.,*** lec., lith., **LYC.,** lycps., mag-m., med., ***merc.,*** **MERC-C.,** ***merc-cy., merc-i-r.,*** methyl-b., mez., morph., mur-ac., myric., **NAT-A., NAT-C.,** ***nat-m.,*** **NAT-P.,** ***nat-s., nit-ac.,*** oci., ol-j., ol-sant., op., osm., ***petr.,*** **PH-AC.,** ***phos., phyt., pic-ac.,*** **PLB.,** polyg., puls., ***pyrog.,*** rad., **RHUS-T.,** ***sabin., sal-ac.,*** sars., ***sec.,*** sil., squil., ***stroph., sulph.,*** sul-ac., tab., ***tarent.,*** tax., **TER.,** thuj., thyr., tub., ***uran-n.,*** urea, valer., vanad., ***visc.,*** zinc.
- alcohol, after abuse of - **ARS.,** aur., bell., ***berb., calc-ar.,*** **CARB-V.,** ***chin., crot-h.,*** cupr., ferr., ***lach.,*** led., merc., ***nat-c., nux-v.,*** sulph.
- amaurosis - ***apis, ars.,*** cann-i., colch., ***gels., hep.,*** kalm., ***merc-c.,*** phos., ph-ac., plb.
- chronic - ***atro., cedr.,*** glon., ***petr., plb.***
- cold and dampness, from exposure to - ***calc., colch., dulc.,*** kali-c., merc-c., nux-v., ***rhus-t.,*** sep.
- diphtheria after - ***ars., apis, carb-ac.,*** hell., hep., kali-chl., lach., lyc., ***merc-c.,*** merc-cy., phyt.
- heart, disease, consecutive to - apis, apoc., ***ars.,*** ars-i., ***aur.,*** **CALC-AR.,** coc-c., ***colch., crot-h., cupr., dig.,*** glon., kali-bi., kali-p., ***kalm., lach.,*** lyc., ***lycps.,*** petr., ph-ac., ***ter.,*** uran.
- hypertension, with - visc.
  - orthostatic - tub.
- insanity, during - phyt.
- menses, during - helon.
- periodical - phos.

ALBUMINOUS, proteinuria
- pregnancy, during - **APIS,** apoc., ***ars.,*** ars-i., ***aur-m.,*** benz-ac., berb., bry., cact., ***calc-ac., canth., chin.,*** cinnb., ***colch., crot-h., cupr-ar.,*** dig., dulc., ferr., ***gels.,*** glon., hell., ***helon.,*** ind., ***kali-ar.,*** kali-br., ***kali-c., kali-chl.,*** kalm., ***lach.,*** led., ***lyc., merc.,*** **MERC-C.,** ***nat-m., ph-ac., phos.,*** rhus-t., sabin., senec., ***sep.,*** sulph., ***ter.,*** thlaspi, thyr., uran., ***verat-v.***
  - and after delivery - ***merc-c.,*** ph-ac., ***pyrog.***
  - kidneys inflammation, with - ***crot-h.***
- scarlet fever, after - **APIS,** ***ars.,*** asc-t., ***aur-m.,*** bell., bry., ***canth.,*** carb-ac., coch., ***colch., con.,*** cop., crot-h., dig., dulc., ***glon., hell.,*** helon., ***hep.,*** kali-c., ***kali-chl., kali-s., lach.,*** **LYC.,** ***merc-c.,*** **NAT-S.,** ***phos.,*** phyt., rhus-t., ***sec.,*** senec., ***stram., ter.,*** uran.
- septic - carb-v., ***crot-h.,*** pyrog.
- syphilitics, in - ***aur.,*** aur-i., **AUR-M.,** ***aur-m-n.,*** kali-bi., kali-i., ***merc-c.,*** nit-ac., sars.

ALKALINE - am-c., am-caust., **BAPT.,** ***benz-ac., canth.,*** **CARB-AC.,** chin-s., chlor., cina, ***ferr., fl-ac., hyos., kali-a., kali-bi., kali-c.,*** kreos., mag-p., med., morph., ***nat-m., ph-ac.,*** plb., stram., uran., xan.

ALTERNATION, copious and scanty urine - ***berb.,*** dig., gels., sang.

BILE, containing - ***acon., card-m.,*** cean., ***chel.,*** **CHION.,** ***con., crot-h.,*** cupr-s., kali-chl., kali-i., ***mag-m., merc., myric., nat-s., nit-ac.,*** osm., phos., ***sang., sep.,*** sulph., uran., valer.

BITING - sel.

BLACK - ang., ***apis,*** arn., ***ars., ars-h., benz-ac., benz-d-n., canth.,*** **CARB-AC.,** chion., cina, **COLCH.,** ***dig.,*** erig., ***hell.,*** kali-ar., ***kali-c., kali-chl.,*** kreos., **LACH.,** merc-c., naphtin., ***nat-m.,*** nicc., ***pareir., phos.,*** sec., **TER.,** verat.
- ink, like - arn., **COLCH.**

BLACKISH - kali-c.

BLOODY - ***acon.,*** aloe, alumn., ambr., am-c., ant-c., ***ant-t.,*** **APIS, ARG-N., ARN., ARS.,** ars-h., aspar., ***aur., bell.,*** benz-ac., ***berb.,*** **BOTH., CACT.,** cadm-s., **CALC.,** ***camph.,*** **CANN-S., CANTH.,** ***caps.,*** carb-s., ***carb-v., caust., chim.,*** chin., ***chin-a.,*** chin-s., cimic., **COC-C.,** ***colch.,*** coloc., ***con., cop.,*** crot-c., **CROT-H.,** cub., cupr., cupr-s., dulc., equis., epig., ***erig.,*** eucal., ferr., ***ferr-ar.,*** ferr-m., ferr-p., gall-ac., ger., **HAM.,** ***hell.,*** hep., hydrang., ***hyper.,*** **IP.,** jatr., ***kali-ar., kali-chl.,*** kali-i., kali-n., kalm., ***kreos., lach., lyc., merc.,*** **MERC-C.,** ***mez.,*** **MILL.,** murx., ***nat-m., nit-ac., nux-v.,*** oci., ol-sant., ***op.,*** ox-ac., pall., pareir., petr., ***ph-ac.,*** **PHOS.,** pic-ac., ***plb.,*** psor., **PULS.,** rhod., ***rhus-a., rhus-t.,*** sabad., ***sabin.,*** sant., ***sars.,*** **SEC.,** ***senec., sep.,*** **SQUIL.,** stigm., ***sulph., sul-ac.,*** tab., tarent., **TER.,** ***thlaspi,*** thuj., tub., urea, uva., vesp., vib., ***zinc.***
- backache, with - kali-bi.
- childbed, in - **BUFO.**

BLOODY, urine
chronic - ***erig.***
clots - ***alumn.,*** apis, ars., ***cact.,*** canth., ***chim.,*** coc-c., colch., ***ip., lyc., mill., ph-ac., plat.,*** puls.
putrid, decomposed blood, of - colch.
constipation, with - lyc.
cramps in bladder, after - mez.
cutting in abdomen and urethra, with - ip.
dysentery in - cop., ***ip., merc-c.***
excitement, after - phos.
first part - con.
hemorrhoidal flow or menses, after sudden stopping of - ***nux-v.***
last part - ***ant-t.,*** canth., ferr-p., **HEP.,** lyc., ***mez., puls., sars.,*** thuj., zinc.
mixed with blood and pus - ***sars.***
violent pain in the bladder, with - ant-t., ***sars.***
menses, suppressed, from - laur., lyc., mez., mill., nux-v., senec.
night - ***caust.***
paraplegia, with - lyc.
pathological cause, without - bell., phos.
sexual excesses, after - ***phos.***
shivering along spine, with - nit-ac.
urination, after, blood flows from urethra - **HEP.,** lmez., puls., sars., sulph., ***thuj.***
frequent - ham.
urging for, with - sabin.
water-like - pall.

BLUISH - nit-ac.
containing indican - pic-ac.

BROWN - ***acon.,*** alum., alumn., ***ambr.,*** ant-c., apis, arg-n., **ARN., ARS.,** ***asaf.,*** bar-c., bell., **BENZ-AC.,** brom., **BRY.,** bufo, calc., camph., ***canth., carb-ac.,*** carb-v., ***card-m.,*** **CHEL.,** chin-s., ***cimx.,*** coc-c., ***colch.,*** coloc., ***con.,*** crot-h., cupr., ***dig.,*** dros., fl-ac., graph., ***hell.,*** hep., ip., kali-bi., kali-c., kali-chl., kali-i., ***kreos.,*** lach., lact., lil-t., lyc., ***manc.,*** merc., **MERC-C.,** ***myric.,*** nat-c., nat-hchls., nat-m., ***nit-ac., nux-v.,*** olnd., op., petr., ph-ac., ***phos.,*** phyt., pic-ac., plb., prun., ***puls., rhus-t., sec.,*** sep., squil., staph., stram., sulph., sul-ac., tarent., ***ter.,*** valer., zinc.
beer, like - ***aspar., benz-ac., bry.,*** **CHEL.,** ***coloc., hyper.,*** phos., puls., stry., **SULPH.**
chestnut - ***kreos.***
cow-dung with water, like - **ARS.**
dark - ***acon.,*** aesc., all-c., ***all-s., ambr.,*** ant-t., ***arn., ars.,*** asaf., ***bar-c., calc.,*** camph., ***carb-ac., caust.,*** **CHEL.,** ***colch., dig., eup-pur., graph.,*** jatr., ***lach., lept., lyc., merc.,*** nit-ac., ***op.,*** osm., petr., phos., ***plb., podo., psor.,*** puls., ***sec.,*** **SEP.,** sulph., tab., valer., zing.
prune juice, like, or prune colored - sec.
fever, during - ***acon.,*** arn., ***bell.,*** bry., carb-v., ip., lyc., ***nux-v.,*** puls., rhus-t., **SEP., VERAT.**
menses, during - eupi., nat-m.

BROWN, urine
perspiration, during - acon., ant-t., arn., **ARS.,** bell., bry., ***calc.,*** canth., carb-v., hep., ip., ***merc.,*** puls., ***sel.,*** **SEP.,** staph., ***sulph.,*** thuj., ***verat.***
reddish - ant-c., bell., **BENZ-AC.,** ***canth.,*** **CHEL.,** dig., iod., lyc., nat-a., phos., plb., sep., sul-ac., verat.
yellowish - ***ambr., dig.,*** lyss., squil.

BURNING, hot urine - ***acon., aesc.,*** agar., agn., **ALOE,** all-c., alum., alumn., ***ambr.,*** am-c., am-m., ang., ***ant-c., ant-t.,*** **APIS,** apoc., arg-m., ***arg-n.,*** arn., **ARS.,** ***asaf.,*** asc-c., aspar., aur., aur-m., bapt., bar-c., bar-m., **BELL.,** ***benz-ac., berb.,*** bov., **BOR.,** ***bry.,*** cact., calad., calc., ***calc-p.,*** **CAMPH., CANN-I., CANN-S., CANTH.,** ***caps.,*** carb-an., carb-s., carb-v., caust., ***cham., chel., chim.,*** chin., chin-a., chin-s., cimic., ***clem.,*** cob., coc-c., ***colch.,*** coloc., ***con.,*** conv., ***cop.,*** cor-r., crot-t., **CUB.,** cupr., cur., ***dig.,*** dulc., erig., ***eup-pur.,*** equis., ery-a., eug., ***ferr.,*** ferr-ar., ferr-p., ***fl-ac.,*** glon., grat., helon., **HEP.,** hydr-ac., ign., indg., ***ip., kali-ar.,*** kali-bi., ***kali-c., kali-i., kali-n.,*** kali-p., kali-s., kalm., kreos., ***lach.,*** lact., laur., ***lil-t., lyc.,*** mag-c., med., **MERC., MERC-C.,** ***mez.,*** mur-ac., mygal., **NAT-A., NAT-C.,** nat-m., nat-p., **NAT-S.,** nicc., **NIT-AC.,** nux-m., **NUX-V.,** olnd., op., ox-ac., pareir., par., petr., ***petros., ph-ac.,*** phos., pic-ac., plb., prun., psor., ***puls.,*** ran-s., rhod., ***rhus-r., rhus-t.,*** sabad., ***sabin.,*** sang., ***sars.,*** sec., senec., seneg., sep., sil., spig., squil., ***staph.,*** stram., **SULPH.,** sul-ac., tab., ***tarent., ter.,*** **THUJ., UVA.,** verat., vesp., viol-t., zinc.
acid, as from - ox-ac.
children - bor.
constipation, with - ferr.
coryza, fluent, with - ran-s.
menorrhagia, with - ferr.
menses, during - nux-v., zinc.
before - apis, ***canth.,*** verat., zinc.
urination, before and after - seneg.

CASTS, containing - ***apis, ars.,*** aur-m., brach., ***canth., carb-ac.,*** chel., crot-h., kali-chl., merc-c., nat-a., nat-hchls, phos., pic-ac., plb., puls-n, rad., sul-ac., uran-n., vanad.
blood - ***plb., ter.***
epithelial - ***apis,*** ant-t., arg-n., **ARS.,** bell., brach., cact., canth., carb-ac., chel., crot-h., ***eran.,*** hep., kali-bi., lycps., **MERC-C.,** ***phos.,*** pic-ac., ***plb.,*** sul-ac., ter.
fat drops, with - ***merc-c.,*** **PHOS.,** ph-ac.
fibrous - cann-s., cimic., ***kalm.,*** phos., ph-ac., sul-ac.
granular - canth., carb-ac., carc., coc-c., ***merc-c.,*** nat-h., ***petr.,*** phos., pic-ac., ***plb.,*** sul-ac.
hyaline - carb-ac., brach., med., ***petr., phos., plb.***
infants, in - bor.
mucous - brach., cann-s., cimic.
pale - sul-ac.

CASTS, containing
tubes, of - ant-c., **APIS,** bism., ***canth., cimic., hep., merc-c.,*** phos., pic-ac., ***plb.,*** sulph., ***ter.***
waxy - brach., morph., ***phos.***
yellowish - sul-ac.

CLAY - agar., anac., berb., cor-r., laur., nat-m., sabad., sars., **SEP.,** sul-ac., zinc.
shaking, on - anac.
standing, on - cham., ferr-m., laur.

CLOUDY - acet-ac., ***acon., aesc.,*** agar., agn., aloe, alum., alumn., ***ambr., anac.,*** am-c., am-m., ***ant-c., ant-t.,*** **APIS,** apoc., arg-m., ***arn., ars.,*** ars-i., aspar., ***aur.,*** aur-m., ***bell.,*** benz-ac., **BERB.,** bov., brom., **BRY.,** ***cact.,*** calad., ***calc.,*** calc-f., camph., ***cann-s.,*** **CANTH.,** carb-an., **CARB-S., CARB-V.,** ***card-m., caust.,*** **CHAM., CHEL., CHIN.,** chin-a., ***chin-s.,*** **CINA,** cinnb., clem., coca, coc-c., ***colch., coloc.,*** com., **CON.,** cop., crot-h., crot-t., ***cupr.,*** cur., cycl., ***daph., dig., dulc.,*** elaps, ferr., ferr-ar., ***gels.,*** **GRAPH.,** ***grat., hep.,*** hyos., hydr-ac., hyper., ign., indg., iod., ***ip.,*** kali-a., kali-ar., kali-bi., ***kali-c.,*** kali-chl., kali-i., ***kali-n., kali-p.,*** kali-s., kreos., ***lac-c., lach.,*** laur., lith., ***lyc.,*** lyss., mag-c., ***mag-m.,*** **MERC.,** ***merc-c.,*** mez., **MYRIC.,** nat-c., ***nat-m.,*** nat-p., ***nit-ac., nux-v.,*** olnd., ***op.,*** pall., par., ***petr.,*** **PH-AC., PHOS.,** plat., ***plb., psor., puls.,*** raph., rat., rhod., rhus-t., rumx., **SABAD.,** sabin., sarr., ***sars.,*** sec., ***seneg.,*** **SEP.,** sil., stram., **SULPH.,** sul-ac., ***thuj.,*** uva., valer., verat., viol-t., zinc., zing.
brown - petr.
chalk had been stirred into it, as if - alum., ***ph-ac., sulph.***
fever, with - ars., bell., berb., bry., lyc., ***phos.,*** ph-ac., puls., rhus-t., sabad., sars., sep.
gray clouds - lyc.
limewater - sep.
morning - berb., cann-s., meph., zinc.
standing, on - chel., chin-a., dig.
night - alum., kali-bi., phos., sulph.
passed, when - ***ambr.,*** anac., ***ars.,*** aspar., **CANTH.,** carb-an., **CHEL.,** colch., dulc., ***hep.,*** hyos., ***merc.,*** mur-ac., nat-a., ***rhus-t.,*** sabin., sant., ***sars., sep.,*** sulph., **TER.,** verat., zinc.
soon after - ang., aspar., bar-c., **BERB.,** ***cham.,*** **CHEL.,** coloc., ***lyc.,*** nat-c., rhus-t., seneg., sil.
perspiration, with - chin., cina, con., dulc., ign., **IP., MERC., PHOS.,** puls., rhus-t., sabad., sep.
reddish clouds - ambr., kali-n.
standing, on - acet-ac., agar., aloe, alum., alumn., ambr., am-c., am-m., ang., ant-t., ***apis,*** arg-n., arn., ***ars.,*** aur., bar-c., **BELL.,** ***berb.,*** bov., brom., **BRY.,** ***calc., carb-s., caust.,*** **CHAM., CHEL., CHIN.,** ***chin-s.,*** cimic., ***cina,*** coc-c., ***coloc., con.,*** crot-t., ***cupr., dig., dulc.,*** equis., ery-a., ferr., ferr-ar., ferr-p., **GRAPH.,** ***grat., hep.,*** kali-n., kreos., lach., ***laur.,*** lob., **LYC.,** mag-m., manc., mang., ***meph., merc., mez.,*** nat-c., ***nit-ac.,*** olnd., ol-an., ***par., petr.,*** **PH-AC.,** phos., ***plat.,*** rat., ***rhus-t.,*** sabad., sang., ***sars., seneg.,*** sep., sil., squil., ***sulph.,*** sul-ac., **TER.,** ***thuj., valer.,*** verat., ***zinc.***
turning cloudy - bell., berb., **BRY.,** ***cham.,*** chel., chin., graph., lyc., ***ph-ac.,*** ter.
white clouds - cina, mur-ac., nat-m., nit-ac., ph-ac., plat., rhus-t., ***sars.***
turbid, which becomes more so as the emission continues so that the last drops look like flocks - rhus-t., ***sars., sep.***

COFFEE, like - apis, berb., cob., kali-n., lac-c., ***lach., nat-m.,*** phyt.
from admixture with blood - kali-n.

COLD - agar., ***nit-ac.***

COLORLESS - ***agar.,*** alum., anac., apis, ang., ***apoc.,*** bar-c., bell., berb., camph., **CANN-I.,** carb-ac., ***caust., cham.,*** coc-c., ***coff.,*** con., crot-h., ***dig.,*** **EQUIS.,** ***ferr.,*** **GELS.,** hyos., kali-c., kali-n., ***kreos.,*** laur., lil-t., lith., ***lycps., mag-p.,*** med., mosch., ***murx.,*** nat-a., **NAT-M.,** ***nux-v., ph-ac., phos., plan., puls.,*** rhus-t., rumx., ***sang.,*** sarr., ***sars.,*** **SEP.,** ***sil.,*** stram., stront-c., squil., ***sulph.,*** verat., vib., ust., zing.
menses, during - ***cham.,*** ph-ac., vib.
morning - kreos.
paroxysms of pain, with - phos.

CONSTITUENTS, where there is diminution of, there is increase of stools - colch.

COPIOUS - **ACET-AC.,** ***acon.,*** aesc., ***aeth., agar.,*** agn., all-c., all-s., **ALOE,** ***alum.,*** alumn., ***ambr.,*** am-c., ***am-m.,*** anac., ang., ***anthr., ant-c.,*** ant-t., ***apis, apoc.,*** **ARG-M., ARG-N.,** arn., ***ars.,*** ars-i., ***arum-t.,*** aster., **ASPAR.,** atro., ***aur., aur-m., aur-m-n., bar-c.,*** bar-m., ***bell.,*** benz-ac., berb., ***bism.,*** bov., brach., brom., bry., bufo, ***cact., cahin., calc.,*** calc-f., ***calc-p., camph.,*** **CANN-I.,** cann-s., ***canth.,*** caps., carb-ac., ***carb-an.,*** carb-s., carb-v., caust., ***chel., chim., chin.,*** chin-a., chin-s., ***chlol.,*** cic., ***cimic., cina,*** cinnb., ***clem.,*** cob., cocc., coc-c., ***coff., colch., coloc., con.,*** conv., cop., ***crot-c., crot-h.,*** crot-t., cub., ***cupr.,*** cur., ***cycl., daph., dig.,*** dros., dulc., ***echi.,*** elaps, elat., erig., **EQUIS.,** ery-a., eup-per., ***eup-pur.,*** euphr., eupi., fago., ***ferr.,*** ferr-ar., ferr-i., ferr-ma., ferr-p., ***fl-ac.,*** form., gamb., **GELS.,** gins., glon., gnaph., graph., grat., guai., ham., ***helon.,*** hell., hep., hyos., ***ign., iod., iris,*** jatr., kali-ar., ***kali-c.,*** kali-chl., ***kali-i., kali-n., kali-p., kali-s., kalm.,*** **KREOS., LAC-C.,** ***lac-d., lach.,*** lact., laur., ***lec.,*** **LED.,** ***lil-t., lith.,*** lob., ***lyc., lycps.,*** lyss., ***mag-c.,*** mag-p., ***mag-s.,*** mang., ***meli.,*** **MERC.,** ***merc-c.,*** merc-i-f., ***merc-i-r.,*** mez., morph., **MOSCH.,** ***murx.,*** **MUR-AC.,** mygal., ***nat-a.,*** **NAT-C.,** nat-m., ***nat-p.,*** **NAT-S.,** nicc., nit-ac., nux-m., ***nux-v.,*** olnd., ***ol-an.,*** op., ***ox-ac.,*** pall., par., ***petros.,*** petr., **PH-AC., PHOS.,** ***phyt.,*** pic-ac., ***plan., plb., podo., prun.,*** psor., **PULS.,** ***raph.,*** rat., rheum, ***rhod.,*** **RHUS-R., RHUS-T.,**

COPIOUS - rumx., ruta., sabad., ***sabin.***, samb., sang., sarr., ***sars.***, sec., sel., ***senec.***, ***seneg.***, sil., **SPIG.**, spong., **SQUIL.**, stann., ***staph.***, stram., stront-c., **SULPH.**, sul-ac., tab., ***tarax.***, ***tarent.***, tax., ***ter.***, ***teucr.***, ***ther.***, ***thuj.***, tril., **URAN.**, valer., ***verat.***, verat-v., **VERB.**, ***viol-t.***, vip., zinc., zing.
afternoon - ***all-c.***, aloe, alum., am-c., bor., bov., dig., laur., nat-m., nat-p., nicc., op., rumx., thuj.
siesta, after - cycl.
alternating with scanty flow - bell., ***berb.***, dig., gels., nit-ac., sang., senec.
amenorrhea with - alum., am-c., caul., ***cham.***, gels., nat-m., sulph.
apyrexis, during - ars., calc., chin., ferr., graph., nux-v., samb., valer.
bleeding, with - calc., gels., ign., lach., mosch., sars., stram., sulph., vib.
bronchitis, in - chin.
chill, during - lec.
coffee, after - cahin., olnd.
coryza, with - ***all-c.***, calc., verat.
daytime - cina, ham., pic-ac., ***sulph.***
delirium, after - ***stram.***
diarrhea - acon., bell., con., puls., spig.
dropsy, in - squil.
drunk, more than is - ambr., apis, aur., aur-m-n., ***bell.***, carb-v., caust., ***coloc.***, kali-i., kali-n., ***lac-ac.***, lac-c., lach., lyc., ***merc.***, nat-c., ***nux-v.***, ph-ac., raph., sars., sep., zinc.
eating, after - puls.
epilepsy, after - caust., ***cupr.***, lach.
evening - am-c., coloc., fl-ac., helon., kali-chl., laur., **LYC.**, lyss., op., ox-ac., pall., sang., sulph., thuj., zinc.
7 p.m. - cic., pic-ac.
8 p.m. - cic.
10 p.m. - phos.
exhaustion, attended with - acet-ac., benz-ac., ***calc-p.***, carb-ac., chin-s., ***cimic.***, dig., ferr., lyc., med.
attended with, and much thirst - chin-s.
fever, during - ant-c., arg-m., ars., ***aur-m-n.***, cedr., ***cham.***, ***colch.***, dulc., ***eup-pur.***, ***lyc.***, med., ***mur-ac.***, ph-ac., ***phos.***, squil., **STRAM.**
forenoon - arg-n., lyc., ***mez.***
headache, with - acon., ***bell.***, bov., ***canth.***, ***chin-s.***, ***cinnb.***, coloc., cupr., eug., ferr-p., ***gels.***, ***glon.***, ***ign.***, iris, kalm., lac-c., **LAC-D.**, ***lil-t.***, ***mosch.***, ***ol-an.***, sang., ***sel.***, sep., sil., uran., ***verat.***, vib., vip.
after - **ASC-C.**, gels., ign., ***iris***, nux-v., sang.
followed by copious limpid urine and vomiting - iris.
heat of body, with - samb.76
hysterical - ol-an.76
hunger and thirst, with - verat.
menses, during - canth., ***cham.***, ***hyos.***, kali-bi., lac-c., med., **PH-AC.**, ***phyt.***, sars., sulph., vib.
before - cinnb., hyos.

COPIOUS, urine
menses, begining of, at - bell.
morning - ambr., am-m., bar-ac., cahin., carb-an., equis., laur., lyc., mag-s., merc., ***mez.***, nat-c., ***nat-p.***, ***op.***, ***sars.***, sul-ac.
6 a.m. - nat-a.
nervous, women - ***ign.***
night - agar., aloe, am-c., ***am-m.***, ***ant-c.***, ant-t., ***apis***, ***arg-m.***, arg-n., ars., ***bapt.***, bar-c., ***bell.***, bov., bry., ***cact.***, calc., **CALC-F.**, ***carb-ac.***, ***carb-an.***, caust., chin., chin-a., chlol., coloc., cop., cupr., cycl., ***dig.***, euphr., ***gels.***, hyper., kali-chl., kali-n., kali-p., ***kreos.***, ***lac-c.***, ***led.***, ***lith.***, **LYC.**, mag-c., mag-p., ***med.***, ***merc.***, mez., ***murx.***, nat-a., nat-c., ***nat-m.***, nat-p., ***nat-s.***, nicc., op., petr., ***ph-ac.***, phyt., plan., prun., rhus-r., ruta., ***sang.***, ***sars.***, ***sil.***, **SPIG.**, ***stram.***, **SULPH.**, ther., ***thuj.***, **URAN.**, zinc.
lying, while - bell.
menses, before - am-m., cann-s., hyos.
menses, during - ph-ac.
midnight - coff., op.
midnight, 4 a.m. - plb.
midnight, 5 a.m. - carb-ac., ox-ac.
midnight, after - carb-ac., ox-ac., plb., **SULPH.**
stool, during - am-c., sulph.
noon - op.
pain in back, which amel. - **LYC.**, ***med.***
with paroxsms of - phos.
pains, during - arg-m., coloc., lac-d., phos., vib.
perspiration, with - **ACON.**, ant-c., bell., cham., **DULC.**, ign., lach., lyc., mag-c., ***mur-ac.***, nat-c., nat-m., **PHOS.**, ***ph-ac.***, **RHUS-T.**, samb., seneg., spig., squil., stann., stram., thuj.
scanty, then, alternating - bell., ***berb.***, dig., eup-per., gels., nit-ac., senec., sul-ac.
vomiting, with - acon., lach., verat.

CUTICLE, forming on the surface of the - agar., ***all-c.***, alum., ***alumn.***, arg-n., aspar., bell., bor-ac., calad., ***calc.***, canth., chin., chin-s., cob., coca, com., crot-t., ***dulc.***, ***graph.***, ***hep.***, iod., kali-ar., kali-bi., lac-ac., laur., ***lyc.***, ***med.***, merc-c., op., **PAR.**, ***petr.***, ph-ac., ***phos.***, pic-ac., plb., ***psor.***, puls., rumx., ***sars.***, **SEP.**, sin-a., sul-ac., sul-i., ***sulph.***, ***sumb.***, thuj., verat., verat-v., zinc.
iridescent - agar., **ALL-C.**, alumn., bapt., bell., canth., chin., coca, ***cycl.***, ***graph.***, ***hep.***, ***iod.***, op., **PAR.**, ***petr.***, **PHOS.** ***puls.***, ***sars.***, sep., sin-a., ***sulph.***, thuj.
bluish - alumn.
pellicle - coloc., ***par.***, phos., psor., puls., sep.
oily - adon., ***crot-t.***, hep., ***iod.***, lyc., petr., phos., sumb.
red - mez.
whitish - arg-n., kali-bi., merc-c., plb., sep.
morning - arg-n.

DARK - **ACON.**, ***aesc.***, agar., agn., ang., all-s., aloe, alum., am-caust., anag., ***ant-c.***, **ANT-T.**, **APIS**, apoc., arg-n., ***arn.***, ***ars.***, ***ars-i.***, asaf., asc-t., bapt., **BELL.**, **BENZ-AC.**, berb., bov., brach., brom., **BRY.**, **CALC.**, calc-f., ***calc-p.***, cann-i., ***canth.***, caps., ***carb-ac.***, carb-s., ***carb-v.***, card-m., cedr., **CHEL.**, chim., ***chin.***, ***chin-a.***, chin-s., cic., cimic., clem., cob., coc-c., **COLCH.**, con., conv., cop., **CROT-H.**, crot-t., cupr., cur., cycl., ***dig.***, echi., ***elat.***, erig., **EQUIS.**, ery-a., eug., ***eup-per.***, ferr., ferr-ar., ferr-i., ferr-p., gels., glon., graph., **HELL.**, ***hep.***, ***hydr.***, hyos., hyper., ***iod.***, ***ip.***, iris, ***jab.***, kali-ar., kali-bi., kali-c., ***kali-i.***, kali-n., kali-p., **LACH.**, **LAC-AC.**, ***lac-d.***, ***lil-t.***, ***lith.***, ***lyc.***, **MERC.**, **MERC-C.**, ***merc-i-f.***, ***merc-i-r.***, mez., mill., ***mur-ac.***, ***myric.***, ***nat-a.***, ***nat-c.***, ***nat-m.***, nat-p., nat-s., nit-ac., ***nux-m.***, ***nux-v.***, op., pall., par., petr., ph-ac., ***phos.***, pic-ac., **PLB.**, ***podo.***, ***ptel.***, ***puls.***, ***rhus-t.***, sabad., sabin., samb., sang., sars., ***sec.***, **SEL.**, senec., seneg., **SEP.**, spig., stann., ***staph.***, stram., stront-c., ***sulph.***, sul-ac., tab., tarax., tell., **TER.**, thuj., uran., valer., **VERAT.**, ***verat-v.***, vip., xan., zinc., zing.
- evening - ruta., sang., thuj.
- menses, during - nat-m., sars.
- morning - **CHEL.**, mez., sang., seneg.

FROTHY - acon., **ALL-C.**, ***apis***, arn., ars., aur., ***berb.***, carb-v., cean., **CHEL.**, ***chin.***, chin-s., clem., con., cop., crot-t., cub., glon., iris, jatr., ***kali-c.***, **LACH.**, laur., lith., **LYC.**, myric., nat-m., ***nat-s.***, op., ***pareir.***, ***phos.***, raph., sars., scop., **SEL.**, **SENEG.**, **SPONG.**, thuj., yohim.
- afternoon - chel.
- albumen, no trace of - yohim.
- greenish-yellow - phos.
- morning - ars-h., crot-t., hyper.
- night - crot-t.
- violet ring - puls.

GELATINOUS, lumpy on standing - cina, ***coloc.***, crot-h., ph-ac.

GREENISH - apis, ***ars.***, ***aur.***, bapt., bell., berb., bov., calc., **CAMPH.**, cann-i., ***carb-ac.***, ***cean.***, ***chel.***, ***chim.***, ***chin.***, ***chin-a.***, chin-s., ***cina***, ***colch.***, ***cop.***, crot-h., dig., ***iod.***, iris, kali-ar., ***kali-c.***, ***mag-c.***, mag-s., mang., merc., **MERC-C.**, nat-m., ***nit-ac.***, ol-an., ped., phel., phos., ***rheum***, ***rhod.***, ***ruta.***, ***sant.***, seneg., sulph., sul-ac., uran., uva., ***verat.***
- afternoon - mag-c.
- black - kali-chl.
- dark - anac., ***carb-ac.***, nat-m., ***sant.***
- grass, as - cyt-l.
- light - bapt., cina
- red sediment, with - mag-s.

INDICAN, containing - nit-ac., nux-m., pic-ac.

LIMPID - bell., carb-ac., chin., cina, coc-c., dig., dulc., elat., eup-per., **GELS.**, hydr., iris, kali-i., merc., plan., sarr., thuj.

MAHOGANY - aesc., ***eup-per.***, plb.

MILKY - ***agar.***, ***alum.***, ambr., **APIS**, arn., **AUR.**, ***aur-m.***, berb., bov., ***calc.***, caj., cann-s., caps., ***carb-v.***, card-m., caust., chel., chin-s., ***cina***, clem., ***coloc.***, con., cop., cycl., ***dulc.***, eup-pur., ***ferr.***, ***ferr-i.***, gels., **HEP.**, ***iod.***, kali-bi., kali-p., lappa-a., ***lil-t.***, **LYC.**, merc., merc-c., ***mur-ac.***, nat-m., ***nit-ac.***, nux-v., petros., ***phos.***, **PH-AC.**, plb., raph., rhus-t., ***sep.***, stann., still., ***sulph.***, ***uran.***, ***viol-o.***, visc.
- afternoon - **AGAR.**
- blood, with - kali-bi.
- chalk had been stirred in it, as if - alum., ***ph-ac.***, sulph.
- cheesy milk had been stirred in, as if - alumn., ***ph-ac.***
- curdled-like - **PH-AC.**, phos.
- emotion, after every, as if stirred up with chalk - ***ph-ac.***
- flour, as if mixed with - ***ph-ac.***
- hydrocephalus, in, very little but frequent discharges of milky urine with unconsciousness and delirium - **APIS.**
- menses, during - berb., nat-m.
  - after - ***nat-m.***
  - before - ***ph-ac.***
- morning - lil-t., nat-m.
- passed, when - mur-ac.
- perspiration, during - phos.
- standing, on - ***cina***, ***ph-ac.***, stann.
- stool, after - iod.
- turbid, and - bry., calc., cann-s., chin., ***cina***, con., cycl., dulc., ***hep.***, psor., rhus-t.
- urination at close of - ***carb-v.***, coff., ph-ac., rhus-t., sars., ***sep.***

MUDDY - ***aesc.***, hyper., ***kali-c.***, lyc., ***nat-m.***, pall., ***rhus-t.***, sabad., uva., zinc.

NEUTRAL - arn., bapt., canth., dig., eup-per., helon., kali-c., hyos., lept., phos., plb.

ODOR, offensive - agar., aloe, ambr., ant-t., **APIS**, ***arg-m.***, **ARN.**, ***ars.***, ars-i., asaf., ***asar.***, ***aspar.***, ***aur.***, aur-m., **BAPT.**, ***bar-m.***, **BENZ-AC.**, ***bor.***, bufo, ***calad.***, **CALC.**, camph., ***carb-ac.***, ***carb-an.***, ***carb-s.***, **CARB-V.**, ***caust.***, ***chim.***, chin., chin-a., clem., colch., coloc., cupr., daph., dig., dros., **DULC.**, fl-ac., ***graph.***, ***guai.***, hell., hep., hydr., hyper., ***ind.***, iod., iris, kali-ar., kali-bi., kali-br., ***kali-c.***, ***kali-i.***, ***kali-p.***, ***kali-s.***, ***kreos.***, lach., ***lyc.***, med., ***meph.***, ***merc.***, ***murx.***, ***nat-a.***, ***nat-c.***, nat-m., nat-p., nat-s., **NIT-AC.**, ***nux-v.***, op., ***petr.***, ***ph-ac.***, ***phos.***, plb., ***puls.***, pyrog., ***rhod.***, sal-ac., sec., **SEP.**, stann., **SULPH.**, tab., tarent., ***ter.***, tril., uran., vario., ***verat-v.***, **VIOL-T.**
- acrid, pungent - am-c., ***asaf.***, **BOR.**, ***calc.***, calc-f., camph., cann-s., caust., clem., ***cob.***, ***fl-ac.***, graph., hep., ***lyc.***, merc., nit-ac., par., ***rhus-t.***, rhod., sep., stram., thuj.
  - fever, during - arg-m., kreos., ***lyc.***, ***merc.***, ***ph-ac.***, rhus-t., squil., staph., sulph.
  - menses, during - ***nit-ac.***, sep.
  - perspiration, during - ars., carb-v., dulc., nit-ac., ph-ac., puls., ***sep.***, thuj., viol-t.
  - sweaty feet, like - sulph.

ODOR, offensive
ammoniacal - aloe, am-caust., am-m., **ASAF.,** ***aur.,*** bell., benz-ac., bor., brom., bufo, cahin., calc., carb-ac., ***carb-v.,*** chel., chin-s., coc-c., cop., dig., ***dulc.,*** equis., ***ferr.,*** ferr-p., graph., **IOD.,** kreos., ***lach.,*** lyc., med., ***merc.,*** **MOSCH.,** naphtin., naphtin., ***nit-ac., pareir., petr., phos.,*** pic-ac., puls., rhod., sil., solid., stigm., stront-c., sumb., tab., ***tub.,*** viol-t.
infants, in - ***calc., iod.***
menses, during - nit-ac.
aromatic - benz-ac., carb-ac., eup-pur., ferr-i., onos., ter., thlaspi.
burnt horn - arum-m.
cat's urine - aspar., bor., caj., vib., ***viol-t.***
changeable - ***benz-ac.***
coffee - berb.
eggs, spoiled, like - ***daph.***
fishy - astac., ol-an., sanic., uran-n.
fish-brine - bufo, ol-an.
garlic, like - cupr-ar., phos.
horrible, on standing - **IND.**
horse's like - absin., ***benz-ac., nat-c.,*** **NIT-AC.,** phos.
mouldy - am-m., camph., phys., sulph.
mousy - bry.
musk - oci.
nutmeg - nux-m.
offensive, dark red at night, normal during day - mosch.
profuse - rhod.
onions - cupr-ar., gamb., phos.
putrid - aloe, ars., aur., ***aur-m.,*** bar-m., ***benz-ac., calad.,*** **CALC.,** carb-an., carb-v., coc-c., coloc., daph., hell., hydr., nat-c., ***ph-ac., sep.***
evening - ***calad.***
fever, during - ph-ac.
menopause, during - **SEP.**
raspberry, like - sul-i.
sourish - ***ambr.,*** benz-ac., ***calc.,*** chel., ***graph.,*** hep., ***merc., nat-c.,*** petr., **SEP.**
strong - ***absin.,*** aesc., aloe, ***am-be.,*** am-m., arg-n., **ASAF.,** ***ant-t., aspar., aur.,*** **BENZ-AC.,** ***bor.,*** bufo, calad., ***calc.,*** calc-f., calc-p., carb-ac., ***carb-v.,*** chel., **CHIN-S.,** cob., conv., dig., dros., ***dulc.,*** erig., ***ferr., fl-ac.,*** hydr., **IOD.,** iris, kali-bi., kreos., ***lach.,*** lil-t., ***lyc.,*** med., ***merc.,*** merc-c., mez., **MOSCH.,** nat-m., **NIT-AC.,** nux-m., ped., ***petr., phos.,*** pic-ac., pin-s., ***sep.,*** stram., sulph., ***sumb., thuj.,*** tub., valer., viol-o., zinc., zing.
intensely urinous - **BENZ-AC.**
menses, before - merc.
menses, during - ***nit-ac.***
sulphur, of - phos.
sweetish - aeth., ***arg-m.,*** arg-n., ***cop.,*** cub., eucal., ferr-i., hyper., ind., ***juni.,*** kali-a., ***lact., nux-m.,*** phos., prim-o., ***ter.,*** thyr.
tobacco, like - nit-ac.
valerian, like - murx.

ODOR, offensive
violets, like - camph., clem., cop., cub., inul., lact., nux-m., osm., phos., sel., ter., thyr.
evening - osm.

ODORLESS - bell., camph., ***cedr.,*** chlol., coc-c., dros., kali-cy., senec., ***spong.***

OLIVE-hue, milky - pic-ac.

OILY - chin-s., merc-c.

OXALIC acid - berb., caust., kali-s., nat-p., nat-s., ***nit-m-ac.,*** ox-ac., ter.

PALE - acet-ac., acon., aeth., ***agar., alum.,*** ambr., ***am-c.,*** anac., ***ang.,*** anthr., ant-c., apis, apoc., ***arg-m.,*** arg-n., ***arn., ars., arum-t.,*** asaf., atro., aur., ***bell., berb.,*** brach., ***bry.,*** bufo, calad., calc., ***calc-f.,*** camph., ***cann-i.,*** canth., caps., carb-ac., carb-s., ***carb-v., caul.,*** cedr., ***cham., chel., chin.,*** chin-a., chin-s., cimic., cina, ***clem.,*** cob., cocc., coc-c., coff., ***colch., coloc.,*** **CON.,** cop., crot-t., cycl., dig., dulc., echi., erig., **EQUIS.,** eup-pur., euphr., ferr., ferr-i., ferr-p., fl-ac., gels., glon., ham., hell., helon., ***hep.,*** hydr., hyos., ***ign.,*** iod., kali-ar., kali-c., kali-i., **KALI-N.,** ***kreos.,*** lach., lac-ac., ***lac-d.,*** laur., **LED.,** lil-t., ***lyc., mag-c.,*** mag-m., mag-s., merc., **MERC-C.,** mez., mosch., ***mur-ac.,*** nat-a., nat-c., **NAT-M.,** nat-p., ***nat-s., nit-ac.,*** nux-m., ***nux-v.,*** ol-an., olnd., op., ox-ac., par., **PH-AC.,** ***phos.,*** phel., phyt., pic-ac., plat., ***plan.,*** plb., ***puls.,*** raph., rheum, ***rhod., rhus-t.,*** **SARS.,** sec., seneg., sep., sil., squil., ***staph., stram., stront-c.,*** sulph., sul-ac., tab., tarax., ter., teucr., thuj., verat., vinc., zinc., zing.
afternoon - sars.
evening - mag-c.
fever, during - cedr., cham.
headache and heart pain - kali-c.
perspiration, during - arn., ***bell.,*** chin., con., ign., **PH-AC.,** phos., puls., rhus-t., stram., thuj.

PHOSPHATES, containing - alf., benz-ac., calc-p., lappa-a., ***ph-ac.,*** phos., pic-ac., solid., stann.

POLYOUS, formation in - calc.

PROTEINURIA, (see Albuminous)

REACHES penis, glans and then urine returns - prun.

RED - ***acon., aesc.,*** aeth., agar., agn., ***all-c.,*** aloe, ***alum.,*** alumn., am-m., ***ant-c., ant-t., apis, arg-n., arn.,*** ars., ars-i., asc-t., aur., bad., ***bapt., bell.,*** **BENZ-AC.,** ***berb., bov.,*** **BRY.,** bufo, ***cact.,*** calad., calc., ***camph.,*** cann-i., cann-s., **CANTH.,** caps., carb-ac., ***carb-an.,*** carb-s., ***carb-v.,*** caust., cedr., ***chel.,*** clem., cocc., coc-c., coff., ***colch.,*** con., ***cop., crot-h.,*** crot-t., cupr., cycl., daph., dig., ***dulc.,*** elaps, equis., ferr., ferr-ar., ferr-p., ***grat., hep., iod.,*** ip., iris, kali-ar., ***kali-bi., kali-c.,*** kali-i., kali-n., kali-s., kreos., lach., lachn., laur., led., ***lept.,*** lil-t., ***lith.,*** lob., ***lyc., merc.,*** merc-c., merc-i-f., merc-i-r., mez., ***mur-ac.,*** nat-m., nat-p., ***nux-v., op.,*** par., petr., phos., phyt., pic-ac., ***plat.,*** plb., podo., puls., rheum, rhus-r., ***rhus-t.,*** sabin., sang., ***sars., sel.,*** senec., seneg., **SEP.,** ***sil.,*** squil., staph., **STRAM.,** ***sulph.,*** sul-ac., sumb., tab., tax., ***ter.,*** thuj., tub., verat., zinc.

RED, urine
blood-red - aesc., apis, bell., ***berb., calc., carb-v., cham.,*** coff., ***crot-h.,*** crot-t., ferr., ***hell., hep., kali-i.,*** merc., petr., pic-ac., rhus-t., ***sep.***
bright red - am-m., bov.
brownish-red - ***ant-c., ant-t.,*** apis, apoc., ***chel.,*** coc-c., ***hep., lac-ac.,*** lyc., merc., plb., puls., rhod., sulph.
clear and - ***acon.,*** chel.
cloud, like a - ambr.
dark-red - ***acon.,*** aesc., aloe, ant-c., ant-t., ***apis, arg-n., bapt.,*** bell., ***benz-ac., bry.,*** canth., ***carb-v.,*** cedr., clem., cob., ***cop., crot-h., cupr.,*** cupr-ac., ***dig., ferr.,*** grat., ***hep.,*** ip., ***kali-bi., lob., lyc., merc., merc-c.,*** merc-d., merc-i-f., merc-i-r., nat-s., nux-v., op., ***pareir.,*** petr., phos., phyt., plb., ***plan.,*** polyg., puls., rheum, sec., sel., **SEP.,** ***squil.,*** staph., sul-ac., tab., tarent., tell., thuj., valer.
dark-night - mosch.
deep-red - ant-c., ant-t., carb-v., cupr., hep., lob., ***merc.,*** phyt., ***rhus-r.,*** sul-ac.
evening - **SEL.,** sulph.
fever, with - ***nux-v.***
fiery red - ars., bell., camph., chin., crot-t., merc., plb., sel.
perspiration, with - cedr.
reddish-yellow - acon., daph.
standing, while - dig.

SALT, deficient in - led.

SCANTY - abrot., ***acon., aesc., agar., ail.,*** all-s., ***aloe,*** alum., alumn., ambr., am-c., am-m., anac., ang., anthr., ant-c., ***ant-t.,*** **APIS,** ***apoc., arg-n., arn.,*** **ARS.,** ***ars-i.,*** **ARUM-T.,** asaf., asc-c., ***aspar., aur., aur-m., bapt., bell.,*** benz-ac., ***berb.,*** bov., brom., ***bry.,*** bufo, cact., calad., calc., calc-ar., calc-f., ***camph.,*** cann-i., cann-s., **CANTH.,** caps., ***carb-ac.,*** carb-an., **CARB-S.,** carb-v., ***card-m.,*** cast., ***caust.,*** cedr., ***cham.,*** chel., chim., ***chin., chin-a., chin-s.,*** cic., cimx., cimic., cina, ***clem., cob., cocc.,*** coc-c., coff., **COLCH.,** coloc., **CON.,** cop., ***corn., croc., crot-h., cupr.,*** cupr-s., cur., ***cycl.,*** **DIG.,** ***dros., dulc.,*** echi., elat., **EQUIS.,** erig., ery-a., eug., eup-per., ***eup-pur.,*** euph., eupi., ***ferr., ferr-ar.,*** ferr-i., ferr-p., ***fl-ac.,*** **GRAPH., GRAT.,** guai., ***ham.,*** **HELL.,** helon., ***hep.,*** hydr., ***hyos.,*** hyper., ign., indg., iod., ***ip.,*** iris, jatr., ***kali-ar., kali-bi., kali-br., kali-c., kali-chl.,*** kali-i., **KALI-N.,** kali-p., ***kali-s., kreos.,*** **LAC-C., LAC-AC.,** ***lach., lac-d.,*** lact., ***laur.,*** lec., ***led.,*** lept., **LIL-T.,** ***lith.,*** lob., ***lyc.,*** lyss., ***mag-m.,*** mag-s., mang., ***meny.,*** **MERC., MERC-C., MERC-D.,** ***mez.,*** morph., mur-ac., ***naja, nat-a., nat-c.,*** nat-m., nat-p., **NAT-S.,** nicc., **NIT-AC.,** ***nux-m.,*** **NUX-V.,** olnd., **OP.,** osm., ox-ac., pall., ***pareir.,*** par., ***petr.,*** ph-ac., ***phos., phyt., pic-ac.,*** **PLB.,** ***podo.,*** prun., ***psor., puls.,*** pyrog., ***rat.,*** rhod., rhus-r., ***rhus-t.,*** **RUTA.,** sabad., sabin., sac-alb., sang., sarr., **SARS.,** sec., **SEL.,** ***seneg.,*** **SEP.,** sil., spong., ***squil.,*** **STAPH.,** stann., ***stram.,*** stront-c., **SULPH.,** sul-ac., ***sumb., syph.,*** tab., tarax., tell., **TER.,** ther., thuj., tub., ***verat.,*** verat-v., ***verb.,*** xan., zinc.
agg. other complaints - benz-ac., oci., solid.
afternoon - hell., rumx., sumb., ***thuj.***
alternating with copious flow - ***berb., dig.,*** gels., sang.
amenorrhea, with - acon., apis, chin., cocc., ham., hell., laur., lil-t., nux-m., xan.
asthma, with - acon.
before - ***apis,*** sil.
brain affection, with - ***apis,*** bell., bry., ***cupr.,*** squil., stram.
daytime - aesc., ***lyc.,*** ther.
evening - arg-n., ferr-i., fl-ac., mag-c., nat-m., sel., zinc.
fever, during - ***apis,*** arn., ars., bell., cact., cann-s., canth., cocc., colch., crot-h., eup-pur., hyos., lyc., nat-m., nit-ac., nux-v., ***op.,*** plb., ***puls.,*** sec., staph., stram.
frequent, and - meny., merc., ol-an.
headache, during, copious after - asc-c., sang.
followed by headache - iod., ol-an.
menses, during - nat-m.
morning - alum., ars-h., coff., dig., fl-ac., mez., ox-ac., sang., sars., sul-ac., zinc.
nervous women - ***agar.***
night - ant-c., carb-an., cic., coc-c., lyc., ***morph.,*** xan.
pain in abdomen, from - arn., graph.
perspiration, during - ant-t., apis, arn., bell., bry., **CALC.,** ***canth.,*** carb-v., caust., cedr., chin., dig., dulc., ***graph.,*** **HELL.,** hep., hyos., ***merc.,*** nit-ac., ***nux-v.,*** **OP.,** puls., rhus-t., ***staph.,*** **SULPH.,** verat.
thirst, with - lith., sep.

SEDIMENT - ***acon.,*** aesc., agar., alum., ambr., am-caust., am-m., ant-c., ant-t., apis, arn., ***ars., benz-ac., berb.,*** bry., calad., calc., **CANTH.,** carb-s., carb-v., caust., cedr., cham., ***chim.,*** chin., chin-a., chin-s., cimx., cina, **COLOC.,** con., ***cop.,*** cupr., dig., dulc., ferr., ferr-p., graph., ip., ***kali-ar.,*** kali-c., kali-i., kali-n., ***kali-p.,*** kali-s., laur., led., **LYC.,** ***mang.,*** **MERC.,** ***mez., naja,*** nat-a., nat-m., ***nit-ac.,*** nux-m., op., par., ***petr.,*** **PH-AC.,** ***phos.,*** plb., **PULS.,** rhus-t., sal-ac., **SARS., SEP.,** ***sil.,*** spong., ***staph., sulph.,*** sul-ac., ***tarent.,*** ter., thuj., **VALER., ZINC.**
adherent - apis, brom., canth., chim., ***chin-s., cimx.,*** coca, coc-c., ***coloc.,*** crot-t., ***cupr., daph., ferr.,*** kali-m., ***lac-c.,*** nat-c., nat-m., nit-ac., ***petr.,*** phos., phyt., plat., polyg., ***puls.,*** pyrog., rad-br., rumx., **SEP.,** stann., sumb., tub.
white - phos.
albuminous, (see Urine, albuminous) - apoc., merc-c., oci.
amorphous - ang., ***hydrang.,*** iod.
black - colch., lach., ter.
bloody - ***acon.,*** ant-t., apis, ***berb.,*** cact., cadm-s., calc., cann-s., **CANTH.,** carb-ac., ***carb-v.,*** colch., coloc., cham., **CHIM.,** con., crot-h., ***dulc., ham.,*** hell., hep., lyc., mez., ***nit-ac.,*** pareir., **PH-AC.,** ***phos.,*** **PULS.,** rad., **SEP.,** sulph., sul-ac., ***ter.,*** uva.

SEDIMENT,

bluish - pic-ac., prun.

bran-like - aloe, ambr., ant-t., berb., cedr., merc., phos., valer.

bright - nit-ac.

brown - **AMBR.**, ***apis, arn.,*** chin-s., crot-t., dig., epig., ***lach.,*** lob., thuj., valer.

and white - coloc.

dark - ***aesc., all-s.,*** plb., spig.

dirty - acon.

light - ***coloc.,*** puls.

pinkish - myric.

reddish - lith.

burnt, as if - sep.

chalk - alum., anan., ant-t., bufo, calc., chel., eup-per., graph., led., ***merc.,*** nat-m., ***ph-ac.,*** phos., phyt., ruta., sulph.

cheesy - alumn., ***ph-ac.,*** **PHOS.**, ***sars., sec.***

chocolate-colored - chin-s.

circles - chin-s., lac-c., sulph.

clay-colored - alum., alumn., ***am-c., am-m., anac.,*** **BERB.**, chin-s., cor-r., mang., phos., ***sars., sep., sulph.,*** thuj., **ZINC.**

adhesive - ***sep.***

adhesive, menses, during, hard to wash off - ***sep.***

clots, yellow-red - cob.

cloudy - alum., alumn., ambr., am-m., anac., **BERB.**, bry., carb-v., caust., cham., chin., crot-t., elaps, hydr-ac., ***kali-n.,*** lach., laur., mag-m., merc., olnd., par., petr., ***ph-ac.,*** phos., plat., rat., ***seneg.,*** sumb., ***thuj.,*** valer., zinc.

coffee, grounds, like - ***ambr.,*** **APIS, HELL.,** ***lach., ter.***

copious - agar., all-s., am-c., arn., ***ars.,*** bell., **BERB.**, calc., carb-an., cham., ***chim.,*** chin., ***coloc.,*** con., ***cop.,*** crot-t., cycl., kali-ar., kali-bi., kali-c., laur., lyc., ***phos., puls.,*** sal-ac., ***tarent.,*** thuj.

crusty - caust., ***nat-c., phos., sars., sep.***

crystals - arg-n., coloc., crot-t., ferr-m., ***lyc.***

dark - ***crot-h.,*** iod., phos., puls.

dirty - anac., chin.

earthy - mang., sul-ac.

fine, deposit - sep.

flocculent - acon., ambr., aspar., agar., ***alum., benz-ac.,*** **BERB.**, brom., calc., calc-p., ***cann-s.,*** **CANTH.**, caust., ***cham., chel.,*** cina, chin., ***clem.,*** cob., coca, coc-c., coloc., crot-t., cycl., eup-pur., ery-a., grat., hell., ***hep.,*** iod., kali-c., kali-i., kali-n., kali-p., laur., lith., merc., merc-c., **MEZ.**, nit-ac., ***petr., ph-ac., phos., plb.,*** rhus-t., rumx., **SARS.**, seneg., squil., sumb., thuj., uran., valer., zinc.

white - calc., merc., phos.

white, standing, on - zinc.

gelatinous - **BERB.**, calad., ***chim., cina, coca,*** coc-c., **COLOC.**, crot-h., ***dulc.,*** hydr., ***oci., pareir.,*** ph-ac., ***puls.***

granular - aloe, berb., chin-s.

SEDIMENT,

gray - agar., ant-t., ***con.,*** hyos., kali-i., led., mang., ph-ac., ***phos.,*** puls., spong.

brownish-gray - chin.

whitish-gray - **BERB.**, calc., canth., ***graph.,*** hyos., merc-c., sars., sep., spong.

hemoglobinuria - ***ars-h.,*** carb-ac., chin-a., chin-s., ferr-p., kali-bi., ***kali-chl.,*** nat-n., ***phos.,*** pic-ac., sant.

kidney stones, from - bell., **BENZ-AC.**, ***berb.,*** **CALC.**, ***canth.,*** coc-c., coloc., equis., hydrang., **LITH., LYC.**, med., mill., morg-g., nat-s., oci., **PAREIR.**, ***phos.,*** **SARS.**, ***sil.,*** **URT-U.**

limy - sabal.

loose - alum., carb-an., ***chin.***

mealy - ***agar.,*** ant-t., apis, **BERB.**, ***calc., canth., cedr., chin.,*** chin-s., cor-r., ***graph., hyos.,*** kali-c., merc., ***nat-m.,*** ph-ac., phos., ***sep.,*** sulph., valer., zinc.

meat, like - merc.

milky - ant-t., coloc., ferr-i., lyc., ox-ac., ***ph-ac.,*** phos., sec.

mucous - aesc., ***aloe, alumn., ant-c.,*** apoc., ***arg-n.,*** ars., asc-t., aspar., ***aur.,*** bals-p., bar-c., ***baros.,*** bell., **BENZ-AC., BERB.**, brach., brom., bry., calc., camph., cann-i., ***cann-s., canth.,*** carb-s., ***carb-v.,*** caust., ***chel.,*** **CHIM.**, chin-s., ***cimic.,*** cina, ***clem., coc-c., colch., coloc.,*** con., cop., crot-t., ***cub.,*** dig., ***dulc.,*** epig., **EQUIS.**, eup-pur., ***ferr.,*** ferr-ar., ferr-p., ***glon., hep., hydr.,*** hydrang., hyos., indg., kali-ar., ***kali-bi., kali-c., kali-chl.,*** kali-n., kali-p., ***lach.,*** lith., lyc., med., menthol, ***merc.,*** **MERC-C.**, naja, nat-a., ***nat-c.,*** **NAT-M.**, nat-p., **NAT-S.**, ***nit-ac., nux-v.,*** op., **PAREIR.**, ***petr.,*** ph-ac., phos., ***pop.,*** **PULS., SARS.**, seneg., **SEP.**, stigm., sulph., sul-ac., tab., ***thuj., til., ter., tritic.,*** tub., uran-n., ***uva.,*** valer., verat.

menses, before - ***lach.***

milky white - ***kali-chl.***

standing, after - crot-t.

tenacious - caust., ***coloc.,*** con., nat-c., ***nux-v., puls.,*** sil.

thick - gall-ac.

ropy bloody mucous great quantity of - **CHIM.**, ***dulc.,*** kali-bi.

uterine displacement, with - senec.

white - phos.

yellow - nat-c.

muddy - ter.

offensive - cupr., lyc.

orange-colored - chin-s.

oxalate of lime - brach., ***caust.,*** coca, ***kali-s.,*** lyc., lycps., ***nat-p.,*** **NIT-AC.**, nit-m-ac., ox-ac., plb., rhus-t., ***ter.,*** zinc.

pasty - ars., **SEP.**

phosphates - agar., ***alf.,*** arn., aspar., aven., bell., ***benz-ac.,*** brach., calc., ***calc-p.,*** cann-s., canth., chel., chin-s., colch., ***ferr-m.,*** graph., gua., guai., helon., hydrang., hydrc., kali-br., kali-chl., kalm., lec., mag-p., med., nat-a., nit-ac., **PH-AC.**, ***phos.,*** pic-ac., ***ptel., raph.,***

SEDIMENT,

phosphates - sang., ***sarr.***, senn., ***stann.***, ter., thlaspi, uran-n.

pink - ***berb.***, **BRY.**, ***chin.***, lith., lob., rheum, rhus-r., ***sep.***, ***sumb.***

purple - ant-c., bov., ***fl-ac.***, mang., ptel.

purulent - **ARN.**, ***ars.***, aspar., bapt., ***baros.***, ***benz-ac.***, berb., bry., cadm-s., calc., ***cann-s.***, **CANTH.**, carb-ac., carb-s., carb-v., cham., chim., **CLEM.**, ***con.***, cop., ***daph.***, ***dulc.***, ***epig.***, eucal., eup-pur., ham., hep., hyos., ip., kali-ar., kali-bi., kali-c., ***kali-s.***, lith., ***lyc.***, ***merc.***, ***merc-c.***, **NAT-S.**, ***nit-ac.***, ***nux-v.***, oci., petr., ***phos.***, polyg., ***pop.***, ***puls.***, sabad., ***sars.***, sabin., sal-ac., sep., ***sil.***, staph., stigm., sul-i., ***sulph.***, ter., thlaspi, tritic., uran-n., **UVA.**

urination, after - hep.

red - ***acon.***, agar., ***alum.***, ambr., am-c., ***ant-c.***, ***apis***, ***arg-n.***, ***arn.***, ars., ars-h., arund., aspar., astac., ***bell.***, ***berb.***, brom., bry., cact., camph., **CANTH.**, carb-v., cham., ***chel.***, ***chin.***, chin-a., ***chin-s.***, cimx., cob., coc-c., coch., ***coloc.***, ***cop.***, cupr., ***daph.***, dig., dulc., ***elaps***, gall-ac., ***graph.***, hydr-ac., iod., ip., kali-ar., kali-c., kali-p., kali-s., kreos., lac-ac., ***lac-c.***, ***lach.***, ***laur.***, led., lil-t., ***lith.***, ***lob.***, ***lyc.***, lyss., mag-s., merc-c., ***mez.***, naja, **NAT-M.**, nat-s., ***nit-ac.***, ***nux-v.***, op., pall., par., pareir., ***petr.***, ph-ac., phos., plat., ***psor.***, ptel., **PULS.**, sang., ***sec.***, sel., senec., seneg., **SEP.**, sil., squil., stann., sulph., sul-ac., tarent., ***ter.***, thuj., **VALER.**, verat-v.

blood-color - am-c., sep.

brick-color - merc-c., nat-s., petr., phos., puls.

bright - **BERB.**, ***lyc.***, nit-ac., osm., phos.

brownish - sul-ac.

circles, in - lac-c.

dark - chin., dor., phyt.

dirty - ***berb.***, dor.

filaments, fibres - ant-c., ant-t.

flocculent or powdery - agar., cob.

grainy - sel.

hard to wash off - ars-i., aspar., brom., ***cimx.***, ***cupr.***, ***daph.***, ***lac-c.***, ***phyt.***, pyrog., **SEP.**

mahogany-colored - chin., laur., phyt.

pepper, like - iod., pyrog.

rosy - am-p.

thick - kali-c.

white - ter.

rings - apis, ***lac-c.***, pyrog.

ropy - ***chim.***, coloc., ***hydr.***, ***kali-bi.***, ***lyc.***, ***ph-ac.***

sand - all-c., ambr., **AM-C.**, ***ant-c.***, arg-n., arn., ars., aspar., arund., aur., aur-m., bell., **BENZ-AC.**, ***berb.***, ***calc.***, canth., carb-v., ***chel.***, chin., chin-a., ***chin-s.***, coc-c., coloc., con., eup-pur., ferr-m., kali-i., kali-p., ***lach.***, **LED.**, **LYC.**, meny., merc., ***nat-m.***, ***nat-s.***, ***nit-ac.***, nux-m., nux-v., **PHOS.**, ***puls.***, raph., ***ruta.***, **SARS.**, ***sec.***, **SEL.**, **SEP.**, **SIL.**, sul-i., tarent., thuj., ***tub.***, **ZINC.**

adherent - ***puls.***

bright colored in concentric layers - chin-s.

brown - sul-i.

SEDIMENT,

sand, in urine

gravel - arg-n., aspar., ***bar-m.***, baros., ***berb.***, ***calc.***, cann-s., ***canth.***, carb-v., chin-s., coc-c., cocc-s., colch., coloc., con., ***dios.***, ***epig.***, erig., ery-a., ***eup-a.***, ***eup-pur.***, ferr-m., gali., graph., ***hedeo,*** hep., hydrang., ipom., kali-i., kreos., ***lith.***, **LYC.**, med., ***nit-ac.***, nit-m-ac., nux-m., ***nux-v.***, onis., op., oxyd., ph-ac., phys., polyg., ***sars.***, senn., **SEP.**, skook., ***stigm.***, ***tab.***, ***thlaspi***, tritic., ***urt-u.***, uva., zinc.

gray - phos.

pale - ***sars.***

red - acon., agar., all-c., alum., ***am-c.***, am-caust., ant-t., apis, arg-n., **ARN.**, **ARS.**, **ARUND.**, ***aspar.***, aur-m., bapt., bell., ***benz-ac.***, ***berb.***, bry., ***cact.***, ***camph.***, ***carb-v.***, ***caust.***, chel., ***chim.***, chin., chin-a., ***chin-s.***, ***cimic.***, cob., coc-c., ***coloc.***, con., ***cop.***, **DIG.**, ***elaps***, ***glon.***, grat., ***hyos.***, ***ip.***, ***kali-c.***, kali-n., ***lach.***, ***led.***, **LOB.**, **LYC.**, ***meph.***, **MERC-C.**, ***mez.***, ***nat-m.***, ***nat-s.***, nit-ac., nux-m., ***nux-v.***, ***oci.***, ***op.***, ox-ac., pall., **PAREIR.**, ***petr.***, **PHOS.**, pic-ac., **PLAN.**, ***psor.***, puls., pyrog., rumx., **SEL.**, **SENEC.**, **SEP.**, ***sil.***, sumb., **TARENT.**, ter., thuj., valer., zinc.

red, fever, during - ***lyc.***, phos.

sticky - pyrog., tub.

white - ***am-c.***, berb., calc., graph., kreos., nat-a., phos., **RHUS-T.**, sars., sep.

white, precipitated by heat - nat-a.

yellow - chin-s., cimic., phos., sant., sep., **SIL.**, thuj., zinc.

yellowish-red crystals - ***berb.***, chel., chin-s., ***lyc.***

straw colored - ***chin-s.***

sugar, like a conglomerate of candied - chin-s.

thick - aesc., ***alum.***, apoc., bell., **BERB.**, ***camph.***, ***coloc.***, ***cop.***, dig., ferr-i., hydr-ac., lach., laur., lob., merc., ph-ac., phos., psor., sabad., sec., ***spong.***, sulph., ***sumb.***, ter., valer.

standing over night, after - bry., crot-t.

thready - cann-s., coc-c., merc., nit-ac.

translucent - ***berb.***, ***coloc.***

uric acid - arg-n., thymol., ***urt-u.***

violet colored - bov., fl-ac., ***mang.***, puls.

white - acon., aesc., aeth., agar., aloe, ***alum.***, alumn., am-c., aspar., bar-m., bell., ***benz-ac.***, **BERB.**, brach., brom., bry., ***calc.***, camph., ***canth.***, caps., carb-s., carb-v., ***chin.***, chin-s., coc-c., colch., ***coloc.***, conv., con., crot-t., dig., dulc., euph., eup-per., eup-pur., ferr., ferr-i., fl-ac., **GRAPH.**, ***hep.***, ign., kali-bi., **KREOS.**, laur., lil-t., lyss., mag-c., murx., nat-m., ***nat-s.***, ***nit-ac.***, ***olnd.***, ox-ac., ***petr.***, ***ph-ac.***, **PHOS.**, phyt., plan., **RHUS-T.**, **SARS.**, sec., seneg., **SEP.**, spig., spong., ***sulph.***, sul-ac., sumb., ter., ***valer.***, zinc.

adhesive - brom., **SEP.**

cloudy - aspar., benz-ac., con., ph-ac., phos., plat., rhus-t., sumb.

SEDIMENT,
white,
fever, during - phos., sep.
filmy, very hard to wash off - **SEP.**
pearly - kali-bi.
snow-white - rhus-t.
yeast-like - caust., mag-m., mosch., raph.
yellow - aesc., ***aloe, bar-c.,*** bufo, ***cham., chin.,*** chin-s., cob., coca, ***cupr.,*** daph., ***kali-chl., kali-i.,*** kali-n., ***lyc., nat-s.,*** **PHOS., SEP.,** sil., spong., sul-ac., ter., zinc.
adhesive - ***ferr.***
dirty - chin., nux-v., ***raph.***
grayish - chel.
pasty - **SEP.**
reddish - all-c., chel., chin., chin-s., cob., coca, ***crot-t., nat-s., sep.***
white - ***carb-an.,*** chin-s., coca, lyss., nat-s., phos., raph., ter.

SHREDDY - seneg.

SHERRY - apoc., squil., sulph.

SMOKE-COLOR - carb-ac., crot-h., nat-h., **TER.**

SOUR - coc-c., graph., petr., ***sep.,*** solid.
whooping cough, during - ambr.

SPECIFIC gravity
decreased - apoc., brach., chlf., cimic., coff., colch., dig., equis., helon., kali-ar., merc., ***merc-c.,*** morph., murx., nat-a., nat-m., ***phos.,*** **PLB.,** sulph., uran., verat-v.
increased - apoc., **ARN.,** aur-m., ***benz-ac.,*** calc., ***calc-p.,*** canth., chim., coc-c., **COLCH.,** coloc., dig., elat., ***eup-pur., ferr.,*** ferr-p., ***helon.,*** iod., ***kali-a., kali-p., merc.,*** morph., mur-ac., nat-a., ***nat-s.,*** onos., ph-ac., ***phos., phyt.,*** nit-ac., ***puls.,*** sarr., senec., sep., sul-ac., tab., tell., uran., zinc.

STAINS diaper, brown - benz-ac.
red - sanic.
yellow - phyt.
dark - chel.

SUGAR, in urine (see Immunity, Diabetes) - ***acet-ac., adren.,*** alf., all-s., alumn., am-c., aml-n., ant-t., ***arg-m.,*** arg-n., arist-m., arn., ***ars., ars-br.,*** ars-i., ***aur.,*** aur-m., bar-c., bell., ***benz-ac., bor-ac.,*** **BOV.,** ***bry., calc., calc-p.,*** camph., caps., ***carb-ac., carb-v.,*** cean., ***cham., chel., chim., chin.,*** chin-a., ***chion., coca, cod.,*** coff., ***colch.,*** con., conv., ***crot-h.,*** cupr., cupr-ar., ***cur., elaps,*** eup-pur., fel., ferr-i., ***ferr-m.,*** fl-ac., glon., glyc., grin., ***hell.,*** **HELON.,** ***hep.,*** iod., ***iris,*** kali-a., kali-br., ***kali-chl.,*** kali-n., ***kali-p., kreos., lac-d., lach., lac-ac., lec.,*** lith., **LYC.,** ***lycps.,*** lyss., mag-s., ***med.,*** mosch., morph., mur-ac., murx., nat-m., nat-p., ***nat-s., nit-ac.,*** nux-v., op., petr., **PH-AC.,** phase., **PHOS.,** ***pic-ac.,*** **PLB.,** ***podo., rat., rhus-a.,*** sal-ac., sec., sep., ***sil.,*** squil., ***sulph., sul-ac.,*** tarax., **TARENT., TER.,** ***thuj.,*** thyr., tub., **URAN-N.,** urea, vanad., zinc., ziz.
debility, with - acet-ac., op., ***ph-ac.***

SUGAR, in urine
gangrene, boils, carbuncles and diarrhea, with - ars.
gastro-hepatic origin - ars., ***ars-i.,*** bry., calc., cham., chel., kreos., ***lac-ac.,*** lept., lyc., ***nux-v., phos., uran-n.***
gouty symptoms, with - ***lac-ac., nat-s.***
impotency, with - coca, mosch.
melancholia, emaciation, thirst and restlessness, with - helon.
motor paralysis, with - cur.
nervous origin - ars., aur-m., calc., ***ign., ph-ac., phos.***
pancreatic origin - iris, phos.
rapid course, with - cur., morph.

THICK - acon., am-be., am-caust., anan., aster., ***apis,*** apoc., ***arn., ars.,*** aur., aur-m., bell., ***benz-ac.,*** berb., bufo, camph., canth., ***carb-v.,*** caust., cina, ***chim.,*** clem., coc-c., ***coloc., con., cop.,*** crot-t., cur., ***daph., dig.,*** dulc., elaps, ***hep.,*** iris, ***ip., iod., lac-d.,*** laur., lil-t., ***merc.,*** **MERC-C.,** ***merc-i-r.,*** mosch., **NUX-V.,** oci., ***ph-ac., phos.,*** plb., ***psor.,*** raph., rheum, rhus-t., ***sabad.,*** seneg., **SEP.,** still., stram., sulph., sul-ac., verat., vesp., zing.
standing, on - ***alum., berb., bry.,*** camph., ***cham., cina,*** **COLOC.,** ***hep., merc.,*** sulph., ter., thuj.

VIOLET - apis, indg., ***mur-ac.,*** nux-m.

VISCID - arg-n., aster., canth., **COLOC.,** ***con.,*** cop., cupr., cur., dulc., kreos., ***nat-s.,*** pareir., ***ph-ac., sep.,*** tub.

URIC acid - thyr.

WATERY, clear as water - ***acet-ac.,*** acon., aeth., agar., alum., alumn., anac., anthr., ant-c., ant-t., arn., arum-m., ars., aster., aur., bapt., bar-c., ***bar-m.,*** bell., berb., ***bism.,*** bry., calc., calc-f., calc-p., cann-s., canth., ***caust.,*** cedr., cham., chin., chin-a., chin-s., ***cimic.,*** cinnb., ***cocc.,*** coc-c., colch., ***coloc.,*** cycl., ***dig.,*** dros., **EQUIS.,** euphr., ***fl-ac.,*** **GELS.,** grat., hell., hipp., hydr-ac., hyos., **IGN.,** iod., kali-a., kali-ar., kali-bi., kali-i., kali-p., ***lac-d.,*** lact., laur., ***lyc., lycps., mag-c.,*** med., meph., merc., mez., ***mosch.,*** murx., **MUR-AC.,** nat-c., ***nat-m., nat-s.,*** nux-m., nux-v., op., ***ph-ac., phos.,*** plat., plb., ***puls.,*** rhus-t., sang., ***sec.,*** **SEP.,** spig., **SQUIL.,** stann., stram., ***staph.,*** sulph., sul-ac., tab., ***ter., teucr., thuj.,*** zinc.
dung, mixed with - ars.
inodorous, with fetid mucous stool - dros.
paroxysms of pain - phos.
typhus, in - **MUR-AC.**

WHEY-like - agar., ***arg-m.,*** hyos., op., ***ph-ac.,*** nat-s.
menses, before - ph-ac.
morning - cann-s.
standing, after - agar.

WHITE - ***all-s.,*** alum., alumn., ambr., am-c., ang., arn., bapt., bell., berb., bry., cann-s., canth., ***caust.,*** cham., ***chel., chin.,*** cina, ***coloc.,*** con., cycl., ***dulc.,*** ferr., lac-ac., lyc., merc., nat-m., phos., plan., ***rhus-t.,*** sec., ***spong., sulph.***

chalk, as if mixed with - merc., **PHOS.,** ***ph-ac.***

close of urination, at - ph-ac., sars.

jelly-like - cina, ***coloc.***

morning - lac-ac.

standing, on - nit-ac.

YEAST-like - ***caust., raph.***

YELLOW, bright - sars.

dark - ***aesc.,*** agar., ***arg-n., ars.,*** berb., bov., bry., camph., ***cedr.,*** **CHEL.,** chen-a., ***con.,*** crot-t., ***hep., iod., kali-c., kali-p.,*** myric., ***nat-c.,*** petr., ***pic-ac.,*** podo., ***sang.,*** staph.

golden - mang., phos.

lemon - agar., ambr., bell., ***chel.,*** coc-c., eupi., ign., nat-c., op., sant., tab., zinc.

light - absin., acon., ***agar., aloe, am-m.,*** ang., ***ant-c.,*** apis, apoc., ars., **AUR.,** bar-m., ***bell.,*** berb., bufo, cact., camph., ***cann-s.,*** carb-an., carb-v., ***card-m.,*** cean., ***cham.,*** chel., chin., colch., ***crot-t., daph.,*** hydr., hydr-ac., ***hyos.,*** ign., iod., jatr., kali-bi., kali-n., kalm., **LACH.,** ***lact.,*** laur., led., mag-m., ***nat-c.,*** nit-ac., oci., op., ped., plb., raph., samb., **SEP.,** uva., verat., zinc.

orange - am-m., ang., carb-an., ***cina,*** crot-t., cupr-ar., lept., lyc., phos., plan., plb., sant., seneg., zinc.

saffron - aloe, ***cina,*** form., kali-p., oci., sang.

straw - alum.

thick and turbid like rotten eggs - daph.

wine - mez.

Vertigo

VERTIGO, general - abies-c., abies-n., absin., acet-ac., **ACON.**, act-sp., ***aesc., aeth.,*** **AGAR.**, agn., **AIL.**, alet., all-c., ***aloe,*** alumn., ***alum., ambr., am-c.,*** am-m., aml-n., anac., anan., ***ant-c.,*** ant-t., **APIS,** apoc., **ARG-M.,** ***arg-n., arn., ars., ars-h.,*** ars-i., arum-t., arund., asaf., asar., asc-c., asc-t., aspar., ***aster., aur., aur-m.,*** bad., **BAPT.,** ***bar-c.,*** bar-m., **BELL.,** benz-ac., ***berb.,*** bism., bor., both., bov., brach., brom., **BRY.,** bufo, ***cact.,*** cahin., calad., **CALC.,** calc-ar., calc-f., ***calc-p.,*** **CALC-S.,** ***camph.,*** **CANN-I.,** ***cann-s., canth.,*** caps., carb-ac., ***carb-an.,*** carb-h., carb-o., **CARB-S.,** ***carb-v.,*** carl., cast-eq., caul., ***caust., cedr., cham.,*** **CHEL.,** chen-a., chim., ***chin.,*** chin-a., **CHIN-S.,** chlol., chlf., chlor., ***cic., cimic.,*** cina, cinnb., cist., clem., cob., coca, **COCC.,** coc-c., ***coff.,*** colch., ***coloc.,*** com., **CON.,** ***cop.,*** corn., croc., ***crot-c.,*** crot-h., crot-t., ***cupr.,*** cupr-ar., **CYCL.,** daph., **DIG.,** dios., dirc., dros., **DULC.,** echi., ***elaps,*** equis., euon., eup-per., eup-pur., euph., euphr., eupi., fago., ***ferr., ferr-ar.,*** ferr-i., ***ferr-p.,*** ferr-ma., fl-ac., form., gamb., **GELS.,** ***glon.,*** goss., gran., ***graph.,*** grat., ***guare.,*** ham., hell., helon., ***hep.,*** hura, hydr-ac., ***hydrc., hyos.,*** hyper., ign., ill., indg., ***iod.,*** ip., iris, jab., jatr., jug-c., jug-r., kali-ar., ***kali-bi., kali-br., kali-c., kali-i., kali-n.,*** kali-p., ***kali-s., kalm.,*** kreos., lac-c., ***lac-d., lach.,*** lachn., lact., laur., ***led.,*** lept., lil-t., lob., **LYC.,** lycps., lyss., mag-c., mag-m., mag-s., maland., ***manc.,*** mang., med., meny., ***merc., merc-c.,*** merc-i-f., merc-i-r., ***mez.,*** mill., ***mosch., mur-ac.,*** murx., ***mygal.,*** naja, ***nat-a., nat-c., nat-h.,*** **NAT-M.,** ***nat-p., nat-s.,*** nicc., ***nit-ac.,*** par., **PETR.,** phel., ***ph-ac.,*** **PHOS.,** ***phyt.,*** pic-ac., plan., ***plat.,*** plb., ***podo., psor.,*** ptel., **PULS.,** ***ran-b.,*** ran-s., raph., rheum, ***rhod.,*** **RHUS-T.,** ***rhus-v.,*** rumx., ruta, sabad., ***sabin.,*** samb., **SANG.,** sanic., sars., **SEC.,** sel., senec., ***seneg., sep.,*** **SIL.,** ***spig., spong.,*** squil., ***stann.,*** staph., ***stram., stront-c., stry.,*** **SULPH.,** sul-ac., sumb., ***syph.,*** **TAB.,** tarent., tarax., tell., ***ter.,*** teucr., ther., ***thuj.,*** uran., ***urt-u.,*** ust., ***valer., verat., verat-v., vesp.,*** vib., ***zinc.,*** zing.

AFTERNOON - ***aesc.,*** agar., alum., ***ambr.,*** anac., benz-ac., ***bry.,*** carb-s., chel., chin., crot-t., cupr., cycl., dios., eupi., ferr., ferr-p., glon., hura, kali-c., kali-p., lyc., merc., nat-m., nicc., nux-v., ph-ac., phos., puls., rhus-t., sabad., sars., ***sep.,*** sil., staph., stront-c., sulph., sul-ac., thuj.

AIR, open, in - acon., act-sp., aeth., ***agar.,*** ambr., anac., anag., ars., aur., bry., calc., canth., ***caust.,*** cocc., crot-t., dros., euph., gins., ***glon.,*** grat., kali-ar., kali-c., ***kreos.,*** lach., laur., Manc., merc-c., ***mur-ac.,*** nicc., ol-an., ***phel.,*** podo., psor., ***ran-b.,*** ruta, sars., senec., ***sep.,*** sil., sulph., tarax.

amel. - ***aeth.,*** agar., ***am-m.,*** aur-m., bell., calc-s., ***camph.,*** carb-s., carl., ***caust.,*** clem., croc., genist., graph., hell., hydr-ac., hyos., ***grat.,*** kali-bi., kali-c., kali-p., ***kali-s.,*** lil-t., ***mag-m.,*** mag-s., manc., merc., mosch., mur-ac., ***nat-s.,*** nicc., oena., ***phel.,*** ph-ac., phos., plb., ***puls., sanic.,***

AIR, open, in

amel. - sol-n., staph., ***sulph., sul-ac.,*** **TAB.**

AGG. of symptoms during - ***acon., calc.,*** cycl., ferr., **GELS., NUX-V.,** ***phos., puls., stram.***

ALTERNATING with, colic - coloc., mag-c., spig.

ALCOHOL, drinks, from - caust., **COLOC., NAT-M., NUX-V.,** verat.

ANEMIA, with - ***chin., ferr.,*** ferr-p., trinit.

anemia of brain, with - arn., bar-m., calc., ***chin.,*** chin-s., con., dig., ***ferr.,*** ferr-c., hydr-ac., nat-m., sil.

ANGER, after - acon., calc.

ANXIETY, during - acon., aloe, alum., arn., asar., bell., ***cact., caust.,*** coff., ***dig.,*** ign., merc., nux-m., nux-v., ***op.,*** rhod., rhus-t., ***sulph.***

ASCENDING, on - bor., con., dirc., sulph.

eminence, an - bor., **CALC.,** dig., phos., ***sulph.***

stairs, on - aloe, ant-c., apoc., ars-h., bor., cahin., **CALC.,** carb-ac., coca, glon., ***kali-bi.,*** merc., par., pic-ac., sulph.

ASCENDING, sensation of - am-m., ***asaf.,*** asar., bor., hep., laur., lyc., ***merc.,*** nat-c., nux-v., ***phos., plat.,*** ran-b., ***spig.,*** sul-ac., valer., ***verat.***

AURA, sees - aur., bry., chen-a., chin., nat-sal., sil.

noises in ear, with - iris.

BACK, comes up the - ***sil.***

BALANCING, sensation - calad., ferr., lact., merc., thuj., zinc.

BATHING, after - phys., samb.

BED, on going to. - nat-m., sabad., stram.

seems as if bouncing up and down in - bell.

turned about, sensation, as if - **CON.,** nux-v., plb., ***puls.,*** sol-n.

BEER, after - kali-n., merc., sulph.

BEGINNING in, nape of neck or occiput - ***gels.,*** iber., petr., ***sil.***

BELCHING, after - hep., nux-v.

during - gymn., nat-m., nux-v., ***puls.,*** sars.

BENDING, head backwards, on - glon., seneg.

amel. - ol-an.

forwards - clem., mag-m., merc., pic-ac., ***sulph.***

BINDING, the hair agg. - sul-i.

BLOWING, the nose - cod., culx., ***sep.***

BREAD, after eating - manc., sec.

BREAKFAST, after - bufo, coc-c., gels., lyc., phos., sel., tarent.

amel. - ***alum.,*** calc., cinnb.

amel. walking rapidly, after - coloc.

during - con., ***sil.***

BREATH, deep, agg. - anac., ***cact.***

amel. - acon.

difficult - cur.

BURDENS carrying on head agg. - tarent.

CEREBRAL diseases, in - bell., ***cocc.,*** gels., sulfon., tab.

CHILD, grasps the nurse when carried - bor., ***gels.***

CHILL, during - alum., ant-t., **CALC.,** caps., ***chin.,*** cocc., ***ferr.,*** ferr-p., ***glon.,*** kali-bi., laur., lyss., nat-m., **NUX-V.,** phos., plb., puls., ***rhus-t.,*** sulph., verat., viol-t.
after - colch., sec.
before - ***ars., bry.,*** nat-m.

CHILLINESS, during - gels., merc-c., rhus-t.

CHRONIC - **AMBR.,** cocc., con., nat-m., ***nux-v.,*** **PHOS.,** ***sec.***
headache one-sided, with - ***nat-m.***

CLOSED, eyes, cannot walk with - alum., arg-n., ars., stram., thuj.

CLOSING, eyes, on - ***alum., alumn.,*** aml-n., ***ant-t., apis, arg-n.,*** **ARN.,** ***ars.,*** calad., cham., **CHEL.,** cycl., ferr., ferr-p., grat., ***hep.,*** **LACH.,** mag-s., pen., petr., ***ph-ac.,*** phos., ***pip-m.,*** rhus-t., sabad., **SEP.,** ***sil., stram.,*** **THER.,** ***thuj.,*** vib., zinc.
amel. - alum., ***con.,*** dig., ferr., ***gels.,*** graph., phel., ***pip-m.,*** sel., sulph., tab., verat-v.
lying, while - ***lac-d.***
focus, when out of - alum.
nausea, with - ***lach., ther.***
opening, or - alum.
sitting, while - thuj.

COFFEE, after - arg-n., ***cham.,*** mosch., **NAT-M.,** ***nux-v.,*** phos.
amel. - cann-i.

COLD, applications amel. - nat-m.
water when overheated - ***ars., kali-c.***
weather, during - ***sang.***

COLIC, alternating with - verat.

COLORED, glass, light shining thro', from - art-v.

CONCUSSION, of brain, from - acon., ***arn., hyper., nat-s.***

CONGESTION of blood to the head, with - ***acon.,*** arn., ***bell.,*** chin., ***cupr.,*** dig., ***glon.,*** hell., hydr-ac., ***iod.,*** merc., ***nux-v.,*** op., stram., ***sulph.,*** verat-v.

CONSCIOUSNESS, with loss of - sep.

CONSTIPATION, during - aloe, ***calc-p.,*** chin., crot-h., nat-s., sulph.

CONTINUOUS - bor., olnd., phos., psor., sil.

CONVULSIONS, with - arg-n., bell., calc., caust., cocc., cupr., hydr-ac., nit-ac., op., sil., stram.
before - ars., ***calc-ar., caust.,*** **HYOS.,** indg., lach., ***plb.,*** sil., ***sulph., tarent.,*** visc.

CORYZA, after amel. - aloe

COUGHING, on - acon., ant-t., calc., ***coff.,*** cupr., ***kali-bi.,*** led., ***mosch.,*** naja, nux-v.

CROSSING, a bridge - bar-c., brom., lyss.
running water - ***ang., arg-m.,*** bell., brom., ferr., hyos., lyss., sulph.

CROWD, in - nux-v.

DAMP, weather - brom., sars.

DARK, room, on entering - agar., alum., ***arg-n.,*** kali-i., pic-ac., ***stram.***

DEAFNESS, with - chin-s., merc-c.

DESCENDING, on - **BOR.,** coff., con., **FERR.,** gels., mag-m., merl., plat., sanic., stann., tarent., vib.
spire, on - sil.
stairs - **BOR.,** carb-ac., chr-ac., ***con.,*** ferr., gins., meph., merl., merc., phys., ***plat., sanic.,*** tarent.

DIARRHEA, before and after - **LYC.**

DILATED, pupils - ***bell.,*** hell., teucr.

DINNER, after - acon., aloe, bell., bufo, coloc., ery-a., ferr., ***hep.,*** mag-s., ***nat-s.,*** **NUX-V.,** petr., phos., ***puls.,*** rhus-t., sel., ***sulph.,*** thuj., ***zinc.***
amel. - ***arg-n.,*** dulc., sabad.
during - arn., calc-p., chel., ***hep., mag-c., mag-m.,*** mag-s., olnd., sil.
on rising from - phos., phys.
while walking after - ***cocc.***

DOUBLE, vision, with - arg-n., bell., **GELS.,** glon., nux-v., olnd., vinc.
when looking down - olnd.

DRAWN up and pitched forward, as if - calc., euon.

DRINKING, while - crot-t., ***lyc.,*** mang., ***sep.***
alcoholics, in - ***phos.***
water amel. - op.
cold amel. - paeon.

EATING, after - aloe, ***alum.,*** ambr., aran., bell., bry., bufo, ***cham.,*** chel., chin., ***cocc.,*** coc-c., cor-r., cycl., gels., graph., **GRAT.,** ***kali-bi., kali-c.,*** kali-i., kali-p., kali-s., ***lach.,*** lyc., mag-s., merc., nat-m., ***nat-s.,*** **NUX-V.,** ***petr.,*** ph-ac., ***phos.,*** plb., **PULS.,** ***rhus-t.,*** sanic., scut., sel., sep., ***sulph., tarent.,*** zinc.
amel. - alum., arg-n., cinnb., cocc., dulc., nux-v., sabad.
while - am-c., arn., calc., chel., con., dios., form., **GRAT.,** hep., mag-c., mag-m., merc., nat-c., ***nux-v.,*** olnd., ***phos.,*** sel., sil.

ELDERLY people, in - **AMBR.,** arn., ***ars-i., bar-c.,*** bar-m., bell-p., bry., calc-p., **CON.,** ***cupr.,*** dig., galph., ***gels.,*** gran., ***iod.,*** op., ***phos., rhus-t., sin-n.,*** sulph.

ELEVATED, as if - aloe, calc., cann-i., hyper., mosch., phos., rhus-t., sil.
eating, after - aloe.
evening - phos.

EMISSION, after - bov., calc., caust., nat-c., sars., sep.

EMOTION, after - acon.

EPILEPTIC - ***apis,*** arg-n., ars., art-v., bufo, calc., ***calc-ar.,*** calc-s., ***caust.,*** crot-h., ***cupr., cur., hyos.,*** ign., kalm., ***nat-m., nux-v.,*** plb., ***sil.,*** tarent., thuj., ***visc.***
after - calc., tarent.
before - ars., calc-ar., caust., **HYOS.,** lach., plb., sulph., tarent.

ERECTIONS, during - tarent.

ERUPTIONS, preceding - cop.
suppressed, from - bell., bry., calc., carb-v., cham., hep., ip., lach., phos., rhus-t., ***sulph.***

EVENING - alum., alumn., ***am-c., apis,*** arn., **ARS.,** asaf., bor., ***calc.,*** calc-s., carb-an., ***carb-s.,*** carb-v., caust., cham., chel., chin., chin-a., coloc., ***cycl.,*** dios., eug., ***graph., hep.,*** hydr., iris, ***kali-ar.,*** kali-bi., ***kali-c., kali-p.,*** kali-s., ***lach.,*** laur., lyc., lycps., mag-c., meph., merc., nat-m., nat-s., nicc., ***nit-ac.,*** nux-m., ***nux-v.,*** petr., ***ph-ac., phos.,*** pic-ac., phys., plat., **PULS.,** raph., ***rhod.,*** rhus-t., rhus-v., sabad., sel., sep., ***sil.,*** spong., staph., stront-c., ***sulph.,*** tarent., thuj., til., zinc.
bed, in - brom., lach., ***mag-c.,*** nit-ac., nux-m., ***nux-v., petr., phos.,*** rhus-t., sep., staph., sulph.

EXERCISING, on - ars., berb., bism., ***cact.,*** chin., cycl., kali-c., nat-c., sol-n.
amel. - phos.
open air, in - coff., ***nat-c.***
the arms - berb., sep.

EXERTION, on - ars., ***cact.,*** cop., nit-ac., sol-n.
vision - all-s., ***cur., graph., mag-p.,*** **NAT-M., PHOS.,** ruta., ***sil.,*** tarent.
violent, on - mill.

FAINT-like - bry., cocc., gels., nux-v., ther.

FAINTING, with - alum., ars., berb., ***bry.,*** canth., ***carb-v., cham.,*** croc., glon., hep., hipp., ign., lach., mag-c., mosch., **NUX-V.,** paeon., phos., sabad., sulph.

FALL, tendency to - ***acon.,*** agar., alum., am-c., anac., ang., apis, arn., ***ars.,*** bar-c., ***bell.,*** berb., bov., ***calc.,*** calc-s., carb-ac., ***carb-an.,*** carb-s., ***carb-v.,*** caust., chin., ***cic., cocc.,*** coloc., ***con.,*** crot-h., ***cupr.,*** dig., dros., euph., ***ferr.,*** ferr-ar., gels., ***glon.,*** graph., ham., hell., ***hyos.,*** kali-c., kali-p., kali-s., kreos., lach., lact., laur., led., ***lyc.,*** mag-c., ***mag-m.,*** mag-s., merc., mez., nat-c., nat-h., nat-m., ***nat-n.,*** nat-p., nit-ac., nux-m., ***phel.,*** ph-ac., phyt., plb., ***psor., puls., ran-b.,*** rheum, rhod., ***rhus-t.,*** ruta., sabad., ***sabin.,*** sars., sep., ***sil.,*** spig., ***spong.,*** squil., ***stram., sulph.,*** tab., tarent., ***ter., zinc.***
as if, high objects leaned forward and would fall on him - arn., sabad.
high walls would fall on him - arg-n., sabad.
backward - agar., anan., bell., bov., brom., ***bry., calc., carb-an., caust., chin.,*** dios., helo., ***kali-c.,*** kali-n., kali-s., led., merc., mill., ***nux-v.,*** oena., phel., ***ph-ac.,*** **RHUS-T.,** sars., ***sil., spong.,*** stram., sulph.
stooping, when - caust.
walking, while - stram.
dark, in the - ***stram.***
fever, during - sep.
forward - agar., ***alum.,*** arn., bov., ***calc-p., camph.,*** carb-s., card-m., ***caust.,*** chel., ***cic.,*** cupr., ***elaps, ferr.,*** ferr-p., ***graph.,*** hell., hyos., iod., kali-n., kali-p., ***lach.,*** led., lyc., lycps., mag-c., mag-m., mag-s., mang., **NAT-M.,** ***nux-v.,*** petr., phel., ***ph-ac.,*** phos., ***podo.,*** puls., ***ran-b.,*** **RHUS-T.,** sars., ***sabin.,*** sec., senec., ***sil.,*** spig., stry., ***sulph.,*** tarax., vip.
left, to - anac., ***aur., bell., bor., calc., caust.,*** cic., dirc., dros., ***eup-per., eup-pur.,*** euph., ***ir-foe., lach.,*** lycps., merl., mez., nat-c., **NAT-M.,** nux-m., sal-ac., spig., stram., ***sulph.,*** vib., vip., ***zinc.***
looking upward - ***caust.***
morning - zinc.
sitting, while - anac.
walking in open air - aur., dros.
looking down, on - **SPIG.**
morning, on waking - ***graph.,*** phos.
motion, on - sec.
right - ***acon.,*** ars., ***calc.,*** camph., carb-an., ***caust.,*** euph., eup-pur., ferr., kali-n., lycps., lyss., mill., nat-s., rhus-t., ruta., ***sil., zinc.***
sitting, while - stram.
rising bed, from - **RHUS-T.**
sideways - acon., am-m., arg-n., ars., ***benz-ac.,*** bov., **CALC.,** cann-s., ***caust.,*** **COCC.,** ***con.,*** dros., euph., led., mez., **NUX-V.,** phel., puls., rheum, sil., squil., staph., sulph., valer., zinc.
walking, while - sul-ac.
sleep, after - ferr.
stooping, on - merl.

FALLING, sensation of, from a height - ***caust., gels.,*** mosch.
rising, and falling - bar-c., **BELL.,** lach., thuj.

FALLING, with - dig.

FASTING, agg. - sul-i.
sensation as if rouse - ph-ac.

FEET, higher than the head, sensation as if - spig.

FEVER, during the - acon., arg-m., bell., bry., ***carb-an.,*** carb-v., chin., ***cocc.,*** croc., ***gels.,*** ign., ***kali-c.,*** laur., led., mag-m., merc., mosch., nux-v., phos., ***puls.,*** sep., stram., verat., urt-u.

FLOATING, as if - acon., arg-n., **ASAR.,** bell., ***calc., calc-ar.,*** calc-s., camph., cann-i., cocc., coff., hyos., ***hyper., lac-c., lach.,*** lact., ***manc., mez.,*** mosch., nat-m., ***nux-m., op., ph-ac.,*** phos., phys., rhus-t., ***sep.,*** spig., stict., stram., tell., thuj., ***valer.,*** xan., zinc-i.
body feels - mez.
onanism from or hysterical - gels.
left, to - eup-per.
lying down, on - ox-ac.
sitting, while - xan.
vision, of, with - stroph.
waking, on - phos.

FLOWERS, smell, from the - ***hyos.,*** **NUX-V., PHOS.**

FLUIDS, loss of - ***chin.,*** **PHOS.,** ***sep.***

FOREHEAD, felt in - arn., croc., euon., gels., phos., sulph.

FORENOON - acon., agar., ambr., atro., bry., calc., camph., carb-v., ***caust.,*** cham., chin-s., eup-pur., fl-ac., ***lach.,*** lact., ***lyc.,*** lycps., ***nat-m., phos.,*** samb., sars., stann., ***sulph.,*** viol-t., ***zinc.***

FRIGHT, after - ***acon.,*** crot-h., gels., ign., ***op.***

FULLNESS, and aching, in vertex - **CIMIC.**

GARGLING, while - carb-v.

GASLIGHT, from - ***caust.***

GASTRO-enteric derangements, with - aloe, ***bry.,*** chin., ***cocc.,*** ip., kali-c., ***nux-v., puls., tab.***

GLIDING, in the air sensation, as if feet did not touch the ground, while walking in the open air - agar., ***asar.,*** **CALC-AR.,** ***camph., chin.,*** coff., cop., hura, **LAC-C.,** nat-m., nux-m., op., ***rhus-t.,*** sep., ***spig.,*** stram., ***thuj.,*** valer.

HEAD, holding perfectly still amel. - con.
pushed forward as if - ferr-p.
sinks forward - cupr.

HEAD, injuries, after - arn., cic., ***hell.,*** **NAT-S.,** op., ruta.

HEADACHE, during - acet-ac., ***acon.,*** aeth., agar., ail., alumn., anac., anthr., ant-t., **APIS,** ***arg-n., arn., ars.,*** asaf., ***aur., bar-c.,*** **BELL.,** brom., bry., ***bov.,*** **CALC.,** calc-ar., calc-p., carb-s., carb-v., ***caust., chel.,*** cimic., coca, cocc., ***coff., cupr.,*** **CON.,** crot-h., cycl., dulc., eug., ferr., ferr-ar., ferr-p., fl-ac., form., ***gels., glon.,*** grat., ***hep.,*** kali-ar., ***kali-bi., kali-br., kali-c.,*** kali-n., kali-p., kali-s., ***kalm.,*** lach., laur., lob., mag-c., mag-m., ***merc.,*** nat-c., ***nat-m., nat-s., nux-m.,*** **NUX-V.,** ox-ac., ***phos.,*** pic-ac., plb., ***psor., puls.,*** rhus-t., ***sang.,*** sec., sep., **SIL.,** ***spig.,*** stram., ***stront-c.,*** sulph., ***tab., verat-v.,*** xan., zinc.
after - merc., merl., ***phos.***
before - ***aran.,*** berb., calc., plat., til.
morning - bov.
one-sided, with - ***nat-m.***

HEART, symptoms, with - kali-c., lach., phos., verat.

HEAT, from - con., ptel.
after - aeth.
before - chin., sep.
room, of - grat., ***lyc.,*** paeon., phos., ***puls.***
sun, of - ***agar.,*** cast-v., gels., glon., nat-c.

HEAT, sensation of, after - chin., sep.
chest, in, and about heart, with - lachn.

HIGH, places, in - **ARG-N.,** aur., **CALC.,** gels., ***nat-m.,*** phos., puls., staph., **SULPH.,** ***zinc.***
as if falling from a - caust., gels.

HOUSE, in - agar., am-m., arg-m., bell., ***croc.,*** crot-t., ***lyc., mag-m.,*** merc., mur-ac., nat-c., par., phos., ***puls.,*** stann., sil., staph., sul-ac.
amel. in - ***agar.,*** caust., ***cycl.,*** grat., kreos., merc., sulph.
entering, on - acon., ars., carb-ac., merc., pall., ***phos.,*** plat., ***puls.,*** ran-b., sil., tab.
entering, on, after walking - arg-m., plat., tab.

HUNGRY, when - dulc., ***kali-c., phos.***

HYSTERICAL - ***asaf.,*** gels., ***ign.,*** valer.

INSPIRATION, deep, on - ***cact.***

INTOXICATED, as if - acet-ac., ***acon.,*** act-sp., ail., agar., ***alum.,*** am-c., ***anac.,*** anan., ***arg-m., arg-n.,*** ars., asar., ***aur., bell.,*** berb., ***bry.,*** caj., ***camph.,*** cann-i., ***carb-ac.,*** carb-s., caust., ***cham.,*** chel., ***chin.,*** chin-s., ***cic.,*** clem., **COCC.,** ***con.,*** cori-r., croc., crot-h., cur., dig., ***ferr.,*** ferr-p., ***gels.,*** glon., ***graph.,*** grat., ham., ***hydr., hyos., kali-br.,*** kali-c., kreos., lact., laur., ***led., lil-t.,*** lyc., mag-c., ***med.,*** merc., merl., ***mez.,*** mosch., nat-m., ***nux-m.,*** **NUX-V.,** oena., ***op.,*** petr., phel., ***ph-ac.,*** phos., **PULS.,** rhod., ***rhus-t.,*** sabad., sars., ***sec.,*** sel., sep., ***sil., spig., spong.,*** stram., ***tab.,*** tarax., tep., ***thuj.,*** til., valer.

KNEADING, bread or making similar motions - sanic.

KNEELING, when - mag-c., **SEP.,** stram., ther.

LEANING, against anything - cycl., ***dig.***
head - verb.
left cheek against hand - verb.

LEFT, swaying toward - anac., arg-n., ***aur.,*** bell., ***bor.,*** calc., cic., dirc., dros., ***eup-per.,*** eup-pur., euph., ir-foe., lycps., merl., mez., myris., nat-c., nux-m., sol-n., spig., ***sulph., zinc.***
evening - nux-m.
lying, while - merl., ox-ac.
morning on waking - myris.
sitting, while - anac., merl.
standing - merl.
walking in open air - aur., bor., nux-m., sol-n., sulph.

LIFTING, a weight - ant-t., **PULS.**

LIGHTNING, from - crot-h.

LIGHTS, from being in a room, with many - nux-v.
bright, in - agar.

LIVER, problems, with - bry., card-m., chel., mur-ac.

LOOKING, general
colored lights, at - art-v.
downward - alum., ars., calad., calc., camph., cham., cina, con., ferr., ferr-ar., ferr-p., graph., ***kalm.,*** mag-m., merc., nat-c., nit-ac., nux-v., olnd., ox-ac., petr., **PHOS.,** puls., rhod., rhus-t., salam., sep., **SPIG.,** staph., **SULPH.,** thuj.
downward, as if - phos.
either way, right or left - ***con.,*** lec., olnd., op., sabad., ***spig.,*** sulph., sumb., thuj.
eyes turned, with - **SPIG.**
large plain, at a - sep.
mirror, into a - kali-c.
moving object, at, nausea, with - piloc.
object, at a moving - ***agar.,*** anac., ***con., cur.,*** graph., ***jab.,*** laur., mosch., nat-m., olnd., sep., ***sulph.***
revolving objects, at - lyc.
right, to - lec.
sideways - thuj.

LOOKING, general
steadily - all-s., am-c., ars., ***caust.,*** colch., con., ***cur., kali-c., lach.,*** manc., **NAT-M.,** olnd., ***phos.,*** sars., ***sil.,*** **SPIG.,** sulph., tarent.
amel. - con., ***dig.,*** sabad.
straight ahead, amel. - olnd.
upwards - ***calc.,*** carb-v., ***caust.,*** chin-a., crot-t., ***cupr.,*** dig., ***graph.,*** iod., kali-p., kali-s., ***lach.,*** mur-ac., nat-h., ***nux-v., petr.,*** **PHOS.,** plat., plb., **PULS.,** ***sang.,*** sep., ***sil.,*** stram., ***tab., thuj.***
high buildings, at - ***arg-n.***
light, at a - cupr., plb., thuj., zinc.
walking in open air, while - ***arg-n.,*** ox-ac., ***sep.***
water, at running - arg-m., brom., ***ferr., verat.***
window, out, a - camph., ***carb-v.,*** **NAT-M.,** ox-ac.

LYING, while - alum., am-c., ***apis,*** ars., aur., bar-c., brom., calad., calc., ***carb-v., caust., cham.,*** coca, **CON.,** ***crot-c.,*** cycl., dig., ham., iod., lac-d., ***lach.,*** lact., kali-m., mag-c., merc., merl., nat-c., nat-s., ***nit-ac.,*** nux-v., ox-ac., petr., phel., phos., pic-ac., ***puls.,*** rhod., ***rhus-t.,*** sang., sep., sil., spig., staph., stry., sulph., ***sumb., thuj.***
amel. - acon., alum., alumn., ***arn.,*** aur-m., ***carb-an., chin.,*** cic., ***cina,*** cocc., crot-h., cupr., grat., ham., kalm., lach., nat-m., nit-ac., olnd., op., petr., phel., phos., rhus-t., sil., stann., sul-ac., tell., thuj.
as if, feet were going up - ***ph-ac.,*** stict.
he did not touch the bed - **LAC-C.**
sinking down through or with the bed - bell., benz-ac., **BRY.,** ***calc-p.,*** chin-s., dulc., kali-c., ***lach., lyc.,*** mosch., nat-c., rhus-t., sac-alb.
back, on - ***alum.,*** alumn., anan., ***merc.,*** merc-sul., mur-ac., nux-v., ***puls., sil.,*** sulph.
amel. - stram.
cool room, in a, amel. - cast-v.
down, on, in the act of - ***bell.,*** brom., caust., ferr., kalm., nit-ac., ***nux-v.,*** olnd., ox-ac., ***rhus-t.,*** sabad., sang.
face, on, while - phos.
amel. - ***coca.***
head high, with amel. - nat-m., ***petr.***
left, agg. - alumn., ***iod.,*** lac-d., onos., ***phos., sil.,*** zinc-j.
necessary - ***ambr.,*** ant-t., ***aran.,*** asaf., ***aur.,*** chel., **COCC.,** crot-h., cupr., ***graph., kali-c.,*** kali-p., kali-s., kalm., kreos., laur., merc., mosch., nat-c., nat-m., ***nit-ac.,*** op., **PHOS., PULS.,** sabin., sec., ***sil., sul-ac.,*** zinc.
opening eyes - lac-d.
right agg. - eup-per., gels., hell., ***mur-ac., phos.,*** rhus-t., tub.

MEDITATING, on - agar., arg-n., coff., gran., ***ph-ac., puls.,*** sil.
amel. - phos.

MEDITATING, on
thinking of something else amel. - agar., pip-m., sep.
walking in open air, while - agar., sil.

MENIERE'S disease, noises in ear with vertigo - alum., arg-m., ***arg-n.,*** arn., ars., bar-m., bell., benz-ac., bry., calc., ***camph.,*** carb-v., carb-s., ***caust.,*** chen-a., chin., **CHIN-S.,** ***chin-sal., cic., cocc.,*** colch., com., con., crot-h., crot-t., ***dig.,*** eucal., ferr-p., gels., ***glon.,*** gran., hell., kali-c., kali-i., kali-m., kali-p., kalm., laur., mag-c., myric., nat-a., nat-c., nat-m., nat-p., nat-s., nat-sal., nux-v., onos., op., petr., ph-ac., **PHOS.,** pic-ac., piloc., psor., puls., rad-br., ***sal-ac., sang.,*** seneg., sep., ***sil.,*** stann., tab., ***ther.,*** zinc.
seasick, as if - tab.

MENOPAUSE, during - con., ***crot-h., glon.,*** lach., ***sang.,*** tril., ***ust.***
after - con.

MENSES, during - ***acon.,*** am-c., ant-t., arg-n., bor., bov., brom., cact., ***calc.,*** calc-p., carb-s., carb-v., caul., ***caust., con., croc.,*** cub., ***cycl.,*** elaps, ferr., ***ferr-p., gels.,*** graph., ***iod., kali-bi., lach.,*** lyc., mosch., nux-v., ***ph-ac.,*** phos., plat., **PULS.,** ***sec., sulph.,*** thuj., tril., uran., ust.
amel. - all-s., lach.
stooping, on - calc., caust.
stooping, on, and rising again - ***calc.***
walking, while - phos.
after - agar., ant-t., con., nat-m., puls., ust.
before - acon., agn., bor., bov., bry., calc., ***calc-p., caul.,*** chel., ***con., lach.,*** nux-m., phos., ***puls., verat., zinc.***
suppressed - ***acon.,*** bry., calc., cimic., con., **CYCL.,** gels., lach., nux-v., phos., plat., **PULS.,** sabin., sep., sil., sulph., verat., zinc.

MENTAL, exertion, from - ***agar.,*** agn., am-c., arg-m., ***arg-n.,*** arn., bar-c., ***bor.,*** calc., cham., coff., cupr., gran., grat., kalm., merc-i-f., **NAT-C., NAT-M.,** nat-p., **NUX-V.,** ***ph-ac.,*** pic-ac., ***puls.,*** sep., sil., ***staph.***
exertion, amel. - phos.

MIRROR, after looking into - kali-c.

MORNING - acon., ***agar.,*** ail., ***alum., am-c.,*** am-m., ***arg-n.,*** bell., bism., ***bov., bry.,*** bufo, calad., ***calc.,*** calc-s., **CARB-AN.,** ***carb-s., cast-eq.,*** caust., cham., ***chel., chin.,*** chin-s., ***cinnb.,*** coc-c., dig., dios., ***dulc.,*** eup-per., eup-pur., form., ***gels.,*** glon., ***graph., hep.,*** hyper., iod., kali-bi., ***kali-c.,*** kali-n., kali-p., kali-s., kreos., **LACH.,** lact., **LYC.,** lyss., ***mag-c., mag-m.,*** mag-s., manc., ***nat-m., nat-p.,*** nicc., ***nit-ac., nux-v.,*** olnd., ox-ac., ***petr., ph-ac., phos.,*** psor., ***puls.,*** ran-b., rhus-t., ruta., sabin., sang., sars., sel., seneg., sep., ***sil.,*** sol-n., squil., stront-c., ***sulph.,*** tell., verat., verat-v., ***zinc.***
bed, in - alum., bor., ***carb-v., calc.,*** con., chel., form., gels., graph., lach., lyc., nat-m., ol-an., ph-ac., phos., pip-m., sep., sil., ***zinc.***
breakfast, after - bufo, cocc., gels., lyc., phos., sel., tarent.

MORNING,
breakfast, during - con., ***sil.***
amel. - ***alum.,*** calc., cinnb.
before, worse - alum., ***calc.***
lie down, compelled to - ***nit-ac.,*** **PULS.**
rising, on - acon., ***ambr.,*** am-c., aml-n., asar., atro., **BELL.,** bov., **BRY.,** calc., carb-an., carb-s., caul., ***caust.,*** cham., cimic., ***con., dulc.,*** fl-ac., ***gamb.,*** glon., gran., graph., guai., hell., iod., kali-bi., lach., **LYC.,** mag-c., ***mag-m.,*** mag-s., manc., **NAT-M.,** nat-s., nicc., ***nit-ac.,*** ph-ac., **PHOS., PULS., RHUS-T.,** ruta., sabad., samb., sep., sil., sol-n., ***spig.,*** squil., sulph., thuj., tril., verat., verat-v.
after - am-c., bar-c., calc., chel., hep., lach., **LYC.,** mag-c., mag-m., mur-ac., nat-m., ***nit-ac.,*** **PHOS.,** sabad., sil., stram., sulph., **TELL.**
amel - caust., rhus-t.
waking, on - acon., atro., brom., bry., calc., caps., ***carb-v., chin., dulc.,*** euphr., fago., fl-ac., ***graph.,*** hell., hyper., iris, ***kali-bi.,*** **LACH.,** merc-i-f., myris., ***nat-m.,*** rhus-t., stann., til., tarent., zinc.

MOTION, from - ***agar.,*** ail., aloe, ***am-c.,*** am-m., arn., ***aur.,*** aur-m., bar-c., ***bell.,*** **BRY.,** ***calc-p.,*** carb-ac., ***carb-v., chin., cocc., coff., con.,*** crot-h., crot-t., cupr., ferr-i., fl-ac., gels., ***glon., graph.,*** grat., ***hep.,*** hydr-ac., ***kalm.,*** laur., lycps., ***mag-c., med.,*** nat-a., nat-c., nat-m., nux-v., paeon., phel., ***phos.,*** phys., ***puls.,*** sabad., sang., sec., sel., ***sil.,*** sin-n., sol-n., spong., staph., sumb., tab., tell., ther.
amel. - coff., cycl., mag-m., rhod.
arms, of - bar-c., berb., sep.
eyelids, of - alum., mosch.
eyes, of - bell., chel., cocc., ***con.,*** mur-ac., petr., plat., puls., spig.
floor, as from motion of - sulph.
least, from - morph., ther., zinc.
neck, of - verat.
rapid, from - sang.
shaking - hep.
sudden - ferr., gels., lact., ptel., sumb.
vomiting and nausea - sel., ***ther.***

MOVING, the head - acon., ***agar.,*** aloe, am-c., ***arn.,*** atro., aur., ***bar-c., bell.,*** **BRY.,** ***calc.,*** calc-ar., carb-an., ***carb-v.,*** caust., clem., cocc., **CON.,** cupr., echi., ***glon., hep., ign.,*** ip., kali-bi., kali-c., lac-d., meph., mosch., nat-m., paeon., ***phos., ptel.,*** rhus-t., samb., sang., sep., sel., spig., tell., ther., thuj.
quickly - am-c., atro., bar-c., ***bry.,*** **CALC.,** calc-s., ***carb-v., coloc., gels.,*** helo., ***kali-c.,*** lac-ac., sang., spig., ***staph.,*** sulph., verat.
quickly, amel. - agar.

NAUSEA, with - **ACON.,** agar., ail., ***alum., alumn., am-c.,*** amyg., aml-n., ***ant-c.,*** ant-t., apis, arg-n., ***arn.,*** ars., ***bapt., bar-c., bell.,*** bor., brom., ***bry.,*** calad., cahin., ***calc., calc-p., calc-s., camph., carb-an., carb-v., caust., cham., chel.,*** chin., chin-a., **CHIN-S.,** cimic., ***cinnb.,***

NAUSEA, with - coca, **COCC.,** coloc., ***con., cycl.,*** crot-h., crot-t., **FERR.,** ***ferr-ar.,*** ferr-p., fl-ac., gels., ***glon.,*** gran., ***graph.,*** gymn., ***ham., hell., hep.,*** hyos., ***ind.,*** kali-ar., ***kali-bi.,*** kali-br., kali-c., kali-p., kali-s., ***kalm., lac-c., lach., lob., lyss., lyc.,*** mag-c., ***merc.,*** mill., ***mosch.,*** mur-ac., myric., ***nat-m., nat-s.,*** nicc., ***nit-ac., nux-m., nux-v.,*** **PETR.,** ***phos.,*** pic-ac., plat., ***puls., rhus-t.,*** rumx., sabad., ***sang.,*** sanic., sars., sel., senec., ***sep., sil., spig.,*** spong., squil., ***staph.,*** stram., stront-c., ***sulph., tab.,*** tarent., tell., ***ter.,*** ther., ***verat., verat-v.,*** vip., ***zinc.***
after - calc., cimic., gran., lyss., ***zinc.***
closing eyes, on - ***lach., ther.***
evening - zinc.
looking long at one object - sars.
lying, while - ars.
on right side of back - ***mur-ac.***
with the head low - ***petr.***
middle of chest - bry., phos.
morning - ***calc.,*** nit-ac., sabad., squil., stront.
motion, on - sel.
periodic - **NAT-M.**
raising the head - ***merc.***
rising in bed, on - bry., **COCC.,** ***verat-v.***
stooping amel. - ***petr.***
vomiting, and nausea - ***chin-s.,*** cocc., ferr., lappa-a., lob., petr., sel., ***tab., ther.***
waking, on - ***spong.***

NERVOUS origin, of - ambr., arg-n., ***cocc.,*** con., ***gels., ign.,*** nux-v., ***phos.,*** rhus-t., ther.

NIGHT - ***am-c.,*** bar-c., bell., calc., caust., chin., clem., croc., cycl., dig., fago., ham., hyper., lac-c., lach., nat-c., nux-v., phos., phys., pic-ac., rhod., rhust-t., sang., sarr., sep., sil., ***spong.,*** stram., sulph., tarent., ther., ***thuj.,*** zinc.
bed, in - am-c., ***arg-m.,*** bar-c., ***caust., con.,*** ind.
on going to, amel. - aur-m., carb-an.
waking, on - ***chin.,*** dig., lac-c., lyc., phos., sabad., sil., ***spong.,*** stront-c., sulph., thuj.
him from sleep - **NUX-V.**

NIGHT-watching, and loss of sleep, from - **COCC.,** coff., **NUX-V.**

NOISE, from - asar., nux-v., ***ther.***

NOISES, in ear, with vertigo - alum., arg-m., ***arg-n.,*** arn., ars., bar-m., bell., benz-ac., bry., calc., ***camph.,*** carb-v., carb-s., ***caust.,*** chen-a., chin., **CHIN-S.,** ***chin-sal., cic., cocc.,*** colch., com., con., crot-h., crot-t., ***dig.,*** eucal., ferr-p., ***gels., glon.,*** gran., hell., iris, kali-c., kali-i., kali-m., kali-p., kalm., laur., mag-c., myric., nat-a., nat-c., nat-m., nat-p., nat-s., nat-sal., nux-v., onos., op., petr., ph-ac., **PHOS.,** pic-ac., piloc., psor., puls., rad-br., ***sal-ac., sang.,*** seneg., sep., ***sil.,*** stann., ***stry.,*** tab., ***ther.,*** valer., zinc.
after vertigo - chin.
seasick, as if - tab.

NOON - aeth., arn., ***calc-p., caust.,*** chin., dulc., ham., kali-c., kalm., lyc., mag-m., mag-s., manc., merc., nat-s., nux-v., ***phos.,*** stram., stront-c., sulph., zinc.

NOSEBLEEDS, with - bell., bor., bry., carb-an., ferr-p., vip.
amel. - brom

OBJECTS, seem, to, approach and then recede - cic.
are inverted - bufo. gels.
too far off - anac., gels., **PULS.,** stann., stram.
large - caust.
move - ***cocc.,*** hydr-ac., kali-cy., mosch., sep., thuj.
reel - anac., ***bell., bry.,*** glon.
run into each other - ir-fl.
the seat on which he sat - zinc.
to the left and downward - tab.
to the right - ***lac-d.,*** nat-s., sal-ac.
vibrate - ***carb-v.***
stand still - dulc.
turn in a circle - ***agar.,*** agn., ***alum.,*** am-c., anac., arn., bar-c., bar-m., bov., ***bry.,*** cadm-s., **CHEL.,** ***cic.,*** coca, cocc., colch., con., **CYCL.,** hell., kali-c., kali-n., kali-p., kali-s., laur., ***lyc.,*** mag-c., merc., merc-i-r., morph., mosch., ***mur-ac.,*** **NAT-M.,** nat-p., nat-s., olnd., ***nux-v.,*** op., ph-ac., ***psor.,*** rhus-t., sabad., sel., sep., sil., sol-n., sul-ac., zinc.
on looking at running water - ferr.
room whirls - ***calc., caust.,*** cann-s., cod., dub., grat., kali-bi., **NUX-V.,** ***phos.,*** tab.
turn in a circle, sensation - ***agar.,*** agn., ***alum.,*** am-c., anac., arn., bar-c., bar-m., bov., ***bry.,*** cadm-s., **CHEL.,** ***cic.,*** coca, cocc., colch., con., **CYCL.,** hell., kali-c., kali-p., kali-s., laur., ***lyc.,*** mag-c., merc., merc-i-r., morph., mosch., ***mur-ac.,*** **NAT-M.,** nat-p., nat-s., olnd., ***nux-v.,*** op., ph-ac., ***psor.,*** rhus-t., sabad., sel., sep., sil., sol-n., sul-ac.
room whirls, sensation - alum., ***calc., caust.,*** cann-s., cod., dub., grat., kali-bi., merc., **NUX-V.,** ***phos.,*** sil., tab.

OCCIPITAL - ang., bell., bry., carb-v., chin., con., crot-t., fl-ac., **GELS.,** gins., glon., iber., led., med., **PETR.,** pic-ac., ran-b., senec., **SIL.,** spig., sulph., tab., thuj., verat., ***zinc.***

ODOR, of flowers - ***hyos.,*** **NUX-V., PHOS.**

PAIN, agg. - cimic.
before - ran-b.
spleen, of, with - urt-u.
stomach, of - cic.

PAINFUL - phos., tab., tarent.

PALPITATIONS, during - plat.
heart, from, or with heart symptoms - aeth., bell., ***cact.,*** dig., plat., spig.
vertigo of head, with palpitations - glon., sec.

PAROXYSMAL - agar., aloe, ant-t., ***arg-m.,*** bell., bor., calc., camph., caul., cupr., graph., kali-bi., morph., ***nat-m., nux-v.,*** phos., plat., ptel., sep., tab., til., verb.

PELVIC troubles, with - aloe, con.

PERIODICAL - agar., ang., ***arg-m., camph., cocc.,*** cycl., ***ign., kali-c.,*** **NAT-M., PHOS.,** ***tab.,*** ust.
every two weeks - cocc.

PERSPIRATION, with - merc-c., tab., verat.
amel. - nat-s.

PREGNANCY, during - alet., ars., bell., cocc., ***gels.,*** **NAT-M.,** nux-v., phos.

PRESSURE of root of nose, with - bapt.

PULSE, with slow - ther.

PUSHED, forward, as if - calc., euon.

RAILWAY, travelling - kali-i.

RAISING, hands above head - onos.

RAISING, head - acon., aeth., ant-t., ***arn.,*** bar-c., **BRY.,** cact., ***calc.,*** carb-an., ***carb-v., chin.,*** clem., coloc., croc., hell., jatr., laur., mag-s., merc., merc-c., ***nux-v.,*** op., ***phos.,*** pic-ac., sel., spig., stann., stram.
bed, on waking from - spig.

REACHING, up, on - ars., bar-c., cupr., lac-d., ***lach.,*** sep., sil., sulph.

READING, while - ***am-c.,*** ang., arg-m., arn., cupr., ***cur.,*** gran., ***graph.,*** grat., ham., merl., merc-i-f., par., phys., stann.
after - kali-c., ph-ac.
aloud - manc., par.
too long - arn.
walking amel. - am-c.

RED face, with - anan., ***bell., cact., cocc., stram.***

REELING - acon., ***agar., alum.,*** anac., arg-n., ***ars., bell.,*** bruc., bry., camph., ***caps., caust., cic.,*** cann-s., cimic., croc., cupr., ferr., ***gels., glon.,*** graph., hell., hydr-ac., hyos., kali-i., kali-n., lach., lol., ***lyc.,*** mag-c., mag-m., nat-c., nat-m., ***nux-m., nux-v.,*** ol-an., op., paeon., ph-ac., ***phos.,*** plat., prun., puls., rhod., rhus-t., ruta, sabad., sanic., ***sec.,*** seneg., spong., ***stram.,*** sulph., ***tab.,*** tarax., ter., teucr., thuj., verat., verb., viol-t.
amel. - carb-an.
sex, after - bov.
standing - plat., stram.
walking - agar., alum., am-c., bel., bruc., carb-an., caust., cocc., dros., mag-m., nat-m., petr., ph-ac., prun., rhod., rhus-t., ruta., sabad., stram., teucr., verat., verb.

RELAXATION, after - calc., lach.

REST, agg. - acon., bell., ***calc.,*** cycl., ***lach.,*** manc., nat-c., puls., rhus-t., sil.
amel. - arn., cann-i., coca, colch., ***con.,*** cycl., eupi., nat-m., nux-m., nux-v., spig.

RESTING, head on the table amel. - sabad.

RIDING, while - ant-t., dig., grat.
boat, in a - apom., ***cocc.,*** petr., staph., tab.
carriage, in a - acon., calc., ***cocc., hep.,*** lac-d., lyc., petr., sel., ***sil.***
amel. - glon., sil.
carriage, as from, in a - cycl., ferr., grat., hep.
horseback, while - cop., rhus-t.

RIDING, while
horseback, while, amel. - tarent.
railroad - kali-i.

RIGHT, swaying toward - **ACON.,** ars., berb., calc., carb-an., caust., dios., euph., ferr., grat., kali-n., lac-d., lycps., lyss., mill., nat-s., rhus-t., ruta., sars., sil., ***zinc.***
circle, in a - berb., ***caust.***

RISING, on - absin., **ACON.,** acon-c., aeth., ***ail.,*** aml-n., apoc., ***arn.,*** ars., arund., atro., ***bar-c., bell.,*** berb., bov., **BRY.,** ***calc., cann-i., carb-an.,*** carb-o., ***caust.,*** cedr., chel., ***chin.,*** chin-s., ***cic.,*** cina, cocc., colch., con., cupr., ***dig.,*** **FERR.,** ferr-ar., ferr-p., form., genist., ***glon.,*** grat., ***guai., ham.,*** hell., hep., hyos., ind., kali-bi., kali-c., kali-p., kali-s., lac-ac., ***lac-d., lach.,*** laur., lyss., manc., meny., merc., morph., **NAT-M.,** nat-s., nux-v., olnd., op., ***petr.,*** **PHOS.,** pic-ac., plat., ptel., ***puls.,*** **RHUS-T.,** sabin., seneg., sil., sul-ac., sulph., **TAB.,** thuj., trom., ***verat-v.,*** vip., zinc.
after - apoc., bar-c., ***bell.,*** bry., calc., cocc., dig., eug., ***form.,*** gnaph., ***lyc.,*** lyss., ***mag-c.,*** ph-ac., ***phos.,*** sabad., stann.
amel. - ars., ***aur.,*** caust., hell., mosch., nat-m., phos., ***rhus-t.***
bed, from, on - ***agar., arn.,*** ars., bar-c., ***bell., bry., cact.,*** caust., cham., **CHEL.,** ***chin.,*** chin-s., cic., ***cimic.,*** cinnb., **COCC.,** con., cupr., dulc., **FERR.,** ***ferr-p., fl-ac., glon.,*** graph., ind., iod., kali-bi., kali-s., lach., lyc., mag-m., mag-s., ***merc-c.,*** **NAT-M.,** nat-s., nicc., ***nit-ac.,*** **NUX-V.,** olnd., ***op., petr., ph-ac.,*** **PHOS., PHYT.,** ***pic-ac.,*** puls., ***rhus-t.,*** ruta., sabin., ***sep., sil., stram.,*** sul-ac., ***sulph.,*** verat-v.
kneeling, from, on - cer-b., sep.
seat, from, on - ***acon.,*** aesc., aeth., all-s., asar., bov., **BRY.,** ***calc., calc-p., carb-an.,*** cham., coca, ***con.,*** dig., **FERR.,** grat., hell., ind., iod., kali-bi., kali-c., kali-s., kalm., laur., ***lyc.,*** lyss., merc., merc-i-f., nicc., nit-ac., **NUX-V.,** ox-ac., ***petr.,*** ph-ac., **PHOS.,** pic-ac., ptel., **PULS., RHUS-T.,** sabad., ***sang.,*** sel., sep., spig., staph., ***sulph.,*** sumb., thuj., verat., verat-v.
seat, from, after - apoc., bry., cocc., dig., phos.
seat, from, after, long lasting - laur.
seat, from, after, sitting bent - merc.
seat, from, after, sitting bent, long - cham., laur., ph-ac.
stooping, from - acon., ***anac.,*** apoc., ***arn.,*** ars., bar-c., **BELL.,** berb., bov., ***bry., calc., carb-an.,*** cic., cocc., con., **FERR.,** ***graph.,*** ham., hell., laur., lyss., meny., merc., nat-m., nicc., ***nit-ac.,*** nux-v., ***op.,*** petr., phos., pic-ac., ***puls., sang.,*** sanic., sep., sil., sulph., thuj., zinc.
stooping, from, after - laur., zinc.
stooping, from, after, amel. - aur., ***hell.***
stooping, from, quickly - ***ferr.,*** sang.
stooping, from, supine position - croc., merc-c., olnd., petr., puls., sel., sil.

ROCKING, as if - bell., calad.
amel. - sec.
from - bor., ***coff.***

ROOM, in, with a high ceiling - cupr-ac.

RUBBING, the eyes amel. - alum.

SCRATCHING skin agg. - calc.

SEWING, while - graph., lac-d., lact., mag-c., phel., sul-ac.

SEX, after - ph-ac., sep.

SHAKING, the head - acon., calc., ***con.,*** corn., genist., glon., hep., kali-c., ***morph.,*** nat-a., sep., spig.
quickly - sep.
involuntary - lyc.

SHAVING, after - ***carb-an.***

SINKING, as if - ***bry.,*** lach., ***lyc.,*** nat-m., ph-ac.
bed, down through or with the bed when lying - bell., benz-ac., **BRY.,** ***calc-p.,*** chin-s., dulc., kali-c., ***lach., lyc.,*** mosch., nat-c., rhus-t., sac-alb.

SITTING, while - aeth., aloe, alum., am-c., anac., ***apis,*** arg-n., ars., bell., calc., ***camph.,*** carb-ac., ***carb-an., carb-s., carb-v., caust., cham.,*** chin., cic., coca, ***cocc.,*** colch., coloc., cop., crot-h., crot-t., ***cupr.,*** dig., eug., euon., fl-ac., ***glon.,*** grat., hell., ind., kali-bi., ***kali-c.,*** kali-s., lach., lycps., mang., meph., ***merc.,*** merc-cy., nat-c., nat-m., nat-p., nit-ac., par., ***petr.,*** phel., ph-ac., **PHOS.,** pic-ac., ***plat.,*** **PULS.,** ran-s., rhod., ***rhus-t.,*** ruta., sabad., sabin., sanic., sars., ***sep., sil., spig., spong.,*** stann., staph., stram., sul-ac., ***sulph.,*** tab., tell., ***thuj., viol-o., zinc.***
amel. - ***acon.,*** ars., aur., bry., ***cycl.,*** form., lach., puls., ***sil.***
bed, up in - acon., ars., ***bry.,*** caust., **CHEL.,** chin-s., **COCC.,** croc., ***cupr.,*** euph., eupi., ind., kali-br., merc., nat-m., nit-ac., op., ***phos., phyt., puls.,*** sep., ***sil.,*** thuj., ***zinc.***
bed, up in amel. - hell., ***lac-d.,*** phos., puls.
eating, before - kali-c.
erect - ***cham., hydr.***
erect, high, as if too - aloe, ***phos.***
walk, after a - caust., colch., lach.
writing, while - kali-bi., merc.

SLEEP, during - aeth., crot-h., ***lyc., sang.,*** **SEP.,** ***sil.,*** ther.
agg., after - ambr., ant-t., apis, ars., atro., ***calc., carb-v., chin.,*** cimic., ***dulc., graph.,*** hep., ***kali-c.,*** kali-i., **LACH.,** ***lact., med.,*** merc., nat-m., **NUX-V.,** op., ***sep., spong.,*** stann., stict., stram., stront-c., tarent., ***ther.,*** thuj., zinc.
amel. - bell., ferr., grat., pall.
half asleep., while - arg-m., ***sil.***
night, at - caust.
on going to - arg-n., hep., nat-m., tell., ***ther.***

SLEEPINESS, with - aeth., arg-m., crot-t., gels., laur., nat-m., ***nit-ac.,*** nux-m., puls., sarr., ***sil.,*** zinc.
alternating with - ***ant-t.***

SMOKING, from - alum., asc-t., bor., brom., calad., clem., ***gels.,*** **NAT-M.,** op., seneg., sil., **NUX-V.,** ***tab.,*** zinc.
as from - zinc.

SNEEZING, from - bar-c., benz-ac., nux-v., ***seneg.***

SPASMS, of muscles, convulsions, vertigo before - cic.

SPRING, in spells of - apis.

STAGGERING, with - acon., agro., ***ail.,*** agar., am-c., anan., ang., ***arg-n.,*** asar., aster., astra-m., atro., ***aur., bell.,*** bry., ***calc.,*** calc-p., ***camph.,*** caps., carb-ac., ***carb-an., carb-s., carb-v., caust., cham.,*** chen-a., ***chin., cic., cocc.,*** colch., coloc., ***con.,*** cupr-ar., dub., ***ferr.,*** ferr-ar., ferr-p., fl-ac., **GELS.,** helo., hydr-ac., ign., ip., kali-br., kali-c., kali-s., kreos., lac-ac., ***lath.,*** lil-t., lol., lyc., lyss., mag-arct., mag-aust., mang., med., merc., morph., mur-ac., ***mygal.,*** nat-c., nicc., ***nux-m.,*** **NUX-V.,** olnd., onos., oxyd., ***oxyt.,*** paeon., petr., ph-ac., **PHOS.,** ***phyt.,*** rhus-t., sars., ***sec., sep.,*** sil., ***stram.,*** sulfon., sulph., tab., tarax., teucr., til., thuj., trio., ***zinc.***
eyes closed, with, or in the dark when walking - ***alum.,*** apis, ***arg-n.,*** carb-s., dub., ***gels.,*** iodof., ***stram.,*** zinc.
incoordination, muscular, with - alum., arag., arg-n., aster., astra-m., ***bar-m.,*** bell., cocc., ***gels.,*** kali-br., med., onos., ph-ac., ***phys.,*** pic-ac., plb., sec., sil., trio., zinc.
uneven ground, walking on, when - lil-t.

STANDING, while - ***acon.,*** aeth., aloe, am-c., apis, arg-m., ***arn.,*** aur., bar-c., bor., ***bov., bry., calc., cann-s., caust.,*** cham., ***cocc.,*** coff., cop., crot-t., cycl., euph., euphr., fl-ac., gels., glon., kali-bi., kali-br., kali-c., kali-n., kali-p., kali-s., ***lach.,*** laur., led., lyc., mag-c., mang., ***merc.,*** merc-sul., merl., nux-m., ***olnd.,*** petr., ***ph-ac., phos.,*** phyt., plat., ***puls.,*** rheum, rhus-t., ***sabin.,*** sars., sec., sel., sil., sol-n., ***spig.,*** stram., ***sulph.,*** ter., valer., zinc.
against something - dig.
air, in open - euph., ***podo.***
amel. - nux-v., ph-ac.
height, on a - ***zinc.***
room, in - cupr., stram.
walking, after - bry., ***calc.***
window, near - nat-m.

STARS, white, before eyes - alum., ant-t.

STOMACH, proceeding from - ***kali-c.***
empty, from - nux-v.
weakness in, compelled to lie down, accompanied by - ambr.

STOOL, during - ***caust.,*** cham., cob., ***cocc.,*** colch., ptel., stram., zinc.
after agg. - apoc., carb-an., ***caust.,*** cupr., gran., lach., ***nat-m.,*** petr., phos., zinc.
amel. - ***cupr.,*** phos., zinc.
before - alum., calc-p., carb-v., caust., chel., cocc., colch., ***cupr.,*** glon., lach., mag-m., mang., nat-c., oena., ***phos.,*** ptel., zinc.

STOOPING, on - acon., act-sp., ail., ***alum., anac.,*** aran-s., ***arg-n., aur.,*** aur-m., bapt., ***bar-c.,*** **BELL.,** berb., ***bry., cact., calc., calc-p.,*** calc-s., ***camph.,*** cann-i., carb-s., ***carb-v., caust., cham.,*** chin., chin-s., cic., cimic., cinnb., coff., con., corn., dig., **GELS.,** ***glon., graph., guare., ham.,*** helon., ***hell., ign.,*** ind., ***iod., kali-bi., kali-c.,*** kali-n., kali-p., kali-s., ***kalm.,*** lac-ac., ***lach.,*** led., ***lyc.,*** mang-m., med., meny., meph., ***merc., merc-c.,*** merl., mill., mosch., myric., nat-m., nat-s., nicc., ***nit-ac.,*** **NUX-V.,** ol-an., op., ***petr.,*** ph-ac., ***phos.,*** pic-ac., plb., ptel., **PULS.,** rhus-t., sant., sep., ***sil.,*** sol-n., ***staph.,*** **SULPH.,** sumb., ther., thuj., valer., verat.
amel. - carb-an., petr.
long, stooping, after - cham.
supper, after - sep.

STRETCHING, on - apoc.

STUPEFACTION, with, as if there was a barrier between his organs of sense and external objects - aeth.

SUDDEN - aeth., agar., apoc., ***arg-m.,*** ars., asar., aster., ***bov.,*** bry., calc-ar., camph., carb-s., chen-a., chin-a., coloc., iris, kali-bi., meph., mosch., sec., senec., sep., stann., stram., sulph., tarent., thuj., tub., verb.

SUMMER, spells of, in - phos., ***psor.***

SUNLIGHT, and heat - acon., ***agar.,*** brom., ***glon.,*** kali-p., ***nat-c.,*** nux-v.

SUPPORTING, head amel. - sabad.

SUPPRESSED, foot sweat, from - sil., zinc.

SUSPENSION, of the senses - ant-t., ***camph., nat-m., nux-m., stram.,*** verat.
as if there were a barrier between his organs of sense and external objects - aeth.

SWINGING, like - calad., ferr., ***merc., sulph.,*** thuj., zinc.
here and there, like - petr.

SYPHILITIC - **AUR.**

TALKING, while - alum., bor., cham., cocc., par., sol-n.
animated, after - bor., cham., lyc., nat-c., par., thuj.
long - thuj.

TEA, after - **NAT-M., SEP.**
tea, after, amel. - glon.

TEMPLES, in felt - coloc.

THINKING, about it, on - pip-m., plb.

THROAT, with choking in - iber.

TOBACCO, poisoning - con., zinc.

TOUCH, agg. - cupr.

TREMBLING - am-c., ***arg-n.,*** ars., bell., ***camph.,*** carb-v., crot-h., ***dig., dulc., gels., glon.,*** nat-m., nux-v., ph-ac., phos., puls., stram., zinc.
internal - cupr.

TURNED, as if bed turned about - **CON.,** nux-v., plb., ***puls.,*** sol-n.

TURNED,
and whirled as if, renewed by thinking about it - plb.

TURNING, on - ***agar.***, am-c., calc., ***con.***, genist., glon., ind., ip., ***kali-c.***, merc., nat-m., phos., rhus-t., tell., ther.
amel. - staph.
left, to - coloc., con., gran.
looking at revolving objects - lyc.
right, to the - lach.
bed, in - **BELL.**, ***cact.***, carb-v., cean., **CON.**, ***graph.***, ind., kalm., ***lac-d.***, meph., ***phos.***, rhus-t., sulph.
left, to - bor., calc-p.
right side, amel. - ***alumn.***
circle, sensation, as if turning in a - acon., ***alum.***, aloe, am-c., anac., ***arg-n.***, ***arn.***, asaf., ***aur.***, ***bell.***, bar-m., berb., ***bism.***, **BRY.**, camph., calad., ***calc.***, caust., chel., ***chin-s.***, ***cic.***, cocc., **CON.**, cupr., **CYCL.**, euph., euon., eup-per., eup-pur., eupi., ferr., grat., hell., hep., hydr-ac., kali-bi., kreos., lact., laur., ***lyc.***, mosch., ***mur-ac.***, nat-m., nat-s., ***nux-v.***, olnd., op., par., ***phos.***, plat., **PULS.**, ran-b., rhod., rhus-t., ruta., sabad., spig., staph., sulph., tab., til., valer., verat., viol-o.
he turns in a circle - bell., berb., ***calc.***, carb-o., caust.
headache, followed by - rhus-t.
left - bell.
right, to - berb., ***caust.***
moving the head, or turning - acon., ***agar.***, aloe, am-c., ***arn.***, atro., aur., ***bell.***, **BRY.**, ***calc.***, calc-ar., carb-an., ***carb-v.***, caust., clem., cocc., **CON.**, cupr., echi., ***glon.***, ***graph.***, hep., ***ign.***, ip., ***kali-bi.***, ***kali-c.***, kali-p., kalm., ***lac-d.***, lec., meph., mosch., nat-c., nat-m., paeon., ***phos.***, ptel., rhus-t., samb., sang., sep., spig., sel., tell., ther., thuj.
quickly - aloe, am-c., atro., bar-c., ***bry.***, **CALC.**, ***carb-v.***, ***coloc.***, **CON.**, ***gels.***, ***kali-c.***, kreos., lac-ac., merc., ***phos.***, ***sang.***, spig., ***staph.***, ***verat.***
amel. - ***agar.***

TWITCHING eyelids, with - chin-s.

UNCONSCIOUSNESS, followed by - acon., alet., berb., ***bry.***, camph., ***carb-v.***, glon., ***nux-v.***, phos., sabad., sil., tab.

URINATION, during - acon.
copious, amel. - gels.
urging, when - ***hyper.***

VERTEX, from - berb., calc., chel., kreos., lyc., lyss., med., merc-i-f., phos., scop., ***scroph-n.***

VEXATION, after - calc., ign., nux-v.

VIOLENT - meph.

VISION obscuration, with - ***acon.***, act-sp., agar., alum., amyg., ***anac.***, ant-t., apis, arg-m., arg-n., ars., asaf., ***bell.***, ***calc.***, ***camph.***, canth., carb-an., carb-v., cham., cic., cimic., ***cupr.***, **CYCL.**, dulc., euon., **FERR.**, ***ferr-ar.***, ferr-p., graph., **GELS.**, gins., ***glon.***, gran., gymn., hell., hep., hyos., ***kali-bi.***, kalm., lach., lact., laur., ***merc.***, mosch., mur-ac., nat-m., ***nit-ac.***, **NUX-V.**, olnd., par., ***phos.***, ***phyt.***, plat., puls., raph., sabad., ***sabin.***, seneg., ***stram.***, ***stront-c.***, ***sulph.***, tep., ter., til., zinc.

VOMITING, with - ail., aloe, ***ars.***, ***bry.***, calc., ***canth.***, ***chel.***, chin., cimic., ***cocc.***, crot-h., crot-t., ***glon.***, gran., ***graph.***, ***hell.***, ip., kali-bi., kali-c., ***lach.***, mag-c., ***merc.***, mosch., ***nat-s.***, ***nux-v.***, oena., ***petr.***, ***puls.***, rham-cal., sabad., ***sang.***, sars., sel., sep., ***tab.***, tell., ***ther.***, **VERAT.**, ***verat-v.***, vip.
after - aeth.
amel. - aeth., eup-per., nat-s., op., tab.
before - nat-s., phos.
nausea, and vomiting - ***chin-s.***, cocc., ferr., lappa-a., lob., petr., sel., ***ther.***

WALKING, while - acon., agar., agn., aloe, alum., am-m., anac., ant-t., ***apis***, ***arg-n.***, ***arn.***, ***ars.***, ars-i., asar., aster., atro., aur-m., bar-c., bar-m., ***bell.***, berb., bism., bor., ***bry.***, calad., ***calc.***, calc-ar., calc-p., calc-s., camph., cann-i., cann-s., carb-an., carb-s., ***carb-v.***, caust., ***chin.***, chin-a., ***cic.***, coca, cocc., coff., colch., ***con.***, cop., cycl., daph., dig., dirc., ***dulc.***, ***ferr.***, ***ferr-i.***, fl-ac., ***gels.***, graph., ***hell.***, hura, hyos., hyper., ign., iod., ip., kali-ar., kali-bi., kali-br., kali-c., kali-n., kali-p., kali-s., lac-c., laur., led., lil-t., lycps., mag-m., merc., merl., mill., ***mur-ac.***, nat-a., ***nat-c.***, **NAT-M.**, nat-p., ***nat-s.***, ***nit-ac.***, ***nux-m.***, **NUX-V.**, op., ox-ac., paeon., ***petr.***, ***phel.***, ***ph-ac.***, **PHOS.**, phys., ***phyt.***, pic-ac., ***psor.***, ptel., **PULS.**, ran-b., ***rhus-t.***, ruta., sars., ***sec.***, sel., ***sep.***, ***sil.***, ***spig.***, stann., staph., ***stram.***, sul-ac., ***sulph.***, sumb., tab., tarax., tarent., tell., thuj., valer., verat., viol-t., ***zinc.***
across an open place - ***ars.***
after - acon., arg-m., bry., calad., ***calc.***, caust., colch., laur., lyss., phos., rhus-t.
after, long - merl., nat-m.
air, open, in the - acon., ***agar.***, ***ambr.***, ang., arn., ***ars.***, aur., aur-m., bry., ***calc.***, calc-ar., ***calc-p.***, canth., carb-s., ***chin.***, chin-a., clem., coff., crot-t., ***cycl.***, ***dros.***, euph., gels., graph., ip., kali-ar., ***kali-c.***, kali-p., kreos., ***lach.***, laur., ***led.***, ***lyc.***, merc., ***mur-ac.***, nicc., ***nux-m.***, ***nux-v.***, olnd., phel., ***phos.***, phys., **PULS.**, rhod., rhus-t., ruta., sars., senec., ***sep.***, sil., spig., stann., stram., stry., **SULPH.**, tab., tarax., tell., thea., thuj., til.
after - anac.
amel. - am-m., ***carb-ac.***, crot-h., kali-c., mag-c., mag-m., ***nat-c.***, par., ***puls.***, rhod., ***rhus-t.***, tab.
elevation, on an - **SULPH.**
sensation of gliding in the air, as if feet did not touch the ground - dub.
amel. - ***acon.***, am-c., bry., lil-t., mag-c., sil., ***staph.***, sulph., ***zinc.***
backward sensation, of - sil.
bridge, over a high - puls., staph., ***sulph.***
bridge, over a narrow - bar-c., ferr., sulph.
dark, while, in - stram.

WALKING, while
eating, after - ***nux-v.***
gliding, sensation of in the air, as if feet did not touch the ground, while - agar., ***asar.,*** calc., **CALC-AR.,** ***camph., chin.,*** coff., cop., hura, **LAC-C.,** nat-m., nux-m., op., ***rhus-t.,*** sep., ***spig.,*** stram., ***thuj.,*** valer.
narrow path, along - bar-c.
near a declivity - sulph.
rapidly - ***ferr.,*** grat., ***puls.,*** sulph.
room, in a - iris, mag-m., manc., merc., nat-c., nit-ac., paeon.
sideways - kali-c.
slowly, but not when taking violent exercise - mill.
water, near - ang.
water, over - ang., brom., ***ferr., sulph.,*** verat.
running - ***arg-m., brom., ferr., sulph.***

WALLS, of house seem to be falling in on her - arg-n., sabad.

WARM, amel. - mang., sil., stront-c.
bed amel. - cocc.
room, from - acon., brom., ***croc., grat.,*** kali-s., lact., lil-t., ***lyc., merc.,*** **NAT-C.,** ph-ac., phos., ***ptel.,*** **PULS.,** ***sanic.,*** sars., tab.
entering, on - arg-m., ars., ***iod., phos.,*** plat., tab.
soup amel. - kali-bi.

WARMTH, rose from chest to throat, sensation as if - merc.

WASHING, feet - merc.
warm water, in - sumb.

WATER, crossing running - ang., ***arg-m.,*** bar-c., ***bell.,*** brom., ***ferr., hyos.,*** stram., ***sulph.,*** verat.

WEAKNESS, with - ***acet-ac., arg-n., chin.,*** colch., con., crot-h., cupr-s., dulc., echi., ***gels.,*** graph., hell., nux-v., ph-ac., phos., sel., ***sil.,*** stram., uran-n.

WILL, exerting, the, amel. - pip-m.

WINDY, weather - ***calc-p.***

WINE, after - ***alum.,*** bell., bov., cocc., ***con., nat-c.,*** nat-m., ***nux-v.,*** petr., sumb., ***zinc.***
amel. - arg-n., coca, gels., phos.

WIPING, eyes amel. - ***alum.***

WORM affections, in - cina, spig.

WRITING, while - arg-m., form., ***graph., kali-bi.,*** kali-c., merc., ph-ac., ptel., rhod., ***sep.,*** stram., thuj.

YAWNING, when - agar., apoc., petr.

Vision

ACCOMMODATION, defective
action too great - phys.
defective - ail., ***agar., arg-n.,*** aur-m., ***hydr., morph., nat-m.,*** nit-ac., onos., ***phys.,*** spig.
diminished - morph., phys., tab.
disturbed - ip., phys., ruta.
headaches - ***mag-p.***
over-exertion, from - ***nux-v.,*** ruta,
slow - ***aur-m., cocc.,*** **CON., GELS.,** ***nat-m., onos., plat., psor.***
tension - ***jab.***

ACUTE, sensitive - acon., ang., aspar., **BELL.,** ***bufo, chin.,*** colch., cycl., fl-ac., hyos., lach., ***nux-v.,*** ph-ac., sars., seneg., viol-o.
hysterical persons in, at night - ***ferr.***

AMAUROSIS, (see Blindness) - acon., anac., anan., ***arg-m.,*** arg-n., ***ars.,*** aur., ***aur-m., aur-m-n.,*** bar-c., **BELL.,** ***bov.,*** both., bry., bufo, **CALC.,** caps., ***caust., chel., chin.,*** chin-s., cic., cocc., **CON.,** croc., dig., dros., dulc., ***elaps,*** euphr., ***ferr.,*** ferr-ar., fl-ac., **GELS.,** guai., ***hyos.,*** kali-ar., kali-c., **KALI-I.,** kali-p., ***kali-s.,*** laur., ***lyc., meny., merc.,*** nat-a., nat-c., **NAT-M.,** nat-p., nit-ac., ***nux-v.,*** olnd., ***op.,*** petr., ***ph-ac.,*** **PHOS.,** ***plb., psor.,*** **PULS.,** ***rhus-t., ruta.,*** **SEC.,** ***sep.,*** **SIL.,** spig., staph., **STRAM., SULPH.,** syph., ***thuj.,*** verat., verat-v., vib., ***zinc.***
anemia, from - ***verat-v.***
appeared and ceased with the appearance and cessation of albuminuria - plb.
beginning, in - ***ant-s.***
could not distinguish large objects, with paresis of legs - rhus-t.
cold, from a - ***bell.***
congestive - ***gels.***
diplopia, with or without, from suppressed eruption - ***sulph.***
eruption, after a sudden disappearance of an, on head - sulph.
with scabby, on occiput and ears - ***psor.***
fever, from nervous - ***bell.***
gutta serena - aur-m-n.
early stage - ***hell.***
headache, during - ***zinc.***
violent, after - ***sep.***
hemorrhage, especially from, debility and exhaustion - crot-h.
incipient, especially of left eye - ***phos.***
left - ***arg-m.,*** phos., thuj.
losses, by debilitating - ***ph-ac.***
masturbation, from - **GELS.**
nerve, from congestion or irritation of optic - ***verat-v.***
pupils, with contracted - ***sep., zinc.***
dilatation of - ***gels., phos.***
quinine, from - ***bell., gels.***
rheumatic, from, troubles - ***chel.***
right - ***bov.***
right then left - ***chin.***
ringworm, after suppression of - ***chel.***

AMAUROSIS,
scarlatina, after suppression of rash in - ***bell.***
sexual, excesses, associated with fatty liver - **PHOS.**
spinal irritation, first right, then left eye, with - ***chin.***
stroke, after - ***gels.***
threatened - ***caust.***
confinement, during - ***caust.***
scrofulous children, in - dulc.
tobacco, from - ***nux-v.***
transient, complicating motor palsy - plb.
typhoid fever, after - ***lyc.***
years, of seven, duration - **PHOS.**

AMBLYOPIA, (see Dim, vision) - ***ammc.,*** anag., atro., caps., chin-s., **CHIN.,** con., crot-h., ***dros.,*** euph., **GELS.,** hyos., ign., ***merc., nat-m.,*** nux-v., ***op.,*** **PHOS.,** ***ph-ac.,*** puls., ***ruta.,*** sil., ***stram.***
alcoholics, in - ***chin.,*** ter.
blow to head, after a - arn.
blurring of, better by rubbing - thuj.
brightii, morbus, in - ***phos.***
cloudy day amel., or when it begins to grow dark - nux-v.
deafness, with - ***puls.***
diphtheria, after - ***sil.***
discharge, from suppression of any bloody - ***puls.***
emotion, following strong - ant-t.
epilepsy, in - ***hyos.***
eruption, after suppression of an - cycl.
with or without diplopia - ***sulph.***
eyes, from overexertion of - **RUTA.**
hysterical, from onanism or ciliary neuralgia - ***ign.***
fluids, after loss of - **CHIN.,** crot-h., **PHOS.**
gastric, from, derangement with heart disease - ***puls.***
gout, from metastasis of, or rheumatism - ***puls.***
grief, caused by - ***crot-h.***
heart, with, affections - ***lach.***
hemiplegia, in - ***caust.***
hemorrhage, from - crot-h.
hydrocephalus, acute, in - ***lyc., merc.***
lung, affections, with - ***lach.***
masturbation, after - ***chin., phos.***
meningitis, in - ant-t.
menses, caused by stoppage of - bell., cycl.
mistiness of sight, with complete obscuration at a distance - ***ruta.***
morning, amel. - ***chin.***
nervous, sensitive persons - ign., ***sil.***
refraction, dependent upon anomalies of - ***ruta.***
retinitis, apoplectica, in - chel.
sewing, overuse of eyes, from - ***crot-h.***
stimulants, from abuse of - nux-v., ***sil.***
sweat, from checked foot - ***sil.***
venereal, consequent upon, excesses and intoxication - ***chin.***
vomiting, and coma, with - chel.
weaver, in a - ***ruta.***

APPROACH, objects seem to approach and then recede - ***cic.***

ASTHENOPIA, (see Eyestrain) - agar., ***arn.,*** asar., ***cinnb., con., croc., hydr.,*** **KALM.,** ***lach.,*** merl., nicc., **PHOS., RUTA, SULPH.,** ***tab.***
accommodative - ***sulph.***
aching in eye after using - puls.
anemia of optic nerve, from excessive tea drinking, with neuralgia or slight retinitis - ***spig.***
diplopia, from muscular - ***nux-v.***
exhaustion, with, dependent upon loss of semen - sep.
eyeball, with dull pain behind, as if it would be forced out - ***led.***
females, in hysterical, from onanism or ciliary neuralgia - ***ign.***
headache, with chronic - ***iris.***
hypermetropia, in - ***arg-n.***
hysterical, weak - ***lil-t.***
measles, sequel to - ***caust.***
motes, with black, before eyes - ***lith.***
neuralgia, causes ciliary - com.
object, shining, worse from looking at any bright, better in twilight - phos.
pale, flabby subjects inclined to grow fat - calc.
prostration, from general - puls.
stitches in sewing run together - **NAT-M.**
uterus, dependent upon reflex irritation from - ***sep.***

asthenopia, muscular - am-c., ***chin., mur-ac.,*** **NAT-M., RHOD.,** sulph.
ciliary weakness of - ***ruta***
focal distance unequal - ***chin.***
general weakness, spinal irritation and overuse of eyes, or reflex irritation from uterus - **NAT-M.**
inability to keep eyes fixed on reading - ***agar.***
insufficiency of external recti - ***gels.***
internal recti - rhod.
paresis of accommodation - phys.
spinal anemia, from - agar.
uterine disorders, from - agar.

ASTIGMATISM - ***phys., gels., lil-t., tub.***
granular lids, from - sep.
returning in spite of glasses, causing dull pain in back of neck and head - pic-ac.
turns head to left when reading, trying to look with left eye out of right glass of spectacles, to see whole of letters b and d - ***lil-t.***

BALLS, (see Colors) - verat-v.
fire, of - stram.
floating - kali-c.
luminous - cycl.

BLACK, colors before the vision - agar., ***arn., atro.,*** bell., ***carb-s., carb-v.,*** chin., cina, ***clem.,*** cycl., dig., ***lach.,*** lyc., mag-c., mag-p., ***merc.,*** **NAT-M.,** ***phos.,*** phys., sep., stront-c., ***tab.,*** thuj., zinc.
animals - nat-a.
balls - ***bell.,*** cund., ***kali-c.***

BLACK, colors before the vision
disk - elaps
figures - cocc., petr.
floating before eyes - cocc.
flickering - **LACH.**
flies, floating - sulph.
floating - ***chel.,*** chin., chlf., cop., daph., gins., led., petr., **PHOS.**
halo - phos.
horns - cund.
letters change to points - ***calc-p.***
lightning - staph.
looking down, when - ***kalm.***
motes - merc-i-f.
moving - thuj.
objects - caps., ***cic.,*** sol-n., stram., sul-ac.
turning, on - cocc., sarr.
plate - kali-bi.
reading, while - cic., kali-c., sol-n.
accompanying letter - calc.
rising, from stooping - mez.
serpents - cund.
sparks - stry.
veil - aur., phos.
before the right eye - ***phos.***

black, points - anan., ant-c., calc., ***caust.,*** chin., con., elaps, ***gels.,*** jatr., ***kali-c., merc.,*** mosch., nat-m., nit-ac., ***nux-v., phos.,*** sol-n., tab., thuj.
candlelight, by - carb-an.
dinner, before - thuj.
morning - bell.
reading, while - calc., ***kali-c.***

black, rings - hell., nit-s-d., psor., sol-n.
fever, during - dig.
floating - dig.
headache, before - ***psor.***
reading - kali-c.
waving - dig.

black, spots - agar., am-c., arg-n., asc-t., ***aur., bar-c.,*** bell., ***calc., camph.,*** carb-an., chel., chin-s., chlor., ***cimic.,*** cocc., ***con.,*** cupr-ar., cur., dulc., elaps, **GLON.,** hell., ***lil-t., lyc., mag-c.,*** med., meli., nat-c., **NAT-M.,** ***nit-ac.,*** petr., ***phos., psor.,*** **SEP.,** ***sil.,*** stram., stront-c., syph., tab., thuj., verat.
eating, after - lyc.
exertion, physical - ***calc.***
eyes are closed, when - ***con.,*** elaps
floating, amel. by fixing eye on an object - aesc.
brown - agar.
left - agar., calc., ***caust.,*** merc., ***sulph.***
right - chin-s., cimic., sel., ***sil.***
spots, (see Floaters)
headache, during - ***glon.,*** **MELI.**
before a - ***psor.***
morning, waking, on - dulc.
moving in all directions - ***chin-s., sep.,*** stram.
reading, after - cocc., ***cur.***
rising from a seat, on - verat.
sewing, after - am-c.
turning quickly - ***glon.***
vertigo, with - ***con., glon.***
writing, while - ***nat-c.***

black, stripes - con., ph-ac., ***sep.,*** sol-n., sulph.
morning - bell.
reading, while - kali-c., sol-n.

BLINDNESS, (see Amaurosis) - **ACON.,** ***agar.,*** all-c., alum., ant-c., ant-t., apis, arg-m., arg-n., arn., ars., aster., ***aur., aur-m.,*** **BELL.,** berb., ***both., bov.,*** bufo, cact., ***calc.,*** camph., cann-i., caps., carb-an., carb-o., ***carb-s., caust.,*** cham., chel., ***chin., chin-s.,*** chlf., chlol., cic., clem., ***con.,*** croc., crot-c., crot-h., crot-t., cupr-ac., cycl., ***dig.,*** elaps, eug., eupi., ***euphr.,*** eup-per., ferr., ferr-p., ***gels.,*** glon., hell., hep., hura, hydr-ac., **HYOS.,** ip., kali-ar., kali-bi., kali-br., kali-cy., ***kali-i.,*** kali-n., kalm., kreos., lach., lac-ac., lact., lam., led., ***lith., lyc., lyss.,*** meny., meph., **MERC.,** morph., mosch., naja, **NAT-M.,** nat-s., nit-ac., nux-m., ***nux-v.,*** olnd., ***op.,*** ph-ac., ***phos., plb.,*** **PULS.,** raph., rhus-t., rhus-v., sars., ***sec., sep.,*** **SIL.,** sol-n., spig., **STRAM., SULPH.,** ***tab.,*** ter., ***ther.,*** thuj., verat., ***verat-v.,*** vip., zinc., zinc-m.
abdominal, pain, with - crot-t., plb.
afternoon - indg.
4 p.m. - ***lyc.***
air, open - nit-ac.
amel. - merc., phos.
alcohol, from - ter.
alternates with headaches - ***kali-bi.***
anus, in prolapsus - ***arn.***
ascending, stairs - coca.
attacks, in - mosch.
concussion of brain, in - ***arn.***
day, during - ***hep.***
typhoid, in - ***gels.***
bed, after getting out of, for a minute or two - colch.
bleeding, retinal, from - both., crot-h., ***phos.***
bright, objects, by - grat., ph-ac.
camphor, odor of, at - kali-n.
cause, without - tab.
childbirth, during - aur-m., caust., cocc., cupr.
chill, during - cann-i.
cold, after catching - acon.
convulsions, after - dig., sec.
before - ***cupr.***
cornea, from obscuration of - ***apis.***
damp, weather - crot-h.
daytime - acon., ***both.,*** cast., con., lyc., phos., ran-b., ***sil.,*** **STRAM.,** sulph.
light, caused by - merl., nat-m., nit-ac., ***phos.,*** sep.
delirium, during - phos.
dinner, after - ***calc.,*** zinc.
eating, after - ***calc., crot-t.,*** sil.
eclampsia, in puerperal - cocc.
emotion, sudden, from - jug-c.
epileptiform, in, spasms - ***chin-a.***
evening - bell., calc., camph., ferr., nat-c., phos., psor., til.
light, caused by - lyc., mang., thuj.
menses, during - ***sep.***
reading, while - brom.
sitting down during vertigo, on - coloc.

BLINDNESS,
evening,
sunset, at - bell.
twilight - both., lyc., psor.
exerting, them - chin., helon., lyc., nat-m., ruta.
sewing, from - berb., ***nat-m., ruta.***
fainting, as from - ***agar.,*** aur., bell., ***calc., caust.,*** chel., ***chen-a., cic.,*** cycl., dros., ferr., ferr-p., ***graph.,*** hep., ***hyos.,*** kali-n., ***mang.,*** merc., ***nat-m.,*** olnd., ***phos., puls., sep.,*** spig., stram.
faintness, and nausea, with - ***glon.***
fixing, eyes - ant-t., euphr., kali-bi., mag-c., ***nat-m.,*** nit-ac., spig.
fluids, loss of, after - nat-m.
forenoon - thuj.
gastralgia, in - ***camph.***
grief, after - crot-h., gels., nat-m.
head, on turning - sec.
pain in head and eyes, after - ***con.***
rush of blood to, during - grat.
suddenly - helon.
headache, with - atro., ***bell., caust.,*** cupr-m., ***ferr-p., gels.,*** iris, ***lac-d.,*** **MELI.,** ***nat-m., sep., stram., zinc.***
after - sil.
amel. with upcoming - ***iris,*** lac-d., nat-m.
at beginning of - kali-bi., sars.
heart, disease, in - tub.
hemicrania, in - ***chen-a., gels.***
hemeralopia - anac., cadm-s., **CHIN.,** ***hyos.,*** **LYC.,** stram.
afternoon, 4 p.m., must stop work at - ***lyc.***
menstrual disturbances, with, as if eyes were tightly bound - ***puls.***
myopic eye, in a - ***hyos.***
nightly diarrhea, with - ***verat.***
pregnancy, during - ran-b.
sudden - ran-b., **SULPH.**
6 or 8 days before menses, every afternoon, toward sundown, increases as night comes on - verat.
severe cutting pains, with - ***lyc.***
swelling of eyes, with - petros.
hemorrhage, in - ***chin.***
hepatitis, in, eyes open, but cannot see - ***bell.***
hydrocephalus, in - apis, ***apoc., dig.,*** hell., ***kali-i.***
hysteria, in - ferr., gels.
grief, from - ***gels.***
inflammation, from - manc.
injury to eye, after - ***arn., calen.,*** manc.
head, to - ***nat-s.***
left eye, of
awaking, on - tarent.
can see but faint glimmer of light with - ***com.***
complete, in, for three years, nearly so in right - ***elaps***
could not see anything by day with, while at night could distinguish a light - sulph.
could not see from - cund.

BLINDNESS, general

left, eye, of

suppressed itch, after - sulph.

light, by - calc., ***graph.,*** mang., phos.

artificial light - aur-m., chin., ***lyc.,*** mang., ***nux-m.,*** phos.

entering from dark - dig.

eyes, does not affect - cocc.

sun, of - ***lith.***

lightning, strike, after - phos.

looking, at near objects - mag-m.

downward - kalm.

object, on looking long at an - mang.

sideways - olnd.

upwards - ***cupr.***

lying, down amel. - cina, phos., sep.

when quietly - verat-v.

masturbation, from - ph-ac.

meningitis, in - ***glon.***

after - ***hell.,*** phos.

cerebrospinal - ***glon., hydr.***

menses, during - ***graph.,*** lyc., puls., ***sep.***

amel. - ***sep.***

before - dict.

mental, derangement, in - stram.

mental, exertion, from - arg-n., meny.

momentary - hyos., ***nux-m.,*** olnd., sil.

fainting, as from - ***phos.***

grasps head, it feels strangely - ***nux-m.***

morning, in hypochondriasis - ***arg-n.***

ophthalmia, in - ***cic.***

second for a - ***lach.***

uterine affections, in pregnancy - ***sil.***

vertigo, with - ***merc.***

morning - bell., ign., sulph.

fasting - ***calc.***

rising - puls.

motion, agg. - grat.

sudden, from - verat-v.

nausea, during - ***sep.***

neuralgia, from - ***arg-n.***

neuritis, from retro-bulbair - chin-s., iodof.

night-blindness - bell., cadm-s., chel., chin., hell., ***hyos.,*** lyc., meph., merc., ***nit-ac.,*** nux-v., petros., psor., puls., ***ran-b.,*** stram., verat., zinc.

flickering by day, blind at night - anac.

noon - am-c.

eating, before - dulc.

nosebleed, with - ox-ac.

nyctalopia - ***hell.***

hysteria, in - ***ferr.***

paroxysms, in - ***phos.***

sudden appearance of furuncles, with - ***sil.***

ophthalmia, in - ***apis.***

chronic, in - vario.

scrofulous, in - ***sulph.***

overuse of eye, from - crot-h.

paroxysmal - acon., con., kali-n., mang., nit-ac., nux-v., phos., sil., stram., sulph.

paralysis, in - **GRAPH.,** bell.

partial - **AMMC.,** ***phys.***

BLINDNESS, general

periodic - ***ant-t., chel.,*** chin., ***dig., euphr.,*** hyos., merc., ***nat-m., phos., puls., sep., sil., sulph.***

blackness - **BELL.,** caps., cic., ***con.,*** cycl., glon., graph., hyos., merc., nat-m., olnd., ***phos., puls.,*** sep., ***sil.,*** sulph.

menses, during - graph., puls., sep.

pregnancy, during - ran-b.

progressive, central scotoma, with - carb-s., iodof., plb., tab., thyr.

pupils, with dilated - ***gels.,*** stram.

ptosis, with - ***gels.***

reading, while - agar., arg-n., aur-m., caust., clem., crot-h., dros., haem., lachn., lyc., nat-c., nat-m., ***phos.,*** ruta, staph.

letters disappear - cic., cocc.

standing posture, in a - glon.

types, small - cadm-s.

right eye, in, during pain - ***kali-bi.***

all seemed smoke and mist, while walking through fields covered with snow - ***kali-m.***

contracted pupil, with - verat-v.

inflammatory rheumatism, with - puls.

paralysis of optic nerve, with - ***bov.***

rising - cedr., glon., ***hep.,*** olnd.

and standing after sitting bent over - ***hep.***

bed, from - bell., ***cina,*** colch., com., sec.

eating, after - merc.

sleep, after, on - ferr.

scarlet fever, after - ***bell., hep.***

sitting, while - kalm., merc., phos.

bent over, after - ***hep.***

sleep, amel. - calc., grat.

sleeping, in the sun, after - con.

snow-blindness - calc-p., cic., ***kali-m., merl.,*** sol.

sore throat, after - ***gels.***

soup, while eating - nat-s.

standing, on - colch.

amel. - merc.

stooping, when - apis., bell., coff., com., elaps, ***ferr-p.,*** graph., nat-m., phos., ther., upa.

stool, after - petr.

amel. - apis

strength, with loss of, can only distinguish light - ***lac-d.***

stupefaction, with, dizziness and vacancy in head - kreos.

sudden - acon., aur-m., calc., chin., cupr., mosch., ***nat-m.,*** phos., psor., sec.

childbed, in - aur-m.

complicating motor palsy - plb.

night, in lead colic - op.

photopsia, after - ***bell.***

scarlet fever, after - aur-m.

upper half of visual field, in - verat-v.

violent pain in occiput to eyes, with - chin.

sunlight, sleeping in - con.

sunset, at - bell.

BLINDNESS, general
- **temporary,** frequent, in amblyopia - ***merc.***
  - cerebrospinal meningitis, in - ***glon.***
- **tobacco** - ars., ***nux-v.,*** phos.
- **transient** - kali-c., merc., phos.
  - pain from occiput over head to forehead and eyes, with - ***petr.***
- **typhus** fever, in - ***stram.***
- **vertigo,** with - anac., apis, arg-n., asaf., ***bell.,*** chen-a., crot-t., ***gels.,*** hep., ***kalm.,*** merc., morph., nux-v., rhus-t., ter., thea., ***verat.***
  - and dilated pupils - ***gels.***
  - evening - **PULS.**
  - ophthalmia, in - ***cic.***
- **waking,** on - bell., oena.
- **walking,** while - dor., ferr., hell., lachn., nat-m., sulph., ***verat-v.***
  - air, in open - merc.
  - brought on by, with fainting - ***verat-v.***
- **warm,** room agg. - merc.
- **white,** objects, looking at - graph., tab.
- **wink,** with frequent desire to - ph-ac.
- **writing** - arg-n., grat., kali-c., nat-m., phys., zinc.

BLUE, colors before the vision - acon., act-sp., aml-n., ***aur., bell., bry.,*** **CHIN.,** coff., ***crot-c.,*** crot-h., cycl., dig., elaps, piloc., kali-c., kreos., ***lach., lyc.,*** nicc., ***stram.,*** stront-c., sulph., thuj., tril., ***tub.,*** valer., xan., zinc.
  - blindness for - carb-s.
  - circles - zinc.
  - closed, when eyes are - thuj.
  - dark blue - cycl., kreos.
  - distance, in the - ***iod.***
  - evening - am-br.
  - flashes - xan.
  - halo around candle - ***ip., lach.***
  - haze - ***bry.***
  - lace, as through blue - xan.
  - light around - ***lach.***
    - the candle - hipp.
  - objects - tril.
  - points - sec.
  - reading - bell.
  - right eye - nicc.
  - rubbing, on - stront.
  - sparks - ars.
  - stars - psor.
  - stars, during headache - ***psor.***
- **blue,** spots - acon., ***kali-c.***
  - dark room, in a - hep., stram.
  - morning on rising - thuj.
  - night, when lying on right side in a dark room - stram.

BLURRED - ***acon.,*** aeth., arn., ***ars., aur.,*** cact., calc., calc-f., chel., chin., ***con., crot-c.,*** dros., fago., **GELS.,** ***glon.,*** iris, jab., kali-p., **LAC-C.,** ***lil-t.,*** lyc., med., merl., nat-a., **NAT-M.,** nat-s., ***nux-v.,*** onos., ***phos., phys., plat., psor., rhus-t., ruta.,*** sec., stram., ter., ***teucr.,*** thuj., tril.
  - aching in and over eyes, after using eyes and straining them at fine work, with - **RUTA.**

BLURRED, vision,
- body arose, as if, which impeded sight - am-m.
- closing, eyes amel. - calc-f.
- confused spots - **CON.**
- deafness, after - ***glon.***
- distant, objects - chel., jab.
- emissions, after - ***calc., chin., lil-t.,*** **PHOS.**
- endless strings of white and transparent globules were in eye - upa.
- evening - ruta.
- figures - ail.
  - and letters - ail.
- fine work at night, after - pic-ac.
- fog, as from looking through a - pic-ac.
- gaslight - calc.
- headache, at beginning of sick - **IRIS**
  - before - ***gels.,*** hyos., **IRIS,** ***kali-bi.,*** lac-d., podo., ***psor., sep., sulph.***
  - sudden, in - podo.
  - chronic, in - psor.
- heat in lids and eyes, with - ***lil-t.***
- holding eyes to left for some time, on - ***merc-i-f.***
- irritable, when, in anemia of brain - ***con.***
- irritated, when - con.
- letters - ail., arg-m., arg-n., ***ars., bell.,*** cann-i., cann-s., carb-ac., ***chel.,*** cina, cob., ferr., graph., piloc., kali-c., lyc., meph., ***nat-m.,*** ox-ac., phys., ***ruta, sil.,*** staph., stram., sulph., thlaspi.
  - letters run together, in asthenopia - **RUTA.**
- looking a short time - nat-a.
- morning - ***merl.,*** nat-s.
- muscae volitantes, with - ***lil-t.***
- objects look as if one had been looking at sun for a moment, or the part at which the eyes are directed appears clearly and the rest blurred and indistinct - podo.
  - seem running together - berb., ***calc.***
  - when he looks at them a short time - nat-a.
- only noticed when looking to left - ***kali-i.***
- outlines of objects uneven, wavering, trembling - phos.
- overheated - ***nux-v.***
- paralysis of accommodation - ***arg-n.***
- parenchymatous metritis - lac-c.
- pressure, amel. - calc-f.
- prolapsus uterus - ***lil-t.***
- reading on, in tobacco amaurosis - ***nux-v.***
- reading, sudden, after - phos.
- rubbing, amel. - thuj.
- seminal emissions, after - ***lil-t.***
- turning eyes - gels.
- winking, amel. - ***euph.***
- wiping, amel. - ***euph.***
- writing, after, with aching, better closing eyes and pressing tightly - calc-f.
- writing, while - calc-f.

BRIGHT, colors before the vision - aloe, alum., am-c., anan., ***ant-t.,*** ars., ***aur.,*** bar-c., ***bell., bor.,*** bry., ***camph.,*** cann-s., caust., chel., cic., **CINA,** coloc., ***con.,*** croc., ***dig.,*** dros., dulc., euphr., fl-ac., ***graph., hyos.,*** ign., ***iod., ip., kali-bi., lyc.,*** mang., meny., mez., nat-m., **NUX-V.,** olnd., op., phos., plat., ***puls.,*** rhus-t., sabin., sec., seneg., spig., stram., stront-c., ***valer.,*** verat., viol-o., zinc.

BRIGHTER, objects seem - agar., carb-an., camph., dig., hyos., nat-c., nux-v., valer.
dark room, in - valer.

BROWN, colors before the vision - agar., atro., lac-c., med.
gloomy, weather in - agar.
spot, on closing other eye - agar.

CHANGING, (see Moving, Vanishing) - gels.

CIPHERS - phos., ph-ac., sulph.

CIRCLES, (see Colors) - calc., ***calc-p., carb-v.,*** caust., elaps., hell., iod., ***kali-c.,*** phos., plb., ***psor.,*** stront-c., zinc.
about light - cycl.
around an internal brighter field - carb-v.
colored, around white objects - hyos.
around a bright center - ammc.
bands - con.
fever, during - dig.
letters seem - bell.
objects move in a circle on closing eyes - hep.
reading, while - kali-c.
semicircles - ***con.***
turning - ***kali-c.***
yellow and white rays, with - kali-c.
zigzags - viol-o.
color, of - sep.
flickering - ign.

CLEARER - aspar., ***bell.,*** **CHIN.,** ***colch.,*** fl-ac., ***hyos.,*** viol-o.
air, in open - coff.
enjoyment, a luxurious, in looking at some things he sees daily - fl-ac.
oversensitive - ***bell.***
reads fine print easier - **COFF.**
rubbing, after, eyes - ***cina.***

CLOUDY - ***cycl., lac-d., plb.***
albuminuria, in - ***ars.***
before left eye, in twilight and cloudy weather - ***arg-n.***
candlelight, by - all-c.
dark clouds, pass - lac-ac.
itching and sticking in inner canthi, with - ***zinc.***
menses, before - ***bell.***
morning - nicc.
myelitis, in - ***stram.***
over outer half of field of vision of left eye, due to sub retinal effusion - ***gels.***

COLOR, blindness - bell., carb-s., chlol., cina, sant.
fast motions, when making - stram.
rubbing, after - stront.

COLORS, before the vision - agar., am-c., anac., arn., arund., aur., bar-c., ***bell., bry., calc., camph.,*** caust., chin., chin-s., ***cic., cina,*** cocc., **CON.,** ***cycl., dig.,*** euph., hep., ip., ***iod.,*** kali-ar., ***kali-bi., kali-c.,*** kali-n., kali-p., mag-c., ***mag-p.,*** merc., nat-c., ***nat-m.,*** nat-p., nit-ac., ph-ac., **PHOS.,** psor., puls., ruta, sars., sep., sil., spong., stram., stront-c., sulph., thuj.
evening - agar., kali-n., sars.

CONFUSED, vision - acon., aeth., amyg., atro., ***aur.,*** bapt., bell., cann-i., cedr., ***con.,*** croc., dig., eug., **GELS.,** ***glon.,*** kali-bi., lil-t., lyc., **NAT-M.,** ***phys.,*** pic-ac., ***plat., psor., rhus-t.,*** sec., stram., stry.
anxiety, after - ***psor.***
colors, of - ***bell.,*** calc., croc., merc., puls., ruta, staph., stram.
delirium, with, in diphtheria - ***bapt.***
distant objects look as if anterior lines were shaded with same colors - ***gels.***
dots, as if black, filled visual field, worse after stimulants - tab.
down, on looking - ***camph.***
head, in congestion to - ***chin.***
hysteria, in - ther., valer.
menses, dysmenorrhea, in - verat-v.
object, on looking at an, sees only that part upon which eye is fixed, everything else seems to swim around that point - ***nux-v.***
objects appear flowing into one another, at three to four inches distance, in strabismus - ***calc.***
window, on looking through, everything in street appears in tumult - camph.

CROOKED, lines, while reading - ***bell.,*** bufo.
objects appear - ***bell.,*** bufo, nux-m., stram.

DANCING - all-c., ***bell.,*** calc., ***cic., glon.,*** nux-m., ***psor.,*** sant.
headache, before - ***psor.***
letters appear - bell., lyss.

DARK, colors before the vision - acon., agar., ambr., am-m., ***anac.,*** arn., ars., asaf., ***bell.,*** berb., ***calc.,*** carb-v., ***caust.,*** cham., ***chin., cocc., con.,*** cupr., dig., dros., ***euphr.,*** ferr., hep., ***kali-c.,*** kali-p., kali-s., laur., lyc., mag-c., mang., meny., ***merc.,*** mosch., mur-ac., nat-a., nat-c., nat-m., nat-p., ***nit-ac.,*** nux-v., olnd., op., petr., ph-ac., ***phos.,*** plb., ruta, sabad., sec., ***sep., sil.,*** squil., staph., ***stram.,*** **SULPH.,** thuj., verat., verb.
circles - ***iod.,*** kali-c.
with points of light - caust.
clouds - coca, lac-ac., ol-an., tarent.
objects - ant-t., ign., ***nat-m.,*** phos., sulph.
moving - carb-h.
seem dark - bell., berb., hep., nit-ac., thuj.
points - chlf., cic., ***con.,*** **SULPH.**
floating - aur., hyos., phos.
serpent-like waves - phys.
specks - ***calc.,*** con., cupr-ar., ***kali-c.,*** mag-c., nat-m., nit-ac., **PHOS.,** sep., **SIL.,** sulph.

DARK, colors before the vision,
spots - agar., anac., asc-t., cact., carb-ac., carb-an., chlol., ***cimic., cocc.,*** con., elaps, fl-ac., hell., jatr., ***kali-c.,*** med., ***merc., phos.,*** **SULPH.,** thuj.
floating - agar., cocc., phos., **SULPH.**
reading agg. - fl-ac., ***kali-c.,*** lachn.
white margins, with - con.
stripes - cic., ***sulph.,*** zinc.
worms - phys.

DARKNESS, before eyes - eug., ***psor.,*** puls.
attempting to fix thoughts, on - ***arg-n.***
to rise, in paralysis of bladder, on - ***cic.***
complained of, wanted a light - ***stram.***
could not read or see thread when spinning - stram.
evening, with aching pains and slight epistaxis - ferr.
faintness, with, following pressing in cardiac region and hard heart-beats - manc.
giddy - ***ferr.***
heaviness of head, with - phos.
looking sideways, when - ***olnd.***
menses, during - cycl., ***graph.***
morning, on rising from bed - com., ***puls.***
vertigo, with - dulc., ***op.,*** ox-ac.
hemiplegia , in - ***elaps***
menses, before - puls.
stooping, on - ***calc.***
waking, on - ***dulc.***
warm room agg., before menses - ***puls.***

DAZZLING - acon., am-m., anan., ant-c., ars., **BAR-C.,** bell., ***calc., camph.,*** **CON.,** crot-c., **DROS.,** ***euphr.,*** **KALI-C.,** kali-s., lach., ***lyc., merc.,*** nat-c., olnd., ph-ac., ***phos.,*** plat., plb., ***psor., seneg.,*** sep., **SIL.,** stram., ***sulph., valer.,*** verat-v.
candlelight - lyc.
distant objects - all-c.
looking long - **SULPH.**
morning - sulph.
near objects - ph-ac.
reading, while - ***seneg.***
snow - ant-c., ***ars.,*** olnd., sep.
spot before eyes - ***chel.***
sunlight - euphr., lith., ***sep., stram.***
urination, after - eug.

DIM, vision (see Amblyopia) - absin., **AGAR.,** ail., ***alum.,*** alumn., ambr., ***ammc., am-c., anac.,*** ang., ***apis, arg-m., arg-n., ars., ars-i., arum-t.,*** arund., asaf., ***asar.,*** astac., atro., **AUR.,** ***aur-m., bar-c., bar-m.,*** **BELL.,** berb., bism., bry., bufo, ***cact.,*** cadm-s., **CALC.,** ***calc-f.,*** calc-s., camph., cann-i., **CANN-S.,** canth., caps., carb-ac., ***carb-an.,*** **CARB-S.,** ***carb-v.,*** **CAUST.,** cedr., ***cham., chel.,*** **CHIN.,** ***chin-a., chin-s., chlol., cic., cimic., cina, cinnb., clem., cob., cocc., colch., coloc., com.,*** **CON.,** ***croc., crot-c., crot-h., crot-t.,*** cupr., cupr-ar., **CYCL.,** dig., ***dulc., elaps,*** **EUPH.,** euphr., fago., ferr-ar., ***form.,*** **GELS.,** ***glon.,*** graph., ham., hell., helon., **HEP.,** hura, ***hydr., hyos.,*** hyper., ***ign., iod., ip.,*** jab., ***kali-ar., kali-bi., kali-br., kali-c.,*** kali-cy., ***kali-i., kali-p.,*** kali-s., ***kalm., kreos., lac-c., lac-d.,*** **LACH.,** lachn., ***laur., led., lil-t., lith.,*** **LYC.,** lyss., ***mag-c., mag-m., mang.,*** meph., **MERC.,** ***merl., mur-ac., nat-a., nat-c., nat-m.,*** nat-p., ***nat-s.,*** nicc., **NIT-AC.,** nux-m., ***nux-v.,*** oena., olnd., ol-an., onos., **OP.,** osm., par., ***petr.,*** phel., **PH-AC.,** ***phos., phys., phyt.,*** pic-ac., ***plb., psor.,*** **PULS.,** raph., rhod., ***rhus-t.,*** rhus-v., **RUTA.,** ***sabad.,*** sang., ***sars., sec.,*** sel., ***seneg.,*** **SEP., SIL.,** sol-n., ***spig., staph., stram.,*** stry., **SULPH.,** ***sul-ac.,*** sumb., tab., ***tarent.,*** tax., ***teucr., ther., thuj.,*** til., upa., ***verat., verat-v.,*** verb., viol-o., viol-t., vip., zinc.
afternoon, while reading - ol-an.
air, open - alum., asar., con., merl., **PULS.,** thuj., upa.
fresh, amel. - ***asar.,*** nat-s.
alcoholics, in - **NUX-V.**
alternating, with
clearness - anac., euphr.
cramps in hands and feet - bell.
deafness - cic.
anxiety, during - chel.
asthenopia, in - phos.
awaking, on - **CYCL., LACH.**
black, everything turns, when stooping - ***graph.***
blackness, and - dor.
head, when shaking - ***hep.***
menses, before and during - ***graph.***
blowing, nose - ***caust.***
blue, as if looking through dark, glass - cycl.
brain, affections, in - ***zinc.***
congestion of blood to base of, from - ***verat-v.***
inflammation of, from - ***merc.***
bright, light - bell., caust., sol-n.
bright's, disease in - phos.
bulimia, in - ***lyc.***
candle, light - all-c., arg-n., aur-m., bar-c., ***euphr., hep.***
catarrh, in - ***cast.,*** sec.
chronic, in - ***alum.***
suppressed, in, after - ***ars.***
chill, during - bell., chin., nat-m., sabin.
chilliness, with - cham.
cholera, in - ***cupr-ac.***
chorioretinitis, in, of right eye - ***kali-m.***
cold, bathing amel. - **ASAR.,** glon., nicc.
head becoming, from - ***calc.***
confused, dim and, with vertigo - ***kali-bi.***
cornea, as if, had lost its transparency - **SULPH.**
morning - ang.
coryza, in - ***anac.***
cough, during - coff., ign., kali-m.
damp, weather - ***calc.,*** crot-h.
dark, all being, could not sew for a week - eup-per.
daytime, amel. - ***euph.,*** sep.
daytime - apis, both., mang., sep.
descending, stairs - phys.
diabetes, in - tarent.
diarrhea, in - **ANT-T.**

DIM, vision,
dilatation, of pupils, holding hand before eyes amel., with - ph-ac.
dinner, after - bell., calc., peti.
diphtheria, after - apis, gels., **LACH.,** nux-v., phys., **PHYT.,** ***sil.***
dissolved, things seem as if - ***stram.***
distance, cannot see at a - ***cact.***
distant, objects - ***cact.,*** euphr., ***gels., jab.,*** mang., nat-a., nat-c., nat-m., nat-p., ol-an., ph-ac., phos., phys., rat., spong., **STRAM.,** ***sulph.***
dimness of objects, followed by contraction of pupil - phys.
distinguish, inability to, objects at a short distance - **STRAM.**
dots, as if black, filled visual field, worse after stimulants - tab.
drowsiness, with frequent - mag-s.
dysmenorrhea, in - ***laur.***
dull - bism., **GELS.**
diabetes, in - sul-ac.
optic nerve, from weakness of - mag-p.
pupils, with dilatation of - lyss.
writing, when, sees only one half of objects clearly - ***sep.***
eating, while - bufo, nat-s., ***nux-v.***
after - ***calc., kali-c., nux-v.***
edema, in - ***ars.***
elderly, people - ***bar-c.***
erect, on becoming - ***verat-v.***
evening - alum., ***ammc.,*** anac., ***apis,*** asar., bor., ***euphr.,*** ind., ***kalm.,*** lachn., merl., nicc., nit-ac., ***puls., ruta.,*** sulph., tarent.
9 p.m. - stram.
firelight agg. - merc.
lying down, amel. - sep.
menses, during - ***sep.***
reading - **APIS,** croc., ***hep.,*** mez., rhod., ***ruta.***
by light - mez.
room, agg., in - nat-c.
twilight - arg-n.
walking, while - kali-bi., ***puls.***
after, on entering a room - dros.
fast - **PULS.**
warm from exertion, when - **PULS.**
exertion, of body, after - ***calc.,*** **PULS.**
evening - nicc.
exertion, of eyes, after - ***calc.,*** mang., ***nat-m.,*** nit-ac., ***petr.***
on fine work - agar., ***calc., nat-m.,*** **RUTA.**
eyelids, with heavy, and drowsiness - ***kali-br.***
eyes, with inflammation of - ***mag-c.***
fainting, spells, in - ***lac-d.***
feathery, with, appearance - ***calc.,*** lyc.
fever, during - bell., sabin.
film, as if caused by a - ***aml-n.,*** lac-c., ***phys.***
firelight, agg. - ***merc., nat-s.***
forenoon - carb-v., sulph., ***tarent.***
7 until 10 a.m. - tarent.
11 a.m. - ***sulph.***

DIM, vision,
forenoon,
reading, while - op.
giddiness, with - ***sulph.***
glass, as looking through a dim - nat-m.
head, blow after a - ammc., nat-s.
cold, after getting - ***calc.***
lightness of, worse by sudden movement of head and walking - ***gels.***
pressure in - ***caust.***
tearing in, and right eye, and sensation as if air were rushing through eye - croc.
headache, during - ***ars.,*** asar., aster., ***bell.,*** caul., ***caust.,*** **CYCL.,** ferr-p., ***gels.,*** hyos., ign., **IRIS,** lil-t., mur-ac., ***nat-m.,*** nit-ac., ***petr.,*** ph-ac., ***phos.,*** podo., ***psor., puls., sil., stram.,*** **SULPH.,** til., tub., verat-v., ***zinc.***
after - ***sil., lach.***
before - ***gels.,*** glon., graph., hyos., **IRIS,** ***kali-bi., lac-d.,*** lach., ***nat-m., phos.,*** podo., ***psor., sep.,*** sil., stram., ***sulph.,*** ther., ***tub.***
one-sided - chen-a.
pregnancy, during - ***caust.***
heat, from - asar., carb-v., ***gels.***
hemicrania, in - ***chen-a.***
hemiplegia, in - ***elaps***
hysterical - euph.
lachrymation, with, in open air - ***puls.***
profuse, with - cupr-ar.
lattice, as if one were looking through a fine - ***lyc.***
left, eye - bor., ***com.,*** sars.
pain in, then in right eye - ***lac-c.,*** merc-i-f., sars.
right-sided headache, with - arg-n.
light, can scarcely distinguish, from dark - elaps
can only see, not objects - ***lac-d.***
green halo around - ***caust.***
shunned the - rhus-t.
looking, intently - nit-ac.
long - agar., mang., nat-a.
sideways, amel. - chin-s.
steadily, amel. - ***aur.,*** mang.
white objects, at - cham.
luminosities, after - ther.
lustre, without - bov.
masturbation, from - gels.
measles, sequel to - ***caust.***
membrane, as though, were over eyes - caust., ***daph.***
menses, during - ***graph.,*** cycl., nat-m., ***puls., sep., sil.***
after - ***caust., euphr.,*** **KALI-C.,** ***puls.***
before - agn., bell., cinnb.
mental, exertion - arg-n.
momentary, spells - cadm-s., caust., euphr., ***lyc.***

DIM, vision,

morning - asar., caps., carb-an., cham., chel., cycl., calc., ***carb-v., caust.,*** chel., ***croc.,*** daph., gels., ***hep.,*** elaps, hell., ***kali-c.,*** mag-s., nat-m., ***nux-v., puls.,*** ruta., stram., sul-ac., valer.

amel. - ***chin., phos.***

rising, after - ang.

waking, after - zinc.

waking, on - ***caust.,*** dulc., ***kali-c.,*** mag-c., raph., zinc.

washing, amel. - caust.

motion, from uneven - con.

moving, objects - con., ***gels.***

mucus, as if covered with - nat-m.

nausea, with - kalm., mygal., tub.

near, for, objects - all-c.

and distant - **SULPH.**

nebulous - caust., ***mill.***

net, as from a, in typhus - ***chin-s.***

night - anac., **CHIN.,** hell., ***hyos., puls., ran-b., stram.,*** zinc.

better at night than by day - apis

menses, during - ***puls.***

night-watching, and mental disturbance, after - puls.

noon - bell., nat-a.

rising on, from a seat - nat-a.

nose, on blowing - ***caust.***

occiput, with pain in, extending to eye - ery-a.

outlines, can only distinguish, of distant objects - **CHIN.**

can only see rude, of objects, after typhoid - ***lyc.***

ill defined, in retinitis - ***sulph.***

indistinct - bell., kali-bi.

outer, portions of visual field, in - puls.

overheating - ***nux-v.***

pneumonia, in - ***ant-t.***

pregnancy, during - ***gels.,*** ran-b.

pupils, with dilated - atro., ***lyss., verat-v.***

read, cannot - ***bar-c.***

cannot, nor write - ***gels.,*** sil.

reading, with - agar., alum., am-c., ***apis, arg-m., asar.,*** atro., calc., ***carb-v., caust., croc.,*** daph., gels., ***hep., ign.,*** jab., merl., **NAT-M., NIT-AC.,** op., ph-ac., ***phos.,*** rhod., rhus-v., **RUTA., SENEG.,** sep., **SIL., SULPH.,** vinc.

and writing - rhod.

evening by candlelight - ***hep.***

focal distance changes while, first longer then shorter - agar.

recognize, fails to, those near him or does so but slowly - ***verat.***

recurrent - cact.

rheumatism, during - puls.

right - agar., ars-h., chel., form., iris, ***kali-c.,*** osm., plb., ***puls.,*** rhod., ruta., tarent., teucr., vesp.

rising, from a seat - con., laur., verat-v.

bed, from - ars., sec.

stooping, from - lyss., nat-m.

DIM, vision,

room, amel., in - alum., con.

rubbing, agg. - caust.

amel. - caps., cina, ph-ac., ***puls.,*** sulph.

scale, like a, before eye, with shooting along left orbital arch to external angle of eye - ***kali-bi.***

scotoma, with, of right eye, after a fall - ***merc.***

seminal, emission, after - gels., kali-c., ***lil-t.,*** nat-m., **SEP.**

sex, after - ***chin.,*** gels., **KALI-C.,** ***kali-p.,*** nat-p., **PHOS., SEP.,** ***sil.***

shadow, as if a, were flitting before eyes - ruta.

sharp pain, in eye, with - thuj.

sideways - cham., ruta.

can only see objects when looking at them - ***chin-s.,*** lil-t.

sieve, as if looking through a - puls.

skin, as if a, were drawn over eye - ***apis.***

sleepy, when getting - ***all-c.***

small, unable to discern, things, as point of a pin - stram.

could not see, objects and larger ones appeared as if enveloped in smoke or mist - sulph.

looking at, things, when - eup-per.

smoking - asc-t.

sparks, with fiery - ***cycl.***

standing - dig., verat-v.

stimulants, from - kali-br., **NUX-V.**

straining, eyes - agar., ***calc.,*** **RUTA.**

sunlight, agg. - asar., ***both.,*** cic., ***merc., nat-m.***

suppressed, discharge or eruption, after - cupr.

foot-sweat, after - **SIL.**

itch, after - cycl.

sweat, after suppressed foot - ***sil.***

syphilis, in - ***lyc.***

thinking, from - arg-n.

thick, it seems, before eyes - viol-o.

thirst, with - ***stram.***

thinking, from - arg-n.

tobacco, poisoning, from - nux-v., ***phos.***

twilight, amel. - bry., lyc., ***phos.***

typhoid fever, from - phos.

uncovering, head, from - ***calc.***

urination, amel. - ***gels.***

uterine, derangement, in - ***caul.***

hemorrhage at menopause - ***tril.***

vertigo, during - ***acon.,*** act-sp., agar., amyg., ***anac.,*** ant-t., apis, arg-m., arg-n., ars., asaf., ***bell.,*** calc., ***camph.,*** canth., carb-an., cham., cic., cimic., ***cupr.,*** **CYCL.,** dulc., euon., **FERR.,** graph., **GELS.,** gins., ***glon.,*** gran., gymn., hell., hep., hyos., ***kali-bi.,*** kalm., lach., lact., laur., ***merc.,*** mosch., mur-ac., ***nit-ac.,*** **NUX-V.,** olnd., par., ***phos., phyt.,*** puls., raph., sabad., ***sabin.,*** seneg., ***stram., stront-c., sulph.,*** tep., ter., til., zinc.

before - stram.

dimness improves as, gets worse - ***camph.***

reading or when sitting, after - par.

DIM, vision,
vertigo, with
sitting up in bed, when - cham.
typhoid, in - ***cic.***
vexation, on - iris.
vomit, with inclination to, face pale - ***puls.***
vomiting, with - **KREOS.**
waking, on - **CYCL.,** ***puls.***
walking, while - dor., gels., ***puls.,*** sanic., sin-a.
air, in open - agar., con., gels., nat-m., sulph., til.
amel. - lachn.
warm, especially on getting, from exercise - ***puls.***
warmth - calc., **PULS.**
washing, in water, after - kali-c.
water, as full of - **ACON.,** arg-n., chin., **EUPHR.,** iod., ***merc.,*** nux-v., phyt., **PULS.,** ***rhus-t.,*** squil., ***spig., staph.,*** stram., verb.
like seeing through a glass of turbid - agar., ***stram.***
could scarcely recognize an object a yard away - verb.
white, objects, when fixing eyes upon - cham.
winking, amel. - anac., anan., ***euphr.***
wiping, eyes amel. - ***alum.,*** arg-n., carl., ***cina,*** croc., ***euphr., lyc., nat-a., nat-c., puls., sil.***
work, after fine - ***calc.***
writing, while - aloe, calc-f., chel., con., lyc., **NAT-M.,** ol-an., phys., rhod., sep., thuj., zinc.

DIPLOPIA, (see Double, vision)

DISTANT, objects, seem - ***all-c., anac.,*** atro., ***aur.,*** bell., calc., cann-i., carb-an., ***carb-s.,*** **GELS.,** glon., merc-c., nat-m., ***nux-m.,*** ox-ac., ***phos., plb., stann., stram.,*** **SULPH.**
dark, in the - nux-m.
waking, on - anac.
yawning, when - all-c.

DISTORTED - bell., nux-v., stram.

DISTURBANCES of, convulsions, before - bell., calc., hyos., lach., sulph.
headache, before or during - anh., ***ars.,*** asar., aster., ***bell., caust.,*** **CYCL.,** dys-co., epip., ferr-p., ***gels.,*** hyos., ign., **IRIS,** ***kali-bi.,*** kali-c., lac-c., ***lac-d., nat-m.,*** nicc., nux-v., ***petr., phos.,*** pic-ac., podo., ***psor., sang., sep., sil.,*** spig., ***stram.,*** **SULPH.,** ***ther.,*** tub., verat-v., ***zinc.,*** zinc-s.
amel. when headache comes on - ***iris,*** lac-d., nat-m.

DROPS, before the eyes - kali-c.

DOUBLE, vision - aeth., ***agar., alumn.,*** am-c., anag., apis, arag., ***arg-n.,*** art-v., atro., **AUR.,** arn., bar-c., ***bell.,*** bry., calc., cann-i., cann-s., carb-s., ***caust., chel.,*** chlf., ***cic.,*** clem., ***con.,*** crot-h., cupr., ***cycl., daph., dig.,*** eug., euph., **GELS.,** ger., gins., ***graph.,*** **HYOS.,** ***iod.,*** kali-bi., kali-c., ***kali-cy.,*** kali-i., ***lyc., lyss.,*** mag-p., med., merc., ***merc-c., morph.,*** **NAT-M.,** ***nicc.,*** **NIT-AC.,** nux-m., ***nux-v., olnd.,*** onos., op., par.,

DOUBLE, vision - petr., phos., phys., phyt., ***plb.,*** psor., ***puls.,*** raph., rhus-t., sec., ***seneg.,*** sep., ***spong.,*** stann., ***stram.,*** sulfon., ***sulph.,*** syph., tab., ter., ther., ***thuj.,*** tub., ust., ***verat.,*** verat-v., visc., zinc.
alternating with deafness - cic.
amaurosis, in - sulph.
asthenopia, in muscular - ***nux-v.***
bending head backwards amel. - seneg.
blowing nose, on - caust.
candlelight, by - ***alum.,*** alumn.
convulsions, with - ***bell.,*** cic., ***hyos., nux-v., stram.***
diphtheria, after - lach.
distant objects - am-c., bell., nit-ac., plb.
eating, amel. after breakfast - ***camph.***
dinner, half hour after - ***stram.***
evening - agar., con., nit-ac., phyt.
eyes, using, after - ***camph.***
figures on carpet - atro.
headache, with - ***gels.***
with giddiness and - phyt.
heart affections, with - lach.
horizontal objects, of - gels., mag-p., **NIT-AC.,** olnd.
inclining head to either side - gels.
head towards shoulders or looking sideways - ***gels.***
injuries, to eye, after - arn.
lachrymation, with - ***morph.***
left eye more affected - zinc.
inability to turn, eye upward - ***caust.***
on holding eyes to - ***merc-i-f.***
only noticed when looking to - ***kali-i.***
lens, in opacity of - ***chel.***
letters, when writing - graph.
light, when looking at - ther.
looking, downward - ***arn.,*** olnd.
intensely - am-c., con., gins.
upward - ***caust.***
looking, sideways - gels.
right - caust., dig.
right, amel. - caust.
lower, one image seems, than another - syph.
lying down amel. - spong.
masturbation, from - cina, sep.
measles, after - caust., ***kali-c.***
meningitis, after - ***apis***
morning - cycl., gels.
motes, with black, or specks before eyes, worse rising from bed or chair - verat.
multiplied, as if objects would be, slight - phys.
muscles, with spasm of various, throughout body - ***gels.***
nausea, with - crot-t.
causing fluttering - ther.
near objects - aur., bell., cic., con., nit-ac., phyt., stann., verat-v.
night - nit-ac.
occiput, followed by burning in, better by pressure on vertex - ***gels.***
ophthalmia, in - ***cic.***
overwork at the desk - ***agar.***

DOUBLE, vision,
perpendicular - atro.
persons, more in young and strong - **MAG-P.**
point, sees, of pin double - kali-bi.
pregnancy, during - bell., cic., ***gels.***
ptosis, with - gels., syph.
reading - agar., ant-t., arg-n., ***camph., graph.,*** stram., thuj.
retina, in hyperaemia of - puls.
riding in the cars, after - cupr.
railroad cars, after - ***cupr-ac.***
right, image obliquely above real one, with - seneg.
images to, and downward - sulph.
rubbing eyes, amel. - carb-an.
sexual excess, from - sep.
sleep, after - chlol., gels.
squint, especially if dependent on convergent, from helminthiasis, convulsions, falls, etc. - ***cycl.***
standing erect and looking down - olnd.
strabismus - zinc.
paralytic, in - ***nux-v.***
stroke, in - ***plb.***
sunstroke, in - ***verat-v.***
tobacco, in, poisoning - nux-v.
turning eyes to right, on - dig.
uterine affections, from - sep.
vertical - atro., cic., kali-bi., lith., rhus-t., seneg., stram., syph.
menses, during - lith.
vertigo, after - bell., olnd.
will, controllable by force of - ***gels.***
work, from over, at desk - ***agar.***
writing - coca, ***graph.***
letters appear double - ***graph.***
yellow fever, in - ***gels.***

DOWNCAST - kali-c., stann., verat.

EXERTION, physical, amel. - ***aur.***

EYESTRAIN, general, agg. (see Asthenopia) - agar., alum., ***am-c.,*** am-m., anac., ***apis,*** arg-m., **ARG-N.,** ***asaf.,*** asar., ***aur.,*** bar-c., bar-m., bell., bor., bry., **CALC.,** cann-i., canth., ***carb-v., caust.,*** chlol., ***cic.,*** **CINA,** cocc., coff., con., **CROC.,** cupr., dros., dulc., ferr., ***graph.,*** hep., ign., ***jab.,*** **KALI-C.,** kali-p., kali-s., kreos., led., **LYC.,** mag-c., mag-m., mang., merc., mez., mur-ac., ***naja,*** nat-a., ***nat-c.,*** **NAT-M.,** ***nat-p.,*** nicc., nit-ac., nux-m., ***nux-v.,*** olnd., **ONOS.,** par., petr., ***ph-ac., phos.,*** phys., ***phyt.,*** puls., ran-b., **RHOD.,** ***rhus-t.,*** **RUTA.,** sabad., ***sars.,*** sel., **SENEG.,** ***sep.,*** **SIL.,** ***spig., spong.,*** staph., stram., stront-c., sulph., sul-ac., ther., thuj., valer., verb., viol-o., zinc.
back, pain, of eyes on looking at near objects - ***aml-n.***
bones, aggravates feeling as if, were scraped - ***par.***
brain, produces, fag - **PHOS.**
agg. tense feeling in, eyes and skin - ***par.***
dread of - apis.
eyesight, causes weak - bell., ***carb-v.,*** **RUTA.**
worse from exerting better in dark - ***nux-m.***

EYESTRAIN, general
headache, from - ***agar.,*** arg-n., ***aur.,*** bell., ***bor., cact., calc., carb-v., caust., cimic., cina,*** gels., ***ham.,*** jab., **KALI-C.,** kali-p., kali-s., **LYC.,** mag-p., mur-ac., ***nat-c.,*** **NAT-M.,** ***nat-p., onos.,*** par., **PH-AC.,** ***phos.,*** phys., **RHOD.,** ***rhus-t.,*** **RUTA.,** sep., **SIL.,** ***spong.,*** staph., sulph., ***tub.,*** valer., zinc.
intense, over eyes - sep.
looking, downward - alum., kalm., nat-m., olnd., phyt., spig., sulph.
fixedly at anything - anac., ***aur.,*** cadm-s., calc., caust., cina, gent-c., glon., helon., ***ign.,*** lac-c., lith., mur-ac., ***nat-m.,*** nux-v., olnd., **ONOS.,** par., ***puls., ruta.,*** sabad., sars., ***spig., spong.,*** sulph., tarent.
upward - acon., aeth., arn., arum-t., bapt., bell., ***calc.,*** calc-s., caps., caust., coca, colch., cupr., glon., gran., graph., ***ign.,*** lach., ***lac-c.,*** plat., plb., **PULS.,** sep., sil., stram., ***sulph., thuj.***
school children, in - ***ph-ac., ruta.***
light, after excessive use by insufficient, loss of use of left eye, vision of right incomplete - ***lith.***
needle, eye worse from looking fixedly at an object, cannot thread a - croc.
pain, as if strained - **RUTA.**
artificial light, using eyes by, after - cina, ***lith.,*** sep.
nausea, with - ***jab.***
objects, when trying to look at - ruta.
overexertion, as from - meph., ***phys.,*** **RUTA.**
vertigo, causes - all-s., ***graph., mag-p.,*** **NAT-M., PHOS.,** ***sil.***
looking fixedly, from - ***caust., kali-c., lach.,*** olnd., tarent.

FADE, away, then reappear, objects - gels.

FARSIGHTED, hypermetropia - acon., ***aesc.,*** alum., sang., **ARG-N.,** ***bell.,*** bry., **CALC.,** ***carb-an.,*** caust., chel., ***chin., coloc., con.,*** dios., ***dros.,*** grat., ***hyos., lil-t., lyc.,*** mag-m., mez., morph., nat-c., ***nat-m., nux-v., onos., petr.,*** phos., phys., phyt., psor., raph., **SEP., SIL.,** spig., stram., sulph., tab., valer.
asthenopia, with - ***jab.***
choroiditis, in - ***coloc.***
distant objects appear more distant - ***con.***
eating, after - mez.
evening - hyper.
long lasting - stram.
overuse of eyes, in fine work - ***arg-n.***
pupils dilated - carb-an.
reads fine print without glasses - petr.
right, commencing in, eye - sulph.

FEATHERY - ***alum., calc.,*** kreos., **LYC.,** mag-c., ***merc., nat-c.,*** nat-m., seneg., spig.

FIELD of vision, sees objects beside - calc., camph., cann-s., coloc., graph., ign., lac-c., nux-m., nux-v., stram., thuj.

FIERY - **BELL.**, ***bry.***, ***dig.***, dulc., ***hyos.***, iod., **KALI-C.**, ***lach.***, ***nat-m.***, ***nux-v.***, ***phos.***, ***psor.***, ***sep.***, **SPIG.**, stram., viol-o., zinc.
balls - ***cycl.***, stram.
bodies - arg-n., zinc.
circles - anan., calc-p., ***camph.***, carb-v., ip., ***puls.***, ***zinc.***
disks - thuj.
points - ammc., ***aur.***, merl., merc., ***nat-m.***, petr., sec., zinc.
falling - ph-ac.
moving with the eyes - am-c., nat-m.
rays about the light - ***kali-c.***, **LACH.**
rising from seat, on - verat.
shimmerings - ***calc-p.***
showers - plb.
spots - ***alum.***, coca, elaps
surface - ph-ac.
zigzags - con., ign., ***graph.***, **NAT-M.**, ***sep.***
around objects - graph., ***nat-m.***

FIRE, a sea of, on closing the eyes - **PHOS.**, spig.

FLAMES - **BELL.**, calc., cann-s., ***carb-v.***, ***chin-s.***, cinch-b., cycl., dulc., myric., ***puls.***, sant., spong., staph., ther., ***thuj.***
night in bed - spong., staph.
waking, on - cycl.
various colored flames - ***crot-h.***, ***phos.***, thuj.

FLASHES - agar., aloe, **BELL.**, benz-n., brom., calc., calc-f., carb-s., caust., ***cedr.***, chlf., clem., coca, ***croc.***, cycl., dig., fl-ac., ***glon.***, hep., ign., iris, lyc., merc., merc-i-f., ***nat-c.***, op., **PHOS.**, **PHYS.**, ***puls.***, sec., seneg., ***sil.***, spong., stram., sulph., tab., tarent., ***valer.***, viol-o.
awake, while - ***nat-c.***
closing the eyes, on - ail., ***nat-c.***, phos., sep., spong., sulph.
coughing, on - kali-c., kali-chl.
dark, in the - arg-n., **PHOS.**, stram., ***valer.***
electric shocks, like - ***croc.***
evening on falling asleep - nat-c.
morning in the dark - arg-n.
waking, on - ***nat-c.***
sleep, on going to - ***phos.***
streaks - nat-c., nux-v.

FLICKERING - acon., ***aesc.***, ***agar.***, all-c., aloe, alum., ***am-c.***, anac., ***ant-t.***, ***aran.***, ***ars.***, ***ars-i.***, bar-c., bar-m., **BELL.**, ***bor.***, bry., calc., calc-f., calc-s., camph., cann-i., cann-s., caps., **CARB-S.**, ***carb-v.***, carb-o., carl., ***caust.***, ***cham.***, ***chel.***, ***chin.***, chin-a., chlf., clem., coca, coff., con., croc., cupr-ac., **CYCL.**, dig., ***gels.***, **GRAPH.**, hell., ***hep.***, ***hyos.***, ***ign.***, ***iod.***, ***kalm.***, **LACH.**, ***led.***, ***lyc.***, med., meny., merc., merl., mez., mur-ac., nat-a., nat-c., **NAT-M.**, nat-p., ***nux-v.***, op., paeon., ***petr.***, ph-ac., **PHOS.**, phys., ***plat.***, plb., ***psor.***, ***puls.***, sant., sars., sec., ***seneg.***, **SEP.**, ***sil.***, sol-n., ***staph.***, stram., stront-c., **SULPH.**, sumb., tab., ther., ***thuj.***, ***zinc.***
afternoon after nap - ***lyc.***
around outside the range of vision - ***graph.***
ascending stairs - dig.
borders, with black - cimic.
breakfast, after - sulph.
candlelight - bar-c.

FLICKERING,
chill, during - cham., led., lyc., sep., ther.
circles - calc-p.
closing eyes, when - nat-a., ther.
colors, various - **CYCL.**
daytime - anac., phos.
dinner, during - ***thuj.***
after - bry.
eating amel. - phos.
entering a house, on - dig.
evening - merc., plat., til.
read, on attempting to - ***cycl.***
exercise, after - dig.
headache, during - **CHIN.**, chin-a., chin-s., ***coloc.***, con., **CYCL.**, graph., ***lach.***, **NAT-M.**, ***phos.***, sars., ***sil.***, ***sulph.***
at beginning of - ***sars.***
before - aran., ***graph.***, iris, ***nat-m.***, ***plat.***, ***psor.***, ***sars.***, sep., ***sulph.***, ther.
left - ***chin-a.***, nat-p.
light, when looking at - anac., ***sep.***
looking, intently - led., tab.
long - caust., ph-ac., psor.
lying, while - ***cham.***
morning - am-c., ***bor.***, calc., kali-c.
morning, 5 a.m. - nat-p.
headache, with - **CYCL.**
rising, on - carb-v., **CYCL.**, nat-p.
waking - calc., dulc.
writing - ***bor.***
moving to the right - bor.
night agg. - cycl.
paroxysmal - ***ther.***
reading, while - aran., arn., cob., ***cycl.***, merc., ph-ac., ***seneg.***
by light - ph-ac.
right - bry., lach.
rising, on - acon., verat.
sewing, while - iod.
sleep, on going to - lyc.
sudden - zing.
vertigo, with - alum., aran., ***bell.***, ***calc.***, dig., ***glon.***, mez., ***stram.***, thuj., vinc.
wiping eyes agg. - seneg.
writing, while - agar., ***aran.***, arn., ***bor.***, nat-m., ***seneg.***

FLOATERS, muscae volitantes - acon., aesc., ***agar.***, ***arg-n.***, am-c., anan., ant-t., arn., asaf., ***aur.***, ***bar-c.***, ***bell.***, ***calc.***, ***carb-v.***, ***carl.***, ***caust.***, chel., **CHIN.**, chlol., cob., **COCC.**, coff., ***con.***, ***crot-h.***, cupr-ar., ***cycl.***, ***daph.***, dig., ***gels.***, glon., hyos., ***kali-c.***, kali-p., kali-s., lact., ***lil-t.***, ***lyc.***, mag-c., ***merc.***, mez., morph., nat-c., **NAT-M.**, ***nit-ac.***, ***nux-m.***, ***nux-v.***, par., **PHOS.**, **PHYS.**, ***psor.***, ***rhus-t.***, **SEP.**, **SIL.**, sol-n., ***stram.***, **SULPH.**, ***tab.***, ter., thuj., verat., zinc.
eating, after - lyc., ***phos.***
reading, while - ***kali-c.***
sewing, after - am-c.
walking in open air - ter.
writing, while - ***nat-c.***

FOCAL, distance, changes, headache, during - aster., ***cycl.***, sulph.

FOCAL, distance,
changes while reading - agar., carb-ac., jab., lyc.
unequal - ***chin.***

FOGGY, vision - acon., ***agar., alum.,*** ambr., am-c., am-m., ammc., ***ant-t., apis,*** aran., ***arg-m., arg-n.,*** **ARS.,** ***ars-i.,*** arum-t., arund., asaf., atro., ***aur., bar-c., bell.,*** berb., bism., bruc., bry., bufo, cahin., **CALC.,** calc-f., ***calc-p.,*** calc-s., ***camph.,*** cann-i., carb-an., carb-s., carl., ***cast.,*** **CAUST.,** cedr., ***cham., chel.,*** **CHIN.,** ***chin-s., cina,*** clem., ***cocc.,*** coff-t., coloc., ***con.,*** **CROC.,** crot-t., cund., **CYCL.,** dig., ***dros., dulc.,*** elaps, euphr., eupi., form., gamb., **GELS.,** gent-c., ***glon., graph.,*** grat., haem., ***hep.,*** hydr-ac., ***hyos., iod.,*** ip., jab., kali-ar., ***kali-c., kali-i.,*** kali-p., kali-s., kalm., ***kreos.,*** lach., lac-ac., ***laur., lil-t., lith., lyc.,*** mag-c., **MERC.,** merl., ***mill., morph.,*** nat-a., ***nat-m.,*** nat-p., nit-ac., nux-m., ol-an., op., osm., ***petr., ph-ac.,*** **PHOS.,** pic-ac., plan., ***plat., plb.,*** podo., psor., **PULS.,** ***ran-b.,*** raph., ***rhod., rhus-t., ruta.,*** sabad., sang., ***sars., sec., sep., sil.,*** sol-n., spig., staph., ***stram.,*** stry., **SULPH.,** tab., ***tarent., ther., thuj.,*** til., upa., **ZINC.**
afternoon - ***cycl.,*** mag-c., nat-m.
3 to 4 p.m. - bufo.
4 p.m. after sleep - cahin., lyc.
air, open agg. - alum., am-m., thuj.
bright light agg. - am-m.
candlelight, around - osm., tell.
by candlelight - nit-ac.
cataract, incipient - **CAUST.**
circles - merl.
closing, and pressing eyeballs, when - bar-c.
closing, eyes amel. - nit-ac.
colors caused by - tarent.
daytime - bar-c.
dinner, after - bar-c., lyc.
distant objects - phos.
eating, after - ***bar-c.,*** calc., zinc.
evening - alum., cina, euphr., ind., lyc., phos., rhus-t., **SULPH.,** tab.
candlelight, in - sulph.
faintness, with - petr.
fever, with - sep.
headache, during - aster., ***cycl.,*** sulph.
mist before the eyes - podo.
hemiopia, in - **AUR.**
iritis, in - ***euph.***
lachrymation, amel. - calc.
looking, intently - calc.
luminous yellow, quivering - kali-c.
lying, on left side - merc-i-f.
melancholy, after mortification - ***ign.***
morning - alum., am-m., ***bar-c.,*** bov., bry., caust., ***lyc.,*** nicc., nit-ac., stram., zinc.
10 a.m. to 3 p.m. - nat-m.
motion, during - con.
of eyes amel. - nit-ac..
prosopalgia, in - verb.
reading, while - arn., ***ars.,*** calc., camph., cina, croc., gent-c., grat., ***kali-c.,*** lyc., nat-m., ph-ac., ***sulph.,*** vinc.
looking at a bright light, while - ***kali-c.***
walking, while - vinc.

FOGGY, vision
right, before - sep.
rising, from a seat - puls.
room, in - lac-ac., osm.
rubbing, agg. - caust., spig.
amel. - cina, **PULS.**
seminal emissions, after - sars.
sewing - ph-ac.
sitting, after long - sars.
sleep, after - stram.
standing - ***caust.,*** nat-m.
stupefaction, with - bism.
sunlight, agg. - am-m., ***tarent.***
tremulous - kali-c.
typhoid, after - ***lyc.***
typhus, in - chin-s.
vertigo, in - canth.
walking - phys., puls., vinc.
air, in open - caust.
washing, amel. - alum., am-m., caust.
white - ars.
wiping amel. - alum.
writing - asaf., calc-f., grat., lyc., ph-ac.

GAUZE, as if looking through - ***calc., caust., dros., dulc.,*** hydr-ac., ***kreos., nat-m., sep., sulph.***
left eye - sars.
looking steadily or reading, better by wiping eyes, when - cina
morning and after a meal - bar-c.
vertigo, with - ***nat-m.***
white - **ARS.**

GLIMMERING, (see flickering)

GLITTERING, bodies on blowing nose - alum., nat-s.
bodies on blowing nose, bright, luminous appearances - calc., ***hep., phos.***
outside, the range of vision - ***nux-v.***
candlelight, in - anag.
circles - calc-p.
gaslight, in - aur.
needles - **CYCL.**
objects - aran., arund., ***calc-p., camph., cycl., graph.,*** iod., lach., ***nux-v.,*** ol-an., phos., stroph., syph., ***ther.***
points - chel.
reading, while - aran.
stars - con.
stooping, on - ther.
vertigo with - calc.
zigzags - ign.

GOLDEN, colors before the vision
chain dangling before eyes - ***chin.***
everything looks - hyos.
letters seem - bell.

GRAY, colors before the vision
as if looking through a gray cover - sil.
black objects seem gray - ***stram.***
bluish-gray circles around light - lach.
circles - lachn.
covering before eyes - phos.
distance, at a - nit-ac.
fog - cic.

GRAY, colors before the vision,
halo - phos., sep.
letters - stram.
change to round gray spots - calc-p.
objects seem - ammc., arg-n., ***ars.,*** brom., calc-p., camph., chelin., elaps, guare., lachn., nit-ac., ***nux-v.,*** phal., ***phos.,*** sep., ***sil., stram.***
point before right eye moving with eye - brom.
points - ***nux-v.***
reddish gray border around white things - ***stram.***
serpent-like bodies - **ARG-N.**
spots - ***arg-n.,*** calc-p., chlf., cic., lachn.
veil - ***apis,*** elaps

GREEN, colors before the vision - aml-n., **ARS.,** bry., calc., cann-i., canth., carb-s., caust., **CINA,** ***cycl., dig.,*** hep., kali-ar., kali-c., ***lac-c.,*** mag-m., merc., osm., **PHOS.,** phyt., ***ruta,*** **SANT.,** sep., stram., ***stront-c.,*** stry., sulph., ***tub.,*** vario., verat-v., zinc.
blindness for - carb-s.
circles - zinc.
around light - verat-v.
dinner, during - mag-m.
amel. by belching - mag-m.
halo around light - ammc., anag., atro., calc., ***caust.,*** chin., com., mag-m., **PHOS.,** ruta, ***sep.,*** sil., ***sulph.,*** zinc.
letters - canth.
pea green, saw herself on looking in the glass - cina.
radiations - bell., con., ign., ph-ac.
rising, on - vario.
sparks - kali-c.
spots - ***caust., kali-c., lac-c.,*** nit-ac., stram., stront.
walking in the dark, while - ***stront.***
stripes - thuj.
vomiting - tab.
yellow-green - sant.

HAIR, as if a, hung before the sight and must be wiped away - alum., ars-h., colch., dig., ***euphr.,*** kali-c., lach., plan., sang., spig., staph.

HALO, of, around the light - alum., ***anac.,*** bar-c., **BELL.,** ***bry., calad.,*** calc., ***carb-v.,*** cham., chim., ***cic., cycl., dig.,*** gels., ***hep., ip.,*** kali-c., kali-n., kali-p., kali-s., ***lach.,*** mag-m., merl., nat-p., ***nicc.,*** nit-ac., **OSM.,** ***ph-ac.,*** **PHOS., PULS.,** ran-b., ***ruta., sars., sep.,*** stann., ***staph.,*** **SULPH.,** ***tub.,*** zinc.
around the letters while reading - alum., cic.

HAZY - gels., ***phos.***
bluish, in hyperaemia of optic nerve and retina - ***bry.***
everything at a distance is - ***jab.***
left - verat-v.
vision good for fixed objects, but when put in motion before eyes there is a haze and dull producing vertigo - con.

HEMERALOPIA, (see Blindness, night-blindness)

HEMIOPIA - ***ars., aur.,*** aur-m., ***bov.,*** cahin., ***calc.,*** calc-s., cann-s., caust., chion., cic., ***cocc.,*** cycl., dig., gels., ***glon.,*** lach., ***lith.,*** lob., ***lyc.,*** morph., mur-ac., nat-a., nat-c., ***nat-m.,*** plb., psor., rhus-t., ***sep.,*** staph., ***stram.,*** sulph., titan., zinc.
as if upper part of field of, were covered by dark cloud, evenings while walking - ***dig.***
evening - calc-s., dig.
eyestrain, from - aur.
headache, followed by - nat-m.
hemicrania, with - lyc.
horizontal - **ARS.,** ***aur., lith., lyc.,*** sep., sulph., ***tub.***
can see no trace of upper half - ***aur.***
hydrocephalus, acute, in - ***lyc.***
left eye, of - ***aur.***
left, only, half is visible - cycl., ***lyc., lith.***
lower half covered with black veil - ***aur.***
left half, lost - calc., cic., lyc., nat-c.
lower, lost - ***aur.,*** cahin., sulph.
menses, during - lith.
perpendicular - bov., calc., lith., ***mur-ac., nat-m.***
pregnancy, during - ran-b.
right half, lost - ***calc., cocc.,*** cycl., glon., iod., **LITH.,** ***lyc.***
sees only below axis, and not clear - ***ars.***
upper, lost - ***ars.,*** **AUR.,** ***camph., dig.,*** gels.
vertical - aur., bov., calc., ***caust.,*** cic., gels., glon., **LITH.,** ***lyc.,*** morph., ***mur-ac., nat-m.,*** op., plb.
visible, upper portion of large object not - ***camph.***
walking, while - dig.
writing, can see only left half of line while reading or - ***cocc.***

HYPERMETROPIA, (see Farsighted)

ILLUSIONS, of - ***absin., agar.,*** aesc., ambr., anac., anh., ***antipyrin.,*** ars., ***atro., bell.,*** bry., calc., camph., ***cann-i.,*** carb-s., chel., cimic., cocaine, dig., eup-per., ***hyos.,*** kali-bi., kali-br., lach., lact., ***merc., morph.,*** nat-sal., ***onos., op.,*** past., **PHOS.,** plat., plb., puls., sang., sant., sec., sep., spig., ***stram.,*** sulph., thuj., valer., verat.
falling asleep, when - **PHOS.**
insects - caust., dig., merc.
objects passing - glon.
surgery, after - stront-c.

IMAGES, too long retained - alum., anan., gels., piloc., ***lac-c., nat-m.,*** nicc., phos., tab., tub.

INDISTINCT - **ANAC.,** ***caust., kali-i.,*** sil., verb.
dilated pupils, from - amyg.
distant objects seem, riding or walking - ***gels.***
faintness, with - ***calc.***
headache and nausea, with - ***coca.***
ophthalmia, in - apis.
catarrhal, in - phos.
prosopalgia, in - ***chel.***
raving, in - amyg.
reading, after - ***apis***
straining body, mind or eyes, from - ***calc.***
using eyes, after - ***camph.***

INDISTINCT,
weakness, from - ***calc.***
yellow fever, in - ***gels.***

INVERTED, objects seem - bell., gels., guare., kali-c.

JUMP, words when reading - bell., lyss.

LARGE, field of vision - fl-ac., stry.
flame of light - dig., osm.

LARGE, objects, seem - aeth., apis, atro., berb., cann-i., cann-s., caust., con., euph., **HYOS.,** ***laur., nat-m., nicc.,*** **NUX-M.,** ***onos.,*** op., ox-ac., phys., verb.
cerebral congestion - aeth.
elongated - bell., zinc.
linear - ox-ac.
raises his foot unnecessarily high in stepping over small objects when walking - euph., **ONOS.**
rising from a seat, on - staph.
twilight, in - ***berb.***

LIGHTNINGS - ***bell.,*** brom., ***caust.,*** croc., cycl., dig., fl-ac., ***glon., kali-c., nat-c., nux-v.,*** olnd., op., ***phos.,*** phys., ***puls.,*** sant., sec., sep., ***sil., spig.,*** staph., stram., valer., zinc.
dark, in - ***phos.,*** stram., valer.
night, distant, sheet lightning in the dark, 11 p.m. - coca.
noon - dig.
asleep, on falling - nat-c., **PHOS.,** sulph.
waking, on - ***nat-c.***

LIGHTS - calc., ***caust., chin-s., phos.,*** spong.
insensibility, to - agar., kali-br.
points - nat-m.
dark circle, in a - caust.
spots - con.
streaks of - **NAT-M.**
pass downward, seen to one side of eye in dark - thuj.
waves of - bor.

LINE, the lower seems above the upper - kali-c.

LOSS, of vision, (see Blindness)

LUMINOUS, objects jumping, covering eyes - dig.
dark, in - valer.
surgery, after - zinc.

MENSES, during agg. - cycl., graph., puls., sep.
before agg. - dict.

MIRAGE - lyc.

MISTAKES - bell., bov., euph., hyos., kali-c., ***plat.***

MISTY - ***agar.,*** ambr., ammc., ***arg-m., arg-n.,*** asaf., ***bell.,*** bism., cahin., ***caust.,*** cycl., form., ***gels., glon., graph.,*** lact., ***petr., ran-b.,*** sil., spig., thuj.
afternoon, when writing - ol-an.
amaurosis, or cataract, in - ***calc-p.***
amblyopia, obscuration at a distance, in - ***ruta***
as if enveloped in a halo or, objects look in ophthalmia tarsi - ***merc-c.***
asthenopia, in morning - merl.
attacks of vanishing of sight - ***phos.***

MISTY, vision
bright light, after a - phos.
cataract, in - ***chel.,*** sec.
distance, at a - mill., phos.
evening - ind.
injury to eye, after - ***arn.***
looking intently at anything, or reading - ***calc.***
long - cann-s.
mercury, after abuse of - ***kali-i.***
morning, after waking - zinc.
objects seemed enveloped in, and to move, then burning - euph.
read, cannot, worse after seminal emissions - ***sars.***
reading or writing, when - grat.
scrofulous ophthalmia, after - ***kali-i.***
whitish-gray, in staphyloma - ***apis***

MOONLIGHT, amel. - ***aur.***

MOVING - ***agar., aloe,*** am-c., **ARG-N.,** ***bell., bor., calc.,*** calc-p., ***cann-i., cic., con., euphr., glon.,*** ign., ***lach.,*** laur., lyc., meny., merc., mosch., ***nux-v., olnd.,*** par., petr., ***psor.,*** sabad., ***sep.,*** stram.
evening, reading, while - merc.
letters - ***agar.,*** am-c., con., ***hyos.,*** iod., merc., phys.
towards noon - am-c.
something moving - lyss., psor.

moving, objects seem to be - ***arg-n.,*** bapt., bell., carb-ac., cic., cocc., con., euphr., glon., hydr-ac., ign., nux-m., petr., psor.
backward - ***bell.,*** calc., cic., sep.
and forward - carb-ac., ***cic.***
slowly - sep.
fine motion - petr.
floating - nux-m.
jumping - meny.
revolving - ***bell.***
side to side - cic.
to and fro, towards noon - elaps
float, to - anag., lyss.
up and down - ars., ***cocc.,*** con., sil., spong.
pulsation in ear, from - sil.

MYOPIA, (see Nearsighted)

NEARER, objects seem - ***bov.,*** phys., rhus-t., stram.
to each other - ***nux-m.***
eyes, to - valer.

NEARSIGHTED, myopia - acon., ***agar., am-c., anac., ang.,*** apis, ***arg-n.,*** ars., aur-m., bell., ***calc.,*** carb-s., ***carb-v., chin.,*** cimic., coff-t., ***con., cycl.,*** dig., euph., ***euphr., gels., graph.,*** grat., ***hyos., jab., lach.,*** lil-t., ***lyc., mang., meph.,*** mez., nat-a., ***nat-c., nat-m.,*** nat-p., **NIT-AC.,** ***petr., ph-ac.,*** **PHOS., PHYS.,** ***piloc., pic-ac.,*** plb., psor., **PULS.,** raph., ***ruta.,*** sel., spong., ***stram., sulph., sul-ac.,*** syph., ***thuj., tub.,*** viol-o., ***valer.,*** verb., viol-t.
burning, with, heat in face - grat.
candlelight, sight worse by, than by daylight - arg-n.
diarrhea, with, typhus, after - ***chin.***
exerting, the eyes, after - ***carb-v.***

NEARSIGHTED, myopia
increasing - ***phos.***
looking, away from work amel. - ph-ac.
objects seem too large, left eye, after a blow - ***phys.***
reading, while - agar., grat., lyc.
sleepy feeling, with - eup-pur.
spasm, from ciliary - **PHYS.**
and twitching of lids - ***agar.***
touch, nose has to, paper to read - ***calc.***
turns head sideways to see clearly - lil-t.

NET, before eyes - anac., ***carb-an., chin-s.,*** hyos.
swimming - ***carb-an.***

NYCTALOPIA - bell., ***chin.,*** hell., ***lyc.,*** nux-v., phys., sil., stram., sulph.

OBJECTS, in vision
blurred outlines - phos.
color, changing in - stront-c.
half in light, half in dark - glon.
high, lean forward and about to fall - arn.
ill defined in retinitis - **SULPH.**
indistinct - bell., kali-bi.
move, right, to - nat-sal.
move, to and fro - cic.
persons seem - bell., calc., nat-p., stram.
shade, as if in - seneg.
turning in circle, as if - chel., cycl., nat-m.
vibrating - carb-v.
dark, then become - psor.
whirling around each other - chlol., grat.

OBLIQUITY - ***nux-m., stram.***

PALE, vision - ***sil.***
objects become, after looking long - ***agar.***

PERCEPTIVE power lost - kali-p.

POLYOPSIA - gels., iod.

PRESBYOPIA, (see Farsighted)

PURPLE, colors before the vision - ***verat-v.***

RAIN, seems looking through - nat-m.

RAINBOW - ***bell., bry., con.,*** dig., ip., ph-ac., puls.
beaming light of - bell.
circles - dig., ip.
strip on closing one eye - bry.

RANGE, of vision (see Focal)

RAYS, curved, shooting, from visual axis - iod.
around light - kali-c.
light seems broken up into - bell.

READING, inability from weak eyes - asar., ***cann-i., kali-c.***
black, everything becomes - meny.
candlelight, inability by - ***phos.***
darkening, of sight, causes - ***calc.***
difficult, worse by candlelight - phos., puls.
eyes, give out, while - **NAT-M.,** ***phos.***
film over, from reading or looking closely - lac-c.
eye, if one is used longer than a minute, words and letters become blurred - chlol.
fatigues - ***ammc., jab.,*** sep., ***sulph.***
flickering, causes - cob.

READING,
glimmering, causes, and glittering - aran.
gray, black seemed - sep.
light, cannot read with, worse by bright light - ***asar.***
letters, on blackboard, cannot see - lac-ac.
blend and dance - **STRAM.**
blurred, look - aml-n., cund., cob., meph., oxal., sulph.
change into little black points - ***calc-p.***
change into small round gray spots - ***calc-p.***
colors of rainbow around them, or disappear - ***cic.***
disappear in evening by candlelight, paper white as if not printed on - aur-m.
distinguish, cannot - ***chel.***
double, appear - ***graph.***
reading, after - ***lyss.***
exertion to distinguish, must make - ***carb-v.***
go up and down - ***cic.***
fade and appear as a black line - ***daph.***
large, cannot be distinguished, seem only something black on white ground - ***aur.***
pale, appear - **SIL.**
and blurred, look - dros.
surrounded by white borders - ***chin.***
red, outline undefined, look - ***phos.***
by gaslight, flashing of lights before vision - phos.
run together - ***art-v.,*** bry., calc-ar., ***camph.,*** cann-i., carb-ac., chel., coca, ***con., ferr., graph., lyc., merl.,*** ruta, seneg., **SIL.,** viol-o.
asthenopia, in - **NAT-M.**
black spots on white ground - ***chin.***
diphtheria, after - lac-c.
mental disturbance - **STAPH.**
mental labor, after - ***arg-n.***
smaller, appear - ***glon., kali-m.***
coryza, in - ***all-c.***
lines, appear crooked - ***bell.***
page, appeared covered with letters, in great confusion - bell.
seems covered with pale spots of red, yellow, green and other colors - ***lac-c.***
pain, in eyes, cannot read much - ars-m., ruta.
paper, looking at piece of, pain in right eye - calc-s.
looks red, eyes pain by candlelight - sars.
looks red or rose color - croc.
shines on reading - croc.
dances in a fog and vanishes - arn.
inability to read fine - cadm-s., meph., ***nat-c.***
printed matter is spelled out with difficulty, cannot take in the whole word at a glance - ***nux-v.***
sight, objects seem to swim before - **NAT-M.**
as if strained too much by reading - ***ruta.***
weak, must wipe eyes which aggravates - seneg.
spots, black or brown, dancing over her book, - med.

READING,
spots,
if he looks at a, for some time it becomes quite dark, also if he reads any length of time - lachn.
tears, brings - carb-s.
temples, contractive pain above - agn.
type, seems to move - agar.
could hardly see large, when held close to eyes during daylight - ***phos.***

RED, colors before the vision - antipyrin., apis, atro., **BELL.,** bry., ***cact.,*** carb-s., cedr., com., **CON.,** croc., cund., ***dig.,*** ***dub.,*** elaps, fl-ac., ***hep.,*** ***hyos.,*** iodof., ip., ***kali-bi.,*** lac-c., mag-m., ***nux-m.,*** nux-v., **PHOS.,** ruta, sars., sep., spong., stram., ***stront-c.,*** ***sulph.,*** tarent., verat-v., zinc.
blindness for - carb-s.
circles - cact.
light seems to be - ***sulph.***
on rubbing - stront.
closing eyes - elaps
dinner, during - mag-m.
evening, while reading by light - sars.
fiery spots - elaps
halo - ***bell.,*** com., ***ip.,*** sil., verat-v.
around the lamplight - com.
letters - phos.
luminous appearance - ***phos.,*** spong.
masses - spig.
night - cedr., chin., elaps, mag-m., spong.
and yellow during day - cedr.
objects seem - atro., **BELL.,** carb-s., **CON.,** ***dig.,*** ***hep.,*** ***hyos.,*** iodof., ***nux-m.,*** **PHOS.,** ***stront.***
obstructions on looking at the light - cund.
paper looks red - croc., sars.
points - elaps
sparks - fl-ac., stry.
spots - dub., elaps, hyos., lac-c., lyc., verat-v.
wheel, candlelight seems to be a red wheel - sulph.

RINGS - calc., calc-p., carb-v., elaps, kali-c., phos., psor.
turning - kali-c.

RISING, body obscuring vision - am-m.

ROUND, objects rise before eyes while lying - caust.

RUN, together, letters - arg-n., ***art-v.,*** atro., bell., berb., bry., calc., calc-ar., ***camph.,*** **CANN-I.,** ***chel.,*** ***chin.,*** clem., coca, ***con.,*** ***dros.,*** elaps, euphr., ***ferr.,*** gels., gins., ***graph.,*** iris, ***lac-c.,*** ***lyc.,*** meph., ***merl.,*** **NAT-M.,** op., osm., **RUTA.,** ***seneg.,*** **SIL.,** **STAPH.,** **STRAM.,** ***tub.,*** viol-o.
after a little while - ***con.***
evening - merl.
reading in bed, while - bell.
exertion, of vision, from fine work - nat-c.
mental exertion, after - ***arg-n.***
morning - bry.
writing, while - carb-ac., ***chel.,*** clem., ***ferr.,*** gels., lyc., ***merl.,*** op., sil.

run, together, objects - berb., sil.
sewing, while - berb., ***calc.***
stitches while sewing - **NAT-M.**

SCOTOMA, central - aloe, carb-s., tab., thyr.
central - carb-s., tab.

SHADE, amel. - con., phos.

SHADOWS - ***ruta.,*** ***seneg.***
look shaded - ***seneg.***
objects, on one side of - ***calc.***

SMALL, objects seem - ***all-c.,*** ***aur.,*** benz-d-n., berb., camph., carb-v., cycl., ***glon.,*** ***hyos.,*** ***kali-chl.,*** ***lyc.,*** med., ***merc.,*** ***merc-c.,*** nat-c., nit-ac., op., petr., ***plat.,*** ***plb.,*** ***staph.,*** stram., thuj.

SMOKY, (see Foggy) - **CHIN.,** **GELS.,** lac-ac., ***phos.***

SNAKE, before the vision - arg-n., ***gels.***

SNOW, falling - plb.
flakes - bell., jab.
morning, on waking, objects seem covered with - dig.
surface - ph-ac.

SPARKS - acon., ammc., am-c., ant-t., arn., ars., ars-i., ***aur.,*** ***bar-c.,*** **BELL.,** bufo, calc., ***calc-f.,*** ***camph.,*** ***caust.,*** ***chel.,*** **CHIN.,** chin-a., ***chin-s.,*** chlf., coff., coloc., con., cupr., cupr-ar., ***cycl.,*** dulc., ferr-i., ***glon.,*** hyos., iod., kali-ar., ***kali-bi.,*** ***kali-c.,*** kali-s., ***lach.,*** lyc., lyss., mag-p., ***merc.,*** mez., nat-a., nat-c., nat-p., nit-ac., ***nuph.,*** ***nux-v.,*** ***op.,*** petr., phos., pic-ac., ***plat.,*** ***psor.,*** sec., ***sep.,*** ***sil.,*** sol-n., ***spig.,*** staph., stram., stront-c., stry., ***sulph.,*** thuj., valer., verat., zinc.
air, open, on going into - con., lyc.
black, when looking at light - mang.
blowing the nose, on - alum., cod.
breakfast, after - ferr-i.
closing eyes, on - ***hydr.,*** mang.
coughing, when - bell., kali-c., nuph., par.
dark, in - ***bar-c.,*** calc., lyc., ***phos.,*** thuj., valer.
daytime - croc.
dinner, during - thuj.
epileptic fit, before - ***hyos.***
evening - ammc.
like rays - mang.
exertion of mind - ***aur.***
headache, before - carb-ac., chin-s., coca, cycl., eug., lach., phos., ***plat.,*** psor., sars., spong., viol-o.
headache, during - am-c., ars., ***chel.,*** **MAG-P.**
morning - calc., ferr-i.
motion of eyelids, on - bell.
night - ***am-c.,*** ***staph.***
on falling asleep - **PHOS.**
on waking - ***am-c.,*** ***calc.***
noon - dig., verat.
outside the field of either side - thuj.
rest, during, agg. - dulc.
sewing, while - iod.
sitting, while - hura
streaks in, after writing - ***carl.***

SPARKS,
vertigo, during - ars., ***camph.,*** psor.
waking, on - ***calc.***
walking, while - hura.
air, in open - con.
winking, on - ***caust.***
writing - kali-bi.

SPOTS - act-sp., alum., carb-s., ***caust.,*** colch., ***con.,*** **CYCL.,** elaps, ***jab.,*** kali-bi., **KALI-C., PHOS.,** sil., sol-n., **SULPH.,** verat-v.
bright - con.
closing eyes, on - ***hydr.***
colored - astac.
floating - am-m., cann-i., dig., hell., phos., ruta.
luminous, undulating - arund.
green in dark - stront-c.
headache, before - ***psor.***
headache, with - cycl.
jumping up and down - ***croc.***
looking steadily - act-sp.
luminous - ***hyos.***
reading - astac., jab., kali-c.
round - dig.
sewing, after - am-c.
waking, on - **CYCL.**
wooly - dys-co.
writing - kali-bi.

STARS - alum., ***ammc.,*** atro., ***aur., calc.,*** cast., con., hyos., ***kali-c.,*** nat-c., puls., sec., tarent., verat-v.
artificial light, in - puls.
dancing - croc.
drowsy feeling in head, with - ign.
right side of field of vision - ***calc.***
sneezing agg. - nat-c.
starry halo round light - puls.
white, (see Colors)
writing, when - ***kali-c.***

STRIPED, colors before the vision - ***am-c.,*** bell., **CON.,** ***nat-m.,*** puls., ***sep.,*** sol-n., sulph., thuj.

STRIPES - **CON.,** ***sep., sulph.,*** thuj.

SWIMMING, of, letters - bell., coca
objects - carb-ac., ***carl.,*** coloc., merl., mez., **NAT-M.,** par., sumb., thuj., til., zinc.
afternoon, 5 p.m. - thuj.

THREAD, before - con.

TREMBLING, objects - alum., bell., camph., ***cann-i.,*** carb-s., ***con., cur.,*** kali-c., ***lyc., petr.,*** ph-ac., ***phos.,*** phys., ***plat.,*** plb., ***psor.,*** sabad., sumb., thuj., viol-o.
artificial light, in - **LYC.**
evening by light - **LYC.,** petr.
morning on waking - phos.
yellow shining tremulous mist - ***kali-c.***

TRIPLOPIA - ***bell.,*** con., ***gels.,*** sec.
turning eyes to right - dig.

TWILIGHT, and morning amel. - phos.

UNSTEADY - ***nat-m., verat-v.,*** polyg.

VANISHING of sight, (see Blindness) - ant-t., ***arg-m., arg-n., carb-s., chel., chen-a., cic., crot-t., cycl., gels.,*** graph., ***grat.,*** kali-bi., ***kali-c.,*** kali-n., ***laur.,*** lyc., lyss., ***nat-m., nux-m.,*** nux-v., ***ox-ac., puls., sep., sil.,*** spig., thuj., ***zinc.***
cough, inability to, from - sulph.
evenings, in - asaf.
giddiness, with, and sweat - ***ox-ac.***
head, with stitches in one side of, generally in one temple or in back part - ***puls.***
hemicrania, in - ***chen-a.***
intoxication, after, on previous day, worse after dinner and in sun - **NUX-V.**
lachrymation, with burning, after dinner, and frequently when writing - zinc.
lid, with aching and stitches as from a splinter in upper - sil.
menses, during - ***graph.***
mind, with absence of - zinc.
misty, appearance, with - ***phos.***
momentary, with profuse lachrymation - crot-h.
nausea, with, worse after eating - ***crot-t.***
nosebleed, with - ***ox-ac.***
reading, while - crot-h.
especially when, frequent - dros.
rising, from a seat - hep.
sitting, when, up in bed - bell.
stooping, from - ***kali-bi.***
transient, with vertigo - ***chen-a.***
vertigo, with - ***bell.,*** **NUX-V.,** ***sulph.***
writing, while - ***kali-c.***

VARIEGATED, colors before the vision - ***bell., bry., cic.,*** **CON.,** dig., kali-c., kali-n., kali-s., mag-p., nicc., ***ph-ac., phos., sep.,*** stram., sulph.
wheels - kali-n.

VARIES, from day to day, or from hour to hour, sometimes fever with thirstlessness - ***gels.***

VEIL, as if looking through a - acon., ant-t., arum-t., arund., berb., bufo, ***caust., croc.,*** crot-t., ***hyos., iod., laur., lith.,*** lyc., ***nat-m.,*** nat-p., ***petr., phos., rhus-t., stram.,*** **SULPH.,** thuj.
amaurosis or cataract, in - ***calc-p.***
asthenopia, in - sep.
bed, after getting out of - ***stram.***
better from rubbing or wiping - **PULS.**
black, as if a, were before right - phos.
dark, passes from right to left every morning at 10 a.m. - ***nat-m.***
evening - ***euph.,*** tab.
hysteria, in - ***lyc., ther.***
objects appear covered with a gray - elaps, ***phos.***
rheumatic ophthalmia, in - ***cocc.***
scarlet fever, after - ***hep.***

VIBRATION, as of heated air - ***lyc.***

VIOLET, colors before the vision - **CINA.**

VISIONS, sees, on closing eyes (see Delusions) - ***calc.,*** spong.

WATER, of, causes desire for stool, urination, etc. - **LYSS.**

WAVERING - bell., chlor., con., lyc., mag-p-a., manc., morph., ***nat-m.,*** sant., sumb., ***verat-v.,*** zinc-chr.
luminous openings, he sees - arund.

WEAK, vision (see Eyes, Weak) - acet-ac., acon., ***agar.,*** alum., ***am-c., anac., apis, arg-m., arg-n., ars.,*** ars-i., asaf., ***asar., aur-m.,*** bar-c., bell., cact., cann-i., cann-s., ***caust.,*** chel., **CHIN.,** ***chin-a.,*** cic., ***cina, cinnb.,*** coc-c., **CON.,** croc., ***crot-h.,*** dig., **GELS.,** ***ham.,*** hura, hyos., hyper., ***iod.,*** kali-ar., kali-bi., kali-br., ***kali-c.,*** kali-i., ***kali-p.,*** kali-s., ***kalm., lach.,*** lact., ***led., lil-t., lith., lyc., mang.,*** meph., ***merc.,*** merl., ***morph.,*** nat-a., ***nat-m., nat-s.,*** nicc., ***nux-v.,*** **OP.,** par., ***petr.,*** **PHOS.,** ***ph-ac.,*** **PHYS.,** plb., ***puls.,*** raph., rhus-t., **RUTA,** sal-ac., sec., ***seneg., sep., sil.,*** sol-n., ***spig.,*** stann., ***stram., sulph.,*** sul-ac., tab., ***tarent.,*** thuj., til., upa., verat., zing.
alcoholism, in - ***kali-br.,*** **NUX-V.**
bright light agg. - bell., sol-n.
burning, with, and lachrymation - seneg.
catarrhal fever, in - ***kali-c.***
chronic, result of onanism - ***cina***
coryza, in - ***anac.***
diminished - chr-ac., lyss., ***plb.***
vertigo, with, before vomiting - ***sang.***
diphtheria, after - **GELS., LACH.,** lac-c., ***phyt.***
elderly, people, in - ***bar-c.***
evening - euphr., tarent.
candlelight, by - bar-c., ***hep.***
twilight - arg-n.
using agg. - **APIS.**
eye, with twitching in - nicc.
eyeballs, with drawing and pressure in - seneg.
eyes, with pressure above, goes off after vomiting - raph.
worse from excitement and using - par.
facial, with contortion of, muscles - ***mill.***
failed for near objects - ***arg-n.***
failing for one year - ***merc.***
failure, gradual, after fine work at night - pic-ac.
with dull pain in left eye - verat-v.
gaslight, worse from - ars-m., nat-p.
gland, with diseased submaxillary - ***kali-i.***
glaucoma, in - osm.
gradual failure, with violent pains involving eyeball, extend to orbit and head, worse at approach of storm - rhod.
grief, after - ***ign.***
headache, with - ***glon.,*** sulph.
and pain in eyes - meph.
and swollen eyelids - croc., ferr., ***nat-m., piloc., ruta,*** seneg., zinc.
chronic sick, with - ***zinc.***
dull, with, pressive - ***phyt.***
mental work, from - ***phos.***
health, from his condition of - nat-a.
hoarseness, with - ***nicc.***
imperfect, with tendency to stagger - ***gels.***
lachrymation, with, weak - ***ferr.***

WEAK, vision
left, could scarcely see with - atro.
gradually weaker from month to month - ***kali-m.***
locomotor ataxia, in - ***arg-n.***
liver, with, complaint - acet-ac.
long distances, for - nat-a.
look, cannot bear to, at one object for any length of time - bar-c.
looking, when, carefully at small objects - dros.
intently at an object - rheum
lost, nearly, in serous choroiditis - ***gels.***
masturbation, from - cina.
measles, after - ***euph.,*** **KALI-C.,** ***puls.***
menopause, during - ***tril.***
menses, before - ***cinnb.***
miscarriage, after - **KALI-C.**
morning, as if the eyes were strained - ruta.
myelitis, in - ***phos.***
nerve, from exhausted condition of optic - kali-p., **PHOS.**
periodic - cact.
pupils, with dilated - ***verat.***
right, in, eye - ***atro.,*** euph.
sex, after - ***chin.,*** **KALI-C., PHOS.**
smoking, after - asc-t., tab.
strained, as if eyes were - ***ruta.***
stroke, in - ***anac.***
sunstroke, from - ***verat-v.***
tire easily - ***apis.***
transient - ***phos.***
twice, must look, to be sure of seeing an object - vib.
typhus fever, in - ***lach.***
using, eyes agg. - agar., alum., ***am-c.,*** **APIS,** ***arg-m., carb-v.,*** caust., gels., ***piloc.,*** **NAT-M.,** par., ***phos.,*** **RUTA, SENEG.,** sulph.
vertigo, with - ***aran.***

WRITING, darker, letters become - asaf.
eyes give out - **NAT-M.,** zinc.
glimmering and glittering before eyes - aran.
inability from weak sight - ***arg-n.***
letters run together - clem.
worse from - asaf.

WHIRLING - apis, atro., eug., ***glon.,*** kali-c., pic-ac., ust., verat.

WHITE, colors before the vision - alum., am-c., apis, ars., atro., bell., caust., chlol., chlor., coca, ***dig.,*** elaps, grat., ***kali-c., ph-ac.,*** sulph., thuj., ust.
blindness for - carb-s.
bottles of water - thuj.
candlelight seems - dig.
clouds, wandering from left to right - bell.
falling drops on looking at snow - ***kali-c.***
flames - chlf.
flickering - ***ign.,*** sep.
flies - atro., dig.
globules - upa.
green, objects look - grat.
margin around letters - ***chin.***
pale, faces appear white - dig., ind.

WHITE, colors before the vision,
points - ars., rat., ust.
rays, flaming - cann-s.
sparks - alum., croc., rat., stry., ust.
spots - acon., ars., ***caust.,*** coca, con., gins., mez., sol-n., ***sulph.,*** ust.
floating - piloc., ust.
green, then - ***caust.***
waving - dig.
stars - alum., am-c., bell., caust., kali-c., nat-c.
blowing nose, on - alum.
sneezing - am-c.
writing, while - kali-c.
stripes - sol-n.
wheels - kali-c.
zigzags in a circle - ign.
white, glistening points falling - ph-ac.

YELLOW, colors before the vision - agar., aloe, alum., am-c., am-m., aml-n., ars., aur., ***bell.,*** bry., calen., cann-i., ***canth.,*** cedr., chin., **CINA,** coff., coloc., ***crot-h., cycl., dig.,*** hyos., ind., irid., kali-ar., ***kali-bi., kali-c.,*** kali-s., lac-c., lachn., osm., petr., phos., plb., sant., ***sep.,*** sil., stront-c., sulph., zinc.
attacks of blindness, after - bell.
border around all objects - bell., hyos.
circle around light - alum., ***kali-c., osm.,*** zinc.
moving - ***aloe.***
cloud - kali-c.
crescent-shaped bodies floating obliquely upwards - ***aur.***
day, and red at night - cedr.
flames - sant., thuj.
halo around the light - **ALUM.,** sarr.
letters - canth.
points - carb-an.
red things look yellow - bell.
shiny tremulous mist - kali-c.
spots - agar., am-c., am-m., carb-an., plb.
before left eye - agar.
looking at white objects - am-c.
reading, while - phos.
veil - kali-bi.
vomiting, while - tab.
wheels - kali-c., zinc.

ZIGZAGS - cann-i., coloc., ***con.,*** fl-ac., ***graph.,*** ign., kali-bi., lach., lyc., **NAT-M.,** phos., ***sep., sul-i.***
circles of colors - ***sep.,*** viol-o.
fiery - con., graph., ign., nat-m., sep.
flickering - ***graph.,*** ign., ***lach.,*** phos.
fluttering - thuj.
headache, during - ign.
outside the range of vision - ***graph.***
wavy - thuj.
writing, while - thuj.

PAIN, wrists - act-sp., am-c., anag., ***ant-c.,*** ant-t., ***arg-n.,*** ars., arund., asc-t., bell., brach., bry., buf-s., ***calc.,*** calc-p., calc-s., camph., cann-i., carb-s., carb-v., cast-eq., ***caul.,*** cham., chel., cimic., cina, cist., clem., cob., cocc., colch., coloc., cop., cor-r., crot-c., cub., dios., dulc., ***eup-per.,*** euph., ferr., ferr-ar., fl-ac., form., gels., grat., ***guai., hep.,*** hipp., hura, hyos., jug-c., ***kali-bi., kali-n., kalm.,*** lach., lac-ac., led., lil-t., ***lyc.,*** lycps., mag-s., manc., mang., merc., merc-i-f., mez., nat-s., osm., ***ox-ac.,*** pall., phys., plan., plb., podo., ptel., ***puls., rhod.,*** **RHUS-T.,** rhus-v., ***ruta.***, sabad., ***sabin.,*** sal-ac., sars., sol-n., squil., stann., still., stry., **SULPH.,** sul-ac., tab., tarent., tep., trom., urt-u., ***viol-o.,*** xan., zinc.

afternoon - calc-s., lycps., nux-v., sulph.
alternately in one or the other - arund., ***lac-c.***
back of - agar., all-c.
evening - all-c.
bending, on - arg-n.
dislocation, as of - ***arn., eup-per.,*** phos.
evening - dios., ***led.,*** nat-s., phys., pip-m., rhod., sars., verat-v.
exertion, after - alum., berb., kali-n., sulph.
extending into,
arm - arn., jug-c., plb.
elbow - kali-n., lach.
forearm - ferr-p., pall., stann.
forearm, writing, while - ferr-p.
hand - fago., rhod.
index finger - asaf.
knuckles - kali-n.
front of - com., plb., tarent.
motion agg. - plb.
sudden - com.
walking in open air, after - com.
grasping anything - bov., **RHUS-T.**
jerking - anac., rhus-t.
left - asc-t., brach., camph., cop., crot-c., dios., ferr., ***guai.,*** kalm., mag-s.
and right ankle - lach.
lifting - alum., ***rhus-t.***
lying down, after - nat-s.
morning - am-c., calc-p., carb-v., cupr., dios., dulc., hura, iod., kali-c., mag-m., merc-i-f., nux-v., osm., plb., puls., staph., sulph., zinc.
bed, in - calc., hyper., nat-c.
twisting, on - merc-i-f.
waking, on - dulc., merc-i-f.
motion, on - act-sp., arn., ***bry.,*** calo., carb-v., euph., ***guai.,*** hep., hyper., kali-c., ***kalm.,*** merc., ***mez.,*** ox-ac., plb., rhod., ruta., sabad., sil., staph., still., sulph., tarent.
amel. - ***arg-m.,*** aur-m-n., bism., hyos., nat-s., prun., ***rhod.,*** **RHUS-T.,** sulph.
violent, amel. - sulph.
night - kali-n., sil., tab., tarent.
waking, on - mez.
outer side - calc., chel., ferr-p., phys., rumx., sulph.
rheumatic - ferr-p.
writing, while - ferr-p.

PAIN, wrists
paralytic - acon., agn., arg-m., asar., carb-v., cham., coc-c., con., euph., kali-c., ***kalm.,*** mez., nat-p., rhus-v.
paroxysmal - ***anac., aur.,*** bov., spig.
pressure, on - mag-c., merc.
pulsating - brach., kali-n., polyg.
when at dinner - kali-n.
radial side - arg-m., calc., sabin., stann.
right - act-sp., arund., buf-s., calc-p., chin., chin-s., cimic., colch., lac-c., ***lyc.,*** nat-p., ***ox-ac.,*** petr., plb., ***rhus-t.,*** sulph., **VIOL-O.**
sewing, while - kali-c., lach.
stormy weather - rhod.
string, as from - manc.
touch - dros., merc., sil.
turning, hand - agn.
twisting, agg. - dros., merc-i-f.
twitching, with - arund., calc., carb-s., kali-n.
wandering - ***kalm.,*** polyg., ***puls.***
warmth, agg. - ***guai., puls.***
wind, in - carb-v.
writing, while - ferr-p., lyc., **MAG-P.**
as after much rapid writing - cor-r.

PARALYSIS - ***acon.,*** hipp., merc., **PLB.,** ruta.
extensors - carb-s., cur., **PLB.,** rhus-t.
from piano playing - cur., ***plb.,*** rhus-t.
morning - hipp.
right and left ankle - nat-p.
paralysis, sensation of - agar., bism., bov., carb-v., kali-c., merc., mez., petr., thuj.
extending to elbow - euphr.
morning - sil.
right - euphr., laur., lyc., nat-p., ox-ac.

PEMPHIGUS - sep.

PERSPIRATION - petr., syph.

PINCHING, pain - nat-m., nit-ac., ph-ac., stann.
back of - caust., dig.

PRESSING, pain - aloe, ang., arg-m., arg-n., aur., aur-m-n., bell., berb., ***bism.,*** brom., calc-p., camph., cann-i., card-m., coloc., dig., ***guai.,*** hell., hep., jatr., ***led.,*** lil-t., meny., ***mez.,*** nat-s., nit-ac., ***sars., spig.,*** stann., viol-o.
asunder - aloe
cramp-like - bar-c., meny.
drawing - coloc., hyos., spong., staph.
evening - ang., led., nat-s.
after lying down - nat-s.
left - camph.
motion, agg. - ruta., staph.
amel. - aur-m-n.
right - ang., led., nit-ac.
sitting, while - aur-m-n., coloc., led.
sleep, nap, during - nit-ac.
tearing - bism., ruta.
ulnar side - zinc.
walking, while - nat-s.

PULSATION - bov., brach., grat., hura, ***lach.,*** merc., phos.
evening - bov.

RASH - calad., elaps, hydr., led.
burning, after scratching - calad.
itching - calad., led.

RESTLESSNESS - calc., rhus-t.

RHEUMATIC - ***act-sp.,*** aesc., ammc., asc-t., ***caul.,*** chel., clem., ***colch.,*** crot-c., ery-a., ferr-p., form., grat., ***guai., jug-c., kali-bi.,*** kalm., lac-ac., ***lach.,*** mag-s., nat-a., nat-p., ptel., ***puls.,*** **RUTA., RHUS-T.,** stict., urt-u., ***vac., viol-o.***
writing, after - chin-s.

ROUGHNESS - rhus-t.

SCRAPING, pain - cist.

SHARP, pain - ***acon.,*** alum., anac., ang., apis, arg-m., arn., ars., ars-i., aster., aur., aur-m., bapt., bar-c., bell., berb., ***bov.,*** brach., ***bry.,*** calc., calc-ar., canth., caust., carb-s., cham., chel., chin., chin-s., clem., cob., colch., com., con., corn., dulc., euphr., ferr., graph., ham., ***hell.,*** hura, hyper., indg., inul., iod., kali-bi., kali-c., kali-n., kalm., laur., ***led.,*** lyc., lycps., mang., meny., ***merc.,*** merc-sul., ***nat-m.,*** op., ox-ac., phos., plat., rhod., ruta., sabin., samb., sars., ***sep., sil.,*** sol-n., spig., spong., squil., staph., ***sulph.,*** tarent., thuj., trom., zinc.
acute - arn., bov., phos.
afternoon - canth., lyc.
alternating in each - lyc.
back of - chin-s., dig., led.
bringing thumb and index finger together - bov.
drawing - clem.
evening - euphr., rhod., tarent.
walking in open air - hell.
extending, to
finger - lyc., sep.
shoulder - staph.
upwards - bell., bry., canth., cham., mang., sabin., sars., sil., staph.
front surface - arg-m., colch.
grasping anything - aur-m., bov., iod., nat-m.
left - sep.
lifting anything - iod.
morning - lyc.
motion - arn., calc., indg., kali-c., sep.
amel - bar-c., dulc., samb., spong.
motion, of index finger - spig.
night - calc., sil.
pulsating - canth.
radial side - arg-m., dig., sars.
rhythmical with pulse - samb.
right - canth.
rubbing amel. - laur.
sudden - lyc.
tearing - calc., mang., rhus-t., sabin.
twitching - ***bry.,*** carb-s.
ulnar side - anac., bell., berb., calc., samb.
walking in the open air - clem.
warm, when hands become - ***bry.***
washing, while - alum.
work, at - alum., caust.
writing, while - lyc., ox-ac., sil.

SHOOTING, pain - ***acon.,*** bell., brach., ferr., **HYPER.,** merc-sul., sol-n., tarent., trom.
evening - tarent.
extending along ulnar to elbow - acon., bell.

SHORT, wrist, sensation as if - carb-v.

SORE, pain - alumn., ammc., arg-m., ***arn.,*** asaf., aur-m-n., bov., brach., ***calc.,*** camph., caust., cham., ***dros.,*** **EUP-PER.,** led., lyss., mez., nat-m., nat-p., nit-ac., pip-m., podo., **RUTA.,** sep., tanac., thuj., zinc.
rest, during - aur-m-n.
wet, cold weather - ruta.

SPRAINED, as if - agar., alumn., ambr., ***am-c.,*** arg-n., **ARN.,** ***bov., bry.,*** **CALC., CARB-AN.,** carb-v., cast-eq., ***caust., cina,*** cist., dios., ferr., graph., hep., jug-c., kali-n., ***lach.,*** laur., ***lyc.,*** mag-c., mez., nat-m., nux-v., ***ox-ac.,*** petr., phos., puls., ***rhod.,*** **RHUS-T., RUTA.,** sabin., sars., seneg., sil., stann., ***stront-c., sulph.,*** tep., thuj., ***verb.,*** zinc.
bent - ferr-m.
evening - lach.
on exertion - lach.
extending into fourth and fifth fingers hanging arm down - cast-eq.
forenoon - ox-ac.
grasping anything - **RHUS-T.**
left - ***agar., rhus-t.***
morning - lyss.
motion, on - bov., ***bry.,*** hyper., mez.
amel. - prun., rhod.
fast, amel. - sulph.
night - arg-n.
noon - alumn.
paralytic - mez.
right - **CALC.,** gels., ***lyc.,*** mez., ***ox-ac.***
rough weather - ***rhod.***
work, during - caust.
writing, while - lyc.

STIFFNESS - ***apis,*** arg-n., ars., ***bell.,*** calc., ***chel.,*** cub., dios., ham., ign., kali-c., lact., ***led., lyc.,*** merc., merl., nat-a., nat-c., nat-s., ph-ac., ***phos.,*** plb., ***puls.,*** rhod., **RHUS-T.,** rhus-v., ***ruta., sabin.,*** sel., ***sep.,*** staph., ***sulph.,*** thuj., wye., zinc.
evening - chel., sep.
amel. - arg-n.
holding a glass - nat-c.
morning - plb., sel., ***sulph.***
motion, agg. - ph-ac.
paralytic - ruta.
wet, cold weather - **RHUS-T.,** ruta.

SWELLING - ***act-sp.,*** am-c., am-m., ***apis,*** aur., aur-m., ***bufo, calc.,*** carb-v., ***crot-h.,*** cub., dulc., euphr., kali-bi., kreos., ***lac-ac., lach.,*** mag-c., ***merc.,*** phos., plb., rhod., **RHUS-T.,** ***rhus-v.,*** sabin., sec., sep., stry., sul-ac., tarent., tep., vip.
alternate, and knee - kreos.
bursa-like - ***aur.***
evening - sep.
morning - lac-ac.
motion, on - merc., phos.
nodular swellings - stann.

SWELLING,
pain, after - cub.
painful, soft and watery - ***sec.***
palmar surface of - carb-v., rhus-t.
red - mag-c.
rheumatic - act-sp.
spots, in - kali-bi.
sudden - rhod.

TEARING, pain - ***acon.,*** agar., alum., am-c., am-m., ammc., anac., ***arg-m.,*** arn., ars., **AUR.,** bar-c., bell., berb., ***bism.,*** bor., bov., ***calc., calc-p.,*** carb-s., **CARB-V.,** caust., chel., chin., chin-a., colch., cycl., euphr., gran., grat., ***guai.,*** inul., kali-ar., kali-bi., ***kali-c.,*** kali-chl., kali-i., ***kali-n.,*** lach., lact., laur., led., lyc., ***mag-m.,*** mag-s., meny., ***merc.,*** merl., mez., mur-ac., nat-c., nat-m., **NAT-S.,** nit-ac., ol-an., ***ph-ac.,*** phos., plb., ran-b., ***rat.,*** rhod., **RHUS-T.,** ruta., sabin., ***sars.,*** sep., ***sil.,*** **STANN.,** staph., **STRONT-C.,** ***sulph.,*** tarax., teucr., thuj., ***zinc.***
afternoon - am-m., lyc., mag-s.
2 p.m. - sars.
alternating with the same in hand - berb.
back of - berb., caust., merl.
extending to middle finger - caust.
bed, on going to - stront.
bones - ***arg-m., aur.,*** bell., bism., chin., cupr., lach., lact., nat-c., sabin., spig., teucr.
chill, during - ph-ac.
convulsive - ph-ac.
cramp-like - aur.
drawing - guai., kali-bi., mez., **RHUS-T.**
dull - lyc.
evening - bov., lyc., phos., stront.
7 p.m. - lyc.
extending to,
dorsum of hand - ran-b.
finger, ring - kali-c.
fingers - am-c., bar-c., caust., phos., plb., tarax., zinc.
fingers, little - am-c.
fingers, tips of two smaller - chel.
knuckles - kali-n.
shoulder - sep., ***sil.***
upwards - sars.
forenoon - ran-b., sil., sulph.
grasping anything, when - ***carb-v.***
hanging down - ***sabin.***
jerking - chin.
knitting, while - kali-c.
left - am-m., bism., sep.
morning - lyc.
motion, on - ***calc.,*** kali-bi., meny., ***merc.,*** merl., ***sil.,*** stann.
amel. - arg-m., ***bism.,*** mur-ac., rhod., **RHUS-T.,** sulph.
of wrist - phos., sep.
night - am-c., **ARS.,** ***aur.,*** kali-n., ***merc.,*** sep.
11 p.m. - nat-s.
bed, in - **ARS.,** ***merc.,*** nat-m.
paralytic - bell., ***bism.,*** meny., stann.
pressive - arg-m., guai., stann.
resting on hand - merl.

TEARING, pain
rheumatic - gran., zinc.
right - bism., calc-p., caust., ***rat.***
sticking - ***arn.,*** calc., sep., staph.
sudden - bar-c.
transversely - ph-ac.
twitching - colch., laur., **RHUS-T.**
ulnar side - kali-c., kali-n., lach., merl., zinc.
extending to tips of both outer fingers - lach.
walking, open air, in - rhod.
warmth, of bed amel. - am-c., ***ars.,*** calc-p., **RHUS-T.,** ***sil.***
writing, while - arn.

TENSION - am-c., am-m., aml-n., arg-n., aur-m., bar-c., carb-an., carb-v., kali-c., lach., lyc., mang., ***merc.,*** nat-p., phos., puls., spong., thuj., verb., zinc.
bending, on - arg-n., aur-m.
evening amel. - arg-n.
morning, in bed - lyc.
motion, on - am-c., carb-an., spong.

TIED, sensation as if - glon.

TREMBLING - acon., chel., glon., olnd., plb.
emotion, from - plb.
headache, during - glon.
motion, from - acon., plb.

TUBERCLES - am-c., am-m., crot-h., mag-c.

TUMORS - calc-f., ***cupr-ar., led., ruta.***

TWISTING, sensation - plb.

TWITCHING - agar., ***bar-c.,*** calc., eupi., nat-c., pall., rhus-t., sulph., verat.
electric shocks, like - agar.
flexor tendons - am-m., anac.
motion, on - ***rhus-t.***
sudden - pall.
ulnar side - plat.

ULCERS - dor., kali-bi., lac-c., mez., psor.

VESICLES - am-m., bufo, calad., calc-p., ***crot-h.,*** hep., iris, kali-i., merc., ***mez.,*** nat-m., ***rhus-t.,*** rhus-v., sars., ***sulph.***
burning - am-m., bufo, ***mez.,*** sars.
when scratched - am-m.
erysipelatous - rhus-t., rhus-v.
front surface - rhus-t.
hard base - am-m.
itching - am-m., bufo, calc-p., kali-i., nat-m., sars.
radial side - ant-c., merc., nat-m., sars.
scratching, after - nat-m.
scurfy from scratching - am-m.
water, limpid, containing - rhus-t.
yellow - rhus-t., ***sulph.***
white - calad.

WARTS - ferr-ma.

WEAKNESS - aloe, arn., ars., brach., calc., ***calc-p., carb-v., caust., cur.,*** dig., dor., ***glon.,*** hura, kali-c., kalm., lil-t., lyc., ***merc.,*** mez., nat-m., nat-p., phos., phys., ***plb.,*** podo., rhod., ***rhus-t.,*** **RUTA,** sep., ***sil.,*** spong., sulph., sul-ac.
evening - phos.

WEAKNESS, of
hand, using - ruta, sep.
menses, after - nat-p.
morning - lil-t.
motion, agg. - bry., dig.
amel. - rhod., rhus-t.
paralytic - ***carb-v.,*** caust., phos.
right - ***sil.***
and left ankle - nat-p.
sprained, as if - arn., bry., kali-c., ruta.
writing, while - calad., ***kali-br., ruta.***

A

abel. abelmoschus (= hibiscus abelmoschus)
abies-c. abies canadensis, (pinus) **Hemlock Spruce**
abies-n. abies nigra, Black Spruce
abr. abrus precatorius (= jequirity)
abrot. abrotanum (= artemisia abrotanum), **Southernwood**
absin. absinthium (= artemisia absinthium), **Common Wormwood**
acal. acalypha indica, Indian Nettle
acanthia lectularia = cimx.
acarus = trom.
acer negundo = neg.
acet-ac. aceticum acidum
acetan. acetanilidum (= antifebrinum)
achillea millefolium = mill.
achy. achyranthes calea
acokanthera schimperi = car.
acon. aconitum napellus, Monkshood
acon-a. aconitum anthora
acon-c. aconitum cammarum
acon-f aconitum ferox
acon-l. aconitum lycoctonum
acon-s. aconitum septentrionale
aconin. aconitinum
actaea racemosa = cimic.
act-sp. actaea spicata, Baneberry
adel. Adelheid aqua
adeps-s. adeps suis
adlu. adlumia fungosa
adon. adonis vernalis, Pheasant's eye
adonin. adonidinum
adox. adoxa moschatellina
adren. adrenalinum
adrenocorticotropinum = cortico.
aesc. aesculus hippocastanum, Horse Chesnut
aesc-g. aesculus glabra, Ohio Buckeye
aethanolum = alco.
aeth. aethusa cynapium, Fool's Parsley
aether = ether
aethi-a. aethiops antimonialis
aethi-m. aethiops mineralis (= mercurius sulphuratus niger = mercurius cum kali)
aethylium nitrosum = nit-s-d.
aethyl-n. aethylium nitricum
agar. agaricus muscarius (= amanita muscaria), **Fly agaric**
agar-cit. agaricus citrinus
agar-cpn. agaricus campanulatus
agar-cps. agaricus campestris
agar-em. agaricus emeticus
agar-pa. agaricus pantherinus
agar-ph. agaricus phalloides (= amanita phalloides)
agar-pr. agaricus procerus
agar-se. agaricus semiglobatus
agar-st. agaricus stercorarius
agar-v. agaricus vernus (= amanita verna)
agarin. agaricinum
agav-a. agave americana, Century Plant
agav-t. agave tequilana
agn. agnus castus, Chaste Tree
agra. agraphis nutans, Bluebell
agre. agremone ochroleuc
agri. agrimonia eupatoria, Cockleburr
agropyrum repens = tritic.
agro. agrostema githago
ail. ailanthus glandulosa, Tree of Heaven, Chinese Sumach
alco. alcoholus (= aethanolum)
ald. aldehydum
alet. aletris farinosa, Stargrass
alf. alfalfa (= medicago sativa)
alkekengi = physal.
all-c. allium cepa (= cepa), **Red Onion**
all-s. allium sativum, Garlic
allox. alloxanum

aln. alnus rubra (serrulata), **Red alder**
aloe aloe socotrina
alst. alstonia constricta, Bitter Bark
alst-s. alstonia scholaris
alth. althaea officinalis, Marshmallow
alum. alumina (= argilla)
alum-p. alumina phosphorica
alum-sil. alumina silicata
(= bolus alba = kaolinum)
alumin. aluminium metallicum
alumin-a. aluminium aceticum
alumin-m. aluminium muriaticum
alumn. alumen
alumen chromicum = kali-s-chr.
amanita muscaria = agar.
amanita phalloides = agar-ph.
amanita verna = agar-v.
am-a. ammonium aceticum
ammonium auricum = aur-fu.
am-be. ammonium benzoicum
am-br. ammonium bromatum
am-c. ammonium carbonicum
am-caust. ammonium causticum (hydratum)
am-i. ammonium iodatum
am-m. ammonium muriaticum,
Ammonium Chloride
am-n. ammonium nitricum
am-p ammonium phosphoricum
am-pic. ammonium picricum
am-t. ammonium tartaricum
am-val. ammonium valerianicum
am-van. ammonium vanadinicum
ambr. ambra grisea,
Morbid Secretion of the Whale
ambro. ambrosia artemisiae folia, Ragweed
amgd-p. amygdalus persica
(= persica amygdalus), **Peach tree**
aml-ns. amylenum nitrosum
ammc. ammoniacum gummi
amn-l. amnii liquor
amor-r. amorphophallus rivieri
ampe-qu. ampelopsis quinquefolia
ampe-tr. ampeiopsis trifoliata
amph. amphisbaena vermicularis
amyg. amygdalae amarae aqua
amylam. amylaminum hydrochloricum
anac. anacardium orientale,
Marking Nut, Malacca Bean
anac-oc. anacardium occidentale
anag. anagallis arvensis, Scarlet Pimpernel
anagy. anagyris foetida
anan. anantherum muricatum (= cuscus)
ancistrodon mokeson = cench.
andira inermis = geo.
andromeda arborea = oxyd.
andr. androsace lactea
ane-n. anemone nemorosa
anemone pratensis = puls.
ane-r. anemone ranunculoides
anemps. anemopsis californica (= yerba mansa)
ang. angustura vera (= galipea cusparia)
ange. angelica atropurpurea
ange-s. radix angclicae sinensis
ango. angophora lanceolata
angustura spuria = bruc.
anh. anhalonium lewinii
(= lophophora williamsii = peyotl)
anil. anilinum, Amidobenzene
anil-s. anilinum sulphuricum
anis. anisum stellatum
(= illicium stellatum), **Star Anise**
antifebrinum = acetan.
ant-ar. antimonium arsenicosum
ant-c. antimonium crudum
(= antimonium sulphuratum nigrum)
ant-i. antimonium iodatum
ant-m. antimonium muriaticum
ant-o. antimonium oxydatum
ant-s-aur. antimonium sulphuratum auratum
(aureum, aurantiacum)

antimonium sulphuratum nigrum = ant-c.
ant-t. antimonium tartaricum
(= tartarus emeticus)
anth. anthemis nobilis (= chamomilla romana)
antho. anthoxanthum odoratum
anthr. anthraci. anthracinum, Anthrax Nosode
anthraco. anthracokali
antip. antipyrinum
ap-g. apium graveolens, Common Celery
ap-v. apium virus, Honey-Bee
aphis, aphis chenopodii glauci
(= chenopodii glauci aphis)
apiol. apiolum
apis, apis mellifica, Honey-Bee
apisin. apisinum (= apium virus)
apoc. apocynum cannabinum, Indian Hemp
apoc-a. apocynum androsaemifolium, Dogbane
apom. apomorphinum hydrochloricum
aq-calc. aqua calcarea
aq-chl. aqua chlorata
aqua glandium quercus = querc.
aq-mar. aqua marina, Sea water
aq-pet. aqua petra
aqua regia = nit-m-ac.
aq-sil. aqua silicata
aqui. aquilegia vulgaris
arag. aragallus lamberti
aral. aralia racemosa, Spikenard
aral-h. aralia hispida
aralia quinquefolia = gins.
aranea avicularia = mygal.
aran. aranea diadema (= diadema aranea), **Papal-Cross Spider**
aran-ix. aranea ixobola
aran-sc. aranea scinencia
araneae tela = tela
aranin. araninum
arb. arbutus andrachne
arbin. arbutinum
arctium lappa = lappa
arec. areca catechu
aren. arenaria glabra
arg-cy. argentum cyanatum, Silver Cyanide
arg-i. argentum iodatum
arg-m. argentum metallicum, Silver Metal
arg-mur. argentum muriaticum
arg-n. argentum nitricum, Silver Nitrate
arg-o. argentum oxydatum
arg-p. argentum phosphoricum
arge. argemone mexicana
argilla = alum.
arist-cl. aristolochia clematitis
arist-co. aristolochia colombiana
arist-m. aristolochia milhomens
aristolochia serpentaria = serp.
armoracia sativa = coch.
arn. arnica montana, Lepord's Bane
ars. arsenicum album
ars-br. arsenicum bromatum
ars-h. arsenicum hydrogenisatum
ars-i. arsenicum iodatum
ars-met. arsenicum metallicum
ars-n. arsenicum nitricum
ars-s-f. arsenicum sulphuratum flavum
ars-s-r. arsenicum sulphuratum rubrum
artanthe elongata = mati.
artemisia abrotanum = abrot.
artemisia absinthium = absin.
artemisia maritima (cina) = cina
art-v. artemisia vulgaris, Muwort
arum-d. arum dracontium, Green Dragon
arum-dru. arum dracunculus
arum-i. arum italicum
arum-m. arum maculatum
arum-t. arum triphyllum, Jack-in-the-Pulpit
arund. arundo mauritanica
arund-d. arundo donax
asaf. asafoetida, Gum of the Stinkasand
asagraea officinalis = sabad.
asar. asarum europaeum

asar-c. asarum canadense
asc-c. asclepias cornuti (syriaca), **Milkweed, Silkweed**
asc-i. asclepias incarnata
asc-t. asclepias tuberosa, Pleurisy-root
asclepias vincetoxicum = vince.
asim. asimina triloba (= papaya vulgaris), **American Papaw**
ask. askalabotes laevigatus
aspar. asparagus officinalis, Garden Asparagus
asper. asperula odorata
aspidium filix-mas = fil.
aspidium panna = pann.
aspidosperma quebracho = queb.
assaku = hura
astac. astacus (cancer) **fluviatilis, Crawfish**
aster. asterias rubens, Red Starfish
astra-e. astragalus excapus
astra-m. astragalus menziesii
atha. athamanta oreoselinum
atra-r. atrax robustus
atri. atriplex hortensis
atropa belladonna = bell.
atro. atropinum purum aut sulphuricum
aur. aurum metallicum, (foliatum) **aut aurum colloidale, Metallic Gold**
aur-ar. aurum arsenicicum, Arseniate of Gold
aur-br. aurum bromatum
aur-fu. aurum fulminans (= ammonium auricum)
aur-i. aurum iodatum, Iodide of Gold
aur-m. aurum muriaticum, Chloride of Gold
aur-m-k. aurum muriaticum kalinatum
aur-m-n. aurum muriaticum natronatum
aur-s. aurum sulphuratum
auran. aurantii cortex
aurantium = cit-v.
aven. avena sativa, Common Oat
aza. azadirachta indica (= melia azadirachta indica)

B

bac. bacillinum Burnett
bac-t. baccillinum testium
bach, bacillus Bach-Paterson
bacillus Calmette-Gue'rin = v-a-b.
bad. badiaga, Fresh water Sponge
baj. baja
balsamum copaivae = cop.
bals-p. balsamum peruvianum
bals-t. balsamum tolutanum
bapt. baptisia tinctoria, Wild Indigo
bapt-c. baptisia confusa
bar-a. baryta acetica
bar-c. baryta carbonica
bar-i. baryta iodata
bar-m. baryta muriatica
bar-p. baryta phosphorica
bar-s. baryta sulphurica
barb. barbae cyprini ova
baros. barosma crenulatum (= buchu)
bart. Bartfelder aqua
basaka = just.
bell. belladonna (= atropa belladonna), **Deadly Nightshade**
bell-p. bellis perennis, Daisy
ben. benzinum
ben-d. benzinum dinitricum
ben-n. benzinum nitricum
benz-ac. benzoicum acidum
benzo. benzoinum oderiferum
benzol. benzolum
berb. berberis vulgaris, Barberry
berb-a. berberis aquifolium (= mahonia), **Mountain grape**
berbin. berberinum
beryl. beryllium metallicum
beta, beta vulgaris
betin. betainum muriaticum

beto. betonica aquatica
betu. betula alba
bism. bismuthum subnitricum
(oxidum " Hahnemann, Kent)
bism.met. bismuthum metallicum
bism-o. bismuthum oxydatum
bism-val. bismuthum valerianicum
bix. bixa orellana
blatta, blatta orientalis, Indian Cockroach
blatta-a. blatta americana, American Cockroach
bol-la. boletus laricis (= polyporus officinalis)
bol-lu. boletus luridus
bol-s. boletus satanas
bold. boldo (= peumus boldo)
bolus alba = album-sil.
bomb-chr. bombyx chrysorrhea
bomb-pr. bombyx processionea
bond. Bondonneau aqua
bor. borax veneta
bor-ac. boricum acidum, Boracic Acid
both. bothrops lanceolatus
(= lachesis lanceolatus), **Yellow Viper**
botul. botulinum
bounafa = ferul.
bov. bovista lycoperdon, Puff Ball
brach. brachyglottis repens,
New Zealand "Puka Puka"
bran. branca ursina
brass. brassica napus
brayera anthelmintica = kou.
brom. bromium
bruc. brucea antidysenterica,
(= angustura spuria)
brucel. brucella melitensis
brucin. brucinum
brugmansia candida = dat-a.
bry. bryonia alba (dioica), **Wild Hops**
buchu = baros.
bufo, bufo rana (= rana bufo), **Poison of the Toad**
bufo-s. bufo sahytiensis, The Toad
bung. bungurus fasciatus
buni-o. bunias orientalis
bursa pastoris = thlas.
but-ac. butyricum acidum
buth-a. buthus australis (= prionurus australis)
buth-af. buthus afer
buth-oc. buthus occitanus
bux. buxus sempervirens

C

cac. cacao (= theobroma cacao)
cact. cactus grandiflorus, (selenicereus)
Night-blooming Cereus
cadm-br. cadmium bromatum
cadm-i. cadmium iodatum
cadm-m. cadmium muriaticum
cadm-met. cadmium metallicum
cadm-o. cadmium oxydatum
cadm-s. cadmium sulphuratum
cael. caela zacatechichi
caes. caesium metallicum
caffeinum = coffin.
cain. cainca racemosa, Brazilia Chiococca
(= chiococca racemosa),
caj. cajuputum, Cajuput Oil
(= oleum cajuputi = oleum wittnebianum),
calabar = phys.
cal-ren. calculus renalis (lapis), **Kidney stone**
calad. caladium seguinum, American Arum
calag. calaguala
calam. calamus aromaticus
calc. calcarea carbonica Hahnemanni
(= calcarea ostrearum = conchae praeparatae)
calc-a. calcarea acetica
calc-ar. calcarea arsenicosa
calc-br. calcarea bromata
calc-caust. calcarea caustica
calc-chln. calcarea chlorinata
calc-f. calcarea fluorica naturalis

calc-hp. calcarea hypophosphorosa
calc-i. calcarea iodata
calc-lac. calcarea lactica
calc-m. calcarea muriatica
calcarea ostrearum = calc.
calc-o-t. calcarea ovi testae
(= ovi testa = testa praeparata)
calc-ox. calcarea oxalica
calc-p. calcarea phosphorica, Phosphate of Lime
calc-pic. calcarea picrica
calc-s. calcarea sulphurica, Plaster of Paris
calc-sil. calcarea silicata
calcarea silico-fluorica = lap-a.
calc-st-sula. calcarea stibiato-sulphurata
calcarea sulphurata Hahnemanni = hep.
calen. calendula officinalis
calli. calliandra houstoni (= pambotano)
calomel = merc-d.
calo. calotropis gigantea (= madar)
calth. caltha palustris, Cowslip
camph. camphora (= laurus camphora),
camph-ac. camphoricum acidum
camph-br. camphora bromata
cancer fluviatilis = astac.
canch. canchalagua (= erythraea chilensis),
Venusta-Centaury
cann-i. cannabis indica, Hashish, Marijuana
cann-s. cannabis sativa, Hemp, Marijuana
canna canna angustifolia
canth. cantharis vesicatoria, (lytta), **Spanish Fly**
canthin. cantharidinum
capp. capparis coriaccea
capsella bursa pastoris = thlas.
caps. capsicum annuum, Cayenne Pepper
carbamidum = urea-n.
car. carissa schimperi, (acokanthera)
carb-ac. carbolicum acidum (= phenolum)
carb-an. carbo animalis, Animal Charcoal
carb-v. carbo vegetabilis, Vegetable Charcoal
carbn. carboneum
carbn-chl. carboneum chloratum
carbn-h. carboneum hydrogenisatum
carbn-o. carboneum oxygenisatum
carbn-s. carboneum sulphuratum
carc. carcinosinum Burnett
card-b. carduus benedictus
card-m. carduus marianus, St. Mary's Thistle
cardam. cardamine pratensis
carl. Carlsbad aqua, (Karlsbad)
caru. carum carvi
cary. carya alba
cas-s. cascara sagrada (= rhamnus purshiana),
Sacred bark
casc. cascarilla, Sweet Bark
cass. cassada (= manihot utilissima)
cassia acutifolia = senn.
cast. castoreum canadense aut sibiricum
cast-eq. castor equi,
Rudimentary Thumbnail of the Horse
cast-v. castanea vesca, Chestnut Leaves
caste. castella texana
catal. catalpa bignonoides, Cigar tree
catar. cataria nepeta
caul. caulophyllum thalictroides, Blue Cohosh
caust. causticum Hahnemanni
cean. ceanothus americanus,
Red root, New Jersey Tea
cean-r. ceanothus thrysiflorus
cecr. cecropia mexicana
cedr. cedron (= simaruba ferroginea),
Rattlesnake Bean
celt. celtis occidentalis
cench. cenchris contortrix
(= ancistrodon mokeson), **Copperhead Snake**
cent. centaurea tagana
cepa = all-c.
ceph. cephalanthus occidentalis
cer-ox. cerium oxalicum
cere-b. cereus bonplandii
cere-s. cereus serpentinus

cerv. cervus brasilicus (campestris)
ceto. cetonia aurata
cetr. (cet.) **cetraria islandica**
(= lichen islandicus), **Iceland Moss**
cham. chamomilla, German Chamomile
chamomilla romana = anth.
chamae. chamaedrys (= teucrium chamaedrys)
chap. chaparro amargoso, Goat-bush
chaul. chaulmoogra
chei. cheiranthus cheiri
chel. chelidonium majus, Celandine
chel-g. chelidonium glaucum
chelin. chelidoninum
chelo. chelone glabra
chenopodii glauci aphis = aphis
chen-a. chenopodium anthelminticum,
Jerusalem Oak
chen-v. chenopodium vulvaria
chim. chimaphila umbellata, Pipsissewa
chim-m. chimaphila maculata
chin. china officinalis (regia), **Peruvian Bark**
(= cinchona calisaya aut cinchona succirubra),
chin-ar. chininum arsenicosum
chin-b. china boliviana, (cinchona)
chin-m. chininum muriaticum
chin-s. chininum sulphuricum
chin-val. chininum valerianicum
chinid. chinidinum hydrochloricum
chiococca racemosa = cain.
chion. chionanthus virginica (americana),
Fringe-tree
chlf. chloroformium
chlol. chloralum hydratum, Choral Hydrate
chlor. chlorum, Chlorine Gas in Water
chloram. chloramphenicolum
chlorpr. chlorpromazinum
cho. cholas terrapina
chol. cholesterinum
cholin. cholinum
chr-met. chromium metallicum
chr-ac. chromicum acidum, Chromic Acid
chr-o. chromium oxydatum
chr-s. chromium sulphuricum
chrys-ac. chrysophanicum acidum
chrysan. chrysanthemum leucanthemum
chrysar. chrysarobinum
cic. cicuta virosa, Water Hemlock
cic-m. cicuta maculata
cice. cicer arietinum
cich. cichorium intybus
cimic. cimicifuga racemosa
(= actaea racemosa = macrotys racemosa),
Black Cohosh, Snake-root
cimx. cimex lectularius
(= acanthia lectularia), **Bedbug**
cina, cina maritima, Wormseed
(= artemisia maritima aut cina),
cinchona boliviana = chin-b.
cinchona calisaya = chin.
cinchona succirubra = chin.
cinch. cinchoninum sulphuricum
cine. cineria maritima
cinnb. cinnabaris
(= mercurius sulphuratus ruber)
cinnm. cinnamomum ceylanicum, Cinnamon
cist. cistus canadensis, Rock Rose
cit-ac. citricum acidum
citrullus colocynthis = coloc.
cit-d. citrus decumana
cit-l. citrus limonum, Lemon
cit-v. citrus vulgaris (= aurantium),
Bitter Orange
clem. clematis erecta, Virgin's Bower
clem-vir. clematis virginiana
clem-vit. clematis vitalba
cloth. clotho arictans
cob. cobaltum metallicum
cob-n. cobaltum nitricum
coc-c. coccus cacti, Cochineal
coca, coca (= erythroxylon coca), **cocaine**

cocain. cocainum hydrochloricum
cocc. cocculus indicus, Indian Cockle
cocc-s. coccinella septempunctata, Lady Bug
coch. cochlearia armoracia
(= armoracia sativa), **Horse Radish**
coch-o. cochlearia officinalis
cod. codeinum purum aut phosphoricum aut sulphuricum, Alkaloid from Opium
coff. coffea cruda (arabica), **unroasted Coffee**
coff-t. coffea tosta, roasted Coffee berries
coffin. coffeinum (= caffeinum)
colch. colchicum autumnale, Meadow Saffron
colchin. colchicinum
coli. colibacillinum
coll. collinsonia canadensis, Stone-root
coloc. colocynthis, Bitter Cucumber
(= cucumis colocynthis = citrullus colocynthis)
colocin. colocynthinum
colos. colostrum, Milk first secreted after childbirth
com. comocladia dentata (= guao)
condurango = cund.
con. conium maculatum, Poison Hemlock
conchae praeparatae = calc.
conch. conchiolinum
(= mater perlarum = perlarum mater)
conin. coniinum
conin-br. coniinum bromatum
conv. convallaria majalis, Lily of the Valley
convo-a. convolvulus arvensis
convo-d. convolvulus duartinus
(= ipomoeabona-nox)
convo-s. convolvulus stans (= ipomoea stans)
cop. copaiva (= balsamum copaivae)
cor-r. corallium rubrum, Red Coral
corh. corallorhiza odontorhiza
cori-m. coriaria myrtifolia
cori-r. coriaria ruscifolia
corn. cornus circinata, Round-leaved Dogwood
corn-a. cornus alternifolia
corn-f. cornus florida, Dogwood
corn-s. cornus sericea
cortico. corticotropinum
(= adrenocorticotropinium)
cortiso. cortisonum
cory. corydalis formosa (= dicentra canadensis)
cot. cotyledon umbilicus, Pennywort
coto, coto
crat. crataegus oxyacantha et monogyna, Hawthorn Berries
cresolum = cresylolum = kres.
croc. crocus sativus, Saffron
crot-c. crotalus cascavella, Brazilian Rattle-snake
crot-chlol. croton chloralum
crot-h. crotalus horridus, Rattlesnake
crot-t. croton tiglium, Croton-oil Seed
cryp. cryptopinum
cub. cubeba officinalis
cucumis colocynthis = coloc.
cuc-c. cucurbita citrullus
cuc-p. cucurbita pepo
culx, culex musca, Mosquito
cumin. cumarinum
cund. cundurango (= condurango), **Condor Plant**
cuph. cuphea viscosissima
cupr. cuprum metallicum, Copper
cupr-a. cuprum aceticum
cupr-am-s. cuprum ammoniae sulphuricum
cupr-ar. cuprum arsenicosum
cupr-c. cuprum carbonicum
cupr-cy. cuprum cyanatum
cupr-m. cuprum muriaticum
cupr-n. cuprum nitricum
cupr-o. cuprum oxydatum nigrum
cupr-s. cuprum sulphuricum
cupre-au. cupressus australis
cupre-l. cupressus lawsoniana

cur. curare, Arrow-poison
curc. curcuma javanensis
cuscus = anan.
cycl. cyclamen europaeum, Sow-bread
cyd. cydonia vulgaris
cymin. cymarinum
cynanchum = vince.
cyn-d. cynodon dactylon
cyna. cynara scolymos
cyno. cynoglossum officinale
cypr. cypripedium pubescens, Yellow Lady's Slipper
cyt-l. cytisus laburnum (= laburnum anagyroides)
cytin. cytisinum
cytisus scoparius = saroth.

D

dam. damiana (= turnera aphrodisiaca)
daph. daphne indica, Spurge Laurel
daphne mezereum = mez.
dat-a. datura arborea (= brugmansia candida)
dat-f. datura ferox
dat-m. datura metel
dat-s. datura sanguinea
datura stramonium = stram.
datin. daturinum
datis. datisca cannabina
del. delphinus amazonicus
delphin. delphinium staphysagria = staph.
dema. dematium petraeum
der. derris pinnata
dextrum lacticum acidum = sarcol-ac.
diadema aranea = aran.
dicentra canadensis = cory.
des-ac. desoxyribonucleinicum acidum
dicha. dichapetalum
dict. dictamnus albus
dig. digitalis purpurea, Foxglove
digin. digitalinum
digox. digitoxinum
dios. dioscorea villosa, Wild Yam
diosm. diosma lincaris
dip. dipodium punctatum
diph. diphtherinum, Diphtheria Nosode
diphtox. diphtherotoxinum
dipterix odorata = tong.
dirc. dirca palustris, Leatherwood, Moosewood
ditin. ditainum (= echitaminum)
dol. dolichos pruriens, (mucuna), **Cowhage**
dor. doryphora decemlineata, Colorado Potato-bug
dracontium foetidum = ictod.
dros. drosera rotundifolia, Round-leaved Sundew
dub. duboisinum
dubo-h. duboisia hopwoodi
dubo-m. duboisia myoporoides
dulc. dulcamara (= solanum dulcamara), **Bitter-sweet**
durum = scir.
dys. bacillus dysenteriae

E

eaux, Eaux bonnes aqua
eberth. eberthinum
ecballium elaterium = elat.
echi. echinacea angustifolia, (rudbeckia) **Purple Cone-flower**
echi-p. echinacea purpurea
echitaminum = ditin.
echit. echites suberecta
elae. elaeis guineensis
elaps, elaps corallinus, Coral-snake
elat. elaterium officinarum (= ecballium elaterium = momordica elaterium), **Squirting Cucmber**
elem. elemuy gauteria
emetin. emetinum

enteroc. enterococcinum
eos. eosinum
ephe. ephedra vulgaris
epig. epigaea repens, Gravel weed
epih. epihysterinum
epil. epilobium palustre, Willow herb
epiph. epiphegus virginiana (= orobanche), **Beechdrop**
equis. equisetum hyemale Horse-tail, Scouring-rush
equis-a. equisetum arvense
eran. eranthis hymnalis
erech. erechthites hieracifolia, Fire-weed
ergot. ergotinum
erig. erigeron canadensis (= leptilon canadense), **Fleabane**
erio. eriodyction californicum (glutinosum) (= yerba santa)
erod. erodium cicutarium
ery-a. eryngium aquaticum, Button Snake-root
ery-m. eryngium maritinum
erythraea chilensis = canch.
eryt-j. erythrophlaeum judiciale
eryth. erythrinus
erythroxylon coca = coca
esch. eschscholtzia californica
escoba amargo = parth.
esin. eserinum (= physostigminum)
esp-g. espeletia grandiflora
esponjilla = luf-op.
ether, ether (aether)
eucal. eucalyptus globulus, Blue Gum-tree
eucal-r. eucalyptus rostrata
eucal-t. eucalyptus tereticortis
eucol. eucalyptolum
eugenia cheken = myrt-ch.
eug. eugenia jambosa (= jambosa vulgaris), **Rose-apple**
euon. euonymus europaea, Wahoo, Spindle-tree
euon-a. euonymus atropurpurea
euonin. euonyminum
eup-a. eupatorium aromaticum
eup-per. eupatorium perfoliatum, Bone-set, Thoroughwort
eup-pur. eupatorium purpureum, Queen of the Meadow
euph. euphorbium officinarum (= euphorbia resinifera)
euph-a. euphorbia amygdaloides
euph-c. euphorbia corrolata
euph-cy. euphorbia cyparissias
euph-he. euphorbia heterodoxa
euph-hy. euphorbia hypericifolia
euph-ip. euphorbia ipecacuanhae
euph-l. euphorbia lathyris
euph-m. euphorbia marginata
euph-pe. euphorbia peplus
euph-pi. euphorbia pilulifera
euph-po. euphorbia polycarpa (= golondrina)
euph-pr. euphorbia prostata
euph-re. euphorbia resinifera = euph.
euphr. euphrasia officinalis, Eyebright
eupi. eupionum
exogonium purga = jal.
eys. eysenhardtia polystachia, (= orteaga)

F

fab. fabiana imbricata (= pichi-pichi)
faec. bacillus faecalis
fago. fagopyrum esculentum, Buckwheat
fagu. fagus silvatica farfara = tus-fa.
fel, fel tauri, Ox bile
ferr. ferrum metallicum, Iron
ferr-a. ferrum aceticum
ferr-ar. ferrum arsenicosum
ferr-br. ferrum bromatum
ferr-c. ferrum carbonicum
ferr-cit. ferrum citricum

ferr-cy. ferrum cyanatum
ferr-i. ferrum iodatum
ferr-lac. ferrum lacticum
ferr-m. ferrum muriaticum (sesquichloratum)
ferr-ma. ferrum magneticum
ferr-o-r. ferrum oxydatum rubrum
ferr-p. ferrum phosphoricum
ferr-pern. ferrum pernitricum
ferr-p-h. ferrum phosphoricum hydricum
ferr-pic. ferrum picricum
ferr-prox. ferrum protoxalatum
ferr-py. ferrum pyrophosphoricum
ferr-r. ferrum reductum
ferrum sesquichloratum = ferr-m.
ferr-s. ferrum sulphuricum
ferr-t. ferrum tartaricum
ferul. ferula glauca (= bounafa)
ferula sumbul = sumb.
ficus indica = opun-f.
fic. ficus religiosa (= pakur)
fic-v. ficus venosa
fil. filix-mas (= aspidium filix-mas), **Male Fern**
fl-ac. fluoricum acidum
flav. flavus (= neisseria flava)
foll. folliculinum
flor-p. flor de piedra (= lophophytum leandri)
foen. foeniculum sativum
form. formica rufa, Crushed Live Ants
form-ac. formicicum acidum
formal. formalinum
frag. (frag-v.) **fragaria vesca, Wood-strawberry**
fram. framboesinum
franc. franciscaea uniflora (= manaca)
frangula = rham-f.
franz. Franzensbad aqua
frax. fraxinus americana
fuc. fucus vesiculosus, Kelp-ware
fuch. fuchsinum
fuli. fuligo ligni

G

gad. gadus morrhua, Cod Fish
gaert. bacillus Gaertner
gal-ac. gallicum acidum
gala. galanthus nivalis
galeg. galega officinalis
galeo. galeopsis ochroleuca
galipea cusparia = ang.
gali. galium aparine, Goose grass
galin. galinsoga parviflora
galph. galphimia glauca
gamb. gambogia
(= gummi gutti = garcinia morella)
gardenalum = phenob.
gast. Gastein aqua
gaul. gaultheria procumbens, Wintergreen
gels. gelsemium sempervirens,
Yellow Jasmine
genist. genista tinctoria, Dyer's Greenweld
gent-c. gentiana cruciata, Cross-leaved Gentian
gent-l. gentiana lutea, Yellow Gentian
gent-q. gentiana quinquefolia
geo. geoffroya vermifuga (= andira inermis)
ger. geranium maculatum, Wild Cranesbill
gerin. geraninum
get. Gettysburg aqua
geum, geum rivale
gink-b. ginkgo biloba
gins. ginseng, Wild Ginseng
(= panax quinquefolia = aralia quinquefolia),
glanderinum = hippoz.
glandula thyreoidea = thyr.
glech. glechoma hederacea
glon. glonoinum, Nitro-glycerine
glyc. glycerinum, Glycerine
gnaph. gnaphalium polycephalum,
Cud-weed - Old Balsam
golondrina = euph-po.
gonotox. gonotoxinum

goss. gossypium herbaceum,
Cotton-plant
gran. granatum, Pomegranate root bark
graph. graphites naturalis,
Black Lead-Plumbago
grat. gratiola officinalis, Hedge Hyssop
grin. grindelia robusta aut squarrosa,
Rosin-wood
gua. guaco (= mikania guaco),
Climbing Hemp Weed
guai. (guaj.) **guaiacum officinale,**
Resin of Lignum Vitae
guajol. guajacolum
guan. guano australis
guao = com.
guar. guarana (= paullinia sorbilis),
Brazilian Coca
guare. guarea trichiloides, Ballwood
guat. guatteria gaumeri
gummi gutti = gamb.
gunp. gunpowder
gymne. gymnema silvestre
gymno. gymnocladus canadensis,
American Coffee-tree

H

haem. haematoxylum campechianum,
Logwood
hall, Hall aqua
halo. haloperidolum
ham. hamamelis virginiana, Witch-hazel
harp. harpagophytum procumbens
hecla, hecla (Hekla) **lava** = lava Heclae (Heklae),
Volcanic ash from Mount Hecla
hed. hedera helix
hedeo. hedeoma pulegioides, Pennyroyal
hedy. hedysarum ildefonsianum
helia. helianthus annuus
helin. heloninum
helio. heliotropinum peruvianum
hell. helleborus niger,
Black Hellebore, Christmas rose
hell-f. helleborus foetidus
hell-o. helleborus orientalis
hell-v. helleborus viridis
helm. helminthochortos
helo. heloderma suspectum, Gila Monster
helon. helonias dioica, Unicorn-root
helx. helix tosta
hep. hepar sulphuris calcareum
(= calcarea sulphurata Hahnemanni)
hepar sulphuris kalinum = kali-sula
hepat. hepatica triloba
hera. heracleum sphondylium
heuch. heuchera americana
hibiscus abelmoschus = abel.
hippomane mancinella = manc.
hip-ac. hippuricum acidum
hipp. hippomanes
hippoz. hippozaeninum
(= glanderinum = malleinum)
hir. hirudo medicinalis (= sanguisuga officinalis)
hist. histaminum muriaticum
hoang-nan = strych-g.
hoit. hoitzia coccinea
holarrhena antidysenterica = kurch.
hom. homarus, Digestive Fliud of Live Lobster
home. homeria collina
hume. humea elegans
humulus lupulus = lup.
hura, hura brasiliensis (= assaku)
hura-c. hura crepitans
hydr. hydrastis canadensis, Golden Seal
hydr-ac. hydrocyanicum acidum, Prussic Acid
hydrang. hydrangea arborescens, Seven-barks
hydrc. hydrocotyle asiatica, Indian Pennywort,
Gotu kola
hydrin-m. hydrastinum muriaticum
hydrin-s. hydrastinum sulphuricum

hydro-v. hydrophyllum virginicum
hydrobr-ac. hydrobromicum acidum
hydroph. hydrophis cyanocinctus
hydrophobinum = lyss.
hyos. hyoscyamus niger, Henbane
hyosin. hyoscyaminum bromatum aut sulphuricum
hyper. hypericum perforatum, St. John's-wort
hydropiper = polyg-h.
hypo. hypophyllum sanguineum
hypophysis posterior = pitu.
hypoth. hypothalamus

I

iber. iberis amara, Bitter candytuft
ichth. ichthyolum
ichthyotoxinurn = ser-ang.
ictod. ictodes foetida (= pothos foetidus = dracontium foetidum)
ign. ignatia amara, St. Ignatia's bean
ikshugandha = trlb.
ille. illecebrum verticillatum
ilx-a. ilex aquifolium
ilx-c. ilex casseine
ilex paraguariensis = mate
illicium stellatum = anis.
imp. imperatoria ostruthium
ind. indium metallicum
indg. indigo tinctoria
indol. indolum
influ. influenzinum
ins. insulinum, Insulin
inul. inula helenium, Scabwort
iod. iodium purum, Iodine
iodof. iodoformium
iodothyrinum = thyr.
ip. ipecacuanha, Ipec root
ipom. ipomoea purpurea
ipomoea bona-nox = convo-d.
ipomoea stans = convo-s.
irid. iridium metallicum
irid-m. iridium muriaticum
iris, iris versicolor, Blue flag
iris-fa. iris factissima
iris-fl. iris florentina
iris-foe. iris foetidissima
iris-g. iris germanica
iris-ps. iris pseudacorus
iris-t. iris tenax (minor)
itu, itu (= resina itu)

J

jab. jaborandi (= pilocarpus pennatifolius aut microphyllus)
jac. jacaranda gualandai
jac-c. jacaranda caroba, Brazilian caroba tree
jacea = viol-t.
jal. jalapa (= exogonium purga)
jambosa vulgaris = eug.
jasm. jasminum officinale
jatr. jatropha curcas, Purging nut
jatr-u. jatropha urens
jequirity = abr., **Crab's eye vine**
joan. joanesia asoca (= saraca indica)
jug-c. juglans cinerea (cathartica), **Butternut**
jug-r. juglans regia (= nux juglans), **Walnut**
junc-e. juncus effusus, Common rush
junc-p. juncus pilosus
juniperus sabina = sabin.
juni. junlperus vlrglmana
juni-c. juniperus communis, Juniper berries
just. justicia adhatoda (= basaka) **Singhee**

K

kali-a. kali aceticum
kali-ar. kall arsenicosum, Fowler's solution

kali-bi. kali bichromicum
kali-biox. kali-bioxalicum
kali-bit. kali bitartaricum (= tartarus depuratus)
kali-br. kali bromatum
kali-c. kall carbonicum, Carbonate of potassium
kali-caust. kali causticum
kali-chls. kali chlorosum
kali-chr. kali chromicum
kali-cit. kali citricum
kali-cy. cyanatum, Potassium cynaide
kali-f. kali fluoratum
kali-fcy. kali ferrocyanatum
kali-hp. kali hypophosphoricum
kali-i. kali iodatum, Potassium iodide
kali-m. kali muriaticum, Potassium chloride
kali-n. kali nitricum (= nitrum), **Saltpetre**
kali-ox. kali oxalicum
kali-p. kali phosphoricum
kali-perm. kali permanganicum
kali-pic. kali picricum
kali-s. hali sulphuricum, Potassium sulphate
kali-s-chr. kali sulphuricum
chromicum (= alumen chromicum)
kali-sal. kali salicylicum
kali-sil. kali silicicum
kali-sula. kali sulphuratum
(= hepar sulphuris kalinum)
kali-sulo. kali sulphurosum
kali-t. kali tartaricum
kali-tel. kali telluricum
kali-x. kali xanthogenicum
kalm. kalmia latifolia, Mountain laurel
kam. kamala
kaolinum = alum-sil., **Chinese clay**
kara. karaka
karw-h. karwinskia humboldtiana
Karlsbad aqua = carl.
kava-kava = pip-m.
kerose. kerosenum
keroso. kerosolenum
kino, kino australiensis
kiss. Kissingen aqua
kola, kola (= nux colae)
kou. kousso (= brayera anthelmintica)
kreos. kreosotum
krameria triandra = rat.
kres. kresolum (= cresolum = cresylolum),
Beechwood kreosote
kurch. kurchi
(= holarrhena aut wrightia antidysenterica)

L

laburnum anagyroides = cyt-l.
lacticum acidum dextrum = sarcol-ac.
lac-ac. lactis acidum
lac-c. lac caninum, Dog's milk
lac-d. lac vaccinum defloratum, Skimmed milk
lac-f. lac felinum, Cat's milk
lac-v. lac vaccinum, Cow's milk
lac-v-c. lac vaccinum coagulatum
lac-v-f. lactis vaccini flos
lacer. lacerta agilis
lachesis lanceolatus = both.
lach. lachesis muta (trigonocephalus),
Bushmaster, Surucucu
lachn. lachnanthes tinctoria, Spirit-weed
lact. lactuca virosa, Acrid Lettuce
lact-s. lactuca sativa, Garden Lettuce
lactrm. lactucarium thridace
lam. lamium album, White nettle
lap-a. lapis albus (= calcarea silico-fluorica)
lapis renalis = cal-ren.
lapa. lapathum acutum (= rumex obtusifolius)
lappa lappa arctium (major) (= arctium lappa),
Burdock
laps. lapsana communis
latrodectus curassavicus = ther.
lat-h. latrodectus hasselti
lat-k. latrodectus katipo

lat-m. latrodectus mactans, Spider
lath. lathyrus sativus aut cicera, Chickpea
laur. laurocerasus, Cherry laurel
laurus camphora = camph.
lava Heclae (Heklae) = hecla
lec. lecithinum
led. ledum palustre, Marsh tea
lem-m. lemna minor, Duckweed
leon. leonurus cardiaca, Motherwort
lepi. lepidium bonariense, Brazilian cress
lept. leptandra virginica, Culver's root
leptilon canadense = erig.
lesp-c. lespedeza capitata
lesp-s. lespedeza sieboldii
lev. Levico aqua
levist. levisticum officinale
levo. levomepromazinum
liat. liatris spicata (= serratula), **Colic root**
lichen islandicus = cetr.
lil-a. lilium album
lil-s. lilium superbum
lil-t. lilium tigrinum, Tiger lily
lim. limulus cyclops, Horse foot, King crab
limx. limex ater
lina. linaria vulgaris, Snap dragon
linu-c. linum catharticum
linu-u. linum usitatissimum, Common Flax
lip. lippia mexicana
lipp. Lippspringe aqua
lith-be. lithium benzoicum
lith-br. lithium bromatum
lith-c. lithium carbonicum
lith-lac. lithium lacticum
lith-m. lithium muriaticum
lith-sal. lithium salicylicum
loa. loasa tricolor
lob. lobelia inflata, Indian tobacco, Puke weed
lob-a. lobelia acetum
lob-c. lobelia cardinalis, Red lobelia
lobelia coerulea = lob-s.
lob-d. lobelia dortmanna
lob-e. lobelia erinus
lob-p. lobelia purpurascens, Purple lobelia
lob-s. lobelia syphilitica (coerulea)
lobin. lobelinum
lol. loleum temulentum, (lolium), **Darnel**
lon-c. lonicera caprifolium
lon-p. lonicera pericylmenum
lon-x. lonicera xylosteum, Fly woodbine
lophophora williamsii = anh.
lophophytum leandri = flor-p.
luesinum = syph.
luf-act. luffa actangula
luf-op. luffa operculata (= esponjilla)
luna, luna (moonlight)
lup. lupulus humulus (= humulus lupulus), **Hops**
lupin. lupulinum
lyc. lycopodium clavatum, Club moss
lycpr. lycopersicum esculentum (= solanum lycopersicum), **Tomato**
lycps. lycopus virginicus, Bugle-weed
lycps-eu. lycopus europaeus
lysi. lysimachia nummularia
lyss. lyssinum (= hydrophobinum)
lytta vesicatoria = canth.

M

macro. macrotinum
macrotys racemosa = cimic.
macroz. macrozamia spiralis
madar = calo.
mag-aust. (m-aust.) **magnetis polus australis**
mag-arct. (m-arct.) **magnetis polus arcticus**
mag-c. magnesia carbonica
mag-bcit. magnesia borocitrica
mag-f. magnesia fluorata
mag-i. magnesia iodata
mag-m. magnesia muriatica

mag-p. magnesia phosphorica
mag-s. magnesia sulphurica, Epsom salt
mag-u. magnesia usta
magn-gl. magnolia glauca
magn-gr. magnolia grandiflora, Magnolia
mahonia = berb-a.
majeptilum = thiop.
maland. malandrinum, Grease of horses
malar. malaria officinalis
malatox. malariatoxinum
malleinum = hippoz.
manaca = franc.
manc. mancinella, Manganeel apple
(= hippomane mancinella)
mand. mandragora officinarum
mang. manganum aceticum aut carbonicum
mang-coll. manganum colloidale
mang-m. manganum muriaticum
mang-o. manganum oxydatum nativum
mang-s. manganum sulphuricum
mangi. mangifera indica, Mango tree
manihot utilissima = cass.
manz. manzanita
mapato = rat.
marr. marrubium album
marum verum = teucr.
mate, mate (= ilex paraguariensis)
mater perlarum = conch.
mati. matico
(= piper angustifolium = artanthe elongata)
matth. matthiola graeca
mec. meconium
medicago sativa = alf.
med. medorrhinum, Gonorrhea nosode
medus. medusa, Jellyfish
mela. melastama ackermanni
melal. melaleuca hypericifolia
melia azadirachta indica = aza.
meli. melilotus officinalis,
Yellow clover, Sweet clover
meli-a. melilotus alba, White clover
melis. melissa officinalis
melit. melitagrinum
melo. melolontha vulgaris
meningoc. meningococcinum
menis. menispermum canadense, Moonseed
menth. mentha piperita, Peppermint
menth-pu. mentha pulegium
menth-v. mentha viridis
mentho. mentholum
meny. menyanthes trifoliata, Buckbean
meph. mephitis putorius, Skunk secretion
merc. mercurius solubilis, Quicksilver
Hahnemanni aut mercurius vivus,
merc-a. mercurius aceticus
merc-aur. mercurius auratus
mercurius biniodatus = merc-i-r.
merc-br. mercurius bromatus
merc-c. mercurius corrosivus (sublimatus)
mercurius cum kali = aethi-m.
merc-cy. mercurius cyanatus
merc-d. mercurius dulcis, Calomel
merc-i-f. mercurius iodatus flavus
(= mercurius protoiodatus)
merc-i-r. mercurius iodatus ruber
(= mercurius bi(n)iodatus)
merc-k-i. mercurius biniodatus cum kali iodato
merc-meth. mercurius methylenus
merc-ns. mercurius nitrosus
(= mercurius nitricus oxydulatus)
mercurius oxydatus = merc-pr-r.
merc-p. mercurius phosphoricus
merc-pr-a. mercurius praecipitatus albus
merc-pr-f. mercurius praecipitatus flavus
merc-pr-r. mercurius praecipitatus ruber
(= mercurius oxydatus)
mercurius protoiodatus = merc-i-f.
mercurius sublimatus = merc-c.
merc-s-cy. mercurius sulphocyanatus
mercurius sulphuratus niger = aethi-m.

mercurius sulphuratus ruber = cinnb.
merc-sul. mercurius sulphuricus
(= turpethum minerale)
merc-tn. mercurius tannicus
mercurius vivus = merc.
merl. mercurialis perennis, Dog mercury
mesp. mespillus germanica
meth-ae-ae. methylium aethylo-aethereum
meth-sal. methylium salicylicum
methyl. methylenum coeruleum
methys. methysergidum
mez. mezereum (= daphne mezereum),
Spurge olive
micr. micromeria douglasii, Yerba buena
mikania guaco = gua.
mill. millefolium, Yarrow (= achillea millefolium)
millipedes = onis.
mim-h. mimosa humilis
mim-p. mimosa pudica
mit. mitchella repens, Partridge berry
moly-met. molybdaenum metallicum
mom-b. momordica balsamica, Balsam apple
mom-ch. momordica charantia
momordica elaterium = elat.
monar. monarda didyma
moni. monilia albicans
mono. monotropa uniflora
mons. monsonia ovata
morb. morbillinum
morg. bacillus Morgan
morph. morphinum aceticum aut
muriaticum aut sulphuricum, Alkaloid of Opium
mosch. moschus, Musk
muc-u. mucuna Ilrens
mucor, mucor mucedo
mucot. mucotoxinum
mucuna pruriens = dol.
mur-ac. muriaticum acidum
muru. murure leite
murx. murex purpureus, Purple fish
musa, musa sapientum
muscin. muscarinum
mut. bacillus mutabilis
mygal. mygale lasiodora (avicularia)
(= aranea avicularia), **Black cuban spider**
myos-a. myosotis arvensis
myos-s. myosotis symphytifolia
myric. myrica cerifera, Bayberry
myris. myristica sebifera, Brazilian ucuba
myrrha, myrrha
myrtillus = vacc-m.
myrt-c. myrtus communis, Myrtle
myrt-ch. myrtus cheken (= eugenia cheken)
myrt-p. myrtus pimenta
mytil. mytilus edulis

N

nabal. nabalus serpentaria
naja, naja tripudians, Cobra
napht. naphta
naphtin. naphtalinum
narc-po. narcissus poeticus, Daffodil
narc-ps. narcissus pseudonarcissus
narcin. narceinum
narcot. narcotinum
narz. Narzan aqua
nast. nasturtium aquaticum
nat-a. natrum aceticum
nat-ae-s. natrum aethylosulphuricum
nat-ar. natrum arsenicosum
nat-be. natrum benzoicum
nat-br. natrum bromatum
nat-bic. natrum bicarbonicum
nat-c. natrum carbonicum
nat-cac. natrum cacodylicum
nat-ch. natrum choleinicum
nat-f. natrum fluoratum
nat-hchls. natrum hypochlorosum
nat-hsulo. natrum hyposulphurosum

nat-i. natrum iodatum
nat-lac. natrum lacticum
nat-m. natrum muriaticum, Salt, Sodium chloride
nat-n. natrum nitricum
nat-ns. natrum nitrosum
nat-p. natrum phosphoricum
nat-s. natrum sulphuricum, Glauber's salt
nat-s-c. natrum sulphocarbolicum (sulphophenolicum)
nat-sal. natrum salicylicum
nat-sel. natrum selenicum
nat-sil. natrum silicicum
nat-sil-f. natrum silicofluoricum
nat-suc. natrum succinicum
nat-sula. natrum sulphuratum
nat-sulo. natrum sulphurosum
nat-taur. natrum taurocholicu
nat-tel. natrum telluricum
nect. nectandra amare
nectrin. nectrianinum
neg. negundium americanum (= acer negundo)
neisseria flava = flav.
nep. nepenthes distillatoria
nepet. nepeta cataria, Catnip
nerium oleander = olnd.
neur. neurinum
nicc. niccolum carbonicum aut metallicum
nicc-s. niccolum sulphuricum
nicotiana tabacum = tab.
nicot. nicotinum
nid. nidus edulis
nig-d. nigella damascena
nig-s. nigella sativa
nit-ac. nitri acidum
nit-m-ac. nitromuriaticum acidum (= aqua regia)
nit-s-d. nitri spiritus dulcis, (= aethylium nitrosum) (= spiritusnitrico-aethereus)
nitro-o. nitrogenium oxygenatum
nitrum = kali-n.
nuph. nuphar luteum (= nymphaea lutea), **Yellow pond lily**
nux-a. nux absurda
nux colae = kola
nux juglans = jug-r.
nux-m. nux moschata, Nutmeg
nux-v. nux vomica, Poison nut
nyct. nyctanthes arbor-tristis, Paghala tree, Sad tree
nymphaea lutea = nuph.
nymph. nymphaea odorata

O

oci. ocimum canum, Brazilian alfavaca
oci-s. ocimum sanctum
oena. oenanthe crocata, Water dropwort
oeno. oenothera biennis
oestronum = foll.
oest. oestrus cameli
okou. okoubaka aubrevillei
ol-an. oleum animale aethereum Dippeli, Dipple's Animal oil
oleum cajuputi = caj.
ol-car. oleum caryophyllatum
ol-j. oleum jecoris aselli, Cod liver oil
ol-myr. oleum myristicae
ol-sant. oleum santali, Sandalwood oil
ol-suc. oleum succinum
oleum wittnebianum = caj.
olnd. oleander (= nerium oleander), **Rose laurel**
onis. oniscus asellus (= millipedes), **Wood louse**
onon. ononis spinosa (arvensis)
onop. onopordon acanthium
onos. onosmodium virginianum, False cromwell
oophorinum = ov., **Ovarian extract**
op. opium, Poppy (dried latex)

oper. operculina turpenthum, Nishope
opl. oplia farinosa
opop. opopanax chironium
opun-f. opuntia ficus (= ficus indica), **Prickly pear**
opun-v. opuntia vulgaris
orch. orchitinum
oreo. oreodaphne californica,California laurel
orig. origanum majorana, Sweet marjoram
orig-cr. origanum creticum
orig-v. origanum vulgare
orni. ornithogalum umbellatum, Star of Bethlehem
orobanche = epiph.
orteaga = eys.
oscilloc. oscillococcinum
osm. osmium metallicum
ost. ostrya virginica, Ironwood
ouabin. ouabainum
ov. ovininum (= oophorinum), **Ovarian extract**
ovi-p. ovi gallinae pellicula, Egg shell membrane
ovi testa = calc-o-t.
ox-ac. oxalicum acidum, Sorrel acid
oxal. oxalis acetosella
oxyd. oxydendron arboreum (= andromeda arborea), **Sorrel tree**
oxyg. oxygenium (= ozonum)
oxyt. oxytropis lamberti, Loco-weed
ozonum = oxyg.

P

paeon. paeonia officinalis, Peony
pakur = fic.
pall. palladium metallicum
palo. paloondo
pambotano = calli.
pana. panacea arvensis
panax quinquefolia = gins.
pann. panna (= aspidium panna)
papin. papaverinum
papaya vulgaris = asim.
par. paris quadrifolia, One berry
paraf. paraffinum
paraph. paraphenylendiaminum
parathormonum = parathyr.
parat. paratyphoidinum
parathyr. parathyreoidinum, (= parathormonum)
pareir. pareira brava, Virgin vine
pariet. parietaria officinalis
paro-i. paronychia illecebrum
parot. parotidinum
parth. parthenium hysterophorus (= escoba amargo), **Bitter broom**
passi. passiflora incarnata, Passion flower
past. pastinaca sativa
paull. paullinia pinnata
paullinia sorbilis = guar.
pect. pecten jacobaeus
ped. pediculus capitis
pedclr. pedicularis canadensis
pelarg. pelargonium reniforme
pelias berus = vip.
pellin. pelletierinum
pen. penthorum sedoides, Virginia stone crop
penic. penicillinum
perlarum mater = conch.
persica amygdalus = amgd-p.
perh. perhexilin
peri. periploca graeca
pers. persea americana
pert. pertussinum, Whooping cough nosode
pest. pestinum
petasites officinalis = tus-p.
peti. petiveria tetrandra
petr. petroleum, Crude Rock oil
petros. petroselinum sativum, Parsley
peumus boldus = bold.
peyotl = anh.

ph-ac. phosphoricum acidum
phal. phallus impudicus
phase. phaseolus nanus, Dwarf bean
phel. phellandrium aquaticum,Water dropwort
phenac. phenacetinum
phenob. phenobarbitalum, (= gardenalum)
phenolum = carb-ac.
phila. philadelphus coronarius
phle. phleum pratense
phlor. phlorizinum
phos. phosphorus
phos-h. phosphorus hydrogenatus
phos-pchl. phosphorus pentachloratus
phys. physostigma, Calabar bean
physostigminum = esin
physal. physalis alkekengi
(= alkekengi = solanum veslcarium)
physala-p. physalia pelagica
phyt. phytolacca decandra, Poke root, weed
phyt-b. phytolacca berry
pichi-pichi = fab.
pic-ac. picricum (picronitricum) **acidum**
(= trinitrophenolum)
picro. picrotoxinum
pilo. pilocarpinum hydrochloricum
aut nitricum aut purum
pilocarpus pennatifolius aut
microphyllus = pilo., **Jaborandi**
pime. pimenta officinalis
pimp. pimpinella saxifraga (alba)
pinus canadensis = abies-c.
pin-c. pinus cupressus
pin-l. pinus lambertiana
pin-s. pinus silvestris, Scotch pine
piper angustifolium aut elongatum = mati.
pip-m. piper methysticum Kava-kava
pip-n. piper nigrum, Black pepper
pipe. piperazinum
pisc. piscidia erythrina, Jamaica dogwood
pitu. pituitarium posterium
(= hyophysis posterior)
pitu-gl. pituitaria glandula
pituin. pituitrinum
pix. pix liquida, Pine tar
planifolia = vanil.
plan. plantago major, Plantain
plan-mi. plantago minor
plat. platinum metallicum
plat-m. platinum muriaticum
plat-m-n. platinum muriaticum natronatum
platan. platanus occidentalis,
Sycamore buttonwood
plb. plumbum metallicum, Lead
plb-a. plumbum aceticum
plb-c. plumbum carbonicum
plb-chr. plumbum chromicum
plb-i. plumbum iodatum
plb-n. plumbum nitrlcum
plb-p. plumbum phosphoricum
plect. plectranthus fruticosus
plumbg. plumbago litteralis
plume. plumeria celinus
pneu. pneumococcinum venenosum
(= pneumococcus)
podo. podophyllum peltatum,
Mandrake, May apple
pole. polemonium coeruleum
poll. pollen
polygala senega = seneg.
polyg-a. polygonum aviculare
polyg-h. polygonum punctatum
(= hydropiper), **Smartweed**
polyg-m. polygonum maritimum
polyg-pe. polygonum persicaria
polyg-s. polygonum sagittatum
polym. polymnia uvedalia
polyporus officinalis = bol-la.
polyp-p. polyporus pinicola, Pine agaric
polytr. polytrichum juniperinum

scolo-v. scolopendrium vulgare
scop. scopolia carniolica
scopin. scopolaminum bromatum
scor. scorpio europaeus
scroph-m. scrophularia marylandica
scroph-n. scrophularia nodosa, Knotted figwort
scut. scutellaria laterifolia, Skull cap
sec. secale cornutum, Ergot
sed-ac. sedum acre, Small houseleek
sed-r. sedum repens (alpestre)
sed-t. sedum telephium
sedi. sedinha
selenicereus grandiflorus = cact.
sel. selenium
seli. selinum carvifolium
sem-t. semen tiglii
semp. sempervivum tectorum, Houseleek
senec. senecio aureus,Golden ragwort
senec-j. senecio jacobaea
senecin. senecinum
seneg. senega (= polygala senega), **Snakewort**
senn. senna (= cassia acutifolia)
sep. sepia succus, Cuttlefish juice
septi. septicaeminum
serratula = liat.
ser-ang. serum anguillae
(= ichthyotoxinum), **Eel serum**
serp. serpentaria aristolochia
(= aristolochia serpentaria)
sieg. siegesbeckia orientalis
sil. silicea terra (= silica), **Flint**
sil-mar. silica marina
silpho. silphion cyrenaicum
silphu. silphium laciniatum, Rosin weed
sima. simaruba amara, (officinalis) **aut glauca**
simaruba ferroginea = cedr.
sin-a. sinapis alba, White mustard
sin-n. sinapis nigra, Black mustard
sisy. sisyrinchium galaxoides
sium, sium latifolium
skat. skatolum
skook. Skookum chuck aqua
slag, slag
smilax officinalis = sars.
sol, sol (sunlight)
sol-a. solanum arrebenta
sol-c. solanum carolinense
solanum dulcamara = dulc.
solanum lycopersicum = lycpr., **Tomato**
sol-m. solanum mammosum
sol-n. solanum nigrum, Black nightshade
sol-o. solanum oleraceum
sol-ps. solanum pseudocapsicum
sol-t. solanum tuberosum
sol-t-ae. solanum tuberosum aegrotans
solanum vesicarium = physal.
solid. solidago virgaurea, Goldenrod
solin. solanium aceticum aut purum
soph. sophora japonica
spartium scoparium = saroth., **Broom**
sphingurus martini, (spiggurus)
spig. spigelia anthelmia
(anthelmintica), **Pinkroot**
spig-m. spigelia marylandica
spiggurus martini = sphing.
spil. spilanthes oleracea
spiritus nitrico-aethereus = nit-s-d.
spir-sula. spiritus sulphuratus
spira. spiranthes autumnalis, Lady's tresses
spirae. spiraea ulmaria, Hardhack
spong. spongia tosta, Roasted Sponge
squil. squilla maritima, (scilla), **Sea onion**
stach. stachys betonica
stann. stannum metallicum, Tin
stann-i. stannum iodatum
stann-m. stannum muriaticum
stann-pchl. stannum perchloratum
staph. staphysagria
(= delphinium staphysagria), **Stavesacre**
staphycoc. staphylococcinum

staphytox. staphylotoxinum
stel. stellaria media, Chickweed
stict. sticta pulmonaria, Lungwort
stigm. stigmata maydis = zea maydis, **Corn silk**
still. stillingia silvatica, Queen root
stram. stramonium (= datura stramonium), **Jimson weed, Thornapple**
strept-ent. bacillus strepto-enterococcus
streptoc. streptococcinum
stront-br. strontium bromatum
stront-c. strontium carbonicum
stront. strontium metallicum = stront-c.
stront-i. strontium iodatum
stront-n. strontium nitricum
stroph-h. strophantus hispidus, Kombe seed
stroph-s. strophantus sarmentosus
stry. strychninum purum
stry-ar. strychninum arsenicosum
stry-n. strychninum nitricum
stry-p. strychninum phosphoricum
stry-s. strychninum sulphuricum
stry-val. strychninum valerianicum
strych-g. strychnos gaultheriana (= hoang-nan)
strychnos tieute = upa.
stryph. stryphnodendron barbatimam
succ. succinum thal.
succ-ac. succinicum acidum
sul-ac. sulphuricum acidum
sul-h. sulphur hydrogenisatum
sul-i. sulphur iodatum
sulphur sublimatum = sulph.
sul-ter. sulphur terebinthinatum
sulfa. sulfanilamidum
sulfon. sulfonalum
sulfonam. sulfonamidum
sulo-ac. sulphurosum acidum
sulph. sulphur lotum (sublimatum)
sumb. sumbulus moschatus (= ferula sumbul), **Musk root**
syc. bacillus sycoccus
sym-r. symphoricarpus racemosus, Snowberry
symph. symphytum officinale, Comfrey, Knitbone
syph. syphilinum (= luesinum), **Syphilis nosode**
syr. syringa vulgaris
syzyg. syzygium jambolanum (cumini), **Jambol seeds**

T

tab. tabacum (= nicotiana tabacum), **Tobacco**
tam. tamus communis
tama. tamarix germanica
tanac. tanacetum vulgare, Tansy
tang. tanghinia venenifera
tann-ac. tannicum acidum (= tanninum)
tarax. taraxacum officinale, Dandelion
tarent. tarentula hispanica, Spanish tarentula
tarent-c. tarentula cubensis, Cuban tarentula
tart-ac. tartaricum acidum
tartarus depuratus = kali-bit.
tartarus emeticus = ant-t.
tax. taxus baccata, Yew
tela, tela araneae (= araneae tela), **Spider's web**
tell. tellurium metallicum
tell-ac. telluricum acidum
tep. Teplitz aqua
ter. terebinthiniae oleum, Turpentine
tere-ch. terebinthina chios
terebe. terebenum
testa praeparata = calc-o-t.
tet. tetradymitum
tetox. tetanotoxinum
teucrium chamaedrys = chamae.
teucr. teucrium marum verum (= marum verum), **Cat-thyme**
teucr-s. teucrium scorodonia
thallium metallicum aut aceticum
thal-s. thallium sulphuricum
thala. thalamus

thaspium aureum = ziz., **Meadow parsnip**
thea, thea chinensis, Tea
thebin. thebainum
theobroma cacao = cac.
ther. theridion curassavicum
(= latrodectus curassavicus), **Orange spider**
thev. thevetia nerifolia
thiop. thioproperazinum
thiosin. thiosinaminum (= rhodallinum),
Mustard seed oil
thlas. thlaspi bursa pastoris, Shepherd's purse
(= bursa pastoris = capsella bursa pastoris)
thuj. thuja occidentalis, Arbor vitae
thuj-l. thuja lobii
thym-gl. thymi glandulae extractum
thymol. thymolum, Thyme-camphor
thymu. thymus serpyllum, Wild thyme
thyr. thyroidinum, Sheep's thyroid gland
(= glandula thyreoidea = iodothyrinum)
thyreotr. thyreotropinum (= thyreostimulinum)
til. tilia europaea, Linden
tinas. tinaspora cordifolia
titan. titanium metallicum
tol. toluidinum
tong. tongo (= dipterix odorata = tonca)
tor. torula cerevisiae (= saccharomyces),
Yeast plant
torm. tormentilla erecta
tox-th. toxicophloea thunbergi
toxi. toxicophis pugnax
trach. trachinus draco
trad. tradescantia diuretica
trib. tribulus terrestris (= ikshugandha)
trich. trichosanthes amara
trif-p. trifolium pratense, Red clover
trif-r. trifolium repens
tril. trillium pendulum, White beth root
tril-c. trillium cernuum
trimethylaminum = prop.
trinitrophenolum = pic-ac.
trinit. trinitrotoluenum, T.N.T
trios. triosteum perfoliatum, Fever root
tritic. triticum repens, (agropyrum)
Couch grass
trito. trito
trom. trombidium muscae domesticae
(= acarus), **Red acarus of the fly**
trop. tropaeolum majus
tub. tuberculinum bovinum Kent,
Tuberculosis nosode of cows
tub-a. tuberculinum avis,
Tuberculosis nosode of birds
tub-d. tuberculinum Denys
tub-k. tuberculinum Koch
tub-m. tuberculinum Marmoreck
tub-r. tuberculinum residuum Koch
tub-sp. tuberculinum Spengler
turnera aphrodisiaca = dam. **Damiana**
turpethum minerale = merc-sul.
tus-fa. tussilago farfara (= farfara), **Coltsfoot**
tus-fr. tussilago fragans
tus-p. tussilago petasites
(= petasites officinalis), **Butterburr**
typh. thypha latifolia

U

ulm. ulmus campestris (fulva), **Slippery elm**
upa. upas tieute (= strychnos tieute), **Upas tree**
upa-a. upas antiaris
ur-ac. uricum acidum
uran. uranium metallicum
uran-n. uranium nitricum
uranoth. uranothorium
urea, urea pura, Carbamide
urea-n. urea nitrica (= carbamidum)
urt-c. urtica crenulata
urt-g. urtica gigas
urt-u. urtica urens, Stinging nettle
usn. usnea barbata, Tree moss

ust. ustilago maydis, Corn smut
uva, uva ursi, Bearberry
uvar. uvaria triloba
uza, uzara

V

v-a-b. vaccin attenue bilie
(= bacillus Calmette-Guerin)
vac. vaccininum (= vaccinotoxinum),
Nosode from vaccine matter
vacc-m. vaccinium myrtillus (= myrtillus)
valer. valeriana officinalis, Valerian
vanad. vanadium metallicum
vanil. vanilla aromatica (= planifolia), **Vanilla**
vario. variolinum, Smallpox nosode
ven-m. venus mercenaria
verat. veratrum album, White hellebore
verat-n. veratrum nigrum
verat-v. veratrum viride, American hellebore
verb. verbascum thapsus (thapsiforme) **Mullein**
verb-n. verbascum nigrum
verbe-h. verbena hastata, Vervain
verbe-u. verbena urticaefolia
verin. veratrinum
vero-b. veronica beccabunga
vero-o. veronica officinalis
vesi. vesicaria communis
vesp. vespa crabro, Wasp
vib. viburnum opulus, High Cranberry
vib-od. viburnum oderatissinum
vib-p. viburnum prunifolium
vib-t. viburnum tinus
vichy-g. Vichy aqua, grande grille
vichy-h. Vichy aqua, hopital
vinc. vinca minor, Lesser periwinkle
vince. vincetoxicum officinale
(= asclepias vincetoxicum = cynanchum)
viol-o. viola odorata, Violet
viol-t. viola tricolor (= jacea), **Pansy**
vip. vipera berus (torva) (= pelias berus)
vip-a. vipera aspis
vip-l-f. vipera lachesis fel
vip-r. vipera redi
vipera torva = vip.
visc. viscum album, Mistletoe
visc-q. viscum quercinum
vit. vitex trifolia
vitr. vitrum antimonii
voes. Voeslau aqua
vulpis pulmo = pulm-v.

W

wies. Wiesbaden aqua
wildb. Wildbad aqua
wildu. Wildungen aqua
wrightia antidysenterica
wye. wyethia helenoides, Poison weed

X

x-ray x-ray
xan. xanthoxylum fraxineum (americanum),
Prickly ash
xanrhi. xanthorrhiza apifolia
xanrhoe. xanthorrhoea arborea
xanth. xanthium spinosum
xero. xerophyllum, Tamalpais lily
xiph. xiphosura americana

Y

yerba buena = micr.
yerba mansa = anemps.
yerba santa = erio.
yohim. yohimbinum
yuc. yucca filamentosa, Bear grass

Z

zea-i. zea italica

zea maydis = stigm.

zinc. zincum metallicum

zinc-a. zincum aceticum

zinc-ar. zincum arsenicosum

zinc-br. zincum bromatum

zinc-c. zincum carbonicum

zinc-cy. zincum cyanatum

zinc-fcy. zincum ferrocyanatum

zinc-i. zincum iodatum

zinc-m. zincum muriaticum

zinc-o. zincum oxydatum

zinc-p. zincum phosphoricum

zinc-pic. zincum picricum

zinc-s. zincum sulphuricum

zinc-val. zincum valerianicum

zing. zingiber officinale, Ginger

ziz. zizia aurea (= thaspium aureum), **Meadow parsnip**

Word Index

A

B

D

E

F

G

H

I

N

O

P

Q

R

S

T